C000282890

Butterworths
Medical Dictionary

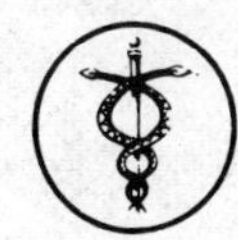

Butterworths
Medical Dictionary

Second Edition

Editor-in-Chief
Macdonald Critchley

First Edited by Sir Arthur Salusbury MacNalty

Complete and unabridged

Butterworths
London · Boston
Sydney · Wellington · Durban · Toronto

The Butterworth Group

United Kingdom
Butterworth & Co (Publishers) Ltd
London: 88 Kingsway, WC2B 6AB

Australia
Butterworths Pty Ltd
Sydney: 586 Pacific Highway, Chatswood, NSW 2067
Also at Melbourne, Brisbane, Adelaide and Perth

South Africa
Butterworth & Co (South Africa) (Pty) Ltd
Durban: 152–154 Gale Street

New Zealand
Butterworths of New Zealand Ltd
Wellington: 26–28 Waring Taylor Street, 1

Canada
Butterworth & Co (Canada) Ltd
Toronto: 2265 Midland Avenue, Scarborough, Ontario, M1P 4S1

USA
Butterworth (Publishers) Inc
Boston: 10 Tower Office Park, Woburn, Mass. 01801

First published in 1961 by the Caxton Publishing Co Ltd as The British Medical Dictionary, edited by Sir Arthur Salusbury MacNalty.

Revised Edition 1963
Revised Edition 1965 as Butterworths Medical Dictionary
Second Edition 1978
Reprinted 1980, in reduced format, complete and unabridged

ISBN 0 407 00193 X

British Library Cataloguing in Publication Data

Butterworths medical dictionary—2nd ed.
1. Medicine—Dictionaries
I. MacNalty, *Sir* Arthur Salusbury
I. Critchley, Macdonald
610'.3 R125 77-30154

ISBN 0 407 00193 X

Printed in the United States of America
by the George Banta Company, Inc., Menasha, Wis.

Contents

Preface to the Second Edition

The duties of a lexicographer are arduous and exacting, but at the same time seductive, especially to one who nurses a curious fascination for words in all their vagaries. Dr. Johnson defined a lexicographer as a writer of dictionaries; a harmless drudge. Drudge he may be, and certainly harmless. Indeed he is in many ways as vulnerable as an unwinged housefly. His duties entail the coaxing and cajoling of co-operating co-authors many of them eager, others reluctant. Among the former some prove infirm of purpose. To quote Johnson again—for he was in a position to know—"the promises of authors are like the vows of lovers; made in moments of careless rapture, and subject, during the long process of fulfilment, to all kinds of unforeseen dangers and difficulties".

Reference has been made to wordlore or the collecting of words for their aesthetic, euphonious or allusive qualities. No one has expressed this urge better than Dylan Thomas, who explained this obsession in that he liked to treat them as a craftsman does his wood or stone or what-have-you, to hew, carve, mould, coil, polish and plane them into patterns, sequences, sculptures, figures of sound. . . . But whoever embarks upon the editorship of a medico-scientific lexicon has a rather different task. Avoiding all sensitivity to their alluring colour, he now finds himself confronted by the power of words, the tyranny of words, their not infrequent falsity and fickleness, their imposture and their force. At times the lexicographer has to assume the mantle of metalanguage and to sit in judgement outside the arena of word-spinning.

To begin with he faces the fundamental question of what constitutes a dictionary. Is it a catalogue of synonyms? Linguists tell us that dictionary definitions are but verbal equivalents. Does a dictionary supply a "meaning" of a given word? At once we are up against the ambiguity inherent in the term "meaning". In what way does the meaning of a word differ from the sense of a word? This kind of philosophical quibbling could go on and on but without satisfying anyone in the end. There comes a time when semeiological jargon has to yield to common sense.

The chief aim of a constructor of definitions is to endeavour, difficult though it be, to bring precision to a discipline which is not yet a Science nor even an Art. Only too often medical men in their writings, their thinking, and in their practice, are hamstrung by muddled ideas. Over 450 years ago Tyndale said that 20 doctors may expound one single text in 20 different ways—as children make descent upon plainsong. It is the duty of the medical purist to promote professional plainsong.

The compiler of a dictionary should, I submit, feel warmly towards out-worn, old-fashioned, archaic terms that are but seldom used. To reject them from his lexicon would be a grievous error. It is just those expressions which most often baffle the contemporary research-worker or student, should he ever deem it worth while to consult the older literature or the original sources. How many undergraduates today are clear about what is understood by pithiatism, sialism, megrims, ague, a clyster, a cupping, a seeton? No one refers to them any longer, but they must have meant something, sometime, to our learned but bygone teachers. The lexicographer's duty is fulfilled if he includes these terms, explains them, and then proceeds to establish them as obsolete. He then becomes a terminological fossilizer, but important for all that.

The other secret pleasure of the dictionary-monger is to seek out, appraise, and preserve eponymous terms. They are unfashionable today, but the rejection of eponyms is a rather ugly reaction against what has been dubbed ancestor-worship. Sometimes an eponym is face-saving. To speak nowadays of mongolism runs the risk of offending race-relationships: but to refer to Down's syndrome is respectable; to speak of Langdon–Down's syndrome would be even better. Eponyms are lasting tributes to the resourcefulness and originality of our elders. Of course, difficulties continually arise. The Germans speak of Horner's syndrome, the French of *le symptome de Claude Bernard*. Others compromise and refer to the Horner–Bernard phenomenon. Should we speak of the manifestations associated with port-wine staining of the face as the Sturge syndrome? the Sturge–Weber syndrome? the Parkes Weber–Sturge syndrome? or the Sturge–Weber–Kalischer syndrome? The Argyll-Robertson phenomenon is the product of an individual endowed with a double-barrelled name, and not of two authors——as I have seen in print. Warren–Tay Sachs were two men, not three. And so on. The struggle for priorities is, however, a worthy but teasing one.

We come now to the vexed question of new words. Like new tools, new words and neologisms in the rapidly expanding discipline of medical science are unavoidable, and indeed, imperative. As exemplified by Boiardo, who—out hunting—suddenly conceived a highly appropriate new term, galloped home and caused all the village bells to be rung to celebrate the happy invention. Sir William Gowers was always chary of additions to medical terminology but even he had to admit that if there exists a conception for which no name exists, and which we need frequently to speak of, it is not wise to shrink from an attempt to give it a name. But it behoves the would-be verbal coiner who aspires to be the creator of novel terms, to express in black and white and in the simplest terminology, precisely what he has in mind when he dares to inject something new into the ocean of language: otherwise it is mere verbal pollution. Despite the cynicism of John Hunter on this matter, remember that Voltaire—an even greater man—insisted that if you would converse, first define your terms.

The coinage of neologisms lends itself to abuse. It can be overdone. The basic vocabulary of the medic profession, according to Dr. Manuila of the Wor Health Organization, already consists of 50,0 terms. A chaotic, even dangerous situation is liab to arise in some specialities where, for example, t same drug may be known by as many as 80 differe names. Some disciplines, outside of medicine and al within it, are offenders in this respect. Unless care taken there may spring up a veritable jargon, pr sumably understood by initiates but not by tho outside the clique. The lexicographer may deplore b he cannot ignore the overgrowth of jargon. It is h duty, however, to ensure that each novel term is ful and clearly defined. If not, the result is chaos, wh Americans call gobbledygook. Ivor Brown h spoken of barnacular; pudder; or jargantuan, but so doing has created three new words to describe t new words of others, and is thereby himself a offender.

As Editor-in-chief of this Second Edition I a particularly indebted to my predecessor and o colleague, Arthur MacNalty. The First Edition is tribute to his industry and scholarship, and to h team of contributors.

The compilation of this dictionary stands as monument to the cooperative achievement of scor of medical and scientific workers in the Unite Kingdom; behind the footlights on both occasior have been legions of highly experienced and highl efficient men and women who have been responsib for the publishing and printing of this book. It believed that it will represent for some decades medical source-book of world-wide value.

We regret to announce that prior to publicatio two of our distinguished contributors have die namely Sir Rowan Boland and Mr. D. H. Patey.

Macdonald Critchley
1978

From the Preface to the First Edition

Medicine has a language of its own, and from earliest times practitioners of the healing art have been compelled to invent new words to describe their discoveries. This practice inevitably led to the need for a medical dictionary for students and practitioners of medicine. Galen wrote such a dictionary, and his example has been followed by many others. The coinage of new medical words has proceeded apace, most of them based on Greek or Latin derivations. Some coined words where the assistance of classical scholars has not been invoked are hybrids or of doubtful etymology. New sciences, the offspring of chemistry and physics, for example, biochemistry and radiology, have come into being each demanding a new vocabulary. The revolutionary advances in medical science which have been made between the two world wars, during the Second World War and subsequently have added copiously to the English language. Many of these advances and discoveries have been made by British scientists and members of the British medical profession, so that this British medical dictionary is both appropriate and desirable.

Dr. Samuel Johnson at first hoped to complete his *Dictionary* in three years. When reminded by Dr. Adams that the French Academy took forty years to compile their dictionary, he made light of the prodigious labour on which he was embarking. In the end, Dr. Johnson took nearly eight years over his task, from 1747 to 1755. The preparation of this *Dictionary* has taken over fourteen years, which cannot be regarded as excessive when it is remembered that the whole range of modern medicine had to be surveyed before the actual work could be begun.

It is worth noting here that, in 1743, Dr. Johnson himself participated in the preparation of *A Medicinal Dictionary* in three volumes folio, by Robert James, M.D., inventor of the celebrated "fever powders", which bear his name. To oblige James, his old school fellow, Johnson, "an amateur of Physick", wrote some of the articles as well as the sonorous dedication to Dr. Mead. This dictionary, however, resembles our encyclopaedias and dictionaries of treatment rather than the key to terminology connoted by the word "dictionary". In Johnson's day the most popular dictionary of terms was John Quincy's, a book which went into many editions and was not entirely superseded when Dr. R. G. Mayne published in 1836 a "Medical Vocabulary" for the use of students. The author worked for a further twenty-four years enlarging and improving this work and the result of his labours was published in 1860 as "An expository lexicon of the terms, ancient and modern, in medical and general science" in a single volume of 1506 double-columned pages. Mayne's dictionary was the prototype of the medical dictionary as we know it today and it was used as the basis of the Sydenham Society's "Lexicon" published in five volumes between 1879 and 1899. It can be claimed that with *The British Medical Dictionary* we are returning to the great tradition of English lexicography.

A comprehensive medical dictionary does not emerge ready-made like Athena from the brain of Zeus. Several years were occupied in organizing an administrative staff at headquarters, in the consultation of many dictionaries, textbooks and medical treatises both British and foreign; and in preparing a scheme of work and a classification of subjects which are included in the art and science of medicine, and under which entries were to be made. Also, a number of words which are obsolete and seldom if ever referred to in modern practice were eliminated. In doing this the importance of retaining definitions of such archaic words as "humours" and reference to schools or systems of medicine which concern the historical aspect of medicine was not forgotten. A cardinal feature of the scheme was that the information supplied by the *Dictionary* should be made readily available to the busy general practitioner.

Arthur S. MacNalty
1961

Contributors and Consultants

Second Edition

Stanley Alstead CBE, MD, FRCP, FRSE
Formerly Regius Professor of Materia Medica, University of Glasgow; Consultant Physician, Stobhill General Hospital, Glasgow.

Alec W. Badenoch MA, MD, ChM, FRCS
Honorary Civilian Consultant in Urology to the Royal Air Force; Consulting Surgeon, Royal Hospital of St. Bartholomew, and St. Peter's Hospital, London; Consulting Urologist, King Edward VII's Hospital for Officers, London; Past President of the British Association of Urological Surgeons.

Sir Geoffrey Hirst Bateman MA, BM, BCh(Oxon), FRCS(Eng)
Editor, *Journal of Laryngology and Otology*; Honorary Consulting Ear Nose and Throat Surgeon, St. Thomas' Hospital, London; Formerly Member of Council of the Royal College of Surgeons; Adviser in Otolaryngology to the Chief Medical Officer of the Department of Health; President of the British Association of Otolaryngologists.

Sir John Henry Biggart CBE, DSc, MD, FRCP, FRCPath, LLD(QUB), MD(Dub), DSc(NUI), FRCPI, FRCGP, FIMLT
Pro-Chancellor, Queen's University of Belfast; Formerly Professor of Pathology, Queen's University of Belfast; Dean of the Medical Faculty, Queen's University of Belfast.

Peter Maxwell Farrow Bishop DM, FRCP, FRCOG
Endocrinologist Emeritus, Guy's Hospital, London; Consulting Endocrinologist, Chelsea Hospital for Women, London; Formerly Consulting Medical Officer to the Family Planning Association; Past Master, Worshipful Society of Apothecaries of London.

Norman M. Bleehen MA, BSc, BM, BCh, FRCP, FRCR
Cancer Research Campaign Professor of Clinical Oncology, and Honorary Director of MRC Clinical Oncology and Radiotherapeutics Unit, Cambridge; Honorary Consultant, Addenbrooke's Hospital, Cambridge.

Sir Rowan Boland Kt 1964, CBE 1945, OBE 1941, MD, FRCP
Formerly Physician Emeritus, Guy's Hospital, London; Consulting Physician, Hospital of St. John and St. Elizabeth, London; Honorary Consulting Physician to the Army, 1945–1970, Emeritus 1971.

J. W. D. Bull CBE, MD, FRCP, FRCR
Honorary Consultant Radiologist, National Hospital for Nervous Diseases, Queen Square, London.

E. H. Burrows MRad, FRCR
Consultant Neuroradiologist, Wessex Neurological Centre, Southampton; Honorary Senior Lecturer in Neuroradiology, Southampton University.

J. H. Chamberlain MB, BS, MRCP, DIC
Consultant Clinical Physiologist, Guy's Hospital, London.

Macdonald Critchley CBE, MD, FACP, FRCP (*Editor-in-Chief*)
Emeritus President World Federation of Neurology; Honorary Consulting Physician, National Hospital for Nervous Diseases, Queen Square, London; Honorary Consulting Neurologist, King's College Hospital, London; Formerly Consulting Neurologist, Royal Masonic Hospital, London; Consultant in Neurology to the Royal Navy 1939–1977.

Robert Cruickshank CBE, MD, FRCP, FRCP(Edin), DPH, FRSE
Formerly Emeritus Professor of Bacteriology, University of Edinburgh.

Howard Dickson Darcus BSc(Oxon), MA, BM, BCh
Formerly 1st Assistant Department of Physical Medicine, Hospital for Sick Children, Great Ormond Street, London; Physical Medicine Adviser, Wolfson Centre, Institute of Child Health, London.

Dennis C. Deuchar MD, FRCP
Consultant Cardiologist, Guy's Hospital, London.

G. P. Deutsch MBBS, MRCP, DMRT, FRCR
Consultant in Radiotherapy and Oncology, Royal Sussex County Hospital, Brighton, Sussex.

Philip R. Evans CBE, MD, MSc, FRCP
Consultant Physician Emeritus, The Children's Department, Guy's Hospital, London, and The Hospital for Sick Children, Great Ormond Street, London.

John Godfrey Fairer TD, LLB, MB, BS, FFARCS, Barrister, Inner Temple
Formerly Consultant Anaesthetist, Charing Cross Hospital, London, and Royal National Orthopaedic Hospital, London; Civilian Consultant Anaesthetist to the Army; Honorary Archivist, Faculty of Anaesthetists, Royal College of Surgeons of England.

J. A. Fraser Roberts CBE, MA, MD, DSc, FRCP, FRCPsych, FRS
Geneticist, Paediatric Research Unit, Guy's Hospital Medical School, London; Honorary Consultant in Medical Genetics, Guy's Hospital, London.

F. Giannelli MD, PhD
Reader in Cytogenetics and Cell Biology, Paediatric Research Unit, Guy's Hospital Medical School, London.

M. Harris MD, BChD, FDSRCS
Consultant, Department of Oral and Maxillo-Facial Surgery, King's College Hospital and Dental School, London.

F. Dudley Hart MD, FRCP
Consulting Physician, Westminster Hospital, Chelsea Hospital for Women, and The Hospital of St. John and St. Elizabeth, London.

William Hayes MB, DSc, FRCP(I), FAA, FRS
Professor and Head of the Department of Genetics, Research School of Biological Sciences, The Australian National University, Canberra.

Thomas Hunt CBE, DM(Oxon), FRCP
Consulting Physician, St. Mary's Hospital, London, and King Edward VII's Hospital for Officers, London; Honorary President, International Society of Gastroenterology.

Sir Norman Jeffcoate MD, FRCSE, FRCOG, LLD, FACOG, FRCSC, FCOG(SA)
Emeritus Professor of Obstetrics and Gynaecology, University of Liverpool.

H. Gwynne Jones BSc, FBPsS
Professor of Psychology and Pro-Vice Chancellor, University of Leeds.

Basil Kiernander MB, BS, FRCP, DMRE, DPhysMed
Director of Department of Physical Medicine, Hospital for Sick Children, Great Ormond Street, London, and the Royal National Throat, Nose and Ear Hospital, London; Honorary Civilian Consultant in Physical Medicine to the Royal Air Force; Honorary Consultant Physician, Charterhouse Rheumatism Clinic, London; Honorary Medical Adviser, Leonard Cheshire Foundation; Past President, Section of Physical Medicine, Royal Society of Medicine.

Sylvia D. Lawler MD, MRCP, FRCPath
Senior Lecturer, Recognized Teacher in Immunogenetics, Department of Cytogenetics and Immunogenetics, Institute of Cancer Research; Honorary Consultant in Cytogenetics and Immunology, Royal Marsden Hospital, London.

J. Alfred Lee FFA, RCS, FFA RCSI, DA
Honorary Consulting Anaesthetist (formerly Senior Consultant Anaesthetist), General Hospital, Southend-on-Sea.

H. Lehmann MD, ScD, FRCP, FRIC, FRCPath, FRS
Professor of Clinical Biochemistry, University of Cambridge; University Professor of Clinical Biochemistry to Addenbrooke's Hospital, Cambridge.

W. Linford Rees MD, FRCP, PRCPsych, DPM, FACP
Professor of Psychiatry, University of London; Physician in Charge, Department of Psychological Medicine, St. Bartholomew's Hospital, London.

C. R. Madeley MD
Senior Lecturer in Clinical Virology, University of Glasgow, Ruchill Hospital, Glasgow.

W. B. Matthews DM, FRCP
Professor of Clinical Neurology, University of Oxford.

Stephen J. H. Miller MD, FRCS
Surgeon-Oculist to Her Majesty The Queen; Surgeon, Moorfields Eye Hospital, London; Ophthalmic Surgeon, King Edward VII's Hospital for Officers, St. George's Hospital and The National Hospital for Nervous Diseases, Queen Square, London; Civil Consultant in Ophthalmology to the Royal Navy.

D. B. Moffat VRD, MD, FRCS
Professor of Anatomy, University College, Cardiff.

C. S. Nicol TD, MD, FRCP
Adviser in Genito-Urinary Medicine, Department of Health and Social Services; Honorary Consultant in Genito-Urinary Medicine, St. Thomas' Hospital, London; Adviser in Genito-Urinary Medicine to the Ministry of Defence (Army).

Air Vice-Marshal P. J. O'Connor CB, OBE, QHP, MD, FRCP(E), FRCPsych
The Senior Consultant RAF, Central Medical Establishment, Royal Air Force.

David Patey MS(London), FRCS(Eng)
Formerly Surgeon Emeritus, Middlesex Hospital, London; late Director of Surgical Studies, Middlesex Hospital Medical School, London.

C. I. Pogson BA, PhD
Lecturer in Biochemistry, University of Kent at Canterbury.

Joan M. E. Quixley SRN, RNT
Formerly Gynaecological, Medical and Surgical Ward Sister, St. Thomas' Hospital, London; Nurse Tutor, The Nightingale School, St. Thomas' Hospital, London.

Philip J. Randle PhD, MD, FRCP
Professor of Clinical Biochemistry, University of Oxford.

Dame Kathleen A. Raven DBE, SRN, SCM, OOSt.J, FRSA
Nursing Consultant to Allied Medical Group (London); Vice-President of the Royal College of Nursing; Formerly Chief Nursing Officer to the Ministry of Health and Matron of the General Infirmary at Leeds.

Ronald W. Riddell MD, FRCP, FRCP(Edin), FRCPath, Dipl Bact
Consultant Microbiologist, National Heart and Chest Hospitals (Brompton Hospital, London Chest Hospital, National Heart Hospital), London; Senior Lecturer, Department of Medicine, Cardiothoracic Institute, University of London.

Brian Fitzgerald Russell MD, FRCP, DPH
Consulting Dermatologist, London Hospital; Honorary Consulting Physician to St. John's Hospital for Diseases of the Skin, London.

Keith Simpson CBE, MD, LLD, FRCP, FRCPath
Emeritus Professor of Forensic Medicine, University of London; Home Office Pathologist; Member of the European, American and Spanish Academies of Legal Medicine.

Francis Vella MD, MA(Oxon), PhD, FRIC, FCIC, FRCPath
Professor of Biochemistry, University of Saskatchewan, Saskatoon, Canada.

J. H. Walters MD, FRCP, FRCP(Edin)
Consulting Physician, Hospital for Tropical Diseases, London, and University College Hospital, London; Lately Consultant Physician, Tropical Unit, Queen Mary's Hospital, Roehampton, London; Lately Lecturer in Tropical Medicine, King's College Hospital, London.

W. E. Waters MB, BS, FFCM, DIH
Professor of Community Medicine, University of Southampton; Honorary Specialist in Community Medicine, Wessex Regional Health Authority and the Hampshire Area Health Authority.

Peter C. Wilkinson MD
Senior Lecturer in Bacteriology and Immunology, University of Glasgow; Honorary Consultant in Bacteriology and Immunology, Western Infirmary, Glasgow.

E. S. Williams MD, PhD, BSc, MRCP
Director, Department of Nuclear Medicine, Middlesex Hospital Medical School, London; Honorary Consultant in Nuclear Medicine, Middlesex Hospital, London; Professor of Nuclear Medicine in the University of London.

J. N. Wilson ChM, FRCS
Consultant Orthopaedic Surgeon, Royal National Orthopaedic Hospital, London and Stanmore, Middlesex, and the National Hospital for Nervous Diseases, Queen Square, London.

C. N. Young BSc, PhD, MIBiol
Medical Mycologist, South African Institute for Medical Research; Lecturer in Medical Mycology, School of Pathology, University of the Witwatersrand, Johannesburg, South Africa.

First Edition

Ian Aird ChM, FRCS, FRCSE, FACS
V. D. Allison DSc, MD, DPH
Stanley Alstead CBE, MD, FRFPS, FRCP, FRCP(Edin), FRSE
David Band MB, FRCS(Edin), FRSE
C. H. Barnett MA, MB, BChir, FRCS
J. N. Barron MB, ChB, FRCS
W. W. Binns BSc, BPharm, FPS
W. J. Bishop FLA
M. J. Blunt PhD, MB, BS, LMSSA
A. S. Breathnach MSc, MD, BAO
A. J. Bridge FDSRCS, MRCS, LRCP
Sir Hugh Cairns KBE, MA, DSc, DM, FRGS
Sir Roy Cameron DSc, LLD, MB, BS, FRCP, FRS
Frances E. Camps MD, DTM
E. H. P. Cave MB, BS, MRCS, LRCP, DMRE
D. L. Chadwick MD, FRCS, DLO
Arthur R. G. Chamings BPharm, FPS
Patrick Collard MD, MRCP
Michael Connaughton MB, BS, DGO, MRCOG
K. E. Cooper BSc, PhD, MRCS, LRCP
W. S. C. Copeman OBE, MA, MD, FRCP
G. R. M. Cordiner CVO, MB, ChB, DMRE
E. J. Crisp BA, MD, DPhysMed
P. L. H. Davey MB, BS, MRCS, LRCP
D. V. Davies MA, MB, BS, MRCS, LRCP
P. R. Davis PhD, MB, BS, MRCS, LRCP
E. W. Dorrell MA, MB, BChir, FRCS, DOMS
George Edwards MRCS, LRCP, FFARCS, DA
S. D. Elek MD, DSc, PhD, DPH
Sir Charles Lovatt Evans DSc, LLD, FRCP, MRCS, FRS
Maurice R. Ewing MSc, MB, ChB, FRCS, FRCS(Edin), FRACS, FACS
W. C. Fowler MD
R. B. Freeman MBE, MA
J. S. Frew BSc, MB, ChB, MRCP
Frank Goldby MA, MD, MRCP, MRCS
J. F. Goodwin MD, FRCP
H. S. Grainger FPS
Raymond Greene MA, DM, FRCP
A. L. Gregg MA, MD, MCh, DTM&H, BAO
George Hall CMG, BSc, MD, FRCP
Leslie J. Harris ScD, DSc, PhD, FRIC
G. W. Hayward MD, FRCP
F. J. Hebbert, MD, FRFPS
I. S. Hodgson-Jones MA, MD, MRCP, MRCS
F. W. Holdsworth MA, MB, MChir, FRCS
R. B. Hunter MBE, MB, ChB, FRCP(Edin), MRCP
Betty P. Jackson PhD, BSc, BPharm, FPS, FRMS
G. A. Jackson MRCP, MRCS
W. P. Kennedy BSc, PhD, FRFPS, FRIC, FRSE
Basil Kiernanader MB, BS, MRCP, DMRE, DPhysMed

H. F. W. Kirkpatrick PhD, ARCS, DIC, FRIC
Robert Knox MA, MD, FRCP
V. F. Lambert MD, ChM, FRCS, FRCS(Edin)
A. Dennis Leigh BSc, MD, FRCP
V. M. Leveaux MD, MRCP
V. E. Lloyd MC, MB, BS, MRCS, LRCP
J. F. Loutit CBE, DM, FRCP
Alan Maberly MA, MB, BCh, MRCS, LRCP
R. M. B. MacKenna MA, MD, BCh, FRCP
Sir Arthur MacNalty KCB, MA, MD, FRCP, FRCS
Sir George R. McRobert CIE, MD, FRCP, DTM&H
Sir Phillip Manson-Bahr CMG, DSO, MA, MD, FRCP, DTM&H
J. D. Martin MD, MRCS, LRCP, MRCOG
R. T. Martin MB, ChB, MRCOG
E. L. Middleton OBE, MD, DPH, DIH
Henry Miller MD, FRCP, DPM
E. W. T. Morris FRCS, LRCP
C. R. Murdock MD, BCh
J. R. Napier MRCS, LRCP
L. Everard Napier CIE, FRCP
P. A. Nasmyth PhD, BPharm
G. J. Neary MA, PhD
J. A. Nixon CMG, MD, FRCP
W. C. W. Nixon MD, FRCS, FRCOG
Edwin A. Owen MA, ScD, DSc, MSc, FInstP
H. J. Parish MD, FRCP, DPH
J. Hamilton Paterson MD, FRCP
Mary Pickford DSc, MSc, MRCS, LRCP, FRSE
Phyllis M. Piper SRN, SCM
F. N. L. Poynter BA, PhD, FRSL, FLA
R. T. C. Pratt MA, DM, MRCP, DPM
J. J. Pritchard MA, BSc, DM, MRCS, LRCP
J. Douglas Robertson DSc, PhD, MD, FRCP, FRIC, DPH, FRSE
Derrick Rowley BSc, PhD, MD
Sir William Savage BSc, MD, DPH
D. Hay Scott MB, ChB
L. K. Sharp BSc, PhD, FPS, FRIC
Ursula Shelley MD, FRCP
H. A. B. Simons MA, PhD
Eliot T. O. Slater MA, MD, FRCP, DPM
D. W. Smithers MD, FRCP, FFR
G. F. Somers BSc, PhD, FPS, MIBiol
W. P. Stamm CBE, MB, BS, DCP, FRCP, DTM&H
J. B. Stenlake DSc, PhD, FPS, FRIC
H. C. Stewart MA, PhD, MD, MRCP
M. J. Stewart CBE, LLD, MB, ChB, FRCP
Sir Charles P. Symonds KBE, CB, MD, FRCP
Selwyn Taylor DM, MCh, FRCS
Sir Geoffrey S. Todd KCVO, OBE, MB, ChM, FRCP, FRACP
W. J. Tulley BDS, FDS, DOrthRCS
Jacqueline Walker BSc, PhD
F. S. Warner FDSRCS, MRCS, LRCP
Sir Lionel E. H. Whitby CVO, MC, MA, MD, FRCP, DPH
C. W. M. Whitty MA, BSc, DM, FRCP
J. F. Wilkinson MSc, PhD, MD, FRCP, FRIC
F. A. Williamson-Noble BA, MB, BCh, FRCS
W. H. Wynn MSc, MD, FRCP

Explanatory Notes

Main Entries

The main term (headword) is printed in **bold** type flush with the left-hand margin of each column and followed, where appropriate, by a guide to its pronunciation in round brackets. The material in light type that follows on the same line and on succeeding indented lines explains and defines the term. Where the term has more than one distinct meaning, the individual definitions are introduced by arabic numbers. Derivations normally terminate the entries, but precede eponymous cross references relevant to the headword.

Sub-entries

Subsidiary terms relative to the headword are printed in the same **bold** type and run-on after the main definition in alphabetical order according to the adjective. Sub-entries have thus been grouped under the governing headword. For example, **iopanic acid** is defined as a sub-entry under the main headword, **acid**; **typhoid fever** under the main headword, **fever**; and **zone of polymorphous cells** under **zone**. Exceptions to this rule are anatomical entries, eponymous entries and entry for the headword TEST.

Anatomical Entries

Specific arteries, bones, muscles, nerves and veins do not appear under their nouns but separately as main headwords in their appropriate alphabetical position according to the operative qualifying adjective, or, in the case of arteries, nerves and veins, the organ or structure supplied or drained. This method reduces the number of large entries in the text, obviates large tabular statements, and brings closer together structures that are anatomically associated.

Terms that constitute part of a structure, ANGLE, APEX, AREA, BASE, BED, BODY, BORDER, BRANCH, CIRCUMFERENCE, COAT, DORSUM, FLOOR, FUNDUS, HEAD, HILUM, INLET, LIP, LOBE, MASS, NECK, NUCLEUS, OPENING, OUTLET, PART, ROOF, ROOT, SHAFT, SURFACE, TRIBUTARY, WALL, are defined under the structure concerned. However, in some instances, when otherwise qualified, such terms may be descriptive of a separate anatomical structure or concept, e.g. **geniculate body**, **costophrenic angle**, and in such cases they are defined, as sub-entries under the headwords, **body**, **angle**.

Eponymous Entries

The surname constitutes the headword and, where identity has been established, is followed by brief biographical details. The diseases, syndromes, operations, tests, anatomical structures, etc., with which proper names are associated, appear as sub-entries, arranged in alphabetical order according to the noun. In cases where identity has not been established, the qualified terms are treated as part of the headwords. In the entries DISEASE, SYNDROME, etc., cross-references to appropriate eponymous entries are included.

The abbreviations, b. for born, or d. for died, fl. for flourished and c. for circa, have been used in the biographical details.

The Entry TEST

This calls for special mention in that it has been divided into two parts. In the first section following the main definitions are qualified entries of the most important clinical, biochemical, chemical, physiological and psychological tests, arranged in alphabetical order of the ordinary names by which they are known. Eponymous tests are defined under the eponymous entry, but cross-references are given in the entry TEST.

The second section consists of comprehensive cross-references to all tests for specific substances or purposes. Where tests are ambiguously named, this method has the advantage of eliminating confusion as to whether it is a test in which the named substance is used, or a test *for* that substance, e.g. antimony test could be a test in which a preparation of antimony is used as the reagent, or a test to determine the quantitative or qualitative presence of antimony. An additional advantage is that for reference purposes the entry becomes considerably less cumbersome.

Abbreviations and Symbols

These are listed on p. xxi for ease of reference. In appropriate cases further definitions of the words for which they stand will be found in their alphabetical place in the dictionary.

In the selection of these abbreviations, the most favoured practice in British journals and other publications has been the criterion, and several "suggestions to contributors" issued by such journals have been consulted. There is, however, in many instances little unanimity among these—especially with reference to the choice between capitals and small letters, and a decision has had to be made; in some cases alternative forms have been given.

Alphabetical Order

The rules of the British Standards Institution *Alphabetical Arrangement* have been adopted as follows:

In instances where one or more eponymous entries are identical with an ordinary single-word main entry, the order shall be: eponymous entries, the single-word entry, entries consisting of more than one separate or hyphenated words, and lastly the compound words, thus:

EYE, ADAM	EYE-SHIELD
EYE, THOMAS	EYE WASH
EYE	EYEBROW
EYE FLY	EYELID

The umlaut in German and other names (ä, ö, ü) has been rendered as a diphthong (ae, oe, ue) where it occurs in the first syllable, e.g. LOEFFLER and not LÖFFLER, with consequent effect on alphabetical place.

In chemical entries (see below), certain prefixes, for example *m*-, *o*-, and *p*-, D-, L-, and *dl*-, α-, β-, and γ-, are ignored in the alphabetical arrangement, but where it has been considered suitable to spell out the prefixes, e.g. meta, dextro, alpha, the words take their natural place under M, D, and A.

Pronunciation

The guide to pronunciation compiled in relation to this dictionary has been based on a simple phonetic interpretation dictated by common usage. For many reasons, variation in medical pronunciation exists, giving rise to controversy, and the intention here is to assist rather than to dogmatize.

Pronunciations follow the headword in round brackets. The stressed syllable is printed in small bold type, and where there are two or more stressed syllables in a word, the stronger is marked with an accent, e.g. **as**·id·o·**jen**′·ik (acidogenic). For simplicity only the main vowel sounds are differentiated, in accordance with the following key:

vowels	*example*
a as in make	**a**·jent (agent), ab·**rade** (abrade)
a as in mat	**ab**·ses (abscess)
a as in father	bahm (balm)
e as in meet	**he**·mo·site (haemocyte), am·e·bah (amoeba)
e as in met	ap·**en**·dix (appendix)
i as in mite	**si**·klo·tron (cyclotron), re-**fine** (refine)
i as in mit	par·al·**it**·ik (paralytic)
o as in note	ab·**do**·men (abdomen), **bone**·set (boneset)
o as in cot	ab·**dom**·in·al (abdominal)
u as in mute	al·**bew**·min (albumin)
u as in but	ab·**duk**·tor (abductor)
oo as in boot	ak·**oos**·tik (acoustic)
aw as in bawl	**awl**·der (alder)
oi as in boil	**goi**·ter (goitre)
ow as in how	**kown**·ter (counter)
ow as in bowl	**gro**·th (growth)

consonants	*example*
c as in cot	**kos**·tal (costal)
c as in face	**as**·id (acid)
g as in got	mal·**ig**·nant (malignant)
g as in wager	aje (age)
s as in lesson	**as**·pir·in (aspirin)
s as in poison	an·**oz**·me·ah (anosmia)
ng as in finger	**ang**·gl (angle)
wh as in when	hweet (wheat)

suffixes	*example*
-age as in message	**ban**·dij (bandage)
-age as in fuselage	bros·**ahzh** (brossage)
-sion as in fusion	ab·**ra**·zhun (abrasion)
-sion as in obsession; -tion as in attention	**ak**·shun (action)
-tion as in exhaustion	kom·**bust**·yun (combustion)
-ture as in picture	**kul**·tcher (culture)
-ture as in signature	**sew**·tewr (suture)
-ure as in cure	**fish**·ewr (fissure)

Derivations

The etymological derivation of the headword appears in square brackets at the end of each entry. Greek terms are transliterated into the Roman alphabet. In the case of anatomical terms which are adjectivally qualified, e.g. TEMPORAL NERVE, the derivation of the adjective and noun will be found under the main entries of the adjective and noun, respectively.

In compound words no derivation is given when the elements of the compound are mentioned in the definition. Otherwise, either derivations are given or reference is made to the main headword(s) where derivations are to be found.

Derivations are given for chemical terms where they are in common lay use or give the key to a whole group of terms, or are intrinsically of interest as throwing light on the historical origin of the term. No attempt has been made to cover the many chemical prefixes, suffixes and combining forms; to do so would entail a treatise on chemical nomenclature which, when split up into separate entries scattered throughout the dictionary, would be so complex as to render it valueless.

The meaning of prefixes in common use, e.g. ab-, ad-, epi-, are explained in separate main entries, and are not repeated in individual derivations.

The following abbreviations are used in the derivations:

abbr.	abbreviated
Amer.	American
Ar.	Arabic
AS	Anglo-Saxon
class.	classical
D	Dutch

Dan.	Danish	ME	Middle English
dial. E.	dialect of English	Mex.	Mexican
dim.	diminutive	MHG	Middle High German
etym. dub.	etymology dubious	mythol.	mythological
Finn.	Finnish	O Fr.	Old French
foll.	following (entry)	OHG	Old High German
Fr.	French	onomat.	onomatopoeic
G	German	O Sp.	Old Spanish
Gael.	Gaelic	Pers.	Persian
Gk	Greek	Peruv.	Peruvian
HG	High German	Port.	Portuguese
Hind.	Hindustani	prec.	preceding (entry)
Ind.	Indian	prob.	probably
It.	Italian	S.	South
Jap.	Japanese	Scand.	Scandinavian
L	Latin	Scot.	Scottish
LG	Low German	Sp.	Spanish
lit.	literally	W. Afr.	West African
LL	Late Latin		

Spelling

British spelling has been used throughout this Dictionary, except that where American usage affects the first letter of the word (e.g. aetiology, oedema, oestrius) the headword appears in both places, but the definition is placed with the British spelling. Where the meaning of an American spelt word is required little difficulty will be experienced when the difference occurs towards the end of the word. For example, diarrhea for *diarrhoea*; goit*er* for goitre. When the difference occurs at or near the beginning of a word, the required entry will be elusive since it is far removed from the alphabetical area which is being searched. In cases of difficulty try the following: *ae* or *oe* for *e*; *ei* for *i*; *c* for *k*; *ph* for *f*; *-tre* for- *ter*; *our* for *or*.

Units

Although the change to SI Units is gaining momentum there are still many areas where these are unfamiliar, so in appropriate cases the traditional nomenclature has been shown in parentheses.

In fact, the adoption of SI Units has left basically unchanged many measurement units used in practice, as the SI includes the metre (m), kilogram (kg), second (s) and the degree Celsius (°C) while the litre (l) is accepted as an alternative name for the cubic decimetre (dm^3). Thus the units for volume, the litre and millilitre (ml), have been used. Concentrations in the SI are expressed in molar terms, but as the change-over to SI is rather slow conventional descriptions in terms of weight per volume have been retained. Units which are coming into general use include the "pascal" (Pa) as a unit of pressure and the "joule" (J) as a unit for energy. The pascal has been introduced alongside the measures of pressure in mmHg; 150 mmHg is equivalent to 20 kilopascals (kPa). The joule has been introduced in calorie measures; 2000 kilocalories is equivalent to 8.4 megajoules (MJ).

Anatomical Nomenclature

The primary nomenclature used in this dictionary is that usually known as the Birmingham Revision (the BR); this nomenclature was drawn up by a Committee appointed by the Anatomical Society of

Great Britain and Ireland, and was published in 1933, as the *Final Report of the Committee appointed by the Anatomical Society of Great Britain and Ireland on June 22nd* 1928. The terms appearing in the second column of this publication, headed "English Equivalent, or Latin Form where no English Equivalent is suggested", have been taken as the vocabulary terms. However, the Sixth International Congress of Anatomists, held in Paris in July 1955, unanimously adopted the nomenclature of the *Nomina Anatomica*, the revision of the International Anatomical Committee appointed by the Fifth International Congress of Anatomists held at Oxford in 1950. This new terminology—the NA (Paris)—is now used in anatomical and other textbooks but, since it has only been in widespread use for some 10–12 years, the great majority of medical practitioners will use the BR terminology. For this reason, the dictionary has not yet adopted the NA as a primary nomenclature, although NA terms, including those added at subsequent Congresses in 1960 and 1965, have been incorporated in the anatomical entries. It is anticipated that in future editions, when the majority of doctors will have been educated in the newer terminology, this dictionary will use NA nomenclature throughout.

For the present, in the anatomical entries each BR term is followed in square brackets by the equivalent NA term, e.g. CANAL [CANALIS (NA)], but where the BR and NA terms are identical, the latter is denoted by [NA], e.g. CEREBELLUM [NA]. From each of these publications there have been omissions; where a valid anatomical term has been omitted from the BR, the appropriate term has been taken from a British anatomical textbook, and where such a term has been omitted from the NA nomenclature, the BNA (Basle Nomina Anatomica of 1895, an earlier quasi-international anatomical nomenclature) term, where such occurs, has been used, but in the latter instance, with the initials BNA placed beside it in round brackets within the square brackets. There are, however, some BR terms that have no NA or BNA equivalent.

Widely used obsolete terms, some of which are of historical interest, have been included; certain of these have been briefly defined, but more usually there are cross-references to the appropriate NA term.

Finally, the Anatomical Appendix gives a list of NA terms in alphabetical order in the first column, the corresponding BR term in the second column and in the third column a cross-reference is given to the term under which the definition is to be found.

Chemical Nomenclature and Formulae

The nomenclature used in chemical and biochemical entries conforms largely to the nomenclature recommended by IUPAC.

Systematic names have been run together without the use of hyphens as, for example, DIHYDRODIETHYLSTILBOESTROL. Exceptions have been made in the case of acids, esters, ethers, glycosides, ketones, and salts, e.g. acetylene carboxylic acid, ethyl aminobenzoate, methyl phenyl ketone, etc. Hyphens have been introduced to separate prefixes that distinguish isomers and are represented by symbols, e.g. *m*-, *o*-, and *p*-, D-, L-, and *dl*-; the Greek letters α-, β-, and γ-; atoms carrying substituents, e.g. *N*-, and for positional numbering, e.g. 1,3-dimethyl-4-methyl-4-propionoxy-piperidine. (Such prefixes have been ignored in the alphabetical arrangement of the entries and *N*-METHYL-α-PHENYLSUCCINAMIDE will be found under M, not under N.) In certain cases, however, the hyphen has been resorted to where its use has made for easier reading; thus, the prefix di- has been hyphened in the di-iodo compounds, e.g. di-iodohydroxypropane, to separate the two identical vowels, and phenyl-lactosazone has been hyphened to separate the two identical consonants.

Owing to the frequent practice of using the prefix iso- in contemporary medical publications as part of the name of the isomer, unhyphenated and unitalicized, e.g. isopropyl alcohol, such isomers have been treated as one word throughout the text and the principal iso compounds will be found under I. For similar reasons, the systematic names of important alpha- and beta-acids are given in the entry ACID prefixed by the word alpha- or beta-, e.g. alpha-oxynaphthoic acid, beta-hydroxybutyric acid, and other compounds commonly referred to as alpha- or beta-, e.g. ALPHANAPHTHOL, BETANAPHTHOL, will accordingly be found under the letters A and B respectively.

All chemical formulae are written in linear form, and care has been taken to show the substituent radicals in their correct position in the molecule, as far as this is possible without the use of structural formulae. In the case of cyclic compounds, a horizontal bond has been printed wherever practicable to show linkage of the atoms composing the ring.

Pharmaceutical Nomenclature

Drugs listed in the *British Pharmacopoeia* and the *British Pharmaceutical Codex* are included, in addition to the many other drugs, both old and new, among them new drugs that have been given "approved" names by the British Pharmacopoeia Commission, and others which, though not included in these official publications, are in common use today.

Prior to 1953 the *British Pharmacopoeia* used the Latin name as the "official" name and gave the English equivalent, but in 1953 and subsequently the Commission adopted the English name as the "official" name supported by its Latin equivalent; other publications such as the *British Pharmaceutical Codex* adopted the same procedure for conformity. Consequently the definitions of preparations for which the English "official" names were adopted are to be found under the main English terms whereas those not officially "approved" which still retain their Latin names are defined under the main Latin terms, e.g. Peppermint Oil BP 1958 will be found under OIL, and Oleum Betulae BPC 1949 under OLEUM.

Abbreviations and Symbols

A

A. 1. The chemical symbol for the element argon. 2. Ampere.
Å. Ångström unit.
A. In parasitology, *Acanthocheilonema Achorion, Aëdes, Amblyomma, Ancylostoma, Anopheles, Ascaris, Aspergillus.*
A or a. In anatomy, *angulus*—angle; *arteria*—artery.
α. Alpha, the first letter of the Greek alphabet.
a. In cardiology, the venous wave produced by atrial contraction.
a-. In chemistry, denoting an asymmetric isomer.
A_2. In cardiology, used to denote the second sound in the aortic region.
A.A. Achievement age.
$\overline{AA}$, $\overline{aa}$. In prescribing, an abbreviation used at the end of a group of two or more substances, to indicate that equal quantities of each are to be used.
AAV. Adenovirus-associated virus.
A.B. *Artium Baccalaureus*—Bachelor of Arts.
ABO. *See* Blood GROUP.
abs. Absolute.
abs. feb. In prescriptions, *absente febre*—when fever is absent.
abst. Abstract.
Ac. 1. The chemical symbol for the element actinium. 2. The conventional symbol for the acetyl radical, CH_3CO-. 3. Used also to denote the acyl group.
ac. 1. In electricity, alternating current. 2. In prescriptions, *ante cibum*—before food.
ACC. Anodal closure contraction.
ACCl. Anodal closure clonus.
ACh. Acetylcholine.
ACS. Anticytotoxic serum.
ACTH. Adrenocorticotrophic hormone.
ACTH.R.H. ACTH-releasing hormone.
ad aur. *Ad aurem*—to the ear.
ADC. Analogue to digital converter. Apparatus which receives data in analogue form and converts this to digital form.
add. *Adde*—add (thou).
ADH. Anti-diuretic hormone.
ad lib. *Ad libitum*—at pleasure, freely.
ADMS. Assistant Director of Medical Services.
ADP. Adenosine diphosphate.
adst. feb. *Adstante febre*—in the presence of fever.
AEG. Air encephalogram.
Aero. ***Aerobacter.***
AF. In cardiology, atrial fibrillation.
AFB. Acid-fast bacillus.
Ag. The chemical symbol for the element silver (argentum).
a.h. *Alternis horis*—every other hour.
AHA. 1. Associate Institute of Hospital Administrators. 2. Area Health Authority.
A.H.G. Antihaemophilic globulin.
AI. In cardiology, aortic incompetence.
AIMLT. Associate of the Institute of Medical Laboratory Technology.
Al. The chemical symbol for the element aluminium.
altern. d. *Alternis diebus*—every other day.
A.M. Actomyosin.
Am. 1. Used to denote the ammonium radical, NH_4, in formulae. 2. The chemical symbol for the element americium.
AMA. American Medical Association.
AMP. Adenosine 5′-phosphate.
AMS. Army Medical Service.
amu. Atomic mass unit.
anhydr. Anhydrous.
AOC. Anodal opening contraction.
AOCl. Anodal opening clonus.
AP. Artificial pneumothorax.
a.p. *Ante prandium*—before dinner.
APE. Anterior pituitary extract.
APF. Animal protein factor.
A.P.H. In obstetrics, ante-partum haemorrhage.
approx. Approximately.
APT. Alum-precipitated toxoid.
AQ. Achievement quotient.
aq. ad. *Aquam ad*—water to (e.g. ℥ ii).
aq. dest. *Aqua destillata*—distilled water.
Â QRST. In cardiology, manifest mean QRST axis. *See* GRADIENT, VENTRICULAR.
AR. Analytical reagent.
ARIC. Associate of the Royal Institute of Chemistry.
ARM. 1. In obstetrics, artificial rupture of the membranes. 2. Annual Representative Meeting of the British Medical Association.
ARSH. Associate of the Royal Society for the Promotion of Health.
AS. In cardiology, aortic stenosis.
As. The chemical symbol for the element arsenic.
ASD. In cardiology, atrial septal defect.
ASF. A mounting material in microscopy; composed of aniline, sulphur, and formaldehyde.
At. The chemical symbol for the element astatine.
atm. Atmosphere (pressure).
ATP. Adenosine triphosphate.
ATPase. Adenosine triphosphatase.
at. wt. Atomic weight.
A.U. 1. Alternative abbreviation for Ångström unit. 2. Antitoxic unit; antitoxic serum unit.
Au. The chemical symbol for the element gold (aurum).
AV. In cardiology, atrioventricular or auriculoventricular.
awu. Atomic weight unit.

B

B. The chemical symbol for the element boron.
B. In bacteriology and parasitology, ***Bacillus, Balantidium, Bertiella*** (also ***Bert.***), ***Boophilus.***
β. Beta, the second letter of the Greek alphabet.
BA. 1. Bachelor of Arts. 2. Bromo-acetone.
Ba. The chemical symbol for the element barium.
Bact. ***Bacterium.***
BAL. British Anti-Lewisite.
BAO. Bachelor of the Art of Obstetrics.
BAPN. Beta-aminopropionitrile.

Bart. *Bartonella.*
B.B.A. In obstetrics, born before arrival (of doctor or midwife).
BBC. Bromobenzylcyanide.
B.C., B.Ch., or **B.Chir.** Bachelor of Surgery.
B.C.G. Bacille Calmette-Guérin.
bcg. Ballistocardiogram.
B.Ch.D. Bachelor of Dental Surgery.
b.d. *Bis die*—twice a day.
B.D.A. British Dental Association.
BDS. Bachelor of Dental Surgery.
BDSc. Bachelor of Dental Science.
Be. The chemical symbol for the element beryllium.
Bert. *Bertiella.*
BHyg. Bachelor of Hygiene.
Bi. The chemical symbol for the element bismuth.
b.i.d. *Biduum*—two days.
Bk. The chemical symbol for the element berkelium.
BM. Bachelor of Medicine.
B.M.A. British Medical Association.
BMedSc. Bachelor of Medical Science.
BMR, b.m.r. Basal metabolic rate.
BNA. *Basle* (*Basel*) *Nomina Anatomica.*
BNF. *British National Formulary.*
BP. 1. Blood pressure. 2. *British Pharmacopoeia.*
bp. Boiling point.
BPC. *British Pharmaceutical Codex.*
BPharm. Bachelor of Pharmacology.
BR. Birmingham Revision (of anatomical nomenclature).
Br. The chemical symbol for the element bromine.
Br. *Brucella.*
BS. 1. Bachelor of Surgery. 2. British Standard.
BSc. Bachelor of Science.
BSR. Blood sedimentation rate.
BTU. Board of Trade Unit.
BThU. British thermal unit.
Bz. In chemical formulae, benzoyl.

C

C. 1. Coulomb. 2. The chemical symbol for the element carbon. 3. Congius (gallon measure).
C or **c.** In anatomy, condyle.
C. In bacteriology and parasitology, ***Ceratophyllus, Cimex, Corynebacterium, Culex, Culicoides.***
°C. Degree Celsius (or centigrade).
c. 1. *Circa*—about. 2. In cardiology, the venous wave occurring early in systole.
C 5. Pentamethonium.
C 6. Hexamethonium.
C 10. Decamethonium.
Ca. 1. The chemical symbol for the element calcium. 2. Cathode.
CAH. 1. Cyanacetic acid hydrazine. 2. Congenital adrenal hyperplasia.
Cal. Large calorie; always expressed with capital initial letter.
cal. Small calorie; always expressed without capital initial letter.
calc. In table headings, calculated.
CAP. Chloro-acetophenone.
cc. Cubic centimetre or cubic centimetres (ml preferred).
CCC. Cathodal closure contraction.
CCCl. Cathodal closure clonus.
CCF. In ward notes, congestive cardiac failure.
Cd. The chemical symbol for the element cadmium.
cd. Candela.
Ce. The chemical symbol for the element cerium.
Cf. The chemical symbol for the element californium.
CFT. Complement-fixation test.
cg. Centigram.
CG. Chorionic gonadotrophin.
CGI. Carbimazole.
cgm. Centigram.
CG—P. Chorionic growth hormone prolactin.
C.G.S., cgs. Centimetre-gram-second.
Ch. *Chrysops.*
CH. cH. The symbol for the concentration of hydrogen ion, i.e. the number of grams ionized of hydrogen per litre of a solution. The logarithm of its reciprocal is the pH value.
ChB. Bachelor of Surgery.
ChE. Cholinesterase.
ChM. Master of Surgery.
CI. Colour index (of the blood).
Ci. Curie.
c.i.s. Central inhibitory state.
Cl. The chemical symbol for the element chlorine.
Cl. *Clostridium.*
Clon. *Clonorchis.*
Cm. The chemical symbol for the element curium.
cm. Centimetre.
cm². Square centimetre.
CMA. Canadian Medical Association.
CMB. Central Midwives Board.
CNAA. Council for National Academic Awards.
CNS, cns. Central nervous system.
Co. 1. In prescriptions, *compositus*—compound. 2. The chemical symbol for the element cobalt.
Co 60. Cobalt 60.
CoA. Co-enzyme A.
COC. Cathodal opening contraction.
COCl. Cathodal opening clonus.
Coeff. Coefficient.
CON. Cyclopropane, oxygen and nitrogen, a non-flammable mixture of anaesthetic gases.
c.p. Candle power.
CPB. Cetyl pyridinium bromide.
CPH. Certificate in Public Health.
Cr. The chemical symbol for the element chromium.
CRCP. Certificant Royal College of Physicians.
CRCS. Certificant Royal College of Surgeons.
C.R.H. Corticotrophin releasing hormone.
CRM. Cross-reacting material.
C.R.P. C-reative protein. *See* PROTEIN.
C.S. In obstetrics, caesarian section.
Cs. The chemical symbol for the element caesium.
c/s. Cycles per second (hertz, Hz).
CSF, c.s.f. Cerebrospinal fluid.
C.T. In ward notes, coronary thrombosis or cerebral tumour.
Ct. *Ctenocephalides, Ctenocephalus.*
CTAB. Cetrimide.
ct/min. Counts per minute.
Cu. The chemical symbol for the element copper. [L *cuprum.*]
cu. Cubic.
c.μm. Cubic micron.
C.V. In obstetrics, conjugate vera, the true conjugate.
C.V.P. Central venous pressure.
CWR. Cardiolipin Wassermann reaction.
Cy. The chemical symbol for the element cyclonium.
Cyl. In ophthalmology, cylinder.

D

D. 1. In optics, dioptre. 2. The chemical symbol for the hydrogen isotope, deuterium.
D. In parasitology, *Dientamoeba, Dinopsyllus, Diphyllobothrium, Dirofilaria, Dracunculus.*
d. Density.
Δ or δ. Delta.
DA. Diphenylchlorarsine.
DA. Diploma in Anaesthetics.
DADPS. Dapsone; 4,4-diaminodiphenyl-sulphone.
D.A.H. Disordered action of the heart.
DAPT. Amiphenazole; 2,4-diamino-5-phenylthiazole.
DAvMed. Diploma in Aviation Medicine.
dB. Decibel.
DBA. Dibenzanthracene.
DC. Diphenylcyanarsine.
dc. Direct current.
DCA. Deoxycortone acetate.
DCH. Diploma in Child Health.
DCh. Doctor of Surgery.
DCP. Diploma in Clinical Pathology.
DCTMA. Deoxycortone trimethyl acetate.
d.d. In prescriptions, *de die*—daily.
DDMS. Deputy Director of Medical Services.
DDO. Diploma in Dental Orthopaedics.
DDS. Doctor of Dental Surgery.
DDSc. Doctor of Dental Science.
DDST. Denver Developmental Screening Test.
DDT. Dicophane; dichlorodiphenyltrichloro-ethane.
deg. Degree.
dest. *Destillatus*—distilled.
DFP. Dyflos; di-isopropylfluorophosphonate.
DGO. Diploma in Gynaecology and Obstetrics.
DHA. Dehydroepiandrosterone.
1,25DHcc. 1,25-Dihydroxycholecalciferol.
DHO 180. Dihydroergocornine.
DHyg. Doctor of Hygiene.
DIH. Diploma in Industrial Health.
dil. Dilute.
Dip. Bact. Diploma in Bacteriology.
Dip. Microbiol. Diploma in Microbiology.
***dl*-.** In chemistry, prefix denoting a racemic compound.
DLO. Diploma in Laryngology and Otology.
DM. Diphenylaminechlorarsine.
DM. Doctor of Medicine.
dm. Decimetre.
DMJ. Diploma of Medical Jurisprudence.
DMR. Diploma in Medical Radiology.
DMRD. Diploma in Medical Radio-Diagnosis.
DMRE. Diploma in Medical Radiology and Electrology.
DMRT. Diploma in Medical Radio-Therapy.
DMS. Director of Medical Services.
DNA. Deoxyribonucleic acid.
DNTP. Dinitrothiophosphate. *See* ORGANOPHOSPHATES.
DO. Diploma in Ophthalmology.
DObstRCOG. Diploma in Obstetrics of the Royal College of Obstetrics and Gynaecology.
DOCA. Deoxycortone acetate.
DOMS. Diploma in Ophthalmology, Medicine, and Surgery.
DOPA. Dihydroxyphenylalanine.
DOrth. Diploma in Orthodontics.
DP. Diploma in Pathology.
DPD. Diploma in Public Dentistry.
DPH. Diploma in Public Health.
DPh. Doctor of Philosophy.
DPhysMed. Diploma in Physical Medicine.
DPM. Diploma in Psychological Medicine.
DPsych. Diploma in Psychiatry.
DR. Diploma in Radiology.
dr. Drachm or drachms.
DRCPath. Diploma of the Royal College of Pathologists.
DRM. Diploma in Radiation Medicine.
DS. Doctor of Surgery.
DSc. Doctor of Science.
d. seq. In prescriptions, *die sequente*—on the following day.
DSM. Diploma in Social Medicine.
DSSc. Diploma in Sanitary Science.
DTCD. Diploma in Tuberculous and Chest Diseases.
DTCH. Diploma in Tropical Child Health.
DTD. Diploma in Tuberculous Diseases.
DTH. Diploma in Tropical Hygiene.
DTM. Diploma in Tropical Medicine.
DTM & H. Diploma in Tropical Medicine and Hygiene.
DTPH. Diploma in Tropical Public Health.
dur. In prescriptions, *durus*—hard.
Dy. The chemical symbol for the rare-earth element, dysprosium.
dyn. Dyne.

E

E. Emmetropia.
E or e. In anatomy, epicondyle.
E. 1. In parasitology, *Echinococcus, Echinostoma, Eimeria, Endamoeba* (in USA), *Endolimax, Entamoeba, Enterobius, Enteromonas.* 2. Electrode potential.
E3. Lachesine chloride.
EC. Electron capture.
ECF, ecf. Extracellular fluid.
ECG, ecg. Electrocardiogram.
ECoG. Electrocorticogram.
ECT, ect. Electroconvulsive therapy.
E.D. Erythema dose.
ED_{50}. Median effective dose.
E.D.D. In obstetrics, expected date of delivery.
EDTA. Ethylenediamine tetra-acetic acid.
EEG, e.e.g. Electro-encephalogram.
Emb. In parasitology, *Embadomonas.*
EMF. Endomyocardial fibrosis.
emf. Electromotive force.
EMAS. Employment Medical Advisory Service.
EMG, e.m.g. Electromyogram.
EMS. Emergency Medical Service.
emu. Electromagnetic unit.
ENT. Ear, nose, and throat.
EP. *Extra Pharmacopoeia.*
eqn. Equation.
equiv. Equivalent.
Er. The chemical symbol for the element erbium.
ERG, e.r.g. Electroretinogram.
ERPF. Effective renal plasma flow.
Ery. In bacteriology, *Erysipelothrix.*
Es. The chemical symbol for the element einsteinium.
Esch. In bacteriology, *Escherichia.*
esp. Extrasensory perception.
ESR. Erythrocyte sedimentation rate.
e.s.r. Electron spin resonance.
esu. Electrostatic unit.
Et. In chemical formulae, ethyl.
Eu. The chemical symbol for the element europium.
EUA. In obstetrics, examination under anaesthetic.
eV. Electron volt.
EVA. Extravehicular activity. *See* ACTIVITY.
ex aq. In prescriptions, *ex aqua*—in water.
ext. In prescriptions, *extractum*—extract.

F

F. 1. Fahrenheit. 2. Farad. 3. The chemical symbol for the element fluorine.
F or f. In anatomy, fascia, facies, fontanelle and fossa.
F. In bacteriology and parasitology, *Fasciola, Fasciolopsis, Fusiformis.*
F_1. In genetics, the first filial generation, the offspring of the parental generation (P_1).
F_2. In genetics, the second filial generation, the offspring of members of F_1.
F.A. Fluorescent antibody.
FACA. Fellow of the American College of Anaesthetists.
FACC. Fellow of the American College of Cardiology.
FACDS. Fellow of the Australian College of Dental Surgeons.
FACG. Fellow of the American College of Gastroenterology.
FACMA. Fellow of the Australian College of Medical Administrators.
FACO. Fellow of the American College of Otolaryngology.
FACOG. Fellow of the American College of Obstetricians and Gynaecologists.
FACP. Fellow of the American College of Physicians.
FACR. Fellow of the American College of Radiology.
FACS. Fellow of the American College of Surgeons.
FBPsS. Fellow of the British Psychological Society.
FCAP. Fellow of the College of American Pathologists.
FCCP. Fellow of the American College of Chest Physicians.
FCMS. Fellow of the College of Medicine & Surgery.
FCPath. Fellow of the College of Pathologists.
FCPS. Fellow of the College of Physicians and Surgeons.
FCRA. Fellow of the College of Radiologists, Australasia.
FCS. Fellow of the Chemical Society.
FCSP. Fellow of the Chartered Society of Physiotherapy.
FDNB. Fluorodinitrobenzene.
FDS. Fellow in Dental Surgery.
FDS RCS Ed. Fellow in Dental Surgery of the Royal College of Surgeons of Edinburgh.
FDS RCS Eng. Fellow in Dental Surgery of the Royal College of Surgeons of England.
Fe. The chemical symbol for the element iron.
feb. dur. In prescriptions, *febris durante*—during fever.
FFA. Fatty acids, free.
FFA RCS. Fellow of the Faculty of Anaesthetists, Royal College of Surgeons.
FFD. In radiology, focus–film distance.
FFHom. Fellow of the Faculty of Homoeopathy.
FFR. Fellow of the Faculty of Radiologists.
F.H. In obstetrics, fetal heart as heard through the abdominal wall by auscultation.
FIBiol. Fellow of the Institute of Biology.
FICS. Fellow of the International College of Surgeons.
figlu. Formiminoglutamic acid.
FIMLS. Fellow of the Institute of Medical Laboratory Sciences.
FLA. In obstetrics, frontolaeva anterior position of the brow presentation. *See* PRESENTATION.
flav. In prescriptions, *flavus*—yellow.
fl.dr. In prescriptions, fluid drachm.
fl.oz. In prescriptions, fluid ounce.
FLS. Fellow of the Linnean Society.
fm. 1. Fathom. 2. The chemical symbol for the element fermium.
FMC. Fellow of the Medical Council.
fort. In prescriptions, *fortis* or *forte*—strong.
f.p. Freezing point.
FPS. Fellow of the Pharmaceutical Society.
f.p.s. Foot-pound second.
Fr. The chemical symbol for the element francium.
FRACDS. Fellow of the Royal Australasian College of Dental Surgery.
FRACGP. Fellow of the Royal Australian College of General Practitioners.
FRACP & S. Fellow of the Royal Australian Colleges of Physicians and Surgeons.
FRAI. Fellow of the Royal Anthropological Institute.
FRCD. Fellow of the Royal College of Dentists.
FRCGP. Fellow of the Royal College of General Practitioners.
FRCOG. Fellow of the Royal College of Obstetricians and Gynaecologists.
FRCP. Fellow of the Royal College of Physicians.
FRCPA. Fellow of the Royal College of Pathologists, Australasia.
FRCPath. Fellow of the Royal College of Pathologists.
FRCPC. Fellow of the Royal College of Physicians of Canada.
FRCPEd. Fellow of the Royal College of Physicians of Edinburgh.
FRCPI. Fellow of the Royal College of Physicians of Ireland.
FRCPsych. Fellow of the Royal College of Psychiatrists.
FRCR. Fellow of the Royal College of Radiology.
FRCS. Fellow of the Royal College of Surgeons.
FRCSC. Fellow of the Royal College of Surgeons of Canada.
FRCSEd. Fellow of the Royal College of Surgeons of Edinburgh.
FRCSI. Fellow of the Royal College of Surgeons in Ireland.
FRCVS. Fellow of the Royal College of Veterinary Surgeons.
FRES. Fellow of the Royal Entomological Society.
FRFPS. Fellow of the Royal Faculty of Physicians and Surgeons.
FRIC. Fellow of the Royal Institute of Chemistry.
FRIPHH. Fellow of the Royal Institute of Public Health and Hygiene.
FRMS. Fellow of the Royal Microscopical Society.
FRS. Fellow of the Royal Society.
FRSC. Fellow of the Royal Society of Canada.
FRSE. Fellow of the Royal Society of Edinburgh.
FRSH. Fellow of the Royal Society of Health.
F.S.D. In radiology, focus–skin distance.
f.s.d. Full-scale deflection.
FSH. Follicle-stimulating hormone.
FSH R.H. FSH releasing hormone.
FSS. Fellow of the Royal Statistical Society.
FT. Formol toxoid.
FT_4I. Free thyroxine index.
ft. 1. In prescriptions, *fiat*—let it be made. 2. Foot.
ft.c. Foot-candle.
ft.lb. Foot-pound.
ft/min. Feet per minute.
ft/sec. Feet per second.
F.U.O. Fever of unknown (or uncertain) origin.
FZS. Fellow of the Zoological Society.

G

G. 1. In magnetism, gauss. 2. In the *British Pharmacopoeia*, the abbreviation for gram (when stating doses). 3. Giga-, $10^9\times$.
G. In parasitology, *Gastrodiscus, Gastrophilus, Giardia, Glossina, Gnathostoma, Gordius.*
g. Gram.
g. The symbol for the acceleration due to the earth's gravity.
γ. 1. Gamma, the third letter of the Greek alphabet. 2. Microgram.
$\gamma\gamma$. Micro-microgram.
Ga. The chemical symbol for the element gallium.
gal. Gallon.
gal/min. Gallons per minute.
g-cal. Gram-calorie or small calorie.
GCFT. Gonococcal complement-fixation test.
Gd. The chemical symbol for the element gadolinium.
Ge. The chemical symbol for the element germanium.

GFR, g.f.r. Glomerular filtration rate.
GH. Growth hormone.
GHRF. Growth hormone releasing factor.
g-ion. Gram-ion.
Glc. Glucose.
g.l.c. Gas-liquid chromatography.
GMC. General Medical Council.
g-mol. Gram-molecule.
GNC. General Nursing Council.
GO-T. Glutamic-oxalacetic transaminase.
GP. General practitioner.
GPB. Glossopharyngeal breathing.
GPI. General paralysis of the insane.
GP-T. Glutamic-pyruvic transaminase.
gr. Grain.
gt. In prescriptions, *gutta*—drop.
GTP. Guanosine triphosphate.
gtt. In prescriptions, *guttae*—drops.
guttat. In prescriptions, *guttatum*—drop by drop.

H

H. 1. Henry. 2. The chemical symbol for the element hydrogen. 3. The symbol for dose equivalent.
H. In bacteriology and parasitology, *Haemagogus, Haemaphysalis, Haemophilus, Heterodera, Heterophyes, Hippelates, Hymenolepis, Hypoderma.*
h. 1. In prescriptions, *hora*—hour, at the hour of. 2. Hecto- ($10^2\times$).
h. The symbol for Planck's constant.
H^+. The symbol for the hydrogen ion.
$[H^+]$. The symbol for the concentration of hydrogen ion.
H^2. The symbol for the hydrogen isotope, heavy hydrogen or deuterium.
Ha. In ophthalmology, absolute hypermetropia.
haust. In prescriptions, *haustus*—draught.
Hb. Haemoglobin.
H.C.C. 25-Hydroxychole calciferol.
HCG. Human chorionic gonadotrophin.
h.d. In prescriptions, *hora decubitus*—at bediime.
HDD. Higher Dental Diploma.
HE. Haematoxylin and eosin.
He. The chemical symbol for the element helium.
HETP. Hexa-ethyltetraphosphate.
Hf. 1. The chemical symbol for the element hafnium. 2. In ophthalmology, facultative hypermetropia.
h.f. In electricity, high frequency.
Hg. The chemical symbol for the element mercury (hydrargyrum).
HGH. Human growth hormone.
5-HIAA. 5-Hydroxyindole acetic acid.
His. Histidine.
Hl. In ophthalmology, latent hypermetropia.
Hm. In ophthalmology, manifest hypermetropia.
H.M.G. Human menopausal gonadotrophin.
H.M.M.A. 4-Hydroxy-3-methoxy mandelic acid.
Ho. The chemical symbol for the element holmium.
HPC. Hydroxyphenylcinchoninic acid.
HPL. Human placental lactogen.
h.s. In prescriptions, *hora somni*—at bedtime.
HSA. Human serum albumin.
hst. In prescriptions, *haustus*—draught.
5-HT. 5-Hydroxytryptamine.
Ht. In ophthalmology, total hypermetropia.
ht. Height.
h.t. In electricity, high tension.
H.V.A. Homovanillic acid.
Hz. Hertz.

I

I. 1. The chemical symbol for the element iodine. 2. *See* Blood GROUP.
I. In parasitology, *Iodamoeba, Isospora, Ixodes.*
i.a. Intra-arterial.
IB. In immunology, immune body.
IC. Internal conversion.
ICF, i.c.f. Intracellular fluid.
ICN. International Council of Nurses.
ICRP. International Commission on Radiological Protection.
ICRU. International Committee on Radiological Units and Measurements.
ICSH. Interstitial-cell-stimulating hormone.
IF. In haematology, intrinsic factor.
Il. The chemical symbol for the element illinium.
i.m. Intramuscular.
In. The chemical symbol for the element indium.
in. Inch.
INI. Intranuclear inclusion.
IP. *International Pharmacopoeia.*
IPL. *Indian Pharmacopoeial List.*
IPPR. Intermittent positive-pressure respiration.
IPPV. Intermittent positive-pressure ventilation.
IQ. Intelligence quotient.
i.r. Infrared.
Ir. The chemical symbol for the element iridium.
i.s.q. *In statu quo.*
IT. Isomeric transition. *See* TRANSITION.
iu. 1. International unit, e.g. for vitamins. 2. Immunizing unit.
IUD. In obstetrics, intra-uterine death.
IV. Intravenous.
iv. Iodine value.
IVP, i.v.p. Intravenous pyelogram.
IZS. Insulin zinc suspension.

J

J. Joule.
JNA. *Jena Nomina Anatomica.*
JVP. Jugular venous pressure.

K

K. 1. The chemical symbol for the element potassium (*kalium*). 2. The symbol for the kelvin, the unit of thermodynamic temperature. 3. In chemistry and physics the usual symbol for a constant, in particular the equilibrium constant in mass action, the dissociation or ionization constant and the solubility product. 4. Kappa.
K. In parasitology, *Katayama*.
k. Kilo, a prefix signifying $\times 10^3$.
keV. One thousand electron volts $= 10^3$ eV.
Kf. An immunological symbol used for indicating the speed of flocculation in antigen–antibody reactions.
kg. Kilogram.
kg-cal. Kilogram calorie or large calorie.
kg.m. Kilogram-metre.
km. Kilometre.
km.h. Kilometres per hour.
kΩ. Kilohm.
K.P. In ophthalmology, keratitic precipitates.
Kr. The chemical symbol for the element krypton.
17-KS. 17-Ketosteroids.
kV. Kilovolt.
kW. Kilowatt.
kWh. Kilowatt hour.

L

L. 1. Latin. 2. In ophthalmology, signifying light sense.
L. In bacteriology and parasitology, *Lactobacillus, Leishmania, Leptomonas, Leptopsylla, Leptospira, Leuconostoc, Liponyssus, Loa, Lucilia, Lymnaea*.
L-. A prefix in chemistry denoting a laevorotatory compound, also expressed by prefix (−).
l. Left, litre, length.
λ. The symbol for wavelength.
L_0. Immunological symbol (Ehrlich's) for *limes nul*.
L_+. Immunological symbol for *limes* (or *limit*) of *death*: Ehrlich's *limes tod*.
L. and A. In ophthalmology, light and accommodation.
La. The chemical symbol for the element lanthanum.
LAA. LATS absorbing activity.
LAH. Licentiate of Apothecaries Hall, Dublin.
LATS. Long-acting thyroid stimulator.
lb. A pound (*libra*) in weight.
LCPS. Licentiate College Physicians & Surgeons.
LD. In pharmacology, lethal dose.
LD_{50}. Literally, lethal dose 50 per cent. That dose of radiation which, when absorbed by members of a population, will result in the death of 50 per cent of that population.
LDA. In obstetrics, left dorso-anterior position of the fetus *in utero* or at delivery. *See* PRESENTATION.
LDP. In obstetrics, left dorsoposterior position of the fetus *in utero* or at delivery. *See* PRESENTATION.
LDS. Licentiate in Dental Surgery.
LDSc. Licentiate in Dental Science.
LE. Left eye.
L_f. Immunological symbol for *limes* (or *limit*) of *flocculation*.
lf. In electricity, low frequency.
LFA. In obstetrics, left fronto-anterior position of the brow presentation. *See* PRESENTATION.
LFD. In pharmacology, least fatal dose.
LFL. In obstetrics, left frontolateral position of the brow presentation. *See* PRESENTATION.
LFP. In obstetrics, left frontoposterior position of the brow presentation. *See* PRESENTATION.
LH. Luteinizing hormone. *See* HORMONE.
Li. The chemical symbol for the element lithium.
Lig. or **lig.** In anatomy, *ligamentum*—ligament.
Ligg. or **ligg.** In anatomy, *ligamenta*—ligaments.
LLCO. Licentiate of the London College of Osteopathy.
LM. Licentiate in Midwifery.
LMA. In obstetrics, the left mento-anterior position of the brow presentation. *See* PRESENTATION.
LMCC. Licentiate of the Medical Council of Canada.
LML. In obstetrics, left mentolateral position of the brow presentation. *See* PRESENTATION.
LMP. In obstetrics, (*a*) last menstrual period (1st day of); (*b*) left mentoposterior position of the fetus *in utero* or at delivery. *See* PRESENTATION.
LMS. Licentiate in Medicine and Surgery.
LMSSA. Licentiate in Medicine and Surgery, Society of Apothecaries.
LOA. In obstetrics, the left occipito-anterior position of the vertex presentation. *See* PRESENTATION.
LOL. In obstetrics, left occipitolateral position of the vertex presentation. *See* PRESENTATION.
LOP. In obstetrics, the left occipitoposterior position of the vertex presentation. *See* PRESENTATION.
Lr. The chemical symbol for the element lawrencium.
L_r. Immunological symbol for *limes* (or *limit*) of *reaction*.
LRCP. Licentiate of the Royal College of Physicians of London.
LRCPEd. Licentiate of the Royal College of Physicians, Edinburgh.
LRCPI. Licentiate of the Royal College of Physicians, Ireland.
LRCSEd. Licentiate of the Royal College of Surgeons, Edinburgh.
LRCSI. Licentiate of the Royal College of Surgeons, Ireland.
LRFPS. Licentiate of the Royal Faculty of Physicians and Surgeons.
LSA. 1. In obstetrics, the left sacro-anterior position of the breech presentation. *See* PRESENTATION. 2. Former abbreviation for the Licentiateship of the Society of Apothecaries, now LMSSA (see above).
LSCS. In obstetrics, lower segment caesarean section.
LSD. Lysergic acid diethylamide; lysergide.
LSL. In obstetrics, left sacrolateral position of the breech presentation. *See* PRESENTATION.
LSP. In obstetrics, the left sacroposterior position of the breech presentation. *See* PRESENTATION.
LTH. Luteotrophic hormone.
Lu. The chemical symbol for the element lutetium.
lx. Lux.

M

M. 1. Molar concentration. 2. In chemical formulae, the symbol for any unspecified metal. 3. In ophthalmology, media, myopia. 4. Mega-, denoting one million.
M. In bacteriology and parasitology, *Mansonia, Mansonioides, Melania, Micrococcus, Moniliformis, Moraxella, Multiceps, Musca, Mycobacterium*.

♏. In prescriptions, minim.
M or m. In anatomy, *musculus*—muscle; *margo*—border.
m. 1. Metre. 2. Milli-; denoting one thousandth part of a unit. 3. In prescriptions, *mane*—in the morning; *misce*—mix.
μ. 1. The Greek letter mu. 2. Micron (preferably use micrometre, μm). 3. Muon; magnetic permeability; refractive index. 4. Micro-, denoting one millionth part of a unit.
***m*-.** In chemistry, a prefix denoting the meta-position.
***μ*-.** In chemistry, a prefix denoting the meso-position.
M_1. Mitral first sound.
M_2. Mitral second sound.
mA. Milliampere.
MACD. Member of the Australasian College of Dermatology.
MACGP. Member of the Australasian College of General Practitioners.
MACO. Member of the Australian College of Ophthalmologists.
MACR. Member of the American College of Radiology.
mAm. Milliampere minute.
MAO. Master in Obstetrics.
mAs. Milliampere second.
max. Maximum.
MB. Bachelor of Medicine.
mc. Millicurie (now mCi).
μc. Microcurie (now μCi).
mcD. Millicurie-destroyed (now mCiD).
MC. Master of Surgery.
MCB. Master of Clinical Biochemistry.
MCD. In haematology, mean corpuscular diameter.
MCFP. Member of the College of Family Physicians.
MCh. Master of Surgery.
MCH. In haematology, mean corpuscular haemoglobin.
MCHC. In haematology, mean corpuscular haemoglobin concentration.
MChD. Master of Dental Surgery.
MChir. Master of Surgery.
MChOrth. Master of Orthopaedic Surgery.
MChOtol. Master of Otology.
MCommH. Master of Community Health.
MCPath. Member of the College of Pathologists.
MCPA. Member of the College of Pathologists, Australasia.
MCPS. Member of the College of Physicians & Surgeons.
MCRA. Member of the College of Radiologists, Australasia.
MCSP. Member of the Chartered Society of Physiotherapy.
M.C.V. In haematology, mean corpuscular volume.
MD. Doctor of Medicine.
Md. The chemical symbol for the element mendelevium.
m.d. In prescriptions, *more dicto*—(use) as directed.
MDD. Doctor of Dental Medicine.
MDentSc. Master in Dental Science.
MDS. Master of Dental Surgery.
Me. A purely conventional symbol for the methyl radical, CH_3.
MEA. Multiple endocrine adenopathy.
MED. Minimal erythema dose.
mEq or m.equiv. Milli-equivalent.
m. et v. In prescriptions, *mane et vespere*—morning and evening.
MeV. Million electron volts = 10^6 eV.
MF. Megafarad.
Mf or mf. In parasitology, microfilaria.
μF. Microfarad.
MFA. Methyl fluoroacetate.
MFCM. Member of the Faculty of Community Medicine.
MFHom. Member of the Faculty of Homoeopathy.
Mg. 1. The chemical symbol for the element magnesium. 2. A recently discovered antigen sub-grouped to the MNSs system.
mg. Milligram.
μg. Microgram.
MHD. Minimum haemolytic dose.
MHyg. Master of Hygiene.
MI. In cardiology, mitral incompetence.
MIBiol. Member of the Institute of Biology.
m.i.c. Minimal inhibitory concentration.
MID. Minimum infective dose.
m.i.d. Minimal inhibitory dose.
MIH. Master of Industrial Health.
mil. Millilitre (now ml).
min. Minimum; minute; minim.
MIO. Minimum identifiable odour.
mist. *Mistura*—a mixture.
mitt. In prescriptions, *mitte*—send.
ml. Millilitre.
μl. Microlitre.
MLA. In obstetrics, mentolaevo anterior position of the face presentation. *See* PRESENTATION.
MLD. Minimum lethal dose.
Mm or mm. In anatomy, *musculi*—muscles.
mM. Millimol (now mmol).
mmHg. Millimetres of mercury pressure.
mmol. Millimol.
mm. Millimetre.
MMed. Master of Medicine.
μμ. Micromicron (preferably use picometre, pm).
μμF. Micromicrofarad (now picofarad, pF).
μmg. Micromilligram (now nanogram, ng).
μμg. Micromicrogram (now picogram, pg).
MMSA. Master of Midwifery of the Society of Apothecaries.
Mn. The chemical symbol for the element manganese.
MNSs. *See* Blood GROUP.
MO. Medical officer.
Mo. The chemical symbol for the element molybdenum.
MΩ. Megohm.
μΩ. Microhm.
MO & G. Master of Obstetrics & Gynaecology.
MOH. Medical Officer of Health.
mol. Mole, molecule, molecular.
mol/l. Moles per litre.
mol.wt. Molecular weight.
m.p. 1. Melting point. 2. In prescriptions, *mane primo*—early in the morning.
mpc. Maximum permissible concentration.
MPH. Master of Public Health.
MPharm. Master in Pharmacy.
MPS. Member of the Pharmaceutical Society.
MPsyMed. Master of Psychological Medicine.
MR. In cardiology, mitral regurgitation.
mR or mr. Milliroentgen.
μR or μr. Microroentgen.
MRACGP. Member of the Royal Australasian College of General Practitioners.
MRACP. Member of the Royal Australasian College of Physicians.
MRACR. Member of the Royal Australasian College of Radiologists.
MRad. Master of Radiology.
MRCP. Member of the Royal College of Physicians.
MRCPath. Member of the Royal College of Pathologists.
MRCS. Member of the Royal College of Surgeons.
MRCVS. Member of the Royal College of Veterinary Surgeons.
MRD. Minimum reacting dose.
MRIH. Melanocyte-stimulating-hormone-release-inhibiting hormone.
MRSH. Member of the Royal Society of Health.
MS. 1. Master of Surgery. 2. In cardiology, mitral stenosis.
MSc. Master of Science.
MSH. Melanocyte-stimulating hormone.
μs, μsec. Microsecond.
mu. Mouse unit.
MV. Megavolt.
mV. Millivolt.
μV. Microvolt.
Myco. *Mycobacterium.*

N

N. 1. The chemical symbol for the element nitrogen. 2. Newton. 3. The symbol for *normal* as it refers to solutions used in volumetric analysis.
N. In bacteriology and parasitology, *Necator, Neisseria, Nitrobacter, Nocardia.*
N or **n.** In anatomy, *nervus*—nerve.
N-. In chemical nomenclature, denoting that the radical which follows is attached to the nitrogen atom.
n. Nano- ($10^{-9}\times$).
n. 1. The symbol for refractive index. 2. In prescriptions, *nocte*—at night. 3. In cytogenetics, the symbol used to indicate a chromosome set. It is usually preceded by a number which indicates the degree of ploidy, for example 2n (diploid), 3n (triploid), and so on.
***n*-.** In organic chemistry, a prefix denoting the normal form of several isomers.
N/1. In volumetric analysis, normal, normal solution, and with a figure, fractions of normal, e.g. N/10 = one-tenth of normal.
NA. 1. In optics, numerical aperture. 2. Nomina Anatomica.
Na. The chemical symbol for the element sodium. [L *natrium.*]
NAD. Accepted abbreviations for the oxidized and reduced forms of nicotinamide adenine dinucleotide (coenzyme I) are NAD and $NADH_2$ or NAD^+ and NADH.
NAD. No appreciable disease—no abnormality discovered.
NADP. Accepted abbreviations for the oxidized and reduced forms of nicotinamide adenine dinucleotide phosphate (coenzyme II) are NADP and $NADPH_2$ or $NADP^+$ and NADPH.
NAPT. National Association for the Prevention of Tuberculosis.
Nb. The chemical symbol for the element niobium.
nCi. Nanocurie.
Nd. The chemical symbol for the element neodymium.
Ne. The chemical symbol for the element neon.
neb. In prescriptions, *nebula*—a spray.
NEFA. Non-esterified fatty acids.
NEM. Nahrungs Einheit Milch. *See* NEM.
n. et m. In prescriptions, *nocte et mane*—night and morning.
ng. Nanogram.
NHI. National Health Insurance.
NHS. National Health Service.
Ni. The chemical symbol for the element nickel.
NIH. National Institute of Health (USA).
NK. Nomenklatur Kommission, a committee of the Anatomy Society of Germany that has recommended certain anatomical names.
nm. Nanometre.
nmol. Nanomol.
n.m.r. Nuclear magnetic resonance.
Nn or **nn.** In anatomy, *nervi*—nerves.
NND. In vital statistics, neonatal death.
NNN. In parasitology, Novy–Nicolle–McNeal culture medium.
N.N.R. *New and Nonofficial Remedies.*
No. 1. Number. 2. The chemical symbol for the element nobelium.
nov. sp. In entomology, *nova species*—new species.
Np. The chemical symbol for the element neptunium.
NPL. National Physics Laboratory.
NPN. In biochemistry, non-protein nitrogen.
NSD. Nominal standard dose.
NTP. Normal temperature and pressure.
NYD. Not yet diagnosed.

O

O. 1. In prescriptions, *octarius*—a pint. 2. The chemical symbol for the element oxygen.
O. In parasitology, *Onchocerca, Oncomelania, Opisthorchis, Ornithodorus.*
***o*-.** In chemistry, the symbol for the ortho-position.
Ω. Ohm.
o.alt.hor. In prescriptions, *omnibus alternis horis*—every other hour.
OD or **o.d.** *Oculus dexter*—right eye.
OE. In parasitology, *Oesophagostomum.*
OER. Oxygen enhancement ratio.
17-OHCS. 17-Hydroxycorticosteroids.
OL or **o.l.** *Oculus laevus*—left eye.
ol. *Oleum*—oil.
o.m. In prescriptions, *omni mane*—every morning.
omn. bid. In prescriptions, *omni biduo*—every 2 days.
OMPA. Octamethyl pyrophosphoramide.
o.n. In prescriptions, *omni nocte*—every night.
OPD. Outpatients' Department.
Os. The chemical symbol for the element osmium.
OT. Old tuberculin.
ov. *Ovum*—an egg.
OX_2. A strain of *Proteus* used in the diagnosis of tick-borne typhus.
OX_{19}. A strain of *Proteus* agglutinated by the blood of patients with classical (louse-borne) typhus.
oz. In prescriptions, *uncia*—an ounce.

P

P. 1. The chemical symbol for the element phosphorus. 2. In cardiology, the electrocardiographic wave produced by atrial depolarization.
P. 1. In parasitology and bacteriology, *Paragonimus, Pasteurella, Pediculus, Penicillium, Pfeifferella, Phlebotomus, Physopsis, Planorbis, Plasmodium, Propionibacterium, Proteus, Pseudomonas, Pulex.* 2. In statistics, the probability of an event being due to chance alone.
***p*-.** In chemistry, para-.
p. Pico- ($10^{-12}\times$).
P_1. In cardiology, pulmonary first sound.
P_2. In cardiology, pulmonary second sound.
Pa. 1. Pascal. 2. The chemical symbol for the element protactinium.
PABA. Para-aminobenzoic acid.
p.aeq. In prescriptions, *partes aequalis*—equal parts.
PAPS. Phosphoadenosine phosphosulphate.
part. vic. In prescriptions, *partitis vicitus*—in divided doses.
PAS. 1. Para-aminosalicylic acid. 2. A histochemical method of staining necrotic heart muscle affected by infarction, by periodic acid–Schiff stain.
Past. In bacteriology, *Pasteurella.* [Obsolete.]
past. In prescriptions, *pasta*—a paste.
PAT. In cardiology, paroxysmal atrial tachycardia.
Pb. The chemical symbol for the element lead (plumbum).
PBE. Perlsucht bacillen-emulsion.
PCG. Phonocardiogram.
P_{CO_2}, pCO_2. Carbon-dioxide pressure.

PCS. Postcardiotomy syndrome.
PCV, p.c.v. In haematology, packed-cell volume.
PD. Pupillary distance.
Pd. The chemical symbol for the element palladium.
PDA. In cardiology, persistent ductus arteriosus.
PEEP. Positive end-expiratory respiration.
per bid. In prescriptions, *per biduum*—for a period of 2 days.
pess. In prescriptions, *pessus*—a pessary.
PET. In obstetrics, pre-eclamptic toxaemia.
PETN. Penta-erythritol tetranitrate.
Pf. In bacteriology, *Pfeifferella.* [Obsolete.]
pF. Picofarad.
PFO. In cardiology, patent foramen ovale.
pg. Picogram.
Ph. In chemical formulae, phenyl.
pH, *p*H, $P_{\bar{H}}$, p_H. Symbols used to denote the acidity or alkalinity of a solution expressed in a scale ranging from 0 for maximum acidity to 14 for the opposite extreme of alkalinity, true neutrality being midway, 7. It is defined as the negative value of the power to which the numerical base 10 must be raised to equal the concentration of hydrogen ions in grams per litre.
PhC. Pharmaceutical Chemist.
PhD. Doctor of Philosophy.
Phe. In chemistry, phenylaniline.
PhG. *Pharmacopoeia Germanica.*
PI. 1. In cardiology, pulmonary incompetence. 2. *Pharmacopoeia Internationalis.*
PID. Prolapsed intervertebral disc.
PIF. Prolactin-inhibiting factor.
pig. In prescriptions, *pigmentum*—a paint.
PIH. Protein-inhibiting hormone.
***p*K.** A symbol used to indicate the degree of ionic dissociation of an electrolyte. It is the logarithm to the base 10 of the reciprocal of K, the dissociation constant: strong acids have a low *p*K value and strong bases in common notation have a high *p*K value, K for the base being calculated as an acidic dissociation constant pK_a where $pK_a = 14\text{-}pK_b$ (the basic dissociation constant).
PL. In ophthalmology, light perception.
pl. Plate.
PLA. Procaine and lactic acid.
Pm. The chemical symbol for the element promethium.
PMB. In obstetrics, postmenopausal bleeding.
PMI. In cardiology, point of maximum impulse.
pmol. Picomole.
PMP. In obstetrics, persistent mentoposterior position of the face presentation. *See* PRESENTATION.
PMSG. Pregnant mare's serum gonadotrophin.
PN. In clinical medicine, percussion note.
PNA. 1. Pentose nucleic acid. 2. *Paris Nomina Anatomica.*
PNed. *Nederlandsche Pharmacopee.*
PNF. Proprioceptive neuromuscular facilitation.
Po. The chemical symbol for the element polonium.
Poly. Polymorphonuclear leucocyte, or neutrophil granulocyte.
pond. In prescriptions, *ponderosus*—heavy.
POP. In obstetrics, persistent occipitoposterior position of the vertex presentation. *See* PRESENTATION.
post. Posterior.
post prand. In prescriptions, *post prandium*—after dinner.
PPD. Purified protein derivative (of tuberculin).
p.p.m. Parts per million.
ppt. Precipitate.
Pr. The chemical symbol for the element praseodymium.
Pr. In bacteriology, *Propionibacterium.* [Obsolete.]
p.r. In clinical medicine, *per rectum.*
praep. In prescriptions, *praeparatus*—prepared.
p.r.n. In prescriptions, *pro re nata*—occasionally, when required.
pro rat. aet. In prescriptions, *pro ratione aetatis*—according to age.
PS. In cardiology, pulmonary stenosis.
Ps. In bacteriology, *Pseudomonas.* [Obsolete.]
Pt. The chemical symbol for the element platinum.
pt. Pint.
PTAP. Purified toxoid aluminium phosphate.
PTC. Plasma thromboplastin component.
PTO. Perlsucht-tuberculin original.
PTR. Perlsucht-tuberculin rest.
Pu. The chemical symbol for the element plutonium.
pulv. In prescriptions, *pulvis*—a powder.
PUO. Pyrexia of unknown or uncertain origin.
PVP. Polyvidone (polyvinylpyrrolidone).
PZI. Protamine zinc insulin.

Q

Q. In cardiology, a negative electrocardiographic wave occurring at the commencement of the wave complex produced by ventricular depolarization.
Q. Quality factor. *See* FACTOR.
q.d. In prescriptions, *quater die*—4 times a day.
q.dx. In prescriptions, *quantitas duplex*—double quantity.
q.l. In prescriptions, *quantum libet*—as much as you please.
q.p. In prescriptions, *quantum placet*—as much as you please.
qq.h. In prescriptions, *quaque hora*—every hour.
q.q.h. In prescriptions, *quarta quaque hora*, every fourth hour.
q.s. In prescriptions, *quantum sufficiat*—sufficient.
qt. Quart.
Qu. In chemical formulae, the quinine molecule, $C_{20}H_{24}N_2O_2$.
quot. mane. In prescriptions, *quolibet mane*—any morning.

R

R. 1. In bacteriology, rough variant. 2. A measurement on the Réaumur thermometer. 3. In cardiology, a positive electrocardiographic wave occurring during the wave complex produced by ventricular depolarization.
R or r. In anatomy, *ramus*—branch.
R. In parasitology, *Rhinosporidium, Rhipicephalus, Rickettsia.*
℞. In prescriptions, *recipe*—take.
r. 1. The symbol for roentgen. 2. The symbol for rad.
***r*-.** In organic chemistry, racemic.
Ra. The chemical symbol for the element radium.
rad. In prescriptions, *radix*—a root.
RADC. Royal Army Dental Corps.
RAMC. Royal Army Medical Corps.
ras. In prescriptions, *rasurae*—shavings.
Rb. The chemical symbol for the element rubidium.
RBC, rbc. Red blood corpuscle, also red blood (corpuscle) count.
RBE. Relative biological effectiveness.
RCAMC. Royal Canadian Army Medical Corps.
RCOG. Royal College of Obstetricians and Gynaecologists.
RCP. Royal College of Physicians (London).
RCS. Royal College of Surgeons (England).
RCSE. Royal College of Surgeons of Edinburgh.
RCSI. Royal College of Surgeons of Ireland.
RDA. In obstetrics, right dorso-anterior position of the fetus *in utero* or at delivery. *See* PRESENTATION.

RDE. In immunology, receptor-destroying enzyme.
RDP. In obstetrics, right dorsoposterior position of the fetus *in utero* or at delivery. *See* PRESENTATION.
Re. The chemical symbol for the element rhenium.
REM. 1. Rapid eye movement. 2. Roentgen-equivalent man, the unit of dose equivalent. The absorbed dose in rads multiplied by the quality factor of the type of radiation.
REP. 1. In prescriptions, *repetatur*—let it be repeated. 2. Roentgen-equivalent physical, a unit used for a few years only and now obsolete.
RES. Reticulo-endothelial system.
R_F. Rate of flow (chromatography).
RFA. In obstetrics, the right fronto-anterior position of the brow presentation. *See* PRESENTATION.
RFL. In obstetrics, the right frontolateral position of the brow presentation. *See* PRESENTATION.
RFP. In obstetrics, the right frontoposterior position of the brow presentation. *See* PRESENTATION.
RH or **rh.** Relative humidity.
Rh. 1. The chemical symbol for the element rhodium. 2. Rhesus factor. *See* Rh AGGLUTINOGEN.
RIHSA. Radio-iodinated human serum albumin.
Rhod. *Rhodococcus.*
RIF. Right iliac fossa.
R. in pulv. In prescriptions, *redactum in pulverem*—reduced to powder.
RIPH. Royal Institute of Public Health and Hygiene.
RMA. In obstetrics, the right mento-anterior position of the face presentation. *See* PRESENTATION.
RML. In obstetrics, the right mentolateral position of the face presentation. *See* PRESENTATION.
RMO. 1. Resident Medical Officer of a hospital or institution. 2. Regional Medical Officer in the National Health Service (Great Britain).
RMP. In obstetrics, the right mentoposterior position of the face presentation. *See* PRESENTATION.
rms. Root mean square.
RN. 1. Registered nurse (USA). 2. Royal Navy (UK).
Rn. The chemical symbol for the element radon, or radium emanation.
RNA. Ribonucleic acid.
RNase. Ribonuclease.
ROA. In obstetrics, the right occipito-anterior position of the vertex presentation. *See* PRESENTATION.
ROL. In obstetrics, the right occipitolateral position of the vertex presentation. *See* PRESENTATION.
ROP. In obstetrics, the right occipitoposterior position of the vertex presentation. *See* PRESENTATION.
RP2224. Melarsen.
RP3177. Melarsen oxide.
RPF, r.p.f. Renal plasma flow.
rpm. Revolutions per minute.
RPS. Renal pressor substance.
RQ, r.q. Respiratory quotient.
Rr or **rr.** In anatomy, *rami*—branches.
RS, r.s. Respiratory system.
RSA. In obstetrics, the right sacro-anterior position of the breech presentation. *See* PRESENTATION.
RSH. Royal Society of Health.
RSL. In obstetrics, the right sacrolateral position of the breech presentation. *See* PRESENTATION.
RSM. Royal Society of Medicine.
RSP. In obstetrics, the right sacroposterior position of the breech presentation. *See* PRESENTATION.
RT. Reaction time.
Ru. The chemical symbol for the element ruthenium.
ru. Rat unit.

S

S. 1. The chemical symbol for the element sulphur. 2. In cardiology, a negative electrocardiographic wave following an R wave during the wave complex produced by ventricular depolarization. 3. Siemens.
S or **s.** In anatomy, *sutura*—suture.
S. Svedburg unit.
S. In parasitology, *Saccharomyces, Sarcocystis, Sarcoptes, Schistosoma, Schizotrypanum, Siphunculina, Sparganum, Stomoxys, Strongyloides.*
s. 1. In bacteriology, smooth variant. 2. In prescriptions, *sumat* or *sumendus*—let him take, or to be taken.
σ. Lower case Greek sigma. Standard deviation.
Σ. Capital Greek sigma. 1. Sum. 2. Euphemistic abbreviation for syphilis.
s-. In chemistry, denoting a symmetric isomer.
Salm. *Salmonella.*
sat. Saturated.
SB. Stillbirth.
Sb. The chemical symbol for the element antimony (stibium).
SBE. Subacute bacterial endocarditis.
Sc. The chemical symbol for the element scandium.
s.c. Subcutaneous.
SCD. Subacute combined degeneration (of the cord).
ScD. Doctor of Science.
s.d. Standard deviation.
SDC. Succinyldicholine.
s.e. Standard error.
Se. The chemical symbol for the element selenium.
Sec. Second (of time).
sec. Secondary.
S.E.D. Skin erythema dose.
SEN. State Enrolled Nurse.
seq. luc. In prescriptions, *sequenti luce*—the following day.
S.G. or **sp. gr.** Specific gravity.
SGOT. Serum glutamic oxalo-acetic transaminase.
SGPT. Serum glutamic pyruvic transaminase.
Sh. *Shigella.*
SI. 1. Soluble insulin. 2. International System of Units.
Si. The chemical symbol for the element silicon.
sig. In prescriptions, *signa*—label.
sing. aur. In prescriptions, *singulis auroris*—every morning.
sing. hor. quad. In prescriptions, *singulis horae quadrantibus*—every quarter of an hour.
SLA. In obstetrics. sacrolaevo-anterior position of the breech presentation. *See* PRESENTATION.
SLE. Systemic lupus erythematosus.
Sm. The chemical symbol for the element samarium according to European custom, and the one most frequently used.
SMC. Succinylmonocholine.
SMR. 1. Submucous resection. 2. Standardized mortality ratio.
Sn. The chemical symbol for the element tin (stannum).
sol. Soluble.
soln. Solution.
sp. Species (singular).
Sp. *Spirillum.*
sp. act. Specific activity.
Sph. In ophthalmology, sphere.
sp. ht. Specific heat.
spp. Species (plural).
SPR. Society for Psychical Research.
sq. Square.
Sr. The chemical symbol for the element strontium.
SR. In cardiology, sinus rhythm.
SRN. State Registered Nurse.

Ss., ss. 1. In prescriptions, *semis*—one-half. 2. A blood antigen present in some 55 per cent of white people and related to the MN groups in which the proportions are higher in the M (75 per cent) than in N.
Staph. *Staphylococcus.*
Stat. 1. *Statim*—at once. 2. A prefix signifying a unit in the electrostatic cgs system.
S.T.D. In serology, skin test dose.
Stet. Let it stand.
s.t.p. Standard temperature and pressure.
Str. *Streptococcus.*
S.T.U. In serology, skin test unit.
suff. In prescriptions, *sufficiens*—sufficient.
supp. In prescriptions, *suppositorium*—suppository.
SV40. Simian virus type 40.
Syn. In anatomy, *synchondrosis*—joint.
syr. In prescriptions, *syrupus*—syrup.

T

T. 1. In ophthalmology, intra-ocular tension. 2. In cardiology, the electrocardiographic wave produced by ventricular repolarization. 3. Tera- ($\times 10^{12}$).
T or **t.** In anatomy, *tuberculum*—tuberosity.
T. 1. In physics and chemistry, the symbol for temperature. 2. In parasitology, *Tabanus, Taenia, Taeniorhynchus, Tinea, Trapa, Triatoma, Trichinella, Trichomonas, Trichostrongylus, Trichuris, Trombidium, Trypanosoma, Tunga.*
t. In chemistry and physics, the symbol for temperature on the Centigrade or Fahrenheit scales, also the symbol for time. 2. In prescriptions, *ter*—thrice. 3. Ton (weight).
$T_{\frac{1}{2}}$. Symbol denoting half-life.
T_2. Di-iodotyrosine.
T_3. Tri-iodothyronine.
T_4. Thyroxine.
T_4I. Thyroxine iodine.
T_3RU. Tri-iodothyronine resin uptake.
Ta. The chemical symbol for the element tantalum.
TAB. Typhoid-paratyphoid A and B vaccine.
tab. In prescriptions, *tabella*—tablet.
TABC. Typhoid-paratyphoid A, B, and C vaccine.
TABT. Combined TAB vaccine and tetanus toxoid.
TABTD. Combined TAB vaccine, tetanus toxoid, and diphtheria toxoid.
TACE. Trianisylchloroethylene chlorotrianisene.
TAF. 1. Toxoid–antitoxin floccules. 2. Abbreviation for the German *Tuberculin Albumose Frei*, meaning albumin-free tuberculin.
TAM. Toxoid–antitoxin mixture. [Obsolete term.]
TAPV. In cardiology, totally anomalous pulmonary venous drainage.
TAT. 1. Thematic apperception test. 2. A common, very undesirable, abbreviation for tetanus antitoxin, and for toxin–antitoxin mixtures formerly used for diphtheria immunization.
Tb. The chemical symbol for the element terbium.
Tb. Tubercle bacillus (*Mycobacterium tuberculosis*); also loosely extended to denote tuberculosis.
Tc. The chemical symbol for the element technetium.
TCA. Trichloroacetic acid.
TDD. Tuberculosis Diseases Diploma.
t.d.d. In prescriptions *ter de die*—thrice a day.
t.d.s. In prescriptions, *ter die sumendum*—to be taken thrice a day.
Te. The chemical symbol for the element tellurium.
TEAB. Tetraethylammonium bromide.
TEAC. Tetraethylammonium chloride.
TED. Threshold erythema dose.
temp. Temperature.
TEPA. Triethylenephosphoramide.
TEPP. Tetraethylpyrophosphate.
tert. Tertiary.
TF. Tuberculin filtrate; applied to a method of preparing a purified tuberculin by precipitation and filtration.
TGV. In cardiology, transposition of the great vessels.
Th. The chemical symbol for the element thorium.
Thio-TEPA. Triethylenethiophosphoramide.
TI. In cardiology, tricuspid incompetence.
Ti. The chemical symbol for the element titanium.
t.i.d. In prescriptions, *ter in die*—thrice a day.
Tl. The chemical symbol for the element thallium.
t.l.c. Thin layer chromatography.
Tm. 1. The chemical symbol for the element thulium. 2. Tubular maximum.
TNT. Trinitrotoluene.
TPN. Triphosphopyridine nucleotide.
tr. In prescriptions, *tinctura*—tincture.
Trep. *Treponema.*
TRH. Thyrotrophin-releasing hormone.
TS. In cardiology, tricuspid stenosis.
TSH. Thyroid-stimulating hormone.
tuss. In prescriptions, *tussis*—a cough.
tuss. urg. In prescriptions—when the cough is troublesome.

U

U. 1. Unit. 2. The chemical symbol for the element uranium. 3. In cardiology, the electrocardiographic wave produced by terminal ventricular repolarization.
U 235. The chemical symbol for the fissile isotope of uranium.
UDP. Uridine diphosphate.
UHHA. Unstable haemoglobin haemolytic anaemia.
Ult. praescript. In prescriptions, *ultimo praescriptus*—the last ordered.
Ung. In prescriptions, *unguentum*—an ointment.
USAN. United States Adopted Name. The objectives of the USAN Council resemble those of the British Pharmacopoeia Commission in allocating to suitable proprietary pharmaceutical preparations *Official Names* and *Approved Names.*
USP. *United States Pharmacopeia.*
Ut dict. In prescriptions, *ut dictum*—as stated.
Ut direct. In prescriptions, *ut directum*—as directed.
Ut supr. In prescriptions, *ut supra*—as above.
u.v. Ultraviolet.

V

V. 1. The chemical symbol for the element vanadium. 2. In electricity, volt. 3. In ophthalmology, vision.
V. In bacteriology, *Vibrio.*
V or v. In anatomy, *vena*—vein.
v. 1. In physics, velocity. 2. In prescriptions, *vespere*—in the evening. 3. In cardiology, the venous wave occurring towards the end of systole.
v-. In chemistry, denoting a vicinal isomer.
vac. Vacuum.
var. In zoological and botanical nomenclature, variety.
VD. Venereal disease.
v.d. Vapour density.
VDG. Venereal disease—gonorrhoea.
VDH. Valvular disease of the heart.
VDRL. Venereal Disease Reference Laboratory.
VDS. Venereal disease—syphilis.
vel. Velocity.
VF. 1. In cardiology, ventricular fibrillation. 2. In clinical medicine, vocal fremitus.
Vi. 1. In bacteriology, virulent (e.g. antigen). 2. The chemical symbol for the element virginium.
vit. In prescriptions, *vitellus*—yolk.
VMA. Vanilmandelic acid. *See* ACID.
VOD. Venous occlusive disease.
vol. Volume.
vos. In prescriptions, *vitello ovi solutus*—suspended in the yolk of egg.
v.p. Vapour pressure.
VR. In clinical medicine, vocal resonance.
vs. *Venae sectio*—bleeding.
VSD. In cardiology, ventricular septal defect.
VT. In cardiology, ventricular tachycardia.
Vv or vv. In anatomy, *venae*—veins.
v/v. Volume in volume.
Vx. In obstetrics, vertex.

W

W. 1. The chemical symbol for the element tungsten. 2. In electricity, watt.
W. In parasitology, *Watsonius, Wohlfahrtia, Wuchereria.*
Wb. Weber.
WBC, w.b.c. In haematology, white blood-cell count or white blood cell.
WHO. World Health Organization.
W.R. Wassermann reaction.
wt. Weight.
w/v. Weight in volume.
w/w. Weight in weight.

X

x. In cardiology, the descent in the venous pulse occurring after the A wave.
X. In homoeopathy a symbol for the decimal scale of potencies or dilutions of drugs or other preparations.
X. In parasitology, *Xenopsylla.*
X_2. A *Proteus* antigen that reacts with the serum in tick-borne typhus.
X_{19}. A *Proteus* antigen that reacts with the serum in epidemic typhus.
Xe. The chemical symbol for the element xenon.
Xg. *See* Blood GROUP.
X K. A *Proteus* antigen that reacts with the serum in scrub typhus.
Xyl. Xylose.

Y

y. In cardiology, the descent of the venous pulse occurring after the V wave.
Y. The chemical symbol for the element yttrium.
Yb. The chemical symbol for the element ytterbium.
yd. Yard.
yr. Year.
Yt. *See* Blood GROUP.

Z

Z. The symbol for atomic number or net positive charge on the nucleus of the atom of an element.
Z. In bacteriology, *Zopfius.*
Z.N. In bacteriology, Ziehl–Neelsen.
Zn. The chemical symbol for the element zinc.
Zr. The chemical symbol for the element zirconium.

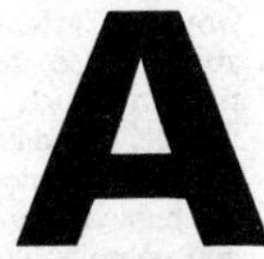

a-. Greek *alpha privativum.* As a non-hyphenated prefix it indicates a negative, *not, without*; equivalent to the Latin *non.*

a tergo (a **ter**·go). The face to back position during sexual intercourse. [L from the back.]

Aalsmeer, William Charles (b. 1889). Dutch physician.

Aalsmeer's test. For beriberi: the administration of 1 mg of adrenaline will bring down the diastolic pressure, as indicated by the point of disappearance of the auscultatory bruit, to zero; in other words, the bruit will not disappear on complete relaxation of the arterial pressure immediately after 1 mg of adrenaline has been administered in a patient with beriberi.

Aaron, B. J. 20th century Australian anaesthetist.

Aaron's clamp. A clamp for controlling the rate of intravascular transfusions.

aasmus (a·as·mus). Asthma. [Gk *aasmos.*]

ab-. Prefix, from the Latin *ab,* meaning *from, away.*

abacterial (a·bak·**teer**·e·al). Indicative of a state in which bacteria are absent.

abactio (ab·**ak**·she·o). Artificially induced abortion or labour. [L *abigere* to drive out.]

abactus venter (ab·**ak**·tus **ven**·ter). Artificially induced abortion. [L *abigere* to drive out, *venter* belly.]

Abadie, Charles (b. 1842). Paris ophthalmologist.

Abadie's sign. Von Graefe's sign; spasm of the levator palpebrae superioris muscle, seen frequently in thyrotoxicosis and occasionally in normal people. [Obsolete term.]

abaissement (ah·base·**mahn**). 1. A depressing or a lowering. 2. In ophthalmology, a term synonymous with lenticular displacement (couching). [Fr. falling; couching.]

abalienated (ab·a·le·en·a·ted). 1. Deranged mentally. 2. In reference to serious disease or injury of a limb, when the affected part is so grossly interfered with as to require amputation. [L *ab, alienare* to alienate.]

abalienatio mentis (ab·a·le·en·a'·she·o **men**·tis). Insanity; mental derangement. [L.]

abalienation (ab·a·le·en·a'·shun). Abalienatio mentis.

abaptiston (ab·ap·**tis**·ton). A trephine made of a certain shape so that when it is in use penetration of the brain is prevented. [Gk *a, baptistos* plunged.]

abarognosis (a·bar·og·**no**'·sis). Inability to recognize the quality of weight; absence of weight sense. [Gk *a,* barognosis.]

abarthrosis (ab·ar·**thro**·sis). 1. Diarthrosis (ball and socket joint). 2. Abarticulation. [L *ab,* arthrosis.]

abarticular (ab·ar·**tik**·ew·lar). Not applicable to a joint; away from a joint. [L *ab, articulus* joint.]

abarticulation (ab·ar·tik·ew·**la**'·shun). Dislocation of a joint. [see prec.]

abasia (ab·a·ze·ah). Loss of power of walking, the result of motor inco-ordination. **Abasia astasia.** Loss of ability to stand or walk normally because of defective will power. **Abasia atactica.** A form of abasia in which there is uncertainty and awkwardness of movement. **Choreic abasia.** Abasia associated with chorea of the legs. **Paralytic abasia.** Inability to walk because the legs give way under the weight of the body. **Paroxysmal trepidant abasia, Spastic abasia.** A form of abasia astasia in which the legs become stiffened in spasm when an attempt is made to stand. **Trembling abasia, Abasia trepidans.** Inability to walk owing to gross degree of tremor of the legs. [Gk *a, basis* step.]

abasic (ab·a·sik). Associated with, referring to or affected by abasia. [see prec.]

abatardissement (ab·at·ar·dees·**mahn**). The slow degeneration or deterioration of a race or breed. [Fr. deterioration.]

abatic (ab·**at**·ik). Abasic.

abaxial, abaxile (ab·**ax**·e·al, ab·**ax**·ile). Situated away from the line of axis of the body, part or organ. [L *ab,* axis.]

Abbé, Ernst Karl (b. 1840). German physicist.

Abbé apertometer. An instrument for measuring microscope apertures.

Abbé camera lucida. An optical device for sketching objects in microscopy.

Abbé condenser. A combination of lenses beneath a microscope that intensifies the illumination of the specimen.

Abbé homogeneous immersion. The inclusion of both specimen and front face of the objective in a medium of cedarwood oil for high-power microscopy.

Abbé apochromatic lens. An arrangement of lenses in a microscope to correct chromatic aberration.

Abbé test-plate. A micrometer slide for gauging the spherical and chromatic aberration of a microscope objective.

Abbé theory. A formula giving the limit of visual resolution in terms of the wavelength of the light used to illuminate the specimen.

Abbé-Zeiss apparatus, or counting cell. An instrument for counting blood corpuscles; Thoma-Zeiss counting cell.

Abbe, Robert (b. 1851). New York surgeon.

Abbe's operation. Section within the skull of the second and third divisions of the trigeminal nerve, for neuralgia.

Abbe's operation, or string method. A method of treatment seldom practised in modern times which involves the passage of a string through an oesophageal stricture as a preliminary to its division.

Abbot's paste. Arsenic trioxide and morphine massed with creosote and used in dentistry to destroy the nerve of a tooth.

Abbott, Alexander Crever (b. 1860). Philadelphia bacteriologist.

Abbott's method. To demonstrate spores in bacteria. The spores are stained blue by Loeffler's alkaline methylene blue, and the bacilli are stained red by eosin or fuchsin.

Abbott, Edville Gerhardt (b. 1871). Portland (Maine) orthopaedic surgeon.

Abbott's method. A method of correction of scoliosis by the use of a frame and bandages, the correction being followed by the application of a plaster jacket.

Abbott, William Osler (b. 1902). Philadelphia physician.

Miller-Abbott tube. A long rubber tube with a double lumen one of which passes to an inflatable bag at the leading end of the tube, the second being used for suction. It is passed through the mouth or nose and guided into the intestine to relieve intestinal obstruction.

abdomen [NA] (ab·**do**·men). The cavity of the body which extends from the diaphragm to the floor of the pelvis. The cavity is bounded by the abdominal walls, the vertebral column and the ilia, and contains the viscera. **Accordion abdomen.** Swelling of the abdomen which suddenly appears and suddenly goes, especially under anaesthesia. Respiration rate is increased and the diaphragmatic arch is flattened. No physical basis such as tumour or gas has been found, and the condition is generally accepted as one of pseudotympany of nervous origin. **Acute abdomen.** A slang expression in universal use indicating that an acute abdominal disturbance is present, generally requiring urgent operation. **Boat-shaped abdomen.** Scaphoid abdomen (see below). **Burst abdomen.** Internal abdominal injury caused by blast or falling wreckage, but without associated external wound. **Carinate abdomen, Navicular abdomen.** Scaphoid abdomen (see below). **Abdomen obstipum.** A congenital condition in which there is shortening of the rectus abdominis muscle. **Pendulous abdomen.** A condition in which the anterior part of the abdominal wall is so relaxed that it hangs down over the pubic region. **Scaphoid abdomen.** A state caused by wasting and commonly seen in patients with much emaciation and in children with cerebrospinal fever; there is hollowing of the anterior abdominal wall, producing a boat-shaped concavity. [L etym. dub.]

abdominal (ab·**dom**·in·al). Associated with or relating to the abdomen.

abdominalgia (**ab**·dom·in·**al**′·je·ah). Abdominal pain or discomfort; rarely used. [abdomen, Gk *algos* pain.]

abdomino-anal (ab·**dom**·in·o·a′·nal). Referring to the abdomen and anus.

abdomino-anterior (ab·**dom**·in·o·an·**teer**′·e·or). Referring to a position of the fetus *in utero*; having the abdomen towards the maternal front. [abdomen, anterior.]

abdominocentesis (ab·**dom**·in·o·sen·**te**′·sis). Puncture of the abdominal cavity, for diagnostic or therapeutic purposes. [abdomen, Gk *kentesis* puncture.]

abdominocystic (ab·dom·in·o·**sis**′·tik). Referring to the abdomen and bladder. [abdomen, Gk *kystis* bladder.]

abdominogenital (ab·**dom**·in·o·**jen**′·it·al). Referring to the abdomen and reproductive organs. [abdomen, genital.]

abdominohysterectomy (ab·**dom**·in·o·his·ter·**ek**′·to·me). Excision of the uterus by the abdominal route. [abdomen, hysterectomy.]

abdominohysterotomy (ab·**dom**·in·o·his·ter·**ot**′·o·me). An incision of the uterus made after preliminary abdominal section. [abdomen, hysterotomy.]

abdominoperineal (ab·**dom**·in·o·per·in·e′·al). In surgery, describing an operative route through the abdomen and the perineum for the removal of pelvic organs, especially of the rectum or bladder; a similar route is employed for the removal of the contents of the pelvis in cases of widespread cancer. The abdominal and perineal parts of the operation may be performed by 2 surgeons separately (synchronous combined abdomino-perineal excision).

abdominoposterior (ab·**dom**·in·o·pos·**teer**′·e·or). A position of the fetus *in utero*; having the abdomen towards the maternal back. [abdomen, posterior.]

abdominoscopy (ab·**dom**·in·**os**′·ko·pe). Examination of the abdomen, especially by endoscopy. *See* PERITONEOSCOPY. [abdomen, Gk *skopein* to view.]

abdominoscrotal (ab·**dom**·in·o·**skro**′·tal). Referring to the abdomen and scrotum.

abdominothoracic (ab·**dom**·in·o·thor·**as**′·ik). Referring to the abdomen and thorax.

abdomino-uterotomy (ab·**dom**·in·o·ew·ter·**ot**′·o·me). Abdomino-hysterotomy. [abdomen, uterotomy.]

abdominovaginal (ab·**dom**·in·o·**vaj**′·in·al). Referring to the abdomen and vagina.

abdominovesical (ab·**dom**·in·o·**ves**′·ik·al). Referring to the abdomen and bladder.

abducent (ab·**dew**·sent). 1. Effecting abduction. 2. Causing separation. [L *abducens* drawing away.]

abducent nerve [nervus abducens (NA)]. The 6th cranial nerve. It is a motor nerve arising from a nucleus in the pons and supplying the lateral rectus muscle. It enters the orbit through the superior orbital fissure.

nucleus [nucleus nervi abducentis (NA)]. A nucleus in the dorsal part of the lower end of the pons, close to the midline.

abduct (ab·**dukt**). To draw outwards away from the middle line of the body. [L *abducere* to draw away.]

abduction (ab·**duk**·shun). 1. Drawing away of any part of the body from the median axis. 2. Used to describe the position of a limb or part of a limb when it has been abducted; the act of abducting. 3. The separation or the drawing away from each other of the edges of a wound or of the portions of a fractured bone. [see prec.]

abductor (ab·**duk**·tor). A muscle which tends to pull a limb away from the middle line, or one part from another. [L *abducere* to draw away.]

abductor digiti minimi muscle of the foot [musculus abductor digiti minimi (NA)] (ab·**duk**·tor **dij**·it·i **min**·im·i). A muscle lying along the lateral side of the sole of the foot from the heel to the base of the first phalanx of the 5th toe.

abductor digiti minimi muscle of the hand [musculus abductor digiti minimi (NA)] (ab·**duk**·tor **dij**·it·i **min**·im·i). The most medial and superficial of the hypothenar muscles. It extends from the ulnar side of the wrist to the base of the 1st phalanx of the 5th finger.

abductor hallucis muscle [musculus abductor hallucis (NA)] (ab·**duk**·tor **hal**·oo·sis). A muscle on the inner side of the sole, extending from the region of the heel to the inner side of the 1st phalanx of the big toe.

abductor ossis metatarsi quinti muscle (ab·**duk**·tor **os**·is met·at·**ar**·si **kwin**·ti). Occasional muscle fibres derived from the abductor digiti minimi muscle, passing to the base of the 5th metatarsal bone.

abductor pollicis brevis muscle [musculus abductor pollicis brevis (NA)] (ab·**duk**·tor **pol**·is·is **brev**·is). The most lateral and superficial of the short muscles of the thumb; it arises on the radial side of the wrist and inserts on the lateral side of the base of the 1st phalanx.

abductor pollicis longus muscle [musculus abductor pollicis longus (NA)] (ab·**duk**·tor **pol**·is·is **long**·gus). A long muscle of the thumb arising deeply in the forearm from both bones and inserted into the base of the 1st metacarpal bone.

Abe, Nakao. 19th–20th century Kyoto bacteriologist.

Abe's culture medium. A low-temperature (0°C) peptone and meat-extract medium for gonococci.

Abegg, Richard (b. 1869). German chemist.

Abegg's rule. Hypothesis based on the Periodic Table that each element possesses normal and contra-valencies numerically totalling 8.

abenteric (ab·en·**ter**·ik). Relating to or involving organs or parts other than those of the intestine; situated outside the intestine. [L *ab*, Gk *enteron* intestine.]

abepithymia (**ab**·ep·e·**thi**′·me·ah). 1. Paralysis of the coeliac (solar) plexus. 2. The word epithymia is based on the Greek *thymos*, the soul, which was believed by the ancient Greeks to be seated in the diaphragm; here also desires took origin. The term has therefore been used to describe pathological or abnormal desires. [L *ab*, Gk *epithymia* desire.]

Abercrombie, John (b. 1780). Edinburgh physician.

Abercrombie's degeneration. Amyloid degeneration. *See* DEGENERATION.

Abercrombie's syndrome. Amyloid disease affecting a number of organs.

Abernethy, John (b. 1764). London surgeon.

Abernethy's fascia. The connective tissue separating the peritoneum from the fascia covering the iliacus muscle.

Abernethy's operation. Ligation of the external iliac artery through an incision above the lateral part of the inguinal ligament.

Abernethy's sarcoma. A circumscribed, slow-growing, fatty sarcoma found chiefly on the trunk.

aberrans (ab·er·anz). One of the 2 ductuli aberrantes of the epididymis. [L wandering.]

aberrant (ab·er·ant). Deviating from the normal; applied to a vessel or nerve which follows any unusual course. It sometimes refers to abnormality of structure or appearance. [see prec.]

aberratio (ab·er·a·she·o). **Aberratio humorum.** Abnormality of the direction of flow of any body fluid. **Aberratio lactis.** The metastatic occurrence of milk in a situation away from the normal mammary glands. **Aberratio mensium, Aberratio menstruorum.** Vicarious menstruation. **Aberratio testis.** The presence of the testis outside its normal path of descent. [see foll.]

aberration (ab·er·**a**·shun). 1. Deviation from the normal course; a deviation from the normal. 2. Malformation of the fetus. 3. Intellectual disorder or derangement. 4. In cardiology, conduction of an excitatory impulse around the ventricles by an abnormal pathway so that the QRS complex has a form different from that occurring with normal conduction. The use of the term is normally restricted to those instances where normal conduction and aberrant conduction are both occurring in the same patient. 5. In optics, a condition in a lens in which refraction or focalization, or both, are defective. **Chromatic aberration.** A display of colours produced by an unequal refraction of rays of different wavelengths. **Chromatid aberration.** Abnormality involving the whole of one and only one chromatid of a chromosome. Distinct from subchromatid and chromosome aberrations, where a subunit of a chromatid or both chromatids are involved, respectively. **Dioptric aberration.** Spherical aberration (see below). **Distantial aberration.** Blurred vision due to presence of the object at a distance. **Lateral aberration.** Deviation of a ray in any direction from the focus measured on a line perpendicular to the axis at the focus. **Longitudinal aberration.** The deviation of a ray from the focus measured along the axis. **Mental aberration.** A degree of mental instability which is not marked enough to constitute insanity and is temporary. **Meridional aberration.** Variation of the power of refraction in different parts of the same meridian of a lens. **Newtonian aberration.** Chromatic aberration (see above). **Spherical aberration.** The natural property intrinsic to a convex lens whereby there is excessive refraction from the periphery; rays of light cannot be brought to a single focus, and this gives rise to blurred images. **Zonal aberration.** Aberration exhibited by a lens composed of zones of different refractive index, each zone having its own focal length so that the lens is multifocal. [L *aberrare* to wander.]

See also: NEWTON (I.).

aberrometer (ab·er·**om**·et·er). An instrument for the measurement of errors in fine observations or delicate experiments. [aberration, meter.]

abetalipoproteinaemia (a·**be**·tah·lip·o·pro·te·in·**e**′·me·ah). Defect in synthesis of beta-lipoprotein with acanthocytosis, steatorrhoea, ataxia and retinitis pigmentosa. [Gk *a, beta,* lipoprotein, *haima* blood.]

abevacuation (**ab**·e·vak·ew·**a**′·shun). 1. Abnormal or morbid evacuation; a deficient or an excessive discharge. 2. Metastasis.

abiatrophy (a·bi·**at**·ro·fe). Premature loss of intrinsic vital power; early decay because of weak resistance to environment. [Gk *a, bios* life, *trophe* nutrition.]

abient (**ab**·e·ent). Tending to go away from the source in responding to a stimulus; negative. Cf. ADIENT. [L *abire* to go away.]

Abies (**ab**·e·eez). A group of coniferous trees and plants amongst which are the firs, spruces and hemlock. **Abies balsamea.** Balsam fir; it yields Canada balsam. **Abies canadensis.** The hemlock spruce; it furnishes Canada pitch, also the astringent extract and volatile oil of hemlock. **Abies excelsa.** Norway spruce, the source of Burgundy pitch. **Abies pectinata.** The silver fir of Europe; it has resinous balsamic buds which are sudorific. **Abies sibirica.** This gives the oil of Siberian fir (oil of pine) used in inhalations and perfumery. [L silver fir.]

abietate (ab·i·et·ate). A salt of abietic acid.

abietene (ab·i·et·een). 1. A colourless aromatic liquid distilled from the resin of *Pinus sabiniana* and consisting of a mixture of hydrocarbons, principally heptane. 2. $C_{19}H_{30}$, a colourless hydrocarbon distilled from pine resin. [L *abies* silver fir.]

abietin (ab·i·et·in). A resinous crystalline substance, $C_{53}H_{76}O_8$, extracted from the pitch of the silver fir, *Abies pectinata.*

abietite (ab·i·et·ite). A sugar, $C_4H_8O_6$, related to mannose, occurring in the needles of the silver fir, *Abies pectinata.*

abiochemistry (a·bi·o·**kem**′·is·tre). Inorganic chemistry. *See* CHEMISTRY. [GK *a, bios* life, chemistry.]

abiogenesis (a·bi·o·**jen**′·es·is). The origination of living matter from lifeless matter; formerly referred to as spontaneous generation. [Gk *a, bios* life, *genein* to produce.]

abiogenetic, abiogenous (a·**bi**·o·jen·**et**′·ik, a·bi·**oj**·en·us). Characterized by, or referring to, abiogenesis.

abiogeny (a·bi·**oj**·en·e). Abiogenesis.

abiologic, abiological (a·bi·o·**loj**′·ik, a·bi·o·**loj**′·ik·al). 1. Not relating or belonging to the science of living things. 2. Relating or belonging to the science of inanimate things. [see foll.]

abiology (a·bi·**ol**·o·je). The science of inanimate things. [Gk *a, bios* life, *logos* science.]

abionarce (a·bi·o·**nar**′·se). Inactivity caused by weakness of mind and body, the result of infirmity, especially in old age. [Gk *a, bios* life, *narke* stupor.]

abionergy (a·bi·on·**er**′·je). Abiotrophy. [Gk *a, bios* life, *ergon* work.]

abiophysiology (a·**bi**·o·fiz·e·**ol**′·o·je). The science of inorganic activities in living organisms. [Gk *a, bios* life, physiology.]

abiosis (a·bi·**o**·sis). 1. The condition of being lifeless. 2. Abiotrophia. [Gk *a, bios* life.]

abiotic (a·bi·**ot**·ik). Characterized by, or relating to, absence of life; incapable of being alive; incompatible with, or opposed to, life. [see prec.]

abiotrophia, abiotrophy (a·bi·o·**tro**′·fe·ah, a·bi·**ot**′·ro·fe). Nutritional defect causing a degree of loss of vitality with consequent diminution or failure of resistance, so that endurance is lost. [Gk *a, bios* life, *trophe* nutrition.]

abirritant (ab·**ir**·it·ant). 1. Having a soothing effect, with the property of relieving or diminishing irritation. 2. In relation to decreased sensitiveness. 3. An agent which tends to relieve irritation. [L *ab,* irritant.]

abirritation (**ab**·ir·it·**a**′·shun). Asthenia or atony; lessened responsiveness to stimulation. [see prec.]

abiuret (a·**bi**·ewr·et). Not giving the biuret reaction. [Gk *a,* biuret.]

abiuretic (a·**bi**·ewr·**et**′·ik). 1. Not reacting to the protein copper (biuret) test. 2. Not possessing the peptide linkage. [see prec.]

ablastemic (a·blas·**te**·mik). Non-germinal; not referring to germination. [Gk *a,* blastema.]

ablastin (a·**blas**·tin). An antibody present in rats harbouring *Trypanosoma lewisi,* whose sole effect is to prevent reproduction of the parasites by inhibiting cell division. [Gk *ablastos* sterile.]

ablastous (a·**blas**·tus). In biology, producing neither germ nor bud. [see prec.]

ablate (ab·**late**). To cut off or to remove. [L *ab, latus* carried.]

ablatio (ab·**la**·she·o). Removal; detachment. **Ablatio placentae.** Premature detachment of a normal placenta. **Ablatio retinae.** Detachment of the retina. [L carrying away.]

ablation (ab·**la**·shun). Cutting away, especially with regard to removal of tumours, gangrenous areas and damaged tissues. [see prec.]

ablepharia, ablepharon (a·blef·**a**·re·ah, a·**blef**·ar·on). A congenital defect characterized by total absence of the eyelids or of the interpalpebral fissure; in some cases the defect is partial. [Gk *a, blepharon* eyelid.]

ablepharous (a·**blef**·ar·us). Not having any eyelids. [Gk *a, blepharon* eyelid.]

ablepharus (a·**blef**·ar·us). A person who is congenitally affected with ablepharia. [see prec.]

ablephary (a·**blef**·ar·e). Ablepharia.

ablepsia, ablepsy (a·**blep**·se·ah, a·**blep**·se). Blindness; loss or lack of sight. [Gk *a, blepein* to see.]

abluent (**ab**·loo·ent). 1. A detergent, or cleansing agent. 2. Describing any substance which has the ability to cleanse or wash out. [L *abluere* to wash away.]

ablutomania (ab·loo·to·**ma**·ne·ah). A compulsion to wash oneself frequently and repeatedly. [L *abluere* to wash away, Gk *mania* madness.]

abmortal (ab·**mor**·tal). Of electric currents, those passing from dead or moribund tissues to living tissues. Cf. ADMORTAL. [L *ab,* mortal.]

abnerval, abneural (ab·nerv·al, ab·newr·al). 1. Away from the central nervous system; referring to a region apart from the dorsal region; ventral. 2. Designating an electric current passing from a nerve ending to and through a muscle. Cf. ADNERVAL. [L *ab*, Gk *neuron* nerve.]

Abney, Sir William De Wiveleslie (b. 1843). British scientist.

Abney's law. The luminosity of the recombined spectrum is equal to the sum of the luminosities of its parts.

abnormal (ab·nor·mal). Deviating from type or normality; contrary to the usual system, structure or condition. [L *ab*, *norma* rule.]

abnormalism, abnormality (ab·nor·mal·izm, ab·nor·mal·it·e). 1. A malformation or deformity. 2. The state or quality of being abnormal. [L *ab*, *norma* rule.]

abnormity (ab·nor·mit·e). Any irregularity from the normal. [see prec.]

abocclusion (ab·ok·loo·zhun). In dentition, the relation of the teeth in which the mandibular teeth do not make contact with the maxillary teeth. [L *ab*, occlusion.]

aboral (ab·or·al). At some distance from the mouth; opposite to the mouth. Cf. ADORAL. [L *ab*, oral.]

abort (ab·ort). 1. To give birth, as in miscarriage, before the fetus is viable. 2. To check or stop the usual course of a disease. 3. Not to reach full development, on account of some check. [L *ab*, *oriri* to be born.]

aborticide (ab·or·tis·ide). 1. The killing of a fetus. 2. An agent which destroys the fetus and causes abortion. [L *abortus* an aborted fetus, *caedere* to kill.]

abortient (ab·or·she·ent). 1. Giving rise to abortion. 2. Abortifacient.

abortifacient (ab·or·te·fa·shent). An agent or a drug which may bring about abortion. [abort, L *facere* to make.]

abortin (ab·or·tin). An extract from cultures of *Brucella abortus*, analogous to tuberculin, and employed in the treatment of infectious abortion in cows. **Abortin reaction.** *See* REACTION. [*Brucella abortus*.]

abortion (ab·or·shun). 1. Premature or untimely expulsion of the fetus: in law, at any period; in obstetrics, before the 28th week—whether natural or induced by some means, medical or other. 2. A term applied to the actual product of an abortion. **Accidental abortion.** Abortion resulting from accident. **Afebrile abortion.** Abortion in which the temperature is only seldom above 37.4°C (99.4°F). **Ampullar abortion.** A tubal abortion which takes place from the ampulla of the uterine tube. **Artificial abortion.** Abortion produced deliberately. **Cervical abortion.** Abortion caused by the continued resistance of the external os uteri to dilatation; the fetus is trapped in the neck of the uterus. **Complete abortion.** Abortion in which the products of conception are expelled in an intact condition. **Criminal abortion.** That procured by illegal methods, or the attempt to bring this about; an abortion for which there is no proper medical reason. **Embryonic abortion.** One which takes place before the 4th month. **Epidemic abortion.** In times of acute suffering or starvation in a community, the occurrence of an unusually high rate of abortion so as to constitute an epidemic; poisoning such as ergotism can also give rise to this. **Fetal abortion.** An abortion which occurs after the 4th month. **Habitual abortion.** Abortion occurring in 3 (some say 2) successive pregnancies. **Imminent abortion.** A stage characterized by certain signs indicating that abortion is about to occur. These signs are haemorrhage, a dilated soft cervix and cramp-like pains due to uterine contractions. **Incipient abortion.** The commencing stage of abortion following on imminent abortion. **Incomplete abortion.** That in which the membranes or the placenta are not expelled. **Induced abortion.** Artificial abortion (see above). **Inevitable abortion.** A term that embraces both the imminent and incipient stages. **Infectious abortion.** An infectious disease of pregnant animals, due to inflammation of the uterine mucosa and fetal membranes, which gives rise to premature expulsion of the fetus. Cf. UNDULANT FEVER, BRUCELLOSIS, where the infection is conveyed from animal to man usually through cow's milk infected with *Brucella* organisms. **Intermediate abortion.** That taking place during the second 6 weeks of pregnancy. **Justifiable abortion.** Therapeutic abortion (see below). **Late abortion.** Abortion taking place after the placenta is completely formed and before the 28th week has been reached. **Lawful abortion.** In accordance with the provisions of law, e.g. therapeutic, under the 1968 Abortion Act. **Missed abortion.** An abortion in which the embryo or fetus is dead, and is retained in the uterine cavity. **Natural abortion.** Any except an induced abortion. **Ovular abortion.** Abortion which takes place within the first 3 weeks. **Partial abortion.** When there is multiple pregnancy, the loss of one fetus prematurely. **Septic abortion.** Abortion from an infected uterus. **Spontaneous abortion.** Naturally occurring abortion. **Therapeutic abortion.** Abortion brought about deliberately to protect the life or health (physical or mental) of the mother. Some would add other circumstances such as a substantial risk that the child, if born, would suffer serious physical or mental disability. **Threatened abortion.** The presence of signs of the premature expulsion of the fetus. **Tubal abortion.** The termination of a tubal pregnancy on account of rupture of the uterine tube. **Unlawful abortion.** Not in accordance with the provisions of the law. [L *ab*, *oriri* to be born.]

Abortion Act 1968. Under this Act a woman may have a pregnancy terminated legally if two doctors certify that, in their opinion, one of the following conditions applies: (*a*) continuance of the pregnancy would involve risk to the life of the pregnant woman greater than if the pregnancy was terminated; (*b*) continuance of the pregnancy would involve risk of injury to the physical or mental health of the pregnant woman greater than if the pregnancy was terminated; (*c*) continuance of the pregnancy would involve risk of injury to the physical or mental health of an existing child or children of the family of the pregnant woman greater than if the pregnancy was terminated; (*d*) there is a substantial risk that if the child was born, it would suffer from such physical or mental abnormalities as to be seriously handicapped. All abortions must be notified to the Department of Health and Social Security.

abortionist (ab·or·shun·ist). Strictly, any person who procures an abortion, but the term is often used to denote a person who procures an abortion illegally. [L *ab*, *oriri* to be born.]

abortive (ab·or·tiv). 1. Incompletely developed or rudimentary. 2. Prematurely born. 3. Abortifacient. 4. Term applied to treatment which cuts short an attack of a disease. 5. Of a disease, subsiding before it has run its full course. 6. Of abortive transduction of phage, indicating transfer and expression of donor genes without formation of stable recombinants; the transduced donor fragment of DNA is neither replicated nor integrated into the recipient chromosome, but is inherited unilinearly among the recipient progeny. [L *abortivus* born prematurely.]

abortus (ab·or·tus). An abortion. [L.]

abouchement (ah·boosh·mahn). The ending of a small vessel in a larger one. [Fr.]

aboukine (ab·oo·keen). Yaws. [African name.]

aboulia (ab·ool·e·ah). Abulia. [Gk *a*, *boule* will.]

aboulomania (ab·ool·o·ma·ne·ah). Abulomania. [Gk *a*, *boule* will, mania.]

abrachia (ah·bra·ke·ah). Lacking arms, especially congenitally in monsters. [Gk *a*, *brachion* arm.]

abrachiatism (ah·bra·ke·at·izm). Abrachia.

abrachiocephalia (ah·bra·ke·o·kef·a'·le·ah). A condition in monsters in which both head and arms are lacking. [Gk *a*, *brachion* arm, *kephale* head.]

abrachiocephalus (ah·bra·ke·o·kef'·al·us). A monster without arms and head. [see prec.]

abrachius (ah·bra·ke·us). An armless fetus. [abrachia.]

abradant (ab·ra·dant). Abrasive. [abrade.]

abrade (ab·rade). 1. To excoriate the skin. 2. To injure or to rub away the superficial layer or surface of a part. [L *ab*, *radere* to scrape.]

Abrahams, Robert (b. 1861). New York physician.

Abrahams' sign. An impaired percussion note over the acromion process in early apical tuberculosis.

Abrami, Pierre (b. 1879). Paris physician.

Abrami's disease, Widal-Abrami disease. Acquired haemolytic jaundice.

Abrams, Albert (b. 1863). San Francisco physician.

Abrams' box. An electrical contrivance which was reputed to have both diagnostic and therapeutic properties. There was no accepted scientific basis for the claims made for it.

Abrams' reflex. Reflex contraction of the underlying lung on stimulation of the skin over the chest.

abrasio (ab·ra·ze·o). **Abrasio corneae.** A scraping off of the superficial epithelium of the cornea. **Abrasio dentium.** The wearing away of the hard structures of the teeth. [L a scraping.]

abrasion (ab·ra·zhun). 1. Attrition. 2. A portion of surface from which the skin or mucous membrane has been removed by rubbing. 3. In dentistry, the wearing away of the substance of the teeth by the process of friction. [see prec.]

abrasive (ab·ra·ziv). 1. Any substance used for rubbing away or grinding down. 2. Causing abrasion. [L *ab, radere* to scrape.]

abrasor (ab·ra·zor). An instrument used for abrading; a rasp. [see prec.]

abreaction (ab·re·**ak**·shun). In psychoanalysis the working off, in speech and action, of a repressed disagreeable experience (psychocatharsis, catharsis). **Motor abreaction.** An abreaction arrived at by means of muscular or motor expression. [L *ab*, reaction.]

Abrikosov, Aleksei Ivanovich (b. 1875). Russian pathologist.

Abrikosov's tumour. Myoblastoma.

abrin (a·brin). A mixture of 2 poisonous proteins obtained from the seeds of jequirity, *Abrus precatorius*; it resembles snake venom in physiological action, and is used as an ophthalmic irritant.

abrine (a·breen). A poisonous alkaloid, *N*-methyltryptophane, $C_{12}H_{14}O_2N_2$, extracted from jequirity. [abrus.]

abrism (a·brizm). Poisoning by abrine, derived from the seed of jequirity, *Abrus precatorius*.

Abroma (ab·ro·mah). A genus of sterculiaceous trees occurring in Southern Asia; the viscid juice of *Abroma augusta* is used in the treatment of dysmenorrhoea.

abrosia (a·bro·ze·ah). The condition induced by lack of food. [Gk fasting.]

abrotanum (ab·rot·an·um). *Artemisia abrotanum*, southernwood; a plant used as a vermifuge, healing agent, stimulant and tonic. [Gk *abrotonon*.]

abrotine (ab·rot·een). An alkaloid, $C_{21}H_{22}ON_2$, obtained from *Artemisia abrotanum*, southernwood. Used as a stimulant and anthelminthic. [see prec.]

abruptio placentae (ab·**rup**·she·o plas·**en**·te). Premature separation of the placenta. [L *ab, rumpere* to rupture, placenta.]

abruption (ab·**rup**·shun). 1. A sudden breaking off or tearing apart. 2. A transverse fracture. [L *ab, rumpere* to rupture.]

Abrus (a·brus). A genus of leguminous plants. **Abrus precatorius.** A species occurring in India, yielding poisonous seeds (jequirity) the infusion of which is violently irritant to mucous surfaces and is used therefore in the treatment of trachoma. [Gk *habros* delicate.]

abscess (ab·ses). A collection of pus circumscribed in a cavity produced by tissue disintegration and displacement. **Actinomycotic abscess.** An abscess in which the causative organism is an actinomycete (*Actinomyces, Nocardia, Streptomyces*). **Acute abscess.** An abscess of short course characterized by great pain, local inflammation and swelling, with pyrexia. **Acute apical abscess, Acute periapical abscess.** An acute inflammatory condition occurring around the apex of a tooth whose pulp has become necrotic; acute periapical infective periodontitis. **Alveolar abscess.** Inflammation of a dental alveolus with the formation of pus. **Amoebic abscess.** 1. An abscess of the liver consequent on hepatitis produced by *Entamoeba histolytica*. 2. A cerebral abscess due to *Entamoeba histolytica* secondary to an amoebic liver abscess, or due to *Hartmanella* (*Naegleria*) species of amoebae. These are small, free-living amoebae present in water, which may gain entry into the brain via the cribriform plate of the ethmoid bone. **Anorectal abscess.** An abscess in the celluloadipose tissue of the perianal region. **Apical abscess.** An abscess at the apex of the root of a tooth. **Appendiceal abscess, Appendicular abscess, Appendix abscess.** An abscess localized around an inflamed and perforated vermiform appendix. **Arthritic abscess.** Any abscess in the intestinal wall occurring as the result of the arthritis of podagra. **Atheromatous abscess.** One which arises in the wall of a vessel softened by sclerotic endarteritis. **Axillary abscess.** An abscess arising in the armpit from infection of a modified sweat gland. **Bartholinian abscess.** An abscess of the greater vestibular gland (Bartholin's gland). **Bicameral abscess.** An abscess with 2 pockets. **Bile-duct abscess.** Cholangitic abscess (see below). **Bilharziasis abscess.** An abscess in the intestinal wall resulting from infection by *Schistosoma mansoni*. **Biliary abscess.** An abscess affecting any part of the biliary tract or the gall bladder itself. **Blind abscess.** An abscess which has no external opening, such as a dental granuloma, or periapical abscess (see below). **Bone abscess.** An abscess excavated in the bone marrow by the inflammation of osteomyelitis. **Canalicular abscess.** A mammary abscess which communicates with and discharges into a milk duct. **Carniform abscess.** A term applied to a hard sarcoma of a joint. **Caseous abscess.** An abscess, typically a tuberculous one, that contains yellowish, semisolid material not unlike cheese. **Cerebellar abscess.** Cerebral abscess (see following). **Cerebral abscess.** An abscess of the brain; it occasionally complicates chronic suppurative middle ear or lung disease. **Cheesy abscess.** Caseous abscess (see above). **Cholangitic abscess.** An abscess of the liver due to ascending bile-duct infection. **Chronic abscess.** An abscess which develops slowly and persists over a long period of time. **Chronic apical abscess, Chronic periapical abscess.** A chronic abscess forming at the apex of a tooth due to the breaking down of an apical granuloma; chronic periapical infective periodontitis. **Circumscribed abscess.** An abscess shut off from related tissues by a wall of fibroblasts. **Circumtonsillar abscess.** Peritonsillar abscess (see below). **Cold abscess.** An abscess, usually tuberculous, which is slow in development and shows little redness, pain or local warmth. **Collar-stud abscess.** A double abscess in which the 2 main cavities are connected by a narrow channel. The classical mode of presentation of a caseating lymph node in the neck, the narrow channel perforating the deep fascia and expanding into a cavity containing the caseous material in the subcutaneous tissue. **Consecutive abscess.** Critical abscess (see below). **Constitutional abscess.** An abscess arising out of constitutional weakness or disease. **Critical abscess.** One which marks the crisis in an illness or the end of an acute infection. **Dental abscess.** An abscess lying alongside a carious tooth which destroys bone and may spread into the adjoining soft tissues; often close to the root of a tooth. **Dentoalveolar abscess.** Alveolar abscess (see above). **Diffuse abscess.** An abscess that is unrestricted by a fibrous wall and extends widely into the adjacent tissues. **Dry abscess.** An abscess which disperses without pointing or bursting. **Embolic abscess.** An abscess forming around organisms that are transported from a distant part by the blood. **Emphysematous abscess.** Tympanitic abscess (see below). **Encysted abscess.** An abscess occurring in a serous cavity and localized by adhesions. **Endamoebic abscess, Entamoebic abscess.** Amoebic abscess (see above). **Epidural abscess.** Extradural abscess (see below). **Epiploic abscess.** An abscess occurring in the omentum. **Extradural abscess.** An abscess between the dura mater of the brain and the skull, or between the dura mater of the spinal cord and the vertebral canal. It occurs especially as a complication of mastoiditis, frontal sinusitis or tuberculous spondylitis (Pott's disease). **Faecal abscess.** An abscess of the rectum or large intestine which contains pus and faecal matter. **Filarial abscess.** An abscess due to filarial infection. **Fixation abscess.** An abscess artificially produced with a view to the attraction of the circulating bacteria of an infection to the chosen site, with stimulation of the antibacterial defences of the patient. **Folli-**

cular abscess. An abscess of a hair follicle. **Frontal abscess.** An abscess arising in the frontal lobe of the cerebrum. **Fungal abscess.** An abscess attributable to infection by a fungus. **Gas abscess.** Tympanitic abscess (see below). **Gastric abscess.** Another name for phlegmonous gastritis. **Gingival abscess.** An abscess under the mucosal covering of the gum and arising in relation to the neck of a tooth. **Glandular abscess.** An abscess of a lymph node. **Gluteal abscess.** An abscess of the buttock. **Gravitation abscess, Gravity abscess.** Hypostatic abscess (see below). **Haematic abscess.** An abscess arising out of the infection of extravasated blood. **Heart abscess.** A small abscess of the myocardium, usually multiple. **Helminthic abscess.** An abscess attributed to an intestinal worm. **Hepatic abscess.** Abscess of the liver due to *Entamoeba histolytica* or to various colonic bacteria. **Hypostatic abscess.** An abscess which extends from its original site towards a more dependent part. **Iliac abscess.** An abscess located in the iliac region. **Intracranial abscess.** An abscess within the skull, in the brain, or in relation to the brain and its meninges. **Intradural abscess.** Subdural abscess (see below). **Intramammary abscess.** Parenchymatous abscess of the breast. **Intramastoid abscess.** Mastoid abscess (see below). **Intraspinal abscess.** An abscess within the vertebral canal, usually extradural. **Ischiorectal abscess.** A suppurative lesion in the ischiorectal fossa, often associated with fistula. **Lacrimal abscess.** An abscess resulting from infection of the lacrimal sac. **Lacunar abscess.** An abscess in a urethral lacuna. **Lateral abscess, Lateral alveolar abscess.** Paradental abscess (see below). **Liver abscess.** An abscess in the liver substance due to a variety of causes, e.g. amoebiasis, portal pyaemia or cholangitis. **Lumbar abscess.** Any abscess located in the lumbar region, particularly a tuberculous abscess pointing in the loin. **Lung abscess.** Pulmonary abscess (see below). **Lymphatic abscess.** A typical cold abscess of a lymphatic gland with the gradual breaking down of tissue, usually resulting from tuberculous infection. **Mammary abscess.** Abscess of the breast, usually in the lactation period or on weaning. **Marginal abscess.** An abscess situated at the anal orifice. **Mastoid abscess.** Suppurative inflammation in the cells of the mastoid process of the temporal bone. **Mediastinal abscess.** An abscess located in the space between the lungs. **Mesenteric abscess.** An abscess between the layers of the mesentery. **Metastatic abscess.** A secondary abscess arising at a distance from the primary site of inflammation as the result of transportation of the micro-organisms in the blood. **Migrating abscess.** Wandering abscess (see below). **Miliary abscesses.** Abscesses not larger than millet seeds, widespread and multiple as the outcome of blood infection. **Milk abscess.** An abscess of the breast arising during the lactation period. **Multiple abscess.** One of the small collections of abscesses which occur in great numbers in pyaemia. **Mural abscess.** An abscess in the wall of a hollow organ or of a cavity, as in the abdominal wall after operation. **Myocardial abscess.** An abscess of the myocardium. **Orbital abscess.** A suppurative abscess located in the eye socket or upon the eyelids. **Ossifluent abscess.** An abscess in bone tissue. **Otic abscess, Otic cerebral abscess.** Abscess of the brain consequent on otitis media. **Otogenic abscess.** Otic abscess (see above). **Palatal abscess.** An abscess affecting an upper incisor and extending towards the palate. **Palmar abscess.** An abscess in the palm of the hand. **Paradental abscess.** An abscess formed alongside a tooth. **Parafrenal abscess.** An abscess on one or other side of the preputial frenulum. **Parametric abscess, Parametritic abscess.** An intraligamentous suppuration of the broad ligament of the uterus. **Paranephric abscess, Paranephritic abscess.** Perinephric abscess (see below). **Parapancreatic abscess.** An abscess in the neighbourhood of the pancreas. **Paravertebral abscess.** An abscess lying in relation to the bodies of the vertebrae. **Parietal abscess.** An abscess occurring in any part of the periodontal tissue except that investing the foramen at the apex of the root of a tooth. **Parotid abscess.** An abscess arising in the parotid salivary gland. **Pelvic abscess.** A suppurative condition arising in the pelvic peritoneum, particularly in the recto-uterine pouch. **Pelvirectal abscess.** An abscess between the rectum and the levator ani muscle; it may follow appendicitis, more rarely Crohn's disease or cancer of the rectum, and usually forms a sinus into the rectum. **Perianal abscess.** An abscess in the perianal space, close to the anal margin. **Periapical abscess.** An abscess occurring in the periodontal tissue investing the apex of the root of a tooth. **Peribronchitic abscess.** An abscess of the lung associated with peribronchitis. **Pericaecal abscess.** An abscess around the caecum, often originating from the appendix. **Pericemental abscess.** Parietal abscess (see above). **Pericolic abscess.** An abscess in direct relation with the colon and usually the result of infection from the lumen. **Pericoronal abscess.** An abscess arising in the tissue investing the crown of an unerupted molar. **Peridental abscess.** Periodontal abscess (see below). **Perimetric abscess, Perimetritic abscess.** An abscess related to an inflamed uterus. **Perinephric abscess, Perinephritic abscess.** An abscess arising in the fatty tissue investing the kidney; probably the result of rupture of a cortical abscess. **Periodontal abscess.** An abscess of the periodontal tissue which may be parietal or apical, but which does not open out through the gum. **Peripleuritic abscess.** An abscess situated between the pleura and the chest wall. **Periproctic abscess, Periproctitic abscess.** Perirectal abscess (see following). **Perirectal abscess.** An abscess arising in the loose tissue around the rectum. **Perisinuous abscess, Perisinus abscess.** An abscess round the lateral sinus, commonly due to a spread of infection from the mastoid cavity. **Peritoneal abscess.** An abscess in the peritoneal cavity walled-in by adhesions and the direct result of peritonitis. **Peritonsillar abscess.** Suppuration of the lax tissues surrounding a tonsil; a quinsy. **Perityphlitic abscess.** A pericaecal abscess, and therefore commonly an appendicular abscess. **Peri-ureteral abscess.** An abscess round the ureter; an uncommon complication of a stone or of an operation on the ureter. **Peri-urethral abscess.** An abscess close to the urethra, often a complication of gonorrhoea. It is occasionally complicated by the development of a perineal or urethral sinus or fistula. **Perivesical abscess.** An abscess occurring in the alveolar tissue investing the urinary bladder. **Pharyngeal abscess.** An abscess in relation to the wall of the pharynx. **Phlegmonous abscess.** An acute abscess in connective tissue which is not provided with a localizing wall; cellulitis. **Pneumococcal abscess.** An abscess attributable to infection by a pneumococcus. **Postcaecal abscess.** Retrocaecal abscess (see below). **Postileal abscess.** An abscess, usually the result of appendicitis, lying behind the termination of the ileum. **Postmammary abscess.** Retromammary abscess (see below). **Postpharyngeal abscess.** An abscess behind the pharynx. **Post-typhoid abscess.** An abscess which may appear in the course of typhoid fever, often when the acute phase of the disease is abating, in the spleen or thyroid. **Pre-ileal abscess.** An abscess, usually consequent upon appendicitis, lying in front of the terminal ileum. **Prelacrimal abscess.** An abscess produced in the region of the inner canthus by disease of the underlying bone. **Premammary abscess.** An abscess superficial to the breast, and due usually to a skin infection. **Primary abscess.** An abscess occurring at the initial point of infection by a pyogenic micro-organism. **Protozoal abscess.** Amoebic abscess (see above). **Psoas abscess.** An abscess, usually tuberculous, arising out of disease of the thoracic or lumbar spine and spreading in the sheath of the psoas muscle sometimes as far as the thigh. **Pulmonary abscess.** A complication of inflammation of the lung; especially liable to follow aspiration of infected material from the mouth, e.g. during operation on the mouth. **Pulp abscess.** 1. A suppurating abscess developing in the pulp of a tooth. 2. An abscess arising in the pulp of a finger. **Pyaemic abscess.** A secondary abscess produced at some distance from the primary site of infection in pyaemia by the transportation of the organisms in the blood stream. **Radicular abscess.** Dental abscess (see above). **Residual abscess.** An abscess appearing near the site of an earlier abscess and caused by pyogenic organisms remaining from the latter. **Retrocaecal abscess.** Suppuration in the tissues lying posterior to the caecum, usually attributable to appendicitis. **Retromammary abscess.** An abscess located between the glandular tissue of the breast and the underlying tissues of the chest wall. **Retroperitoneal abscess.** An abscess located between the peritoneum and the posterior abdominal wall. **Retropharyngeal abscess.** Inflammation of the tissues between the pharynx and the spine, due either, in the acute form, to pyogenic infection of the lymph nodes in the posterior pharyngeal wall or, chronically, to a forward extension of infection from a tuberculous cervical spine. **Retrovesical abscess.** Pelvic abscess (see above). **Ring abscess.** Peripheral annular infiltration, an inflammation of the corneal periphery marked by a ring of pus around the site. **Root abscess.** Granuloma at the root of a tooth. **Satellite abscess.** One of the secondary abscesses close to and surrounding the primary abscess from which they have arisen. **Scrofulous abscess.** An abscess produced by infection of a lymph node by *Mycobacterium tuberculosis.* **Secondary abscess.** An embolic abscess arising apart from a primary abscess and due to the transportation of micro-organisms from the latter by the blood stream. **Septal abscess.** An abscess occurring at the root of a tooth on the proximal surface. **Serous abscess.** An abscess containing a clear, serum-like fluid; usually applied to the collection of fluid between a mildly inflamed bone and its periosteum. **Shirt-stud abscess.** Collar-stud abscess (see above). **Solitary abscess.** Amoebic abscess (see above). **Spermatic abscess.** An abscess occurring in the seminiferous tubules. **Spinal abscess.** An abscess in relation to a tuberculous spine. **Spleen abscess, Splenic abscess.** An abscess within the substance of the spleen; common in Africa. **Stercoraceous abscess, Stercoral abscess.** Faecal abscess (see above). **Sterile abscess.** An abscess from the contents of which it is impossible to culture micro-organisms. **Stitch abscess.** An abscess which develops in or around a suture. **Strumous abscess.** Cold abscess (see above). **Subaponeurotic abscess.** An abscess occurring beneath a fascial layer or aponeurosis. **Subareolar abscess.** An abscess arising beneath the epithelium of the areola of the nipple. **Subcutaneous abscess.** An abscess lying directly beneath the skin. **Subdiaphragmatic abscess.** Subphrenic abscess (see below). **Subdural abscess.** An abscess situated between the dura mater and the brain or spinal cord, usually in the subarachnoid space. **Subgaleal abscess.** An abscess situated beneath the epicranial aponeurosis. **Submammary abscess.** An abscess occurring immediately beneath the mammary gland. **Submucous abscess.** An abscess situated between the mucous lining and the muscular wall of a hollow organ or structure such as the rectum. **Subperiosteal abscess.** An abscess which develops between an infected bone and its periosteum in osteomyelitis. **Subperitoneal abscess.** An abscess located between the peritoneum and the abdominal wall. **Subphrenic abscess.** An abscess which develops in relation to the under surface of the diaphragm, usually after peritonitis or by extension from an intra-abdominal infected site. **Subscapular abscess.** An abscess which occurs between the scapula and the chest wall, usually in relation to the deeper aspect of the serratus anterior muscle. **Subungual abscess.** An abscess between a nail and the nail bed. **Sudoriparous abscess.** An abscess arising in a sweat gland. **Suprahepatic abscess.** An abscess located between the liver and the diaphragm. **Sweat gland abscess.** Sudoriparous abscess (see above). **Sympathetic abscess.** A secondary abscess appearing in some other part than that at which infection has entered, but due to the latter. **Syphilitic abscess.** An abscess of tertiary syphilis arising out of the liquefaction of a gumma. **Thecal abscess.** An abscess of a tendon sheath. **Thymus abscess.** An abscess of the thymus gland, such as that occurring in congenital syphilis. **Tonsillar abscess.** A suppurative condition of the parenchyma of a tonsil. **Tooth abscess.** Dental abscess (see above). **Traumatic abscess.** An abscess arising in tissue damaged by wound or injury. **Tropical abscess.** Amoebic abscess (see above). **Tuberculous abscess.** An abscess due to a tuberculous infection; a not uncommon and usually unfavourable sequel of tuberculosis. It may occur in bone, in lymph nodes, in joints and in the intestine. **Tubo-ovarian abscess.** An abscess involving the uterine tube and the ovary; commonly a sequel of salpingitis. **Tympanitic abscess.** An abscess in which air or gas is present. **Tympanomastoid abscess.** An abscess which involves both the tympanic antrum and the mastoid air cells. **Umbilical abscess.** An abscess developing in relation to, or pointing at, the umbilicus. **Urachal abscess.** An abscess of the abdominal wall below the navel due to infection of the urachal remnants. **Urethral abscess.** An abscess in the submucous tissue of the urethra or in a mucosal depression of the latter. **Urinary abscess.** An abscess communicating with a urinary passage. **Urinous abscess.** An abscess relating to the urinary system and containing pus and urine. **Verminous abscess.** An abscess in which animal parasites are present. **Wandering abscess.** An abscess which passes through the tissues, eventually coming to a point at some distance from the original site. **Web-space abscess.** An abscess of the areolar tissue at the base of the fingers. **Worm abscess.** Verminous abscess (see above). [L *abscedere* to go away.]

See also: BARTHOLIN (C.), BEZOLD (F.), BRODIE (B. C.), DELPECH, DOUGLAS (J.), DUBOIS (P.), FOCHIER, MÔNRO (I.), PAGET, POLITZER.

abscess root (ab·ses root). The root of the Greek valerian, *Polemonium reptans,* used as a stimulant and expectorant.

abscessus (ab·ses·us). **Abscessus flatuosus.** Tympanitic abscess, the result of the presence of gas liberated in the process of putrefaction. **Abscessus per fluxum.** An acute abscess. **Abscessus gangraenescens, Abscessus gangraenosus.** Anthrax. **Abscessus siccus corneae.** A term applied by von Arlt to keratitis disciformis; he attributed the condition to the presence of inspissated pus in the cornea. [L.]

abscissa (ab·sis·ah) (pl. *abscissae*). In a graph, the length cut off along the *x*-axis (horizontal axis) by a perpendicular dropped on the axis from a point. Cf. ORDINATE. [L a cut.]

abscission (ab·sish·un). 1. Removal by cutting away; the process of being cut off. 2. Suppression of a physiological function. **Corneal abscission.** Excision of the prominent part of the cornea in staphyloma. [L *abscindere* to cut away.]

absconsio (ab·skon·she·o). A fossa or cavity. [L hidden.]

absence (ab·sens). 1. Inattention to existing surroundings. 2. Temporary mental abstraction (absence of mind). [L *absentia.*]

Absidia (ab·sid·e·ah). A genus of fungi belonging to the class Phycomycetes and occurring in soil. **Absidia corymbifera.** A species which may cause pulmonary and generalized mycosis or otosclerosis in man. **Absidia ramosa** (Lindt) Lendner 1908. A pathogenic species which has been isolated from the human ear, from lesions in horses and swine, and from cases of abortion in cows. [Gk *apsis* vault.]

absinthate (ab·sin·thate). A salt of absinthic acid, the acid derived from wormwood, *Artemisia absinthium.*

absinthe (ab·sinth). A French liqueur containing, in addition to anise and other aromatic oils, oil of thuja, a cerebral convulsant with a marked cumulant effect. [Gk *apsinthion* wormwood.]

absinthiin (ab·sin·the·in). $C_{15}H_{20}O_4$. A poisonous crystalline compound derived from wormwood. [see prec.]

absinthin (ab·sin·thin). A yellowish-brown glucoside, $C_{20}H_{28}O_4$, obtained from *Artemisia absinthium,* wormwood. A narcotic poison, soluble in alcohol; used as a gastric tonic.

absinthism (ab·sin·thizm). A diseased condition which results from the excessive or continued use of absinthe. [Fr. *absinthe* wormwood.]

absinthium (ab·sin·the·um). Wormwood, being the dried leaves and tops of *Artemisia absinthium*; used as a tonic and anthelmintic. [Gk *apsinthion.*]

absinthol (ab·sin·thol). Thujone, $C_{10}H_{16}O$, the alcohol derived from oil of thuja. A cerebral convulsant with cumulative action. [see prec.]

absolute (ab·sol·ewt). Unrestricted; independent of arbitrary standards; unconditional; real. **Absolute cell increase.** An increase in the actual number of cells of a certain type in a fixed volume of fluid, irrespective of the number of cells of other types present [L *absolutus* set loose.]

absorbefacient (ab·zor·be·fa·shent). 1. Any agent which causes or promotes absorption. 2. Producing or promoting absorption. [absorb, L *facere* to make.]

absorbent (ab·zor·bent). 1. Any agent which attracts and sucks up gases or secretions from a wound. 2. Any vessel or organ which can draw material into the tissues, e.g. a lymph vessel. 3. Capable of sucking up liquids or gases. [L *absorbere* to suck up.]

absorptio (ab·**sorp**·she·o). **Absorptio morbosa.** Excrementitial absorption. **Absorptio pulmonalis.** Pulmonary absorption. **Absorptio sana.** Physiological absorption. [L absorption.]

absorptiometer (ab·sorp·she·**om**·et·er). 1. An apparatus for measuring the absorption of a gas by a liquid. 2. An arrangement for regulating the thickness of liquid drawn up by capillary attraction between a pair of glass plates; used in haematoscopy.

absorption (ab·**sorp**·shun). 1. The taking-in or abstraction of material, selectively or as a whole, e.g. of fluid by its passage into pores of any size in a solid or semisolid; of gases, by liquids or solids; of water and other materials from the alimentary canal, into the blood or lymph. 2. The transfer of any substance into the blood stream or lymphatic circulation from any of the body surfaces or tissues. 3. Intense mental concentration. 4. Of radiation: (*a*) the retention in a material of energy removed from radiation passing through it; (*b*) the removal of radiation or the reduction of its energy on passing through water; (*c*) the process whereby a neutron (or other particle) is captured by a nucleus. Cf. ADSORPTION. **Apparent absorption.** Absorption occurring by scattering, in which the apparent decrease in intensity of the beam is due to the scattered radiation no longer entering the detector. **Broad-beam absorption.** Absorption measured with a broad beam of radiation and a large absorber. **Buccal absorption.** Sublingual absorption (see below). **Carbon dioxide absorption.** Absorption of carbon dioxide by soda lime in an anaesthetic circuit. **Chylous absorption.** Absorption of chyle, i.e. fat-holding lymph, from the intestine. **Cutaneous absorption.** Absorption through the skin. **Disjunctive absorption.** The process of sloughing over a necrosed area through the removal of its zone of attachment to its tissue of origin. **Enteral absorption.** Absorption from the intestine. **Excrementitial absorption.** Pathological absorption (see below). **Interstitial absorption.** Absorption into interstices. **Intestinal absorption.** Enteral absorption (see above). **Lymphatic absorption.** The removal of fluid or cells by means of the lymphatics. **Narrow-beam absorption.** Absorption measured with a narrow parallel beam of radiation. **Nuclear absorption.** Absorption by interaction with an atomic nucleus: for example, production of neutrons by a (γ, n) process. **Parenteral absorption.** Absorption from a site other than the alimentary tract, as following intramuscular injection. **Pathological absorption.** The removal by natural physical or enzymological forces, or through cell action, of fluids, deposits or cells from a tissue, cavity or surface to which these may be foreign. **Percutaneous absorption.** Penetration of chemical substances from the exterior through the entire thickness of the skin. Permeability is greatest through epidermal cells and pilosebaceous units, less through sweat ducts and glands. Any break in the surface of the skin increases permeability. **Progressive absorption.** Slow but continuous absorption of a tissue, as in pressure atrophy, or the disappearance of scar tissue. **Purulent absorption.** A variety of pathological absorption (see above). **Self absorption.** Absorption of radiation within the radiation source itself. **Sublingual absorption.** Absorption from the mucous membrane of the mouth, and thus directly into the systemic circulation. **Total absorption.** Absorption due to true disappearance of the absorbed radiation and to scattering. **True absorption.** Absorption by disappearance of the absorbed radiation only, not by scattering. **Ulcerative absorption.** The extension of an ulcer. **Venous absorption.** Absorption by the veins. **Wall absorption.** Absorption of x- or γ-radiation in the wall of an ionization chamber used for measurement. It is significant if the wall thickness is too great for the type of radiation measured. [L *absorbere* to suck up.]

See also: COMPTON.

abstergent (ab·**ster**·jent). 1. Cleansing, purifying. 2. A detergent remedy or application. [L *abstergere* to cleanse.]

abstersion (ab·**ster**·shun). 1. The act or process of cleansing or purging. 2. A purgative. [see prec.]

abstersive (ab·**ster**·siv). Abstergent.

abstraction (ab·**strak**·shun). 1. The withdrawal of blood. 2. In pharmacy, the separation of any one ingredient from the others of a mixture. 3. In psychology, the focusing of attention on one quality of a complex object to the exclusion of other qualities. [L *abstrahere* to draw off.]

abterminal (ab·**term**·in·al). Of an electrical current, passing through muscular substance from the end towards the centre. [L *ab, terminus* end.]

abtorsion (ab·**tor**·shun). A condition in which, as a result of divergence outwards at the upper ends of the normally parallel vertical meridians of the eyeballs, there is a tendency towards extorsion in each eye. Disclination. [L *ab, torquere* to twist.]

abulia (a·**bew**·le·ah). Impairment or loss of will power. **Cyclic abulia.** Periodic recurrence of abulia. [Gk *a, boule* will.]

abulic (a·**bew**·lik). Referring to or affected with abulia. [see prec.]

abulomania (a·**bew**·lo·**ma'**·ne·ah). A form of mental disorder marked by indecision or impairment of will power. An obsolescent term, little used. [abulia, mania.]

abundance (ab·**un**·dans). **Isotopic abundance.** The number of atoms of a particular isotope in a mixture of the isotopes of an element, expressed as a fraction of all the atoms of the element. **Relative abundance.** The mass percentage of an individual isotope of an element in a mixture of isotopes; most commonly used for naturally occurring mixtures, e.g. ${}_{11}Na^{23}$ 100 per cent, but ${}_{6}C^{12}$ 98.9 per cent and ${}_{6}C^{13}$ 1.1 per cent. [L *abundare* to abound.]

abuse (ab·**ewz**). 1. Wrong use, especially excessive use, of anything. 2. Violation. [L *abuti* to misuse.]

abutment (ab·**ut**·ment). 1. A support against sideways pressure. 2. A tooth or root of a tooth which retains or supports a bridge or denture that is connected to it by a retainer or clasp. [O Fr. *abouter* place end to end.]

acacanthrax (a·kak·**an**·thrax). Non-malignant anthrax. [Gk *a, kakos* bad, anthrax.]

Acacia (ak·a·she·ah). 1. A genus of widely distributed leguminous trees, embracing many species, and from which are obtained black catechu (cutch) and certain gums including gum arabic. 2. Acacia BP 1973, gum acacia. The dried exudate from the branches and stem of *Acacia senegal* and several other species of *Acacia*; gum arabic. It is used in pharmacy as a pill excipient and as a suspending and emulsifying agent. **Acacia bark.** The dried bark of *Acacia arabica*, a native of India, Arabia and Africa, and of *Acacia decurrens*, which occurs in Australia; used in the form of a decoction as an astringent. **Acaciae Gummi.** *European Pharmacopoeia* name for Acacia BP 1973. [Gk *akakia*.]

acalculia (a·kal·**kew**·le·ah). Lack of mental power to do simple arithmetic; inability to calculate. [Gk *a*, L *calculare* to reckon.]

Acalypha (ak·**al**·e·fah). 1. A large group of euphorbiaceous plants native to warm regions. 2. The plant *Acalypha indica* of Southern Asia which yields the Acalypha of the BPC 1934, an expectorant, emetic and gastro-intestinal irritant. [Gk *akalyphes* uncovered.]

acamathesia (a·kam·ah·**theez'**·e·ah). Acatamathesia.

acampsia (a·**kamp**·se·ah). Inflexibility of limbs or joints to the point of rigidity. [Gk *a, kampsein* to bend.]

acantha (ak·**an**·thah). 1. The vertebral column. 2. The spinous process of a vertebra. 3. Spina bifida. [Gk thorn.]

acanthaceous (ak·an·**tha**·shus). In botany, armed with prickles. [see prec.]

acanthaesthesia (ak·**an**·thes·**the'**·ze·ah). A perverted sensation of being pricked with sharp points. [Gk *akantha* thorn, aesthesia.]

acanthamoebiasis (ak·**anth**·am·e·**bi'**·as·is). Acute meningo-encephalitis, usually fatal, due to acanthamoeba (Hartmanella), acquired by bathing in stagnant water. [Gk *akantha* thorn, amoebiasis.]

acanthia (ak·**an**·the·ah). *Cimex.* [Gk *akantha* thorn.]

acanthial (ak·**an**·the·al). Referring to the acanthion. [Gk *akanthion* little thorn.]

acanthion (ak·**an**·the·on). In craniology, the point in the medial plane of the skull at the tip of the anterior nasal spine. [see prec.]

Acanthobdellidea (ak·**an**·tho·del·**id'**·e·ah). A family of leeches belonging to the class Hirudinea and noted for the spines they bear on the surface of the body. [Gk *akantha* thorn, *bdella* leech.]

Acanthocephala (ak·**an**·tho·**kef'**·al·ah). A phylum of parasitic worms characterized by a spiny eversible proboscis with which they attach themselves to their hosts. *Macracanthorhynchus hirudinaceus* of pigs and *Moniliformis dubius* of rats have both been observed in the human intestine. [Gk *akantha* thorn, *kephale* head.]

acanthocephaliasis (ak·**an**·tho·kef·al·**i'**·as·is). The state of being infested by any species of the thorn-head worm (phylum Acanthocephala). [Gk *akantha* thorn, *kephale* head.]

Acanthocheilonema perstans (ak·**an**·tho·ki·lo·**ne'**·mah **per**·stanz). A filarial threadworm very common in Africa. The larvae are found in the peripheral blood stream; the adult inhabits various parts of the abdomen; and the microfilariae, which are unsheathed, are present in the blood day and night. It may cause a tropical eosinophilia-like syndrome, Calabar swelling, arthritis and arthralgia, and various neurological and psychological syndromes. The larvae have been found in the cerebrospinal fluid. **Acanthocheilonema streptocerca.** A filarial worm closely resembling *Acanthocheilonema perstans,* common in Africa and transmitted by the midge *Culicoides grahami.* The microfilariae occur in the skin of the limbs in man and chimpanzees. An irritant rash may be caused. [Gk *akantha* thorn, *cheilos* lip, *nema* thread, L *perstare* to persist.]

acanthocheilonemiasis (ak·an·tho·ki·lo·ne·**mi'**·as·is). Infection with the filarial worm *Acanthocheilonema perstans.* The infection causes no symptoms or pathogenic lesions.

acanthocyte (ak·**an**·tho·site). An erythrocyte with thorn-like projections. [Gk *akantha* thorn, *kytos* cell.]

acanthocytosis (ak·**an**·tho·si·**to'**·sis). A condition of the blood in which there are intrinsically abnormal erythrocytes having an unusual distorted, crenated or thorny appearance when examined in wet preparations and films. The condition is said to be associated with coeliac disease in earlier life, later with progressive diffuse ataxic neuropathy due to damage to the posterior columns and cerebellar pathways, and is reported in those with consanguineous parents; some patients have an atypical retinitis pigmentosa. It may be due to a mutant recessive allelomorph for a gene controlling normal red cell architecture. [Gk *akantha* thorn, *kytos* cell, *-osis* condition.]

acanthoid (ak·**an**·thoid). 1. Spinous. 2. Shaped like a spine. [Gk *akantha* thorn, *eidos* form.]

acanthokeratodermia (ak·an·tho·ker·at·o·**derm'**·e·ah). Thickening of the epidermal layers, especially the palm of the hand and the sole of the foot. [Gk *akantha* thorn, *keras* horn, *derma* skin.]

acantholysis (ak·an·**thol**·is·is). Separation of epidermal cells resulting from breakage of desmosomes. Intra-epidermal blistering results, as in pemphigus chronicus, pemphigus foliaceus, and familial benign chronic pemphigus (Hailey–Hailey disease). **Acantholysis bullosa.** Epidermolysis bullosa. [Gk *akantha* thorn, *lysis* a loosing.]

acanthoma (ak·an·**tho**·mah). A tumour associated with hypertrophy of the prickle-cell layer of the epidermis. Formerly applied to both benign and malignant lesions, the term has come to mean only benign epithelial tumours. **Acanthoma adenoides cysticum.** Epithelioma adenoides cysticum. **Malignant acanthoma.** Epithelioma. **Pale cell acanthoma.** Acanthoma of Degos. **Acanthoma papilloma.** Epithelioma adenoides cysticum. **Pigmented acanthoma.** An epithelioma of the skin that shows much pigmentation. **Acanthoma tropicum.** Pinkish, papillomatous warty growths in the inguinal region, of unknown aetiology. It has been reported from Colombia. [Gk *akantha* thorn, *-oma* tumour.]

acanthopelvis, acanthopelyx (ak·**an**·tho·**pel'**·vis, ak·**an**·tho·**pel'**·ix). A pelvis on the pubic crest of which there are sharp exostoses, sometimes causing disturbance of neighbouring structures. [Gk *akantha* thorn, *pelyx* pelvis.]

Acanthophis (ak·**an**·tho·fis). A genus of elapid snakes. **Acanthophis antarctica.** The death adder of Australia and New Guinea. [Gk *akantha* thorn, *ophis* snake.]

acanthorrhexis (ak·**an**·tho·**rex'**·is). Rupture of the intercellular bridges of the prickle cells of the epidermis, as seen in vesicular eczema. [Gk *akantha* thorn, *rhexis* a breaking.]

acanthosis (ak·an·**tho**·sis). Proliferation of the prickle-cell layer of the epidermis without destruction of the intercellular fibrils and often associated with a downward projection of the interpapillary processes; the condition is seen typically in psoriasis and eczema. **Acanthosis nigricans.** Keratosis nigricans, hypertrophy and pigmentation occurring usually in the flexures, the perianal area and other sites, with the development of papillary growths; the buccal and other mucosae may be affected. In the adult, the condition is usually symptomatic of visceral carcinoma. **Acanthosis papulosa nigra.** Dermatitis papulosa nigra, a papular eruption peculiar to the Negro race. **Acanthosis seborrhoeica.** Seborrhoeic wart. *See* WART. [Gk *akantha* thorn, *-osis* condition.]

acanthotic (ak·an·**thot**·ik). Referring to or affected with acanthosis. [see prec.]

acanthulus (ak·**an**·thew·lus). An instrument employed to remove penetrating foreign bodies, such as thorns, from small puncture wounds. [Gk *akantha* thorn.]

acapnia (a·**kap**·ne·ah). 1. An abnormal condition of the blood, in which the amount of carbon dioxide is diminished. 2. The functional disturbance due to a diminution of carbon dioxide in the blood. [Gk *a, kapnos* smoke.]

acapnial (a·**kap**·ne·al). Affected with or referring to acapnia. [see prec.]

acarbia (a·**kar**·be·ah). A condition in which the amount of sodium bicarbonate of the blood is lessened. [Gk *a,* carbonate.]

acardia (a·**kar**·de·ah). Congenital absence of the heart. [Gk *a, kardia* heart.]

acardiac (a·**kar**·de·ak). 1. Not having a heart. 2. An acardiacus. [see prec.]

acardiacus (a·kar·**di**·ak·us). A fetal monster without a heart and usually parasitic. **Acardiacus acephalus.** A monster having no head and consisting chiefly of pelvis and lower limbs. **Acardiacus amorphus, Acardiacus anceps.** A fetal monster with only rudimentary head, heart and extremities. [Gk *a, kardia* heart.]

acardiohaemia (a·**kar**·de·o·**heem'**·e·ah). A condition in which there is too little blood in the heart. [Gk *a, kardia* heart, *haima* blood.]

acardionervia (a·**kar**·de·o·**nerv'**·e·ah). Diminished nerve stimulus to the heart. [Gk *a, kardia* heart, nerve.]

acardiotrophia (a·**kar**·de·o·**tro'**·fe·ah). An atrophied condition of the heart. [Gk *a, kardia* heart, *trophe* nutrition.]

acardius (a·**kar**·de·us). Acardiacus. **Acardius anceps.** Acardiacus anceps.

Acari (**ak**·ar·i). 1. An order of the class Arachnida containing mites and ticks; Acarina. 2. A general term for all mites, but not ticks. [Gk *akari* mite.]

acarian (ak·**ar**·e·an). Referring or relating to the mites or acarids. [see prec.]

acariasis (ak·ar·**i**·as·is). The condition of being infested with mites. [Obsolete term.] **Chorioptic acariasis.** A misnomer for chorioptic sarcoptidosis (i.e. infestation with *Chorioptes*); it is more usually referred to as *chorioptosis.* **Demodectic acariasis.** An infection of the follicles of human hair by *Demodex folliculorum.* **Psoroptic acariasis.** A misnomer for psoroptic sarcoptidosis or psoroptosis, a form of scabies affecting sheep, horses and cattle, but almost unknown in man. **Pulmonary acariasis.** Infestation of the bronchi and bronchioles by mites; it occurs rarely in man, and has been associated, probably wrongly, with tropical eosinophilia. **Sarcoptic acariasis.** Infestation produced by the mite *Sarcoptes.* The eggs are deposited in channels burrowed in the skin. Cf. SCABIES. [Gk *akari* mite.]

acaricide (**ak**·ar·is·ide). An agent destructive to acarids or mites. [Gk *akari* mite, L *caedere* to kill.]

acarid (**ak**·ar·id). A mite. [Gk *akari* mite.]

acaridiasis (ak·ar·id·i′·as·is). Acariasis.

Acarina (ak·ar·i·nah). An order of the class Arachnida, comprising the mites and ticks, the bites of which may set up serious symptoms and introduce infection. [Gk *akari* mite.]

acarinosis, acariosis (ak·ar·in·o′·sis, ak·ar·e·o′·sis). Any one of the diseases due to acarids; acariasis. [Gk *akari* mite, *-osis* condition.]

Acariscus masoni (ak·ar·is·kus ma·son·i). *Trombicula masoni.* [Gk *akari* mite.]

acarodermatitis (ak·ar·o·der·mat·i′·tis). An inflammatory condition of the skin caused by acari. **Acarodermatitis urticarioides.** Grain itch. *See* ITCH. [Gk *akari,* mite, dermatitis.]

acaroid (ak·ar·oid). Having resemblance to a mite. [Gk *akari* mite, *eidos* form.]

acarophobia (ak·ar·o·fo′·be·ah). 1. An unreasoning fear of becoming infested with mites or other insects. 2. The delusion of parasitosis. [Gk *akari* mite, *phobein* to fear.]

acarotoxic (ak·ar·o·tox′·ik). Poisoning or destroying mites. [Gk *akari* mite, toxic.]

acarpia (a·karp·e·ah). 1. The condition of being sterile or barren. 2. The quality of unfruitfulness. [Gk *akarpia* unfruitfulness.]

acarpous (a·karp·us). 1. Barren or sterile; not producing fruit. 2. Without nodules or prominences. [see prec.]

Acarus (ak·ar·us). 1. In loose medical usage, any mite. 2. A genus of mites not containing species of medical importance: used as a genus in old literature for all small mites and thus including *Demodex, Dermanyssus, Pediculoides* and *Sarcoptes.* **Acarus folliculorum.** *Demodex folliculorum.* **Acarus scabiei.** *Sarcoptes scabiei.* [Gk *akari* mite.]

acaryote (a·kar·e·ot). Not nucleated. [Gk *a, karyon* nucleus.]

acatalasia (a·kat·al·a′·ze·ah). Autosomal recessive defect of catalase in all tissues, asymptomatic in the Swiss variety, associated with oral gangrene in Japanese variants. [Gk *a,* catalysis.]

acatalepsia, acatalepsy (a·kat·al·ep′·se·ah, a·kat·al·ep′·se). 1. Inability to understand; feeblemindedness. 2. Uncertainty of diagnosis or prognosis. [Obsolete term.] [Gk *a, katalepsis* understanding.]

acataleptic (a·kat·al·ep′·tik). 1. Deficient in understanding or comprehension; mentally deficient. 2. In diagnosis or prognosis, uncertain or doubtful. 3. Referring to or marked by acatalepsy. [Obsolete term.] [see prec.]

acatamathesia (a·kat·am·ah·theez′·e·ah). 1. Impairment or loss of perception, or of power to understand speech. 2. Abnormal blunting of the powers of perception, such as that seen in mental deafness or blindness. [Obsolete term.] [Gk *a, katamathesis* thorough knowledge.]

acataphasia (a·kat·ah·fa′·ze·ah). As a result of cerebral lesion, loss of power of orderly verbal expression, with abnormal syntax. [Obsolete term.] [Gk *a, kataphasis* affirmation.]

acataposis (a·kat·ah·po′·sis). Dysphagia. [Gk *a, kata, posis* swallowing.]

acatastasia (a·kat·as·ta′·ze·ah). 1. Of disease, deviation from type. 2. Of excretion, lack of regularity. [Gk *a, katastasis* stability.]

acatastatic (a·kat·as·tat′·ik). 1. Abnormal in nature. 2. Irregular in type. 3. Referring to or marked by acatastasia. [see prec.]

acatharsia, acatharsis (a·kath·ar·se·ah, a·kath·ar·sis). 1. A condition in which there is need of purgation. 2. Failure to obtain natural or artificial purgation. 3. Foulness. [Gk *a, katharsis* a cleansing.]

acathectic (a·kath·ek·tik). Referring to acathexia; marked by deficiency of the normal power of retention of the bodily secretions.

acathexia (a·kath·ex·e·ah). A condition in which there is failure normally to retain excretions or secretions. [Gk *a, kathexis* retention.]

acathexis (a·kath·ex·is). The stage in which certain things or ideas have no emotional charge attached to them. [see prec.]

acathisia (a·kath·iz·e·ah). Akathizia. [Gk *a, kathizein* to sit.]

acaudal, acaudate (a·kaw·dal, a·kaw·date). Tail-less. [Gk *a,* L *cauda* tail.]

acaulinosis (ak·aw·lin·o′·sis). A fungous disease of the skin caused by *Acaulium vagnoli-lutatii,* marked by erythema with formation of pus and crusts. [Gk *a,* L *caulis* stem, Gk *-osis* condition.]

Acaulium (ak·aw·le·um). A genus of fungi which are stemless or imperfect. *Acaulium vignoli-lutatii* is the fungus responsible for the disease, acaulinosis. [Gk *a,* L *caulis* stem.]

accelerant (ak·sel·er·ant). A catalytic agent. [L *accelerans* hastening.]

acceleration (ak·sel·er·a′·shun). 1. Quickening of movement or of rate. 2. In chemistry, an alteration in the speed of a chemical reaction. **Centripetal acceleration.** The acceleration towards the centre of curvature of a body moving with uniform velocity in a curved path. **Negative acceleration.** A decrease in the speed of a chemical reaction. **Positive acceleration.** An increase in the speed of a chemical reaction. [L *accelerare* to hasten.]

accelerator (ak·sel·er·a·tor). 1. Any nerve or muscle which increases the rate of performance of a function. 2. A device, such as a cyclotron, for accelerating charged particles so that they will take part in nuclear reactions. **Accelerator nerve.** *See* NERVE. **Accelerator partus.** An agent with ecbolic or abortifacient properties. **Linear accelerator.** A device for accelerating electrons to a high energy for use directly in radiotherapy or for the production of high energy x-rays, also for radiotherapy. **Serum accelerator.** *See* CONVERTIN. **Accelerator urinae.** The bulbospongiosus muscle. [see prec.]

accelerin (ak·sel·er·in). *See* CONVERTIN. [L *accelerare* to hasten.]

accelerometer (ak·sel·er·om′·et·er). An electrical or mechanical instrument for the measurement of acceleration.

accentuation (ak·sen·tew·a′·shun). Increase in loudness or distinctness. Generally applied to the heart sounds, and refers to increase of sound volume of the beats or extraordinary distinctness. [L *accentus* accent.]

accentuator (ak·sen·tew·a·tor). Any agent or substance which intensifies the action of a stain on tissues. [see prec.]

acceptor (ak·sep·tor). 1. A body or substance which receives and becomes unified with another. 2. In oxidation–reduction systems, the substance which unites with the active oxygen or hydrogen as the case may be. **Hydrogen acceptor.** In the oxidation of a substrate by an enzyme, the substance which combines with the hydrogen and is reduced. **Oxygen acceptor.** In the above type of reaction, the substance which combines with the oxygen and is oxidized. [L *accipere* to receive.]

access (ak·ses). 1. The onset of a disease. 2. A recurrence of an attack of a disease, or of a paroxysm or fit. 3. Legal cohabitation. [L *accedere* to approach.]

accessiflexor (ak·ses·e·flex·or). An accessory flexor muscle. [L *accessorius* supplementary, *flectere* to bend.]

accession (ak·sesh·un). The invasion or beginning of a disease or of a stage of a disease. The term is applied particularly to the recurrence of a periodical disease. [L *accedere* to approach.]

accessorius (ak·ses·or·e·us). Any accessory muscle or nerve. **Accessorius ad accessorium.** The flexor digitorum accessorius muscle. **Accessorius ad iliocostalem.** The costalis muscle. [L supplementary.]

accessory (ak·ses·or·e). A term descriptive of an organ or structure which aids in a secondary way a similar more important organ or structure. **Accessory muscle.** *See* MUSCLE. **Accessory pancreas.** *See* PANCREAS. **Accessory process of a lumbar vertebra.** *See* PROCESS. **Accessory spleen.** *See* SPLEEN. [see prec.]

accessory nerve [nervus accessorius (NA)]. The 11th cranial nerve. It is composed of 2 portions, the cranial and spinal, arising from the medulla oblongata and cervical part of the spinal cord respectively.

Branch to the sternomastoid muscle [ramus externus (NA)]. Fibres from the spinal root to the sternomastoid and trapezius muscles.

Branch to the vagus nerve, accessory [ramus internus (NA)]. A few filaments from the bulbar part to the superior vagal ganglion.

Nucleus [nucleus nervi accessorii (NA)]. The nucleus comprising the nucleus ambiguus and the spinal nucleus. **Spinal nucleus [nucleus spinalis nervi accessorii (NA)].** The column of grey cells at the base of the anterior grey column of the upper 6 cervical segments of the spinal medulla, giving origin to the axons of the spinal part of the nerve. **Cranial root [radix cranialis (NA)].** A division of the accessory nerve arising from the medulla oblongata and joining the vagus nerve below the skull. It is distributed mainly through the pharyngeal and laryngeal branch of the nerve. **Spinal root [radix spinalis (NA)].** A division of the accessory nerve arising from the spinal cord down to the 5th cervical segment. After a short union with the cranial portion in the skull it separates from it to supply the sternomastoid and trapezius muscles.

accident (ak·sid·ent). 1. An unexpected and sudden event or contingency, especially one of a harmful character. 2. An unforeseen occurrence which complicates the normal course of a disease. **Cerebral accident.** Any sudden disturbance of cerebral function. **Cerebral vascular accident.** A cerebral accident due to disease of blood vessels; the term covers spontaneous (non-traumatic) cerebral and subarachnoid haemorrhage, thrombosis and embolism. **Radiation accident.** An unplanned exposure to potentially harmful radiation. **Serum accident.** A haemolytic crisis due to the intravenous injection of heterologous serum. [L *accidere* to happen.]

accidentalism (ak·sid·**ent**·al·izm). A system of medicine founded on symptoms only, without regard to aetiology or pathology. [see prec.]

accipiter (ak·**sip**·it·er). A tailed bandage which resembles the claw of a hawk, for application over the nose. [L hawk.]

acclimatation, acclimation (ak·li·mat·**a**′·shun, ak·lim·**a**·shun). Acclimatization.

acclimatization (ak·**li**·mat·i·**za**′·shun). The process whereby the body adapts to a novel environment, e.g. high altitude, tropical conditions. **Altitude acclimitization.** Physiological adaptation to reduced atmospheric pressure and oxygen content; hypoxia may cause hypernoea and result in altitude alkalosis and altitude alkaluria. [L *ad*, climate, Gk *klima* region.]

accoine (**ak**·o·een). A mixture of sodium benzoate and carbonate used to preserve milk.

Accolé (ak·o·**la**). Term applied to a particular form of the malarial parasite, *Plasmodium falciparum*, appearing as a thin attachment to the erythrocyte; appliqué form. [Fr. embraced.]

accommodation (ak·om·o·**da**·shun). Adjustment, e.g. in ophthalmology, applied to the mechanism by which the focus of the eye is shortened through contraction of the ciliary muscle, increasing the convexity of the lens. **Absolute accommodation.** The amount in dioptres by which each eye, separately, is able to change its focus. **Amplitude of accommodation.** A term similar in meaning to absolute accommodation, except that it can be applied to uniocular or binocular vision. **Binocular accommodation.** The act, or the amount, by which the two eyes, working together, alter their focus when looking from a far to a near object. **Dynamic accommodation.** A term sometimes employed for the act of accommodation, to emphasize the fact that work is done in shortening the focus of the eye. **Excessive accommodation.** Accommodation in excess of what is needed. **Histological accommodation.** Modulation; change in the morphological characteristics of a cell or tissue, associated with altered functional activity. **Negative accommodation.** The amount by which accommodation can be reduced below that which would be associated with a given degree of convergence. **Nerve accommodation.** The rise in the threshold of excitability of a nerve that occurs with a slowly increasing strength of electrical stimulation, as contrasted with a rapidly increasing current. With the former, high values may be obtained without eliciting a response. **Pelvic accommodation.** The space available in the pelvic cavity. **Positive accommodation.** The amount by which accommodation can be increased beyond that which would be associated with a given degree of convergence. **Range of accommodation.** The distance between the far point and the near point. **Reflex accommodation.** A term formerly applied to the Argyll Robertson pupil, in which the pupil is inactive to light but contracts on near vision. The contraction is, however, due to the act of convergence and not to that of accommodation. **Relative accommodation.** The total amount of accommodation (positive plus negative) which can be exercised without altering the degree of convergence. **Static accommodation.** The state of the eye when the ciliary body is at rest. **Subnormal accommodation.** Amplitude of accommodation below the normal for the patient's age. **Supernormal accommodation.** Amplitude of accommodation above the normal for the patient's age. [L *accommodatio* adjustment, adaptation.]

accommodometer (ak·om·o·**dom**·et·er). In ophthalmology, an instrument by which the accommodative capacity of the eye can be measured.

accouchement (ah·koosh·**mahn**). Childbirth; delivery in childbed; confinement. **Accouchement forcé.** Quick and forcible delivery with the hand or by means of instruments. [Fr. delivery.]

accoucheur, accoucheuse (ah·koosh·**er**, ah·koosh·**erz**). A male or female professional obstetrician. [see prec.]

accrementitial (**ak**·re·men·**tish**′·al). Referring or belonging to accrementition. [L *accrescere* to increase, increment.]

accrementition (**ak**·re·men·**tish**′·un). In biology, increase by interstitial development, and by reproduction of cells by fission; gemmation. [see prec.]

accretio cordis, accretio pericardii (ak·**re**·she·o **kor**·dis, per·e·**kar**·de·i). Adhesive pericarditis; especially applied to a variety of adhesive pericarditis in which extensive adhesions have been formed, from the pericardium to the diaphragm, the pleurae and the wall of the chest. [L accretion of the heart.]

accretion (ak·**re**·shun). 1. Organic growth. 2. Growth by external addition. 3. A growing together of parts naturally separate. 4. A collection of foreign matter in a cavity. [L *accrescere* to increase.]

accrochage (**ak**·ro·chaje). Isorhythmic atrioventricular dissociation. *See* DISSOCIATION.

accubation (ak·ew·**ba**·shun). 1. The posture adopted when a person lies on his side in bed or on a couch. 2. Parturition. [L *accubatio*, a reclining.]

ace-. Prefix indicating the presence of the ethylene radical, $—CH_2CH_2—$, in a molecule.

Acebutolol (as·e·**bew**·to·lol). BP Commission approved name for (±) - 1 - (2 - acetyl - 4 - butyramidophenoxy) - 3 - isopropylaminopropan - 2 - ol; an adrenergic beta-receptor blocking agent.

Acedapsone (as·e·**dap**·sone). BP Commission approved name for di-(4-acetamidophenyl)sulphone; an antimalarial and antileprotic.

acedia (a·**se**·de·ah). A form of mental disorder marked by great depression, with lack of interest in surrounding persons and things; melancholia. [Gk *akedia* apathy.]

acenaphthene (as·e·**naf**·theen). Ethylene naphthalene, $C_{10}H_6(CH_2)_2$. A hydrocarbon derived from coal-tar, crystallizing in colourless needles. Insoluble in water, it is used in organic synthesis and dye manufacture.

acentric (a·**sen**·trik). 1. Away from the centre; eccentric. 2. In cytogenetics, of chromosome or chromosome regions without a centromere. **Acentric fragment.** *See* FRAGMENT. [Gk *a*, L *centrum* centre.]

aceognosia (**as**·e·og·**no**′·se·ah). A knowledge of remedies for diseases. [Gk *akos* remedy, *gnosis* knowledge.]

acephalia, acephalism (a·kef·**a**·le·ah, a·**kef**·al·izm). Acephaly.

acephalobrachia (a·**kef**·al·o·**bra**′·ke·ah). The condition of being without head and arms. [Gk *a*, *kephale* head, *brachion* arm.]

acephalobrachius (a·**kef**·al·o·**bra**′·ke·us). A monster without head and arms. [see prec.]

acephalocardia (a·**kef**·al·o·**kar**′·de·ah). The condition of being without head and heart. [Gk *a*, *kephale* head, *kardia* heart.]

acephalocardius (a·**kef**·al·o·**kar**′·de·us). A monster without head and heart. [see prec.]

acephalocheiria, acephalochiria (a·**kef**·al·o·**ki**′·re·ah). The condition of being without head and hands. [Gk *a, kephale* head, *cheir* hand.]

acephalocheirus, acephalochirus (a·**kef**·al·o·**ki**′·rus). A monster without head and hands. [see prec.]

acephalocyst (a·**kef**·al·o·sist). A sterile hyatid cyst without a scolex. [Gk *a, kephale* head, cyst.]

acephalocystis (a·**kef**·al·o·**sis**′·tis). **Acephalocystis plana.** A term for certain kinds of mineral aggregations met with in muscles or the sheaths of tendons (Laënnec). **Acephalocystis racemosa.** A hydatidiform mole found in the uterus. [see prec.]

acephalogaster (a·**kef**·al·o·**gas**′·ter). A fetus without head, thorax and upper abdomen. [Gk *a, kephale* head, *gaster* belly.]

acephalogasteria, acephalogastria (a·**kef**·al·o·gas·**teer**′·e·ah, a·**kef**·al·o·**gas**′·tre·ah). The condition of being without head and abdomen. [see prec.]

acephalophorous (a·kef·al·**of**·or·us). Lacking a completely formed head. [Gk *a, kephale* head, *pherein* to bear.]

acephalopodia (a·**kef**·al·o·**po**′·de·ah). The condition of being without head and feet. [Gk *a, kephale* head, *pous* foot.]

acephalopodius (a·**kef**·al·o·**po**′·de·us). A monster without head and feet. [see prec.]

acephalorachia (a·**kef**·al·o·**ra**′·ke·ah). The condition of being without head and vertebral column. [Gk *a, kephale* head, *rhachis* spine.]

acephalorachus (a·**kef**·al·o·**ra**′·kus). A monster without head and vertebral column. [see prec.]

acephalostomia (a·**kef**·al·o·**sto**′·me·ah). A teratomic condition in which the head is absent, but in which there is a mouth-like opening on the superior aspect. [Gk *a, kephale* head, *stoma* mouth.]

acephalostomus (a·**kef**·al·**os**′·to·mus). A monster with the characteristics of acephalostomia. [see prec.]

acephalothoracia (a·**kef**·al·o·thor·**as**′·e·ah). The condition of being without head and chest. [Gk *a, kephale* head, thorax.]

acephalothorax, acephalothorus (a·**kef**·al·o·**thor**′·ax, a·**kef**·al·o·**thor**′·us). A monster without head and thorax. [see prec.]

acephalus (a·**kef**·al·us). A monster without a head. **Acephalus dibrachius.** A monster with upper limbs in an undeveloped state. **Acephalus dipus.** A monster in which there is an undeveloped condition of the lower extremities. **Acephalus monobrachus.** A monster with only one upper limb, the rest of the body being extremely rudimentary. **Acephalus monopus.** A monster with only one of the lower limbs. **Acephalus paracephalus.** A monster without a brain and with a defective skull. **Acephalus sympus.** A monster in which there is fusion of the lower limbs, the latter together forming a long cone. [Gk *a, kephale* head.]

acephaly (a·**kef**·al·e). Absence of the head. [see prec.]

Acepifylline (as·**e**·pe·**fi**′·leen). BP Commission approved name for piperazine theophyllin-7-ylacetate; a spasmolytic.

Acepromazine (as·e·**pro**·maz·een). **Acepromazine Maleate BPC 1968.** The hydrogen maleate; a drug with a tranquillizing action similar to that of chlorpromazine, but stated to be less toxic.

acerate (as·er·ate). A salt of aceric acid, which occurs in the juice of the maple. [L *acer* maple.]

acerbity (as·er·bit·e). Sourness combined with bitterness and astringency. [L *acerbitas* sharpness.]

acercus (as·er·kus). A monster lacking a coccyx. [Gk *a, kerkos* tail.]

aceric (as·**er**·ik). Relating to the maple tree. [L *acer* maple.]

aceride (as·er·ide). Term applied to an ointment or plaster which contains no wax. [Gk *a*, L *cera* wax.]

acerin (as·er·in). The active principle of a substance obtained from the seeds of the Norway maple (*Acer platanoides*); this substance inactivates the phage of several bacterial species and also vaccinia virus, *in vitro.* [L *acer* maple.]

acerotous (as·**er**·o·tus). Waxless, denoting ointments and plasters made up without wax. [Gk *a*, L *cera* wax.]

acervuline (as·er·vew·leen). Aggregated in a small mass; refers commonly to groups of glands. [acervulus.]

acervuloma (as·**er**·vew·**low**·mah). Psammoma. [acervulus, Gk *-oma* tumour.]

acervulus, acervulus cerebri (as·**er**·vew·lus **ser**·e·bri). The mass of gritty matter present at the base of the pineal body in persons over the age of 16. It consists of phosphatic and carbonate concretions, and is often referred to as *brainsand.* [L little heap of the brain.]

acescence (as·**es**·ens). 1. The process of becoming acid. 2. Sourness. [L *acescere* to turn sour.]

acescent (as·**es**·ent). Acidulous. [see prec.]

acesodyne (as·**es**·o·dine). Anodyne. [Gk *akeisthai* to cure, *odyne* pain.]

acestoma (as·es·**to**·mah). Granulation tissue, especially the active mass which is the basis of a cicatrix. [Gk *akestos* curable, *-oma* tumour.]

acetabular (as·et·**ab**·ew·lar). Referring or belonging to the acetabulum. **Acetabular notch.** *See* NOTCH.

acetabulectomy (**as**·et·ab·ew·**lek**′·to·me). The surgical removal of the acetabulum as well as the remainder of the hip joint. [acetabulum, Gk *ektome* a cutting out.]

acetabuloplasty (as·et·**ab**·ew·lo·**plas**′·te). A plastic operation performed on the acetabulum. [acetabulum, Gk *plassein* to form.]

acetabulum [NA] (as·et·**ab**·ew·lum). The socket, shaped like a cup, on the outer aspect of the innominate bone into which the head of the femur is set and moves. **Acetabulum humeri.** The glenoid cavity. [L a little saucer for vinegar.]

acetal (**as**·et·al). Diethyl acetal, $C_2H_4(OC_2H_5)_2$. Ethereal colourless liquid, slightly soluble in water, readily in alcohol. It is used medicinally as a hypnotic. Cf. METHYLAL.

acetaldehyde (as·et·**al**·de·hide). Acetic aldehyde, CH_3CHO. *See* ALDEHYDE.

acetals (**as**·et·alz). A group of substances similar in structure to acetal, and formed by the condensation of aldehydes with alcohols.

acetamide (as·et·**am**·ide). CH_3CONH_2. White crystals, readily soluble in water or alcohol. They are deliquescent and form crystalline compounds with sodium and magnesium halides, also unstable combinations with Na, K, Mg, Zn, Hg, and with mineral acids. **Phenyl acetamide.** Acetanilide.

acetamidine (as·et·**am**·id·een). $CH_3C(NH)NH_2$. The amidine of acetic acid. A crystalline base forming stable salts.

acetamido-antipyrin (as·et·**am**·id·o·an·te·**pi**′·rin). A crystalline compound used as an antipyretic and analgesic.

***p*-acetamidobenzene sulphonamide** (**par**·ah·as·et·**am**·id·o·**ben**′·zeen sul·**fon**·am·ide). Acetyl sulphanilamide, $CH_3CONHC_6H_4SO_2NH_2$. In detoxication, one of the forms in which sulphonamides are modified and excreted.

***p*-acetamidobenzoyleugenol** (**par**·ah·as·et·**am**·id·o·**ben**·zo·il·**ew**′·jen·ol). Acetaminol.

acetamidophenol (as·et·**am**·id·o·**fe**′·nol). $C_6H_4OHNHCOCH_3$, an acetyl derivative of *p*-aminophenol, less toxic than acetanilide, and used as an antipyretic.

acetamidosalol (as·et·**am**·id·o·**sal**′·ol). $C_6H_4(OH)COOC_6H_4NHCOCH_3$, white crystalline scales, soluble in hot water, alcohol or ether. Of value medicinally as an antirheumatic, antipyretic and intestinal antiseptic. Acetylparamidosalol.

acetaminofluorene (as·et·**am**·in·o·**floo**′·or·een). $C_6H_4CH_2C_6H_3NHCOCH_3$. A derivative of fluorene, $C_{13}H_{10}$, a coal-tar hydrocarbon; it has carcinogenic properties.

acetaminol (as·et·**am**·in·ol). *p*-Acetamidobenzoyleugenol, $C_{18}H_{23}NO_4$. A crystalline compound derived from eugenol. Insoluble in water, soluble in alcohol; used in pulmonary tuberculosis.

acetaminotoluene (as·et·**am**·in·o·**tol**′·ew·een). Acetoluide.

acetanilide (as·et·**an**·il·ide). Acetylaminobenzene, phenyl acetamide, $C_6H_5NHCOCH_3$. An acetyl derivative of aniline. Lustrous white scales which sublimate easily; odourless, with a burning taste. Soluble in water and alcohol. Antipyretic, analgesic, antirheumatic; continued administration is likely to produce methaemoglobinaemia. **Ammoniated acetanilide.** A mixture of acetanilide, ammonium carbonate, sodium bicarbonate and sugar of milk; it causes less depression than acetanilide alone. **Methoxy acetanilide.** Acetanisidin. **Methyl acetanilide.** Acetaminotoluene, acetyl toluidine. **Methylated acetanilide.** Acetanisidin. **Monobromated acetanilide.** Acetbromanilide, acetobromanilide.

acetanisidin (as·et·an·**is'**·id·in). Methoxy acetanilide, methylated acetanilide, $C_6H_4(OCH_3)NHCOCH_3$. *ortho* form, colourless crystals soluble in water. *meta* form, only slightly soluble in water but readily in alcohol or ether; an antipyretic and analgesic. *para* form, colourless needles slightly soluble in water; methacetin.

acetannin (as·e·**tan**·in). Acetyltannic acid, acetyltannin, $C_{14}H_8O_7(COOCH_3)_2$. Greyish powder, odourless and tasteless. Insoluble in water or alcohol, but soluble in ethyl acetate. Used medicinally in chronic diarrhoea and intestinal catarrh.

acetarct (as·et·arkt). Acet-extract. Extraction of drugs with acetic acid.

Acetarsol BP 1973, acetarsone (as·et·**ar**·sol, as·et·**ar**·sone). 3-Acetamido-4-hydroxyphenylarsonic acid, $C_6H_3OHAsO(OH)_2NHCOCH_3$. White crystals, almost insoluble in water or alcohol; readily soluble in alkalis. A form of treatment now entirely superseded in amoebiases or any form of syphilis. Used locally in treatment of Vincent's angina, and leucorrhoea, especially that due to *Trichomonas vaginalis.* The sodium salt, acetarsol sodium, a more soluble form, is injected for yaws and general paralysis. **Diethylamine acetarsol.** The diethylamine salt of acetarsol; a water-soluble organic arsenical used for cardiovascular and hepatic syphilis.

acetate (as·et·ate). A salt of acetic acid. Most acetates are soluble in water, with the exception of Hg and Ag. Decomposed by heat or strong acids.

Acetazolamide BP 1973 (as·et·ah·**zol'**·am·ide). 5-Acetamido-1,3,4-thiadiazole-2-sulphonamide. An oral diuretic used mainly for congestive heart failure. It has also been used with favourable results in glaucoma and epilepsy.

acetbromanilide (as·et·bro·**man'**·il·ide). $BrC_6H_4NHCOCH_3$, colourless needles, sparingly soluble in water. It has antipyretic, antiseptic and antineuralgic properties.

acetenyl (as·**et**·en·il). Ethinyl. The monovalent radical, $HC{\equiv}C-$, derived from acetylene.

aceteugenol (as·et·**ew**·jen·ol). 1-Ethyl-3-methoxy-4-acetoxy-benzene, obtained from oil of cloves. *See* EUGENOL.

acethaemin (as·et·**he**·min). A biological pigment formed during the breakdown of haemoglobin, the red colouring matter of blood.

acetic (as·**e**·tik). 1. Relating to, or having the properties of, vinegar or acetic acid; sour. 2. Compounds containing the acetyl radical, CH_3CO-. **Acetic acid.** *See* ACID. **Acetic aldehyde.** *See* ALDEHYDE. **Acetic anhydride.** *See* ANHYDRIDE. **Acetic ester.** Ethyl acetate. **Acetic ether.** Ethyl acetate. **Acetic oxide.** Acetic anhydride. **Acetic peracid.** Peracetic acid. *See* ACID. [L *acetum* vinegar.]

aceticoceptor (as·e·tik·o·**sep'**·tor). A molecular side-chain with a preferential affinity for the acetyl group. [acetic, L *recipere* to receive.]

aceticoseptor (as·e·tik·o·**sep'**·tor). Ehrlich's name for the point in a trypanosome that has become arsenic-resistant at which an arsenic drug containing an acetyl group can still be attached. Cf. ARSENOCEPTOR. [see prec.]

acetidin (as·**et**·id·in). Ethyl acetate, $CH_3COOC_2H_5$. An inhalant in laryngeal catarrh; also used internally as an antispasmodic and diaphoretic.

acetification (as·e·tif·ik·**a'**·shun). The production of vinegar from fermented liquids by atmospheric oxidation catalysed by the presence of bacterial organisms such as *Acetobacter aceti.* [L *acetum* vinegar, *facere* to make.]

acetify (as·**e**·tif·i). To carry through the process of making vinegar; to add acetic acid. [see prec.]

acetimeter (as·e·**tim**·et·er). A device for measuring the amount of acetic acid in vinegar.

acetimetry (as·e·**tim**·et·re). Determination, by measuring with an acetimeter, of the amount of acetic acid in vinegar.

acetin (as·et·in). One of the 3 esters produced by the reaction of glycerol with acetic acid, which occur naturally in cod-liver oil and butter fats.

aceto-acetate (as·et·o·**as'**·et·ate). A salt or ester of aceto-acetic acid, an acid which occurs in diabetic urine.

aceto-acetic esters (as·et·o·as·**e'**·tik **es**·terz). A series of ethereal-smelling liquids of the general formula RC_3H_4OCOOR', synthesized by the action of metallic sodium upon various alkyl esters. They are insoluble in water and can be distilled easily. Each may occur in 2 isomeric forms, enolic and ketonic.

aceto-arsenite (as·et·o·**ar'**·sen·ite). A double salt composed of the acetate and arsenite of the same metal. Schweinfurt green, an important pigment prepared from verdigris, is cupric aceto-arsenite, $Cu(C_2H_3O_2)_23Cu(AsO_2)_2$.

Acetobacter (as·e·to·**bak**·ter). A genus of non-pathogenic bacteria of the family Bacteriaceae which are rod-shaped cells, aerobic, and able to oxidize alcohol into acetic acid in the course of their metabolism; the differentiation of this genus from the genus *Bacterium* is not accepted by many British bacteriologists. **Acetobacter aceti.** The organism responsible for the conversion of wine into vinegar, forming a scum on the surface known as *mother of vinegar.* [L *acetum* vinegar, bacterium.]

acetobromanilide (as·et·o·bro·**man'**·il·ide). Acetbromanilide.

acetobromide (as·et·o·**bro'**·mide). A salt in which the acetate and bromide radicals are attached to the same metallic atom, as in lead acetobromide, $BrPb(C_2H_3O_2)$.

acetocarmine (as·et·o·**kar'**·mine). A valuable chromatin stain incorporating acetic acid.

acetochloral (as·et·o·**klor'**·al). A hypnotic derived from chloral.

acetochloride (as·et·o·**klor'**·ide). A salt of acetic and hydrochloric acids, analogous to the acetobromide.

acetoform (as·e·to·form). Hexamethylenetetramine, $(CH_2)_6N_4$. Colourless crystals, soluble in water. A powerful urinary antiseptic.

acetoglycocoll (as·et·o·**gli'**·ko·kol). Acetamido-acetic acid, $CH_3CONHCH_2COOH$. Colourless crystals, soluble in water and alcohol, but insoluble in ether. It is a substance related to the amino acid glycine, and is involved in the protein metabolism.

Acetohexamide (as·et·o·**hex**·am·ide). BP Commission approved name for *N*-4-acetylbenzenesulphonyl-*N'*-cyclohexylurea; an oral hypoglycaemic agent.

acetoin (as·et·o·in). Acetylmethylcarbinol, $CH_3COCHOHCH_3$. A colourless liquid formed during the fermentation of glucose by *Aerobacter aerogenes.* It is oxidized to diacetyl, the substance which imparts the characteristic odour to butter.

aceto-iodide (as·et·o·**i'**·o·dide). A salt containing acetate and iodide radicals, analogous to an acetobromide.

acetol (as·e·tol). Acetyl carbinol, CH_3COCH_2OH, a ketol obtained from fused cane sugar.

acetoluide (as·et·**ol**·ew·ide). Acetotoluidine, acetyl toluidine, acetaminotoluene, methyl acetanilide $CH_3C_6H_4NHCOCH_3$. An antipyretic, similar to acetanilide but less toxic. *ortho* and *para* forms only slightly soluble in water, but freely in alcohol.

acetolysis (as·et·**ol**·is·is). 1. The removal of acetyl groups from organic compounds with alkalis. 2. The breaking-up of an organic molecule by the action of acetic acid. [acetic, Gk *lysis* a loosing.]

acetomel (as·**et**·o·mel). Oxymel. Honey medicated with acetic acid. (acetic, L *mel* honey.]

Acetomenaphthone BP 1973 (as·et·o·men·**af'**·thone). 1,4-Diacetoxy-2-methylnaphthalene, $C_{15}H_{14}O_4$. A white crystalline compound derived from menaphthone (menadione). It is almost insoluble in water, but is given orally, either as tablets or in oily solution, in the last days of pregnancy, or in the newborn child, to prevent haemorrhagic disease.

acetometer (as·e·**tom**·et·er). Acetimeter.

acetometry (as·e·**tom**·et·re). Acetimetry.

acetomorphine (as·et·o·**mor'**·feen). Diacetylmorphine, $C_{21}H_{23}O_5N$, diamorphine hydrochloride. A compound of morphine and acetic anhydride; better known as *heroin.* It is a colourless crystalline powder readily soluble in water. More effective than morphine in the relief of pain, and not as constipating, though the danger of addiction is greater.

acetonaemia (as·e·ton·**e'**·me·ah). The condition in which there are acetone bodies in the blood. [acetone, Gk *haima* blood.]

acetonaemic (as·e·ton·**e'**·mik). Characterized by or referring to acetonaemia. [see prec.]

acetonal (as·**et**·o·nal). A double acetate of aluminium and sodium.

acetonaphthone (as·et·o·**naf'**·thone). Naphthylmethyl ketone, $C_{10}H_7COCH_3$. The acetyl derivative of naphthalene. It exists in 2 isomeric forms; the α-form consists of colourless crystals soluble in alcohol.

acetonasthma (as·e·ton·**as'**·mah). Asthma combined with acetonuria, the symptoms and signs being those of headache, vomiting, defective vision of temporary character and general restlessness of mind and body, with shortness of breath, and acetone in the urine.

acetonation (as·e·ton·**a'**·shun). The process of being combined with acetone.

Acetone (as·e·tone). Dimethylketone, CH_3COCH_3. A colourless limpid liquid with an ethereal odour and an acrid taste. It is highly inflammable, and is present in crude wood-spirit. Traces are to be found in the blood and normal urine; the quantity is very much increased in the urine of diabetics. It mixes with water, alcohol, or ether, in all proportions, and is an anaesthetic, anthelmintic, and is also used in dyspnoea (BPC 1968). It forms the starting point of many important synthetic drugs. **Acetone acid.** *See* ACID. **Acetone alcohol.** Acetol, acetyl carbinol, CH_3COCH_2OH, a ketol obtained from fused cane sugar. **Acetone bodies.** Aliphatic ketones and hydroxy ketones found in the blood and urine of severe diabetics as the result of the incomplete breakdown of fatty and amino acids, a condition known as *ketosis.* **Acetone bromoform.** Brometone, $CBr_3COH(CH_3)_2$, a sedative. **Acetone chloroform.** $CCl_3COH(CH_3)_2$, white crystals soluble in water, more readily in alcohol; used as a hypnotic, as an anaesthetic and for seasickness and hay fever. **Acetone compounds.** Acetone bodies (see above). **Acetone diethysulphone.** The hypnotic, sulphonal, $(CH_3)_2C(SO_2C_2H_5)_2$. **Monochlorated acetone.** $CH_2ClCOCH_3$, a colourless liquid with a pungent odour. **Acetone resorcinol.** $C_{15}H_{16}O_4$, insoluble in water, alcohol or ether, but soluble in alkalis; used as an antiseptic and bactericide.

acetones (as·e·to·nz). The series of compounds analogous to acetone, the first member, all containing 2 alkyl radicals joined by a CO= group.

acetonglycosuria (as·e·tone·gli·ko·**zewr'**·e·ah). Glycosuria resulting from acetone poisoning. [acetone, glucose, urine.]

acetonin (as·e·to·nin). A complex condensation product of acetone and ammonia.

acetonitrate (as·e·to·**ni'**·trate). A salt of acetic and nitric acids with the same base, in similar manner to an acetobromide.

acetonitrile (as·e·to·**ni'**·trile). Methyl cyanide, carbamine, CH_3CN. A colourless liquid with a pleasant odour, occurring in coal tar and molasses. Used in organic synthesis and the manufacture of perfumery.

acetonoresorcin, acetonoresorcinol (as·e·**to**·no·rez·**or'**·sin, as·e·to·no·rez·**or'**·sin·ol). Acetone resorcinol.

acetonumerator (as·e·to·**new'**·mer·a·tor). An instrument with which the amount of acetone in urine can be determined. [acetone, numerator.]

acetonuria (as·e·to·**newr'**·e·ah). The presence of an excess quantity of acetone bodies in the urine. [acetone, urine.]

acetonyl (as·**et**·o·nil). The monovalent radical, CH_3COCH_2—.

aceto-orthotoluide (as·et·o·or·tho·**tol'**·ew·ide). $CH_3C_6H_4NHCOCH_3$, an isomeric form of acetaminotoluene, or acetoluide, occurring in colourless crystals slightly soluble in water; used as an antipyretic.

acetoparatoluide (as·et·o·par·ah·**tol'**·ew·ide). $CH_3C_6H_4NHCOCH_3$, the *para* form of acetaminotoluene, or acetoluide; an antipyretic, insoluble in water.

Acetophenetidin (as·et·o·fen·**et'**·id·in). Phenacetin BP 1958, $CH_3CONHC_6H_4OC_2H_5$, an acetyl compound of phenetidin. White laminar crystals, tasteless, and only sparingly soluble in water but soluble in alcohol or ether. It is an analgesic and antirheumatic, similar to acetanilide, but heavy and prolonged dosage may cause renal papillary necrosis.

acetophenone (as·et·o·fe·**none'**). Phenylmethyl ketone, $C_6H_5COCH_3$. A colourless liquid with an odour of bitter almonds; insoluble in water, but soluble in alcohol and oils. It is used in perfumery, and medicinally as a hypnotic.

acetophenone-ortho-oxyquinoline (as·et·o·fe·**none**·or·tho·ox·e·**kwin'**·ol·een). A compound of acetophenone and quinoline, useful as a hypnotic; tasteless and non-irritating.

acetophenonephenetidin (as·et·o·fe·**none**·fen·**et'**·id·in). $C_2H_5OC_6H_4NC(CH_3)(C_6H_4)CH_3$, a compound formed from acetophenone and phenetidin; used as an antipyretic and antineuralgic.

acetopyrin, acetopyrine (as·et·o·**pi'**·rin, as·et·o·**pi'**·reen). Antipyrin acetylsalicylate. A compound of antipyrine, or phenazone, with acetylsalicylic acid, that is soluble in hot water or alcohol. It is an analgesic and antirheumatic; used in sciatica and influenza. Antipyrin is a notorious cause of agranulocytosis.

Acetorphine (as·et·**or**·feen). BP Commission approved name for 5-acetoxy-1,2,3,3a,8,9-hexahydro-2α-[1(*R*)-hydroxy-1-methylbutyl]-3-methoxy-12-methyl-3,9a-etheno-9,9b-iminoethanophenanthro[4,5-*bcd*]furan; a narcotic analgesic.

acetorthotoluide (as·et·or·tho·**tol'**·ew·ide). Aceto-orthotoluide.

acetosal (as·et·o·sal). Acetylsalicylic acid. *See* ACID.

acetosalicylate (as·et·o·**sal'**·is·il·ate). A salt of acetylsalicylic acid.

acetosoluble (as·e·to·**sol'**·ewbl). Applied to any substance which dissolves in acetic acid. [acetic, soluble.]

acetotoluide, acetotoluidine (as·et·o·**tol'**·ew·ide, as·et·o·tol·**ew'**·id·een). Acetoluide.

acetous (as·et·us). 1. Having the qualities of vinegar; sour. 2. Containing vinegar or acetic acid. [L *acetum* vinegar.]

acetparamidotoluol (as·et·par·**am'**·id·o·**tol**·ew·ol). Acetoparatoluide, $CH_3C_6H_4NHCOCH_3$. The *para* form of acetaminotoluene, or acetoluide; an antipyretic, insoluble in water.

acetparaphenetidin (as·et·par·ah·fen·**et'**·id·in). Acetophenetidin.

acetparatoluide (as·et·par·ah·**tol'**·ew·ide). Acetoparatoluide.

acetphenetidin (as·et·fen·**et'**·id·in). Acetophenetidin.

acetract (as·e·trakt). An extraction of a drug made with acetic acid.

acet-toluide (as·et·**tol**·ew·ide). Acetoluide.

acetum (as·e·tum). 1. Vinegar, an impure and dilute solution of acetic acid prepared by percolating a weak solution of alcohol over beech shavings or birch twigs previously moistened with vinegar which contains the necessary bacteria to catalyse the process of atmospheric oxidation. 2. Denoting any drug that is dissolved in a menstruum of acetic acid. **Acetum aromaticum.** Aromatic vinegar, acetic acid in an alcoholic solution of fragrant oils, used as a cooling lotion. **Acetum Cantharidini BPC 1949.** Vinegar of cantharidin, a solution of cantharidin in acetic acid. **Acetum cantharidis.** Vinegar of cantharides, cantharides extracted with an acetic acid menstruum. **Acetum Ipecacuanhae BPC 1949.** Vinegar of ipecacuanhae, a liquid extract of ipecacuanha with water, alcohol and acetic acid. **Acetum plumbi.** An aqueous solution of lead subacetate. **Acetum scillae.** Vinegar of Squill BPC 1959. [L.]

acetyl (as·et·il). The monovalent radical CH_3CO-, entering into compounds of acetic acid. Denoted in formulae by the symbol Ac. **Acetyl anhydride.** Acetic anhydride. *See* ANHYDRIDE. **Acetyl arsenate.** The arsenical spirochaetocide, arsacetin, a derivative of arsonic acid. **Acetyl benzene.** Acetophenone. **Acetyl bromide.** A fuming liquid, CH_3COBr, important in organic synthesis. **Acetyl carbamide.** Acetylurea. **Acetyl carbinol.** Methyl ketol, CH_3COCH_2OH, obtained from fused cane sugar and known as pyroracemic alcohol or acetol. Soluble in water, alcohol or ether; used in organic synthesis. **Acetyl chloride.** CH_3COCl, a highly refracting volatile liquid with a pungent smell. **Acetyl dioxide.** $(C_2H_3O)_2O_2$, a strong oxidizing agent. **Acetyl ethylphenylhydrazine.** $C_{14}H_{22}N_4O_2$, colourless crystals, used as an antipyretic. **Acetyl formyl.** Pyroracemic aldehyde, CH_3COCHO.

See ALDEHYDE. **Acetyl hydrate.** Acetic aldehyde. *See* ALDEHYDE. **Acetyl iodide.** CH_3COI, a brown fuming liquid used in organic substitutions. **Acetyl isocyanide.** Cyanacetyl, CH_3COCN. **Acetyl isoeugenol.** A substance used in the manufacture of artificial vanillin. **Acetyl leucomethylene blue.** A colourless derivative of methylene blue, used as an internal antiseptic. **Acetyl methyl.** Acetone. **Acetyl methyl carbinol.** Acetylmethylcarbinol, acetoin. **Acetyl number.** *See* NUMBER. **Acetyl oxide.** Acetic anhydride. *See* ANHYDRIDE. **Acetyl peroxide.** A powerful oxidizing agent; insoluble in water, and unstable. **Acetyl sulphanilamide,** $CH_3CONHC_6H_4SO_2NH_2$, an inactive form in which sulphanilamide is excreted. **Acetyl toluidine.** Acetaminotoluene, acetoluide. **Acetyl urethane.** *See* URETHANE. **Acetyl value.** Acetyl number. *See* NUMBER.

acetylaminobenzene (as·et·il·am·in·o·**ben**′·zeen). Acetanilide.

acetylation (as·et·il·**a**′·shun). The replacement of another radical by the acetyl group in organic synthesis.

acetylatoxyl (as·et·il·at·**ox**′·il). Arsacetin.

acetylbetamethylcholine (as·et·il·**be**·tah·meth·il·**ko**′·leen). A derivative of acetylcholine, it occurs in the form of the chloride, $(CH_3)_3NClCH_2CH(CH_3)OCOCH_3$, deliquescent white crystals highly soluble in water and alcohol. More stable than acetylcholine, it is a much more powerful parasympathetic stimulant. Administered orally or subcutaneously, it lowers blood pressure, increases peristaltic movements and promotes the activity of the sweat and salivary glands; used in tachycardia.

acetylcholine (as·et·il·**ko**′·leen). $(CH_3)_3N(OH)C_2H_4COOCH_3$. An acetic ester of choline, occurring in ergot and the tissues of higher animals. The most powerful depressor base known; intravenous injection of the chloride causes a sharp fall in blood pressure. It is also responsible for certain physiological functions, principally fat accumulation in the liver. A chemical transmitter of nerve impulses at certain sites in the central nervous system, at parasympathetic nerve terminals and at the neuromuscular junction. *See also:* CHOLINESTERASE.

Acetylcysteine (as·et·il·**sis**′·te·een). BP Commission approved name for *N*-acetyl-L-cysteine; it is used in the liquefaction of bronchial secretion.

acetyldimethylodihydrothebaine (as·et·il·di·**meth**·il·o·di·hi·dro·**the**′·bane). A derivative of thebaine, used like morphine.

acetylene (as·**et**·il·een). Ethine, C_2H_2. A colourless gas with an unpleasant odour; burns with a bright smoky flame, and is used therefore as an illuminant. Generated by the hydrolysis of calcium carbide, it is an unsaturated hydrocarbon with the formula HC≡CH. It has value as a general anaesthetic. The name is also applied to the tetravalent radical =CH=CH=. **Acetylene acids.** A series of acids containing the -C≡C- group. **Acetylene alcohols.** A series of alcohols derived from the above acids. **Acetylene dichloride.** CHCl=CHCl, a colourless liquid used as a solvent for rubber, and also for iodine in the surgical sterilization of the skin. **Acetylene series.** The series of unsaturated hydrocarbons of which acetylene is the first member. **Acetylene tetrachloride.** Tetrachlorethane, $C_2H_2Cl_4$, a solvent for oils, sulphur and phosphorus; it is also an insecticide.

acetylgalactosamine (as·et·il·gal·ak·**to**′·zam·een). $CH_3CONHC_6H_{11}O_5$. An acetyl derivative of galactosamine which occurs in cartilage.

acetylglucosamine (as·et·il·gloo·**ko**′·zam·een). $CH_3CONHC_6H_{11}O_5$. An acetyl derivative of glucosamine which occurs in the chitin of insects and crustacea.

acetylglycocoll (as·et·il·**gli**′·ko·kol). Acetoglycocoll, acetamidoacetic acid, $CH_3CONHCH_2COOH$. Colourless crystals, soluble in water and alcohol, but insoluble in ether. A substance related to the amino acid glycine, and involved in the protein metabolism.

acetylization (as·et·il·i·**za**′·shun). Acetylation.

acetylmethylcarbinol (as·et·il·meth·il·**kar**′·bin·ol). Acetoin, $CH_3COCHOHCH_3$. A colourless liquid formed during the fermentation of glucose by *Aerobacter aerogenes.* It is oxidized to diacetyl, the substance which imparts the characteristic odour to butter.

acetyloxyphenol (as·et·il·ox·e·**fe**′·nol). Resorcinol monoacetate, a reddish viscid liquid used in the treatment of acne.

acetylparamidophenyl salicylate (as·et·il·par·am·id·o·**fe**′·nil sal·is·il·ate). Acetylparamidosalol.

acetylparamidosalol (as·et·il·par·**am**·id·o·**sal**′·ol). Acetamidosalol, $C_6H_4(OH)COOC_6H_4NHCOCH_3$. White crystalline scales, soluble in hot water, alcohol or ether. Used medicinally as an antirheumatic, antipyretic and antiseptic.

acetylphenylhydrazine (as·et·il·fe·nil·**hi**′·draz·een). Hydracetin, $C_6H_5NHNHCOCH_3$. Colourless crystals, soluble only slightly in water but readily in alcohol. Used as an antipyretic, as an analgesic and in the treatment of polycythaemia because of its destructive effect upon erythrocytes. It is less toxic than the parent substance, phenylhydrazine.

acetylsalicylamide (as·et·il·sal·**is**′·il·am·ide). $CH_3COOC_6H_4CONH_2$. A white compound used in the treatment of rheumatism.

acetysalicylate (as·et·il·sal·**is**′·il·ate). A salt of acetylsalicylic acid.

acetylsulphadiazine (as·et·il·sul·fah·**di**′·az·een). Acetylated sulphadiazine; a compound forming a proportion of the urinary excretion of the drug, sulphadiazine. It does not respond directly to colour tests but will do so after hydrolysis.

acetylsulphaguanidine (as·et·il·sul·fah·**gwan**′·id·een). Acetylated sulphaguanidine; a compound forming a proportion of the urinary excretion of the drug, sulphaguanidine. It does not respond directly to colour tests but will do so after hydrolysis.

acetylsulphanilamide (as·et·il·sul·fah·**nil**′·am·ide). Acetylated sulphanilamide; a compound forming a proportion of the urinary excretion of the drug, sulphanilamide, It does not respond directly to colour tests but will do so after hydrolysis.

acetylsulphathiazole (as·et·il·sul·fah·**thi**′·az·ole). Acetylated sulphathiazole; a compound forming a proportion of the urinary excretion of the drug, sulphathiazole. It does not respond directly to colour tests, but will do so after hydrolysis.

acetyltannin (as·et·il·**tan**′·in). Acetannin, acetyltannic acid, $C_{14}H_8O_7(COOCH_3)_2$. A greyish powder, odourless and tasteless, it is insoluble in water or alcohol, but soluble in ethyl acetate; used medicinally in chronic diarrhoea and intestinal catarrh.

acetylthymol (as·et·il·**thi**′·mol). $C_{12}H_{16}O_2$, a colourless pungent liquid; it is used as an antiseptic.

acetyltribromsalol (as·et·il·tri·**brom**′·sal·ol). Fine white needles, soluble in alcohol; a hypnotic, analgesic, antispasmodic and intestinal antiseptic.

acetylurea (as·et·il·ewr·**e**′·ah). $CH_3CONHCONH_2$. The parent of a number of safe hypnotics of moderate strength useful as sedatives in nervous insomnia, Cf. CARBROMAL.

achalasia (ak·al·**a**·ze·ah). 1. Failure of relaxation in an opening of the body such as the oesophagus. 2. So-called cardiospasm. **Anal achalasia.** Megacolon. **Achalasia of the cardia.** Cardiospasm; neuromuscular dysfunction of the cardiac sphincter of the oesophagus, with failure of its normal relaxation and dilatation of the oesophagus itself. **Pelvirectal achalasia.** Congenital hypertrophic dilatation of the colon. Cf. MEGACOLON. **Achalasia of the pharyngo-oesophageal sphincter.** Usually a reflex spasm resulting from obstruction further down in the oesophagus. **Sphincteral achalasia.** Failure of relaxation of one or more of the sphincters of the colon. [Gk *a, chalasis* relaxation.]

Achard, Emile Charles (b. 1860). Paris physician.

Achard-Castaigne test. A test of kidney function: a solution of methylene blue is injected intramuscularly and the time of appearance of the dye in the urine is noted. Normally, this occurs in about 30 minutes. This was one of the first substances used as a test of renal function by ingestion or injection. It has for long been superseded by other substances such as phenolsulphonephthalein (the phthalein test of Rowntree and Geraghty) or by indigo carmine.

Achard-Thiers syndrome. Diabetes and hypertrichosis in women, a form of adrenal cortical overactivity.

acheilia (a·**ki**·le·ah). A congenital condition in which one or both lips are absent. [Gk *a, cheilos* lip.]

acheilous (a·**ki**·lus). Lipless. [see prec.]

acheilus (a·**ki**·lus). A person lacking congenitally in lip or lips. [Gk *a*, *cheilos* lip.]
acheiria (a·**ki**·re·ah). A condition of congenital lack of hand or hands. [Gk *a*, *cheir* hand.]
acheiropodia (a·**ki**·ro·**po**′·de·ah). Having no hands or feet. [Gk *a*, *cheir* hand, *pous* foot.]
acheirous (a·**ki**·rus). A condition in which the individual has lacked one hand or both from birth. [Gk *a*, *cheir* hand.]
acheirus (a·**ki**·rus). A fetus without hand or hands; it also applies to those born with such defect. [see prec.]
achibromine (ak·e·**bro**·meen). Monobromoisovalerianyl glycolurea, $CH_2(OH)CONHCONHC_4H_8Br$. A crystalline glycol formed from bromoisovalerianylurea, a mild hypnotic or sedative.
achi-iodine (ak·e·**i**·o·deen). Mono-iodisovalerianyl glycolurea. The iodine analogue of achibromine, also used as a sedative.
achilia (a·**ki**·le·ah). Acheilia.
Achillea (ak·il·**e**·ah). A genus of plants of the order Compositae; *Achillea millefolium*, yarrow, was formerly used as a bitter tonic. [Gk hero *Achilles*.]
achillein (ak·il·e·in). $C_{20}H_{38}N_2O_{15}$. A glucoside extracted from milfoil, or yarrow, *Achillea millefolium*. A brownish substance with a very bitter taste. It is soluble in water and is used as an antiperiodic.
Achilles. Greek mythological hero who was vulnerable only in the heel.
Achilles bursa. The bursa lying between the Achilles tendon and the calcaneum; bursa of the tendo calcaneus.
Achilles bursitis. Inflammation of the bursa under the Achilles tendon.
Achilles reflex. The stretch reflex elicited by tapping the Achilles tendon.
Achilles tendon. Tendo calcaneus, the common tendon of insertion of the calf muscles.
achillobursitis (ak·il·o·ber·**si**′·tis). Inflammation and thickening of the bursae associated with, and especially the bursae between, the tendo calcaneus and the posterior surface of the calcaneum. [Achilles tendon, bursitis.]
achillodynia (ak·**il**·o·**din**′·e·ah). 1. The pain attendant on achillobursitis. 2. A sensation of pain in the tendo calcaneus, especially at the heel. [Achilles tendon, Gk *odyne* pain.]
achillorrhaphy (ak·il·**or**·af·e). Suture of the tendo calcaneus, with the object of increasing its length (Bayer's operation). [Achilles tendon, Gk *rhaphe* a sewing.]
achillotenotomy, achillotomy (ak·il·o·ten·**ot**′·om·e, ak·il·**ot**·o·me). Division of the tendo calcaneus, especially subcutaneous division by tenotome. **Plastic achillotenotomy, Plastic achillotomy.** A plastic operation undertaken for the purpose of lengthening the tendo calcaneus. [Achilles tendon, Gk *temnein* to cut.]
achilous (a·**ki**·lus). Acheilous.
achilus (a·**ki**·lus). Acheilus.
achiria (a·**ki**·re·ah). Acheiria.
achirous (a·**ki**·rus). Acheirous.
achirus (a·**ki**·rus). Acheirus.
achlorhydria (a·klor·**hi**·dre·ah). Complete lack of free hydrochloric acid in the gastric juice. [Gk *a*, chlorhydria.]
achloroblepsia, achloropsia (a·**klor**·o·**blep**′·se·ah, a·klor·**op**·se·ah). Lack of ability to recognize or to distinguish green colours. [Gk *a*, *chloros* green, *blepein* to see, *opsis* vision.]
Achlya (**ak**·le·ah). A genus of fungi belonging to the Thallophyta, and found growing in colonies on fish and insects.
achlys (**ak**·lis). A corneal opacity of mild degree. [Gk mist.]
acholia (a·**ko**·le·ah). 1. Deficiency or lack in the secretion of bile. 2. Any condition that obstructs the flow of bile into the small intestine. 3. A gentle or mild attitude of mind. 4. Coeliac disease; the name acholia was given to this disease by Cheadle in 1903, now seldom used in this sense. 5. Asiatic chlolera; obsolete use. **Pigmentary acholia.** A state in which, although jaundice is not present, the faeces are pale and the secretion of bile is insufficient. [Gk *a*, *chole* bile.]
acholic (a·**ko**·lik). 1. Without bile. 2. Referring to, caused by or affected with acholia. [see prec.]
acholuria (a·ko·**lewr**·e·ah). Complete lack of bile pigment in the urine. [Gk *a*, *chole* bile, urine.]
acholuric (a·ko·**lewr**·ik). Pertaining to acholuria. [see prec.]
achondrodystrophy (a·kon·dro·**dis**′·tro·fe). *See* ACHONDROPLASIA.
achondroplasia (a·kon·dro·**pla**′·ze·ah). A hereditary disease of the skeleton in which there is faulty endochondral ossification, resulting in dwarfism. The epiphyses and diaphyses are prematurely united and growth of the normally long bones does not occur. The long bones are thickened and stout. Also known as *chondrodystrophia fetalis*. [Gk *a*, chondroplasty.]
achondroplastic (a·kon·dro·**plas**′·tik). Affected with or referring to achondroplasia. [see prec.]
achondroplasty (a·kon·dro·**plas**′·te). Achondroplasia.
achor (a·kor). 1. A papular eruption which occurs on the hairy parts of the body; when it occurs in infants it is popularly known as milk crust. 2. A sharply pointed pustule. **Achor barbatus.** Tinea barbae. [Gk dandruff.]
achordal (a·**kor**·dal). Not developed from, or destitute of, the notochord. [Gk *a*, *chorde* cord.]
achoresis (a·kor·e·sis). Diminution of the capacity of a hollow organ. [Gk *a*, *chorein* to make room.]
Achorion (ak·**o**·re·on). Obsolete synonym for *Trichophyton* species causing favus in man and animals. [Gk *achor* dandruff.]
achreocythaemia (a·kre·o·si·**the**′·me·ah). Achroiocythaemia. [Gk *achroios* colourless, *kytos* cell, *haima* blood.]
achrestic (a·**kres**·tik). Indicating failure of utilization. [Gk *a*, *chresis* use.]
achroa (a·**kro**·ah). Achromia.
achroacyte (a·**kro**·ah·site). Lymphocyte. [Gk *achroios* colourless, *kytos* cell.]
achroacytosis (a·**kro**·ah·si·**to**′·sis). Excessive development of lymph cells in the blood. [Gk *achroios* colourless, cytosis.]
achrochordon (ak·ro·**kor**·don). Soft warts or skin tags. [Gk *achroios* colourless, *chorde* string.]
achroglobin (ak·ro·**glo**·bin). A colourless protein occurring in certain molluscs and tunicates and believed to be concerned in respiratory processes. [Gk *achroios* colourless, globin.]
achroia (a·**kroi**·ah). Achromia.
achroiocythaemia (a·**kroi**·o·si·**theem**′·e·ah). 1. Lack or deficiency of haemoglobin in the erythrocytes. 2. The state of health relative to haemoglobin deficiency. [Gk *achroios* colourless, *kytos* cell, *haima* blood.]
achroiocytosis (a·**kroi**·o·si·**to**′·sis). Achroacytosis.
achroma (a·**kro**·mah). Achromia. [Gk *a*, *chroma* colour.]
achromachia (a·kro·**ma**·ke·ah). Loss of normal coloration of the hair; the development of whiteness or greyness. [Gk *a*, *chroma* colour.]
achromacyte (a·**kro**·mah·site). An erythrocyte which has lost its pigmentary character. A phantom corpuscle. [Gk *a*, *chroma* colour, *kytos* cell.]
achromasia (a·kro·**ma**·ze·ah). 1. Lack of normal colouring in the skin; type of pallor. 2. Absence of the usual colour reaction in a tissue or cell subjected to a staining agent. [see foll.]
achromata (a·**kro**·mat·ah). Total colour blindness. [Gk *a*, *chroma* colour.]
achromate (a·**kro**·mate). An individual who is colour blind. [see prec.]
achromatia (a·kro·**ma**·she·ah). Achromia.
Achromatiaceae (**ak**·ro·mat·e·**a**′·se·e). A family of bacteria belonging to the order Thiobacteriales; they are saprophytic and occur in brackish water and marine muds. [Gk *a*, *chroma* colour.]
achromatic (a·kro·**mat**·ik). 1. Not readily coloured by staining agents. 2. Free from colour. 3. Containing achromatin. 4. In optics, transmitting light without decomposing it into its constituent colours. 5. Colour blind. [see foll.]

achromatin (a·kro·mat·in). The obsolete term for the parts of a cell nucleus which will not readily stain with basic dyes. [Gk *a, chroma* colour.]

achromatinic (a·kro·mat·**in**′·ik). 1. Containing achromatin. 2. Referring to achromatin. [see prec.]

achromatism (a·**kro**·mat·izm). The quality or state of being achromatic. [see foll.]

achromatistous (a·kro·mat·**is**′·tus). Signifying a condition in which colouring matter or pigment is defective. [Gk *a, chroma* colour.]

Achromatium (ak·ro·**ma**·she·um). A genus of bacteria in the family Achromatiaceae; they are unicellular water organisms varying in shape from spherical to short rods, and contain both sulphur granules and calcium-carbonate crystals. [see prec.]

achromatocyte (a·kro·**mat**·o·site). Achromacyte.

achromatolysis (a·kro·mat·**ol**·is·is). Disintegration of the achromatin of a cell. [Gk *a, chroma* colour, *lysis* a loosing.]

achromatophil (a·kro·**mat**·o·fil). 1. An organism or histological element which does not readily take up stains. 2. Entirely lacking in affinity for stains. [see foll.]

achromatophilia (a·kro·mat·o·**fil**′·e·ah). The state or quality of being resistant to the action of a stain. [Gk *a, chroma* colour, *philein* to love.]

achromatopsia (a·kro·mat·**op**′·se·ah). 1. Total colour blindness due to disease or trauma of the retina, optic nerve or visual pathways. 2. Some older books used the word to indicate acquired colour blindness, as opposed to congenital colour blindness. [Gk *a, chroma* colour, *opsis* sight.]

achromatosis (a·kro·mat·**o**′·sis). Deficiency of pigmentation, especially in the integumentary tissues. [Gk *a, chroma* colour.]

achromatous (a·**kro**·mat·us). Without colour. [see prec.]

achromaturia (a·kro·mat·**ewr**′·e·ah). A condition in which the urine is almost or entirely colourless. [Gk *a, chroma* colour, urine.]

achromia (a·**kro**·me·ah). 1. Absence or disappearance of normal pigmentation. 2. Paleness. **Acquired achromia.** Vitiligo. **Congenital achromia.** Albinism. **Consecutive achromia.** Achromia resulting from maladies such as leprosy, syphilis, psoriasis and tinea versicolor. **Cortical achromia.** Achromia of the cerebral cortex in which, within a certain area, the ganglion cells have disappeared. **Achromia parasitica.** Tinea versicolor in pigmented skin, whether racial or sun-tanned. **Achromia unguium.** Leuconychia. [Gk *a, chroma* colour.]

See also: JEANSELME.

achromic (a·**kro**·mik). 1. Without colour. 2. Referring to or marked by achromia. **Achromic point.** *See* POINT. [see prec.]

achromin (a·**kro**·min). Achromatin.

Achromobacteriaceae (a·**kro**·mo·bak·teer·e·**a**′·se·e). A family of bacteria found chiefly in water and soil. They are saprophytic, and form no pigment. [see foll.]

Achromobacterium (a·**kro**·mo·bak·**teer**′·e·um). A genus of the family Bacteriaceae; occurring in soil, milk and animal manure, they consist of motile or non-motile Gram-negative rods which are saprophytic, non-pathogenic and do not form any pigment on agar. [Gk *a, chroma* colour, bacterium.]

achromoderma, achromodermia (a·kro·mo·**der**′·mah, a·kro·mo·**der**′·me·ah). Albinism; leucoderma. [Gk *a, chroma* colour, *derma* skin.]

achromophil, achromophilia (a·**kro**·mo·fil, a·kro·mo·**fil**′·e·ah). Achromatophil; achromatophilia. [Gk *a, chroma* colour, *philein* to love.]

achromotrichia (a·kro·mo·**trik**′·e·ah). Absence of pigment in, or greying of, the hair. [Gk *a, chroma* colour, *thrix* hair.]

achromous (a·**kro**·mus). Achromatous.

achronizoic (**ak**·ron·iz·**o**′·ik). A term applied to a drug which is chemically unstable and therefore liable to change its pharmacological action within a short time. [Gk *a, chronizein* to hold out.]

achroo-amyloid (ak·ro·o·**am**′·il·oid). Referring to amyloid substance when it is in its primary stage of inability to hold a stain. [Gk *achroios* colourless, amyloid.]

achroocytosis (ak·**ro**·o·si·**to**′·sis). Achroacytosis.

achroodextrin (**ak**·ro·o·**dex**′·trin). α-Dextrin. Formed during the ptyalin digestion of starch and subsequently converted into maltose by the amylopsin of the pancreatic juice, it is a yellow amorphous substance, readily soluble in water, and gives no colour reaction with iodine. Cf. ERYTHRODEXTRIN. [Gk *achroios* colourless, dextrin.]

Achucarro, Nicolas (b. 1881). Spanish histologist.

Achucarro's method. A tannic acid–silver method for demonstrating astrocytes in tissue sections. With modifications it can be used to impregnate connective tissues generally.

achylanaemia (a·**ki**·lan·e′·me·ah). Anaemia characterized by achylia gastrica. [Gk *a,* chyle, anaemia.]

achylia, achylosis (a·**ki**·le·ah, a·ki·**lo**·sis). Absence of chyle: the word is sometimes used unqualified to mean achylia gastrica. **Achylia gastrica.** Absence of acid and pepsin from the gastric juice. **Achylia gastrica haemorrhagica.** A condition of the stomach in which both hydrochloric acid and pepsin are absent but occult blood is present. **Achylia pancreatica.** A state in which the external secretion of the pancreas is absent. [Gk *a,* chyle.]

achylous (a·**ki**·lus). Having an insufficient amount of chyle. [see prec.]

achymia, achymosis (a·**ki**·me·ah, a·ki·**mo**·sis). A state in which there is insufficient or abnormal chyme. [Gk *achymos* juiceless.]

achymous (a·**ki**·mus). Having an insufficient amount of chyme. [see prec.]

acicular (as·**ik**·ew·lar). Needle-shaped; having sharp points like needles. [L *aciculus* little needle.]

acid (as·id). 1. Biting to the taste; tart; not alkaline, A substance possessing a sour taste. 2. A substance capable of neutralizing bases with the formation of salts; exhibiting properties the opposite of those exhibited by alkalis. 3. A combination of electronegative elements with one or more hydrogen atoms each of which is replaceable by electro-positive elements (metals) or basic radicals; the acid is said to be accordingly mono-, di-, tri-, or tetra-basic. 4. A chemical compound which, in solution, dissociates in such a way that there is an excess of hydrogen ions over hydroxyl ions. 5. A substance which dissociates in water to form H^+ ions, causing an increase in $[H^+]$ and a fall in pH below 7. 6. A solution that turns blue litmus red, and affects similar indicators in a recognized fashion. **Abienic acid, Abiennic acid.** A resin acid, $C_{12}H_{19}COOH$, occurring in the silver fir, *Abies pectinata.* **Abietic acid.** An acid occurring as a complex anhydride in colophony which is obtained from crude turpentine; it is a resin acid, $C_{19}H_{29}COOH$, and a derivative of the pine-tar hydrocarbon, retene. Used in soap and varnish manufacture. **Abietinic acid.** A resin acid, similar to abietic acid, also present in colophony. **Abietinolic acid.** A resin found in the pitch of the silver fir. **Abietolic acid.** An acid of the resin family, $C_{19}H_{27}COOH$, constituting a small proportion of certain crude turpentines. **Abric acid.** A crystalline substance, $C_{21}H_{24}NO_3$, extracted from the seeds of *Abrus precatorius,* jequirity. **Absinthic acid.** An acid derived from wormwood, *Artemisia absinthium.* **Aceric acid.** An acid occurring in the juice of the maple, *Acer campestre.* **Acetamido-acetic acid.** Acetoglycocoll, $CH_3CONHCH_2COOH$, an acetyl derivative of the amino acid, glycine, concerned in protein metabolism. **Acetamido-ethylsalicylic acid.** Benzacetin, an antipyretic similar to phenacetin in action. **Acetic Acid BP 1973.** A saturated fatty acid, CH_3COOH, produced commercially by the oxidation of ethyl alcohol with aerobic bacteria (vinegar), or, in a crude form, during the destructive distillation of wood (pyroligneous acid). It is a colourless liquid, or clear crystals (glacial), soluble in water or alcohol. A strong caustic, it is used as such to remove corns and warts; also an important solvent for oils, resins and gums. **Acetic acid anhydride.** *See* ANHYDRIDE. **Acetic acid, aromatic.** Aromatic vinegar, used as a restorative; it consists of glacial acetic acid with fragrant additives. **Acetic Acid, Dilute BP 1973.** A 6 per cent solution of pure acetic acid in water used as an antidote for alkali poisons and as a lotion. **Acetic Acid, Glacial**

BP 1958. The 99 per cent acid in crystalline form; used as a reagent, solvent, vesicant and escharotic. **Aceto-acetic acid.** Diacetic acid, CH_3COCH_2COOH, a fat metabolite occurring excessively during diabetes and giving rise to acetone bodies in the urine. **Acetone acid, Acetonic acid.** Butyl-lactic acid, $(CH_3)_2C(OH)COOH$, a hydroxy derivative of isobutyric acid. **Acetopropionic acid.** Acetylpropionic acid (see below). **Acetrizoic Acid BP 1973.** $C_9H_6I_3NO_3$, a white, odourless, tasteless powder, slightly soluble in water, more readily so in alcohol and in solutions of alkali hydroxides. In the form of sodium acetrizoate it is used as an intravenous and retrograde contrast medium for visualizing the urinary tract radiologically, for cholangiography and for arteriogaphy. **Acetylaminohydroxybenzisoxazine arsonic acid.** A substance related to acetarsone and used in the treatment of disseminated sclerosis and neurosyphilis. **Acetylaminohydroxyphenylarsonic acid.** Acetarsol, $C_6H_3OHAsO(OH)_2NHCOCH_3$, white crystals, insoluble in water but easily in alkalis; an amoebacide and antisyphilitic. **Acetylbromosalicylic acid.** $CH_3COOC_6H_3BrCOOH$, an analgesic and antipyretic, with sedative properties conferred by the bromine atom. **Acetylcresotinic acid.** Acetyl methyl salicylic acid, an antipyretic. **Acetylene acid.** One of the series of unsaturated fatty acids containing the group, -C=C-; such acids are distinguished by the termination, *-olic.* **Acetylenecarboxylic acid.** Propiolic acid (see below). **Acetyliodosalicylic acid.** $CH_3COOC_6H_3ICOOH$, an acid used in rheumatism and arteriosclerosis. **Acetylorthocresotinic acid.** Acetylcresotinic acid (see above). **Acetylpropionic acid.** Laevulinic acid (see below). **Acetylsalicylic Acid BP 1973.** Acetosal, aspirin, $CH_3COOC_6H_4COOH$, colourless crystals not very soluble in water but readily in alcohol. Hydrolysed by alkalis, and, slowly, by exposure to air. The best anodyne of the salicylates, it depresses the optic thalamus and is useful therefore in the treatment of nervous headache, neuralgia and the pain of rheumatic affections. **Acetyltannic acid.** Acetannin, acetyltannin, $C_{14}H_8O_7(COOCH_3)_2$, a grey powder, odourless and tasteless. Insoluble in water or alcohol but soluble in ethyl acetate, it is used medicinally in chronic diarrhoea and intestinal catarrh. **Achilleic acid.** An acid occurring in yarrow, or milfoil, *Achillea millefolium,* it is identical with aconitic acid. **Aconitic acid.** Propenetricarboxylic acid, $C_3H_3(COOH)_3$, a crystalline substance, occurring in aconite, *Aconitum napellus,* the *Adonis* and *Achillea* families, and in sugar-cane and beetroot. **Acrolactic acid.** Glucic acid (see below). **Acroleic acid.** $CH_2{=}CHCOOH$, an olefinic acid obtained from acrolein; a colourless pungent liquid. **Acrylic acid.** 1. Acroleic acid (see above). 2. One of a series of unsaturated aliphatic acids occurring in animal and vegetable tissues. **Adenosine diphosphoric acid.** ADP, the nucleoside diphosphate composed of the purine base adenine linked to ribose with a diphosphate group attached at the 5′-position. A precursor of ATP in oxidative phosphorylation and formed from it during synthetic activity, muscular contraction, etc. **Adenosine monophosphoric acid.** AMP, the nucleoside monophosphate composed of the purine base adenine linked to ribose with a single phosphate group attached at the 5′-position. It occurs as an intermediate in ATP synthesis *de novo* and as a result of ATP participation in certain activation processes, i.e. fatty acid and amino acid activations. Held in equilibrium with ATP and ADP by the action of adenylate kinase. **Adenosine triphosphoric acid.** ATP; a nucleoside triphosphate containing the purine base adenine linked to ribose with a triphosphate group attached at the 5′-position, The major energy source in all organisms. In animals and plants it is primarily synthesized in the mitochondrion as a result of oxidative phosphorylation. Its functions involve participation in synthetic reactions, in muscle contraction, maintenance of body temperature and production of light and electrical energy in lower organisms and specialized tissues. **Adenyl pyrophosphoric acid.** An adenine derivative which is involved in the building up of polysaccharides in plants and animals, and also, as the phosphate carrier in muscle, acts in conjunction with actomyosin, the contractile protein; it supplies phosphoric acid during the contraction, becoming adenosine diphosphate, and later recovers the phosphate when the muscle relaxes. **Adenylic acid.** Adenosine monophosphoric acid (see above), the nucleotide formed from adenosine by esterification with a phosphoric acid molecule. **Adipic acid, Adipinic acid.** $COOH(CH_2)_4COOH$, a dibasic acid, slightly soluble in water, formed by the oxidation of oleic and other fatty acids. **Agaric acid, Agaricic acid.** $C_{19}H_{36}(OH)(COOH)_3$, a white tasteless and odourless powder extracted from the fungus, *Formes officinalis,* that grows on larches. It is used to check night sweats and diarrhoea, and to reduce bronchial secretions; agaricin. **Ailanthic acid, Ailantic acid.** A bitter principle derived from the bark of the tree of heaven, *Ailanthus excelsa;* used as a tonic. **Alantic acid, Alantolic acid.** Inulic acid, an acid distilled from the root of elecampane, *Inula helenium;* it is an antiseptic administered in bronchitis. **Acid albumin.** *See* ALBUMIN. **Acid albuminate.** Metaprotein formed during the hydrolysis of protein in acid solution. **Albuminic acid, ferrated.** A compound of albumin, iron and phosphate; a light brown powder used as a tonic. **Alcohol acids.** A series of organic acids which contain both hydroxyl, -OH, and carboxyl, -COOH, groups. **Aldehyde acids.** Organic acids which have both aldehyde, -CHO, and carboxyl, -COOH, radicals. **Aldepalmitic acid.** $C_{15}H_{29}COOH$, an acid found in butter fat. **Aldobionic acid.** $C_{11}H_{19}O_{10}COOH$, an oxidized disaccharide containing a uronic acid grouping and found in certain bacteria. **Alepric acid, Aleprylic acid.** Acids occurring in chaulmoogra oil; they are alicyclic acids homologous with chaulmoogric acid used in the treatment of leprosy. **Alginic Acid BPC 1968.** A polysaccharide obtained from seaweeds and kelps (algae); the iron salt is used in the treatment of anaemia, the sodium salt as a substitute for tragacanth. **Alicyclic acids.** A family of acids, aliphatic in nature, but with a saturated ring structure. **Aliphatic acids.** Organic acids derived from the aliphatic hydrocarbons, having an open chain; fatty acids. **Alkannic acid.** A red colouring matter occurring in alkanna, the root of *Alkanna tinctoria.* **Allanic acid.** $C_3H_4O_3N_5COOH$, an oxidation product of allantoin. **Allantoic acid.** Dicarbamidoacetic acid, $(NH_2CONH)_2CHCOOH$, derived from allantoin. **Allanturic acid.** NH(CO)(CONH)CHOH, glyoxalylurea, a heterocyclic compound produced by the hydrolysis of allantoin. **Allanuric acid.** A purine compound formed from alloxan and urea. **Allonic acid.** $CH_3(CHOH)_4COOH$, a tetrahydroxy caproic acid obtained from the hexose, allose. **Allophanic acid.** Urea carbonic acid, $NH_2CONHCOOH$, occurring only in the form of esters. **Allotelluric acid.** H_6TeO_6, obtained by heating telluric acid; it forms organic esters. **Alloxanic acid.** NH_2CONH COCOCOOH, a derivative of alloxan. **Alloxyproteic acid.** A nucleoprotein breakdown product which occurs in the urine. **Allylarsonic acid.** $AsO(C_3H_3)(OH)_2$, used in the form of salts, for the treatment of skin diseases. **Aloetic acid, Aloitinic acid.** Tetranitro-anthraquinone, $C_6H_2(NO_2)_2COCOC_6H_2(NO_2)_2$, an orange-coloured substance formed by the nitration of aloin. **Alpha-aminobetahydroxypropionic acid.** Serine. **Alpha-glucoheptonic acid.** $CH_2OH(CHOH)_5COOH$, a hexahydroxy acid from vomitol, an alcohol occurring in the roots of the cowslip, *Primula officinalis.* **Alpha-hydroxypropionic acid.** Lactic acid (see below). **Alpha-oxynaphthoic acid.** Carbonaphthoic acid, $C_{10}H_6(OH)COOH$, colourless crystals, insoluble in water but soluble in alcohol, ether and chloroform; a disinfectant, surgical antiseptic, inhibiting enzyme action. **Alpharsonic acid.** An arsonic acid with alphyl groupings in its structure. **Alphatoluic acid.** Phenylacetic acid, $C_6H_5CH_2COOH$, a crystalline acid produced during the bacterial decomposition of certain proteins. **Altronic acid.** An isomer of allonic acid. **Amalic acid, Amalinic acid.** Tetramethylalloxantin, $C_8(CH_3)_4N_4O_7$, a purine derivative. **Ambrettolic acid.** $C_{16}H_{30}O_3$, an acid occurring in musk. **Amfonelic Acid.** BP Commission approved name for 7-benzyl-1-ethyl-4-oxo-1,8-naphthyridine-3-carboxylic acid; a CNS stimulant. **Amic acid.** Amido acid (see below). **Acid amide.** An organic compound containing the radical, $-CONH_2$. **Amido acid.** Strictly, an acid containing the group $-CONH_2$, but the term is applied also to amino acids. Cf. AMINO ACID (below). **Amido-acetic acid.** Amino-acetic acid (see below). **Amido-**

benzoic acid. Aminobenzoic acid (see below). **Amidobutyric acid.** Aminobutyric acid (see below). **Amidocaproic acid.** Aminocaproic acid (see below). **Amido-ethylsulphonic acid.** Amino-ethylsulphonic acid (see below). **Amidoformic acid.** Aminoformic acid (see below). **Amidohydrocumaric acid.** Tyrosine, $C_6H_4(OH)CH_3CH(NH_2)COOH$, a cyclic amino acid highly important in animal metabolism. **Amido-isethionic acid.** Amino-ethylsulphonic acid (see below). **Amido-oxyphenylpropionic acid.** Amidohydrocumaric acid (see above). **Amidopropionic acid.** Aminopropionic acid (see below). **Amidosuccinic acid.** Aspartic acid (see below). **Amidothiolactic acid.** Aminothiolpropionic acid (see below). **Amidothiolpropionic acid.** Aminothiolpropionic acid (see below). **Amidovalerianic acid.** Homopiperidinic acid (see below). **Aminic acid.** Formic acid (see below). **Amino acid.** One of a class of compounds which contain both an amino and a carboxylic acid grouping. **Amino acid, alternative.** The different amino acid which appears in corresponding positions of related proteins when their amino acid sequences are aligned. **Amino acid, C-terminal.** The amino acid at the free carboxyl end of a polypeptide chain. **Amino acid, invariant.** An amino acid residue at a given point in a polypeptide chain which, during the course of evolution of a protein, has remained unchanged. **Amino acid, N-terminal.** The amino acid at the free amino end of a polypeptide chain. **Radical amino acid change.** *See* CHANGE. **α-Amino acid.** One of a class of compounds obtained by hydrolysis of proteins; a compound which contains an amino and a carboxyl group attached to the α-carbon. **Amino-acetic acid.** Amido-acetic acid, glycine, NH_2CH_2COOH, the simplest amino acid which is found as a protein unit. **Aminobenzenesulphonic acid.** Sulphanilic acid. **Aminobenzoic acid.** Amidobenzoic acid, $NH_2C_6H_4COOH$: *ortho* form, anthranilic acid; *meta* form, benzaminic acid; *para* form, dracilic acid. **Aminobenzoylformic acid.** Isatic acid (see below). **Aminobutyric acid.** Butyrine, $CH_3CH_2CHNH_2COOH$, an α-amino acid which occurs in protein. **Aminocaproic Acid BP 1973.** 6-Aminohexanoic acid, $C_6H_{13}NO_2$, an antifibrinolytic agent which inhibits plasminogen activators. It is used in the treatment of haemorrhage due to excessive fibrinolysis. **Amino-ethylsulphonic acid.** Taurine; $NH_2(CH_2)_2SO_3H$, derived from the amino acid, cysteine; it is produced by hydrolysis of the bile acids. **Aminoformic acid.** Carbamic acid (see below). **Aminoglutaric acid.** Glutaric acid (see below). **Aminoguanidinevalerianic acid.** Arginine, $NH{=}C(NH_2)NH(CH_2)_3CH(NH_2)COOH$, an amino acid occurring in albumen and vegetable seeds, most probably a constituent of all proteins; it plays an essential part in nutrition, growth and urea formation; it is also contained in insulin. **Amino-indolepropionic acid.** Tryptophane, C_8H_6N $CH_2CH(NH_2)COOH$, an aromatic amino acid formed during the bacterial decomposition of protein in the intestine, and responsible for the putrefaction products, indole and skatole; essential in the animal diet. **Amino-isocaproic acid.** Leucine. **Amino-isovalerianic acid, Amino-isovaleric acid.** Valine. **Aminolaevulinic acid.** An intermediate in porphyrin synthesis, formed from succinyl CoA and glycine in a reaction catalysed by aminolaevulinate synthetase. **6-Aminopenicillanic acid.** An amino acid isolated from a culture of *Penicillium chrysogenum.* It can be regarded as the parent of the penicillins and is a possible intermediate in the synthesis of new penicillins. **Aminophenylarsonic acid.** Arsanilic acid (see below). **Aminophenylglyoxylic acid.** Isatic acid (see below). **Aminophenylstibinic acid.** An antimony compound used, in combination with urea, in the treatment of kala-azar. **Aminopropionic acid.** Alanine, CH_3 $CH(NH_2)COOH$, an α-amino acid which can be regarded as the parent of the polypeptides; it is glycogenic and acts as such in diabetic animals. **Aminosuccinic acid.** Aspartic acid (see below). **Aminosulphonic acid.** Sulphaminic acid (see below). **Aminothiolactic acid.** Aminothiolpropionic acid (see following). **Aminothiolpropionic acid.** Cysteine. $HSCH_2CH(NH_2)COOH$, an α-amino acid derived from cystine and forming in turn taurine; an intermediate in the sulphur metabolism. **Aminovalerianic acid.** Homopiperidinic acid (see below). **Aminovaleric acid.** Norvaline, $CH_3(CH_2)_2CH(NH_2)COOH$, an α-amino acid occurring in protein. **Amygdalic acid.** 1. $C_{20}H_{28}O_{13}$, a glucoside obtained from almond oil. 2. Mandelic acid (see below). **Anacardic acid.** $C_{22}H_{32}O_3$, a brown substance obtained from cashew nuts, the seeds of *Anacardium occidentale*; used as an anthelmintic. **Anchusic acid.** A red colouring matter occurring in anchusa, the root of *Anchusa tinctoria.* **Angelic acid, Angelicic acid.** $CH_3CH{=}C(CH_3)COOH$, an unsaturated acrylic acid occurring, with isomeric acids, as esters in chamomile oil and angelica root; used as a diuretic and diaphoretic. **Acid anhydride.** An acid which has given up hydrogen and oxygen in the form of a molecule or molecules of water. **Anilic acid.** Any of the monobasic half-anilides formed by aniline with dibasic acids. **Aniline parasulphonic acid.** Sulphanilic acid (see below). **Anisic acid.** $CH_3OC_6H_4COOH$, an acid obtained from anethole, the phenolic ether contained in anise and fennel oils; it is used in medicine as a carminative, antiseptic and antipyretic. **Anisidin citric acid.** A more soluble form of anisidine for use as an analgesic. **Anisuric acid.** $C_{10}H_{11}NO_2$, an acid formed from anisic acid, and occurring under certain conditions in the urine. **Anthranilic acid.** *o*-Aminobenzoic acid, $NH_2C_6H_4COOH$, yellow crystals used in the manufacture of dyestuffs and perfumes. **Anticyclic acid.** A phenazone preparation used as an antipyretic. **Antimonic acid.** An acid of pentavalent antimony; *ortho,* H_3SbO_4, from which is derived phenylstibinic acid, the parent of a number of antispirochaetal drugs; *meta,* $HSbO_3$; *para,* $H_4Sb_2O_7$. **Antimonious acid, Antimonous acid.** An acid of trivalent antimony; *meta,* $HSbO_2$, from which is prepared tartar emetic; *ortho,* H_3SbO_3; *para,* $H_4Sb_2O_5$. **Antiscorbic acid, Antiscorbutic acid.** Ascorbic acid (see below). **Antitartaric acid.** The optically-inactive form of tartaric acid. **Antoxyproteic acid.** An acid derived from urine. **Apiolic acid.** $C_{10}H_{10}O_6$, an acid prepared from apiol, an aromatic substance occurring in oil of parsley and celery oil. **Apocrenic acid.** $C_{24}H_{12}O_{12}$, formed by the action of certain moulds on soil humus, and appearing therefore in natural spring waters. **Aposorbic acid.** $C_5H_8O_7$, an acid produced by the oxidation of sorbose, a monosaccharide occurring in the berries of the mountain ash, *Sorbus.* **Arabic acid, Arabitic acid.** CH_2OH $(CHOH)_3COOH$, tetrahydroxyvaleric acid, an acid extracted from gum acacia. **Arabonic acid.** An isomer of arabic acid, prepared from the pentose gum sugar, arabinose. **Arachic acid, Arachidic acid.** $CH_3(CH_2)_{18}COOH$, a saturated fatty acid occurring as a glyceride in arachis oil and butter fats. **Arachidonic acid.** An unsaturated (polyene) fatty acid, $CH_3(CH_2)_4$ $(CH{=}CHCH_2)_4(CH_2)_2COOH$, which occurs in animal fats; as a glycerol ester it is present in lecithin and cephalin. It is necessary for normal growth, and plays an important part in hepatic fat metabolism. **Argentic acid.** Applied to silver oxide, Ag_2O; used as an antiseptic. **Aristic acid, Aristidic acid, Aristolic acid, Aristolochic acid.** Acids of undetermined constitution, derived from serpentary, the rhizome and roots of various plants of the *Aristolochiaceae* family. **Aromatic acids.** Organic acids containing one or more benzene rings or other closed and saturated rings; they occur naturally in balsams and resins. The term is also applied, in pharmacy, to a mineral acid flavoured with an aromatic substance. **Arsanilic acid.** $NH_2C_6H_4AsO(OH)_2$, a derivative arsonic acid, and itself the parent of many important arsenical spirochaeticides. **Arsellic acid.** An acrylic acid, $C_{16}H_{31}$ COOH, obtained from cod-liver oil. **Arsenic acid.** An acid of pentavalent arsenic: *ortho,* H_3AsO_4, from which are formed the arsenates useful in medicine, and the older arsenical spirochaeticides; *meta,* $HAsO_3$; *para,* $H_4As_2O_7$. **Arsenous acid.** An acid in which arsenic is trivalent, the most effective form for the destruction of trypanosomes, and the basis of the more recent arsenical spirochaeticides; *ortho,* H_3AsO_3; *meta,* $HAsO_2$. **Arsinic acid.** An organic compound containing the radical $-As(OH)_2$, (arsenic trivalent). **Arsinosalicylic acid.** An arsenical spirochaeticide. **Arsonic acid.** An organic compound containing the radical $-AsO(OH)_2$, (arsenic pentavalent). **Arylarsonic acid.** A compound consisting of one or more arsonic acid radicals joined to aryl groups. **Ascorbic Acid BP 1973.** Cevitamic acid, antiscorbutic acid, vitamin C; $C_6H_8O_6$, a lactone of tetrahydroxyketohexanoic acid, known as 3-keto-L-gulofuranolactone.

It occurs in citrus fruits and raw vegetables, also in liver and fresh milk; it is identical with hexuronic acid from the suprarenal cortex, and can be synthesized. It is a colourless compound, dextrorotatory, soluble in water but unstable, and is believed to be concerned in the synthesis of chlorophyll and carotenoids in plants; in animals it is essential for the formation and maintenance of bone, collagen, and teeth. It is a necessary factor in wound repair, and also functions in the protein metabolism; a deficiency leads to scurvy. **Aseptic acid.** Term applied to an antiseptic solution of boric acid in hydrogen peroxide. **Asparacemic acid.** An optically-inactive form of aspartic acid (see following). **Asparagic acid, Asparaginic acid, Asparamic acid, Aspartic acid.** Aminosuccinic acid, $COOHCH_2CH(NH_2)COOH$, an α-amino acid embodied in many proteins and found as the amide, asparagine, in the seeds of cereals. It is important as an amino-carrier for the synthesis of amino acids in the metabolism. **Aspergillic acid.** An antibiotic secreted by species of *Aspergillus*, a genus of parasitic moulds. **Atractylic acid.** A poisonous glucoside obtained from the essential oil of *Atractylis.* **Atrolactic acid, Atrolactinic acid.** Phenyllactic acid, $CH_3C(OH)(C_6H_5)COOH$, a white crystalline acid formed from acetophenone. **Atropic acid.** α-Phenylacrylic acid, $CH_2{=}C(C_6H_5)COOH$, colourless crystals insoluble in water; prepared from atropine. **Auric acid.** 1. H_3AuO_3, a yellow insoluble powder forming aurates with alkalis. 2. Also applied, incorrectly, to auric oxide, Au_2O_3. **Avivitellinic acid.** An acid found in vitellin, the chief protein of the yolk of birds' eggs. **Axinic acid.** $C_{18}H_{28}O_2$, an oily acid obtained from axin, the fat of the Mexican cochineal, *Lacus axinus.* **Azelaic acid, Azelainic acid.** $(CH_2)_7(COOH)_2$, an acid of the oxalic acid series, used as a standard in the analysis of fats. **Azotic acid.** Nitric acid (see below).

Barbituric acid. Malonyl urea, $CH_2(CONH)_2CO$, a cyclic ureide with acidic properties, forming stable and more soluble sodium and potassium salts. By the substitution of different organic radicals for the 2 hydrogens in $CH_2{=}$, a large family of important hypnotics, the barbiturates, has been synthesized. **Behenic acid.** $C_{21}H_{43}COOH$, a monobasic saturated fatty acid similar to stearic acid and occurring in the roots of *Centaurea behen* and ben oil. **Benzamic acid, Benzaminic acid.** *m*-Aminobenzoic acid, $NH_2C_6H_4COOH$, yellow crystals insoluble in water. **Benzaminoacetic acid.** Hippuric acid (see below). **Benzenedicarboxylic acid.** Phthalic acid (see below). **Benzenehexacarboxylic acid.** Mellitic acid (see below). **Benzenesulphonic acid.** $C_6H_5SO_2OH$, colourless crystals soluble in water; used in organic synthesis. **Benzoboric acid.** A mixture of benzoic and boric acids used as a preservative and antiseptic. **Benzoglycollic acid.** Mandelic acid (see below). **Benzoic Acid BP 1973.** C_6H_5COOH, white crystals, almost insoluble in water but soluble in alcohol, chloroform, ether, fats and oils. It occurs with cinnamic acid in gum benzoin, and synthesized from the coal-tar hydrocarbon, toluene. It is used as a preservative and antiseptic; also in the treatment of ringworm and as an expectorant in bronchitis. **Benzoylaminoacetic acid.** Hippuric acid (see below). **Beta-acetylpropionic acid.** Laevulinic acid, $CH_3COCH_2CH_2COOH$, an acid occurring in the nucleic acid of the thymus. **Beta-aminobutyric acid.** $CH_3CH(NH_2)CH_2COOH$, an isomer of butyrine; it is a narcotic. **Beta-hydroxybutyric acid.** $CH_3CH(OH)CH_2COOH$, an acid occurring as the principal acetone body in ketonuria. **Beta-ketobutyric acid.** Diacetic acid, CH_3COCH_2COOH, a fat metabolite which appears in the urine as an acetone body in diabetes. **Beta-ketopalmitic acid.** $CH_3(CH_2)_{12}COCH_2COOH$, a keto acid derived from palmitic acid by oxidation. **Beta-naphtholsulphonic acids.** $C_{10}H_6(OH)SO_2OH$, 3 isomeric acids, intermediates in the synthesis of drugs and dyestuffs. They are narcotic in action; the calcium salt of one, having the property of precipitating albumen, is used in urinary analysis. **Beta-oxybutyric acid.** Beta-hydroxybutyric acid (see above). **Beta-parahydroxyphenylaminopropionic acid.** Tyrosine, $C_6H_4(OH)CH_2CH(NH_2)COOH$, a cyclic amino acid considered essential for higher animal life. **Beta-phenylpropionic acid.** Hydrocinnamic acid, $C_6H_5CH_2CH_2COOH$, an acid occurring in the body during the decomposition of proteins containing aromatic nuclei; it has been used in the treatment of tuberculosis. **Bichloracetic acid.** Dichloracetic acid, $CHCl_2COOH$, a colourless liquid, soluble in water; used to remove corns and warts. **Bile acid.** A number of closely-related acids present in the bile as sodium salts. They consist principally of glycocholic and taurocholic acids with several other derivatives of cholanic acid. By reducing surface tension they facilitate the emulsification of fats, whilst exerting a solvent (hydrotropic) effect upon otherwise insoluble fatty acids and lipides in intestinal digestion. **Bilianic acid.** $C_{24}H_{34}O_8$, a cholane derivative formed from dehydrocholic acid, a bile acid, by oxidation and opening of the sterol-ring structure. **Bilic acid.** $C_{16}H_{22}O_6$, an acid derived from cholic acid (see below). **Bilirubic acid, Bilirubinic acid.** $C_{16}H_{22}O_3N_2$, a monobasic acid constituted of 2 pyrrole rings; it is derived from the red bile pigment, bilirubin, and from the haemin of haemoglobin. **Biliverdic acid, Biliverdinic acid.** $C_8H_9O_4N$, a derivative of biliverdin, the green bile pigment. **Binary acids.** Acids which contain no oxygen and, for the most part, are comprised of 2 elements only, of which hydrogen is one. Their names terminate, like the majority of acids, in *-ic*, but they are to be distinguished by the prefix, *hydro-*; their salts end in *-ide.* **Bioluric acid.** A derivative of uric acid. **Bionic acid, Biotic acid.** Biotin, vitamin H, $C_{10}H_{16}O_3N_2S$, an acid occurring naturally in yeasts, the outer coating of seeds, green leaves and, to a very small extent, in animal tissue; deficiency leads to pallor of the skin and dermatitis. **Bismuthic acid.** $HBiO_3$, an acid best known in the form of the sodium salt, sodium bismuthate, $NaBiO_3$, used in the preparation of soluble bismuth antisyphilitics. **Blattic acid.** A diuretic. **Blue acid.** Prussic acid, hydrocyanic acid, HCN, so called from its use in the manufacture of Prussian blue. **Boheic acid.** $C_7H_{10}O_6$, an acid occurring in the extract of tea. **Boracic acid, Acid of borax.** Boric Acid BP 1973 (see below). **Acid Bordeaux.** A red food-dye; the sodium salt of naphthalene azonaphthol disulphonic acid. **Boric Acid BP 1973.** H_3BO_3, white crystals soluble in water, alcohol, and glycerin. A mild antiseptic used in urinary infections, eczemas and dry skin diseases; also as a wound dressing, eye wash and food preservative. **Borobenzoic acid.** $B(OH)_2C_6H_4COOH$, an acid used as an antiseptic and preservative. **Boroboracic acid, Boroboric acid.** A mixture of boric acid and borax. **Borocitric acid.** A compound of boric and citric acids, best known as the magnesium salt; it is a urinary antiseptic and a solvent for urates, and is of value in the treatment of gout, stone and rheumatism. **Borophenylic acid.** Phenylboric acid, $C_6H_5OB(OH)_2$, an acid soluble in water and used as an antiseptic. **Borosalicylic acid.** A heterocyclic compound, $(C_6H_4COOOB)_2$, used in the treatment of skin diseases. **Borussic acid.** Hydrocyanic acid (see below). **Boswellic acid, Boswellinic acid.** $C_{32}H_{52}O_4$, an acid obtained from olibanum, an oleo gum resin exuded by the African species of *Boswellia.* **Botulinic acid.** An acid appearing during the putrefaction of meat, and attributed to *Clostridium botulinum.* **Brassic acid, Brassidic acid.** $C_{21}H_{41}COOH$, an unsaturated acrylic acid, stereo-isomeric with erucic acid. **Brassylic acid.** $COOH(CH_2)_{11}COOH$, a dibasic acid of the oxalic acid series. **Brenzcatechin sulphuric acid.** $C_6H_4(OH)OSO_2OH$, a derivative of catechol, *o*-dihydroxybenzene, appearing in the urine as the result of the detoxication of phenolic substances in the body. **Brom- acid.** An acid into whose molecule bromine has been introduced elsewhere than in the acid, -COOH, group. **Bromacetic acid.** $CH_2BrCOOH$, colourless crystals soluble in water; it has an escharotic action. **Bromauric acid.** $HAuBr_4$, an acid that has been used with arsenic oxide and mercuric bromide in the treatment of syphilis. **Bromebric Acid.** BP Commission approved name for *cis*-3-bromo-3-(4-methyoxybenzoyl)-acrylic acid; a cytotoxic agent. **Bromhydric acid.** Hydrobromic acid (see below). **Bromic acid.** $HBrO_3$, colourless crystals only slightly soluble in water, but readily in alkalis forming bromates. **Bromo- acid.** Brom- acid (see above). **Bromo-acetic acid.** Bromacetic acid (see above). **Bromphenylmercapturic acid.** Bromphenylacetyl cysteine, $C_6H_4BrSCH_2CH(NHCOCH_3)COOH$, an acid that has been found excreted in the urine in certain metabolic experiments on dogs. **Bursic acid, Bursinic**

acid. An acid derived from shepherd's purse, *Capsella bursapastoris*; an emmenagogue and vasoconstrictor. **Butadiene carboxylic acid.** Muconic acid (see below). **Butic acid, Butinic acid.** Arachic acid (see above). **Butylacetic acid.** Caproic acid (see below). **Butylcarboxylic acid.** Normal valeric acid, $CH_3(CH_2)_3COOH$. **Butylethylbarbituric acid.** $CO(NHCO)_2C(C_2H_5)(C_4H_9)$, one of the disubstituted derivatives of barbituric acid used as a hypnotic. **Butyl-lactic acid.** Acetone acid (see above). **Butyric acid.** $CH_3CH_2CH_2COOH$, a saturated fatty acid; a colourless liquid with an unpleasant smell, formed during fermentation and the putrefactive breaking-down of protein; it appears in cheese, butter and the excretions.

Caffeic acid. Dihydroxycinnamic acid, $C_6H_3(OH)_2(CH)_2COOH$, an acid obtained from the resin of the black fir; it is also present in the clematis and in certain tannins. **Caffeotannic acid.** Chlorogenic acid (see below). **Caffuric acid.** Trimethyluric acid, $C_8H_{10}O_3N_4$, an acid obtained from caffeine; a diuretic. **Cahincic acid, Cahinic acid, Caincic acid.** $C_{40}H_{64}O_{18}$, a glucoside obtained from cahinca root, *Chiococca racemosa*; a purgative and diuretic. **Calumbic acid.** Columbic acid, a yellow amorphous acid prepared from the bitter principle of calumba root, *Jateorhiza palmata*. **Cambogic acid.** Gambogic acid (see below). **Camphoglycuronic acid.** $C_{16}H_{24}O_8$, the form in which camphor is excreted in the urine after partial oxidation and subsequent combination with glycuronic acid. **Campholic acid.** $C_9H_{17}COOH$, a cyclopentane carboxylic acid derived from camphor. **Camphoric acid.** $C_8H_{14}(COOH)_2$, a cyclopentane dicarboxylic acid produced from camphor and used as a laryngeal antiseptic; also as a urinary and intestinal disinfectant. **Camphoronic acid.** $C_6H_{11}(COOH)_3$, a butane tricarboxylic acid formed by oxidizing camphor; an antiseptic. **Camphosulphonic acid.** $C_{10}H_{15}OSO_3H$, an acid used in the form of sodium, quinine, calcium or magnesium salts, as a cardiac and respiratory stimulant. **Canadinic acid.** $C_{19}H_{34}O_2$, a constituent of Canada turpentine, the oleoresin of *Abies balsamea*. **Canadinolic acids.** $C_{19}H_{30}O_2$, 2 isomeric acids constituting the largest proportion of Canada turpentine. **Canadolic acid.** $C_{19}H_{28}O_2$, an acid occurring as a very small percentage in Canada turpentine. **Cantharic acid.** A dibasic acid occurring with the lactone, cantharidin, in cantharides, *Cantharis vesicatoria*; a vesicant, rubefacient and counter-irritant, it has been used internally as a diuretic and externally as a stimulant to promote the growth of hair. **Cantharidic acid.** $C_8H_{12}O(COOH)_2$, the acid of which cantharidin is the anhydride; used as a diuretic and stimulant. **Capric acid, Caprinic acid.** $CH_3(CH_2)_8COOH$, a saturated fatty acid found in butter and other animal fats. **Caprilic acid.** Caprylic acid (see below). **Caproic acid, Capronic acid.** Butylacetic acid, $CH_3(CH_2)_4COOH$, a saturated liquid fatty acid occurring in animal fats, and the basis of a number of important and essential natural amino acids. **Caprylic acid.** $CH_3(CH_2)_6COOH$, a saturated solid fatty acid in butter; it is used as a fungicide. **Capsic acid.** A substance extracted from the volatile oil of pimenta, *Pimenta officinalis*. **Carbamic acid.** NH_2COOH, aminoformic acid, the simplest of the amino acids, whose esters, the urethanes, are important as hypnotics. **Carbaminocarboxylic acid.** $COOHNHCH_2COOH$, a dibasic acid prepared from glycine. **Carbaminophenylarsonic acid.** Carbarsone. $NH_2CONHC_6H_4AsO(OH)_2$, a white substance, soluble in alkalis, and used as an amoebacide. **Carbazotic acid.** Picric acid (see below). **Carbolic acid.** Phenol, C_6H_5OH, colourless crystals slightly soluble in water, but much more soluble in alcohol, chloroform, ether or glycerin. It is obtained from coal tar and is used widely as an antiseptic and disinfectant. **Carbolic acid, camphorated.** Carbolic camphor, a mixture of camphor and phenol used as an antiseptic and local anaesthetic in dentistry. **Carbolic acid, chlorinated.** Chlorophenisic acid, trichlorophenol, $C_6H_2(OH)Cl_3$, colourless crystals used as an antiseptic and disinfectant. **Carbolic acid, iodized.** 10 to 25 per cent iodine in phenol; it has been found useful for ringworm, also intra-uterine and sinus disinfection. **Carbolic acid, liquefactum.** Liquefied Phenol BP 1958, 80 per cent phenol, employed in the treatment by injection of varicose veins and haemorrhoids. **Carbonaceous acid.** Carbonic acid (see below).

Carbonaphthoic acid. Alpha-oxynaphthoic acid (see above). **Carbonic acid.** Incorrectly applied to carbon dioxide, CO_2, it is more accurately the extremely unstable acid formed by the solution of carbon dioxide in water which gives rise to important salts, the carbonates. **Carboxylic acid.** An organic acid containing one or more carboxyl, -COOH, groups. **Carlic acid, Carlosic acid.** Acids formed in the metabolism of *Penicillium charlesii*. **Carmic acid.** A glucoside obtained from cochineal, *Dactylopius coccus*. **Carminic acid.** $C_{22}H_{20}O_{13}$, an anthropurpurin compound prepared from cochineal and used as a stain in microscopy; it is also a pH indicator. **Carnaubic acid.** $CH_3(CH_2)_{22}COOH$, a saturated fatty acid found in carnauba wax, from the Brazilian wax palm, *Copernicia cerifera*, wool fat and beef kidney. **Carnic acid.** An amino acid derivative related to carnosine, and occurring as the phospho- compound in muscle. **Carolic acid, Carolinic acid.** Acids formed in the metabolism of *Penicillium charlesii*. **Caronic acid.** $(CH_3)_2C(CHCOOH)_2$, a derivative of the hydrocarbon, carane, found in certain essential oils. **Carthamic acid.** $C_{14}H_{16}O_7$, the red dye from the safflower, *Carthamus tinctorius*. **Caryophyllinic acid.** $C_{20}H_{32}O_8$, an acid prepared from caryophyllin contained in oil of cloves. **Caseanic acid.** $C_9H_{16}O_7N_2$, an acid from the milk protein, casein. **Caseinic acid.** $C_{12}H_{24}O_5N_2$, an acid derived from casein. **Catechinic acid.** Catechin, $C_{15}H_{14}O_6$, an acid obtained from gambir, the extract of *Uncaria gambier*, or from cutch, the extract of *Acacia catechu*; white crystals used as an astringent in diarrhoea, leucorrhoea and haemorrhages. **Catechutannic acid.** The anhydride of catechuic acid; an amorphous red phlobatannin which yields catechu red. **Cathartic acid, Cathartinic acid.** A laxative glucoside in senna. **Cephalinic acid.** An unsaturated aliphatic acid whose glycerol ester is to be found in cephalin, the brain phospholipide. **Cephalylphosphoric acid.** An acid formed during the disintegration of the cephalin molecule. **Cerebric acid, Cerebrinic acid.** An aliphatic acid occurring in brain substance. **Cerebronic acid.** The name given to the mixture of 2 aliphatic acids produced, with glycerol, phosphoric acid and the amine base, by the hydrolysis of cephalin. **Cerosic acid.** Tetracosanic acid, a saturated fatty acid occurring in cerosin. **Cerotic acid, Cerotinic acid.** $CH_3(CH_2)_{25}COOH$, a saturated fatty acid occurring in beeswax and, as a myricyl ester, in carnauba. **Cetoleic acid.** An unsaturated acid, $CH_3(CH_2)_9CH{=}CH(CH_2)_9COOH$, found in fish oils. **Cetraric acid.** An acid with a bitter taste, found in Iceland moss, *Cetraria islandica*, and other lichens. **Cevitamic acid.** Vitamin C, $C_6H_8O_6$. *See* ASCORBIC ACID (above). **Acid characteristic.** The radical which confers acid properties upon an organic compound, usually the carboxyl group, -COOH. **Chaulmoogric acid.** $C_5H_7(CH_2)_{12}COOH$, an unsaturated cyclic fatty acid obtained from hydnocarpus and chaulmoogra oils; used in the prolonged treatment of leprosy. **Chelidonic acid.** Pyronedicarboxylic acid, $CO(CH{=}CCOOH)_2O$, from the greater celandine, *Chelidonium majus*. **Chenocholalic acid, Chenocholic acid.** $C_{27}H_{44}O_4$, a steroid compound occurring as chenotaurocholic acid in goose bile. **Chenotaurocholic acid.** $C_{29}H_{49}O_6NS$, a derivative of taurine and chenocholic acid, found in goose bile. **Chinovic acid.** Quinovic acid, $C_{30}H_{48}O_6$, an acid found in small quantities in cinchona barks. **Chitonic acid.** $CH_2OHCHO(CHOH)_2CHCOOH$, a substance related to glucosamine and contained in chitin, the polysaccharide of lobster shell. **Chloracetic acid.** Monochloracetic acid, $CH_2ClCOOH$, colourless crystals soluble in water, alcohol or ether, and used to remove corns and warts. **Chlorauric acid.** $HAuCl_4$, yellow crystals soluble in water; the sodium salt, chloride of gold, has been used in the treatment of cirrhosis of the liver and to arrest the progress of locomotor ataxia. **Chlorhydric acid.** Hydrochloric acid (see below). **Chloric acid.** $HClO_3$, best known in the form of chlorates, especially potassium chlorate, $KClO_3$, which is used as a mouth-wash and gargle. **Acid chloride.** A compound containing the radical -COCl. **Chlorocarbonic acid, Chloroformic acid.** $ClCOOH$, a very unstable acid which forms esters that are used in organic synthesis and in chemical warfare as tear gases. **Chlorogenic acid.** Caffeotannic acid, $C_{16}H_{18}O_9$; a condensation of caffeic and quinic acids, it is found in maté, coffee, and nux vomica.

Chloropeptic acid. A solution of pepsin, obtained from pig's stomach, in dilute hydrochloric acid; used as a digestive. **Chlorophenisic acid.** Chlorinated carbolic acid (see above). **Chloroplatinic acid.** H_2PtCl_6, an acid useful as a reagent for nicotine, quinine and other alkaloids. **Chlorosulphonic acid.** HSO_3Cl, an acid used to generate fog screens and chemical smoke. **Chlorous acid.** $HClO_2$, an acid important for the salts it forms, chlorites, which readily yield chlorine and are used therefore as disinfectants. **Cholalic acid.** Cholic acid (see below). **Cholanic acid.** $C_{23}H_{39}COOH$, a saturated acid of sterol structure from which all the bile acids are derived. **Choleic acid.** One of a number of complexes formed by the hydrotropic combination of desoxycholic acid in the bile with fats, alcohols and similar substances, thereby rendering the latter soluble and more easily absorbed in the intestines. **Choleocamphoric acid.** $C_{10}H_{16}O_4$, a compound isomeric with camphoric acid, resulting from the oxidation of cholic acid. **Cholesteric acid.** $C_{12}H_{10}O_7$, an oxidation product of cholic acid. **Cholesterinic acid.** $C_8H_{10}O_5$, a substance prepared by oxidizing cholesterol. **Cholic acid.** Cholalic acid, trihydroxycholic acid, $C_{23}H_{39}O_3COOH$, an acid occurring in bile combined with glycine and taurine, respectively, as the peptides, glycocholic and taurocholic acids. **Cholodinic acid.** $C_{24}H_{38}O_4$, an acid produced from cholic acid by dehydration. **Choloidanic acid.** $C_{16}H_{24}O_7$, an acid obtained as an oxidation product of cholic acid. **Choloidic acid.** An oxidation product of cholic acid. **Cholonic acid.** $C_{26}H_{41}O_5N$, an anhydride of glycocholic acid (see below). **Chondroitic acid, Chondroitinsulphuric acid.** Chondroitin sulphate, $C_{18}H_{27}O_{17}NS$, a mucopolysaccharide built of uronic-acid molecules combined with acetylgalactosamine and esterified with sulphuric acid; it occurs in cartilage. **Chromic acid.** Strictly, H_2CrO_4, an acid which forms chromates as salts, but commonly applied to chromium trioxide, CrO_3; deliquescent red crystals soluble in water, used as an oxidizing agent and, because of its caustic and astringent properties, in the treatment of warts, lupus and ulcers of the mouth and pharynx. **Chrysenic acid.** Phenylnaphtholcarboxylic acid, $C_{16}H_{11}OCOOH$, an acid derived from the coal-tar hydrocarbon, chrysene. **Chrysophanic acid.** Dihydroxymethylanthraquinone, $C_6H_3(OH)(CO)_2C_6H_2CH_3(OH)$, an acid occurring as a glucoside in rhubarb, as a rhamnoside in cascara and in chrysarobin; used in skin diseases, especially psoriasis and eczema. **Cinchomeronic acid.** Pyridinedicarboxylic acid, $C_5H_3N(COOH)_2$, an acid derived from cinchona bark. **Cinchonic acid.** $C_8H_9(OH)_3(COOH)_3$, an acid obtained by reducing cinchomeronic acid. **Cinchoninic acid.** Quinolinemonocarboxylic acid, C_9H_6NCOOH, an oxidation product of cinchonine. **Cinchotannic acid.** $C_{14}H_{16}O_9$, a phlobatannin found in cinchona bark. **Cinnamic Acid BPC 1968, Cinnamylic acid.** β-Phenylacrylic acid, $C_6H_5CH{=}CHCOOH$, an acid occurring free, and as esters, in benzoin, tolu, storax, and, with cocaine, in coca leaves; it has been used to bring about leucocytosis in cancer and tuberculosis. **Citraconic acid.** Methylmaleic acid, $CH_3(COOH)C{=}CHCOOH$, an acid that can be synthesized from citric acid. **Citric Acid BP 1973.** $(OH)(COOH)C(CH_2COOH)_2$, an acid found in the juice of citrus fruits; colourless crystals soluble in water, it is used (and as citrates) as a diuretic, diaphoretic, febrifuge and anticoagulant. **Clamidoxic Acid.** BP Commission approved name for 2-(3,4-dichlorobenzamido) phenoxyacetic acid; an antirheumatic. **Clorazepic Acid.** BP Commission approved name for 7 - chloro - 2,3 - dihydro - 2,2 - dihydroxy - 5 - phenyl - 1*H* - 1,4 - benzodiazepine - 3 - carboxylic acid; a sedative. **Clupadonic acid.** $C_{17}H_{27}COOH$, an acid found in cod-liver oil and other fish oils. **Clupanodonic acid.** $C_{22}H_{34}O_2$, an unsaturated fatty acid found, with other similar acids, in cod-liver oil and fish blubber. **Cocatannic acid.** $C_{17}H_{22}O_{10}$, from coca, the leaves of *Erythroxylon coca.* **Cocceric acid.** Tetracosanic acid, $C_{24}H_{28}O_2$, a saturated fatty acid occurring in brain tissue, and also as an ester in sugar cane. **Cochinealic acid.** $CH_3C_6H(OH)(COOH)_3$, an acid produced by the oxidation of carminic acid and by the breakdown of kermic acid. **Cocinic acid.** $C_{10}H_{21}COOH$, a fatty acid found as an ester, cocinin, in coconut oil. **Colchicinic acid.** $C_{16}H_{15}O_5N$, an acid obtained during the hydrolysis of colchicine, the extract of the corms of the autumn crocus, *Colchicum autumnale.* **Colopholic acid, Colophonic acid.** A constituent of colophony; a bitter-tasting acid used in soap manufacture. **Columbic acid.** Calumbic acid (see above). **Comanic acid.** Pyronecarboxylic acid, $C_5H_3O_2(COOH)$ obtained from chelidonic acid (see above) by reduction. **Comenic acid.** Oxypyrone carboxylic acid, $OHC_5H_2O_2COOH$, produced by the oxidation of comanic acid. **Convolvulic acid, Convolvulinic acid.** $CH_3(CH_2)_3CHOH(CH_2)_9COOH$, an acid occurring as a glucoside in jalap. **Copaibic acid.** $C_{19}H_{29}COOH$, an acid isomeric with abietic acid; it occurs in the resin of copaiba, the balsam from various species of *Copaifera.* **Coumaric acid, Coumarinic acid.** $C_6H_4(OH)(CH)_2COOH$, an acid occurring in aloes, wild cherry and, as a lactone, in tonka seeds; a vasodilator, also used as a flavouring agent. **Coumarilic acid.** C_8H_5OCOOH, an acid that can be prepared from coumarin, the anhydride of coumaric acid (see above). **Creatine phosphoric acid.** Creatine phosphate. **Crenic acid.** $C_{24}H_{12}O_{16}$, a substance related to apocrenic acid, and found in soil humus. **Cresolsulphonic acid.** $C_6H_3(CH_3)(OH)(SO_2OH)$, one of a series of acids derived from cresol and used as antiseptics. **Cresolsulphuric acid, Cresosulphuric acid.** $CH_3C_6H_4SO_2OH$, toluenesulphonic acid, an acid occurring in the urine as the result of the bacterial breakdown of phenylalanine and tyrosine in the intestine. **Cresotic acid, Cresotinic acid.** $C_6H_3(CH_3)(OH)COOH$, a group of isomers, some of which have value as antiseptics and antipyretics. **Cresylic acid.** Cresol, $CH_3C_6H_4OH$, a mixture of isomers constituting the major proportion of crude carbolic acid; it is less poisonous than phenol, if somewhat less effective as a disinfectant. **Crocic acid, Croconic acid.** $CO(COCOH)_2$, a ketonic acid derived from crocin, the pigment of saffron, *Crocus sativus.* **Cromoglycic Acid.** BP Commission approved name for 1,3-di-(2-carboxy-4-oxochromen-5-yloxy)propan-2-ol; it is used in the treatment of allergic airway obstruction. **Crotonic acid.** $CH_3CH{=}CHCOOH$, one of the isomers occurring in the group of unsaturated acids from croton oil; a violent purgative and vesicant. **Crotonoleic acid, Crotonolic acid.** $C_8H_{13}COOH$, an acid derived from croton oil, the oil of the seeds of *Croton tiglium*; a purgative. **Cryptophanic acid.** $C_3H_7NO(COOH)_2$, an acid present in urine. **Cubebic acid.** $C_{13}H_{14}O_7$, an acid obtained from cubebs, the fruits of *Piper cubeba*; it stimulates mucous membrane and has been used in bronchitis and gonorrhoea, also as a purgative. **Cumaric acid.** Coumaric acid (see above). **Cumic acid, Cuminic acid.** Isopropylbenzoic acid, $C_3H_7C_6H_4COOH$, an acid occurring as the aldehyde in oil of cumin from the fruits of *Cuminum cyminum.* **Cuminuric acid.** $C_3H_7C_6H_4CONHCH_2COOH$, a compound of glycine and cumic acid excreted in the urine. **Cyanhydric acid.** Hydrocyanic acid (see below). **Cyanic acid.** HCNO, an unstable acid which forms cyanates; it is poisonous and a vesicant. **Cyanuric acid.** Pyrolithic acid, tricyanic acid, $C_3H_3O_3N_3$, a colourless substance synthesized by heating urea. **Cyclamic Acid BP 1968.** Cyclohexylsulphamic acid; used as a sweetening agent. **Cyclohexenylethylbarbituric acid.** Cyclobarbitone BP 1958. **Cyclohexylsulphamic acid.** Cyclamic Acid BP 1968 (see above). **Cyclopentenylundecyclic acid.** Hydnocarpic acid (see below). **Cynurenic acid.** Kynurenic acid, $C_9H_6ONCOOH$, a breakdown product of tryptophane, appearing in the urine of dogs. **Cysteic acid.** $CH_2(SO_2OH)CH(NH_2)COOH$, an oxidation product of the amino acid, cysteine; it forms taurine on further oxidation.

Damalic acid. $C_{12}H_{22}O_2$, an acid that has been found in urine. **Damaluric acid.** $C_7H_{12}O_2$, an acid occurring in cows' urine. **Decanoic acid, Decatoic acid.** Capric acid (see above). **Decenedicarboxylic acid.** Traumatic acid (see below). **Decenoic acid.** $CH_2{=}CH(CH_2)_7COOH$, an olefine unsaturated acid of the oleic (acrylic) series. **Decoic acid.** Capric acid (see above). **Dehydroascorbic acid.** $C_6H_6O_6$, a diketohexonic acid formed by the oxidation of ascorbic acid. **Dehydrochaulmoogric acid.** Gorlic acid (see below). **Dehydrocholalic acid.** Dehydrocholic acid (see below). **Dehydrocholeic acid.** An acid resulting from the oxidation of the corresponding choleic acid. **Dehydrocholic Acid.** BP Commission approved name for $C_{23}H_{36}O_3COOH$; it is formed by the oxidation of cholic acid with replacement of three hydroxyl groups by oxygen atoms; a powerful cholagogue. "Decholin", "Dehydrocholin". **Dekacrylic acid.** $C_9H_{17}COOH$, an unsaturated olefine acid produced by the distillation of cork. **Deoxyribonucleic acid, Deoxyribosenucleic acid.** DNA; the basic genetic material. Of high molecular weight ($>10^6$), it is a nucleotide polymer containing bases, deoxyribose residues and phosphate groups in the ratio 1:1:1. The bases are adenine, guanine, thymine and cytosine. The molecule in higher organisms consists of a double helix of 2 antiparallel chains with hydrogen bonding between opposing bases, adenine with thymine and guanine with cytosine. **Desoxalic acid.** Dihydroxyethanetricarboxylic acid, $COOHCHOHC(OH)(COOH)_2$, a colourless liquid slightly soluble in water. **Desoxycholeic acid.** An acid produced by the reduction of one of the complexes of desoxycholic acid with aliphatic acids of the bile. **Desoxycholic acid.** $C_{23}H_{37}(OH)_2COOH$, an acid occurring naturally in the bile of man, sheep, ox and goat; it is formed by the reduction of cholic acid. **Desoxyribonucleic acid, Desoxyribose nucleic acid.** Deoxyribonucleic acid (see above). **Dextropimaric acid.** Pimaric acid (see below). **Dextrotartaric acid.** $(CHOHCOOH)_2$, ordinary tartaric acid, a constituent of grapejuice which is dextrorotatory, rotating in a clockwise direction the plane of a beam of polarized light passed through its solution. **Diacetic acid.** 1. Aceto-acetic acid, CH_3COCH_2COOH, a fat metabolite produced excessively during diabetes, and responsible for the acetone bodies in the urine. 2. Diacetylacetic acid, $(CH_3CO)_2CHCOOH$, an acid which can be prepared from ethyl aceto-acetate; it also occurs in ketonuria. **Diacetyltannic acid.** Acetannin, acetyltannin, $C_{14}H_8O_7(COOCH_3)_2$, the acetic ester of digallic acid; a grey powder insoluble in water and used in chronic diarrhoea and intestinal catarrh. **Diallylbarbituric acid.** $(C_3H_5)_2C{=}(CONH)_2{=}CO$, allobarbitone, a sedative and hypnotic used in cases of nervous insomnia. **Dialuric acid.** Hydroxybarbituric acid, $CO(NHCO)_2CHOH$, a dibasic cyclic ureide formed from alloxan; on oxidation it yields alloxantin. **Diamino acid.** One of the group of basic amino acids which contain 2 NH_2 groups; they include the hexone bases, arginine and lysine. **Diamino-acetic acid.** $(NH_2)_2CHCOOH$, an acid formed from the protein casein, by hydrolysis. **Diaminocaproic acid.** Lysine, $NH_2(CH_2)_4CHNH_2COOH$, an amino acid indispensable to animal nutrition and occurring in casein, gelatin and certain protamines. **Diaminocarboxylic acid, Diaminotrihydroxydodecanoic acid.** $(NH_2)(CH_2)_7(CHOH)_3CHNH_2COOH$, an amino acid contained in casein. **Diaminovaleric acid.** $NH_2(CH_2)_3CHNH_2COOH$, an α-amino acid occurring in bird excrement; it is believed to be responsible for the formation of urea in the liver, and is itself produced from arginine by the enzyme arginase. It decomposes to the ptomaine putrescine. **Diatomic acid.** Dibasic acid (see below). **Diatrizoic Acid.** BP Commission approved name for 3,5-diacetamido-2,4,6-tri-iodobenzoic acid, a radio-opaque substance. **Diazobenzenesulphonic acid.** $C_6H_4(N_2OH)(SO_2OH)$, a substance used in the manufacture of dyestuffs; formed from sulphanilic acid and sodium nitrite, it is the reagent in the diazo test for free bilirubin. **Dibasic acid.** An acid which offers 2 hydrogen atoms for replacement by a metal or by basic radicals. **Dibromgallic acid.** $C_6Br_2(OH)_3COOH$, a brown substance soluble in hot water, alcohol or ether; used in the treatment of epilepsy and neurasthenia. **Dibromobarbituric acid.** $CBr_3(CONH)_2CO$, a disubstituted derivative of barbituric acid, used as a hypnotic with a more sedative effect. **Dicarbamidoacetic acid.** Allantoic acid (see above). **Dichloracetic acid.** $CHCl_2COOH$, an acid prepared from chloral hydrate; a heavy colourless liquid, used as an escharotic to remove corns, warts, calluses and venereal sores. **Dichromic acid.** $H_2Cr_2O_7$, an acid derived from chromium trioxide and forming dichromates. **Diethylbarbituric acid.** Diethylmalonylurea, barbital, malonal, $(C_2H_5)_2C(CONH)_2CO$, white crystals, slightly soluble in water, more soluble in alcohol, ether or chloroform; used as a sedative and hypnotic, but, being cumulative, likely to cause chronic poisoning with serious mental changes. **Digallic acid.** $C_6H_2(OH)_3COOC_6H_2(OH)_2COOH$, a white substance, only slightly soluble in water, occurring in gallotannic acid, extracted from the galls of the oak and other plants, as a pentadigalloylglucose or condensation of glucose and digallic acid; used as a reagent for iron, in the manufacture of ink, and as an astringent and coagulant, especially in the treatment of burns. **Digentisic acid.** A gallotannic acid of depside structure which is found in lichens. **Diglycoldisalicylic acid.** $O(CH_2COOC_6H_4COOH)_2$, diglycollic acid with 2 molecules of salicylic acid substituted; an analgesic and antipyretic similar in effect to aspirin. **Diglycollic acid.** $O(CH_2COOH)_2$, an acid formed from 2 molecules of monochloracetic acid by the action of lime; it is a dibasic acid with the properties of an ether. **Dihydro-ambrettolic acid.** Juniperic acid (see below). **Dihydroxy acid.** An acid containing, in addition to one or more carboxyl, -COOH, groups, two hydroxyl, -OH, groups. **Dihydroxyacetic acid.** Glyoxylic acid (see below). **Dihydroxyanthraquinonecarboxylic acid.** Rheinic acid (see below). **Dihydroxybenzoic acid.** Gentisic acid (see below). **Dihydroxycinnamic acid.** Caffeic acid (see above). **Dihydroxydimethylbutyric acid.** $(CH_3)_2C(CH_2OH)CHOHCOOH$, an acid which occurs in pantothenic acid. **Dihydroxyethanetricarboxylic acid.** Desoxalic acid (see above). **Dihydroxymalonic acid.** Mesoxalic acid (see below). **Dihydroxymethylbenzoic acid.** Orsellic acid (see below). **Dihydroxyphenylacetic acid.** Homogentisic acid (see below). **Dihydroxyphenylpropionic acid.** Hydrocaffeic acid (see below). **Dihydroxypropionic acid.** Glyceric acid (see below). **Dihydroxyquinolinecarboxylic acid.** Xanthurenic acid (see below). **Dihydroxystearic acid.** $CH_3(CH_2)_{14}(CHOH)_2COOH$, an acid occurring as a glyceride in castor oil, obtained from the seeds of *Ricinus communis.* **Dihydroxysuccinic acid.** Tartaric acid (see below). **Dihydroxytartaric acid.** $[(OH)_2CCOOH]_2$, a reagent for the detection of sodium, which it precipitates as an insoluble salt. **Dihydroxytoluic acid.** Dioxyphenylacetic acid (see below). **Di-iodochelidamic acid.** $C_5HI_2ON(COOH)_2$, a derivative of chelidonic acid (see above). **Di-iodoparaphenolsulphonic acid, Di-iodophenolsulphonic acid.** Sozo-iodolic acid (see below). **Di-iodophenylaminopropionic acid.** Thyroxine, $C_6H_2I_2(OH)OC_6H_2I_2CH_2CHNH_2COOH$, an acid occurring in the form of a peptide, with di-iodotyrosine, as the hormone of the thyroid gland. The sodium salt is used in the treatment of simple goitre, cretinism and myxoedema. **Di-iodopyridoneacetic acid.** $C_5H_2ONI_2CH_2COOH$, an acid used in excretion pyelograph. **Di-iodosalicylic acid.** $C_6H_2I_2(OH)COOH$, an iodine derivative of salicylic acid; it is antipyretic, analgesic and antirheumatic. **Dilactic acid.** Lactolactic acid, $CH_3CH(OH)COOCH(CH_3)COOH$, one of the anhydrides of lactic acid. **Dimethoxybenzoic acid.** Veratric acid (see below). **Dimethoxyphthalic acid.** Hemipic acid (see below). **Dimethylacetic acid.** Isobutyric acid (see below). **Dimethylarsenic acid, Dimethylarsonic acid.** Cacodylic acid (see above). **Dimethylbenzoic acid.** Mesitylenic acid (see below). **Dimethylcolchicinic acid.** $C_{18}H_{19}O_5N$, an acid obtained from colchicine, the alkaloid in meadow saffron, *Colchicum autumnale.* **Dimethylcyclobutane dicarboxylic acid.** Norpinic acid (see below). **Dimethylketoheptoic acid.** Geronic acid (see below). **Dimethyllaevulinic acid.** Mesitonic acid (see below). **Dimethylmaleic acid.** Pyrocinchonic acid (see below). **Dimethylpentenic acid.** Teracrylic acid (see below). **Diolefinic acid.** One of the unsaturated monobasic fatty acids of the general type $C_nH_{2n-3}COOH$ (linoleic series), which contain 2 double bonds. **Diolic acid.** $C_{10}H_{18}O_3$, an acid obtained from buchu oil, extracted from the leaves of *Barosma (Diosma) betulina.* **Dioxydiaminosuberic acid.** $(CH_2CHOHCHNH_2COOH)_2$, a diaminocarboxylic acid found in casein. **Dioxyphenylacetic acid.** Dihydroxytoluic acid, homogentisic acid, $(OH)_2C_6H_3CH_2COOH$, an intermediate in the metabolism of the phenylalanine and tyrosine of the diet, which makes its appearance in the urine in the condition known as alkaptonuria; the urine turns black on exposure to air. **Dioxysalicylic acid.** Trihydroxybenzoic acid, gallic acid, $C_6H_2(OH)_3COOH$, an acid occurring in oak galls; yellowish crystals slightly soluble in water, used like tannic acid as an astringent. **2,3-Diphosphoglyceric acid.** Glyceric acid diphosphate, a metabolite produced mainly in red blood cells, where it functions as an important regulator of haemoglobin function. **Dithioaminolactic acid.**

Cystine, dicysteine, $S_2(CH_2CHNH_2COOH)_2$, an α-amino acid present in the human hair. In the diet it provides the main source of sulphur for the metabolism; it is excreted in the urine in the abnormal condition known as cystinuria. **Dithiocarbamic acid.** Thiocarbamic acid (see below). **Dithiochloralsalicylic acid.** $C_6HS_2Cl(OH)COOH$, an acid prepared by the action of sulphur dichloride on salicylic acid; an antiseptic. **Dithiodiamino-ethylene lactic acid.** Dithioaminolactic acid (see above). **Dithionic acid.** Hyposulphuric acid (see below). **Dithionous acid.** Hyposulphurous acid, $H_2S_2O_4$, an unstable acid which forms hyposulphites as salts. **Dithiosalicylic acid.** $C_6H_2S_2(OH)COOH$, a yellowish powder, slightly soluble in water; the lithium and sodium salts are used in place of salicylic acid. Bismuth dithiosalicylate is a dental antiseptic. **Djenkolic acid.** Jenkolic acid, $CH_2(SCH_2CH(NH_2)COOH)_2$, an amino acid closely related to cystine, and found in the protein of djenkol beans, *Pithecolobium lobatum.* **Doeglic acid.** $C_{18}H_{35}COOH$, an unsaturated aliphatic acid of the acrylic series, obtained from doegling oil, the oil of the bottle-nosed whale. **Dracic acid.** Anisic acid (see above). **Dracilic acid, Dracylic acid.** Para-aminobenzoic acid, $NH_2C_6H_4COOH$, an acid that occurs in yeast, and is part of the vitamin B complex; a vital factor in bacterial growth. **Draconic acid, Draconylic acid.** Anisic acid (see above). **Durylic acid.** Trimethylbenzoic acid, $(CH_3)_3C_6HCOOH$, a derivative of durene, tetramethylbenzene.

Edetic Acid. BP Commission approved name for ethylene-diamine-*N,N,N',N*-tetra-acetic acid. As sodium salts this is a powerful sequestering agent for metallic ions. It is used in the treatment of lead poisoning. **Elaeostearic acid.** $C_{17}H_{29}COOH$; this constitutes the major portion of the acids from tung oil, and half that from *Aleurites trisperma.* **Elaidic acid.** $C_{17}H_{33}COOH$, an unsaturated acid of the acrylic series, which is a stereo-isomer of oleic acid. **Ellagic acid.** $C_{14}H_6O_8$, a yellow crystalline substance soluble in alkalis, which occurs in certain tannins. **Embelic acid.** $C_{18}H_{28}O_4$, an acid found in the berries of the Indian plant, *Embelia ribes,* and used as an anthelmintic, especially against tapeworm. **Emulcic acid.** $C_{23}H_{42}O_{10}N_6$, an acid obtained from emulsin, an albuminous enzyme present in almonds. **Enanthic acid, Enanthylic acid.** Oenanthylic acid (see below). **Episaccharic acid.** A dibasic saccharic acid of the formula, $COOH(CHOH)_4COOH$, which has undergone epimerization, or the change-over of the -H and -OH attached to the last asymmetric carbon atom of the chain. **Ergotic acid.** Sclerotic acid, $C_{15}H_{30}O_{15}(NH_2)SO_3H$, an acid found in ergot. **Erucic acid.** $C_{21}H_{41}COOH$, an unsaturated acid of the acrylic series, found in rape and mustard-seed oils; isomeric with brassidic and cetoleic acids. **Acid esters.** Esters of organic acids in which at least one carboxyl group remains unaltered, -COOH. **Ethacrynic Acid BP 1973.** 2,3-Dichloro-4-(2-ethylacryloyl)phenoxy acetic acid, a diuretic; it acts by inhibiting tubular reabsorption of sodium and chloride. Action may be intense, serious loss of potassium being a potential hazard. Administered orally or (in emergencies) intravenously. **Ethamal acid.** Glyoxalic acid, CHOCOOH, an aldehyde acid found in unripe fruits such as grapes and gooseberries; it is the anhydride of glyoxylic acid. **Ethanedicarboxylic acid.** Succinic acid (see below). **Ethanethiolic acid.** Thio-acetic acid (see below). **Ethanoic acid.** Acetic acid (see above). **Ethionic acid.** Ethylene sulphonic acid, $SO_3HCH_2CH_2SO_3H$, a dibasic acid of which taurine is the amino derivative. **Ethoxyphenylcarbamic acid.** $C_2H_5OC_6H_4NHCOOH$, an acid closely related to phenacetin; combined with quinine it yields the drug quinaphenin. **Ethylenediaminetetra-acetic acid.** EDTA, $(COOHCH_2)_2NCH_2CH_2N(CH_2COOH)_2$, a preparation combining preferentially with metal ions to form water soluble complexes more readily excreted; it is used for the treatment of lead poisoning. **Ethylenedicarboxylic acid.** Fumaric acid (see below). **Ethylenelactic acid.** Hydracrylic acid, CH_2OHCH_2COOH, an alcohol acid, isomeric with ethylidene lactic acid; it forms acrylic acid on heating. **Ethylenephenylhydrazinesuccinic acid.** $C_{20}H_{22}N_4O_6$, an antipyretic resulting from the combination of ethylenephenylhydrazine and succinic acid. **Ethylene sulphonic acid.** Ethionic acid (see above). **Ethyloxydithiocarbonic acid.** Xanthic acid (see below). **Ethylsulphonic acid.** $C_2H_5SO_3H$, an acid that appears in the urine when sulphonal is given. **Eugenic acid, Eugenitic acid.** Eugenol, $C_6H_3(OCH_3)(OH)C_3H_5$, a constituent of oil of cloves, it is used as an antiseptic, and by dentists to reduce sensitivity.

Fatty acids, non-esterified (NEFA). The free fatty acids of plasma which are carried in association with plasma albumin and which represent the non-esterified transport form of fatty acids in plasma. They are added to albumin by adipose tissue and removed for utilization by muscle, liver and other tissues. (*a*) Acetic or Stearic series; saturated acids of the general formula, $C_nH_{2n}O_2$: (*b*) Acrylic or Oleic series; unsaturated acids, $C_nH_{2n-2}O_2$, with 1 double bond in their chain: (*c*) Acetylene or Propiolic series; unsaturated acids, $C_nH_{2n-4}O_2$, with 1 triple bond: (*d*) Linoleic series; unsaturated acids, $C_nH_{2n-4}O_2$, with 2 double bonds: (*e*) Linolenic series; unsaturated acids, $C_nH_{2n-6}O_2$, with 3 double bonds: (*f*) Arachidonic series; unsaturated acids, $C_nH_{2n-8}O_2$, with 4 double bonds: (*g*) Clupadonic series; unsaturated acids, $C_nH_{2n-10}O_2$, with 5 double bonds: (*h*) Cyclic acids, consisting of 2 members only, hydnocarpic and chaulmoogric acids. **Fellanic acid.** $C_{50}H_{72}O_6$, a complex bile acid. **Fellic acid.** $C_{23}H_{40}O_4$, a constituent of human bile closely allied to cholic acid. **Fenclozic Acid.** BP Commission approved name for 2-(4-chlorophenyl)thiazol-4-ylacetic acid; an anti-inflammatory agent. **Ferulic acid.** Methyl caffeic acid, hydroxy-methoxycinnamic acid, $CH_3OC_6H_3(OH)(CH)_2COOH$, an acid occurring as an ester of the phenolic substance, asaresinol, in asafoetida, the oleo gum resin of *Ferula asafoetida.* **Fibril acid.** An acid that has been identified in the cytoplasm of nerve cells. **Filicic acid.** $C_{14}H_{14}O_5$, an insoluble substance isolated from the extract of the rhizomes of male fern, *Dryopteris filix mas*; its anhydride, filicin, is used as a vermifuge. **Filicinic acid.** $(CH_3)_2CCO(CHCOH)_2$, a cyclic derivative of phloroglucinol, formed by the reduction of filmarone, a complex dibasic acid in filix mas. **Filixic acid.** $C_{35}H_{38}O_{12}$, an acid occurring in the extract of filix mas; reduction yields filicinic acid. **Flavaspidic acid.** One of the acids isolated from filix-mas extract; it is a derivative of butyric acid and phloroglucinol. **Flufenamic Acid.** BP Commission approved name for *N*-(α,α,α-trifluoro-*m*-tolyl) anthranilic acid; an anti-inflammatory agent. **Fluoric acid.** Name applied, incorrectly, to hydrofluoric acid; the fluorine analogue of chloric acid, HFO_3, is unknown. **Fluosilicic acid.** Hydrofluosilicic acid (see below). **Folic Acid BP 1973.** Vitamin B_c, a polypeptide of glutamic and pteroic acids found in green leaves, fungi, yeasts, liver, and kidney; part of the vitamin B complex, and essential for the growth of rats, chicks, yeasts and certain micro-organisms. It has been identified as an anti-anaemic factor. It is absorbed in the upper small intestine and is essential for maintaining the integrity of the jejunal mucosa. **Formic acid.** Methanoic acid, aminic acid, HCOOH, an acid prepared by the oxidation of methyl alcohol or formaldehyde, and by the partial decomposition of oxalic acid; it is the offensive irritant in the stings of ants, bees and nettles; a colourless pungent liquid which has been used in the treatment of influenza, gout and rheumatism, and to reduce muscular tremor. It is also a vesicant. **Formiminoglutamic acid.** $HOOCCH(NHCH{=}NH)CH_2CH_2COOH$, an intermediate product in the metabolism of histidine. In folic acid deficiency it is excreted in the urine. **Frangulic acid.** Dihydroxyanthraquinone, $C_{14}H_6O_2(OH)_3$, a laxative and aperient, obtained from the bark of the alder buckthorn, *Rhamnus frangula.* **Acid fuchsine.** A derivative of pararosaniline used as a stain in microscopy. **Fulminic acid.** C=NOH, an acid that is isomeric with cyanic acid; a very unstable and poisonous substance. The mercurous salt explodes violently, and is used in the manufacture of detonators, percussion caps and cartridges. **Fulminuric acid.** $CNCH(NO_2)CONH_2$, an isomer of cyanuric acid; an explosive compound. **Fumaric acid.** Ethylene dicarboxylic acid, $COOHCH{=}CHCOOH$, an acid found in combination with cetraric acid in the lichen acid from Iceland moss, *Cetraria islandica,* and in the common fumitory, *Fumaria officinalis*; an isomeric form of maleic acid. **Fumaric acid series.** A family of dibasic acids containing 1 double bond,

with the general formula $C_nH_{2n-4}O_4$; the most important representatives of the series are fumaric, maleic and citraconic acids. **Furane carboxylic acid.** Paramucic acid, C_4H_3OCOOH, a derivative of the cyclic compound furane; prepared by the distillation of mucic acid (see below). **Fusidic Acid.** BP Commission approved name for an antibiotic produced by a strain of *Fusidium*; it inhibits bacterial protein synthesis by interfering with the translocation mechanism.
Gadelaidic acid. An unsaturated fatty acid of the formula $CH_3(CH_2)_7CH{=}CH(CH_2)_9COOH$, isomeric with gadoleic acid, and also found in cod-liver oil. **Gadoleic acid.** An unsaturated acid of the oleic series, found in cod-liver oil, sardine oil, herring oil and blubber; its formula is $CH_3(CH_2)_9CH{=}CH(CH_2)_7(COOH)$. **Gaidic acid.** $C_{15}H_{29}COOH$, an isomer of hypogaeic acid, with which it exists in arachis oil as a glyceride. **Galactonic acid.** A lactonic acid, pentahydroxycaproic acid, $CH_2OH(CHOH)_4COOH$, formed by the oxidation of galactose. **Galacturonic acid.** $CHO(CHOH)_4COOH$, a hexuronic acid derived from galactose, and occurring naturally, combined with sugars, in mucilages and pectins. **Gallhumic acid.** Melanogallic acid (see below). **Gallic acid.** Trihydroxybenzoic acid, $C_6H_2(OH)_3COOH$, fine white silky needles, soluble in water, alcohol and ether; it occurs free in nutgalls, tea, mangoes, rhubarb, witch hazel, and, as a decomposition product of tannic acid, in certain tannins. It is used in the manufacture of ink, as a reagent for ferric salts and, in medicine, as an astringent. **Gallotannic acid.** $C_{76}H_{52}O_{46}$, so-called tannic acid; a tannin extracted from fermented nutgalls, and consisting of pentadigalloylglucose, glucose condensed with 5 molecules of digallic acid. It is used in tanning, dyeing and the manufacture of ink. A powerful astringent and coagulant, it is employed in medicine for throat infections, to check superficial bleeding and to provide a coagulum in the treatment of burns. **Gambogic acid.** Cambogic acid, $C_{29}H_{23}O_4$, an acid that comprises the major proportion of the gum resin, gamboge, secreted by *Garcinia hanburyi*, a tree in Vietnam; it emulsifies with water, and is used as a purgative, and against tapeworm. **Gamma hydroxybutyric acid.** Sodium oxybate, an anaesthetic agent derived from gamma aminobutyric acid, a naturally occurring neurohormone. **Gamolenic Acid.** BP Commission approved name for *cis,cis,cis*-octadeca-6,9,12-trienoic acid; it is used in the treatment of hypercholesterolaemia. **Garcinolic acids.** Three isomeric acids which have been isolated from the resin of gamboge. **Gaultheric acid.** Methyl salicylate, $C_6H_4(OH)COOCH_3$, an odorous liquid from oil of wintergreen, *Gaultheria procumbens*; used as a liniment. **Geic acid.** Ulmic acid (see below). **Gentianic acid.** Gentisic acid (see below). **Gentiotannic acid.** $C_{14}H_{10}O_5$, a tannin occurring in the root of the yellow gentian, *Gentiana lutea*; it is used to promote gastric secretion. **Gentisic acid, Gentisinic acid.** Dihydroxybenzoic acid, hydroquinone carboxylic acid, $C_6H_3(OH)_2COOH$, an acid prepared from the bitter principle of gentian root. **Geranic acid.** $C_9H_{15}COOH$, an unsaturated acid, produced by the oxidation of citral, derived from oil of lemons, oil of oranges, or of geraniol, the alcohol in roses, lemongrass and geraniums. **Geronic acid.** Dimethylketoheptoic acid, $CH_3CO(CH_2)_3C(CH_3)_2COOH$, an acid that has been obtained by the oxidation of vitamin A, β-carotene, and β-ionone, thereby affording valuable evidence as to the structure of the carotenoids. **Glucic acid.** Acrolactic acid, hydroxyacrylic acid, $CH(OH){=}CHCOOH$, a colourless liquid, soluble in water, obtained by the hydrolysis of cane sugar. **Glucoascorbic acid.** $\overline{COC(OH){=}(COH)CH}CH(OH)CH(OH)CH_2OH$ (ring closed through O), a synthetic compound which acts as a metabolic antagonist to ascorbic acid; thus mice fed with it develop scurvy-like symptoms which are not curable by ascorbic acid but disappear when gluco-ascorbic acid is withdrawn from the diet. **Gluconic acid.** $CH_2OH(CHOH)_4COOH$, a typical saccharinic acid, produced by the oxidation of glucose or cane sugar; it occurs in the oxidative changes brought about in glucose by strains of bacteria and by moulds, such as *Aspergillus niger* and *Penicillium purpurogenum*. **Glucothionic acid.** A sugar acid containing sulphur, which occurs in nucleoproteins and has been observed in the mammary gland. **Glucuronic acid.** Glycuronic acid, $CHO(CHOH)_4COOH$, the most important of the uronic acids; it appears in the urine combined with camphors, phenols or higher alcohols, when the latter are administered, thus acting as a detoxication agent. It also occurs in the prosthetic group of the glycoproteins, usually linked to hexosamine units. **Glutamic acid, Glutaminic acid.** $HOOC(CH_2)_2CH(NH_2)COOH$. An amino acid, a common constituent of protein and an important metabolic intermediate. **Glutaric acid.** $COOH(CH_2)_3COOH$, an isomer of pyrotartaric acid, occurring naturally in sheep-wool, lanolin, and pus. It gives rise to important amino acids and amines. **Glyceric acid.** Dihydroxypropionic acid, $CH_2OHCHOHCOOH$, an acid prepared by the careful oxidation of glycerol; it also arises during alcoholic fermentation, and plays an intermediate part in the phosphate cycle of muscle contraction, **Glycerinphosphoric acid.** Glycerophosphoric acid (see below). **Glycerinsulphuric acid.** Glycerosulphuric acid (see below). **Glyceroarsenic acid.** $(CH_2OH)_2CHO_2As(OH)_2$, an arsonic acid derivative of glycerol. **Glycerophosphoric Acid BPC 1963.** An acid that occurs in 2 forms, $CH_2OHCHOHCH_2OPO(OH)_2$ and $CH_2OHCHO[PO(OH)_2]CH_2OH$, giving rise respectively to α- and β-lecithins, in which they are combined with fatty acids and choline. The glycerophosphates are given as nerve tonics. **Glycerosulphuric acid.** $CH_2OHCHOHCH_2OHSO_3$, a sulphuric ester of glycerol which saponifies easily. **Glycerylphosphoric acid.** Glycerophosphoric acid (see above). **Glycerylsulphuric acid.** Glycerosulphuric acid (see above). **Glycocholeic acid.** $C_{27}H_{45}O_5N$, a complex occurring in the bile. **Glycocholic acid.** $C_{23}H_{39}O_3CONHCH_2COOH$; this predominates in human bile as a sodium salt; it is derived from glycine and cholic acid into which it hydrolyses. The sodium salt is a cholagogue and aids pancreatic digestion. **Glycollic acid.** Hydroxyacetic acid, $CH_2OHCOOH$, the simplest of the monohydroxy fatty acids; formed by the reduction of oxalic acid, and found in unripe grapes and vine leaves. **Glycoluric acid.** Hydantoic acid, uramino-acetic acid, $NH_2CONHCH_2COOH$, the ureide of glycollic acid; derived from allantoin. **Glycosuric acid.** An acid that has been observed in minute quantities in the urine. **Glycuronic acid.** Glucuronic acid (see above). **Glycyrrhetic acid, Glycyrrhetinic acid.** An acid of which glycyrrhizinic acid is a glucuronic ester; it has haemolytic properties. **Glycyrrhizic acid, Glycyrrhizinic acid.** $C_{44}H_{64}O_9$, an acid that occurs as the potassium and calcium salts in liquorice root, *Glycyrrhiza glabra*; a demulcent and expectorant. **Glyoxalic acid.** HCOCOOH, the simplest aldehyde acid; it occurs in unripe fruits and, dissolved in water, it forms glyoxylic acid. **Glyoxylic acid.** Dihydroxyacetic acid, $CH(OH)_2COOH$, an acid responsible for the characteristic purple reaction in the Hopkins-Cole test for tryptophan. **Gorlic acid.** Dehydrochaulmoogric acid, $C_5H_7(CH_2)_6CH{=}CH(CH_2)_4COOH$, an acid contained in gorli oil, from *Oucoba echinata*. **Granatotannic acid.** $C_{20}H_{16}O_{13}$, a tannic acid obtained from the rind of the pomegranate, *Punica granatum*, and also the root bark; it is very astringent. **Acid group.** The carboxyl radical, -COOH, which is characteristic of all organic acids. **Guaiacolcarbonic acid, Guaiacolcarboxylic acid.** $C_6H_3(OH)(OCH_3)COOH$, white crystals, insoluble in water but soluble in alcohol and ether; used to reduce cough and expectoration in phthisis and bronchitis, also to relieve pain and swelling in rheumatoid arthritis. **Guaiacolsulphonic acid.** $C_6H_3(OH)(OCH_3)SO_3H$, an acid, the calcium salt of which, guaiacyl, is used subcutaneously as a local anaesthetic, and intravenously in lung affections. **Guaiaconic acid.** $C_{20}H_{24}O_5$, a mixture of 2 isomeric acids comprising the bulk of guaiacum resin, from *Guaiacum officinale*; an amorphous brown powder, it is used as a diaphoretic, laxative and diuretic. On oxidation it gives blue compounds, and is used for this reason to detect blood. **Guaiaretic acid.** $C_{20}H_{26}O_4$, an acid that forms, with guaiac resin, the lesser proportion of guaiacum. **Guanylic acid.** A purine mononucleotide, built of guanine, phosphate and the pentose ribofuranose; it occurs in yeast, liver, pancreas and spleen. **Gulonic acid.** $CH_2OH(CHOH)_4COOH$, an isomer of gluconic acid, obtained from gulose by oxidation.

Gummic acid. $CH_2OH(CHOH)_3COOH$, an acid formed from the pentose arabinose, in gum arabic, by oxidation. **Gurjunic acid.** $C_{22}H_{34}O_4$, an acid occurring in the oleo gum resin, gurjun, obtained from the *Dipterocarpus turbinatus* of India. **Gymnemic acid.** $C_{32}H_{55}O_{12}$, a constituent of the extract of the leaves of *Gymnema sylvestre*, a shrub of India and Africa; it has an acrid taste and suspends temporarily the ability to savour sweet or bitter things. **Gynocardic acid.** $C_{18}H_{34}O_2$, an oily liquid extracted from the seeds of *Gynocardia adorata*. The name sodium gynocardate is applied to the mixture of sodium salts of the fatty acids contained in chaulmoogra oil, which is used in the treatment of leprosy.

Acid halide. An organic compound with a halogen substituted for the -OH in the acid group. **Halogen acid, Haloid acid.** An inorganic acid consisting of hydrogen and a halogen element only; a hydrogen halide. **Helvellic acid.** $C_{12}H_{20}O_7$, a poisonous substance, occurring in the fungus *Helvella esculenta*, which causes haemolysis. **Helvolic acid.** An antibiotic secreted by certain species of *Aspergillus*, a parasitic mould. **Hemipic acid, Hemipinic acid.** Dimethoxyphthalic acid, $C_6H_2(CH_3O)_2(COOH)_2$, an acid produced by the oxidation of narcotine. **Hepta-iodic acid.** Periodic acid, HIO_4, colourless crystals, soluble in water; derived from the heptavalent oxide, I_2O_7, and of variable constitution. **Heptoic acid.** Oenanthylic acid (see below). **Hexabasic acid.** Hexatomic acid (see below). **Hexadecanoic acid.** Palmitic acid (see below). **Hexadecenoic acid.** Palmitoleic acid (see below). **Hexadecynoic acid.** Palmitolic acid (see below). **Hexadienic acid.** Sorbic acid (see below). **Hexahydrotetrahydroxybenzoic acid.** Quinic acid (see below). **Hexamethylenaminesalicylsulphonic acid.** $(CH_2)_6N_4SO_3HC_6H_3(OH)COOH$, an acid used as a urinary and intestinal antiseptic especially for affections of the urinary tract. **Hexanoic acid.** Caproic acid (see above). **Hexatomic acid.** An acid offering 6 hydrogens for replacement by metals or basic radicals. **Hexonic acid.** An acid applied to the isomers of pentahydroxycaproic acid. They arise from the oxidation of the hexoses, have the formula $CH_2OH(CHOH)_4COOH$, and are represented chiefly by gluconic, galactonic and mannonic acids. **Hexosediphosphoric acid.** Fructose 1,6-diphosphate. **Hexuronic acid.** One of the acids, $CHO(CHOH)_4COOH$, formed from the various hexoses by oxidation of the primary alcohol group; represented in nature chiefly by glucuronic, galacturonic and mannuronic acids. **Hidrolic acid, Hidrotic acid.** Sudoric acid (see below). **Hippuric acid.** Benzoyl glycine, benzamino acetic acid, $C_6H_5CONHCH_2COOH$, a detoxication product in the urine of herbivorous animals and, to a much less extent, in the urine of man. White crystals, soluble in hot water, and used in the treatment of gout and rheumatism. **Hircic acid.** Derived from hircine, the principle in goat fat; it occurs also in goats' milk. **Homogentisic acid.** Dihydroxyphenylacetic acid, hydroquinone acetic acid, $C_6H_3(OH)_2CH_2COOH$, a normal intermediate in the metabolism of tyrosine and phenylalanine. In the condition known as alkaptonuria, it appears unchanged in the urine; the characteristic blackening is due to the formation of melanins. **Homophthalic acid.** Phenylaceto-orthocarboxylic acid, $C_6H_4(COOH)CH_2COOH$, an acid produced from gamboge. **Homopiperidic acid, Homopiperidinic acid.** $NH_2(CH_2)_4COOH$, an amino acid which appears in protein undergoing decomposition. **Humic acid.** One of the many acids which form in soil and humus, and appear subsequently in natural waters. **Humulotannic acid.** $C_{25}H_{24}O_{13}$, a tannin obtained from hops, the strobiles of *Humulus lupulus*. **Hyaluronic acid.** An acid that occurs in the prosthetic group of the mucoproteins which exist in saliva, vitreous humour, the skin and cartilage; it is built of acetylglucosamine units combined with glucuronic acid. **Hydantoic acid.** Glycoluric acid (see above). **Hydnocarpic acid.** Cyclopentenylundecylic acid, $C_5H_7(CH_2)_{10}COOH$, an acid that occurs, with chaulmoogric acid, in the hydnocarpus oil expressed from the seeds of *Hydnocarpus wightiana*; it is used subcutaneously or intramuscularly in the treatment of leprosy. **Hydracrylic acid.** Ethylene lactic acid (see above). **Acid hydrazide.** A compound containing the radical $-CONHNH_2$. **Hydrazoic acid.** Triazoic acid, hydronitric acid, HN_3, an explosive compound which forms salts known as hydrozoates, hydronitrides or azides (lead azide, used as a detonator); an intense protoplasmic poison. **Hydriodic acid.** Hydrogen iodide, HI, a colourless gas, soluble in water (57 per cent solution); used as a reducing agent and reagent. The dilute solution (10 per cent), and the syrup, are used in the treatment of arthritic conditions, tertiary syphilis, aneurysm and exophthalmic goitre. **Hydrobromic acid.** Hydrogen bromide, HBr, a colourless pungent gas, forming a 34.5 per cent solution in water; a reagent in organic synthesis. The 10 per cent solution is used in medicine for its effect on the central nervous system; it allays cerebral excitement, controls epileptic fits and has a sedative action. **Hydrocaffeic acid.** Dihydroxyphenylpropionic acid, $C_6H_3(OH)_2(CH_2)_2COOH$, a derivative of caffeic acid. **Hydrochloric Acid BP 1973.** Hydrogen chloride, HCl, a colourless gas forming a concentrated solution (32 per cent) in water; used as an escharotic. The dilute solution (10 per cent) (BP 1973) is of value in achlorhydria and hypochlorhydria. **Hydrochloroplatinic acid.** H_2PtCl_6; a reddish-brown crystalline substance, soluble in water, and used in platinization. **Hydrocinnamic acid.** $C_6H_5(CH_2)_2COOH$, an acid produced during the decay of albuminous matter; it has been used in the treatment of tuberculosis. **Hydrocoumaric acid, Hydrocumaric acid.** Hydroparacoumaric acid, hydroxyphenylpropionic acid, $OHC_6H_4(CH_2)_2COOH$, an acid that results from the deamination of tyrosine, and appears therefore in the products of the bacterial decomposition of protein. Cf. MELILOTIC ACID (below). **Hydrocyanic acid.** Prussic acid, HCN, a colourless gas, dissolving readily in water (4 per cent solution); it has an almond odour, and occurs free in bitter almonds, in the leaves of the wild cherry and the peach. It is a deadly poison, checking cellular respiration; the dilute solution (2 per cent) (BPC 1954) is used as a gastric sedative and antispasmodic to allay vomiting. It is a fumigant and insecticide. **Hydroferricyanic acid.** $H_3Fe(CN)_6$, a complex iron compound which forms ferricyanides; brown needle-like crystals. **Hydroferrocyanic acid.** $H_4Fe(CN)_6$, a complex iron compound which forms ferrocyanides, and from which the Prussian blues are derived. **Hydrofluoric acid.** Hydrogen fluoride, HF, a highly poisonous gas, readily soluble in water, forming a 40 per cent solution which is used to etch glass. The gas, much diluted with air, has been tried as an inhalant in pulmonary tuberculosis. **Hydrofluosilicic acid.** Fluosilicic acid, H_2SiF_6, an acid that decomposes in water into silicon tetrafluoride and hydrofluoric acid; it forms salts, of which sodium fluosilicate is best known as an insecticide. **Acid hydrogen.** The hydrogen of the -COOH group in organic acids which is replaceable by metals or basic radicals. **Hydronitric acid.** Hydrazoic acid (see above). **Hydroparacoumaric acid.** Hydrocoumaric acid (see above). **Hydroquinone acetic acid.** Homogentisic acid (see above). **Hydroquinone carboxylic acid.** Gentisic acid (see above). **Hydrosulphuric acid.** Hydrogen sulphide, sulphuretted hydrogen, H_2S, a colourless gas with an odour of rotten eggs; it is poisonous. Formed by the action of acids on sulphides, it is found in natural waters; it also occurs as the result of the decomposition of sulphur-containing proteins. The gas has been used as an inhalant in tuberculosis. **Hydroxy acid.** An organic acid containing, in addition to one or more carboxyl, -COOH, groups, one hydroxyl, -OH, group. **Hydroxyacetic acid.** Glycollic acid (see above). **Hydroxyacrylic acid.** Glucic acid (see above). **Hydroxyaminopropionic acid.** Serine, $CH_2(OH)CH(NH_2)COOH$, an amino acid occurring in protein hydrolysates. **Hydroxybarbituric acid.** Dialuric acid (see above). **Hydroxybutyric acid.** An important biological acid which occurs in 3 forms: α-, $CH_3CH_2CHOHCOOH$; β-, $CH_3CHOHCH_2COOH$; γ-, $CH_2OHCH_2CH_2COOH$. The β- form results from abnormal fat metabolism, and can be detected in the blood and urine of diabetics. **Hydroxycapric acid.** Hydroxydecanoic acid (see below). **Hydroxycoumaric acids.** Acids of the formula $C_6H_3(OH)_2(CH_2)COOH$, including caffeic and umbellic acids. **Hydroxydecanoic acid.** Hydroxycapric acid, $CH_3(CH_2)_7CHOHCOOH$, an acid that occurs, esterified, in the compound lipides of the brain. **Hydroxydi-iodophenylpropionic acid.** Iodoalphionic acid (see below). **Hydroxydodecanoic acid.** Sabinenic acid (see below). **Hydroxyethylsulphonic acid.** Isethionic acid (see below). **Hydroxyformobenzoylic acid.** Hydroxymandelic acid, hydroxyphenylglycollic acid, $C_6H_4(OH)CHOHCOOH$, an acid found in the urine in cases of acute atrophy of the liver. **Hydroxyglutamic acid.** $COOHCH_2CHOHCHNH_2COOH$, an acid found in the seeds of cereals. **Hydroxyhexadecanoic acid.** Jalapinolic acid (see below). **Acid hydroxyl.** The hydroxyl of the acid group COOH. **Hydroxylaminopropionic acid.** β-Hydroxy alanine, serine, $OHCH_2CH(NH_2)COOH$, an amino acid which occurs in cephalin. **Hydroxymalonic acid.** Tartronic acid (see below). **Hydroxymandelic acid.** Hydroxyformobenzoylic acid (see above). **Hydroxymethoxybenzoic acid.** Vanillic acid (see below). **Hydroxymethoxycinnamic acid.** Ferulic acid (see above). **Hydroxynaphthoic acid.** $C_{10}H_6(OH)COOH$, colourless crystals, slightly soluble in water, and used as a disinfectant. **Hydroxyoleic acid.** Ricinoleic acid (see below). **Hydroxypalmitic acid.** Juniperic acid (see below). **Hydroxypentacosanic acid.** $C_{24}H_{48}(OH)COOH$, one of the fatty acids yielded by the hydrolysis of the phrenosin of brain substance, and making up the so-called cerebronic acid. **Hydroxyphenylacetic acid.** OH $C_6H_4CH_2COOH$, an isomer of mandelic acid, formed by the decomposition of tyrosine, and appearing in the urine. **Hydroxyphenylcinchoninic acid.** HPC, a drug that has been used with some success in rheumatoid arthritis; its action is somewhat similar to that of ACTH. **Hydroxyphenylglycollic acid.** Hydroxyformobenzoylic acid (see above). **Hydroxyphenylpropionic acid.** Hydrocoumaric acid (see above). **Hydroxypropionic acid.** Lactic acid (see below). **Hydroxystearic acid.** $CH_3(CH_2)_7$ $CHOH(CH_2)_8COOH$, a saturated hydroxy acid derived from castor oil. **Hydroxytetracosanic acid.** $C_{23}H_{46}(OH)COOH$, a fatty acid produced, with hydroxypentacosanic acid, by the hydrolysis of brain substance, and constituting the so-called cerebronic acid. **Hydroxytoluic acid.** Cresotinic acid (see above). **Hydurilic acid.** $C_8H_7N_4O_6$, a derivative of alloxantin. **Hygric acid, Hygrinic acid.** $(CH_2)_3N(CH_3)CHCOOH$, an acid prepared from hygrine, one of the alkaloids present in coca leaves. **Hyodesoxycholic acid.** $C_{23}H_{37}(OH)_2COOH$, a natural acid occurring in pig bile. **Hyoglycocholic acid.** $C_{27}H_{45}O_5N$, an acid present as a sodium salt in hog bile. **Hyotaurocholic acid.** $C_{26}H_{45}O_6NS$, an acid associated with hyoglycocholic acid in hog bile. **Hypobromous acid.** HBrO, an unstable compound, the salts of which, particularly sodium hypobromite, are used to liberate nitrogen in the estimation of urea in the urine. **Hypochlorous acid.** HClO, an acid that readily yields free chlorine, and is valuable therefore as a bleaching agent. The hypochlorites have been for a long time used as disinfectants and antiseptics in surgery. **Hypogaeic acid.** $CH_3(CH_2)_7CH{=}CH$ $(CH_2)_5COOH$, an unsaturated acid of the oleic series, occurring in tallow, and in peanut oil, from *Arachis hypogaea*. **Hyponitrous acid.** HNO, an acid that is useful both as an oxidizing and reducing agent, in organic synthesis. **Hypophosphoric acid.** $H_4P_2O_6$, an acid of pentavalent phosphorus, which gives rise to the hypophosphates. **Hypophosphorous Acid BPC 1973.** H_3PO_2, an acid in which phosphorus is trivalent; it forms hypophosphites which are prescribed as nerve tonics in neurasthenia and anaemia. **Hyposulphuric acid.** Dithionic acid, $H_2S_2O_6$; an acid that forms hyposulphates. **Hyposulphurous acid.** Dithionous acid, $H_2S_2O_4$; an acid that forms hyposulphites, not to be confused with photographers' "hypo", which is sodium thiosulphate, $Na_2S_2O_3$. **Hypoxanthylic acid.** Inosinic acid (see below). **Ichthulinic acid.** An acid that exists in the glycoprotein of fish eggs, ichthulin. **Ichthyolsulphonic acid.** $C_{28}H_{38}O_6S_3$, an acid obtained as an ammonium salt, ichthammol, by the distillation of bituminous shale; it is used as an intestinal antiseptic, and externally in skin diseases. **Idonic acid.** $CH_2OH(CHOH)_3$ $C(OH)_2COOH$, an oxidation product of the hexose idose, also obtained by the reduction of ascorbic acid. **Igasuric acid.** An acid that occurs in nux vomica, the seeds of *Strychnos nuxvomica*, also in Ignatius beans, *Strychnos ignatii*. **Iminazoleacrylic acid.** Urocanic acid (see below). **Imino acid.** An organic acid containing in its structure the imino group =NH. Such acids occur in the deamination of amino acids in the metabolism; 2, proline and hydroxyproline, appear among the products of protein hydrolysis. **Indigodisulphonic acid.** $C_{16}H_8N_2O_2(SO_3H_2)$, a soluble form of indigo obtained by treating it with fuming sulphuric acid; the sodium salt, known as indigo carmine, is injected intravenously in the cytoscopic examination for kidney function. **Indole-acetic acid.** Hetero-auxin, indolyl β-acetic acid, $C_6H_4C(NHCH)(CH_2)_2COOH$, an acid that occurs during the bacterial decomposition of tryptophane. **Indole pyruvic acid.** $C_8H_6NCH_2COCOOH$, an oxidation product of tryptophane which is assumed to occur as an intermediate compound in tryptophane metabolism. Its production from tryptophane has been shown to be reversible since it can replace tryptophane as an essential amino acid in the diet. **Indolylacetic acid.** Indole-acetic acid (see above). **Indoxylic acid.** $C_6H_4(COH)NHCCOOH$, an acid derived from indoxyl; can be oxidized to indigo. **Indoxylsulphonic acid, Indoxylsulphuric acid.** $C_6H_4(NHCH)CO$ SO_3H, an acid that arises from the bacterial decomposition of tryptophane in the intestine, and appears as an ethereal sulphate of potassium, urinary indican, in the urine. **Inorganic acid.** An acid, usually mineral, composed of hydrogen combined with elements other than carbon. **Inosinic acid.** A nucleoside monophosphate composed of the purine hypoxanthine linked to ribose with a phosphate group at the 5′-position; it is formed by deamination of AMP by adenylate deaminase. **Inositol phosphoric acid.** Phytic acid, $C_6H_6[OPO(OH)_2]_6$, an acid that occurs, combined with Mg and Ca, in the outer coat of cereals; it is of no value in nutrition, and the existence of free phytic acid in the diet may even reduce seriously the Ca available for the metabolism. Cf. INOSITOL. **Inulic acid.** Alantic acid (see above). **Iobenzamic Acid.** BP Commission approved name for *N*-(3 - amino - 2,4,6 - tri - iodobenzoyl) - *N* - phenyl - β - alanine; a diagnostic aid. **Iocarmic Acid.** BP Commission approved name for 5,5′-(adipoyldiamino)bis - (2,4,6 - tri - iodo - *N* - methylisophthalamic acid); a radio-opaque substance. **Iocetamic Acid.** BP Commission approved name for 3 - (*N* - 3 - amino - 2,4,6 - tri - iodophenyl) - acetamido - 2 - methylpropionic acid; a contrast medium. **Iodic acid.** HIO_3, white crystals, very soluble in water; used as a deodorant and antiputrefactive, also, internally, as an antiseptic. The sodium salt has been injected in articular rheumatism. **Iodoalphionic acid.** 3-(4-hydroxy-3,5-di-iodo)-phenylpropionic acid, $C_6H_2I_2(OH)CH_2CH(C_6H_5)COOH$, Pheniodol BP 1958. A contrast medium used in cholecystography. **Iodogorgoic acid.** Di-iodotyrosine, $C_6H_2I_2(OH)CH_2$ $(CHNH_2)COOH$, an acid that has been found only in the protein of sponges and corals; it is closely related to thyroxine, the amino acid of the thyroid. **Iodohydroxyquinolinesulphonic acid.** Iodoxyquinolinesulphonic acid (see below). **Iodophenylarsonic acid.** $C_6H_4IAsO(OH)_2$, a substance closely resembling arsanilic acid, and used similarly as a spirochaeticide. **Iodosalicylic acid.** $C_6H_3I(OH)COOH$, an antipyretic and analgesic compound, and the parent of important antiseptics for internal and external use. **Iodosobenzoic acid.** $C_6H_4(IO)COOH$, used as an antiseptic in surgery. **Iodoxamic Acid.** BP Commission approved name for *N,N′*-(1,16-dioxo - 4,7,10,13 - tetraoxahexadecane - 1,16 - diyl)di - (3 - amino - 2,4,6 - tri - iodobenzoic acid; a contrast medium. **Iodoxybenzoic acid.** $C_6H_4(IO_2)COOH$, in which iodine has the higher valency; used in arthritic conditions. **Iodoxyquinolinesulphonic acid.** $C_9H_4INOHSO_3H$, a compound, the sodium salt of which constitutes Chiniofon Sodium BP 1958, a pale yellow powder which dissolves in water with effervescence to give a deep orange solution. It is used as an amoebacide, preferably in the form of enteric-coated tablets, but also in solution. It may be administered rectally in solution. **Ioglycamic Acid.** BP Commission approved name for α,α′-oxydi-(3-acetamido-2,4,6-tri-iodobenzoic acid; a radio-opaque substance. **Acid ion.** An electronegative atom or radical produced by the dissociation of an acid in solution. **Iopanoic Acid BP 1973.** β-(3-amino-2,4,6-tri-iodophenyl)-α-ethylpropionic acid, $C_6HI(NH_2)CH_2CH(C_2H_5)COOH$; a contrast medium used in the x-ray examination of the biliary tract. **Iothalamic Acid BP**

1973. 5-Acetamido-2,4,6-tri-iodo-*N*-methylisophthalamic acid, a contrast medium used in diagnostic radiology in the form of its meglumine and sodium salts. **Iridic acid.** $C_{16}H_{12}O_5$, an acid that occurs as a glucoside, iridin, in orris root, *Iris florentina*; it has the properties of a cholagogue. **Isanic acid.** $C_{13}H_{19}COOH$, a fatty acid with a purgative action, derived from oil of tsana. **Isatic acid, Isatinic acid.** Aminophenylglyoxylic acid, aminobenzoylformic acid, $C_6H_4(NH_2)COCOOH$, an acid that yields isatin on heating. **Isethionic acid.** $CH_2(OH)CH_2SO_3H$, hydroxyethylsulphonic acid; an acid, the amino derivative of which, taurine, occurs in bile. **Iso-amylethylbarbituric acid.** $C_5H_{11}(C_2H_5)C(CONH)_2CO$, white crystals, insoluble in water, soluble in alcohol or ether; a valuable hypnotic, "Amytal", which is not excreted unchanged in the urine. The sodium salt is very soluble, and is used for basal narcosis. **Iso-anemonic acid.** An acid derived from species of *Anemone*; it is an alterative and depressant, and is useful in treating inflammation, **Isobarbituric acid.** Hydroxy uracil, CO(NHCO)(NHCH)COH, a derivative of urea, and isomeric with barbituric acid. **Isobilianic acid.** $C_{24}H_{34}O_8$, a cholane substance, and an isomer of bilianic acid; both are produced by rupture of the sterol ring when the bile acid, dehydrocholic acid, is oxidized, **Isobutylamino-acetic acid.** Leucine, $(CH_3)_2CHCH_2CH(NH_2)COOH$, an amino acid found in maize, and considered essential for animal growth. **Isobutylcarbonic acid, Isobutylcarboxylic acid.** Isovaleric acid (see below). **Isobutyric acid.** Dimethylacetic acid, $(CH_3)_2CHCOOH$, an acid occurring free in carob beans, *Ceratonia siligua*, and arnica root; it may appear in the urine as the result of protein breakdown. **Isocitric acid.** $HOOCCH_2CH(COOH)CHOHCOOH$, an isomer of citric acid occurring in the citric acid cycle of the metabolism. It is formed from aconitic acid, and is in turn converted into α-ketoglutaric acid. **Isocyanic acid.** HN=CO, an acid which occurs as a tautomeric isomer with cyanic acid; it gives rise to the isocyanates. **Isodialuric acid.** CO(NHCO)(NHCOH)COH, a derivative of barbituric acid, and an isomer of tartronyl urea. **Iso-erucic acid.** Brassidic acid (see above). **Isonicotinic acid.** 3-Pyridinecarboxylic acid, pyridine α-carboxylic acid, $C_5H_4N(COOH)$; an isomer of nicotinic acid. **Isonitrosobarbituric acid.** Violuric acid (see below). **Isopentoic acid.** Isovaleric acid (see below). **Isopropylacetic acid.** Isovaleric acid (see below). **Isopropylamino-acetic acid.** Amino-isovaleric acid, valine, $(CH_3)_2CHCHNH_2COOH$, an α-amino acid existing in the protein of seeds, and regarded as essential to nutrition. **Isopropylbenzoic acid.** Cumic acid (see above). **Isosaccharic acid.** $COOH(CHOH)_4COOH$, one of the stereo-isomers of saccharic and mucic acids, prepared from glucosamine by oxidation. **Isosulphocyanic acid.** Isothiocyanic acid (see following). **Isothiocyanic acid.** Sulphocarbimide, S=C=NH, an acid that forms stable esters, the mustard oils, the most important of which is allyl isothiocyanate, derived from mustard seed, *Sinapis nigra*. **Iso-uracylcarboxylic acid.** Orotic acid (see below). **Iso-uric acid.** $CNCH(CONH)_3$, an acid prepared from alloxantin. **Isovaleric acid.** $(CH_3)_2CHCH_2COOH$, the common, optically-inactive valeric acid, found in valerian and angelica; it also occurs in decomposed cheese and the perspiration of the feet, and in the urine in certain diseases. It is used in hysteria as a sedative, and in neurotic states. **Itaconic acid.** $CH_2C(COOH)CH_2COOH$, an acid produced by the fungus *Aspergillus terreus* (*itaconicus*).

Jalapinolic acid. Hydroxyhexadecanoic acid, $CH_3(CH_2)_3CHOH(CH_2)_{10}COOH$, an acid occurring as a glycoside in orizaba jalap root (*Ipomoea*). **Japonic acid.** A tannin occurring in catechu. **Jecoleic acid.** $C_{18}H_{35}COOH$, an acid occurring as the glyceride in cod-liver oil; it is an isomer of doeglic acid. **Jenkolic acid.** Djenkolic acid (see above). **Jervic acid.** An acid of uncertain constitution, which is obtained from white hellebore, *Veratrum album*. **Juglandic acid.** An acid prepared from the bark of the butternut, *Juglans cinerea*; it is a cathartic, hepatic stimulant and antispasmodic. **Juniperic acid.** Dihydroambrettolic acid, hydroxypalmitic acid, $C_{15}H_{30}(OH)COOH$, an acid found in oil of savin, from *Juniperus sabina*.

Kephalophosphoric acid. An acid formed by the breaking-up of the complex molecule of the brain phospholipide, cephalin. **Kermesic acid, Kermic acid.** An acid occurring in the red dye extracted from kermes, the dried insect, *Coccus ilicis*. **Keto acid.** An organic acid having in its structure both the carboxyl group, -COOH, and the divalent ketone group, =CO. **Ketocholanic acid.** An acid obtained by the oxidation of the saturated bile compound, cholanic acid. **Ketoglutaric acid.** $COOHCOCH_2CH_2COOH$, an intermediate compound formed in the citric acid cycle. **Ketomethoxymethylenehexenoic acid.** Penicillic acid (see below). **Ketostearic acid.** $CH_3(CH_2)_{11}CO(CH_2)_4COOH$, an acid that occurs in mushrooms; the γ-form, $CH_3(CH_2)_{13}CO(CH_2)_2COOH$, is obtained by hydrogenation of the seed-fat of *Licania rigida*. **Kinic acid.** Quinic acid (see below). **Kinotannic acid.** The astringent tannin which is found in Malabar kino, the dried juice of *Pterocarpus marsupium*; it forms kino red on decomposition. **Kojic acid.** Hydroxy-hydroxymethyl pyrone, CO=(COHCH)[CH=C(CH_2OH)]=O, a cyclic compound, closely related to ascorbic acid; it is produced by a species of the mould *Aspergillus* in mono- and polysaccharides, and is highly toxic. **Kombic acid.** An acid that occurs as a glucoside in *Strophanthus kombé*; it is a diuretic and cardiac stimulant. **Krameric acid.** Rhatanytannic acid, the tannin in the root of *Krameria*; an astringent and tonic. **Kynurenic acid.** Cynurenic acid, $C_9H_6ONCOOH$, a decomposition product of tryptophane, which appears in the urine of dogs.

Laccaic acid, Laccainic acid, Laccic acid. $C_{16}H_{12}O_8$, the red colouring matter in lac, the secretion of the insect, *Laccifer lacca*. **Lactamic acid.** Alanine; aminopropionic acid (see above). **Lactic acid.** $CH_3CHOHCOOH$; L-lactic acid formed from pyruvate by the action of lactate dehydrogenase present in all tissues, an important end-product of muscle glycolysis and an intermediate of the Cori cycle. **Lactic acid series.** A family of monobasic hydroxy-saturated acids of the general formula, $C_nH_{2n}(OH)COOH$; glycollic and lactic acids are the most important representatives of the series. **Lactolactic acid.** Dilactic acid, $CH_3CH(OH)COOCH(CH_3)COOH$, the anhydride of lactic acid. **Lactonic acid.** One of the so-called saccharinic acids, resulting from the bacterial oxidation of the aldehyde group in the hexoses; they are crystallizable, and have the formula, $CH_2OH(CHOH)_4COOH$; examples are gluconic and galactonic acids. **Lactucic acid.** An acid found in the juice of lettuce opium, *Lactuca virosa*; it is a mild sedative, and is useful for troublesome coughs. **Laevotartaric acid.** $(CHOHCOOH)_2$, a form of tartaric acid, identical with ordinary tartaric acid except that it rotates in a counter-clockwise direction the plane of a beam of polarized light passed through its solution. **Laevulic acid, Laevulinic acid.** Acetylpropionic acid, $CH_3COCH_2CH_2COOH$, an acid formed from cane sugar, laevulose, gum and starch, by the action of strong acids; it has also been found in the products of the breakdown of the nucleic acid of the thymus. **Lanoceric acid.** $CH_2(CH_2)_{26}(CHOH)_2COOH$, a saturated dihydroxy fatty acid, which, combined with higher unsaturated alcohols, occurs in crude lanolin. **Lanopalmitic acid.** $CH_3(CH_2)_{13}(CHOH)COOH$, a saturated monohydroxy acid obtained from crude lanolin. **Laricic acid.** Larixin, $C_{10}H_{10}O_5$, a principle extracted from the bark of the larch, *Larix europaea*; used as an expectorant. **Laricinolic acid.** $C_{20}H_{30}O_2$, a resinous acid obtained from the turpentine of the larch. **Larinolic acid.** $C_{18}H_{26}O_2$, the chief resin acid to be found in larch turpentine. **Larixinic acid.** Laricic acid (see above). **Lauric acid, Laurostearic acid.** $C_{11}H_{23}COOH$, a saturated fatty acid contained in oil of laurels, *Laurus nobilis*, and palm kernels; also in spermaceti. **Lecanoric acid.** $C_{16}H_{14}O_7$, a lichen acid occurring in certain species of *Roccella*, which, on hydrolysis, gives orcin. **Leucamic acid.** Leucine, amino-isocaproic acid, $(CH_3)_2CHCH_2CHNH_2COOH$, an acid that occurs in maize, and is essential for life in higher animals. **Leuconic acid.** $(CO)_5$, a pentaketocyclopentane, obtained by the strong oxidation of crocic acid. **Licanic acid.** $C_{18}H_{28}O_3$, an unsaturated ketonic acid, obtained from *Licania rigida*. **Lignoceric acid.** Tetracosanic acid, $C_{23}H_{47}COOH$, a saturated acid found in the oil of *Adenanthera pavonina*. It is the fatty acid which, combined with sphingosine and galactose, makes up the cerebroside, cerasine. **Lignulmic acid.** $C_{54}H_{28}O_6$, a dark-brown substance found in elm trees. **Linoleic acid.** Linolic acid, $CH_3(CH_2)_4(CH=CHCH_2)_2(CH_2)_6COOH$, an unsaturated fatty acid which is present as a glyceride in the drying oils, linseed, hemp and poppy; also in cod-liver oil. **Linoleic acid series.** A family of unsaturated fatty acids, with 2 double bonds and the general formula, $C_nH_{2n-4}O_2$; it includes linoleic and palmitolic acids. **Linolenic acid.** $CH_3(CH_2CH=CH)_3(CH_2)_7COOH$, an unsaturated fatty acid with 3 double bonds, occurring, as a glyceride, in linseed oil, from *Linum usitatissimum.* **Linolenic acid series.** A family of unsaturated fatty acids, with 3 double bonds and the general formula, $C_nH_{2n-6}O_2$; linolenic and elaeostearic acids are in this family. **Linolic acid.** Linoleic acid (see above). **Lithic acid.** Uric acid (see below). **Lithocholic acid.** $C_{23}H_{38}(OH)COOH$, an acid that occurs in the bile acids of ox and man. **Lithofellic acid.** $C_{20}H_{36}O_4$, insoluble crystals which occur in the calculi of cattle. **Lupamaric acid.** A bitter principle in the lupulin of hops, *Humulus lupulus.* **Luteic acid.** A polysaccharidic acid, resulting from the oxidative changes brought about in a sugar medium by *Penicillium luteum.* **Lymphokentric acid.** A specific substance said to be excreted in urine, excess of which in the body is supposed to cause acute lymphatic leukaemia. **Lysalbic acid.** An acid produced by the effect of caustic alkalis on albumin. **Lysergic acid.** $C_{16}H_{16}N_2O_2$, a monobasic acid in the ergot of rye, where it is combined to form both inert and active alkaloids. **Lysuric acid.** $C_6H_5CONHCH(COOH)(CH_2)_4NHCOC_6H_5$, a derivative of lysine, the amino acid of many proteins. **Lyxonic acid.** $CH_2OH(CHOH)_3COOH$, a tetrahydroxyvaleric acid, produced by the oxidation of lyxose, a pentose isomeric with arabinose.

Acid magenta. Acid fuchsine, a mixture of pararosaniline di- and tri- sulphonic acids, used as a harmless food-dye and also as an indicator. **Maizenic acid.** An acid that occurs in maize, *Zea mays.* **Maleic Acid BP 1973.** Ethylenedicarboxylic acid, $(CHCOOH)_2$, an olefine acid formed by the dehydration of malic acid; a stereo-isomer of fumaric acid. **Malic acid.** $COOHCH_2CHOHCOOH$, an alcohol acid, occurring widely in sour apples, rhubarb, unripe berries of the mountain-ash, grapes and quinces; it is used as a spray in throat affections. It exists in 2 optically-active forms, and a racemic form. **Malonic acid.** Methane dicarboxylic acid, $COOHCH_2COOH$, one of the saturated oxalic acid series; occurs, as a calcium salt, in beetroot. **Mandelic Acid BPC 1959.** Amygdalic acid, benzoglycollic acid, phenylglycollic acid, $C_6H_5CH(OH)COOH$, an acid obtained by the hydrolysis of the glucoside, amygdalin; it is used in the treatment of infecting organisms in the urine, and in gastro-intestinal affections. The mydriatic homatropine is an ester with tropine. **Manganic acid.** H_2MnO_4, an acid that does not exist free, but as salts, the manganates: not to be confused with permanganates. **Mannitic acid.** $CH_2OH(CHOH)_4COOH$, an acid that has been prepared by the careful oxidation of the hexahydric alcohol, mannitol. **Mannonic acid.** $CH_2OH(CHOH)_4COOH$, one of the 2 isomeric saccharinic acids produced by the oxidation of mannose; a stereo-isomer of gluconic acid. **Mannosaccharic acid.** $COOH(CHOH)_4COOH$, an acid that results from the further oxidation of mannose; a stereo-isomer of saccharic acid. **Mannuronic acid.** $CHO(CHOH)_4COOH$, a uronic acid formed by the oxidation of the terminal alcohol group of mannose with the aldehyde group protected; it is found in certain seaweeds associated with polysaccharides. **Margaric acid.** Originally applied to the mixture of palmitic and stearic acids obtained by the hydrolysis of animal fats, it is, in fact, $CH_3(CH_2)_{15}COOH$, a saturated fatty acid found among the lichen acids. **Margosic acid.** $C_{22}H_{40}O_2$, an unsaturated fatty acid obtained from the oil of Indian lilac, *Azadirachta indica*; it is used as a bitter. **Marine acid.** Hydrochloric acid (see above). **Meclofenamic Acid.** BP Commission approved name for *N*-(2,6-dichloro-*m*-tolyl)anthranilic acid; an anti-inflammatory agent. **Meconic acid.** Oxypyronedicarboxylic acid, $C_5HO_2(OH)=(COOH)_2$, the acid with which the opium alkaloids are combined in nature. **Medullic acid.** $C_{21}H_{41}COOH$, an unsaturated fatty acid occurring in bone marrow. **Mefenamic Acid BP 1973.** *N*-2,3-Xylylanthranilic acid; an analgesic, anti-inflammatory and antipyretic agent chemically unrelated to morphine, given to relieve pain of mild or moderate severity. Low toxicity is claimed with recommended doses, but rashes, diarrhoea and blood dyscrasias have been reported. **Melanogallic acid.** Gallhumic acid, $C_6H_4O_2$, an amorphous substance produced, with pyrogallol, by heating gallic acid. **Melassic acid.** An insoluble compound resulting from the action of caustic alkalis on cane sugar. **Melilotic acid.** $C_6H_4(OH)(CH_2)_2COOH$, an acid found naturally in sweet yellow clover, *Melilotus officinalis.* **Melissic acid.** $CH_3(CH_2)_{28}COOH$, a saturated fatty acid which, combined with palmitic and stearic acids, is to be found in beeswax. **Mellitic acid.** Benzenehexacarboxylic acid, $C_6(COOH)_6$, an acid that occurs as an aluminium salt in peat, and is obtained by the oxidation of lignite and graphite. **Mercapturic acid.** A sulphur-containing acid in the urine as the result of detoxication by cystine or cysteine; bromobenzene, administered to dogs, appears subsequently as bromphenylmercapturic acid. **Mersalyl Acid BP 1973.** $C_{13}H_{17}O_6NHg$, a white, odourless powder, slightly soluble in water, readily soluble in a solution of sodium hydroxide; a diuretic. **Mesitic acid.** Uvitic acid (see below). **Mesitonic acid.** Dimethyl-laevulinic acid, $CH_3CO(CHCH_3)_2COOH$, a ketonic acid, homologous with laevulinic acid. **Mesitylenic acid.** Dimethylbenzoic acid, $C_6H_3(CH_3)_2COOH$, an acid isomeric with the phenylpropionic acids; it is prepared from mesitylene. **Mesityluric acid.** $C_6H_3(CH_3)_2CONHCH_2COOH$, a combination of mesitylene and glycine; it is observed during certain urinary experiments. **Mesotartaric acid.** Inactive tartaric acid, $COOH(CHOH)_2COOH$; unlike racemic acid, this acid cannot be resolved into optically-active constituents, as the active groups within the molecule have neutralized one another. **Mesoxalic acid.** Dihydroxymalonic acid, $C(OH)_2(COOH)_2$, a dibasic ketonic acid which is prepared by the hydrolysis of alloxan; it decomposes on heating into glyoxylic acid. **Meta acid.** 1. An inorganic acid of a trivalent non-metal, like boron or phosphorus, which has only 1 replaceable hydrogen to offer. 2. An organic aromatic acid with its carboxyl radical in the *meta* position in the benzene ring relative to another radical. **Meta-arsenic acid.** $HAsO_3$, a white substance which forms salts, the meta-arsenates, but is itself converted into ortho-arsenic acid in solution. **Metaphosphoric acid.** HPO_3, an acid that precipitates albumin from urine and is used in the analysis of the latter. **Metasaccharic acid.** $COOH(CHOH)_4COOH$, a dibasic acid isomeric with mannosaccharic acid and produced by the oxidation of mannitol. **Metastannic acid.** H_2SnO_3, an acid derived from stannic oxide, SnO_2, and forming metastannates of varying constitution. **Metavanadic acid.** HVO_3, an acid that exists only as metavanadates, which are used as reagents. **Methane-arsenic acid.** Methylarsenic acid (see below). **Methanedicarboxylic acid.** Malonic acid (see above). **Methanedisulphonic acid.** Methionic acid (see below). **Methanoic acid.** Formic acid (see above). **Methionic acid.** Methanedisulphonic acid, $CH_2(SO_3H)_2$, an acid that is of importance in organic synthesis. **Methoxyquinolinecarboxylic acid.** Quininic acid (see below). **Methylamino-acetic acid.** Methylglycine, sarcosine, CH_3NHCH_2COOH, an amino acid which results from the hydrolysis of creatine. **Methylarsenic acid.** Methane-arsenic acid, $CH_3AsO(OH)_2$, a primary arsenic compound, related to cacodylic acid. **Methylbenzoic acid.** Toluic acid (see below). **Methylcaffeic acid.** Ferulic acid (see above). **Methylcrotonic acid.** Tiglic acid (see below). **Methylenecitrylsalicylic acid.** $C_3H_2O_3(CH_2COOC_6H_4COOH)_2$, a white powder, insoluble in water, soluble in alcohol; it is an antirheumatic and antiseptic. **Methylenedioxyphenylpentadienoic acid.** Piperic acid (see below). **Methylenehippuric acid.** A derivative of hippuric acid which decomposes into formaldehyde, and is employed therefore as an antiseptic. **Methylethylacetic acid.** $(C_2H_5)(CH_3)CHCOOH$, the isomer of valeric acid which is optically active. **Methylguanidine-acetic acid, Methylguanido-acetic acid.** Guanidine methyl glycine, creatine. $NH_2CN(NH)(CH_3)CH_2COOH$, an amino acid metabolite which occurs as phosphagen in muscle tissue and is involved in the cycle of muscle contraction; it is normally excreted as creatinine, but itself appears in the urine of pregnant women and of childen (creatinuria). **Methylhydantoic acid.** $NH_2CON(CH_3)CH_2COOH$, an acid formed by the hydrolysis of creatinine. **Methylhydroxybenzoic acid.** Cresotic acid (see above). **Methylisophthalic acid.** Xylidic acid (see below). **Methylmaleic acid.** Citraconic acid (see above). **Methylphenylquinolinecarboxylic acid.** $C_6H_5C_9H_4CH_3NCOOH$, a methyl derivative of cinchophen, and used similarly as an analgesic antipyretic, and in the treatment of gout, lumbago and sciatica. **Methylprotocatechuic acid.** Vanillic acid (see below). **Methylstearic acid.** Tuberculostearic acid (see below). **Methylsuccinic acid.** Pyrotartaric acid (see below). **Methyltoluic acid.** Xylic acid (see below). **Methyltrihydroxyglutaric acid.** Saccharonic acid (see below). **Mineral acid.** An inorganic acid, particularly those acids used as reagents. **Molybdic acid.** H_2MoO_4, an acid, the ammonium salt of which, ammonium molybdate, is an important reagent in testing for phosphates. **Monatomic acid.** Monobasic acid (see below). **Mono-amino acid.** An organic acid containing one $-NH_2$ group only. **Mono-aminodicarboxylic acid.** An organic dibasic acid, possessing two carboxyl, -COOH, groups, and an amino, $-NH_2$, group, usually attached to the carbon atom next to one of the carboxyls. **Mono-aminomonocarboxylic acid.** An organic monobasic acid, possessing one carboxyl, -COOH, group, and one amino, $-NH_2$, group, both attached, in the case of the amino acids which occur in nature, to the same carbon atom. **Monobasic acid.** An acid which offers only 1 hydrogen atom for replacement by a metal or by a basic radical. **Monobromacetic acid.** Bromacetic acid, $CH_2BrCOOH$, colourless crystals, soluble in water; it has an escharotic action. **Monochloracetic acid.** Chloracetic acid, $CH_2ClCOOH$, colourless crystals, soluble in water, and used to remove corns and warts. **Mono-iodomethanesulphonic acid.** CH_2ISO_3H, an acid, the sodium salt of which, sodium mono-iodomethane sulphonate, is used intravenously in pyelography. **Mono-iodosalicylic acid.** $C_6H_3I(OH)COOH$, an acid that has been used in the treatment of rheumatic arthritis. **Mononitrosalicylic acid.** $C_6H_3(OH)(NO_2)COOH$, an acid obtained by the nitration of indigo. **Moritannic acid.** $C_{13}H_{19}O_6$, the tannin of fustic wood, *Morus tinctoria*, used in dyeing wool. **Morphoxylacetic acid.** $C_{17}H_{16}(NO_3)CH_2COOH$, a derivative of morphine, and a useful narcotic, much less toxic than the parent alkaloid. **Morrhuic acid.** $C_9H_{13}O_3N$, an acid occurring to a small extent in cod-liver oil; it has been used in the treatment of varicose veins. **Mucic acid.** $COOH(CHOH)_4COOH$, one of the stereo-isomeric acids of this formula; it is formed by the oxidation of gums, mucilages and milk sugar. It is optically inactive, and readily changes into furane compounds. **Mucoitinsulphuric acid.** The prosthetic group of the nucleoprotein that is found in saliva, the vitreous humour, mucous membrane and cartilage. It is composed of 2 acetylated glucosamine units and two glucuronic acid units, combined with sulphuric acid. **Muconic acid.** Butadiene carboxylic acid, $COOH(CH)_4COOH$, an acid excreted in dogs' urine if benzene is administered. **Muscle adenosine phosphoric acid, Muscle adenylic acid.** *See* ADENYLIC ACID (above). **Myelokentric acid.** A specific substance said to be excreted in the urine, excess of which in the body is supposed to cause acute myeloblastic leukaemia. **Mycotonic acid.** A poisonous narcotic substance from the extract of *Palicourea marcgraphii.* **Myristic acid.** Tetradecanoic acid, $CH_3(CH_2)_{12}COOH$, a saturated fatty acid occurring in spermaceti, oil of iris, nutmeg butter (*Myristica fragrans*), myrtle wax and human subcutaneous fat. **Myronic acid.** $C_{10}H_{17}O_9NS_2$, an acid that occurs as a glucoside in sinigrin, from black mustard, *Brassica nigra*, and horseradish, *Cochlearia armoracia*; it is hydrolysed by the enzyme myrosin into allyl isothiocyanate, mustard oil.

Nalidixic Acid. BP Commission approved name for 1-ethyl-7-methyl-4-oxo-1,8-naphthyridine-3-carboxylic acid; an antibacterial agent. **Naphthalene carboxylic acid.** Naphthoic acid (see below). **Naphthalene dicarboxylic acid, Naphthalic acid.** $C_{10}H_6(COOH)_2$, one of the isomers of importance in organic synthesis. **Naphthalinsulphonic acid.** Naphtholsulphonic acid (see below). **Naphthionic acid.** Naphthylaminemonosulphonic acid, $NH_2C_{10}H_6SO_3H$, an acid obtained by the sulphonation of α-naphthylamine; it is used in the manufacture of dyestuffs, also in the treatment of urinary affections. **Naphthoic acid.** Naphthalene carboxylic acid, $C_{10}H_7COOH$, an acid occurring in 2 isomeric forms, of importance in organic synthesis. **Naphtholcarboxylic acid.** $C_{10}H_6OHCOOH$, an acid used as an antiseptic, also as an anthelmintic. **Naphtholdisulphonic acid.** $C_{10}H_5(OH)(SO_3H)_2$, one of a number of isomeric-named acids used in the manufacture of dyestuffs and synthetic drugs. **Naphtholsulphonic acid.** $C_{10}H_6(OH)(SO_3H)$, one of a number of isomeric-named monosulphonic acids used as dyestuffs intermediates, and in the preparation of synthetic drugs; calcium β-naphthol sulphonate is a sensitive reagent for albumin in acid solutions. **Naphthylaminemonosulphonic acid, Naphthylaminosulphonic acid.** Naphthionic acid (see above). **Naphthylmercapturic acid.** The particular mercapturic acid which is produced in the urine by the administration of naphthalene. **Nervonic acid.** Selacholeic acid, $CH_3(CH_2)_7CH{=}CH(CH_2)_{13}COOH$, an unsaturated fatty acid found in fish-liver oils, and, in combination with sphinosine and galactose, in the cerebroside, nervone, of brain tissue. **Neuraminic acid.** Sialic acid, $CH_2OH(CHOH)_3CHNH_2CHOHCH_2COCOOH$; an important constituent of mucopolysaccharides, gangliosides and blood group substances. Its synthesis involves the precursors *N*-acetylglucosamine 6-phosphate and phosphoenolpyruvate. **Neurostearic acid.** Phrenosinic acid, $CH_3(CH_2)_{21}CHOHCOOH$, an acid that occurs in brain substance; it is combined with sphingosine and galactose to form the cerebroside, phrenosin. **Nicotinic Acid BP 1973.** Pyridine β-carboxylic acid, β-carboxypyridine, niacin, C_5H_4NCOOH, the pellagra-preventing (P-P) factor. It occurs in milk, meat, wheat, liver, kidney, yeast and bread; lack of it in the diet leads to the food-deficiency disease, pellagra. Its amide is a vitamin substance in the vitamin B_2 complex. It is involved in the maintenance of the integrity of the alimentary mucosa. **Nitric acid.** Azotic acid, aqua fortis, HNO_3, a colourless fuming liquid, used as a caustic, escharotic and cauterizing agent, when concentrated (BP 1953) (68 per cent). The dilute acid (10 per cent solution) is an astringent, tonic and bile stimulant. *Fuming nitric acid* consists of the concentrated acid with oxides of nitrogen in solution; it is a strong caustic. Aqua regia, 1 part HNO_3 to 4 parts HCl, is a solvent for gold. **Nitro acid.** An organic acid containing both carboxyl, -COOH, and nitro, $-NO_2$, radicals. **Nitroferricyanic acid.** $H_2Fe(NO)(CN)_6$, an acid used as the sodium salt, sodium nitroprusside, to detect metaproteins, and other compounds containing the thiol group, -SH; it also reacts with aceto-acetic acid and acetone in ketonuric urine. **Nitrohydrochloric acid, Nitromuriatic acid.** Aqua regia, a mixture of 1 part concentrated nitric acid and 4 parts concentrated hydrochloric acid, which dissolves gold; diluted, it has been administered for liver disorder. **Nitroprussic acid, Nitrosoferricyanic acid.** Nitroferricyanic acid (see above). **Nitrosonitric acid.** Fuming nitric acid, a solution of the oxides of nitrogen in concentrated nitric acid. **Nitrospiroylic acid.** Mononitrosalicylic acid (see above). **Nitrous acid.** HNO_2, an unstable acid derived from nitrogen trioxide, N_2O_3, and forming nitrites, which have a vasodilator action. **Nonanoic acid.** Pelargonic acid (see below). **Nordhausen acid.** Name given to the fuming acid formed by dissolving sulphur trioxide in concentrated sulphuric acid; it is of great importance in the manufacture of drugs and dyestuffs. **Normal acid.** 1. Normal fatty acid (see following). 2. Ortho acid (see below). 3. A solution containing the gram-equivalent weight of an acid in a litre of distilled water. Designated N/1, solutions containing other proportions are expressed as fractions of N; they are used to titrate against solutions whose alkali content is to be ascertained volumetrically. **Normal fatty acid.** A fatty acid whose chain of carbon atoms in its molecule is straight and unforked. **Norpinic acid.** Dimethylcyclobutane dicarboxylic acid, $COOHCH{=}(CH_2)C(CH_3)_2{=}CHCOOH$, a derivative of the hydrocarbon pinene from oil of turpentine. **Nucleic acid.** One of the acids which occur, combined with proteins, as nucleoproteins in cell nuclei and protoplasm. They are built of the molecules of 2 purines and 2 pyrimidines, together with 4 molecules of a pentose combined with 4 molecules of phosphoric acid; though the arrangement of these units in chains gives rise to great variety, it seems likely that there may be only 2 distinct types of nucleic acid: (*a*) thymonucleic acid found in thymus, spleen and other glandular tissue, and composed of cytosine, thymine, adenine, guanine and the sugar deoxyribose, combined with phosphoric acid: (*b*) yeast-nucleic acid (pentose nucleic acid, PNA), found in yeast, wheat germ and similar sources, and made up of cytosine, uracyl, adenine, guanine and ribose with phosphoric acid. Hydrolysis of the nucleic acids yields nucleotides, which are themselves phosphoric esters of nucleoside units. **Nucleic acid, genetic.** The class of nucleic acid which is the hereditary material; in eukaryotes and prokaryotes this is DNA, in viruses and bacteriophages it is RNA or DNA. **Nucleothymic acid, Nucleothyminic acid, Nucleotinphosphoric acid.** Thymonucleic acid (*see* NUCLEIC ACID, above), an acid that is prepared from calf pancreas; a yellowish-brown powder, soluble in water, it dissolves uric acid, and is of value in the treatment of gout. **Acid number.** *See* NUMBER.

Octadecenic acid. Petroselinic acid (see below). **Octadecynoic acid.** Stearolic acid (see below). **Octanedicarboxylic acid.** Sebacic acid (see below). **Octanedioic acid.** Suberic acid (see below). **Octanoic acid.** Caprylic acid (see above). **Octodecylic acid.** Stearic acid (see below). **Octoic Acid BPC 1954.** Caprylic acid (see above). **Oenanthylic acid.** Enanthylic acid, heptoic acid, $C_6H_{13}COOH$, a saturated fatty acid of unpleasant smell, produced by the oxidation of oenanthal, the aldehyde obtained from castor oil. **Olefine acids.** A family of unsaturated acids derived from the olefine hydrocarbons, and having the general formula, $C_nH_{2n-2}O_2$, with 1 double bond in the chain; the principal members of this series are acrylic and oleic acids. **Oleic Acid BP 1973, Oleinic acid.** $CH_3(CH_2)_7CH{=}CH(CH_2)_7COOH$, the most widely occurring fatty acid, present in nearly all fats and oils, especially olive and almond oils, as olein, the glycerol ester; a pale oily liquid, insoluble in water, but readily soluble in alcohol, ether, chloroform and essential oils. It is easily absorbed by the skin. **Oleophosphoric acid.** A mixture of oleic and phosphoric acids, found among the products of the hydrolysis of lecithins. **Opianic acid.** $C_6H_2(CHO)(CH_3O)_2COOH$, an acid prepared from hydrastine, the alkaloid of *Hydrastis canadensis*, by oxidation; also from narcotine. **Organic acid.** A carbon compound which displays the properties of an acid. Such compounds usually contain one or more carboxyl, -COOH, groups, a fact denoted by the prefix, *carboxy-*, or the inclusion in their names of *carboxylic*. **Ornithuric acid.** $C_6H_5CONH(CH_2)_3CH(COOH)NHCOC_6H_5$, a derivative of ornithine, excreted by birds in their detoxication of phenolic compounds. **Orotic acid.** Iso-uracylcarboxylic acid, $(CONHCH)_2(OH)COOH$, an acid derived from nucleoprotein; it has been observed in milk. **Orsellic acid, Orsellinic acid.** Dihydroxymethylbenzoic acid, $C_6H_2(CH_3)(OH)_2COOH$, an acid obtained from species of the lichen, *Roccella*. **Ortho acid.** 1. An inorganic acid of a trivalent element, such as phosphorus, which has 3 hydrogen atoms to offer for replacement by metals or by basic radicals. 2. An organic aromatic acid which has its carboxyl, -COOH, group in the *ortho*, or adjacent, position in the benzene ring. **Ortho-aminosalicylic acid.** $CH_3(NH_2)OHCOOH$, an insoluble grey derivative of salicylic acid, used in the treatment of chronic rheumatism. **Ortho-arsenic acid.** H_3AsO_4, an acid from which are formed the arsenates, useful in medicine, and the basis of the earlier, pentavalent arsenic spirochaeticides. **Orthoboric acid.** Boric acid, boracic acid, H_3BO_3, a mild antiseptic used in urinary infections and dry skin diseases, and as a wound dressing and food preservative. **Orthohydroxybenzoic acid, Ortho-oxybenzoic acid.** Salicylic Acid BP 1958 (see below). **Orthophenolsulphonic acid.** Sozolic acid, $C_6H_4(OH)SO_3H$; an antiseptic, **Orthophosphoric acid.** Ordinary phosophoric acid, H_3PO_4; it occurs in bone, tissue and tissue fluids, as salts, phosphoproteins, nucleoproteins, phosphagens and phospholipides; used medicinally, in dilute solution, in dyspepsia and bone-deficiency diseases. **Orthophosphorous acid.** Phosphorous acid (see below).

Oshaic acid. An expectorant, obtained from osha root, *Ligusticum filicinum*. **Osmic acid.** H_2OsO_4, the hypothetical dibasic acid which forms the salts, osmates; the term is more commonly applied to osmium tetroxide, used to fix and stain fats in histological work. **Oxalic acid.** Ethane diacid, $(COOH)_2$, found in many plants, such as woodsorrel, *Oxalis acetosella*, and rhubarb. An important reagent, it is used in bleaching and dyeing, photography, and in organic synthesis; it is poisonous. **Oxalic acid series.** A family of dibasic acids having the general formula, $C_nH_{2n-2}O_4$; oxalic, malonic and succinic acids are representative of this series. **Oxalo-acetic acid.** $COOHCOCH_2COOH$, an acid which plays a considerable part in transamination and tissue respiration. **Oxalosuccinic acid.** $COOHCOCH(COOH)CH_2COOH$, an intermediate in the citric-acid cycle. **Oxaluric acid.** Oxalic monoureide, $NH_2CONHCOCOOH$, a derivative of urea, which appears in normal urine. **Oxamic acid.** $NH_2COCOOH$, an acid prepared from ammonium hydrogen oxalate. **Oxolinic Acid.** BP Commission approved name for 5 - ethyl - 5,8 - dihydro - 8 - oxo - 1,3 - dioxolo[4,5-*g*]quinoline - 7 - carboxylic acid; an antiproteus agent. **Oxy acid.** 1. An inorganic acid containing oxygen, usually in -OH groups, as distinct from binary acids. The names of such acids end in *-ic*, and the salts are known as *-ates*, except where there are 2 oxy acids, when the lower one is denoted by the termination *-ous*, and the salts by *-ites*. 2. An organic acid containing, in addition to the carboxyl, -COOH, group, the group, =O. **Oxyacetic acid.** Glycollic acid (see above). **Oxyamygdalic acid.** Hydroxyformobenzoylic acid (see above). **Oxybenzoic acid.** Salicylic acid (see below). **Oxybutyric acid.** Hydroxybutyric acid (see above). **Oxycarnic acid.** Formed by the oxidation of the carnic acid in muscle, **Oxyformobenzoylic acid.** Hydroxyformobenzoylic acid (see above). **Oxygen acid.** Oxy acid (see above). **Oxyiodopyridone-acetic acid.** $C_5H_3ONICH_2COOH$, an acid used, as the sodium salt, in excretion pyelography. **Oxymandelic acid.** Hydroxyformobenzoylic acid (see above). **Oxynaphthoic acid.** Hydroxynaphthoic acid (see above). **Oxynaphthylortho-oxytoluylic acid.** $OHC_{10}H_6CH_2C_6H_3(OH)COOH$, a phenol derivative used in the treatment of skin diseases. **Oxynervonic acid.** $C_{24}H_{45}(OH)O_2$, an unsaturated hydroxy acid found associated with nervonic acid in brain tissue. **Oxyphenylacetic acid.** Hydroxyphenylacetic acid (see above). **Oxyphenylaminopropionic acid.** Parahydroxyphenylaminopropionic acid (see below). **Oxyphenylquinolinedicarboxylic acid.** A substance closely related to cinchophen, and used in the treatment of gout, rheumatism and lumbago. **Oxypropionic acid.** Lactic acid (see above). **Oxypyronecarboxylic acid.** Comenic acid (see above). **Oxypyronedicarboxylic acid.** Meconic acid (see above). **Oxytoluic acid.** Cresotic acid (see above).

Palmitic acid. Hexadecanoic acid, $CH_3(CH_2)_{14}COOH$, a saturated fatty acid which occurs widely, usually associated with stearic and oleic acids, in animal and vegetable fats and oils, in the form of glycerides; it is used in the manufacture of soap and candles. **Palmitoleic acid.** Zoomaric acid, hexadecenoic acid, $CH_3(CH_2)_5CH{=}CH(CH_2)_7COOH$, an unsaturated fatty acid occurring in cod-liver oil, and in the oil of whales, seals and certain fish. **Palmitolic acid.** Hexadecynoic acid, $C_{16}H_{28}O_2$, an unsaturated acid of the linoleic series, found in oils, and japan wax, from *Rhus succedanea*. **Pantothenic acid.** $COOH(CH_2)_2NHCOCHOHC(CH_3)_2CH_2OH$, a substituted amide, pantoyl β-alanine formed from pantoic acid and β-alanine and an intermediate in the biosynthesis of coenzyme A. It is a member of the B group of vitamins. **Para-aminobenzenesulphonic acid.** Sulphanilic acid (see below). **Para-aminobenzoic acid.** $C_6H_4(NH_2)COOH$, an acid present in yeast and liver; it is a member of the *Bios* complex, and believed essential for the growth of micro-organisms. It can be regarded as a bacterial vitamin, in which respect it is inhibited by sulphonamides. **Para-aminosalicylic acid.** *See* PAS. **Parabanic acid.** Oxalylurea, $(CONH_2)_2CO$, a derivative of urea; it forms salts which are easily converted into those of oxaluric acid. **Paracreosotic acid, Paracresotic acid.** *p*-Hydroxytoluic acid, $C_6H_3(CH_3)(OH)COOH$, an acid

acid

used as an antiseptic, and, in the form of the sodium salt, in the treatment of rheumatism in children. **Paraffinic acid.** $C_{24}H_{48}O_2$, an acid, isomeric, but not identical with carnaubic acid, formed by the oxidation of paraffin wax. **Parafumaric acid.** Maleic Acid BP 1958. **Parahydroxybenzoic acid.** $C_6H_4(OH)COOH$, the *para* isomer of salicylic acid; anisic acid is the methyl ether. **Parahydroxyhydratropic acid.** Hydrocoumaric acid (see above). **Parahydroxyphenylacetic acid.** Hydroxyphenylacetic acid (see above). **Parahydroxyphenylaminopropionic acid.** Tyrosine, $C_6H_4(OH)CH_2CH(NH_2)COOH$, an α-amino acid considered essential for animal life, providing, as it does, the chief source of the aromatic ring which cannot be synthesized in the body. During metabolism it breaks down into hydroxyphenylacetic acid, aceto-acetic acid, and, in alkaptonurics, into homogentisic acid. It occurs in many proteins. including old cheese, and is found in the pancreas. **Parahydroxyphenylglycollic acid.** $OHC_6H_4CHOHCOOH$, an acid that occurs in the urine as a product of tyrosine metabolism. **Parahydroxyphenylpropionic acid.** $OHC_6H_4(CH_2)_2COOH$, an acid produced by the deamination of tyrosine in the body; it is subsequently oxidized to phenol, detoxicated and thus excreted. **Para-iodophenylarsenic acid.** $C_6H_4IAsO(OH)_2$, a derivative of arsanilic acid, used as a spirochaeticide. **Paralactic acid.** Dextrolactic acid (see above). **Para-oxyphenylacetic acid.** Hydroxyphenylacetic acid (see above). **Paraphenolsulphonic acid.** Sulphocarbolic acid, $C_6H_4(OH)SO_3H$, the most stable of the phenolsulphonic acids; it is readily soluble in water, and a strong disinfectant. **Pararosolic acid.** Trihydroxytriphenylmethane, $CH(C_6H_4OH)_3$, an acid derived from pararosaniline; it yields aurin, the dye, on oxidation, and is used as a pH indicator. **Parasaccharic acid.** $COOH(CHOH)_4COOH$, an isomer of saccharic acid. **Paratartaric acid.** The optically-inactive racemic form of tartaric acid. **Parillic acid.** $C_{40}H_{70}O_{18}$, a glucoside found in the root and rhizomes of sarsaparilla, *Smilax omata.* **Pectic acid.** $C_{35}H_{50}O_{33}$, a complex uronic acid containing galactose and arabinose, which occurs in ripe fruit, beets, turnips and other vegetables; pectin is the methoxyester. It is by virtue of the formation of a jelly-like calcium pectate that jams and preserves are able to set. **Pectinic acid.** An acid intermediate between pectic acid and pectin in the degree of methoxy esterification. **Pelargonic acid.** Nonanoic acid, $CH_3(CH_2)_7COOH$, a normal saturated fatty acid which occurs in the geranium oil of *Pelargonium roseum.* **Penicillic acid.** Keto-methoxymethylenehexenoic acid, $CH_3C{=}(CH_2)COC(OCH_3){=}CHCOOH$, an antibiotic secreted by *Penicillium puberulum.* **Penicilloinic acids.** Name given to a series of complex acids produced from the penicillins by the ferment, penicillinase. **Pentacosanic acid.** $C_{25}H_{50}O_2$, the saturated fatty acid that is combined with sphingosine and galactose in the phrenosin of brain tissue. **Pentahydroxycaproic acid.** Galactonic acid (see above). **Pentanedicarboxylic acid.** Pimelic acid (see below). **Pentanoic acid.** Valerianic acid (see below). **Pentenic acid.** Name given to any of the isomers of formula C_4H_7COOH; angelic and tiglic acids are examples. **Pentonic acid.** One of the numerous acids of the general formula, $CH_2OH(CHOH)_3COOH$, isomeric with tetrahydroxyvaleric acid, and produced by the oxidation of pentoses; arabonic and ribonic acids are representative. **Penturonic acid.** One of the aldehyde acids, $CHO(CHOH)_3COOH$, produced from pentoses by oxidation of the alcohol group; xylosic acid is an example. **Peptohydrochloric acid.** A hypothetical acid resulting from the combination of the enzyme pepsin, in the gastric juice, with hydrochloric acid. **Peracetic acid.** CH_3COOOH, an acid derived from acetic anhydride. **Perboric acid.** HBO_3, (*meta*), or $H_2B_4O_8$, an unstable acid, the salts of which, perborates, are strong oxidizing agents used as bleaches and disinfectants. Sodium perborate is effective in tonsillitis and Vincent's angina. **Perchloric acid.** $HClO_4$, a powerful oxidizing agent used in organic synthesis; also a qualitative and quantitative reagent for potassium. **Performic acid.** HCOOH, used to disrupt disulphide bridges in proteins by oxidation, thereby to separate peptide chains linked through disulphide bridges and thus to facilitate structural analysis. **Periodic acid.** An acid of variable constitution, obtained by dissolving I_2O_7 in water; it is a strong oxidizing agent. **Permanganic acid.** $HMnO_4$, an unstable acid, readily decomposing into MnO_2 and free oxygen; the permanganates are important oxidizing agents and disinfectants. **Perosmic acid.** The name ordinarily applied to osmium tetroxide, OsO_4, which stains fats, and is used in histological work for this purpose; it has also been found of value as an antineuralgic. **Acid peroxide.** A compound containing the radical -COO-OCO-. **Peroxymonosulphuric acid.** H_2SO_5; Caro's acid, an oxidizing agent. **Persulphuric acid.** $H_2S_2O_8$, an acid formed by the electrolysis of sulphuric acid; it is a strong oxidizing agent. **Petroselinic acid.** Octadecenic acid, $CH_3(CH_2)_{10}CH{=}CH(CH_2)_4COOH$, an unsaturated fatty acid, isomeric with oleic acid, and found in oil of coriander, *Coriandrum satirum*, and oil of parsley, *Petroselinum satirum.* **Phenaceturic acid.** Phenylaceturic acid, phenyl acetyl glycine, $C_6H_5CH_2CONHCH_2COOH$, an acid that occurs in the urine of dogs and other animals, as the result of their detoxication of phenylacetic acid by glycine. **Phenic acid.** Carbolic acid (see above). **Phenoldisulphonic acid.** $C_6H_3(OH)(SO_3H)_2$, an acid prepared from benzene disulphonic acid; it is a disinfectant. **Phenolsulphonic acid.** $C_6H_4(OH)(SO_3H)$; the *ortho* form, sozolic acid, is a strong disinfectant. The sodium salt is given for flatulence and the zinc salt is injected for gonorrhoea; it is also used as a nasal spray. **Phenylacetic acid.** Alpha-toluic acid, $C_6H_5CH_2COOH$, an acid that occurs, in the hydroxy form, as the result of tyrosine decomposition in the metabolism. **Phenylaceto-orthocarboxylic acid.** Homophthalic acid (see above). **Phenylaceturic acid.** Phenaceturic acid (see above). **Phenylacrylic acid.** An acid that occurs in 2 forms: α-, atropic acid; β-, cinnamic acid. **Phenylaminobenzoic acid.** Phenylanthranilic acid (see below). **Phenylaminopropionic acid.** Phenylalanine, $C_6H_5CH_2CH(NH_2)COOH$, an α-amino acid which provides, with tyrosine, a source of the aromatic benzene ring which the metabolism is unable to synthesize for itself. It is essential for nutrition; forms aceto-acetic acid in glycosuria, and homogentisic acid in alkaptonuria. **Phenylanthranilic acid.** Phenylaminobenzoic acid, $C_6H_5NHC_6H_4COOH$, an acid used as an indicator in the estimation of ferrous iron in organic mixtures. **Phenylboric acid.** $C_6H_5OB(OH_2)$, a germicidal compound. **Phenylcincholincarbonic acid, Phenylcinchoninic acid.** Cinchophen, $C_6H_5C_9H_5NCOOH$, a yellowish powder, soluble in alkalis, and used as an analgesic and antipyretic, It promotes the excretion of uric acid, and is of value therefore in the treatment of gout. **Phenylcyclopentanecarboxylic acid.** $CH_2CH_2CH_2CH_2C(C_6H_5)COOH$, an acid, the diethylaminoethyl derivative of which is a parasympatholytic agent of possible value for the relief of muscular spasm and tremor in parkinsonism. **Phenylethylbarbituric acid.** Phenobarbitone, $(C_6H_5)(C_2H_5)C(CONH)_2CO$, a hypnotic and sedative of particular merit in epilepsy; it forms a soluble sodium salt with NaOH. **Phenylglucuronic acid.** $C_6H_5OCH{=}O(CHOH)_3{=}CHCOOH$, the conjugated form in which phenol is detoxicated by glucuronic acid in the system. **Phenylglycinamide-*p*-arsonic acid.** $NH_2COCH_2NHC_6H_4AsO(OH)_2$, an acid, the sodium salt of which, tryparsamide, is used in the treatment of trypanosomes and spirochaetal infections. **Phenylglycollic acid.** Mandelic acid (see above). **Phenylhydracrylic acid.** Tropic acid (see below). **Phenylhydrazinelaevulinic acid.** $C_{11}H_{14}O_2N_2$, an analgesic and antiseptic. **Phenylhydroxypropionic acid.** Tropic acid (see below). **Phenylic acid.** Carbolic acid (see above). **Phenyl-lactic acid.** Atrolactic acid (see above). **Phenylmercapturic acid.** $C_6H_5SCH_2CH(NHCOCH_3)COOH$, phenylacetylcysteine, an acid observed in the urine as a detoxication product. **Phenylmethylbarbituric acid.** $(C_6H_5)(CH_3)C(CONH)_2CO$, a hypnotic and sedative of special importance in epilepsy. **Phenylnaphtholcarboxylic acid.** Chrysenic acid (see above). **Phenylpropionic acid.** Hydrocinnamic acid (see above). **Phenylpyruvic acid.** $C_6H_5CH_3COCOOH$, a deamination derivative of phenylalanine, and an intermediary in the metabolism of the latter. It is excreted, unchanged, in the inherited condition, phenylketonuria. **Phenylquinolinecarboxylic acid.** Phenylcincholincarbonic acid (see above). **Phenylsalicylic**

acid. $C_6H_3(OH)C_6H_5COOH$, an antiseptic powder. **Phenylsulphonic acid, Phenylsulphuric acid.** Paraphenolsulphonic acid (see above). **Phloretic acid.** $C_6H_4OHCH(CH_3)COOH$, an isomer of hydrocoumaric acid, produced by the oxidation of phloretin. **Phocenic acid.** Valeric acid (see below). **Acid phosphatase.** Secreted by the prostate. **Phosphatidic acid.** L-glycerol 3-phosphate in which the 2 hydroxyls have been esterified with fatty acids. Important intermediate in the synthesis of triglycerides and phospholipids. **Phosphocarnic acid.** The phospho-compound of carnic acid, which occurs in muscle. **Phosphoglyceric acid.** Glycerophosphoric acid (see above). **Phosphomolybdic acid.** $H_3PO_412MoO_2$, an acid, the sodium salt of which, dissolved in nitric acid (Sonnenschein's reagent), gives a yellow precipitate with the alkaloids. **Phosphoric Acid BP 1973.** Orthophosphoric acid, H_3PO_4, a white crystalline solid, soluble in water to give an 89 per cent solution, which forms phosphates, and acid (hydrogen) phosphates, of the types, Na_3PO_4, Na_2HPO_4 and NaH_2PO_4, all diuretics. Dilute solution of the acid (10 per cent) (BP 1958) is used as a nerve tonic, and the calcium salt is of value in bone formation and general nutrition. **Phosphoric acid, glacial.** The reagent for albumen in the urine; it consists of metaphosphoric acid, HPO_3. **Phosphorous acid.** Orthophosphorous acid, H_3PO_3, a yellow substance, soluble in water, and used as a reducing agent; it forms phosphites. **Phosphotungstic acid.** $2H_3PO_4WO_3$, an acid employed, in the form of the sodium salt, to detect alkaloids (Scheibler's reagent), also for albumose in urine (Salkowski's reagent). **Phrenosinic acid.** Neurostearic acid (see above). **Phthalic acid.** Benzenedicarboxylic acid, $C_6H_4(COOH)_2$, an acid prepared by the catalytic oxidation of naphthalene; crystals, slightly soluble in water, used in the manufacture of dyestuffs and in organic synthesis. **Phthalic acid series.** A family of aromatic dibasic acids of the general formula, $C_nH_{2n-8}(COOH)_2$. **Phthioic acid.** $C_{26}H_{52}O_2$, a saturated fatty acid which occurs in tubercle bacilli. **Phyllocyanic acid.** A porphyrin compound, obtained by the hydrolysis of chlorophyll. **Physetoleic acid.** An unsaturated acid, $C_{16}H_{30}O_2$, occurring in tallow and seal oil, and perhaps identical with hypogaeic acid. **Phytic acid.** Inositol phosphoric acid (see above). **Phytomonic acid.** $C_{20}H_{40}O_2$, a crystalline saturated fatty acid derived from *Phytomonas tumefaciens.* **Picolinic acid.** An isomer of nicotinic acid. **Picramic acid.** $C_6H_2(NH_2)(NO_2)_2OH$, a derivative of picramide, which appears in the blood in the case of picric acid poisoning. **Picric acid.** Trinitrophenol, carbazotic acid, $C_6H_2(NO_2)_3OH$, yellow crystals, only slightly soluble in water, and used as an explosive, as a yellow dye and as a stain in microscopy; it is employed to precipitate albumen (Esbach's reagent), and to detect glucose in urine. Medicinally, it is no longer employed in malaria owing to toxicity; it is a strong antiseptic and has been used in burn dressings, but there is the danger of absorption. **Picricnitric acid.** A histological fixative. **Picricsulphuric acid.** A histological fixative. **Picrolonic acid.** Methylnitro-nitrophenylpyrazoline, $NO_2C_6H_4C_4H_3N_3O_2(OH)$, an acid used in microchemistry as a reagent for calcium; also as a precipitant for alkaloids. **Picropodophyllic acid.** An acid obtained from podophyllum, the rhizome and roots of *Podophyllum peltatum.* **Pimaric acid.** Dextropimaric acid, $C_{20}H_{30}O_2$, an isomer of abietic acid; it is obtained from the resin, French galipot, *Pinus maritima*; it also occurs in Burgundy pitch. **Pimarinic acid.** $C_{12}H_{20}O_2$, an acid that occurs with pimaric acid in Burgundy pitch, the oleoresin from the spruce, *Picea excelsa.* **Pimarolic acid.** $C_{18}H_{28}O_2$, an acid that occurs in Burgundy pitch with pimaric and pimarinic acids. **Pimelic acid.** Pentanedicarboxylic acid, $COOH(CH_2)_5COOH$, homologous with oxalic acid, of interest as an aliphatic acid obtained by the splitting of the aromatic ring of hydroxybenzoic acid with metallic sodium. **Piperic acid, Piperinic acid.** Methylenedioxyphenylpentadienoic acid, $CH_2O_2C_6H_3(CH)_4COOH$, an acid found, in combination with piperidine in the alkaloid, piperine, of black pepper, *Piper nigrum.* **Pipitzahoic acid, Pipitzahoinic acid.** Aurum vegetable, $C_{15}H_{20}O_3$, a yellow substance obtained from the roots of the Mexican *Perezia adnata*; it is used as a vegetable indicator in volumetric analysis, and, medicinally, as a purgative. **Pivalic acid.** $(CH_3)_3CCOOH$, one of the isomers of valeric acid. **Plasminic acid.** Name applied to the split products of the hydrolysis of nucleic acids. **Platinochloric acid.** Hydrochloroplatinic acid (see above). **Plumbic acid.** A hypothetical acid, H_4PbO_4, derived from lead peroxide, PbO_2, which forms orthoplumbates. **Plumbodithiopyridinecarboxylic acid.** A heterocyclic compound which has been used in cancer treatment. **Podophyllic acid.** $C_{15}H_{16}O_7$, an acid obtained by the hydrolysis of podophyllin, the resin extracted from the roots of *Podophyllum peltatum.* **Polyadenylic acid.** A polynucleotide made up solely of adenylic acid units. Such polynucleotides are found attached at both ends of several, if not all, messenger RNAs. **Polyatomic acid, Polybasic acid.** An acid which offers 2 or more hydrogen atoms for replacement by metals or by basic radicals. **Polygalic acid.** Polygalin, $C_{32}H_{54}O_{18}$, an acid obtained from the dried root of *Polygala senega*; it is an expectorant used in chronic bronchitis. **Polyglycolic Acid.** BP Commission approved name for poly(oxycarbonylmethylene); used as a synthetic absorbable suture. **Propanoic acid.** Propionic acid (see below). **Propargylic acid.** Propiolic acid (see below). **Propenetricarboxylic acid.** Aconitic acid (see above). **Propiolic acid.** Carboxyacetylene, acetylene carboxylic acid, propargylic acid, CH≡CCOOH, a powerful acid, the sodium and copper salts of which are explosive. **Propiolic acid series.** A family of organic unsaturated acids of the general formula $C_nH_{2n-4}O_2$, with 1 triple bond; propiolic and tetrolic acids are representative. **Propionic acid.** Propanoic acid, CH_3CH_2COOH, a saturated fatty acid resulting from the reduction of lactic acid; it occurs also in fermentation, and in the conversion of glycogen to lactic acid in muscle. It is used as a fungicide in ointments and dusting-powders (BPC 1954). **Propionylsalicylic acid.** $CH_3CH_2COOC_6H_4COOH$, an acid used as an antirheumatic, and in the treatment of gout. **Propylacetic acid.** Normal valeric acid (see below). **Protocatechuic acid.** $C_6H_3(OH)_2COOH$, an acid obtained by fusing catechu, or benzoin, with alkalis, or from alizarin; it occurs in oil of shepherd's purse, *Capsella bursapastoris.* It is an isomer of gentisic acid. **Prussic acid.** Hydrocyanic acid (see above). **Pteroic acid.** $NH_2C_4N_2(OH)N_2C_2HCH_2NHC_6H_4COOH$, an acid occurring in the wing pigments of butterflies, from which is also derived vitamin B_c (pteroylglutamic acid) and the anti-anaemia factor, folic acid. **Pteroylglutamic acid.** Folic acid (see above). **Puberulic acid.** $C_8H_4O_6$, an acid that results from the growth of *Penicillium puberulum*; it is an antibiotic. **Puberulonic acid.** $C_8H_4O_6$, an acid that occurs in the metabolism of *Penicillum puberulum*; it is an antibiotic. **Punicotannic acid.** A tannin obtained from the root of the pomegranate, *Punica granaum.* **Purpuric acid.** $CO(NHCO)_2CNCH(CONH)_2(COOH)$, a derivative of alloxantin which does not exist as a free acid. The ammonium salt, murexide, is responsible for the characteristic purple colour which develops in the murexide test for uric acid. **Pyridine α-carboxylic acid.** Isonicotinic acid (see above). **Pyridine β-carboxylic acid.** Nicotinic acid (see above). **Pyridinedicarboxylic acid.** Cinchomeronic acid (see above). **Pyridine-3-sulphonic acid.** $C_5H_4NSO_3H$, an analogue of nicotinic acid which inhibits the growth of certain micro-organisms, its effect being overcome by nicotinic acid. **Pyridinetricarboxylic acid.** $C_5H_2N(COOH)_3$, an acid that occurs in several isomers; it is related to cinchomeronic acid, and has been used in malaria. **Pyridoxic acid.** 2-Methyl-3-hydroxy-5-hydroxymethylpyridine-4-carboxylic acid, $C_5HN(CH_3)(OH)(COOH)(CH_2OH)$, a compound excreted in human urine after the ingestion of pyridoxine (vitamin B_6). Heating with strong nitric acid converts it into a lactone that is highly fluorescent. **Pyro acid.** An acid produced by heating an ortho acid, with the elimination of a molecule of water. **Pyro-arsenic acid.** $H_4As_2O_7$, an acid produced by heating ortho-arsenic acid; it is $As_2O_3(OH)_4$. **Pyroboric acid.** $H_2B_4O_7$; an acid produced by heating orthoboric acid; the sodium salt is borax, $Na_2N_4O_7$. **Pyrocholesteric acid.** $C_{11}H_{16}O_7$, an acid obtained during the oxidation of cholic acid by the rupture of the sterol-ring structure. **Pyrocinchonic acid.** Dimethylmaleic acid, $(CH_3CCOOH)_2$, an acid produced by heating cinchonic acid. **Pyrocitric acid.** Citraconic acid (see above). **Pyrogallic acid.** Pyrogallol, trihydroxybenzene, $C_6H_3(OH)_3$, an acid obtained by heating gallic acid; white crystals, soluble in water, forming a powerful reducing agent; it is used in photography, and as an absorbent for oxygen in gas analysis. It is of value, medicinally, as a caustic in lupus, ringworm and other parasitic skin diseases; it is toxic, causing methaemoglobinuria. **Pyroligneous acid.** Wood vinegar, mainly crude acetic acid, produced by distilling wood. **Pyrolithic acid.** Cyanuric acid (see above). **Pyromucic acid.** Furane carboxylic acid (see above). **Pyronecarboxylic acid.** Comanic acid (see above). **Pyronedicarboxylic acid.** Chelidonic acid (see above). **Pyrophosphoric acid.** $H_4P_2O_7$, an acid formed by heating orthophosphoric acid. **Pyroracemic acid.** Pyruvic acid (see below). **Pyrosulphuric acid.** $H_2S_2O_7$, so-called disulphuric acid; it is prepared from Nordhausen acid. **Pyrotartaric acid.** Methylsuccinic acid, $CH_3CH(COOH)CH_2COOH$, an acid formed, with pyruvic acid, by distilling tartaric acid. **Pyrrolidine carboxylic acid.** α-Carboxypyrrolidine, proline, $(CH_2)_3(NH)$=CHCOOH, an amino acid which is glycogenetic. **Pyruvic acid.** Pyroracemic acid, $CH_3COCOOH$, an acid formed by heating tartaric acid; it is an intermediate product in the formation of alcohol from glucose by fermentation, and also appears in the phosphate cycle of muscular contraction. It accumulates in the blood, urine and cerebrospinal fluid in beriberi, but is immediately reduced by the administration of vitamin B_1.

Quercitannic acid. $C_{28}H_{28}O_{14}$, an amorphous phlobatannin obtained from oak bark; hydrolysed to the brownish phlobaphene, oak-red. **Quillaic acid.** $C_{19}H_{30}O_{10}$, a saponin present in quillaia bark, *Quillaja saponaria*; it is used as an emulsifier for oils, and to produce copious froth. It has a haemolytic effect if taken orally. **Quinaldic acid.** Quinolinecarboxylic acid, C_9H_6N (COOH), an isomer of cinchoninic acid. **Quinic acid.** Kinic acid, hexahydrotetrahydroxybenzoic acid, $C_6H_7(OH)_4COOH$, an acid present in cinchona bark, combined with the alkaloids, and in coffee beans; a white crystalline substance, soluble in water, and used in the treatment of gout and rheumatism. **Quininic acid.** Methoxyquinolinecarboxylic acid, $CH_3OC_9H_5NCOOH$, an acid obtained from quinine and quinidine by oxidation and splitting of the ring systems; it is used in organic synthesis. **Quinizarinsulphonic acid.** Rufianic acid (see below). **Quinolinecarboxylic acid.** Quinaldic acid (see above). **Quinolinemonocarboxylic acid.** Cinchoninic acid (see above). **Quinolinic acid.** α-, β-Pyridine dicarboxylic acid, $C_5H_3N(COOH)_2$, an isomer of cinchomeronic acid formed during the biodegradation of tryptophan; an inhibitor of phosphoenolpyruvate carboxykinase. **Quinotannic acid.** $C_{14}H_{16}O_9$, the tannin obtained from cinchona bark; it decomposes into cinchona red. **Quinovic acid.** $C_{30}H_{48}O_6$, an acid that occurs, to a small extent, in cinchona bark.

Racemic acid. 1. The optically-inactive form of tartaric acid, $COOH(CHOH)_2COOH$, which can be separated into the dextro and laevo forms, of which it is a mixture; it is found in grape juice. 2. Term applied to an equal mixture of dextro- and laevorotatory isomers which exhibits no optical activity. **Acid radical.** The group remaining when the acid hydrogen is subtracted from the molecule of an organic acid. **Reductic acid.** A compound, known also as a *reductone*, that develops in carbohydrate treated with alkali, or dehydrated; it has a strongly reducing action. **Resin acids.** A family of related acidic substances which are extracted from the resins and balsams. **Rhatanytannic acid.** Krameric acid (see above). **Rheic acid.** $C_{20}H_{16}O_9$, a red substance obtained from rhubarb. **Rheinic acid.** Dihydroxyanthraquinonecarboxylic acid, rhein, $C_{15}H_8O_6$, an acid found as a glucoside in senna leaves, *Cassia acutifolia*, and rhubarb. **Rheotannic acid.** $C_{26}H_{26}O_{11}$, the tannin occurring in rhubarb. **Rheumic acid.** $C_{20}H_{16}O_9$, an acid that can be prepared from rheotannic acid. **Rhodanic acid.** Thiocyanic acid (see below). **Ribonic acid.** $CH_2OH(CHOH)_3COOH$, an acid obtained by oxidizing the pentose, ribose. **Ribonucleic acid, Ribose nucleic acid.** RNA. Polymers of the monophosphate of adenosine, guanosine, cytidine and uridine: *messenger RNA*, formed by transcription from the nuclear DNA, codes for the synthesis of proteins in the process of translation; *ribosomal RNA*, of high molecular weight, associated with ribosomal structure, the slowest of all RNAs within the cell to turn over; *soluble* or *transfer RNA*, molecular weight approximately 80 000, the final amino acid acceptor before peptide bond synthesis during translation. **Ricinoleic acid, Ricinolic acid.** Hydroxyoleic acid, $CH_3(CH_2)_5CHOHC$ $H_2CH=CH(CH_2)_7COOH$, an acid that occurs in castor oil, free, and as a glyceride; it is considered to be responsible for the purgative action of the oil. The sodium salt is a strong detoxifier, and is used as a mouthwash and spray, also in the treatment of varicose veins. **Roccellic acid.** $C_{20}H_{20}O_7$, a lichen acid from a species of Roccella. **Rosacic acid.** Purpurin, $C_{14}H_8O_5$, a trihydroxyanthraquinone which forms part of the red dye extracted from madder root, *Rubia tinctorium*. **Rosolic acid.** Dihydroxyphenyloxytolylmethane, $CH_3C_6H_3(O)C(C_6H_4OH)_2$, an acid dye, used as a pH indicator. **Ruberythric acid, Rubianic acid.** $C_{26}H_{28}O_{14}$, the glucoside of dihydroxyanthraquinone, which occurs in the red dye of madder root. **Rufianic acid.** Quinizarinsulphonic acid, $C_{14}H_7O_4SO_3H$, a reagent employed in the analysis of the amino acids. **Rufigallic acid.** Hexahydroxyanthraquinone, $C_{14}H_2O_2(OH)_6$, an orange dyestuff. **Rutic acid.** $C_{10}H_{20}$ O_2, a saturated fatty acid occurring in oil of rue from *Ruta graveolens*. **Rutinic acid.** $C_{25}H_{28}P_{15}$, a colouring matter found in rue.

Sabinenic acid, Sabinic acid. Hydroxydodecanoic acid, $(OH)(CH_2)_{11}COOH$, an acid that occurs in both oil of savin from *Juniperus sabina*, and oil of juniper from *Juniperus communis*. **Saccharic acid.** 1. One of the dibasic acids of the general formula, $COOH(CHOH)_nCOOH$, obtained by the oxidation of both alcohol and aldehyde groups of the aldoses. 2. The dibasic acid, $COOH(CHOH)_4COOH$, formed by the oxidation of dextrose. **Saccharide acid.** General term for the dibasic acids produced by oxidation of the terminal groups of simple sugars. **Saccharinic acid.** One of the monobasic acids of general formula $CH_2OH(CHOH)_nCOOH$, formed from an aldose by the oxidation of the aldehyde group. **Saccharonic acid.** Methyltrihydroxyglutaric acid, $COOHC(CH_3)(OH)(CHOH)_2$ COOH, an acid produced by oxidizing sucrose. **Salicylacetic acid.** $OHC_6H_4COOCH_2COOH$, a condensation product of sodium salicylate and sodium monochloracetate, used as an antiseptic. **Salicylic Acid BP 1973.** Orthohydroxybenzoic acid, $C_6H_4(OH)COOH$, an acid found free in *Spiraea ulmaria*, species of the willow, *Salix*, and, as methyl salicylate, in wintergreen, *Gaultheria procumbens*. Colourless, odourless crystals, only slightly soluble in water, but readily in alcohol or ether, it is used as a preservative, as a bactericide and, in concentrated solutions, to remove warts and corns; also in the treatment of ringworm, and skin diseases. **Salicylosalicylic acid.** $OHC_6H_4COOC_6H_4$ COOH, an antipyretic used like aspirin. **Salicylous acid.** Salicylic aldehyde, $C_6H_4(OH)CHO$, a colourless fragrant liquid, with the properties of a phenol, and used in perfumery. **Salicylsulphonic acid.** Sulphosalicylic acid, $C_6H_3(OH)(SO_3H)COOH$, a reagent employed in testing urine for the presence of albumin. **Salicyluric acid.** $CH_2NH_2COOC_6H_4COOH$, a condensation product which appears in the urine when salicylic acid is given as a urinary disinfectant. **Acid salt.** A compound in which the acid hydrogen is only partially replaced by basic radicals. **Santalenic acid, Santalic acid.** $C_{15}H_{24}O_5$, an acid derived from oil of sandal wood (santalwood), *Pterocarpus santalinus*; a red colouring matter. **Santonic acid, Santoninic acid.** $C_{15}H_{20}O_4$, an acid extracted from the flower heads of santonica, *Artemisia cina*; the lactone (internal anhydride), santonin, is an anthelmintic for round- and thread-worms. **Sapocholic acid.** $C_{29}H_{46}O_3$, an acid prepared from ox bile. **Sarcolactic acid.** Lactic acid (see above). **Sarcylic acid.** Inosinic acid (see above). **Sclerotic acid, Sclerotinic acid.** Ergotic acid (see above). **Scoparic acid.** Scoparin, $C_{20}H_{20}O_{10}$, a yellow flavone obtained from broom, *Cytisus scoparius*, and used as a diuretic. **Sebacic acid.** Octanedicarboxylic acid, $COOH(CH_2)_8COOH$, a saturated acid of the oxalic series, which occurs in olein and has been observed in urine as the product of the metabolic oxidation of the food fatty acids. **Secale-aminosulphonic acid.** Ergotic acid (see above). **Selacholeic acid.** Nervonic acid (see above). **Selenic**

acid. H_2SeO_4, the selenium analogue of sulphuric acid; it forms selenates. **Selenious acid.** H_2SeO_3, an acid analogous with sulphurous acid; it forms salts and selenites, and is derived from selenium dioxide, SeO_2. **Sialic acid.** Neuraminic acid (see above). **Silicic acid.** One of a number of acids formed of varying proportions of water and silicon dioxide, SiO_2; almost insoluble in water, they are principally, *ortho,* H_4SiO_4, and *meta,* H_2SiO_3, which together give rise to a large number of silicate minerals. **Silicotungstic acid.** $SiO_2 \cdot 12WO_3 \cdot 26H_2O$, yellowish crystals, soluble in water, and employed as a reagent in the analysis of alkaloids. **Sinapic acid, Sinapinic acid.** $(CH_3O)_2C_6H_2(OH)CH{=}CHCOOH$, an acid obtained from the alkaloid, sinapine, of white mustard, *Sinapis alba.* **Skatolecarboxylic acid.** $C_6H_4(NH)(CCH_3)CCOOH$, an acid that results from the decomposition of tryptophane in the intestine, and appears in the faeces. **Skatoleglucuronic acid.** A conjugation of skatole with glucuronic acid in detoxication. **Skatoxylsulphonic acid.** $C_9H_8ONSO_3H$, believed to be an oxidation product of skatole; it has been observed in the urine. **Sorbic Acid BPC 1968.** Hexadienic acid, $CH_3(CH)_4COOH$, an acid that occurs in the unripe berries of the mountain ash, *Sorbus aucuparia.* **Sozo-iodolic acid.** $C_6H_2I_2(OH)SO_3H$, an antiseptic used similarly to iodoform. **Sozolic acid.** Orthophenolsulphonic acid, $C_6H_4(OH)SO_3H$, a strong disinfectant and antiseptic. **Spermanucleic acid.** A nucleic acid occurring in the spermatozoa of certain animals. **Sphacelic acid, Sphacelinic acid.** A toxic substance obtained from ergot. **Sphingomyelinic acid.** A mixture of acids produced by the hydrolysis of the brain phospholipide, sphingomyelin. **Sphingostearic acid.** A form of stearic acid, $C_{17}H_{35}COOH$, which is found in the products of the hydrolysis of sphingomyelin. **Stannic acid.** One of the number of acids of variable composition formed by tin dioxide, SnO_2; the most important, H_2SnO_3, forms stannates, which are used in the treatment of staphylococcal infections. **Stannous acid.** A hypothetical acid, H_2SnO_2, from which the stannites are derived. **Stearic acid.** Octodecylic acid, $CH_3(CH_2)_{16}COOH$, an acid that occurs very widely, accompanied by palmitic and oleic acids, as a glyceride in vegetable and animal fats; it forms the basis of soaps (BPC 1959). **Stearinsulphuric acid.** Sulpholeic acid (see below). **Stearolic acid.** Octadecynoic acid, $CH_3(CH_2)_7C{=}C(CH_2)_7COOH$, an unsaturated acid of the propiolic series, obtained from oleic acid. **Stibanilic acid.** $NH_2C_6H_4SbO(OH)_2$, an antimony compound that has been used in protozoal diseases. **Stibinic acids.** Antimonic acids, the acids of pentavalent antimony: *ortho,* H_3SbO_5; *meta,* $HSbO_3$; and *para,* $H_4Sb_2O_7$. They form the basis of the organic antimony preparations, similar to the arsenicals, which have been used in the treatment of protozoal infections. **Stibious acids.** Antimonous acids, the acids of trivalent antimony: *ortho,* H_3SbO_3; *meta,* $HSbO_2$; and *para,* $H_4Sb_2O_5$. **Suberic acid.** Octanedioic acid, $COOH(CH_2)_6COOH$, an acid of the oxalic series; it is produced by the oxidation of cork. **Succinic acid.** Ethanedicarboxylic acid, butane diacid, $COOH(CH_2)_2COOH$, a saturated acid of the oxalic series found in amber succinum, resins and lignites; it also occurs during alcoholic fermentation and in animal tissues. It is used as a diuretic. **Succinylsalicylic acid.** An antipyretic. **Sudoric acid.** $C_5H_9O_7N$, an acid thought to have been identified in perspiration. **Sulphaloxic Acid.** BP Commission approved name for 2-{4-(hydroxymethylureidosulphonyl) phenylcarbamoyl}-benzoic acid; a sulphonamide. **Sulphaminic acid.** Aminosulphonic acid, NH_2SO_3H; an acid that forms important sulphamino compounds. **Sulphanilic acid.** Para-aminobenzenesulphonic acid, aniline parasulphonic acid, $NH_2C_6H_4SO_3H$, an acid prepared from aniline; colourless crystals, soluble in water, alcohol and ether, and used in the manufacture of dyes, drugs and organic chemicals. It is the reagent in the van den Bergh (Ehrlich) test for bile pigments. The sodium salt is used in the treatment of throat and ear infections; the zinc salt is an astringent and antiseptic. **Sulphazotized acid.** A mixture of nitrous and sulphurous acids. **Sulphichthyolic acid.** Ichthyolsulphonic acid (see above). **Sulphindigotic acid.** Indigodisulphonic acid (see above). **Sulphinic acid.** An organic acid containing the monovalent radical, $-SO_2H$; derivatives are denoted by the prefix, *sulphino-*. **Sulpho acid.** Term applied to a sulphonic acid (see below). **Sulpho-aminolactic acid.** Aminothiolpropionic acid, cysteine, $HSCH_2CH(NH_2)COOH$, an α-amino acid which is found in proteins, and is the principal source of sulphur for the body. It breaks down in the metabolism into taurine. **Sulphocarbolic acid.** Paraphenolsulphonic acid (see above). **Sulphocarbonic acid.** Thiocarbonic acid (see below). **Sulphocyanic acid.** Thiocyanic acid (see below). **Sulpho-ichthyolic acid.** Ichthyolsulphonic acid (see above). **Sulpho-indigotic acid, Sulpho-indylic acid.** Indigodisulphonic acid (see above). **Sulpholeic acid.** $CH_3(CH_2)_{15}CH(SO_3H)COOH$, a derivative of stearic (not oleic) acid, produced by the action of strong sulphuric acid upon fats and oils. **Sulphondichloro-aminobenzoic acid.** Halazone, $C_6H_4(SO_2NCl_2)COOH$, a white substance with a smell of chlorine, used as a disinfectant and antiseptic. **Sulphonic acid.** One of the numerous organic acids containing the monovalent radical $-SO_3OH$. They are formed usually by the action of fuming sulphuric acid upon hydrocarbons; soluble in water, and decomposed by fusing with caustic potash. They are of great importance in the manufacture of drugs and dyestuffs. **Sulphophenic acid, Sulphophenolic acid.** Paraphenolsulphonic acid (see above). **Sulphoricinic acid, Sulphoricinoleic acid.** A mixture of acids obtained by the sulphonation of castor oil; the mixture of the sodium salts, known as turkey red oil, or alizarin oil, is used as a detergent and emulsifier, and in dyeing as a fixative; with phenol, it forms a pharyngeal antiseptic. **Sulphosalicylic acid.** Salicylsulphonic acid (see above). **Sulphovanadic acid.** A solution of sodium vanadate in concentrated sulphuric acid used in the detection of alkaloids. **Sulphovinic acid.** Ethyl hydrogen sulphate, $C_2H_5HSO_4$, an acid prepared from ethyl alcohol and sulphuric acid; a thick oily liquid. **Sulphuric Acid BPC 1968.** Oil of vitriol, a highly corrosive liquid, not less than 95 per cent H_2SO_4, of great importance in industry and chemical manufacture. Fuming sulphuric acid, Nordhausen acid, consists of sulphur trioxide dissolved in concentrated sulphuric acid. Aromatic sulphuric acid, elixir of vitriol, contains 10 per cent H_2SO_4, in chloroform and alcohol. Dilute Sulphuric Acid BPC 1954 (10 per cent) is used as an astringent and antiseptic in diarrhoea; also in staphylococcal infections. **Sulphurous acid.** The term usually applied to sulphur dioxide, SO_2, is more correctly the solution of the gas in water, H_2SO_3, a powerful reducing and bleaching agent; it is used in medicine as a lotion in skin affections, and as a throat and nasal spray. It forms sulphites which are valuable antiseptics, antifermentatives and antizymotics. **Sulphydric acid.** Hydrosulphuric acid (see above). **Sumbulic acid, Sumbulonic acid.** An acid found in musk root, *Ferula sumbul*; it is used as a nerve sedative and antispasmodic. **Talonic acid.** $CH_2OH(CHOH)_4COOH$, a saccharinic acid formed by the oxidation of the syrupy hexose, talose. **Tannic acid.** 1. The name given to the tannin which occurs in oak galls and sumach, which is more properly gallotannic acid, a pentagalloylglucose, or glucose esterified with digallic acid; used in tanning, dyeing and in the manufacture of ink. It is a powerful astringent and coagulant, and has been employed medicinally in throat affections, to check superficial bleeding, and to provide a coagulum in the treatment of burns (BP 1973). 2. Digallic acid, $C_6H_2(OH)_3COOC_6H_2(OH)_2COOH$, a white astringent substance, slightly soluble in water, and occurring as a glucoside in oak galls, tan bark, sumach and other plants; used as a reagent for ferric salts. **Tariric acid.** $CH_3(CH_2)_{10}C{\equiv}C(CH_2)_4COOH$, an unsaturated higher acid of the propiolic series, found naturally in *Picramnia.* **Tartaric Acid BPC 1973.** Butane diol diacid, dihydroxysuccinic acid, $COOH(CHOH)_2COOH$, an acid found in the crust that forms on grape juice, as potassium hydrogen tartarate. It exists in 4 isomeric forms, distinguished by their effect on the plane of a beam of polarized light passed through their solutions: (*a*) dextrotartaric acid, the ordinary natural form, which rotates the plane of polarized light in a clockwise direction: (*b*) laevotartaric acid, identical with (*a*) but rotating the plane counter-clockwise: (*c*) racemic acid, which is formed from ordinary tartaric acid, and consists of a mixture of equal proportions of (*a*) and (*b*), displaying therefore no optical activity: (*d*) mesotartaric acid, which is optically inactive by reason of the active groups neutralizing one another within the molecule. The tartrates (BP 1958) reduce the acidity of the urine, and are used consequently as diuretics and in the treatment of infections of the urinary tract; they also have a cathartic action. **Tartronic acid.** Hydroxymalonic acid, propanol diacid, $(CHOH)(COOH)_2$, an acid obtained by oxidizing glycerol, or by reducing mesoxalic acid. **Tartronic acid series.** The series of dibasic hydroxy acids of the general formula COOH $(CHOH)_nCOOH$, produced by the oxidation of the carbohydrates; tartronic, tartaric and saccharic acids are representative of the series. **Taurocarbamic acid.** $NH_2CONHCH_2CH_2SO_3H$, the conjugated form of taurine, detoxicated, and subsequently excreted in the urine. **Taurocholeic acid.** $C_{27}H_{47}O_6NS$, one of the bile acids, which hydrolyses to taurine and choleic acid. **Taurocholic acid.** $C_{26}H_{45}O_7NS$, one of the bile acids which, on hydrolysis, yields taurine and cholic acid. **Taurylic acid.** $C_7H_{14}O_2$, an acid that occurs in the urine under certain conditions. **Telluric acid.** H_2TeO_4, an acid formed from tellurium trioxide, TeO_3. **Tellurious acid, Tellurous acid.** H_2TeO_3, an acid formed by hydrolysis of tellurium tetrachloride. **Teracrylic acid.** Dimethylpentenic acid, $(CH_3)_2(CH)_3CH_2COOH$, a derivative of the corresponding unsaturated pentenic acid. **Terebic acid, Terebinic acid.** $C_5H_8O_2CHCOOH$, an acid produced by the oxidation of pinene, the hydrocarbon of turpentine. **Terpenylic acid.** $C_5H_8O_2CHCH_2COOH$, an acid produced, with terebic acid, by the oxidation of pinene. **Terrestric acid.** A substance which occurs during the growth of the mould *Penicillium terrestre.* **Tetrabasic acid.** An acid which offers 4 hydrogen atoms for replacement by a metal or by a basic radical. **Tetraboric acid.** Pyroboric acid (see above). **Tetracosanic acid.** $C_{24}H_{48}O_2$, a saturated fatty acid which occurs, with pentacosanic acid, in the phrenosin of the brain tissue. **Tetradecanoic acid.** Myristic acid (see above). **Tetrahydrofolic acid.** The metabolically active form of folic acid which constitutes coenzyme F, the coenzyme for the formylation reactions or so-called *active one carbon transfer.* These reactions are of considerable importance in the biosynthesis of amino acids, pyrimidines and purines, etc. **Tetramethyluric acid.** $C_5O_3N_4(CH_3)_4$, a purine derivative which occurs in tea. **Tetrathionic acid.** $H_2S_4O_6$, a fairly stable acid which forms salts, tetrathionates, which are employed in enrichment media for paratyphoid and typhoid organisms in faeces. **Tetratomic acid.** Tetrabasic acid (see above). **Tetrazotic acid.** $(CH_2)N_4$, a heterocyclic compound, not existing free, but forming many derivatives. **Tetrodonic acid.** An acid prepared from tetrodonine, a poisonous substance extracted from the roe of the Japanese fish, *Tetrodon.* **Tetrolic acid.** $CH_3C{\equiv}CCOOH$, an unsaturated acid of the propiolic series. **Thapsic acid.** A fatty acid found in *Thapsia garganica.* **Thebolactic acid.** An acid which occurs in opium. **Therapic acid.** $C_{17}H_{26}O_2$, an unsaturated acid which is found in cod-liver oil. **Thio-acetic acid.** Ethanethiolic acid, CH_3COSH, an acid prepared by the action of phosphorus pentasulphide on acetic acid. **Thio-aminopropionic acid.** Aminothiolproprionic acid (see above). **Thio-arsenic acid.** A hypothetical acid, H_3AsS_4, which forms thio-arsenates as salts. **Thio-arsenious acids.** Hypothetical acids, H_3AsS_3 (*ortho*), $H_4As_2S_5$ (*para*), and $HAsS_2$ (*meta*), which form the corresponding thio-arsenites. **Thiocarbamic acid.** Dithiocarbamic acid, NH_2CSSH, an acid formed from carbon disulphide and ammonia. **Thiocarbonic acid.** H_2CS_3, a red oily liquid obtained from the sodium thiocarbonate formed when carbon disulphide combines with sodium sulphide. **Thiocyanic acid.** Sulphocyanic acid, $N{\equiv}CSH$, a volatile pungent liquid that is unstable and polymerizes on heating, but its salts and esters are numerous and important; potassium and sodium thiocyanates are used to relieve hypertension, also in testing for ferric salts, with which they give a red coloration. **Thioglycollic acid.** $CH_2SHCOOH$, an acid employed as a delicate reagent for the detection of iron salts. **Thiolactic acid.** $CH_3CH(SH)COOH$, an acid produced by the breaking-down of keratin; the β-form (thiol), $CH_2(SH)CH(OH)COOH$, results from the deamination of cystine in the body. **Thiopyruvic acid.** $CH_2(SH)COCOOH$, an acid produced by the breaking-down of cysteine in the metabolism. **Thiosalicylic acid.** $(SH)C_6H_4COOH$, an acid best known in the form of the sodium salt. **Thiosulphuric acid.** $H_2S_2O_3$, an acid that does not occur free, but in the form of salts known as thiosulphates; sodium thiosulphate is used in papermaking, dyeing, and in photography ("hypo"); it is employed medicinally in the treatment of eczema and scabies, and in cases of metallic poisoning. **Thiuretic acid.** Thio-acetic acid (see above). **Thymic acid.** The name given to the mixture of nucleotides obtained by the careful hydrolysis of the thymonucleic acid. **Thyminic acid.** A pyrimidine derivative; it is one of the end-products of the hydrolysis of the thymonucleic acid. **Thymonucleic acid, Thymus nucleic acid.** An acid found in the thymus, the spleen and other glandular tissue; it is a polynucleotide, each nucleotide consisting of phosphoric acid, the sugar deoxyribose and one of the bases thymine, adenine, cytosine or guanine. **Tibric Acid.** BP Commission approved name for 2-chloro-5-(*cis*-3,5-dimethylpiperidinosulphonyl)benzoic acid; used in the treatment of hyperlipaemia. **Tiglic acid.** Methylcrotonic acid, $CH_3CH{=}C(CH_3)COOH$, a stereo-isomer of angelic acid which occurs in croton oil, from *Croton tiglium,* and in chamomile oil; it is an unsaturated acid, violently purgative and a vesicant. **Toluenesulphonic acid.** Cresolsulphuric acid (see above). **Toluic acid.** Methylbenzoic acid, $CH_3C_6H_4COOH$, an acid that exists in 3 isomeric forms, and is itself isomeric with phenylacetic acid; used in organic synthesis. **Toluric acid.** A conjugation of glycine and toluic acid which arises in the detoxication of xylene. **Toxicodendric acid.** An acid that occurs in poison ivy, *Rhus toxicodendron.* **Tranexamic Acid.** BP Commission approved name for *trans*-4-aminomethylcyclohexanecarboxylic acid; an antiplasminic agent. **Traumatic acid.** Decenedicarboxylic acid, $COOHCH{=}CH(CH_2)_8COOH$, a plant autocoid, or phytohormone, which takes part in the repair of damaged vegetable tissue. **Triatomic acid.** Tribasic acid (see below). **Triazoic acid.** Hydrazoic acid (see above). **Tribasic acid.** An acid which offers 3 hydrogen atoms for replacement by a metal or by a basic radical. **Trichlorethylglucuronic acid.** Urochloralic acid, $CCl_3CH_2CO(CHOH)_4COOH$, the form in which chloral is detoxicated by conjugation with glucuronic acid; it is formed in the liver and excreted thus in the urine. **Trichloro-acetic Acid BP 1973.** CCl_3COOH, an acid obtained by the oxidation of chloral hydrate; deliquescent crystals, soluble in water, alcohol or ether. It is used as an escharotic for venereal and other warts, corns and leprotic lesions, and also as an astringent and caustic in throat affections. It precipitates albumin and is employed as a reagent in urinary analysis. **Tricyanic acid.** Cyanuric acid (see above). **Trihydroxybenzoic acid.** Gallic acid (see above). **Trihydroxycholic acid.** Cholic acid (see above). **Triketocholanic acid.** An acid produced by the oxidation of the OH groups at positions 3, 7 and 12 in cholic acid to ketone, CO, groups. **Trimethylacetic acid.** *See* VALERIC ACID, below. **Trimethylaminoacetic acid.** $(CH_3)_3(OH)NCH_2COOH$, an acid that forms, as anhydride, the cyclic base, betaine, which occurs in beetroot. **Trimethylbenzoic acid.** Durylic acid (see above). **Trimethyluric acid.** Caffuric acid (see above). **Triosephosphoric acids.** Glyceraldehyde 3-phosphate and dihydroxyacetone phosphate; glycolytic intermediates formed by the cleavage of fructose diphosphate by aldolase, and themselves interconvertible in the presence of triosephosphate isomerase. **Triticonucleic acid.** An acid occurring in wheat germ. **Tropic acid.** Phenylhydracrylic acid, phenylhydroxypropionic acid, $CH_2(OH)CH(C_6H_5)COOH$, a hydroxy saturated acid; it is prepared from atropine, which is its tropine ester. **Tropinecarboxylic acid.** Ecgonine, $C_9H_{15}O_3N$, a crystalline substance derived from coca leaves. **Tuberculinic acid.** A nucleic acid found in tubercle bacilli. **Tuberculostearic acid.** Methylstearic acid, $CH_3(CH_2)_7CH(CH_3)(CH_2)_8COOH$, an acid that occurs in bovine tubercle bacilli. **Tungstic acid.** An acid, H_2WO_4, formed by the trioxide of tungsten. The name is sometimes applied to the trioxide itself.

Ulmic acid. Geic acid, $C_{20}H_{14}O_6$, an acid obtained from peat, and the sap and bark of certain species of elm, *Ulmus.* **Umbellic**

acid. $(OH)_2C_6H_3(CH)_2COOH$, an acid present in galbanum, the gum resin of *Ferula galbaniflua*, and in species of *Daphne*; umbelliferone is the lactone. **Undecenoic Acid BP 1973.** Undecylenic acid, $CH_2{=}CHCH_2(CH_2)_7COOH$, an unsaturated acid produced by the heating of castor oil. It is used as a fungicide. **Undecylenic acid.** Undecenoic acid (see above). **Undecylinic acid.** $CH_3(CH_2)_9COOH$, a straight-chain carboxylic acid which is used as a topical therapeutic agent in ringworm infections. **Uramino-acetic acid.** Glycoluric acid (see above). **Uraminobenzoic acid.** $NH_2CONHC_6H_4COOH$, an acid that appears in the urine as the result of the conjugation of carbamic acid with aminobenzoic acid when the latter is administered. **Urea carbonic acid.** Allophanic acid (see above). **Ureido acid.** An acid formed by the union of urea with a dibasic acid, 1 carboxyl group of which is retained. **Ureous acid.** Name given to the purine base, xanthine, which occurs in the blood and urine. **Uric acid.** Lithic acid, trihydroxypurine, $C_5H_4N_4O_3$, a white crystalline substance, slightly soluble in water, but soluble in alkalis; it exists in 2 tautomeric forms, keto and enol. It is a constituent of the urine of carnivorous animals and, to a smaller extent, of human urine, as the result of the breakdown of the purines of the nucleic acids and nucleoproteins. In the condition known as gout, uric acid and urates are deposited in the joints; they also appear in calculi and urinary sediments, and can be detected there by the murexide test. **Uridylic acid.** Uridine-3′-phosphate, $C_4H_3N_2O_2C_5H_8O_4PO(OH)_2$, a nucleotide obtained from yeast-nuclei acid by alkaline hydrolysis. It is a combination of uracil, D-ribose and phosphoric acid. **Urine acid.** Name applied to the acid constituents of the urine, mainly phosphoric and uric acids. **Urobenzoic acid.** Hippuric acid (see above). **Urocanic acid.** Iminazole-acrylic acid, $C_3H_3N_2CH{=}CHCOOH$, a ptomaine in dogs' urine, derived from histidine. **Urochloralic acid, Urochloric acid.** Trichlorethylglucuronic acid (see above). **Uroferric acid.** A protein in urine. **Uroleucic acid, Uroleucinic acid.** $C_9H_{10}O_5$, a constituent of alkaptonuric urine. **Uronic acids.** The series of polyhydroxy-aldehyde monobasic acids of the general formula, $CHO(CHOH)_nCOOH$, produced by the oxidation of the terminal alcohol group of monosaccharides whilst the aldehyde group remains protected; glucuronic and galacturonic acids are representative. **Uroproteic acid.** A complex acid observed in dogs' urine. **Uroxanic acid.** $C(NHCONH_2)_2(COOH)_2$, a urinary pigment derived from uric acid. **Ursolic acid.** $C_{29}H_{46}(OH)COOH$, an acid extracted from the bearberry, *Arctostaphylos uva-ursae*, the wild cherry, *Prunus serotina*, and the apple, *Pyrus malus*. **Uvitic acid.** Mesitic acid, $CH_3C_6H_3(COOH)_2$, an oxidation product of mesitylene, which forms crystals insoluble in water.

Valerianic acid, Valeric acid. Pentanoic acid, C_4H_9COOH, an acid that exists in 4 forms: (*a*) propylacetic acid, normal valeric acid, $CH_3(CH_2)_3COOH$, does not occur in nature: (*b*) isovaleric acid, isopropyl acetic acid, $(CH_3)_2CHCH_2COOH$, is found free in valerian root, *Valeriana officinalis*, angelica root, *Angelica archangelica*, decomposed cheese, the perspiration of the feet, and in certain diseases in the urine; used as a sedative in hysteria and in neuroses: (*c*) methylethylacetic acid, methyl butane acid, active valeric acid, $(CH_3)(C_2H_5)CHCOOH$, occurs with (*b*) in nature, and is in 3 isomers, dextro, laevo and racemic, the latter being a mixture of the 2 former: (*d*) trimethylacetic acid, pivalic acid, $(CH_3)_3CCOOH$, has a smell of acetic acid, which it resembles. **Acid value.** 1. A measure of the acidity of a solution expressed as a fraction of normality. *See* NORMAL ACID (above). 2. Acid number. *See* NUMBER. **Vanadic acids.** Acids derived from vanadium pentoxide, V_2O_5; *meta*, HVO_3; *ortho*, H_3VO_4; *para*, $H_4V_2O_7$. The salt, ammonium vanadate, is used as a reagent for salicylates. **Vanillic acid.** Hydroxymethoxybenzoic acid, methylprotocatechuic acid, $CH_3OC_6H_3(OH)COOH$, an acid prepared from vanilla pods, *Vanilla planifolia*. **Vanilmandelic acid (VMA).** 3-Methoxy-4-hydroxymandelic acid, a metabolite of adrenaline and of noradrenaline. *See* EXCRETION, CATECHOLAMINE. **Valproic acid.** 2-Propylpentanoic acid; an anticonvulsant. **Veratric acid.** Dimethoxybenzoic acid, $(CH_3O)_2C_6H_3COOH$, an acid occurring in the seeds of *Veratrum sabadilla*. **Violuric acid.** Oxime alloxan, isonitrosobarbituric acid, $C_4H_2N_2O_3NOH$, an acid prepared from hydroxylamine and alloxan. **Vitriolic acid.** Sulphuric acid (see above); an obsolete name. **Vulpic acid, Vulpinic acid.** $C_{19}H_{14}O_5$, an acid found in the lichen *Cetraria vulpina*.

Xanthic acid, Xanthogenic acid, Xanthonic acid. Ethyloxydithiocarbonic acid, $S{=}C(OC_2H_5)SH$, is an unstable oil, insoluble in water; the copper salt is used in indigo dyeing. **Xanthoproteic acid.** The yellow coloration produced in protein by concentrated nitric acid. **Xanthurenic acid.** 4,8-Dihydroxyquinoline-2-carboxylic acid, $C_6H_3(OH)C_3N(OH)(COOH)$. A yellow pigment excreted in the urine after ingestion of tryptophane in pyridoxine deficiency in man and animals. **Xanthylic acid.** A nucleic acid which yields a nucleoside containing xanthine. **Xylic acid.** $(CH_3)_2C_6H_3COOH$, an acid that occurs in 6 isomers. **Xylidic acid.** Methylisophthalic acid, $C_6H_3(CH_3)(COOH)_2$, an acid isomeric with uvitic acid. **Xylosic acid.** $CH_2OH(CHOH)_3COOH$, a penturonic acid obtained by the oxidation of the pentose, xylose.

Yeast-nucleic acid. A type of nucleic acid found in yeast, wheat and other similar substances. *See* NUCLEIC ACID (above). **Yohimbic acid.** $C_{20}H_{24}N_2O_3$, an acid obtained from the alkaloid yohimbine, extracted from the bark of *Corynanthe johimbe*. **Zincic acid.** H_2ZnO_2, an acid formed from the amphoteric zinc hydroxide; it gives rise to salts, zincates. **Zoomaric acid.** $CH_3(CH_2)_5CHCH(CH_2)_7COOH$, an unsaturated acid which has been identified with palmitoleic acid, and is found in whale oil, seal oil and cod-liver oil. [L *acidus* sour.]

See also: NISSL, REINECKE, SCHEELE.

acid-fast, acid-proof (as·id·fahst, as·id·proof). Terms descriptive of a substance which when stained is not easily decolorized by acids or other similar agents. [acid, AS *faest*, OFr. *prueve*.]

acidaemia (as·id·e·me·ah). An increase of $[H^+]$ in the blood. **Butyric and hexanoic acidaemia.** A fatal familial disease of infants in which breath, blood and urine smell of sweaty feet. **Isovaleric acidaemia.** Defect in oxidation of isovaleric acid to beta-methyl-crotonic acid, leading to accumulation of isovaleric acid which causes acidosis, vomiting, coma and an odour of sweaty feet. **Methylmalonic acidaemia.** A congenital condition of recurrent acidosis due to methylmalonic acid, in some cases responsive to massive cyanocobalamin dosage. [acid, Gk *haima* blood.]

acidaminuria (as·id·am·in·**ewr**′·e·ah). A condition in which there is an excessive amount of amino acids in the urine.

acidification (as·**id**·e·fik·**a**′·shun). 1. The process of converting into an acid, or making acid. 2. The process or act of becoming acid. [acid, L *facere* to make.]

acidify (as·**id**·e·fi). 1. To make acid. 2. To undergo the process of becoming acid. [see prec.]

acidimeter (as·id·**im**·et·er). An apparatus used to determine how much free acid a solution contains. [acid, meter.]

acidimetry (as·id·**im**·et·re). The process of determining the proportion of free acids contained in a solution. [see prec.]

acidism, acidismus (as·id·izm, as·id·**iz**·mus). A condition of acid intoxication caused by taking acids into the body. [L *acidus* sour.]

acidity (as·**id**·it·e). 1. Sourness, or sharpness of taste. 2. The state of being acid, or containing an excess of acid. 3. In chemistry, the capacity of a compound to yield hydrogen ions in aqueous solution, or a state of dissociation in which the concentration of hydrogen exceeds 10^{-7} g/l. **Free acidity.** The amount of uncombined acid present. **Total acidity.** The total amount of acid present, both ionized and undissociated. [see prec.]

acidocyte (as·**id**·o·site). An acidophil cell, e.g. eosinophil. [acid, Gk *kytos* cell.]

acidocytopenia (as·**id**·o·si·to·**pe**′·ne·ah). A condition in which there is pathological reduction in the eosinophil leucocytes in the blood. [acidocyte, Gk *penia* poverty.]

acidocytosis (as·**id**·o·si·**to**′·sis). A condition in which there is an abnormally large number of eosinophil leucocytes in the blood. Eosinophilia is a better name. [acidocyte, Gk *-osis* condition.]

acidogenic (as·id·o·**jen'**·ik). Giving rise to acidity, particularly in the urine. [acid, Gk *genein* to produce.]
acidology (as·id·**ol**·o·je). The science or formulated knowledge of surgical appliances. [Gk *akis* pointed instrument, *logos* science.]
acidometer (as·id·**om**·et·er). Acidimeter.
acidometry (as·id·**om**·et·re). Acidimetry.
acidopenia (as·**id**·o·**pe'**·ne·ah). Acidocytopenia.
acidophil, acidophile (as·**id**·o·fil, as·**id**·o·file). 1. A substance capable of absorbing acid stains or having an affinity for them. 2. An acid-staining cell of the anterior lobe of the hypophysis cerebri. Eosinophil cell. 3. The name applied to any organism that flourishes in any medium of strongly acid reaction. **Amphophilic acidophil.** A cell which has greater affinity for acid dyes, but which takes the stain also of basic dyes; amphophilic oxyphil. [acid, Gk *philein* to love.]
acidophilic (as·**id**·o·**fil'**·ik). 1. A term descriptive of micro-organisms which thrive in strongly acid media. 2. Readily taking the stain of an acid dye. [see prec.]
acidophilous (as·id·**of**·il·us). Acidophilic.
acidoproteolytic (as·id·o·**pro**·te·o·**lit'**·ik). Acid-producing and protein-digesting. [acid, protein, Gk *lysis* a loosing.]
acidoresistance (as·id·o·re·**zis'**·tans). Acid resistance; the property possessed by some bacteria, after staining, of resisting decolorization with acid.
acidoresistant (as·id·o·re·**zis'**·tant). A term descriptive of those bacteria which cannot be decolorized by acids. [acid, resistant.]
acidosic (as·id·o·sik). Referring to or affected with acidosis.
acidosis (as·id·**o**·sis). An increase in the [H^+] in body fluids above the normal range. Usually defined as a decrease in pH of the blood below 7.36. It may be confined to a fluid compartment. **Carbon dioxide acidosis.** A condition in which there is retention of carbon dioxide in the blood caused by lack of air in the lungs, as in drowning. **Compensated acidosis.** A condition in which the pH of the blood has been kept within its proper limits, although the blood bicarbonate usually is lower than normal. **Gaseous acidosis.** Carbon dioxide acidosis (see above). **Metabolic acidosis.** Acidosis arising from an accumulation of H^+ ions in body fluids either because of excessive production (e.g. diabetic coma, hypoxia) by metabolic process, or failure of normal elimination by the kidney (renal failure) or excessive administration of acids. The excess H^+ ions are buffered by HCO_3^- ions in the blood and tissues, thus reducing [HCO_3^-]. The excess CO_2 so formed leads to a rise in $PaCO_2$ and this stimulates respiration to promote elimination of CO_2. **Respiratory acidosis.** Acidosis resulting from inadequate elimination of CO_2 from the lungs. Retained CO_2 combines with water to form carbonic acid which dissociates into H^+ and HCO_3^- ions resulting in a rise in the concentration of both ions in blood. **Uncompensated acidosis.** A form of acidaemia in which, usually, the blood bicarbonate is lowered. [acid, Gk *-osis* condition.]
acidosteophyte (as·id·**os**·te·o·fite). An osteophyte with a sharp point. [Gk *akis* point, osteophyte.]
acidotic (as·id·**ot**·ik). Characterized by acidosis.
acidoxyl (as·id·**ox**·il). The negative group of an organic acid which remains when the hydrogen of the acid hydroxyl is removed.
acidulate (as·**id**·ew·late). To acidify. [see foll.]
acidulous (as·**id**·ew·lus). Having acid characteristics; mildly acid. [L *acidulus* slightly sour.]
acidulum (as·**id**·ew·lum). Acid salt. *See* SALT. [see prec.]
acidum (**as**·id·um). Acid. **Acidum Acetylsalicylicum.** *European Pharmacopoeia* name for Aspirin BP 1973. **Acidum Ascorbicum.** *European Pharmacopoeia* name for Ascorbic Acid BP 1973. **Acidum Boricum.** *European Pharmacopoeia* name for Boric Acid BP 1973. **Acidum Hydrochloricum Concentratum.** *European Pharmacopoeia* name for Hydrochloric Acid BP 1973. **Acidum Hychrochloricum Dilutum.** *European Pharmacopoeia* name for Dilute Hydrochloric Acid BP 1973. **Acidum Phosphoricum Concentratum.** *European Pharmacopoeia* name for Phosphoric Acid BP 1973.
aciduria (as·id·**ewr**·e·ah). The condition in which the urine is acid. **Arginosuccinic aciduria.** An error of amino acid metabolism due to defect of the enzyme arginosuccinase, causing hair-loss due to monilethrix. **Orotic aciduria.** Urinary excretion of orotic acid, an intermediate metabolite in pyrimidine synthesis, with megaloblastic anaemia.
aciduric (as·id·**ewr**·ik). Acidophilic. [acid, L *durare* to endure.]
acidyl (**as**·id·il). The acid radical which remains when the acid hydroxyl OH group is removed from the formula of an organic acid.
acidylated (as·id·il·a·ted). Having had an acidyl or acyl group introduced into the molecule.
acidylation (as·id·il·a·shun). The introduction of an acid radical into the molecule of an organic compound.
acies (a·se·eez). A margin or border. **Acies thalami optici.** The auditory striae. *See* STRIA. [L edge.]
acinar (**as**·in·ar). Associated with or affecting an acinus. [L *acinus* grape.]
acinetic (a·sin·**et**·ik). Referring to acinesia.
acinic (as·**in**·ik). Referring to an acinus.
aciniform (as·**in**·e·form). Shaped like a grape or a bunch of grapes, and generally referring to glands. [acinus, form.]
acinitis (as·in·**i**·tis). Glandular inflammation affecting the acini. [acinus, Gk *-itis* inflammation.]
Acinitrazole (as·in·i·traz·ole). BP Commission approved name for 2-acetamido-5-nitrothiazole, an orally-administered treatment for trichomoniasis.
acinose (**as**·in·oze). 1. Composed of acini. 2. Having a resemblance to an acinus or a grape.
acinotubular (**as**·in·o·**tew'**·bew·lar). Descriptive of a gland or similar tissue in which the acini are tubular.
acinous (**as**·in·us). Acinose.
acinus [NA] (**as**·in·us). The tube leading to the smallest lobule of a compound gland; it is characterized by a narrow lumen. **Acinus lienis.** A corpuscle of the kidney. [L grape.]
Acipenser (a·si·**pen**·ser). A genus of fish; sturgeons. **Acipenser huso.** One of the species from which isinglass is obtained. [L.]
ackee (ak·**ee**). *Blighia sapida*, a plant found in Jamaica, eating the unripe fruit of which gives rise to sickness, vomiting and symptoms of poisoning of the nervous system. Two polypeptides, hypoglycin 1 and 2, cause profound hypoglycaemia, which is the basis of the symptomatology.
Ackermann, Conrad Theodor (b. 1825). German physician. **Ackermann's angle.** The inclination of the base of the skull defined by a special method, useful in the diagnosis of kyphosis and hydrocephalus.
aclasis, aclasia (a·**kla**·sis, a·**kla**·se·ah). A pathological process which follows a consistent pattern of development. **Diaphysial aclasis.** A condition in which the bone structure in the cartilage between the epiphysis and the diaphysis is abnormal or imperfect; a particular form is dyschondroplasia, in which bone fails to develop in the fetal cartilage and a dwarf with short limbs is produced. **Tarso-epiphyseal aclasis.** Trevor's disease. [Gk *a*, *klasis* a breaking.]
aclastic (a·**klas**·tik). In optics, not capable of refracting light. [see prec.]
acleistocardia (a·kli·sto·**kar**·de·ah). Patent foramen ovale. *See* FORAMEN. [Gk *a*, *kleistos* closed, *kardia* heart.]
aclinic (a·**klin**·ik). In physics, denoting absence of dipping or inclination. [Gk *a*, *klinein* to lean.]
acmaesthesia (ak·mes·**the**·ze·ah). A condition in which there is a sensation as of a sharp point in contact with the skin. [Gk *akme* highest point, aesthesia.]
acmastic (ak·**mas**·tik). Referring to the acme of a disease. [Gk *akmastikos* at the height.]
acme (**ak**·me). In reference to disease, the height or crisis with precedent epacmastic phase and subsequent paracmastic phase. [Gk *akme* highest point.]
acmon (**ak**·mon). The incus. [Gk *akmon* anvil.]
acne (**ak**·ne). A generic term denoting an inflammatory disease occurring in or around the sebaceous glands, generally affecting

the face, chest and back, the eruption being characterized by papules and pustules, or by cysts and other more specific lesions. **Adolescent acne, Acne adolescentium.** Acne vulgaris (see below). **Acne aggregata seu conglobata.** Acne conglobata (see below). **Acne agminata.** Acnitis. **Acne albida.** Milium. **Amputation stump acne.** Acneiform pustules and nodules at an amputation stump. **Apocrine acne.** Name given to certain forms of hidradenitis suppurativa. **Acne artificialis.** A papular or pustular eruption produced by the internal administration of iodides, iodized salt or bromides, or by the external application of irritants such as tar. **Acne atrophica.** 1. A term formerly employed to describe the small scars and pits in the skin left by acne vulgaris. 2. Acne varioliformis (see below). **Acné boutonneuse.** Acne vulgaris (see below). **Bromide acne.** A characteristic eruption due to intolerance to bromides. *See also* ACNE COAGMINATA (below). **Bromine acne.** An eruption due to exposure to bromine. *See also* ACNE COAGMINATA (below). **Acne cachecticorum.** 1. Furuncular or sluggish abscess-like lesions occurring as a variety of acne vulgaris. 2. Acne scrofulosorum (see below). 3. An acneiform eruption in which comedones are not formed; the lesions are indolent purple-red papules or nodules, develop mainly on the legs and trunk in wasting diseases, and ultimately become replaced by scars. **Acné chéloidienne, Acné chéloidique.** Dermatitis papillaris capillitii. **Chloric acne, Chlorine acne.** An acne of bizarre distribution due to exposure to chlorine or to chlorinated hydrocarbons. **Acne ciliaris.** An affection of the margins of the eyelids. **Acne coagminata.** A term occasionally employed to denote the variety of bromine or bromide acne in which the lesions consist of groups of large pustules. **Colloid acne.** Scattered yellow transparent papules developing on the face at the sites of acneic lesions, from which on puncture a yellow jelly can be extruded; colloid milium. **Common acne.** Acne vulgaris (see below). **Acne conglobata.** A severe eruption characterized by numerous comedones, deep nodules, suppurating plaques, torpid abscesses, canalizing sinuses and large papillomata, occurring almost exclusively in men considerably after puberty, and most severely on the lumbar area, buttocks and thighs; healing takes place by the formation of scars, many of which show characteristic bands or bridges of fibrous tissue. **Cystic acne.** A form of acne in which sebaceous cysts are present. **Acné décalvante.** Folliculitis decalvans. **Acne dorsalis.** Acne vulgaris of the back. **Acne ephebica.** Acne vulgaris in adolescents. **Epidemic acne.** Keratosis follicularis contagiosa of Brook; cystic acne affecting a group of individuals in which contact with, or ingestion of, chlorinated naphthalenes may be suspected. **Acne erythematosa.** Rosacea. **Acné excorié des jeunes filles, Excoriated acne.** An acneiform eruption in nervous subjects who constantly squeeze and scratch the lesions; it may equally affect males, in which case the eruption is termed *excoriated acne.* **Acne frontalis.** Acne varioliformis affecting the forehead. **Halogen acne.** Acne due to contact with halogens, e.g. chlorine or bromine acne. Cf. PERNA. **Honeycomb acne.** Folliculitis ulerythematosa reticulata. **Acne hypertrophica.** A name formerly used to denote hypertrophic or cheloidal scarring following acne vulgaris. **Acne indurata.** Chronic acne vulgaris in which the lesions are pustular and deeply seated, with inflammatory thickening of the underlying tissues; much disfigurement may ensue. **Infantile acne.** Acne occurring between 3 months and 2 years of age. **Iodine acne.** An eruption caused by the use of iodine-containing substances. **Acne keloid.** Dermatitis papillaris capillitii. **Acne keratosa.** A variety of acne vulgaris characterized by the development on the face of red nodules with suppurating apices, and the formation of crusts enclosing horny plugs which must be removed before the lesions will heal. **Lupoid acne, Acne luposa.** Acne varioliformis (see below). **Acne medicamentosa.** Acne resulting from the medicinal use of iodine, bromine, camphor, tar and certain other substances. **Acne mentagra.** Coccogenic sycosis. *See* SYCOSIS. **Acne miliaris.** Acne with multiple milia. **Acne molluscoidea, Acne molluscum.** Molluscum contagiosum. **Necrotic acne, Acne necrotica.** Acne varioliformis (see below). **Acne necrotica miliaris.** A pustular folliculitis or perifolliculitis of the scalp associated with much itching. It is probably staphylococcal in origin; the lesions leave scars, and alopecia cicatrisata may ensue. **Acne neonatorum.** Acne of the newborn and up to 3 months of age. **Occupational acne.** Acne resulting from occupational exposure to oils, tar or chlorinated products. **Oil acne.** Acne resulting from external exposure to oil. **Pancreatic acne, Acne pancreatica.** A condition of the pancreas in which enlargement of the minute lobules of the pancreatic duct gives rise to small cysts. **Acne papulosa.** A variety of acne vulgaris in which the lesions are small papules with but little inflammation. **Petroleum acne.** An acneiform eruption occurring among those who work with crude petroleum. **Acne picealis.** A type of acne caused by exposure to or contact with coal tar, heavy coal-tar distillates or coal-tar pitch. **Acne punctata.** A variety of acne vulgaris in which the lesions are all small conical papules, each having a comedo at its apex. **Acne punctata albida.** Milium. **Acne pustulosa.** A type of acne vulgaris in which the majority of lesions are pustular; serious disfigurement may ensue. **Acne rodens.** Acne varioliformis (see below). **Acne rosacea.** Rosacea. **Acne scorbutica.** The eruption of follicular papules which occurs in scurvy. **Acne scrofulosorum.** Lichen scrofulosorum, an eruption characterized by small indolent papulopustular or acneiform lesions, particularly on the hips and buttocks; it occurs in infants or children suffering from tuberculosis of a surgical type. **Acne sebacea.** Seborrhoea. **Acne sebacea cornea, Acné sébacée cornée.** Keratosis follicularis contagiosa. **Acne sebacea molluscum.** Sebaceous cysts. *See* CYST. **Acne simplex.** Acne vulgaris (see below). **Steroid acne.** Acne caused by corticosteroid drugs, either taken internally or applied externally. **Syphilitic acne, Acne syphilitica.** An eruption of scattered sharply-pointed pustules occurring in secondary syphilis. **Tar acne.** Acne picealis (see above). **Acne tarsi.** A type of acne which affects the sebaceous glands of the eyelids. **Acne telangiectodes.** Acnitis. **Trade acne.** Any acneiform eruption caused by exposure to an industrial hazard; examples are chlorine and halogen acne. **Tropical acne.** Acne caused or aggravated by high temperature with high humidity. **Acne urticata.** A malady affecting neurotic persons in which papules and weals develop associated with rubbing and scratching. **Acne varioliformis.** A chronic inflammatory eruption characterized by the development of moderately superficial papulopustular lesions, discrete or grouped, occurring most commonly on the forehead and the adjacent part of the scalp, particularly at the temples. It has been regarded as a hybrid of pustular folliculitis and seborrhoea, with the forehead and the middle facial and mid-thoracic regions as the sites of election. The lesions leave pitted scars. **Acne venenata.** Acne of external, chemical origin. **Acné vermoulante.** Folliculitis ulerythematosa reticulata. **Acne vulgaris.** A common malady which commences in adolescence, involving the pilosebaceous glands, particularly of the face, chest and back, and notorious for its chronicity. The lesions consist of comedones, papules, pustules, miliary sebaceous cysts (*whiteheads*) and steatoid or colloid cysts. The primary cause is probably endocrine, but many other factors are also involved. [corruption of Gk *akme* point.]

acneform, acneiform (ak·ne·form, ak·ne·e·form). Having a resemblance to acne. [acne, form.]

acnegen (ak·ne·jen). A substance which causes, or aggravates, acne. [acne, Gk *genein* to produce.]

acnemia (ak·ne·me·ah). 1. A condition in which the calf of the leg is atrophied. 2. Congenital lack of both lower extremities. [Gk *a*, *kneme* lower leg.]

acnemous (ak·ne·mus). 1. With defective calves of the legs. 2. With legs entirely missing. [see prec.]

acnitis (ak·ni·tis). A name used to denote an eruption of round, red-brown papules protruding somewhat from the skin, in which they are firmly embedded; the lesions undergo necrosis and leave scars. The face is the site of election, but occasionally the trunk and limbs are affected. Of uncertain aetiology, most authorities regard it as a variety of papulonecrotic tuberculide, but many consider that the eruption can be caused by organisms other than the tubercle bacillus; others have stated that the malady is a variety of disseminated follicular lupus. [acne, Gk *-itis* inflammation.]

acoasma (ak·o·**az**·mah). A hallucination of sound in which auditory sensations of an indefinite character are experienced. [Gk *akouein* to hear.]

Acocanthera (ak·o·**kan**·ther·ah). A group of mainly tropical herbs, shrubs, or trees belonging to the family Apocynaeceae; the dogbanes. **Acocanthera schimperi.** A species used in Africa as an arrow poison, from which ouabain is obtained. [Gk *akoke* point, *antheros* blooming.]

acoelia (a·**se**·le·ah). The absence of a natural body cavity. [Gk *a koilia* cavity.]

acoelious (a·**se**·le·us). Without a coelom. The term is applied to conditions of extreme emaciation. [see prec.]

acoelomate (a·**se**·lo·mate). One lacking a natural body cavity. [acoelia.]

acoelosis (a·se·**lo**·sis). Acoelia.

acoelous (a·**se**·lus). In biology, devoid of intestines. [acoelia.]

acoenaesthesia (a·sen·es·**the**′·ze·ah). 1. Lack of the normal consciousness of being alive or of bodily function. 2. In physical disorders, loss of the sense of well-being. [Gk *a, koinos* common, aesthesia.]

acognosia, acognosy (ak·og·**no**·ze·ah, ak·**og**·no·se). Knowledge of remedies; the study of remedies. [Gk *akos* cure, *gnosis* knowledge.]

Acokanthera (ak·o·**kan**·ther·ah). Acocanthera.

acology (ak·**ol**·o·je). Therapeutics; knowledge of curative drugs. [Gk *akos* cure, *logos* science.]

acolous (a·**kol**·us). Destitute of limbs. [Gk *a, kolon* limb.]

acomia (a·**ko**·me·ah). 1. The state of being bald. 2. The state in which hair on other parts of the body is diminished or lacking. [Gk *a, kome* hair.]

acomous (a·**ko**·mus). Without hair; bald. [see prec.]

aconative (a·**kon**·at·iv). Destitute of conation, i.e. without desire to act or impulsion to make an effort of any kind whether psychical or physical; loss of the striving instinct. [Gk *a*, L *conari* to attempt.]

aconine (**ak**·on·een). $C_{25}H_{41}O_9N$. A virtually non-poisonous alkaloid of aconite.

aconitase (ak·**on**·it·aze). Aconitate hydratase.

aconitate hydratase (ak·**on**·it·ate **hi**·drat·aze). The enzyme catalysing the interconversion of citrate and isocitrate; *in vitro cis*-aconitate is a third product. The enzyme occurs in both cytoplasmic and mitochondrial compartments.

Aconite (**ak**·on·ite). 1. A genus of plants of the family Ranunculaceae. 2. (BPC 1968) Aconite root, aconiti tuber, aconiti radix, the tuberous root of the monkshood, or wolfsbane, *Aconitum napellus* Linn., collected in the autumn and dried. It contains the important alkaloids aconitine, picraconitine and aconine. Applied to the tongue it produces a characteristic tingling sensation followed by local anaesthesia; in toxic doses this tingling occurs first in the throat and stomach and later in the skin, with a copious flow of saliva, a feeling of warmth and some muscular weakness. Death may result from cardiac or respiratory failure, sometimes preceded by convulsions. The drug is excreted in the urine, but small quantities have been found in the saliva and bile. Externally the liniments are useful in the treatment of neuralgia; internally aconite is an antipyretic but should not be used in preference to other less toxic drugs. [Gk *akoniton.*]

aconitina (ak·on·it·e·nah). Aconitine.

aconitine (ak·**on**·it·een). $C_{34}H_{47}O_{11}N$, a poisonous alkaloid derived from *Aconitum napellus,* the common monkshood. It stimulates sensory nerve-endings, producing a tingling sensation, and is accordingly included in some liniments.

Aconitum (ak·on·**i**·tum). A genus of plants of the family Ranunculaceae. **Aconitum ferox.** A species from which acraconitine or pseudo-aconitine is obtained. **Aconitum heterophyllum.** The source of a non-toxic bitter alkaloid, atisine. **Aconitum napellus** Linn. The species from which aconite is obtained. [Gk *akoniton.*]

aconuresis (ak·on·ewr·**e**′·sis). Involuntary passing of urine. [Gk *akon* unwilling, uresis.]

acopia (a·**ko**·pi·ah). Difficulty in making a copy on paper from printed or written text. [Gk *a* not, L *copia* transcript.]

acoprosis (a·kop·**ro**·sis). Lack of faeces in the bowel or deficiency of formation of faeces. [Gk *a, kopros* excrement.]

acoprous (a·**kop**·rus). Devoid of faecal residue. [see prec.]

acopyrine (**ak**·o·**pi**′·reen). Acetopyrin; a compound of antipyrin and acetylsalicylic acid that is soluble in hot water or alcohol. It is analgesic and antirheumatic, and is used in sciatica and influenza.

acor (**a**·kor). Acidity, e.g. gastric acidity. [L a sour taste.]

acorea (ak·o·**re**·ah). The condition in which the pupil of the eye is absent. [Gk *a, kore* pupil.]

acoria (a·**ko**·re·ah). A nervous condition in which there is a feeling of hunger, although food may have been taken; an insatiable craving for food of all kinds. [Gk *a, koros* satiety.]

acormus (a·**kor**·mus). A monster without any or with only a rudimentary body. [Gk *a, kormos* trunk.]

Acorus (**ak**·o·rus). A group of rush-like plants belonging to the arum family. *See* CALAMUS. [Gk *akoros* yellow flag.]

acosmia (a·**koz**·me·ah). 1. Deviation from the normal course of a disease. 2. Ill health. 3. Deformity with associated irregularity of the features. 4. Loss of hair and resultant alopecia. [Gk *a kosmos* order.]

acostate (a·**kos**·tate). Without ribs. [Gk *a*, L *costa* rib.]

acouaesthesia (ak·**oo**·es·**the**′·ze·ah). The faculty of being able to hear well; normal function of hearing. [Gk *akouein* to hear aesthesia.]

acouasm (ak·**oo**·azm). Hallucination of sound of simple type. [Gk *akouein* to hear.]

aculalion (ak·oo·**la**·le·on). A microtelephonic instrument used in teaching deaf-mutes to speak. [Gk *akouein* to hear, *lalia* speech.]

acoumeter (ak·**oo**·me·ter). 1. An instrument used in the determination of the degree of acuteness as well as the accuracy of hearing. 2. An apparatus which produces a typical vowel sound to be used, in comparison, as the standard of that sound. [see foll.]

See also: POLITZER.

acoumetric (ak·oo·**met**·rik). Referring to the acuity of the hearing. [Gk *akouein* to hear, meter.]

acoumetry (ak·**oo**·met·re). The testing of the extent or of the acuteness of the sense of hearing. [see prec.]

acouometer (ak·oo·**om**·et·er). Acoumeter.

acouoxylon (ak·oo·**ox**·il·on). A stethoscope made of pine-wood. [Gk *akouein* to hear, *xylon* wood.]

acousia (ak·**oo**·se·ah). 1. Hearing, or the ability to hear. [Gk *akouein* to hear.] 2. Action performed independently of the will. [Gk *akousos* unwilling.]

acousma (ak·**oos**·mah). Hallucination of hearing; hearing of imaginary sounds. [Gk *akousma* something heard.]

acousmatagnosis (ak·**oos**·mat·ag·**no**′·sis). In certain mental diseases, inability to recognize sounds; also inability to carry sounds in the memory. [acousma, Gk *a, gnosis* knowledge.]

acousmatamnesia (ak·**oos**·mat·am·**ne**′·ze·ah). A defect of memory resulting in inability to recall sounds. [acousma, amnesia.]

acousmetric (ak·oos·**met**·rik). Acoumetric.

acoustic (ak·**oos**·tik). Relating to the organs or to the sense of hearing, or to the science of sound. [Gk *akouein* to hear.]

acousticophobia (ak·oos·tik·o·**fo**′·be·ah). A functional disorder in which there is a morbid fear of loud sounds. [Gk *akouein* to hear, *phobein* to fear.]

acoustics (ak·**oos**·tix). In physics, the science, in general, of sound, e.g. production, transmission, effects. [Gk *akouein* to hear.]

acoutometer (ak·oo·**tom**·et·er). Acoumeter.

acquired (ak·**wi**·rd). A term used to describe a condition, habit or other characteristic which is not present at birth, but which is developed in the individual by reaction to environment. [L *acquirere* to obtain.]

acquisitus (ak·**wiz**·it·us). Acquired. [L.]

acra (**ak**·rah). The distal portion of the limbs. [Gk *akron* extremity.]

acracholia (ak·rah·**ko**·le·ah). The state of being in a passion; a paroxysm of passion. [Gk *a*, *krasis* moderation, *chole* bile.]

acraconitine (ak·rah·**kon**·it·een). Pseudo-aconitine, $C_{36}H_{51}O_{12}N$. A crystalline alkaloid obtained from *Aconitum ferox*; it has the same action as aconitine, but is more potent.

acragnosis (ak·rag·**no**·sis). Acro-agnosis.

acral (**ak**·ral). Referring to or affecting the extremities. [Gk *akron* extremity.]

acrania (a·**kra**·ne·ah). A teratomatous condition in which the skull is incomplete or partial; in extreme cases the skull is absent. [Gk *a*, *kranion* skull.]

acranial (a·**kra**·ne·al). Affected with acrania; lacking a skull.

acranius (a·**kra**·ne·us). A monster with an incomplete or only partial skull or without a skull at all. [Gk *a*, *kranion* skull.]

acrasia (a·**kra**·ze·ah). Intemperance of behaviour; absence of self-control. [Gk *akrasia* excess.]

acratia (a·**kra**·she·ah). A condition of being destitute of power or strength; the state of impotence. [Gk *a*, *kratos* power.]

acraturesis (ak·**rat**·ewr·**e**'·sis). Inability to pass or difficulty in passing urine because of lack of muscular tone in the bladder. [Gk *a*, *kratos* power, uresis.]

Acrel, Olof (b. 1717). Stockholm surgeon.

Acrel's ganglion. The gangliform enlargement of the posterior interosseous nerve on the back of the carpus.

acribometer (ak·rib·**om**·et·er). An instrument used for measuring extremely small objects. [Gk *akribes* exact, meter.]

acrid (**ak**·rid). Pungent; irritating. [L *acer* pungent.]

acridine (**ak**·rid·een). $C_6H_4CHNC_6H_4$. A coal-tar hydrocarbon with a pungent smell and an intensely irritant effect upon the skin and mucous membrane. It is the parent of a number of yellow and orange fluorescent dyes; the diamino derivatives, acriflavine and proflavine, are antiseptics and bactericides used in surgery, and in the treatment of burns, gangrene and gonorrhoea. [see prec.]

Acriflavine (ak·re·**fla**·veen). Flavine; a mixture of the hydrochloride of diaminomethylacridine chloride, acriflavine base, $C_6H_3NH_2CHN(CH_3)ClC_6H_3NH_2$ and diamino-acridine dihydrochloride. Reddish-brown crystals, soluble in water, slightly in alcohol; a non-irritant antiseptic used for burns, urinary disinfection and also, intravenously, in gonorrhoea and glandular infections (BPC 1963). **Acriflavine hydrochloride.** The hydrochloride of acriflavine base; soluble in water or alcohol, and of value in ophthalmic surgery, and ear, nose and throat work generally. **Neutral acriflavine.** Euflavine, a mixture of acriflavine base and diamino-acridine monohydrochloride, which is particularly suitable for intravenous injection. [L *acer* pungent, *flavus* yellow.]

acrinia (a·**kri**·ne·ah). Any lowering of the rate or amount of secretion or excretion; a state of total cessation of these functions. [Gk *a*, *krinein* to separate.]

acrinyl (**ak**·ri·nil). The parahydroxybenzyl radical, $OHC_6H_4CH_2$–. **Acrinyl isothiocyanate.** $OHC_6H_4CH_2NCS$, a product of the hydrolysis of sinalbin, the glucoside contained in white mustard seeds, *Sinapis alba*. **Acrinyl sulphocyanate.** $OHC_6H_4CH_2CNS$, an isomer of acrinyl isothiocyanate, which also occurs in white mustard seeds.

acrisia (a·**kriz**·e·ah). 1. A condition in certain diseases in which there is no critical point; absence of crisis. 2. Crisis in which the patient becomes worse instead of better. 3. Doubtful course in any disease. [Gk want of judgement.]

acritical (a·**krit**·ik·al). Having no crisis or critical phase. [Gk *a*, *krisis* crisis.]

acritochromacy (a·**krit**·o·**kro**'·mas·e). Colour blindness. *See* BLINDNESS. [Gk *akritos* indistinguishable, *chroma* colour.]

acro-aesthesia (**ak**·ro·es·**the**'·ze·ah). 1. Extraordinary sensitiveness [Gk *akros* extreme, aesthesia.] 2. Sensation of pain in the hands or feet. [Gk *akron* extremity, aesthesia.]

acro-agnosis (**ak**·ro·ag·**no**'·sis). 1. Loss of sense of position, weight or shape of a limb or limbs, or even of the existence of them. 2. Sensory defect in a limb. [Gk *akron* extremity, *a*, *gnosis* knowledge.]

acro-agonines (ak·ro·**ag**·on·eenz). Substances formed or released in the tissues when the body is violently stimulated. [Gk *akros* extreme, *agonia* contest.]

acro-anaesthesia (**ak**·ro·an·es·**the**'·ze·ah). Anaesthesia of the hands or feet, or both. [Gk *akron* extremity, anaesthesia.]

acro-arthritis (**ak**·ro·ar·**thri**'·tis). An arthritic condition of the extremities. [Gk *akron* extremity, arthritis.]

acroasia (ak·ro·a·se·ah). Lack of comprehension of what is actually heard. [Gk *akroasis* a listening.]

acro-asphyxia (**ak**·ro·as·**fix**'·e·ah). A vasomotor neurosis which is an early symptom of Raynaud's disease. The condition of the toes and fingers alternates between that of coldness and pallor and that of heat and redness. [Gk *akron* extremity, *a*, *sphyxis* pulse.]

acro-ataxia (**ak**·ro·at·**ax**'·e·ah). Irregularity or impairment of action in the intrinsic muscles of the hands and feet, affecting mainly fingers and toes. [Gk *akron* extremity, *ataxia* lack of order.]

acroblast (**ak**·ro·blast). A body in the spermatid, derived from the Golgi apparatus and centrosphere, which gives rise to the acrosome and an acroblastic remnant in spermatogenesis. [Gk *akron* extremity, *blastos* germ.]

acrobrachycephaly (**ak**·ro·brak·e·**kef**'·al·e). An abnormal shortening of the head in the anteroposterior diameter resulting from fusion of the coronal suture. [Gk *akros* extreme, *brachys* short, *kephale* head.]

acrobystia (ak·ro·**bis**·te·ah). 1. The prepuce. 2. Removal of the prepuce by circumcision. [Gk prepuce.]

acrobystiolith (ak·ro·**bis**·te·o·lith). A calculus in the prepuce. [acrobystia, Gk *lithos* stone.]

acrobystitis (**ak**·ro·bis·**ti**'·tis). An inflammatory condition of the prepuce. [acrobystia, Gk *-itis* inflammation.]

acrocentric (ak·ro·**sen**·trik). Of chromosomes with centromere very close to one end and having, therefore, very unequal arms. [Gk *akron* extremity, *kentron* centre.]

acrocephalia (**ak**·ro·kef·**a**'·le·ah). A deformity of the head, more commonly termed oxycephaly, in which the crown rises to a blunt point. [Gk *akron* extremity, *kephale* head.]

acrocephalic (**ak**·ro·kef·**al**'·ik). Referring to acrocephalia.

acrocephalosyndactylia, acrocephalosyndactylism, acrocephalosyndactyly (ak·ro·**kef**·al·o·sin·dak·**til**'·e·ah, ak·ro·**kef**·al·o·sin·**dak**'·til·izm, ak·ro·**kef**·al·o·sin·**dak**'·til·e). Congenital defect of the head and extremities in which the former rises to a point and the latter show syndactylism. [acrocephalia, syndactylism.]

acrocephalous (ak·ro·**kef**·al·us). Referring to acrocephalia.

acrocephaly (ak·ro·**kef**·al·e). Acrocephalia.

acrochordon (ak·ro·**kor**·don). Neurofibromatosis. [Gk *akron* extremity, *chorde* string.]

acrocinesis (**ak**·ro·sin·**e**'·sis). Acrokinesis.

acrocinetic (**ak**·ro·sin·**et**'·ik). Acrokinetic.

acrocontracture (**ak**·ro·kon·**trak**'·tcher). A shortening or distortion of the hand or the foot, or of its joints. [Gk *akron* extremity, contracture.]

acrocyanosis (**ak**·ro·si·an·**o**'·sis). A vasomotor defect of the hands and feet as a result of which there is a variable blue tinge in these regions. **Chronic progressive acrocyanosis.** A condition marked by a blue or a bright-red colour of the hands or feet, which are also enlarged and soft. [Gk *akron* extremity, *kyanos* blue.]

acrodermatitis (**ak**·ro·der·mat·**i**'·tis). Inflammation of the skin of the extremities. **Acrodermatitis chronica atrophicans.** A term used loosely to denote any form of diffuse idiopathic atrophy of the skin of the limbs; correctly employed, the name indicates a localized cutaneous atrophy characterized by a prodromal stage of erythematous infiltration affecting the extensor surfaces of the extremities, particularly at the knees, elbows and finger joints, and often associated with infiltrations extending down the arms (ulnar bands). The affected skin eventually becomes glazed and atrophic, and scleroderma-like changes occur in many cases. The face, palms and soles are not affected, and the trunk only rarely. **Acrodermatitis continua.** Acrodermatitis perstans (see below). **Acrodermatitis enteropathica.** A rare, severe and often fatal congenital disease due to enzyme defect occurring in infancy, with vesicles, ulcers and erythema of the skin, loss of hair and sometimes with diarrhoea due to steatorrhoea. **Acrodermatitis hiemalis.** Lupus pernio, or a tuberculide selectively affecting the chilblain areas of the fingers. **Acrodermatitis perstans.** A rare condition which usually commences in the peri-ungual area of a digit, extending slowly to involve the finger and palm, eventually invading larger areas. The lesions are vesicles, bullae and pustules, and ulceration may ensue. **Acrodermatitis pustulosa.** Acrodermatitis perstans (see above). **Acrodermatitis pustulosa hiemalis.** 1. A form of folliclis. 2. Used incorrectly as a synonym for lupus pernio. **Acrodermatitis urticarioides.** Grain itch. *See* ITCH. **Acrodermatitis vesiculosa tropica.** A symmetrical painful malady occurring in Sri Lanka, in which the skin of both hands becomes tense and glossy; the fingers taper and ulceration may occur, but the hands eventually become normal again. [Gk *akron* extremity, *derma* skin, *-itis* inflammation.]

acrodermatosis (**ak**·ro·der·mat·**o**′·sis). A skin affection in the form of an eruption which occurs on the hands and feet. [Gk *akron* extremity, *derma* skin, *-osis* condition.]

acrodolichomelia (ak·ro·**do**·lik·o·**me**′·le·ah). A condition in which the hands and feet are disproportionately or abnormally long. [Gk *akron* extremity, *dolichos* long, *melos* limb.]

acrodynia (ak·ro·**din**·e·ah). syn.: Pink disease. An allergic reaction of infants to mercury in teething powders, lotions, ointments or napkin rinses. The child is restless, irritable and feverish. There is flabbiness and tachycardia, and the hands and feet are red and swollen although cold and painful. There is usually a generalized erythema, also hyperhidrosis, stomatitis, and dystrophy of hair and nails. Gangrene may occur and there is a mortality of about 10 per cent, but other cases recover completely. [Gk *akron* extremity, *odyne* pain.]

acrodystrophy (ak·ro·**dis**·tro·fe). Any dystrophy mainly or solely involving the extremities. [Gk *akron* extremity, dystrophy.]

acrogeria (ak·ro·**jeer**·e·ah). A condition in which the skin of the hands and feet shows signs of premature old age. [Gk *akron* extremity, *geron* old man.]

acrognosis (ak·rog·**no**·sis). The position sense; a state of being conscious of the limbs as a whole and of one part of a limb relative to another part. [Gk *akron* extremity, *gnosis* knowledge.]

acrohyperhidrosis, acrohyperidrosis (**ak**·ro·**hi**·per·hid·**ro**′·sis, **ak**·ro·**hi**·per·id·**ro**′·sis). Abnormal exudation of sweat from the hands and feet. [Gk *akron* extremity, hyperhidrosis.]

acrohypothermia, acrohypothermy (**ak**·ro·hi·po·**ther**′·me·ah, **ak**·ro·hi·po·**ther**′·me). Abnormally reduced temperature of the hands and feet. [Gk *akron* extremity, hypothermia.]

acrohysterosalpingectomy (**ak**·ro·**his**·ter·o·sal·pin·**jek**′·to·me). An operation which consists in the excision of a part of the fundus of the uterus and of both the attached uterine tubes. [Gk *akron* extremity, hysterosalpingectomy.]

acrokerato-elastoidosis (ak·ro·**ker**·at·o·e·las·toid·**o**′·sis). Collagenous plaques on the hands of outdoor workers who are habitually exposed to the sun. [Gk *akron* extremity, *keras* horn, *elaunein* to drive, *-osis* condition.]

acrokeratosis verruciformis (**ak**·ro·ker·at·**o**′·sis **ver**·ew·se·**for**′·mis). An epithelial papular naevus transmitted dominantly and characterized by warty lesions on the backs of the hands and feet, with some involvement of the palms, the palmar surfaces of the fingers, the wrists and the forearms; the knees may also be affected. [Gk *akron* extremity, keratosis, L *verruca* wart, form.]

acrokinesis (**ak**·ro·kin·**e**′·sis). A state which may be the result of psychoneurotic disturbance, in which there is excessive freedom of action or range of movement of the limbs. [Gk *akros* extreme, kinesis.]

acrokinetic (**ak**·ro·kin·**et**′·ik). Referring to or marked by acrokinesis.

acrolein (ak·**ro**·le·in). Acrylic aldehyde, CH_2=CHCHO. A pungent liquid prepared from glycerol, with an irritant effect on the eyes, and used in chemical warfare; it is the starting point for the preparation of synthetic sugars.

acromacria (ak·ro·**mak**·re·ah). Abnormal length and thinness of the bones of the fingers or toes, so that they resemble spider's legs (also called *arachnodactyly*). [Gk *akron* extremity, *makros* long.]

acromania (ak·ro·**ma**·ne·ah). Extreme degree of mania characterized by motor activity in excessive amount. [Gk *akros* extreme, mania.]

acromastitis (**ak**·ro·mas·**ti**′·tis). Inflammation of the nipple. [Gk *akron* extremity, *mastos* breast, *-itis* inflammation.]

acromastium (ak·ro·**mas**·te·um). The nipple. [Gk *akron* extremity, *mastos* breast.]

acromegalic (ak·ro·**meg**·al·ik). Referring to or having the characteristics of acromegaly.

acromegalogigantism (ak·ro·**meg**·al·o·ji·**gant**′·izm). Excessive size of the bones caused by the onset of acromegaly during adolescence. [acromegaly, Gk *gigas* giant.]

acromegaly (ak·ro·**meg**·al·e). A chronic disease which is marked by gradual enlargement of the hands and feet and of the bones of the head and chest. It is caused by excessive secretion of, or sensitivity to, growth hormone developing in adult life, in contrast to gigantism, which develops before puberty. Excessive growth hormone influence may continue after puberty, producing signs of acromegaly superimposed on the gigantism. The excessive growth hormone is characteristically due to a tumour of the acidophil (eosinophil) cells of the pituitary (eosinophil adenoma), though it may occur in cases of chromophobe adenoma. **Fugitive acromegaly.** A type of acromegaly which ceases to progress. **Localized acromegaly, Partial acromegaly.** A condition in which the acromegalic changes occur in only one part of the body, and are possibly due to localized hypersensitiveness of the growth hormone rather than to hypersecretion of this hormone. [Gk *akron* extremity, *megas* great.]

acromelalgia (**ak**·ro·mel·**al**′·je·ah). A condition in which there is severely painful swelling and redness of the feet and toes and, less commonly, of the hands and fingers, aggravated by warmth and standing. The disorder, the origin of which is uncertain, is intractable and may persist for many years. There may be accompanying general weakness, headache, vertigo and tachycardia, among other symptoms; erythromelalgia. [Gk *akron* extremity, *melos* limb, *algos* pain.]

acromelic (ak·ro·**mel**·ik). Affecting or referring to the end of an arm or leg. [Gk *akron* extremity, *melos* limb.]

acrometagenesis (**ak**·ro·met·ah·**jen**′·es·is). Abnormal growth of the hands and feet. [Gk *akron* extremity, *meta*, *genein* to produce.]

acromial (ak·**ro**·me·al). Relating to the acromion process of the scapula.

acromiale os (ak·ro·me·**a**·le os). A false joint formed of the spine of the scapula and the adjacent and movable epiphyseal portion of the acromion. **Acromiale os secondarium.** In a skiagram, a rounded structure apparent immediately above the greater tuberosity of the humerus. [acromion, L *os* bone.]

acromicria (ak·ro·**mik**·re·ah). 1. Excessive smallness of the hands and feet. 2. A condition of facies characterized by smallness of the face, nose and ears, in association with abnormal smallness of the hands and feet. [Gk *akron* extremity, *mikros* small.]

acromioclavicular (ak·**ro**·me·o·klav·**ik**′·ew·lar). Concerning the acromion and the clavicle. **Acromioclavicular joint.** *See* JOINT.

acromiocoracoid (ak·**ro**·me·o·**kor**′·ak·oid). Concerning the acromion and the coracoid process.

acromiohumeral (ak·**ro**·me·o·**hew**′·mer·al). Concerning the acromion and the humerus.

acromion [NA] (ak·**ro**·me·on). A flat plate of triangular shape which is continuous with and projects beyond the outer end of the spine of the scapula. Its free borders are placed medially and laterally, the 3rd border being at its attachment to the spine. Near the spine the lateral border bears a well-marked angle, the acromial angle [angulus acromialis], near its junction with the spine, whilst the medial border carries an articular facet [facies articularis acromii (NA)] for the lateral end of the clavicle. [Gk *akron* extremity, *omos* shoulder.]

acromionectomy (ak·ro·me·on·ek′·to·me). An operation to remove the whole or part of the acromion, used infrequently for the treatment of derangements of the rotator cuff of the shoulder. [acromion, Gk *ektome* a cutting out.]

acromioscapular (ak·ro·me·o·skap′·ew·lar). Concerning the acromion and the scapula.

acromiothoracic (ak·ro·me·o·thor·as′·ik). Concerning the acromion and the thorax.

acromiothoracic artery [arteria thoracoacromialis (NA)]. A short wide trunk from the 2nd part of the axillary artery which pierces the clavipectoral fascia and sends branches to the pectoral [rami pectorales (NA)], deltoid and subclavius muscles [ramus deltoideus (NA)], the breast and the sternoclavicular joints [ramus clavicularis (NA)], and the skin over the acromion [ramus acromialis (NA)].

acromiothoracic vein [vena thoraco-acromialis (NA)]. The vein accompanying the artery of the same name.

acromphalus (ak·rom·fal·us). 1. The central point of the umbilicus. 2. Undue proturberance of the umbilicus, generally indicative of hernial development. 3. The few inches of the umbilical cord left in contact with the infant's navel. [Gk *akron* extremity, *omphalos* navel.]

acromycosis (ak·ro·mi·ko′·sis). Mycotic disease of the limbs. [Gk *akron* extremity, *mykes* fungus, *-osis* condition.]

acromyle (ak·rom·il·e). The patella. [Gk *akron* extremity, *myle* patella.]

acromyotonia, acromyotonus (ak·ro·mi·o·to′·ne·ah, ak·ro·mi·ot′·o·nus). Myotonia affecting the hands or feet, or both; contractions occur, with subsequent deformities of spastic type. [Gk *akron* extremity, myotonia.]

acronarcotic (ak·ro·nar·kot′·ik). 1. Having a sharp and bitter character as well as sleep-producing and pain-relieving properties. 2. Any drug or agent which possesses both stringent and blunting propensities. [L *acer* sharp, narcotic.]

acroneuropathy (ak·ro·newr·op′·ath·e). Any neuropathic disorder whose manifestations are most evident in the periphery of the extremities; polyneuritis is an example. [Gk *akron* extremity, *neuron* nerve, *pathos* disease.]

acroneurosis (ak·ro·newr·o′·sis). 1. A functional nervous disorder affecting the hands and feet. 2. A condition which affects airmen and is caused by exposure to the upper atmosphere. There are digestive and nervous disturbances, emotional stress and restlessness. [Gk *akron* extremity, neurosis.]

cronyx (ak·ron·ix). A nail which, at its edges, grows downwards into the flesh of the finger or toe. [Gk *akron* extremity, *onyx* nail.]

cro-oedema (ak·ro·e·de′·mah). Chronic oedema of the hand or foot. The condition may be the result of an injury or may occur in neurotic individuals. [Gk *akron* extremity, oedema.]

cro-osteolysis (ak·ro·os·te·ol′·is·is). A familial condition in which osteolysis of (usually) all 4 extremities occurs without preceding ulceration or subsequent spontaneous amputation, in otherwise well-developed young children. The toes are eventually reduced to mere nipples. [Gk *akron* extremity, osteolysis.]

cropachy (ak·rop·ak·e). Clubbing of the fingers, with enlargement in certain cases, giving an acromegalic character to the condition. **Thyroid acropachy.** Clubbing of the fingers associated with pretibial myxoedema and thyrotoxicosis. [Gk *akron* extremity, *pachys* thick.]

cropachyderma (ak·ro·pak·e·der′·mah). A condition in which there is clubbing of the fingers, deformity of the long bones, and areas of thickened skin on the scalp, the face, the hands and the feet. [acropachy, Gk *derma* skin.]

croparaesthesia (ak·ro·par·es·the′·ze·ah). Tingling or other abnormal spontaneous sensations in the extremities. Often due to nerve compression but sometimes associated with vascular disease, either mild or severe. [Gk *akron* extremity, paraesthesia.]

See also: NOTHNAGEL, SCHULTZE (F.).

acroparalysis (ak·ro·par·al′·is·is). Paralysis of the hands and feet. [Gk *akron* extremity, paralysis.]

acropathology (ak·ro·path·ol′·o·je). The pathology of diseases which attack the hands and feet. [Gk *akron* extremity, pathology.]

acropathy (ak·rop·ath·e). Any one of the diseases which attack the hands and feet. [Gk *akron* extremity, *pathos* suffering.]

acropetal (ak·rop·et·al). Growth or development from below upwards. [Gk *akron* extremity, L *petere* to seek.]

acrophobia (ak·ro·fo·be·ah). Overwhelming fear of being at a great height. [Gk *akron* extremity, phobia.]

acropigmentation (ak·ro·pig·men·ta′·shun). Hereditary diffuse hyperpigmentation of the dorsa of the hands and feet. [Gk *akron* extremity, pigmentation.]

acroposthia (ak·ro·pos·the·ah). The distal portion of the prepuce; the turned fold of the skin which covers the glans penis. [Gk *akros* extreme, *posthe* foreskin.]

acroposthitis (ak·ro·pos·thi′·tis). Inflammation of the prepuce. [acroposthia, Gk *-itis* inflammation.]

acropustulosis (ak·ro·pus·tew·lo′·sis). Acrodermatitis perstans. [Gk *akron* extremity, L *pustula* pustule, Gk *-osis* condition.]

acrorrheuma (ak·ro·roo·mah). Acute rheumatic infection of the hands and feet. [Gk *akron* extremity, *rheuma* flux.]

acroscleriasis (ak·ro·skler·i′·as·is). Acrosclerosis.

acroscleroderma, acrosclerodermia (ak·ro·skler·o·der′·mah, ak·ro·skler·o·derm′·e·ah). Sclerodermia involving the fingers, toes, face or chest; sclerodactyly. [Gk *akron* extremity, sclerodermia.]

acrosclerosis (ak·ro·skler·o′·sis). A variety of sclerodermia, characterized by Raynaud's phenomenon, associated with sclerodermatous changes in the distal parts of the extremities, the face and neck, with muscular and visceral involvement. The malady chiefly affects women. [Gk *akron* extremity, sclerosis.]

acrose (ak·rose). A synthetic hexose formed by the polymerization of formaldehyde; it is obtained in 2 isomeric forms from which other hexoses can be synthesized.

acrosome (ak·ro·some). The minute organ situated at the head of a spermatozoon and therefore sometimes referred to as the *apical body.* [Gk *akron* extremity, *soma* body.]

acrosphacelus (ak·ro·sfas·el·us). Gangrene of a finger or toe. [Gk *akron* extremity, *sphakelos* gangrene.]

Acrostalagmus cinnabarinus (ak·ro·stal·ag′·mus sin·ah·bar·i′·nus) Corda 1838. An orange-red mould belonging to the family Moniliaceae. It has been found as a saprophyte of human skin. [Gk *akron* extremity, *stalagmos* a dripping, *kinnabarinos* vermilion.]

acrostealgia (ak·ro·ste·al′·je·ah). A painful inflammation of the bones of the hands and feet. [Gk *akron* extremity, *osteon* bone, *algos* pain.]

acroteric (ak·ro·ter·ik). 1. Referring to the outermost parts of the periphery. 2. Referring to the conditions chiefly affecting the extremities. [Gk *akron* extremity.]

Acrotheca pedrosoi (ak·ro·the·kah ped·ro·so·i). *Hormodendrum pedrosoi,* a fungus identified in cases of dermatitis verrucosa (chromoblastomycosis). *Phialophora pedrosoi,* isolated from cases of chromomycosis. [Gk *akron* extremity, *theke* case.]

acrothymion, acrothymiosis, acrothymum (ak·ro·thi·me·on, ak·ro·thi·me·o′·sis, ak·ro·thi·mum). A rough wrinkled wart the top of which is relatively broad. [Gk *akron* extremity, *thymion* cutaneous wart.]

acrotic (ak·rot·ik). 1. Affecting or referring to the surface. 2. Referring to the glands of the skin. [Gk *akrotes* an extreme.] 3. In reference to the pulse, indicating absence or imperceptibility of pulsation. [Gk *a*, *krotos* a beating.]

acrotism (ak·rot·izm). Absence or imperceptibility of pulsation. [see prec.]

acrotrophodynia (ak·ro·trof·o·din′·e·ah). A painful condition of the feet with trophic, neuritic and vascular changes, occurring as a result of immersion; immersion foot, trench foot. [Gk *akron* extremity, *trophe* nutrition, *odyne* pain.]

acrotrophoneurosis (ak·ro·trof·o·newr·**o**′·sis). Trophic disorders of the extremities secondary to organic nervous disease. [Gk *akron* extremity, *trophe* nutrition, neurosis.]

acrylaldehyde (ak·ril·**al**·de·hide). Acrolein.

acrylic (ak·**ril**·ik). Referring to synthetic plastics resins derived from acrylic acid and used in the manufacture of medical and dental prostheses.

acrylonitrile (ak·ril·o·**ni**′·trile). Vinyl cyanide, CH_2=CHCN. A compound prepared from acetylene and hydrocyanic acid. It is used in the manufacture of synthetic rubber and fibre (polyacrylonitrile). As such it constitutes a serious industrial risk.

act (akt). The performance of a deed; the fulfilling of a function. **Compulsive act.** An act performed by an individual which is accompanied by a subjective impulse which he tries to resist but without success. **Imperative act.** In mental illness, the performance of an act in response to a dominant abnormal impulse. **Imperious act.** Compulsive act (see above). **Impulsive act.** Imperative act (see above). **Isometric muscular act.** In stimulation of a muscle, change in tension without change in length. **Purposive act.** An act carried out because it is willed by the individual. **Reflex act.** Reflex action. *See* ACTION. **Sexual act.** Coitus. [L *agere* to do.]

Actaea (ak·**te**·ah). A genus of plants of the Crowfoot family, many of which are used in therapeutics. **Actaea racemosa.** *Cimicifuga racemosa*, or black cohosh, the roots of which are used in chorea, rheumatism and neuralgia. **Actaea rubra, Actaea spicata.** Baneberry. [L baneberry.]

actidione (ak·te·**di**·one). An antibiotic isolated from streptomycin-producing strains of *Streptomyces griseus*. It shows activity against certain fungi.

actin (**ak**·tin). A protein which, combined with myosin, forms actomyosin, the contractile constituent of muscle. [see foll.]

actinic (ak·**tin**·ik). 1. In physics, a term used with reference to the ultra-violet rays of the spectrum. 2. Referring to light or to radiations which give rise to chemical change. [Gk *aktis* ray.]

actinicity (ak·tin·**is**·it·e). Actinism.

actiniform (ak·**tin**·e·form). Having the form of a ray. [Gk *aktis* ray, form.]

actinine (**ak**·tin·een). $(CH_3)_3NO(CH_2)_3CO$, a cyclic base found in the coral, *Actinia equina*.

actinism (**ak**·tin·izm). The ability of light and other forms of radiant energy to bring about chemical changes. [Gk *aktis* ray.]

Actinium (ak·**tin**·e·um). 1. The radioactive element of atomic number 89 and chemical symbol Ac. It occurs in pitchblende, and, by radioactive distintegration, is the precursor of a series of related elements. 2. One of the genera of Actiniaria, sea anenome, a member of which causes dermatitis in sponge divers. [see prec.]

actinobacillosis (ak·tin·o·bas·il·**o**′·sis). A disease of cattle and sheep which can affect man also. It is caused by *Actinobacillus lignieresi* and spreads usually by way of the lymph vessels. [Gk *aktis* ray, bacillus, Gk *-osis* condition.]

Actinobacillus (ak·tin·o·bas·**il**′·us). There are 4 members of the genus *Actinobacillus* all of which are pathogenic for various animals and one of which, *Actinobacillus actinomycetemcomitans*, is found in human cases of actinomycosis either alone or, more usually, along with *Actinomyces israelii*. Actinobacilli are small, Gram-negative, non-motile rods which rarely grow into filaments; they are aerobic and facultatively anaerobic although preferring micro-aerophilic conditions for primary isolation. **Actinobacillus actinoides.** An organism which has been isolated from epizootic pneumonia in calves. **Actinobacillus lignieresi.** The cause of slowly developing granulomata, especially in the soft tissues of the lower jaw and neck in cattle; lesions also develop in the tongue muscle—so-called "woody-tongue" disease. Unlike actinomycosis, there is little tendency to invade bones and spread is usually by lymphatics. Strains identical with those isolated from pathological material have been isolated from bovine ruminal contents and from the tongues of normal cattle, and it would appear that infection is endogenous in origin. [Gk *aktis* ray, bacillus.]

actinochemistry (ak·tin·o·**kem**′·is·tre). The chemistry which investigates and explains the effect of light on substances and the subsequent disintegration of them. [Gk *aktis* ray, chemistry.]

Actinocladothrix (ak·tin·o·**klad**′·o·thrix). *Actinomyces bovis.* [Gk *aktis* ray, *klados* branch, *thrix* hair.]

actinocongestin (ak·tin·o·kon·**jes**′·tin). A name given by Richet to a toxic substance obtained from the tentacles of some sea anemones (actinia) which causes congestion of the viscera of animals into which it has been injected. [Gk *aktis* ray, congestion.]

actinocutitis (ak·tin·o·kew·**ti**′·tis). Actinodermatitis. [Gk *aktis* ray, cutitis.]

actinodaphnine (ak·tin·o·**daf**′·neen). An alkaloid, $C_{18}H_{17}NO_4$, resembling strychnine, and found in species of *Actinodaphne*.

actinodermatitis (ak·tin·o·der·mat·**i**′·tis). X-ray dermatitis; excessive skin reactions, generally in the form of inflammation and destruction, as a result of accidental or deliberate exposure to x-rays. [Gk *aktis* ray, dermatitis.]

actinogen (ak·**tin**·o·jen). Any material capable of producing radiation. [Gk *aktis* ray, *genein* to produce.]

actinogenesis (ak·tin·o·**jen**′·es·is). The origination or the production of rays of light. [see foll.]

actinogenic (ak·tin·o·**jen**′·ik). 1. Radiogenic. 2. Producing rays of any kind. 3. Referring to an actinogen. [Gk *aktis* ray, *genein* to produce.]

actinogenics (ak·tin·o·**jen**′·ix). The study or the science of the origination or production of rays of light. [see prec.]

actinogram (ak·**tin**·o·gram). The record made by the actinograph. [Gk *aktis* ray, *gramma* mark.]

actinograph (ak·**tin**·o·graf). An instrument which is used for measuring and recording changes in the action of light rays of different kinds on a sensitized surface. [Gk *aktis* ray, *graphein* to record.]

actinographema (ak·tin·o·graf·**e**′·mah). Actinogram.

actinography (ak·tin·**og**·raf·e). The measuring and recording of changes in the action of light rays on a sensitized surface. [Gk *aktis* ray, *graphein* to record.]

actinokymography (ak·tin·o·ki·**mog**′·raf·e). Cinematographic recording of radiographs. [Gk *aktis* ray, *kyma* wave, *graphein* to record.]

actinolite (ak·**tin**·o·lite). A natural silicate of calcium, magnesium and iron, green in colour and of monoclinic structure (specific gravity 3); a variety of it is asbestos. [Gk *aktis* ray, *lithos* stone.]

actinology (ak·tin·**ol**·o·je). The science which is concerned with light rays and their chemical effects, as well as with radiant energy. [Gk *aktis* ray, *logos* science.]

actinolyte (ak·**tin**·o·lite). 1. An apparatus for producing ultra-violet rays. 2. Any substance which is affected by light. [Gk *aktis* ray, *lyein* to loosen.]

actinometer (ak·tin·**om**·et·er). 1. An instrument by which the penetrative effect of light rays can be measured. 2. An instrument by which the degree of intensity of actinic rays can be determined. [Gk *aktis* ray, meter.]

actinometry (ak·tin·**om**·et·re). The measurement and assessment of the photochemical effects of light. [see prec.]

actinomycelial (ak·tin·o·mi·**se**′·le·al). 1. Actinomycetic. 2. Relating to the mycelium of actinomyces.

Actinomyces (ak·tin·o·**mi**′·seez). One of the genera of the family Actinomycetaceae, the other being *Nocardia*. The family is closely related to the Streptomycetaceae, of which the genus *Streptomyces* is entirely saprophytic but is important as the source of numerous antibiotics. Of the 3 main species within the genus, *Actinomyces israelii*, although primarily a commensal of man, is occasionally pathogenic as the cause of actinomycosis; *Actinomyces bovis* behaves similarly in cattle, and *Actinomyces baudetii* is the causal organism of actinomycosis in dogs and cats. **Actinomyces (Streptothrix) antibioticus.** The source of the antibiotic actinomycin. **Actinomyces asteroides.** *Nocardia asteroides.* **Actinomyces farcinicus.** An acid-fast type causing farcy in cattle. **Actinomyces graminis.** An aerobe, saprophytic on grain and grasses, and devoid of pathogenicity to animals. **Actinomyces gypsoides.** A species which has been found in sputum. **Actinomyces lavendulae.** A source of the antibiotic streptothricin. **Actinomyces madurae.** *Nocardia madurae.* **Actinomyces muris.** A parasite inhabiting the nasopharynx of rats. It causes in man a type of rat-bite fever called infectious erythema or Haverhill fever; also called *Streptobacillus moniliformis.* **Actinomyces necrophorus.** *Fusiformis necrophorus,* an organism responsible for some necrotic lesions in animals and occasionally in man. It has been isolated from lung abscesses and noted in chronic ulcerative colitis. It consists of Gram-negative, highly pleomorphic forms varying from coccobacilli to long filaments. **Actinomyces somaliensis.** *Nocardia somaliensis.* [see foll.]

Actinomycetaceae (**ak**·tin·o·mi·se·**ta'**·se·e). One of the 5 families constituting the order Actinomycetales. The organisms are filamentous, often branching, and occasionally form true mycelia. The family includes *Actinomyces* and *Leptotrichia.* [Gk *aktis* ray, *mykes* fungus.]

Actinomycetales (**ak**·tin·o·mi·se·ta'·leez). An order of the class Schizomycetes, consisting of 5 families: Actinomycetaceae, Mycobacteriaceae, Streptomycetaceae and Actinophoceae. The cells are rigid and rod-shaped or filamentous, with a tendency to branch; they may grow as a mycelium which may develop aerial conidia, oidiospores or sporangiospores, and so give mould-like colonies. They are mostly non-motile, usually Gram-positive, and some species are acid-fast. [Gk *aktis* ray, *mykes* fungus.]

actinomycetes (**ak**·tin·o·**mi'**·set·eez). Members of the order Actinomycetales.

actinomycetic (**ak**·tin·o·mi·**se'**·tik). Referring to or caused by *Actinomyces.* [Gk *aktis* ray, *mykes* fungus.]

actinomycetin (**ak**·tin·o·**mi'**·se·tin). An antibiotic isolated from *Streptomyces albus.* It lyses killed bacteria and is of no therapeutic importance. [see prec.]

actinomycetoma (**ak**·tin·o·mi·se·**to'**·mah). Mycetoma caused by species of *Nocardia* and *Streptomyces.* White-grain mycetoma may be caused by *Nocardia brasiliensis, Streptomyces madurae* and *Streptomyces somaliensis,* and red-grain mycetoma by *Streptomyces pelletieri.* [*Actinomyces,* Gk *mykes* fungus, *-oma* tumour.]

Actinomycin (ak·tin·o·**mi**·sin). BP Commission approved name for antimicrobial substances with antitumour activity produced by *Streptomyces antibioticus* and *Streptomyces chrysomallus.* It has a markedly bacteriostatic effect on Gram-positive organisms but its activity is less in the case of Gram-negative organisms. It is antagonistic to certain fungi and *in vitro* is inhibitory to the growth of *Mycobacterium tuberculosis.* Mixtures of specific substances are designated by a terminal letter or number, e.g. Actinomycin C, C_1, IV, etc.

actinomycoma (**ak**·tin·o·mi·**ko'**·mah). A tumour which forms in the tissues as a result of the presence of the actinomyces. [*Actinomyces,* Gk *-oma* tumour.]

actinomycosis (**ak**·tin·o·mi·**ko'**·sis). A chronic infective disease transmitted from cattle. In man due to *Actinomyces israelii,* in cattle due to *Actinomyces bovis.* Many granulated tumours are to be found on the tongue and jaws, and pus-containing tumours may occur locally; there may be irregular pyrexia. [*Actinomyces,* Gk *-osis* condition.]

actinomycotic (**ak**·tin·o·mi·**kot'**·ik). Affected with, related or referring to actinomycosis.

actinon (**ak**·tin·on). Actinium emanation: a gaseous radioactive element, Radon-219, produced by the disintegration of actinium, and of very short life. [Gk *aktis* ray.]

actinoneuritis (**ak**·tin·o·newr·**i'**·tis). The neuritis which is an effect of the prolonged or repeated exposure to radium or x-rays. [Gk *aktis* ray, neuritis.]

actinophage (**ak**·tin·o·faje). A virus (phage) which infects and grows in Actinomycetaceae. [*Actinomyces,* Gk *phagein* to eat.]

actinophor (ak·**tin**·o·for). A mixture of cerium and thorium oxides applied as a coating to fluorescent screens in x-ray work. [Gk *aktis* ray, *pherein* to carry.]

actinophytosis (**ak**·tin·o·fi·**to'**·sis). Botryomycosis. [Gk *aktis* ray, *phyton* plant.]

actinopraxis (**ak**·tin·o·**prax'**·is). The use of the rays which emanate from radioactive substances, for the purposes of diagnosis and treatment. [Gk *aktis, praxis* doing.]

actinoscopy, actinostereoscopy (ak·tin·**os**·ko·pe, **ak**·tin·o·steer·e·**os'**·ko·pe). The use of x-rays for examination of the body. [Gk *aktis* ray. *stereos* solid, *skopein* to watch.]

actinotherapeutics (**ak**·tin·o·ther·ap·**ew'**·tix). The branch of medicine that is concerned with the curative properties of light rays. [Gk *aktis* ray, therapeutics.]

actinotherapy (**ak**·tin·o·**ther'**·ap·e). The application of violet and ultra-violet rays for curative purposes, especially in diseases of the skin. [Gk *aktis* ray, therapy.]

actinotoxaemia (**ak**·tin·o·tox·**e'**·me·ah). A state of toxaemic reaction caused by the destruction of tissues resulting from the therapeutic application of rays. [Gk *aktis* ray, toxaemia.]

action (**ak**·shun). 1. Activity; the carrying out of a function, or the production of an effect. 2. The application of any force. **Antagonistic action.** The counter action caused by an opposing principle or agent, which may be a drug, muscle, etc. **Bactericidal action.** The lethal effect which many antibiotics and disinfectants have on bacteria. **Bacteriostatic action.** The action of certain drugs in preventing or arresting bacterial growth. **Ball-valve action.** 1. A pedunculated thrombus in the left auricle of the heart in mitral stenosis, which may produce intermittent obstruction of the mitral valve ring by acting in a "ball valve" fashion. It is also known as *ball thrombus,* or *pseudomyxoma;* very rarely a true myxoma may occur in the left auricle and act in the same way. 2. The action of any round object within a hollow viscus in causing intermittent obstruction to the outlet. **Buffer action.** The action of weak acids and salts (or weak bases) in solution, which allows only gradual change in the pH upon addition of further acids or alkalis. **Calorigenic action.** Specific dynamic action; in physiology, the liberation of heat which results from the metabolism in the body of a food or food constituent. **Capillary action.** A general term for phenomena observed with liquids, due to the force of attraction between the molecules, e.g. the rise or depression of a liquid in a capillary tube. **Catalytic action.** The effect upon a chemical reaction of the introduction of a substance (catalyst) which accelerates the reaction without itself being affected. **Chemical action.** Any process resulting in a change in the arrangement of the atoms within the molecule of a substance. **Concentric action.** The action of muscles when they produce a movement by shortening. **Contact action.** Catalytic action (see above) at a surface, e.g. of platinized asbestos. **Cumulative action.** The effect which results from the repeated administration of a drug which is slowly excreted or broken down by the body, and thus accumulates in the tissues. **Diastatic action.** The action of a group of enzymes, termed *amylases* or *diastases,* in breaking down starch and glycogen to less complex compounds, the end-product being maltose. **Disordered action of the heart.** D.A.H., soldier's heart, effort syndrome; a condition characterized by palpitation, dyspnoea on exertion, stabbing left inframammary pain, dizziness, syncope and easy fatigability, symptoms which are due to imbalance of the autonomic nervous system so that the normal co-ordination between the vagus and the sympathetic systems controlling the heart is disturbed. It is the result of emotional factors acting on the hypothalamus, is a manifestation of an anxiety state and may occur in any individual who has been subjected to considerable mental or physical stress. The terms cardiac neurosis or neurocirculatory asthenia are to be preferred, since the heart is perfectly healthy. **Eccentric action.** The action of muscles when they actively lengthen or "pay out". They thus enable a prime mover (or the force of gravity) to produce a controlled movement. **Electrocapillary action.** Electrical effect, e.g. surface tension alteration, at the interface formed by the junction of 2 liquids in a capillary tube; advantage is taken of it in the capillary electrometer. **Hydrotropic action.** The action of hydrotropic substances, such as the cholic acids in bile, which by the reduction of surface forces render otherwise insoluble substances, such as fat, soluble and diffusible through a membrane. **Mass action.** The influence upon a chemical reaction of the molecular concentration of the reacting substances. **Opsonic action.** The effect which opsonins exert on bacteria, i.e. to increase their liability to phagocytosis. **Physical action.** Any process resulting in a change in the physical state of a substance, e.g. melting, vaporization, without affecting the arrangement of the atoms within the molecule. **Reflex action.** The sequence of events in which an effector organ is thrown into action through the intermediation of the lower parts of the central nervous system in response to a stimulus applied to an afferent nerve or sensory nerve-ending. **Safety-valve action.** Any compensatory mechanism acting in the manner of a safety valve. An example is the relief of the pulmonary congestion in mitral stenosis which may result if compensatory incompetence of the tricuspid valve develops. **Specific action.** The particular or predominant action of a drug or chemical substance, either on another substance or on a micro-organism. **Specific dynamic action.** The augmentation of the basal metabolic rate due to the heat set free in the body by the combustion of foodstuffs, especially protein. **Synergistic action.** The additive action caused by a co-operative principle or agent, which may be a drug, muscle, etc. **Thermogenic action.** The action of any chemical or food that raises body temperature. **Trigger action.** A stimulus that initiates any vital process which may be wholly unlike the original action. [L *agere* to do.]

action-tremor (ak′·shun·trem·or). Tremor continuing during voluntary movement (syn: intention tremor). [action, tremor.]

activation (ak·tiv·a·shun). 1. In enzymology, the promotion or protection of enzyme activity occurring in the presence of certain more or less specific substances termed activators. 2. In chemistry, the increasing of the activity of a catalyst by the addition of another substance, or the regeneration of a catalyst by appropriate treatment. **Activation analysis.** *See* ANALYSIS. **Amino acid activation.** The first step in protein synthesis whereby amino acids react with ATP in reactions catalysed by amino-acid-specific enzymes to yield amino-acyl-AMP derivatives. **Embryonic activation.** 1. The liberation of evocators from inactive precursors. 2. The stimulation of egg development by artificial means. **Plasma activation.** The stimulation of cellular activity following the intravenous injection of non-specific substances such as proteins or colloids. (L *activus* active.]

activator (ak·tiv·a·tor). 1. Any substance which induces or prolongs the activity of an enzyme. It may be an essential factor in the enzyme system, or it may render the action optimal. This term is now largely restricted to the simpler ions or substances, e.g. metallic ions, which have such action as distinct from the more complex co-enzymes. 2. In embryology, an inductor, organizer or evocator; a substance which initiates local cellular differentiation in the course of development. 3. In chemistry, a catalyst. 4. In dentistry, an upper and lower appliance joined together in the form of a monobloc but constructed to a postural bite and activated by the muscles of mastication to produce intermaxillary traction. **Allosteric activator.** A compound which, when bound to an allosteric site of an allosteric enzyme, produces an increase in the catalytic activity; a positive allosteric effector. [see prec.]

active (ak·tiv). 1. Causing change. 2. Producing rapid action. 3. In optics, possessing the power to turn the plane of polarization. 4. Dynamic or working. [L *activus.*]

activity (ak·tiv·it·e). **Equivalent activity.** Of a radiation source, the activity of a point source of the same radionuclide which will give the same exposure rate at the same distance from the centre of the source. **Extravehicular activity (EVA).** When astronauts leave their space vehicle outside the earth's atmosphere, they need artificial atmospheric pressure, respiratory facilities, temperature control and signalling capability. For short journeys a flexible line from the spacecraft may provide these facilities (*umbilical EVA*); for more prolonged EVA it is necessary to include a portable pack within the pressure suit; this combination of portable pack and pressure suit is more correctly termed a *space suit.* **Gamma-ray activity.** A relative measure of th strength of a radioactive source in terms of the number o intensity of the gamma-rays emitted, usually referred to th corresponding quantity for a standard source, e.g. radium **Optical activity.** The rotation of the plane of vibration of a bea of polarized light when passed through certain substances o their solutions. It is associated with the presence of one or mo asymmetric atoms in the molecule of the compound. **Specif activity.** The activity per unit mass of an element or compour containing a radioactive nuclide.

actomyosin (ak·to·mi·o·sin). A.M. A combination of the protei actin and myosin which is found in voluntary muscle; in slight modified form it may also occur in smooth muscle. It exists muscle cells, probably as parallel micelles (long threads) whic on stimulation shorten without change of volume, and so cau muscle contraction.

actuation (ak·tew·a·shun). The mental faculty which translat volition into action. [L *actuatio* an acting.]

acuaesthesia (ak·ew·es·the′·ze·ah). Acouaesthesia.

acuclosure (ak·ew·klo·zher). The arresting of haemorrhage by t method of acupressure and acutorsion. [L *acus* needle, closure.]

acuductor (ak·ew·duk·tor). A holder or carrier for a needle. *acus* needle, *ducere* to lead.]

acufilopressure (ak·ew·fi·lo·presh·er). A method of closure whi combines ligation with acupressure. [L *acus* needle, *filum* threa pressure.]

acuity (ak·ew·it·e). In optics, sharpness or clearness of visio **Displacement threshold acuity.** Vernier acuity (see below). **Li acuity.** Ability to detect the presence of a single line on uniform background; resolving powers of ½ s can be achieve **Minimal separable acuity.** The smallest distance between points so that the eye can just differentiate them as 2. It measured by the visual angle subtended by this distance, a normally equals 1 min. **Vernier acuity.** The minimal distance displacement of contours or lines that can be appreciated by t eye. It is measured by the visual angle subtended by th displacement, and is in the region of 10 s. Used in verniers, ran finders, etc. **Visual acuity.** *See* VISUAL. [L *acuitas* sharpness.]

aculeate (ak·ew·le·ate). 1. In zoology, one of the Aculeata, sub-order of Hymenoptera which includes ants, wasps and be 2. Having a sting. 3. In botany, having sharp points or prick technically known as aculei. [L *aculeus* little needle.]

acumeter (ak·ew·me·ter). Acoumeter.

acuminate (ak·ew·min·ate). Tapering to a sharp point. *acuminare* to sharpen.]

acupressure (ak·ew·presh·er). A method of stopping bleed from a lacerated vessel by inserting needles into the surround tissues in such a way as to compress the vessel. [L *acus* need pressure.]

acupuncture (ak·ew·pungk·tcher). The puncturing of the skin tissues with needles so as to relieve pain or to allow the escape fluid, or for the purpose of counter-irritation. Used in China the relief of pain during surgical operations. Aneurysms may treated by acupuncture of the cavity with a view to coagulation of the contained blood. [L *acus* needle, puncture.]

acus (ak·us). 1. A needle used in surgery. 2. A needle-like proc [L needle.]

acusection (ak·ew·sek·shun). The use of an electrosurgical nee in cutting or sectioning. [L *acus* needle, section.]

acusector (ak·ew·sek·tor). An electric needle which is used lik knife to divide tissues. [see prec.]

acusia (ak·ew·ze·ah). Acousia.

acusticus (ak·oos·tik·us). The auditory nerve. [Gk *akousti* relating to hearing.]

acute (ak·ewt). 1. In disease, referring to symptoms, signs course of intense character, with early resolution in a cer direction—convalescence, chronicity or mortality. 2. Keen or sharpness of sensation. [L *acutus* sharp.]

acutenaculum (ak·ewt·en·ak′·ew·lum). A holder for a surg needle. [L *acus* needle, *tenaculum* holder.]

acuteness (ak·ewt·nes). 1. The state or quality of being acute, clear, sharp or quick; not chronic. 2. In optics, acuity or keenness of sight. [L *acutus* sharp.]

acuticostal (ak·ewt·e·kos'·tal). Descriptive of a condition in which the thorax is enlarged, the ribs projecting beyond usual limits and showing prominently. [acute, L *costa* rib.]

acutorsion (ak·ew·tor·shun). The using of a needle to twist a vessel in order to control bleeding. [L *acus* needle, *torsio* a twisting.]

acutumine (ak·ew·tum·een). $C_{20}H_{27}O_8N$. An isoquinoline alkaloid obtained from the roots of *Sinomenium acutum.*

acyanoblepsia (a·si·an·o·blep'·se·ah). The state of being unable to distinguish the colour blue or shades of blue. [Gk *a*, *kyanos* blue, *blepsis* sight.]

acyanobleptic (a·si·an·o·blep'·tik). Referring to or affected with acyanoblepsia.

acyanopsia (a·si·an·op'·se·ah). Acyanoblepsia. [Gk *a*, *kyanos* blue, *opsis* sight.]

acyclia (a·si·kle·ah). A state in which the circulation of the body fluids is interfered with so that movement is stopped. [Gk *a*, *kyklein* to circulate.]

acyclic (a·si·klik). 1. In botany, not arranged spirally. 2. In chemistry, a term applied to organic compounds with an open-chain structure; aliphatic. 3. Not limited by, or occurring within, the menstrual cycle. [see prec.]

acyesis (a·si·e·sis). 1. The state of being non-pregnant. 2. Sterility in the female. [Gk *a*, *kyesis* pregnancy.]

acyeterion (a·si·et·eer'·e·on). A contraceptive. [see prec.]

acyetic (a·si·e·tik). Referring to acyesis.

acyl (as·il). The acid radical remaining when the acid-hydroxyl group is separated from the formula of an organic acid; it is known also as the *acidyl group.*

acylation (as·il·a·shun). The introduction of an acyl group into the molecule of an organic compound.

acystia (a·sis·te·ah). Absence of the bladder. [Gk *a*, *kystis* bag.]

acystinervia, acystineuria (a·sis·tin·erv'·e·ah, a·sis·tin·ewr'·e·ah). Absence of nerve stimulus in, or paralysis of, the bladder. [Gk *a*, *kystis* bag, L *nervus* (Gk *neuron*) nerve.]

Acystosporidia (a·sis·to·spor·id'·e·ah). An order of Sporozoa closely related to the Haemosporidia. [Gk *a*, *kystis* bag, *sporos* seed.]

acytotoxin (a·si·to·tox·in). A crystalline toxin.

ad-. Prefix, from the Latin *ad*, meaning *to.*

adacrya (a·dak·re·ah). Deficiency or entire absence of the secretion of tears. [Gk *a*, *dakryon* tear.]

adactyl (a·dak·til). Adactylous.

adactylia, adactylism (a·dak·til·e·ah, a·dak·til·izm). The condition of being without fingers or toes, or without both, from birth. [see foll.]

adactylous (a·dak·til·us). Lacking either fingers or toes or both; it may also refer to monsters born without fingers or toes. [Gk *a*, *daktylos* finger.]

adactylus (a·dak·til·us). A monster born lacking fingers or toes, or both. [see prec.]

adactyly (a·dak·til·e). Adactilia.

adamantine (ad·am·an·teen). Appertaining to dental enamel. [Gk *adamas* very hard.]

adamantinocarcinoma (ad·am·an·tin·o·kar·sin·o'·mah). An adamantinoma in which signs of malignancy have appeared. [Gk *adamas* very hard, carcinoma.]

adamantinoma (ad·am·an·tin·o'·mah). Ameloblastoma; a monocystic or more commonly polycystic tumour occurring in the jaws, especially the lower molar region in males. It is derived from tooth-forming epithelial cells or the basal layer of the oral epithelium, and is treated by radical excision. **Pituitary adamantinoma.** An ectopic adamantinoma that has arisen from epithelial remnants, most likely of Rathke's pouch, in the region of the sella turcica or in the pituitary stalk. **Adamantinoma polycysticum.** A slow-growing adamantinoma in which cystic degeneration has taken place. [Gk *adamas* very hard, *-oma* tumour.]

adamantoblast (ad·am·an·to·blast). An enamel-forming cell; an ameloblast. [Gk *adamas* very hard, *blastos* germ.]

adamantoblastoma (ad·am·an·to·blas·to'·mah). Adamantinoma. [adamantoblast, Gk *-oma* tumour.]

adamantoma (ad·am·an·to'·mah). Adamantinoma.

adamas dentis (ad·am·as den·tis). The dental enamel. [Gk *adamas* very hard, L *dens* tooth.]

Adami, John George (b. 1862). Montreal and Liverpool pathologist.

Adami's theory. An explanation of heredity based on the hypothesis that cells possess side-chains or receptors which give them special functional characteristics.

Adamkiewicz, Albert (b. 1850). Cracow and Vienna pathologist.

demilune of Adamkiewicz. A neurilemmal cell.

Adamkiewicz's reaction, or test. For tryptophan, and proteins containing tryptophan: 3 ml of solution is mixed with 2 ml glacial acetic acid which has been exposed to sunlight and layered with H_2SO_4. A deep purple forms at the junction of the liquids. *See also* HOPKINS-COLE TEST.

adam's apple (ad·amz ap·l). The laryngeal prominence, a subcutaneous projection of the thyroid cartilage, visible on the front of the neck and movable on swallowing.

Adams, James A. (b. 1857). Glasgow gynaecologist.

Alexander-Adams operation. Extraperitoneal shortening of the round ligaments for the correction of uterine retroversion. The ligaments are shortened by dividing them in their course through the inguinal canal, pulling on the proximal ends and then securing them to the external oblique aponeurosis.

Adams, Robert (b. 1791). Dublin surgeon.

Adams-Stokes attack, disease or syndrome, Morgagni-Adams-Stokes disease or syndrome, Stokes-Adams syndrome. Disturbance of consciousness due to inadequate cerebral blood flow, accompanying extreme slowing of the heart or ventricular standstill; in severe cases complete loss of consciousness and even epileptiform convulsions may result. As soon as ventricular beating is resumed, consciousness is rapidly regained, followed by a widespread flush (reactive hyperaemia). It occurs not infrequently when partial atrioventricular heart block is becoming complete, and less frequently in cases of established complete heart block. Ventricular asystole may sometimes follow an episode of ventricular paroxysmal tachycardia with a similar clinical syndrome, but this is not strictly the Morgagni-Adams-Stokes syndrome. Originally described by Morgagni in 1700, it is usually called the *Stokes-Adams syndrome.*

Adams, Sir William (b. 1783). London ophthalmic surgeon.

Adams' operation. 1. For glaucoma: the original iridotasis operation. 2. For ectropion: a through-and-through resection of a wedge-shaped portion of the eyelid, the base being along the central part of the lid margin. One of the first of this type of operation.

Adams, William (b. 1820). London surgeon.

Adams' operation. 1. Subcutaneous division of palmar fascia for Dupuytren's contraction. 2. Subcutaneous osteotomy of the upper part of the femur.

Adams' saw. A small narrow saw used for linear division of a bone through a small skin wound.

Adams' method. For fat in milk; 5 ml of milk is dried on filter paper which is then coiled and extracted with ether in a Soxhlet's apparatus. The ether is removed by distillation and the residual fat dried and weighed.

Adams' position. A forward-bending position with the heels together and the body well stretched.

adamsite (ad·amz·ite). Diphenylaminechlorarsine, $NH(C_6H_4)_2AsCl$. A yellow substance, the vapour of which irritates the nasal mucous membrane, and is used therefore in chemical warfare.

Adamson, Horatio George (b. 1865). London dermatologist.

Adamson's fringe. In tinea capitis infection, the terminal growing hyphae within the hair and near its root.

Kienboeck-Adamson method, or technique and points. In epilation of the scalp, the hair is cut very short all over the scalp, and 5 points are then marked as follows: Point A, 3.8 to 5 cm (1½ to 2 in) behind the frontal margin of the hair; Point B, 2.5 to 3.8 cm (1 to 1½ in) above the centre of the flat area which forms the upper part of the occiput; Point C, 2.5 cm (1 in) above the lower border of the scalp at the lower part of the occiput; Point D, on the right side just above and in front of the ear; Point E, on the left side just above and in front of the ear. Points A, B and C are in the mid-sagittal plane of the scalp: the distance between any 2 of the points is 13 cm (5 in). An x-ray beam is focused on each of the points in turn and a sufficient exposure is given (about 400 R) to cause epilation. During the exposures, the glabrous skin is protected by lead.

Adansonia (ad·an·**so**·ne·ah). A genus of sterculaceous trees. **Adansonia digitata.** The Indian and African baobab tree, the leaves of which are febrifugal. [Michel *Adanson,* 1727–1806, French naturalist.]

adaptation (ad·ap·**ta**·shun). 1. The process of modification which an animal or a plant undergoes in order to adapt itself to novel environmental conditions. The process is opposed to the influence of heredity. 2. The ability possessed by the normal eye to adjust itself to alterations in the intensity of light. 3. Immunization. 4. In reflex activity, a condition in which the repetition of sensory stimuli has induced a lowering of the frequency of impulses. **Dark adaptation.** The power of the eye to adjust itself to seeing in the dark. General adaptation syndrome (GAS). *See* SELYE SYNDROME. **Light adaptation.** Adaptation of the eyes to an abnormally bright or dim light; adaptation to a normal light after being in darkness. **Retinal adaptation.** The changes in sensitivity which take place in the retina so that the eyes may adjust themselves completely to alterations in intensity of the surrounding light. [L *adaptatio* process of adapting.]

adaptometer (ad·ap·**tom**·et·er). An instrument used to detect night blindness; it measures the time required for the visual purple to be renewed. [L *adaptare* to fit to, meter.]

adarticulartion (ad·ar·tik·ew·**la′**·shun). In anatomy, a form of joint in which the articular surfaces are flat and glide over or against each other in movement; arthrodia. [L *ad, articulare* to divide into joints.]

adatom (**ad**·at·om). An atom absorbed at a surface and remaining in the plane of the interface. [L *ad,* atom.]

adaxial (ad·**ax**·e·al). Directed towards or situated to the side of an axis. [L *ad,* axis.]

adder (**ad**·er). A poisonous snake of North Europe (*Vipera berus*), distinguished from the non-poisonous British snakes by the vertical elliptical pupil and, usually, a zigzag dark line down the back. **Adder bite.** A bite by the adder, *Vipera berus.* Its bite may be fatal in children and small adults. This causes local haemorrhages and cardiovascular failure that may amount to severe collapse; in the absence of antivenene the latter should be treated by immobilization and hydrocortisone injection. [AS *naedre* serpent.]

addict (**ad**·ikt). An individual who has surrendered himself to a habit; generally used in reference to alcohol or dangerous drugs such as morphine, cocaine, heroin. [L *addicere to devote.]*

addiction (ad·**ik**·shun). The state of having surrendered to a habit. [see prec.]

addiment (**ad**·e·ment). Complement. [L *addere* to add.]

addimentary (ad·e·**ment**·ar·e). Referring or belonging to addiment.

Addis, Thomas (b. 1881). San Francisco physician.

Addis count, or method. A test for renal disease based upon the principle that the nature and extent of kidney disease gives rise to different numbers of cells and casts in the urine. The count is made in an aliquot of a 12-h specimen collected under rigidly defined conditions.

Addis and Shevsky test. For kidney function: the patient abstains from fluid for 24 h; the urine is collected during the second 12 h of this period and the specific gravity determined. Normal function is shown by a specific gravity of more than 1.026.

Addison, Christopher, 1st Viscount (b. 1869). London statesman, formerly anatomist.

Addison's transpyloric plane. An imaginary transverse plane lying halfway between the suprasternal notch and the pubic symphysis. It passes through the tips of the 9th costal cartilages and the lower border of the 1st lumbar vertebra.

Addison's point. The midpoint of the epigastric region.

Addison, Thomas (b. 1793?). London physician.

Addison's anaemia. Pernicious anaemia. *See* ANAEMIA.

Addisonian crisis. Acute failure of the adrenal glands, as occurs in Addison's disease, characterized by hypoglycaemia and sodium deficiency.

Addison's disease. A disease due to atrophy or tuberculosis of the adrenal cortex leading to deficiency or absence of cortisol (*see* AUTOIMMUNE ADRENALITIS and CARD-ADDISON'S DISEASE).

Addison's keloid. Sclerodermia circumscriptum.

additamentum (ad·it·ah·**men′**·tum). Any outgrowth or appendage. An obsolete anatomical term not found in any modern nomenclature. [L addition.]

addition (ad·**ish**·un). In chemistry, the union of 2 or more whole molecules to form another molecule. [L *additio* something added.]

adducens oculi (ad·**ew**·senz **ok**·ew·li). The medial rectus muscle of the orbit. *See* RECTUS MUSCLES OF THE ORBIT. [L *adducere* to bring to, *oculus* eye.]

adducent (ad·**ew**·sent). In physiology, adducting; causing adduction.

adduct (ad·**ukt**). In physiology, to draw towards the median line or the axis of the body. [L *adducere* to bring to.]

adduction (ad·**uk**·shun). The act of adducting or of drawing, especially towards the median line of the body. **Convergence-stimulus adduction.** The power of adduction of the eyes brought into play when the gaze is fixed on an object at the near point. [see prec.]

adductor (ad·**uk**·tor). Any muscle which adducts or draws a part towards the median line or the axis of the body. **Adductor tubercle.** *See* TUBERCLE. [L *adducere* to bring to.]

adductor brevis muscle [musculus adductor brevis (NA)] (ad·**uk**·tor **brev**·is). One of the adductors of the thigh, placed behind the pectineus and the adductor longus muscles. It is attached to the inferior pubic ramus and the upper part of the shaft of the femur.

adductor hallucis muscle [musculus adductor hallucis (NA)] (ad·**uk**·tor **hal**·oo·sis). A deep muscle of the sole of the foot arising by 2 heads, an oblique [caput obliquum] at the bases of the middle 3 metatarsal bones, and a transverse [caput transversum] from the plantar metatarsal and phalangeal ligaments, and inserted into the outer side of the base of the first phalanx of the big toe.

adductor longus muscle [musculus adductor longus (NA)] (ad·**uk**·tor **long**·gus). The most anterior of the adductor muscles of the thigh. It stretches from the front of the body of the pubis to the middle third of the linea aspera.

adductor magnus muscle [musculus adductor magnus (NA)] (ad·**uk**·tor **mag**·nus). The largest of the adductor muscles of the thigh with extensive origin from the inferior rami of the ischium and the pubis, and the ischial tuberosity. It is attached to the whole length of the shaft of the femur. **Opening [hiatus tendineus (adductorius)].** The opening in the lower part of the adductor magnus muscle through which pass the femoral vessels into the popliteal fossa.

adductor minimus muscle (ad·**uk**·tor **min**·im·us). An occasional separate upper portion of the adductor magnus muscle.

adductor pollicis muscle [musculus adductor pollicis (NA)] (ad·**uk**·tor **pol**·is·is). One of the deep muscles of the thenar eminence arising by an oblique head [caput obliquuum (NA)] from the capitate and neighbouring bones and a transverse head [caput transversum (NA)] from the 3rd metacarpal bone. It is inserted into the base of the 1st phalanx of the thumb. It approximates the thumb to the index finger.

Adelmann, Georg Franz Blasius (b. 1811). Dorpat surgeon.

Adelmann's manoeuvre. Forcible flexion of a limb to control haemorrhage by impeding the arterial flow.

Adelmann's operation. Amputation of the finger together with the metacarpal head.

adelomorphic, adelomorphous (ad·el·o·**mor'**·fik, ad·el·o·**mor'**·fus). In biology, having an obscure or not clearly defined form. The term is applied specifically to the central cells of the gastric glands. [Gk *adelos* not apparent, *morphe* form.]

adelphia (ad·el·fe·ah). A form of monstrosity in which the upper portions of 2 organisms are united and the lower portions are separate. [Gk *adelphos* brother.]

adelphotaxis, adelphotaxy (ad·el·fo·**tax'**·is, ad·el·fo·**tax'**·e). In biology, the assuming of a particular arrangement and position by motile cells. [Gk *adelphos* brother, *taxis* arrangement.]

adenalgia (ad·en·**al**·je·ah). A painful condition of a gland. [Gk *aden* gland, *algos* pain.]

adenase (**ad**·en·aze). An enzyme which exists in the liver and spleen and plays an important part in purine metabolism, deaminating, as it does, adenine into hypoxanthine. [Gk *aden* gland.]

adenasthenia (ad·en·as·**the'**·ne·ah). Functional deficiency in a gland. **Adenasthenia gastrica.** Functional deficiency in the gastric glands so that there is diminished secretion from them. [Gk *aden* gland, asthenia.]

adendric, adendritic (a·**den**·drik, a·den·**drit**·ik). Referring to the condition in neural cells when dendrites are absent. [Gk *a*, dendrite.]

adenectomy (ad·en·**ek**·to·me). 1. Removal of a gland by surgical means. 2. Surgical removal of growths in the nasopharyngeal tonsil. [Gk *aden* gland, *ektome* a cutting out.]

adenectopia (ad·en·ek·**to'**·pe·ah). A condition in which a gland is displaced either because of simple malposition or because of disease or accident. [Gk *aden* gland, ectopia.]

adenectopic (ad·en·ek·**top'**·ik). Referring to adenectopia.

adenemphratic (ad·en·em·**frat'**·ik). Referring to adenemphraxis.

adenemphraxis (ad·en·em·**frax'**·is). Obstruction in a gland or glands. [Gk *aden* gland, emphraxis.]

adenia (ad·e·ne·ah). A state of chronic adenitis in which the lymph glands are greatly enlarged. **Angiobromic adenia.** Any disease which attacks the glands in the region of the alimentary canal. **Leukaemic adenia.** A leukaemic state of the blood associated with adenia. **Simple adenia.** 1. Adenia in which there is no leucocytosis. 2. Hodgkin's disease [obsolete term.] [Gk *aden* gland.]

adenic (ad·e·nik). Having a resemblance or referring to a gland. [see prec.]

adeniform (ad·e·ne·form). Gland-like; having the shape of a gland. [Gk *aden* gland, form.]

adenine (**ad**·en·een). An amino purine base, $C_5H_5N_5$, which is found widely distributed in plant and animal nucleoproteins. It is produced by the decomposition of the nucleic acids, in which it occurs combined with phosphoric acid and ribose (or deoxyribose), and is deaminated in the metabolism to hypoxanthine. The urine of leukaemic patients contains large quantities of adenine. **Adenine hypoxanthine.** Adenine with its corresponding oxypurine, hypoxanthine. **Adenine nucleotide.** Any nucleotide containing adenine as the base. Common examples are ATP, ADP, AMP, cyclic 3′,5′-AMP, NAD^+ and FAD. **Adenine sulphate.** $C_5H_5N_5(SO_4)$, prepared from yeast-nucleic acid, and given intravenously in cases of agranulocytosis.

adenitis (ad·en·i·tis). A state of acute or chronic inflammation in a gland. The term may be qualified anatomically, such as *cervical, axillary, cubital,* or according to the infecting organism, as in the case of *pyogenic* or *tuberculous adenitis,* or according to the pathological character or stage, e.g. *hyperplastic adenitis.* **Acute salivary adenitis.** The name given to an epidemic that occurred in Naples, in which the parotid and other salivary glands, the axillary lymphatic glands and the spleen were enlarged and painful. **Lymphatic adenitis.** Lymphadenitis; adenitis in a lymph node. **Mesenteric adenitis.** Inflammation of the mesenteric lymph nodes which may simulate acute appendicitis. It may be due to adenovirus infection. **Salivary adenitis.** Sialadenitis; adenitis in a salivary gland. [Gk *aden* gland, *-itis* inflammation.]

adenization (**ad**·en·i·**za'**·shun). 1. Glandular or adenoid degeneration. 2. Assuming the appearance of glands. [Gk *aden* gland.]

adeno-acanthoma (ad·en·o·ak·an·**tho'**·mah). Squamoglandular tumour of the uterus. [Gk *aden* gland, acanthoma.]

adeno-ameloblastoma (ad·en·o·am·**el**·o·blas·**to'**·mah). A benign non-recurrent neoplasm of the maxilla. [Gk *aden* gland, ameloblastoma.]

adeno-angiosarcoma (ad·en·o·**an**·je·o·sar·**ko'**·mah). An angiosarcoma involving glandular structures. [Gk *aden* gland, angiosarcoma.]

adenoblast (**ad**·en·o·blast). 1. Any embryonic animal cell in which glandular tissue has its origin. 2. Any cell the activity of which is secretory or glandular. [Gk *aden* gland, *blastos* germ.]

adenocancroid (ad·en·o·**kan'**·kroid). Adeno-acanthoma. [Gk *aden* gland, cancroid.]

adenocarcinoma (ad·en·o·kar·sin·**o'**·mah). A malignant or carcinomatous adenoma. **Papillary adenocarcinoma, Polypoid adenocarcinoma.** An adenocarcinoma of clearly malignant character. **Scirrhous adenocarcinoma.** A malignant tumour of gland-like structure in which the supporting connective tissue has grown copiously and threatens to overwhelm the malignant cells. **Adenocarcinoma sudorificum.** Carcinoma arising in sweat glands. [Gk *aden* gland, carcinoma.]

adenocele (**ad**·en·o·seel). A cystic tumour in which there are adenomatous structures. [Gk *aden* gland, *kele* hernia.]

adenocellulitis (ad·en·o·**sel**·ew·**li'**·tis). Inflammation of a gland with inflammation of the surrounding cellular tissue. [Gk *aden* gland, cellulitis.]

adenochondroma (ad·en·o·kon·**dro'**·mah). A tumour involving glandular and cartilaginous tissues. [Gk *aden* gland, chondroma.]

adenochondrosarcoma (ad·en·o·**kon**·dro·sar·**ko'**·mah). A sarcomatous tumour involving glandular and cartilaginous tissues. [Gk *aden* gland, chondrosarcoma.]

adenochrome (**ad**·en·o·krome). The colouring matter contained in the adrenal glands. [Gk *aden* gland, *chroma* colour.]

adenocyst (**ad**·en·o·sist). Adenocystoma.

adenocystoma (ad·en·o·sis·**to'**·mah). Adenoma in association with cystic growths. **Papillary adenocystoma lymphomatosum.** A cystic tumour involving the submandibular and the parotid glands. [Gk *aden* gland, cystoma.]

adenocyte (**ad**·en·o·site). Any fully developed secretory cell contained in a gland. [Gk *aden* gland, *kytos* cell.]

adenodermia (ad·en·o·**derm'**·e·ah). Disease affecting the skin glands. [Gk *aden* gland, *derma* skin.]

adenodiastasis (ad·en·o·di·**as'**·tas·is). 1. A condition of a gland in which it is separated into 2 or more distinct parts. 2. Displacement of a gland. [Gk *aden* gland, *diastasis* separation.]

adenodynia (ad·en·o·**din'**·e·ah). Adenalgia. [Gk *aden* gland, *odyne* pain.]

adeno-epithelioma (ad·en·o·**ep**·e·the·le·**o'**·mah). A tumour consisting of both glandular and epithelial cells. [Gk *aden* gland, epithelioma.]

adenofibroma (ad·en·o·fi·**bro'**·mah). A tumour consisting of glandular and connective tissue. **Adenofibroma oedematodes.** A nasal polypus largely consisting of glandular elements. [Gk *aden* gland, fibroma.]

adenofibrosarcoma (ad·en·o·**fi**·bro·sar·**ko'**·mah). A malignant tumour that is a sarcomatous degeneration of an adenofibroma. [adenofibroma, sarcoma.]

adenofibrosis (ad·en·o·fi·**bro'**·sis). Glandular degeneration of fibroid character. [Gk *aden* gland, fibrosis.]

adenogenesis (ad·en·o·**jen'**·es·is). The origin and growth of a gland. [Gk *aden* gland, *genein* to produce.]

adenogenous (ad·en·**oj**·en·us). Having origin in a gland or in glandular tissue. [see prec.]

adenohypersthenia (ad·en·o·**hi**·per·**sthe'**·ne·ah). Over-activity of the glands. **Adenohypersthenia gastrica.** A state in which the glands of the stomach are overactive, or in which there is an excessive quantity of hydrochloric acid in the gastric juice. [Gk *aden* gland, hypersthenia.]

adenohypophysis (**ad**·en·o·hi·**pof**′·is·is). The anterior lobe (glandular portion) of the hypophysis cerebri. Also referred to as the pars glandularis of the pituitary. [Gk *aden* gland, hypophysis.]

adenoid (**ad**·en·oid). 1. Having resemblance or relating to a gland. 2. Resembling or relating to lymphoid tissue. [Gk *aden* gland, *eidos* form.]

adenoidectomy (**ad**·en·oid·**ek**′·to·me). An operation for excision of adenoids. [adenoids, Gk *ektome* excision.]

adenoidism (**ad**·en·oid·izm). A term which describes the general condition of persons with adenoids: adenoid face, mouth breathing, facial pallor.

adenoiditis (**ad**·en·oid·**i**′·tis). An inflamed condition of adenoids. [adenoid, Gk *-itis* inflammation.]

adenoids (**ad**·en·oidz). Hypertrophy of the pharyngeal tonsil in the nasopharynx in children. The name generally given to the adenoid syndrome. *See* ADENOIDISM. [Gk *aden* gland, *eidos* form.]

adenoleiomyofibroma, adenoliomyofibroma (**ad**·en·o·li·o·mi·-o·fi·**bro**′·mah). A leiomyofibroma in which there are glandular elements. [Gk *aden* gland, leiomyofibroma.]

adenolipoma (**ad**·en·o·li·**po**′·mah). A glandular tumour in which there is a large amount of adipose tissue. [Gk *aden* gland, lipoma.]

adenolipomatosis (**ad**·en·o·**lip**·o·mat·**o**′·sis). A disease marked by painless symmetrical fatty infiltrations containing small hard nodules of lymphatic tissue. The masses form in the subcutaneous tissues and occur mainly in the groin, the axillae and the neck. [Gk *aden* gland, lipomatosis.]

adenologaditis (**ad**·en·o·log·ad·**i**′·tis). Inflammation of conjunctival glands, an old term for ophthalmia neonatorum. [Gk *aden* gland, *logades* whites of the eyes, *-itis* inflammation.]

adenology (ad·en·**ol**·o·je). The complete science of the glandular system. [Gk *aden* gland, *logos* science.]

adenolymphitis (**ad**·en·o·lim·**fi**′·tis). Lymphadenitis.

adenolymphocele (**ad**·en·o·**lim**′·fo·seel). Cystic degeneration of the lymph glands, often with glandular hyperplasia and dilatation of the lymph vessels. [Gk *aden* gland, lymphocele.]

adenolymphoma (**ad**·en·o·lim·**fo**′·mah). An encapsulated tumour formed of abundant irregular papillary processes projecting into cystic spaces. The epithelium consists of tall columnar cells with a copious finely granular cytoplasm. The stroma consists of lymphoid tissue containing well-formed follicles. It is usually found in the salivary glands, particularly the parotid. [Gk *aden* gland, lymphoma.]

adenoma (ad·en·**o**·mah). A simple tumour of glandular epithelium and connective tissue. either of which may predominate; it often reproduces the structure and function of the parent tissue. **Acidophilic adenoma.** An adenoma of the eosinophil (acidophil) cells of the hypophysis. **Adamantine adenoma.** Adamantinoma. **Alveolar adenoma.** An adenoma the basic structure of which is that of the alveolar gland. **Basophil adenoma.** A hypophyseal tumour the cells of which take basophil dyes. **Adenoma carcinomatodes renis.** Malignant renal adenoma (see below). **Chromophobe adenoma.** A hypophyseal tumour associated with hypopituitarism; the cells do not take up eosinophil or basophil dyes. **Cortical adenoma.** An adenoma of the adrenal cortex. **Cylindricellular adenoma.** Cystoma. **Destructive adenoma.** A malignant adenoma which destroys as it grows. **Diffuse adenoma.** Glandular hyperplasia of the mucous membrane. **Eosinophil adenoma.** A tumour, associated with gigantism and acromegaly, which arises in the eosinophilic cells of the anterior lobe of the pituitary gland. **Fibrous adenoma, Adenoma fibrosum.** Fibro-adenoma. **Heteropodous adenoma.** A metastatic adenoma the origin of which is in normal glandular tissue. **Hidradenoid adenoma.** Syringocystadenoma. **Islet cell adenoma.** Insuloma. **Lupiform adenoma.** Lupus erythematosus. **Malignant adenoma.** Adenocarcinoma. **Malignant renal adenoma.** Adenoma carcinomatodes renis, a hypernephroma with unusually prominent glandular structure, or a cystic adenoma which has undergone complete or partial malignant change. **Adenoma of the nipple.** Benign papillomatosis of the nipple, a naevoid tumour probably arising from lactiferous ducts. **Papillary adenoma.** An adenoma in which the glandular lining membrane projects into the alveoli, or one growing out from the surface of a cavity. **Papillary cystic adenoma.** A form of adenoma in which outgrowths of tissue or cystic collections of fluid distend the alveoli. **Pleomorphic salivary adenoma.** The commonest of salivary-gland tumours, most frequently found in the parotid. It appears to be encapsulated but in focal areas neoplastic tissue may be seen in direct contact with salivary-gland tissue. The epithelial tissues of the tumour may show acinar formation or may be arranged as irregular sheets of cells. Mucoid changes often occur in the stroma, as may areas of chondroid or cartilaginous tissue. **Racemose adenoma.** One resembling a racemose gland in structure. **Renal adenoma.** A simple glandular tumour of the kidney. **Sebaceous adenoma.** A slow overgrowth of the sebaceous glands of the face, accompanied by oversecretion and sometimes cyst formation; it occurs in middle-aged or old persons and is very rarely malignant. **Simple adenoma.** A gland which has undergone simple hyperplasia. **Sudoriparous adenoma.** Adenoma of the sweat glands; spiradenoma. **Toxic adenoma of the thyroid gland.** Adenoma which gives rise to hyperthyroidism. **Tubular adenoma.** A type which presents the pattern of a tubular gland. **Umbilical adenoma.** A tiny cystic glandular tumour arising from remnants of the allantois in the navel. [Gk *aden* gland, *-oma* tumour.]

See also: GETSOWA, HUERTHLE.

adenomalacia (**ad**·en·o·mal·**a**′·she·ah). Morbid or unnatural softness of a gland. [Gk *aden* gland, malacia.]

adenomammectomy (**ad**·en·o·mam·**ek**′·to·me). Removal of the breast substance leaving the covering integuments, including the nipple. [Gk *aden* gland, mammectomy.]

adenomatoid (ad·en·**o**·mat·oid). Having a resemblance to adenoma. [adenoma, Gk *eidos* form.]

adenomatome (ad·en·**o**·mat·ome). An instrument for the excision or removal of adenomatous growths; it may be in the form of scissors or forceps. [adenoma, Gk *temnein* to cut.]

adenomatosis (**ad**·en·o·mat·**o**′·sis). A condition in which excessive adenomatous growth occurs in a gland or a group of glands. **Adenomatosis of the colon.** Benign polyps of the colon, usually in the sigmoid colon, which often bleed and sometimes cause intussusception. They may be multiple or single and are of frequent occurrence, especially in man. If large, they may become malignant. **Multiple endocrine adenomatosis.** A combination of adenomas which may be present in the pancreas, parathyroids, anterior pituitary or adrenals. **Pancreatic-islet adenomatosis.** An adenomatous overgrowth of the islets associated clinically with hypoglycaemic episodes; a rare condition. **Polyendocrine adenomatosis.** Multiple tumours of several endocrine glands, especially the parathyroids, often causing peptic ulcer, as in the Zollinger–Ellison syndrome. [adenoma, Gk *osis* condition.]

adenomatous (ad·en·**o**·mat·us). 1. Relating to or characteristic of adenoma. 2. Relating to general hyperplasia of gland tissue. [adenoma.]

adenomere (**ad**·en·o·meer). The functional portion of a gland, generally situated at the blind end of the developing cavity. [Gk *aden* gland, *meros* part.]

adenomesenteritis (**ad**·en·o·**mes**·en·ter·**i**′·tis). An inflammatory condition of the mesenteric glands. [Gk *aden* gland, mesenteritis.]

adenomyofibroma (**ad**·en·o·**mi**·o·fi·**bro**′·mah). A fibroma in which there are hyperplastic glandular and muscular tissues. [Gk *aden* gland, myofibroma.]

adenomyoma (**ad**·en·o·mi·**o**′·mah). A tumour formed from muscular and glandular tissue, and occurring in the uterus (endometrioma) and the stomach. **Branchiogenic adenomyoma.** A tumour arising from remnants of the gill clefts in the neck, and sometimes malignant. **Mesonephric adenomyoma.** Wilms' tumour; a mixed tumour containing embryonic renal and mesenchymal elements, including muscle and sometimes cartilage. It arises in the kidneys of young children. **Psammo-papillary adenomyoma.** A multiple papillary tumour which occurs in the broad ligament of the uterus. [Gk *aden* gland, *mys* muscle, *-oma* tumour.]

adenomyomatosis (ad·en·o·mi·o·mat·o′·sis). A condition of primary adenomyoma, with considerable extension into the surrounding tissues. [adenomyoma, Gk *-osis* condition.]

adenomyometritis (ad·en·o·mi·o·met·ri′·tis). An inflammatory condition of the uterus in which there is hyperplasia with characters of adenomyoma. [Gk *aden* gland, myometritis.]

adenomyosarcoma (ad·en·o·mi·o·sar·ko′·mah). Adenosarcoma characterized by the inclusion of striped muscle. **Embryonal adenomyosarcoma.** Wilms' tumour; mesonephric adenomyoma. [Gk *aden* gland, myosarcoma.]

adenomyosis (ad·en·o·mi·o′·sis). Endometriosis; growth of endometrial type of tissue outside the endometrium. **Adenomyosis externa.** Endometriosis occurring in a situation other than that of the uterus. **Adenomyosis of the gall bladder.** A condition in which, in a localized area of the gall bladder wall, there is a combination of gross muscular hypertrophy and multiple diverticula from the mucous membrane; cholecystitis glandularis proliferans. **Adenomyosis interna.** Internal endometriosis to be found in the wall of the uterus. **Stromal adenomyosis.** Endometriosis. [Gk *aden* gland, *mys* muscle, *-osis* condition.]

adenomyositis (ad·en·o·mi·o·si′·tis). A condition of the uterus which resembles that of adenomyoma; there is inflammation and pathological enlargement. [Gk *aden* gland, *mys* muscle, *-itis* inflammation.]

adenomyxoma (ad·en·o·mix·o′·mah). A tumour which consists partly of mucous and partly of glandular tissue. [Gk *aden* gland, *myxa* mucus, *-oma* tumour.]

adenomyxosarcoma (ad·en·o·mix·o·sar·ko′·mah). A malignant tumour, beginning as an adenoma and undergoing sarcomatous degeneration with accompanying myxomatous changes. [Gk *aden* gland, myxoma, sarcoma.]

adenoncosis (ad·en·ong·ko′·sis). A swollen condition of a gland. [Gk *aden* gland, *ogkosis* swelling.]

adenoncus (ad·en·ong·kus). A tumour of a gland. [Gk *aden* gland, *ogkos* tumour.]

adenoneural (ad·en·o·newr′·al). Involving gland and nerve. [Gk *aden* gland, *neuron* nerve.]

adenoneure (ad·en·o·newr). A neurone which controls the action of a gland. [see prec.]

adenopathy (ad·en·op·ath·e). Any disease affecting a gland, more particularly a lymph gland. **Angiobromic adenopathy.** Angiobromic adenia. *See* ADENIA. **Multiple endocrine adenopathy.** A syndrome in which 2 or more endocrine glands secrete excessive amounts of hormone, especially involving parathyroid glands, islet cells of the pancreas, and anterior pituitary glands. **Primary adenopathy.** An inflammation of the lymph glands occurring after primary syphilis. **Syphilitic adenopathy.** A condition, symptomatic of syphilitic infection, in which the supratrochlear, inguinal or cervical lymph glands, or all 3 groups, are hardened and enlarged to a variable extent. **Tracheobronchial adenopathy, Tracheobronchic adenopathy.** A condition which causes spasmodic cough and is the result of enlargement of the lymph glands in the neighbourhood of the bronchus. **Tracheolaryngeal adenopathy.** Inflammation and enlargement of the lymph glands of the trachea and the larynx. [Gk *aden* gland, *pathos* suffering.]

adenopharyngeal (ad·en·o·far·in′·je·al). Involving the tonsils and the pharynx. [Gk *aden* gland, pharynx.]

adenopharyngitis (ad·en·o·far·in·ji′·tis). An inflammatory condition of the tonsils and the pharynx. [Gk *aden* gland, pharynx, Gk *-itis* inflammation.]

adenophlegmon (ad·en·o·fleg′·mon). Phlegmonous adenitis, with sepsis and pus formation; septic invasion of lymph glands, with formation of abscess or ulcer. [Gk *aden* gland, *phlegmone* inflammation.]

adenophthalmia (ad·en·of·thal′·me·ah). Inflammation of the tarsal (meibomian) glands of the eyelid. [Gk *aden* gland, *ophthalmos* eye.]

adenophyma (ad·en·o·fi′·mah). A glandular swelling, e.g. bubo. [Gk *aden* gland, *phyma* a growth.]

adenosarcoma (ad·en·o·sar·ko′·mah). 1. A tumour of mixed adenomatous and sarcomatous tissue. 2. Sarcoma of a gland. **Embryonal adenosarcoma.** A complex sarcoma-like growth which occurs congenitally in the adrenal gland or kidney. [Gk *aden* gland, sarcoma.]

adenosarcorhabdomyoma (ad·en·o·sar·ko·rab·do·mi·o′·mah). A tumour in which there are elements of adenoma, sarcoma and rhabdomyoma.

adenoscirrhus (ad·en·o·skir′·rus). An adenoma composed of scirrhous or hard cancerous constituents. [Gk *aden* gland, *skirrhos* hard.]

adenosclerosis (ad·en·o·skler·o′·sis). Induration of a gland, with or without enlargement. [Gk *aden* gland, sclerosis.]

adenose (ad·en·oze). With excessive glandular elements. [Gk *aden* gland.]

adenosinase (ad·en·o·sin·aze). A hydrolytic enzyme which breaks down adenosine.

adenosine (ad·en·o·seen). The nucleoside, adenine D-ribose, obtained by the acid hydrolysis of the mononucleotide adenylic acid; it is considered the chief source of ammonia in the blood. **Adenosine 3′5′-cyclic monophosphate.** Cyclic AMP; the nucleotide which acts as the intracellular mediator of the action of several hormones, including glucagon, adrenaline, ACTH, parathyroid hormone and vasopressin. It is formed from ATP by the action of adenylyl cyclase and is broken down by a specific phosphodiesterase. Its action has in some cases been shown to be primarily an activation of intracellular protein kinases by combination with, and consequent neutralization of, the inhibitory "regulatory" subunit of the kinase. **Adenosine deaminase.** The enzyme which accomplishes the deamination of adenosine into inosine. **Adenosine diphosphate.** Adenosine diphosphoric acid. *See* ACID. **Adenosine hydrolase.** The enzyme which brings about the hydrolysis of adenosine into adenine and ribose. **Adenosine monophosphate.** (CYCLIC) ADENOSINE MONOPHOSPHATE activates phosphorylase to break down glycogen to glucose. Adenylic acid. *See* ACID. **Adenosine phosphosulphate.** Active sulphate, the sulphur-containing precursor of certain structural mucopolysaccharides, e.g. keratin sulphate, chondroitin sulphate. It is formed from inorganic sulphate and ATP. **Adenosine triphosphatase.** An enzyme found in voluntary muscle, able to split the high energy-giving substance adenosine triphosphate, and thus restore the potential energy of muscle. Myosin has this enzymatic property. **Adenosine triphosphate (ATP).** The substance formed during oxidative phosphorylation which acts as a major source of energy. Hydrolysis of the terminal high energy phosphate bond results in release of energy. **Adenosine triphosphatase (ATPase).** The enzyme which catalyses the hydrolysis of the high energy phosphate bond of ATP.

adenosis (ad·en·o·sis). 1. Any disease or chronic disorder of the glands, particularly of the lymph glands. 2. The process of formation or the development of glandular tissue. **Fibrosing adenosis.** An innocent histological finding in the breast resulting from atypical involution of a breast lobule which may simulate a carcinoma. **Adenosis scrofulosa.** Glandular disease of tuberculous origin. [Gk *aden* gland, *-osis* condition.]

adenositis (ad·en·o·si′·tis). A condition in which the reaction of the body to inflammation has been the development of glandular tissue. [Gk *aden* gland, *-itis* inflammation.]

adenosynchitonitis (ad·en·o·sin·ki·ton·i′·tis). 1. Inflammation of the tarsal glands of the eyelids. 2. A term sometimes used for ophthalmia neonatorum. [Gk *aden* gland, *syn, chiton* tunic, *-itis* inflammation.]

adenotome (ad·en·o·tome). An instrument used for excising glands or more particularly for removing adenoids. [Gk *aden* gland, *temnein* to cut.]

adenotomy (ad·en·ot·o·me). 1. The dissection or incision of glands. 2. The operation of removal of the adenoid growths by excision. [see prec.]

adenotonsillectomy (ad·en·o·ton·sil·ek′·to·me). Excision of the adenoids and tonsils. [Gk *aden* gland, tonsil, Gk *ektome* a cutting out.]

adenous (**ad**·en·us). 1. Like a gland. 2. With glandular characteristics. [Gk *aden* gland.]

adenovarix (ad·en·o·**va**·rix). A varicose condition of a lymphatic gland or group of lymphatic glands caused by back pressure due to lymphatic obstruction, e.g. in filariasis, where it is often situated in the axilla or groin. [Gk *aden* gland, L *varix* a dilated vein.]

adenovirus (**ad**·en·o·**vi**′·rus). A DNA-containing virus, 65 nm in size. There are 33 serotypes of which types 1–7 are most commonly associated with disease in man. Adenoviruses cause mild upper respiratory tract infections and/or conjunctivitis in adults but can cause a more severe or fatal pneumonia in infants. Adenoviruses may be found in the stools of children by culture and electron microscopy. Although sometimes found in association with enteritis the significance of these observations has yet to be established. Morphologically identical but serologically distinct viruses are found in monkeys, cats, dogs, mice and chickens. Some less common human strains (types 7, 12 and 18) have been found to cause tumours in suckling hamsters but are not known to be oncogenic in man. [Gk *aden* gland, L *virus* poison.]

adenyl (**ad**·en·il). Adenylyl.

adenylyl (ad·**en**·il·il). The monovalent radical $C_5H_4N_5$–, which enters into combination to form adenosine and AMP. **Adenylyl cyclase.** The enzyme responsible for the production of cyclic AMP from ATP; its activity is associated with the cell membrane and is responsive to the presence of several hormones (*see* ADENOSINE 3′,5′-CYCLIC MONOPHOSPHATE). **Adenylyl pyrophosphatase.** Adenosine triphosphoric acid (ATP).

adephagia (ad·e·**fa**·je·ah). Extreme hunger; gluttony. [Gk *haden* to repletion, *phagein* to eat.]

adeps (**ad**·eps). Adeps praeparatus, Lard BPC 1959; the purified fat obtained from the omentum of the hog and used in making ointments. **Adeps benzoinatus.** Benzoinated lard, lard containing 3 per cent of benzoin, the balsamic acids of the latter acting as a preservative. It is used as an ointment base. **Adeps lanae.** Wool Fat BP 1958, anhydrous lanolin; a brownish-yellow fat from sheep's wool. It contains cholesterol and will act as an emulsifying agent. **Adeps lanae hydrosus.** Hydrous Wool Fat BP 1958, lanolin; consisting of 7 parts adeps lanae melted and mixed with 3 parts distilled water. It is yellowish-white in colour with a creamy consistency, used as an ointment base, particularly when a solution is to be incorporated into the ointment. The addition of olive oil or soft paraffin renders it less sticky and more easily absorbable by the skin. **Adeps myristicae.** Nutmeg oil. *See* OIL. [L fat.]

adermia (a·**der**·me·ah). Defect or lack of skin, of congenital origin. [Gk *a, derma* skin.]

adermin (ad·**er**·min). Pyridoxine, or vitamin B_6.

adermogenesis (a·**der**·mo·**jen**′·es·is). A condition in which the skin is imperfectly developed. [Gk *a, derma* skin, *genein* to produce.]

adermotrophia (a·**der**·mo·**tro**′·fe·ah). An atrophic condition of the skin. [Gk *a, derma* skin, *trophe* nutrition.]

adesmosis (a·des·**mo**·sis). An atrophied condition of the connnective tissue of the skin. [Gk *a, desmos* band, *-osis* condition.]

Adhatoda BPC 1949 (ad·**hat**·o·dah). Adhatodae folia; the leaves of *Adhatoda vasica* Nees, the Malabar nut tree, of the family Acanthaceae. It is an expectorant in small doses, but an emetic in large. [Tamil name.]

adhesiectomy (ad·**he**·ze·**ek**′·to·me). The cutting away of adhesions. [adhesion, Gk *ektome* a cutting out.]

adhesiolysis (ad·**he**·ze·**ol**′·is·is). The freeing of adhesions. [adhesion, Gk *lysis* a loosing.]

adhesion (ad·**he**·zhun). 1. The union of normally separate parts by new tissue produced as a result of inflammation. 2. Any band of tissue uniting parts which normally are separate. **Attic adhesions.** Adhesions which form in the region of the pylorus and gall bladder. **Lenticular adhesion.** A posterior synechia which binds the anterior lens capsule to the posterior surface of the iris. **Primary adhesion.** Healing by first intention or primary union. **Secondary adhesion.** Healing by second intention or granulation. [L *adhesio* a sticking to.]

adhesiotomy (ad·**he**·ze·**ot**′·o·me). The operation of dividing or cutting adhesions. [adhesion, Gk *temnein* to cut.]

adhesive (ad·**he**·ziv). 1. Of the nature of adhesion. 2. Marked by or resulting in adhesion. [L *adhesio* a sticking to.]

adiabatic (a·di·ah·**bat**′·ik). In thermodynamics, a term descriptive of a change in volume or pressure which takes place without loss or gain of heat. [Gk *a, dia, bainein* to go.]

adiactinic (a·di·ak·**tin**′·ik). Incapable of absorbing or transmitting actinic rays. [Gk *a, dia, aktis* ray.]

adiadochokinesia, adiadochokinesis (a·**de**·ad·o·ko·kin·**e**′·se·ah, a·**de**·ad·o·ko·kin·**e**′·sis). Lack of power to arrest one movement and rapidly to substitute for it an alternative movement. [Gk *a, diadochos* succeeding, kinesis.]

adiaemorrhysis (a·di·em·**or**′·is·is). Stoppage, on account of obstruction of the veins, of the circulation of the blood. [Gk *a, dia, haima* blood, *rhysis* flow.]

Adiantum (ad·e·**an**·tum). A large genus of ferns, mainly tropical; the maidenhair ferns. *Adiantum capillus-veneris* and *Adiantum pedatum,* species occurring in North America, are serviceable in coughs as demulcents. [Gk *a, diainein* to moisten.]

adiaphoresis (a·di·af·or·**e**′·sis). Deficiency or absence of sweat. [Gk *a, diaphoresis* sweat.]

adiaphoretic (a·di·af·or·**et**′·ik). 1. Preventing or diminishing sweat. 2. An anhidrotic agent. [see prec.]

adiaphoria (a·di·af·**or**′·e·ah). Absence of response to stimulation as a result of the previous application of similar stimulation. [Gk *a, dia, pherein* to carry.]

adiaphorous (a·di·**af**·or·us). Neither beneficial nor harmful; neutral. [Gk *a, diaphoros* different.]

adiapneustia (a·di·ap·**new**′·ste·ah). Anhidrosis. [Gk *a, diapnein* to breathe through.]

adiaspiromycosis (a·di·ah·**spi**·ro·mi·**ko**′·sis). A pulmonary mycosis of rodents and other small animals which live or dig in the ground or are aquatic. Eight cases have been reported in man. It is caused by *Emmonsia crescens* and *Emmonsia parva.* [Gk *a, dia,* L *spirare* to breathe, Gk *mykes* fungus, *-osis* condition.]

adiaspirosis (a·di·ah·spi·**ro**′·sis). Adiaspiromycosis.

adiaspore (a·**di**·ah·spor). A fungus which, when introduced into an animal or inoculated *in vitro* at elevated temperatures, increases in size without eventual reproduction or replication. [Gk *a, dia, sporos* seed.]

adiastole (a·di·**as**·to·le). Absence of the stage of dilatation of the heart. [Gk *a,* diastole.]

adiathermance, adiathermancy (a·di·ah·**ther**′·mans, a·di·ah·**ther**′·man·se). The condition of being impervious to the penetration of radiant heat. [Gk *a, dia, therme* heat.]

adiathermic, adiathermous (a·di·ah·**ther**′·mik, a·di·ah·**ther**′·mus). Impervious to penetration of radiant heat. [see prec.]

adiathesia (a·di·ah·**the**′·ze·ah). A term applied to a state of the body which is non-congenital or to an acquired disease. [Gk *a, diathesis* disposition.]

adiathesic, adiathetic (a·di·ah·**the**′·zik, a·di·ah·**thet**′·ik). Without relation to or connection with diathesis.

Adicillin (ad·e·**sil**·in). BP Commission approved name for 6-[D(+)-5-amino-5-carboxyvaleramido] penicillanic acid; an antibiotic.

adicity (ad·**is**·it·e). The combining power, or valency, of an element or radical. *See* VALENCY.

Adie, William John (b. 1886). London physician.

Adie's pupil. A pupil that is usually larger than its fellow and reacts poorly to light. On convergence, it reacts slowly but eventually develops a sustained contraction. Usually unilateral and found in young women; also called *pseudo- or non-luetic Argyll Robertson pupil, tonic pupil, myotonic pupil,* Syn.: Myotonic pupil [*See also* ADIE'S SYNDROME.]

Adie's syndrome, Holmes-Adie syndrome. Adie's pupil

associated with absent tendon reflexes. Also called *pseudotabes, tonic pupils with absent tendon reflexes.*

adient (ad·e·ent). Moving towards a stimulus. Cf. ABIENT. [L *adire* to go towards.]

adietetic (a·di·et·et'·ik). 1. Indicating an unwholesome character of food. 2. Denoting a disregard of dietetic requirements. [Gk *a,* dietetic.]

Adinida (ah·din·id·ah). A family of Flagellata of the order Protozoa, in which the flagella are free. [Gk *a, dine* a whirling.]

adipectomy (ad·ip·ek·to·me). Excision of adipose tissue, generally in considerable mass. [L *adeps* fat, Gk *ektome* a cutting out.]

adipic (ad·ip·ik). 1. Relating to adipose tissue. 2. In chemistry, derived from or relating to oily or fatty substances. [L *adeps* fat.]

adipocele (ad·ip·o·seel). A hernia the sac of which contains fat or adipose tissue. [L *adeps* fat, Gk *kele* hernia.]

adipocellular (ad·ip·o·sel'·ew·lar). Made up of connnective tissue and fat. [L *adeps* fat, cellula.]

adipoceration (ad·ip·o·ser·a'·shun). The conversion into adipocere.

adipoceratous (ad·ip·o·ser'·at·us). Like or belonging to adipocere.

adipocere (ad·ip·o·seer). A white or yellowish wax-like substance to which body fat is converted after death by hydrogenation into higher fatty acids and calcium soaps. [L *adeps* fat, *cera* wax.]

adipochrome (ad·ip·o·krome). A pigment arising directly from the body fat. In certain diseases there is increased production of adipochrome. [L *adeps* fat, Gk *chroma* colour.]

adipofibroma (ad·ip·o·fi·bro'·mah). A tumour in which there are both fatty and fibrous constituents; a fibrous lipoma. [L *adeps* fat, fibroma.]

adipogenesis (ad·ip·o·jen'·es·is). The process of producing fat. [L *adeps* fat, Gk *genein* to produce.]

adipogenic, adipogenous (ad·ip·o·jen'·ik, ad·ip·oj·en·us). Forming fat or fatty tissue. [see prec.]

adipohepatic (ad·ip·o·hep·at'·ik). Relating to fatty degeneration of the liver, or having it as a characteristic in any disease. [L *adeps* fat, *hepar* liver.]

adipoid (ad·ip·oid). Having the characters of fat; lipoid. [L *adeps* fat, Gk *eidos* form.]

adipolysis (ad·ip·ol·is·is). The digestion (hydrolysis) of fats by the action of a fat-splitting enzyme. [L *adeps* fat, Gk *lysis* a loosing.]

adipolytic (ad·ip·o·lit'·ik). In chemistry, capable of decomposing fats; causing the digestion or splitting up of fats. [see prec.]

adipoma (ad·ip·o·mah). 1. A fatty tumour (lipoma). 2. A mass of fat present in the interior of the body. [L *adeps* fat, Gk *-oma* tumour.]

adipometer (ad·ip·om·et·er). An instrument which measures the thickness of the integument; by this means an estimation of the subcutaneous fat may be made. [L *adeps* fat, meter.]

adiponecrosis (ad·ip·o·nek·ro'·sis). Necrosis affecting the fatty tissue of the body. **Adiponecrosis e frigore.** Firm plaques of fat necrosis on the cheeks of children after exposure to cold, clearing up spontaneously without scarring. **Adiponecrosis subcutanea neonatorum.** In the newborn or young infant, hard fat lying beneath the skin. [L *adeps* fat, necrosis.]

adipopectic, adipopexic (ad·ip·o·pek'·tik, ad·ip·o·pex'·ik). Storing or stabilizing fat. [L *adeps* fat, Gk *pexis* fixation.]

adipopexia, adipopexis (ad·ip·o·pex'·e·ah, ad·ip·o·pex'·is). A condition in which fat is stabilized or stored. [see prec.]

adiposalgia (ad·ip·oze·al'·je·ah). A neurosis in which there is a sensation of pain in areas of the subcutaneous fat. [L *adeps* fat, Gk *algos* pain.]

adiposclerosis subcutanea neonatorum (ad·ip·o·skler·o'·sis sub·kew·ta·ne·ah ne·on·at·or'·um). A disease of fat metabolism, probably slightly different from Underwood's disease. Isolated irregular areas of thickened subcutaneous tissue develop in an otherwise healthy infant a few days after birth, usually on the thighs, buttocks, calves and cheeks. Recovery is the rule, but fatal cases have been reported. [L *adeps* fat, sclerosis, L *sub, cutis* skin, Gk *neos* new, L *natus* born.]

adipose (ad·ip·oze). 1. Of or belonging to animal fat. 2. Fatty to an abnormal degree. [L *adeps* fat.]

adiposis (ad·ip·o·sis). A condition in which fat exists in excess in the body, more especially when such obesity is of a pathological type. **Adiposis cerebralis.** Cerebral adiposity. *See* ADIPOSITY. **Adiposis dolorosa.** Decum's disease; a disease chiefly affecting the female sex and characterized by the presence of nerve lesions and painful local accumulations of fat. It is doubtful whether this is a true clinical entity. **Adiposis hepatica.** Infiltration of fat into, or fatty degeneration of, the liver. **Adiposis orchalis, Adiposis orchica.** A condition of excessive fatness which develops when there is a tumour of the brain; in association with it there is imperfect development of the genital organs. **Adiposis universalis.** Depositions of fat over and throughout the entire body. [L *adeps* fat, Gk *-osis* condition.]

adipositis (ad·ip·os·i'·tis). An inflammatory condition of the fatty tissue beneath the skin. [L *adeps* fat, Gk *-itis* inflammation.]

adiposity (ad·ip·os·it·e). The quality or state of being too fat; obesity. **Cerebral adiposity.** Obesity as the result of disease of the cerebrum, particularly of the hypophysis. Cf. DYSTROPHY, ADIPOSOGENITAL. **Pituitary adiposity.** Excessive fatness caused by hyposecretion of the hypophysis cerebri. A rare condition. [L *adeps* fat.]

adiposogenital (ad·ip·o·so·jen'·it·al). Referring to obesity associated with (apparent) small size of the external genital organs; the term is especially applied to Fröhlich's syndrome. [L *adeps* fat, *genitalis* concerned with generation.]

adiposuria (ad·ip·o·sewr'·e·ah). A condition of the urine in which fat is present; lipuria. [L *adeps* fat, urine.]

adipsia, adipsy (a·dip·se·ah, a·dip·se). 1. Abnormal abstinence from drinking. 2. Complete lack of thirst. [Gk *a, dipsa* thirst.]

adipsous (a·dip·sus). Capable of quenching thirst. [see prec.]

aditus [NA] (ad·it·us). In anatomy, an opening or passage. **Aditus ad aquaeductum cerebri.** The inlet to the aqueduct of the midbrain. **Aditus glottidis.** Any one of the cavities of the glottis. **Aditus to the tympanic antrum [aditus ad antrum].** The inlet to the tympanic antrum. [L approach.]

adjunction (ad·jungk·shun). In treatment, the use of a combination of remedies. [L *adjungere* to join to.]

adjuster (ad·just·er). An instrument for holding together the ends of a silver wire suture so that the edges of the parts may be brought together without strain being put on the tissues. [L *adjuxtare* to bring together.]

adjustment (ad·just·ment). 1. In biology, the phases through which an organism goes for the purpose of adapting itself to altering external conditions. 2. The mechanical means by which the tube of a microscope is raised and lowered. **Absolute adjustment.** Absolute accommodation. *See* ACCOMMODATION. **Coarse adjustment.** A device which quickly raises or lowers the tube of a microscope so as to approximately to focus the lens. **Fine adjustment.** The mechanism by which the tube of a microscope can be raised or lowered slowly so as to obtain accurate focusing. [see prec.]

adjustor (ad·just·or). In a reflex nerve arc, the name given to the ganglion concerned. [L *adjuxtare* to bring together.]

adjuvant (ad·jew·vant). A substance mixed and injected with an antigen which non-specifically enhances or modifies the antibody response to that antigen, e.g. aluminium hydroxide in diphtheria toxoid, oil-emulsion adjuvant, bacterial adjuvant. **Adjuvant disease.** Clinical abnormality seen in animals injected with Freund's adjuvant (mycobacteria in water-in-oil emulsion), and characterized by inflammation of joints and particular tissues. [L *ad, juvare* to help.]

Adler, Alfred (b. 1870). Vienna psychiatrist.

Adler's theory. An approach to psychiatry in which emphasis is laid particularly on the will to power and on the feeling of organ and biological inferiority, as determining mental mechanisms.

Adlerius (ad·leer·e·us). A sub-genus of *Phlebotomus.*

adlumidine (ad·loo·mid·een). $C_{19}H_{15}O_6N$. An alkaloid found in *Adlumia cirrhosa.*

adlumine (ad·loo·meen). An alkaloid, $C_{21}H_{21}NO_6$, found in species of *Adlumia.*

admedial, admedian (ad·**me**·de·al, ad·**me**·de·an). In biology, situated in proximity to the median plane. [L *ad, medius* middle.]

adminiculum (ad·min·**ik**·ew·lum). An adminicle or support. **Adminiculum lineae albae [NA].** In the abdomen, the triangular fibrous lamella attached behind the rectus abdominis muscle to the posterior surface of the pubic crest; it gives extra strength to the pectineal ligament (ligament of Cooper). [L support.]

admortal (ad·**mor**·tal). Of electric currents, a term applied to those which pass from living to moribund or dead tissue. Cf. ABMORTAL. [L *ad, mors* death.]

adnata (ad·**na**·tah). The tunica adnata; the fibrous layer of the conjunctiva in contact with the eyeball. [L *ad, nasci* to grow.]

adnerval, adneural (ad·**nerv**·al, ad·**newr**·al). 1. In physiology, placed near or towards a nerve. 2. A term applied to any nervous disease which is present at the point at which the symptoms are apparent. 3. Of electric currents, a term applied to those which pass through muscle towards a nerve or nerve-ending. Cf. ABNERVAL. [L *ad, nervus* (Gk *neuron*) nerve.]

adnexa (ad·**nex**·ah). Appendages; conjoined parts. **Adnexa bulbi.** The accessory structures of the eyeball. **Adnexa oculi.** The accessory organs of the eye. **Adnexa uteri.** The ovaries and the uterine tubes. [L *adnectere* to tie to.]

adnexal (ad·**nex**·al). Relating to accessory structures or organs, particularly those of the uterus. [see prec.]

adnexectomy (ad·nex·**ek**·to·me). Removal of accessory structures or organs (adnexae) by excision. [adnexa, Gk *ektome* a cutting out.]

adnexitis (ad·nex·**i**·tis). An inflamed condition of the accessory organs of the uterus, generally ovaries and uterine tubes. [adnexa, Gk *-itis* inflammation.]

adnexogenesis (ad·**nex**·o·**jen**'·es·is). The fetal development of accessory structures and organs. [adnexa, Gk *genein* to produce.]

adnexopexy (ad·**nex**·o·**pex**'·e). The operation in which the uterine tubes and ovaries are raised and sutured to the abdominal wall. [adnexa, Gk *pexis* fixation.]

adnexorganogenic (ad·**nex**·or·gan·o·**jen**'·ik). Originating in the accessory organs of the uterus. [adnexa, organogenesis.]

adolescence (ad·ol·**es**·ens). The process of developing from childhood to adulthood; youth; the years between the onset of puberty and the attainment of maturity. In males the period extends from 14 to 25 years; in females, from 12 to 21 years. [L *adolescere* to grow up.]

adonidin (ad·**on**·id·in). A hygroscopic glucoside, $C_{24}H_{42}O_9$, with a bitter taste, found in *Adonis vernalis.* It has an action similar to that of digitalin, and has been employed as a local anaesthetic and diuretic.

adonin (ad·o·nin). A glucoside, $C_{20}H_{40}O_9$, obtained from species of *Adonis*, and used like digitalin as a heart stimulant.

Adonis (ad·o·nis). A genus of poisonous plants, family Ranunculaceae. **Adonis vernalis.** A species whose glucosides, adonidin and adonin, have a digitalis-like action. [Gk Adonis-flower.]

adonite, adonitol (ad·**on**·ite, ad·**on**·it·ol). $C_5H_7(OH)_5$. A pentahydric alcohol which occurs in *Adonis vernalis*; it is oxidized to ribose.

adoptive transfer. Passive transfer of lymphocytes from an antigen-reactive donor to a non-immune recipient.

adoral (ad·**or**·al). 1. In the proximity of the mouth. 2. Directed towards the mouth. Cf. ABORAL. [L *ad,* oral.]

adorbital (ad·**or**·bit·al). Relating to the orbit. [L *ad,* orbit.]

adosculation (ad·**os**·kew·**la**'·shun). 1. In zoology, the act of fecundation by external contact only. 2. A form of joint in which one part is lodged within a cavity in the other part. [L *adosculari* to kiss.]

adrenal (ad·**re**·nal). 1. Pertaining to or produced by the adrenal (suprarenal) glands. 2. An adrenal gland. Adrenal is now more often referred to than suprarenal. **Adrenal rest cells.** Similar to luteal cells, give rise to tumours of the ovary that secrete androgens and cortisol. [L *ad, ren* kidney.]

See also: MARCHAND.

adrenalectomize (ad·**re**·nal·**ek**'·tom·ize). To remove the adrenal glands by excision. [adrenal, Gk *ektome* a cutting out.]

adrenalectomy (ad·**re**·nal·**ek**'·to·me). Removal of the adrenal glands. [see prec.]

adrenalinaemia (ad·**ren**·al·in·**e**'·me·ah). The presence in the blood of adrenaline. [adrenaline, Gk *haima* blood.]

Adrenaline (ad·**ren**·al·een, ad·**ren**·al·in). Epinephrine, $(OH)_2C_6H_3CH(OH)CH_2NHCH_3$. A white or pale-brown crystalline odourless substance, one of the active principles of the adrenal medulla. It is mainly secreted by the adrenal medulla, whereas noradrenaline is chiefly found released from the sympathetic nerve endings. Its pharmacological actions resemble in many respects the effects of stimulation of the sympathetic nervous system; the heart is stimulated, increasing its output and generally its rate, and arrhythmias may occur. The effect on blood vessels varies: those of the skin and mucous membranes, the splanchnic, cerebral, retinal, pulmonary and renal vessels tend to be constricted, while the vessels in skeletal muscle, and probably the coronary arteries, are dilated. The blood pressure is increased at first, but this may be followed by a fall. The bronchial muscle is relaxed, as is the muscle of the gastro-intestinal tract, except for the sphincters, which are closed; the capsule of the spleen is contracted; the bladder retrusor is relaxed, and the sphincter closed. It raises the metabolic rate and increases the blood-sugar level. It does not affect the pupil size in normal individuals, and has very little stimulant effect on the central nervous system, though occasionally apprehensive feelings, restlessness and tremor may occur with therapeutic doses. It is an important therapeutic drug, but has no general action when given by mouth. After absorption from parenteral routes, the drug is rapidly destroyed in the body and its actions are transient. It is employed locally to arrest haemorrhage, and together with local anaesthetics to prolong their action and limit bleeding. It may be used in syncope due to heart block or in cardiac arrest due to anaesthesia, etc.; in the latter case it may be administered directly into the myocardium. It is a valuable drug in treating the paroxysms of bronchial asthma, when it may be given subcutaneously, by inhalation or, rarely, intravenously. It is used also in other allergic disorders such as urticaria and angio-neurotic oedema, particularly where oedema of the glottis occurs. (BP 1973.) **Adrenaline Acid Tartrate BP 1973.** A soluble salt used in solutions for injection. [L *ad, ren* kidney.]

Adrenalinii Tartras. *European Pharmacopoeia* name for Adrenaline Acid Tartrate BP 1973.

adrenalitis (ad·**re**·nal·**i**'·tis). An inflammatory condition of the adrenal glands. [adrenal, Gk *-itis* inflammation.]

adrenalone (ad·**ren**·al·one). $(OH)_2C_6H_3COCH_2NHCH_3$. The ketone of adrenaline; it is used like the latter as a vasoconstrictor, and is especially valuable, by injection, in the treatment of glaucoma.

adrenarche (ad·ren·**ar**·ke). Signs of puberty, sometimes including menstruation but characteristically consisting of growth of pubic and axillary and, sometimes, other body hair as the result of adrenal hyperplasia or tumour-producing adrenogenic hormone before the normal age of puberty. [L *ad, ren* kidney, Gk *arche* beginning.]

adrenergic (ad·ren·**er**·jik). 1. Referring to the sympathetic nerve fibres. 2. Stimulated by adrenaline. [adrenal, Gk *ergon* work.]

adrenitis (ad·re·**ni**·tis). Adrenalitis.

adrenochrome (ad·**ren**·o·krome). Red oxidation product of adrenaline, having an indole structure and without pressor activity. **Adrenochrome monosemicarbazone dihydrate.** A derivative of adrenaline used to prevent and cure all types of capillary bleeding, and hence of great use in surgical operations. [adrenaline, Gk *chroma* colour.]

adrenocortical (ad·re·no·**kor**·tic·al). Appertaining to the adrenal cortex. *See* CORTICOTROPHIN. RELEASING FACTOR (RF).

Adrenocorticotrophin (ad·re·no·kor·tik·o·**tro**'·fin). Adrenocorticotrophic hormone. *See* HORMONE.

adrenocorticotropic (ad·re·no·kor·tik·o·**tro**'·pik). Exerting a hormonal influence upon the growth or action of the cortex of the adrenal gland. [adrenal cortex, Gk *tropos* a turning.]

adrenogenital (ad·re·no·**jen′**·it·al). Referring to the adrenal glands and the organs of generation. [adrenal, genitalia.]

adrenoglomerulotropin (ad·re·no·glom·er·ew·lo·**trop′**·in). A hormone secreted by the hypothalamus which releases aldosterone from the zona glomerulosa of the adrenal cortex. [adrenal cortex, L *glomerulus* small ball, Gk *trophe* nutrition.]

adrenogram (ad·**re**·no·gram). The radiograph made during adrenography. [adrenal, Gk *gramma* record.]

adrenography (ad·ren·**og**·raf·e). Radiographic visualization of the suprarenal gland, including angiographic and retroperitoneal gas insufflation. [adrenal, Gk *graphein* to record.]

adrenolytic (ad·re·no·**lit′**·ik). Arresting or restraining the activity of adrenergic nerves; arresting the reaction to stimulation with adrenaline. [adrenal, Gk *lysis* a loosing.]

adrenomedulloblastoma (ad·re·no·med·**ul**·o·blas·**to′**·mah). A malignant tumour composed of the cells of origin of the adrenal medulla or of the sympathetic nerve cells. **Metastatic adrenomedulloblastoma.** A secondary tumour resulting from the bloodstream spread of a malignant primary tumour in the medullary portion of the adrenal gland. [adrenal medulla, Gk *blastos* germ, *-oma* tumour.]

adrenomegaly (ad·re·no·**meg′**·al·e). Enlargement of the adrenal gland or glands. [adrenal gland, Gk *megas* large.]

adrenopathy (ad·re·**nop**·ath·e). Any disease of the adrenal glands. [adrenal, Gk *pathos* disease.]

adrenostatic (ad·re·no·**stat′**·ik). Inhibiting adrenal activity. [adrenal, Gk *statikos* causing to stand.]

adrenosterone (ad·re·no·**steer′**·one). $C_{19}H_{24}O_3$, a steroid with androgenic properties which has been identified in the lipoid of the adrenal cortex.

adrenotrophic (ad·re·no·**trof′**·ik). Having a special relation to or stimulating effect upon the adrenal glands. [adrenal, Gk *trophe* nutrition.]

adromia (ad·**ro**·me·ah). Failure of conduction in a motor nerve. [Gk *a*, *dromos* course.]

Adson, Alfred Washington (b. 1887). Rochester, Minnesota, surgeon.

Adson's operation. 1. Division of the sensory root of the trigeminal nerve, for neuralgia. 2. Division of the anterior roots of spinal nerves, intrathecally, for hypertension.

adsorbate (ad·**sor**·bate). Any substance which is adsorbed. [L *ad*, *sorbere* to suck in.]

adsorbent (ad·**sor**·bent). Any substance, such as suitably prepared charcoal, which is employed for adsorption. [see prec.]

adsorption (ad·**sorp**·shun). The phenomenon of a surface removing a substance from solution and concentrating it upon the interface. The process is complicated, depending upon surface tension, the interfacial area and the electric charges involved. It is particularly important in colloidal solutions, and many biological reactions are attributed to the close contact brought about by adsorption on cellular surfaces. Cf. ABSORPTION. [L *ad*, *sorbere* to suck in.]

adsternal (ad·**stern**·al). Adjacent to the sternum. [L *ad*, sternum.]

adstrictio (ad·**strik**·she·o). 1. Retention of faeces or urine, or of both. 2. Ligation of a blood vessel. 3. Astringent action. **Adstrictio alvei.** Constipation. [L *adstringere* to draw together.]

adstringent (ad·**strin**·jent). Astringent.

adterminal (ad·**ter**·min·al). Of an electric current, passing in the direction of muscle or nerve-endings or the extremity of a structure. [L *ad*, terminus.]

adtorsion (ad·**tor**·shun). A condition in which both eyes turn inwards and their vertical meridians converge above instead of being parallel; conclination. [L *ad*, *torquere* to twist.]

adulteration (ad·ul·ter·**a′**·shun). The addition of inferior and usually cheaper substitutes to a product. There are various statutes regulating the sale of food and drugs aimed at preventing adulteration. [L *adulterare* to defile.]

adultery (ad·**ul**·ter·e). Sexual intercourse by a married person other than with the legal partner. [see prec.]

advance (ad·**vahns**). In surgery, to bring forward a tendon or a muscle, as in the operation of advancement in cases of strabismus. [Fr. *avancer* to move forward.]

advancement (ad·**vahns**·ment). The operation of detaching at the point of its insertion a muscle or tendon and reattaching it at a point further forward; in the case of muscles this procedure is carried out in order to correct the action of the muscle, e.g. in strabismus or uterine retroversion. **Capsular advancement.** A method of reattaching the fascial sheath of the eyeball (Tenon's capsule) so that the insertion of a muscle of the eye is brought forward. **Tendon advancement.** The procedure of advancement carried out on a tendon. [Fr. *avancer* to move forward.]

adventitia (ad·ven·**tish**·e·ah). The adventitious coat of an artery. [L *adventitius* coming from abroad.]

adventitious (ad·ven·**tish**·us). 1. Accidental, or acquired; not hereditary. 2. In anatomy, belonging or referring to the adventitious coat. 3. Occurring in an abnormal place. [see prec.]

adynamia (a·di·**nam**·e·ah). Asthenia, sometimes to a degree of prostration; loss of vital powers, or lack of them, caused by disease. **Adynamia episodica hereditaria.** Periodic muscular weakness with increased serum potassium starting in childhood; it is an autosomal dominant. [Gk *a*, *dynamis* strength.]

adynamic (a·di·**nam**·ik). 1. Asthenic. 2. Showing the characteristics of or referring to adynamia.

adynamico-ataxic (a·di·**nam**·ik·o·at·**ax′**·ik). Referring to or showing the characteristics of adynamia and ataxy.

adynatus (a·**di**·nat·us). Debilitated; sickly; vitally depleted. [Gk *a*, *dynamis* strength.]

Aeby, Christoph Theodor (b. 1835). Swiss anatomist.

Aeby's muscle. A muscle found in the upper and lower lip. The slender fibres, which are better developed in the infant than in the adult, are directed anteroposteriorly.

Aeby's plane. A plane passing through the basion and the nasion at right angles to the sagittal plane.

Aëdes (a·e·deez). A genus of mosquito in which the females have palpi much shorter than the proboscis, a trilobed scutellum and an abdomen that is pointed and usually marked with light bands, as are the legs. It lays eggs separately and not clumped. **Aëdes aegypti.** An important species, being the carrier of yellow fever and dengue. It probably transmits equine encephalitis and is a potential vector of filariasis and tularaemia. It is distinguished by a lyre-shaped marking on the thorax and white-tipped hind legs. It breeds in or near houses, and any puddle is suitable, for, should it dry up, the eggs can remain fertile for months and develop when rewetted. **Aëdes africanus.** A vector of yellow fever. **Aëdes albopictus.** A species that transmits dengue in Japan, and also yellow fever. **Aëdes cantator.** A vector of equine encephalitis. **Aëdes cinereus.** A potential vector of tularaemia. **Aëdes dorsalis.** A vector of equine encephalitis. **Aëdes esoensis.** A vector of autumn and Japanese encephalitides. **Aëdes fluviatilis.** A vector of yellow fever. **Aëdes furcifer.** A species which probably transmits yellow fever. **Aëdes geniculatus.** A vector of yellow fever. **Aëdes lateralis.** A vector of St. Louis encephalitis. **Aëdes leucocelaenus, Aëdes luteocephalus, Aëdes metallicus.** A vector of yellow fever. **Aëdes scapularis.** A potential vector of yellow fever. **Aëdes scutellaris hebrideus.** A species that transmits dengue. **Aëdes scutellaris pseudoscutellaris.** A species that transmits the Pacific diurnal form of filariasis. **Aëdes simpsoni.** A species that transmits yellow fever. **Aëdes sollicitans.** A vector of equine encephalitis. **Aëdes stokesi.** A vector of yellow fever. **Aëdes taeniorhyncus.** A species that transmits equine and St. Louis encephalitides, and can transmit yellow fever and filariasis under laboratory conditions. **Aëdes taylori.** A species that transmits yellow fever. **Aëdes togoi.** A species that transmits autumn and Japanese encephalitides and can transmit filariasis under laboratory conditions. **Aëdes triseriatus.** A vector of equine encephalitis and yellow fever. **Aëdes variegatus.** *Aëdes scutellaris pseudoscutellaris* (see above). **Aëdes vexans.** A species that transmits St. Louis and equine encephalitides. **Aëdes vittatus.** A vector of yellow fever. [Gk *aedes* annoying.]

aegilops (e·jil·ops). An ulcer, with fistula, at the inner canthus of the eye. [Gk *aix* goat, *ops* eye.]

aegobronchophony (e·go·bron·**kof'**·on·e). The quality of voice which is characteristic of pleuropneumonia; bronchial and bleating. [Gk *aix* goat, *brogchos* air passage, *phone* voice.]

aegonia (e·**go**·ne·ah). A condition of slight aegophony. [L.]

aegophony (e·**gof**·on·e). The bleating quality of voice heard on auscultation which is characteristic of certain lung conditions, e.g. pleurisy with effusion. [Gk *aix* goat, *phone* voice.]

aeipathy (a·i·path·e). A condition of being in constant and irremediable pain. [Gk *aei* always, *pathos* disease.]

aelurophobia (e·**lewr**·o·**fo'**·be·ah). Ailurophobia. [Gk *ailouros* cat, phobia.]

aeluropsis (e·lewr·**op**·sis). Ailuropsis; a condition of the palpebral fissures so that the opening is oblique and narrowed, like that of a cat. [Gk *ailouros* cat, *opsis* appearance.]

aeolipile, aeolipyle (e·**ol**·ip·ile). A kind of spirit lamp used for the heating of cautery irons. [L *Aeoli pila* ball of Aeolus (god of the winds).]

aequator (e·**kwa**·tor). Equator. [L.]

aequum (**e**·kwum). A term applied by von Pirquet to the minimum number of calories sufficient to maintain weight at a constant level while a person does a specific amount of work. [L level.]

aer (a·er). Atmos; an obsolete unit of air pressure, one degree being equal to the weight of a column of 760 mm of mercury on 1 cm^2. [Gk air.]

aeraemia (a·er·e·me·ah). Caisson disease. *See* DISEASE. [Gk *aer* air, *haima* blood.]

aerasthenia (a·er·as·**the'**·ne·ah). In air pilots especially, a psychoneurosis marked by worry and lack of self-confidence. [Gk *aer* air, asthenia.]

aerated (a·er·a·ted). Artificially impregnated or charged with air, oxygen or carbon dioxide. [Gk *aer* air.]

aeration (a·er·a·shun). 1. The process of artificially impregnating or charging with oxygen or carbon dioxide. 2. Arterialization. 3. Exposing to the action of air. [see prec.]

aerator (a·er·**a**·tor). An apparatus for charging liquids with oxygen or carbon dioxide. [Gk *aer* air.]

aerendocardia (a·er·en·do·**kar'**·de·ah). A condition of the heart in which air or gas is present inside it. [Gk *aer* air, *endon* in, *kardia* heart.]

aerenterasic (a·er·en·ter·**a'**·sik). Flatulent; of the intestine, setting up a tympanic note on abdominal percussion. [Gk *aer* air, *enteron* intestine.]

aerenterectasia (a·er·**en**·ter·ek·**ta'**·ze·ah). Tympanites; intestinal distension by gas or air so that the abdomen is swollen and tympanitic. [Gk *aer* air, *enteron* intestine, *ektasis* distension.]

aerhaemoctonia (a·er·he·mok·**to'**·ne·ah). Death as a result of the entrance of air into the veins. [Gk *aer* air, *haima* blood, *ktonos* killing.]

aericolous (a·er·**ik**·ol·us). Living out of doors. [Gk *aer* air, L *colere* to inhabit.]

aerification (a·er·if·e·**ka'**·shun). 1. Filled or being filled with air. 2. Emphysema of the lung. [Gk *aer* air, L *facere* to make.]

aeris (a·er·is). Nitrous oxide.

aero-anaerobic (a·er·o·an·a·er·**o'**·bik). Able to live and multiply equally well in the presence or absence of free oxygen. [aerobe, anaerobe.]

aeroarthrosis (a·er·o·ar·**thro'**·sis). Perceptible and usually painless accumulation of gas within a joint as a result of lowered atmospheric pressure (*See* DECOMPRESSION SICKNESS). [Gk *aer* air, *arthron* joint.]

aero-asthenia (a·er·o·as·**the'**·ne·ah). Aerasthenia.

Aerobacter (a·er·o·**bak'**·ter). Term, now discarded, for a genus within the family Enterobacteriaceae; species previously included in this genus are now allocated to other genera, e.g. *Aerobacter aerogenes* is now *Klebsiella aerogenes*, and *Aerobacter cloacae* is *Cloaca cloacae*. [Gk *aer* air, *bakterion* a small staff.]

aerobe, aerobian (a·er·obe, a·er·**o**·be·an). A micro-organism which utilizes and assimilates atmospheric oxygen during growth and multiplication. Cf. ANAEROBE. **Facultative aerobe.** A micro-organism which normally grows best in the absence of free oxygen, but has acquired the power of living and multiplying in its presence. **Obligate aerobe.** A micro-organism for the growth and multiplication of which free oxygen is essential. [Gk *aer* air, *bios* life.]

aerobic (a·er·**o**·bik). Requiring gaseous oxygen in order to live. [see prec.]

aerobiology (a·er·o·bi·**ol'**·o·je). The science dealing with the occurrence, transportation and effects of airborne micro-organisms or biological objects (viruses, pollen or plant spores). [Gk *aer* air, biology.]

aerobion (a·er·o·be·on). Aerobe.

aerobioscope (a·er·o·**bi'**·o·skope). An apparatus used for the investigation of bacteria filtered from samples of air. [Gk *aer* air. bioscope.]

aerobiosis (a·er·o·bi·**o'**·sis). Existence in oxygen or air. [Gk *aer* air, *bios* life.]

aerocele (a·er·o·seel). A tumour formed when a small natural cavity or an acquired sac becomes distended with air or gas. [Gk *aer* air, *kele* hernia.]

aerocolia (a·er·o·**ko'**·le·ah). Gaseous distension of the colon. [Gk *aer* air, colon.]

aerocolic (a·er·o·**kol'**·ik). Referring to aerocolia.

aerocolpos (a·er·o·**kol'**·pos). Gaseous distension of the vagina. [Gk *aer* air, *kolpos* vagina.]

aerocoly (a·er·o·ko·le). Aerocolia.

aerocystography (a·er·o·sis·**tog'**·raf·e). Injection of air into the bladder, with immediate x-ray examination. [Gk *aer* air, cystography.]

aerocystoscope (a·er·o·**sis'**·to·skope). An instrument for examination of the inside of the bladder after it has been distended with air. [Gk *aer* air, cystoscope.]

aerocystoscopy (a·er·o·sis·**tos'**·ko·pe). Examination of the bladder by means of an aerocystoscope.

aerodermectasia (a·er·o·**derm**·ek·**ta'**·se·ah). A condition of infiltration of air into the loose subdermal tissues; surgical emphysema. [Gk *aer* air, *derma* skin, *ektasis* a stretching.]

aerodontalgia (a·er·o·don·**tal'**·je·ah). Pain, often acute, in a tooth brought on by reduction in ambient pressure and thought to be due to expansion of gas trapped in the tooth. [Gk *aer* air, *odous* tooth, *odyne* pain.]

aerodontia (a·er·o·**don'**·she·ah). That subdivision of the science of dentistry associated with aviation. [Gk *aer* air, *odous* tooth.]

aerodontics (a·er·o·**don'**·tix). The study of the effects of reduced atmospheric pressure on teeth. [Gk *aer* air, *odous* tooth.]

aerodromophobia (a·er·o·dro·mo·**fo'**·be·ah). Pathological fear of travelling by air-borne transport. [Gk *aer* air, *dromos* course, phobia.]

aeroductor (a·er·o·**duk'**·tor). An apparatus for the prevention of asphyxiation of the fetus in cases of breech or other abnormal presentation when delivery of the head is delayed. [Gk *aer* air, L *ducere* to lead.]

aerodynamics (a·er·o·di·**nam'**·ix). The study of gases in motion, particularly air; also applied to bodies moving in air. [Gk *aer* air, *dynamis* power.]

aero-embolism (a·er·o·**em'**·bol·izm). (*See* DECOMPRESSION SICKNESS.) [Gk *aer* air, *emballein* to put in.]

aero-emphysema (a·er·o·em·fi·**se'**·mah). Emphysema generally occurring in aviators who have been flying at great heights; air bubbles form in various parts of the body. [Gk *aer* air, emphysema.]

aero-enterectasia (a·er·o·**en**·ter·ek·**ta'**·se·ah). A condition in which the bowels are distended with gas. [Gk *aer*, enterectasis.]

aerogastria (a·er·o·**gas'**·tre·ah). A condition in which the stomach is distended with gas or air. [Gk *aer* air, *gaster* stomach.]

aerogastrocolia (a·er·o·gas·tro·**ko'**·le·ah). Distension of the stomach and colon by gas or air. [Gk *aer* air, *gaster* stomach, colon.]

aerogen (a·er·o·jen). Any micro-organism which is capable of producing gas during growth in a suitable substrate, *in vitro* or *in vivo*. [see foll.]

aerogenesis (a·er·o·**jen**′·es·is). Production of gas. [Gk *aer* air, *genein* to produce.]

aerogenic, aerogenous (a·er·o·**jen**′·ik, a·er·**oj**·en·us). Giving rise to gas. [see prec.]

aerogram (a·er·o·gram). An x-ray photograph taken of an organ or part after it has been distended with air. [Gk *aer* air, *gramma* mark.]

aerohydropathy, aerohydrotherapy (a·er·o·hi·**drop**′·ath·e, a·er·o·**hi**·dro·**ther**′·ap·e). The use of air and water in treatment of disease. [Gk *aer* air, *hydor* water, *pathos* suffering, therapy.]

aero-ionization (a·er·o·i·on·i·**za**′·shun). The charging electrically of particles (e.g. oil drops) suspended in the air, for use therapeutically by inhalation. [Gk *aer* air, ionization.]

aero-ionotherapy (a·er·o·i·on·o·**ther**′·ap·e). A method of treatment of respiratory conditions by the inhalation of electrified air. [Gk *aer* air, ion, therapy.]

aeromammography (a·er·o·mam·**og**′·raf·e). Mammography carried out after the space behind the mammary gland has been distended with carbon dioxide. [Gk *aer* air, mammography.]

aeromedicine (a·er·o·**med**′·is·in). Aviation medicine. *See* MEDICINE. [Gk *aer* air, medicine.]

aerometer (a·er·**om**·et·er). An instrument used in determining the weight or the density of air or gases. [Gk *aer* air, meter.]

aeromicrobe, aeromicrobion (a·er·o·**mi**·krobe, a·er·o·mi·**kro**′·be·on). Any aerobic micro-organism. [Gk *aer* air, microbe.]

aeroneurosis (a·er·o·newr·**o**′·sis). An obsolete term used when it was thought that flying caused a specific neurosis. (Shell shock and soldier's heart were similarly inappropriate terms.) Flying entails a number of stresses (responsibility, risk of accident, separation from home, etc.). In susceptible individuals flying may be a factor in causing neurosis of any form. It is incorrect to associate a specific aeroneurosis with a set pattern of symptoms. [Gk *aer* air, neurosis.]

aero-odontalgia (a·er·o·o·don·**tal**′·je·ah). Aerodontalgia. [Gk *aer* air, *odous* tooth, *algos* pain.]

aero-odontodynia (a·er·o·o·don·to·**din**′·e·ah). Aerodontalgia. [Gk *aer* air, *odous* tooth, *odyne* pain.]

aero-otitis externa (a·er·o·o·ti′·tis ex·**ter**·nah). Irritation of the external auditory meatus, occasionally with haemorrhage, as a result of flying. [Gk *aer* air, otitis externa.]

aero-otitis media (a·er·o·o·**ti**′·tis **me**·de·ah). An inflamed condition of the middle ear, seen in airmen; aviator's ear. The cause is trauma due to a difference in pressure between the air in the tympanic cavity and the atmospheric air; there is congestion associated with discomfort or pain in the middle ear and a temporary impairment of hearing, and sometimes tinnitus. The condition may be acute, lasting less than 48 h, or chronic, lasting for variable longer periods and increasing temporarily during flights. Also called *otitic barotrauma.* [Gk *aer* air, otitis media.]

aeropathy (a·er·**op**·ath·e). Disease arising as a result of a person undergoing changes of atmospheric pressure, e.g. caisson disease, air sickness. [Gk *aer* air, *pathos* suffering.]

aeroperitoneum, aeroperitonia (a·er·o·**per**·e·ton·**e**′·um, a·er·o·**per**·e·**to**′·ne·ah). The presence of gas or air in the peritoneum. [Gk *aer* air, peritoneum.]

aerophagy (a·er·**of**·aj·e). The excessive swallowing of air. **Rectal aerophagy.** The indrawing of air *per rectum.* [Gk *aer* air, *phagein* to eat.]

aerophile, aerophilous (a·er·o·file, a·er·**of**·il·us). Referring to bacteria, air-loving; requiring air for life and growth. [Gk *aer* air, *philein* to love.]

aerophobia (a·er·o·**fo**′·be·ah). Morbid fear of fresh air or draughts. [Gk *aer* air, phobia.]

aerophore (a·er·o·for). 1. A portable apparatus containing compressed air for the resuscitation of apparently stillborn children by inflating their lungs. 2. An apparatus for trapping poisonous gases and purifying the air for breathing. [Gk *aer* air, *phoros* bearing.]

aerophyte (a·er·o·fite). Any vegetable organism, from the bacterium upwards, living in and feeding on air. [Gk *aer* air *phyton* plant.]

aeropiesotherapy (a·er·o·pi·e·so·**ther**′·ap·e). The use of rarefied air or of compressed air as a therapeutic measure. [Gk *aer* air, *piesis* pressure, therapy.]

aeroplethysmograph (a·er·o·pleth·**iz**′·mo·graf). An apparatus for recording by means of a graph the quantity of air expired. [Gk *aer* air, *plethysmos* enlargement, *graphein* to record.]

aeropleura (a·er·o·**ploor**′·ah). Pneumothorax. [Gk *aer* air, *pleura* side.]

aeroporotomy (a·er·o·por·**ot**′·o·me). Artifical introduction of air into the lungs, in order to relieve obstruction to breathing, by tracheotomy or by insertion of a tube into the air passage. [Gk *aer* air, *poros* passage, *temnein* to cut.]

aeroscope (a·er·o·skope). 1. In biology, a glass apparatus for the collection of bacteria from the air. 2. An apparatus for estimating the purity of the air by microscopical examination of it. [Gk *aer* air, *skopein* to watch.]

aerosialophagy (a·er·o·si·al·**of**′·aj·e). Sialo-aerophagy; the habit of swallowing frequently, causing saliva and air to be taken into the stomach. [Gk *aer* air, *sialon* saliva, *phagein* to eat.]

aerosinusitis (a·er·o·si·nus·**i**′·tis). An inflammatory condition of the sinuses which occurs in aviators; it is comparable to aero-otitis media. The frontal sinus is most frequently affected. [Gk *aer* air, sinusitis.]

aerosis (a·er·**o**·sis). A condition in which gas is formed in the organs or in the tissues of the body. [Gk *aer* air, *-osis* condition.]

aerosol (a·er·o·sol). 1. Finely divided particles of a virus hanging or floating in the air. 2. A colloidal system in which solid particles are dispersed in a continuous phase of gas, as in smoke. 3. Any solution in the form of a fine spray in which the droplets approximate colloidal size. [Gk *aer* air, hydrosol.]

aerosolization (a·er·o·sol·i·**za**′·shun). The formation of an aerosol.

aerosome (a·er·o·some). A hypnotic body once held to be present in tropical air which makes acclimatization of Europeans difficult. (Obsolete term.) [Gk *aer* air, *soma* body.]

aerostatics (a·er·**stat**′·ix). The study of gases at rest or in equilibrium. [Gk *aer* air, *statikos* causing to stand.]

aerostatotherapy (a·er·o·stat·o·**ther**′·ap·e). The treatment of respiratory ailments by taking the patient up into rarefied air. It has been used in the cure of whooping-cough by means of an aeroplane flight to a high altitude. [Gk *aer* air, *statikos* causing to stand, therapy.]

aerotaxis (a·er·o·**tax**′·is). The term used to describe the positive or negative influence exerted by oxygen on bacteria, attractive in the case of aerobes and repellent in the case of anaerobes. [Gk *aer* air, *taxis* arrangement.]

aerotherapy (a·er·o·**ther**·ap·e). 1. Fresh-air treatment. 2. The treatment of disease by causing the patient to breathe air that is rarefied or compressed, or medicated. 3. Artificial respiration. [Gk *aer* air, therapy.]

aerothermotherapy (a·er·o·ther·mo·**ther**′·ap·e). Treatment of disease by the use of currents of hot air. [Gk *aer* air, *therme* heat, therapy.]

aerothorax (a·er·o·**thor**′·ax). Pneumothorax. [Gk *aer* air, thorax.]

aerotitis media (a·er·o·**ti**′·tis **med**·de·ah). Aero-otitis media.

aerotonometer (a·er·o·ton·**om**′·et·er). An instrument used for the measurement of the pressure of gases in the blood. [Gk *aer* air, *tonos* tone, meter.]

aerotonometry (a·er·o·ton·**om**′·et·re). The process of measuring the pressure of gases in the blood. [see prec.]

aerotropism (a·er·**ot**·ro·pizm). 1. In botany, the deviation of roots and other parts of plants which, because of the actions of gases, have grown in other than normal directions. 2. A term that refers to the direction of growth of organisms—towards or away from air. [Gk *aer* air, *tropos* a turning.]

aerotympanal (a·er·o·**tim**′·pan·al). Referring to the relation of air to the middle ear. [Gk *aer* air, tympanum.]

aero-urethroscope (a·er·o·ewr·e′·thro·skope). The instrument with which aero-urethroscopy is carried out; it allows of dilatation of the urethra with air. [Gk *aer* air, urethroscope.]

aero-urethroscopy (a·er·o·ewr·e·**thros**'·kop·e). Instrumental examination of the urethra after it has been dilated with air. [see prec.]

aertryckosis (a·er·trik·**o**'·sis). The condition of being infected with *Bacillus aertrycke* (*Salmonella typhimurium*), one of the food-poisoning group of bacteria which causes acute gastro-enteritis. [*Bacillus aertrycke*, Gk *-osis* condition.]

aerumna (e·**rum**·nah). Mental distress, with or without associated physical distress. [L.]

aeschrolalia (es·kro·**la**·le·ah). Coprolalia; the involuntary utterance of digusting and obscene words mainly concerning the excretions, a symptom encountered in some diseases and in certain states of insanity. [Gk *aischros* shameful, *lalein* to babble like a child.]

aescorcin (es·**kor**·sin). Escorcin, $C_9H_8O_4$. A derivative of esculetin; a brownish powder used to stain and thereby identify corneal defects.

Aesculapius (es·kew·**la**·pe·us). The Latin name for Asklepios, the Greek god of medicine, whose cult was introduced into Roman religion about 203 B.C. as the result of a Sibylline oracle promising relief from plague then raging in Rome. He was associated with the goddess Hygeia and the temples of his cult was called Asklepieia.

Staff of Aesculapius. The staff, a rough stick, or a rod, with a snake entwined around it, always associated with Aesculapius. This symbol is included in the crests of many medical services, societies and journals.

aesculin (es·**kew**·lin). A glucoside from the horse chestnut, *Aesculus hippocastanum*. It is fluorescent and has been used to protect the skin from ultra-violet rays and in bacteriological media.

aestates (es·ta·teez). 1. Freckles. 2. Sunburn. [L *aestas* summer.]

aesthema (es·**the**·mah). A sensation or perception. [Gk *aisthema* sensation.]

aesthematology (es·**the**·mat·**ol**'·o·je). The science of the senses and the organs of sense. [Gk *aisthema* sensation, *logos* science.]

aesthesia (es·**the**·ze·ah). 1. Sensibility or feeling; capacity for sensing or perceiving. 2. Any disorder of the nerves, or a neurosis, that affects sensation or perception. [Gk *aisthesis* feeling.]

aesthesic (es·**the**·zik). Aesthetic; 1. Referring or belonging to aesthesia. 2. Referring to sensation. [see prec.]

aesthesioblast (es·**the**·ze·o·blast). Ganglioblast; in embryology, one of the primitive cells from which the spinal ganglion cells develop. [aesthesia, Gk *blastos* germ.]

aesthesiodermia (es·**the**·ze·o·**der**'·me·ah). A skin affection in which there is disordered function so that there may be complete anaesthesia, hypo-aesthesia or hyperaesthesia of the skin. [aesthesia, Gk *derma* skin.]

aesthesiodic (es·**the**·ze·**od**'·ik). Able to convey sense impressions, e.g. to the brain. [aesthesia, Gk *hodos* way.]

aesthesiogen (es·**the**·ze·o·jen). Any material, such as a metal, which produces sensation in hysterical or hypnotic subjects when brought near the body. [see foll.]

aesthesiogenic (es·**the**·ze·o·**jen**'·ik). Relating or belonging to an aesthesiogen. [aesthesia, Gk *genein* to produce.]

aesthesiogeny (es·**the**·ze·**oj**'·en·e). Setting in motion the action of alteration or of perversion of sensation so that abnormal or peculiar nervous responses are elicited. [see prec.]

aesthesiography (es·**the**·ze·**og**'·raf·e). 1. Study or description of the organs of perception and sensation. 2. The procedure of tracing on the skin the position of areas of sensibility, e.g. the tactile area. [aesthesia, Gk *graphein* to record.]

aesthesiology (es·**the**·ze·**ol**'·o·je). The science of sensory phenomena. [aesthesia, Gk *logos* science.]

aesthesiomania (es·**the**·ze·o·**ma**'·ne·ah). Insanity associated with extreme eccentricity or moral perversion. [aesthesia, mania.]

aesthesiometer (es·**the**·ze·**om**'·et·er). **Depth-sense aesthesiometer.** An instrument used for testing spatial sensibility in a plane at right angles to the skin surface. A smooth surface with a central ridge, increasing in height at a measured rate, is drawn across the patient's finger tip until the ridge can be appreciated.

aesthesiometry (es·**the**·ze·**om**'·et·re). The measurement or the estimation of sensibility by an aesthesiometer.

aesthesioneure (es·**the**·ze·o·newr). An afferent (sensory) neurone. [aesthesia, neurone.]

aesthesioneuroblastoma (es·**the**·ze·o·newr·o·blas·**to**'·mah). A glioma containing ganglionic tissue, which is highly sensitive to x-rays and radium; occurs in the nasal cavity in children. [aesthesia, neuroblastoma.]

aesthesioneurosis (es·**the**·ze·o·newr·**o**'·sis). Abnormality or disorder of the sensory nerves. [aesthesia, neurosis.]

aesthesionosus (es·**the**·ze·**on**'·o·sus). Aesthesioneurosis. [aesthesia, Gk *nosos* disease.]

aesthesiophysiology (es·**the**·ze·o·fiz·e·**ol**'·o·je). The physiology of the sensory organs and the faculties of perception. [aesthesia, physiology.]

aesthesioscopy (es·**the**·ze·**os**'·ko·pe). Examination with regard to the degree of tactile and other types of sensibility, or tenderness experienced within certain areas on the skin, and the subsequent mapping of such areas. [aesthesia, Gk *skopein* to watch.]

aesthesis (es·**the**·sis). Aesthesia.

aesthesodic (es·the·**zod**·ik). Aesthesiodic.

aesthetic (es·**thet**·ik). Aesthesic.

aesthetica (es·**thet**·ik·ah). Any disease in which one sense or more may be impaired or lost. [Gk *aisthesis* feeling.]

aestheticokinetic (es·**thet**·ik·o·kin·**et**'·ik). Motor as well as sensory. [aesthesia, Gk *kinesis* movement.]

aesthophysiology (es·tho·fiz·e·**ol**'·o·je). Aesthesiophysiology.

aestivation (es·tiv·a·shun). In biology, the state of torpidity or dormancy in which some animals and plants pass the dry, warm months of the year. [L *aestivare* to pass the summer.]

aestivo-autumnal (es·**ti**·vo·aw·**tum**'·nal). Relating or belonging to the summer and the autumn. The term is applied to a form of tropical malaria (malignant tertian). [L *aestivus* summer, autumn.]

aestuarium (es·tew·a·re·um). A vapour bath. [L *aestuare* to boil up.]

aestuation (es·tew·a·shun). 1. A surging or boiling up; ebullition. 2. Feverish excitement or agitation. [see prec.]

aestus (es·tus). Sudden access of heat to a part, particularly flushing of the face. **Aestus volaticus.** Strophylus, the so-called wildfire rash of children, a type of severe erythema with papules. [L heat.]

aethal (e·thal). Cetyl alcohol. *See* ALCOHOL.

aethanolamina (e·than·ol·am·e'·nah). Ethanolamine BP 1958.

aether (e·ther). Ether. **Aether anaestheticus.** Anaesthetic Ether BP 1958. *See* ETHER. **Aether solvens.** Solvent Ether BP 1958. *See* ETHER. [L the upper air.]

aetherism (e·ther·ism). 1. The condition caused by administration of ether or by the excessive use of ether. 2. Etheromania. [see prec.]

Aethinyloestradiolum (e·thin·il·e·strad·i·**o**'·lum). *European Pharmacopoeia* name for Ethinyloestradiol BP 1973.

aethiopification (e·the·op·if·ik·**a**'·shun). The production of argyria, the permanent ashen darkening of the skin occurring in long-continued use of preparations of arsenic, silver or mercury. [Gk *Aithiops* Negro, L *facere* to make.]

aethisteronum (e·this·ter·**o**'·num). Ethisterone BP 1958.

aethocaine hydrochloride (e·tho·kane hi·dro·**klor**·ide). Procaine Hydrochloride BP 1958.

aethomma (e·**thom**·ah). 1. A pigmented condition of the coats and the humours of the eye. 2. An abnormal condition of the eye in which stabs of light and flame flash before it. [Gk *aithos* of a browned or burnt colour, *omma* eye.]

aethyl (e·thil). Ethyl.

aethylenum (e·thil·**en**·um). The official Latin name for *ethylene* before the BP 1953.

aethylis (e·thil·is). The official Latin name for *ethyl* before the BP 1953. **Aethylis aminobenzoas.** Ethyl aminobenzoate. **Aethylis**

chaulmoogras. Ethyl chaulmoograte. **Aethylis oxidum.** Ethyl oxide.

aethylmorphinae (eth·il·**mor**·fe·ne). Ethylmorphine.

aetiocholanolone (e·te·o·ko·**lan**′·o·lone). Aetiocholane-3(α)-ol-17-one, $C_{19}H_{30}O_2$. A 17-ketosteroid hormone isolated from the urine of both normal men and normal women. It is an isomer of androsterone.

aetiologic, aetiological (e·ti·o·**loj**′·ik, e·te·o·**loj**′·ik·al). 1. Belonging to aetiology. 2. Assigning a cause or origin to a disease. [see foll.]

aetiology (e·te·**ol**·o·je). 1. The science of the investigation of the cause or origin of disease. 2. The science of the origin and development of vital phenomena. [Gk *aitia* cause, *logos* science.]

aetionymous (e·te·**on**·im·us). Applied to a name of a disease which is derived from its cause, e.g. caisson disease. [Gk *aitia* cause, *onyma* name.]

aetiopathogenesis (e·te·o·path·o·**jen**′·es·is). The cause, initiation and development of a disease. [Gk *aitia* cause, *pathos* disease, *genein* to produce.]

aetiopathology (e·te·o·path·**ol**′·o·je). Pathogenesis; the generation or development of morbid or diseased conditions. [Gk *aitia* cause, pathology.]

aetioporphyrin (e·te·o·**por**′·fir·in). Methyl ethyl porphin, $C_{32}H_{38}N_4$, occurring in several isomeric forms; the one prepared from haemoglobin bears a close relationship to another derived from chlorophyll, and is to be regarded as an interesting link.

aetiotropic (e·te·o·**tro**′·pik). Applied to any remedy or treatment which is directed against the cause of a disease. [Gk *aitia* cause, *tropos* a turning.]

afebrile (a·**feb**·rile). Without fever. [Gk *a*, L *febris* fever.]

afetal (a·**fe**·tal). Without a fetus. [Gk *a*, L *fetus* offspring.]

affect (af·**ekt**). 1. The reflection of a mental state in terms of the emotions; the emotional aspect of instinctual life ranging from cognition to conation. 2. Emotional outlet expressed as a feeling; affective attitude, a feeling towards something. 3. The technical term for mood or emotional state. **Affect epilepsy.** A psychosomatic state resulting from the stimulus of strong emotion, characterized by loss of colour, trembling of the lips and hands, and sometimes leading to loss of consciousness. **Affect laden.** Describing an emotionally-charged state associated with an idea or a memory. [L *affectus* state of mind.]

affectability (af·**ek**·tab·**il**′·it·e). The quality or state of being responsive to a stimulus. [see prec.]

affectation (af·ek·**ta**·shun). Artificiality of manner. [L *affectare* to strive after.]

affection (af·**ek**·shun). 1. A morbid process affecting either the whole body or one of its organs or tissues. 2. A kindly feeling towards someone. **Para-infectious affection.** A diseased state associated with an infection, but not directly due to the same causal agent. [L *afficere* to affect.]

affective (af·**ek**·tiv). 1. Exciting emotion. 2. In psychology, relating to emotion or feeling. [L *affectus* state of mind.]

affectivity (af·ek·**tiv**·it·e). 1. The emotional faculty. 2. In psychology, the trend or tension of the emotions or feelings of an individual. [see prec.]

affectomotor (af·**ek**·to·**mo**′·tor). Emotional as well as muscular activity. [L *affectus* state of mind, motor.]

affektepilepsie (af·**ekt**·ep·il·**ep**′·se). A convulsion occurring in cases of obsessive psychosis or psycho-asthenia and having its origin in the disturbed mental state of the patient. [G.]

affenspalte (**af**·en·spahl·te). Ape fissure. *See* FISSURE. [G.]

afferent (**af**·er·ent). In physiology, conducting inwards to, or towards, the centre of an organ, gland or other structure or area, and applying to sensory nerves, arteries and lymph vessels. Cf. EFFERENT. [L *ad*, *ferre* to bear.]

afferentia (af·er·**en**·she·ah). The afferent vessels or nerves.

affiliation (af·il·e·**a**′·shun). In medical jurisprudence, the decision as to, and the legal fixation of, the paternity of a child for the purpose of providing for maintenance. [L *ad*, *filius* son.]

affinity (af·**in**·it·e). 1. Resemblance, or relationship. 2. Mutual attraction. **Chemical affinity.** The attraction that causes atoms to combine into molecules. **Elective affinity.** The tendency of a chemical element to prefer combination with certain elements rather than others. **Electro affinity.** The force with which atoms retain their ionic charges. **Genetic affinity.** The kinship of individual organisms. **Haemoglobin oxygen affinity.** A measure of the degree to which oxygen is bound by haemoglobin at different partial pressures of oxygen. It is expressed as the P_{50} value, the partial pressure of oxygen at which a solution of haemoglobin has 50 per cent oxygen saturation. **Affinity label.** In enzymology and protein chemistry, a compound resembling the natural substrate which is able to bind at the active site and subsequently react with neighbouring residues to form covalent compounds; these enable irreversible modification of protein activities and identification of active site amino-acid residues. **Morbid affinity.** Synchronism or close association of certain pathological conditions. **Residual affinity.** The attraction that binds molecules into aggregates. **Vital affinity.** The idea that tissues possess the power of selecting their special nutritive requirements. [L *affinis* related.]

affirmation (af·er·**ma**·shun). 1. In autosuggestion, the point at which a tendency towards a positive reaction is obtained. 2. A solemn declaration without taking an oath. [L *affirmare* to make firm.]

afflux, affluxion (af·**lux**, af·**luk**·shun). A sudden flow of blood or other liquid to any part of the body. [L *affluere* to flow to.]

affuse (af·**ewz**). To shower or sprinkle upon. [L *affundere* to pour out.]

affusion (af·**ew**·zhun). A form of treatment for pyrexia or for nervous symptoms which consists in the pouring or sprinkling of water on to the affected part or on to the body. **Cold affusion.** The pouring of cold water over a patient in order to lower the temperature. [see prec.]

afibrinogenaemia (a·fi·brin·o·jen·**e**′·me·ah). A congenital or constitutional haemorrhagic disease due to absence or great reduction of blood fibrinogen rendering the blood incoagulable. [Gk *a*, fibrinogen, Gk *haima* blood.]

afibrinogenopenia (**a**·fi·brin·**oj**·en·o·**pe**′·ne·ah). Pseudohaemophilia. [Gk *a*, fibrinogen, Gk *penia* poverty.]

aflatoxicosis (**af**·lah·tox·ik·**o**′·sis). The disease caused by the ingestion of foodstuffs contaminated with aflatoxins. A fatal disease in ducklings and young turkeys, and carcinogenic for rats and possibly man. [aflatoxin, Gk *-osis* condition.]

aflatoxin (af·lah·**tox**·in). A toxic metabolite of the fungus *Aspergillus flavus* which grows on stored grain and groundnuts under conditions of damp heat. It is carcinogenic on the liver cells of mammals, birds and fish, especially in early life. Its role as a cause of human hepatoma is not yet established. [Gk *a*, L *flavus* yellow, Gk *toxikon* poison.]

after-birth (**ahf**·ter·berth). The placenta, umbilical cord and membranes by which the fetus was connected to the mother and which are expelled from the uterus shortly after the birth of the child. [AS *aefter*, ME *burth*.]

after-brain (**ahf**·ter·brane). The hind-brain or rhombencephalon, which consists of 2 parts: (*a*) metencephalon (cephalic); (*b*) myelencephalon (caudal). [AS *aefter*, *bragen*.]

after-care (**ahf**·ter·kare). The treatment of those who have recovered from mental or physical illness and who, although not in need of active curative treatment, require to be kept under observation and given guidance, e.g. in the rehabilitation period. [AS *aefter*, *caru*.]

after-cataract (**ahf**·ter·**kat**′·ar·akt). 1. Secondary cataract (1st def.). 2. An opacity in or adherent to the capsule of the lens of the eye which recurs after operation for cataract and is frequently due to regeneration of lens fibres left behind after extra-capsular extraction. 3. Any membrane in the area of the pupil after the lens has been absorbed or removed. [AS *aefter*, Gk *kataraktes* waterfall.]

after-current (**ahf**·ter·**kur**′·ent). A current produced in a nerve or muscle after the flow of an electric current through it has ceased. [AS *aefter*, L *currere* to run.]

after-damp (ahf·ter·damp). An irrespirable mixture of gases occurring in a coal mine after the explosion of firedamp. It consists chiefly of carbon dioxide and nitrogen, but carbon monoxide which is also present is responsible for most of the deaths. [AS *aefter*, ME *damp*.]

after-discharge (ahf·ter·dis·charj'). 1. Of sensory nerves, persistence of response to stimulation after the stimulation has ceased. 2. Continued electrical activity of muscle after cessation of voluntary contraction in myotonia. [AS *aefter*, OFr. *deschargier*.]

after-gilding (ahf·ter·gil'·ding). Gold-toning; in histology, the treatment of silver-impregnated sections with solutions of gold salts in order to replace the silver by gold and so improve contrast. [AS *aefter*, *gyldan*.]

after-glow (ahf·ter·glo). A phosphorescent glow that persists after phosphors have been excited to fluorescence by radiation. In modern fluorescent and intensifying screens used in radiology, a degree of after-glow which might interfere with diagnosis has been eliminated. [AS *aefter*, *glowan*.]

after-hearing (ahf·ter·heer'·ing). A neurosis in which there is a continuance of sound impressions after the actual stimulus which produced them has ceased to act. [AS *aefter*, *hieran*.]

after-image (ahf·ter·im'·ij). 1. After-sensation. 2. The visual impression which remains after the stimulation of the retina has ceased. **Complementary after-image.** An after-image in which the complementary colour of that seen in the original impression is visualized. **Negative after-image.** One when light is substituted for dark, and dark for light. **Positive after-image.** One in which light and dark remain as they were in the original impression. **Transferred after-image.** One which is visible in the eye to which the original stimulation was not applied. [AS *aefter*, L *imago*.]

after-impression (ahf·ter·im·presh'·un). After-sensation. [AS *aefter*, L *impressio*.]

after-load (ahf·ter·lode). Placement of a radio-active source into a previously located applicator. [AS *aefter*.]

after-movement (ahf·ter·moov'·ment). Involuntary continued muscular contraction causing persistent movement of the part after cessation of strong exertion against resistance, usually elicited in abduction of the arm; Kohnstamm's phenomenon. [AS *aefter*, L *movere* to move.]

after-nystagmus (ahf·ter·nis·tag'·mus). A nystagmus occurring on cessation of rotation, due to the labyrinthine fluid continuing to move for a short time after the head movement has stopped; also called *secondary nystagmus*. [AS *aefter*, nystagmus.]

after-pains (ahf·ter·pa'·nz). The cramp-like abdominal pains which are felt after the birth of a child, caused by the contracting of the uterus. [AS *aefter*, Gk *poine* penalty.]

after-perception (ahf·ter·per·sep'·shun). The continued perception of a sensation after the removal of the stimulus which gave rise to it. [AS *aefter*, L *perceptio*.]

after-potential (ahf·ter·po·ten'·shl). Either of the smaller waves, positive or negative, which follow the main deviation or spike potential in the oscillograph tracing of the action-potential wave passing along a nerve fibre. [AS *aefter*, L *potentia* power.]

after-pressure (ahf·ter·presh'·er). The sensation of pressure continuing for a short time after the force has been removed. [AS *aefter*, L *premere* to press.]

after-sensation (ahf·ter·sen·sa'·shun). A sense impression which remains after the removal of the stimulus which produced the primary sensation. **Auditory after-sensation.** After-sound. [AS *aefter*, L *sensus* sense.]

after-sound (ahf·ter·sownd). The continuance of a sound impression after the vibrations which produced the primary sound have stopped. [AS *aefter*, L *sonus* sound.]

after-stain (ahf·ter·stane). Counterstain; a stain used in histology to bring out further detail or to heighten contrast already produced by another stain. [AS *aefter*, OFr. *desteindre* to take away colour.]

after-taste (ahf·ter·ta·st). A taste which persists after the removal of the substance which caused it. [AS *aefter*, OFr. *taster* to feel.]

after-treatment (ahf·ter·treet'·ment). 1. General care of a patient in the convalescent phase, including periodical examinations to ascertain, for example, whether a formerly active lesion is in a quiescent state; rehabilitation. 2. Postoperative treatment. [AS *aefter*, L *tractare* to treat.]

after-vision (ahf·ter·vizh'·un). Awareness of an after-image. [AS *aefter*, L *visio*.]

afunction (a·fungk·shun). A state of being without function or of having lost the power to function. [Gk *a*, function.]

agalactia, agalactosis (a·gal·ak'·she·ah, a·gal·ak·to·sis). A condition in which there is complete or partial failure to secrete milk after childbirth. [Gk *a*, *gala* milk.]

agalactosuria (a·gal·ak·to·zewr'·e·ah). Lack of galactose in the urine. [Gk *a*, *gala* milk, urine.]

agalactous (a·gal·ak·tus). Lacking the secretion of milk. [Gk *a*, *gala* milk.]

agamete (a·gam·eet). In biology, a unicellular organism which reproduces asexually. [Gk *a*, *gamos* marriage.]

agamic (a·gam·ik). 1. In biology, asexual. 2. Reproducing unisexually. [see prec.]

agammaglobulinaemia (a·gam·ah·glob·ew·lin·e'·me·ah). Synonym for hypogammaglobulinaemia. [Gk *a*, gamma-globulin, Gk *haima* blood.]

agamobium (a·gam·o·be·um). In zoology, the asexually-reproducing generation in species in which there is alternation of generation. [Gk *a*, *gamos* marriage, *bios* life.]

agamodistomum ophthalmobium (a·gam·o·dis'·to·mum of·thal·mo·be·um). A non-specific name for immature trematode flukes in their migratory phase, which have occasionally been found in the eye. [Gk *a*, *gamos* marriage, *Distomum*, Gk *ophthalmos* eye, *bios* life.]

agamofilaria (a·gam·o·fil·a'·re·ah). A non-specific term for immature round nematode worms of the family Filariidae, occasionally found in superficial ulcers. [Gk *a*, *gamos* marriage, filaria.]

agamogenesis (a·gam·o·jen'·es·is). Reproduction by asexual means; parthenogenesis. [Gk *a*, *gamos* marriage, *genein* to produce.]

agamogony (a·gam·og·on·e). Parthenogenesis. [Gk *a*, *gamos* marriage, *gonos* offspring.]

agamomermis (a·gam·o·mer'·mis). A non-specific term for immature round nematode worms of the family Mermithidae. Normally parasites of invertebrates, they have been observed in the mouth and in urine, but their occurrence there is probably accidental. [Gk *a*, *gamos* marriage, Mermithidae.]

agamonema (a·gam·o·ne'·mah). A non-specific term for immature round nematode worms which cannot be further identified. Such forms may occur in urine. [Gk *a*, *gamos* marriage, nematode.]

Agamonematodum migrans (a·gam·o·nem·at·o'·dum mi·granz). The larva of *Ancylostoma brasiliense*, producing a dermatitis in man. [Gk *a*, *gamos* marriage, nematode, L migrating.]

agamont (a·gam·ont). Schizont; a protozoan which gives rise to isospores, these developing independently of any conjugative process. [Gk *a*, *gamos* marriage, *on* being.]

agamospore (a·gam·o·spore). A spore asexually reproduced. [Gk *a*, *gamos* marriage, *sporos* seed.]

agamous (a·gam·us). 1. In botany, cryptogamous. 2. In biology, without sexual organs, asexual, reproducing independently of impregnation. [Gk *a*, *gamos* marriage.]

aganglionosis (a·gang·le·on·o'·sis). Absence of parasympathetic ganglion cells, a condition found in Auerbach's plexus in a distal segment of the colon in congenital megacolon (Hirschsprung's disease). [Gk *a*, *gagglion* knot, *-osis* condition.]

Agar (a·gar). 1. General name given to species of seaweed of the genus *Gelidium*. 2. A polysaccharide obtained by drying the aqueous decoctions of certain seaweeds and other closely allied Rhodophyceae, e.g. *Gelidium corneum*. It occurs in the form of translucent strips, flakes or sheets, or as a coarse powder, and is widely used in the preparation of solid bacteriological media, in the manufacture of certain foods and drugs, and in industry in silk and paper manufacture. Medicinally it is employed to soften and provide bulk to the faeces in the treatment of constipation (BPC 1954). Also known as *agar-agar.* When used as the solidifying agent in bacteriological culture media to which growth-promoting or selectively inhibitory substances are added, identifying names are used, e.g. nutrient agar, blood agar, desoxycholate citrate agar, malt agar, milk agar, salt agar, etc. **Aesculin agar.** A nutrient agar containing 0.1 per cent aesculin, 0.5 per cent sodium taurocholate and 0.05 per cent ferric chloride. **Alkaline-blood agar.** Dieudonné's medium; defibrinated blood steamed with caustic soda, aged 10 days, and added to 3 per cent agar. **Ascitic agar, Ascitic-fluid agar.** Nutrient agar to which has been added 10-20 per cent sterile ascitic fluid. **Beerwort agar.** A medium prepared from sterile beerwort and 1.5 per cent agar. **Bile-salt agar.** A 2 per cent peptone solution solidified with agar to which bile salt 0.5 per cent and lactose 1 per cent are added, with neutral red as indicator. **Blood agar.** A nutrient agar to which a proportion of fresh sterile citrated or defibrinated blood has been added. This medium is of great value for the culture of demanding organisms, and for the study of haemolysis in certain genera, particularly the streptococci. **Blood-smeared agar.** Washbourn's blood agar; nutrient agar slopes or plates over which fresh sterile blood has been spread. **Agar bouillon.** Nutrient agar (see below). **Brilliant-green agar.** Nutrient agar containing beef extract 0.3 per cent, sodium chloride 0.5 per cent, peptone 1 per cent, Andrade's indicator 1 per cent, lactose 1 per cent, glucose 0.1 per cent and brilliant green (from 1 in 330 000 to 1 in 500 000). **Brilliant-green eosin agar.** A nutrient agar containing peptone 1 per cent, sodium chloride 0.5 per cent, lactose 1 per cent, sucrose 1 per cent, yellow eosin 0.06 per cent and brilliant green 0.0032 per cent. **Chocolate agar.** Nutrient agar containing 5-10 per cent defibrinated rabbit or horse blood, which is heated to 75°C before pouring; the heating produces methaemoglobin from the blood. It is valuable for the culture of *Neisseria* and *Haemophilus.* **Cholera agar.** Dieudonné's agar; a medium prepared by the addition to 7 parts of nutrient agar of 3 parts of a mixture containing equal parts of defibrinated blood and normal sodium hydroxide solution. **Cornmeal agar.** A medium containing 4 per cent cornmeal extract. **Crystal-violet blood agar.** A medium containing crystal violet, used for the isolation of streptococci. **Cystine blood agar.** A preparation of peptone 1 per cent, sodium chloride 0.5 per cent, glucose 1 per cent, cystine 0.1 per cent, and rabbit or horse blood 5 per cent. **Desoxycholate citrate agar.** A medium prepared from pork or beef infusion 1 litre, peptone 10 g, agar 20 g, lactose 10 g, sodium citrate 25 g, sodium desoxycholate 5 g, ferric ammonium citrate 2 g and neutral red 20 mg. **Dextrose agar.** A nutrient agar containing 1 per cent dextrose. **Egg-yolk agar.** A preparation made from the yolks of 4 eggs, normal saline 30 ml (or 25.5 ml normal saline and 4.5 ml glycerin), and 5 ml of 2 per cent aqueous malachite green. It is used for the culture of tubercle bacilli and *Pasteurella tularensis.* **EMB agar, Eosin methylene blue agar.** A preparation used for the isolation of non-lactose fermenting bacteria from faeces, made from peptone 10 g, dipotassium hydrogen phosphate 20 g, agar 15 g, lactose 1 g, yellowish eosin 0.04 g, methylene blue 0.01 g and distilled water to 1 litre. **Fish-gelatin agar.** A medium prepared by boiling 500 g of the flesh of whiting for 30 min, filtering through paper and adding sufficient gelatin to render it solid. **Gelatin agar.** A medium prepared from chopped meat 500 g, agar 10 g, gelatin 20 g, peptone 20 g, sodium chloride 5 g and distilled water 1 litre. **Glucose agar.** Dextrose agar (see above). **Glucose formate agar.** A nutrient agar containing 2 per cent glucose and 0.4 per cent sodium formate. **Glycerin agar.** Nutrient agar containing 5-8 per cent glycerin. **Heated-blood agar.** Chocolate agar (see above). **Lactose-litmus agar.** Conradi's agar; a nutrient agar containing peptone 1 per cent, nutrose 1.9 per cent, calcium chloride 0.5 per cent, lactose 1.5 per cent, crystal violet 0.001 per cent and litmus solution 15 per cent. It is an indicator medium used to test the ability of organisms to ferment lactose. **Lead acetate agar.** Nutrient agar containing 0.05 per cent lead acetate. **Liver-infusion agar.** A medium prepared from liver infusion 500 ml, peptone 5 g, sodium chloride 5 g, agar 20 g and water 500 ml. It is used for the isolation of *Brucella.* **Malachite-green agar.** A nutrient agar containing 10 g of dextrose and 8-12 ml of a 2 per cent aqueous solution of malachite green. **Meat-extract agar.** Meat-extract broth solidified with 1-1.5 per cent agar. **Meat-infusion agar.** Meat-infusion broth solidified with 1-1.5 per cent agar. **Nutrient agar.** A nutrient broth containing 1-2 per cent agar. **Nutrose agar.** A medium containing nutrose 10 g, sodium chloride 5 g, agar 15 g and water to 1 litre. **Plain agar.** Nutrient agar (see above). **Potato agar.** A watery extract of potato solidified with agar. **Potato-blood agar.** Bordet-Gengou agar; a nutrient agar containing potato extract, peptone, glycerol, and 20-50 per cent of fresh defibrinated horse or sheep blood. **Saccharose-mannitol agar.** A nutrient agar containing sucrose 1 per cent and mannitol 0.1 per cent, with Andrade's indicator. **Salt agar.** A medium prepared from yeast extract 2.5 g, tryptone 10 g, mannitol 10 g, lactose 2 g, dipotassium hydrogen phosphate 5 g, sodium chloride 75 g, gelatin 30 g, agar 15 g and water 1 litre. **Serum agar.** Nutrient agar with 10 per cent horse serum; of this Heiman's, Kanthack and Stephens', and Wertheimer's serum agars are variants. **Serum-tellurite agar.** A nutrient agar containing 15 per cent trypsinized horse serum, and 0.04 per cent potassium tellurite. **Sodium oleate agar.** A nutrient agar containing 2 per cent sodium oleate. **Starch agar.** A nutrient agar containing 1 per cent soluble starch. **Tryp agar.** A nutrient agar prepared from trypsin digest broth. **Whey agar.** Milk whey containing 0.5 per cent peptone solidified with 1.5 per cent agar. **Wort agar.** Beerwort agar (see above). [Malay.]

See also: BAILEY (S. F.), BORDET, CHAPMAN, CLURMAN, CONRADI (H.), DIEUDONNÉ, DOUGLAS (S. R.), DRIGALSKI, ENDO, GARROD, GENGOU, GUY, HEIMAN, HITCHENS, HOLT-HARRIS, HYNES, JORDAN, KANTHACK, KITASATO, KRUMWEIDE, LEIFSON, MACCONKEY, MCLEOD, MOOR, RUSSELL (F. F.), SIMMONS, STEPHENS, TEAGUE, VEDDER, WASHBOURN, WASSERMANN, WEIL (E.), WERTHEIMER, WILSON (W. J.), WURTZ.

agar-agar (a·gar·a′·gar). Agar. [Malay.]

Agaric (ag·ar·ik). 1. A genus of mushrooms, particularly the *Agaricus* species. Other species, e.g. *Psilocybe,* are noted for their hallucinogenic properties. 2. The touchwood or spunk obtained by drying mushrooms. **Fly agaric.** *Amanita muscaria.* **Larch agaric, Purging agaric.** *Polyphorus officinalis,* or *Boletus laricis,* a species found on larch trees and containing agaricin. **Surgeon's agaric.** *Agaricus chirurgorum,* a species of agaric which, when dried, has been used as a haemostatic. **White agaric.** Larch agaric (see above). [Gk *agarikon,* fungus.]

agaricin (ag·ar·is·in). A poisonous principle from the mushroom *Polyphorus officinalis* (purging agaric), said to be useful in the treatment of night sweats of tuberculosis.

Agaricus (ag·ar·ik·us). A variety of fungus of the family Agaricaceae. **Agaricus campestris.** The edible field mushroom. **Agaricus chirurgorum.** Surgeon's agaric. *See* AGARIC. **Agaricus muscarius.** *Amanita muscaria.* [Gk *agarikon* fungus.]

agaster, agastria (a·gas·ter, a·gas·tre·ah). The condition of being without a stomach. [Gk *a, gaster* stomach.]

agastric (a·gas·trik). Being without a stomach or digestive canal. [see prec.]

agastroneuria (a·gas·tro·newr′·e·ah). Defective or deficient nervous action in the stomach; the stimuli reaching the organ are weak. [Gk *a, gaster* stomach, *neuron* nerve.]

Agave (ag·a·ve). A genus of American plants of the family Amaryllidaceae. The plants bear fleshy leaves which yield certain important fibres such as sisal (from *Agave sisalana*). **Agave americana.** The American aloe, yielding a juice (pulque) which is diuretic, alterative and laxative. [Gk *agauos* noble.]

age (aje). **Achievement age.** The age at which, according to an accepted standard of capability, any particular young person should be able to carry out any particular task with success. **Anatomical age.** Age determined by the stage of development which the body has reached. **Bone age.** The stage of development of the bones, seen in x-ray examination, when compared with the development normal for the chronological age.

Chronological age. Age measured by years lived. **Climacteric age.** The menopause. **Age of consent.** In medical jurisprudence, the age at which, on the part of a minor, consent to sexual intercourse is held to be valid. **Critique age.** The climacteric. **Emotional age.** Age determined by the stage of emotional development reached. Lacks objective criteria. **Fertilization age.** The age of an embryo or fetus calculated from the time of fertilization. **Functional age.** Age determined by a combined assessment of stages reached in mental, emotional and physiological development. **Marriageable age.** Nubility. **Menstrual age.** The age of an embryo or fetus calculated from the first day of the last normal menstruation preceding pregnancy. **Mental age.** In intelligence testing, the measurement of an individual's mental power by his ability to amass scores graded for different years according to normal mental capacity. **Ovulational age.** The age of an embryo or fetus calculated from time of ovulation. **Physiological age.** Age determined by the stage of development at which the body has arrived and by the capability of its functions. [L *aetas.*]

See also: BINET.

ageing (a·jing). 1. The process of growing old; maturing. 2. A property of silver-tin alloy used in conservative dentistry and induced by heat; it has the effect of retarding the initial stages of amalgamation when the alloy is mixed with mercury. [see prec.]

agene (a·jeen). The commercial name for the gas, nitrogen trichloride, used in a process for the bleaching and improvement of the baking qualities of wheat flour. The protein of the flour is altered to give a dough more suitable for mechanical handling and a loaf that is better in colour and texture and in keeping properties. The flour, however, produces severe toxic symptoms in dogs and certain other animals, though it has not been shown to affect human beings in the same way. The use of agene has been discontinued in favour of chlorine dioxide which is believed free of toxicity.

agenesis (a·**jen**·es·is). Imperfection or lack of development. **Callosal agenesis.** Defective development of the corpus callosum. **Agenesis corticalis.** Failure of development in the fetus of the cortical cells, particularly those of the cerebral cortex; such failure may result in the child being born an idiot or affected with cerebral paralysis. **Agenesis of gastric muscles.** Congenital muscle-defect causing perforation of the stomach in newborn infants. **Nuclear agenesis.** Nuclear aplasia. *See* APLASIA. **Ovarian agenesis.** Congenital absence of functional ovarian tissue, causing failure of development of secondary female sexual characteristics, short stature and sometimes webbing of the neck (Turner's syndrome), diffuse osteoporosis, coarctation of the aorta and dental maldevelopment. **Testicular agenesis.** Congenital absence of testicular tissue with consequent failure of development of secondary male sexual characteristics and exaggerated length of the long bones. The Wolffian duct derivatives end in a small nodule of tissue which is assumed to be an "atrophied" testis. This atrophy presumably occurred after the stage at which the male phenotype had been determined at the 10th week of fetal life. Used to be referred to as "prepubertal testicular failure" and thought to be due to some undetected post-natal event giving rise to testicular atrophy. [Gk *a, genein to produce.]*

agenetic (a·jen·**et**·ik). Descriptive of factors which in the general consideration of racial development tend to interrupt or delay progress, so that degenerative influences are allowed to become too active. [see prec.]

agenization (a·jen·i·za′·shun). The process of treating flour with agene (NCl_3). *See* AGENE.

agenized flour (a·jen·i·zd flowr). Wheat flour treated with agene (nitrogen trichloride) to bleach it and alter its protein in such a way that its baking properties and colour are improved. *See* AGENE.

agent (a·jent). Any substance or force which brings about a change. Cf. REAGENT. **Amphipathic agents.** Substances with molecules or ions, some of which have an affinity and some a repulsion for the medium in which they are dissolved. They are emulsifying agents, anionic, cationic, non-ionic (not dissociating in water), or ampholytic (with activity depending on the pH of the solution). **Chelating agents.** Substances which form complexes with metal ions and bind them, so rendering them inactive. **Clearing agent.** Any substance used in histology to clear sections. *See also* DUNHAM (E.K.). **Competitive blocking agents.** Myoneural blocking agents (see below) of the non-depolarizing type, e.g. tubocurarine. **I.N.I. (intranuclear inclusion) agent.** A virus obtained from pigeons, usually but not always associated with the psittacosis virus. It differs from the psittacosis virus in its smaller size, its more rapid growth on the chorio-allantoic membrane, its greater resistance to storage at 20°C, its ability to give rise in the parenchymatous tissues of the liver to intranuclear inclusion bodies of the herpetic type, and its lack of pathogenicity for rabbits, guinea-pigs or mice. Its relation to the virus producing intranuclear inclusions in parrots is uncertain. **Mammary-tumour agent, Mouse mammary-tumour agent.** The milk factor, thought by some to be a virus, which is transmitted to certain mouse strains from mother to offspring during suckling. **Marburg agent.** Marburg virus. *See* VIRUS. **Myoneural blocking agent.** A drug which prevents the transmission of nervous impulses across the myoneural junction, resulting in the relaxation and paralysis of voluntary muscles. They include curare and the curare-like compounds which block by competition with acetylcholine (competitive block) and decamethonium and related compounds including suxamethonium which block by a prolonged depolarization of the muscle end plate (depolarization block). **Simian vacuolating agent.** Simian virus type 40. *See* VIRUS. [L *agere* to do.]

agerasia (a·jer·**a**·se·ah). In an old person, the quality of being of youthful appearance and of being hale and hearty in body. [Gk *a, geras* old age.]

ageusia, ageustia (a·**gew**·se·ah, a·**gew**·ste·ah). Impairment or lack of the taste sense. **Central ageusia.** Ageusia caused by a lesion in the cerebral centres of the nerves of taste. **Conduction ageusia.** Ageusia caused by a lesion affecting the nerves of taste at some point on their course, between their origin and distribution. **Peripheral ageusia.** Ageusia caused by disturbance of function at the ends of the gustatory nerves. [Gk *a, geusis* taste.]

Aggazzotti, Alberto (b. 1877). Modena physiologist.

Aggazzotti's mixture. A mixture of oxygen (87 parts) and carbon dioxide (13 parts) which has been used in aviation sickness.

agger (aj·er). A mound or eminence. **Agger auriculae.** The ponticulus of the auricle. **Agger nasi [NA].** A curved elevation above the atrium of the nose, running downward and forward from the anterior free border of the middle concha; the anterior part of the ethmoidal crest. **Agger perpendicularis.** The eminence of the triangular fossa. **Agger valvae venae.** The knot-like expansion of the wall of a vein on the cardiac side over a valve. [L mound.]

agglutinable (ag·**loo**·tin·abl). Susceptible to the action of specific agglutinins. [see foll.]

agglutinant (ag·**loo**·tin·ant). 1. Bringing about adhesion; agglutinative. 2. An antibody produced in the serum *in vivo* stimulated by the injection of an antigen; agglutinin. 3. Any material used to maintain divided structures in apposition, e.g. a thrombin clot in the repair of small nerves. [L *agglutinare* to glue.]

agglutination (ag·**loo**·tin·a′·shun). 1. The clumping together of cells dispersed in a fluid; the action of an agglutinant. 2. The phenomenon of aggregation into clumps of homogeneous suspensions of bacteria, or other antigenic particulate substances, under the influence of specific antisera, or solutions of acids, salts or certain dyes. As bacterial agglutination with specific antisera is easily visible, it forms the basis of many serological reactions, e.g. Widal's test. 3. The adhesion of wound edges in the process of natural healing. **Acid agglutination.** Agglutination of micro-organisms occurring at certain hydrogen ion concentrations. **Bacteriogenic agglutination.** The clumping of erythrocytes due to bacterial contamination. **Cross agglutination.** The agglutination of related organisms or corpuscles by one antiserum, due to the possession by the organisms of a common antigen. **Group agglutination.** Agglutination of members of a group of related organisms by the serum of an animal immunized against one member of the group. The phenomenon is due to the presence in the organisms of an antigen common to the species in the group. **Immediate agglutination.** The healing of a wound by first intention, the divided edges adhering directly with each other. **Intravascular agglutination.** Agglutination of the red cells within the vascular lumen, which interferes with the local circulation and causes local anoxia. **Macroscopic agglutination.** Agglutination which is visible to the naked eye. **Microscopic agglutination.** Agglutination which is visible only with the aid of a magnifying lens or microscope. **Salt agglutination.** Agglutination of micro-organisms occurring in particular concentrations of certain salts. **Specific agglutination.** The clumping of a microbial culture by a specific antiserum, indicating the presence in the organism of a certain specific antigen. **Spontaneous agglutination.** Agglutination of organisms in a fluid which does not contain known agglutinating substances. **Vi agglutination.** Agglutination by specific antisera of certain species of Enterobacteriaceae (e.g. *Salmonella typhi*) possessing Vi antigen. [see prec.]

agglutinative (ag·**loo**·tin·at·iv). Agglutinant; bringing about or promoting adhesion. [see foll.]

agglutinator (ag·**loo**·tin·a·tor). 1. An agglutinin; that which causes agglutination. 2. Applied to a micro-organism that is agglutinated by specific antiserum, in contrast to a morphologically and biochemically-similar micro-organism that is not agglutinated by this serum (i.e. *a non-agglutinator*). [L *agglutinare* to glue.]

agglutinin (ag·**loo**·tin·in). An antibody which reacts with, and agglutinates, particles which carry antigens on their surfaces (cells, bacteria or inert particles coated with antigen). The antibody causes the particles to adhere in visible clumps. This aggregation of particles is used to detect specific antibodies and for the identification of bacteria. Most blood agglutinins are of IgM type. **Albumin agglutinin.** Blocking or incomplete antibody; important in the Rhesus system developing later in the immune response than saline agglutinating antibodies. The reaction with red cells carrying the corresponding agglutinogen is not visible in saline suspensions but agglutination does occur if the cells are suspended in protein media, e.g. albumin. Incomplete antibodies have only a single combining site and with cells suspended in saline cannot make the cross-linkages between cells necessary for agglutination. Because of their small molecular size, sedimentation coefficient in the ultracentrifuge, 7 *S*, they can cross the placental barrier (cf. SALINE AGGLUTININ below). **Anti-A, or α, agglutinin.** Antibody found in the serum of people of groups O and B, absent in people of groups A and AB, that corresponds to the agglutinogen A, combination of antibody and red cells results in agglutination. **Anti A_1, or α_1, agglutinin.** Antibody that reacts only with red cells carrying the A_1 agglutinin. **Anti-B, or β, agglutinin.** Antibody found in the serum of people of groups O and A, absent in people of groups B and AB, that corresponds to the agglutinogen B. **Anti-M, N and S agglutinins.** Antibodies corresponding to the red cell antigens of the MNS system. **Anti P_1 agglutinin.** Cold agglutinin corresponding to the P_1 agglutinogen. **Anti-Rhesus agglutinins.** Antibodies corresponding to the agglutinogens of the Rhesus system. There are many specificities controlled by a single complex genetic locus. The most important specificity clinically is anti-D (Rh_0) which reacts with red cells called Rhesus positive because they carry the D (Rh_0) agglutinogen. **Cold agglutinins.** Agglutinins that are reactive only at low temperatures. They occur in the sera of patients with atypical pneumonia, and in certain pathological blood conditions. **Cross agglutinin.** Group agglutinin (see below). **Flagellar agglutinin.** An agglutinin specific for the flagellar substance of motile bacteria. **Group agglutinin.** An antibody to an antigen that is possessed by several related bacterial species and which agglutinates them all. **H-agglutinin.** Flagellar agglutinin (see above). **Natural agglutinin, Normal agglutinin.** An agglutinin contained in the serum of normal animals that have never had disease. **O-agglutinin.** Somatic agglutinin (see below). **Platelet agglutinin.** An antibody produced in the recipient after multiple platelet transfusions; there are probably several groups of these platelet agglutinins which differ antigenically and are globulins adsorbed on to the affected platelets. **Saline agglutinin.** Antibody formed in the early stages of immunization, particularly in Rhesus sensitization. It agglutinates red cells suspended in saline because the antibody molecules, having 2 or more combining sites, can form cross-linkages between the cells. Saline agglutinins do not usually cross the placental barrier; they are macroglobulins, sedimentation coefficient 19 *S*. **Somatic agglutinin.** An agglutinin produced by both a non-motile and a motile organism in response to the antigenic material in the body of the bacterium, but particularly by the former. **Vi agglutinin.** One produced against an antigen associated with virulence in typhoid bacilli and acting on antigens on the surface of the body of freshly isolated virulent strains. [see prec.]

agglutinogen (ag·**loo**·tin·o·jen). 1. Any substance that, injected into the blood stream, can lead to the production of specific antibodies (agglutinins) which have the power of combining with the original agglutinogen. 2. A specific substance (haemagglutinogen) present in erythrocytes, characterizing particular blood group systems, which has the property of combining with its corresponding agglutinin often resulting in agglutination of the red cells. An agglutinogen and the corresponding agglutinin are not normally present together in the same individual. The agglutinogens at present known include those belonging to the following red cell blood group systems: ABO, MNSs, P, Rhesus, Lutheran, Kell, Lewis, Duffy, Kidd, Diego, Yt, I and Xg. Blood group substances of the ABO and Lewis systems may be found in other tissues and secretions. **Agglutinogen A.** A substance, discovered by Landsteiner, characterizing the red cells of individuals belonging to group A. The cells agglutinate in the presence of anti-A (α) antibody. The A antigen is subdivided, the chief subdivisions being A_1 and A_2. Red cells carrying the A_1 antigen are agglutinated by anti-A but not by anti-A_1 antibody. **Agglutinogen B.** A substance discovered by Landsteiner, characterizing the red cells of people belonging to group B. These cells agglutinate in the presence of anti-B (β) antibody. **Agglutinogens M and N.** Discovered by Landsteiner and Levine, antibodies to M and N antigens, unlike α and β, are rarely present in normal sera. The MN system was complicated by the subsequent discovery of two genetically associated antigens, S and s. **Agglutinogen P_1.** A blood group substance, cells carrying which agglutinate when exposed to anti-P_1 agglutinin at low temperatures. **Rhesus agglutinogens.** Belong to the blood group system discovered by Landsteiner and Wiener in 1940, using an antibody prepared by immunizing rabbits and guinea-pigs with the blood of the monkey *Macacus rhesus*. The antibody agglutinated not only the red cells of the monkey but also the cells of 85 per cent of Caucasians who were called Rhesus (Rh) positive. Wiener and Peters then showed that antibody of the same specificity could be found in the serum of people who had reacted against ABO compatible blood transfusions. A large number of Rh antigens have now been identified. There are at least 2 nomenclatures, the CDE of Fisher and Race, and the Rh-Hr of Wiener. The most important antigen, clinically, is the D (Rh_0). Rhesus positive cells have the D (Rh_0) antigen, rhesus negative cells do not. A Rhesus negative mother can be immunized by a Rhesus positive fetus and form anti-D antibody which may cross the placental barrier and damage the fetal red cells, and the child subsequently suffers from haemolytic disease of the newborn. [agglutinin, Gk *genein* to produce.]

agglutinogenic (ag·**loo**·tin·o·**jen**′·ik). Producing agglutinin; of or relating to the production of agglutinin. [see prec.]

agglutinoid (ag·**loo**·tin·oid). A non-agglutinating agglutinin that still retains its ability to combine with its own agglutinogen. [agglutin, Gk *eidos* form.]

agglutinometer (ag·**loo**·tin·**om**′·et·er). Agglutometer.

agglutinophilic (ag·**loo**·tin·o·**fil**′·ik). Agglutinating easily or readily. [agglutination, Gk *philein* to love.]

agglutinophore (ag·**loo**·tin·o·fore). The part or grouping in an agglutinin that is responsible for its agglutinogenic powers. [agglutinin, Gk *pherein* to bear.]

agglutinoscope (ag·**loo**·tin·o·skope). An instrument with which the process of agglutination in a test tube may be watched and the results read. [agglutination, Gk *skopein* to watch.]

agglutinum (ag·**loo**·tin·um). That part of a bacterium responsible for agglutination.

agglutinumoid (ag·loo·**tin**·ew·moid). An agglutinin in which the agglutinating power still remains after the serum containing it has been exposed to a temperature of more than 50°C for a specified time.

agglutogenic (ag·**loo**·to·**jen**′·ik). Agglutinogenic.

agglutometer (ag·loo·**tom**·et·er). A type of apparatus used in the performance of the Widal or agglutination test, which obviates the need of a microscope; it can be used at the bedside or in the field. [agglutination, meter.]

aggregate (ag·re·gate). 1. To unite, accumulate or clump together. 2. A clump, e.g. of molecules. [L *ad, gregare* to collect into a flock.]

aggressinogen (ag·res·**in**·o·jen). A hypothetical antigen, produced *in vivo* by certain pathogenic bacteria, which stimulates the production of aggressin. [aggressin, Gk *genein* to produce.]

aggressins (ag·**res**·inz). Diffusible substances produced by pathogenic bacteria which, although not themselves toxic, interfere with normal mechanisms of the host, e.g. capsular polysaccharide of pneumococci. [L *aggressio* an attack.]

aggression (ag·**resh**·un). The first attack in a dispute; an unprovoked or inadequately provoked attack. [L *aggressio* an attack.]

aggressivity (ag·res·**iv**·it·e). The characteristic activity shown by invading bacteria in maintaining their integrity and at the same time striving to overcome the body's defences. [see prec.]

agitation (aj·it·**a**·shun). 1. Mental disturbance causing physical excitement and restlessness. 2. Tremor. 3. Shaking a tube or other container so that the contents are moved about rapidly, or mixed. [L *agitatio* shaking.]

agitographia (aj·it·o·**graf**′·e·ah). A condition in which writing is abnormally rapid and illegible, with omission of letters, syllables and words. Cf. AGITOPHASIA, with which agitographia generally is found in association. [L *agitare* to shake, Gk *graphein* to write.]

agitolalia (aj·it·o·**la**′·le·ah). Agitophasia. [L *agitare* to shake, Gk *lalein* babble like a child.]

agitophasia (aj·it·o·**fa**′·ze·ah). A condition in which speaking is abnormally rapid and syllables or words are indistinctly run together or are omitted. Cf. AGITOGRAPHIA, which is generally found in association with agitophasia. [L *agitare* to shake, Gk *phasis* speech.]

Agkistrodon (ag·**kis**·tro·don). A genus of Asiatic and American poisonous snakes of the family Crotalidae, all the species being dangerously venomous. **Agkistrodon contortrix.** The copperhead, a native of North America. **Agkistrodon piscivorus.** Water moccasin, a native of North America. **Agkistrodon rhodostoma.** The pit viper, a native of Malaya. [Gk *agkistron* fish hook, *odous* tooth.]

aglandular (a·**glan**·dew·lar). Being without glands. [Gk *a*, glandular.]

aglaucopsia (a·glaw·**kop**·se·ah). Inability to see the colour green; green blindness. [Gk *a, glaukos* green, *opsis* vision.]

aglia (**ag**·le·ah). A spot or a mark on the sclera or cornea. [Gk *aglie* speck.]

aglobulia, aglobuliosis, aglobulism (a·glob·**ew**′·le·ah, a·glob·ew·le·**o**′·sis, a·**glob**·ew·lizm). A condition in which the number of erythrocytes in a given volume of blood is decreased. [Gk *a*, L *globula* globule.]

aglomerular (a·glom·**er**·ew·lar). Descriptive of a type of kidney which is characterized by absence of glomeruli, the latter having been absorbed. [Gk *a*, glomerulus.]

aglossia (a·**glos**·e·ah). 1. Lack of the power to speak. 2. The congenital condition of being without a tongue. [Gk *a, glossa* tongue.]

aglossostomia (a·glos·o·**sto**′·me·ah). A congenital condition of being without a tongue and of having a (usually closed) mouth. [Gk *a, glossa* tongue, *stoma* mouth.]

aglossus (a·**glos**·us). An individual who does not have a tongue. [Gk *a, glossa* tongue.]

aglucone (a·**gloo**·kone). The portion of a glucoside which remains when the glucose is removed. [Gk *a, glykys* sweet.]

aglutition (a·gloo·**tish**·un). Absence of the power to swallow; difficulty in swallowing. [Gk *a*, L *glutire* to swallow.]

aglycaemia (a·gli·**se**·me·ah). Lack of sugar in the blood. [Gk *a, glykis* sweet, *haima* blood.]

aglycone (a·**gli**·kone). The compound which remains when a glycoside is hydrolysed and the sugar, or mixture of sugars, abstracted; also known as a *genin.* [Gk *a, glykys* sweet.]

aglycosuric (a·**gli**·ko·**zewr**′·ik). 1. Non-glycosuric; applied to the urine which is entirely free of sugar. 2. It may be applied to the patient as indicating that he is free of sugar in the urine after having been glycosuric for a period. [Gk *a, glykys* sweet, urine.]

aglypha (**ag**·lif·ah). A term applied to those snakes of the families Colubridae and Viperidae that are non-poisonous and in which the fangs, as such, are absent. Cf. OPISTHOGLYPHA, PROTEROGLYPHA, SOLENOGLYPHA. [Gk *a, glyphe* a carving.]

agmatine (**ag**·mat·een). Aminobutyl guanidine, $NH_2(CH_2)_4NHNHCNH_2$, found in ergot and herring spawn; also occurs in protein decomposition as a break-down product of arginine. It is a pressor base, and induces uterine contractions.

agmatology (ag·mat·**ol**·o·je). That branch of surgery which is centred upon the study and the treatment of fractures. [Gk *agma* fragment, *logos* science.]

agmen (**ag**·men) (pl. *agmina*). A collection or aggregation. **Agmen peyerianum.** The aggregated lymphatic nodules to be found in the ileum, jejunum and duodenum (Peyer's patches). [L a multitude.]

agminated (**ag**·min·a·ted). Grouped or clustered together. **Agminated follicles, glands and nodules.** The aggregated lymphatic nodules which are to be found mainly in the ileum (Peyer's patches) but also in the jejunum and duodenum. [agmen.]

agmination (ag·min·**a**·shun). A state of being clustered together, as is to be found in certain glands. [agmen.]

agnail (**ag**·nale). 1. Hangnail. 2. Inflammation round or under the nail; whitlow. [AS *angnaegl.*]

agnate (**ag**·nate). According to Scots law, that relative of a certified insane individual who is appointed guardian by virtue of being the nearest relative on the male, or spear, side. [L *ad, natus* born.]

agnathia (ag·**na**·the·ah). Without a jaw or jaws, or with only imperfect development of jaws. [Gk *a, gnathos* jaw.]

agnathus (ag·**na**·thus). A monster without a lower jaw. [see prec.]

Agnew, David Hayes (b. 1818). Philadelphia surgeon.

Agnew's splint. 1. A splint used for fracture of the patella. 2. One used for fracture of the wrist.

agnoea (ag·ne·ah). A condition in which the affected individual does not show any recognition of persons or things. [Gk *agnoia* lack of perception.]

agnogenic (ag·no·**jen**·ik). Unknown as far as origin or aetiology is concerned. [Gk *a, gnosis* knowledge, *genein* to produce.]

agnosia (ag·**no**·se·ah). In this condition there is inability to recognize objects and lack of the perceptive faculty in general. Agnosia is found in relation with the senses: auditory agnosia, gustatory agnosia, olfactory agnosia, optic agnosia and tactile agnosia. **Auditory agnosia.** Failure to recognize sounds in the absence of deafness. **Body-image agnosia.** Autotopagnosia. **Finger agnosia.** Failure to identify individual fingers of one's own or another person's hand. **Ideational agnosia.** Loss of that function of the mind by which ideas are entertained and are related one with and to another. **Tactile agnosia.** Failure to recognize objects by touch, in the absence of sensory loss.

Visual agnosia. Failure to recognize objects by sight in spite of normal vision. [Gk *a*, *gnosis* knowledge.]

agnosiac (ag·**no**·se·ak). A person suffering from agnosia.

agnosic (ag·**nos**·ik). Affected with agnosia.

agnosterol (ag·no·**steer**·ol). $C_{30}H_{48}O$. A sterol found in wool wax or lanolin.

agomphiasis, agomphosis (a·gom·**fi**′·as·is, a·gom·**fo**′·sis). 1. Absence of teeth. 2. A loose condition of the teeth. [Gk *a*, *gomphios* tooth.]

agomphious (a·**gom**·fe·us). Toothless; without teeth. [see prec.]

agonad (a·**gon**·ad). An individual lacking sex glands. [Gk *a*, gonad.]

agonadal (a·**gon**·ad·al). 1. Pertaining to absence of gonads or sex glands. 2. Having no gamete-producing glands. [see prec.]

agonal (**ag**·on·al). Of or pertaining to death; terminal. [see foll.]

agonia (ag·**o**·ne·ah). 1. Anguish, or distress of mind. 2. The pangs of death. [Gk *agon* a struggle.]

agonist (**ag**·on·ist). Of muscles, one which by contraction, and against its opposing muscle, causes movement. Cf. ANTAGONIST. [see prec.]

agonous (**ag**·on·us). Sterile or impotent. [Gk *agonos* unfruitful.]

agony (**ag**·on·e). Agonia.

agoraphobia (ag·or·ah·**fo**′·be·ah). Morbid dread of large open spaces. Cf. CLAUSTROPHOBIA. [Gk *agora* market place, *phobos* fear.]

agraffe (ah·**graf**). An instrument used for clasping together the edges of a wound whilst they are joined by suture. [Fr. *agrafe* hook.]

agrammaphasia (a·**gram**·af·**a**′·ze·ah). A form of dysphasia in which the power of grammatical and syntactical expression is lost. [Gk *a*, *gramma* letter, *phasis* speech.]

agrammatism, agrammatologia (a·**gram**·at·izm, a·**gram**·at·o·**lo**′·je·ah). Agrammaphasia. [Gk *agrammatos* illiterate, *logos* word.]

agranulaemia (a·gran·ew·**le**′·me·ah). Agranulocytosis. [Gk *a*, granule, Gk *haima* blood.]

agranulocyte (a·**gran**·ew·lo·site). A leucocyte which on being stained does not show any granules in the cytoplasm. [Gk *a*, granulocyte.]

agranulocythaemia, agranulocytopenia (a·**gran**·ew·lo·si·**the**′·me·ah, a·**gran**·ew·lo·si·to·**pe**′·ne·ah). Agranulocytosis. [agranulocyte, Gk *haima* blood, *penia* poverty.]

agranulocytosis (a·**gran**·ew·lo·si·**to**′·sis). Agranulocytic angina, malignant leucopenia; a severe, acute, usually fatal disease with marked diminution or absence of granular leucocytes from the bone marrow and peripheral blood. It occurs as an idiopathic type with no obvious aetiology, but is more commonly seen, probably as an idiosyncrasy, after taking various toxic or therapeutic synthetic drugs, such as the derivatives of sulphonamides, thiouracil and organic compounds of the heavy metals. It may be a secondary feature of certain blood diseases, especially acute leukaemia, thrombocytopenic purpura, aplastic anaemia and pernicious anaemia. [agranulocyte, Gk *-osis* condition.]

agranuloplastic (a·**gran**·ew·lo·**plas**′·tik). Not able to form granular cells, although capable of forming non-granular cells. [Gk *a*, granule, Gk *plassein* to form.]

agranulosis (a·**gran**·ew·**lo**′·sis). Agranulocytosis.

agraphia (a·**graf**·e·ah). A special form of apraxia in which there is a loss of power, or complete absence of power, to express ideas in a written form. Cf. PARAGRAPHIA. **Absolute agraphia.** A type in which the separate letters of the alphabet, even, cannot be written. **Acoustic agraphia.** Acquired inability to take down in writing anything which is being read aloud. **Agraphia amnemonica.** A type of agraphia in which the letters and words which are written down are not arranged so as to convey any idea or to make sense. **Agraphia atactica.** Absolute agraphia (see above). **Cerebral agraphia.** Mental agraphia (see below). **Jargon agraphia.** A type in which, although writing can be carried on, only fortuitous combinations of letters appear. **Literal agraphia.** Absolute agraphia (see above). **Mental agraphia.** A type in which there is inability to write down ideas in phrases or sentences. **Motor agraphia.** Loss of all faculty of forming letters. **Musical agraphia.** Inability or loss of power to write musical notation. **Optic agraphia.** A type in which there is inability to copy writing. **Verbal agraphia.** Inability to write words although there is ability to form letters. [Gk *a*, *graphein* to write.]

agraphic (a·**graf**·ik). Affected with or relating to agraphia; resembling agraphia.

agravic (a·**grav**·ik). Weightless (zero-*G*); a condition of a system in which no acceleration can be detected by observers inside the system. This state can be produced in a spacecraft orbiting the earth where the centrifugal force exactly counteracts the earth's gravitational force, or in free fall in a vacuum where the acceleration ($-1G$) cancels the $+1G$ force of the earth's gravity. [Gk *a*, L *gravis* heavy.]

agria (**ag**·re·ah). A persistent malignant or severe pustular eruption, sometimes of herpetic character. [Gk *agrios* fierce.)

agrimony (**ag**·rim·on·e). Any plant of the rosaceous genus *Agrimonia*. The common European agrimony (*Agrimonia eupatoria*) was at one time used in various forms as an astringent and tonic, and in relaxed conditions of the respiratory and urinary systems. [Gk *argemone* poppy.]

agriothymia (ag·re·o·**thi**′·me·ah). Severe mania of active type. The patient is menacing, fierce and dangerous. [Gk *agrios* fierce, *thymos* mind.]

agrippa (ag·**rip**·ah). A child delivered with the feet as the presenting parts. [L.]

agrius (**ag**·re·us). Skin eruptions of an angry appearance or very severe in form. [Gk *agrios* fierce.]

agromania (ag·ro·**ma**·ne·ah). Morbid love for or delight in being alone, or for wandering in open country. [Gk *agros* field, mania.]

agron (**ag**·ron). A disease encountered in India and characterized by a fissured and roughened tongue. [Indian name.]

agropyrum (ag·ro·**pi**·rum). Couch grass; the dried rhizome of *Agropyron repens* Beauvois. It is used for making a decoction that has a demulcent diuretic action. [Gk *agros* field, *pyr* fire.]

Agrostemma githago (ag·ro·**stem**·ah gith·**a**·go). The corn cockle, the seeds of which contain toxic saponins and cause the disease githagism. It is a weed which is common in cornfields in Europe and in Asia. [Gk *agros* field, *stemma* wreath, L *gith* coriander.]

agrypnetic (a·grip·**net**·ik). 1. Of agrypnotic tendency (causing wakefulness). 2. Wakeful, sleepless. [see foll.]

agrypnia (a·**grip**·ne·ah). Insomnia. **Agrypnia excitata.** Insomnia associated with restlessness, confusion or mental excitability. **Agrypnia pertaesa.** Sleeplessness due to physical disease. **Agrypnia senilis.** Insomnia of old age. [Gk *agrypnos* sleepless.]

agrypnocoma (a·**grip**·no·**ko**′·mah). A state of coma in which wakefulness is a feature; sometimes the condition is one of extreme lethargy, marked by delirious muttering and lack of sleep. [Gk *agrypnos* sleepless, coma.]

agrypnode (a·**grip**·node). A drug or stimulus which induces wakefulness. [Gk *agrypnos* sleepless.]

agrypnotic (a·grip·**not**·ik). 1. An agrypnode. 2. Having the power to induce wakefulness. [see prec.]

ague (**a**·gew). A term originally used for a chill or fever, but in more modern times restricted to the initial fever or relapses of malaria, especially that encountered in the fen districts of East Anglia, and today rarely used in medical literature though it persists colloquially. It is also applied to localized painful symptoms, e.g. face ague, and to any attack of shaking or shivering. **Aden ague.** Aden fever; sandfly or dengue fever. *See* FEVER. **Brassfounder's ague.** Metal-fume fever. *See* FEVER. **Brow ague.** Neuralgia of the forehead. **Ague cake.** An old term used to designate the enlarged hard spleen of chronic malaria. **Catenating ague.** A complex fever. **Face ague.** Trigeminal neuralgia. *See* NEURALGIA. **Ague fit.** A colloquial expression for a malaria-like attack with shivering followed by fever. **Quartan ague.** The paroxysms, caused by *Plasmodium malariae*, recurring every fourth day, that is at 72 h intervals, in quartan malaria. **Quotidian ague.** A daily fever, found in association with double infections of subtertian malaria, and more rarely with benign tertian. **Shaking ague.** An acute attack of fever, with pronounced shivering. **Spelter-workers' ague.** Metal-fume fever. *See* FEVER. **Tertian ague.** A fever occurring every 3rd day, which was the commonest form of indigenous malaria in England, the benign tertian form. **Zinc-smelters' ague.** Metal-fume fever. *See* FEVER. [Fr. *aigu* sharp.]

agyiophobia (aj·e·o·**fo**'·be·ah). Fear of streets; reluctance to cross the road. [Gk *agyia* street, *phobein* to fear.]

agyria (a·**ji**·re·ah). Congenital absence of gyri or convolutions of the cerebral cortex. [Gk *a*, gyrus.]

Ahlfeld, Friedrich (b. 1843). Marburg obstetrician.

Ahlfeld's method. For measurement of the fetal head with a pelvimeter: one arm is placed against the child's head and the other on the fundus uteri.

Ahlfeld's sign. Irregular contractions of the uterus after the first trimester of pregnancy.

ahypnia, ahypnosis (a·**hip**·ne·ah, a·hip·**no**·sis). Absolute insomnia; the term implies sleeplessness of a morbid mental character. [Gk *a*, *hypnos* sleep.]

aichmophobia (ike·mo·**fo**·be·ah). A fear of sharp-pointed objects which amounts to an obsession. [Gk *aichme* spearpoint, phobia.]

aidoitis (a·do·**i**'·tis). Vulvitis. [Gk *aidoion* vulva, *-itis* inflammation.]

aidoiomania (a·**doy**·o·**ma**'·ne·ah). Morbid increase in sex drive. [Gk *aidoion* vulva, mania.]

Ailanthus glandulosa (a·**lan**·thus glan·dew·**lo**·sa). The tree of heaven (family Simarubaceae). The leaves are used as a substitute for belladonna leaf. [Moluccan *ai lanit*, tree of heaven, L *glandulosus* glandulous.]

ailurophilia (a·lewr·o·**fil**'·e·ah). Excessive fondness for cats. [Gk *ailouros* cat, *philein* to love.]

ailurophobia (a·lewr·o·**fo**'·be·ah). Fear of cats exaggerated to a morbid degree; aelurophobia. [Gk *ailouros* cat, phobia.]

ailuropsis (a·lewr·**op**'·sis). Obliquity of the palpebral fissure or of the eyes; aeluropsis. [Gk *ailouros* cat, *opsis* appearance.]

ainhum (**ine**·hum). The African name for the trophic condition, symptomless and usually painless, in which a linear depression develops at the digitoplantar fold of, usually, the 5th toe, and gradually progresses until the toe falls off. It is confined to the black races, particularly to the males, in the tropics. [Yoruba (Nigeria) name.]

Ainsworth's punch. An instrument used for punching a hole in a rubber dam, used in conservative dentistry.

air (a·er). 1. The old name for a gas, e.g. *inflammable air* (hydrogen). 2. The mixture of gases constituting the earth's atmosphere. At sea-level the average composition by volume is 78.08 per cent nitrogen, 20.95 per cent oxygen, 0.93 per cent argon, 0.03 per cent carbon dioxide, 0.0018 per cent neon, 0.0005 per cent helium, 0.0001 per cent krypton and 0.00001 per cent xenon. Normally there is in addition water vapour, with varying amounts of hydrocarbons, ammonia, oxides of sulphur and nitrogen, organic matter (spores, etc.) and inorganic matter (dust). Air exerts a pressure at sea-level and at 0°C and latitude 45° of 101.325 kPa (14.72 lb/in^2), equivalent to a column of mercury 760 mm (29.92 in) high, and has a density of 0.081 lb/ft^3. It is the oxygen of the air that renders respiration possible, the nitrogen and other gases merely acting as a diluent. **Alveolar air.** The air in contact with the pulmonary capillaries. **Arterial alveolar air.** Alveolar air in equilibrium with arterial blood. **Complemental air.** The volume of air that can be drawn into the lungs over and above that of normal tidal inspiration. **Compressed air.** Air compressed to a pressure of several atmospheres; it is used to operate tools. **Dead-space air.** The volume of air (usually 100–150 ml) which fills the upper respiratory passages and air tubes, and which is last to enter at inspiration. **Functional residual air.** Residual air plus supplemental air (see below). **Inspired air.** The general atmosphere which is breathed. **Liquid air.** Air liquefied by pressure; on evaporation it causes a very great lowering of temperature (-190°C). **Pendulum air.** The air which passes from lung to lung when there is spontaneous breathing with an open pneumothorax; it is the result of internal paradoxical respiration. **Reserve air.** Supplemental air (see below). **Residual air.** The air remaining in the lungs at the end of a maximal expiratory effort. **Supplemental air.** The volume of air which can be expelled by maximal effort after completion of a normal expiration. **Tidal air.** The air normally drawn in at a breath. **Venous alveolar air.** Alveolar air in equilibrium with the mixed venous blood of the pulmonary artery. [Gk *aer*].

airbrasive (a·er·**bra**·siv). A mixture of sand and aluminium oxide projected under pressure to remove decayed tooth substance and thereby save the use of a burr. [air, abrasive.]

airway (a·er·way). 1. The passage from the outer air to the alveolar space of the lungs, i.e. nose or mouth, pharynx, larynx, trachea, bronchi and bronchioles. 2. A rubber or metal tube employed in anaesthesia which passes through either nose or mouth and ensures a free passage of air or gases to the pharynx. **Nasopharyngeal airway.** An artificial airway passed from the nose into the hypopharynx and used in anaesthesia. **Oropharyngeal airway.** A curved breathing tube which passes from the mouth to the hypopharynx, used in unconscious patients to maintain a free airway. **Pharyngeal airway.** A curved breathing tube passed from the mouth into the pharynx to prevent airway obstruction. [air, AS *weg*.]

ajacine (aj·a·seen). $C_{34}H_{46}O_9N_2$. An alkaloid obtained from larkspur, *Delphinium ajacis*.

ajaconine (aj·**ak**·o·neen). $C_{21}H_{31}O_3N$. An alkaloid obtained from larkspur, *Delphinium ajacis*.

ajellomyces (a·jel·o·**mi**'·seez). Ajellomyces dermatitidis, the ascomycetous (sexual) state of *Blastomyces dermatitidis*, the causative organism of blastomycosis.

akanthocytosis (ak·**an**·tho·si·**to**'·sis). Erythrocytosis involving akanthocytes. [akanthocyte, Gk *-osis* condition.]

akaryocyte (a·**kar**·e·o·site). A non-nucleated cell, e.g. an erythrocyte. [Gk *a*, karyocyte.]

akaryota, akaryote (a·kar·e·**o**'·tah, a·**kar**·e·ote). A cell without a nucleus; a non-nucleated cell. [Gk *a*, *karyon* nucleus.]

akathisia (ak·ath·**iz**·e·ah). A form of restlessness in which the subject is unable to remain seated for any length of time. It is a not uncommon symptom of Parkinson's disease. [Gk *a*, *kathizein* to sit.]

akembe (ak·**em**·be). Onyalai. [African word.]

akeratosis (a·ker·at·**o**'·sis). Imperfection or lack of horny tissue. [Gk *a*, *keras* horn, *-osis* condition.]

Åkerlund, Ake Olof (b. 1887). Stockholm radiologist.

Åkerlund deformity. A deformity of the duodenal cap, due to ulcer. A niche is present on one surface, and an incisura on the other.

Aker-tuba (**ah**·ker·tu'·bah). Derris BPC 1949.

akidogalvanocautery (ak·id·o·gal·van·o·**kaw**'·ter·e). The process of cauterizing with a needle electrode. [Gk *akis* needle, galvanocautery.]

akidopeirastic (ak·id·o·pi·**ras**'·tik). Relating to or characterized by puncture with a needle as an exploratory procedure. [Gk *akis* needle, *peirastikos* testing.]

akidopeirastica (ak·id·o·pi·**ras**'·tik·ah). Puncture or incision as an exploratory measure. [see prec.]

akinaesthesia (a·kin·es·**the**'·ze·ah). Lack or loss of muscular sense; loss of the sense of perception of moving and movement. [Gk *a*, kinesis, aesthesia.]

akinesia, akinesis (a·kin·e·se·ah, a·kin·e·sis). 1. Paralysis of the motor nerves. 2. Loss of facility of movement, whether voluntary or automatic, without actual paralysis, as in Parkinson's disease. 3. Temporary muscular paralysis as a result of injection of a local anaesthetic solution. **Akinesia algera.** A neurotic condition characterized by voluntary refraining on the part of the patient from movement which he thinks will cause pain; the condition may also occur in cases of organic muscular defect or disease. **Akinesia amnestica.** Loss of motor function through disuse of muscles. **Cerebral akinesis.** Motor paralysis caused by a lesion in the cerebrum. **Crossed akinesia.** Loss of the power of movement on the side opposite to that on which there is a lesion. **Akinesis iridis.** Rigidity of the iris. **Reflex akinesia.** Weakness or loss of reflex action. **Spinal akinesis.** Motor paralysis caused by a lesion of the spinal cord. [Gk *a*, kinesis.]

akinetic (a·kin·et·ik). 1. An agent which lessens muscular power. 2. Affected with or relating to akinesia. 3. Amitotic. [see prec.]

Akis (a·kis). A genus of tenebrionid beetles. **Akis spinosa.** A secondary host of the tapeworm *Hymenolepis diminuta.* [Gk a point.]

akiyami (ak·e·yah·me). Nanukayami, a fever of short duration marked by enlargement of the lymph glands, pain and dyspepsia. It occurs in Japan, usually in the autumn, and is believed to be caused by *Leptospira hebdomadis* transmitted by the bites of field rodents. [Japanese.]

aknephascopia (ak·nef·as·ko′·pe·ah). Defective vision in twilight or in inadequate artificial lighting; twilight blindness. [Gk *a*, *knephas* twilight, *skopein* to watch.]

akrencephalon (ak·ren·kef·al·on). Telencephalon; the anterior portion of the forebrain, from which are developed the cerebral hemispheres, the lateral ventricles, the anterior parts of the 3rd ventricle and hypothalamus and the interventricular foramen. [Gk *akros* extreme, encephalon.]

akromikrie (ak·ro·mik·re). A disease the characteristic signs of which are thirst, less than normal growth, thin hands and feet, alopecia, acrocyanosis and amenorrhoea. [Gk *akros* extreme, *mikros* small.]

ala [NA] (a·lah) (pl. *alae*). A wing, or a process expanded like a wing. **Ala auris.** The auricle, or pinna of the external ear. **Ala of the central lobule [ala lobuli centralis (NA)].** The lateral extensions of the central lobule on to the cerebellar hemispheres. **Ala of the crista galli [ala cristae galli (NA)].** *See* CRISTA GALLI. **Ala of the ilium [ala ossis ilii (NA)].** The wing-like expansion of the ilium. **Ala of the nose [ala nasi (NA)].** The wing of the nostril, the lateral part of the external nose supported by cartilage. **Ala sacralis, Ala of the sacrum.** The upper end of the lateral mass on either side of the first sacral vertebra. **Ala temporalis.** Greater wing of the sphenoid bone. *See* WING. **Ala of the vomer [ala vomeris (NA)].** Either of the lateral eversions of the superior border of the vomer where it articulates with the body of the sphenoid bone. [L.]

alabaster (al·ab·as·ter). A white gypsum, $CaSO_4{\cdot}2H_2O$, of particularly fine and compact grain, and used ornamentally. [Gk *alabastos* alabaster box.]

alabastrine (al·ab·as·treen). 1. Pertaining to alabaster. 2. A name for naphthalene.

alalia (al·a·le·ah). 1. Impairment of speech, or lack of the power to speak, because of loss of control or defect of the muscles of articulation or other parts of the vocal organs. 2. Aphasia resulting from a psychosis. **Alalia cophica.** Deaf-mutism. **Logographic alalia.** Inability to express thoughts in written words. **Mental alalia.** Inability to speak because of an extreme degree of stammering—a condition found in children. **Alalia organica.** Alalia caused by an organic disease. **Alalia physiologica.** Deaf-mutism. **Alalia prolongata.** Delay in speaking. **Relative alalia.** Mental alalia (see above). [Gk *a*, *lalein* to babble like a child.]

alalic (a·lal·ik). Resembling, affected with or relating to alalia.

alangine (al·an·jeen). $C_{19}H_{25}O_2N$. An alkaloid derived from the bark of *Alangium lamarckii,* and used as an antipyretic and emetic.

Alangium lamarckii (al·an·je·um lam·ar·ke·i). A plant native to Indonesia, the root of which may be used for emetic, antipyretic and diuretic purposes.

alanine (al·an·een). CH_3CHNH_2COOH, 2-aminopropionic acid. An amino acid which is a common constituent of proteins; produced as a major product of nitrogen metabolism in peripheral tissues, it is utilized as a gluconeogenic source by the liver.

Alanson, Edward (b. 1747). Liverpool surgeon.

Alanson's amputation. A circular amputation to give a conical stump.

alant camphor (al·ant kam·for). Helenin; a constituent of elecampane, the root of *Inula helenium.* [G *Alant* elecampane.]

alantic (al·an·tik). Relating to elecampane, *Inula helenium.* **Alantic anhydride.** $C_{15}H_{20}O_2$, a terpene extracted from the roots of elecampane, and given in the treatment of bronchitis. [see prec.]

alantin (al·an·tin). Alant starch, inulin, $(C_6H_{10}O_5)_x$. A complex carbohydrate built of fructofuranose units, and found in the roots and rhizomes of elecampane, *Inula helenium,* and other plants; used as a culture medium in bacteriology. [G *Alant* elecampane.]

alanyl (al·an·il). The monovalent radical $CH_3CH(NH_2)CO-$, derived from alanine; it enters largely into the building of synthetic polypeptides.

alar (a·lar). 1. Having alae or wings; relating to wings; wing-like. 2. Relating to the axilla or the shoulder. [L *ala* wing.]

alare (a·lar·e) (pl. *alaria*). An anthropometric point; the external border of an ala of the nose. [see prec.]

alastrim (al·as·trim). Variola minor; a mild form of smallpox. The virus is slightly different in having a lower maximum growth temperature, although antigenetically identical with the major form. The disease carries a low case-mortality ($<$ 1 per cent) and may be confused with chickenpox. [Port. *alastrar* to spread.]

alastrimic, alastrinic (al·as·trim·ik, al·as·trin·ik). Relating to alastrim.

alate (a·late). Having wings. [L *ala* wing.]

alatus (a·la·tus). 1. An individual whose shoulder blades project markedly backward. 2. Having wings. [see prec.]

albaras, albarras (al·bar·as). An old term that probably included both leucoderma and the depigmented lesions of leprosy. [Ar.]

Albarran, y Dominguez, Joaquin (b. 1860). Cuban urogenital surgeon in Paris.

Albarran's disease. *Bacterium coli* bacilluria.

Albarran's gland. The part of the median lobe of the prostate that lies immediately under the uvula of the bladder.

Albarran's test. For renal inadequacy; a simple physical and clinical test of renal function, known as the *polyuria test.* The night urine is normally more concentrated than the day urine; in renal inadequacy this difference may disappear. Accordingly the night urine is collected at 10 p.m., in the morning at 5 a.m., followed by a light breakfast with 600 ml of water. The urine is then collected hourly for a number of hours. The specimens may be analysed for urea, freezing point, etc., but simple determination of volume and specific gravity is satisfactory.

Albarran's tubules. A small group of prostatic glands opening into the posterior aspect of the upper part of the prostatic urethra.

albaspidin (al·bas·pid·in). A substance obtained from the male fern, *Dryopteris filix-mas,* and used as a remedy for worms, particularly for taeniae. [L *albus* white, aspidium.]

albedo (al·be·do). 1. A whiteness. 2. In a special case of a reflection coefficient, e.g. for neutrons entering a medium across a boundary, the albedo is the number of particles that leave the medium after diffusion divided by the number entering the medium. **Albedo retinae.** Oedema of the retina. **Albedo unguis, Albedo unguium.** The lunula of a nail. [L *albus* white.]

Albee, Fred Houdlett (b. 1876). New York surgeon.

Albee's operation. Fusion of the spine by insertion of a tibial graft into a split in the vertebral spinous processes.

Albee's saw. An electrically-driven saw with a circular blade, or double blade, rotating on a central spindle, for cutting bone-grafts.

Albee-Delbet operation. An operation for fractured femoral neck; the fracture is fixed to a bone graft driven up a hole drilled in the neck of the femur.

Albers-Schoenberg, Heinrich Ernst (b. 1865). Hamburg radiologist.

Albers-Schoenberg disease, or marble bone. Osteopetrosis; a dystrophy of bone associated with apparent increased density and obliteration of the distinction between cortex and medulla.

Albert, Eduard (b. 1841). Vienna surgeon.

Albert's disease. Achillobursitis.

Albert's operation. A method of arthrodesis of the knee.

Albert, Henry (b. 1878). Iowa City physician.

Albert's stain. For *Corynebacterium diphtheriae*: the cells are stained with a mixture of toluidine blue and methyl green and, after washing, treated with a solution of iodine in potassium iodide. The cells stain green and the metachromatic granules bluish-black.

Albert's position. The semi-recumbent position used to x-ray the pelvic brim.

Albertini, Ippolito Francisco (b. 1662). Bologna physician.

Albertini's treatment. Bed rest, and abstinence from food, once advised as treatment for aortic aneurysm. (Although rest is still important, more effective additional treatment is now available.)

albescent (al·**bes**·ent). Moderately white; becoming whitish. [L *albescere* to grow white.]

albiduria (al·bid·**ewr**·e·ah). 1. The secretion and passing of white or pale urine. 2. Chyluria. [L *albidus* whitish, urine.]

albine (**al**·been). A phosphorus compound found in egg-yolk. [L *albus* white.]

Albini, Giuseppe (b. 1830). Italian physiologist.

Albini's nodules. Small nodules on the edges of auriculoventricular valves of infants; not pathological.

albinic (al·**bin**·ik). Affected with or relating to albinism.

albinism (**al**·bin·izm). 1. The condition of being an albino; characterized by the absence of pigment in the skin, hair, eyes or feathers. 2. Congenital leucoderma, either partial or total. **Acquired albinism.** Vitiligo. **Localized albinism.** Naevus anaemicus. **Piebald albinism.** An inherited type of partial albinism. [L *albus* white.]

albinismus (al·bin·**iz**·mus). Albinism. **Albinismus acquisita.** Vitiligo. **Albinismus universalis.** Total albinism; nystagmus and astigmatism as well as photophobia can usually be demonstrated in this state.

albino (al·**be**·no). 1. An individual, who may belong to any race, in whom there is a marked deficiency of pigment in eyes, hair and skin. 2. A Mexican octoroon. 3. In zoology, an animal in which there is abnormal deficiency of colouring matter in the skin of part or of the whole of the body. 4. In botany, a plant in which the pigment cells remain colourless. [Port. from L *albus* white.]

albinoidism (al·**be**·noid·izm). Incomplete albinism, usually dominant, sometimes recessive. The skin and hair are slightly darker than in total albinism. The eyes may appear normal, apart from photophobia. [albino, Gk *eidos* form.]

albinoism (al·**be**·no·izm). Albinism.

albinotic (al·bin·**ot**·ik). 1. Marked by albinism. 2. Relating to albinos.

albinuria (al·bin·**ewr**·e·ah). Albiduria. [L *albus* white, urine.]

Albinus, Bernhard Siegfried (b. 1697). Leyden anatomist.

Albinus' muscle. 1. A triangular-shaped muscle passing from the side of the nose to the nasolabial furrow; also known as the *musculus anomalus of Albinus.* 2. Scalenus minimus muscle; also known as *scalenus pleuralis of Sibson.*

Albl's ring. The calcified shadow of an intracranial aneurysm.

albocinereous (al·bo·sin·**eer**′·e·us). Neural tissue consisting of or containing both white and grey matter. [L *albus* white, *cinereus* grey.]

albomycin (al·bo·**mi**·sin). An antibiotic obtained from a species of *Actinomyces.* It is very active against staphylococci, including the strains that are resistant to other antibiotics; it is of great value in pneumonia, especially in young children, and in septic complications of many conditions such as measles and dysentery. It was originally developed in the USSR. [L *albus* white, Gk *mykes* fungus.]

Albrecht, Karl Martin Paul (b. 1851). Brussels anatomist.

Albrecht's bone. An unpaired ossicle found between the basisphenoid and basi-occipital in abnormal skulls.

Albright, Fuller (b. 1900). Boston physician.

Albright's disease. Polyosteotic fibrous dysplasia with pigmentation of the skin and, in the female, precocious puberty.

Albright's syndrome. A syndrome occurring mainly in females, consisting of polyosteotic fibrous dysplasia with pigmental areas overlying the bone lesions and sometimes associated with precocious puberty and hypothyroidism.

albugineotomy (al·bew·jin·e·**ot**′·o·me). Incision into the tunica albuginea of the testis; one of the ways in which pressure is relieved in chronic orchitis. [tunica albuginea, Gk *temnein* to cut.]

albugineous (al·bew·**jin**·e·us). Like or relating to the white of the eye; referring to the tunica albuginea.

albuginitis (al·bew·jin·**i**′·tis). An inflammatory condition of the tunica albuginea of the testis or of any other similar structure elsewhere. [tunica albuginea, Gk *-itis* inflammation.]

albugo (al·**bew**·go). 1. Any white spot, especially one causing corneal opacity; leucoma. 2. Eruption of greyish-white scaly type on the skin. [L whiteness.]

albukalin (al·bew·**ka**·lin). $C_8H_{16}N_2O_6$, a substance that occurs in the blood in leukaemia.

albumen (al·**bew**·men). 1. Obsolescent name for protein and for albumin. 2. Protein-rich material of egg white or of vegetable seeds. [L *albus* white.]

albumimeter (al·bew·**mim**·et·er). Albuminimeter.

albumin (al·**bew**·min). One of a class of simple proteins, soluble in water and dilute salt solutions and coagulable by heating, occurring widely in animals and plants. Albumins may be distinguished from globulins by their non-precipitation from solutions saturated with magnesium or sodium sulphate or half-saturated with ammonium sulphate. In animals the more important albumins are serum albumin in blood, lactalbumin in milk, ovalbumin in egg white and myo-albumin in muscle, whilst typical vegetable albumins are legumelin in the seeds of leguminous plants, and leucosin in the seeds of wheat, barley and rye. **Acid albumin.** Acid metaprotein. A substance formed by the action of dilute acids on albumin: on neutralization *denatured albumin* is precipitated. **Dried Human Albumin BP 1973.** A cream-coloured powder prepared by freeze-drying Human Albumin BP 1973 of protein concentration not exceeding 10 per cent w/v. **Human Albumin BP 1973.** A solution of human albumin in water. **Albumin tannate.** An insoluble brown powder prepared from albumin and tannic acid; it is used in diarrhoea. [L *albus* white.]

albuminaemia (al·bew·min·**e**′·me·ah). The existence of albumin in the blood in quantity in excess of the normal amount (3.4–6.7 g per 100 ml). [albumin, Gk *haima* blood.]

albuminate (al·**bew**·min·ate). A salt-like derivative of albumin, in which the protein forms the anion, e.g. sodium albuminate.

albuminaturia (al·**bew**·min·at·**ewr**′·e·ah). The presence in the urine of an unusually large quantity of albuminates. [albuminate, urine.]

albuminid (al·**bew**·min·id). 1. Obsolete name for the proteins of connective tissues, e.g. collagen, elastin. 2. Albuminoid. [albumin, Gk *eidos* form.]

albuminiferous (al·**bew**·min·**if**′·er·us). Yielding or producing albumin. [albumin, L *ferre* to bear.]

albuminimeter (al·**bew**·min·**im**′·et·er). An instrument with which can be determined the quantity of albumin present in a fluid. [albumin, meter.]

albuminimetry (al·**bew**·min·**im**′·et·re). Determination of the quantity of albumin present in a fluid. [see prec.]

albuminiparous (al·**bew**·min·**ip**′·ar·us). Albuminiferous. [albumin, L *parere* to produce.]

albuminocholia (al·**bew**·min·o·**ko**′·le·ah). The presence in the bile of albumin or similar protein. [albumin, Gk *chole* bile.]

albuminogenous (al·**bew**·min·**oj**′·en·us). Albumin-producing. [albumin, Gk *genein* to produce.]

albuminoid (al·**bew**·min·oid). 1. Possessing similar properties to those of albumin; related to albumin. 2. The term applied to the scleroproteins which resemble albumin, but are insoluble and much more stable; they form the skeletal and connective tissue of animals, and constitute hair, horns and claws. [albumin, Gk *eidos* form.]

albuminolysin (al·bew·min·ol'·is·in). A lysin which splits albumins. [albumin, Gk *lysis* a loosing.]

albuminolysis (al·bew·min·ol'·is·is). The breaking-down of albumins and the splitting of them into various simple constituents; proteolysis. [see prec.]

albuminometer (al·bew·min·om'·et·er). Albuminimeter.

albuminometry (al·bew·min·om'·et·re). Albuminimetry.

albuminone (al·bew·min·one). A constituent of certain albuminoids that is soluble in alcohol, and uncoagulable by heat.

albuminoptysis (al·bew·min·op'·tis·is). A condition of the sputum in which albumin is present. [albumin, Gk *ptyein* to spit.]

albumino-reaction (al·bew·min·o·re·ak'·shun). *See* LESIEUR-PRIVEY TEST.

albuminorrhoea (al·bew·min·or·e'·ah). The discharge of an abnormally large quantity of albumin. [albumin, Gk *rhoia* flow.]

albuminose (al·bew·min·oze). Albumose.

albuminosis (al·bew·min·o'·sis). An abnormally excessive amount of albumin in the blood; the morbid condition which is the result of such excess. [albumin, Gk *-osis* condition.]

albuminous (al·bew·min·us). Having the properties of or resemblance to albumin; relating to or charged with albumin.

albuminuretic (al·bew·min·ewr·et'·ik). 1. Inducing or aggravating a condition of albuminuria. 2. Any drug which causes excretion of albumin in the urine. [albumin, Gk *ouretikos* diuretic.]

albuminuria (al·bew·min·ewr'·e·ah). The presence of serum albumin and serum globulin in the urine. It may be due to functional causes, or to renal disease. **Accidental albuminuria.** Adventitious albuminuria (see below). **Acetone albuminuria.** Anoxaemic albuminuria (see below). **Albuminuria of adolescence.** Cyclic albuminuria (see below). **Adventitious albuminuria.** The variety which is not due to disease of the kidneys. **Alimentary albuminuria.** That which occurs after a meal rich in proteins has been taken. **Anoxaemic albuminuria.** That which is caused by asphyxiation. **Athletic albuminuria.** A functional variety which occurs in athletes or those who have been engaging in hard exercise. **Cardiac albuminuria.** A type caused by disease of the valves of the heart. **Cicatricial albuminuria.** The type in which it is believed that the tissue which has replaced lost epithelium is incapable of preventing the seepage of albumin from the blood. **Colliquative albuminuria, Consumptive albuminuria.** A form in which the albuminuria attendant on a disease is slight at first, but during convalescence suddenly and noticeably increases. **Cyclic albuminuria.** A form in which a small quantity of albumin is found in the urine at only certain times during the day; it is not connected with renal disease. **Dietetic albuminuria, Digestive albuminuria.** That caused by the eating of particular foods. **Dystrophic albuminuria.** Albuminuria resulting from faulty formation of the erythrocytes and leucocytes in the blood. **Emulsion albuminuria.** A form in which the urine has a milky appearance. **Essential albuminuria.** A functional form of albuminuria which is not connected with disease of the kidneys. **Exudative albuminuria.** That which is due partly to the presence in the urine of the products of an inflammatory condition, and partly to albumin seeping through the renal membrane. **False albuminuria.** Adventitious albuminuria (see above). **Febrile albuminuria.** That caused by a condition of pyrexia, or associated with acute infective disease. **Functional albuminuria.** Any form of albuminuria which is not caused by disease of the kidneys. **Globular albuminuria.** A form caused by blood in the urine, or by the destruction of erythrocytes. **Gouty albuminuria.** The albuminuria of old age, in which an excessive quantity of urea is also excreted. **Haematogenous albuminuria, Haemic albuminuria.** A form which occurs during the course of any disease producing changes in the blood proteins. **Hypostatic albuminuria.** A form of postural albuminuria which is present only when the patient is supine. **Intermittent albuminuria.** Cyclic albuminuria (see above). **Intrinsic albuminuria.** True albuminuria (see below). **Lordotic albuminuria.** A form of orthostatic albuminuria caused by lordosis of the spine. **Mixed albuminuria.** Concurrent true and adventitious albuminuria. **Nephrogenous albuminuria.** Albuminuria which is the result of disease of the kidneys. **Neurotic albuminuria.** That form which is associated with neuroses and psychoses. **Orthostatic albuminuria, Orthotic albuminuria.** Albuminuria which is present when the patient is ambulatory but which disappears when he is at rest in bed. **Palpatory albuminuria.** A temporary manifestation of albuminuria which is caused by bimanual palpation of the kidneys. **Paroxysmal albuminuria.** Cyclic albuminuria (see above). **Partial albuminuria.** A type in which only certain of the renal tubules appear to be involved. **Physiological albuminuria.** The fortuitous occurrence of albuminuria when there is an absence of any condition of disease. **Postrenal albuminuria.** Albuminuria which has its origin at some point in the urinary system other than the renal tubules. **Postural albuminuria.** Orthostatic albuminuria (see above). **Prerenal albuminuria.** A type which is caused primarily by disease of an organ other than the kidney. **Pretuberculous albuminuria.** A variety which is found in incipient pulmonary tuberculosis. **Recurrent albuminuria.** Cyclic albuminuria (see above). **Regulatory albuminuria.** A temporary condition in which albumin is discharged in the urine after violent exertion or muscular work. **Renal albuminuria.** Albuminuria caused by disease of the kidneys. **Residual albuminuria.** The continued appearance of albumin in the urine after an attack of acute nephritis has cleared. **Serous albuminuria.** True albuminuria (see below). **Transient albuminuria.** Cyclic albuminuria (see above). **True albuminuria.** A form in which certain albuminous constituents of the blood are discharged during the excretion of urine.

See also: BAMBERGER (H.), BENCE-JONES.

albuminuric (al·bew·min·ewr'·ik). Related to, associated with, or characterized by albuminuria.

albuminurophobia (al·bew·min·ewr·o·fo'·be·ah). Undue fear of the significance of an albumin reaction in the urine. Particular fear of acquiring albuminuria. [albuminuria, phobia.]

albumoid (al·bew·moid). Albuminoid.

albumone (al·bew·mone). Albuminone.

albumosaemia (al·bew·mo·se'·me·ah). The presence in the blood of albumose. [albumose, Gk *haima* blood.]

albumoscope (al·bew·mo·skope). An instrument by which the presence in the urine of albumin can be detected and the amount determined. [albumin, Gk *skopein* to watch.]

albumose (al·bew·mose). A non-coagulable intermediate formed during the pepsin digestion of protein, also by the hydrolysis of syntonins and albuminates.

See also: BENCE-JONES.

albumosuria (al·bew·mo·sewr'·e·ah). A condition in which albumoses are present in the urine. **Enterogenic albumosuria.** That due to decomposition in the intestine. **Haematogenic albumosuria.** Albumosuria caused by toxic substances in the blood. **Myelopathic albumosuria.** Bence-Jones proteinuria. **Pyogenic albumosuria.** That caused during certain diseases by absorption of pus or of exudates.

See also: BENCE-JONES, BRADSHAW.

albutannin (al·bew·tan·in). Albumin tannate.

Alcaligenes (al·kal·ij·en·eez). A bacterial genus of the family Achromobacteriaceae. They are Gram-negative, usually motile, do not produce acid or gas from carbohydrates, and turn litmus milk alkaline. They are of doubtful pathogenicity. **Alcaligenes abortus.** *Brucella abortus.* **Alcaligenes bronchisepticus.** *Brucella bronchisepticus.* **Alcaligenes faecalis.** A motile Gram-negative organism, resembling *Bacterium coli* except that no sugars are fermented nor is indole formed. It occurs in the intestinal canal of normal people, more commonly in diarrhoea. **Alcaligenes melitensis.** *Brucella melitensis.* **Alcaligenes viscosus.** An organism similar to *Alcaligenes faecalis* in appearance; it produces "ropiness" in milk and is found in water and around dairies. [alkali, Gk *genein* to produce.]

alcaptonuria (al·kap·ton·ewr'·e·ah). Alkaptonuria.

alcarsin (al·kar·sin). Alkarsin.

alchemist (al·kem·ist). One who practised alchemy.

alchemy (al·kem·e). The chemistry of the middle ages; it was mainly confined to the search for a means of converting the baser metals into gold. [Ar. *al* the, Gk *Chemia* Egypt.]

Alclofenac (al·klo·fen·ak). BP Commission approved name for 4-allyloxy-3-chlorophenylacetic acid; an analgesic.

Alcock, Thomas (b. 1784). London surgeon.

Alcock's canal. The pudendal canal. *See* CANAL.

alcogel (al·ko·jel). A gel in which alcohol is the liquid medium.

Alcohol (al·ko·hol). 1. The official (BP 1973) preparation of ethyl alcohol or ethanol, containing 95 per cent ethyl alcohol and 5 per cent water. 2. A series of derivatives of hydrocarbons containing 1 or more hydroxyl OH groups, and known accordingly as mono-, di- or poly-hydroxy alcohols. They are saturated or unsaturated, depending upon the nature of the parent hydrocarbon, and are classified primary, secondary or tertiary alcohols in accordance with the nature of the group containing the hydroxyl, these latter being, respectively, $-CH_2OH$, $=CHOH$, and $\equiv COH$. They are more active than hydrocarbons, forming alkyl salts or esters with acids, and alcoholates with the alkali metals. **Absolute alcohol.** Ethyl alcohol containing not more than 1 per cent weight of water. **Acetophenone alcohol.** Phenacyl alcohol, benzoyl carbinol, $C_6H_5COCH_2OH$, a white crystalline aromatic alcohol. **Acid alcohol.** Ethyl alcohol containing a small percentage of hydrochloric acid. **Allyl alcohol.** Propenol, $CH_2=CHCH_2OH$, a colourless liquid with a pungent smell used in chemical warfare and, in dilute solution, as a disinfectant. **Amyl alcohol, Amylic alcohol.** $CH_3(CH_2)_4OH$, an alcohol occurring in a mixture of isomeric alcohols prepared from fusel oil, and used as a solvent in industry; the tertiary, dimethyl ethyl carbinol, $(CH_3)_2C_2H_5\equiv COH$, is a hypnotic more powerful than paraldehyde. **Anisyl alcohol.** *p*-Methoxybenzyl alcohol, $CH_3OC_6H_4CH_2OH$, a pungent substance used in the manufacture of perfumes. **Arachyl alcohol.** Eicosyl alcohol, $C_{20}H_{41}OH$, a colourless substance found in palm wax. **Aromatic alcohol.** 1. An aromatic compound with an alcoholic OH radical substituted in a side chain. 2. An aliphatic alcohol with an aromatic ring substituted for a hydrogen atom in the hydrocarbon chain. **Batyl alcohol.** $C_{18}H_{37}O C_3H_5(OH)_2$, a glyceryl ether found in shark-liver oil. **Benzyl Alcohol BP 1973.** Phenylmethyl alcohol, $C_6H_5CH_2OH$, a colourless liquid with aromatic odour, occurring in Peru and Tolu balsams; used in perfumery, and as a local anaesthetic and anodyne. **Bornyl alcohol.** Camphyl alcohol (see below). **Butyl alcohol.** A normal butyl alcohol, $CH_3(CH_2)_2CH_2OH$, is obtained during the fermentation of maize, and is used as a solvent. **Camphyl alcohol.** Borneol, Borneo camphor, $C_{10}H_{18}O$, a terpene alcohol occurring in oil of Siberian fir, the camphor of *Dryobalanops officinalis* and certain essential oils. It is used as a stimulant and antiseptic. **Carnaubyl alcohol.** $CH_3(CH_2)_{23}OH$, an alcohol that occurs in carnauba wax and lanolin. **Caustic alcohol.** Sodium ethoxide, C_2H_5ONa, used in organic synthesis. **Ceryl alcohol.** Cerotin, $CH_3(CH_2)_{25}OH$, an alcohol that occurs as an ester in Chinese wax. **Cetostearyl Alcohol BP 1973.** A mixture of solid aliphatic alcohols, principally stearyl and cetyl. It is used as an ingredient of the emulsifying wax employed in the manufacture of non-greasy creams and ointments. **Cetyl alcohol.** Cetol, aethal, ethal, $CH_3(CH_2)_{15}OH$, an alcohol that occurs as a cetic ester in spermaceti; used in ointments for the treatment of eczema and pruritus, and as a base for cosmetics. **Chlorethyl alcohol.** CH_2ClCH_2OH, a derivative of ethyl alcohol. **Cinnamic alcohol, Cinnamyl alcohol, Cinnamylic alcohol.** Styryl alcohol, $C_6H_5(CH)_2CH_2OH$, found as a cinnamate, styracin, in styrax, and in certain other balsams; used as a deodorant and antiseptic. **Coniferyl alcohol.** $C_6H_3(OH)(OCH_3)CH=CHCH_2OH$, white crystals obtained from the glucoside, coniferin. **Dehydrated Alcohol BP 1973.** Absolute alcohol (see above). **Denatured alcohol.** Ethyl alcohol used for industrial purposes, to which substances have been added to render it unfit for human consumption. **Deodorized alcohol.** Ethyl alcohol which has been freed of contaminating odorous impurities. **Di-acid alcohol, Diatomic alcohol, Dibasic alcohol, Dihydric alcohol, Dihydroxy alcohol.** An alcohol which contains 2 hydroxyl OH groups. **Dilute Alcohols BP 1973.** To be used in pharmacy, are prepared by diluting alcohol 95 per cent with water to the desired proportion. **Eicosyl alcohol.** Arachyl alcohol (see above). **Ethyl alcohol.** Ethanol, spirit of wine, ethyl hydroxide, C_2H_5OH, obtained by the fermentation of starches and sugars, as in wine making; it also occurs in coal tar, bone oil and wood spirit. It is a colourless liquid which mixes with water or ether, and is used as a solvent and reagent in industry. Medicinally it is of value as a general anaesthetic and, by injection, in the treatment of neuralgia; also administered as a stimulant, and applied locally as an antiseptic and astringent. **Fatty alcohol.** An alcohol of the aliphatic series. **Glyceryl alcohol.** Glycerol, glycerin, $CH_2OH CHOHCH_2OH$, a trihydroxy alcohol obtained as a by-product in the manufacture of soap. It is a thick, colourless liquid, with a sweet taste, hygroscopic and soluble in water; used as a sweetening agent and emollient, and, in suppositories, to relieve constipation. **Glycide alcohol.** $CH_2OHC_2H_3O$, a cyclic alcohol prepared by dehydrating glycerol; it combines with HCl to give chlorhydrin, and yields esters known as *glucides*. **Heptyl alcohol.** The alcohol $C_7H_{15}OH$. The isomeric alcohol is formed in the catalytic production of methyl alcohol. **Hexabasic alcohol, Hexacid alcohol, Hexahydric alcohol, Hexahydroxy alcohol, Hexatomic alcohol.** An alcohol which contains 6 hydroxyl OH groups; the hexoses are the corresponding aldehydes and ketones. **Iso-alcohol.** 1. An alcohol which is an isomer of a normal alcohol. 2. An alcohol derived from a hydrocarbon containing a branched chain of carbon atoms. **Iso-amyl alcohol.** $(CH_3)_2CHCH_2CH_2OH$, an alcohol that forms the largest proportion of the fusel oil of sugar fermentation; it is optically inactive. **Isopropyl Alcohol BP 1973.** Secondary propyl alcohol, dimethylcarbinol, $CH_3CH(OH)CH_3$, a petroleum by-product, used as a solvent and denaturant, and in perfume manufacture; also as a surgical antiseptic. **Ketone alcohol.** Ketol, an alcohol which contains, in addition to its hydroxyl group, the ketone group, CO. **Lauryl alcohol.** $C_{12}H_{25}OH$, an alcohol obtained by the hydrolysis and subsequent hydrogenation of coconut oil. **Melissyl alcohol.** $CH_3(CH_2)_{29}OH$, an alcohol that occurs as a palmitic ester in beeswax and carnauba wax. **Methoxybenzyl alcohol.** Anisyl alcohol (see above). **Methyl alcohol.** Methanol, carbinol, wood alcohol, CH_3OH, prepared commercially by the destructive distillation of wood, or by catalysis from carbon monoxide and hydrogen (water-gas). It is used as a solvent to denature ethyl alcohol, and as a fuel. **Monacid alcohol, Monatomic alcohol, Monobasic alcohol, Monohydric alcohol, Monohydroxy alcohol.** An alcohol which contains only 1 hydroxyl OH group. **Myricyl alcohol.** Melissyl alcohol (see above). **Nicotinyl Alcohol.** BP Commission approved name for 3-pyridyl-methanol. It is used as a vasodilator in peripheral vascular diseases. **Octadecyl alcohol.** Stearyl alcohol (see below). **Oleyl alcohol.** Obtained by the hydrolysis of olein and subsequent hydrogenation; it is a mixture of higher alcohols, principally $C_{18}H_{35}OH$, which, when sulphonated, yields a detergent used in industry and domestically as a soapless cleanser. **Pantothenyl alcohol.** An alcohol with an action similar to that of pantothenic acid; it is used in the treatment of paralytic ileus. **Phenacyl Alcohol BPC 1973.** Acetophenone alcohol (see above). **Phenethyl Alcohol.** BP Commission approved name for 2-phenylethanol; an antiseptic. **Phenylethyl alcohol.** Benzyl carbinol, $C_6H_5CH_2CH_2OH$, an alcohol that occurs in the oils of rose and geranium; used in perfumery. **Phenylmethyl alcohol.** Benzyl alcohol (see above). **Phytyl alcohol.** Phytol, $CH_3[(CH_3)CH(CH_2)_3]_3CCH_3=CHCH_2OH$, an ester in chlorophyll; it is the precursor of the carotenoids and a unit in the composition of vitamin K. **Polyacid alcohol, Polyatomic alcohol, Polybasic alcohol, Polyhydric alcohol, Polyhydroxy alcohol.** An alcohol containing several hydroxyl OH groups. **Polyvinyl alcohol.** $(CH_2=CHOH)_2$, a substance obtained by the polymerization of vinyl acetate and subsequent hydrolysis. It is used in the manufacture of size, and in the production of polyvinyl resins. **Primary alcohol.** An alcohol containing the primary alcohol group, $-CH_2OH$; oxidation yields an acid. **Propargyl alcohol,**

Propinyl alcohol. $CH{\equiv}CCH_2OH$, a liquid with a pleasant smell which is an alcohol related to acetylene; it yields both esters and metallic compounds. **Propyl alcohol.** Propanol, normal propyl alcohol, $CH_3CH_2CH_2OH$, obtained from fusel oil; a colourless liquid similar in properties to ethyl alcohol. **Pyroligneous alcohol.** Methyl alcohol (see above). **Pyroracemic alcohol.** Acetyl carbinol. **Saccharide alcohol.** One formed by the reduction of the aldehyde or ketone group of a simple sugar. **Salicyl alcohol, Salicylic alcohol, Salicylyl alcohol.** Saligenin, $C_6H_4(OH)CH_2OH$, an alcohol obtained by the acid or enzymic hydrolysis of salicin. **Secondary alcohol.** An alcohol containing the secondary alcohol group, =CHOH; oxidation yields a ketone. **Sorbic alcohol.** 2,4-Hexadienol, $CH_3CH{=}CHCHCH_2OH$; an amber-coloured semisolid, once used in the treatment of burns, but now employed to isolate anhidrotic areas of skin and to assess intensity of sweating after administration of drugs, etc. **Stearyl alcohol.** Octadecyl alcohol, $CH_3(CH_2)_{17}OH$, prepared by hydrogenation of stearic acid; used in ointments. **Styryl alcohol.** Cinnamic alcohol (see above). **Sugar alcohol.** A polyhydric alcohol obtained by the reduction of the aldehyde or ketone group of a monosaccharide; mannitol is an example. **Sulphonated alcohols.** Name given to a mixture of sulphonated higher aliphatic alcohols obtained from natural fats and oils; used as detergents, wetting agents and cleansers, and as the basis of domestic soapless preparations. **Tertiary alcohol.** An alcohol containing the tertiary alcohol group, ≡COH; oxidation disrupts the carbon chain. **Thujyl alcohol.** $(CH_3)_2CHC_6H_7OHCH_3$, a derivative of the terpene, sabinene, found in wormwood, *Artemisia absinthium*. **Triacid alcohol, Triatomic alcohol, Tribasic alcohol, Trihydric alcohol, Trihydroxy alcohol.** An alcohol which contains 3 hydroxyl OH groups. **Tribromoethyl Alcohol BP 1953.** Bromethol, tribromoethanol, CBr_3CH_2OH; dissolved in amyl alcohol, it is used as a basal anaesthetic and in twilight sleep, also to control convulsive states such as tetanus. **Trichlorobutyl alcohol.** Chlorbutol, $(CH_3)_2C(CCl_3)OH$, a local anaesthetic and antiseptic; used as a hypnotic, being less toxic than chloral hydrate. **Unsaturated alcohol.** An alcohol derived from an unsaturated hydrocarbon. **Vinyl alcohol.** Ethenol, $CH_2{=}CHOH$, an unsaturated alcohol which is unstable, only derivatives being known. **Wood alcohol.** Methyl alcohol (see above). **Wool Alcohols BP 1973.** *See* WOOL. [Ar. *alkohl* essence.]

See also: RANVIER.

alcoholaemia (al·ko·hol·**e**'·me·ah). The presence of alcohol in the blood. [alcohol, Gk *haima* blood.]

alcoholase (al·ko·hol·aze). A zymase, or fermenting enzyme, which converts monosaccharides into alcohol.

alcoholate (al·ko·hol·ate). 1. Any preparation made up with alcohol. 2. A compound of an alcohol in which the hydrogen of the hydroxyl group is replaced by a metal or base; an ethoxide.

alcoholature (al·ko·**hol**·at·ewr). A tincture made with alcohol as solvent.

alcoholia lanae (al·ko·**hol**·e·ah **lan**·e). Wool Alcohols BP 1973. *See* WOOL. [alcohol, L *lana* wool.]

alcoholic (al·ko·**hol**·ik). 1. A person who is dependent on alcohol and shows personality and behavioural changes as a result. 2. Relating to alcohol or its qualities; caused by, containing or derived from alcohol.

alcoholica (al·ko·**hol**·ik·ah). A term used in pharmacy for preparations containing alcohol.

alcoholism (al·ko·hol·izm). Poisoning and disease caused by taking alcoholic drinks to excess. **Acute alcoholism.** Drunkenness; transient disorder caused by excess of alcoholic drinks. **Chronic alcoholism.** A physical degeneration of body-tissues, especially the liver (fatty change or cirrhosis), the heart (cardiomyopathy) and central nervous system (Korsakoff's disease), or peripheral nerves (neuritis and degeneration) due to prolonged drinking of alcoholic fluids.

alcoholist (al·ko·hol·ist). The term usually reserved for an individual who is accustomed to take large quantities of alcohol regularly and does not show any sign of inebriation—the so-called "sober alcoholist".

alcoholization (al·ko·hol·i·**za**'·shun). Treatment by the use of alcohol as an application or as an injection.

alcoholomania (al·ko·hol·o·**ma**'·ne·ah). A morbid craving for alcohol. [alcohol, mania.]

alcoholometer (al·ko·hol·**om**'·et·er). In chemistry, an instrument with which the proportion of alcohol in any preparation or substance, or the percentage of pure alcohol in spirits, may be determined. [alcohol, meter.]

alcoholometry (al·ko·hol·**om**'·et·re). The estimation of the alcohol content of a liquid. [see prec.]

alcoholophilia (al·ko·hol·o·**fil**'·e·ah). Pathological craving for alcoholic drinks or intoxicants. [alcohol, Gk *philein* to love.]

alcoholuria (al·ko·hol·**ewr**'·e·ah). The presence of alcohol in voided urine.

alcoholysis (al·ko·**hol**·is·is). The breaking-up of an ester or other compound by alcohol, an action comparable with hydrolysis. [alcohol, Gk *lysis* a loosing.]

alcolene (al·ko·leen). A mixture of ethyl and methyl alcohols.

alcometrical (al·ko·**met**·rik·al). Concerned with the measurement of the alcohol contained in a liquid. [alcohol, meter.]

alcosol (al·ko·sol). A colloidal solution in which alcohol is the liquid phase. [alcohol, sol.]

Alcuronium Chloride (al·kew·**ro**·ne·um **klor**·ide). BP Commission approved name for diallyldinortoxiferin dichloride; a muscle relaxant, used as an adjuvant in anaesthesia.

aldactone (al·dac·ton). A spironolactone that leads to a fall in blood pressure and a rise in plasma potassium in cases of aldosteronism.

aldamine (al·dam·een). A certain type of stable oxidase.

aldebaranium (al·de·bar·**a**'·ne·um). Name given to a rare earth element, proved subsequently to be identical with thulium. [Aldebaran, name of a star.]

aldehydase (al·de·**hi**·daze). An oxidase occurring in the liver, which converts aldehydes into acids.

aldehyde (al·de·hide). 1. Acetic aldehyde (see below). 2. A series of compounds obtained by the oxidation of the primary alcohols, the $-CH_2OH$ group becoming $-CHO$ characteristic of the aldehydes; further oxidation converts them into the corresponding acids. They are both oxidizing and reducing agents, and combine with themselves or other compounds to produce either condensation or addition products. **Acetic aldehyde.** Acetaldehyde, acetyl hydrate, CH_3CHO, one that occurs in the first runnings in the distillation of spirits; also prepared by the oxidation of ethyl alcohol. A colourless liquid, producing irritation when inhaled; used in catarrh and ozaena, also as an anaesthetic and antiseptic. **Acrylic aldehyde.** Acrolein, $CH_2{=}CHCHO$, a pungent liquid prepared from glycerol, with an irritant effect on the eyes, and used in chemical warfare. **Aldehyde alcoholate.** An additive product formed from acetaldehyde and ethyl alcohol. **Aldehyde ammonia.** 1. $(CH_3CHONH_3)_3$ an addition compound formed by acetaldehyde with ammonia gas. 2. One of the series of compounds formed by the different aldehydes with ammonia. **Amyl aldehyde, Amylic aldehyde.** Valeric aldehyde (see below). **Anisic aldehyde.** Anisaldehyde, $CH_3OC_6H_4CHO$, found in oil of anise, fennel oil and vanilla; also prepared from anisole. It is used in perfume manufacture. **Aromatic aldehyde.** An aldehyde obtained by the oxidation of an aromatic alcohol. **Benzoic aldehyde.** Benzaldehyde, oil of bitter almonds, C_6H_5CHO, obtained by hydrolysing amygdalin, the glucoside in bitter almonds. It is a colourless oil with characteristic odour, used in perfumery, and in the manufacture of drugs and dyestuffs. **Butyl aldehyde.** Butaldehyde, butyraldehyde, $CH_3CH_2CH_2CHO$, an aldehyde formed by the hydrogenation of croton aldehyde, or from normal butyl alcohol; used in the manufacture of rubber. **Cinnamic aldehyde.** Cinnamaldehyde, $C_6H_5CH{=}CHCHO$, the main constituent of cinnamon oil from *Cinnamonum zeylanicum*; a flavouring, and useful medicinally as an inhalant. **Croton aldehyde.** $CH_3CH{=}CHCHO$, produced by the polymerization of acetaldehyde and dehydration of the aldol so formed; a solvent for waxes and resins. **Cumic aldehyde.** $(CH_3)_2CHC_6H_4CHO$, an aldehyde contained in cumin oil from *Cuminum cyminum*; used as a stimulant and sedative. **Formic aldehyde.** Formaldehyde, methanol, HCHO, prepared by the oxidation of methyl alcohol. A colourless gas, soluble in water, alcohol or ether; a strong antiseptic and disinfectant, used to preserve specimens and to sterilize instruments. It is applied in skin and throat affections, and is the basis of certain plastics. **Glyceric aldehyde.** Glyceraldehyde, glycerose, $CH_2OHCHOHCHO$, a synthetic triose which polymerizes to form a hexose similar to fructose. It plays a part in the sugar metabolism. **Glycollic aldehyde.** CH_2OHCHO, a very simple monosaccharide, diose, formed from tartaric acid in ripening grapes. **Glyoxylic aldehyde.** Glyoxal, CHOCHO, a dialdehyde prepared by the oxidation of ethyl alcohol or acetaldehyde. **Heptyl aldehyde.** Heptaldehyde, oenanthal, $CH_3(CH_2)_5CHO$, an aldehyde obtained by distilling castor oil; used in organic synthesis. **Isobutyl aldehyde.** $(CH_3)_2CHCHO$, a highly refracting liquid. **Isovaleric aldehyde.** $(CH_3)_2CH$ CH_2CHO, an aldehyde prepared from fusel oil; it has a smell of apples. **Keto-aldehyde.** An aldehyde formed by the reduction of a keto-acid; contains both the keto =CO group and the aldehyde -CHO group. **Palmitic aldehyde.** $C_{15}H_{31}CHO$, the aldehyde corresponding to palmitic acid. **Phenyl aldehyde.** Benzoic aldehyde (see above). **Propiolic aldehyde.** $CH{\equiv}CCHO$, a derivative of propargyl alcohol and related to acetylene; a liquid with an intensely irritant odour. **Pyroracemic aldehyde, Pyruvic aldehyde.** Acetyl formyl, methyl glyoxal, CH_3COCHO, an aldehyde derived from the corresponding aldoxime. **Salicylic aldehyde.** A hydroxybenzaldehyde, $C_6H_4(OH)CHO$, extracted from the glucoside salicin, obtained from willow bark; used as an astringent and in perfumery. **Thio-aldehyde.** A compound containing the group -CHS, which is an aldehyde group with the oxygen replaced by sulphur. **Tiglic aldehyde.** $CH_3CH{=}C(CH_3)$ CHO, an unsaturated aldehyde derived from croton oil. **Toluic aldehyde.** $C_6H_5CH_2CHO$, a substance isomeric with methylbenzaldehyde, and prepared directly from toluene. **Trichloracetic aldehyde.** Chloral, CCl_3CHO, produced by the action of chlorine on ethyl alcohol; a pungent oily liquid, forming a crystalline hydrate which is used as a hypnotic and antiseptic. **Valeric aldehyde.** Valeraldehyde, amyl aldehyde, $CH_3(CH_2)_2CHO$, an aldehyde obtained from normal valeric acid. **Vanillic aldehyde.** Vanillin. [abbv. for *al*cohol, *dehyd*rogenatum deprived of hydrogen.]

alder (awl·der). Correctly, a tree or shrub of the genus *Alnus*, though the name is also applied to other plants. **Alder buckthorn bark.** *See* FRANGULA. **Black alder.** *Alnus glutinosa*, the bark of which has astringent properties. [AS *alor*.]

aldin (al·din). One of a series of organic compounds with basic properties, produced from aldehydes by the action of ammonia.

aldohexose (al·do·hex·oze). One of the isomeric hexoses, CH_2OH $(CHOH)_4CHO$, which display reducing properties by virtue of the aldehyde group, -CHO, at the end of the chain of carbon atoms; glucose is an exammle.

aldol (al·dol). $CH_3CHOHCH_2CHO$, a condensation of 2 molecules of acetaldehyde; used as a hypnotic and sedative. **Aldol condensation.** The combination of 2 aldehyde molecules in the presence of catalysts to form a hydroxyaldehyde.

aldolase (al·do·laze). An enzyme of glycolysis. Muscle and most other tissues contain *aldolase A*, whose primary function is to cleave fructose 1,6-diphosphate with the production of triose phosphates. *Aldolase B* in liver also catalyses fructose 1,6-diphosphate cleavage, but in addition acts on fructose 1-phosphate with production of dihydroxyacetonephosphate and glyceraldehyde.

aldopentose (al·do·pen·toze). One of the isomeric pentoses, $CH_2OH(CHOH)_3CHO$, which display reducing properties by virtue of the aldehyde group, -CHO, at the end of the chain of carbon atoms; arabinose is an example.

aldose (al·doze). General term applied to monosaccharides which possess an aldehyde group, -CHO, at the end of their chain of carbon atoms. Cf. KETOSE.

aldoside (al·do·side). Any glycoside formed by the union of an aldose with an alcohol, phenol or other compound containing an OH group.

Aldosterone (al·do·steer'·one). BP Commission approved name for 11β,21-dihydroxy-3, 20-dioxopregn-4-en-18-al, a compound which has been isolated from extracts of the adrenal gland. It has sodium-retaining properties when administered to patients with Addison's disease, and is at least 10 times as active as deoxycortone acetate. It is administered intramuscularly in oil, being effective in 2 h and lasting 8 h. Unlike cortisone, it has not corrected the abnormality in water excretion in Addison's disease, and it has only 1/100 its activity in carbohydrate effects. It affords a substitution therapy in Addison's disease as regards metabolism of electrolytes.

aldosteronism (al·do·steer'·on·izm). A syndrome characterized by excessive amounts of the salt-retaining corticoid, aldosterone, in the blood and urine, a disturbance of sodium-potassium metabolism, alkalosis and deficient absorption of water in the renal tubules produced by a cortico-adrenal tumour. Clinically, there is intermittent tetany, severe muscular weakness occasionally amounting to paralysis, polyuria, and polydipsia, hypertension, but not usually oedema.

aldosteronoma (al·do·steer·on·o'·mah). A tumour secreting aldosterone. [aldosterone, Gk *-oma* tumour.]

aldosteronopenia (al·do·steer·on·o·pe'·ne·ah). A deficiency of aldosterone. [aldosterone, Gk *penes* poor.]

aldosteronuria (al·do·steer·on·ewr'·e·ah). The presence of excessive aldosterone in the urine. [aldosterone, Gk *ouron* urine.]

aldotetrose (al·do·tet·roze). One of the isomeric tetroses, CH_2OH $(CHOH)_2CHO$, which display reducing properties by virtue of the aldehyde group, -CHO, at the end of the chain of carbon atoms; erythrose is an example.

aldoxime (al·dox·ime). A condensation of an aldehyde with hydroxylamine in which the bivalent group =NOH replaces the oxygen of the aldehyde group; they form salts with metal hydroxides, and also with mineral acids.

Aldrich, Charles Anderson (b. 1888). Rochester, Minnesota, paediatrician.

McClure-Aldrich test. A biological test for the rate of absorption of fluid from the skin. An 0.8 per cent solution of sodium chloride is injected into the skin. The rate of disappearance of the resulting weal is noted.

Aldrich, Martha. 20th century Rochester, Minnesota, physician.

Hench-Aldrich salivary urea index, or test. A measure of the salivary urea obtained by titrating saliva with 5 per cent mercuric chloride solution. The index is the number of millilitres of the latter solution required by 100 ml saliva, and normally lies between 30 and 50.

Aldrich, Robert Henry (b. 1902). Boston surgeon.

Aldrich's mixture. A 1 per cent solution of gentian violet for the treatment of burns.

Aldridge, Albert Herman (b. 1893). New York gynaecologist.

Aldridge's operation. 1. A method of treatment for stress incontinence of urine, wherein a fascial sling for the bladder neck is fashioned from the abdominal aponeurosis. 2. An operation for reversible sterilization: the fimbriated ends of the fallopian tubes are buried in the broad ligaments.

aldrin (al·drin). One of the more toxic insecticides of the chlorinated hydrocarbon type. There is evidence to show that it causes pathological changes in certain organs, and hence it should be used with care on foodstuffs.

ale (ale). A fermented liquor made from malt and flavoured with hops; a beer containing roughly 5 per cent of alcohol. [AS *alu*.]

alecithal (a·les·ith·al). In biology, a term used to describe eggs which do not have any food yolk in the protoplasm, or very little of it. [Gk *a*, *lekithos* yolk.]

alegar (a·leg·ar). Malt vinegar; vinegar which has been made from sour ale. [ale, Fr. *aigre* sour.]

aleipsis (al·ipe·sis). A general increase of fatty tissue; fatty degeneration. Steatosis. [Gk *aleiphein* to anoint.]

alembic (al·**em**·bik). An obsolete form of still, or more particularly the inverted cup-shaped removable head which served the function now performed by a condenser. [Ar. *al* the, *ambig* cup.]
alembroth (al·**em**·broth). An antiseptic dressing, composed of mercury and ammonium chlorides; $(NH_4Cl)_2HgCl_2{\cdot}2H_2O$.
alemmal (a·**lem**·al). Of a nerve fibre, one that does not have a neurolemma. [Gk *a*, *lemma* sheath.]
alethia (a·**le**·the·ah). Lacking the power to forget. [Gk *a*, *lethe* forgetfulness.]
Aletris (**al**·et·ris). In botany, a genus of bitter-rooted liliaceous plants. **Aletris farinosa.** The colic root of North America, from which diuretic, tonic and anthelmintic preparations are made. [Gk corn-grinder.]
aleucaemia (a·lew·**se**·me·ah). Aleukaemia.
aleucaemic (a·lew·**se**·mik). Aleukaemic.
aleucaemoid (a·lew·**se**·moid). Aleukaemoid.
aleucia (a·**lew**·se·ah). Aleukia.
aleucocytic (a·**lew**·ko·**sit**'·ik). Not having any leucocytes. [Gk *a*, leucocyte.]
aleucocytosis (a·lew·ko·si·**to**'·sis). A condition of the blood in which the proportion of leucocytes to other cells is abnormally small. [Gk *a*, leucocytosis.]
aleukaemia (a·lew·**ke**·me·ah). Aleukaemic leukaemia; an acute blood disease in which there is a low or diminished total white-cell count in the peripheral blood due to gross impairment of bone-marrow function. Its aetiology is unknown; it is sometimes thought to be a special type of acute leukaemia, but is really only an earlier aleukaemic phase of acute leukaemia. [Gk *a*, leukaemia.]
aleukaemic (a·lew·**ke**·mik). 1. Having the characteristics of aleukaemia. 2. Not marked by or associated with leukaemia. [see prec.]
aleukaemoid (a·lew·**ke**·moid). Having resemblance to aleukaemia. [aleukaemia, Gk *eidos* form.]
aleukia (a·**lew**·ke·ah). A condition of the blood in which there are no leucocytes. **Aleukia haemorrhagica.** Aplastic anaemia. *See* ANAEMIA. [Gk *a*, *leukos* white.]
aleukocytic (a·**lew**·ko·**sit**'·ik). Aleucocytic.
aleukocytosis (a·lew·ko·si·**to**'·sis). Aleucocytosis.
aleuriospore (al·**ewr**·e·o·spor). A terminal or lateral spore attached by a wide base to the conidiophore and detached by fracture of the wall below the spore. [Gk *aleuron* flour, *sporos* seed.]
Aleurisma (al·ew·**riz**·mah). *Paracoccidioides.* [Gk *aleuron* flour.]
aleuron, aleurone (**al**·ewr·on, al·ewr·**one**). The collective term applied to minute grains of protein, which probably contain vitamins, found in the seeds of many plants. [Gk *aleuron* flour.]
aleuronoid (al·**ewr**·on·oid). Of the nature of flour, or having the appearance of flour. [Gk *aleuron* flour, *eidos* form.]
Alexander, William (b. 1844). Liverpool surgeon.

Alexander's incision. An incision above and parallel with the left inguinal ligament.

Alexander-Adams operation. Extraperitoneal shortening of the round ligaments for the correction of uterine retroversion. The ligaments are shortened by dividing them in their course through the inguinal canal, pulling on the proximal ends and then securing them to the external oblique aponeurosis.

Alexander test. *Haemophilus influenzae* antibody test. *See* TEST.
Alexanderism (al·ex·**ahn**·der·izm). A form of insanity in which the patient is obsessed by the idea that he is a conqueror of the calibre of Alexander the Great.
alexeteric (al·**ex**·e·**ter**'·ik). Antidotal to and prophylactic against poisoning and infection. [Gk *alexeter* defender.]
alexia (a·**lex**·e·ah). 1. Lack of ability, because of a disease of the brain, to understand printed or written words, although they are visible. 2. Lack of ability, because of disease of the brain, to read aloud. **Cortical alexia.** A variety of sensory aphasia which is caused by lesions of the left angular gyrus. **Literal alexia.** Inability to recognize letters. **Motor alexia.** Inability to read aloud written or printed matter although the content is understood. **Musical alexia.** Music blindness; inability to read musical notation. **Optical alexia, Sensory alexia.** Inability to understand what is seen to be written or printed. **Subcortical alexia.** A variety caused by disrupted connection between the angular gyrus and the optical centre. **Verbal alexia.** Inability to recognize words although isolated letters are identified. **Visual alexia.** Optical alexia (see above). [Gk *a*, *lexis* speech.]
alexin (al·**ex**·in). Synonym for complement (q.v.). [Gk *alexein* to ward off.]
alexipharmac (al·ex·e·**far**·mak). 1. Antidotal. 2. A counter-poison; a remedy for or an antidote to poisonous substances. The terms are no longer in common usage. [Gk *alexein* to ward off, *pharmakon* poison.]
alexipharmacon (al·ex·e·**far**·mak·on). An antidotal medicine; a term now obsolete. [see prec.]
alexipyretic (al·ex·e·pi·**ret**'·ik). 1. An agent which prevents the occurrence of fevers; febrifuge. 2. Descriptive of such remedies. [Gk *alexein* to ward off, *pyretos* fever.]
alexofixagen, alexofixagin, alexofixogen (al·ex·o·**fix**·aj·en, al·ex·o·**fix**·aj·in, al·ex·o·**fix**·o·jen). An antigen, which stimulates *in vivo* the production of complement-fixing antibodies in the serum. [alexin, fixation, Gk *genein* to produce.]
alexofixin (al·ex·o·**fix**·in). The complement-fixing antibody resulting from the injection of alexofixagen.
Alezzandrini, Arturo Alberto (b. 1932). Argentine ophthalmologist.

Alezzandrini's syndrome. Unilateral impairment of vision from degenerative retinitis followed by facial vitiligo and poliosis on the same side, inclusive of the brows and eyelashes. Bilateral perceptive deafness may also develop.

Alfalfa (al·**fal**·fah). Lucerne. [Sp.]
Algae (**al**·je). A class of lower unicellular or multicellular plants which contain chlorophyll and reproduce cryptogamically, often with motile gametes. There are several orders: the Red (Rhodophyceae) and the Brown (Phaeophyceae) are marine seaweeds; the Green (Chlorophyceae) are often microscopic, and occur also in fresh water and on land. [L *alga* seaweed.]
algaesthesia, algaesthesis (al·jes·**the**·ze·ah, al·jes·**the**·sis). 1. The state of being able to perceive pain and to register it accurately among sensory stimuli. 2. Experience of painful sensation. [Gk *algos* pain, aesthesia.]
algal (**al**·gal). Relating or belonging to algae, or caused by algae.
alganaesthesia (**al**·gan·es·**the**'·ze·ah). Analgesia. [Gk *algos* pain, anaesthesia.]
algedonic (al·je·**don**·ik). Relating to or characterized by sensations or emotions of pain and of pleasure. [Gk *algos* pain, *hedone* pleasure.]
algefacient (al·je·**fa**·shent). 1. Tending to make colder. 2. An agent which has a cooling effect. [L *algere* to be cold, *facere* to make.]
algeoscopy (al·je·**os**·ko·pe). 1. The use of pressure in physical examination for the purpose of ascertaining whether or not pain is so produced. [Gk *algos* pain, *skopein* to watch.] 2. Cryoscopy; the determination of the freezing point of a fluid (in medicine, urine, blood, etc.) as compared with that of distilled water. There is depression of the freezing point as the content of solids increases. [L *algere* to be cold, Gk *skopein* to watch.]
algesia (al·**je**·ze·ah). 1. Pain or suffering of any kind. 2. Excessive sensitiveness to painful stimuli. [Gk *algesis* pain.]
algesic (al·**je**·zik). 1. Painful. 2. Affected with or relating to sensitiveness to pain; hyperaesthetic. [see prec.]
algesichronometer (al·je·ze·kro·**nom**'·et·er). An instrument to record the time which elapses between the application of a painful stimulus and the response of the nerve centre. [algesia, chronometer.]
algesimeter (al·je·**zim**·et·er). An instrument for measuring sensitivity to deep or superficial pain. [algesia, meter.]

See also: BJÖRNSTRÖM, BOAS.

algesiogenic (al·**je**·ze·o·**jen**'·ik). Pain-producing. [algesia, Gk *genein* to produce.]

algesiometer (al·je·ze·**om**'·et·er). Algesimeter.
algesis (al·**je**·sis). Algesia.
Algestone Acetonide (**al**·jes·tone as·**e**·ton·ide). BP Commission approved name for 16α,17α-isopropylidenedioxypregna-4-ene-3,20-dione; a progestational steroid.
algetic (al·**jet**·ik). Producing or relating to pain. [Gk *algesis* pain.]
algicide (**al**·jis·ide). Any substance which destroys algae. [L *alga* seaweed, *caedere* to kill.]
algid (**al**·jid). Chilly; cold. [L *algere* to be cold.]
algidism, algidity (**al**·jid·izm, al·**jid**·it·e). Feeling of excessive coldness or chilliness. **Progressive algidism.** Sclerema neonatorum. [see prec.]
algin (**al**·jin). Alginic acid; a compound of units of mannuronic acid linked with glycosides. It occurs in the protein of the brown alga, bladderwrack, *Fucus vesiculosus*, and other seaweeds, and is obtained as a by-product in the extraction of iodine from kelp; used as a textile dressing, and to thicken jellies. The sodium salt is a substitute for tragacanth.
alginate (**al**·jin·ate). Any salt of alginic acid, e.g. sodium alginate.
alginuresis (**al**·jin·ewr·**e**'·sis). Pain on passing urine. [Gk *algos* pain, uresis.]
algioglandular (al·je·o·**glan**'·dew·lar). Relating to glandular activity as a result of application of a painful stimulus. [Gk *algos* pain, glandular.]
algiometabolic (al·je·o·met·ah·**bol**'·ik). Relating to changes in metabolism which occur as a result of painful stimulation. [Gk *algos* pain, metabolism.]
algiomotor, algiomuscular (al·je·o·**mo**'·tor, **al**·je·o·**mus**'·kew·lar). Causing painful spasm of the muscles, also pain on movement; applies to painful peristalsis. [Gk *algos* pain, motor, muscle.]
algiovascular (**al**·je·o·**vas**'·kew·lar). Relating to changes in blood vessels as the result of the stimulus of pain. [Gk *algos* pain, vascular.]
algogenesia, algogenesis (**al**·go·jen·**e**'·ze·ah, al·go·**jen**·es·is). The origin of pain, or the production of it. [Gk *algos* pain, *genein* to produce.]
algogenic (al·go·**jen**·ik). 1. Setting up pain. [Gk *algos* pain, *genein* to produce.] 2. Producing cold or chill, or lowering of the temperature. [L *algor* cold, Gk *genein* to produce.]
ALGOL (al·gol). A computer language.
algolagnia (al·go·**lag**·ne·ah). Sexual perversion in which in intercourse there is an urge, in the case of the male, to inflict pain (active algolagnia; sadism), or in the case of the female, to suffer pain or discomfort (passive algolagnia; masochism). [Gk *algos* pain, *lagneia* lust.]
algomenorrhoea (al·go·men·o·**re**'·ah). Painful menstruation. [Gk *algos* pain, menorrhoea.]
algometer (al·**gom**·et·er). An instrument for measuring the sensitiveness of any particular part to pain by pressure. [Gk *algos* pain, meter.]
algometry (al·**gom**·et·re). The testing of sensitiveness to pain. **Electric algometry.** A method of estimating pain comparatively by induction of a current of electricity. [see prec.]
algophilia, algophily (al·go·**fil**·e·ah, al·**gof**·il·e). 1. Strong urge to suffer pain during sexual intercourse, applicable to one or both partners. 2. Desire to undergo pain inflicted, for example by flagellation, as a sexual stimulant. [Gk *algos* pain, *philein* to love.]
algophobia (al·go·**fo**·be·ah). Excessive horror of witnessing pain or dread of experiencing it. [Gk *algos* pain, phobia.]
algopsychalia (**al**·go·si·**ka**'·le·ah). Psycho-algalia; a melancholic state which on occasion leads to suicide, characterized by distorted visual and auditory sensations and producing fear and hopelessness. [Gk *algos* pain, *psyche* mind.]
algor (**al**·gor). 1. A sensation of chilliness or a rigor occurring during the first stage of a fever. 2. Coldness. **Algor mortis.** The chill of death. [L cold.]
algos (**al**·gos). A painful attack of disease; pain. [Gk pain.]
algoscopy (al·**gos**·ko·pe). Cryoscopy. [L *algere* to be cold, Gk *skopein* to view.]
algosis (al·**go**·sis). A condition in which the body is harbouring algae. *See* PROTOTHECOSIS.
algospasm (**al**·go·spazm). Cramp or spasm of muscles, with acute pain. [Gk *algos* pain, spasm.]
algospastic, algospasticus (al·go·**spas**·tik, al·go·**spas**·tik·us). Having a resemblance or relating to algospasm.
algovascular (al·go·**vas**·kew·lar). Algiovascular.
Alibert, Jean Louis Marc (b. 1768). Paris dermatologist.
Alibert's eburnated carcinoma. Cancer en cuirasse, in which hard plaques are formed in the skin so that the upper part of the trunk may become almost immobile.
Alibert's disease. Mycosis fungoides.
Alibert–Bazin disease. Psoriasis arthropathica.
alible (**al**·ibl). Of value as a food; nourishing. [L *alere* to nourish.]
alices (**al**·is·eez). The red spots which constitute the prodromal rash in smallpox. [L.]
alicyclic (al·e·**si**·klik). Term applied to organic compounds which are aliphatic in character, but composed of rings, or closed chains of carbon atoms, similar to benzene and its derivatives. [aliphatic, cyclic.]
alienatio partis (a·le·en·**a**'·she·o **par**·tis). Gangrene. [L *alienare* to estrange, *pars* part.]
alienation (a·le·en·**a**'·shun). State or quality of being mentally deranged; insanity. [L *alienare* to estrange.]
alienia (a·li·**e**·ne·ah). Absence of the spleen. [Gk *a*, L *lien* spleen.]
alienism (**a**·le·en·izm). 1. The study and the treatment of insanity or mental derangement. [Obsolete term.] 2. Alienation. [L *alienare* to estrange.]
alienist (**a**·le·en·ist). A psychiatrist; a specialist in the treatment of mental diseases. [Obsolete term.] [see prec.]
aliform (**al**·e·form). Wing-shaped. **Aliform process.** Wing of the sphenoid bone. [L *ala* wing, form.]
alignment (al·**ine**·ment). 1. Arranged in a straight line; more specifically, the regular parabolic arches formed by the upper and lower teeth when occupying their normal positions. 2. A display of related protein or nucleic acid sequences so that corresponding amino-acid residues or nucleotide units appear in vertical register. [L *ad*, *linea* kine.]
aliment (**al**·im·ent). Nutrient material; food. [L *alimentum* nourishment.]
alimentary (al·im·**en**·tar·e). Relating or referring to food. [see prec.]
alimentation (**al**·im·en·**ta**'·shun). The process of providing or of taking nourishment. **Artificial alimentation.** The giving, by mechanical or other means, of food or nourishment to individuals who are incapacitated from taking it by mouth. **Forced alimentation.** 1. Forced feeding. 2. The giving to an individual of food beyond the stage at which his appetite is satisfied. **Iodic alimentation.** Providing of food with added iodine. **Rectal alimentation.** The giving of nourishment in concentrated form by means of injection into the rectum. **Voluntary alimentation.** The feeding of persons desiring food but unable for any reason to feed themselves. [L *alimentum* nourishment.]
alimentology (**al**·im·en·**tol**'·o·je). The study of nutrition. [L *alimentum* nourishment, Gk *logos* science.]
alimentotherapy (**al**·im·en·to·**ther**'·ap·e). Treatment by dieting; feeding according to a system of giving nourishment. [L *alimentum* nourishment, therapy.]
Alipamide (al·**ip**·am·ide). BP Commission approved name for *N*-(4-chloro-3-sulphamoylbenzoyl)-*N'*,*N'*-dimethylhydrazine; a diuretic.
aliphatic (al·if·**at**·ik). Fatty; acyclic. Term applied to organic compounds which are constituted of open chains of carbon atoms. Fats and their derivatives are of this type, and have thus given their name to the group. [Gk *aleiphar* oil.]
alipogenetic (a·**lip**·o·jen·**et**'·ik). Not having fat-forming properties. [Gk *a*, lipoid, Gk *genein* to produce.]
alipoidic (a·lip·**oid**·ik). Not containing lipoids. [Gk *a*, lipoid.]
alipotropic (a·lip·o·**trop**'·ik). Not affecting the metabolism of fat. [Gk *a*, *lipos* fat, *trope* a turning.]

aliptic (al·ip·tik). 1. An ointment. 2. Concerned with inunction. 3. Relating to gymnastics or physical culture. [Gk *aleiptos* anointed.]

aliquot (al·e·kwot). A part; a factor. A solid or solution may be divided into a number of equal parts, each part being called an *aliquot*. [L so many.]

alisphenoid (al·e·sfe·noid). 1. In the fetus, that part of the greater wing of the sphenoid bone on the side of the basisphenoid which is preformed in cartilage. 2. Relating to the greater wings of the sphenoid bone. [L *ala* wing, sphenoid.]

Alivisatos, Gerasimus P. (b. 1889). Athens hygienist.

Alivisatos' vaccine. A prophylactic rabies vaccine in which the virus is modified by ether.

alizaramide (al·iz·ar·am·ide). Aminohydroxyanthraquinone, $C_6H_4(CO)_2C_6H_2(NH_2)OH$. A derivative of alizarin, produced by the action of ammonia; brown crystals.

alizarimide (al·iz·ar·im·ide). Imino-anthraquinone, $C_6H_4(CO)_2$ C_6H_2=NH. Formed from alizarin by hot ammonia solution; a violet-red compound.

alizarin (al·iz·ar·in). Dihydroxyanthraquinone, $C_6H_4(CO)_2$ $C_6H_2(OH)_2$. The chief constituent of madder, the ancient dye of the East, in which it occurs as a glucoside, ruberythric acid; now prepared synthetically. A red crystalline compound, insoluble in water, but soluble in alkalis, from which metal hydroxides precipitate insoluble coloured lakes, a property made use of in fast dyeing with mordants; gives rise to a long series of important dyestuffs, many of which are also useful as indicators over different ranges of pH value. **Alizarin X.** Flavopurpurin. [Ar. *al* the, *asara* extract.]

alizarinopurpurin (al·iz·ar·in·o·per′·pewr·in). Trihydroxyanthraquinone, $C_6H_4(CO)_2C_6H(OH)_3$. The particular purpurin that is found associated with alizarin in madder; also prepared synthetically from phthalic anhydride.

alkadiene (al·kah·di·een). An aliphatic hydrocarbon possessing 2 double bonds; allene and diallyl are examples.

alkalaemia (al·kah·le·me·ah). A state in which there is an increase in the hydrogen-ion concentration in the blood without changes in the bicarbonate content of the blood. [alkali, Gk *haima* blood.]

alkalescence (al·kal·es·ens). A condition of slight alkalinity.

alkalescent (al·kal·es·ent). Slightly alkaline; tending towards alkalinity.

alkali (al·kal·i). 1. A caustic substance, like soda-lye or potash, used to saponify fats in soap-making. 2. A basic hydroxide which is soluble in water and neutralizes acids to form salts. 3. A base which dissociates in solution in such a way that there is an excess of hydroxyl OH^- ions over hydrogen H^+ ions. 4. A solution in which the concentration of hydrogen ions is less than 10^{-7} g/l; a solution with a pH value greater than 7. 5. A solution that turns red litmus blue, and appropriately affects other indicators. 6. A solution of a hydroxide of the so-called alkali metals, or of the hypothetical ammonium radical. **Alkali albuminate.** Water-soluble culture medium formed by the action of an alkali on albumin. **Alkali blue.** Sodium triphenylrosaniline sulphonate, a synthetic indicator which changes from blue to red at pH 12–13. **Caustic alkali.** The hydroxide of potassium or sodium. **Alkali disease.** 1. Tularaemia. 2. Selenium poisoning. **Alkali earths.** Lime and baryta, the oxides of calcium and barium respectively. **Fixed alkali.** The alkali hydroxides, except that of ammonium. **Alkali metals.** The family of monovalent elements, lithium, sodium, potassium, rubidium and caesium. **Alkali metaprotein.** A product of protein cleavage dissolved in alkali. **Alkali reserve.** The base held in combination in blood plasma; it is expressed in terms of CO_2 liberated by an acid. **Alkali tolerance test.** *See* TEST. **Volatile alkali.** Ammonium hydroxide or ammonia. [Ar. *al* the, *qaliy* wood ashes.]

alkalify (al·kal·e·fi). To change into an alkali; to make alkaline.

alkaligenous (al·kal·ij·en·us). Producing or yielding an alkali. [alkali, Gk *genein* to produce.]

alkalimeter (al·kal·im·et·er). An instrument by which the strength of an alkali can be determined or the quantity contained in any substance or mixture ascertained. [alkali, Gk *metron* measure.]

alkalimetry (al·kal·im·et·re). The estimation of the alkali content of a substance. [see prec.]

See also: ENGEL.

alkaline (al·kal·ine). Relating to or having the properties of alkalis; reacting as an alkali.

alkalinity (al·kal·in·it·e). The property of being alkaline; the quality of an alkali. **Actual alkalinity.** The amount of hydroxyl ions present. **Total alkalinity.** The total amount of alkali present, both ionized and undissociated.

alkalinization (al·kal·in·i·za′·shun). 1. The process or act of rendering alkaline. 2. The administration of alkalis, or substances such as citrates or tartrates which produce alkalis, by mouth or by injection, for the purpose of counteracting acidity in the stomach, in the urine or in the body generally.

alkalinize (al·kal·in·ize). To make alkaline.

alkalinuria (al·kal·in·ewr′·e·ah). An alkaline condition of recently passed urine.

alkalion (al·kal·i·on). The hydroxyl ion, OH^-, an excess of which confers alkaline properties upon a solution.

alkalipenia (al·kal·i·pe′·ne·ah). A condition marked by a poor alkali reserve in the body. [alkali, Gk *penes* poor.]

alkalitherapy (al·kal·i·ther′·ap·e). Treatment in which alkalis are mainly used, and generally for a specific purpose. [alkali, therapy.]

alkalization (al·kal·i·za′·shun). Alkalinization.

alkalize (al·kal·ize). To make alkaline.

alkalizer (al·kal·i·zer). Any agent which, administered internally, causes general alkalinization of the tissues. It may be either a soluble alkali such as sodium bicarbonate, or a soluble salt such as a citrate, acetate or tartrate which can be oxidized in the body to increase the alkali reserve.

alkalogenic (al·kal·o·jen′·ik). Giving rise to alkalinity; specifically, of the urine. [alkali, Gk *genein* to produce.]

alkaloid (al·kal·oid). Name given to a group of drugs, mostly of plant origin. They are basic organic compounds containing nitrogen, weakly alkaline in solution and forming salts with acids, which salts are soluble in water, the free base being usually soluble only in organic solvents. They all have a characteristically bitter taste, and though most are solids, a few, such as nicotine, are liquids. Morphine and atropine are 2 of the commonest alkaloids used therapeutically. Many of the naturally-occurring alkaloids have been successfully synthesized, and numerous other synthetic compounds can be classified under this heading on chemical grounds. [alkali, Gk *eidos* form.]

alkaloidal (al·kal·oid·al). Having the nature of, or relating to, alkaloids.

alkalosis (al·kal·o·sis). 1. A decrease in the $[H^+]$ of the body tissues. Usually defined as an increase in the pH of the blood above 7.44. 2. An increase in the blood bicarbonate above the normal range. **Acapnial alkalosis, Carbon dioxide alkalosis.** That caused by diminished carbon dioxide in the blood. **Compensated alkalosis.** A condition in which the blood bicarbonate usually is increased, but buffering mechanism keeps the pH within the normal range. **Gaseous alkalosis.** A carbon dioxide deficiency in the blood caused by over-breathing, and remaining uncompensated. **Metabolic alkalosis.** Alkalosis arising from administration of alkalis which combine with H^+ ions or increased elimination of H^+ ions from the gastro-intestinal tract or kidney. $[HCO_3^-]$ is usually elevated. **Respiratory alkalosis.** Alkalosis resulting from excessive elimination of CO_2 from the lungs (e.g. artificial ventilation, hysterical over-breathing). Blood $[HCO_3^-]$ tends to decrease. **Tropical alkalosis.** An alkalosis of small degree which the European tends to exhibit during the hot weather months in a tropical climate. **Uncompensated alkalosis.** A condition in which there is alkalaemia, usually with raised blood bicarbonate. [alkali, Gk *-osis* condition.]

alkalotherapy (al·kal·o·ther′·ap·e). Alkalitherapy.

alkalotic (al·kal·ot·ik). Marked by or relating to alkalosis.

alkaluria (al·kal·**ewr**·e·ah). The passing of alkaline urine.

alkamine (al·kam·een). An amino alcohol; an alcohol containing an NH_2 group, and possessing the properties of both alcohol and amine: an example is ethanolamine, $NH_2CH_2CH_2OH$.

alkane (**al**·kane). The name applied to any hydrocarbon of the methane series, with general formula C_nH_{2n+2}; a paraffin.

alkanet root (**al**·kan·et root). Anchusa BPC 1949. [Ar. *alhinna* henna.]

alkanin (al·**kan**·in). Alkannin.

alkanna (al·**kan**·ah). Anchusa BPC 1949. [Ar. *alhinna* henna.]

alkannin (al·**kan**·in). $C_{16}H_{16}O_5$. A red substance extracted from alkanna, the root of *Anchusa tinctoria*, and soluble in alcohol or acetone; used to stain wood, colour fats and oils, and as an indicator. **Alkannin paper.** A paper impregnated with alkannin, and used to detect acids (red) or alkalis (green). [see prec.]

alkapton, alkaptone (al·**kap**·ton, al·**kap**·tone). Homogentisic acid. *See* ACID. [alkali, Gk *haptein* to possess.]

alkaptonuria (al·**kap**·ton·**ewr**′·e·ah). The excretion of homogentisic acid in the urine. This condition arises from an inborn error in the metabolism of the tyrosine and phenylalanine of the diet which normally progresses by oxidation through homogentisic acid to aceto-acetic acid, and thence to carbon dioxide and water. The urine darkens on standing owing to oxidation of the homogentisic acid to melanins. [alkapton, urine.]

alkargen (al·**kar**·jen). Cacodylic acid, dimethylarsonic acid, $(CH_3)_2AsOOH$. It is prepared from alkarsin. [alkarsin, Gk *genein* to produce.]

alkarsin (al·**kar**·sin). Cadet's fuming liquid, a mixture of cacodyl and cacodyl oxide, produced by the distillation of potassium acetate and arsenious oxide; a brown liquid, intensely poisonous, fuming in air and liable to ignite spontaneously.

alkatriene (al·kah·**tri**·een). Name applied to an aliphatic hydrocarbon which possesses 3 double bonds.

alkein (al·ke·in). Term given to an ether derived from an alkine.

alkene (**al**·keen). Name applied to any hydrocarbon of the ethylene series, with general formula C_nH_{2n}; an olefine.

alkermes (al·**ker**·meez). Kermes. An insect, *Coccus ilicis*, of the family Coccidae, found on the leaves of the kermes-oak, *Quercus coccifera*; the dried bodies furnish a red dye of great antiquity, and at one time were used in medicine. [Ar. *alqirmiz*.]

alkine (**al**·kine). Name applied to any hydrocarbon of the acetylene series, with general formula C_nH_{2n-2}.

alkone (**al**·kone). Name applied to any hydrocarbon of the terpene series, with general formula C_nH_{2n-4}.

alkyl (**al**·kil). The monovalent radical obtained by subtracting 1 hydrogen atom from an aliphatic or aromatic hydrocarbon. Cf. ARYL, ALPHYL.

alkylamine (al·kil·**am**′·een). General term applied to an ammonia base formed by the introduction of 1 or more alkyl radicals into the molecule of ammonia to replace the hydrogen atoms. *See* AMINE.

alkylate (**al**·kil·ate). A compound of an alcohol in which the hydrogen of the hydroxyl group is replaced by a metal or base; an alcoholate.

alkylation (al·kil·a·shun). 1. The process of introducing an alkyl radical into a compound in place of a hydrogen atom. 2. The addition of a side-chain to an aromatic ring.

alkylene (**al**·kil·een). 1. The divalent radical obtained by subtracting 2 hydrogen atoms from an aliphatic hydrocarbon. 2. A hydrocarbon of the ethylene series; an alkene; an olefine.

alkylogen (**al**·kil·o·jen). An alkyl halide, so called from its use as a source of the alkyl radical in organic syntheses. [alkyl, Gk *genein* to produce.]

allachaesthesia, allaesthesia (al·ak·es·**the**′·ze·ah, al·es·**the**·ze·ah). Touch sensation referred to a place distant from the point at which stimulus has been applied, but on the same side of the body. Cf. ALLOCHEIRIA. **Optical allachaesthesia.** Transfer of an image by illusion from its proper quadrant in the visual field to the quadrant in a diagonal line opposite. [Gk *allache* elsewhere, aesthesia.]

allantiasis (al·an·**ti**·as·is). Poisoning caused by sausages harbouring active bacterial toxins. Cf. BOTULISM. [Gk *allas* sausage.]

allantochorion (al·**an**·to·**kor**′·e·on). The single structure formed by fusion of the allantois and the primitive chorion; the true chorion.

allantogenesis (al·**an**·to·**jen**′·es·is). A term which covers the laying-down of the allantois and the subsequent development of it. [allantois, Gk *genein* to produce.]

allantoic (al·an·**to**·ik). Relating to the allantois, or contained in it. **Allantoic circulation.** The circulation passing to the fetus through the umbilical cord and vessels.

allantoid, allantoidal (al·**an**·toid, al·an·**toi**·dal). 1. Relating to or resembling the allantois. 2. Sausage-shaped. [Gk *allantoeides*, sausage-shaped.]

allantoidean (al·an·**toi**·de·an). Describing those vertebrates in the embryo of which a complete allantois develops. [see prec.]

allantoides (al·an·**toi**·deez). 1. Allantoid. 2. The allantois. 3. The big toe. [Gk *allantoeides* sausage-shaped.]

allantoido-angiopagus (al·an·**toi**·do·an·je·**op**′·ag·us). A term referring to enzygotic twins, which show the characteristic linkage formed by the umbilical vessels; omphalo-angiopagus. [allantois, Gk *aggeion* vessel, *pagos* fixed.]

allantoin (al·**an**·to·in). $NH_2CONHCH{=}(CONH)_2$. A diureide of glyoxylic acid, produced by oxidation of uric acid, present in allantoic fluid and in trace amounts in urine. It is used to stimulate epithelialization, especially of chronic suppurating wounds and ulcers.

allantoinuria (al·an·to·in·**ewr**′·e·ah). The excretion in the urine of allantoin.

allantois (al·**an**·to·is). One of the extra-embryonic membranes of amniotes. Typically it has the form of a hollow sac connected with the urinary bladder, lined with epithelium of entodermal origin, and covered with vascular mesoderm. In reptiles and birds it fuses with the chorion and has both a respiratory and excretory function; in most mammals it takes part in the formation of the placenta, and its blood vessels become the umbilical arteries and vein. In man the entodermal part is vestigial, but the mesodermal part, or body stalk, is the basis of the umbilical cord. [Gk *allas* sausage, *eidos* form.]

Allarton, George (fl. 1876). London surgeon.

Allarton's operation. Median lithotomy. *See* LITHOTOMY.

allassotherapy (al·**as**·o·**ther**′·ap·e). Treatment, the principle of which is to effect a change in the general condition or the metabolism of the body. [Gk *allassein* to alter, therapy.]

allaxis (al·**ax**·is). Metamorphosis. [Gk *allassein* to alter.]

allegorization (al·eg·or·i·**za**′·shun). In psychiatry, the process of describing something under the guise of some other thing resembling it in some appropriate way. [Gk *allegorein* to speak of others.]

allele (**al**·eel). Allelomorph.

allelic (al·e·lik). Relating to an allelomorph.

allelism (**al**·e·lizm). Allelomorphism.

allelocatalysis (al·e·lo·kat·**al**′·is·is). The mutual and beneficial effect upon each other's growth exhibited by 2 or more protozoan cells in a drop of nutrient medium. It is most likely due to catalytic stimulation. [Gk *allelon* of one another, catalysis.]

allelocatalytic (al·e·lo·kat·al·**it**′·ik). Causing mutual stimulation of growth; inducing allelocatalysis.

allelomorph (al·**e**·lo·morf). 1. One of a pair of differing but related genes derived from the 2 parents, or one of a pair of mendelian characters resulting from the action of such genes. 2. More generally, one of a group of related genes which can replace one another at a particular locus on a chromosome, or one of a group of inherited characters resulting from the action of such genes. *See also* HETEROALLELES, HOMOALLELES. **Multiple allelomorphs.** A series of genes that are allelomorphs, i.e. occupying the same relative positions on the chromosomes of different individuals. Only 2 of such a series can be present in normal diploid somatic cells. Individual members are changed to others by mutation. [Gk *allelon* of one another, *morphe* form.]

allelomorphism (al·e·lo·**mor**·fizm). The existence or the hereditary transmission of allelomorphic genes or the mendelian characteristics dependent on them. [see prec.]

allelotaxis, allelotaxy (al·e·lo·**tax'**·is, al·e·lo·**tax'**·e). The development of an organ from more than 1 embryonal tissue or structure. [Gk *allelon* of one another, *taxis* arrangement.]

allelotrope (al·e·lo·trope). An isomer that exists in equilibrium with another. [Gk *allelon* of another, *trepein* to turn.]

Allen, Frederick Madison (b. 1879). New York physician.

Allen's paradoxical law. The more sugar taken by a normal person the more is utilized. With diabetics the reverse is the case; the more sugar taken the less is utilized.

Allen's treatment. A dietetic treatment for diabetes, now superseded.

Allen, Willard Myron (b. 1904). St. Louis gynaecologist.

Corner–Allen test. A method of assaying progesterone based on the effects of progesterone on the uterus of the rabbit which has been mated and had the ovaries removed 18 h later. *See also:* MACPHAIL TEST.

Allen's test. For occlusive lesions of the ulnar and/or radial arteries. The patient holds both hands in front of him and opens and closes them rapidly for 15 s to reduce the circulating blood to a minimum; both radial arteries are then rapidly compressed and the patient extends his hands. If the ulnar artery is intact, colour rapidly returns to the hand; if it is occluded the flush is delayed and patchy. The same manoeuvre may be carried out to test the radial artery (compresses the ulnar), and to test the dorsalis pedis and posterior tibial arteries at the ankle.

Allen, tract of. Tractus solitarius.

allene (al·een). Propadiene, $CH_2{=}C{=}CH_2$. A gaseous diolefine which readily forms additive compounds.

allenthesis (al·**en**·the·sis). The introduction of foreign substances by various means into the body. [Gk *allos* other, *enthesis* insertion.]

allergen (al·er·jen). Any substance capable of producing specific hypersensitivity in a suitable animal. **Bacterial allergen.** The factors present in bacteria or bacterial cultures to which certain individuals can become hypersensitive, e.g. tuberculin. **Pollen allergen.** The factors present in various pollens which cause hypersensitivity reactions in certain people; they may sometimes be quite specific and form the basis of diagnostic skin testing for allergic states. [allergy, Gk *genein* to produce.]

allergenic (al·er·**jen**·ik). Referring to a substance giving rise to allergic manifestations in a susceptible person; having the properties and activities of an allergen. [see prec.]

allergia (al·er·je·ah). Allergy.

allergic (al·**er**·jik). Caused by or affected with allergy; relating to or of the nature of allergy; anaphylactic.

allergization (al·er·ji·**za'**·shun). The process of introducing allergens into the body; sensitization.

allergodermia (al·er·go·**der'**·me·ah). A skin disease or affection with an allergic basis. [allergy, Gk *derma* skin.]

allergometry (al·er·**gom**·et·re). Determination, by testing with particular allergens, of the reactive state of the body so far as these allergens are concerned. [allergy, Gk *metron* measure.]

allergosis (al·er·**go**·sis). One of the syndromes associated with the allergic diathesis. [allergy, Gk *-osis* condition.]

allergy (al·er·je). An imprecisely used synonym for hypersensitivity, usually used of immediate hypersensitivity. Term introduced by von Pirquet (1906) for altered host reactivity to an antigen, but it is no longer used in this sense. It is now used either to refer to immune states associated with tissue damage, i.e. hypersensitivity states, or to mean heightened reactivity to an antigen, i.e. synonymously with immunity. **Bacterial allergy.** Hypersensitivity to the action of a particular bacterium; it is contingent on present or previous infection, or prior contact of the tissues with a similar organism or its products. Usually used as a synonym for delayed hypersensitivity. **Bronchial allergy.** Asthma. **Contact allergy.** Hypersensitivity manifested by the occurrence of a cutaneous reaction after the skin has been in contact for some time with the particular allergen. **Food allergy.** Hypersensitivity to the proteins of foods, especially fish and meat. **Hereditary allergy.** Allergy due to the existence of certain hereditary factors. **House dust allergy.** Respiratory hypersensitivity, usually allergic rhinitis or asthma following inhalation of house dust. Often due to antigens from the mite *Dermatophagoides pteronyssimus.* **Induced allergy.** An allergic condition caused by contact with or the injection of an antigen, or by bacterial infection. **Latent allergy.** Allergy which is detectable when tests are made but which is otherwise symptomless. **Polyvalent allergy.** Allergy to more than one antigen. [Gk *allos* other, *ergein* to work.]

Allescheria (al·e·**sheer**·e·ah). A genus of fungi belonging to the family Eurotiaceae. *Allescheria boydii* may cause mycetoma and otomycosis in man. **Allescheria boydii.** A species which may cause subcutaneous pyogenic lesions in man.

Alletorphine (al·et·**or**·feen). BP Commission approved name for *N* - allyl - 7,8 - dihydro - 7α - (1(*R*) - hydroxy - 1 - methylbutyl) - O^6 - methyl - 6 - 14 - *endo* - ethenonormorphine; an analgesic.

alliaceous (al·e·a·shus). 1. Of or relating to the plant family Allium. 2. Like garlic. [L *allium* garlic.]

alligation (al·ig·a·shun). 1. In pharmacy, a method whereby one may determine the various amounts of solutions of different strengths which must be taken or put together to form a final mixture of a given strength. 2. Determination of the cost of a mixture when the proportions and prices of the different ingredients are known. [L *ad, ligare* to bind.]

alligator skin (**al**·ig·a·tor skin). Ichthyotic skin; hyperkeratosis marked by rough scaliness of the skin. *See* ICHTHYOSIS. [Sp. *el lagarto* the lizard.]

Allingham, Herbert William (b. 1862). London surgeon.

Allingham's operation. Inguinal colostomy just above and parallel to the inguinal ligament.

Allis, Oscar Huntington (b. 1836). Philadelphia surgeon.

Allis' forceps. A mouse-tooth peritoneal forceps.

Allis's sign. In fracture of the neck of the femur, the trochanter is displaced upwards, relaxing the fascia lata and allowing the finger to be sunk deeply between the trochanter and the iliac crest.

alliteration (al·it·er·**a'**·shun). A type of dysphasia in which the patient uses in close connection words beginning with the same consonant or containing the same consonantal sound. [L *ad, litera* letter.]

Allium (**al**·e·um). 1. A genus of plants of the family Liliaceae, including the onion and garlic. 2. (BPC 1949) Garlic, the fresh bulb of *Allium sativum.* It contains a volatile oil with a disagreeable pungent odour, chiefly due to the presence of allyl disulphide and allyl-propyl disulphide; used principally in pulmonary complaints such as bronchitis. [L garlic.]

alloaesthesia (al·o·es·**the'**·ze·ah). Allocheiria. Touch sensation referred to the other side of the body in a mirror-opposite fashion. [Gk *allos* other, aesthesia.]

allo-antibody (al·o·**an**·te·bod·e). Iso-antibody. [Gk *allos* other, antibody.]

allo-antigen (al·o·**an**·te·jen). Iso-antigen. [Gk *allos* other, antigen.]

allobarbital (al·o·**bar**·bit·al). Allobarbitone.

Allobarbitone BPC 1959 (al·o·**bar**·bit·one). Diallylbarbituric acid, $(C_3H_5)_2C{=}(CONH)_2{=}CO$, "Dial". A sedative and hypnotic used in cases of nervous insomnia.

allobiosis (al·o·bi·**o'**·sis). The change in response which is produced in an organism by altered circumstances or modification of physiological conditions. [Gk *allos* other, *bios* life.]

allocentric (al·o·**sen**·trik). Having ideas and interests centred on other people, not self-centred. [Gk *allos* other, centre.]

allochaesthesia (al·o·kes·**the'**·ze·ah). Allachaesthesia.

allocheiral (al·o·**ki**·ral). Affected with or relating to allocheiria.

allocheiria (al·lo·**ki**·re·ah). Alloaesthesia. [Gk *allos* other, *cheir* hand.]

allochetia, allochezia (al·o·**ke**·she·ah, al·o·**ke**·ze·ah). The passing of faeces through an abnormal channel such as a fistula or artificial anus, or the passing of non-faecal matter through the anus. [Gk *allos* other, *chezein* to defaecate.]

allocholesterol (al·o·kol·**es′**·ter·ol). $C_{27}H_{46}O$. An isomer of cholesterol, differing from the latter only in the position of the double bond in the steroid ring system.
allochroic (al·o·**kro**·ik). Relating to allochroism; changeable or diversified in colour.
allochroism (al·o·**kro**·izm). Variation, change or diversity in colour. [Gk *allos* other, *chroma* colour.]
allochromasia (al·o·kro·**ma′**·ze·ah). 1. Change in colour of hair or skin. 2. Colour blindness. [Gk *allos* other, *chroma* colour.]
allocinesia (al·o·sin·**e′**·ze·ah). Wrong movement made by a patient in response to a command or request in that the limb or part opposite to that mentioned is moved. [Gk *allos* other, kinesis.]
allocinetic (al·o·sin·**et′**·ik). Allokinetic.
allocolloid (al·o·**kol**·oid). A colloidal solution in which each of the phases consists of the same element in different allotropic forms; plastic sulphur is an example. [Gk *allos* other, colloid.]
allocortex (al·o·**kor**·tex). The non-laminated part of the cerebral cortex usually representing the less developed areas. [Gk *allos* other, cortex.]
allocrine (**al**·o·krine). Secreting more than 1 specific juice; heterocrine. [Gk *allos* other, *krinein* to separate.]
allocycly (al·o·**si**·kle). A phenomenon resulting from differences in the state and/or the time of contraction of chromosomes or chromosomal regions. In man, the X chromosome forming the Barr body shows a typical allocyclic behaviour. [Gk *allos* other, *kyklos* circle.]
allocymarin (al·o·si·mar·in). $C_{30}H_{44}O_9$. An isomeric form of the glucoside cymarin, which occurs in the seeds of species of *Strophanthus,* and also in Canadian hemp, *Apocynum cannabinum.*
Allodermanyssus (al·o·der·man·**e′**·sus). A genus of mites of the superfamily Parasitoidea. **Allodermanyssus sanguineus.** A vector of *Rickettsia akari* to man in eastern North America. [Gk *allos* other, *derma* skin, *nyssein* to prick.]
allodesmism (al·o·**dez**·mizm). An allomerism resulting from a difference in linkage within the molecule, rather than in chemical composition. [Gk *allos* other, *desmos* ligament.]
allodiploid (al·o·**dip**·loid). *See* ALLOPLOID. [Gk *allos* other, *diploos* double, *eidos* form.]
allodromy (al·o·**dro**·me). Disturbance of the cardiac rhythm. [Gk *allos* other, *dromos* running.]
alloeosis (al·e·**o**·sis). 1. Alteration in the character of a constitution or a disease. 2. Recovery from illness. 3. Disorder of the mind. 4. Alterative effect. [Gk *alloiosis* change.]
allo-eroticism, allo-erotism (al·o·er·**ot′**·is·izm, al·o·**er**·ot·izm). Sexual desire, urge and action stimulated by and directed towards another person; hetero-eroticism. Cf. AUTO-EROTICISM. [Gk *allos* other, eroticism.]
allogamy (al·**og**·am·e). Cross fertilization. [Gk *allos* other, *gamos* marriage.]
allogeneic (al·o·gen·**e′**·ik). Of different genetic constitution. In grafts, applied to those between one individual and another of the same species but different genetic constitution; homograft. [Gk *allos* other, *genein* to produce.]
allogotrophia (al·o·go·**tro′**·fe·ah). Growth or building up of one part of the body at the expense of another part. [Gk *allos* other, *trophe* nutrition.]
allograft (**al**·o·graft). Graft exchanged between genetically dissimilar individuals of the same species, i.e. in clinical practice, all grafts from any human donor who is not an identical twin of the recipient. [Gk *allos* other, graft.]
alloheteroploid (al·o·**het′**·er·o·ploid). Of cells or individuals, with additional chromosomes characteristic of a different species. [Gk *allos* other, *heteros* different, *ploos* times, *eidos* form.]
allo-isomerism (al·o·i·**som′**·er·izm). An isomerism resulting from a difference in the spatial arrangement within the molecules of compounds otherwise identical in chemical constitution. *See* STEREO-ISOMERISM. [Gk *allos* other, isomerism.]
allokeratoplasty (al·o·**ker**·at·o·**plas′**·te). Repair of the cornea with synthetic transparent material. [Gk *allos* other, kerato-plasty.]
allokinesis (al·o·kin·**e′**·sis). 1. Generally applied to passive movement or even forcible movement. 2. Reflex action of muscle. [Gk *allos* other, kinesis.]
allokinetic (al·o·kin·**et′**·ik). Referring to non-voluntary action of muscles; involving reflex action or passive movement. [see prec.]
allolactose (al·o·**lak**·toze). $C_{12}H_{22}O_{11}$. A stereo-isomer of lactose, or milk sugar.
allolalia (al·o·**la**·le·ah). 1. With regard to the power to speak, any impairment which is of central nervous origin. 2. A form of aphasia in which the speaker utters words he had not any intention of uttering, or substitutes for the relevant word one totally irrelevant. [Gk *allos* other, *lalein* to babble like a child.]
allomerism (al·**om**·er·izm). The phenomenon of substances which, though differing in chemical composition, have the same crystalline form. [Gk *allos* other, *meros* part.]
allomethadione (al·o·meth·ah·**di′**·one). Aloxidone.
allometropia (al·o·met·**ro′**·pe·ah). Refraction of the eye in indirect vision. [Gk *allos* other, meter, *ops* eye.]
allometry (al·**om**·et·re). The comparison between the proportional relationship of a part of an organism to the whole, and the same relationship at a later stage in development of the individual or in the evolution of the species. [Gk *allos* other, *metron* measure.]
allomorphic (al·o·**mor**·fik). Affected with allomorphism.
allomorphism (al·o·**mor**·fizm). 1. In chemistry, a difference in crystalline form although the chemical constitution is identical. 2. In biology, change in the shape of cells owing to pressure or to metaplasia. [Gk *allos* other, *morphe* form.]
allomorphosis (al·o·**mor**·fo·sis). Differential growth-rate of parts of organisms in relation to the growth-rate of the whole. [Gk *allos* other, *morphe* form, *-osis* condition.]
allomorphous (al·o·**mor**·fus). Allomorphic.
allongement (al·onzh·**mon**). A plastic procedure for lengthening a structure, e.g. a tendon. [Fr. lengthening.]
allonomous (al·**on**·om·us). Regulated by external stimuli. [Gk *allos* other, *nomos* law.]
allopath (**al**·o·path). Term used commonly by homoeopathists to designate the orthodox practitioner of medicine. [Gk *allos* other, *pathos* suffering. Coined by Hahnemann.]
allopathic (al·o·**path**·ik). Relating to or exhibiting the characteristics of allopathy.
allopathist (al·**op**·ath·ist). Allopath.
allopathy (al·**op**·ath·e). Treatment by the induction in the body of a different reaction from that which is produced by the disease, as opposed to that of homoeopathists, who treat like by like. The word is wrongly applied to modern scientific medicine by homoeopathists and others. Cf. ENANTIOPATHY; HOMOEOPATHY. [Gk *allos* other, *pathos* suffering.]
allophanamide (al·o·**fan**·am·ide). Biuret, $NH_2CONHCONH_2$. A crystalline substance obtained by heating urea at 160°C. It is used as a reagent, giving a violet coloration with copper salts in alkaline solution (biuret test).
allophasis (al·**of**·as·is). Delirium; confused, incoherent speech. [Gk *allos* other, *phasis* speech.]
allophemy (al·**of**·em·e). 1. A variety of aphasia in which terms and words are habitually or often incorrectly used; heterophasia; heterolalia. 2. Saying one thing and meaning another. [Gk *allos* other, *pheme* speech.]
allophone (al·o·fon). A minor variation of a phoneme.
allophthalmia (al·of·**thal**·me·ah). Difference between the two eyes, usually with respect to direction of gaze or iris colour. [Gk *allos* other, *ophthalmos* eye.]
alloplasia (al·o·**pla**·ze·ah). 1. The development of abnormal tissue; a condition in which normal cells are in the wrong place or position; heteroplasia. 2. Dysplasia. [Gk *allos* other, *plassein* to form.]
alloplasmatic (al·o·plaz·**mat′**·ik). Evolved from basic protoplasm by differentiation into cell groups. [Gk *allos* other, protoplasm.]
alloplasty (**al**·o·plas·te). A system of plastic surgery which makes use of materials foreign to the human body, e.g. glass, ivory, silver. Cf. AUTOPLASTY; HETEROPLASTY. [Gk *allos* other, *plassein* to form.]

alloploid (al·o·ploid). Of cells or individuals, produced by crosses between partners belonging to different species and therefore containing chromosome sets characteristic of different species. If such cells or individuals have 2 sets of chromosomes they are *allodiploid*; if they have more they are *allopolyploid.* [Gk *allos* other, *ploos* times, *eidos* form.]

alloploidy (al·o·**ploid**·e). The state characteristic of alloploids.

allopolyploid (al·o·**pol**·ip·loid). Of chromosome complements, cells or organisms with more than 2 sets of non-homologous chromosomes. [Gk *allos* other, *polyplous* many times, *eidos* form.]

allopregnanediol (al·o·preg·nane·**di**′·ol). The short name for the reduction derivative of progesterone, 17(β)-[1(α)-hydroxyethyl]-androstane-3(β)-ol, which occurs in the urine of male cattle, and that of pregnant cows, mares and women; also applied to the isomeric 17(β)-[1(β)-hydroxyethyl]-androstane-3(β)-ol, which occurs in the urine of pregnant mares. It is used as a standard in the determination of urinary pregnanediol.

allopsyche (al·o·**si**·ke). The psyche of another. [Gk *allos* other, psyche.]

allopsychic (al·o·**si**·kik). Referring to the attitude of the mind towards the environment, near and distant, and not to the personality. [see prec.]

allopsychosis (al·o·si·**ko**′·sis). A psychosis in which the perception of things is illusory and hallucinatory, although the motor system is unaffected. [Gk *allos* other, psychosis.]

Allopurinol BP 1973 (al·o·**pewr**·in·ol). 1*H*-pyrazolo[3,4-*d*]pyrimadin-4-ol; a xanthine oxidase inhibitor used in the treatment of hyperuricaemia.

allorrhythmia (al·o·**rith**·me·ah). Irregular cardiac rhythm. [Gk *allos* other, rhythm.]

allorrhythmic (al·o·**rith**·mik). Relating to or affected with allorrhythmia.

allose (**al**·oze). $CH_2OH(CHOH)_4CHO$. An aldohexose, isomeric with glucose, and prepared synthetically.

allosome (**al**·o·some). 1. A chromosome, particularly one of the sex chromosomes, possessing characteristics which make it readily distinguishable from ordinary chromosomes, or autosomes. 2. Less commonly, any unusual or abnormal cellular constituent. [Gk *allos* other, *soma* body.]

allosteatodes (al·o·ste·at·**o**′·deez). A condition in which there is morbid or abnormal secretion of sebum. [Gk *allos* other, *steatodes* fat-like.]

allosteric (al·o·**ster**·ik). Having the property of allostery. [Gk *allos* other, *stereos* solid.]

allostery (al·**os**·ter·e). The name given to the phenomenon of the binding of effector molecules (activators or inhibitors) to an enzyme protein at sites distinct from those which bind the substrate. The effector is usually chemically distinct from the substrate. The binding of effector molecules results in intramolecular conformational changes such that the substrate-binding capacity and/or the catalytic effectiveness is/are modified. [Gk *allos* other, *stereos* solid.]

allotopia (al·o·**to**·pe·ah). Malposition or displacement of any organ; dystopia; heterotopia. [Gk *allos* other, *topos* place.]

allotopic (al·o·**to**·pik). Referring to allotopia; dystopic.

allotoxin (al·o·**tox**·in). Any antitoxin, or other substance formed in the blood or tissues, which neutralizes or checks toxins. [Gk *allos* other, toxin.]

allotransplantation (al·o·tranz·plan·**ta**′·shun). Transplantation of an allograft. [Gk *allos* other, transplantation.]

allotriodontia (al·ot·re·o·**don**′·she·ah). 1. The presence of teeth in any abnormal situation. 2. The transplanting of teeth from one individual to another. [Gk *allotrios* strange, *odous* tooth.]

allotriogeustia (al·**ot**·re·o·**gew**′·ste·ah). Perverted gustation; abnormality of appetite. [Gk *allotrios* strange, *geusis* taste.]

allotriolith (al·o·**tri**·o·lith). A calculus the composition of which is unusual, or one found in an unusual place. [Gk *allotrios* strange, *lithos* stone.]

allotriolithiasis (al·o·tri·o·lith·**i**′·as·is). The existence or the forming of an allotrolith.

allotriophagia, allotriophagy (al·**ot**·re·o·**fa**′·je·ah, al·o·tri·**of**′·aj·e). The craving for, or the habit of eating, improper or unnatural food; depraved appetite. [Gk *allotrios* strange, *phagein* to eat.]

allotriosmia (al·**ot**·re·**oz**′·me·ah). A condition in which the sense of smell is perverted so that odours are wrongly interpreted; heterosmia. [Gk *allotrios* strange, *osme* smell.]

allotriuria (al·**ot**·re·**ewr**′·e·ah). An abnormal condition of the urine. [Gk *allotrios* strange, urine.]

allotrope (**al**·o·trope). One of the forms of an element that displays allotropy.

allotrophic (al·o·**trof**·ik). Altered by digestion so as to lose nutritive value. [Gk *allos* other, *trophe* nutrition.]

allotropic (al·o·**trop**·ik). 1. In chemistry, showing or relating to allotropism. 2. Denoting an individual who is not self-centred but is preoccupied with other people and their affairs. [see foll.]

allotropism (al·**ot**·rop·izm). 1. The phenomenon of allotropy. 2. A tropism, or directive urge, of an organism towards another of different form. [Gk *allos* other, *tropos* a turning.]

allotropy (al·**ot**·rop·e). The peculiarity possessed by certain elements, such as carbon, sulphur and phosphorus, of existing in several forms, each differing in physical and chemical properties. [see prec.]

allotrylic (al·o·**tril**·ik). Relating to, or caused by, the presence of a foreign agent or substance. [Gk *allotrios* strange, *hyle* matter.]

alloxamide (al·**ox**·am·ide). A derivative of alloxan formed by ammonia.

alloxan (al·**ox**·an). Mesoxalyl urea. $CO(NHCO)_2CO$. Obtained by oxidizing uric acid; a crystalline compound, soluble in water, with acidic properties. It stains the skin red, forms a deep blue coloration with ferrous salts, and is reduced to alloxantin by sulphuretted hydrogen. It occurs in the intestine during diarrhoea, and injection of it into the body produces diabetes by destruction of the islet tissue of the pancreas.

alloxantin (al·ox·**an**·tin). $[CO{=}(NHCO)_2{=}C(OH)]_2$. A diureide produced by the reduction of alloxan; a colourless compound which yields the purple dye, murexide, with ammonia, a fact made use of in the sensitive test for uric acid.

alloxazine (al·**ox**·az·een). $C_{10}H_6N_4O_2$. A heterocyclic constituent of certain plant pigments; related to the flavins and to vitamin B_2.

alloxin (al·**ox**·in). A general term applied to any one of the purines, adenine, guanine, xanthine and hypoxanthine, which are derived from the nucleic acids.

alloxur (al·**ox**·ewr). **Alloxur bases, Alloxur bodies.** The purines derived from the nucleic acids, and so called because of the alloxan and urea groups of which they are constructed.

alloxuraemia (al·**ox**·ewr·**e**′·me·ah). A toxic condition caused by the presence in the blood of alloxur bodies. [alloxur, Gk *haima* blood.]

alloxuria (al·ox·**ewr**·e·ah). The presence in the urine of alloxur bodies.

alloxuric (al·ox·**ewr**·ik). Pertaining to the alloxur bases or bodies.

alloy (**al**·oi). A combination, fusion, or mixture of 2 or more metals. **Amalgam alloy.** An alloy composed mainly of silver and tin in the form of filings, which, when triturated with mercury, forms a plastic mass. It is inserted in a cavity prepared in a tooth and sets to form a watertight filling. **Cobalt-chrome alloy.** An alloy composed mainly of cobalt, chromium and nickel, used widely in the manufacture of the plates and other prosthetic implants used in orthopaedic surgery. **Eutectic alloy.** An alloy of such proportions that it melts at a lower temperature than any other alloy of the same metals. **Gold alloy.** An alloy, containing a high percentage of gold, which is used as a base for artificial dentures and for restorations in the mouth, such as inlays, crowns, and bridges. **Submarine alloy.** An amalgam alloy which when combined with mercury sets under water. **Tungsten alloy (heavy metal alloy).** An alloy of tungsten, copper and nickel having greater density and less malleability than lead. Used as a protective shield against radiation, especially in telecurietherapy units and supervoltage x-ray apparatus. [OFr. *aleier* to combine.]

allspice (**awl**·spise). The dried fruit of *Pimenta officinalis*, an evergreen of the West Indies and Central America. [AS *all*, L *species* sort.]

Allworden's reaction. The appearance of blister formation on the edges of hair or wool fibres acted upon by chlorine in watery solution.

allyl (al·il). The monovalent unsaturated organic radical, CH_2=$CHCH_2$-, isomeric with propenyl and isopropenyl. **Allyl alcohol.** CH_2=$CHCH_2OH$, a colourless liquid with a pungent smell, found in wood spirit and employed in dilute solution as a disinfectant. **Allyl aldehyde.** Acrolein, CH_2=$CHCHO$, a pungent liquid prepared from glycerol, with an irritant effect on the eyes and used in chemical warfare; it is the starting point for the preparation of synthetic sugars. **Allyl chloride.** CH_2=$CHCH_2Cl$, a highly toxic liquid with an irritant vapour. **Allyl cyanamide.** CH_2=$CHCH_2NHCN$, a compound derived from black mustard seed. **Allyl cyanide.** CH_2=$CHCH_2CN$, a minor constituent of volatile oil of mustard. **Allyl iodide.** CH_2=$CHCH_2I$, a yellow liquid used in the synthesis of allyl isothiocyanate. **Allyl isopropyl barbituric acid.** Alurate, a hypnotic derivative of barbituric acid; with amidopyrine it constitutes "Allonal". **Allyl isothiocyanate.** CH_2=$CHCH_2NCS$, a colourless liquid which occurs as the glucoside sinigrin, in black mustard seed and horseradish; it has a pungent odour and is highly vesicant. **Allyl morphine.** A morphine derivative at one time considered as effective as morphine but without its disadvantages. **Allyl mustard oil.** Volatile oil of mustard; allyl isothiocyanate (see above). **Allyl sulphide.** $(CH_2$=$CHCH_2)_2S$, a pale yellow oil with a garlic smell, present in oil of garlic but usually prepared synthetically. It is considered to have germicidal properties and was formerly used in the treatment of pulmonary tuberculosis. **Allyl sulphocarbamide, Allyl thiocarbamide.** Thiosinamine, CH_2=$CHCH_2$ $NHCSNH_2$, a compound prepared from volatile oil of mustard and used as a resolvent in the treatment of scar tissue though of doubtful efficacy. **Allyl thiocyanate.** CH_2=$CHCN_2SCN$, a colourless liquid with a leek-like odour, converted on heating into allyl isothiocyanate. **Allyl thiourea.** Allyl sulphocarbamide (see above). **Allyl tribromide.** $CH_2BrCHBrCH_2Br$, a pale yellow liquid which has been used as an antispasmodic in coughs and chest diseases. [L *allium* garlic, Gk *hyle* matter.]

allylamine (al·il·**am**·een). CH_2=$CHCH_2NH_2$, a yellow liquid with an ammoniacal smell and caustic properties; prepared from mustard oil.

allylestrenol (**al**·il·es·tren·ole). A progestogen that stimulates secretion of endogenous placental hormones essential for the maintenance of pregnancy and is given in cases of habitual abortion, threatened abortion and failure of nidation. Virilization of the fetus has not been reported.

allylguaiacol (al·il·**gwi**·ak·ol). Chavibetol.

allylisopropylacetylurea (**al**·il·i·so·pro·pil·**as**·et·il·ewr·e′·ah). $(C_3H_5)(C_3H_7)CHCONHCONH_2$. A sedative and hypnotic structurally related to the barbiturates, but milder in its action.

allylisopropylbarbiturate (**al**·il·i·so·**pro**·pil·bar·bit·**ewr**′·ate). Any salt of allylisopropylbarbituric acid. The amidopyrine salt is a well-known proprietary hypnotic.

N-allylnormorphine hydrobromide (**en**·al·il·nor·**mor**′·feen hi·dro·**bro**·mide). Nalorphine hydrobromide; a substance that inhibits the effect of an excess of narcotic analgesics, morphine, pethidine, etc.

Allyloestrenol (al·il·e·stren·ol). BP Commission approved name for 17α-allyloestr-4-en-17β-ol; it is used in sex-hormone therapy.

Allylprodine (al·il·**pro**·deen). BP Commission approved name for 3-allyl-1-methyl-4-phenyl-4-propionyloxypiperidine, an analgesic.

Almeida, Floriano Paulo de (b. 1898). São Paulo physician.

Lutz-Splendore-Almeida disease. Paracoccidioidomycosis.

Almén, August Theodor (b. 1833). Upsala physiologist.

Almén's reagent. For nucleoprotein in urine: to 5 g of tannic acid dissolved in 240 ml of 50 per cent alcohol add 10 ml of 25 per cent acetic acid.

almond (**ah**·mond). The seed of the tree *Prunus amygdalus* Batsch. (*Prunus communis* Arcang), family Rosaceae. There are 2 varieties, bitter almond and sweet almond. **Bitter almond.** The seed of *Prunus amygdalus* var. *amara*. **Almond Oil BP 1973.** Oleum amygdalae, the fixed oil expressed from both types of almond; it is demulcent and mildly laxative and is also used in toilet preparations. **Sweet almond.** The seed of *Prunus amygdalus* var. *dulcis*. **Volatile Bitter Almond Oil BP 1953.** Prepared by distillation of the cake left after expressing the fixed oils from bitter almonds, and peach or apricot kernels, followed by removal of the hydrocyanic acid. It consists of not less than 95 per cent benzaldehyde, and is used as a flavouring agent. [Fr. *amande*.]

almoner (**ah**·mon·er). A trained social worker attached to a hospital or municipality who investigates the domestic and social circumstances of patients in relation to their illnesses so that aid can be given when necessary. [Gk *eleemosyne* compassionateness.]

alochia (a·**lo**·ke·ah). Lack of secretion of lochia after childbirth. [Gk *a*, lochia.]

Aloe (**al**·o). A genus of plants of the family Liliaceae; they are mostly indigenous to Africa. They are xerophytes with fleshy leaves which yield the drug, aloes. **Aloe africana.** An arborescent species of South Africa. **Aloe barbadensis.** A West Indian strain of *Aloe vera* (see below). **Aloe chinensis.** A species of the West Indies which with *Aloe vera* provides Curaçao or Barbados aloes. **Aloe ferox.** A South African species which yields Cape aloes. **Aloe officinalis.** *Aloe vera* (see below). **Aloe perryi.** A species from the island of Socotra, and Arabia, which is the source of Socotrine aloes. **Aloe spicata.** A South African species. **Aloe vera, Aloe vulgaris.** A species indigenous to Africa and cultivated in the West Indies. [Gk.]

Aloes BP 1973 (**al**·oze). A dark-brown or olive-brown resinous drug obtained from the leaves of a xerophyte which grows in Africa and the West Indies. It has a purgative action by virtue of its containing a glycoside, aloin, which after absorption slowly hydrolyses, producing emodin. This is excreted in the large intestine, where it causes irritation and purgation; the hydrolysis is so slow that it may be several hours before purgation is produced. Some of the active principle is converted into yellow chrysophanic acid by the liver and excreted in the urine, where it behaves as an indicator, turning red if the urine is rendered alkaline. Aloes should not be used as a laxative during pregnancy. [see prec.]

aloetic (al·o·**et**·ik). 1. Of the nature of aloes, or containing aloes. 2. An aloetic medicine.

alogia (a·**lo**·je·ah). 1. Lack of the power to speak because of a lesion of a nerve centre, or because of mental defect. 2. Foolish or stupid behaviour. [Gk folly, dumbness.]

alogotrophy (al·og·**ot**·ro·fe). Irregular morbid nutrition causing deformity, especially of the bones, as in rickets. [Gk *alogos* not according to reason, *trophe* nutrition.]

Aloin BP 1953 (**al**·o·in). $C_{20}H_{20}P_8$. A glycoside found in aloes, being a derivative of aloe-emodinanthrol and D-arabinose. It has itself no purgative action, but after absorption in the small intestine is hydrolysed and the irritant emodin produced is secreted into the large intestine, where it produces a purgative effect. It exercises a similar irritant action on uterine muscle and should therefore be avoided as a purgative during pregnancy.

alopecia (al·o·**pe**·she·ah). Loss of hair; baldness. **Alopecia acquisita.** Baldness arising from any but congenital causes. **Alopecia adnata.** Congenital baldness. **Alopecia areata.** A malady of unknown cause in which the hair falls from one or more circumscribed round or oval areas, leaving the skin smooth and white. The scalp is the site of predilection, but any area of the body may be involved. At the periphery of an early lesion, "note of exclamation" or club-shaped hairs may usually be found. **Cachectic alopecia.** Alopecia associated with general debility. **Alopecia capitis totalis.** Baldness of the entire scalp. **Alopecia celsi.** Alopecia areata (see above). **Chignon alopecia.** Alopecia caused by a chignon (mass of hair at the back of the head).

Alopécie cicatricielle miliare. Scarring and baldness of the scalp occurring particularly in elderly seborrhoeic women. The vertex is the site of election, upon which appear numerous small scars each involving 3 or 4 follicles. **Alopecia cicatrisata.** Baldness associated with scarring, and causing permanent alopecia. Whilst many authors use the term as a synonym for pseudopelade, others employ it to mean *cicatricial baldness* and include permanent baldness due to injury, infection, disease such as lupus erythrematosus, and maladies peculiar to the scalp. **Alopecia circumscripta.** Alopecia areata (see above). **Alopecia congenita, Congenital alopecia, Alopecia congenitalis.** This may be complete or partial. Congenital absence of hair (atrichosis congenitalis or alopecia adnata) has been noted in certain families in which the hair is absent at birth or falls out in early childhood. Another variety is associated with defects of the nails and teeth, and is part of the syndrome known as *congenital ectodermal defect.* Localized congenital alopecia may be due to adherence of membranes to the scalp *in utero*, or to naevoid abnormalities of the hairy skin. **Alopecia disseminata.** Loss of hair in patches at various places on the body. **Alopécie dite du chignon, Alopecia dynamica.** Permanent baldness due to destruction of hair follicles by disease, trauma or ulceration. **Alopecia follicularis.** Baldness following inflammation of pilosebaceous follicles. **Frontal alopecia of women.** Alopecia liminaris frontalis (see below). **Alopecia furfuracea.** Alopecia pityroides (see below). **Alopecia generalisata.** Alopecia universalis (see below). **Alopecia hereditaria.** Premature hereditary alopecia in which, without visible disease of the scalp, the hair commences to fall soon after the age of 20 years, leaving the frontal area and vertex completely bald. The malady is not uncommon in men, but is seldom seen in women. **Alopecia hippocratica.** Alopecia seborrhoeica (see below). **Alopecia indurata atrophica.** A rare, possibly familial, malady affecting women of middle age. The back-hair is involved (whence the name chignon alopecia), the hair falling from the vertex and occipital area of the scalp whilst the skin becomes atrophic and bound down to the underlying aponeurosis. It is suggested that the malady is symptomatic of vascular disease (Sutton). **Alopecia liminaris frontalis.** A form of alopecia affecting women between the ages of 15 and 20 years who also suffer from seborrhoea of the face. An eruption combining features of keratosis pilaris, pityriasis steatoides and seborrhoea, develops on the whole of the frontal border of the hair-scalp and extends from one temple to the other, involving a band about 2.4 cm (1 in) in width; within a few months permanent alopecia develops. **Alopecia localis.** A form which occurs in irregular-shaped patches along the course of a nerve. **Male pattern alopecia.** Common baldness in males in a pattern which results from androgenic stimulation, genetic influences and ageing. A similar condition may develop in women, sometimes alone and without detectable endocrine disorder, sometimes with hirsutism, after the menopause, or sometimes with virilism and due to endocrine disorder. **Alopecia maligna.** Severe and persistent alopecia. **Marginal alopecia.** Baldness of the margins of the scalp due to endocrine causes, particularly hypothyroidism. **Mechanical alopecia.** Traumatic alopecia (see below). **"Moth-eaten" alopecia.** Patchy temporoparietal and occipital loss of hair in secondary syphilis. **Neonatal alopecia.** Traumatic alopecia (see below). **Alopecia neurotica.** A form of alopecia localis which is caused by trauma or disease of the nervous system, psychic disturbances or insanity, or in association with neuralgia. **Occipital alopecia.** Traumatic alopecia often seen on the occipital area in infants. **Ophiasic alopecia.** A variety of alopecia areata in which the bald area extends round the margin of the scalp. **Alopecia orbicularis.** Alopecia cicatrisata (see above). **Alopecia parvimaculata.** An epidemic form of pseudopelade of undetermined cause. **Peroneal alopecia.** Baldness of the peroneal areas of the legs. **Alopecia pityroides.** A diffuse loss of hair considered paroxysmal (Sabouraud), and associated with pityriasis steatoides; though the hair becomes more and more scanty, no region develops complete baldness. It is most severe on the temples and frontal area. **Alopecia pityroides capillitii.** Baldness associated with pityriasis or dandruff. **Alopecia pityroides universalis.** A discarded term indicating loss of hair from the scalp and other areas due to debility. **Alopecia praesenilis, Alopecia prematura.** Acquired baldness occurring in individuals who are not elderly. **Pressure alopecia.** Temporary focal loss of hair from trauma at birth or, in women, from prolonged pressure on the occiput during operations in the Trendelenburg position. **Reflex alopecia.** Jacquet's disease; alopecia associated with dental abnormality. **Alopecia seborrhoeica.** Slowly-developing and progressive alopecia of the scalp, associated in the earlier stages with seborrhoea. The baldness commences by thinning of the hair on the temples and on the vertex, and extends until the dome of the scalp is wholly or partially denuded of hair; the progress is more rapid in young persons. **Alopecia senilis.** The baldness or falling out of hair which is normal in old age. **Alopecia serrata.** Narrow and elongated areas of baldness occurring in folliculitis decalvans. **Alopecia simplex.** Idiopathic premature alopecia. **Sutural alopecia.** Alopecia tending to occur along the cranial sutures, as in dyscephalia mandibulo-oculofacialis. **Alopecia symptomatica.** Baldness occurring during the course of a febrile illness, in maladies such as syphilis, and possibly after severe mental stress; baldness due to trauma or diseases of the scalp may also be included in this category. **Alopecia syphilitica.** Baldness occasioned by syphilis; the term is usually applied to the temporary baldness of secondary syphilis. **Thallium alopecia.** Baldness following the administration of thallium salts, particularly of thallium acetate. **Alopecia totalis.** Alopecia in which the whole body is involved; pelade décalvante. **Alopecia toxica.** Baldness due to toxic causes. **Traction alopecia.** Sparseness of hair caused by traction from hair-curlers, rubber bands, over-vigorous combing, nylon brushes, habitual manipulation, etc. **Traumatic alopecia.** The breaking-off of hairs due to friction or other forms of injury. **Traumatic marginal alopecia.** Baldness due to traction, as seen in some negresses. **Alopecia triangularis congenitalis.** A triangular hairless patch of skin at the junction of the temporal and frontal regions. **Trichophytic alopecia.** Baldness due to trichophytic infection. **Alopecia ungualis.** Onychomadesis; shedding of the nails (an obsolete term). **Alopecia universalis.** Complete baldness of all parts of the head and body. [Gk *alopex* fox, the disease resembling the mange of foxes.]

See also: JONSTON.

alopecic (al·o·**pe**·sik). Having the characteristics of or relating to alopecia.

Alouette's amputation, or operation. Amputation at the hip, with the use of a short outer and long inner flap.

aloxanthin (al·o·**zan**·thin). $C_{15}H_{10}O_6$. A yellow pigment derived from *Aloe vera.* [aloe, Gk *xanthos* yellow.]

Aloxidone (al·**ox**·id·one). BP Commission approved name for 3-allyl-5-methyloxazolidine-2,4-dione; allomethadione. An anticonvulsant, used in epilepsy and petit mal. It may cause agranulocytosis and skin rashes, and is contraindicated in kidney and liver disease and when the leucocyte count is low.

Aloxiprin (al·**ox**·e·prin). BP Commission approved name for a polymeric condensation product of aluminium oxide and *O*-acetylsalicylic acid; an analgesic.

alpenstich (**al**·pen·shtik). Epidemic pneumonia in Alpine valleys. [G.]

alpha (**al**·fah). 1. A or α, the first letter of the Greek alphabet. 2. In chemistry, α-, denoting the isomer in which substitution has taken place at the alpha position (see below). **Alpha angle.** *See* ANGLE. **Alpha block.** *See* BLOCK. **Alpha cell.** *See* CELL. **Alpha fibre.** *See* FIBRE. **Alpha globulin.** *See* GLOBULIN. **Alpha granule.** *See* GRANULE. **Alpha helix.** *See* HELIX. **Alpha particle.** *See* PARTICLE. **Alpha position.** In an organic compound comprising a straight chain of carbon atoms, the carbon atom to which the characteristic group is attached; in a dicyclic compound, the carbon atoms numbered 1, 4, 5 and 8. In a heterocyclic compound, the alpha position is that of the carbon atom nearest to the heterocyclic atom. **Alpha ray.** A stream of alpha particles (*see* PARTICLE). **Alpha rhythm.** *See* RHYTHM. **Alpha thalassaemia.** *See* THALASSAEMIA. **Alpha wave.** *See* WAVE.

Alphacetylmethadol (al·fah·se·til·meth'·ad·ol). BP Commission approved name for the α-3-acetoxy derivative; the alcohol of methadone. An analgesic with morphine-like properties.

Alphadolone (al·fad·o·lone). BP Commission approved name for 3α,21-dihydroxy-5α-pregnane-11,20-dione; an anaesthetic component.

alphahypophamine (al·fah·hi·pof'·am·een). Oxytocin.

alphalobeline (al·fah·lo·bel·een). Lobeline.

Alphameprodine (al·fah·mep·ro·deen). BP Commission approved name for the 3-ethyl derivative of the "reversed ester" of pethidine. It has similar properties to the latter and is used in the same way as alphaprodine.

Alphamethadol (al·fah·meth·ad·ol). BP Commission approved name for the alcohol of which methadone is the compounding ketone; it has similar morphine-like properties.

alphanaphthol (al·fah·naf·thol). α-Hydroxynaphthalene, $C_{10}H_7OH$, occurring in coal-tar with the β-isomer; colourless crystals with a phenolic odour and insoluble in water. A strong antiseptic.

Alphaprodine (al·fah·pro·deen). Prisilidene hydrochloride. BP Commission approved name for the 3-methyl derivative of the "reversed ester" of pethidine. It is used as a narcotic and analgesic, primarily in obstetrics.

alphatocopherol (al·fah·to·kof'·er·ol). Tocopherol.

alphatropeine (al·fah·tro·pe·een). One of a set of esters of tropine which are used as drugs, as distinct from those derived from pseudotropine which have no therapeutic value.

alphavirus (al·fa·vi·rus). The official generic name for the Group A arboviruses. The members of the genus either do not infect man or cause a mild encephalitis without permanent sequelae (e.g. O'nyong n'yong, Chikungunya, etc.). (Gk *alpha*, the letter a).

Alphaxalone (al·fax·al·one). BP Commission approved name for 3α-hydroxy-5α-pregnane-11,20-dione; an anaesthetic component.

alphelasma (al·fel·az·mah). A condition in which white patches of irregular shape form on the mucous membrane of the gums, tongue or cheeks. Thickening of the epithelium results and there may be hypertrophy of the papillae; leucoplakia. [Gk *alphos* vitiligo, *elasma* metal plate.]

alphenols (al·fe·nolz). Phenols which exhibit definite alcoholic characteristics.

alphitomorphous (al·fit·o·mor'·fus). Having the appearance of barley meal; a term used to describe certain fungi. [Gk *alphiton* barley meal, *morphe* form.]

alphodeopsoriasis (al·fo·de·o·so·ri'·as·is). A form of psoriasis which resembles leprosy in appearance. [Gk *alphodes* leprous, psoriasis.]

alphodermia (al·fo·der·me·ah). A condition in which there is no pigment in the skin. [Gk *alphos* vitiligo, *derma* skin.]

alphos (al·fos). 1. A harmless blemish on the skin (Hippocrates); later the word was used to denote leprosy associated with cutaneous depigmentation. 2. Psoriasis. [Gk.]

alphosis (al·fo·sis). Alphodermia. [Gk *alphos* vitiligo.]

alphus (al·fus). Alphos.

alphyl (al·fil). An alkyl radical derived from an aliphatic hydrocarbon.

Alpinia (al·pin·e·ah). A genus of plants with aromatic root-stocks and belonging to the family Zingiberaceae. **Alpinia officinarum.** Lesser galangal, a Chinese species, the rhizomes of which are used like ginger. [Prospero *Alpini*, 1553-1616?, Padua physician and botanist.]

Alport, Arthur Cecil (b. 1880). South African physician.

Alport's syndrome. Congenital glomerulo-nephritis associated with deafness. Albuminuria of long-standing, leading inevitably to chronic nephritis and death before middle age, occurs in families where there is an inheritance of a partially sex-linked dominant trait; early perceptive deafness begins in some members, both male and female; occasionally, ocular abnormalities such as lenticonus, cataract and Drüsen are also found. No satisfactory pathological explanation is available. Treatment, as well as aetiology, is still unknown. First described as a syndrome in December 1961.

Alprenolol (al·pren·o·lol). BP Commission approved name for (±) - 1 - (2 - allylphenoxy) - 3 - isopropylaminopropan - 2 - ol. **Alprenolol Hydrochloride BP 1973.** The hydrochloride, a beta-receptor adrenergic blocking agent.

Alsberg's angle. Angle of elevation of Alsberg's triangle.

Alsberg's triangle. An equilateral triangle formed by lines passing through the long axis of the femoral shaft, the long axis of the neck of the femur and the base of the head of the femur.

alseroxylon (al·ser·ox·il·on). An alkaloidal extract of *Rauwolfia serpentina*, a tropical plant (family Apocyanaceae). The alkaloids present include reserpine. It is used in the treatment of hypertension.

Alsever, John Bellows (b. 1908). USA Public Health Service.

Alsever's solution. A solution used in the preservation of sheep's red blood corpuscles used in the complement-fixation test.

Alstonia (al·sto·ne·ah). A genus of tropical trees or shrubs of the family Apocynaceae, the barks of which contain alkaloids, and are used in the East in the treatment of diarrhoea and malaria. **Alstonia constricta** F. Muell. The Australian fever-tree, a species yielding a bitter tonic bark. It has been found to be a source of reserpine. **Alstonia scholaris** R. Br. The devil-tree of Indonesia, from which is obtained dita bark. [Charles *Alston*, 1683-1760, Edinburgh botanist and pharmacologist.]

alstonine (al·sto·neen). An alkaloid of *Alstonia constricta*: $C_{21}H_{20}N_2O_3$. It has been used in diarrhoea and in malaria in India without any convincingly good results.

altauna (al·taw·nah). An Arabic term which includes bubos, endemic ulcers and malignant carbuncles.

alterant (awl·ter·ant). A drug which corrects, or is presumed to correct, disordered bodily function. The term is now obsolete. [L *alterare* to change.]

alterative (awl·ter·at·iv). Alterant; the term is obsolete.

alteregoism (awl·ter·eg'·o·izm). An altruistic feeling for an individual in a similar situation to oneself. [L *alter* other, *ego* I.]

alternans (awl·ter·nanz). Alternation. **Alternans of the electrocardiogram.** Electrical alternation; regular variation of the height of the R wave of the electrocardiogram in alternate ventricular complexes, sometimes, but not invariably, associated with alternans of the pulse (see below). **Alternans of the heart.** Alternation of the force of the heart beat (pulsus alternans). Also applied to alternation in the ventricular complex of the electrocardiogram. **Alternans of the pulse, Pulsus alternans.** Regular rhythm in which strong beats alternate with weak beats, occurring in severe left ventricular failure and occasionally in auricular tachycardia or flutter; the sum of 1 weak beat and 1 strong beat equals 2 normal beats. The cardiac impulse, as well as the arterial pulse, may alternate in force. The explanation is uncertain, the phenomenon being due either to a state of unequal refractoriness of all the muscle fibres, fewer fibres contracting with the weaker than with the stronger beats, or to abnormal relaxation of the ventricular muscle, more blood being expelled from the ventricles during the stronger beats than during the weaker. [L *alternare* to alternate.]

Alternaria (awl·ter·na·re·ah). A genus of fungi which may be present in flour; one species has caused asthma and eczema in man by inhalation and contact. [see prec.]

alternation (awl·ter·na·shun). In neurology, with particular application to the auditory nerve, the phenomenon whereby at stimulus frequencies above 900-1000 Hz a given fibre, owing to its refractory period, can respond only to every other stimulus. Since the refractory period of all the fibres does not begin and end at the same instant, the nerve as a whole continues to conduct. **Electrical alternation.** Alternans of the electrocardiogram. [L *alternare* to alternate.]

alternator (awl·ter·na'·tor). A dynamo so constructed that it generates electric current which changes polarity a predetermined number of times per second. [see prec.]

Althaea BPC 1949 (al·the·ah). Marshmallow, marshmallow root, the root of *Althaea officinalis*, from which a mucilaginous demulcent solution may be made; useful in the symptomatic treatment of coughs and inflammation of the membrane of the mouth and throat. It is not, however, commonly used nowadays. [Gk *althaia* marshmallow.]

althein (al·the·in). The active principle found in marshmallow roots (*Althaea*), which has been found to be identical with asparagine, α-aminosuccinic acid. It is found in many other plants, but it is of no medicinal importance today.

Altmann, Richard (b. 1852). German histologist.

Altmann's fluid. A fixative compounded of osmic acid and potassium bichromate.

Altmann's granule. Mitochondrion.

Altmann's theory. The hypothesis that the mitochondria are the essential living constituents of cells.

Altmann–Gersh method. The preparation of tissues for sectioning by freezing followed by dehydration *in vacuo*.

altofrequent (al·to·fre·kwent). Possessing a high frequency. [L *altus* high, frequency.]

altrigenderism (al·tre·jen·der·izm). The state of being attracted to the other sex. [L *alter* other, *genus* race.]

altroketoheptose (al·tro·ke·to·hep′·toze). $CH_2OH(CHOH)_4COCH_2OH$, a heptose found naturally in the leaves and stem of *Sedum spectabile*.

altrose (al·troze). An aldohexose, $CH_2OH(CHOH)_4CHO$, which exists in 2 optically-active forms, and is isomeric with glucose.

Alum (al·um). 1. The general name given to members of a group of double salts of formula $M'[M'''(SO_4)_2]\cdot 12H_2O$, which crystallize in the cubic system; also includes analogous compounds in which selenium replaces sulphur. 2. (BP 1958). Potassium alum or ammonium alum (see below). **Ammonioferric alum.** Iron ammonium alum, $NH_4Fe(SO_4)_2\cdot 12H_2O$, pale-violet crystals used as a reagent and indicator; a styptic and astringent. **Ammonium alum.** Ammonia alum, $NH_4Al(SO_4)_2\cdot 12H_2O$, white crystals used like potash alum; heating leaves a residue of pure alumina. **Ammonium chrome alum.** Ammonium chromium sulphate, $NH_4Cr(SO_4)_2\cdot 12H_2O$, violet crystals used for the same purposes as the potassium chrome alum. **Burnt alum.** Anhydrous potash alum made by calcining the latter; an astringent used as a dressing, also in water-softening. **Chrome alum.** Potassium chromium sulphate, $KCr(SO_4)_2\cdot 12H_2O$, deep-violet crystals used in tanning, and as a mordant in dyeing. **Common alum.** Potassium alum (see below). **Copper alum.** A mixture of potassium and copper sulphates with camphor and potassium nitrate, used as a caustic in ophthalmology. **Exsiccated alum.** Burnt alum (see above). **False alum.** Pseudo alum (see below). **Ferric alum.** Ammonioferric alum (see above). **Alum haematoxylin.** A solution of haematoxylin in potassium or ammonium alum, used as a stain in microscopy. **Iron alum.** Ammonioferric alum (see above). **Official alum.** Either potassium or ammonium alum. **Potassium alum.** Potash alum, common alum, $KAl(SO_4)_2\cdot 12H_2O$, colourless crystals with astringent properties; it precipitates colloids, and is used therefore as a styptic to check bleeding; also an antidote and emetic in lead-poisoning. **Potassium chrome alum.** Chrome alum (see above). **Pseudo alum.** A double sulphate of monovalent and divalent metals, such as ferrous ammonium sulphate, $FeSO_4(NH_4)_2SO_4\cdot 6H_2O$; not a true alum. **Roman alum.** A sulphate of iron and aluminium found free in Italy. **Sodium alum.** $NaAl(SO_4)_2\cdot 12H_2O$, similar to potash alum. **Alum whey.** An astringent and styptic made by the addition of alum to milk. [L *alumen*.]

alum-root (al·um root). Name applied to 2 roots, *Heuchera americana*, family Saxifragaceae, and *Geranium maculatum*, family Geraniaceae, both of which possess strongly astringent properties attributable to their tannin content. [alum, root.]

Alumen (al·ew·men). *European Pharmacopoeia* name for Alum BP 1973. **Alumen exsiccatum.** Burnt alum. *See* ALUM. [L.]

alumil (al·ew·mil). Aluminium hydroxide in acid solution.

alumina (al·ew·min·ah). Aluminium oxide, Al_2O_3. It occurs pure, as corundum, sapphire, ruby and topaz; also as the mineral bauxite. Used as an abrasive and refractory.

aluminated (al·ew·min·a′·ted). Charged or combined with alum.

aluminiferous (al·ew·min·if′·er·us). A substance productive of aluminium. [aluminium, L *ferre* to bear.]

aluminium (al·ew·min·e·um). An element of atomic weight 26.98, atomic number 13 and chemical symbol Al. It is a ductile and malleable white metal of low specific gravity, used for its lightness in domestic cooking ware, aircraft parts, artificial dentures, and surgical appliances and instruments; it forms light-weight alloys of high tensile strength. Occurring abundantly on the surface of the earth as silicates in rocks, slates and clays, it is rarely found in animal tissues, though all plants, especially mosses, contain minute amounts of the element. The metal remains unchanged in air but is rapidly affected by sea-water or alkalis; it is trivalent, forming salts which are mostly astringent. It is known in the USA as *aluminum*. **Aluminium acetate.** $(CH_3COO)_3Al$, an amorphous powder used in aqueous solution as an astringent. **Aluminium ammonium sulphate.** Ammonium alum, $(NH_4)Al(SO_4)_2\cdot 12H_2O$, a white powder with a sweet but astringent taste; 0.5–1.0 per cent solutions in water are used as astringent lotions or as haemostatics, stronger solutions being employed to harden the skin of tender feet and in the treatment of soft corns. **Aluminium carbonate.** $Al_2(CO_3)_3$, a chalk-like compound with mild antiseptic properties. **Aluminium chloride.** $AlCl_3$, a white hygroscopic powder which has been used in locomotor ataxia and also in dentistry. **Aluminium Clofibrate.** BP Commission approved name for di[2-(4-chlorophenoxy)-2-methylpropionato]-hydroxyaluminium; it is used in the treatment of arteriosclerosis. **Aluminium hydrate, Aluminium hydroxide.** $Al(OH)_3$, an odourless and tasteless white powder used as an antacid, particularly in peptic ulcer. It can be prepared in a colloidal state, in which form it acts as an antacid more by adsorption than by neutralization, with the advantage that it does not produce systemic alkalosis and is to some extent a protective and demulcent for the mucous membranes of the alimentary tract; its limited reaction with gastric juice results in the formation of aluminium chloride which is astringent and limits gastric secretion. It adsorbs toxins, gases and bacteria, but does not appear to affect enzymes as digestive processes are not inhibited. **Aluminium Hydroxide Gel BP 1973.** *See* GEL. **Aluminium Magnesium Silicate BPC 1968.** A native colloidal hydrated aluminium magnesium silicate (saponite), used pharmaceutically for its suspending, thickening and emulsion-stabilizing properties. **Aluminium oxide.** Alumina. **Aluminium phosphate.** $AlPO_4$, a compound used in the form of a gelatinous suspension for the treatment of peptic ulcers. Complete drying of the precipitated compound yields a fine insoluble powder which has no medicinal value. **Aluminium potassium sulphate.** Potassium alum, $KAl(SO_4)_2\cdot 12H_2O$, colourless crystals with astringent and styptic properties, used as an emetic in lead poisoning. **Aluminium silicate.** $Al_2O_3\cdot 2SiO_2\cdot 2H_2O$, occurs naturally as *kaolin*. It is a good adsorbent, and given internally will adsorb toxins and bacteria, also forming a protective coat over the gastric mucous membranes. Mixed with glycerin, methyl salicylate and certain volatile oils, it forms a stiff paste that is employed as a heat-retaining poultice. **Aluminium Sulphate BPC 1968.** $Al_2(SO_4)_3\cdot 18H_2O$, a very soluble salt of aluminium used in the preparation of aluminium hydroxide; its solution is more powerfully astringent than that of the alums. [L *alumen* alum.]

aluminoferric (al·ew·min·o·fer′·ik). A mixture of aluminium and ferrous sulphates used in the precipitation method of dealing with sewage.

aluminon (al·ew·min·on). Aurin tricarboxyllic acid. *See* AURIN.

aluminosis (al·ew·min·o′·sis). Fibrosis of the lungs caused by inhalation of aluminium dust. [aluminium, Gk *-osis* condition.]

aluminous (al·ew·min·us). 1. Pertaining to alum, alumina or aluminium. 2. Containing aluminium, as applied to minerals or chalybeate waters.

alundum (al·un·dum). Alumina fused in an electric furnace, and made into laboratory ware; also an abrasive powder.

alurate (al·ewr·ate). A barbiturate which has a moderate duration of action and is therefore suitable for the treatment of insomnia. It is more commonly used in the USA than in the UK. Mixed with amidopyrine it constitutes an analgesic hypnotic. **Sodium alurate, Soluble alurate.** The sodium salt employed as a pre-anaesthetic.

alusia (al·**ew**·se·ah). Hallucination. [Gk *alysis* wandering.]

alvearium, alveary (al·ve·a·re·um, al·ve·ar·e). The external auditory meatus. [L hollow vessel.]

alveated (al·ve·a·ted). Vaulted; honeycombed. [L *alveatus* hollowed out.]

alveo-algia (al·ve·o·**al**′·je·ah). Pain in the socket of a tooth after extraction of the tooth. Cf. SOCKET, DRY. [alveolus, Gk *algos* pain.]

alveobronchiolitis (al·ve·o·**brong**·ke·o·**li**′·tis). Inflammatory condition of the terminal bronchioles and alveoli; bronchopneumonia. [alveolus, bronchiolitis.]

alveola (al·**ve**·o·lah). In botany, a small depression on the surface of an organ. [L *alveolus* a little hollow.]

alveolar (al·**ve**·o·lar). Relating or belonging to an alveolus, or resembling an alveolus. **Alveolar air.** *See* AIR. **Alveolar arteries.** *See* MAXILLARY ARTERY. **Alveolar juga.** *See* JUGUM. **Alveolar process.** *See* PROCESS. **Alveolar structure.** *See* STRUCTURE.

alveolarium (al·ve·o·**la**′·re·um). The external auditory meatus. [L *alveolus* a little hollow.]

alveolate (al·**ve**·o·late). In botany, pitted in structure like a honeycomb. [see prec.]

alveolectomy (al·ve·o·**lek**′·to·me). Surgical excision of the whole or a part of the alveolar process. [alveolus, Gk *ektome* a cutting out.]

alveolingual (al·ve·o·**ling**′·gwal). Appertaining to the alveolar processes of the jaws and the tongue. [alveolus, L *lingua* tongue.]

alveolitis (al·ve·o·**li**′·tis). A condition of inflammation of an alveolus, as of a tooth. [alveolus, Gk *-itis* inflammation.]

alveoloclasia (al·ve·o·lo·**kla**′·ze·ah). Alveolar absorption, alveolar resorption; the resorption of the alveolar bone of the jaws. It may occur pathologically when teeth are present, producing looseness, but is a normal physiological process after their extraction. [alveolus, Gk *klasis* a breaking.]

alveolocondylean (al·ve·o·lo·kon·**di**′·le·an). 1. In craniometry, term applied to the plane passing through the alveolar point and the occipital condyles. 2. Belonging to the alveolus and condyle.

alveolodental (al·ve·o·lo·**den**′·tal). Relating or belonging to the teeth and the sockets of the teeth. [alveolus, L *dens* tooth.]

alveololabial (al·ve·o·lo·**la**′·be·al). Referring to the relation between the alveolar process and the lip. [alveolus, L *labium* lip.]

alveololabialis (al·ve·o·lo·la·be·**a**′·lis). The buccinator muscle. [see prec.]

alveololingual (al·ve·o·lo·**ling**′·gwal). Alveolingual.

alveolomaxillary (al·ve·o·lo·max·**il**′·ar·e). The buccinator muscle. [alveolus, maxilla.]

alveolomerotomy (al·ve·o·lo·mer·**ot**′·o·me). Surgical excision of a part of the alveolar process. [alveolus, Gk *meros* part, *temnein* to cut.]

alveolonasal (al·ve·o·lo·**na**′·zal). In craniometry, relating or belonging to the alveolar point and the nasion.

alveolopalatal (al·ve·o·lo·**pal**′·at·al). Relating or belonging to the palatal surface of the alveolar process of the maxilla.

alveolosubnasal (al·ve·o·lo·sub·**na**′·zal). In craniometry, relating or belonging to the alveolar point and the acanthion (subnasal point).

alveolotomy (al·ve·o·**lot**′·o·me). The surgical process of incising the alveolus of a tooth. [alveolus, Gk *temnein* to cut.]

alveolus [NA] (al·**ve**·o·lus). 1. That part of the bone of the jaw to which the teeth are attached; the alveolar bone. 2. A glandular acinus. 3. Any one of the air cells of the lungs. 4. Any one of the shallow depressions on the inner surface of the mucous coat of the stomach. **Pulmonary alveoli [alveoli pulmonis (NA)].** *See* 3rd def. above. [L a little hollow.]

alveolysis (al·ve·**ol**·is·is). The resorption of the alveolar bone supporting a tooth. [alveolus, Gk *lysis* a loosing.]

Alvergniat's pump. A mercurial blood-gas pump made about 1870 by Alvergniat Frères of Paris. Now of historical interest only.

Alves, William. 20th century London and Rhodesia parasitologist.

Alves' skin test. An intradermal test for schistosomiasis with a cercarial extract for antigen.

alveus (al·ve·us). A channel or groove. **Alveus cornu ammonis, Alveus hippocampi.** The layer of white fibres on the ventricular surface of the hippocampus; they form a groove or channel in which the hippocampus lies, and constitute its efferent pathway, continued as the fimbria and fornix. **Alveus urogenitalis.** The prostatic utricle. *See* UTRICLE. [L trough.]

alvine (al·vine). Of, from or relating to the abdomen or its contents. [L *alvus* belly.]

alvinolith (al·vi·no·lith). A concretion formed in the intestine from various debris, including lime salts, oatmeal and other food constituents. [L *alvus* belly, Gk *lithos* stone.]

alvus (al·vus). The abdomen together with the organs contained in its cavity. [L.]

alymphia (a·**lim**·fe·ah). Entire lack or deficient quantity of lymph. [Gk *a*, lymph.]

alymphocytosis (a·**lim**·fo·si·**to**′·sis). A condition of the blood in which only a very few lymphocytes, or none at all, are present. [Gk *a*, lymphocytosis.]

alymphopotent (a·lim·fo·**po**′·tent). Not able to form lymphocytes. [Gk *a*, lymph, L *potens* able.]

alysmus (a·**lis**·mus). The feeling of anxiety and restlessness which naturally accompanies physical diseases. [Gk *alysmos* disquiet.]

alysosis (al·is·o·sis). Boredom. [Gk *alys* boredom, *-osis* condition.]

alyssous (a·**lis**·us). Against rabies; applied to prevention and supposed cures. [Gk *a*, *lyssa* raging madness.]

Alzheimer, Alois (b. 1864). Breslau neurologist.

Alzheimer's baskets. In senile dementia, any one of the concentrations of intracellular neurofibrils.

Alzheimer's cell. A degenerated astrocyte.

Alzheimer's dementia, Alzheimer's disease. A form of presenile dementia. It is characterized by memory failure for recent events, and lack of spontaneous activity and initiative. Extrapyramidal and akinetic hypertonic symptoms occur. Loss of spatial orientation is common. After 2 or 3 years dementia becomes well established and focal symptoms, such as aphasia, apraxia and agnosia, occur. The average duration of the disease is about 7 years.

Alzheimer's sclerosis. Degeneration of the smaller cerebral blood vessels with mental symptoms.

Alzheimer stain. A methyl blue, eosin mixture used for the demonstration of certain types of cytoplasmic granules.

Alzheimer's syndrome. Alzheimer's disease (see above).

ama (a·mah). A distension of a semicircular canal in the bony labyrinth of the ear at the end away from the ampulla. [L vessel.]

amaas (**ah**·mahs). Alastrim or variola minor. [Kaffir sour milk.]

amacrinal (a·**mak**·rin·al). Having the nature of an amacrine.

amacrine (am·ak·rin). In histology, pertaining to nerve cells without processes, such as have been thought to exist in the retina. [Gk *a*, *makros* long, *is* fibre.]

amalgam (am·al·gam). 1. An alloy of mercury with a metal. 2. A combination of one or more metals with mercury. Such an amalgam may vary in consistency from a buttery mass to metallic hardness, and is used in dentistry to fill prepared cavities. **Amalgam carrier.** An instrument for conveying mixed amalgam to a cavity prepared in a tooth. **Copper amalgam.** An amalgam of copper used in the restoration of deciduous teeth affected by caries. It is considered to have some bacteriostatic effect. **Dental amalgam.** A combination of a silver-tin alloy, together with traces of other metals such as copper and zinc, which are amalgamated to a rapidly setting plastic mass by trituration with a measured quantity of mercury; commonly used to restore the effects of caries in posterior teeth. **Amalgam die.** The model made in amalgam of a cavity prepared in a tooth, on which an inlay which is to be fixed in the tooth is constructed.

Amalgam matrix band. A thin metal strip held in position around a tooth by a matrix band holder while a cavity involving the interstitial surface of a tooth is being filled with amalgam. **Amalgam mixer.** A pestle and mortar or an electrically-operated apparatus in which a dental amalgam is combined with mercury prior to insertion in a cavity prepared in a tooth. **Amalgam plugger.** A flat-faced serrated instrument used for condensing amalgam in a cavity prepared in a tooth. **Amalgam tattoo.** Blue-black pigmentation within the mouth, usually of the gums, from particles of silver amalgam deposited in the subepithelial connective tissue during filling of a tooth or during the extraction of a filled tooth. [Gk *malagma* emollient.]

amalgamable (am·al·gam·abl). Describing any metal that can be combined with mercury to form an amalgam.

amalgamate (am·al·gam·ate). To form an amalgam; to triturate a metal with mercury causing them to combine and produce an amalgam.

amalgamation (am·al·gam·a·shun). The combination of a metal or metals with mercury to form an amalgam.

amalgamator (am·al·gam·a·tor). A mechanical apparatus for facilitating the amalgamation of a metal or metals with mercury.

amandin (am·an·din). A globulin, obtained from the kernels of fruits such as the sweet almond. [Fr. *amande* almond.]

Amanita (am·an·e·tah). A large genus of fungi, some species of which are edible. **Amanita muscaria.** The fly agaric; a mushroom which is poisonous, containing muscarine. **Amanita phalloides.** The death-head; a very poisonous mushroom. **Amanita rubescens.** A species of mushroom held to be edible. **Amanita verna.** The fool's mushroom; a poisonous mushroom. **Amanita virosa.** The destroying angel; a poisonous mushroom. [Gk *amanitai* a fungus.]

amanitine (am·an·it·een). 1. A poisonous alkaloid, $(CH_3)_3N(OH)CHOHCH_3$, closely related to neurine, and obtained from species of the fungus *Amanita.* 2. A poisonous alkaloid, $(CH_3)_3N(OH)CH_2CH_2OH$, isomeric with choline, and occurring in fly agaric, *Amanita muscaria*; oxidized, it yields muscarine.

amanitotoxin (am·an·it·o·tox'·in). A poisonous protein in the death-head fungus, *Amanita phalloides.* [*Amanita,* Gk *toxikon* poison.]

amantadine (am·an·tad·een). 1-Adamantanamine hydrochloride, $C_{10}H_{17}NHCl$; a compound which has been used in prophylaxis against influenza A virus. Some reduction in the severity of symptoms has been observed and also in incidence after prophylactic administration of the drug. It is also used in Parkinsonism.

Amaranth BPC 1954 (am·ar·anth). A harmless red dye synthesized from naphthionic acid; it is $NaSO_3C_{10}H_6N{=}NC_{10}H_4(SO_3Na)_2OH$, and is used to colour foodstuffs and medicines. [Gk *a, marainein* to wither.]

amaril (am·ar·il). Yellow fever. *See* FEVER. [Sp. *amarillo* yellow.]

amarilla (am·ar·il·ah). The international nomenclature for yellow fever. *See* FEVER. [Sp. yellow.]

amarine (am·ar·een). Dihydrotriphenyliminazole, $C_6H_5CH{=}(NHCC_6H_5)_2$. A poisonous substance found in bitter almonds. [L *amarus* bitter.]

amaroid (am·ar·oid). General term applied to bitter substances occurring in plants; it does not include the alkaloids, glucosides, or tannins. [L *amarus* bitter, Gk *eidos* form.]

amaroidal (am·ar·oi·dal). 1. Rather bitter. 2. Of the nature of a bitter principle (amaroid). [see prec.]

amarthritis (am·ar·thri·tis). A condition of inflammation affecting several joints at the same time; polyarthritis. [Gk *ama* together, arthritis.]

amasesis (am·as·e·sis). Inability to masticate food. [Gk *a, masesis* chewing.]

amastia (a·mas·te·ah). The condition in which the breasts or nipples are lacking. [Gk *a, mastos* breast.]

amathophobia (am·ath·o·fo'·be·ah). Morbid fear of dust. [Gk *amathos* sand, phobia.]

amativeness (am·at·iv·nes). Propensity to love. [L *amare* to love.]

Amato, Alessandro (b. 1879). Italian pathologist.

Amato bodies. Cytoplasmic degenerations or particles occurring as small irregular blue clumps in the cytoplasm of polymorphonuclear leucocytes as a result of scarlet fever; they were once thought to be inclusion bodies. Also known as *Amato inclusion bodies.*

amatol (am·at·ol). An explosive, consisting of a mixture of trinitrotoluene and ammonium nitrate.

amaurosis (am·aw·ro·sis). Blindness, without any demonstrable lesion of the eye. **Albuminuric amaurosis.** Amaurosis caused by renal disease. **Amaurosis arthritica.** Amaurosis caused by gout. **Amaurosis atonica.** Amaurosis which is the result of physical debility. **Cat's-eye amaurosis.** Blindness of the eye with bright reflection from the pupil due to a white mass in the vitreous which may be inflammatory or neoplastic, the latter usually arising from retinoblastoma. **Central amaurosis.** That caused by disease of the central nervous system. **Cerebral amaurosis.** Amaurosis caused by disease of the cerebrum. **Compression amaurosis.** Amaurosis resulting from pressure on the optic nerve. **Congenital amaurosis.** Amaurosis present from birth. **Congestive amaurosis.** That caused by or associated with cerebral congestion. **Diabetic amaurosis.** Amaurosis occurring in diabetes mellitus. **Dimidiate amaurosis.** Amaurosis which occurs in only one half of the visual field. **Eclamptic amaurosis.** That coming on in pregnancy and associated with eclampsia. **Epileptiform amaurosis, Epileptoid amaurosis.** Blindness following an epileptic attack, and lasting for a few days or weeks. It is commoner in children and is ascribed to postepileptic exhaustion or anaesthesia of the cortex. Also blindness associated with attacks not truly epileptic. **Amaurosis with excavation.** Pseudoglaucoma. **Amaurosis fugax.** Fleeting blindness due to vascular insufficiency of the retina or optic nerve, usually due to carotid disease. **Amaurosis ex haemorrhagia.** Sudden incurable blindness that occurs after harmorrhages, especially of the stomach, commonly bilateral; rare. **Hysterical amaurosis.** Amaurosis associated with a condition of hysteria. **Amaurosis intermittens larvata.** Unilateral blindness associated with intermittent fever of mild type and often resulting in atrophy of the optic nerve. **Intermittent amaurosis.** Bilateral amaurosis associated with intermittent fever. **Intoxication amaurosis.** That caused by systemic poisoning due to drug addiction or to alcohol. **Amaurosis partialis fugax.** Sudden attacks of transitory blindness with vertigo, headache, scintillations, nausea and scotomas. **Progressive amaurosis.** Gradually increasing blindness as in cases of chronic glaucoma. **Quinine amaurosis.** Blindness resulting from the taking of excessive amounts of quinine; it has occurred on rare occasions in sensitive persons, taking quinine in pharmacopoeial doses. **Rachialgic amaurosis.** Spinal amaurosis (see below). **Reflex amaurosis.** Amaurosis caused by the reflex action of some distant stimulus on the retina, the optic nerve or its connections. **Saburral amaurosis.** Transient blindness which occurs suddenly during an attack of acute gastritis. **Simulation amaurosis.** The blindness that is put on by malingerers. **Spasmodic amaurosis.** Amaurosis originating in convulsions. **Spinal amaurosis.** That due to atrophy of the optic nerve caused by an affection originating in the spine, such as lateral or disseminated sclerosis. **Sympathetic amaurosis.** The end result of sympathetic ophthalmitis. **Toxic amaurosis.** Blindness due to poisons which may be endogenous, e.g. diabetes, or exogenous, e.g. tobacco, or alcohol. **Uraemia amaurosis of pregnancy.** Eclamptic amaurosis (see above). **Uraemic amaurosis.** Blindness of fairly rapid onset in cases of uraemia, due to a cortical origin and not to any retinopathy which may be present. [Gk *amauroein* to darken.]

See also: BURNS (J.).

amaurotic (am·aw·rot·ik). 1. Of the nature of or relating to amaurosis. 2. Suffering from amaurosis. **Amaurotic family idiocy.** *See* IDIOCY and TAY, WARREN.

amaxophobia (am·ax·o·fo'·be·ah). Morbid dread of riding in a vehicle or of meeting one. [Gk *amaxa* wagon, phobia.]

amazia (a·ma·ze·ah). Amastia. [see foll.]
amazon (am·az·on). An individual without breasts. [Gk *a*, *mazos* breast.]
Ambazone (am·bah·zone). BP Commission approved name for 1,4-benzoquinone amidinohydrazine thiosemicarbazone hydrate; it is used in the treatment of infections of the mouth.
Ambenonium Chloride (am·ben·o·ne·um·klor·ide). BP Commission approved name for *N,N′*-di-(2-diethylaminoethyl)oxamide bis-2-chlorobenzylochloride; a cholinesterase inhibitor.
Ambenoxan (am·ben·ox·an). BP Commission approved name for 2-(2-methoxyethoxyethylaminomethyl)-1,4-benzodioxan; a muscle relaxant.
amber (am·ber). Amber succinum; a fossilized resin. **Oil of amber.** Oleum Succini BPC 1949. [Ar. *'anbar* ambergris.]
Amberg, Emil (b. 1868). Detroit surgeon.
Amberg's line. A surface marking which outlines an approach to the lateral sinus; it is a line dividing the angle formed by the anterior border of the mastoid process and the temporal line.
ambergris (am·ber·gris). An opaque, grey, waxlike mass of biliary or intestinal origin, obtained from the sperm whale; it is sometimes ejected and is then found floating in the sea. Formerly used as a stimulant in low fevers and in nervous affections, now only of value in perfumery manufacture. [Ar. *'anbar* ambergris, Fr. *gris* grey.]
ambidexter (am·be·dex·ter). An individual who can use one hand as effectively as the other. [L *ambo* both, *dexter* right.]
ambidexterity (am·be·dex·ter′·it·e). The faculty of being ambidextrous.
ambidextrous (am·be·dex·trus). Able to use both hands with equal facility. [L *ambo* both, *dexter* right.]
ambilaevous (am·be·le·vus). Unable to use either hand effectively. [L *ambo* both, *laevus* left.]
ambilateral (am·be·lat·er·al). Affecting or relating to both sides. [L *ambo* both, lateral.]
ambiocularity (am·be·ok·ew·lar·it·e). The condition of having equal use of both eyes. [L *ambo* both, *oculus* eye.]
ambiopia (am·be·o·pe·ah). A disorder of sight in which a single object is seen either as double or as 2 single objects; diplopia. [L *ambo* both, Gk *ops* eye.]
ambisexual (am·be·sex·ew·al). Affecting or relating to both sexes; bisexual. [L *ambo* both, sex.]
ambisinister, ambisinistrous (am·be·sin·is·ter, am·be·sin·is·trus). Clumsy. Not having skilled use of either hand; ambilaevus. [L *ambo* both, *sinister* left.]
ambitendency (am·be·ten·den·se). The state in which a tendency is accompanied by a corresponding counter-tendency. [L *ambo* both, *tendere* to direct a course.]
ambivalence, ambivalency (am·biv·al·ens, am·biv·al·en·se). In psychology, the property of being able to respond equally well to 2 opposing impulses. [L *ambo* both, *valentia* strength.]
ambivalent (am·biv·al·ent). 1. Having equal power in opposite directions. 2. *Genetic.* Genes with both advantageous and disadvantageous action. **Ambivalent emotions.** In psychology, emotions of opposite character felt for the same person, e.g. love and hate. [see prec.]
ambiversion (am·be·ver·shun). The property of being midway between extroversion and introversion in personality type. [L *ambo* both, *vertere* to turn.]
ambivert (am·be·vert). In psychology, an individual who is as much introverted as extroverted; an intermediate type. [see prec.]
ambloma (am·blo·mah). 1. An abortion. 2. An aborted fetus. [see foll.]
amblosis (am·blo·sis). Abortion. [Gk.]
amblotic (am·blot·ik). An agent or a drug which brings about abortion; abortifacient. [see prec.]
amblyacousia, amblyacusia (am·ble·ak·oo′·se·ah, am·ble·ak·ew′·ze·ah). Blunted or dulled auditory sense. [Gk *amblys* dull, *akousis* hearing.]
amblyaphia (am·ble·af·e·ah). Lack of acuteness in the sense of touch. [Gk *amblys* dull, *haphe* touch.]
amblychromasia (am·ble·kro·ma′·ze·ah). A condition of cells in which, since there is little chromatin, they stain only faintly. [Gk *amblys* dull, *chroma* colour.]
amblychromatic (am·ble·kro·mat′·ik). Staining only faintly. [see prec.]
amblygeustia (am·ble·gew·ste·ah). Lack of acuteness of the sense of taste. [Gk *amblys* dull, *geusis* taste.]
amblykusis (am·ble·kew·sis). Dulled auditory sense; amblyacousia. [Gk *amblys* dull, *akousis* hearing.]
Amblyomma (am·ble·om·ah). Acarina; a genus of ticks, several species of which are carriers of rickettsial fevers. Some species can transmit tularaemia under laboratory conditions. **Amblyomma americanum.** The lone-star tick of southern United States, a vector of tick-borne typhus and possibly of Bullis fever. **Amblyomma brasiliense.** A vector of tick-borne typhus. **Amblyomma cajennense.** Of tropical Africa, a vector of Rocky Mountain spotted fever and other tick-borne rickettsioses. **Amblyomma hebraeum.** The bont tick of South Africa, a vector of tick-borne typhus. **Amblyomma longirostrum.** A potential vector of American trypanosomiasis. **Amblyomma maculatum.** Of Florida and the Gulf states, an important carrier of screw-worm eggs, may also transmit Q fever. **Amblyomma ovale.** A South American species suspected as a vector of mucocutaneous leishmaniasis. **Amblyomma striatum.** A species found in South America, a vector of Rocky Mountain spotted fever and other tick-borne rickettsioses. [Gk *amblys* dull, *omma* eye.]
amblyope (am·ble·ope). An individual suffering from amblyopia.
amblyopia (am·ble·o·pe·ah). Diminished visual form sense, without structural abnormality of the visual pathway and uncorrectable by optical means. **Alcoholic amblyopia.** Deterioration of vision resulting from alcoholic poisoning. **Amblyopia ex anopsia.** An old term which includes stimulus deprivation amblyopia and strabismic amblyopia (see below). **Ammetropic amblyopia.** Bilateral amblyopia due to uncorrected refractive error. **Anisometropic amblyopia.** Uni-ocular amblyopia due to unequal refractive errors of the two eyes. **Arsenic amblyopia.** Impairment of vision occasioned by arsenical poisoning. **Astigmatic amblyopia.** Dimness of vision resulting from astigmatism. **Colour amblyopia.** Colour blindness. *See* BLINDNESS. **Crapulous amblyopia.** Alcoholic amblyopia (see above). **Hysterical amblyopia.** Amblyopia associated with a condition of hysteria. **Nocturnal amblyopia.** Diminished ability to see after dark. **Postmarital amblyopia.** That due to debilitation caused by sexual excess (Burns' amaurosis). **Quinine amblyopia.** Dimness of vision as a result of taking large amounts of quinine, which causes anaemia of the retina. **Reflex amblyopia.** A form caused by peripheral irritation. **Stimulus deprivation amblyopia.** Amblyopia due to inadequate visual stimuli and which is unrelieved by the correction of any optical error. **Strabismic amblyopia.** Amblyopia due to squint. **Tobacco amblyopia.** That due to tobacco smoking in a highly susceptible person. **Toxic amblyopia.** Partial loss of sight due to the action of toxins, which may be endogenous, e.g. diabetes, or exogenous, e.g. tobacco, or alcohol. **Traumatic amblyopia.** That resulting from an injury. **Uraemic amblyopia.** Partial blindness which may occur during an attack of uraemia. [Gk *amblys* dull, *ops* eye.]
amblyopiatrics (am·ble·o·pe·at′·rix). The system of treatment of amblyopia. [amblyopia, Gk *iatrikos* healing.]
amblyoscope (am·ble·o·skope). An instrument for training an amblyopic eye so that it may share equally with the other eye in binocular vision; it is a form of reflecting stereoscope. Two pictures are presented to the 2 eyes, by 2 tubes; the angle between these tubes can be varied both horizontally and vertically. By this means, the subjective angle of squint can be measured, the state of the binocular vision investigated and exercises carried out to improve the binocular vision. The original instrument was invented by Claud Worth in 1901: the modern counterpart is very much more complex and the types in common use are the *major amblyoscope*, the *synoptophore* and the *synoptoscope*. They are the main instruments used in orthoptic treatment. [amblyopia, Gk *skopein* to watch.]

Amblystoma (am·**blis**·to·mah). A genus of salamanders of America and Asia; the neotenous forms are called *axolotl.* [Gk *amblys* blunt, *stoma* mouth.]

ambo (**am**·bo). Ambon.

amboceptoid (am·bo·**sep**·toid). A modified amboceptor which has lost one of its elements, the cytophil group, whilst retaining the complementophil group. [amboceptor, Gk *eidos* form.]

amboceptor (am·bo·**sep**·tor). Obsolete term for complement-fixing antibody whose reaction with antigen results in lysis of target cells. **Bactericidal amboceptor.** Bactericidin, an amboceptor concerned in killing bacteria. **Bacteriolytic amboceptor.** Bacteriolysin, an amboceptor taking part in the lysis of bacteria. **Haemolytic amboceptor.** Haemolysin, an amboceptor taking part in the lysis of red blood corpuscles. [L *ambo* both, *capere* to take.]

See also: BORDET.

amboceptorgen (am·bo·**sep**·tor·jen). An antigen which causes *in vivo* the production of amboceptor. [amboceptor, Gk *genein* to produce.]

ambomalleal (am·bo·**mal**·e·al). Relating to the incus and the malleus of the ear. [Gk *ambos* anvil, malleus.]

ambon (**am**·bon). The fibrocartilaginous ring which surrounds an articular cavity occupied by the head of a long bone. [Gk a raised stage.]

ambos (**am**·bos). The incus. [Gk anvil.]

ambosexual (am·bo·**sex**·ew·al). Affecting or relating to both sexes; bisexual. [L *ambo* both, sex.]

ambotoxoid (am·bo·**tox**·oid). An immunizing agent prepared by the admixture of killed bacteria, e.g. staphylococci, with the toxin produced by them, after the latter has been rendered non-poisonous. [L *ambo* both, Gk *toxikon* poison, *eidos* form.]

ambrain, ambrein (**am**·bra·in, **am**·bre·in). Ambrin.

ambrin (**am**·brin). A sterol, closely related to cholesterol, and found in ambergris.

Ambrosia (am·**bro**·ze·ah). The ragweeds, a genus of composite-flowered plants, the airborne pollens of which may give rise to hay fever, also dermatitis on exposed areas and around the collar line, waist and ankles. The common ragweed and the giant ragweed (*Ambrosia artemisiaefolia* and *Ambrosia trifida*) are used as febrifuges and anthelmintics. [Gk *ambrotos* immortal.]

ambrosin (am·**bro**·sin). The substance present in ragweed pollens (*Ambrosia*) which causes hay fever in the autumn.

ambrosterol (am·bro·**steer**·ol). A sterol, $C_{20}H_{34}O$, in the pollen of species of *Ambrosia*, and perhaps responsible for the hay fever caused by the latter.

Ambucetamide (am·bew·**set**·am·ide). BP Commission approved name for α-dibutylamino-4-methoxyphenylacetamide; an antispasmodic.

ambulant, ambulatory (**am**·bew·lant, am·bew·**la**·tor·e). Walking; not confined to bed. [L *ambulare* to walk about.]

Ambuside (**am**·bew·side). BP Commission approved name for 5 - allylsulphamoyl - 2 - chloro - 4 - (3-hydroxybut - 2 - enylidene-amino)benzenesulphonamide; a diuretic.

Ambutonium Bromide (am·bew·**to**·ne·um **bro**·mide). BP Commission approved name for (3-carbamoyl-3,3-diphenylpropyl) ethyldimethyl-ammonium bromide.

ameiosis (a·mi·o·sis). Nuclear division replacing the 2 divisions characteristic of meiosis and failing to produce chromosome reduction. [Gk *a*, *meiosis* diminution.]

ameleia (am·el·i·ah). A state of indifference or apathy as part of a psychosis. [Gk indifference.]

amelia (a·**me**·le·ah). 1. Absence of the limbs. 2. Complete absence of the distal part of a limb. [Gk *a*, *melos* limb.]

amelification (am·el·if·ik·a′·shun). The process by which ameloblasts form dental enamel. [OFr. *amel* enamel, L *facere* to make.]

ameloblast (am·**el**·o·blast). A tall columnar epithelial cell of ectodermal origin which secretes dental enamel, and is derived from the inner layer of the enamel organ. Each cell is responsible for the formation of 1 enamel prism. [OFr. *amel* enamel, Gk *blastos* germ.]

ameloblastoma (am·**el**·o·blas·**to′**·mah). Adamantinoma; a monocystic or more commonly polycystic tumour occurring in the jaws, especially the lower molar region. It is derived from tooth-forming epithelial cells or the basal layer of the oral epithelium, and is treated by radical excision. **Melanotic ameloblastoma.** A benign tumour occurring in infancy, usually in the anterior part of the maxilla as a pigmented mass. It has also been reported in the anterior fontanelle, shoulder, mediastinum and epididymis. It is probably derived from the neural crest. [ameloblast, Gk *-oma* tumour.]

amelodentinal (**am**·el·o·**den′**·tin·al). Appertaining to enamel and dentine. [OFr. *amel* enamel, dentine.]

amelogenesis (**am**·el·o·**jen′**·es·is). The production of tooth enamel. **Amelogenesis imperfecta.** Either hereditary enamel hypoplasia, in which much of the enamel is missing and the teeth are rapidly worn down, or hereditary enamel hypocalcification, where there are areas of confluent pitting or complete loss of enamel. [OFr. *amel* enamel, Gk *genein* to produce.]

amelus (a·**me**·lus). A monster lacking legs or arms. [Gk *a*, *melos* limb.]

amenia (am·**e**·ne·ah). Amenorrhoea. [Gk *a*, *men* month.]

amenorrhoea (am·en·or·**e**·ah). The pathological absence or stoppage of the menstrual discharge from the uterus for reasons other than pregnancy, lactation or the menopause, all of which are purely physiological. **Absolute amenorrhoea.** Primary amenorrhoea (see below). **Emotional amenorrhoea.** That due to psychological disturbance. **Ovarian amenorrhoea.** Amenorrhoea due to ovarian disease or abnormality. **Pathological amenorrhoea.** Amenorrhoea due to disease. **Physiological amenorrhoea.** The normal state of freedom from the menses, such as before puberty, during pregnancy and lactation, and after the menopause. **Pituitary amenorrhoea.** Amenorrhoea due to pituitary disease or dysfunction. **Primary amenorrhoea.** The non-appearance of the menses, an uncommon condition usually due to congenital defect in the organs connected with menstruation. **Secondary amenorrhoea.** The suspension of the menses after they have once been established; it may be caused by illness, change in environment, or the removal or irradiation of the uterus or ovaries. [Gk *a*, *men* month, *rhoia* to flow.]

amenorrhoeal (am·en·or·**e**·al). Caused or accompanied by, or relating to, amenorrhoea.

ament (**a**·ment). An individual suffering from amentia; an imbecile.

amentia (a·**men**·she·ah). An arrest of the development of the mind from birth to early age. It is synonymous with gross mental deficiency, mental retardation and subnormality. **Naevoid amentia.** Weber's disease; amentia associated with a naevoid condition of the face and scalp, cerebral calcification and glaucoma. **Phenylpyruvic amentia.** A specific form of inherited imbecility, due to an autosomal recessive gene, which is characterized by the appearance of phenylpyruvic acid in the urine. [Gk *a*, L *mens* mind.]

americium (am·er·**is**·e·um). A transuranic element of atomic number 95 and chemical symbol Am. It was synthesized in 1944 by the cyclotronic bombardment of uranium-238 with high energy α-particles, and has a half-life of 500 years. [America.]

amerisia (a·mer·**iz**·e·ah). A form of aphasia in which there is difficulty in enunciation or in forming letters or words in writing. [see foll.]

amerism (**am**·er·izm). The quality of being unable to split into fragments or segments. [Gk *a*, *meros* part.]

ameristic (am·er·**is**·tik). Undifferentiated; not split into fragments. [see prec.]

amesiality (am·e·ze·**al′**·it·e). The impulsion of a part of the body to one side of the mesial line, with resultant asymmetry. [Gk *a*, *mesos* middle.]

ametabolic (a·met·ab·**ol′**·ik). Not causing metabolism and not due to it. [Gk *a*, metabolism.]

ametabolon (a·met·**ab**·o·lon). An animal in which the adult form differs from the newly-born young only in size and sexual maturity; more usually applied to an insect such as the silver fish, which does not undergo metamorphosis. [Gk *a, metabole* change.]

ametabolous (a·met·**ab**·ol·us). Ametabolic.

ametachromophil (a·met·a·**kro**′·mo·fil). Staining normally with neutral dyes; orthochromophil. [Gk *a*, metachromophil.]

ametamorphosis (a·met·a·**mor**′·fo·sis). 1. A state of abstraction and absorption due to excessive mental activity. 2. The condition in which the shape, structure or function remains unchanged. [Gk *a*, metamorphosis.]

ametaneutrophil, ametaneutrophile (a·met·ah·**new**·tro·fil, a·met·ah·**new**·tro·file). Staining normally with neutral dyes, e.g. normal neutrophil leucocytes. [Gk *a*, metaneutrophil.]

Ametazole (a·met·ah·zole). BP Commission approved name for 3-(2-aminoethyl)pyrazole; it is used to stimulate gastric secretion in diagnostic tests.

Amethocaine Hydrochloride BP 1973 (**am**·eth·o·kane hi·dro·**klor**·ide). Tetracaine hydrochloride, $C_4H_9NHC_6H_4COO(CH_2)_2N(CH_3)_2HCl$. A synthetic local analgesic of the procaine type.

ametria (a·**met**·re·ah). Congenital absence of the uterus. [Gk *a, metra* womb.]

ametrohaemia (a·met·ro·**he**′·me·ah). Absence or defect of the blood supply to the uterus. [Gk *a, metra* womb, *haima* blood.]

ametrometer (a·met·**rom**·et·er). An instrument with which the degree of ametropia can be measured.

ametrope (a·met·rope). A person suffering from ametropia.

ametropia (a·met·**ro**·pe·ah). A condition in which there is abnormality of the refractive powers of the eye; parallel rays are not correctly focused on the retina, but either behind it (hypermetropia), in front of it (myopia) or diffused over an area (astigmatism). **Axial ametropia.** That caused by lengthening of the eyeball on the optic axis. **Curvature ametropia.** Ametropia resulting from inequalities in the curvature of the eye's surface. **Index ametropia.** That caused by changes in the refracting media. **Position ametropia.** Ametropia resulting when the lens is in an abnormal position. **Refractive ametropia.** That caused by a faulty dioptric system of the eye. [Gk *ametros* irregular, *opsis* sight.]

ametropic (a·met·**ro**·pik). Affected with or relating to ametropia.

ametrous (a·**met**·rus). Being without a uterus. [Gk *a, metra* womb.]

Amfecloral (am·fe·**klor**·al). BP Commission approved name for α-methyl-*N*-(2,2,2-trichloroethylidene)-phenethylamine; an appetite suppressant.

amianthinopsy (**am**·e·an·thin·**op**′·se). Lack of ability to distinguish the colour violet; violet-ray blindness. [Gk *a, ianthinos* violet, *opsis* sight.]

amianthoid (am·e·**an**·thoid). Descriptive of degenerated fibres found in broken-down laryngeal and costal cartilage; these fibres resemble asbestos. [Gk *amiantos* asbestos, *eidos* form.]

amianthosis (**am**·e·an·**tho**′·sis). A form of pneumoconiosis affecting those who work with asbestos; it is caused by breathing-in minute particles of the substance, which lodge in the respiratory passages, particularly the lungs; asbestosis. [Gk *amiantos* asbestos.]

amic (**am**·ik). Having the characteristics of ammonia; derived from ammonia.

Amici, Giovanni Battista (b. 1784). Italian astronomer and microscopist.

Amici's disc, line or stria. The dark band hemisecting the light isotropic band of a striated muscle fibre and separating adjacent sarcomeres. Also known as *Krause's membrane.*

amicrobic (a·mi·**kro**·bik). Not caused by or related to microbes. [Gk *a*, microbe.]

amicron, amicrone (a·**mi**·kron, a·**mi**·krone). A particle which is beyond the range of the ultramicroscope, of the order of 10^{-8} mm. [Gk *a*, micron.]

amicroscopic (a·mi·kro·**skop**′·ik). Too small to be visible with the highest power of a microscope. [Gk *a*, microscope.]

amidase (**am**·id·aze). A hydrolytic and deamidizing enzyme which opens C–N linkages and usually, as in the case of urease, splits off ammonia.

amide (**am**·ide). A compound formed from an organic acid by the substitution of an amido group, NH_2, for the hydroxyl of the carboxyl COOH group; ammonia in which an acyl group has replaced a hydrogen atom; a primary amide. **Nicotinic acid amide.** Nicotinamide. **Secondary amide.** Ammonia in which 2 acyl groups have replaced 2 hydrogen atoms; an imide. **Tertiary amide.** Ammonia with all 3 hydrogen atoms replaced by acyl groups. Cf AMINE. [sal *am*moniac, ox*ide*.]

Amidephrine (am·id·**ef**·reen). BP Commission approved name for 3-(1-hydroxy-2-methylaminoethyl)-methanesulphonanilide; a vasoconstrictor and nasal decongestant.

amidin (**am**·id·in). The soluble carbohydrate within the starch granule, and released when the starch is treated with boiling water; it is the precursor of maltose. Also known as *granulose, soluble-starch* or *amylose*. Cf. AMYLIN. [Fr. *amidon* starch.]

amidine (**am**·id·een). A compound containing both amino $-NH_2$ and imino =NH groups, attached to the same carbon atom; an amide in which the oxygen of the acid group is replaced by an imino =NH group.

amido group (**am**·id·o groop). The monovalent radical, NH_2, when replacing the hydroxyl of the carboxyl COOH group in an organic acid to form an amide; the group $-CONH_2$. Cf. AMINO GROUP. [sal *am*moniac, ox*ide*.]

amidoazotoluene (**am**·id·o·az·o·**tol**′·ew·een). Aminoazotoluene.

amidobenzene (**am**·id·o·**ben**′·zeen). Aminobenzene.

amidocephalin (**am**·id·o·**kef**′·al·in). An aminated cephalin found in brain and nerve tissue.

amidogen (**am**·id·o·jen). The monovalent radical NH_2, which enters into combination to form amides. [amide, Gk *genein* to produce.]

amidoguaiacol (**am**·id·o·**gwi**′·ak·ol). $C_6H_3(OH)(NH_2)OCH_3$. Prepared from acetanisidin, it is used in medicine as an antiseptic.

amidohexose (**am**·id·o·**hex**′·oze). An aldohexose into which an amido group has been introduced.

amidol (**am**·id·ol). $(NH_2)_2C_6H_3OHHCl$, used as a photographic developer, and also as a hair-dye.

amidomyelin (**am**·id·o·**mi**′·el·in). A lipoid substance containing amino nitrogen, and occurring in nerve tissue.

amidone hydrochloride (**am**·id·one hi·dro·**klor**·ide). Methadone hydrochloride.

amidopurine (**am**·id·o·**pewr**′·een). Aminopurine.

Amidopyrine BPC 1954 (**am**·id·o·**pi**′·reen). Aminopyrine, dimethylaminophenyldimethylpyrazolone, dimethylamino-antipyrine, $C_{13}H_{17}N_3O$. A white compound, fairly soluble in water, used as an analgesic and antipyretic in acute pyrexial conditions, and in the treatment of sciatica, neuralgia and migraine; continued use may lead to agranulocytosis. **Amidopyrine poisoning.** *See* POISONING.

amidoxime (am·id·**ox**·ime). One of a number of organic compounds formed by the replacement of the hydrogen of the imino group NH, of an amidine, with a hydroxyl OH group; a compound containing the group $-C(NOH)NH_2$.

amidoxyl (am·id·**ox**·il). Any compound derived from hydroxylamine, and containing the group –NHOH.

amidulin (am·**id**·ew·lin). Soluble starch, formerly called *granulose*; a tasteless granular substance liberated from the starch envelope by cold mineral acids. It is soluble in water, forming a dextrorotatory non-reducing solution that produces a characteristic blue additive compound with iodine. [Fr. *amidon* starch.]

Amiloride (am·il·or·ide). BP Commission approved name for *N*-amidino-3,5-diamino-6-chloropyrazinamide; a diuretic.

amimia (a·**mim**·e·ah). Loss of the power of imitation and of that of expression by the medium of sign and gesture. **Amnesic amimia.** A condition in which, although gestures or signs can be made, their meaning has been forgotten. **Ataxic amimia.** Complete loss of the power to make gestures and signs. [Gk *a, mimos* mimic.]

Aminacrine Hydrochloride BP 1968 (am·**in**·ak·reen hi·dro·**klor**·ide). 5-Aminoacridine hydrochloride monohydrate, $C_{13}H_{10}N_2HCl·H_2O$. A bacteriostatic derived from acridine and equalling proflavine in activity, with the advantage of being non-staining.

aminase (am·in·aze). A hydrolytic enzyme which attacks the amino NH_2 group, or the imino linkage =CH–NH–, in amino acids and purines.
amine (am·een). One of a series of important organic compounds which may be regarded as an ammonia molecule in which 1 or more of the hydrogen atoms have been replaced by alkyl radicals; they are known as primary, secondary, tertiary or quaternary amines, according to the number of hydrogen atoms so affected, the last-mentioned being derived from the hypothetical ammonium, NH_4. Cf. AMIDE. [sal *am*moniac, suffix *-ine*.]
amino group (am·in·o groop). The monovalent radical NH_2, which replaces a hydrogen atom in organic compounds to form amines. Cf. AMIDO GROUP. [see prec.]
aminoacetophenetidin (am·in·o·as·et·o·fen·et′·id·in). Phenocoll, $C_6H_4(C_2H_5O)NHCOCH_2NH_2$. A compound derived from phenacetin and formerly used as an antipyretic.
amino-acidaemia (am·in·o·as·id·e′·me·ah). A condition of the blood in which amino acids are present. [amino acid, Gk *haima* blood.]
amino-aciduria (am·in·o·as·id·ewr′·e·ah). A condition in which amino acids are present in urine.
aminoacyl (am·in·o·as′·il). **Aminoacyl adenylate.** A class of adenylic acid derivatives in which an amino-acid residue is attached through an acid-anhydride linkage to the adenylate molecule. **Aminoacyl tRNA.** A class of transfer RNA charged with a residue of an amino acid; each tRNA molecule can bind only the amino acid for which it is specific. Formation of aminoacyl tRNA in living cells is catalysed by an aminoacyl tRNA synthetase. **Aminoacyl tRNA synthetase.** A class of enzymes which catalyse the transfer of the aminoacyl moiety from an aminoacyl adenylate to the 3′-hydroxyl group of the ribose of a terminal adenylic acid residue of a transfer RNA molecule. [amino acid.]
aminoarsonoethanol (am·in·o·ar·son·o·eth′·an·ol). An arsenical spirochaeticide derived from ethyl alcohol, which has been used in the treatment of syphilis and trypanosomiasis.
aminoazotoluene (am·in·o·az·o·tol′·ew·een). Orthoaminoazotoluene, amidoazotoluene, non-staining scarlet, $CH_3C_6HN{=}NC_6H_3(NH_2)CH_3$. A scarlet dye, related to Scarlet Red BPC 1954, and used in ointment to promote the regeneration of epithelium in the treatment of ulcers; carcinogenic.
aminobenzene (am·in·o·ben′·zeen). Amidobenzene, phenylamine, aniline, $C_6H_5NH_2$. An oily liquid, only slightly soluble in water, obtained from coal tar or by the distillation of indigo; used in plastics manufacture, the rubber industry and the synthesis of dyestuffs. It is poisonous to heart muscle, causing arrhythmia and heart-block.
aminobutanoic methylsulphone (am·in·o·bew·tan·o′·ik meth·il·sul·fone). α-Aminobutanoic-γ-methyl sulphone, 191 RB. A sulphone which has been used in the treatment of tuberculosis and leprosy.
aminofructose (am·in·o·fruk′·toze). Fructosamine.
aminoglutethimide (am·in·o·gloo·teth·im·ide). A compound that blocks the circulation of adrenal cortical hormones. It has been used in the treatment of Cushing's syndrome.
aminoguanidine (am·in·o·gwan′·id·een). Arginine.
aminolipide, aminolipin (am·in·o·lip′·ide, am·in·o·lip′·in). One of a class of complex lipides, consisting of aliphatic acids combined with substituted amines, and containing no phosphorus.
aminolysis (am·in·ol·is·is). The process of splitting a metabolite by detachment of amino groups. [amino-, Gk *lysis* a loosing.]
Aminometradine (am·in·o·met′·rad·een). BP Commission approved name for 1-allyl-6-amino-3-ethyl-pyrimidine-2,4-dione, a non-mercurial diuretic for oral administration, especially useful when mercurials are contra-indicated.
aminomyelin (am·in·o·mi′·el·in). A lipoid substance containing aminonitrogen, which occurs in nerve tissue.
aminonitrogen (am·in·o·ni′·tro·jen). The nitrogen of protein combined in the form of amino acids; the expression of the amino acid content of blood plasma in terms of combined nitrogen.
amino-oxyacetate (am·in·o·ox·e·as′·et·ate). NH_2OCH_2COOH, carboxymethoxylamine, a potent inhibitor of pyridoxal-phosphate containing enzymes, e.g. transaminases.
aminopeptidase (am·in·o·pep′·tid·aze). An enzyme which catalyses the breakdown of a peptide, removing the amino acid at the amino end of the chain; it is found in intestinal juice. [amino acid, Gk *peptein* to digest, *-ase* enzyme.]
Aminophylline BP 1973 (am·in·of·il·een). Theophylline with ethylenediamine, $C_7H_8N_4O_2C_2H_4(NH_2)_2$. A double salt used as diuretic in the same way as theophylline, with the added advantage of greater solubility. It is of value in the relief of paroxysmal dyspnoea of cardiac origin, and in spasmodic asthma. It can be taken by mouth or given by injection.
aminopolypeptidase (am·in·o·pol·e·pep′·tid·aze). Aminopeptidase; an enzyme which acts on polypeptides to liberate a terminal amino acid having a free amino-group; it is a constituent of the enzyme complex, erepsin, the other constituent being carboxypeptidase.
***p*-aminopropiophenone** (par·ah·am·in·o·pro·pe·o·fen·one′). $CH_3CH_2COC_6H_4NH_2$. A substance which has been used in the experimental production of methaemoglobin in animals.
aminoprotease (am·in·o·pro′·te·aze). An aminopeptidase acting on proteoses, i.e. on high polypeptides.
aminopterin (am·in·op·ter·in). The sodium salt of 4-aminopteroyl glutamic acid. A synthetic derivative of folic acid which reverses the effects of the latter by competitive antagonism. It has been employed in acute leukaemia for its action on leukaemic bone marrow; it decreases the leukaemic cells and causes a reversion to normal of the peripheral white-cell count. Its effects, however, are only temporary, and the compound is toxic. The BP Commission approved name, Aminopterin Sodium, is the sodium salt.
aminopurine (am·in·o·pewr′·een). 1. Term applied to any one of the purine bases which enter into the composition of nucleic acids. 2. Adenine, $C_5H_5N_5$, a base found widely in plant and animal nucleoproteins, and produced by the decomposition of nucleic acids.
aminopyrine (am·in·o·pi′·reen). Amidopyrine.
Aminorex (am·in·or·ex). BP Commission approved name for 2-amino-5-phenyl-2-oxazoline; an appetite suppressant.
aminosaccharide (am·in·o·sak′·ar·ide). A sugar in which an amino NH_2 group has replaced a hydroxyl; those occurring in nature are known as hexosamines, and have the general formula $CH_2OH(CHOH)_3CHNH_2CHO$.
aminosis (am·in·o·sis). 1. Excess of amino acids in the body as a result of pathological overproduction. 2. The production in the body of amino acids. [amino acid, Gk *-osis* condition.]
aminostiburea (am·in·o·stib·ewr·e′·ah). A pentavalent antimony preparation used in the treatment of kala-azar.
aminosuria, aminuria (am·in·oze·ewr′·e·ah, am·in·ewr·e·ah). The presence of amines in urine.
aminotoluene (am·in·o·tol·ew·een). Toluidine.
Amiphenazole (am·e·fen·az·ole). The BP Commission approved name for 2,4-diamino-5-phenylthiazole, a mild respiratory stimulant. This compound also antagonizes heroin, and the synthetic analgesics pethidine and methadone. It has itself a respiratory stimulant action and a high therapeutic ratio. It has no analgesic properties of its own. This compound has also been used effectively in combination with β,β-methylethylglutarimide in the treatment of barbiturate poisoning.
Amisometradine (am·i·so·met′·rad·een). BP Commission approved name for 6-amino-1-methallyl-3-methylpyramidine-2,4-dione, a non-mercurial diuretic for oral administration.
amitosis (a·mi·to·sis). Simple or direct division of a cell by cleavage of the nucleus only. [Gk *a*, *mitos* thread.]
amitotic (a·mi·tot·ik). Marked by or relating to amitosis; not taking place by mitosis.
Amitriptyline (am·e·trip·ti·leen). BP Commission approved name for 3 - (3 - dimethylaminopropylidene) - 1,2:4,5 - dibenzocyclohepta - 1,4 - diene. **Amitriptyline Hydrochloride BP 1973.**

An antidepressant drug used in depressive disorders. Chemically and pharmacologically, it is closely related to imipramine.

ammeter (am·et·er). An instrument for measuring in amperes the strength of an electric current; in medical electricity the scale is graded in milliamperes. [ampere, meter.]

Ammi majus (am·i ma·jus). A plant the extract of the seeds of which has been used in the treatment of vitiligo by Arabs for centuries. There is good evidence to suggest that it may be of some value in this condition. [Gk *ammi* an African plant, L *major* greater.]

ammic (am·ik). Pertaining to or having the characteristics of ammonia.

ammine (am·ine). One of a series of complex metallic salts in which ammonia, as such, enters into combination.

ammism (am·izm). Ammotherapy.

Ammon. A ram-headed deity of ancient Egypt.

Ammon's horn. The hippocampus.

Ammon, Friedrich August von (b. 1799). Dresden ophthalmic surgeon.

filament of Ammon. One of the hair-like processes of the ciliary body of the eye.

Ammon's fissure. A slit-like gap in the early embryonic sclera.

Ammon's operation. 1. Canthoplasty; the suturing of the skin and conjunctiva after canthotomy to widen the palpebral fissure. 2. For epicanthus: excision of a vertical fold of skin over the nose. 3 For ectropion: resection of a triangle of skin from the outer part of the lower lid.

Ammon's scleral prominence or protuberance. A prominence on the posterior aspect of the eyeball which appears transiently in the fetus, usually during the third month.

Ammon's staphyloma. Protrusion of the sclera below the posterior pole of the eye, in association with a coloboma of the choroid.

Ammon's triangle. The triangle of skin resected in Ammon's operation No. 3 (above).

ammonaemia (am·on·e·me·ah). Ammoniaemia.

ammonal (am·on·al). An explosive consisting of trinitrotoluene and ammonium nitrate.

ammonaldehyde (am·on·al·de·hide). Hexamine.

Ammonia (am·o·ne·ah). NH_3. A colourless gas with a pungent smell, dissolving readily in water to form ammonium hydroxide. It is a normal product of animal metabolism, and is converted to urea in the liver; it may also form ammonium salts in the body which are excreted in the urine. Its presence in smelling salts and sal volatile produces irritation of the mucous membrane of the nose and throat, thereby reflexly stimulating the medulla and promoting a rise in blood pressure that combats the fainting attack. As most insect stings are acid, a solution of ammonia may be applied locally to allay the pain (BP 1958). **Ammonia base.** Name applied to an amine, in which the hydrogen atoms of ammonia have been replaced by one or more alkyl radicals. **Ammonia haemate.** A stain used in histology. **Ammonia water.** A dilute or strong solution of ammonia gas in water. [*Ammon*, near whose temple in Libya ammonium chloride was found.]

Ammoniacum BPC 1949 (am·on·i·ak·um). A gum resin obtained from the flowering and fruiting stems of the Persian plant *Dorema ammoniacum* Don. of the family Umbelliferae. It was formerly used for chronic bronchitis as it facilitates expectoration. [*Ammon*, near whose temple in Libya the tree grew.]

ammoniaemia (am·o·ne·e′·me·ah). A pathological condition in which there is ammonia or its compounds in the blood. [ammonia, Gk *haima* blood.]

ammoniagenesis (am·o·ne·a·jen′·es·is). The production of ammonia in the kidney. Glutamine is the major precursor. [ammonia, Gk *a*, *genein* to produce.]

ammoniameter (am·o·ne·am′·et·er). An apparatus for determining the ammonia content of a solution.

ammoniated (am·o·ne·a·ted). Combined with or containing ammonia.

ammonification (am·o·nif·ik·a′·shun). The formation of ammonia from proteins or from their cleavage products by the action of bacteria. [ammonia, L *facere* to make.]

Ammonii Chloridum. *European Pharmacopoeia* name for Ammonium Chloride BP 1973.

ammonin (am·on·in). A soda used in soap manufacture.

ammonioferric sulphate (am·o·ne·o·fer′·ik sul·fate). Ammonioferric alum, iron ammonium alum, $NH_4Fe(SO_4)_2 \cdot 12H_2O$. Violet crystals, used as a reagent and indicator; styptic and astringent.

ammonionitrometry (am·o·ne·o·ni·trom′·et·re). Analysis of a substance in such a way that the ammonia, nitric acid, and nitrogen otherwise combined, are separately determined. [ammonia, nitrogen, meter.]

ammonirrhoea (am·o·ne·re′·ah). Excretion of ammonia in the urine or sweat. [ammonia, Gk *rhoia* flow.]

ammonium (am·o·ne·um). The alkaline monovalent radical NH_4– present in aqueous solutions of ammonia and forming salts in the same way as an alkali metal, but never itself isolated. The ion stimulates the central nervous system, producing a rise in blood pressure, and has an action on heart and voluntary muscle similar to that of potassium. **Ammonium acetate.** CH_3COONH_4, a very soluble white crystalline substance employed medicinally in the form of Strong Solution of Ammonium Acetate BP 1953 (57.5 per cent) or Dilute Solution of Ammonium Acetate BP 1953 (7.2 per cent), made by neutralizing glacial acetic acid with ammonium carbonate and ammonia. It must be stored in lead-free glass bottles, and is used as a diaphoretic and expectorant. **Ammonium benzoate.** $C_6H_5COONH_4$, colourless crystals used as an expectorant. **Ammonium Bicarbonate BP 1953.** $(NH_4)HCO_3$, a white powder formed on exposing ammonium carbonate to air; a cardiac and respiratory stimulant. **Ammonium Bromide BPC 1963.** NH_4Br, very soluble colourless crystals; a sedative acting like other bromides and used as such in medicine. **Ammonium carbamate.** NH_2COONH_4, a white compound forming a proportion of ammonium carbonate. **Ammonium carbonate.** $(NH_4)_2CO_3$, white translucent lumps, usually consisting, after exposure to air, of a mixture of ammonium carbamate, ammonium bicarbonate and free ammonia. It has an expectorant action and is used in cough mixtures. **Ammonium Chloride BP 1973.** Sal ammoniac, NH_4Cl, white crystals freely soluble in water. It may be used as an expectorant, but is most important for its diuretic action and for its ability to render the urine acid and to produce acidosis. **Ammonium citrate.** $C_3H_4(OH)(COONH_4)_3$, a water-soluble salt used as a mild expectorant and diuretic. **Ammonium ichthosulphonate.** Ichthammol BP 1958, a brown viscous substance obtained by sulphonating the distillate of certain bituminous schists and neutralizing the product with ammonia. It has emollient and antiseptic properties and is used, usually in the form of an ointment, to treat skin conditions such as erysipelas and psoriasis. **Ammonium mandelate.** $C_6H_5(CH)OHCOONH_4$, a hygroscopic salt of mandelic acid, used as a urinary antiseptic. Mandelic acid itself, in order to exert an antiseptic effect in the urinary tract, must be in the form of the free acid; giving the ammonium salt achieves this, as the metabolism of the latter produces an acid urine. **Ammonium molybdate.** $(NH_4)_6Mo_7O_{24}$, a compound used in the detection and estimation of phosphates. **Ammonium nitrate.** NH_4NO_3, a white hygroscopic powder which has a diuretic action and is also of importance in promoting the excretion of lead in lead poisoning. **Ammonium phosphate.** $(NH_4)_2HPO_4$, a diuretic used in the treatment of gout and rheumatism. **Ammonium sulphate.** $(NH_4)_2SO_4$, a compound produced in the manufacture of coal gas and used as a fertilizer. A mild aperient. **Ammonium urate.** Ammonium dihydrogen urate, $NH_4C_5H_3N_4O_3$, a compound deposited in sediments from acid urine. **Ammonium valerate, Ammonium valerianate.** $C_4H_9COONH_4$, an antispasmodic compound. [ammonia.]

ammoniuria (am·o·ne·ewr′·e·ah). An excessive quantity of ammonia in the urine.

ammonolysis (am·on·ol·is·is). 1. The splitting up of an organic compound by the action of ammonia in a manner analogous to hydrolysis. 2. Chemical action brought about by hot ammonia gas under pressure. 3. The ionic dissociation of ammonia. [ammonia, Gk *lysis* a loosing.]

ammotherapy (am·o·**ther**·ap·e). The use of hot sand baths as a form of treatment. [Gk *ammos* sand, therapy.]

amnalgesia (am·nal·**je**·ze·ah). A state of relative freedom from pain, e.g. during light anaesthesia with nitrous oxide and oxygen. [Gk *amnesia* forgetfulness, *algesis* pain.]

amnemonic (am·ne·**mon**·ik). Referring to any defect of memory; amnesic. [Gk *a*, mnemonic.]

amnesia (am·**ne**·ze·ah). Loss of memory of varying degree attributable to organic or psychological causes. **Anterograde amnesia.** Loss or impairment of the memory for events which have occurred since the onset of the causative disorder and after consciousness has been regained. **Infantile amnesia.** Inability to remember the first 5 or 6 years of life. **Lacunar amnesia.** Loss of memory for patches or areas of past experience. **Localized amnesia.** Circumscribed loss of memory for a particular experience, situation or thing. **Obstetric amnesia.** Drug-induced loss of memory for the discomfort of labour. **Olfactory amnesia.** Loss of ability to recognize smells. **Post-hypnotic amnesia.** Inability to remember experiences occurring spontaneously or by suggestion during hypnosis. **Post-traumatic amnesia.** Anterograde amnesia following cerebral trauma; usually measured back to the time of actual injury and not to the time when consciousness has apparently been regained. **Retroactive amnesia, Retrograde amnesia.** Loss of memory for events preceding the causal illness or injury. **Transient global amnesia.** A condition affecting the middle-aged, usually as an isolated event, in which there is total amnesia, with or without confusion, for a varying period but with full recovery. Cerebral ischaemia is a possible cause. **Visual amnesia.** Word blindness; inability to recognize objects previously seen, including words. [Gk forgetfulness.]

amnesiac (am·**ne**·ze·ak). An individual affected with amnesia.

amnesic, amnestic (am·**ne**·zik, am·**nes**·tik). Forgetful; affected with or relating to amnesia.

amnestia (am·**nes**·te·ah). Amnesia.

amnial (**am**·ne·al). Amniotic.

amniocentesis (**am**·ne·o·sen·**te**'·sis). Transabdominal or trans-vaginal puncture of the amniotic sac to drain or sample amniotic fluid, often employed for the diagnosis of certain biochemical or chromosomal disorders. [amnion, Gk *kentesis* a pricking.]

amnioclepsis (**am**·ne·o·**klep**'·sis). The gradual, unnoticed escape of amniotic fluid. [amnion, Gk *kleptein* to steal away.]

amniocleptic, amnioclepticous (**am**·ne·o·**klep**'·tik, **am**·ne·o·**klep**'·tik·us). Descriptive of the unnoticed escape of amniotic fluid. [see prec.]

amniogenesis (**am**·ne·o·**jen**'·es·is). The formation and development of the amnion. [amnion, Gk *genein* to produce.]

amniography (am·ne·**og**·raf·e). A radiological method formerly used to confirm pregnancy or to diagnose placenta praevia. It consists of the administration by mouth of potassium iodide, or the injection of radio-opaque substances such as strontium iodide directly into the amniotic sac, in order that the latter may be clearly outlined in the subsequent skiagram. [amnion, Gk *graphein* to record.]

amnioma (am·ne·**o**·mah). A dermal tumour the result of adhesion of amniotic elements to some part of the fetal skin. [amnion, Gk *-oma* tumour.]

amnion (**am**·ne·on) (pl. *amnia*). A thin, strong, translucent, and smooth membrane which covers the whole of the fetal surface of the placenta. It contains liquor amnii, which separates it from the fetus, and can be peeled from the placenta and detached from the chorion. [Gk the fetal membrane.]

See also: PANDER.

amnionic (am·ne·**on**·ik). Amniotic.

amnionitis (**am**·ne·on·**i**'·tis). An inflammatory condition of the amnion. [amnion, Gk *-itis* inflammation.]

amniorrhexis (**am**·ne·or·**ex**'·is). Rupture of the amnion. [amnion, Gk *rhexis* rupture.]

amniorrhoea (**am**·ne·or·**e**'·ah). Discharge or escape of liquor amnii from the sac of the amnion. [amnion, Gk *rhoia* flow.]

amnios (**am**·ne·os). 1. The amnion. 2. The amniotic fluid.

amniota (am·ne·**o**·tah). Vertebrate animals in which an amnion is formed during development, i.e. reptiles, birds and mammals.

amniotic (am·ne·**ot**·ik). Relating to the amnion; characterized by having an amnion.

amniotitis, amnitis (**am**·ne·o·**ti**'·tis, am·**ni**·tis). Amnionitis.

amniotome (**am**·ne·o·tome). An instrument used for puncturing the fetal membranes. [amnion, Gk *temnein* to cut.]

amniotomy (am·ne·**ot**·o·me). Artificial puncture of the fetal membranes to induce labour. [see prec.]

amobarbital (am·o·**bar**·bit·al). USA name for Amylobarbitone BP 1958.

amobarbitalum (am·o·bar·bit·a·lum). **Amobarbitalum Natricum.** *European Pharmacopoeia* name for Amylobarbitone Sodium BP 1973.

Amodiaquine (am·o·**di**·ah·kween). BP Commission approved name for 7-chloro-4-(3-diethylaminomethyl-4-hydroxy-anilino) quinoline. An antimalarial drug with an action very similar to that of chloroquine. The official preparation is Amodiaquine Hydrochloride BP 1973.

Amoeba (am·**e**·bah). 1. A genus of rhizopod Protozoa of the family Amoebidae. The species are relatively large, with single nuclei and more than 1 pseudopodium; they live in fresh water, particularly where there is much organic material, and occasionally in stale faeces. *Amoeba proteus* is the best-known species, and a name given indiscriminately to laboratory teaching material. 2. Amoebae (pl.). A general term for any member of the rhizopod order Amoebida. **Artificial amoeba.** Combinations of certain chemicals which behave like living amoebae, e.g. in dilute nitric acid, mercury will move towards a crystal of potassium dichromate. **Amoeba buccalis.** *Entamoeba gingivalis.* **Amoeba coli.** *Entamoeba histolytica.* **Amoeba coli mitis.** *Entamoeba coli.* **Amoeba dentalis.** *Entamoeba gingivalis.* **Amoeba dysenteriae.** *Entamoeba histolytica.* **Amoeba histolytica.** *Entamoeba histolytica.* **Amoeba limax.** *Endolimax nana.* **Amoeba proteus.** See MAIN DEFINITION 1 (above). **Shelled amoeba.** Any member of the rhizopod order Testacea; they are sometimes coprozoic, occurring in stale faeces. **Amoeba urogenitalis.** *Entamoeba histolytica.* [Gk *amoibe* change.]

amoebacidal (am·e·bah·**si**'·dal). Referring to a substance with the power of destroying amoebae. [amoeba, L *caedere* to kill.]

amoebacide (am·e·bah·side). An agent which is capable of destroying amoebae. [see prec.]

amoebadiastase (am·e·bah·**di**'·as·taze). An intracellular enzyme formed by amoebae. [amoeba, diastase.]

amoebaism (am·**e**·bah·izm). The intrinsic property of being able to move in amoeboid fashion.

amoebiasis (am·e·**bi**·as·is). The condition of being infected with amoeba. **Amoebiasis cutis.** Infection of the skin by *Entamoeba histolytica.* **Hepatic amoebiasis.** Metastatic infection of the liver by *Entamoeba histolytica.* **Intestinal amoebiasis.** Infection of the intestinal canal by *Entamoeba histolytica.* **Parenteral amoebiasis.** Any infection by *Entamoeba histolytica* other than of the intestinal canal. **Perianal amoebiasis.** Perianal abscesses, fistulae or ulcers caused by *Entamoeba histolytica.* **Thoracic amoebiasis.** Amoebic abscess of the lung or mediastinum, or rupture of an amoebic abscess of the liver into the lung, pleura, pericardium or mediastinum.

amoebic (am·**e**·bik). Having the nature of or relating to an amoeba.

amoebicidal (am·e·be·**si**'·dal). Amoebacidal.

amoebicide (am·**e**·be·side). Amoebacide.

Amoebida (am·**e**·bid·ah). An order of the protozoan subclass Rhizopoda, characterized by the presence of lobular pseudopodia and absence of test. Members of the families Amoebidae and Entamoebidae are of medical interest. [see foll.]

Amoebidae (am·**e**·bid·e). A family of the rhizopod order Amoebida. It contains no genera of medical interest, but species of *Amoeba* and other genera may be coprozoic. [amoeba, *Gk eidos* form.]

amoebiform (am·e·be·form). Having resemblance to or being shaped like an amoeba. [amoeba, form.]
amoebina (am·e·bin·ah). Amoebida.
amoebiosis (am·e·bi·**o**′·sis). Amoebiasis.
amoebism (am·e·bizm). 1. The actual movements characteristic of an amoeba. 2. The state of being infected with amoebae.
amoebocyte (am·**e**·bo·site). A granular cell, with amoeboid properties, generally to be found in invertebrates. [amoeba, Gk *kytos* cell.]
amoebodiastase (am·e·bo·**di**′·as·taze). Amoebadiastase.
amoeboid (am·e·boid). Having the characteristics of or resembling an amoeba; able to assume different shapes, like an amoeba. [amoeba, Gk *eidos* form.]
amoeboma (am·e·**bo**·mah). Amoebic granuloma; a condition relatively frequent in countries where amoebiasis is common. It may occur in any part of the large intestine, more especially in the caecum, rectum and ileosigmoid colon, where it may cause obstruction and be mistaken clinically and radiologically for a neoplasm; the granulomatous tissue, in which amoebae may be seen, infiltrates the whole thickness of the bowel wall. Emetine usually causes an early and obvious shrinkage, and eventually almost complete, if not quite complete, disappearance of the filling defect. [amoeba, Gk *-oma* tumour.]
amoebula (am·e·bew·lah). Any spore, particularly of the Sporozoa, which moves by means of pseudopodia. [dim. of amoeba.]
amoeburia (am·e·**bewr**·e·ah). A condition in which there are amoebae in the urine.
amoenomania (am·e·no·**ma**′·ne·ah). 1. A form of insanity characterized by cheerful delusions and morbid gaiety. 2. A condition of deliriously high spirits. [L *amoenus* delightful, mania.]
amok (ah·**mok**). Amuck; a nervous or psychic malady seen in Asiatics, particularly in Malays, marked by periods of depression followed by frenzied desire to kill any individual encountered. [Malay *amoq* furious.]
Amomum (ah·**mo**·mum). A large genus of plants of the family Zingiberaceae, from several species of which are obtained aromatic seeds, such as cardamoms and grains of paradise. [Gk *amomon* Indian spice.]
amor (**am**·or). **Amor insanus.** Erotomania. **Amor lesbicus.** Sapphism. **Amor sui.** Self-love or vanity. **Amor veneris.** The clitoris. [L love.]
amoralia (a·mor·a·le·ah). Moral imbecility. [Gk *a*, moral.]
amoralis (a·mor·a·lis). A moral imbecile. [see prec.]
amorph (ah·**morf**). Digitalin BPC 1954.
amorphia, amorphism (a·**mor**·fe·ah, a·**mor**·fizm). The quality or state of being amorphous; not having any powers of crystallization. [Gk *a*, *morphe* shape.]
amorphinism (a·**mor**·fin·izm). The condition produced in a morphine addict when he is deprived of the drug. [Gk *a*, morphinism.]
amorphous (a·**mor**·fus). 1. Without visible form or definite structural shape. 2. In chemistry, not crystalline. [Gk *a*, *morphe* shape.]
amorphus (a·**mor**·fus). A shapeless acardiac monster without limbs. **Amorphus globulus.** Anideus. [see prec.]
amotio retinae (a·**mo**·she·o **ret**·in·e). Detachment of the retina; ablatio retinae. [L.]
Amoxycillin (am·**ox**·e·**sil**′·in). BP Commission approved name for 6-[(−)-α-amino-4-hydroxyphenylacetamido]-penicillanic acid; an antibiotic.
Ampelopsis (am·pel·**op**·sis). A genus of polypetalous plants of the family Vitaceae. **Ampelopsis quinquefolia.** The Virginia creeper, the leaves of which have tonic, astringent and expectorant properties. [Gk *ampelos* grape, *opsis* appearance.]
ampelotherapy (**am**·pel·o·**ther**′·ap·e). The grape cure; grapes are used exclusively, in various dishes. [Gk *ampelos* grape, therapy.]
amperage (**am**·per·ij). The strength of an electric current expressed in amperes.
Ampère, André Marie (b. 1775). French physicist and mathematician.

Ampère's law. An empirical rule for the motion of a magnet in an electrical field: the north pole will move in a direction at right angles and clockwise to that of the current producing the field.
ampere (**am**·pare). The unit of electric current. One of the base units of the SI system having the following definition. The ampere is that constant current which, if maintained in 2 straight parallel conductors of infinite length, of negligible circular cross-section, and placed 1 m apart in vacuum, would produce between these conductors a force equal to 2×10^{-7} newton per metre of length. [André Marie *Ampère*.]
amperemeter (**am**·pare·me·ter). Ammeter; an instrument, commonly used in medical electricity, for measuring in milliamperes the strength of an electric current.
amph-. Amphi-.
amphamphoterodiplopia (amf·am·**fo**·ter·o·dip·**lo**′·pe·ah). Amphodiplopia. [Gk *amphi*, *amphoteros* both together, diplopia.]
ampharkyochrome (am·**far**·ke·o·krome). Amphiarkyochrome.
ampheclexis (am·fek·**lex**·is). Sexual selection by both male and female. [Gk *amphi*, *eklexis* selection.]
amphemeros, amphemerus (am·**fem**·er·os, am·**fem**·er·us). 1. Quotidian. 2. A quotidian fever. [Gk *amphi*, *hemera* day.]
amphemerous (am·**fem**·er·us). Occurring daily; quotidian. [see prec.]
Amphetamine (am·**fet**·am·een). Racemic 2-aminopropylbenzene, $C_6H_5CH_2CH(NH_2)CH_3$. A volatile liquid used as a sympathomimetic drug, usually in the form of an inhalant, for the relief of catarrh, etc. (BP 1958). **Amphetamine Sulphate BP 1973.** A colourless salt of amphetamine, readily soluble in water. It is administered in tablet form for catarrh and coryza and also for decreasing the appetite in obesity. It stimulates the central nervous system and has been used to lessen fatigue; also in the treatment of narcolepsy.
amphi-. Prefix, from the Greek *amphi*, meaning *both, on both sides, of both kinds, around.*
amphiarkyochrome (am·fe·**ar**·ke·o·krome). A nerve cell, the body of which contains a pale network, the nodal points being joined by a network which stains readily and intensely. [Gk *amphi*, *arkys* net, *chroma* colour.]
amphiarthrodial (**am**·fe·ar·**thro**′·de·al). Relating to amphiarthrosis.
amphiarthrosis (**am**·fe·ar·**thro**′·sis). A joint which has only limited movement, and of which the surfaces are connected by synovial membranes or by fibrocartilaginous discs; there is an incomplete cavity in the centre of the joint. [Gk *amphi*, *arthrosis* joint.]
amphiaster (am·fe·**as**·ter). In mitosis, the achromatic figure formed shortly before nuclear division. It consists of paired asters and their connecting spindle, composed of gelled cytoplasm, and resembling in appearance the lines of force between opposite magnetic poles. [Gk *amphi*, *aster* star.]
Amphibia (am·**fib**·e·ah). A class of the phylum Chordata which contains frogs, toads, newts and salamanders. [Gk *amphi*, *bios* life.]
amphiblastic (am·fe·**blas**·tik). 1. Forming unequal segments. 2. Relating to that form of complete but unequal segmentation which produces an amphiblastula. [Gk *amphi*, *blastos* germ.]
amphiblastula (am·fe·**blas**·tew·lah). A type of blastula, common in sponges, in which the cells of one hemisphere are strikingly different from those of the other. [Gk *amphi*, blastula.]
amphiblestritis (**am**·fe·bles·**tri**′·tis). Inflammation of the retina. [Gk *amphiblestron* net, *-itis* inflammation.]
amphiblestrodes (**am**·fe·bles·**tro**′·deez). The retina. [see foll.]
amphiblestroid (am·fe·**bles**·troid). Like a net. [Gk *amphiblestron* net, *eidos* form.]
amphibolia (am·fe·**bo**·le·ah). The stage in the course of a disease at which the prognosis is in doubt. [Gk *amphiballein* to doubt.]
amphibolic, amphibolous (am·fe·**bol**·ik, am·**fib**·ol·us). Ambiguous; doubtful; of uncertain prognosis. [see prec.]
amphicentric (am·fe·**sen**·trik). In anatomy, a term used of a plexus of blood vessels with 1 afferent and 1 efferent trunk; converging at both ends. [Gk *amphi*, *kentron* centre.]

amphichroic, amphichromatic (am·fe·**kro**·ik, **am**·fe·kro·**mat**′·ik). Describing substances which in the colour test turn blue litmus paper red and red litmus paper blue. Cf. AMPHOTERIC. [Gk *amphi, chroma* colour.]

amphicoelous (am·fe·**se**·lus). Biconcave; descriptive of a vertebra the centre of which is concave anteriorly and posteriorly, as in fishes. [Gk *amphi, koilos* hollow.]

amphicrania (am·fe·**kra**·ne·ah). Pain affecting both sides of the head, particularly neuralgia. [Gk *amphi, kranion* skull.]

amphicreatine (am·fe·**kre**·at·een). A leucomaine formed in muscle and derived from creatine. [Gk *amphi,* creatine.]

amphicreatinine (**am**·fe·kre·**at**′·in·een). A leucomaine formed in muscle and derived from creatinine. [Gk *amphi,* creatinine.]

amphicyte (**am**·fe·site). One of the cells which surround the cerebrospinal ganglionic neurone. [Gk *amphi, kytos* cell.]

amphicytula (am·fe·**si**·tew·lah). 1. In mammals, the impregnated ovum. 2. The parent cell of an amphiblastic egg. [Gk *amphi,* cytula.]

amphidesmic, amphidesmous (am·fe·**dez**·mik, am·fe·**dez**·mus). Having a double ligament. [Gk *amphi, desmos* bond.]

amphidiarthrosis (**am**·fe·di·ar·**thro**′·sis). A form of joint which combines amphiarthrosis with diarthrosis; the articulation of the lower jaw is an example. [Gk *amphi,* diarthrosis.]

amphierotism (am·fe·**er**·ot·izm). A mental condition in which a person is able to regard himself as of either sex separately or simultaneously. [Gk *amphi, eros* love.]

amphigastrula (am·fe·**gas**·troo·lah). In mammals, the ovum in the late gastrula stage. [Gk *amphi,* gastrula.]

amphigenesis (am·fe·**jen**·es·is). The condition in which a homosexual is also able to have sexual relations with the opposite sex. [Gk *amphi, genein* to produce.]

amphigenetic (**am**·fe·jen·**et**′·ik). Term descriptive of reproduction by means of the union of the two sexes. [see prec.]

amphigony (am·**fig**·on·e). 1. Sexual reproduction. 2. Burlesque writing devoid of meaning. [Gk *amphi, gonos* generation.]

amphikaryon (am·fe·**kar**·e·on). A nucleus containing 2 haploid sets as the result of fertilization. [Gk *amphi, karyon* nucleus.]

amphikreatine (am·fe·**kre**·at·een). Amphicreatine.

amphikreatinine (**am**·fe·kre·**at**′·in·een). Amphicreatinine.

amphimicrobian (**am**·fe·mi·**kro**′·be·an). Anaerobic as well as aerobic; term descriptive of organisms able to sustain life with or without oxygen. [Gk *amphi,* microbe.]

amphimixis (am·fe·**mix**·is). 1. The union of maternal and paternal gametes in sexual reproduction. 2. Interbreeding. 3. In psychosexual development, the centring of the early manifestations of energy in the sexual organs. [Gk *amphi, mixis* a mingling.]

Amphimonas caudata (am·fe·**mo**·nas kaw·**da**·tah). A highly motile, flagellate protozoon, found in polluted water and occasionally in human faeces; non-pathogenic. Also known as *Bodo caudatus.* [Gk *amphi, monas* unit, L *caudatus* tailed.]

amphimorula (am·fe·**mor**·ew·lah). Morula in the mammalian ovum which are composed of cells of unequal size. [Gk *amphi,* morula.]

amphinucleolus (**am**·fe·new·kle·**o**′·lus). A nucleolus having affinities for both acidic and basic dyes. [Gk *amphi,* nucleolus.]

amphinucleus (am·fe·**new**·kle·us). A nucleus that is made up of a single body composed of centrosome and spindle fibres, with the chromatin massed round it; a karyosome. [Gk *amphi,* nucleus.]

Amphioxus (am·fe·**ox**·us). A genus of primitive marine chordates, fish-shaped but tapering at each end. They show characters, such as the notochord and pharyngeal gill slits, which were probably present in the ancestors of the vertebrates. [Gk *amphi, oxys* sharp.]

amphipyrenin (am·fe·**pi**·ren·in). The substance composing the nuclear membrane in a cell. [Gk *amphi, pyren* fruit stone.]

Amphistomata (am·fe·**sto**·mah·tah). Paramphistomoidea; a sub-order of the trematode order Prostomata. The families Gastrodiscidae and Paramphistomatidae are of medical interest. [Gk *amphi, stoma* mouth.]

amphistomiasis (**am**·fe·sto·**mi**′·as·is). Infestation with trematode worms of the sub-order Amphistosomata.

Amphistomum (am·fe·**sto**·mum). Gastrodiscus; a genus of parasitic trematode worms belonging to the family Gastrodiscidae. **Amphistomum hominis.** Normally a parasite of pigs, it has been described as a parasite of man; especially common in North India. It lives in the caecum and large intestine, giving rise to inflammatory changes and causing diarrhoea. [Gk *amphi, stoma* mouth.]

amphitene (**am**·fe·teen). Relating to or indicating the synaptic stage of miosis; zygotene. [Gk *amphi, tainia* ribbon.]

amphithymia (am·fe·**thi**·me·ah). A mental state in which there is both elation and depression. [Gk *amphi, thymos* mind.]

amphitrichate, amphitrichous (am·**fit**·rik·ate, am·**fit**·rik·us). Possessing a flagellum at each end. [Gk *amphi, thrix* hair.]

amphitropic (am·fe·**trop**·ik). Entering a cavity of the body, e.g. the abdomen, from the side. [Gk *amphi, tropos* a turning.]

amphixenosis (**am**·fe·zen·**o**′·sis). Infections transmissible between man and vertebrates where the maintenance host can be either man or animal, e.g. *Trypanosoma cruzi* or *Schistosoma japonicum.* [Gk *amphi, xenos* stranger, *-osis* condition.]

amphocyte (**am**·fo·site). A cell which stains readily with either acid or basic dyes. [Gk *ampho* both, *kytos* cell.]

amphodiplopia (**am**·fo·dip·**lo**′·pe·ah). The condition of having double vision in each eye; also called *bilateral uniocular diplopia.* [Gk *ampho* both, diplopia.]

amphogenic (am·fo·**jen**·ik). Producing offspring of both sexes. [Gk *ampho* both, *genein* to produce.]

amphogenous (am·**foj**·en·us). Amphoteric. [see prec.]

ampholyte (**am**·fo·lite). A substance which, dissolved in water, behaves as an acid or base according to whether the pH of the solution was above or below iso-electric point; an amphoteric electrolyte. [Gk *ampho* both, electrolyte.]

Amphomycin (am·fo·**mi**·sin). BP Commission approved name for an antibiotic produced by *Streptomyces canus.*

amphophil, amphophile (**am**·fo·fil, **am**·fo·file). 1. A cell which stains readily with either acid or basic dyes. 2. Amphophilic. [Gk *ampho* both, *philein* to love.]

amphophilic, amphophilous (am·fo·**fil**·ik, am·**fof**·il·us). Of tissues and cells, having equal affinity for basic and acid dyes. [see prec.]

amphoric (am·**for**·ik). A term used to denote quality of resonance or respiration; descriptive of the sound produced when one blows over the mouth of an empty bottle. [Gk *amphoreus* two-handled jar.]

amphoricity (am·for·**is**·it·e). Describing the state in which amphoric sounds are produced by auscultation or percussion.

amphoriloquy (am·for·**il**·o·kwe). The producing of the amphoric sound in speaking. [Gk *amphoreus* two-handled jar, L *loqui* to speak.]

amphorophony (am·for·**of**·on·e). Amphoric resonance of voice. [Gk *amphoreus* two-handled jar, *phone* sound.]

amphoteric (am·fo·**ter**·ik). In chemistry, combining opposite characters; able to act with both bases and acids, or as a base or an acid; having effect on both red and blue litmus. Cf. AMPHICHROIC. **Amphoteric elements.** Elements some of the oxides of which combine with water to form bases and others to form acids. [Gk *amphoteros* both.]

Amphotericin BP 1973 (am·fo·**ter**·is·in). A mixture of antifungal substances produced by the growth of certain strains of *Streptomyces nodosus* or by any other means. **Amphotericin B.** A relatively broad-spectrum fungistatic agent.

amphotericity, amphoterism (**am**·fo·ter·**is**′·it·e, am·**fot**·er·izm). The condition of having basic as well as acid properties. [see prec.]

amphoterodiplopia (am·**fot**·er·o·dip·**lo**′·pe·ah). Amphodiplopia. [Gk *amphoteros* both, diplopia.]

amphoterous (am·**fot**·er·us). Amphoteric.

amphotony (am·**fo**·to·ne). Existence of tone in both the parasympathetic and the sympathetic nervous systems (vagus and sympathetic). [Gk *ampho* both, *tonos* tone.]

Ampicillin BP 1973 (am·pe·**sil**·in). 6-[D(−)-α-aminophenylacetamido] penicillanic acid, a white, microcrystalline powder, almost odourless with a bitter taste; an antibiotic. **Ampicillin Sodium BP 1973.** The sodium salt of ampicillin with action similar to that of benzylpenicillin against Gram-positive organisms. Its action more closely resembles that of the tetracyclines and chloramphenicol. **Ampicillin Trihydrate BP 1973.** The trihydrate of ampicillin, with similar actions and uses.

amplexatio (am·plex·**a**·she·o). Sexual intercourse. [L an embrace.]

amplexation (am·plex·**a**·shun). A method of treating a fractured clavicle by the use of an apparatus which holds the shoulder rigid and encircles the chest and the neck. [see prec.]

amplexus (am·**plex**·us). In species in which fertilization of the eggs takes place externally, as in the frog, the pairing of male and female at the time when the eggs and the sperm are discharged. [L embrace.]

ampliation (am·ple·**a**·shun). Distension or dilatation of a cavity or part. [L *ampliare* to make wider.]

amplification (**am**·plif·ik·**a**′·shun). 1. Increase of effect, enlargement of scope or extension of boundary. 2. In radio, the increase of incoming signal by means of the thermionic valve. 3. In optics, the widening of the visual field of a microscope. [see foll.]

amplifier (**am**·plif·i·er). Device for controlling power from a source so that more is delivered at the output than is supplied at the input. Source of power may be mechanical, hydraulic, pneumatic, electric etc. **Image amplifier.** A form of static imaging device for recording the distribution of a radionuclide within an organ or part of the body. Used alone, it is suitable for recording only low energy gamma radiation. **Magnetic amplifier.** An electronic amplifier employing magnetic couplings, used as a power amplifier for signals of very low frequency. **Pulse amplifier.** An electronic instrument used for the amplification of electrical pulses of potential. [L *amplificare* to make wider.]

amplitude (**am**·plit·ewd). Width, fullness, range; the maximum displacement of an oscillating point. **Amplitude of accommodation.** The amount in dioptres by which the refractive power of the eye can be increased through action of the ciliary muscle; a value showing a steady decrease with age. **Amplitude of convergence.** The maximum amount by which the angle between the visual axes can be altered through the action of convergence; the measurement may be made in degrees, metre angles or prism dioptres. [L *amplus* wide.]

ampoule (**am**·pool). Ampule.

ampule (**am**·pewl). A glass vessel of characteristic shape varying in capacity from 1 to 50 ml and sealed at the neck by melting in a flame. It is used to contain sterile drugs either in powder form or in solution. [Fr. *ampoule.*]

ampulla [NA] (am·**pul**·ah) (pl. *ampullae*). A flask-shaped or spherical dilatation of a canal, usually near its beginning or ending. **Ampulla of the bile duct [ampulla hepatopancreatica (NA)].** Ampulla of Vater, the dilatation at the end of the common bile duct where it is joined by the pancreatic duct before opening into the second part of the duodenum. **Bony ampullae [ampullae osseae (NA)].** The dilated ends of a semicircular canal of the bony labyrinth of the ear where it opens into the vestibules: namely, the dilatation [ampulla ossea anterior (NA)] of the superior osseous semicircular canal which accommodates the superior membranous ampulla; the dilatation [ampulla ossea lateralis (NA)] of the lateral osseous semicircular canal which accommodates the lateral membranous ampulla; and the dilatation [ampulla ossea posterior (NA)] of the posterior osseous semicircular canal which accommodates the posterior membranous ampulla. **Ampulla of the lacrimal canaliculus [ampulla canaliculi lacrimalis (NA)].** The dilatation at the angle of a lacrimal canaliculus. **Ampulla lactifera.** Lactiferous sinus, the distension of a milk duct at its entrance into the nipple. **Membranous ampullae [ampullae membranaceae (NA).** Dilatations at the lateral end of the superior semicircular duct [ampulla membranacea anterior (NA)], the inferior end of the posterior duct [ampulla membranacea posterior (NA)] and the anterior end of the lateral duct [ampulla membranacea lateralis (NA)], each containing a transverse elevation, the septum transversum, the most prominent part of which is the ampullary crest. The depression on each side of the crest is the ampullary sulcus [sulcus ampullaris (NA)]. **Ampulla of the rectum [ampulla recti (NA)].** The dilatation near the end of the rectum immediately above the anal canal, and behind the prostrate gland. **Ampulla of the uterine tube [ampulla tubae uterinae (NA)].** The thin-walled, tortuous portion of the tube, between the infundibulum and the isthmus. **Ampulla of the vas deferens [ampulla ductus deferentis (NA)].** Henle's ampulla, a dilatation at the base of the bladder near the end of the vas deferens. [L jug.]

See also: BRYANT, GALEN, HENLE, THOMA, VATER.

ampullaceous (am·pul·**a**·shus). 1. Shaped like a flask or bladder. 2. Describing a condition in which blebs form. [see prec.]

ampullar (am·**pul**·ar). Ampullary.

Ampullaria luteosoma (am·pul·a·re·ah **lew**·te·o·**so**′·mah). The intermediate snail host of *Paragonimus ringeri* in Venezuela. [L *ampulla* jug, *luteus* yellow, Gk *soma* body.]

ampullary (am·**pul**·ar·e). Resembling or relating to an ampulla, and in particular to the ampulla of the bile duct.

ampullary nerves. Anterior ampullary nerve [nervus ampullaris anterior (NA)]. A branch of the vestibular nerve to the superior semicircular canal. **Lateral ampullary nerve [nervus ampullaris lateralis (NA)].** A branch of the vestibular nerve to the lateral semicircular canal. **Posterior ampullary nerve [nervus ampullaris posterior (NA)].** A branch of the vestibular nerve to the posterior semicircular canal.

ampullate (am·**pul**·ate). 1. Having an ampulla. 2. Shaped like a flask. [L *ampulla* jug.]

ampullitis (am·pul·**i**·tis). An inflammatory condition of an ampulla, particularly that of the vas deferens. [L *ampulla* jug, Gk *-itis* inflammation.]

ampullula (am·**pul**·ew·lah). Any minute dilatation such as is present in the lymph and blood vessels and the lactiferous ducts. [L little ampulla.]

amputation (am·pew·**ta**·shun). The removal of a limb or portion of a limb, or of any other appendage. **Above-elbow amputation.** Amputation through the arm approximately 20 cm (8 in) below the tip of the acromion process. **Above-knee amputation.** Amputation through the thigh approximately 25–30 cm (10–12 in) below the tip of the great trochanter. **Accidental amputation.** Loss of a limb or other part as a result of an accident. **Amniotic amputation.** The separation of an extremity of a fetus within the uterus, formerly thought to be due to the tightening around it of a band of amnion. **Aperiosteal amputation.** One in which the end of the severed bone is denuded of periosteum. **Below-elbow amputation.** Amputation through the forearm approximately 18 cm (7 in) below the tip of the olecranon process. **Below-knee amputation.** Amputation through the leg approximately 13 cm (5 in) below the knee joint. **Bloodless amputation.** One in which the circulation is mechanically controlled so that there is only slight loss of blood. **Breast amputation.** Mastectomy; removal of the breast. **Central amputation.** One after which the scar runs across the middle of the end of the stump. **Cervix amputation.** Removal of the cervix, which is often done at the same time as repair of the perineum in genital prolapse. **Chop amputation.** Guillotine amputation (see below). **Cinematic amputation, Cineplastic amputation.** One where the stump muscles are used to activate the artificial limb by direct attachment to skin tunnels. **Circular amputation.** One in which a single tubular flap is made by a circular cut through skin and muscles directly across the limb, the bone being divided at a higher level. **Circular skin-flap amputation.** A modified form of the circular amputation; the skin flap is dissected and the muscles are divided at a higher level. **Coat-sleeve amputation.** A modification of the circular amputation; the skin flap is made very long, and is tied over the stump by ligature. **Complete amputation.** One in which the whole limb or the complete part of a limb is amputated. **Congenital amputation.** Amputation *in utero* by the pressure of constricting bands or because of intrinsic deficiency of embryonic tissue. **Conservative amputa-**

tion. An amputation which aims at sacrificing as little tissue as possible. **Cutaneous amputation.** One in which the flaps consist only of skin. **Definitive amputation.** Final amputation (see below). **Double-flap amputation.** One in which 2 flaps are made from the soft tissues. **Dry amputation.** Bloodless amputation (see above). **Eccentric amputation.** Excentric amputation (see below). **Elliptical amputation.** A modified circular amputation in which the cut is made obliquely to the long axis of the limb to give a single flap. **End-bearing amputation.** An amputation designed for subsequent weight-bearing upon the end of the stump. **Excentric amputation.** An amputation the scar of which is not centrally placed on the end of the stump. **Final amputation.** Amputation performed late, at a desirable level, when the stump of a provisional amputation has healed. **Flap amputation.** An amputation in which the flaps, made of the soft tissues, cover the stump. **Flapless amputation.** One without flaps, healing being by granulation. **Forequarter amputation.** Interscapulothoracic amputation (see below). **Galvanocaustic amputation.** One in which a galvanocautery is used for dividing the soft tissues. **Guillotine amputation.** A rapid through-and-through flapless circular amputation in which knife and saw are used, and bone and soft tissues are divided at the same level; seldom practised now except in the direst emergency. **Hindquarter amputation.** Interpelvi-abdominal amputation (see below). **Immediate amputation.** One performed during the period of shock, within 12 h of the injury. **Interinnomino-abdominal amputation.** Interpelvi-abdominal amputation (see below). **Intermediary amputation, Intermediate amputation.** Amputation performed after recovery from shock, and before infection can become established. **Interpelvi-abdominal amputation.** Amputation of the thigh, together with the innominate bone. **Interscapulothoracic amputation.** Amputation of the whole arm, together with the scapula and the lateral portion of the clavicle. **Intrapyretic amputation.** Intermediary amputation (see above). **Intra-uterine amputation.** Congenital amputation (see above). **Kineplastic amputation.** Cineplastic amputation (see above). **Linear amputation.** This consists of straightforward division of all tissues. **Major amputation.** Removal of a limb above the ankle or wrist. **Mammary amputation.** Surgical excision of a breast. **Mediate amputation.** Intermediary amputation (see above). **Mediotarsal amputation.** Amputation of the foot at the midtarsal joint, leaving only the talus and the calcaneum; the soft parts of the sole of the foot cover the stump. **Metacarpal amputation.** Removal of a finger together with its metacarpal bone. **Metacarpophalangeal amputation.** Disarticulation of a whole finger or toe. **Midtarsal amputation.** Mediotarsal amputation (see above). **Minor amputation.** Amputation of a toe or a finger or of any other small part. **Mixed amputation.** That in which both flap and circular methods are used together. **Multiple amputation.** Amputation of more than one part or member at one time. **Musculocutaneous amputation, Musculotegmentary amputation.** One in which the flap is of both muscle and skin. **Myoplastic amputation.** One in which muscle flaps are fashioned to cover the end of the bone. **Natural amputation.** Congenital amputation (see above). **Oblique amputation.** Elliptical amputation (see above). **Osteoplastic amputation.** One in which the raw surface of the severed bone is covered by a fragment from below the line of section hinged on periosteum, or by apposition with the cut surface of another bone. **Oval amputation.** Elliptical amputation (see above). **Partial amputation.** 1. Amputation of a segment or part only, of a limb. 2. Incomplete congenital amputation. **Pathological amputation.** Amputation made necessary because of a diseased condition of the part and not because of injury. **Penis amputation.** Partial or total resection of the penis, commonly for cancer. **Periosteoplastic amputation.** Subperiosteal amputation (see below). **Phalangophalangeal amputation.** Disarticulation of a finger or a toe at an interphalangeal joint. **Primary amputation.** Amputation performed early after injury, the wound of the stump being closed to obtain primary healing. **Provisional amputation.** Amputation performed early to remove damaged or infected tissues, and with the intention of subsequent amputation at a higher and usually preferable level. **Quadruple amputation.** Amputation of all 4 extremities. **Racket amputation.** Amputation in which a single incision made in the axis of a limb meets a circular or oval amputation, to give the stump a linear scar. **Rectal amputation.** Resection of the rectum with sacrifice of the sphincter mechanism; a term used most frequently on the Continent. **Rectangular amputation.** An amputation with 2 equal or unequal rectangular flaps. **Root amputation.** In dentistry, the operation of removal by burr of the carious root of a tooth. **Scapulohumeral amputation.** Disarticulation of the arm at the shoulder joint. **Secondary amputation.** Amputation performed late, for the removal of a suppurating extremity. **Semicircular-flap amputation.** Amputation with the use of convex flaps. **Spontaneous amputation.** Congenital amputation (see above). **Subastragaloid amputation.** Subtalar amputation (see below). **Submalleolar amputation.** Amputation of the foot at the ankle joint. **Subperiosteal amputation.** A method by which a flap of periosteum is left distal to the line of bone section, and replaced over the bone end. **Subtalar amputation.** Amputation of the foot with retention of the talus only. **Supracondylar amputation.** Of a leg; amputation at a level above the femoral condyles. **Synchronous amputation.** Multiple amputation, particularly that performed by several operators working simultaneously. **Tarsometatarsal amputation.** Lisfranc's amputation. **Tertiary amputation.** Amputation delayed until suppuration has subsided. **Through knee amputation.** An end-bearing amputation through the knee joint. **Amputation by transfixion.** Amputation in which the flaps are fastened by piercing the limb with a knife and cutting from within outward. **Traumatic amputation.** Accidental amputation (see above). **Triple amputation.** Amputation of 3 extremities. [L *amputare* to cut away.]

See also: ALANSON, ALOUETTE, BÉCLARD, BIER, BUNGE, CARDEN, CHOPART, DIEFENBACH, FARABEUF, FORBES, GRITTI, GUYON, HANCOCK, HEY (W.), JABOULAY, KRUKENBERG (H.), LAGENBECK (B. R. K.), LARREY, LE FORT, LISFRANC, MACKENZIE (R. J.), MAISONNEUVE, MALGAIGNE, MIKULICZ-RADECKI, PIROGOFF, RICARD, SKEY, SMITH (N.), STOKES (SIR WILLIAM), SYME, TEALE, TRIPIER, VLADIMIROFF.

Amsler, Marc. 20th century Swiss ophthalmologist.

Amsler charts. Grid charts used for subjective plotting of field defects or localized metamorphopsia.

Amsler's marker. An instrument for marking the sclera; employed principally in operation for the cure of retinal detachment.

amuck (ah·**muk**). Amok.

amusia (a·**mew**·ze·ah). A form of aphasia in which the faculty of musical expression or reception is lost. **Instrumental amusia.** Loss of ability to play a musical instrument. **Motor amusia.** Lack of ability to produce musical sounds. **Sensory amusia.** Inability to understand musical sounds. **Vocal motor amusia.** Lack of ability to sing in tune. [Gk *amousos* unmusical.]

Amussat, Jean Zuléma (b. 1796). Paris surgeon.

Amussat's operation. Lumbar colostomy at the outer border of the quadratus lumborum muscle.

Amussat's valves. Heister's valves.

amyasthenia (a·mi·as·**the'**·ne·ah). Amyosthenia; the muscular weakness to which neurotic or hysterical patients are prone. [Gk *a, mys* muscle, *sthenos* strength.]

amyasthenic (a·mi·as·**then'**·ik). 1. Referring or belonging to amyasthenia. 2. Descriptive of a person suffering from amyasthenia.

amychophobia (am·i·ko·**fo'**·be·ah). An excessive fear of claws or nails or of being scratched by a clawed animal. [Gk *amyche* scratch, phobia.]

amyctic (am·**ik**·tik). 1. Causing abrasion; excoriative. 2. A drug which has corrosive or caustic properties. [Gk *amyche* scratch.]

amyelencephalia (a·mi·el·en·kef·**a'**·le·ah). The condition in which spinal cord and brain are lacking. [Gk *a, myelos* marrow, *egkephalos* brain.]

amyelencephalus (a·mi·el·en·kef′·al·us). A monster without brain or spinal cord. [see prec.]
amyelia (a·mi·e·le·ah). The condition of lacking the spinal cord. [Gk *a*, *myelos* marrow.]
amyelic (a·mi·el·ik). Relating to amyelia; being without a spinal cord.
amyelineuria (a·mi·el·in·ewr′·e·ah). Amyelonervia. [Gk *a*, *myelos* marrow, *neuron* nerve.]
amyelinic (a·mi·el·in·ik). Having no medullary sheath. [Gk *a*, *myelos* marrow.]
amyeloidaemia (a·mi·el·oid·e′·me·ah). A condition in which there are no myelocytes in the blood. [Gk *a*, myelocyte, Gk *haima* blood.]
amyelonervia, amyeloneuria (a·mi·el·o·nerv′·e·ah, a·mi·el·o·newr′·e·ah). Partial paralysis or defective function of the spinal cord. [Gk *a*, *myelos* marrow, *neuron* (L *nervus*) nerve.]
amyelonic (a·mi·el·on·ik). 1. Amyelic. 2. Without bone marrow.
amyelotrophy (a·mi·el·ot′·rof·e). Atrophy of the spinal cord; myelatrophy. [Gk *a*, *myelos* marrow, *trophe* nutrition.]
amyelous (a·mi·el·us). Amyelic.
amyelus (a·mi·el·us). A fetus lacking a spinal cord. [Gk *a*, *myelos* marrow.]
amyencephalus (a·mi·en·kef′·al·us). Amyelencephalus.
amygdala (am·ig·dal·ah). 1. The almond; the seed of *Prunus communis* (fam. Rosaceae). 2. An obsolete name for the tonsil. 3. Amygdaloid nucleus. *See* NUCLEUS. **Amygdala amara.** Bitter almond. **Amygdala cerasorum.** The dried kernels of cherry stones; may be used as an adulterant of almond seeds. **Amygdala dulcis.** Sweet almond. *See* ALMOND. [Gk *amygdale* almond.]
amygdalase (am·ig·dal·aze). An enzyme contained in bitter almonds which activates the first hydrolysis of amygdalin into prunasin and glucose. [see prec.]
amygdalectomy (am·ig·dal·ek′·to·me). Tonsillectomy. Resection or destruction of the amygdaloid nucleus of the brain. [Gk *amygdale* almond, *ektome* a cutting out.]
amygdalin (am·ig·dal·in). $C_{20}H_{27}O_{11}$, a glucose which occurs in oil of almonds, the leaves of the cherry-laurel, *Prunus laurocerasus*, apricot, peach and cherry kernels. It is hydrolysed by the enzyme emulsin, which is found with it, first to the isomeric prunasin, then to glucose, benzaldehyde and hydrocyanic acid. Used as an expectorant, and in toilet preparations. [see foll.]
amygdaline (am·ig·dal·een). 1. Resembling an almond. 2. Belonging to the tonsils. [Gk *amygdale* almond.]
amygdalitis (am·ig·dal·i′·tis). Tonsillitis. [Gk *amygdale* almond, *-itis* inflammation.]
amygdaloglossus (am·ig·dal·o·glos′·us). A muscle arising from the aponeurosis external to the tonsil and inserted with the palatoglossus into the tongue. [Gk *amygdale* almond, *glossa* tongue.]
amygdaloid (am·ig·dal·oid). 1. Almond-shaped. 2. Resembling a tonsil. **Amygdaloid nucleus.** *See* NUCLEUS. [Gk *amygdale* almond, *eidos* form.]
amygdalolith (am·ig·dal·o·lith). Tonsillolith; a tonsillar calculus. [Gk *amygdale* almond, *lithos* stone.]
amygdaloncus (am·ig·dal·ong′·kus). Any tumour or swelling occurring in a tonsil. [Gk *amygdale* almond, *ogkos* mass.]
amygdalopathy (am·ig·dal·op′·ath·e). Tonsillopathy; any disease or pathological condition of the tonsils. [Gk *amygdale* almond, *pathos* suffering.]
amygdalophenin (am·ig·dal·of′·en·in). Salicyl *p*-phenetidin, $C_2H_5OC_6H_4NHCOC_6H_4(OH)$. A derivative of phenetidin employed in the treatment of rheumatism.
amygdalose (am·ig·dal·oze). The disaccharide in amygdalin, in which it is combined with benzaldehyde cyanohydrin; it hydrolyses into glucose.
amygdalothrypsis (am·ig·dal·o·thrip′·sis). Excision of an enlarged tonsil after it has been crushed in a forceps. [Gk *amygdale* almond, *thrypsis* a crushing.]
amygdalotome (am·ig·dal·o·tome). Tonsillotome; an instrument used for incising and removing enlarged tonsils. [see foll.]
amygdalotomy (am·ig·dal·ot′·o·me). Tonsillotomy. [Gk *amygdale* almond, *temnein* to cut.]
amygdalo-uvular (am·ig·dal·o·ew′·vew·lar). Relating to or including the tonsil and uvula. [Gk *amygdale* almond, uvula.]
amygdophenin (am·ig·dof·en·in). Phenylglycolphenetidine, phenetidin amygdalate, $C_2H_5OC_6H_4NHCOCH(OH)C_6H_5$. A phenetidin derivative employed as an analgesic.
amygmus (am·ig·mus). Scarification. [Gk *amyche* scratch.]
amyl (am·il). The monovalent organic radical, C_5H_{11}-, derived from amyl alcohol. **Amyl acetate.** $C_5H_{11}OCCH_3$, banana oil, a liquid with the odour of pears, used as a flavouring and a solvent for lacquers. **Amyl alcohol.** *See* ALCOHOL. **Amyl chloride.** $C_5H_{11}Cl$, a liquid used as an anaesthetic. **Amyl iodide.** $C_5H_{11}I$, a liquid employed as an inhalation in dyspnoea and cardiac affections. **Amyl Nitrite BP 1953.** $C_5H_{11}NO_2$, a pale-yellow volatile liquid used as an inhalation to give relief in angina pectoris; it is a vasodilator. **Amyl salicylate.** $C_5H_{11}OOC C_6H_4OH$, a liquid used as an analgesic and in the treatment of rheumatism. **Amyl valerate.** $C_5H_{11}OOCC_4H_9$, apple oil, a synthetic flavouring, used medicinally as a solvent for gallstones. [Gk *amylon* starch, *hyle* matter.]
amylaceous (am·il·a·shus). Starchy; of the nature of, containing or relating to starch. [Gk *amylon* starch.]
amylaemia (am·il·e·me·ah). The presence of starch in the circulating blood. [Gk *amylon* starch, *haima* blood.]
amylase (am·il·aze). An amylolytic or starch-splitting enzyme which hydrolyses polysaccharides to dextrin and maltose. **Pancreatic amylase.** Amylopsin. **Salivary amylase.** Ptyalin. **Vegetable amylase.** Diastase. [Gk *amylon* starch.]
amylate (am·il·ate). 1. An alcoholate of amyl alcohol with a metal or base. 2. A compound of starch. [see foll.]
amylatic (am·il·at·ik). Marked by conversion of starch into sugar. [Gk *amylon* starch.]
amylene (am·il·een). C_5H_{10}. A liquid hydrocarbon of the olefine series, with an anaesthetic effect which is too dangerous to permit its clinical use. **Amylene Hydrate BP 1953.** Dimethylethylcarbinol, $(CH_3)_2{=}C{=}(C_2H_5)(OH)$, a tertiary alcohol used to dissolve tribromethanol; the resultant solution injected rectally is a very good basal narcotic.
amylenization (am·il·een·i·za′·shun). Anaesthesia produced as a result of administration of amylene.
amylic (am·il·ik). Containing or relating to the radical, amyl.
amylin (am·il·in). Starch-cellulose, amylopectin. The insoluble outer layer of the starch granule. Cf. AMIDIN. [Gk *amylon* starch.]
amylism (am·il·izm). The state of having been poisoned by amyl alcohol.
Amylobarbitone (am·il·o·bar·bit·one). 5-Iso-amyl-5-ethyl-barbituric acid, $CO(NHCO)_2C(C_2H_5)(CH_2CH_2CH(CH_3)_2)$; a hypnotic and sedative used for insomnia (BP 1973). **Amylobarbitone Sodium BP 1973, Soluble amylobarbitone.** The sodium salt of amylobarbitone, administered in capsules or by injection.
amylocaine hydrochloride (am·il·o·kane hi·dro·klor·ide). $C_6H_5C OOC(CH_3)(C_2H_5)(CH_2N(CH_3)_2)$, a local analgesic of the procaine type.
amylocellulose (am·il·o·sel′·ew·loze). Amylopectin; starch-cellulose. [Gk *amylon* starch, cellulose.]
amyloclast (am·il·o·klast). A starch-splitting enzyme. [Gk *amylon* starch, *klastikos* breaking up.]
amyloclastic (am·il·o·klas′·tik). Descriptive of enzymes capable of splitting up or digesting starch. [see prec.]
amylocoagulase (am·il·o·co·ag′·ew·laze). An enzyme in starch which thickens starch paste after a time, producing a deposit of amyloses. [Gk *amylon* starch, coagulase.]
amylodextrin (am·il·o·dex′·trin). A dextrin, or starch-gum, appearing at an early stage in the hydrolysis of starch by diastase or ptyalin; it gives a blue coloration with iodine. [Gk *amylon* starch, dextrin.]
amylodyspepsia (am·il·o·dis·pep′·se·ah). Impairment or lack of the power to digest starch-containing foods. [Gk *amylon* starch, dyspepsia.]

amylogen (**am**·il·o·jen). The portion of the starch granule that is rendered soluble in water by the action of mild acids or enzymes. [see foll.]

amylogenesis (**am**·il·o·**jen**'·es·is). The formation or production of starch. [Gk *amylon* starch, *genein* to produce.]

amylogenic (**am**·il·o·**jen**'·ik). 1. Forming starch. 2. Relating to amylogen. [see prec.]

amylohemicellulose (**am**·il·o·hem·e·**sel**'·ew·loze). A polysaccharide, insoluble in water, which is present in the cell wall of plants. It differs from cellulose in that it may be hydrolysed with dilute mineral acids to give soluble monosaccharides. [Gk *amylon* starch, hemicellulose.]

amylohydrolysis (**am**·il·o·hi·**drol**'·is·is). Amylolysis. [Gk *amylon* starch, hydrolysis.]

amylohydrolytic (**am**·il·o·hi·dro·**lit**'·ik). Amylolytic. [see prec.]

amyloid (**am**·il·oid). 1. Pertaining to starch; having the characteristics of starch. 2. A protein compound of albumin and chondroitin sulphuric acid which is deposited abnormally in certain tissues and which resembles starch in appearance; lardacein. 3. A horny substance produced by the action of sulphuric acid upon cellulose; parchment paper is manufactured by surfacing paper in this way; it forms a blue iodide, like starch, whence its name. 4. An intermediate starchy substance formed in wood tissues. [Gk *amylon* starch, *eidos* form.]

amyloidaemia (**am**·il·oid·e'·me·ah). A condition where there is amyloid in the blood. [amyloid, Gk *haima* blood.]

amyloidosis (**am**·il·oid·**o**'·sis). Amyloid degeneration. *See* DEGENERATION. **Amyloidosis cutis.** Amyloid degeneration of the skin with characteristic pigmented itching eruption. **Familial amyloidosis.** A genetically-determined form of systemic amyloidosis (see below) due to disturbed protein synthesis in plasma cells. **Primary amyloidosis.** The process of amyloid formation in tissues as a primary degeneration; it is a rare disease and affects mainly muscle, bone and cartilage. **Secondary amyloidosis.** Amyloid formation secondary to prolonged suppuration; it is more common and affects first the vascular system in an organ. **Systemic amyloidosis.** A rare disorder of protein metabolism, presumed to be a dysplasia of the plasma cells. There is a characteristic macroglossia, waxy amber papulation of the skin and involvement of one or more of the heart, kidneys, liver, gastro-intestinal tract, spinal ganglia or peripheral nerves. [amyloid, Gk *-osis* condition.]

amylolysis (am·il·**ol**·is·is). The conversion of starch into sugar by the action of enzymes or by hydrolysis; amylohydrolysis. [Gk *amylon* starch, *lysis* a loosing.]

amylolytic (**am**·il·o·**lit**'·ik). Capable of transforming starch into sugar, as by the process of digestion. [see prec.]

amylon (**am**·i·lon). 1. Greek for starch. 2. Glycogen. 3. Name applied to a constituent of grape juice.

amylopectin (**am**·il·o·**pek**'·tin). β-Amylose. The starch cellulose of the envelope of the starch granule. It is a calcium salt of a phosphoric acid complex, insoluble in water, and is the cause of starch gelatinizing when boiled; it gives a variable colour reaction with iodine. [Gk *amylon* starch, pectin.]

amylophagia (**am**·il·o·**fa**'·je·ah). An abnormal appetite or craving for starch. [Gk *amylon* starch, *phagein* to eat.]

amyloplast (**am**·il·o·plast). A chromatophore, or cytoplasmic organ of plant cells, which forms starch by photosynthesis. [Gk *amylon* starch, *plassein* to form.]

amyloplastic (**am**·il·o·**plas**'·tik). Starch-forming. [see prec.]

amyloprolamine (**am**·il·o·**pro**'·lam·een). The gliadin present in wheat and rye. It is rich in proline, whence the name, and confers on flour the adhesive property necessary for bread-making. [Gk *amylon* starch, prolamine.]

amylopsin (am·il·**op**·sin). Pancreatic amylase; an enzyme secreted by the pancreas which converts starch to dextrins and maltose. [Gk *amylon* starch, *opsis* appearance.]

amylorrhexis (**am**·il·o·**rex**'·is). The hydrolysis of starch by enzyme action. [Gk *amylon* starch, *rhexis* rupture.]

amylorrhoea (**am**·il·or·**e**'·ah). A condition in which an excessive amount of undigested starch is found in the stools. [Gk *amylon* starch, *rhoia* flow.]

amylose (**am**·il·oze). **α-Amylose.** The granulose or soluble starch within the starch granule; it is soluble in water, gives a blue reaction with iodine and is converted into maltose by amylase. **β-Amylose.** Amylopectin. **Crystalline amyloses.** General name given to the crystalline compounds formed from starch solution with a species of *Bacillus.* They include α-tetramylose, β-hexamylose, and α-octamylose. [Gk *amylon* starch.]

amylosis (am·il·o·sis). Albuminoid degeneration of cells. [Gk *amylon* starch, *-osis* condition.]

amylosuria (**am**·il·o·**zewr**'·e·ah). The presence of amylose in urine.

amylosynthease (**am**·il·o·**sin**'·the·aze). An enzyme which plays an important part in the synthesis of starch. [see foll.]

amylosynthesis (**am**·il·o·**sin**'·thes·is). The building-up of the starch molecule from glucose units. [Gk *amylon* starch, synthesis.]

amylum (**am**·il·um). Starch BP 1973. **Amylum Maydis, Amylum Oryzae, Amylum Solani, Amylum Tritici.** *European Pharmacopoeia* names for maize starch, rice starch, potato starch and wheat starch, respectively. [L from Gk *amylon* starch.]

amyluria (am·il·**ewr**·e·ah). The presence of starch in urine. [Gk *amylon* starch, urine.]

amynology (am·in·**ol**·o·je). Immunology; that branch of science which is concerned with immunity and its phenomena. [Gk *amyna* defence, *logos* science.]

amyo-aesthesia, amyo-aesthesis (a·**mi**·o·es·**the**'·ze·ah, a·**mi**·o·es·**the**'·sis). Lack of awareness of the position, weight and movement of the muscles; lack of muscle sense. [Gk *a, mys* muscle, aesthesis.]

amyocardia (a·mi·o·**kar**·de·ah). A condition in which the strength of the heart muscle is impaired so that the contractions are feeble; myasthenia cordis. [Gk *a, mys* muscle, *kardia* heart.]

amyoplasia (a·**mi**·o·**pla**'·ze·ah). A condition in which there is absence of muscle formation. **Amyoplasia congenita.** A condition marked by congenital rigidity of the joints. [Gk *a, mys* muscle, *plassein* to form.]

amyostasia (a·**mi**·o·**sta**'·ze·ah). Muscular tremor due to lack of co-ordination, as in tabes dorsalis, so that it is difficult for the sufferer to stand. [Gk *a, mys* muscle, *stasis* a standing.]

amyostatic (a·**mi**·o·**stat**'·ik). Affected with amyostasia; referring to amyostasia.

amyosthenia (a·**mi**·o·**sthe**'·ne·ah). Amyasthenia.

amyosthenic (a·**mi**·o·**sthen**'·ik). Amyasthenic.

amyotaxia, amyotaxy (a·**mi**·o·**tax**'·e·ah, a·**mi**·o·**tax**'·e). Ataxia: irregularity of or inability to control voluntary muscular movements. [Gk *a, mys* muscle, *taxis* arrangement.]

amyotonia (a·**mi**·o·**to**'·ne·ah). Myatonia: atony of the muscles. **Amyotonia congenita.** Myatonia congenita (syn.: Werdnig-Hoffmann's disease). [Gk *a, mys* muscle, *tonos* tone.]

amyotrophia, amyotrophy (a·**mi**·o·**tro**'·fe·ah, a·mi·**ot**·ro·fe). Myatrophy; a condition of atrophy affecting a muscle or muscles; muscular atrophy. **Neuralgic amyotrophia.** An acute neuritis of spinal roots characterized by severe pain, muscular wasting and weakness, and often some sensory impairment in the distribution of affected segments. It usually affects the muscles of the shoulder girdle, and may follow injections of serum, or trauma; it is possibly allergic, perhaps due to a virus. Also called *shoulder girdle neuritis, neuralgic amyotrophy.* **Amyotrophia spinalis progressiva.** Progressive muscular atrophy. *See* ATROPHY. **Pseudomyopathic neurogenic amyotrophy.** Kugelberg-Welander syndrome. **Syphilitic amyotrophia.** A muscular atrophy of syphilitic origin that may be arrested by antisyphilitic treatment. [Gk *a, mys* muscle, *trophe* nourishment.]

amyotrophic (a·**mi**·o·**trof**'·ik). Relating to or marked by muscular atrophy. [see prec.]

amyous (a·**mi**·us). Indicating that there is deficiency of muscular tissue or lack of muscular strength. [Gk *a, mys* muscle.]

Amyris (**am**·e·ris). A genus of trees or shrubs of the family Rutaceae, from which certain elemi are obtained. **Amyris balsamifera.** A species which yields West Indian sandalwood

oil. **Amyris plumierii.** The species from which Yucatan elemi is extracted. [Gk *a, myron* balsam.]
amyrol (**am**·e·rol). An isomeric camphor obtained from sandalwood, *Santalum album.* [see prec.]
amyxia (a·**mix**·e·ah). Deficiency or entire lack of mucus. [Gk *a, myxa* mucus.]
amyxis (am·**ix**·is). Scarification. [Gk *amyssein* to scarify.]
amyxorrhoea (a·**mix**·or·e'·ah). A condition in which there is deficiency or lack of mucous secretion. **Amyxorrhoea gastrica.** A condition in which an abnormally small quantity of mucus is present in the gastric secretion. [Gk *a, myxa* mucus, *rhoia* flow.]
ana (**an**·ah). In prescriptions, so much of each; abbreviated usually to $\overline{AA}$ or $\overline{aa}$. [Gk of each.]
ana-. Prefix, from the Greek *ana,* meaning *up, back, again.*
anabacteria (an·ah·bak·**teer'**·e·ah). An autolysate obtained from aqueous suspensions of bacteria macerated and treated with formalin; it is used for prophylactic and therapeutic vaccination against bacterial infections. [Gk *ana,* bacterium.]
Anabaena (an·**ab**·e·nah). A genus of fresh-water algae, blue-green in colour and of the family Nostocaceae. They contaminate reservoirs, emit a faecal odour and sometimes impart a cloudy appearance to the water. [Gk *anabainein,* to go up.]
anabasine (an·**ab**·as·een). $C_{10}H_{14}N_2$. An alkaloid very similar to nicotine, with which it is isomeric; extracted from *Anabasis aphylla,* and used as an insecticide.
anabasis (an·**ab**·as·is). The first period, or augmentation, in the course of a disease. [Gk a mounting.]
anabatic (an·ab·**at**·ik). Augmenting; growing more intense; relating to anabasis. [see prec.]
anabiosis (an·ah·bi·**o'**·sis). Reanimation or resuscitation of an organism after apparent death. [Gk revival.]
anabiotic (an·ah·bi·**ot'**·ik). 1. Resuscitating. 2. A restorative agent. 3. Apparently without life but capable of being reanimated. [see prec.]
anabole (an·**ab**·ol·e). 1. Vomit; expectoration. 2. A throwing-up. [Gk something heaped up.]
anabolergy (an·ah·**bol**·er·je). The amount of energy expended in the process of anabolism. [Gk *anaballein* to build up, *ergon* work.]
anabolic (an·ah·**bol**·ik). Relating to, or promoting, anabolism. [Gk *anaballein* to build up.]
anabolism (an·**ab**·ol·izm). The process of making new living tissue from nutrient material. [Gk *anaballein* to build up.]
anabolistic (an·ah·bol·**is'**·tik). Relating or belonging to the process of anabolism.
anabrosis (an·ah·**bro**·sis). Superficial ulceration of the soft tissues. [Gk an eating up.]
anabrotic (an·ah·**brot**·ik). Relating to or characterized by anabrosis; corrosive.
anacampsis (an·ah·**kamp**·sis). 1. A flexure. 2. In acoustics or optics, reflection. [Gk a bending back.]
anacamptic (an·ah·**kamp**·tik). In acoustics, reflected or reflecting. [see prec.]
anacamptics (an·a·**kamp**·tix). Name applied at one time to the branch of natural philosophy that dealt with light or sound reflected from surfaces. [Gk *anakamptein* to bend back.]
anacamptometer (an·ah·kamp·**tom'**·et·er). An apparatus for measuring the intensity of deep reflexes. [Gk *anakampsis* a bending back, meter.]
Anacardiaceae (an·ah·kar·de·**a'**·se·e). A family of mainly tropical trees and shrubs which includes *Pistacia lentiscus* Linn., the source of mastic, and *Anacardium occidentale* Linn., the seeds of which are known as *cashew nuts.* [Gk *ana, kardia* heart.]
Anacardium (an·ah·**kar**·de·um). A genus of tropical American trees of the family Anacardiaceae, the juice of which is poisonous. **Anacardium occidentale.** The cashew tree, the fruit of which is the cashew nut; the pericarp of the nut contains an acrid oil which has vesicant and anthelmintic properties. [see prec.]
anacatadidymous (an·ah·kat·ah·**did'**·im·us). Term applied to a twin monster the bodies of which are fused centrally. [see foll.]
anacatadidymus (an·ah·kat·ah·**did'**·im·us). A twin monster the bodies of which are united at the waist but separate above. [Gk *ana, kata, didymos* twin.]
anacatharsis (an·ah·kath·**ar'**·sis). 1. Severe and persistent vomiting. 2. Expectoration. [Gk *ana, katharsis* purgation.]
anacathartic (an·ah·kath·**ar'**·tik). 1. Emetic; causing anacatharsis. 2. An agent which causes vomiting or expectoration.
anachlorhydria (an·ah·klor·**hi'**·dre·ah). Achlorhydria. [Gk *ana,* chlorhydria.]
anacholia (an·ah·**ko**·le·ah). The condition in which there is diminution in the secretion of bile. [Gk *ana, chole* bile.]
anachoresis (an·ah·kor·**e'**·sis). The attraction of micro-organisms to certain local lesions, e.g. tuberculous or syphilitic, in which they establish themselves, while the rest of the body of the host appears to enjoy some immunity. [Gk *ana, choresis* a retiring.]
anachoretic, anachoric (an·ah·kor·**et'**·ik, an·ah·**kor**·ik). 1. Marked by or relating to anachoresis. 2. Indicating a condition caused by anachoresis.
anachromasis (an·ah·kro·**ma'**·sis). A synonym for *prophase,* the first stage in mitosis, in which chromosomes become visible. [Gk *ana, chroma* colour.]
anacidity (an·as·**id**·it·e). Lack of the normal amount of acidity; subacidity. **Gastric anacidity.** Achlorhydria. [Gk *a,* acidity.]
anaclasis (an·**ak**·las·is). 1. Refraction or reflection of light. 2. Refraction of light in the media of the eye. 3. Reflex action. 4. The forcible breaking up of fibrous ankylosis. [Gk *anaklan* to bend back.]
anaclastic (an·ah·**klas**·tik). Produced by or relating to anaclasis or refraction.
anaclisis (an·**ak**·lis·is). 1. The reclining posture; decubitus. 2. In psychology, a term denoting dependence upon, and applied to the first object of love because of the original dependence upon the mother for food and care. [Gk *ana, klisis* a leaning.]
anacmesis (an·**ak**·me·sis). The arrest of maturation of the early or primitive granular white cells, although these may be increased in number. [Gk *a, akmenos* fully grown.]
anacobra (an·ah·**ko**·brah). Cobra venom after it has been subjected to treatment with formaldehyde and to heat.
anacousia (an·ak·**oos**·e·ah). Total deafness. [Gk *a, akouein* to hear.]
anacroasia (an·ah·kro·**a'**·ze·ah). Lack of comprehension of spoken words as a result of disease of the cerebrum; the patient can understand words when he sees them written down. [Obsolete term.] [Gk *a, akroasis* hearing.]
anacrotic (an·ah·**krot**·ik). Marked by anacrotism.
anacrotism (an·**ak**·rot·izm). Abnormality of the pulse wave consisting in a secondary expansion seen in the upstroke of the sphygmogram. [Gk *ana, krotos* stroke.]
anaculture (an·ah·**kul**·tsher). A broth culture of bacteria treated with weak formalin solution and incubated until sterile.
anacusia, anacusis (an·ak·**ews**·e·ah, an·ak·**ew**·sis). Anacousia.
Anacyclus pyrethrum (an·ah·**si**·klus pi·**re**·thrum). Pellitory, Spanish chamomile; the root of a plant of the family Compositae, which has a pungent taste and when chewed increases salivation. It contains an irritant organic base, pyrethrine, and may cause gastro-enteritis when swallowed. It should not be confused with the insecticide known as *pyrethrum.*
anadenia (an·ah·**de**·ne·ah). 1. Deficiency of glandular function. 2. Lack of glands. **Anadenia gastrica.** Achylia gastrica. **Anadenia ventriculi.** Destruction or absence of the glands of the stomach. [Gk *a, aden* gland.]
anadesma (an·ah·**dez**·mah). A fascia or a band of tissue. [Gk *anadesme* fillet.]
anadicrotic (an·ah·di·**krot'**·ik). Marked by anadicrotism.
anadicrotism (an·ah·**di**·krot·izm). A condition in which the pulse curve obtained with a sphygmograph exhibits 2 notches in the ascending portion of the wave. [Gk *ana, dis* twice, *krotos* stroke.]
anadidymous (an·ah·**did**·im·us). Term descriptive of the teratism in which there are twin fetuses the lower limbs of which are fused into one. [Gk *ana, didymos* twin.]

anadidymus (an·ah·**did**·im·us). An anadidymous monster.

anadiplosis (**an**·ah·dip·**lo'**·sis). The reduplication of a paroxysm of fever. [Gk *ana, diploun* to double.]

anadipsia (an·ah·**dip**·se·ah). Excessive or intense thirst. [Gk *ana, dipsa* thirst.]

anadrenalism (an·ad·**re**·nal·ism). Lack of failure of function of the adrenal glands; the constitutional result of such defect. [Gk *a*, adrenalism.]

anadrenia (an·ad·**re**·ne·ah). The state resulting from failure or lack of function of the adrenal glands. [see prec.]

anaedeous (an·e·de·us). Without genitalia. [Gk *a, aidoia* genitalia.]

anaematopoiesis (an·e·mat·o·poi·e'·sis). A condition in which blood is produced in insufficient quantity. [Gk *a, haima* blood, *poiein* to make.]

anaemia (an·e·me·ah). A condition of the blood in which there are quantitative and qualitative changes in the red cells (erythrocytes) and haemoglobin in the circulating blood and bone marrow: there may also be a reduction in the total amount of blood (*oligohaemia*) temporarily, as in a severe acute haemorrhagic condition. Defective red-cell formation due to deficiency conditions produces macrocytic megaloblastic or microcytic normoblastic anaemias according to the deficiency; inhibition or aplasia of the haemopoietic tissues causes aplastic and hypoplastic anaemias. Excessive red-cell destruction occurs in the haemolytic anaemias, while acute or chronic blood loss is followed by posthaemorrhagic, secondary or hypochromic normocytic normoblastic anaemias. **Achlorhydric anaemia.** A hypochromic microcytic anaemia found in association with achlorhydria gastrica. **Achrestic anaemia.** A hyperchromic, macrocytic megaloblastic anaemia the cause of which is considered to be a failure to mobilize from the tissue stores, or to utilize, the anti-anaemic principle which is necessary for the normal formation of normoblasts. **Anaemia achylica, Achylic anaemia.** Usually a macrocytic anaemia or pernicious anaemia (see below). **Acute anaemia.** A severe sudden anaemia usually due to blood loss or to toxic or haemolytic causes. **Acute febrile anaemia.** A disease which progresses rapidly and is marked by pyrexia, cardiac weakness and the occurrence of hyaline thromboses. **Acute haemolytic anaemia.** A disease that occurs most commonly in the first 3 decades of life; there is usually a severe normoblastic normocytic anaemia with many immature erythrocytes and reticulocytes in the peripheral blood, and a variable degree of leucocytosis, pyrexia and jaundice. Various causes include severe bacterial, protozoal and other parasitic infections, chemical poisons such as derivatives of the heavy metals, benzene and aniline, haemolytic agents such as lysolecithin, saponin, snake venoms and fava (broad bean), incompatible blood transfusions, and haemolysins and agglutinins of various types. **Addisonian anaemia.** Pernicious anaemia (see below). **African anaemia.** Sickle-cell anaemia (see below). **Agastric anaemia.** Anaemia occurring after a considerable part of the stomach has been removed. **Alimentary anaemia.** Deficiency or nutritional anaemia (see below). **Angiospastic anaemia.** Anaemia caused by spasm occurring locally in the blood vessels. **Anhaematopoietic anaemia, Anhaemopoietic anaemia.** Anaemia caused by deficiency in the formation of erythrocytes. **Aplastic anaemia.** Severe, fatal, normocytic, normochromic anaemia in which the bone marrow, having ceased partially or completely to function, becomes fatty, and aplastic. Owing to the inability of the primitive reticuloendothelial cells to divide normally there are also low leucocyte and platelet counts. It may be idiopathic in type, or due to toxic drugs and other factors of many kinds. **Aregenerative anaemia, Aregeneratory anaemia.** Aplastic anaemia (see above). **Asiderotic anaemia.** Hypochromic microcytic anaemia (see below). **Atrophic anaemia.** A form in which anaemia is associated with bone marrow atrophy. **Atrophic aplastic anaemia.** Myelophthisic anaemia (see below). **Baghdad anaemia.** A seasonal haemolytic anaemia due to pollens. **Bartonella anaemia.** Oroya fever. *See* FEVER. **Blind-loop anaemia.** A megaloblastic anaemia usually associated with a steatorrhoea and multiple diverticuloses of the small intestine, usually the jejunum, or with isolated loops of the intestine caused by stricture or anastomoses of sections of the small intestine. These blind loops become infected stagnant areas in which bacteria multiply and remove or destroy cyanocobalamin in the gut contents, so causing a deficiency of this vitamin and consequently a megaloblastic anaemia which may be relieved by treatment with parenteral cyanocobalamin and antibiotic therapy or by removal of the blind loops. **Bothriocephalus anaemia.** Diphyllobothrium anaemia (see below). **Brickmakers' anaemia.** Ancylostomiasis. **Cameloid anaemia.** Elliptocytotic anaemia (see below). **Cerebral anaemia.** Deficiency in the supply of blood to the brain. **Chloritic anaemia, Chlorotic anaemia.** Chlorosis. **Chronic anaemia.** A hypochromic anaemia caused by the constant drain on the blood-forming tissues by recurrent bleeding or oozing of blood, particularly from the alimentary, genito-urinary and pulmonary systems. **Chronic haemolytic anaemia.** Acholuric jaundice; chronic spherocytic anaemia. *See* HAEMOLYTIC ANAEMIA (below). **Chronic hypochromic anaemia.** Microcytic anaemia; an anaemia caused by deficient supply, absorption or utilization of iron to maintain normal formation and haemoglobinization of the red cells. It is nearly always associated with achylia gastrica, dysphagia and, very frequently, koilonychia. **Chronic infective anaemia.** Anaemia due to or associated with long-standing infections. **Congenital haemolytic anaemia.** A haemolytic anaemia often with a familial incidence, of chronic nature characterized by a normocytic, normochromic and normoblastic anaemia, undue fragility of the red cells, persisting reticulocytosis in the circulating blood, recurrent haemolytic crises and considerable relief of the condition after splenectomy. **Congenital hypoplastic anaemia.** A familial type of hypoplastic anaemia (see below). **Congenital, or familial, microcytic anaemia.** Cooley's anaemia; a familial, haemolytic, erythroblastic anaemia which occurs usually in families of Mediterranean stock. It is seen in major and minor forms, and may be overt or mild in adults but more marked in children, who often show developmental retardation, splenomegaly and skeletal changes, with a hypochromic microcytic anaemia and sometimes mongoloid facies. **Cow's-milk anaemia.** A form of anaemia occurring in infants when fed solely on cow's milk and due to a deficiency of iron. **Crescent-cell anaemia.** Sickle-cell anaemia (see below). **Cytogenic anaemia.** Pernicious anaemia (see below). **Deficiency anaemia.** Any anaemia caused by ineffective formation of normal red cells and haemoglobin and which may be due to a deficiency in hormones or vitamins, to deficiency or error in diet, to feeding, or to the inadequate absorption of iron, vitamins, mineral elements or anti-pernicious anaemia factors. **Dimorphic anaemia.** Anaemia in which there is a combined macrocytic and microcytic hypochromic anaemia on account of multiple deficiencies. The marrow is not megaloblastic and there is reputed to be poor response to liver extracts, folic acid and vitamin B_{12}. A very questionable entity. **Diphyllobothrium anaemia.** Megaloblastic anaemia, very like addisonian pernicious anaemia, that occurs in a percentage of persons infected by the fish tapeworm *Diphyllobothrium latum.* There is still some uncertainty about the exact mechanism of this anaemia, but there is evidence that the worm intercepts vitamin B_{12} in the proximal portion of the small intestine before it is absorbed; when the worm happens to be located in the distal portion of the small intestine, anaemia does not occur. **Drepanocytic anaemia.** Sickle-cell anaemia (see below). **Dyshaematopoietic anaemia.** One of a group of anaemias caused by a defect in haemopoiesis; they include the deficiency anaemias, metabolic anaemias, the toxic anaemias and the aplastic anaemias. **Dyspoietic anaemia.** Anaemia due to a diminished red-cell formation, although marrow biopsy shows a hyperplastic condition. **Egyptian anaemia.** Ancylostomiasis. **Elliptocytary anaemia, Elliptocytotic anaemia.** Elliptocytosis; an anaemia characterized by oval-shaped (cameloid) cells (elliptocytes) in the blood. **Erythroblastic anaemia.** An anaemia usually characterized by a megaloblastic (erythroblastic) bone marrow and a macrocytic anaemia; occasionally there may be a haemolytic anaemia, of which there are many types, with sometimes a leucocytosis of leukaemoid type. **Erythroblastic anaemia of childhood.** 1. Thalassaemia. 2. Anaemia pseudoleukaemia infantum (see below). **Erythronoclastic anaemia.** Haemolytic anaemia (see below). **Erythronormoblastic anaemia.** Hypochromic anaemia (see below). **Essential anaemia.** Pernicious anaemia (see below). **Experimental anaemia.** A macrocytic anaemia produced in rats by feeding on goat's milk only (goat's-milk anaemia; see below), or any other anaemia experimentally produced. **Familial erythroblastic anaemia.** Congenital, or familial, microcytic anaemia (see above). **Familial haemolytic anaemia.** Acholuric jaundice or chronic haemolytic anaemia (see above); sometimes refers to Cooley's anaemia. **Familial microcytic anaemia.** Cooley's anaemia; congenital, or familial, microcytic anaemia (see above). **Familial splenic anaemia.** Gaucher's disease. **Febrile pleiochromic anaemia.** A form of anaemia in which thrombi composed of agglutinated erythrocytes or platelets block the terminal arterioles and the capillaries. **Globe-cell anaemia, Globular anaemia.** A haemolytic anaemia (usually chronic, often familial) in which the red cells are spherical or spherocytes; congenital haemolytic jaundice. **Glossitic anaemia.** Pernicious anaemia (see below). **Goat's-milk anaemia.** A macrocytic anaemia, associated with dyspepsia, in infants or produced in rats fed on goat's milk. **Ground-itch anaemia.** Ancylostomiasis. **Haemolytic anaemia.** Any one of a number of different kinds of anaemia characterized by crises of severe anaemia often with intermittent chronic phases due to excessive red-cell destruction, severe haemolytic phenomena, and variable degrees of jaundice. The anaemia is usually normocytic but may be hyperchromic and macrocytic, while the hyperplastic marrow is usually normoblastic in type. There are acute and chronic forms with special features, e.g. acute haemolytic anaemia (see above) and acute Lederer's anaemia; the chronic forms include such as achloluric jaundice, chronic spherocytic anaemia, sickle-cell anaemia, thalassaemia and erythroblastosis. **Haemolytic anaemia of pregnancy.** Macrocytic anaemia of pregnancy (see below). **Haemorrhagic anaemia.** Anaemia caused directly by acute or chronic loss of blood from whatever cause, in adults or the newborn. **Haemotoxic anaemia.** A haemolytic anaemia due to destruction of red cells by toxic substances, drugs or haemolytic toxins. **Hookworm anaemia.** Ancylostomiasis. **Hyperchromic anaemia.** An anaemia characterized by a greater reduction in the number of red cells in comparison with the haemoglobin so that the cells are more highly coloured or haemoglobinized; they are frequently larger in size than normal and usually associated with a hyperplastic and megaloblastic or normoblastic bone marrow. **Hypochromic anaemia, Hypochromic microcytic anaemia.** Hypochromaemia; an anaemia in which the haemoglobin is very greatly reduced in proportion to the number of red cells, so that the latter are pale, containing less than the normal amount of haemoglobin. The cells are smaller than normal, but the marrow is usually normoblastic; achylia, dysphagia and koilonychia are commonly seen in this anaemia, in which there is an iron deficiency. It may be idiopathic, or secondary to neoplasms or ulceration of the alimentary tract or to phthisis, or arising from prolonged milk diets. **Hypoferric anaemia.** Anaemia caused by deficiency of iron in the blood. **Hypoplastic anaemia, Hyporegenerative anaemia.** An anaemia, essentially an incomplete aplastic anaemia, caused by depression of marrow function from various causes such as inhibition by toxic drugs, severe infections or congenital weakness of marrow function. **Icterohaemolytic anaemia.** Haemolytic jaundice. *See* JAUNDICE. **Idiopathic anaemia.** Anaemia arising through disease of the blood-forming organs of unidentified cause. **Idiopathic hypochromic anaemia.** A benign, iron-deficiency, hypochromic, microcytic anaemia caused by inadequate iron intake or iron absorption; it is often associated with achylia, dysphagia and koilonychia, and cured by massive iron therapy. **Idiopathic microcytic anaemia.** Hypochromic anaemia (see above). **Intertropical anaemia.** Ancylostomiasis. **Isochromic anaemia.** An anaemia in which the number of erythrocytes is diminished proportionately to the fall in haemoglobin content. **Leuco-erythroblastic anaemia.** Leucoerythroblastosis; a fatal, acute anaemic condition in which the peripheral blood contains many immature leucocytes, megaloblasts, normoblasts and reticulocytes, reflecting the picture seen in the active hyperplasia of the bone marrow; there may be splenomegaly and lymphadenopathy, and it is often associated with space-occupying disturbances of the bone marrow (myelopathic anaemia). **Local anaemia.** Anaemia limited to certain parts of the body, caused by mechanical interference with the supply of blood or from permanently low pressure in local blood channels. **Lymphatic anaemia.** Lymphadenoma; Hodgkin's disease. **Lysolecithin haemolytic anaemia.** Cooley's anaemia; congenital, or familial, microcytic anaemia (see above). **Macroblastic anaemia, Macrocytic anaemia.** An anaemia in which the red cells are diminished in number in the peripheral blood to a greater extent than the haemoglobin; the red-cell volume is increased, and so the red cells contain more haemoglobin per cell; there is usually, but not always, a megaloblastic marrow. Macrocytic anaemia is seen in pernicious anaemia, in some cases of steatorrhoea and in macrocytic anaemia of pregnancy. **Macrocytic anaemia of pregnancy.** A macrocytic anaemia seen in pregnant women, with which there may be a megaloblastic or mixed megaloblastic-normoblastic marrow; treatment with folic acid is better than with liver extracts or vitamin B_{12}. It clears up rapidly after parturition, but may be very severe before. **Malignant anaemia.** Pernicious anaemia (see below). **Mediterranean anaemia.** Cooley's anaemia; congenital, or familial, microcytic anaemia (see above). **Megaloblastic anaemia.** A macrocytic anaemia with megaloblastic hyperplasia of the marrow; there are often megaloblasts in the peripheral blood. **Megaloblastic anaemia of infancy.** A severe macrocytic anaemia with megaloblastic marrow, occasionally seen in young infants. **Megalocytic anaemia.** Macrocytic anaemia (see below). **Meniscocytic anaemia.** Sickle-cell anaemia (see below). **Microcytic anaemia, Microcytic hypochromic anaemia.** Any of the idiopathic or hypochromic anaemias. **Micro-elliptopoikilocytic anaemia.** Thalassaemia; Cooley's anaemia. **Milk anaemia.** An iron-deficiency anaemia produced in young children, patients on long-standing uncompensated milk diets for peptic ulceration or faddists on special diets, caused by keeping them for too long on an exclusively milk diet without supplementary vitamins and iron (hypochromic anaemia). **Miners' anaemia.** Ancylostomiasis. **Myelogenous anaemia.** An anaemia in which there is hyperplasia of myeloid cells in blood and marrow, such as occurs in myeloid leukaemia. **Myelopathic anaemia, Myelophthisic anaemia.** A chronic refractory anaemia secondary to the mechanical or toxic inhibition of bone marrow or its destruction by the infiltrations of secondary carcinomatosis, myelomata, Gaucher cells, or due to the mechanical restriction imposed by such bone diseases as Albers-Schoenberg disease, myelosclerosis and Hodgkin's disease. **Anaemia neonatorum.** Erythroblastosis neonatorum. **Normocytic anaemia.** An anaemia having diminished numbers of normal sized and normally haemoglobinated erythrocytes. **Nutritional anaemia.** Any deficiency anaemia (see above). **Nutritional macrocytic anaemia.** Anaemia due to a specific dietary deficiency; curable by folic acid. **Occult anaemia.** An anaemia that is not apparent owing to haemoconcentration, such as occurs in severe shock. **Osteosclerotic anaemia.** A myelopathic anaemia in which the bone-marrow function is depressed by osteosclerosis. **Ovalocytary anaemia, Ovalocytic anaemia.** Ovalocytosis; elliptocytotic anaemia (see above). **Paludal anaemia.** Usually a haemolytic anaemia caused by or associated with malaria. **Pernicious anaemia.** A severe, progressive, ultimately fatal (if untreated), macrocytic, hyperchromic, megaloblastic anaemia which can be relieved and maintained under full control by adequate treatment. It is associated with achylia gastrica, clear-cut changes in the blood and bone marrow, typical symptoms due to the gastro-intestinal deficiencies, and frequently with changes in the central nervous system; spontaneous temporary remissions occur sometimes but relapses follow unless treated. It is due to the absence of an essential anti-pernicious anaemia factor necessary to enable the proerythroblasts to produce normoblasts in the marrow. **Physiological** anaemia. An anaemia of varying severity that develops in babies in the first 6 months of life; it is due to iron deficiency of milk feeds (maternal or cow). It usually disappears after weaning, but promptly when small supplements of iron salts are given. **Pleiochromic anaemia.** Acute febrile anaemia (see above). **Primary anaemia.** Pernicious anaemia (see above) [obsolete term]. **Primary erythroblastic anaemia.** Cooley's anaemia; congenital, or familial, microcytic anaemia (see above). **Anaemia pseudoleukaemia infantum.** An anaemia of children under 3 years of age in which there is a splenomegaly with many nucleated red cells (megaloblasts, normoblasts), and leucocytosis in the peripheral blood. It may be associated with tuberculosis, syphilis and other infections, and with nutritional deficiencies. **Puerto Rican anaemia.** A severe anaemia associated with ancylostomiasis and possibly nutritional deficiencies. **Refractory anaemia, Refractory macrocytic anaemia.** A severe, sometimes chronic anaemia usually macrocytic in type that does not respond to ordinary anti-anaemic therapy. There may be megaloblastic or normoblastic marrow and the condition is often associated with an obvious or overt steatorrhoea. Treatment is not very satisfactory in most cases; other cases have hypoplastic non-responding marrows. **Scorbutic anaemia.** An anaemia, usually macrocytic in type, associated with a deficiency of ascorbic acid in the diet. **Secondary anaemia.** An anaemia that is secondary to a chronic disease such as cancer, tuberculosis, gross sepsis, or to other blood diseases, and also following traumatic haemorrhage. The older meaning, when all anaemias were classified as primary and secondary, is now obsolete. **Semi-aplastic anaemia.** A hypoplastic anaemia (see above). **Septic anaemia.** An anaemia secondary to severe sepsis or infection. **Sickle-cell anaemia.** A familial haemolytic anaemia, found most commonly in patients of negro origin and associated with chronic ulcers of the leg. It is a severe, often fatal, anaemia, in which the erythrocytes are sickle-shaped or crescentic as a result of the presence in them of an abnormal haemoglobin (haemoglobin S). **Spherocytic anaemia.** Haemolytic anaemia (see above). **Splenic anaemia, Anaemia splenetica.** Banti's anaemia; a chronic mild anaemia in which there is enlargement of the spleen with or without hepatomegaly, said to be due to portal thrombosis or portal hypertension. In the early stages either the spleen or the liver may be the first to enlarge. The anaemia is usually mildly hypochromic, normocytic or slightly microcytic, and non-characteristic. **Splenic anaemia of infants.** Anaemia pseudoleukaemia infantum (see above). **Symptomatic anaemia.** Secondary anaemia (see above). **Symptomatic haemolytic anaemia.** Cooley's anaemia; congenital, or familial, microcytic anaemia (see above). **Target-cell anaemia.** Cooley's anaemia, characterized by erythrocytes with a dark centre and concentric light and dark zones. **Thrombocytopenic anaemia, Thrombopenic anaemia.** A purpuric anaemia due to acute or chronic thrombocytopenia. **Thrombotic micro-angiopathic haemolytic anaemia.** A severe febrile disease in which there is haemolytic anaemia, purpura and neurological disturbances. It is associated pathologically with a widespread thrombosis of the smallest-calibre blood vessels, especially in the myocardium, adrenals and renal cortex. Also called *thrombotic thrombocytopenic purpura.* **Toxic anaemia.** Anaemia due to exposure to poisons or toxins destroying or affecting the formation of the red cells or haemoglobin (haemolytic anaemias, aplastic anaemia). **Traumatic anaemia.** Haemorrhagic anaemia (see above). **Trophoneurotic anaemia.** Anaemia induced by severe nervous shock. **Tropical anaemia.** A vague and undesirable term. There is no physiological anaemia in hot countries, but, if anything, a slight tendency to polycythaemia; there are, however, more causes of anaemia-producing parasitic infections, and nutritional deficiencies are commoner. The term has been applied to the anaemia of ancylostomiasis. **Tropical macrocytic anaemia.** A mixed group of macrocytic hyperchromic anaemias resembling pernicious anaemia in some respects and occurring in tropical or sub-tropical regions. They are probably associated with specific nutritional deficiencies, pregnancy, malaria and other parasitic infections; there is no nervous involvement and achlorhydria is uncommon. **Tropical megalocytic anaemia.** Tropical macrocytic anaemia (see preceding). **Tunnel anaemia.** Ancylostomiasis. **Unstable haemoglobin haemolytic anaemia (UHHA).** Anaemia caused by unstable haemoglobin. *See* HAEMOGLOBIN. [GK *a, haima* blood.]

See also: ADDISON (T.), BANTI, BIERMER, CHVOSTEK (FRANZ), COOLEY, CZERNY (A.), DI GUGLIELMO, DRESBACH, EDELMANN, EHRLICH, FABER, FANCONI, HAYEM, HERRICK, JAKSCH, LEDERER, LEISHMAN, LUZET, PLUMMER, VINSON, WIDAL, WILKINSON (J. F.), WILLS, WITTS.

anaemic (an·**e**·mik). Relating to anaemia; caused by or suffering from anaemia.

anaemotrophy (an·e·**mot**·rof·e). A state of impoverishment of the blood. [Gk *a, haima* blood, *trophe* nutrition.]

anaeretic (an·e·**ret**·ik). Term descriptive of substances which tend to destroy animal tissue. [Gk *anairesis* destruction.]

anaerobe (an·**a**·er·obe). A micro-organism which is able to exist and multiply although deprived of either free oxygen or air. Cf. AEROBE. **Facultative anaerobe.** A micro-organism which is not dependent upon gaseous oxygen but prefers an atmosphere containing oxygen. **Obligatory anaerobe.** A micro-organism which cannot live in an atmosphere containing oxygen. [Gk *a, aer* air, *bios* life.]

anaerobian (an·a·er·**o**'·be·an). 1. An anaerobe. 2. Able to live without air.

anaerobiase (an·a·er·o·**bi**'·aze). A proteolytic enzyme which is active in anaerobic conditions; it is produced by *Clostridium welchii* and other anaerobes.

anaerobic (**an**·a·er·**o**'·bik). 1. Growing most vigorously in an atmosphere which is free from oxygen. 2. Able to sustain life without free oxygen. 3. Referring or belonging to an anaerobe. [Gk *a, aer* air, *bios* life.]

anaerobion (an·a·er·**o**'·be·on). Anaerobe.

anaerobiosis (an·a·er·o·bi·**o**'·sis). The state of existing or the power of living in an atmosphere which is devoid of free oxygen. [Gk *a, aer* air, *bios* life.]

anaerobiotic, anaerobious (an·a·er·o·bi·**ot**'·ik, **an**·a·er·**o**'·be·us). Anaerobic.

anaerobism (an·a·er·o·bizm). The state of an organism which is able to live without oxygen or air. [Gk *a, aer* air, *bios* life.]

Anaeromyces bronchitica (an·a·er·o·**mi**'·seez brong·**kit**·ik·ah). A branching diphtheroid-like bacillus which has been claimed as a cause of bronchitis in the tropics; an obligate anaerobe, Gram-positive and non-motile. [Gk *a, aer* air, *mykes* fungus, bronchitis.]

anaerophyte (an·a·er·o·fite). A plant or micro-organism which grows in the absence of free oxygen. [Gk *a, aer* air, *phyton* plant.]

anaeroplastic (an·a·er·o·**plas**'·tik). Relating to anaeroplasty.

anaeroplasty (an·a·er·o·**plas**'·te). The treatment of wounds by the application of water or wet bandages, or by immersion of the part in water, to exclude the air. The method is obsolete but the principle is still applied in the modern treatment of wounds by "closed plaster", and the wrapping of leg ulcers with adhesive bandage. [Gk *a, aer* air, *plassein* to mould.]

anaerosis (**an**·a·er·**o**'·sis). A state in which respiratory function is interrupted. The term is applied particularly to such a state in newborn infants. [Gk *a, aer* air, *-osis* condition.]

anaesthecinesia, anaesthecinesis, anaesthekinesia, anaesthekinesis (an·es·**the**·sin·e'·ze·ah, an·es·**the**·sin·e'·sis, an·es·**the**·kin·e'·ze·ah, an·es·**the**·kin·e'·sis). Lack of the powers of moving and feeling. [Obsolete term.] [Gk *a*, aesthesia, *kinesis* movement.]

anaesthesia (an·es·**the**·ze·ah). Loss of feeling or sensation in some part of the body due to nervous lesion, or a local anaesthetic agent, or loss of consciousness produced by some general anaesthetic inhaled or injected. **Angiospastic anaesthesia.** Denoting the loss of all forms of tactile sensation in an area as the result of ischaemia produced by the reduction in the blood vessels supplying that area. It may occur in Raynaud's phenomenon, in which the digital arteries contract as a result of cold, and the digits become numb and blue; also in ischaemia from any cause, such as arterial embolism or thrombosis, and in ischaemic neuritis when the peripheral nerves are damaged by an impaired blood supply as a result of occlusive arterial disease. Spasm is not necessary for its development. **Balanced anaesthesia.** A combination of several agents such as premedication, regional analgesia and general anaesthesia, nicely balanced so as to avoid the excessive administration of any one agent. A term first used by John S. Lundy, of the Mayo Clinic, in 1926. **Basal anaesthesia.** Basal narcosis. *See* NARCOSIS. **Block anaesthesia.** *See* BLOCK, ANAESTHETIC. **Bulbar anaesthesia.** That due to a lesion of the pons or mid-brain. **Carbon dioxide absorption anaesthesia.** A form of general anaesthetic administration in which the gases and vapours are inhaled by the patient over and over again, the oxygen needs being maintained by a continuous flow of that gas and the carbon dioxide produced by metabolism being prevented from accumulating by absorption in a cannister of soda lime. **Caudal anaesthesia.** Caudal analgesia. *See* ANALGESIA. **Central anaesthesia.** That due to a lesion of nerve centres or tracts. **Cerebral anaesthesia.** That due to a cerebral lesion. **Closed anaesthesia.** Inhalational anaesthesia in which the expired gases are totally re-breathed after suitable modification. **Closed-circuit anaesthesia.** A form of carbon dioxide absorption anaesthesia (see above) in which the gases and vapours are rebreathed. **Colonic anaesthesia.** Rectal anaesthesia (see below). **Compression anaesthesia.** Anaesthesia produced by pressure on a nerve or artery; pressure anaesthesia, Javanese anaesthesia (see below). **Conduction anaesthesia.** *See* BLOCK, ANAESTHETIC. **Continuous spinal anaesthesia.** Continuous spinal analgesia. *See* ANALGESIA. **Crossed anaesthesia.** Anaesthesia found on the opposite side of the body to that of the causal lesion. **Dissociated anaesthesia, Dissociation anaesthesia.** Loss of sensation for painful and thermal stimuli while tactile sensation persists; seen in syringomyelia. **Anaesthesia dolorosa.** A tactile pain in an anaesthetic area. **Draw-over anaesthesia.** A method of vaporizing volatile anaesthetic agents by the patient drawing air over their surface, as in the EMO ether inhaler. **Endoneural anaesthesia.** Anaesthetic block by injecting a solution into the covering of a nerve. **Endotracheal anaesthesia.** Inhalational or insufflation anaesthesia with a tube passed into the trachea, either through a tracheotomy opening or via the nose or mouth. **Epidural anaesthesia.** Epidural analgesia. *See* ANALGESIA. **Facial anaesthesia.** That due to lesions of the 5th cranial nerve. **Field-block anaesthesia.** Field-block analgesia. *See* ANALGESIA. **Gas-ether anaesthesia.** General anaesthesia induced by the inhalation of nitrous oxide and maintained by ether vapour. **Gas-oxygen anaesthesia.** General anaesthesia by the inhalation of a mixture of nitrous oxide and oxygen. **Gas-oxygen-ether anaesthesia.** The same as gas-oxygen anaesthesia (preceding) but with ether vapour added to the mixture. **Gauntlet anaesthesia.** Anaesthesia of the hand in the area covered by the gauntlet or glove; a hysterical phenomenon. **General anaesthesia.** The administration of chemical agents to produce reversible unconsciousness and depression of reflex response to afferent stimuli. **Girdle anaesthesia.** Diminution or loss of sensation around the body, in segmental distribution, seen in spinal-cord lesions, e.g. tabes dorsalis. **Glove anaesthesia.** Gauntlet anaesthesia (see above). **Gustatory anaesthesia.** Absence or loss of the sense of taste. **Hysterical anaesthesia.** Anaesthesia of the skin and/or mucous membranes as a result of hysteria. **Ice anaesthesia.** Refrigeration anaesthesia (see below). **Infiltration anaesthesia.** Infiltration analgesia. *See* ANALGESIA. **Infusion anaesthesia.** General anaesthesia by infusing into a vein a solution of some appropriate anaesthetic agent. **Inhalation anaesthesia.** The state produced by the inhalation of gaseous or volatile anaesthetic agents. **Insufflation anaesthesia.** A form of anaesthesia administration in which a continuous positive flow of anaesthetic gas or vapour is delivered into the air passages. **Intercostal anaesthesia.** Intercostal analgesia. *See* ANALGESIA. **Intradural anaesthesia.** Intradural analgesia. *See* ANALGESIA. **Intra-oral anaesthesia.** Anaesthesia produced by the injection of solution into the tissues inside the mouth. **Intra-osseous anaesthesia.** Intra-osseous analgesia. *See* ANALGESIA. **Intraspinal anaesthesia.** Subarachnoid analgesia. *See* ANALGESIA. **Intratracheal anaesthesia.** Endotracheal anaesthesia (see above). **Intravenous anaesthesia.** Induction of anaesthesia by the intravenous injection of general anaesthetic drugs, e.g. thiopentone. **Javanese anaesthesia.** Unconsciousness produced by pressure on the carotid arteries. **Levels of anaesthesia.** The stages and planes of anaesthesia from full consciousness to death. Systematized by A. E. Guedel in the years following 1920. **Local anaesthesia.** Local analgesia. *See* ANALGESIA. **Mental anaesthesia.** Failure of the mind to respond to appropriate stimuli. **Mixed anaesthesia.** The simultaneous use of varied anaesthetic methods and drugs with the aim of achieving the minimum physiological disturbance. **Morphine-hyoscine anaesthesia.** Deep narcosis produced by injecting large or repeated doses of these drugs; twilight sleep. **Muscular anaesthesia.** Loss of deep (or muscle) sensation, e.g. in tabes dorsalis. **Nasotracheal anaesthesia.** Endotracheal anaesthesia in which the carrying tube traverses the nose. **Nerve-blocking anaesthesia.** Nerve-blocking analgesia. *See* ANALGESIA. **Neural anaesthesia.** Regional anaesthesia (see below). **Neurolept anaesthesia.** Anaesthesia produced by the injection of a butyrophenone derivative, e.g. droperidol with a narcotic analgesic. A neologism introduced in 1959 by De Castro and Mundeleer. **Nitrous oxide anaesthesia.** General anaesthesia by the inhalation of "gas", which is nitrous oxide; it must be of short duration as air (oxygen) is excluded. **Nitrous oxide-oxygen anaesthesia.** Gas-oxygen anaesthesia (see above). **Oil-ether anaesthesia.** General anaesthesia produced by running a mixture of olive oil and ether through the rectum into the colon; the ether is absorbed into the blood stream. **Olfactory anaesthesia.** Loss of the sense of smell. **Open anaesthesia.** A form of administration in which a volatile anaesthetic liquid is dropped on to cotton gauze stretched on a frame (or mask) held over the patient's face. If there is complete approximation between the mask and the face, the term *perhalation* is used. **Optic anaesthesia.** Temporary loss of function of the optic nerve. **Orotracheal anaesthesia.** Endotracheal anaesthesia with the carrying tube traversing the mouth. **Paraneural anaesthesia.** Nerve block by injecting a solution around a nerve. **Parasacral anaesthesia.** Nerve block of the sacral nerves as they leave the sacral canal. **Paravertebral anaesthesia.** Paravertebral block. *See* BLOCK. **Perhalation anaesthesia.** Open anaesthesia (see above). **Peridural anaesthesia.** Peridural analgesia. *See* ANALGESIA. **Perineural anaesthesia.** Paraneural anaesthesia (see above). **Peripheral anaesthesia.** Anaesthesia produced by nerve block. **Pharyngeal anaesthesia.** Anaesthesia of the pharyngeal mucosa. **Plexus anaesthesia.** Plexus analgesia. *See* ANALGESIA. **Pressure anaesthesia.** Pressure analgesia. *See* ANALGESIA. **Rectal anaesthesia.** General anaesthesia produced by absorption through the mucous membrane of anaesthetic drugs placed in solution or mixture in the rectum, e.g. Gwathmey's oil-ether anaesthesia. **Refrigeration anaesthesia.** Refrigeration analgesia. *See* ANALGESIA. **Regional anaesthesia.** Regional analgesia. *See* ANALGESIA. **Rehalational anaesthesia.** Closed or semi-closed inhalational anaesthesia. **Sacral anaesthesia.** Sacral analgesia. *See* ANALGESIA. **Saddle-block anaesthesia.** Saddle-block analgesia. *See* ANALGESIA. **Segmental anaesthesia.** Segmental analgesia. *See* ANALGESIA. **Semi-closed anaesthesia.** Inhalational anaesthesia in which a proportion of the vapours and gases breathed out are allowed to escape whilst the remainder is re-breathed. **Sexual anaesthesia.** Absence of physical sexual feelings. **Sleeved-jacket anaesthesia.** Sensory loss over the thorax and both arms, as in syringomyelia. **Spinal anaesthesia.** Subarachnoid analgesia. *See* ANALGESIA. **Splanchnic anaesthesia.** Splanchnic analgesia. *See* ANALGESIA. **Spraying anaesthesia.** Local anaesthesia by the freezing effect of spraying a volatile liquid such as ether or ethyl chloride on to a small area of skin. **Stocking anaesthesia.** Stocking analgesia. *See* ANALGESIA. **Subarachnoid anaesthesia.** Subarachnoid analgesia. *See* ANALGESIA. **Submucous anaesthesia.** Submucous analgesia. *See* ANALGESIA. **Surface anaesthesia.** Surface analgesia. *See* ANALGESIA. **Surgical anaesthesia.** Implies not only analgesia and unconsciousness but also abolition of reflex activity and complete relaxation of the voluntary muscles. **Tactile anaesthesia.** Loss or diminution of the sense of touch. **Terminal anaesthesia.** Terminal analgesia. *See* ANALGESIA. **Thalamic hyperaesthetic anaesthesia.** That associated with lesions of the thalamus. **Thermic anaesthesia.** Loss of sensation of stimuli by heat and cold, seen in central lesions of the spinal cord. **Total spinal anaesthesia.** Total spinal analgesia. *See* ANALGESIA. **Trans-sacral anaesthesia.** Trans-sacral analgesia. *See* ANALGESIA. **Traumatic anaesthesia.** Anaesthesia which is the result of direct injury to a nerve. **Twilight anaesthesia.** Twilight sleep; obstetrical hypnosis and amnesia produced by injections of morphine and scopolamine. **Unilateral anaesthesia.** Hemianaesthesia. **Visceral anaesthesia.** The absence of sensations from the viscera. [Gk *anaisthesia* lack of feeling.]

See also: ARNOTT (J.), BIER, CORNING, GWATHMEY, JONNESCO.

anaesthesimeter (an·es·the·**zim**'·et·er). 1. An apparatus for measuring the quantity of anaesthetic administered by inhalation in a given time. 2. An instrument with which degrees of insensitiveness in a part may be determined.

anaesthesiology (an·es·the·ze·**ol**'·o·je). The study of anaesthesia and of its induction and the complications attendant on it, and of anaesthetics and their administration. [anaesthesia, Gk *logos* science.]

anaesthesiometer (an·es·the·ze·**om**'·et·er). Anaesthesimeter.

anaesthesiophore (an·es·**the**·ze·o·for). That part of the molecule of an anaesthetic to which it owes its physiological action. [Obsolete term.] [anaesthesia, Gk *pherein* to bear.]

anaesthetic (an·es·**thet**·ik). 1. Without sensitivity. 2. Any drug or chemical used to produce anaesthesia. 3. Appertaining to or causing anaesthesia. **General anaesthetic.** A drug that produces general anaesthesia. **Local anaesthetic.** More properly local *analgesic.* Any substance applied locally or by injection to produce freedom from the sensation of pain, limited to the part. **Volatile anaesthetic.** A liquid anaesthetic agent which is inspired after conversion into a vapour, e.g. halothane. [Gk *anaisthesia* lack of feeling.]

anaesthetist (an·**ees**·thet·ist). An expert in the administration of anaesthetics.

anaesthetization (an·ees·thet·i·**za**'·shun). The process of anaesthetizing.

anaesthetize (an·**ees**·thet·ize). To place under the influence of anaesthetics; to induce a state of anaesthesia in a person.

anaesthetizer (an·**ees**·thet·i·zer). A person who administers an anaesthetic.

anaesthetometer (an·**ees**·thet·**om**'·et·er). An apparatus with which anaesthetic gases and vapours can be measured and mixed; anaesthesimeter.

anaetiological (an·e·te·o·**loj**'·ik·al). Contrary to aetiological principles. [Gk *a*, aetiology.]

anagen (**an**·ah·jen). The active stage in the hair-growth cycle. In humans each follicle acts independently of its neighbours (mosaic pattern). On the human scalp anagen lasts for 3 years or more; elsewhere it is of shorter duration. At any one time 75-95 per cent of the hairs on the scalp are in the anagen phase. *See also* CATAGEN and TELOGEN. [Gk *ana*, genein to produce.]

anagenesis (an·ah·**jen**·es·is). Repair or reconstruction of tissue or of lost parts taking place within the organism. [Gk *ana*, genesis.]

anagenetic (an·ah·jen·**et**'·ik). Producing or relating to the process of anagenesis.

anaglyph (**an**·ah·glif). A picture of two images of which one in red and one in green are not accurately superimposed, giving a blurred effect. When the picture is looked at through an anaglyphoscope, the object appears clear, uncoloured and in relief, because the image printed in green corresponds with what the right eye would see, and that in red with what the left eye would see, if together they were viewing the picture normally. [Gk *ana*, *glyphein* to engrave.]

anaglyphoscope (an·ah·**glif**·o·skope). Goggles with green transparent material before the right eye and red before the left, through which specially prepared anaglyphs can be viewed to obtain the stereoscopic effect of solidity. [Gk *ana*, *glyphein* to engrave, *skopein* to view.]

anagnosasthenia (an·ag·no·zas·**the**'·ne·ah). 1. Inability to read although the printed words are apparent to the eye. 2. A form of neurasthenia in which any attempt to read gives rise to symptoms of distress. [Gk *anagnosis* reading, asthenia.]

Anagnostakis, André (b. 1826). Greek ophthalmologist.

Anagnostakis' operation, Hotz-Anagnostakis operation. For entropion, usually upper lid: excision of orbicularis fibres along the length of the lid, followed by suture of the skin margin to the tarsal plate high up, so everting the lid margin and straightening out the deformed tarsus.

anagocytic (an·ag·o·**sit**'·ik). Inhibiting or retarding the growth of cells. [Gk *ana*, *agein* to lead, *kytos* cell.]

anagoge (an·ag·o·je). 1. Vomiting. 2. In psychology, the upward striving of the unconscious. **Anagoge haematis, Anagoge sanguinis.** A rush of blood to the head. [Gk *anagoge* a leading up.]

anagogic (an·ag·o·jik). Relating to anagoge.

anagogy (an·ag·o·je). Anagoge.

anagotoxic (an·ag·o·**tox**'·ik). Counteracting the action of a toxin. [Gk *ana*, *agein* to lead, toxin.]

anahaematopoiesis (an·ah·**he**·mat·o·poi·**e**'·sis). A condition of the bone marrow in which there is decreased functional activity. [Gk *ana*, *haima* blood, *poiein* to make.]

anakinetomere (an·ah·**kin**·et·o·meer). Matter possessing a high degree of energy. [Gk *ana*, *kinesis* motion, *meros* a part.]

anakinetomeric (an·ah·**kin**·et·o·mer'·ik). Possessing a high degree of energy. [see prec.]

anakroasia (an·ah·kro·**a**'·ze·ah). Anacroasia.

anakusis (an·ah·**kew**·sis). Anacousia. [Gk *a*, *akouein* to hear.]

anal (**a**·nal). Situated near or relating to the anus. **Anal sinus.** *See* SINUS. **Anal valve.** *See* VALVE.

analepsia, analepsis (an·al·**ep**·se·ah, an·al·**ep**·sis). Recovery of strength after illness. [Gk a repairing.]

analeptic (an·al·**ep**·tik). An agent which causes arousal. Previously used to improve the conscious level of comatose or drowsy patients. [Gk *analepsia* a repairing.]

analgecize (an·**al**·je·size). To make insensitive to pain. [see foll.]

analgesia (an·al·**je**·ze·ah). A state of insensitivity to painful stimuli; a preliminary stage in the induction of surgical anaesthesia. **Analgesia algera.** Acute pain in a part with loss of sensibility. **Caudal analgesia.** Analgesia resulting from the injection of a local analgesic solution into the sacral extradural space; used in surgery and obstetrics. **Continuous caudal analgesia.** A method of pain relief used in obstetrics and surgery in which a catheter is introduced and left in the caudal canal for repeated injection of an anaesthetic solution. **Continuous spinal analgesia.** Regional analgesia of the lower part of the body by continuous intrathecal injection, through a specially adapted spinal needle, of appropriate quantities of analgesic solution. **Analgesia dolorosa.** Analgesia algera (see above). **Epidural analgesia, Extradural analgesia.** Analgesia produced by injecting appropriate solutions into the space surrounding the spinal cord external to the dura mater. **Gas-air analgesia.** A method of pain relief produced by inhalation of a mixture of nitrous oxide and air, used in obstetrics and dentistry. **Infiltration analgesia.** Injection of local analgesic solution into tissues so that they become insensitive to painful stimuli. **Intercostal analgesia.** Analgesia of the thoracic and abdominal walls produced by injection of analgesic solution around the intercostal nerves. **Intradural analgesia.** Injection of local analgesic solution into the intradural or subarachnoid space. **Intra-osseous analgesia.** In dentistry, analgesia of a tooth obtained by injecting the analgesic solution into the surrounding alveolar bone. **Intraspinal analgesia.** Subarachnoid analgesia (see below). **Local analgesia.** Application or injection of local analgesic solution in order to remove painful sensation from the part or parts so treated. **Nerve-blocking analgesia.** Regional analgesia (see below). **Obstetrical analgesia.** Relief of pain in childbirth by nerve block (caudal analgesia) or by the inhalation of appropriate dilutions of anaesthetic vapours or gases (e.g. nitrous oxide). **Analgesia panaris.** Painless whitlow seen in syringomyelia. **Parasacral analgesia.** The injection of a local analgesic solution into the tissues close to the hollow of the sacrum to block the sacral nerves. **Paravertebral analgesia.** Paravertebral block. *See* BLOCK. **Paretic analgesia.** Loss of sense of pain associated with paresis. **Peridural analgesia.** Injection of local analgesic solution into the peridural or extradural space. **Perineural analgesia.** Analgesia produced by injection of an analgesic substance into the tissues around a nerve. **Plexus analgesia.** A form of nerve-block in which an analgesic solution is applied to a nerve-plexus, such as the brachial. **Presacral analgesia.** Parasacral analgesia (see above). **Pressure analgesia.** 1. Nerve-block caused by pressure of a conducting nerve. 2. Unconsciousness caused by pressure on carotid arteries (Javanese anaesthesia). 3. In dentistry, analgesia of the pulp of a tooth by forcing cocaine into it. **Refrigeration analgesia.** A method of pain relief produced by artificial lowering of the temperature, e.g. of a limb, about 5°C. **Regional analgesia.** The removal of the perception of pain from one area, rather than from the whole body, by the application of local analgesic drugs. **Sacral analgesia.** Analgesia of the region supplied by the sacral nerves produced by subarachnoid or epidural block. **Saddle-block analgesia.** Restricted spinal analgesia affecting only the buttocks, perineum and inner aspects of the thighs, i.e. the areas in contact with the saddle when sitting a horse. **Spinal analgesia.** The production of analgesia and muscular relaxation in the areas supplied by spinal nerves, resulting from the injection of local analgesic solution into either the intradural (subarachnoid) or the extradural (epidural, peridural) spaces. **Splanchnic analgesia.** Splanchnic nerve-block by the injection of analgesic solution into the region of the splanchnic ganglia. **Stocking analgesia.** Analgesia of the leg in the area covered by a stocking; a hysterical phenomenon. **Subarachnoid analgesia.** Analgesia of the lower part of the body by injection of analgesic solution into the subarachnoid space. **Submucous analgesia.** The analgesia obtained by the injection of a local analgesic solution beneath the mucous membrane of the mouth. **Surface analgesia.** Local analgesia produced by the absorption of an analgesic drug from a solution applied to the body surface. **Terminal analgesia.** Local analgesia produced by injecting analgesic solution at the exact site of operation, thereby anaesthetizing nerve-endings. **Topical analgesia.** Analgesia produced by placing a local analgesic solution on a tissue, e.g. a mucous membrane. **Total spinal analgesia.** An extended subarachnoid block in which all the sympathetic outflow is affected and widespread analgesia is achieved with an accompanying fall in blood pressure. **Trans-sacral analgesia.** Analgesia of the perineal region by blocking the sacral nerves as they traverse the sacral foramina. [Gk *a, algos* pain.]

analgesic (an·al·**je**·zik). 1. A remedy or agent which deadens pain. 2. Producing or relating to analgesia. [see prec.]

analgesin (an·al·**je**·zin). Antipyrin. [see foll.]

analgesist (an·al·**je**·zist). Anaesthetist. [Gk *a, algos* pain.]

analgetic (an·al·**jet**·ik). Analgesic.

analgia (an·**al**·je·ah). Absence of pain. [Gk *a, algos* pain.]

analgic (an·**al**·jik). Insensitive to pain, analgesic. [see prec.]

analgin (an·**al**·jin). Creolin.

anallergic (an·al·**er**·jik). Not producing hypersensitiveness; not allergic. [Gk *a*, allergic.]

analogous (an·**al**·o·gus). 1. Having a similar function, though derived from different embryological structures, e.g. the wing of a bird and that of an insect. 2. In chemistry, of the nature of an analogue. Cf. HOMOLOGOUS. [see foll.]

analogue (**an**·al·og). 1. An organ, or part of an organism, which is different in structure and origin from another but has a similar function. 2. In chemistry, any compound which has similar structure to another but differs in respect of a particular element, the differing element being usually of the same valency and group in the Periodic Table as the other; thus, NaCl and NaBr, H_2O and H_2S. 3. The representation of a system to be studied in an analogous but more manipulative form than the original. **Analogue computer.** *See* COMPUTER. **Analogue recording.** Data recording by such means as diagrams or graphs, the changes in which are analogous to the changes in the data being recorded. **Homologous analogue.** An organ or part which has both similar structure and function to that of another. [Gk *analogos* proportionate.]

analogy (an·**al**·o·je). 1. A resemblance; a correspondence between 2 things to a certain degree; a reasoning from similar cases. 2. Biologically, resemblance in function or form of organs which differ structurally or in origin. [Gk *analogia* proportion.]

analosis (an·al·**o**·sis). Atrophy; wasting. [Gk, expenditure.]

analyser (**an**·al·i·zer). 1. Name applied to that part of the nervous system which governs an organism's reaction to changing environment, especially the cerebral cortex. 2. A sensory nerve terminal and its central connections which allow differentiation of sensitivity to stimulation. 3. An instrument in electro-encephalography for determining the amount of each component frequency in a record which is a mixture of frequencies. **Pulse-height analyser.** An electronic device for recording separately detected radiation of differing energies. The energy spectrum of the radiation can thus be determined. *Kick sorter.* [Gk *analysis* a loosing.]

analysis (an·**al**·is·is). 1. The separation of a mixture into its components. 2. The resolution of a complex substance into simpler substances; the opposite of synthesis. 3. The chemical examination of a substance; the determination or assay of its constituents. 4. *See* PSYCHOANALYSIS. **Activation analysis.** The elemental analysis of a specimen by exposing it to irradiation by neutrons, thus converting many elements to a radioactive form, hence making it possible to assay them by measuring the radiation emitted. This method can also be applied to a limited extent to intact man and animals. **Blowpipe analysis.** The detection of metallic salts by the coloration of a borax bead in a blowpipe flame. **Bradycinetic analysis.** The study of growth by means of the slow-motion film. **Chromatographic analysis, Chromographic analysis.** The estimation of the constituents of a substance by their selective adsorption in a column of suitable material. **Clinical analysis.** The examination of tissues in the diagnosis of disease. **Colorimetric analysis.** The estimation of a substance by comparison of the colour of its solution with other coloured solutions of known strength. **Colour analysis.** Ehrlich's method of identifying leucocytes, based upon the staining of the protoplasmic granules. **Compartment analysis.** The analysis of the movement of ions and other diffusible materials in and through physiological compartments. The use of radioactive tracers in the determination of the size and dynamic characteristics of these compartments. **Competitive inhibition analysis, Competitive protein-binding analysis.** Saturation analysis (see below). **Densimetric analysis.** The estimation of the amount of a substance in a solution by determination of the density of the latter. **Derivative analysis.** A method of chemical analysis depending upon causing the compound of interest to react with a radioactive reagent so that a radioactive derivative of the compound is formed which can be assayed by measurement of the radiation it emits. **Diffusion analysis.** The separation of constituents by taking advantage of their differing rates of diffusion. **Dilution analysis.** The measurement of the amount of a material present by diluting with it a known amount of a radioactive form of the material. A sample is then taken and assayed both for the material of interest and for its radioactive content. The ratio of the radioactivity to the material in the sample is the same as the ratio of the radioactivity diluted in the unknown quantity to that quantity, and, hence, this can be calculated. **Displacement analysis.** A term not in general use but occasionally employed as a synonym for *saturation analysis.* **Distributive analysis.** Psychological treatment during which information about the patient is distributed along the lines which are indicated by the patient's complaints. **Electrometric analysis.** Potentiometric analysis (see below). **Elementary analysis.** The estimation of the amount of any particular element in a compound or mixture. **Eudiometric analysis.** Gasometric analysis (see below). **Fluorescence analysis.** The recognition of chemical compounds by their fluorescence in ultra-violet light. **Gas analysis.** Quantitative estimation of gases in a mixture by absorbing them successively in suitable agents. **Gasometric analysis.** Estimation of the amount of any substance present in a mixture by the liberation of a gas from it and measurement of the volume of the latter, e.g. urea in urine by the liberation of nitrogen. **Gravimetric analysis.** Determination of the composition of a mixture by separation of its constituents and weighing them. **Inorganic analysis.** The analysis of inorganic substances. **Micro-analysis.** 1. The recognition of constituents by means of their appearance under the microscope. 2. Analysis of minute quantities of materials by a specially modified technique. **Microchemical analysis.** Chemical analysis of minute quantities by ordinary qualitative or quantitative methods in miniature. **Nephelometric analysis.** Estimation of an insoluble constituent by comparison of the cloudiness it produces in a given quantity of liquid with a known standard. **Neutron activation analysis.** Activation analysis (see above). **Organic analysis.** The analysis of organic substances. **Peptide map analysis.** *See* PEPTIDE. **Polarimetric analysis, Polariscopic analysis.** Analysis of an optically-active solution by measurement of the rotation of the axis of a beam of polarized light passed through it. **Polarographic analysis.** Analysis of a solution by recording the current-voltage curve (polarogram) at the dropping mercury electrode. **Positive-ray analysis.** The separation of mixed ions of different weights or charges by means of the mass spectrograph. It is used to determine the masses of individual atoms or molecules. **Potentiometric analysis.** Determination of end-points in titrations involving neutralization or oxidation-reduction reactions, by means of a potentiometer. **Proximate analysis.** The recognition of the main types of compounds present in a sample. **Qualitative analysis.** The investigation of the constituents of a sample according to their kind. **Quantitative analysis.** The investigation of a sample in order to determine the proportions of its constituents. **Radioactivation analysis.** The radioactivation of the elements in a specimen by some form of particle or photon bombardment. Subsequently, the quantity of the elements of interest present can be deduced from measurement of the characteristic radiations emitted by the corresponding radio-isotopes to which they give rise. The particles usually used are neutrons. **Rational analysis.** The expression of a mixture in terms of the compounds which it contains rather than the elements comprising the latter. **Saturation analysis.** A method for the analysis of compounds based upon the binding equilibrium between the compound of interest and another compound with which it associates. The distribution of the compound to be assayed between such a specific binding agent and the free or non-specifically bound state is determined by the distribution of radioactivity when a radioactively-labelled tracer quantity of the compound is added during the assay procedure. **Sequence analysis.** The methods whereby the sequence of the different monomers of a polymer, e.g. of amino acids in polypeptides or of nucleotide bases in polynucleotides, may be analysed. **Spectrophotometric analysis.** The recognition and estimation of compounds by measuring the amount of light they absorb in the infra-red, visible or ultra-violet regions of the spectrum. **Spectroscopic analysis, Spectrum analysis.** The recognition of elements through their emission spectra. **Statistical analysis.** A term denoting the detailed examination of collected figures (vital statistics) relating to a problem of health or disease, in an attempt to determine the underlying factors producing such causes and effects and, if possible, to identify those specially requiring correction. **Thermometric analysis.** Estimation of any constituent of a mixture by measuring the heat liberated or absorbed in a chemical reaction in which it is made to take part. **Ultimate analysis.** The analysis of a substance in order to determine the elements of which it is composed. **Volumetric analysis.** Determination of the quantities of substances in solution by titration with standard solutions of reagents. **Wet analysis.** The separation of constituents by precipitation from solution and filtering. **X-ray diffraction analysis.** A method of analysis by which the diffraction by a substance of a narrow beam of x-rays is photographed and forms a characteristic pattern. It is especially useful in crystallography. [Gk a loosing.]

analyzer (**an**·al·i·zer). In polarimetry, the portion of a polariscope containing the Nicol prism, rotation of which measures the angle that the axis of polarized light has been turned through by the solution under examination. Cf. POLARIZER. [see prec.]

Anamirta (an·am·**er**·tah). A genus of plants of the family Menispermaceae. **Anamirta paniculata.** A climbing shrub of South-east Asia; furnishes a fruit which, when dried, constitutes cocculus indicus, the source of picrotoxin. [Sanskrit immortal.]

anamirtin (an·a·**mer**·tin). A narcotic glyceride, $C_{18}H_{24}O_{16}$, extracted from Levant berries, cocculus indicus. [see prec.]

anamnesia, anamnesis (an·am·**ne**·ze·ah, an·am·**ne**·sis). 1. The faculty of recollecting. 2. The act of recalling to mind. 3. The past medical history of a patient. [Gk *anamimneskein* to recall to memory.]

anamnestic (an·am·**nes**·tik). 1. Relating to anamnesia. 2. Serving to recall to mind. 3. Aiding memory. **Anamnestic response.** Immune response to an antigen to which the patient has previously been sensitized, provoked by entry of an unrelated antigen into the body. Term also sometimes used to mean a secondary immune response. [see prec.]

anamnionic, anamniotic (**an**·am·ne·**on**′·ik, **an**·am·ne·**ot**′·ik). Not having an amnion. [Gk *a*, amnion.]

anamniota (an·am·ne·**o**′·tah). A classificatory grouping of all those vertebrates in whose eggs the amnion and other extra-embryonic membranes are not present, particularly fish and Amphibia. [see prec.]

anamorphosis (an·ah·**mor**·fo·sis). 1. An ascending or progressive development of a species in the animal or vegetable kingdom. 2. The use of an anamorphote lens. [Gk *ana*, *morphe* form.]

ananabasia (**an**·an·ab·**a**′·se·ah). The condition of being unable to go up to high places or to ascend heights. [Gk *a*, *anabasis* ascent.]

ananaphylaxis (**an**·an·ah·fil·**ax**′·is). Anti-anaphylaxis. [Gk *a*, anaphylaxis.]

ananastasia (**an**·an·as·**ta**′·ze·ah). The condition in which the sufferer lacks the ability either to rise from a sitting position or to stand up on his feet. [Gk *a*, *anastasis* standing up.]

anancastia (an·an·**kas**·te·ah). The obsessive compulsive type of personality. [Gk *anagkastos* forced.]

anandria (an·**an**·dre·ah). 1. In a male, the loss of male characters and the development of female characters. 2. Lack of masculinity or virility. 3. Impotence. [Gk *a*, *aner* man.]

anangioplasia (an·**an**·je·o·**pla**′·ze·ah). A congenital condition in which there is imperfect development of the blood vessels, so that their calibre is abnormally small and too little blood is carried to the tissues. There may be entire non-development of the vessels. [Gk *a*, *aggeion* vessel, *plassein* to form.]

anangioplasm (an·**an**·je·o·plazm). Imperfect development of the blood vessels. [see prec.]

anapausis (an·ah·**paw**·sis). The allaying of excitement by hypnosis in order to induce quiet sleep. [Gk rest.]

anapeiratic (**an**·ah·pi·**rat**′·ik). Describing the condition caused by the excessive or repeated use of a muscle, or by the prolonged exercise of a part. [Gk *anapeirasthai* to try again.]

anapepsia (an·ah·**pep**·se·ah). Entire lack of pepsin in the stomach secretion. [Gk *ana*, *a*, pepsin.]

anaphase (**an**·af·aze). In mitosis and meiosis, the stage between metaphase and telophase during which chromosomes move away from each other towards the poles of the spindle. [Gk *ana*, *phainein* to appear.]

anaphia (an·**af**·e·ah). Absence or loss of the sense of touch. [Gk *a*, *haphe* touch.]

anaphora (**an**·af·or·ah). The repetition of the same word or phrase in several successive clauses.

anaphoretic (**an**·af·or·**et**′·ik). 1. An agent which causes decrease in the secretion of sweat. 2. Inhibiting sweating. [Gk *ana*, diaphoresis.]

anaphoria (an·af·**or**·e·ah). Double hyperphoria; a condition in which the axes of the eyes are parallel as long as they remain open together but, if one eye is covered, the other immediately turns upward. [Gk *ana, phorein* to bear.]

anaphrodisia (**an**·af·ro·**diz**'·e·ah). A condition in which there is impairment of sexual feeling, or entire lack of it. [Gk *a, Aphrodite* goddess of love.]

anaphrodisiac (**an**·af·ro·**diz**'·e·ak). Antaphrodisiac: 1. Having the power to lessen or inhibit sexual feeling. 2. An agent which produces anaphrodisia.

anaphrodite (an·**af**·ro·dite). A person with impaired sexual feeling, or without any at all. [Gk *a, Aphrodite* goddess of love.]

anaphylactia (**an**·ah·fil·**ak**'·te·ah). An anaphylactic attack. [Gk *ana,* phylaxis.]

anaphylactic (**an**·ah·fil·**ak**'·tik). Relating to anaphylaxis. **Anaphylactic shock.** Generalized and often severe anaphylaxis characterized in man by hypotension, peripheral circulatory failure, with perhaps asthma and urticaria. It follows injection of allergen by any route which disseminates it widely and results from generalized histamine release.

anaphylactin (**an**·ah·fil·**ak**'·tin). Reagin; an antibody produced in response to an anaphylactogen; a substance reacting specifically with an agent which can cause anaphylaxis.

anaphylactogen (an·ah·fil·**ak**·to·jen). Any substance which causes anaphylaxis. [see foll.]

anaphylactogenesis (**an**·ah·**fil**·ak·to·**jen**'·es·is). The production of anaphylaxis. [anaphylaxis, Gk *genein* to produce.]

anaphylactogenic (**an**·ah·fil·ak·to·**jen**'·ik). A term descriptive of substances which produce anaphylaxis. [see prec.]

anaphylactoid (**an**·ah·fil·**ak**'·toid). Pseudo-anaphylactic. [anaphylaxis, Gk *eidos* form.]

anaphylatoxin (**an**·ah·fil·ah·**tox**'·in). The non-specific toxic substance which is supposed to be liberated in the tissues during anaphylactic shock. [anaphylaxis, Gk *toxikon* poison.]

anaphylatoxis (**an**·ah·fil·ah·**tox**'·is). The reaction which is the result of the presence of an anaphylatoxin.

anaphylaxin (**an**·ah·fil·**ax**'·in). Anaphylactin.

anaphylaxis (**an**·ah·fil·**ax**'·is). A condition of hypersensitiveness to certain foreign proteins, e.g. horse serum, induced by the injection of 2 doses with an interval of not less than 10 days between them. The first or sensitizing dose renders an animal hypersusceptible to a subsequent injection, and the sensitization is specific. The guinea-pig is the animal most susceptible to anaphylaxis, the rabbit and the dog much less so, while man is very slightly susceptible. It is characterized by a symptom complex, constant for a given animal, with onset a few minutes after administration of the second dose of antigen, and a fatal termination regularly in guinea-pigs, frequently in rabbits and less commonly in dogs. The anaphylactic response is probably the result of an antigen–antibody reaction occurring on or in tissue cells that have removed the antibody from the blood and fixed it to themselves, as there is absence of circulating antibody in the anaphylactic state. The syndrome of anaphylactic shock is due to liberation of histamine from cells injured by the second or "assault" dose of antigen. Hypersensitiveness in man, e.g. serum sickness, food and drug idiosyncrasies, and hay fever, presents reactions with analogies to the anaphylactic reaction in experimental animals. Substances producing the syndrome of anaphylaxis include horse serum, egg albumin, milk, bacterial antigens, peptone and histamine. **Acquired anaphylaxis, Active anaphylaxis.** The state produced by administration of a foreign protein. **Local anaphylaxis.** A reaction peculiar to the rabbit, whereby repeated subcutaneous injections of horse serum give rise to local swellings and localized areas of necrosis of the skin and subcutaneous tissues. **Passive anaphylaxis.** Hypersensitiveness produced by the injection of serum from a sensitized animal or individual. **Passive cutaneous anaphylaxis.** *In vivo* passive transfer technique for recognizing homocytotropic antibody responsible for immediate hypersensitivity reactions. It depends on the release of histamine at the site where antigen (injected intravenously) reacts with cell-fixed antibody (previously injected intradermally) and is demonstrated by a blue spot on the skin due to the leak of the dye, Evans' blue, through the now permeable capillaries. **Reverse passive anaphylaxis.** Anaphylaxis after injection of the antigen followed by injection at the same site of serum from a sensitized individual. [Gk *ana, phylaxis* protection.]

anaphylodiagnosis (**an**·ah·**fil**·o·di·ag·**no**'·sis). Anaphylactic reactions used as a means of diagnosis of disease.

anaphylotoxin (**an**·ah·fil·o·**tox**'·in). Anaphylatoxin.

anaplasia, anaplase (an·ah·**pla**·ze·ah, **an**·ah·plaze). Dedifferentiation; in biology, a change in a cell which prevents complete growth and function; reversion of a cell to a less differentiated and more primitive and embryonic type. **Monophasic anaplasia.** A change of cell character to the embryonic type, characteristic of malignancy and associated with an increased capacity for multiplication. **Polyphasic anaplasia.** A change of a cell into one which is more complex. [Gk *ana, plassein* to mould.]

anaplasis, anaplasm (an·ah·**pla**·zis, **an**·ah·plazm). Plastic surgery or any reparative surgical procedure. [see prec.]

Anaplasma (an·ah·**plaz**·mah). A genus of sporozoan organisms found in the red blood cells of cattle. [Gk *ana, plasma* something formed.]

anaplasmosis (**an**·ah·plaz·**mo**'·sis). Infection with *Anaplasma.* [*Anaplasma,* Gk *-osis* condition.]

anaplastia (an·ah·**plas**·te·ah). Anaplasia.

anaplastic (an·ah·**plas**·tik). 1. A term applied to cells which are affected with anaplasia or are imperfect in development. 2. Relating to the plastic restoration of a part that has been lost or to the plastic formation of an absent part. [Gk *ana, plassein* to mould.]

anaplasty (**an**·ah·plas·te). Anaplasis.

anaplerosis (**an**·ah·pler·**o**'·sis). Repair of tissues, but especially with regard to regrowth or replacement of losses or making good of defects. [Gk *ana, plerosis* filling.]

anaplerotic (**an**·ah·pler·**ot**'·ik). 1. Any agent which promotes the formation of granulation tissue and thus stimulates repair. 2. Relating to anaplerosis; making good a defect. [see prec.]

anapneometer (**an**·ap·ne·**om**'·et·er). An apparatus used to determine the sum of the tidal, complemental or supplemental air (vital capacity) of the lungs. [Gk *ana, pnoia* breath, meter.]

anapnoeic, anapnoic (an·ap·**ne**·ik, an·ap·**no**·ik). 1. Relating to respiration. 2. Re-establishing respiration; relieving dyspnoea. [Gk *ana, pnoia* breath.]

anapnograph (an·**ap**·no·graf). A form of spirometer which records the rate and the force of respiration. [Gk *anapnon* respiration, *graphein* to record.]

anapnometer (**an**·ap·**nom**'·et·er). Anapneometer.

anapnotherapy (an·**ap**·no·**ther**'·ap·e). Resuscitative treatment by inhalation of a gas. [Gk *anapnein* to inhale, therapy.]

anapophysis (an·ap·**of**·is·is). An accessory process of the spinal vertebrae, particularly of a thoracic or lumbar vertebra. [Gk *ana, apophysis* offshoot.]

anaptic (an·**ap**·tik). Characterized by or relating to anaphia (lack of the sense of touch). [Gk *a, haphe* touch.]

anarithmia (an·ar·**ith**·me·ah). A disease in which there is inability to use numbers or to count; it is caused by a lesion of the central nervous system. [Gk *a, arithmos* numeration.]

anarrhexis (an·ar·**ex**·is). The surgical procedure of refracturing a bone, e.g. in cases in which there is deformity because of faulty union. [Gk *ana, rhexis* fracture.]

anarrhoea (an·ar·**e**·ah). A flux or a flowing to an upper part, causing suffusion, such as a rush of blood to the head. [Gk *ana, rhoia* flow.]

anarthria (an·**ar**·thre·ah). 1. The loss of the power of articulating words. Cf. DYSARTHRIA. 2. Lack of vigour. 3. A condition of being without joints. **Anarthria centralis.** Defective power of speaking caused by a lesion of the central nervous system. **Anarthria literalis.** Stuttering. [Gk *a, arthron* joint.]

anasarca (an·ah·**sar**·kah). A more or less generalized oedema of the subcutaneous tissues often associated with transudation of fluid into the serous sacs. It may be due to cardiac, renal or, occasionally, hepatic disease, and to starvation. **Anasarca hystericum.** Transient anasarca in a hysteric. [Gk *ana, sarx* flesh.]

anasarcous (an·ah·sar·kus). Dropsical, of the nature of anasarca.

anascitic (an·as·it·ik). Not showing ascites. [Gk *a*, ascites.]

anaspadia, anaspadias (an·ah·spa·de·ah, an·ah·spa·de·as). Epispadias; a congenital deformity in which the urethra opens on the top of the glans penis or the dorsum of the penis. [Gk *ana, spadon* a rent.]

anaspadiac (an·ah·spa·de·ak). 1. Referring to anaspadia. 2. An individual who is affected with anaspadia.

anastalsis (an·ah·stal·sis). 1. Antiperistalsis; an upward-moving wave of contraction without a preceding wave of inhibition, occurring in the intestine in addition to peristalsis. 2. Styptic action. [Gk *ana, stalsis* constriction.]

anastaltic (an·ah·stal·tik). 1. Styptic. 2. An astringent medicine or remedy. [Gk *anastaltikos* able to contract.]

anastasis (an·as·tas·is). Return to health. [Gk a rising up.]

anastate (an·as·tate). Any substance formed from simpler substances by an anabolic process. [Gk *anastatos* raised up.]

anastatic (an·as·tat·ik). 1. Tending towards recovery. 2. Restorative. [see prec.]

anastigmatic (an·as·tig·mat′·ik). In optics, not astigmatic. [Gk *a*, astigmatic.]

anastole (an·as·tol·e). Retraction or gaping of the edges of a wound. [Gk retraction.]

anastomat (an·as·to·mat). A device by which an anastomosis may be made between the pelvic colon and the lower end of the rectum, after conservative excision of the latter.

anastomose (an·as·to·moze). 1. To communicate by channels or to open directly one into another, as of veins and arteries. 2. To effect an anastomosis. [see foll.]

anastomosis (an·as·to·mo′·sis). 1. Direct or indirect inter-communication between vessels. 2. The surgical establishment of a communication, shunt or fistula, between two conduits or cavities which normally are separate, in order to short-circuit the intervening portion, or to effect a repair after its removal. **Antiperistaltic anastomosis.** A short circuit between 2 segments of gut so apposed that the peristaltic wave in one proceeds in a direction opposite to that in the other part. **Aorticopulmonary anastomosis, Aortopulmonary anastomosis.** A communication created between the aorta and the pulmonary artery used to palliate various forms of cyanotic congenital heart disease in which the blood supply to the lungs is diminished. **Arteriovenous anastomosis [anastomosis arteriovenosa (NA)].** A communication, anatomically present or surgically produced, between an artery and a vein. **Aseptic anastomosis.** A method of excising the colon by a technique designed to prevent soiling of the peritoneum by the escaping content. **Button anastomosis.** Anastomosis by the use of Murphy's button [obsolete term]. **Crucial anastomosis.** An anastomosis in the upper part of the thigh formed between the first perforating branch of the profunda femoris artery, the inferior gluteal artery, and the lateral and medial circumflex arteries. **Direct transperitoneal ureterocolic anastomosis.** An operation carried out within the peritoneal cavity by joining the proximal ends of the divided ureters to the colon, in order to divert the flow of urine from the bladder into the large bowel. **End-to-end anastomosis.** The union to each other of divided ends of a hollow viscus or of a nerve, the intervening portion having been usually removed. **End-to-side anastomosis.** A union of one hollow viscus to another, the divided end of one being united to an opening in the side of the other. **Heterocladic anastomosis.** Anastomosis between branches of different arteries. **Homocladic anastomosis.** Anastomosis between branches of the same artery. **Hypoglossal-facial-nerve anastomosis.** Suture of the proximal end of the hypoglossal nerve to the distal end of the facial nerve in facial paralysis. **Intersubcardinal anastomosis.** An important transverse connection between the subcardinal veins of the embryo, from which the greater part of the left renal vein is derived. **Intestinal anastomosis.** Any operation which involves the joining together of any 2 portions of the intestinal tract, e.g. in by-passing an obstruction or in restoring continuity after removal of a length of bowel. It is named according to the segments of bowel used, e.g. gastrojejunal, duodenojejunal, ileocolic, colocolic, etc. **Isoperistaltic anastomosis.** A short circuit between two segments of gut so performed in the same direction. **Lateral anastomosis.** A union of hollow viscera by suture of the edges of openings made in their sides. **Nerve anastomosis.** 1. Anatomical connection between nerves. 2. The surgical union of 2 nerves, or 2 segments of the same nerve, after loss of the intervening portion. **Oesophagogastric anastomosis.** An anastomosis between the upper oesophagus and the stomach, which is mobilized and drawn up into the chest, to short-circuit a cancer of the oesophagus or to replace a malignant oesophagus which has been surgically removed. **Oesophagojejunal anastomosis.** An anastomosis between the oesophagus and the jejunum, drawn up through the diaphragm to reach it, to short-circuit a cancer or stricture of the oesophagus, or to reconstitute the alimentary canal after the removal of a malignant segment of oesophagus. **Portacaval anastomosis.** 1. Schmiedel's anastomosis. 2. A surgical communication established between the portal and inferior caval veins, or their tributaries, to relieve portal hypertension or short-circuit a cirrhotic liver. **Portal-systemic anastomosis.** Portacaval anastomosis (see preceding). **Postcostal anastomosis.** A longitudinal connection between the posterior divisions of the intersegmental arteries of the embryo, lying between the ribs and vertebral transverse processes. Part of the vertebral artery is derived from such an anastomosis. **Post-transverse anastomosis.** A longitudinal connection between the posterior divisions of the intersegmental arteries of the embryo, lying behind the transverse processes of the vertebrae. The deep cervical artery is derived from such an anastomosis. **Precapillary anastomosis.** Anastomosis between the small branches of an artery just before they are transformed into capillaries. **Precostal anastomosis.** A longitudinal connection between the intersegmental arteries of the embryo, lying in front of the necks of the ribs, e.g. the superior intercostal artery. **Primary anastomosis.** Anastomosis undertaken at the same time as resection, e.g. in restoring continuity after resection of a colon cancer. **Side-to-end anastomosis.** Anastomosis when the side of the proximal divided end of a structure is anastomosed to the cut end of the distal portion. **Side-to-side anastomosis.** Anastomosis of 2 structures lying side by side: this may be used either as a by-pass or to restore continuity after closing each end of the divided structure (especially bowel). **Splenorenal anastomosis.** A surgical communication established between splenic and renal veins; a form of portacaval anastomosis. **Stirrup anastomosis.** The arterial loop which joins the lateral plantar and the dorsalis pedis arteries. **Subclavian-pulmonary anastomosis.** A communication created between the proximal end of a subclavian artery and the pulmonary artery on the same side for the palliation of various forms of cyanotic congenital heart disease in which the blood supply to the lungs is diminished. **Sutureless anastomosis.** Of nerves, especially small nerves; the divided ends are glued together by fibrin. **Triple anastomosis.** The treatment of hourglass stomach by anastomosis of a loop of jejunum to each gastric pouch in turn, with anastomosis to each other of the limbs of the jejunal loop. **Uretero-intestinal anastomosis.** Implantation of the ureters into the bowel, usually into the colon, to divert the urinary stream and permit excision of the bladder; also performed in the treatment of extroversion of the bladder. **Vena caval-pulmonary anastomosis.** A communication created between the superior vena cava and the right pulmonary artery to conduct venous blood to the lungs, used for the palliation of tricuspid atresia (Glenn's operation). [Gk *anastomoein* to provide with a mouth.]

See also: BRAUN (H.), CLADO, GALEN, HOYER, HYRTL, MAYLARD-SONNENBURG, SCHMIEDEL, SUCQUET.

anastomotic (an·as·to·mot′·ik). Relating to or of the nature of an anastomosis; characterized by anastomosis. **Anastomotic vessel.** *See* VESSEL.

anastomotic veins. Inferior anastomotic vein [vena anastomotica inferior (NA)]. An anastomosis connecting the superficial middle cerebral vein with the transverse sinus. **Superior anastomotic vein [vena anastomotica superior (NA)].** An irregular connection between the superficial middle cerebral veins and the superior sagittal sinus.

anastomotica magna (an·as·to·**mot**·ik·ah **mag**·nah). 1. The ulnar collateral artery arising from the brachial artery and joining the anastomosis round the elbow joint. 2. The descending genicular artery arising from the femoral artery, supplying the knee, and anastomosing with adjacent arteries.

anatabine (an·**at**·ab·een). An alkaloid, $C_{10}H_{12}N_2$, extracted from tobacco.

anatherapeusis (an·ah·ther·ap·**ew**′·sis). A method of treatment according to which dosage is continually increased. [Gk *ana*, therapeutics.]

anathrepsis (an·ah·**threp**·sis). The putting on of flesh after recovery from illness. [Gk a fresh growth.]

anathreptic (an·ah·**threp**·tik). 1. Nutritive. 2. Serving to form flesh that has been lost. [see prec.]

anatomical, anatomic (an·at·**om**·ik·al, an·at·**om**·ik). 1. Having to do with the structure of the body. 2. Concerned with dissection or anatomy. **Anatomical neck.** *See* HUMERUS.

anatomist (an·**at**·o·mist). One experienced in the science of anatomy.

anatomy (an·**at**·o·me). 1. Dissection or cutting apart. 2. The study of the structure of living organisms, vegetable or animal, or the description of the parts of any organized structure. 3. In medical literature, the macroscopic structure of the adult human body. 4. In general scientific literature it is virtually synonymous with morphology, the scientific study of the shape and structure of organisms, and of the way in which shape and structure change in evolution (comparative anatomy) or in the development of the individual (morphogenesis), and including microscopic as well as macroscopic methods of study. The various kinds of anatomy are defined by their limitation to some particular aspect of structure (e.g. surface anatomy) or to the use of some particular technique (e.g. radiological anatomy). **Applied anatomy.** Anatomy studied in relation to some practical problem, such as the diagnosis and treatment of disease (medical or surgical anatomy). **Descriptive anatomy.** Anatomy limited to the verbal description of the parts of an organism; usually applied only to human anatomy. **Gross anatomy, Macroscopic anatomy.** The study of structure so far as it can be seen with the naked eye. **Microscopic anatomy.** The study of the minute structure of organisms; histology. **Morbid anatomy, Pathological anatomy.** The study of the structural changes which can be seen in diseased organs, tissues or parts of the body. **Regional anatomy.** The study of the structure of a particular region of an organism, e.g. of the upper limb, or of the abdomen, including all the systems which may be represented in it, and their relationship to each other. **Surface anatomy.** The study of the form and marking of the surface of the body, especially in their relation to underlying structures. **Systematic anatomy.** The separate study of the structure of particular systems, e.g. the nervous system or the vascular system, without limitation to any one region of the organism. **Topographical anatomy.** Regional anatomy (see above). **Transcendental anatomy.** The study of the structure of organisms to show how any particular organism may be a variant from some ideal or hypothetical type, from which all similar organisms can be derived as different variants. [Gk *ana*, *temnein* to cut.]

anatopism (an·**at**·op·izm). A mental state which constrains the patient to go against the social observance and customs of the level of society to which he belongs. [Gk *ana*, *topos* place.]

anatoxic (an·ah·**tox**·ik). 1. Relating to anatoxin. 2. Anaphylactic.

anatoxin (an·ah·**tox**·in). A toxin which has been rendered non-toxic by the action of formalin, but still retains the power to stimulate the production of antitoxin; also called *toxoid.* [Gk *ana*, toxin.]

anatresis (an·ah·**tre**·sis). 1. Trephining; the removing of discs of bone, particularly from the skull, with a circular saw (trephine). 2. Perforation, as with a trephine. [Gk.]

anatricrotic (an·ah·tri·**krot**′·ik). Marked by anatricrotism, in which the ascending curve of the sphygmogram is broken by 3 notches. [Gk *ana*, *treis* three, *krotos* stroke.]

anatricrotism (an·ah·**tri**·krot·izm). Abnormality of the pulse wave shown by the presence of 3 expansions in the upstroke as traced on the sphygmogram. [see prec.]

anatripsis (an·ah·**trip**·sis). 1. The employment of rubbing or friction as a remedy. 2. Inunction. [Gk friction.]

anatriptic (an·ah·**trip**·tik). A remedy applied by inunction or friction. [see prec.]

anatrophic (an·ah·**trof**·ik). 1. Nourishing. 2. Correcting or preventing atrophy. 3. A remedy by means of which wasting of the tissue can be prevented. [Gk *ana*, *trophe* nutrition.]

anatropia (an·ah·**tro**·pe·ah). Anaphoria. [Gk *ana*, *trepein* to turn.]

anautinum (an·**aw**·tin·um). Dimenhydrinate.

anavenin (an·ah·**ven**·in). Venom modified by the addition of formaldehyde but still retaining its antigenic properties. [Gk *ana*, L *venenum* poison.]

anaxon (an·**ax**·on). A neuron, such as an amacrine cell of the retina, which is apparently axonless. [Gk *a*, axon.]

anazotic (an·az·**o**·tik). Existing without nitrogen; containing no nitrogen. [Gk *a*, azote.]

anazoturia (an·az·o·**tewr**′·e·ah). Deficiency or lack of nitrogen or nitrogenous compounds in the urine. [Gk *a*, azoturia.]

anchilops (ang·kil·ops). Anchylops.

anchone (an·ko·ne). In hysterical conditions, a spasmodic constriction of the throat. [Gk *agchein* to strangle.]

anchorage (ang·kor·ij). 1. The surgical fixation of a movable or displaced organ. 2. In dentistry, points of retention of fillings and artificial restorations and appliances; they may be intra-oral, i.e. within the mouth, or extra-oral, i.e. from outside the mouth, as in fixation of fractures of the jaw. **Reciprocal anchorage.** Deliberate use of forces of action and reaction to produce reciprocal movement of two segments. [Gk *agkyra* anchor.]

Anchusa BPC 1949 (an·**kew**·zah). Alkanna or alkanet root, the dried root of *Alkanna tinctoria*, family Boraginaceae. It contains red colouring matters, and the tincture of alkanet is used in microscopy to stain fixed oils and fats. [Gk *agchousa* alkanet.]

anchusin (an·**kew**·sin). $C_{35}H_{40}O_8$. A red dye obtained from the root of *Alkanna tinctoria* (anchusa). [see prec.]

anchyloblepharon (ang·kil·o·**blef**′·ar·on). Ankyloblepharon.

anchyloglossia (ang·kil·o·**glos**′·e·ah). Ankyloglossia.

anchylops (ang·kil·ops). An abscess present at the medial angle of the palpebral fissure. [Gk *agchi* near, *ops* eye.]

anchylosis (ang·kil·o·sis). Ankylosis.

anchylostomiasis (an·kil·os·to·**mi**′·as·is). Ancylostomiasis.

ancipital (an·**sip**·it·al). Two-edged; two-headed. [L *anceps* two-headed.]

Ancistrodon piscivorus (an·**sis**·tro·don pis·e·**vor**·us). The water moccasin. [Gk *agkistron* fish hook, *odous* tooth, L fish-eating.]

ancistroid (an·**sis**·troid). Shaped like a hook. [Gk *agkistron* fish hook, *eidos* form.]

ancistrum (an·**sis**·trum). A surgical hook used to displace or retract tissue. [Gk *agkistron* fish hook.]

anconagra (an·kon·**ag**·rah). Pain in the elbow, such as that of gout. [Gk *agkon* elbow, *agra* a catching.]

anconal, anconeal (an·kon·al, an·**ko**·ne·al). Relating or belonging to the elbow. [Gk *agkon* elbow.]

anconeus muscle [musculus anconeus (NA)] (an·**ko**·ne·us). A small triangular muscle at the back of the elbow joint, attached to the lateral epicondyle of the humerus and to the ulna; it assists in extension of the elbow joint. [Gk *agkon* elbow.]

anconitis (an·kon·**i**·tis). Inflammation of the elbow joint. [Gk *agkon* elbow, *-itis* inflammation.]

anconoid (**an**·kon·oid). Having resemblance to the elbow; shaped like an elbow. [Gk *agkon* elbow, *eidos* form.]

Ancrod (**an**·krod). BP Commission approved name for an active principle obtained from the venom of the Malayan pit viper

Agkistrodon rhodostoma, acting specifically on fibrinogen. It is used as an anticoagulant.

ancyloglossia, ancyloglossum (an·sil·o·glos′·e·ah, an·sil·o·glos′um). Ankyloglossia.

ancylomele (an·sil·o·me′·le). Ankylomele.

Ancylostoma (an·sil·os·to·mah). A genus of nematode roundworms. **Ancylostoma americanum.** *Necator americanus.* **Ancylostoma braziliense.** A true parasite of dogs and cats in tropical America; its larvae cause a creeping dermatitis in man but do not mature. **Ancylostoma caninum.** A parasite of dogs and cats, and doubtfully of man. **Ancylostoma duodenale.** The most important hookworm, which is widespread in the tropics and sub-tropics. The adults inhabit the small intestine, where the females lay eggs which are passed in the faeces. The larvae first live free in the soil, then later penetrate the intact skin, causing ground itch, and subsequently migrate to the intestine, via the lungs. **Ancylostoma malayanum.** A parasite of bears, rarely found in man. [Gk *agkylos* crooked, *stoma* mouth.]

ancylostomatic (an·sil·os·to·mat′·ik). Applied to disease caused by a nematode worm of the genus *Ancylostoma* (hookworm).

Ancylostomatidae (an·sil·os·to·mat′·id·e). Ancylostomidae.

ancylostomiasis (an·sil·os·to·mi′·as·is). An acute or chronic disease caused by *Ancylostoma duodenale* or *Necator americanus,* nematode worms which resemble each other closely. The disease, commonly called *hookworm disease,* is prevalent in many tropical and sub-tropical countries. It occurs among miners and other workmen in Europe, especially when conditions of work (e.g. underground) with regard to temperature and moisture are similar to those of the tropics. Predisposing factors are bad sanitation, damp earth and contact of the bare skin (particularly of the feet) with the latter. **Ancylostomiasis cutis.** Ground itch. *See* ITCH.

Ancylostomidae (an·sil·os·to·mid·e). A family of the nematode super-family or sub-order Strongyloidea; hookworms. The genera *Ancylostoma* and *Necator* are of medical importance. [Gk *agkylos* crooked, *stoma* mouth, *eidos* form.]

ancyra (an·sir·ah). Ankyra; a hook. [Gk *agkyra* anchor.]

ancyroid (an·sir·oid). Ankyroid; shaped like a hook. [Gk *agkyra* anchor, *eidos* form.]

Anda (an·dah). A genus of euphorbiaceous trees; they are of wide distribution and yield medicinal oils. **Anda assu, Anda gomesii.** Brazilian species from which purgative oils are obtained.

Andernach, Johann Winther (or Guenther) von (b. 1487). German physician.

Andernach's ossicles. The wormian bones of the skull.

Anders, James Meschter (b. 1854). Philadelphia physician.

Anders' disease. Nodular circumscribed lipomatosis. *See* LIPOMATOSIS.

Andersch, Carol Samuel (fl. 1797). Gottingen anatomist.

Andersch's ganglion. The inferior ganglion of the glossopharyngeal nerve.

Andersch's nerve. The tympanic branch of the glossopharyngeal nerve.

Andersen, Dorothy Hansine (b. 1901). New York paediatrician.

Andersen's disease. Glycogen-storage disease *Type IV* associated with hepatic cirrhosis.

Andersen's syndrome. Cystic fibrosis. *See* FIBROSIS.

Anderson, James (b. 1891). London pathologist.

Anderson's stain. A mixture of ammonia, alum, calcium chloride and carmine, used for counterstaining Weigert-Pal sections of nervous tissue.

Anderson, Roger (b. 1891). Seattle, Washington, orthopaedic surgeon.

Anderson's operation. A method of tendon lengthening.

Anderson's splint. A splint for external fixation of fractures of long bones. The fragments above and below the fracture are transfixed by pins which are then attached to rods.

Roger Anderson well-leg traction. Traction on the femur by incorporating both legs in plaster. The feet are then connected by an apparatus which forces the affected leg into full abduction and the well leg into full adduction, thus producing traction on the abducted leg.

Anderson, Rose G. (b. 1893). American psychologist.

Kuhlmann-Anderson tests. A series of intelligence tests for children.

Anderson and MacSween silica-gel medium. A sodium silicate broth sterilized by filtration and poured into plates after an aseptic pre-adjustment with bromthymol-blue indicator.

Andira (an·di·rah). A genus of leguminous trees of tropical regions; poisons are derived from some species and anthelmintics from others. **Andira araroba.** A Brazilian species the trunk of which yields araroba, or Goa powder, from which in turn chrysarobin is obtained for use in ointments as a parasiticide. **Andira retusa.** A tree, the bark of which is known as *Surinam bark.* It is the source of methyltyrosine.

andirine (an·di·reen). Methyltyrosine.

Andrade, Eduardo Penny (b. 1872). Florida bacteriologist.

Andrade's indicator. An indicator used to demonstrate the production of acid in bacterial cultures. It is a mixture of 100 ml of an aqueous 0.5 per cent solution of acid fuchsine and 16 ml N sodium hydroxide. It is colourless at pH 7.2, but turns pink in the presence of acid.

Andral, Gabriel (b. 1797). Paris physician.

Andral's decubitus, or sign. The position assumed by a patient in lying down, in the early stages of pleurisy, on the sound side.

andreioma, andreoblastoma (an·dri·o·mah, an·dre·o·blas·to′·mah). Arrhenoblastoma; an androma. [Gk *aner* man, *-oma* tumour; blastoma.]

Andrews, Edward Wyllys (b. 1856). Chicago surgeon.

Wyllys Andrews' operation. 1. The repair of inguinal hernia by enclosing the spermatic cord in a tunnel of external oblique aponeurosis. 2. An operation for hydrocele with eversion of the tunica vaginalis.

Andrews, George Clinton (b. 1891). New York dermatologist.

Andrews' disease. Pustular bacteride. *See* BACTERIDE.

andriatrics, andriatry (an·dri·at·riks, an·dri·at·re). The science of the treatment of diseases of men, particularly of the male genital organs. [Gk *aner* man, *iatreia* healing.]

androcyte (an·dro·site). A spermatoblast. [Gk *aner* man, *kytos* cell.]

androgalactozemia (an·dro·gal·ak·to·ze′·me·ah). Secretion and excretion of milk of the male breast due to faulty glandular function. [Gk *aner* man, *gala* milk, *zemia* loss.]

androgen (an·dro·jen). The general name given to the group of steroids, both natural and artificial, which promote growth in, and maintain the functions of, the secondary sexual structures in the male. The natural androgens, which are found in the male urine or in the testis, include androsterone, dehydro-androsterone, testosterone and androstanedione. They are responsible for the beard and hair, deeper voice and heavier muscles, among other things characteristic of the male, and they also exercise a masculinizing psychological effect. Though in many ways opposed to the female sex hormones, androgens resemble the oestrogens in causing vaginal cornification and testicular atrophy, and the progestogens in activating progestational changes in the endometrium. [Gk *aner* man, *genein* to produce.]

androgenesis (an·dro·jen·es·is). The development of an individual from an ovum in which only paternal chromosomes are present owing to the destruction of the female pronucleus. [see prec.]

androgenic (an·dro·jen·ik). 1. Productive of male characteristics. 2. Term denoting that the offspring are habitually male. [Gk *aner* man, *genein* to produce.]

androgenous (an·droj·en·us). Tending towards the production of male rather than of female offspring. [see prec.]

androglossia (an·dro·glos·e·ah). Masculine quality in a woman's voice. [Gk *aner* man, *glossa* tongue.]

androgone (an·dro·gone). A spermatogenous cell. [Gk *aner* man, *gone* seed.]

andrographis (an·dro·graf·is). Kalmegh; the dried plant *Andrographis paniculata.* A simple bitter used in India.

andrographolide (an·dro·**graf**·o·lide). The bitter principle from *Andrographis paniculata.*

androgyne (**an**·dro·jine). 1. A male whose secondary genital organs are like those of a female; a male pseudo-hermaphrodite. 2. An individual who is genetically male, but in whom influences, believed to be hormonal, have produced a partial inversion towards the female sex. [see foll.]

androgyneity (**an**·dro·jin·**e'**·it·e). 1. Hermaphroditism. 2. Feminism. [Gk *aner* man, *gyne* woman.]

androgynism (an·**droj**·in·izm). Hermaphroditism in the female. [see prec.]

androgynoid (an·**droj**·in·oid). A male hermaphrodite whose female characteristics are marked enough to cause him to be mistaken for a woman. [Gk *aner* man, *gyne* woman, *eidos* form.]

androgynous (an·**droj**·in·us). 1. Hermaphroditic. 2. Physically or mentally characteristic of both sexes. 3. Of doubtful sex. [Gk *aner* man, *gyne* woman.]

androgynus (an·dro·**ji**·nus). Androgyne.

androgyny (an·**droj**·in·e). Androgyneity.

android, androidal (**an**·droid, an·**droi**·dal). 1. In physical structure and mental capacity resembling a man; manlike. 2. An automaton with human form. [Gk *aner* man, *eidos* form.]

andrology (an·**drol**·o·je). Medical science concerned with the constitution of the male sex and the diseases peculiar to men, particularly diseases of the generative organs. [Gk *aner* man, *logos* science.]

androma (an·dro·mah). Arrhenoblastoma; an ovarian adenoma which causes the development of secondary male sex characteristics in the female. The tumour contains imperfectly developed elements of gonadal character and male hormones. [Gk *aner* man, *-oma* tumour.]

andromania (an·dro·**ma**·ne·ah). Nymphomania; ungovernable sexual desire in women. [Gk *aner* man, mania.]

Andromeda (an·**drom**·ed·ah). A genus of trees and shrubs of the family Ericaceae, of which certain species contain poisonous narcotics. [Gk mythological heroine.]

andromimetic (**an**·dro·mim·**et'**·ik). Productive of the characteristics of a male; simulating man. [Gk *aner* man, mimetic.]

andromorphous (an·dro·**mor**·fus). Having a male appearance or form; having the physical structure of a man. [Gk *aner* man, *morphe* form.]

andropathy (an·**drop**·ath·e). Any disease peculiar to the male sex. [Gk *aner* man, *pathos* suffering.]

androphany (an·**drof**·an·ee). Virilism: 1. Adrenogenital syndrome. 2. Hermaphroditism in which there are male external genitalia although the individual concerned is a female. [Gk *aner* man, *phainein* to appear.]

androphilism (an·**drof**·il·izm). A liking for men, as opposed to women. In entomology, the term is wrongly used to indicate a preference for human blood, anthropophilism. [see foll.]

androphilous (an·**drof**·il·us). A term applied to parasitic organisms which preferably infest individuals of the male sex. [Gk *aner* man, *philein* to love.]

androphobia (an·dro·**fo**·be·ah). Repugnance to the male sex; morbid fear or dislike of men. [Gk *aner* man, phobia.]

androphonomania (**an**·dro·fo·no·**ma'**·ne·ah). Homicidal mania. *See* MANIA. [Gk *androphonos* man-slaying, mania.]

androsome (**an**·dro·some). A chromosome occurring only in the male germ line. [Gk *aner* man, *soma* body.]

androstane (**an**·dro·stane). $C_{19}H_{32}$. A saturated hydrocarbon with the cyclopentenophenanthrene (steroid) structure peculiar to the sterols and bile acids; it must be regarded as the parent of the testicular hormones, or androgens. **Androstane ring.** Cholane ring. *See* RING.

androstanediol (**an**·dro·**stane'**·di·ol). $C_{19}H_{32}O_2$. A hormone with chiefly male characters, not found in the tissues but prepared by the reduction of androsterone, than which it is 3 times more potent.

androstanediolone (**an**·dro·stane·**di'**·o·lone). A 17-ketosteroid hormone isolated from the urine of both normal men and normal women.

androstanedione (**an**·dro·**stane'**·di·one). $C_{19}H_{28}O_2$. A sex hormone, steroid in structure, which occurs in nature with the male hormone, androsterone, and is isomeric with testosterone.

androstanolone (an·dro·**stan**·o·lone). An androgenic substance isomeric with androsterone.

androstendion (an·dro·**sten**·di·on). A synthetic androgen.

androstene (**an**·dro·steen). $C_{19}H_{30}$. An unsaturated hydrocarbon of steroid structure with a double linkage in a certain position; for this reason it is the parent of the sex hormones testosterone, androstenediol and androstenedione.

androstenediol (**an**·dro·**steen'**·di·ol). $C_{19}H_{30}O_2$. A bisexual hormone related structurally to androstene.

androstenedione (**an**·dro·**steen'**·di·one). $C_{19}H_{26}O_2$. A sex hormone with definite male characters, related structurally to androstene.

androsterone (an·dro·**steer**·one, an·**dros**·ter·one). Androstane-3(α)-ol-17-one, $C_{19}H_{30}O_2$. An androgen or male sex hormone occurring naturally in the urine of men, male cattle, women with adrenal tumours and pregnant women. It is less effective than testosterone in causing growth of the seminal vesicles, but its influence on the prostate is greater. [Gk *andros* male, steroid.]

anebous (an·e·bus). Immature. Below the age of puberty. [Gk *anebos.*]

anecpyetous (**an**·ek·pi·**e'**·tus). 1. Preventing the formation of pus. 2. Not suppurating. [Gk *a, ek, pyein* to suppurate.]

anectasin (an·**ek**·tas·in). A substance, produced by bacteria, which causes vasoconstriction. [Gk *a, ektasis* a stretching.]

Anel, Dominique (b. 1679). Toulouse surgeon.

Anel's operation. Ligation of an artery just proximal to an aneurysm.

Anel's probe. The original probe used for passing down the lacrimal passages by Anel in 1713. Not used now.

Anel's syringe. The original lacrimal syringe, a modification of which is still used. It is all metal and fitted with a special cannula.

anelectrotonus (**an**·el·ek·tro·**to'**·nus). The reduction of conductivity and excitability of a nerve in the vicinity of the anode when an electric current is applied. [Gk *a*, electric, Gk *tonos* tone.]

anemometer (an·em·**om**·et·er). An instrument for measuring the volume of the flow of gases, e.g. the tidal exchange. [Gk *anemos* wind, *metron* measure.]

Anemone (an·**em**·o·ne). 1. A large genus of ranunculaceous plants growing widely throughout sub-arctic and temperate regions. From *Anemone pulsatilla, Anemone ludoviciana* (American pulsatilla) and *Anemone pratensis* (European pulsatilla), anemonin and iso-anemonic acid are derived; they are alteratives and depressants and are of use in treating inflammation. 2. *Anemone sculteus,* sea anemone; the source of thalassin. [Gk wind-flower.]

anemonism (an·**em**·on·izm). The state of having been poisoned by a plant of the genus *Anemone* (pulsatilla).

anemopathy (an·em·**op**·ath·e). 1. Aerotherapy; treatment by inhalation. 2. Disease associated with life in a district in which high winds prevail. [Gk *anemos* wind, *pathos* suffering.]

anemophobia (**an**·em·o·**fo'**·be·ah). Excessive or morbid fear of draughts or of being out in a high wind. [Gk *anemos* wind, phobia.]

anempeiria, anempiria (an·em·**pi**·re·ah). Lack of practical knowledge or experience; want of ability to apply principles already learned. [Gk *a, empeiria* experience.]

anencephalia (**an**·en·kef·**a'**·le·ah). Lack of the brain. [Gk *a, egkephalos* brain.]

anencephalic (**an**·en·kef·**al'**·ik). 1. Not having any brain. 2. Relating to anencephalia.

anencephaloid (an·en·**kef**·al·oid). Resembling anencephalia. [anencephalia, Gk *eidos* form.]

anencephaloneuria (**an**·en·kef·al·o·**newr'**·e·ah). A condition in which there is imperfect functioning of the nerves of the brain. [Gk *a, egkephalos* brain, *neuron* nerve.]

anencephalotrophia, anencephalotrophy (an·en·kef·al·o·**tro**′·fe·-ah, an·en·kef·al·**ot**′·rof·e). A state of atrophy of the brain due to lack of nutrition. [Gk *a, egkephalos* brain, *trophe* nutrition.]
anencephalous (an·en·**kef**·al·us). Anencephalic.
anencephalus (an·en·**kef**·al·us). A monster without a brain. [Gk *a, egkephalos* brain.]
anencephaly (an·en·**kef**·al·e). Anencephalia.
anenergia (an·en·**er**·je·ah). A state of inactivity; a state in which there is a lack of power or vigour. [Gk *a, energeia* energy.]
anenteraemia (an·**en**·ter·e′·me·ah). A condition in which there is lack of deficiency of supply of blood to the bowels. [Gk *a, enteron* intestine, *haima* blood.]
anenteroneuria (an·**en**·ter·o·**newr**′·e·ah). Lack of normal intestinal tonicity. [Gk *a, enteron* intestine, *neuron* nerve.]
anenterotrophia (an·**en**·ter·o·**tro**′·fe·ah). A condition in which there is deficient or defective nutrition of the intestine. [Gk *a, enteron* intestine, *trophe* nutrition.]
anenterous (an·**en**·ter·us). Not having an intestine. The term is applied to certain parasites. [Gk *a, enteron* intestine.]
aneosinophilia (an·e·o·sin·o·**fil**′·e·ah). Eosinopenia; the condition in which there is an abnormally small number of eosinophil leucocytes in the blood. [Gk *a*, eosinophilia.]
anepia (an·**ep**·e·ah). Lack of power of speaking. [Gk *a, epos* word.]
anepiploic (an·ep·e·**plo**′·ik). Not having an omentum. [Gk *a, epiploon* caul.]
anepithymia (an·ep·e·thi′·me·ah). A condition in which natural desires or appetites are deficient, lacking, or have been lost. [Gk *a, epithymia* desire.]
anerethisia (an·er·eth·**iz**′·e·ah). Impairment or deficiency of sensitiveness to stimulation; lack of usual irritability. [Gk *a, erethizein* to excite.]
anergasia, anergasis (an·er·**ga**·ze·ah, an·er·**ga**·sis). 1. Deficiency or lack of functional activity. 2. Impairment of mental activity or function. [Gk *a, ergon* work.]
anergastic (an·er·**gas**·tik). Relating to anergasia, or characterized by it.
anergic (an·**er**·jik). 1. Characterized by or relating to anergy. 2. Lethargic. 3. Extremely inactive. [see foll.]
anergy (**an**·er·je). 1. Asthenia. 2. In immunology, absence of reaction of cell-mediated immunity in a primed animal. Loss of tuberculin hypersensitivity in patients with diseases of lymphoid tissue has been described as anergic. 3. Sluggishness. [Gk *a, ergon* work.]
anerythroblepsia (an·er·ith·ro·**blep**′·se·ah). Anerythropsia. [Gk *a, erythros* red, *blepsis* sight.]
anerythrocyte (an·er·**ith**·ro·site). Lympho-erythrocyte; a non-nucleated erythrocyte without haemoglobin. [Gk *a*, erythrocyte.]
anerythroplasia (an·er·ith·ro·**pla**′·ze·ah). A condition in which erythrocytes are not formed. [Gk *a, erythros* red, *plassein* to form.]
anerythroplastic (an·er·ith·ro·**plas**·tik). 1. Relating to anerythroplasia. 2. Characterized by lack of erythrocyte formation.
anerythropoiesis (an·er·**ith**·ro·poi·e′·sis). Deficiency in the production of erythrocytes by the bone marrow. [Gk *a*, erythropoiesis.]
anerythropsia (an·er·ith·**rop**′·se·ah). 1. Blindness to the colour red. 2. Deficient perception of shades of red. [Gk *a, erythros* red, *opsis* sight.]
anerythroregenerative (an·**er**·ith·ro·re·**jen**′·er·a·tiv). Failing to show erythrocyte regeneration, aplastic or hypoplastic. [Gk *a*, erythrocyte, regeneration.]
anesis (**an**·es·is). A lessening in severity of symptoms. [Gk remission.]
Anethii fructus (an·e·the·i **fruk**·tus). Anethum. [Gk *anethon* anise, L fruit.]
anethole (**an**·e·thole). $CH_3OC_6H_4CH{=}CHCH_3$, a solid phenolic ether which is the main constituent of anise oil and the oil of fennel; it is used as a flavouring and carminative. [Gk *anethon* anise.]
anethopathy (an·eth·**op**·ath·e). Psychopathy. [Gk *a, ethos* character, *pathos* disease.]
anethum (an·e·thum). The dried ripe fruits of *Anethum graveolens*, family Umbelliferae. It contains 3–4 per cent of volatile oil, the main constituent of which is carvone. It is used mainly in the form of dill water (prepared from the oil), as a carminative for infants. **Anethum sowa.** The source of Indian dill, which is sometimes supplied in place of dill, but is an undesirable substitute as it contains a toxic substance. [Gk *anethon* anise.]
anetic (an·**et**·ik). Soothing; causing relaxation, as of nerves or muscles. [Gk *anetos* relaxed.]
anetoderma, anetodermia (an·et·o·**der**′·mah, an·et·o·**der**′·me·-ah). 1. Dermatolysis; a condition in which there are soft fibromata of the skin and mucous membranes, these forming large misshapen and pendulous masses, which may be pedunculated. 2. Atrophy of the skin. [Gk *anetos* relaxed, *derma* skin.]
aneuploid (an·**ew**·ploid). Term describing the chromosome complement of cells or individuals whose karyotype differs from that characteristic of their species by the presence of 1, 2 or few chromosomes rather than complete chromosomal sets. Monosomic, trisomic, double trisomic, tetrasomic, pentasomic, etc., are different types of aneuploids. [Gk *a, eu* good, *ploos* fold, *eidos* form.]
aneuploidy (an·ew·**ploid**·e). The state of aneuploids.
aneuria (a·**newr**·e·ah). Neurasthenia, lack of nerve force. [Gk *a, neuron* nerve.]
aneuric (a·**newr**·ik). Deficient in nervous energy; affected with aneuria.
aneurine, aneurin (**an**·ewr·een, **an**·ewr·in). Thiamine, an essential vitamin forming part of an enzyme system in the biochemistry of carbohydrate, by catalysing the oxidation and decarboxylation of pyruvic acid. The richest natural sources are whole grains, yeast and pork; deficiency results in fatigue, alimentary disturbances, irritability, depression and, if severe, beriberi. **Aneurine Hydrochloride BP 1958.** Thiamine hydrochloride, vitamin B_1, $C_{12}H_{17}ON_4SClHCl{\cdot}H_2O$, the hydrochloride of aneurine, administered orally in tablets or by supplementation in food substances, or by injection. **Aneurine phosphate.** Thiamine pyrophosphate.
aneuros (a·**newr**·os). Relaxed; inelastic; weak. [Gk without sinews.]
aneurosis (a·newr·**o**·sis). Absence of nerves. [Gk *a, neuron* nerve.]
aneurysm (**an**·ewr·izm). A localized dilatation of the walls of a blood vessel, usually an artery, due to weakening through infection, injury, degenerative conditions or congenital defects. **Abdominal aneurysm.** An aneurysm of the abdominal aorta. **Acute aneurysm.** One formed by the sudden weakening of the wall of an artery or of a chamber of the heart resulting in localized dilatation. **Ampullary aneurysm.** A small aneurysm often found in the arteries of the brain. **Aneurysm by anastomosis, Anastomotic aneurysm.** An aneurysm formed by the dilatation of several vessels under the skin. **Aortic aneurysm.** Aneurysm of the aorta. **Arteriovenous aneurysm.** A condition in which there is abnormal communication between an artery and a vein, often associated with a false aneurysm (see below). **Arteriovenous aneurysm of the orbit.** A form of aneurysm caused by the development of an anastomosis between the cavernous sinus and the internal carotid artery, the eyeball being displaced and visibly pulsating, and a loud roaring sound being audible at any point over the head. The condition is, as a rule, a result of fracture of the base of the skull. **Axial aneurysm.** One in which the whole circumference of the blood vessel is involved. **Axillary aneurysm.** An aneurysm affecting the axillary artery. **Bacterial aneurysm.** Mycotic aneurysm (see below). **Berry aneurysm.** A small aneurysm of the branches of the internal carotid artery or basilar artery at the base of the brain, caused by congenital weakness of the wall. **Bone aneurysm.** A tumour of bone containing many vessels which cause pulsation. **Branching aneurysm.** Cirsoid aneurysm (see below). **Cardiac aneurysm.** Dilatation of a circumscribed part of the wall of the heart as a result of its becoming thin through disease. **Circumscribed aneurysm.** True aneurysm (see below). **Circumscribed saccular aneurysm.** A common form of aneurysm of the aorta. **Cirsoid**

aneurysm. A condition in which as a result of an abnormal arteriovenous communication, congenital or acquired, a group of veins becomes lengthened, dilated and tortuous, to form a pulsatile swelling. **Compound aneurysm.** One in which 1 or more coats of an artery are dilated while others are ruptured. **Consecutive aneurysm.** False aneurysm (see below). **Cylindroid aneurysm.** Dilatation of an artery of uniform dimensions extending for a considerable length. **Diffuse aneurysm.** False aneurysm (see below). **Dissecting aneurysm.** One in which there is splitting of the media, usually of the aorta, and a new tube is formed for a considerable length; finally, there is rupture either outward through the remaining coat, or inward into the lumen. **Ectatic aneurysm.** An aneurysm formed without rupture of any of the coats of an artery but with uniform dilatation over a certain length of it. **Embolic aneurysm.** Aneurysm resulting from the presence of an embolus. **Embolomycotic aneurysm.** Mycotic aneurysm (see below). **Endogenous aneurysm.** One which arises as the result of disease of the coats of a blood vessel. **Erosion aneurysm, Erosive aneurysm.** One formed by the weakening of the wall of the aorta or other large artery by extension of an infective lesion, often tuberculous, or as the result of external trauma. **Exogenous aneurysm.** Aneurysm forming in a normal artery as a result of a wound or injury. **External aneurysm.** An aneurysm which forms in parts of the body other than the thorax or abdomen. **False aneurysm.** That which occurs after the wounding or the rupturing of an artery or after the rupture of a true aneurysm, so that a haematoma is formed in the surrounding tissues, which may be circumscribed or diffuse. **Fusiform aneurysm.** A spindle-shaped and elongated dilatation of an artery. **Hernial aneurysm.** An aneurysm of an inner coat of a blood vessel protruding through a ruptured outer coat. **Internal aneurysm.** An aneurysm arising in any of the cavities of the body. **Intracranial aneurysm.** One formed within the cranium. **Intramural aneurysm.** One in which the blood-filled sac remains within the wall of the vessel. **Intrathoracic aneurysm.** Aneurysm of the intrathoracic part of the aorta, or of large major intrathoracic branches. **Lateral aneurysm.** A dilatation of one side of an artery. **Leaking aneurysm.** The early stage in the rupture of an aneurysm when the opening is small and the blood exuding is also small in amount. **Miliary aneurysm.** One affecting one of the tiny arteries, particularly within the cranium. **Mixed aneurysm.** Compound aneurysm (see above). **Mycotic aneurysm.** Aneurysm caused by an infected embolus weakening the walls of a blood vessel; the embolus usually arises from bacterial endocarditis, but other sources are the lungs and the bones. **Orbital aneurysm.** An aneurysm situated within the orbit of the eye. **Osteoid aneurysm.** Bone aneurysm (see above). **Partial aneurysm.** Lateral aneurysm (see above). **Passive aneurysm, Passive cardiac aneurysm.** Cardiac aneurysm (see above). **Peripheral aneurysm.** 1. Lateral aneurysm (see above). 2. An aneurysm of a smaller branch of an artery. 3. Axial aneurysm (see above). **Phantom aneurysm.** A condition in which there is throbbing of the aorta and the vessel can be palpated. **Popliteal aneurysm.** Aneurysm of the popliteal artery. **Racemose aneurysm.** Cirsoid aneurysm (see above). **Renal aneurysm.** An aneurysm arising in the renal branch of the abdominal aorta. **Saccular aneurysm, Sacculated aneurysm.** An arterial aneurysm connected with the artery by a narrow mouth. **Secondary aneurysm.** One which forms again after apparent cure. **Serpentine aneurysm.** A condition of certain arteries which is present in senility; they become tortuous and elongated. **Silent aneurysm.** One without signs or symptoms. **Spongy aneurysm.** Angioma. **Spontaneous aneurysm.** Endogenous aneurysm (see below). **Spurious aneurysm.** False aneurysm (see above). **Subclavicular aneurysm.** An aneurysm forming too high up in the axillary artery to allow a ligature to be applied below the clavicle. **Subclinoid aneurysm.** Aneurysm of the circle of Willis below the level of the sella turcica. **Supraclinoid aneurysm.** Aneurysm of the circle of Willis above the level of the sella turcica. **Traction aneurysm.** One produced by traction on the wall of an artery. **Traumatic aneurysm.** Exogenous aneurysm (see above). **True aneurysm.** One in which the wall of the aneurysm is formed by one or more coats of the blood vessel. **Tubular aneurysm.** Cylindroid aneurysm (see above). **Varicose aneurysm.** An aneurysm lying between an artery and an adjacent vein and forming a sac-like communication between them. **Ventricular aneurysm.** Strictly, a localized dilatation of part of the wall of the cardiac ventricle, but the term is also applied to a thinned non-contractile part of the wall of a ventricle, which will usually show paradoxical bulging in systole but which does not protrude significantly from the normal contour of the ventricle. The cause is nearly always previous full-thickness myocardial infarction. [Gk *aneurysma* a widening.]

See also: POTT, RASMUSSEN.

aneurysmal (an·ewr·iz·mal). Relating to or of the nature of aneurysm; resembling aneurysm.

aneurysmatic (an·ewr·iz·**mat**'·ik). 1. Characterized by the formation of aneurysms. 2. Suffering from aneurysm. 3. Having the character of aneurysm, or resembling it; aneurysmal.

aneurysmectomy (an·ewr·iz·**mek**·to·me). Removal of an aneurysm by cutting out the sac. [aneurysm, Gk *ektome* a cutting out.]

aneurysmograph (an·ewr·iz·mo·graf). An x-ray photograph of an aneurysm. [aneurysm, Gk *graphein* to record.]

aneurysmoplasty (an·ewr·**iz**·mo·plas·te). Endo-aneurysmorrhaphy; an operation for the radical cure of aneurysm. The aneurysmal sac is opened, the contents are evacuated, and the internal openings closed by continuous sutures (Matas' operation). [aneurysm, Gk *plassein* to form.]

aneurysmorrhaphy (an·ewr·iz·**mor**'·af·e). The process of repairing an aneurysm. **Obliterative aneurysmorrhaphy (Matas).** Obliteration of an aneurysmal sac by suture of its walls to each other. **Reconstructive aneurysmorrhaphy (Matas).** Surgical closure of the communication between the sac of an aneurysm and the lumen of the artery from which it arises. **Reparative aneurysmorrhaphy (Matas).** Removal of an aneurysmal sac with repair of the artery from which it arises. [aneurysm, Gk *rhaphe* suture.]

See also: MATAS.

aneurysmotomy (an·ewr·iz·**mot**'·o·me). An incision into an aneurysm. [aneurysm, Gk *temnein* to cut.]

aneurysmus (an·ewr·**iz**·mus). 1. Aneurysm. 2. Dilatation.

aneuthanasia (an·**ew**·than·**a**'·ze·ah). A state in which the act of dying is attended with pain and difficulty. [Gk *an*, *euthanasia* easy death.]

anfractuosity (an·frak·tew·**os**'·it·e). The sinuous depressions separating the convolutions of the brain; the cerebral sulci. [Fr. *anfractuosité* sinuosity, windings.]

anfractuous (an·**frak**·tew·us). Tortuous; sinuous or winding. [see prec.]

angeial (an·je·e·al). Vascular. [Gk *aggeion* vessel.]

angeielcus (an·je·**el**·kus). Angielcus.

angeiochalasis (an·je·o·**kal**'·as·is). Angiochalasis.

angeiorrhagia (an·je·o·**ra**'·je·ah). Angiorrhagia.

angeitis (an·je·**i**·tis). Angiitis.

angel's wing (**ane**·jlz wing). Winged scapula. *See* SCAPULA.

angelica (an·**jel**·ik·ah). The umbelliferous plant *Angelica archangelica* (garden angelica), a perennial widely distributed in Europe and Asia. All parts of the plant contain volatile oil, and the dried fruits, root and rhizome, or the distilled oil, have been used in medicine for their tonic, stimulant and diaphoretic properties. Confectionery angelica is prepared by steeping the young stems in syrup. [Gk *aggelikos*, angelic.]

Angelucci, Arnaldo (b. 1854). Italian ophthalmologist.

Angelucci's syndrome. Tachycardia, vasomotor instability and lymphoid hyperplasia, with particular susceptibility to infective or allergic condition, hence sometimes associated with spring catarrh.

angialgia (an·je·**al**·je·ah). Pain felt in a blood vessel. [Gk *aggeion* vessel, *algos* pain.]

angiasthenia (an·je·as·**the**'·ne·ah). Angio-asthenia.

angiectasia, angiectasis (an·je·ek·**ta**'·ze·ah, an·je·**ek**·tas·is). Angio-ectasia.

angiectatic (an·je·ek·tat'·ik). Angio-ectactic.
angiectaticus (an·je·ek·tat'·ik·us). Indicating the presence of enlarged blood vessels. [Gk *aggeion* vessel, *ektasis* a stretching.]
angiectomy (an·je·ek·to·me). Angio-ectomy.
angiectopia (an·je·ek·to'·pe·ah). Angio-ectopia.
angielcosis (an·je·el·ko'·sis). Angio-elcosis.
angielcus (an·je·el·kus). An ulcer within the walls of a vessel. [Gk *aggeion* vessel, *elkos* ulcer.]
angiemphraxis (an·je·em·frax'·is). Angio-emphraxis.
angiitis (an·je·i·tis). A state of inflammation in a blood vessel or lymph vessel. Cf. PHLEBITIS; LYMPHANGITIS. **Allergic granulomatous angiitis.** A hypersensitivity angiitis affecting the skin and other tissues (heart, lungs, kidneys, spleen). In the *acute* form there are skin necrosis, asthma, fever and eosinophilia. Henoch–Schoenlein purpura is an example of the *subacute* form. **Consecutive angiitis.** Inflammation extended to a vessel from surrounding tissues. **Leucocytoclastic angiitis.** Allergic vasculitis in which a polymorphonuclear infiltrate and fibrinoid changes occur in the small arteries of the skin and sometimes in other organs. **Necrotizing angiitis.** Fibrinoid necrosis of the skin of allergic nature occurring in arteries in collagen diseases. **Visceral angiitis.** A term which includes a number of disorders showing lesions of the smaller arteries, e.g. lupus erythematodes disseminatus. [Gk *aggeion* vessel, *-itis* inflammation.]
angileucitis (an·je·lew·si'·tis). Angioleucitis.
angina (an·jin·ah, an·ji·nah). 1. A tight strangling or oppressive sensation, discomfort, or pain. 2. A disease which produces spasmodic attacks of suffocation; the term is used, in Continental literature particularly, to imply choking and suffocation associated with diseases of the throat. **Abdominal angina.** Abdominal pain following eating, due to stenosis of the superior mesenteric artery and consequent ischaemia of the small intestine. **Angina acuta.** A simple sore throat. **Agranulocytic angina.** Progressive ulceration of the pharynx and soft palate associated with severe diminution of granular white cells in the blood, and also a degree of anaemia. It results from damage to the blood-forming elements of the bone marrow, and is found in overdoses of, or sensitivity to, the sulphonamides and amidopyrine drugs. **Aphthous angina.** An infection of the throat resulting from multiple ulceration of the mucous membrane, of previously unknown aetiology. **Angina arthritica.** A gouty pharyngitis. **Benign croupous angina.** Pharyngitis herpetica. **Angina capitis.** Headache due to errors of refraction and/or muscle balance; it is curable by wearing correct glasses. **Cardiac angina.** Angina pectoris (see below). **Angina catarrhalis.** Catarrhal pharyngitis. *See* PHARYNGITIS. **Crescendo angina.** Angina increasing in severity or frequency of occurrence provoked by lessening effort so that it may occur at rest, and which may be followed by myocardial infarction. **Angina crouposa.** Angina associated with membrane, or false membrane, development. **Angina cruris.** Intermittent claudication; a cramp-like pain occurring in the calves of the legs on effort, relieved by rest and due to insufficient blood supply to the calf muscles owing to occlusive arterial disease of the arteries to the lower extremity. It may be precipitated by severe anaemia. **Angina decubitus.** Angina pectoris (see below) occurring when the sufferer lies flat, seen in severe myocardial ischaemia; the increase in cardiac output in the supine position may induce coronary insufficiency. **Diphtheritic angina, Angina diphtheritica.** Ulceration of the throat due to the diphtheria bacillus. **Angina dyspeptica.** Pain and a sense of oppression resembling angina pectoris, but of gastric origin. **Angina of effort.** Angina pectoris (see below) produced by effort and relieved by rest; the available coronary-artery blood flow is inadequate for the increased demands of the myocardium. It may also occur on exposure to cold or after a heavy meal. **Angina epiglottidea.** Acute oedema of the epiglottis, of inflammatory origin. **Angina erysipelatosa.** Angina resulting from an acute inflammatory infection of streptococcal origin. **Exudative angina.** Angina associated with the formation of an exudate or membrane. **Fibrinous angina.** Fibrinous exudate in the pharynx. **First-effort angina.** Angina pectoris (see below) which occurs on first effort, but passes if the exertion is continued; the augmented cardiac output on effort increases the coronary flow just enough to meet the myocardial demand after the degree of exertion has become stabilized. The initial onset of pain is probably due to failure of the coronary arterioles to dilate quickly enough. **Angina follicularis.** Follicular tonsillitis. *See* TONSILLITIS. **Fusospirochaetal angina.** Angina resulting from infection of the Vincent's type. **Gangrenous angina.** A fulminating destructive inflammation of the throat. **Angina of the heart.** Angina pectoris (see below). **Herpetic angina.** Angina associated with herpetic blebs, and now regarded as of virus origin. **Hippocratic angina.** Angina associated with an acute retropharyngeal infection. **Hypercyanotic angina.** Angina pectoris (see below) which occurs in patients with grossly reduced arterial oxygen saturation, particularly in those forms of congenital heart disease in which venous blood is shunted across an abnormal communication in the heart into the systemic circulation; diminution in oxygen content of the blood perfusing the coronary arteries rather than disease of the latter is the cause. **Hypoleucocytic angina.** Hypogranulocytosis; a less severe and often more chronic type of agranulocytosis. **Lacunar angina.** Follicular tonsillitis. *See* TONSILLITIS. **Angina laryngea.** Inflammation of the larynx associated with oedema. **Angina ludovici.** Acute septic pharyngitis associated with a brawny swelling of the neck; Ludwig's angina. **Angina lymphomatosa.** Enlargement of the lymph tissue of the buccal cavity or throat; part of a lymph hypertrophy. **Malignant angina.** An acute, rapidly fatal angina. **Angina membranacea.** A membranous angina, most commonly due to diphtheria. **Monocytic angina.** Angina from a lesion which is usually associated with monocytic anaemia but does not occur in mononucleosis. **Nerve angina.** Pain in the distribution of a nerve. **Neutropenic angina.** Agranulocytosis. **Angina nosocomii.** An acute and ulcerative pharyngitis. **Angina parotidea.** An uncommon term for mumps or other form of parotitis. **Angina pectoris.** Literally angina of the chest; a substernal pain, or sense of constriction or oppression, often radiating into the neck or arms and sometimes into the back, produced by insufficient blood-supply to the myocardium to meet its oxygen demand at the time. The principal cause is atheromatous disease of the coronary arteries, but severe anaemia, aortic valve disease, hypertension, hypertrophic cardiomyopathy or disorders of thyroidal function may be precipitating or aggravating factors; syphilitic aortitis producing coronary ostial narrowing may also be a cause. The discomfort is commonly brought on by exertion, but emotional tension may also precipitate it and, and in some cases, pain occurs at rest or during sleep. *See* Crescendo angina, Angina decubitus (above) and Pre-infarction angina, Variant angina (below). **Phlegmonous angina.** An acute severe inflammation of the mouth or pharynx. **Pre-infarction angina.** Crescendo angina (see above); the frequent occurrence of myocardial infarction as the climax of the condition, but this event is not invariable and the term is therefore best used only in retrospect. **Pseudomembranous angina.** Vincent's angina. **Pultaceous angina.** The formation of white patches in the throat, not due to true exudate. **Angina at rest.** Attacks of angina pectoris (see above) when at rest. In persons with extremely severe myocardial ischaemia they may follow excitement, but often are premonitory to cardiac infarction. **Rheumatic angina.** Pharyngitis associated with a rheumatic tendency. **Angina scarlatinosa.** The pharyngitis or sore throat associated with scarlet fever. **Serous angina.** Sore throat with a serous exudate. **Angina simplex.** Simple sore throat. **Streptococcal angina.** Acute sore throat of streptococcal origin. **Angina suffocativa.** Angina with a pronounced feeling of suffocation, due to any cause, e.g. in severe faucial angina or in angina pectoris. The term has also been used for diphtheria of the pharynx or larynx. **Thymic angina.** A generic term used for anginal attacks of suffocation in childhood, including laryngismus stridulus, bronchial asthma, and dyspnoea due to enlarged thymus gland. **Angina tonsillaris.** Peritonsillar infection, or quinsy. **Angina trachealis.** Acute infection of the trachea; the term would probably now include acute tracheobronchitis. **Ulceromem-**

branous angina. Vincent's angina. **Angina ulcerosa, Angina ulcerosa benigna.** A condition with an ulcer on the anterior part of the faucial pillar, just above the tonsil. **Variant angina.** Angina pectoris occurring at rest and typically at night, being associated with elevation of ST segments in the electrocardiogram (as opposed to the depression usually seen in angina pectoris) and often having a serious prognosis (Prinzmetal's angina). [L *angina* quinsy.]

See also: BRETONNEAU, LUDWIG (W. F.), PLAUT, SCHULTZ, VINCENT.

anginal (an·jin·al, an·**ji**·nal). Relating to angina.

anginiform (an·jin·e·form, an·**ji**·ne·form). Having resemblance to angina. [angina, form.]

anginoid (an·jin·oid). Resembling one of the anginas, particularly angina pectoris. [angina, Gk *eidos* form.]

anginophobia (an·jin·o·**fo**'·be·ah). Excessive fear of falling a victim to angina pectoris. [angina, phobia.]

anginose, anginous (an·jin·oze, an·jin·us). Relating to or affected with angina, particularly angina pectoris.

anginosis (an·jin·**o**·sis). Any form of angina. [angina, Gk *-osis* condition.]

angio-asthenia (an·je·o·as·**the**'·ne·ah). Instability, or loss of vigour or tone, of the vascular system. [Gk *aggeion* vessel, asthenia.]

angio-ataxia (an·je·o·at·**ax**'·e·ah). A condition in which there is spasmodic variability in the tonicity of the blood vessels. [Gk *aggeion* vessel, ataxia.]

angioblast (an·je·o·blast). 1. One of the cells, or collections of cells, of mesenchymal origin, from which the primitive blood vessels and blood cells of the embryo are derived. 2. That part of the mesoderm which is supposedly destined from an early stage in development to give rise to the blood vessels and blood cells. [Gk *aggeion* vessel, *blastos* germ.]

angioblastoma (an·je·o·blas·**to**'·mah). A tumour of the blood vessels which has its origin in the cerebral spinal meninges. [Gk *aggeion* vessel, blastoma.]

angiocardiogram (an·je·o·**kar**'·de·o·gram). A series of x-ray films of the heart taken in rapid succession during and immediately after the intravenous injection of a radio-opaque substance; by this procedure the cavities of the heart and the great vessels are very clearly outlined. [Gk *aggeion* vessel, *kardia* heart, *gramma* record.]

angiocardiography (an·je·o·kar·de·**og**'·raf·e). The x-ray examination of the great vessels and the chambers of the heart immediately following a rapid injection of a radio-opaque substance into the venous system. [Gk *aggeion* vessel, *kardia* heart, *graphein* to record.]

angiocardiokinetic (an·je·o·kar·de·o·kin·**et**'·ik). 1. A drug or other agent which affects the movement of the heart and of the blood vessels. 2. Having an effect on the heart movement and on that of the blood vessels. [Gk *aggeion* vessel, cardiokinetic.]

angiocardiopathy (an·je·o·kar·de·**op**'·ath·e). Any disease involving the blood vessels or the heart. [Gk *aggeion* vessel, cardiopathy.]

angiocarditis (an·je·o·kar·**di**'·tis). An inflammatory condition of the large blood vessels and of the heart. [Gk *aggeion* vessel, carditis.]

angiocavernous (an·je·o·kav·**ern**'·us). Having the characteristics of an angioma cavernosum. [Gk *aggeion* vessel, L *cavernosus* full of hollows.]

angioceratoditis (an·je·o·ser·at·o·**di**'·tis). Angiokeratoditis.

angiochalasis (an·je·o·**kal**'·as·is). Dilatation of the blood vessels, caused by lack of tonicity. [Gk *aggeion* vessel, *chalasis* relaxation.]

angiocheiloscope (an·je·o·**ki**'·lo·skope). An instrument with a magnifying attachment, with which the circulation of the blood in the lips may be observed. [Gk *aggeion* vessel, *cheilos* lip, *skopein* to watch.]

angiocholecystitis (an·je·o·**ko**·le·sis·**ti**'·tis). An inflammatory condition of the gall bladder and the bile duct and biliary ductules. [Gk *aggeion* vessel, *chole* bile, cystitis.]

angiocholitis (an·je·o·ko·**li**'·tis). Cholangitis; a condition of inflammation of the bile ducts. **Angiocholitis proliferans.** A condition of inflammatory proliferation of the biliary ductules. [Gk *aggeion* vessel, *chole* bile, *-itis* inflammation.]

angiochondroma (an·je·o·kon·**dro**'·mah). A type of chondroma in which there is abnormal development of the blood vessels surrounding it. [Gk *aggeion* vessel, chondroma.]

angioclast (an·je·o·klast). An instrument resembling and put to the same use as artery forceps. [Gk *aggeion* vessel, *klestes* a breaker.]

angiocrine (an·je·o·krine). Indicating vasomotor disorders caused by abnormality of the endocrine glands. [Gk *aggeion* vessel, endocrine.]

angiocrinosis (an·je·o·krin·**o**'·sis). Any vasomotor disorder caused by abnormality of the endocrine glands. [angiocrine, Gk *-osis* condition.]

angiocyst (an·je·o·sist). Blood island; in embryology, a dilated capillary whose endothelium is actively engaged in manufacturing blood cells. [Gk *aggeion* vessel, *kystis* bag.]

angioderm (an·je·o·derm). Angioblast, 2nd def. [Gk *aggeion* vessel, *derma* skin.]

angioderma pigmentosum (an·je·o·**der**'·mah pig·men·**to**·sum). Xeroderma pigmentosum. [Gk *aggeion* vessel, *derma* skin, pigment.]

angiodermatitis (an·je·o·der·mat·**i**'·tis). An inflammatory condition involving the vessels of the skin. **Pruritic angiodermatitis.** An orange-coloured itchy purpura caused by carbromal and other drugs, or by chemicals in clothing or other, unknown, factors. [Gk *aggeion* vessel, dermatitis.]

angiodiascopy (an·je·o·di·**as**'·ko·pe). Naked-eye examination of the blood vessels of the hands or feet. A light is placed behind the part being examined, so that the course of the vessels may be followed. [Gk *aggeion* vessel, diascopy.]

angiodiastasis (an·je·o·di·**as**'·tas·is). 1. Retraction of the cut ends of a blood vessel. 2. Dilatation or displacement of a vessel. [Gk *aggeion* vessel, diastasis.]

angiodiathermy (an·je·o·di·ah·**ther**'·me). Diathermy of the long posterior ciliary arteries, formerly used in glaucoma. [Gk *aggeion* vessel, diathermy.]

angiodystrophia, angiodystrophy (an·je·o·dis·**tro**'·fe·ah, an·je·o·**dis**'·tro·fe). A condition in which the blood vessels are receiving insufficient nourishment. **Angiodystrophia ovarii.** Increase in the number of the blood vessels of the ovary, combined with disease of the ovary. [Gk *aggeion* vessel, dystrophy.]

angio-ectasia, angio-ectasis (an·je·o·ek·**ta**'·ze·ah, an·je·o·**ek**'·tas·is). Angiectasia: 1. A condition in which the blood vessels are more than normally dilated. 2. Vascular dilatation due to tortuosity, enlargement, aneurysm or other morbid condition. [Gk *aggeion* vessel, *ektasis* a stretching.]

angio-ectatic (an·je·o·ek·**tat**'·ik). Characterized by dilatation of the blood vessels. [see prec.]

angio-ectomy (an·je·o·**ek**'·to·me). Angiectomy; resection or excision of a blood vessel. [Gk *aggeion* vessel, *ektome* a cutting out.]

angio-ectopia (an·je·o·ek·**to**'·pe·ah). Angiectopia; a condition in which a blood vessel is present in an abnormal situation, or has been displaced. [Gk *aggeion* vessel, ectopia.]

angio-elcosis (an·je·o·el·**ko**'·sis). Angielcosis; the presence of an ulcer within the walls of a vessel. [Gk *aggeion* vessel, *elkos* ulcer.]

angio-elephantiasis (an·je·o·el·ef·an·**ti**'·as·is). A widespread angiomatosis of the subcutaneous tissue. [Gk *aggeion* vessel, elephantiasis.]

angio-emphraxis (an·je·o·em·**frax**'·is). Angiemphraxis; obstruction involving a vessel or vessels. [Gk *aggeion* vessel, emphraxis.]

angio-endothelioma (an·je·o·en·do·the·le·**o**'·mah). An endothelioma in which there is a large number of blood vessels. [Gk *aggeion* vessel, endothelioma.]

angiofibroma (an·je·o·fi·**bro**'·mah). An angioma which contains connective tissue, often in profusion. **Angiofibroma contagiosum tropicum.** A form of dermatosis occurring in Brazil, in the course of which there is an eruption of bright-red papules which change later into nodules of a bluish colour. [Gk *aggeion* vessel, fibroma.]

angiogenesis (an·je·o·**jen**′·es·is). The origin or development of the blood vessels and the lymph vessels. [Gk *aggeion* vessel, genesis.]

angiogenic (an·je·o·**jen**′·ik). 1. Developing into blood vessels or lymph vessels. 2. Originating in the vascular system. [see prec.]

angioglioma (an·je·o·gli·**o**′·mah). A glioma in which there are a large number of blood vessels. [Gk *aggeion* vessel, glioma.]

angiogliomatosis (an·je·o·gli·om·at·**o**′·sis). The presence of multiple vascular gliomas. [Gk *aggeion* vessel, glioma, Gk *-osis* condition.]

angiogliosis (an·je·o·gli·**o**′·sis). A condition in which there is formation of angiogliomata. **Angiogliosis retinae.** Haemangioblastoma retinae. [angioglioma, Gk *-osis* condition.]

angiogram (an·je·o·gram). Arteriogram. [Gk *aggeion* vessel, *gramma* a writing.]

angiograph (an·je·o·graf). A type of sphygmograph which records the character and rhythm of successive pulse waves. [Gk *aggeion* vessel, *graphein* to record.]

angiography (an·je·**og**·raf·e). 1. Sphygmography; the recording of the movements of the arterial pulse by means of a sphygmograph. 2. The study of blood vessels or lymph vessels by radiological means after the injection of an opaque contrast medium into the lumen of the vessel. *See also* LYMPHOGRAPHY, VENOGRAPHY. **Cerebral angiography.** Visualization of the vascular system of the brain—arteries, capillaries and veins—by injection of a contrast substance into a supplying artery. **Fluorescein angiography.** The study of vessels rendered visible by the fluorescence of an intravascular injection of sodium fluorescein. It is used particularly to study the circulation of the eye in health and disease. [see prec.]

angiohyalinosis (an·je·o·hi·al·in·**o**′·sis). Hyaline degeneration of the blood-vessel musculature. **Angiohyalinosis haemorrhagica.** Angiohyalinosis associated with haemorrhagic manifestations that may be congenital and resemble haemophilia. [Gk *aggeion* vessel, hyalin, Gk *-osis* condition.]

angiohydrography (an·je·o·hi·**drog**′·raf·e). Hydroangiography.

angiohypertonia (an·je·o·hi·per·**to**′·ne·ah). Vasoconstriction; a constriction or narrowing of the internal diameter of the blood vessels. [Gk *aggeion* vessel, hypertonia.]

angiohypotonia (an·je·o·hi·po·**to**′·ne·ah). Vasodilatation; abnormal dilatation of the blood vessels. [Gk *aggeion* vessel, hypotonia.]

angioid (an·je·oid). Having resemblance to a blood vessel. [Gk *aggeion* vessel, *eidos* form.]

angiokeratoditis (an·je·o·ker·at·o·**di**′·tis). Vascular keratitis. *See* KERATITIS. [Gk *aggeion* vessel, *keras* horn, *eidos* form, *-itis* inflammation.]

angiokeratoma (an·je·o·ker·at·**o**′·mah). Kerato-angioma; a rare condition affecting particularly the fingers and toes of those who suffer from chilblains. The lesions are telangiectases on which warty excrescences develop. **Angiokeratoma circumscriptum.** An angiomatous naevus with hyperkeratosis of the overlying epidermis. **Angiokeratoma corporis diffusa.** Fabry's disease. **Angiokeratoma corporis diffusum.** An inherited, sex-linked recessive trait with lipid deposits in small blood-vessels of the skin and viscera, causing oedema, small cutaneous angiokeratomata, corneal opacities, left ventricular hypertrophy, vasomotor disturbances, glomerulitis, cerebrovascular episodes, coronary disease and muscle involvement. The prognosis is grave. **Angiokeratoma of the scrotum.** A condition in which, clinically, the lesions are similar to angiokeratomata elsewhere, but differ in aetiology and histopathology; it has been suggested that scrotal angiokeratomata may be a manifestation of Osler's disease. [Gk *aggeion* vessel, *keras* horn, *-oma* tumour.]

angiokeratosis (an·je·o·ker·at·**o**′·sis). A condition in which multiple angiokeratomata are present. [angiokeratoma, Gk *-osis* condition.]

angiokinesis (an·je·o·kin·**e**′·sis). A state of activity or stimulation of the blood vessels. [Gk *aggeion* vessel, *kinesis* movement.]

angiokinetic (an·je·o·kin·**et**′·ik). Relating to vascular activity. [see prec.]

angioleucitis, angioleukitis (an·je·o·lew·**si**′·tis, an·je·o·lew·**ki**′·tis). Lymphangitis; an inflammatory condition of the lymph vessels. [Gk *aggeion* vessel, *leukos* white, *-itis* inflammation.]

angiolipoleiomyoma (an·je·o·**lip**·o·li·o·mi·**o**′·mah). A non-capsulated tumour of the kidney associated with the syndrome of tuberous sclerosis. [Gk *aggeion* vessel, *lipos* fat, leiomyoma.]

angiolipoma (an·je·o·lip·**o**′·mah). An angioma in which there is fatty tissue. It often forms in the subcutaneous tissues. [angioma, lipoma.]

angiolith (an·je·o·lith). A calcareous deposit in the wall of a blood vessel. [Gk *aggeion* vessel, *lithos* stone.]

angiolithic (an·je·o·**lith**′·ik). Relating to an angiolith.

angiology (an·je·**ol**·o·je). The science of the blood vessels and lymph vessels. [Gk *aggeion* vessel, *logos* science.]

angiolupoid (an·je·o·**loo**′·poid). A cutaneous sarcoid of the Boeck type usually affecting the upper part of the sides of the nose or the adjacent areas. [Gk *aggeion* vessel, L *lupus* wolf, Gk *eidos* form.]

See also: BROCQ, PAUTRIER.

angiolymphangioma (an·je·o·**limf**·an·je·**o**′·mah). An angioma composed of both dilated lymph vessels and dilated blood vessels. [angioma, lymphangioma.]

angiolymphitis (an·je·o·limf·**i**′·tis). Lymphangitis.

angiolymphoma (an·je·o·limf·**o**′·mah). A tumour which is chiefly formed of dilated lymph vessels. [Gk *aggeion* vessel, lymphoma.]

angiolysis (an·je·**ol**·is·is). The degeneration and obliteration of a blood vessel such as is found, for example, in the embryogenetic state. [Gk *aggeion* vessel, *lysis* a loosing.]

angioma (an·je·**o**·mah). A simple tumour composed of blood vessels or of lymphatic vessels. **Angioma arteriale racemosum.** A condition in which capillaries and other small vessels, by means of proliferation, change and dilatation, are formed into an intricate mass and eventually involve other vessels. **Angioma of bone.** A benign vascular tumour of bone. **Capillary angioma.** A benign tumour composed of capillaries. **Cavernous angioma, Angioma cavernosum, Angioma circumscriptum.** A common tumour of the skin and subcutaneous tissue in which there are large spaces filled with blood, these giving the tumour erectile properties. **Cutaneospinal angioma.** Angiomatosis of the cervical cord with a telaniectatic naevus. **Cutaneous angioma.** A form of hypertrophic naevus composed of widely dilated blood vessels in the form of a network. **Encephalic angioma.** A mass in the brain composed of dilated arteries. **Encephalotrigeminal angioma.** A developmental abnormality of the intracranial, ocular and cutaneous vessels. The cutaneous angiomatosis is of port-wine-stain type in part, or all, of the trigeminal area. The oral mucosa may be affected. Epilepsy and mental retardation are common. (Syn.: Sturge-Weber-Kalischer syndrome.) **Fissural angioma.** One which occurs on sites corresponding to the embryonal fissures of the face, the lips and the neck. **Hereditary haemorrhagic angioma.** Hereditary haemorrhagic telangiectasia. *See* TELANGIECTASIA. **Hypertrophic angioma.** An angioma composed of capillary vessels and a solid substance which is based on hyperplasia of the endothelium. **Infective angioma.** Serpiginous angioma (see below). **Angioma lymphaticum.** Lymphangioma. **Multiple progressive angioma.** Multiple cavernous subcutaneous haemangiomata, which may disappear spontaneously. **Angioma pigmentosum atrophicum.** Xeroderma pigmentosum. **Plexiform angioma.** A tumour occurring usually in the skin and consisting of enlarged tortuous capillary vessels. **Sclerosing angioma.** A pigmented lesion of the skin showing histologically histiocytes, fibrous tissue and granules of haemosiderin. **Scrotal angioma.** Angiokeratoma of the scrotum. **Senile angioma.** The angioma that commonly arises in the skin of old people. **Serpiginous angioma.** A skin affection in which there are present rings of red dots which have a tendency towards expansile proliferation; there is subsequent atrophy of the surface capillaries. **Simple angioma.** A vascular naevus. **Spider angioma, Stellate angioma.** Naevus araneus. **Telangiectatic angioma.** One composed of dilated blood vessels. **Tuberose angioma, Tuberous angioma.** Angiolipoma; a tumour of the subcutaneous tissue which may be present in association with a fatty growth, or which may by degrees absorb the adipose tissue. **Angioma venosum racemosum.** The swellings associated with superficial varicose veins of advanced state. [Gk *aggeion* vessel, *-oma* tumour.]

angiomalacia (an·je·o·mal·**a**'·she·ah). Pathological softening of the walls of blood vessels or lymph vessels. [Gk *aggeion* vessel, malacia.]

angiomatosis (an·je·o·mat·**o**'·sis). A congenital condition characterized by the formation of multiple angiomata, most commonly in the skin. **Haemorrhagic familial angiomatosis.** Hereditary haemorrhagic telangiectasia. *See* TELANGIECTASIA. **Angiomatosis of the retina.** A rare disease of the retinal blood vessels which may produce varying ophthalmoscopic appearances. In general, there are 4 stages: (*a*) dilatation of the vessels and formation of angiomata; (*b*) formation of haemorrhagic exudates; (*c*) massive exudation and retinal detachment; (*d*) glaucoma and loss of the eye. If the changes are limited to the eye, it is called *von Hippel's disease*; if associated with cysts in other parts of the body, *von Hippel-Lindau disease.* [Gk *aggeion* vessel, *-oma* tumour, *-osis* condition.]

angiomatous (an·je·**o**·mat·us). Resembling, relating to or of the nature of angioma.

angiomegaly (an·je·o·**meg**'·al·e). A condition of enlargement of the blood vessels, particularly of the eyelid. [Gk *aggeion* vessel, *megas* large.]

angiometer (an·je·**om**·et·er). An apparatus used in measuring the diameter and tension of blood vessels. [Gk *aggeion* vessel, meter.]

angiomyocardiac (an·je·o·mi·o·**kar**'·de·ak). Relating to or affecting the cardiac muscle and the blood vessels. [Gk *aggeion* vessel, *mys* muscle, *kardia* heart.]

angiomyoma (an·je·o·mi·**o**'·mah). A myoma which contains a large number of blood vessels; mixed angioma and myoma. **Angiomyoma cutis.** A form of cutaneous myoma in which the tumour arises from the muscular elements of the wall of a blood vessel. Usually the lesions are circumscribed, solitary and deeply seated.

angiomyoneuroma (an·je·o·mi·o·newr·**o**'·mah). A glomus tumour. [Gk *aggeion* vessel, *mys* muscle, *neuron* nerve, *-oma* tumour.]

angiomyopathy (an·je·o·mi·**op**'·ath·e). Any disorder of the blood vessels that involves the muscular apparatus. [Gk *aggeion* vessel, myopathy.]

angiomyosarcoma (an·je·o·mi·o·sar·**ko**'·mah). A composite tumour consisting of angiomatous, myomatous and sarcomatous elements in varying proportions. [angioma, myoma, sarcoma.]

angionecrosis (an·je·o·nek·**ro**'·sis). The condition in which the walls of blood vessels are necrotic. [Gk *aggeion* vessel, necrosis.]

angioneoplasm (an·je·o·**ne**'·o·plazm). A neoplasm the main structure of which consists of blood vessels or, in some cases, lymph vessels. [Gk *aggeion* vessel, neoplasm.]

angioneurectomy (an·je·o·newr·**ek**'·to·me). 1. The cutting out of the vessels and nerves of any part of the body. 2. Resection of the spermatic-cord elements with the exception of the vas deferens and its vessels. [Gk *aggeion* vessel, neurectomy.]

angioneuroedema (an·je·o·newr·e·**de**'·mah). Angioneuro-oedema.

angioneuromyoma (an·je·o·newr·o·mi·**o**'·mah). Glomus tumour; a minute and painful tumour arising from arteriovenous anastomoses in the fingers and toes. [Gk *aggeion* vessel, *neuron* nerve, *mys* muscle, *-oma* tumour.]

angioneuro-oedema (an·je·o·newr·o·e·**de**'·mah). Angioneurotic oedema. *See* OEDEMA. [Gk *aggeion* vessel, *neuron* nerve, oedema.]

angioneurosis (an·je·o·newr·**o**'·sis). A neurosis affecting the blood vessels; it may be the result of vascular disease or of injury to the vasomotor nerves or nerve centre, and may take the form of paralysis (angioparalysis) or spasm (angiospasm). Vasomotor neurosis. [Gk *aggeion* vessel, neurosis.]

angioneurotic (an·je·o·newr·**ot**'·ik). Pertaining to angioneurosis.

angioneurotomy (an·je·o·newr·**ot**'·o·me). The operation of dividing nerves and vessels. [Gk *aggeion* vessel, *neuron* nerve, *temnein* to cut.]

angionoma (an·je·o·**no**'·mah). Ulceration of a blood vessel or lymph vessel. [Gk *aggeion* vessel, *-oma* tumour.]

angionosis (an·je·o·**no**'·sis). Angiopathy. [Gk *aggeion* vessel, *nosos* disease.]

angiopancreatitis (an·je·o·**pan**·kre·at·**i**'·tis). An inflammatory condition of the vascular tissue of the pancreas or of the pancreatic vessels. [Gk *aggeion* vessel, pancreatitis.]

angioparalysis, angioparesis (an·je·o·par·**al**'·is·is, an·je·o·par·**e**'·sis). Vasomotor paralysis. *See* PARALYSIS. [Gk *aggeion* vessel, paralysis, paresis.]

angiopathology (an·je·o·path·**ol**'·o·je). The pathology of diseases of the blood and lymph vessels. [Gk *aggeion* vessel, pathology.]

angiopathy (an·je·**op**·ath·e). Any disease of the vessels, especially the blood vessels. [Gk *aggeion* vessel, *pathos* suffering.]

angiophacomatosis (an·je·o·fak·o·mat·**o**'·sis). Single or multiple haemangiomata of the retina usually associated with haemangiomata and cysts in the central nervous system, the kidneys and suprarenal glands, the pancreas and the ovaries. It is of congenital origin but persists and grows through life; von Hippel–Lindau disease. [Gk *aggeion* vessel, phacomatosis.]

angiophorous (an·je·**of**·or·us). Term applied to the supporting tissue which surrounds vessels. [Gk *aggeion* vessel, *pherein* to bear.]

angioplania, angioplany (an·je·o·**pla**'·ne·ah, an·je·o·**pla**'·ne). Angio-ectopia. [Gk *aggeion* vessel, *plane* a straying.]

angioplasty (an·je·o·plas·te). Plastic reconstruction of a diseased or injured blood vessel. [Gk *aggeion* vessel, *plassein* to mould.]

angiopneumography (an·je·o·new·**mog**'·raf·e). Radiography of the vessels of the lungs. [Gk *aggeion* vessel, pneumography.]

angiopoietic (an·je·o·poi·**et**'·ik). Descriptive of those cells from which the blood vessels in new tissues are built up. [Gk *aggeion* vessel, *poiein* to make.]

angiopsathyrosis (an·je·o·sath·ir·**o**'·sis). A condition of fragility of the blood vessels. [Gk *aggeion* vessel, *psathyros* friable, *-osis* condition.]

angioreticuloma (an·je·o·ret·ik·ew·**lo**'·mah). Haemangioma, particularly haemangioma of the brain. The tumour is composed of newly-formed blood vessels. [Gk *aggeion* vessel, reticuloma.]

angiorrhagia (an·je·o·**ra**'·je·ah). A haemorrhage from a vessel. [Gk *aggeion* vessel, *rhegnynein* to gush forth.]

angiorrhaphy (an·je·**or**·af·e). The suturing of any type of vessel; arteriorrhaphy. **Arteriovenous angiorrhaphy.** The suturing of artery to vein for the purpose of allowing the arterial blood to flow through the vein. [Gk *aggeion* vessel, *rhaphe* suture.]

angiorrhexis (an·je·o·**rex**'·is). Rupture of a blood vessel or a lymph vessel. [Gk *aggeion* vessel, *rhexis* rupture.]

angiorrhigosis (an·je·o·ri·**go**'·sis). A condition in which the walls of a blood vessel are rigid. [Gk *aggeion* vessel, *rhigos* rigor.]

angiorrhoea (an·je·o·**re**'·ah). A condition in which there is oozing of blood from the vessels. [Gk *aggeion* vessel, *rhoia* flow.]

angiosarcoma (an·je·o·sar·**ko**'·mah). A vascular sarcoma. **Angiosarcoma myxomatodes.** One in which there is mucous degeneration of the walls of the blood vessels. [Gk *aggeion* vessel, sarcoma.]

angiosclerosis (an·je·o·skler·**o**'·sis). Abnormal thickening and hardening of the walls of the vessels throughout the entire vascular system. [Gk *aggeion* vessel, sclerosis.]

angiosclerotic (an·je·o·skler·**ot**'·ik). Relating to angiosclerosis.

angioscope (an·je·o·skope). A particular type of microscope through which the capillary vessels may be studied. [Gk *aggeion* vessel, *skopein* to watch.]

angioscotoma (an·je·o·sko·**to**'·mah). A scotoma caused by shadows of the blood vessels of the retina falling across the visual field. The shadows appear as extensions of the blind spot and require special methods of examination for their detection. [Gk *aggeion* vessel, scotoma.]

angioscotometry (an·je·o·sko·**tom**'·et·re). The method employed for the detection and plotting of angioscotomata. [angioscotomata, Gk *metron* measure.]

angiosialitis (an·je·o·si·al·i′·tis). An inflammatory condition of a salivary duct. [Gk *aggeion* vessel, *sialon* saliva, *-itis* inflammation.]

angiosis (an·je·o·sis). Angiopathy; any disease of the vessels, particularly the blood vessels. [Gk *aggeion* vessel, *-osis* condition.]

angiospasm (an·je·o·spazm). A condition of spasmodic contraction of the blood vessels, causing intermittent claudication or cramping of the muscles. [Gk *aggeion* vessel, spasm.]

angiospastic (an·je·o·spas′·tik). Pertaining to angiospasm.

angiostaxis (an·je·o·stax′·is). 1. The haemorrhagic diathesis; haemophilia. 2. Any oozing of blood. [Gk *aggeion* vessel, *staxis* a trickling.]

angiostenosis (an·je·o·sten·o′·sis). Abnormal narrowing of the internal diameter of a vessel. [Gk *aggeion* vessel, stenosis.]

angiosteogenic, angiosteogenous (an·je·os·te·o·jen′·ik, an·je·os·te·oj′·en·us). Associated with or belonging to the process of calcification in a blood vessel. [Gk *aggeion* vessel, *osteon* bone, *genein* to produce.]

angiosteosis (an·je·os·te·o′·sis). Calcareous degeneration of the walls of a blood vessel or lymph vessel. [Gk *aggeion* vessel, *osteon* bone.]

angiosthenia (an·je·os·the′·ne·ah). Tension within an artery. [Gk *aggeion* vessel, *sthenos* strength.]

angiostomy (an·je·os·to·me). The opening of a blood vessel by surgical methods, generally with a view to repair by implantation. [Gk *aggeion* vessel, *stoma* mouth.]

angiostrongylus (an·je·o·stron′·jil·us). **Angiostrongylus cantonensis.** The rodent lung worm, which has an intermediate host in slugs and snails (especially the giant snail *Schatina fulica*). If these are eaten raw by man, the larvae may pass to the brain causing an eosinophilic meningitis. The human disease may occur in the Pacific islands. [Gk *aggeion* vessel, *stroggylos* round.]

angiostrophe, angiostrophy (an·je·os·tro·fe). The twisting of the cut end of a blood vessel for the purpose of arresting haemorrhage. [Gk *aggeion* vessel, *strophe* twist.]

angiosynizesis (an·je·o·sin·iz·e′·sis). Term denoting that the walls of a blood vessel have collapsed and adhered together. [Gk *aggeion* vessel, synizesis.]

angiotelectasia, angiotelectasis (an·je·o·tel·ek·ta′·ze·ah, an·je·o·tel·ek′·tas·is). A state of dilatation of the capillary vessels and of the terminal arterioles and venules. Telangiectasis. [Gk *aggeion* vessel, *telos* end, *ektasis* a stretching.]

angiotenic (an·je·o·ten′·ik). Caused by distension of the blood vessels. [Gk *aggeion* vessel, *teinein* to stretch.]

angiotensin (an·je·o·ten·sin). A substance, also known as *hypertensin,* responsible for the occurrence of renal hypertension and produced from angiotensinogen by the action of renin. [Gk *aggeion* vessel, L *tendere* to stretch.]

Angiotensin Amide (an·je·o·ten′·sin am·ide). BP Commission approved name for val$_5$-hypertensin II-asp-β-amide; it is used in the treatment of severe shock and collapse.

angiotensinogen (an·je·o·ten·sin·o·jen). The inactive precursor of angiotensin.

angiotitis (an·je·o·ti′·tis). An inflammatory condition of the blood vessels of the ear. [Gk *aggeion* vessel, otitis.]

angiotomy (an·je·ot·o·me). Section of a blood vessel or lymph vessel. [Gk *aggeion* vessel, *temnein* to cut.]

angiotonia (an·je·o·to′·ne·ah). Vasotonia; the tonus of a blood vessel. [Gk *aggeion* vessel, *tonos* tone.]

angiotonic (an·je·o·ton′·ik). 1. Relating to angiotonia. 2. Descriptive of an agent that increases the tension of the vascular system.

angiotonin (an·je·o·to′·nin). Angiotensin. [Gk *aggeion* vessel, *tonos* tone.]

angiotribe (an·je·o·tribe). A powerful forceps with screw attachment formerly employed to arrest haemorrhage by crushing an artery together with the tissue around it; now superseded by ligation. [Gk *aggeion* vessel, *tribein* to crush.]

angiotripsy (an·je·o·trip′·se). The production of haemostasis by the use of an angiotribe.

angiotrophic (an·je·o·trof′·ik). Relating to or promoting the nutrition of the blood vessels or lymph vessels. [Gk *aggeion* vessel, *trophe* nutrition.]

angiotrophoneurosis (an·je·o·tro·fo·newr·o′·sis). Any functional nervous disease due to failure of nutrition, resulting from defective nerve influence and an affection of vascular tissue, such as a spasm. [Gk *aggeion* vessel, *trophe* nourishment, neurosis.]

angitis (an·ji·tis). Angiitis.

Angle, Edward Hartley (b. 1855). St. Louis dentist.

Angle's arch. An appliance used in orthodontics; a continuous wire fixed to the teeth, which on account of its elasticity moves malplaced teeth into their correct positions.

Angle's band. An adjustable anchor band devised by Angle.

Angle's classification. A classification of the malocclusion of teeth based upon the anteroposterior relationship of the first permanent molar teeth. *Class* 1. The first permanent molar teeth are in normal anteroposterior relationship to each other, associated with overcrowding of anterior teeth. *Class* 2. The mandibular 1st permanent molar tooth is in postnormal occlusion with the corresponding upper tooth. *Division* 1: the arches are narrowed; the upper incisor teeth are protrusive, and the mandibular arch is postnormal to the maxillary arch. *Division* 2: a small upper arch in which there is crowding of the anterior teeth, the central incisors lying in a plane posterior to the lateral incisors. *Class* 3. The mandibular 1st permanent molar tooth is in prenormal occlusion with the corresponding upper tooth; the mandibular incisor teeth are in labial occlusion to the maxillary incisor teeth.

Angle's splint. A metallic splint held in position by bands cemented to the teeth, used for immobilizing a fractured mandible by fixation to the maxilla.

angle (ang·gl). 1. The degree of inclination of 2 intersecting lines or planes. 2. [Angulus (NA).] A bend, or corner. 3. The form produced by any sharp change in direction of a surface or line. 4. In dentistry, a restoration in a tooth fits accurately into the angles of a cavity in order to provide for its retention. **Angle of aberration.** The angle subtended at the eye of the observer between the apparent and true positions of a star or other heavenly body. **Acromial angle [angulus acromialis (NA)].** *See* ACROMION. **Alpha angle.** The angle at the nodal point of the eye between the visual and optic axes. **Angle of altitude.** Angle of elevation (see below). **Angle of anomaly.** That found in certain cases of squint with abnormal retinal correspondence; it equals the difference between the angle of deviation of the squint, measured objectively, and the angle of deviation of the projected image as measured subjectively. **Angle of anterior chamber.** Filtration angle (see below). **Angle of aperture.** The angle subtended at the focus of a lens by 2 lines drawn from the extremities of its diameter. **Axial angle.** The angle formed by the meeting of 2 planes, one which lies parallel to the long axis of a tooth. **Angle of azimuth.** The amount of lateral rotation round a vertical axis performed by the eye when it moves from its primary position to view an object at one side or the other. **Basal angle.** An anthropological measurement, an angle of the skull base; formed when one line is drawn from the glabella to the middle of the hypophyseal fossa, and the other from the latter point to the basion. In modern man it varies between 123 and 152 degrees. **Beta angle.** The angle made by the radius fixus with a line joining the bregma and the hormion. **Buccal angle.** Any angle formed by the buccal surface with another surface of a tooth. **Cardiohepatic angle.** The angle between the right border of the heart and the upper surface of the right lobe of the liver. **Carrying angle.** The obtuse angle at the elbow between the arm and forearm when the upper limb is hanging extended at the side of the body. **Cavity angle.** Any angle formed by the distal wall of a cavity prepared in a tooth, and designed to provide for the retention of a restoration. **Cavosurface angle.** The angle in a cavity prepared in a tooth, which is formed by the wall of the cavity with the surface of the tooth. **Cerebellopon-**

tine angle. The angular depression below the lateral extremity of the lower border of the pons in which the roots of the 7th and 8th cranial nerves are found. (Syn.: lateral recess.) **Colic angle.** The junction between the mid-gut and the hind-gut of the embryo. **Angle of convergence.** When the eye is looking at an object, the angle between its visual axis and a line drawn from the centre of rotation parallel to the meridian plane. **Coronary angle.** The angle between the coronal and sagittal sutures. **Costal angle.** Posterior angle of a rib. *See* RIBS. **Costophrenic angle.** The angle between the upper surface of the diaphragm and the inner surface of the ribs and costal cartilages; both surfaces are covered with pleura. **Critical angle.** The angle of total internal reflection; the angle at which a ray of light passing from a denser to a lighter medium (i.e. from one of higher to one of lower refractive index) becomes totally reflected at the interface. **Angle of declination.** 1. The angle between the neck of the femur and the femoral shaft. 2. In physics, the angle between the geographical and magnetic meridians at any point on the earth's surface. **Angle of deviation.** The angle between the incident and emergent ray when light is refracted by a glass prism. **Angle of direction.** The angle through which the eye must move in order to see a given object. **Distal angle.** Any angle formed by the distal wall of a cavity prepared in a tooth with another surface of the tooth. **Distobuccal angle.** The angle formed by the junction of the distal and buccal surfaces of a tooth. **Distobucco-occlusal angle.** The angle formed by the junction of the distal, buccal and occlusal surfaces of a tooth. **Distobuccopulpal angle.** The angle formed by the junction of the distal and buccal walls with the pulpal surface of a cavity prepared in a tooth. **Distocervical angle.** The angle formed by the junction of the distal and cervical walls of a cavity prepared in a tooth. **Disto-incisal angle.** The angle formed by the distal surface with the incisive edge of a tooth. **Distolabial angle.** The angle formed by the junction of the distal and labial surfaces of a tooth. **Distolabiopulpal angle.** The angle formed by the junction of the distal and labial walls with the pulpal surface of a cavity prepared in a tooth. **Distolingual angle.** The angle formed by the junction of the distal and lingual surfaces of a tooth. **Distolinguo-occlusal angle.** The angle formed by the junction of the distal, lingual and occlusal surfaces of a tooth. **Distolinguopulpal angle.** The angle formed by the junction of the distal and lingual walls with the pulpal surface of a cavity prepared in a tooth. **Disto-occlusal angle.** The angle formed by the junction of the distal and occlusal surfaces of a tooth. **Distopulpal angle.** The angle formed by the junction of the distal wall with the pulpal surface of a cavity prepared in a tooth. **Angle of elevation.** The angle between the normal plane of vision and that assumed by the eye when looking upwards or downwards. **Ethmocranial angle.** The angle between the basicranial axis and the plane of the cribriform plate of the ethmoid. **Angles of the eye.** *See* EYE. **Facial angle.** The angle that a line pssing through the nasion and the prosthion makes with Reid's base line. **Filtration angle.** The angle at the periphery of the anterior chamber of the eye between the sclerocorneal junction, the root of the iris and the most anterior portion of the ciliary body. It is important in glaucoma, as the aqueous drains through this angle to the canal of Schlemm. **Frankfort-mandibular-plane angle.** The angle between the Frankfort and mandibular planes. **Frontal angle.** The anterosuperior angle of the parietal bone; it occurs at the bregma where the sagittal and coronal sutures meet. **Gamma angle.** The angle between the fixation and optic axes. **Gastric angle.** The angular notch of the stomach. **Gonial angle.** The angle between the posterior border of the ascending ramus and the horizontal border of the mandible, usually 110–120 degrees. **Angle of incidence.** The angle which an incident ray of light makes with the normal to the reflecting surface at the point of incidence. **Incisal angle.** The angle formed by a surface of the tooth with the incisive edge. **Infrasternal angle of the thorax.** *See* THORAX. **Iridocorneal angle [angulus iridocornealis (NA)].** Filtration angle (see above). **Angle of the iris, Iritic angle.** Filtration angle (see above). **Kappa angle.** The angle between the visual axis and one perpendicular to the cornea through the centre of the pupil. **Limiting angle.** Critical angle (see above). **Line angle.** The angle formed at the line where 2 planes meet. **Lumbosacral angle.** The angle between the anterior surfaces of the 5th lumbar and the 1st sacral vertebrae; the promontory of the sacrum. **Angle of the mandible.** *See* MANDIBLE. **Manubriosternal angle.** Angle of the sternum. *See* STERNUM. **Mastoid angle of the parietal bone.** *See* PARIETAL BONE. **Mesial angle.** Any angle formed by the mesial wall of a cavity prepared in a tooth with another surface of the tooth. **Mesiobuccal angle.** The angle formed by the junction of the mesial and buccal surfaces of a tooth. **Mesiobucco-occlusal angle.** The angle formed by the junction of the mesial, buccal and occlusal surfaces of a tooth. **Mesiobuccopulpal angle.** The angle formed by the junction of the mesial and buccal walls with the pulpal surface of a cavity prepared in a tooth. **Mesiocervical angle.** The angle formed by the junction of the mesial and cervical walls of a cavity prepared in a tooth. **Mesio-incisal angle.** The angle formed by the mesial surface wth the incisive edge of a tooth. **Mesiolabial angle.** The angle formed by the junction of the mesial and labial surfaces of a tooth. **Mesiolabiopulpal angle.** The angle formed by the junction of the mesial and labial walls with the pulpal surface of a cavity prepared in a tooth. **Mesiolingual angle.** The angle formed by the junction of the mesial and lingual surfaces of a tooth. **Mesiolinguo-occlusal angle.** The angle formed by the junction of the mesial, lingual and occlusal surfaces of a tooth. **Mesiolinguopulpal angle.** The angle formed by the junction of the mesial and lingual walls with the pulpal surface of a cavity prepared in a tooth. **Mesio-occlusal angle.** The angle formed by the junction of the mesial and occlusal surfaces of a tooth. **Mesiopulpal angle.** The angle formed by the junction of the mesial wall with the pulpal surface of a cavity prepared in a tooth. **Metre angle.** Devised by Nagel so that the convergence shall correspond with the dioptres of accommodation: 1 m.a. represents the angle between the meridian plane and a line joining the centre of rotation of the eye to an object 1 m away, in the median plane. The convergence needed to see an object 2 m away is 0.5 m.a., that to see one 0.5 m away 2 m.a., i.e. the m.a. is the reciprocal of the distance of the object in metres. **Minimal visual angle.** The smallest angle subtended at the nodal point of the eye by 2 points which can just be distinguished as 2. **Minimum cognoscible angle.** The smallest angle subtended by an object which will allow of its recognition. **Angle of minimum deviation.** The least possible change in the direction of a light ray when passing through a glass prism. **Minimum legible angle.** The smallest angle subtended by a letter which will allow of its recognition by the eye. **Minimum separable angle.** The minimum angular separation of 2 objects which will allow of their being discriminated by the eye. **Angle of the mouth.** *See* MOUTH. **Nasal angle of the eye.** The inner canthus. *See* CANTHUS. **Occipital angle.** The angle formed between the plane of the foramen magnum and the line from the nasion to the opisthion. **Occlusaldistal angle.** Disto-occlusal angle (see above). **Ocular angle.** Canthus. **Ophryospinal angle.** The angle formed between lines drawn from the glabella in the midline and the centre of the external auditory meatus to the nasal spine. **Optic angle.** The angle subtended at the nodal point of the eye by the extremities of the object looked at. **Parietal angle.** The angle between a line on both sides of the skull drawn tangential to the maximum curve of the zygomatic arch and the end of the maximum frontal diameter. Such lines when parallel give an angle of zero, and when divergius give a negative angle. **Angles of the parietal bone.** *See* PARIETAL BONE. **Phrenicopericardial angle.** The angle between the heart and the pericardium and the upper surface of the diaphragm. **Point angle.** The angle at a point where three planes meet. **Angle of polarization, Polarizing angle.** The angle at which light reflected from a transparent medium is almost completely plane-polarized in the plane of incidence. **Prism angle.** The angle formed at the apex of the prism; used in grading prisms. **Pubic angle.** The junction of the rami of the pubes. **Angle of reflection.** The angle which a reflected ray of light makes with the normal to the reflecting surface at the point of incidence. **Angle of refraction,**

Refracting angle. The angle between the refracted ray and the normal to the surface of the refracting medium at the point of incidence of the light ray. **Angles of a rib.** *See* RIBS. **Rolandic angle.** The angle between the central sulcus and the line of the sagittal suture. **S angle, Σ angle.** The angle between the radius fixus (the line from the hormion to the inion) and a line from the staphylion and hormion. **Sacrolumbar angle, Sacrovertebral angle.** Lumbosacral angle (see above). **Angles of the scapula.** *See* SCAPULA. **Scattering angle.** The angle between the initial direction of a particle and its direction after scattering of the particle has occurred. **Sigma angle.** S angle (see above). **Solid angle.** The angle formed at a point where 3 or more planes meet; it is measured by the area cut off the surface of a sphere of unit radius described with the point as centre. **Somatosplanchnic angle.** The junction of the somatopleural and splanchnopleural mesodermal layers of the early embryo, posterolateral to the root of the mesentery of the alimentary canal. **Angle of squint.** The angle between the visual axes of the squinting and fixing eyes, positive for convergence and negative for divergence. **Sternoclavicular angle.** The angle between the clavicle and the sternum. **Angle of the sternum.** *See* STERNUM. **Subcostal angle.** Infrasternal angle of the thorax. *See* THORAX. **Subpubic angle [angulus subpubicus (NA)].** The angle below the symphysis between the inferior rami of the 2 pubic bones. **Tooth angle.** A line at which 2 surfaces of a tooth meet, or a point at which more than 2 surfaces meet. **Angle of torsion.** The deviation of the primary vertical meridian of the eye when out of the primary position. **Angle of torsion of the humerus.** The angle between the transverse axes of the upper and lower ends of the humerus. **Tympanic angle.** The angle of the basilar membrane to the wall of the cochlea. **Uterine angle.** That part of the uterus immediately surrounding the opening of the fallopian tube. **Venous angle.** The angle between the internal jugular and the subclavian veins. **Visual angle.** Optic angle (see above). **Y angle.** In craniology, the angle between the radius fixus and a line drawn from the inion to the lambda. [L *angulus.*]

See also: ACKERMANN, ALSBERG, BROCA, CAMPER, DAUBENTON, EBSTEIN, FLOWER, FUCHS (E.), JACQUART, LOUIS, MIKULICZ-RADECKI, PIROGOFF, QUATREFAGES, RANKE (J.), SYLVIUS, TOPINARD, VIRCHOW, VOGT (K.), WEISBACH, WELCKER.

angophrasia (ang·go·**fra**·ze·h). The drawling type of speech, periodically interrupted by spasms of choking, as described by Kussmaul, and typical of dementia paralytica. [Gk *agchein* to choke, *phrasis* a saying.]

angor (**ang**·gor). 1. Angina. 2. Extreme distress. **Angor abdominis.** Abdominal angina. *See* ANGINA. **Angor animi.** Severe distress of mind with a sensation as if death were impending. **Angor nocturnus.** Pavor nocturnus. **Angor ocularis.** A condition characterized by sudden attacks of mistiness of vision and by fear of impending blindness. **Angor pectoris.** Angina pectoris. [L anguish.]

angostura (an·gos·**tewr**·ah). Cusparia bark; the bark of *Galipea officinalis* Hancock, family Rutaceae, from South America. It contains a bitter substance angosturin, and several bitter alkaloids; used medicinally as an aromatic bitter tonic in the form of an infusion, and is one of the constituents of Angostura bitters. [*Angostura,* a town in Venezuela.]

angosturin (ang·gos·**tewr**·in). $C_9H_{12}O_5$. A crystalline bitter principle obtained from cusparia bark.

angosturine (an·gos·**tewr**·een). A crystalline alkaloid mixture obtained from angostura, the bark of *Galipea cusparia*; a tonic stimulant, used in the treatment of diarrhoea and dysentery.

Ångström, Anders Jonas (b. 1814). Swedish physicist.

Ångström's law. The wavelength of the light absorbed by any substance equals that of the light that would be emitted by the substance if it were rendered incandescent.

Ångström's unit. *See* ANGSTROM.

ångstrom (**ang**·strom). A unit of length for the measurement of the wavelengths of light: one ten thousand millionth of a meter (10^{-10}m). [see prec.]

Anguillula (ang·gwil·**ew**′·lah). A genus of round nematode worms. **Anguillula aceti.** The vinegar worm, a species occasionally found in stale urine, and in vaginal exudate where it occurs by accident. **Anguillula stercoralis.** *Strongyloides stercoralis.* [L little eel.]

anguilluliasis (ang·gwil·ew·**li**′·as·is). Strongyloidiasis: infestation with *Strongyloides* (*Anguillula*) *stercoralis,* a genus of intestinal nematode worms found in man in the tropics and sub-tropics. Gastric disturbance and intermittent diarrhoea may result.

Anguillulina (ang·gwil·ew·**li**′·nah). A genus of nematode worms. **Anguillulina putrefaciens.** A species which is a round worm of the onion, and hence occasionally seen in human faeces; a pseudoparasite. [L *anguillula,* little eel.]

anguillulosis (ang·gwil·ew·**lo**′·sis). Anguilluliasis.

angular (**ang**·gew·lah). Forming an angle; sharply bent. **Angular notch.** *See* NOTCH.

angular artery [arteria angularis (NA)]. The terminal part of the facial artery from the angle of the mouth to the medial canthus.

angular vein [vena angularis (NA)]. A vein of the anterior angle of the orbit. It is a tributary of the anterior facial vein.

angustura (ang·**gus**·**tewr**·ah). Angostura.

anhaematopoiesis (an·**he**·mat·o·poi·**e**′·sis). Anhaematosis. [Gk *a, haima* blood, *poiein* to make.]

anhaematopoietic (an·**he**·mat·o·poi·**et**′·ik). 1. Relating to anhaematosis. 2. Caused by impairment of the blood-forming quality of the bone marrow owing to defect in the latter. [see prec.]

anhaematosis (**an**·he·mat·**o**′·sis). Defect of the bone marrow leading to deficient formation of blood cells. [Gk *a,* haematosis.]

anhaemolytic (**an**·he·mo·**lit**′·ik). Incapable of destroying blood cells; not haemolytic. [Gk *a,* haemolytic.]

anhalamine (an·**hal**·am·een). $(CH_3O)_2C_9H_7OHNH$. A crystalline alkaloid obtained from mescal buttons, the buds of *Anhalonium lewinii*; used as a cardiac stimulant.

anhaphia (an·**haf**·e·ah). Anaphia.

anhedonia (an·he·**do**·ne·ah). In psychology, an incapacity to feel normal happiness or pleasure. [Gk *a, hedone* pleasure.]

anhelation (an·hel·**a**·shun). Panting in association with dyspnoea. [L *anhelare* to pant.]

anhelose, anhelous (an·**he**·loze, an·**he**·lus). Panting respiration or shortness of breath. [see prec.]

anhepatic, anhepatogenic (an·hep·**at**·ik, an·**hep**·at·o·**jen**′·ik). Not arising in, or caused by, the liver or by any condition of the liver. [Gk *a, hepar* liver, *genein* to produce.]

anhidrosis (an·hid·**ro**·sis). Marked deficiency in the secretion of sweat, or entire lack of it. **Congenital anhidrosis.** Absence of or defective sweating as a result of a congenital defect. **Heat anhidrosis, Postmiliarial anhidrosis, Tropical anhidrosis.** A sequel to prickly heat in which the sweat glands involved in the latter disease are blocked by small keratin plugs so that the sweat cannot escape. If only small and scattered areas are affected little is noticed, but if large areas are involved there is marked lethargy and exhaustion (anhidrotic exhaustion), with grave risk of heat stroke. An area of skin showing complete tropical anhidrosis is dry, devoid of sweat, deficient in sebum, and stippled with small grey, shining macules which lie flush with its surface and which are the top of the keratin plugs. After exertion deep-seated vesicles may be noted under the macules; these disappear if the subject rests in a cool place. The affected areas are immune from prickly heat. [Gk *a, hidros* sweat]

anhidrotic (an·hid·**rot**·ik). 1. Relating to anhidrosis. 2. Inhibiting the secretion of sweat. 3. Any agent which prevents the secretion of sweat. [see prec.]

anhydraemia (an·hi·**dre**·me·ah). A condition of the blood in which the watery constituent is diminished. [Gk *a, hydor* water, *haima* blood.]

anhydrase (an·**hi**·draze). An enzyme which promotes the elimination of molecules of water from a compound. **Carbonic anhydrase.** An enzyme containing zinc, which occurs in the red corpuscles; by dehydrating carbonic acid, or alternatively hydrating carbon dioxide, it controls the amount of the latter in the blood and its rate of excretion in the lungs. [see foll.]

anhydration (an·hi·**dra**·shun). 1. The state of not being hydrated. 2. Dehydration. [Gk *a, hydor* water.]

anhydric (an·**hi**·drik). The state of a compound from which water has been eliminated, especially water of crystallization; anhydrous. [see prec.]

anhydride (an·**hi**·dride). A compound obtained by the elimination of 1 or more molecules of water from another compound. **Abietic anhydride.** $C_{44}H_{62}O_4$, a complex anhydride of abietic acid, forming, with its isomers, the chief constituent of colophony. **Acetic anhydride.** $(CH_3CO)_2O$, a pungent liquid prepared from acetic acid and used in acetylation reactions, especially those required in artificial-silk manufacture. **Acid anhydride.** A non-metallic oxide which dissolves in water to form an acid; an organic compound obtained by the elimination of a molecule of water from 2 molecules of an organic acid. **Arsenious anhydride.** Arsenic trioxide, white arsenic, As_2O_3, a highly poisonous white substance which dissolves in water to form arsenious acid, H_3AsO_3. **Basic anhydride.** A metallic oxide which dissolves in water to form a basic hydroxide. **Cantharidic anhydride.** Cantharidin, $C_8H_{12}O(CO)_2O$, the lactone of cantharidic acid; a strong vesicant. It occurs in Spanish flies and other insects. **Chromic anhydride.** Chromium trioxide, CrO_3, deep-red crystals, soluble in water, and in alkalis giving rise to chromates and di-, tri- and tetra-chromates. **Inner anhydride, Internal anhydride.** An organic compound which has a ring structure due to its chain of carbon atoms having joined ends with the elimination of water. **Mixed anhydride.** A compound formed from 2 different organic acids by the elimination of a molecule of water between them. **Osmic anhydride.** Osmium tetroxide, OsO_4, usually called *osmic acid,* a yellowish crystalline substance used as a stain for fats in histology. [Gk *a, hydor* water.]

anhydrite (an·**hi**·drite). A natural form of calcium sulphate, $CaSO_4$, containing no water of crystallization. Cf. GYPSUM. [see prec.]

anhydrochloric (an·hi·dro·**klor**′·ik). A state in which the usual hydrochloric acid is absent. [Gk *a,* hydrochloric.]

anhydrohydroxyprogesterone (an·**hi**·dro·hi·drox·e·pro·**jes**′·ter·one). Pregneninolone, Ethisterone BP 1958, 17(*β*)-ethinyl-Δ^4-androstene-3-one-17(*α*)-ol, $C_{21}H_{28}O_2$. A synthetic steroid which is orally active, with the pharmacological actions of progesterone.

anhydromyelia (an·**hi**·dro·mi·**e**′·le·ah). A condition in which the normal fluid in the central canal of the spinal cord is reduced in quantity. [Gk *a, hydor* water, *myelos* marrow.]

anhydrosugar (an·**hi**·dro·**shug**′·ar). A powdery form of cane sugar produced by drying the latter in vacuum pans; being pure disaccharide, it is not fermentable, and is useful in cases of diabetes. [Gk *a, hydor* water, sugar.]

anhydrous (an·**hi**·drus). In chemistry, not containing any water. [Gk *a, hydor* water.]

anhypnosis (an·hip·**no**·sis). Insomnia. [Gk *a, hypnos* sleep.]

aniacinamidosis (an·i·as·in·am·id·**o**′·sis). A disorder caused by lack of nicotinic acid (niacin) amide in the diet. The lesions of the skin, mucous membranes and nervous system, characteristic of pellagra, are due to this deficiency. It is usually associated with deficiency of the other members of the B_2 complex. [Gk *a,* niacin, amide, Gk *-osis* condition.]

aniacinosis (a·**ni**·as·in·**o**′·sis). The state of deficiency of niacin or nicotinic acid. [Gk *a,* niacin, Gk *-osis* condition.]

anianthinopsy (an·e·**an**·thin·**op**′·se). Lack of the power to recognize the colour purple or violet; violet blindness. [Gk *a, ianthinos* violet, *opsis* sight.]

anicteric (an·ik·**ter**·ik). Occurring without the accompaniment of icterus; not having any taint of jaundice. [Gk *a,* icteric.]

anidean (an·**id**·e·an). 1. Relating to an anideus. 2. Amorphous.

anideation (an·**i**·de·**a**′·shun). The state of not being able to form an idea of an object; non-ideation. [Gk *a,* ideation.]

anideus (an·**id**·e·us). A double monster of which the parasite is represented by a shapeless mass with a dermal covering. [Gk *a, eidos* form.]

anidous (an·**i**·dus). Applied to teratisms which are without form because of arrested development. [see prec.]

Anidoxime (an·e·**dox**·eem). BP Commission approved name for 3-diethylaminopropiophenone *O*-(*p*-methoxyphenylcarbamoyl)-oxime; an analgesic.

anidrosis (**an**·id·**ro**·sis). Anhidrosis.

anidrotic (an·id·**rot**·ik). Anhidrotic.

anile (**an**·ile). 1. Like an old woman. 2. Senile; imbecile. [L *anus* old woman.]

Anileridine (an·il·**er**·id·een). BP Commission approved name for ethyl 1,4′-aminophenethyl-4-phenylpiperidine-4-carboxylate, a narcotic analgesic.

anilide (**an**·il·ide). Any derivative of aniline in which one or both of the hydrogen atoms of the NH_2 group are replaced by acyl groups.

anilinction, anilinctus (a·ne·**lingk**·shun, a·ne·**lingk**·tus). Licking of the anus. [anus, L *lingua* tongue.]

aniline (**an**·il·een). Phenylamine, $C_6H_5NH_2$. A colourless liquid with a characteristic odour, derived from coal tar, and the parent of many synthetic drugs and dyestuffs. Pharmacologically it has an antipyretic action, but its use is liable to cause methaemoglobinaemia and other symptoms of the condition known as *anilism.* It has therefore been replaced by derivatives such as *p*-phenetidin and phenacetin. **Aniline antimonyl tartrate.** $COOH(CHOH)_2COO(OSb)C_6H_5NH_2$, a trypanocide. **Aniline poisoning.** *See* POISONING. [Ar. *alnil,* indigo.]

anilinism (**an**·il·in·izm). A condition of poisoning caused by inhalation by workers of the vapours which arise during the manufacture of aniline; the main signs are weakness, fainting, cyanosis, gastric disturbances and sometimes collapse.

anilinophil, anilinophile, anilinophilous (an·il·**in**·o·fil, an·il·**in**·o·file, an·il·in·**of**′·il·us). Denoting a cell or structure which stains readily with aniline dyes. [aniline, Gk *philein* to love.]

anilism (**an**·il·izm). Anilinism.

anility (an·**il**·it·e). The state of being an old woman. 2. The state of being senile or imbecile. [L *anus* old woman.]

anilquinoline (an·il·**kwin**·ol·een). Name used to distinguish the synthetic quinoline prepared by the oxidation together of aniline and glycerol.

anima (**an**·im·ah). The archetypal figure of the soul image, as the representation of the other sex, that each individual is postulated to carry within himself. Thus, *anima* in the male and *animus* in the female. **Anima aloes.** An old name for the active principle of aloe, aloin. **Anima brutalis.** The blood. **Animae deliquium.** Syncope. **Animae gravitas.** Offensiveness of the breath. **Anima mundi.** Paracelsus' term for vital force which is responsible for the continuity of life of the individual and of the world. [L soul.]

animal (**an**·im·al). 1. A living organism which feeds holozoically, that is by the breakdown of organic substances to soluble form, followed by synthesis. The distinction between an animal and a plant cannot be made in certain acellular organisms. 2. In general use, as a synonym for a mammal excluding man, or any tetrapod except a bird. 3. Pertaining to or derived from an animal. **Control animal.** In animal experiments designed to elucidate the efficiency of a certain procedure, e.g. immunization, a series of animals also tested to ensure that various nonspecific parts of the procedure have not influenced the result. **Decerebrate animal.** One in which the brain stem above the midbrain has been removed or disconnected. **Experimental animal.** One on which experiments are performed. **Animal heat.** *See* HEAT. **Immune animal.** An animal which by virtue of an immunization with specific toxin or antigen is rendered immune to the effects of that particular bacterial poison at a later date. **Laboratory animal.** Experimental animal (see above). **Normal animal.** An animal, used for experiments, which as far as can be ascertained is healthy and free from the effects of past infection. **Spinal animal.** One in which the spinal cord has been severed in the cervical region. **Thalamic animal.** One in which the brain stem has been severed just above the thalamus. [L.]

See also: HOUSSAY.

animalcule (an·im·**al**·kewl). Any minute microscopical animal organism; a protozoon. **Slipper animalcule.** Paramoecium. [L *animalculum* little animal.]

animalized (**an**·im·al·i·zd). A term applied to bacteria which have been cultivated on animal secretions or in an animal's body.

animism (**an**·im·izm). The theory that the vital principle is the soul and that it is responsible for every organic development whether normal or pathological. It now has very few supporters. [L *anima* soul.]

animus (**an**·im·us). In psycho-analysis, the image of the perfect man which is present in the subconscious of a woman. Cf. ANIMA. [L soul.]

anincretinosis (**an**·in·kre·tin·**o**'·sis). A disease which is caused by the functional breakdown of an endocrine organ or by deficiency of hormonal output. [Gk *a*, incretion, Gk *-osis* condition.]

anion (an·i·on). A negatively charged ion. [Gk *ana, ion* going.]

anionic (an·i·**on**·ik). 1. Having the properties of an anion. 2. Term applied to a disinfectant which exercises a detergent action on a surface by reason of the active negatively-charged chemical group it contains; soap and the bile salts are examples.

aniridia (an·ir·**id**·e·ah). 1. Lack of the iris, in whole or in part. 2. Irideremia; congenital absence of the iris. [Gk *a, iris.*]

anisakiasis (**an**·is·ak·**i**'·as·sis). Gastro-intestinal infection with the parasite *Anisakis marina,* usually acquired by eating raw or undercooked herring, causing eosinophilic gastro-enteritis. [*Anisaklis,* Gk *-osis* condition.]

anisal (an·**is**·al). The divalent radical $CH_3OC_6H_4CH=$ which occurs in anisic aldehyde.

anisalcohol (**an**·is·**al**'·ko·hol). Anisyl alcohol. *See* ALCOHOL.

anisaldehyde (**an**·is·**al**'·de·hide). Anisic aldehyde. *See* ALDEHYDE.

anisalyl (an·**is**·al·il). The monovalent radical $CH_3OC_6H_4CH_2$–, which occurs in anisyl alcohol; also called *anisyl.*

anisamide (an·**is**·am·ide). Anisyl amine, anisidine, $CH_3OC_6H_4NH_2$. A base used like aniline in the manufacture of dyestuffs.

anisate (**an**·is·ate). Any salt of anisic acid, e.g. sodium anisate; they have antiseptic and antipyretic properties.

anisated (**an**·is·a·ted). Flavoured with or containing anise.

anischuria (an·is·**kewr**·e·ah). Enuresis; incontinence of urine; the involuntary passing of urine. [Gk *a,* ischuria.]

Anise BPC 1954 (**an**·ees). The dried ripe fruits of *Pimpinella anisum* (family Umbelliferae), which is cultivated in many European countries. The carminative and expectorant properties of the drug are due to the volatile oil, present to the extent of 1.5–4 per cent and consisting largely of anethole. **Anise oil.** *See* OIL. [L *anisum.*]

aniseed (**an**·is·eed). Anise.

aniseikometer (**an**·is·i·**kom**'·et·er). An instrument for measuring the size of the images of the two eyes in cases of aniseikonia. Also called *eikonometer.* [Gk *anisos* unequal, *eikon* image, *metron* measure.]

aniseikonia (**an**·is·i·**ko**'·ne·ah). A defect of vision in which the form and size of the objective image is different in the two eyes; aniso-iconia. **Meridional aniseikonia.** That in which one of the images is larger than the other in one meridian. **Overall aniseikonia.** That in which one of the images is larger than the other in all meridians. [Gk *anisos* unequal, *eikon* image.]

aniseikonic (**an**·is·i·**kon**'·ik). Relating to or correcting aniseikonia.

anisergy (**an**·is·er·je). Inequality of blood pressure as between different sections of the cardiovascular system. [Gk *anisos* unequal, *ergon* work.]

anisidine (an·is·id·een). Anisamide, anisyl amine, $CH_3OC_6H_4NH_2$. A base occurring in 3 isomeric forms, and used like aniline in the manufacture of dyestuffs. The acetyl derivative, *p*-acetanisidin, is an antipyretic and analgesic. **Anisidine citrate.** An analgesic.

Anisindione (an·is·**in**·di·one). BP Commission approved name for 2-*p*-methoxyphenylindane-1,3-dione; an anticoagulant.

aniso-accommodation (an·i·so·ak·om·o·**da**'·shun). A difference between the two eyes as regards accommodative capacity. [Gk *anisos* unequal, accommodation.]

anisochromasia (an·i·so·kro·**ma**'·ze·ah). An anaemic condition in which there is colour in only the peripheral zone of the erythrocytes. [Gk *anisos* unequal, *chroma* colour.]

anisochromatic (an·i·so·kro·**mat**'·ik). A term descriptive of solutions used in testing for colour blindness; there are in them 2 pigments which can be detected by the colour-blind as well as the normal eye. [see prec.]

anisochromia (an·i·so·**kro**'·me·ah). An anaemic condition in which the haemoglobin content of the erythrocytes varies so that they are not all equally red. [Gk *anisos* unequal, *chroma* colour.]

anisocoria (an·i·so·**ko**'·re·ah). Inequality of diameter of the pupils of the two eyes. [Gk *anisos* unequal, *kore* pupil.]

anisocytosis (an·i·so·si·**to**'·sis). An abnormal condition in which the erythrocytes are not all of the same size. [Gk *anisos* unequal, *kytos* cell.]

anisodactylous (an·i·so·**dak**'·til·us). In zoology, descriptive of certain birds and animals which have unsymmetrically divided feet, some toes being directed forwards and others (usually only 1) backwards. [Gk *anisos* unequal, *daktylos* finger.]

anisodont (an·i·so·dont). Having teeth unequal in length and set irregularly in the jaw. [Gk *anisos* unequal, *odous* tooth.]

anisogamy (an·i·**sog**·am·e). Among the protozoa, fusion of 2 gametes of different size and form. [Gk *anisos* unequal, *gamos* marriage.]

anisognathous (an·i·**sog**·na·thus). Having an upper jaw abnormally wide in relation to the size of the lower jaw. [Gk *anisos* unequal, *gnathos* jaw.]

anisogynaecomastia (**an**·i·so·gi·ne·ko·**mas**'·te·ah). Unequal enlargement of the breast in males. [Gk *anisos* unequal, *gyne* woman, *mastos* breast.]

anisohypercytosis (an·i·so·hi·per·si·**to**'·sis). A condition of the blood in which there is first an increase in the number of leucocytes, and secondly abnormal proportion as between one form of neutrophil cell and another. [Gk *anisos* unequal, *hyper* over, cytosis.]

anisohypocytosis (an·i·so·hi·po·si·**to**'·sis). A condition of the blood in which there is, in addition to leucopenia, abnormal proportion as between one form of neutrophil cell and another. [Gk *anisos* unequal, *hypo* below, cytosis.]

anisoic (an·iz·o·ik). Relating to anise.

aniso-iconia (an·i·so·i·**ko**'·ne·ah). Aniseikonia.

Anisolabis (**an**·is·o·**la**'·bis). A genus of earwigs. **Anisolabis annulipes.** A commensal earwig in which the cysticercoids of the tapeworm *Hymenolepis diminuta* develop. [Gk *anisos* unequal, *labis* forceps.]

anisole (**an**·is·ole). Phenylmethyl ether, $C_6H_5OCH_3$. A liquid with a fragrant odour, obtained by heating anisic acid with lime; used as an insecticide, especially against lice.

anisoleucocytosis (an·i·so·lew·ko·si·**to**'·sis). A condition in which, although there is a normal number of leucocytes in the blood, the proportional relation between the different kinds of neutrophil cells is abnormal. [Gk *anisos* unequal, *leukos* white, cytosis.]

anisomastia (an·i·so·**mas**'·te·ah). The state in which one breast is larger than the other. [Gk *anisos* unequal, *mastos* breast.]

anisomelia (an·i·so·**me**'·le·ah). The state in which one of a pair of corresponding limbs is larger than the other. [Gk *anisos* unequal, *melos* limb.]

anisomelous (an·i·**so**·mel·us). Said of one of a pair of corresponding limbs that is longer or larger than the other. [see prec.]

anisomeria (an·i·so·**meer**'·e·ah). With unequal organs. [Gk *anisos* unequal, *meros* part.]

anisomeric (**an**·i·so·**mer**'·ik). Not isomeric. [see prec.]

anisometrope (an·i·so·**met**'·rope). Term for anyone suffering from anisometropia.

anisometropia (an·i·so·met·**ro**'·pe·ah). A condition in which there is marked inequality of refractive power of the two eyes. [Gk *anisos* unequal, *metron* measure, *ops* eye.]

anisometropic (an·i·so·met·**rop**'·ik). 1. Relating to anisometropia. 2. Having eyes markedly unequal in refraction.

anisophoria (**an**·i·so·**for**'·e·ah). A latent deviation of the visual axes, which is unequal in the two eyes. It becomes evident when one or other eye is covered and constitutes an asymmetrical form of heterophoria. [Gk *anisos* unequal, *pherein* to carry.]

anisopia (an·i·**so**·pe·ah). Inequality of power of vision as between one eye and the other. [Gk *anisos* unequal, *ops* eye.]

anisopiesis (an·i·so·pi·**e**′·sis). The condition in which the blood pressure is not the same all over the body but varies as between part and part. [Gk *anisos* unequal, *piesis* pressure.]

anisorrhythmia (an·i·so·**rith**′·me·ah). An abnormal state of cardiac rhythm in which the rate of atrial systole is not the same as that of ventricular systole. The heart therefore beats irregularly. [Gk *anisos* unequal, rhythm.]

anisosphygmia (an·i·so·**sfig**′·me·ah). Inequality of some kind in the pulse in any 2 symmetrical arteries. The volume, the force or the rate may be affected. [Gk *anisos* unequal, *sphygmos* pulse.]

anisospore (an·i·so·spore). In biology, the fusion of a cell of one sex with a cell of the other sex. Cf. ISOSPORE. [Gk *anisos* unequal, spore.]

anisosthenic (an·i·so·**sthen**′·ik). A term applied to a pair or group of muscles when the agonist unit and the antagonist unit are of unequal strength. [Gk *anisos* unequal, *sthenos* strength.]

anisotonic (an·i·so·**ton**′·ik). Term applied in comparison of solutions with a normal or with each other, and indicating that one is not isotonic with the other, i.e. either below (hypotonic) or above (hypertonic). [Gk *anisos* unequal, *tonos* tone.]

anisotropic (an·i·so·**tro**′·pik). Having the property of anisotropy.

anisotropy (an·i·**sot**·ro·pe). 1. The peculiarity of certain substances which do not display the same physical attributes in all directions, as when the refractive index of a crystal varies with the axis. 2. Of living things, responding unequally to the same stimulus applied to different parts of the organism. [Gk *anisos* unequal, *tropos* turning.]

anisuria (an·i·**sewr**·e·ah). A state in which urine is passed alternately in large quantity (polyuria) and in small (oliguria). [Gk *anisos* unequal, urine.]

anisyl (**an**·is·il). The monovalent radical $CH_3OC_6H_4CH_2$– which occurs in anisyl alcohol; sometimes called *anisalyl.*

anitin (**an**·it·in). Anytin.

anitol (**an**·it·ol). Anytol.

Anitschkow, Nikolay Nikolaevich (b. 1885). Russian pathologist.

Anitschkow's cell, or myocyte. A phagocytic cell of the myocardium, found aggregated in rheumatic Aschoff's nodes.

Anjesky's method. A spore stain for bacteria; the spores are stained red by carbolfuchsin, and the bacterial bodies blue by methylene blue.

ankle (**ang**·kl). 1. The ankle joint. 2. [Talus (NA)], the part of the leg immediately above the ankle joint. **Ankle bone.** Talus. **Deck ankle.** Swelling and oedema of the ankles that is very common among troops on board ship. It is probably due to the jarring of the joint through running and playing games on hard decks, aggravated by the wearing of tennis shoes, without heels. There is little or no pain associated and the condition is rapidly reversible. **Footballer's ankle.** Arthritic changes in the anterior margin of the tibia due to repeated plantar flexion strain. **Ankle jerk.** Achilles reflex. Ankle clonus. Clonic jerkings of the foot of alternate flexion and extrusion elicited by the stimulus of stretch. **Ankle joint.** *See* JOINT. **Tailors' ankle.** A form of chronic bursitis over the lateral malleolus of the ankle owing to the adoption of the sitting posture on the floor with crossed legs. **Weak ankle.** Instability of the ankle joint due to stretching of the ligaments of the joint, and often associated with weakness of the muscles of the leg. [AS *ancleow.*]

ankyloblepharon (**ang**·ki·lo·**blef**′·ar·on). Adhesion of the edge of one eyelid to that of the other. **Ankyloblepharon filiforme adnatum.** A congenital condition in which the edges of the eyelids are joined together by bands of filament. [Gk *agkylos* crooked, *blepharon* eyelid.]

ankylocheilia, ankylochilia (**ang**·kil·o·**ki**′·le·ah). Adhesion of one lip to the other. [Gk *agkylos* crooked, *cheilos* lip.]

ankylocolpos (**ang**·kil·o·**kol**′·pos). 1. Imperforate state of the vagina. 2. Vulvar or vaginal atresia. [Gk *agkylos* crooked, *kolpos* vagina.]

ankylodactylia, ankylodactyly (**ang**·kil·o·dak·**til**′·e·ah, **ang**·kil·o·**dak**′·til·e). A condition in which there is adhesion between 2 or more fingers or toes. [Gk *agkylos* crooked, *daktylos* finger.]

ankylodontia (**ang**·kil·o·**don**′·she·ah). Eruption of the teeth in an irregular pattern. [Gk *agkylos* crooked, *odous* tooth.]

ankyloglossia, ankyloglossum (**ang**·kil·o·**glos**′·e·ah, **ang**·kil·o·**glos**′·um). 1. Abnormal shortness of the frenulum of the tongue. 2. Adhesion of the tongue to some part of the walls of the mouth cavity. [Gk *agkylos* crooked, *glossa* tongue.]

ankylokolpos (**ang**·kil·o·**kol**′·pos). Ankylocolpos.

ankylomele (**ang**·kil·o·**me**′·le). 1. The growing together of limbs or of parts of limbs, as fingers or toes, to make a single limb or part. [Gk *agkylos* crooked, *melos* limb.] 2. An angular or curved probe. [Gk *mele* probe.]

ankylomerism (ang·kil·**om**·er·izm). A condition in which there is adherence of parts which normally are separate. [Gk *agkylos* crooked, *meros* part.]

ankylophobia (**ang**·kil·o·**fo**′·be·ah). In persons who have suffered a fracture or whose joints are diseased, an excessive fear that ankylosis will occur. [ankylosis, phobia.]

ankylopoietic (**ang**·kil·o·poi·**et**′·ik). 1. Characterized by ankylosis. 2. Causing or producing ankylosis. [ankylosis, Gk *poiein* to make.]

ankyloproctia (**ang**·kil·o·**prok**′·she·ah). A condition in which the opening of the anus is closed on account of atresia or stricture. [Gk *agkylos* crooked, *proktos* anus.]

ankylose (**ang**·kil·oze). 1. To become fixed by ankylosis. 2. To become solidly united or fused. [Gk *agkyloun* to stiffen.]

ankylosis (ang·kil·**o**·sis). Complete immobility of a joint resulting from pathological changes in that joint or of the structures associated with it. **Artificial ankylosis.** Arthrodesis, the surgical procedure of fixing the parts of a joint together so that the whole structure is immovable. **Bony ankylosis.** True ankylosis (see below). **Central ankylosis.** Ankylosis originating from causes within the joint itself. **Extra-articular ankylosis.** Extracapsular ankylosis (see following). **Extracapsular ankylosis.** That resulting from abnormal inflexibility of parts outside the joint. **False ankylosis.** Extracapsular ankylosis (see preceding). **Fibrous ankylosis.** Ankylosis resulting from the formation of fibrous adhesions within the joint. **Generalized ankylosis.** The tendency towards the formation of ankyloses in a number of joints, or the actual formation of them. **Sound ankylosis.** A fixed joint from any cause in which there is no tendency to further deformity whatever strain is put upon the joint. **Spurious ankylosis.** Extracapsular ankylosis (see above). **Tooth ankylosis.** The pathological process whereby the cementum of the root of a tooth is united with surrounding alveolar bone. **True ankylosis.** The abnormal fusion or union of the bones composing a joint. **Unsound ankylosis.** Spurious ankylosis; apparent firm immobility of a joint which, however, will deform when subjected to prolonged strain. [Gk *agkylosis* stiffness of a joint.]

ankylostomatic (**ang**·kil·os·to·**mat**′·ik). Ancylostomatic.

ankylostomiasis (**ang**·kil·os·to·**mi**′·as·is). Ancylostomiasis.

ankylotia (ang·kil·**o**·she·ah). A condition in which the external auditory meatus is closed on account of union of the walls. [Gk *agkylos* crooked, *ous* ear.]

ankylotic (ang·kil·**ot**·ik). 1. Marked by ankylosis. 2. Characterized by the condition of ankylotia.

ankylotome (ang·**kil**·o·tome). A special kind of surgical knife for separating surfaces which normally are not adherent; in particular, an instrument for cutting the frenulum of the tongue in cases of ankyloglossia. [Gk *agkylos* crooked, *temnein* to cut.]

ankylotomy (ang·kil·**ot**·om·e). The operation of separating the frenulum of the tongue for the cure of ankyloglossia. [see prec.]

ankylo-urethria, ankylurethria (**ang**·kil·o·ewr·**e**′·thre·ah, **ang**·kil·ewr·**e**′·thre·ah). 1. Imperforation of the urethra. 2. Urethral stricture. [Gk *agkylos* crooked, urethra.]

ankyra (**ang**·kir·ah). A hook. [Gk *agkyra* anchor.]

ankyrism (ang·kir·izm). 1. An articulation by the hooking of one bone on another. 2. A suture shaped like a hook. [Gk *agkyra* anchor.]

ankyroid (ang·kir·oid). Shaped like a hook. [Gk *agkyra* anchor, *eidos* form.]

anlage (ahn·lah·ge) (pl. *anlagen, anlages*). In embryology, that area in the embryo at which the first traces of the various structures appear; the first undifferentiated grouping of cells from which any organ or part will develop. **Lateral thyroid anlage.** A small mass of epithelium derived from the last pharyngeal pouch of the embryo. It may contribute to the function of the thyroid. Also known as the *ultimobranchial body.* **Vesico-urethral anlage.** The ventral subdivision of the entodermal cloaca from which the bladder and urethra are derived. It is separated from the rectum by the cloacal septum. [G foundation.]

Annandale, Thomas (b. 1838). Scottish surgeon.

Annandale's operation. 1. Fixing the semilunar cartilages of the knee by sutures. 2. Correction of genu valgum by reshaping the femoral condyles.

annatto (an·at·o). A red colouring material prepared from the aril of the seeds of *Bixa orellana* (family Bixaceae), which is cultivated in many tropical countries; the main constituent is the carotenoid bixin. Annatto is used for colouring varnishes, lacquers, soaps, textiles, etc., and particularly butter and cheese, but it has been largely replaced by substitutes. [Galibi (South America) name.]

anneal (an·eel). The treatment of metals and alloys by heat to render them malleable and ductile. [AS *aelan* to burn.]

annelid (an·el·id). 1. Composed of annular segments. 2. In zoology, one of the Annelida. [L *annellus* little ring, Gk *eidos* form.]

Annelida (an·el·id·ah). A phylum of coelomate invertebrate animals, the segmented worms. It contains the class Hirudinea, the leeches. [see prec.]

annelism (an·el·izm). 1. The state of being ringed structurally. 2. A ringed structure. [L *annellus* a little ring.]

annotta (an·ot·ah). Annatto.

annulate (an·ew·late). 1. Composed of or surrounded by rings. 2. Characterized by a ring-like structure. [L *annulus* ring.]

annuloplasty (an'·ew·lo·plas·te). An operation for narrowing dilated annulus of the left atrioventricular (mitral) valve. [L *annulus* ring, Gk *plassein* to mould.]

annulorrhaphy (an·ewl·or·af·e). The surgical procedure of suturing together the edges of a hernial sac or ring. [L *annulus* ring, Gk *rhaphe* suture.]

annulose (an·ew·loze). Having rings or ring-like segments; composed of rings. [L *annulus* ring.]

annulus [anulus (NA)] (an·ew·lus). A ring; hence, any ring-shaped structure. **Annulus abdominalis.** An obsolete term for either the deep or superficial inguinal ring. **Annulus conjunctivae [anulus conjunctivae (NA)].** The region of junction between the conjunctiva and the periphery of the cornea. **Annulus fibrosus [anulus fibrosus (NA)].** The peripheral part of an intervertebral disc. In cardiology, this term is sometimes applied to the fibrous skeleton of the heart to which the atria and ventricles are attached and which forms the valve rings. **Annulus migrans.** Geographical tongue; an affection of the tongue, mainly occurring in children, in which small circular red patches, due to hypertrophy of the filiform papillae, appear on the dorsum. These spread peripherally in widening circles which may intersect or coalesce and pass on to the undersurface. The centre of the circles is smooth and red and the margins slightly raised and yellowish. The condition is harmless but may be recurrent. **Annulus ovalis [limbus fossae ovalis].** The raised margin which bounds the fossa ovalis on the interatrial septum of the heart; Vieussens' annulus. [L.]

See also: HALLER, VIEUSSENS, ZINN.

anocavernosus (an·o·kav·er·no'·sus). The bulbospongiosus muscle. [Gk *ano* upwards, cavernosus.]

anocheiloschisis, anochiloschisis (an·o·ki·los·kis·is). The operative repair of hare-lip. [Gk *ano* upwards, *cheilos* lip, *schizein* to split.]

anochlesia (an·o·kle·ze·ah). 1. Catalepsy. 2. Quietness of mind. [Gk *a, ochlesis* disturbance.]

anochromasia (an·o·kro·ma'·ze·ah). 1. Poor or negligible staining of red cells so that they appear pale or unstained centrally, but some coloration may be noted peripherally. 2. Achromasia. [Gk *ano* upwards, *chroma* colour.]

anoci-association (an·o·se·as·o·se·a'·shun). An anaesthetic routine devised to obviate surgical shock. The latter being considered due to exhaustion of the vasomotor centre by excessive stimuli arising from pre-operative apprehension, operative trauma and postoperative pain, the patient is kept free from fear by management and narcotics, remains in ignorance of the time of the operation, and is anaesthetized in such a way that no adaptive response is excited. The field of operation is completely blocked by local anaesthetics so that traumatic impulses do not reach the brain, and in closing the wound, nerve impulses are cut off for a period by another local anaesthetic to prevent after-pains. The method is used nowadays only in such cases as "stealing the thyroid", where the absence of apprehension is to be desired. The term originated with G. W. Crile, a Cleveland, Ohio, surgeon in 1913. [Gk *a,* L *nocere* to injure, *ad, socius* fellow.]

anociated (an·o·se·a·ted). In a state of anoci-association.

anociation (an·o·se·a'·shun). Anoci-association.

anocithesia (an·o·se·the'·ze·ah). Anoci-association. [anoci-association, anaesthesia.]

anococcygeal (a·no·kok·sij'·e·al). Indicating involvement of the anus and the coccyx. **Anococcygeal body.** *See* BODY.

anococcygeal nerves [nervi anococcygei (NA)]. A few fine filaments from the coccygeal plexus which pierce the sacrotuberous ligament to supply the skin in the region of the coccyx.

anodal (an·o·dal). Emanating from an anode; relating to an anode; electropositive.

anode (an·ode). 1. The positive pole of a battery. 2. The positive electrode of an electrical apparatus, as in an x-ray tube. 3. The conductor by which electric current enters an electrolyte, nerve, or other substance. Cf. CATHODE. **Soluble anode.** In electrodeposition processes such as plating, the rod or sheet of metal used as an anode, which is dissolved by the electrolyte and carried over to the objects forming the cathode. [Gk *ana, hodos* way.]

anoderm (a·no·derm). The lining of the proctodaeum, or ectodermal portion of the anal canal. [anus, Gk *derma* skin.]

anodermous (an·o·der·mus). Devoid of any evidence of having an epidermis. [Gk *a, derma* skin.]

anodic (an·o·dik). Pertaining to the anode; electropositive. In the general sense it refers to an element below hydrogen in the electrochemical series; in a relative sense it signifies a more positive electrode potential.

anodinia (an·o·din·e·ah). The absence of pains during labour. [Gk *a, odis* pains of childbirth.]

anodinous (an·o·din·us). Term applied to a birth in which the pains of labour are lacking. [see prec.]

anodmia (an·od·me·ah). Anosmia; loss of the sense of smell. [Gk *a, odme* odour.]

anodont (an·o·dont). Lacking teeth. [see foll.]

anodontia (an·o·don·she·ah). The absence of teeth. **Senile anodontia.** As a result of natural or extractive loss of teeth, the toothlessness of old age. **Anodontia vera.** Absence of teeth because of lack of development. [Gk *a, odous* tooth.]

anodontism (an·o·don·tizm). Complete absence of the tooth-forming and tooth-developing organs. [see prec.]

anodontous, anodous (an·o·dont·us, an·od·us). Anodont.

anodyne (an·o·dine). 1. Any drug or medicine which stills pain or quiets disturbed feelings. 2. Soothing; serving to allay pain. [Gk *a, odyne* pain.]

anodynia (an·o·din·e·ah). 1. The state of being free from pain. 2. State of being without sensation. Cf. ANODINIA. [see prec.]

anoesia (an·o·e·ze·ah). A condition in which the power of comprehension is lacking; imbecility; idiocy. [Gk want of understanding.]

anoestrum, anoestrus (an·e·strum, an·e·strus). The period of sexual quiescence in the female of monoestrous mammals. [Gk *a*, *oistros* rut.]

anoetic (an·o·e·tik). 1. Relating or belonging to, or characterized by, anoesia. 2. In psychology, indicative of the margin of consciousness, that is to say referrring to sentience as fundamentally distinct from thought.

anoia (an·**oi**·ah). Amentia. [Gk want of understanding.]

anolobine (an·ol·**o**·been). $C_{17}H_{17}O_3N$. An alkaloid obtained from the bark of *Anona triloba* L. (*Asimina triloba* Dun.).

anomalopia (an·om·al·**o**·pe·ah). Incomplete colour blindness. It may take the form of one of 3 types: (*a*) *protanomalopia*, in which there is subnormal appreciation of red, and a person with such would add too much red in matching yellow with a mixture of red and green in a test with the anomaloscope; (*b*) *deuteranomalopia*, in which there is subnormal appreciation of green, and too much green would be added; and (*c*) *tritanomalopia*, in which there is subnormal appreciation of blue, prompting the addition of too much blue in matching green with a mixture of blue and yellow. [Gk *anomalos* irregular, *ops* eye.]

anomaloscope (an·**om**·al·o·skope). An instrument for the detection of colour blindness by examining the eye. A circular field is presented, the lower half illuminated by yellow (sodium lime) light, and the upper by red and green lights, the relative amounts being controlled by variable slits until the colours in the two halves match. [Gk *anomalos* irregular, *skopein* to view.]

anomalotrophy (an·om·al·**ot**·ro·fe). Anomaly or abnormality in the nutritive processes. [Gk *anomalos* irregular, *trophe* nutrition.]

anomalus (an·**om**·al·us). Musculus anomalus of Albinus; a muscular slip which may be present beneath the levator labii superioris alaeque nasi muscle; it is attached to the maxilla at each end and follows the line of the nasolabial furrow. [Gk *anomalos* irregular.]

anomaly (an·**om**·al·e). A deviation from the normal. **Alder anomaly.** Autosomal recessive leucocytic anomaly with large deeply-staining neutrophil granules. [Gk *anomalia* irregularity.]

See also: ARISTOTLE, FREUND, HÜET, PELGER.

anomia (a·**no**·me·ah). Inability to put a name to an article the identity of which is recognized. [Gk *a*, *onoma* name.]

anomous (an·o·mus). Not having shoulders. [Gk *a*, *omos* shoulder.]

anonychia (an·on·**ik**·e·ah). A congenital condition characterized by absence of one or more nails. [Gk *a*, *onyx* nail.]

anonyma (an·**on**·im·ah). Name for innominate artery. [Gk *a*, *onoma* name.]

anoperineal (a·no·per·in·e′·al). Involvement of the anus and perineum.

Anopheles (an·**of**·el·eez). A genus of the family Culicidae (mosquitoes), which includes over 160 species, of which some 64 act as definitive hosts for the malaria parasites. The species of this genus are distinguished from other commoner genera (e.g. *Culex*) by several well-marked characteristics. Of these the resting position is the most conspicuous: they hold the proboscis, head and abdomen nearly in a straight line, giving the impression of a splinter lifted at an angle from a surface; the back pair of legs is usually held at an elevation. Exceptionally, as in *Anopheles culicifacies*, the stance is horizontal as in *Culex*. The wings are usually spotted with dark-brown or yellow scales. In the females the palpi, usually banded, are equal in length to the proboscis and are usually closely applied; in the male the 2 terminal joints of the palpi are club-shaped. There are sets of stiff hairs, or setae, arranged in definite groups on the thorax and abdomen: the scutellum is arcuate. The eggs are boat-shaped and are laid simply on the surface of water. When the anopheles larvae lie on the surface the dorsal aspects of the thorax and abdomen face upwards and the head is rotated 180° so that its ventral surface lies upwards. There is no respiratory syphon. The larva maintains itself on the surface in a horizontal position by a row of dorso-abdominal plaques, palmate hairs and a series of scales in rosette form on its back. Several species of *Anopheles* are capable of transmitting *Wuchereria bancrofti* and some arboviruses as well as the malaria parasites. **Anopheles aconitus, Anopheles albimanus, Anopheles albitarsis.** Important vectors of malaria and potential vectors of filariasis. **Anopheles algeriensis.** A potential vector of filariasis and a minor vector of malaria. **Anopheles amictus.** A potential vector of filariasis. **Anopheles annularis.** An important vector of malaria and a potential vector of filariasis. **Anopheles annulipes.** An important vector of malaria. **Anopheles aquasalis.** An important vector of malaria and a potential vector of filariasis. **Anopheles argyritarsis.** A minor vector of malaria. **Anopheles austeni, Anopheles baezai.** Minor vectors of malaria. **Anopheles balabacensis.** A vector of malaria in Borneo; it breeds only in dense jungle shade. **Anopheles bancrofti.** An important vector of malaria and a potential vector of filariasis. **Anopheles barbirostris.** A vector of filariasis and a minor vector of malaria. **Anopheles bellator.** An important vector of malaria. **Anopheles brunnipes.** A minor vector of malaria. **Anopheles claviger.** A species which breeds in wells and passes the winter months in the larval stage; an important vector of malaria. **Anopheles coustani tenebrosus, Anopheles crucians, Anopheles cruzi.** Minor vectors of malaria. **Anopheles culicifacies.** An important vector of malaria. **Anopheles darlingi.** An important vector of malaria and a potential vector of filariasis. **Anopheles d'thali, Anopheles dureni, Anopheles eiseni.** Minor vectors of malaria. **Anopheles fluviatilis.** An important vector of malaria. **Anopheles funestus.** A species that is widespread in the Middle East: an important vector of malaria and a potential vector of filariasis. **Anopheles gambiae.** The most widespread and dangerous malaria-carrier in Africa and a potential vector of filariasis. **Anopheles goeldii, Anopheles grabhamii.** Minor vectors of malaria. **Anopheles hancocki, Anopheles hargravesi.** Important vectors of malaria. **Anopheles hectoris, Anopheles hyrcanus.** Minor vectors of malaria. **Anopheles hyrcanus nigerrimus.** An important vector of malaria and a potential vector of filariasis. **Anopheles hyrcanus sinensis.** A vector of filariasis and an important vector of malaria. **Anopheles hyrcanus X.** An important vector of malaria and a vector of filariasis. **Anopheles jeyporiensis, Anopheles jeyporiensis candidiensis.** Important vectors of malaria. **Anopheles karwari, Anopheles kochi, Anopheles koliensis.** Minor vectors of malaria. **Anopheles leucosphyrus.** An important vector of malaria. **Anopheles lindesayi japonicus.** A minor vector of malaria. **Anopheles maculatus.** An important vector of malaria and a potential vector of filariasis. **Anopheles maculipennis.** A species with a world-wide distribution, and divided into several varieties which breed in different localities and lay different-coloured eggs: these are *atriparvus, freeborni, labranchiae* and *messae. Atroparvus* is the important malarial carrier in Europe; others also carry malaria and *freeborni* is also a vector of equine encephalitis. **Anopheles mangyanus, Anopheles marshalli gibbinsi.** Minor vectors of malaria. **Anopheles melas, Anopheles minimus, Anopheles minimus flavirostris, Anopheles moucheti, Anopheles moucheti nigeriensis.** Important vectors of malaria. **Anopheles multicolor.** A minor vector of malaria. **Anopheles neomaculipalpus.** A vector of equine encephalitis. **Anopheles nili, Anopheles novumbrosus.** Important vectors of malaria. **Anopheles oswaldoi guarujaensis, Anopheles oswaldoi metcalfi.** Minor vectors of malaria. **Anopheles oswaldoi oswaldoi, Anopheles pallidus.** Minor vectors of malaria and potential vectors of filariasis. **Anopheles pattoni, Anopheles pharoensis.** Important vectors of malaria. **Anopheles philippinensis.** An important vector of malaria and a potential vector of filariasis. **Anopheles plumbeus, Anopheles pretoriensis.** Minor vectors of malaria. **Anopheles pseudojamesi.** *Anopheles ramsayi* (see below). **Anopheles pseudopunctipennis, Anopheles pseudopunctipennis rivadeneirai.** Important vectors of malaria. **Anopheles pulcherrimus.** A minor vector of malaria. **Anopheles punctimacula.** An important vector of malaria. **Anopheles punctulatus.** An important vector of malaria and a potential vector of filariasis. **Anopheles punctulatus farauti,**

Anopheles quadrimaculatus. Important vectors of malaria. **Anopheles ramsayi (pseudojamesi), Anopheles rhodesiensis.** Minor vectors of malaria and potential vectors of filariasis. **Anopheles rufipes.** A minor vector of malaria. **Anopheles sacharovi.** An important vector of malaria. **Anopheles separatus.** A minor vector of malaria. **Anopheles sergenti.** An important vector of malaria. **Anopheles smithi, Anopheles splendidus.** Minor vectors of malaria. **Anopheles squamosus.** A potential vector of filariasis. **Anopheles stephensi.** An important vector of malaria and a potential vector of filariasis. **Anopheles stephensi mysorensis.** An important vector of malaria. **Anopheles strodei.** A minor vector of malaria. **Anopheles subpictus.** An important vector of malaria and a potential vector of filariasis. **Anopheles subpictus malayensis.** A minor vector of malaria. **Anopheles sundaicus.** An important vector of malaria and a potential vector of filariasis. **Anopheles superpictus.** An important vector of malaria. **Anopheles tessellatus.** A minor vector of malaria. **Anopheles triannulatus.** A minor vector of malaria and a potential vector of filariasis. **Anopheles turkhudi.** A minor vector of malaria. **Anopheles umbrosus.** An important vector of malaria. **Anopheles vagus.** A minor vector of malaria. **Anopheles varuna.** An important vector of malaria and a potential vector of filariasis. **Anopheles vestitipennis.** A minor vector of malaria. **Anopheles walkeri.** An important vector of malaria. [Gk *anopheles* harmful.]

anophelicide (an·**of**·el·is·ide). Any agent which destroys mosquitoes of the genus *Anopheles.* [anopheles, L *caedere* to kill.]

anophelifuge (an·**of**·el·e·fewj). Any agent which drives away or prevents the bite of an anopheles mosquito. [anopheles, L *fugare* to chase away.]

anopheline (an·**of**·el·een). 1. Caused by or referring to mosquitoes of the sub-family Anophelinae. 2. Any agent which destroys the anopheles mosquito.

Anophelini (an·**of**·el·**e**′·ne). A tribe of the mosquito sub-family Culicinae; it contains the genera *Anopheles* (world-wide), *Chagasia* (New World) and *Bironella* (New Guinea). Many, particularly in *Anopheles,* are important intermediate hosts of malarial parasites. [Gk *anopheles* harmful.]

anophelism (an·**of**·el·izm). A term applied to infestation of any geographical region with mosquitoes of the genus *Anopheles.*

anophoria (an·o·**for**·e·ah). Upward strabismus; anotropia; hyperphoria. [Gk *ano* upwards, *pherein* to bear.]

anophthalmia (an·of·**thal**·me·ah). Congenital absence of one or both eyes. **Anophthalmia cyclopica.** A condition in which the eyes remain rudimentary and are fused together. [Gk *a, ophthalmos* eye.]

anophthalmos, anaphthalmus (an·of·**thal**·mos, an·af·**thal**·mus). 1. A person who has never had any eyes or who has always had only one eye. 2. The state of always having been without eyes; congenital absence. [see prec.]

anopia (an·o·pe·ah). 1. Defection or lack of the power of seeing; anopsia. **Quadrantic anopia.** A defect of a quarter of the visual field bounded by vertical and horizontal radii. [Gk *a, ops* eye.]

anoplasty (a·no·plas·te). Plastic repair of the anus. [anus, Gk *plassein* to form.]

Anoplocephalidae (an·o·plo·kef·**al**′·id·e). A family of the cestode order Cyclophyllidea. The genera *Bertiella* and *Inermicapsifer* are of medical interest. [Gk *anoplos* unarmed, *kephale* head, *eidos* form.]

Anoplura (an·o·**ploor**·ah). An order of insects which includes the Siphunculata or blood-sucking lice: they are dorsoventrally flattened, wingless, external parasites. The genera of medical interest are *Pediculus* and *Phthirus.* [Gk *anoplos* unarmed, *oura* tail.]

anoproctitis (a·no·prok·**ti**′·tis). Inflammation of the anus and rectum. [anus, Gk *proktos* rectum, *-itis* inflammation.]

anopsia (an·**op**·se·ah). Anopia. [Gk *a, opsis* vision.]

anorchia, anorchidism, anorchism (an·**or**·ke·ah, an·**or**·kid·izm, an·**or**·kizm). The state in which the testes are congenitally lacking or have failed to descend. [Gk *a, orchis* testis.]

anorchous (an·**or**·kus). A term signifying that the testes are lacking. [Gk *a, orchis* testis.]

anorchus (an·**or**·kus). An individual in whom the testes are congenitally lacking or have failed to descend. [see prec.]

anorectal (a·no·**rek**·tal). Involving the anus and the rectum.

anorectum (a·no·**rek**·tum). The rectum and anus viewed as a single viscus.

anorexia (an·or·**ex**·e·ah). The condition of being without, or of having lost, the appetite for food. **Anorexia nervosa.** Aversion to food due to psychological causes, leading to severe loss of weight. It occurs usually in young women, associated with amenorrhoea but with very little complaint of loss of strength. [Gk *a, orexis* appetite.]

anorgasmy (an·or·**gaz**·me). Failure to achieve an orgasm during coitus. [Gk *a,* orgasm.]

anormal (a·**nor**·mal). Abnormal. [Gk *a,* normal.]

anorthography (an·or·**thog**·raf·e). Motor agraphia; loss of the faculty of forming letters or of writing in orthodox fashion. [Gk *a, orthos* straight, *graphein* writing.]

anorthopia (an·or·**tho**·pe·ah). 1. A distortion of vision which causes straight lines to appear as curves or angles; there is also diminished perception of symmetry. 2. Strabismus; heterophoria. [Gk *a, orthos* straight, *ops* eye.]

anorthoscope (an·**or**·tho·skope). An optical arrangement of rotating discs designed to present to the eye, in one complete picture, a number of separate component pictures. [Gk *a, orthos* straight, *skopein* to look at.]

anorthosis (an·or·**tho**·sis). Lack of erectility. [Gk *a, orthos* straight.]

anoscope (a·no·skope). Proctoscope. [anus, Gk *skopein* to view.] *See also:* BACON.

anoscopy (a·**nos**·ko·pe). The use of the anoscope in examination of the anus and lower part of the rectum.

anosmatic (an·os·**mat**·ik). 1. Being altogether without or having only an imperfect sense of smell. 2. In zoology, applied to toothed cetaceans (whales, dolphins) which have only rudimentary olfactory organs. [see foll.]

anosmia (an·**oz**·me·ah). Loss of the sense of smell. There are 2 main types: (*a*) *obstructive,* where loss of function depends on the inability of scent particles to be deposited in the olfactory region of the nose, due to some form of nasal obstruction; and (*b*) *essential,* where the nervous mechanism responsible for this special sensation is damaged. **Afferent anosmia.** Anosmia where the olfactory nerves are damaged. **Central anosmia.** That resulting from destruction of the central mechanism. **Anosmia gustatoria.** Loss of the sense of smell associated with food ingestion. **Obstructive anosmia.** That due to obstruction of the nasal fossae. **Organic anosmia.** Anosmia due to organic disease, and not to some hysterial disorder. **Peripheral anosmia.** The opposite of central anosmia (see above), where the cause is in the peripheral mechanism. **Respiratory anosmia, Anosmia respiratoria.** Obstructive anosmia (see above). [Gk *a, osme* smell.]

anosmic, anosmous (an·**oz**·mik, an·**oz**·mus). 1. Lacking the sense of smell. 2. Odourless. [see prec.]

anosognosia (an·o·sog·**no**′·se·ah). Lack of awareness of an illness, symptom or disability, e.g. for blindness or paralysis of limbs. The term was first used by Babinski and referred to a hemiplegia, usually of the left side. [Gk *a, nosos* disease, *gnosis* knowing.]

anosphrasia, anosphresia (an·os·**fra**·ze·ah, an·os·**freez**·e·ah). Anosmia. [Gk *a, osphrasia* smell.]

anospinal (a·no·**spi**·nal). Referring to the anus and the spinal cord.

anosteoplasia (an·os·te·o·**pla**′·ze·ah). A condition in which there is defect in bone formation. [Gk *a, osteon* bone, *plasis* formation.]

anostosis (an·os·**to**·sis). A condition in which there is defective development of bone. [Gk *a,* ostosis.]

anotia (an·o·she·ah). Congenital absence of the ears or of the pinnae. [Gk *a, ous* ear.]

anotous (an·o·tus). Without ears. [see prec.]

anotropia (an·o·**tro**·pe·ah). A variation from equilibrium of the visual axes, affecting both eyes though not always equally, and causing them to turn above the point of regard upon the least innervation of the extra-ocular muscles. [Gk *ano* upward, *trepein* to turn.]

anotus (an·o·tus). A fetal monster without either internal or external organs of hearing. [Gk *a, ous* ear.]

anovaria, anovarism (an·o·vare·e·ah, an·o·var·izm). Congenital absence of ovaries. [Gk *a*, ovary.]

anovesical (a·no·ves·ik·al). Relating or belonging to the anus and the bladder. [anus, L *vesicula* small bladder.]

anovular (an·o·vew·lar). Applied to uterine haemorrhage occurring independent of and at a time other than that of ovulation. [Gk *a*, ovulum.]

anovulation (an·o·vew·la'·shun). The interruption of the process of ovulation, or its complete cessation. [see prec.]

anovulatory (an·o·vew·la'·tor·e). Anovular.

anovulia (an·o·vew·le·ah). Anovulation.

anoxaemia (an·ox·e·me·ah). Blood with zero O_2 content (incorrectly used to mean blood with low O_2 content). *See* HYPOXAEMIA. Cf. ANOXIA. [Gk *a*, oxygen, Gk *haima* blood.]

anoxaemic (an·ox·e·mik). Caused or marked by too small an amount of oxygen in the blood. [see prec.]

anoxhaemia (an·ox·he·me·ah). Anoxaemia.

anoxia (an·ox·e·ah). Without oxygen (incorrectly used to indicate inadequate oxygenation). *See* HYPOXIA. **Anaemic anoxia.** A state in which the oxygen tension in the blood is normal, but the total amount of oxygen is diminished owing to reduction or alteration of the haemoglobin such as occurs in anaemia, or carbon monoxide poisoning. **Anoxic anoxia.** A condition in which the oxygen tension in the arterial blood is reduced and the haemoglobin is therefore incompletely oxidized. It occurs at high altitudes and in any disease of the lung which prevents the normal diffusion of oxygen from the alveoli into the blood capillaries. **Cerebral anoxia.** Anoxia of the brain due to a fall in pressure in the cerebral arteries, with resultant syncope. **Fulminating anoxia.** Anoxia of very rapid onset, in which unconsciousness can occur without any warning. **Histotoxic anoxia.** The situation in which the tissue protoplasm is poisoned, and although the oxygen tension in the blood is normal, it cannot be utilized by the tissues owing to interference with the respiratory enzyme necessary for tissue oxidation, e.g. in cyanide poisoning. **Stagnant anoxia.** Anoxia in which the oxygen in the blood is of normal tension and amount, but the supply to the tissues is deficient owing to the decreased rate of blood flow through the capillaries, as in congestive heart failure. [Gk *a*, oxygen.]

anoxoluin, anoxolyin (an·ox·ol'·ew·in, an·ox·ol'·e·in). A constituent of albumins and globulins that is insoluble in acetic acid. [Gk *a, oxys* acid, *lyein* to dissolve.]

anoxyaemia (an·ox·e·e'·me·ah). Anoxaemia.

anoxybiosis (an·ox·e·bi·o'·sis). Anaerobiosis; the state of existing or the power of living in an atmosphere which is devoid of free oxygen. [Gk *a*, oxygen, *bios* life.]

anoxycausis (an·ox·e·kaw'·sis). The process of burning in an atmosphere containing no oxygen. [Gk *a, oxys* sharp, *kausis* burning.]

ansa [NA] (an·sah) (pl. *ansae*). In anatomy, a loop. **Ansa hypoglossi [ansa cervicalis (NA)].** A loop of communication formed by a superior branch [ramus superior] and an inferior branch [ramus inferior]. **Ansa hypoglossi, inferior branch [ramus inferior (NA)].** The lower root of the ansa cervicalis, derived from the 2nd and 3rd cervical nerves and joining the ramus superior in front of the carotid sheath. **Ansa hypoglossi, superior branch [ramus superior (NA)].** The descending branch of the hypoglossal nerve. It is from the 1st cervical nerve which joins the hypoglossal nerve and then leaves it on the carotid artery and descends in front of this to join the ramus inferior. **Ansa hypoglossi, thyrohyoid branch [ramus thyrohyoideus (NA)].** A branch of the hypoglossal nerve which derives its fibres from the 1st cervical nerve by the communicating branch. **Ansa lenticularis [NA].** A bundle of efferent fibres from the globus pallidus of the lentiform nucleus which pass to the thalamus, subthalamic region and tegmentum of the midbrain. **Ansae nervorum spinalium [NA].** Loop-like connections between neighbouring spinal nerves. **Ansa peduncularis [NA].** Fibres which are said to pass from the thalamus below the lentiform nucleus to the claustrum and insula. **Ansa subclavia [NA].** A loop of fibres which passes round the subclavian artery and joins the middle with the inferior cervical sympathetic ganglion; it is additional to the usual interganglionic trunk; Vieussens' ansa. [L handle.]

See also: GRATIOLET, HALLER, HENLE, REIL, VEIUSSENS, WRISBERG.

ansate (an·sate). 1. Shaped like a loop. 2. Having a handle. [see prec.]

anserine (an·ser·een). β-Alanyl-methyl-histidine, a basic constituent of goose muscle. [L *anserinus* like a goose.]

ansiform (an·se·form). Shaped like a loop. **Ansiform lobule.** *See* LOBULE. [L *ansa* handle, form.]

ansotomy (an·sot·o·me). Division of the ansa lenticularis in the treatment of tremor and rigidity of Parkinson's disease and other similar syndromes, either by open operation or by the method of stereotactic surgery. [L *ansa* handle, Gk *temnein* to cut.]

antacid (an·tas·id). 1. Acting as a corrective or neutralizer of acidity. 2. Any remedy or substance which neutralizes or reduces acidity in the gastric juice or other bodily secretion. [Gk *anti*, acid.]

antagonism (an·tag·on·izm). Opposition in action as between diseases, medicines, muscles or physiological processes. **Bacterial antagonism.** The inhibiting action exercised by one micro-organism on another. **Induced bacterial antagonism.** The interaction of 2 bacteria, induced or selected by growing one strain on a medium containing killed cells of the other bacterium. [Gk *antagonisma* struggle.]

antagonist (an·tag·on·ist). 1. Any organ or muscle which neutralizes the effect of another organ or muscle. 2. In dentistry, a tooth in one jaw which meets one in the other jaw on closure of the mouth. 3. A drug which opposes the action of another drug. **Associated antagonists.** Opposing muscles or groups of muscles which pull in different, but not opposite, directions. When they contract simultaneously the resulting movement is in a direction between the 2 lines of action. **Competitive antagonist.** Antimetabolite. **Direct antagonists.** Muscles or groups of muscles which pull in exactly opposite directions. When they contract simultaneously the result is either no movement at all, or movement in the direction of the line of action of the stronger muscles. **Enzyme antagonist, Metabolic antagonist, Metabolite antagonist.** Antimetabolite. **Narcotic antagonist.** A drug which specifically antagonizes the depressant effects of the narcotic analgesics, e.g. nalorphine. **Sulphonamide antagonist.** *p*-Aminobenzoic acid. The antagonism has been suggested to arise from the fact that both substances exert their effect upon the same essential enzyme system. [Gk *antagonisma* struggle.]

antagonization (an·tag·on·i·za'·shun). In dentistry the act of being opposed by, or articulating with, as a tooth. [see prec.]

antagonizer (an·tag·on·i'·zer). 1. A substance which will reverse the effect of either an inhibitor or a growth factor on micro-organisms. 2. In dentistry, a tooth which opposes and articulates with a tooth in the other jaw. [Gk *antagonisma* struggle.]

antalgesic, antalgic (ant·al·je·zik, ant·al·jik). 1. Any remedy or other agent, or circumstance such as a particular posture or position of the body, which results in the relief or the alleviation of pain. 2. Having the effect of relieving or easing pain. [Gk *anti*, *algos* pain.]

antalkaline (ant·al·kal·ine). Any substance administered to reduce alkalinity, such as acetic or hydrochloric acids. [Gk *anti*, alkaline.]

antaphrodisiac (ant·af·ro·diz'·e·ak). Anaphrodisiac. [Gk *anti*, aphrodisiac.]

Antazoline (an·ta·zo·leen). BP Commission approved name for 2-*N*-benzylanilinomethyliminazoline. **Antazoline Hydrochloride BP 1973.** The hydrochloride of antazoline; an antihistamine drug of relatively low toxicity. **Antazoline Mesylate BPC 1968.** The mesylate of antazoline, with actions and uses similar to those of the hydrochloride.

ante-. Prefix, from the Latin preposition *ante*, meaning *before*.

ante mortem (**an**·te **mor**·tem). Before death. [L.]

ante natal (an·te **na**·tal). The period between conception and birth. [L *ante, natus* born.]

ante partum (an·te **part**·um). Before parturition; before childbirth. [L.]

antebrachial (an·te·**bra**·ke·al). In anatomy, relating or belonging to the forearm. [see foll.]

antebrachium [NA] (an·te·**bra**·ke·um). The forearm. [L *ante, brachium* arm.]

antecardium (an·te·**kar**·de·um). Precordium. [L *ante*, Gk *kardia* heart.]

antecornu (an·te·**korn**·ew). The anterior horn of the lateral ventricle of the brain. [L *ante, cornu* horn.]

antecubital (an·te·**kew**·bit·al). 1. Situated in the front of the forearm. 2. In front of the elbow; at the bend of the elbow. [L *ante, cubitum* elbow.]

antecurvature (an·te·**ker**·vat·ewr). A slight degree of antiflexion. [L *ante*, curvature.]

antefebrile (an·te·**fe**·brile). Antepyretic; occurring before the beginning of the period of pyrexia. [L *ante, febris* fever.]

anteflect (**an**·te·**flekt**'). To bend, or to cause to bend, forwards. [L *ante, flectere* to bend.]

anteflexion (an·te·**flek**·shun). 1. An abnormal forward curve or angular turn. 2. A bending forwards of the upper part of an organ. **Anteflexion of the uterus, Anteflexio uteri.** An angular forward bend of the uterus at the region of the internal os. [see prec.]

antegrade (**an**·te·grade). Anterograde. [L *ante, gredi* to go.]

antehelix (an·te·**he**·lix). Antihelix.

antehypophysis (**an**·te·hi·**pof**'·is·is). The anterior lobe of the hypophysis cerebri. [L *ante*, hypophysis.]

antelocation (an·te·lo·**ka**'·shun). The displacement forwards of an organ or part, especially of the uterus when there is neither version nor flexion. [L *ante, locus* place.]

antemetic (ant·em·**et**·ik). 1. Any remedy which tends to arrest or prevent vomiting. 2. Controlling or preventing vomiting. [Gk *anti*, emetic.]

antenarial (an·te·**nare**·e·al). In front of the nostrils. [L *ante, nares* nostrils.]

antenna (an·**ten**·ah) (pl. *antennae*). A sensory organ of arthropods; in the form of lateral paired appendages at the side of the anterior segment of the head. [L sail-yard.]

antephialtic (**ant**·ef·e·**al**'·tik). Anti-ephialtic: 1. Any remedy which is efficacious in preventing nightmare. 2. Conducive to the prevention of nightmare. [Gk *anti, ephialtes* nightmare.]

antepileptic (**ant**·ep·il·**ep**'·tik). Affording relief in epilepsy. [Gk *anti*, epilepsy.]

antepituitary (**an**·te·pit·**ew**'·it·ar·e). Referring to the anterior lobe of the pituitary gland (hypophysis cerebri). [L *ante*, pituitary.]

anteposition (**an**·te·po·**zish**'·un). Displacement forwards of any part or organ. [L *ante*, position.]

anteprandial (an·te·**pran**·de·al). Before the midday meal; before meals. [L *ante, prandium* dinner.]

anteprostate (an·te·**pros**·tate). One of the bulbo-urethral (Cowper's) glands. [L *ante*, prostate.]

anteprostatic (**an**·te·pros·**tat**'·ik). In a position in front of the prostate gland. [see prec.]

anteprostatitis (**an**·te·pros·tat·**i**'·tis). A condition of inflammation of the bulbo-urethral (Cowper's) glands. [L *ante*, prostate, Gk *-itis* inflammation.]

antepyretic (**an**·te·pi·**ret**'·ik). Antefebrile; occurring before the beginning of the period of pyrexia. [L *ante*, Gk *pyretos* fever.]

anterethic (**ant**·er·**eth**·ik). Any remedy which tends to allay irritation or has a soothing effect. [Gk *anti, erethismos* irritation.]

anterior [NA] (an·**teer**·e·or). 1. Descriptive of the front of the body or limbs, and of the relation of one structure within the body to another. 2. Referring to the forward part of any organ. 3. Towards the head. [L foremost.]

anterodorsal (**an**·ter·o·**dor**'·sal). In embryology, referring to the dorsal aspect of the head. [anterior, L *dorsum* back.]

antero-external (**an**·ter·o·ex·**ter**'·nal). Denoting a position in front and to the outer or lateral side.

anterograde (**an**·ter·o·grade). 1. Moving or proceeding forwards. 2. Extending towards the front. [anterior, *gredi* to go.]

antero-inferior (**an**·ter·o·in·**feer**'·e·or). Denoting a position in front and at a lower level.

antero-internal (**an**·ter·o·in·**ter**'·nal). Denoting a position in front and to the inner or medial side.

anterolateral (**an**·ter·o·**lat**'·er·al). Denoting a position or direction in front and to the lateral side or to either side. **Anterolateral sulcus.** *See* SULCUS.

anteromedian (**an**·ter·o·**me**'·de·an). Denoting a position in front and towards the median plane.

antero-occlusion (**an**·ter·o·ok·**loo**'·zhun). Mesio-occlusion; that form of malocclusion in which the lower teeth bite anterior to the normal position of occlusion with corresponding upper teeth. The mandibular incisor teeth bite outside those in the maxilla. [anterior, L *occludere* to shut.]

anteroparietal (**an**·ter·o·par·**i**'·et·al). Denoting a position in front and on the wall of a cavity. [anterior, L *paries* wall.]

anteroposterior (**an**·ter·o·pos·**teer**'·e·or). 1. Extending from the front to the back. 2. Referring to the front and the back.

anterosuperior (**an**·ter·o·sew·**peer**'·e·or). Denoting a position in front and above.

anteroventral (**an**·ter·o·**ven**'·tral). Denoting a position in front and towards the anterior surface. [anterior, L *venter* belly.]

anteversion (an·te·**ver**·zhun). The tipping or inclining forwards of an organ; forward displacement without angulation. [L *ante, versio* a turning.]

antevert (an·te·**vert**). To incline or turn forwards, or to cause to do so. [see prec.]

antexion (ant·**ek**·shun). Flexion of the spine. [L *ante, flectere* to bend.]

anthaemorrhagic (**ant**·hem·or·**aj**'·ik). Antihaemorrhagic.

anthelicine (ant·**hel**·is·een). Antihelicine.

anthelminthic, anthelmintic (an·hel·**min**·thik, ant·hel·**min**·tik). 1. A remedy for infestation with worms. 2. Having the power to destroy worms. [Gk *anti, helmins* worm.]

anthelone (**an**·the·lone). A substance, probably not a true hormone, which stimulates healing processes in the stomach.

anthelotic (ant·hel·**ot**·ik). 1. Any agent which is efficacious against corns or callosities. 2. Effective against corns and callosities. [Gk *anti, helos* nail.]

anthema (**an**·them·ah). Exanthem. [Gk *anthein* to bloom.]

Anthemis BPC 1949 (**an**·the·mis). Chamomile, the dried double or semi-double flowerheads of cultivated varieties of *Anthemis nobilis*, family Compositae. The main constituents are volatile oil, a bitter principle and a flavone. It is a popular domestic remedy for indigestion, taken as an infusion, and for certain inflammatory conditions; also as a fomentation or poultice. [Gk camomile.]

antheridium (an·ther·**id**·e·um). The male gametangium. [Gk *antheros* flowery.]

antherozoid (**an**·ther·o·zoid). Spermatozoid. [Gk *antheros* flowery, *zoon* living thing, *eidos* form.]

anthocyan (an·tho·**si**·an). Relating to the red, blue or purple colouring matters of plants. **Anthocyan pigment.** Anthocyanin. [see foll.]

anthocyanidin (**an**·tho·si·**an**'·id·in). Any one of the bases produced by the hydrolysis of anthocyanin glycosides. They are cyanidin, delphinidin or pelargonidin, according to the number of hydroxyl groups present, or the methyl derivatives of these. [Gk *anthos* flower, *kyanos* blue.]

anthocyanin (an·tho·**si**·an·in). General term for members of a family of soluble glycosidic pigments which form the vivid red, blue or purple colouring matters of certain flowers, fruits and autumnal leaves. They are derivatives of chromone, constituted of the chloride of a flavylium base united to sugars, and are closely related to vitamins E and P. [see prec.]

anthocyaninaemia (an·tho·**si**·an·in·e′·me·ah). The presence of anthocyanin in the blood. [anthocyanin, Gk *haima* blood.]

anthocyaninuria (an·tho·**si**·an·in·**ewr**′·e·ah). The presence in urine of anthocyanin.

anthophobia (**an**·tho·**fobe**′·e·ah). Excessive dislike of flowers, or fear that they are harmful. [Gk *anthos* flower, phobia.]

anthorism, anthorisma (**an**·thor·izm, an·thor·**iz**·mah). An uncircumscribed diffuse swelling; a swelling with ill-defined boundaries. [Gk *anti, horisma* boundary.]

anthoxanthin, anthoxanthine (an·tho·**zan**·thin, an·tho·**zan**·theen). An anthocyanin which occurs as a yellow pigment in certain flowers. [Gk *anthos* flower, *xanthos* yellow.]

anthracaemia (an·thrah·**se**·me·ah). 1. The presence in the blood of *Bacillus anthracis.* 2. A condition of asphyxia caused by poisoning with carbon monoxide. [Gk *anthrax* carbuncle, coal, *haima* blood.]

anthracene (**an**·thras·een). Paranaphthalene, $C_{14}H_{10}$. A solid hydrocarbon, colourless but with a blue fluorescence, obtained during the fractional distillation of coal tar. It is insoluble in water, slightly in ether or alcohol, but readily in hot benzene; used in the manufacture of dyestuffs. **Anthracene oil.** The distillate of coal tar above 270°C, which contains carbazole and phenanthrene in addition to anthracene. [Gk *anthrax* coal.]

anthracia (an·**thra**·she·ah). A condition which is marked by carbuncular eruptions. **Anthracia pestis.** Plague. **Anthracia rubula.** Yaws or framboesia. [Gk *anthrax* carbuncle.]

anthracic (an·**thras**·ik). 1. Term applied to an infection resembling that caused by the anthrax bacillus. 2. Referring to anthrax.

anthracin (**an**·thras·in). A hypothetical chemical agent which in the view of Fokker and Osol was the cause of anthrax. They claimed that the bacillus cultured by Pasteur occurred only as a consequence of the disease produced by this substance. [Gk *anthrax* carbuncle.]

anthracina (an·thrah·**se**·nah). Melanotic carcinoma; a cancer which produces dark pigment as it spreads. [Gk *anthrax* coal.]

anthracoid (**an**·thrah·koid). 1. Resembling a carbuncle or a pustule. 2. Resembling anthrax. [anthrax, Gk *eidos* form.]

anthracoma (an·thrah·**ko**·mah). Carbuncle. [anthrax, Gk *-oma* tumour.]

anthracometer (an·thrah·**kom**·et·er). An instrument for estimating the amount of carbon dioxide present in air and other gaseous mixtures. [Gk *anthrax* coal, meter.]

anthracometry (an·thrah·**kom**·et·re). The measurement of the carbon dioxide present in gaseous mixtures or air. [see prec.]

anthraconecrosis (**an**·thrah·ko·nek·**ro**′·sis). The degeneration of tissue into a dry black mass by the action of necrosis. [Gk *anthrax* coal, necrosis.]

anthracosilicosis (**an**·thrah·ko·sil·e·**ko**′·sis). A type of pneumoconiosis consisting in co-existent anthracosis and silicosis; miner's asthma. [Gk *anthrax* coal, silicosis.]

anthracosis (an·thrah·**ko**·sis). 1. A term used to describe the blackening of the lungs due to deposit of carbon particles, especially in city dwellers. 2. A form of pneumoconiosis found in coal workers, and characterized by increased fibrous-tissue formation and focal emphysema; the pathological changes are probably due to associated silicosis. **Anthracosis linguae.** Black tongue; an affection of the tongue in which dark-brown or greenish-black patches form on the dorsum. The patches consist of hypertrophied filiform papillae with moulds and other microorganisms. [Gk *anthrax* coal, *-osis* condition.]

anthracotherapy (**an**·thrah·ko·**ther**′·ap·e). A method of treatment based on the use of charcoal. [Gk *anthrax* coal, therapy.]

anthracotic (an·thrah·**kot**·ik). 1. Affected by or suffering from anthrax. 2. Referring to anthrax.

anthraflavin (an·thrah·**fla**·vin). $C_6H_3OH(CO)_2C_6H_3OH$, an isomer of alizarin, in the form of yellow crystals with the properties of a dibasic acid; used in the synthesis of dyestuffs. Cf. ALIZARIN.

anthragallol (an·thrah·**gal**·ol). Anthracene brown, trihydroxyanthraquinone, $C_6H_4(CO)_2C_6H(OH)_3$. A condensation of benzoic and gallic acids; brown crystals dissolving in alkalis with a green colour, and used as a dye.

anthraglucorhamnin (**an**·thrah·gloo·ko·**ram**′·nin). A glucoside obtained from *Rhamnus fragula,* the alder buckthorn, which on hydrolysis yields rhamnose, glucose and an emodin, trihydroxymethylanthraquinone; it is cathartic.

anthraglucorhein (**an**·thrah·gloo·ko·**re**′·in). A glucoside obtained from rhubarb (*Rheum*) which has a cathartic effect.

anthrapurpurin (an·thrah·**per**·pewr·in). A trihydroxy derivative of anthraquinone which is the basis of certain dyes.

anthraquinone (an·thrah·**kwin**·one). $C_6H_4(CO)_2C_6H_4$, a glycosidic derivative in many vegetable drugs, principally aloes, araroba, cascara, frangula and senna; synthesized by the oxidation of anthracene. Yellow crystals, insoluble in water, but soluble in alcohol, ether or hot benzene; used in the manufacture of dyestuffs.

anthrarobin (an·thrah·**ro**·bin). Dihydroxyanthranol, $C_6H_4=CHC(OH)=C_6H_2(OH)_2$. A yellowish compound derived from alizarin and sometimes used in skin diseases.

anthrax (**an**·thrax). A fatal disease of cattle and sheep, due to infection by *Bacillus anthracis,* and transmissible to man by infected animal carcasses, hides, furs, wool and brushes. In man it appears as a malignant pustule, a little papule which blisters, ulcerates, sloughs and develops around it a brownish swelling; constitutional disturbance may be severe. **Cerebral anthrax.** Anthrax with cerebral symptoms from the invasion of the brain by bacilli. **Intestinal anthrax.** A lethal form of anthrax in which the intestinal tract is mainly affected. **Malignant anthrax.** A form common in sheep and cattle, which may occur also in untreated human subjects; the local lesion is accompanied by anthrax septicaemia, produced by the bacilli circulating in the blood. It is a very fatal form. **Anthrax oedema.** *See* OEDEMA. **Pulmonary anthrax.** Woolsorters' disease, caused by circulating bacilli which produces a severe pneumonia. **Skin anthrax.** Malignant pustule. *See* MAIN DEF. (above). [Gk carbuncle.]

anthropobiology (**an**·thro·po·bi·**ol**′·o·je). The study, from the point of view of biology, of the anthropoid apes and of man. [Gk *anthropos* human being, biology.]

anthropogenesis, anthropogeny (**an**·thro·po·**jen**′·es·is, an·thro·**poj**·en·e). The science of the racial and individual origin and development of man. [Gk *anthropos* human being, genesis.]

anthropography (an·thro·**pog**·raf·e). That branch of anthropology which is concerned with the distribution of the human race according to physical character, language, customs and institutions. Cf. ETHNOGRAPHY. [Gk *anthropos* human being, *graphein* to record.]

anthropoid (**an**·thro·poid). Term applied to those apes which most nearly resemble man in form and structure, e.g. the chimpanzee and gorilla. Used incorrectly to designate the family Pongidae. [Gk *anthropos* human being, *eidos* form.]

Anthropoidea (an·thro·**poi**·de·ah). A sub-order of the Primates. It includes monkeys, apes and man. [see prec.]

anthropology (an·thro·**pol**·o·je). The whole science of the human being and of all branches of knowledge of which he is the subject; the study of man as an animal. The science of the human organism. **Criminal anthropology.** The science of the habitual criminal in all his relations to the outside world and to his own mentality. **Cultural anthropology.** The scientific investigation of the intellectual and moral qualities of man in comparison with those of his fellow beings, and in relation to his racial, social and environmental conditions. **Physical anthropology.** Anthropography. [Gk *anthropos* human being, *logos* science.]

anthropometer (an·thro·**pom**·et·er). An instrument used in anthropometry for measuring the human body and its parts. [see foll.]

anthropometry (an·thro·**pom**·et·re). That branch of anthropology which is concerned with the comparative measurement of the human body and of its parts. [Gk *anthropos* human being, meter.]

anthropomorphic (**an**·thro·po·**mor**·fik). Resembling man in form or character; having the figure of a man. [Gk *anthropos* human being, *morphe* shape.]

anthropomorphism (**an**·thro·po·**mor'**·fizm). The attributing of human characteristics and affections to things not human. [see prec.]

anthroponomy (an·thro·**pon**·o·me). That branch of anthropology which is concerned with the development of the human organism with regard to its environment and its relations to other organisms. [Gk *anthropos* human being, *nomos* law.]

anthropopathy (an·thro·**pop**·ath·e). The ascription of human passions or feelings to something which is not human. [Gk *anthropos* human being, *pathos* suffering.]

anthropophagy (an·thro·**pof**·aj·e). Cannibalism. [Gk *anthropos* human being, *phagein* to eat.]

anthropophile (an·**thro**·po·file). One with a liking for man; in entomology, a blood-sucking insect with a preference for human blood rather than that of other mammals, or of reptiles or birds. [Gk *anthropos* human being, *philein* to love.]

anthropophilic (**an**·thro·po·**fil'**·ik). Of the nature of an anthropophile.

anthropophilism (an·thro·**pof**·il·izm). A liking for man. [Gk *anthropos* human being, *philein* to love.]

anthropophobia (**an**·thro·po·**fo'**·be·ah). Excessive or morbid reluctance to be in the society of other people. [Gk *anthropos* human being, phobia.]

anthroposcopy (an·thro·**pos**·ko·pe). The classifying of human beings by the study of their type of body build and not by use of the anthropometric method. [Gk *anthropos* human being, *skopein* to view.]

anthroposomatology (**an**·thro·po·so·mat·**ol'**·o·je). That branch of anthropology which is concerned with the human body. [Gk *anthropos* human being, *soma* body, *logos* science.]

anthroposophy (an·thro·**pos**·of·e). The knowledge of man and his natural characteristics. [Gk *anthropos* man, *sophos* wise.]

anthropotomy (an·thro·**pot**·o·me). The anatomy of the human body. [Gk *anthropos* human being, *temnein* to cut.]

anthropozoonoses (**an**·thro·po·zo·on·**o'**·seez). Infections of man naturally acquired from vertebrate maintenance hosts, e.g. rabies, trichinosis. [Gk *anthropos* human being, zoonosis.]

anthydropic (ant·hi·**drop**·ik). Antihydropic.

anthypnotic (ant·hip·**not**·ik). Antihypnotic.

anti-. Prefix, from the Greek preposition *anti*, meaning *against, instead of.*

anti-abrin (an·te·a·brin). An antibody which is formed in the blood as a result of the injection of abrin, the irritant protein from black and red jequirity beans. Its activity in the blood can be measured.

anti-achromotrichia (**an**·te·a·kro·mo·**trik'**·e·ah). Anticanitic; any remedy employed against greying of the hair [Gk *anti, a, chroma* colour, *thrix* hair.]

anti-aditis (**an**·te·ad·**i'**·tis). Tonsillitis. [Gk *anti, aden* gland, *-itis* inflammation.]

anti-adrenocorticotrophin (**an**·te·ad·re·no·kor·tik·o·**tro'**·fin). An antihormone which may develop in experimental animals and intercept the action of adrenocorticotrophin.

anti-agglutinating (an·te·ag·**loo'**·tin·a·ting). 1. The property of being able to prevent agglutination. 2. Preventing agglutination. [Gk *anti*, agglutinate.]

anti-agglutinin (**an**·te·ag·**loo'**·tin·in). A specific antibody which counteracts the effect of the agglutinin to which it corresponds.

anti-aggressin (**an**·te·ag·**res'**·in). An antibody to an aggressin.

anti-albumate (an·te·**al**·bew·mate). An albumin incompletely digested. [see foll.]

anti-albumid, anti-albumide (**an**·te·al·**bew'**·mid, an·te·**al**·bew·mide). A product formed from albumin by pancreatic and gastric digestion. [Gk *anti*, albumin.]

anti-albumin (an·te·**al**·bew·min). 1. A constituent of albumin which is converted into anti-albumose by the process of gastric digestion. 2. An antibody for albumin. [see prec.]

anti-albuminate (**an**·te·al·**bew'**·min·ate). Anti-albumate.

anti-albumose (an·te·**al**·bew·moze). An antibody for albumose.

anti-amboceptor (**an**·te·am·bo·**sep'**·tor). Anti-immune body: an antibody to an immune body produced by injection of the serum containing the immune body into an animal of a different species. [Gk *anti*, amboceptor.]

anti-analgesic (**an**·te·an·al·**je**·zik). A drug reducing the effectiveness of analgesic agents, e.g. hyoscine, barbiturates, promethazine, halothane. [Gk *anti, a, algos* pain.]

anti-anaphylaxis (**an**·te·an·ah·fil·**ax'**·is). The abolition of anaphylactic phenomena. It may be achieved by the administration of a small sensitizing dose, and, before anaphylaxis is established (i.e. before the 10th day), another larger injection of the same antigen, so that the animal becomes non-susceptible to anaphylactic shock although its serum is capable of conferring passive anaphylaxis. A similar state of non-susceptibility occurs for a time when an animal recovers from anaphylactic shock, or can be brought about by desensitization which involves the repeated injection of small but increasing doses of anaphylactogen in amounts insufficient to produce symptoms. Insensitiveness can also be attained by ether anaesthesia at the time when the assaulting dose is given, or by administering drugs such as adrenaline or atropine. [Gk *anti*, anaphylaxis.]

anti-antibody (an·te·**an**·te·bod·e). Antibody which combines with immunoglobulin molecules which have reacted with antigen but not with unreacted immunoglobulin. May react with determinants revealed by the change in conformation which an immunoglobulin shows on reacting with antigen. [Gk *anti*, antibody.]

anti-antitoxin (**an**·te·an·te·**tox'**·in). A substance formed in the body during the process of immunization with an antitoxin, and which has a neutralizing effect on the latter. [Gk *anti*, antitoxin.]

anti-arachnolysin (**an**·te·ar·ak·**nol'**·is·in). An antitoxic serum to control or counteract the effects of a spider bite. [Gk *anti, arachne* spider, lysin.]

anti-arrhythmic (**an**·te·a·**rith'**·mik). Applied to drugs which are used to control or correct abnormal rhythms of cardiac action. [Gk *anti, rhythmos* rhythm.]

antibacterial (**an**·te·bak·**teer'**·e·al). 1. Any substance which destroys bacteria or inhibits their growth. 2. Checking the growth of bacteria. [Gk *anti*, bacterium.]

antibacteriolytic (**an**·te·bak·**teer**·e·o·**lit'**·ik). Inhibiting the action of bacteriolysis. [Gk *anti*, bacteriolysis.]

antibechic (an·te·**bek**·ik). 1. A remedy for cough. 2. Having the property of curing or relieving cough. [Gk *anti, bex* cough.]

antibiosis (**an**·te·bi·**o'**·sis). A relationship between 2 organisms, or among the members of a group of organisms, which results in harm to one of them owing to the production of an antibiotic by the other. [Gk *anti, bios* life.]

antibiotic (**an**·te·bi·**ot'**·ik). 1. Characterized by antibiosis. 2. Inimical to life. 3. Any of the specific substances produced *in vitro* by certain bacteria and fungi which are capable of killing or inhibiting the growth of certain other bacteria and viruses *in vitro* and *in vivo.* Penicillin, produced from *Penicillium notatum*, was the first antibiotic used successfully to combat certain bacterial infections in man; others are streptomycin, chloramphenicol, aureomycin, oxytetracycline and polymyxin. Many antibiotics can now be reproduced synthetically. **Broad-spectrum antibiotics.** Agents with a lethal or growth-inhibiting action on a wide variety of pathogenic bacteria. The term usually refers to agents acting on both Gram-positive and Gram-negative species. [see prec.]

antiblastic (an·te·**blas**·tik). 1. Denoting the slowing down of bacterial growth. 2. Marked by reduction in speed of bacterial growth. [Gk *anti, blastos* germ.]

antiblennorrhagic (**an**·te·blen·o·**ra'**·jik). 1. Preventive or curative of gonorrhoea. 2. A remedy for the prophylaxis or treatment of gonorrhoea. 3. Checking or curing any discharge of mucus. [Gk *anti, blennos* mucus, *rhegnynein* to gush forth.]

antibody (**an**·te·bod·e). Serum protein with the molecular properties of an immunoglobulin. Antibodies are produced in the body by cells of the lymphoid series, especially plasma cells in response to stimulation by an antigen. Antibodies are usually referred to according to the method used for their demonstration, e.g. precipitating, agglutinating or complement-fixing, and as they react specifically with their corresponding antigens their specificity makes them useful laboratory reagents for the recognition of the latter. **Antinuclear antibody.** An antibody reacting with various components of cell nuclei. **Artificial antibody.** One claimed to be prepared *in vitro.* There is no evidence that a real antibody has ever been made artificially. **Blocking antibody.** 1. Incomplete antibody which does not agglutinate the corresponding antigen but which attaches and prevents agglutination by normal complete antibody. 2. Antibody formed during specific desensitization in atopy, capable of blocking the harmful reaction of a reagin with an allergen. **Complete antibody.** That part of an antibody which is precipitable by addition of an antigen. **Cytophilic antibody.** A globulin component of immune serum which binds to the surface of cells *in vitro* in such a way that these cells are still capable of binding to other antigens in the vicinity. **Duffy antibody.** An agglutinin of the Duffy (Fy^a, Fy^b) human blood group system, described by Cutbush, Mollison and Parkin, 1950, different from the ABO, MN, Rh–Hr and other systems. **Fluorescent antibody (FA).** The labelled specific reagent used in the immunofluorescence technique. **Heterogenetic antibody, Heterophil antibody.** An antibody produced when a heterophil antigen is injected. **Incomplete antibody, Inhibiting antibody.** An antibody that will not form a precipitate with its corresponding antigen, but will add on to a precipitate formed from the corresponding complete antibody with the antigen. **Lipoidotropic antibody.** An alcoholic extract of normal animal tissues, such as ox heart, with the addition of cholesterol as a sensitizing agent. This substance identifies reagin by complement fixation and precipitation tests (Wassermann and V.D.R.L. slide tests). **Natural antibody.** One produced in the absence of environmental stimulus and in accordance with the laws of heredity. [Gk *anti*, AS *bodig.*]

See also: FORSSMAN.

antibromic (an·te·**bro**·mik). 1. Any deodorizing agent. 2. Deodorant. [Gk *anti*, *bromos* stench.]

anticanitic (**an**·te·kan·**it'**·ik). 1. Counteracting greying of the hair. 2. Any remedy employed against the greying of the hair. [Gk *anti*, L *canities* grey hair.]

anticarcinogen (**an**·te·kar·**sin'**·o·jen). A substance that neutralizes the effect of a carcinogen. [Gk *anti*, carcinogen.]

anticardium (an·te·**kar**·de·um). Praecordium. [Gk *anti*, *kardia* heart.]

anticatalase (an·te·**kat**·al·aze). A serum inhibitor of catalase. [Gk *anti*, catalase.]

anticatalyser, anticatalyst (an·te·**kat**·al·i·zer, an·te·**kat**·al·ist). A substance that slows or prevents a chemical action by inhibiting, or even poisoning, the catalyst. [Gk *anti*, catalyst.]

anticataphylactic (an·te·**kat**·ah·fil·**ak'**·tik). A substance able to prevent cataphylaxis. [see foll.]

anticataphylaxis (**an**·te·kat·ah·fil·**ax'**·is). The inhibition of the movement of phagocytes and antibodies towards the site of an infection. [Gk *anti*, *kata*, *phylax* guard.]

anticathexis (**an**·te·kath·**ex'**·is). The removal of an emotional charge from an impulse to an impulse of opposite nature; counter-investment. [Gk *anti*, *kathexis* retention.]

anticathode (an·te·**kath**·ode). An inclined surface, or target, of high-melting-point metal enclosed in an x-ray tube opposite the cathode. It is bombarded by the stream of electrons from the latter, and emits penetrating rays of extremely short wavelength. [Gk *anti*, cathode.]

anticaustic (an·te·**kaw**·stik). 1. Any agent which prevents or checks the action of a caustic substance. 2. Preventing or checking the action of a caustic agent. [Gk *anti*, caustic.]

anticephalalgic (**an**·te·kef·al·**al'**·jik). 1. Any remedy for headache. 2. Preventing or curing headache. [Gk *anti*, cephalalgia.]

anticheirotonus (**an**·te·ki·**rot'**·o·nus). A strong inflection of the thumb, generally a prodromal sign of epilepsy, but also noted sometimes during the fit. [Gk *anti*, *cheir* hand, *tonos* tension.]

antichlor (**an**·te·klor). Name given to a reagent such as sodium thiosulphate, which neutralizes the excess chlorine after bleaching. [Gk *anti*, chlorine.]

anticholagogue (an·te·**ko**·lag·og). A substance that reduces the secretion of bile. [Gk *anti*, cholagogue.]

anticholinergic (**an**·te·ko·lin·**er'**·jik). A substance that antagonizes acetylcholine. [Gk *anti*, *chole* bile, *ergein* to work.]

anticholinesterase (**an**·te·ko·lin·**es'**·ter·aze). Any substance inhibiting cholinesterase, e.g. physostigmine. [Gk *anti*, cholinesterase.]

antichoromanic (**an**·te·kor·o·**man'**·ik). 1. Controlling or preventing spasm and choromania. 2. Any remedy effective in the treatment of choromania and spasm. [Gk *anti*, choromania.]

antichymosin (an·te·**ki**·mo·sin). An antibody which checks the action of rennin (chymosin) on milk.

anticlinal (an·te·**kli**·nal). Applied to surfaces which incline in opposite directions, as in a pyramid. [Gk *anti*, *klinein* to slope.]

anticnemion (an·te·**ne**·me·on). The shin. [Gk *anti*, *kneme* leg.]

anticoagulant (**an**·te·ko·**ag'**·ew·lant). 1. A substance which prevents clotting in blood or milk. 2. Preventing clotting. [Gk *anti*, L *coagulare* to curdle.]

anticoagulin (**an**·te·ko·**ag'**·ew·lin). A substance formed in the body which inhibits the clotting of blood. It has the opposite effect to that of coagulin. [see prec.]

anticodon (an·te·**ko**·don). The triplet sequence of bases on a molecule of transfer ribonucleic acid (tRNA) which recognizes, by hydrogen bonding, the corresponding codon triplet on messenger-RNA. [Gk *anti*, L *caudex* book.]

anticollagenase (**an**·te·kol·**aj'**·en·aze). Any substance inhibiting collagenase. [Gk *anti*, collagenase.]

anticolloidoclastic (**an**·te·kol·oid·o·**klas'**·tik). 1. Term applied to any measure taken to control a haemoclastic crisis. 2. Any remedy used in the attempt to control haemoclastic crises. [Gk *anti*, colloidoclasia.]

anticomplement (an·te·**kom**·ple·ment). Descriptive of a substance, other than antigen-antibody, which activates serum complement, thus causing complement fixation in the absence of a specific antigen-antibody reaction. [Gk *anti*, complement.]

anticomplementary (**an**·te·kom·ple·**ment'**·ar·e). Descriptive of a substance which is able to diminish or destroy the action of complement, or of serum containing such a substance. [see prec.]

anticonceptive (**an**·te·kon·**sep'**·tiv). Contraceptive. [Gk *anti*, conception.]

anticreatinine (**an**·te·kre·**at'**·in·een). A creatinine-type leucomaine formed in muscle. [Gk *anti*, creatinine.]

anticritical (an·te·**krit**·ik·al). Preventing or easing of the crisis of a disease. [Gk *anti*, crisis.]

anticytolysin (**an**·te·si·**tol'**·is·in). A substance which inhibits cytolytic action in the destruction of living cells. [Gk *anti*, cytolysis.]

anticytotoxin (**an**·te·si·to·**tox'**·in). An antibody which has a specific action against cytotoxins and prevents cell damage and death. [Gk *anti*, cytotoxin.]

antidiarrhoeal (**an**·te·di·ar·**e'**·al). Efficacious against diarrhoea. [Gk *anti*, diarrhoea.]

antidiastase (an·te·**di**·as·taze). An antibody, formed in the blood serum following the injection of diastase, and opposing its action. [Gk *anti*, diastase.]

antidinic (an·te·**din**·ik). 1. A remedy which relieves vertigo or prevents its occurrence. 2. Preventing or relieving vertigo. [Gk *anti*, *dinos* a whirling.]

antidiuresis (**an**·te·di·ewr·**e'**·sis). The reduction of urine formation resulting from an increased reabsorption of fluid in the distal convoluted tubule of the kidney. [Gk *anti*, diuresis.]

antidotal (**an**·te·do·tal). Acting as an antidote.

antidote (**an**·te·dote). Any agent which neutralizes or opposes the action of a poison on an organism. **Arsenical antidote.** A preparation of hydrated iron oxide and magnesia used formerly to counteract the effect of arsenic but now replaced by dimercaprol for this purpose. **Chemical antidote.** Any substance which alters or precipitates a poison in such a way as to render it harmless. **Mechanical antidote.** 1. Any means for ridding the system of a poison, e.g. a stomach pump. 2. Any agent which mechanically prevents the absorption of a poison, e.g. by coating the stomach. **Physiological antidote.** A drug that has the opposite effect on the organism to that produced by a poison and therefore counteracts the latter. **Universal antidote.** 1. A mixture of 1 part magnesium oxide, 1 part tannic acid, and 2 parts charcoal, administered when the nature of the poison is unknown. 2. A solution of 1 part ferrous sulphate in 2 parts of magnesia water, given for the same purpose. [Gk *anti, dotos* that which is given.]

See also: BIBRON, FANTUS.

antidromic (an·te·**drom**·ik). Applied to those nerve fibres along which impulses pass in an opposite direction to that in which they normally pass, or to the nerve impulses so flowing. [Gk *anti, dromos* course.]

antidysuric (**an**·te·dis·**ewr'**·ik). 1. A remedy for the relief or prevention of pain or difficulty in passing urine. 2. Preventing or relieving dysuria. [Gk *anti,* dysuria.]

anti-emetic (**an**·te·em·**et'**·ik). A drug which reduces the incidence and severity of nausea and vomiting. [Gk *enti, emesis* vomiting.]

anti-emulsin (**an**·te·e·**mul'**·sin). An antibody which interferes with the action of emulsin.

anti-enzyme (an·te·**en**·zime). 1. An antibody to an enzyme. 2. Less strictly, any substance or agent which prevents or hinders the action of an enzyme.

anti-ephialtic (**an**·te·ef·e·**al'**·tik). Antephialtic.

antifebrile (an·te·**fe**·brile). Applied to any remedy or form of treatment which ends pyrexia or has the effect of lessening it; antipyretic; febrifugal. [Gk *anti,* L *febris* fever.]

antifibrinolysin (**an**·te·fi·brin·**ol'**·is·in). A substance which is held to be produced as an immune allergic reaction to infection by a streptococcus, and which is capable of preventing fibrinolysis by streptococcal cultures. [Gk *anti,* fibrinolysis.]

antigalactic (**an**·te·gal·**ak'**·tik). Any agent which suppresses the secretion of milk. [Gk *anti, gala* milk.]

antigelatinase (**an**·te·jel·**at'**·in·aze). A substance which forms in the serum of animals inoculated with gelatinase or gelatinase-producing organisms, and prevents the digestion of gelatin. [Gk *anti,* gelatinase.]

antigen (**an**·te·jen). A substance which, under suitable circumstances, can stimulate a specific immune response (immunogenicity) and can react specifically with the antibody or cells associated with that response (reactivity). For an antigen to realize its potential immunogenicity it must be introduced in the proper quantity into a responsive animal or tissue. **Artificial antigen.** 1. An antigen prepared by coupling an aromatic organic compound with a protein, e.g. azoprotein. 2. An antigen whose specificity has been modified by chemical means. **Australia antigen.** Also known as *Australia serum hepatitis* (Au/SH) and *hepatitis-associated antigen* (H.A.A.). Australia antigen is more correctly and unambiguously referred to as *type B hepatitis antigen* to distinguish it from any antigens found in association with type A infective hepatitis. The antigen consists of small (20 nm), spherical or bacillary bodies found in the serum of those who have, or have had, serum hepatitis. Occasional larger, 42 nm, forms (Dane particles) may also be found. The presence of the antigen in the patient's serum is diagnostic of serum hepatitis. It appears shortly after the onset of the disease and may persist for some time after the symptoms regress, though the frequency and duration of positive findings depend on the type of assay used. Chronic carriage of the antigen is found in a proportion of cases, usually in association with continuing active liver disease, but apparently healthy carriers also occur, and in some tropical areas carriage rates can reach 15-20 per cent without widespread liver damage in the population. Antibody to the antigen also develops and may make the antigen difficult to detect. It may be demonstrated in the blood by immunodiffusion, immune electro-osmophoresis, complement fixation, radio-immunoassay, latex agglutination, electron microscopy and other tests. Of these, the most commonly used are immune electro-osmophoresis and complement fixation. The exact relationship of the antigen to the virus of serum hepatitis has yet to be determined but it may be self-assembled coat protein. It is called *Australia antigen* because it was originally identified in the serum of an Australian aborigine, but its distribution is world-wide and the name implies no geographical localization. Small amounts of RNA are said to be associated with the antigen. **Be antigen.** Be blood factor. *See* FACTOR. **Blood-group antigen.** Substances in red blood cells determining the blood group specificities (*see* AGGLUTINOGEN). **Boivin antigen.** Endotoxin. **Capsular antigens.** The antigens of bacterial capsules, usually polysaccharide but may be polypeptide. **Carbohydrate antigen.** The pure polysaccharide components of certain encapsulated bacterial cells which can act as complete or partial antigens. **Chick-embryo antigen.** An artificial antigen used in the intradermal test for lymphopathia venereum. **Conjugated antigen.** An antigen in which one of the reactive groups has been modified chemically, e.g. by acylation. **Fimbrial antigens.** Antigens associated with the fine hair-like outgrowths (fimbriae or pili) found on some Gram-negative bacteria. **Flagellar (H) antigens.** The thermolabile protein antigens of bacterial flagella. The abbreviation *H* (G *Hauch,* breath or emanation) derives from the spreading behaviour of colonies of some flagellated bacteria. **Hepatitis-associated antigen.** Particulate antigen found in the serum of patients with viral hepatitis. *See also* Australia antigen (above). **Heterogenetic antigen, Heterophile antigen.** Antigen which stimulates formation of antibody which will react with phylogenetically unrelated antigens as well as with the homologous antigen. **Histocompatibility antigens.** H antigens; transplantation antigens: the antigens of animal cells which determine the immune reactions to grafts. Their nature and location are controversial, but they appear to be lipoproteins of the cell membranes, controlled by dominant genes (strong or weak). **Inaccessible antigen.** A hidden antigenic determinant which is sequestered in some part of the body (e.g. lens protein) so that it is not accessible for recognition by lymphocytes and does not stimulate an antibody response unless some change or disease causes the hidden antigen to be revealed. **K antigens.** Envelope or capsular antigens on *Escherichia* which mask the O antigens. **M antigen.** A surface protein antigen of *Streptococcus pyogenes* associated with the pathogenicity of the organism. **Mouse-brain antigen.** An artificial antigen used in the intradermal test for lymphopathia venereum. **O antigens.** *See* SOMATIC (O) ANTIGENS (below). **Organ specific antigen.** A characteristic antigenic substance which can be isolated from a particular organ of several different species of animal, e.g. lens protein of the eye. **Pollen antigen.** A saline extract from defatted pollen, used in the diagnosis, prophylaxis and desensitization of hay fever. **Rh antigen.** *See* RH CLASSES. **SH antigen.** Australia antigen (see above). **Somatic (O) antigens.** Antigens of the cell body (soma), especially the lipopolysaccharide-protein complexes of Gram-negative bacterial cell walls. The abbreviation *O* (G *ohne Hauch,* without emanation) derives from non-flagellated or non-motile bacteria. **Synthetic antigen.** Artificial antigen, 1st def. (see above). **T antigens.** Tumour antigens (see below). **Therapeutic antigen.** Any antigenic material used to stimulate antibody formation for therapeutic purposes. **Tumour antigens.** Antigens of tumour cells which are not detectable in normal cells of the same origin. Other tumour antigens may be present in the parent tissue and are therefore not tumour-specific. **V.D.R.L. antigen.** Veneral Disease Reference Laboratory standard antigen for use in the Wassermann test. **Vi antigen.** An antigen of the typhoid bacillus distinct from the O and H antigens. Like the O antigen it is situated on the surface of the bacillary body. It is associated with virulence, hence the name. [antibody, Gk *genein* to produce.]

See also: FORSSMAN, FREI, MEINICKE, SACHS (H.), STEIN.

antigenic (an·te·**jen**·ik). Referring to or having the properties of an antigen.

antigenicity (**an**·te·jen·**is'**·it·e). The state of potency inherent in any particular antigen.

antigenophil (an·te·**jen**·o·fil). Relating to the receptor group of an amboceptor which unites with the antigen for which it is specific, and for which therefore it has an affinity. [antigen, Gk *philein* to love.]

antigenotherapy, antigentotherapy (**an**·te·jen·o·**ther'**·ap·e, **an**·te·jent·o·**ther'**·ap·e). Vaccine therapy. *See* THERAPY. [antigen, therapy.]

antigerminal (an·te·**jer**·min·al). Referring to the pole of an ovum that is opposite to the germinal pole. [Gk *anti*, germinal.]

antiglobulin (an·te·**glob**·ew·lin). An antibody against a serum globulin or globulins. [Gk *anti*, globulin.]

antiglyoxalase (**an**·te·gli·**ox'**·al·aze). A substance formed in the pancreas which is an antagonist of glyoxalase. [Gk *anti*, glyoxalase.]

antigonadotrophin (**an**·te·gon·ad·o·**tro'**·fin). A substance that appears in the serum of a subject who has received repeated injections of a gonadotrophic hormone, and neutralizes the action of that hormone. [Gk *anti*, gonadotrophin.]

antigonadotropic (**an**·te·gon·ad·o·**trop'**·ik). Neutralizing the action of a specific gonadotropin [see prec.]

antihaemagglutinin (**an**·te·he·mah·**glew'**·tin·in). A substance the action of which is opposed to that of haemagglutinin. [Gk *anti*, haemagglutinin.]

antihaemolysin (**an**·te·he·**mol'**·is·in). Any agent which prevents or hinders the action of a haemolysin, or prevents destruction of the blood components. [Gk *anti*, haemolysin.]

antihaemolytic (**an**·te·he·mo·**lit'**·ik). 1. Any agent which hinders or prevents the breakdown of erythrocytes and the liberation of haemoglobin. 2. Hindering or preventing haemolysis. [Gk *anti*, haemolysis.]

antihaemorrhagic (**an**·te·hem·or·**aj'**·ik). 1. A remedy for haemorrhage, or for a haemorrhagic diathesis or syndrome. 2. Tending to arrest or to prevent bleeding. [Gk *anti*, haemorrhage.]

antihelicine (an·te·**hel**·is·een). Belonging to the antihelix.

antihelix [anthelix (NA)] (an·te·**he**·lix). A curved prominence in front of and parallel with the prominent rim of the auricle of the ear. [Gk *anti*, helix.]

antiheterolysin (**an**·te·het·er·**ol'**·is·in). Any substance which counterbalances the action of heterolysin. [Gk *anti*, heterolysin.]

antihidrotic (**an**·te·hid·**rot'**·ik). Anhidrotic: 1. Relating to anhidrosis. 2. Inhibiting the secretion of sweat. 3. Any agent which prevents the secretion of sweat. [Gk *anti*, *hidros* sweat.]

antihistamine (an·te·**his**·tam·een). Any drug that counteracts the effect of histamine. [Gk *anti*, histamine.]

antihormone (an·te·**hor**·mone). A substance said to be secreted in the body which, when circulating in the blood, antagonizes the effect of a hormone. Cf. COLYONE. [Gk *anti*, hormone.]

antihydropic (**an**·te·hi·**drop'**·ik). 1. A remedy for the relief of dropsy or dropsical conditions. 2. Relieving dropsy. [Gk *anti*, hydropic.]

antihypnotic (**an**·te·hip·**not'**·ik). 1. Any agent which is intended to prevent sleep. 2. Hindering sleep. [Gk *anti*, *hypnos* sleep.]

anti-infectious (**an**·te·in·**fek'**·shus). Term denoting an agent which counteracts infection. [Gk *anti*, infection.]

anti-infective (**an**·te·in·**fek'**·tiv). 1. Anti-infectious. 2. Any substance or agent which prevents or hinders infection.

anti-isolysin (**an**·te·i·**sol'**·is·in). A substance the effect of which is to work against an isolysin. [Gk *anti*, isolysin.]

antikenotoxin (**an**·te·ke·no·**tox'**·in). A hypothetical antitoxin said to be produced in response to the presence of an equally hypothetical toxin which is supposed to develop in active tissues and cause their fatigue. [Gk *anti*, *kenos* empty, *toxikon* poison.]

See also: WEICHARDT.

antiketogen (an·te·**ke**·to·jen). A substance which produces antiketogenesis.

antiketogenesis (**an**·te·ke·to·**jen'**·es·is). The prevention of ketone formation; a property attributed to substances, principally carbohydrates, the utilization of which by the liver does not result in the production of ketones, or takes place in preference to that of substances, such as fatty acids, the increased metabolism of which would produce ketonaemia and ketonuria. [Gk *anti*, ketogenesis.]

antiketogenic (**an**·te·ke·to·**jen'**·ik). 1. Referring to antiketogenesis. 2. Reducing the number or preventing the formation of ketone (acetone) bodies.

antiketoplastic (**an**·te·ke·to·**plas'**·tik). Restrictive of the number of ketone (acetone) compounds which are excreted in the breath or the urine. Antiketogenic. [Gk *anti*, ketone, *plassein* to form.]

antikinase (an·te·**kin**·aze). An antibody which is held to counteract or stop the action of kinase. [Gk *anti*, kinase.]

antikinesis (**an**·te·kin·**e'**·sis). The tendency of organisms to resist and to lean back against the drag of rotatory motion. [Gk *anti*, *kinesis* movement.]

antilactase (an·te·**lak**·taze). A substance which is antagonistic to lactase. [Gk *anti*, lactase.]

antileptic (an·te·**lep**·tik). 1. Revulsive, or derivative. 2. Aiding or supporting. [Gk *antilepsis* a receiving in return.]

antilethargic (**an**·te·leth·**ar'**·jik). 1. Any agent which is used to counteract lethargy or somnolence. 2. Preventing sleep or overcoming lethargy. [Gk *anti*, lethargy.]

antileucocidin (**an**·te·lew·ko·**si'**·din). A serum antibody which inhibits or neutralizes leucocidin. [Gk *anti*, leucocidin.]

antileucotoxin (**an**·te·lew·ko·**tox'**·in). An antibody to a leucocytotoxin. [Gk *anti*, leucotoxin.]

anti-lewisite (an·te·**loo**·is·ite). Dimercaprol BP 1958, BAL; 2,3-dimercaptopropanol, $CH_2SHCHSHCH_2OH$. An antidote for the war gas, lewisite; it is also of value as an antidote in cases of poisoning by the compounds of other metals such as mercury and arsenic.

antilipase (an·te·**lip**·aze). Any substance which inhibits the action or counteracts the effects of a lipase. [Gk *anti*, lipase.]

antilipoid (an·te·**lip**·oid). An antibody which is capable of reacting with a lipoid. [Gk *anti*, lipoid.]

antilithic (an·te·**lith**·ik). Any agent which prevents the formation of a calculus or stone, particularly urinary calculus, by hindering the deposit of sediment, supposedly by dissolving it. [Gk *anti*, *lithos* stone.]

antilobium (an·te·**lo**·be·um). The tragus; a small curved flap of fibrocartilaginous tissue projecting backwards over the orifice of the external auditory meatus. [Gk *antilobion*.]

antilogia (an·te·**lo**·je·ah). In diagnosis, a term used to describe a combination of symptoms of contradictory significance so that it is not possible to establish the diagnosis. [Gk *anti*, *legein* to speak.]

antiluetic (**an**·te·loo·**et'**·ik). Antisyphilitic. [Gk *anti*, L *lues* syphilis.]

antiluetin (**an**·te·loo·**et'**·in). Potassium ammonium antimonyl tartrate; an antisyphilitic. [see prec.]

antilysin (an·te·**li**·sin). An antibody that forms in the blood and destroys bacterial lysins.

antilysis (an·te·**li**·sis). The process of destruction of lysins by antilysins.

antilyssic (an·te·**lis**·ik). Antirabic. [Gk *anti*, *lyssa* frenzy.]

antilytic (an·te·**lit**·ik). 1. A substance which prevents the destruction of cells by a lysin. 2. Referring to antilysis. [Gk *anti*, lysis.]

antimere (an·te·meer). 1. One of the halves of a bilaterally symmetrical part or organism. 2. A segment of the body formed by planes cutting the body at right angles to the long axis. [Gk *anti*, *meros* part.]

antimetabolite (**an**·te·met·**ab'**·ol·ite). A substance which, owing to chemical relationship, can replace an essential metabolite in any system, but does not confer the same physiological benefit; a competitive metabolite. [Gk *anti*, metabolite.]

antimetropia (**an**·te·met·**ro'**·pe·ah). A condition in which the refractive error in one eye is of a different kind from the refractive error in the other eye. For example, there may be myopia in one eye and hypermetropia in the other. [Gk *anti*, *metron* measure, *ops* eye.]

antimicrobic (**an**·te·mi·**kro'**·bik). Antibacterial: 1. Any substance which destroys bacteria or inhibits their growth. 2. Checking the growth of bacteria. [Gk *anti*, microbe.]

antimitotic (an·te·mi·**tot**·ik). Of factors, interfering with the normal process of mitosis. [Gk *anti, mitos* thread.]

antimongolism (an·te·**mon**·gol·izm). A term coined to denote a syndrome of mental retardation and congenital abnormalities (downward sloping palpebral fissures, prominent nasal bridge, low-set malformed ears, microcephaly, hand with normal palmar creases and long fingers, iliac index increased, congenital heart disease, renal agenesis, and so on) somewhat antithetic to mongolism and due to the deficiency of part, or of the whole, of one G group chromosome thought to be a No. 21. As it is easy to distinguish chromosomes 21 and 22, this term should be restricted to cases where it is clear that the former chromosome is involved. [Gk *anti, Mongol* an Asian race.]

antimonial (an·te·**mo**·ne·al). 1. In pharmacy, a preparation containing antimony. 2. Referring to antimony.

antimonic (an·te·**mo**·nik). 1. Relating to or containing antimony. 2. A compound of antimony in which the latter is pentavalent.

antimonide (an·te·mon·ide). A compound of antimony with hydrogen or a metal.

antimonious (an·te·**mo**·ne·us). 1. Having the properties of or resembling antimony. 2. A compound of antimony in which the latter is trivalent.

antimonium (an·te·**mo**·ne·um). Antimony.

antimony (an·te·mo·ne). An element of atomic weight 121.76, atomic number 51 and chemical symbol Sb (*stibium*). It is a silvery-white metal, crystalline and brittle, and expands on solidifying from the molten state, for which reason it is alloyed in type metals. It occurs free in nature and as the mineral stibnite, a native sulphide Sb_2S_3, found in France, Italy and China. There are several allotropic forms, all of which are unstable. The inorganic salts are not used in medicine because they are irritant and toxic, but the organic compounds are of considerable value in the treatment of protozoal diseases. Of the latter, potassium or sodium antimonyl tartrate, antimony thioglycollamide, antimony sodium thioglycollate and stibophen, all containing trivalent antimony, have been used in schistosomiasis, filariasis, leishmaniasis and lymphopathia venerea, but they are liable to produce vomiting, a dry cough leading to pneumonia, pain in the abdomen and shoulder, acute arthritis of the wrists and ankles, and bradycardia. The compounds of pentavalent antimony are less toxic, and are most effective in the treatment of leishmaniasis and trypanosomiasis. **Antimony aniline tartrate.** $C_6H_5NH_2(SbO)C_4H_4O_6$, a yellow compound less toxic than tartar emetic and used against trypanosomes. **Butter of antimony, Antimony chloride.** $SbCl_3$; forms a fuming solution which could be used as a caustic. **Antimony oxide.** Antimony trioxide, Sb_2O_3, a white compound dissolving in alkalis to form the antimonious acids. **Antimony oxychloride.** Antimonyl chloride. **Antimony oxysulphide.** Kermes mineral. **Antimony pentasulphide.** Golden sulphuret of antimony, Sb_2S_5, a yellow precipitate used in vulcanizing rubber. **Antimony poisoning.** *See* POISONING. **Antimony Potassium Tartrate BP 1963.** Tartar emetic, $2K(SbO)C_4H_4O_6{\cdot}H_2O$, a colourless compound, readily soluble in water, with a highly irritant effect on the cells surrounding the cutaneous glands, producing redness followed by pustules which coalesce and result in scarring and necrosis. It may be given intravenously, the intima of the vein resisting the irritation, but produces vomiting, headache and pain in the joints; taken orally it irritates the gastric mucosa, and stimulates the vomiting centre in the medulla so that emesis results within a short time. **Antimony Sodium Tartrate BP 1973.** $2Na(SbO)C_4H_4O_6{\cdot}H_2O$, a compound used in the same way as tartar emetic. **Antimony sodium thioglycollate.** $NaOOCCH_2SSbS{=}COOCH_2$, a compound used intramuscularly or intravenously in the treatment of schistosomiasis, leishmaniasis and granuloma inguinale. **Sulphurated antimony.** Kermes mineral. **Tartrated antimony.** Sodium or potassium antimony tartrate. **Antimony thioglycollamide.** $Sb(SCH_2CONH_2)_3$, a compound used similarly to antimony sodium thioglycollate (above) but considered more toxic. **Antimony trichloride.** Antimony chloride (see above). **Antimony trioxide.** Antimony oxide (see above). **Trisulphide antimony.** Sb_2S_3, a compound used in vulcanizing, an industrial risk. [L *antimonium.*]

antimonyl (**an**·te·mo·nil). The monovalent radical SbO–, forming a series of compounds in which antimony is trivalent. **Antimonyl chloride.** Antimony oxychloride, basic antimony chloride, SbOCl; a white substance used as an emetic and purgative. **Antimonyl potassium tartrate.** Antimony Potassium Tartrate BP 1963.

antimosan (**an**·te·mo·san). A trivalent antimony preparation, potassium pyrocatechol sulphonate of antimony. It never had an important place in the treatment of tropical infections as it was soon replaced by a closely allied and less toxic preparation Stibophen BP 1958.

antimycin (an·te·**mi**·sin). An antibiotic; an inhibitor of mitochondrial electron transport. [Gk *anti* against, *mykes* fungus.]

antimycotic (an·te·mi·**kot**'·ik). Applied to any substance which destroys or prevents the growth of fungi. [Gk *anti, mykes* fungus.]

antimydriatic (an·te·mi·dri·**at**'·ik). Of a drug, one that counteracts the mydriatic action. [Gk *anti,* mydriatic.]

antinarcotic (an·te·nar·**kot**'·ik). 1. Any agent which is of use in combating the action of narcotics. 2. Counteracting the action of narcotics. [Gk *anti,* narcotic.]

antinial (an·**tin**·e·al). Relating or belonging to the antinion.

antinion (ant·**in**·e·on). The most prominent point in the median line of the glabella, i.e. that farthest from the inion. [Gk *anti,* inion.]

anti-obesic (an·te·o·**be**'·sik). 1. Any remedy given for the purpose of preventing or curing obesity. 2. Correcting obesity. [Gk *anti,* obesity.]

anti-odontalgic (an·te·o·dant·**al**'·jik). 1. A remedy for toothache. 2. Term applied to treatment which is effective against toothache. [Gk *anti,* odontalgia.]

anti-ophidica (an·te·o·**fid**'·ik·ah). Sera or other remedies used for the purpose of counteracting snake bite. [Gk *anti, ophis* snake.]

anti-otomy (an·te·**ot**·o·me). Tonsillectomy. [Gk *antias* tonsil, *temnein* to cut.]

anti-oxidant (an·te·**ox**·id·ant). A substance used to delay or prevent oxidation. [Gk *anti,* oxidation.]

anti-oxidase (an·te·**ox**·id·aze). A substance which hinders the action of an oxidase. [Gk *anti,* oxidase.]

anti-oxidation (an·te·ox·id·**a**'·shun). Prevention of oxidation. [Gk *anti,* oxidation.]

anti-oxygen (an·te·**ox**·e·jen). Anti-oxidant.

antipaludean, antipaludian (an·te·pal·**ew**'·de·an). Applied to any remedy administered or measure taken to prevent malaria. [Gk *anti,* L *palus* swamp.]

antiparastata (an·te·par·**as**'·tah·tah). The bulbo-urethral (Cowper's) glands. [Gk *anti, parastates* testis.]

antiparastatitis (an·te·par·as·tah·**ti**'·tis). An inflamed condition of the bulbo-urethral (Cowper's) glands. Ante-prostatitis. [Gk *anti, parastates* testis, *-itis* inflammation.]

antipathogen (an·te·**path**·o·jen). Any substance which inhibits the action of or destroys a virus or other disease-producing organism. [Gk *anti,* pathogen.]

antipathy (an·**tip**·ath·e). 1. Natural incompatibility of qualities or properties. 2. Strong constitutional aversion to particular substances or objects. 3. Excessive dislike, which may be unreasoning, directed towards particular individuals. [Gk *anti, pathos* suffering.]

antiperiodic (an·te·peer·e·**od**'·ik). 1. Antimalarial. 2. Acting against the periodic recurrence of a disease. [Gk *anti,* period.]

antiperistalsis (an·te·per·is·**tal**'·sis). Anastalsis; contrary contractions which force the contents of the digestive tube upwards. **Oesophageal antiperistalsis.** Regurgitation of food before it has reached the stomach. [Gk *anti,* peristalsis.]

antiperistaltic (an·te·per·is·**tal**'·tik). 1. Arresting or diminishing peristalsis. 2. Referring to antiperistalsis. [see prec.]

antiphagocytic (an·te·fag·o·**sit**'·ik). Impeding or affording protection against the action of phagocytes. [Gk *anti,* phagocytes.]

antiphlogistic (an·te·flo·**jis'**·tik). 1. Any agent or therapeutic measure which serves to check or counteract inflammation. 2. Preventing or counteracting inflammation, or relieving a febrile condition. [Gk *anti, phlogosis* inflammation.]

antiphone (an·te·fone). An appliance worn in the external auditory meatus for the purpose of reducing sound. [Gk *anti, phone* voice.]

antiphrynolysin, antiphrynolysine (an·te·frin·**ol'**·is·in, an·te·frin·ol'·is·een). An antitoxic serum for toad venom. [Gk *anti, phryne* toad, lysin.]

antiphtheiriac, antiphthiriac (an·te·**thi**·re·ak). 1. Any agent which destroys lice or prevents infestation with lice. 2. Conducing to the destruction of lice. [Gk *anti, phtheir* louse.]

antiplastic (an·te·**plas**·tik). Any agent which checks or prevents the process of healing, inhibiting the development of granulation tissue or of plastic exudation. [Gk *anti, plassein* to mould.]

antipneumococcal (an·te·new·mo·**kok'**·al). Having power to check the growth of or destroy the pneumococcus (*Streptococcus pneumoniae*). [Gk *anti*, pneumococcus.]

antipneumotoxin (an·te·new·mo·**tox'**·in). An antitoxin which counteracts the poison of pneumotoxin. [Gk *anti*, pneumotoxin.]

antipodagric (an·te·pod·**ag'**·rik). 1. Applied to a remedy which conduces to the relief of gout. 2. A remedy for gout. [Gk *anti, podagra* gout.]

antipraxia (an·te·**prax**·e·ah). Applied to conditions in which symptoms appear to be in opposition to each other or in which there is lack of harmony in various functions. [Gk *anti, praxis* a doing.]

antipraxy (an·te·**prax**·e). The theory that the effect of a large dose of a drug is exactly the opposite of that of a small dose, and vice versa. [see prec.]

antiprostate (an·te·**pros**·tate). Anteprostate.

antiprostatitis (an·te·pros·tat·**i'**·tis). Anteprostatitis.

antiprotease (an·te·**pro**·te·aze). A substance found in bacteria and capable of arresting proteolysis. [Gk *anti*, protease.]

antiprothrombin (an·te·pro·**throm'**·bin). An anticoagulant which slows or inhibits the conversion of prothrombin into thrombin. The substance may be derived from the liver and other organs of the body. [Gk *anti*, prothrombin.]

antiprotozoal, antiprotozoan (an·te·pro·to·**zo'**·al, an·te·pro·to·**zo'**·an). Having the power to stop the growth of protozoa, or to destroy them. [Gk *anti*, protozoa.]

antipruriginous (an·te·proor·**ij'**·in·us). Applied to substances which are conducive to the lessening of itching. [Gk *anti*, L *prurire* to itch.]

antipruritic (an·te·proor·**it'**·ik). 1. Any remedy which relieves the sensation of itching or prevents its occurrence. 2. Descriptive of a substance which allays or prevents itching. [see prec.]

antipsoric (an·te·**so**·rik). 1. A remedy for scabies (itch). 2. Applied to any agent useful in preventing or curing scabies. [Gk *anti, psora* itch.]

antipyic, antipyogenic (an·te·**pi**·ik, an·te·pi·o·**jen'**·ik). Term applied to any remedy or other treatment which prevents the formation of pus or decreases the quantity produced. [Gk *anti, pyon* pus, *genein* to produce.]

antipyresis (an·te·pi·**re'**·sis). The treatment of feverish conditions or the reduction of the degree of fever by administration of antipyretics. [see foll.]

antipyretic (an·te·pi·**ret'**·ik). 1. A drug or other remedy for the allaying of fever. 2. Descriptive of substances or a form of treatment by the use of which fever is reduced. Cooling; antifebrile. [Gk *anti, pyretos* fever.]

antipyrin (an·te·**pi**·rin). Phenazone, 1-phenyl-2,3-dimethyl pyrazolone, $CHCO[=C(CH_3)N(CH_3)]NC_6H_5$. A white crystalline compound, soluble in water, and used as a reagent for ferric chloride and nitrous acid. Medicinally its action is more rapid than that of phenacetin but of shorter duration. Antipyrin itself is now obsolescent and has been dropped from the *British Pharmacopoeia*, but its salts are still used in certain proprietary preparations. [Gk *anti, pyr* fire.]

antipyrinomania (an·te·pi·rin·o·**ma'**·ne·ah). 1. A state of insanity resulting from excessive or too long continued use of antipyrin. 2. Addiction to antipyrin. [antipyrin, mania.]

antipyrotic (an·te·pi·**rot'**·ik). 1. An application for the relief of burns or scalds. 2. Antiphlogistic. 3. Applied to any medicament which relieves the sensation of burning. [Gk *anti, pyr* fire.]

antirabic (an·te·**rab**·ik). Antilyssic: 1. A remedy or drug used in the treatment of suspected cases of rabies and for its cure. 2. Conducive to the prevention or cure of rabies. [Gk *anti*, rabies.]

antirennet, antirennin (an·te·**ren**·et, an·te·**ren**·in). A substance present in blood serum which counteracts the enzymic effects of rennin and prevents the curdling of milk. [Gk *anti*, rennet.]

antirheoscope (an·te·**re**·o·skope). An apparatus used in the investigation of vertigo of visual origin. [Gk *anti, rhoia* flow, *skopein* to view.]

antiricin (an·te·**ri**·sin). An antitoxin which forms in the blood as the result of the injection of ricin into the body.

antirobin (an·te·**ro**·bin). An antitoxin which forms in the blood after the injection of robin, a poisonous principle from the bark of *Robinia pseudacacia.*

antiscorbutic (an·te·skor·**bew'**·tik). 1. A remedy for scurvy or minor degrees of vitamin C deficiency. 2. Term denoting that a substance is effective in the treatment of scurvy. [Gk *anti*, L *scorbutus* scurvy.]

antisensitization (an·te·sen·sit·i·**za'**·shun). The condition produced by Ehrlich in the serum of a goat by injecting the animal with inactivated haemolytic serum of a rabbit which had been immunized with red cells of an ox. The goat's serum when mixed with red ox cells and haemolytic serum prevents sensitization of the cells by the haemolysin. [Gk *anti*, sensitize.]

antisensitizer (an·te·**sen**·sit·i·zer). Anti-amboceptor. [see prec.]

antisepsis (an·te·**sep**·sis). The prevention of infection in tissues, particularly skin and mucous membranes, by causing the exclusion or destruction of harmful microbes. **Physiological antisepsis.** The degree of immunity from infection which prevails in the body as the result of the combined efforts of the various protective mechanisms to preserve health by destroying harmful organisms. [Gk *anti, sepsis* decay.]

antiseptic (an·te·**sep**·tik). A chemical sterilizing substance sufficiently non-toxic for superficial application to living tissues in order to kill pathogenic microbes or prevent their growth. The antiseptics belong to a variety of chemical substances, e.g. alcohols, metallic salts, phenols, acridine dyes, etc., and are commonly applied to the intact skin before surgical operation or injections, or they are applied to broken skin after wounds, burns, etc., or to certain mucous membranes, e.g. conjunctiva, bladder, to prevent or treat superficial infections. [Gk *anti, sepsis* decay.]

See also: DAKIN, LISTER (J.).

antiserum (an·te·**seer**·um). A general term for serum (human or animal) containing antibodies, produced naturally or artificially, to pathogenic microbes or their products, e.g. bacterial toxins (antitoxin). It may be used in the prevention, treatment or amelioration of specific infections, e.g. diphtheria, tetanus, measles. The antibodies or immunoglobulins in the serum are often concentrated by the removal of unwanted proteins such as albumin. **Antilymphocytic antiserum.** An antiserum used to facilitate tissue grafting. **Diagnostic antisera.** Antisera used in the identification of micro-organisms, blood groups, etc. **Rabies Antiserum BP 1973.** An antiserum prepared from native serum containing antiviral globulins or their derivatives with neutralizing effect on the rabies (fixed) virus. **Therapeutic antisera.** Antisera containing antibodies to pathogenic bacteria or their products, used in the treatment or prevention of specific infections. [Gk *anti*, L *serum* whey.]

antisialic (an·te·si·**al'**·ik). 1. Checking the secretion of saliva. 2. An antisialogogue. [Gk *anti, sialon* saliva.]

antisialogogue (an·te·si·**al'**·o·gog). 1. Any agent which lessens or stops the flow of saliva. 2. Term descriptive of a drug or other substance which checks the secretion of saliva. [Gk *anti, sialon* saliva, *agogos* leading.]

antisideric (an·te·sid·er·ik). In chemistry, a substance which is incompatible with iron and inhibits its action. [Gk *anti, sideros* iron.]

antisocial (an·te·so·shal). Not companionable; not complying with the ordinary rules of the society in which the subject is living. [Gk *anti*, L *socius* comrade.]

antispasmodic (an·te·spaz·mod′·ik). 1. Able to prevent or relieve spasm or convulsion. 2. Any substance which lowers the tonus of plain muscle, usually by direct action on the muscle itself. In some cases they exert their effect by interfering with the passage of nervous impulses either in the ganglia or at the neuromuscular junctions of the nerves which are stimulating the muscle concerned. The most important are belladonna, the volatile oils and papaverine, which may be used to relieve the spasm of the intestinal musculature in colic. The nitrites are particularly effective in relieving the spasm of the coronary arteries in angina pectoris; they also help to relieve biliary and renal colic. Atropine, adrenaline and papaverine are particularly effective in the treatment of the bronchiolar spasm of asthma. [see foll.]

antispastic (an·te·spas·tik). 1. Any drug or other agent which allays or prevents convulsion or spasm, or soothes excitement; an antispasmodic. 2. A counter-irritant. 3. Term applied to a drug which has a sedative effect on the nervous system. [Gk *anti*, spasm.]

antisplenetic (an·te·splen·et′·ik). 1. A medicine of use in diseases of the spleen. 2. Term applied to such medicines. [Gk *anti*, spleen.]

antistalsis (an·te·stal·sis). Movement of the faeces upwards instead of progression downwards. [Gk *anti, stalsis* contraction.]

antistaphylococcal, antistaphylococcus (an·te·staf·il·o·kok′·al, an·te·staf·il·o·kok′·us). Destructive of the staphylococcus; checking staphylococcal infection. [Gk *anti*, staphylococcus.]

antistaphylohaemolysin, antistaphylolysin (an·te·staf·il·o·he·mol′·is·in, an·te·staf·il·ol′·is·in). A substance found in healthy blood serum and antagonistic to the toxic properties of the staphylococcus. [Gk *anti*, staphylococcus, Gk *haima* blood, lysin.]

antistatic (an·te·stat·ik). Materials treated so that they conduct electricity, so avoiding the accumulation of static charges which might cause an explosion. [Gk *anti, statikos* causing to stand.]

antisteapsin (an·te·ste·ap′·sin). An enzyme which inhibits the action of the fat-splitting ferment (steapsin) present in the pancreatic juice. [Gk *anti*, steapsin.]

antistreptococcal (an·te·strep·to·kok′·al). A drug or other substance which has an adverse effect on, or prevents the poisonous action of, the streptococcus. [Gk *anti*, streptococcus.]

antistreptokinase (an·te·strep·to·kin′·aze). An agent that antagonizes streptokinase. [Gk *anti*, streptokinase.]

antistreptolysin (an·te·strep·tol′·is·in). A drug or other substance which inhibits the action of the haemolytic streptolysin. **Antistreptolysin-O.** An antibody against streptolysin O. Serum titre is elevated in patients suffering from infections due to Lancefield group A streptococci or the sequelae (e.g. rheumatic fever) of such infections. [Gk *anti*, streptolysin.]

antistrumous (an·te·stroo·mus). Term applied to remedies efficacious in the treatment of tuberculous adenitis and goitre. [Gk *anti*, L *struma* scrofulous tumour.]

antisudoral, antisudorific (an·te·sew·dor·al, an·te·sew·dor·if′·ik). Anhidrotic. [Gk *anti*, L *sudor* sweat, *facere* to make.]

antisyphilitic (an·te·sif·il·it′·ik). A remedy which is specific in curing syphilis. [Gk *anti*, syphilis.]

antitabetic (an·te·tab·et′·ik). An agent that is of use in the cure of tabes dorsalis, or is effective in arresting its progress or relieving its symptoms. [Gk *anti*, tabes.]

antitetanic (an·te·tet·an′·ik). An agent which conduces to the relaxing of muscular contraction in tetanus. [Gk *anti*, tetanus.]

antithenar (an·te·the·nar). 1. In a position opposite to the palm or the sole. 2. Hypothenar. [Gk *anti, thenar* palm, sole.]

antithermic (an·te·ther·mik). 1. Cooling. 2. Term applied to any remedy for feverishness; antifebrile. [Gk *anti, therme* heat.]

antithrombin (an·te·throm·bin). A substance present in blood plasma. It prevents coagulation of the blood in the vessels by inhibiting the action of thrombin. [Gk *anti*, thrombin.]

antithromboplastin (an·te·throm·bo·plas′·tin). A substance that antagonizes thromboplastin. [Gk *anti*, thromboplastin.]

antithyroid (an·te·thi·roid). An agent which counteracts the influence exerted by the thyroid gland. [Gk *anti*, thyroid.]

antithyrotrophin (an·te·thi·ro·tro′·fin). A substance that appears in the serum after repeated administration of thyrotrophic hormone and produces the opposite effect to that of the hormone when injected into another individual. [Gk *anti*, thyrotrophin.]

antithyrotropic (an·te·thi·ro·trop′·ik). Opposing or inhibiting the action of the thyrotropic hormone; counteracting the effects of excessive secretion of the hormone. [Gk *anti*, thyrotropic.]

antitonic (an·te·ton·ik). 1. Diminishing tonicity or tone. 2. Diminishing or checking the action of a tonic. [Gk *anti, tonos* tone.]

antitoxic (an·te·tox·ik). 1. An antidote. 2. Term applied to any treatment which counteracts the effect of a poison; referring to antitoxin. [Gk *anti*, toxin.]

antitoxigen (an·te·tox·e·jen). Any substance that induces or stimulates the formation of antitoxin in animal organisms. [antitoxin, Gk *genein* to produce.]

antitoxin (an·te·tox·in). An antibody produced against a toxin, especially a bacterial exotoxin. When appropriate amounts of toxin and the corresponding antitoxin are mixed together, the mixture is non-toxic. This neutralization occurs in fixed multiple proportions and can be demonstrated both *in vitro* and *in vivo.* Immunity against certain diseases depends on the presence of circulating antitoxins in the blood. Certain bacteria produce disease solely by means of their toxin, e.g. *Corynebacterium diphtheriae*, and against these a relatively low concentration of antitoxin in the blood confers protection against natural infection. Such small amounts of antitoxin can be demonstrated in human beings by means of injecting intradermally a minute amount of toxin: a skin reaction signifies lack of antitoxin, whilst no reaction shows the presence of enough antitoxin to neutralize the test dose of toxin; this is the basis of the Schick test for immunity to diphtheria and the Dick test for scarlet fever. In active immunization, antitoxin is formed by the patient. Antitoxic sera are sera obtained from animals actively immunized against bacterial toxins. Such sera contain relatively large amounts of antitoxin and can be used for short-term prophylaxis or for the treatment of disease. In treatment, the function of the antitoxin is to neutralize the toxin before it can affect the cells, and it must therefore be administered early. The estimation of antitoxic potency, or standardization of antitoxic sera, is achieved by comparing them with "standard sera". Antitoxic units are calculated on the basis of neutralizing a certain amount of toxin when tested in animals. Antitoxins, like other antibodies, are associated with the globulin fraction of the serum. Commercially-prepared horse antitoxins, after concentration of the antibodies or immunoglobulins by ammonium sulphate precipitation or treatment with proteolytic enzymes and then standardized in units, are, or may be, used in the treatment and prophylaxis of toxic infections, e.g. diphtheria, tetanus, botulism and gas gangrene. For individuals sensitized to horse protein, antitoxin produced in other animals, e.g. ox, ass, may be used. Human immunoglobulins derived from immunized individuals are replacing horse antitoxins in the prophylaxis and treatment of tetanus in some countries. **Alpha antitoxin.** An antitoxin specific for the alpha toxin of *Clostridium perfringens.* **Avidity of antitoxin.** The ability to form a firm union with toxin. **Botulinum Antitoxin BP 1973.** An antitoxic serum obtained from animals injected with botulinus toxin; usually a bivalent serum containing antitoxins to both types A and B. **Bovine antitoxin.** One prepared in the cow. Commercial antitoxins unless otherwise specified are generally obtained from the horse. In case of sensitization to horse serum, antitoxin obtained from another species should be used, or the patient desensitized. **Concentrated antitoxin.** An antitoxin prepared by ammonium sulphate precipitation of the globulins, removal of the ammonium sulphate by dialysis, and redissolving the precipitate in a smaller amount of physiological salt solution. **Diphtheria Antitoxin BP 1973.** One prepared by immunizing horses with diphtheria toxoid: the serum used therapeutically is standardized as regards strength and quality. **Mixed Gas-gangrene Antitoxin BP 1973.** Polyvalent gas-gangrene antitoxin (see below). **Natural antitoxin.** An antitoxin which occurs in the sera of normal individuals. **Perfringens antitoxin.** Welchii antitoxin (see below). **Polyvalent gas-gangrene antitoxin.** A serum which is available for prophylactic use in cases where the causative agent cannot be determined. It contains *Clostridium welchii* antitoxin as well as antitoxin prepared against the toxins of *Clostridium septicum* and *Clostridium oedematiens*: it can also be used as a curative agent in gas gangrene in conjunction with antibiotic therapy. **Refined antitoxin globulin.** A globulin prepared by treating the material with proteolytic enzymes: this method also results in considerable concentration, and by removal of non-essential proteins lessens the likelihood of serum reactions. Gamma globulin, obtained from normal human sera by electrophoresis, is used for prophylaxis against measles. **Scarlet Fever Antitoxin BP 1963.** Streptococcus antitoxin (see below). **Snake venom antitoxin.** Venom antiserum, antivenin, antitoxin obtained from animals immunized against the particular venom. **Staphylococcus Antitoxin BP 1968.** An antitoxin prepared against staphylococcal toxoid; seldom used now. **Streptococcus antitoxin.** One prepared against the erythrogenic toxin of streptococci, and used in the treatment of toxic cases of scarlet fever. **Tetanus Antitoxin BP 1973.** An antitoxin obtained by immunizing horses with tetanus toxoid and toxin: the serum is of great value in the prophylaxis of tetanus if given immediately after sustaining a wound likely to be infected with tetanus; as a curative agent it is less reliable. **Welchii antitoxin BP 1968.** A serum prepared against the toxins of *Clostridium welchii*, and used for the prophylaxis and treatment of gas gangrene produced by this organism. [Gk *anti, toxikon* poison.]

antitoxinogen (an·te·tox·**in**'·o·jen). Antitoxigen.

antitragicus muscle [musculus antitragicus (NA)] (an·te·**tra**·je·kus). An intrinsic muscle of the auricle on the lateral surface; it covers the antitragus and extends on to the antihelix and the tail of the helix.

antitragus [NA] (an·te·**tra**·gus). A small tubercle on the auricle of the ear, above the lobule and opposite the tragus. [Gk *anti*, tragus.]

antitrismus (an·te·**triz**·mus). A condition of tonic muscular spasm in which the mouth is forced open and cannot be closed. [Gk *anti, trismos* gnashing of the teeth.]

antitrope (an·te·trope). 1. Antibody. 2. One of a pair of bilaterally symmetrical parts of an organism. [Gk *anti, trepein* to turn.]

antitrypsic (an·te·**trip**·sik). Antitryptic.

antitrypsin (an·te·**trip**·sin). An antiferment which inhibits the action of trypsin. **Alpha$_1$ antitrypsin.** A protein which inhibits tryptic activity; deficiency may be associated with pulmonary emphysema in young adults or with hepatitis in infants. [see foll.]

antitryptic (an·te·**trip**·tik). Any agent which counteracts the digestive action of trypsin. [Gk *anti*, trypsin.]

antituberculin (an·te·tew·**ber**'·kew·lin). An antibody to the tubercle bacillus which forms in the blood and other body fluids as a result of injections of tuberculin. [Gk *anti*, tuberculin.]

antituberculous (an·te·tew·**ber**'·kew·lus). Applied to any agent which is efficacious in checking the progress or hindering the spreading throughout the body of tuberculosis. [Gk *anti*, tuberculosis.]

antitulase (an·te·**tew**·laze). A serum used for immunization against tuberculosis; it was prepared from the blood of animals which had been injected with tulase. [Obsolete term.] [Gk *anti*, tulase.]

antitussive (an·te·**tus**·iv). 1. A remedy for cough. 2. Term applied to any preparation which relieves or checks cough. [Gk *anti*, L *tussis* cough.]

antityphoid (an·te·**ti**·foid). Preventing or curing typhoid fever. [Gk *anti*, typhoid.]

antityrosinase (an·te·ti·**ro**'·sin·aze). An anti-enzyme the action of which counteracts that of tyrosinase. [Gk *anti*, tyrosinase.]

antiuratic (an·te·ewr·**at**'·ik). 1. An agent which prevents the precipitation of urates. 2. Term applied to substances which restrict or prevent the formation of urates. [Gk *anti*, urate.]

antiurease (an·te·**ewr**·e·aze). An antiferment which hinders or suppresses the action of urease. [Gk *anti*, urease.]

antivenene (an·te·**ven**·een). Antivenom serum prepared by injecting into suitable animals at intervals gradually increasing amounts of the venom of snakes or poisonous insects; the serum may be monovalent or polyvalent according to whether the venom of a single species or of several species is used. Therapeutically, the serum is injected intravenously in large doses, e.g. 20–30 ml. **Bothropic antivenene.** Serum prepared against the venom of vipers of the genus *Bothrops*. **Crotalus antivenene.** Serum prepared against the venom of vipers of the genus *Crotalus*. [Gk *anti*, L *venenum* poison.]

See also: CALMETTE.

antivenereal (an·te·ven·**eer**'·e·al). 1. Term applied to any drug or system of treatment administered for the prophylaxis or cure of venereal disease. 2. Referring to any drug or measure of anaphrodisiac character. [Gk *anti*, venereal.]

antivenin (an·te·**ven**·in). The active principle in antivenomous sera against snake or insect bite. [Gk *anti*, L *venenum* poison.]

antivenom (an·te·**ven**·om). An antitoxic serum against snake venom; antivenene. [see foll.]

antivenomous (an·te·**ven**·om·us). Applied to any drug or other substance which acts as an antidote to or counteracts the effects of snake or other venom. [Gk *anti*, L *venenum* poison.]

antivermicular (an·te·ver·**mik**'·ew·lar). 1. A remedy for infestation with intestinal worms. 2. Having the power to destroy worms. 3. Antiperistaltic. [Gk *anti*, L *vermis* worm.]

antiverminous (an·te·**ver**·min·us). 1. Antivermicular. 2. Any remedy for or form of treatment directed against the condition of being infested with body lice or other parasite. [Gk *anti*, L *vermis* worm.]

antiviral (an·te·**vi**·ral). Applied to any substance which inhibits the growth of a virus either by direct action on the virus or indirectly by acting on the host or host cells. [Gk *anti*, virus.]

antivirus (an·te·**vi**·rus). Killed broth-cultures of staphylococci or streptococci used to produce local immunity by application to the skin; the term is now obsolete. [Gk *anti*, virus.]

antivitamins (an·te·**vi**·tam·inz). Substances which exert metabolic effects antagonistic to those of the vitamins. They are synthetic analogues of the vitamins, obtained by modification of the vitamin molecule, chiefly by substitution. Examples are pyrithiamine, gluco-ascorbic acid, pyridine-3-sulphonic acid, isoriboflavin and pantoyl taurine, which are antagonistic respectively to aneurine, ascorbic acid, nicotinic acid, riboflavin and pantothenic acid. [Gk *anti*, vitamin.]

antixenic (an·te·**zen**·ik). Referring to the reaction set up in living tissue by the introduction of a foreign substance. [Gk *anti, xenos* foreign.]

antixerophthalmic (an·te·zer·of·**thal**'·mik). Preventing or counteracting xerophthalmia: the term is applied most commonly to vitamin A. [Gk *anti*, xerophthalmia.]

antixerotic (an·te·zer·**ot**'·ik). Preventing the condition of abnormal dryness (xerosis), as of the skin. [Gk *anti*, xerosis.]

antizymohexase (an·te·zi·mo·**hex**'·aze). A substance neutralizing zymohexase. [Gk *anti*, zymohexase.]

antizymotic (an·te·zi·**mot**'·ik). 1. Applied to any agent or form of treatment directed against infectious (zymotic) diseases. 2. Denoting any substance or process which hinders the development of, or checks, fermentation, or the action of which is opposed to that of ferments. [Gk *anti*, zymosis.]

antodontalgic (ant·o·dont·**al**'·jik). Anti-odontalgic.

Anton, Gabriel (b. 1858). Czech neurologist and psychiatrist.

Anton's symptom. Failure on the part of a patient who is blind to recognize the fact; it may occur in disease of both parieto-occipital lobes.

antophthalmic (ant·of·**thal**·mik). 1. Referring to the prevention, relief or cure of ophthalmia. 2. Any substance that has these properties. [Gk *anti*, ophthalmia.]

antorgastic (ant·or·**gas**·tik). Anaphrodisiac. [Gk *anti*, *orge* passion.]

antozone (**ant**·o·zone). Name given to atomic oxygen, O, produced when a high-voltage electric discharge is passed through oxygen at low pressure; an extremely active oxidizing agent. [Gk *anti*, ozone.]

antracele (an·trah·seel). Antrocele.

antral (ant·ral). Referring to an antrum.

antrectomy (an·**trek**·to·me). Surgical excision of the walls of an antrum, more especially those of the tympanic (mastoid) antrum. [antrum, Gk *ektome* a cutting out.]

antritis (an·**tri**·tis). An inflamed condition of an antrum, particularly the maxillary sinus. [antrum, Gk *-itis* inflammation.]

antro-atticotomy (an·tro·at·ik·**ot**'·o·me). The surgical operation of making an opening into and removing the contents of the tympanic antrum and the epitympanic recess (attic). [antrum, Gk *temnein* to cut.]

antrocele (**an**·tro·seel). A collection of fluid in an antrum, particularly the maxillary sinus. [antrum, Gk *kele* hernia.]

antrochoanal (an·tro·**ko**'·an·al). Relating to the antrum and nasal cavity. [Gk *antron* cave, *choane* funnel.]

antroduodenectomy (**an**·tro·dew·o·de·**nek**'·to·me). The surgical removal of the first part of the duodenum together with the gastric antrum, followed by an end-to-end anastomosis. [antrum, duodenum, Gk *ektome* excision.]

antrodynia, antronalgia (an·tro·**dine**·e·ah, an·tron·**al**·je·ah). Pain felt in an antrum or sinus, generally the maxillary sinus. [antrum, Gk *odyne* pain.]

antronasal (an·tro·**na**·zal). Referring to the maxillary sinus and the nose. [Gk *antron* cave, nose.]

antrophose (**an**·tro·foze). A subjective sensation in the line of vision, as of colour, the origin of which lies in the central ocular mechanism. [Gk *antron* cave, *phos* light.]

antropyloric (an·tro·pi·**lor**'·ik). Belonging to or involving the pyloric part of the stomach. [Gk *antron* cave, pylorus.]

antrorse (ant·**rors**). In biology, having an upward or forward direction. [L *ante*, *versus* turned.]

antroscope (**an**·tro·skope). 1. An instrument for the ocular examination of a cavity. 2. An instrument for the illuminated examination of the maxillary sinus. [Gk *antron* cave, *skopein* to view.]

antroscopy (an·**tros**·ko·pe). Inspection of an antrum or sinus by means of an antroscope.

antrostomy (an·**tros**·to·me). The making of a surgical incision into an antrum or sinus so that the contents may be drained away. [antrum, Gk *temnein* to cut.]

antrotome (**an**·tro·tome). An instrument for making an opening into an antrum or sinus. [see prec.]

antrotomy (an·**trot**·o·me). Surgical incision through the wall of an antrum or sinus. [antrum, Gk *temnein* to cut.]

antrotonia (an·tro·**to**·ne·ah). Increased tension of the wall of the pyloric antrum. [antrum, Gk *tonos* a stretching.]

antrotympanic (**an**·tro·tim·**pan**'·ik). Referring to the tympanic antrum and the tympanic cavity.

antrotympanitis (**an**·tro·tim·pan·**i**'·tis). An inflammatory condition involving the tympanic cavity and the tympanic antrum. It may be either acute or chronic, and catarrhal or suppurative in character. [antrum, tympanum, Gk *-itis* inflammation.]

antrum [NA] (**an**·trum). A cavity or hollow; commonly used for a cavity surrounded by bone. **Cardiac antrum.** An unusual dilatation of the oesophagus, above the diaphragm but near the cardiac orifice of the stomach. **Dental antrum.** The pulp cavity of a tooth. **Antrum folliculi.** The cavity of an ovarian follicle. **Mastoid antrum.** Tympanic antrum (see below). **Maxillary antrum.** Antrum of Highmore; the maxillary air sinus. **Pyloric antrum [antrum pyloricum (NA)].** The part of the cavity of the stomach immediately preceding the pylorus. **Tympanic antrum [antrum mastoideum (NA)].** An extension backward and upward from the middle ear with which the mastoid air cells communicate. [Gk *antron* cave.]

See also: HIGHMORE.

antuitarism (an·**tew**·it·ar·izm). The condition of which gigantism or acromegaly is a symptom; the cause is hyperfunction of the anterior lobe of the hypophysis cerebri. [anterior, pituitary.]

Antyllus. 2nd century A.D. Greek physician and surgeon.

Antyllus' method, or operation. Ligation of an artery just proximal and just distal to an aneurysm, with evacuation of the aneurysm.

Antyllus-Kuhnt operation. Kuhnt's operation, 1st def.

anuclear (a·**new**·kle·ar). Without nuclei; applied to non-cellular tissues. [Gk *a*, nucleus.]

anuresis (an·ewr·e·sis). Inability to pass urine. [Gk *a*, uresis.]

anuria (an·ewr·e·ah). Complete cessation of the secretion and excretion of urine. **Angioneurotic anuria.** The anuria associated with circulatory interference that is present in necrosis of the cortex of the kidney. **Calculous anuria.** Anuria resulting from obstruction or blockage by a calculus or calculi. [Gk *a*, urine.]

anuric (an·**ewr**·ik). Affected with or having the characteristics of anuria.

anurous (an·**ewr**·us). Term used in zoology to indicate a tail-less state. [Gk *a*, *oura* tail.]

anus [NA] (**a**·nus). The opening of the terminal part of the alimentary canal (the anal canal) in the posterior part of the perineum. **Artificial anus.** An opening made in the colon through the abdominal wall by the operation of colostomy above the diseased area, in the lower colon or rectum. **Covered anus.** An anus covered by the excessive fusion of embryological structures. **Ectopic anus.** A normal anal opening that is abnormally placed, e.g. side by side with the vaginal opening. **Entero-uterine anus.** A condition in which faecal matter is discharged from the uterus following rupture or perforation of that organ. [Obsolete term.]. **Fissure of anus.** A painful ulcer of the anal margin caused by a tear during defaecation. It is accompanied by spasms of the external sphincter muscle and much pain on defaecation. It may become chronic and indurated, and small abscesses or fistulae may develop. **Fistula of anus.** A sinus resulting from the bursting of an ischiorectal abscess. The sinus may open through the skin (a blind external fistula), into the anal canal (a blind internal fistula), or into both positions (a complete fistula in ano). **Ileovaginal anus.** A condition in which the ilium discharges its contents into the vagina. **Imperforate anus.** One where there is no opening from the rectum to the exterior owing to failure of the cloacal membrane to break down. There may be a slight depression in the anal region or the anus may be well formed but separated from the rectum by a thin membrane. **Infundibuliform anus.** A relaxed condition of the anus with flattening of the usual folds. **Preternatural anus.** An anus situated in some abnormal site; a colostomy. **Umbilical anus.** An opening of the bowel at the umbilicus. **Anus vestibularis, Vulvovaginal anus.** A condition in which there is no true anus and the rectum opens into the vulva. [L.]

See also: BARTHOLIN (T.), RUSCONI.

anusitis (a·nus·**i**·tis). Inflammation of the anus. [anus, Gk *-itis* inflammation.]

anvil (**an**·vil). The incus. [AS *anfilt*.]

anxietas (ang·**zi**·et·as). The Latin for *anxiety*. **Anxietas praesenilis.** A form of involutional melancholia in which anxiety is the predominant feature. **Anxietas tibiae, Anxietas tibiarum.** 1. A sensation of malaise and tiredness in the muscles of the legs, accompanied by twitching, so that the sufferer has continually to change the position of the limbs. 2. A restless moving of the legs; fidgeting. Cf. ASTHENIA CRURUM PARAESTHETICA.

anxiety (ang·**zi**·et·e). An emotional condition in which feelings of fear, dread and mental agitation predominate. **Castration anxiety.** Castration complex. *See* COMPLEX. **Anxiety neurosis.** *See* NEUROSIS. **Situation anxiety.** A sensation of nervous apprehension which affects a person at the beginning of a new enterprise. **Anxiety state.** Anxiety neurosis. *See* NEUROSIS. [L *anxietas*.]

anytin (an·it·in). Anitin. A dark-brown substance prepared from ichthyol; it has germicidal properties.
anytol (an·it·ol). Anitol. One of the group of germicides formed by phenols, cresols and alcohols, with anytin.
aochlesia (a·ok·le·ze·ah). 1. Catalepsy. 2. A state of quietness or restfulness. [Gk *a*, *ochlesis* disturbance.]
aorta [NA] (a·or·tah). The main arterial trunk of the body, beginning at the left ventricle of the heart and ending opposite the body of the 4th lumbar vertebra by dividing into the 2 common iliac arteries. It is a typical "elastic" artery, as opposed to a "muscular" one. For descriptive purposes it is divided as follows: *ascending aorta* [aorta ascendens (NA)], passing from the left ventricle upwards and slightly to the right to end in the *arch of the aorta* [arcus aortae (NA)], which curves downwards (*descending aorta* [aorta descendens (NA)]) and to the left to become the *descending thoracic aorta* [aorta thoracica (NA)]; the latter passes downwards, at first to the left of the bodies of the thoracic vertebrae, and leaves the thorax anterior to the body of the 12th thoracic vertebra through the aortic opening in the diaphragm. Here it becomes the *abdominal aorta* [aorta abdominalis (NA)], anterior to the bodies of the upper 4 lumbar vertebrae. **Aorta angusta.** A narrow aorta. **Branches of the thoracic aorta, mediastinal [rami mediastinales (NA)].** Branches to the lymph glands and tissue of the mediastinum. **Branches of the thoracic aorta, oesophageal [rami esophagei (NA)].** Four or five small branches to the wall of the oesophagus from the descending thoracic aorta. They anastomose with oesophageal branches of the inferior thyroid, left phrenic and left gastric arteries. **Branches of the thoracic aorta, pericardial [rami pericardiaci (NA)].** Branches of the descending thoracic aorta to the posterior surface of the pericardium. **Branches of the thoracic aorta, phrenic [arteriae phrenicae superiores (NA)].** Small branches from the lower end of the descending thoracic aorta to the back of the diaphragm. **Aorta chlorotica.** A small aorta described in some cases of chlorosis. **Dorsal aortae.** Two, right and left, in the early embryo, running longitudinally beneath the notochord. At an early stage they fuse caudal to the heart to form a single channel, the descending thoracic and abdominal aorta of the adult; cranially they remain bilateral as the common and internal carotid arteries. **Dynamic aorta.** The markedly pulsating abdominal aorta seen in some neurotic persons. **Left aorta.** The left dorsal aorta (see above). **Palpable aorta.** The abdominal aorta that is easily felt owing to thinness and laxness of the abdominal wall. **Pericardiac aorta.** The ascending aorta which is included within the pericardium. **Pulsating aorta.** Visible pulsation of the abdominal aorta. **Right aorta.** The right dorsal aorta (see above). **Throbbing aorta.** Forcible pulsations of the abdominal aorta which are easily seen and felt. **Ventral aorta.** The single arterial trunk which springs from the heart in fishes and from which the branchial arterial arches are derived; it is represented in the human embryo by the aortic sac, subsequently divided into the pulmonary trunk and the ascending aorta. [Gk *aerein* to raise.]
aortal (a·or·tal). Aortic.
aortalgia (a·or·tal·je·ah). A sensation of pain round about or in the region of the aorta. [aorta, Gk *algos* pain.]
aortarctia (a·or·tark·she·ah). A condition in which there is stenosis of the aorta; aortostenosis. *See also* COARCTATION, AORTIC. [aorta, L *arctare* to narrow.]
aortectasia, aortectasis (a·or·tek·ta′·ze·ah, a·or·tek·tas·is). A state of dilatation of the aorta. [aorta, Gk *ektasis* a stretching.]
aortectomy (a·or·tek·to·me). Resection of a segment of the aorta, e.g. in the operation for the relief of coarctation. [aorta, Gk *ektome* excision.]
aortic (a·or·tik). Referring to the aorta, or aortic valve. **Aortic lymph gland.** *See* GLAND. **Aortic opening.** *See* OPENING. **Aortic orifice.** *See* ORIFICE. **Aortic plexus.** *See* PLEXUS. **Aortic valve.** *See* VALVE.
aorticopulmonary (a·or·tik·o·pul′·mon·ar·e). Aortopulmonary.
aorticorenal (a·or·tik·o·re′·nal). Term denoting that both the aorta and the kidneys are involved. [aorta, L *ren* kidney.]
aortism (a·or·tizm). 1. Hodgson's disease; dilatation due to aneurysm of the proximal part of the aorta. In addition, the heart may be enlarged or dilated. 2. The state of being constitutionally prone to disease of the aorta.
aortismus abdominalis (a·or·tiz·mus ab·dom·in·a·lis). Phantom aneurysm. *See* ANEURYSM. [aorta, L of the stomach.]
aortitis (a·or·ti·tis). A condition of inflammation affecting the aorta. **Nummular aortitis.** Aortitis in which, post mortem, white patches of circular shape are to be found on the inner coat of the vessel. **Syphilitic aortitis.** Syphilitic inflammation of the outer and middle coats of the first part and arch of the aorta, leading to a typical clinical syndrome, and sometimes to development of an aneurysm. **Aortitis syphilitica obliterans.** A form of syphilitic aortitis in which branches of the aorta or the aorta itself become greatly thickened and narrowed. [aorta, Gk *-itis* inflammation.]
See also: DOEHLE, HELLER (A. L. G.), WELCH (F. H.).
aortoclasia, aortoclasis (a·or·to·kla′·ze·ah, a·or·to·kla′·sis). Rupture of the aorta. [aorta, Gk *klasis* a breaking.]
aortography (a·or·tog·raf·e). The injection of an opaque medium into the blood and subsequent x-ray examination of the aorta. **Retrograde aortography.** Radiography of the abdominal aorta opacified by contrast medium forcefully injected into the femoral artery after temporary occlusion of the artery distal to the needle. **Translumbar aortography.** Aortography by means of direct injection of the contrast medium into the abdominal aorta through the lumbar region. [aorta, Gk *graphein* to record.]
aorto-iliac (a·or·to·il′·e·ak). Pertaining to the aorta and the iliac arteries; commonly applied to atheromatous disease concentrated in this area or to operations for such disease. [Gk *aerein* to raise, L *ilia* flank.]
aortolith (a·or·to·lith). A deposit of calcareous material in the wall of the aorta. [aorta, Gk *lithos* stone.]
aortolithia (a·or·to·lith′·e·ah). A condition in which calcareous deposits or calculi are formed in the aorta. [see prec.]
aortomalacia (a·or·to·mal·a′·she·ah). A condition in which the walls of the aorta have become abnormally soft. [aorta, Gk *malakia* softness.]
aortomesenteric (a·or·to·mes·en·ter′·ik). Relating to the aorta and a mesenteric artery, e.g. a by-pass operation. [aorta, mesentery.]
aortopathy (a·or·top·ath·e). Any disease involving the aorta. [aorta, Gk *pathos* disease.]
aortoptosis (a·or·top·to′·sis). Displacement downwards of the abdominal aorta in association with visceroptosis. [aorta, Gk *ptosis* fall.]
aortopulmonary (a·or·to·pul′·mon·ar·e). Pertaining to the aorta and the pulmonary artery, and used to describe congenital communications between their origins (aortopulmonary septal defect) or surgical anastomoses made between them. [aorta, L *pulmoneus* relating to the lungs.]
aortorrhaphy (a·or·tor·af·e). In surgery, the suturing of the aorta. [aorta, Gk *rhaphe* seam.]
aortosclerosis (a·or·to·skler·o′·sis). A condition in which the walls of the aorta have become abnormally hard. [aorta, Gk *skleros* hard.]
aortostenosis (a·or·to·sten·o′·sis). A condition in which the lumen of the aorta is narrowed or in which stricture occurs; aortarctia. *See also:* COARCTATION, AORTIC. [aorta, Gk *stenosis* a narrowing.]
aortotomy (a·or·tot·o·me). The operation of making an incision into the aorta. [aorta, Gk *temnein* to cut.]
aosmic (a·oz·mik). Devoid of odour. [Gk *a*, *osme* odour.]
apallaesthesia (a·pal·es·the′·ze·ah). Pallanaesthesia; a condition in which the power to receive vibrations is lacking or has been lost, or in which the vibrations of a tuning-fork cannot be appreciated. [Gk *a*, *pallein* to quiver, aesthesia.]
apancrea (a·pan·kre·ah). The state of being without a pancreas. [Gk *a*, pancreas.]
apancreatic (a·pan·kre·at′·ik). 1. Caused by lack of the pancreas. 2. Term denoting that the pancreas is not involved. [see prec.]
apandria (ap·an·dre·ah). Excessive and morbid aversion to the male sex. [Gk *apo*, *aner* man.]

apanthropia, apanthropy (ap·an·**thro**·pe·ah, ap·**an**·thro·pe). 1. Apandria. 2. Pathological aversion to or dread of the society of human beings; abnormal desire for solitude. [Gk *apo, anthropos* man.]

aparalytic (a·par·al·it′·ik). Not affected by paralysis. [Gk *a*, paralysis.]

aparathyreosis (a·par·ah·thi·re·**o**′·sis). Aparathyrosis.

aparathyroidism (a·par·ah·**thi**′·roid·izm). The state obtaining when the parathyroid glands are inactive or are not functioning properly. [Gk *a*, parathyroid.]

aparathyrosis (a·par·ah·thi·**ro**′·sis). The physical condition resulting from disordered function of the parathyroid glands or from their surgical removal. [Gk *a*, parathyroid, Gk *-osis* condition.]

apareunia (a·par·ew·ne·ah). Absence of or inability to perform coitus. [Gk *a, para, eune bed.]*

aparthrosis (ap·ar·**thro**·sis). 1. In anatomy, a term applied to a joint, e.g. the shoulder joint, which moves freely in any direction; diarthrosis. 2. A state of dislocation of a joint. [Gk *apo*, arthrosis.]

apastia (ap·**as**·te·ah). The refusal to take food as a feature of certain mental disorders. [Gk fasting.]

apastic (ap·**as**·tik). Referring to apastia.

apathic (ap·**ath**·ik). Referring to a state of apathy; apathetic.

apathism (**ap**·ath·izm). A state in which stimulation of any kind elicits only a slow response. [Gk *a, pathos* suffering.]

apathy (**ap**·ath·e). Indifference to surroundings and to anything that would excite interest in normal circumstances. [see prec.]

apatite (**ap**·at·ite). Native tricalcium orthophosphate, of the general formula $3Ca(PO_4)_2CaX_2$, where X is usually chlorine or fluorine; found in Canada and Norway, and used as fertilizers. **Carbanato apatite.** The phosphate of bone and teeth which appears to be $3Ca(PO_4)_2CaCO_3$, related in composition to the mineral apatites. [Gk *apate* deceit, because easily misidentified.]

apatropine (ap·**at**·ro·peen). Apo-atropine.

ape (ape). Properly, a member of the family Pongidae, that includes the gibbon, chimpanzee, gorilla and orang-utan. **Anthropoid ape.** Used incorrectly to designate the family Pongidae. **Barbary ape.** A monkey of the genus *Macaca.* **Black ape, Celebes ape.** A monkey of the genus *Cynopithecus.* **Ape fissure.** *See* FISSURE. **Ape hand.** *See* HAND. [AS *apa.*]

apectomy (a·**pek**·to·me). Apicectomy.

apeidosis (ap·i·**do**·sis). Progressive modification or disappearance of the clinical and histological characteristics of a disease so that in form or aspect or both it becomes atypical. [Gk *apo, eidos* form.]

apella (a·**pel**·ah). An individual who has been circumcised, or who has a short prepuce. [Gk *a, pella* skin.]

apellous (a·**pel**·us). 1. Term applied to a penis from which the prepuce is lacking or of which it is short. 2. Term applied to a wound lacking cicatrix or skin. [see prec.]

Apelt, Friedrich (b. 1877). Hamburg physician.

Nonne–Apelt reaction. Equal volumes of cerebrospinal fluid and saturated ammonium sulphate are shaken together and allowed to stand for at least 3 min. If globulin is present the liquid becomes opalescent or turbid, or a precipitate forms, depending upon the amount present. Normal fluids remain clear or faintly opalescent.

apenteric (ap·en·**ter**·ik). Abenteric. [Gk *apo, enteron* intestine.]

apepsia (a·**pep**·se·ah). Complete cessation of the digestive function. **Achlorhydria apepsia.** Failure of the stomach to produce digestive secretions. **Hysterical apepsia, Apepsia nervosa.** Anorexia nervosa. [Gk *a, pepsis* digestion.]

apepsinia (a·pep·**sin**·e·ah). A condition in which there is deficiency in or failure of the peptic secretion by the stomach. [see prec.]

apeptic (a·**pep**·tik). Affected with or appertaining to apepsia.

aperient (ap·**eer**·e·ent). 1. Describing drugs which have a laxative action. 2. A purgative of a mild nature. [L *aperire* to open.]

aperiodic (a·peer·e·**od**′·ik). 1. Descriptive of membranes which can take up any vibrations to which they are subjected since they have not any intrinsic vibrations. 2. In physics, denoting absence of periodic vibrations. [Gk *a*, periodic.]

aperistalsis (a·per·is·**tal**′·sis). A condition in which the peristaltic movement of the intestine is not occurring. [Gk *a*, peristalsis.]

aperitive (ap·**er**·it·iv). 1. A stimulant of the appetite. 2. Aperient, or stimulating. **Hygienic aperitive.** Any hygienic measure which has a beneficial effect on the appetite. [L *aperire* to open.]

Apert, Eugène (b. 1868). Paris paediatrician.

Apert's disease, or syndrome. Acrocephalosyndactyly.

apertometer (ap·er·**tom**·et·er). An instrument for measuring microscope apertures.

See also: ABBÉ.

aperture (**ap**·er·tewr). 1. [Apertura (NA)] A hole or opening. 2. In an optical instrument, the size of the opening admitting light. 3. In dentistry, the foramen at the apex of the root of a tooth. **Angular aperture.** The angle included between the 2 limiting rays entering an optical system in a meridian plane; the angle which the entrance-pupil of an optical system subtends at the object. **Bony aperture of the nose, anterior [apertura piriformis (NA)].** The pear-shaped anterior opening in the skull which leads into the nasal cavities. **Bony aperture of the nose, posterior, right and left [choanae (NA)].** The openings which lead from the nasal cavity to the nasopharynx. **Aperture of the fourth ventricle, lateral [apertura lateralis ventriculi quarti (NA)].** Foramen of Luschka; the opening of the lateral recess of the 4th ventricle into the cerebellomedullary cisterna. **Aperture of the fourth ventricle, median [apertura mediana ventriculi quarti (NA)].** Foramen of Magendie; the medial foramen in the tela chorioidea of the 4th ventricle, which opens into the cisterna cerebello-medullaris. **Aperture of the frontal sinus [apertura sinus frontalis (NA)].** The opening of the frontonasal duct into the middle meatus of the nose at the anterior end of the hiatus semilunaris. **Aperture of the larynx.** The opening which leads into the larynx from above; it lies behind the epiglottis and between the aryepiglottic folds. **Aperture of a lens.** The angle between 2 lines from the focus of the lens to opposite ends of one of its diameters. **Numerical aperture.** N.A. Of an optical instrument, the product of the sine of half the angular aperture and the refractive index of the medium between the object and the objective. The quantity of light entering an instrument is proportional to the square of its numerical aperture. In the case of a microscope, its limit of resolution is inversely proportional to its N.A. **Palpebral aperture.** The gap between the eyelids when the eyes are open. **Aperture ratio.** *See* RATIO. **Aperture of the sphenoidal sinus [apertura sinus sphenoidalis (NA)].** The opening from the sinus into the spheno-ethmoidal recess of the nose. **Tympanic aperture of the canaliculus for the chorda tympani [apertura tympanica canaliculi chordae tympani (NA)].** A small aperture at the lower part of the anterior wall of the tympanum, just above the petrotympanic fissure (gasserian fissure). [L *apertura.*]

apex (a·pex). 1. Summit; top; point, as of a cone. 2. [Apex (NA)] In anatomy, the more or less pointed or conical extremity of an organ or part of the body; often, but not always, its highest point. **Apex of the arytenoid cartilage [apex cartilaginis arytenoideae (NA)].** *See* CARTILAGE, ARYTENOID. **Apex of the auricle.** *See* AURICLE. **Apex of the bladder [apex vesicae (NA)].** *See* URINARY BLADDER. **Apex of the heart [apex cordis (NA)].** *See* HEART. **Apex height.** The size of contraction of a summated muscle twitch. **Apex of the lung [apex pulmonis (NA)].** *See* LUNG. **Apex of the nose [apex nasi (NA)].** The tip of the nose. **Orbital apex.** The posterior conical extremity of the orbital cavity where the optic foramen is situated. **Apex of the patella [apex patellae (NA)].** *See* PATELLA. **Apex of the petrous part of the temporal bone [apex partis petrosae (NA)].** *See* TEMPORAL BONE. **Apex of the prostate [apex prostatae (NA)].** *See* PROSTATE. **Root apex [apex radicis dentis (NA)].** The pointed extremity of the root of a tooth. **Apex of the sacrum [apex ossis sacri (NA)].** *See* SACRUM. [L summit.]

Apgar, Virginia (b. 1909). American anaesthetist.

Apgar score. A system, described in 1953, by which the

condition of a newly-born infant can be assessed one (or more) minutes after its birth. A score of 0, 1 or 2 is given in each of 5 variables—heart rate, respiratory effort, muscle tone, colour and reflex irritability. The maximum score is 10.

aphacia (af·a·se·ah). A condition in which the lens of the eye is absent. [Gk *a, phakos* lens.]

aphacic (af·a·sik). Term applied to an eye devoid of the lens. [see prec.]

aphagia (af·a·je·ah). A condition in which the power to swallow is lacking. **Aphagia algeria.** Refusal to take food because it causes pain. [Gk *a, phagein* to eat.]

aphakia (af·a·ke·ah). Aphacia.

aphakic (af·a·kik). Aphacic.

aphalangia (a·fal·**an**·je·ah). Absence of the fingers or toes or both; the condition may be congenital or acquired. [Gk *a, phalagx* a finger bone.]

aphalangiasis (a·fal·an·**ji**'·as·is). A condition of absence of fingers or toes, because of disease, as in leprosy. [see prec.]

Aphaniptera (af·an·**ip**·ter·ah). Siphonaptera; an order of insects, the fleas, characterized by the absence of wings, lateral flattening and hind legs modified for jumping. The larvae are apodal. Members of the genera *Ctenocephalides, Oropsylla, Pulex, Tunga* and *Xenopsylla* are of medical importance. [Gk *aphanizein* to abolish, *pteron* wing.]

aphanisis (a·**fan**·is·is). A state of apprehension lest sexual potency be lost. [Gk *aphanizein* to abolish.]

aphanozoa (af·an·o·**zo**'·ah). Name given by Kruse (1914) to the ultramicroscopic and filter-passing agents of infection, now known as *viruses.* [Gk *aphanes* invisible, *zoon* animal.]

aphantobiont (a·**fan**·to·**bi**'·ont). Any one of the ultramicroscopical particles that constitute a filtrable virus. [Gk *aphantos* invisible, *bion* a living thing.]

aphasia (af·a·ze·ah). Defect or loss of the power to produce or to understand spoken or written speech, due to pathological interference with the speech centre or speech region in the brain. This is situated on both sides of the brain, but in right-handed people predominantly on the left side, in an area including the posterior end of the inferior frontal convolution (Broca's speech area), and the posterior end of the first temporal convolution (hearing). The visual centre, it must be noted, is situated in the angular gyrus. The cause of the symptoms is damage in the cortical and subcortical regions of these areas, and also in the fibres linking them and so preventing either proper reception or production of spoken or written speech. According to the predominant defect on either the motor or the sensory side, the symptom complexes are varied. **Acoustic aphasia.** Auditory aphasia (see below). **Ageusic aphasia.** Inability to express in words ideas connected with the sense of taste. **Amnemonic aphasia, Amnesic aphasia, Amnestic aphasia.** Incapacity to remember words. **Amnosmic aphasia.** Inability to use the right words for ideas connected with the sense of smell. **Associative aphasia.** Commissural aphasia (see below). **Ataxic aphasia.** Motor aphasia (see below). **Auditory aphasia.** Word deafness: aphasia due to disease of the auditory centre of the brain; sounds are heard but their meaning is not understood. **Central aphasia.** That caused by an injury of the cerebral cortex. **Combined aphasia.** Two or more forms of aphasia present in the same individual. **Commissural aphasia.** That due to defective connection between the motor and the sensory speech centres, due to a lesion interrupting the path between motor and sensory centres. **Complete aphasia.** Total inability to communicate in any way with other people; the condition is caused by a lesion of all the centres concerned with language and the phenomena associated with language. **Conduction aphasia.** Commissural aphasia (see above). **Cortical aphasia, Cortical motor aphasia.** Typical motor aphasia, due to a cortical lesion. **Cortical sensory aphasia.** Typical sensory aphasia, due to a cortical lesion. **Expressive aphasia.** Motor aphasia (see below). **Expressive-receptive aphasia.** Global aphasia (see below). **Frontocortical aphasia.** Motor aphasia (see below). **Frontolenticular aphasia.** Commissural aphasia (see above). **Functional aphasia.** That due to excitement either in hysterical individuals or in those suffering from severe constitutional disorders. **Gibberish aphasia.** Use of meaningless phrases in a state of aphasia. **Global aphasia.** A form involving all the functions of speech. **Graphomotor aphasia.** Agraphia. **Impressive aphasia.** Sensory aphasia (see below). **Inchoate, Incipient, Ingravescent aphasia.** Latent aphasia. **Intellectual aphasia.** True aphasia (see below). **Isolated aphasia.** Subcortical aphasia (see below). **Jargon aphasia.** A form in which several words are expressed in a jumbled form as one word, with wrong placing of accent. **Latent aphasia.** A speech defect which is so very subtle as to elude superficial testing but can be discerned by sufficiently deep probing. **Lenticular aphasia.** Commissural aphasia (see above). **Aphasia lethica.** Amnemonic aphasia (see above). **Mixed aphasia.** Co-existent motor and sensory aphasia (see below). **Motor aphasia.** A form in which the individual, because of disease of the speech centre and consequent inco-ordination of muscles, cannot utter in words what he wishes to say. **Musical aphasia.** Amusia. **Nominal aphasia.** That characterized by the calling of objects by wrong names. **Optic aphasia.** Ability to perceive objects without the ability to name them or to recognize and remember names; anomia. **Parieto-occipital aphasia.** Co-existent alexia and apraxia. **Pathematic aphasia.** That due to fear or anger. **Pictorial aphasia.** Global aphasia (see above). **Psychosensory aphasia.** Inability to understand any form of the faculty of language or any phenomenon associated with language. **Puerperal aphasia.** That occuring during the puerperium or during pregnancy. **Pure aphasia.** Subcortical aphasia (see below). **Receptive aphasia.** Sensory aphasia (see below). **Residual aphasia.** The slight speech impairment of a person recovering from a cerebral lesion. **Semantic aphasia.** That form in which there is forgetfulness of words and inability to recognize their significance. **Sensory aphasia.** A type which is the result of injury to the receptive mechanism; the meaning of words both written and spoken is not understood. **Subcortical aphasia.** Aphasia due to the interruption of the subcortical nerve fibres between the centres. **Subcortical motor aphasia.** Pure word dumbness, attributed to a lesion of white matter beneath Broca's area. **Subpictorial aphasia.** Aphasia due to interference with the passage of impulses towards the afferent tracts to the auditory special centre. **Supracortical aphasia, Suprapictorial aphasia.** A form of aphasia due to interruption between the auditory and cortical centres, the auditory speech centre remaining intact, and the tracts proceeding to or from the motor speech centre being maintained. **Syntactical aphasia.** Inability to arrange words in correct order, so that what is spoken becomes nonsense. **Tactile aphasia.** Inability to name objects which have been touched. **Temporoparietal aphasia.** Cortical sensory aphasia (see above). **Total aphasia.** Mixed aphasia (see above). **Transcortical aphasia.** Mixed aphasia (see above) caused by a lesion interrupting the paths between the centres. **Transcortical motor aphasia.** Motor aphasia (see above) attributed to a lesion between Broca's area and a hypothetical central speech centre. **True aphasia.** Aphasia caused by injury to any one of the speech centres. **Aphasia universalis, Verbal aphasia.** Only slight ability to form words in the mind or to utter them. **Visual aphasia.** Alexia. [Gk *a, phasis* speech.]

See also: BROCA, GRASHEY, KUSSMAUL, LICHTHEIM, WERNICKE.

aphasiac (af·a·ze·ak). A person suffering from aphasia.

aphasic (af·a·zik). Affected with aphasia.

aphasiologist (af·a·ze·ol·o·gist). One who studies the pathology of language.

aphasiology (af·a·ze·ol·o·gy). The study of the phenomena of central disorders of language.

Aphasmidia (a·fas·**mid**·e·ah). A class of the phylum Nematoda, or sub-class when Nematoda are treated as a class, characterized by the absence of phasmids. The order Enoplata is of medical interest. [Gk *a*, phasmid.]

aphelotic (af·el·**ot**·ik). Denoting a state of being withdrawn or absent in mind; characterized by day dreaming. [Gk *aphelkein* to draw away.]

aphelxia (af·elx·e·ah). The state of being absent-minded or withdrawn into a dream and oblivious of external circumstances. [see prec.]

aphemaesthesia (af·em·es·the′·ze·ah). A condition of combined alexia and auditory aphasia; inability to hear spoken words and see written words. [Gk *a*, *pheme* speech, aesthesis.].

aphemia (af·e·me·ah). A name given by Bastian to motor aphasia. *See* APHASIA. [Gk *a*, *pheme* speech.]

aphemic (af·e·mik). Affected with or characterized by aphemia.

aphephobia (af·e·fo·be·ah). Pathological dread of being touched by other people or of coming in contact with objects. [Gk *aphe* touch, phobia.]

apheter (af·et·er). A hypothetical trigger substance, probably a catastate, which is held to decompose inogen and thus cause contraction of the muscles. [Gk sender.]

aphilanthropy (a·fil·an·thro·pe). A state in which antisocial feeling is manifested; it is evident often in incipient melancholia. [Gk *a*, *philein* to love, *anthropos* man.]

aphilopony (a·fil·op·on·e). A condition in which dislike or dread of physical exertion or work is so excessive as to be morbid. [Gk *a*, *philein* to love, *ponos* bodily exertion.]

aphonia (af·o·ne·ah). The inability to produce sound by means of the laryngeal mechanism. **Aphonia clericorum.** Clergyman's sore throat. *See* SORE THROAT. **Hysterical aphonia.** A form of aphonia due to hysteria. **Aphonia paranoica.** A state of obstinate silence maintained in mental disease. **Spastic aphonia.** Spasmodic contraction of the adductor muscles producing firm apposition of the true vocal cords during phonatory effort. It may result from a purely functional condition, or may sometimes be due to organic disease of the nervous system. [Gk *a*, *phone* voice.]

aphonic (a·fon·ik). Characterized by or referring to aphonia.

aphonogelia (a·fon·o·je′·le·ah). A condition in which the power to laugh out loud is lacking. [Gk *a*, *phone* voice, *gelos* laughter.]

aphoresis (a·for·e·sis). 1. Lack of the power to endure, e.g. pain. 2. The removal of a part, by excision or amputation. [Gk *a*, *pherein* to bear.]

aphoria (a·for·e·ah). Sterility in the sense of barrenness, and therefore referring to females. **Aphoria impercita.** That caused by physical aversion to coitus. **Aphoria impotens.** Aphoria due to lessened power of conception. **Aphoria incongrua.** Sterility held to be due to the failure of the seminal fluid to fertilize the ovum. **Aphoria paramenica.** Aphoria caused by disorders of menorrhoeal origin. **Aphoria polyposa.** Aphoria resulting from obstruction by a uterine polypus. [Gk *a*, *pherein* to bear.]

aphose (a·foze). A subjective sensation of a dark or shadowy patch in the line of vision. Cf. PHOSE. [Gk *a*, *phos* light.]

aphosphagenic (a·fos·fah·jen′·ik). A condition which is the result of lack or deficiency of phosphorus. [Gk *a*, phosphorus, Gk *genein* to produce.]

aphosphorosis (a·fos·for·o′·sis). The condition resulting from lack of phosphorus in the diet. Various manifestations are to be found in different countries. [Gk *a*, phosphorus.]

aphotaesthesia (a·fot·es·the′·ze·ah). A condition of reduced retinal sensitivity to light following undue exposure. [Gk *a*, *phos* light, *aisthesis* feeling.]

aphraenous (a·fre·nus). Demented. [Gk *a*, *phren* mind.]

aphrasia (a·fra·ze·ah). 1. Dumbness. 2. A language disorder in which words are understood and can be uttered but not in orderly sequence as in a phrase. **Aphrasia paralytica.** Aphrasia caused by paralysis of the faculty to form mental concepts. **Aphrasia paranoica.** In the insane, voluntary dumbness. **Superstitious aphrasia.** Prudery in speech occasioned by primness or religious scruples. [Gk *a*, *phrasis* a speaking.]

aphrenia (a·fre·ne·ah). The state of being demented or mad. Not having a mind. [Gk *a*, *phren* mind.]

aphrenic, aphrenous (a·fren·ik, a·fren·us). Demented. [see prec.]

aphrodisia (af·ro·diz·e·ah). 1. Sexual desire, particularly when it is immoderate or pathological. 2. Sexual indulgence. [Gk venery.]

aphrodisiac (af·ro·diz·e·ak). 1. Any drug which stimulates sexual desire. 2. Capable of stimulating sexual impulse. [see prec.]

aphrodisiomania (af·ro·diz·e·o·ma′·ne·ah). Erotomania; sexual madness. [aphrodisia, mania.]

aphronesia, aphronesis (af·ron·e·ze·ah, af·ron·e·sis). The state of being silly or mad. [Gk *a*, *phronesis* good sense.]

aphronia (a·fro·ne·ah). Impairment of the mental faculty, with faulty discernment. [Gk *a*, *phronein* to understand.]

aphthae (af·thee). Shallow, painful erosions of the oral mucosa and occasionally involving the external genitalia. They may occur singly or in crops and are usually recurrent. **Aphthae anginosae.** Minute ulcers which accompany a sore throat, with associated redness and swelling of the fauces. They may be on the mucosa of the mouth, throat and tongue, and scrapings from these areas may demonstrate Vincent's organisms. **Cachectic aphthae.** Riga's aphthae; aphthous ulcers which occur on the tongue, inner cheeks, palates, oesophagus and gastro-intestinal tract in a rare syndrome seen among children who are severely under-nourished and whose oral hygiene is bad. Antibiotic therapy is sometimes successful, but the outcome is usually fatal. **Chronic intermittent recurrent aphthae.** Mikulicz's aphthae; recurrent ulcers on the tongue and oral mucosa, associated with leucopenia, and which disappear with improvement in the blood picture. The granulocytes are most severely affected, and secondary infection may retard the usual return to normality. Sulphonamides should be avoided in treatment. **Contagious aphthae, Epizootic aphthae.** Foot and mouth disease. *See* DISEASE. **Aphthae febriles.** Aphthae occurring in a feverish condition where local infection has produced ulceration of the oral mucosa. **Major aphthae.** Periadenitis mucosa necrotica recurrens; deep, painful ulcers which tend to persist and leave a scar on healing. Occasionally a feature of Behçet's syndrome. **Minor aphthae.** Mikulicz's aphthae; idiopathic in origin, aphthae which may rarely be a manifestation of cyclical neutropenia and coincide with the fall in the neutrophil count. **Aphthae resistentiae.** Periadenitis mucosa necrotica recurrens, 2nd def. **Aphthae tropicae.** Ulceration of the mouth which frequently accompanies many disorders encountered in the tropics. Those affections which are associated with gross vitamin deficiency are most likely to demonstrate the aphthous areas in the mouth, and vitamin B_2 (riboflavine or lactoflavine) helps to cure the condition, with the appropriate specific and anti-infective therapy. [Gk *aphtha* eruption.]

See also: BEDNAR, CARDARELLI, MIKULICZ-RADECKI, RIGA, VALLEIX.

aphthargia (af·thar·ge·ah). Lingual spasm. *See* SPASM.

aphthenxia (af·thenx·e·ah). A form of aphasia in which there is inability to enunciate. [Gk *aphthegtos* voiceless.]

aphthoid (af·thoid). Any eruption resembling that of thrush. [Gk *aphtha* eruption, *eidos* form.]

aphthongia (af·thon·je·ah). A form of aphasia caused by spasmodic contraction of the muscles controlling speech. [Gk *a*, *phthoggos* sound.]

aphthosis (af·tho·sis). Any condition of which aphthae are a sign. [aphthae, Gk *-osis* condition.]

aphthous (af·thus). Affected with, characterized by or resembling thrush or aphthae.

aphylactic (a·fil·ak·tik). Denoting a condition characterized by aphylaxis.

aphylaxis (a·fil·ax·is). A state in which there is non-immunity to a disease. Lack of bodily defence against infection. [Gk *a*, *phylax* guard.]

aphytria retinae (a·fit·re·ah ret·in·e). A state of the eyes in which the retina loses its pigment; the cause is held to be toxaemia, the result of infective disease.

apical (a·pik·al). Located at, or appertaining to the apex of any structure.

apicectomy (a·is·ek·to·me). 1. Root resection; the operation of resection of the apex of the root of a dead tooth to eradicate infection; it is usually accompanied by curettage of surrounding infected alveolar bone. 2. Excision of the apex of the petrous part of the temporal bone. [apex, Gk *ektome* excision.]

apicilar (a·pis·il·ar). Situated on or attached to an apex.

apicitis (a·pis·i·tis). An inflammatory condition of the apex of any structure, e.g. the root of a tooth or the apex of the lung. [apex, Gk *-itis* inflammation.]

apicolysis (a·pik·ol·is·is). The therapeutic measure of incising the anterior wall of the thorax so that the upper portion of the lung is collapsed and the apex obliterated. [apex, Gk *lysis* a loosing.]

apicostome (a·pik·os·tome). An instrument with which apicostomy is carried out, consisting of cannula with trocar.

apicostomy (a·pik·os·to·me). The surgical procedure of cutting through the mucoperiosteum and bone to reach the apex of the root of a tooth. [apex, Gk *stoma* mouth.]

apicotomy (a·pik·ot·o·me). Incision into the apex of the petrous part of the temporal bone. [apex, Gk *temnein* to cut.]

Apidae (a·pid·e). A family of the order Hymenoptera that includes the honey bee. [L *apis* bee.]

apiin (a·pe·in). $C_{26}H_{28}O_{14}$. A glycoside found in parsley, *Apium petroselinum*; a yellow crystalline substance, insoluble in water, used as an aperient and diuretic, and in the treatment of amenorrhoea and dysmenorrhoea.

apinealism (a·pin·e·al·izm). The symptoms which appear after excision of the pineal body and the resultant state. [Gk *a*, pineal.]

apinoid (a·pin·oid). Clean; free from extraneous matter. [Gk *a*, *pinos* dirt, *eidos* form.]

Apiochaeta (a·pe·o·ke·tah). A genus of small dark hump-back flies belonging to the family Phoridae and found in the tropics. **Apiochaeta ferruginea** (*Megaselia scalaris*). A species which lays its eggs in putrefying meat, and which may cause wound myiasis. The larvae are frequently found in intestinal myiasis, especially in Burma. [L *apis* bee, Gk *chaite* hair.]

apiol (a·pe·ol). An extract of parsley used as a diuretic; also as an abortifacient. [L *apium* parsley.]

apiole (a·pe·ole). Parsley camphor, $C_3H_5C_6H(OCH_3)_2CH_2O_2$. An ether which occurs in parsley and celery.

apiophobia (a·pe·o·fo′·be·ah). Pathological fear of bees and of being stung by bees; melissophobia. [L *apis* bee, phobia.]

apiose (a·pe·oze). $(CH_2OH)_2C(OH)CH(OH)CHO$. A pentose found in apiin, the glycoside of parsley.

apiotherapy (a·pe·o·ther′·ap·e). A type of treatment in which bees are used to sting a particular part with a view to reactionary betterment or in which bee venom is administered, e.g. in the form of ointment; melissotherapy. [L *apis* bee, therapy.]

apiphobia (a·pe·fo′·be·ah). Apiophobia.

Apis mellifica (a·pis mel·if·ik·ah). The common honeybee, from which bee venom is obtained. It produces honey and beeswax, both of which are used in pharmacy. [L *apis* bee, *mel* honey, *facere* to make.]

apisin (a·pis·in). Bee venom. *See* VENOM. [L *apis* bee.]

apisination (a·pis·in·a′·shun). The condition of poisoning resulting from being stung by a bee or bees. [see prec.]

apitoxin (a·pe·tox·in). A toxic protein constituent of bee sting. [L *apis* bee, Gk *toxikon* poison.]

apituitarism (a·pit·ew·it·ar·izm). The condition in which there is absence or total arrest of the functional activity of the hypophysis cerebri (pituitary gland), on account of its removal or total atrophy. Dwarfism or hypophyseal cachexia results. [Gk *a*, pituitarism.]

Apium (a·pe·um). 1. A genus of plants including celery and parsley. 2. Apium BPC 1949 (Celery, Celery fruit, Celery seed), consists of the dried ripe fruits of cultivated plants of *Apium graveolens* (family Umbelliferae). It contains a volatile oil composed mainly of terpenes. Apium is used as a domestic remedy for rheumatism, but its therapeutic properties are doubtful. [L parsley.]

aplacental (a·plas·en·tal). In zoology, descriptive of mammals which have no placenta, e.g. the kangaroo. [Gk *a*, placenta.]

aplanasia (a·plan·a·ze·ah). Aplanatism.

aplanatic (a·plan·at·ik). 1. In optics, a term applied to a focus or lens to indicate its freedom from spherical aberration. 2. Term indicating a condition of aplanasia. [Gk *a*, *planan* to wander.]

aplanatism (a·plan·at·izm). In optics, complete or almost complete absence of spherical aberration. [Gk *a*, *planan* to wander.]

aplasia (a·pla·ze·ah). 1. A congenital state in which there is atrophy or absence of a part or organ. 2. A condition of the tissues in which they are defective or incomplete in development. **Aplasia axialis corticalis congenita.** Diffuse sclerosis. *See* SCLEROSIS. **Aplasia axialis extracorticalis congenita.** Merzbacher-Pelizaeus disease. **Dental aplasia.** Imperfect development of the teeth. **Germinal aplasia.** Defective development of the germinal tissues of the gonads. **Nuclear aplasia.** Imperfect development of the nuclei of the cranial nerves. **Aplasia pilorum intermittens.** Virchow's term for a condition in which the hairs are spindle-shaped. [Gk *a*, *plassein* to form.]

aplasmic (a·plaz·mik). Without protoplasm or sarcoplasm; a term applied to cells which are represented by their envelopes only. [see prec.]

aplastic (a·plas·tik). Referring to aplasia; unable to form, or not tending to develop new tissue.

apleuria (a·ploor·e·ah). A condition in which ribs are absent, generally congenitally, but the term may also be applied to acquired conditions. [Gk *a*, *pleura* rib.]

aplotomy (ap·lot·o·me). Simple incision. [Gk *aploos simple*, *temnein* to cut.]

apneumatic (ap·new·mat·ik). 1. Any part of a lung that is collapsed and uninflatable. 2. Denoting any surgical or other procedure during which air is excluded from the part being operated on. [Gk *a*, *pneuma* air.]

apneumatosis (ap·new·mat·o′·sis). Imperfect expansion or partial collapse of the lungs in the newly-born child; a collapsed state of the air cells of the lungs. [Gk *a*, *pneuma* air, *-osis* condition.]

apneumia (ap·new·me·ah). Congenital absence of the lungs. [Gk *a*, *pneumon* lung.]

apneusis (ap·new·sis). A condition which is the result of the removal of the upper part of the pons. There is extraordinary activity of inspiration, each breath drawn in being long and spasmodic. [Gk *a*, *pneusis* breathing.]

apnoea (ap·ne·ah). The cessation of breathing. 1. The state of being unable to draw breath; asphyxia. 2. The temporary pause in breathing which occurs after forced respiration. **Cardiac apnoea.** The temporary cessation of breathing characteristic of Cheyne-Stokes respiration. **Controlled apnoea.** Deliberate abolition of respiration, e.g. by an anaesthetist. First described by A. E. Guedel of Los Angeles in 1934. **Deglutition apnoea.** The temporary cessation of breathing which takes place during the act of swallowing. **Narcotic-induced controlled apnoea.** Intermittent positive pressure ventilation in a patient made apnoeic by the injection of a narcotic analgesic. **Apnoea neonatorum.** Asphyxia of the newborn. **Nervous apnoea.** Cessation of breathing caused by a disorder of the centres of respiration. **Traumatic apnoea.** Traumatic asphyxia. *See* ASPHYXIA. **Apnoea vagi.** The suspension of inspiration caused by stimulation of the vagus. **Apnoea vera.** The absence of respiratory movements as a result of acapnia and the failure of stimulation of the respiratory centres. **Voluntary apnoea.** Deliberate holding of the breath. [Gk *a*, *pnein* to breathe.]

apo-. Prefix, from the Greek preposition *apo*, meaning *from, away.*

apo-atropine (ap·o·at·ro·peen). Atropamine, $C_{17}H_{21}O_2N$. The anhydride of atropine formed by the elimination of water from the latter; also occurring naturally along with atropine in belladonna root. It is optically inactive and has no mydriatic properties. [Gk *apo*, atropine.]

apobiosis (ap·o·bi·o′·sis). 1. In physiology, death of a part of an organism. 2. Diminution of the vital activity of protoplasm. [Gk *apo*, *bios* life.]

apobiotic (ap·o·bi·ot′·ik). Applied to a change which lessens the vital activity of tissue. [see prec.]

apoblema (ap·o·ble·mah). The mass extruded in the process of abortion; any conglomeration of aborted matter. [Gk *apo*, *ballein* to throw.]

apocamnosis (ap·o·kam·no′·sis). 1. A condition in which a person quickly becomes very greatly fatigued. 2. A sensation of heaviness and numbness in a limb while it is in motion. 3. In myasthenia, an exceptional tendency to feel fatigued. [Gk *apokamnein* to grow very weary.]

apocarteresis (ap·o·kar·ter·**e**'·sis). Suicide by starvation. [Gk *apokarteresis*.]

apocatastasis (ap·o·kat·**as**'·tas·is). 1. Of an abscess or tumour, the stage during which it subsides and the surrounding area returns to a normal condition. 2. The process of restoration to a previous condition. [Gk *apokatastasis* restoration.]

apocatharsis (ap·o·kath·**ar**'·sis). Catharsis; purgation. [Gk *apo*, catharsis.]

apocathartic (ap·o·kath·**ar**'·tik). Cathartic. [see prec.]

apochromatic (ap·o·kro·**mat**'·ik). The term applied to an improved form of achromatic lens in which chromatic aberration is fully corrected, and spherical aberration is corrected completely for 2 colours. [Gk *apo*, *chroma* colour.]

apocleisis (ap·o·**kli**·sis). Aversion to eating. [Gk *apokleisis* a shutting up.]

apocodeine (ap·o·**ko**·deen). $C_{18}H_{19}O_2N$. An alkaloid derived from codeine by the elimination of a molecule of water. It blocks the responses of sympathetically innervated tissues. **Apocodeine hydrochloride.** $C_{18}H_{19}O_2NHCl$, a soluble form of apocodeine used as a hypodermic purgative because of its paralysing effect on the splanchnic nerves, resulting in increased peristalsis, but without vomiting. [Gk *apo*, codeine.]

apocope (ap·**ok**·o·pe). Amputation or abscission. [Gk *apokope* a cutting away.]

apocoptic (ap·o·**kop**·tik). Applied to a condition occurring as a result of amputation. [Gk *apokope* a cutting away.]

apocrine (**ap**·o·krine). 1. A term descriptive of a gland cell which loses part of its protoplasmic substance when it is secreting. 2. Applied to sweat glands which differ from ordinary (eccrine) sweat glands in that they occur only in hairy areas, especially the axilla, mons veneris, anus and mammary regions, are red instead of yellow, extend into the subcutaneous tissue and open usually into hair follicles. They are better developed in women than in men, are best developed in the Negro race and do not appear before puberty. The secretion contains cellular granules, not merely fluid droplets, and differs from the eccrine secretion also in containing iron; it is responsible for the characteristic odour of the body. [Gk *apo*, *krinein* to separate.]

apocynamarin (ap·o·sin·**am**'·ar·in). A crystalline aglycone found in Canadian hemp, the root of *Apocynum cannabinum*; used as a tonic, alterative, and cathartic.

apocynum (ap·o·**si**·num). Black Indian hemp; Canada hemp; dogbane; wild cotton; consists of the dried rhizome and roots of *Apocynum cannabinum* or of *Apocynum androsaemifolium* (family Apocynaceae). It contains apocynamarin, probably identical with the aglycone of cymarin, which is the most important cardio-active principle. Its therapeutic effects are related to digitalis. It is a powerful diuretic, making it particularly useful in dropsy. In the treatment of heart disease it is inferior to digitalis, being more irritant to mucous membranes and causing nausea, vomiting and even purgation. [Gk *apokynon* dogbane.]

apodactylic (ap·o·dak·**til**'·ik). Indicative of a state in which there is deprivation of the use of the fingers or the touch of the fingers. [Gk *apo*, *daktylos* finger.]

apodal (a·**po**·dal). 1. Characterized by the condition of apodia. 2. In zoology, term applied to an organism which is without feet. [Gk *a*, *pous* foot.]

apodemialgia (ap·o·de·me·**al**'·je·ah). A state of overpowering longing to travel or to leave home. The opposite of nostalgia. [Gk *apodemia* journey, *algos* pain.]

Apodemus (ap·o·**de**·mus). A genus of rodents, the long-tailed field or wood mice. **Apodemus agrarius.** A species which has been suspected as the rodent reservoir of the causal organism of acute haemorrhagic fever. **Apodemus speciosus.** A host of *Leptospira autumnalis* in the temperate Far East. **Apodemus sylvaticus.** The British species. [Gk *apodemein* to be away from home, *mys* mouse.]

apodia (a·**po**·de·ah). Congenital absence of feet. [Gk *a*, *pous* foot.]

apodous (a·**po**·dus). Apodal.

apoenzyme (ap·o·**en**·zime). The protein component of an enzyme which is dependent on the presence of coenzyme for its activity. The active complex of apoenzyme and coenzyme is known as the *holoenzyme*. [Gk *apo*, enzyme.]

apoferment (ap·o·**fer**·ment). Apozymase. [Gk *apo*, L *fermentum* leaven.]

apoferritin (ap·o·**fer**·it·in). A colourless protein of the globulin class, molecular weight about 460 000, obtained by removal of iron from ferritin by the action of a reducing agent in acid solution. Free apoferritin has not been detected in the body, and it would appear that iron is necessary either to initiate its synthesis or to prevent its breakdown in the tissues. [Gk *apo*, L *ferrum* iron.]

apogamia, apogamy (ap·o·**gam**·e·ah, ap·**og**·am·e). Non-sexual reproduction occurring in place of normal sexual reproduction; parthenogenesis. [Gk *apo*, *gamos* marriage.]

apogee (**ap**·o·je). The climax of a disease, involving the most severe aspects; often followed by crisis. [Gk *apo*, *ge* earth.]

apohaemoglobin (ap·o·he·mo·**glo**'·bin). The protein moiety of haemoglobin. [Gk *apo* from, haemoglobin.]

apokamnosis (ap·o·kam·**no**'·sis). Apocamnosis.

apolar (a·**po**·lar). In anatomy, without poles; commonly applied to nerve cells which are devoid of processes. [Gk *a*, pole.]

apolegamic (ap·**ol**·e·**gam**'·ik). In evolution, referring to selection, especially to sexual selection. [Gk *apolegein* to pick out, *gamos* marriage.]

apolepsis (ap·o·**lep**·sis). 1. The cessation of a natural function. 2. Retention of an excretion. 3. The arresting of secretion. [Gk a leaving off.]

apomixia, apomixis (ap·o·**mix**·e·ah, ap·o·**mix**·is). Non-sexual reproduction; parthenogenesis. [Gk *apo*, *mixis* a mingling.]

apomorphine (ap·o·**mor**·feen). $C_{17}H_{17}O_2N$. An artificial alkaloid prepared by the removal of water from the molecule of morphine. It has little narcotic action but stimulates the chemoreceptor trigger zone and causes vomiting when given subcutaneously and is used therefore as an emetic in acute poisoning. It should not be used, however, in cases of poisoning by depressants of the central nervous system, as it is apt to reinforce the depression. In small doses it increases the mucus in the respiratory tract and is a useful expectorant. **Apomorphine Hydrochloride BP 1973.** The soluble hydrochloride.

apomorphosis (ap·o·**mor**·fo·sis). A chemical change brought about in a compound by the removal of part of it. [Gk *apomorphosis* a changing of form.]

apomyoglobin (ap·o·mi·o·**glo**'·bin). The protein moiety of myoglobin. [Gk *apo* from, *mys* muscle, globin.]

apomyttosis (ap·o·mit·**o**'·sis). Any disease of which sneezing or stertorous breathing is a characteristic sign. [Gk *apomyssein* to blow the nose.]

aponal (ap·**on**·al). $CH_3CH_2C(CH_3)_2OOCNH_2$. The carbamate of dimethylethylcarbinol; a urethane derivative used as a hypnotic.

aponeurectomy (ap·o·newr·**ek**'·to·me). Surgical removal of the aponeurosis of a muscle. [aponeurosis, Gk *ektome* a cutting out.]

aponeurorrhaphy (ap·o·newr·**or**'·af·e). The suturing together of cut or torn aponeuroses or fasciae. [aponeurosis, Gk *rhaphe* seam.]

aponeurosis [NA] (ap·**on**·ewr·**o**'·sis). A sheet of collagenous fibres to which a muscle is attached and which takes the place of a cord-like tendon. Muscles with aponeurotic attachments usually have their fibres arranged in a flat sheet (e.g. the oblique muscles of the abdomen) but this is not always so, as in the case of the palmaris longus, where a fusiform muscle is inserted into the palmar aponeurosis. The term may be applied to any fascial thickening to which muscle fibres are attached, but it is usually limited in its application to more strictly defined structures. **Abdominal aponeuroses.** The aponeuroses of the oblique and transverse muscles. **Bicipital aponeurosis [aponeurosis musculi bicipitis brachii (NA)].** A flat, fibrous band passing from the tendon of the biceps muscle medially across the brachial artery to an attachment on the dorsal border of the ulna, essentially a thickening in the deep fascia of the forearm through which the biceps gains an accessory attachment to the ulna. **Epicranial aponeurosis [galea aponeurotica (aponeurosis epicranialis) (NA)].** The fibrous sheet which covers the vault of the skull and connects the occipital and frontal bellies of the occipitofrontalis muscle. **Palatal aponeurosis.** The expanded tendon of the tensor palati in the soft palate; all the other palatal muscles are attached to it. **Palmar aponeurosis [aponeurosis palmaris (NA)].** Deep fascia of the palm covering the muscles, palmar arterial arches, and terminal parts of the median and ulnar nerves. This fascia is thin over the thenar and hypothenar muscles but much thickened centrally. The central portion receives the tendon of the palmaris longus muscle and divides into 4 slips distally, 1 to each of the lateral 4 digits. **Plantar aponeurosis [aponeurosis plantaris (NA)].** The deep fascia of the sole of the foot, highly developed centrally [fasciculi transversi (NA)], and giving partial origin to some of the muscles in the sole. **Aponeurosis of the tongue [aponeurosis linguae (NA)].** A thin fibrous lamina attaching the root of the tongue to the hyoid bone. [Gk *apo, neuron* tendon.]

See also: PETIT (P.), ZINN.

aponeurositis (ap·**on**·ewr·o·**si**'·tis). An inflammatory condition of an aponeurosis. [aponeurosis, Gk *-itis* inflammation.]

aponeurotic (ap·**on**·ewr·**ot**'·ik). Of the same kind as, or referring to, an aponeurosis.

aponeurotome (ap·**on**·ewr·o·tome). A scalpel used for dividing aponeuroses. [aponeurosis, Gk *temnein* to cut.]

aponeurotomy (ap·**on**·ewr·**ot**'·o·me). Surgical division of aponeuroses. [see prec.]

aponia (a·**pon**·e·ah). 1. A state of absence of pain. 2. A state of non-exertion. [Gk *a, ponos* pain, bodily exertion.]

aponic (a·**pon**·ik). 1. Analgesic. 2. Descriptive of anything which relieves fatigue. [see prec.]

aponoea, aponoia (ap·o·**ne**·ah, ap·o·**noi**·ah). Amentia. [Gk *apo, nous* mind.]

apopathetic (ap·o·path·**et**'·ik). A term descriptive of a form of behaviour in which an individual noticeably modifies his conduct according to the presence or absence of other people. [Gk *apo, pathos* feeling.]

apophlegmatic (ap·o·fleg·**mat**'·ik). Expectorant; giving rise to a mucoid discharge from the air passages. [Gk *apo, phlegma* phlegm.]

apophylactic (ap·o·fil·**ak**'·tik). Pertaining to apophylaxis.

apophylaxis (ap·o·fil·**ax**'·is). Decrease in the protective or phylactic power of the blood, exemplified in the so-called negative phase of vaccine therapy. [Gk *apo, phylax* guard.]

apophysary (ap·**of**·iz·ar·e). Apophyseal.

apophysate (ap·**of**·is·ate). Term indicating the presence of an apophysis, or that a structure bears an apophysis.

apophyseal (ap·of·**iz**·e·al). Having reference to an apophysis.

apophysectomy (ap·**of**·is·**ek**'·to·me). Removal of an apophysis. [apophysis, Gk *ektome* excision.]

apophyseopathy (ap·o·**fiz**·e·**op**'·ath·e). 1. Any diseased condition of an apophysis. 2. Osteochondrosis of the tubercle of the tibia. [apophysis, Gk *pathos* disease.]

apophysial, apophysiary (ap·of·**iz**·e·al, ap·of·**iz**·e·ar·e). Apophyseal.

apophysis [NA] (ap·**of**·is·is). A process, outgrowth or projection of small size, most commonly of a bone. **Basilar apophysis.** The basilar part of the occipital bone. **Cerebral apophysis.** The pineal body. **Lenticular apophysis.** The lentiform nodule on the incus. **Zygomatic apophysis.** The zygomatic process of the temporal bone. [Gk a growing away.]

See also: INGRASSIA, RAU.

apophysitis (ap·**of**·is·**i**'·tis). 1. An inflammatory condition of an apophysis. 2. Osteochondrosis of the calcaneum. 3. Appendicitis. **Apophysitis tibialis adolescentium.** Osteochondrosis of the tubercle of the tibia. [apophysis, Gk *-itis* inflammation.]

apoplasmia (ap·o·**plaz**·me·ah). Deficiency of the plasma constituents of the blood. [Gk *apo*, plasma.]

apoplectic (ap·o·**plek**·tik). 1. A person affected with apoplexy or prone to attacks of apoplexy. 2. Of or pertaining to apoplexy.

apoplectiform, apoplectoid (ap·o·**plek**·te·form, ap·o·**plek**·toid). Having a resemblance to apoplexy. [apoplexy, L *forma*, Gk *eidos* form.]

apoplexia (ap·o·**plex**·e·ah). Apoplexy. **Apoplexia febricosa.** Febrile apoplexy. *See* APOPLEXY. **Apoplexia uteri.** A sudden effusion of blood into the uterus because of arterial degeneration or haemorrhagic infarction. [Gk stroke.]

apoplexy (ap·o·**plex**·e). 1. A sudden loss of consciousness (a "stroke"), the result of an acute vascular disturbance caused by the rupture of an intracerebral artery or its occlusion by thrombosis or embolism. The rupture of an extracerebral artery causing subarachnoid haemorrhage may also be a cause. 2. A sudden severe haemorrhage into any organ. [Obsolete term.] **Abdominal apoplexy.** Overwhelming abdominal bleeding due, for example, to a ruptured aneurysm of the abdominal aorta. **Adrenal apoplexy.** 1. Massive bleeding into the adrenal gland. 2. The clinical condition resulting from such bleeding. **Atherosclerotic apoplexy.** That due to atherosclerosis of the cerebral blood vessels. **Cerebellar apoplexy.** A form of apoplexy usually the result of thrombosis of the posterior inferior cerebellar artery; haemorrhage into the cerebellum may also be a cause. The patient has sudden intense vertigo and falls to the ground, but consciousness is not usually lost. **Delayed apoplexy.** Apoplexy occurring a few days or weeks after injury to the head in cases where cerebral vascular disease exists. **Febrile apoplexy.** Apoplexy with fever. **Fulminating apoplexy.** A form of very sudden onset in which the patient falls, passes into deep coma and dies. **Heat apoplexy.** Unconsciousness due to syncope in heat exhaustion or to coma in heat hyperpyrexia. **Ingravescent apoplexy.** An apoplexy of slow onset caused by the gradual escape of blood from a ruptured vessel. **Neonatal apoplexy.** Intracranial haemorrhage in the newborn. **Ovarian apoplexy, Placental apoplexy.** Respectively refer to sudden apoplectic haemorrhages into the organ or organs designated. **Pontine apoplexy.** One due to haemorrhage into the pons; it may commence with convulsions followed by deepening coma, pin-point pupils and hyperpyrexia. **Pulmonary apoplexy.** The result of embolism or thrombosis of a branch of the pulmonary artery. **Renal apoplexy, Retinal apoplexy.** Ovarian apoplexy (see above). **Spinal apoplexy.** Haemorrhage from a spinal blood vessel, causing symptoms of compression of the cord. **Uterine apoplexy, Uteroplacental apoplexy.** Ovarian apoplexy (see above). [Gk *apoplexia* stroke.]

apopnixis (ap·op·**nix**·is). Globus hystericus. [Gk *apopnigein* to choke.]

apopsychia (ap·o·si·ke·ah). Syncope; temporary loss of consciousness. [Gk *apo, psyche* spirit.]

apoptosis (ap·op·to·sis). The loosening or falling off of a dermal crust or scab, e.g. in disease or injury of the skin; also applied to falling scalp hair. [Gk *apo, ptosis* fall.]

apoquinamine (ap·o·**kwin**·am·een). $C_{19}H_{22}ON_2$. The anhydride of quinamine, an alkaloid found in cinchona bark.

apoquinine (ap·o·**kwin**·een). $C_{19}H_{22}O_2N_2$. An alkaloid found in cinchona bark, and isomeric with cupreine.

aporeine (ap·o·re·een). $C_{18}H_{16}O_2N$. An alkaloid obtained from a species of *Papaver*.

aporepressor (ap·o·re·**pres**'·or). A protein, synthesized under the direction of a regulator gene, which is only functional when bound with one or more specific small molecular weight compounds (called co-repressors). [Gk *apo* from, L *reprimere* to press back.]

aporetin (ap·o·**ret**·in). A brown resinous substance in rhubarb; it has purgative properties. [Gk *apo, rhetine* resin.]

aporia (ap·**or**·e·ah). Anxiety of a type shown especially by fevered patients. [Gk doubt.]

aporinosis (ap·o·rin·**o**'·sis). A term for any disease due to deficiency of an element in the diet. [Gk *aporos* scarce, *-osis* condition.]

aporioneurosis (ap·or·e·o·newr·o′·sis). Anxiety neurosis. *See* NEUROSIS. [Gk *aporia* doubt, neurosis.]

aporocephalus (ap·o·ro·kef′·al·us). A monster with a head which cannot easily be distinguished from the trunk. [Gk *aporos* indistinguishable, *kephale* head.]

aporrhipsis (ap·or·ip·sis). The action of discarding clothes or of throwing off bedclothes, generally associated with states of delirium or with conditions of insanity. [Gk *apo, rhiptein* to throw.]

aposepsis (ap·o·sep·sis). A term applied to matter which has become completely putrefied. [Gk putrefaction.]

aposia (ap·o·ze·ah). Adipsia: 1. Abnormal abstinence from drinking. 2. Complete lack of thirst. [Gk *a, posis* drinking.]

apositia (ap·o·sish·e·ah). A state of strong aversion to the taking of food; loathing inspired by the idea of food [Gk *apo, sitos* food.]

apositic (ap·o·sit·ik). Affected with apositia; giving rise to a strong aversion to food.

aposome (ap·o·some). A cytoplasmic inclusion originating by the activity of the cell itself. [Gk *apo, soma* body.]

apospory (ap·os·por·e). In botany, the lack of power to produce spores; applied to ferns and mosses which produce prothallia directly from the sporophyte. [Gk *apo*, spore.]

apostasis (ap·os·tas·is). The crisis or the end of an illness. [Gk a departure from.]

apostatic (ap·os·tat·ik). Pertaining to an apostasis.

apostem, apostema (ap·os·tem, ap·os·te·mah). An abscess. [Gk.]

aposthia (ap·os·the·ah). The state in which the prepuce is congenitally lacking. [Gk *a, posthe* foreskin.]

Apostoli, Georges (b. 1847). French physician.

Apostoli's treatment. The treatment of fibroids with electrotherapy.

apothanasia (ap·o·than·a′·ze·ah). The employment of measures to prolong life or delay death. [Gk *apo, thanatos* death.]

apothecary (ap·oth·e·kar·e). A pharmaceutical chemist [obsolete term]. [Gk *apotheke* a store.]

apothem, apothema, apotheme (ap·o·them, ap·o·them·ah, ap·o·theem). A dark-coloured precipitate seen in vegetable infusions exposed to the air, or in decoctions. [Gk *apo, thema* deposit.]

apothesis (ap·oth·es·is). The reduction of a fracture or dislocation. **Apothesis funculi umbilicalis.** During labour, the putting back of a protruded umbilical cord, generally by use of the apotheter. [Gk a putting back.]

apotheter (ap·oth·et·er). An appliance with which to replace a prolapsed umbilical cord during childbirth. [Gk *apo, tithenai* to place.]

apotripsis (ap·o·trip·sis). The removal of an opacity of the cornea. [Gk *apo, tribein* to rub.]

apotrophic (ap·o·trof·ik). Refers to any protoplasmic group, e.g. cells, growing at the extremity of some supporting tissue and away from the source of nutrition. [Gk *apo, trophe* nutrition.]

apous (a·pus). Apodal. [Gk *a, pous* foot.]

appalaesthesia (ap·al·es·the′·ze·ah). Pallanaesthesia.

apparatus (ap·ar·a·tus). 1. A single instrument or collection of instruments, appliances and material, used together to accomplish some purpose, operation or experiment. 2. In anatomy, a collection of structures or organs which serve a common function, e.g. the lacrimal apparatus [apparatus lacrimalis (NA)], consisting of the lacrimal gland, its ducts, the conjunctival sac, the lacrimal punctae and canaliculi, the lacrimal sac and the nasolacrimal duct. Occasionally the term is used in a specialized sense, e.g. the juxtaglomerular apparatus, for a cuff of cells, possibly contractile, surrounding the afferent arteriole to a renal glomerulus. **Absorption apparatus.** An apparatus used in gas analysis by means of which a constituent of the gas under examination is absorbed by a suitable reagent and its quantity determined through the reduction in volume. **Acoustic apparatus, Auditory apparatus.** Various component parts which, combined, produce the organ of hearing. **Canalicular apparatus.** Golgi apparatus. **Central apparatus.** The cell centre, which forms the asters and spindle during cell division. **Chromidial apparatus.** A basophilic mass of nucleoprotein in the cytoplasm of actively growing and protein-secreting cells. **CON apparatus.** An anaesthetic apparatus for use under field conditions, described in 1960, consisting of a mixture (non-flammable) of cyclopropane 40 parts, oxygen 30 parts and nitrogen 30 parts. **EMO apparatus.** An anaesthetic thermocompensated device for enabling a patient to inhale a controlled percentage of ether vapour in air (H. G. *E*pstein, R. R. *M*acintosh, *O*xford, 1956). **Emotril apparatus.** A thermocompensated anaesthetic apparatus for the self-administration of trichloroethylene vapour in air, used in obstetrics (*E*pstein, H. G., *M*acintosh, R. R., *T*richloroethylene, 1949). **Falling-plate apparatus.** An apparatus for determining the frequency of a tuning fork. **Fixed apparatus.** In dentistry, an orthodontic appliance which cannot be removed from the mouth by the patient. **Internal reticular apparatus.** Golgi apparatus. **Juxtaglomerular apparatus of the nephron.** A complex consisting of the granular juxtaglomerular cells in relation to the afferent arteriole, the efferent arteriole, some non-granular lacis cells and the macula densa of the distal convoluted tubule. The apparatus produces renin and may act as a sensor for the sodium concentration in the distal tubule. **Kite apparatus.** An apparatus for exercising the arm and hand. **Apparatus major.** The instruments used for median lithotomy. **Mental apparatus.** A general term embracing the available functions of the mind. **Apparatus minor.** The instruments used for lateral lithotomy. **Mitotic apparatus.** The complex of transient structures which appear at mitosis and are responsible for the movement and segregation of chromosomes during mitosis. It consists of asters, which in some cells surround a centriole, the spindle and a matrix in which the spindle fibres are formed. **Removable apparatus.** In dentistry, an orthodontic appliance which can be removed and inserted at will. **Sound-conducting apparatus.** The part of the auditory mechanism by which airborne sounds are conducted to the internal ear. This, therefore, will include the external and middle ear. **Sound-perceiving apparatus.** The part of the auditory mechanism which actually picks up and appreciates the sound waves. It includes the internal ear and its central connections. **Sucker apparatus.** Sucker foot; any of the numerous sucker-like terminal expansions of the processes of astrocytes which are applied to the walls of capillaries within the central nervous system. **Vocal apparatus.** The structures, particularly the larynx, which are used in the production of sound. [L *ad, parare* to prepare.]

See also: ABBÉ, BARCROFT, BECKMANN, BENEDICT (F. G.), BOYLE (H. E. G.), BOYLE (R.), CARREL, CLAYTON, CLOVER, COXETER, ESBACH, FELL, FINSEN (N. R.), FISCHER (M. H.), FLOSDORF, GOLGI, GUTHRIE-SMITH, HALDANE, HAMILTON IRVING, HARE (R.), HEIDBRINK, HEMPEL, JANKER, JUNKER, KEKWICK, KIRSCHNER, KJELDAHL, KROGH, LINDBERGH, LINDEMANN, LUNGE, MCKESSON, MARRIOTT (H. L.), MINNITT, MUDD, MUSHIN, O'DWYER, ORSAT, PERRONCITO, PFEIFFER, POTAIN, PRANA, REICH, RICHES, ROTH (P.), SAYRE, SHIPWAY, SOXHLET, TALLERMAN, TIMOFEEW, TISELIUS, TWINING, VAN SLYKE, WANGENSTEEN, WARBURG (O. H.), ZANDER, ZEISS, ZÜND-BURGUET.

apparition (ap·ar·ish·un). An illusory or hallucinatory experience, usually visual, relating to the phantom appearance of a person. [L *aparere* to come in sight.]

appearance (ap·eer·ans). **Beaten-silver appearance.** A neuroradiological term describing the inner wall of the skull vault, seen almost entirely in children, often indicating raised intracranial pressure. Also known as *digital markings*; the markings are an imprint of the cerebral convolutions. **Faded-leaf appearance.** In pernicious anaemia, the dark speckled appearance of the cardiac muscle. **Gross appearance.** The appearance of tissue regarded with the naked eye. **Ground-glass appearance.** In asbestosis, the filmy appearance of the lung caused by fibrosis. [L *aparere* to come in sight.]

Appelbaum, Leo. 19th–20th century physician.

Recklinghausen-Appelbaum disease. Haemochromatosis.

appendage (ap·en·daje). A part or outgrowth from the body or from an organ, small relative to the whole; used collectively for the accessory structures associated with a particular organ. **Auricular appendage.** 1. The auricle of each atrium of the heart. 2. A term for the antitragus. **Caecal appendage.** The vermiform appendix. *See* APPENDIX. **Cutaneous appendages, Dermal appendages.** Appendages of the skin (see below). **Epiploic appendages.** Appendices epiploicae. *See* APPENDIX. **Appendages of the eye.** The conjunctiva, eyebrows, eyelashes and lacrimal apparatus. **Appendages of the fetus.** The placenta, membranes and umbilical cord. **Ovarian appendages.** The epoöphoron and paroöphoron. **Pineal appendage.** The pineal body. *See* BODY. **Pituitary appendage.** The hypophysis cerebri. **Appendages of the skin.** Sebaceous glands, sweat glands and nails. **Testicular appendage.** Small vestigial structures occurring in relation to the testis or epididymis. **Uterine appendages.** The ovaries, uterine tubes and the ligaments of the uterus. **Vermicular appendage.** The vermiform appendix. *See* APPENDIX. [L *appendere* to hang upon.]

appendalgia (ap·en·**dal**·je·ah). A sensation of pain in the neighbourhood of the vermiform appendix. [appendix, Gk *algos* pain.]

appendectomy (ap·en·**dek**·to·me). Appendicectomy.

appendekthlipsia (ap·en·dek·**thlip'**·se·ah). Removal of the appendix, a clamp being left on the stump and the wound closed around it. [appendix, Gk *thlipsis* compression.]

appendical, appendiceal (ap·en·dik·al, ap·en·dis·e'·al). Referring to an appendix, in most cases the vermiform appendix.

appendicealgia (ap·en·dis·e·**al'**·je·ah). Appendalgia.

appendicectasis (ap·en·dis·**ek'**·tas·is). A condition of dilatation of the vermiform appendix. [appendix, Gk *ektasis* a stretching.]

appendicectomy (ap·en·dis·**ek'**·to·me). 1. Surgical removal of the vermiform appendix. 2. The operation of cutting away an appendage. [appendix, Gk *ektome* a cutting out.]

appendices (ap·en·dis·eez). Plural of appendix. *See* APPENDIX.

appendicism (ap·en·dis·izm). A condition in which there are symptoms in the neighbourhood of the vermiform appendix suggestive of appendicitis or of other abnormality.

appendicitis (ap·en·dis·**i'**·tis). An inflamed condition of the vermiform appendix, with or without obstruction of its lumen. **Acute appendicitis.** Rapid development, over hours or a few days, of inflammation in the appendix. **Bilharzial appendicitis.** Appendicitis due to invasion of the appendix wall by *Schistosoma* (*Bilharzia*) *mansoni*. **Catarrhal appendicitis.** A mild inflammation of the mucous membrane of the appendix with excess mucus production but without the formation of pus. **Chronic appendicitis.** A condition in which there is a long-continued slight or recurrent inflammation of the organ. Correctly applied by the morbid anatomist to describe the appendix which is scarred by previous attacks of acute appendicitis. Widely used by surgeons who believe that inflammation may persist with exacerbations in the appendix for a very long time. **Concomitant appendicitis.** Appendicitis occurring as an integral lesion in another infective disease. **Extraperitoneal appendicitis.** Subperitoneal appendicitis (see below). **Follicular appendicitis.** Hypertrophy of the lymphoid tissue of the appendix wall. **Foreign-body appendicitis.** Inflammation due to a foreign body in the lumen. **Fulminating appendicitis.** An acute, sudden and severe attack with rapid development of peritonitis and fatal ending. **Gangrenous appendicitis.** A condition in which there is gangrene of the appendix caused by interruption of its circulation, usually a result of obstruction of its lumen. **Helminthic appendicitis.** Appendicitis as a result of invasion by worms. **Intramural appendicitis.** Inflammation of the wall of the appendix without obstruction or suppuration in its lumen. **Appendicitis larvata.** A quiescent condition which at any moment may become active. **Left-side appendicitis.** Appendicitis when the appendix is on the left side of the abdomen, e.g. in transposition of the viscera. **Masked appendicitis.** Appendicitis proceeding without overt symptoms. **Non-obstructive appendicitis.** Appendicitis when the lumen of the appendix is not blocked. **Obliterative appendicitis.** A subacute inflammatory condition of the mucosa which leads to adhesion of the walls with obliteration of the lumen, or an intramural inflammation healing with constriction. **Obstructive appendicitis.** Inflammation associated with obstruction of the lumen by faecal concretion, foreign body or mucosal oedema, distension of the obstructed organ, interference with its circulation, and early gangrene and rupture. **Pelvic appendicitis.** Inflammation of an appendix lying low in the pelvic basin. **Perforating appendicitis, Perforative appendicitis.** An inflammation of the appendix, usually preceded by obstruction of the lumen, which has resulted in distension, gangrene of the wall, rupture of the appendix and local or generalizing peritonitis. **Protective appendicitis.** Obliterative appendicitis (see above). **Purulent appendicitis.** Suppurative appendicitis (see below). **Recurrent appendicitis.** Repeated attacks of mild appendicitis, usually without the complete obstruction of the lumen. **Relapsing appendicitis.** Recurring appendicitis in which the attacks are sharp and recur at short intervals. **Retrocaecal appendicitis.** Inflammation in an appendix situated behind the caecum, commonly intraperitoneal but occasionally extraperitoneal in position. **Segmental appendicitis.** Appendicitis limited to a particular portion of the vermiform appendix. **Skip appendicitis.** A condition in which circumscribed areas of inflammation are separated by healthy appendiceal tissue. **Stercoral appendicitis.** Appendicitis occurring in an organ which is the seat of faecal concretion. **Subacute appendicitis.** Appendicular inflammation of mild degree, especially in the cases where there is no obstruction of the lumen of the appendix. **Subperitoneal appendicitis.** Inflammation of an appendix which, by abnormal anatomical situation or as a result of previous disease, does not lie free in the peritoneal cavity. **Suppurative appendicitis.** An inflammation of the appendix associated with the presence of pus in the appendix, or the development of pus around it. **Syncongestive appendicitis.** Involvement of the appendix in a congestive and non-infective lesion of adjacent tissues. **Traumatic appendicitis.** Appendicitis caused by direct external injury. **Verminous appendicitis.** That caused by the presence of a worm in the appendix; helminthic appendicitis. [appendix, Gk *-itis* inflammation.]

appendiclausis (ap·en·de·**klaw'**·sis). A condition of obstruction of the vermiform appendix in which the symptoms are like those of acute appendicitis. [appendix, L *clausis* closure.]

appendicocaecostomy (ap·en·dik·o·se·**kos'**·to·me). The operation of draining the caecum by a large-bore catheter inserted through the appendix. [appendix, caecum, Gk *stoma* mouth.]

appendicocele (ap·en·dik·o·seel). Hernia of the vermiform appendix. [appendix, Gk *kele* hernia.]

appendico-enterostomy (ap·en·dik·o·en·ter·**os'**·to·me). 1. The surgical establishment of an anastomatic opening between the appendix and the small intestine; obsolete. 2. Appendicostomy. [appendix, enterostomy.]

appendicolithiasis (ap·en·dik·o·lith·**i'**·as·is). A condition in which concretions are present in the vermiform appendix. [appendix, Gk *lithos* stone.]

appendicolysis (ap·en·dik·**ol'**·is·is). A method of removing the vermiform appendix when adhesions are present. The adherent seromuscular coat round the base is divided by a circular incision and the mucosa with its submucosa is gradually withdrawn from the outer walls. [appendix, Gk *lysis* a loosing.]

appendicopathia, appendicopathy (ap·en·dik·o·**path'**·e·ah, ap·en·dik·**op'**·ath·e). Any unhealthy condition of the vermiform appendix. **Appendicopathia oxyurica.** Appendicitis caused by the presence of a nematode worm of the genus *Enterobius* (*Oxyuris*). [appendix, Gk *pathos* suffering.]

appendicosis (ap·en·dik·**o'**·sis). Any non-infective condition of the vermiform appendix. [appendix, Gk *-osis* condition.]

appendicostomy (ap·en·dik·**os'**·to·me). The operation of making an opening through the tip of the vermiform appendix and using the latter as a tube through which the caecum and the colon may be flushed. [appendix, Gk *stoma* mouth.]

appendicular (ap·en·**dik**·ew·lar). 1. Referring to any condition in which the vermiform appendix is involved. 2. Belonging to an appendix.

appendicular artery [arteria appendicis vermiformis]. *See* MESENTERIC ARTERY, SUPERIOR.

appendicular vein [vena appendicularis (NA)]. A tributary of the ileocolic vein. It accompanies the corresponding artery in the free margin of the mesentery of the vermiform appendix.

appendiculoradiography (ap·en·dik·ew·lo·ra·de·og′·raf·e). X-ray photography of the vermiform appendix after the administration of contrast medium. [appendix, radiograph.]

appendix (ap·en·dix) (pl. *appendices, appendixes*). 1. An appendage; a subsidiary to a main body. 2. [NA] In anatomy, a small accessory part which is attached to the main part of an organ. **Auricular appendices.** The auricles of the atria, right and left. **Ensiform appendix.** Xiphoid process. *See* PROCESS. **Appendix of the epididymis [appendix epididymidis (NA)].** A small pedunculated body attached to the head of the epididymis; it is probably a vestige of the upper end of the mesonephros. **Appendices epiploicae [NA].** Small nodules of fat projecting under the serous coat of the large intestine, particularly in the transverse colon. **Appendices epoöphori.** Remnants of the mesonephros found in the broad ligaments near the ovary. **Appendix fasciolae.** Term applied to extensions of the pellagrous rash round the neck known as *Casal's collar* or *necklace.* **Fibrous appendix of the liver [appendix fibrosa hepatis (NA)].** An occasionally-occurring fibrous sheet connecting the extremity of the left lobe to the diaphragm and lying in the left triangular ligament. **High appendix.** An appendix lying, usually with a high caecum, above its normal position and in relation to the lower surface of the liver. **Pelvic appendix.** A vermiform appendix (see below) which hangs over the pelvic brim into the cavity of the pelvis. **Appendix testis [NA].** A small pedunculated body attached to the upper pole of the testis; it is probably a vestige of the paramesonephric (muellerian) duct. **Undescended appendix.** High appendix (see above). **Uterine appendices.** Uterine appendages. *See* APPENDAGE. **Appendices of the ventricles of the larynx.** Saccules of the larynx; diverticula from the anterior part of the ventricles of the larynx which lead upwards between the false vocal folds and the thyroid cartilages; many mucous glands open into them. **Vermiform appendix [appendix vermiformis (NA)].** A blind tubular structure which springs from the posteromedial aspect of the caecum, 2.5-5 cm (1-2 in) below the ileocaecal junction. Its mucous lining is similar to that of the large intestine, and the submucosa contains many lymph nodules. **Vermiform appendix, opening of the [ostium appendicis vermiformis (NA)].** The communication between the cavities of the caecum and the appendix vermiformis. **Appendices vesiculosae [NA].** One or more small pedunculated vesicles attached to the fimbriae of the uterine tube or the adjacent broad ligament. **Xiphoid appendix.** Xiphoid process. *See* PROCESS. [L *appendere* to hang upon.]

See also: MORGAGNI.

appendolithiasis (ap·en·do·lith·i′·as·is). Appendicolithiasis.

appendotome (ap·en·do·tome). A special instrument for the removal of the vermiform appendix. [appendix, Gk *temnein* to cut.]

apperception (ap·er·sep·shun). 1. In psychology, perception with the addition of self-consciousness. 2. The ability to perceive and interpret sensory stimuli or impressions. [L *ad, percipere* to perceive.]

apperceptive (ap·er·sep·tive). Referring to or having powers of apperception.

appersonification (ap·er·son·if·ik·a′·shun). 1. The process by which one person becomes identified with another emotionally. 2. A psychical disorder in which the sufferer regards himself as someone else and lives as if he were that person. [L *ad, persona* mask, *facere* to make.]

appet (ap·et). A term for the sensation experienced in anticipatory thought corresponding to the sensation experienced by the sight of a desired object. [L *appetere* to long for.]

appetite (ap·et·ite). A natural or instinctive need, as for food or sexual relations. [L *appetere* to long for.]

appetition (ap·et·ish·un). The objective focusing of longing or desire. [L *appetitio* desire.]

appetizer (ap·et·i·zer). Anything that whets the appetite or induces hunger.

applanate (ap·lan·ate). In botany, term signifying flattened or expanded horizontally, as the thallus of a seaweed. [L *ad, planus* flat.]

applanation (ap·lan·a·shun). The condition of being abnormally flattened or flat; term applied to structures or parts of an organ. **Corneal applanation.** Undue flatness of the cornea. [see prec.]

apple (ap·l). The fruit of *Pyrus malus* (family Rosaceae); it contains protein, oil, malic acid, sugars, pectin and cellulose, together with vitamins A and C. Apple pulp and powder have been used in the treatment of diarrhoea in infants, and are also of value because of their pectin content in gastro-intestinal disease in adults. **Adam's apple.** The laryngeal prominence. **Balsam apple.** The fruit of *Mormordica balsamina* (family Cucurbitaceae); it has purgative properties. **Apple eye.** Proptosis. **May apple.** Podophyllum. **Thorn apple.** The fruit of *Datura stramonium* (family Solanaceae); the seeds contain the same alkaloids as stramonium. [AS *aeppel.*]

appliance (ap·li·ans). 1. Anything that is applied or worn for a particular purpose; an apparatus. 2. In orthodontics, an apparatus worn in the mouth which moves misplaced teeth to their normal occlusion and alignment. **Fixed appliance.** An appliance which is fixed in the mouth and cannot be removed by the patient. **Removable appliance.** An appliance which can be removed from the mouth by the patient. [L *applicare* to apply.]

applicator (ap·lik·a·tor). 1. An instrument used for the local application of remedies. 2. A hermetically-sealed appliance containing radium or other radioactive material and designed to be placed in a known relationship to the part of the patient to be treated. The term may be qualified to indicate the type of radiation, e.g. *β-ray applicator, γ-ray applicator,* the nature of the source, e.g. *radium applicator, radiophosphorus applicator,* or the site of use, e.g. *intracavitary applicator, lip applicator, cervix applicator.* When such an applicator is moulded to fit the contour of the patient it is usually called a *mould applicator.* **Beam-therapy applicator.** An attachment to an x-ray therapy tube head or telecurie therapy unit designed so that it defines the cross-section of the radiation beam. It may also help to prescribe the distance between the x-ray target and the skin of the patient. It is sometimes called a *telecurie therapy nozzle* or *treatment cone.* **Sandwich-mould applicator.** A surface applicator made in two halves, placed on either side of the lesion being treated. **Surface applicator.** Radioactive sources distributed in any medium applied or moulded to the surface of a patient. **X-ray therapy applicator.** In x-ray therapy, a fitting on the x-ray tube which limits the radiation falling on the patient to a definite area. It consists of a lead-lined box of approximately conical shape, open at one end and closed at the other end, with a Perspex sheet which is placed in contact with the patient. [L *applicare* to apply.]

See also: CHAOUL.

appliqué (ap·le·ka). Term applied to a particular form of the malarial parasite *Plasmodium falciparum* appearing as a thin attachment to the erythrocyte; accolé form. [Fr. *appliqué* applied.]

apposition (ap·o·zish·un). 1. Of adjacent organs or parts, the state of being in contact. 2. The placing in contact of 2 substances. 3. The process of developing by means of accretion. 4. The adding of other parts to a group of parts. [L *apponere* to put to.]

approach (ap·ro·ch). The steps in an operation concerned with the division of the parietes and the exposure of the operation site, e.g. transthoracic, thoraco-abdominal, transdiaphragmatic approach. [L *ad, propiare* to draw near.]

See also: BLALOCK, MCLAUGHLIN.

approximator (ap·rox·im·a·tor). An instrument for drawing together the edges of divided tissues thereby facilitating the closure of wounds. **Rib approximator.** A hinged screw tractor for drawing together the ribs on each side of a wound in the chest wall while pleura and intercostal muscles are sutured. **Skin-edge approximator.** A toothed dissecting forceps used to appose skin edges for the insertion of sutures or clips. [L *ad, proximare* to approach.]

apraxia (ap·rax·e·ah). A disorder of voluntary movement characterized by inability to perform, command or imitate a familiar action, the nature of which is understood, in the absence of severe inco-ordination or paralysis of the parts concerned. **Agnostic apraxia.** Apraxia due to agnosia. **Amnesic apraxia, Amnestic apraxia.** A condition in which actions can be imitated but not performed to command. **Articulatory apraxia.** Inability to perform the movements required to reproduce sounds accurately (in isolation or combination) when hearing and perception are normal, and in the absence of actual paralysis of the organs of articulation. **Congenital apraxia.** A congenital childhood difficulty for learning complex motor patterns; often associated with congenital word blindness or deafness. **Constructional apraxia, Constructive apraxia.** Inability to arrange objects or lines in accordance with a two- or three-dimensional plan; usually associated with visual agnosia. **Cortical apraxia.** Limb-kinetic apraxia (see below). **Dressing apraxia.** Inability to put on garments the right way round; commonly encountered with agnosic difficulties. **Finger apraxia.** Inability to move a specific finger in the absence of finger agnosia or motor paralysis; often an early feature of a more widespread apraxia. **Ideational apraxia.** A disorder resulting from defective mental representation (engram) of the action as a whole, the component features of which may be correctly executed but, for example, combined in the wrong order. **Ideokinetic apraxia, Ideomotor apraxia.** Apraxia through dissociation of the intact mental representation of an action from the kinaesthetic processes necessary for its execution. **Innervation apraxia, Kinetic apraxia.** Limb-kinetic apraxia (see following). **Limb-kinetic apraxia, Motor apraxia.** Apraxia attributed to defective motor kinaesthetic functions; often restricted to part of a limb, such as the hand. **Optical apraxia.** Constructional apraxia (see above). **Reflexive apraxia.** Apraxia for actions directed towards the subject's own body. **Sympathetic apraxia, Transcortical apraxia.** Ideokinetic apraxia (see above). **Trunk apraxia.** Apraxia for trunk movements with inability to sit, lie down or stand up. [Gk *a, prassein* to do.]

See also: LIEPMANN, PICK (A.).

aprication (ap·re·ka·shun). 1. Sunstroke. 2. Sun-bathing; the use of solar rays in therapeutics. [L *apricatio* basking in the sun.]

Aprindine (a·prin·deen). BP Commission approved name for 3-[*N*-indan-2-yl)-*N*-phenylamino] propyldiethylamine; an anti-arrhythmic agent.

aproctia (a·prok·she·ah). A condition in which the anus is imperforate or absent. [Gk *a, proktos* anus.]

aproctous (a·prok·tus). Indicating the state of being without an anus or of having an imperforate anus. [see prec.]

apron (a·pron). The omentum. **Hottentot apron.** Pudendal apron (see below). **Lead-rubber apron.** A protective shield of lead rubber. It may be a flap suspended from the fluorescent screen of an x-ray couch or stand, or a garment to be worn by the operator. In the latter case it may be called a *body apron.* **Mackintosh apron.** A waterproof apron. **Masonic apron.** A term given to an appliance which fastens round the waist and supports the male genitalia in cases of gonorrhoea. **Protective apron.** Lead-rubber apron (see above). **Pudendal apron.** Elongation, either abnormal or artificially produced, of the labia minora. [Fr. *napperon.*]

aprophoria (a·pro·for·e·ah). Aphasia with agraphia. [Gk *a, propherein* to present.]

aprosexia (a·pro·sex·e·ah). Inattention, or inability to concentrate the attention, with lack of ability to think clearly or to comprehend readily; the condition may be present as a result of disorders of the eyes, the throat or the ears, or of mental weakness. **Aprosexia nasalis.** The mental changes which may develop in association with adenoids or other disorder of the nasopharynx. [Gk *a, prosexein* to heed.]

aprosopia (a·pro·so·pe·ah). In teratology, denoting entire absence or imperfect development of the face. [Gk *aprosopos,* without a face.]

aprosopus (ap·ro·so·pus). A monster the head of which lacks a face. [Gk *aprosopos* without a face.]

Aprotinin (a·pro·tin·in). BP Commission approved name for a polypeptide proteinase inhibitor, used in the treatment of acute pancreatitis and of fat embolism.

apselaphesia (ap·sel·af·e′·ze·ah). Absence or loss of the sense of touch. [Gk *a, pselaphesis* touch.]

apsithurea, apsithyria (ap·sith·ewr·e·ah, ap·sith·i·re·ah). Aphonia in association with hysteria. There is loss even of the power to whisper. [Gk *a, psithyros* whispering.]

apsychia (a·si·ke·ah). 1. Loss of consciousness. 2. The state of being in a faint or swoon. [Gk *a, psyche* mind.]

apsychical (a·si·kik·al). 1. Not psychical. 2. Without involvement of consciousness. [see prec.]

apsychosis (a·si·ko·sis). Loss or lack of the functions of the mind; absence of thinking power. [Gk *a, psyche* mind, *-osis* condition.]

apterous (ap·ter·us). Wingless. [Gk *a, pteron* wing.]

Aptocaine (ap·to·kane). BP Commission approved name for *N*-[2-(pyrrolidin-1-yl) propionyl]-*o*-toluidine; a local anaesthetic.

aptyalia, aptyalism (ap·ti·a·le·ah, ap·ti·al·izm). Arrest or diminution of the secretion of saliva, resulting in xerostomia. [Gk *a, ptyalizein* to spit.]

apudoma (ap·ud·o·mah). A tumour of apud cells, such as insulinoma. A gastrin-secreting apudoma causes the Zollinger-Ellison syndrome (q.v.). [amine precursor uptake and D-carboxylation, Gk *-oma* tumour.]

apulmonism (a·pul·mon·izm). The state in which a lung or a part of a lung is lacking. [Gk *a,* L *pulmo* lung.]

apulosis (ap·ew·lo·sis). 1. A cicatrix. 2. The process of cicatrization. [Gk *apo, oulein* to cicatrize.]

apulotic (ap·ew·lot·ik). Term applied to any agent which aids cicatrization; promoting apulosis.

apus (a·pus). A footless monster or fetus. [Gk *a, pous* foot.]

apyetous (a·pi·et·us). Non-suppurating; not resulting in formation of pus or purulent matter. [Gk *a, pyon* pus.]

apyknomorphous (a·pik·no·mor′·fus). Applied to a cell or similar structure signifying that its staining elements are poor or loosely aggregated. [Gk *a, pyknos* compact, *morphe* form.]

apyogenous (a·pi·oj·en·us). Not originating in pus; not resulting from a suppurative condition. [Gk *a, pyon* pus, *genein* to produce.]

apyous (a·pi·us). Apyetous.

apyrene (a·pi·reen). Being without a nucleus or nuclear matter. [Gk *a, pyren* kernel.]

apyretic (a·pi·ret·ik). Afebrile. [Gk *a, pyretos* fever.]

apyrexia (a·pi·rex·e·ah). Absence or a temporary cessation of fever. [Gk *a, pyrexis* fever.]

apyrexial (a·pi·rex·e·al). Characterized by the absence of fever. [see prec.]

apyrogenetic, apyrogenic (a·pi·ro·jen·et′·ik, a·pi·ro·jen′·ik). Not productive of fever. [Gk *a, pyr* fire, *genein* to produce.]

aqua (ak·wah). 1. The Latin for *water.* 2. In pharmacy, a medicated solution of an aromatic substance such as a volatile oil in water. **Aqua amnii.** The liquor amnii. **Aqua anethi concentrata.** Concentrated Dill Water BP 1958. *See* WATER. **Aqua anisi concentrata.** Concentrated Anise Water BPC 1959. *See* WATER. **Aqua Aurantii Floris Concentrata BPC 1949.** A solution of 1 in 170 of oil of neroli in dilute alcohol. It is about 40 times the strength of the orange-flower water of commerce and is used in perfumery. **Aqua aurantii floris triplex.** The triple orange-flower water of commerce used in perfumery, and a constituent of eau de Cologne. **Aqua bulliens.** Boiling water; a term used in prescription writing. **Aqua calcis.** Lime water. *See* WATER. **Aqua camphorae.** Camphor Water BP 1958. *See* WATER. **Aqua Camphorae Concentrata BPC 1949.** A solution of camphor in dilute alcohol. It is 40 times the strength of Camphor Water BP 1958. **Aqua cari (carui) concentrata.** Concentrated Caraway Water BPC 1959. *See* WATER. **Aqua caryophylli concentrata.** A solution of 2 per cent v/v of oil of clove in dilute alcohol. Diluted 1 to 40 with distilled water it gives a preparation which is used as a carminative and flavouring agent. **Aqua chlori.** A solution of about 0.5 per cent w/v of chlorine gas in water. **Aqua chloroformi.** Chloroform Water BP 1958. *See* WATER. **Aqua chloroformi concentrata.** Concentrated Chloroform Water BPC 1959. *See* WATER. **Aqua cinnamomi concentrata.** Concentrated Cinnamon Water BP 1958. *See* WATER. **Aqua coloniensis.** Spiritus Coloniensis BPC 1949. **Aqua destillata.** Distilled water. *See* WATER. **Aqua destillata sterilisata.** Water distilled from a glass still, the first of the distillate being excluded, and collected in a neutral glass container and autoclaved. **Aqua foeniculi concentrata.** A solution of 2 per cent v/v of the essential oil of fennel in dilute alcohol. Diluted with 39 parts of distilled water it yields a preparation used as a flavouring agent. **Aqua fortis.** Concentrated nitric acid. **Aqua pro injectione.** Water for Injection BP 1958. *See* WATER. **Aqua Laurocerasi BPC 1949.** A preparation made from the cherry-laurel, *Prunus laurocerasus* (family Rosaceae), and containing 0.1 per cent of hydrocyanic acid. **Aqua levico.** A natural mineral water from Italy containing arsenic and iron. **Aqua marina.** Sea-water. **Aqua menthae piperitae concentrata.** Concentrated Peppermint Water BP 1958. *See* WATER. **Aqua menthae viridis concentrata.** A solution of 2 per cent v/v of oil of spearmint in dilute alcohol. It is diluted 1 to 40 with distilled water for use as a flavouring agent. **Aqua mentholis.** A 1 in 1000 solution of menthol in water, used as a carminative. **Aqua oculi.** The aqueous humour of the eye. **Aqua pericardii.** The small quantity of serous fluid normally found in the pericardial cavity. **Aqua phenolata.** A 2 per cent solution of phenol. **Aqua pimentae concentrata.** A 1 in 50 solution of oil of pimento in dilute alcohol. **Aqua Purificata.** *European Pharmacopoeia* name for Purified Water BP 1973. **Aqua regia.** A mixture of 4 parts of concentrated hydrochloric acid with 3 parts of concentrated nitric acid. **Aqua rosae.** Equal parts of triple rose water and distilled water. **Aqua Rosae Concentrata BPC 1949.** 1 per cent oil of rose in dilute alcohol; it is approximately 40 times stronger than aqua rosae. **Aqua rosae triplex.** Triple rose water, the undiluted rose water of commerce. **Aqua Sambuci BPC 1949.** Equal parts of triple elder-flower water and distilled water mixed immediately before use. **Aqua Sambuci Triplex BPC 1949.** A saturated solution of the oil of elder flowers in water. **Aqua tepida.** Tepid water; a term used in prescription writing. **Aqua vitae.** Brandy.

aquacapsulitis (ak·wah·kap·sew·li′·tis). Serous iritis. *See* IRITIS. [L *aqua* water, capsule of the lens, Gk *-itis* inflammation.]

aquapuncture (ak·wah·pungk·tcher). 1. Injection of water underneath the skin, as a placebo. 2. The playing of a very fine jet of water on the skin as a form of counter-irritant. [L *aqua* water, puncture.]

aqueduct (ak·we·dukt). A canal containing a clear colourless fluid. **Aqueduct of the cochlea [ductus perilymphaticus (aqueductus cochleae) (NA)].** A bony canal from near the beginning of the scala tympani to an opening in the jugular fossa of the petrous part of the temporal bone; it forms a communication between the perilymphatic and subarachnoid spaces. **Aqueduct of the cochlea, vein of the [vena aqueductus cochleae (NA)].** A small vein which drains the perilymphatic duct into the internal jugular vein. **Aqueduct of the mid-brain [aqueductus cerebri (NA)].** Cerebral aqueduct, aqueduct of Sylvius, the canal connecting the 3rd and 4th ventricles. **Aqueduct of the vestibule [aqueductus vestibuli (NA)].** Aqueduct of Cotunnius, a canal from the bony labyrinth opening on the posterior surface of the petrous part of the temporal bone; it contains the endolymphatic duct. **Aqueduct of the vestibule, external opening of the [apertura externa aqueductus vestibuli (NA)].** An opening posterior to the orifice of the internal auditory meatus in the petrous temporal bone. [L *aqueductus.*]

See also: COTUGNO (COTUNNIUS), FALLOPIUS, SYLVIUS.

aqueduct of the vestibule, vein of the [vena aqueductus vestibuli (NA)]. A small vein accompanying the endolymphatic duct.

aqueous (ak·we·us). 1. The aqueous humour of the eye. *See* HUMOUR. 2. Made by the addition of water, as a preparation; watery. [L *aqua* water.]

aquiducous (ak·we·dew·kus). Producing water or a watery discharge. [L *aqua* water, *ducere* to lead.]

aquiferous (ak·wif·er·us). Conveying or carrying watery lymph or water. [L *aqua* water, *ferre* to carry.]

aquiparous (ak·wip·ar·us). Secreting water, or producing a watery secretion. [L *aqua* water, *parere* to produce.]

aquocapsulitis (ak·wo·kap·sew·li′·tis). Aquacapsulitis.

aquocobalamin (ak·wo·ko·bal′·am·in). *See* VITAMIN B_{12}.

aquosity (ak·wos·it·e). 1. Moisture. 2. A watery condition or state. [L *aquositas.*]

aquozon (ak·wo·zone). A dilute and unstable solution of ozone in distilled water, used as an antiseptic. [L *aqua* water, ozone.]

aquula (ak·woo·lah). **Aquula externa.** The perilymph. **Aquula interna.** The endolymph. [L small stream.]

Ara, Kiyosha. Contemporary Japanese pathologist.

Takata-Ara test. For liver function: place 1 ml of normal saline in each of 8 small tubes. To the first add 1 ml of serum, mix, and transfer 1 ml of the diluted serum to tube 2. Continue the serial dilution, discarding 1 ml from tube 8. To each tube add with mixing 0.25 ml of 10 per cent sodium carbonate followed by 0.15 ml of 0.5 per cent mercuric chloride. Allow the tubes to stand 24 h. A positive reaction is shown by a thick flocculent precipitate in at least 3 tubes, 1 of which should be the 1:32 dilution or higher. Any fine granular precipitate is disregarded. Positive results are usually obtained in advanced liver disease, especially in cirrhosis.

araban (ar·ab·an). A polymeric pentosan, $(C_5H_8O_4)_n$, found in gum arabic, various other gums and mucilages, bran and pectin; hydrolysed to L-arabinose.

arabate (ar·ab·ate). A salt of arabic acid.

arabin (ar·ab·in). $(C_5H_{10}O_5)_2$. A carbohydrate in gum arabic and other gums, which is soluble in water but insoluble in alcohol; sometimes called, erroneously, *arabic acid.* **Arabin water.** A solution of arabin in hydnocarpus oil.

arabinosazone (ar·ab·in·o′·zaz·one). The diphenylhydrazone of arabinose, formed from the latter by reaction with phenylhydrazine; it has the formula $CH_2OH(CHOH)_3C(NNHC_6H_5)CH{=}NNHC_6H_5$.

arabinose (ar·ab·in·oze). Gum sugar, pectinose, L-arabinose, laevo-arabinose, $CH_2OH(CHOH)_3CHO$. An aldopentose derived from gum arabic, cherry gum, beet pulp, pectin and bran. The dextro-isomer occurs in nature as the glycoside, aloin, and in tubercle bacilli. Laevo-arabinose appears in the urine during the pathological condition known as pentosuria.

arabinosuria (ar·ab·in·o·zewr′·e·ah). A condition in which there is arabinose in the urine.

arabinulose (ar·ab·in·ew·loze). $CH_2OH(CHOH)_2COCH_2OH$. The keto-pentose isomeric with arabinose.

arabite, arabitol (ar·ab·ite, ar·ab·it·ol). $CH_2OH(CHOH)_3CH_2OH$. The pentahydroxy alcohol corresponding to arabinose and derived from it by reduction with sodium amalgam.

arabopyranose (ar·ab·o·pir′·an·oze). The more scientific name for arabinose in the nomenclature of sugars, which proclaims its 6-membered ring structure and relationship to pyran.

arachanol (ar·ak·an·ol). $C_{20}H_{41}OH$. An alcohol which occurs in dermoid cysts.

arachidic (ar·ak·id·ik). Resulting from the eating of peanut kernels, e.g. arachidic bronchitis. [Gk *arachos* leguminous plant.]

arachin (ar·ak·in). A globulin which occurs in peanuts, *Arachis hypogaea.*

arachine (ar·ak·een). $C_5H_{14}N_2O$. An alkaloid found in peanuts, *Arachis hypogaea.*

Arachis (ar·ak·is). A genus of leguminous plants. **Arachis hypogaea.** An annual plant cultivated chiefly in the tropical regions of India, Africa and South America. The seeds, peanut, groundnut or earthnut, contain fixed oil, protein and starch. **Arachis Oil BP 1958.** *See* OIL. [Gk *arachos* leguminous plant.]

arachnephobia (ar·ak·ne·fo′·be·ah). Dread and horror of spiders. [Gk *arachne* spider, phobia.]

Arachnida (ar·ak·nid·ah). A class of the phylum Arthropoda, to which belong scorpions, spiders, mites and ticks. [Gk *arachne* spider.]

arachnidism (ar·ak·nid·izm). Spider poisoning; systemic poisoning after having been bitten by a spider. [see prec.]

arachnitis (ar·ak·ni·tis). Arachnoiditis.

arachnodactyly (ar·ak·no·dak′·til·e). Abnormal length of the bones of the hands and feet. The condition may be accompanied by relaxed joint ligaments and general muscular dystrophy, but there is no paralysis; acromacria. Cf. MARFAN'S SYNDROME. [Gk *arachne* spider, *dactylos* finger.]

arachnogastria (ar·ak·no·gas′·tre·ah). The uniform enlargement of the abdomen seen in ascites; the condition is accentuated when there is wasting of the rest of the body, hence the term, *spider belly.* [Gk *arachne* spider, *gaster* stomach.]

arachnoid (ar·ak·noid). 1. Like a spider's web. 2. Applied to the pulse, a term signifying thread-like or feeble. 3. The arachnoid mater or membrane, which lies under the dura mater and over the pia mater of the cerebrospinal system. 4. Referring to any membranous structure. **Arachnoid granulations.** *See* GRANULATION. [Gk *arachne* spider, *eidos* form.]

arachnoid mater (arachnoidea encephali (NA)) (ar·ak·noid ma·ter). A delicate membrane enveloping the brain [arachnoidea encephali (NA)] and spinal cord [arachnoidea spinalis (NA)] and extending beyond the end of the latter to the level of the 2nd sacral vertebra. It is separated from the dura, which it follows closely, by the subdural space, and from the pia mater by the subarachnoid space and its contained cerebrospinal fluid. [arachnoid, L *mater* mother.]

arachnoidal (ar·ak·noi·dal). Referring to the arachnoid mater.

arachnoidea (ar·ak·noi·de·ah). The arachnoid mater of the brain.

arachnoiditis (ar·ak·noi·di′·tis). Inflammation of the arachnoid mater of the brain. **Chiasmal arachnoiditis.** A questionable entity, but described as a local thickening of the arachnoid in close relation to the optic nerves and chiasma. Unilateral or bilateral progressive failing of vision occurs. **Rachidian arachnoiditis, Spinal arachnoiditis.** Spinal meningitis. *See* MENINGITIS. [arachnoid mater, Gk *-itis* inflammation.]

arachnolysin (ar·ak·nol·is·in). The haemolysin in spider venom. [Gk *arachne* spider, lysin.]

arachnopia (ar·ak·no·pe·ah). The pia-arachnoid; it is customary in certain cases to consider the pia mater, the arachnoid and the subarachnoid space as one. [arachnoid, pia.]

arack (ar·ak). Arrack.

araeometer (ar·e·om·et·er). Areometer; hydrometer. [Gk *araios* thin, meter.]

Aragão, Henrique de Beaurepaire. 19th–20th century Brazilian physician.

Aragão's vaccine. A vaccine used formerly for protection against yellow fever.

araiocardia (ar·a·o·kar′·de·ah). Bradycardia. [Gk *araios* thin, *kardia* heart.]

Aralia (ar·a·le·ah). A genus of the Araliaceae; aromatic plants including spikenard. **Aralia nudicaulis.** Wild sarsaparilla; it has been used as a tonic. **Aralia quinquefolia.** A North American species the root of which affords ginseng. **Aralia racemosa.** American spikenard, the rhizome and roots of which contain volatile oil, resin and tannin. It has stimulant and diaphoretic properties. [Iroquois name.]

aralkyl (ar·al·kil). An alkyl radical which contains both aryl and alphyl groups.

Aran, François Amilcar (b. 1817). Paris physician.

Aran's green cancer. A rapidly-growing yellowish-green malignant tumour of the orbit, associated with leukaemia and arising from leukaemic deposits. More usually called *chloroma.* **Aran's law.** Basal skull fractures result from injuries to the vault, and tend to occur along the line of the shortest circumference from the original site of injury to the base; largely obsolete.

Aran–Duchenne atrophy, disease or type. Progressive spinal muscular atrophy; motor neurone disease of the progressive muscular atrophy type.

Aranea (ar·a·ne·ah). An order of the arthropod class Arachnida; spiders. Members of many genera bite man. *Latrodectus* and *Lycosa* are of medical interest. [L spider.]

araneism (ar·a·ne·izm). Spider poisoning; systemic poisoning from the bites of certain spiders. That of the black-widow spider, *Latrodectus mactans,* causes dilatation of the pupils, cyanosis, oedema of the face and extremities, and neurotoxic and peritoneal signs. [L *aranea* spider.]

araneous (ar·a·ne·us). Resembling a cobweb. [see prec.]

Aranzio (Arantius), Giulio Cesare (b. 1530). Italian anatomist and physician.

body, corpus or nodule of Arantius. Minute fibrocartilaginous nodules found in the centre of the free margin of the semilunar cusps of the aortic and pulmonary valves.

canal, or duct of Arantius. The ductus venosus.

Arantius' ligament. The ligamentum venosum.

ventricle of Arantius. A depression in the posterior extremity of the 4th ventricle.

araroba (ar·ar·o·bah). Goa powder; a powder deposited in the wood of the tree *Andira araroba* (family Leguminosae). When extracted with benzene it yields chrysarobin. [Port. bark.]

arbacin (ar·ba·sin). A protein found in the spermatozoa of the sea-urchin.

arbor (ar·bor). A tree-like structure. **Arbor alveolaris.** The ramifications of the air passages of the lung distal to the terminal bronchiole, into which the alveoli open directly; a term now rarely used. **Arbor vitae.** 1. Of the cerebellum [Arbor vitae cerebelli (NA)]: the tree-like outline of the white matter of the cerebellum, seen on the cut surface of a median section. 2. Of the cervix of the uterus [plicae palmatae]: *see* CANAL OF THE CERVIX. 3. The popular name for the coniferous tree *Thuja occidentalis.* [L tree.]

arborescent (ar·bor·es·ent). Branching; tree-like. [L *arborescere* to grow into a tree.]

arborization (ar·bor·i·za′·shun). 1. The ramification present at the termination of certain nerve cells or fibres, and at the ending of a motor nerve fibre on a muscle fibre. 2. The interlacing of venule, capillary vessels and arterioles. 3. The branched appearance of capillary vessels when inflammation is present. [L *arbor* tree.]

arboroid (ar·bor·oid). Applied to a colony of protozoa, signifying a branching or dendritic figure like a tree. [L *arbor* tree, Gk *eidos* form.]

arbovirus (ahr·bo·vi·rus). A large heterogeneous group of RNA-containing viruses, whose common property is that they are transmitted by blood-sucking insects. To be classed as an arbovirus the virus must multiply in both the vertebrate and invertebrate hosts. About 200 arboviruses are known, not all of which are known to cause disease in man. Terminology of the viruses is inconsistent, some being named after the disease caused, some after the locality of first isolation and some after the host or vector. Of those that have been characterized some serological and morphological groups have been found: *Alphaviruses (syn: Group A arboviruses).* Enveloped RNA viruses 40–80 nm in diameter with surface projections. Serologically related by haemagglutination inhibition tests, the principal members of the group associated with human diseases are the equine encephalitides (Eastern, Western and Venezuelan), O'Nyong Nyong and Chikungunya. *Flaviviruses (syn: Group B arboviruses).* Enveloped RNA viruses 20–50 nm in diameter with less well defined surface projections than Group A viruses. Serologically related by haemagglutination inhibition the members of the group associated with human disease are transmitted either by mosquitoes (yellow fever, dengue, and Japanese B, St. Louis and Murray Valley encephalitides) or ticks (louping-ill, Russian Spring–Summer encephalitis, Central European tick-borne encephalitis, Omsk haemorrhagic fever and Kyasanur Forest disease). Members of the group are called flaviviruses after yellow fever virus. Alphaviruses and flaviviruses collectively form the togaviruses. *Bunyamwera supergroup.* Enveloped RNA-containing viruses 90–100 nm in size, serologically related though not as closely as in Groups A and B. May cause febrile illnesses in man but they are not important human pathogens. *Colorado tick-fever group.* Morphologically and serologically distinct from other arboviruses, these viruses are members of the orbivirus genus. Other arboviruses, including those of Naples and Sicilian sandfly fevers, do not fit readily into the above groupings, being serologically distinct or because insufficient evidence is yet available. [*ar*thropod-*bo*rne-*virus*.]

arbutin (ar·bew·tin). A crystalline glucoside found in bearberry leaves (*Arctostaphylos uva-ursi*). On hydrolysis it yields hydroquinone and dextrose. It is responsible for the diuretic action of bearberry, being mainly absorbed unchanged and excreted by the kidneys, whence it exerts an antiseptic action on the urinary tract. [L *arbutus* wild strawberry-tree.]

arc (ark). 1. A part of the circumference of a circle. 2. In anatomy, a part of a curved line which may not be strictly circular; the term is most commonly used in craniometry. 3. A luminous discharge of electricity between electrodes in a gas or vapour when the material of one or both of the electrodes is volatilized and conducts the current whether direct or alternating. **Auricular arc.** The curved line over the vertex of the skull from one external auditory meatus to the other. **Bigonial arc.** The curved line between the angles of the jaw which passes around the symphysis menti. **Binauricular arc.** Auricular arc (see above). **Bregmaticolambdoid arc.** The line of the sagittal suture between the parietal bones, from the bregma to the lambda. **Carbon arc.** A maintained electric arc between 2 carbon electrodes. **Arc de cercle.** Opisthotonos; emprosthotonos, extreme arching of the body forwards or backwards in the convulsions of tetanus or hysteria. **Electric arc.** A low-voltage, high-current discharge usually between carbon electrodes, giving an intense light from the incandescent electrodes and gas between them. In engineering, an electric discharge used in welding. **Enclosed arc.** A carbon arc maintained in a glass enclosure not air-tight but designed to restrict access of air so that the arc burns in an atmosphere of its own products of combustion. **Frontal arc.** The curved line on the surface of the skull from the nasion to the bregma. **Mercury arc.** An electric discharge through a vacuum tube with mercury electrodes, giving light rich in ultra-violet radiation. **Metallic arc.** An arc formed between 2 similar metallic electrodes. **Nasobregmatic arc.** Frontal arc (see above). **Naso-occipital arc.** The curved line from the nasion to the external occipital protuberance (inion). **Neural arc.** Any complete nervous pathway beginning at a receptor and ending at an effector organ. **Occipital arc.** The curved line from the lambda to the most posterior point on the margin of the foramen magnum (opisthion). **Open arc.** A carbon arc burning in free air. **Parietal arc.** Bregmaticolambdoid arc (see above). **Reflex arc.** The nervous pathway for a reflex action. The path consists of at least 2 neurones, the ingoing, or afferent, arising in the receptor organ, and the outgoing, or efferent, ending in the effector organ. Any number of internuncial neurones may be interposed between these 2. **Sensorimotor arc.** Neural arc (see above). **Singing arc.** A carbon arc connected in circuit with inductance and capacitance, generating continuous oscillations of audible frequency. **Voltaic arc.** Early term used for the electric arc formed between 2 carbon electrodes connected to the terminals of a powerful voltaic battery. [L *arcus* bow.]

arcade (ar·kade). Anatomically, an arch or series of arches. **Arterial arcades.** The communications between the jejunal and ileal branches of the superior mesenteric artery. **Inferior temporal arcade.** The zygomatic arch. *See* ARCH. [L *arcus* bow.]

See also: FLINT, RIOLAN.

arcaine (ar·ka·een). $NH_2(NH)CNH(CH_2)_4NHC(NH)NH_2$, a base found in the mussel, Noah's ark, *Arca noae*; administration of this base lowers the blood sugar.

arcanum (ar·ka·num). An elixir; a secret remedy or nostrum. [L secret.]

arceine (ar·se·een). Arecoline hydrobromide, $C_8H_{13}O_2NHBr$; a myotic, and also a veterinary anthelmintic.

arcesis (ar·se·sis). Any drug or article of diet which sustains or increases the resistance to disease of the individual. [Gk *arkesis* a warding off.]

arch (arch). 1. A structure or structures having a regular curved form; in anatomy [arcus (NA)], any structure curved like an arch or bow. 2. One of the 3 fundamental dermatoglyphic patterns of the fingertips. This is characterized by the presence of dermal ridges running across the fingertip without forming triradii and cores. Such a pattern is rare in normal individuals. **Abnormal arch.** In dentistry, the irregular form of the curve made by the teeth. **Alveolar arch [arcus alveolaris (NA)].** The arch or arcade formed by the alveolar margins of the jaws. **Arch of the aorta [arcus aortae (NA)].** The curved part of the aorta which joins the ascending to the descending parts of the aorta in the thorax. **Arterial arch.** Bilateral arched arteries present in the embryo which run round the side of the pharynx and join the aortic sac to the right and left dorsal aortae; there are 6 arterial arches on each side. **Arch of the atlas, anterior [arcus anterior (NA)].** The short, curved bar of bone uniting the lateral masses of the atlas in front and articulating with the odontoid process of the axis. **Arch of the atlas, posterior [arcus posterior (NA)].** The curved bar of bone uniting the lateral masses of the atlas behind the spinal canal. **Arch of the foot, anterior.** The shallow, transverse arch formed by the heads of the metatarsal bones. **Axillary arch.** A variable slip of muscle, sometimes present in the axilla, which may join the pectoralis major and latissimus dorsi muscles; it may have attachments to the ribs or fasciae of the region. **Branchial arches.** Arched structures in the wall of the embryonic pharynx which bear gills in aquatic vertebrates; the term is also applied to similar structures in the pharyngeal wall present in the embryos of air-breathing vertebrates, including man, which do not, however, bear gills or branchiae. Each arch has a core of mesoderm and is lined by endoderm and covered externally by ectoderm, and is separated from its neighbour by endodermal pouches and ectodermal grooves or clefts. **Carpal arch, anterior.** An anastomosis across the front of the carpus deep to the flexor tendons formed by branches from the radial, ulnar and anterior interosseous arteries and a recurrent branch from the deep palmar arch. **Carpal arch, posterior [rete carpi dorsale (NA)].** The arterial arch on the back of the carpus formed from the small posterior carpal branches of the radial and ulnar arteries and the anterior and posterior interosseous arteries. **Cortical arch of the kidney.** Part of the cortex of the kidney which joins the 2 renal columns round the base of a renal pyramid. **Costal arch [arcus costalis (NA)].** The arch formed by the shafts of the ribs. **Arch of the cricoid cartilage [arcus cartilaginis cricoideae (NA)].** The U-shaped anterior part of the cricoid cartilage. **Crural arch, deep.** A thickening in the transversalis fascia in the anterior wall of the femoral sheath; the iliopubic tract. **Dental arches.** The curves made by the upper [arcus dentalis superior (NA)] and lower [arcus dentalis inferior (NA)] teeth. **Epiphyseal arch.** That part of the roof of the 3rd ventricle of the embryonic brain from which the pineal and associated structures develop. **Expansion arch.** An orthodontic appliance made of wire which is employed to increase the size of the dental arch. **Fallen arch.** Flattening of the arches of the foot, chiefly of the medial longitudinal arch. **Arch of the foot [arcus pedis longitudinalis (NA)].** The arched form of the tarsal and metatarsal bones, divided for descriptive purposes into medial [pars medialis (NA)] and lateral [pars lateralis (NA)] longitudinal arches and a transverse arch [arcus pedis transversalis (NA)]. **Glossopalatine arch.** Palatoglossal arch (see below). **Haemal arches.** Processes which extend laterally from a vertebra and in the caudal region of many vertebrates fuse ventrally to enclose an artery and vein; they may be represented by the costal processes in man. **Hyoid arch.** The 2nd visceral or pharyngeal arch. In man and other air-breathing vertebrates it is present in typical form only in the embryo; its skeletal elements are found in the adult as the stapes, styloid process of the temporal bone, stylohyoid ligament and the lesser horn of the hyoid bone. **Hypochordal arch.** A transverse mesenchymal band connecting the costal processes in front of the centrum of a cervical vertebra. The anterior arch of the atlas develops from the first of the series; the other arches are transitory. **Iliopectineal arch [arcus iliopectineus (NA)].** The fascial partition separating the lacuna musculorum and the lacuna vasorum. **Ischiopubic arch.** The bone which forms the lateral boundary of the urogenital triangle in the perineum, formed by the inferior ramus of the pubis and the ramus of the ischium. **Jugular arch [arcus venosus juguli (NA)].** A vessel joining the right and left anterior jugular veins in the lower part of the neck. **Lingual arch.** An orthodontic appliance made of wire which conforms to the inner aspects of the teeth. **Lumbocostal arch, lateral [arcus lumbocostalis lateralis (NA)].** A tendinous arch over the quadratus lumborum muscle to which some fibres of the diaphragm are attached; the lateral arcuate ligament. **Lumbocostal arch, medial [arcus lumbocostalis medialis (NA)].** A tendinous arch over the psoas muscle, to which some fibres of the diaphragm are attached; the medial arcuate ligament. **Malar arch.** Zygomatic arch (see below). **Mandibular arch.** The first visceral arch from which the lower jaw and much of the face is developed. **Mesencephalic arch.** The mid-brain flexure of the embryo. **Metatarsal arch.** Anterior arch of the foot (see above). **Neural arch.** Vertebral arch (see below). **Palatal arch.** The concave roof of the mouth. **Palatoglossal arch [arcus palatoglossus (NA)].** The fold of mucous membrane covering the palatoglossus muscle anterior to the tonsil; the anterior pillar of the fauces. **Palatopharyngeal arch [arcus palatopharyngeus (NA)].** The fold of mucous membrane covering the palatopharyngeus muscle posterior to the tonsil; the posterior pillar of the fauces. **Palmar arch, deep [arcus palmaris profundus (NA)].** A transverse artery in the palm formed mainly by the radial artery, and completed by the deep branch of the ulnar artery. It lies between the flexor tendons and the metacarpal bones. **Palmar arch, superficial [arcus palmaris superficialis (NA)].** A transverse artery in the palm superficial to the flexor tendons, formed mainly by the termination of the ulnar artery. It may be completed by a branch from the radialis indicis artery [arteria radialis indicis], passing from the radial artery to the lateral side of the index finger, the arteria princeps pollicis or the superficial palmar branch of the radial artery, which arises as the main artery is winding around the wrist. Four palmar digital arteries [arteriae digitales, palmares, propriae et communes] pass distally from the arch towards the webs of the fingers, where they anastomose with the palmar metacarpal arteries. **Palpebral arches, inferior [arcus palpebralis inferior (NA)] and superior [arcus palpebralis superior (NA)].** *See* OPHTHALMIC ARTERY. **Paraphyseal arch.** A part of the roof of the 3rd ventricle, from which a thin-walled sac, the paraphysis, is developed in many vertebrates. **Parieto-occipital arch.** An arched gyrus surrounding the end of the parieto-occipital sulcus. **Pelvic arch, anterior.** That formed by the pubic bones and their superior rami. **Pelvic arch, posterior.** That formed by the upper 3 sacral vertebrae and the thickened part of the ilium, which extends from the sacro-iliac joint to the acetabulum. **Pharyngeal arches.** A series of arched structures present in the wall of the embryonic pharynx. *See* BRANCHIAL ARCHES (above). **Pharyngopalatine arch.** Palatopharyngeal arch (see above). **Plantar arch [arcus plantaris (NA)].** The arterial arch in the sole of the foot, placed over the metatarsal bone and interossei formed by the anastomosis of the lateral plantar and dorsalis pedis arteries. **Postvelar arch.** The part of the roof of the embryonic 3rd ventricle immediately behind the velum transversum. **Pubic arch [arcus pubis (NA)].** The arch formed below the symphysis between the 2 inferior rami of the pubic bones. **Pulmonary arch.** The 6th arterial arch of the embryo which forms the left pulmonary artery and ligamentum arteriosum on the left, and the right pulmonary artery only on the right. **Rhinencephalic arch.** The gyrus fornicatus. **Ribbon arch.** An orthodontic appliance made of a flattened wire which conforms to the dental arch and moves malposed teeth into the correct position. **Right aortic arch.** The presence of the arch of the aorta passing to the right side of the trachea and oesophagus instead of to the left; it occurs rarely as an isolated abnormality but is frequent in patients with Fallot's tetralogy. **Superciliary arch [arcus superciliaris (NA)].** The bony upper margin of the orbit. **Supraorbital arch.** Superciliary arch (see preceding). **Tarsal arches.** Palpebral arches (see above). **Tendinous arch [arcus tendineus (NA)].** A fibrous-tissue arch, usually stretching between 2 bony points, and affording partial attachment to a muscle. **Tendinous arch of the fascia of pelvic muscles [arcus tendineus fasciae pelvis (NA)].** A thickening in the fascia of the upper surface of the pelvic diaphragm which extends from the lower part of the symphysis pubis to the spine of the ischium over the surface of the obturator internus muscle; it gives origin to part of the levator ani muscle. **Tendinous arch of the levator ani muscle [arcus tendineus musculi levatoris ani (NA)].** Arcus tendineus or white line of the pelvic fascia. **Tendinous arch of the soleus muscle [arcus tendineus musculi solei (NA)].** A fibrous band in the upper part of the calf giving origin to part of the soleus muscle and arching from the tibia to the fibula over the popliteal vessels and medial popliteal nerve. **Venous arch of the foot, dorsal [arcus venosus dorsalis pedis (NA)].** Veins joining the beginnings of the great and small saphenous veins on the dorsum of the foot. **Venous arch of the hand, dorsal [arcus venosus dorsalis manus (NA)].** *See* BASILIC VEIN. **Venous arch, palmar [arcus venosus palmaris (NA)].** Veins accompanying the deep [profundus (NA)] and superficial [superficialis (NA)] palmar arterial arches. **Venous arch, plantar [arcus venosus plantaris (NA)].** *Cutaneous:* superficial veins at the roots of the toes in the sole of the foot. *Deep:* veins which accompany the plantar arterial arch. **Vertebral arch [arcus vertebrales (NA)].** The arch formed on the posterior aspect of the body of a vertebra by the pedicles and laminae. **Visceral arch.** Branchial arches (see above). **Volar arches.** Palmar arches (see above). **V-shaped arch.** A dental arch which is angular rather than parabolic in form. **Wire arch.** An orthodontic appliance made of rounded or oval wire which conforms to the dental arch and moves malposed teeth into the correct position. **Zygomatic arch [arcus zygomaticus (NA)].** The arch formed by the junction of the zygomatic process of the temporal bone with the zygomatic bone. [L *arcus* bow.]

See also: ANGLE, CORTI, HALLER, LANGER, PARKER (W. K.), SHENTON, TREITZ, ZIMMERMANN (K. W.).

archaeocyte (ar·ke·o·site). A free or wandering amoeboid cell. [Gk *archaios* ancient, *kytos* cell.]

archaeus (ar·**ke**·us). The anima mundi or vital force which, according to Paracelsus, is responsible for the continuity of life in the universe and for the maintenance of life in the individual. [Gk *archaios* ancient.]

archaic (ar·**ka**·ik). Belonging to an earlier period. [see prec.]

archamphiaster (**ark**·am·fe·**as**'·ter). In biology, an amphiaster which produces polar globules. [Gk *arche* beginning, *amphi*, *aster* star.]

archangelica (**ark**·an·**jel**'·ik·ah). *Archangelica officinalis* (*Angelica archangelica*). *See* ANGELICA. [Gk *arche* beginning, *aggelos* angel.]

archebiosis (**ar**·ke·bi·**o**'·sis). Abiogenesis. [Gk *arche* beginning, *bios* life.]

archecentric (ar·ke·**sen**·trik). A term applied to the primitive type of organism or organ, the basic pattern on which all modifications of type in other members of the same group are made. [Gk *arche* beginning, centre.]

archegenesis (ar·ke·**jen**·es·is). Abiogenesis. [Gk *arche* beginning, genesis.]

archegony (ark·**eg**·on·e). The scientific doctrine of abiogenesis. [Gk *arche* beginning, *gone* seed.]

archelogy (ark·**el**·o·je). The study of the science of principles. [Gk *arche* beginning, *logos* science.]

archencephalon (ark·en·**kef**·al·on). The embryonic primitive structure from which the forebrain and the mid-brain grow. [Gk *arche* beginning, *kephale* head.]

archenteric (ark·en·**ter**·ik). Referring to the archenteron.

archenteron (ark·en·ter·on). In zoology, the primitive cavity which forms at the conversion of an ovum into a gastrula, and from which the alimentary cavity develops; the coelenteron. [Gk *arche* beginning, *enteron* intestine.]

archeocinetic (ar·ke·o·sin·**et'**·ik). Archeokinetic.

archeocyte (ar·ke·o·site). Archaeocyte.

archeokinetic (ar·ke·o·kin·**et'**·ik). A primitive and low type of motor nerve mechanism such as is shown in the ganglionic and the peripheral nervous systems. [Gk *archaios* ancient, kinesis.]

archepyon (ark·**ep**·e·on). Pus of thick or cheesy consistency. [Gk *arche* beginning, *pyon* pus.]

Archer, Henry Edwards. 20th century London chemical pathologist.

Archer and Robb method. For urea in blood: oxalated blood (0.2 ml) is added to 2.2 ml water, a knife-point of soya or jack-bean meal is added and the mixture incubated at 55°C for 15 min. 0.3 ml of 2/3 N sulphuric acid, 0.3 ml of 10 per cent sodium tungstate and 5 ml of water are added; the mixture is shaken and centrifuged. To 5 ml of filtrate is added 5 ml of water and 2 ml of Nessler reagent. The colour is compared with that given by standard ammonium sulphate solutions.

archespore, archesporium (ar·ke·spore, ar·ke·**spo**·re·um). In biology, the layer of cells from which the mother cells of pollen or of spores arise. [Gk *arche* beginning, *sporos* seed.]

archetype (**ar**·ke·tipe). 1. A prototype. 2. An ideal anatomical type which serves as a standard for the measuring or comparing of other individuals or classes. [Gk *arche* beginning, *typos* type.]

archiblast (ar·ke·blast). 1. In zoology, the protoplasm of the egg. 2. A term applied to the fundamental part of the primary mesoderm as contrasted with the peripheral part. [Gk *arche* beginning, *blastos* germ.]

archiblastic (ar·ke·**blas**·tik). Having reference to or derived from the archiblast.

archiblastoma (ar·ke·blas·**to'**·mah). Any parenchymatous tumour. [Gk *arche* beginning, blastoma.]

archiblastula (ar·ke·**blas**·tew·lah). A hypothetical hollow spherical stage in animal evolution which is recapitulated in the embryonic blastula. [Gk *arche* beginning, blastula.]

archicarp (ar·ke·karp). Ascogonium. [Gk *arche* beginning, *karpos* fruit.]

archicentre (ar·ke·**sen**·ter). 1. Archetype; prototype. 2. A primitive organism or organ from which another organism or organ has arisen. [Gk *arche* beginning, centre.]

archicentric (ar·ke·**sen**·trik). Referring to an archicentre.

archicerebellum (ar·ke·ser·e·**bel'**·um]. The phylogenetically oldest portion of the cerebellum, represented by the flocculonodular lobe. [Gk *arche* beginning, cerebellum.]

archicoele (ar·ke·seel). Blastocoele. [Gk *arche* beginning, *koilia* cavity.]

archicortex (ar·ke·**kor**·tex). Archipallium. [Gk *arche* beginning, cortex.]

archicyte (**ar**·ke·site). An egg which has been fertilized but in which the process of segmentation has not yet begun. [Gk *arche* beginning, *kytos* cell.]

archicytula (ark·e·**si**·tew·lah). An egg cell which has been fertilized and in which the nucleus is just beginning to form. [Gk *arche* beginning, cytula.]

archigaster (ar·ke·**gas**·ter). Archenteron. [Gk *arche* beginning, *gaster* belly.]

archigastrula (ar·ke·**gas**·troo·lah). In zoology, a typical gastrula at its first stage of development from an archiblastula. [Gk *arche* beginning, gastrula.]

archigenesis (ar·ke·**jen**·es·is). Abiogenesis. [Gk *arche* beginning, *genein* to produce.]

archigonocyte (ar·ke·**gon**·o·site). The primary germ cell produced when the fertilized ovum divides. [Gk *arche* beginning, gonocyte.]

archikaryon (ar·ke·**kar**·e·on). The nucleus of a fertilized ovum. [Gk *arche* beginning, *karyon* nucleus.]

archil (**ar**·kil). Orchil, orseille; a violet colouring matter obtained from lichens of the *Roccella* and *Lecanora* species by boiling with water, treating with ammonia and exposing to the air. It contains orcein, and was at one time used as a dye; now employed to colour pharmaceutical preparations. The name was originally applied to the plants themselves. [Gk *orchilos* wren.]

Archimedes (b. 287 BC). Greek mathematician.

Archimedes principle. The upthrust on a body immersed in a fluid equals the weight of fluid it displaces; that is to say, a body immersed in a fluid loses a part of its weight equal to the weight of the displaced fluid.

archimonerula (ar·ke·mon·**er'**·ew·lah). In embryology, the egg in the monerula stage while the process of first and total division is going on. [Gk *arche* beginning, monerula.]

archimorula (ar·ke·**mor**·ew·lah). In embryology, the mulberry-like mass of cells which arises between the segmentation of the archicytula and the formation of the archigastrula. [Gk *arche* beginning, morula.]

archinephric (ar·ke·**nef**·rik). Referring to the archinephron.

archinephron (ar·ke·**nef**·ron). The mesonephros; a structure developing in the embryo after the pronephros, extending from the 6th cervical segment to the 3rd lumbar segment and consisting of numerous tubules and a like number of unsegmented internal glomeruli. The primitive kidney or renal system; commonly referred to as the wolffian body. [Gk *arche* beginning, *nephros* kidney.]

archineuron (ar·ke·**newr**·on). 1. A primitive neuron. 2. The neuron at which the activity of an efferent impulse begins, thus putting into train the sequence of actions which characterize physiological function. [Gk *arche* beginning, *neuron* nerve.]

archipallial (ar·ke·**pal**·e·al). Referring to the archipallium or involving it.

archipallium (ar·ke·**pal**·e·um). The cortex of the hippocampal formation on the medial side of the cerebral hemisphere, including that of the dentate gyrus, the hippocampus and the subiculum. [Gk *arche* beginning, pallium.]

archiplasm (ar·ke·plazm). The most primitive living substance; the substance of the fertilized egg. [Gk *arche* beginning, *plasma* something formed.]

archisome (**ar**·ke·some). The substance of the fertilized egg. [Gk *arche* beginning, *soma* body.]

archispore (**ar**·ke·spore). Archespore.

archistriatum (**ar**·ke·stri·**a'**·tum). The primitive striatum the representative of which in the human subject is the amygdaloid nucleus in the cerebrum. [Gk *arche* beginning, striatum.]

architectonic (ar·ke·tek·**ton'**·ik). 1. Referring to the systematizing of knowledge. 2. Referring to the structural pattern. [Gk *arkitekton*, chief artificer.]

architis (ar·**ki**·tis). Proctitis, or an inflammatory condition of the anus. [Gk *archos* anus, *-itis* inflammation.]

archocele (**ar**·ko·seel). Rectal hernia. *See* HERNIA. [Gk *archos* anus, *kele* hernia.]

archocystocolposyrinx (ar·ko·**sis**·to·kol·po·**sir'**·inx). Fistula of rectum, bladder and vagina. [Gk *archos* anus, *kystis* bag, *kolpos* vagina, *syrigx* pipe.]

archocystosyrinx (**ar**·ko·sis·to·**sir'**·inx). A fistula between the rectum and the bladder. [Gk *archos* anus, *kystis* bladder, *syrigx* pipe.]

archoplasm, archoplasma (ar·ko·plazm, ar·ko·**plaz**·mah). In mitotic cell division, the substance of which the attraction spheres, the astral rays and the spindles consist, and from which they are derived. [Gk *arche* beginning, plasma.]

archoptoma (ar·kop·**to**·mah). A part of the rectum affected by prolapse. [Gk *archos* anus, *ptosis* fall.]

archoptosis (ar·kop·**to**·sis). Prolapse of the lower part of the rectum. [see prec.]

archoptotic (ar·kop·**tot**·ik). 1. Referring to archoptoma. 2. Affected with archoptosis.

archorrhagia (ar·ko·**ra**·je·ah). Haemorrhage from the rectum. [Gk *archos* anus, *rhegnynein* to gush forth.]

archorrhoea (ar·ko·re·ah). A discharge of blood or pus or other pathological fluid from the rectum. [Gk *archos* anus, *rhoia* flow.]
archos (ar·kos). The anus. [Gk.]
archosome (ar·ko·some). Archiplasm. [Gk *arche* beginning, *soma* body.]
archostenosis (ar·ko·sten·o'·sis). Stricture of the rectum. [Gk *archos* anus, stenosis.]
archosyrinx (ar·ko·sir·ingx). 1. A fistula of the rectum or anus. 2. A rectal syringe. [Gk *archos* anus, *syrigx* pipe.]
archusia (ar·kew·ze·ah). A hypothetical substance, assumed to be present in the body cells and to be the same as vitamin B; it is supposed to stimulate activity and growth. [Gk *arche* beginning, *ousia* essence.]
archyl, archyle (ar·kil, ar·kile). Protyle; the postulated fundamental form of matter from which all the chemical elements are believed to have been built up. [Gk *arche* beginning, *hyle* matter.]
arciform (ar·se·form). Bowshaped. [L *arcus* bow, form.]
arciform arteries. Arcuate arteries.
arciform veins. Arcuate veins.
arctation (ark·ta·shun). Stricture; narrowing of an opening or channel. [L *arctare* to press together.]
Arctium (ark·she·um). A genus of the Compositae. **Arctium lappa.** European burdock, yields a root that is diuretic and antirheumatic. [Gk *arktion* burdock.]
Arctomys (ark·to·mis). The tarabagan *Arctomys bobac*, a large marmot, which is an important reservoir of plague in Manchuria. Its usual vector flea is *Oropsylla silantiewi*. [Gk *arktos* bear, *mys* rat.]
Arctostaphylos (ark·to·staf·e·los). A large genus of evergreen shrubs of the family Ericaceae; some species have diuretic properties. **Arctostaphylos uva-ursi.** A species found in Europe and North America which yields bearberry leaves (uva ursi). [Gk *arktos* bear, *staphyle* grape.]
arcuate (ar·kew·ate). Arched; bow-shaped. **Arcuate line.** *See* LINE. [L *arcuare* to bow.]
arcuate artery [arteria arcuata (NA)]. 1. A branch of the dorsalis pedis artery which passes laterally across the metatarsal bones on the dorsum of the foot. 2. One of the major branches of the interlobar arteries of the kidney. The arcuate arteries run in the region of the corticomedullary junction and give off a series of interlobular arteries.
arcuate veins [venae arcuatae (NA)]. Veins which accompany the arcuate arteries of the kidney. They receive interlobular veins and a series of veins which drain the renal medulla.
arcuation (ar·kew·a·shun). 1. A bending. 2. An abnormal curvature. [L *arcuare* to bow.]
arcula (ar·kew·lah). The orbit. **Arcula cordis.** The pericardium. [L casket.]
arculus (ar·kew·lus). Bed cradle. *See* CRADLE. [L little bow.]
arcus (ar·kus). The Latin for *arch*. **Arcus corneae.** Arcus senilis (see below). **Arcus juvenilis.** Premature formation of arcus senilis (see below). **Arcus lipoides corneae.** Arcus senilis (see below). **Arcus lipoides myringis.** Fatty deposits in the ear-drum; usually regarded as degenerative change. **Arcus lipoides tympani.** Fatty deposits in the tympanum; usually regarded as degenerative change. **Arcus pinguiculus.** Arcus senilis (see below). **Arcus presenilis.** Premature formation of arcus senilis (see following). **Arcus senilis.** A ring of opacity in the peripheral part of the cornea, separated from the limbus by a narrow, clear zone. It develops constantly in later life and is a simple senile degeneration characterized by lipoid infiltration of the stroma of the cornea. **Arcus senilis lentis.** Formation of an opaque ring in the periphery of the lens with age.
ardanaesthesia (ar·dan·es·the'·ze·ah). Thermo-anaesthesia; loss of sensibility to heat; inability to distinguish between heat and cold. [L *ardor* heat, anaesthesia.]
ardor (ar·dor). A sensation of heat or of burning. Cf. CALOR; DOLOR; FERVOR. **Ardor urinae.** A sensation of scalding while urine is being passed. **Ardor ventriculi.** Heartburn. [L heat.]
area (a·re·ah). 1. A plane surface; a measure of a plane surface. 2. [NA] In anatomy, a term used for a part of the whole of any surface. **Acoustic area.** A triangular area in the floor of the lower and intermediate parts of the 4th ventricle overlying the vestibular nuclei. **Aortic area, Aortic-valve area.** The approximate precordial surface marking of the aortic valve and the site at which sounds and murmurs arising from the aortic valve are usually best heard. It lies in the 2nd intercostal space, just to the right of the sternum; sometimes, however, aortic-valve murmurs are better heard down the left sternal border and at the apex of the heart. **Association area.** An area of the cerebral cortex concerned with the association or integration of stimuli from several different sources, in contrast to a projection area (see below). **Asthmagenic area.** The posterior third of the nasal septum; sometimes referred to as the trigger area of the nose. **Auditopsychic area.** That part of the temporal cortex concerned with the association and correlation of auditory impulses; Brodmann's area 22. **Auditory area, Auditory-projection area, Auditosensory area.** The cortex in the superior temporal gyrus and the upper surface of the temporal operculum which receives the auditory radiations from the medial geniculate body; also called the *auditory cortex*, Brodmann's areas 41 and 42. **Auscultatory areas.** The precordial areas at which sounds and murmurs arising from each of the 4 valves of the heart respectively are best heard with the stethoscope. They correspond approximately with the surface markings of the valves concerned. **Bare area of the liver [area nuda (NA)].** The large triangular area, not clothed with peritoneum, on the back of the liver, between the upper and lower layers of the coronary ligament. It is grooved by the inferior vena cava and is in contact with the right suprarenal gland. **Bleeding area.** A highly vascular portion of the anterior part of the nasal septum where the varicosities frequently rupture; also called *Little's area*. **Buccopharyngeal area.** A mesoderm-free portion of the embryonic disc in front of the notochord, from which the buccopharyngeal membrane is derived. **Calcarine area.** Striate area. *See* CORTEX, CALCARINE. **Cardiogenic area.** A portion of the splanchnic mesoderm at the front end of the embryonic disc, from which the heart is derived. **Catchment area.** The complete area from which water drains to a river, lake, reservoir or other source of water supply. **Area celsi.** Alopecia areata. **Area centralis.** The fovea centralis. **Cochlear area.** *See* MEATUS, INTERNAL AUDITORY. **Cord area.** Parts of the cortex of the cerebrum, lesions of which are associated with tract degenerations of the cord, e.g. motor cortex. **Cortical area.** Any part of the cerebral cortex that can be differentiated structurally or functionally from neighbouring parts. **Cribriform area [area cribrosa (NA)].** 1. The area round the renal papillae where the vessels and nerves of the kidney enter. 2. The apex of a renal papilla pitted with openings of the ducts of Bellini. **Area of critical definition.** The clear portion of an image formed by a lens. **Dangerous area.** The portion of the sclera which overlies the ciliary body. Penetrating injuries of this area are liable to cause blindness of both eyes from sympathetic ophthalmitis. **Dangerous area of the scalp.** The loose tissue beneath the epicranial aponeurosis. In cellulitis of the scalp if infection extends to this region suppuration may spread and separate the scalp from the skull, with great risk of fatal septic sinus thrombosis. **Dermatomic areas.** The areas of body surface which are innervated by individual spinal nerve roots; also called *dermatomes, segmental areas*. **Area diffluens.** Alopecia areata. **Diffraction area.** The lighter area seen round the image of an object under a microscope, caused by the diffraction of light at its edges. **Donor area.** Any area from which skin, bone or other tissue is taken for grafting elsewhere in the body. **Area embryonalis, Embryonic area.** That part of the developing ovum from which the embryo proper will be formed, as distinct from the extra-embryonic membranes. **Excitable area.** That part of the cerebral cortex from which movements can be produced by electrical stimulation. **Extra-pyramidal motor areas.** The areas of the cerebral cortex, other than the prerolandic motor area, that produce motor activity when stimulated, and loss of activity

when excised. Brodmann's areas 5, 6, 19 and 22 may be considered to fall into this group, particularly area 6, the premotor cortex. These observations lack confirmation, and other functions are attributed to these areas. **Eye area.** Cortical areas in the frontal and occipital lobes from which eye movements can be elicited by stimulation, **Flush area.** The centre of the face and the upper part of the chest to which emotional flushing is usually limited. **Gastric areas [areae gastricae (NA)].** The areas on the mucous membrane of the stomach bearing the gastric pits. **Germinal area, Area germinativa.** The germinal disc on the surface of the yolk in large-yolked eggs from which development starts. **Glove area.** The skin area covered by a glove or gauntlet. Anaesthesia that is confined to the glove area or stocking area is usually hysterical in origin. **Hyaline area.** The area of cartilage matrix within a mass of fibro- or elastic cartilage. **Hysterogenic area.** Hysterogenic point, pressure on which produces a hysterical attack. **Intercondylar area of the tibia.** *See* TIBIA. **Interfacial area.** The area at the interface between 2 liquids or a liquid and a gas. **Interglobular area.** The area of the dentine of a tooth which contains interglobular spaces. **Intermediate area of the iliac crest [linea intermedia].** A rough area between the outer and inner lips of the iliac crest. **Area jonstoni.** Alopecia areata. **Mirror areas.** Areas of specular reflection (see below). **Mitral area, Mitral-valve area.** The region of the cardiac apex, and the point at which murmurs arising from the mitral valve are best heard. Diastolic murmurs are usually localized to the apex; systolic murmurs arising from mitral-valve incompetence are best heard at the apex but are usually conducted into the left auricle. **Motor area.** Pyramidal area (see below). **Oculomotor area.** Brodmann's area 8. This is situated in the posterior parts of the frontal gyri immediately in front of Brodmann's area 6. The parts of the areas 6 and 8 lying in the middle frontal gyrus are concerned with eye movements. **Olfactory area.** That part of the cerebral cortex which is presumed to have olfactory function; the piriform area. The surface of the olfactory tubercle in the anterior perforated space may be included. **Area opaca.** A whitish region surrounding the germinal area in the early development of large-yolked eggs where the cellular layer is adherent to the underlying yolk. **Optic area.** The site of the future eye in early embryos. **Parastriate area.** The portion of the occipital cortex surrounding the calcarine area, and concerned with visual association; Brodmann's area 18. **Parolfactory area [area subcallosa (NA)].** *See* CORTEX, CEREBRAL. **Pectinated area.** The area of mucosa in the anal canal between the valves and the mucocutaneous junction. **Area pellucida.** The central transparent part of the embryonic disc in large-yolked eggs where the cellular layer is separated from the underlying yolk by fluid. **Area perforata.** The anterior or posterior perforated space. **Peristriate area.** A second concentric zone of occipital cortex, surrounding the parastriate area (see above) and also concerned with visual association; Brodmann's area 19. **Piriform area.** The cortex of the uncus of the hippocampal gyrus which receives fibres from the lateral olfactory tract. **Placental area.** That part of the ectoderm of the ovary that is associated with the wall of the uterus. **Postcentral area.** The area of the cerebral cortex posterior to the central sulcus; the sensory area. This includes the whole of the postcentral gyrus and part of the paracentral lobule. The anterior part of this area corresponds to Brodmann's area 3, and in it are received the exteroceptive and proprioceptive impulses from the opposite half of the body. The remainder of the postcentral area corresponds to Brodmann's areas 1 and 2. The function of these areas is to relate the impulses received in area 3 to past experience. **Posterior hypothalamic area.** A region of the hypothalamus above and behind the mamillary bodies from which efferent fibres pass to the brain stem. **Area postrema.** A very small highly vascular area in the extreme caudal part of the floor of the 4th ventricle. **Postrolandic area.** Postcentral area (see above). **Precentral area.** The precentral gyrus or so-called *motor* or *pyramidal area* of the cerebral cortex. **Precordial area.** The area of the anterior chest wall which overlies the heart. **Premotor area.** The portion of frontal cortex immediately anterior to the true motor cortex; the main extrapyramidal motor area; Brodmann's area 6. **Pre-optic area.** The region lateral to the lamina terminalis in which the pre-optic hypothalamic nuclei are situated. **Prerolandic motor area.** Precentral area (see above). **Pretectal area.** The area which receives fibres from the optic tract and lies lateral to the posterior commissure, and rostral to the superior colliculus. **Projection area.** An area of cortex, the main connections of which are to subcortical structures. Projection areas may be motor, e.g. the precentral gyrus, connected to motor nuclei of the brain stem and cord, or sensory, e.g. the visual area, receiving connections from the lateral geniculate body. **Psychoauditory area.** The auditopsychic area (see above). **Psychomotor area.** An indefinite term sometimes applied to the cortex immediately anterior to the motor area; it is thought to be concerned with the integration of single movements into patterns. **Pulmonary area, Pulmonary-valve area.** The approximate precordial surface marking of the pulmonary valve and the site at which sounds and murmurs arising from the valve are best heard. It lies in the 2nd intercostal space, just to the left of the sternum. **Pulse area.** The area on the front of the wrist at which the pulse is most easily felt. **Pyramidal area.** The area of cerebral cortex lying immediately anterior to the rolandic fissure and encroaching upon it; it is concerned with voluntary-muscle activity, and is characterized histologically by the presence of large pyramidal or Bétz cells; also called the *motor cortex, motor area, Brodmann's area 4.* **Recipient area.** Any area of the body which receives a surgical graft. **Rolandic area.** Precentral area (see above). **Segmental area.** Dermatomic area (see above). **Sensory area.** The general sensory area. *See* POSTCENTRAL AREA (above). **Septal area.** The surface of the brain anterior to the lamina terminalis and below the rostrum and genu of the corpus callosum. It includes the septum lucidum, and corresponds approximately with the parolfactory area (see above). **Silent area.** An area of cortex where stimulation or injury seems to produce no effect, sensory or motor. **Somaesthetic area.** Postcentral area (see above). **Somaesthetopsychic areas.** Not generally recognized but described as the areas of parietal cortex lying posterior to the sensory area, and concerned with the association and correlation of somaesthetic stimuli; Brodmann's areas 5 and 7. **Areas of specular reflection.** The anterior and posterior surfaces of the cornea and lens, by observing light reflected from which it is possible to see surface changes not otherwise visible. They are best seen through the corneal microscope with a slit lamp, but the anterior surface of the cornea can be examined by the naked eye by observing the reflection of a source of light, e.g. lamp or window. **Stocking area.** *See* GLOVE AREA (above). **Striate area.** *See* CORTEX, CALCARINE. **Tricuspid area, Tricuspid-valve area.** The approximate precordial surface marking of the tricuspid valve and the site at which murmurs and sounds arising at the tricuspid valve are best heard with the stethoscope. It lies at the left lower part of the sternum, opposite the 4th and 5th costal cartilages. **Trigger area.** That area which, on stimulation, is the site of a trigger action. **Trigger area of the nose.** Asthmagenic area (see above). **Vagus area.** Trigone of the vagus. **Area vasculosa.** That part of the wall of the yolk sac which is well supplied with blood vessels; the extra-embryonic splanchnopleure. **Vestibular area.** *See* MEATUS, INTERNAL AUDITORY *and* VENTRICLE, FOURTH. **Visual area.** Striate area. *See* CORTEX, CALCARINE. **Visual-projection area.** Striate area. *See* CORTEX, CALCARINE. **Visuopsychic area.** The cortex surrounding the striate area which is concerned in the integration and interpretation of visual stimuli. **Visuosensory area.** Striate area. *See* CORTEX, CALCARINE. **Area vitellina.** That part of the surface of the yolk which is not yet covered by embryonic cells; it lies peripheral to the area opaca (see above). **Vocal area.** The area of the glottis between the vocal folds. [L a space.]

See also: BAMBERGER (H.), BETZ, BROCA, BRODMANN, CAMPBELL (A. W.), COHNHEIM, FLECHSIG, HEAD, KIESSELBACH, KROENIG, LAIMER-HAECKERMANN, LITTLE (J. L.), MARTEGIANI, OBERSTEINER, PANUM, PITRES, REDLICH, ROLANDO, SMITH (G. E.), SPENCER (W. G.), STROUD, WERNICKE (K.).

areatus (a·re·a·tus). Occurring in circumscribed areas; patchy. [L.]

Areca (ar·e·kah). 1. A genus of palms, occurring in India and southern Asia. 2. Areca BPC 1949 (areca nut, betel nut), the dried ripe seeds of *Areca catechu*, which is cultivated in many Eastern countries. It contains the volatile liquid alkaloid arecoline, tannin and fat, and has been used as a decoction and enema to expel tapeworm in humans, but is employed mainly in veterinary medicine as a vermifuge. Considerable quantities are used in the East in conjunction with fresh betel leaf (*Piper betel*), lime and catechu, as a masticatory. **Areca nut.** The seed of the betel palm, *Areca catechu*; arecae semina. [Malayan.]

arecaidine, arecaine (ar·ek·a·id·een, ar·ek·a·een). *N*-methylguvacine, $CH_3C_5H_7NCOOH$. One of the less important alkaloids present in areca nut (betel nut), resembling muscarine in pharmacological properties. Arecoline is its methyl ester.

arecaline (ar·**ek**·al·een). Arecoline.

arecin (ar·es·in). Areca red. A red colouring matter occurring in betel nuts, *Areca catechu*.

arecoline (ar·**ek**·o·leen). $C_8H_{13}O_2N$, the principal alkaloid obtained from *Areca catechu* (betel nut). Pharmacologically it simulates the postganglionic parasympathetic fibres. The drug is not used in modern therapeutics, but is occasionally employed as a vermifuge in veterinary medicine because it causes a marked increase of peristalsis which promotes the expulsion of the worms. **Arecoline hydrobromide.** $C_8H_{13}O_2NHBr$, a soluble white compound with a cholinergic action similar to that of pilocarpine.

areflexia, areflexion (a·re·**flex**·e·ah, a·re·**flek**·shun). A condition in which reflexes cannot be elicited, or are absent, generally as a result of breakdown in the reflex arc. [Gk *a*, reflex.]

aregenerative (a·re·**jen**·er·a·tiv). Marked by absence of regeneration. [Gk *a*, regeneration.]

arenaceous (ar·en·a·shus). Gritty or sandy; like gravel or sand. [L *arena* sand.]

arenation (ar·en·a·shun). Ammotherapy; the use of hot sand baths as a form of treatment. [see prec.]

Arenavirus (ar·en·ah·**vi**·rus). A genus of enveloped RNA-containing viruses, about 100 nm in diameter. The members include the lymphocytic choriomeningitis virus and the viruses of South American haemorrhagic fevers and lassa fever. The name is due to electron-dense granules in the virions giving a sandy appearance by electron microscopy. [L *arena* sand, *virus* poison.]

arenobufagin (ar·e·no·**boof**'·aj·in). A particular bufagin, with digitalis-like effect, obtained from the skin of certain toads.

arenoid (ar·en·oid). Having the appearance, colour and consistence of sand. [L *arena* sand, Gk *eidos* form.]

areocardia (ar·e·o·**kar**'·de·ah). Bradycardia. [Gk *araios* thin, *kardia* heart.]

areola (ar·e·o·lah). 1. An interstice in areolar or other tissue. 2. [Areola mammae (NA)]. The brownish ring surrounding the nipple of the breast. 3. The reddish ring around any inflammatory lesion of the skin. 4. The part of the iris of the eye which surrounds the pupil. **Areola of the breast [areola mammae].** The pigmented area surrounding the mammary papilla, or nipple. **Areola papillaris.** The areola of the breast. **Primary areola.** In the matrix of cartilage which is becoming ossified, those cell spaces which are occupied by cartilaginous cells. **Secondary areola.** A darkish ring which during pregnancy is present round the areola papillaris. **Umbilical areola, Areola umbilicalis, Areola umbilicaris.** The area of pigmentation around the umbilicus which is present in pregnancy. **Vaccinal areola.** The circle of angry red which surrounds the pustule of the vaccinated area. [L little space.]

See also: CHAUSSIER.

areolar (ar·e·o·lar). 1. Referring to or resembling an areola. 2. Of or pertaining to tissue or other structure in which there are many interstices.

areolate (ar·e·o·late). Characterized by areolae.

areolitis (ar·e·o·**li**'·tis). A condition of inflammation of the areola of the breast. [areola, Gk *-itis* inflammation.]

areometer (ar·e·**om**·et·er). Hydrometer; used in the determination of the specific gravity of liquids. [see foll.]

areometric (ar·e·o·**met**'·rik). Referring to or involving hydrometry. [Gk *araios* thin, meter.]

areometry (ar·e·**om**·et·re). Hydrometry. [see prec.]

areosis (ar·e·**o**·sis). The process of being diluted or of becoming less concentrated. [Gk *araios* thin.]

arevareva (ar·e·var·**e**'·vah). A disease of the skin characterized by the occurrence of scales and found in association with general debility; it is caused by addiction to the drug kava. [Tahitian.]

argal (ar·gal). Argol.

argamblyopia (arg·am·ble·**o**'·pe·ah). Amblyopia occurring as a result of the eyes not having been used for a long time. [Gk *argos* idle, amblyopia.]

Argand, Aimé (b. 1755). Swiss physicist.

Argand burner. A type of oil or gas burner which is fitted with a chimney and has a regulated supply of air. It is used in the laboratory.

Argas (ar·gas). A genus of ticks, mostly bird parasites. **Argas mianensis.** A suspected vector of human relapsing fever in Persia. Also called *Argas persicus*. [Gk *argos* idle.]

Argasidae (ar·gas·id·e). A family of ticks (Acari) containing the vector genera *Argas* and *Ornithodorus*. The adults, unlike Ixodoidae, remain on the hosts for short feeding periods only. [see prec.]

argema (ar·je·mah) (pl. *argemata*). A white ulcer of the corneal margin, usually the sequel to phylyctenular ulceration. [Gk ulcer.]

argentaffin, argentaffine (ar·**jen**·taf·in, ar·**jen**·taf·een). Having an affinity for silver salts; taking the stain of solutions of silver. [L *argentum* silver, *affinitas* affinity.]

argentaffinoma (ar·jen·taf·in·**o**'·mah). A tumour, either benign or malignant, of the gastro-intestinal tract; it is derived from the chromargentaffin cells of Kultchitzky found in the intestinal canal. [L *argentum* silver, *affinitas* affinity, Gk *-oma* tumour.]

argentation (ar·jen·**ta**·shun). 1. The state of being stained with a salt of silver. 2. Argyria. [L *argentum* silver.]

Argenti Nitras. *European Pharmacopoeia* name for Silver Nitrate BP 1973.

argentic (ar·**jen**·tik). 1. Having the characteristics of silver. 2. Denoting a compound containing silver, particularly the rare compounds of bivalent silver with pyridine or fluorine. [L *argentum* silver.]

argentine (ar·jen·tine). Referring to and including silver. Resembling silver; silvery. [see prec.]

argentocyanide (ar·jen·to·**si**'·an·ide). A complex salt formed by silver cyanide with other metallic cyanides. [L *argentum* silver, cyanide.]

argentophil, argentophile (ar·**jen**·to·fil, ar·**jen**·to·file). Argyrophil; taking silver stain readily or easily becoming impregnated with silver. [L *argentum* silver, *philein* to love.]

argentoproteinum (ar·**jen**·to·pro·te·**i**'·num). Colloidal silver proteinate in an excess of denatured protein, and dried *in vacuo*. An antiseptic for especial use on mucous membrane, and in the treatment of conjunctivitis, corneal ulcers and ophthalmia neonatorum; also in throat and nose affections. It has been largely replaced by sulphonamides and penicillin in gonorrhoea, urinary infections and gynaecological work. **Argentoproteinum forte.** Silver Protein BP 1958. **Argentoproteinum mite.** Mild Silver Protein BPC 1959. [L *argentum* silver, protein.]

argentous (ar·**jen**·tus). Containing silver. 2. Denoting a compound of monovalent silver. [see foll.]

argentum (ar·**jen**·tum). Latin for *silver*, whence the symbol, Ag; genitive *argenti*. **Argentum credé.** Colloidal silver. *See* SILVER.

argiamblyopia (ar·je·am·ble·**o**'·pe·ah). Argamblyopia.

argilla (ar·jil·ah). Kaolin, china clay, potters' clay, Al_2O_3 $2SiO_2·2H_2O$. A hydrated aluminium silicate found naturally, and used in the making of porcelains and earthenwares; also as a filler for paper. Purified, it is employed in medicine as an absorbent, a protective, a dusting powder and a constituent of poultices. It is also used for filtering and clarifying liquids. [L white clay.]

argillaceous (ar·jil·a·shus). Clay-like in character; composed of clay. [see prec.]

arginase (ar·jin·aze). An enzyme which occurs in the liver of animals that excrete their nitrogen in the form of urea.

arginine (ar·jin·een). Aminoguanidine valerianic acid, δ-guanidino-α-aminovaleric acid, $NHC(NH_2)NH(CH_2)_3CH(NH_2)COOH$. An α-amino acid considered essential for animal life, which occurs widely in proteins and can be synthesized by the body to a limited degree. It forms a link in the excretion of nitrogen, being hydrolysed into ornithine and urea by the enzyme, arginase. It is a constituent of insulin, and is itself glucogenetic. **Arginine Glutamate.** BP Commission approved name for the L-arginine salt of L-glutamic acid; a nutrient. **Suberyl arginine.** A compound of suberic acid and arginine, which forms a unit in the chemical structure of toad poisons.

Argipressin (ar·je·pres·in). BP Commission approved name for 8-argininevasopressin; an antidiuretic hormone.

argol (ar·gol). Argal. An impure form of potassium hydrogen tartrate, $KH(C_4H_4O_6)$, in grape juice, which separates as a crystalline crust in wine-making. It is known as *cream of tartar* when purified, and is the commercial source of tartaric acid and tartar emetic.

argon (ar·gon). An inert gas existing in the air and the gases of certain mineral springs; produced commercially by the fractional distillation of liquid air. It is an element of atomic weight 39.948, atomic number 18 and chemical symbol A. It forms no compounds, and is used to fill electric lamps, radio valves and vacuum tubes. [Gk *argos* idle.]

Argyll Robertson, Douglas Moray Cooper Lamb (b. 1837). Scottish physician.

Argyll Robertson's operation. 1. For ectropion: removal of a triangle of skin near the outer canthus combined with a strap-like pedicle flap of skin cut parallel to the lid margin and swung upwards and outwards. 2. For glaucoma: trephining of the sclera. Of historical interest.

Argyll Robertson pupil. Rigidity of the pupil to light, with retained convergence activity. The condition is usually bilateral and is most commonly associated with syphilis of the central nervous system and with miosis.

Argyll Robertson reflex. *See* ARGYLL ROBERTSON PUPIL.

pseudo- or non-leutic Argyll Robertson pupil. Adie's pupil.

argyraemia (ar·ji·re·me·ah). A condition of the blood in which silver or salts of silver are present. [Gk *argyros* silver, *haima* blood.]

argyria, argyriasis (ar·ji·re·ah, ar·ji·ri·as·is). A condition induced by the prolonged use of salts of silver. The skin, the conjunctiva and the internal organs take on a leaden-grey colour. **Argyria nasalis.** Argyria affecting the nasal mucosa. [Gk *argyros* silver.]

argyric (ar·ji·rik). 1. Caused by the therapeutic use of silver. 2. Having relation to silver. [see prec.]

argyrism (ar·ji·rizm). Argyria.

argyrophil, argyrophile (ar·ji·ro·fil, ar·ji·ro·file). Taking silver stain readily or easily becoming impregnated with silver, a characteristic of certain cells, especially those of the gut; argentophil. [Gk *argyros* silver, *philein* to love.]

argyrosiderosis (ar·ji·ro·sid·er·o′·sis). A condition produced by exposure to a mixture of silver and iron, as occurs in the polishing of silver with rouge. There are heavy deposits of metal in the lungs and associated lymphatics, but no clear pathological changes. [Gk *argyros* silver, *sideros* iron, *-osis* condition.]

argyrosis (ar·ji·ro·sis). Argyria.

arhigosis (a·ri·go·sis). Lack of a feeling for cold; inability to feel the cold; insensitiveness to cold. [Gk *a*, *rhigos* cold.]

arhinencephalia (a·ri·nen·kef·a′·le·ah). Congenital lack of the rhinencephalon. [Gk *a*, rhinencephalon.]

ariboflavinosis (a·ri·bo·fla·vin·o′·sis). A condition caused by a lack of riboflavin in the diet, of which the symptoms include fissuring of the angles of the mouth, local stomatitis, granulation in the nasolabial folds and seborrhoeic dermatitis. There are also changes in the eye. [Gk *a*, riboflavin, Gk *-osis* condition.]

aristogenesis (ar·is·to·jen′·es·is). The development in the organism of new and more serviceable powers through continuous slow adaptation of existing mechanisms. [Gk *aristos* best, genesis.]

aristogenics (ar·is·to·jen′·ix). Eugenics. [Gk *aristos* best, *genein* to produce.]

Aristolochia (ar·is·to·lo′·ke·ah). A genus of the family Aristolochiaceae consisting of about 180 species, mostly herbs or climbing plants, many of which have been used in medicine. **Aristolochia indica.** (Indian birthwort), a species the root and stem of which have tonic properties. **Aristolochia reticulata.** Texan snake root or serpentary. **Aristolochia serpentaria.** Virginian snake root or serpentary; American species with stimulant and tonic properties. [Gk *aristos* best, lochia.]

aristolochine (ar·is·to·lo′·keen). $C_{17}H_{19}O_3N$. A crystalline alkaloid obtained from species of *Aristolochia.*

aristoquinine (ar·is·to·kwin′·een). Quinine carbonate, diquinine carbonic ester, $(C_{20}H_{23}O_2N_2)_2CO$. A white powder insoluble in water, but soluble in alcohol, ether, or chloroform; used as a substitute for quinine in malaria.

Aristotle (b. 384 B.C.). Greek philosopher.

Aristotle's anomaly. When the first and second fingers are crossed and a small object such as a pencil is placed between them the false impression is gained that there are 2 objects.

arithmomania (ar·ith·mo·ma′·ne·ah). A pathological compulsion to count or repeat numbers. It may occur as an obsessional symptom in a variety of psychiatric disorders, but is characteristically a symptom of obsessive compulsive states proper. [Gk *arithmos* number, mania.]

Arkövy's mixture. A mixture containing phenol, camphor and oil of eucalyptus used in the treatment of the infected root canals of a tooth.

arkyochrome (ar·ke·o·krome). Any kind of nerve cell the stainable substance of which is in the form of a network. [Gk *arkys* net, *chroma* colour.]

arkyostichochrome (ar·ke·o·stik′·o·krome). Any cell which presents the combination of an arkyochrome and a stichochrome. [Gk *arkys* net, *stichos* row, *chroma* colour.]

Arloing, Saturnin (b. 1846). French pathologist.

Arloing-Courmont test. An agglutination reaction similar to that of Widal's typhoid test, in which a dilute emulsified culture of *Mycobacterium tuberculosis* is mixed with a patient's serum and examined macroscopically and microscopically after incubation for a few hours. Clumping is said to indicate the presence of the specific antigen. Its reliability is questioned.

Arlt, Carl Ferdinand Ritter von (b. 1812). Vienna ophthalmologist.

Arlt's operation. 1. For cicatricial entropion: the grey line at the lid margin is split, an elliptical area of skin is excised 5 mm above the lid margin, and the flap of skin bearing the lashes is then stitched to the upper edge of the raw area. 2. Tarsorrhaphy; useful for the inner canthal angle. A horseshoe-shaped strip of skin including the lash margin is excised from the upper and lower lid margins and into the inner canthal angle. The raw area is united. 3. For symblepharon; a double-armed suture is passed through the head or the bulbar end of the adhesion, which is then separated and the suture passed to the bottom of the conjunctival fornix, brought through, and tied on the skin of the lid. The conjunctival wound is repaired. 4. For pterygium: the pterygium is excised from the inner canthus to the head which is torn off the cornea. The conjunctiva is mobilized and sutured in a crucial fashion.

Arlt's recess, or sinus. An inconstant recess in the lower reaches of the lacrimal sac.

Arlt's stratum. The deeper layer of the corium of the skin.

Arlt's trachoma. Trachoma folliculare.

Arlt-Blaskovics operation. A modification of Dieffenbach's blepharoplasty; a pedicle flap shaped like a hatchet with a narrow base is fashioned from the nearby area to fill the lid defect.

Gaillard-Arlt sutures. For ectropion: 2 double-armed sutures passed through the conjunctiva at the edge of the tarsus nearest the lid margin and then brought out through the skin well below the lid, and tied over a roll of gauze.

Jaesche-Arlt operation. For trichiasis; the lid margin is split just behind the lash margin; a crescentic area of skin is excised from the lid about 3-4 mm from the margin. This is sutured, so pulling the lash margin up, and the excised skin is trimmed and inserted into the gaping raw area below the lash margin where the lid was originally split. Of historical interest.

arm (arm). Term commonly used for the whole upper extremity. It is more strictly the part of the upper extremity between the shoulder and the elbow [brachium (NA)], in contrast to the forearm between the elbow and the wrist. There are 4 named surfaces; medial [facies medialis (NA)]; lateral [facies lateralis (NA)]; anterior [facies anterior (NA)]; and posterior [facies posterior (NA)]. **Bird arm.** A condition in which the forearm is shrunken from atrophy of the muscles. **Brawny arm.** A swollen hard oedematous condition of the arm from pressure on the axillary veins and lymphatics. **Chromosome arm.** *See* CHROMOSOME. **Golf arm.** A muscular sprain in the neighbourhood of the shoulder or elbow joint in golfers. **Lawn-tennis arm.** Tennis elbow; a painful condition of the tissues in the region of the external epicondyle, at or near to the origin of the extensor muscles of the wrist and fingers. The exact cause is uncertain. **Arm of a microscope.** The shaped metal carrying the tube in which is mounted the optical system, and supported on a swivel at the top of the pillar. It is by means of this that the instrument is handled. **Milk arm.** A chronic oedema of the arm from venous obstruction; a phlegmasia alba of the arm. [AS].

See also: KRUKENBERG (H.).

arm, nerves of the. Lower lateral cutaneous nerve of the arm [nervus cutaneus brachii lateralis inferior (NA)]. A branch of the radial nerve to the skin on the lateral and posterior aspect of the arm. **Medial cutaneous nerve of the arm [nervus cutaneus brachii medialis (NA)].** A branch of the medial cord of the brachial plexus, arising in the axilla and carrying fibres from the 8th cervical and 1st thoracic roots to supply the skin on the medial side of the arm. **Posterior cutaneous nerve of the arm [nervus cutaneus brachii posterior (NA)].** A branch of the radial nerve, supplying a small area of skin over the back of the arm. **Upper lateral cutaneous nerve of the arm [nervus cutaneus brachii lateralis superior (NA)].** A branch of the circumflex nerve, supplying the skin over the deltoid muscle.

Armadillo (ar·mad·il·o). A South American mammal that is a reservoir of *Trypanosoma cruzi*, the causal organism of American trypanosomiasis. [Sp. dim, of *armado* armed one.]

Armanni, Luciano (b. 1839). Italian pathologist.

Armanni-Ebstein cells. Terminal convoluted renal cells filled with glycogen in diabetes mellitus.

Armanni-Ehrlich degeneration. Hyaline change in the epithelial cells of Henle's loops in the diabetic kidney.

armature (arm·ah·tewr). 1. In biology, a structure which serves as an offensive or defensive weapon, e.g. a sting. 2. In magnetism, a bar of soft steel or iron which connects the poles of a magnet or of adjacent magnets. [L *armatura* a piece of armour.]

Armenian bole (ar·me·ne·an bole). An impure form of iron oxide, used in tooth powders because of its red colour.

armepavine (ar·mep·av·een). $C_{19}H_{23}O_3N$. An alkaloid obtained from *Papaver armeniacum.*

Armigeres obturbans (ar·mig·er·eez ob·ter·bans). *Armigeres (Desvoidea) obturbans*, a mosquito of Japan which is the transmitter of dengue. In New Guinea the vector of dengue is probably a related species, *Armigeres breinli.* [L troublesome armour-bearer.]

armilla (ar·mil·ah). The annular enlargement of the wrist dependent in part on the annular ligament of the superior radio-ulnar joint. [L bracelet.]

Armillifer (ar·mil·if·er). A genus of Pentastomida. **Armillifer armillatus.** A species which occurs in tropical Africa. **Armillifer moniliformis.** A species of China, the Philippines and Sumatra. The adults of both are found in the lungs of snakes, but the larvae have been found in human retroperitoneal or retropleural tissues, where they cause no symptoms but die and calcify in the form of crescents. [L *armilla* bracelet, *ferre* to bear.]

armoracia (ar·mor·a·se·ah). Horseradish, the fresh root of the cultivated cruciferous plant *Cochlearia armoracia.* It contains a glycoside, sinigrin, and an enzyme, myrosin, which in the presence of water hydrolyses the glycoside to give allyl isothiocyanate, a volatile oil with a pungent odour. The pulped root has been used for its rubefacient and vesicant properties, and a compound spirit was formerly employed as a carminative. [L.]

armpit (arm·pit). The axilla. [AS *armpytt.*]

Armstrong, Arthur Riley (b. 1904). Hamilton, Ontario, physician.

King and Armstrong method. For serum alkaline phosphatase: equal volumes of a sodium barbitone buffer (pH 9.0) and disodium phenylphosphate substrate solution are mixed and incubated at 37°C, 0.5 ml of serum is added, and, after exactly 30 min, diluted Folin-Ciocalteau's reagent, and the mixture filtered. Sodium carbonate solution is added to the filtrate and the blue colour developed by incubating at 37°C for 15 min. A control is prepared by omitting incubation to determine preformed phenol. The reading of the control is subtracted from that of the test and the result is compared with the reading of a standard phenol and reagent mixture. 1 unit of phosphatase activity is defined by King and Armstrong as 1 mg of phenol liberated by 100 ml of serum. Normal range, from 3 to 13 units.

King-Armstrong unit. A phosphatase (alkaline) activity of 1 unit per 100 ml of serum or plasma liberates 1 mg of phenol at 37°C in 30 min from a substrate of disodium phenylphosphate at pH 9.

Armstrong, Charles (b. 1886). US Public Health Service.

Armstrong's disease. Benign lymphocytic choriomeningitis. *See* CHORIOMENINGITIS.

Arndt, Rudolf (b. 1833). German psychiatrist.

Arndt-Schulz law. A weak stimulus increases physiological activity, but a strong one abolishes or diminishes it.

Arneth, Joseph (b. 1873). German physician.

Arneth's classification, count, formula or index. A slightly complex classification of the leucocytes of the myeloid series (from myeloblasts to polymorphonuclear leucocytes) suggested by Arneth, according to the shape and number of lobes in their nuclei. These granular cells are divided into 5 classes according to the number of segments of the nuclei, and a number of subdivisions according to their shape, making a total of 20 placing the more immature cell with a single-lobed nucleus to the left of the table and the most mature cell with a multi-lobed nucleus to the right. Thus, *shift to the left* or *shift to the right* are terms implying a greater proportion of cells being immature or mature respectively.

Arnica (ar·nik·ah). 1. A genus of flowering plants of the family Compositae. 2. The compositous herb *Arnica montana*, indigenous to central Europe. The dried flowerheads (Arnicae Flos BPC 1949) and the dried rhizome roots are sometimes used in the form of tinctures for sprains and bruises.

arnicin (ar·nis·in). $C_{20}H_{30}O_4$. A bitter glucoside found in the roots and flowers of arnica, *Arnica montana.*

arnicine (ar·nis·een). $C_{35}H_{54}O_7$. A resinous base found in the flowers of arnica, *Arnica montana.*

Arnold, Friedrich (b. 1803). Heidelberg anatomist.

Arnold's bundle, or fasciculus. The frontopontine fibres in the medial part of the cerebral peduncle.

Arnold's canal. The mastoid canaliculus. *See* CANALICULUS.

Arnold's innominate canal. A canal near the foramen spinosum of the sphenoid for the lesser superficial petrosal nerve.

Arnold's fold. The opercula of the insula.

Arnold's ganglion. The otic ganglion. *See* GANGLION.
Arnold's auricular nerve. The auricular branch of the vagus; the so-called *alderman's nerve.*
Arnold's recurrent nerve. An anastomotic connection between the ophthalmic nerve and the trochlear nerve and distributed to the tentorium cerebelli.
Arnold's operculum. The operculum of the insula.
Arnold's nerve reflex cough syndrome. Reflex cough produced by irritation of Arnold's nerve, the auricular branch of the vagus, in the external auditory meatus.

Arnold, Julius (b. 1835). Heidelberg pathologist.
Arnold's bodies. Small fragments of erythrocytes, or erythrocyte "ghosts", in blood.
Arnold-Chiari deformity, disease, malformation or syndrome, Chiari-Arnold syndrome. Congenital elongation and caudal displacement of the brain stem and cerebellar tonsils, with herniation of the cerebellum and medulla through the foramen magnum; usually associated with meningocele or meningomyelocele and lumbosacral spina bifida. It commonly produces hydrocephalus.

Arnold and Gunning method. A modification of Kjeldahl's method, designed to determine the total nitrogen in urine.

Arnott, James (b. 1797). Brighton surgeon formerly in the Indian Medical Service.
Arnott's anaesthesia. Insensitivity produced by packing a part with ice.

Arnott, Neil (b. 1788). Scottish physician in London.
Arnott's dilator. An inflatable tube of oiled silk for the dilatation of urethral strictures.

Arnoux, Émile (b. 1871). French gynaecologist.
Arnoux's sign. The sound said to be heard in twin pregnancy and produced by the double heart beat.

aromatic (ar·o·**mat**·ik). 1. Possessing a spicy odour or taste, e.g. cinnamon, nutmeg. 2. In organic chemistry, referring to a compound which has a benzene or quinonoid ring, as distinct from an aliphatic or open-chain compound. [Gk *aroma* spice.]

aromine (ar·o·meen). Name given to an aromatic constituent observed in urine; it has the characteristics of an alkaloid.

Aron, Max. 20th century French histologist.
Aron's test. *See* TEST FOR CANCER.

Aronson, Hans (b. 1865). German bacteriologist.
Aronson's culture medium. An alkaline peptone medium for *Vibrio cholerae.*

arrachement (ar·ahsh·**mahn**). In membranous cataract, the removal of the capsule by pulling it through an incision made in the cornea. [Fr. extraction.]

arrack (ar·ak). An Eastern name for any native liquor distilled from rice and sugar, dates, palm sap and similar substances. [Ar. *araq* juice.]

arrectores pilorum muscles [musculi arrectores pilorum (NA)] (ar·ek·**tor**·eez pi·**lo**·rum). Small involuntary muscles running from the superficial part of the corium to the hair follicle below the sebaceous gland. They may help to expel the secretion from the gland; their contraction also erects the follicles and produces the appearance known as *goose flesh* (cutis anserina). [L hair raisers.]

arrest (ar·est). **Auricular arrest.** Auricular standstill. *See* STANDSTILL. **Cardiac arrest.** Cessation of the action of the heart. The term is generally used to describe sudden ventricular asystole such as may occur in subjects with variable atrioventricular block, or after a paroxysm of ventricular arrhythmia, or in acute myocardial failure. It may occur as a result of sudden vagal over-action, occasionally during the induction of anaesthesia. **Circulatory arrest.** Cessation of the normal circulation of the blood due to cardiac arrest or ventricular fibrillation, It leads to loss of consciousness in a few seconds and death ensues from permanent cerebral anoxic damage if cardiac activity is not resumed, or some circulation restored by cardiac massage, within 2 or 3 min. **Deep transverse arrest.** In obstetrics, arrest of the head at the level of the ischial spines, with the sagittal suture in the transverse diameter of the pelvis. **Epiphyseal arrest.** Diaphyseal–epiphyseal fusion. *See* FUSION. **Maturation arrest.** In erythrocytes, the stoppage at a certain level of the process of maturation. **Pelvic arrest.** Arrest of the head in the pelvis. [L *ad, restare* to withstand.]

arrhenic (ar·e·nik). Referring to arsenic or involving the use of it. **Arrhenic medication.** Treatment with arsenic. [Gk *arrhenikon,* yellow orpiment.]

Arrhenius, Svante August (b. 1859). Swedish physical chemist.
Arrhenius' doctrine, hypothesis or theory. The theory of ionization: a theory propounded in 1887, that acids, bases and salts in aqueous solution are dissociated to a greater or lesser extent into positively and negatively charged particles or *ions,* and that the increase in the number of units in solution which arises from this dissociation is responsible for the abnormally high osmotic activity of these substances. The theory also furnishes an intelligible interpretation of various other phenomena.
Arrhenius' law. Solutions of high osmotic pressure are good conductors of electricity.

arrhenoblastoma (ar·e·no·blas·**to**'·mah). An ovarian adenoma which causes the development of secondary male sex characteristics in the female. The tumour contains imperfectly developed elements of gonadal character and male hormones. [Gk *arrhen* male, blastoma.]

arrhenogenic (ar·e·no·**jen**'·ik). Producing male offspring only. [Gk *arrhen* male, *genein* to produce.]

arrhenokaryon (ar·e·no·**kar**'·e·on). An organism which is the product of androgenesis. [Gk *arrhen* male, *karyon* nucleus.]

arrhenoma (ar·e·**no**·mah). Arrhenoblastoma.

arrhenomimetic (ar·e·no·mim·**et**'·it). A term applied to secondary male sex characteristics when they appear in the female. [Gk *arrhen* male, *mimetikos* imitative.]

arrhenoplasm (ar·e·no·plazm). The male element in the germ plasm. [Gk *arrhen* male, plasm.]

arrhenotocia, arrhenotoky (ar·e·no·**to**'·se·ah, ar·e·not·o·ke). In zoology, the production of only male offspring in parthenogenesis. [Gk *arrhen* male, *tokos* birth.]

arrhinencephalia (a·ri·nen·kef·a'·le·ah). Deficiency of the forebrain; common is trisomy 13-15 and 17-18. [Gk *a, rhis* nose, *egkephalos* brain.]

arrhinia (a·**ri**·ne·ah). The state in which the nose is lacking congenitally. [Gk *a, rhis* nose.]

arrhoea (a·**re**·ah). The suppression, stoppage, or cessation of the flow of a body fluid. [Gk *a, rhoia* flow.]

arrhythmia (a·**rith**·me·ah). 1. Absence of rhythm; irregularity. 2. Any variation in either the force or the rate of the heart beat, such as tachycardia, auricular fibrillation, extrasystole or heart block. **Cardiac arrhythmia.** Any abnormal cardiac rhythm, whether the abnormality is one of rate, regularity or origin of the impulse initiating each heart-beat. **Continuous arrhythmia.** A permanent form of abnormality of the heart beat. **Juvenile arrhythmia.** Sinus arrhythmia (see below). **Nodal arrhythmia.** Nodal rhythm, contraction of the atria before or at the same time as the ventricles, the contraction originating in the atrioventricular node. **Perpetual arrhythmia.** Atrial fibrillation, inco-ordinate contraction of the individual muscle fibres of the atrium. **Phasic sinus arrhythmia.** Alteration in the heart rate as a result of rhythmical waxing and waning of vagal influence; deep inspiration causes acceleration, and expiration causes deceleration, of the heart. **Respiratory arrhythmia.** Sinus arrhythmia (see following). **Sinus arrhythmia.** An irregularity of heart rhythm caused by changes in the vagus control of the sinu-atrial node during respiration. It is commonly met with in children and young adults, the rate increasing with inspiration and decreasing during expiration. **Vagal arrhythmia.** Any irregular rhythm caused by stimulation of the vagus nerve. [Gk *a, rhythmos* rhythm.]

arrhythmic (a·**rith**·mik). Characterized by arrhythmia.

arrhythmokinesis (a·**rith**·mo·kin·e'·sis). Inability to carry out voluntary rhythmic movements in sequence. [Gk *a, rhythmos* rhythm, kinesis.]

arrosion (ar·o·zhun). Wasting of the wall of a vessel due to pressure or ulceration. [L *ab, rodere* to gnaw.]

Arrowroot BPC 1968 (ar·o·root). A starchy product from the rhizomes of *Maranta arundinaceae* Linn. (family Marantaceae) grown in the West Indies and certain subtropical countries. It is used in place of starch in tablet making, also in the preparation of barium meals. [AS *arwe, roote.*]

Arroyo, Carlos F. (b. 1892). Florida physician.

Arroyo's sign. Sluggishness of the pupillary light reflex.

Arruga, Hermenegildo (b. 1886). Barcelona ophthalmologist.

Arruga's eye speculum. A speculum with screw adjustments for each arm specifically designed to prevent pressure on the globe.

arsacetin (ars·as·et·in). Acetylatoxyl, $CH_3CONHC_6H_4AsO(OH)ONa$. The sodium salt of *p*-acetaminophenylarsonic acid, at one time used in the treatment of trypanosome infections. It was found to have high toxicity, and has now been replaced by other organic preparations of arsenic.

arsanilate (ar·san·il·ate). A salt of arsanilic acid.

arsenamide (ar·sen·am·ide). *p*-bis-(Carboxymethylmercapto)-arsino-benzamide. An efficient anti-filarial drug, but it is too toxic for general use.

arsenate (ar·sen·ate). A salt of arsenic acid.

arseniasis (ar·sen·i·as·is). A condition of chronic arsenical poisoning.

arsenic (ar·sen·ik). An element of atomic weight 74.9216, atomic number 33, and chemical symbol As. It is a greyish metalloid which also exists in several allotropic forms; it occurs in nature free, and in minerals, principally the sulphides orpiment (As_2S_3) and realgar (As_2S_2). Its presence in iron pyrites used for the manufacture of sulphuric acid may lead to its appearance in articles intended for human consumption. Marine crustacea and certain fish absorb arsenic from sea-water and the element is passed on to fish-eaters, who accumulate it in the skin and hair. In acute poisoning there is difficulty in swallowing, vomiting, diarrhoea, suppression of urine and thirst; death from exhaustion may occur in 2 or 3 days. The symptoms of chronic poisoning are milder, with peripheral neuritis of both motor and sensory nerves, nephritis, irritation of the nasal mucous membrane and skin changes. Excretion is slow, and the retention of arsenic may act as a preservative of persons who have died from arsenical poisoning. Few of the inorganic compounds of arsenic are used in medicine owing to their toxicity, but the organic compounds were employed in the treatment of syphilis until largely replaced by penicillin and bismuth derivatives; they are still used in cases of sleeping sickness. The organic arsenicals in which arsenic is trivalent include acetarsol and tryparsamide, employed in amoebiasis and trypanosomiasis, whilst it is believed that organic compounds of pentavalent arsenic such as arsphenamine, neoarsphenamine, mapharside and sulpharsphenamine are reduced in the body to the trivalent form before becoming effective. **Arsenic 74.** A radio-isotope used in detecting brain lesions. **Arsenic bromide.** $AsBr_3$, a yellow compound used in diabetes. **Arsenic disulphide.** As_2S_2. Realgar. **Arsenic iodide.** Arsenic tri-iodide (see following). **Arsenic tri-iodide.** AsI_3, a yellow compound, soluble in water and used as an antiseptic in skin diseases. **Arsenic Trioxide BP 1963.** White arsenic, commonly known as *arsenic*, As_2O_3, a white compound slightly soluble in water, more so in potassium carbonate solution (liquor arsenicalis or Fowler's solution), used in the treatment of various skin diseases for its stimulant action, externally as a caustic, and in chronic myelogenous leukaemia to raise the red blood cell count and lower the white. **Arsenic trisulphide.** Orpiment As_2S_3, used as a pigment. **White arsenic.** Arsenic trioxide (see above). [Gk *arsen* strong.]

arsenic-fast (ar·sen·ik·fahst). Resistant to arsenic; it may be due to immunity acquired by repeated administration of the drug. This occurs in man and in other mammals and in infecting parasites; *arsenoresistant* is the word frequently used. Cf. ARSENORESISTANT.

arsenical (ar·sen·ik·al). 1. Term applicable to any drug or medicament that contains arsenic or the effects of which are dependent upon its arsenious content. 2. Referring to or containing arsenic.

arsenicalism (ar·sen·ik·al·izm). Arseniasis.

arsenicophagy (ar·sen·ik·of'·aj·e). The habitual eating of arsenic, a form of drug addiction. [arsenic, Gk *phagein* to eat.]

arsenicum (ar·sen·ik·um). Arsenic. [L.]

arsenide (ar·sen·ide). A binary compound of arsenic with a metal or hydrogen, in which arsenic behaves as a trivalent negative element; dilute acids acting on metallic arsenides generate arsine.

arsenionization (ar·sen·i·on·i·za'·shun). The diffusion in the tissues of arsenic ions as a measure against diseases due to the presence of protozoa. [arsenic, ionization.]

arsenious (ar·sen·e·us). 1. Containing arsenic, or possessing the characteristics of arsenic. 2. A compound in which arsenic is trivalent. **Arsenious iodide.** Arsenous iodide.

arsenism (ar·sen·izm). Chronic arsenical poisoning.

arsenite (ar·sen·ite). 1. A salt of arsenous acid. 2. Any one of a series of complex salts formed by different proportions of arsenic trioxide with alkalis.

arsenium (ar·sen·e·um). The element, arsenic.

arseniuretted (ar·sen·e·ewr·et'·ed). United with arsenic in a binary combination. **Arseniuretted hydrogen.** Arsine.

arsenization (ar·sen·i·za'·shun). Arsenotherapy.

arsenobenzene (ar·sen·o·ben'·zeen). 1. Name applied in general to arsphenamine derivatives used as spirochaeticides. 2. The compound of trivalent arsenic, $C_6H_5As{=}AsC_6H_5$, which may be regarded as the parent of arsphenamine and related compounds.

arsenoblast (ar·sen·o·blast). The male element in a sexual cell. [Gk *arsen* male, *blastos* germ.]

arsenoceptor (ar·sen·o·sep'·tor). Ehrlich's name for the point in the body of a trypanosome at which an arsenic drug attaches itself. Cf. ACETICOSEPTOR. [arsenic, L *recipere* to receive.]

arsenophagy (ar·sen·of·aj·e). Arsenicophagy.

arsenoresistant (ar·sen·o·re·zist'·ant). A term applied to cases of syphilis and other diseases in which resistance to arsphenamine is encountered. Cf. ARSENIC-FAST.

arsenotherapy (ar·sen·o·ther'·ap·e). The therapeutic use of arsenic and arsenicals.

arsenous (ar·sen·us). Arsenious. **Arsenous acid.** *See* ACID. **Arsenous iodide.** Arsenious iodide, arsenic tri-iodide, AsI_3, a yellow crystalline compound, soluble in water, with an action similar to that of arsenic trioxide; it is used for its iodine in skin diseases, and as an antiseptic.

arsenoxide (ar·sen·ox·ide). A partial oxidation product of the arsphenamines, containing the group $RAs{=}O$. The arsphenamines are converted to arsenoxide in the body, and it is this compound which is responsible for their trypanocidal activity. Experiments *in vitro* show that the arsphenamines do not affect motility or growth of trypanosomes, whereas arsenoxide or compounds containing the $RAs{=}O$ group are trypanocidal in low concentrations.

arsine (ar·seen). 1. Arsenic hydride, arseniuretted hydrogen, AsH_3. A colourless gas with unpleasant odour, and extremely poisonous even when diluted largely with air. It is a reducing agent, and is decomposed by heat into metallic arsenic and hydrogen, this latter being the basis of the delicate Marsh test for arsenic. 2. Name given to any one of a series of organic derivatives of arsine in which one or more of its hydrogen atoms are replaced by alkyl radicals.

arsonate (ar·son·ate). A salt of arsonic acid.

arsonium (ar·son·e·um). The monovalent radical AsH_4, in which arsenic behaves like the nitrogen in ammonium. **Arsonium compounds.** Addition compounds formed by arsine. **Arsonium hydroxide.** AsH_4OH, giving rise to a number of organic quaternary salts in which the hydrogen atoms of arsonium are replaced by alkyl radicals.

arsonvalization (ar·son·val·i·za'·shun). D'Arsonvalization.

arsphenamine (ars·fen·am·een). 1. Diaminodihydroxyarsenobenzene hydrochloride. Ehrlich's first successful arsenobenzene derivative for the treatment of syphilis. It has now been largely replaced by the arsenoxides and by neoarsphenamine. 2. Used in a wider sense, the term means any arsphenamine derivative. **Arsphenamine glucoside.** A condensation product of arsphenamine and glucose. It is more stable and more soluble than arsphenamine itself, but has the same physiological action. It is supplied in solution in ampules ready for injection and is thus more convenient than other arsphenamines, which have to be dissolved immediately prior to use. **Arsphenamine poisoning.** *See* POISONING. **Silver arsphenamine.** The sodium salt of the silver derivative of arsphenamine base, once thought to combine the effects of silver and arsphenamine but now obsolescent.

arsthinol (**ars**·thin·ol). Cyclic-3-hydroxypropylene ether of 3-acetamido-4-hydroxydithiobenzene-arsenous acid; a trivalent arsenical used in amoebiasis and yaws.

artefact (**ar**·te·fact). 1. Anything made or introduced artificially; a man-made article, e.g. in archaeology, a flint chipped by prehistoric man. 2. In histology, a misleading appearance in a preparation caused by some form of contamination or by physical or chemical changes induced by manipulation or the reagents employed in making the preparation. 3. In electroencephalography, any wave that has its origin elsewhere than in the brain. 4. In dermatology, a self-induced lesion. 5. In radiology, a fault on the radiograph, not a true shadow of the structure being x-rayed. [L *ars* art, *facere* to make.]

artefactitious (**ar**·te·fak·**tish**'·us). Having the quality of an artefact.

Artemisia (ar·tem·e·ze·ah). A genus of plants of the order Compositae. *Artemisia absinthium* Linn. yields the herb, wormwood. *Artemisia cina* Berg yields wormseed (santonica), which with other species of *Artemisia* is used as a source of santonin. [Gk *Artemis* the goddess Diana.]

arterectomy (ar·ter·**ek**·to·me). Arteriectomy.

arteriagra (ar·teer·e·**ag**'·rah). Any gouty condition affecting an artery. [artery, Gk *agra* a catching.]

arterial (ar·teer·e·al). Referring to the arterial system or to a particular artery.

arterialization (ar·teer·e·al·i·**za**'·shun). The transforming of venous into arterial blood by exposure to oxygen in the respiratory organs.

arteriarctia (ar·teer·e·**ark**'·she·ah). Arterio-arctia.

arteriasis (ar·ter·i·as·is). A degenerative condition of the walls of an artery.

arteriectasia, arteriectasis (ar·**teer**·e·ek·**ta**'·ze·ah, ar·**teer**·e·**ek**'·tas·is). Arterial dilatation. [artery, Gk *ektasis* a stretching.]

arteriectomy (ar·teer·e·**ek**'·to·me). The cutting away of a portion of an artery. [artery, Gk *ektome* a cutting out.]

arteriectopia (ar·teer·e·ek·**to**'·pe·ah). Displacement of an artery. [artery, Gk *ektopos* out of place.]

arterio-arctia (ar·teer·e·o·**ark**'·she·ah). Stenosis or contraction of an artery. [artery, L *arctare* to contract.]

arterio-atony, arteriochalasis (ar·**teer**·e·o·**at**'·on·e, ar·**teer**·e·o·**kal**'·as·is). Atony of arterial walls.

arteriodiastasis (ar·teer·e·o·di·**as**'·tas·is). 1. Arteriectopia. 2. Of 2 arteries which normally are placed near together, the divergence of the one from the other. 3. Retraction of the cut ends of an artery. [artery, diastasis.]

arteriofibrosis (ar·teer·e·o·fi·**bro**'·sis). Fibrosis of inflammatory type, causing thickening of the arteries and arterioles and consequent narrowing of the lumina of the vessels concerned.

arteriogenesis (ar·teer·e·o·**jen**'·es·is). The natural development of the arteries. [artery, Gk *genein* to produce.]

arteriogram (ar·**teer**·e·o·gram). 1. An x-ray picture of an artery produced by arteriography. 2. Sphygmogram. [artery, Gk *gramma* a writing.]

arteriograph (ar·**teer**·e·o·graf). 1. An arteriogram. 2. To make an arteriogram. 3. Sphygmogram. [artery, Gk *graphein* to record.]

arteriography (ar·teer·e·**og**'·raf·e). The visualization of arteries by means of x-rays after injection of radio-opaque material. 2. Sphygmography. [see prec.]

arteriolar (ar·teer·e·**o**'·lar). 1. Having resemblance to an arteriole. 2. Referring to or involving an arteriole or the arterioles.

arteriole [arteriola (NA)] (ar·**teer**·e·ole). A tiny arterial branch. **Precapillary arteriole.** One which ends in a capillary vessel. **Preglomerular arteriole.** The afferent arteriole supplying the capillary loops of a renal glomerulus. **Arteriola recta [NA].** Descending vas rectum. [L *arteriola* little artery.]

See also: ISAACS, LUDWIG (K. F. W.).

arteriolith (ar·**teer**·e·o·lith). Arterial concretion; formation of chalky stones in an artery. [artery, Gk *lithos* stone.]

arteriolitis (ar·**teer**·e·o·**li**'·tis). Necrotic or inflammatory changes in the arteriolar wall. **Necrotizing arteriolitis.** Arteriolar necrosis, arteriolonecrosis; hyperplasia of the intima, with narrowing of the lumen of arterioles, to which is added necrosis and loss of structure of the entire wall with red-cell infiltration and often haemorrhage and aneurysm formation. The condition is the characteristic systemic arteriolar lesion of malignant hypertension, but has also been described in the pulmonary arterioles in cases of mitral stenosis with pulmonary hypertension. [arteriole, Gk *-itis* inflammation.]

arteriology (ar·teer·e·**ol**'·o·je). The science of the arterial system; the anatomy of the arteries. [artery, Gk *logos* science.]

arteriolonecrosis (ar·**teer**·e·o·lo·nek·**ro**'·sis). Destruction of arterioles by disease. [arteriole, necrosis.]

arteriolosclerosis (ar·**teer**·e·o·lo·skler·**o**'·sis). Narrowing of the lumen of arterioles due to duplication of the internal elastic lamina and fibrosis of the media; it is the arteriolar lesion found in essential hypertension. **Hypertensive arteriolosclerosis.** Hypertensive arteriosclerosis. *See* ARTERIOSCLEROSIS. [arteriole, sclerosis.]

arteriomalacia, arteriomalacosis (ar·**teer**·e·o·mal·**a**'·se·ah, ar·**teer**·e·o·mal·ak·**o**'·sis). Excessive softness of the arterial walls. [artery, Gk *malakia* softness.]

arteriometer (ar·**teer**·e·**om**'·et·er). An instrument with which changes in the size of an artery during pulsation, or the diameter of an artery, can be measured.

arteriomotor (ar·**teer**·e·o·**mo**'·tor). 1. Causing changes in the calibre of an artery. 2. Belonging to arterial constriction and dilatation. [artery, L *motor* mover.]

arteriomyomatosis (ar·**teer**·e·o·mi·o·mat·**o**'·sis). A state of thickening of the arterial wall due to an irregular overgrowth of muscle fibres. [artery, myomatosis.]

arterionecrosis (ar·**teer**·e·o·nek·**ro**'·sis). The process of destruction of an artery or arteries by disease. [artery, necrosis.]

arteriopalmus (ar·**teer**·e·o·**pal**'·mus). Throbbing or palpitation of an artery or arteries. [artery, Gk *palmos* palpitation.]

arteriopathy (ar·**teer**·e·**op**'·ath·e). Any disease of an artery or arteries. [artery, Gk *pathos* suffering.]

arteriophlebotomy (ar·**teer**·e·o·fleb·**ot**'·o·me). Scarification of the skin in a certain area in order to cause bleeding and thus to reduce pressure. [artery, Gk *phlebs* vein, *temnein* to cut.]

arterioplania (ar·**teer**·e·o·**pla**'·ne·ah). A term describing the deviation of an artery from its accustomed course; it may also comprise arterial tortuosity. [artery, Gk *planan* to wander.]

arterioplasty (ar·**teer**·e·o·**plas**'·te). Endo-aneurysmorrhaphy. *See* MATAS' OPERATION. A method of cure in certain cases of substantial aneurysm, in which the walls of the sac are fashioned into new vessels. [artery, Gk *plassein* to form.]

arterioplegmus, arterioploce (ar·**teer**·e·o·**pleg**'·mus, ar·**teer**·e·o·**plo**'·se). Perplication; the operation of drawing the free end of a divided artery through an incision made in its wall immediately above the cut, for the purpose of arresting haemorrhage. [artery, Gk *plegma* something twined, *ploke* complication.]

arteriopressor (ar·**teer**·e·o·**pres**'·or). Causing an increase of blood pressure in the arteries. [artery, L *premere* to press.]

arteriopuncture (ar·teer·e·o·**pungk**'·tcher). The obtaining of blood from an artery by means of a hypodermic syringe. [artery, L *pungere* to prick.]

arteriorenal (ar·teer·e·o·re'·nal). Referring to or involving the arteries of the kidney. [artery, L *ren* kidney.]

arteriorrhagia (ar·**teer**·e·o·**ra**'·je·ah). Haemorrhage from arteries or an artery. [artery, Gk *rhegnynein* to gush forth.]

arteriorrhaphy (ar·teer·e·or′·af·e). Suture of an artery. [artery, Gk *rhaphe* seam.]

arteriorrhexis (ar·teer·e·o·rex′·is). Rupture of an artery. [artery, Gk *rhexis* rupture.]

arteriosclerosis (ar·teer·e·o·skler·o′·sis). A condition found mainly in elderly people in which there are degenerative changes in the arterial system often resulting in interference with blood supply and functional disturbance in organs and tissues. There is pathological thickening and loss of elasticity of the walls of the arteries, which may become calcified. **Cerebral arteriosclerosis.** Arteriosclerosis of cerebral vessels. **Coronary arteriosclerosis.** Arteriosclerosis of coronary vessels. **Decrescent arteriosclerosis.** Senile arteriosclerosis (see below). **Diffuse arteriosclerosis.** A condition in which the walls of arteries and capillary vessels in general are thickened, especially the intima of the smaller vessels; usually associated with chronic nephritis and essential hypertension. **Hypertensive arteriosclerosis.** Diffuse thickening of the arterial wall, with proliferation of connective tissue both in the intima and media: there is reduplication of the internal elastic lamina. In the small vessels the intima shows the most change. In malignant hypertension, the arterioles show great intimal stretching, with hyaline and fatty changes and fibrinoid necrosis. **Infantile arteriosclerosis.** Diffuse arteriosclerosis (see above) affecting infants and young children; it is the result of congenital syphilis or chronic nephritis. **Intimal arteriosclerosis.** Arteriosclerosis with main changes in the intima. **Medial arteriosclerosis.** Moenckeberg's arteriosclerosis. **Nodose arteriosclerosis, Nodular arteriosclerosis.** A disease of the arteries of which the formation of flat nodules or plaques involving the tunica intima is characteristic. **Arteriosclerosis obliterans.** A slow narrowing of the arteries with intimal degeneration and thrombosis leading to complete occlusion and infarction, or gangrene. **Peripheral arteriosclerosis.** Arteriosclerosis affecting the hands or feet. **Senile arteriosclerosis.** A form met with in the elderly in which the smaller vessels become rigid and the larger dilated and tortuous. **Syphilitic arteriosclerosis.** Arteriosclerosis of syphilitic origin. [artery, Gk *skleros* hard.]

See also: MOENCKEBERG.

arteriosclerotic (ar·teer·e·o·skler·ot′·ik). 1. A person affected with arteriosclerosis. 2. Pertaining to arteriosclerosis.

arteriospasm (ar·teer·e·o·spazm). Spasm affecting an artery.

arteriostenosis (ar·teer·e·o·sten·o′·sis). Narrowing or contraction of an artery. [artery, Gk *stenosis* a narrowing.]

arteriosteogenesis (ar·teer·e·os·te·o·jen′·es·is). Calcification affecting an artery. [artery, Gk *osteon* bone, *genein* to produce.]

arteriosteosis, arteriostosis (ar·teer·e·os·te·o′·sis, ar·teer·os·to′·sis). A condition of ossification of an artery or arteries. [artery, Gk *osteon* bone, *-osis* condition.]

arteriostrepsis (ar·teer·e·o·strep′·sis). The act of twisting the severed end of an artery for the purpose of arresting bleeding. [artery, Gk *strepsis* a twisting.]

arteriosympathectomy (ar·teer·e·o·sim·path·ek′·to·me). Periarterial sympathectomy. *See* SYMPATHECTOMY.

arteriotome (ar·teer·e·o·tome). A lancet used in the performance of arteriotomy. [artery, Gk *temnein* to cut.]

arteriotomy (ar·teer·e·ot′·o·me). 1. The surgical procedure of opening or cutting through an artery. 2. Blood-letting from an artery. 3. Dissection or anatomy of the arteries. [artery, Gk *temnein* to cut.]

arteriotony (ar·teer·e·ot′·on·e). Blood pressure; the degree of tension of the blood throughout the arterial system. [artery, Gk *tonos* tension.]

arteriotrepsis (ar·teer·e·o·trep′·sis). Arteriostrepsis.

arterious (ar·teer·e·us). Arterial.

arteriovasodilator (ar·teer·e·o·va·zo·di·la′·tor). A drug that causes dilatation of the arteries. [artery, vasodilator.]

arteriovenous (ar·teer·e·o·ve′·nus). Venous as well as arterial; affecting or referring to an artery as well as a vein.

arterioversion (ar·teer·e·o·ver′·shun). In surgical operations, the eversion of the walls of an artery in order to arrest bleeding. [artery, L *versio* a turning.]

arterioverter (ar·teer·e·o·ver′·ter). An instrument with which arterioversion is performed.

arteritis (ar·ter·i·tis). An inflammatory condition of the wall of an artery or arteries. **Arteritis deformans.** A chronic form of endarteritis with calcification of the arterial tissues; endarteritis deformans. **Giant-cell arteritis.** Thickening of the intima of the smaller arteries, consisting of new connective tissue and fibroblasts infiltrated with inflammatory cells, lymphocytes and macrophages. Multinucleate giant cells can be seen at the junction of the intima and media, and the internal elastic lamina is fragmented; thrombosis is common. It is often localized in the temporal arteries, and is accompanied by fever, loss of weight, leucocytosis and tenderness along the affected parts. Sudden blindness may occur due to involvement of retinal vessels. **Arteritis hyperplastica.** Arteritis associated with the formation of connective tissue in the media or intima. **Necrosing arteritis.** Periarteritis nodosa. **Arteritis nodosa.** Nodular swellings in the walls of small arteries throughout the body which may cause rupture or thrombosis of the artery. It is usually associated with peripheral neuritis. **Arteritis obliterans.** Endarteritis obliterans; arterial inflammation ultimately causing complete closure of the arterial lumen. **Suppurative arteritis.** Pyogenic infection of an artery as the result of septicaemia, pyaemia or involvement in an acute abscess. **Temporal arteritis.** Giant-cell arteritis affecting predominantly the extracranial vessels, particularly the superficial temporal arteries. **Arteritis umbilicalis.** A condition met with in newborn infants in which there is septic inflammation of the umbilical arteries. [artery, Gk *-itis* inflammation.]

artery [arteria (NA)] (ar·ter·e). A vessel carrying blood from the heart to the different parts of the body. Arteries all arise directly or indirectly from 2 great arterial trunks, the aorta and the pulmonary artery, which take origin from the left and right ventricles of the heart respectively. Their walls are thick compared with veins in order to withstand the greater pressure of blood on the arterial side of the circulation, and are composed of elastic tissue, smooth muscle and collagenous connective tissue arranged, from within outwards, in 3 layers, the intima, the media and the adventitia. Each layer may contain more or less of any of these 3 tissues, and the intima is lined by a layer of vascular endothelium. In the walls of the larger arteries near the heart, elastic tissue predominates (elastic arteries); in tracing the arterial system peripherally it is found that the amount of elastic tissue diminishes, and smooth muscle increases to form muscular arteries such as the radial or ulnar arteries. The smallest branches of arteries recognizable as such are known as *arterioles*, and just before the latter become continuous with the capillary network, as *precapillary arterioles*. (For specific arteries, see under regional qualifying adjective or the organ or region supplied.) **Coiled arteries.** Arteries which pass through the myometrium into the basal layers of the endometrium, where they become coiled before branching into the rich capillary bed of the more superficial parts of the endometrium. **Collateral artery.** 1. An artery which follows the course of another structure, e.g. ulnar collateral artery, an artery which follows the same course as the ulnar nerve in the arm. 2. An artery additional to the main artery supplying an organ or region of the body. **Conducting artery.** A large artery of the elastic type (e.g. the aorta) from which arteries of distribution arise. **Copper-wire artery.** Exaggeration of the normal linear reflex of the retinal arteries which occurs when they are sclerosed. **Corkscrew artery.** Tortuosity of small arteries in the region of the macula, occurring in retinal arteriosclerosis. **Distributing artery.** An artery of the muscular type concerned with the distribution of blood received from a conducting artery to the tissues and organs. **Elastic artery.** One in which there is a large proportion of elastic tissue, as is the case with most of the large arteries, such as the aorta. **End artery.** One which has no anastomosis. **Hybrid arteries.** Short regions of transition between elastic conducting arteries and muscular arteries of distribution. **Muscular artery.** An artery in which the greater part of the wall is composed of circularly-disposed smooth muscle contained in the tunica media. Most medium and small arteries are of this type. **Nutrient artery.** An artery of supply to a bone and to the marrow it may contain. **Sheathed artery.** The terminal penicillate branches of the splenic artery in the splenic pulp; they are surrounded by a sheath of elongated reticular cells, the Schweigger-Seidel sheath, which may be contractile. The artery with its sheath is known as an *ellipsoid.* **Silver-wire arteries.** Thickened arteries that under the light of the ophthalmoscope glisten like a silver wire; seen on the retinae of hypertensive subjects. [Gk *arteria* windpipe.]

See also: CHARCOT, CHAUSSIER, COHNHEIM, DURET, GUIDI, KONSTANTINOWICH, NEUBAUER (J. E.), SYLVIUS, VIDIUS, WEBER (M. I.), ZINN.

arthraemia (ar·**thre**·me·ah). A congested state of a joint. A condition of suffusion of the blood vessels supplying a joint so that swelling and congestion result. [Gk *arthron* joint, *haima* blood.]

arthraesthesia (ar·thres·**the**·ze·ah). The subjective perception of the movements of a joint. [Gk *arthron* joint, aesthesis.]

arthragra (ar·**thrag**·rah). An attack of gout in a joint or joints. **Arthragra anomala.** So-called gout affecting the viscera. [Gk *arthron* joint, *agra* a catching.]

arthral (**ar**·thral). Referring to or involving a joint or joints. [Gk *arthron* joint.]

arthralgia (ar·**thral**·je·ah). Pain of any kind affecting a joint. **Gonorrhoeal arthralgia.** Arthralgia of gonococcal origin. **Arthralgia hysterica.** Arthralgia of hysterical origin. **Arthralgia saturnina.** Arthralgia caused by lead poisoning. [Gk *arthron* joint, *algos* pain.]

arthrectomy (ar·**threk**·to·me). Surgical excision of a joint. [Gk *arthron* joint, *ektome* a cutting out.]

arthrempyesis (**ar**·threm·pi·**e**′·sis). Arthro-empyesis.

arthrifuge (**ar**·thre·fewj). Any drug or other measure for the relief or cure of gout. [arthritis, L *fugare* to drive away.]

arthritic (ar·**thrit**·ik). 1. A person suffering from arthritis. 2. Of or pertaining to arthritis.

arthritide (**ar**·thrit·eed). An inflammatory process or lesion of arthritic or gouty origin affecting the skin; a rare usage. [Fr.]

arthritis (ar·**thri**·tis) (pl. *arthritides*). Inflammation of a joint. **Acute arthritis.** Acute joint inflammation; acute serous arthritis. **Acute gouty arthritis.** Acute joint inflammation due to gout; it may subside completely between attacks, or become chronic. **Acute rheumatic arthritis.** Rheumatic fever. *See* FEVER. **Allergic arthritis.** 1. Joint swelling following the ingestion of food allergens. 2. Serum sickness; swelling of joints occurring 7–10 days after injection of horse serum. Generally accompanied by fever and urticaria. **Atrophic arthritis.** Rheumatoid arthritis (see below). **Blenorrhagic arthritis.** Gonococcal arthritis (see below). **Chronic arthritis.** A general term for chronic joint disease of any type. **Chronic infective arthritis.** A general term for polyarthritis believed to be of infective aetiology; often used as a synonym for rheumatoid arthritis (see below), especially in European countries. **Chronic villous arthritis.** Any chronic arthritis with marked synovial proliferation. **Climacteric arthritis.** Menopausal arthritis (see below). **Arthritis deformans.** Any form of crippling arthritis of unknown causation. [Obsolete term.] **Degenerative arthritis.** Osteo-arthritis. **Dysenteric arthritis.** A form of arthritis occurring as a sequel to an attack of dysentery. It is often polyarticular and may become chronic. **Formalin arthritis.** Arthritis induced by the injection of formaldehyde solution into the feet of rats; this method of producing an artificial arthritis has been used in screening substances proposed for the treatment of arthritis, but recent work has indicated it is unsuitable for this purpose. **Gonococcal arthritis, Gonorrhoeal arthritis.** A specific blood-borne gonococcal infection of the joints. It may be acute or chronic, monarticular or polyarticular, and can lead to bony ankylosis. The organism can often be recovered from the joint fluid, which may become purulent. **Gouty arthritis.** The form of arthritis which is associated with gout. It may be acute or chronic in onset and course, and may affect many joints. **Guinea worm arthritis.** Arthritis due to the presence of adult female *Dracunculus medinensis* within, or in close proximity to, a joint. **Haemophilic arthritis.** Arthritis occurring in a haemophilic subject. It is due to bleeding into the joint cavities, and may become chronic, leading to inflammatory changes, and even ankylosis. **Hypertrophic arthritis.** Osteo-arthrosis. **Intervertebral arthritis.** Arthritis of the intervertebral joints; it may occur in the course of either rheumatoid arthritis or ankylosing spondylitis. If it occurs in association with a generalized condition of osteo-arthrosis, it is often symptomless. It may occur in localized form as the result of trauma. **Juvenile rheumatoid arthritis.** Still's disease. **Arthritis maxillaris.** An arthritic condition affecting the temporomaxillary joint; generally an episode in the course of rheumatoid arthritis. **Menopausal arthritis.** An arthritis occurring in women in or around the menopause. It is most commonly either a generalized osteo-arthropathy or rheumatoid arthritis. The knees are often affected. These joints often later develop degenerative changes if the process is progressive. It may be relieved by oestrogen therapy. **Mixed arthritis.** A combination of rheumatoid arthritis and osteo-arthritis in the same joints, or in the same patient. **Neurogenic arthritis, Neuropathic arthritis, Arthritis neuropathica, Neurotrophic arthritis.** A trophic disease of one or more joints, seen in disorders of the central nervous system such as tabes dorsalis and syringomyelia, and in leprosy. There is little pain, but hypermotility and joint enlargement due to disorganization of the articular structures is present. Also called *Charcot's disease.* **Palindromic arthritis.** A rare form of acute recurrent arthritis of the large joints. It is of unknown aetiology, and disappears ultimately without leaving residual joint damage. **Pericapsular arthritis.** A term sometimes used to describe an inflammatory condition of a joint which does not involve joint surfaces, e.g. frozen shoulder. **Arthritis podagra.** Gouty arthritis affecting the great toe. **Proliferating arthritis.** Rheumatoid arthritis. [Obsolete term.] **Pyaemic arthritis.** An acute suppurative arthritis. **Rheumatoid arthritis.** A polyarthritis of unknown aetiology which is accompanied by severe constitutional disturbances such as malaise, loss of weight and weakness. Pathologically the joint lesions are inflammatory, and may lead to gross deformity or ankylosis. The disease is most common in women and may run a very chronic course, although remissions are not unusual. It tends to affect the smaller peripheral joints early and the larger joints later in its course. There is a juvenile form generally known as *Still's disease.* **Scarlatinal arthritis.** Painful swelling of joints which occurs in association with scarlet fever, generally at the end of 10 days. It usually subsides completely; scarlatinal synovitis. **Septic arthritis.** A pyogenic infection of a joint cavity. **Serum arthritis.** An arthritis that may follow serum injections; it is an anaphylactic phenomenon. *See* ALLERGIC ARTHRITIS (above). **Arthritis sicca.** Perichondritis. **Strumous arthritis.** Tuberculous arthritis. [Obsolete term.] **Suppurative arthritis.** Arthritis resulting from invasion of the joint space by pyogenic organisms; pus in the articular cavity. **Syphilitic arthritis.** Swollen joints due to syphilitic proliferation of the joint membrane and capsule during secondary or tertiary stages of syphilis. **Tuberculous arthritis.** Invasion of the joint structures by the tuberculosis bacillus, generally from a primary focus elsewhere in the body, often the chest. It causes slow painful swelling of one or more joints, and may result in great disorganization and ankylosis. **Uratic arthritis, Arthritis urica.** Gouty arthritis.; implies a deposition of sodium biurate crystals in the joint. **Vertebral arthritis.** Arthritis affecting the intervertebral joints. **Villous arthritis.** A synonym for chronic menopausal arthritis as it affects the knees. It leads to considerable hypertrophy of the villi of the synovium, which limits joint movement. [Gk *arthron* joint, *-itis* inflammation.]

See also: BECHTEREW, BRODIE (B. C.), CHARCOT, HEBERDEN, MARIE, REITER, STRUEMPELL.

arthritism (**ar**·thrit·izm). A term referring to a particular type of constitution which predisposes to gouty disease or inflammatory processes in the joints and skin; the gouty diathesis. Many of the manifestations are of allergic nature. [see prec.]

arthritolith (ar·thrit·o·lith). A calculus of gouty origin in a joint. [arthritis, Gk *lithos* stone.]

arthrobacterium (ar·thro·bak·teer′·e·um). A bacterium in which the reproductive process is carried out by fission or segmentation, with the formation of joints or arthrospores. [Gk *arthron* joint, bacterium.]

arthrocace (ar·throk·as·e). 1. Complete decay of a joint. 2. Strumous arthritis. *See* ARTHRITIS. **Arthrocace coxarum.** Coxalgia. **Senile arthrocace.** The natural changes which occur in the joints as age increases. [Gk *arthron* joint, *kake* badness.]

arthrocele (ar·thro·seel). 1. Hernia of a part of the synovial membrane of a joint through the articular capsule. 2. A swelling of a joint. [Gk *arthron* joint, *kele* hernia.]

arthrocentesis (ar·thro·sen·te′·sis). Arthrotomy. [Gk *arthron* joint, *kentesis* a pricking.]

arthrochondritis (ar·thro·kon·dri′·tis). A state of inflammation of the articular cartilages. [Gk *arthron* joint, chondritis.]

arthroclasia, arthroclasis (ar·thro·kla·ze·ah, ar·thro·kla·sis). The procedure of achieving free movement in a joint by the breaking-down of ankylosis. [Gk *arthron* joint, *klasis* a breaking.]

arthroclisis (ar·thro·kli·sis). 1. Ankylosis. 2. Surgical ankylosis. [Gk *arthron* joint, *kleisis* closure.]

Arthroderma (ar·thro·der·mah). The generic name of the perfect (sexual) state of the dermatophytes of the genus *Trichophyton.* [Gk *arthron* joint, *derma* skin.]

arthrodesis, arthrodesia (ar·thro·de·sis, ar·thro·de·ze·ah). Creation of ankylosis by surgical treatment. The ends of adjacent bones are freshened and made suitable for fusion, and by subsequent splinting the bones are united, a completely stiff joint resulting. **Compression arthrodesis.** A surgical technique using compression clamps to fix the excised joint surfaces. **Extra-articular arthrodesis.** The operation of fixing a joint by means of bone grafts which do not traverse the articular cavity. **Ischiofemoral arthrodesis.** An extra-articular arthrodesis of the hip obtained by inserting a graft between the upper end of the femur and the ischium (*see* BRITTAIN's ischiofemoral graft). **Pantalar arthrodesis.** An arthrodesis of the subtaloid and midtarsal joints. [Gk *arthron* joint, *desis* a binding together.]

See also: DUNN, WATSON-JONES.

arthrodia (ar·thro·de·ah). In anatomy, a form of joint in which the articular surfaces are flat and glide over or against each other in movement. [Gk *arthrodes* well articulated.]

arthrodial (ar·thro·de·al). Having the characters of, or with reference to, an arthrodia.

arthrodynia (ar·thro·din·e·ah). Arthralgia. [Gk *arthron* joint, *odyne* pain.]

arthrodysplasia (ar·thro·dis·pla′·ze·ah). A hereditary condition of deformity of the joints. [Gk *arthron* joint, dysplasia.]

arthroedema (ar·thre·de·mah). A state of oedema surrounding or associated with a joint. [Gk *arthron* joint, *oidema* swelling.]

arthro-empyesis (ar·thro·em·pi·e′·sis). A suppurative condition within a joint. [Gk *arthron* joint, *empyesis* suppuration.]

arthro-endoscopy (ar·thro·en·dos′·ko·pe). Endoscopic examination of a joint. [Gk *arthron* joint, endoscopy.]

arthro-ereisis (ar·thro·er·i′·sis). A surgical procedure undertaken for the purpose of limiting the abnormal extent of movement possible in a joint affected by paralysis. [Gk *arthron* joint, *ereisis* a raising up.]

arthrogenous (ar·throj·en·us). 1. Forming a separate joint or an articulation. 2. Originating in a joint. [Gk *arthron* joint, *genein* to produce.]

arthrogram (ar·thro·gram). Radiograph of a joint; term often used to describe the radiograph after arthrography. [Gk *arthron* joint, *gramma* record.]

arthrography (ar·throg·raf·e). Radiography of a joint after injection of air or oxygen or of a fluid contrast medium into the joint space in order to visualize cartilage and the limits of the joint cavity. [Gk *arthron* joint, radiography.]

arthrogryposis (ar·thro·gri·po′·sis). 1. Retention of a joint in a contracted or flexed position. 2. Spasm of tetanic origin. 3. Ankylosis. **Arthrogryposis multiplex congenita.** General fibrotic ankylosis of the joints of the hands and feet; congenital. [Gk *arthron* joint, *gryposis* curve.]

arthrokatadysis (ar·thro·kat·ad′·is·is). A condition in which there is subsidence of the acetabular fossa and protrusion of the head of the femur through it into the pelvis. [Gk *arthron* joint, *katadysis* a falling down.]

arthrolith (ar·thro·lith). Any calculus or stone which forms in a joint as the result of outgrowth of the synovial membrane or cartilage. [Gk *arthron* joint, *lithos* stone.]

arthrolithiasis (ar·thro·lith·i′·as·is). Gout. [see prec.]

arthrology [syndesmologia (NA)] (ar·throl·o·je). The branch of medical science which is concerned with joints and their diseases and deformities. [Gk *arthron* joint, *logos* science.]

arthrolysis (ar·throl·is·is). The operative procedure of loosening an ankylosed joint by breaking down the adhesions around it; arthroclasia. [Gk *arthron* joint, *lysis* a loosing.]

arthromeningitis (ar·thro·men·in·ji′·tis). Synovitis. [Gk *arthron* joint, meningitis.]

arthrometer (ar·throm·et·er). An instrument used to determine the range of mobility in a joint by measuring the angles of movement. [Gk *arthron* joint, meter.]

arthrometry (ar·throm·et·re). The measurement by means of an arthrometer of the range of movement in a joint.

arthronalgia (ar·thron·al·je·ah). Arthralgia. [Gk *arthron* joint, *algos* pain.]

arthronosos (ar·thro·no·sos). Any disease of the joints. **Arthronosos deformans.** Rheumatoid arthritis. *See* ARTHRITIS. [Gk *arthron* joint, *nosos* disease.]

arthropathia (ar·thro·path·e·ah). Arthropathy. **Arthropathia psoriatica.** A disease of the joints associated with psoriasis.

arthropathology (ar·thro·path·ol′·o·je). The pathology of articular disease. [Gk *arthron* joint, pathology.]

arthropathy (ar·throp·ath·e). 1. Any disease affecting a joint. 2. Trophic disease of the joints to be found in certain degenerative nervous conditions. **Inflammatory arthropathy.** Arthritis. **Neurogenic arthropathy, Neuropathic arthropathy.** A destructive type of joint disease which occurs when deep sensation is impaired. The condition was first described by Charcot in tabes dorsalis (Charcot's joint, q.v.) but occurs in a number of other conditions, particularly diabetes mellitus and syringomyelia, the pattern of joint involvement depending on the distribution of sensory loss. **Osteopulmonary arthropathy.** The swelling and enlargement of the ends of the long bones and clubbing of toes and fingers, typical of certain cardiac and pulmonary affections. **Psoriatic arthropathy.** A type of polyarthritis resembling rheumatoid arthritis, which occurs in about 10 per cent of patients with psoriasis. The serological tests for rheumatoid arthritis, for example, the latex test, are negative and there is a tendency for distal interphalangeal joints to be involved. **Pyrophosphate arthropathy.** Deposition of calcium pyrophosphate dihydrate crystals into synovial membrane and fluid, causing either recurrent acute arthritis or chronic degenerative arthritis, or both. These are often associated with the radiological appearance of calcification of joints. **Static arthropathy.** Changes occurring in joints of a limb secondary to immobilization of the limb. **Syphilitic arthropathy.** Charcot's joints (q.v.). **Tabetic arthropathy.** A modification of neurogenic arthropathy (see above) which is met with in patients with tabes dorsalis. [Gk *arthron* joint, *pathos* disease.]

See also: CHARCOT.

arthroplastic (ar·thro·plas·tik). Referring to arthroplasty. [Gk *arthron* joint, *plassein* to form.]

arthroplasty (ar·thro·plas·te). 1. In bony ankylosis, the formation of an artificial joint by plastic surgery. 2. An operation for the restoration of the functional part of a joint, either by reconstruction or by prosthetic replacement. **Cup arthroplasty.** Smith-Petersen mould arthroplasty.

See also: CHARNLEY, KELLER (W. L.), SMITH-PETERSEN.

arthropneumography (ar·thro·new·mog′·raf·e). Radiography of a joint after injection of air or oxygen into the joint space in order to visualize cartilage and the limits of the joint cavity. The more comprehensive term *arthrography* is usually used in the UK. [Gk *arthron* joint, *pneuma* air, radiography.]

arthropod (ar·thro·pod). An animal organism belonging to the Arthropoda. [Gk *arthron* joint, *pous* foot.]

Arthropoda (ar·throp·o·dah). The largest of the invertebrate phyla, characterized by the bilaterally symmetrical, segmented body, with a thickened exoskeleton and jointed appendages, and the absence of cilia. The classes Arachnida, Crustacea, Insecta, Myriapoda and Pentastomida are of medical interest. [Gk *arthron* joint, *pous* foot.]

arthropodan, arthropodic, arthropodous (ar·throp·od·an, ar·throp·od·ik, ar·throp·od·us). Caused by or referring to arthropods.

arthropyosis (ar·thro·pi·o′·sis). Arthro-empyesis. [Gk *arthron* joint, *pyosis* suppuration.]

arthrorisis (ar·thro·ri·sis). Arthroereisis.

arthrorrhagia (ar·thro·ra·je·ah). Haemorrhage into a joint. [Gk *arthron* joint, *rhegnynein* to gush forth.]

arthrosclerosis (ar·thro·skler·o′·sis). A condition in which the joints are inflexible or hard. [Gk *arthron* joint, *sklerosis* hardening.]

arthroscope (ar·thro·skope). A type of endoscope used for arthro-endoscopy. [Gk *arthron* joint, *skopein* to watch.]

arthroscopy (ar·thros·ko·pe). Arthro-endoscopy; the use of an endoscope for examination of a joint. [see prec.]

arthrosis (ar·thro·sis). 1. Degenerative disease of a joint; arthritis. 2. An articulation. [Gk joint.]

See also: CHARCOT.

arthrospore (ar·thro·spor). A term used in bacteriology to describe fragments, derived by the fission of the original cell, which have become surrounded by a resistant coat. Found in soil bacteria. [Gk *arthron* joint, *sporos* spore.]

arthrostenosis (ar·thro·sten·o′·sis). Contraction affecting a joint. [Gk *arthron* joint, stenosis.]

arthrosteopaedic (ar·thros·te·o·pe′·dik). Referring to the bony structure of the body and to the hands and feet. [Gk *arthron* joint, *osteon* bone, *pous* foot.]

arthrostomy (ar·thros·to·me). The surgical procedure of making a temporary opening into a joint cavity, especially for the insertion of a drainage tube. [Gk *arthron* joint, *stoma* mouth.]

arthrosynovitis (ar·thro·si·no·vi′·tis). An inflammatory condition of the synovial membrane of a joint. [Gk *arthron* joint, synovitis.]

arthrosyrinx (ar·thro·sir·ingx). Fistula of a joint. [Gk *arthron* joint, *syrigx* pipe.]

arthrotome (ar·thro·tome). A large strong scalpel used in operations on joints. [Gk *arthron* joint, *temnein* to cut.]

arthrotomy (ar·throt·o·me). The surgical procedure of cutting into or puncturing a joint; arthrocentesis. [see prec.]

arthrotropia (ar·thro·tro·pe·ah). A twisted condition of a limb. [Gk *arthron* joint, *trope* a turning.]

arthrotropic (ar·thro·trop·ik). With a tendency to settle in, or likely to affect joints. [Gk *arthron* joint, *tropos* turning towards.]

arthrous (ar·thrus). Jointed; having the properties of a joint. [Gk *arthron* joint.]

arthroxesis (ar·throx·e·sis). The procedure of scraping diseased tissue from a joint. [Gk *arthron* joint, *xesis* a scraping.]

Arthus, Nicholas Maurice (b. 1862). Paris physiologist.

Arthus' phenomenon, or reaction. An inflammatory reaction characterized by oedema, haemorrhage and necrosis, which follows repeated injection of antigen into an animal that possesses precipitating antibody to the antigen. Caused by local release of inflammatory and neutrophil-attracting substances generated by complement-fixing immune complexes.

artiad (ar·te·ad). Term used formerly to denote an element with an even-number valency. [Gk *artios* even.]

article (ar·tikl). In zoology, an articulated segment. [L *articulus* little joint.]

articular (ar·tik·ew·lar). Having reference to a joint; indicating that the joints are involved. **Articular disc.** *See* DISC. **Articular facet.** *See* FACET. **Articular fossa.** *See* FOSSA. **Articular process of a vertebra.** *See* PROCESS. **Articular surface.** *See* SURFACE. [L *articulare* to divide into joints.]

articularis cubiti muscle [musculus articularis cubiti (NA)] (ar·tik·ew·la′·ris kew·bit·i). A small muscle of the elbow.

articularis genu muscle [musculus articularis genu (NA)] (ar·tik·ew·la′·ris jen·ew). A small muscle under the lower end of the quadriceps mass. It is attached to the shaft of the femur and the synovial membrane of the knee, which it pulls up during extension.

articulate (ar·tik·ew·late). 1. To enunciate clearly and connectedly. 2. Of speech, distinct and connected. 3. Jointed. 4. United so as to form a joint. 5. To unite in a joint, or to divide so as to form a joint. [see foll.]

articulation (ar·tik·ew·la′·shun). 1. [Articulatio (junctura ossium) (NA)] A joint between 2 skeletal elements, bones or cartilages. 2. The enunciation of words and sentences in the form of speech. 3. In dentistry, the meeting of natural or artificial teeth in opposing jaws. **Ambomalleal articulation.** The articulation between the incus and the malleus. **Capitular articulation.** The articulation between a vertebra and the head of a rib. **Confluent articulation.** Speech in which the syllables are run together or slurred. **False articulation.** False joint; a joint occurring in an abnormal position as the result of disease or injury. **Supplementary articulation.** A pseudarthrosis in which a capsule of fibrous tissue has grown over the fragments of broken bone. [L *articulare* to divide into joints.]

articulator (ar·tik·ew·la·tor). An appliance used in prosthetic dentistry for registering the natural relationship between the upper and lower jaw. **Anatomical articulator.** One of the various types of articulator which records normal movements of the mandible as well as the vertical relationship of the jaws; it has a double hinge representing the temporomandibular joints. **Guy's articulator.** A simple type of anatomical articulator used at Guy's Hospital Dental School. **Plain-line articulator.** A simple, hinged type of articulator which records only the vertical relationship of the jaws. [see prec.]

articulatory (ar·tik·ew·la′·tor·e). 1. Having reference to the articulation of bones. 2. Qualifying utterance.

Artyfechinostomum (ar·te·fek·in·os′·to·mum). A genus of flukes. **Artyfechinostomum sufrartyfex.** A species the true host of which is the hog, though instances have been recorded of human infestation in north India.

aryepiglottic, aryepiglottidean (ar·e·ep·e·glot′·ik, ar·e·ep·e·glot·id′·e·an). Referring to the arytenoid cartilage and the epiglottis. [Gk *arytaina* ladle, epiglottis.]

aryepiglottic muscle [musculus aryepiglotticus (NA)]. A prolongation of the oblique arytenoid muscle into the aryepiglottic fold.

aryl (ar·il). An alkyl radical derived from an aromatic hydrocarbon. **Aryl arsonate.** A salt of an organic acid containing one or more arsonic acid radicals joined to aryl groups.

arytaenoideus (ar·e·te·noid′·e·us). One of the arytenoid muscles of the larynx. [Gk *arytainoeides* shaped like a ladle.]

aryteno-epiglottic (ar·e·te·no·ep·e·glot′·ik). Aryepiglottic.

arytenoid (ar·e·te·noid). 1. The arytenoid muscles. 2. Shaped like a ladle or pitcher. [Gk *arytainoeides* shaped like a ladle.]

arytenoid muscles. Oblique arytenoid muscle [musculus arytenoideus obliquus (NA)]. A slender muscle running from the back of the muscular process of one arytenoid to the apex of the other, prolonged into the aryepiglottic fold as the aryepiglottic muscle. It helps to close the inlet of the larynx. **Transverse arytenoid muscle [musculus arytenoideus transversus (NA)].** A small muscle between the 2 arytenoid cartilages; it helps to close the glottis by drawing them together.

arytenoidectomy (ar·e·te·noid·ek′·to·me). Surgical excision of one or both of the arytenoid cartilages. [arytenoid, Gk *ektome* a cutting out.]

arytenoiditis (ar·e·te·noid·i′·tis). An inflammatory condition of the arytenoid muscles or cartilages. [arytenoid, Gk *-itis* inflammation.]

arytenoidopexy (ar·e·te·**noid**′·o·pex·e). The fixing in position by surgical means of the arytenoid muscle or cartilage. [arytenoid, Gk *pexis* fixation.]

Arzberger, Friedrich (b. 1833). Vienna engineer.
Arzberger's pear. A pear-shaped hollow instrument for insertion in the rectum. It acted as a cooling agent when cold water was passed through it. Used in haemorrhoids, rectal prolapse, etc.

asacria (a·sa·kre·ah). Congenital absence of the sacrum. [Gk *a*, sacrum.]

Asafoetida BPC 1949 (as·af·e·tid·ah). The oleo gum resin obtained by incising the living rhizome and root of umbelliferous plants of species of *Ferula* growing in eastern Iran and western Afghanistan. The constituents are gum, resin and a volatile oil containing disulphides to which the strong alliaceous odour of the drug is due. It is used as a carminative in intestinal flatulence, and in hysterical conditions. [Persian *aza* gum, L *foetidus* stinking.]

asaphia (as·af·i·ah). Indistinctness of enunciation. [Gk *asapheia* obscurity.]

asaprol (as·ap·rol). Calcium β-naphthol α-monosulphonate, $Ca(SO_3C_{10}H_6OH)_2$. A white powder with a bitter taste; it has mild antiseptic properties.

asarcia (a·sar·se·ah). Emaciation. [Gk *a*, *sarx* flesh.]

asarin, asarone (as·ar·in, as·ar·one). Asarum camphor, propenyl trimethoxybenzene, $(CH_3O)_3C_6H_2CH{=}CHCH_3$. A constituent of the essential oil of snakewood, or asarabacca, *Asarum europaeum*; crystals with a camphor smell, used as an antiseptic and stimulant.

Asarum (as·ar·um). 1. A genus of aristolochiaceous plants. 2. The dried rhizome and roots of *Asarum canadense*, wild ginger or Canada snake root. It contains a bitter acrid resin and a volatile oil. **Asarum europaeum.** Asarabacca or wild nard; the dried rhizome and roots have a local irritant action. [Gk *asaron* hazelwort.]

asbestosis (as·bes·**to**·sis). A form of pneumoconiosis affecting those who work with asbestos. This appears to be the agent responsible for the development of mesothelioma. [asbestos, Gk *-osis* condition.]

ascariasis (as·kar·i·as·is). Infestation of the gastro-intestinal canal with the common human parasite, *Ascaris lumbricoides* (roundworm), and the state of general ill-health and debilitation characteristic of such infestation. [Gk *askaris* intestinal worm.]

ascaricide (as·kar·is·ide). 1. A drug or agent which is destructive of roundworms. 2. Destructive of roundworms. [Gk *askaris* intestinal worm, L *caedere* to kill.]

Ascaridae (as·kar·id·e). A family of the nematode super-family or sub-order Ascaroidea. The genera *Ascaris, Lagochilascaris, Toxascaris* and *Toxocara* are of medical interest. [Gk *askaris* intestinal worm, *eidos* form.]

Ascaridata (as·kar·id·a′·tah). An order or sub-order of the nematode class or sub-class Phasmidia. The super-families Ascaroidea and Oxyuroidea are of medical interest. [Gk *askaris* intestinal worm.]

ascaridiasis (as·kar·id·i′·as·is). Ascariasis.

ascaridole (as·kar·id·ole). $C_{10}H_{16}O_2$. A terpene dioxide related to cineole, and the active principle of oil of chenopodium, of which it constitutes about 65 per cent.

ascaridosis (as·kar·id·**o**′·sis). Ascariasis.

ascariosis (as·kar·e·**o**′·sis). Ascariasis.

Ascaris (as·kar·is) (pl. *Ascarides*). A genus of very large round nematode worms. **Ascaris lumbricoides.** A species parasitic in man. The adults live in the small intestine and lay eggs which pass in the faeces. There is no free-living larva, infection being due to ingested eggs; the first larvae migrate through various tissues to the lungs, and thence via the trachea back to the intestine. **Ascaris lumbricoides suum.** The pig ascaris, a species morphologically identical with the preceding but the eggs do not develop in man. [Gk *askaris* intestinal worm.]

Ascaroidea (as·kar·**oi**·de·ah). A super-family or sub-order of the nematode sub-order or order Ascaridata. The family Ascaridae is of medical interest. [Gk *askaris* intestinal worm, *eidos* form.]

Asch, Morris Joseph (b. 1833). American otolaryngologist.
Asch's forceps. A forceps designed for the atraumatic manipulation of the nasal septum in corrective rhinoplasty.
Asch's operation. One of the early methods employed for the correction of deviations of the nasal septum.

Ascherson, Ferdinand Moritz (b. 1789). German physician.
Ascherson's membrane. The protein layer surrounding the fat globules of milk.

ascheturesis (as·ket·ewr·**e**′·sis). The compulsive passing of urine; uncontrollable desire to pass urine. [Gk *aschetos* resistless, *ouresis* urination.]

Aschheim, Selmar (b. 1878). Berlin biochemist and gynaecologist.
Aschheim–Zondak test. For pregnancy: a female immature mouse is injected subcutaneously with the urine of a pregnant women 6 times in 2 days; 0.2 ml of urine is used for the first injection and the dose gradually increased to 0.4 ml; 96 h after the first injection the mouse is killed, and the ovaries will show haemorrhagic spots and yellowish protrusions, indicating pregnancy in the patient. This test can reach a high degree of accuracy but is time-consuming.

aschistodactylia, aschistodactylism (a·skis·to·dak·**til**′·e·ah, a·skis·to·**dak**′·til·izm). Syndactylia; a congenital condition in which the fingers are joined or fused together. [Gk *a*, *schistos* cleft, *dactylos* finger.]

aschistodactylous (a·skis·to·**dak**′·til·us). Characterized by webbing of fingers or toes, or both, or by their fusion. [see prec.]

Aschiza (a·ski·zah). A classificatory division of the insectan order Diptera; used for those Cyclorrhapha in which the ptilinum is absent. The families Phoridae and Syrphidae are of medical interest. [Gk *a*, *schizen* to split.]

Aschner, Bernhard (b. 1883). Austrian gynaecologist in USA.
Aschner's phenomenon, reflex or sign. Oculocardiac reflex; a reflex slowing of the heart due to pressure on the eyeball. It is mediated through the connection of the sensory nucleus of the trigeminal nerve with the nucleus of the vagus, stimulation of which slows the heart, and is sometimes deliberately induced to terminate attacks of paroxysmal supraventricular tachycardia.

Aschner, Karl W. (b. 1887). American ophthalmologist.
Aschner's phenomenon. Bradycardia following pressure on the globe of the eye.

Aschoff, Karl Albert Ludwig (b. 1866). Berlin pathologist.
Aschoff's body, cell, node or nodule. The specific lesion of rheumatic fever; a microscopic rounded or spindle-shaped nodule consisting of multinucleated giant cells, fibroblasts and basophilic cells with irregular edges, found in subcutaneous nodules, in joints and tendons, in the aorta and pleura, and in the heart, where they may be scattered throughout the pericardium, endocardium and myocardium including the conducting system. They are rarely found in the lungs.
Rokitansky–Aschoff sinuses. Hernia-like pouches or diverticula of the gall bladder mucosa into and through the muscular coat.

ascia (as·e·ah). Name applied to the reverse spiral bandage, the folds of which are supposed to resemble an axe. [L.]

ascites (as·i·teez). An abnormal accumulation of fluid in the peritoneal cavity. **Ascites adiposus.** A form of ascites in which the fluid is clouded by cells in which fatty degeneration has taken place. **Bloody ascites.** Haemorrhagic ascites (see below). **Chyliform ascites, Ascites chylosus.** Chyle in the peritoneal cavity, the result of rupture of a chyliferous vessel. **Fatty ascites.** Ascites adiposus (see above). **Haemorrhagic ascites.** A form in which blood is present in the fluid. **Hydraemic ascites.** A form of ascites which is associated with a severe anaemia. **Ascites intermuscularis.** Oedema of the abdominal muscles. **Malignant ascites.** Ascites resulting from the presence of a malignant growth in the abdominal cavity. **Mechanical ascites.** Ascites the cause of which is a slowing of the rate of flow of the blood in the portal vein. **Milky ascites.** Ascites adiposus (see above). **Ascites oleosus.** Ascites adiposus (see above). **Pre-**

agonal ascites. A serous effusion into the cavity of the abdomen just before death and as the result of intestinal congestion. **Pseudochylous ascites.** A form of ascites in which there is no fatty substance in the fluid although in other respects it resembles chyle. **Ascites saccatus.** 1. Ovarian cystoma. 2. Ascites in which adhesions form loculi, and prevent the free movement of the fluid in the cavity of the abdomen. **Ascites vaginalis.** A collection of fluid inside the sheath of the rectus abdominis muscle. [Gk *askos* bag.]

ascitic (as·it·ik). Pertaining to or characterized by ascites.

ascitogenous (as·it·**oj**·en·us). Productive of or causing ascites. [ascites, Gk *genein* to produce.]

Asclepias (as·**kle**·pe·as). A genus of herbs of the family Asclepiadaceae. **Asclepias curassavica.** A species of the West Indies which has diuretic properties but is only important as a source of a filling material consisting of the hairs from the seeds. **Asclepias incarnata.** Yellow milk-weed, a species which yields white Indian hemp rhizome, a potent diuretic. **Asclepias syriaca.** Wild cotton, used as a filling material. **Asclepias tuberosa** (pleurisy root). A species the root of which is diuretic and expectorant. [Gk swallow-wort.]

asclepion (as·**kle**·pe·on). $C_{20}H_{34}O_3$. A balsam extracted from *Asclepias syriaca.*

ascocarp (**as**·ko·karp). The developed fruit-body in the mycelium of fungi belonging to the Ascomycetes. [Gk *askos* bag, *karpos* fruit.]

Ascococcus (as·ko·**kok**·us). Former name for a group of bacteria now known as *Leuconostoc.* They consist of spherical or ovoid cocci surrounded by a gelatinous envelope, which unites them into zoogloeal masses. **Ascococcus mesenterioides.** *Leuconostoc mesenterioides,* a species found in fermenting vegetable material; it is non-pathogenic. [Gk *askos* bag, *kokkos* kernel.]

ascogonium (as·ko·**go**·ne·um). The female gametangium in Ascomycetes. A spiral organ from which are formed the asci after fertilization by the antheridium. [Gk *askos* bag, *gone* seed.]

Ascoli, Alberto (b. 1876). Italian serologist.

Ascoli test. A precipitation (ring) test used for the diagnosis of anthrax in carcasses, hides, etc., of infected animals by detecting anthrax antigens in these tissues.

Ascoli, Maurizio (b. 1876). Italian pathologist.

Ascoli treatment. A treatment for chronic malaria by intravenous injection of minute (0.01 ml) but rapidly increasing doses of adrenaline (epinephrine). The rationale is to cause repeated contractions of the spleen.

Ascomycetes (**as**·ko·mi·**se**'·teez). One of the 3 main divisions of Fungi, characterized by the inclusion of the sexually formed spores within structures known as *asci.* They include the yeasts and moulds. [Gk *askos* bag, *mykes* fungus.]

ascorbate (as·**kor**·bate). A salt formed by ascorbic acid with its tertiary hydroxyl groups.

ascorburia (as·kor·**bewr**'·e·ah). A condition in which ascorbic acid is present in the urine.

ascospore (**as**·ko·spor). In botany, a fungal spore contained in a membranous sac or ascus. [Gk *askos* bag, spore.]

ascus (**as**·kus) (pl. *asci*). A structure in the Ascomycetes division of the fungi which contains the sexually-formed spores. A sac-like cell in which ascospores are borne by free cell formation. [Gk *askos* bag.]

Aselli, Gaspare (b. 1581). Italian anatomist.

Aselli's glands, or pancreas. Lymphatic glands related to the pancreas in the dog.

asemasia (a·sem·a·ze·ah). Absence or loss of the power to communicate by word of mouth or by means of signs. [Gk *a, semasia* sign.]

asemia (a·**se**·me·ah). A form of aphasia in which the sufferer cannot understand or use words or signs. The condition is due to a lesion of the central nervous system. **Asemia graphica.** Lack of power to write or to understand what is written, owing to a lesion of the central nervous system. **Asemia mimica.** Lack of power to understand or to carry out any action expressing emotion or thought. **Asemia verbalis.** Lack of power to understand or to use words. [Gk *a, sema* sign.]

asepsis (a·**sep**·sis). The condition of being free from infection or from the presence of living pathogenic organisms. **Integral asepsis.** A surgical technique which renders sterile the entire space in which an operation is to be performed, and everyone and everything within that space, including the air. [Gk *a, sepsis* decay.]

aseptic (a·**sep**·tik). Free from sepsis or septic matter. [see prec.]

asepticism (a·**sep**·tis·izm). The principles of aseptic methods.

aseptol (a·**sep**·tol). Sozolic acid, orthophenolsulphonic acid, $C_6H_4OHHSO_3$. A strong antiseptic and disinfectant prepared by the sulphonation of phenol; also a reagent for albumin.

asequence (a·**se**·kwens). A term signifying that the atrial and ventricular contractions of the heart do not follow each other in the normal order. [Gk *a,* L *sequi* to follow.]

asexual (a·**sex**·ew·al). 1. Not sexual. 2. In biology, signifying that a process or organ is independent of sexual action, e.g. generation. [Gk *a,* sex.]

asexualization (a·**sex**·ew·al·i·**za**'·shun). The process of sterilization as applied to both sexes: in the male by castration or vasectomy; in the female by removal of ovaries or ligation of the uterine tubes. [see prec.]

ash (ash). 1. The residue obtained by the complete incineration of plant or animal matter. It consists of the inorganic constituents of the original material (lime, phosphates, etc.). 2. Any tree or species of the genus *Fraxinus* (family Oleaceae) including the European ash, *Fraxinus excelsior.* Manna is obtained from *Fraxinus ornus* and other species. **Bone ash.** The ash produced by the incineration of bones, consisting principally of calcium phosphate and carbonate. **Flowering ash.** The root bark of *Chionanthus virginicus* (family Oleaceae). **Pearl ash.** Crude potassium carbonate obtained by leaching wood ash. **Prickly ash.** Toothache tree, suterberry, yellow wood; the trees *Xanthoxylum carolinianum* (*americanum*) and *Fagara clavaherculis* (family Ranunculaceae). The berries contain no active substance other than a volatile oil and hesperidin, and have no therapeutic value; the bark appears to contain small quantities of alkaloids, but is of no medicinal value. **White ash.** American ash, *Fraxinus americana*; the bark is used deprived of its corky layer. **Wood ash.** The ash from the incineration of wood. It contains potassium carbonate (pearl ash). [AS *asce.*]

ashing (**ash**·ing). In chemistry, the conversion of anything to ash, especially in analysis. **Dry ashing.** The removal of organic material by the agency of heat alone. **Wet ashing.** The removal of organic material by heat in the presence of a liquid oxidizing agent.

asialia (a·si·a·le·ah). Arrest of the secretion of saliva, or diminished secretion of it, commonly resulting in xerostomia. [Gk *a, sialon* saliva.]

asiderosis (a·sid·er·**o**'·sis). An abnormally low state of the iron reserve of the body. [Gk *a, sideros* iron.]

asitia (a·**sish**·e·ah). Loathing of food. [Gk *a, sitos* food.]

Askenstedt's method. A method for the determination of indican in urine by conversion to indigo and extraction with chloroform.

asoma (a·**so**·mah). A monster with only the vestiges of a trunk and with an imperfectly developed head. [Gk *a, soma* body.]

asomatophyte (a·**so**·mat·o·fite). In botany, low organisms such as bacteria in which there is no distinction between somatic and reproductive cells. [Gk *a, soma* body, *phyton* plant.]

asomnia (a·**som**·ne·ah). Insomnia. [Gk *a,* L *somnus* sleep.]

asonia (a·**so**·ne·ah). Tone-deafness; a form of amusia in which there is inability to understand or hear the difference between one tone in music and another, so that it is impossible to sing or to play a stringed instrument in tune. [Gk *a,* L *sonus* sound.]

aspalasoma (as·pal·as·**o**'·mah). An autositic monster with, among other deformities, lateral or median eventration at the lower part of the abdomen. The 3 external orifices, urinary, genital, and anal, are distinct. [Gk *aspalax* mole, *soma* body.]

asparaginase (as·**par**·aj·in·aze). An enzyme catalysing the hydrolysis of the amide asparagine with the production of aspartic acid and ammonia.

asparagine (as·par·aj·een). Ammosuccinic acid, $CONH_2CH_2CHNH_2COOH$, the half amide of aspartic acid; a natural constituent of protein.

Asparagus (as·par·ag·us). A genus of plants of the order Liliaceae. **Asparagus officinalis.** An edible vegetable the shoots of which contain asparagine (althein), a diuretic used in cardiac dropsy and gout. [Gk *aspharagos.*]

aspartase (as·par·taze). An enzyme which catalyses the deamination of aspartic acid with production of fumarate and ammonia.

aspastic (a·spas·tik). Not spastic nor characterized by spasm. [Gk *a*, spastic.]

aspecific (a·spes·if·ik). Non-specific; applied to a disease or infection that is not due to the action of any particular micro-organism. [Gk *a*, specific.]

aspect (as·pekt). 1. The particular appearance or look, as of the face. 2. The part of a surface which fronts a particular direction, e.g. *dorsal aspect*, facing towards the dorsum, or back, or *medial aspect*, facing towards the median sagittal plane of the body. [L *aspicere* to look at.]

aspen (as·pen). *Populus tremula*, a tree of the family Salicaceae, the bark of which contains the glucosides salicin and populin. [AS *aespae.*]

Aspergillaceae (as·per·jil·a′·se·e). A family of common moulds which includes a number of species used in industry in the production of citric acid and digestive enzymes and a few species which are potentially pathogenic to animals, birds and man, e.g. *Aspergillus fumigatus.* [L *aspergere* to sprinkle.]

aspergillin (as·per·jil·in). A black pigment found in the mould *Aspergillus niger.* It is also used for skin-testing reagents from *Aspergillus* species in the diagnosis of allergic and pulmonary aspergillosis. [*Aspergillus.*]

aspergillomycosis (as·per·jil·o·mi·ko′·sis). Aspergillosis.

aspergillosis (as·per·jil·o′·sis). A disease caused by a fungus of the genus *Aspergillus.* **Aural aspergillosis.** Otomycosis. **Pulmonary aspergillosis.** A disease of the nature of broncho-pneumonia, or secondary to a chronic affection of the lungs, due to infection with a species of *Aspergillus.* [*Aspergillus*, Gk *-osis* condition.]

Aspergillus (as·per·jil·us). A genus of fungi belonging to the family Ascomycetes. They are characterized by a felted, septate, branching mycelium having the conidial apparatus developed on specialized hyphae, sporophores, which terminate in a vesicle on which are borne chains of conidia. Many species cause otomycoses, maduromycetoma, pulmonary mycetomas, allergic and disseminated aspergillosis; identification may be difficult. **Aspergillus candicus.** A common saprophyte occurring in soil and on grain. **Aspergillus chevalieri.** A fungus that has been claimed as a cause of mycetoma. **Aspergillus clavatus** Desmazieres 1834. A species commonly isolated from soil and dung: probably of no medical importance. **Aspergillus concentricus** Castellani 1907. *Trichophyton concentricum* Blanchard 1896, the cause of tinea imbricata (Tokelau ringworm). **Aspergillus flavus** Link 1809. A species isolated on several occasions from the human ear. It is also a parasite of certain insects, and is used in industry in the production of Chinese sauce (Koji). **Aspergillus fumigatus** Fresenius 1775. The common cause of aspergillosis in man and birds. **Aspergillus giganteus** Wehmer 1907. A species isolated from a case of bronchomycosis in Zaire. It is frequently found in nature. **Aspergillus glaucus** Link 1824. A group of common saprophytes. The name has been used loosely, and includes several species of *Aspergillus* which produce green spores. **Aspergillus itaconicus.** *Aspergillus terreus* (see below). **Aspergillus nidulans** (Eidam) Wint. 1884. A common saprophyte in soil and dust, frequently encountered in cultures made at autopsy. It has also been isolated from cases of otomycosis, and from a case of mycetoma with white grains. **Aspergillus niger** van Tieghem 1867. A common species group characterized by the black colour of the sporing heads. It has caused otomycosis and bronchomycosis in man, and is used in industry in the production of citric acid. **Aspergillus ochraceous** Wilhelm 1877. A common saprophyte, recorded on one occasion from a case of otitis media. **Aspergillus oryzae.** A species that occurs commonly as a saprophyte but has been isolated from otomycosis and sometimes attacks insects. **Aspergillus pictor** R. Blanchard 1895. The species of *Aspergillus* which has been found as a contaminant in the violet variety of pinta. **Aspergillus repens** (Corda) De Bary 1870. A species isolated by Siebenmann 3 times from the human ear, but its pathogenic rôle is doubtful. **Aspergillus terreus** Thom 1916. A species used in the production of itaconic acid from sugar. Isolated from a case of otomycosis in Brazil. **Aspergillus unguis** (Weil and Gaudin) Dodge 1935. A species isolated once from a toe nail. [L *aspergere* to sprinkle.]

aspermatic (a·sper·mat·ik). Referring to aspermia. [Gk *a*, *sperma* seed.]

aspermatism (a·sper·mat·izm). Aspermia.

aspermatogenesis (a·sper·mat·o·jen′·es·is). Non-functioning of the process by which spermatozoa are produced. [Gk *a*, *sperma* seed, genesis.]

aspermia (a·sper·me·ah). A condition in which there is inability to secrete or ejaculate seminal fluid. [Gk *a*, *sperma* seed.]

aspersion (as·per·shun). 1. A form of hydrotherapy in which the body is sprinkled with water of a particular temperature. 2. The sprinkling of the body with any medicinal agent. [L *aspersio* a sprinkling.]

aspersus (as·per·sus). Descriptive of a surface that is sprinkled over with punctures or dots. [L sprinkled.]

asphalgesia (as·fal·je·ze·ah). A condition present during hypnosis in which sensations of burning pain are felt when certain objects are touched. [Gk *asphi* one's own, *algos* pain.]

asphyctic, asphyctous (as·fik·tik, as·fik·tus). Affected with or referring to asphyxia. [Gk *a*, *sphyxis* pulse.]

asphygmia (a·sfig·me·ah). A condition in which the beat of the pulse is temporarily undetectable. [Gk *a*, *sphyxis* pulse.]

asphyxia (as·fix·e·ah). An inability to breathe, resulting from obstruction to air-flow at the mouth and nose. **Blue asphyxia.** Asphyxia livida (see below). **Asphyxia carbonica.** Asphyxia resulting from the inspiration of water gas, carbon monoxide, or coal gas. **Asphyxia cataphora.** Asphyxia interrupted by short periods of incomplete respiration. **Asphyxia cyanotica.** Traumatic asphyxia (see below). **Fetal asphyxia.** Asphyxia of the fetus *in utero* resulting from interference with the circulation. **Lethargic asphyxia.** Coma with depression of respiration. **Asphyxia livida.** Asphyxia with cyanosis. **Local asphyxia.** Capillary congestion and cyanosis occurring in severe cases of Raynaud's disease. **Asphyxia neonatorum.** A form of asphyxia occurring in newborn infants before breathing has become properly established. **Asphyxia pallida.** Asphyxia combined with pallid skin, faint pulse and absence of reflexes. **Asphyxia reticularis.** Livedo reticularis. **Secondary asphyxia.** Asphyxia recurring after there has been apparent recovery from suffocation. **Asphyxia sideratorum.** Suspended animation as a result of being struck by lightning. **Solar asphyxia, Asphyxia solaris.** Sunstroke. **Traumatic asphyxia.** Discoloration of head and neck caused by strong compression of the thorax or the upper part of the body generally. **White asphyxia.** Asphyxia pallida (see above). [Gk *a*, *sphyxis* pulse.]

asphyxial (as·fix·e·al). Referring to a state of asphyxia; characterized by the presence of, or involving, asphyxia.

asphyxiant (as·fix·e·ant). 1. Anything which produces asphyxia, particularly a gas. 2. Asphyxiating.

asphyxiate (as·fix·e·ate). To induce asphyxia or suffocation, partial or complete.

asphyxiation (as·fix·e·a′·shun). 1. A state of asphyxia or suffocation. 2. The action of causing asphyxia or suffocation.

Aspiculuris tetraptera (as·pe·kul·ewr·is tet·rap·ter·ah). The threadworm of the mouse: useful in comparative therapeutic trials.

aspidin (as·pid·in). $C_{23}H_{32}O_7$. A substance derived from male fern, *Dryopteris* (*Aspidium*) *filix-mas.* It paralyses the muscle of the tapeworm and so assists in its expulsion from the alimentary tract. Though toxic to invertebrates it does not seem to affect mammals, except when introduced into a vein, in which case it causes death by paralysing the respiratory centre.

aspidinol (as·**pid**·in·ol). Methylmethoxybutyrylphloroglucinol, $CH_3(CH_3O)(CH_3CH_2CH_2CO)C_6H(OH)_2$. A dihydroxy alcohol isolated from the extract of male fern, *Dryopteris* (*Aspidium*) *filix-mas*. **Aspidinol filizinol.** A solution of 10 per cent filicin in vegetable oil; used as a taenicide.

Aspidium (as·**pid**·e·um). 1. A genus of ferns of the family Polypodiaceae. 2. The rhizome and leaf bases of *Dryopteris* (*Aspidium*) *filix-mas*, the male fern. It contains filicic acid and aspidinol, which are effective in the treatment of worms, particularly against taeniae. [Gk *aspidion* small shield.]

aspidosamine (as·pid·o·sam·een). $C_{22}H_{28}O_2N_2$. One of the alkaloids obtained from the bark of Quebracho blanco (*Aspidosperma quebracho*). All these alkaloids are nauseating, but only aspidosamine causes actual vomiting, and it is used therefore as an emetic.

Aspidosperma (as·pid·o·**sper**'·mah). 1. A genus of trees of the family Apocynaceae. 2. Quebracho, Quebracho blanco, the dried bark of *Aspidosperma quebracho*, an evergreen tree indigenous to Argentina. It contains alkaloids, chiefly aspidospermine, yohimbine and quebrachamine, and is used in the form of a tincture as a tonic and febrifuge. [Gk *aspis* shield, *sperma* seed.]

aspidospermine (as·pid·o·**sper**'·meen). $C_{22}H_{30}O_2N_2$. An alkaloid obtained from the bark of Quebracho blanco (*Aspidosperma quebracho*). It produces nausea and salivation, but not vomiting.

aspirate (as·pir·ate). 1. To treat by the method of aspiration. 2. To draw away by suction. [L *aspirare* to breathe upon.]

aspiration (as·pir·a·shun). 1. The act of drawing in the breath. 2. The act of withdrawal by suction of fluid or gas from any of the cavities of the body. [see foll.]

aspirator (as·pir·a·tor). An apparatus for removing fluid from a cavity by suction. [L *aspirare* to breathe upon.]

See also: DIEULAFOY, POTAIN, SENORAN.

Aspirin (as·pir·in). An official synonym for Acetylsalicylic Acid BP 1968, $CH_3COOC_6H_4COOH$. A white crystalline powder only slightly soluble in water, the calcium, sodium and lithium salts being much more soluble. It is usually dispensed in tablet form, but a mixture of aspirin can be made with tragacanth as a suspending agent. Because of the rapidity with which the mixture hydrolyses it should be freshly prepared; it has the advantage that it is absorbed much more quickly than the tablet, and higher blood levels can thus be obtained. Aspirin is less irritant than salicylic acid and has a more powerful analgesic effect; the calcium salt is even less irritant. The drug achieves the same effect as salicylic acid in the treatment of rheumatic fever at lower dose levels, but idiosyncrasy occurs more commonly with aspirin than with other compounds of salicylic acid. The symptoms are localized oedemas and urticarial rashes. Aspirin has an antipyretic as well as an analgesic action owing to its effect on the heat centre and, because it depresses the optic thalamus, it is also employed as an anodyne in neuralgia and nervous headache.

Aspis (as·pis). A genus of snakes of the family Viperidae. **Aspis cornutus.** The horned viper found in Africa. [Gk asp.]

asplenia (a·**sple**·ne·ah). Absence of the spleen, congenital or acquired. [Gk *a*, spleen.]

asplenic (a·**splen**·ik). Referring to asplenia.

Asplenium (as·**ple**·ne·um). A genus of ferns of the family Polypodiaceae. **Asplenium filix-foemina** Bernh. (*Athyrium filix-foemina* Roth.). A species which has anthelminthic properties. [Gk *asplenon* spleen wort.]

asporogenic, asporogenous (a·spor·o·**jen**'·ik, a·spor·**oj**'·en·us). 1. Not bearing spores. 2. Not producing spores. 3. Not reproduced by spores. [Gk *a*, sporogenic.]

asporous (a·**spor**·us). Descriptive of micro-organisms which do not have any true spores. [Gk *a*, *sporos* seed.]

asporulate (a·**spor**·ew·late). Asporogenic; not producing spores. [Gk *a*, *sporos* seed.]

Assalini, Paolo (b. 1759). Italian surgeon.

Assalini's operation. For iridodialysis: detachment of the iris through an opening in the cornea; obsolete.

assanation (a·san·a·shun). The application of sanitary methods; sanitation. [L *ad*, *sanitas* health.]

assault (as·**awlt**). A violent attack. **Common assault.** 1. A threatened assault not including actual blows, e.g. shaking by the lapel or arms. 2. The delivery of blows (actual battery) or some other damage, e.g. throwing corrosive or a missile. **Criminal assault.** A lay term indicating rape. **Indecent assault.** An assault with indecent intent (mere touching may constitute this). [L *assilire* to leap upon.]

assay (as·a). 1. The estimation of the purity of precious metals. 2. The analysis of ores, metals or alloys; the term has been extended to the quantitative determination of the constituents, purity or activity of drugs and biological substances. **Biological assay.** The estimation of a substance possessing a specific biological activity, by observations upon animals or isolated living tissues, and comparison of the activity observed with that of a standard preparation. **Dry assay.** Assay by dry gravimetric analysis. **Microbiological assay.** The assay of vitamins or other nutritional factors by measurement of the growth of specific bacteria. **Radio-enzymatic assay.** A form of saturation analysis where the specific binding agent is an enzyme. **Wet assay.** Analysis by precipitation from solution, or by volumetric methods. *See* ANALYSIS. [Fr. *essayer* to try.]

Assézat, Jules (b. 1832). French anthropologist.

Assézat's triangle. A triangle used as an index in physical anthropology, comprised by the nasion, the basion and the alveolar point.

assident (as·id·ent). A term applied to symptoms, indicating that they are usually, but not invariably, present. [L *assidere* to sit by.]

assideration (as·id·er·a·shun). In medical jurisprudence, causing death by immersion in ice-cold water thereby concealing how it was effected. (Mediaeval law.) [L *ad*, *sideratio* evil intent.]

assimilation (as·im·il·a·shun). In physiology, constructive metabolism; the incorporation of nutritive material into the body substance and fluids, the last series of stages in the digestive process. **Assimilation limit.** The amount of sugary or starchy food which can be ingested before glycosuria occurs. **Mental assimilation.** The conscious appreciation of impressions received and their relegation to the proper spheres. **Assimilation pelvis.** *See* PELVIS. **Primary assimilation.** The absorption of nutritive substances from the intestinal canal in a relatively unchanged state. **Secondary assimilation.** The conversion of absorbed food into organized tissue. [L *assimilare* to make like.]

Assmann, Herbert (b. 1882). German pathologist.

Assmann's focus, or infiltrate. A primary focus of tuberculous infection in the lung parenchyma that in due course usually undergoes healing, shrinkage and calcification. In the radiograph, at first this does not show at all, but later it appears as a soft shadow and finally, if healing occurs, as a hard circumscribed, usually rounded or bean-shaped, lesion. At no stage is it recognizable clinically, but in children it may be associated with malaise and slight fever. When this lesion occurs in the subapical region, it is called an Assmann's focus. It is often associated with secondary glandular foci in the hilar region.

Assmann's psychrometer. A psychrometer in which air is driven past the bulb by a fan.

association (as·o·se·a'·shun). 1. In chemistry, the aggregation of molecules, such as occurs when steam (H_2O) condenses to water (H_6O_3). 2. The connection of things, in particular of the contents of the mind according to some principle or law, especially the primary laws of association, those of contiguity and similarity. **Clang association.** The association of words from the similarity of their sounds. **Colour association.** Encephalopsy. **Controlled association.** The process adopted when responses to stimulus words are restricted to a predetermined category, e.g. synonyms. **Dream association.** A patient's association to items of reported dream-content; a psycho-analytic technique. **Association fibre.**

See FIBRE. **Free association.** The process adopted when the content of the mind is allowed to range, undirected and uncriticized, from a given starting point. **Association of ideas.** The mechanism by which one idea is associated in the mind with another. **Word association.** The study of the word responses made to the giving of a stimulus word. [L *ad, socius* fellow.]

assonance (as·on·ans). An abnormal tendency to use alliterative words. [L *assonare* to correspond to in sound.]

assortment (as·**ort**·ment). In meiosis, the segregation of chromosomes or chromatids resulting in genically different gametes. [O Fr. *assorter* to sort.]

assuetude (as·we·tude). 1. The state of having become accustomed to unpleasant or disturbing influences. 2. Drug tolerance. [L *assuetudo* custom, habit.]

astacin (as·tas·in). $C_{40}H_{48}O_4$. A compound which occurs in crabs and lobster shells, produced by the oxidation of astaxanthin.

Astacus (as·ta·kus). Crayfish, a genus of crustaceans. **Astacus similis.** A species which is the secondary host to flukes of the genus *Paragonimus* in Korea: man is infected by eating the crayfish. [Gk *astakos* lobster.]

astasia (as·**ta**·ze·ah). Inability to stand or to sit erect because of inco-ordination of muscles. **Astasia abasia.** Abasia astasia; loss of ability to stand or walk normally because of defective will power. [Gk *a, stasis* a standing still.]

astatic (a·**stat**·ik). Not static. [Gk *a, stasis* a standing still.]

astatine (as·tat·een). A radioactive element of atomic number 85 and chemical symbol At. It was prepared in 1940 by the bombardment of bismuth with high energy α-particles in the cyclotron and is a member of the halogen group. [see prec.]

astaxanthin (as·tah·**zan**·thin). ($C_{40}H_{52}O_4$). A carotenoid pigment obtained from the crayfish (genus *Astacus*); it oxidizes to astacin.

asteatodes, asteatosis (a·ste·at·**o**′·deez, a·ste·at·**o**′·sis). 1. Arrested or diminished action of the sebaceous glands. 2. Any cutaneous disease characterized by arrest or diminished action of the sebaceous glands. **Asteatosis cutis.** A condition in which absence or deficiency of sebaceous secretion has caused the skin to become dry, scaly and fissured. [Gk *a, stear* tallow, *eidos* form, *-osis* condition.]

aster (as·ter). The star-like structure which, in mitosis and meiosis, surrounds the centrosome. **Aster of fertilization, Sperm aster.** In the fertilized ovum, the radial arrangement of the granules of cytoplasm in the immediate neighbourhood of the male pronucleus. [Gk star.]

astereocognosy, astereognosis (a·steer·e·o·**kog**′·no·se, a·**steer**·e·og·**no**′·sis). Inability to recognize objects by the feel of them or by touching them. Lack of the stereognostic sense. [Gk *a, stereos* solid, *gnosis* knowledge.]

asterion (as·ter·e·on). In craniometry, the point on the skull at which the occipital, parietal, and temporal bones meet. [Gk star-like.]

Asterionella (as·**ter**·e·on·**el**′·ah). A genus of diatoms which occur in fresh-water reservoirs and emit an aromatic odour due to an essential oil produced by the living organisms. [Gk *aster* star.]

asterixis (a·ster·**ix**·is). A form of irregular tremor of the outstretched fingers and hands seen in hepatic failure and other metabolic diseases. [Gk *a, sterixis* fixed position.]

asternal (a·**ster**·nal). 1. Not joined or related to the sternum. 2. Lacking a sternum. [Gk *a*, sternum.]

asternia (a·**ster**·ne·ah). Absence of the sternum. [see prec.]

asterococcus (as·ter·o·**kok**′·us). A generic name for certain organisms of the pleuropneumonia group, which are as yet imperfectly worked out. They are pathogenic to cattle and a number of other animals. They are closely related to *Actinomyces muris* (*Streptobacillus moniliformis,* which has been given the name *Asterococcus muris* by some writers). **Asterococcus mycoides.** The causal organism of pleuropneumonia of cattle, it is said to have been recovered from man. [Gk *aster* star, *kokkos* berry.]

asteroid (as·ter·oid). Resembling the aster in mitosis; star-shaped. [Gk *aster* star, *eidos* form.]

asterubin (as·ter·**oo**·bin). A sulphonic acid derivative of guanidine (not a pigment) obtained from certain starfish.

asthenia (as·**the**·ne·ah). Debility; loss of vital forces. **Asthenia crurum paraesthetica.** Painful weakness of the lower limbs, symptomatic of a variety of psychiatric and neuralogic illnesses. **Asthenia gravis hypophyseogenea.** Severe weakness with wasting and premature senility caused by destruction of the pituitary gland in Simmonds' disease. **Neurocirculatory asthenia.** Effort syndrome. *See* SYNDROME. **Periodic asthenia.** A condition in which phases of loss of strength and general debility recur periodically. **Asthenia pigmentosa.** Addison's disease. **Asthenia of the retina.** Retinal asthenopia. *See* ASTHENOPIA. **Tropical anhidrotic asthenia.** Enfeeblement consequent to absence of sweating in miliaria rubra. **Asthenia universalis.** Constitutional visceroptosis with gastro-intestinal atony and vasomotor weakness combined with a tendency towards neurasthenia. [Gk *a, sthenos* strength.]

asthenic (as·**then**·ik). Feeble, weak, lacking strength, debilitated. [see prec.]

asthenobiosis (as·**then**·o·bi·**o**′·sis). In biology, a state of activity in which temperature and atmospheric conditions play no direct part but in which there is resemblance to a condition of aestivation or hibernation. [Gk *a, sthenos* strength, *bios* life.]

asthenocoria (as·**then**·o·**kor**′·e·ah). A condition met with in states of adrenal insufficiency; the pupil reacts slowly to the stimulus of light. [Gk *a, sthenos* strength, *kore* pupil.]

asthenogenesis, asthenogenia (as·**then**·o·**jen**′·es·is, as·**then**·o·**je**′·ne·ah). The inducing of a condition of asthenia; the production of asthenia. [asthenia, Gk *genein* to produce.]

asthenope (as·then·ope). A person affected by asthenopia.

asthenophobia (as·**then**·o·**fo**′·be·ah). Pathological fear of weakness. [Gk *a, sthenos* strength, phobia.]

asthenopia (as·then·**o**·pe·ah). The symptoms produced by ocular muscle fatigue due to errors of refraction, upset of accommodation or muscle imbalance. They include headache, pain, tiredness, watering and congestion of the eyes, twitching of the lids and blurring of vision. **Accommodative asthenopia.** That caused by refractive errors and weakness or spasm of accommodation, and resulting in strain of the ciliary muscle. **Convergence asthenopia.** That due to fatigue of the internal recti muscles, due to a weakness or deficiency of convergence, occasionally due to spasm of convergence. **Asthenopia dolorosa.** That due to spasm of the ciliary muscle. **Glare asthenopia.** Asthenopia due to the glare of the sun, usually the indirect glare reflected, e.g. from snow. **Muscular asthenopia.** Asthenopia caused by strain or inco-ordination of the extrinsic muscles of the eye. **Myopic asthenopia.** That found in myopes, often caused by the disturbance of the accommodation. **Nervous asthenopia.** A form of asthenopia due to functional causes. **Retinal asthenopia.** That caused by glare. **Tarsal asthenopia.** Eye strain caused by excessive pressure of the eyelids on the cornea. [Gk *a, sthenos* strength, *ops* eye.]

asthenopic (as·then·**o**·pik). Referring to or characterized by asthenopia.

asthenospermia (as·then·o·**sper**′·me·ah). In spermatozoa, reduction in or loss of motility. [Gk *a, sthenos* strength, *sperma* seed.]

asthenoxia (as·then·**ox**·e·ah). A condition in which there is insufficient oxygenation of waste products. [Gk *a, sthenos* strength, oxygen.]

asthenozoospermia (as·then·o·zo·o·**sper**′·me·ah). Asthenospermia. [Gk *asthenes* weak, *zoon* animal, *sperma* seed.]

asthma (**as**·mah). The term used for a syndrome characterized by paroxysmal attacks of dyspnoea of expiratory type. These are caused by a narrowing of the smaller bronchi and bronchioles due to spasmodic contraction of the circular muscles of the bronchi together with swelling of the mucous membrane and later an exudation of mucus. It is a manifestation of the allergic state, and occurs in persons who have become sensitized to some foreign substance usually of protein nature or a bacterial toxin. The predisposition to become sensitized is in many cases, if not in all, inherited. The offending substances or allergens may enter by inhalation, ingestion or injection, the first being the most important. Infection or trauma, e.g. by operation, of the upper respiratory or bronchial tract may aid entrance. The possible allergens are innumerable, but air-borne dusts such as the hairs of animals, finely powdered vegetable matter such as flour, face powder, pollens of grasses and trees, and mixed house dust are among the commonest. Ingested and injected allergens are more likely to cause other allergic symptoms, such as urticaria, than asthma. Respiratory infections play an important part either as a primary cause, as opening the path for the entrance of other substances, or as secondary infections after repeated paroxysms. An individual attack may be excited reflexly by, for instance, stimulation of nerve-endings in the nose or stomach, or by psychological disturbances. *Status asthmaticus* is a more or less continuous state of asthma in which paroxysms occur with very little intermission maybe for days. *Bronchial asthma* and *spasmodic asthma* are unnecessary synonyms for asthma, as all asthma is bronchial and spasmodic. Asthma due to certain causes has been dignified by special names such as *cat asthma, horse asthma, food asthma, rye asthma, flour asthma, hay asthma*, and so on, but all these differ in no way except the cause. **Bronchitic asthma.** Asthma associated with bronchitis; there is usually some expiratory wheezing with bronchitis due to obstruction by sticky mucus but in some cases there may be a spasmodic element. True asthma may of course be associated with bronchitis. **Cardiac asthma.** Paroxysmal cardiac dyspnoea. *See* DYSPNOEA. **Extrinsic asthma.** Asthma caused by some environmental factor. **Melanodermic asthma.** Darkening of the skin before an attack of asthma through increased activity of melanocytes. **Miners' asthma.** Anthracosis. **Platinum asthma.** A nasal and bronchial irritation with dyspnoea occurring in workers refining platinum salts when the concentration of dust exceeds 5 $\mu g/m^3$. **Printers' asthma.** Asthma following exposure to a spray of gum acacia and isopropyl alcohol among printers. **Renal asthma.** Uraemic asthma (see below). **Strippers' asthma.** Byssinosis; a fibroid condition of the lungs occurring in workers in cotton factories who are exposed to the inhalation of cotton dust. **Thymic asthma.** A form of asthma associated with enlargement of the thymus, usually in childhood; severe paroxysms occur and death has been reported. **Uraemic asthma.** Paroxysmal dyspnoea occurring in chronic nephritis; it has no relation to true asthma. [Gk panting.]

See also: KOPP, ROSTAN.

asthmagenic, asthmogenic (as·mah·**jen**·ik, as·mo·**jen**·ik). Giving rise to asthma; term applied to substances, materials and climate. [Gk *asthma* panting, *genein* to produce.]

astigmagraph (as·tig·mah·graf). An instrument employed in the investigation of astigmatic eyes. [astigmatism, Gk *graphein* to record.]

astigmatic (as·tig·**mat**·ik). 1. A person affected with astigmatism. 2. Pertaining to astigmatism.

astigmatism (as·**tig**·mat·izm). A condition in which a point source of light cannot be brought to a point focus on the retina by the use of spherical lenses. It is caused by unequal refraction in different meridians of the eye. In regular astigmatism, the refraction is unequal in only 2 meridians, which are perpendicular to each other; in irregular astigmatism, the meridians are more numerous and the condition cannot be corrected by cylindrical lenses, e.g. conical cornea. **Acquired astigmatism.** That resulting from local injury or disease. **Astigmatism against the rule.** Astigmatism correctable by a convex cylinder approximately in the horizontal meridian, or by a concave one approximately vertical. **Compound astigmatism.** Astigmatism complicated by myopia or hypermetropia in all meridians. **Compound hypermetropic astigmatism, Compound hyperopic astigmatism.** That in which both meridians are hypermetropic, each coming into focus behind the retina. **Compound myopic astigmatism.** Astigmatism in which both meridians are myopic with anteretinal focus. **Congenital astigmatism.** A type present at birth. **Corneal astigmatism.** That due to irregularity of the refractive surfaces of the cornea. **Direct astigmatism.** Astigmatism with the rule (see below). **Hypermetropic astigmatism, Hyperopic astigmatism.** Astigmatism in which one meridian comes to a focus on the retina, the other behind it. **Inverse astigmatism.** Astigmatism against the rule (see above). **Irregular astigmatism.** Astigmatism in which the refraction is unequal in more than 2 meridians and cannot be corrected by cylindrical lenses. **Lenticular astigmatism.** Astigmatism which is the result of defect of the lens. **Mixed astigmatism.** Astigmatism in which one principal meridian is myopic and the other hypermetropic. **Myopic astigmatism.** Astigmatism in which one principal meridian is in focus on the retina, the other in front of it. **Oblique astigmatism.** Astigmatism in which the axes of the correcting cylinders are oblique, i.e. not vertical or horizontal. **Physiological astigmatism.** The small amount of astigmatism present in almost all eyes. **Regular astigmatism.** Astigmatism in which the refraction is unequal in only 2 meridians, which are at right angles. **Simple hypermetropic astigmatism, Simple hyperopic astigmatism.** Hypermetropic astigmatism (see above). **Simple myopic astigmatism.** Myopic astigmatism (see above). **Astigmatism with the rule.** A form of astigmatism which can be corrected by a convex cylindrical lens with axis approximately vertical, or a concave one with axis approximately horizontal. [Gk *a*, *stigma* point.]

astigmatometer (as·tig·mat·**om**′·et·er). An instrument with which the variety of astigmatism present may be determined and the degree measured.

astigmatoscope (as·tig·**mat**·o·skope). An instrument for detecting the presence of astigmatism and measuring its degree. [astigmatism, Gk *skopein* to watch.]

astigmatoscopy (as·tig·mat·**os**′·ko·pe). The measuring of astigmatism by means of the astigmatoscope.

astigmia (as·**tig**·me·ah). Astigmatism.

astigmic (as·**tig**·mik). Astigmatic.

astigmometer (as·tig·**mom**·et·er). Astigmatometer.

astigmometry (as·tig·**mom**·et·re). Determination of the variety of astigmatism present and of its degree.

astigmoscope (as·**tig**·mo·skope). Astigmatoscope.

astigmoscopy (as·tig·**mos**·ko·pe). Astigmatoscopy.

astomatous (a·**sto**·mat·us). 1. In biology, without a mouth. 2. In botany, without breathing pores. [Gk *a*, *stoma* mouth.]

astomia (a·**sto**·me·ah). In biology, the condition of being without a mouth opening. [see prec.]

astomous (a·**sto**·mus). Astomatous.

astragalar (as·**trag**·al·ar). Talar; relating to the talus, or belonging to it. [astragalus.]

astragalectomy (as·**trag**·al·**ek**′·to·me). Talectomy; surgical excision of the talus. [astragalus, Gk *ektome* a cutting out.]

astragalocalcanean (as·**trag**·al·o·kal·**ka**′·ne·an). Talocalcanean; involving both the talus and the calcaneum. [astragalus, calcaneum.]

astragalocrural (as·**trag**·al·o·**kroo**′·ral). Talocrural; involving both the talus and the bones of the leg. [astragalus, L *crus* leg.]

astragalofibular (as·**trag**·al·o·**fib**′·ew·lar). Talofibular; involving both the talus and the fibula. [astragalus, fibula.]

astragaloscaphoid (as·**trag**·al·o·**ska**′·foid). Talonavicular (taloscaphoid); concerned with the articulation of the talus and the navicular (scaphoid) bone. [astragalus, scaphoid.]

astragalotibial (as·**trag**·al·o·**tib**′·e·al). Talotibial; relating to the talus and the tibia. [astragalus, tibia.]

Astragalus (as·**trag**·al·us). 1. An obsolete term for the talus, the bone of the tarsus with which the tibia and fibula articulate. 2. A genus of plants of the family Leguminosae, including the milk vetch, many of which yield gums. **Astragalus gummifer.** A species of Asia Minor, Kurdistan, Syria, and Armenia, which is a source of tragacanth. **Astragalus mollissimus.** A species of North America, the locoweed, with toxic properties. [Gk *astragalos* ball of ankle joint.]

astral (as·tral). Belonging to an aster or star-shaped body. [Gk *aster* star.]

astraphobia, astrapophobia (as·trah·**fo**·be·ah, as·trah·po·**fo**′·be·ah). Excessive fear of lightning or of being struck by lightning. [Gk *astrape* lightning, phobia.]

astrict (as·**trikt**). 1. To confine, constrict or compress. 2. To cause to contract, as by application of an astringent. 3. To cause to become constipated. [see foll.]

astriction (as·**trik**·shun). 1. Constipation. 2. The contraction of parts by application of an astringent. [L *astringere* to draw tight.]

astringent (as·**trin**·jent). 1. Arresting secretion or discharge. 2. Causing contraction of tissues. 3. A drug, usually a tannic-acid-containing vegetable product, a mineral salt or a salt of a metal, which has these properties. [see prec.]

astroblast (**as**·tro·blast). The primitive stage of a cell before it develops into an astrocyte. [Gk *aster* star, *blastos* germ.]

astroblastoma (**as**·tro·blas·**to′**·mah). A tumour the cells composing which are astroblasts. [astroblast, Gk *-oma* tumour.]

astrochemistry (as·tro·**kem**·is·tre). The study of the composition and reactions of the matter composing astronomical bodies. [Gk *aster* star, chemistry.]

astrocyte (**as**·tro·site). A type of neuroglial cell, consisting of a cell body and a large number of branching processes. Astrocytes are of ectodermal origin and function as specialized supporting cells within the central nervous system. It is possible that they are also concerned with the nutrition of the nerve cells in their vicinity. **Fibrous astrocyte.** A neuroglial cell found chiefly in the white matter. **Protoplasmic astrocyte.** One found in the grey matter. [Gk *aster* star, *kytos* cell.]

astrocytoma (**as**·tro·si·**to′**·mah). A glioma; a tumour the cells of which are astrocytes. **Astrocytoma diffusum.** A widespread astrocytoma of the brain, which resembles very closely an area of gliosis or scarring. **Astrocytoma fibrillare.** An astrocytoma composed of fibrous astrocytes. **Gemistocytic astrocytoma.** Astrocytoma protoplasmaticum (see below). **Pilocytic astrocytoma.** Astrocytoma fibrillare (see above). **Astrocytoma protoplasmaticum.** An astrocytoma the cells of which are protoplasmic astrocytes. [astrocyte, Gk *-oma* tumour.]

astroglia (as·**trog**·le·ah). Macroglia; a type of neuroglia in which the cells are multipolar. [Gk *aster* star, neuroglia.]

astroid (**as**·troid). 1. An astrocyte. 2. Stellate; shaped like a star. [Gk *aster* star, *eidos* form.]

astrokinetic (**as**·tro·kin·**et′**·ik). Referring to the movements of the asters during cell division. [aster, Gk *kinesis* movement.]

astroma (as·**tro**·mah). Astrocytoma.

astronaut (**as**·tro·nawt). A person who travels in a space vehicle. [Gk *aster* star, *nautes* sailor.]

astrophobia (as·tro·**fo**·be·ah). Fear of universal space and the stars. [Gk *aster* star, phobia.]

astrophorous (as·**trof**·or·us). Having stellate processes. [Gk *aster* star, *phoros* bearing.]

astrosphere (**as**·tro·sfeer). The figure formed by the threads of protoplasm arranged radially round the centrosome in mitosis. [Gk *aster* star, *sphaira* sphere.]

astrostatic (as·tro·**stat**·ik). A term applied to the centrosome when it is in the resting stage. [Gk *aster* star, *statikos* standing.]

astrovirus (**as**·tro·**vi**·rus). A small 28 nm virus probably containing RNA, it is associated with enteritis in infants. The virus has yet to be grown in cell cultures but its unique morphology with five or six pointed stars superimposed on a circular outline distinguish it clearly from other viruses of similar size. It is not yet known to be related to other human or animal viruses, and its role in disease has yet to be established. (Gk *astron*, a star.)

Astrup, P. 20th century Scandinavian physiologist.

micro-Astrup method. An interpolation technique for estimating the acid–base state of the blood, using a very small sample of blood.

astyphia (a·**stif**·e·ah). Inability to cause erection of the penis; impotence. [Gk *a*, *styein* to stiffen.]

astysia (a·**stiz**·e·ah). Impairment of power to erect the penis. [Gk *a*, *styein* to make erect.]

asuerotherapy (as·oo·**er**·o·**ther′**·ap·e). A therapeutic measure consisting in treatment by suggestion and cauterization of the sphenopalatine ganglion. [Fernando *Asuero*, Spanish physician, fl. 1929.]

asulphurosis (a·sul·fewr·**o′**·sis). The bodily condition resulting from loss or absence of sulphur in the body. [Gk *a*, sulphur, Gk *-osis* condition.]

asuprarenalism, asurrenalism (a·sew·prah·**re′**·nal·izm, a·ser·**e**·nal·izm). Anadrenalism. [Gk *a*, suprarenal.]

asyllabia (a·sil·**a**·be·ah). A form of word blindness in which, although single letters can be recognized, the sufferer cannot group them to make syllables. [Gk *a*, *syllabe* taken together.]

asylum (as·**i**·lum). 1. An institution in which destitute, afflicted and unfortunate persons are cared for. 2. A name formerly in use for a mental hospital. **Asylum dysentery.** *See* DYSENTERY. **Asylum ear.** Haematoma auris. [Gk *asylon* inviolable.]

asymbolia (a·sim·**bo**·le·ah). Asemia; a form of aphasia in which the sufferer cannot understand or use words or signs. The condition is due to a lesion of the central nervous system. **Pain asymbolia.** Inability to understand pain symbolism or to make signs of feeling pain. [Gk *a*, symbol.]

asymmetry (a·**sim**·et·re). 1. The condition of being without symmetry in relation to any point, line or plane. The term is especially used in morphology when the left and right sides of an organism are not mirror images of one another. 2. In anatomy, lack of correspondence between the right and left halves of an organ or of regions of the body. 3. In chemistry, the arrangement of atoms or radicals about a central atom in a molecule in such a way as to exhibit no symmetry in any direction. Such an arrangement in respect of a carbon atom gives rise to stereoisomerism and optical activity. **Chromatic asymmetry.** Difference in colour of the two irides. **Meridional asymmetry.** Difference in refractive power of 2 meridians in the eye, which produces astigmatism. **Unilateral asymmetry.** Hemihypertrophy; enlargement of one half of the body, usually of congenital origin. [Gk *a*, *symmetria* commensurableness.]

asymphytous (a·**sim**·fit·us). Distinct and separate; not fused. [Gk *a*, *syn*, *phyein* to grow.]

asymptomatic (a·simp·to·**mat′**·ik). Without symptoms; not giving rise to symptoms. [Gk *a*, symptom.]

asynapsis (a·sin·**ap**·sis). The lack of pairing of chromosomes at meiosis. [Gk *a*, *synaptein* to join.]

asynaptic (a·sin·**ap**·tik). Of chromosomes, failing to pair at meiosis. [Gk *a*, *synaptein* to join.]

asynchronism (a·**sin**·kron·izm). 1. A condition in which occurrences normally coinciding in time do so no longer. 2. Inco-ordination. [Gk *a*, synchronism.]

asynclitism (a·**sin**·klit·izm). In parturition, oblique presentation of the head. **Anterior asynclitism.** Naegele's obliquity. **Posterior asynclitism.** Litzmann's obliquity. [Gk *a*, *synklinein* to lean together.]

asyndesis (a·**sin**·des·is). A defect of mentality on account of which related thoughts or ideas cannot be assembled to make a coherent concept. [Gk *a*, *syn*, *desis* a binding.]

asyndromic (a·sin·**dro**·mik). Of signs or symptoms, indicating that they are not those classically associated with the infection or disease in question. [Gk *a*, syndrome.]

asynechia (a·sin·**ek**·e·ah). A term signifying that there is absence of continuity of structure in a part or organ. [Gk *a*, *synecheia* a holding together.]

asynergia (a·sin·**er**·je·ah). Asynergy.

asynergy (a·**sin**·er·je). Lack of co-ordination or co-operation of parts the normal function of which is to act in unison. As applied to the nervous system, inco-ordination of muscular action so that a movement is incorrectly carried out because its component parts are inaccurately timed and in incorrect sequence. **Appendicular asynergy.** Asynergy affecting the hands and feet only. **Axial asynergy.** That affecting the musculature of the head and trunk. **Axio-appendicular asynergy.** Asynergy affecting the extremities as well as the head and trunk. **Asynergy major.** Severe muscular inco-ordination the sign of which is a staggering gait. **Asynergy minor.** Slight inco-ordination the sign of which is failure to point at a fixed object with eyes open and closed alternately. **Motorial asynergy, Progressive locomotor asynergy.** Locomotor ataxia. *See* ATAXIA. **Truncal asynergy.** That affecting the musculature of the trunk. **Ventricular asynergy.** Inco-ordinate contraction of the wall of a cardiac ventricle, usually the left. **Verbal asynergy.** Inco-ordination of the laryngeal musculature caused by chorea. [Gk *a, synergia* co-operation.]

asynesia (a·sin·e·ze·ah). Stupidity; intellectual dullness. Disturbance or defect of intellectual power. [Gk *asynesia* stupidity.]

asynodia (a·sin·o·de·ah). In sexual intercourse non-coincidence in orgasm. [Gk *a, synodia* a journeying together.]

asynovia (a·sin·o·ve·ah). Deficiency or absence of synovial secretion. [Gk *a*, synovial.]

asyntaxia dorsalis (a·sin·tax·e·ah dor·sa·lis). A congenital abnormality due to partial failure of the closing of the neural tube. [Gk *a, syntaxis* a putting together, L of the back.]

asyntrophy (a·sin·tro·fe). Asymmetrical development or growth. [Gk *a, syn, trophe* nutrition.]

asystematic (a·sis·tem·at′·ik). In nervous disease, not limited to one system or set of organs or structures; a general or diffuse nervous disease. [Gk *a*, system.]

asystole, asystolia, asystolism (a·sis·to·le, a·sis·to·le·ah, a·sis·to·lizm). The condition when the heart stops contracting. Usually distinguished from fibrillation, where electrical activity persists but effective mechanical activity ceases. **Cardiataxic asystole.** A condition caused by acceleration in the heart rate setting up a brief spell of asystole. **Cardioplegic asystole.** Amyocardia. **Ventricular asystole.** Asystole (see main def. above). [Gk *a*, systole.]

atactic (at·ak·tik). 1. Ataxic. 2. Inco-ordinated; irregular. 3. Referring to aphasic muscular inco-ordination, or involving it. [Gk *ataktos* irregular.]

atactiform (at·ak·te·form). 1. Like ataxia. 2. Showing a mild form of ataxia.

atactilia (a·tak·til·e·ah). Absence or loss of the sense of touch. [Gk *a*, L *tactus* touch.]

ataractic (a·tar·ak·tik). Term used to describe tranquillizing drugs. [Gk *a, taraktos* disturbed.]

ataralgesia (a·tar·al·je′·ze·ah). Tranquillity of mind and insensitivity to pain, a state produced by the injection of a narcotic analgesic, a phenothiazine and a respiratory stimulant; used in minor surgery. [Gk *a, taraktos* disturbed, *algos* pain.]

ataraxia, ataraxy (a·tar·ax·e·ah, a·tar·ax·e). A state of complete mental tranquillity. [Gk *a, taraktos* disturbed.]

atavic (at·av·ik). Atavistic.

atavism (at·av·izm). 1. In general, the recurrence in an individual of a characteristic or of a tendency towards a particular diathesis or disease which was latent in the more immediate forebears but present in a remote ancestor. 2. In genetics, inheritance from a grandparent of a trait or characteristic which is dissimilar from the corresponding characteristic in the parent. Cf. REVERSION. [L *atavus* ancestor.]

atavistic (at·av·is·tik). Characterized by, referring to or involving atavism.

ataxaphasia (at·ax·af·a′·ze·ah). Inability to arrange words in proper sequence in sentences although single words can be spoken. [ataxia, aphasia.]

ataxia (at·ax·e·ah). Loss of control over the voluntary movements of everyday life, which depend upon the various groups of muscles involved being completely balanced with each other. This state of balance is determined by various factors, the most important of which are the afferent impulses coming from the muscles via the afferent nerves. Any condition which interferes with the passage of these impulses either in peripheral nerves, spinal-cord tracts or centrally in the cerebellar regions will to a varying extent allow symptoms of unsteadiness in the movements concerned. **Acute ataxia.** Ataxia due to multiple lesions of the spinal cord associated with acute infectious disease. **Alcoholic ataxia.** Ataxia seen in cases of peripheral neuritis due to alcoholism. Similar symptoms are associated with neuritis due to other toxic agents, e.g. diphtheria. **Central cerebellar ataxia.** A form of muscular inco-ordination due to lesions of the higher centres and the cerebellum. **Diphtheritic ataxia.** Symptoms arising out of diphtheria infection, due to neuritis caused by the diphtheria toxin. **Hereditary ataxia.** Friedreich's disease, a familial affection beginning in childhood and characterized by unsteadiness of gait, and other movements, absent reflexes, and extensor plantar response, all due to sclerosis of posterior and lateral columns in the spinal cord. **Intrapsychic ataxia.** A lack of co-ordination between affect and thinking; incongruity of affect. **Locomotor ataxia.** Tabes dorsalis, ataxic symptoms due to degeneration of the posterior columns of the spinal cord. **Noöthymopsychic ataxia.** Intrapsychic ataxia (see above). **Ocular ataxia.** Nystagmus. **Sensory ataxia.** A disturbance of muscular co-ordination resulting from defective sensory information; usually found with nerve root or spinal-cord disorder. **Ataxia telangiectasia.** A type of infantile cerebellar ataxia with telangiectases of the conjunctiva (syn.: Le Bar syndrome). **Truncal ataxia, Trunkal ataxia.** Ataxia affecting the movements necessary for maintaining the posture of the trunk, as in sitting or standing. **Vestibular ataxia.** Muscular inco-ordination due to vestibular disease. [Gk lack of order.]

See also: BROWN (S.), FRIEDREICH, MARIE.

ataxiadynamia (at·ax·e·ah·di·nam′·e·ah). Weakness as well as inco-ordination of the muscles. [ataxia, Gk *a, dynamis* force.]

ataxiagram (at·ax·e·ah·gram). 1. The curve drawn by an ataxiagraph. 2. The line drawn, with the eyes closed or open, by a patient with ataxia. The degree of its deviation from the straight is held to be of value in diagnosis. [ataxia, Gk *gramma* a writing.]

ataxiagraph (at·ax·e·ah·graf). An instrument which records the degree and direction of movements of the head, and thus can be used as a method of estimating the degree of static ataxia when the patient stands with the eyes closed. [ataxia, Gk *graphein* to record.]

ataxiamnesia (at·ax·e·am·ne′·ze·ah). Impairment or loss of memory in association with muscular inco-ordination. [ataxia, Gk *amnesia* forgetfulness.]

ataxiamnesic (at·ax·e·am·ne′·zik). Characterized by amnesia as well as ataxia. [see prec.]

ataxiaphasia (at·ax·e·af·a′·ze·ah). A state in which disconnected words may be used with understanding but there is inability to form a connected sentence. [ataxia, aphasia.]

ataxic (at·ax·ik). Referring to ataxia.

ataxiophemia (at·ax·e·o·fe′·me·ah). A state of inco-ordination of the muscles controlling utterance. [ataxia, Gk *phemi* to speak.]

ataxiophobia (at·ax·e·o·fo′·be·ah). Morbid or excessive dread of untidiness or disorder. [ataxia, phobia.]

ataxo-adynamia (at·ax·o·a·di·nam′·e·ah). Ataxiadynamia.

ataxophemia (at·ax·o·fe′·me·ah). Ataxiophemia.

ataxophobia (at·ax·o·fo′·be·ah). Ataxiophobia.

ataxy (at·ax·e). Ataxia.

atelectasis (at·el·ek·tas·is). Collapse of the lung. The alveolar walls become apposed, preventing ventilatory exchange of respiratory gases. **Absorption atelectasis.** Pulmonary collapse resulting when the absorption of gas from the pulmonary alveoli exceeds the ventilatory inflow; one cause is breathing 100 per cent oxygen during rapid acceleration which dilates the dependent alveolar capillaries. **Compression atelectasis.** Atelectasis induced by pressure, e.g. from a tumour outside the lungs. **Obstructive atelectasis.** A form of absorption atelectasis caused by the blocking of a bronchial tube. [Gk *ateles* incomplete, *ektasis* a stretching.]

atelectatic (at·el·ek·tat′·ik). Affected with or pertaining to atelectasis.

ateleiosis (at·el·e·o′·sis). Hypophyseal dwarfism (Lorain, Lorain-Lévi or Paltauf type); due to insufficiency or destruction of the eosinophil cells of the anterior pituitary. The frame and facies are childlike and the muscles poorly developed; sexual development may or may not be delayed. In cases due to a destructive lesion of the pituitary, panhypopituitarism may occur. [Gk *ateles* incomplete, *-osis* condition.]

atelencephalia, atelencephaly (at·el·en·kef·a′·le·ah, at·el·en·kef′·al·e). A state of imperfect development of the brain. [Gk *ateles* incomplete, *egkephalos* brain.]

atelia (at·e·le·ah). Continuance in the adult of the characteristics of childhood; infantilism. [Gk *ateleia* incompleteness.]
atelic (at·el·ik). Without function. [see foll.]
ateliotic (at·el·e·ot'·ik). 1. Characterized by atelia. 2. Incomplete in development. [Gk *ateles* incomplete.]
atelocardia (at·el·o·kar'·de·ah). An incompletely developed state of the heart. [Gk *ateles* incomplete, *kardia* heart.]
atelocephalous (at·el·o·kef'·al·us). Having a skull that is incompletely developed. [Gk *ateles* incomplete, *kephale* head.]
atelocheilia (at·el·o·ki'·le·ah). Imperfect development of a lip or the lips. [Gk *ateles* incomplete, *cheilos* lip.]
atelocheiria (at·el·o·ki'·re·ah). Defective development of a hand. [Gk *ateles* incomplete, *cheir* hand.]
atelo-encephalia (at·el·o·en·kef·a'·le·ah). Atelencephalia.
ateloglossia (at·el·o·glos'·e·ah). A condition in which the tongue is imperfectly developed or formed. [Gk *ateles* incomplete, *glossa* tongue.]
atelognathia (at·el·og·na'·the·ah). Structural defect of the jaw, particularly of the mandible. [Gk *ateles* incomplete, *gnathos* jaw.]
atelomyelia (at·el·o·mi·e'·le·ah). A condition in which there is incomplete or imperfect development of the spinal cord. [Gk *ateles* incomplete, *myelos* marrow.]
atelopodia (at·el·o·po'·de·ah). A condition of defective structure of the foot (congenital). [Gk *ateles* incomplete, *pous* foot.]
ateloprosopia (at·el·o·pro·so'·pe·ah). Incomplete development, or defect in structure, of the face. [Gk *ateles* incomplete, *prosopon* face.]
atelorrhachidia (at·el·o·rak·id'·e·ah). Defective formation of the vertebral column. [Gk *ateles* incomplete, *rhachis* spine.]
atelostomia (at·el·o·sto'·me·ah). Defective development or structure of the mouth. [Gk *ateles* incomplete, *stoma* mouth.]
Atenolol (at·en·o·lol). BP Commission approved name for 4-(2-hydroxy-3-isopropylaminopropoxy)phenylacetamide, a beta-adrenergic blocking agent.
athalposis (a·thal·po·sis). Insensitiveness to warmth. [Gk *a*, *thalpos* warmth.]
athelia (a·the·le·ah). Lack of nipples. [Gk *a*, *thele* nipple.]
athermal (a·ther·mal). A term applied to cool springs the water of which is below 15°C (59°F). [Gk *a*, *therme* heat.]
athermancy (a·ther·man·se). The condition of being athermanous.
athermanous (a·ther·man·us). Able to absorb and retain heat rays; impermeable by radiant heat. [Gk *a*, *therme* heat.]
athermic (a·ther·mik). 1. Afebrile. 2. Athermanous. [see prec.]
athermosystaltic (a·ther·mo·sis·tal'·tik). A term applied to striped muscle and signifying that it does not contract or expand under the action of cold or of heat. [Gk *a*, *therme* heat, *systaltikos* drawing together.]
atherocheuma (ath·er·o·kew'·mah). Atheromatous abscess. *See* ABSCESS. [Gk *athere* meal, *cheuma* melting.]
atheroma (ath·er·o·mah). The process affecting blood-vessels involving the formation of sub-intimal plaques which start as lipid (cholesterol) deposits and which later become fibrotic or calcified. The surface may ulcerate and superimposed thrombosis occur. It is the basis of the commonest form of arterial disease. **Capillary atheroma.** A condition affecting the capillary walls causing the formation of fatty granules. **Atheroma cutis.** Sebaceous cyst. *See* CYST. [Gk *athere* meal, *-oma* tumour.]
atheromasia (ath·er·o·ma'·ze·ah). 1. The condition in which atheroma tends to develop. 2. Atheromatous degeneration. *See* DEGENERATION.
atheromatosis (ath·er·o·mat·o'·sis). A generalized atheromatous condition of the arteries. **Atheromatosis cutis.** Sebaceous cyst. *See* CYST. [atheroma, Gk *-osis* condition.]
atheromatous (ath·er·o·mat·us). Affected with or pertaining to atheroma.
atheronecrosis (ath·er·o·nek·ro'·sis). The degenerative alteration of physical condition which is an accompaniment of atherosclerosis. [Gk *athere* meal, necrosis.]
atherosclerosis (ath·er·o·skler·o'·sis). Nodular arteriosclerosis; the outer coat is hyperplastic, and there is fatty degeneration of the middle coat. **Atherosclerosis obliterans.** Arteriosclerosis obliterans, atheroma, endarteritis deformans; thickening of the intima, with patchy degenerative changes in which fat crystals may be seen and in which calcium may be deposited. It involves mainly the large arteries. [Gk *athere* meal, sclerosis.]
atherosis (ath·er·o·sis). Arteriosclerosis. [Gk *athere* meal, *-osis* condition.]
athetoid (ath·e·toid). 1. Having a resemblance to athetosis. 2. Affected with athetosis.
athetosic (ath·e·to·sik). Referring or pertaining to athetosis.
athetosis (ath·e·to·sis). Slow, writhing involuntary movements mainly affecting the distal segments of the upper limbs (syn.: mobile spasm). Most commonly occurring as a form of infantile cerebral palsy but also in hemiplegia from any cause. Bilateral athetosis is a juvenile form of dytonic movement disorder. **Bilateral acquired athetosis, Double athetosis.** Vogt's syndrome. **Pupillary athetosis.** Hippus. [Gk *athetos* not fixed.]
athetotic (ath·e·tot·ik). Athetosic.
athrepsia, athrepsy (a·threp·se·ah, a·threp·se). 1. Marasmus. 2. Malnutrition. 3. A name given by Ehrlich to a state of immunity to tumour inoculation which he held to be due to absence of specific nutritive material essential for tumour growth. [Gk *a*, *threpsis* nutrition.]
athreptic (a·threp·tik). Pertaining to athrepsia.
athrombia (a·throm·be·ah). Imperfect clotting of the blood. [Gk *a*, *thrombos* clot.]
athrophagocytosis (ath·ro·fag·o·si·to'·sis). The ingestion by a cell of non-nutritive material. [Gk *athroos* in masses, phagocytosis.]
athymia, athymism, athymismus (a·thime·e·ah, a·thime·izm, a·thime·iz·mus). 1. Lack of the thymus gland. 2. The condition brought about by the lack of the secretions of the thymus gland. 3. Amentia. 4. A state of unconsciousness. 5. Morbid impassivity or despondency. [Gk *a*, *thymos* mind.]
athyrea (a·thi·re·ah). 1. Myxoedema. 2. Deficiency of secretion in the thyroid gland. 3. Lack of the thyroid gland. [Gk *a*, thyroid.]
athyreosis (a·thi·re·o'·sis). The pathological condition consequent upon removal of the thyroid gland or interference with its powers of secretion. [Gk *a*, thyroid, Gk *-osis* condition.]
athyroidaemia (a·thi·roid·e'·me·ah). The condition of the blood caused by deficiency or absence of the thyroid secretion. [Gk *a*, thyroid, Gk *haima* blood.]
athyroidation (a·thi·roid·a'·shun). Athyroidism.
athyroidea (a·thi·roid·e·ah). Lack of the thyroid gland. [Gk *a*, thyroid.]
athyroidism, athyroidosis, athyrosis (a·thi·roid·izm, a·thi·roid·o'·sis, a·thi·ro'·sis). The clinical condition present because of deficient secretion in the thyroid gland or absence of the gland. [see prec.]
athyrotic (a·thi·rot·ik). Referring to athyreosis.
atisine (at·is·een). $C_{22}H_{33}O_2N$. An amorphous bitter and non-toxic alkaloid obtained from *Aconitum heterophyllum*.
Atkinson, Isaac Edmundson (b. 1846). Baltimore dermatologist.
Atkinson's depilatory. A depilatory consisting of 6 parts of quicklime, 1 part of arsenic trisulphide, and flour.
atlantal (at·lan·tal). Referring to the atlas.
atlanto-axial (at·lan·to·ax'·e·al). Referring to the atlas and the axis. **Atlanto-axial joints.** *See* JOINT.
atlantodidymus (at·lan·to·did'·e·mus). A double-headed monster with one body and one neck. [atlas, *didymos* twin.]
atlantomastoid (at·lan·to·mas'·toid). Referring to the atlas and the mastoid part of the temporal bone.
atlanto-occipital (at·lan·to·ok·sip'·it·al). Referring to the atlas and the occipital bone. **Atlanto-occipital joint.** *See* JOINT. **Atlanto-occipital membrane.** *See* MEMBRANE.
atlanto-odontoid (at·lan·to·o·dont'·oid). Referring to the atlas and the odontoid process of the axis.
atlas [NA] (at·las). The 1st cervical vertebra, which supports the globe of the head; above, it articulates with the occipital bone, below with the axis. [from Gk *thenai* to bear.]
Lateral mass [massa lateralis (NA)]. The irregular bony part at each side of the atlas vertebra.

atlo-axoid (at·lo·**ax**·oid). Atlanto-axial.

atlodidymus, atlodymus (at·lo·**did**·e·mus, at·lo·**di**·mus). Atlantodidymus.

atloido-occipital (at·**loid**·o·ok·**sip**′·it·al). Atlanto-occipital.

atmiatria, atmiatrics, atmiatry (at·mi·**at**·re·ah, at·mi·**at**·rix, at·mi·at·re). Treatment of disease of the respiratory tract by means of medicated sprays or vapours. [Gk *atmos* vapour, *iatreia* healing.]

atmidalbumin (at·mid·al·**bew**′·min). A protein substance formed from albumin by superheated steam. [Gk *atmos* vapour, albumin.]

atmidalbumose (at·mid·al·**bew**′·moze). The albumose corresponding to atmidalbumin and derived from it by hydrolytic cleavage.

atmocausis (at·mo·**kaw**·zis). The direct application, by means of a two-way catheter, of superheated steam. The method is used in affections of the mucous membrane, especially of the uterus, and is a substitute for curettage. [Gk *atmos* vapour, *kausis* burning.]

atmocautery (at·mo·**kaw**·ter·e). An instrument with which atmocausis is performed. [Gk *atmos* vapour, cautery.]

atmograph (at·mo·graf). An instrument for making continuous records of the respiratory movements. [Gk *atmos* vapour, *graphein* to record.]

atmokausis (at·mo·**kaw**·zis). Atmocausis.

atmolysis (at·**mol**·is·is). 1. The separation of mixed gases of unequal diffusibility by passing them through porous walls, the lighter gas diffusing more readily. 2. The submitting of organic tissues, for the purpose of disintegrating them, to the action of fumes from volatile fluids. [Gk *atmos* vapour, *lysis* a loosing.]

atmometer (at·**mom**·et·er). An apparatus used in ascertaining the humidity of the atmosphere. It measures the amount of water which passes into the air by evaporation from a particular surface in a certain length of time. [Gk *atmos* vapour, meter.]

atmos (at·mos). A unit of atmospheric pressure, defined as the weight at 0°C of a column of mercury 760 mm high on each square centimetre of surface and equal to 101 325 pascal. Cf. ATMOSPHERE. [Gk vapour.]

atmosphere (at·mos·feer). 1. The gases or air surrounding the earth. 2. The state of the air in any particular locality. 3. In chemistry, a gaseous envelope or medium. 4. The pressure upon the earth exerted by the air at sea-level, about 101 kilopascal (15 lb/in^2). [Gk *atmos* vapour, *sphaira* sphere.]

atmospherization (at·mos·fer·i·**za**′·shun). The conversion, by the absorption of oxygen, of venous blood into arterial blood. Cf. DEARTERIALIZATION. [see prec.]

atmotherapy (at·mo·**ther**·ap·e). 1. Treatment of disease of the respiratory tract by means of medicated sprays or vapours; atmiatria. 2. The treatment of neurotic spasm by the therapeutic reduction of respiration. [Gk *atmos* vapour, therapy.]

atocia (a·to·se·ah). Nulliparity; female sterility. [Gk *a*, *tokos* birth.]

atom (at·om). The smallest particle of a chemical element which retains the characteristics of that element; further subdivision would destroy its identity. It consists of a positively-charged nucleus composed of protons and neutrons surrounded by negatively-charged electrons, although theories differ as to the nature and arrangement of both. Chemical reactions are the result of interplay between individual atoms, and chemical compounds are produced by the union of integral numbers of atoms with atoms of other elements to form molecules. **Excited atom.** Activated atom. **Ionized atom.** An atom which has relinquished valency electrons and is therefore positively charged, or an atom which has accepted valency electrons and become negatively charged. **Labelled atom.** An atom the nucleus of which has been made radioactive. **Radiating atom.** An atom emitting energy in quanta. **Tagged atom.** Labelled atom (see above). [Gk *atomos* indivisible.]

See also: BOHR, LANGMUIR, LEWIS (G. N.), RUTHERFORD, SCHROEDINGER.

atomic (at·**om**·ik). Referring to an atom.

atomicity (at·om·**is**·it·e). 1. The combining power of an element; valency. 2. The number of atoms in the molecule of an element. [atom.]

atomism (**at**·om·izm). 1. The doctrine of the independent action of individual atoms. 2. The science of atoms. 3. In philosophy, the doctrine that the universe, both physical and mental, is composed of indivisible atoms.

atomistic (at·om·**is**·tik). 1. Referring to atomism. 2. Referring to or consisting of an atom or atoms.

atomization (**at**·om·i·**za**′·shun). The breaking-up of a liquid so that a fine spray is formed, consisting of minute drops. [Gk *atomos* indivisible.]

atomizer (**at**·om·i·zer). An instrument or device for producing a jet of spray or for breaking up a liquid into a fog or spray. [see prec.]

atonia (a·**to**·ne·ah). Atony. **Choreatic atonia.** The hypotonia of skeletal muscles seen in rheumatic chorea. [Gk *a*, *tonos* tone.]

atonic (a·**ton**·ik). Of muscles, relaxed; lacking in normal tone. [see prec.]

atonicity (a·ton·**is**′·it·e). Atony; the quality of being atonic.

atony (**at**·on·e). 1. Lack of tone or tension, as of a muscle. 2. Systemic weakness or weakness of an organ. 3. Absence of normal energy or strength. [Gk *a*, *tonos* tone.]

atopen (a·to·pen). Allergen. [atopy, Gk *genein* to produce.]

atopic (a·**top**·ik). 1. Referring to or characterized by atopy. 2. Misplaced; out of place. [Gk *a*, *topos* place.]

atopognosia, atopognosis (a·top·og·**no**′·ze·ah, a·top·og·**no**′·sis). Inability to indicate the exact place at which a sensation or stimulus is felt. [Gk *a*, *topos* place, *gnosis* knowledge.]

atopomenorrhoea (a·**top**·o·men·or·e′·ah). Vicarious menstruation. *See* MENSTRUATION. [Gk *a*, *topos* place, menorrhoea.]

atopy (**at**·o·pe). A constitutional tendency in certain persons to develop immediate hypersensitivity states such as asthma or hay fever. [Gk *a*, *topos* place.]

atoxic (a·**tox**·ik). 1. Not caused by a poison or venom. 2. Not poisonous. [Gk *a*, *toxikon* poison.]

atrabiliary (at·rah·**bil**·e·ar·e). Melancholic. [L *ater* black, *bilis* bile.]

atrachelia (a·trah·**ke**·le·ah). Abnormal shortness of the neck, amounting to near absence. [Gk *a*, *trachelos* neck.]

atrachelocephalus (a·**trak**·el·o·**kef**′·al·us). 1. Atrachelia. 2. A monster with abnormal shortening of the neck. [Gk *a*, *trachelos* neck, *kephale* head.]

atractoid (at·**rak**·toid). Spindle-shaped. [Gk *atraktos* spindle, *eidos* form.]

atractylate (at·**rak**·til·ate). An inhibitor of the adenine nucleotide translocating system in the mitochondrial membrane. [Gk *atraktos* spindle.]

atractyloside (at·**rak**·til·o·side). Atractylate.

atraumatic (a·traw·**mat**·ik). Not causing traumatism. Applied to instruments and needles, and indicating that damage or destruction of tissues is reduced to the minimum. [Gk *a*, trauma.]

Atrax (a·trax). A genus of poisonous spiders found in Australia. **Atrax formidabilis.** A venomous spider found in Australia. **Atrax robustus.** A poisonous species; also called the *funnelweb spider.*

atremia (a·**tre**·me·ah). 1. Inability to walk owing to hysterical paralysis. 2. Absence of tremor. [Gk *a*, *tremein* to tremble.]

atrepsy (a·**trep**·se). Athrepsia.

atreptic (a·**trep**·tik). Athreptic.

atresia (at·**re**·ze·ah). Congenital imperforation of a normal channel or opening of the body, or pathological closure of it. **Atresia ani.** Imperforation or an abnormal closed condition of the anus. **Aortic atresia.** A congenital anomaly of the heart in which the whole of the left side of the heart is hypoplastic and, in most cases, there is true atresia of the aortic valve. The systemic circulation is dependent upon patency of the ductus arteriosus. It presents as heart failure in the first week or two of life, and survival rarely exceeds 1 month. **Congenital atresia of the oesophagus.** Most common of the congenital abnormalities; it is due to failure of the pharyngeal and gastric pouches to unite or to develop a continuous lumen. Defects in the septum dividing the oesophagus and the trachea may arise from mechanical flaws or from altered cellular growth. Four principal types are recognized clinically: 1. With an upper blind pouch at the level of the bifurcation of the trachea, and a lower pouch arising from the stomach and connected with the trachea by a fistula; it constitutes from 70 to 80 per cent of the total cases. 2. With an upper and a lower pouch each ending blindly and neither having any connection with the air passages. 3. With an upper pouch opening into the trachea and a lower one ending blindly. 4. With both segments opening into the air passages, usually the trachea. Symptoms arise as soon as fluid is ingested by the newborn child and depend upon the position of the upper pouch in relation to its distal end, although vomiting accompanies each variation. The first mouthful or two is swallowed successfully, but is then followed by immediate return of fluids, clear or mixed with air. Coughing, struggling and cyanosis quickly supervene and the child refuses to suck any more. The stomach may become distended with air or it may remain flat. **Congenital atresia of the small intestine.** Complete obstruction occurring in any part of the small intestine due to defective development of the alimentary tract in the fetus. **Atresia folliculi.** Death of a vesicular ovarian (graafian) follicle because of abortion of the ovum. **Atresia iridis.** Atretopsia. **Mitral atresia.** True atresia of the mitral valve occurring as part of the syndrome of aortic atresia. **Pulmonary atresia.** A congenital anomaly of the heart characterized by atresia of the right ventricular outflow. There are 2 forms, of which the commoner represents an extreme form of Fallot's tetralogy in which the atresia of the outflow tract may be extensive; less common is that with an intact ventricular septum, in which form the atresia is characteristically confined to the valve, and in which there is always an interatrial communication and persistence of the ductus arteriosus. **Tricuspid atresia.** A congenital anomaly of the heart in which true atresia of the tricuspid valve is present; septal defects are obligatory to allow for continuing circulation of the blood, but the other associated lesions are variable. The clinical picture and severity of the condition are largely determined by the volume of the pulmonary blood flow. **Atresia tubalis.** Closure of one of the uterine tubes. **Atresia uteri.** An imperforate os uteri. **Atresia vaginae, Vaginal atresia.** Often a form of reflex spasm. [Gk *a, tresis* a boring.]

atresic, atretic (at·**re**·sik, at·**ret**·ik). Characterized by atresia.

atretoblepharia (at·ret·o·blef·**a**'·re·ah). Symblepharon; pathological adhesion of the eyelids to the eyeball, as occurs after a burn. [Gk *atretos* imperforate, *blepharon* eyelid.]

atretocephalus (at·ret·o·**kef**'·al·us). A monster lacking mouth or nostrils or having an imperforate condition of mouth or nostrils. [Gk *atretos* imperforate, *kephale* head.]

atretocormus (at·ret·o·**kor**'·mus). A fetus in which one of the body openings is imperforate. [Gk *atretos* imperforate, *kormos* trunk.]

atretocystia (at·ret·o·**sis**'·te·ah). An atresic condition of the bladder. [Gk *atretos* imperforate, *kystis* bag.]

atretogastria (at·ret·o·**gas**'·tre·ah). Atresia of the stomach. [Gk *atretos* imperforate, *gaster* stomach.]

atretolaemia (at·ret·o·**le**'·me·ah). The condition of having an imperforate oesophagus or larynx. [Gk *atretos* imperforate, *laimos* gullet.]

atretometria (at·ret·o·**met**'·re·ah). Atresia of the uterus. [Gk *atretos* imperforate, *metra* uterus.]

atretopsia (at·ret·**op**·se·ah). Imperforation of the circular opening of the pupil. [Gk *atretos* imperforate, *ops* eye.]

atretorrhinia (at·ret·o·**ri**'·ne·ah). Absence or closure of the nostrils. [Gk *atretos* imperforate, *rhis* nose.]

atretostomia (at·ret·o·**sto**'·me·ah). The state of being without a mouth opening. [Gk *atretos* imperforate, *stoma* mouth.]

atreturethria (at·ret·ewr·**e**'·thre·ah). A closed or imperforate condition of the urethra. [Gk *atretos* imperforate, urethra.]

atria (a·tre·ah). *See* ATRIUM.

atrial (a·tre·al). Referring to an atrium. **Atrial septum.** *See* SEPTUM.

atricha (a·trik·ah). A group of bacteria which do not possess flagella. [Gk *a, thrix* hair.]

atrichia (a·**trik**·e·ah). Not having hair. [see prec.]

atrichosis (a·trik·o·sis). Atrichia. **Atrichosis congenitalis.** Congenital lack of hair. [atrichia, Gk *-osis* condition.]

atrichous (a·**trik**·us). Applied to bacteria which have no flagella. [Gk *a, thrix* hair.]

atriofemoral (a·tre·o·**fem**'·or·al). Relating to the atrium of the heart and the femoral artery, e.g. atriofemoral by-pass. [L *atrium* hall, femur *thigh.*]

atrionector (a·tre·o·**nek**'·tor). The sinu-atrial node. *See* NODE. [L *atrium* hall, *nector* connector.]

atrioseptal (a·tre·o·**sep**'·tal). Relating to the septum between the atria of the heart.

atriotome (a·tre·o·tome). A specially devised knife introduced through the auricle of the heart to divide the edges of a mitral orifice narrowed by mitral stenosis. [atrium, Gk *temnein* to cut.]

atrioventricular (a·tre·o·ven·**trik**'·ew·lar). Belonging to an atrium and a ventricle of the heart. **Atrioventricular node.** *See* NODE. **Atrioventricular orifice.** *See* ORIFICE. **Atrioventricular valve.** *See* VALVE.

atrioventricularis communis (at·re·o·ven·trik·ew·**la**'·ris kom·**ew**·nis). Persistence of the common atrioventricular canal.

Atriplex (a·**trip**·lex). A genus of plants. **Atriplex littoralis.** A poisonous species that causes a series of skin lesions known as *atriplicism.* **Atriplex serrata.** A species of plant resembling spinach which may cause photodermatitis after ingestion. [L the herb orach.]

atriplicism (a·**trip**·lis·izm). Poisoning or intoxication caused by eating certain species of atriplex, e.g. *Atriplex littoralis,* a plant of the spinach variety. The fingers swell, ulcers and bullae may form on them, and they can subsequently become gangrenous. The condition has been known to spread to the forearm.

atrium (a·tre·um) (pl. *atria*). 1. Literally, an entrance hall or vestibule; in anatomy, a cavity into which one or more other cavities open. 2. The site of entrance of pathogenic micro-organisms. **Atria glottidis.** That part of the laryngeal cavity immediately below the superior aperture of the larynx and above the false vocal folds. **Atria of the heart [atria cordis (NA)].** The 2 thin-walled cavities of the heart. **Infection atrium.** The point of entrance of the organisms of an infectious disease. **Atria laryngis.** Atria glottidis (see above). **Left atrium [atrium sinistrum (NA)].** The left atrium of the heart, which receives arterial blood from the lungs via the openings of the 4 pulmonary veins [ostia venarum pulmonalium (NA)] and which opens into the left ventricle by means of the left atrioventricular orifice. **Atrium of the middle meatus [atrium meatus medii].** The part of the nasal cavity immediately anterior to the middle meatus. **Atrium of the nose.** The vestibule of the nasal cavity. **Respiratory atria.** Cavities into which alveoli of the lung open, and which lead to the alveolar ducts and respiratory bronchioles. **Right atrium [atrium dextrum (NA)].** The right atrium of the heart, which receives venous blood from the body via the openings for the superior venae cavae [ostium venae cavae inferioris et ostium venae cavae superioris (NA)] and from the heart itself via the coronary sinus, etc. The atrium opens into the right ventricle by means of the right atrioventricular orifice. **Atrium vaginae.** The vestibule of the vagina. [L hall.]

atrolactyl (at·ro·**lak**·til). The monovalent acyl radical $CH_3C(OH)(C_6H_5)CO-$ derived from atrolactic acid. **Atrolactyl tropeine.** An alkaloid isomeric with atropine.

Atropa (a·**tro**·pah). A genus of the Solanaceae of which 2 species are important medicinally, viz: *Atropa belladonna* (deadly nightshade) of Europe, and *Atropa acuminata* (Indian belladonna) of India and Pakistan. Both plants are used as a source of belladonna. [Gk *Atropos* Fate.]

atropanine (at·tro·pan·een). Apo-atropine.

atrophia (at·**ro**·fe·ah). The Latin for *atrophy.* **Atrophia cachochymica.** Wasting which is the result of the ingestion of unsuitable food. **Atrophia choroideae et retinae.** Atrophy of the choroid and retina, in association with night blindness. **Atrophia cordis.**

Atrophy of the heart. **Atrophia cutis.** Atrophoderma. **Atrophia cutis idiopathica.** Diffuse idiopathic atrophy of the skin; dermatitis chronica atrophicans; erythromelia. **Atrophia cutis reticularis cum pigmentatione.** Poikiloderma vascularis atrophicans. **Atrophia cutis senilis.** Senile atrophy of the skin. *See* ATROPHY. **Atrophia dolorosa.** Painful paroxysmal atrophy of the eyeball. **Atrophia gyrata of the choroid and retina.** A hereditary primary degenerative condition of the choroid and retina of the eye, starting usually in early adult life and slowly progressing. It was first described by Fuchs. **Atrophia infantum.** Tabes mesenterica. **Atrophia maculosa cutis.** Circumscribed wasting of the skin. **Atrophia mesenterica.** Tabes mesenterica. **Atrophia musculorum lipomatosa.** Pseudohypertrophic muscular dystrophy. *See* DYSTROPHY. **Atrophia nervea.** Neuropathic atrophy. *See* ATROPHY. **Atrophia nervosa.** A gradual wasting, with disinclination to eat, the result of living in unhealthy or depressing surroundings or conditions. **Atrophia pilorum propria.** Atrophy of the hair. **Atrophia senilis.** Senile physiological atrophy of the alveolar margin. **Atrophia striata et maculosa.** Atrophic striae and small macular atrophic areas in the skin. The striae may be due to overdistension as in pregnancy (striae gravidarum), rapid growth, obesity, ascites, or to the stretching caused by an internal tumour or cyst. Whilst the striae caused by pregnancy are noted in the abdomen and breasts, those caused by obesity are mostly found on the upper arms, hips and thighs; striae produced by rapid growth in adolescence run transversely across the thighs, hips and lumbar areas. Occasionally they may develop on the lower parts of the thighs after typhoid fever, dysentery or other infections. The lesions are formed by atrophy or structural alteration of the elastic fibres in the deeper layers of the corium. **Atrophia testiculi.** Wasting of the testis. **Atrophia unguium.** Atrophy affecting the nails. **Atrophia verminosa.** Wasting caused by the presence of worms in the intestine. [Gk *a, trophe* nourishment.]

atrophic (at·**rof**·ik). Characterized by atrophy.

atrophied (at·ro·fid). Shrunken or wasted away. [see foll.]

atrophite (at·ro·fite). A cell which does not have any food substance in reserve. [Gk *a, trophe* nourishment.]

atrophoderma, atrophodermia (at·ro·fo·**der**·mah, at·ro·fo·**der**·me·ah). Atrophy of the whole or part of the skin. **Atrophoderma albidum.** Symmetrical thinning of the skin, usually affecting the legs. It begins early in childhood and is probably a congenital defect. **Atrophoderma biotripticum.** Senile atrophy of the skin. **Atrophoderma diffusum.** Acrodermatitis chronica atrophicans. **Atrophoderma erythematodes reticulare.** Poikiloderma vascularis atrophicans. **Follicular atrophoderma.** A hereditary condition with atrophic depressions at follicular orifices. **Atrophoderma maculatum.** Macular atrophy of the skin. **Atrophoderma neuriticum.** Glossy skin associated with neuritis; commencing with erythema, the skin eventually assumes a shiny grey colour. **Atrophoderma pigmentosum.** Xeroderma pigmentosum. **Atrophoderma reticulatum symmetricum faciei.** Folliculitis ulerythematosa reticulata. **Atrophoderma senile.** Senile atrophy of the skin. *See* ATROPHY. **Atrophoderma striatum et maculatum.** Linear and small circumscribed areas of atrophy in the skin due to alterations in the elastic tissue of the corium. **Atrophoderma vermiculatum.** Folliculitis ulerythematosa reticulata. [Gk *a, trophe* nourishment, *derma* skin.]

atrophodermatosis (at·**ro**·fo·der·mat·**o**′·sis). Any disease of the skin which is marked by atrophoderma. [atrophoderma, Gk *-osis* condition.]

atrophoedema (at·**rof**·e·**de**′·mah). Angioneurotic oedema. *See* OEDEMA. [atrophy, oedema.]

atrophy (**at**·ro·fe). 1. To waste away. 2. A condition of general malnutrition from whatever cause, the signs of which are wasting or shrinking of the tissues of the whole body or of a part of it. 3. Wasting of a tissue or organ. **Accidental atrophy.** Atrophy of a part as the result of failure of its blood supply because of arterial compression or stoppage of the flow. **Acute yellow atrophy.** Acute diffuse necrosis of the liver cells, with shrinkage of the liver, jaundice and intoxication. It is rare in civil life but often epidemic during wars; the causes are dietary, infective, and toxic. **Adipose atrophy.** Wasting caused by lack of fatty tissue. **Angibromic atrophy.** Narrowing of the lumen of the alimentary canal. **Arthritic atrophy.** Atrophy of the muscles in the neighbourhood of a joint, the result of injury or disease. **Benign spinal muscular atrophy.** Slowly progressive or stationary muscular atrophy with onset in childhood or adolescence, due to degeneration of lower motor neurons and transmitted by autosomal recessive inheritance. (Syn.: Kugelberg-Welander disease.) **Brown atrophy.** Pigmentary atrophy affecting usually the liver, spleen and heart, and caused by natural wear and tear. **Cardiac atrophy.** Wasting of the heart as a result of cachexia, pressure by a mediastinal tumour or senile changes. **Cerebral atrophy.** Loss of brain substance from degeneration or scarring. **Chronic spinal muscular atrophy.** Progressive muscular atrophy (see below). **Cicatricial atrophy.** Atrophy of the skin, with sclerosis. **Circumscribed atrophy of the brain.** Lobar sclerosis. *See* SCLEROSIS. **Compression atrophy.** Wasting of an organ or a part as a result of continued pressure. **Concentric atrophy.** Wasting of a hollow organ leading to reduction of its capacity. **Convolutional atrophy.** Lobar sclerosis. *See* SCLEROSIS. **Correlated atrophy.** Atrophy of a part after a correlated part has been removed or destroyed. **Cortical atrophy.** Atrophy of the cerebral cortex due to loss of neurons. *See also* PICK'S DISEASE. **Cyanotic atrophy.** Destruction and atrophy of the parenchyma in tissue as a result of venous congestion of long standing. **Cyanotic atrophy of the liver.** Nutmeg liver. *See* LIVER. **Degenerative atrophy.** Atrophy caused by degeneration of the cells of a part or organ. **Denervated-muscle atrophy.** Atrophy of a muscle as a result of the division of its motor nerve. **Dental atrophy.** Wearing away of the substance of a tooth. **Diffuse idiopathic atrophy of the skin.** A form of atrophy of the skin in which, in the final stages, there is partial atrophy of the prickle-cell layer of the epidermis as well as of the collagenous and elastic tissue of the corium. There are at least 3 varieties: the first, *dermatitis atrophicans diffusa vel universalis,* in which large areas or the whole body are involved; the second, *dermatitis atrophicans maculosa,* in which small circumscribed areas of skin are affected; the third, *acrodermatitis chronica atrophicans,* is characterized by cutaneous atrophy affecting particularly the extensor surfaces of the limbs. **Atrophy of disuse.** That caused in a part by excessive immobility, or because it is not exercised sufficiently. **Eccentric atrophy.** In a hollow organ, atrophy of the walls so that the size of the cavity increases. **Facial atrophy.** Progressive facial atrophy (see below). **Familial spinal muscular atrophy.** Progressive wasting of the muscles as the result of spinal degeneration in infants, often occurring in several members of one family; benign spinal muscular atrophy (see above), infantile spinal muscular atrophy (see below). **Fatty atrophy.** Infiltration with fat cells, secondary to atrophy of the tissue elements of an organ or part. **General atrophy.** Marasmus; emaciation. **Granular atrophy of the kidney.** A state of chronic fibrotic inflammation of the tissues of the kidney so that the parenchyma becomes compressed and then atrophies. **Granuloproteic atrophy.** The replacement of the ordinary structural elements of a cell by granular elements. **Grey atrophy.** A term applied to a degenerative state of the optic disc in which it becomes of a smoky colour. **Halisteretic atrophy.** A degenerative condition of bone in which the lamellae of the spongy substances gradually become thinned. **Hemifacial atrophy.** Atrophy affecting one side of the face. **Hemilingual atrophy.** Wasting of one side of the tongue. **Hereditary sex-linked optic atrophy.** A hereditary type of retrobulbar neuritis. **Honeycomb atrophy.** Atrophoderma vermiculatum. **Hypoglossal atrophy.** Wasting of the tongue caused by a lesion of the hypoglossal nerve. **Ichthyosiform atrophy.** A form of acquired cutaneous atrophy associated, particularly, with Hodgkin's disease. **Idiopathic muscular atrophy.** Progressive wasting of groups of muscles caused by primary changes in the muscles themselves. **Inanition atrophy.** Wasting caused by continued diarrhoea. **Individual atrophy.** Atrophy of specific muscles in different regions. **Infantile atrophy.** Marasmus. **Infantile spinal muscular atrophy.** A progressive and fatal muscular atrophy in infants due to degeneration of lower motor neurons, and transmitted by recessive autosomal inheritance (syn.: *Werdnig–Hoffman atrophy*). **Inflammatory atrophy.** Wasting of a tissue as the result of prolonged inflammation. **Insulin fat atrophy.** Atrophic depressions or sometimes granulomatous nodules in the skin at sites of repeated injections of insulin. **Interstitial atrophy.** A degeneration which causes absorption of the mineral elements of bone leaving only the reticular framework. **Ischaemic muscular atrophy.** Volkmann's contracture. **Juvenile muscular atrophy.** Pseudohypertrophic muscular paralysis; pseudohypertrophic muscular dystrophy. *See* DYSTROPHY. **Lactation atrophy.** Superinvolution of the uterus which sometimes occurs in the post-partum period. **Leaping atrophy.** A form of progressive muscular dystrophy which affects first the muscles of the hand and then those of the shoulder, leaving the arm muscles untouched. **Macular atrophy.** Primary or secondary varioliform atrophy of the skin; it may be secondary to syphilis, lupus erythematosus and other conditions. **Muscular atrophy.** Degeneration of the muscles of whatever kind and from whatever cause. **Myelopathic muscular atrophy.** Wasting of the muscles which usually begins in the small muscles of the hand or upper arm and shoulder and progresses slowly to the muscles of the leg. The cause is anterior-horn degeneration of the spinal cord (Aran-Duchenne type). **Myopathic atrophy.** Muscular degeneration caused by disease of the muscle tissue. **Myotonic atrophy.** Dystrophia myotonica. **Necrobiotic atrophy.** Atrophy affecting a part together with a varying amount of necrosis. **Neural atrophy.** Neuropathic atrophy (see below). **Neuritic muscular atrophy.** Muscle-wasting which results from neuritis. **Neuropathic atrophy.** Degeneration of muscle tissue as a result of systemic nervous disease. **Neurotic atrophy.** Atrophy based on functional disease of the central nervous system. **Neurotrophic atrophy.** That due to malnutrition of tissue caused by disease of the peripheral neurones which supply it. **Numerical atrophy.** Atrophy of some of the elements of a part. **Olivopontocerebellar atrophy.** A slowly progressive systematized degeneration occurring in the middle-aged or elderly and involving the cortex of the cerebellum, the peduncles of the middle lobe and the olivary nucleus of the medulla oblongata. **Olivorubrocerebellar atrophy.** A hereditary and degenerative disease of the central nervous system, involving particularly the olivary and red nuclei and the superior cerebellar peduncle. Coarse static tremor of the limbs and trunk may develop, and ataxia and hypotonia occur; sometimes dementia and evidence of pyramidal tract involvement are superadded. **Optic atrophy.** A condition of atrophy affecting the optic nerve. **Pathological atrophy.** Atrophy due to disease, in contrast to that due to physiological causes. **Peroneal atrophy, Peroneal muscular atrophy.** A hereditary and slowly progressive disease causing atrophy of the distal muscles of the extremities usually beginning in the peroneal group and due to peripheral nerve degeneration (syn.: Charcot-Marie-Tooth disease). **Physiological atrophy.** That which occurs at certain ages, e.g. of the thymus. **Pigmentary atrophy, Pigmented atrophy.** A form in which the atrophied cells show a brownish coloration. **Pressure atrophy.** Compression atrophy (see above). **Primary macular atrophy of the skin.** Atrophia maculosa cutis. **Progressive atrophy of the skin.** Senile atrophoderma; the wasting of the skin which accompanies senility. **Progressive facial atrophy.** A condition of unknown origin in which there is progressive wasting of the skin of the face. **Progressive muscular atrophy.** A fatal disease of adults of unknown cause with degeneration of lower and upper motor neurons, characterized by varying degrees of muscular wasting, fasciculation and spasticity; *motor neuron disease* (syn.: Aran–Duchenne's disease). **Progressive nervous atrophy.** A name given to atrophy of the spinal nerve roots caused by pressure of fibrous deposits on the spinal arachnoid mater. **Progressive neuromuscular atrophy.** Progressive neuropathic (peroneal) muscular atrophy (see following). **Progressive spinal muscular atrophy.** Muscular atrophy, Benign spinal muscular atrophy, Progressive muscular atrophy (see above). **Progressive spinal muscular atrophy of infants.** Familial spinal muscular atrophy (see above). **Progressive unilateral facial atrophy.** Atrophy affecting the bone, connective tissue, fat and skin of one side of the face, and sometimes involving the muscles as well. **Pseudohypertrophic muscular atrophy.** Pseudohypertrophic muscular dystrophy. *See* DYSTROPHY. **Qualitative atrophy.** Degeneration. **Quantitative atrophy.** Simple atrophy (see below). **Receptoric atrophy.** A name for a condition held to be due to atrophy of the receptor neurones of the cell. **Red atrophy.** A form met with in an organ in which there is chronic passive congestion, e.g. in the liver. **Remitting spinal atrophy.** Progressive muscular atrophy (see above). **Reversionary atrophy.** Anaplasia. **Rheumatic atrophy.** Muscular atrophy occurring after rheumatic infection. **Roentgen atrophy of the skin.** Chronic x-ray dermatitis. **Sclerotic atrophy.** A term for a condition in which after myocarditis there are found to be deposits of connective tissue in the cardiac muscle. **Senile atrophy.** The normal physiological atrophy of certain organs in old age. **Senile circumpapillary choroidal atrophy.** A ring of choroidoretinal atrophy seen around the optic disc in old age. **Senile atrophy of the skin.** The shrinkage of the skin present in general senile degeneration. **Serous atrophy.** Infiltration of serous fluid into atrophied tissue. **Simple atrophy.** Shrinkage in size of individual cells leading to atrophy of the tissues. **Simple brown atrophy.** A heart condition in which the cells of the muscles are decreased in size and are yellow in colour. **Spinal atrophy.** Wasting of portions of the spinal cord, as in tabes dorsalis. **Spinoneural atrophy.** Muscular atrophy with impairment of motor function caused by a lesion of the motor tract of the lower part of the spinal cord. **Sympathetic atrophy.** Atrophy occurring in the second of a pair of organs, as a sequel to disease of the first. **Syphilitic spinal muscular atrophy.** A condition resembling progressive muscular atrophy and amyotrophic lateral sclerosis, in which muscular wasting in the upper limbs is often accompanied by spastic paraplegia; due to syphilitic hypertrophic meningitis in the cervical region. **Toxic atrophy.** Atrophy caused by the poison of an infection. **Trophoneurotic atrophy.** That caused by disease of the nerves or of a nerve centre supplying a part. **Unilateral facial atrophy.** Progressive unilateral facial atrophy (see above). **White atrophy.** Nervous degeneration leaving only white connective tissue. [Gk *a, trophe* nourishment.]

See also: ARAN, BROSSARD, BUCHWALD, CHARCOT, CRUVEILHIER, DÉJÉRINE, DUCHENNE, FAZIO-LONDE, GOWERS, HUNT (J. R.), KIENBOECK, LANDOUZY, LEBER, MARIE, PARROT, PICK (A.), SCHNABEL, SOTTAS, SUDECK, TOOTH, VULPIAN.

atropic (at·**rop**·ik). 1. Referring to belladonna or atropine. 2. Referring to the genus of plants, *Atropa*.

Atropine (**at**·ro·peen). $C_{17}H_{23}O_3N$. A poisonous alkaloid found in traces in solanaceous plants (e.g. *Atropa belladonna*), where it occurs with the laevorotatory isomer, hyoscyamine. It is a tropine ester of tropic acid, optically inactive when pure, and formed by the racemization of L-hyoscyamine. It blocks the effects of acetylcholine on structures in effector organs supplied by post-ganglionic cholinergic nerves. Its effect on the central nervous system is to stimulate the motor areas, producing inco-ordination of movements, restlessness, and even convulsions preceded by delirium; respiration becomes deeper by excitation of the medulla, and paralysis of the peripheral terminations of the vagus gives rise to quickening of the heart with increased blood pressure attributable also to vasoconstriction. Glands stimulated by cholinergic fibres, e.g. salivary, those of the stomach, pancreas and intestine, bronchial and sweat glands, have their secretions diminished, and its effect on plain muscle is to produce dilatation of the pupil of the eye (mydriasis) with paralysis of accommodation (cycloplegia), and also dilatation of the bronchioles. It is used in ophthalmology as a mydriatic and to abolish accommodation in refraction, to diminish secretions, e.g. salivation and bronchial secretions prior to general anaesthesia and night sweats in phthisis, as an antispasmodic to relieve asthma and emphysema, and as an antidote in cases of poisoning by drugs of the muscarine group.

(BP 1968). **Atropine hydriodate.** $C_{17}H_{23}NO_3HIO_3$, a drug used in ophthalmology. **Atropine Methonitrate BP 1973.** "Eumydrin", $C_{17}H_{23}O_3NCH_3NO_3$, a drug with an action similar to that of atropine but less toxic; it is used especially as an antispasmodic in the treatment of congenital pyloric stenosis. **Atropine methylbromide.** Mydriasine, $C_{17}H_{23}O_3NCH_3Br$, a compound used as a mydriatic since its action is less prolonged than that of atropine. **Atropine methylnitrate.** Atropine Methonitrate BP 1973 (see above). **Atropine salicylate.** $C_{17}H_{23}O_3NC_7H_6O_3$, a crystalline compound, soluble in water and alcohol, and used as is the sulphate. **Atropine Sulphate BP 1973.** $(C_{17}H_{23}O_3N)_2 H_2SO_4$, a crystalline powder soluble in water, and the salt used most frequently in solution. [Gk *Atropos* Fate.]

atropini (at·ro·pin·i). **Atropini Sulfas.** *European Pharmacopoeia* name for Atropine Sulphate BP 1973.

atropinism (at·ro·pe·nizm). General poisoning of the system caused by excessive use of belladonna or atropine.

atropinization (at·ro·pe·ni·za′·shun). 1. Atropism. 2. The state of being under the influence of atropine or belladonna.

atroscine (at·ro·seen). $C_{17}H_{21}O_4N$. An optically-inactive alkaloid obtained from the rhizomes of species of *Scopolia.* It is the racemic form of hyoscine with the same central action but less powerful in peripheral effect.

attachment (at·ach·ment). In dentistry, a wire around a natural tooth to retain an artificial denture; an inlay cemented in a tooth to which a bridge is attached. **Epithelial attachment.** The attachment of the gingiva to a tooth, formed during eruption of the tooth by the fusion of the remains of cells of the enamel organ lying on the surface of the enamel with the deep layers of cells of the oral epithelium; initially attached to the crown, it later moves down to become attached to the root during process of continuous eruption of the tooth. [Fr. *attachement.*]

See also: GOTTLIEB.

attack (at·ak). An access of illness or an episode in the course of a disease, usually of an acute or distressing nature. **Anxiety attack.** An attack characterized essentially and primarily by the mental experience of anxiety. **Breath-holding attacks.** Brief spells of unconsciousness occurring in infants or young children following breath-holding induced by fear or temper. **Drop attacks.** Abrupt falls without warning, usually in the elderly, without loss of consciousness or subsequent amnesia, often recurrent but with good prognosis. There are no abnormal physical signs and no specific treatment. **Oculogyral attack.** Oculogyral crisis. *See* CRISIS. **Uncinate attack.** An epileptic variant characterized by olfactory hallucinations, movements of tongue and lips, and a dreamy state; it is usually due to a lesion of the uncinate gyrus. **Vagal attack, Vasovagal attack.** Terms used to describe a paroxysmal symptom complex due to disturbance of the vagus nerves. The attack begins with a sensation of fullness in the epigastrium which spreads to the precordium. It is associated with dyspnoea, disturbance of the heart beat and occasionally a sense of impending death. The attacks last from a few minutes to half an hour and are followed by a feeling of weakness and tremulousness. [Fr. *attaquer.*]

See also: ADAMS (R.), STOKES (W.).

attar (at·ar). 1. Name given to any essential oil distilled from a plant. 2. Otto of rose, ottar of rose, the volatile oil distilled from the fresh flowers of *Rosa damascena* (the damask rose), cultivated in Bulgaria and used as a perfume. [Pers. essence or perfume.]

attention (at·en·shun). 1. The state of giving heed to an object or objective. 2. In psychology, cognition of the object thought of, as distinct from the act of thinking; the taking possession of the mind by a single train of thought. **Central attention.** The formation by and in the mind of the image of an object which is no longer present to the visual attention; imagination. **Compound synchronous attention.** The recognition and correlation by the mind of different stimuli, such as light and sound, occurring at the same time. **Multiple synchronous auditory attention.** The mental recognition of the co-existence of more than one sound or variation of sound, as when listening to an orchestra. **Multiple synchronous central visual attention.** A state in which multiple co-existent visual images are formed in the mind without the actual presence of the objects themselves; an imaginative visual composite. **Multiple synchronous visual attention.** The mental recognition of more than one individually-distinct set of co-existent visual images, actually produced on the retina by external objects. **Single-stream auditory attention.** A state of picking out and giving heed to only one sound—it may be a single note or a series of single sounds—occurring amongst other sounds or notes. **Single-stream central attention.** A state of attention in which the mind imagines and passes in review, one after the other, single successive images without the stimuli of the actual objects themselves. **Single-stream central auditory attention.** The imagination of a sound without actually hearing it objectively. **Single-stream visual attention.** A state of attention in which there is selection and exclusive visual observation of a linked line of single successive images from among a number of images produced by real objects upon the retina. **Visual attention.** That state in which the eyes and the mind are aware of an actual external object. [L *attendere* to stretch.]

attenuant (at·en·ew·ant). A substance that attenuates.

attenuate (at·en·ew·ate). 1. To weaken the toxicity or virulence of a poison or drug, or of a micro-organism or virus. 2. To make thin, as, for example, by disease or starvation, or in the case of fluids by dilution. 3. To increase fluidity. [L *attenuare* to make thin.]

attenuation (at·en·ew·a′·shun). The process of attenuating.

attic (at·ik). The epitympanic recess; the part of the middle ear which is above the level of the tympanic membrane, and which contains part of the malleus and most of the incus. [Gk *attikos* of Athens; so called because it is the upper part of the structure.]

atticitis (at·ik·i·tis). A state of inflammation in the epitympanic recess. [attic, Gk *-itis* inflammation.]

attico-antrostomy (at·ik·o·an·tros′·to·me). The making of an opening for drainage purposes into the epitympanic recess and tympanic antrum. [attic, antrum, Gk *stoma* mouth.]

attico-antrotomy (at·ik·o·an·trot′·o·me). Incision of the epitympanic recess and the tympanic antrum. [attic, antrum.]

atticomastoid (at·ik·o·mas′·toid). Referring to the epitympanic recess and the mastoid part of the temporal bone. [attic, mastoid.]

atticotomy (at·ik·ot·o·me). Incision of the epitympanic recess. **Transmeatal atticotomy.** Removal of the outer wall of the epitympanic recess by way of the external auditory meatus. [attic, Gk *temnein* to cut.]

atticotympanotomy (at·ik·o·tim·pan·ot′·o·me). An operation carried out in cases of chronic suppurative otitis media in which the pathogeny is mainly confined to the attic; the diseased area is eradicated and drained transmeatally. The ear becomes dry and safe, and any residual hearing is usually preserved. [attic, tympanum, Gk *temnein* to cut.]

attitude (at·e·tewd). 1. Posture, stance; the position taken up by the body. 2. A set, or disposition of the mind in preparation for an experience or response. **Attitude of combat.** The posture in which bodies become fixed, with elbows, knees and fingers flexed, and ankles extended, like a boxer, as a result of exposure to intense heat by burning or immersion in hot fluid. It is due to coagulation of albuminates in the muscles with contraction, and persists until putrefaction occurs. **Crucifixion attitude.** The attitude of the body in imitation of the crucifixion posture. **Discobolus attitude.** A posture like that of the discus thrower, produced by stimulation of the semicircular canals, as by rotation of the body. **Attitude of the fetus.** The position of the fetus in the uterus; normally one of flexion. **Forced attitude.** An abnormal position of the whole or part of the body which develops as a result of disease and cannot be overcome by voluntary effort. **Frozen attitude.** A stiff, spastic type of gait due to pyramidal-tract disease, said to occur most commonly in amyotrophic lateral sclerosis. **Illogical attitude.** Strange posture assumed during convulsive hysteria. **Pugilistic attitude.** The fighting attitude developing in the arms owing to the contraction of muscles upon exposure to great heat as in fire. **Stereotyped attitude.** Bizarre and enduring postures assumed during catatonic states and associated with waxy flexibility. [L *attitudo* posture.]

See also: DEVERGIE, DUCHENNE.

attollens (at·**ol**·enz). A term applied to muscles and indicating the action of raising or lifting up. [L.]

attraction (at·**rak**·shun). 1. The force that draws 2 bodies together. 2. The tendency of 2 bodies under some influence to draw closer together. **Capillary attraction.** 1. The force of attraction between molecules of a liquid, effective only at very small distances. 2. The force which causes a liquid to rise or fall in a capillary tube of very narrow bore. **Chemical attraction.** The tendency which an atom of one element has for combining chemically with an atom of another element. **Electrical attraction.** The force which draws 2 oppositely-charged bodies together. **Gravitational attraction.** The inherent tendency in bodies, owing to their mass, to approach one another. **Magnetic attraction.** The force between a magnetic body and some other magnetic substance, tending to draw them together. **Molecular attraction.** The force existing between 2 molecules in the interior of a substance, tending to draw them together, and acting over small distances. **Sphere of attraction.** The sphere beyond the boundary of which a molecule at the centre exerts no influence. [L *attrahere* to draw to.]

attrahens (**at**·rah·henz). A term applied to muscles and indicating drawing towards. [L.]

attraxin (at·**rax**·in). The radical of a compound which is held to have a chemotactic effect on the epithelial cells of the body. [L *attrahere* to draw to.]

attrition (at·**rish**·un). Abrasion; the wearing away of anything by friction, e.g. the natural process of wearing down the biting surfaces of the teeth by mastication. [L *atterere* to rub away.]

Atwater, Wilbur Olin (b. 1844). American physiologist.

Atwater's calorimeter. A combined calorimeter and respiration chamber in which heat production and respiratory exchange can be measured over given periods, on men or animals. In the closed type, oxygen is circulated, CO_2 absorbed, and the utilization of oxygen made good by addition of measured volumes of oxygen: the chamber is well insulated and surrounded by radiators through which water circulates; the heat production is measured from the volume of water circulated and its rise of temperature.

atylosis (a·til·o·sis). An atypical form of tuberculosis.

atypia (a·**tip**·e·ah). The condition of not corresponding to a standard type or of being irregular in type. [Gk *a*, *typos* type.]

atypical (a·**tip**·ik·al). Not corresponding to a normal form; non-typical; irregular. [see prec.]

Aub, Joseph Charles (b. 1890). Boston physician.

Aub–Du Bois standards. Tables of calories per square metre of body surface per hour, for different ages.

Aubert, Herman (b. 1826). German physiologist.

phenomenon of Aubert. A vertical line of light is viewed in darkness: the head is tilted to one side and the line will appear to tilt to the opposite side; if the movement of the head is sudden, there is a lapse of a few seconds before the line tilts. When the room is suddenly lit the line immediately returns to its vertical position.

Auchmeromyia luteola (awk·mer·o·**mi**·e·ah lew·te·o·lah). A sarcophagid fly which is widely distributed through tropical Africa. In general colour it is orange-buff, but small hairs give it a smoky appearance. The larva, which is known as the Congo floor-maggot, is dirty-white, semi-transparent, and about 1.5 cm (0.5 in) in length. It causes myiasis in man. It emerges at night from holes and cracks in the floor of native huts and attacks man by scraping the skin with mouth hooks until it reaches a blood vessel. [Gk *auchmeros* dirty, *myia* fly, L *luteolus* yellow.]

audibility (aw·dib·**il**·it·e). The capability of being appreciated by the hearing mechanism of the human. **Range of audibility.** As applied to the human ear, is between 16 and 20 000 hertz (cycles per second). Some living creatures have the ability to appreciate sound waves of higher and lower frequencies than those which mark the limit of human audibility. [L *audire* to hear.]

audiclave (**aw**·de·klave). An instrument the use of which aids hearing. [L *audire* to hear, *clavis* key.]

audile (**aw**·dile). 1. Referring to hearing. 2. In psychology, an individual whose ideas take the form of mental sounds or speech, not of motor or visual images. 3. Indicating the mentality which remembers sounds more easily than images. [L *audire* to hear, *mutus* dumb.]

audimutism (aw·de·**mewt**·izm). Mutism without deafness. [L *audire* to hear, *mutus* dumb.]

audimutitas (aw·de·**mewt**·it·as). An individual who is dumb but not deaf. [see prec.]

audioanalgesia (aw·de·o·an·al·**je**'·ze·ah). Alleviation of pain by an auditory stimulus, e.g. *white sound.* [L *audire* to hear, analgesia.]

audiogenic (aw·de·o·**jen**'·ik). Having origin in sound. [L *audire* to hear, Gk *genein* to produce.]

audiogram (**aw**·de·o·gram). The graph plotted by an audiometer. [L *audire* to hear, Gk *gramma* mark.]

audiology (aw·de·**ol**·o·je). The study and measurement of hearing, including the detection and definition of hearing defects. [L *audire* to hear, Gk *logos* science.]

audiometer (aw·de·**om**·et·er). An instrument for measuring hearing capacity. The ones in modern use are electrical and of 2 main types, the *pure-tone audiometer*, capable of producing pure tones of varying, and known, frequency and intensity, which means that the hearing of a patient can be compared with that of the established normal threshold of hearing, and the *speech audiometer*, which reproduces phonetically balanced words at known and variable intensity whereby the threshold of intensity for reception of speech can be determined. [L *audire* to hear, meter.] *See also:* BEKESY.

audiometry (aw·de·**om**·et·re). Evoked response. A method of testing the hearing without active co-operation from the patient; the threshold of hearing is determined by recording a reflex response of the person being tested. [see prec.]

audiphone (**aw**·de·fone). A device for aiding deafness, by means of which the bones of the head are used as sounding-boards to carry vocal sounds to the labyrinth. [L *audire* to hear, Gk *phone* sound.]

audition (aw·**dish**·un). 1. The faculty or sense of hearing. 2. The act of listening or hearing. **Chromatic audition.** Individual involuntary or natural association of a certain colour with a certain sound; one of the forms of chromaesthesia. **Gustatory audition.** A form of synaesthesia in which there is individual involuntary or natural association of a certain taste with a certain sound. [L *audire* to hear.]

auditive (**aw**·dit·iv). 1. An individual who learns and remembers more easily through hearing than through sight. 2. Auditory. [see prec.]

auditognosis (aw·dit·og·**no**'·sis). 1. The faculty of perceiving, understanding, and interpreting sound. 2. The use of auscultation and percussion in diagnosis. [L *audire* to hear, Gk *gnosis* knowledge.]

auditopsychic (aw·dit·o·**si**'·kik). Concerned with or pertaining to the auditopsychic area of the temporal cortex. [L *audire* to hear, Gk *psyche* soul.]

auditory (**aw**·dit·or·e). 1. Belonging to the sense or organs of hearing. 2. Belonging to the perception of sound. **Auditory ganglion.** *See* GANGLION. **Auditory meatus.** *See* MEATUS. **Auditory radiation.** *See* RADIATION. **Auditory stria.** *See* STRIA. [L *auditorius* hearing.]

auditory artery, internal [arteria labyrinthi (NA)]. A branch of the anterior inferior cerebellar artery (or the basilar). Accompanied by the facial and auditory nerves and a companion vein, the internal vein, it enters the internal auditory meatus to reach the internal ear, to which it gives cochlear [ramus cochleae] and vestibular [rami vestibulares (NA)] branches.

auditory nerve [nervus vestibulocochlearis (nervus octavus (NA))]. The 8th cranial nerve. It arises from the brain stem at the junction of the pons and medulla, and passes through the internal auditory meatus to supply the internal ear. It consists of 2 main portions, the vestibular and cochlear divisions with communicating filaments [fila anastomotica (NA)].

nuclei [nuclei nervi stato-acustici]. *See* COCHLEAR NERVE, and VESTIBULAR NERVE.

roots [radix inferior et radix superior]. Two roots, the vestibular and the cochlear, forming the vestibular and cochlear nerves respectively.

auditory vein, internal [vena labyrinthi (NA)]. The companion vein to the internal auditory artery; the main venous drainage of the internal ear, entering the inferior petrosal sinus.

auditosensory (aw·dit·o·**sen'**·sor·e). Concerned with or pertaining to the auditosensory area of the temporal cortex. [L *audire* to hear, *sentire* to feel.]

Auenbrugger, Leopold Joseph (b. 1722). Austrian physician. The inventor of percussion, e.g. of the chest and abdomen, as a diagnostic procedure.

Auenbrugger's sign. A bulging of the epigastrium seen with large pericardial effusions.

Auer, John (b. 1875). American physiologist.

Auer's bodies. Peroxidase-positive bar-shaped structures or large granules staining red with Leishman's stain, sometimes found in the cytoplasm of monocytes, myelocytes and myeloblasts but not in lymphocytes or lymphoblasts; their significance is unknown but they are seen in the blood in acute myeloblastic leukaemia and myelomatosis.

Auerbach, Leopold (b. 1828). Breslau anatomist and neuropathologist.

Auerbach's ganglia. Ganglia in the myenteric plexus.

Auerbach's plexus. The myenteric plexus. *See* PLEXUS.

Aufrecht, Emanuel (b. 1844). German physician.

Aufrecht's disease. Infectious jaundice, with parenchymatous changes in the liver and kidneys.

Aufrecht's sign. Feeble breath sounds heard just above the jugular fossa suggest tracheal obstruction.

augmentor (awg·**men**·tor). 1. A substance which, although alone it cannot cause cell division, is held to increase the action of a kinetic or auxetic. 2. Term descriptive of nerve cells or of nerves the action of which is to increase the rapidity and force of the heart beat. [L *augmentare* to increase.]

augnathus (awg·**na**·thus). A monster with a double lower jaw. [Gk *au* again, *gnathos* jaw.]

Aujeszky, Aladár (b. 1869). Budapest pathologist.

Aujeszky's disease. Psuedorabies; a bulbar palsy of infective origin occurring in Brazil and Hungary, and colloquially referred to as *the scratching pest.*

aula (aw·lah). The inflammatory flush or areola surrounding the vesicle of the vaccination lesion. [Gk *aule* hall.]

aura (aw·rah). A premonitory, subjective sensation preceding an attack of epilepsy or other paroxysmal disorder. It may take numerous forms, simple, or more specialized, e.g. auditory, visual, olfactory or taste. **Aura asthmatica.** A sensation of tightness in the chest which precedes an attack of asthma. **Auditory aura.** A simple noise or buzzing, or more specialized, e.g. sound of bells, etc. **Cephalic aura.** Aura associated with head sensation. **Electric aura.** A sensation of breeze experienced when receiving a discharge of static electricity. **Epigastric aura.** A vague sensation in the epigastrium. **Aura hysterica.** An aura (of various sensations) which may occasionally precede an hysterical attack. **Intellectual aura.** A dreamy state which may precede an epileptic attack. **Kinaesthetic aura.** Retrograde or forward movements just before an attack of epilepsy. **Motor aura.** Kinaesthetic aura (see preceding). **Olfactory aura.** Aura associated with sensation of smell. **Aura procursiva.** Forward movement of the patient before an attack. **Reminiscent aura.** Intellectual aura (see above). **Somatosensory aura.** Aura associated with body sensation. **Aura vertiginosa.** A sensation of giddiness preceding an attack of epilepsy, or a momentary sensation of unsteadiness in patients with functional nervous disorders. **Visual aura.** Aura associated with vision, e.g. flashing. [L breath.]

aural (aw·ral). 1. Belonging to the sense of hearing; involving the sense of hearing. [L *auris* ear.] 2. Belonging to or having the characteristics of an aura. [L *aura* breath.]

auramine (aw·ram·een). Tetramethyldiamido-imidobenzophenone, tetramethyldiaminodiphenylketonimine, $N(CH_3)_2C_6H_4C(NH)C_6H_4N(CH_3)_2$. A yellow dye used for textiles, paper and leather. **Auramine hydrochloride, Auramine O.** A soluble yellow dye used as a food colouring and as an antiseptic for sterilizing the skin prior to operation. [L *aurum* gold, amine.]

aurantia (aw·**ran**·she·ah). Ammonium hexanitrodiphenylamine, $(NO_2)_3C_6H_2N{=}C_6H_2(NO_2)_2NOONH_4$. An orange dye used as a food colouring and a biological stain.

aurantiamarin (aw·**ran**·she·**am'**·ar·in). A bitter glucoside found in orange peel; related to hesperidin.

aurantiasis cutis (aw·ran·**ti**·as·is **kew**·tis). A yellowish pigmentation of the skin which results from eating an excessive number of carrots and oranges. [L *aurantium* orange, *cutis* skin.]

aurantine (aw·**ran**·teen). An extract of the bitter orange, *Citrus aurantium.*

aurantium (aw·**ran**·she·um). The specific name for orange. **Citrus aurantium** var. **amara.** The bitter or Seville orange, the peel of which is used as a flavouring agent, bitter, and carminative. Fresh Bitter-orange Peel BP 1958 (aurantii cortex recens) is used as a tincture and syrup, and Dried Bitter-orange Peel BP 1958 (aurantii cortex siccatus) as an infusion. **Citrus aurantium** var. **dulce.** The sweet orange. [L.]

aurate (aw·rate). A salt of auric acid.

aureolin (aw·**re**·o·lin). Primuline yellow; a dyestuff derived from *p*-toluidine. It is a sulphonated mixture of *p*-amino-benzo di- and tri- thiazoles. [L *aurum* gold.]

aureomycin (aw·re·o·**mi'**·sin). A mixture of several antimicrobial substances produced by the growth of *Streptomyces aureofaciens.* It is an antibiotic of wide range, and hence finds use as a prophylactic against a number of infections. Its activity is not restricted to bacteria, and it is effective in virus pneumonia and rickettsial diseases. **Aureomycin Hydrochloride BP 1953.** The mixture of the hydrochlorides of the several substances comprising aureomycin. [L *aurum* gold, Gk *mykes* fungus.]

auriasis (aw·**ri**·as·is). Chrysiasis: 1. The condition in which grey patches appear on the skin after administration of gold. 2. Impregnation of the tissues by gold. [L *aurum* gold.]

auric (aw·rik). Containing, derived from, or referring to gold. [L *aurum* gold.]

auricle [auricula (NA)] (aw·rikl). 1. The expanded portion of the external ear. The apex [apex auriculae] is the highest point on the ear of an animal: in man it is the tubercle of the auricle; Darwin's tubercle. 2. One of the auricles of the atria [auricula atrii (NA)]; pyramidal appendages arising from the anterior and upper parts of the atria [auricula sinistra, auricula dextra (NA)], and lying on either side of the emerging arterial trunks which their apices overlap anteriorly. 3. One of the chambers of the embryonic heart. 4. Term commonly used as synonymous with an atrium of the heart. **Cervical auricle.** An appendage of yellow cartilage and skin which may be attached at the external opening of a persisting branchial cleft. [L *auricula* little ear.]

See also: DARWIN.

auricle, muscles of the. Oblique muscle of the auricle [musculus obliquus auriculae (NA)]. An intrinsic muscle of the auricle on the medial surface; it stretches across the transverse sulcus of the antihelix. **Transverse muscle of the auricle [musculus transversus auriculae (NA)].** An intrinsic muscle of the medial surface, stretching from the eminence of the concha to the concavity of the helix.

auricular (aw·**rik**·ew·lar). 1. Belonging to the ear or to an auricle. 2. Atrial.

auricular arteries. Deep auricular artery [arteria auricularis profunda (NA)]. *See* MAXILLARY ARTERY. **Posterior auricular artery [arteria auricularis posterior (NA)].** A small branch of the external carotid artery supplying the back of the ear and adjoining region of the scalp [ramus auricularis, ramus occipitalis (NA)], the tympanic cavity [arteria stylomastoidea, ramus stapedius (NA)], tympanic membrane [arteria tympanica posterior (NA)] and the mastoid air cells [rami mastoidei (NA)].

auricular nerves. Great auricular nerve [nervus auricularis magnus (NA)]. A large sensory branch of the cervical plexus, deriving its fibres from the 2nd and 3rd cervical nerves and supplying the skin on both surfaces of the auricle [ramus posterior (NA)] and on the face immediately in front of the auricle [ramus anterior (NA)]. **Posterior auricular nerve [nervus auricularis posterior (NA)].** A motor branch of the facial nerve at its exit from the stylomastoid foramen, supplying the auricular muscles and the occipital belly of the occipitofrontalis muscle [ramus occipitalis (NA)].

auricular veins. Anterior auricular veins [venae auriculares anteriores (NA)]. Tributaries of the posterior facial vein. **Posterior auricular vein [vena auricularis posterior (NA)].** A superficial vein draining the back of the auricle and posterior part of the scalp and uniting with the posterior division of the posterior facial vein to form the external jugular vein.

auriculare (aw·**rik**·ew·**la'**·re). The auricular point; the centre of the orifice of the auditory meatus.

auricularis anterior muscle [musculus auricularis anterior (NA)] (aw·**rik**·ew·**la'**·ris). A thick sheet continuous with the auricularis superior muscle, attached to the epicranial aponeurosis and temporal fascia and running posteriorly to the helix.

auricularis posterior muscle [musculus auricularis posterior (NA)]. A thin sheet of muscle attached to the mastoid process of the temporal bone and the cranial surface of the auricle.

auricularis superior muscle [musculus auricularis superior (NA)]. A pale, fan-shaped muscle attached to the epicranial aponeurosis and temporal fascia and the cranial surface of the auricle.

auriculate (aw·**rik**·ew·late). 1. Having auricles. 2. In botany and zoology, having ears or lobes or appendages shaped like ears.

auriculocranial (aw·**rik**·ew·lo·**kra'**·ne·al). Referring to or involving the auricle of the ear and the cranium.

auriculo-occipital (aw·**rik**·ew·lo·ok·**sip'**·it·al). Referring to the ear and the occipital region. [auricle, occiput.]

auriculotemporal (aw·**rik**·ew·lo·**tem'**·por·al). Referring to the auricle of the ear and the region of the temple.

auriculotemporal nerve [nervus auriculotemporalis (NA)]. A sensory branch of the mandibular nerve to the skin of the temple [rami temporales superficiales (NA)], auricle [nervi auriculares anteriores (NA)] and external auditory meatus [nervus meatus acustici externi (NA)], the ear-drum [ramus membranae tympani (NA)] and the jaw joint. It also carries parasympathetic nerve supply to the parotid gland [rami parotidei (NA)]. The latter and temporal branches communicate with the facial nerve [rami communicantes cum nervo faciali (NA)].

auriculoventricular (aw·**rik**·ew·lo·ven·**trik'**·ew·lar). Atrioventricular. [auricle, ventricle.]

auride (aw·ride). A dermatitis resulting from the use of gold salts. [L *aurum* gold.]

auriform (aw·re·form). Shaped like an ear. [L *auris* ear, form.]

auriginous (aw·**rig**·in·us). 1. Having the colour of gold. 2. Icteric; jaundiced. [L *auriginosus* golden.]

aurilave (aw·re·lave). An instrument or apparatus used to wash out or clean out the ear. [L *auris* ear, *lavare* to wash.]

aurin (aw·rin). $OC_6H_4{=}C(C_6H_4OH)_2$. An acid phenol dye crystallizing in dark-red needles with a metallic lustre; used to a limited extent in textile printing, and as an indicator, being yellow in acids and magenta in alkalis (pH 7–8). **Aurin R.** Corallin, a red dye used as an indicator for weak bases. **Aurin tricarboxyllic acid.** Aluminon, an extremely delicate reagent for aluminium, giving a vivid red coloration.

aurinarium (aw·rin·a·re·um) (pl. *aurenaria*). Aural bougie; a form of suppository for the outer ear, usually prepared with a cocoa-butter base, and weighing about 300 mg. [L *auris* ear.]

aurine (aw·reen). Aurin.

auriphone (aw·re·fone). An ear trumpet fitted with an amplifier. [L *auris* ear, Gk *phone* voice.]

auripuncture (aw·re·pungk·tcher). The surgical procedure of puncturing the tympanic membrane. [L *auris* ear, puncture.]

auris (aw·ris). Ear. [L.]

auriscalp, auriscalpium (aw·re·skalp, aw·re·**skal**·pe·um). An instrument with which foreign bodies in the ear may be scraped away or picked out. [L *auris* ear, *scalpere* to scrape.]

auriscope (aw·re·skope). A form of otoscope. [L *auris* ear, Gk *skopein* to watch.]

aurist (aw·rist). A specialist in ear diseases. [L *auris* ear.]

auristillae (aw·ris·**til**·e). Ear-drops. [L.]

aurobromide (aw·ro·**bro**·mide). A double bromide of monovalent gold, such as potassium aurobromide, $KAuBr_2$.

aurochloride (aw·ro·**klor**·ide). A double chloride of monovalent gold, such as sodium aurochloride, $NaAuCl_2$.

aurochromoderma (aw·ro·kro·mo·**der'**·mah). A green-blue stain which is permanent in the skin as the result of injections of certain gold compounds. [L *aurum* gold, Gk *chroma* colour, *derma* skin.]

Aurococcus (aw·ro·**kok**·us). A synonym (USA) for *Staphylococcus aureus.* [L *aurum* gold, Gk *kokkos* berry.]

aurocyanide (aw·ro·si·an·ide). A double salt containing aurous cyanide: potassium aurocyanide, $KAu(CN)_2$, has been used in the treatment of lupus and syphilis.

aurometer (aw·**rom**·et·er). An apparatus by which the power of hearing and the extent of deafness may be determined. It consists of a metal bar along which a watch suspended from it may be moved towards and away from the external auditory meatus of the ear. [L *auris* ear, meter.]

aurosol (aw·ro·sol). Colloidal gold. *See* GOLD. [L *aurum* gold, sol.]

aurotherapy (aw·ro·**ther**·ap·e). Chrysotherapy. [L *aurum* gold, therapy.]

aurothioglucose (aw·ro·thi·o·**gloo'**·koze). $C_6H_{11}O_5SAu$, an organic compound of gold.

aurothiosulphate (aw·ro·thi·o·**sul'**·fate). A double thiosulphate of monovalent gold: sodium aurothiosulphate, $Na_3Au(S_2O_3)_2$, has been used intravenously in tuberculosis and in the treatment of lupus erythematosus; also intramuscularly in rheumatoid arthritis.

aurous (aw·rus). 1. In chemistry, indicating a compound of monovalent gold. 2. Referring to gold and the compounds of gold. [L *aurum* gold.]

aurum (aw·rum). Latin for *gold*, whence the symbol Au; genitive *auri.* **Aurum vegetabile.** Pipitzahoic acid, $C_{15}H_{20}O_3$, a bright-yellow substance found in the Mexican *Perezia adnate*; used as an indicator (acids, yellow; alkalis, red), and medicinally as a purgative.

auscult, auscultate (aws·**kult**, aws·kul·tate). To practise auscultation. [L *auscultare* to listen.]

auscultation (aws·kul·**ta**·shun). The art of listening to and interpreting the meaning of sounds produced within the body. Invented by René Laënnec in 1819. **Direct auscultation.** Auscultation performed by applying the unaided ear directly to the chest wall. **Immediate auscultation.** Direct auscultation (see above). **Mediate auscultation.** Auscultation by means of a stethoscope. The sounds can be magnified and made audible to a large class by the use of a microphone, radio amplifier and loudspeaker. Though principally for examining sounds produced in the chest, a stethoscope is also used in the auscultatory method of determining blood pressure, and for the auscultation of sounds produced in the larger arteries and veins, in arthritic joints and in the abdomen. **Obstetric auscultation.** Auscultation of the fetal heart sounds or placental souffle through a stethoscope placed on the abdominal wall. **Oral auscultation.** Listening to breath sounds through a stethoscope held just in front of the open mouth. **Rod auscultation.** Auscultation by listening with the stethoscope to the sound vibrations set up by scratching the upper end of a short wooden or ivory rod placed vertically on the body surface. **Vibratory auscultation.** Auscultation with the stethoscope and a tuning fork applied to the surface. [L *auscultare* to listen.]

auscultatory (aws·kul·ta·tor·e). Referring to or used in auscultation.
auscultoscope (aws·kul·to·skope). Phonendoscope. [L *auscultare* to listen, Gk *skopein* to watch.]
Auspitz, Heinrich (b. 1835). German physician.
Auspitz's sign. Pin-point bleeding from a lesion of psoriasis when it is rubbed with a spatula to remove loose scales. It indicates the patchy thinning of the epidermis overlying papillary processes of the dermis.
Australia antigen (aws·tra·li·a an·te·jen). *See* Hepatitis B antigen.
Australian blight (aws·tra·le·an blite). Angioneurotic oedema. *See* OEDEMA.
australoids (aws·tral·oidz). Aboriginals, Melanesians, Papuans, Negritos, tribal folk of India. [L *australis* southern, Gk *eidos* form.]
Australorbis (aws·tral·or·bis). A genus of ram's-horn snails, some species of which act as intermediary hosts of *Schistosoma mansoni*, e.g. *Australorbis centrimetalis olivaceus, Australorbis glabratus.* This genus is now merged into the genus *Biomphalaria* by some writers. [L *australis* southern, *orbis* country.]
autacoid (awt·ak·oid). 1. An organic substance produced in one organ and carried by the blood to other organs upon which its effect is similar to that of drugs. 2. Any internal secretion. **Chalonic autacoid.** A colyone. **Duodenal autacoid.** Secretin. **Excitatory autacoid, Hormonic autacoid.** A hormone. **Inhibitory autacoid, Restraining autacoid.** A colyone. [Gk *autos* self, *akos* remedy, *eidos* form.]
autarcesiology (awt·ar·se·ze·ol'·o·je). The science of immunology based on autarcesis. [Gk *autos* self, *arkesis* warding off, *logos* science.]
autarcesis (awt·ar·se·zis). Natural or inherent immunity as distinguished from immunity due to administration of antibodies. [Gk *autos* self, *arkesis* warding off.]
autarcetic (awt·ar·se·tik). Referring or belonging to autarcesis.
autechoscope (awt·ek·o·skope). An instrument for self-auscultation. [Gk *autos* self, *echos* sound, *skopein* to watch.]
autecology (awt·ek·ol·o·je). The study of the relationships of a particular species of organism to its environment. [Gk *autos* self, ecology.]
autemesia (awt·em·e·ze·ah). Vomiting which has no apparent cause; spontaneous vomiting. [Gk *autos* self, *emesis* vomiting.]
autism (awt·izm). 1. Anthropophobia; excessive and morbid dislike of the society of others. 2. A condition in which the individual tends to be morbidly self-centred. 3. A rare syndrome of early childhood involving a failure to develop normal relationships with parents, unresponsiveness and delay of language. [Gk *autos* self.]
auto-activation (awt·o·ak·tiv·a'·shun). The activation of a gland by its own secretions. [Gk *autos* self, activation.]
auto-agglutination (awt·o·ag·loo·tin·a'·shun). Agglutination of the blood corpuscles by the serum of the same individual or of the sperms of a male by auto-agglutinins. [Gk *autos* self, agglutination.]
auto-agglutinin (awt·o·ag·loo'·tin·in). A substance formed in the blood that causes the agglutination of the erythrocytes of the same individual. [see prec.]
auto-allergy (awt·o·al·er·je). Autosensitization. [Gk *autos* self, *allos* other, *ergein* to work.]
auto-analyser (awt·o·an·al·i·zer). A machine for the automatic analysis of tissues or fluids, registering results by graph. [Gk *autos* self, analysis.]
auto-analysis (awt·o·an·al'·is·is). A method of treatment of nervous disorders by which the patient is led to analyse his own condition and interpret his symptoms and thus become aware of the state of mind which is the cause of the illness. [Gk *autos* self, analysis.]
auto-anamnesis (awt·o·an·am·ne'·sis). In psychiatry, the process by which the entire history of a case is obtained from the patient himself. [Gk *autos* self, *anamnesis* a recalling.]
auto-anaphylaxis (awt·o·an·ah·fil·ax'·is). Anaphylaxis brought about by the injecting of the patient's own serum, blood or secretions. [Gk *autos* self, *ana, phylaxis* protection.]
auto-antibiosis (awt·o·an·te·bi·o'·sis). The self-limitation of cultures grown in artificial media, resulting from exhaustion of certain factors or the accumulation of a toxic metabolite. [Gk *autos* self, *anti, bios* life.]
auto-antibody (awt·o·an·te·bod·e). An antibody, present in the serum of some patients with acquired haemolytic anaemia, that is capable of reacting even *in vitro* with the patient's own erythrocytes, causing haemolysis. Auto-antibodies to other tissues are occasionally found in the serum and are thought to be responsible for the degenerative changes in the specific tissue, e.g. Hashimoto's thyroiditis. [Gk *autos* self, antibody.]
auto-anticomplement (awt·o·an·te·kom'·ple·ment). An anticomplement which is formed in the organism itself. [Gk *autos* self, anticomplement.]
auto-antigen (awt·o·an·te·jen). *See* AUTO-IMMUNITY. [Gk *autos* self, antibody, Gk *genein* to produce.]
auto-antisepsis (awt·o·an·te·sep'·sis). Spontaneous antisepsis. [Gk *autos* self, antisepsis.]
auto-antitoxin (awt·o·an·te·tox'·in). An antitoxin which, produced by the body itself, induces self-protection against disease. [Gk *autos* self, antitoxin.]
autobacteriophage (awt·o·bak·teer'·e·o·faje). A bacteriophage which is obtained from the patient himself. [Gk *autos* self, bacteriophage.]
autoblast (awt·o·blast). In biology, an independent elementary micro-organism. [Gk *autos* self, *blastos* germ.]
autocatalysis (awt·o·kat·al'·is·is). Catalysis hastened or modified by certain of the products of the process themselves acting as catalysts. [Gk *autos* self, catalysis.]
autocatalyst (awt·o·kat·al·ist). A factor in autocatalytic reaction.
autocatalytic (awt·o·kat·al·it'·ik). Producing or referring to autocatalysis.
autocatharsis (awt·o·kath·ar'·sis). A method of psychiatric treatment which consists in the encouraging of the patient to rid his mind of its agitations and troubles by writing them out himself. [Gk *autos* self, *katharsis* a cleansing.]
autocatheterism (awt·o·kath·et·er·izm). The habit of passing of a catheter by the patient himself. [Gk *autos* self, catheter.]
autocerebrospinal (awt·o·ser·e·bro·spi'·nal). Referring to cerebrospinal fluid derived from the patient himself. [Gk *autos* self, cerebrospinal.]
autocholecystectomy (awt·o·ko·le·sis·tek'·to·me). A condition in which there is invagination of the gall bladder so that the latter is turned inside out through the common bile duct and forms a tumour in the intestine. This tumour is eventually eroded and cast off, being finally expelled *per anum.* [Gk *autos* self, cholecystectomy.]
autochthonous (awt·ok·thon·us). 1. A term used to describe a disease or other morbid condition which originated in the same part of the body in which it is encountered. 2. In psychiatry, an adjective denoting delusions which appear suddenly out of the blue and carry intense conviction. 3. Indigenous. [Gk *autos* self, *chthon* earth.]
autocinesis (awt·o·sin·e'·sis). Autokinesis.
autocinetic (awt·o·sin·et'·ik). Autokinetic.
autoclasis (awt·o·kla·sis). Rupturing or destruction of a part as a result of an intrinsic or internal condition. [Gk *autos* self, *klasis* a breaking.]
autoclave (awt·o·klave). An automatically regulated apparatus which produces steam under pressure for the purposes of sterilization. [Gk *autos* self, L *clavis* key.]
autocondensation (awt·o·kon·den·sa'·shun). A modified method of general diathermy therapy in which the patient acts as one plate of a condenser. The other condenser plate and the condenser dielectric are incorporated in the autocondensation treatment couch. [Gk *autos* self, condenser.]
autoconduction (awt·o·kon·duk'·shun). A method of electrotherapy in which the patient is surrounded by a solenoid in a high-frequency alternating-current circuit; the whole body is

thus subjected to an induced high-frequency current. [Gk *autos* self, conduction.]

autocystoplasty (awt·o·**sis**·to·plas·te). Plastic repair of the bladder, the grafts being obtained from the patient's own body (autoplasty). [Gk *autos* self, cystoplasty.]

autocytolysin (awt·o·si·**tol**'·is·in). A haemolysin in the blood plasma which brings about the self-disintegration of the erythrocytes of the same individual. [Gk *autos* self, cytolysis.]

autocytolysis (awt·o·si·**tol**'·is·is). Autolysis. [see prec.]

autocytolytic (awt·o·si·to·**lit**'·ik). Autolytic.

autocytotoxin (awt·o·si·to·**tox**'·in). 1. A cytotoxin which destroys cells of the organism in which it is made. 2. Term referring to cytotoxins which have arisen in the body on account of the presence of dead and dying cells, which produce degeneration products. [Gk *autos* self, cytotoxin.]

autodermic (awt·o·**der**·mik). A term used to describe a skin graft made by taking skin from another part of the patient's own body. [Gk *autos* self, *derma* skin.]

autodesensitization (awt·o·de·**sen**·sit·i·**za**'·shun). A method of desensitizing a patient by giving him an intramuscular injection of blood aspirated from one of his own veins. [Gk *autos* self, desensitize.]

autodestruction (awt·o·des·**truk**'·shun). Applied particularly to the phenomenon of self-destruction of enzymes occurring when the latter are in solution. [Gk *autos* self, destruction.]

autodiagnosis (awt·o·di·ag·**no**'·sis). 1. Autognosis. 2. The diagnosis by an individual of his own disease. [Gk *autos* self, diagnosis.]

autodiagnostic (awt·o·di·ag·**nos**'·tik). Referring or giving rise to autodiagnosis.

autodigestion (awt·o·di·**jes**'·chun). 1. Autolysis. 2. A condition found in disease of the stomach; the stomach wall is digested by the gastric juice. [Gk *autos* self, digestion.]

autodrainage (awt·o·**dra**·nij). The draining away of the fluid in a body cavity by means of a channel made through the patient's tissues. [Gk *autos* self, drainage.]

autodyne (awt·o·dine). $CH_2OHCHOHCH_2OC_6H_5$. The monophenyl ester of glycerol, reported to have analgesic properties. [Gk *autos* self, *odyne* pain.]

auto-echolalia (awt·o·ek·o·**la**'·le·ah). Meaningless repetition by an individual of sentences he himself has spoken. [Gk *autos* self, echolalia.]

autoecic, autoecious (awt·e·sik, awt·e·shus). In biology, a term applied to parasites which pass their entire life cycle in the same host. [Gk *autos* self, *oikos* house.]

autoecology (awt·ek·**ol**·o·je). The individual life history and environment of an organism. Cf. SYNOECOLOGY. [Gk *autos* self, *oikos* house, *logos* science.]

auto-epilation (awt·o·ep·il·**a**'·shun). Spontaneous falling out of the hair. [Gk *autos* self, epilation.]

auto-erotic (awt·o·er·**ot**'·ik). Characterized by auto-eroticism.

auto-eroticism, auto-erotism (awt·o·er·**ot**'·is·izm, awt·o·**er**·ot·izm). 1. Satisfaction of sexual drives by self-stimulation of the body. 2. Sexual emotion in association with self-admiration. [Gk *autos* self, *eros* love.]

auto-erythrophagocytosis (awt·o·er·**ith**·ro·fag·o·si·**to**'·sis). Phagocytosis of the erythrocytes brought about by phagocytes of the same organism. [Gk *autos* self, erythrophagocytosis.]

auto-eczema (awt·o·**ek**·ze·mah). A local, later widespread, and symmetrical eczematous reaction caused by sensitization to cutaneous breakdown products, topical remedies or organisms on the skin. It may originate from a wound, ulcer or localized patch of eczema. [Gk *autos* self, *ekzein* to boil over.]

autofluorescence (awt·o·floo·or·**es**'·ens). The ability of certain tissues to exhibit fluorescence in the absence of any special treatment. [Gk *autos* self, fluorescence.]

autofluoroscope (awt·o·**floo**·or·o·skope). A form of static imaging device used in nuclear medicine. Although based on a different principle, it performs a function similar to that of a gamma camera. [Gk *autos* self, L *fluere* to flow, Gk *skopein* to view.]

autofundoscope (awt·o·**fun**·do·skope). An instrument the working of which is based on the fact that faint pictures of the retinal vessels may be seen by the observer when a lighted empty space is gazed at through a pin-point hole. [Gk *autos* self, L *fundus* base, Gk *skopein* to watch.]

autofundoscopy (awt·o·fun·**dos**'·ko·pe). Examination of the fundus of the observer's eye by means of an autofundoscope.

autogamous (awt·**og**·am·us). 1. In biology, having autogamy as a characteristic. 2. Referring to autogamy.

autogamy (awt·**og**·am·e). 1. In zoology, a form of reproduction or rejuvenation in some species of Protozoa where the unicellular organism divides into 2 daughter gametes which undergo a period of nuclear maturation before fusing with each other. 2. In botany, self-fertilization. [Gk *autos* self, *gamos* marriage.]

autogenesis (awt·o·**jen**·es·is). Abiogenesis. [see foll.]

autogenetic, autogenous (awt·o·jen·**et**'·ik, awt·**oj**·en·us). 1. Abiogenetic. 2. Self-producing; self-produced. [Gk *autos* self, genesis.]

autognosis (awt·og·**no**·sis). Autodiagnosis; in psychiatry, a method of self-diagnosis in which the patient, through his own statements, is led to appreciate and understand the mental processes which have caused his symptoms. [Gk *autos* self, *gnosis* knowledge.]

autognostic (awt·og·**nos**·tik). Referring to autognosis (autodiagnosis).

autograft (**awt**·o·grahft). A graft of tissue or skin taken from one part of a patient's body to make good a defect in another part. Autoplast. [Gk *autos* self, graft.]

autografting (**awt**·o·grahft·ing). The operation of removing a piece of healthy tissue from one part of the patient's body and using it to repair lesions in another part. Autoplasty. [see prec.]

autogram (**awt**·o·gram). A mark caused by superficial pressure with a blunt instrument in dermatographism. [Gk *autos* self, *gramma* mark.]

autographic (awt·o·**graf**·ik). Pertaining to autographism.

autographism (awt·**og**·raf·izm). The condition in which superficial pressure applied with a blunt instrument causes raised marks to appear and linger on the skin. Dermatographism. [Gk *autos* self, *graphein* to record.]

autohaemagglutination (awt·o·he·mag·loo·tin·**a**'·shun). Autoagglutination. [Gk *autos* self, haemagglutination.]

autohaemagglutinin (awt·o·he·mag·**loo**'·tin·in). *See* HAEMAGGLUTININ. [see prec.]

autohaemic (awt·o·**he**·mik). Descriptive of treatment in which the patient's own blood is used. [Gk *autos* self, *haima* blood.]

autohaemolysin (awt·o·he·**mol**'·is·in). A circulating haemolysin present in the blood of the individual or organism concerned, which causes haemolysis of its own erythrocytes in that blood. A haemolysin which, when introduced into the organism from which it was derived, destroys the erythrocytes in the blood of that organism. [Gk *autos* self, haemolysin.]

autohaemolysis (awt·o·he·**mol**'·is·is). Destruction or haemolysis of the erythrocytes in the blood of an individual by haemolytic agents in his own blood serum. [see prec.]

autohaemolytic (awt·o·he·mo·**lit**'·ik). Referring to or characterized by autohaemolysis.

autohaemopsonin (awt·o·he·**mop**'·son·in). An opsonin which so affects the erythrocytes in an individual's blood that they can be destroyed by other of the body cells. [Gk *autos* self, haemopsonin.]

autohaemotherapy (awt·o·he·mo·**ther**'·ap·e). A method of treatment in which the patient's own blood is administered to him. [Gk *autos* self, haemotherapy.]

autohistoradiograph (awt·o·his·to·**ra**'·de·o·graf). An autoradiograph from a histological slide, used to demonstrate the distribution of radio-active material within minute tissue structure. [Gk *autos* self, historadiograph.]

autohydrolysis (awt·o·hi·**drol**'·is·is). Spontaneous hydrolysis; a decomposition reaction occurring in proteins in neutral solutions. [Gk *autos* self, hydrolysis.]

autohypnosis (awt·o·hip·**no**'·sis). The self-induction of hypnosis by mental concentration on one particular object or thought; or, in a susceptible subject who has been often hypnotized, by concentration on the fact of hypnosis. [Gk *autos* self, hypnosis.]

autohypnotic (awt·o·hip·**not**′·ik). 1. An individual who is able to induce hypnosis in himself. 2. Referring to or characterized by autohypnosis. [see prec.]
autohypnotism (awt·o·**hip**·not·izm). Autohypnosis.
auto-immune (awt·o·im·**ewn**). Relating to an immune reaction developing in response to antigens from the subject's own tissues. [Gk *autos* self, L *immunis* free from.]
auto-immunity (awt·o·im·**ewn**′·it·e). Specific humoral or cell-mediated immunity to constituents of the body's own tissues (auto-antigens). If reactions between auto-antigen and auto-antibody cause tissue damage and clinical manifestations, the result is an auto-immune disease. [Gk *autos* self, L *immunis* free from.]
auto-immunization (awt·o·**im**·ew·ni·**za**′·shun). Immunization against a disease produced naturally within the body as a result of reaction to invasion by the same or associated micro-organisms. [Gk *autos* self, immunity.]
auto-infection (awt·o·in·**fek**′·shun). Re-infection by agents already present in the body, but usually in a different part. [Gk *autos* self, infection.]
auto-inflation (awt·o·in·**fla**′·shun). Self-ventilation of the pharyngotympanic tube in order to equalize intra- and extra-tympanic pressures during sudden changes of pressure. It is usually carried out by swallowing, with lips and nostrils tightly closed. [Gk *autos* self, inflation.]
auto-infusion (awt·o·in·**few**′·zhun). A measure undertaken when there has been excessive loss of body fluids. It consists in the bandaging of the extremities in order to compel the blood to flow towards the heart. [Gk *autos* self, infusion.]
auto-inoculation (awt·o·in·ok·ew·**la**′·shun). Inoculation of a virus from a lesion in one's own body, by contact (e.g. yaws, oriental sore) or otherwise. [Gk *autos* self, inoculation.]
auto-intoxicant (awt·o·in·**tox**′·ik·ant). Any agent responsible for auto-intoxication.
auto-intoxication (awt·o·in·tox·ik·**a**′·shun). A state of poisoning resulting from absorption of waste or decomposition products which act as toxins. **Dyscratic auto-intoxication.** Metabolic disturbance causing a pathological condition of the body fluids. **Endogenous auto-intoxication.** That due to poisons generated within the body. **Exogenous auto-intoxication.** A pathological state caused by absorption in the body of poisons entering through one of the tracts. **Indirect auto-intoxication.** That which results from the absorption from unvoided excreta. **Intestinal auto-intoxication.** The absorption of toxin from the faecal matter in the intestinal tract. [Gk *autos* self, intoxication.]
auto-isolysin (awt·o·i·**sol**′·is·in). An antibody which lyses the cells of the organism from which it is derived and also those of other organisms of the same species. [Gk *autos* self, isolysin.]
autokeratoplasty (awt·o·**ker**·at·o·plas·te). The operation of using a graft which has been taken from the tissue of one eye for repair of a lesion of the cornea of the other eye. [Gk *autos* self, keratoplasty.]
autokinesis (awt·o·kin·**e**′·sis). Voluntary movement. [Gk *autos* self, *kinesis* movement.]
autokinetic (awt·o·kin·**et**′·ik). 1. Moving spontaneously. 2. Referring to or characterized by autokinesis.
autolaryngoscope (awt·o·lar·**in**′·go·skope). A special kind of laryngoscope with which a person can examine his own larynx. [Gk *autos* self, laryngoscope.]
autolaryngoscopy (awt·o·lar·in·**gos**′·ko·pe). The examination of one's own larynx with a laryngoscope. [see prec.]
autolavage (awt·o·**lav**·ahzh). Irrigation performed by an individual on himself, for instance of the stomach or bowel. [Gk *autos* self, Fr. *lavage* washing.]
autolesion (awt·o·**le**·zhun). An injury inflicted by anyone on himself. [Gk *autos* self, lesion.]
autoleucocytotherapy (awt·o·**lew**·ko·si·to·**ther**′·ap·e). A method of treatment by which leucocytes derived from the patient's own blood are administered to him. [Gk *autos* self, leucocytotherapy.]
autologous (awt·**ol**·og·us). Describing that which is normal to, or occurs naturally in a part, or which is normally present in the body tissues or fluids. **Autologous transplantation.** *See* TRANSPLANTATION. [Gk *autos* self, *logos* ratio.]
autology (awt·**ol**·o·je). The knowledge or the science of one's self. [Gk *autos* self, *logos* science.]
autolysate (awt·**ol**·is·ate). Any substance produced by autolysis.
autolyse (**awt**·o·lize). To produce autolysis or to undergo autolysis.
autolysin (awt·**ol**·is·in). A lysin or ferment responsible for autolysis.
autolysis (awt·**ol**·is·is). The process of spontaneous disintegration of cells and tissues resulting from the action of intracellular enzymes; it may occur locally in certain conditions and is generalized after death. It results chiefly from the action of catheptic enzymes, and is favoured by diminished oxygen supply and increased acidity. **Post-mortem autolysis.** A change which occurs shortly after death, affecting many tissues and consisting of a kind of cloudy swelling. [Gk *autos* self, *lysein* to loosen.]
autolysosome (awt·o·**li**·so·some). A membrane-bound body within a cell resulting from the fusion of a lysosome and an autophagosome so that the contents of the latter are exposed to the enzymes of the former. [Gk *autos* self, *lysis* a loosing, *soma* body.]
autolytic (awt·o·**lit**·ik). Causing or referring to autolysis.
automallet (awt·o·**mal**·et). An automatic mallet used in dentistry, which is energized manually or mechanically for use with chisels and amalgam or gold-foil pluggers. [Gk *autos* self, mallet.]
automaticity (**awt**·o·mat·**is**′·it·e). The property of automatic repetitive activity as exemplified by the sino-atrial node of the heart, but which can also at times occur in other cardiac tissue. [Gk *automatismos* self-action.]
automatism (awt·**om**·at·izm). 1. The performance of actions not the consequence of conscious effort. 2. In psychology, a state in which an individual is impelled to perform some particular act without the will or the intention to perform it. 3. The belief that activity of the brain lies at the root of all mental processes. **Ambulatory automatism.** A condition in which the patient, unconscious of what he is doing, moves about and wanders away from home (poriomania). **Command automatism.** A psychopathic state in which there is extreme sensitiveness on the part of the patient to mental suggestions made by those around him that he should perform a certain act on which they have decided and of which he is himself ignorant. **Motor automatism.** A condition in which movements are made without conscious effort of will and without objective stimulation; the power of motion without external stimulation, or resulting from external stimulation but lacking conscious control. **Postepileptic automatism.** Automatic acts performed after an attack of epilepsy that may have no relation to the patient's normal life; they are usually of a constant type. **Sensory automatism.** Hallucination. [Gk *automatismos* self-action.]
automatization (awt·o·mat·i·**za**′·shun). The rendering automatic of frequently repeated actions such as walking, riding a bicycle, or even playing the piano, which actions, however, still remain under conscious control. [Gk *automatismos* self-action.]
automatogen (awt·o·**mat**·o·gen). Automatinogen.
automatograph (awt·o·**mat**·o·graf). An apparatus used for the recording of involuntary movements. [Gk *automatos* self-acting, *graphein* to record.]
automaton (awt·**om**·at·on). An individual who acts involuntarily or mechanically, particularly one who goes on following a monotonous routine. [Gk *automatos* self-acting.]
automixis (awt·o·**mix**·is). Autogamy, 1st def. [Gk *autos* self, *mixis* mixture.]
automnesia (awt·om·**ne**·ze·ah). The recollection by a person of his past experiences. [Gk *autos* self, *mneme* memory.]
automonosexualism (awt·o·mon·o·**sex**′·ew·al·izm). A form of sexual perversion in which narcissism is associated with masturbation. [Gk *autos* self, *monos* alone, sexualism.]
automysophobia (awt·o·mi·so·**fo**′·be·ah). A morbid obsession with personal cleanliness; the patient is convinced that he is dirty and malodorous. [Gk *autos* self, *mysos* filth, phobia.]

autonarcosis (awt·o·nar·**ko**'·sis). A state of insensitiveness induced by autosuggestion. [Gk *autos* self, narcosis.]

autonephrectomy (awt·o·nef·**rek**'·to·me). A condition in which the kidney is atrophied and the ureter completely constricted. It is generally the result of renal tuberculosis. [Gk *autos* self, nephrectomy.]

autonephrotoxin (awt·o·nef·ro·**tox**'·in). A substance in an organism which has a poisonous effect on the kidney cells of that organism. [Gk *autos* self, *nephros* kidney, toxin.]

autonomasia (awt·on·o·**ma**'·ze·ah). Amnesic aphasia. *See* APHASIA. [Gk *autos* self, *onoma* name.]

autonomic (awt·o·**no**·mik). 1. Spontaneous. 2. Existing independently; being functionally independent. **Autonomic nervous system** (syn.: sympathetic and parasympathetic nervous system). *See* SYSTEM. [Gk *autos* self, *nomos* law.]

autonomotropic (awt·o·no·mo·**tro**'·pik). Having an inherent relation to or attraction for the autonomic nervous system. [Gk *autos* self, *nomos* law, *trope* a turning.]

autonomous (awt·**on**·om·us). Autonomic, 2nd def.

autonomy (awt·**on**·om·e). Functional independence. [Gk *autos* self, *nomos* law.]

auto-ophthalmoscope (awt·o·of·**thal**'·mo·skope). An ophthalmoscope used by the subject in examination of his own eye. [Gk *autos* self, ophthalmoscope.]

auto-ophthalmoscopy (awt·o·of·thal·**mos**'·ko·pe). Examination by an individual of his own eye with an auto-ophthalmoscope.

auto-oxidation (awt·o·ox·id·**a**'·shun). 1. Oxidation caused by the effect of the atmosphere alone. 2. An oxidation reaction induced by the presence of an inductor. [Gk *autos* self, oxidation.]

autopath (awt·o·path). An allergically sensitive individual. [Gk *autos* self, *pathos* suffering.]

autopathic (awt·o·**path**·ik). 1. Idiopathic. 2. Referring to an autopath.

autopathography (awt·o·path·**og**'·raf·e). An account of the disease written by a patient. [Gk *autos* self, *pathos* suffering, *graphein* to record.]

autopathy (awt·**op**·ath·e). Idiopathy. [Gk *autos* self, *pathos* suffering.]

autopepsia (awt·o·**pep**·se·ah). Autolysis. [Gk *autos* self, *peptein* to digest.]

autophagia, autophagy (awt·o·**fa**·je·ah, awt·**of**·aj·e). 1. The consumption of its own tissues by the body, as in fasting. 2. The biting or the eating by an individual of his own flesh; a state encountered in mental disorder. [Gk *autos* self, *phagein* to eat.]

autophagosome (awt·o·**fag**·o·some). A membrane-bound body within a cell, containing degenerating cell organelles. [Gk *autos* self, *phagein* to eat, *soma* cell.]

autopharmacology (awt·o·far·mah·**kol**'·o·je). The regulation of the functions of the body by the action of the natural chemical constituents of the tissues. [Gk *autos* self, pharmacology.]

autophil (awt·o·fil). 1. Any subject who is prone to develop manifestations of allergy (hay fever, urticaria, asthma, etc.). 2. A person subject to autophilia. [see foll.]

autophilia (awt·o·**fil**·e·ah). Self-admiration amounting to an obsession; narcissism. [Gk *autos* self, *philein* to love.]

autophobia (awt·o·**fo**·be·ah). Morbid dread of solitude. [Gk *autos* self, phobia.]

autophonia (awt·o·**fo**·ne·ah). Autophony.

autophonomania (awt·o·fo·no·**ma**'·ne·ah). Insanity in which suicidal tendencies are present. [Gk *autos* self, *phonos* murder, mania.]

autophonometry (awt·o·fon·**om**'·et·re). The use of a vibrating tuning-fork laid on a patient's body in order to arrive, through his description of them, at the kinds of sensation produced. [Gk *autos* self, *phone* voice, meter.]

autophonous (awt·**of**·on·us). Having the quality of autophony.

autophony (awt·**of**·on·e). 1. In auscultation, observation of the tone of the examiner's own voice when he is speaking with his head against the patient's chest. 2. Increased resonance, of which the individual himself is aware, of the vocal passages and cords and of the arteries, a condition present in diseases of the nasal passages and the middle ear. [Gk *autos* self, *phone* voice.]

autophthalmoscope (awt·of·**thal**·mo·skope). Auto-ophthalmoscope.

autophthalmoscopy (awt·of·thal·**mos**'·ko·pe). Auto-ophthalmoscopy.

autophyte (awt·o·fite). In botany, a plant which can live on inorganic matter alone. Cf. SAPROPHYTE. [Gk *autos* self, *phyton* plant.]

autoplasmotherapy (awt·o·plaz·mo·**ther**'·ap·e). The use of the patient's own blood plasma in treatment. [Gk *autos* self, plasmotherapy.]

autoplast (awt·o·plast). A piece of healthy tissue or skin taken from one part of a patient's body to make good a defect in another part. Autograft. [Gk *autos* self, *plassein* to form.]

autoplastic (awt·o·**plas**·tik). Pertaining to autoplasty.

autoplasty (awt·o·plas·te). 1. The repair of a diseased or injured tissue or organ by material taken from another part of the body. Autografting. 2. The process of adaptation by intrapsychic modification. [Gk *autos* self, *plassein* to mould.]

autoploids (awt·o·ploidz). Of chromosome complements, cells or individuals having homologous chromosome sets (that is, of one species only). [Gk *autos* self, *ploos* times, *eidos* form.]

autoplugger (awt·o·**plug**·er). An automatic plugger energized by compressed air for use in condensing gold foil or amalgam in a cavity prepared in a tooth.

autopolyploid (awt·o·**pol**'·e·ploid). Of chromosome complements, cells or organisms with more than 2 sets of homologous chromosomes. [Gk *autos* self, *polyplous* many times.]

autoprecipitin (awt·o·pre·**sip**'·it·in). A precipitin which has the power of acting on the substances of the animal in which it was formed. [Gk *autos* self, precipitin.]

autoprotection (awt·o·pro·**tek**'·shun). A condition in which the organism is protected from disease and infection because it has been able to form auto-antitoxins. [Gk *autos* self, protection.]

autoproteolysis (awt·o·pro·te·**ol**'·is·is). Autolysis.

autopsia (awt·**op**·se·ah). Autopsy. **Autopsia in vivo.** Examination of the organs of a living person by means of an exploratory incision or operation.

autopsy (awt·**op**·se). Post-mortem examination of a body, including its organs, in order to establish the cause of death; necropsy. **Medico-legal autopsy.** An examination by a pathologist of the body and its organs after death for medico-legal purposes, e.g. in criminal investigation, or for the purpose of civil litigation. [Gk *autos* self, *opsis* view.]

autopsyche (awt·o·si·ke). The psyche of oneself. [Gk *autos* self, psyche.]

autopsychic (awt·o·**si**·kik). Referring or belonging to the state of being conscious of one's own personality. [see prec.]

autopsychorrhythmia (awt·o·si·ko·**rith**'·me·ah). A pathological rhythmic activity of the brain which is a feature of severe forms of insanity. [Gk *autos* self, *psyche* mind, *rhythmos* rhythm.]

autopsychosis (awt·o·si·**ko**'·sis). Mental disorder in which the patient's own ideas about himself are confused and unreal. [Gk *autos* self, psychosis.]

autopsychotherapy (awt·o·si·ko·**ther**'·ap·e). Psychotherapy administered by a person to himself. [Gk *autos* self, psychotherapy.]

autoptysotherapy (awt·o·tiz·o·**ther**'·ap·e). A form of treatment in which the patient's own sputum is injected subcutaneously. [Gk *autos* self, *ptysma* spittle, therapy.]

autopunition (awt·o·pew·**nish**'·un). The morbid habit of inflicting punishment on oneself because of real or imaginary wrong-doing. It may take the form of childish penalties or severer measures up to whipping. The habit is characteristic of certain forms of religious mania. [Gk *autos* self, L *punire* to punish.]

autopyotherapy (awt·o·pi·o·**ther**'·ap·e). Administration, as a treatment, of the patient's own pathological excretions or exudations; for example, the use of a subcutaneous injection of pus from an abscess active in the body. [Gk *autos* self, *pyon* pus, therapy.]

autoradiograph (awt·o·**ra**·de·o·graf). A radiograph produced by the radiation emitted from within an object so as to record the distribution and relative concentration of the radio-active material it contains. It is used extensively for histological specimens with thin films of specially prepared emulsion. [Gk *autos* self, radiograph.]

autoradiography (awt·o·ra·de·**og**′·raf·e). The process of making autoradiographs.

autoreduction (awt·o·re·**duk**′·shun). The process whereby a hernia spontaneously returns to the abdomen, or is returned by the patient; also applied to the spontaneous disappearance of an intussusception of bowel. **Autoreduction en masse.** The autoreduction of a strangulated hernia, together with its sac, through the abdominal wall. [Gk *autos* self, reduction.]

autoregulation (awt·o·reg·ew·**la**′·shun). Self-adjustment. **Heterometric autoregulation.** The intrinsic adaptive mechanisms controlling the cardiac output which involve changes in myocardial fibre length. **Homoeometric autoregulation.** The intrinsic adaptive mechanisms controlling the cardiac output which are independent of changes of myocardial fibre length. [Gk *autos* self, L *regula* rule.]

autoreinfusion (awt·o·re·in·**few**′·zhun). Reinfusion into a patient, by the method of intravenous injection, of blood or lymph effused into his body cavities. [Gk *autos* self, reinfusion.]

autorrhaphy (awt·**or**·af·e). In the suturing of a wound, the use of strands of tissue excised from the flaps of the wound. [Gk *autos* self, *rhaphe* suture.]

autosensitization (awt·o·sen·sit·i·**za**′·shun). Sensitization of an individual by humoral antibody or a delayed cellular-type reaction, or both, to constituents of his own tissues. [Gk *autos* self, L *sentire* to feel.]

autosensitized (awt·o·**sen**·sit·i·zd). Descriptive of an individual in whom sensitization to his own body cells has been developed, usually spontaneously. [Gk *autos* self, sensitize.]

autosepticaemia (awt·o·sep·te·**se**′·me·ah). Septicaemia which originates from an infection within the body. [Gk *autos* self, septicaemia.]

autoserobacterin (awt·o·seer·o·**bak**′·ter·in). An autogenous vaccine which has been sensitized *in vitro* with the patient's own serum. [Gk *autos* self, serobacterin.]

autoserodiagnosis (awt·o·seer·o·di·ag·**no**′·sis). Diagnosis in which the patient's own blood serum is made use of. [Gk *autos* self, serodiagnosis.]

autoserotherapy (awt·o·seer·o·**ther**′·ap·e). A method of treatment in which blood serum derived from the patient himself is used. [Gk *autos* self, serum, therapy.]

autoserum (awt·o·**seer**·um). A therapeutic serum derived from the subject's own blood. [Gk *autos* self, serum.]

autosexualism (awt·o·**sex**·ew·al·izm). The direction of sexual interest or activity to oneself. [Gk *autos* self, sexualism.]

autosite (**awt**·o·site). 1. A teratism that is capable of maintaining independent life. 2. A fetal monster which bears a parasitic monster either within its body or outside it, and nourishes both. [Gk *autos* self, *sitos* food.]

autositic (awt·o·**sit**·ik). Referring to or having the character of an autosite.

autosmia (awt·**oz**·me·ah). Awareness on the part of an individual of his own body odour. [Gk *autos* self, *osme* smell.]

autosomal (awt·o·**so**·mal). Pertaining to autosomes. [Gk *autos* self, *soma* body.]

autosomatognosis (awt·o·so·mat·og·**no**′·sis). A sensation of still possessing a part or member which has been removed or amputated. Cf. LIMB, PHANTOM. [Gk *autos* self, *soma* body, *gnosis* knowledge.]

autosomatognostic (awt·o·so·mat·og·**nos**′·tik). Referring to or possessing the property of autosomatognosis.

autosome (**awt**·o·some). Any chromosome other than the sex chromosomes. [Gk *autos* self, *soma* body.]

autospermatoxin, autospermotoxin (awt·o·sper·mah·**tox**′·in, awt·o·sper·mo·**tox**′·in). A spermicidal substance formed in the blood serum of an animal, capable of agglutinating the animal's own spermatozoa. [Gk *autos* self, *sperma* seed, *toxikon* poison.]

autosterilization (awt·o·ster·il·i·**za**′·shun). Destruction of viruses in the body by the normal action of the body fluids, so that they finally disappear. This is a characteristic of some, probably many, viral infections. [Gk *autos* self, sterilization.]

autosuggestibility (awt·o·suj·est·ib·**il**′·it·e). Abnormal receptivity to autosuggestion.

autosuggestion (awt·o·suj·**est**′·yun). 1. The spontaneous reproduction in the mind of impressions or ideas previously received by the brain so that they become the source of new ideas or actions, in the same way as suggestions from an external source. 2. A mental condition which is encountered in individuals who have suffered physical trauma, and is related to a state of hypnosis. By the constant dwelling upon an idea or fact, for example, a minor injury to a part, the subject produces paralysis, contracture or other disability of that part. [Gk *autos* self, suggestion.]

autosynnoia (awt·o·sin·**oi**′·ah). Self-centredness to the point of obsession, so that all objective and external interests become non-existent. [Gk *autos* self, *syn*, *nous* mind.]

autotemnous (awt·o·**tem**·nus). In biology, term denoting that an organism is capable of dividing spontaneously. [Gk *autos* self, *temnein* to divide.]

autotherapy (awt·o·**ther**·ap·e). 1. Self-treatment. 2. Autoserotherapy. 3. Autopyotherapy. 4. Spontaneous cure. [Gk *autos* self, therapy.]

autotomy (awt·**ot**·om·e). 1. Fission. 2. Any surgical procedure carried out by an individual on himself. [Gk *autos* self, *temnein* to cut.]

autotopagnosia (awt·o·top·ag·**no**′·ze·ah). Loss of the sense or power of localization or orientation so far as bodily regions or parts are concerned. [Gk *autos* self, *topos* place, *a*, *gnosis* knowledge.]

autotoxaemia, autotoxicosis (awt·o·tox·**e**′·me·ah, awt·o·tox·e·**ko**′·sis). A type of blood poisoning caused by the activities of toxins which have arisen in the individual himself. [Gk *autos* self, *toxikon* poison, *haima* blood, *-osis* condition.]

autotoxin (awt·o·**tox**·in). Any poisonous principle which forms within the body as the result of pathological alteration of tissue. [Gk *autos* self, *toxikon* poison.]

autotoxis (awt·o·**tox**·is). Auto-intoxication.

autotransformer (awt·o·trans·**form**′·er). In electricity, a transformer, part of the coils of which are common to the primary and secondary circuits. [Gk *autos* self, transformer.]

autotransfusion (awt·o·trans·**few**′·zhun). 1. Reinfusion into a patient's body of his own blood. 2. Auto-infusion. [Gk *autos* self, transfusion.]

autotransplant (awt·o·**trans**·plant). Isogeneic or syngeneic graft. [Gk *autos* self, transplant.]

autotransplantation (awt·o·trans·plan·**ta**′·shun). Autoplasty. [see prec.]

autotrepanation (awt·o·trep·an·**a**′·shun). Eating away of the skull by a tumour of the brain. [Gk *autos* self, *trepanon* auger.]

autotroph, autotrophe (**awt**·o·trof, **awt**·o·trofe). An autotrophic bacterium. [Gk *autos* self, *trophe* nutrition.]

autotrophic (awt·o·**trof**·ik). Capable of self-nourishment. The term is applied to saprophytic bacteria which, like plants, derive their energy from inorganic nitrogen and salts and atmospheric carbon dioxide. [see prec.]

autotrophy (awt·o·**tro**·fe). The ability of certain micro-organisms to grow with inorganic salts and carbon dioxide as their sole sources of energy. [Gk *autos* self, *trophe* nourishment.]

autotuberculin (awt·o·tew·**ber**′·kew·lin). 1. Tuberculin or a similar product which is absorbed in a patient's body from some lesion or focus of the disease. 2. Tuberculin derived from cultures prepared from a patient's own sputum. [Gk *autos* self, tuberculin.]

autotuberculinization (awt·o·tew·**ber**·kew·lin·i·**za**′·shun). The absorption by an individual of the products of disintegration or metabolism of *Mycobacterium tuberculosis*; such a condition was sometimes induced by making a patient work until he was febrile. The procedure, which was also called *auto-inoculation*, is not favoured today. [Gk *autos* self, tuberculinization.]

auto-urotherapy (awt·o·ewr·o·**ther'**·ap·e). Urotherapy; treatment consisting in injecting his own urine into the patient's subcutaneous tissues. [Gk *autos* self, urine, therapy.]

autovaccination (awt·o·vak·sin·**a'**·shun). 1. A second vaccination in which virus from the first vaccine sore is used. 2. Vaccination of an individual with an autovaccine. 3. Treatment to induce the formation of antibodies by causing the release of antigens from diseased tissue or from the micro-organisms present. [Gk *autos* self, vaccination.]

autovaccine (awt·o·**vak**·seen). A bacterial vaccine made from cultures prepared from the subject's own tissues or secretions. [see prec.]

autovaccinotherapy (awt·o·vak·sin·o·**ther'**·ap·e). Treatment by autovaccination. [autovaccination, therapy.]

autoxaemia (awt·ox·e·me·ah). Autotoxaemia.

autoxidation (awt·ox·id·**a'**·shun). Auto-oxidation.

autoxidator (awt·**ox**·id·a·tor). A substance obtainable from any cell which, on the addition of water, gives rise to hydrogen peroxide. [Gk *autos* self, oxide.]

Auvard, Pierre Victor Alfred (b. 1855). French gynaecologist.

Auvard's speculum. A perineal self-retaining retractor, useful in the lithotomy position. On an arm coming from the blade is a mass of lead which retracts the perineal body, making the cervix easily visible.

Auvray, Maurice (b. 1868). Paris surgeon.

Auvray's incision. For splenectomy: vertically along the outer border of the left rectus muscle and then angled upwards and backwards over the lower ribs to the 8th intercostal space.

auxanodifferentiation (awx·an·o·dif·er·en·she·**a'**·shun). The appearance of specific function in a developing organ as it nears adult proportion and structure. [Gk *auxanein* to grow, L *differentia* difference.]

auxanogram (awx·**an**·o·gram). Plate culture used in auxanography. [Gk *auxanein* to grow, *gramma* mark.]

auxanographic (awx·an·o·**graf'**·ik). Referring to auxanography, or belonging to its practice.

auxanography (awx·an·**og**·raf·e). A method of discovering the medium in which a bacterium grows best by placing drops of various nutrient solutions on a simple gelatin or agar plate. The microbe will reach its most luxuriant growth in the drop of that solution which suits it best. [Gk *auxanein* to grow, *graphein* to record.]

auxanology (awx·an·**ol**·o·je). The scientific study of growth. [Gk *auxanein* to grow, *logos* science.]

auxesis (awx·e·sis). Natural increase or normal growth in size or bulk. [Gk.]

auxetic (awx·**et**·ik). 1. Having reference or belonging to auxesis; characterized by auxesis. 2. Stimulating proliferation of cells. 3. A hypothetical chemical substance the action of which is held to excite proliferation of cells. [Gk *auxetikos* growing.]

auxiliary (awx·**il**·e·ar·e). 1. Helpful, supporting, complementary. 2. One who helps. **Medical auxiliary.** One who, without being qualified in medicine, assists a doctor or undertakes independently work that helps in the diagnosis and treatment of disease, e.g. a laboratory technician, a masseur. [L *auxilium* aid.]

auxiliomotor (awx·il·e·o·**mo'**·tor). 1. Stimulating or adding movement. 2. In psychology, kinaesthetic. [L *auxilium* aid, motor.]

auxilytic (awx·il·**it**·ik). Intensifying the power to destroy or to bring about lysis. [Gk *auxein* to increase, *lysis* a loosing.]

auxin (**awx**·in). A hormone, produced naturally in higher plants, which controls plant growth and which will promote growth in seedlings when applied in low concentrations. **Auxins A and B.** The auxins present in oat and maize, respectively. [Gk *auxein* to increase.]

auxiometer (awx·e·**om**·et·er). 1. An instrument with which the magnifying power of a lens or a system of lenses can be measured. 2. A dynamometer. [Gk *auxein* to increase, meter.]

auxo-action (awx·o·**ak**·shun). The stimulating effect of a substance on the growth of a micro-organism. [Gk *auxein* to increase, action.]

auxo-amylase (awx·**o**·**am**·il·aze). An agent which quickens the rate of action of amylase. [Gk *auxein* to increase, amylase.]

auxobaric (awx·o·**bar**·ik). Descriptive of the action of the contraction pressure force which causes the cavities of the heart to empty. [Gk *auxein* to increase, *baros* weight.]

auxocardia (awx·o·**kar**·de·ah). Enlargement of the heart: (*a*) physiologically, e.g. during diastole, (*b*) pathologically. Cf. MIOCARDIA. [Gk *auxein* to increase, *kardia* heart.]

auxochrome (**awx**·o·krome). A chemical group, such as NH_2 (basic), or SO_3H (acidic), which confers dyeing properties upon a compound already coloured (chromogenic) by reason of its containing chromophores. [Gk *auxein* to increase, *chroma* colour.]

auxochromous (awx·o·**kro**·mus). In chemistry, term applied to a chemical group with the properties of an autochrome. [see prec.]

auxocyte (**awx**·o·site). A cell the presence of which is material to reproduction or growth. [Gk *auxein* increase, *kytos* cell.]

auxoflore (**awx**·o·flor). A substance which increases the intensity of fluorescence in a compound. Cf. BATHOFLORE. [Gk *auxein* to increase, fluorescence.]

auxogluc (**awx**·o·glook). Any radical or atom which in combination with a glucophore produces sweet-tasting compounds. [Gk *auxein* to increase, *glykys* sweet.]

auxohormone (awx·o·**hor**·mone). A substance with a property, as possessed by vitamins, by which hormonic activity can be increased. [Gk *auxein* to increase, hormone.]

auxology (awx·**ol**·o·je). The scientific study of the growth of organisms. [Gk *auxein* to increase, *logos* science.]

auxometer (awx·**om**·et·er). An instrument with which the magnifying power of a lens or a system of lenses can be measured; auxiometer. [Gk *auxein* to increase, meter.]

auxoneurotropic (**awx**·o·newr·o·**tro'**·pik). 1. An agent which strengthens the neurotropic properties of a substance. 2. Descriptive of the action referred to. [Gk *auxein* to increase, neurotropic.]

auxospore (**awx**·o·spor). The large spore which is a morphological feature of the sporing bacteria, the Bacillaceae, when they are growing in artificial culture. It divides into smaller daughter cells which themselves enlarge into new auxospores. [Gk *auxein* to increase, spore.]

auxotherapy (awx·o·**ther**·ap·e). Substitution therapy; the giving of endocrine preparations or other hormonic substances. [Gk *auxein* to increase, therapy.]

auxotonic (awx·o·**ton**·ik). Contracting with greater force as increasing resistance is encountered (e.g. in muscle). [Gk *auxein* to increase, *tonos* strain.]

auxotox (**awx**·o·tox). A chemical group which renders a compound toxic; thus the methylimine radical $CH_3N=$ introduced into the structure of a drug makes it liable to cause liver degeneration. [Gk *auxein* to increase, *toxikon* poison.]

auxotroph (**awx**·o·trofe). An organism requiring an organic nitrogen-containing substance for growth, derived by mutation from a parent strain with no such complex requirement. [Gk *auxein* to increase, *trophe* nourishment.]

ava, ava-kava (**ah**·vah, ah·vah·**kah**·vah). Kava, Kava-kava, the dried rhizome of *Piper methysticum* (family Piperaceae). *See* KAVA. [see foll.]

avaism (**ah**·vah·izm). Kavaism; the morbid condition resembling absinthism which is the result of addiction to kava, an intoxicating drink made from the root of *Piper methysticum.* [Polynesian *kava.*]

avalanche (av·al·ansh). **Avalanche conduction.** *See* CONDUCTION. **Avalanche theory.** *See* THEORY. [Fr. *à val* to the valley.]

See also: TOWNSEND (J. S. E.).

avalvular (a·**val**·vew·lar). Being without valves. [Gk *a*, L *valva* valve.]

avascular (a·**vas**·kew·lar). Not vascular; not containing many blood vessels, in some cases not containing any vessels. [Gk *a*, L *vasculum* vessel.]

avascularization (a·vas·kew·lar·i·za′·shun). 1. The cutting-off of the blood supply or the expelling of blood from any part, for instance by means of tight bandaging. 2. The removal of blood from any part; devascularization. [see prec.]

Aveling, James Hobson (b. 1828). London obstetrician.

Aveling's repositor. An instrument by which pressure is applied continuously on the fundus of an inverted uterus to reduce its inversion.

Avellis, Georg (b. 1864). German otolaryngologist.

Avellis' symptom complex, or syndrome. Ipsilateral paralysis of palatal and intrinsic laryngeal muscles due to a lesion of the nucleus ambiguus, with contralateral hemianaesthesia to pain and temperature. Also called *syndrome of nucleus ambiguus and spinal fillet* and *ambiguospinothalamic paralysis.*

Avena (av·e·nah). Oat, a large genus of the Gramineae. **Avena decorticata.** Groats. **Avena fatua.** The wild oat. **Avena sativa.** The cultivated oat. [L oats.]

avenin (av·e·nin). A nitrogenous substance obtained from oats (*Avena sativa*), which resembles legumin.

avenolith (av·e·no·lith). A calculus formed in the intestine by the deposition of salts on the surface of undigested grains of oats. [L *avena* oats, Gk *lithos* stone.]

Avery, Oswald Theodore (b. 1877). New York bacteriologist.

Dochez-Avery reaction. Typing of the causal pneumococcus by precipitin test on the patient's urine, using the type-specific antisera.

avian (a·ve·an). Associated with birds, especially with reference to pathogenic micro-organism. [L *avis* bird.]

avidin (av·id·in). A crystalline protein occurring in raw egg-white. It combines with biotin, thus depriving all systems of the latter.

avidity (av·id·it·e). 1. Eagerness; having a strong desire for a thing. 2. Originally applied to chemical affinity or activity, the term is now restricted to a physical sense, such as the attraction of water by hygroscopic substances. [L *avidus* eager.]

avirulent (a·vir·ew·lent). Not virulent. [Gk *a*, virulence.]

avitaminosis (a·vi·tam·in·o′·sis). Any disease or condition which is caused by lack or insufficiency of vitamins in the diet. Cf. DISEASE, DEFICIENCY. [Gk *a*, vitamin, Gk *-osis* condition.]

avitaminotic (a·vi·tam·in·ot′·ik). Affected with or having the character of avitaminosis.

avivement (ah·veev·mahn). The surgical trimming and freshening of the edges of a wound. [Fr. *aviver* to give freshness to.]

avocalia (a·vo·ka·le·ah). Inability to produce musical tones. [Gk *a*, L *vox* voice.]

Avogadro, Count Amedeo (b. 1776). Italian physicist.

Avogadro's constant, or number. The number of molecules in a gram-molecule of gas at 0°C and 101 325 pascal (760 mmHg) pressure: $N_A = 6.06 \times 10^{23}$.

Avogadro's hypothesis, law, postulate or theory. Equal volumes of gases or vapours, at the same temperature and pressure, contain the same number of molecules.

avulsion (av·ul·shun). The forcible separation of 2 parts. **Nerve avulsion.** The operative procedure of forcibly drawing away a nerve from its central origin or of removing a portion of it. **Phrenic avulsion.** Avulsion of the phrenic nerve at the root of the neck so that the diaphragm on that side is paralysed and thus raised, and there is partial collapse of the corresponding lung. [L *avulsio* a pulling away.]

awareness (ah·wa·er·nes). A state of partial pain-free consciousness, occasionally seen during surgical operations under very light anaesthesia. [AS *gewaer* knowing.]

awl (awl). A strong-handled needle for the passage of suture material through a rigid tissue such as bone. [AS *ael.*]

axanthopsia (ax·an·thop·se·ah). Blindness to the colour yellow or to shades of yellow. [Gk *a*, *xanthos* yellow, *opsis* sight.]

Axenfeld, Karl Theodor Paul Polykarpos (b. 1867). Freiburg ophthalmologist.

Axenfeld's anomaly. A prominent Schwalbe's line (q.v.) with adherent processes passing across the angle of the anterior chamber of the eye. It may predispose to infantile glaucoma.

Axenfeld's operation. 1. For lagophthalmos: a silk suture is passed completely round the whole palpebral fissure, starting at the internal canthal ligament and finishing at the periosteum lateral to the outer canthus. 2. For repair of upper lid: the damaged upper lid is given a clean straight edge, the complete lash line of the lower lid is removed, and this is stitched to the cut border of the upper. Before sutures are tied the skin of the lower lid is incised and this gap filled with free skin graft. Later, new openings are made for a palpebral fissure at the necessary level.

Axenfeld's lagophthalmos suture. *See* AXENFELD'S OPERATION, 1st def.

Axenfeld-Krukenberg spindle. A vertical narrow fusiform deposition of pigment on the corneal endothelium. bilateral and occurring mainly in myopic females of middle age and over. It is thought to be degenerative in nature.

Morax-Axenfeld bacillus, or diplococcus. A bacilliary organism that is responsible for subacute angular conjunctivitis. Also called *Moraxella lacunata.*

axerophthol (ax·er·of·thol). Vitamin A; so called because it prevents xerophthalmia. [Obsolete term.] [Gk *a*, xerophthalmia.]

axial (ax·e·al). 1. Lying in or closely related to the axis of a part of the body or of an organ. 2. Appertaining to the axis of a structure, such as the long aixs of a tooth.

axiation (ax·e·a·shun). The development of structures which lie along a body axis; e.g. the notochord, or the neural tube. [L *axis* axle.]

axifugal (ax·if·ew·gal). Centrifugal. [L *axis* axle, *fugere* to flee.]

axilemma (ax·il·em·ah). The covering sheath of an axon. [L *axis* axle, Gk *lemma* husk.]

axilla [NA] (ax·il·ah). The armpit. The pyramidal space between the upper part of the medial side of the upper arm and the upper part of the outer wall of the thorax. [L a wing.]

axillary (ax·il·ar·e). Referring to, situated in or involving the axilla. **Axillary fold.** *See* FOLD. **Axillary lymph gland.** *See* GLAND.

axillary artery [arteria axillaris (NA)]. A continuation of the subclavian artery. It ends at the lower border of the teres major muscle, becoming the brachial artery. It is divided into 3 parts which lie respectively proximal to, behind and distal to the pectoralis minor muscle.

axillary vein [vena axillaris (NA)]. The main venous drainage of the upper limb in the axilla. It is continuous with the subclavian vein.

axio-axial (ax·e·o·ax′·e·al). Pertaining to those parts of a cavity which are parallel to a surface which is itself parallel to the long axis of the tooth in which the cavity is prepared. [L *axis* axle.]

axiobuccal (ax·e·o·buk′·al). Pertaining to the line angle formed by the axial and buccal walls of a cavity prepared in a tooth.

axiobuccocervical, axiobuccogingival (ax·e·o·buk·o·ser′·vik·al, ax·e·o·buk·o·jin′·jiv·al). Relating to the point angle formed by the axial, buccal and cervical or gingival walls of a cavity prepared in a tooth.

axiocervical (ax·e·o·ser′·vik·al). Relating to the line angle formed by the axial and cervical or gingival walls of a cavity prepared in a tooth; axiogingival.

axiodistal (ax·e·o·dis′·tal). Pertaining to the line angle formed between the axial and the distal walls of a cavity prepared in a tooth.

axiodistocclusal (ax·e·o·dist·ok·loo′·sal). Describing the point angle formed by the axial, distal and occlusal walls of a cavity prepared in a tooth.

axiodistocervical, axiodistogingival (ax·e·o·dist·o·ser′·vik·al, ax·e·o·dist·o·jin′·jiv·al). Appertaining to the point angle formed by the axial, distal and cervical or gingival walls of a cavity prepared in a tooth.

axiodisto-incisal (ax·e·o·dist·o·in·si′·zal). Concerning the point angle formed between the axial, distal and incisal walls of a cavity prepared in a tooth.

axiogingival (ax·e·o·**jin'**·jiv·al). Axiocervical. [axis, gingival.]
axio-incisal (ax·e·o·in·**si'**·zal). Pertaining to the line angle formed between the axial and incisal walls of a cavity prepared in a tooth.
axiolabial (ax·e·o·**la'**·be·al). Relating to the line angle formed between the axial and labial walls of a cavity prepared in a tooth.
axiolemma (ax·e·o·**lem'**·ah). Axilemma.
axiolingual (ax·e·o·**ling'**·gwal). Relating to the line angle formed by the axial and lingual walls of a cavity prepared in a tooth.
axiolinguocclusal (ax·e·o·ling·gwok·**loo'**·zal). Concerning the point angle formed by the axial, lingual and occlusal walls of a cavity prepared in a tooth.
axiolinguocervical, axiolinguogingival (ax·e·o·ling·gwo·**ser'**·vik·al, ax·e·o·ling·gwo·**jin'**·jiv·al). Describing the point angle formed by the axial, lingual and cervical or gingival walls of a cavity prepared in a tooth.
axiomesial (ax·e·o·**me'**·ze·al). Pertaining to the line angle formed by the axial and mesial walls of a cavity prepared in a tooth.
axiomesiocervical, axiomesiogingival (ax·e·o·me·ze·o·**ser'**·vik·al, ax·e·o·me·ze·o·**jin'**·jiv·al). Concerning the line angle formed between the axial, mesial and cervical or gingival walls of a cavity prepared in a tooth.
axiomesio-incisal (ax·e·o·me·ze·o·in·**si'**·zal). Describing the point angle formed between the axial, mesial and incisal walls of a cavity prepared in a tooth.
axion (ax·e·on). The brain and the spinal cord; rarely used term. [L *axis* axle.]
axio-occlusal (ax·e·o·ok·**loo'**·zal). Pertaining to the line angle formed between the axial and occlusal walls of a cavity prepared in a tooth.
axioplasm (ax·e·o·plazm). Axoplasm.
axiopodium (ax·e·o·**po'**·de·um). Axopodium.
axiopulpal (ax·e·o·**pul'**·pal). Describing the line angle formed between the axial and pulpal walls of a cavity prepared in a tooth.
axipetal (ax·ip·et·al). Centripetal. [L *axis* axle, *petere* to seek.]
axis (ax·is) (pl. *axes*). 1. A line about which a body rotates; a line through the centre of anything. 2. [NA] The 2nd cervical vertebra. 3. In anatomy, a line on either side of which the parts of the body, or of the organ or region under consideration, are more or less symmetrical; the term is sometimes used for a diameter of a part without reference to its symmetry. **Basibregmatic axis.** The line from the basion to the bregma. **Basicranial axis.** The line of bones from the basion (front margin of foramen magnum) to the nasion (frontonasal suture), including the basioccipital bone, the body of the sphenoid and the ethmoid. **Binauricular axis.** The line joining the centres of the right and left external auditory meatuses. **Cardiac axis.** Electrical axis of the heart (see below). **Cell axis.** An imaginary line drawn through the longest dimension of a cell, usually passing through the centre of the nucleus and the cell centre (centrosome). In epithelial cells it passes from the attached to the free end. **Cerebrospinal axis.** The brain and spinal cord. **Coeliac axis.** The coeliac artery. **Craniofacial axis.** Basicranial axis (see above). **Cylindrical axis, Axis of a cylindrical lens.** The axis which lies in the meridian parallel to the flat surface of a cylindrical lens and at right angles to the curved surface. **Electric axis.** The straight line joining 2 point charges of electricity. **Electrical axis of the heart.** The angle which the mean cardiac vector in the frontal plane makes with a horizontal plane drawn through the centre of Einthoven's triangle. The direction of the vector and its axis in the frontal plane can be determined by constructing Einthoven's triangle and finding the sum of the positive and negative deflections in leads I and II. The usual electrical axis lies between $-10°$ and $+100°$ and is found in hearts which are electrically intermediate between the horizontal and vertical positions. **Embryonic axis.** A line running longitudinally in the existing or future plane of bilateral symmetry of an egg or embryo. **Axis of the eye, external [axis bulbi externus (NA)].** A line joining the centre of the cornea in front to the posterior pole of the eyeball. **Axis of the eye, internal [axis bulbi internus (NA)].** An imaginary line joining the 2 poles of the eyeball. **Fixation axis.** The line joining the centre of rotation of the eye with the point of fixation; fixation line. **Frontal axis.** A line passing from side to side of the eyeball, through its centre. **Geometrical axis.** The line joining the central points of the corneal and scleral surfaces, i.e. the anterior and posterior poles of the eyeball. **Axis of the lens [axis lentis (NA)].** 1. *Principal:* a line connecting the central points (or poles) of the anterior and posterior lens surfaces. 2. *Secondary:* the line along which a ray of light suffers no change of direction though striking the lens obliquely. **Magnetic axis.** The straight line joining the 2 poles of a magnet. **Optic axis [axis opticus (NA)].** The line upon which the refracting surfaces of the eye should be centred. In actual fact, the centring of the components being asymmetrical, such a line is not straight but it can be taken as such because the errors more or less cancel out each other. **Axis of the pelvis [axis pelvis (NA)].** The curved central line of the pelvic canal. **Principal axis.** In optics, the line joining the centres of curvature of the 2 surfaces of a lens; a ray of light passing along this line will not be refracted. It also refers to the centre line passing through the schematic eye, on which all the refracting surfaces are centred. **Pupillary axis.** A line perpendicular to the cornea and passing through the centre of the pupil. **Sagittal axis.** The anteroposterior axis of the eyeball, about which it rotates when making torsional movements. **Secondary axis.** Axis of the lens (see above). **Thoracic axis.** The acromiothoracic artery. **Thyroid-pituitary axis.** The endocrine link between the thyroid and pituitary glands. **Axis uteri.** An imaginary line passing through the longest diameter of the uterus. **Vertical axis.** The axis around which horizontal movements and versions or vergences take place. **Visual axis.** A line joining the object of regard and the macula; visual line. **Y axis.** The growth axis as represented by a line drawn from the centre of the sella turcica to the chin point. [L axle.]
See also: FICH.
axis-cylinder (ax·is·**sil**·in·der). An axon; the long process of a nerve cell which with its covering sheath constitutes a nerve fibre. [L *axis* axle, cylinder.]
axite (ax·ite). A terminal filament of an axon. [L *axis* axle.]
axodendrite (ax·o·**den**·drite). Name given to the fibril-like appendages which spring like root-fibrils from the main axon, and which are non-medullated; their function is to convey impulses towards the axon, and they should be carefully differentiated from the cytodendrites. [Gk *axon* axle, *dendron* tree.]
axofugal (ax·**of**·ew·gal). Centrifugal. [Gk *axon* axle, L *fugere* to flee.]
axograph (ax·o·graf). An apparatus for recording axes on a kymographic tracing. [Gk *axon* axle, *graphein* to record.]
axoid, axoidean (ax·oid, ax·**oid**·e·an). Belonging to the axis bone of the vertebral column (2nd cervical vertebra). [Gk *axon* axle, *eidos* form.]
axolemma (ax·o·**lem**·ah). Axilemma. [Gk *axon* axle, *lemma* husk.]
Axolotl (ax·o·lotl). A tailed larval amphibian of the family Ambystomidae. It is used as a laboratory animal for experiments with the thyroid gland. [Mexican.]
axolysis (ax·**ol**·is·is). Degeneration or disintegration of the axon of a nerve cell. [Gk *axon* axle, *lysis* a loosing.]
axometer (ax·**om**·et·er). In optics, a measuring instrument used for the adjusting of a spectacles frame to suit the optic axis. [Gk *axon* axle, meter.]
axon (ax·on). 1. The axis of the body. 2. The long process of a nerve cell which with its covering sheath constitutes a nerve fibre. **Axon degeneration.** Loss of function in an axon. **Axon hill, Axon hillock.** Cone of origin in the nerve cell from which the axis-cylinder emerges. **Naked axon.** One without a medullary sheath, as in the cells in the sympathetic ganglia. [Gk axle.]
axonal (ax·on·al). Belonging to or having effect upon an axon.
axone (ax·on). Axon.
axoneme (ax·on·eem). The gene-string, or filament which forms the permanent structural basis of the chromosome; chromoneme. [Gk *axon* axle, *neme* thread.]

axoneure (ax·o·newr). Axoneuron.

axoneuron (ax·o·**newr**·on). Any nerve cell in the central nervous system, possessing an axon or axis-cylinder process. [Gk *axon* axle, *neuron* nerve.]

axonometer (ax·on·**om**·et·er). In optics, an axometer with which the cylindrical axis of a lens can be measured. [Gk *axon* axle, meter.]

axonotmesis (ax·on·ot·**me**'·sis). Injury to a nerve, such as that caused by crushing or prolonged pressure, which damages the nerve fibres without completely severing the nerve structure. Cf. NEURAPRAXIA; NEUROTMESIS. [Gk *axon* axle, *tmesis* a cutting apart.]

axopetal (ax·**op**·et·al). Centripetal. [Gk *axon* axle, *petere* to seek.]

axoplasm (ax·o·plazm). Cytoplasm of the axon. [Gk *axon* axle, plasma.]

axopodium (ax·o·**po**·de·um). In zoology, a long pseudopodium stiffened by an axostyle. Cf. LOBOPODIUM. [Gk *axon* axle, *pous* foot.]

axospongium (ax·o·**spun**·je·um). The structure in the form of a mesh which constitutes the substance of a nerve axon. [Gk *axon* axle, *spoggos* sponge.]

axostyle (ax·o·stile). The clear axial filament which is the central support of an axopodium. [Gk *axon* axle, *stylos* post.]

ayahuasca (ah·yah·**was**·kah). $C_{13}H_{12}ON_2$. An alkaloid derived from *Banisteria caapi*, dead-man's vine, a plant of Brazil; it is probably identical with harmine. The name is derived from a native drink.

Ayala, Giuseppe (b. 1878). Italian neurologist.

Ayala's disease. Congenital absence of the sternal portion of the pectoralis major muscle.

Ayala's index, or quotient. *See* AYALA'S TEST (below).

Ayala's test. A manometric test used to distinguish between intracranial tumour and communicating hydrocephalus: the pressure of the cerebrospinal fluid in the lumbar theca is recorded; a measured volume of fluid is removed and the pressure is taken again. Ayala's index or quotient is obtained from the formula $(Q \times F)/I$, where Q is the volume of fluid removed in ml, I the original pressure, and F the final pressure. An index of below 5.5 is said to favour tumour, while one above 6.5 favours a diagnosis of communicating hydrocephalus.

Ayer, James Bourne (b. 1882). Boston neurologist.

Ayer's test. For spinal block: in the normal subject lying horizontally, the pressure of the cerebrospinal fluid as measured on cisternal puncture is identical with that recorded from the lumbar theca. If the pressures in these 2 sites are measured simultaneously and there is a significant difference between the 2, particularly if the lumbar pressure is much lower, a block in the spinal subarachnoid space must be suspected.

Tobey-Ayer test. For thrombosis of the lateral cerebral sinus: pressure on one or both jugular veins normally causes a rise in pressure of the cerebrospinal fluid, and this rise can be measured by a manometer connected to a lumbar-puncture needle. In cases of lateral sinus thrombosis, no rise occurs on the affected side.

Ayer, S. Henry (b. 1893). American bacteriologist.

Ayer's casein-agar method. The preparation of a culture medium by dissolving casein in caustic soda and solidifying with agar.

Ayer and Johnson's method. A method of preparing stock culture from gelatin, casein, glucose, peptone, citrate, phosphate and agar.

Ayerza, Abel (b. 1861). Buenos Aires physician.

Ayerza's disease, or syndrome. Chronic pulmonary heart disease, with occlusive changes in the pulmonary arterioles, pulmonary hypertension, intense cyanosis, polycythaemia and right ventricular insufficiency. It is characterized by asthma, bronchitis and dyspnoea; there may be clubbing of the fingers, and sometimes splenomegaly, hepatomegaly and hyperplasia of the bone marrow. Originally thought to be due to syphilitic disease of the pulmonary vasculature, it is now recognized as a syndrome which may arise in connection with a number of different pulmonary diseases. *See* SYNDROME, COR PULMONALE.

Ayre, Philip. 20th century Newcastle-upon-Tyne anaesthetist.

Ayre's tube, or T-piece. A T-shaped tube used particularly in administration of endotracheal anaesthesia to children to reduce rebreathing and resistance to expiration.

ayurvedism (ah·yoor·**va**·dizm). The indigenous system of medicine in India, based on the Hindu Scriptures, or Vedas. [Sansk. *Áyurveda* the science of life.]

Azacyclonol (az·a·si·**klo**'·nol). BP Commission approved name for diphenyl-(4-piperidyl)methanol, a tranquillizing drug used in the treatment of psychotic disorders.

azadirachta (az·ad·e·**rak**·tah). Indian azadirach, neem or nim bark, margosa bark, the bark of *Melia azadirachta* (family Meliaceae) indigenous to and cultivated in India. It contains a bitter alkaloid, margosine, and is used in the East in the form of a tincture or infusion as a tonic. [Pers. *azad* free, *dirakht* tree.]

azafrin (az·af·rin). $C_{27}H_{38}O_4$. A phytoxanthin of carotenoid nature, found in the roots of azafranilla, *Escobedia scrabifolia*; it is oxidized to geronic acid.

Azalomycin (az·al·o·**mi**'·sin). BP Commission approved name for a mixture of related antibiotics produced by *Streptomyces hygroscopicus* var. *azalomyceticus.*

Azamethonium Bromide (az·ah·meth·o'·ne·um **bro**·mide). BP Commission approved name for 3-methyl-3-azapentamethylenebis(ethyldimethyl ammonium) dibromide. It is a ganglion-blocking substance used to produce controlled hypotension, and thus to reduce bleeding in operations.

Azapropazone (a·zah·**pro**·paz·one). BP Commission approved name for 5 - dimethylamino - 9 - methyl - 2 - propyl - 1*H* - pyrazolo[1,2-*a*][1,2,4] - benzotriazine - 1,3(2*H*) - dione; an analgesic and anti-inflammatory agent.

Azaribine (az·ah·**ri**·been). BP Commission approved name for 2 - β - D - ribofuranosyl - *as* - triazine - 3,5 - (2*H*,4*H*) - dione 2',3',5'-triacetate; it is used in the treatment of psoriasis.

azarin (**az**·ar·in). $C_{16}H_{17}O_4N_3S$. A harmless red dye derived from aniline.

Azathioprine BP 1973 (az·ah·**thi**·o·preen). 6 - (1 - Methyl - 4- nitroimidazol - 5 - ylthio)purine; a cytotoxic agent used for immunosuppression.

azedarach (az·**ed**·ar·ak). The root-bark of *Melia azedarach* (family Meliaceae), cultivated in some parts of India and China. A decoction is used as an anthelmintic. [Pers. *azad* free, *dirakht* tree.]

Azepetine (az·a·pet·een). BP Commission approved name for 1-allyl-2,7-dihydro-3,4-5,6-dibenzazepine; the phosphate is used in the treatment of vascular disorders.

Azetepa (az·e·**te**·pah). BP Commission approved name for *P,P* - diaziridin - 1 - yl - *N* - ethyl - 1,3,4 - thiadiazol - 2 - ylphosphinamide; an antimetabolite.

azide (**az**·ide). 1. A salt of hydrazoic acid, NH_3. 2. A compound containing the monovalent triazo or azoimide group $-N_3$.

Azidocillin (az·id·o·**sil**'·in). BP Commission approved name for 6-[D(−)-α-azidophenylacetamido]penicillanic acid; an antibiotic.

azo-. *See* AZO-COMPOUND.

azo-bordeaux (az·o·bor·**do**'). A red dye used to colour foodstuffs.

azo-compound (az·o·**kom**·pownd). One of the organic aromatic compounds containing the divalent azo group -N=N- which is a chromophore. Azo-compounds are produced by the alkaline reduction of nitro-compounds, and are either coloured (chromogenes) or actual dyes. [Fr. *azote* nitrogen.]

azo-itch (az·o·ich). Pruritus which attacks those who work with azo dyes. [Fr. *azote* nitrogen, itch.]

azoamyly (a·zo·**am**·il·e). Defect of the liver cells by which they do not have the capacity to become charged with glycogen in normal amount. [Gk *a*, *zoon* animal, *amylon* starch.]

azobenzene (az·o·**ben**·zeen). Benzene azobenzene, $C_6H_5NNC_6H_5$. Orange crystals prepared by the reduction of nitrobenzene; further reduced to aniline. It forms the starting-point for the azo dyes.

azobenzoid (az·o·**ben**·zo·id). A substance prepared from benzaldehyde or oil of bitter almonds by treatment with ammonia.
azocarmine (az·o·**kar**·mine). A number of azo dyes derived from naphthalene and used as stains in histology.
azoic (a·**zo**·ik). Not containing any living organisms; without organic life. [Gk *a*, *zoe* life.]
azoimide (az·o·**im**·ide). 1. Name given to the monovalent triazo group $-N_3$. *See* AZIDE. 2. Hydrazoic acid. *See* ACID.
azole (**az**·ole). 1. Term applied to any of the heterocylic pentatomic-ring compounds which include a nitrogen atom in the ring. 2. Pyrrole, C_4H_5N, a heterocylic 5-member ring compound which occurs in bone oil; the parent of a number of antiseptics, and itself entering into the construction of the porphin ring of haemoglobin and of chlorophyll.
azolitmin (az·o·**lit**·min). $C_7H_7O_4N$. The principal constituent of litmus, the colouring matter extracted from lichens of the species *Roccella*; a dark-blue solid, soluble in water and used as an indicator (acids, red; alkalis, blue).
azomethane (az·o·**me**·thane). Name applied to hydrocyanic acid HC≡N, being regarded as methane in which nitrogen has replaced 3 of the hydrogen atoms.
azoospermatism, azoospermia (a·zo·o·**sper′**·mat·izm, **a**·zo·o·**sper′**·me·ah). Lack of spermatozoa in the semen or deficiency in their functional activity. [Gk *a*, *zoon* animal, *sperma* seed.]
azoprotein (az·o·**pro**·te·in). In immunology, a protein coupled with a diazonium compound so as to form an azo derivative. This latter gives rise to an immune serum which is specific for the diazonium group introduced, and thereby permits the study of the immunoreactions characteristic of the particular chemical grouping.
azoresorcin (**az**·o·rez·**or′**·sin). $C_6H_3(OH)_2C_6H_2(OH)_2NO_2$. A compound formed by the nitration of resorcinol.
azorubin S (az·o·**roo**·bin **es**). A red azo dye which has been used intravenously as the basis of a test of liver function; its excretion is largely increased in cases of liver disease.
azorubrum (az·o·**roo**·brum). Bordeaux B.
azotaemia (az·o·te·me·ah). The accumulation of nitrogenous compounds, mainly urea, in the blood. The word has almost dropped out of modern terminology; uraemia is now used. **Chloropenic azotaemia.** A condition in which sodium chloride is deficient in amount, and there is azoturia and fixation of chlorine in the tissues. **Extrarenal azotaemia, Non-renal azotaemia, Prerenal azotaemia.** Uraemia due to causes other than renal dysfunction. [Fr. *azote* nitrogen, Gk *haima* blood.]
azotaemic (az·o·**te**·mik). Referring to or showing the characteristics of azotaemia.
azotation (az·o·**ta**·shun). Absorption of nitrogen from the atmosphere. [Fr. *azote* nitrogen.]
azote (**az**·ote). Nitrogen. [Fr.]
azotenesis (**az**·o·ten·**e′**·sis). Any one of those diseases which are caused by the presence in the body of an excess of nitrogenous substances. [Fr. *azote* nitrogen.]
azothermia (az·o·**ther**·me·ah). An increase in temperature caused by the presence of nitrogenous substances in the blood. [Fr. *azote* nitrogen, Gk *therme* heat.]
azotic (az·**ot**·ik). Pertaining to nitrogen. **Azotic acid.** Nitric acid. *See* ACID. [Fr. *azote* nitrogen.]
azotification (az·ot·if·ik·**a′**·shun). Nitrogen fixation. *See* FIXATION. [Fr. *azote* nitrogen, L *facere* to make.]
azotize (**az**·ot·ize). To combine with nitrogen. [Fr. *azote* nitrogen.]
Azotobacter (**az**·o·to·**bak′**·ter). A genus of aerobic nitrogen-fixing bacteria; they are non-pathogenic. They are soil-inhabiting, but are found also in water. Several species have been separated: the type species is *Azotobacter chroococcum* Beijerinck. [Fr. *azote* nitrogen, bacterium.]
azotometer (az·o·**tom**·et·er). An apparatus for measuring the nitrogen content of compounds in solution, e.g. urea or uric acid in urine. [Fr. *azote* nitrogen, meter.]
azotorrhoea (**az**·o·tor·**e′**·ah). Excessive elimination of nitrogenous material in the faeces or urine. [Fr. *azote* nitrogen, Gk *rhoia* flow.]
azoturia (az·o·**tewr**·e·ah). An excess of nitrogenous compounds or of urea in the urine. [Fr. *azote* nitrogen, urine.]
azoturic (az·o·**tewr**·ik). Referring to azoturia.
azoxybenzene (az·ox·e·**ben′**·zeen). $C_6H_5N{=}O{=}NC_6H_5$. The first stage in the reduction of nitrobenzene: it is in turn reduced to azobenzene. Yellow crystals, insoluble in water but soluble in alcohol or ether.
azoxycompound (az·**ox**·e·**kom′**·pownd). One of the organic aromatic compounds containing the divalent radical $-N{=}O{=}N-$ in which oxygen displays 2 extra valencies. Azoxycompounds are prepared by the reduction of nitro-compounds, and are themselves reduced to the corresponding azo-compounds.
azul (**az**·ewl). Pinta.
azulene (**az**·ew·leen). Any of the series of blue sesquiterpene derivatives which occur in essential oils such as cubebs and wormwood; they are produced by dehydrogenation of azulogens, and appear to contain a 7-carbon ring.
azulin (az·ew·lin). A blue dye formed from corallin and aniline.
azulmin (az·**ul**·min). $C_4H_5N_5O$. A complex compound formed as a brown mass by the decomposition of liquid hydrocyanic acid in the presence of traces of water or ammonia.
azulogen (az·**ew**·lo·jen). One of a family of sesquiterpenes with a 7-carbon ring in their structure; they are dehydrogenated to the blue azulenes of essential oils.
azure (**az**·ewr). General name given to the thionine group of basic dyes which are important stains for chromatin and other basophilic cell constituents. They are closely related to methylene blue. **Azure A.** Dimethyl thionine. **Azure B.** Trimethyl thionine. **Azure C.** Monomethyl thionine. **Azure I.** A Giemsa stain containing azure B. **Azure II.** A Giemsa stain containing azure B and methylene blue. **Methylene azure.** One of the components of polychrome methylene blue, containing azure A and azure B. [OF. *azur.*]
Azuresin (az·ew·**rez**·in). BP Commission approved name for a complex of azure A and an acrylic carboxylic acid cationic-exchange resin. It is used as an indicator in the diagnosis of achlorhydria; when free hydrochloric acid is present in the stomach the blue dye (azure A) in the resin is displaced by hydrogen ions, the displaced dye being excreted in the urine. [azure, resin.]
azurin (**az**·ewr·in). A mixture in molecular proportions of the acetate of theobromine and sodium salicylate, used mainly because of its diuretic properties.
azurophil, azurophile (az·ewr·o·fil, az·**ewr**·o·file). Staining readily with blue aniline dye. [azure, Gk *philein* to love.]
azurophilia (**az**·ewr·o·**fil′**·e·ah). A condition in which there are, in the blood, cells containing azurophil granulations.
azyges (**as**·ij·eez). The sphenoid bone. [Gk unwedded.]
azygography (az·ig·**og**·raf·e, az·i·**gog**·raf·e). Contrast radiography of the vena azygos. [Gk *a*, *zygon* yoke, *graphein* to record.]
azygos (**az**·ig·os, az·**i**·gos). 1. Azygous. 2. A part that is single, not paired. **Azygos lobe.** *See* LOBE. **Azygos vein.** Vena azygos. [Gk *a*, *zygon* yoke.]
azygosperm, azygospore (az·**i**·go·sperm, az·**i**·go·spore). A spore which is formed directly from a gamete and without conjugation. [Gk *a*, *zygon* yoke, *sperma*, *sporos* seed.]
azygous (**az**·ig·us, az·**i**·gus). Applied to anatomical structures which are unpaired. Single. [Gk *a*, zygon yoke.]
azymia (a·**zi**·me·ah). Absence of a ferment. [Gk *a*, *zyme* ferment.]
azymic (a·**zi**·mik). Not caused by or causing fermentation. [see prec.]
azymous (a·**zi**·mus). Unfermented. [Gk *a*, *zyme* ferment.]

B

Babbitt, Isaac (b. 1799). Boston inventor.

Babbitt metal. A soft alloy, principally tin, with variable proportions of copper and antimony; it is sometimes used in dentistry. Its chief use is in bearings because of its low coefficient of friction.

Babcock, Harriett. 20th century American psychologist.

Babcock test. A test designed to estimate intellectual impairment or deterioration. The score on the vocabulary test is considered to be relatively resistant to intellectual impairment, and gives an indication of the subject's intellectual level before the onset of the illness. The present intellectual level or "efficiency" is estimated from scores on a variety of tests (information, rote and non-rote memory, motor speed and learning). The discrepancy between the scores on the vocabulary test and on the efficiency tests gives a measure of intellectual impairment.

Babcock, Maclean Jack (b. 1918). American biochemist.

Babcock's method. For fat in milk and milk products: 17.6 ml of milk at 20°C is pipetted into a special bottle with a graduated neck and 17.5 ml of sulphuric acid (sp. gr. 1.823-1.833) is added slowly with shaking. The flask is centrifuged 5 min, water at 60°C is added to fill the bulb and the liquid centrifuged 2 min. Further water at 60°C is added to bring the level of liquid well up in the neck and the bottle is centrifuged 1 min. The fat percentage is read off after standing the bottle in a water-bath at 55-60°C.

Babcock, William Wayne (b. 1872). Philadelphia surgeon.

Babcock's operation. An operation for removal of varicose veins by subcutaneous stripping.

Babcock's probe. An acorn-tipped probe used in Babcock's operation.

Babès, Victor (b. 1854). Rumanian bacteriologist.

Babès' treatment. Preventive inoculation against rabies by injecting a vaccine, prepared from spinal-cord suspensions attenuated to varying degrees by heating to 80, 60 or 45°C for 10 min.

Babès' tubercle. Rabic tubercle. *See* TUBERCLE.

Babès-Ernst body, corpuscle or granule. Metachromatic granule (*see* GRANULE) seen in *Corynebacterium diphtheriae.*

Babesia (ba·be·ze·ah). A genus of blood-inhabiting parasites infecting certain animals (dogs, horses, cattle and pigs); the parasites are found in the red cells, which they eventually destroy. They are transmitted from animal to animal by certain species of several genera of ticks: *Rhipicephalus, Dermacentor* and *Ixodes.* The genus was previously *Piroplasma.* **Babesia bigemina.** The cause of Texas cattle fever. **Babesia canis.** The cause of piroplasmosis in dogs. **Babesia ovis.** The cause of ovine piroplasmosis. [Victor *Babès.*]

babesiasis, babesiosis (ba·be·zi·as·is, ba·be·ze·o'·sis). Infection with babesia.

Babinski, Josef François Félix (b. 1857). Paris neurologist.

Babinski's law. In vertigo produced by electrical stimulation of the labyrinth, a normal subject falls to the side of the positive pole. In disease of the labyrinth, if advanced, there is no reaction; if less severe, falling occurs towards the side to which the subject inclines normally.

Babinski's phenomenon, or reflex. The extensor plantar response which occurs in pyramidal-tract disease: on stroking the lateral aspect of the sole of the foot there is spontaneous dorsiflexion of the great toe with plantar flexion and "fanning" of the other toes.

Babinski's combined flexion phenomenon. A sign seen in hemiplegia of organic origin: the supine patient attempts, with arms folded across the chest, to rise to the sitting position. There is flexion at the hip joint with raising of the heel on the paralysed side, but the unaffected side remains stationary.

Babinski's sign. 1. The extensor plantar response; usually called the Babinski reflex. 2. Absence of the ankle jerk in sciatica. 3. In organic hemiplegia, during the movements of whistling and blowing, contraction of the platysma is more marked on the unaffected side. 4. Gradual separation of the toes occurs as a result of repeated flexion and extension of the trunk upon the thighs in pyramidal-tract disorders. This sign has, however, been noted in hysteria. 5. Babinski's combined flexion phenomenon (see above). 6. The pronation sign: if an arm affected by spastic paralysis is placed in a position of supination, pronation occurs spontaneously.

pseudo-Babinski sign. In certain cases of poliomyelitis, where all muscles to the foot and toes are paralysed save those extending the great toe, a spurious extensor response may be seen when the plantar reflex is elicited.

Babinski's syndrome. The association of luetic aortic incompetence, and possibly aortic aneurysm, with neurosyphilis.

Babinski-Froehlich syndrome. A term for Froehlich's syndrome; not in general use.

syndrome of Babinski-Nageotte, syndrome of Nageotte-Babinski. Multiple medullary lesions of vascular origin, involving the pyramidal tract, medial fillet, restiform body and reticular structures. Clinically, hypotonia, ataxia, lateropulsion, dyssynergia and Horner's syndrome occur on the side of the lesion, and hemiplegia with loss of tactile discrimination and of proprioceptive sensation on the opposite side.

Babinski-Vaquez syndrome. Babinski's syndrome (see above).

Babinski-Weil test. For labyrinthine disease: with eyes closed, the patient walks first forwards and then backwards. In labyrinthine lesions, the patient staggers towards one side going forwards, and to the other going backwards.

babool, babul (bah·**bool**). The bark of *Acacia arabica* (family Leguminosae), growing in India and Africa. The bark and pods are used in tanning, and as an astringent. [Hind. and Pers.]

baby (**ba**·be). An infant; either a newly-born child, or one not yet walking. **Battered baby.** A condition resulting from the repeated subjection of infants, in their first several years, to violence; characterized by variously dated (successive) surface bruises, fractures of skull, ribs or limbs, brain injury, or deep abdominal trauma, often ruptured liver. First described in 1945-1946 as *Caffey's syndrome.* **Blue baby.** A newly-born child with cyanosis due either to congenital atelectasis or to congenital malformation of the heart. In the latter case there may be imperfect development of the septa between the right and left sides of the heart, or hypertrophy of the right ventricle. It may also result from malformation of the great vessels, dextroposition of the aorta or pulmonary stenosis. The cyanosis is caused by the mixing of blood from both sides of the heart and by the lungs receiving an inadequate amount of blood. **Collodion baby.** Lamellar desquamation of the newborn. It may occur with ichthyosis vulgaris and with erythrodermia ichthyosiforme congenitum. [ME.]

bacciform (**bak**·se·form). Like a berry in shape. [L *bacca* berry, form.]

Bacelli, Guido (b. 1832). Rome physician.

Bacelli's method, or treatment. The treatment of tetanus with subcutaneous or intramuscular injections of 2 per cent carbolic acid.

Bacelli's mixture. A mixture containing quinine sulphate, tartaric acid, sodium arsenate and water, which was used in malarial fevers.

Bacelli's operation. Passage of a wire thread into the sac of an aneurysm to induce coagulation.

Bacelli's sign. Whispered pectoriloquy heard over a pleural effusion.

Bach's reagent. A solution of potassium dichromate, aniline and oxalic acid, used for the detection of hydrogen peroxide; it produces a violet coloration.

Bachman, George William (b. 1890). Panama parasitologist.

Bachman test. An intradermal test for trichiniasis: a 1 per cent solution of a dried powder obtained from the *Trichinella spiralis* is injected intradermally. If trichiniasis is present, a circumscribed red swelling appears after an interval of some days.

Bacillaceae (bas·il·a·se·e). A family of the order Eubacteriales, including the genera *Bacillus* and *Clostridium*, which have in common the characteristics of being rod-shaped, spore-bearing and generally Gram-positive.

bacillaemia (bas·il·e·me·ah). The condition in which bacilli are present in the circulating blood. [bacillus, Gk *haima* blood.]

bacillary, bacillar (bas·il·ar·e, bas·il·ar). Pertaining to, of the nature of, or caused by bacilli.

bacillicidal (bas·il·e·si'·dal). Having a destructive action on bacilli. [bacillus, L *caedere* to kill.]

bacillicide (bas·il·e·side). An agent or drug which is destructive to bacilli. [see prec.]

bacilliculture (bas·il·e·kul·tcher). 1. A culture which contains bacilli. 2. The propagation of bacilli in or on artificial media. [bacillus, L *colere* to cultivate.]

bacilliform (bas·il·e·form). 1. Shaped like a bacillus. 2. Resembling a bacillus in any way.

bacilliparous (bas·il·ip·ar·us). Bacillogenic. [bacillus, L *parere* to produce.]

bacillogenic, bacillogenous (bas·il·o·jen'·ik, bas·il·oj·en·us). 1. Producing bacilli. 2. Of bacillary origin. [bacillus, Gk *genein* to produce.]

bacillophobia (bas·il·o·fo'·be·ah). A state of exaggerated fear of becoming infected by bacilli and other micro-organisms. [bacillus, phobia.]

bacilloscopy (bas·il·os·ko·pe). Microscopical examination of material for the presence of bacilli. [bacillus, Gk *skopein* to watch.]

bacillosis (bas·il·o·sis). A condition in which bacilli (*sensu lato*) have invaded the tissues and in which the reactions amount to a disease. [bacillus, Gk *-osis* condition.]

bacillotherapy (bas·il·o·ther'·ap·e). Bacteriotherapy. [bacillus, therapy.]

bacilluria (bas·il·ewr·e·ah). A condition in which bacilli are present in the urine, and the disease to which the condition gives rise.

Bacillus (bas·il·us). 1. A genus of the family Bacillaceae; Gram-positive, aerobic, spore-bearing, rod-shaped organisms, most species of which are motile. The type species is *Bacillus subtilis.* The non-pathogenic species are ubiquitous in habitat, being found in air, soil and the intestines. Important species are *Bacillus anthracis*, anthrax bacillus, the cause of anthrax and the only pathogenic species in the group, distinguished by its being non-motile; *Bacillus cereus*, a non-pathogenic soil bacillus; *Bacillus megatherium; Bacillus mycoides;* and *Bacillus polymyxa*, the source of the antibiotic polymyxin. 2. Formerly, a generic term for any rod-shaped member of the order Eubacteriales; this term is obsolete and the various species are distributed in other genera. 3. Loosely, as a term for the causal organism of any bacterial infection, particularly where the organism is rod-shaped, e.g. colon bacillus (*Escherichia coli*), comma bacillus (*Vibrio cholerae*), diphtheria bacillus (*Corynebacterium diphtheriae*), tubercle bacillus (*Mycobacterium tuberculosis*), typhoid bacillus (*Salmonella typhi*). **Bacillus abortus.** *Brucella abortus.* **Bacillus acidi-lactici.** *Bacterium coli* var. *acidi lactici.* **Bacillus acidophilus.** *Lactobacillus acidophilus.* **Acne bacillus.** *Corynebacterium acnes.* **Bacillus aerogenes.** *Bacterium aerogenes.* **Bacillus aerogenes capsulatus.** *Clostridium welchii.* **Bacillus aertrycke.** *Salmonella typhimurium.* **Bacillus alkalescens.** *Shigella alkalescens.* **Bacillus alkaligenes.** *Bacterium alkaligenes.* **Bacillus ambiguus.** *Shigella schmitzi.* **Bacillus amylobacter.** *Clostridium butyricum.* **Bacillus asiaticus.** *Bacterium asiaticum.* **Bacillus azotobacter.** *Azotobacter chroococcum.* **Bacillus of blue pus.** *Pseudomonas pyocyanea.* **Bottle bacillus.** *Pityrosporon ovale.* **Bacillus bronchisepticus.** *Haemophilus bronchisepticus.* **Bacillus bulgaricus.** *Lactobacillus bulgaricus.* **Bacillus butyricus.** *Clostridium butyricum.* **Bacillus caucasicus.** *Lactobacillus caucasicus.* **Bacillus ceylonensis.** *Shigella dispar.* **Bacillus cholerae.** *Vibrio cholerae.* **Bacillus cholerae-suis.** *Salmonella cholerae-suis.* **Bacillus cloacae.** *Bacterium cloacae.* **Bacillus coli.** *Bacterium coli.* **Bacillus coli communior.** *Bacterium coli communius.* **Bacillus coli communis.** *Bacterium coli commune.* **Bacillus coli mutabilis.** *Bacterium coli mutabile.* **Comma bacillus.** *Vibrio cholerae.* **Bacillus diphtheriae.** *Corynebacterium diphtheriae.* **Bacillus diphtheriae vitulorum.** *Fusiformis necrophorus.* **Bacillus dispar.** *Shigella dispar.* **Drumstick bacillus.** The tetanus bacillus, *Clostridium tetani*, so called because of the terminal position of the spores. **Bacillus dysenteriae.** *Shigella shigae.* **Bacillus el tor** (cholera-like). El Tor vibrio. *See* VIBRIO. **Bacillus enteritidis.** *Salmonella enteritidis.* **Bacillus enteritidis sporogenes.** *Clostridium sporogenes.* **Bacillus faecalis alkaligenes.** *Bacterium alkaligenes.* **Bacillus fluorescens liquefaciens.** *Pseudomonas fluorescens.* **Bacillus friedländeri.** *Bacterium friedländeri.* **Bacillus gärtner.** *Salmonella enteritidis.* **Bacillus haemolyticus.** *Clostridium haemolyticum.* **Bacillus hofmannii.** *Corynebacterium hofmannii.* **Bacillus icteroides.** *Salmonella typhimurium.* **Bacillus influenzae.** *Haemophilus influenzae.* **Bacillus lactis aerogenes.** *Bacterium aerogenes.* **Bacillus leprae.** *Mycobacterium leprae.* **Bacillus mallei.** *Pfeifferella mallei.* **Bacillus manchester.** *Shigella paradysenteriae.* **Bacillus melitensis.** *Brucella melitensis.* **Bacillus mesentericus.** The potato bacillus, an organism resembling *Bacillus subtilis* (see below) and occurring in faeces, dust, soil, water and milk. **Bacillus moniliformis.** *Actinomyces muris.* **Bacillus muris.** *Actinomyces muris.* **Bacillus necrophorus.** *Fusiformis necrophorus.* **Bacillus oedematiens.** *Clostridium oedematiens.* **Bacillus oedematis maligni.** *Clostridium septicum.* **Bacillus paludis.** *Clostridium welchii.* **Para-influenza bacillus.** *Haemophilus para-influenzae.* **Parapertussis bacillus.** An atypical strain of *Haemophilus pertussis.* **Bacillus parashigae.** *Shigella parashigae.* **Bacillus paratyphosus.** *Salmonella paratyphi.* **Bacillus perfringens.** *Clostridium welchii.* **Bacillus pertussis.** *Haemophilus pertussis.* **Bacillus pestis.** *Pasteurella pestis.* **Bacillus phlegmonis emphysematosae.** *Clostridium welchii.* **Bacillus pneumoniae.** *Bacterium friedländeri.* **Bacillus polymyxa.** A non-pathogen; a source of the antibiotic colistin. **Bacillus polymyxa var. collistinus.** The source of the antibiotic colistin. **Bacillus prodigiosus.** *Chromobacterium prodigiosum.* **Bacillus proteus, Bacillus proteus vulgaris.** *Proteus vulgaris.* **Bacillus pseudomallei.** *Pfeifferella whitmori.* **Bacillus psittacosis.** *Salmonella typhimurium.* **Bacillus pyocyaneus.** *Pseudomonas pyocyanea.* **Bacillus pyogenes.** *Corynebacterium pyogenes.* **Bacillus of rat leprosy.** *Mycobacterium lepraemurium.* **Bacillus schmitzi.** *Shigella schmitzi.* **Bacillus shigae.** *Shigella shigae.* **Bacillus sonnei.** *Shigella sonnei.* **Bacillus stanleyi.** *Salmonella stanleyi.* **Bacillus subtilis.** The hay bacillus, a non-pathogenic organism present in soil, faeces, hay dust, milk and water. **Bacillus tetani.** *Clostridium tetani.* **Bacillus of timothy grass.** *Mycobacterium phlei.* **Bacillus tuberculosis.** *Mycobacterium tuberculosis.* **Bacillus tularensis.** *Brucella tularensis.* **Bacillus typhi.** *Salmonella typhi.* **Bacillus typhimurium.** *Salmonella typhimurium.* **Bacillus typhosus.** *Salmonella typhi.* **Bacillus vaginalis.** *Lactobacillus acidophilus.* **Bacillus violaceus.** *Chromobacterium violaceum.* **Vole bacillus.** *Mycobacterium muris.* **Bacillus vulgaris.** *Proteus vulgaris.* **Bacillus welchii.** *Clostridium* *welchii.* **Bacillus whitmori.** *Pfeifferella whitmori.* **Bacillus xerosis.** *Corynebacterium xerosis.* [L *bacillum* a small rod, staff, or stick.]

See also: AXENFELD, BANG (B. L. F.), BOAS, BORDET, CALMETTE, DANYSZ, DAVAINE, DOEDERLEIN, DUCREY, DUVAL (C. W.), FLEXNER, FRIEDLAENDER, GAERTNER (A.), GENGOU, GUÉRIN (C.), HANSEN, HISS, HOFMANN WELLENHOF, JOHNE, KITASATO, KLEBS, KOCH (R.), KRUSE, LOEFFLER (F. A. J.), MASSOL, MORAX, MORGAN, OPPLER, PFEIFFER (R. F. J.), RUSSELL (F. F.), SCHMITZ, SCHUETZ, SHIGA, SONNE, WEEKS, WELCH (W. H.), WHITMORE.

Bacitracin BP 1968 (bas·e·**tra**·sin). An antibacterial basic polypeptide produced by a strain of *Bacillus subtilis.* It is active against Group A haemolytic streptococci, staphylococci and gas-gangrene organisms, and is employed in ointment form for superficial skin diseases, and in lozenges for septic throat infections.

Bacitracin Zinc BP 1973. A zinc salt of bacitracin, an antibiotic for external application.

back [dorsum (NA)] (bak). The posterior part of the trunk. **Bent back.** Forward angulation of the spine, usually in the dorsal region. **Flat back.** Abnormal straightness of the back; absence of the normal vertebral curves. **Functional back.** Painful back following injury and showing no pathological change. **Hollow back.** Abnormal increase in the lumbar curve, producing a hollow above the sacrum. **Old man's back.** Senile kyphosis. **Poker back.** Ankylosis of the back following certain types of arthritis. **Saddle back.** Lordosis. **Sprung back.** Sprain of the back in which 2 or more of the interspinous ligaments have been damaged. **Static back.** Painful back following postural abnormalities. **Sway back.** Increase in the normal curves of the back. [AS *baec.*]

back-cross (**bak**·kros). In biology, the crossing of a hybrid with one of its parental forms. [AS *baec, cruc.*]

back-flow (**bak**·flo). Flowing on a course the reverse of normal. **Pyelovenous back-flow.** That occurring when the intrapelvic pressure is unduly raised and there is drainage from within the renal pelvis to the venous channels. [AS *baec, flowan.*]

back pointer (bak **poin**·ter). A device for beam direction in radiotherapy in which a pointer defines on the patient the exit point of the central axis of the beam employed. [AS *baec,* L *pungere* to prick.]

back-rest (**bak**·rest). A frame for the support of the back in bed; it can be adjusted to the degree of uprightness required. [AS *baec, raest.*]

backing (**bak**·ing). A strip of metal, usually a gold alloy, to which a facing is attached in the replacement of a missing tooth by a crown, bridge or artificial denture. [AS *baec.*]

Baclofen (bak·**lo**·fen). BP Commission approved name for 4-amino-3-(4-chlorophenyl)butyric acid; a muscle relaxant.

Bacon, Harry Ellicott (b. 1900). Philadelphia proctologist.

Bacon's anoscope. A slit proctoscope carrying an electric bulb within it.

Bacon's operation. Rectosigmoidectomy for cancer of the rectum with conservation of the anus.

bacteraemia (bak·teer·e·me·ah). A condition in which there are bacteria in the circulating blood. [bacterium, Gk *haima* blood.]

Bactereae (bak·teer′·e·e). A tribe of the family Bacteriaceae, which includes the genera *Proteus* and *Bacterium.*

bacteria (bak·**teer**·e·ah). *See* BACTERIUM.

Bacteriaceae (bak·**teer**·e·**a**′·se·e). A family of the order Eubacteriales, which includes Chromobacteriae, Erwineae, Zopfeae, Bactereae, Lactobacilleae, Pasteurelleae and Haemophileae; the genera included are *Chromobacterium, Achromobacterium, Erwinia, Zopfius, Proteus, Bacterium, Lactobacillus, Pasteurella, Haemophilus* and *Brucella.* The only features in common to these genera are that they are non-sporing and rod-shaped. [bacterium.]

bacteriaemia (bak·**teer**·e·e′·me·ah). Bacteraemia.

bacterial (bak·**teer**·e·al). Originating in, derived from, belonging to or consisting of bacteria.

bactericholia (bak·**teer**·e·**ko**′·le·ah). Bacteriocholia.

bactericidal (bak·**teer**·e·**si**′·dal). Effecting the destruction of bacteria; often used in describing the antimicrobial activity of chemotherapeutic substances (*see* BACTERIOSTATIC). [bacterium, L *caedere* to kill.]

bactericide (bak·**teer**·e·side). Any agent, physical, chemical or biological, which kills or destroys bacteria. **Specific bactericide.** A bacteriolysin which has a destructive effect upon a particular species or genus of bacteria. [see prec.]

bactericidin (bak·**teer**·e·**si**′·din). A thermostabile substance in the blood serum which, in conjunction with complement, kills bacteria. [bacterium, L *caedere* to kill.]

bacterid, bacteride (**bak**·teer·id, **bak**·teer·ide). Any rash on the skin which is due, directly or indirectly but usually the latter, to bacterial toxins or to bacteria. **Pustular bacterid, Pustular bacteride.** A chronic pustular eruption of the palms and/or soles in which crops of sterile pustules frequently appear; when the latter rupture, the skin becomes scaly. The malady persists for an indefinite period because of the frequent appearance of the pustules. The condition is believed to be an allergic reaction to a circulatory toxin derived from a focus of bacterial infection.

bacteriform (bak·**teer**·e·form). Like a bacterium in shape.

bacterin, bacterine (**bak**·teer·in, **bak**·teer·een). Bacterial vaccine. *See* VACCINE.

bacterinia (bak·teer·**in**·e·ah). A condition in which the bodily system has reacted unfavourably to bacterial inoculation.

bacterio-agglutinin (bak·**teer**·e·o·ag·**loo**′·tin·in). A specific antibody in the serum, which causes the agglutination of bacteria *in vitro.*

bacteriocholia (bak·**teer**·e·o·**ko**′·le·ah). A condition in which there are bacteria in the bile ducts. [bacterium, Gk *chole* bile.]

bacteriocidin (bak·**teer**·e·o·**si**′·din). Bactericidin.

bacteriocine (bak·**teer**·e·o·seen). Naturally-occurring substances, present particularly in members of the family Enterobacteriaceae, with antimicrobial activity mainly against other strains of the same species although members of another genus may also be attacked; tests using indicator strains are useful in identifying particular strains of a species causing outbreaks of infection, e.g. *Shigella sonnei, Pseudomonas pyocyanea* (*see* COLICINE, PYOCINE). [bacterium, L *caedere* to kill.]

bacterioclasis (bak·**teer**·e·**ok**′·las·is). The breaking up of bacteria into fragments. [bacterium, Gk *klasis* a breaking.]

bacteriofluorescein (bak·**teer**·e·o·floo·or·**es**′·e·in). A fluorescent pigment produced by bacteria belonging to the genus *Pseudomonas.*

bacteriogenic, bacteriogenous (bak·**teer**·e·o·**jen**′·ik, bak·**teer**·e·**oj**′·en·us). 1. Productive of bacteria. 2. Derived from or originating in bacteria. [bacterium, Gk *genein* to produce.]

bacteriohaemagglutinin (bak·**teer**·e·o·he·mag·**loo**′·tin·in). A haemagglutinin produced in the body by bacterial action.

bacteriohaemolysin (bak·**teer**·e·o·he·**mol**′·is·in). A haemolysin which is formed in the body by bacterial action.

bacteriological (bak·**teer**·e·o·**loj**′·ik·al). Referring or belonging to bacteriology.

bacteriologist (bak·**teer**·e·**ol**′·o·jist). One who is expert in the science of bacteriology. The term may be used as being synonymous with *microbiologist.* [Gk *bakterion* small staff, *logos* science.]

bacteriology (bak·**teer**·e·**ol**′·o·je). The science which deals with bacteria, i.e. all organisms falling into the class Schizomycetes. The 5 orders of medical and veterinary interest are the Eubacteriales, Actinomycetales, Spirochaetales, Pseudomonales and Mycoplasmatales. They are all microscopic, and vary in morphology, staining reactions, conditions of growth and metabolic powers. Multiplication is by fission or sporulation. **Hygienic bacteriology.** The bacteriology of environmental conditions in relation to the prevention or spread of infection to man via water, milk, food, sewage and fomites. **Medical bacteriology.** The branch of bacteriology which investigates and identifies the bacteria causing disease in the human body. **Pathological bacteriology.** The branch of bacteriology which deals with the effects produced in the human or animal body by pathogenic bacteria or their toxic products. **Sanitary bacteriology.** Hygienic bacteriology (see above). **Systematic bacteriology.** The study of bacteria from the point of view of identification, classification and ecology. [bacterium, Gk *logos* science.]

bacteriolysant (bak·**teer**·e·**ol**′·is·ant). Any agent which is able to destroy bacteria by dissolving them. [bacterium, Gk *lysis* a loosing.]

bacteriolysin (bak·**teer**·e·**ol**′·is·in). 1. A thermostabile substance in serum, usually an immunoglobulin, which, acting along with non-specific and thermolabile complement, kills bacteria by lysis. 2. Lysozyme. [bacterium, Gk *lysis* a loosing.]

bacteriolysis (bak·**teer**·e·**ol**′·is·is). The destroying of bacteria by dissolution, generally through the action of a specific antibody. [bacterium, Gk *lysis* a loosing.]

bacteriolytic (bak·**teer**·e·o·**lit**′·ik). Pertaining to bacteriolysis.

bacteriolyze (bak·**teer**·e·o·lize). To produce bacteriolysis.

bacterio-opsonic (bak·**teer**·e·o·op·**son**′·ik). Having an opsonic influence on bacteria.

bacterio-opsonin (bak·**teer**·e·o·**op**′·son·in). An opsonin which renders bacteria more susceptible to phagocytosis.

bacteriopathology (bak·**teer**·e·o·path·**ol**′·o·je). Pathology in its bearing upon the toxic action of bacteria in the body.

bacteriopexia, bacteriopexy (bak·**teer**·e·o·**pex**′·e·ah, bak·**teer**·e·o·**pex**′·e). The fixation of bacteria by the action of histiocytes. [bacterium, Gk *pexis* fixation.]

bacteriophage (bak·**teer**·e·o·faje). A virus which can only infect bacteria and which is usually both species- and strain-specific. Growth in susceptible bacteria results in their lysis, with the release of new bacteriophage, and shown by the clearing of a growing broth culture or the appearance of plaques in cultures on solid media. Part or all of the viral nucleic acid may become incorporated into the bacterial nucleic acid (the phenomenon of lysogeny) making the bacterium resistant to the virus. The possession of a lysogenic phage may alter the properties of a bacterium, e.g. toxin production by diphtheria bacilli is due to such a phage. Particular strains of bacteria can be identified by the use of known bacteriophages to lyse them (phage-typing). Their ease of handling and rapid growth cycle have made bacteriophages and their host bacteria useful research tools for virologists, geneticists and biochemists. Bacteriophages are of no use in the treatment of disease. [bacterium, Gk *phagein* to eat.]

bacteriophagia (bak·**teer**·e·o·**fa**′·je·ah). Bacteriophagy.

bacteriophagic (bak·**teer**·e·o·**fa**′·jik). Referring to bacteriophagy.

bacteriophagy (bak·**teer**·e·**of**′·aj·e). Bacteriolysis produced by the action of a bacteriophage on its specific bacterium.

bacteriophobia (bak·**teer**·e·o·**fo**′·be·ah). A condition characterized by morbid fear of bacteria and of micro-organisms in general and their effects on health. [bacterium, phobia.]

bacteriophytoma (bak·**teer**·e·o·fi·**to**′·mah). A neoplasm caused by the presence of bacteria in the tissues. [bacterium, Gk *phyton* plant, *-oma* tumour.]

bacterioprecipitin (bak·**teer**·e·o·pre·**sip**′·it·in). A precipitin developed in the body as the result of bacterial action.

bacterioprotein (bak·**teer**·e·o·**pro**′·te·in). The protein which forms a considerable part of the bacterial body. Several classes of protein can be extracted from the bacterial bodies; all are antigenic, some specific for the bacterial species, others specific for the genus. Variations in the protein make-up of strains within a species enable subdivisions to be made into specific serological types; thus, for example, more than 40 serological types based on specific protein precipitations have been identified among strains of *Streptococcus pyogenes*.

bacteriopsonic (bak·**teer**·e·op·**son**′·ik). Bacterio-opsonic.

bacteriopsonin (bak·**teer**·e·**op**′·son·in). Bacterio-opsonin.

bacteriopurpurin (bak·**teer**·e·o·**per**′·pewr·in). A light-purple colouring matter produced by bacteria of the order Thiobacteriales. [bacterium, L *purpura* purple.]

bacterioscopic (bak·**teer**·e·o·**skop**′·ik). Referring to bacterioscopy.

bacterioscopy (bak·**teer**·e·**os**′·ko·pe). The study of bacteria under a microscope. [bacterium, Gk *skopein* to watch.]

bacteriosis (bak·**teer**·e·**o**′·sis). Any disease caused by bacterial infection and the effects on the system of bacterial toxins. [bacterium, Gk *-osis* condition.]

bacteriosolvent (bak·**teer**·e·o·**sol**′·vent). 1. Any agent with the power to dissolve bacteria. 2. Effecting the dissolution or lysis of bacteria. [bacterium, L *solvere* to dissolve.]

bacteriostasis (bak·**teer**·e·o·**sta**′·sis). Inhibition of the growth or propagation of bacteria without causing their immediate destruction. [bacterium, Gk *stasis* a standing still.]

bacteriostat (bak·**teer**·e·o·stat). Any agent which inhibits the growth or propagation of bacteria. [see foll.]

bacteriostatic (bak·**teer**·e·o·**stat**′·ik). 1. A term applied to various chemotherapeutic substances, e.g. sulphonamides, tetracycline. 2. Inhibiting the growth or propagation of bacteria. [bacterium, Gk *statikos* standing.]

bacteriotherapy (bak·**teer**·e·o·**ther**′·ap·e). A method of treating disease by injection of, or inoculation with, bacteria or the products of bacteria. [bacterium, therapy.]

bacteriotoxaemia (bak·**teer**·e·o·tox·**e**′·me·ah). A condition in which the blood is poisoned by the presence of bacteria. [bacterium, toxaemia.]

bacteriotoxin (bak·**teer**·e·o·**tox**′·in). 1. Any poisonous product of bacteria. 2. Any agent which kills or poisons bacteria. [bacterium, Gk *toxikon* poison.]

bacteriotrope (bak·**teer**·e·o·trope). With affinity for bacteria. [see foll.]

bacteriotropic (bak·**teer**·e·o·**trop**′·ik). Applied to antibodies in the blood which are attracted to, and/or cause changes in, bacteria so that the latter become more vulnerable. [bacterium, Gk *tropos* a turning.]

bacteriotropin (bak·**teer**·e·**ot**′·ro·pin). A heat-resisting opsonin which acts on bacteria, and which assists the phagocytes in their work. Also known as *immune opsonin*. [see prec.]

bacteriotrypsin (bak·**teer**·e·o·**trip**′·sin). One of the enzymes formed by the micro-organism *Vibrio cholerae*. [bacterium, Gk *tripsis* a rubbing.]

bacteritic (bak·ter·**it**·ik). Pertaining to, or caused by bacteria.

Bacterium (bak·**teer**·e·um) (pl. *bacteria*). 1. A term formerly used for a genus within the family Enterobacteriaceae, e.g. *Bacterium coli* (now *Escherichia coli*), or more widely applied to different genera of the same family. 2. In a wider, non-technical sense, any micro-organism within the class of Schizomycetes. 3. Formerly applied to all members of the family Enterobacteriaceae, e.g. *Bacterium typhosum* (*Salmonella typhi*), *Bacterium dysenteriae shigae* (*Shigella shigae*). 4. In a wider and non-technical sense, any micro-organism, microbe or germ, not including, at the one extreme, protozoa or algae, and at the other, viruses or rickettsiae. **Bacterium acidi lactici.** A colon bacillus. **Bacterium aerogenes.** A soil organism. **Bacterium alkaligenes.** A normal bowel commensal, but apparently capable of invading the blood and giving rise to a typhoid-like disease. **Bacterium asiaticum.** A species that may cause a typhoid-like disease in man in the tropics. **Bacterium cloacae.** A soil organism, occasionally found in the faeces of mammals. **Bacterium coli** and its varieties, var. **commune**, var. **communius**, var. **mutabile**, var. **neapolitanum.** The colon bacillus; a gut commensal of man and animals. **Bacterium dysenteriae.** *Shigella shigae.* **Bacterium faecalis alkaligenes.** *Bacterium alkaligenes.* **Bacterium flexneri.** *Shigella flexneri.* **Bacterium friedländeri.** An organism that infects the respiratory and intestinal tracts in man, and causes suppuration in other tissues; also known as *Friedlaender's pneumobacillus.* **Bacterium lactis aerogenes.** *Bacterium aerogenes* (see above). **Bacterium morgani.** *Proteus morgani.* **Bacterium mucosum capsulatum.** *Bacterium friedländeri* (see above). **Bacterium paratyphosum A, B and C.** *Salmonella paratyphi* A, B and C. **Bacterium sonnei.** *Shigella sonnei.* **Bacterium suipestifer.** *Salmonella choleraesuis.* **Bacterium tularense.** *Brucella tularensis.* **Bacterium typhosum.** *Salmonella typhi.* [Gk *bakterion* small staff.]

bacteriuria (bak·teer·e·ewr′·e·ah). A condition in which there are bacteria in the urine.

bacteroid (bak·ter·oid). 1. Having resemblance to bacteria. 2. A bacterium which is of degenerate or modified structure. [bacterium, Gk *eidos* form.]

Bacteroides (bak·ter·oid·eez). A genus in the family Bacteroidaceae, mostly commensals in the mammalian intestine; small, Gram-negative bacilli, non-sporing, non-capsulate, non-motile. Generally anaerobes, some species are pathogenic in man and animals, e.g. *Bacteroides fragilis.* Other pathogenic species belong to the related genera *Fusobacterium, Sphaerophorus* and *Streptobacillus.* [bacterium, Gk *eidos* form.]

bacteroidosis (bak·ter·oid·o′·sis). Infection by bacteroides. The word is not used in the UK, since most organisms of the genus are now placed in the genus *Fusiformis.* [bacteroides, Gk *-osis* condition.]

bacteruria (bak·teer·ewr·e·ah). Bacteriuria.

baculiform (bak·ew·le·form). Rod-shaped. [L *baculum* rod, form.]

Badenoch, Alec William. Contemporary British urologist.

Badenoch's bladder neck spreader. For opening the bladder neck during retropubic prostatectomy; pull-through operation for traumatic stricture of the posterior urethra.

badian (ba·de·an). Star anise, the ripe fruit of *Illicium verum* (family Magnoliaceae). [Pers.]

bael (ba·el). Bael fruit, belae fructus, Bengal quince, the fruit of *Aegle marmelos* (family Rutaceae). *See* BELA. [An Indian name.]

Baelz, Erwin von (b. 1849). German physician.

Baelz's disease. Glandular cheilitis. *See* CHEILITIS.

Baer, Karl Ernst von (b. 1792). Russian embryologist and anatomist.

Baer's cavity. The blastocoele of the early developing embryo.

Baer's law. The early stages in the development of an organ in related species resemble each other more closely than the adult stages.

Baer's membrane. The zona striata of the mature graafian follicle; originally termed the *chorionic membrane.*

Baer's plane. A plane passing through the superior margins of the two zygomatic arches.

Baer's vesicle. The mammalian ovum.

Baer, William Stevenson (b. 1872). Baltimore orthopaedic surgeon.

Baer's method. Injection of oil into a joint to prevent the formation of adhesions.

Baerensprung, Friedrich Wilhelm Felix von (b. 1822). Berlin physician.

Baerensprung's disease, or erythrasma. Tinea cruris.

bag (bag). 1. An apparatus incorporating a pouch. 2. A sac (physiological). **Bolus bags.** Bags partly filled with soft powder or other material which has, for x-rays, scattering and absorption characteristics approximately the same as those for soft tissue. They are used to fill in air spaces between applicator and patient in radiotherapy so as to obtain full back scatter. **Cardiff infant inflating bag.** A small bag, described in 1967, for assisting the respiration of a neonate. **Colostomy bag.** A rubber bag used to cover a colostomy opening and receive bowel contents. **Concertina bag.** A reservoir bag on an anaesthetic apparatus shaped like a concertina. On some machines these bags are self-inflating. **Deodorant bag.** A bag, usually containing charcoal, used to absorb the malodour of wound discharge, especially in osteomyelitis. **Ice bag.** A bag to contain ice, for application to any part of the body to produce local cooling. **Ileostomy bag.** A bag, usually of rubber or plastics, which is secured to the abdomen to collect the discharge from an ileostomy. **Nuclear bag.** The collection of nuclei found at the centre of the intrafusal fibres of a muscle spindle. **Reservoir bag.** A bag from which a patient inhales gases from an anaesthetic machine; formerly called a *rebreathing bag.* **Sarcolemmal bag.** Name given to a mass of phagocytic cells found in necrotic areas of deteriorating striped muscle fibres. **Bag of waters.** The fetal membranes containing the liquor amnii. [AS *baelg.*]

See also: BARNES, BUNYAN, CHAMPETIER DE RIBES, CHAPMAN, HAGNER, KOENIG-RUTZEN, PETERSEN, PILCHER, POLITZER, VOORHEES.

bagassosis (bag·as·o·sis). A hypersensitivity reaction of the respiratory system caused by inhaling the dust of sugar-cane waste contaminated with thermophilic actinomycetes. [Fr. *bagasse* sugar-cane refuse, Gk *-osis* condition.]

Bailey, Henry Hamilton (b. 1894). London surgeon.

Bailey's cannula. A silver cannula with contra-angle and butterfly wings, strapped to the skin in intravenous infusion.

Hamilton Bailey's suprapubic catheter introducer. An angled trocar used for the introduction of the stretched Malecot self-retaining catheter to the bladder after the latter has been exposed suprapubically.

Bailey, Sadie F. Pittsburgh bacteriologist.

Bailey's "hormone" agar, broth or gelatin. A culture medium prepared by dissolving agar or gelatin in water, cooling to 60°C and extracting meat with it (or plain water at 60°C may be used). The product is filtered, peptone is added and it is then sterilized by intermittent steaming or low-pressure autoclaving.

Bailey's flask. A box used in dentistry for making dies and counter-dies.

Baillarger, Jules Gabriel François (b. 1806). French physician.

Baillarger's bands, layers, lines, striae or stripes. Striations on the cerebral cortex consisting of 2 white bands, inner and outer, visible to the naked eye. The outer band, also known as *Gennari's line,* is exceptionally prominent in the occipital lobe.

Baillarger's sign. Inequality of the pupils as found in general paralysis of the insane.

Baillie, Matthew (b. 1761). London physician.

Baillie's pill. A pill containing equal parts of squill, digitalis and blue pill; used in cardiac dropsy.

bain-marie (bahn·mah·re). A utensil on the principle of a double saucepan or water-bath, which is used in the kitchen for preparing food, or in the laboratory for heating drugs and other preparations. [Fr.]

Bainbridge, Francis Arthur (b. 1874). London physiologist.

Bainbridge reflex. Increase in heart rate induced by increase in pressure of the blood in the right auricle. The reflex is mediated through afferent vagal nerve endings in the auricular endocardium and walls of the great veins.

bakankosine (bak·an·ko·seen). $C_{16}H_{23}O_8N$, a non-toxic alkaloidal glucoside isolated from the seeds of *Strychnos vacacona* (*bacacona*).

Baker, William Morrant (b. 1839). London surgeon.

Baker's cyst. A cyst arising from a herniation of synovial membrane from a joint, especially from the knee.

Morrant Baker's disease, Baker-Rosenbach disease. Rosenbach's disease.

BAL (bee·a·el). Dimercaprol BP 1958. [*B*ritish *a*nti-*l*ewisite.]

balance (bal·ans). 1. An instrument for comparing the weights and thus the masses of 2 bodies; a weighing machine. 2. That which is needed to produce equilibrium; the sum or quantity required to make the 2 sides of an account equal. 3. Equality of weight or power. 4. A ratio. 5. The relation of intake to output. **Acid-base balance, Anion-cation balance.** The ratio of acid and basic ions in a tissue or body fluid, resulting in a definite hydrogen-ion concentration. **Calcium balance.** The statement of the calcium intake and output of the body. **Electrolyte balance.** The state of the patient when the plasma electrolytes are within normal limits. **Electromagnetic balance.** A balance depending for its action on electromagnetic induction or the reaction of circuits carrying electric currents. **Fluid balance.** Maintaining body fluids at a normal level. **Heat balance.** Balance between heat loss and heat gain, which is physiologically necessary for the maintenance of normal temperatures. **Nitrogen balance.** The balance between the intake and excretion of nitrogen, which may be positive (with the intake higher than the excretion), negative or in equilibrium (when the intake equals the excretion). **Thermal balance.** The state of a hot body in equilibrium with its surroundings, when at any moment it is emitting as much heat as it is receiving. **Torsion balance.** A balance with which quantitative measurements of electric charges can be made by the use of a fine torsion fibre; also a weighing balance depending for its action on the torsion of a fibre (metal, quartz, etc.), used in micro-analysis. **Water balance.** The statement of the water intake, formation and output of the body, shown as a balance sheet. [L *bilanx* having two scales.]

See also: COULOMB, DU NOÜY.

balaneutics (bal·an·**ew**·tix). Balneology. [L *balneum* bath, Gk *therapeutikos* relating to healing.]

balanic (bal·**an**·ik). Belonging to the glans penis or the glans of the clitoris. [Gk *balanos* gland.]

balanism (**bal**·an·izm). The therapeutic use of suppositories or pessaries. [Gk *balanos* suppository.]

Balanites aegyptiaca (bal·an·i·teez e·**jip**·ti·ak·ah). An African plant, the fruits of which have molluscicidal properties. [Gk *balanites* acorn-shaped, L *Aegyptiacus* Egyptian.]

balanitis (bal·an·**i**·tis). A condition of inflammation of the glans penis, usually of a penis the seat of phimosis, or of the glans of the clitoris. **Ammoniacal balanitis.** A form of infantile balanitis due to the presence of urea-splitting organisms in the preputial sac. **Amoebic balanitis.** An erosive or ulcerative condition of the glans penis caused by *Entamoeba histolytica* and thought to be acquired by anal intercourse with a sufferer from amoebic dysentery. **Circinate balanitis.** A form of balanitis seen in Reiter's (Brodie's) disease. **Diabetic balanitis.** A variety of balanitis due to the sugary condition of the urine in diabetes. **Gangrenous balanitis.** An infection, held to be due to the presence of a spirochaete, which causes rapid ulceration and destruction of the glans penis and may affect all the external genital organs. **Monilial balanitis.** Balanitis caused by *Candida* species. **Phagedic balanitis.** Gangrenous balanitis (see above). **Plasma-cell balanitis.** A benign, chronic balanitis with shiny, moist plaques. Histologically there is an intense plasma cell infiltrate and deposits of haemosiderin. **Pseudo-epitheliomatous balanitis.** A keratosic, micaceous balanitis with pseudo-epitheliomatous changes histologically. It is benign and thought to be secondary to chronic infection. **Trichomonal balanitis.** An erosive balanitis caused by *Trichomonas* species. **Balantis xerotica obliterans.** An atrophic and shrinking process which involves the glans penis and prepuce and is associated with stenosis of the urethral meatus. Because of the sclerosing process, the term *kraurosis penis* has also been used. [Gk *balanos* gland, *-itis* inflammation.]

See also: FOLLMAN.

balanoblenorrhoea (**bal**·an·o·blen·or·**e**′·ah). Inflammation of the glans penis of gonorrhoeal origin. [Gk *balanos* gland, *blennos* mucus, *rhoia* flow.]

balanocele (**bal**·an·o·seel). Protrusion of the glans penis through a ruptured prepuce. [Gk *balanos* gland, *kele* hernia.]

balanochlamyditis (**bal**·an·o·klam·id·**i**′·tis). Inflammation of the glans penis and the prepuce. [Gk *balanos* gland, *chlamys* hood, *-itis* inflammation.]

balanoplasty (**bal**·an·o·**plas**′·te). Any plastic operation carried out on the glans penis. [Gk *balanos* gland, *plassein* to mould.]

balanoposthitis (**bal**·an·o·pos·**thi**′·tis). A condition of inflammation of the glans penis and the prepuce. **Specific gangrenous and ulcerative balanoposthitis.** A condition of acute inflammation of the glans penis and the overlying part of the prepuce; there is generally a copious discharge of offensive pus from the ulcerated surfaces. The condition is due to the presence of a spirochaete and there may be gangrene. It is sometimes referred to as the *fourth venereal disease.* [Gk *balanos* gland, *posthe* foreskin, *-itis* inflammation.]

balanoposthomycosis (**bal**·an·o·**pos**·tho·mi·**ko**′·sis). Gangrenous balanitis. *See* BALANITIS. [Gk *balanos* gland, *posthe* foreskin, *mykes* fungus, *-osis* condition.]

balanopreputial (**bal**·an·o·pre·**pew**′·shal). Belonging to the glans penis and the prepuce. [Gk *balanos* gland, L *praeputium* foreskin.]

balanorrhagia (**bal**·an·o·**ra**′·je·ah). Balanitis, the outstanding sign of which is freely flowing pus; generally of gonorrhoeal origin. [Gk *balanos* gland, *rhegnynai* to gush forth.]

balanorrhoea (**bal**·an·o·**re**′·ah). Balanitis with associated copious discharge of pus. [Gk *balanos* gland, *rhoia* flow.]

balantidiasis, balantidiosis (**bal**·an·tid·**i**′·as·is, **bal**·an·tid·e·**o**′·sis). A form of colitis due to infection by the parasite *Balantidium coli.* It may cause diarrhoea and colic or be asymptomatic. [balantidium, Gk *-osis* condition.]

Balantidium (bal·an·**tid**·e·um). A genus of ciliated protozoa belonging to the class of Ciliophora. The only member pathogenic to man is *Balantidium coli,* causing a disease known as balantidiasis which is characterized by ulceration of the intestinal wall and symptoms of diarrhoea, colitis or dysentery. **Balantidium minuta.** A small variety resembling *Balantidium coli.* [Gk *balantidion* little bag.]

balantidosis (**bal**·an·tid·**o**′·sis). Balantidiasis.

balanus (**bal**·an·us). The glans penis. [Gk *balanos* gland.]

balata (bal·**at**·ah). Coagulated latex of *Manilkara bidentata* (*Mimusops balata*), family Sapotaceae, of South America. It is used similarly to gutta-percha, but is non-elastic, and as a substitute for chicle.

Balbiani, Eduard Gérard (b. 1823). French embryologist.

Balbiani's body, or nucleus. A yolk nucleus of the ovum.

balbuties (bal·**bew**·she·eez). Stammering. [L *balbutire* to stammer.]

baldness (**bawld**·nes). Absence or loss of hair, especially in the region of the head. [ME *balled.*]

Baldwin, James Fairchild (b. 1850). Columbus, Ohio, gynaecologist.

Baldwin's operation. An operation for the treatment of congenital absence of the vagina by transplantation of a loop of ileum between the bladder and the rectum.

Baldy, John Montgomery (b. 1860). Philadelphia gynaecologist.

Baldy's operation, Baldy-Webster operation. A seldom-used operation for correction of retrodisplacement of the uterus. The round ligaments are passed through the perforated broad ligaments and fixed to the posterior surface of the uterus.

Balfour, Donald Church (b. 1882). Rochester, Minnesota, surgeon.

Balfour's operation. Anastomosis of the stomach to the second part of the duodenum for duodenal ulcer.

Balfour's cautery resection. For gastric ulcer: a method of destroying a gastric ulcer by cautery, the defect in the stomach being subsequently repaired.

Balfour, George William (b. 1823). Edinburgh physician.

Balfour's test. For death: flagged pins are inserted vertically into the skin of the precordial area. Any movements of the heart will be transmitted to the pins.

Balfour's treatment. Treatment of syphilitic aneurysms with potassium iodide, which stimulates fibrosis in the wall and contraction of the sac. Further and more effective treatment is now available. *See* WIRING.

Ball, Sir Charles Bent (b. 1851). Dublin surgeon.

Ball's operation. Division of the sensory nerves of the anus for the relief of pruritus ani.

Ball's valves. The anal valves.

ball (bawl). Any globe-like part or mass. **Chondrin ball.** One of the round gristly elastic masses seen in hyaline cartilage, and composed of rounded or slightly angular translucent cells. **Food ball.** Phytobezoar. **Ball of the foot.** The widest part of the foot; it is composed of the heads of the metatarsal bones covered with a thick tough fatty fibrous pad. **Hair ball.** Trichobezoar. **Martial ball.** Balls formerly used in the preparation of chalybeate baths and consisting of 1 part of iron filings to 2 parts of potassium acid tartrate. **Sperm ball.** A globe-shaped clump of spermatozoa. **Ball thrombus.** *See* THROMBUS. **Ball of the thumb.** Thenar eminence. *See* EMINENCE. **Wool ball.** A trichobezoar composed of substances such as fibres of plants and wool. [ME *bal.*]

See also: BICHAT, MARCHI.

ball-valve (**bawl**·valv). A sphere set in a tube so that it permits the passage of fluid in one direction only: a type of valve incorporated in pumps. For its medical applications, *see* ACTION, BALL-VALVE. [ME *bal*, L *valva* leaf of a door.]

Ballance, Sir Charles Alfred (b. 1856). London surgeon.

Koerte-Ballance operation. Hypoglossal-facial-nerve anastomosis. *See* ANASTOMOSIS.

Ballet, Gilbert (b. 1853). Paris physician.

Ballet's disease. Paralysis of the extra-ocular muscles with thyrotoxic exophthalmus.

Ballet's sign. Partial or complete paralysis of one or more extra-ocular muscles without internal ophthalmoplegia.

balling (**bawl**·ing). The forming of boluses or balls, particularly those consisting of masses of nuclear matter in the erythrocytes. [ME *bal*.]

Ballingall, Sir George (b. 1780). Edinburgh surgeon.

Ballingall's disease. Mycetoma.

ballism, ballismus (bal·izm, bal·**iz**·mus). A term which essentially implies choreic movements of jerking or twitching type and which may be exemplified in chorea or paralysis agitans. [Gk *ballismos* a dancing.]

ballistocardiogram (bal·**is**·to·**kar**'·de·o·gram). A record of the body's motion which results from the forces generated by the heart when accelerating blood down the aorta and its branches. [Gk *ballein* to throw, *kardia* heart, *graphein* to record.]

ballistocardiograph (bal·**is**·to·**kar**'·de·o·graf). An instrument for recording the movements of the body which occur in reaction to the beating of the heart and the circulation of the blood; there are a variety of types of instrument used, but in most the subject lies on a suitably suspended platform and the movements of the platform are detected and recorded. [Gk *ballein* to throw, *kardia* heart, *graphein* to record.]

ballistophobia (bal·**is**·to·**fo**'·be·ah). A state of excessive fear of missiles. [Gk *ballein* to throw, phobia.]

ballonnement (bal·on·**mahn**). Ballooning. [Fr. distension.]

balloon (bal·**oon**). 1. To puff out like a balloon; to expand a cavity of the body (e.g. vagina) by means of air or water contained in bags. 2. A short-necked round container made of glass, used in chemical experiments. [Fr. *ballon* ball.]

ballooning (bal·**oon**·ing). Distension of a body cavity with air or a water bag. [see prec.]

ballotable (bal·**ot**·abl). Able to show the phenomenon of ballottement.

ballottement (bal·ot·**mahn**). A technique of clinical examination used in diverse circumstances. The movements of any body, or organ, suspended in fluid of approximately the same specific gravity are detected; usually the impact of the fetus on the fingers when it is displaced in the liquor amnii. **Abdominal ballottement.** Ballottement through the abdominal wall. **Cephalic ballottement.** Ballottement of the head. **Direct ballottement.** Ballottement with a finger in the vagina. **Ballottement of the eye.** Ocular ballottement (see below). **Indirect ballottement.** Ballottement through the abdominal wall. **Ocular ballottement.** Applied to the movements of opacities in the vitreous which occur after the eye has been moved. **Renal ballottement.** A method of palpating the kidney in which one hand is placed anteriorly on the abdominal wall below the ribs and the other hand, placed in the lumbar region, makes quick jerks forward so as to throw the kidney against the hand in front. **Vaginal ballottement.** Ballottement through the vagina. [Fr., a shaking about.]

balm (bahm). 1. Balsam. 2. Commonly applied to any soothing application. 3. A plant of the genus *Melissa.* **Balm of Gilead.** 1. Mecca balsam. 2. The balsam fir, the source of Canada balsam. **Lemon balm.** Balm from *Melissa officinalis* Linn. (family Labiatae), an infusion of which has a lemon-like colour and is employed as a diaphoretic and febrifuge. [Gk *balsamon* balsam.]

balneal (**bal**·ne·al). Relating to baths, particularly medicated baths. [L *balneum* bath.]

balneation (bal·ne·**a**·shun). Balneotherapy.

balneology (bal·ne·**ol**·o·je). The study or the science of the therapeutic use of baths. [L *balneum* bath, Gk *logos* science.]

balneophysiology (**bal**·ne·o·fiz·e·**ol**'·o·je). The study or the science of the effect on the system of taking baths. [L *balneum* bath, physiology.]

balneotechnics (**bal**·ne·o·**tek**'·nix). The practical and technical aspects of balneology. [L *balneum* bath, Gk *techne* art.]

balneotherapeutics (**bal**·ne·o·ther·ap·**ew**'·tix). Balneotherapy.

balneotherapy (**bal**·ne·o·**ther**'·ap·e). The use of baths in the treatment of disease. [L *balneum* bath, therapy.]

balneum (**bal**·ne·um). A bath. **Balneum arenae.** Sand bath. **Balneum calidum.** Hot bath. **Balneum coenosum.** Mud bath. **Balneum frigidum.** Cold bath. **Balneum lacteum.** Milk bath. **Balneum luteum.** Mud bath. **Balneum mariae.** Water bath. **Balneum maris.** Sea-water bath. **Balneum pneumaticum.** Air bath. **Balneum tepidum.** Warm bath. *See also* BATH. [L.]

Baló, Jozsef (b. 1896). Budapest neurologist.

Baló's disease. Demyelinating encephalopathy. *See* ENCEPHALOPATHY.

balsam (**bawl**·sam). 1. Balm; a healing ointment. 2. When used in the strict sense, the term applies to oleoresins containing high proportions of benzoic and cinnamic acids (aromatic balsamic acids), e.g. Peru balsam and Tolu balsam. The name has, however, been applied erroneously to certain other oleoresins, e.g. balsam of copaiba, Canada balsam and gurjun balsam. **Canada balsam.** A resin used to mount preparations on glass slides for microscopic examination. **Balsam of copaiba.** Copaiba BPC 1949. **Friars' balsam.** Compound Benzoin Tincture BP 1958. **Gurjun balsam.** Wood oil, an oleoresin derived from *Dipterocarpus laevis,* a species found in India and China. **Mecca balsam.** Balm of Gilead, an oleoresin obtained from *Balsamodendron opobalsamum,* a species of the Orient. **Peru Balsam BPC 1968, Peruvian balsam, St. Thomas' balsam.** A dark liquid obtained from the trunk of *Myroxylon Pereirae* (family Leguminosae) after the bark has been beaten and scorched. It is used externally as an antiseptic and parasiticide, particularly in scabies. **Tolu Balsam BP 1968, Balsam of Tolu.** A yellow substance obtained from the trunk of *Myroxylon balsamum* (family Leguminosae). It has antiseptic and expectorant properties. **West Indian balsam.** *See* CLUSIA. [Gk *balsamon.*]

balsamic (bawl·**sam**·ik). Having the qualities of balsam; a soothing medicine or application.

Balsamodendron (**bal**·sam·o·**den**'·dron). A genus of amyridaceous trees of the family Burseraceae. **Balsamodendron opobalsamum.** A species which yields Mecca balsam (balm of Gilead). [Gk *balsamon* balsam, *dendron* tree.]

balsamum (**bal**·sam·um). Balsam.

Balser, W. 19th–20th century German physician.

Balser's fatty necrosis. White areas of fat necrosis occurring in the fat of the pancreas, omentum, mesentery, retroperitoneal tissue, etc., in cases of acute haemorrhagic pancreatitis.

Bamberger, Eugen (b. 1858). Vienna physician.

Bamberger-Marie disease. Marie's disease, or syndrome (1st def.).

Bamberger, Heinrich von (b. 1822). Würzburg and Vienna physician.

Bamberger's haematogenic albuminuria. Albuminuria occurring during the later stages of severe anaemia.

Bamberger's area. The area of dullness to percussion near the inferior angle of the left scapula found in cases of pericardial effusion; it is due to collapse of the base of the left lung by pressure from the distended pericardial sac, or to pneumonitis.

Bamberger's disease. Saltatory spasm. *See* SPASM.

Bamberger's bulbar pulse. Pulsation seen in the bulb of the jugular vein in cases of tricuspid insufficiency.

Bamberger's sign. 1. On painful stimulation of an extremity, the sensation is referred to a corresponding point on the opposite side of the body; seen in tabes dorsalis, confusion and a variety of cerebral disorders. Also called *allocheiria.* 2.

Consolidation of the lower lobe of the left lung (Bamberger's area) in a patient with a pericardial effusion.

Bamethan (bam·eth·an). BP Commission approved name for 2-*n*-butylamino-1-*p*-hydroxyphenylethanol; the sulphate is used in the treatment of vascular disorders.

Bamifylline (bam·e·fi·leen). BP Commission approved name for 8 - benzyl - 7 - [2 - (*N* - ethyl - 2 - hydroxyethylamino)ethyl] - theophylline; a bronchodilator.

Bamipine (bam·e·peen). BP Commission approved name for 4-(*N*-benzylanilino)-1-methylpiperidine; an antihistamine.

Bancroft, Joseph (b. 1836). English physician and parasitologist in Australia.

Bancroft's filariasis, Bancroftian filariasis. Filariasis caused by *Wuchereria bancrofti. See* FILARIASIS.

bancroftosis (ban·kroft·o·sis). Infestation with *Wuchereria bancrofti* [Joseph *Bancroft*, Gk *-osis* condition.]

band (band). 1. [Tenia (NA).] Any cord or tape-like strand of tissue which binds or connects other structures together; a stripe or stria seen on the cut surface of an organ. The term is seldom used now in anatomy, having been generally replaced by *ligament, stria, tract* or *bundle.* 2. A fibrosed or peritoneal cord compressing or distorting a hollow viscus. 3. In dentistry, a piece of metal which either partially or completely encircles the crown of a natural tooth. 4. Describing a range of frequencies, generally in the electromagnetic spectrum. **A band.** One of the anisotropic bands of a striated muscle fibre which appears light with the polarizing microscope but dark in stained preparations. **Absorption band.** A region of darkness produced in the spectrum of white light which has passed through an absorbing medium. For solid and liquid absorbers, the absorption bands do not have a distinct edge, and cannot be resolved into a series of lines. **Adjustable band.** A prefabricated anchor band which can be adjusted to the size of a tooth by means of a bolt and nut. **Amniotic band.** A fibrous amniotic band passing from the amnion to the fetus, probably the result of local necrosis of fetal tissues. **Anchor band.** A metal band which is fixed around a tooth to provide anchorage for an orthodontic appliance. **Angiomesenteric band.** A tight band which may occlude the third part of the duodenum where it is crossed by the mesenteric vessels. **Bands of the atlanto-axial joint, longitudinal [fasciculi longitudinales (NA)].** The vertical portion of the cruciate ligament, extending from the back of the body of the axis to the upper surface of the occipital bone in front of the foramen magnum. **Atrioventricular band, Auriculoventricular band.** The atrioventricular bundle; the bundle of His. **Axis band.** An obsolete term for the primitive streak. **Belly band.** An abdominal binder. **Cholecystoduodenal band.** A fold of peritoneum continuous with the right edge of the lesser omentum, passing from the gall bladder to the duodenum or the transverse colon and occluding the first portion of duodenum. **Choroid band of the lateral ventricle.** Taenia chorioidea; a fold of pia mater enclosed in arachnoid mater and lying under the fornix of the cerebral hemisphere. **Clamp band.** A band held in place around a tooth by means of a bolt and nut. **Bands of the colon.** The taeniae coli. **Contoured band.** A band which fits accurately around the surface of a tooth to which it is fitted. **Diagonal band (of Broca).** A superficial tract of nerve fibres immediately behind the anterior perforated space, thought to connect the septal region on the medial side with the amygdaloid nucleus laterally. **Enamel bands.** Epithelial strands connecting the dental lamina to the enamel organs during early development of the teeth. **Episternal band.** Tissue immediately cranial to the embryonic sternum from which the interclavicular ligament is developed. **Feto-amniotic band.** Amniotic band (see above). **Band form.** A polymorphonuclear leucocyte with a banded instead of lobulated nucleus. **Genitomesenteric band.** A band passing from the terminal ileum over the posterior abdominal wall to the inguinal ring and sometimes kinking the lower ileum downward. **H band.** Hensen's line, the transverse light area which can be seen traversing the centre of the A band in stained preparations of striated muscle. It corresponds to the central segment of the myosin filaments of the myofibrils. **Head band.** A band for keeping a head mirror in position. **Hepatoduodenal band.** A fold or band of peritoneum that extends from the gall bladder and cystic duct across the transverse colon and mesocolon. It may compress the duodenum near the hepatic flexure of the colon. Also known as *Harris' band.* **I band.** One of the isotropic bands of a striated muscle fibre which appears dark with the polarizing microscope but light in stained preparations. **Iliotibial band.** The iliotibial tract; the thickening in the fascia lata on the lateral aspect of the thigh, through which the gluteus maximus and tensor fasciae latae gain insertion into the tibia. **Intra-uterine constriction bands.** Grooves around the forearm or the leg, sometimes attributed to amniotic bands. **Moderator band [trabecula septomarginalis (NA)].** A bridge passing across the cavity of the right ventricle of the heart from the interventricular septum to the base of the anterior papillary muscle. It contains, besides cardiac muscle, the major portion of the right branch of the atrioventricular bundle (His) of specialized conducting tissue. Also known as *band of Reil.* **Pecten band.** A ring of fibrosed tissue around the pectinate line of the anus causing rigidity of the anal mucous lining in cases of fissure. **Phonatory bands.** The vocal folds. *See* FOLD. **Retention band.** 1. One of the two fibromuscular ligaments fixing the ends of the mid-gut loop to the posterior abdominal wall during the physiological herniation and rotation of the gut in embryonic development. The proximal band becomes the suspensory ligament of the duodenum (muscle or ligament of Treitz). 2. Any fibrous band retaining an organ in position. **Sternal band.** A paired bar of mesenchyme, precursor of the sternum. **Ulnar band.** One of the bands seen in the early infiltrative stages of acrodermatitis chronica atrophicans, extending from the olecranon to the medial surface of the wrist; it is red in colour, firm or like dough on pressure and may disappear as the skin becomes atrophic. Similar lesions occasionally are seen along the radius, and near the knees or ankles. **Ventricular band.** The false vocal cords; folds of mucous membrane in the larynx above the vocal cords. **Z band.** Krause's membrane of the striated muscle fibre. [ME.]

See also: ANGLE, BAILLARGER, BIETT, BROCA, BUENGNER, CLADO, D'AZYR, GENNARI, GIACOMINI, HARRIS (M. La S.), LANE (W. A.), LEONARDO DA VINCI, LIESGANG, MAISSIAT, MATAS, MECKEL, PARHAM, PRINGLE (S. S.), REIL, REMAK (R.), SCHREGER, SEBILEAU, TARIN.

bandage (ban·dij). A binder, usually made of textile material. It is used for keeping dressings and other appliances in position, for the support or immobilization of an injured limb, or for compression purposes in order to limit the exudation of fluid or the circulation of blood to an area. **Adhesive bandage.** One which is composed of adhesive plaster which, adhering to the skin, forms a protective covering, also immobilizing the part. **Ascia bandage.** The reverse-spiral bandage, the folds of which are supposed to resemble an axe. **Barrel bandage.** A bandage, applied either as a roller or a folded triangular, for the support of an injured jaw. **Capeline bandage.** A bandage to cover the head, usually applied by means of a double-headed roller bandage. **Crêpe bandage.** A bandage of wool or other material with an open weave that makes it stretch easily and subsequently return to its original length. **Elastic bandage.** One made of rubber or elastic crêpe material, used to exert continuous mild pressure on varicosed tissues, swollen or sprained joints, etc. **Figure-of-eight bandage.** A roller bandage which is applied in such a way that the turns resemble the figure 8. **Four-tailed bandage.** An oblong piece of material which is split at both ends. It may be used for the support of an injured jaw, or to retain a dressing on a chin. **Jelly bandage.** A bandage prepared with a mixture of gelatin, glycerin, zinc oxide and phenol solution; it is essentially the same as an Unna's-paste boot. **Many-tailed bandage.** A bandage composed of several strips of material which are sewn together lengthwise, each seam covering two-thirds of the previous strip. It is popular as an abdominal or chest binder. **Plaster bandage.** A bandage made of crinoline which is impregnated with plaster of Paris. Its main purpose is for immobilization and splintage. **Pressure bandage.** One which exerts mild continuous pressure, such as that used in the treatment of varicose veins. **Reverse-spiral bandage.** A roller bandage applied round a limb, each turn being given a half twist on the outer side to make the bandage fit comfortably. **Roller bandage.** A long strip of material rolled from one or both ends. **Spica bandage.** A roller bandage applied as a figure of eight in such a way that the finished bandage resembles an ear of wheat. **Spiral bandage.** A roller bandage applied round a limb, without turns or reverses. **"T" bandage.** A bandage composed of 2 strips of material sewn together to form the letter T. It is used to keep dressings on the perineum. **Triangular bandage.** A three-cornered bandage, usually made from a metre of material cut diagonally. It is used extensively in first-aid work. [Fr. *bande* strip.]

See also: BULLER, DESAULT, ESMARCH.

bandelette (ban·del·et'). *See* GIACOMINI, HOCHE, MAISSIAT. [Fr. small strip.]

banderella (ban·der·el·ah). *See* GIACOMINI. [It. small strip.]

Bandi, Ivo (b. 1867). Naples pathologist.

Bandi and Terni vaccine. A prophylactic vaccine against plague, made from the peritoneal exudate of rats and rabbits inoculated with *Pasteurella pestis.*

bandicoot (ban·de·koot). 1. A marsupial of the family Peramelidae; a reservoir of Q fever. 2. A rodent of India and Sri Lanka of burrowing habits, often common in agricultural land but not in houses. The *lesser bandicoot,* lesser bandicoot-rat or Indian mole-rat, is *Bandicota bengalensis* (including *kok*). The *large bandicoot,* or large bandicoot-rat, is *Bandicota indica.* Both are sometimes put in the genera *Nesokia* or *Gunomys.* They are probable reservoirs of plague and hosts of *Spirillum minus.* [Telugu (India) *pandi-kokku* pig-rat.]

banding (band·ing). In cardiology, the surgical procedure of applying a band around a vessel so as to constrict it in order to reduce the transmission to the vascular tree distal to the band of the pressure developed proximal to it. **Pulmonary arterial banding.** The banding procedure applied to the pulmonary artery, usually in infants with large ventricular septal defects where it is desired to protect the pulmonary vascular bed from developing permanent obstructive changes secondary to the high pressure in the main pulmonary artery. [ME.]

Bandl, Ludwig (b. 1842). Vienna gynaecologist.

Bandl's ring. Retraction ring; Lusk's ring; Schroeder's ring: a ridge formed in labour in the uterus at the junction of the upper and lower uterine segments. It marks the lower border of the active uterine muscle.

Bandl's segment. Lower uterine segment; the thinned-out lower portion of the uterus which forms in labour, probably from the isthmus of the cervix, and may become of paper-like thickness in cases of obstructive labour. It is not active in normal labour.

bandolin (ban·do·lin). A mucilage from quince seeds, used in the manufacture of cosmetics. It has been employed as a substitute for glycerin in this connection. [Fr. *bandeau* headband.]

bane (bane). A poison; a cause of ruin. The word occurs nowadays mostly in combination, e.g. wolfsbane. [AS *bana* murder.]

baneberry (bane·ber·e). The rhizome of *Actaea spicata,* formerly used for skin diseases and asthma, and an adulterant for black hellebore. [AS *bana* murder, berry.]

Bang, Bernhard Laurits Frederik (b. 1848). Copenhagen veterinarian.

Bang's bacillus. *Brucella abortus.*

Bang's disease. Brucellosis; infectious abortion of cattle; abortus fever.

Bang's method. A method that aimed at preventing the spread of bovine tuberculosis in a herd by isolating the infected cows, removing their calves from them after birth and bringing the calves up on the milk of healthy cows.

Bang, Ivar Christian (b. 1869). Lund biochemist.

Bang's method. Tests for the estimation of small quantities of urea, sugar, albumin, etc., in the blood and for the identification of dextrose in urine.

bangue (bang). Bhang.

Banisteria (ban·is·teer·e·ah). A genus of plants of the family Malpighiaceae. **Banisteria caapi.** Yagé, a woody climber of South America; it contains an alkaloid, harmine; also known as *banisterine, telepathine* or *vajeine.* A decoction of the stems is taken by the American Indians and produces hallucinations. Harmine has been used in paralysis agitans.

banisterine (ban·is·ter·een). $C_{13}H_{12}ON_2$. An alkaloid obtained from the South American plant, yagé (*Banisteria caapi*), and most probably identical with harmine. It was formerly used in the treatment of paralysis agitans.

bank (bank). **Blood bank.** A collection of different types of blood withdrawn from human beings and stored for use in transfusions. **Bone bank.** A supply of sterile bone tissue stored for future use in bone grafting. **Skin bank.** Storage of split-skin grafts by a refrigeration technique. [It. *banca* bench.]

Bankart, Arthur Sydney Blundell (b. 1879). London orthopaedic surgeon.

Bankart's shoulder-dislocation operation. An operation for recurrent anterior dislocation of the shoulder: the glenoid limbus and the anterior capsule are reattached to the anterior rim of the glenoid fossa of the scapula.

banko-kerende (bahn·kaw ker·en·de). Ainhum.

Bannerman, Robert George (b. 1891). London pathologist.

Cramer and Bannerman solution. A diluting fluid used in an indirect method for enumerating blood platelets; it consists of sodium citrate (0.2 g), sodium chloride (0.8 g), 1 per cent aqueous solution of brilliant cresyl blue (1 ml), formalin (2 ml) and distilled water to 100 ml.

Bannick, Edwin G. (b. 1896). Rochester, Minnesota, physician.

Hines-Bannick syndrome. Intermittent attacks of intense sweating, combined with low temperature.

Bannister, Henry Martyn (b. 1844). Chicago physician.

Bannister's disease. Angioneurotic oedema. *See* OEDEMA.

bant (bant). Colloquially, to diet. *See* BANTINGISM.

Banti, Guido (b. 1852). Florence physician.

Banti's anaemia, disease or syndrome. A chronic anaemia with slight leukopenia characterized by splenomegaly, cirrhotic hepatomegaly, portal hypertension, haemorrhages from gastric and oesophageal varices, with ascites later. It has also been termed *splenic anaemia, chronic congestive splenomegaly, hepatolienal fibrosis.*

bantingism (ban·ting·izm). The cult of dieting for the treatment of obesity by reduction of food intake in general and particularly carbohydrates and fats. [William *Banting,* 1797–1878, London coffinmaker, who invented the diet.]

Bantu (ban·too). Negro races living in South Africa. **Bantu porphyria.** *See* PORPHYRIA. **Bantu siderosis.** *See* SIDEROSIS.

baobab (ba·o·bab). *Adansonia digitata,* family Bombacaceae. [African name.]

Baptisia (bap·tiz·e·ah). A genus of plants of the family Leguminosae. **Baptisia tinctoria.** Wild indigo root; the dried root contains an alkaloid, glycosides and a purgative substance. It has been used in the form of a decoction as a laxative. [Gk *baptizein* to dip.]

baptisin (bap·tiz·in). A glucoside obtained from wild indigo, the dried root of *Baptisia tinctoria.* It is non-toxic and was formerly used as a laxative and in the treatment of fevers.

Bar, Paul (b. 1853). Paris obstetrician.

Bar's incision. A midline subumbilical incision for caesarean section.

bar (bar). 1. A stout piece of metal, round or oval in form, used in dental prosthetics and orthodontics. 2. A unit of pressure, being a pressure of 100 kPa (kilo pascal), i.e. approximately 1 atm, as used in meteorology; a smaller unit is the millibar, one-thousandth of the above. **Bar of the bladder.** The interureteric bar (see below). **Episternal bar.** One of the paired cartilages from which the lateral parts of the manubrium sterni are derived. **Hyoid bar.** The cartilage of the 2nd visceral arch of the embryo. **Hypochordal bar.** A bar of condensed mesenchyme lying ventral to the primitive vertebral centrum and derived from the inner ends of the costal elements. It chondrifies and ossifies to form the anterior arch of the atlas, and may contribute also to the front of the body of the axis; elsewhere it disappears as a distinct structure. **Interureteric bar.** The ridge of muscle forming the base of the trigone between the two intra-ureteric orifices. In certain cases of vesical neck obstruction, particularly with hyperplasia of the subcervical glands, the hypertrophy of the trigonal muscle is reflected in the undue development of the interureteric bar. The division of this bar should be included when a trigonectomy is performed in the relief of bladder-neck obstruction. **Lingual bar.** A bar fitting on the lingual aspect of the gums to which artificial teeth are attached to provide a partial lower denture. **Median bar.** Contractures of the vesical neck, or constriction of the vesical meatus at its median commissure, caused by a combination of benign prostatic hyperplasia and chronic fibrous prostatitis. In certain cases the contracture may be associated with hypertrophy of the muscular vesical neck, as in achalasia of the vesical neck, and certain types of neurogenic vesical dysfunction. In others, the elevation of the posterior commissure may be associated with shrinkage of the prostate from fibrosis due to chronic inflammation. **Palatal bar.** A bar fitting across the palate to which artificial teeth are attached to provide a partial upper denture. **Sternal bar.** One of the bars of pro-cartilage joining the ventral ends of the ribs of the embryo, from which the sternum is formed. **T bar.** A T-shaped bar used in orthodontics. **Talocalcanean bar.** A congenital bony bar between the talus and calcaneus which is an occasional cause of spastic flat foot. **Terminal bar.** A dark area, visible by light microscopy, at the junction between adjacent cells. Electron microscopy shows that it consists of 3 components which, together, form a junctional complex. **Thyroid bar.** An embryonic cartilage which forms one half of the thyroid cartilage. [OFr. *barre.*]

See also: KINGSLEY, MERCIER, PASSAVANT.

bar reading (bar **reed**·ing). The placing of a vertical bar between the patient's eyes and the book. This will obstruct the vision of first one, then the other eye, if the head is kept stationary. Uninterrupted reading can be carried out only in the presence of good binocular vision.

Barach, Alvan Leroy (b. 1895). New York physician.

Barach's index. Systolic and diastolic pressures are added and multiplied by the pulse rate. Normal figures are said to lie between 13 000 and 20 000.

baraesthesia (bar·es·**the**·ze·ah). The faculty of appreciating weight or pressure. [Gk *baros* weight, aesthesia.]

baraesthesiometer (bar·es·the·ze·**om**'·et·er). An instrument with which sensitivity to weight or pressure can be estimated. [Gk *baros* weight, aesthesiometer.]

baraesthesiometric (bar·es·**the**·ze·o·**met**'·rik). Referring or belonging to a baraesthesiometer.

baragnosis (bar·ag·**no**·sis). Abarognosis; lack of power of recognizing weight; absence of weight sense. [Gk *baros* weight, agnosia.]

baralyme (ba·rah·lime). A mixture of barium and calcium hydroxides used to absorb carbon dioxide in anaesthetic circuits. [Gk *barys* heavy, AS *lim* lime.]

Bárány, Robert (b. 1876). Vienna otologist.

Bárány's drum. A striped rotating drum used to elicit optokinetic nystagmus.

Bárány noise box. A device invented by Bárány for producing noise of high intensity. It consists of a clockwork machine which actuates the noise-producing mechanism. The whole is contained within a small, usually metal, case, and the instrument fits comfortably into one hand. When held close to one ear the noise produced makes it impossible for other sounds to be appreciated by the ear. It is, therefore, a form of masking device. It is used to put one ear completely out of action in certain hearing tests.

Bárány's sign. Absence of nystagmus after thermic stimulation of the labyrinth suggests disease.

Bárány's caloric (or water) test. One ear is douched with water at room temperature with the head at an angle of 30 degrees forward. The onset of rotating nystagmus (away from the irrigated ear) is timed from the beginning of the douche. It is delayed beyond 30 s (normal) when there are granulations or a polypus, and it is absent when the labyrinth is not reacting. If the head is then put 120 degrees backward, the rotating nystagmus should change to a horizontal.

Bárány's chair test. A test used in the examination of candidates for the air service. The nystagmus rate and reaction of pulse and blood pressures are tested as follows: the turning chair must have a head-rest which will hold the head 30 degrees forward, a foot rest and a stop pedal: the head is 30 degrees forward so that the tragus of the ear is on a horizontal line with the external canthus of the eye. The examinee is then asked to fix his eyes on a distant point and the chair is turned slowly from side to side in order to note whether or not spontaneous nystagmus is present. Then the examinee is rotated to the right, eyes closed, 10 times in exactly 20 s. The instant the chair is stopped the stop-watch is clicked: the examinee opens his eyes and looks straight ahead at some distant point. There should occur a horizontal nystagmus to the left of 26 s duration. The examinee then closes his eyes and is rotated to the left; there should occur a horizontal nystagmus to the right of 26 s duration. Before the rotation described above, and after the candidate is seated in the chair, the sitting pulse and blood pressures are taken. They are taken again after rotation ceases. For the vestibular tests a nystagmus of 10–34 s should qualify, provided it is approximately the same duration in the two directions. Any variation in the two directions of more than 5 s should disqualify. A marked increase in systolic blood pressure, or fall in diastolic blood pressure, after rotation should also disqualify.

Bárány's pointing test. A clinical test for cerebellar lesions: the patient points at a fixed object and then closes his eyes; he is now asked to move the limb in a given plane and then to return it to its original position. Constant failure of the limb to return to its former site is indicative of a unilateral cerebellar lesion and is most evident when movement takes place in the vertical plane; in this case the arm deviates laterally to the side of the lesion.

barasheh (bar·**ash**·a). Burning feet.

Barasty, P. 20th century French surgeon.

Duval–Barasty operation. Splitting of the sternum and incision of the diaphragm to explore the pericardium.

barb (barb). One of the sharp projections from the surface of a metal broach, used for removing the pulp from a tooth. [L *barba* beard.]

barbaloin (barb·**al**·o·in). $C_{20}H_{20}O_8$. The particular aloin obtained from Barbados aloes (Curacao aloes). It hydrolyses into aloe-emodinanthranol and D-arabinose.

barbaralalia (bar·bar·al·a'·le·ah). An impaired form of utterance present in the speaking of a foreign language because the external organs of speech lack training in the production of the required sounds. [Gk *barbaros* strange, *lalein* to babble like a child.]

barbasco (bar·**bas**·ko). Lonchocarpus.

Barber, Harold Wordsworth (b. 1886). London dermatologist.

Barber's seborrhoeic state. The condition of a person constitutionally subject to seborrhoea who is either fair-complexioned, flushed, active and later plethoric, or dark, coarse-skinned, pallid and indolent, with diffuse hypertrophy of the horny layer of the skin and enlarged pilosebaceous follicles exuding inspissated sebum when pressed.

barberry (**bar**·ber·e). The dried bark of *Berberis vulgaris* (family Berberidaceae), a shrub indigenous to Great Britain. It contains alkaloids, one of which is the yellow crystalline berberine; a bitter tonic. [L *berberis*.]

barbiero (bar·be·a·ro). A name given by the people of Brazil to the bug *Panstrongylus megistus*, which transmits human trypanosomiasis, because the insect often bites the face (beard). [L *barba* beard.]

barbiers (bar·be·a). A paralysis of nervous origin which occurs commonly in India and the island of Réunion. [Eastern Indian.]

barbital (bar·bit·al). The name given to barbitone in the *United States Pharmacopeia*; also synonym for Barbitone BP 1953. **Barbital poisoning.** *See* POISONING, BARBITURATE. **Barbital sodium.** Barbitone Sodium BP 1958.

barbitalism (bar·bit·al·izm). Barbiturism.

barbitone (bar·bit·one). Diethylbarbituric acid, $(C_2H_5)_2=C(CONH)_2CO$. A colourless, odourless, crystalline compound used as a hypnotic (BP 1953). **Barbitone Sodium BP 1973, Soluble barbitone.** The sodium salt of barbitone, which is more soluble and therefore more rapid in action. [see foll.]

barbiturate (bar·bit·ewr·ate). Name given to derivatives of barbituric acid, having the general formula $R_1R_2C=(CONH)_2=CO$, where R_1 and R_2 are organic alphyl radicals. A large number of these have been prepared, varying in strength and duration of action; amongst them are barbitone, phenobarbitone, pentobarbitone and thiopentone. They are effective sedatives and hypnotics, used in insomnia, neurasthenia, hysteria, hyperthyroidism and chorea, and in mental disturbances and all states where depression of the nervous system is desirable. Their analgesic effect is weak. Overdosage is treated by correction of respiratory difficulty, washing out of stomach contents, dialysis and general nursing care, while prolonged administration may lead to habituation and dependence. **Barbiturate poisoning.** *See* POISONING.

barbiturism (bar·bit·ewr·izm). A condition resulting from the ingestion of barbiturates or their derivatives. There is a dermatitis with heightened temperature, headache, and chills.

barbotage (bar·bo·tahzh). In the giving of spinal analgesia, the method of aspirating the cerebrospinal fluid, mixing it with the local analgesic drug, reinjecting and reaspirating several times in an effort to produce a high block. [Fr., dabbling in water.]

barbula hirsi (bar·bew·lah her·se). The hairs which are present on the antitragus, the tragus and the incisura intertragica of the external ear. [L goat's beard.]

Barclay, Alfred Ernest (b. 1876). Manchester radiologist.

Barclay's niche. In radiology, a direct sign of duodenal ulcer: it consists of the protrusion of contrast medium into the ulcer crater.

Barcroft, Sir Joseph (b. 1872). Cambridge physiologist.

Barcroft's apparatus. An apparatus for determining the oxygen and/or carbon dioxide content of blood.

Bard, Louis (b. 1857). Lyons and Strasbourg anatomist, pathologist and physician.

Bard-Parker knife. A knife with a metal handle and detachable renewable blades.

Bard-Pic syndrome. Progressive jaundice with enlargement of the gall bladder and cachexia, due to carcinoma of the head of the pancreas.

bardana (bar·da·nah). Burdock; the root of *Arctium lappa*.

Bardeen, Charles Russell (b. 1871). American anatomist.

Bardeen's primitive disc. The embryonic intervertebral disc.

Bardenheuer, Bernard (b. 1839). German surgeon.

Bardenheuer's extension. Extension (traction) method for the treatment of limb fractures.

Bardenheuer's operation. Interilio-abdominal amputation.

Bardinet, Barthélemy Alphonse (b. 1809). Limoges physician.

Bardinet's ligament. The deep portions of the medial ligament of the elbow joint, supposed by Bardinet to prevent separation of fragments after a transverse fracture of the olecranon.

baregine (bar·e·jeen). Glairin. These terms refer to the gelatinous masses derived from bacteria which are found in sulphurous spas. They are formed by moulds and other lowly vegetable growths (*Beggiatoa alba, Thiothrix linea, Byssus langinosa*) which grow in certain sulphurous waters, and by their coalescence produce jelly-like masses that are used as local applications. [*Barèges*, a Pyrenean spa.]

Baréty, Jean Paul (b. 1887). French surgeon.

Baréty's method. A method of traction used in the treatment of hip disease.

Barfoed, Christen Thomsen (b. 1815). Swedish physician.

Barfoed's reagent. For the detection of monosaccharides: dissolve 13.3 g of crystalline neutral copper acetate in 200 ml of 1 per cent acetic acid.

Barfoed's test. Monosaccharide test: to 5 ml of Barfoed's reagent add 0.5 ml of solution and boil. A red precipitate of cuprous oxide is formed if a monosaccharide is present.

Bargen, Jacob Arnold (b. 1894). Rochester, Minnesota, physician.

Bargen's serum. A serum prepared by inoculating horses with a diplococcus which was thought to be a cause of ulcerative colitis.

Bargen's treatment. The treatment of ulcerative colitis with Bargen's serum.

baric (ba·rik). 1. Referring or belonging to barium. 2. Pertaining to weight, especially that of the atmosphere. [Gk *baros* weight.]

baricity (bar·is·it·e). A term used to describe the specific gravity of a local analgesic solution in relation to that of cerebrospinal fluid when it is injected into the intradural space to produce spinal analgesia. [Gk *baros* weight.]

Barii Sulfas. *European Pharmacopoeia* name for Barium Sulphate BP 1973.

Barilla (bar·il·ah). 1. Originally the name for a species of *Salsola* growing on the Mediterranean shore. 2. Term extended to denote the impure sodium carbonate obtained by burning seaweeds and kelps; used to make soap. [Sp.]

barite (bar·ite). Barytes, heavy spar, $BaSO_4$. A natural barium sulphate used as a filler for paper and in paint manufacture. [Gk *barys* heavy.]

baritosis (bar·it·o·sis). Barytosis.

barium (ba·re·um). An element of the alkaline earth group, with atomic weight 137.36, atomic number 56 and chemical symbol Ba. It is a silvery metal, soft and malleable, which tarnishes readily in air. It occurs naturally in barytes as the sulphate, $BaSO_4$, and has been detected in foraminifera and in certain plants. The salts, especially the soluble ones, are highly poisonous and for this reason are now little used in medicine. The barium ion increases the tone of plain muscle, increases cardiac contractions and prolongs the contraction of voluntary muscle. **Barium acetate.** $(CH_3COO)_2Ba$, a soluble compound used in analysis as a reagent. **Barium aluminate.** $Ba(AlO_2)_2$, a compound used as a water softener. **Barium arsenate.** $Ba_3(AsO_4)_2$, an insoluble black compound formerly used in the treatment of skin diseases. **Barium bromide.** $BaBr_2$, a compound formerly used as a cardiac tonic, but too toxic to find general use in medicine. **Barium carbonate.** $BaCO_3$, a white compound employed in the manufacture of rat poisons, in sugar refining and in water sterilizing. **Barium chloride.** $BaCl_2$, the most important soluble salt; it is highly toxic and stimulates all muscle. It has been used in the treatment of heart block, but is too poisonous for common use. **Barium dioxide.** Barium peroxide (see below). **Barium hydrate, Barium hydroxide.** $Ba(OH)_2$, a soluble crystalline compound used as a reagent, and in the refining of oils and sugar. **Barium iodide.** BaI_2, a compound used at one time in medicine for the same purpose as potassium iodide, but found to be too poisonous. **Barium oxide.** BaO, a basic oxide formed by heating barium carbonate. **Barium peroxide.** BaO_2, an amorphous compound employed as a bleach for plant and animal tissue. **Barium platinocyanide.** $BaPt(CN)_4{\cdot}4H_2O$, a crystalline yellow compound formerly used in the manufacture of fluorescent screens. When excited by x-rays it emits a green fluorescence. **Barium Sulphate BP 1973.** $BaSO_4$, a white compound insoluble in water and opaque to x-rays, for which reason it is administered as a meal or by enema for the examination of the alimentary tract. **Barium sulphide.** BaS, used in the pure form or mixed with barium sulphate as a depilatory paste; it may irritate the skin. [Gk *barys* heavy.]

bariumize (ba·re·um·ize). 1. To add barium to, as in a diet, or for a test-meal. 2. To use barium in treatment.

bark (bark). In pharmacognosy, the tissues of a stem or root external to the cambium, and containing some or all of the following tissues; periderm, cortex, primary and secondary phloem. In the preparation of barks the outer tissues are sometimes removed, e.g. cinnamon and quillaia barks. Medicinally important barks are: cascara sagrada, cinchona, cinnamon and quillaia. [of Scandinavian origin.]

Barkan, Otto (b. 1887). San Francisco ophthalmologist.

Barkan's operation. Goniotomy; most useful in infantile glaucoma. The trabeculae at the angle of the anterior chamber are incised under direct vision through a contact lens with a knife-needle or Barkan's goniotomy knife, and Schlemm's canal is opened.

Barker, Arthur Edward James (b. 1850). London surgeon.

Barker spinal needle. A stiff wide-bore needle with stilette, for thecal puncture; it is no longer popular.

Barker's operation. 1. Excision of the hip by an anterior approach. 2. Excision of the astragalus by an anterolateral incision.

Barker's point. A point 32 mm (1¼ in) above and 32 mm (1¼ in) behind the middle of the external auditory meatus. It is the traditional site for tapping a temporosphenoidal abscess.

Barker's solution. 5 per cent amylocaine hydrochloride and 5 per cent glucose, used for spinal analgesia.

Barker, Samuel Booth. 20th century Tennessee physiologist.

Summerson-Barker method. For lactic acid in blood: protein-free blood filtrate is treated with copper sulphate solution and powdered calcium hydroxide to remove interfering substances. An aliquot of filtrate is heated with concentrated sulphuric acid to convert lactic acid to acetaldehyde and the latter is determined colorimetrically with *p*-hydroxydiphenyl.

Barkman, Ake. 20th century Swedish physician.

Barkman's reflex. Contraction of the homolateral rectus abdominis muscle on pinching or scratching the skin beneath the nipple.

Barkow, Hans Karl Leopold (b. 1798). Breslau anatomist.

Barkow's ligament. Vertical ligamentous strands passing through the fatty pad of the olecranon fossa.

barley (bar·le). The well-known cereal belonging to the order Gramineae, grown in Great Britain and many other parts. The varieties *Hordeum vulgare* and *Hordeum distichon* are chiefly associated with manufactured foodstuffs and with preparation of malt used in brewing and distilling. Several preparations are made. *Pearl barley* is barley the grains of which have been decorticated and polished, fitting them for use in domestic cookery (soups, puddings). **Decoction of barley, Barley water.** A decoction made by adding to 1 litre of water 60 g pearl barley, boiling and straining; or it can be made from "patent barley", a prepared barley flour. The use of barley water as a beverage is a convenient way of increasing the fluid intake, and it has sometimes been recommended as a demulcent drink, e.g. when the gastro-intestinal tract is inflamed. The germ of barley is a good source of vitamin B_1. [AS *baerlic*.]

Barlow, Donald. 20th century British surgeon.

Barlow belt. A belt easily secured round the lower rib cage to facilitate coughing and deep breathing in the postoperative period. Described in 1964.

Barlow, Sir Thomas (b. 1845). London physician.

Barlow's disease. Infantile scurvy. *See* SCURVY.

Barlow, Thomas Geoffrey. 20th century British orthopaedic surgeon.

Barlow's splint. A device used in the early treatment of congenital dislocation of the hip.

barm (barm). Yeast. [ME *berme*.]

barn (barn). A unit of cross section $= 10^{-28}$ m^2, used as a measure of the probability of nuclear reactions.

Barnes, Robert (b. 1817). London obstetrician.

Barnes' bag, or dilator. A rubber bag filled with water, introduced into the cervix to induce labour by dilating the cervix.

baro-agnosis (bar·o·ag·no'·sis). Abarognosis; lack of power of recognizing weight; absence of weight sense. [Gk *baros* weight, *a*, *gnosis* knowledge.]

baroceptor (bar·o·sep·tor). Pressure receptor. *See* RECEPTOR. [Gk *baros* weight, L *recipere* to receive.]

baro-electro-aesthesiometer (bar·o·el·ek·tro·es·the·ze·om'·et·er). An instrument which, when electric sensitivity to pain or prickling is present, can measure the amount of pressure felt. [Gk *baros* weight, electric, aesthesiometer.]

barognosis (bar·og·no·sis). Knowledge or instinct of weight. [Gk *baros* weight, *gnosis* knowledge.]

barograph (bar·o·graf). An apparatus on which pressure changes shown by a barometer can be recorded. [Gk *baros* weight, *graphein* to record.]

baromacrometer (bar·o·mak·rom'·et·er). An instrument with which newly-born infants can be weighed and measured. [Gk *baros* weight, *makros* long, meter.]

barometer (bar·om·et·er). An instrument with which the atmospheric pressure can be measured. **Aneroid barometer.** A portable barometer in which changes of atmospheric pressure cause alterations in thickness of a flat cylindrical evacuated metal box, such alterations being magnified mechanically and causing rotation of a pointer on a scale. **Boiling-point barometer.** A barometer in which observation of the boiling point of water enables the atmospheric pressure to be determined. **Mercury barometer.** A barometer in which atmospheric pressure is measured by the height of a column of mercury, in a sealed tube, which is supported by the pressure. **Plague barometer.** A method used in the prevention of the spread of plague during an epidemic. A watch is kept on guinea-pigs or similar animals, placed in a house for the purpose, and when one dies it is examined for plague; should it be found to have the infection, local prophylaxis against plague is carried out. [Gk *baros* weight, meter.]

barometrograph (bar·o·met·ro·graf). Barograph.

baroreceptors (bar·o·re·sep·torz). Receptors found in the carotid sinus and aortic arch which respond to changes in systemic blood pressure. They form with the vagus nerve the afferent part of a reflex pathway which tends to maintain a stable blood pressure, and respond to distortive forces rather than simply changes in pressure. [Gk *baros* weight, L *recipere* to receive.]

baroscope (bar·os·kope). 1. An instrument which registers changes in the density of the air. 2. A form of balance the beam of which supports 2 balls of very unequal size which balance one another in air but not when the instrument is enclosed in a vacuum or is surrounded by a gas other than air, thus illustrating the principle of Archimedes. [Gk *baros* weight, *skopein* to view.]

barosinusitis (bar·o·si·nus·i'·tis). An inflammatory condition of one or more of the nasal sinuses brought on by changes in barometric pressure; change of volume of air in a sinus with a blocked outlet causes pain and inflammation. [Gk *baros* weight, L *sinus* curve, Gk *-itis* inflammation.]

Barosma (bar·oz·mah). A genus of plants of the family Rutaceae, several species of which yield buchu. [Gk *barys* heavy, *osme* smell.]

barosmin (bar·oz·min). 1. A substance with a diuretic action prepared from the leaves of *Barosma betulina* (buchu), a shrub occurring in South Africa. 2. A rhamnoside, $C_{34}H_{44}O_{21}$, obtained from buchu leaves. [see prec.]

barospirator (bar·o·spi·ra·tor). An apparatus, such as the Drinker respirator, used in artificial respiration. It produces variations in the pressure of air in a closed chamber and thus induces respiration. [Gk *baros* weight, L *spirare* to breathe.]

barotalgia (bar·ot·al·je·ah). Barotitis. [Gk *baros* weight, *algos* pain.]

barotaxis (bar·o·tax·is). The stimulating of living cells by alterations in the pressure under which they exist. [Gk *baros* weight, *taxis* arrangement.]

barotitis (bar·ot·i·tis). Inflammation of the middle ear caused by change in atmospheric pressure. A malfunctioning pharyngo-tympanic tube may trap air in the middle ear; change in volume of the trapped air distorts the tympanic membrane and causes inflammation. [Gk *baros* weight, *-itis* inflammation.]

barotrauma (bar·o·traw·mah). Disturbance of function due to difference of barometric pressure on 2 surfaces of vital organs; it includes *barosinusitis, barotitis* and *bends.* **Otic barotrauma, Otitic barotrauma.** Barotitis. **Sinus barotrauma.** Barosinusitis. [Gk *baros* weight, *trauma* wound.]

barotropism (bar·ot·ro·pizm). Barotaxis. [Gk *baros* weight, *tropos* a turning.]

Barr, Murray Llewellyn (b. 1908). Canadian anatomist and cytologist.

Barr body. Planoconvex, spherical or pyramidal chromocentra visible in the interphase nuclei of most mammalian females. This chromocentra is frequently situated at the periphery of the nucleus and is formed by one, or part of one, condensed (heteropyknotic) X chromosome. In man, the whole of one X chromosome appears to take part in the formation of the Barr body and the following relationship exists between the number of autosomal sets (*A*), X chromosomes (*X*), and the maximum number of Barr bodies visible in the cells of an individual (*B*): $B = X - (A/2)$.

barracuda, barracouta (bar·ah·kewt·ah). A pike-like fish, *Spirometra houghtoni,* that is poisonous when eaten in certain seasons. [Sp.]

Barraquer, Ignacio (b. 1884). Barcelona ophthalmologist.

Barraquer's method, or operation. Of cataract extraction: the extraction of the crystalline lens of the eye, within its capsule, by means of an erisiphake which grips the capsule by suction. It is useful in cases when forceps will not grip the capsule.

Barraquer, José Antonio (b. 1852). Barcelona physician.

Barraquer's disease. Lipodystrophia progressiva.

Barraquer-Simons disease. Partial lipo-atrophy.

Barré, Jean Alexander (b. 1880). Strasbourg neurologist.

Barré's sign. Retardation of reflex pupillary constriction in mental deterioration; obsolete.

Barré's pyramidal sign. A patient lying in the prone position is unable to hold the legs flexed at the knee joints to an angle of 90 degrees if there is disease of the pyramidal tract; a sign of flexor weakness.

Barré-Guillain syndrome, Guillain-Barré syndrome. Acute infective polyneuritis. After non-specific infection, demyelination in spinal roots and peripheral nerves leads to the rapid onset of generalized weakness or paralysis, often ascending to the facial muscles and sometimes causing respiratory paralysis. Tendon reflexes are absent but sensory changes are slight. The cerebrospinal fluid protein is increased with no increase in cells. The prognosis is generally good. Also called acute *polyradiculoneuropathy.*

Landry-Guillain-Barré syndrome. A name adopted for the conditions previously known as *Landry's ascending paralysis* and the *Guillain-Barré syndrome,* which are now recognized as clinically and pathologically identical.

Barrett, Norman Rupert. 20th century London surgeon.

Barrett's ulcer. An ulcer in the lower end of the oesophagus which is lined with gastric mucous membrane, usually associated with hiatus hernia and often stricture.

Barrier, François Marguerite (b. 1813). Lyons physician.

Barrier's vacuole. A peribronchial abscess.

barrier (bar·e·ah). An impediment or obstacle. **Blood-brain barrier.** Some toxins, bacteria, vital dyes and other substances, do not pass through the endothelium of capillaries into direct contact with tissues of the central nervous system as readily as they pass through the capillary endothelium in other tissues: the capillary endothelium in the central nervous system is therefore presumed to constitute a protective "blood-brain barrier". **Blood-liquor barrier.** A term sometimes used to indicate that similar conditions apply between the blood stream and the cerebrospinal fluid. **Fission barrier.** The energy deficit in an atomic nucleus which has to be made good before fission becomes probable. **Haemato-encephalic barrier.** Blood-brain barrier (see above). **Placental barrier.** The epithelial layer of the placenta which prevents the mingling of the fetal and maternal bloods. **Protective barrier.** In radiology, material used for absorbing ionizing radiation for protective purposes. [ME *barrere.*]

Barry, Martin (b. 1802). English physiologist.

Barry's retinacula. Filamentous strands within the graafian follicle.

Barth, Jean Baptiste, Snr (b. 1806). Strasbourg physician.

Barth's hernia. Hernia of the intestine between the abdominal wall and a persistent vitelline duct.

Barthélemy, P. Toussaint (b. 1850). French dermatologist.

Barthélemy's disease. 1. Acnitis. 2. Folliclis.

Bartholin, Caspar, Jnr (b. 1655). Copenhagen anatomist.

Bartholin's abscess, Bartholinian abscess. An abscess forming in Bartholin's gland or duct.

ducts of Bartholin. Sublingual ducts. *See* DUCT.

Bartholin's gland. 1. A gland lying in the substance of the labium majus at the junction of its middle and lower third and 6 mm in diameter with a duct opening into the side of the vestibule. 2. Sublingual gland. *See* GLAND.

Bartholin, Thomas (b. 1616). Copenhagen physician and anatomist.

Bartholin's anus. The commencement of the aqueduct of the mid-brain in the 3rd ventricle.

Bartholin's foramen. The obturator foramen. *See* FORAMEN.

bartholinitis (bar·to·lin·i′·tis). Inflammation of the greater vestibular (Bartholin's) glands. [Caspar *Bartholin,* Jnr, Gk *-itis* inflammation.]

Barton, John Rhea (b. 1794). Philadelphia surgeon.

Barton's fracture. Fracture of the dorsal articular margin of the lower end of the radius with backward displacement of the wrist.

Barton's operation. A method of producing a pseudarthrosis by excision of bone.

Bartonella (bar·ton·el·ah). A genus of bacillus-like micro-organisms. Some authors recognize 2 genera, *Bartonella,* which are able to develop in fixed tissue cells as well as invading the red blood corpuscles, and *Haemobartonella,* which only grow in blood and rarely produce disease except in animals whose spleens have been removed; in these they may cause severe anaemia. **Bartonella bacilliformis.** A small micro-organism which invades the red blood cells and is responsible for Oroya fever and verruga peruana. [Alberto *Barton,* fl. 1909, Peruvian bacteriologist and parasitologist of British descent.]

bartonelliasis, bartonellosis (bar·ton·el·i′·as·is, bar·ton·el·o′·sis). A disease which occurs in the deep valleys of the Andes in South America and is caused by infection with *Bartonella bacilliformis,* a blood parasite the vector of which is a sand fly. There are 2 stages in the course; the first the febrile stage (Carrion's disease, Oroya fever), in which there is marked anaemia, and the second the chronic stage (verruga peruana), in which a miliary or nodular eruption occurs. **Cutaneous bartonellosis.** Verruga peruana. [*Bartonella,* Gk *-osis* condition.]

Baruch, Simon (b. 1840). New York physician.

Baruch's sign. The failure to affect the rectal temperature by placing the patient in a bath at 24°C (75°F) for 15 min; formerly regarded as pathognomonic of enteric fever.

baruria (bar·ewr·e·ah). The state in which urine of a high specific gravity is secreted and excreted. [Gk *baros* weight, urine.]

Barwell, Richard (b. 1826). London surgeon.

Barwell's operation. Correction of genu valgum by osteotomy of the tibia.

baryaesthesia (bar·e·es·the′·ze·ah). Baraesthesia.

baryecoia (bar·e·ek·oi′·ah). Partial deafness. [Gk *barys* heavy, *echo* sound.]

baryencephalia (**bar**·e·en·kef·**a**′·le·ah). Mental or intellectual dullness. [Gk *barys* heavy, *egkephalos* brain.]

baryencephalus (**bar**·e·en·**kef**′·al·us). An individual who is dull of mind or intellect. [see prec.]

baryglossia (bar·e·**glos**·e·ah). A slow and thick kind of speech. [Gk *barys* heavy, *glossa* tongue.]

barylalia (bar·e·**la**·le·ah). Speech that is thick and indistinct because articulation is imperfect. [Gk *barys* heavy, *lalein* to babble like a child.]

baryphonia (bar·e·**fo**·ne·ah). 1. A heavy timbre of voice. 2. Barylalia. [Gk *barys* heavy, *phone* voice.]

baryta (bar·i·tah). Barium oxide, BaO. A highly refractory white powder; basic and poisonous. It is used as a drying agent and as an absorbent for CO_2 in chemical work.

barytes (bar·i·teez). Barite, heavy spar, $BaSO_4$. Natural barium sulphate, used as a filler for paper and in the manufacture of paint.

barytic (bar·**it**·ik). Referring to or indicating the presence of baryta or barium.

barytosis (bar·e·**to**·sis). A benign condition produced by exposure to the dust of barium or barytes that occurs in certain trades, or by the application of certain pharmaceutical preparations containing barium; very dense nodular lung shadows are found in the lungs. [barytes, Gk *-osis* condition.]

barytron (**bar**·e·tron). Yukawa particle. A heavy electron which may be charged either positively or negatively; also called a *yukon* after its discoverer. [Gk *barys* heavy, electron.]

basal (**ba**·sal). 1. Fundamental. 2. Referring to a base. 3. In position near a base. [Gk *basis* foundation.]

basal metabolic rate (BMR). Used as a test of thyroid function. The oxygen consumption is estimated in the resting and fasting patient and expressed as a percentage of the consumption by a normal person of the same sex, age, surface area, etc., which can be obtained by reference to the appropriate tables. Great attention must be paid to the conduct of the estimation, and the patient must attend on two mornings. Nevertheless, it is still employed as one of the standard tests of thyroid function.

basal vein [vena basalis (NA)]. A vein beginning at the anterior perforated substance and draining the deep structures and adjacent basal regions of the brain into the great cerebral vein.

basalia (ba·**sa**·le·ah). A term applied by T. H. Huxley to the metacarpal bones. [Gk *basis* foundation.]

basaloma (ba·sal·**o**·mah). 1. A carcinoma affecting the basal cells. 2. A rodent ulcer. [basal, Gk -oma tumour.]

basculation (bas·kew·**la**·shun). The correction of retroversion of the uterus by drawing the neck of the uterus downwards and pressing the fundus upwards with a swinging movement. [Fr. *basculer* to sway up and down.]

base (base). 1. [Basis (NA).] The bottom or foundation of an object. 2. The principal constituent of a mixture. 3. In dentistry, that part of an artificial denture which supports the teeth. 4. An element, radical or compound which combines with acids to form salts. 5. An organic compound which has exceptional combining power or physiological activity by virtue of the negative chemical groups or radicals it contains. 6. A compound which dissociates into hydroxyl ions in water, or into analogous negative ions in other media. 7. A compound whose molecules are able to absorb hydrogen ions. **Aldehyde base.** An aldehyde ammonia. *See* ALDEHYDE. **Alloxur base, Alloxure base.** One of the purine bodies such as adenine and guanine, derived from the nucleic acids. **Animal base.** A ptomaine or leucomaine; a toxic nitrogenous substance produced by decomposition or metabolism of animal tissue. **Apical base.** A hypothetical area of the basal bone of the maxilla or mandible in the region of the apices of the teeth in which the alveolar bone containing the teeth is superimposed. **Cast base.** The base of an artificial denture or crown produced by forcing molten metal into a mould of the required shape and allowing it to cool. **Depressor base.** An amine such as histamine, which causes vasodilatation and accompanying cardiac and pulmonary effects. **Fixed base.** A base which has been neutralized by an acid. **Heart base.** The upper, wider portion of the heart formed by the auricles into which open the pulmonary veins and venae cavae. **Hexone base.** One of the basic amino acids such as arginine, lysine or histidine, constituted of 6 carbon atoms and resulting from the hydrolysis of proteins. **Histone base.** A hexone base (see preceding); a product of the hydrolysis of the simple basic proteins known as *histones*. **Leuco base.** A colourless compound formed by reduction of a dye, and readily oxidized again to the dye. **Base of the metacarpus.** *See* METACARPUS. **Nitrogenous base.** One of the nitrogen compounds that occur widely in nature as amines, onium derivatives and alkaloids. **Nucleinic base.** Alloxur base (see above). **Base of the patella.** *See* PATELLA. **Base of a phalanx.** *See* PHALANGES. **Pressor base.** An amine with a physiological effect resembling that produced by stimulation of the sympathetic nervous system; examples are tyramine and adrenaline. **Primary base.** Primary amine. *See* AMINE. **Base of the prostate.** *See* PROSTATE. **Purine base.** Any of the amines or alkaloids, such as adenine or caffeine, with a purine-ring structure. **Pyrimidine base.** One of the bases with a pyrimidine structure, produced by the breakdown of nucleotides; cytosine, uracil and thymine are examples. **Quaternary base.** Quaternary amine. *See* AMINE. **Base of the sacrum.** *See* SACRUM. **Secondary base.** Secondary amine. *See* AMINE. **Base of the skull.** *See* SKULL. **Tertiary base.** Tertiary amine. *See* AMINE. **Xanthine base.** One of the oxypurines, xanthine, hypoxanthine, uric acid, caffeine and others, found in animal and vegetable tissues. [Gk *basis* foundation.]

basedoid (**bas**·id·oid). A condition resembling exophthalmic goitre (Basedow's disease) except that there is not thyrotoxicosis. [K. A. von *Basedow*, Gk *eidos* form.]

Basedow, Karl Adolf von (b. 1799). Merseburg physician.

Basedow's disease. Graves' disease; the term commonly used in continental Europe.

Joid-Basedow. Hyperthyroidism developing in a patient with a goitre due to iodine deficiency being treated with iodine.

baseplate (**base**·plate). A plastics material moulded to a model of the mouth; used in the construction of artificial dentures. [Gk *basis* foundation, ME *plate*.]

bas-fond (bah·**fon**). A fundus or base, particularly the base of the urinary bladder. [Fr. bottom (of an organ).]

Basham, William Richard (b. 1804). London physician.

Basham's mixture. A solution of iron and ammonium acetate used as a haematinic and as a diuretic in Bright's disease.

basial (**ba**·se·al). Referring or belonging to, or involving, the basion.

basi-alveolar (**ba**·se·al·**ve**′·o·lar). In craniometry, indicating a line running from the basion to the alveolar point.

basi-arachnitis, basi-arachnoiditis (**ba**·se·ar·ak·**ni**′·tis, **ba**·se·ar·ak·noid·**i**′·tis). A condition of inflammation in that part of the arachnoid mater which invests the base of the brain. [base, arachnoid mater, Gk *-itis* inflammation.]

basibregmatic (**ba**·se·breg·**mat**′·ik). In craniometry, indicating a line running from the basion to the bregma.

basic (**ba**·sik). 1. Referring to a base. 2. Fundamental. 3. In chemistry, relating to a base; containing or having the character of a base, i.e. able to neutralize acids; showing alkaline reaction. 4. A computer language.

basichromatin (ba·se·**kro**·mat·in). The reticular tissue of a nucleus taking a basic dye. [see foll.]

basichromiole (ba·se·**kro**·me·ole). A particle which, with others similar, constitutes the chromatin of the nucleus of a cell. [basis, Gk *chroma* colour.]

basicity (ba·**sis**·it·e). 1. The number of replaceable hydrogen atoms possessed by an acid, which is accordingly said to be mono-, di-, tri- or tetra-basic. 2. Applied on the other hand to the measure of alkalinity of a base, expressed in terms of hydroxyl concentration, pH value or normality of its solution. [Gk *basis* foundation.]

basicranial (ba·se·**kra**·ne·al). Referring or belonging to the basilar part of the skull. [basis, Gk *kranion* skull.]

basicytoparaplastin (ba·se·si·to·par·ah·**plas'**·tin). That part of the cytoplasm of the living cell which takes the stain of basic dyes. [basis, Gk *kytos* cell, paraplastin.]

basidigital (ba·se·**dij**·it·al). Referring or belonging to the base of a digit. [basis, L *digitus* finger.]

basidiobolus (ba·**sid**·e·o·**bo**·lus). **Basidiobolus haptosporus, Basidiobolus meristosporus.** A causative organism of subcutaneous phycomycosis. Infections are prevalent in tropical Africa, Indonesia and South-East Asia, and occur predominantly in males. The disease was previously thought to be caused by *Basidiobolus ranarum,* a saprophyte commonly found on frogs' dung. [basidium, Gk *bolos* lump of earth.]

basidiogenetic (ba·**sid**·e·o·jen·**et'**·ik). Formed on a basidium. [basidium, genesis.]

Basidiomycetes (ba·**sid**·e·o·mi·**se'**·teez). One of the 4 classes of Eumycetes or true fungi. They develop spores, typically 4 in number, from the ends of club-shaped structures (basidia). The class includes mushrooms, toadstools, fungi of trees and fungi causing damage to cereal crops. There are poisonous species, sometimes mistaken for edible mushrooms. [basidium, Gk *mykes* fungus.]

basidiophore (ba·**sid**·e·o·for). Having basidia. [basidium, Gk *pherein* to bear.]

basidiospore (ba·**sid**·e·o·spor). A simple spore produced by a basidium.

basidium (ba·**sid**·e·um). The organ which forms the spores in all fungi of the class Basidiomycetes. [Gk *basis* foundation.]

basifacial (ba·se·**fa**·shal). Referring or belonging to, or involving, the lower portion of the face. [basis, L *facies* face.]

basil (**baz**·il). Any plant of the mint family. **Sweet basil.** *Ocimum basilicum,* a species of the genus *Ocimum,* the leaves of which are used for flavouring. [Gk *basileus* king.]

basilar (**ba**·sil·ar). Referring or belonging to a basal part or the base of a surface, structure, or organ. **Basilar impression.** *See* IMPRESSION. **Basilar part of the occipital bone.** *See* OCCIPITAL BONE. **Basilar sinus.** *See* SINUS. **Basilar sulcus.** *See* SULCUS. [Gk *basis* foundation.]

basilar artery [arteria basilaris]. A large midline artery formed at the lower margin of the pons by the union of the vertebrals, and terminating at its upper margin by dividing into the 2 posterior cerebral arteries. It supplies branches to the pons [rami ad pontem], cerebellum and internal ear.

basilateral (ba·se·**lat**·er·al). Referring or belonging to the base and the side. [basis, L *latus* side.]

basilemma (ba·se·**lem**·ah). 1. A neuroglia. 2. A basement membrane. *See* MEMBRANE. [basis, Gk *lemma* sheath.]

basilic (bas·**il**·ik). Of a part or structure, prominent or important, e.g. basilic vein. [Gk *basilikos* royal.]

basilic vein [vena basilica]. The vein of the postaxial (ulnar) border of the upper limb. It commences at the ulnar side of the dorsal venous arch of the hand [arcus venosus dorsalis manus (NA)] and ends just below the axilla by passing through the deep fascia to become continuous with the axillary vein. **Median basilic vein [vena mediana basilica].** *See* VEIN OF THE FOREARM, MEDIAN.

basilobregmatic (ba·sil·o·breg·**mat'**·ik). Referring or belonging to the occiput and the bregma. [basis, Gk *bregma* front of the head.]

basiloma (ba·sil·**o**·mah). 1. A carcinoma consisting of, and arising in, the basal cells of the epithelium; basal-cell carcinoma. 2. A rodent ulcer. *See* ULCER. [basis, Gk *-oma* tumour.]

basilomental (ba·sil·o·**men'**·tal). Referring or belonging to the base of the skull and the chin. [basis, L *mentum* chin.]

basilopharyngeal (ba·sil·o·far·**in'**·je·al). Referring or belonging to the basilar part of the occipital bone and the pharynx. [basis, Gk *pharygx* gullet.]

basilosubnasal (ba·sil·o·sub·**na'**·zal). Basinasial. [basis, L *sub, nasus* nose.]

basilysis (ba·**sil**·is·is). The crushing of the base or the cutting in pieces of the skull of the fetus in order to assist delivery when it is not possible to deliver the child alive. [basis, Gk *lysis* a loosing.]

basilyst (**ba**·sil·ist). An instrument used for crushing the base of the skull (basilysis) in fetal craniotomy.

basin (**ba**·sin). 1. The pelvis. 2. The 3rd ventricle of the brain. [Fr. *bassin* hollow vessel.]

basinasial (ba·se·**na**·ze·al). Referring or belonging to the basion and the nasion.

basio-alveolar (ba·se·o·al·**ve'**·o·lar). Referring or belonging to the basion and the alveolar point, or involving them.

basi-occipital (ba·se·ok·**sip'**·it·al). Referring or belonging to the basilar part of the occipital bone, or involving it.

basioglossus (ba·se·o·**glos'**·us). That part of the hyoglossus muscle associated with the base of the hyoid bone.

basion (**ba**·se·on). In craniology, the middle point on the anterior margin of the foramen magnum of the occipital bone. [Gk *basis* foundation.]

basiotribe (**ba**·se·o·tribe). A forceps-like instrument with a central point, used in craniotomy. [basis, Gk *tribein* to crush.]

basiotripsy (ba·se·o·**trip'**·se). The crushing and breaking up of the fetal head with a basiotribe.

basiparachromatin, basiparaplastin (ba·se·par·ah·**kro'**·mat·in, ba·se·par·ah·**plas'**·tin). That part of the paraplastin which takes basic dyes. [basis, parachromatin.]

basiphilic (ba·se·**fil**·ik). Basophilic.

basiphobia (ba·se·**fo**·be·ah). A neurotic affection in which there is inability to stand upright or to walk; excessive fear of walking or of not being able to walk; basophobia. [Gk *basis* a stepping, phobia.]

basipresphenoid (ba·se·pre·**sfe'**·noid). Referring to the lower and the anterior parts of the body of the sphenoid bone; involving these parts. [basis, presphenoid.]

basirrhinal (ba·se·**ri**·nal). Belonging to the base of the brain and the nose, or referring to them. [basis, Gk *rhis* nose.]

basis [NA] (**ba**·sis). The lower or fundamental part of an organ or structure. **Basis cerebri, Basis encephali.** The inferior surface of the cerebrum. **Basis pedunculi.** The ventral portion of the cerebral peduncle; it is made up chiefly of longitudinal bundles of efferent fibres and on transverse section is seen to be shaped like a half-moon. **Basis scapulae.** The medial border of the scapula. [Gk foundation.]

basisphenoid (ba·se·**sfe**·noid). A plate of cartilage which ossifies in late adolescence and early adulthood and joins the posterior surface of the body of the sphenoid bone to the basilar part of the occipital bone.

basitemporal (ba·se·**tem**·por·al). Belonging to the lower part of the temporal bone. [basis, temporal.]

basivertebral (ba·se·**ver**·te·bral). In embryology and anatomy, belonging to the centrum of a vertebra. [basis, vertebra.]

basivertebral vein [vena basivertebralis]. A large vein draining the marrow and bone of the vertebral body, leading posteriorly into the internal vertebral plexus.

basket (**bah**·sket). A basket cell or any fibrous network resembling a basket. **Fibre baskets.** The networks of fine sustentacular fibres which unite to form the membrana limitans externa at the bases of the rods and cones in the supporting framework of the retina. [ME.]

See also: ALZHEIMER.

Basle (Basel) nomenclature (bahl, **bah**·zl no·**men**·klah·tcher). The anatomical terminology agreed upon and incorporated in the *Basle (Basel) Nomina Anatomica.* [see foll.]

Basle (Basel) Nomina Anatomica (bahl, **bah**·zl **nom**·in·ah an·at·**om**·ik·ah). B.N.A. or BNA. The anatomical terminology adopted at Basle (Basel), Switzerland, in 1895 by the German Anatomical Society. [L *nomen* name, Gk *anatome* dissection.]

basocyte (**ba**·so·site). A basophil leucocyte.

basocytopenia (ba·so·si·to·**pe'**·ne·ah). Absence of basophilic leucocytes from the peripheral blood; normally there are only about 1.0–0.5 per cent, so that a deficiency means virtual absence in a differential blood count. [basocyte, Gk *penia* poverty.]

basocytosis (ba·so·si·**to'**·sis). Basophilic leucocytosis. *See* LEUCOCYTOSIS. [basocyte, Gk *-osis* condition.]

baso-erythrocyte (ba·so·er·ith′·ro·site). An erythrocyte that takes a diffuse basophilic stain or shows basophilic stippling.

baso-erythrocytosis (ba·so·er·ith·ro·si·to′·sis). Basophilic staining or stippling of the erythrocytes. [baso-erythrocyte, Gk *-osis* condition.]

basograph (ba·so·graf). An instrument which records on a graph abnormalities in the gait. [Gk *basis* a stepping, *graphein* to record.]

basometachromophil, basometachromophile (ba·so·met·ah·kro′·mo·fil, ba·so·met·ah·kro′·mo·file). Capable of taking a basic dye stain so that a different colour from that of the neighbouring structures is obtained. [basis, metachromophil.]

basopenia (ba·so·pe·ne·ah). Basocytopenia.

basophil, basophile (ba·so·fil, ba·so·file). 1. A basophilic granulocyte. 2. Any tissue which takes the stain of basic dyes such as the basophil cells of the anterior pituitary which secrete thyroid-stimulating hormone, follicle-stimulating hormone, luteinizing hormone, adrenocorticotrophic hormone and melanocyte-stimulating hormone. **Amphophilic basophil.** A basophil which takes acid as well as basic stains. [basis, Gk *philein* to love.]

basophilia (ba·so·fil·e·ah). 1. An increase in the number of basophils in the blood; the average normal is 0.5 per cent of the total leucocytes. 2. A condition in which there is blue stippling of stained erythrocytes. The condition is of particular import in lead poisoning. **Diffuse basophilia.** Basophilia where the basic staining is evenly distributed throughout the cell. **Punctate basophilia.** The staining or stippling with basic dyes of the red cells. [see prec.]

basophilic (ba·so·fil·ik). Capable of taking the stain of basic dyes; basiphilic. [basis, Gk *philein* to love.]

basophilous (ba·sof·il·us). Basophilic.

basophobia (ba·so·fo·be·ah). Basiphobia.

basoplasm (ba·so·plazm). Cytoplasm taking a basic dye.

Bass, Charles Cassedy (b. 1875). New Orleans physician.

Bass and Johns culture medium. A semi-solid blood-containing medium for the growth of malaria parasites. This was the first successful medium for this purpose; there are many modifications of it.

Bass-Watkins test. A slide agglutination method for the diagnosis of typhoid fever; now obsolescent.

Basset, Antoine (b. 1882). French surgeon.

Basset's operation. Radical excision of the vulva and the superficial and deep inguinal lymph glands, for vulval carcinoma.

Bassia (bas·e·ah). A genus of deciduous trees found widely distributed in India. **Bassia latifolia.** The Matura tree. An astringent extract is obtained for the medicinal value of which the practitioners of the indigenous system in India claim that it cures such widely differing conditions as diabetes and chronic rheumatism. [Ferdinand *Bassi,* Italian botanist.]

Bassini, Edoardo (b. 1844). Italian surgeon.

Bassini's operation. For inguinal hernia: after ligation and removal of the sac the lower edge of the conjoint tendon is sutured to the deep surface of the inguinal ligament.

bassorin (bas·or·in). The water-insoluble portion of various gums such as tragacanth and karaya; it is also insoluble in alcohol, and swells up in water. It is a complex polysaccharide containing units of arabinose. **Bassorin paste.** A cream made with tragacanth for application to the skin. [*Bassora,* a city in Asia Minor.]

Bastian, Henry Charlton (b. 1837). London neurologist.

Bastian's law, Bastian-Bruns' law, or sign. Tendon reflexes in the lower extremities cannot be elicited if the spinal cord has a complete transverse lesion above the lumbar enlargement.

basyl (ba·sil). Of a substance or salt, the electropositive element or base. [basis, Gk *hyle* stuff.]

basylous (ba·sil·us). In chemistry, referring to substances which act as the basic element in a compound; basic. [see prec.]

Bateman, Thomas (b. 1778). London physician.

Bateman's disease. Molluscum contagiosum.

Bateman's herpes iris. Erythema multiforme.

bath (bahth). 1. The immersion of the body in a liquid (water, etc.) for washing or therapeutic purposes; the term is extended to the therapeutic exposure of the body to air (hot or cold), vapour, the sun, etc. 2. The receptacle or chamber employed for such immersion or exposure; the room in which such a bath is taken. 3. In chemistry, an apparatus for applying controlled heat to an object by surrounding the latter with a heated medium such as water, sand, paraffin, etc. **Abdominal bath.** *See* X-RAY BATH (below). **Acid bath.** A bath medicated with a mineral acid to check excessive sweating. **Acrothermal bath.** A bath prepared from natural mineral waters at high temperature, but in which the gaseous and saline constituents are small. **Air bath.** The exposure of the body to warm air or to air charged with a vapour. **Aix bath.** A flow of warm water passed over the body whilst massage is being given. **Alcohol bath.** The sponging of the body with weak alcohol to reduce temperature in fevers. **Alkaline bath.** A bath containing soda, used in squamous skin diseases and chronic rheumatism. **Alum bath.** A bath containing alum, used in skin diseases and arthritis. **Antimonial bath.** A bath containing tartar emetic, used in skin diseases. **Antipyretic bath.** A bath given to reduce fever. **Antirheumatic bath.** A bath used in the treatment of rheumatism. **Antiseptic bath.** A bath containing an antiseptic. **Aromatic bath.** A medicated bath scented with aromatic substances or essential oils. **Arthritic bath.** A bath containing boric acid or alum, used for arthritis. **Astringent bath.** A bath containing tannic acid, alum or other astringent. **Balsamic bath.** A bath containing tar, turpentine or balsamic resins. **Blanket bath.** A wet pack, the patient being wrapped in blankets. **Body bath.** *See* X-RAY BATH (below). **Bog bath.** A bath of thin peaty mud used therapeutically. **Borax bath.** A bath containing glycerin and borax. **Box bath.** A bath in which the patient is enclosed in a heated cabinet, except for the head. **Bran bath.** A bath in which bran has been boiled, used for the relief of skin irritation. **Brine bath.** A bath in brine given for its tonic and stimulant effect. **Bubble bath.** A bath in which the water is agitated by air bubbles blown through it. **Cabinet bath.** Box bath (see above). **Camphor bath.** An air bath charged with the vapour of camphor. **Carbon dioxide bath.** A bath in water charged with carbon dioxide. **Chemical bath.** Any apparatus designed for the application of heat to a flask, retort, etc., by surrounding it with heated air, water, sand or other medium. **Cold bath.** A bath in cold water. **Colloid bath.** A bath containing gelatin, bran, starch, etc., given for the treatment of toxic exfoliative dermatitis. **Contrast bath.** The immersion of a part of the body alternatively in hot and cold water, usually the hands or feet. **Cool bath.** A bath in water at a temperature of 15-24°C (60-75°F). **Creosote bath.** A bath containing a trace of creosote, used in scaly skin diseases. **Dipolar bath.** Electric bath (see below). **Douche bath.** The application of water to the body in the form of a douche. **Dowsing bath.** A high-temperature hot-air bath employing electric-light bulbs. **Earth bath.** The covering of a part of the body with warmed earth or sand. **Effervescent bath.** A bath containing water charged either naturally or artificially with carbon dioxide gas. **Egyptian bath.** A modified form of the Turkish bath (see below). **Electric bath.** A bath in which the medium forms part of an electric circuit and the patient is subjected to a discharge or current. **Electric-light bath.** A form of box bath in which the interior of the cabinet is heated by electric-light bulbs. **Electrotherapeutic bath.** A form of electric bath. **Electrothermal bath.** An electric bath (see above) in which the medium is at the same time heated. **Emollient bath.** A bath in an emollient liquid, e.g. a colloid bath (see above). **Fan bath.** The passage of cool air over a patient's body to reduce fever. **Faradic bath.** An electric bath in which the current is inductive (faradic). **Finnish bath.** A modified form of Russian bath (see below). **Foam bath.** A bath of foam formed by the aeration of water containing a surface-tension reducing agent. **Foot bath.** A bath for the feet. **Fucus bath.** A bath containing seaweed or seaweed derivatives, given for the benefit of the constituent salts. **Galvanic bath.** An electric bath in which the current is galvanic. **Gas bath.** A bath in which gas is applied to the body in a closed cabinet. **Gas-bubble bath.** A bath in which gases such as carbon dioxide or oxygen are released in bubble form. **Gelatin bath.** A colloidal bath of hot thin gelatin solution given as an emollient. **Glycerin bath.** A warm bath in water containing glycerin and gum acacia, given for emollient purposes. **Graduated bath.** A hot bath in which the temperature is gradually reduced. **Grease bath.** The application of lanolin or other grease to the body in the treatment of psoriasis. **Hafussi bath.** Carbon dioxide bath (see above). **Half bath.** A bath confined to the lower part of the body. **Herb bath.** A medicated bath containing a decoction of herbs. **Hip bath.** Sitz bath (see below). **Hot bath.** One in which the temperature is between 37 and 44°C (98 and 112°F). **Hot-air bath.** A bath in hot air and vapour at 38-54°C (100-130°F). **Hydro-electric bath.** Electric bath (see above). **Hydrostatic bath.** A bath in which the patient is supported without total immersion. **Hyperthermal bath.** Hot bath (see above). **Immersion bath.** The sudden and brief immersion of the patient into a bath of water. **Indian bath.** A form of Turkish bath (see below) involving massage. **Infra-red bath.** A cradle of polished metal containing elements generating infra-red rays, which covers the body or part of it. **Internal bath.** The washing of the stomach or rectum by the injection of water. **Iodine bath.** A bath in a solution of iodine and potassium iodide. **Iron bath.** A bath in a dilute solution of ferrous sulphate. **Kinotherapeutic bath.** A bath in which exercise is also taken. **Light bath.** The exposure of the body to the sun, or to actinic light rays from an artificial source. **Lime bath.** A bath containing slaked lime, used in gout to allay itch. **Linseed bath.** An emollient bath containing linseed mucilage. **Lukewarm bath.** One in which the temperature is between 32 and 36°C (90 and 96°F). **Medicated bath.** A bath containing a medicinal substance. **Mercurial bath.** A bath containing a weak solution of a mercury salt, e.g. mercuric chloride. **Mercury bath.** A shallow vessel containing heated mercury into which is placed a flask or other vessel for gentle heating. **Milk bath.** A bath taken in milk for emollient or cosmetic purposes. **Mineral bath.** A bath in water from a mineral spring or containing mineral salts. **Monopolar bath.** A hydro-electric bath in which the wall of the metal bath is one large electrode; the current is conducted to the entire surface of the body in contact with the water and passes out by means of a metal electrode protected by a rubber pillow to prevent the patient coming into contact with it. **Moor bath.** A bath in water containing earth from a moor as distinct from cultivated soil bearing pathogenic organisms. **Mud bath.** A method of applying moist heat therapeutically, using certain soils heated by thermal springs or artificially. **Mustard bath.** A bath in water containing mustard; used as a counter-irritant in bronchitis, colds and the treatment of infants in convulsions. **Nauheim bath.** Carbon dioxide bath (see above). **Needle bath.** A shower bath with a fine spray. **Nutritive bath.** A bath containing wine, milk, etc. **Oatmeal bath.** A bath used in pruritic and xerodermatous conditions. Boiling water is poured over a muslin containing oatmeal. **Oil bath.** A bath in warm olive oil, usually medicated. **Oxygen bath.** A gas-bubble bath impregnated with oxygen. **Ozet bath.** A bath chemically impregnated with oxygen. **Pack bath.** A bath in which the body is placed in wet cloths. **Peat bath.** A variant of the mud bath. **Peloid bath.** A term applied to any form of bath in which substances such as mud, peat or fango are applied externally. **Pine bath.** A bath in water containing an extract of pine cones. **Plunge bath.** Immersion bath (see above). **Radiant-heat bath.** The application of heat to the whole or part of the body by means of electric lamps placed inside a cabinet in which the subject lies, or places a limb. **Rain bath.** Shower bath (see below). **Reducing bath.** Antipyretic bath (see above). **Russian bath.** A hot vapour bath, with friction, and ending with a plunge in cold water. **Sand bath.** The application of dry heated sand or damp sand to the body. **Sauna bath.** Finnish-style steam bath. **Schwalbach bath.** A bath aerated by carbon dioxide and containing ferrous carbonate. **Scotch bath.** An alternating douche. **Sea bath, Sea-water bath.** A bath in sea-water. **Seaweed bath.** Fucus bath (see above). **Sedative bath.** A warm bath taken for sedative purposes; the patient remains in it for some time. **Sheet bath.** A bath in which the body is placed in wet sheets; it is used in fever. **Shower bath.** A bath in a fine spray of water falling on the body. **Sinusoidal electric bath.** A bath in which a limb is immersed and a surged sinusoidal current passed across it. It is used in peripheral-artery disease to improve the circulation. **Sitz bath.** A bath in which the patient immerses only the buttocks and hips. **Slime bath.** A bath taken in ooze from a river. **Slush bath.** The pouring of water over a patient in bed on a rubber sheet; it is used to reduce temperature. **Sponge bath.** Washing of the body with a wet sponge. **Stimulating bath.** A bath containing a tonic or astringent substance, such as pine extract or alum. **Sulphur bath.** A bath containing sodium sulphide, or sublimed or colloidal sulphur, used in certain skin diseases. **Sulphuretted aerated bath.** A bath usually of natural waters, aerated by hydrogen sulphide. **Sun bath.** The exposure of the body to the sun for therapeutic purposes. **Surprise bath.** The sudden and unexpected immersion of the patient in a cold bath in the treatment of mental disorder. **Sweat bath.** A bath given to induce sweating. **Swedish bath.** Steam bath, the water being poured on heated stone. **Temperate bath.** A bath in water at 24-30°C (75-85°F). **Tepid bath.** A bath in water at 30-35°C (85-95°F). **Thoracic bath.** *See* X-RAY BATH (below). **Trunk bath.** *See* X-RAY BATH (below). **Tub bath.** A bath taken in a large tub. **Turkish bath.** A bath in which the patient passes from room to room of increasing temperature and is then massaged, after which the bath ends with a douche of warm water followed by cold. **Vacuum bath.** The treatment of any part of the body by subjecting it to a partial vacuum. **Vapour bath.** The exposure of the body to a vapour such as steam. **Vichy bath.** The application of a douche and massage at the same time. **Warm bath.** A bath in water at 32-40°C (90-104°F). **Water bath.** In chemistry, a vessel of water heated to a certain temperature; flasks or retorts are either immersed in it or placed on top of it for heating. **Wax bath.** The application of warm wax to a limb or part of the body as an insulation to raise the temperature of the part. **Whirlpool bath.** The immersion of a part of the body in hot water that is agitated by a stream of hot water and air. **X-ray bath.** Large-field x-ray treatment, to the whole body (body bath, total body irradiation), the whole trunk (trunk bath), the thorax (thoracic bath) or the abdomen (abdominal bath). [AS *baeth.*]

See also: FINSEN (N. R.), GREVILLE, HELLER (J. F.), SARASON, SCHNEE.

bathaesthesia (bath·es·**the**·ze·ah). Bathyaesthesia.

bathmic (**bath**·mik). Referring or belonging to bathmism.

bathmism (**bath**·mizm). The vital force which controls growth and the function of nutrition.

bathmophobia (bath·mo·**fo**·be·ah). Excessive fear of looking down or of going down into a deep place. [Gk *bathmos* step, phobia.]

bathmotropic (bath·mo·**trop**·ik). Affecting muscular and nervous response to stimulation. **Negatively bathmotropic.** Lessening muscular and nervous irritability. **Positively bathmotropic.** Increasing muscular and nervous irritability. [Gk *bathmos* step, *tropos* a turning.]

bathmotropism (bath·**mot**·ro·pizm). The quality of affecting muscular and nervous response to stimulation. [see prec.]

bathoflore (**bath**·o·flor). A substance the action of which is to diminish the fluorescent intensity of a compound. [Gk *bathys* deep, L *fluere* to flow.]

bathomorphic (bath·o·**mor**·fik). Term applied to a person who has a myopic eye; the latter often has a sunken appearance, as its surface is flattened. [Gk *bathys* deep, *morphe* form.]

bathophobia (bath·o·**fo**·be·ah). Bathmophobia.

bathyaesthesia (**bath**·e·es·**the'**·ze·ah). Awareness of sensation in the deeper parts of the body, such as the muscles; deep sensibility. [Gk *bathys* deep, aesthesia.]

bathyanaesthesia (**bath**·e·an·es·**the'**·ze·ah). Lack or loss of deep sensibility; that is, of awareness of sensation in the deeper parts of the body. [Gk *bathys* deep, anaesthesia.]

bathycardia (bath·e·**kar**·de·ah). An abnormal anatomical condition in which the heart occupies a lower place in the thorax than is usual. [Gk *bathys* deep, *kardia* heart.]

bathycentesis (bath·e·sen·**te**'·sis). Deep puncture with a surgical instrument; deep acupuncture. [Gk *bathys* deep, *kentesis* a pricking.]

bathygastria, bathygastry (bath·e·**gas**·tre·ah, bath·e·**gas**·tre). Gastroptosis. [Gk *bathys* deep, *gaster* stomach.]

bathyhypaesthesia (bath·e·hi·pes·**the**'·ze·ah). Lack or impairment of sensibility in the deeper structures, such as the muscular tissues. [Gk *bathys* deep, hypo-aesthesia.]

bathyhyperaesthesia (bath·e·hi·per·es·**the**'·ze·ah). Excessive sensibility of the deep structures, such as the muscular tissues. [Gk *bathys* deep, hyperaesthesia.]

bathymetry (bath·**im**·et·re). Anatomically, the process of measuring any cavity of the body. [Gk *bathys* deep, meter.]

batonet (bat·on·**et**). Pseudochromosome. [Fr. *bâton* stick.]

batophobia (bat·o·**fo**·be·ah). 1. Abnormal fear of being among or passing high objects or geological formations, such as buildings or mountains. 2. Acrophobia. [Gk *batos* height, phobia.]

batrachoplasty (bat·rak·o·**plas**'·te). The cure of ranula by plastic surgery. [Gk *batrachos* frog, *plassein* to mould.]

battarism, battarismus (**bat**·ar·izm, bat·ar·**iz**·mus). Stammering or stuttering; impediment in speech. [Gk *battarismos* a stuttering.]

Batten, Frederick Eustace (b. 1865). London neurologist.

Batten's hydrophthalmoscope. An instrument used in ophthalmology, consisting of an appliance like a small watchmaker's glass which can be filled with fluid and worn in front of the eyeball to facilitate examination. *See* HYDROPHTHALMOSCOPE.

Batten-Mayou disease. The juvenile form of cerebromacular degeneration (cerebral lipidosis); usually called *Spielmeyer-Vogt disease.*

battery (**bat**·er·e). A number of similar appliances acting in conjunction, thereby multiplying the effect produced by one. **Dry battery.** Cells of the Leclanché type with electrolyte impregnated in an absorbent medium and made into a pack for convenient transportation. **Electric battery.** An arrangement to produce a continuous electric current from 2 or more voltaic cells connected in series or parallel. **Galvanic battery.** Voltaic battery (see below). **Primary battery.** A number of connected primary cells. **Secondary battery.** A number of connected storage cells. **Storage battery.** An accumulator, consisting of one or more storage cells. **Voltaic battery.** A number of connected voltaic cells each producing a continuous electric current by chemical action between an electrolyte solution and plates of dissimilar metals. *See* CELL: PRIMARY, VOLTAIC; LECLANCHÉ CELL. [Fr. *batterie.*]

Battle, William Henry (b. 1855). London surgeon.

Battle's incision. For appendicectomy: a vertical incision medial to the outer border of the right rectus, with division of the rectus sheath and retraction of the rectus muscle inwards.

Battle's operation. Removal of the appendix through Battle's incision (see above).

Battle's sign. Ecchymosis sometimes seen around the mastoid following fractured base of skull.

Battle-Jalaguier-Kammerer incision. Battle's incision (see above).

Baudelocque, Jean Louis (b. 1746). Paris obstetrician.

Baudelocque's diameter. The external conjugate diameter. *See* DIAMETER.

Bauhin, Caspar (b. 1560). Swiss anatomist.

Bauhin's gland. The anterior lingual gland. *See* GLAND.

Bauhin's valve. The ileocolic valve. *See* VALVE.

Bauhinia (bo·**hin**·e·ah). A genus of plants of the family Leguminosae. **Bauhinia tomentosa.** A species the leaves, buds and young flowers of which are used in India in the treatment of dysentery.

Baumés, Jean Baptiste Timothée (b. 1756). Montpellier physician.

Baumés' sign. Retrosternal pain due to cardiac ischaemia; angina pectoris.

Baumés, Pierre Prosper François, (b. 1791). Lyons physician.

Baumés' law. Colles' law.

Baumgarten, Paul Clemens von (b. 1849). German pathologist.

Baumgarten's glands. Tubular glands in the conjunctiva; Henle's glands.

Baumgarten, Walter (b. 1873). St. Louis, Missouri, physician.

Cruveilhier-Baumgarten cirrhosis, or syndrome. Thrombosis of the portal vein, often within its hepatic course, with cirrhosis of the liver; it occurs in young children.

Baunscheidt, Karl (b. 1809). Bonn inventor.

Baunscheidt's air-puncture treatment. The revulsive treatment of rheumatisms and neuralgias by acupuncture with a *révulseur,* an instrument set with a number of fine needles. These are dipped into an irritant liquid and then applied to the skin over the affected area.

baunscheidtism (**bown**·shi·tizm). Baunscheidt's air-puncture treatment.

bauxite (**bawx**·ite). A naturally-occurring oxide of aluminium, and the source of pure alumina and aluminium. [*Baux,* in France.]

bay (ba). In anatomy, a depression or recess containing liquid. **Lacrimal bay.** The lacus lacrimalis. [L *baia.*]

See also: RIDLEY.

bay laurel (ba **law**·rel). *Laurus nobilis* Linn. [L *baca* berry, *laurus.*]

bay rum (ba **rum**). A reputed hair astringent containing oleum myrciae. [L *baca* berry, rum.]

Bayard, Henri Louis (b. 1812). Paris physician.

Bayard's ecchymoses. The small stains found in the pericardium and pleura of an infant who, through some abnormality in the birth process, has begun to breathe *in utero.* They are due to capillary haemorrhage.

bayberry (**ba**·ber·e). 1. The fruit of the European laurel, *Laurus nobilis* Linn. 2. Bayberry bark, wax myrtle bark, myrica, the dried root-bark of *Myrica cerifera,* family Myricaceae. It contains volatile oil, tannin and an astringent resin; used for its astringent properties. [L *baca* berry, AS *berie.*]

baycuru (ba·koo·**roo**). The root of *Statice braziliensis* (family Plumbaginaceae); used in Brazil for its astringent properties. [local name.]

Bayer's operation. A form of tenotomy used for lengthening the Achilles tendon by a Z-shaped incision.

Bayle, Antoine Laurent Jessé (b. 1799). Paris physician.

Bayle's disease. Dementia paralytica; general paralysis of the insane.

Bayley, Robert Hebard (b. 1906). Oklahoma City cardiologist.

Bayley's triaxial reference system. A method for plotting the QRS vector of the electrocardiogram in the frontal plane. The 3 sides of Einthoven's triangle are arranged so that they intersect at a central point.

Bazett, H. C. 20th century Baltimore physiologist.

Bazett index, or formula. A formula for relating the Q-T interval (duration of ventricular systole) to the heart rate. The Q-T interval varies inversely with the heart rate, and the formula states that $Q\text{-}T = K\sqrt{C}$, where C is the cycle length and K is a constant which varies from 0.38 to 0.39 ± 0.04. Abnormalities of the Q-T may be detected in a given cardiogram by correcting the Q-T for the rate by modifying Bazett's formula, and expressing the corrected Q-T as $Q\text{-}T_c$ thus:

$$Q\text{-}T_c = (Q\text{-}T)/\sqrt{C};\ Q\text{-}T_c$$

is then identical with K. The corrected Q-T may also be expressed as a ratio of 1 by the use of the normogram devised by Goldberger. *See* INTERVAL, Q-T.

Bazin, Antoine Pierre Ernest (b. 1807). French dermatologist.

Bazin's classification. A classification of the fungi, now largely obsolete; it depended on their tissue preference, e.g. trichophyta, epidermophyta.

Bazin's disease. A tuberculous variety of erythema induratum.

Bazin's ulcer. A painful ulcer that occurs in the back of the calf; it is usually symmetrical, indurated and nodular.

Alibert-Bazin disease. Psoriasis arthropathica.

bazin (ba·zin). Molluscum contagiosum; a skin disease caused by a filtrable virus and occurring chiefly on the skin of the face, breast and genital organs. It is characterized by chronic rounded tubercles filled with a caseous substance and very small bodies termed *molluscum corpuscles.* [Antoine Pierre Ernest *Bazin.*]

bdella (del·lah). A leech. [Gk.]

bdellepithecium (del·ep·e·the′·se·um). A cylinder used for the application of leeches to the skin. [Gk *bdella* leech, *epithesis* a putting on.]

bdellium (del·e·um). The name applied to several gum resins resembling myrrh, and of uncertain botanical origin. African and Indian bdelliums occur in commerce. [Gk *bdellion.*]

Bdellonyssus (del·on·is′·us). A genus of mites. **Bdellonyssus bacoti.** The tropical rat mite, a very common parasite of rats in warm regions and in urban areas of temperate regions. It causes intense irritation and rash in man, and infestations are common after rats in buildings have been killed. Also known as *Liponyssus.* [Gk *bdella* leach, *nyssein* to prick.]

bdellotomy (del·ot·o·me). Incision of a sucking leech or the cutting off of the end of it, so that it will continue to suck and the blood drain away at the cut. [Gk *bdella* leech, *temnein* to cut.]

bdelygmia (del·ig·me·ah). Aversion to food. Nausea. [Gk.]

bead (beed). A small globular mass. **Rachitic bead.** One of the nodular enlargements at the junction of the ribs and cartilages which may be present in rickets. [ME *bede,* prayer bead.]

beading (beed·ing). **Beading of the ribs.** The rachitic (rickety) rosary. *See* ROSARY. [see prec.]

beak (beek). 1. The lower portion of the calamus scriptorius. 2. The mandibular part of a pair of forceps. 3. The splenium of the corpus callosum. **Coracoid beak.** The tip of the coracoid process of the scapula. **Beak of the encephalon.** Main def. 3 (above). **Beak of the sphenoid bone.** The rostrum of the sphenoid bone. [LL *beccus.*]

beaker. *See* MARINELLI.

Beale, Lionel Smith (b. 1828). London physician and microscopist.

Beale's ganglion cell. A bipolar nerve cell in which the two processes are spiralled around each other.

Beale's fibre. A spirally-twisted nerve fibre, particularly one from a spinal ganglion.

beam (beem). **Balkan beam.** A frame fitted to the bed for suspension of a splint or for supporting pulleys for weight traction. The apparatus was first used by a volunteer Dutch ambulance unit in the Balkan War of 1903. Also known as *Balkan frame* or *splint.* **Beam direction.** *See* DIRECTION. **Beam therapy.** 1. *See* THERAPY. 2. Chromotherapy, 1st def. [AS, tree.]

bean (been). 1. The seed formed in the pods of certain leguminous plants, e.g. the common bean, *Faba vulgaris.* 2. Applied to any oval flattened body, from its similarity to a bean in shape. **Calabar bean.** Ordeal bean, the seed of *Physostigma venenosum,* containing physostigmine (eserine). **Castor-oil bean.** The seed of *Ricinis communis,* yielding a bland and non-irritant oil; it is the irritant ricinoleates formed from it by saponification in the duodenum that cause purgation. The bean also contains a toxic protein, ricin. **Nux-vomica bean.** *Strychnos nux vomica.* **Ordeal bean.** Calabar bean (see above). **St. Ignatius bean.** *Strychnos ignatii.* **Vanilla bean.** The pods of the epiphyte *Vanilla planifolia* used as a flavouring in confectionery. [AS.]

bearberry (ba·er·ber·e). The dried leaves of *Arctostaphylos uva-ursi,* used as a diuretic. [AS *bera, berie.*]

Beard, George Miller (b. 1839). New York physician.

Beard's disease. Neurasthenia.

Beard's treatment. The treatment of cancer by the injection of trypsin.

Beard-Valleix points. In cases of neuralgia in the distribution of a particular nerve, exquisitely tender points along the crust of the nerve. These are also known as *puncta dolorosa.*

beard [barba (NA)] (be·ard). The hair of the male chin and cheeks. [AS.]

bearsfoot (ba·erz·fut). *Polymnia uvedalia.* [AS *bera, fot.*]

bearsweed (ba·erz·weed). Yerba santa, the dried leaves of *Eriodictyon californicum*; a bitter tonic and expectorant. [AS *bera, weod.*]

beat (beet). 1. To throb. 2. A rhythmic variation in volume produced between notes of slightly different pitch when sounded together: due to interference. 3. A recurring stroke or throb, as of the heart or the pulse. **Apex beat.** The impulse, which may be felt by the hand, occurring on the surface of the chest over the cardiac apex as this thrusts against the chest wall with the heart beat. **Atrial beat.** A heart beat arising from an impulse originating spontaneously in the atrial wall. **Coupled beat.** Bigeminal pulse. *See* PULSE. **Dropped beat.** The occasional loss of a ventricular beat in partial heart block. **Echo beat.** Reciprocal beat (see below). **Ectopic beat.** A cardiac systole which has its origin at some point other than the sinu-atrial node. **Forced beat.** An extrasystole which is produced when the heart is subjected to artificial stimulation. **Fusion beat.** A ventricular contraction which results from more than one advancing excitatory wavefront occurring at the same time, such as may occur when a ventricular ectopic focus discharges shortly after the sinus node. It is a characteristic feature of parasystole. The electrocardiogram shows a QRST complex which combines features of the different complexes that occur when each of the foci activates the ventricles entirely. **Heart beat.** The recurrent throb of the heart as the left ventricle pumps the blood through the aortic valve into the aorta. **Idioventricular beat.** A ventricular contraction produced by an impulse originating spontaneously in the ventricular myocardium. **Junctional beat.** A ventricular contraction produced by an impulse originating spontaneously in the region of the atrioventricular node and His' bundle system between the atria and the ventricles. **Nodal beat.** A ventricular contraction produced by an impulse originating spontaneously in the atrioventricular node. **Premature beat.** A heart beat occurring earlier than predicted from the prevailing heart rhythm and rate, usually an ectopic beat (see above). **Pulse beat.** The visible or palpable throb in an artery at points where the vessel has become superficial. **Reciprocal beat.** A contraction of a cardiac chamber resulting from an impulse which originated in the same chamber but which has been conducted back to it from the other chamber of the heart. An *atrial reciprocal beat* can occur if, after a normal sinus beat, the impulse is conducted back to the atrium from the ventricles via an accessory pathway of conduction; a *ventricular reciprocal beat* can occur if a retrograde atrial beat, following a ventricular ectopic beat, is followed by forward conduction back to the ventricles. **Re-entry beat.** Reciprocal beat (see above). **Retrograde beat.** An atrial contraction produced by an impulse which arises in the atrioventricular node and passes backward to excite the atria in a retrograde fashion. [AS *beatan.*]

Beau, Joseph Honoré Simon (b. 1806). Paris physician.

Beau's line. A transverse line or groove on the finger nails appearing after an illness.

Beau's syndrome. Cardiac asystole; absence of cardiac contraction.

Beaumé, Antoine (b. 1728). French chemist.

Beaumé's hydrometers. Two hydrometers, graduated with Beaumé scales, the one for measuring the specific gravities of liquids heavier than water (called a *salinometer*), the other for measuring the specific gravities of liquids lighter than water (called an *alcoholometer*).

Beaumé scales. Hydrometer scales with equidistant graduations, one for use with liquids heavier than water, graduated from 0° (sp. gr. 1.000) near the top of the stem of the hydrometer, to 66° (sp. gr. 1.860) near the bottom, the other for use mainly with liquids lighter than water graduated from 0° (sp. gr. 1.085) near the bottom to 50° (sp. gr. 0.762) near the top of the stem.

Beauvais, Landré.
Beauvais' disease. Rheumatoid arthritis. *See* ARTHRITIS.

Beaver, R. A. 20th century British anaesthetist.
Beaver ventilator. An artificial ventilating machine, electrically operated. Described in 1956.

bebeerine (be·be·reen). $C_{36}H_{38}O_6N_2$. An alkaloid obtained from bebeeru and used in the form of the soluble sulphate. As it is an aromatic bitter, it is sometimes employed as a stomachic. [see foll.]

bebeeru (be·be·roo). The bark of the greenheart tree, *Nectandra rodiaei* (family Lauraceae), of British Guiana. It yields commercial bebeerine, consisting of about 30 per cent bebeerine with other alkaloids and colouring matter. [Sp. *biburu.*]

Beccari, Nello (b. 1883). Florence anatomist.
Beccari's membrane, or stratum. A hypothetical membrane said to exist at a nerve synapse.

bechic (bek·ik). 1. Anything which relieves or cures cough. 2. Belonging or referring to cough. [Gk *bex* cough.]

Bechterew, Vladimir Mikhailovich von (b. 1857). Leningrad neurologist.
Bechterew's arthritis, or disease. Ankylosing spondylitis, spondylitis ankylopoietica; most correctly used when the disease presents in the cervical spine.
Bechterew's layer. Kaes-Bechterew layer (see below).
Bechterew's accessory lemniscus. Supposedly, a bundle of fibres passing between the peduncle of the superior olive and the medial lemniscus.
Bechterew's nucleus. The superior vestibular nucleus. *See* NUCLEUS.
Bechterew's reaction. In cases of tetany, repetitive electrical stimulation of muscles with the initially minimal effective current for inducing contraction causes a tetanic contraction, unless at each repetition the current strength is reduced.
Bechterew's reflex. 1. Nasal: irritation of the nasal mucosa produces contraction of the facial muscles on the same side. 2. Pupil: the paradoxical pupillary reaction occasionally seen in early cases of tabes dorsalis or dementia paralytica; the pupil dilates on exposure to light. 3. Hypogastric: in normal individuals, stroking of the skin of the medial surface of the thigh produces contraction of the lower abdominal muscles. 4. Plantar: in pyramidal-tract disease, tapping of the dorsum of the foot may induce plantar flexion. 5. Deep: in pyramidal-tract disease, dorsiflexion of the foot with flexion at hip and knee may occur on releasing suddenly a foot which has been firmly though passively plantar-reflexed. 6. Tapping of the extensor tendons of the wrist when it is flexed gives reflex extension; the carpophalangeal reflex.
Bechterew's sign. 1. Bechterew's reflex (see above). 2. Anaesthesia in the popliteal fossa in tabes dorsalis. 3. Paralysis of emotional movements of the face.
Bechterew's test. A clinical test for sciatica: the patient is seated upright in bed with the hips and knees flexed; he is then asked to straighten both legs so that they lie flat upon the bed. A patient with sciatica cannot perform this test, though he may be able to extend each leg independently, through rotation of the pelvis.
Bechterew's tract. Fibres in the tegmentum of the mid-brain connecting the superior olivary nuclei to the medial lemniscus.
Kaes-Bechterew layer. A horizontal layer of fibres found in the cerebral cortex, just deep to the outer granular layer.
Bechterew-Mendel reflex. In normal subjects percussion of the dorsum of the foot may produce dorsiflexion of the 2nd to 5th toes; in pyramidal-tract disease plantar-flexion occurs (Bechterew's reflex, 4th def.). The normal reflex has also been called the *tarsophalangeal reflex, Mendel's dorsal reflex of the foot, dorsocuboidal reflex, cuboidodigital reflex.*
Mendel-Bechterew sign. 1. The paradoxical pupil reaction; dilatation on exposure to light in early cases of tabes dorsalis; Bechterew's reflex, 2nd def. 2. The tarsophalangeal reflex. *See* REFLEX.

Beck, Claude Schaeffer (b. 1894). Cleveland surgeon.
Beck's triad. Three physical signs denoting compression of the heart: rising venous pressure, falling arterial pressure and small quiet heart.

Beck Emil G. (b. 1866). Chicago surgeon.
Beck's gastrostomy. The establishment of a canal from skin surface to stomach by way of a tube formed from the greater curvature.
Beck's method. A method of treatment of bone abscess, especially tuberculous abscess: the cavity is curetted out and filled with Beck's paste.
Beck's paste. Bismuth subnitrate (1 part) and soft paraffin (2 parts).

Becker, Otto Heinrich Enoch (b. 1828). German ophthalmologist.
Becker's sign. Increased pulsation in the retinal arteries, sometimes observed in thyrotoxicosis.

Becker-Lennhoff index. The distance between the top of the sternum and the symphysis pubis in centimetres is multiplied by 100 and divided by the greatest circumference of the abdomen. An index above 75 indicates an atonic habitus.

Beckmann, Ernest Otto (b. 1853). Berlin chemist.
Beckmann's apparatus. An apparatus for determining the molecular weight of a substance by observing the lowering of the freezing point or raising of the boiling point when small quantities of the substance are introduced into a solvent.
Beckmann's formula. $m = Kw/dW$, where w g of solute of molecular weight m is dissolved in W g of solvent, producing a depression d of the freezing point of the solvent. K is a constant for a particular solvent, and the formula may be used for the determination of the molecular weight of solutes which do not dissociate or associate in solution.
Beckmann's thermometer. A mercury thermometer covering a small temperature range which is finely divided. The position of the range of temperature on the Celsius scale may be varied by adjusting the thermometer, which is then calibrated.

Beclamide (bek·lam·ide). BP Commission approved name for *N*-benzyl-β-chloropropionamide; it is used in the treatment of epilepsy.

Béclard, Pierre Augustin (b. 1785). French surgeon.
Béclard's amputation. Amputation at the hip joint, with the use of a posterior flap.
Béclard's hernia. Femoral hernia protruding through the saphenous opening.
Béclard's nucleus. The secondary centre of ossification in the cartilaginous epiphysis at the lower end of the femur.
Béclard's triangle. A triangle bounded by the posterior border of the hyoglossus muscle, the posterior belly of the digastric muscle and the greater cornu of the hyoid bone.

Beclomethasone (be·klo·meth·az·one). BP Commission approved name for 9α - chloro - 11β, 17α, 21 - trihydroxy - 16β - methylpregna - 1, 4 - diene - 3, 20 - dione. **Beclomethasone Dipropionate BP 1973.** 9α - Chloro - 11β - hydroxy - 16β - methyl - 17α, 21 - dipropionyloxypregna - 1 - diene - 3, 20 - dione, a corticosteroid used topically in the treatment of skin diseases. In the form of the dipropionate it is used chiefly in the respiratory system, often by inhalation, in asthma and allergic rhinitis.

Becquerel, Antoine Henri (b. 1852). Paris physicist.
Becquerel's disc. An apparatus devised to measure the difference in temperature between a sound and a paralysed limb.
Becquerel rays. Rays emitted from uranium and capable of affecting a wrapped photographic plate; first noted by Becquerel in 1896; now shown to be gamma rays.

bed (bed). 1. The mattress and bed-clothes, usually supported on a bedstead, designed for repose in sleep or sickness. 2. In anatomy, a supporting base or structure. **Air bed.** A rubber bed which is inflated with air. **Capillary bed.** The network of capillary blood vessels throughout the body or in any particular part or organ. **Cardiac bed.** A bed prepared with several pillows and provided with a bed table, in order that an orthopnoeic patient may be supported from behind and, if necessary, be able to lean forward over the bed table. **Cognate vascular bed.** The normal vascular bed, exclusive of the vessels that may be associated through a collateral circulation. **Emergency bed.** A bed prepared and retained for emergency admissions to hospital. **Fracture bed.** A bed under the mattress of which is arranged a board or series of boards to prevent sagging and consequent displacement of a fractured limb or spine. **Hydrostatic bed.** Water bed (see below). **Nail bed [matrix unguis].** *See* NAIL. **Operation bed.** A prepared, warmed bed, with the bed-clothes turned back lengthwise or folded into a pack to facilitate the return of a patient after an operation. **Plaster bed.** 1. A plaster mould or cast, usually made for the immobilization of the spine. 2. A bed with the clothes so arranged that a limb in plaster is allowed to dry by exposure to the air. **Renal bed.** A bed supplied with thin blankets or flannelette sheets between which the patient lies, intended to induce and absorb perspiration. **Rheumatism bed.** A bed supplied with thin blankets or flannelette sheets between which the patient lies as in a renal bed (see above). One pillow only is allowed in order to avoid heart strain, and a bed cradle is supplied to prevent the weight of the bed-clothes on painful joints. **Ripple bed.** A bed with a mattress subdivided into a series of compartments which can be serially inflated and deflated by an automatic pump so that a recumbent patient's points of maximum pressure are constantly changing. **Vascular bed.** All the blood vessels, including arteries, capillaries, veins and sinuses, of an area or an organ. **Water bed.** A bed with a rubber mattress which is filled with water; it is intended to prevent bedsores. [AS *bedd.*]

See also: BIRMINGHAM.

bedbug (**bed**·bug). Two species of bugs of the genus *Cimex* (Hemiptera) which are commensal with man: the temperate bedbug (*Cimex lectularius*), and the tropical bedbug (*Cimex hemipterus* = *rotundatus*). Both are dorsoventrally flattened, brown and wingless, and live by day in crevices of dwelling-houses, emerging at night to feed on blood. They are not regular vectors of any human disease. [AS *bedd*, bug.]

bedlamism (**bed**·lam·izm). Insanity. [ME *Bedlem*, Bethlehem: the Hospital of St Mary of Bethlehem, London.]

Bednar, Alois (b. 1816). Vienna paediatrician.

Bednar's aphthae. Small ulcerated patches found on the hard palate and gingival margins in cases of marasmus, and caused by local infection of damaged mucosa as a result of sucking infected articles.

bedpan (**bed**·pan). A shallow receptacle made of china, enamel, stainless steel or rubber, designed for the reception of the faeces and urine of a person confined to bed. [AS *bedde, panne.*]

Bedsonia (bed·**so**·ne·ah). A term originally applied to a genus of micro-organisms in the family Rickettsiaceae which is taxonomically intermediate between the bacteria and viruses. The genus is now called *Chlamydia.* [Sir Samuel *Bedson*, 1886–1969, London bacteriologist.]

bedsore (**bed**·sore). Decubitus ulcer; ulceration affecting bed-ridden patients and occurring over the vertebral spines, the sacrum, the heel and other prominent bony points. It is caused by continuous pressure of the part on the mattress. [AS *bedd, sar.*]

bee (be). An insect of the genus *Apis* of the family Apidae (order Hymenoptera). **Hive or honey bee.** *Apis mellifica*; a social insect lending itself readily to domestication and the commercial production of honey. It is also the source of beeswax, a secretion used to build the honeycomb. Bee venom has been employed in the treatment of rheumatism. [AS *beo.*]

Beebe, Silas Palmer (b. 1876). New York physician.

Beebe's serum. A serum which was prepared from the blood of a thyroidectomized animal and used for the treatment of hyperthyroidism.

Beebe loupe. A binocular loupe used in ophthalmic surgery to magnify the field of operation.

Beer, Georg Joseph (b. 1763). Austrian ophthalmologist.

Beer's knife. A knife with a triangular blade, used in ophthalmology.

Beer's operation. 1. For cataract: using his special triangular knife a section was cut through the lower corneal limbus; there was no iridectomy. Of historical interest as one of the earliest successful methods of cataract extraction. 2. Incision is made with a lance and the iris withdrawn through the wound and excised. Original iridectomy, 1798.

Beer's law. The absorption of light by a liquid is proportional to the thickness of liquid through which the light passes.

beerwort (**beer**·wert). A malt infusion in water; a stage in the preparation of beer. This infusion is used also in bacteriological culture media. [AS *beor, wyrt.*]

beeswax (**beez**·wax). A yellow wax obtained from the honeycomb of the bee (Yellow Beeswax BPC 1968). A purified and bleached preparation is more commonly used in medicine (White Beeswax BP 1968). It consists of fatty-acid esters of the higher alcohols, the principal ester being myricin. It is used in ointment bases, particularly those incorporating water, as it acts as an emulsifying agent. [AS *beo, weax.*]

beetles (**bee**·tlz). Coleoptera. Beetles of the genera *Epicauta, Lytta* and *Paederus* produce vesicating substances; several genera including *Caccobius* and *Onthophagus* have caused intestinal canthariasis. [AS *bitula* biter.]

beeturia (beet·**ewr**·e·ah). Pink to deep-red coloration of urine occasionally seen following eating of beetroot; an allergic phenomenon. [beetroot, urine.]

Beevor, Charles Edward (b. 1854). London neurologist.

Beevor's sign. 1. Upward displacement of the umbilicus in paralysis of the lower part of the rectus abdominis muscle. 2. Overaction of antagonistic muscles, a characteristic feature of hysterical weakness.

Begbie, James (b. 1798). Scottish physician.

Begbie's disease. Hysterical pseudochorea; sometimes applied to chorea in which movements are localized.

Beggiatoa (bej·e·at·o′·ah). A genus of the family Beggiatoaceae: filamentous, motile, segmented water organisms occurring singly or in creamy or white felted masses. They are sulphur bacteria, non-pathogenic to man. **Beggiatoa alba.** A species which produces glairin. [Francesco Secondo *Beggiato*, 1806–1883, Italian botanist.]

Beggiatoaceae (bej·e·at·o·a′·se·e). A family of thiobacteria (sulphur bacteria), including *Thiothrix* and *Beggiatoa.* [see prec.]

begma (**beg**·mah). 1. A cough. 2. The sputum or other material ejected in the act of coughing. [Gk sputum.]

behaviour (be·**have**·yer). The act or mode of behaving. **Automatic behaviour.** Automatism. **Crowd behaviour.** That shown by a group of persons, and resulting from the fact that the group shows a certain mental unity. **Invariable behaviour.** Response or activity the form of which is defined by the limitations of structure. **Variable behaviour.** That which is able to be modified by experiences through which the individual passes. [see foll.]

behaviourism (be·**have**·yer·izm). The psychological doctrine which emphasizes the importance of an objective study of actual responses, rather than considerations of consciousness or conscious processes. [AS *bihabban.*]

behaviourist (be·**have**·yer·ist). An adherent of the psychological doctrine of behaviourism. [see prec.]

Behçet, Hulusi (b. 1889). Turkish dermatologist.

Behçet's disease, or syndrome. The association of aphthous lesions of the mouth with ulceration of the genitals and uveitis with iridocyclitis going on to hypopyon. In some cases there is thrombophlebitis and extensive and often fatal involvement of the nervous system due to venous thrombosis. It is caused by a virus.

behen (**be**·hen). 1. Name given to various plants including *Statice, Silene* and *Centaurea* species. 2. Oil of behen. [Fr. *béhen.*]

Béhier, Louis Jules (b. 1813). Paris physician.

Béhier-Hardy sign, or symptom. Aphonia in early gangrene of the lung.

Behla, Robert Franz (b. 1850). Prussian physician.
Behla's body. An intracellular body found in cancer cells and degenerative in origin. Also known as *Plimmer's body.*

Behnken's unit. An obsolete unit of radiation, also known as *R unit,* equal to 1.06 roentgen.

Behr, Carl (b. 1876). German ophthalmologist.
Behr's disease. A form of familial retinal degeneration affecting the macula, usually in patients at about the age of 20.

Behre, Jeanette Allen (b. 1891). American biochemist.
Behre's test. For acetone bodies in urine: to 3 ml of urine in a test tube add 1 drop of 50 w/v sulphuric acid. Place 1 drop of salicylic aldehyde and 2 drops of a saturated solution of potassium hydroxide in the centre of a small square of cotton and when solidified to a yellow disc place over the test tube spot downward. Heat in boiling-water bath for 8 min. A positive reaction is indicated by a pink to red colour. A blank is run at the same time with 3 ml water for comparison.

Behring, Emil Adolf von (b. 1854). Marburg bacteriologist.
Behring's immunity. Passive immunity; that obtained as a result of the transfer of some immune substance (e.g. serum containing antibodies) from another animal.
Behring's law. When whole blood or serum of an immune animal is transferred to a non-immune animal, some protection of that animal occurs.
Behring's serum. Antidiphtheritic serum. *See* SERUM.

Beigel, Hermann (b. 1830). Vienna physician.
Beigel's disease. 1. Small brownish nodules occurring on the hairs of wigs, probably caused by a fungus. 2. Piedra.

Beijerinck, Martinus Willem (b. 1851). Dutch bacteriologist and microbiologist.
Beijerinck's medium. A glucose–salt mixture for the culture of nitrogen-fixing organisms.
Beijerinck's reaction. Cholera reaction, cholera red reaction; a test dependent on the production of indole and nitrites in peptone water. 4–8 drops of pure sulphuric acid are added to a 24-h vibrio culture in peptone broth. The reaction is positive, indicated by the development of a pink coloration, with cultures of vibrios of group A (Heiberg) which include the true cholera vibrios. The reaction is of value for "screening", but is not specific.

bejel (ba·jel). A non-venereal form of syphilis which is endemic among the Arabs (particularly the children) of the valleys along the Middle Euphrates. The infecting organism is morphologically indistinguishable from *Treponema pallidum.* [Arabic term.]

Békésy, Georg von (b. 1899). Hungarian and American physiologist.
Békésy audiometer. An instrument with continuous and automatic variation of frequency; the person being tested controls the intensity and endeavours to keep the sound level at his threshold. It produces a chart with a wavering line about the threshold of hearing.

bel (bel). 1. A unit of intensity of sound, giving a measure of intensity in terms of another fixed intensity; numerically equal to the logarithm to the base 10 of the ratio of the two intensities. A decibel is one-tenth of a bel. It is approximately the smallest perceptible change in sound intensity that can be detected by the human ear. 2. A measure of the amplification of electrical power defined in terms of def. 1 (above). [Alexander Graham *Bell,* 1847–1922, poineer of telephony.]

Bela BPC 1949 (**be**·lah). Bael, Bengal quince, consisting of the fresh, half-ripe fruit of the cultivated tree of *Aegle marmelos* (family Rutaceae). It is astringent and is largely employed in India for diarrhoea and dysentery, especially in children. [Hind. *bael.*]

belae fructus (**be**·le **fruk**·tus). Bael fruit, the fruit of *Aegle marmelos.* [Hind. *bael,* L *fructus* fruit.]

Belascaris (bel·**as**·kar·is). A genus of nematode (ascarid) worms that infect cats and dogs, but rarely man.

belemnoid (bel·**em**·noid). 1. Shaped like a dart. 2. The styloid process. *See* PROCESS. [Gk *belemnon* dart, *eidos* form.]

Belfield, William Thomas (b. 1856). Chicago urologist.
Belfield's operation. Vasotomy for irrigation of the vas and seminal vesicle.

Bell, Sir Charles (b. 1774). Scottish surgeon and physiologist.
Bell's law. In a reflex arc the impulse can be conducted in one direction only.
Bell's muscle. Specialized portions of the internal longitudinal muscular coat of the bladder extending from the ureteric orifices to its attachment to the median lobe of the prostate.
Bell's nerve. The nerve to the serratus anterior muscle.
Bell's palsy, or paralysis. Acute peripheral facial nerve paralysis, generally of unknown cause, but possibly viral in origin.
Bell's phenomenon. The upward and outward rolling movement of the eyes on forced closure of the lids. Most easily seen in a patient with Bell's palsy.
inverse Bell's phenomenon. On closure or attempted closure of the eyelids the eyes turn downwards.
Bell's sign. Bell phenomenon (see above).
Bell's spasm. Facial spasm; usually called *facial hemispasm* or *convulsive tic.*
Bell–Magendie law. Bell's law (see above).

Bell, Luther Vose (b. 1806). Massachusetts physician.
Bell's mania. Acute delirious mania.

belladonna (bel·ah·**don**·ah). The dried leaves (Belladonna Herb BP 1973) or roots (Belladonna Root BPC 1968) of *Atropa belladonna* or of *Atropa acuminata,* the former being commonly known as deadly nightshade, a perennial herb common in Britain and on the Continent. The plant contains the alkaloids L-hyoscyamine and L-hyoscine. The L-hyoscyamine racemizes rapidly and the racemic mixture is known as *atropine.* In addition to the various preparations of the raw drug, the *British Pharmacopoeia* describes the preparation of, and sets standards for, the tincture, the liquid and dry extracts (BP 1958), and the liniment of belladonna. Belladonna as a tincture is used as an antispasmodic in whooping cough and spasmodic affections of the bronchi (asthma), the bladder and the anal sphincter: also employed in enuresis. It suppresses the secretion of saliva and sweat and has a mydriatic action on the iris. The root and liniment are employed externally, especially in the treatment of lumbago, neuralgia and sciatica, where the drug acts as an anodyne. **Belladonna leaf.** Belladonna herb. **Belladonna praeparata, Prepared Belladonna Herb BP 1973.** Belladonna herb reduced to a fine powder. **Belladonnae Folium.** *European Pharmacopoeia* name for Belladonna Herb BP 1973. **Belladonnae Pulvis Normatus.** *European Pharmacopoeia* name for Prepared Belladonna Herb BP 1973. [It. fair lady.]

belladonnine (bel·ah·**don**·een). $C_{17}H_{21}O_2N$. An alkaloid occurring with atropine in belladonna, and formed from it by the removal of a molecule of water. It is a resinous insoluble base isomeric with apoatropine.

Bellini, Lorenzo (b. 1643). Pisa anatomist.
Bellini's ducts, or tubules. Large straight collecting tubules of the kidney.
Bellini's ligament. A part of the ischiofemoral ligament extending to the greater trochanter.

Bellocq, Jean Jacques (Jean Louis Belloc) (b. 1732). Paris surgeon.
Bellocq's cannula, or tube. A form of curved cannula used for the introduction of a plug or sponge into the postnasal space, mostly used to control nasal haemorrhage.

bellows (**bel**·oze). **Inflating bellows.** An apparatus for inflating the patient's lungs with air or anaesthetic gases. It can be used to inflate the lungs when respiration has been suspended during abdominal or thoracic surgery, or for provision of artificial respiration in other circumstances such as suspension of breathing due to nerve paralysis in poliomyelitis and nerve gas poisoning. **Oxford inflating bellows.** A small hand-unit consisting of a bellows, an air intake and a pair of unidirectional valves, used for inflating the lungs. Described by Sir Robert McIntosh in 1953. [AS *belg* bag.]

belly (bel·e). 1. The abdomen. 2. The bulging central portion of a muscle or other structure. **Belly ache.** Colic. **Belly button.** The navel. **Drum belly.** Tympanites. **Frog belly.** A condition occurring in rickety children in which the abdomen is in a semitympanic state. **Muscle belly.** The bulging central part of a muscle; in some muscles there are more than one such, which may be separately named. **Spider belly.** Arachnogastria. [AS *belg* bag.]

Belminus rugulosus (bel·min·us roo·gew·lo·sus). A reduviid bug that is a potential vector of American trypanosomiasis.

belonephobia (bel·o·ne·fo′·be·ah). Overmastering fear of sharp-pointed objects, particularly pins and needles. [Gk *belone* needle, phobia.]

belonoid (bel·on·oid). Styloid; like a needle in shape. [Gk *belone* needle, *eidos* form.]

Belsen drip (bel·sen drip). In severe cases of peptic ulcer a mixture of 100 g of dried milk and 400 g of glucose in 1500 ml of water is given in 24 h with a duodenal tube passed through the nose. [*Belsen*, German prison in World War II.]

belt (belt). A flat strap used as a girdle; anything used as a girdle. **Surgical belt.** *See* BRACE; CORSET. [L *balteus.*]

See also: HAMILTON IRVING, MOMBURG.

Bemegride BP 1968 (bem·e·gride). β - Ethyl - β - methylglutarimide, a barbiturate antagonist used for the relieving of barbiturate anaesthesia and in the treatment of barbiturate coma. Now seldom used.

ben (ben). Behen.

Benactyzine (ben·ak·ti·zeen). BP Commission approved name for 2-diethylaminoethyl benzilate; one of a group known as tranquillizing drugs used in the treatment of psychoneuroses.

Benapryzine (ben·ah·pri·zeen). BP Commission approved name for 2-(*N*-ethylpropylamino)ethyl benzilate; it is used in the treatment of Parkinson's syndrome.

Benario, Jacob. 19th–20th century Frankfurt physician.

Benario's method. A method for fixing a blood film with a 1 per cent alcohol solution of formalin.

Bence-Jones, Henry (b. 1813). London physician.

Bence-Jones albuminuria. Bence-Jones proteinuria (see below).

Bence-Jones protein. Protein found in urine of patients with myelomatosis which consists of light chains (usually dimerized) of myeloma immunologlobulin. It is soluble in water, precipitates when the solution is heated to a temperature of about 55°C, redissolves on boiling and reappears as a precipitate on cooling. It was formerly known as *Bence-Jones albumose* or *Bence-Jones proteose.*

Bence-Jones proteinuria. A condition in which Bence-Jones protein (see above) appears in the urine.

bend (bend). A curve, angle, or turn. **Head bend.** In the embryo, the cephalic flexure. *See* FLEXURE. **Neck bend.** In the embryo, the cervical flexure. *See* FLEXURE. [AS.]

Benda, Carl (b. 1857). German physician.

Benda's methods. 1. A mixture of chromic acid, osmium tetroxide and acetic acid, used to impregnate cell inclusions such as the Golgi apparatus and the mitochondria. 2. A method for staining mitochondria with crystal violet, and counterstaining with alizarin. 3. A modification of the Weigert–Pal method for myelin sheaths.

Benda, Raymond (b. 1896). French physician.

Benda's test. In a patient with aplastic anaemia the subcutaneous injection of adrenaline fails to cause the appearance of large numbers of white blood cells in the peripheral blood from the marrow, but there may sometimes be a monocytosis.

bendee (bend·ee). Okra. [West African name.]

Bender, Lauretta (b. 1897). New York psychiatrist.

Bender visual-motor gestalt test. A test in which the subject copies a series of patterns; the result is said to vary with the specific intellectual or psychiatric disorder of the subject.

Bender's bodies. Degenerative granules sometimes seen in leucocytes in severe anaemia.

Bendien, S. G. T. 19th–20th century Zeist, Holland, physician.

Bendien's test. *See* TEST FOR CANCER.

Bendrofluazide BP 1973 (ben·dro·floo·az·ide). 3 - Benzyl - 3,4 - dihydro - 7 - sulphamoyl - 6 - trifluoromethylbenzo - 1,2,4 - thiadiazine 1,1 - dioxide; a diuretic.

bends (bendz). The first severe symptoms of caisson disease, consisting of neuralgic pain in the joints and limbs, which are maintained in a semiflexed position (hence the name *bends*). The pain affects the knees, ankles and hips most commonly, and may be so severe as to be intolerable. There is also a mild form of which the chief symptoms are pain and a temporary sensation of weakness. A very similar condition occurs in airmen. [AS *bendan* strain.]

beneceptor (ben·e·sep·tor). The type of nervous machinery which receives beneficial stimuli and passes them on to the various nerve centres concerned. Cf. CEPTOR; NOCICEPTOR. [L *bene* well, *capere* to take.]

Benecki, stigmata of. Small petechial haemorrhages and erosions in the mucous membrane of the stomach.

Benedict, Francis Gano (b. 1870). American biochemist and physiologist.

Benedict's apparatus, Benedict-Roth apparatus. An apparatus for determining the metabolic rate. It consists of a tank filled with oxygen and suspended in water: the patient breathes through a tube from the tank, carbon dioxide is removed by soda lime, and the decrease in volume of the gas in the tank gives a direct measure of the oxygen consumed.

Benedict's calorimeter. Oxycalorimeter; a variant of the bomb calorimeter, for determination of the heat of combustion of substances by an indirect method. The substance is ignited in a known volume of oxygen in an enclosed space, the carbon dioxide produced is absorbed by soda lime and the oxygen utilized is measured by observing the reduction of volume. Each litre of oxygen used represents a heat production of 1.96–2.09 kilojoules (4.68–5.0 kg calories) according to the nature of the substance combusted.

Benedict-Talbot standards. Tables of the calorie output per hour of children, based on their weight in kilograms.

Benedict, Stanley Rossiter (b. 1884). Cornell biochemist.

Benedict's method. 1. For glucose in urine: *Qualitative:* to 5 ml of Benedict's solution 1 (see below) add 0.5 ml urine and heat in boiling water for 5 min. The presence of sugar is indicated by reduction giving a green, orange or red precipitate, according to the amount present. *Quantitative:* to 25 ml of Benedict's solution 2 (see below) add 3-4 g anhydrous sodium carbonate, heat to boiling and titrate with urine until the colour has been completely discharged. 2. For total sulphur in urine: to 10 ml urine add 5 ml reagent (crystalline copper nitrate, 200 g; sodium or potassium chlorate, 50 g; water to 1 litre), evaporate to dryness, ignite, dissolve in hydrochloric acid, precipitate sulphate with barium chloride filter, ignite and weigh the barium sulphate.

Benedict's solution, for detection and estimation of glucose. 1. *Qualitative:* 173 g of sodium citrate and 100 g of anhydrous sodium carbonate are dissolved in 600 ml of water. 17.3 g of crystalline copper sulphate is dissolved in 100 ml of water and this solution is added slowly, with constant stirring, to the first solution. The volume is adjusted to 1 litre with water, the solution is well mixed and filtered if necessary. 2. *Quantitative:* 200 g of sodium citrate, 75 g of anhydrous sodium carbonate and 125 g of potassium thiocyanate are dissolved in about 600 ml warm water, cooled and filtered. A solution of exactly 18 g of crystalline copper sulphate in 100 ml water is added slowly with constant stirring. 5 ml of 5 per cent potassium ferrocyanide solution is added, and the volume adjusted to 1 litre with water; 5 ml of this solution is equivalent to 10 mg glucose.

Benedict and Denis method. This is essentially Benedict's method (2nd def.) for total sulphur in urine, except that 25 ml urine is mixed with 5 ml of a reagent made up from copper nitrate, 25 g, sodium chloride, 25 g, ammonium nitrate, 10 g, water to 1 litre.

Benedict and Franke method. For uric acid in urine: the urine is diluted about 1 in 20, and to 10 ml of this solution is added 5 ml of 5 per cent sodium cyanide, followed by 1 ml of arsenophosphotungstic acid reagent. The colour is compared with standards after 5 min.

Benedict and Osterberg method. For sugar in urine: the urine is treated with activated charcoal and filtered. To the filtrate is added saturated picric acid solution, sodium carbonate solution and a few drops of acetone. The red colour is matched against standards.

Benedict and Theis method. For phenols in blood: proteins are precipitated by tungstic acid. 10 ml of filtrate is mixed with 1 ml of 1 per cent gum acacia solution, 1 ml of 50 per cent sodium acetate solution and 1 ml of diazotized *p*-nitraniline reagent (1.5 g *p*-nitraniline, 40 ml conc. HCl, water to 500 ml; to 25 ml add 0.75 ml of 10 per cent sodium nitrite solution). After 2-4 min, compare with standard (10 ml of phenol solution containing 0.0025 mg per ml).

Benedikt, Moritz (b. 1835). Vienna physician.

syndrome of Benedikt. A unilateral 3rd-nerve palsy with contralateral ataxia, hyperkinesis and tremor; contralateral hemianaesthesia and hemiparesis may occur. The syndrome is due to a lesion of the tegmentum of the mid-brain, involving the 3rd-nerve nucleus, red nucleus and medial fillet.

beng (beng). Cannabis indica. [Hind.]

Bengal quince (ben·gawl kwins). Bela. [*Bengal,* Indian province, *Cydonia* ancient town in Crete.]

bengaline (ben·gawl·een). A safranine dyestuff derived from β-naphthol and used in the dyeing of tannined cotton.

benign (ben·ine). 1. Of a disease, slight or non-malignant; favouring recovery. 2. Of a neoplasm, unlikely to recur. [L *benignare* to bless.]

benignancy (ben·i·nen·se). The quality of being benign. In neoplasms the opposite of malignancy. [L *benignare* to bless.]

Béniqué, Pierre Jules (b. 1806). Paris urologist.

Béniqué's sound. A special type of urethral bougie having a wide curve.

Bennet, James Henry (b. 1816). London obstetrician.

Bennet's corpuscles. Fatty epithelial cells found in ovarian cysts.

Bennet's small corpuscles. Tiny transparent cells found in the fluid of ovarian cysts.

Bennett, Edward Hallaran (b. 1837). Dublin surgeon.

Bennett's fracture. Fracture of the base of the first metacarpal bone.

Bennett's operation. An operation for varicocele by partial excision of the pampiniform plexus, followed by suture of the divided ends of the plexus, in order to provide support to the testis.

Bennett, Sir Norman Godfrey (b. 1870). London dental surgeon.

Bennett's classification. Of malocclusion and occlusion. A classification of malocclusion and dentofacial abnormalities: *Class I,* the abnormal position of one or more teeth is due to local causes; *Class II,* the abnormal formation of part or the whole of the maxillary or the mandibular dental arch is due to developmental bony defects; *Class III,* the abnormal relationship between the dental arches, and between either arch and the facial contour, is due to developmental bony defects.

Bennhold, Hans Hermann (b. 1893). Tübingen physician.

Bennhold's test. For amyloidosis and nephrosis: inject 1 ml of 1 per cent aqueous solution of Congo red per 4.5 kg (10 lb) body weight. Take 10 ml blood after 4 min, and again after 1 h, and collect the urine at the end of 1 h. Compare the colours of the sera to obtain the percentage disappearing from the blood. In normal subjects less than 40 per cent disappears in 1 h; in amyloidosis 60-100 per cent usually disappears in 4 min; in lipoid nephrosis 40-60 per cent disappears from the blood in 1 h and the dye is present in the urine.

Benoist, Louis (b. 1856). Paris physicist.

Benoist's scale. A scale for measuring the quality of radiation in terms of the thickness of aluminium required to reduce the intensity of a beam to the same value as a 0.11 mm screen of silver would do.

benorterone (be·nor·ter·on). 17α-Methyl B nortestosterone. An androgen antagonist recently used in acne and virilism.

Benorylate (ben·or·il·ate). BP Commission approved name for 4-acetamidophenyl *O*-acetylsalicylate; an analgesic.

Benperidol (ben·per·id·ol). BP Commission approved name for 1-{1 - [3 - (4 - fluorobenzoyl)propyl] - 4 - piperidyl}benzimidazolin-2 - one; a tranquillizer.

Benserazide (ben·ser·az·ide). BP Commission approved name for DL - 2 - amino - 3 - hydroxy - 2′ - (2,3,4 - trihydroxybenzyl)propionohydrazide; it is used in the treatment of Parkinson's syndrome.

Bensley, Robert Russell (b. 1867). Chicago anatomist.

Bensley's granules. The α- and β-granules in the islets of Langerhans.

Benson, Arthur Henry (b. 1852). Dublin ophthalmologist.

Benson's disease. Numerous small white disc-like and spherical bodies floating in the vitreous of the eye. It is a senile change of no pathological significance. Also called *asteroid hyalitis.*

Bentonite BP 1973 (ben·ton·ite). A native hydrated colloidal aluminosilicate of composition $(Mg,Ca)OAl_2O_35SiO_2{\cdot}nH_2O$, found at Fort Benton USA, and in California. It forms very viscous suspensions with water, and is used as a suspending agent and for clarifying liquids. It resists high temperatures and may be sterilized by heat.

benzacetin (ben·zas·et·in). Acetamido-ethylsalicylic acid. *See* ACID.

benzaconine (ben·zak·on·een). Benzoyl aconine, $C_{32}H_{45}O_{10}N$. An alkaloid derived from *Aconitum napellus* and less toxic than aconitine. It hydrolyses to benzoic acid and aconine.

Benzadon's sign. Retraction of the nipple felt when it is held between the fingers and an underlying tumour is pressed away.

benzal (ben·zal). Benzylidene. The divalent aromatic radical C_6H_5CH=derived from toluene.

Benzaldehyde BPC 1968 (ben·zal·de·hide). C_6H_5CHO. A constituent of oil of bitter almond, and largely responsible for its flavour. It is employed in very small quantities as a flavouring agent in pharmacy; used mainly in the manufacture of drugs and dyestuffs. **Benzaldehyde cyanohydrin.** One of the primary hydrolytic products of certain cyanogenetic glycosides. Further hydrolysis yields benzaldehyde and prussic acid, and oil of bitter almond contains all 3 substances.

benzaldoxime (ben·zal·dox·ime). Benzaldehyde-oxime, $C_6H_5CH{=}NOH$. A substance formed from benzaldehyde with hydroxylamine; it occurs in 2 isomeric forms, α- (anti-) and β- (syn-).

Benzalkonium Chloride (ben·zal·ko·ne·um klor·ide). BP Commission approved name for a mixture of alkyl chlorides of dimethylbenzyl ammonium. It is a cationic detergent with bactericidal properties, used for the irrigation of the bladder and for the disinfection of surgical instruments and theatre equipment.

benzamide (ben·zam·ide). $C_6H_5CONH_2$ prepared from benzaldehyde, or by the oxidation of benzonitrile; colourless plates insoluble in water, but readily in alcohol, ether or ammonia. **Benzamide silver.** A silver derivative existing in 2 tautomeric forms: $C_6H_5CONHAg$ and $C_6H_5C(OAg){=}NH$.

benzamine (ben·zam·een). Beta-eucaine, trimethylbenzoyloxypiperidine, $C_{15}H_{21}O_2N$. A synthetic substitute for cocaine and resembling the latter in chemical structure. It is not much used in medicine nowadays. **Benzamine Hydrochloride BPC 1954.** $C_{15}H_{21}O_2NHCl$, the soluble hydrochloride of benzamine. **Benzamine lactate.** $C_{15}H_{21}NO_2C_3H_6O_3$, betacaine lactate, beta-eucaine lactate; the most widely used salt of benzamine, on account of its solubility and the stability of its solutions.

benzanthracene (ben·zan·thras·een). $C_{18}H_{12}$. A hydrocarbon consisting structurally of a benzene ring attached to an anthracene ring; it forms many derivatives which, having this structure, are strongly carcinogenic.

benzaurin (ben·**zaw**·rin). Phenyldiphenylcarbinol, $(C_6H_5)(C_6H_4OH)C{=}C_6H_4{=}O$. A crystalline substance, closely related to aurin; insoluble in water, but soluble in alkalis with a violet coloration.

Benzbromarone (benz·**bro**·mar·one). BP Commission approved name for 3 - (3,5 - dibromo - 4 - hydroxybenzoyl) - 2 - ethylbenzofuran; it is used in the treatment of hyperuricaemia.

benzene (**ben**·zeen). A colourless liquid hydrocarbon with a pleasant odour, obtained by the fractional distillation of coal tar. It is insoluble in water, miscible with alcohol and ether, and highly inflammable, burning with a luminous, smoky flame. It is used as a solvent for fats, resins, mastic and phosphorus (BPC 1954), as a motor fuel, and in the industrial synthesis of organic compounds, e.g. dyes and drugs. Chemically it is the parent of the large and important group of aromatic compounds. The hydrocarbon is extremely volatile and highly poisonous, the toxic concentration in air being 1 part in 10 000: chronic poisoning causes aplastic anaemia; acute poisoning gives rise to headache, dizziness and convulsions followed by paralysis and death. It was formerly used as a pulmonary antiseptic, as a taeniacide and to destroy pediculi, but its use is not advised in therapeutics. **Acetyl benzene.** Acetophenone. **Benzene compound.** Any one of a large number of compounds derived from the benzene ring by substitution; they include drugs, such as phenol, salicylates, phenacetin, dyestuffs such as indigo and the aniline dyes, and perfumes. **Benzene dichloride.** Dichlorobenzene. **Dimethyl benzene.** Xylene. **Methyl benzene.** Toluene. **Benzene ring.** The diagrammatic representation of the benzene molecule in the form of a hexagon with a carbon atom at each angle linked alternately by double bonds. [Fr. *benjoin* gum benjamin.]

benzenoid (**ben**·zen·oid). 1. Applied to an aromatic compound containing a 6-carbon ring with the benzene linkage, as distinct from the quinone linkage (quinonoid). 2. A theoretical benzene molecule in which the carbon atoms are represented as tetrahedra. [benzene, Gk *eidos* form.]

benzenyl (**ben**·zen·il). The trivalent aromatic radical $C_6H_5C{\equiv}$ related to toluene. **Benzenyl amidothiophenol.** Benzenylamidophenyl mercaptan, $C_6H_5C{\equiv}NS{=}C_6H_4$; a yellow substance with the odour of roses, and used in perfumery.

Benzethidine (ben·**zeth**·id·een). BP Commission approved name for ethyl 1 - (2 - benzyloxyethyl) - 4 - phenylpiperidine - 4 - carboxylate; a narcotic analgesic.

Benzethonium Chloride (ben·zeth·**o**·ne·um **klor**·ide). BP Commission approved name for benzyldimethyl - *p* - (1,1,3,3 - tetramethylbutyl) - phenoxyethoxyethylammonium chloride. A synthetic quaternary ammonium compound belonging to the cationic group of detergents, and a surface-active and anti-infective. It is used as a germicide and antiseptic, but is incompatible with soaps.

Benzhexol (benz·**hex**·ol). BP Commission approved name for 1 - cyclohexyl - 1 - phenyl - 3 - piperidinopropan - 1 - ol. **Benzhexol Hydrochloride BP 1973.** The hydrochloride of the base $(C_6H_{11})(C_6H_5)C(OH)CH_2N{=}C_5H_{10}HCl$. A synthetic spasmolytic drug, used in the treatment of extrapyramidal parkinsonism.

benzhydrol (benz·**hi**·drol). Benzohydrol, diphenylcarbinol, $(C_6H_5)_2CHOH$. A secondary alcohol derived from benzophenone by reduction; related to Michler's ketone used in dyestuffs manufacture.

benzidine (**ben**·zid·een). Paradiaminodiphenyl, $NH_2C_6H_4C_6H_4NH_2$. A basic compound prepared from azobenzene and used in the synthesis of the direct substantive cotton dyes. It forms a very sensitive test for blood, giving blue coloration with the latter in an acetic solution of sodium perborate.

benzil (**ben**·zil). Diphenylglyoxal, dibenzoyl, $C_6H_5COCOC_6H_5$. A diketone produced by the oxidation of phenyl benzoyl carbinol (benzoin); a yellow compound dissolving in alcoholic potash with a violet coloration. Used in organic synthesis.

benzilimide (ben·**zil**·im·ide). $C_{28}H_{20}O_2(NH)_2$. A white substance obtained by the action of ammonia on benzil.

Benzilonium Bromide (ben·zil·**o**·ne·um **bro**·mide). BP Commission approved name for 3 - benziloyloxy - 1,1 - diethylpyrrolidinium bromide; it is used in the treatment of peptic ulcer.

benzin, benzine (**ben**·zin, **ben**·zeen). Petroleum benzine: a mixture of petroleum hydrocarbons, principally hexane and heptane, with various paraffins, oleins, naphthalenes and benzene derivatives, according to origin, distilling below 150°C in the refining of natural petroleum. It is used as a solvent for fats and resins, and for cleaning purposes.

Benziodarone (benz·i·**o**·dar·one). BP Commission approved name for 2 - ethyl - 3 - (4 - hydroxy - 3,5 - di - iodobenzoyl) - coumarone; it is used in the treatment of angina pectoris.

benzoate (**ben**·zo·ate). A salt of benzoic acid.

benzoated (**ben**·zo·a·ted). 1. Mixed with benzoic acid. 2. Having had introduced into its molecule the benzoyl radical C_6H_5CO-.

Benzocaine BP 1973 (**ben**·zo·kane). Ethyl aminobenzoate, $NH_2C_6H_4COOC_2H_5$, a local anaesthetic which is very insoluble in water; it is used in dusting powders to anaesthetize mucous surfaces.

Benzocainum. *European Pharmacopoeia* name for Benzocaine BP 1973.

Benzoctamine (ben·**zok**·tam·een). BP Commission approved name for *N* - methyl - 9,10 - ethanoanthracene - 9(10*H*) - methylamine; a tranquillizer.

benzodiureide (**ben**·zo·di·ewr·**e**′·ide). $C_9H_{12}N_4O_2$. A purine formed from benzaldehyde and urea.

benzoglycollate (ben·zo·**gli**·kol·ate). A salt of benzoglycollic (mandelic) acid.

benzohelicin (ben·zo·**hel**·is·in). Benzoyl helicin, $C_6H_5COC_{13}H_{15}O_7$. A glucoside derived from helicin, an oxidation product of salicin; used as an antipyretic.

benzohydrol (ben·zo·**hi**·drol). Benzhydrol.

benzoin (**ben**·zo·in). Phenyl benzoyl carbinol, $C_6H_5CHOHCOC_6H_5$. A crystalline compound formed by the polymerization of benzaldehyde; used as an antiseptic in ointments. **Benzoin oxime.** Cupron, $C_6H_5CHOHC{=}NOHC_6H_5$, a delicate reagent for the detection or determination of copper, with which it gives a green precipitate.

Benzoin BP 1958 (**ben**·zoin). Gum benjamin, gum benzoin: brittle masses of balsamic resin obtained from the incised stem of various species of styraceous plants. The resin contains a high percentage of cinnamic and benzoic acids, and has some antiseptic action. It is applied to the skin in parasitic skin diseases, and, combined with styrax, aloes and Tolu balsam in the form of a compound tincture, is used as an expectorant. The principal ingredient of friars' balsam. [Fr. *benjoin.*]

benzoinam (ben·**zo**·in·am). $C_{28}H_{24}N_2O$. A substance prepared from phenyl benzoyl carbinol (benzoin) by the action of ammonia.

benzoinum (ben·**zoi**·num). Benzoin BP 1958.

benzol (**ben**·zol). A synonym for benzene.

benzoline (**ben**·zo·leen). Petroleum benzine.

benzolism (**ben**·zol·izm). A toxic condition produced by the use of benzene or the inhalation of its vapour.

Benzonatate (ben·zo·**na**·tate). BP Commission approved name for 2 - (ω - methoxypolyethyleneoxy)ethyl *p* - butylaminobenzoate; a cough suppressant.

benzonitrile (ben·zo·**ni**·trile). Phenyl cyanide, C_6H_5CN. A colourless liquid with an odour of bitter almonds; formed from the hydrocarbon benzene, and a step in the synthesis of artificial benzoic acid. It is used in drug manufacture.

benzophenanthrene (**ben**·zo·fen·**an**′·threen). Chrysene, $C_{18}H_{12}$. A carcinogenic hydrocarbon obtained in the distillation of coal tar, and from some natural fats and oils.

benzophenide, benzophenol (ben·zo·**fen**·ide, ben·zo·**fe**·nol). Phenylbenzoate, benzocarbolic acid, $C_6H_5COOC_6H_5$.White crystals slightly soluble in water.

benzophenone (ben·zo·**fen**·one). Diphenylketone, $(C_6H_5)_2CO$. A compound with hypnotic properties.

benzopurpurine (ben·zo·**per**·pewr·een). Ozamin. A scarlet dyestuff derived from toluidine and naphthionic acid; it dyes unmordanted cotton. It is a useful indicator between pH 3.5 and 4.5, being purple in acid and scarlet in alkali.

benzopyrine (ben·zo·**pi**·reen). Antipyrine benzoate, $C_{11}H_{12}N_2OC_6H_5COOH$. A compound with mild analgesic and antipyretic properties, but little used because of the danger of toxic effects.

benzopyrone (ben·zo·**pi**·rone). Coumarin.

benzopyrrole (ben·zo·**pir**·ole). Benzpyrrole.

benzoresinol (ben·zo·**rez**·in·ol). $C_{16}H_{26}O_2$. An alcohol derived from the resin of benzoin.

benzosulphate (ben·zo·**sul**·fate). Any of the salts of benzene sulphuric acid.

benzosulphimide (ben·zo·**sul**·fim·ide). Saccharin BP 1958, $C_6H_4=CONHSO_2$. A white crystalline powder with a sweetness about 500 times that of sugar, prepared by the oxidation of *o*-toluenesulphonamide. It is moderately soluble in water, but when neutralized with sodium bicarbonate or sodium hydroxide the sodium salt is formed (Saccharin Sodium BP 1958), which dissolves readily. Used as a substitute for sugar, especially in the diet of diabetics.

benzotherapy (ben·zo·**ther**·ap·e). Treatment with a benzoate, particularly the intravenous injection of sodium benzoate in cases of abscess of the lung. [benzoate, therapy.]

benzotrichloride (ben·zo·tri·**klor**'·ide). Trichlorotoluene, benzenyl chloride, phenylchloroform, $C_6H_5CCl_3$. A colourless liquid with a pungent odour, formed from benzoyl chloride and used in the synthesis of dyestuffs.

benzoyl (ben·zo·il). The monovalent radical, C_6H_5CO-, occurring in benzoic acid and the basis of a wide range of important organic compounds. **Benzoyl acetate,** $C_6H_5COOOCCH_3$, a component of several essential oils, and used in perfumery. **Benzoyl acetyl peroxide.** $C_6H_5COOOCOCH_3$, a disinfectant. **Benzoyl aconine.** Benzaconine. **Benzoyl carbinol.** $C_6H_5COCH_2OH$, a compound used as a local anaesthetic. **Benzoyl chloride.** C_6H_5COCl, a colourless liquid with a pungent odour which has been employed hypodermically in the treatment of leprosy, and as a local application; principally used in organic synthesis. **Benzoyl ecgonine.** $C_6H_5COC_9H_{14}O_3N$, an ester of ecgonine found in Peruvian coca leaves and also prepared from cocaine; it resembles caffeine in its action on the central nervous system. **Benzoyl eugenol.** $(CH_2=CHCH_2)C_6H_3(OCH_3)OCOC_6H_5$, a colourless compound soluble in alcohol or ether, which was formerly used to treat tuberculosis. **Benzoyl glycine, Benzoyl glycocoll.** Hippuric acid. *See* ACID. **Benzoyl guaiacol.** Guaiacol benzoate, $C_6H_5COOC_6H_4(OCH_3)$, a compound used as an antiseptic. **Benzoyl morphine.** A weak anaesthetic stated to produce similar local effects to ethyl-morphine. **Benzoyl naphthol.** β-naphthol benzoate, $C_6H_5COOC_{10}H_7$ an intestinal antiseptic. **Benzoyl paracresol.** $C_6H_5COOC_6H_4CH_3$, a compound which has been used as an intestinal antiseptic. **Benzoyl peroxide.** $C_6H_5COOOCOC_6H_5$, a crystalline compound used as a dusting powder, or in oil solution, for application to burns and some forms of dermatitis. **Benzoyl pseudotropeine.** Tropacocaine, $C_{15}H_{19}O_2N$, an alkaloid derived from Java coca leaves or prepared synthetically; it is used as a local anaesthetic, especially in ophthalmology. **Benzoyl quinine.** $C_6H_5COC_{20}H_{24}O_2N_2$, a compound with the properties of a local anaesthetic. **Benzoyl salicin.** Populin, $C_6H_{11}O_5OC_6H_4CH_2OOC_6H_5$, a glucoside occurring in the bark and leaves of species of poplar and willow. **Benzoyl superoxide.** Benzoyl peroxide (see above). **Benzoyl tropeine.** An isomer of tropacocaine employed as a local anaesthetic.

Benzphetamine (benz·**fet**·am·een). BP Commission approved name for (+) - *N* - benzyl - *Na* - dimethylphenethylamine; it is used in the treatment of obesity.

benzpyrene (benz·**pi**·reen). $C_{20}H_{11}$. A complex hydrocarbon, consisting of an anthracene ring fused to a naphthalene ring. It occurs in coal-tar pitch, and with other carcinogenic derivatives of benzanthracene is responsible for cancer among workers in tar-distillation plants.

benzpyrrole (benz·**pir**·ole). Indole, $C_6H_4CH=CHNH$. A colourless compound found in essential oil of jasmine and clover oil; it has a faecal odour and occurs in the body as a decomposition product of tryptophane. It is the parent of indigo, into which it is converted by oxidation. Used in perfumery.

Benzquinamide (benz·**kwin**·am·ide). BP Commission approved name for 2 - acetoxy - 3 - diethylcarbamoyl - 1,3,4,6,7,11b - hexahydro - 9,10 - dimethoxy - 2*H* - benzo [a] quinolizine; a tranquillizer.

Benzthiazide (benz·**thi**·az·ide). BP Commission approved name for 3 - benzylthiomethyl - 6 - chlorobenzo - 1,2,4 - thiadiazine - 7 - sulphonamide 1,1 - dioxide; a diuretic.

Benztropine (benz·**tro**·peen). BP Commission approved name for 3-diphenylmethoxytropane. **Benztropine Mesylate BP 1973.** A white, odourless, crystalline powder with a bitter taste, soluble in water and in alcohol, insoluble in ether. It is an antiparasympathomimetic agent and is used, usually in conjunction with certain other drugs, in the treatment of parkinsonism for the relief of reduction of spasm, tremor, rigidity and sialorrhoea.

Benzydamine (benz·i·dam·een). BP Commission approved name for 1 - benzyl - 3 - (3 - dimethylaminopropoxy)indazole; an anti-inflammatory and analgesic agent.

benzyl (**ben**·zil). The monovalent radical $C_6H_5CH_2-$, derived from toluene and occurring in derivatives of benzyl alcohol. **Benzyl acetate.** $C_6H_5CH_2OCOCH_3$, an aromatic liquid found in oil of jasmin and used in perfumery. **Benzyl alcohol.** *See* ALCOHOL. **Benzyl Benzoate BP 1973.** $C_6H_5CH_2OCOC_6H_5$, a volatile oil present in various balsams (e.g. Tolu and Peru) and prepared synthetically. It possesses antispasmodic properties but is mainly used in the form of a 25 per cent emulsion in the treatment of scabies; also employed as a solvent. **Benzyl bromide.** $C_6H_5CH_2Br$, a compound with a vapour that is irritant to the mucous membrane of the nose and eyes and employed in chemical warfare as a tear gas. **Benzyl carbinol.** Phenylethyl alcohol, $C_6H_5CH_2CH_2OH$, occurring in oil of rose and used in perfumery. It possesses anaesthetic properties. **Benzyl chloride.** $C_6H_5CH_2Cl$, a lacrimatory compound used in chemical warfare and also in the synthesis of oil of bitter almond and of certain dyes. **Benzyl cinnamate.** $C_6H_5CH_2OCOC_8H_7$, a compound which has been used in oil as an intramuscular injection in tuberculosis. **Benzyl fumarate.** $C_6H_5CH_2OCOCH=CH=COOCH_2C_6H_5$, a compound used as an antispasmodic in similar manner to benzyl benzoate with the advantage that it is tasteless. **Benzyl glycocoll.** Hippuric acid. *See* ACID. **Benzyl iodide.** $C_6H_5CH_2I$, a lacrimatory compound used in chemical warfare as a tear gas. **Benzyl mandelate.** $C_6H_5CH_2OCOCH(OH)C_6H_5$, a compound used as a substitute for mandelic acid and reported to have a depressant effect on involuntary muscle. **Benzyl morphine.** $C_6H_5CH_2OC_{17}H_{18}O_2N$, a colourless bitter powder with actions similar to those of codeine and ethylmorphine. **Benzyl penicillin.** Benzylpenicillin. **Benzyl succinate.** $C_6H_5CH_2OCOCH_2CH_2COOCH_2C_6H_5$, a compound which has been used as an antispasmodic.

benzylic (ben·**zil**·ik). Of the nature of a benzyl derivative.

benzylidene (ben·**zil**·id·een). Benzal. The divalent aromatic radical $C_6H_5CH=$ derived from toluene.

Benzylpenicillin BP 1973 (**ben**·zil·pen·is·**il**'·in). Penicillin G (or II). Either the crystalline potassium salt or the crystalline sodium salt. It is the only type of penicillin permitted by the *British Pharmacopoeia*, and must be dispensed when penicillin is prescribed or demanded.

Benzylpenicillinum (**ben**·zil·pen·is·**il**'·in·um). **Benzylpenicillinum Kalicum, Benzylpenicillinum Natricum.** *European Pharmacopoeia* name for Benzylpenicillin BP 1973.

Bephenium Hydroxynaphthoate (bef·**en**·e·um hi·drox·e·**naf**·tho·-ate). BP Commission approved name for benzyldimethylphenoxyethylammonium 3 - hydroxy - 2 - naphthoate; an anthelminthic.

Bérard, Auguste (b. 1802). French surgeon.

Bérard's aneurysm. Arteriovenous aneurysm.

Béraud, Bruno Jean Jacques (b. 1823). Paris anatomist.

Béraud's ligament. The vertebropericardial ligament, a band of fibrous tissue which connects the upper part of the pericardium with the 3rd thoracic vertebra and the disc below it.

valve of Béraud. A fold of mucous membrane guarding the opening of the lacrimal ducts into the lacrimal sac.

berbamine (ber·bam·een). $C_{37}H_{40}O_6N_2$. An alkaloid obtained from the barberry, *Berberis vulgaris.*

berberine (ber·ber·een). $C_{20}H_{19}O_5N$. An alkaloid isolated from *Hydrastis canadensis* (golden seal) and barberry root bark (*Berberis vulgaris*). It has been used as a bitter tonic, usually in conjunction with others such as quassia. **Berberine sulphate.** Berberinae Sulphas BPC 1949; the injection of a 2 per cent solution around oriental sore is sometimes curative.

Berberis (ber·ber·is). A genus of shrubs of the family Berberidaceae. **Berberis aristata.** A species of India and Sri Lanka, the dried root of which contains the alkaloid berberine. It is a bitter tonic and diaphoretic and is used in India to treat intermittent fevers. **Berberis vulgaris.** The main source of berberine sulphate. [L barberry.]

Berchillet-Jourdain, Anselme Louis Bernard (b. 1734). Paris surgeon.

Jourdain's disease. Chronic suppurative periodontitis; pyorrhoea alveolaris.

Berens, Conrad (b. 1889). New York ophthalmologist.

Berens' operation. For chronic glaucoma: a form of iridocorneosclerectomy in which the scleral lip is excised and serrated along its length with a punch, and combined usually with a broad iridectomy; a modification of Lagrange's sclerectomy.

bergamot (ber·gam·ot). The fruit of *Citrus bergamia* Risso (family Rutaceae). **Bergamot camphor.** Bergaptene. **Oil of bergamot.** Oleum Bergamottae BPC 1949 (essence of bergamot), an oil obtained by expression of the fresh rind of the fruit. The fragrant odour of the oil is due mainly to linalyl acetate, and it is used extensively in perfumery. [*Bergamo*, an Italian town.]

bergaptene (ber·gap·teen). $C_{12}H_8O_4$. A constituent of oil of bergamot from the rind of *Citrus bergamia*; also known as *bergamot camphor.*

Bergenhem, Bengt Ludwig (b. 1898). Swedish surgeon.

Bergenhem's operation. For implanting the ureter into the rectum [obsolete].

Berger, Emil (b. 1855). Austrian ophthalmologist.

Berger's sign. An irregular or elliptical pupil, seen in early cases of neurosyphilis.

Berger, Hans (b. 1873). Jena neurologist.

Berger rhythm, or wave. Alpha rhythm; term used in electroencephalography to describe the normal dominant activity of the postcentral cortex. It is a regular waveform with a frequency varying between 8 and 13 Hz (c/s); it is seen most clearly in the occipital regions and varies greatly in amount in different individuals. In some normal subjects it is almost continuous and of high amplitude; in others it is extremely scanty. As a rule, the rhythm is inhibited by visual or mental attention.

Berger, Oskar (b. 1844). Breslau neurologist.

Berger's paraesthesia. Paraesthesia and weakness in the lower limbs of young persons, but with no signs of organic disease.

Berger, Paul (b. 1845). Paris surgeon.

Berger's method. Treatment of transverse fracture of the patella by suture of the fragments.

Berger's operation. Interscapulothoracic amputation. *See* AMPUTATION.

Bergeron, Étienne Jules (b. 1817). Paris physician.

Bergeron's disease, Henoch-Bergeron's disease. The myoclonic form of encephalitis lethargica; electrical chorea; also called *Dubini's disease.*

Bergh, Albert Abraham Hujmans van den (b. 1869). Utrecht physician.

van den Bergh's reaction, or test. For bilirubin in serum: to 1 ml of serum in a centrifuge tube add 0.5 ml of diazo reagent. A "direct" reaction is shown by the development of a red colour. Add 0.5 ml of saturated ammonium sulphate and 3 ml of absolute industrial alcohol. Shake and allow to stand for 15–30 min, centrifuge and compare the colour with a standard methyl red solution to obtain the concentration of bilirubin in the serum. *Standard methyl red: stock solution,* 0.29 g in glacial acetic acid to 100 ml; *working solution,* 1 ml of stock solution + 5 ml of glacial acetic acid + 14.4 g of crystalline sodium acetate made to 1 litre with water. The colour of the working solution is equivalent to 1.6 mg bilirubin per 100 ml serum treated by the above process.

Bergmann, Ernst von (b. 1836). Berlin surgeon.

Bergmann's cell. A type of neuroglial cell in the outer zone of the cerebellar cortex.

Bergmann's fibres. Non-medullated nerve fibres in the molecular layer of the cerebellum.

Bergmann's hernia. A small intermittent form of hiatus hernia of the diaphragm.

Bergmann's incision. For exposure of the kidney, from the outer border of the erector spinae at the level of the 12th rib towards the junction of the outer and middle third of the inguinal ligament.

Bergmann's operation. Incision of the tunica vaginalis, with removal of its parietal layer, performed for hydrocele.

Kuester-Bergmann operation. Radical mastoid for chronic mastoiditis; the mastoid process, mastoid antrum and middle-ear cavity are cleaned of diseased tissue and converted into a single cavity draining the external auditory meatus.

Bergmann, Gottlieb Heinrich (b. 1781). Hildesheim psychiatrist.

Bergmann's conductors, or cords. Auditory striae. *See* STRIA.

Bergmann, Gustav von (b. 1878). Munich physician.

Bergmann's hypopituitarism. Juvenile hypopituitarism.

Bergmeister, Otto (b. 1845). Vienna ophthalmologist.

Bergmeister's papilla. A mass of neuroglial tissue around the bulb of the hyaloid artery situated in the centre of the optic disc in the embryo. Rarely, it remains as a congenital abnormality.

Bergonié, Jean Alban (b. 1857). Bordeaux physicist and radiologist.

Bergonié method, or treatment. The treatment of obesity by faradism (induced electricity) applied to the whole body simultaneously.

law of Bergonié and Tribondeau. A statement about radiosensitivity of tissues in general, evolved from work on the testes. It is stated either as "The biological action of Roentgen rays is greater the higher the reproductive activity of the cell, the longer the period of its mitosis and the less the degree of differentiation of the cell in respect to its morphology and function" or as "The biological effect of x-rays varies directly as the mitotic activity of the cell and inversely as the stage of embryonic development and degree of differentiation".

beriberi (ber·e·ber·e). A deficiency disease associated with imbalance between the intakes of carbohydrate and of vitamin B_1 (aneurine, thiamine). The critical level below which beriberi will occur is 0.4 mg/1000 non-fat calories. It is characterized by multiple neuritis, dropsy and cardiovascular disturbances. It is generally found amongst those living entirely on a diet of highly milled rice. **Alcoholic beriberi.** Vitamin-B_1 deficiency in an alcoholic. **Atrophic beriberi.** A type in which peripheral neuritis is the outstanding feature. **Cardiac beriberi.** Beriberi in which the effect on the heart is severe. **Cerebral beriberi.** A Wernicke's encephalopathy. **Dropsical beriberi.** A type in which oedema (dropsy) is the outstanding feature. **Dry beriberi.** Atrophic beriberi (see above). **Infantile beriberi.** A severe and often fatal form of beriberi with cardiac and laryngeal symptoms due to carbohydrate: aneurine imbalance in the milk of the mother, who may not show signs of the disease. **Paralytic beriberi, Paraplegic beriberi.** Atrophic beriberi (see above). **Ship beriberi.** A form found among fishermen of the Newfoundland Banks and

Norway and due to the use of too highly milled white flour. **Wet beriberi.** Dropsical beriberi (see above). [Singhalese *beri* weakness.]

Berkefeld, Wilhelm (b. 1836). German manufacturer.

Berkefeld filter. A bacterial filter prepared from diatomaceous earth.

berkelium (ber·ke·le·um). A transuranic element of atomic number 97 and chemical symbol Bk. It was obtained in 1949 by bombarding americium with α-particles in the cyclotron, and has a half-life of 4.6 h. [City of *Berkeley*, USA.]

Berkow, Samuel Gordon (b. 1899). New Jersey surgeon.

Berkow's table. A table for estimating the extent of surface burn lesions.

Berlin, Rudolf (b. 1833). Stuttgart ophthalmologist.

Berlin's disease, or oedema. Commotio retinae: oedema affecting the posterior part of the retina involving the macular region, after a blow on the front of the eye; contrecoup effect.

Berlin blue (ber·lin bloo). Prussian blue, $Fe_4(FeC_6N_6)_3$, used for colouring anatomical specimens and, as an injection, for demonstrating blood and lymphatic vascular patterns. [City of *Berlin*, Germany, ME *blew.*]

See also: MUELLER (H. F.).

Bernard, Claude (b. 1813). Paris physiologist.

Bernard's canal, or duct. Accessory pancreatic duct. *See* DUCT, PANCREATIC.

Bernard's granular layer. The inner granular zone of the acinous cells of the pancreas.

Bernard's puncture. Diabetic puncture; the needling of a point in the floor of the 3rd ventricle of the brain in experimental animals, which causes glycosuria; hence *piqûre diabetes.*

Bernard's syndrome, Bernard-Horner syndrome, Horner-Bernard syndrome, Claude Bernard-Horner syndrome. Horner's syndrome.

Bernard, Leon (b. 1872). Paris physician.

Bernard-Sergent syndrome. A term not in general use that has been employed to describe the abdominal symptoms of Addison's disease.

Bernhardt, Martin (b. 1844). Berlin neurologist.

Bernhardt's disease, paraesthesia, paralysis, symptom or syndrome. Meralgia paraesthetica; pain, numbness, and paraesthesia on standing or on exertion, in the distribution of the lateral cutaneous nerve of the thigh. It usually occurs in obese subjects, and is important in differential diagnosis of leprosy. Also called *Roth's disease.*

Bernhardt-Roth symptom complex, or syndrome, Roth-Bernhardt disease. Meralgia paraesthetica; Bernhardt's disease.

Bernhardt formula. The height of an adult is multiplied by the chest circumference in centimetres, and the product divided by 240. The result gives the ideal weight in kilograms.

Bernheim, Alice Rheinstein (b. 1883). New York physician.

Bernheim's icterus index method. A method for the estimation of bilirubinaemia in serum or plasma by comparison of a clear non-haemolysed sample with a 1 in 10 000 solution of potassium dichromate, either in a colorimeter or in a comparator, with suitable dilutions of dichromate as standards.

Bernheim's syndrome. A syndrome consisting of systemic congestive failure, elevated central venous pressure, oedema, clear lungs and absence of orthopnoea, occurring in patients with left ventricular hypertrophy and insufficiency; said to be due to bulging of the hypertrophied intraventricular septum in the right ventricular cavity, and obstructing the outflow tract.

Bernheimer, Stefan (b. 1861). Innsbrück and Vienna ophthalmologist.

Bernheimer's fibres. A fibre tract supposedly connecting the optic tract with the subthalamic nucleus (Luys' nucleus).

Bernreuter test. A personality inventory for older children and adults, scored for 6 traits: neurotic tendency, self-sufficiency, introversion-extroversion, dominance-submission, confidence and sociability. The questions require the answers Yes or No, e.g. "Have you ever crossed the street to avoid meeting a person?"

Berry, Sir George Andreas (b. 1853). Edinburgh ophthalmologist.

Berry's circles. Stereoscopic charts inscribed with circles.

Berry, Sir James (b. 1860). London surgeon.

Berry's ligaments. Suspensory ligaments of the thyroid gland.

berry (ber·e). A succulent fruit with an entirely soft pericarp, and one or more carpels, usually many-seeded. **Bear berry.** Uva ursi. **Fish berry.** Cocculus. **Juniper berry.** Juniper fructus. **Levant berry.** Cocculus. [AS *berie.*]

Berthollet, Claude Louis (b. 1748). French chemist.

Berthollet's law. If one or more products of a chemical reaction are likely to be removed from the sphere of action by reason of their volatility or insolubility, the equilibrium of the reaction will be displaced in that direction.

Bertiella (ber·te·el·ah). A genus of tapeworms, of which *Bertiella studeri* is a large species found occasionally in children around the Indian Ocean. Secondary hosts are probably mites of the family Oribatidae. *Bertiella macronata* is another rare incidental parasite of man. [Paul *Bert*, French physiologist, 1833-1886.]

bertielliasis (ber·te·el·i'·as·is). Infection with tapeworms of the genus *Bertiella.*

Bertillon, Alphonse (b. 1853). French criminologist.

Bertillon system. A system of identification and registration of criminals based upon the characteristics of the individual under 3 headings: *descriptive data*, such as colour of hair, eyes, complexion, shape of nose, chin, ears; *bodily marks,* such as moles, tattoo marks, scars; *body measurements,* 11 in number, including standing and sitting heights, length and breadth of head, arm reach, and certain measurements of the hand and foot.

Bertin, Exupère Joseph (b. 1712). Paris anatomist.

Bertin's bone, or ossicles. Sphenoidal conchae. *See* CONCHA.

Bertin's columns. Renal columns. *See* COLUMN.

Bertin's cornet. Sphenoid cornet. *See* CORNET.

Bertin's ligament. The iliofemoral ligament. *See* LIGAMENT.

Bertolotti's syndrome. Sciatica associated with sacralization of the 5th lumbar vertebra.

Bertram's mixture. A mixture of sodium acetate, sulphate, phosphate and chloride, plus a small quantity of iodophenol, used for intravenous injection.

Bertrand, Gabriel (b. 1867). Paris biochemist.

Bertrand's reagent. A reagent similar to Fehling's solution, used for the detection of reducing sugars.

berylliosis (ber·il·e·o'·sis). Inflammation of the lungs associated with fibrosis, caused by inhalation of particles of beryllium oxide; seen in beryllium workers. **Acute berylliosis.** An acute pneumonic inflammation caused by inhalation of beryllium. **Chronic berylliosis.** A chronic pneumonic condition with formation of nodular granulomata; seen in beryllium workers. [Gk *beryllos* beryl, *-osis* condition.]

beryllium (ber·il·e·um). An element of the alkaline earth group, with atomic weight 9.013, atomic number 4 and symbol Be. Occurs in beryl, an aluminosilicate, in the precious stones emerald, aquamarine and chrysoberyl, and in the minerals euclase, heivite and phenacite. It is a very hard white metal of high melting point, and extremely light; used in aluminium and silver alloys for strength, lightness and untarnishability. It is divalent; forms basic salts and complex compounds. Also known as *glucinum.* Beryllium poisoning is an important industrial risk. **Beryllium acetylacetonate.** $CH(CCH_3O)_2Be(CCH_3O)_2CH$, a chelate compound. **Beryllium nitrate.** $Be(NO_3)_2$, used in the manufacture of gas mantles. **Beryllium oxide.** BeO, a refractory. **Beryllium poisoning.** *See* POISONING. [Gk *beryllos* beryl.]

Berzelius, Baron Jöns Jacob (b. 1779). Swedish chemist.

Marsh-Berzelius test. For arsenic: the arsenic in the prepared solution is reduced to arsine by zinc and dilute sulphuric acid and the gas is passed through a heated tube. A mirror of metallic arsenic is deposited and may be estimated by comparison with standard deposits prepared from known amounts of arsenic. A similar stain is given by antimony, but the latter may be differentiated from arsenic by its insolubility in sodium hypochlorite solution.

besiclometer (bes·e·**klom**·et·er). An instrument which is used in the fitting of spectacles to determine the width appropriate to the particular forehead. [Fr. *besïcles* spectacles, meter.]

Besnier, Ernest (b. 1831). Paris dermatologist.

Besnier's coup d'ongle. A diagnostic sign in tinea versicolor. Scratching the skin produces a desquamative lamella.

Besnier's lupus pernio. A form of sarcoidosis chiefly affecting the nose.

Besnier's prurigo. Diathetic prurigo, a chronic eruption affecting the flexor surfaces of the knees, elbows and wrists, also the back of the neck; it develops usually in early childhood and may be associated with xeroderma. From time to time eczematous reactions occur, which may be widespread. This form of prurigo is often associated with asthma, and is one of the more characteristic manifestations of the atopic state.

Besnier's rheumatism. Chronic synovitis.

Besnier–Boeck disease. Cutaneous sarcoidosis.

Besnier–Boeck–Schaumann disease, or syndrome. Sarcoidosis.

Best, Franz (b. 1878). German physician.

Best's disease. A familial type of retinal degeneration affecting the macula in adolescence.

Best's carmine stain. A mixture of carmine, potassium carbonate, potassium chloride and ammonia, used as a stain for glycogen.

bestiality (bes·te·**al**·it·e). Sexual intercourse with an animal. [L *bestia* beast.]

Bestucheff, Alexei Petrovich (b. 1693). Russian Field-Marshal.

Bestucheff's mixture. An ethereal tincture of ferric chloride.

Beta (be·tah). A genus of plants of the family Chenopodiaceae. *Beta maritima* Linn. is the wild beet from which have been derived the cultivated beets (varieties of *Beta vulgaris* Linn. yielding chard, mangels, sugar beets and common beets). [L beet.]

beta (**be**·tah). 1. β, the second letter of the Greek alphabet. 2. In chemistry, β-, denoting an isomer in which substitution has taken place at the beta position (see below). **Beta angle.** *See* ANGLE. **Beta cell.** *See* CELL. **Beta chain.** *See* CHAIN. **Beta fibre.** *See* FIBRE. **Beta globulin.** *See* GLOBULIN. **Beta granule.** *See* GRANULE. **Beta H.** The abnormal human haemoglobin which contains only beta chains and is characteristic of alpha thalassaemia. **Beta particle.** *See* PARTICLE. **Beta position.** In an organic compound comprising a straight chain of carbon atoms, the second carbon atom from that to which the characteristic group is attached; in a dicyclic compound, the carbon atoms numbered 2, 3, 6 and 7. **Beta ray.** *See* RAY. **Beta rhythm.** *See* RHYTHM. **Beta thalassaemia.** *See* THALASSAEMIA. **Beta wave.** *See* WAVE.

beta-alaninaemia (be·tah·**al**·an·een·**e'**·me·ah). A condition in which β-alanine, beta-aminobutyric acid and taurine are increased in the blood, while β-alanine is increased also in the urine. [β-alanine, Gk *haima* blood.]

beta-albumosease (**be**·tah·al·bew·**mo'**·se·aze). Erepsin; a mixture of enzymes, chiefly polypeptidases, present in intestinal mucosa and capable of converting polypeptides into amino acids.

beta-aminopropionitrile (**be**·tah·**am**·in·o·pro·pe·o·**ni'**·trile). A water-soluble substance derived from the sweet pea (*Lathyrus odoratus*); it is presumed now to be the causative toxic factor of lathyrism.

betacaine (**be**·tah·kane). Beta-eucaine lactate, Benzaminae Lactas BPC 1949, $C_{15}H_{21}NO_2C_3H_6O_3$. A local anaesthetic having about half the toxicity of cocaine, but only about a quarter of the activity of the latter in producing anaesthesia of mucous membranes. It is irritant when injected and may cause hyperaemia; consequently adrenaline is usually incorporated in solution of the drug in order to keep its action local. Its use is now obsolete.

Betacetylmethadol (be·tah·se·til·**meth'**·ad·ol). BP Commission approved name for the beta analogue of alphacetylmethadol; it has similar morphine-like properties.

betacism (**be**·tah·sizm). A speech defect in which the *b* sounds are over-emphasized and the sounds of other consonants are converted into the sound *b*. [Gk *beta* the letter *b*.]

betacyaninuria (be·tah·**si**·an·in·**ewr'**·e·ah). Beeturia. [L *beta* beet, cyanin, urine.]

beta-eucaine (**be**·tah·**ew'**·kane). **Beta-eucaine hydrochloride.** Benzamine Hydrochloride BPC 1954. **Beta-eucaine lactate.** Benzamine lactate, Benzaminae Lactas BPC 1949. Its use is now obsolete.

Betahistine (be·tah·**his**·teen). BP Commission approved name for 2-(2-methylaminoethyl)pyridine; a diamine oxidase inhibitor.

betahypophamine (**be**·tah·hi·**pof'**·am·een). Vasopressin; the pressor constituent of posterior pituitary extracts. It constricts capillaries, stimulates the intestinal movements and has an antidiuretic action.

betaine (**be**·tah·een). Trimethylglycocoll, $(CH_3)_3NCH_2COO$. A nitrogenous base formed by the oxidation of choline, and occurring widely in plants and the animal tissues: beetroot is an important source. It is intimately concerned in the metabolism of the methyl group. **Betaine hydrochloride.** Betaine Hydrochloridum BPC 1949, $[N^+(CH_3)_3CH_2COO^-]HCl$, a compound used as a source of hydrochloric acid in gastric disorders. [L *beta* beet.]

betaines (**be**·tah·eenz). Methylated nitrogenous compounds analogous to betaine, $HO(CH_3)_3NCH_2COOH$, and derived by the methylation of simpler substances, as betaine is derived by the methylation of glycine; several betaines occur in animal and plant tissues.

betalactose (be·ta·**lak**·tose). $C_{12}H_{22}O_{11}$. An isomer of the disaccharide lactose by mutarotation. It occurs with the α-form in the milk of most animals; it is more soluble than α-lactose, but changes into the latter in solution.

betalysin (be·**tal**·is·in). A term applied to relatively thermostable, non-specific bactericidal serum constituents found in normal sera of certain animal species, and not to be confused with the beta haemolysins of certain bacterial species.

Betameprodine (be·tah·**mep**·ro·deen). BP Commission approved name for β-propionoxy - 3 - ethyl - 1 - methyl - 4 - phenylpiperidine, the reversed ester of β-pethidine, resembling the latter in its analgesic action.

Betamethadol (be·tah·**meth**·ad·ol). BP Commission approved name for the beta analogue of alphamethadol; it has similar morphine-like properties.

Betamethasone BP 1973 (be·tah·**meth**·az·one). 9α - Fluoro - 11β,17α,21 - trihydroxy - 16β - methyl - pregna - 1,4 - diene - 3,20 - dione, a white to creamy-white powder with a bitter taste; it is used in corticosteroid therapy. **Betamethasone Acibutate.** BP Commission approved name for 21 - acetoxy - 9α - fluoro - 11β - hydroxy - 16β - methyl - 17 - (2 - methylpropionyloxy) pregna - 1,4 - diene - 3,20 - dione. **Betamethasone Sodium Phosphate BP 1973.** The disodium salt of the 21-phosphate ester of metamethasone, a synthetic glucocorticoid with the general actions of the corticosteroids. Its effect on sodium and water retention is less than that of prednisolone. **Betamethasone Valerate BP 1973.** 9α - Fluoro - 11β,21 - dihydroxy - 16β - methyl - 17α - valeryloxypregna - 1,4 - diene - 3,20 - dione, a synthetic compound with therapeutic effects similar to those of betamethasone, but as it is insoluble in water it is used only as a topical application in an ointment or a cream.

Betamethasonum (**be**·tah·meth·ah·**zo'**·num). *European Pharmacopoeia* name for Betamethasone BP 1973.

betanaphthol (be·tah·**naf**·thol). $C_{10}H_7OH$. A white compound with a faint phenolic odour, insoluble in water but readily in alcohol, and volatile at ordinary temperatures. It occurs in coal tar and is used industrially in the manufacture of dyestuffs; medicinally it has been employed as an internal antiseptic and anthelmintic, externally in skin diseases as a 5–15 per cent ointment. Its internal use is limited by its toxic effects, which resemble those of phenol in character. **Betanaphthol benzoate.** Benzoyl naphthol, $C_6H_5COOC_{10}H_7$; a compound that has been used as an internal antiseptic. **Betanaphthol benzylamine.** A compound employed as a reagent in differentiating between aldoses and ketoses; it forms characteristic crystalline compounds with the former. **Betanaphthol bismuth.** A mixture of bismuth oxide and betanaphthol used like other bismuth preparations for internal antiseptic purposes. **Betanaphthol carbonate.** $(C_{10}H_7O)COOH$, a colourless compound reputed to be an intestinal antiseptic. **Betanaphthol salicylate.** $C_{10}H_7OOCOC_6H_4OH$, a compound used as an intestinal and urinary antiseptic.

betanaphthyl (be·tah·**naf**·thil). The monovalent group $C_{10}H_7$, which is derived from betanaphthol. **Betanaphthyl benzoate.** Benzoyl naphthol. **Betanaphthyl salicylate.** Betanaphthol salicylate.

betanin (be·tan·in). The red colouring matter of beetroot. [L *beta* beet.]

beta-oxybutyria (be·tah·ox·e·bew·**tir**'·e·ah). The occurrence of β-hydroxybutyric acid in the blood and urine of diabetics. It has been suggested that in such cases the liver converts the toxic enolic form of aceto-acetic acid into the less harmful β-hydroxybutyric acid.

Betaprodine (be·tah·**pro**·deen). BP Commission approved name for β-1,3-dimethyl-4-phenyl-4-propionoxypiperidine. A compound almost identical with betameprodine.

betaquinine (be·tah·**kwin**·een). Quinidine, $C_{20}H_{24}O_2N_2$. An alkaloid stereo-isomeric with quinine and obtained from cinchona barks. It is used to treat auricular fibrillation, its main action on the heart muscle being to increase the refractory period and slow the conduction of impulses. The former effect is directed towards stopping auricular fibrillation, while the latter tends to perpetuate it: for this reason its use is only successful in about half of the cases. Where fibrillation has been going on for some time, there is considerable risk of detaching clots if the auricular beat is re-established with quinidine.

betatron (**be**·tah·tron). An electron accelerator in which electrons, travelling in a circular orbit, are accelerated to high energies in a varying magnetic flux. The electron beam may be used directly, or allowed to strike a target and produce penetrating x-rays. [β rays, electron.]

Bête rouge (bate·**roozh**). The six-legged red larva of mites of the family Trombidiidae, in the West Indies and Central America; it is perhaps *Eutrombicula alfreddugèsi.* They cause the usual chigger irritation and dermatitis. [Fr. red creature.]

betel (**be**·tel). 1. The dried leaves of the betel pepper, *Piper betle* Linn. (family Piperaceae) of India, Sri Lanka and Malaysia. They contain a volatile oil, and have stimulant and carminative properties. 2. A masticatory very popular in the East, consisting of fresh betel leaves, areca (betel nut), lime and catechu. Also called *pan.* [Tamil *vettilei.*]

Bethanidine (beth·**an**·id·een). BP Commission approved name for *N*-benzyl-*N'*,*N''*-dimethylguanidine. **Bethanidine Sulphate BP 1973.** The sulphate of bethanidine, an adrenergic blocking agent used in arterial hypertension.

Bethe, Albrecht (b. 1872). Frankfurt physiologist.

Bethe's method. 1. A complicated method employing ammonium molybdate as a mordant, and staining with toluidine blue, for the demonstration of axis cylinders and neurofibrillae. 2. A method for fixing methylene-blue-stained nerve fibres with ammonium molybdate.

Bethe, H. A. German physicist in America.

Bethe's stopping formula. A theoretical quantum mechanical relationship which predicts the stopping-power due to collision processes.

Bethea, Oscar Walter (b. 1878). New Orleans physician.

Bethea's method, or sign. Unilateral deficiency of expansion of a lung, best detected when the examiner standing behind the patient places his hands symmetrically over the upper part of each axillary region of the chest.

bethroot (**beth**·root). The root of *Trillium erectum* Linn. (family Liliaceae).

betol (**be**·tol). Betanaphthol salicylate.

betony (**bet**·on·e). Wood betony, *Stachys betonica* Benth. (family Labiatae), a domestic herbal remedy for dyspepsia and rheumatism. [Fr. *bétoine.*]

Betula (**bet**·ew·lah). A genus of the Betulaceae, comprising the birches. The bark of *Betula lenta* Linn. yields oil of sweet birch (Oleum Betulae BPC 1949), and the bark and wood of *Betula pendula* Roth. and *Betula pubescens* Ehrh., birch-tar oil (Oleum Rusci BPC 1949). [L birch.]

betulase (**bet**·ew·laze). Gaultherase; an enzyme acting on the glucosides of *Gaultheria* and *Betula* species.

betulol (**bet**·ew·lol). $C_{15}H_{24}O$. A dicyclic sesquiterpene alcohol obtained from species of *Betula.*

between-brain (be·**tween**·brane). The diencephalon. [AS *betweon, braegen.*]

Betz, Vladimir Aleksandrovich (b. 1834). Russian anatomist.

Betz's cell area. The posterior part of the precentral gyrus in which the large pyramidal cells of Betz are found; Brodmann's area 4.

Betz's cell. A large pyramidal neurone of the motor cortex. The axons of these cells form part of the pyramidal tract subserving volitional movements.

Beurmann, Charles Lucien de (b. 1851). French dermatologist.

Beurmann's disease, de Beurmann–Gougerot disease. Sporotrichosis.

Beuttner, Oskar (b. 1866). Swiss gynaecologist.

Beuttner's method. Removal of both fallopian tubes, together with cuneiform excision of the fundus of the uterus (to include the intramural portions of the tubes), portions of both ovaries usually being conserved.

Bevan, Arthur Dean (b. 1861). Chicago surgeon.

Bevan's incision. For exposure of the gall bladder: a vertical incision made along the outer border of the right rectus abdominis muscle.

Bevan's operation. 1. Replacement of an undescended testicle in the scrotum. 2. Two-stage drainage of lung abscess.

Bevan-Lewis, William (b. 1847). Leeds physiologist.

Bevan-Lewis cells. Large pyramidal cells of the motor cortex; Betz cells.

bevel (**bev**·el). A definite angle, as in the enamel margins of a cavity in a tooth which is to be filled with gold or gold alloy. **Cavosurface bevel.** In conservative dentistry, the bevel of the enamel prisms made at the junction of the walls of a cavity with the surface of a tooth. [O Fr.]

bevelling (**bev**·el·ing). 1. A bevel. 2. The operation of making a bevel.

Bevonium Methylsulphate (bev·o·ne·um meth·il·**sul**·fate). BP Commission approved name for 2-benziloyloxymethyl-1,1-dimethylpiperidinium methylsulphate; an antispasmodic.

bex (bex) 1. A cough. 2. A disease in which coughing is the predominant characteristic. **Bex convulsiva, Bex theriodes.** Whooping-cough. [Gk.]

bexia (**bex**·e·ah). Brazilian smallpox; a mild and modified form of smallpox also known as *alastrim* or *Kaffir pox.* It is never epidemic like true smallpox, but usually "smoulders", alternately waxing and waning.

Bezitramide (bez·**it**·ram·ide). BP Commission approved name for 1 - (3 - cyano - 3,3 - diphenylpropyl) - 4 - (2 - oxo - 3 - propionyl- 1 - benzimidazolinyl)piperidine; a narcotic analgesic drug.

bezoars (**be**·zo·arz). Concretions of hair, fibres and other substances found in the stomach, and commonly seen in the alimentary tract of animals. They were formerly held to be efficacious against poisons and to have other remarkable medicinal properties. [Ar *bazahr* counter-poison.]

Bezold, Albert von (b. 1836). Würzburg physiologist.

Bezold's ganglia. Nerve ganglia in the atrial septum.

Bezold, Friedrich (b. 1842). Munich otologist.

Bezold's abscess and mastoiditis. A condition where a mastoid abscess spontaneously perforates the mastoid process near its tip, resulting in an abscess formation in the upper part of the neck, under cover of the sternomastoid muscle.

Bezold's perforation. Perforation of the inner surface of the mastoid bone into the digastric fossa. It gives rise to Bezold's abscess of the neck.

Bezold's sign. An inflammatory swelling below the mastoid process, seen in cases of mastoiditis.

Bezold's triad. Three classical signs of early otosclerosis: loss of hearing for lower tones; increase in bone conduction; increase in the ability to hear the tuning fork by bone conduction as compared with hearing by air conduction. This latter is called a *negative Rinne test.*

bhang (bang). The larger leaves and tops of the male or female plants of *Cannabis sativa* Linn., used part dried as a smoking preparation, and sometimes also as a decoction or a chewing gum, in India. The term is also falsely applied to *hashish*, the Egyptian, Arabian and Turkish preparations of the same plant. [Hind.]

Bial, Manfred (b. 1870). Berlin physician.

Bial's reagent. For the detection of pentosuria: a solution of 0.4 g of orcinol in 200 ml of concentrated hydrochloric acid, with 0.5 ml of 10 per cent ferric chloride solution.

Bial's test. To 5 ml of Bial's reagent (see above) add 0.5 ml of urine and bring just to the boil. After standing for 5-20 min, pentose gives a green colour with a greenish-blue precipitate if sufficient is present.

bialuminate (bi·al·ew·min·ate). A salt formed by dissolving aluminium hydroxide in hot alkali.

Bianchi, Giovanni Battista (b. 1681). Turin anatomist.

Bianchi's nodules. The corpora arantii (the bodies of Arantius).

Bianchi's valve. A valve guarding the lower extremity of the nasolacrimal duct.

Bianchi, Leonardo (b. 1848). Italian psychiatrist.

Bianchi's syndrome. Alexia, apraxia and receptive aphasia, in lesions of the left parietal lobe.

biarsenate (bi·ar·sen·ate). An acid salt of arsenic acid of the type MH_2AsO_4, where M is a monovalent metal.

biarticular (bi·ar·**tik**·ew·lar). Referring or belonging to 2 joints; involving 2 joints. [L *bis, articulare* to divide into joints.]

biarticulate (bi·ar·**tik**·ew·late). Provided with a double joint. [see prec.]

biasteric (bi·as·**ter**·ik). In mitosis, referring or belonging to the 2 asters. [L *bis,* Gk *aster* star.]

biastigmatism (bi·as·**tig**·mat·izm). A technique described by Morquer in which the corneal astigmatism and the residual astigmatism are measured separately, and corrected separately by crossed cylinders. [L *bis,* astigmatism.]

biauricular (bi·aw·**rik**·ew·lar). Pertaining to the auricles of both ears. [L *bis, auricula* little ear.]

bib (bib). A corpuscular fragment often attached to a malaria crescent in aestivo-autumnal fever (malignant tertian malaria). [L *bibere* to drink.]

bibasic (bi·**ba**·sik). Dibasic. Term applied to an acid which has 2 replaceable hydrogen atoms. *See* BASICITY. [L *bis,* basic.]

Bibenzonium Bromide (bi·ben·zo·ne·um **bro**·mide). BP Commission approved name for 2-(1,2-diphenylethoxy)ethyltrimethylammonium bromide; a cough suppressant.

Biber-Haab-Dimmer degeneration. A familial type of dystrophy or degeneration of the corneal epithelium, beginning about puberty and characterized by the junction of fine lines which may or may not intersect. *See* DYSTROPHY, RETICULAR-TYPE CORNEAL.

Bibliofilm (bib·le·o·**film**'). A proprietary name used for the method of photostatic reproduction of a book or scientific article in the form of a standard cinematograph film strip which can subsequently be read by the help of a magnifying apparatus. [Obsolete term.] [Gk *biblion* book, film.]

bibliomania (bib·le·o·**ma**·ne·ah). An obsession to acquire or collect books. [Gk *biblion* book, mania.]

bibliophobia (bib·le·o·**fo**'·be·ah). Excessive dislike or dread of books. [Gk *biblion* book, phobia.]

bibliotherapy (bib·le·o·**ther**'·ap·e). The use of books and reading as a form of treatment in disorders of the nervous system. [Gk *biblion* book, therapy.]

biborate (bi·**bor**·ate). Name applied to an acid borate such as a pyroborate or tetraborate, which retains an acid hydrogen atom of the original acid.

bibromide (bi·**bro**·mide). Dibromide. A bromide of a metal or radical, containing 2 bromine atoms. [L *bis,* bromide.]

bicameral (bi·**kam**·er·al). Having 2 divisions or compartments. [L *bis, camera* chamber.]

bicapitate (bi·**kap**·it·ate). Having 2 heads. [L *bis, caput* head.]

bicapsular (bi·**kap**·sew·lar). In botany, term applied to plants which have a double capsule, or 2 capsules. [L *bis, capsula* little box.]

bicarbonataemia (bi·**kar**·bon·ate·**e**'·me·ah). The condition of having bicarbonate in the blood. [bicarbonate, Gk *haima* blood.]

bicarbonate (bi·**kar**·bon·ate). Name applied to any salt of carbonic acid in which only one of the hydrogen atoms has been replaced by a metal or radical; any salt containing the acid group, HCO_3, e.g. sodium bicarbonate, $NaHCO_3$. **Blood bicarbonate, Plasma bicarbonate.** The bicarbonate content of the circulating blood, and a measure of the alkali reserve. **Standard bicarbonate.** The bicarbonate concentration in the plasma of fully oxygenated blood at a CO_2 pressure of 5.3 kPa (40 mmHg) at 38°C. Normal range 22-26 mmol/l. [L *bis,* carbon.]

bicaudal, bicaudate (bi·**kawd**·al, bi·**kawd**·ate). Having 2 tails or appendages. [L *bis, cauda* tail.]

bicellular (bi·**sel**·ew·lar). 1. Having 2 compartments. 2. Made up of 2 cells. [L *bis, cellula* little cell.]

bicephalic, bicephalous (bi·kef·**al**·ik, bi·**kef**·al·us). Having 2 heads; dicephalous. [L *bis,* Gk *kephale* head.]

bicephalus (bi·**kef**·al·us). A fetal monster with 2 heads; dicephalus. [see prec.]

biceps (**bi**·seps). 1. Bicephalous. 2. A muscle that has 2 heads. [L *bis, caput* head.]

biceps brachii muscle [musculus biceps brachii (NA)] (**bi**·seps **bra**·ki·i). A muscle of the upper arm arising by 2 heads, long [caput longum (NA)] and short [caput breve (NA)], from the scapula, and inserted by a single tendon into the tuberosity on the radius. It is one of the main supinators of the forearm and a flexor of the elbow joint.

biceps femoris muscle [musculus biceps femoris (NA)] (**bi**·seps **fem**·or·is). One of the hamstring or flexor muscles of the thigh. Arising by 2 heads, the long [caput longum (NA)] from the ischial tuberosity and the short [caput breve (NA)] from the middle of the linea aspera, it is inserted into the head of the fibula.

biceptor (bi·**sep**·tor). A receptor with 2 complementophil groups. [L *bis, recipere* to receive.]

Bichat, Marie François Xavier (b. 1771). French anatomist and physiologist.

Bichat's canal, or foramen. A communication said to exist between the 3rd ventricle and the cisterna venae magnae cerebri; a very doubtful entity.

Bichat's fat-ball, or fat-pad. The so-called sucking pad of fat found in the cheek outside the buccinator muscle, just in front of the ramus of the mandible. It is best marked in infants.

Bichat's fissure. The transverse fissure below the splenium.

Bichat's fossa. Pterygopalatine fossa. *See* FOSSA.

Bichat's ligament. Part of the sacrotuberous ligament arising from the posterior superior iliac spine.

Bichat's membrane. The fenestrated elastic layer beneath the endothelium of the arterial wall.

Bichat's tunic. The intimal coat of the blood vessels.

bichloride (bi·**klor**·ide). 1. Dichloride; a chloride of a metal or radical, containing 2 chlorine atoms. 2. Bichloride of mercury, $HgCl_2$; corrosive sublimate. [L *bis* chloride.]

bicho (**be**·cho). Epidemic gangrenous proctitis. *See* PROCTITIS.

bichromate (bi·**kro**·mate). Dichromate. A salt of the hypothetical dichromic acid, $H_2Cr_2O_7$.

biciliate (bi·sil·e·ate). Having 2 cilia or hair-like processes. [L *bis, cilium* eyelid.]
bicipital (bi·sip·it·al). 1. Belonging to a biceps muscle. 2. Having 2 origins or heads. **Bicipital groove.** *See* GROOVE. [L *bis, caput* head.]
bicipitoradial (bi·sip·it·o·ra′·de·al). Associated with the biceps brachii muscle and the radius. **Bicipitoradial bursa.** *See* BURSA.
Bickel, Gustav. 19th century Wiesbaden physician.
Bickel's ring. A ring of lymphoid tissue found round the margin of the oropharyngeal isthmus.
biconcave (bi·kon·kave). Concave on 2 surfaces, a term used particularly of lenses. [L *bis*, concave.]
biconvex (bi·kon·vex). Convex on 2 surfaces, a term applied particularly to lenses. [L *bis*, convex.]
bicornate, bicornuate, bicornute (bi·kor·nate, bi·kor·new·ate, bi·kor·newt). Having 2 horns or horn-like processes or projections. [L *bis, cornu* horn.]
bicoudate (bi·koo·date). Having 2 bends or angles. [L *bis*, Fr. *couder* to bend as an elbow.]
bicrescentic (bi·kres·en·tik). Applied to a tooth having 2 ridges in the shape of a double crescent. [L *bis*, crescent.]
bicuspid (bi·kus·pid). 1. A premolar tooth. 2. A valve with 2 cusps. 3. Bicuspidal. [L *bis, cuspis* spear-point.]
bicuspidal, bicuspidate (bi·kus·pid·al, bi·kus·pid·ate). Having 2 points, cusps, or prongs, as a tooth. [see prec.]
bicyanate (bi·si·an·ate). Dicyanate. A cyanate of a metal or radical which contains 2 CNO- groups.
bidactyly (bi·dak·til·e). A congenital abnormality of the hand in which the first and fifth digits only are present. [L *bis*, Gk *daktylos* finger.]
Bidder, Heinrich Friedrich (b. 1810). Dorpat anatomist.
Bidder's ganglion. A ganglionated plexus at the lower end of the atrial septum.
bidental, bidentate (bi·den·tal, bi·den·tate). Relating to, involving or having 2 teeth or tooth-like processes. [L *bis, dens* tooth.]
bidermoma (bi·der·mo·mah). A teratoid growth involving 2 germ layers; didermoma. [L *bis*, Gk *derma* skin, *-oma* tumour.]
bidet (be·da). A basin on a low, narrow stand, which can be bestridden for washing the genital region. [Fr. a little horse.]
Bidimazium Iodide (bid·e·ma·ze·um i·o·dide). BP Commission approved name for 4 - (biphenyl - 4 - yl) - 2 - (4 - dimethylaminostyryl) - 3 - methylthiazolium iodide; an anthelmintic.
biduotertian (bi·dew·o·ter′·shan). A term used to describe a fever, particularly malarial fever, in which the paroxysms recur at intervals so short that they are nearly continuous. [L *bis, dies* day, *tertius* three.]
biduous (bid·ew·us). Of 2 days' duration; applied to fevers. [L *bis, dies* day.]
Biebrich scarlet (be·brik). The sodium salt of *p*-sulphobenzene azo-*o*-sulphobenzene azo-*β*-naphthol; a soluble plasma stain. **Biebrich scarlet R. medicinal.** Scarlet Red BPC 1959.
Biedert, Philipp (b. 1847). Strasbourg paediatrician.
Biedert's cream mixture. A mixture of cream, milk, sugar and water, used as a food for young infants.
Biedl, Artur (b. 1869). Prague physician.
Biedl's disease, or syndrome. Terms for the Laurence-Moon-Biedl dystrophy, or syndrome. Not in general use.
Bardet-Biedl syndrome, Biedl-Bardet syndrome. Terms for the Laurence-Moon-Biedl dystrophy, or syndrome. Not in general use.
Laurence-Biedl syndrome. More generally known as the Laurence-Moon-Biedl syndrome.
Laurence-Moon-Biedl dystrophy, or syndrome. The combination of obesity, sexual underdevelopment, retinitis pigmentosa, mental deficiency and polydactylism or syndactylism. It may be incomplete, and other abnormalities may be present. A familial congenital syndrome.
bielectrolysis (bi·el·ek·trol′·is·is). The simultaneous deposition, by suitable voltage regulation, of 2 metals by the electrolysis of a mixture of 2 electrolytes. It is a method of importance in industrial electrolytic processes. [L *bis*, electrolysis.]
Bielschowsky, Max (b. 1869). Berlin neuropathologist.
Bielschowsky's methods. A number of silver impregnation methods for the demonstration of nerve cells and fibres, neuroglia and reticulin, involving fixation with formalin, impregnation with silver nitrate, then treatment with ammoniacal silver solutions, and reduction with formalin.
Bielschowsky-Jansky disease, Jansky-Bielschowsky disease. The late infantile form of cerebromacular degeneration. *See* DEGENERATION.
Bier, August Karl Gustav (b. 1861). Berlin surgeon.
Bier's amputation, or operation. Amputation through the leg with the use of osteoplastic flaps to cover the raw ends of the tibia and the fibula [obsolete].
Bier's local anaesthesia. Produced by injecting an analgesic solution into the vein of a limb rendered bloodless by elevation and constriction.
Bier's cup. A cupping glass in which a partial vacuum is caused by the suction of a rubber ball.
Bier's passive hyperaemia. *See* BIER'S TREATMENT (below).
Bier's method. 1. Of local analgesia (see above). 2. Of spinal analgesia: by the injection of analgesic solutions into the subarachnoid space.
Bier's spots. Pale areas on engorged erythematous skin which has been deprived of its normal circulation; coalescence of the areas may occur.
Bier's suction. 1. Bier's treatment. 2. Negative pressure applied over snake-bite wounds to withdraw as much poison as possible.
Bier's treatment. Treatment of inflammation by the production of active and passive hyperaemia by means of ligation or of negative pressure.
Biermer, Anton (b. 1827). Zürich physician.
Biermer's anaemia, or disease. Pernicious anaemia. *See* ANAEMIA.
Biermer's change of note. A change of resonance on percussion when the patient changes from the upright to a recumbent position.
Biermer's sign. The metallic bell-like sounds (bruit d'airain) which are heard in the presence of pneumothorax and vary with the position of the patient if fluid is present in the pleural cavity (hydropneumothorax). On shaking the patient the fluid moves freely in these circumstances, so that when the patient's position is such that fluid is interposed between the chest wall and the pneumothorax, the metallic sounds disappear.
Addison-Biermer anaemia. Pernicious anaemia. *See* ANAEMIA.
Biernacki, Edmond Adolfovich (b. 1866). Polish physician.
Biernacki's sign. Ulnar analgesia in syphilis of the central nervous system.
Biesenberger, H. 20th century Austrian surgeon.
Biesenberger's operation. A technique for reduction mammaplasty.
Biesiadecki, Alfred von (b. 1839). Cracow pathologist.
Biesiadecki's fossa. A recess of the peritoneum between the psoas muscle and the iliac crest: also called the *iliacosubfacialis fossa.*
Biett, Laurent Théodore (b. 1781). Swiss dermatologist in Paris.
Biett's band, or collar. A band of papular syphilitic eruption on the neck.
Biett's disease. Lupus erythematodes.
bifacial (bi·fa·shal). 1. With 2 faces or fronts. 2. Having 2 opposite surfaces similar the one to the other. [L *bis, facies* face.]
bifid (bi·fid). Divided into 2 equal parts by a median cleft. [L *bis, findere* to cleave.]
biflagellate (bi·flaj·el·ate). Having 2 flagella or whip-like appendages. [L *bis, flagellum* whip.]
Bifluranol (bi·floor·an·ol). BP Commission approved name for erythro - 4,4′ - (1 - ethyl - 2 - methylethylene)di - (2 - fluorophenol); it is used in treatment of benign hypertrophy of the prostate.
bifocal (bi·fo·kal). Having 2 foci, referring to spectacles in which

the lenses combine distance and reading corrections; *see* BIFOCALS. [L *bis*, focus.]

bifocals (bi·**fo**·kalz). Spectacles in which the lens combines the distance and the reading corrections, the latter being below. They are useful for presbyopes. **Cemented bifocals.** Those in which the reading correction is obtained by cementing a wafer or extra lens on to the surface of the distance lens. **Fused bifocals.** Those in which the reading correction is obtained by making the distance lens of crown glass, and then fusing on an extra lens of flint glass into a hollow ground for it. The difference in refractive index gives the added strength necessary, and there is no line of demarcation in the completed lens. **Solid bifocals.** Those in which the reading correction is obtained by grinding 2 different curves on the same lens, the spherical curve on one side and any cylindrical curve necessary on the other. [see prec.]

See also: FRANKLIN.

biforate (bi·**for**·ate). Having 2 perforations or foramina. [L *bis*, *forare* to pierce.]

biformity (bi·**for**·mit·e). The condition of having 2 forms or bodies, or that in which characteristics of 2 forms are combined. Dimorphism. [L *bis*, *forma* form.]

bifurcate, bifurcated (bi·**fer**·kate, bi·fer·**ka**·ted). Divided into 2 prongs or branches. [L *bis*, *furca* fork.]

bifurcation (bi·fer·**ka**·shun). A division or a forking into 2 branches, as of a blood vessel. **Bifurcation of the trachea [bifurcatio tracheae (NA)].** The division of the trachea into 2 main bronchi. It lies at the level of the sternal angle (the lower border of the 4th thoracic vertebra) in the recumbent cadaver, but may descend to the level of the 6th thoracic vertebra on deep inspiration. [see prec.]

bigaster (bi·**gas**·ter). Biventer; having 2 bellies, as a muscle. [L *bis*, Gk *gaster* stomach.]

Bigelow, Henry Jacob (b. 1818). Boston surgeon.

Bigelow's ligament. Iliofemoral ligament, Y-shaped ligament; a triangular band, the central part of which is thin, giving it the appearance of an inverted Y, attached by its apex to the anterior inferior iliac spine and acetabular margin, and by its base to the intertrochanteric line of the femur.

Bigelow's operation. Litholapaxy by large cannulae which were passed through the urethra to the bladder: by means of an evacuator which incorporated a rubber bulb and a filling tap, fragments of stone were sucked from the bladder and collected in the glass-bottle trap attached to the under part of the bulb.

Bigelow's septum. The calcar femorale; a thickened spur in the cancellous bone of the neck of the femur.

bigemina (bi·**jem**·in·ah). Term applied to a bigeminal pulse, i.e. one which shows 2 beats in rapid succession followed by an appreciable interval before the next pair of beats. [L *bis*, *geminus* a twin.]

bigeminal, bigeminous (bi·**jem**·in·al, bi·**jem**·in·us). Paired, double. [see prec.]

bigeminum (bi·**jem**·in·um). In the embryo, one of the 2 bigeminal (quadrigeminal) bodies of the mid-brain.

bigeminy (bi·**jem**·in·e). The condition of occurring in pairs, a term used particularly of a bigeminal pulse. **Nodal bigeminy.** An arrhythmia in which nodal extrasystoles precede nodal automatic beats. [L *bis*, *geminus* twin.]

bigerminal (bi·**jer**·min·al). Relating or belonging to 2 ova or germs (primitive embryos). [L *bis*, *germen* germ.]

Bignami, Amico (b. 1862). Rome pathologist.

Marchiafava-Bignami disease. Primary degeneration of the corpus callosum, giving rise to mental symptoms, convulsions and variable motor weakness; usually called *Marchiafava's syndrome.*

bigo (**be**·go). An ulcer of the lower lip which is endemic in Somaliland. The condition is contagious.

bigonial (bi·**go**·ne·al). In craniometry, relating to or connecting the 2 gonions. [L *bis*, Gk *gonion* angle.]

bilabe (**bi**·labe). A long narrow instrument with a movable lower jaw used to remove small stones from the bladder by way of the urethra. [L *bis*, *labium* lip.]

bilamellar, bilamellate, bilamellated (bi·lam·**el**·ar, bi·lam·**el**·ate, bi·**lam**·el·a·ted). In botany, composed of 2 plates, as a stigma; or having 2 raised ridges, as the lips of certain flowers. [L *bis*, *lamella* small thin plate.]

bilaminar, bilaminate, bilaminated (bi·**lam**·in·ar, bi·**lam**·in·ate, bi·**lam**·in·a·ted). Having or composed of 2 thin plates or layers. [L *bis*, *lamina* thin plate.]

bilateralism (bi·**lat**·er·al·izm). Bilateral symmetry. *See* SYMMETRY. [L *bis*, *latus* side.]

bilberry (**bil**·ber·e). Whortleberry, blueberry, the fruit of *Vaccinium myrtillus* Linn. (family Ericaceae). It is diuretic and astringent. [AS *blew*, *berie*.]

bile [fel (bilis)] (bile). A greenish-yellow to brown fluid secreted continuously by the liver and stored and concentrated in the gall bladder, whence it is expelled into the duodenum under suitable stimuli. It assists in maintaining an alkaline pH in the intestinal tract, and by bringing fats into a state of emulsification plays an essential part in their splitting and absorption. **A, B and C bile.** Three fractions of bile separable by duodenal intubation after stimulation with olive oil or 25 per cent magnesium sulphate solution. They are from the bile ducts, the gall bladder and the liver, respectively. **Bile acids.** Glycocholic and taurocholic acids present in bile as the sodium salts. **Hepatic bile.** C bile (see above). **Limey bile.** A condition in which there is so much calcium in the bile that the gall bladder shows up on a plain x-ray film. **Ox bile.** The fresh bile of the ox; it contains the bile salts sodium glycocholate and sodium taurocholate as well as the pigments biliverdin and bilirubin. For medicinal purposes the evaporated bile is extracted with alcohol; its main use is as an enema in impacted ileus. **Bile pigments.** The characteristic pigments of bile, chiefly bilirubin and its oxidation product, biliverdin. **Bile salts.** A mixture of the sodium salts of the bile acids, normally occurring in the bile of animals. Solutions of these salts have low surface tension and this property is a primary factor in the emulsifying action of bile upon fats in the intestine. **White bile.** Colourless fluid found distending the bile ducts in cases of chronic obstructive jaundice of very long standing. Formed partly of mucous secretion, partly of transudate from the duct wall. [L *bilis*.]

Bilharzia (bil·**harts**·e·ah). *See* SCHISTOSOMA. [Theodor Maximilian *Bilharz*, 1825–1862, German physician in Cairo.]

bilharzial (bil·**harts**·e·al). Caused by or relating to *Bilharzia* (*Schistosoma*).

bilharziasis (bil·harts·i·as·is). Former term for schistosomiasis, a parasitic disease due to the presence in the blood of the fluke of the genus *Schistosoma*. [*Bilharzia*.]

bilharzioma (bil·**harts**·e·o′·mah). A small neoplasm which forms in the mucous membrane or the skin as the result of the presence of *Bilharzia* (*Schistosoma*). [*Bilharzia*, Gk *-oma* tumour.]

bilharziosis (bil·**harts**·e·o′·sis). Bilharziasis.

biliary (**bil**·e·ar·e). Relating to bile.

biliation (bil·e·**a**·shun). The process of secreting bile.

bilicyanin (bil·e·**si**·an·in). A blue pigment derived by oxidation of biliverdin. [bile, L *cyaneus* blue.]

bilifaction (bil·e·**fak**·shun). Biliation. [bile, L *facere* to make.]

bilifaecia (bil·e·**fe**·se·ah). The condition in which the faeces contain bile.

bilification (**bil**·if·ik·**a**′·shun). Biliation.

biliflavin (bil·e·**fla**·vin). A yellow pigment derivable from biliverdin. [bile, L *flavus* yellow.]

bilifulvin (bil·e·**ful**·vin). A yellow-brown impure form of the bile pigment bilirubin; a pigment of ox bile not normally occurring in human bile. [bile, L *fulvus* tawny.]

bilifuscin (bil·e·**few**·sin). $C_{16}H_{20}N_2O_4$. A dark-brown pigment, occurring in bile and gall-stones. [bile, L *fuscus* brown.]

biligenesis (bil·e·**jen**·es·is). The formation or production of bile. [bile, Gk *genein* to produce.]

biligenetic, biligenic (**bil**·e·jen·**et**′·ik, bil·e·**jen**·ik). Producing or involving the production of bile. [see prec.]

biligulate, biligulatus (bi·lig·ew·late, bi·lig·ew·la′·tus). 1. Resembling 2 tongues in shape. 2. Having 2 processes shaped like tongues. [L *bis, ligula* little tongue.]
bilihumin (bil·e·hew·min). The insoluble residue of gall-stones after treatment with chloroform, alcohol and ether. [bile, humin.]
bilin (bi·lin). Crude mixture of bile salts, sodium glycocholate and taurocholate.
bilineurine (bil·e·newr·een). Choline. [bile, Gk *neuron* nerve.]
bilious (bil·e·us). 1. Biliary. 2. Associated with or characterized by biliousness or an excess of bile. [L *bilis* bile.]
biliousness (bil·e·us·nes). A semi-popular term for a condition attributed to disordered secretion of bile and hepatic dysfunction. The main symptoms are nausea, headache, weariness, constipation and loss of appetite. [see prec.]
biliphein (bil·e·fe·in). Obsolete name for bilirubin, the pigment of bile.
biliprasin (bil·e·pra·sin). A light-green pigment which can be extracted from gall-stones. [bile, Gk *praseos* leek-green.]
bilipurpin, bilipurpurin (bil·e·per·pin, bil·e·per·pewr·in). A form of bilicyanin, obtained by oxidation of the bile pigment bilirubin by nitric acid. [bile, L *purpura* purple.]
bilirachia (bil·e·rak·e·ah). The condition in which bile is present in the spinal fluid. [bile, Gk *rachis* spine.]
bilirubin (bil·e·roo·bin). $C_{33}H_{36}O_6N_4$. A red pigment occurring in human bile, and, as the calcium salt, in gall-stones. It is formed in the reticulo-endothelial system by the breakdown of haemoglobin, and conjugated with glycuronate in the liver cells. Its concentration in blood is greatly increased in jaundice, in which condition it is also excreted in urine. It is reduced in the intestine and excreted mainly in faeces as stercobilinogen. [bile, L *ruber* red.]
bilirubinaemia (bil·e·roo·bin·e′·me·ah). The condition in which bilirubin is present in the blood. [bile, L *ruber* red, Gk *haima* blood.]
bilirubinate (bil·e·roo·bin·ate). A salt of bilirubin.
bilirubinic (bil·e·roo·bin′·ik). Pertaining or referring to bilirubin.
bilirubinuria (bil·e·roo·bin·ewr′·e·ah). The condition in which bilirubin is present in the urine.
bilitherapy (bil·e·ther·ap·e). A system of treatment in which bile or bile salts in solution are administered. [bile, therapy.]
biliuria (bil·e·ewr·e·ah). The condition in which bile or bile salts are to be found in the urine.
biliverdin (bil·e·ver·din). $C_{33}H_{34}O_6N_4$. A green pigment produced by the oxidation of bilirubin. It occurs in bile, in gall-stones and, to a varying extent, in the urine during jaundice. [bile, L *viridis* green.]
bilixanthine (bil·e·zan·theen). Choletelin. [bile, Gk *xanthos* yellow.]
Bill of Health (bil ov helth). An authenticated certificate concerning the health of a ship's company and of the seaport, regarding infectious disease, which the master has to obtain before he may leave the port. The certificate is "clean" when there is not any infectious disease at all, "touched" or "suspected" when there are rumours of infection, and "foul" when infection is certified. [ME *bille*, AS *haelth*.]
Billroth, Christian Albert Theodor (b. 1829). Vienna surgeon.
Billroth's cambric. Prepared cotton fabric which is used for the dressing of wounds, or as a cover for the skin around an operation wound at the time of operation.
Billroth's cord. One of the anastomosing columns of reticular cells and erythrocytes composing the red pulp of the spleen.
Billroth's disease. 1. Malignant lymphoma. *See* LYMPHOMA. 2. Pseudomeningocele.
Billroth I gastrectomy, or operation. The excision of the stomach with end-to-end anastomosis of its remnant to the duodenum. **Billroth II gastrectomy, or operation.** Excision of the stomach with closure of the duodenum, the gastric remnant also being closed and joined side-to-side to the jejunum.
Billroth's mixture. An anaesthetic mixture somewhat like A.C.E. mixture; not now used.
Billroth's strands. Trabeculae of the spleen.
Billroth's tubes. Valentin's tubes.
bilobate (bi·lo·bate). Divided into or having 2 lobes. [L *bis, lobus* lobe.]
bilobular (bi·lob·ew·lar). Having 2 lobules. [L *bis, lobulus* small lobe.]
bilocular, biloculate (bi·lok·ew·lar, bi·lok·ew·late). Divided into 2 compartments or cells. [L *bis, loculus* compartment.]
bimalar (bi·ma·lar). Extending from one zygomatic (malar) bone to the other. [L *bis, mala* cheek.]
bimalate (bi·mal·ate). Of the 2 or more malates of a metal or radical, that which contains twice the number of malic acid radicals, $-COOC_2H_3(OH)COO-$, contained by the lowest.
bimanual (bi·man·ew·al). Done with, or necessitating the use of, both hands. [L *bis, manus* hand.]
bimastic (bi·mas·tik). Having 2 breasts. [L *bis*, Gk *mastos* breast.]
bimastism (bi·mas·tizm). The state of having 2 breasts. [see prec.]
bimastoid (bi·mas·toid). Belonging or relating to the 2 mastoid processes of the temporal bone. [L *bis*, mastoid.]
bimaxillary (bi·max·il·ar·e). 1. Affecting, or relating or belonging to, both the maxilla and the mandible. 2. Extending from the maxilla to the mandible. [L *bis, maxilla* jaw-bone.]
bimodal (bi·mo·dal). Descriptive of a curve in a graph which has 2 peaks. [L *bis, modus* measure.]
bimolecular (bi·mol·ek·ew·lar). Relating to 2 molecules. [L *bis*, molecule.]
bimolybdate (bi·mol·ib·date). Of the 2 or more molybdates formed by a metal or radical, that which contains twice the number of molybdic acid radicals, $=MoO_4$, contained by the lowest.
binary (bi·nar·e). 1. Separating into or consisting of 2 branches or 2 parts. 2. In chemistry, noting a compound of only 2 elements. 3. A scale used in counting or calculating in which only 2 symbols are used. When written, these are 0 and 1 and in a digital computer the 2 symbols are represented by a circuit element being in a state of electrical conduction, or not. [L *binarius* consisting of two.]
binaural (bi·naw·ral). 1. Having 2 ears. 2. Relating to or involving both ears. 3. Used for both ears, e.g. binaural stethoscope. [L *bini* two at a time, *auris* ear.]
binauricular (bi·naw·rik·ew·lar). 1. Biauricular; having reference to or involving the auricles of the 2 ears. [L *bis* auricle.] 2. Binaural.
Binda's sign. Raising of the shoulder when the head is turned quickly to the opposite side; this sign is due to neck stiffness, and was first described in cases of tuberculous meningitis.
Bindazac (bin·daz·ak). BP Commission approved name for 1-benzylindazol-3-yloxyacetic acid; an anti-inflammatory agent.
binder (bine·der). A broad abdominal bandage or girdle. **Obstetric binder.** The broad supporting bandage applied round the abdomen after childbirth for the purpose of supporting the parts until the muscles should have fully recovered their tone. [AS *bindan*.]
bindweb (bine·dweb). 1. Connective tissue or matrix. 2. Neuroglia. [AS *bindan, webb*.]
binegative (bi·neg·at·iv). Doubly negative. [L *bis*, negative.]
Binet, Alfred (b. 1857). French psychologist.
Binet age. The mental age determined by the results of Binet's test.
Binet formula. An estimate of the degree of intellectual function as determined by the Binet intelligence test.
Binet test. A test of intelligence devised by Binet to detect those children in the schools of Paris who were unable to benefit from the usual education. The underlying hypothesis was that it is possible to classify differences in intelligence by comparing individual scores in a series of tests with the scores obtained by average children of different ages, thus obtaining a mental age which could be compared with the chronological age. Initially the test comprised a wide variety of 30 sub-tests. It has been extensively revised, adapted and translated.
Herring-Binet test. A revision (1922) of the Binet test,

including a grouping of tests enabling a short form to be used when required.

Binet-Simon scale, or test. A revision of the Binet test (see above).

Stanford-Binet test. A revision of the Binet test (see above).

Bing, Alfred (b. 1844). Austrian otologist.

Bing's entotic test. For lesions of the incus or malleus: a hearing test to compare hearing by the direct stimulation of sound waves within the middle-ear cavity with hearing by the normal route. A catheter is inserted into the eustachian tube. Externally, it is connected to the ear-piece of a hearing trumpet. The degree of the ability to hear speech by this method is compared with hearing through the ear trumpet placed in the external meatus. If speech is heard better by ways of the eustachian tube, this is said to indicate a conductive lesion affecting the malleus or incus.

Bing's tuning-fork test. For differentiating middle- and inner-ear lesions: the base of a tuning fork is placed over the mastoid process. When the sound ceases to be heard, a finger is placed so as to occlude the meatus. In an impedance deafness due to middle-ear disease the sound will not be heard again, but in labyrinthine disease the note of the tuning fork may again be audible. It is mainly of use in severe degrees of middle-ear deafness.

Bing, Richard John (b. 1909). Birmingham, Alabama, clinical physiologist.

Bing's test. In patients with the tetralogy of Fallot (congenital pulmonary stenosis, ventricular septal defect, overriding aorta) the oxygen consumption per litre of ventilated air falls during exercise, in contrast to normal persons, who consume more oxygen per litre of ventilation during effort. In this test the oxygen consumption per litre of ventilation is measured before and after effort, and the ratio oxygen consumption/ventilation is determined. Unlike the tetralogy of Fallot, subjects with cyanotic congenital heart disease but without pulmonary stenosis (such as the Eisenmenger syndrome) show a rise in the ratio, rather than a fall, and this test may be an indication of the presence or absence of pulmonary stenosis in cyanosed patients.

Taussig-Bing syndrome. A developmental abnormality of the heart, falling within the group of transposition of the great vessels in which the aorta arises from the right ventricles and the pulmonary artery overrides the ventricular system, there being a septal defect present.

biniodide (bin·i·o·dide). Di-iodide. An iodide of a metal or radical, containing 2 atoms of iodine.

binocular (bin·**ok**·ew·lar). 1. Relating to both eyes. 2. Of optical instruments, adapted for use by both eyes together. [L *bini* two at a time, *oculus* eye.]

binoculus (bin·**ok**·ew·lus). An imaginary single eye, centrally situated between the 2 actual eyes. In binocular vision, images received from the corresponding retinal points of each eye give the impression of a single image coming from this central eye. Also called *bi-uniac eye.* [see prec.]

binophthalmoscope (bin·of·**thal**·mo·skope). An ophthalmoscope with which the posterior segments of both eyes of a subject can be examined at the same time. [L *bini* two at a time, ophthalmoscope.]

binoscope (**bin**·o·skope). An instrument used in the correction of squint. The lateral parts of the field of vision are screened off and the object is presented in the centre of the field. [L *bini* two at a time, Gk *skopein* to watch.]

binotic (bin·**ot**·ik). Binaural; relating to or involving both ears. [L *bini* two at a time, Gk *ous* ear.]

binovular (bin·**ov**·ew·lar). Derived from or relating to 2 separate ova. [L *bini* two at a time, *ovum* egg.]

binoxide (bin·**ox**·ide). Dioxide.

Binswanger, Otto (b. 1852). Jena psychiatrist.

Binswanger's encephalitis. Chronic progressive subcortical encephalitis; degeneration of subcortical white matter owing to atherosclerotic changes which are severe in subcortical vessels, the cortical vasculature escaping. It affects particularly the temporal and occipital lobes.

binuclear, binucleate (bi·**new**·kle·ar, bi·**new**·kle·ate). Having 2 nuclei. [L *bis*, nucleus.]

binucleolate (bi·**new**·kle·o·late). Having 2 nucleoli. [L *bis*, *nucleolus* little kernel.]

bio-aeration (bi·o·a·er·**a'**·shun). In the purifying of sewage, a modification of the activated sludge method. [Gk *bios* life, *aer* air.]

bio-analysis (**bi**·o·an·**al'**·is·is). The separation of biological products by the selective action of organisms. [Gk *bios* life, analysis.]

bio-assay (bi·o·**as**·a). A method for determining the concentration of substances such as drugs, hormones, vitamins, sera and antibiotics, of unknown chemical composition, or whose concentration is too low for ordinary chemical or physical analysis. It involves the strictly controlled observation of the effect of the substance upon appropriately chosen living animals or tissues, and the comparison of its activity with that of an internationally agreed standard. [Gk *bios* life, assay.]

bio-astronautics (**bi**·o·as·tro·**nawt'**·ix). The study of the effects of space travel upon living matter. [Gk *bios* life, *aster* star, *nautes* sailor.]

bioblast (**bi**·o·blast). Micelle; one of the hypothetical units of living matter composed of one or a number of molecules, capable of dividing or growing, and stimulative to cell function. [Gk *bios* life, *blastos* germ.]

bioblastic (bi·o·**blas**·tik). Referring to a bioblast (micelle).

biocatalyser (bi·o·**kat**·al·i·zer). Another name for a bacterial growth factor. [see foll.]

biocatalyst (bi·o·**kat**·al·ist). Enzyme. [Gk *bios* life, *katalein* to dissolve.]

biocenosis (**bi**·o·se·**no'**·sis). Association of infection [Gk *bios* life, cenosis.]

biochemical (bi·o·**kem**·ik·al). Belonging to biological chemistry. [see foll.]

biochemistry (bi·o·**kem**·is·tre). The chemistry of living tissues and of the substances that take part in their metabolism. [Gk *bios* life, chemistry.]

biochemorphic (bi·o·kem·**or'**·fik). Referring to biochemorphology.

biochemorphology (**bi**·o·kem·or·**fol'**·o·je). The science which deals with the relationship between the chemical structure of drugs and foods and their action on living organisms. [Gk *bios* life, chemistry, morphology.]

biochemy (bi·o·**kem**·e). The chemical activities associated with life and as exhibited in various organisms. [Gk *bios* life, chemistry.]

biocidal (bi·o·**si**·dal). Lethal to living organisms. [Gk *bios* life, L *caedere* to kill.]

bioclimatology (**bi**·o·kli·mat·**ol'**·o·je). The science which relates to the effects of climate on living organisms and the interactions between the two. [Gk *bios* life, climatology.]

biocoenosis (**bi**·o·sen·**o'**·sis). The relationship which exists between different organisms living in similar conditions and in association with each other. [Gk *bios* life, *koinos* common.]

biocoenotic (**bi**·o·sen·**ot'**·ik). Referring to biocoenosis.

biocolloid (bi·o·**kol**·oid). A colloid which is present in and necessary to the life of animal and vegetable organisms. [Gk *bios* life, colloid.]

bioculate, bioculatus (bi·**ok**·ew·late, **bi**·ok·ew·**la'**·tus). 1. Marked with 2 eye-like spots, such as the wings of certain insects. 2. Describing any structure which resembles 2 eyes. [L *bis*, *oculus* eye.]

biocytoculture (**bi**·o·si·to·**kul'**·tcher). The propagation of living cells by culture. [Gk *bios* life, *kytos* cell, culture.]

biocytoneurology (**bi**·o·si·to·newr·**ol'**·o·je). The science or study of living nerve cells. [Gk *bios* life, *kytos* cell, neurology.]

biodialysate (**bi**·o·di·**al'**·is·ate). The fluid in the bath after biodialysis.

biodialysis (bi·o·di·**al**′·is·is). In experimental physiology, the process of bathing the intestine for an hour in Ringer–Locke solution at body temperature. The fluid in the bath is then the biodialysate. [Gk *bios* life, *dialysis* a separation.]

biodynamics (**bi**·o·di·**nam**′·ix). The study of the effects of dynamic processes (acceleration, radiation, weightlessness) on living matter. [Gk *bios* life, *dynamis* force.]

bio-electricity (**bi**·o·el·ek·**tris**′·it·e). The electricity inherent in the phenomena of living tissue. [Gk *bios* life, electricity.]

bio-element (bi·o·**el**·e·ment). 1. Any element which is essential to life. 2. Any chemical element present in living tissues. [Gk *bios* life, L *elementum* a beginning.]

bio-energetics (**bi**·o·en·er·**jet**′·ix). The study of the energy transformations of organisms. [Gk *bios* life, *energetikos* active.]

biogen (**bi**·o·jen). A hypothetical "living" molecule, the unit of protoplasmic structure. [Gk *bios* life, *genein* to produce.]

biogenesis (bi·o·**jen**·es·is). T. H. Huxley's term for the view that life has its origin only in material already living and cannot be produced artificially. The development of living forms from matter already alive. [Gk *bios* life, *genein* to produce.]

biogenetic (**bi**·o·jen·**et**′·ik). Referring to or characterized by biogenesis.

biogenous (bi·**oj**·en·us). 1. Having origin in life. 2. Producing life. 3. A term applied, for example, to bacteria which grow and propagate on living organisms. [Gk *bios* life, *genein* to produce.]

biogeny (bi·**oj**·en·e). The progressive development and unfolding of individual or tribal organic forms. [see prec.]

biognosis (bi·og·**no**·sis). Biology. [Gk *bios* life, *gnosis* knowledge.]

biohydraulic (**bi**·o·hi·**draw**′·lik). Referring to the action of water and solutions existing in or instilled into living tissues. [Gk *bios* life, *hydor* water.]

bio-instrumentation (**bi**·o·in·stroo·men·**ta**′·shun). The study of techniques of recording, transmitting and processing physiological data. [Gk *bios* life, L *instrumentum* tool.]

biokinetics (**bi**·o·kin·**et**′·ix). That branch of science which deals with the changes undergone by and movements taking place in developing organisms. [Gk *bios* life, *kinetikos* moving.]

biological, biologic (bi·o·**loj**·ik·al, bi·o·**loj**·ik). Belonging or referring to biology.

Biological Standards Act 1975. This Act provides for the establishment in the UK of a National Biological Standards Board to perform functions in relation to the establishment of standards for biological substances, the provision of standard preparations of such substances and the testing of such substances. Biological substances are defined as substances whose purity or potency cannot, in the opinion of the Secretary of State, be adequately tested by chemical means.

biologos (bi·**ol**·og·os). That power of intelligence which appears to be present in the activities of living organisms, e.g. cells. [Gk *bios* life, *logos* science.]

biology (bi·**ol**·o·je). That branch of science which is concerned with living organisms and the phenomena associated with them. **Cell biology.** The study of vital processes at the cellular level. **Dynamic biology.** Bionomy. **Molecular biology.** A branch of biological science which sprang into prominence in the 1960s with the application of physical techniques, especially x-ray crystallography, to the elucidation of the structure of biological macromolecules such as DNA and proteins, and which has provided molecular mechanisms for genetics, enzyme catalysis and enzyme regulation. It forms part of the general science of biochemistry. **Static biology.** Biostatics. [Gk *bios* life, *logos* science.]

bioluminescence (**bi**·o·loo·min·**es**′·ens). The phosphorescent quality of certain living organisms, both animal and vegetable, e.g. bacteria, fungi. [Gk *bios* life, L *luminare* to make light.]

biolysis (bi·**ol**·is·is). The dissolution or disintegration of organic matter resulting from the action on it of living organisms, e.g. bacteria. [Gk *bios* life, *lysis* a loosing.]

biolytic (bi·o·**lit**·ik). Pertaining to biolysis.

biomathematics (**bi**·o·math·em·**at**′·ix). Mathematics in its application to biology. [Gk *bios* life, mathematics.]

biomechanics (**bi**·o·mek·**an**′·ix). The science of the forces acting internally or externally on the living organism or cell. [Gk *bios* life, mechanics.]

biomedical (bi·o·**med**·ik·al). Term usually referring to the engineering aspects of medicine and surgery. [Gk *bios* life, medical.]

biometer (bi·**om**·et·er). 1. A table according to which the expectancy of life of any particular individual can be calculated; it is used in life-insurance work. 2. An apparatus by which the carbon dioxide given off by tissues can be measured. [Gk *bios* life, meter.]

biometrician (**bi**·o·met·**rish**′·an). One whose special subject is biometry.

biometrics, biometry (bi·o·**met**·rix, bi·**om**·et·re). 1. Anthropometry. 2. Statistics as applied to biological science. 3. In life-insurance work, the calculation with the aid of a biometer (1st def.) of the probable duration of life of any individual. 4. The measurement of the carbon dioxide given off by a tissue by means of a biometer (2nd def.). 5. Use of ultrasound to measure the size of the eye and the position of the lens within it. [Gk *bios* life, meter.]

biomicroscope (bi·o·**mi**·kro·skope). A binocular microscope with which living tissue within the body can be examined. [Gk *bios* life, microscope.]

biomicroscopy (**bi**·o·mi·**kros**′·ko·pe). The use of a biomicroscope in examination of living tissue within the body, e.g. the use of a biomicroscope in examination of the anterior segment of the eye, a slit lamp being used also.

biomolecule (bi·o·**mol**·e·kewl). 1. A unit of living substance such as a micelle. 2. A protoplasmic molecule. [Gk *bios* life, molecule.]

biomonad (bi·o·**mon**·ad). A protoplasmic granule. [Gk *bios* life, *monas* a thing alone.]

biomone (**bi**·o·mone). A particle of living substance composed of molecules.

biomore (**bi**·o·mor). Biomolecules arranged in a pattern to constitute an organ of a cell. [Gk *bios* life, L *more* in the manner of.]

biomotor (bi·o·**mo**·tor). An apparatus for inducing respiration artificially. [Gk *bios* life, motor.]

Biomphalaria (**bi**·om·fal·a′·re·ah). A genus of snails of which several species are intermediary hosts of *Schistosoma mansoni*, e.g. *Biomphalaria alexandrina, B. alexandrina choanomphala, B. alexandrina pfeifferi, B. alexandrina stanleyi, B. alexandrina tanganyicensis.* This genus has been separated from *Planorbis.* **Biomphalaria boissyi.** *Biomphalaria alexandrina* (see above). **Biomphalaria pfeifferi.** *Biomphalaria alexandrina pfeifferi* (see above). **Biomphalaria rupelli katangae.** *Biomphalaria alexandrina pfeifferi* (see above). **Biomphalaria smithi.** *Biomphalaria alexandrina stanleyi* (see above). [L *bis*, Gk *omphalos* navel.]

biomutation (**bi**·o·mew·**ta**′·shun). The process whereby an organism injected into the living animal body changes its characteristics. [Gk *bios* life, L *mutare* to change.]

bion (**bi**·on). A physiological individual with definite and independent function. [Gk a living thing.]

Biondi, Adolfo (b. 1846). Italian physician.

Ehrlich-Biondi-Heidenhain triple stain. A mixture of acid fuchsine, orange G and methyl green, used for staining blood films.

bionecrosis (**bi**·o·nek·**ro**′·sis). Necrobiosis: 1. Death of individual cells in the midst of living tissue. 2. Gradual localized death of a part or tissue as the result of retrograde processes or degeneration, e.g. atrophy of an organ. [Gk *bios* life, necrosis.]

bionergy (bi·on·er·je). The vital force which is generated and exercised in the living cell and organism. [Gk *bios* life, *ergon* work.]

bionics (**bi**·on·iks). The science concerned with the application of data about the functioning of biological systems to the solution of engineering problems.

bionomics (bi·on·**om**·ix). Ecology; that branch of biology which deals with the life and habits of organisms and their relations with their environment. [Gk *bios* life, *nomos* law.]

bionomy (bi·**on**·om·e). The sum of the laws regulating the vital processes; assessment of the phenomena of life. [Gk *bios* life, *nomos* law.]

bionosis (bi·o·**no**·sis). Any disease which is the result of the action of living organisms such as bacteria. [Gk *bios* life, *nosos* disease.]

biontic (bi·**on**·tik). Individual as opposed to tribal. [Gk *bion* a living thing.]

bionucleonics (bi·o·new·kle·**on**′·ix). The study of applied nuclear physics in relation to biological systems. [Gk *bios* life, nucleus.]

bio-occlusion (bi·o·ok·**loo**′·zhun). The occlusion of the teeth on both sides of the mouth; bilateral occlusion. [L *bis*, occlusion.]

biophagism (bi·**of**·aj·izm). The obtaining of nourishment from living organisms. [Gk *bios* life, *phagein* to eat.]

biophagous (bi·**of**·ag·us). Feeding like a parasite or a parasitic plant on living matter or organisms. [see prec.]

biophagy (bi·**of**·aj·e). Biophagism.

biophore (**bi**·o·for). Weismann's term for the smallest particle of matter capable of bearing life. It is nearly equivalent to a micelle. [Gk *bios* life, *phoros* bearer.]

biophoric (bi·o·**for**·ik). Referring to a biophore.

biophotometer (bi·o·fo·**tom**′·et·er). An instrument used to assess the degree of dark adaptation of the eye and thus provide a basis for the determination of the amount of vitamin A lacking in the body of the person so examined. [Gk *bios* life, *phos* light, meter.]

biophylactic (bi·o·fil·**ak**′·tik). Any mechanism or other natural defence in the body which preserves or protects life. [see foll.]

biophylaxis (bi·o·fil·**ax**′·is). The condition of defence against infection and poison which is natural to the body. [Gk *bios* life, *phylax* guard.]

biophysics (bi·o·**fiz**·ix). The application of physical laws to the vital processes in the organism, and their manifestations. [Gk *bios* life, *physis* nature.]

biophysiography (bi·o·fiz·e·**og**′·raf·e). The biology of the organs and structures of the living body. [Gk *bios* life, *physis* nature, *graphein* to record.]

biophysiology (bi·o·fiz·e·**ol**′·o·je). In biology, the science of the development, the form and structure, and the functions of living organisms. [Gk *bios* life, physiology.]

bioplasia, bioplasis (bi·o·**pla**·ze·ah, bi·o·**pla**·sis). The converting of energy derived from food into tissue. [Gk *bios* life, *plassein* to form.]

bioplasm (**bi**·o·plazm). 1. Cell protoplasm. 2. Hyaloplasm. 3. Any formative or germinal matter. 4. Any matter that has life. [Gk *bios* life, plasma.]

bioplasmic (bi·o·**plaz**·mik). Referring to bioplasm.

bioplasmin (bi·o·**plaz**·min). A substance held to be present in living cells and necessary to the performance of their proper function. Its gradual exhaustion is supposed to be the cause of the lessening of physical and chemical activity in the body. [Gk *bios* life, plasma.]

bioplast (**bi**·o·plast). Micelle; one of the hypothetical units of living matter, composed of one or a number of molecules, capable of dividing or growing. [Gk *bios* life, *plassein* to form.]

bioplastic (bi·o·**plas**·tik). Referring to bioplasia.

biopsia (bi·**op**·se·ah). Biopsy.

biopsic (bi·**op**·sik). Referring to or involving biopsy.

biopsy (bi·**op**·se). 1. Examination of the living body. 2. Examination for purposes of diagnosis of tissues cut from the living body. These may be normal or diseased. 3. The term is also used, though loosely, to mean the removal of pieces of tissue from the living body for examination. Cf. NECROPSY. **Aspiration biopsy.** Needle, or trocar and cannula, biopsy from lymph nodes or other deep lesion. **Drill biopsy.** Biopsy by means of a large-bore needle attached to a motor driven by compressed air which rotates the needle at high speed. **Punch biopsy.** Biopsy of tissues removed from the body by means of a punch. **Sponge biopsy.** A biopsy obtained by rubbing a sponge over a superficial lesion of the skin or a mucous membrane. Smears may be made, or the sponge and its adherent cells processed *en bloc.* **Sternal biopsy.** Examination of the sternal bone marrow removed by either aspiration or trephining. **Surface biopsy.** Microscopical examination of scrapings from a lesion of the skin or mucous membranes, e.g. from a suspected lesion of the cervix uteri. **Total biopsy.** Histological study of a growth which has been removed in its entirety. [Gk *bios* life, *opsis* view.]

biopsychic, biopsychical (bi·o·**si**·kik, bi·o·**si**·kik·al). Belonging or having reference to psychic phenomena in their application to biology. [Gk *bios* life, *psyche* mind.]

biopsychology (bi·o·si·**kol**′·o·je). That branch of biology which is concerned with the reciprocal actions of mind and body and their effects on personality. [Gk *bios* life, psychology.]

biopyoculture (bi·o·**pi**·o·kul·tcher). A culture made from pus containing living cells. [Gk *bios* life, pyoculture.]

biorbital (bi·**or**·bit·al). Relating or belonging to both orbits. [L *bis*, orbit.]

biorgan (**bi**·or·gan). A physiological in contradistinction to a morphological organ. [Gk *bios* life, *organon* organ.]

bios (**bi**·os). The term applied to factors necessary for the growth of certain strains of yeasts. They have been shown to be members of the vitamin B complex. **Bios I.** Former term for *iso*-inositol. **Bios II.** Former term for biotin. [Gk life.]

bioscopy (bi·**os**·ko·pe). 1. The examination of the body in order to determine whether or not death has taken place. 2. The examination of a dead newly-born child in order to determine its viability when birth took place. [Gk *bios* life, *skopein* to view.]

biose (**bi**·oze). Diose, glycollic aldehyde, CH_2OHCHO. The simplest of the monosaccharides, formed from the tartaric acid in ripening grapes. It is an intermediate in the synthesis of carbohydrates in plants.

bioside (**bi**·o·side). Name applied to a glucoside which consists of 2 sugar units attached to 1 aglucone molecule. [L *bis*, glucoside.]

biosmosis (bi·oz·**mo**·sis). Osmosis taking place through a living membrane. [Gk *bios* life, osmosis.]

biospectrometry (bi·o·spek·**trom**′·et·re). The measuring of the amount of a substance in a living tissue by the use of a spectroscope. [Gk *bios* life, spectrometry.]

biospectroscopy (bi·o·spek·**tros**′·ko·pe). Examination of living tissue by means of a spectroscope. [Gk *bios* life, spectroscopy.]

biostatics (bi·o·**stat**·ix). The science of the relation between function and structure. [Gk *bios* life, *statikos* a standing.]

biostatistics (bi·o·stat·**is**′·tix). Vital statistics. *See* STATISTICS [Gk *bios* life, statistics.]

biostearin, biosterin (bi·o·**ste**·ar·in, bi·**os**·ter·in). Vitamin A, axerophthol, $C_{20}H_{29}OH$. A fat-soluble vitamin occurring in liver fat, fish-liver oils and butter: structurally it is a hydroxy-semi-β-carotene, and is essential for the growth of young animals.

biosterol (bi·o·**steer**·ol). A rare term for vitamin A. [Gk *bios* life, sterol.]

biosynthesis (bi·o·**sin**·thes·is). The formation of a chemical substance, usually under the influence of a ferment or enzyme, within a living organism or cell. [Gk *bios* life, *synthesis* a placing together.]

Biot, Camille (b. 1878). Lyons physician.

Biot's breathing, respiration or sign. A form of irregular breathing with pauses at irregular intervals; between the pauses the breathing may be slow and deep or quick and shallow without any constant relation between the types. It is accompanied by sighing, and is regarded as pathognomonic of meningitis.

biota (bi·o·tah). Combined flora and fauna. [Gk *bios* life.]

biotaxis, biotaxy (bi·o·**tax**·is, bi·o·**tax**·e). 1. The classification of living organisms into systems. 2. The powers of selection and arrangement inherent in living cells. [Gk *bios* life, *taxis* arrangement.]

biotherapy (bi·o·**ther**·ap·e). A form of treatment in which preparations of micro-organisms or of their products, or living organisms such as yeast, or materials such as bile and gastric juice (biological extracts), are used. [Gk *bios* life, therapy.]

biotic (bi·**ot**·ik). Of or pertaining to living matter. [Gk *bios* life.]

biotics (bi·**ot**·ix). The sum of knowledge regarding the attributes and functions which are peculiar to a living organism. [see prec.]

biotin (bi·o·tin). Vitamin H, $C_{10}H_{16}O_3N_2S$; a necessary constituent of the diet and an essential co-factor for certain enzymes catalysing reactions involving carbon dioxide fixation, i.e. pyruvate carboxylase, acetyl CoA carboxylase. It is covalently bound to enzyme protein through a lysine residue. Biotin-containing enzymes are inhibited by the egg-white protein, avidin, due to specific interaction with biotin. Deficiency is associated with dermatitis, loss of appetite and lassitude. [Gk *bios* life.]

biotomy (bi·ot·o·me). 1. Vivisection. 2. The knowledge, gained through dissection, of the structure of vegetable and animal organisms. [Gk *bios* life, *temnein* to cut.]

biotoxin (bi·o·tox·in). One of the toxins formed in living body tissues and juices. [Gk *bios* life, *toxikon* poison.]

biotrepy (bi·ot·rep·e). The study of the body in the light of the reactions induced by various chemical substances. [Gk *bios* life, *trepein* to turn.]

biotripsis (bi·o·trip·sis). The smooth, shining "worn-away" condition of the skin seen in old people on surfaces near the bone, e.g. the backs of the hands, the forehead. [Gk *bios* life, *tripsis* a rubbing.]

biotropical (bi·o·trop·ik·al). Exhibiting biotropism.

biotropism (bi·ot·ro·pizm). A condition in which the bodily resistance is reduced so that a saprophytic germ can cause disease or a quiescent infection become active. **Direct biotropism.** Biotropism in which a drug when administered stimulates a specific organism instead of destroying it or limiting its action. **Indirect biotropism.** Biotropism in which an organism other than the specific one is stimulated but the specific one is not affected. [Gk *bios* life, *tropos* a turning.]

biotype (bi·o·tipe). Genotype, 1st def. [Gk *bios* life, *typos* mark.]

biotypology (bi·o·ti·pol'·o·je). The study of anthropological types and the variations and modifications of the constitutional characteristics. [Gk *bios* life, typology.]

biovular (bi·o·vew·lar). Pertaining to, or from, 2 ova, used particularly in reference to twins the offspring of 2 ova. [L *bis*, *ovulum* small egg.]

bipara (bip·ar·ah). A woman who has borne 2 children at separate births. [L *bis*, *parere* to give birth.]

biparasitic (bi·par·as·it'·ik). Referring to a parasite of a parasite. [L *bis*, parasite.]

biparental (bi·par·en·tal). Derived from both the male and the female parent. [L *bis*, parent.]

biparietal (bi·par·i·et·al). Relating to the 2 parietal bones or eminences. [L *bis*, *paries* wall.]

biparous (bip·ar·us). Giving birth to 2 at a time. [L *bis*, *parere* to give birth.]

bipartite (bi·part·ite). In biology, divided into 2 parts or consisting of 2 subdivisions or parts. [L *bis*, *pars* part.]

biped (bi·ped). An animal with 2 feet. [see foll.]

bipedal (bi·ped·al). 1. Having 2 feet, as a human being. 2. Relating to both feet. 3. Relating to a biped. [L *bis*, *pes* foot.]

bipennate, bipenniform (bi·pen·ate, bi·pen·e·form). Descriptive of muscles the fibres of which spring from each side of a tendon as the barbs spring from the shaft of a feather. [L *bis*, *penna* feather, form.]

biperforate (bi·per·for·ate). Having 2 perforations or foramina. [L *bis*, *perforare* to pierce through.]

Biperiden (bi·per·id·en). BP Commission approved name for 1 - (bicyclo[2,2,1]hept - 5 - en - 2 - yl) - 1 - phenyl - 3 - piperidinopropan - 1 - ol; an anticholinergic.

biplumbic (bi·plum·bik). Referring to a compound of tetravalent lead that contains twice as much lead as a lower compound of the same type. [L *bis*, *plumbum* lead.]

bipocillated (bi·pos·il·a·ted). Describing the condition of having 2 appendages each like a small cup. [L *bis*, *pocillum* little cup.]

bipolar (bi·po·lar). 1. Possessing 2 poles; a structure with opposite extremities or poles, commonly applied to a particular type of nerve cell which forms the link between a peripheral receptor and the central nervous system. 2. Denoting that both poles are employed in an electrotherapeutic treatment. **Cone bipolar.** One of the bipolar nerve cells of the retina, having synaptic connections with the processes of the visual cones. **Giant bipolars.** Large bipolar nerve cells of the retina whose dendrites connect with several rods and cones. **Individual bipolar, Midget bipolar, Monosynaptic bipolar, Mop bipolar.** A small bipolar nerve cell of the retina whose dendrite connects only with cones, and usually only with a single cone. **Rod bipolar.** A bipolar nerve cell of the retina whose dendrite connects with several rods. [L *bis*, *polus* pole.]

Bipolaris septicus (bi·po·la·ris sep·tik·us). An old name for *Pasteurella septica.* [L *bis*, *polus* pole, Gk *septikos* putrid.]

bipositive (bi·poz·i·tiv). Possessing positive divalence. [L *bis*, positive.]

bipotassic (bi·pot·as·ik). Containing 2 atoms of potassium.

bipotentiality (bi·po·ten·she·al'·it·e). The latent capacity of a cell or organ to differentiate along either of 2 distinct pathways. **Bipotentiality of the gonad.** The doctrine that the early embryonic gonad has the capacity to develop into either a testis or an ovary. [L *bis*, *potentia* power.]

bipp (bip). Paste of Bismuth Subnitrate and Iodoform BPC 1954.

bipubiotomy (bi·pew·be·ot'·o·me). Ischiopubiotomy. [L *bis*, pubes, Gk *temnein* to cut.]

biramous (bi·ra·mus). With or consisting of 2 branches. [L *bis*, *ramus* branch.]

birch (berch). Any tree of the genus *Betula* (family Betulaceae). [AS *birce.*]

Birch-Hirschfeld, Arthur (b. 1871). German ophthalmologist.

Birch-Hirschfeld lamp. A lamp used in radiational treatment of eye disease.

Birch-Hirschfeld, Félix Victor (b. 1842). German pathologist.

Birch-Hirschfeld method. A histological staining method for amyloid in tissues. The stain consists of gentian violet and Bismarck brown.

Bircher, Heinrich (b. 1850). Swiss surgeon.

Bircher's operation. An operation to reduce the size of a dilated stomach. Not now performed.

Bird, Golding (b. 1814). London physician.

Bird's disease. Oxaluria.

Bird's treatment. The treatment of bedsores by galvanism.

Bird, Samuel Dougan (b. 1832). Melbourne physician.

Bird's sign. An area of dullness on percussion, with absent breath sounds, over a hydatid cyst of the lung.

birefractive (bi·re·frak·tiv). Having the power of or characterized by double refraction. [L *bis*, *refringere* to break up.]

birefringence (bi·re·frin·jens). The property possessed by certain biological materials of doubly refracting a beam of plane polarized light. **Stream birefringence.** The ability of certain suspensions containing rod- or disc-shaped particles to be orientated by flow, thus causing double refraction. It has been used to characterize virus particles. [L *bis*, *refringere* to break up.]

birefringent (bi·re·frin·jent). Birefractive.

birhinia (bi·rin·e·ah). A congenital facial deformity consisting of a double nose. [L bis, Gk *rhis* nose.]

birimose (bi·ri·moze). Characterized by having 2 rimae or slits, a term applied to an anther. [L *bis*, *rima* chink.]

Birkett, John (b. 1815). English surgeon.

Birkett's hernia. Protrusion of the synovial membrane of a joint through a defect in the joint capsule.

Birkhaug, Konrad Elias (b. 1892). New York bacteriologist.

Birkhaug's test. A skin test for rheumatic fever. No longer used.

Birmingham, Ambrose (b. 1864). Dublin anatomist.

Birmingham's stomach bed. The surface of the organs forming the posterior relations of the stomach.

Birmingham revision (ber·ming·ham re·vizh·un). *See* REVISION.

birotation (bi·ro·ta·shun). Mutarotation: the change in rotation of an optically active compound, a phenomenon exhibited by freshly prepared solutions of sugar which alter in the value of their optical activity until an equilibrium is attained. It is due to the formation of stereo-isomers. [L *bis*, *rotare* to turn.]

birth (berth). 1. The act of being born; the fact of having been born. 2. The process of bringing forth. 3. That which is produced. **Concealment of birth.** Deliberate concealment in some private place of the birth (after 28 weeks' gestation) of a newborn child. Birth is notifiable and must also be registered after the 28th week. **Cross birth.** Transverse presentation. *See* PRESENTATION. **Dead birth.** An infant in whom either before or during the process of birth all indications of antenatal life have disappeared. **Head birth.** Head presentation. *See* PRESENTATION. **Live birth.** Birth in which the child exhibits some signs of life after the birth is completed. **Multiple birth.** Birth of more than one child at one time. **Partial birth.** Incomplete expulsion of the child during labour. **Plural birth.** Multiple birth (see above). **Posthumous birth.** The birth of a child after the father has died. **Post-term birth.** One taking place after the period of 280 days has passed. **Precocious birth.** That occurring in natural labour at the end of a pregnancy of less than the usual duration. **Premature birth.** A birth occurring before the full term has passed but after pregnancy has been established for 6 months. **Still birth.** *See* STILLBIRTH. **Virgin birth.** Parthenogenesis. [ME *burth.*]

birth control (**berth** kon·**trole**). The prevention, limitation, spacing-out or regulation of conception, either by abstention from sexual intercourse, or by the use of contraceptive measures, or by any other means. **Birth-control clinic.** A clinic where advice and instruction are given upon the subject. [ME *burth*, Fr. *contrôler.*]

birthmark (**berth**·mark). A congenital circumscribed neoplasm; naevus pigmentosus. [ME *burth*, AS *meark.*]

bis. Prefix, from the Latin *bis*, meaning *twice, doubly, two.*

bisabolene (bis·ab·ol·een). $C_{15}H_{24}$. A sesquiterpene found in lemon oil and pine-needle oil.

Bisacodyl BP 1973 (bis·a·**ko**·dil). Di - (4 - acetoxyphenyl) - 2 - pyridylmethane, a laxative used in the treatment of chronic constipation. Its action on the small intestine is negligible or absent altogether. It is often used to empty the colon prior to radiological or endoscopic examination. Given as tablets by mouth, or as suppositories.

bisacromial (bis·ak·**ro**·me·al). Relating or belonging to the 2 acromions. [L *bis*, Gk *akros* outermost.]

bisalt (**bi**·salt). A salt in which hydrogen atoms are united with the base to the acid radical; an acid salt, such as sodium biphosphate, Na_2HPO_4, or potassium bisulphate, $KHSO_4$.

bisamylose (bis·**am**·il·oze). Diamylose, $C_{12}H_{20}O_{10}$. The anhydride of maltose, consisting of 2 α-glucopyranose rings, and considered the fundamental unit in the molecular structure of starch.

bisaxillary (bis·**ax**·il·ar·e). Relating to or involving the 2 axillae. [L *bis, axilla* armpit.]

bische (bish). A local name for a severe form of Shiga's dysentery with gangrene of the large intestine, prevalent in Trinidad.

Bischoff, Theodor Ludwig Wilhelm von (b. 1807). German anatomist.

Bischoff's corona, or crown. The corona radiata of the granulosa cells around the ovum.

bisection (bi·**sek**·shun). 1. The cutting or dividing of any structure into 2 parts. 2. One of 2 parts. [L *bis, secare* to cut.]

biseptate (bi·**sep**·tate). Divided into 2 portions by a septum. [L *bis, septum* partition.]

bisexual (bi·**sex**·ew·al). 1. Hermaphrodite. 2. Being sexually attracted to both the male and the female sex. [L *bis*, sex.]

bisexuality (**bi**·sex·ew·**al**'·it·e). Having physical attributes characteristic of both sexes. [see prec.]

bisferious (bis·**fer**·e·us). Marked by having 2 beats. [L *bis, ferire* to beat.]

Bishop, Louis Faugères, Snr. (b. 1864). American physician.

Bishop's sphygmoscope. An instrument for recording the arterial blood pressure.

Bishop Harman. *See* HARMAN.

bisiliac (bis·**il**·e·ak). 1. Referring to or involving the 2 most widely separated corresponding points on the iliac crests. 2. Referring to any 2 corresponding parts of the ilium. [L *bis, ilia* flank.]

Bismarck brown (**biz**·mark **brown**). $C_6H_4[N_2C_6H_3(NH_2)_2]_2$. A bisazo dye derived from metaphenylenediamine. It is used for staining mucin, cartilage matrix and other basophilic substances.

bismuth (**biz**·muth). An element of atomic weight 208.98, atomic number 83 and chemical symbol Bi. It is a reddish-white metal which is used to form low-melting-point alloys. Most of the inorganic salts of bismuth are insoluble or are rendered insoluble in the body; they are therefore used as protectives, particularly of the mucous membranes of the alimentary canal, from the action of irritants. Certain of them, such as the subnitrate, are astringent and antiseptic and are employed as dusting powders. Cases of poisoning have been recorded, characterized by acute stomatitis, gastro-enteritis, with diarrhoea and vomiting; albumin may appear in the urine and death results from collapse. The metal in suspension, the inorganic salts—especially the oxychloride, the organic compounds including the tartrate, salicylate and subgallate, and combinations of bismuth and arsenic—have been tried in the treatment of trypanosomiasis, amoebiasis, relapsing fever, syphilis and yaws, with limited success. They are given intramuscularly, as they are too insoluble for oral or subcutaneous administration, and too toxic to be injected intravenously. The site usually is deep into the buttock with precaution against entering a vein. Bismuth therapy has, however, been replaced by penicillin. **Acid bismuth sodium tartrate.** Bismuthi et Sodii Tartras Acidus BPC 1949, soluble bismuth tartrate, a compound which is acid in reaction and therefore not suitable for injection. It is used for digestive disorders, usually with pepsin. **Bismuth albuminate.** A white compound used in intestinal colic. **Bismuth and ammonium citrate, Bismuthammonium citrate.** Bismuthi et Ammonii Citras BPC 1949, a compound used as an antacid. **Bismuth arsanilate.** $NH_2C_6H_4AsO(OH)OBi(OH)_2$, a compound used in the treatment of syphilis. **Bismuth benzoate.** $(C_6H_5COO)_3BiBi(OH)_3$, an antiseptic. **Bismuth betanaphtholate.** $(C_{10}H_7O)_3Bi{\cdot}3H_2O$, a tasteless compound employed as an intestinal astringent and antiseptic. **Bismuth Carbonate BP 1953.** $(BiO)_2CO_3H_2O$, an insoluble substance with a weak antacid effect reacting slowly with the hydrochloric acid of the stomach and inhibiting the secretion by coating the mucous membrane. With the carbonates of magnesium and calcium it is employed in gastric or duodenal ulcer, also in cases of diarrhoea. Incorporated in ointments and dusting powders it has a protective and sedative effect on inflamed skin. **Bismuth chrysophanate.** $Bi(C_{15}H_9O_4)_3$, a yellow powder of value as an antiseptic in skin diseases. **Bismuth citrate.** Bismuthi Citras BPC 1949, $C_3H_4(OH)(COO)_3Bi$, an insoluble compound used as a stomachic, and compounded with other citrates, e.g. ammonium citrate, to form intestinal astringents. **Bismuth cresolate.** A greyish insoluble powder used as an antiseptic like iodoform. **Bismuth dithiosalicylate.** A yellow substance used as an external antiseptic. **Bismuth ethyl camphorate.** $(C_{12}H_{19}O_4)_3Bi$, an antisyphilitic compound used intramuscularly. **Bismuth glycollylarsanilate.** BP Commission approved name for *N*-glycollylarsanilate. An anti-amoebic drug used also against intestinal flagellate infections and *Trichomonas vaginalis*, for which latter tablets are inserted in the vagina. **Bismuth iodide.** BiI_3, a compound used in combination with emetine in the treatment of amoebic dysentery. **Bismuth lactate.** $BiH(C_3H_4O_3)_2$, a compound administered as an intestinal astringent. **Bismuth oxide.** Bi_2O_3, a yellowish compound used similarly to the subnitrate. **Bismuth oxycarbonate.** Bismuth carbonate (see above). **Bismuth Oxychloride BP 1963.** BiOCl, a compound used in suspension in a 5 per cent dextrose solution for intramuscular injection. **Bismuth oxygallate.** Bismuth subgallate (see below). **Bismuth Oxyiodogallate BPC 1954, Bismuth oxyiodosubgallate.** A compound used as a powder for external application, as an ointment, and in suppositories. **Bismuth oxysalicylate.** Bismuth salicylate (see below). **Precipitated Bismuth BP 1953.** A purified and finely divided preparation of metallic bismuth from which other preparations, including Injection of Bismuth BP 1953, are made. **Bismuth Salicylate BP 1953.** $Bi(C_7H_5O_3)_3Bi_2O_3$, an insoluble compound used as an antiseptic and, suspended in arachis oil, as an injection in the treatment of syphilis. **Bismuth Sodium Tartrate BP 1963.** Sodium bismuthyl tartrate, $BiNa(C_4H_4O_6)_2$, a soluble compound of bismuth used intramuscularly in syphilis. It is rapidly absorbed and injections must be frequent. **Soluble bismuth tartrate.** Acid bismuth sodium tartrate (see above). **Bismuth subcarbonate.** Bismuth carbonate (see above). **Bismuth subchloride.** Bismuth oxychloride (see above). **Bismuth Subgallate BP 1953.** $Bi(OH)_2C_7H_5O_5$, an internal astringent and antiseptic, also used in the treatment of syphilis. **Bismuth Subnitrate BPC 1968.** $BiONO_3{\cdot}H_2O$, an insoluble compound used in cases of gastric ulcer. **Bismuth subsalicylate.** Bismuth salicylate (see above). **Bismuth tetraiodophenolphthalein.** A reddish antiseptic powder employed in enteritis as an antiseptic. **Bismuth tribromphenate.** Bismuthi Tribromphenas BPC 1949, a yellow insoluble powder used internally for dysentery and diarrhoea, and externally for chronic ulcers as an antiseptic. It has the formula $(C_6H_2Br_3O)BiHOHBi_2O_3$. **Bismuth tryparsamide.** $CONH_2CH_2NHC_6H_4AsO(OH)BiO(OH)_2$, a compound injected formerly in the treatment of syphilis. **Bismuth violet.** A derivative of crystal violet used as an antiseptic. [G *Wismut.*]

bismuthal (**biz**·muth·al). Related to or containing bismuth.

bismuthate (**biz**·muth·ate). Any salt of bismuthic acid, $HBiO_3$.

bismuthia (biz·**muth**·e·ah). The condition in which the skin and mucous membranes show a blue tint after the ingestion of bismuth preparations.

bismuthic (**biz**·muth·ik). A compound of bismuth in which the latter is pentavalent; derived from bismuth pentoxide, Bi_2O_5.

bismuthosis (biz·muth·**o**·sis). A condition of chronic bismuth poisoning. [bismuth, Gk *-osis* condition.]

bismuthotartrate (**biz**·muth·o·**tar**′·trate). Bismuthyl tartrate, tartobismuthate. One of a series of neutral compounds, analogous to tartar emetic, of the general formula $C_4H_4O_6$ (BiO)M, where M is a monovalent metal such as potassium or sodium; they are used intramuscularly in the treatment of syphilis and yaws.

bismuthous (**biz**·muth·us). A compound of bismuth in which the latter is trivalent; derived from bismuth trioxide, Bi_2O_3.

bismuthyl (**biz**·muth·il). The monovalent radical -BiO, derived from bismuth trioxide, Bi_2O_3. **Bismuthyl carbonate.** Bismuth carbonate. **Bismuthyl chloride.** Bismuth oxychloride. **Bismuthyl nitrate.** Bismuth subnitrate. **Bismuthyl tartrate.** Bismuthotartrate.

Bisoxatin (bis·**ox**·at·in). BP Commission approved name for 2,3-dihydro - 2,2 - di - (4 - hydroxyphenyl) - 1,4 - benzoxazin - 3 - one; a laxative.

bissa (**bis**·ah). A disease prevalent in lower Egypt, held to be caused by sheep eating the plant bisse, and so tainting their flesh, which in turn affects human beings, in whom the disease is marked by a dropsical condition. [African name.]

bistephanic (bi·stef·**an**·ik). Referring to the 2 stephanions, particularly the distance between them. [L *bis*, Gk *stephanos* crown.]

bistort (**bis**·tort). Snakeweed, *Polygonum bistorta* Linn. (family Polygonaceae); the dried rhizome is used as an astringent. [L *bis, tortus* twisted.]

bistoury (**bis**·too·re). A long narrow curved or straight surgical knife with a sharp or probe point used for opening up sacs or abscesses. **Bistoury caché.** A bistoury the point of which is concealed until the place of incision has been reached when, on pressure being put on the handle, the probe or blade is exposed and the incision made. [Fr. *bistouri.*]

bistratal (bi·**stra**·tal). Having 2 strata or layers. [L *bis, stratum* layer.]

bisulphate (bi·**sul**·fate). One of the series of acid sulphates of general formula $MHSO_4$, where M is a monovalent metal. [see foll.]

bisulphide (bi·**sul**·fide). A binary compound of 2 atoms of sulphur combined with 1 atom of another element, such as carbon bisulphide, CS_2. [L *bis*, sulphur.]

bisulphite (bi·**sul**·fite). 1. One of the acid sulphites of general formula $MHSO_3$, where M is a monovalent metal. 2. One of the additive compounds formed by sodium bisulphite with aldehydes and ketones; useful in the purification of the latter. [see prec.]

bita higoidea (**bi**·tah hi·**goid**·e·ah). Xanthoma.

bitartrate (bi·**tar**·trate). An acid tartrate of the general formula $C_4H_4O_6HM$, where M is a monovalent metal.

bite (bite). 1. To close the teeth forcibly, with the object of wounding, breaking or marking, or, in the case of an insect, usually by the introduction of the proboscis. 2. The result of such action. 3. In dentistry, to bring the teeth together into occlusion. 4. In dentistry, an appliance, made of an easily softened material, which fits the mouth and is used in prosthetic dentistry to register the correct relationship between the jaws. **Check bite.** A thin sheet of wax or other plastic material used to confirm that the relationship of the teeth as registered on an articulator is identical with that existing in the mouth. **Close bite.** A condition in which the biting edges of the lower incisor teeth impinge heavily upon the palatal aspects of the corresponding upper teeth on closure of the mouth. **Closed bite.** A condition in which the jaws are too close together, owing to the wearing-down of the occlusal surfaces of the natural teeth or to the use of artificial dentures whose vertical height is insufficient. **Cross bite.** When one or both buccal segments are in linguo-occlusion. **Dog bite.** A bite by a dog; this may have septic complications, or, in the case of the dog being rabid, cause hydrophobia. **Edge-to-edge bite.** A condition in which there is no overlap of the upper over the lower incisor teeth, the incisal edges meeting when the mouth is closed. **Insect bite.** A puncture made by the proboscis of an insect; such a bite may convey an infection or may only cause pain and swelling. **Open bite.** A condition in which a space exists between upper and lower incisor teeth when the mouth is closed. **Over bite.** The vertical overlap of the upper over the lower incisors. **Raised bite.** A condition in which the jaws are kept too far apart, due to the use of artificial dentures whose vertical height is too great. **Rat bite.** A bite by a rat; this may cause rat-bite fever. **Snake bite.** A bite by a snake; if the snake is of a poisonous variety it actually inoculates venom by means of hollow or grooved fangs (modified teeth) deep into the tissues. **Stork bites.** Capillary flames. *See* FLAME. **Underhung bite.** A condition in which the lower incisor teeth pass in front of the upper on closing the mouth. [AS *bitan.*]

bite-gauge (**bite**·gaje). An instrument used in prosthetic dentistry to ensure the correct recording of the relationship between the upper and the lower jaw. [AS *bitan*, OFr. *gauge.*]

bite-rim (**bite**·rim). A rim used in prosthetic dentistry to ensure that the biting surfaces of the teeth on an artificial denture occupy the same planes as those of the natural teeth which they replace. [AS *bitan, reoma.*]

bite-wing (**bite**·wing). A special dental x-ray film held between the clenched teeth. [AS *bitan*, Old Norse *vaengr.*]

bitemporal (bi·**tem**·por·al). 1. Relating or belonging to both temples. 2. Relating or belonging to both temporal bones, or involving them. [L *bis, tempora* temples.]

biterminal (bi·**ter**·min·al). Relating to the use of both ends of an electric wire or current, or to both terminals of an alternating current. [L *bis*, Gk *terma* limit.]

Bithionol (bi·**thi**·o·nol). BP Commission approved name for 2,2′-thiobis-(4,6-dichlorophenol); an antiseptic agent.

Bitot, Pierre (b. 1822). Bordeaux surgeon.

Bitot's spots. Small white triangular plaques covered with a foam-like discharge, found on the bulbar conjunctiva near the limbus in xerosis of the conjunctiva due to vitamin A deficiency; sometimes called *Bitot's patches.*

bitrochanteric (**bi**·tro·kan·**ter**′·ik). Referring to or involving the 2 greater trochanters. [L *bis*, Gk *trochanter* runner.]

bitter-wood (**bit**·er·wud). Quassia, the wood of *Picroena excelsa* Lind. [AS *biter, wudu.*]

bitters (**bit**·erz). A drug containing a bitter principle and used to stimulate appetite. The most important simple bitters are quassia and calumba; they contain no tannic acid and may therefore be dispensed with iron. The aromatic bitters, gentian and bitter-orange peel, are said to have a more potent effect than the simple bitters; they both contain tannic acid and are incompatible with iron. Bitters stimulate the secretion of saliva and gastric juice reflexly by exciting the taste buds. They are quite valueless if given directly into the stomach, as for example, in the form of a pill, and do not increase the secretions of people with normal appetites. They are, however, very useful for tempting the palates of patients recovering from long illnesses. Mixtures containing bitters should be given about half an hour before meals. Drugs, such as strychnine and quinine, which have a very bitter taste, have been used as bitters, but such use is quite irrational, as they are in no way superior to the drugs already mentioned, and should be reserved for their more important effects. **Aromatic bitters.** Those containing volatile oils in addition to a bitter principle, e.g. orange peel, and used as flavouring agents. **Astringent bitters.** Those containing tannic acid and having astringent properties; they are incompatible with heavy metals, e.g. iron. Examples are gentian, serpentary and cimicifuga. **Simple bitters.** Those practically free from tannin and volatile oils, used solely for their bitter taste, e.g. gentian, calumba, taraxacum. **Styptic bitters.** Astringent bitters (see above). [AS *biter.*]

Bittner, John Joseph (b. 1904). American cancer research worker.

Bittner agent, milk factor or virus. An RNA-containing tumour virus causing a mammary cancer in mice. The virus is frequently latent and is activated by alteration in hormonal balance. Not all strains of mice are susceptible.

Bittorf, Alexander (b. 1876). Leipzig pathologist.

Bittorf's reaction. Referred pain through the genitofemoral nerve, from lesions of the testis or ovary.

bitumen (**bit**·ew·men). The name applied to natural dark-coloured resins found as such, and also produced in the purification of petroleum and the distillation of schists and brown coals. **Sulphonated bitumen.** Bitumen sulphonated and neutralized with ammonia; a thick brown fluid used in the same way as ichthammol. [L.]

bituminosis (bit·ew·min·**o**'·sis). An affection of the lungs caused by the inhalation of the dust from soft coal. [L *bitumen* mineral pitch, Gk *-osis* condition.]

biurate (bi·**ewr**·ate). An acid urate; a salt of uric acid in which only one of the replaceable hydrogen atoms has been exchanged for a metallic atom or basic group.

biuret (bi·**ewr**·et). Carbamide, allophanamide, NH_2CONH $CONH_2$. A crystalline substance produced by heating urea; used as a reagent, giving a violet coloration with copper salts in alkaline solution.

bivalence (bi·**va**·lens). The ability of a chemical element to combine with or replace 2 atoms of hydrogen, chlorine or any other monovalent element; the term also applies to the equivalent combining power of radicals and groups. [see foll.]

bivalent. 1. (bi·**va**·lent) Of an element or radical, possessing a valency of 2, i.e. having the power to replace or combine with 2 atoms of hydrogen; divalent. 2. (**biv**·al·ent) The complex formed by the pairing of 2 chromosomes during the first meiotic division. **Ring bivalent.** Bivalent whose chromosomes are held together by 2 terminal chiasmata. [L *bis, valere* to be powerful.]

biventer (bi·**ven**·ter). Term applied particularly to a muscle indicating that it has 2 bellies; digastric. [L *bis, venter* belly.]

biventral (bi·**ven**·tral). Digastric; with 2 bellies. [see prec.]

Bivine's method. The treatment of strychnine poisoning with chloral hydrate.

bivitelline (bi·vi·**tel**·een). Term applied to an ovum that has 2 yolks. [L *bis, vitellus* yolk.]

bizincic (bi·**zink**·ik). Term applied to a compound of zinc containing 2 atoms of the latter. [L *bis*, zinc.]

bizygomatic (bi·zi·go·**mat**'·ik). Referring to the most prominent point on each zygomatic arch. [L *bis, zygoma* cheekbone.]

Bizzozero, Giulio (b. 1846). Turin physician.

Bizzozero's cells, or corpuscles. Blood platelets. *See* PLATELET.

Bjerrum, Jannik Petersen (b. 1851). Copenhagen ophthalmologist.

Bjerrum's scotoma, or sign. A form of arcuate scotoma, starting from the top or bottom of the blind spot and arching around the fixation point in the shape of a comet; a diagnostic sign in glaucoma.

Bjerrum screen. A black cloth screen, usually 2 m square, with a central small white disc for fixation, placed 2 m from the patient and well illuminated. Round white or coloured targets varying from 1 to 40 mm are moved over this area and the central field of vision thus minutely investigated. It is a form of perimeter, or tangent, screen.

Björnström's algesimeter. A device by which the sensitiveness of the skin can be ascertained.

Black, Douglas Andrew Kilgour (b. 1909). Scottish physician.

Black's formula. The formula $F=(W+C)-H$, used to estimate the stamina of a man; where F is the empirical factor, W is the weight in pounds, C the expanded chest measurement and H the height, both in inches. Over 120 is classed as very strong; below 80, very weak.

Black, Otis Fisher (b. 1867). American chemist.

Black's method. For β-hydroxybutyric acid in urine: urine is concentrated, mixed with plaster of Paris to a stiff paste, allowed almost to set, broken up and extracted with ether. The ether is evaporated, the residue dissolved in water and neutralized with barium carbonate, and to the neutral solution are added two or three drops hydrogen peroxide followed by a few drops of Black's reagent. In the presence of β-hydroxybutyric acid a rose colour is produced which attains a maximum intensity and then fades.

Black's reagent. 5 g $FeCl_3$, 0.4 g $FeCl_2$ in 100 ml water.

black (blak). The property possessed by a body which absorbs light of all wavelengths and reflects none. **Animal black, Bone black.** Animal charcoal. *See* CHARCOAL. **Carbon black.** Lampblack. **Induline black.** Nigrosin; a mixture of induline with a yellow dye, used as a background stain in bacteriology and histology, and also in staining algae and fungi. **Ivory black, Paris black.** Animal charcoal. *See* CHARCOAL. [AS *blac.*]

black corsair (blak **kor**·sa·re). A free-living bug (*Melanolestes picipes*) in the USA. It is sometimes very abundant and its bites are painful. [AS *blac*, Fr. *corsaire.*]

Black Currant BPC 1968 (blak·**kur**·ant). The fresh ripe fruits of *Ribes nigram.* The syrup is used as a flavouring agent and, diluted, as a beverage.

black haw (**blak** haw). Black haw bark, the dried root-bark of *Viburnum prunifolium* Linn. (family Caprifoliaceae), a shrub indigenous to east and central USA; it contains a bitter glycoside, viburnin. It has been used in asthma and dysmenorrhoea, and as a uterine sedative to check threatened abortion and haemorrhage. [AS *blac, haga.*]

black widow (blak **wid**·o). Any spider of the genus *Latrodectus*, especially *Lactrodectus mactans.* They are black with a white ventral spot; the bite of some species produces serious symptoms and sometimes death. [AS *blac, widewe.*]

Blackburn caliper. Metal hooks fitted upon a sliding bar and used for traction on the skull in spinal injuries.

Blackfan, Kenneth Daniel (b. 1883). American physician.

Blackfan-Diamond syndrome. Congenital anaemia due to lack of red blood corpuscle precursors.

blackhead (**blak**·hed). A comedo; a plug of greasy matter blocking the superficial mouth of a sebaceous follicle and tipped by a blackened cap of dust and debris. [AS *blac, heafod.*]

blackout (**blak**·owt). 1. Amaurosis fugax, including temporary loss of vision and consciousness occurring in airmen, caused by lessening of the quantity of blood circulating to the brain and the retina resulting from centrifugal acceleration while flying. 2. A common lay term for brief spells of unconsciousness whether syncopal or epileptic. [AS *blac, ut.*]

bladder [vesica (NA)] (**blad**·er). A distensible sac, containing fluid. **Allantoic bladder.** A diverticulum of the roof of the bladder of congenital origin, and associated with persistence of a cyst of the urachus which, in fact, forms a diverticulum which communicates with the bladder at its lower end. **Atonic bladder.**

A condition in which the bladder capacity is greatly increased and the detrusor muscle has become weakened. It is brought about by incomplete emptying over a long period, due either to an intravesical obstruction or to a defect in the parasympathetic innervation. **Automatic bladder.** A form of neurogenic bladder (see below) associated with interruption of the spinal cord above the bladder centres in the conus medullaris. There is a characteristic and involuntary reflex micturition, which, however, is complete, at short and frequent intervals. There is no residual urine. **Autonomous bladder.** A form of neurogenic bladder (see below) associated with interruption of the parasympathetic innervation by lesions of the lumbosacral segments of the spinal cord. There is a characteristic and involuntary reflex micturition associated with incontinence, dribbling and incomplete emptying, with residual urine. **Bilocular bladder.** A double bladder (reduplication of the bladder). This may be complete or incomplete, and is believed to be due to a splitting of the vesicourethral anlage. The septum may divide the bladder into right and left segments or, when the septum is frontal, into anterior and posterior segments. **Brain bladder.** An obsolete term for an embryonic cerebral vesicle. **Cord bladder.** A neurogenic bladder (see below) associated with interruption of the parasympathetic innervation in lesions of the cauda equina of the spinal cord. The bladder is of poor tone, and there is a high residue urine. There is a dribbling incontinence. **Encysted bladder.** A condition associated with a cyst of the urachus which may be closed at one or other end; thus a blind external fistulous track may communicate with the umbilicus, or a blind internal fistulous track with the bladder. In the latter case, the cyst forms a vesical diverticulum. **Fasciculated bladder.** Trabeculated bladder (see below). **Gall bladder.** *See* GALL BLADDER. **Hypertonic bladder.** A condition in which there is a hypertonicity of the bladder detrusor muscle as a result of an irritant such as a foreign body or stone, inflammation or intravesical obstruction. **Irritable bladder.** A condition in which there is a constant desire to urinate without any obvious cause, such as the presence of stone, inflammation, bladder-neck obstruction, etc.; a condition usually confined to females. **Multilocular bladder.** A condition which occurs in association with obstructions, often congenital, at the bladder neck or in the urethra. The increased intravesical pressure leads to herniations of the bladder wall through separated detrusor-muscle bundles. When situated at the bladder base, the ureteric opening may be drawn into the sac of the diverticulum as it enlarges. **Neurogenic bladder.** A comprehensive term used to describe any disturbance of bladder function associated with lesions of the bladder innervation, whether affecting intrinsic nerves to the bladder, the sacral roots, the cauda equina or the central nervous system. **Sacculated bladder.** A condition accompanying prolonged intravesical obstruction that has led to hypertrophy of the detrusor muscle. The latter becomes trabeculated, and between its muscle fibres pouches of vesical mucosa may herniate as cellules which may be shallow or deep. **Spastic bladder.** A condition in which there is uncoordinated function of the detrusor muscle and the sphincteric mechanism at the bladder neck, as a result of neuromuscular imbalance, or inflammation, or irritation in the posterior urethra, leading to sphincteric spasm. **Spinal-reflex bladder.** Automatic bladder (see above). **Stammering bladder.** A condition in which there is interruption of the urinary stream due to weakness of the detrusor muscle associated with overdistension from intravesical obstruction. Otherwise there may be an intrinsic disorder of the parasympathetic innervation. **Supplementary bladder.** Bilocular bladder; reduplication of the bladder (see above). **Trabeculated bladder.** A term used to describe the characteristic criss-cross appearance of the detrusor muscle when it is hypertrophied as a result of intravesical obstruction. **Urinary bladder.** *See* URINARY BLADDER. [AS *blaedre.*]

bladderwrack (**blad**·er·rak). The brown alga *Fucus vesiculosus* Linn. [AS *blaedre, wraec* damage.]

blade-bone (**blade**·bone). The scapula. [AS *blaed, ban.*]

blaes. *See* BLASIUS.

Blagden, Sir Charles (b. 1748). London physician.

Blagden's law. The lowering of the freezing point of a solvent by the dissolving of a substance in it is proportional to the concentration of the latter, provided the solution remains a dilute one.

blain (blane). 1. A pustule, bulla, blister or blotch. 2. Anthrax. [ME *bleyn* blister.]

Blainville, Henri Marie Ducrotay de (b. 1777). French anthropologist and zoologist.

Blainville's ear. Lack of symmetry of the 2 ears.

Blair, Vilray Papin (b. 1871). St. Louis, Missouri, surgeon.

Blair knife. An unguarded knife with a 23 cm (9 in) soft-steel blade, used for cutting skin grafts.

Blair-Brown graft. A skin graft cut freehand by the Blair alignment knife.

Blair-Brown operation. 1. Plastic repair of hare-lip. 2. Plastic repair of cleft palate.

Blair-Bell, William (b. 1871). Liverpool gynaecologist.

Blair-Bell's treatment. The treatment of cancer by injections of colloidal lead.

Blake, Clarence John (b. 1843). Boston otologist.

Blake's disc. A paper disc used as a prosthesis for repair to a hole in the drum head.

Blakemore, Arthur Hendley (b. 1897). New York surgeon.

Blakemore-Lord operation. Vascular anastomosis with use of a vitallium cuff (the Blakemore-Lord tube), the proximal vascular segment being passed through the cuff, which is then inserted in the distal segment; the method is particularly applicable to venous anastomosis, e.g. portacaval shunt.

Blakemore-Lord tube. A vitallium tube devised to facilitate vascular suture, by approximating intima to intima without any intervening foreign body in the Blakemore-Lord operation.

Blakemore-Sengstaken tube. A triple-lumen tube carrying 2 separately inflatable balloons, passed down the oesophagus and the distal balloon inflated in the stomach. Distension of the proximal balloon is used to stop haemorrhage from oesophageal varices. The third lumen is for aspirating the stomach contents.

Blalock, Alfred (b. 1899). Baltimore surgeon.

Blalock's approach. (Thoracotomy); an angled incision which extends downwards in the paravertebral region, 5 cm (2 in) from the spinous processes, and is then angled forward along the line of the 6th intercostal space.

Blalock clamp. A clamp with angled blades, for controlling large vessels during the performance of an anastomosis between them.

Blalock's operation. 1. Operative establishment of an anastomosis between the pulmonary artery distal to a pulmonary stenosis and a branch of the aorta, e.g. subclavian artery; for the relief of "blue baby" sufferers from the congenital heart lesion known as Fallot's tetralogy. 2. Removal of the thymus in the treatment of myasthenia gravis.

Blalock-Hanlon operation. Atrial septectomy; the surgical creation of an atrial septal defect for the palliation of transposition of the great vessels.

Blalock-Taussig operation. The operation devised by Blalock to achieve, as suggested by Taussig, an increase in the blood flow to the lungs in patients with cyanotic heart disease who had diminished blood flow to the lungs; a systemic artery, usually the subclavian but sometimes the innominate, was divided and the proximal end anastomosed to the side or the distal end of the pulmonary artery on the same side.

Blanc, Georges (b. 1884). French bacteriologist in Morocco.

Blanc vaccine. A bile-treated living typhus vaccine used in Morocco.

blanch (blahnsh). To lose colour or become pale from fear or other strong emotion or as the result of illness. [Fr. *blanchir* to become white.]

Blanchard, Wallace (b. 1857). Chicago surgeon.

Blanchard's treatment. A method of packing tuberculous bone sinuses with a mixture of wax and petroleum jelly, used in the prechemotherapeutic era, and now obsolete.

bland (bland). Non-stimulating; term applied to a medicine or other remedy that has soft and soothing properties. [L *blandus.*]

Blandin, Philippe Frédéric (b. 1798). Paris surgeon.

cyst of Blandin and Nuhn glands. A rare cyst resulting from obstruction to the duct of one of the anterior lingual glands situated beneath the anterior part of the tongue.

Blandin's ganglion. The sublingual ganglion. *See* GANGLION.

Blandin's glands, Blandin and Nuhn glands. Anterior lingual glands. *See* GLAND.

Blandy, John Peter. British urologist.

Blandy's ureteroplasty. A scrotal flap operation for stricture of the urethra.

Blanfordia formosana (blan·for·de·ah for·mo·sah·nah). *Oncomelania formosana,* a snail intermediary host of *Schistosoma japonicum.*

Blaps (blapz). A genus of beetles. **Blaps mucronata.** The cellar beetle, a common commensal of man, and possible secondary host of *Hymenolepsis diminuta.* [Gk injuring.]

Blasius (Blaes), Gerhard (b. 1626). Dutch anatomist.

Blasius duct. The parotid duct. *See* DUCT.

Blasius' operation. For ectropion of the lower lid: a small pedicle flap is swung from the outer temporal region and sutured into the lower lid under a bridge of skin.

Blaskovics, Lazlo de (b. 1869). Budapest ophthalmologist.

Blaskovics' operation. 1. For ptosis: advancement and resection of the levator palpebrae superioris muscle and removal of the upper part of the tarsal plate. The levator is sutured to the skin just above the lash margin. It is performed from the conjunctival surface, and is widely used. 2. Blepharoplasty: (*a*) for use at the outer canthus by utilizing a pedicle flap from the temporal region, (*b*) Arlt–Blaskovics operation. 3. For epicanthus: excision of a semilunar flap of skin in the canthal fold nearer to the nose than to the medial canthus; useful in mild cases. 4. For entropion of the upper lid.

Arlt–Blaskovics operation. A modification of Dieffenbach's blepharoplasty: a pedicle flap shaped like a hatchet with a narrow base is fashioned from the nearby area to fill the lid defect.

Machek–Blaskovics operation. For entropion of the upper lid: a 3 mm wide bridge of skin and orbicularis with the lash margin is dissected off the tarsal plate. A second narrower bridge is dissected off above the first and passed under it, so that it heals in position between the first bridge and the eyelid margin.

blast (blast, blahst). 1. A blast cell, a primitive cell of any group. 2. Any one of the small spindles of fibrils which have their origin in a mere. [Gk *blastos* germ.] 3. The wave or concussion of air produced by an explosion of any kind. [AS *blaest* a blowing.] **Bechic blast.** In coughing, the strong, forced rush of air through the trachea and bronchi. **Blast chest.** Lung blast (see below). **Immersion blast.** The concussion in water produced by the explosion of a depth charge; it is responsible for internal injury to anyone in the water nearby. **Lung blast.** As the result of exposure to the air concussion of an explosion, concussion and haemorrhage affecting the tympanic membranes, the lungs and various other thoracic and abdominal viscera; the nervous system is also involved. **Wind blast.** The effect of exposing an animal to high wind velocity.

blastation (blas·ta·shun). Any variation of the germ plasm which is likely to be passed on to the offspring. [Gk *blastos* germ.]

blastema (blas·te·mah). Rudimentary protoplasm. [Gk bud.]

blastemic (blas·tem·ik). Referring to the blastema.

blastid (blas·tid). In the fertilized ovum, the small, clear space which is the first sign of the development of a nucleus. [Gk *blastos* germ.]

blastin (blas·tin). Any substance which nourishes cells or stimulates their growth, e.g. allantoin. [Gk *blastanein* to cause to grow.]

blastochyle (blas·to·kile). The colourless fluid within the blastocoele. [Gk *blastos* germ, *chylos* juice.]

blastocoele (blas·to·seel). The fluid-filled cavity of a blastula or a morula. [Gk *blastos* germ, *koilos* hollow.]

blastocyst (blas·to·sist). 1. In human embryology, the fluid-filled cavity within the morula, surrounded by the trophoblast and bearing at one place the formative mass. 2. In parasitology, a protozoon of the genus *Blastocystis.* [Gk *blastos* germ, *kystis* bag.]

Blastocystis hominis (blas·to·sis·tis hom·in·is). A unicellular fungus possessing a rounded body and an annular layer of cytoplasm with one or more nuclei and a large central vacuole. It is found in the stools in the tropics, but may be mistaken for protozoal cyst. [blastocyst, L of man.]

blastocyte (blas·to·site). In embryology, a cell which has not yet begun to undergo differentiation. [Gk *blastos* germ, *kytos* cell.]

blastocytoma (blas·to·si·to′·mah). A tumour consisting of blastocytes or undifferentiated tissue. [blastocyte, Gk *-oma* tumour.]

Blastodendrion intermedium (blas·to·den·dre·on in·ter·me·de·um). *Candida tropicalis.* [Gk *blastos* germ, *dendrion* tree, L *inter, medius* middle.]

blastoderm (blas·to·derm). In embryology, the plate of cells at the animal pole of large-yolked eggs, which results from the cleavage of the blastodisc. Analogous cells in small-yolked eggs with total cleavage line the blastodermic vesicle, or blastocyst, comprising an outer layer of trophoblast, and an inner cell mass, both surrounding the central fluid-filled blastocyst cavity or blastocoele. **Bilaminar blastoderm.** The 2-layered blastoderm, consisting of an upper layer of ectoderm and a lower layer of entoderm. **Embryonic blastoderm.** That part of the blastoderm of a large-yolked egg which develops into the embryo proper, as opposed to the fetal membranes. **Extra-embryonic blastoderm.** That part of the blastoderm which develops into the fetal membranes. **Trilaminar blastoderm.** The 3-layered blastoderm, consisting of ectoderm, mesoderm and entoderm. [Gk *blastos* germ, *derma* skin.]

blastodermal, blastodermic (blas·to·der·mal, blas·to·der·mik). Referring or belonging to the blastoderm.

blastodisc (blas·to·disk). The germinal disc. *See* DISC. **Bilaminar blastodisc.** A stage in the development of the blastodisc in which only ectodermal and entodermal layers are recognizable. **Trilaminar blastodisc.** A stage in the development of the blastodisc in which ectoderm, mesoderm and entoderm are all present. [Gk *blastos* germ, *diskos* disc.]

blastogenesis (blas·to·jen·es·is). 1. In biology, reproduction by budding. 2. The inheritance of characteristics transmitted by the germ plasm. [Gk *blastos* germ, *genein* to produce.]

blastogenetic, blastogenic (blas·to·jen·et′·ik, blas·to·jen·ik). 1. Referring to blastogenesis. 2. Having origin in the germ cell or the germ.

blastogeny (blas·toj·en·e). The history of the development of an organism from the ovum. [Gk *blastos* germ, *genein* to produce.]

blastolysis (blas·tol·is·is). The destruction or splitting up of a reproductive cell. [Gk *blastos* germ, *lysis* a loosing.]

blastoma (blas·to·mah) (pl. *blastomas* or *blastomata*). 1. A true tumour or neoplasm in the strictly pathological sense. 2. Blastocytoma. **Adrenal blastoma.** Adrenal neuroblastoma; a malignant adrenal tumour composed of undifferentiated medullary cells. **Autochthonous blastoma.** A neoplasm caused by the proliferation of cells belonging to the body of the person affected. **Heterochthonous blastoma.** Teratogenous blastoma (see below). **Pluricentric blastoma.** A tumour arising simultaneously from a number of foci of scattered cells or clusters of cells. **Teratogenous blastoma.** Teratoma, a tumour composed of one or more tissues derived from the embryonic germinal layers. **Unicentric blastoma.** A neoplasm originating from a single focus of cells or group of cells. [Gk *blastos* germ, *-oma* tumour.]

blastomatoid (blas·to·mat·oid). Showing resemblance to a blastoma. [blastoma, Gk *eidos* form.]

blastomatosis (blas·to·mat·o′·sis). A condition characterized by the development of blastomata. [blastoma, Gk *-osis* condition.]

blastomatous (blas·to·mat·us). 1. Term applied to tumours that have the general characteristics of a blastoma. 2. Belonging to blastoma.

blastomere (blas·to·meer). Any one cell or a group of cells composing the blastoderm; a morula cell. **Formative blastomere.** One of the blastomeres of a segmentary ovum which will be utilized in the formation of the embryonic area, as opposed to the trophoblast. [Gk *blastos* germ, *meros* part.]

blastomerotomy (blas·to·meer·ot′·o·me). The splitting up or destruction of a blastomere. [blastomere, Gk *temnein* to cut.]

blastomogenic, blastomogenous (blas·to·mo·jen′·ik, blas·to·moj′·en·us). 1. Producing neoplasms. 2. Conducing to the production of tumours or new growths. [blastoma, Gk *genein* to produce.]

Blastomyces (blas·to·mi·seez). A dimorphic fungus. **Blastomyces brasiliensis.** *Paracoccidioides brasiliensis*, causing the disease once known as South American blastomycosis, now paracoccidioidomycosis. **Blastomyces dermatitidis.** The cause of North American blastomycosis. In its tissue form this organism appears as rounded, budding, thick-walled yeast-like fungi; no mycelium is present but, *in vitro*, a mycelial phase can be cultured at room temperature. Mice can be infected. Its perfect state is *Ajellomyces dermatitidis* (Ascomycetes). [Gk *blastos* germ, *mykes* fungus.]

blastomycetic (blas·to·mi·se′·tik). Caused by or pertaining to blastomyces or a budding fungus.

blastomycin (blas·to·mi·sin). A sterile filtrate made from cultures of *Blastomyces dermatitidis* for use in an intradermal test.

Blastomycoides (blas·to·mi·koid′·eez). A generic name proposed by Castellani for a group of unrelated fungi. **Blastomycoides dermatitidis** Castellani 1928. A synonym of *Blastomyces dermatitidis* Gilchrist and Stokes 1898, the cause of North American blastomycosis (Gilchrist's disease). **Blastomycoides immitis.** *Coccidioides immitis*; the causal organism of coccidioidosis. [blastomyces, Gk *eidos* form.]

blastomycosis (blas·to·mi·ko′·sis). Syn.: North American blastomycosis; Gilchrist's disease. The term is reserved for the disease caused by *Blastomyces dermatitidis* which has been reported in North America and, more recently, in Africa and Latin America. It is a chronic granulomatous and suppurative disease which usually originates as a respiratory infection and may disseminate, having a predilection for skin and bones. **Brazilian blastomycosis.** Paracoccidioidomycosis. **European blastomycosis.** Cryptococcosis. **North American blastomycosis.** *See* main definition (above). **South American blastomycosis.** Paracoccidioidomycosis (Lutz-Splendore-Almeida disease). [Gk *blastos* germ, *mykes* fungus, *-osis* condition.]

blastomycotic (blas·to·mi·kot′·ik). Referring to blastomycosis.

blastoneuropore (blas·to·newr·o·por). In embryology, an impermanent opening sometimes present as the result of union of the blastopore and the neuropore. [Gk *blastos* germ, *neuron* nerve, *poros* passage.]

blastophore (blas·to·for). The content of a sperm cell other than the spermatid. **Sperm blastophore.** Blastophore. [Gk *blastos* germ, *pherein* to bear.]

blastophthoria (blas·tof·thor·e·ah). A breaking-down of the germ cells which occurs in toxic conditions resulting from metal or drug poisoning or infective diseases such as syphilis. [Gk *blastos* germ, *phthora* corruption.]

blastophthoric (blas·tof·thor·ik). Referring to blastophthoria; destructive of germ cells.

blastophyllum (blas·to·fil·um). One of the primitive germ layers in the embryo. [Gk *blastos* germ, *phyllon* leaf.]

blastophyly (blas·tof·il·e). The history of an individual organism in its relation to the tribe. [Gk *blastos* germ, *phyle* tribe.]

blastopore (blas·to·por). In embryology, the orifice in the ovum through which the archenteron of the gastrula communicates with the exterior. [Gk *blastos* germ, *poros* passage.]

blastosphere (blas·to·sfeer). Blastula. [Gk *blastos* germ, *sphaira* ball.]

blastospore (blas·to·spor). In botany, a spore formed by the budding process as in yeasts. [Gk *blastos* germ, *sporos* seed.]

blastostroma (blas·to·stro·mah). Those cellular constituents of the ovum which are active in forming the blastoderm. [Gk *blastos* germ, *stroma* a covering.]

blastotomy (blas·tot·om·e). Blastomerotomy; the splitting up or destruction of a blastomere. [Gk *blastos* germ, *temnein* to cut.]

blastotoxy (blas·to·tox·e). A condition of toxicity of the germ-cell protoplasm. [Gk *blastos* germ, *toxikon* poison.]

blastula (blas·tew·lah). An early form of embryo found in many animals, in the form of a fluid-filled cavity surrounded by a single layer of cells within the morula; this stage precedes that of the development of the gastrula. **Sperm blastula.** A globe-shaped blastula, the surface of which is a sperm blastoderm. [Gk *blastos* germ.]

blastular (blas·tew·lar). Belonging to the blastula.

blastulation (blas·tew·la·shun). In embryology, the process of formation of the blastula or blastocyst.

Blatella (blat·el·ah). A genus of cockroaches. **Blatella germanica.** The German cockroach, steam fly or croton bug (USA), a small pale species; it is a common household pest and secondary host of the tapeworm *Hymenolepis diminuta.* [L *blatta* an insect of dark places.]

Blatta (blat·ah). A genus of cockroaches. **Blatta orientalis.** The common cockroach or black beetle, which is a commensal of man throughout the world. [see prec.]

Blaud, Pierre (b. 1774). Beaucaire physician.

Blaud's pill. A pill of ferrous carbonate, formerly used in anaemia but now replaced by ferrous sulphate tablets.

Blaxland's test. A method of distinguishing between ascites and a large ovarian cyst. A flat ruler is laid across the abdomen just above the level of the superior iliac spines and pressed firmly backwards. In ovarian cysts the pulsation of the abdominal aorta can be felt.

blaze (blaze). A current of electricity which passes through mechanically-stimulated living tissue. [Obsolete term.] [ME *blase* torch.]

bleb (bleb). A blister or bulla, usually filled with a serous fluid. [Dial. E.]

bleeder (bleed·er). 1. A haemophiliac. 2. Any individual in whom slight cuts and abrasions give rise to profuse bleeding which may be uncontrollable. [ME *blod* blood.]

bleeding (bleed·ing). 1. Venesection. 2. The emitting or flowing of blood. **Functional bleeding.** A flow of blood from the vagina not caused by any organic lesion. **Midcyclical bleeding.** Uterine bleeding, usually slight, occurring at the time of ovulation, sometimes associated with abdominal pain. **Occult bleeding.** A term usually applied to haemorrhage from the bowel, the result of active peptic ulceration but of such small amount that the presence of blood can be established only by use of an instrument such as the microscope or by chemical test; such tests are used extensively as a guide to prognosis. [see prec.]

blemmatrope (blem·at·rope). An apparatus with which all the positions the eye may assume in its orbit may be seen. [Gk *blemma* glance, *tropein* to turn.]

blenna (blen·ah). Mucus. **Blenna narium.** Nasal mucus. [Gk.]

blennadenitis (blen·ad·en·i′·tis). A condition of inflammation of glandular mucosa and follicles. [Gk *blenna* mucus, *aden* gland, *-itis* inflammation.]

blennemesis (blen·em·es·is). Vomiting of mucus. [Gk *blenna* mucus, *emeein* to vomit.]

blennogenic, blennogenous (blen·o·jen·ik, blen·oj·en·us). Giving rise to or producing mucus. [Gk *blenna* mucus, *genein* to produce.]

blennoid (blen·oid). Resembling mucus; mucoid. [Gk *blenna* mucus, *eidos* form.]

blennophthalmia (blen·of·thal·me·ah). 1. Conjunctivitis of catarrhal origin. 2. Gonorrhoeal ophthalmia. [Gk *blenna* mucous, *ophthalmos* eye.]

blennorrhagia (blen·o·ra·je·ah). 1. Gonorrhoea. 2. Profuse blennorrhoea. [Gk *blenna* mucus, *rhegnynai* to burst forth.]

blennorrhagic (blen·o·ra·jik). Referring to blennorrhagia.

blennorrhoea (blen·o·re·ah). 1. Abnormally free secretion and discharge of mucus. 2. Gonorrhoea; a gonorrhoeal discharge from vagina or urethra. **Blenorrhoea adultorum.** Gonococcal or non-specific conjunctivitis (ophthalmia). **Inclusion blennorrhoea.** A condition of inflammation affecting the cervix, urethra or conjunctiva, in the discharge from which large basophilic inclusion bodies are found; the cause is a filtrable virus. **Blenorrhoea neonatorum.** Gonoccocal or non-specific conjunctivitis of the newborn (ophthalmia neonatorum). [Gk *blenna* mucus, *rhoia* flow.]

See also: STOERK.

blennorrhoeal (blen·o·re·al). Referring to blennorrhoea.

blennostasis (blen·os·tas·is). Suppression or diminution of excessive or abnormal secretion from the mucous membranes. [Gk *blenna* mucus, *stasis* a standing still.]

blennostatic (blen·o·stat·ik). 1. Referring to blennostasis. 2. Any remedy used in the achieving of blennostasis.

blennothorax (blen·o·thor·ax). Any condition in which there is a catarrh of the lungs, generally with excess of mucus lodged in tubes or alveoli or both. [Gk *blenna* mucus, thorax.]

blennotorrhoea (blen·o·to·re'·ah). Discharge of mucus from the ear. [Gk *blenna* mucus, *ous* ear, *rhoia* flow.]

blennuria (blen·ewr·e·ah). A condition in which mucus is present in the urine. [Gk *blenna* mucus, urine.]

Bleomycin (ble·o·mi·sin). BP Commission approved name for an antibiotic produced by *Streptomyces verticillus*; an antineoplastic agent.

blepharadenitis (blef·ar·ad·en·i'·tis). A state of inflammation of the tarsal glands of the eyelids. [Gk *blepharon* eyelid, *aden* gland, *-itis* inflammation.]

blepharal (blef·ar·al). Belonging to the eyelids, or involving them. [Gk *blepharon* eyelid.]

blepharectomy (blef·ar·ek·to·me). The surgical excision of a lesion of the eyelid. [Gk *blepharon* eyelid, *ektome* a cutting out.]

blepharelosis (blef·ar·el·o'·sis). Entropion. [Gk *blepharon* eyelid, *eilein* to roll, *-osis* condition.]

blepharism (blef·ar·izm). Spasm of the eyelids producing the effect of continuous winking. [Gk *blepharizein* to wink.]

blepharitic (blef·ar·it·ik). Pertaining to blepharitis.

blepharitis (blef·ar·i·tis). Inflammation of the eyelids. **Blepharitis acarica.** Marginal blepharitis associated with the presence of *Demodex folliculorum* in the region of the eyelashes. **Angular blepharitis.** Ulcerative blepharitis affecting the skin bordering the outer and inner canthi. **Ciliary blepharitis.** Marginal blepharitis (see below). **Gangrenous blepharitis.** An infection so severe as to produce gangrene of the lids, or primary gangrene may occur from some other cause and secondary infection supervene. **Glandular blepharitis.** A form of blepharitis originating in the glands of the lids (sebaceous glands—Zeis's glands, sweat—Moll's glands, or the large modified sebaceous glands—the meibomian glands). **Hypertrophic blepharitis.** Tylosis, 3rd def. **Internal blepharitis.** Inflammation affecting the conjunctiva lining the lids. **Marginal blepharitis.** A chronic inflammation of the margins of the eyelids and of the sebaceous glands and hair follicles. **Phlegmonous blepharitis.** Cellulitis of the eyelids. **Scrofulous blepharitis, Simple blepharitis.** Slight inflammation of the margins of the eyelids with associated viscid crusts on the ciliary edges and consequent gluing together of the lids. **Squamous blepharitis.** Marginal blepharitis (see above) giving rise to scales on the edges of the lids; probably a form of seborrhoea. **Sycotic blepharitis.** Sycosis palpabrae marginalis. **Ulcerative blepharitis.** Inflammation and ulceration of the eyelids at their margins. [Gk *blepharon* eyelid, *-itis* inflammation.]

blepharo-adenoma (blef·ar·o·ad·en·o'·mah). Adenoma of the eyelid. [Gk *blepharon* eyelid, adenoma.]

blepharo-atheroma (blef·ar·o·ath·er·o'·mah). Sebaceous cyst of the eyelids. [Gk *blepharon* eyelid, atheroma.]

blepharoblennorrhoea (blef·ar·o·blen·o·re'·ah). Purulent ophthalmia. *See* OPHTHALMIA. [Gk *blepharon* eyelid, blennorrhoea.]

blepharochalasis (blef·ar·o·kal'·as·is). A condition of relaxation of the skin and subcutaneous tissues of the eyelid. A fold of skin prolapses, in some cases overlapping the tarsal margin when the eye is open. [Gk *blepharon* eyelid, *chalasis* a relaxing.]

blepharochromidrosis (blef·ar·o·kro·mid·ro'·sis). The excretion of a coloured sweat, usually bluish, from the eyelids. [Gk *blepharon* eyelid, *chroma* colour, *hidros* sweat.]

blepharocleisis (blef·ar·o·kli'·sis). 1. Ankyloblepharon. 2. An abnormal state of closure of the eyelids. [Gk *blepharon* eyelid, *kleiein* to shut up.]

blepharoclonus (blef·ar·o·klo'·nus). Clonic muscular spasm of the eyelids. [Gk *blepharon* eyelid, *klonos* tumult.]

blepharocoloboma (blef·ar·o·kol·o·bo'·mah). Coloboma palpebrale. [Gk *blepharon* eyelid, coloboma.]

blepharoconjunctivitis (blef·ar·o·kon·jungk·tiv·i'·tis). A condition of inflammation of the eyelids and the conjunctiva. [Gk *blepharon* eyelid, conjunctivitis.]

blepharodiastasis (blef·ar·o·di·as'·tas·is). 1. Abnormally wide separation of the eyelids when the eyes are open. 2. Inability to close the eyelids completely. [Gk *blenopharon* eyelid, *diastasis* separation.]

blepharodyschroia (blef·ar·o·dis·kroi'·ah). A discoloured state of the eyelids from any cause, e.g. naevus. [Gk *blepharon* eyelid, *dys, chroa* colour.]

blepharoedema (blef·ar·e·de'·mah). Oedema of the eyelids. [Gk *blepharon* eyelid, *oidema* a swelling.]

blepharomelasma (blef·ar·o·mel·az'·mah). The occurrence of a dark-coloured secretion on the eyelids. [Gk *blepharon* eyelid, *melas* black.]

blepharon (blef·ar·on). The eyelid. [Gk.]

blepharoncus (blef·ar·ong·kus). A neoplasm of the eyelid. [Gk *blepharon* eyelid, *ogkos* tumour.]

blepharopachynsis (blef·ar·o·pak·in'·sis). Thickening of the eyelid due to disease. [Gk *blepharon* eyelid, *pachynsis* a thickening.]

blepharophimosis (blef·ar·o·fi·mo'·sis). Abnormal reduction of the palpebral fissure. **Congenital blepharophimosis.** A general diminution of the palpebral fissure; a rare developmental anomaly. **Familial blepharophimosis.** Autosomal dominant ptosis with laterally displaced and inverted medial canthi. [Gk *blepharon* eyelid, *phimosis* a closure.]

blepharophryplasty (blef·ar·of·re·plas·te). The reforming or restoration of eyebrow and eyelid by plastic surgery. [Gk *blepharon* eyelid, *ophrys* eyebrow, *plassein* to mould.]

blepharophthalmia (blef·ar·of·thal'·me·ah). Inflammation of the conjunctiva of the eyeball and the eyelid. [Gk *blepharon* eyelid, ophthalmia.]

blepharoplast (blef·ar·o·plast). An organelle in flagellate protozoa from which the flagellum arises. [see foll.]

blepharoplasty (blef·ar·o·plas·te). A plastic operation for the reforming or restoration of an eyelid or any part of it. **Marginal blepharoplasty.** Plastic surgery involving the edge of an eyelid. [Gk *blepharon* eyelid, *plassein* to mould.]

See also: CELSUS, KNAPP.

blepharoplegia (blef·ar·o·ple'·je·ah). Paralysis affecting the eyelid and both muscles belonging to it. [Gk *blepharon* eyelid, *plege* stroke.]

blepharoptosis (blef·ar·op·to'·sis). The drooping of the upper eyelid consequent upon paralysis of the muscles or nerve. [Gk *blepharon* eyelid, *ptosis* fall.]

blepharopyorrhoea (blef·ar·o·pi·o·re'·ah). Purulent ophthalmia. *See* OPHTHALMIA. [Gk *blepharon* eyelid, pyorrhoea.]

blepharorrhaphy (blef·ar·or·af·e). Tarsorraphy. [Gk *blepharon* eyelid, *rhaphe* suture.]

blepharorrhoea (blef·ar·o·re'·ah). Copious discharge from the eyelids. [Gk *blepharon* eyelid, *rhoia* flow.]

blepharospasm (blef·ar·o·spazm). Tonic contraction of the eyelids, due either to some local lesion of the eye causing reflex spasm, to hysteria, or to some irritative neurological lesion. [Gk *blepharon* eyelid, spasm.]

blepharosphincterectomy (blef·ar·o·sfingk·ter·ek'·to·me). An ophthalmic operation performed in cases of blepharospasm:

when the pressure of the eyelid on the cornea is excessive, certain fibres of the orbicularis oculi muscle are excised together with the associated skin. [Gk *blepharon* eyelid, sphincter, Gk *ektome* excision.]

blepharostat (blef·ar·o·stat). An instrument used in eye surgery for the purpose of holding the eyelids open. [Gk *blepharon* eyelid, *statikos* a standing still.]

blepharostenosis (blef·ar·o·sten·o′·sis). Blepharophimosis. [Gk *blepharon* eyelid, *stenosis* a narrowing.]

blepharosynechia (blef·ar·o·sin·e′·ke·ah). Permanent adhesion of the upper to the lower eyelid. [Gk *blepharon* eyelid, *synecheia* a holding together.]

blepharotomy (blef·ar·ot·o·me). Incision of an eyelid. [Gk *blepharon* eyelid, *temnein* to cut.]

blepsopathia, blepsopathy (bleps·o·path·e·ah, bleps·op·ath·e). A neurasthenic condition caused by prolonged eyestrain. [Gk *blepsis* sight, *pathos* suffering.]

Blessig, Robert (b. 1830). Russian ophthalmologist.

Blessig's cysts, or spaces. Cystic spaces appearing at the extreme periphery of the retina in early adult life and increasing in number with age. Also known as *Iwanoff's retinal oedema,* or *cystoid degeneration.*

Blessig's groove. A groove in the interior of the embryonic optic cup marking the anterior margin of the future retina.

Blighia sapida (bli·e·ah sap·i·dah). The ackee tree.

blight (blite). 1. A slight paralysis of some of the facial nerves caused by sudden exposure to cold or exposure to extreme cold. 2. Any disease of plants due to the presence of a fungus. **Blight of the eye.** Escape of blood into the conjunctiva. **Sandy blight.** Severe inflammation of the eye with associated photophobia and the accumulation of pus in the tarsal glands, which causes a sensation of grit in the eye. [etym. dub.]

blind-gut (bli·nd·gut). The caecum. [AS *blind, guttas.*]

blindness (bli·nd·nes). 1. Absence of sight; loss of vision due to a variety of causes. 2. The word is sometimes applied figuratively to imply want of intellectual or moral perception. Certain types of blindness, e.g. intellectual blindness, letter blindness, mental blindness, are varieties of symptoms met with in aphasic cases, sensory or motor, and the result of various brain lesions. *See* APHASIA. **Amnesic colour blindness.** Inability to name colours, although they can be seen and recognized; always accompanied by homonymous (usually right) hemianopia, and probably due to an occipital-lobe lesion. **Apperceptive blindness.** Inability to distinguish an object by sight although it is clearly seen, occurring in cases of senile dementia. **Blue blindness.** A rare form of colour blindness in which there is inability to distinguish blue; tritanopia. **Cerebral blindness.** Blindness of cerebral origin; the term covers cortical blindness and hysterical blindness. **Colour blindness.** 1. Congenital: classified according to the trichromatic theory of vision and subdivided into anomalies of colour perception, and blindness to certain colours. The anomalies which occur in the trichromats are called: (*a*) protanomaly, or abnormal perception of red; (*b*) deuteranomaly, or abnormal perception of green; (*c*) tritanomaly, or abnormal perception of blue. Dichromats are: (*a*) protanopes who are blind to red; (*b*) deuteranopes who are blind to green; (*c*) tritanopes who are blind to blue. Monochromats are unable to discriminate colours as such and the world is seen in shades of grey. 2. Acquired: caused by disease, trauma (e.g. snow blindness) or toxins (e.g. tobacco amblyopia), and gives rise to disordered perceptions of colour. **Concussion blindness.** Loss of sight following concussion of the globe, usually associated with oedema of the central part of the retina (Berlin's oedema) and capable of complete recovery in some cases. Also applied to hysterical amaurosis occurring after injury. **Cortical blindness.** That due to a lesion in the cortex of the brain, affecting that part which is associated with vision. **Cortical psychic blindness.** That which occurs in lesions of the occipital lobe, characterized by spatial disorientation and loss of memory of images. **Day blindness.** Hemeralopia, i.e. reduced visual efficiency under high illumination. **Eclipse blindness.** Blindness caused by viewing a partial eclipse of the sun without adequate protective glasses, which produces a burn in the macula. **Economic blindness.** Lack of sight sufficient to debar the patient from work for which sight is essential. **Educational blindness.** Insufficient sight to allow of the patient being educated by methods depending on vision. **Electric-light blindness.** Photo-ophthalmia, snow blindness, Klieg eye, glare asthenopia; the result of exposure to ultra-violet rays, e.g. from an unshaded arc lamp. No permanent damage results, but the symptoms, usually coming on after a latent period of a few hours, may be severe and comprise photophobia, blepharospasm, burning pain, redness of the eye and swelling of the conjunctiva. A minor degree of snow blindness is characterized by erythropia. **Flight blindness.** That which occurs during sudden turns in a fast-moving aeroplane when, owing to centripetal force, an insufficient amount of blood reaches the eyes or brain. **Functional blindness.** Hysterical blindness (see below). **Green blindness.** Defective perception of green; deuteranopia. **Homolateral blindness.** Blindness on the side of the lesion. **Hysterical blindness.** Blindness produced by hysteria, the eyes and nerves being intact. **Lactation blindness.** Loss of sight usually developing about the seventh week of lactation. Rapid improvement is the rule. **Letter blindness.** A condition in which the individual letters can be distinguished but are without meaning. **Mind blindness.** Failure to recognize objects. **Monocular blindness.** Blindness in one eye. **Moon blindness.** A term applied to periodic ophthalmia occurring most commonly in horses but sometimes affecting other animals. It is a severe form of iridocyclitis of doubtful aetiology, with a marked tendency to recurrence which may be monthly, hence the term "moon". **Nervous blindness.** Amaurosis. **Night blindness.** A disturbance of vision in which the individual cannot see as well at night or in a dim light as during daylight; it may be due to a deficiency of vitamin A, but is more commonly seen in diseases destroying the peripheral parts of the retina, e.g. retinitis pigmentosa or pigmentary degeneration of the retina. **Note blindness.** Failure to recognize musical notation. **Object blindness.** Mind blindness (see above). **Psychic blindness.** Sight without recognition. **Red blindness.** Defective perception of red; protanopia. **Red-green blindness.** The commonest form of colour blindness, in which red and green are distinguished imperfectly or not at all. **River blindness.** Onchocerciasis. **Snow blindness.** Weakness of vision with conjunctivitis and photophobia, which are normally temporary conditions only, caused by exposing the eyes to the glare of the sun on snow. **Space blindness.** Visual agnosia; inability to appreciate the positions of objects. **Syllabic blindness.** Inability to form syllables. **Total blindness.** Inability to perceive light. **Twilight blindness.** A stage of night blindness (see above) due to defective dark adaptation. **Vocational blindness.** Loss of sight sufficient to prevent the patient from following his normal occupation. **Word blindness.** Dyslexia. **Yellow blindness.** Tritanopia, a rare form of colour blindness. [AS *blind.*]

See also: BRIGHT.

blister (blis·ter). 1. A vesicle occurring between the epidermis and the corium; the fluid it contains is serous. 2. Any agent which induces the formation of a blister. **Ambulant blister.** One which alters its situation. **Blood blister.** A vesicle filled with blood; these blisters may be the result of long-continued friction or of bruising. **Fever blister.** Herpes labialis. **Fly blister.** The vesicle raised by the application of cantharides to the skin, or as a result of contact with a vesicating fly or other flying arthropod. **Flying blister.** A blistering agent applied to the skin for a length of time sufficient only to redden it without producing vesication. **Pus blister.** One in which the serous contents have become infected. **Water blister.** A vesicle containing watery serous fluid; a semi-popular term. [Old Norse *blästr.*]

See also: MAROCHETTI.

blistering (blis·ter·ing). The forming of a vesicle between the epidermis and the corium. [see prec.]

Bloch, Bruno (b. 1878). Swiss dermatologist.

Jadassohn–Bloch test. *See* PATCH TEST (under TEST).

block (blok). 1. A stoppage. 2. Obstruction to the passage of a nervous impulse either from one neurone to another, as in ganglia, or from a nerve-ending to an effector organ. It may result from a number of causes, e.g. fatigue, or as the outcome of the administration of drugs. 3. In dentistry, a mass of material. 4. To block, *see* present participle BLOCKING. **Air block.** Interstitial emphysema of the lungs causing interference with their expansion during inspiration. **Alpha block.** Block of alpha-adrenergic sympathetic receptors. **Analgesic block.** The interruption of nervous conduction, (*a*) by the introduction of an analgesic solution in or around a nerve, or (*b*) by new growth or other pathological lesion. **Ankle block.** Block of nerves supplying the skin and muscles of the foot by the injection of a local analgesic solution near the ankle. **Arborization block.** Term used to denote light or moderate degrees of conduction defect in the finer ramifications of the bundle branches. (*See* main entry HEART BLOCK.) **Atrioventricular block.** Impairment of conduction between auricles and ventricles. (*See* main entry HEART BLOCK.) **Axillary block.** A method of blocking the brachial plexus with a solution of local analgesic injected from the axilla. **Beta block.** Block of the beta-adrenergic sympathetic receptors. **Biphasic block.** The type of myoneural block which results from the injection of large doses of depolarizing muscle relaxants, when a non-depolarizing type of block eventually appears. **Bite block.** A rim of wax or other suitable material mounted on a baseplate to form a bite plate. **Bundle-branch block.** Interference with conduction down one or other of the main divisions of the bundle of His. (*See* main entry HEART BLOCK.) **Cerebrospinal-fluid block.** Interruption of normal circulation of cerebrospinal fluid. **Cervical nerve block.** Block of cervical nerves by local analgesic solution. **Cervicothoracic sympathetic block.** Block of the cervical, stellate and upper thoracic sympathetic ganglia by local analgesic solution. **Comparator block.** A simple instrument designed for the visual comparison of coloured solutions. It consists of a block holding test tubes, and a row of horizontal holes through which the tubes may be viewed in section; used largely for determining the pH of tinted solutions, e.g. bacteriological media. **Costo-iliac block.** Block by local analgesic solution of the lower thoracic nerves between the 11th and 12th ribs and the iliac crest. **Desensitization block.** A type of non-depolarizing myoneural block which may be produced by the injection of large or repeated doses of a depolarizing relaxant. Also known as *dual* or *biphasic block*. **Digital-nerve block.** Block of the digital nerves by local analgesic solution. **Dynamic block.** An obstruction in the spinal subarachnoid space. *See* SUBARACHNOID BLOCK (below). **Ear block.** Otic barotrauma. *See* BAROTRAUMA. **Epidural block.** Analgesia produced by injecting an analgesic solution into the space between the vertebral canal and the dura mater. **Extradural block.** Injection of a local analgesic solution into the lumbar or sacral extradural space, to inhibit the reception of painful impulses and to produce motor paresis. **Field block.** The injection of local analgesic solution so as to create an area of analgesia around the operative field, e.g. in the anterior abdominal wall. **Ganglionic block.** Paralysis of nerve-impulse transmission across synapses of autonomic ganglia; usually deliberately produced by means of specific drugs, e.g. in the treatment of hypertension. **Heart block.** Depression of the specialized conducting tissue of the heart resulting in delay in or obstruction to the normal passage of the impulses through the heart. (*See* main entry HEART BLOCK.) **Iliac crest block.** Block, by local analgesic solution, of the 12th thoracic, iliohypogastric and ilio-inguinal nerves, near the anterior superior iliac spine. **Infra-orbital nerve block.** Block of the infra-orbital nerve near the infra-orbital foramen to produce local analgesia of the side of the nose, lower eyelid and upper lip. **Intercostal nerve block.** Injection of a local analgesic solution into the intercostal nerves to produce analgesia in the areas supplied by these nerves. **Intradural block.** Injection of a solution of a local analgesic into the intradural or subarachnoid space; spinal analgesia. **Intraventricular block.** A defect of intraventricular conduction due to ventricular hypertrophy, ischaemia or myocarditis. **Lumbar extradural block.** Injection of a solution of local analgesic into the extradural space. **Lumbar sympathetic nerve block.** Block of the ganglia of the lumbar paravertebral sympathetic chain with local analgesic solution. **Mandibular nerve block.** Injection of local analgesic solution near the 3rd division of the trigeminal nerve, on the inner aspect of the ramus of the mandible, to produce analgesia in all the teeth of the lower jaw except the central incisor. **Manometric block.** An obstruction to the free circulation of cerebrospinal fluid in the spinal canal as demonstrated by manometry. *See* QUECKENSTEDT'S TEST. **Maxillary nerve block.** Injection of local analgesic solution into the maxillary division of the trigeminal nerve in the pterygomaxillary fissure; useful for operations on the antrum, upper lip, palate, etc. **Median nerve block.** Injection of local analgesic solution into the median nerve at the elbow or wrist. **Mental nerve block.** Infiltration of local analgesic solution into the mental nerve as it emerges from the ramus of the mandible, to produce analgesia of the lower lip. **Mixed block.** The type of myoneural block resulting from the simultaneous injection of depolarizing and non-depolarizing muscle relaxants. **Myoneural block.** The state of muscle paralysis produced by depolarizing and non-depolarizing muscle relaxants. **Nerve block.** 1. The application or injection of a local analgesic solution into, or near, a nerve in order to make the parts it supplies unresponsive to pain stimuli and/or to remove muscular tone. **Neuromuscular block.** Paralysis of impulse transmission from motor nerve-endings to voluntary muscle fibres, usually without loss of excitability of either nerve or muscle. The condition is induced clinically by means of the so-called muscle relaxants, and is an aid to surgery. **Paracervical block.** Injection of local analgesic solution into the loose cellular tissue at the sides of the cervix uteri for the purpose of obtunding painful sensations in the early stages of labour. Of doubtful utility and safety because of its effect on the fetus. **Parasacral block.** Presacral block (see below). **Paravertebral block.** 1. *Somatic*—block of the spinal nerves by local analgesic solution, near their point of emergence from the intervertebral foramina. 2. *Sympathetic*—blocking of the paravertebral sympathetic chain (or its ganglia) as it lies anterolateral to the vertebral bodies. **Phase 2 block.** A state of non-depolarizing block which may develop in a motor end-plate following the injection of large or repeated doses of a depolarizing myoneural blocking agent. **Physiological branch block.** Pre-excitation syndrome. *See* SYNDROME. **Plexus block.** The anaesthetizing of part of the body by applying analgesic solutions to the plexus of nerves supplying that part; commonly *brachial-plexus block* whereby the arm is anaesthetized by injections at the base of the neck. **Portal block.** Obstruction of the portal vein. **Presacral block.** The injection of local analgesic solution into the region of the hollow of the sacrum so as to block the anterior roots of the sacral nerve. **Regional block.** Analgesia of a limited region produced by either field block or nerve block. **Retrograde block.** Blockage of conduction in a retrograde manner to the auricles in nodal rhythm in which the auriculo-ventricular node is acting as pacemaker. **Sacral-nerve block.** The injection of local analgesic solution into the sacral extradural space or near the nerves in the hollow of the sacrum. **Saddle block.** Intradural injection of local analgesic solution to block the 2nd, 3rd and 4th sacral nerves, and so to produce an area of analgesia corresponding to the saddle area; used in surgery and obstetrics. **Sciatic-nerve block.** Injection, near or into the sciatic nerve, of a local analgesic solution to remove the reception of pain impulses in the area of its distribution. **Sino-auricular block, Sinu-auricular block.** Missing of a beat at regular or irregular intervals by the whole heart. (*See* main entry HEART BLOCK.) **Sinus block.** Sinus barotrauma. *See* BAROTRAUMA. **Spinal block, Spinal-subarachnoid block.** Obstruction of the circulation of cerebrospinal fluid in the spinal canal; the former is the better term as the latter might be taken to include *epidural block*. **Splanchnic-nerve block.** The injection into the splanchnic (or coeliac) plexus of a solution of local analgesic drug, causing analgesia of the upper abdominal viscera. **Stellate ganglion**

block. The injection of a volume of local analgesic solution into the stellate ganglion and, sometimes, the upper thoracic ganglia. **Subarachnoid block.** 1. An obstruction to the free flow of cerebrospinal fluid within the subarachnoid space, either within the skull or in the spinal canal. 2. Block of spinal nerve roots by the intradural or subarachnoid injection of a local analgesic solution. **Supraclavicular brachial plexus block.** Injection of local analgesic solution into the trunks of the brachial plexus as they cross the superior surface of the 1st rib, to make the upper limb analgesic. **Sympathetic block.** Interruption of nervous impulses carried along sympathetic nerves by local analgesic or pharmacological agents. **Thoracic-nerve block.** Injection of local analgesic solution into the thoracic nerves just below the ribs to produce analgesia and muscular relaxation in their areas of distribution. **Tibial-nerve block.** The injection of local analgesic solution into, or near, the anterior or posterior tibial nerves. **Total spinal block.** A high intradural (subarachnoid) block designed to provide total blockade of the sympathetic vasomotor fibres; sometimes used by anaesthetists. **Trans-sacral block.** The method whereby local analgesic solution is injected into the posterior sacral foramena to block the posterior divisions of the sacral nerves. **Tubal block.** Blockage of the eustachian tube from any cause. **Ulnar-nerve block.** Injection of local analgesic solution into the ulnar nerve, either at the elbow or at the wrist. **Ventricular block.** Obstruction of the flow of cerebrospinal fluid by closure of the foramina of Magendie or Luschka, resulting in distension of the brain ventricles. **Block vertebra.** *See* VERTEBRA. **Wrist block.** The injection of local analgesic solution into the main nerves at the level of the wrist. [O Fr. *bloc.*]

See also: KOHS.

Block-Stenger test. For simulated unilateral deafness: the patient is blindfolded; a vibrating tuning fork is placed near the ear under test; hearing is usually denied by malingerers. A tuning fork of the same frequency is approximated closer and closer to the normal ear; a malingerer continues to deny that anything is heard.

blockade, blockage (**blok**·ade, **blok**·ij). Overloading of the reticulo-endothelial system by the intravenous injection of large amounts of Indian ink or other material with the object of engaging for phagocytosis as many cells as possible, and so rendering the reticulo-endothelial system functionally impaired, and less able to deal with a subsequent injection of antigenic material. Blockage is usually combined with splenectomy. **Beta blockade.** Pharmacological inhibition of the response of the beta receptors in organs supplied by the autonomic nervous system. **Cholinergic blockade.** Pharmacological inhibition of transmission of nerve impulses by acetyl choline, notably in autonomic ganglia. **Myoneural blockade.** The pharmacological prevention of conduction at the neuromuscular junction. **Virus blockade.** Virus interference; the action of one virus in establishing itself to the detriment of another. [OFr. *bloc.*]

blocking (**blok**·ing). 1. The inducing of temporary paralysis in the peripheral distribution of a nerve by the injecting of an analgesic solution, so that it infiltrates into a nerve trunk. 2. The process when a person's flow of thought is brought to a stop without a cause apparent either to the observer or to the person. 3. In clinical pathology, the fixing of a specimen embedded in celloidin or other substance to a piece of material such as wood so that it may be held in the microtome. **Adrenergic blocking agent.** α-Adrenergic blocking agents are phentolamine and piperoxan. β-Anadrenergic blocking agent is, for example, propanolol. **Blocking of thought.** A condition in which the patient cannot get beyond a certain point in a process of thought because there seems to be an "obstruction", with the result that he is unable to give clear expression to his ideas. [see prec.]

Blocq, Paul Oscar (b. 1860). Paris physician.

Blocq's disease. Astasia abasia; hysterical inability to walk or stand.

Blondlot, Prosper René (b. 1849). French physicist.

Blondlot's rays. A form of radiation said to be of shorter wavelength than light rays and to have the property of rendering bodies luminous; they are also said to have the effect of diminishing luminosity. They may also be given off from magnetic fields and luminous bodies, but their existence has not been fully established.

blood [sanguis (NA)] (blud). The fluid medium that circulates through the vascular system. It consists of a liquid portion, or plasma, in which are suspended the various red and white blood cells and platelets; dissolved in it are salts of different kinds, organic substances, hormones, vitamins, products of anabolism and catabolism, antibodies and enzymes. It is the means whereby oxygen, as haemoglobin, is transported from the lungs to all the tissues, and carbon dioxide removed therefrom. Other products of the body's metabolic processes are also transported in this medium. Complex mechanisms normally maintain its fluidity, hydrogen-ion concentration (pH value) and normal range of constituents, in the intact vascular system. **Banked blood.** Blood that has been collected from donors and stored, after the addition of a suitable anticoagulant, in a refrigerator at 4°C until required for transfusion purposes. **Citrated blood.** Whole blood treated with citrate or citric acid mixtures to prevent coagulation. **Cord blood.** The blood present in and extractable from the umbilical cord. **Defibrinated blood.** Whole blood from which the fibrin has been removed extravascularly. **Laked blood.** Blood that has been diluted or treated with water, alkali or other agent, to cause destruction of the red cells, thereby liberating the haemoglobin. **Occult blood.** Usually refers to the presence of blood in the faeces, due to haemorrhage from the alimentary tract and mucous membrane, in quantity insufficient to be obvious macroscopically but readily detected by appropriate chemical or microscopical tests. **Oxalated blood.** Whole blood treated with oxalate or an oxalate mixture to prevent coagulation. **Sludged blood.** A condition in which the blood cells mass together in the smaller blood vessels, slowing the blood flow and thus forming a kind of sludge. **Strawberry-cream blood.** Describing the appearance of blood taken from a lipaemic patient; it is due to the excessive quantity of fat in the blood. **Whole blood.** The natural blood as circulating in the vascular system, containing all its normal cellular and chemical constituents. **Whole Human Blood BP 1973.** Blood which has been mixed with a suitable anticoagulant. [AS *blod.*]

blood-chlorides (blud·**klor**·ides). 1. The chlorides in the blood. 2. The concentration of chlorides in blood, expressed as sodium chloride or sometimes as chlorine. Chief significance attaches to the plasma chlorides, the concentration of which is normally from 96 to 106 mmol/l (560 to 620 mg per 100 ml) plasma, as NaCl. Plasma chlorides may be decreased in conditions where there is severe vomiting or diarrhoea, in intestinal obstruction, pneumonia and Addison's disease. [AS *blod,* chloride.]

blood donor (blud **do**·nor). One who gives blood for therapeutic purposes. *See* DONOR. [AS *blod,* L *donare* to give.]

blood group (blud groop). *See* GROUP. [AS *blod,* Fr. *groupe.*]

blood-letting (blud·**let**·ing). In therapeutics, the act of bleeding, e.g. by the opening of an artery or vein. **General blood-letting.** The allowing of blood to escape by the process of venesection. **Local blood-letting, Topical blood-letting.** The withdrawal of blood from a particular area by means of leeches, or by scarification or cupping. [AS *blod, laetan.*]

blood picture (blud **pik**·tcher). Generally, the full blood and differential leucocyte counts of an individual; more specifically, the counts as obtained by the Arneth or similar techniques. [AS *blod,* L *pictura.*]

blood pressure (blud **presh**·er). The pressure of the column of circulating blood within the vascular system. **Arterial blood pressure.** The pressure of the column of blood in the arterial system. It depends upon the pumping action of the heart, the peripheral resistance, the amount of blood in the system, the viscosity of the blood and the elasticity of the arterial walls. **Capillary blood pressure.** The pressure of the blood in the capillary area of the vascular system. **Casual blood pressure.** A reading of arterial blood pressure taken at random. **Diastolic**

blood pressure. The minimal arterial pressure, coinciding with ventricular diastole and resulting from the resistance of the arterial walls. **Mean blood pressure.** The average arterial pressure throughout the cardiac cycle; often stated as the arithmetic mean of the systolic and diastolic pressures, though the geometric mean is more accurate. **Resting blood pressure.** A reading of arterial blood pressure taken with the subject at rest and under basal conditions. **Systolic blood pressure.** The maximal arterial pressure, corresponding to the contraction of the ventricle. **Venous blood pressure.** The pressure of the circulating blood within the venous system: *central venous blood pressure* is the pressure in the great veins and right auricle; *peripheral venous blood pressure* is the pressure in the peripheral veins and is normally higher than the central. *Effective venous blood pressure* is the sum of the positive pressure in the venous system and the suction pressure exerted by the thorax tending to draw blood into the heart. [AS *blod*, L *premere* to press.]

blood shunting (blud shunt·ing). A condition occurring in some forms of congenital heart disease when the blood is short-circuited from the right to the left side of the heart without passing through the lungs, as in pulmonary stenosis with patent interventricular septum or in patent ductus arteriosus. [AS *blod*, ME *shunten.*]

blood substitute (blud sub·stit·ewt). Any substance used for transfusion in the place of blood. [AS *blod*, L *substitutio.*]

blood-urea (blud·ewr·e′·ah). 1. The urea in the blood. 2. The concentration of urea in the blood. This is normally from 2.5 to 7.5 mmol/l (15 to 45 mg per 100 ml) blood. In chronic or acute nephritis the concentration may be increased to very high values, especially in the terminal stages. It may also be raised in conditions such as intestinal obstruction, enlarged prostate and cardiac failure, where renal function is impaired.

Bloodgood, Joseph Colt (b. 1867). Baltimore surgeon.

Bloodgood's operation. Repair of direct inguinal hernia by a triangular flap of anterior rectus sheath hinged on its outer border and turned down to be stitched to the inguinal ligaments.

bloodless (blud·les). 1. Term applied to any part that is actually or apparently destitute of blood. 2. Anaemic. 3. Attended with little loss of blood or no loss at all. [AS *blod.*]

bloodroot (blud·root). Sanguinaria, the dried rhizome of *Sanguinaria canadensis* Linn. (family Papaveraceae). It contains alkaloids of the isoquinoline group (chiefly sanguinarine and chelerythrine), and a red resin. It is used in the form of a tincture as an expectorant in asthma and bronchitis, and in atonic dyspepsia. [AS *blod*, *root.*]

bloodshot (blud·shot). Suffused or congested with blood; term applied to the eyes. [AS *blod*, *sceotan* to shoot.]

bloody (blud·e). 1. Containing blood. 2. Resembling or of the nature of blood. 3. Attended with loss of blood.

Bloor, Walter Ray (b. 1877). Rochester, New York, biochemist.

Bloor's method. For cholesterol. *See* SACKETT'S METHOD.

Bloor, Pelkan and Allen's method. For cholesterol in blood: the blood is treated with alcohol-ether to precipitate proteins and extract the cholesterol. The filtrate is evaporated, the residue is dissolved in chloroform, and the cholesterol determined by the Liebermann–Burchard reaction.

Blot, Claude Philbert Hippolyte (b. 1822). French obstetrician.

Blot's perforator. A pointed instrument used in craniotomy; the fetal skull is pierced and then cut by opening the blades.

blotch (bloch). 1. An area of discoloration on the skin. 2. An eruption of coarse pustules. 3. A large pustule or blister. **Palpebral blotch.** Pinguecula. [etym. dub.]

Blount, Walter Putnam (b. 1900). American orthopaedic surgeon.

Blount's disease. Tibia vara causing genu varum because the upper medial part of the tibia grows too slowly.

blow flies (blo flize). Household flies, particularly of the genus *Calliphora*, whose larvae feed on decaying meat. [AS *blawan*, *flyge.*]

blue (bloo). A colour lying in the visible spectrum between green and violet, with a wavelength about 450 nm (4500 Å). **Afridol blue.** A sulphonated azo dye closely related to trypan blue and used similarly at one time as a trypanocide. **Alizarin blue.** $C_6H_4(CO)_2C_6(OH)_2{=}C_3H_3N$, a blue dye derived from anthraquinone. It can be employed as a pH indicator over the range 9–13, the colour change being brown-green-violet. **Alkali blue.** A triphenylmethane dye, the sodium salt of the monosulphonic acid of aniline blue. **Aniline blue.** Triphenylfuchsine hydrochloride, $C_6H_5NH{=}C_6H_4{=}C(C_6H_4NHC_6H_5)_2Cl$, a triphenylmethane dye slightly soluble in water, soluble in alcohol. Water-soluble forms which consist of the sodium salts of the sulphonic acids, singly or in mixture, are more commonly used (alkali blue, water blue). **Azidine blue 3B.** Trypan blue (see below). **Azovan Blue BP 1958.** Tetra-sodium salt of 4,4′-bis[7-(1-amino-8-hydroxy-2,4-disulpho)naphthylazo]-3,3′-bitolyl; Evans' blue. A non-toxic dye used in estimating total blood and plasma volumes. **Benzamine blue 3B.** Trypan blue (see below). **Benzo blue.** Trypan blue (see below). **Brilliant blue C.** Brilliant cresyl blue (see following). **Brilliant cresyl blue.** An oxazine dye used in the staining of reticulocytes and platelets. **Bromphenol blue.** Tetrabromophenolsulphonephthalein, an indicator used for the measurement of pH over the range 2.8 (yellow) to 4.6 (blue-violet). **Bromthymol blue.** Dibromothymolsulphonephthalein, an indicator used for the measurement of pH over the range 6.0 (yellow) to 7.6 (blue). **Chlorazol blue 3B.** Trypan blue (see below). **Congo blue 3B.** Trypan blue (see below). **Cresyl blue 2RN or BBS.** Brilliant cresyl blue (see above). **Diamine blue.** A sulphonated azo dye derived from benzidine and related to trypan blue. It was used as a trypanocide. **Dianil blue H 3G.** Trypan blue (see below). **Helvetia blue.** Methyl blue (see below). **Indigo blue.** Indigotin, a blue vegetable dye occurring as the glucoside indican in the *Indigoferae* and in woad. It is now mostly obtained synthetically. **Indonaphthol blue.** Indophenol blue (see following). **Indophenol blue.** An amino derivative of naphthylquinone-imine, also known as α-naphthol blue. **Isamine blue.** A triphenylmethane dye, closely related to alkali blue and used in vital staining. **Leucomethylene blue.** A colourless reduced form of methylene blue produced when the latter is employed as a hydrogen acceptor. It is the formation of this compound that renders methylene blue useful as an oxidation-reduction indicator. **Medicinal methylene blue.** Methylene blue which has been freed of zinc, as with the commercial compound, and is less toxic. **Methyl blue.** A phenylated rosaniline dye used as a counterstain in histology, and in bacteriology. It is also an indicator of pH range 10.5–11,0. **Methylene Blue BP 1973.** Tetramethylthionine chloride dihydrate, $C_{16}H_{18}ClN_3S{\cdot}2H_2O$ (not to be confused with commercial methylene blue). A bacteriological staining reagent formerly used as a mild urinary antiseptic and in a renal function test. Now employed in the treatment of drug-induced methaemoglobinaemia. **Methylene blue NN.** New methylene blue N (see below). **Methylene blue O.** Toluidine blue O (see below). **Naphthamine blue 3BX.** Trypan blue (see below). **New methylene blue N.** 1,9-dimethyl-2,8-diethylamino-thiazonium chloride, $N(C_2H_5)HC_6H_2(CH_3)(NS)C_6H_2(CH_3)N(C_2H_5)HCl$, a dye employed like methylene blue. **Niagara blue 3B.** Trypan blue (see below). **Nile blue A, Nile blue sulphate.** An oxazine dye prepared from nitrosodiethyl-*m*-aminophenol and α-naphthylamine. It is used as a fat stain in histology and also for the vital staining of embryos. It is an oxidation-reduction and pH indicator (7.0–8.0). **Polychrome methylene blue.** A mixture of methylene blue and a variety of oxidation products formed by allowing solutions of methylene blue to stand for some time, or, more rapidly, by heating with alkalis. It is used as a blood stain. **Prussian blue.** The deep blue compound formed when a solution of a ferric salt is added to a solution of potassium ferrocyanide. **Pyoktanin blue.** Methyl violet. *See* VIOLET. **Quinoline blue.** Cyanin. **Spirit blue.** Aniline blue (see above). **Sulphan Blue.** BP Commission approved name for the sodium salt of 4,4-di(diethylamino)-4,6-disulphotriphenylmethanol anhydride. **Swiss blue.** Methylene blue (see above).

Thymol blue. Thymosulphonephthalein, an indicator used for the measurement of pH over the ranges 1.2 (red) to 2.8 (yellow), and 8.0 (yellow) to 9.6 (blue). **Toluidine blue O.** A blue dye widely used as a nuclear stain, as a stain for Nissl substance of nerve cells and for the metachromatic staining of mucopolysaccharides. **Trypan Blue BPC 1954.** Sodium ditolyldisazo-bis-8-amino-naphthol-3,6-disulphonate, $(NaSO_3)_2C_{10}H_3(NH_2)(OH)N{=}NC_6H_3(CH_3)C_6H_3(CH_3)N{=}NC_{10}H_3(OH)(NH_2)(NaSO_3)_2$, a dye used chiefly in vital staining. While it has been suggested for the treatment of protozoal infections, it is not so employed in humans. **Victoria blue.** A fuchsine dye, $C_6H_5NHC_{10}H_6C[C_6H_4N(CH_3)_2]_2Cl$, prepared from tetramethyldiaminobenzophenone and phenyl-α-naphthylamine. It has certain bacteriostatic properties. **Water blue.** A term applied to soluble forms of aniline blue (see above). They consist of the sodium salts of the various sulphonic acids. [ME *blew.*]

See also: BONNEY, EVANS, KUEHNE (H.), LOEFFLER (F. A. J.), NISSL, SAHLI, TURNBULL.

blue bottle (bloo botl). A household fly, particularly of the genus *Calliphora,* whose larvae feed on decaying meat. [ME *blew,* OFr. *bouteille.*]

blue drum (bloo drum). A blue cast of the drum head, said to be due to the presence of the bulb of the jugular vein projecting into the tympanum. [ME *blew,* D *trom.*]

Bluemel's treatment. The treatment of morphine addiction by rest in bed, withholding the drug and drastic purgation.

Blum's syndrome. Increase of non-protein nitrogen with reduction of the chlorides in the blood.

Blumberg, Moritz (b. 1873). Berlin surgeon.

Blumberg's sign. Release sign. *See* SIGN.

Blumenau, Leonid Vasilyevich (b. 1862). Russian neurologist.

Blumenau's nucleus. The lateral part of the cuneate nucleus.

Blumenau's test. A form of patch test in which a drop of Koch's old tuberculin is dried on the skin of the forearm and covered with adhesive plaster. A positive reaction is indicated by a reddened swelling or collection of reddened papules.

Blumenbach, Johann Friedrich (b. 1752). Göttingen physiologist.

Blumenbach's clivus. The clivus of the sphenoid bone.

Blumenbach's plane. The plane on which a skull can be placed after the mandible has been removed.

Blumenbach's process. The uncinate process of the ethmoid bone.

Blumer, George Alder (b. 1857). San Francisco physician.

Blumer's shelf, or sign. The ridge of hard tissue felt per rectum and caused by metastases (usually transcoelomic, and commonly from a stomach cancer) in the peritoneum at the bottom of the rectovesical pouch or of the pouch of Douglas (recto-uterine).

blunt-hook (blunt·**huk**). A dissecting instrument used chiefly in embryotomy. [blunt, etym. dub., AS *hoc.*]

blush (blush). 1. An involuntary flow of colour to the face and neck owing to temporary stoppage of the action of local vasomotor nerves so that the capillaries become dilated with blood; sudden emotion is usually the cause. 2. To exhibit such reaction; hence *blushing.* [ME *blosche.*]

Blyth, Alexander Wynter (b. 1845). London public analyst.

Blyth's test. For the detection of lead in drinking water: on the addition of a 1 per cent alcoholic tincture of cochineal a white precipitate forms if lead is present.

Boari, Achille. 19th-20th century Italian surgeon.

Boari's operation. An operation for re-implantation of the ureter into the bladder using a flap from the anterior wall of the bladder as a substitute for the lower part of the ureter.

Boas, Ismar Isidor (b. 1858). Berlin gastro-enterologist.

Boas' algesimeter. An instrument by which sensitiveness over the epigastric region can be determined.

Boas' point. A tender spot to the left of the 12th thoracic vertebra observed in patients with gastric ulcer.

Boas' sign. The presence of lactic acid and large non-motile bacilli in cases of carcinoma of the stomach causing obstruction and dilatation; of historical interest only.

Boas' test-meal. A meal consisting of oatmeal gruel without salt or milk, but with the addition of sugar if so desired. It is used to test the secretory function of the stomach.

bacillus of Boas-Oppler, lactobacillus of Boas-Oppler. A species observed by Oppler in the stomach contents in gastric cancer: not cultivated and therefore not properly identified; of historical interest only. It is generally believed to be identical with *Lactobacillus acidophilus.*

Bobbs, John Stough (b. 1809). Indianapolis surgeon.

Bobbs' operation. The operative removal of gall-stones from the gall bladder.

Bochdalek, Vincenz Alexander (b. 1801). Prague anatomist.

Bochdalek's canal. A minute canal which passes obliquely through the tympanic membrane to open on its external surface.

Bochdalek's duct. The thyroglossal duct. *See* DUCT.

Bochdalek's foramen, or gap. A pleuroperitoneal canal between the diaphragm and upper lumbar vertebrae in the fetus: when this opening connecting the pleural and peritoneal cavities remains unclosed, the abdominal contents may herniate into the chest.

Bochdalek's ganglion. A small plexiform ganglion said to be present at the point of communication of the 3 superior dental nerves.

Bochdalek's gland. Thyroglossal cyst (*see* CYST) in the tongue.

Bochdalek's sinus. An opening connecting the developing pleural and peritoneal cavities.

Bochdalek's tube. One of the cavities connected with the embryonic thyroglossal duct.

Bochdalek's valve. A fold in the wall of the lacrimal canaliculi close to the puncta lacrimalia.

Bock, August Carl (b. 1782). Leipzig anatomist.

Bock's ganglion. A ganglion of the internal carotid artery in the cavernous sinus.

Bock's pharyngeal nerve. The pharyngeal branch of the sphenopalatine ganglion.

Bockhart, Max (b. 1883). German physician.

Bockhart's impetigo. Superficial pustular folliculitis; folliculitis of staphylococcic origin giving rise to small pustules round the sebaceous glands of the hair follicles.

Bodansky, Aaron (b. 1887). New York biochemist.

Bodansky's method. For serum alkaline phosphatase: serum is incubated with a buffered substance of sodium β-glycerophosphate for 1 h at 37°C and the total inorganic phosphate is determined by acid molybdate and stannous chloride. The inorganic phosphate of the serum is determined at the same time by omitting the incubation. Subtraction of the latter value from the total gives the phosphatase activity of the serum in Bodansky units. Normal range for adults is 1.5-4.0 units per 100 ml, and for children 5-12 units.

Bodansky unit. A phosphatase activity of 1 unit per 100 ml serum or plasma liberates 1 mg of phosphorus as phosphate in 1 h at 37°C from the substrate sodium β-glycerophosphate at pH 8.6.

Bodecker index. The ratio of the number of surfaces of teeth attacked by caries to the number of surfaces of all the teeth in the same mouth which could be involved.

Bodian, David (b. 1910). American anatomist.

Bodian method. A method for the demonstration of nerve-endings and axis cylinders in paraffin sections, employing a silver protein ("Protargol") containing metallic copper, and a hydroquinone-sodium sulphite reducer.

bodily harm (bod·e·le harm). Actual bodily harm. In the law, this includes any hurt or injury calculated to interfere with the health or comfort of another person. It need not be of a permanent or dangerous nature, or amount to grievous bodily harm. **Grievous bodily harm.** Bodily harm becomes grievous when it seriously interferes with health or comfort. The effects need neither be dangerous nor permanent, nor need it entail a wound. Whether or not a particular injury amounts to grievous bodily harm is a matter for the jury. [AS *bodig, haerm.*]

bodily injury (**bod**·e·le **in**·jur·e). **Appreciable bodily injury.** Any bodily injury or effect that the person involved would regard as objectionable and/or that competent medical authorities would regard as being deleterious to the health and well-being of the individual. [AS *bodig,* L *injuria.*]

Bodo (**bo**·do). A genus of flagellate protozoa in the intestinal tract; non-pathogenic. **Bodo caudatus.** A flagellate frequently found living coprozoically in human faeces. **Bodo saltans.** A flagellate found in ulcers. **Bodo urinaria.** A flagellate found in the urine. [invented name.]

Bodonidae (bo·**don**·id·e). A family of protozoa of which *Bodo* is a genus. [*Bodo,* Gk *eidos* form.]

body (**bod**·e). 1. The whole of an animal organism. 2. [Truncus (NA)] The trunk or main part of an animal, excluding appendages such as the limbs or tail. 3. [Corpus (NA)] The main, largest or most central part of a structure, e.g. the body of the uterus. 4. Any more or less rounded discrete mass, microscopic or macroscopic. 5. A substance of any kind. **Accessory body.** A particle in the cytoplasm of a spermatid which helps to form the neck of the spermatozoon. **Acetone body.** General name for the compounds acetone, aceto-acetic acid and β-hydroxybutyric acid, appearing in the blood and urine of diabetics as a result of the incomplete breakdown of fatty acids. The condition is known as *ketosis,* and may also occur in starvation, in normal pregnancy, after ether administration and in alkalosis. **Adrenal bodies.** The suprarenal or adrenal glands. *See* GLAND. **Amyloid bodies.** Prostatic concretions, thought to resemble starch grains. The term has also been applied to concretions of similar appearance in other tissues. **Anococcygeal body [ligamentum anococcygeum (NA)].** A mass of fibromuscular tissue between the anal canal and the coccyx to which some of the fibres of the levator ani muscle are attached. **Anti-immune body.** Anti-amboceptor. **Aortic bodies.** The aortic paraganglia, recognizable only in the infant. They are situated anterior to the aorta, near the superior mesenteric artery, and consist of chromaffin tissue resembling the medulla of the suprarenal gland. **Apical body.** *See* ACROSOME. **Asbestos body.** The microscopic drumstick-like mass found within the lungs of workers inhaling asbestos products. **Bacillary bodies.** Pappenheimer's bodies, Pappenheimer's inclusion bodies; iron-containing granules which are Feulgen-negative, seen in mature and immature erythrocytes, and in normoblasts and other red-cell precursors in the bone marrow, usually in patients with haemolytic anaemia but also after splenectomy in certain haemolytic anaemias. They are said to indicate haemoglobin anabolism and to be related to punctate basophilia, apparently being formed in the bone marrow and removed by the spleen. **Bartonian body.** The organism causing Oroya fever, first described by Barton and now known as *Bartonella bacilliformis.* **Basal body.** Acytoplasmic granule to which a cilium or flagellum is attached. **Bigeminal bodies.** The superior pair of the corpora quadrigemina of the mid-brain. **Bird's-nest body.** Cell nest, epithelial pearl; concentrically arranged epithelial cells found in epithelioma, some forming keratin as in normal epidermis. **Brassy body.** A dark, contracted erythrocyte sometimes seen in patients suffering from infection with *Plasmodium falciparum*; it has the appearance of old brass. **Cancer body.** A hyaline degeneration occurring within many cancer cells and imitating parasites. **Carotid body [glomus caroticum (NA)].** A small mass of epithelioid tissue lying in the fork where the common carotid artery divides into its internal and external branches. It has a rich blood and nerve supply, and is a chemoreceptor concerned in certain cardiovascular reflexes. **Catalytic body.** A catalyst. **Cavernous bodies.** The corpora cavernosa of the penis or clitoris. **Cell body.** That portion of a nerve cell which surrounds the nucleus and from which the axon and dendrites arise. **Central body.** The centre of the aster during cell division. **Chromaffin body.** Paraganglion; a body associated with a sympathetic ganglion, staining brown with chromic acid. **Chromatin bodies.** Discrete granules, stained by basic dyes, which are found in all bacteria and which represent the bacterial genetic material. **Chromophilous body.** Nissl substance. **Ciliary body [corpus ciliare (NA)].** The structures by which the choroid of the eye is continued forward to the margin of the iris; it consists of the ciliary ring, processes and muscle. **Coccoid bodies.** Bacillary bodies (see above). **Coccygeal body [corpus coccygeum (NA)].** A small mass of fibromuscular tissue anterior to the apex of the coccyx which contains numerous arteriovenous anastomoses. **Colloid bodies.** Drüsen bodies (see below). **Colostrum bodies.** Large, frequently degenerate, amoeboid cells found in the colostrum; their cytoplasm contains fat droplets. **Crescent bodies.** Large fine discoid bodies having pink crescentic margins, seen in the blood in some anaemia conditions. **Crystalloid body.** A crystalline inclusion within the cytoplasm of certain cells. **Cytoid bodies.** Oval, globulin structures resembling cells and seen at the dermo-epidermal junction in systemic lupus erythematosus. **Demilune body.** A degenerated erythrocyte, sometimes seen after malaria or typhoid fever, having its haemoglobin concentrated at its edge like a crescent, the rest of the cell being transparent and free of haemoglobin. **Drüsen bodies.** Small, discrete, yellowish-white spots seen scattered over the fundus of the eye, consisting of hyaline material situated in Bruch's membrane. They are found usually as a degenerative change in old age and following disease of the retina. Also called *colloid bodies.* It is rarely a primary hereditary degenerative condition, but is then called *Doyne's familial honeycombed choroiditis* or *familial colloid degeneration.* **Elementary body.** A virus particle as seen in the light microscope. Since virus particles are generally too small to be seen except when heavily loaded with stain, the appearance of elementary bodies does not give a reliable guide to either the size or the shape of the virus particles. **Epithelial bodies.** Small masses of epithelium which grow from the dorsolateral wall of the 3rd and 4th pharyngeal pouches of the embryo; they form the parathyroid glands. **Falciform body.** The sporozoite stage of a malarial parasite. **Fatty body of the orbit [corpus adiposum orbitae (NA)].** The fat in the orbit in which the eyeball is embedded. **Filling body.** A degenerated neuroglial cell. **Flagellated body.** A male gametocyte which has extruded its flagella. **Foreign body.** Anything found in a wound or tissue not normally present. **Body of the fornix.** *See* FORNIX. **Fuchsine body.** A rounded hyaline mass, found in cancer cells and occasionally in the renal tubules and mucosa of the nose and stomach, which stains brightly with fuchsine. **Geniculate body, lateral [corpus geniculatum laterale (NA)].** The mass of nerve cells on the lateral aspect of the pulvinar of the thalamus; it receives visual impulses from the optic tract and relays to the visual cortex. **Geniculate body, lateral, nucleus of the [nucleus corporis geniculati lateralis (NA)].** Grey matter arranged in 6 layers separated by intervening layers of white fibres; fibres of the optic tract synapse around the cells of the grey layers. **Geniculate body, medial [corpus geniculatum mediale (NA)].** The mass of nerve cells which forms a prominence beneath the pulvina of the thalamus; it receives auditory impulses from the lateral lemniscus and relays to the auditory cortex. **Geniculate body, medial, nucleus of the [nucleus corporis geniculati medialis (NA)].** A collection of medium-sized neurones in the centre of the body. **Globoid body.** A structure observed by Flexner and Noguchi in poliomyelitis, and thought to be the causal microbe. **Habenular body.** The habenular ganglia or epithalamus. **Haematoxylin bodies.** Typical appearance seen in tissues (especially in the kidneys) in disseminated lupus erythematosus. Believed to be the result of antigen-antibody reactions. **Hyaloid body.** Vitreous body (see below). **Immune body.** Amboceptor. **Inclusion body.** A cellular inclusion in a virus infection; an aggregate or collection of elementary bodies. **Infrapatellar fatty body.** Infrapatellar pad of fat; the collection of fat in the synovial membrane deep to the ligamentum patellae. **Inner body.** A granule seen in an erythrocyte, and includes various types of bodies such as Ehrlich's, Heinz's, etc. **Intercarotid body.** Carotid body (see below). **Ketone body.** Another name for an acetone body (see above) because of the ketonic nature of the compounds concerned. **LCL body.** A minute body in infected tissues in psittacosis, and named after Levinthal, Coles and Lillie. It resembles the Paschen granule. **Lentiform bodies.** Minute, refractile, lens-shaped, transparent masses between the inner and outer segments of the rods of the retina; they are not present in man. **Lyssa body.** A structure resembling the Negri body but showing less definition. **Malpighian body.** Bowman's capsule and the contained glomerulus in the kidney. **Mamillary bodies [corpora mamillaria (NA)].** Nipple-like projections in the interpeduncular fossa of the brain; they form part of the hypothalamus. **Mamillary body, nuclei of the [nuclei corporis mamillaris (NA)].** Cells of grey matter the axons of which form the mamillothalamic, mamillotegmental and mamillopeduncular tracts. **Body of the mandible.** *See* MANDIBLE. **Body of the maxilla.** *See* MAXILLA. **Melon-seed body.** A button-like mass of firm fibrin found free within the joint cavities after chronic inflammation or trauma. **Metachromatic bodies.** Granules or material seen in bacteria, which stain differently from the rest of the cell. **Molluscous body.** An oval hyaline body found within the papule cells of molluscum contagiosum (epitheliale). **Body of a nail.** *See* NAIL. **Olivary bodies.** The olives or olivary nuclei of the medulla oblongata. **Onion body.** Bird's-nest body (see above). **Pacchionian bodies.** Arachnoid granulations; masses of fibrous tissue covered by arachnoid mesothelium which project into the superior sagittal sinus and into the lateral lacunae. They are frequently calcified in old age and are probably hypertrophied and degenerate arachnoid villi. **Body of the pancreas.** *See* PANCREAS. **Para-aortic bodies [corpora para-aortica (NA)].** Zuckerkandl or aortic chromophil bodies. **Parabasal body.** A chromatin-staining body, usually closely associated with the blepharoplast, in the flagellated protozoa. Its function is not known; kinetoplast. **Paranephric body.** A quantity of fat outside the renal fascia, especially posteriorly. **Paranuclear body.** The centrosome. **Para-olivary bodies.** The medial and dorsal accessory olivary nuclei. **Paraterminal body.** The medial wall of the cerebral hemisphere immediately anterior to the lamina terminalis. **Parathyroid bodies.** Parathyroid glands. *See* GLAND. **Pearly body [centrum tendineum perinei (NA)].** Bird's-nest body (see above). **Body of the penis.** *See* PENIS. **Perineal body.** The mass of tissue composed of muscle and fascia between the vagina and rectum in the female and between the urethra and rectum in the male. **Pineal body [corpus pineale].** A small cone-shaped mass attached by a stalk to the posterior end of the roof of the 3rd ventricle of the brain. **Pituitary body.** The hypophysis cerebri. **Polar body.** 1. One of the "non-functional" products of meiosis in the female; these are usually expelled from the ovum and do not take part in fertilization. 2. Metachromatic material to be seen at one or both ends of some bacteria; it is of uncertain significance. **Postbranchial body.** Ultimobranchial body (see below). **Psammoma body.** A calcareous microconcretion found within the brain substance and the prostate, and in some cancers. **Body of the pubis.** *See* PUBIS. **Purine body.** Any of the group of substances of biological importance termed purines, derivatives of the parent substance purine, which does not itself occur in nature. **Quadrigeminal bodies [colliculus superior et inferior (NA)].** Four rounded projections forming the roof or tectum of the mid-brain; the superior [colliculus superior (NA)] and inferior [colliculus inferior (NA)] colliculi. **Quadrigeminal body, inferior, nucleus of the [nucleus colliculi inferioris (NA)].** An oval mass of grey matter in the centre of the inferior quadrigeminal body; it forms a relay station for some of the fibres in the auditory pathway. **Quadrigeminal body, superior, nucleus of the [stratum griseum colliculi superioris (NA)].** The second of the 4 layers forming the body of the superior quadrigeminal body; synapsing with the cells of this layer are the mesencephalic fibres of the optic tract concerned with visual reflexes. **Restiform body.** The inferior cerebellar peduncle. *See* PEDUNCLE. **Reticular body of the skin [stratum reticulare (NA)].** The deeper of the 2 layers of the dermis, composed mainly of interwoven collagenous fibres with elastic fibres, especially around the hair follicles and glands. There are few connective-tissue cells. **Rickettsia body.** One of a group of very small organisms, which include the specific agents of typhus fever, Rocky Mountain spotted fever, trench fever and Q fever. **Sand bodies.** Corpora aranacea; granular material sometimes found in masses of papilloma. **Body of the sphenoid bone.** *See* SPHENOID BONE. **Spiculated bodies.** Spiny granules sometimes seen with leucocytes or giant cells in the spleen. **Spongy body.** The corpus spongiosum penis. **Body of the sternum.** *See* STERNUM. **Body of the stomach.** *See* STOMACH. **Striate body.** The corpus striatum, consisting of the caudate nucleus and the lentiform nucleus. **Suprarenal bodies.** The suprarenal or adrenal glands. **Body of the talus.** *See* TALUS. **Telobranchial body.** Ultimobranchial body (see below). **Threshold body.** Any substance present in blood plasma that is only excreted by the kidneys when it reaches a minimal threshold concentration. **Trachoma body.** A body found within the conjunctival epithelial cell in trachoma. It is regarded as being a virus which causes the disease. **Trapezoid body.** Corpus trapezoideum. **Ultimobranchial body.** A small mass of epithelium derived from the last pharyngeal pouch of the embryo; there is evidence that it gives rise to the parafollicular cells of the thyroid gland. **Body of the uterus.** *See* UTERUS. **Body of a vertebra.** *See* VERTEBRA. **Vitreous body [corpus vitreum (NA)].** A transparent jelly permeated by fine fibrils which fills the eyeball between the lens and the retina. **Wolffian body.** The mesonephros; the second of the 3 kidneys of the reptilian and mammalian embryo, and the permanent kidney of some fish and amphibia. It is functional in those mammalian embryos in which the placental membrane is many-layered (e.g. the pig), rudimentary in those with a more efficient placental membrane, such as man. Some of the mesonephric tubules of the mammal are transformed into the efferent ductules of the testes, as well as into such vestigial structures as the appendix of the epididymis of the male and the epoöphoron and paroöphoron of the female. The mesonephric duct becomes the epididymis and vas deferens of the male. **Xanthine body.** A former term for purine body (see above). **Y body.** A nuclear body visible in cells stained with some fluorescent dyes and indicating the presence of a Y chromosome. Such a body is visible in species such as man and *Drosophila melanogaster,* where a segment of the Y chromosome stains very intensely. **Yellow body.** The corpus luteum of the ovary. [AS *bodig.*]

See also: AMATO, ARANZIO, ARNOLD (J.), ASCHOFF, AUER, BABÈS, BALBIANI, BEHLA, BENDER, BOLLINGER, BORREL, BRACHT, BUIST (J. B.), CABOT, CALL, CESARIS-DEMEL, COUNCILMAN, DEETJEN, DOEHLE, DONNÉ, DONOVAN (C.), EHRLICH, EIMER, ELSCHNIG, ELZHOLZ, ERNST, EXNER, FLEMMING, GIANNUZZI, GOLGI, GREEFF, GUARNIERI, GUTMANN, HALBERSTAEDTER, HARTING, HASSALL, HEINZ, HENDERSON (W.), HENSEN, HERRING, HIGHMORE, HOWELL, JAWORSKI, JOLLY (J. M. J.), KOHN (A.), KURLOV, LALLEMAND, LANDOLT, LANGERHANS, LEISHMAN, LEVINTHAL, LINDNER, LIPSCHUETZ, LUYS (J. B.), MALLORY, MARAGLIANO, MAZZONI, MICHAELIS (L.), MOOSER, MUELLER (J.), NEGRI, NEILL (M. H.), NISSL, NOTHNAGEL, OKEN, PACCHIONI, PAPPENHEIMER, PASCHEN, PATERSON (R.), PERLS, PLIMMER, PROWAZEK, RENAUT, RETZIUS (M. G.), ROSENMUELLER, RUFFINI, RUSSELL (W.), SANDSTRÖM, SAVAGE, SCHMORL, SEIDELIN, SYMINGTON, TORRES-TEIXEIRA, TROUSSEAU, WAECHTER, WOLFF (K. F.), ZUCKERKANDL.

body type (**bod**·e tipe). **Hippocratic body type.** An assessment of a patient's general bodily form, ranging between the extremes of the apoplectic and the phthisic types. [AS *bodig,* Gk *typos* impression.]

Boeck, Caesar Peter Moeller (b. 1845). Oslo dermatologist.

Boeck's disease, mal de Boeck. Sarcoidosis.

Boeck's lupoid. A granulomatous lesion of the skin which, under glass pressure, shows grey-yellow specks similar to the "apple-jelly" of the nodules of lupus vulgaris. There may be only a solitary lesion, or large numbers which can appear as papules, nodules or plaques; all forms are sarcoid.

Boeck's sarcoid. A cutaneous eruption of nodules, papules or plaques, occurring singly or in large numbers: all 3 forms can co-exist. The lesions are composed predominantly of epitheloid infiltrate; after a period of months or years they undergo involution.

Besnier-Boeck disease. Cutaneous sarcoidosis.

Besnier-Boeck-Schaumann disease, or syndrome. Sarcoidosis.

Hutchinson-Boeck disease. Cutaneous sarcoidosis.

Boeck, Carl Wilhelm (b. 1808). Oslo dermatologist.

Boeck's itch. Scabies.

Boeck's scabies. Norwegian scabies; severe scabies associated with crusting and scaling; the affected skin is densely infested. Itching may not be a prominent feature, and possibly the causal mite is not identical with *Sarcoptes scabiei* var. *hominis.*

Boeck, William Charles (b. 1894). Baltimore scientist.

Boeck and Drbohlav medium. Coagulated egg and serum covered with salt-albumin (egg or serum) mixture. It is employed for amoebae.

Boehler, Lorenz (b. 1885). Vienna surgeon.

Boehler clamp. A metal clamp used to restore alignment in fractures of the calcaneum.

Boehler's frame. 1. A metal frame for the reduction of leg fractures. 2. A metal frame for the reduction of arm fractures.

Boehler's iron. A walking appliance used with lower limb plaster immobilization.

Boehler's traction. The operation of a powerful pull upon the limb by means of an apparatus incorporating a powerful screw. The traction is applied to the bone by means of a transfixing pin.

Boehmer, F. 19th century German physician.

Boehmer's haematoxylin. A general nuclear stain made from haematoxylin and alum.

Boerhaave, Hermann (b. 1668). Dutch physician.

Boerhaave's glands. The sweat glands. *See* GLAND.

Boettcher, Arthur (b. 1831). Dorpat pathologist.

Boettcher's canal. The utriculosaccular duct. *See* DUCT.

Boettcher's cells. Dark polyhedral epithelial cells found on the basilar membrane of the cochlea.

Boettcher's ganglion. A small ganglion on the branch of the cochlear nerve to the vestibule.

Boettger, Rudolf Christian (b. 1806). Frankfurt chemist.

Boettger's test. A chemical test for carbon monoxide: paper treated with a solution of palladium chloride (0.0002 g in 100 ml) darkens if exposed to carbon monoxide.

bog bean (bog been). Buckbean; the herb *Menyanthes trifoliata* Linn. (family Gentianaceae). It has tonic and stomachic properties. [Gael. *bogach,* AS *bean.*]

Bogros, Annet Jean (b. 1786). Paris anatomist.

Bogros' space. A space between the peritoneum and the transversalis fascia in the iliac fossa, through which the external iliac artery can be approached extraperitoneally.

Bogros, Antoine (fl. 1848). French physician.

Bogros' serous membrane. A serous membrane lining Tenon's space.

Bogrow, Sergei Livovich (b. 1878). Russian anatomist.

Bogrow's fibres. Fibres running from the optic tract to the thalamus.

Bogue's operation. Multiple ligation of testicular veins in varicocele.

bohemium (bo·he·me·um). Name given by independent discoverers to the element with atomic number 75, now known as *rhenium.* [*Bohemia.*]

Bohn's epithelial pearls. Minute retention cysts, found in the mouth of healthy infants.

Bohn's exercise test. A fall in diastolic arterial pressure on exercise in patients with patent ductus arteriosus. It is probably fallacious, since exercise in normal subjects often produces a fall in diastolic pressure.

Bohr, Christian (b. 1855). Scandinavian physiologist.

Bohr effect. The shift in the oxygen dissociation curve of haemoglobin induced by change in the hydrogen concentration.

Bohr, Niels (b. 1885). Danish physicist.

Bohr atom. The hypothetical atom in which the electrons are visualized rotating about the nucleus in orbits, the radii of which depend upon the energy quanta possessed by the atom.

Bohr magneton. A unit of magnetic moment, being the increase in magnetic moment for each quantum increase in magnetic moment of the electron orbit in the hydrogen atom.

Bohun upas (bo·hun ew·pas). The tree *Antiaris toxicaria* (Pers.) Lesch. (family Moraceae), of tropical Asia. It contains an extremely toxic latex, and is the source of an arrow-poison. The bark is made into a bark cloth used in Sri Lanka and Malaysia.

boil (boil). A furuncle. **Aleppo boil, Baghdad boil, Biskra boil.** Cutaneous leishmaniasis. *See* LEISHMANIASIS. **Blind boil.** A furuncle which resolves with absorption of the central necrotic core without forming an abscess and discharging. **Bolama boil.** A sore occurring in West Africa, chronic in character and held to be caused by the larva of a burrowing insect. (Bolama is an island off West Africa.) **Cat boil.** A small common furuncle. **Delhi boil.** Cutaneous leishmaniasis. *See* LEISHMANIASIS. **Gafsa boil.** Cutaneous leishmaniasis endemic in Tunisia. **Godovrick boil.** Cutaneous leishmaniasis. *See* LEISHMANIASIS. **Gum boil.** Parulis. **Jericho boil.** Cutaneous leishmaniasis. *See* LEISHMANIASIS. **Madura boil.** Mycetoma. **Oriental boil, Penjdeh boil, Rain boil.** Cutaneous leishmaniasis. *See* LEISHMANIASIS. **Salt-water boil.** A papular and pustular eruption occurring on the forearms and wrists of fishermen. **Scinde boil.** Cutaneous leishmaniasis. *See* LEISHMANIASIS. **Shoe boil.** A hygroma affecting the elbow. **Tropical boil.** Cutaneous leishmaniasis. *See* LEISHMANIASIS. [AS *byle* sore.]

Bojanus, Ludwig Heinrich (b. 1776). Vilna, Lithuania, anatomist.

Bojanus' organ. The molluscan kidney.

Boldenone (bol·den·one). BP Commission approved name for 17β-hydroxyanstrosta-1,4-dien-3-one; an anabolic steroid.

boldine (bol·deen). $C_{19}H_{21}O_4N$, an alkaloid derived from the South American evergreen shrub boldo (*Peumus boldus* Molina). It has a lowering effect on blood pressure, and may produce clonic convulsions; formerly used in liver disease and as an antiseptic.

boldo (bol·do). The dried leaves of *Peumus boldus* Molina (family Monimiaceae) of Chile. It contains a volatile oil, boldine (an alkaloid) and boldoglucin (a glucoside). It has been used in the form of a tincture as a diuretic and liver stimulant. [Sp. *boldu.*]

boldoin (bol·do·in). A glucoside occurring in boldo.

Boletus (bo·le·tus). A genus of fungi with both edible and poisonous species. **Boletus laricis.** Agaric; the dried fungus *Fomes officinalis* Faull. [L mushroom.]

Boley gauge (bo·le gaje). An instrument incorporating a vernier scale, used in dentistry for precise and accurate measurement.

Bolk, Louis (b. 1866). Amsterdam anatomist.

Bolk's retardation theory. The theory that man reaches sexual maturity in his ontogenic development at a stage which corresponds to a fetal stage in a higher ape.

Boll, Franz Christian (b. 1849). Genoa and Rome physiologist.

Boll's cells. 1. Basket cells, basal in position, found in the acini of the lacrimal gland. 2. *Cellules à panier* of the acini of the mammary gland.

Boll's passages. Minute ducts connecting the excretory passages of salivary glands with the acini. They are especially prominent in the parotid gland.

Bollinger, Otto von (b. 1843). Munich pathologist.

Bollinger bodies, or granules. Inclusion bodies of fowl-pox.

Bollman, Jesse Louis (b. 1896). Rochester, Minnesota, pathologist.

Mann-Bollman fistula. Experimental diversion of duodenal tissue into the ileum for the production of peptic ulcer in animals.

Bolmantalate (bol·man·tal·ate). BP Commission approved name for 17β-hydroxyoestr-4-en-3-one adamantane-1-carboxylate; an anabolic steroid.

bolometer (bo·**lom**·et·er). An instrument for measuring quantity of radiation. [Gk *bole* ray, meter.]

boloscope (**bo**·lo·skope). An instrument for detecting the presence and finding the exact position in the tissues of a metal foreign body. [Gk *bole* stroke, *skopein* to watch.]

Bolton, Joseph Shaw (b. 1867). Yorkshire neurologist.

Bolton nasion plane. A plane joining the Bolton point to the nasion.

Bolton point. A landmark used in orientating lateral skull x-rays. It is the highest point in the profile of the notches posterior to the occipital condyles.

bolus (**bo**·lus). 1. A lump of food masticated and ready to be swallowed. 2. A mass of food when it is passing along the intestines. 3. In pharmacy, a spherical mass. **Alimentary bolus.** Main def. 1 (above). **Bolus bags.** *See* BAG. [Gk *bolos* lump of earth.]

bomb (bom). A colloquial term for a teletherapy unit with an isotope source. **Cobalt bomb.** A teletherapy apparatus containing cobalt. **Freon bomb.** A vessel containing Freon, used in the dispersion of insecticidal mists. **Radium bomb.** A teletherapy apparatus containing radium [obsolete term]. [Gk *bombos* hum.]

bombard (bom·**bard**). To attack with radiant energy as to attack with bombs or shells; to direct electromagnetic radiation (particularly x-rays and gamma rays) or a stream of particles (alpha rays, beta rays, neutrons, protons) towards some object to the irradiated. [see prec.]

Bonain, Aristide (b. 1860). Brest otologist.

Bonain's liquid, or mixture. A local anaesthetic and antiseptic used for aural operations, consisting of phenol, menthol and cocaine; now obsolete.

bond (bond). A conventional system to indicate the linkages between atoms or groups of atoms in structural and constitutional formulae. *See* LINKAGE. **Peptide bond.** The peptide linkage, -CO-NH-, which joins amino acids into a protein chain. [ME.]

bonduc (**bon**·duk). Bonduc seeds; the seed of *Guilandina bonduc* Linn. and *Guilandina bonducella* Linn. (family Leguminosae). A bitter tonic and antiperiodic. [Ar. *bunduq* hazel-nut.]

bonducin (bon·**dew**·sin). $C_{14}H_{15}O_5$. A bitter compound obtained from bonduc seeds. It is insoluble in water and is used in India as a febrifuge; its value is doubtful.

bone [os (NA)] (bone). A hard form of connective tissue which contains specialized cells (osteocytes) and a calcified collogenous intercellular substance generally arranged in lamellae. A bone often bears an articular surface [facies articularis (NA)]. (For specific bones, see under qualifying adjective.) **Accessory bone.** An inconstant supernumerary bone, found commonly in various positions in the carpus and tarsus, also occasionally in other sites (os acetabuli), and recognized radiographically. **Bone age.** Determined by the appearance of centres of ossification particularly in the bones of the wrist and closure of epiphyses of long bones. The bone age is retarded, compared with the patient's age, in hypopituitarism and increased by androgen and oestrogen. **Alveolar bone.** The bone of the margin of the mandible and maxilla which contains the alveoli in which the teeth are set. **Astragaloscaphoid bone.** An occasional ossicle dorsal to the head of the talus. **Breast bone.** Sternum. **Bundle bone.** A type of bone containing numerous Sharpey's fibres as found near tendinous or ligamentous attachments. **Cancellous bone.** Bone arranged as a network of bony plates and trabecula resembling a sponge. Such bone is characteristic of the ends of long bones; spongy bone. **Cartilage bone.** Bone which is developed by endochondral ossification in a pre-existing cartilage. **Compact bone.** Dense bone in which vascular canals are not visible to the unaided eye; it forms the cortex of all bones, and is characteristically composed of lamellar bone arranged in haversian systems. **Cortical bone.** The layer of compact bone which forms the outer surface of nearly all bones. **Dentary bone.** One of several bones forming the skeleton of the lower jaw in lower vertebrates. It enlarges at the expense of the others to form the whole mandible in mammals. **Dermal bone.** Strictly, bone which is developed by direct ossification of the connective tissue of the dermis; such bones are present only in primitive vertebrates. More loosely, it is used as a synonym for membrane bone (see below). **Endochondrial bone.** Cartilage bone (see above). **Exercise bone.** Ossification in a bone; said to be due to excessive use. **Flat bone [os planum (NA)].** Any of the flat protective bones, such as the tables of the skull, consisting of spongy substance between 2 layers of compact bone. **Intrachondrial bone.** Cartilage bone (see above). **Lamellar bone.** Fine-fibred bone arranged in parallel or concentric sheets (lamellae); it is the usual type of bone found in the adult skeleton of higher vertebrates. **Long bone [os longum (NA)].** Any of the elongated bones of the upper or lower limb. It contains marrow within an outer compact bone shaft. **Marble bone.** A bone in which there has been an increase in the density of a tissue with obliteration of the medullary cavity; Albers-Schoenberg disease. **Membrane bone.** Bone which develops by direct ossification in connective tissue without the preformation of cartilage. **Mosaic bone.** Bone which displays a mosaic pattern through accentuation of growing lines, as seen in Paget's disease. **Non-lamellar bone.** Primary bone (see below). **Bone onlay.** A method of bone grafting where the graft is fixed to a prepared bed on the surface of the host bone. **Periosteal bone.** Bone formed by deposition on the surface immediately beneath the periosteum. The osteoblasts of the deeper layers of the periosteum are responsible for its formation. **Pneumatic bone [os pneumaticum (NA)].** A bone containing air cells, e.g. the ethmoid. **Primary bone.** Coarse-fibred bone usually in the form of an irregular network of anastomosing trabeculae. It is found in the embryo of higher vertebrates, in the adult skeleton of lower vertebrates and wherever bone is being rapidly formed, as in fracture callus, bony tumours, etc. **Replacement bone.** Bone which replaces the primary non-lamellar bone of the embryonic skeleton. **Rider's bone.** Calcification of the tendon of either the adductor longus or the adductor magnus muscles. **Scroll bone.** A nasal concha. **Secondary bone.** Lamellar bone (see above). **Sesamoid bone.** A small discrete bone formed by ossification within a tendon. **Short bone [os breve (NA)].** Any of the compact bones of the carpus or tarsus consisting of spongy bone tissue within a compact bone covering. **Spongy bone.** Cancellous bone (see above). **Subperiosteal bone.** Periosteal bone (see above). **Tabular bone.** Compact bone in the form of a thin flat plate; it is found characteristically in the bones of the cranial vault. **Wormian bone.** *See* SUTURAL BONES. **Woven bone.** Young bone laid down after fracture and not yet differentiated into a mature lamellar pattern. [AS *ban.*]

See also: ALBERS-SCHOENBERG, ALBRECHT, BERTIN, BRESCHET, EYSSON, FLOWER, GOETHE, KRAUSE (W. J. F.), PIRIE, RIOLAN, ROUSSEAU, VESALIUS.

bone-chips (**bone**·chipz). 1. Senn's bone plates. 2. Chips of cancellous bone used in plastic operations on bones. [AS *ban*, ME *choppen.*]

bone-scanning (**bone**·skan·ing). The technique of scanning using various radioactive nuclides for demonstrating particularly bone metastases. [AS *ban*, L *scandere* to climb.]

bone-setter (**bone**·set·er). A person (usually unqualified) who practises in the reduction of fractures and dislocations, and carries out manipulation of stiff joints. [AS *ban, settan.*]

bonelet (**bone**·let). An ossicle. [AS *ban.*]

boneset (**bone**·set). The compositous herb *Eupatorium perfoliatum* Linn. It has diaphoretic and tonic properties.

Bonfil's disease. Lymphadenoma.

bongkrek (bong·**krek**). A Javanese dish that is occasionally poisonous and gives rise to vomiting, sweating, cramps, and coma. [Javanese name.]

Bonjean, Joseph (b. 1810). Chambéry pharmacist.

Bonjean's ergotine. An aqueous extract of ergot [obsolete term].

Bonnaire, Erasme (b. 1858). Paris obstetrician.

Bonnaire's method. A method of dilatation of the cervix uteri by the fingers with one hand pressing down above the pubic symphysis.

Bonnet, Amadée (b. 1802). Lyons surgeon.

Bonnet's capsule. The anterior portion of the episcleral space.

Bonnet's sign. Pain on adduction of the affected thigh, in all cases of sciatica.

Bonney, William Francis Victor (b. 1872). London gynaecologist.

Bonney's blue, or dye. A combination of crystal violet and brilliant green used for the sterilization of the skin and other surfaces.

Bonnier, Pierre (b. 1861). Paris physician.

Bonnier's syndrome. Vertigo with associated nystagmus, and sometimes somnolence and contralateral hemiparesis, due to a lesion of Deiters' nucleus and of vestibular pathways; the 3rd, 5th, 9th and 10th cranial nerves may sometimes be involved.

Bonnot, Edmond. 19th-20th century St. Louis anatomist.

Bonnot's gland. Interscapular gland. *See* GLAND.

Bonwill, William Gibson Arlington (b. 1833). American dentist.

Bonwill triangle. A triangle formed by the 2 heads of the mandible and the centre of the alveolar margin of that bone.

Böök, Jan Arvid (b. 1915). Swedish geneticist.

Böök's syndrome. Premature canities, palmoplantar hyperhidrosis and premolar hypodontia.

boomslang (boom·slang). A colubrid snake of southern Africa, *Dispholidus typus.* It is rear-fanged, but the poison is dangerous. [D *boom* tree, *slang* snake.]

Boophilus (bo·of·il·us). A genus of Acarina; cattle ticks. **Boophilus annulatus.** A cattle tick of the USA, possibly involved in transmission of Q fever. **Boophilus decoloratus.** A species of South Africa, possibly involved in transmission of tick typhus. [Gk *bous* ox, *philein* to love.]

boopia (bo·o·pe·ah). The uninterested, cow-like gaze seen in the eyes of individuals suffering from hysteria. [Gk *bous* ox, *ops* eye.]

booster (boos·ter). 1. A generator or transformer connected in series in a circuit for the purpose of increasing or decreasing the voltage. It may be used also to make up for the voltage drop in a long transmission line, or to charge one or more cells in an accumulator battery, or keep them from discharging independently of the remainder. 2. In immunology, use of second or later dose of antigen given after the priming dose to stimulate formation of large quantities of antibody. [American slang.]

boot (boot). *See* BROWNE (D.), UNNA. [ME *bote.*]

boracite (bor·as·ite). 1. A naturally occurring mineral, magnesium borate. 2. A mixture of 1 part magnesium borocitrate and 2 parts cane sugar, used internally as a urinary antiseptic in cases of gout and rheumatism. [Ar. *bauraq* nitre.]

borage (bor·ij). The plant *Borago officinalis* Linn. (family Boraginaceae). It is used as a herbal remedy for its diuretic and other properties, but is mainly employed as a flavouring agent for certain beverages. [OFr.]

boral (bo·ral). Aluminium borotartrate.

borate (bo·rate). A salt of boric acid.

borated (bo·ra·ted). Impregnated or combined with boric acid or borax.

borax (bo·rax). The common name for sodium pyroborate, $NA_2B_4O_7·10H_2O$, also known as *sodium biborate.* It occurs naturally in California and is a colourless compound, odourless, with a sweetish taste, and soluble in water and glycerin. It is used in glass-making. Medically, it is a weak antiseptic, employed as a mouth wash or gargle in aqueous solution or as a 12 per cent solution in glycerin, or 10 per cent in glycerin and honey (BP 1973). **Borax bead.** Borax fused with a metallic oxide into a small bead, the colour of which serves to identify the metal in analysis. **Borax carmine.** A stain for nuclei, composed of an alkaline solution of borax and carmine in water. [Ar. *bauraq* nitre.]

borborygmus (bor·bo·rig·mus). The rumbling or gurgling sound made by movement of flatus in the intestines. [Gk *borborizein* to rumble in the bowels.]

Borchardt, Leo (b. 1879). Königsberg chemist.

Borchardt's reaction, or test. For fructose (laevulose) in urine: 5 ml of urine is mixed with an equal volume of 25 per cent hydrochloric acid, and a few crystals of resorcinol are added. The mixture is heated to boiling for 1½ min, cooled under the tap, made alkaline with solid potassium hydroxide, and shaken with 3 ml of ethyl acetate. A yellow colour in the ethyl acetate indicates fructose.

Bordeaux B (bor·do be). Azorubrum, fast red B, $C_{10}H_7N{=}NC_{10}H_4(OH)(SO_3H)_2$. An azo dye derived from α-naphthylamine. It is water-soluble, and has largely replaced cochineal as a colouring for pharmaceutical preparations, as it is unaffected by acids, alkalis or sunlight.

border [margo (NA)] (bor·der). The edge or boundary of an organ or mass of tissue. **Brush border.** A collection of large numbers of microvilli found on the free surfaces of certain cells, particularly those concerned with absorption. **Border of the iris.** *See* IRIS. **Border of a nail.** *See* NAIL. **Postaxial border.** The caudal border of a fetal limb which becomes the medial border of the upper limb and (approximately) the lateral border of the lower limb. **Pre-axial border.** The cranial border of a fetal limb which becomes the lateral border of the upper limb and (approximately) the medial border of the lower limb. **Borders of the shaft of the fibula.** *See* FIBULA. **Borders of the shaft of the humerus.** *See* HUMERUS. **Borders of the shaft of the radius.** *See* RADIUS. **Borders of the shaft of the tibia.** *See* TIBIA. **Borders of the shaft of the ulna.** *See* ULNA. **Striated border.** A layer of modified cytoplasm on the free surface of a columnar epithelial cell in the intestine. It shows striations perpendicular to the surface, and may have an absorptive function. **Vermilion border.** The lips; the red external part of the mouth. [OFr. *bordure.*]

See also: MERCK.

Bordet, Jules Jean Baptiste Vincent (b. 1870). Brussels bacteriologist.

Bordet's amboceptor. The antibody present in blood which takes part in the fixation of complement.

Bordet's law. When erythrocytes are added to a haemolysing liquid in bulk, lysis is more rapid than when the same corpuscles are added in small portions.

Bordet's test. Serum test; immunological test for blood, meat or sperms: the suspected material is treated with physiological saline to dissolve some of the protein and added to a specific rabbit antiserum prepared against the substance in question. The mixture will become cloudy if the suspected specimen is of the same species as the antigen used to prepare the antiserum.

Bordet-Gengou agar, or culture medium. A potato, glycerin and plain agar medium with a high proportion of defibrinated bone blood added at 55°C. It is used for the growth of *Bordetella pertussis.*

Bordet-Gengou bacillus. *Bordetella pertussis.*

Bordet-Gengou phenomenon. Complement-fixation test. *See* TEST.

Bordetella (bor·det·el·ah). A genus of bacteria in the family Brucellaceae; it contains 3 species: *Bordetella pertussis, B. parapertussis* and *B. bronchiseptica.* The first 2 are pathogenic to man, causing whooping cough; *Bordetella bronchiseptica* is found in various animal species and may be associated with respiratory infections in them. *Bordetella pertussis* was formerly linked with *Haemophilus* because a blood-containing medium was needed for its primary isolation. [Jules Jean Baptiste Vincent *Bordet.*]

Bordier, Leonard Henri (b. 1863). Paris physician.

Bordier-Frenkel sign. An outward and upward rolling movement of the eye on attempted lid closure, in facial paralysis of lower motor neurone type; also called *Bell's phenomenon, Bell's sign.*

bordoresin (bor·do·rez·in). A resinous substance found in turpentine.

boricin (bo·ris·in). A preparation of borax and boric acid.

boride (bo·ride). A compound of the element boron with another element or radical, having the formula M_3B, where M is a monovalent element or radical.

borism (bo·rizm). The condition of being poisoned with a boron compound.

borneene (bor·ne·een). $C_{10}H_{16}$. An unsaturated hydrocarbon isomeric with bornylene.

borneol (bor·ne·ol). Borneo camphor, bornyl alcohol, camphyl alcohol, $C_{10}H_{17}OH$. A secondary terpene alcohol obtained by the reduction of common camphor. It occurs naturally in 2 stereo-isomeric optically-active forms in the oil of Siberian fir, the camphor of *Dryobalanops officinalis* and other essential oils, e.g. lavender, rosemary. The laevorotatory isomer is obtained from valerian oil. Borneol resembles camphor in its therapeutic properties, but its esters tend to display properties associated with the particular acid radical, e.g. the salicylate used in rheumatic complaints, the valerate in nervous conditions.

bornite (bor·nite). A naturally occurring copper ore; it is a copper iron sulphide, $Cu_2SCuSFeS$.

bornyl (bor·nil). The monovalent organic radical, $C_{10}H_{17}$–, occurring in esters of borneol. **Bornyl alcohol.** Borneol.

bornylene (bor·ne·leen). $C_{10}H_{16}$. A hydrocarbon derived from borneol.

borocalcite (bo·ro·kal·site). A mineral calcium borate, $CaB_4O_7{\cdot}4H_2O$.

borocarbide (bo·ro·kar·bide). Boron carbide, B_4C.

borocitrate (bo·ro·sit·rate). A salt of borocitric acid: magnesium borocitrate is used as a solvent for uric acid in the treatment of gout, stone and rheumatism.

boroglyceride, boroglycerin (bor·o·glis·er·ide, bor·o·glis·er·in). Glyceryl borate; a soft substance prepared by heating boric acid and glycerin together at a temperature between 140 and 150°C. In common with other preparations of boric acid, it is used in the treatment of certain skin and mucosal lesions.

boroglycerol (bor·o·glis·er·ol). Boroglycerin; a term sometimes applied to similar preparations of boric acid and glycerol in different proportions.

boron (bo·ron). An element of atomic weight 10.81, atomic number 5 and chemical symbol B. It is a light metalloid, very hard and unreactive, or an allotropic brown powder. It is not found free, but occurs as borates in certain minerals, and as boric acid in the volcanic steam-jets of Tuscany. Compounds of boron are important in medicine as antiseptics. **Boron carbide.** B_4C, a hard black substance formed by heating boron oxide and carbon in an electric furnace. It is used as an abrasive. **Boron oxide.** B_2O_3, the oxide formed when boron burns in oxygen. It combines with water to form boric acids. [borax, carbon.]

borotartrate (bo·ro·tar·trate). A salt of boric and tartaric acids; potassium borotartrate, soluble cream of tartar, has been used in the treatment of epilepsy.

Borrel, Amédée (b. 1867). Strasbourg bacteriologist.

Borrel body. The elementary body in fowl-pox.

Borrelia (bor·e·le·ah). One of the genera of Spirochaetales. They are large, motile, refractile spirochaetes with relatively few irregular wide and open coils, easily stained and Gram-negative. Species pathogenic to man include *Borrelia recurrentis (obermeieri)* and *B. duttoni,* the causal organisms of relapsing fever; *B. vincenti* is associated with *Fusobacterium fusiforme* in Vincent's angina. Some British bacteriologists do not recognize *Borrelia* as a valid genus and classify all these species in the genus *Treponema.* Since nearly all USA bacteriologists use the genus *Borrelia,* a modified Bergey's classification is given below. **Borrelia buccalis.** An organism found in the mouth. **Borrelia carteri.** Indian strains causing louse-borne relapsing fever. **Borrelia duttoni.** The causal organism of tick-borne relapsing fever. **Borrelia gallinarum.** A species infecting geese and fowls. **Borrelia hermsi.** Probably identical with *Borrelia duttoni.* **Borrelia hispanica.** Probably identical with *Borrelia recurrentis.* **Borrelia kochi.** Probably identical with *Borrelia recurrentis.* **Borrelia novyi.** A louse-borne spirochaete causing North American relapsing fever. It is immunologically different from *Borrelia obermeieri.* **Borrelia obermeieri.** *Borrelia recurrentis.* **Borrelia persica.** Probably identical with *Borrelia recurrentis.* **Borrelia recurrentis.** The causal organism of European relapsing fever. It occurs in the peripheral blood during the febrile stage and can be seen in the blood film. Infection is transmitted from one person to another by the body louse, the excreta of which are infective. Monkeys, white mice and white rats can be infected. **Borrelia refringens.** A species occurring on the body surfaces; non-pathogenic. **Borrelia sogdiana.** Probably identical with *Borrelia recurrentis.* **Borrelia theileri.** A tick-borne organism causing disease in cattle, sheep and horses in Africa. **Borrelia turicatae.** Probably identical with *Borrelia duttoni.* **Borrelia usbekistanica.** Probably identical with *Borrelia recurrentis.* **Borrelia venezuelensis.** Probably identical with *Borrelia recurrentis.* **Borrelia vincenti.** A species generally associated with a large fusiform bacillus and occurring in Vincent's angina, a pseudomembranous condition of the mouth. [Amédée *Borrel.*]

borsal (bor·sal). An antiseptic dusting powder made with equal parts of boric acid and salicylic acid.

Borsieri De Kanilfeld, Giovanni Battista (b. 1725). Italian physician.

Borsieri's line, or sign. An obsolete term for the blanching produced by stroking the skin in the early stages of scarlet fever.

borsten (bor·sten). A disease occurring in Finland among newly-born infants, characterized by the presence of fever and the appearance of cutis anserina. It is caused by an irritation of the sebaceous glands. [Fin. bristles.]

Borthen, Johan. 19th–20th century Norwegian ophthalmologist.

Borthen's operation. For chronic glaucoma: iridotasis; 2 radial cuts through the iris and sphincter; the tongue so formed is left in the wound.

boss (bos). A round protuberant part as, for instance, on a tumour or a bone. **Parietal boss.** The parietal eminence. *See* EMINENCE. **Sanguineous boss.** 1. Caput succedaneum. 2. A swelling caused by a bruise or blow and containing extravasated blood. [ME *boce* a swelling.]

See also: POTT.

Bossalino's operation. For tarsorrhaphy: the upper and lower lids are split at the grey line; double-armed sutures are passed from the conjunctival surface of the lower lid through the posterior layer out through the split, into the split upper lid, and finally out through the skin of the upper lid and tied.

bosselated (bos·el·a·ted). Covered with small protuberances or nodules, or characterized by their presence. [boss.]

bosselation (bos·el·a·shun). 1. The condition of being or the process of becoming bosselated. 2. A boss or a group of bosses.

Bossi, Luigi Maria (b. 1859). Genoa gynaecologist.

Bossi's dilator. An instrument used to dilate the cervix forcibly.

Bostock, John (b. 1773). Liverpool and London physician.

Bostock's catarrh, or disease. Hay fever. *See* FEVER.

Boston, Leonard Napoleon (b. 1871). Philadelphia physician.

Boston's sign. The jerky and uneven movement downwards of the upper lid when the eye looks downwards, as seen in thyrotoxic exophthalmos.

Boston's vertebral circulation. The blood flow through the vertebral plexus of veins by which malignant cells may travel to metastases.

Boswellia (boz·wel·e·ah). A genus of shrubs and trees of the family Burseraceae. *Boswellia carterii* Birdw. of Arabia and Somaliland yields the oleo-gum-resin olibanum (frankincense). *Boswellia frereana* Birdw. is the source of East African elemi and *Boswellia serrata* Roxb. yields Indian frankincense.

Botallo, Leonardo (b. 1530). Italian surgeon and anatomist in Paris.

Botallo's duct. Ductus arteriosus.

Botallo's foramen. The foramen ovale.

Botallo's ligament. Ligamentum arteriosum.

Botelho, C. Brazilian physician.

Botelho's test. *See* TEST FOR CANCER.

botflies (bot·flize). Flies of the families Oestridae and Gastrophilidae whose larvae, "bots", are internal parasites of mammals.

Species of the genera *Dermatobia*, *Hypoderma* and *Oestrus* of the former family, and *Gastrophilus* of the latter, are of medical interest. [etym. dub.]

Both, E. T. 20th century British engineer.

Both respirator. An artificial respirator somewhat similar to the Drinker, but mainly made of wood.

bothridium (both·rid·e·um). Bothrion.

bothriocephaliasis (both·re·o·kef·al·i'·as·is). Diphyllobothriasis; the condition of being infested with a tapeworm belonging to the genus *Diphyllobothrium.* It is due to the eating of raw or partially-cooked fish. [see foll.]

Bothriocephalus (both·re·o·kef'·al·us). The old generic name of a tapeworm now known as *Diphyllobothrium.* [Gk *bothrion* little trench, *kephale* head.]

bothrioid (both·re·oid). Pitted; covered with small depressions. [Gk *bothrion* little trench, *eidos* form.]

bothrion, bothrium (both·re·on, both·re·um). A sucker shaped like a groove borne by some intestinal worms. [Gk *bothrion* little trench.]

Bothrops (both·rops). The name of a genus of South and Central American poisonous snakes: they include *Bothrops atrox* (the fer-de-lance) and *Bothrops jararacussu.* [Gk *bothros* trench.]

botryoid (bot·re·oid). Having resemblance to a bunch of grapes. [Gk *botrys* cluster of grapes, *eidos* form.]

botryomycome (bot·re·o·mi·ko'·me). Granuloma telangiectaticum. [Gk *botrys* cluster of grapes, *mykes* fungus, *-oma* tumour.]

botryomycosis (bot·re·o·mi·ko'·sis). A Gram-positive staphylococcal granuloma; it must be differentiated from actinomycotic granuloma. Stained granules from pus exudates contain only cocci, whereas granules from actinomycotic granuloma are composed of Gram-positive filaments. [Gk *botrys* cluster of grapes, *mykes* fungus, *-osis* condition.]

botryotherapy (bot·re·o·ther'·ap·e). A type of therapy which consists of a diet of grapes (the grape cure), these being prescribed for every meal, only very small amounts of other foodstuffs being allowed. [Gk *botrys* cluster of grapes, therapy.]

Bottini, Enrico (b. 1837). Pavia surgeon.

Bottini's operation. An endoscopic operation devised some 50 years ago, in which the cautery knife was used to incise the prostatic lobes.

bottle (botl). A narrow-necked vessel, usually made of glass. **Wash bottle.** A glass flask fitted with a cork pierced by 2 glass tubes, from one of which a stream of water can be directed by blowing down the other tube. It is employed in chemical analysis to wash filtered precipitates. [OFr. *bouteille.*]

See also: JUNKER, MARRETT, SENORAN, WOULFE.

bottom (bot·om). **Hottentot bottom.** Steatopyga. **Lightermen's bottom, Weavers' bottom.** Ischial bursitis, a condition of chronic inflammation of the bursa over the ischial tuberosity caused by prolonged pressure of the bone during long spells of sitting on a hard thwart or bench, or of standing at the tiller with the end of the latter pressed against the ischial tuberosity. [AS *botm.*]

botuliform (bot·ew·le·form). Shaped like a sausage. [L *botulus* sausage, form.]

botulin (bot·ew·lin). The toxin produced by *Clostridium botulinum* growing under anaerobic conditions in imperfectly sterilized canned meats, fish or vegetables: a cause of food-poisoning (botulism) in man, occurring especially in the USA, due to consumption of home-canned food, and highly lethal. The toxin is not destroyed by the gastric or intestinal juices. [L *botulus* sausage.]

botulinum toxin (bot·ew·li·num tox·in). A group of powerful bacterial poisons produced by strains of *Clostridium botulinum.* Different types (A, B, C, D and E) produce different toxins.

botulinus (bot·ew·li·nus). *Clostridium botulinum.* [see foll.]

botulism (bot·ew·lizm). A rare and fatal form of food poisoning due to the ingestion of preformed botulinum toxin, usually Type A or B, or, more uncommonly, E, which is found in foods or imperfectly canned and preserved vegetables, meat and fish that had been contaminated by *Clostridium botulinum,* a motile spore-bearing bacillus. The symptoms include vomiting, constipation, ocular pareses, pharyngeal paralysis, thirst and sometimes aphonia. There is no fever, and consciousness remains intact till near the end. Death may occur within 24 h or may be delayed for a week. The disease is an intoxication without bacterial multiplication in the body. The term botulism was formerly used as a synonym of allantiasis, but the latter term is strictly confined to sausage poisoning, whereas botulism may be caused as described above. [L *botulus* sausage.]

bouba (boo·bah). Buba.

Bouchard, Charles Jacques (b. 1837). Paris physician.

Bouchard's disease. Atonic dilatation of the stomach.

Bouchard's node, or nodule. A nodular enlargement of the mid-phalangeal joint described in patients with gastric dilatation, but also found in other conditions.

Bouchardat, Apollinaire (b. 1806). Paris physician, chemist, and hygienist.

Bouchardat's treatment. A dietetic treatment for diabetes, now superseded.

bouche de tapir (boosh de tah·peer). Tapir mouth. As seen in facio-scapulo-humeral muscle-dystrophy. *See* MOUTH. [Fr.]

Boucheron's operation. For blind, painful eyes and as a precaution against sympathetic ophthalmia: cutting of the optic and ciliary nerves behind the globe. Also called *opticociliary neurotomy.* [Obsolete.]

Bouchet, Henri (b. 1873). Cruseilles, Haute-Savoie, physician.

Bouchet's disease. Swineherds' disease; pseudotyphoid meningitis: an acute non-fatal disease affecting pigkeepers and pork dealers. It is due to a virus transmitted from swine to man by the hog louse. It first causes intestinal disorder, followed by a remission period and then meningeal symptoms.

bouchon (boo·shon). An internal clot. [Fr. a cork.]

Bouchut, Jean Antoine Eugene (b. 1818). Paris physician.

Bouchut's method. A method of inserting a tube into the larynx; intubation.

Bouchut's respiration. Respiration in which the inspiratory phase is shorter than the expiratory. It occurs in children with bronchopneumonia, and in asthma.

Bouchut's tubes. A set of intubation tubes of varying size used for the larynx.

Boudin, Jean Christian Marie François Joseph (b. 1806). French army physician.

Boudin's law. Tuberculosis and malaria are mutually antagonistic. Not now accepted.

Bouffard's mycetoma. A mycetoma with black grains which was found in Somaliland. The causative fungus was named *Aspergillus bouffardi* by Brumpt in 1906, but it has never been isolated in culture. **Bouffard's white mycetoma.** *See* MYCETOMA, WHITE.

Bougard, Jean Joseph (b. 1815). Brussels physician.

Bougard's paste. A mixture of poisonous metallic salts massed with starch and flour and used for cancer. [Obsolete.]

bougie (boo·zhe). 1. A solid cylindrical bulb for stretching the urethra or other canal. 2. A medicated pointed rod of cocoa butter or glycogelatin base for application to the urethra, ear or nostril, prepared in the same way as a suppository. **Acorn-tipped bougie.** A bougie with a bulbous tip. **Armed bougie.** A bougie carrying a caustic material at its tip. **Bellied bougie.** A bougie tapering to its tip. **Bougie à boule, Bulbous bougie.** A bougie with a bulbous tip. **Caustic bougie, Cauterizant bougie.** Armed bougie (see above). **Conic bougie.** A bougie with a coned tip. **Cylindrical bougie.** A bougie of uniform diameter throughout its length. **Dilatable bougie.** A bougie whose diameter can be increased by the turning of a screw or by some similar mechanical device. **Ear bougie.** A bougie for use in the external auditory meatus. **Elbowed bougie.** A bougie with an angle near its tip. **Exploring bougie.** A bougie used as a probe. **Filiform bougie.** A slender bougie of whalebone. **Fusiform bougie.** A bougie with an expanded segment in its shaft. **Gum-elastic bougie.** A malleable flexible bougie. **Olive-tipped bougie.** A bougie with a bulbous tip. **Whip bougie.** A bougie with a filiform extension at its tip. [Fr. candle.]

bougienage (boo·zhe·**nahzh**). The operation of dilatation of the urethra with a bougie. **Oesophageal bougienage.** Dilatation of an oesophageal stricture by bougie. [Fr.]

Bouillaud, Jean Baptiste (b. 1796). Paris physician.

Bouillaud's disease, or syndrome. Acute rheumatic carditis.

Bouillaud's tinkle. A clicking noise heard during auscultation at a point just medial to the apex beat in cardiac hypertrophy.

bouillon (boo·**yon**). A nutrient broth prepared from various materials for the growth of micro-organisms. The base for most special variations is nutrient bouillon, which is a soup prepared from the lean meat of animals. There are many bouillons associated with the name of their introducer, with their main constituent or with the organism for which they are most suitable. *See* BROTH. **Ascitic bouillon.** A bouillon containing 5-10 per cent of sterile human ascitic fluid. **Dextrose bouillon.** Sugar bouillon (see below). **Fish bouillon.** A nutrient bouillon in which fish meat has been substituted for animal meat. **Glycerin bouillon.** A nutrient broth containing 6 per cent glycerin. **Glycerin-potato bouillon.** 1000 g of washed, peeled and ground potato soaked in water for 24 h and filtered; 3-5 per cent glycerol is added to the filtrate prior to sterilization. **Lactose-litmus bouillon.** A nutrient bouillon to which has been added 1 per cent lactose, and litmus as indicator. **Litmus bouillon.** A nutrient bouillon to which litmus has been added as an indicator. **Malachite-green bouillon.** A nutrient bouillon to which malachite green has been added in the proportion of 1 per cent of a 1 per cent watery solution. **Malt-extract bouillon.** A medium prepared from malt extract 100 g, water to 1 litre. **Meat-extract bouillon.** A nutrient medium similar to bouillon in which commercial meat extract is substituted for the meat infusion. **Nitrate bouillon.** A nutrient bouillon to which 0.02-0.5 per cent potassium nitrate has been added. **Serum bouillon.** Nutrient bouillon to which sterile serum is added in varying amounts (from 1 to 20 per cent). **Sugar bouillon.** A nutrient bouillon to which has been added 0.5-2 per cent of the desired sugar. [Fr. broth.]

See also: KITASATO, MACCONKEY, REDDISH.

Bouin, Paul (b. 1870). Strasbourg histologist.

Bouin's fluid. An important fixative containing picric acid, acetic acid and formaldehyde.

boulimia (boo·**lim**·e·ah). *See* BULIMIA.

bound (bownd). Held in chemical combination. [AS *bindan* to bind.]

bouquet (boo·**ka**). 1. In anatomy, a number of structures such as blood vessels or fibres grouped together. 2. In synapsis, the junction of collateral branches of central nerve processes with the terminals of the nerve fibres. 3. In clinical medicine, the particular recognizable odour of a disease. [Fr.]

See also: RIOLAN.

bourdonnement (boor·don·**mahn**). The murmur or buzzing sound heard on direct or stethoscopic auscultation at any part of the body and held to be caused by the contracting of muscular fibrils; the term also applies to the subjective sensation of humming which may be experienced in certain conditions. [Fr. a droning.]

Bourgery, Marc-Jean (b. 1797). Paris surgeon and anatomist.

Bourgery's ligament. The oblique posterior ligament of the knee joint.

Bourneville, Désiré-Magloire (b. 1840). French neurologist.

Bourneville's disease. Epiloia or tuberous (tuberose) sclerosis.

Bourquin, Anne (b. 1897). Syracuse, New York, chemist.

Bourquin-Sherman unit. A unit of measurement of riboflavine; now obsolete.

boussarolle (boos·ar·ol). A local name for *pinta.*

bouton (boo·ton). Button. **Bouton de Baghdad, Bouton de Biskra, Bouton d'Orient.** Cutaneous leishmaniasis. **Terminal bouton.** The expanded end of an axon which is applied to the dendrite or cell-body of another neuron to form a synapse. *See* LEISHMANIASIS. [Fr.]

boutonneuse (boo·ton·**erz**). Boutonneuse fever. *See* FEVER. [Fr. *bouton* pustule.]

boutonnière (boo·ton·**yare**). 1. Buttonhole operation. 2. A buttonhole incision into a membrane. [Fr.]

Bouveret, Leon (b. 1850). Lyons physician.

Bouveret's disease. Paroxysmal tachycardia. *See* TACHYCARDIA.

Bouveret's sign. A distended caecum felt in the right iliac fossa in obstruction of the colon.

Bouveret's syndrome. Paroxysmal auricular tachycardia.

Bouveret ulcer, or ulceration. An ulcer above and lateral to the tonsillar region, in typhoid fever.

Bovidae (**bo**·vid·ee). A zoological family of ruminants that includes the sheep. [see foll.]

bovine (**bo**·vine). Belonging to or associated with cattle; caused by the milk from diseased cows, e.g. bovine tuberculosis. [L *bos* ox.]

bovinoid (**bo**·vin·oid). A term descriptive of a tubercle bacillus in human beings which is like the bacillus of bovine tuberculosis. [L *bos* ox, Gk *eidos* form.]

Bovril (bov·ril). An extract of meat that stimulates growth hormone secretion in children and women. A positive response to the Bovril test rules out hypopituitarism but a negative test does not necessarily indicate hypopituitarism.

Bowditch, Henry Pickering (b. 1840). Boston physiologist.

Bowditch's law. In given conditions the force of contraction of cardiac muscle cannot be increased by increasing the strength of the stimulus applied.

bowel (**bow**·el). The intestine: a common colloquial usage. **Loose bowels.** Diarrhoea. [OFr. *boel.*]

Bowen, John Templeton (b. 1857). Boston dermatologist.

Bowen's dermatosis, Bowen's precancerous dermatosis. A precancerous condition of later life consisting of chronic round or oval somewhat papular lesions that form crusts which cover a red oozing papilliferous surface. This is later the site of a carcinoma.

Bowen's disease. A variety of endo-epidermal carcinoma in which dyskeratosis and intracellular vacuolation occur.

Bowen, R. A. London anaesthetist.

Bowen-Jackson laryngoscope blade. A long, curved blade occupying little room in the mouth.

Bowman, Sir William (b. 1816). London ophthalmic surgeon.

Bowman's capsule. Capsule of the malpighian glomerulus. *See* GLOMERULUS.

Bowman's discs. Thin plates into which striated muscle fibres may split after treatment with various reagents, e.g. acids, alkalis, gastric juice; the cleavage occurs at Hensen's line.

Bowman's sarcous elements. An obsolete term for Bowman's discs.

Bowman's glands. Glands in the olfactory mucous membrane.

Bowman's lamina, layer or membrane. Anterior elastic lamina; a thin tough membrane immediately beneath the corneal epithelium.

Bowman's muscle. Meridional fibres of the ciliary muscle.

Bowman's operation. 1. For glaucoma: broad iridectomy by 3 cuts to the iris, 2 at each end of the wound forming the 2 pillars, and finally 1 along the base. 2. For ptosis: resection of a portion of the levator palpebrae superioris muscle with the upper edge of the tarsal plate; performed on the everted lid from the conjunctival surface. Blaskovic's operation is now usually used. 3. For discission of after-cataract: using 2 needles. 4. For conical cornea: iridesis or fixing the iris out through a small incision at the limbus and tying it with a purse-string suture. This acted as a stenopaeic slit and improved the vision, but there was marked risk of sympathetic ophthalmia. Of historical interest.

Bowman's probe. A means of bridging the nasal duct in cases of narrowing or stenosis.

Bowman's lacrimal probe. A double-ended, fine, metal probe, slightly curved and with bulbous ends, designed for passing down the lacrimal passages.

Bowman's theory. Bowman (1842) recognized the fact that the capsules surrounding the glomerular tufts are the extended extremities of the renal tubule. He believed the glomerulus filtered water, but that the solids of the urine were secreted by the cells of the tubules.

Bowman-Mueller capsule. Bowman's capsule (see above).

box (box). A receptacle or case. **Black box.** A method or technique whereby a study is made of the output resulting from a specified input without considering the intermediate phenomena. **Fracture box.** A long open case, without ends, used to support a limb the bone or bones of which have been fractured. **Stockholm box.** An intracavitary radium source used for radiotherapy of gynaecological cancer. [etym. dub.]

See also: ABRAMS, HAMILTON IRVING, MORRIS (H.).

box-note (box·note). In emphysema, the hollow sound in the chest heard on percussion. [etym. dub., OFr. *note*.]

Boyce position. The position of the patient employed for the passage of a bronchoscope. The head is supported on a mechanical head-rest and the shoulders project beyond the end of the operating table sufficiently to allow half the scapula to be unsupported.

Boyce's sign. A gurgling sound heard in cases of oesophageal diverticulum when the hand presses on the side of the neck.

Boyd, John Smith Knox. London bacteriologist.

Boyd's types. *See* SHIGELLA.

Boyden, Edward Allen (b. 1886). Minnesota anatomist.

Boyden meal. A meal for testing the emptying of the gall bladder. The main ingredients are egg yolks added to milk.

Boyer, Alexis, Baron de (b. 1757). Paris surgeon.

Boyer's bursa. A bursa lying between the hyoid bone and the thyrohyoid membrane.

Boyle, Henry Edmund Gaskin (b. 1875). London anaesthetist.

Boyle's apparatus. An apparatus for giving mixtures of nitrous oxide and oxygen, and adding to them ether and chloroform or trichloro-ethylene vapour.

Boyle-Davis gag. A specially designed gag to hold the mouth open in an upside-down position and particularly useful in operations on the pharynx, e.g. in tonsillectomy.

Boyle, Robert (b. 1627). English scientist.

Boyle's law. The volume of a given mass of gas is inversely proportional to the pressure upon it, provided the temperature remains constant. The relationship is only true for a perfect gas.

Boyle's-law apparatus. An apparatus for proving Boyle's law, consisting of a U-tube with limbs of unequal length, the shorter being closed, the longer open. Mercury poured into the long limb encloses a definite mass of gas in the closed limb which is subjected to different pressures by varying the length of the mercury column in the open limb.

Bozeman, Nathan (b. 1825). New York gynaecologist and surgeon.

Bozeman's position. The knee-elbow position (genucubital position) with the patient supported by straps.

Bozeman's speculum. A bivalve vaginal speculum with blades which remain parallel when opened.

Bozeman-Fritsch catheter. A double-channel uterine catheter.

Bozzi, Luigi Maria (b. 1859). Genoa gynaecologist.

Bozzi's foramen. The macula lutea.

brace (brase). Any form of splint or appliance used to support the limbs or trunk. [OFr. *bracier* to embrace.]

See also: HUDSON (W. H.).

bracelet (brase·let). Any one of the transverse lines across the palmar surface of the wrists. [OFr. *bracel* armlet.]

See also: NAGEOTTE.

Brachet, Jean Louis (b. 1789). Lyons physician.

Brachet's mesolateral fold. The right part of the dorsal mesentery of the embryonic foregut, cut off by the development of the upper recess of the lesser sac and containing part of the inferior vena cava.

brachial (bra·ke·al). Referring or relating to the arm; arm-like. **Brachial plexus.** *See* PLEXUS. [Gk *brachion* arm.]

brachial artery [arteria brachialis (NA)]. A continuation of the axillary artery. It begins at the lower margin of the teres major muscle and ends 1.5 cm below the elbow joint, in the cubital fossa, by dividing into the radial and ulnar arteries. **Superficial brachial artery [arteria brachialis superficialis (NA)].** A variant of the brachial artery passing anterior to the median nerve in the arm.

brachial veins [venae brachiales (NA)]. Veins, usually 2, accompanying the brachial artery and draining into the axillary vein.

brachialgia (bra·ke·al·je·ah). Severe pain in the arm or arms, generally neuralgic in character and sometimes proceeding from the region of the brachial plexus. **Brachialgia statica paraesthetica.** Brachial paraesthesia occurring during sleep. [L *brachium* arm, Gk *algos* pain.]

brachialis muscle [musculus brachialis (NA)] (bra·ke·a·lis). A muscle arising from the front of the humerus in its lower half and inserted into the coronoid process of the ulna. It flexes the elbow joint.

brachiform (bra·ke·form). Shaped like an arm, i.e. with elbows or bends. [Gk *brachion* arm, form.]

brachiocephalic (bra·ke·o·kef·al′·ik). Referring to or affecting the arm and the head. [Gk *brachion* arm, *kephale* head.]

brachiocrural (bra·ke·o·kroo′·ral). Relating or referring to the arm and the thigh, or involving them. [Gk *brachion* arm, L *crus* leg.]

brachiocubital (bra·ke·o·kew′·bit·al). Relating or referring to or involving the upper arm and the forearm. [Gk *brachion* arm, L *cubitus* elbow.]

brachiocyllosis (bra·ke·o·sil·o′·sis). 1. Curvature of the arm. 2. The paralysis which is associated with crookedness or curvature of the arm. [Gk *brachion* arm, *kyllosis* a bending.]

brachiocyrtosis (bra·ke·o·ser·to′·sis). Deformity of the arm. [Gk *brachion* arm, *kyrtos* bent.]

brachiofacial (bra·ke·o·fa′·shal). Pertaining to the arm and face. [Gk *brachion* arm, L *facies* face.]

brachiofaciolingual (bra·ke·o·fa·she·o·ling′·gwal). Affecting or relating to the arm, the face and the tongue. [Gk *brachion* arm, L *facies* face, *lingua* tongue.]

brachiogram (bra·ke·o·gram). A record of the arterial pulse from the brachial artery. [Gk *brachion* arm, *gramma* record.]

brachioncus (bra·ke·ong·kus). Any persistent hard swelling of the arm. [Gk *brachion* arm, *ogkos* a swelling.]

brachioradialis muscle [musculus brachioradialis (NA)] (bra·ke·o·ra·de·a′·lis). A superficially placed muscle on the radial side of the forearm. It extends from the lower end of the shaft of the humerus to the lower end of the radius, and is a flexor of the elbow joint, especially when the forearm is in the mid-prone position.

brachiostrophosis (bra·ke·o·stro·fo′·sis). Deformity with twisting of the arm. [Gk *brachion* arm, *strephein* to turn.]

brachiotomy (bra·ke·ot·om·e). 1. Surgical cutting or amputation of an arm. 2. In obstetrics, the section or the cutting off of an arm of the fetus. [Gk *brachion* arm, *temnein* to cut.]

brachiplex (bra·ke·plex). The brachial plexus. [Gk *brachion* arm, L *plexus* braid.]

brachistocephalic, brachistocephalous (brak·is·to·kef·al′·ik, brak·is·to·kef′·al·us). Term applied to a person who has a very short and broad head. [Gk *brachistos* shortness, *kephale* head.]

brachium [NA] (bra·ke·um). 1. The arm as a whole. 2. The upper arm. 3. Any process or structure resembling an arm. **Brachium cerebelli.** One of the cerebellar peduncles. *See* PEDUNCLE. **Brachium cerebri.** The cerebral peduncle. *See* PEDUNCLE. **Brachium copulativum.** The superior cerebellar peduncle. *See* PEDUNCLE. **Brachium of the mid-brain, inferior [brachium colliculi inferioris (NA)].** Fibres of the auditory pathway connecting the inferior quadrigeminal body to the medial geniculate body. **Brachium of the mid-brain, superior [brachium colliculi superioris (NA)].** A band of fibres connecting the optic tract and lateral geniculate body with the superior quadrigeminal body. It contains fibres from the optic radiation and tract. **Brachium opticum.** The connections between the quadrigeminal bodies and the thalamus. [L arm.]

Bracht, Erich Franz Eugen (b. 1882). Berlin pathologist.

Bracht-Waechter body. Focal collections of round cells and polymorphonuclear leucocytes found in the myocardium in subacute bacterial endocarditis; they probably represent miliary abscesses but do not suppurate.

brachybasia (brak·e·**ba**·se·ah). The gait that is seen in certain cases of cerebral haemorrhage, such as bilateral hemiplegia, in which short shuffling steps are taken and progress is slow. [Gk *brachys* short, *basis* a stepping.]

brachycardia (brak·e·**kar**·de·ah). Bradycardia. [Gk *brachys* short, *kardia* heart.]

brachycephalia, brachycephalism (brak·e·kef·**a'**·le·ah, brak·e·**kef**·al·izm). Brachycephaly.

brachycephalic, brachycephalous (brak·e·kef·**al'**·ik, brak·e·**kef'**·al·us). 1. Having a head disproportionately short, with a cephalic index of over 80. 2. An individual with such a head. [see foll.]

brachycephaly (brak·e·**kef**·al·e). The state of having a disproportionately short head. [Gk *brachys* short, *kephale* head.]

Brachycera (brak·e·**seer**·ah). A classificatory division of the insectan order Diptera, used either as a sub-order for all Diptera with a free pupa and, usually, 3 segmented antennae, or as a group in the sub-order Orthorrhapha. The families Stratiomyidae and Tabanidae are of medical interest. [Gk *brachys* short, *keras* horn.]

brachycheilia (brak·e·**ki**·le·ah). The condition of having an abnormally short lip or lips. [Gk *brachys* short, *cheilos* lip.]

brachycheirous (brak·e·**ki**·rus). Descriptive of the condition in which the hands are unusually short. [Gk *brachys* short, *cheir* hand.]

brachychronic (brak·e·**kron**·ik). Acute; term applied to disease. [Gk *brachys* short, *chronos* time.]

brachycnemic (brak·e·**ne**·mik). A term applied to a lower limb when the length below the knee is too short in proportion to that above it; brachyknemic. [Gk *brachys* short, *kneme* leg.]

brachydactylia (brak·e·dak·**til'**·e·ah). A condition in which there are abnormally short fingers or toes. [Gk *brachys* short, *daktylos* finger.]

brachydactylous (brak·e·**dak**·til·us). Referring or relating to brachydactylia.

brachydactyly (brak·e·**dak**·til·e). Brachydactylia.

brachyfacial (brak·e·**fa**·shal). 1. Characterized by having a short broad face; brachyprosopic. 2. Having reference to a broad short face. [Gk *brachys* short, L *facies* face.]

brachyglossal (brak·e·**glos**·al). Descriptive of the condition in which the tongue is abnormally short. [Gk *brachys* short, *glossa* tongue.]

brachygnathia (brak·e·**nath**·e·ah). The condition in which an abnormally short or recessive mandible is present. [Gk *brachys* short, *gnathos* jaw.]

brachygnathous (brak·e·**nath**·us). Having an abnormally short or recessive mandible. [see prec.]

brachykerkic (brak·e·**ker**·kik). Having a forearm that is abnormally short in proportion to the upper arm. [Gk *brachys* short, *kerkis* shuttle.]

brachyknemic (brak·e·**ne**·mik). Brachycnemic.

brachymetapody (brak·e·met·**ap'**·o·de). Shortness of metatarsal and/or metacarpal bones. [Gk *brachys* short, metapodalia.]

brachymetropia (brak·e·met·**ro'**·pe·ah). Myopia. [Gk *brachys* short, *metron* measure, *opsis* sight.]

brachymetropic (brak·e·met·**ro'**·pik). Myopic. [see prec.]

brachymorphic (brak·e·**mor**·fik). Brevilineal; characterized by a stature that is abnormally short and broad. [Gk *brachys* short, *morphe* shape.]

brachyoesophagus (brak·e·e·**sof'**·ag·us). A congenitally short oesophagus with the stomach in the thorax. [Gk *brachys* short, *oisophagos* gullet.]

brachyphalangia (brak·e·fal·**an'**·je·ah). A condition in which a bone of a finger or toe is abnormally short. [Gk *brachys* short, phalanx.]

brachypodous (brak·**ip**·od·us). In biology, short-footed; short-stalked. [Gk *brachys* short, *pous* foot.]

brachyprosopic (brak·e·pro·**so'**·pik). Characterized by the existence of a short broad face. [Gk *brachys* short, *prosopon* face.]

brachyrrhinia (brak·e·**rin**·e·ah). The state in which there is an abnormally short nose. [Gk *brachys* short, *rhis* nose.]

brachyskelic, brachyskelous (brak·e·**skel**·ik, brak·e·**skel**·us). Characterized by having abnormally short legs. [Gk *brachys* short, *skelis* leg.]

brachystaphyline (brak·e·**staf**·il·een). Referring or relating to a palate which is abnormally short. [Gk *brachys* short, *staphyle* palate.]

brachystasis (brak·**is**·tas·is). A condition of muscle fibres in which, while relatively shortened, they nevertheless display normal physiological reactions. [Gk *brachys* short, *stasis* a standing.]

brachytypical (brak·e·**tip**·ik·al). Brachymorphic. [Gk *brachys* short, *typos* mark.]

brachyuranic (brak·e·ewr·**an'**·ik). Referring or relating to an abnormally short and wide palate. [Gk *brachys* short, *ouranos* roof of mouth.]

Brackett, Charles Albert (b. 1850). American dentist.

Brackett's probe. A malleable silver-wire probe used for exploring sinuses and fistulae.

Brackett, Elliott Gray (b. 1860). Boston surgeon.

Brackett's operation. A reconstructive procedure after fracture of the neck of the femur (now obsolete).

Bradford, Edward Hickling (b. 1848). Boston orthopaedic surgeon.

Bradford's frame. A rectangular frame, usually made of metal piping, to which a firm canvas sling is laced, the whole forming a firm splint for the nursing of tuberculosis of the spine.

Bradshaw, Thomas Robert (b. 1857). Liverpool physician.

Bradshaw's albumosuria. Bence-Jones proteinuria.

bradyacousia, bradyacusia (brad·e·ak·**oos'**·e·ah, brad·e·ak·**ew'**·se·ah). Abnormal dullness of hearing. [Gk *bradys* slow, *akouein* to hear.]

bradyaesthesia (brad·e·es·**the'**·ze·ah). General dullness of the intellect with diminution of perceptive sense. [Gk *bradys* slow, aesthesia.]

bradyarrhythmia (brad·e·a·**rith'**·me·ah). A slow abnormal cardiac rhythm. [Gk *bradys* slow, *a*, *rhythmos* rhythm.]

bradyarthria (brad·e·**arth**·re·ah). Bradylalia. [Gk *bradys* slow, *arthroun* to articulate.]

bradyauxesis (brad·e·awx·**e'**·sis). The relative slowness of growth of one part of an organism with respect to the whole, or to another faster-growing part. [Gk *bradys* slow, *auxesis* increase.]

bradycardia (brad·e·**kar**·de·ah). Slowing of the heart rate. **Cardiomuscular bradycardia.** Bradycardia as the result of disease of the cardiac muscle. **Central bradycardia.** That resulting from disease of the central nervous system and from an increase in intracranial pressure. **Essential bradycardia.** Bradycardia occurring without any evidence of organic heart disease. **Nodal bradycardia.** Bradycardia due to control of the heart beat by the atrioventricular node instead of the sinu-atrial node. **Pathological bradycardia.** The bradycardia associated with various diseases, heart block and convalescence from severe fevers. **Physiological bradycardia.** 1. That due to the advancement of age. 2. A form occurring in athletes. 3. Bradycardia present in the puerperal state. 4. Bradycardia which is an individual peculiarity. **Postinfective bradycardia.** That present in convalescence after an infective disease. **Sinus bradycardia.** Slowness of the sinus rhythm resulting from disturbance of the sinu-atrial node. **True bradycardia.** A normal slow action of the heart which may be a familial characteristic. **Vagal bradycardia.** That resulting from abnormal tone of the vagus. [Gk *bradys* slow, *kardia* heart.]

bradycardic (brad·e·**kar**·dik). Characterized by or referring to bradycardia.

bradycinesis (brad·e·sin·**e'**·sis). Bradykinesis.

bradycrotic (brad·e·**krot**·ik). Characterized by or relating to slowness of the pulse. [Gk *bradys* slow, *krotos* pulsation.]

bradydactylia, bradydactyly (**brad**·e·**dak**·**til**'·e·ah, brad·e·**dak**·-til·e). Brachydactylia. [Gk *bradys* slow, *daktylos* finger.]

bradydiastalsis (**brad**·e·di·as·**tal**'·sis). A condition in which the movement of the bowel is delayed or slow. [Gk *bradys* slow, diastalsis.]

bradydiastole (**brad**·e·di·**as**'·tol·e). Prolongation of the diastolic phase beyond normal limits, associated generally with myocardial affections of the heart. [Gk *bradys* slow, diastole.]

bradyecoia (**brad**·e·e·**koi**'·ah). A condition of difficulty in hearing; a moderate degree of deafness. [Gk *bradys* slow, *akouein* to hear.]

bradyglossia (brad·e·**glos**·e·ah). Unusual deliberation in verbal expression; slowness in speech. [Gk *bradys* slow, *glossa* tongue.]

bradykinesis (**brad**·e·kin·e'·sis). 1. Extreme slowness of mental processes and responses; increased reaction time. 2. Abnormal sluggishness of physical movement. [Gk *bradys* slow, kinesis.]

bradykinetic (**brad**·e·kin·**et**'·ik). 1. Referring to or characterized by bradykinesis. 2. Descriptive of a method of studying motor action by taking cinematographic pictures of movement very rapidly and showing them very slowly so that the detail can be seen in slow motion.

bradykinin (brad·e·**ki**·nin). Polypeptides produced by the action of enzymes on protein. They affect capillary permeability and are responsible for some of the manifestations of inflammation. [Gk *bradys* slow, *kinesis* movement.]

bradylalia (brad·e·**la**·le·ah). The slow speech which is the result of a lesion of the central nervous system. [Gk *bradys* slow, *lalein* to babble like a child.]

bradylexia (brad·e·**lex**·e·ah). Reading which is abnormally slow, the reduction in rate not being due to lack of knowledge of the alphabet or to lack of good vision or intelligence. [Gk *bradys* slow, *lexis* word.]

bradylogia (brad·e·**lo**·je·ah). Slowness of speech which is caused essentially by mental impairment. [Gk *bradys* slow, *logos* word.]

bradymetapody (**brad**·e·met·**ap**'·o·de). Brachymetapody. [Gk *bradys* slow, metapodalia.]

bradypepsia (brad·e·**pep**·se·ah). A condition in which the digestive process is abnormally slow or is delayed. [Gk *bradys* slow, *pepsis* digestion.]

bradypeptic (brad·e·**pep**·tik). 1. Referring to or involving bradypepsia. 2. An individual affected with bradypepsia.

bradyphagia (brad·e·**fa**·je·ah). Habitual slowness of eating. [Gk *bradys* slow, *phagein* to eat.]

bradyphalangia (**brad**·e·fal·**an**'·je·ah). Brachydactylia. [Gk *bradys* slow, phalanx.]

bradyphasia, bradyphemia (brad·e·**fa**·ze·ah, brad·e·**fe**·me·ah). Bradylalia. [Gk *bradys* slow, *phasis* speech, *pheme* speech.]

bradyphrasia (brad·e·**fra**·ze·ah). Slow speech based on mental disease. [Gk *bradys* slow, *phrasein* to utter.]

bradyphrenia (brad·e·**fre**·ne·ah). A condition present after epidemic encephalitis, in which psychomotor activity, initiative and interest rapidly flag and the mentality in general is sluggish. [Gk *bradys* slow, *phren* mind.]

bradypnoea (brad·e·**ne**·ah). An abnormally slow rate of breathing. [Gk *bradys* slow, *pnein* to breathe.]

bradypragia, bradypraxia (brad·e·**pra**·je·ah, brad·e·**prax**·e·ah). Sluggishness of action. [Gk *bradys* slow, *prassein* to act.]

bradypsychia (brad·e·**si**·ke·ah). Sluggishness of mental reaction. [Gk *bradys* slow, *psyche* mind.]

bradyrhythmia (brad·e·**rith**·me·ah). Bradycardia. [Gk *bradys* slow, *rhythmos* measured motion.]

bradysphygmia (brad·e·**sfig**·me·ah). Abnormal slowness of the pulse rate. [Gk *bradys* slow, *sphygmos* pulse.]

bradystalsis (brad·e·**stal**·sis). A state in which peristalsis is slowed and the bowel contents thus passed on at a very much reduced rate. [Gk *bradys* slow, *stalsis* contraction.]

bradyteleokinesia, bradyteleokinesis (brad·e·tel·e·o·kin·e'·se·ah, brad·e·**tel**·e·o·kin·e'·sis). A sign of disease of the cerebellum which consists in the sudden and unexpected arrest of a movement as it is about to be normally completed, followed, after a pause, by its slow completion in a jerky fashion. [Gk *bradys* slow, *teleos* end, kinesis.]

bradytocia (brad·e·**to**·se·ah). Abnormally slow parturition. [Gk *bradys* slow, *tokos* childbirth.]

bradytrophia (brad·e·**tro**·fe·ah). A condition in which the processes of metabolism are sluggish. [Gk *bradys* slow, *trophe* nutrition.]

bradytrophic (brad·e·**tro**·fik). Referring to bradytrophia; affected with bradytrophia.

bradyuria (brad·e·**ewr**·e·ah). A condition in which urine is passed very slowly. [Gk *bradys* slow, urine.]

Bragada picta (brag·a·dah **pik**·tah). A blood-sucking bug, the young stages of which are believed to transmit spirochaetal relapsing fever in the East Indies.

Bragard's sign. A sign used to distinguish between a pulled hamstring muscle and sciatica: with the knee extended the hip joint is flexed passively until pain occurs, and the foot is then dorsiflexed; no increase in pain suggests that the disturbance is muscular, while an increase suggests that it is of sciatic origin.

Bragg, Sir William Henry (b. 1862). London physicist.

Bragg curve. Of specific ionization: a graph of the specific ionization, i.e. the number of ions per unit length of path, plotted against the distance travelled by an ionizing particle in standard air. The graph shows an increase near the end of the range of the particle.

Bragg reflection. The phenomenon of reflection of x-rays from a crystalline material, reflection occurring at an angle θ to the crystal surface such that $n\lambda = 2d \sin \theta$, where n is a whole number (the order of the spectrum), λ the wavelength of the x-rays and d the crystal-grating constant.

Bragg-Gray principle. If J is the number of ion pairs per unit volume formed in a gas-filled cavity in an extended medium irradiated by γ rays, and W is the energy required to form an ion pair in the gas, the energy absorption per unit volume in the medium is equal to JWS, where S is the relative stopping power of the medium and the gas for electrons.

Bragg-Paul pulsator. An apparatus consisting of a rubber bag wrapped round the chest wall; by means of a pump the air pressure within the bag is increased and released at a given frequency. It is used to provide artificial respiration in cases of respiratory failure.

Brahmachari, Sir Upendranath (b. 1875). Calcutta physician.

Brahmachari's test. A serum test for visceral leishmaniasis similar to Sia's test.

braidism (**bra**·dizm). Hypnotism. [James *Braid*, 1795–1860, British physician.]

Brailey, William Arthur (b. 1845). London ophthalmologist.

Brailey's operation. For glaucoma: stretching of the supratrochlear nerve [obsolete].

braille (brale). A system of embossed printing or writing for the blind, in which the characters are represented by tangible dots. [Louis *Braille*, 1809–1852, French teacher of the blind; himself sightless.]

Brailsford, James Frederick (b. 1888). Birmingham radiologist.

Brailsford's disease. Osteochondrosis of the epiphysis of the head of the radius.

Brailsford-Morquio disease. Morquio's disease.

Brailsford-Morquio syndrome. Collapse of the 1st lumbar vertebra.

Brain, Lord (Walter Russell) (b. 1895). London neurologist.

Brain's reflex. When a patient with a hemiplegia assumes the "all-fours" position, the flexed paralysed arm extends reflexly. Also called the *quadripedal extensor reflex.*

brain [encephalon (NA)] (brane). The cranial part of the central nervous system which is contained in the cavity of the skull. It consists of 3 primary subdivisions: the forebrain [prosencephalon], from which the cerebral hemispheres and the diencaphalon or between-brain are formed; the mid-brain [mesencephalon), around the aqueduct, and containing the tectum, tegmentum and basis pedunculi; and the hind-brain [rhombencephalon] forming the pons, cerebellum and medulla oblongata. The medulla, pons, mid-brain and diencephalon may together be referred to as the brain stem or brain axis, from which the cerebral hemispheres and cerebellum may be regarded as outgrowths. **Base of the brain.** The inferior surface of the cerebrum. **Cyclopean brain.** An abnormal brain in which the optic rudiments have failed to separate at an early stage of development, giving rise to abnormalities in the optic nerves and olfactory tracts and fusion of the eyes (cyclopia). **Electronic brain.** A name once given to computers on account of their appearing to possess many supposedly rational properties of mind. **Great brain.** The cerebral hemispheres. *See* HEMISPHERE. **Little brain.** The cerebellum. **Brain mantle.** The part of the cerebral hemispheres from which the cerebral cortex or pallium is developed. **Railway brain.** Nervous disturbance following injury in a railway accident; formerly described as traumatic neurasthenia or railway spine. **Smell brain.** The rhinencephalon, or those parts of the brain thought to be concerned functionally with smell. **Walnut brain.** Sclerosis and shrinking of brain tissue, giving the appearance of a walnut. **Wet brain.** Oedema of the brain tissues. [AS *bragen.*]

See also: ROBINSON (F. B.).

brain-scan (**brane**·skan). The demonstration of various intracranial and intracerebral masses by isotope scanning. [AS *bragen,* L *scandere* to climb.]

brain-stones (**brane**·stonz). Dense calcifications which replace tuberculomata in the brain. [AS *bragen, stan.*]

brainsand (**brane**·sand). Small calcified granules found in the pineal body in adult life. [AS *bragen, sand.*]

brainstorm (**brane**·storm). Semi-popular description of paroxysms of nervous disturbance. [AS *bragen, storm.*]

brakeroot (**brake**·root). The dried rhizome and roots of *Polypodium vulgare* (family Polypodiaceae). [ME *braken,* AS *rot.*]

bran (bran). The coat of a cereal grain broken and separated from the meal or flour. [OFr. *bren.*]

branch (brahnsh). 1. [Ramus (NA).] A bifurcation of nerves or blood and lymph vessels from the main stem or trunk. 2. In zoology, a primary division of the animal kingdom. **Communicating branch [ramus communicans (NA)].** 1. A branch connecting a sympathetic ganglion with a spinal nerve. 2. A branch connecting adjacent cranial or spinal nerves. **Communicating branches, grey [rami communicantes (NA)].** Filaments passing from the ganglia on the sympathetic trunk to all spinal nerves, consisting mainly of motor postganglionic non-medullated (hence grey) nerve fibres arising in the cells of the ganglia and distributed to the blood vessels, muscles of the hair and sweat glands along the anterior and posterior primary rami. Accompanying these fibres are a few fine medullated fibres, possibly sensory in nature. **Communicating branches, white [rami communicantes (NA)].** Short nerve filaments passing from the spinal nerve trunks or anterior primary rami from the 1st dorsal to the 2nd lumbar nerves to the corresponding ganglia on the sympathetic trunks, and consisting mostly of medullated (hence white) preganglionic motor fibres. Their cells of origin lie in the lateral column of the corresponding part of the spinal cord and relay in the corresponding or more distant sympathetic ganglia. A single fibre may send branches to several ganglia. White communicating branches also carry sensory fibres passing from blood vessels and viscera to the spinal cord. **Lateral and medial branches of the posterior primary ramus.** *See* SPINAL NERVES. **Muscular branch [ramus muscularis (NA)].** The branch of a nerve to a muscle, carrying efferent impulses to produce muscle contraction and afferent proprioceptive impulses from the muscle. **Recurrent meningeal branch.** *See* OPHTHALMIC ARTERY. **Vascular branch [nervus vascularis (NA)].** A branch of an autonomic nerve that supplies a blood vessel. [Fr. *branche* branch.]

branchia (**brang**·ke·ah). In embryology, the arches and clefts of the fetus. [Gk *bragchia* gills.]

branchial (**brang**·ke·al). Relating to the branchia; having resemblance to gills.

branchiogenic, branchiogenous (**brang**·ke·o·**jen**'·ik, brang·ke·**oj**·en·us). Originating in a branchial arch or cleft. [Gk *bragchia* gills, *genein* to produce.]

branchioma (brang·ke·**o**·mah). A tumour deriving from the remains of a branchial arch or cleft, or occurring in relation to embryonal rests of the branchial organs. [Gk *bragchia* gills, *-oma* tumour.]

branchiomere (**brang**·ke·o·meer). In embryology, the portion of mesodermal tissue which exists between 2 branchial clefts and which gives rise to the visceral arches. [Gk *bragchia* gills, *meros* part.]

branchiomerism (brang·ke·**om**·er·izm). In embryology, the arrangement of the entoderm into branchiomeres.

Brand, Ernst (b. 1827). Stettin physician.

Brand method. A system of baths used in the treatment of typhoid fever. Of historical interest.

Brand, Paul Wilson. British surgeon whose main work was carried out at Vellore, India.

Brand's operation. An operation for alleviation of deformity of leprous hands.

Brandt, Thure (b. 1819). Swedish gynaecologist.

Brandt's method. Expression of pus from a pyosalpinx by massage of the fallopian tubes.

brandy (**bran**·de). An amber-coloured alcoholic liquid distilled from the fermented juice of ripe grapes, and having a characteristic odour and taste. It contains between 48 and 54 per cent of ethyl alcohol. It is sometimes used to treat fainting attacks, which it relieves by stimulating the vasomotor centre in the medulla via the tingling sensation which it produces in the mucous membranes of the mouth. After absorption it causes peripheral vasodilatation which antagonizes this beneficial effect. If prescribed, it should always be diluted with, at least, an equal quantity of water before administration. It is contra-indicated in hepatic and renal disease, in ulceration of the gastro-intestinal tract, in epileptics, in acute infections of the urinary tract or for people who may become addicted to it. [D *branden* to burn.]

Branham, Henry H. 19th century American physician.

Branham's phenomenon, or sign. Compression of the artery supplying an arteriovenous aneurysm causing a slowing of the pulse, a rise in diastolic blood pressure and disappearance or diminution of the murmur.

Braquehaye, Jules Pic Louis (b. 1865). French surgeon.

Braquehaye's operation. An operation for vesicovaginal fistula by freshening and invaginating the mucous membrane of the bladder and vagina.

Brasdor, Pierre (b. 1721). Paris surgeon.

Brasdor's operation. Distal ligation for aneurysm.

brash (brash). Any disorder of the digestive system, with a burning sensation in the oesophagus. **Water brash.** An acid eructation. **Weaning brash.** Infantile diarrhoea occurring during the weaning period. [Dan. *braaken* to vomit.]

Brassica (**bras**·ik·ah). A genus of the Cruciferae including the cabbage, turnip and mustard. The seeds of *Brassica alba* Boissier (white mustard) and *Brassica nigra* Koch. (black mustard) are both used for the preparation of bath mustard, mustard flour and mustard bran. The seeds of *Brassica nigra* are the source of volatile oil of mustard (Oleum Sinapis Volatile BPC 1949), and Expressed Mustard Oil BPC 1954. The seeds of *Brassica napus* var. *oleifera* Linn. and certain other species yield Rape Oil BPC 1954. *Brassica juncea* Hooker and Thoms, cultivated in Russia and India, yields Indian mustard. [L cabbage.]

brassy-eye (bras·e·i). Chalkitis; an inflammatory condition of the eyes which may occur after they have been rubbed with fingers that have been handling brass. [AS *braes, eage.*]

Bratton, Andrew Calvin (b. 1912). Baltimore pathologist.

Bratton and Marshall method. For sulphonamides in blood and urine: blood is deproteinized with trichloro-acetic acid and the filtrate treated successively with sodium nitrite, ammonium sulphamate (to destroy excess nitrite) and *N*-(1-naphthyl)-ethylenediamine dihydrochloride. The red colour produced is compared with standards: this gives free sulphonamide. Total sulphonamide is determined similarly after hydrolysis of the blood filtrate by heating with hydrochloric acid in boiling water for 1 h. Urine is diluted 1 to 25 and the dilution treated in the same way as blood.

Brauer, Ludolph (b. 1865). Hamburg physician.

Brauer's method. The use of nitrogen instead of air in the production of artificial pneumothorax, on account of its slower absorption.

Brauer's operation. Removal of ribs and costal cartilages to relax an adherent pericardium.

Braun, Christopher Heinrich (b. 1847). German physician.

Braun's test. A test for glucose in urine based on the reduction of yellow picric acid to red picramic acid when the urine is boiled with picric acid and potassium hydroxide. Also known as *Johnson's test.*

Braun, Gustav August von (b. 1829). Austrian gynaecologist.

Braun's hook. An instrument designed for decapitation of the fetus.

Braun, Heinrich (b. 1847). German surgeon.

Braun's anastomosis. In gastro-enterostomy, an anastomosis formed between the afferent and the efferent intestinal loops.

Roser-Braun sign. Absence of pulsation of the dura mater; a sign of underlying tumour, abscess or cyst.

Braun, Heinrich Friedrich Wilhelm (b. 1862). German surgeon.

Braun's frame. A metal frame for fractures of the femur or of the tibia and fibula.

Braun's splanchnic block. Infiltration of the coeliac or splanchnic sympathetic plexus with local analgesic solution from the anterior approach.

Braun, Maximilian Gustav Christian Carl (b. 1850). Prussian anatomist and zoologist.

Braun's canal. The archenteric canal.

Braun's cord. One of the columns of cells composing the embryonic kidney.

Braune, Christian Wilhelm (b. 1831). Leipzig anatomist.

Braune's canal. The uterine cavity and vagina at full dilatation of the cervix.

Braune's muscle. The puborectalis muscle.

Braune's valvule. A small epithelial fold found at the level of the cardiac sphincter and believed to act independently of it.

Braunia jassyensis (braw·ne·ah yas·e·en·sis). A small tapeworm of the family Diphyllobothriidae, rarely parasitic in man.

Braunitzer, Gerhard. German protein chemist.

Braunitzer gap. A space introduced into the amino acid sequence of a protein to increase the degree of similarity between it and related proteins.

Bravais, L. F. (fl. 1827). French physician.

Bravais-Jackson epilepsy. Jacksonian epilepsy; epilepsy beginning unilaterally with clonic muscular contractions limited to one limb or portion of a limb or of the face, sometimes spreading to other structures on the same side, but without loss of consciousness unless the attack becomes generalized.

Braxton Hicks, John (b. 1825). London obstetrician.

Braxton Hicks' contractions, or sign. Irregular, painless contractions of the uterus during pregnancy, stronger and more frequent towards term when the woman may be aware of them. Dilatation of the cervix does not occur.

Braxton Hicks' version. Bipolar version in which the breech is made to present; a method of treatment for placenta praevia.

Bray, Charles William (b. 1904). Princeton psychologist.

Wever-Bray phenomenon. When sounds fall upon the ear, the auditory nerve shows changes of potential directly and closely related to the incident sound.

Brayera (bra·e·rah). A genus of the family Rosaceae. ***Brayera anthelmintica*** Kunth. yields Cusso BPC 1949.

brayerin (bra·e·rin). $C_{31}H_{38}O_{10}$. The active principle of *Brayera anthelmintica* Kunth. used in the treatment of tapeworm.

bread (bred). An article of food made from different kinds of flour mixed with water and kneaded, with or without the addition of yeast, and baked. **Brown bread.** A vague term indicating only that the loaf has a brown colour. This may have been produced by making the bread from wholemeal flour, that is flour from which the pericarp (bran) and germ have not been extracted, or from flour to which these substances have been added. Such bread is richer in vitamins and minerals. Graham wholemeal and wheatmeal breads are usually considered to be brown bread. **Bread crumb.** The inner part of the loaf; it is used as a pharmaceutical vehicle, especially as a mass for pills. **Diabetic bread.** That made of flour with the least possible quantity of carbohydrate. **Enriched bread.** White or other bread to which has been added nicotinic acid, aneurine hydrochloride and iron or other vitaminic preparations or minerals in order to increase its nutritive qualities. **Geril bread.** A bread prescribed in diabetes mellitus and constipation; it contains 7½ per cent of protein and 9½ per cent of reducing sugar. **Pulled bread.** Bread pulled apart longitudinally when freshly baked and rebaked so that it becomes brittle. **Wheatmeal bread.** Bread made from flour that has undergone about 85 per cent extraction. The percentage is not constant and the distinction from wholemeal is arbitrary. **White bread.** That made with grain from which all the bran and germ have been removed before it is ground, so that it has lost much of the vitamins and minerals. **Wholemeal bread.** Bread made with flour which has undergone only about 92 per cent extraction. [AS.]

See also: GRAHAM (S.).

breadth-feeling (bredth·feel·ing). In vision, the perception of lateral extension. [AS *braedu, felan.*]

break (brake). 1. In surgery, a fracture. 2. The interruption of an electric current. Cf. MAKE. **Break shock.** In electrotherapeutics, the shock produced when the electric current passing through the body is broken or opened. [AS *brecan.*]

breast (brest). 1. [Pectus (NA).] The anterior aspect or surface of the thorax. 2. [Mamma (NA).] The mammary gland; the accessory organ of the female reproductive system concerned with lactation. It consists of glandular tissue [corpus mammae (NA)] covered with a fatty layer. **Broken breast.** A mammary abscess. **Caked breast.** Stagnation mastitis. *See* MASTITIS. **Chicken breast.** Pigeon breast (see below). **Cystic breast.** Chronic cystic mastitis. *See* MASTITIS. **Funnel breast.** A deformity of the lower part of the thorax caused by backward displacement of the xiphoid process. **Gathered breast.** Broken breast (see above). **Hysterical breast.** Enlargement of and severe pain in the breast due to hysteria. **Irritable breast.** Neuralgic pain affecting the mammary gland, as a rule occurring in association with intercostal neuralgia or with some abnormal state of the uterus. **Keeled breast.** Pigeon breast (see following). **Pigeon breast.** A condition of abnormal prominence of the sternum caused either by rickets or some obstruction to the breathing in infants (pectus carinatum). **Proemial breast.** The condition of the female breast which foreshadows the appearance of pathological changes. **Shoemakers' breast.** A backward displacement of the lower part of the thorax caused by pressure of tools against the sternum and xiphoid process. **Shotty breast.** Schimmelbusch's disease. **Supernumerary breast.** Polymastia. **Thrush breast.** In fatty degeneration of the heart, the speckling of the myocardium. [AS *braest.*]

breastings (brest·ings). Colostrum. [see prec.]

breath (breth). The air inhaled or exhaled in respiration. **Lead breath, Saturnine breath.** The sweet-smelling metallic breath which is characteristic of lead poisoning. [see foll.]

breathing (bre·thing). For definition and types of breathing not given below, *see* RESPIRATION. **Abdominal breathing.** Breathing in which full use of the diaphragm is made. **Assisted breathing.** Augmentation of spontaneous inspiration. **Bronchial breathing.** During auscultation, a blowing sound in which the inspiratory and expiratory notes are about equal in duration and pitch, and distinctly divided. The sound is normally heard over the trachea, but elsewhere it suggests lung consolidation. **Controlled breathing.** Reversible abolition of spontaneous respiration, used in anaesthesia. **Glossopharyngeal breathing.** GPB, a method of breathing or gulping air that has been adopted spontaneously by some patients with weakness of the respiratory muscles, and has been taught to others. It often allows a paralysed person to dispense with the respirator. **Luxus breathing.** Breathing in excess of that required by the system. **Mouth breathing.** The habit of breathing through the mouth instead of through the nose. **Mouth-to-mouth breathing.** Expired air resuscitation. **Paradoxical breathing.** Inflation of part of the lung during expiratory chest movements and deflation during inspiratory. *Internal paradoxical breathing* may be seen in the spontaneously breathing patient who has an open chest or severe damage to the rib cage; the lung on the affected side expands during expiration and collapses during inspiration. *External paradoxical breathing* is due to very deep general anaesthesia or respiratory obstruction; during spontaneous respiration the abdomen and the chest move synchronously. **Periodic breathing.** Cheyne–Stokes phenomenon. **Pressure breathing.** The breathing of air or other mixture of gases at pressures higher than ambient atmospheric pressure. The gas is delivered through a tight-fitting mask. To prevent overdistension of the lungs, counter-pressure is made on the thorax and abdomen by a waistcoat or jerkin containing an airtight bladder. It is one method of maintaining adequate alveolar oxygen tension at altitudes in excess of 12 000 m (40 000 ft). **Suppressed breathing.** That which is carried on with complete absence of breath-sounds as in pleural effusion and in consolidation of the lung. **Thoracic breathing.** That in which chest movements predominate. **Transitional breathing.** Vesiculobronchial breathing (see below). **Vesicular breathing.** The respiratory sounds heard normally over healthy air-containing lung. The inspiratory sound has a rustling character and a relatively low pitch; it is audible during the whole of the inspiratory phase. The expiratory sound follows the inspiratory without a pause, is less intense and has lost the rustling character. It is audible only during the first half of the expiratory phase or less. **Vesiculobronchial breathing.** Breathing intermediate between vesicular and bronchial breathing, and containing elements of both, the vesicular element predominating over the bronchial. It is heard over areas where the main bronchi are separated from the surface by air-containing lung or over areas of small or incomplete consolidation. [AS *braeth.*]

See also: BIOT, GRANCHER, KUSSMAUL.

Breda, Achille (b. 1850). Padua dermatologist.

Breda's disease. A name variously attributed to yaws and espundia.

bredouillement (bred·we·**mahn**). A defect in speaking in which the utterance is rapid and thick so that only a part of each word is pronounced. [Fr. spluttering.]

breech (breech). The buttocks. **Frank breech.** Frank breech presentation. *See* PRESENTATION. [ME *brech.*]

breeze (breez). A steady movement of air. **Electric breeze.** Static breeze (see below). **Head breeze.** A static electric breeze applied to the scalp by means of a series of parallel rods attached at right angles to a plate electrode (in the form of a hair-brush). **Static breeze.** In therapeutics, a current of electrified air which can be directed to any particular area. It is set in motion by the discharge from a static electricity machine. [OSp. *briza* NE wind.]

bregma (**breg**·mah). In craniometry, the meeting point on the surface of the skull of the sagittal and coronal sutures. [Gk front of the head.]

bregmatic (breg·**mat**·ik). Referring to the bregma or the region of the bregma.

bregmatodymia (**breg**·mat·o·**di**′·me·ah). A monster consisting of twins joined together at the bregmas. [bregma, Gk *didymos* twin.]

Brehmer, Gustav Adolf Robert Herman (b. 1826). German physician.

Brehmer's method, or treatment. The employment of open-air treatment at moderate altitudes, 900–1200 m (3000–4000 ft) elevation, in cases of tuberculosis unsuitable for higher altitudes.

brei (bri). Pulped tissue. [G.]

Breisky, August (b. 1832). German gynaecologist.

Breisky's disease. A pseudonym for kraurosis vulvae, a condition characterized by atrophy of the skin of the vulva and contracture of the introitus.

Breisky's method. A method to determine the anterior-posterior diameter of the pelvic outlet.

Bremsstrahlung (brem·**shtrah**·lung). The electromagnetic radiation resulting from the retardation of charged particles. [G braking radiation.]

Brenner, Alexander (b. 1859). Austrian physician.

Brenner's operation. An operation for inguinal hernia.

Brenner, Fritz (b. 1887). German pathologist.

Brenner tumour. An ovarian tumour described by Brenner as *oöphoroma folliculare.* The tumour is seen histologically to consist of islands of cells resembling stratified epithelium embedded in a fibrous tissue stroma. The cells immediately around the epithelial islands may show the characters of thecal cells and an occasional tumour secretes oestrin. Generally benign but a malignant form does occur rarely.

brenzcatechinuria (**brentz**·kat·ek·in·**ewr**′·e·ah). Pyrocatechinuria; the excretion in the urine of pyrocatechin (catechol), a dihydroxybenzene used in medicine as an antipyretic. [brenzcatechin (pyrocatechin), Gk *ouron* urine.]

brephic (**bref**·ik). Referring to a very early stage of fetal development. [Gk *brephos* embryo.]

brephoplastic (bref·o·**plas**·tik). Formed during embryonic life or from embryonic tissue. [Gk *brephos* embryo, *plassein* to form.]

brephotrophic (bref·o·**trof**·ik). Referring to the nutrition of infants. [Gk *brephos* infant, *trophe* nutrition.]

Breschet, Gilbert (b. 1784). Paris anatomist.

Breschet's bones. Suprasternal bones.

Breschet's canal, or vein. A diploic vein.

Breschet's helicotrema, or hiatus. Communication between the scala vestibuli and scala tympani at the apex of the modiolus.

Breschet's sinus. The sphenoparietal sinus.

Bretonneau, Pierre Fidèle (b. 1778). French physician.

Bretonneau's angina, diphtheria or disease. Diphtheria (of the pharynx), first recognized as a separate entity by Bretonneau in 1821.

Bretylium Tosylate (bret·**il**·e·um **tos**·il·ate). BP Commission approved name for *N*-*o*-bromobenzyl-*N*-ethyl-*NN*-dimethylammonium tosylate; it is used in the treatment of hypertension.

Breuer, Josef (b. 1842). Vienna psychiatrist.

Hering-Breuer reflex. A reflex regulating respiration, the act of inspiration reflexly exciting expiration, and vice versa.

Breus, Carl (b. 1852). Austrian obstetrician.

Breus' mole. Aborted products of conception characterized by haematomata beneath the amnion lining the fetal surface of the placenta, an avascular chorion and an embryo smaller than it should be for the period of gestation. Also called *carneous* or *blood mole.*

brevicollis (brev·e·**kol**·is). Shortness of the neck. Cf. DYSTROPHIA BREVICOLLIS. [L *brevis* short, *collum* neck.]

breviductor (brev·e·**duk**·tor). The adductor brevis muscle of the lower limb. [L *brevis* short, *ductor* leader.]

breviflexor (brev·e·**flex**·or). Term applied to all muscles which are short and have a flexor action. [L *brevis* short, *flexor* bender.]

brevilineal (brev·e·**lin**·e·al). Brachymorphic; characterized by a stature that is abnormally short and broad. [L *brevis* short, *linea* line.]

breviradiate (brev·e·**ra**·de·ate). A term descriptive of a particular type of neuroglia cell the elongated processes of which are short. [L *brevis* short, *radiare* to emit rays.]

Brewer, George Emerson (b. 1861). New York surgeon.

Brewer's point. An area of tenderness over the costovertebral angle of the lowest ribs, pressure upon which elicits tenderness in some cases of renal disease.

Brewer, John H. 20th century Baltimore bacteriologist.

Brewer's thioglycollate medium. A liquid medium for the

culture of anaerobic organisms; the thioglycollate gives reducing conditions suitable for the growth of anaerobes. Prepared from nutrient broth to which are added pork infusion solids 1 per cent, peptone 1 per cent, sodium chloride 0.5 per cent, sodium thioglycollate 0.1 per cent, agar 0.05 per cent, dextrose 1 per cent and methylene blue 0.0002 per cent.

Brewer's thioglycollate serum medium. Thioglycollate medium with 10 per cent serum, for the growth of treponemata.

Brewster, Sir David (b. 1781). British physicist.

Brewster's law. In reflection from a medium such as glass, in which light is polarized, the tangent of the angle of polarization equals the refractive index of the medium.

Briareus (bri·a·re·us). A generic name for a group of viruses, used in the USA but not generally accepted in Great Britain. The group includes the causal viruses of measles (*Briareus morbillorum*), varicella (*Briareus varicellae*) and herpes zoster. [Gk *briaros* strong.]

Bricker, Eugene. American surgeon.

Bricker procedure. Pelvic clearance, including total cystectomy, using an ileal loop conduit.

Brickner, Richard Max (b. 1896). New York neurologist.

Brickner's sign. In facial paresis, diminution of oculo-auricular associated movements.

bridge (brij). 1. The pons. 2. An appliance, either attached to or abutting on natural teeth, which replaces missing teeth in function and resembles them in appearance; bridgework. **Arteriolovenular bridge.** The main capillary interposing between an arteriole and a venule. **Cell bridge.** Cement substance between each cell. **Cytoplasmic bridge.** The strip of protoplasm which holds together 2 blastomeres. **Fixed bridge.** A bridge which is fixed permanently by inlays or crowns to the adjacent teeth. **Intercellular bridge.** Cell bridge (see above). **Jugal bridge.** The zygomatic arch. *See* ARCH. **Kidney bridge.** A device used on an operating table for the lateral flexion of the vertebral column to facilitate the surgeon's exposure of the kidney. **Bridge of the nose.** *See* NOSE. **Removable bridge.** A bridge which can be removed and replaced by the wearer. [AS *brycg.*]

See also: GASKELL, VAROLIO, WHEATSTONE.

Bridges, James Winfred (b. 1885). Montreal psychiatrist.

Yerkes-Bridges test. A revision of the Binet-Simon test.

Bridgett's line. A surface marking of the facial nerve as traced on the mastoid bone.

bridgework (brij·werk). In dentistry, the same as bridge. [AS *brycg, wyrcan.*]

bridle (bri·dl). 1. In anatomy, a frenum. 2. A fibrous band or loop across the surface of an ulcer or other lesion. 3. A ligament or membranous fold forming an abnormal adhesion. [AS *bridel.*]

bridou (bre·doo). Perlèche. [Fr. *bride* frenum.]

Brieger, Ludwig (b. 1849). Berlin physician.

Brieger's cachexia reaction. An increase in the antitryptic power of the blood which is said to occur in malignant and other cachexias.

Bright, Richard (b. 1789). English physician.

Bright's blindness. Rapid loss of sight, going on to complete blindness, occurring in some cases of approaching uraemia and of cortical origin. Recovery is possible if the uraemia is abated.

Bright's disease. Nephritis.

Bright's granulation. The granular surface of the kidney in chronic nephritis.

Bright's murmur, or friction sound, Beatty-Bright friction sound. A creaking noise produced by 2 dry surfaces rubbing together. It is heard in dry pleurisy and pericarditis.

Brill, Nathan Edwin (b. 1860). New York physician.

Brill's disease. A form of typhus fever occurring in the USA, possibly a recrudescence of latent typhus, in immigrants from countries in which epidemic typhus is or was prevalent. The causal organism is indistinguishable from *Rickettsia prowazeki.*

follicular lymphoblastoma of Brill. Giant follicular lymphadenopathy. *See* LYMPHADENOPATHY.

Brill-Symmers' disease. Giant follicular reticulosis. *See* RETICULOSIS.

Brill-Zinsser disease. Sporadic recurrence of typhus in a previously affected individual.

brim (brim). The rim or margin of a structure. **Brim of the pelvis.** The inlet of the pelvis. [ME edge.]

brimstone (brim·stone). An old name for sulphur. [AS *brinnan* to burn, *stan.*]

Brinton, William (b. 1823). English physician.

Brinton's disease. Diffuse hypertrophy of the submucous coat of the stomach; leather-bottle stomach.

Brion, Albert (b. 1874). Strasbourg physician.

Brion-Kayser disease. Paratyphoid fever. *See* FEVER.

Briquet, Paul (b. 1796). French physician.

Briquet's syndrome. Dyspnoea and sometimes aphonia as a result of hysterical diaphragmatic paralysis.

brisement (breez·mahn). The breaking up, e.g. of adhesions in ankylosis. **Brisement forcé.** The forcible breaking up of a bony ankylosis. [Fr. a breaking.]

Brissaud, Edouard (b. 1852). Paris neurologist.

Brissaud's disease. Tic; habit spasm.

Brissaud's reflex. Contraction of the tensor fasciae latea muscle on stroking the sole of the foot; part of the extensor plantar response.

Brissaud-Marie sign, or syndrome. Unilateral spasm of lips and tongue due to hysteria.

Bristowe, John Syer (b. 1827). London physician.

Bristowe's syndrome. A complex of symptoms and signs which is said to be pathognomonic of a tumour of the corpus callosum: slow insidious onset of hemiplegia, frank hemiplegia on one side, often with a contralateral hemiparesis, drowsiness, apathy, stupidity, often with dysphasia and/or apraxia, absence of cranial nerve signs, terminal coma.

Britannia metal (brit·an·e·ah met·al). An alloy made of tin (80 per cent), antimony (10 per cent); the rest copper, zinc, bismuth and lead. It is used for metalware and utensils. [Gk *Brettania, metallon* mine.]

British anti-lewisite (brit·ish ante·loo·is·ite). BAL, 2,3-dimercaptopropanol, $CH_2SHCHSHCH_2OH$, Dimercaprol BP 1958. An antidote for the war gas lewisite. It is also of value an antidote in cases of poisoning by the compounds of other metals such as mercury, in addition to arsenic and copper.

Brittain, Herbert Alfred (b. 1904). Norwich orthopaedic surgeon.

Brittain's ischiofemoral graft, or operation. A bone graft placed between the ischium and the upper end of the femur for the purpose of extra-articular arthrodesis of the hip.

broach (bro·ch). A fine, pliable piece of steel used for instrumentation in the root canals of the teeth. **Barbed broach.** A broach with fine barbs, used for removing the contents of a root canal; also known as *Donaldson's broach.* **Smooth broach.** A broach used for exploring a root canal. [OFr. *broche.*]

See also: DONALDSON.

Broadbent, Walter (b. 1868). Brighton physician.

Broadbent's sign. Retraction of the posterolateral chest wall in the region of the 11th and 12th ribs and intercostal spaces on the left side during cardiac systole, due to fixation of the visceral pericardium to the diaphragm as a result of adhesive pericarditis.

Broadbent, Sir William Henry (b. 1835). English physician.

Broadbent's inverted sign. Pulsations over the left posterolateral chest wall synchronous with ventricular systole, said to occur in aneurysmal dilatation of the left auricle. These pulsation are probably due to left ventricular hypertrophy (which occurs in mitral incompetence) rather than to the aneurysmal left auricle. The aneurysmal left auricle itself may produce pulsation to the right of the sternum, and dullness to percussion at the base of the right lung.

Broca, Pierre Paul (b. 1824). Paris surgeon and anthropologist.

Broca's angle. The angle between the nasobasilar line and the plane of the foramen magnum.

Broca's aphasia. Motor aphasia. *See* APHASIA.
Broca's area. The posterior part of the 3rd frontal convolution, a lesion of which causes motor aphasia.
band of Broca. Diagonal band; a strip of white matter running diagonally across the anterior perforated substance of the brain, connecting the paraterminal body to the uncus.
Broca's centre. The motor speech centre.
Broca's convolution, or gyrus. The inferior frontal gyrus. *See* GYRUS.
Broca's fissure. The fissure surrounding Broca's convolution.
alveolocondyloid plane of Broca. A plane through the alveolar point and the line tangential to the lower surfaces of the occipital condyles; alveolocondylear plane. Used in anthropology.
Broca's point. The mid-point of the external auditory meatus lying on Reid's base line.
Broca's pouch. A pocket-like cavity said to occur in the tissues of the labia majora.
Broca's region. Broca's convolution (see above).
Broca's space. An ependymal space within the olfactory bulb, common in lower vertebrates, rare in man.

Brock, Lord (Russell Claude) (b. 1903). London surgeon.
Brock's operation. Closed transventricular pulmonary valvotomy and infundibular resection used for the relief of isolated pulmonary valve stenosis and the palliation of Fallot's tetralogy.

Brockman, Edward Phillimore. London orthopaedic surgeon.
Brockman's club-foot operation. Operative correction of club-foot by incision of all the tight soft tissues on the inner and under surfaces of the midtarsal joint.

Brocq, Louis Anne Jean (b. 1856). French dermatologist.
Brocq's disease. 1. Parapsoriasis en plaques. 2. Pseudopélade.
Brocq's eczema. Ringworm of the feet.
Brocq's erythrose peribuccale pigmentaire. A diffuse pigmentation of the face probably caused by a photodynamic substance in a cosmetic.
Brocq's geometric phagadena. Pyoderma gangraenosum.
Brocq's method. Of grattage: an aid to the diagnosis of various skin lesions, particularly psoriasis, by noting the changes produced by scratching their surface.
Duhring-Brocq disease. Dermatitis herpetiformis.
angiolupoid of Brocq and Pautrier. A cutaneous sarcoid of the Boeck type, characterized by bluish-red, round and oval nodules and plaques about ½-2 cm in diameter. The lesions are few in number and occur especially on the upper parts of the sides of the nose, near the inner canthi of the eyes, and on the cheeks adjacent to these parts.
Wilson-Brocq disease. Dermatitis exfoliativa.

Brocresine (bro·kres·een). BP Commission approved name for *O*-(4-bromo-3-hydroxybenzyl)hydroxylamine; a histidine decarboxylase inhibitor.

Brödel, Max (b. 1870). Baltimore medical artist.
Brödel's bloodless line. A linear area around the convex border of the kidney which is said to lie between the areas supplied by the anterior and posterior branches of the renal arteries. In fact, there is considerable overlap and the line is by no means bloodless.

Broders, Albert Compton (b. 1885). Minnesota pathologist.
Broders' grading, or index. A grading of malignant tumours according to the percentage of undifferentiated cells present in representative microscopical fields, e.g. Grade I tumours show fields with 25 per cent undifferentiated cells; Grade IV tumours are composed of completely undifferentiated cells.

Brodie, Sir Benjamin Collins (b. 1783). London surgeon.
Brodie's abscess, or circumscribed abscess of bone. A chronic bone abscess with acute exacerbations, caused by continuing staphylococcal infection, usually of the head of the tibia.
Brodie's bursa. The bursa of the semimembranosus tendon; the bursa between the semimembranous and the medial head of the gastrocnemius.
Brodie's disease. First described in 1818, a polyarthritis often based on venereal infection (*see* REITER'S DISEASE). The typical triad of conjunctivitis, urethritis and arthritis is not always present. It may follow dysentery.
Brodie's sign. Ominous gangrenous patches on the penis associated with the fulminating infections of urinary extravasation.
Brodie's tumour. Giant cystadenoma of the breast.
Brodie-Trendelenburg test. A test to determine the integrity of the saphenous and deep veins of the lower limb. The subject lies recumbent, and the leg is elevated to drain the venous blood. Pressure is applied over the upper part of the saphenous vein in order to occlude it, then the patient stands up, and the pressure is released suddenly. The procedure is repeated, but pressure is maintained for 35 s. The test is positive, and indicates incompetence of the valve of the deep saphenous vein, if the veins (or varices) fill rapidly when pressure is released as soon as the patient stands, fill slowly when the pressure is maintained and are not fully distended at the end of 35 s. The test is negative if they fill slowly when the pressure is maintained, and do not fill more rapidly when it is immediately released.

Brodie, Charles Gordon (b. 1860). London surgeon.
Brodie's ligament. Transverse humeral ligament, that portion of the capsule of the shoulder joint beneath which the long tendon of the biceps emerges to enter the bicipital groove.

Brodie, Thomas Gregor (b. 1866). London physiologist.
Brodie reaction. The fall in blood pressure induced in cats by doses of foreign proteins that are too small to affect other animals such as rabbits and guinea-pigs.

Brodmann, Korbinian (b. 1868). German anatomist.
Brodmann's areas. Forty-seven subdivisions of the cerebral cortex, differentiated by Brodmann on cyto-architectural grounds and assumed to subserve different functions. The most important are: *Areas* 1, 2 *and* 3. Sensory area, postcentral area of the cerebral cortex. *See* AREA. *Area* 4. Motor area, precentral area, pyramidal area. *See* AREA. *Area* 5. *See* AREA, SOMAESTHETOPSYCHIC and AREA, EXTRAPYRAMIDAL MOTOR. *Area* 6. Premotor area. *See* AREA, EXTRAPYRAMIDAL MOTOR. *Area* 7. *See* AREA, SOMAESTHETOPSYCHIC *Area* 8. The oculomotor area. *See* AREA. *Area* 9. An area on the lateral surface of the prefrontal region of the frontal cortex extending on to the medial surface. It occupies the anterior part of the superior frontal gyrus and the middle part of the middle frontal gyrus. *Area* 10. An area on the lateral surface of the prefrontal region of the frontal cortex extending on to the medial surface. It occupies the anterior part of the middle frontal gyrus. *Area* 17. *See* CORTEX, CALCARINE. *Area* 18. Parastriate area. *See* AREA. *Area* 19. Peristriate area. *See* AREA. *Area* 22. Auditopsychic area. *See* AREA. *Area* 24. This occupies the anterior half of the gyrus cinguli. It is believed by some that the benefits of prefrontal lobotomy are due to destruction of the connections of this area. *Areas* 41 *and* 42. Auditosensory area. *See* AREA. *Areas* 44 *and* 45. Motor speech area, Broca's area.

Broesike, Gustave (b. 1853). Berlin anatomist.
Broesike's fossa. A parajejunal peritoneal fossa which is infrequently found.

Brofezil (bro·fe·zil). BP Commission approved name for 2-(4-*p*-bromophenylthiazol-2-yl)propionic acid; an anti-inflammatory agent.

Broglie, Louis Victor de (b. 1892). French physicist.
de Broglie wavelength. The wavelength, λ, associated with the motion of a particle of mass m with a velocity v, given by $\lambda = h/mv$, where h is Planck's constant. The properties of matter, such as particle scattering, can be theoretically derived by the assumption of a "wave" nature of matter.

bromacetone (brom·as·e·tone). Bromo-acetone, acetylbromomethane, $BrCH_2COCH_3$. A colourless volatile liquid, toxic and lacrimatory; used in chemical warfare.

bromal (bro·mal). Tribromacetaldehyde, CBr_3CHO. The bromine analogue of chloral. **Bromal hydrate.** Tribromoethylidene glycol,

$CBr_3CH(OH)_2$, a crystalline irritant compound used as a hypnotic in the belief that the bromide ion would aid narcosis. The molecule does not, however, ionize and the compound is more toxic than chloral hydrate.

bromaldehyde (bro·**mal**·de·hide). Bromal.

bromalin (**bro**·mal·in). Bromethylformin.

bromate (**bro**·mate). A salt of bromic acid, $HBrO_3$.

bromated (bro·**ma**·ted). Brominated.

bromatherapy (bro·mah·**ther**·ap·e). Dietetics and the use of special foods as a measure against disease. [Gk *broma* food, therapy.]

bromatology (bro·mat·**ol**·o·je). The science of dietetics and nutrition. [Gk *broma* food, *logos* science.]

bromatometry (bro·mat·**om**·et·re). The calculation of the amount of food required daily by an individual. [Gk *broma* food, meter.]

bromatotherapy (**bro**·mat·o·**ther**'·ap·e). Bromatherapy.

bromatotoxin (**bro**·mat·o·**tox**'·in). A poison which develops in spoiled food as the result of the presence of bacteria and of fermentative processes. [Gk *broma* food, toxin.]

bromatotoxismus, bromatoxism (**bro**·mat·o·tox·**iz**'·mus, bro·-mah·**tox**·izm). Poisoning by eating tainted food. [see prec.]

bromazine (**bro**·maz·een). Bromodiphenhydramine.

brombenzoyl (brom·**ben**·zo·il). Benzoyl bromide, bromobenzaldehyde, C_6H_5COBr. Colourless liquid prepared by the bromination of benzaldehyde.

bromdiethylacetylcarbamide, bromdiethylacetylurea (brom·-di·**eth**·il·as·et·il·**kar**'·bam·ide, brom·di·**eth**·il·as·et·il·ewr·**e**'·ah). Carbromal BP 1958, $(C_2H_5)_2CBrCONHCONH_2$. A monoureide with a mild sedative and hypnotic action. Its depressant effect is rather feeble, and the diureides derived from barbituric acid are to be preferred.

bromelains (bro·**mel**·anes). A concentrate of proteolytic enzymes derived from the pineapple plant (*Ananas comosus* Merr.).

bromelin (bro·**mel**·in). An intracellular proteolytic enzyme present in tissues and juice of the pineapple; probably a mixture of peptidases.

brom-ergocryptine (**brom**·**erg**·o·cript·en). Reduces plasma prolactin levels and consequent galactorrhoea, amenorrhoea or impotence.

Bromethol BP 1953 (brom·**eth**·ol). A concentrated solution of tribromoethyl alcohol in amylene hydrate. It is appropriately diluted and instilled into the rectum to produce basal narcosis as a preliminary to anaesthesia. "Avertin."

bromethyl (brom·**eth**·il). Ethyl bromide, C_2H_5Br. A volatile liquid which can be used to induce anaesthesia, but which causes dangerous depression of the respiratory centre.

bromethylformin (**brom**·eth·il·**for**'·min). $(CH_2)_6N_4C_2H_5Br$. An additive compound of hexamine with ethyl bromide, formerly used in epilepsy as a sedative.

brometone (**bro**·me·tone). $CBr_3COH(CH_3)_2$, a compound used as a sedative.

Bromhexine (brom·**hex**·een). BP Commission approved name for *N* - (2 - amino - 3,5 - dibromobenzyl) - *N* - cyclohexylmethylamine; a bronchial mucolytic.

bromhidrosiphobia (**brom**·hid·ro·se·**fo**'·be·ah). Dread of exhaling bodily odours, sometimes in association with a hysterical conviction that they are present when they are not, and with hallucinations that others are repelled by them. [Gk *bromos* stench, *hidros* sweat, phobia.]

bromhidrosis (brom·hid·**ro**·sis). A condition in which the perspiration is foul-smelling. [Gk *bromos* stench, *hidros* sweat.]

bromhydric (brom·**hi**·drik). Hydrobromic.

bromhydrin (brom·**hi**·drin). 1. One of a series of compounds of the general formula BrROH formed from the unsaturated olefine hydrocarbons by bromine water. 2. Glycol bromhydrin, $BrCH_2CH_2OH$, formed by bromine from ethylene.

bromic (**bro**·mik). Resembling or containing bromine.

bromide (**bro**·mide). Any salt of hydrobromic acid. In medicine, the term is usually applied to the inorganic binary compounds of bromine with a metal or a basic radical. Potassium and sodium bromides are the ones most commonly used, but ammonium bromide and strontium bromide are also of value. They are depressants of the central nervous system and produce sedation rather than hypnosis: a patient treated with bromide becomes somewhat indifferent to his surroundings, which makes it a useful drug in anxiety states. Since body tissues are unable to distinguish between chlorine ions and bromine ions, a person receiving bromides begins to replace the body chloride with bromide. Thus bromides have a cumulative effect and should not be administered for long periods, particularly if the salt intake is low. Bromides were formerly used in the treatment of epilepsy, but, being generally less effective than phenobarbitone or phenytoin, have been largely replaced by the latter. **Basic bromide.** A compound formed by the oxide and bromide of the same base. **Bromide intoxication, Bromide poisoning.** Brominism. [Gk *bromos* stench.]

bromidrosis (brom·id·**ro**·sis). Bromhidrosis.

bromidum (**bro**·mid·um). Bromide. [L.]

brominated (**bro**·min·a·ted). 1. Treated with, or mixed with, bromine. 2. A compound that has had bromine atoms introduced into its molecule.

Bromindione (bro·min·**di**·one). BP Commission approved name for 2-(4-bromophenyl)indane-1,3-dione; an anticoagulant.

bromine (**bro**·meen). An element of atomic weight 79.904, atomic number 35 and chemical symbol Br. A dark-red heavy liquid with a pungent irritating smell, fuming in air and causing severe burns on the skin; it occurs in nature as bromides, and in sea-water, mineral waters and a few mineral ores. It is a halogen, resembling chlorine in activity and compounds, and forms salts which are of value in medicine as sedatives. **Bromine blocks.** Porous blocks impregnated with bromine and used for fumigation. **Bromine chloride.** BrCl, pale-brown crystals very soluble in water. **Bromine fluorides.** BrF, BrF_3, and BrF_5, from pale-yellow to colourless crystals. **Bromine iodide.** BrI, dark-red crystals. **Bromine monoxide.** Br_2O, a dark-brown gas; very unstable. **Bromine water.** A solution of 3 per cent bromine in water; used as a reagent. [Gk *bromos* stench.]

brominism (**bro**·min·izm). A chronic condition of ill-health or disease due to the excessive or prolonged taking of bromine, its salts or its compounds. The symptoms are headache, muscular weakness, mental inertia, coldness of hands and feet, and acneiform eruption, foul breath, cardiac depression and loss of sexual potency.

brominized (**bro**·min·i·zd). Treated, containing or saturated with bromine.

bromiodide (brom·i·o·dide). A halide containing atoms of both bromine and iodine united to the same metal or radical.

bromiodoform (brom·i·**o**·do·form). $CHIBr_2$, iodoform in which 2 iodine atoms have been replaced by bromine.

bromism (**bro**·mizm). Brominism.

bromite (**bro**·mite). 1. A salt of bromous acid, $HBrO_2$. 2. Bromyrite, a mineral silver bromide, AgBr.

bromization (bro·mi·**za**·shun). The process of saturating with bromine, its salts or compounds, by the administration of large quantities of the element. The impregnating with bromine or its compounds.

bromized (**bro**·mi·zd). 1. Suffering from the effects of bromine or bromides. 2. Treated with bromine or bromides.

bromo-acetone (bro·mo·**as**·e·tone). Bromacetone, acetyl-bromomethane, $BrCH_2COCH_3$. A colourless liquid, toxic and lacrimatory; used in chemical warfare.

bromo-acetophenone (bro·mo·**as**·et·o·**fe**'·none). $C_6H_5COCH_2Br$. A volatile lacrimatory liquid used in chemical warfare.

bromobenzylcyanide (**bro**·mo·ben·zil·**si**'·an·ide). Bromophenylacetonitrile, $C_6H_4BrCH_2CN$. A colourless liquid used in chemical warfare as a tear gas.

bromocamphor (bro·mo·**kam**·for). Monobromated camphor, $C_{10}H_{15}OBr$. A colourless crystalline substance with a camphor smell; soluble in alcohol and used as a hypnotic and antispasmodic in chorea, hysteria, whooping-cough and asthma.

bromoderma (bro·mo·**der**·mah). The acneiform eruption caused by prolonged or excessive ingestion of bromine or its compounds. [bromine, Gk *derma* skin.]

Bromodiphenhydramine (bro·mo·di·fen·**hi**′·dram·een). BP Commission approved name for 2 - (4 - bromodiphenyl - methoxy) ethyldimethylamine; an anti-allergic used in hay fever, urticaria and atopic eczema.

Bromoform BPC 1959 (bro·mo·form). Tribromomethane, $CHBr_3$. The bromine analogue of chloroform and iodoform, used in syrups for whooping-cough. It is also a sedative and has been used in mania.

bromoformism (bro·mo·**form**·izm). The condition of being poisoned with bromoform.

bromohaematin (bro·mo·**he**·mat·in). Haematin hydrobromide, $C_{34}H_{32}O_4N_4FeBr$. A compound analogous to haemin.

bromohydric (bro·mo·**hi**·drik). Hydrobromic.

bromohyperhidrosis, bromohyperidrosis (bro·mo·**hi**·per·hid·**ro**′·sis, bro·mo·**hi**·per·id·**ro**′·sis). Excessive secretion and excretion of foul-smelling perspiration. [Gk *bromos* stench, *hyper* excessive, *hidros* sweat.]

bromo-iodism (bro·mo·i·od·izm). A condition of poisoning with bromine and iodine or their compounds.

bromo-isovalerianylurea (bro·mo·i·so·val·**eer**·e·an·il·ewr·**e**′·ah). Bromvaletone.

bromoketone (bro·mo·**ke**·tone). Bromomethylethyl ketone.

bromol (**bro**·mol). Tribromphenol, $C_6H_2Br_3OH$. An insoluble crystalline compound which has been used as an intestinal antiseptic.

bromolecithin (bro·mo·**les**·ith·in). A compound obtained by the action of bromine on lecithin.

bromomania (bro·mo·**ma**·ne·ah). Mental disorder or delirium resulting from the excessive ingestion of bromine or its compounds. [bromine, mania.]

bromomenorrhoea (bro·mo·men·o·**re**′·ah). A foul-smelling menstrual discharge. [Gk *bromos* stench, menorrhoea.]

bromomethylethyl ketone (bro·mo·**meth**·il·**eth**′·il ke·tone). $CH_2BrCOC_2H_5$. A halogenated ketone with lacrimatory properties; used in chemical warfare.

bromophenol (bro·mo·**fe**·nol). Orthomonobromphenol, phenol monobromate, C_6H_4BrOH; a dark-yellow oily liquid with a strong odour which has been used as a 2 per cent ointment in the treatment of erysipelas.

bromophenylacetonitrile (bro·mo·**fe**·nil·as·et·o·**ni**′·trile). Bromobenzylcyanide, $C_6H_4BrCH_2CN$. A colourless liquid used in chemical warfare as a tear gas.

bromophenylmethyl ketone (bro·mo·**fe**·nil·**meth**·il **ke**·tone). Bromo-acetophenone, $C_6H_5COCH_2Br$. A volatile lacrimatory liquid used in chemical warfare.

bromopnoea (bro·mo·**ne**·ah). A condition in which the breath has a disagreeable fetid odour; halitosis. [Gk *bromos* stench, *pnoe* breath.]

bromopropane (bro·mo·**pro**·pane). Propyl bromide, $CH_3CH_2CH_2Br$, or its isomer, isopropyl bromide, $CH_3CHBrCH_3$, both of which have been used as anaesthetics.

bromopropene (bro·mo·**pro**·peen). Propenyl bromide, $CH_3CH{=}CHBr$, or its isomer, isopropenyl bromide, CH_2CBrCH_3, both of which have been used as anaesthetics.

bromopropylene (bro·mo·**pro**·pil·een). 1. Propylene dibromide, $CH_3CHBrCH_2Br$. A colourless liquid used as a fumigating insecticide. 2. Allyl bromide, CH_2CHCH_2Br. A colourless lacrimatory liquid.

bromotolunitrile (bro·mo·**tol**·ew·**nite**′·rile). Bromobenzylcyanide, $C_6H_4BrCH_2CN$. A colourless liquid used in chemical warfare as a tear gas.

bromouracil (bro·mo·**ewr**·as·il). An analogue of the pyrimidine base, thymine, in which the methyl group at the 5-position is substituted by an atom of bromine. It can replace thymine in the DNA of living cells and is mutagenic. Also used as a density label for newly-synthesized DNA.

bromous (**bro**·mus). Containing the radical $-BrO_2$.

Brompheniramine (brom·fen·i·ram·een). BP Commission approved name for 1 - (4 - bromophenyl) - 3 - dimethylamino - 1 - (2 - pyridyl) - propane; an antihistaminic agent.

bromphenols (brom·**fe**·nolz). Brominated phenols which are formed by the addition of bromine to phenols; they are precipitated when bromine water is added to urine containing phenol or phenolic compounds.

bromphenylacetyl cysteine (brom·fe·nil·**as**′·et·il sis·te·een). Bromphenylmercapturic acid, $C_6H_4BrSCH_2CH(NHCOCH_3)COOH$. A substance excreted in the urine of dogs under certain metabolic conditions.

bromsulphthalein (brom·sulf·**thal**·e·in). Phenoltetrabromphthalein sodium sulphonate, a non-toxic, non-irritant dye used as an indicator of liver function. Injected intravenously, the amount left in circulation after a given interval of time affords a measure of hepatic sufficiency.

bromum (**bro**·mum). Bromine. [L.]

bromurated (**brom**·ewr·a·ted). Bromated; containing bromine or bromine derivatives either in mixture or in combination.

bromuret (**brom**·ewr·et). Term for a bromide or bromurated compound.

bromvaletone (brom·**val**·e·tone). Bromovaletonum BPC 1949, 2-monobromo-isovalerianylurea, $NH_2CONHCOCHBrCH(CH_3)_2$. A hypnotic and sedative of the carbromal type; it is less potent than the barbiturates.

bromyrite (**brom**·e·rite). Bromite, a mineral silver bromide, AgBr.

bronchadenitis (**brongk**·ad·en·**i**′·tis). Broncho-adenitis.

bronchi (**brong**·ki). *See* BRONCHUS.

bronchia (**brong**·ke·ah). Bronchial tubules generally.

bronchial (**brong**·ke·al). Relating to the pulmonary bronchi, as a whole or in part.

bronchial arteries [rami bronchiales (NA)]. Variable arteries to the non-respiratory tissues of the lungs; usually 1 right, from the 3rd posterior intercostal artery, and 2 left, from the thoracic aorta direct.

bronchial blocker (**brong**·ke·al **blok**·er). A long catheter with inflatable balloon used in thoracic anaesthesia to isolate a part of a lung. [Gk *brogchos* windpipe, O Fr. *bloc* block.]

bronchial veins [venae bronchiales (NA)]. Veins draining the larger bronchi, lymph glands and connective tissue of the roots of the lungs; tributaries of the vena azygos, or superior vena hemiazygos, or superior intercostal vein.

bronchiarctia (brong·ke·**ark**·she·ah). Bronchostenosis. [Gk *brogchos* windpipe, L *arctus* narrow.]

bronchiectasia (**brong**·ke·ek·**ta**′·ze·ah). Bronchiectasis.

bronchiectasic (**brong**·ke·ek·**ta**′·zik). Bronchiectatic.

bronchiectasis (brong·ke·**ek**·tas·is). A condition of dilatation of a bronchus or bronchi, secondary to structural changes in the bronchial walls which are predominantly inflammatory in origin. The main clinical signs are chronic cough with purulent, often foul-smelling, sputum, characteristically produced by alterations in posture. Clubbing of the fingers is often associated with this condition. The various forms of bronchiectasis can be most clearly demonstrated in life by bronchography. **Capillary bronchiectasis.** Bronchiolectasis. **Cylindrical bronchiectasis.** That in which a bronchus or bronchial tube is uniformly and symmetrically dilated. **Cystic bronchiectasis.** That in which the dilatations take a roughly circular form, seen especially in children and therefore thought by some to be congenital in origin. **Fusiform bronchiectasis.** That in which there is saccular dilatation of the ends of the bronchi. **Moniliform bronchiectasis.** That in which the bronchiectasis is infected with *Candida albicans* (Monilia). **Postinfective bronchiectasis.** Bronchiectasis after a lung or bronchial infection. **Saccular bronchiectasis, Sacculated bronchiectasis.** That in which sacs of varying size and shape occur along the course of the bronchus. [Gk *brogchos* windpipe, *ektasis* a stretching.]

bronchiectatic (**brong**·ke·ek·**tat**′·ik). Referring to, affected with or characterized by bronchiectasis.

bronchiloquy (brong·**kil**·o·kwe). Bronchophony or pectoriloquy. [Gk *brogchos* windpipe, L *loqui* to speak.]

bronchiocele (**brong**·ke·o·seel). A circumscribed swelling or dilatation of a bronchiole. [Gk *brogchos* windpipe, *kele* hernia.]

bronchiocrisis (**brong**·ke·o·**kri**'·sis). Bronchial crisis. *See* CRISIS. [Gk *brogchos* windpipe, *krisis* separation.]

bronchiogenic (**brong**·ke·o·**jen**'·ik). Originating in or emanating from the bronchi; bronchogenic. [Gk *brogchos* windpipe, *genein* to produce.]

bronchiole [bronchiolus (NA)] (**brong**·ke·ole). One of the smaller subdivisions of the bronchial branches. **Alveolar bronchiole, Respiratory bronchiole.** Terminal bronchiole (see following). **Terminal bronchiole [bronchiolus respiratorius (NA)].** The last and smallest subdivision of a bronchial branch; it does not contain any cartilage and its ciliated epithelial cells are cube-shaped; it ends in an alveolus. [L *bronchiolus* little bronchus.]

bronchiolectasis (**brong**·ke·o·**lek**'·tas·is). A form of bronchiectasis affecting the bronchioles. [bronchiole, Gk *ektasis* a stretching.]

bronchiolith (**brong**·ke·o·lith). Broncholith.

bronchiolitis (**brong**·ke·o·**li**'·tis). Inflammation of the bronchioles; capillary bronchitis. **Acute bronchiolitis.** Acute inflammation of the bronchioles often due to respiratory syncytial virus. **Acute obliterating bronchiolitis.** Pulmonary cirrhosis or fibroid pneumonia caused by hardening of the walls of the bronchioles. **Asthmatic bronchiolitis, Bronchiolitis exudativa, Exudative bronchiolitis.** Inflammation of the bronchioles with accompanying fibrinous exudation, a condition which may pass into bronchitic asthma. **Bronchiolitis fibrosa obliterans, Bronchiolitis obliterans, Obliterating fibrous bronchiolitis.** Bronchiolitis in which plugs of connective tissue obliterate the lumen of the terminal bronchioles. **Vesicular bronchiolitis.** Bronchopneumonia. [bronchiole, Gk *-itis* inflammation.]

bronchiolus (brong·ke·o·lus). A bronchiole.

bronchiospasm, bronchiospasmus (**brong**·ke·o·spazm, **brong**·ke·o·**spaz**'·mus). Spasmodic contraction of the walls of the bronchial tubes; bronchospasm. [Gk *brogchos* windpipe, *spasmos* a drawing.]

bronchiostenosis (**brong**·ke·o·sten·o'·sis). Narrowing or stricture of the bronchi; bronchostenosis. [Gk *brogchos* windpipe, stenosis.]

bronchiotetany (**brong**·ke·o·**tet**'·an·e). A condition of spasm of the bronchial muscles which prevents the passage of air to the lungs and causes severe dyspnoea; bronchotetany. [Gk *brogchos* windpipe, tetany.]

bronchisepticin (brong·ke·**sep**·tis·in). The antigen from *Haemophilus bronchisepticus.*

bronchismus (brong·**kis**·mus). Bronchiospasm.

bronchitic (brong·**kit**·ik). Referring to, of the nature of or affected with bronchitis.

bronchitis (brong·**ki**·tis). An inflammation of the mucous membrane of the larger and medium-sized bronchi. **Acute bronchitis.** More accurately described as acute tracheobronchitis, an acute condition of fairly short duration. This may follow an acute catarrhal infection of the nose and pharynx caused by the virus of the common cold or be due to an exacerbation of a persistent catarrhal infection caused by such organisms as the pneumococcus, streptococcus, *Haemophilus influenzae, Neisseria catarrhalis.* It may be a part of the upper respiratory infection of a specific infectious disease such as measles, whooping-cough, influenza, smallpox, cerebrospinal fever, typhoid fever or typhus fever. The inhalation of irritant gases such as ammonia, chlorine, phosgene, ether, nitrous fumes or mustard gas may cause very intensive acute bronchitis. The inspiration of a foreign body into a bronchus, e.g. an infected tooth or vegetable matter such as a bean or nut containing irritating fatty acids, may similarly cause intense inflammation and oedema. **Acute capillary bronchitis.** Inflammation of the finer bronchi or bronchioles (bronchiolitis) usually due to an extension downward of an acute bronchitis, and a characteristic lesion of influenza. It causes collapse of the alveoli and becomes indistinguishable from a secondary bronchopneumonia. **Acute fibrinous bronchitis.** An inflammation of the bronchi in which firm mucinous casts of a portion of the bronchial tree are coughed up. **Acute suffocative bronchitis.** Acute suppurative bronchitis (see following). **Acute suppurative bronchitis.** Bronchitis characterized by abundant purulent sputum, often blood-streaked, and associated with very rapid laboured breathing and cyanosis; it was epidemic among troops in England and France in 1917, *Haemophilus influenzae* being present in 90 per cent of cases. **Arachidic bronchitis.** The intense reaction to the inhalation of peanut particles, a condition common in America from eating peanut candy. **Chronic bronchitis.** A chronic inflammation of the bronchial mucous membrane. It may follow repeated attacks of acute bronchitis, but probably never occurs without other associated conditions such as a chronic infection of the upper respiratory tract, or of the lung itself in connection with fibrosis or bronchiectasis. It is favoured by general conditions such as rickets, gout, obesity, chronic heart disease, chronic renal disease and alcoholism, and is aggravated by dusty occupations and tobacco smoking. It may lead to and become associated with chronic vesicular emphysema and the diagnosis of chronic bronchitis with emphysema then becomes appropriate. **Fetid bronchitis, Putrid bronchitis.** A condition in which the sputum is offensive from infection with anaerobic bacteria, especially fusiform bacilli and spirilla derived from septic conditions of the mouth. Probably all cases are examples of abscess of the lung or bronchiectasis. [Gk *brogchos* windpipe, *-itis* inflammation.]

See also: CASTELLANI, HOFFMAN (F. L.).

bronchium (**brong**·ke·um) (pl. *bronchia*). One of the ramifications of a bronchus. [L.]

broncho-adenitis (**brong**·ko·ad·en·i'·tis). A condition in which the bronchial glands are inflamed. [Gk *brogchos* windpipe, adenitis.]

broncho-alveolar (**brong**·ko·al·**ve**'·o·lar). Bronchovesicular. [Gk *brogchos* windpipe, alveolus.]

broncho-alveolitis (**brong**·ko·al·ve·o·**li**'·tis). Bronchopneumonia. [Gk *brogchos* windpipe, alveolitis.]

broncho-aspergillosis (**brong**·ko·**as**·per·jil·**o**'·sis). Secondary bronchitis as the result of infection with *Aspergillus.* [Gk *brogchos* windpipe, aspergillosis.]

bronchoblastomycosis (**brong**·ko·blas·to·mi·**ko**'·sis). Blastomycosis affecting the lungs. [Gk *brogchos* windpipe, blastomycosis.]

bronchoblennorrhoea (**brong**·ko·blen·o·**re**'·ah). Chronic bronchitis producing a copious discharge of thin and mucopurulent sputum. [Gk *brogchos* windpipe, blennorrhoea.]

bronchocandidiasis (**brong**·ko·kan·did·**i**'·as·is). A disease of the bronchi caused by infection with *Candida* species and showing signs of bronchitis or bronchopneumonia. [Gk *brogchos* windpipe, *Candida.*]

bronchocavernous (**brong**·ko·kav·**er**'·nus). Bronchial and cavernous; descriptive of a type of breathing.

bronchocele (**brong**·ko·seel). Goitre. **Aerial bronchocele.** Aerocele. **Cystic bronchocele.** Cystic goitre. *See* GOITRE. [Gk *brogchos* windpipe, *kele* hernia.]

bronchocephalitis (**brong**·ko·kef·al·**i**'·tis). Whooping-cough. [Gk *brogchos* windpipe, *kephale* head, *-itis* inflammation.]

bronchoclysis (brong·**kok**·lis·is). The slow gravitational instillation of liquid remedies into the bronchi and bronchioles; any injection into the bronchi. [Gk *brogchos* windpipe, *klyein* to wash out.]

bronchoconstriction (**brong**·ko·kon·**strik**'·shun). Constriction of the bronchial tubes so that the lumen is narrowed.

bronchoconstrictor (**brong**·ko·kon·**strik**'·tor). A spasmodic; an agent which narrows the lumen of the bronchial tubes. [Gk *brogchos* windpipe, L *constringere* to draw together.]

bronchodilatation (**brong**·ko·di·lat·**a**'·shun). 1. The procedure of dilating a constricted bronchus. 2. Bronchiectasis.

bronchodilator (**brong**·ko·di·**la**'·tor). An antispasmodic; an agent which dilates a bronchus or bronchiole.

bronchogenic (brong·ko·**jen**·ik). Arising in or from a bronchus. [Gk *brogchos* windpipe, *genein* to produce.]

bronchogram (**brong**·ko·gram). The x-ray photograph of the bronchial tubes after an opaque medium has been injected into them. [Gk *brogchos* windpipe, *gramma* a writing.]

bronchography (brong·**kog**·raf·e). Examination by x-rays of the bronchial tubes after an opaque medium has been injected into them. [Gk *brogchos* windpipe, *graphein* to record.]

broncholith (**brong**·ko·lith). A bronchial calculus or stone, e.g. calcium from a previously healed lesion in the lung. [Gk *brogchos* windpipe, *lithos* stone.]

broncholithiasis (**brong**·ko·lith·**i**'·as·is). The condition in which calculi occur in the lumena of bronchial tubes. [see prec.]

bronchological (brong·ko·**loj**·ik·al). Referring to bronchology. [Gk *brogchos* windpipe, *logos* science.]

bronchology (brong·**kol**·o·je). The science of bronchial diseases and their treatment. [Gk *brogchos* windpipe, *logos* science.]

bronchomoniliasis (**brong**·ko·mon·il·**i**'·as·is). A disease of the bronchi caused by infection with *Candida* species and showing signs of bronchitis and bronchopneumonia. Now usually termed *bronchopulmonary candidiasis* or *bronchocandidiasis*. [Gk *brogchos* windpipe, *Monilia* (*Candida*).]

bronchomotor (brong·ko·**mo**·tor). Altering the calibre of the bronchial tubes. [Gk *brogchos* windpipe, L *motor* mover.]

bronchomycosis (brong·ko·mi·**ko**'·sis). Bronchial affection or disease resulting from the presence of a fungus. [Gk *brogchos* windpipe, *mykes* fungus, *-osis* condition.]

bronchonocardiasis, bronchonocardiosis (**brong**·ko·no·kar·**di**'·as·is, **brong**·ko·no·kar·de·**o**'·sis). An infected condition of the bronchi due to the presence of *Nocardia*. [Gk *brogchos* windpipe, nocardia, Gk *-osis* condition.]

broncho-oesophageal muscle [musculus broncho-esophageus (NA)] (**brong**·ko·e·sof·ah·**je**'·al). Slips of the muscle coat of the oesophagus which pass on to the left bronchus.

broncho-oesophagology (**brong**·ko·e·sof·ah·**gol**'·o·je). The sum of the diseases associated with the oesophagus and the bronchial tubes. [Gk *brogchos* windpipe, oesophagology.]

broncho-oesophagoscopy (**brong**·ko·e·sof·ah·**gos**'·ko·pe). Examination or inspection of the interior of the oesophagus and the bronchi. [Gk *brogchos* windpipe, oesophagoscopy.]

broncho-oidosis (**brong**·ko·o·id·**o**'·sis). Bronchomoniliasis. [Gk *brogchos* windpipe, *Oidium*.]

bronchopathy (brong·**kop**·ath·e). Any disease or affection of the air passages of the lungs. [Gk *brogchos* windpipe, *pathos* suffering.]

bronchophonic (brong·ko·**fon**·ik). Referring to broncophony.

bronchophony (brong·**kof**·on·e). The laryngeal vibrations of the voice as heard in stethoscopic auscultation over any large bronchus and in some subjects at the root of the neck, anteriorly and posteriorly. In cases of consolidation of lung tissue the sound is exaggerated. **Accidental bronchophony.** Bronchophony caused by disease and not associated with normal manifestations (see above). **Pectoriloquous bronchophony.** Bronchophony with associated pectoriloquy. **Sniffling bronchophony.** Bronchophony with which there is associated a sniffling sound as of air inspired through the nose. **Whispered bronchophony.** That produced when the patient is instructed to whisper. [Gk *brogchos* windpipe, *phone* sound.]

bronchoplasty (**brong**·ko·plas·te). The surgical procedure of closing a fistula in a bronchus or the trachea; any plastic surgical operation on a bronchus. [Gk *brogchos* windpipe, *plassein* to mould.]

bronchoplegia (brong·ko·**ple**·je·ah). A paralysed condition of the bronchial tubes, affecting the muscular fibres of the walls, and altering the tonus. [Gk *brogchos* windpipe, *plege* stroke.]

bronchopleuropneumonia (**brong**·ko·**ploor**·o·new·**mo**'·ne·ah). The condition in which there is co-existence of bronchitis, pleurisy and pneumonia. [Gk *brogchos* windpipe, pleuropneumonia.]

bronchopneumonia (**brong**·ko·new·**mo**'·ne·ah). Infectious inflammation of the lungs and the bronchioles, the condition affecting first the terminal bronchioles, which become filled with tenacious purulent mucus and surrounded by areas of consolidation. The disease is usually secondary in character, occurring as a complication after a specific infection, a debilitating disease or a disease of the upper respiratory tract. The primary form is chiefly a disease of children. **Aspiration bronchopneumonia.** That resulting from the inspiration of fluid or small solid particles from the upper respiratory passages. **Confluent bronchopneumonia.** Bronchopneumonia in which the patches of lobular consolidation have fused into considerable areas which may occupy the whole of a lobe. **Deglutition bronchopneumonia.** That resulting from the drawing in of food particles into the bronchi. **Hypostatic bronchopneumonia.** Bronchopneumonia in the most dependent parts of the lungs, following hypostatic congestion. It occurs as a terminal event in aged or debilitated bedridden patients. **Influenzal bronchopneumonia.** A pulmonary lesion caused by infection with the virus of influenza, especially the epidemic types. Secondary invaders are always present, especially streptococci, *Haemophilus influenzae*, staphylococci, and the type and severity of the lung lesions depend upon the organism which predominates and its virulence. The pathological changes comprise varying degrees of bronchiolitis, congestion, consolidation, haemorrhage, oedema and collapse. Actual consolidation may be only a minor incident. **Inhalation bronchopneumonia.** Aspiration bronchopneumonia (see above). **Subacute bronchopneumonia.** Peribronchitis. **Unresolved bronchopneumonia.** The condition resulting when resolution is delayed and the alveoli are invaded by fibroblasts. The affected parts of the lung become fibrosed, airless and converted into a fleshy mass (carnification). **Virus bronchopneumonia.** Atypical pneumonia caused by a virus. [Gk *brogchos* windpipe, pneumonia.]

bronchopneumonic (**brong**·ko·new·**mon**'·ik). Referring to, affected with, or resulting from bronchopneumonia.

bronchopneumonitis (**brong**·ko·new·mon·**i**'·tis). Bronchopneumonia. [bronchopneumonia, Gk *-itis* inflammation.]

bronchopulmonary (brong·ko·**pul**·mon·ar·e). Affecting or relating to the bronchial tubes and the lungs. **Bronchopulmonary lymph gland.** *See* GLAND, LYMPH. [Gk *brogchos* windpipe, L *pulmonis* lung.]

bronchoradiography (**brong**·ko·ra·de·**og**'·raf·e). X-ray examination or inspection of the bronchi and bronchioles. [Gk *brogchos* windpipe, radiography.]

bronchorrhagia (brong·ko·**ra**·je·ah). Haemorrhage from the bronchial tubes. [Gk *brogchos* windpipe, *rhegnynai* to burst forth.]

bronchorrhaphy (brong·**kor**·af·e). The suturing of torn or incised edges of a bronchus. [Gk *brogchos* windpipe, *rhaphe* suture.]

bronchorrhoea (brong·ko·**re**·ah). An abnormally copious discharge of mucus from the bronchial tubes. **Bronchorrhoea serosa, Serous bronchorrhoea.** A profuse bronchial expectoration like diluted unboiled white of egg. [Gk *brogchos* windpipe, *rhoia* flow.]

bronchoscope (**brong**·ko·skope). 1. An instrument with which the inside of the bronchial tubes can be examined. 2. To make such an examination. [Gk *brogchos* windpipe, *skopein* to watch.]

See also: BRUENINGS, HASLINGER.

bronchoscopic (brong·ko·**skop**·ik). Referring or relating to a bronchoscope or to bronchoscopy.

bronchoscopy (brong·**kos**·ko·pe). The examination of the inside of a bronchial tube with a bronchoscope or through an incision made in the trachea.

bronchosinusitis (**brong**·ko·si·nus·**i**'·tis). An inflammatory condition of the paranasal sinuses and the lower part of the trachea and upper bronchi. [Gk *brogchos* windpipe, sinusitis.]

bronchospasm (**brong**·ko·spazm). Bronchiospasm.

bronchospirochaetosis (**brong**·ko·spi·ro·ke·**to**'·sis). Chronic bronchitis with haemoptysis caused by the activities of a spirochaete (*Treponema*), which infects the larger bronchial tubes. Also called *Castellani's bronchitis*; *haemorrhagic bronchitis*. [Gk *brogchos* windpipe, spirochaete, Gk *-osis* condition.]

bronchospirography (**brong**·ko·spi·**rog**'·raf·e). The graphic recording by means of a revolving drum of the excursions of the levered arm of the bronchospirometer showing the volume of inspired and expired air in the two lungs separately or simultaneously. [Gk *brogchos* windpipe, spirography.]

bronchospirometer (brong·ko·spi·**rom**'·et·er). A bronchoscope with two separate channels, through each of which a catheter with an inflatable rubber cuff is passed into the two main bronchi. By inflating one or other of the cuffs the volume of air inspired by each lung can be measured separately and a gaseous analysis made of the expired air. A more convenient form has a single-channel metal bronchoscope, down which a double-channelled rubber catheter with inflatable cuffs on each of the bifurcations at the end is passed, one into each main bronchus. [Gk *brogchos* windpipe, spirometer.]

bronchospirometry (brong·ko·spi·**rom**'·et·re). The estimation of the volume and rate of gaseous exchange in each lung or both lungs simultaneously by means of a bronchospirometer. The practical value of such measurements to the surgeon is much in doubt and there are contra-indications to its use such as excess of sputum, or oronasal infections, but it is useful for normal physiological investigations.

bronchostaxis (brong·ko·**stax**·is). Acute haemorrhage from the walls of the bronchi. [Gk *brogchos* windpipe, *staxis* a dropping.]

bronchostenosis (brong·ko·sten·**o**'·sis). Abnormal constriction of a bronchus or bronchiole; stricture of the bronchial tubes. **Spasmodic bronchostenosis.** Bronchiospasm. **Tuberculous bronchostenosis.** Stenosis of a bronchus, of tuberculous origin. [Gk *brogchos* windpipe, stenosis.]

bronchostomy (brong·**kos**·to·me). Making an opening into the bronchus through the thoracic wall. [Gk *brogchos* windpipe, *temnein* to cut.]

bronchotetany (brong·ko·**tet**'·an·e). Bronchiotetany.

bronchotome (brong·ko·tome). An instrument used in bronchotomy and tracheotomy. [Gk *brogchos* windpipe, *temnein* to cut.]

bronchotomy (brong·**kot**·o·me). Incision of a bronchus or the trachea. [see prec.]

bronchotracheal (brong·ko·**trak**·e·al). Relating to the bronchi and the trachea, or involving them.

bronchovesicular (brong·ko·ves·**ik**'·ew·lar). Relating to the bronchial tubes and the lung alveoli. [Gk *brogchos* windpipe, L *vesicula* small bladder.]

bronchus (brong·kus) (pl. *bronchi*). Any part of the air passages between the bifurcation of the trachea and the bronchioles in the lungs. The trachea divides into the right and left bronchi [bronchi principales, dexter et sinister (NA)], without any other change in structure. The intrapulmonary bronchi [bronchi lobares et segmentales (NA)] have irregular plates of cartilage in their walls instead of the incomplete rings characteristic of the trachea; they have also a more complete muscular coat [tunica muscularis (NA)]. The right bronchus gives off the eparterial bronchus [bronchus lobaris superior dexter (NA)] and continues as the hyparterial bronchus [rami bronchiales hyparteriales], which lie above and below the pulmonary artery respectively. The eparterial bronchus supplies the upper lobe and divides into (1) bronchus segmentalis apicalis, (2) bronchus segmentalis posterior and (3) bronchus segmentalis anterior. The hyparterial bronchus gives off the bronchus lobaris medius dexter, which divides into (4) bronchus segmentalis lateralis and (5) bronchus segmentalis medialis and is then distributed to the lower lobe [bronchus lobaris inferior dexter]. This, having given off the (6) bronchus segmentalis apicalis superior, ends by dividing into (7) bronchus segmentalis basalis medialis (cardiacus), (8) bronchus segmentalis basalis anterior, (9) bronchus segmentalis basalis lateralis, (10) bronchus segmentalis basalis posterior. The left bronchus divides into a bronchus lobaris superior sinister and bronchus lobaris inferior sinister. The former divides into a superior and inferior division. From the superior division arises bronchus segmentalis apicoposterior and (3) bronchus segmentalis anterior. The former subdivides into (1) bronchus segmentalis apicalis and (2) bronchus segmentalis posterior. The inferior (lingule) division gives rise to (4) bronchus lingularis superior and (5) bronchus lingularis inferior. The bronchus lobaris inferior sinister gives off (6) the bronchus segmentalis apicalis (superior) and ends by dividing into (8) bronchus segmentalis basalis anterior, (9) bronchus segmentalis basalis lateralis, (10) bronchus segmentalis basalis posterior. The following 3 bronchi with their segments occasionally occur: bronchi segmentales subapicales (sub-superiores) dexter et sinister and (7) bronchus segmentalis basilis medialis (cardiacus) sinister. Each segmental bronchus is numbered according to an international agreement of thoracic surgeons and is distributed to a segment of the same name. Within the segment the segmental bronchus divides into intersegmental branches [rami bronchiales segmentorum (NA)]. [Gk *brogchos* windpipe.]

Bronner clamp. A curved clamp with rubber-covered blades, for controlling intestine during anastomosis.

Bronopol (bro·no·pol). BP Commission approved name for 2 - bromo - 2 - nitropropane - 1,3 - diol; an antiseptic and preservative.

brontophobia (bron·to·**fo**·be·ah). Abnormal fear of thunder. [Gk *bronte* thunder, phobia.]

Brooke, Henry Ambrose Grundy (b. 1854). Manchester dermatologist.

Brooke's disease. 1. Epithelioma adenoides cysticum. 2. Keratosis follicularis contagiosa.

Brooke's ointment, or paste. A mixture of equal parts of ointment of oleated mercury and Lassar's paste, containing salicylic acid (6 per cent) and ichthammol (12 per cent).

Brooke's tumour. Epithelioma adenoides cysticum.

broom (broom). Broom tops, scoparium, consisting of the dried tops of *Sarothamnus scoparius* (L.) Koch (family Leguminoseae), a shrub indigenous to temperate Europe. It contains the liquid alkaloid sparteine, amongst other alkaloids, and is employed as a mild diuretic in cardiac dropsy in the form of a decoction, infusion or juice. The infusion is often prescribed with other diuretics. [AS *brom.*]

Brophy, Truman William (b. 1848). American oral surgeon.

Brophy operation. An operation for cleft palate.

brossage (bros·**ahzh**). Scraping with a stiff brush in order to remove granulations, as in trachoma, or to induce adhesive inflammation. [Fr. a brushing.]

Brossard, Jules (fl. 1860–1890). French physician.

Brossard's type of progressive muscular atrophy. Progressive muscular atrophy with predominant involvement of the lower limbs.

broth (broth). Nutrient broth or bouillon; the basis for the media ordinarily employed in the cultivation of pathogenic bacteria. In its simplest form it is a watery extract of meat which has been heated to remove the proteins. **Bile-salt broth.** A broth containing sodium taurocholate bile. **Blood-serum broth.** Serum collected aseptically or sterilized by filtration, and added to broth. **Carbohydrate broth.** A broth to which has been added a solution of a single carbohydrate, e.g. dextrose broth. **Digest broth.** A medium useful for the production of bacterial toxins formed by digesting minced meat with proteolytic enzymes. **Glycerol broth.** A medium made by adding a small percentage of glycerol to an ordinary or digest broth. **Infusion broth.** An extract of meat to which is usually added commercial peptone and salt. **Tetrathionate broth.** A medium prepared from sodium thiosulphate solution, iodine solution, nutrient broth and chalk, with phenol red as an indicator. [AS.]

See also: BAILEY (S. F.), HARTLEY, MACCONKEY, TODD (J. L.), USCHINSKY.

Broussaisism (broo·**sa**·izm). The out-of-date theory that the cause of all disease is a state of abnormal irritability of the alimentary tract. [François Joseph Victor *Broussais*, 1772–1838, Paris physician.]

brow (brow). 1. The forehead; the right or the left half of the forehead. 2. The superciliary arch. **Brow ache, Brow ague.** Neuralgic pain commonly occurring in malaria and affecting the first division of the 5th cranial nerve. **Olympic brow.** The abnormal development of the forehead noticeable in case of congenital syphilis. **Brow pang.** Hemicephalia. [AS *bru.*]

Brown, Arthur Ivor Parry. 20th century London anaesthetist.

Parry Brown position. The patient undergoing thoracotomy is prone with the table tilted head down so that pulmonary secretions can run freely into the tracheal tube, from which they can be sucked as required. Described in 1948.

Brown, Charles Leonard (b. 1899). Boston physician.

Brown-Symmers disease. Serous encephalitis in childhood.

Brown, George Elgie (b. 1885). Rochester, Minnesota, physician.

Brown's vasomotor index. The increase of the skin temperature of the extremities over increase of mouth temperature after an intravenous injection of TAB vaccine in Brown's fever test.

Brown's fever test. A toxiconeurological test for lesions of the sympathetic nervous system: intravenous TAB vaccine is given to induce fever, and skin temperature is measured at half-hour intervals with a skin thermometer. Absence of a rise in temperature over any area of skin indicates a lesion of its sympathetic nerve supply.

Hines and Brown test. Cold pressor test; a test to detect subjects who may be likely to develop persistent hypertension in the future: the basal blood pressure is recorded at rest, and then the other hand of the subject is plunged into water at 3-5°C for 1 min, the blood pressure being recorded at half-minute intervals. A rise of more than 20/15 mmHg (2700/2000 Pa) constitutes a hyper-reaction, and is shown by persons with essential hypertension or by those individuals who are likely to develop it ultimately. The test has also been suggested as a method of differentiating "essential" from "renal" and other forms of hypertension, but some doubt has been cast upon its validity.

Brown, James Barrett (b. 1899). St. Louis surgeon.

Blair-Brown graft. A skin graft cut freehand by the Blair knife.

Blair-Brown operation. 1. Plastic repair of hare-lip. 2. Plastic repair of cleft palate.

Brown, John (b. 1735). Scottish physician.

brunonian theory. A system of medicine devised by John Brown, who regarded all diseases as either sthenic, depending on an excess of stimulation, or asthenic, lacking in stimulation. The former were to be treated by sedative medicines, e.g. opium, and the latter by stimulants (wine or brandy). For a time this theory gained considerable support, especially in Germany and Italy.

Brown, Robert (b. 1773). English botanist.

Brown's phenomenon. Brownian movement.

Brownian movement, Brownian-Zsigmondy movement. The oscillation of minute particles suspended in a liquid, e.g. the movement of non-motile bacteria in a fluid when examined microscopically.

Brown, Sanger (b. 1852). American neurologist.

Sanger Brown's ataxia. A familial disease with similar symptoms to those of Friedreich's ataxia but with less involvement of pyramidal tracts and greater tendency to optic atrophy.

Brown-Séquard, Charles Edouard (b. 1817). French physiologist.

Brown-Séquard disease, paralysis or syndrome. The syndrome of hemisection of the spinal cord: lower motor neuron paralysis and sensory loss in the muscles and skin areas respectively supplied by the affected segment, homolateral pyramidal signs and loss of position and vibration sense and tactile discrimination, and contralateral loss of appreciation of pain and temperature, with an upper level in the skin area corresponding to a few segments below the level of the lesion.

Brown-Séquard injection. The injection of testicular extract.

Browne, Sir Denis John Wolko (b. 1892). London surgeon.

Denis Browne boot. A boot fitted to a Denis Browne splint and used in the treatment of congenital talipes equinovarus.

Denis Browne needle. A full-circle needle used in cleft-palate operation.

Denis Browne's operation. 1. An operation for hare-lip. 2. An operation for cleft palate, with narrowing of the nasopharynx.

Denis Browne's splints. Metal splints for the correction of talipes equinovarus.

Browne, Sir James Crichton (b. 1840). Scottish physician and psychologist.

Browne's sign, Crichton Browne's sign. Facial tremor as found in general paralysis of the insane.

Browne-Pearce tumour. Transmissible metastasizing carcinoma of the rabbit, originally arising in the testicle.

Brownian (brown·e·an). Associated with Robert Brown.

Browning, Carl Hamilton (b. 1881). Glasgow bacteriologist.

Browning's brilliant-green enrichment medium. Tubes of peptone water with 1/400 000, 1/250 000, and 1/150 000 dilution of brilliant green. It is used for the isolation of typhoid or paratyphoid from faeces.

Browning, William (b. 1855). American anatomist.

Browning's vein. The upper portion of the superior anastomotic vein (the great anastomotic vein of Trolard).

Bruce, Alexander (b. 1854). Scottish neurologist.

Bruce's column. The lateral column of grey matter containing cells of origin of autonomic fibres constituting the thoracic outflow.

Bruce's tract, Bruce and Muir tract. Part of the septomarginal tract in cervical and thoracic regions of the spinal cord. Also known as *Muir's tract.*

Bruce, Sir David (b. 1855). British Army pathologist.

Bruce's septicaemia. Undulant fever. *See* FEVER.

Brucella (broo·sel·ah). The generic name of a group of small Gram-negative coccobacilli that are primary pathogens of animals, mainly goats, sheep, cattle and pigs. Infection in pregnant animals, particularly cows, may lead to abortion; involvement of the mammary glands leads to excretion of the *Brucellae* in milk. Man becomes infected by contact with infected animals or their carcases, or by ingesting infected milk or milk products. The 3 main species are *Brucella melitensis,* which infects goats and sheep; *Brucella abortus,* which infects cattle; and *Brucella suis,* which infects pigs. There are biotypes within each species. **Brucella abortus.** Morphologically identical with *Brucella melitensis* (see below), occurs in cow's milk and causes bovine contagious abortion; it may also be responsible for undulant fever in human subjects. Varieties occur in pigs, sheep and horses. **Brucella bronchisepticus.** *Haemophilus bronchisepticus.* **Brucella melitensis.** The causal organism of undulant fever in the Mediterranean littoral and islands (Malta fever) but also occurring in other parts of the world. It is a small coccobacillus. Infection usually results from ingestion of infected goat's milk, sheep and goats being the reservoirs of infection. **Brucella para-abortus.** Former name for a variant of *Brucella abortus.* **Brucella paramelitensis.** A variant of *Brucella melitensis.* **Brucella suis.** A variety of *Brucella abortus* occurring in pigs. **Brucella tularensis.** The cause of tularaemia, a plague-like disease, in man. Its habitat is the ground squirrel and other rodents, especially in the USA and Western Europe. It is found in the liver, blood, spleen and lymph nodes of infected man and animals, and is transmitted via the broken or unbroken skin, by contact with infected animals, by blood-sucking insects and by contaminated food and water. [Sir David *Bruce.*]

brucellaemia (broo·sel·e·me·ah). Undulant fever. *See* FEVER. [*Brucella,* Gk *haima* blood.]

brucellar (broo·sel·ar). Caused by the presence of, or relating to *Brucella.*

brucelliasis (broo·sel·i·as·is). Undulant fever. *See* FEVER. [*Brucella.*]

brucellin (broo·sel·in). The intradermal injection of a killed suspension of *Brucella* species or of a purified extract, which may elicit a delayed tuberculin-like allergic reaction (minimum diameter 5 mm induration) and may mean past or present infection. Non-specific positive reactions may occur, however, so that this test should not *per se* be accepted as diagnostic. [Sir David *Bruce.*]

brucellosis (broo·sel·o·sis). Undulant fever. *See* FEVER. [*Brucella,* Gk *-osis* condition.]

Bruch, Karl Wilhelm Ludwig (b. 1819). Giessen anatomist.

Bruch's glands. Lymphatic follicles of the conjunctiva of the lower lid.

Bruch's membrane. The inner layer of the choroid of the eye. The outer part is called the elastic lamina, and the inner the cuticular lamina, which is really part of the pigment epithelium of the retina. The term is less commonly used for the front layer of the dilator muscle of the iris of the eye. Also called *Henle's membrane.*

brucine (broo·seen). Dimethoxystrychnine, $C_{21}H_{20}O_2N_2(OCH_3)_2 \cdot 4H_2O$. An alkaloid found along with strychnine in nux vomica, the seed of the Indian tree, *Strychnos nux-vomica.* It resembles strychnine in its pharmacological actions, but is less potent. [James *Bruce,* 1730–1794, African traveller.]

Bruck-Lange disease. Congenital muscular dystrophy with extrapyramidal distribution and mental deficiency.

Brudzinski, Josef (b. 1874). Warsaw physician.

Brudzinski's sign. 1. In irritation or inflammation of the basal meninges (the sign was described in meningococcal meningitis), flexion of the neck produces flexion of arms, hips and knees. 2. Passive flexion of one knee joint in a case of meningitis evokes a similar movement on the opposite side; also called the *contralateral reflex.*

Bruecke, Ernst Wilhelm von (b. 1819). Königsberg and Vienna physiologist.

Bruecke's line. The anisotropic dark band of a striated muscle fibre.

Bruecke's muscle. Meridional fibres of the ciliary muscle.

Bruecke's tunic, or tunica. The layers of the retina deep to the layer of rods and cones.

Bruenings, Wilhelm (b. 1876). German otorhinolaryngologist.

Bruenings' bronchoscope. A form of bronchoscope with a slit mirror set at 45 degrees in the handle so that the operator looks downwards instead of along the line of the bronchoscopic tube.

Bruenninghausen, Hermann J. (b. 1761). German physician.

Bruenninghausen's method. A method of inducing labour by dilatation of the cervix.

Brug, S. L. (b. 1879). Parasitologist, one-time Director of Army Medical Institute, Batavia, Netherlands Indies.

Brug's filariasis. Infection with *Wuchereria malayi* Brug; the rural form of filariasis.

Bruggisser, Anton (b. 1835). Swiss physician.

Bruggisser's hernia. Kroenlein's hernia.

Brugsch, Karl Louis Theodor (b. 1878). Berlin physician.

Brugsch's disease. A condition in which marked thinning of the extremities is associated with acrocyanosis, subnormal growth, thirst and scanty hair.

Brugsch's test. A test for iron in the skin, with an intracutaneous injection of potassium ferrocyanide.

Brugsch's syndrome. Thickening of the skin of the face, scalp and extremities, with clubbing of the fingers and toes, and enlargement of long bones.

bruise (brooz). An accumulation of blood in the connective tissues in the vicinity of an injury, usually visible as a discoloration of, or swelling under, the skin; also from bleeding into injured viscera such as the brain, lungs, heart or abdominal viscera. **Stone bruise.** A contused injury; the term is used particularly of injuries of the bare feet of children, caused by walking on or hitting against stones. [ME *brusen.*]

bruissement (broo·eez·**mon**). A humming or purring sound heard during auscultation. [Fr. rustling.]

bruit (**broo**·e). A sound heard on auscultation, particularly an abnormal sound. It may be used as a synonym for murmur, e.g. the systolic bruit of mitral disease. Although no longer in general use it is retained in certain time-honoured expressions. **Bruit d'airain.** The bell sound sometimes heard with the stethoscope over a pneumothorax or large cavity when a coin placed on the opposite wall is struck with another coin. **Aneurysmal bruit.** Blowing murmur of aneurysm. **Bruit de cuir neuf.** A sound like the creaking of new leather heard over fibrinous pericarditis or pleurisy. **Bruit de diable.** A continuous humming murmur heard over the jugular veins during systole and diastole; sometimes detected in hyperthyroidism and severe anaemias, particularly chlorosis. **False bruit.** Bruit due to an artefact, e.g. pressure of stethoscope. **Bruit de galop.** An expressive term for the 3 heart sounds heard with gallop rhythm. **Bruit de moulin.** The succussion splash sometimes heard with pneumohydropericardium, pneumohydrothorax, or in the stomach. **Ocular bruit.** A murmur sometimes heard in the eye in exophthalmic goitre: Snellen's sign. **Bruit placentaire.** Murmur heard over the placenta. **Bruit de pot fêle.** The "cracked-pot" sound heard on percussion which forces air out of a cavity through a narrow opening. Also heard on percussing the chest of a crying child. **Bruit de rape.** The rough presystolic murmur of mitral stenosis, likened to the noise of a grater or saw. **Bruit de rappel.** Reduplication of the second heart sound, resembling a drum. **Bruit de la roue hydraulique.** The metallic tinkling or "mill-wheel sound" heard with pneumopericardium. **Bruit de scie.** Bruit de rape (see above). **Bruit de soufflet.** The "bellows murmur", the systolic murmur of mitral regurgitation. **Systolic bruit.** Heart murmur during systole. [Fr. noise.]

See also: ROGER (H. L.).

Brumpt, Emile (b. 1877). Paris parasitologist.

Brumpt's white mycetoma. *See* MYCETOMA, WHITE.

Brumptius (**brum**·te·us). A sub-genus of *Phlebotomus.*

Brumptomyia (brum·to·**mi**·e·ah). A sub-genus of *Phlebotomus.*

Brun's glucose. A mixture of glucose, camphor and glycerin in aqueous solution, used for clearing biological specimens.

Brunati's sign. Opacities of the cornea appearing during pneumonia or typhoid fever. They are regarded as a sign of impending death.

Brunhilde (**broon**·hild). The name of the chimpanzee from which the Brunhilde strain of poliomyelitis virus was recovered. *See also* STRAIN; VIRUS.

Brunn, Albert von (b. 1849). Gottingen anatomist.

Brunn's membrane. The olfactory epithelium.

Brunn's cell nests. Nests of intra-epithelial glandular cells in the male urethra.

Brunner, Johann Conrad (b. 1653). Swiss anatomist at Heidelberg.

Brunner's glands. Duodenal glands. *See* GLAND.

brunonianism (broo·no·ne·an·izm). Brunonian theory. *See* BROWN, JOHN.

Bruns, Ludwig (b. 1858). Hanover neurologist.

Bruns' law. Bastian-Bruns' law or sign (see below).

Bruns' sign, or syndrome. Paroxysmal headache, vertigo and vomiting on alteration in head posture. First described in cysticercosis of the 4th ventricle, the sign is equally applicable to other cysts in the region, which, by giving intermittent obstruction to the circulation of cerebrospinal fluid, give rise to attacks of hydrocephalus. Vertigo is due to irritation of vestibular pathways in the ventricular floor.

Bastian-Bruns' law, or sign. Tendon reflexes in the lower extremities cannot be elicited if the spinal cord has a complete transverse lesion above to the lumbar enlargement.

Brunschwig, Alexander (b. 1901). Chicago surgeon.

Brunschwig's operation. Pelvic evisceration; the removal of malignant pelvic viscera with ablation of bladder and rectum after establishment of a "wet colostomy", i.e. colostomy of the colon into which the ureters have been transplanted.

Brunton, John (b. 1836). London physician.

Brunton's otoscope. An otoscope with a specially designed light attachment.

brush (brush). 1. An appliance consisting of tufts of hairs, bristles, glass fibres or metal wire, fixed firmly to a handle. 2. A discharge of static electricity in the form of a brush. **Electrical brush.** A device for collecting electric current from a generator of electricity or for supplying electric current to an electric motor; the brushes usually employed are of compact carbon. Wire brushes are used for the collection of static electricity, as in the Wimshurst machine. **Static brush.** A brush-shaped wire electrode used to apply static electricity to the body. **Stomach**

brush. A brush once used for cleansing the stomach. [AS *byrst* bristle.]

See also: HAIDINGER, RUFFINI.

Bruton, Ogden Carr (b. 1908). American paediatrician.

Bruton's disease. Congenital hypogammaglobulinaemia in males (X-linked heredity).

bruxism (**broox**·izm). The grinding or gnashing of the teeth during sleep. [Gk *brychein* to gnash the teeth.]

bruxomania (broox·o·**ma**·ne·ah). A form of neurosis in which the patient grinds the teeth. [Gk *brychein* to gnash the teeth, mania.]

Bryant, Thomas (b. 1828). London surgeon.

Bryant's ampulla. The obvious distension of an artery above a ligature.

Bryant's line. *See* BRYANT'S SIGN, OR TRIANGLE.

Bryant's operation. Lumbar colostomy through an oblique incision between the last rib and the iliac crest.

Bryant's sign, or triangle. The triangle marked on the skin of a supine patient by dropping a vertical line from the anterior superior iliac spine to a horizontal directed cranially from the upper margin of the greater trochanter. It is used to detect, clinically, a shortening of the femoral neck.

Bryce, Thomas Hastie (b. 1862). Glasgow anatomist.

Bryce–Teacher ovum. One of the classical early human embryos.

Bryce-Smith, Roger. Oxford anaesthetist.

Bryce–Smith tube. A double-lumen endobronchial tube used in thoracic anaesthesia. Described in 1959.

brygmus (**brig**·mus). Odontoprisis; grinding of the teeth. [Gk *brygmos* bite.]

bryonin (**bri**·o·nin). A bitter glucoside obtained from the root of bryonia, or *Bryonia dioica* Jacq., a species of vine common in British hedgerows; formerly used as a drastic purgative.

bryony (**bri**·o·ne). English mandrake, white bryony, the root of *Bryonia dioica* Jacq. (England and Europe), or of *Bryonia alba* Linn. (not wild in England) (family Cucurbitaceae). It has been used as a tincture to allay cough, but larger doses are purgative and may cause poisoning. **Black bryony root.** The root of *Tamus communis* Linn. (family Dioscoreaceae), a diuretic and rubefacient. [Gk *bryonia.*]

buaki (boo·**ak**·e). A protein-deficiency disease found in the Congo valley, characterized by dermatoses, anaemia and oedema.

buba (**boo**·bah). American mucocutaneous leishmaniasis: espundia; uta. The name is also used for yaws. **Buba braziliana.** Buba. **Buba madre.** Primary yaws.

bubble (bubl). A sound heard in auscultation as of a bubble bursting. **Amphoric bubble.** A sound like that of liquid being poured from a bottle; it is heard in auscultation in hydropneumothorax. [onomat.]

bubble-oxygenator (bubl·**ox**′·e·jen·a·tor). An apparatus for bubbling oxygen through blood during cardiopulmonary by-pass, thus ensuring adequate arterial oxygenation. [onomat., Gk *oxys* sharp, *genein* to produce.]

bubide (**boo**·bide). Secondary hypochromic macular yaws.

bubo (**bew**·bo). A subacute or chronic inflammatory swelling of a lymph gland with a tendency to slow suppuration; a localized adenitis, usually in the groin. **Bullet bubo.** The characteristic small, hard, indolent swelling of the lymphatic glands associated with a syphilitic chancre. **Chancroidal bubo.** The subacute inflammatory swelling of the inguinal lymph glands, variable in size, associated with a chancroid ulcer; it is liable to suppuration and sinus formation. **Climatic bubo.** The name formerly given to the lymphadenitis associated with lymphopathia venereum. **Gonorrhoeal bubo.** The slight tender swelling of the inguinal glands associated with the early stage of gonorrhoeal urethritis. **Indolent bubo.** Bullet bubo (see above). **Malignant bubo.** A plague bubo. **Non-venereal bubo.** Adenitis of a lymphatic gland from any non-venereal cause. **Parotid bubo.** Inflammation and swelling of the lymph node overlying the parotid salivary gland. **Pestilential bubo.** The glandular enlargement in plague. **Primary bubo.** Bullet bubo unassociated with a visible primary chancre. **Prurigo buboes.** Lymphadenopathy associated with prurigo. **Simple bubo, Sympathetic bubo.** A non-infective bubo caused by friction or other injury. **Syphilitic bubo.** Bullet bubo (see above). **Tropical bubo.** Lymphopathia venereum. **Venereal bubo.** A bubo associated with a venereal disease. [Gk *boubon* groin.]

bubon d'emblée (bew·**bohn** dahm·**bla**). A bubo which appears as the first sign of venereal infection, there being absence of any premonitory lesion. [Fr. tumour, at first onset.]

bubonadenitis (**bew**·bon·ad·en·**i**′·tis). An inflamed condition of the inguinal gland. [Gk *boubon* groin, adenitis.]

bubonalgia (bew·bon·**al**·je·ah). Pain in the groin, generally arising from inguinal adenitis. [Gk *boubon* groin, *algos* pain.]

bubonic (bew·**bon**·ik). Referring or relating to a bubo.

bubonocele (bew·**bon**·o·seel). An inguinal hernia, direct or indirect but usually the former, confined to the groin and showing no tendency to descend into the scrotum. [Gk *boubon* groin, *kele* hernia.]

bubonulus (bew·**bon**·ew·lus). An abscess or nodule of virus origin occurring anywhere in a lymph vessel, particularly on the dorsum of the penis. [L a small bubo.]

bucardia (bew·**kar**·de·ah). Cor bovinum. [Gk *bous* ox, *kardia* heart.]

bucca (**buk**·ah). 1. General term for the cheek. 2. The outer or inner aspect of the fleshy part of the cheek. 3. The buccal cavity; the mouth. [L.]

buccal (**buk**·al). Relating or belonging to the cheek; involving the cheek or mouth. **Buccal pad.** *See* PAD. **Buccal smear.** Shows the presence or absence of a chromatin mass (Barr body), the former indicating the typical female pattern of XX chromosomes, the latter being due to only one X chromosome—a male characteristic. [L *bucca* cheek.]

buccal artery [arteria buccalis (NA)]. *See* MAXILLARY ARTERY.

buccal nerve [nervus buccalis (NA)]. A sensory branch from the mandibular nerve to the skin and mucous membrane of the cheek.

buccal veins. *See* FACIAL VEIN, POSTERIOR.

buccally (**buk**·al·e). Towards the cheek. [L *bucca* cheek.]

buccellation (buk·sel·**a**·shun). The arresting of haemorrhage by a lint compress applied at the site. [L *buccella* morsel.]

buccilingual (buk·se·**ling**·gwal). Buccolingual.

buccinator muscle [musculus buccinator (NA)] (**buk**·sin·a·tor). The thin flat muscle at the side of the face between the maxilla and the mandible. [L *buccina* trumpet.]

bucco-axial (buk·o·**ax**·e·al). Describing the line angle formed by the buccal and axial walls of a cavity prepared in a tooth.

bucco-axiocervical (buk·o·**ax**·e·o·**ser**′·vik·al). The point angle formed by the buccal, axial and cervical walls of a cavity prepared in a tooth.

buccobranchial (buk·o·**brang**·ke·al). Buccopharyngeal. [L *bucca* cheek, Gk *brogchos* windpipe.]

buccocervical (buk·o·**ser**·vik·al). Relating to the buccal surface and the cervical margin of a tooth.

buccodistal (buk·o·**dis**·tal). Relating to the buccal and the distal surfaces of a tooth.

buccogingival (buk·o·**jin**·je·val). Relating to the cheek and the gums. [L *bucca* cheek, *gingiva* gum.]

buccolabial (buk·o·**la**·be·al). Relating to the cheek and the lip. [L *bucca* cheek, *labium* lip.]

buccolingual (buk·o·**ling**·gwal). Relating to the cheek and tongue. [L *bucca* cheek, *lingua* tongue.]

buccolingually (buk·o·**ling**·gwal·e). In a direction from the cheek towards the tongue. [see prec.]

buccomesial (buk·o·**me**·ze·al). Relating to the buccal and the mesial surfaces of a tooth.

bucconasal (buk·o·**na**·zal). Of or pertaining to the mouth and nasal cavity. [L *bucca* cheek, *nasus* nose.]

bucconasopharyngeal (buk·o·na·zo·far·**in**′·je·al). Of or pertaining to the mouth, nasal cavity, and upper part of the pharynx. [L *bucca* cheek, *nasus* nose, pharynx.]

bucco-occlusal (**buk**·o·**ok**·**loo**′·zal). Relating to the buccal and occlusal surfaces of a tooth.

buccopharyngeal (**buk**·o·far·**in**′·je·al). Relating to the mouth and the pharynx. [L *bucca* cheek, pharynx.]

buccopulpal (buk·o·**pul**·pal). Relating to the buccal wall and the floor adjacent to the pulp in the cavity in a tooth.

buccoversion (buk·o·**ver**·shun). The twisting in a buccal direction, as in the case of a tooth. [L *bucca* cheek, *vertere* to turn.]

buccula (**buk**·ew·lah). The puffy fold of flesh or fat beneath the chin; the swelling known popularly as double chin. [L little cheek.]

Bucetin (**bew**·set·in). BP Commission approved name for *N*-3-hydroxybutyryl-*p*-phenetidine; an analgesic.

Buchanan's operation. A form of external urethrotomy. *See* URETHROTOMY.

Buchanan and Schryver test. For formaldehyde: to 10 ml of aqueous extract or distillate add 2 ml of freshly prepared 1 w/v phenylhydrazine hydrochloride, 1 ml of 5 w/v potassium ferricyanide and 5 ml of concentrated hydrochloric acid. A bright magenta colour indicates formaldehyde.

Buchman, Joseph (b. 1899). New York orthopaedic surgeon.

Buchman's disease. Osteochondrosis of the epiphysis of the iliac crest.

Buchner, Hans Ernst August (b. 1850). Munich bacteriologist.

Buchner's tube. An apparatus used for the anaerobic cultivation of bacteria.

Buchner's zymase. The term zymase was first used by Buchner, and refers to the zymase of alcoholic fermentation.

buchu (**boo**·koo). The name applied to the dried leaves of several species of *Barosma*, family Rutaceae. Buchu BPC 1963 consists of the dried leaves of *Barosma betulina* Bartl. & Wendl. ("short" or "round" buchu). It contains volatile oil, mucilage and diosmin. It is a diuretic and genito-urinary antiseptic, best administered as a fresh infusion, usually with other diuretics. *Barosma crenulata* Hooker, a species yielding "oval" buchu, and *Barosma serratifolia* Willd., from which is obtained "long" buchu; both have properties similar to those of *Buchu betulina*, but are not so highly esteemed. [Hottentot.]

Buchwald, Alfred (b. 1845). Breslau physician.

Buchwald's atrophy. Progressive atrophy of the skin.

Buck, Gurdon (b. 1807). New York surgeon.

Buck's extension. Traction on a leg by a weight suspended from the leg, the body being used as countertraction.

Buck's fascia. The deep fascia of the penis.

buckbean (**buk**·bean). Bog bean; the herb *Menyanthes trifoliata* Linn. (family Gentianaceae). It has tonic and stomachic properties. [Flemish *bocks boonen* goats' beans.]

bucket (**buk**·et). 1. A small bucket at one time used for lowering into the stomach to obtain a sample of the contents for examination. 2. The part of an artificial limb into which the amputation stump fits. [O Fr. *buket* tub.]

Buckley, John Peter (b. 1873). New York dentist.

Buckley's paste. A trioxymethylene paste used in dentistry.

buckthorn (**buk**·thorn). The shrub *Rhamnus cathartica* Linn. (family Rhamnaceae); the fresh ripe berries are laxative. **Alder buckthorn.** The shrub *Rhamnus frangula* Linn., the bark of which is mildly purgative. [AS *buc* he-goat, thorn.]

buckwheat (**buk**·wheet). The grain of a species of *Polygonum*, used mainly for feeding cattle and horses, but also as human food. It occasionally gives rise to a form of poisoning. [D *bockweit*.]

Bucky, Gustav (b. 1880). Berlin and New York radiologist.

Bucky diaphragm. A moving grid consisting of thin lead strips alternating with strips of wood or wax, arranged radially to the x-ray beam. The grid is placed between the part to be x-rayed and the film. Its function is to absorb scattered radiation which would otherwise obliterate fine detail.

Bucky's rays. Very soft x-rays of voltage up to 10 kV and wavelength about 0.2 nm (2 Å), intermediate between ultraviolet rays and conventional x-rays. They are also known as *Grenz rays* or *W rays*.

Bucky-Potter diaphragm, Potter-Bucky diaphragm. Bucky diaphragm.

Buclizine (**bew**·kliz·een). BP Commission approved name for a substituted piperazine with antihistaminic actions; it is used to prevent nausea and vomiting of pregnancy and motion sickness.

Buclosamide (bew·**clo**·sam·ide). BP Commission approved name for *N*-butyl-4-chlorosalicylamide; an antimycotic agent.

bucnemia (buk·**ne**·me·ah). 1. Any large tense swelling of the leg. 2. Elephantiasis. [Gk *bous* ox, *kneme* leg.]

bud (bud). 1. The nascent state of a flower, leaf or branch. 2. Any part or structure resembling a plant bud; any small outgrowth. **Alveolar buds.** At the distal ends of the lactiferous ducts. These buds differentiate into the mammary alveoli. **Appendage bud.** Limb bud (see below). **Bronchial bud.** One of the hollow branches of the embryonic bronchial tree. **Cassia bud.** The unripe fruit of various species of *Cinnamomum*. **Farcy buds.** Small tumours, varying in size from that of a pea to that of a walnut, in the skin in glanders. They may be multiple, single or in chains along a lymphatic vessel. **Limb bud.** The earliest stage in the embryonic development of an arm or leg. **Lung bud.** A hollow outgrowth from the floor of the hinder part of the embryonic pharynx which develops into the trachea, bronchi and lung alveoli. **Tail bud.** A solid outgrowth representing the earliest stage in the development of the tail in the embryo. **Taste bud [calculus gustatorius (NA)].** A collection of specialized richly innervated sensory cells forming a flask-like structure lying amongst the epithelial cells of the surface of the tongue and related oral structures, and subserving the sensation of taste. **Ureteric bud.** A diverticulum from the lower end of the mesonephric duct which gives rise to the ureter, renal pelvis and collecting tubules of the kidney. [ME *budde*.]

Budd, George (b. 1808). London physician.

Budd's disease. Cirrhosis of the liver caused by intestinal toxins.

Budd-Chiari disease, or syndrome. Thrombosis of the hepatic veins or of the inferior vena cava in its intrahepatic course, leading to enlargement of the liver, pain and ascites with portal hypertension.

Budde, E. 19th-20th century Danish chemical engineer.

Budde milk. Milk to which hydrogen peroxide has been added to sterilize it.

budding (**bud**·ing). 1. Gemmation. 2. The formative process of a vascular bud. [ME *budde* bud.]

Budge, Julius Ludwig (b. 1811). Bonn anatomist.

Budge's centre. The ciliospinal centre. *See* CENTRE.

budgerigar (**buj**·er·ig·ar). A parakeet of Australia, *Melopsittacus undulatus*, domesticated and used in psittacosis research. [Australian aboriginal name, pretty bird.]

Budin, Pierre-Constant (b. 1846). Paris gynaecologist.

Budin's obstetrical joint. A primary cartilaginous joint between the squamous and condylar portions of the occipital bone.

Budin rule. In healthy babies, after the neonatal period, the required quantity of milk in 24 h should be one-tenth of the body weight. This quantity should not exceed 600 g.

Buedinger, Konrad (b. 1867). Swiss surgeon in Vienna.

Buedinger-Ludloff-Laewen disease. Osteomalacia of the patella.

Buelau, Gotthard (b. 1835). Hamburg physician.

Buelau's method, or treatment. Siphon drainage of an empyema.

Buengner, Otto von (b. 1858). Hanau surgeon.

Buengner's band, or cell cordons. Protoplasmic bands formed from sheath cells in which the neurofibrils and neuroplasm of regenerating peripheral nerves lie embedded and grow.

Buerger, Leo (b. 1879). New York and Los Angeles urologist.

Buerger's disease. Thrombo-angiitis obliterans.

Buerger's exercises. Special exercises to maintain the circulation of the limb.

Buerger's symptom. Pain occurring at rest in a severely ischaemic limb which may be somewhat relieved by hanging the leg downwards to increase the arterial inflow.

Buerger's test. Normal persons retain the colour in the foot when it is elevated to 90 degrees. When the circulation is impaired, blanching of the foot on elevation occurs.

Buergi, Emil (b. 1872). Swiss pharmacologist.

Buergi's theory. The synergistic effect of 2 drugs having identical pharmacological actions.

Buetschli, Otto (b. 1848). Heidelberg zoologist.

Buetschli's spindle. Achromatic spindle. *See* SPINDLE.

bufagin (**boof**·aj·in). $C_{24}H_{32}O_5$. One of the toxic substances of steroid structure found in the skin of certain toads, particularly the tropical toad *Bufo agua.* Physiologically their action resembles that of the cardiotoxic (digitalis) glycosides.

Bufexamac (bew·**fex**·am·ak). BP Commission approved name for 4-butoxyphenylacetohydroxamic acid; an anti-inflammatory agent.

buffer (**buf**·er). 1. A combination of substances present in a solution which tends to control the concentration of hydrogen ions in that solution and maintain it at a level in spite of the addition of comparatively large amounts of acid or alkali; a shock absorber against changes in pH value, usually a mixture of a weak base and its salt with a strong acid, or a weak acid and its salt with a strong base. 2. Anything that slows or inhibits the immediate action of a chemotherapeutic agent. **Buffer action.** The neutralizing of acids or alkalis without affecting the pH value of the solution. **Buffer capacity.** The measure of buffer action expressed in hydrogen ions neutralized. **Buffer index.** Buffer value (see below). **Buffer pair.** A weak acid and its salt, or a weak base and its salt, which act together as a buffer system. **Buffer salt.** A salt of a low dissociation acid, such as a carbonate, acetate or phosphate, which acts as a buffer. **Buffer solution.** A solution of buffers which maintains a desired pH value; a specially prepared buffer solution to produce required pH values. **Buffer system.** A mixture of buffers designed to produce a determined buffer action. **Buffer value.** The buffer action of a solution measured in terms of the standard acid or alkali necessary to effect a change in the pH value of the solution. [ME *buffet.*]

buffering (**buf**·er·ing). The change or action brought about by a buffer. **Secondary buffering.** Hamburger interchange.

Bufo (**boo**·fo). A genus of toads. **Bufo melanostictus.** A toad found throughout South-east Asia that is used in pregnancy tests. **Bufo vulgaris.** The common toad. [L.]

bufotenin (boo·**fo**·ten·in). Indoxylethyldimethylamine, $OHC_8H_5N CH_2CH_2N(CH_3)_2$. An alkaloid obtained from the skin of the common toad. It has the power of paralysing the central nervous system. [L *bufo* toad.]

bufotherapy (boo·fo·**ther**·ap·e). Treatment by use of toxins derived from toads. [L *bufo* toad, therapy.]

bufothionine (boo·fo·**thi**·o·neen). A poisonous derivative of indole extractable from the skin of the common toad. [L *bufo* toad.]

Bufuralol (bew·**fewr**·al·ol). BP Commission approved name for 2 - *tert* - butylamino - 1 - (7 - ethylbenzofuran - 2 - yl)ethanol; a beta-adrenergic blocking agent.

Bufylline (bew·**fi**·leen). BP Commission approved name for theophylline 2-amino-2-methylpropan-1-ol; a bronchodilator.

bug (bug). Colloquially, any small insect or mite; more specifically, insects of the order Hemiptera, which have sucking mouth parts in a long rostrum. Many will bite man if handled, some causing great pain, and are of medical interest as disease vectors or commensals. **Assassin bug.** A bug of the family Reduviidae which preys on other insects. **Barbiero bug.** *Panstrongylus* (*Triatoma*) *megistus,* occurring in Brazil and transmitting *Trypanosoma cruzi.* **Bat bug, Bed bug.** *Cimex.* **Big bed bug.** *Reduvius personatus.* **Cone-nosed bug.** A bug of the family Reduviidae which includes the genus *Triatoma,* species of which transmit South American trypanosomiasis. **Croton bug.** The German cockroach, *Blatella germanica.* **Harvest bug.** The larval form of a trombidiid mite, *Trombicula autumnalis.* **Kissing bug.** The black corsair, *Melanolestes picipes,* a biting bug of the family Reduviidae. **Persian bug.** *Ornithodorus tholozani.* **Pigeon bug.** *Cimex.* **Pito bug.** *Dysodius lunatus* of South America. **Poultry bug.** *Haematosiphon inodora.* **Red bug.** *Eutrombicula alfreddugèsi,* a larval Trombidiid mite which causes an erythematous itch in man. **Swallow bug.** *Oeciacus.* **Unchuca bug, Vinchuca bug.** *Triatoma infestans,* the black bug of South America which transmits *Trypanosoma cruzi.* [probably Welsh *bwg* hobgoblin.]

buggery (**bug**·er·e). Sodomy. [L *Bulgarus* Bulgarian, a race at one time reputed to be given to sodomy.]

Buhl, Ludwig von (b. 1816). Munich pathologist.

Buhl's disease. Acute haemorrhagic sepsis.

Buhl–Dittrich law. The presence of acute miliary tuberculosis always has as an antecedent a caseous focus somewhere in the body.

Buist, John Brown (b. 1846). Edinburgh physician.

Buist–Paschen body. Paschen body or granule; the elementary body in skin lesions in smallpox and vaccinia.

Buist, Robert Cochrane (b. 1860). Dundee gynaecologist.

Buist's method. For resuscitation of an asphyxiated newborn child; the child is held alternately on the stomach and the back.

bulb (bulb). 1. Any rounded organ, mass or part. 2. A rounded enlargement of the end of an organ or part. 3. The medulla oblongata, to which the terms rachidian bulb, spinal bulb and bulb of the spinal marrow are also occasionally applied. In the spinal cord the term has been used for the cervical enlargement which gives origin to the nerve roots of the brachial plexus (brachial bulb; brachiorachidian bulb) and for the lumbosacral enlargement (crural bulb), but these uses are largely obsolete. **Bulb of the aorta [bulbus aortae (NA)].** The dilatation where the ascending aorta unites with the arch of the aorta. **Arterial bulb.** The embryological bulbus cordis, the right limb of the bulboventricular loop. **Bulb of the corpus spongiosum.** Bulb of the penis (see below). **Duodenal bulb.** The duodenal cap. *See* CAP. **Bulb of the eye.** The eyeball. **Gustatory bulb.** Taste bud. *See* BUD. **Bulb of a hair [bulbus pili (NA)].** The deepest part of the hair follicle which is expanded into a bulb-like structure. **Bulb of the jugular vein.** One of the dilatations of the internal jugular vein: the upper bulb [bulbus venae jugularis superior (NA)] lies at the origin of the vein and the lower bulb [bulbus venae jugularis inferior (NA)] near its termination. **Bulb of the lateral ventricle.** Bulb of the posterior horn (see below). **Nerve bulb.** End-bulb. **Olfactory bulb [bulbus olfactorius (NA)].** The name given to that part of the forebrain in which the olfactory nerves (primary olfactory neurones) terminate and the olfactory tracts arise. **Bulb of the penis [bulbus penis (NA)].** The enlarged oval proximal part of the corpus spongiosum penis which lies between the two crura of the penis; it is connected to the lower surface of the perineal membrane. **Bulb of the posterior horn [bulbus cornus posterioris (NA)].** A swelling in the medial wall of the posterior horn of the lateral ventricle caused by the fibres from the splenium of the corpus callosum (forceps major). **Bulb of the urethra.** Bulb of the penis (see preceding). **Vaginal bulb.** Epithelial masses formed in the embryo by proliferation at the caudal end of the uterovaginal canal. **Bulb of the vestibule [bulbus vestibuli (NA)].** Either of 2 elongated masses of erectile tissue within the orifice of the vagina joined in front by the commissure. **Vestibulovaginal bulb.** Bulb of the vestibule (see preceding). [L *bulbus* a swollen root.]

See also: KRAUSE (W. J. F.).

bulbar (**bul**·bar). 1. Relating to a bulb. 2. Relating to the medulla oblongata, or involving it.

bulbiform (**bul**·be·form). Shaped like a bulb.

bulbitis (bul·**bi**·tis). Inflammation of the urethra at the bulbous portion of the penis. [bulb, Gk *-itis* inflammation.]

bulbocapnine (bul·bo·**kap**·neen). $C_{19}H_{19}O_4N$. An alkaloid derived from *Corydalis cava,* and chemically allied to apomorphine. It has been used for the treatment of muscular tremors, especially in chorea, but its clinical value is doubtful. Its action is probably central, inducing prolonged catalepsy in animals with recovery and no after-effects, but large doses lead to convulsions and death.

bulboid (bul·boid). Bulbiform. [bulb, Gk *eidos* form.]

bulbonuclear (bul·bo·**new**·kle·ar). Relating to the medulla oblongata and the nuclei of the nerves associated with it. [bulb, nucleus.]

bulbopontine (bul·bo·**pon**·tine). Descriptive of the part of the brain composed of the pons and the area of the medulla oblongata situated behind and below it and continuous with it. [bulb, L *pons* bridge.]

bulbospongiosus muscle [musculus bulbospongiosus (NA)] (**bul**·bo·spun·je·**o**'·sus). A median muscle arising from the perineal body and median raphe and partially or completely encircling the back of the penis and adjacent parts of the corpus spongiosum and cavernosum.

bulbo-urethral (**bul**·bo·ewr·**e**'·thral). Relating to the bulb of the penis (bulb of the urethra).

bulbous (**bul**·bus). Like a bulb in nature or form; containing a bulb or bulbs; originating in a bulb.

bulboventricular (bul·bo·ven·**trik**'·ew·lar). Pertaining to the bulbus cordis and the ventricular part of the heart in the embryo.

bulbus (**bul**·bus). A bulb or swelling. **Bulbus arteriosus.** The distal part of the bulbus cordis (see following) which becomes subdivided to form the ascending aorta and pulmonary trunk. **Bulbus cordis.** The anterior subdivision of the primitive heart tube of the early embryo. It becomes partly absorbed into the right ventricle (proximal bulbus) and partly subdivided into the ascending aorta and pulmonary trunk (distal bulbus, bulbus arteriosus, or aortic bulb). [L.]

bulesis (bew·**le**·sis). 1. The will. 2. An act initiated by the will. [Gk *boulesis.*]

bulimia (bew·**lim**·e·ah). Perpetual and voracious appetite for food in large quantities, as a result of increased hunger sense, to a morbid degree. [Gk *bous* ox, *limos* hunger.]

bulimiac (bew·**lim**·e·ak). An individual suffering from bulimia.

Bulinus (bew·**li**·nus). A genus of African snails of which one species, *Bulinus truncatus*, is the intermediate snail host of *Schistosoma haematobium* and *S. bovis*; other species have now been reclassified in other genera. **Bulinus africanus.** *Physopsis africana.* **Bulinus contortus.** *Bulinus truncatus* (see main def.). **Bulinus dysbowskii.** *Bulinus truncatus* (see main def.). **Bulinus forskalii.** *Pyrgophysa forskalii.* **Bulinus innesii.** *Bulinus truncatus* (see main def.). **Bulinus strigosus.** *Physopsis africana.* **Bulinus truncatus.** See main def. [L *bulla* bubble.]

bulkage (**bulk**·ij). Any foodstuff which will increase the aggregate of the contents of the intestine and so induce or give added stimulus to peristalsis. [ME *bulke* heap.]

Bull, Carroll Gideon (b. 1884). Baltimore physician.

Bull's serum, Bull and Pritchett serum. A serum used for gas gangrene.

Bull, James William Douglas (b. 1911). London neuroradiologist.

Bull's angle. The angle between the plane of the atlas vertebra and the hard palate in lateral x-ray of the skull, increased from normal zero in basilar impression.

bulla (**bool**·ah). A blister; a collection of clear fluid in the epidermis or just beneath it. **Bulla dolentissima.** A small chronic and tender ulcer of the skin. **Ethmoidal bulla [bulla ethmoidalis (NA)].** A rounded elevation on the upper part of the middle nasal concha. **Bulla a frigore.** A vesicle occurring as the result of exposure to cold. **Bulla gangraenosa.** A bleb which forms in moist gangrene of the skin. **Bulla ossea.** The lateral dilatation of the bony part of the external auditory meatus of the ear. [L bubble.]

Bullard's haematoxylin. A modification of Harris' haematoxylin.

bullate (**bool**·ate). 1. Characterized by the presence of bullae. 2. Inflated; like a bladder. 3. A term descriptive of those bacterial cultures which develop as rounded elevations so that the surface of the medium has the appearance of a cluster of small blisters.

bullation (bool·a·shun). 1. The state of being inflated. 2. The state of being covered with bullae. 3. The state of being marked off in small divisions. [L *bulla* bubble.]

Buller, Frank (b. 1844). Montreal ophthalmic surgeon.

Buller's bandage, or shield. A watch glass surrounded by adhesive plaster or rubber, placed over the eye and carefully stuck down to the skin all round, except at the lower and outer edge; designed to prevent infection spreading to the opposite eye. Seldom used now.

bullous (**bool**·us). Characterized by the presence of or belonging to bullae.

bulpiss (**bool**·pees). A contagious dermatitis endemic in Nicaragua. It is characterized by an itching papular eruption which when it fades leaves areas of dirty white or thick black pigmentation. [Mex. Ind. *buluy* spotted, *piss* grey.]

bultos (**bool**·tose). A form of abdominal tumour occurring in Peru, of uncertain aetiology. [Sp. *bulto* tumour.]

Bumetanide (bew·**met**·an·ide). BP Commission approved name for 3 - butylamino - 4 - phenoxy - 5 - sulphamoyl - benzoic acid; a diuretic.

Bumke, Oswald Conrad Edward (b. 1877). German neurologist.

Bumke's pupil. Absence of psychosensory reflex dilatation of the pupil in catatonia.

bundelhaar (**bundl**·hahr). Trichostasis spinulosa. [G matted hair.]

bundle (bundl). A collection of fibres all running in the same direction; most commonly applied to nerve fibres. The term is practically synonymous with fasciculus or tract. **Aberrant bundle.** Fibres which enter the anterior commissure of the forebrain from the internal capsule; it is present in some marsupial mammals. **Atrioventricular bundle, Auriculoventricular bundle, A-V bundle [fasciculus atrioventricularis (NA)].** The bundle of His; the bundle of modified cardiac muscle fibres which conducts the impulse causing contraction from the atrioventricular node to the muscle of the ventricles of the heart. **Basis bundle.** The anterior and posterior intersegmental tracts of the spinal cord. **Circumolivary bundle of the pyramid.** Fibres from the cerebrum which pass with the main pyramidal fibres to the level of the olive then sweep laterally below the olive on the surface of the medulla to terminate in the nucleus of the circumolivary bundle. **Circumolivary bundle of the pyramid, nucleus of.** A nucleus forming an oblique ridge on the posterolateral surface of the inferior cerebellar peduncle. It receives impulses from the cerebrum via the circumolivary bundle and transmits them to the cerebellum; probably its cells correspond functionally to those of the nuclei pontis. **Cornucommissural bundle.** Intersegmental fibres, mostly descending, in the posterior columns of the spinal cord. **Forebrain bundle, lateral.** Fibres connecting the corpus striatum with the thalamus and with nuclei in the subthalamus and tegmentum of the mid-brain, represented in the main by the ansa lenticularis of mammals. **Forebrain bundle, medial.** A somewhat diffuse collection of fibres which is thought to connect olfactory centres in the cerebral hemisphere with the hypothalamus and tegmentum of the mid-brain; its olfactory function is uncertain. **Fronto-occipital bundle.** Fibres parallel to the superior longitudinal fasciculus on a deeper plane, just lateral to the caudate nucleus. **Fundamental bundle, Ground bundle.** Basis bundle (see above). **Longitudinal bundle, dorsal [fasciculus longitudinalis dorsalis (NA)].** A longitudinal bundle of fine, mostly unmyelinated fibres in the central grey matter of the mid-brain extending into the floor of the 4th ventricle and possibly to lower levels of the nervous system; they are said to arise in the hypothalamus. **Longitudinal bundle, inferior [fasciculus longitudinalis inferior (NA)].** A bundle running from the temporal lobe towards the occipital cortex. **Longitudinal bundle, medial [fasciculus longitudinalis medialis (NA)].** Nerve fibres which run longitudinally in the brain stem in close relationship with the somatic motor nuclei of the 3rd, 4th, 6th and 12th cranial nerves; many of them connect the vestibular with the oculomotor nuclei, and some are continued down into the anterior columns of the spinal cord. **Longitudinal bundle, posterior.** Medial longitudinal bundle (see preceding). **Longitudinal bundle, superior [fasciculus longitudinalis superior (NA)].** The largest of the association bundles, arching from the frontal cortex above the insula to reach the occipital pole, and spreading forward to enter the temporal lobe. **Marginal bundle.** Fibres in the surface of the spinal cord immediately superficial to the gelatinous matter of the posterior horn of grey matter; the dorsolateral fasciculus of Lissauer. **Papillomacular bundle.** The nerve fibres from the macula of the retina which pass to the outer side of the optic disc, where they enter the optic nerve. **Bundles of the pons, longitudinal [fasciculi longitudinales (NA)].** The pyramidal (corticospinal) fibres broken up in the basilar part of the pons into small bundles, together with the corticopontine fibres, derived from the cerebral cortex and terminating in the nuclei pontis. **Bundle of the pons, oblique.** An occasional bundle of fibres running downwards and backwards on the surface of the pons from a point ventral to the trigeminal root towards the lateral side of the inferior cerebellar peduncle. **Respiratory bundle.** The solitary bundle (see below); the justification for the term "respiratory" is doubtful. **Sinu-atrial bundle.** The modified cardiac muscle fibres which convey the impulse to contraction from the sinu-atrial node to the atrioventricular; these fibres are in the form of a network rather than a bundle. **Solitary bundle.** The tractus solitarius; a bundle of fibres in the medulla derived from the 7th, 9th and 10th cranial nerves, and concerned principally with taste. **Bundle of the tegmentum, medial longitudinal [fasciculus longitudinalis medialis (NA)].** The mid-brain portion of a tract linking the vestibular nuclei with the ocular and other nuclei in the brain stem. **Uncinate bundle [fasciculus uncinatus (NA)].** A bundle connecting gyri on the orbital surface of the frontal lobe with the anterior part of the temporal lobe. **Vascular bundle.** One of a number of collections of descending and ascending vasa recta in the outer medulla of the kidney. The vessels are so closely applied to each other that counter-current exchange can easily take place between them. [D *bondel.*]

See also: ARNOLD (F.), CLARKE, D'AZYR, EDINGER, FOREL, GANTZER, GIERKE (H. P.), GOMBAULT, GRATIOLET, HELD, HELIE, HELWEG, HIS (W. JNR), HOEVE, KENT (A. F. S.), KILLIAN, KRAUSE (W. J. F.), LOEWENTHAL, MEYNERT, MONAKOW, MUNZER, PHILIPPE, PICK (A.), SCHULTZE (M. J. S.), SCHUTZ, SPITZKA (E. C.), STILLING, THOREL, TUERCK, WALLENBERG, WEISMANN, WENCKEBACH.

Bungarus (**bung**·gar·us). A genus of very poisonous elapid snakes of the Old World. **Bungarus candidus.** The common krait of India, South China and Malaysia. **Bungarus fasciatus.** The banded krait of the same regions. [Telegu *bangaru* golden.]

Bunge, Richard (b. 1870). Bonn surgeon.

Bunge's amputation. A periosteal amputation. *See* AMPUTATION.

Bunge's mordant. A mixture of tannin, ferric chloride and fuchsin, partially decolorized with hydrogen peroxide.

bungpagga (bung·**pag**·ah). Tropical pyomyositis; myositis purulenta tropica: deep-seated abscesses in muscles in widely separated sites. The disease if often, but not always, associated with filariasis, and is common in Samoa, the West Indies and West Africa.

buninoid (**boo**·nin·oid). Descriptive of tumours which are round in shape. [Gk *bounos* hill, *eidos* form.]

Buniodyl (bew·**ni**·o·dil). BP Commission approved name for 3 - (3 - butyramido - 2,4,6 - tri - iodophenyl) - 2 - ethylacrylic acid; a radio-opaque contrast medium.

bunion (**bun**·yun). An inflammatory swelling of the bursa of the metatarsophalangeal joint of the big toe with abduction of the toe. [Gk *bounion* turnip.]

bunionectomy (bun·yun·**ek**·to·me). Surgical removal of a bunion from the metatarsophalangeal joint of the big toe and plastic repair and straightening of the contour of the toe. [Gk *bounion* turnip, *ektome* a cutting out.]

Bunnell, Sterling (b. 1882). San Francisco surgeon.

Bunnell's operation. An operation for cut flexor tendons of the fingers when the cut is actually in the finger and thus involving the fibrous tendon sheath. The injured tendon is removed and replaced by a tendon graft which runs from above the level of the fibrous sheath to the base of the terminal phalanx, thus avoiding fixation between the tendon and the fibrous sheath at the point of injury.

Bunnell suture. A removable stainless suture used in repair of divided tendons in the hand.

Bunnell, Walls Willard (b. 1902). Connecticut physician.

Paul-Bunnell reaction, or test. A laboratory test used to confirm a clinical diagnosis of infective mononucleosis (glandular fever): dilutions of the patient's serum are mixed with a suspension of washed sheep's corpuscles and incubated, and the degree of agglutination is noted. The test depends on the presence of sheep "heterophile" antibodies (agglutinins) in the blood in glandular fever, and is almost specific.

Bunsen, Robert Wilhelm Eberhard von (b. 1811). German chemist and physicist.

Bunsen burner. The standard laboratory gas burner in which air is drawn in and burnt with gas; this allows more complete combustion and gives a smokeless flame.

Bunsen's coefficient. Coefficient of absorption of gases in liquids.

Bunsen-Roscoe law. In a photochemical reaction, the amount of the products is directly proportional to the energy absorbed. Thus, in the decomposition of silver salts by light, the amount of silver produced depends upon the intensity of light and the length of exposure.

Bunyan, John. London dental surgeon.

Bunyan bag, or envelope. A bag introduced during World War II for the treatment of burns of the extremities. It is waterproof and transparent, and so adjusted as to allow irrigation of the burned surfaces with hypochlorite solution.

Bunyan-Stannard treatment. For burns. *See* BUNYAN BAG (above).

Buphane (**bew**·fane). A genus of plants of the Amaryllidaceae. The bulb of *Buphane disticha* (*Buphane toxicaria*) Herb. contains alkaloids such as buphanine and toxic bases. It is used as an arrow poison in South Africa.

buphanine (**bew**·fan·een). An alkaloid of uncertain composition occurring in *Buphane disticha* (family Amaryllidaceae). It has weak hyoscine-like effects.

Buphenine (**bew**·fen·een). BP Commission approved name for 1-*p*-hydroxyphenyl-2-(1-methyl-3-phenyl-propylamino)propanol; it causes peripheral dilatation by direct action on arterioles. It mobilizes blood from blood depots, and increases cardiac output. It is used in the treatment of intermittent claudication.

buphthalmia, buphthalmos, buphthalmus (buf·**thal**·me·ah, buf·**thal**·mos, buf·**thal**·mus). Increased intra-ocular pressure occurring in infancy, causing enlargement of the eyeball and particularly of the cornea. It arises out of a congenital defect in the mechanism for drainage of the aqueous. [Gk *bous* ox, *ophthalmos* eye.]

Bupivacaine (bew·**piv**·ak·ane). BP Commission approved name for 1-butyl-2-(2,6-xylylcarbamoyl)piperidine. **Bupivacaine Hydrochloride BP 1973.** The monohydrate, a long-acting local analgesic with an amine-linked molecule, first used in 1963.

Buprenorphine (bew·**pren**·**or**·feen). BP Commission approved name for *N* - cyclopropylmethyl - 7α - (1 - (*S*) - hydroxy - 1,2,2 - trimethylpropyl) - 6,14 - *endo* - ethano - 6,7,8,14 - tetrahydronororipavine; an analgesic.

bur (ber). Burr.

Burchardt, Max (b. 1831). Berlin physician.

Burchardt's corpuscles. Yellowish corpuscles described as being present in the conjunctival secretion of cases of trachoma.

Burckhardt's operation. Evacuation of a retropharyngeal (tuberculous) abscess through an open incision in the neck.

Burckhardt-Merian test. For feigned bilateral total deafness: disparaging remarks about the patient are made to a third party behind his back. Frequently, the malingerer's change of expression is sufficient to detect his imposture.

Burdach, Karl Friedrich (b. 1776). Königsberg physiologist.

column or fasciculus of Burdach. The fasciculus cuneatus; fibres which ascend in the lateral part of the posterior columns of the spinal cord, and which arise from the cells in the spinal ganglia from the level of the 6th thoracic upwards, ending in the nucleus cuneatus.

Burdach's fibres. Fibres arising from the cuneate nucleus.

Burdach's fissure. A fissure between the island of Reil (insula) and the operculum.

Burdach's nucleus. The cuneate nucleus of the medulla, continuous below with the fasciculus cuneatus.

Burdach's operculum. The operculum of the island of Reil (insula).

Burdach's tract. Fasciculus cuneatus.

Burdick lamp. A lamp for ultra-violet-ray treatment in dentistry.

burdock (ber·dok). A plant, *Actium lappa. See* LAPPA. [ME *burre*, AS *docce.*]

buret, burette (bew·ret). A graduated glass tube, usually fitted with a stop-cock and having a small aperture; it is used in volumetric analysis for measuring definite quantities of liquids. [Fr. small jug.]

Burger's sign. The absence of recognition of illumination on the side of a diseased maxillary antrum when a light is placed in the mouth.

Burghart, Hans Gerny (b. 1862). Berlin physician.

Burghart's sign. The presence of fine râles heard in front of the lower margin of the lung. They were regarded as an early sign of tuberculosis.

Burkitt, Denis Parsons. East African and London surgeon.

Burkitt's lymphoma. A central African malignant tumour usually involving the maxilla on one side but which may also involve the mandible and, in girls, the ovaries. It is unusually sensitive to cytotoxic drugs with rapid remission and often cure following treatment. Spontaneous remissions also occur. In about 5 per cent of cells cultured from tumour tissue a herpesvirus, EB virus, can be demonstrated. The virus, which is the cause of glandular fever, probably plays some part in the aetiology of the tumour but its exact role has yet to be determined. It is very unlikely that the virus is the sole cause of the tumour.

burn (bern). 1. An injury caused by heat or by chemical or physical agents having an effect similar to heat. For the classification of burns see below. 2. To cauterize. 3. To give rise to the sensation of heat. **Acid burn.** A burn produced by contact with an acid. **Brush burn.** A lesion caused by friction against the skin. **Cement burn.** Corrosive action of this substance upon tissue. **Chemical burn.** A burn produced by caustic or other chemical irritants, including gases. **Classification of burns.** *Dupuytren's classification:* 1st degree, reddening of skin; 2nd degree, blistering of skin; 3rd degree, partial skin destruction; 4th degree, total skin destruction; 5th degree, charring of muscle; 6th degree, charring of bone. *Modern classification:* superficial burn or partial thickness skin destruction; deep burn or whole thickness skin destruction. **Concrete burn.** Cement burn (see above). **Deep burn.** Destruction by heat or similar agent of the whole thickness of the skin. **Electric burn.** A lesion caused by contact with a live electric current. **Flash burn.** A burn from electric flash. **Friction burn.** Brush burn (see above). **Kangri burn.** A burn of the abdomen caused by heat from the kangri stove carried by Kashmiris under their clothes; it may cause carcinoma. **Light burn.** A burn from over-exposure to light rays, natural or artificial, direct or reflected (snow). **Lightning burn.** A burn from lightning stroke. **Radiation burn, Radium burn.** That resulting from exposure to any type of radiant energy, e.g. sunlight, ultra-violet rays, radium or x-rays. **Superficial burn.** A burn which nowhere destroys the whole thickness of the skin. **Thermal burn.** A burn caused by direct contact with a flame or hot surface. **X-ray burn.** Radiation burn (see above). [AS *baernan.*]

burner (bern·er). The part of a lamp that controls the nature of the flame, or in the case of a gas burner usually the whole lamp. [see prec.]

See also: ARGAND, BUNSEN.

Burney Yeo, Isaac. *See* YEO.

burning feet (bern·ing feet). A well-recognized condition, especially among Indian and African women. It is now thought to be due to a dietary deficiency of pantothenic acid of the vitamin B_2 group. The symptom of burning of the sole is usually accompanied by an angular cheilitis. The condition has long been regarded by the people of these countries as a specific affliction, and has been given various names. [AS *baernan, fot.*]

burnisher (ber·nish·er). A smooth-headed instrument for imparting a polished surface to wax or gold in conservative dentistry. [OFr. *burnir* to polish.]

Burns, Allan (b. 1781). Glasgow anatomist.

Burns' ligament. The falciform ligament of the fascia lata at the saphenous opening.

Burns' space. Suprasternal space. *See* SPACE.

Burns, Bryan Hartop. London orthopaedic surgeon.

Burns' disease. Osteochondrosis of the distal ulnar epiphysis.

Burns' procedure. Surgical reposition of the tibial tubercle.

Burns, John (b. 1774). Glasgow physician.

Burns' amaurosis. Postmarital amblyopia. *See* AMBLYOPIA.

Burns, John William. Liverpool gynaecologist.

Burns–Marshall manoeuvre, or method. Delivery of the aftercoming head by allowing the child to hang from the vulva by its own weight. When the head has entered the pelvis the legs are lifted downward and then forward; thus gradually the head is delivered.

Burow, Karl August von (b. 1809). Königsberg surgeon.

Burow's operation. A blepharoplasty for lower-lid defects or cicatricial ectropion: 2 triangular areas of skin are removed, one apex down with the lower-lid margin as base, the other apex up with base extending outwards from the outer canthus. It is not used now, except in the form of Burow's triangles, small triangular excisions of skin at the base of sliding flaps to stop puckering.

Burow's triangle. *See* BUROW'S OPERATION (above).

Burow's veins. Renal veins.

burr (ber). A rotatory instrument made of steel or tungsten carbide, fitting into a handpiece or brace and used for cutting tooth or bone. Various sizes and shapes are made according to the nature of their use. [ME *burre.*]

burrow (ber·o). 1. Any abnormally-placed fistula or sinus. 2. The channel made through the tissues by the passage of pus. 3. The furrow made in the skin or tissues by parasitic insects or their larvae. [AS *burg.*]

bursa [NA] (ber·sah). A term generally applied to a closed cavity in the connective tissue between two structures which move relative to one another, e.g. between a tendon and an adjacent bone. The cavity is lined by a synovial membrane, and contains a small amount of synovial fluid, hence the name synovial or mucous bursa. It may be multilocular. The term is also applied to certain pockets or recesses in the peritoneum, e.g. ovarian bursa (see below). Most bursae take their names from their anatomical situation, or from the tendons and muscles with which they are associated. **Acromial bursa, subcutaneous [bursa subcutanea acromialis (NA)].** A small bursa overlying the acromion. **Adventitious bursa.** An abnormal bursa developed over a prominence as a result of continual friction. **Anserine bursa [bursa anserina (NA)].** A compound bursa related to the tendons of insertion of sartorius, gracilis and semitendinosus muscles in the medial surface of the tibia. **Bursa of the biceps femoris muscle, lower [bursa subtendinea musculi bicipitis femoris inferior (NA)].** A small bursa between this tendon and the lateral ligament of the knee joint. **Bursa of the biceps femoris muscle, upper [bursa musculi bicipitis femoris superior (NA)].** The bursa under the tendon of origin of this muscle. **Bicipitoradial bursa [bursa bicipitoradialis (NA)].** A constant synovial sac between the tendon of insertion of the biceps muscle and the anterior part of the radial (bicipital) tuberosity. **Calcanean bursa, subcutaneous [bursa subcutanea calcanea (NA)].** An occasional small bursa lying between the lower part of the posterior surface of the calcaneus and the skin. **Bursa of**

the coracobrachialis muscle [bursa musculi coracobrachialis (NA)]. An occasional bursa of the upper part of the arm. **Bursa of the extensor carpi radialis brevis tendon [bursa musculi extensoris carpi radialis brevis (NA)].** A small synovial sac occasionally present between the tendon of this muscle and the styloid process on the base of the 3rd metacarpal bone. **Bursa of Fabricius.** Gut-associated lymphoid organ in birds which acts as a source of the cells which mediate humoral immunity. Not found in mammals but there may be an analogous lymphoid tissue controlling humoral immunity in them. **Bursa of the gastrocnemius muscle, lateral [bursa subtendinea musculi gastrocnemii lateralis (NA)].** A bursa under the tendon of origin of the lateral head of the gastrocnemius. **Bursa of the gastrocnemius muscle, medial [bursa subtendinea musculi gastrocnemii medialis (NA)].** A small cavity under the tendon of origin; it occasionally communicates with the knee joint. **Gluteofemoral bursa [bursae intermusculares musculorum gluteorum (NA)].** A synovial sac between the tendon of insertion of the gluteus maximus and the vastus lateralis muscles. **Iliac bursa, subtendinous [bursa subtendinea iliaca (NA)].** A bursa lying deep to the tendon of the iliacus muscle just above the hip joint. **Infracardiac bursa.** A cyst-like transient structure found in the mediastinum near the diaphragm, representing the upper cut-off part of the pneumato-enteric recess (upper recess of the lesser sac) of the embryonic peritoneal cavity. **Infrahyoid bursa [bursa infrahyoidea (NA)].** A small bursa deep to the body of the hyoid bone lying between this and the upper end of the thyrohyoid ligament. **Infrapatellar bursa, deep [bursa infrapatellaris profunda (NA)].** A bursa between the ligamentum patellae and the upper part of the front of the tibia. **Infrapatellar bursa, subcutaneous [bursa subcutanea infrapatellaris (NA)].** A bursa between the skin and the ligamentum patellae. **Bursa of the infraspinatus muscle [bursa subtendinea musculi infraspinati (NA)].** A small synovial bursa which occurs between the tendon of the infraspinatus muscle and the capsule of the shoulder joint. It may communicate with the cavity of this joint. **Interosseous cubital bursa [bursa cubitalis interossea (NA)].** An occasional bursa situated between the tendon of the biceps brachii and the depression on the ulna anterior to the supinator crest. **Ischial bursa of the gluteus maximus muscle [bursa ischiadica musculi glutei maximi (NA)].** A bursa usually found between the lower fibres of this muscle and the ischial tuberosity. **Bursa of the laryngeal prominence [bursa subcutanea prominentiae laryngeae (NA)].** A small subcutaneous bursa sometimes found over the prominence of the thyroid cartilage. **Bursa of the lateral epicondyle, subcutaneous.** A small synovial sac which very occasionally occurs over this bony prominence. **Bursa of the lateral malleolus, subcutaneous [bursa subcutanea malleoli lateralis].** An unusual bursa over the lateral malleolus. **Bursa of the latissimus dorsi muscle [bursa subtendinea musculi latissimi dorsi (NA)].** An elongated bursal synovial sac which may occur deep to the tendon of insertion of this muscle. **Bursa of the medial epicondyle, subcutaneous.** A small synovial sac which very occasionally occurs over this bony prominence. **Bursa of the medial malleolus, subcutaneous [bursa subcutanea malleoli medialis (NA)].** An unusual bursa over the medial malleolus. **Bursa of the obturator externus muscle.** A bursa communicating with the hip joint which often occurs between the tendon of the obturator externus muscle and the capsule of the hip joint and neck of the femur. **Bursa of the obturator internus muscle.** 1. [bursa ischiadica musculi obturatorii interni (NA)], a well-developed synovial sac constantly present deep to and partially encircling the tendon of this muscle as it emerges from a lesser sciatic foramen. 2. [bursa subtendinea musculi obturatorii interni (NA)], a bursa usually present between the tendon of the obturator internus muscle and the capsule of the hip joint. It may communicate with the bursa ischiadica musculi obturatorii interni. **Olecranon bursa, intratendinous [bursa intratendinea olecrani (NA)].** An occasional small bursa lying in the tendon of insertion of the triceps muscle. **Olecranon bursa, subcutaneous [bursa subcutanea olecrani (NA)].** A synovial sac which is frequently present over the olecranon. **Bursa omentalis (NA).** The lesser sac of the peritoneum. **Ovarian bursa.** A peritoneal recess between the ovary and the mesosalpinx. **Pharyngeal bursa [bursa pharyngea (NA)].** A recess found at the lower pole of the nasopharyngeal tonsil and which often continues for some distance upward and backward deep to the tonsillar mass. It is more easily recognized in the fetus and in infants, and is regarded as a remnant of the degenerated end of the notochord. **Bursa of the piriformis muscle [bursa musculi piriformis (NA)].** A small sac sometimes present under the tendon of insertion of this muscle. **Bursa of the popliteus tendon [recessus subpopliteus (NA)].** A tubular extension of the synovial cavity of the knee joint around the tendon of the popliteus. It may also communicate with the superior tibiofibular joint. **Premental bursa.** A small subcutaneous bursa sometimes found on the front of the chin. **Prepatellar bursa, subcutaneous [bursa subcutanea prepatellaris (NA)].** The bursa anterior to the patella and between it and the skin. **Prepatellar bursa, subfascial [bursa subfascialis prepatellaris (NA)].** An occasional bursa between the deep fascia and the tendinous fibres on the front of the patella. **Prepatellar bursa, subtendinous [bursa subtendinea prepatellaris (NA)].** An occasional bursa between the tendinous fibres in front of the patella and the bone itself. **Bursa of the psoas major tendon [bursa iliopectinea (NA)].** A large and constant synovial sac, occasionally in communication with the hip joint, between the tendon on the one hand and the pubis and capsule of the joint on the other. **Bursa of the rectus femoris muscle.** An uncommon and small synovial sac between the reflected tendon and the margin of the acetabulum. **Retrohyoid bursa [bursa retrohyoidea (NA)].** A small synovial sac between the body of the hyoid bone and the thyrohyoid ligament. **Sacral bursa, subcutaneous.** An adventitious subcutaneous bursa situated over the sacrococcygeal joint and the lower sacral spines. **Bursa of the semimembranous tendon [bursa musculi semimembranosi (NA)].** A bursa separating the flattened tendon of the semimembranosus muscle from the medial head of the gastrocnemius muscle. **Bursa of the sinus tarsi.** An occasional bursa between the fibres of the interosseous talocalcaneal ligaments. **Subacromial bursa [bursa subacromialis (NA)].** A large synovial sac between the acromion and the tendon of the supraspinatus muscle. Its upward extension is often called the *subdeltoid bursa.* **Subcutaneous bursa.** *See* SYNOVIAL BURSA (below). **Subcutaneous bursa of the tuberosity of the tibia [bursa subcutanea tuberositatis tibiae (NA)].** A subcutaneous bursa situated over the tuberosity of the tibia and the lower part of the ligamentum patellae. **Subdeltoid bursa [bursa subdeltoidea (NA)].** A bursa between the deltoid muscle and the supraspinatus tendon. It may be continuous with the subacromial bursa. **Subfascial bursa.** *See* SYNOVIAL BURSA (below). **Submuscular bursa.** *See* SYNOVIAL BURSA (below). **Subscapular bursa [bursa subtendinea musculi subscapularis (NA)].** A bursa beneath the tendon of the subscapularis muscle which communicates with the cavity of the shoulder joint. **Subtendinous bursa.** *See* SYNOVIAL BURSA (below). **Subtendinous bursa of the trapezius muscle [bursa subtendinea musculi trapezii (NA)].** A bursa between the tendinous part of this muscle and the medial end of the spine of the scapula. **Bursa of the superior oblique muscle of the orbit [vagina synovialis musculi oblique superioris (NA)].** A small synovial sheath around the tendon of the superior oblique muscle of the orbit, where this passes through the pulley at the upper and medial angle of the orbit. **Suprapatellar bursa [bursa suprapatellaris (NA)].** Suprapatellar synovial pouch; a bursa between the lower end of the femur and the quadriceps femoris muscle, communicating freely with the knee joint. **Synovial bursa [bursa synovialis (NA)].** A sac lined by synovial membrane and moistened by a small amount of fluid (synovial fluid) found where structures rub together or are subjected to pressure. They may be subcutaneous [bursa synovialis subcutanea (NA)], submuscular [bursa synovialis submuscularis (NA)], subtendinous [bursa synovialis subtendinea (NA)] or subfascial [bursa synovialis subfascialis]. **Bursa of the tendo calcaneus [bursa tendinis calcanei (Achillis) (NA)].** A bursa between this tendon and the back of the calcaneum. **Bursa of the tendon of the**

triceps muscle [bursa subtendinea musculi tricipitis brachii (NA)]. A synovial sac which occurs between the tendon of the triceps and the olecranon. **Bursa of the tensor palati muscle [bursa musculi tensoris veli palatini (NA)].** A small sac partly encircling the tendon of the tensor palati muscle, where this turns around the medial ptyergoid hamulus. **Bursa of the teres major muscle [bursa subtendinea musculi teretis majoris (NA)].** A small synovial sac which may be present deep to the tendon of insertion of this muscle. **Tibial intertendinous bursa [bursa subtendineae musculi sartorii (NA)].** A bursa under the tendon of insertion of the sartorius muscle and in front of the gracilis and semitendinosus muscles. **Bursa of the tibialis anterior tendon [bursa subtendinea musculi tibialis anterioris (NA)].** A small bursa which may occur under the portion of the tendon inserted into the first metatarsal bone. **Bursa of the tibialis posterior tendon.** A small bursa which may occur between this tendon and the plantar calcaneonavicular ligament. **Trochanteric bursa, subcutaneous [bursa subcutanea trochanterica (NA)].** The synovial sac over the greater trochanter of the femur. **Trochanteric bursa of the gluteus maximus muscle [bursa trochanterica musculi glutei maximi (NA)].** A small synovial sac, often double, between the tendon of this muscle and the greater trochanter of the femur. **Trochanteric bursa of the gluteus medius muscle [bursa trochanterica musculi glutei medii (NA)].** A bursa between the tendon of this muscle and the lateral surface of the greater trochanter of the femur. **Trochanteric bursa of the gluteus minimus muscle [bursa trochanterica musculi gluei minimi (NA)].** A bursa between the tendon of this muscle and the anterior surface of the greater trochanter of the femur. **Trochlear bursa, synovial [vagina synovialis musculi obliqui superioris (NA)].** A small bursa related to the tendon of the superior oblique muscle of the orbit at the fibrous cartilaginous pulley attached to the trochlear fossa of the frontal bone. [Gk *byrsa* wineskin.]

See also: ACHILLES, BOYER, BRODIE (B. C.), CALORI, CHASSAIGNAC, CODMAN, FLEISCHMANN, LUSCHKA.

bursal (ber·sal). Relating to a bursa.

bursalis (ber·sa·lis). The obturator internus muscle. [bursa.]

bursectomy (ber·**sek**·to·me). The surgical amputation or excision of a bursa. [bursa, Gk *ektome* a cutting out.]

bursine (**ber**·seen). An alkaloid obtained from *Herba capsellae* (*Capsella bursa*, shepherd's purse); it has astringent properties.

bursitis (ber·si·tis). An inflammatory condition affecting a bursa. All the bursae (*sensu restricto*) included in the entry *bursa* are subject to bursitis and the name of the bursa affected usually precedes the word *bursitis*, e.g. *olecranon bursitis, prepatellar bursitis* (see below), but there are exceptions. **Olecranon bursitis.** Inflammation in the subcutaneous bursa which overlies the olecranon. **Omental bursitis.** Seropurulent inflammation of the lesser sac of the peritoneum. **Pharyngeal bursitis.** A cystic condition of the nasopharyngeal tonsil with chronic secretion of mucopus. **Popliteal bursitis.** Inflammation of the bursa in relation to the medial head of the gastrocnemius muscle in the popliteal space. **Prepatellar bursitis.** Housemaids' knee; a state of acute or chronic inflammatory swelling of the prepatellar bursa which lies superficial to the knee cap and its tendon. **Radiohumeral bursitis.** One form of tennis elbow; inflammation in an adventitious bursa said to develop, as a result of forcible pronation, over the origin of the brachioradialis muscle from the lateral epicondyle of the humerus. **Retrocalcaneal bursitis.** Acute inflammation of the bursa overlying the insertion of the Achilles tendon at the heel. **Subacromial bursitis.** Inflammation of the subacromial bursa. **Subdeltoid bursitis.** Inflammation of the subdeltoid bursa. [bursa, Gk *-itis* inflammation.]

See also: ACHILLES, CODMAN, DUPLAY, THORNWALDT.

bursolith (**ber**·so·lith). A concretion or calculus formed in a bursa. [bursa, Gk *lithos* stone.]

bursopathy (ber·**sop**·ath·e). 1. Any disease or pathological condition affecting a bursa. 2. A collection of serous fluid in a bursa as the result of a general disease, e.g. dropsy. **Luetic bursopathy.** Bursitis caused by syphilis. [bursa, Gk *pathos* suffering.]

bursotomy (ber·**sot**·o·me). Incision of a bursa through its wall. [bursa, Gk *temnein* to cut.]

burst size (berst size). The mean number of bacteriophage particles liberated per infected bacterium, when lysis is complete.

bursula (ber·sew·lah). A small bag or sac. **Bursula testium.** The scrotum. [LL, small purse.]

Burton, Henry (b. 1799). London physician.

Burton's line, or sign. Blue line; a dark-blue stippled line within the tissues of the gums near their margin, occurring with chronic lead absorption.

Bury, Judson Sykes (b. 1852). Manchester physician.

Bury's disease. One of the varieties of erythema elevatum diutinum.

Buschke, Abraham (b. 1868). Berlin dermatologist.

Buschke's disease. Cryptococcosis (torulosis or European blastomycosis).

Buschke's scleroedema. Scleroedema adultorum; rapidly spreading, non-pitting oedema, which commences on the head or cervical area, thence involving wide areas and terminating after 8–12 months, leaving no sequelae. The malady usually follows general infections or toxaemias, and may also be a complication of pyoderma.

Busse-Buschke disease. Buschke's disease (see above).

bushmaster (**bush**·mas·ter). A large and very poisonous crotaline snake of tropical Central and South America and Trinidad, *Lachesis mutus.* [ME *busk*, L *magister.*]

Busquet, G. Paul (b. 1866). French physician.

Busquet's disease. Exostosis of the metatarsals, usually of the 1st metatarsal.

Busse, Otto (b. 1867). German physician in Zürich.

Busse's saccharomyces. *Cryptococcus neoformans.*

Busse-Buschke disease. Cryptococcosis (torulosis or European blastomycosis).

Busulphan BP 1973 (bew·**sul**·fan). 1,4-Dimethanesulphonyloxybutane. It has a specific depressant action on granulocytes and has been used in the treatment of leukaemia.

Butacaine Sulphate BP 1953 (bew·tah·kane **sul**·fate). $[NH_2C_6H_4COO(CH_2)_3N(C_4H_9)_2]_2H_2SO_4$. A local anaesthetic similar to cocaine but more rapid and more prolonged in its action.

Butalamine (bew·**tal**·am·een). BP Commission approved name for 3 - phenyl - 5 - (2 - dibutylaminoethyl)amino - 1,2,4 - oxadiazole; a vasodilator.

butalanine (bewt·al·an·een). Norvaline, α-aminovaleric acid, $CH_3CH_2CH_2CH(NH_2)COOH$. An α-amino acid occurring in protein.

butaldehyde (bewt·al·de·hide). Butyl aldehyde. *See* ALDEHYDE.

Butamyrate (bewt·**am**·e·rate). BP Commission approved name for 2-(2-diethylaminoethoxy)ethyl 2-phenylbutyrate; a cough suppressant.

butane (**bew**·tane). Normal butane, methylethylmethane, $CH_3CH_2CH_2CH_3$. A colourless gas occurring naturally with petroleum; a saturated hydrocarbon of the methane or paraffin series, of which it is the fourth member.

Butanilicaine (bewt·an·**il**·e·kane). BP Commission approved name for *N*-butylaminoacetyl-6-chloro-*o*-toluidine; a local anaesthetic.

butanol (**bew**·tan·ol). Normal butyl alcohol. *See* ALCOHOL.

butanone (**bew**·tan·one). Methylethyl ketone, $CH_3COC_2H_5$. A colourless inflammable liquid found in crude wood spirit; used as a solvent and in the manufacture of colourless plastics.

butaprobenz (bew·tah·**pro**·benz). *p*-Aminobenzoyldibutylaminopropanal sulphate, $(C_{18}H_{30}N_2O_2)_2H_2SO_4$. A local anaesthetic having approximately the same activity as cocaine. It does not potentiate the action of adrenaline, and does not therefore dilate the pupil when used to anaesthetize the eye. When given by subcutaneous injection it is usual to incorporate adrenaline in the solution, in order to produce local vasoconstriction and localize the anaesthetic.

Butcher, Richard George Herbert (b. 1819). Dublin surgeon.

Butcher's saw. A saw with an adjustable blade.

Butea (bew·te·ah). A genus of trees of the family Leguminosae. The Indian *Butea frondosa* Roxb. yields butea gum, the inspissated juice from the stem, which is astringent, and butea seeds, the oil of which is used as an aperient and anthelmintic (moodooga oil). [John Stuart, 3rd Earl of *Bute*, 1713–1792, British politician and amateur botanist.]

Butethamate (bewt·eth·am·ate). BP Commission approved name for 2-diethylaminoethyl 2-phenylbutyrate; an antispasmodic.

butethanol (bewt·eth·an·ol). Amethocaine Hydrochloride BP 1958.

Buthalitone Sodium (bew·thal·e·tone so·de·um). BP Commission approved name for a mixture of 100 parts by weight of the monosodium derivative of 5-allyl-5-isobutyl-2-thiobarbituric acid and 6 parts by weight of exsiccated sodium carbonate used intravenously for the production of brief anaesthesia.

Buthus (bew·thus). A genus of scorpions. **Buthus maurus.** A poisonous scorpion. **Buthus occidentalis.** A fairly poisonous species; both this and the preceding species occur in Southern Europe. **Buthus quinquistriatus.** A poisonous species of North Africa.

Butirosin Sulphate (bew·tir·o·zin sul·fate). BP Commission approved name for a mixture of O^4 - (2,6 - diamino - 2,6 - dideoxy - α - D - glucopyranosyl) - O^5 - (β - D - xylofuranosyl) - N^1- (4 - amino - 2 - hydroxybutyryl) - 2 - deoxystreptamine sulphate (1:2)(salt)dihydrate with O^4 - (2,6 - diamino - 2,6 - dideoxy - α - D- glucopyranosyl) - O^5 - (β - D - ribofuranosyl) - N^1 - (4 - amino - 2 - hydroxybutyryl) - 2 - deoxystreptamine sulphate (1:2)(salt)dihydrate; an antibacterial agent.

Butler, Allan Macy (b. 1894). American biochemist.

Butler and Tuthill method. For sodium in blood: organic matter of serum is destroyed by wet oxidation and the sodium precipitated with zinc uranyl acetate. The precipitate is washed with alcohol and ether, dried in a desiccator and weighed as $(VO_2)_3ZnNa(CH_3COO)_9{\cdot}6H_2O$.

Butlin, Sir Henry Trentham (b. 1845). London surgeon.

Butlin's operation. Hemiglossectomy for carcinoma of the tongue.

Butobarbitone BP 1973 (bew·to·bar·be·tone). 5-n-Butyl-5-ethylbarbituric acid $(C_4H_9)(C_2H_5)C(CONH)_2CO$. A sedative and hypnotic of the barbiturate group, also used as a preliminary to general anaesthesia.

Butoxamine (bew·tox·am·een). BP Commission approved name for (±) - *erythro* - 1 - (2,5 - dimethoxyphenyl) - 2 - *tert* - butylamino - propan - 1 - ol; an inhibitor of fatty acid mobilization.

Butriptyline (bew·trip·til·een). BP Commission approved name for DL - 3 - (10,11 - dihydro - 5*H* - dibenzo[*a,d*]cyclohepten - 5 - yl) - 2 - methylpropyldimethylamine; an antidepressant.

butter (but·er). 1. A solid fatty mass resulting from the churning of cream, the fat globules running together leaving the protein, lactose and mineral salts to constitute buttermilk in the bulk of water. It contains approximately 85 per cent of fats (mainly mixed glycerides of even-carbon fatty acids) bearing fat-soluble vitamins (mainly A, with a little D), and owes its colour to carotene; the vitamin and carotene content varies with the winter and summer diets of the cattle. It also contains about 12 per cent of water, and some caseinogen and lactose. The fats are the most palatable and easily digested; rancidity is due to the liberation of butyric and caproic acids. 2. Term applied to certain vegetable fats which resemble butter (above) in consistency; it is also applied to certain chemical salts which present a similar appearance. **Butter of antimony.** Antimony trichloride, $SbCl_3$, a colourless buttery mass a solution of which in chloroform is used as a test for vitamin A. **Butter of cacao.** Cocoa butter. **Butter of tin.** Stannic chloride, $SnCl_4$, used as a mordant in dyeing. **Butter of zinc.** Zinc chloride, $ZnCl_2$, a powerful caustic, but astringent in dilute solution. It also has deodorant properties and has been used for ulcers and wounds, and in eye-drops. [Gk *boutyron.*]

butterfly (but·er·fli). 1. A uterine tampon with wing-like additions or appendages. 2. A skin-flap with double wings. 3. Any lesion resembling a butterfly with wings outstretched. **Butterfly needle.** *See* NEEDLE. **Butterfly patch.** *See* PATCH. **Butterfly shadow.** A characteristic brain scan appearance associated with a malignant glioma in both hemispheres joined through the corpus callosum. **Butterfly vertebra.** A radiological sign where the two lateral halves of a vertebral body do not fuse (congenital). [AS *buttorfleoge.*]

buttermilk (but·er·milk). The fluid containing casein and lactic acid which remains after milk or cream has been churned into butter. [butter, AS *meoluc.*]

butternut (but·er·nut). The white walnut tree *Juglans cinerea* Linn. (family Juglandaceae), of North America and Canada. The root-bark is mildly cathartic. [butter, AS *hnutu.*]

buttock (but·ok). The prominent part of the body at the back of the hip composed of the glutei muscles and other structures; the two buttocks are known as the nates or the clunes [nates (clunes)]. [ME *but*, end.]

button (butn). 1. Term applied to any lesion shaped like a button. 2. Any appliance shaped like a button, used in medicine or surgery. **Aleppo button, Baghdad button, Biskra button, Cretan button.** Oriental button (see below). **Dog button.** Nux vomica. **Mescal button.** Mescal. **Oriental button.** Cutaneous leishmaniasis, oriental sore; a chronic localized skin lesion caused by infection with *Leishmania tropica.* **Peritoneal button.** A glass tube which was introduced at operation through the parietal peritoneum in an attempt to relieve ascites by draining fluid into the tissues of the abdominal wall. This operation is never practised now. **Quaker button.** Nux vomica. [OFr. *boton.*]

See also: CORRIGAN, MURPHY (J. B.).

button-bush (butn·bush). Buttonwood, cranewillow; the bark of *Cephalanthus occidentalis* (family Rubiaceae), containing a glycosidal saponin, cephalanthin. [OFr. *boton*, ME *busk.*]

buttonhole (butn·hole). A short straight cut into the wall of an organ or cavity. **Mitral buttonhole.** A condition of the mitral orifice of the heart when stenosis is advanced. [OFr. *boton*, AS *hol.*]

buttonwood (butn·wud). Button-bush. [OFr. *boton*, AS *wudu.*]

butyl (bew·til). Normal butyl: an organic radical comprising a saturated straight chain of 4 carbon atoms, $CH_3CH_2CH_2CH_2$–. **Butyl alcohol.** C_4H_9OH, a colourless liquid used mainly as a solvent, particularly in the plastics industry. **Butyl aldehyde.** *See* ALDEHYDE, BUTYL. **Butyl Aminobenzoate BP 1953.** $NH_2C_6H_4COOC_4H_9$, a white crystalline powder, practically insoluble in water, and with local anaesthetic properties. Diluted with sterile talc it is applied as a dusting powder. Being soluble in oil it may be incorporated in ointments and suppositories; it also reacts with picric acid to form a yellow amorphous picrate, which combines local anaesthetic and antiseptic actions. **Butyl chloral hydrate.** Butylchloral hydrate. **Butyl formate.** $HCOO(CH_2)_3CH_3$, a liquid with lacrimatory properties. **Butyl hydride.** Butane. **Butyl parahydroxybenzoate.** $C_4H_9OOCC_6H_4(OH)$, a compound used as a preservative, especially for emulsions and creams. **Butyl phenate.** Butyl phenyl ether, $CH_3(CH_2)_3OC_6H_5$, a colourless liquid used as an antiseptic. [Gk *boutyron* butter, *hyle* matter.]

butylchloral hydrate (bew·til·klor·al hi·drate). Trichlorobutylidene glycol, $CH_3CHClCCl_2CH(OH)_2$. A colourless compound resembling chloral hydrate in hypnotic action, and with some value as an analgesic.

butylene (bew·til·een). 1. α-Butylene, ethylethylene, CH_2=$CHCH_2CH_3$. A gaseous hydrocarbon of the olefine series, of which it is the third member. β-Butylene, dimethylethylene, CH_3CH=$CHCH_3$, is used as an anaesthetizing gas. 2. The organic divalent radical C_4H_8=.

butylethylmalonyl urea (bew·til·eth·il·mal′·on·il ewr·e·ah). Butylethylbarbituric acid, $CO(NHCO)_2C(C_2H_5)(C_4H_9)$. A disubstituted derivative of barbituric acid used as a hypnotic.

butylmercaptan (bew·til·mer·kap′·tan). Thiobutyl alcohol, $CH_3(CH_2)_2CH_2SH$. An odorous substance secreted by the skunk.

butyraceous (bew·tir·a·shus). Referring to a consistency like that of butter or having the appearance of butter. [Gk *boutyron* butter.]

butyraldehyde (bew·tir·al·de·hide). Butyl aldehyde. *See* ALDEHYDE.

butyrase (bew·tir·aze). A lipolytic enzyme which splits butyric esters.

butyrate (bew·tir·ate). A salt of butyric acid.

butyric (bew·tir·ik). Derived from or relating to butter. [Gk *boutyron* butter.]

butyrin (bew·tir·in). Tributyrin, $(CH_3CH_2CH_2COO)_3C_3H_5$. A yellow liquid glyceride found in butter.

butyrinase (bew·tir·in·aze). Butyrase.

butyrine (bew·tir·een). α-Aminobutyric acid, $CH_3CH_2CH(NH_2)COOH$. An α-amino acid occurring in protein.

butyroid (bew·tir·oid). Resembling butter; containing buttery elements. [Gk *boutyron* butter, *eidos* form.]

butyrometer (bew·tir·om·et·er). An instrument with which may be measured the quantity of butter fat in milk. [Gk *boutyron* butter, meter.]

butyrone (bew·tir·one). Dipropylketone, $(CH_3CH_2CH_2)_2CO$. A pleasant-smelling colourless liquid, used as a solvent.

butyroscope (bew·tir·o·skope). An apparatus with which milk may be examined in order to estimate the ratio of butter fat. [Gk *boutyron* butter, *skopein* to watch.]

butyrous (bew·tir·us). Butyraceous.

buxine (bux·een). An alkaloid obtained from the box shrub, *Buxus sempervirens.* It is perhaps identical with bebeerine. [L *buxus*, box-tree.]

buyo (boo·yo). A local name for betel. [Philippine Islands.]

Buzzard, Thomas (b. 1831). London neurologist.

Buzzard's manoeuvre, or reflex. The patellar reflex, modified by voluntary pressure of the patient's toes upon the floor at the time when the quadriceps tendon is struck.

Bychowski, Zygmunt (d. 1935). Warsaw physician.

Grasset-Bychowski sign. Grasset's phenomenon.

by-pass (bi·pas). A method of providing artificial circulation and oxygenation, by-passing the heart and lungs, employed in thoracic and cardiac surgery. **Cardiopulmonary by-pass.** The technique whereby the heart and lungs are excluded from the circulation, oxygenated blood being circulated artificially. [AS *bi* near or alongside, Fr *passer.*]

bysma (biz·mah). A plug or tampon. [Gk stopper.]

byssaceous (bis·a·shus). Composed of filaments; fine, like threads of flax. [Gk *byssos* flax.]

byssinosis (bis·in·o·sis). A chronic bronchitis and emphysema with fibrosis resulting from exposure to cotton- or linen-fibre dust. An allergic reaction to the fibre dust and probably to associated fungal components contaminating the dust. [Gk *byssos* flax, *-osis* condition.]

byssocausis (bis·o·kaw·sis). Cauterizing by the use of a moxa. [Gk *byssos* flax, *kausis* a burning.]

byssoid (bis·oid). 1. Byssaceous. 2. Composed of a fringe of filaments of unequal length. [Gk *byssos* flax, *eidos* form.]

byssophthisis (bis·of·thi·sis). Pulmonary tuberculosis occurring as a result of the inhalation of cotton dust. [Gk *byssos* flax, phthisis.]

byssus (bis·us). 1. Material used for surgical dressings—ling, cotton, charpie (prepared cotton lint). 2. The pubic hair. [Gk *byssos* flax.]

Bythinia (bith·in·e·ah). A genus of freshwater snails. **Bythinia leachii.** A species which is an intermediate host of the fluke *Opisthorchis felineus* in Eastern Europe. **Bythinia striatula.** *Parafossarulus striatulus.* [*Bithynia*, a country of Asia Minor.]

bythium (bith·e·um). A missing element of the sulphur group in the Periodic Table, believed to have been identified in sulphur, but the claim has proved to be unfounded. Cf. POLONIUM. [see foll.]

bythus (bith·us). The lower abdomen. [Gk *bythos* depth.]

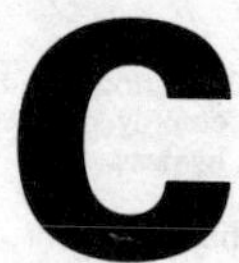

cabbage (**kab**·ij). The cultivated cabbage, *Brassica oleracea* var. *capitata* Linn. (family Cruciferae), the common and important vegetable of the dietary. **Cabbage oil.** The name given to olive oil in which elder leaves have been boiled. [ME *caboche* head.]

CABBS. Computer assisted blood background renography. *See* RENOGRAPHY.

cabinet (**kab**·in·et). *See* SAUERBRUCH. [ME *cabane* cabin.]

Cabot, Richard Clarke (b. 1868). Boston physician.

Cabot's rings, or ring bodies. Nuclear remnants seen in erythrocytes, usually in haemolytic or toxic anaemias, having the appearance of bluish thread-like rings or convolutions; these may be indications of cellular degeneration.

cacaerometer (kak·a·er·**om'**·et·er). An instrument with which the degree of impurity in air can be measured. [Gk *kakos* bad, *aer* air, meter.]

cacaesthesia (kak·es·**the**·ze·ah). Disordered sensibility. [Gk *kakos* bad, aesthesia.]

cacaine (kak·a·een). Theobromine.

cacanthrax (kak·**an**·thrax). Malignant anthrax. *See* ANTHRAX. [Gk *kakos* bad, *anthrax* carbuncle.]

cacao (kak·a·o). The cocoa tree *Theobroma cacao* Linn. (family Sterculiaceae), cultivated in tropical countries. The seeds (cacao seeds, cocoa seeds, theobroma seeds) contain the alkaloids theobromine and caffeine, and a fat (cocoa butter). They are fermented, roasted and separated into kernels (nibs) and husks. The nibs are used in the preparation of cocoa powder and chocolate, and when expressed give cocoa butter (cacao butter, Theobroma Oil BP 1958). The husks yield theobromine, which is a diuretic. [Mexican *caca.*]

cacation (kak·a·shun). Defaecation. [L *cacare* to go to stool.]

cacatory (**kak**·at·or·e). Attended with excessive diarrhoea; term applied to certain illness or diseases. [see prec.]

Caccobius (kak·**o**·be·us). A genus of small dung beetle, species of which, particularly *Caccobius vulcanus* (=*mutans*), cause intestinal canthariasis in South India and Sri Lanka, especially in children. The adult form of the insect may be passed in faeces. [Gk *kakke* excrement, *bios* life.]

cacergasia (kak·er·**ga**·ze·ah). Merergasia. Applied to bodily or mental function, or both, a term indicating output of subnormal character. [Gk *kakos* bad, *ergasia* work.]

cacergastic (kak·er·**gas**·tik). Pertaining to cacergasia.

cachectic (kak·**ek**·tik). Referring to or characterized by the presence of cachexia.

cachet (kash·**a**). A flat capsule made of rice paper, and used to contain powders having an unpleasant taste. The cachet is swallowed intact. [Fr. a seal.]

cachexia (kak·ex·e·ah). An extreme state of general ill-health with malnutrition, wasting, anaemia, and circulatory and muscular weakness. **African cachexia.** Ancylostomiasis. **Aphthous cachexia.** Sprue. **Cachexia aquosa.** Ancylostomiasis. **Bronze cachexia.** Addison's disease. **Cancerous cachexia, Carcinomatous cachexia.** The result of advanced malignant disease. **Cachexia exophthalmica.** That due to thyrotoxicosis. **Fluoric cachexia.** Chronic poisoning with fluorine; fluorosis. **Cachexia hypophyseopriva.** Simmonds' disease. **Lymphatic cachexia.** Hodgkin's disease. **Malarial cachexia.** Chronic ill-health following repeated attacks of malaria. **Cachexia mercurialis.** Chronic mercurial poisoning. **Miners' cachexia.** 1. Ancylostomiasis, better known as *miners' anaemia.* 2. An erythrocytosis sometimes amounting to polycythaemia vera which has been reported in miners working at high altitudes, as in the Peruvian Andes. **Negro cachexia.** Ancylostomiasis. **Osteal cachexia.** Scurvy. **Cachexia ovariopriva.** That following loss of both ovaries. **Pachydermic cachexia.** Myxoedema. **Paludal cachexia.** That due to malaria. **Pituitary cachexia.** Simmonds' disease. **Saturnine cachexia.** That caused by chronic lead poisoning. **Splenic cachexia.** Splenic anaemia. *See* ANAEMIA. **Cachexia strumipriva.** Myxoedema following total ablation of the thyroid as a therapeutic measure in heart disease, or a subtotal thyroidectomy for thyrotoxicosis. **Cachexia suprarenalis.** Addison's disease. **Cachexia thymopriva.** Cachexia attributed to loss of the thymus. **Cachexia thyreopriva.** Myxoedema. **Thyroid cachexia.** Thyrotoxicosis. **Urinary cachexia.** Chronic uraemia. **Cachexia venerea.** Chronic syphilis. **Verminous cachexia.** Cachexia due to infestation with parasitic worms, especially ancylostomiasis. **Cachexia virginum.** Chlorosis. [Gk *kakos* bad, *hexis* state.]

See also: GRAWITZ.

cachexy (kak·**ex**·e). Cachexia.

cachinnation (kak·in·a·shun). The immoderate and loud laughter which is a feature of hysteria or insanity. [L *cachinnare* to laugh loudly.]

cachou (kash·**oo**). A pill or tablet, aromatically flavoured, which can be chewed or sucked for the purpose of sweetening the breath, e.g. after smoking. [Fr. *acajou* cashew.]

cacidrosis (kak·id·**ro**·sis). 1. Bromhidrosis. 2. Any abnormal condition of the sweat. [Gk *kakos* bad, *hidros* sweat.]

cacocholia (kak·o·**ko**·le·ah). An abnormal state of the bile; the condition of ill-health resulting from this. [Gk *kakos* bad, *chole* bile.]

cacochylia (kak·o·**ki**·le·ah). Indigestion; an abnormal state of the gastric juice. [Gk *kakos* bad, *chyle* juice.]

cacodontia (kak·o·**don**·she·ah). An unhealthy or pathological condition of the teeth. [Gk *kakos* bad, *odous* tooth.]

cacodyl (**kak**·o·dil). Dicacodyl, tetramethyldiarsine, $(CH_3)_2AsAs(CH_3)_2$. A colourless liquid insoluble in water, with a disgusting odour that causes vomiting. The vapour is spontaneously inflammable and poisonous. **Cacodyl cyanide.** Dimethylarsenic cyanide, $As(CH_3)_2CN$, colourless crystals with a poisonous vapour. **Cacodyl oxide.** Dimethylarsenious oxide, $As_2(CH_3)_4O$, a liquid with an overpowering odour and an extremely irritant vapour. [Gk *kakodes* evil-smelling.]

cacoethes (kak·o·e·theez). 1. A malignant ulcer. 2. A bad quality in a disease. 3. A bad habit or disposition. 4. Mania. **Cacoethes operandi.** An insatiable desire to operate. [Gk *kakos* bad, *ethos* characteristic.]

cacoethic (kak·o·e·thik). 1. Malignant. 2. Applied to a person whose health is bad. 3. Referring to cacoethes. [see prec.]

cacogastric (kak·o·**gas**·trik). Dyspeptic. [Gk *kakos* bad, *gaster* stomach.]

cacogenesis (kak·o·**jen**·es·is). 1. A monstrosity. 2. Any abnormal structure or formation. 3. The production of unhealthy or recessive types of organism. [Gk *kakos* bad, *genein* to produce.]

cacogenic (kak·o·**jen**·ik). 1. Tending towards deterioration of the human race because of the sexual selection of bad types. 2. Referring to cacogenesis. [see prec.]

cacogenics (kak·o·**jen**·ix). The aggregation of factors which, because of bad sexual selection, tend towards deterioration of the human race. [Gk *kakos* bad, *genein* to produce.]

cacogeusia (kak·o·**gew**·ze·ah). Bad taste, apart from the presence or influence of food, drug or other matter; a constant condition,

usually arising from disturbance of the general metabolism. [Gk *kakos* bad, *geusis* taste.]
cacoglossia (kak·o·**glos**·e·ah). Gangrene or disease of the tongue. [Gk *kakos* bad, *glossa* tongue.]
cacolet (kak·o·**la**). A contrivance in the form of a chair or pannier for transportation of wounded by mule or horse. [Fr.]
cacomelia (kak·o·**me**·le·ah). 1. Congenital deformity of a limb. 2. A pathological condition of a limb originating in fetal life. [Gk *kakos* bad, *melos* limb.]
caconychia (kak·on·**ik**·e·ah). Any defect of a nail. [Gk *kakos* bad, *onyx* nail.]
cacophonia (kak·o·**fo**·ne·ah). The condition in which the normal timbre of the voice is impaired or otherwise abnormal. [Gk *kakos* bad, *phone* voice.]
cacophony (kak·**of**·o·ne). Any discordant sound. [see prec.]
cacoplasia (kak·o·**pla**·ze·ah). 1. A state of morbid growth. 2. A state of defective structure or formation. [Gk *kakos* bad, *plassein* to mould.]
cacoplastic (kak·o·**plas**·tik). 1. Of a low or imperfect grade of organization. 2. Referring to cacoplasia. [see prec.]
cacorrhythmic (kak·o·**rith**·mik). Characterized by, or involving, irregularity of rhythm. [Gk *kakos* bad, *rhythmos* measured motion.]
cacosmia (kak·**oz**·me·ah). A stench or an unpleasant odour. [Gk *kakos* bad, *osme* odour.]
cacostomia (kak·o·**sto**·me·ah). 1. Severe stomatitis. 2. A gangrenous or diseased condition of the mouth. [Gk *kakos* bad, *stoma* mouth.]
cacotheline (kak·o·thel·een). $C_{21}H_{21}O_5N_2(NO_2)$, a red alkaloid substance obtained by treating brucine with nitric acid; used as a reagent for the detection of tin, with which it forms green and violet compounds.
cacothenic (kak·o·**then**·ik). Referring to cacothenics.
cacothenics (kak·o·**then**·ix). Deterioration of the human race because of the bad effects of insanitary conditions and unfavourable surroundings. [Gk *kakos* bad, *thenia* state of being.]
cacothymia (kak·o·**thi**·me·ah). Disordered function of the thymus. [Gk *kakos* bad, thymus.]
cacotrophy (kak·**ot**·rof·e). Malnutrition; disordered or defective nutritive processes. [Gk *kakos* bad, *trophe* nutrition.]
cacumen (kak·**ew**·men). 1. The top or apex of an anatomical structure or a plant. 2. The lobulus culminis of the anterior superior surface of the cerebellum. [L summit.]
cacuminal (kak·**ew**·min·al). Relating to the cacumen.
cadaver (kad·**av**·er). A corpse; a lifeless human body used for dissection. [L.]
cadaveric (kad·**av**·er·ik). Belonging or relating to, or simulating a cadaver. **Cadaveric spasm.** *See* SPASM.
cadaverine (kad·**av**·er·een). Pentamethylenediamine, $NH_2CH_2(CH_2)_3CH_2NH_2$. A foul-smelling, syrupy, fuming liquid soluble in water and alcohol. It is produced during the bacterial decomposition of proteins, being derived from lysine by decarboxylation. By reason of its presence in putrefying tissue it was formerly classed as a ptomaine. It occurs in the urine in some cases of cystinuria. [see foll.]
cadaverous (kad·**av**·er·us). Corpse-like: pale or ghastly in appearance. [L *cadaver* corpse.]
caddis (**kad**·is). The case of the larva of a fly of the order Trichoptera. In susceptible persons, the hairs covering the wings have been reported to set up an allergic reaction of an asthmatic or coryzal nature. [etym. dub.]
Cadet, Louis Claude (b. 1731). French chemist.
Cadet's fuming liquid. Alkarsin; a mixture of cacodyl and cacodyl oxide obtained by distilling potassium acetate with arsenious oxide. It is an extremely poisonous brown liquid which fumes in air, and is liable to ignite spontaneously.
Cadham, Fred Todd (b. 1881). Winnipeg bacteriologist.
Cadham's serum. The serum of rabbits injected with streptococci and staphylococci from septicaemia.
cadinene (**kad**·in·een). $C_{15}H_{24}$, a dicyclic sesquiterpene containing a reduced naphthalene skeleton, and found in oil of cubebs, cade oil, oil of savin and camphor.
cadmium (**kad**·me·um). An element of atomic weight 112.41, atomic number 48 and chemical symbol Cd, found in small amounts in the ores of zinc, which it resembles in chemical properties. It is a soft, bluish metal incorporated in fusible alloys, and now of considerable importance as a moderator in atomic piles. The salts of cadmium are poisonous and are no longer used clinically. **Cadmium oxide.** CdO, a brown compound the fumes of which have caused metal-fume fever (brassfounders' ague). **Cadmium sulphide.** CdS, a yellow precipitate employed as a pigment. [Gk *kadmeia* zinc ore.]
caduca (kad·**ew**·kah). The decidua. [L *cadere* to fall.]
caecal (**se**·kal). 1. Relating to the caecum. 2. A cavity open at one end only. [L *caecus* blind.]
caecectomy (se·**sek**·to·me). The operation of cutting away a part of the caecum. [caecum, Gk *ektome* a cutting out.]
caecitis (se·**si**·tis). Inflammation of the caecum. [caecum, Gk *-itis* inflammation.]
caecocele (**se**·ko·seel). A hernia involving part of the caecum. [caecum, Gk *kele* hernia.]
caecocolon (se·ko·**ko**·lon). For anatomical and physiological considerations, the colon and caecum regarded as a single unit of the intestinal system.
caecocoloplicopexy (se·ko·ko·lo·**pli**′·ko·pex·e). Surgical fixation of the caecum and of the ascending colon. [caecum, colon, L *plica* fold, Gk *pexis* fixation.]
caecocolostomy (se·ko·kol·**os**′·to·me). The formation by surgical means of an anastomosis between the caecum and the colon. [caecum, colon, Gk *stoma* mouth.]
caecocystoplasty (se·ko·**sist**·o·plas·te). The using of the caecum to form a urinary bladder. [caecum, Gk *kystis* bag, *plassein* to mould.]
caecofixation (se·ko·fix·**a**′·shun). Caecopexy. [caecum, L *figere* to fix.]
caecograph (**se**·ko·graf). Special apparatus devised for the blind with the object of enabling them to write in longhand. [L *caecus* blind, Gk *graphein* to record.]
caeco-ileostomy (se·ko·i·le·**os**′·to·me). 1. Ileocaecostomy. 2. Abdominal incision and opening of the ileocolic valve so as to drain the ileum. [caecum, ileum, Gk *stoma* mouth.]
caecopexy (**se**·ko·pex·e). In the case of an abnormally mobile caecum, the surgical fixation of it to the abdominal wall. [caecum. Gk *pexis* fixation.]
caecoplication (se·ko·plik·**a**′·shun). The making of a fold or folds in the wall of the caecum in order to counteract dilatation and ptosis. [caecum, L *plica* fold.]
caecoptosis (se·kop·**to**·sis). Ptosis or downward displacement of the caecum. [caecum, Gk *ptosis* fall.]
caecorrhaphy (se·**kor**·af·e). The surgical procedure of suturing the caecum. [caecum, Gk *rhaphe* suture.]
caecosigmoidostomy (se·ko·sig·moid·**os**′·to·me). The surgical formation of an anastomosis between the caecum and the pelvic colon (sigmoid flexure). [caecum, sigmoid, Gk *stoma* mouth.]
caecostomy (se·**kos**·to·me). The plastic operation of forming an opening in the caecum that communicates with the surface. [caecum, Gk *stoma* mouth.]
caecotomy (se·**kot**·o·me). The surgical incision of the caecum. [caecum, Gk *temnein* to cut.]
caecoureterocele (se·ko·ewr·e′·ter·o·seel). A rare deformity of the intravesical segment of the ureter with an incompetent bladder orifice and a long, submucosal trigonal and urethral extension in the female. [caecum, ureter, Gk *kele* hernia.]
caecum [cecum (NA)] (**se**·kum). The blind pouch in the right iliac fossa which forms the beginning of the large intestine; the vermiform appendix is attached to it. **Caecum cupulare** [cecum cupulare (NA)]. The blind upper end of the duct of the cochlea. **Hepatic caecum.** One of a number of tubular outgrowths of the upper alimentary canal in invertebrates which are functionally equivalent to the liver of vertebrates. **High**

caecum. A caecum situated at a higher level than the right iliac fossa. **Caecum vestibulare** [cecum vestibulare (NA)]. The lower or vestibular end of the duct of the cochlea which forms a small blind pouch beyond its junction with the ductus reuniens. [L *caecus* blind.]

caecus minor ventriculi (se·kus mi·nor ven·trik·ew·li). The cardiac end of the stomach. [L.]

caenogenesis (se·no·jen·es·is). The non-repetition in an individual of phylogenetic processes. [Gk *kainos* new, *genein* to produce.]

caenopsychic (se·no·si·kik). Relating to a factor that is of later expression in mind development. [Gk *kainos* new, *psyche* mind.]

caenotophobia. (se·no·to·fo′·be·ah). Neophobia; abnormal fear of any new or unaccustomed thing or to new circumstances and surroundings. [Gk *kainos* something new, phobia.]

caeruloplasmin (seer·ew·lo·plaz′·min). Ceruloplasmin.

Caesalpinia (se·zal·pin·e·ah). A genus of trees of the Caesalpinioideae (subfamily of the Leguminosae). Certain species yield dye-woods, e.g. *Caesalpinia sappan* Linn. (sappan wood), *Caesalpinia braziliensis* Linn. (Brazil wood) and *Caesalpinia echinata* Lamarck (peach wood). The pods of *Caesalpinia coriaria* Willd. constitute divi-divi, which is used in tanning. [Andrea *Cesalpino*, 1519–1603, Italian botanist and physician.]

caesarean, caesarotomy (se·zare·e·an, se·zar·ot·om·e). Caesarean section. *See* SECTION. [According to Pliny, Julius Caesar was born in this way, the fact giving origin to his name and, traditionally, to the method of delivery. More likely the term is derived from the Latin verb meaning *to cut*, or from the fact that the Roman law (the law of the Caesars) required, in the event of a pregnant woman dying, that the child be cut from her uterus before she was buried.]

caesium (se·ze·um). A comparatively rare element of atomic weight 132.9054, atomic number 55 and chemical symbol Cs. It is a soft white metal of the alkali family, very similar to sodium in properties and even more highly reactive. It occurs in certain natural waters and in some rare minerals such as the silicate pollux; it does not constitute any proportion of plant or animal tissue. [L *caesius* sky blue, from the colour of its spectral lines.]

cafard (kaf·ahr). A form of subacute melancholia in which the sufferer is subject to attacks of severe depression and worry. [Fr. military slang; *lit.* black-beetle or cockroach.]

Cafedrine (kaf·ed·reen). BP Commission approved name for L-7-[2-(β-hydroxy-α-methylphenethylamino)ethyl]theophylline; an analeptic.

caffeidine (kaf·e·id·een). $C_7H_{12}N_4O$, a purine alkaloid derived from caffeine.

caffeine (kaf·e·een). 1,3,7-Trimethylxanthine, $C_8H_{10}O_2N_6 \cdot H_2O$. An alkaloid related to purine, found naturally in the leaves of the tea plant *(Thea sinensis)*, in coffee, the seeds of *Coffea arabica*, in maté, a South American beverage, and in the kola nut. It is employed clinically as a stimulant of the central nervous system, chiefly as an antidote to poisoning with hypnotic drugs (BP 1973). It has a stimulant effect on the myocardium, and is a mild vasodilator with a slight diuretic effect. **Caffeine Citrate BPC 1959.** A white powder with a bitter taste prepared in the form of effervescent granules. **Caffeine Hydrate BP 1973.** A white, odourless powder with a bitter taste; the monohydrate of caffeine. **Caffeine salicylate.** $C_8H_{10}O_2N_4HOOCC_6H_4(OH)$, a molecular compound of caffeine and salicylic acid formerly used in migraine. It is less soluble than caffeine. **Caffeine and Sodium Benzoate BPC 1954.** A white powder with a slightly bitter taste, soluble readily in water. It is a mixture of caffeine and sodium benzoate in equal parts. **Caffeine and Sodium Iodide BPC 1968.** A mixture of caffeine and sodium iodide. Prepared as an elixir, sometimes with the addition of ephedrine; used as a diuretic, and in the treatment of cardiorespiratory failure. **Caffeine and sodium salicylate.** A highly soluble white powder with a bitter taste, containing equal parts of caffeine and sodium salicylate; used for subcutaneous injection as a 50 per cent solution. [Ar. *qahwah* coffee.]

caffeinism, caffeism (kaf·e·in·izm, kaf·e·izm). A state of toxic poisoning brought on by the taking of an excessive amount of coffee. [see prec.]

caffeol, caffeone (kaf·e·ol, kaf·e·one). $C_8H_{10}O_2$, an oil obtained by roasting coffee and believed to be the cause of the characteristic aroma. It is the methyl ether of saligenin. [Ar. *qahwah* coffee.]

Caffey, John (b. 1895). American paediatrician.

Caffey's disease. Infantile cortical hyperostosis; an overgrowth of the cortical bone and resembling osteomyelitis.

Caffey's syndrome. The battered baby syndrome, first recognized by Caffey in 1946.

cage (kaje). **Resuscitation cage.** An electrically heated "cage" in which the patient is placed to counteract shock. **Thoracic cage.** The bony framework that surrounds the thoracic viscera. [L *cavus* hollow.]

Cagot (kag·o). A member of a gypsy tribe of the Pyrenees among which cretinism is rife. **Cagot ear.** An ear without a lobule of the auricle, erroneously thought to be a peculiarity of the Cagots. [Fr.]

cainotophobia (ki·no·to·fo′·be·ah). Caenotophobia.

Cairns, Sir Hugh William Bell (b. 1896). Oxford neurosurgeon.

Cairns' artery forceps. The haemostatic forceps.

Cajal. *See* RAMON Y CAJAL.

cajeput (kaj·e·put). Cajuput.

cajuput (kaj·ew·put). The tree *Melaleuca leucadendron* Linn. of the myrtle family (East Indies). The leaves yield a yellowish or colourless volatile oil (Cajuput Oil BPC 1959) with the odour of camphor and containing cineole, employed in the treatment of rheumatism, some intestinal disturbances and toothache. [Malay *cajuputi* white wood.]

cajuputene (kaj·ew·put·een). $C_{10}H_{16}$, a dipentene contained in cajuput oil; an aromatic liquid used as an anthelmintic, and externally in rheumatism.

cajuputol (kaj·ew·put·ol). Cineole, $C_{10}H_{18}O$. The anhydride of *p*-menthane-1,8-diol, also known as *eucalyptol*. It is a colourless liquid with an aromatic odour resembling camphor, obtained from cajuput oil, from wormseed oil *(Artemesia maritima)* and by distillation of the leaves of various species of eucalyptus. It is employed in the symptomatic treatment of upper respiratory infections, either incorporated in tablets or pastilles or inhaled with steam or in the form of a spray. It is used also as an antiseptic in toothpaste and, combined with zinc oxide, as a temporary dental filling.

caked (ka·kd). Compressed into a solid mass. [Old Norse *kaka*.]

calabarine (kal·ab·ar·een). An alkaloid of uncertain composition obtained from the Calabar bean, *Physostigma venenosum* Balf.; it differs in its pharmacological actions from physostigmine.

calabashcurarine (kal·ab·ash·kew·rah′·reen). *See* CURARINE. [Pers. *kharbuz* melon, curarine.]

calage (kah·lahzh). A measure for the relief of seasickness; the patient lies on his side facing the wall of the cabin and is wedged with pillows placed between the abdomen and the wall and between the back and the edge of the berth. By these measures the viscera are immobilized. [Fr. wedging.]

calamine (kal·am·ine). 1. A native carbonate of zinc, $ZnCO_3$. 2. Calamine BP 1973, an amorphous powder, pink or reddish-brown in colour, composed of basic zinc carbonate with the addition of a variable amount of ferric oxide. It is insoluble in water, has a weak astringent action on the skin and is soothing to inflamed areas; used in the treatment of dermatitis as a dusting powder or lotion, or incorporated in a cream or ointment base. **Compound cream of calamine.** A cream containing 10 per cent of calamine, weight to volume. **Compound Ointment of Calamine BPC 1959.** A preparation containing 12.5 per cent of calamine, with zinc oxide, coal tar, hydrous wool fat and white soft paraffin. **Calamine Lotion BP 1958.** A preparation composed of 15 per cent calamine with zinc oxide and glycerin in distilled water. **Oily Lotion of Calamine BPC 1959.** An oily preparation containing 5 per cent of calamine by weight per volume of arachis oil. **Ointment of Calamine BPC 1959.** A preparation containing 16.7 per cent of calamine in white soft paraffin. **Prepared calamine.** Calamine BP 1958 (see above). [Gk *kadmeia* zinc ore.]

calamus (**kal**·am·us). The dried rhizome of the plant *Acorus calamus*, used as a stomachic. [L a reed.]

calamus scriptorius (**kal**·am·us skrip·**tor**·e·us). The lower (caudal) part of the 4th ventricle, in the floor of which the vagal and hypoglossal triangles are found; it is pointed, and in general shape like the nib of a pen. [L a writing pen.]

calcaemia (kal·**se**·me·ah). The condition in which the blood contains an abnormally large amount of calcium; the effect of such a condition on the general health. [L *calx* lime, Gk *haima* blood.]

calcaneal (kal·**ka**·ne·al). Calcanean.

calcanean (kal·**ka**·ne·an). Relating or belonging to the calcaneum. **Calcanean facet.** *See* FACET.

calcanean arteries. Branches, medial [rami calcanei mediales] and lateral [rami calcanei laterales], of the posterior or peroneal tibial arteries to the tissues of the heel.

calcaneitis (kal·**ka**·ne·**i**'·tis). Inflammation of the calcaneum. [calcaneum, Gk *-itis* inflammation.]

calcaneo-apophysitis (kal·**ka**·ne·o·ap·of·iz·**i**'·tis). A painful inflammatory condition affecting the back of the calcaneum at the insertion of the tendo calcaneus (Achilles tendon) and associated with swelling of the soft parts. [calcaneum, apophysitis.]

calcaneo-astragaloid (kal·**ka**·ne·o·as·**trag**'·al·oid). Relating to the calcaneum and the talus (astragalus).

calcaneocavus (kal·**ka**·ne·o·**ka**'·vus). A form of club-foot in which talipes calcaneus and talipes cavus are combined.

calcaneocuboid (kal·**ka**·ne·o·**kew**'·boid). Relating to the calcaneum and the cuboid bone. **Calcaneocuboid joint.** *See* JOINT.

calcaneodynia (kal·**ka**·ne·o·**din**'·e·ah). Calcanodynia.

calcaneofibular (kal·**ka**·ne·o·**fib**'·ew·lar). Relating to the calcaneum and the fibula, or involving both.

calcaneonavicular (kal·**ka**·ne·o·nav·**ik**'·ew·lar). Relating to the calcaneum and the navicular (scaphoid) bone.

calcaneoplantar (kal·**ka**·ne·o·**plan**'·tar). Relating to the calcaneum and the sole of the foot. [calcaneum, L *planta* sole.]

calcaneoscaphoid (kal·**ka**·ne·o·**skaf**'·oid). Calcaneonavicular. **Calcaneoscaphoid coalition.** *See* COALITION. [calcaneum, scaphoid.]

calcaneotibial (kal·**ka**·ne·o·**tib**'·e·al). Relating to the calcaneum and the tibia.

calcaneovalgocavus (kal·**ka**·ne·o·val·go·**ka**'·vus). A form of club-foot combining talipes calcaneum, talipes valgus and talipes cavus.

calcaneum [calcaneus (os calcis)(NA)] (kal·**ka**·ne·um). The large strong bone which projects backwards beyond the bones of the leg to form the heel. It is roughly cuboidal in shape with upper, lower, medial, lateral, anterior and posterior surfaces. It articulates above with the talus and in front with the cuboid bone. [L *calx* heel.]

anterior surface. The concavoconvex surface which in the articulated foot articulates with the posterior surface of the cuboid bone.

lateral surface. A flat surface bearing the peroneal tubercle.

lower surface. The plantar surface. It carries 2 bone tubercles at its posterior margin, the medial giving origin to the abductor hallucis and flexor digitorum brevis muscles and the lateral to the abductor digiti minimi. Close to its anterior margin is the anterior tubercle, to which the short plantar ligament is attached. The remainder of the lower surface gives attachment to the long plantar ligament and the flexor digitorum accessorius muscle.

medial surface. A concave surface from which projects the sustenaculum tali.

posterior surface [tuber calcanei (NA)]. The back surface of the heel bone giving attachment in its central part to the tendo calcaneus. Above it is related to a pod of fat and occasionally a bursa, and below to the subcutaneous tissue of the heel.

upper surface. The surface related to the under-surface of the talus in the articulated foot. Centrally it bears an oval facet, the posterior articular facet for the talus [facies articularis talaris posterior], and in front of this a groove which in the articulated foot forms the floor of the sinus tarsi. In front of the groove are 2 facets, often partially fused, for the head of the talus.

calcanodynia (kal·**ka**·no·**din**'·e·ah). Pain in the heel or in the region of the calcaneum. [calcaneum, Gk *odyne* pain.]

calcar (**kal**·kar). A spur-like process. **Calcar avis [NA].** A projection in the medial wall of the posterior horn of the lateral ventricle caused by the calcarine sulcus. **Calcar femorale.** A thin vertical plate of bone which arises in the shaft of the femur in front of the lesser trochanter and extends into the spongy substance of the neck, which it strengthens. **Calcar pedis.** The calcaneum. [L a spur.]

calcarea (kal·**ka**·re·ah). Lime; the term is used in homoeopathic prescribing for calcium oxide or hydroxide. **Calcarea carbonica.** A homoeopathic preparation of oyster shells. **Calcarea chlorinata.** Chloride of lime; a disinfectant. **Calcarea fluorica.** A homoeopathic preparation of fluorspar. **Calcarea hydrica.** Lime water. *See* WATER. **Calcarea ostrearum.** Calcarea carbonica (see above). **Calcarea phosphorica.** Precipitated calcium phosphate. **Calcarea usta.** Quicklime. [L.]

calcareous (kal·**ka**·re·us). 1. Chalky. 2. Containing or consisting of lime or calcium. 3. Like lime or chalk. [L *calcarea* lime.]

calcarine (**kal**·kar·een). 1. Relating to the calcar avis. 2. Spur-shaped. **Calcarine sulcus.** *See* SULCUS. [L *calcar* lime.]

calcariuria (**kal**·kar·e·**ewr**'·e·ah). A condition in which lime salts are present in the urine. [L *calcarea* lime, urine.]

calcaroid (**kal**·kar·oid). 1. A term used to describe deposition in the brain of a substance resembling lime salts, although a specific reaction for calcium cannot be demonstrated. 2. Like calcium. [L *calcarea* lime, Gk *eidos* form.]

calcibilia (kal·se·**bil**·e·ah). A condition of the bile in which it contains calcium.

calcic (**kal**·sik). Referring or relating to lime or calcium.

calcicosis (kal·sik·**o**·**sis**). Chronic pneumonic inflammation resulting from the constant inhalation of calcium carbonate dust, especially marble. It affects monumental masons and is commonly referred to as marble-cutters' phthisis. [L *calx* lime, Gk *-osis* condition.]

calciferol (kal·**sif**·er·ol). Vitamin D_2, $C_{28}H_{43}OH$. A colourless crystalline substance prepared by the ultra-violet irradiation of ergosterol, obtained from yeast. It is antirachitic, and 1 mg has approximately 40 000 international units of activity. Calciferol promotes the absorption of calcium and phosphorus from the bowel, and so is essential for the normal development of bone and tooth; deficiency is associated with rickets in children, and osteomalacia in adults. Some vitamin D is formed in the skin by the action of sunlight, and so the adult daily requirement from food is not known with certainty, and in fact must vary widely. Increased amounts are necessary in infancy and childhood, and during pregnancy and lactation, when up to about 1000 units above the usual daily intake are advisable; larger doses are needed if there is evidence of deficiency (BP 1973). Much bigger doses have been used successfully in the treatment of lupus vulgaris, tuberculous lymphadenitis, and in osteoporosis associated with parathyroid deficiency. Toxic symptoms may occur with such doses, including anorexia, loss of weight and alimentary-tract disturbances. Excessive amounts of calcium also may be deposited in various tissues, particularly the kidneys and blood vessels. **Calciferol Solution BP 1973.** A solution of calciferol in a vegetable oil; 1 g contains 3000 units of antirachitic activity. **Calciferol Tablets BP 1973.** Each contains generally 1.25 mg of calciferol, equivalent to 50 000 units of anti-rachitic activity. [see foll.]

calciferous (kal·**sif**·er·us). Producing or containing chalk, lime or calcium. [L *calx* lime, *ferre* to bear.]

calcific (kal·**sif**·ik). 1. Forming lime. 2. Calciferous. [see foll.]

calcification (kal·sif·ik·**a**'·shun). 1. The deposition of calcareous matter within organic tissue so that it becomes hardened. 2. In physiology, the depositing of lime salts in cartilage, one of the first steps in the formation of true bone. **Dystrophic calci-**

fication. Calcium deposition in the dermis or hypoderm with no detectable abnormality of metabolism, as in sclerodermia and dermatomyositis. **Egg-shell calcification.** A thin layer of calcification, e.g. the calcification in the walls of an empyema. **Metastatic calcification.** The process of calcification affecting one part or tissue at the same time that decalcification is taking place in the bones from osteomalacia. **Periarticular calcification.** The deposition of calcified plaques in the capsule or tendons around joints. **Supraspinatus calcification.** Calcification in the supraspinatus tendon immediately superior to the shoulder joint. [L *calx* lime, *facere* to make.]

See also: MOENCKEBERG.

calcigerous (kal·sij·er·us). In biology, containing or producing lime salts. [L *calx* lime, *gerere* to bear.]

calcii (kal·se·i). Calcium. **Calcii Aminocalicylas.** *European Pharmacopoeia* name for Calcium Aminosalicylate BP 1973. **Calcii Carbonas.** *European Pharmacopoeia* name for Calcium Carbonate BP 1973. **Calcii Chloridum.** *European Pharmacopoeia* name for Calcium Chloride BP 1973. **Calcii Gluconas.** *European Pharmacopoeia* name for Calcium Gluconate BP 1973. [L *calx* lime.]

calcination (kal·sin·a·shun). 1. Roasting or calcining. 2. Drying or reducing to a powder consisting of non-volatile inorganic matter, by exposure to intense heat. [L *calcinare* to burn lime.]

calcine (kal·seen). 1. To carry out the process of calcination. 2. To subject to intense dry heat.

calcinosis (kal·sin·o·sis). A condition in which deposits of calcium salts occur in subcutaneous tissue and muscle and in various organs. **Calcinosis circumscripta.** Calcium gout, a condition in which calcification is localized to the skin of the upper extremities, especially that of the fingers. **Interstitial calcinosis.** Calcinosis universalis (see below). **Intervertebral calcinosis.** Calcification of the invertebral disc; a common ageing effect, but occasionally a pathological process in young people. **Subcutaneous postphlebitic calcinosis.** Calcinosis occurring in about 10 per cent of patients with venous stasis; it may interfere with healing. **Calcinosis universalis.** Calcification in the skin tendons, fascia, muscles and nerves. [calcium, Gk *-osis* condition.]

calciorrhachia (kal·se·o·rak′·e·ah). The condition in which there is calcium in the spinal fluid. [L *calx* lime, Gk *rhachis* spine.]

calcipectic (kal·se·pek·tik). Calcipexic.

calcipenia (kal·se·pe·ne·ah). A state in which the tissues and body fluids are deficient in lime salts. [L *calx* lime, *penes* poor.]

calcipenic (kal·se·pe·nik). Referring to calcipenia; having insufficient calcium.

calcipexic (kal·se·pex·ik). Able to fix calcium in the tissue. [see foll.]

calcipexis, calcipexy (kal·se·pex·is, kal·se·pex·e). The fixation of calcium within the tissues during metabolic processes. [L *calx* lime, Gk *pexis* fixation.]

calciphilia (kal·se·fil·e·ah). A condition in which certain structures or organs have an affinity for the lime salts circulating in the blood, and so tend to absorb them and become calcified. [L *calx* lime, Gk *philein* to love.]

calcipyelitis (kal·se·pi·el·i′·tis). Calculus pyelitis. *See* PYELITIS. [L *calx* lime, pyelitis.]

calcite (kal·site). A naturally occurring, crystalline form of calcium carbonate.

calcitonin (kal·se·to·nin). A polypeptide which can be extracted from the thyroid and is probably produced by the parafollicular cells. It helps to regulate the level of calcium in the blood. (Calcitrophic hormone also covers parathyroid hormone.) Salmon and human calcitonin have been synthesized and are used clinically in conjunction with porcine calcitonin. It inhibits osteoclastic bone resorption, preventing calcium and phosphorus from leaving bone but not from entering it, and is used in the treatment of Paget's disease. It is produced in the thyroid parafollicular cells. [calcium, Gk *tonos* tone.]

calcium (kal·se·um). An element of atomic weight 40.08, atomic number 20 and chemical symbol Ca. It is a reactive metal of the alkaline-earth group which does not occur free but is abundantly distributed in nature as compounds, principally the carbonate (limestone), the phosphates and the silicates. It is present in nearly all plants, where it is essential for growth, and in all animals, in whom it constitutes a large proportion of the bone or skeletal tissue. In the human body it is found in the blood and extracellular fluid either ionized or bound to the plasma protein, and is necessary for the normal functioning of cardiac muscle, the phenomena of blood coagulation and milk-clotting, and the regulation of cell permeability. It also plays an important part in nerve-impulse transmission and in the mechanism of the neuromuscular system. **Calcium acetylsalicylate.** A more soluble compound than aspirin and used for the same purposes. **Calcium acid phosphate.** Calcium hydrogen phosphate (see below). **Calcium Alginate BPC 1968.** A precipitate formed when sodium alginate solution is applied to raw surfaces: it exerts a haemostatic effect, and is slowly absorbed. **Calcium Aminosalicylate BP 1973.** A yellowish-white powder used in the treatment of tuberculosis. **Calcium Benzamidosalicylate.** BP Commission approved name for calcium 4-benzamido-2-hydroxybenzoate; it is used in the treatment of tuberculosis. **Calcium benzoate.** A colourless crystalline substance, formerly used as an internal antiseptic. **Calcium bicarbonate.** A form of diffusible calcium found in the serum. **Calcium bromide.** A white deliquescent substance, formerly used in the treatment of epilepsy. **Calcium carbide.** CaC_2, a compound prepared from lime and coke. It generates acetylene when treated with water. **Calcium Carbonate BP 1973.** Precipitated calcium carbonate, precipitated chalk, $CaCO_3$, a white powder, used as an antacid; it has a mild constipating effect. **Calcium caseinate.** A yellowish-white powder used as a food in cases of diarrhoea, especially in children, and to supplement protein intake. **Calcium Chloride BP 1973.** $CaCl_2$, a deliquescent white granular substance with an unpleasant taste, sometimes used in haemorrhagic states, lead poisoning and tetany. **Calcium Cyclamate BP 1968.** The dihydrate of calcium cyclohexylsulphamate, a synthetic sweetening agent; used as an alternative to sodium cyclamate when it is important to avoid excess of sodium in the diet. In dilute solution (0.1–0.15 per cent) these cyclamates are about 30 times as sweet as sugar. **Calcium fluoride.** CaF_2, a white powder, insoluble in water, found in teeth and bones. **Calcium Folinate.** BP Commission approved name for calcium-*N*-[4-(2-amino-5-formyl-5,6,7,8-tetrahydro-4-hydroxypteridin-6-ylmethyl)amino-benzoyl]-L-4-glutamate; an antidote to folic acid antagonists. **Calcium Gluconate BP 1973.** A tasteless white powder, given by mouth or by intramuscular or intravenous injection in calcium-deficient states, e.g. after massive blood transfusion. **Calcium Glycerophosphate BPC 1963, Calcium glycerylphosphate.** A whitish powder, and a frequent constituent of so-called nerve tonics. **Calcium hydrogen phosphate.** A white crystalline powder used in prevention and treatment of calcium deficiency. **Calcium Hydroxide BP 1973.** $Ca(OH)_2$, a white powder with a slightly bitter taste; used as solution of lime (lime water) in the treatment of diarrhoea in infants. **Calcium Hydroxide Solution BP 1968.** Lime water, a clear colourless liquid used as an alkali and antidote. **Calcium Hypophosphite BPC 1963.** $Ca(H_2PO_2)_2$, a white crystalline powder, used sometimes in the treatment of calcium-deficient states. **Calcium iodobehenate.** Calcium monoiodobehenate, $(C_{21}H_{42}ICOO)_2Ca$, a compound used for the same purposes as potassium iodide; it is non-irritant. **Ionized calcium.** Regulates the secretion of parathyroid hormone. **Calcium Lactate BP 1973.** $Ca(C_3H_5O_3)_2$, a white powder with only a slight taste and odour; used wherever calcium therapy is indicated, as in tetany, lead poisoning and rickets. It is probably the most satisfactory oral preparation. **Calcium lactophosphate.** A little-used mixture of the lactate, acid lactate and acid phosphate of calcium; a white granular powder, used where calcium therapy is indicated. **Calcium laevulate, Calcium laevulinate.** A white crystalline powder, readily soluble and stable in solution; used for intramuscular injection when calcium therapy is indicated. **Calcium Mandelate BPC 1954.** A white crystalline powder with only a slight taste and odour; before the advent of antibiotics it was widely used in the treatment of urinary infections. **Calcium monohydrogen phosphate.** Calcium hydrogen phosphate (see above). **Calcium nitrate.** A diffusible form found in the serum. **Calcium oxide.** Lime, quicklime, CaO; a compound obtained by the calcination of chalk or marble. It is used for making caustic pastes. **Calcium Phosphate BP 1953.** $Ca_3(PO_4)_2$, a white powder, almost without taste or odour. **Calcium saccharosates.** A number of compounds formed when calcium hydroxide is dissolved in sugar solutions. **(Total) Serum calcium.** Is equivalent to the sum of the protein-bound (non-diffusible) and the diffusible (bicarbonate, nitrate and phosphate) ionized calcium. **Calcium Sodium Lactate BPC 1968.** A white powder or colourless granules; more soluble than calcium lactate and used for the same purposes. **Calcium Sulphate, Dried, BPC 1968.** $CaSO_4$, a white hygroscopic powder, plaster of Paris, used to make plaster bandages and splints, and for dental casts. **Calcium sulphide.** CaS, the chief constituent of sulphurated lime: a greyish-white powder with an unpleasant odour and taste; formerly used internally in the treatment of boils and carbuncles. **Calcium thiosulphate.** $CaS_2O_3{\cdot}6H_2O$, a soluble compound used for the same purposes as sodium thiosulphate. **Calcium Trisodium Pentetate.** BP Commission approved name for the calcium chelate of the trisodium salt of diethylenetri-amine-*NNN′N″N″*-penta-acetic acid; a chelating agent. [L *calx* lime.]

calciuria (kal·se·**ewr**·e·ah). The presence of calcium in the urine.

calcoid (**kal**·koid). A calcified mass occurring in the dental pulp; a pulp stone. [L *calx* lime, Gk *eidos* form.]

calcospherite (kal·ko·**sfer**·ite). One of the many spherical masses composed of calcium salts (mainly phosphate and carbonate) and organic matter, found in regions in which calcification is progressing. [L *calx* lime, sphere.]

calcspar (**kalk**·spar). A hard crystalline mineral form of calcium carbonate, $CaCO_3$; it is transparent and doubly refracting. [calcium, LG *spar* gypsum.]

calculary (**kal**·kew·lar·e). Relating to calculus.

calculifragous (kal·kew·**lif**·rag·us). Lithotritic; referring to the crushing of a bladder calculus. [calculus, L *frangere* to break.]

calculosis (kal·kew·**lo**·sis). The condition in which a number of calculi are present in the body. [calculus, Gk *-osis* condition.]

calculous (**kal**·kew·lus). 1. Hard like a stone. 2. Caused by a calculus or calculi. 3. Characterized by the presence of calculi. [see foll.]

calculus (**kal**·kew·lus)(pl. *calculi*). A solid pathological concretion, usually of inorganic matter in a matrix of protein and pigment, formed in any part of the body, especially in reservoir organs and their passages. **Alternating calculus.** A urinary calculus built up in alternate layers of mineral substances. **Alvine calculus.** An intestinal stone composed of hardened faecal matter. **Arthritic calculus, Articular calculus.** Chalk stone; a foreign body occurring near a joint as the result of detachment of an osteophyte; a calcified mass of cartilage detached from a damaged articular cartilage and remaining in or near the joint. **Aural calculus.** A hard mass of wax lodged in the external auditory meatus of the ear. **Biliary calculus.** Gall-stone; a rounded or faceted mass consisting of bile constituents, especially cholesterol and bile pigment, precipitated in a protein matrix. It occurs usually in the gall bladder or in the biliary passages and may be single or multiple. **Blood calculus.** 1. Phlebolith. 2. Haematolith. **Bronchial calculus.** A concretion formed on the wall of an air passage. **Calcium oxalate calculus.** A hard stone composed of insoluble calcium oxalate crystals and the most usual source of urinary calculi. **Cardiac calculus.** Cardiolith; a calcified mass of fibrin or of necrotic cardiac muscle located within the heart. **Chalky calculus.** A urinary calculus the main constituents of which are calcium carbonate and calcium phosphate built up with other substances and formed usually round a foreign body or nucleus. **Cholesterol calculus.** A stone composed of cholesterol. **Combination calculus.** Alternating calculus (see above). **Coral calculus.** A large calculus lodged in the pelvis of the kidney and taking its shape with branches extending into the calyces, the whole resembling coral. **Cutaneous calculus.** A hard yellowish-white chalky nodule up to 1 cm in diameter, usually occurring on the face of a child. **Cystic calculus.** 1. Gall-stone. 2. Vesical calculus (see below). **Cystine calculus.** A variety of soft stone composed of cystine and found in the urinary tract, where it occurs as an abnormal metabolite. **Dendritic calculus.** Coral calculus (see above). **Dental calculus.** Subgingival calculus (see below). **Encysted calculus.** A vesical calculus lodged in a sac that has developed from the wall of the bladder. **Essential calculus.** A stone originating in and developing from organic tissue without the nucleus of a foreign body. **Fatty calculus.** A vesical calculus the nucleus of which is composed of fatty matter. **Calculus felleus.** Gall-stone. **Fibrin calculus, Fibrinous calculus.** One of the urinary tract made up of clotted blood or albumin. **Fusible calculus.** One largely composed of calcium carbonate or of the phosphates of calcium, magnesium and ammonium, which fuse characteristically when tested in the blowpipe flame. **Gastric calculus.** Gastrolith; a calcified lymph gland situated in the wall of the stomach; occasionally also a calcified thrombus of the blood vessels supplying the stomach wall. **Gonecystic calculus.** Spermatic calculus (see below). **Haematogenic calculus.** A calculus originating in the blood. **Haemic calculus.** Blood calculus (see above). **Hemp-seed calculus.** A small calculus of calcium oxalate, smooth and round and about the size of a hemp-seed, and occurring as a urinary deposit. **Hepatic calculus.** A gall-stone originating in the liver and remaining embedded in its substance. **Incarcerated calculus.** Encysted calculus (see above). **Indigo calculus.** A dark-blue crystalline or amorphous concretion formed by oxidation of the indican in urine. **Intestinal calculus.** Enterolith; a mass of inspissated faeces lodged in the large intestine. **Joint calculus.** Arthritic calculus (see above). **Lacrimal calculus.** Dacryolith; a tear stone or calculus in a lacrimal duct. **Lacteal calculus.** Mammary calculus (see below). **Laminated calculus.** A stone built up of different materials layer upon layer. **Lung calculi.** Stones formed in the bronchi either around a nucleus of inorganic matter or from indurated pieces of tissue. **Mammary calculus.** A nodule formed in one of the lactiferous ducts of the breast. **Metabolic calculus.** Cholesterol calculus (see above). **Mulberry calculus.** A gall-stone composed mainly of bile pigment with a distinct resemblance to a mulberry; an oxalate urinary calculus. **Nasal calculus.** Rhinolith; a concretion in the nasal cavity. **Nephritic calculus.** Renal calculus (see below). **Organic calculus.** A calculus the nucleus of which is blood or epithelium. **Ovarian calculus.** The corpus luteum in an indurated calcified and enlarged state. **Oxalate calculus.** A round pitted stone composed of calcium oxalate. **Pancreatic calculus.** A stone built up in the pancreatic duct from calcium carbonate or other calcium salts, and organic substances. **Phosphate calculus, Phosphatic calculus.** A soft calculus composed mainly of phosphate, found in the genito-urinary tract. **Pineal calculus.** A small calcified protein mass found within the substance of the pineal gland. **Pocketed calculus.** Encysted calculus (see above). **Podagric calculus.** Arthritic calculus (see below). **Preputial calculus.** Preputial concretion. *See* CONCRETION. **Prostatic calculus.** One formed in the prostate gland, and mainly composed of calcium carbonate and calcium phosphate. **Renal calculus.** Stone in the kidney, a calculus formed in the pelvis of the kidney and composed of calcium urate, oxalate, and phosphate. **Salivary calculus.** 1. Tartar. 2. A stone formed in a duct of the salivary glands. **Scrotal calculus.** 1. A stone which has passed into the scrotum from the prostate gland or the urinary bladder. 2. A stone originating in the scrotum itself from chalky degeneration of the tissue. **Secondary calculus.** A vesical calculus arising out of disease affecting the mucus of the urinary tract. **Seruminal calculus.** Subgingival calculus (see below). **Shellac calculus.** A gastrolith formed as a result of drinking shellac varnish. **Spermatic calculus.** A stone formed in a seminal vesicle. **Staghorn calculus.** An exaggerated coral calculus of the ureteral pelvis with many branches resembling antlers. **Stomachic calculus.** A gastrolith or bezoar located in the stomach. **Subgingival calculus.** Calculus deposited on the teeth beneath the gingival margins. **Supragingival calculus.** Calculus deposited upon those parts of the teeth which are not covered by the gingivae. **Tonsillar calculus.** A chalky deposit in the pits of the tonsil. **Urate calculus.** A calculus composed of urates and affecting mainly young infants. **Uric acid calculus.** One formed from uric acid and occurring in the form of a hard reddish stone in the urinary tract. **Urinary calculus.** A term applied to a calculus occurring in any part of the urinary tract. It may consist of urates or uric acid, calcium oxalate, calcium phosphate or a mixture with triple phosphates, calcium carbonate, or metabolic products such as cystine or xanthine. **Urostealith calculus.** Urostealith; a urinary calculus formed mainly of fatty substances. **Uterine calculus.** Womb stone; a calcified fibroid resulting from degeneration of the uterine wall. **Vesical calculus.** A calculus formed in the urinary bladder. **Vesicoprostatic calculus.** A calculus formed in the prostate with extension into the urinary bladder. **Xanthic calculus.** A urinary calculus the main constituent of which is xanthine, derived from the uric acid metabolism. [L a pebble.]

Caldani, Leopoldo Marco Antonio (b. 1725). Padua anatomist.
Caldani's ligament. The coracoclavicular ligament. *See* LIGAMENT.

Caldwell, George Walter (b. 1834). New York otolaryngologist.
Caldwell-Luc operation. A radical operation on the maxillary antrum carried out through an incision in the gingivolabial fold; the antral cavity is then explored after removal of the bone in the region of the canine fossa.

Caldwell, William Edgar (b. 1880). New York obstetrician.
Caldwell-Moloy classification. A valuable contribution to the classification of the human female pelvis into 4 main types; the types are assessed by clinical and radiological examination.

calefacient (kal·e·fa·shent). 1. A remedy or medicament which gives rise to a sensation of warmth. 2. Making warm. [L *calere* to be warm, *facere* to make.]

Calendula (kal·en·dew·lah). A group of plants with composite flower formation. The pot marigold, *Calendula officinalis* Linn., has resolvent and stimulant properties. [L *Calendae*, first day of the month, when the plant was supposed to flower.]

calenture (kal·en·tewr). 1. Any feverish condition occurring in the tropics caused by excessive heat. 2. Heat stroke. *See* STROKE. [Sp. *calentura* fever.]

calf [sura (NA)] (kahf). The bulky prominence at the back of the leg below the knee formed mainly by the gastrocnemius muscles. **Bull-dog calf.** The bowed appearance of the calf in cases of hereditary achondroplasia. **Gnome's calf.** The rounded, very full calf seen in pseudohypertrophic paralysis affecting the gastrocnemius muscles. **Tennis calf.** Sudden rupture of some fibres of the gastrocnemius or of the plantaris tendon, which typically produces a sensation as of a hard hit by a ball or racket on the back of the leg. [Old Norse *kalfi.*]

calf bone (kahf·bone). The fibula. [Old Norse *kalfi*, AS *ban.*]

calibrate (kal·e·brate). 1. In surgery, to determine the exact size of an opening for the purpose, for instance, of anastomosis of bowel parts. 2. To determine the inside diameter of a tube. 3. To graduate an instrument by means of a standard, or to determine the error in graduations already marked. [Fr. *calibre* the bore of a gun.]

calibration (kal·e·bra·shun). The process or act of calibrating; standardization of an unknown against a known, e.g. mass or length. Similarly, standardization of an instrument by application of a known signal.

calibrator (kal·e·bra·tor). 1. A dilator for urethral stricture. 2. An instrument with which the lumen of a passage can be measured. **Bone calibrator.** An instrument for measuring the diameter and depth of drill holes in bone. [Fr. *calibre* the bore of a gun.]

caliche (kal·e·che). The name given in Chile to the crude sodium nitrate found in deposits there; contains also a proportion of sodium iodate. Chile saltpetre. [Sp. a flake of lime.]

Calicivirus (cay·li·see·vi·rus). A genus of RNA- containing viruses 33 nm in diameter, with cup-shaped surface units. Pathogens of cats, pigs, sea-lions and fur seals have recently been observed in the stools of some young children by direct electron microscopy. The significance of this finding has yet to be established, but they may play a role in causing enteritis. [L *calyx* a cup-like cavity.]

caliculus (kal·ik·ew·lus). Calyculus.

caliectasis (kal·e·ek·tas·is). The process of dilating a calyx of the ureter. [calyx, Gk *ektasis* a stretching.]

Californian buckthorn (kal·if·or·ne·an buck·thorn). *Rhamnus californica* Eschscholz (family Rhamnaceae). The bark has purgative properties and has been used as a substitute for cascara [State of *California*, USA, buckthorn.]

californium (kal·if·or·ne·um). A transuranic element of atomic number 98 and chemical symbol Cf. It was obtained in 1949 by bombarding curium with α-particles in the cyclotron, and has a half-life of 45 min. **Californium-252.** A neutron emitting a radioactive isotope. [State of *California*, USA.]

caligation (kal·ig·a·shun). Caligo.

caligo (kal·i·go). Obscurity or dimness of sight generally the result of corneal, lenticular or vitreous opacity. **Caligo corneae.** Dim sight because of opacity of the cornea. **Caligo lentis.** Cataract. **Caligo pupillae.** Synizesis. [L *caligo* darkness.]

caliper (kal·ip·er). A splint made of 2 iron rods secured to a padded ring into which a limb is placed for the pupose of exerting tension on it; it is especially used for fractures of the femur. Thomas' splint is a form of caliper. **Walking caliper.** Same as above, with distal ends fitting into the heel of the boot so that the weight of the body is carried on the tuber ischii and not on the thigh or leg. Also called *caliper splint.* [corruption of *calibre.*]
See also: BLACKBURN, THOMAS (H. O.).

calipers (kal·ip·erz). A pair of compasses with 2 curved legs linked together by a spring or hinge; they are used for measuring the diameter or thickness of an opening or object, being commonly employed in female pelvic measurements. [see prec.]

calisaya bark (kal·is·a·yah bark). The bark of *Cinchona calisaya* Wedd. (family Rubiaceae) one of the varieties of "yellow" cinchona bark. [South American name.]

calisthenics (kal·is·then·ix). Callisthenics.

calix (ka·lix). Calyx.

Call, Friedrich von (b. 1844). Vienna physician.
Call-Exner bodies. 1. Round dark masses among the follicular cells of a developing ovarian follicle; probably centres of secretion of follicular fluid. 2. Ova-like cells, the result of hydropic degeneration, around which other cells are arranged in rosettes in granulosa-cell tumours of the ovary.

Callahan's test. For simulated unilateral deafness: each ear is connected by rubber tubing to a central mouthpiece. Word repetition is carried out, and the length of the tubes is altered by the addition or removal of further detachable tubes. Normal hearing is loudest in the ear connected to the shortest tube. Improbable responses, therefore, lead to the detection of malingering.

Callander, C. Latimer (b. 1892). San Francisco surgeon.
Callander's amputation. A tenoplastic amputation through the femur at the knee.

Callaway, Thomas (b. 1791). London surgeon.
Callaway's test. For dislocation of the shoulder: the vertical measurement round the axilla and over the outer part of the clavicle is greater on the dislocated side.

Calleja y Sanchez, Camilo (d. 1913). Madrid anatomist.
Calleja's cells, islands or islets. Clumps of small nerve cells found near the surface of the olfactory tubercle of the brain.

Callender, George William (b. 1830). London anatomist and surgeon.
Callender's maxillary clips. The nasal and incisor processes of the maxilla that overgrow the facial aspect of the premaxilla in man.

callicrein (kal·ik·re·in). Kallikrein.

calliper (kal·ip·er). Caliper.

Calliphora (kal·if·or·ah). A genus of flies that may act as a mechanical vector of infection; the larva may cause myiasis in man. The two important species are *Calliphora erythrocephala* and *Calliphora vomitoria* [Gk *kallos* beauty, *pherein* to bear.]

Calliphoridae (kal·if·**or**·id·e). A family of flies which includes flesh flies (*Sarcophaga* and *Wohlfahrtia*), bluebottle flies (*Calliphora* and *Phormia*), greenbottle flies (*Lucilia* and *Chrysomyia*), tumbu flies *(Cordylobia)* and the Congo floor maggot *(Auchmeromyia)*. [see prec.]

callisection (kal·e·**sek**·shun). The vivisection of anaesthetized animals. [L *callere* to be insensible, *secare* to cut.]

Callison, James George (b. 1873). New York otolaryngologist.

Callison's fluid, or solution. A diluting solution containing Loeffler's methylene blue 1 g, formaldehyde 1 g, glycerine 10 g, ammonium oxalate 1 g, sodium chloride 5 g, water 90 g, used in the counting of red blood corpuscles.

callisthenics (kal·is·**then**·ix). Gymnastics in which effort and power are mainly eliminated and in which movements of muscle groups are devised with a view to the development of gracefulness and beauty. [Gk *kallos* beauty, *sthenos* strength.]

callomania (kal·o·**ma**·ne·ah). A state in which a person deludes himself or herself into the belief that he or she is beautiful. [Gk *kallos* beauty, mania.]

Callophis (kal·o·fis). A genus of snakes that includes the coral snakes. [Gk *kallos* beauty, *ophis* snake.]

callosal (kal·o·sal). Relating to the corpus callosum. **Callosal sulcus.** *See* SULCUS. [L *callosus* hard.]

callositas (kal·**os**·it·as). Callosity.

callosity (kal·**os**·it·e). 1. A circumscribed thickening of the horny layers of the skin as the result of intermittent pressure or friction or some other kind of irritation. 2. Keratoma. [L *callosus* hard.]

callosomarginal (kal·o·so·**mar**′·jin·al). Relating to the corpus callosum and the superior frontal gyrus, denoting the superior frontal sulcus which lies between them. [L *callosus* hard, *margo* margin.]

callous (**kal**·us). 1. Indurated. 2. Like a callosity. [L *callosus* hard.]

callus (**kal**·us). 1. A callosity or hard, thick skin. 2. The bone-like reparative substance that is formed round the edges and fragments of broken bone. **Central callus.** The temporary callus formed within the medullary cavity of a bone that is mending after fracture. **Definitive callus.** The permanent reparative exudate that develops into true bone between the broken fragments of a fractured bone. **Ensheathing callus.** The temporary and reabsorbable callus that forms around broken fragments of bone until repair is effected. **Inner callus, Interior callus, Internal callus.** Central callus (see above). **Intermediate callus.** Definitive callus (see above). **Medullary callus, Myelogenous callus.** Central callus (see above). **Permanent callus.** Definitive callus (see above). **Pin callus.** Central callus (see above). **Provisional callus, Temporary callus.** The ensheathing and central callus around and within a broken bone which forms during the first few weeks after fracture, serves as a natural splint during repair and is reabsorbed when the bone is mended. [L hard skin.]

Calmette, Léon Charles Albert (b. 1863). Paris bacteriologist.

Calmette's antivenene. Antivenene prepared from a mixture of 80 per cent cobra venom (predominantly neurotoxic) and 20 per cent Russell's viper venom (predominantly haemolytic), used in India.

Calmette reaction. A diagnostic test for tuberculosis in which a dilute solution of tuberculin is dropped into the conjunctival sac, giving rise in tuberculous people to a severe local reaction. Rarely, if ever, used nowadays.

Calmette's serum. Antivenene.

Calmette vaccine. B.C.G. vaccine. *See* VACCINE.

bacillus of Calmette-Guérin. The bacillus from which the antituberculosis (B.C.G.) vaccine is made.

Calmette-Guérin test. A test for the potency of smallpox vaccine lymph. An eruption of isolated vesicles numbering 3-4 per square centimetre should appear after distributing 1 ml of 1:1000 dilution of lymph over a prepared area of the skin of a rabbit.

Percutaneous Bacillus Calmette-Guérin Vaccine BP 1973. A suspension of living cells of an authentic strain of the bacillus of Calmette-Guérin with a higher viable bacterial count than the latter. A prophylactic against tuberculosis, administered by percutaneous inoculation.

calomel (**kal**·o·mel). Mercurous Chloride BP 1953, HgCl. An insoluble white compound employed in medicine as a purgative. It passes through the stomach unchanged, but in the intestine a small amount is converted to the more soluble oxide. The irritant mercury ion produced causes increased peristalsis, which results in purgation about 12 h after the drug is taken. The stools are semifluid and greenish-yellow in colour owing to their high content of biliverdin. For this reason it was once thought to have a choleretic effect; this is not due to increased bile secretion but to the antiseptic nature of the drug, checking bacterial action in the gut, and the increased speed with which the food passes along the alimentary tract, both of which prevent the conversion of biliverdin to bilirubin. Most of the drug is excreted unchanged but some mercury is absorbed, normally insufficient to cause any systemic effects, but if purgation is not produced, more of the calomel is converted to the soluble oxide and toxic effects may result. Children tolerate the drug very well. It derives its name from the black mixture it forms on the addition of ammonia. [Gk *kalos* beautiful, *melas* black.]

calor (**kal**·or). 1. Animal heat; the natural heat of the body. 2. Moderate fever heat, one of the classical signs of inflammation. Cf. ARDOR, FERVOR. **Calor animalis.** Animal heat. **Calor febrilis.** Fever heat. **Calor fervens.** 1. Fervor. 2. Boiling heat. **Calor innatus.** Animal heat. **Calor internus.** Feverishness which cannot be detected on the surface of the body. **Calor mordax, Calor mordicans.** 1. The rosy skin of scarlet fever. 2. Biting or stinging heat. **Calor nativus.** Animal heat. [L heat.]

calor gas (**kal**·orgas). Butane, used for domestic heating and illumination. **Calor gas poisoning.** *See* POISONING. [L *calor* heat, gas.]

calorescence (kal·or·es·ens). In physics, the conversion to incandescence of invisible or non-luminous rays of heat. [L *calor* heat.]

Calori, Luigi (b. 1807). Bologna anatomist.

Calori's bursa. An inconstant serous sac separating the trachea and the aortic arch.

caloric (kal·**or**·ik). Relating to a calorie or heat. [L *calor* heat.]

caloricity (kal·or·**is**·it·e). In physiology, the faculty possessed by the animal body of producing and maintaining heat. [see prec.]

calorie (**kal**·or·e). A unit of heat approximately equal to 4.2 joules. The *medical* or kilocalorie is equal to 4186.8 joules. [L *calor* heat.]

calorifacient (kal·or·e·**fa**′·shent). A term applied to those foods which are heat-producing. [L *calor* heat, *facere* to make.]

calorific (kal·or·**if**·ik). 1. Heat-producing. 2. Thermal. 3. Holding or carrying warmth. **Calorific value.** *See* VALUE. [see prec.]

calorigenetic, calorigenic (kal·or·e·jen·**et**′·ik, kal·or·e·**jen**′·ik). 1. Producing energy or heat. 2. Increasing the production of energy or heat. [L *calor* heat, Gk *genein* to produce.]

calorimeter (kal·or·**im**·et·er). 1. An instrument for measuring the quantity of heat liberated or absorbed in a chemical or physical change or by the animal body in specified conditions. 2. An apparatus for measuring any systematic heat change. **Bomb calorimeter.** A calorimeter for the determination of the heat of combustion of any substance, e.g. chemical compounds, foods or excreta. A weighed amount of the substance is burnt in oxygen (sometimes under pressure) in the hermetically-sealed bomb, and the heat set free is measured by the rise in temperature of the weighed quantity of water in which the bomb is immersed. **Compensating calorimeter, Differential air calorimeter.** A calorimeter for determining the heat production of animals, in which the loss of heat by conduction and radiation from the calorimeter is compensated by a similar loss from a dummy instrument of identical size and design, in which hydrogen is burnt at an appropriate rate. The heat produced is calculated from the known heat of combustion of hydrogen. **Respiration calorimeter.** A combined calorimeter and respiration chamber in which heat production and respiratory exchange can be measured over given periods, on men or animals. In the closed type, oxygen is circulated, CO_2 absorbed and the utilization of oxygen made good by addition of measured volumes of oxygen; the chamber is well insulated and surrounded by radiators through which water circulates. The heat production is measured from the volume of water circulated and its rise of temperature. [L *calor* heat, meter.]

See also: ATWATER, BENEDICT (F. G.).

calorimetric (kal·or·im·et'·rik). Referring or relating to calorimetry.

calorimetry (kal·or·im·et·re). The measurement of heat production or absorption. **Direct calorimetry.** The actual measurement of heat produced, usually in calories, by observing the rise of temperature produced in a known mass of water. **Indirect calorimetry.** The calculation of heat production by the observation of some phenomenon other than rise of temperature, e.g. by measuring oxygen usage or CO_2 production. **Partitional calorimetry.** The determination and allocation of the different fractions of heat loss of the body according to their respective factors, such as convection, radiation and evaporation. [L *calor* heat, meter.]

caloripuncture (kal·or·e·pungk'·tcher). Ignipuncture: the cauterizing of tissues by the insertion of needles at red heat. [L *calor* heat, *pungere* to prick.]

caloriscope (kal·or·e·skope). 1. An instrument with which the calorific values of various infant-feeding mixtures can be ascertained. 2. An instrument with which the liberation of heat in the breathing of an organism can be noted. [L *calor* heat, Gk *skopein* to watch.]

caloritropic (kal·or·e·trop'·ik). Thermotropic; term applied to bacteria which are sensitive to changes in temperature or are stimulated by them. [L *calor* heat, Gk *tropos* a turning.]

calorization (kal·or·i·za'·shun). The process of applying heat. [L *calor* heat.]

Calot, Jean François (b. 1861). French surgeon.

Calot's operation. Forcible correction of a gibbus under anaesthesia [obsolete].

Calot treatment. Correction of the deformity in Pott's disease by pads applied to a window in a plaster jacket.

Calot's triangle. A triangle formed by the cystic and hepatic ducts, closed inferiorly by the line of the cystic artery.

Calotropis (kal·ot·ro·pis). A genus of plants of the Asclepiadaceae. *Calotropis procera* Ait. and *Calotropis gigantea* Ait. yield a root-bark which has properties similar to ipecacuanha, and is used in India. [Gk *kalos* beautiful, *tropis* keel.]

calotte (kal·ot). 1. Any part that has the shape of a skull-cap. 2. The sinciput. [Fr. flat cap.]

calumba (kal·um·bah). The dried sliced root of *Jateorhiza palmata* (Lamarck) Miers (family Menispermaceae), a climbing plant indigenous to Mozambique. It contains alkaloidal quaternary bases and non-alkaloidal bitter principles; used as a bitter tonic (BPC 1954). **Ceylon calumba.** The stem of *Coscinium fenestratum* Colebr. which contains berberine. [local name.]

calumbin (kal·um·bin). $C_{21}H_{24}O_9$, a non-alkaloidal bitter principle derived from calumba root; it is the glucoside of the lactone of calumbic acid.

calvaria [NA] (kal·va·re·ah). The skull-cap; the cranial portion of the skull—that which lies above the level of the plane which passes through the supra-orbital margins and the superior nuchal lines of the occiput. Its upper surface is smooth, whilst its inner surface is marked by the superior sagittal sinus (sagittal groove), the meningeal vessels, arachnoid granulations and the cerebral gyri (impressions for the cerebral gyri). [L bare skull.]

calvarial, calvarian (kal·va·re·al, kal·va·re·an). Relating to the calvaria, or belonging to it.

Calvé, Jacques (b. 1875). French orthopaedic surgeon.

Calvé's cannula. A cannula for draining an intraspinal abscess by way of the intervertebral foramen in Pott's paraplegia.

Calvé's disease. Osteochondrosis of a vertebral body.

Legg-Calvé disease, Legg-Calvé-Perthes disease, Legg-Calvé-Waldenström disease, Calvé-Perthes disease. Coxa plana; osteochondritis of the upper femoral epiphysis.

calvities, calvitium (kal·vish·e·eez, kal·vish·e·um). Baldness; a term applied particularly to baldness on the crown and occiput. [L baldness.]

calvous (kal·vus). Bald. [L *calvus.*]

calx (kalx). Lime; calcium oxide. Sometimes used also to describe chalk or calcium carbonate. **Calx avis.** Bird lime. **Calx chlorinata.** Chlorinated Lime BP 1958. *See* LIME. **Calx hydrargyri alba.** Ammoniated mercury. *See* MERCURY. **Calx sodica.** Soda Lime BP 1958. *See* LIME. **Calx Sulphurata BPC 1949.** A mixture of calcium sulphide and lime made by boiling quicklime and sublimed sulphur in water. The diluted solution is useful in the treatment of scabies. **Calx usta, Calx viva.** Quicklime. [L.]

calyceal (kal·is·e·al). Pertaining to a calyx.

calycectasis (kal·lis·ek·tas·is). Incomplete or delayed emptying of a calyx or group of calyces, as a result of stricture or achalasia at the neck of the calyx. [calyx, Gk *ektasis* extension.]

calycectomy (ka·lis·ek·to·me). A partial nephrectomy performed in order to remove an isolated calyx, or group of calyces, in which there has been recurrent stone formation or persistent calyceal dilatation. [calyx, Gk *ektome* excision.]

calyciform (kal·is·e·form). Like a calyx, cup-shaped. [Gk *kalyx* shell, form.]

calycine (kal·is·een). Like or relating to a calyx.

calyculus (kal·ik·ew·lus). A cup-shaped or bud-shaped structure resembling a closed calyx. [L dim. from Gk *kalyx* shell.]

calymmatobacterium granulomatis (kal·im·at·o·bak·teer'·e·um gran·ew·lo·mat·is). *Donovania granulomatis;* the intracellular bodies (Donovan bodies) occurring in the mononuclear cells scraped from the granulomatous ulcers of granuloma inguinale. [Gk *kalymma* hood, bacterium, granuloma.]

calyx (ka·lix) (pl. *calyces*). Any cavity or organ shaped like a cup. **Renal calyces [calices renales majores et minores (NA)].** The divisions of the pelvis of the ureter. The pelvis divides first into 2 or 3 major calyces which in turn divide into minor calyces, 12 or more in number, the cup-shaped terminations of which receive the apices of the cone-shaped segments of the medulla. [Gk *kalyx* shell.]

Camallanata (kam·al·an·a'·tah). A sub-order of the nematode class or sub-class Phasmidia. The super-family Dracunculoidea is of medical interest.

Cambarus (kam·bar·us). A genus of Crustacea, several crayfish of which are intermediate hosts of lung flukes of the genus *Paragonimus* in North America. [Gk *kammaros* lobster.]

cambium (kam·be·um). 1. A nutritive juice formerly held to be produced in the blood and to be used for systemic repair and to promote general well-being. 2. A layer of soft formative tissue from which new wood and bark are formed in exogenous trees and shrubs. [L *cambire* to exchange.]

cambogia (kam·boje·e·ah). Gamboge.

cambric (kam·brik). *See* BILLROTH. [*Cambrai*, France.]

camelpox (kam·el·pox). A disease of camels caused by a virus which is very similar antigenically and in other ways to the virus of human smallpox. It is not known whether it can cause disease in man. [camel, AS *pocc.*]

camera (kam·er·ah). 1. A closed compartment or chamber. 2. In anatomy, any chamber, cavity or open space, e.g. the fornix of the rhinencephalon, or the hollow of the auricle of the ear. **Camera aquosa.** The anterior aqueous chamber of the eye. **Camera cordis.** The pericardium. **Electron diffraction camera.** A camera by which a photographic record is obtained of the diffracted beams of electrons produced by irradiating a specimen with electrons. **Gamma camera.** A form of static imaging device used in nuclear medicine which provides a pictorial or diagrammatic representation of the distribution of a radionuclide within an organ, a part of the body, or the whole body. *See* SCAN. **Gastric camera.** A flexible instrument of Japanese manufacture which is passed into the stomach and a series of photographs taken of the interior of the stomach. **Camera lucida.** A prism-attachment fixed to the eyepiece of a microscope so that the image of the object in the field of vision of the microscope is thrown upon drawing-paper, thus enabling its structure to be traced with a pencil. **Moving-film camera.** An x-ray camera developed from the single crystal camera, in which the movement of the film is synchronized with the crystal rotation or oscillation, thus simplifying the interpretation of the diffraction pattern obtained. Also known as the *Weissenberg camera.* **Camera oculi.** Either one of the two chambers of the eye. **Powder camera.** An x-ray camera for revealing photographically the diffraction haloes produced by a powdered specimen. **Camera pulpi.** The cavity of a tooth. **Recording camera.** Photokymograph. **Camera septi lucidi, Camera septi pellucidi.** The cavity of the septum lucidum. **Single-crystal camera.** An x-ray camera in which diffraction beams are produced by a single crystal. If monochromatic x-rays are used, the crystal is oscillated or rotated and the film is placed cylindrically coaxial with the axis of rotation. In the Laue method, heterogenous x-rays are used and the crystal is stationary. **X-ray camera.** An apparatus for the production of a photographic record of the positions and intensities of x-ray beams coherently scattered by a material the atoms of which are arranged in a regular structure. [L vault.]

See also: ABBÉ, NORDENSEN, WEISSENBERG.

Camerer, Johann Friedrich Wilhelm (b. 1842). Württemberg paediatrician.

Camerer's law. The same food requirements are shared by children of the same weight irrespective of their ages.

camisia fetus (kam·is·e·ah **fe**·tus). The chorion. [LL shirt, L offspring.]

camisole (**kam**·e·sole). A strait jacket put on a violently insane person for the purpose of restraining movement and preventing injury to himself or other people. The analogous term in France is *camisole de force.* [Fr. sleeved jacket.]

Cammann, George Philip (b. 1804). New York physician.

Cammann's stethoscope. The binaural stethoscope, first designed by Cammann.

camomile (kam·o·mile). Chamomile.

Campbell, Alfred Walter (b. 1868). British anatomist.

Campbell's area. The precentral area of the cerebral cortex.

Campbell De Morgan. *See* DE MORGAN, CAMPBELL GREIG.

Campbell, William Francis (b. 1867). Brooklyn surgeon.

Campbell's ligament. The suspensory ligament of the axilla.

Campbell, Willis Cohoon (b. 1880). Memphis, Tennessee, orthopaedic surgeon.

Campbell's bone-block operation. An operation for paralytic pes calcaneocavus or pes equinus where a block of bone is used to maintain the normal position of the foot.

campeachy, campechy (kam·pe·che). Logwood, the heartwood of *Haematoxylon campechianum* Linn. (family Leguminosae). [*Campeche,* Mexico.]

Camper, Pieter (b. 1722). Dutch anatomist and physician.

Camper's facial angle. The angle formed at the base of the anterior nasal spine by the intersection of 2 lines running from that point, one to the external auditory meatus (Camper's line), the other to the most prominent median portion of the frontal bone. In anthropometry, a measure of the slope of the forehead.

Camper's chiasm. Chiasma tendinum.

Camper's fascia. *See* FASCIA OF THE ABDOMINAL WALL, SUPERFICIAL.

Camper's line. A line from the external auditory meatus to the median part of the base of the anterior nasal spine.

campesterol (kam·pes·ter·ol). $C_{28}H_{48}O$. A sterol derived from rape oil *(Brassica campestris)* and believed to be identical with that occurring in wheat germ oil.

camphane (**kam**·fane). 1. A member of a family of terpenes, derived from borneol, which contain a 6-carbon ring bridged in the *para* position. 2. $C_{10}H_{18}$, a saturated terpene hydrocarbon prepared from bornyl iodide, and regarded as the parent of the camphors; a white crystalline substance.

camphene (**kam**·feen). $C_{10}H_{16}$, an unsaturated terpene hydrocarbon isomeric with bornylene, and existing in 2 optically-active forms. It is prepared from pinene and occurs naturally in oil of turpentine.

camphin (**kam**·fin). $C_{10}H_8$, a reduction product of camphor occurring as a colourless oil.

camphol (**kam**·fol). Borneol.

camphor (**kam**·for). 1. The general name for a group of dicyclic terpenes found in plants. They are alcoholic or ketonic in structure and members of the camphane family. 2. A colourless crystalline substance, $C_{10}H_{16}O$, obtained from the wood of *Cinnamomum camphora,* a tree found in Taiwan, Japan and China. It has a strong aromatic taste and odour, with an irritant action on the skin and mucous membranes producing local vasodilatation and subsequent slight analgesia. It is frequently incorporated in cough mixtures (BP 1973) for its supposed expectorant action; used as a 10 or 20 per cent solution in arachis oil for subcutaneous injection to produce, by local irritation, reflex stimulation of the medullary centres. Camphor is the main constituent of moth-balls, and the eating of these by children has caused poisoning. **Ammoniated Liniment of Camphor BP 1953.** A preparation composed of camphor (12.5 per cent), lavender oil, ammonia and alcohol; used as a rubefacient in the treatment of non-articular rheumatism. **Borneo camphor.** Camphyl alcohol, obtained from the wood of *Dryobalanops aromatica,* a tree found in Borneo. **Carbolic camphor.** A preparation composed of 3 parts of camphor to 1 part of phenol. **Cedrene camphor.** Camphor from palm kernel oil. **Compound syrup of camphor.** A preparation which includes camphor and tincture of opium, employed as a sedative cough mixture. **Compound tincture of camphor.** Camphorated Opium Tincture BP 1958, a preparation composed of tincture of opium, benzoic acid, camphor, anise oil and alcohol; it contains 0.05 per cent of anhydrous morphine and is employed as a sedative cough mixture. **Concentrated camphor water.** An aqueous preparation containing 4 per cent of camphor; employed as a carminative. **Essence of camphor.** Rubini's essence, a preparation composed of 1 part of camphor and 2½ parts of alcohol; employed formerly for its carminative action. **Hard ointment of camphor.** Camphor ice, a preparation composed of camphor and a mixture of hard and soft paraffin. **Camphor Liniment BP 1973.** Camphorated oil, a preparation containing 20 per cent of camphor in arachis oil. It is given by injection as a reflex stimulant of the central nervous system, and as a counter-irritant in non-articular rheumatism and bronchitis. **Parsley camphor.** Apiole. **Rectified Camphor Oil BPC 1959.** The lighter fraction of the oil obtained as a by-product in the manufacture of natural camphor. **Spirit of Camphor BPC 1959.** A preparation composed of camphor, 10 per cent in 90 per cent alcohol; used as a carminative. **Sumatra camphor.** Borneo camphor (see above). **Camphor Water BP 1958.** An aqueous preparation containing 0.1 per cent of camphor; employed as a carminative. [Malay *kapur* chalk.]

camphoraceous (kam·for·a·shus). Having the qualities of camphor.

camphorate (**kam**·for·ate). A salt of camphoric acid.

camphorated (**kam**·for·ate·ed). Impregnated with camphor, or containing camphor.

camphoric (kam·**for**·ik). Pertaining to, or mixed with, camphor.

camphorism (**kam**·for·izm). The state of being poisoned by the excessive ingestion of camphor or its preparations. Gastroenteritis, convulsions and other cerebral symptoms, and coma mark the condition.

camphorogenol (kam·for·**oj**·en·ol). $C_{10}H_{18}O_2$. A substance found in natural camphor.

camphoromania (**kam**·for·o·**ma**'·ne·ah). Camphor addiction. [camphor, mania.]

camphorquinone (kam·for·**kwin**·one). Diketocamphane, $C_{10}H_{14}O_2$. Yellow needles occurring as an oxidation product of camphor.

camphoryl (**kam**·for·il). The monovalent radical $C_{10}H_{15}O$–, present in camphor compounds.

camphrene (**kam**·freen). $C_9H_{14}O$, a volatile substance formed by the action of sulphuric acid on camphor.

camphyl (**kam**·fil). The divalent radical $C_{10}H_{16}=$, occurring in camphor derivatives.

campimeter (kam·**pim**·et·er). Perimeter. [L *campus* field, meter.]

campimetry (kam·**pim**·et·re). Perimetry. [see prec.]

campospasm (**kam**·po·spazm). Camptocormia. [Gk *kampe* a bending, *spasmos* a drawing.]

camptocormia, camptocormy (kamp·to·**kor**·me·ah, kamp·to·**kor**·me). A hysterical condition in which the back is habitually inclined forwards although the spine remains flexible; there is always compensatory extension of the head. [Gk *kamptos* bent, *kormos* trunk.]

camptodactylia, camptodactylism, camptodactyly (**kamp**·to·dak·**til**′·e·ah, kamp·to·**dak**·til·izm, kamp·to·**dak**·til·e). A state of permanent immobility of one or more flexed joints of a finger. [Gk *kamptos* bent, *daktylos* finger.]

camptospasm (**kamp**·to·spazm). Camptocormia. [Gk *kamptos* bent, *spasmos* a drawing.]

campylognathia (**kam**·pil·o·**nath**′·e·ah). Deformity of the jaw or lip to a degree in which it resembles that of a rabbit. [Gk *kampylos* bent, *gnathos* jaw.]

campylorrhinus (**kam**·pil·o·**ri**′·nus). A fetal monster with deformed nose. [Gk *kampylos* bent, *rhis* nose.]

Canada fleabane (**kan**·ad·ah **fle**·bane). The dried leaves and flowering tops of *Erigeron canadense.* It was at one time used as a diaphoretic and expectorant. [*Canada,* AS *fleah, bana* death.]

canadine (**kan**·ad·een). Tetrahydroberberine, $C_{20}H_{21}O_4N$. An alkaloid present in hydrastis, the dried rhizome and roots of *Hydrastis canadensis.* It causes depression followed by paralysis of the central nervous system.

canal [canalis (NA)] (kan·**al**). An elongated or tubular space or channel which permits the passage of substances such as air, food, blood, excretory material and glandular secretions, or anatomical structures such as nerves or blood vessels. **Adductor canal.** Subsartorial canal (see below). **Alimentary canal [canalis alimentarius (NA)].** The passage from the mouth to the anus. **Alisphenoid canal.** A canal in the greater wing of the sphenoid which transmits the external carotid artery; it is present in dogs and certain other animals, but not in man. **Alveolar canal, Alveolodental canal.** Dental canals, superior (see below). **Anal canal [canalis analis (NA)].** The last 4 cm (1½ in) of the alimentary canal, between the ampulla of the rectum and the anal orifice. **Archenteric canal.** A canal in the head process which projects forwards from the primitive node beneath the ectoderm in the early embryo; when its floor breaks down an opening is left from the primitive node to the entodermal vesicle; the neurenteric canal. **Atrial canal.** The cavity of an atrium of the heart; usually applied to the embryonic heart before the right and left atria are separated. **Atrioventricular canal, common.** A developmental abnormality of the heart in which division of the common atrioventricular canal in the embryo, to form the separate tricuspid and mitral valve canals, fails to occur; the dominant features are those of the atrial septal defect and of atrioventricular valve regurgitation. **Atrioventricular canals, right and left.** The passages from the respective atria to the corresponding ventricles. **Auditory canal, external.** The external auditory meatus. *See* MEATUS. **Auditory canal, internal.** The internal auditory meatus. *See* MEATUS. **Auricular canal.** 1. The external auditory meatus. *See* MEATUS. 2. The atrioventricular canal of the embryonic heart. **Basipharyngeal canal.** The vomerovaginal canal (see below). **Birth canal.** The canal through which the fetus passes during delivery, namely the uterus, vagina and vulva. **Blastoporic canal.** The archenteric canal (see above). **Calciferous canals.** Canals in ossifying cartilage. **Caroticotympanic canals.** Caroticotympanic canaliculi. *See* CANALICULUS. **Cartilage canals.** Vascular canals present in large masses of cartilage, e.g. in the epiphyses of human long bones after the third month of intra-uterine development. **Caudal canal.** Sacral canal (see below). **Central canal of the modiolus.** A canal in the centre of the modiolus of the cochlea, transmitting the fibres of the cochlear nerve which go to the apical turn of the cochlea. **Central canal of the spinal cord [canalis centralis (NA)].** A small canal lined by ependyma which extends throughout the length of the spinal cord. It represents the cavity of the tubular nervous system of the embryo, and is partially obliterated in the adult. **Cerebrospinal canal.** The space within which the brain and spinal cord are contained. **Canal of the cervix [canalis cervicis uteri (NA)], Cervical canal, Cervico-uterine canal.** The canal of the cervix of the uterus, between the internal and external os. It is spindle-shaped and widest in the middle. The mucous membrane is thrown into an anterior and a posterior longitudinal fold from which numerous minor folds run obliquely [plicae palmatae (NA)]. **Cochlear canal.** The duct of the cochlea, or the spiral canal [canalis spiralis cochleae (NA)] in which it lies. **Condylar canal, anterior [canalis hypoglossi (NA)].** A canal above the condyle of the occipital bone, transmitting the hypoglossal nerve. **Condylar canal, posterior [canalis condylaris (NA)].** A canal sometimes present above the posterior part of the occipital condyle, transmitting an emissary vein. **Craniopharyngeal canal.** The transient canal through the developing sphenoid bone occupied by the stalk connecting the anterior lobe of the pituitary with the root of the buccal cavity. **Craniovertebral canal.** The cavity of the cranium and the canal under the neural arches of the vertebrae, which contain the brain, spinal cord, meninges, etc. **Crural canal.** Femoral canal (see below). **Cystic canal.** The cystic duct. *See* DUCT. **Deferent canal.** The vas deferens. **Dental canal, inferior.** The mandibular canal (see below). **Dental canals, superior [canales alveolares (NA)].** Small canals in the maxillary bone which transmit nerves and vessels to the molar and premolar teeth; they may be divided into anterior and posterior. **Dentinal canals.** Dental canaliculi. *See* CANALICULUS. **Descending palatine canals.** Palatine canals (see below). **Digestive canal.** Alimentary canal (see above). **Diploetic canal [canalis diploicus (NA)].** A channel in the diploë for a diploic vein. **Drainage canal.** An artifical channel made for the drainage of a wound or abscess. **Ejaculatory canal.** The ejaculatory duct. *See* DUCT. **Canal of the epididymis [ductus epididymidis (NA)].** The canal into which open the efferent ductules of the testis; it continues as the vas deferens. **Ethmoidal canals.** Canals between the frontal bone and the labyrinth of the ethmoid which open into the medial wall of the orbit and transmit anterior and posterior ethmoidal nerves and arteries. **Eustachian canal.** The canal of the pharyngotympanic tube (see below). **Canal for the facial nerve [canalis facialis (NA)].** The canal in the petrous part of the temporal bone through which passes the facial nerve. The canal has a sharp bend [geniculum canalis facialis (NA)] corresponding to the position of the genu (geniculum) of the facial nerve. **Femoral canal [canalis femoralis (NA)].** The part of the femoral sheath medial to the femoral vein; it usually contains a lymph gland. **Flexor canal.** The carpal tunnel, transmitting the long flexor tendons and the mèdian nerve from the forearm to the hand. **Gastric canals [canales ventriculi (NA)].** Longitudinal furrows between folds of the gastric mucosa which lead from the cardiac to the pyloric orifice along the lesser curvature. **Gubernacular canals.** Small canals in the maxilla and mandible present immediately behind the milk incisor and canine teeth; they transmit the gubernacula of the permanent teeth. **Haemal canal.** The canal formed by the series of haemal arches on the ventral aspects of the bodies of vertebrae in some animals. **Haversian canals.** The fine canals in bone which transmit blood vessels and are surrounded by concentric lamellae of bone. **Hyaloid canal [canalis hyaloideus (NA)].** A canal passing through the vitreous body of the eye from the optic disc to the posterior surface of the lens; the hyaloid artery passes through it in the embryo. **Hypoglossal canal.** The anterior condylar canal (see above). **Incisive canals [canales incisivi (NA)].** 1. Of the maxilla: the canals which pierce the hard palate and transmit the terminal branches of the long sphenopalatine nerve and the greater palatine arteries. 2. Of the mandible; the branch of the mandibular canal which carries nerves to the incisor teeth. **Incisor canal.** The incisive canal of the mandible (see preceding). **Infra-orbital canal [canalis infra-orbitalis (NA)].**

The bony canal in the floor of the orbit, transmitting the infra-orbital nerve and artery. **Inguinal canal [canalis inguinalis (NA)].** The canal which transmits the spermatic cord in the male from the deep to the superficial inguinal ring, lying immediately above the medial part of the inguinal ligament. In the female it transmits the round ligament of the uterus. **Innominate canal.** A canal near the foramen spinosum of the sphenoid, for the lesser superficial petrosal nerve. **Intestinal canal.** The part of the alimentary canal between the pyloric end of the stomach and the anus. **Intracytoplasmic canal.** One of a system of fine canals in the cytoplasm of many cells. **Lacrimal canal.** Nasolacrimal canal (see below). **Longitudinal canals of the modiolus [canales longitudinales modioli (NA)].** Many small canals which pierce the modiolus and transmit filaments of the cochlear nerve. **Malar canal.** A canal in the zygomatic (malar) bone for the zygomaticotemporal branch of the maxillary nerve. **Mandibular canal [canalis mandibulae (NA)].** A canal in the mandible, transmitting the inferior dental nerve. **Medullary canal.** The medullary or marrow cavity of a long bone. **Membranous semicircular canals.** The semicircular ducts of the membranous labyrinth of the ear. **Musculotubal canal [canalis musculotubarius (NA)].** A canal in the petrous part of the temporal bone. It carries the pharyngotympanic tube and the tensor tympani muscle separated by a septum [septum canalis musculotubarii (NA)]. **Nasolacrimal canal [canalis nasolacrimalis (NA)].** The canal in the lateral wall of the nasal cavity which transmits the nasolacrimal duct. **Neural canal.** Vertebral canal (see below); the term may also be used for the cavity of the tubular central nervous system of the embryo. **Neurenteric canal.** The archenteric canal (see above). **Notochordal canal.** The archenteric canal (see above). **Nutrient canal [canalis nutricius (NA)].** The canal through which passes the artery supplying the marrow of a bone. **Obstetric canal.** The birth canal (see above). **Obturator canal [canalis obturatorius (NA)].** A groove in the under-surface of the superior ramus of the pubis through which pass the obturator vessels and nerves. **Omphalomesenteric canal.** The vitello-intestinal duct, connecting the yolk sac with the intestine in the embryo. **Optic canal.** Optic foramen. *See* FORAMEN. **Palatine canals, greater, or anterior [canales palatini majores (NA)].** Canals in the lateral wall of the nasal cavity which transmit the greater palatine nerves and arteries; they lie between the palatine bone and the maxilla. **Palatine canals, lesser, or posterior [canales palatini minores (NA)].** Small branches from the greater palatine canals which transmit the lesser palatine vessels and nerves. **Palatinovaginal canal [canalis palatovaginalis (NA)].** The canal between the vaginal process of the medial pterygoid plate and the palate bone; it transmits the pharyngeal artery and nerve. **Parturient canal.** The birth canal (see above). **Pelvic canal.** The canal enclosed by the two hip bones and the sacrum. **Pharyngeal canal.** The palatinovaginal canal (see above). **Canal of the pharyngotympanic tube [semicanalis tubae auditivae (NA)].** A canal in the petrous part of the temporal bone, running from the middle-ear cleft forward and inward to the anterior border. **Pleuroperitoneal canal.** The temporary communication between the embryonic pleural and peritoneal cavities. **Portal canal.** The spaces in the perilobular connective tissue of the liver which transmit branches of the portal vein, hepatic artery and bile duct. **Pterygoid canal [canalis pterygoideus (NA)].** A canal piercing the root of the pterygoid process of the sphenoid and transmitting the pterygoid nerve and artery. **Pterygopalatine canal.** Palatine canal, greater (see above). **Pudendal canal [canalis pudendalis (NA)].** The fibrous sheath enclosing the internal pudendal artery, the perineal nerve and the dorsal nerve of the penis or clitoris in the lateral wall of the ischiorectal fossa. **Pulp canal.** Root canal of a tooth (see below). **Pyloric canal [canalis pyloricus (NA)].** The lumen of the pyloric part of the stomach. **Root canal of a tooth [canalis radicis dentis (NA)].** The canal in the root of a tooth through which nerves and blood vessels pass to the pulp cavity. **Sacculocochlear canal.** The ductus reuniens. **Sacculo-utricular canal.** The utriculosaccular duct. *See* DUCT. **Sacral canal [canalis sacralis (NA)].** The continuation of the vertebral canal into the sacrum. **Semicircular canals [canales semicirculares ossei (NA)].** The semicircular canals, superior, posterior and lateral (see following). **Semicircular canals, superior, posterior and lateral [canales semicircularis, anterior, posterior et lateralis (NA)].** Canals of the bony labyrinth which enclose the semicircular ducts of the membranous labyrinth. **Spermatic canal.** The male inguinal canal (see above). **Sphenopalatine canal.** Palatine canal, greater (see above). **Spinal canal.** Vertebral canal (see below). **Spiral canal of the cochlea [canalis spiralis cochleae (NA)].** *See* COCHLEAR CANAL (above). **Spiral canal of the modiolus [canalis spiralis modioli (NA)].** The spiral made up by the canals in the modiolus, which transmit filaments of the cochlear nerve; the term may also be applied to the cochlear duct, or to the spiral cavity of the petrous bone which contains the cochlear duct. **Subsartorial canal [canalis adductorius (NA)].** The space in the thigh beneath the sartorius muscle and between the vastus medialis and the adductor muscles, through which the femoral artery and other structures pass. **Supra-orbital canal.** The supra-orbital foramen. *See* FORAMEN. **Temporomalar canal.** Malar canal (see above). **Canal for the tensor tympani [semi-canalis musculus tensoris tympani (NA)].** A small canal in the anterior border of the petrous temporal bone, separated from the pharyngotympanic tube below by a thin bony plate. **Tubotympanal canal.** The first pharyngeal pouch of the embryo which becomes the eustachian tube and middle-ear cavity. **Urinary canal.** A primitive urinary passage. **Urogenital canal.** The urogenital sinus. *See* SINUS. **Uterovaginal canal.** The channel formed by the fused lower ends of the muellerian ducts of the embryo. **Utriculosaccular canal.** The utriculosaccular duct. *See* DUCT. **Vaginal canal.** The cavity of the vagina which leads from the vulva to the external os of the uterus. **Vertebral canal [canalis vertebralis (NA)].** The canal formed anterior to the neural arches and posterior to the bodies of the vertebrae, which contains the spinal cord, meninges, etc. **Vidian canal.** Pterygoid canal (see above). **Vomerovaginal canal [canalis vomerovaginalis (NA)].** A small vascular canal between the vaginal process of the sphenoid and the ala of the vomer. **Wolffian canal.** The wolffian duct; the duct of the mesonephros. **Zygomatic canal, Zygomaticotemporal canal.** Malar canal (see above). [L *canalis* channel.]

See also: ALCOCK, ARANZIO, ARNOLD (F.), BERNARD (C.), BICHAT, BOCHDALEK, BOETTCHER, BRAUN (M. G. C. C.), BRAUNE, BRESCHET, CIVININI, CLOQUET (J. G.), CORTI, COTUGNO (COTUNNIUS), CUVIER, DORELLO, DUPUYTREN, EUSTACHIO, FALLOPIUS, FERREIN, FONTANA (F.), GARTNER, GOLGI, GUIDI, HANNOVER, HAVERS, HENLE, HENSEN, HERING (K. E. K.), HIRSCHFELD (I.), HIS (W. SNR.), HOLMGREN (E. A.), HOVIUS, HOYER, HUGUIER, HUNTER (J.), HUSCHKE, JACOBSON (L. L.), KOVALEVSKI, KUPFFER, LANDZERT, LAUTH (E. A.), LEUCKART, LOEWENBERG, MUELLER (J.), NUCK, PETIT (F. P.), RECKLINGHAUSEN, REICHERT (K. B.), REISSNER, RICHET, RIVINUS, ROSENTHAL (I.), SAVIOTTI, SANTORINI, SCHLEMM, STENSEN (STENO), STILLING, SUCQUET, THEILE, TOURTUAL, VOLKMANN (A. W.), WALTHER, WIRSUNG.

canalicular (kan·al·ik·ew·lar). Pertaining to a canaliculus.

canaliculization (kan·al·ik·ew·il·za'·shun). The formation, in osseous and other tissue, of canaliculi.

canaliculus [NA] (kan·al·ik·ew·lus). A small canal; generally applied to the very fine canals in bone which contain fine processes of bone cells or osteocytes. **Bile canaliculi.** Minute bile capillaries between the liver cells. **Caroticotympanic canaliculi [canaliculi caroticotympanici (NA)].** Minute passages in the petrous bone which transmit tympanic branches of the internal carotid artery and sympathetic nerves. **Canaliculus for the chorda tympani, anterior [canaliculus chordae tympani (NA)].** A canal in the medial end of the squamotympanic fissure. **Canaliculus for the chorda tympani, posterior.** The passage through the petrous bone for the part of the chorda tympani from its origin from the facial nerve to the posterior border of the tympanic membrane. **Cochlear canaliculus [canaliculus cochleae (NA)].** A narrow canal in the petrous bone which conducts a small vein from the cochlea to the inferior petrosal sinus. Its external opening [apertura externa canaliculi cochleae (NA)] lies at the apex of the notch for the glossopharyngeal nerve. **Dental canaliculi [canaliculi dentales (NA)].** Channels in the dentine of the tooth, believed by some to contain prolongations of the odontoblasts. They communicate with the pulp cavity. **Haversian canaliculus.** One of the enormous number of fine canals containing the processes of the bone corpuscles. **Canaliculus innominatus.** Innominate canal. *See* CANAL. **Lacrimal canaliculi [canaliculi lacrimales (NA)].** The ducts which lead from the lacrimal punctae to the lacrimal sac. **Mastoid canaliculus [canaliculus mastoideus (NA)].** A small canal in the temporal bone for the auricular branch of the vagus. **Pseudobile canaliculi.** Duct-like structures which are found in the portal spaces of the liver during hepatic regeneration. **Canaliculus for the tympanic nerve [canaliculus tympanicus (NA)].** A small canal in the temporal bone for the tympanic branch of the glossopharyngeal nerve. **Canaliculus vasculosus.** An obsolete term for a haversian canal. [L dim. of *canalis* channel.]

canaliculus, vein of the cochlear [vena canaliculi cochleae (NA)]. A small vein accompanying the aqueduct of the cochlea, joining the internal jugular vein.

canaline (kan·al·een). $NH_2OCH_2CH_2CH(NH_2)COOH$, a diamino-monocarboxylic acid. It is not an essential constituent of the diet and is formed in the body by the action of the liver enzyme canavanase on canavanine.

canalization (kan·al·i·za′·shun). 1. The process of formation of either natural or pathological channels. 2. The draining of wounds by channels surgically made in the tissues instead of by the insertion of tubes. 3. The making of new paths in the central nervous system by the constant passage of nerve impulses. 4. The development of new channels, such as blood vessels in recently formed tissue, as for instance in a blood clot or in granulation tissue. [L *canalis* channel.]

canavallin (kan·av·al·in). A globulin occurring in jack beans, the seeds of species of *Canavalia.*

canavanase (kan·av·an·aze). A liver enzyme which activates the conversion of canavanine into canaline.

canavanine (kan·av·an·een). $NH_2C(NH)NHOCH_2CH_2CH(NH_2)COOH$, an amino acid originally isolated from the jack bean, and possibly taking part in the hepatic synthesis of urea.

cancellate, cancellated (kan·sel·ate, kan·sel·a·ted). Having a reticular structure; term applied to bone. [L *cancellare* to make like a lattice.]

cancellous (kan·sel·us). Being porous or spongy or reticular in structure, as in the bones. [see foll.]

cancellus (kan·sel·us). The lattice-like structure of cancellous bone. [L lattice.]

cancer (kan·ser). 1. A malignant tumour arising from epithelial cells. 2. More loosely, any malignant growth. **Acinous cancer.** Medullary carcinoma. *See* CARCINOMA. **Acute cancer.** Rapidly growing medullary carcinoma. **Adenoid cancer.** A cancer which retains a glandular pattern as it grows. **Alveolar cancer.** A cancer which retains an alveolar pattern as it grows. **Aniline cancer.** Cancer of the urinary bladder in aniline workers. **Cancer anthracinus.** A cancer which begins as a black speck and develops into a mass like a mulberry; probably a form of melanotic cancer. **Apinoid cancer.** A scirrhous cancer with a sharply defined cut surface. **Apiois cancer.** A scirrhous cancer which resembles an unripe pear on section. **Cancer aquaticus.** Gangrenous stomatitis. *See* STOMATITIS. **Areolar cancer.** Colloid cancer (see below). **Cancer atrophicans.** Scirrhous cancer (see below). **Betel cancer.** Oral carcinoma induced by betel chewing. **Black cancer.** Melanotic cancer (see below). **Branchiogenous cancer.** Cancer arising in a branchial cleft. **Branchogenic cancer.** A cancer arising from the living cells (or their derivatives) of the bronchi. **Buyo cancer.** Betel cancer (see above). **Cavernous cancer.** Colloid carcinoma with large spaces formed by the fusion of colloid clefts. **Cellular cancer.** Medullary carcinoma. *See* CARCINOMA. **Cerebriform cancer.** Medullary cancer (see below). **Chimney-sweeps' cancer.** Epithelioma of the scrotum or thighs in chimney-sweeps. **Chondroid cancer.** Carcinoma resembling cartilage, or containing cartilage. **Clay-pipe cancer.** Epithelioma of the lip or mouth, occurring in smokers. **Colloid cancer.** Carcinoma which produces a large amount of mucus. **Comedo cancer.** A form of cancer of the breast in which, on cutting the tumour, plugs of cancer cells can be seen distending the ducts. **Contact cancer.** The origin of a second cancer in tissue adjacent to a primary cancer. **Corset cancer.** Carcinoma of the liver arising in the furrow resulting from pressure exerted by a corset. **Cancer en cuirasse.** A scirrhous carcinoma of the breast, producing great distortion as its fibrous tissue contracts. **Cystic cancer.** A variety of adenocarcinoma. **Dendritic cancer.** Papillary carcinoma. *See* CARCINOMA. **Dermoid cancer.** A malignant teratoma. **Duct cancer.** Cancer arising in ducts of glands, especially of the breast. **Dye-workers' cancer.** Aniline cancer (see above). **Eburneous cancer.** Sclerodermia. **Embolic cancer.** Secondary carcinoma spreading by embolism. **Encephaloid cancer.** Medullary cancer (see below). **Endothelial cancer.** Endothelioma. **Epidermal cancer, Epithelial cancer.** Epithelioma. **Fasciculated cancer.** Fusocellular sarcoma. *See* SARCOMA. **Fungous cancer.** A descriptive term applied to any form of tumour which resembles a mushroom. **Glandular cancer.** Adenocarcinoma. **Green cancer.** Chloroma. **Hard cancer.** Scirrhous cancer; one containing large amounts of connective tissue. **Jacket cancer.** Cancer which infiltrates extensively the superficial tissue. **Kang cancer, Kangri cancer.** Localized epithelioma developing in scars of burns on the abdomen or thighs, induced by carrying fire-bowls under the clothes in Kashmir. **Lung cancer.** Most often bronchogenic; there is statistical evidence that one of the causes is smoking. **Medullary cancer.** A soft, rapidly-growing cancer that often looks like a piece of brain tissue. **Melanotic cancer.** A pigmented cancer which forms melanin. **Mule-spinners' cancer.** Cancer arising in those parts of the body contaminated with oil during cotton spinning. **Osteolytic cancer.** A cancer which destroys the bone that it has invaded. **Osteoplastic cancer.** A cancer that forms new bony tissue in its substance by metaplasia. **Paraffin cancer.** Cancer due to certain paraffins. **Pitch-workers' cancer.** Cancer due to coal-tar products. **Primary cancer.** Cancer at the primary site, in contrast to metastatic cancer. **Radiologists' cancer.** X-ray cancer (see below). **Retrograde cancer.** A cancer which atrophies and is replaced by fibrous tissue. **Rodent cancer.** A variety of cancer of the skin which is slow-growing and sensitive to x-rays. **Roentgenologists' cancer.** X-ray cancer (see below). **Scirrhous cancer.** A hard cancer rich in fibrous tissue. **Shale-workers' cancer.** A squamous-celled epithelioma of the skin caused by exposure of hands and scrotum to crude shale oil. **Smokers' cancer.** 1. Clay-pipe cancer (see above). 2. Bronchogenic cancer caused by smoking. **Soft cancer.** Medullary carcinoma. *See* CARCINOMA. **Solanoid cancer.** Cancer which resembles a potato on section. **Soot cancer.** Chimney-sweeps' cancer (see above). **Spider cancer.** Naevus. **Spiroptera cancer.** A gastric cancer in rats caused by a nematode worm transmitted by cockroaches. **Tar cancer.** Squamous-celled epithelioma of the skin resulting from continued exposure to tar. **Tar-oil cancer.** Squamous-celled epithelioma of the skin resulting from continued exposure to tar oil. **Tubular cancer.** Duct cancer (see above). **Villous duct cancer.** Papilloma of ducts. **Water cancer.** Gangrenous stomatitis. *See* STOMATITIS. **Withering cancer.** Retrograde cancer (see above). **X-ray cancer.** Squamous-celled epithelioma of the skin resulting from repeated exposure to x-rays. [L crab.]

See also: ARAN, LOBSTEIN.

canceration (kan·ser·a·shun). Malignant degeneration. [see prec.]

cancerigenic (kan·ser·e·jen′·ik). Carcinogenic. [cancer, Gk *genein* to produce.]

cancerism (kan·ser·izm). The constitution which lends itself to the development of carcinoma. [cancer.]

cancerocidal (kan·ser·o·si′·dal). Having lethal effect on cancer cells. [cancer, L *caedere* to kill.]

canceroderm (kan·ser·o·derm). Naevus-like patches which may be present on the thorax and abdomen of certain persons; also referred to as De Morgan's spots. The relationship to carcinoma is very much in doubt. [cancer, Gk *derma* skin.]

cancerogenic (**kan**·ser·o·**jen'**·ik). Carcinogenic. [cancer, Gk *genein* to produce.]

cancerology (kan·ser·**ol**·o·je). The science and the study of cancer. [cancer, Gk *logos* science.]

cancerophobia (**kan**·ser·o·**fo'**·be·ah). Carcinomatophobia. [cancer, phobia.]

cancerous (**kan**·ser·us). Carcinomatous. [cancer.]

cancerphobia (kan·ser·**fo**·be·ah). Carcinomatophobia. [cancer, phobia.]

cancriform (**kang**·kre·form). Having resemblance to a carcinoma. [cancer, form.]

cancrine (**kang**·kreen). Carcinomatous. [cancer.]

cancrocirrhosis (**kang**·kro·sir·**o'**·sis). Carcinoma of the lung associated with pulmonary cirrhosis. [cancer, cirrhosis.]

cancroid (**kang**·kroid). 1. Carcinomatoid. 2. Epithelioma. 3. A neoplasm of a mild degree of malignancy. 4. A kind of keloid. **Dermic cancroid.** Epithelioma involving the whole skin. **Follicular cancroid.** Epithelioma originating in the glands of the skin or the hair follicles. **Papillary cancroid.** Epithelioma involving the papillae of the corium and eventually the other layers of the skin. [cancer, Gk *eidos* form.]

cancrology (kang·**krol**·o·je). The science and the study of cancer. [cancer, Gk *logos* science.]

cancrum (**kang**·krum). Canker. **Cancrum nasi.** The gangrenous rhinitis observed in children. **Cancrum oris.** Gangrenous stomatitis. *See* STOMATITIS. **Cancrum pudendi.** Ulceration of the pudenda. [L *cancer* crab.]

candela (kan·**de**·lah). 1. The unit of luminous intensity; defined as the luminous intensity, in the perpendicular direction, of a surface of 1/600 000 square metres of a black body at the temperature of freezing platinum under a pressure of 101 325 pascals (one atmosphere). 2. A bougie made of wax. 3. A candle containing medicaments, intended to be used in fumigation. [L light.]

Candicidin (kan·de·**si**·din). BP Commission approved name for a mixture of heptaenes with antifungal activity produced by *Streptomyces griseus* and other *Streptomyces* species.

Candida (**kan**·did·ah). A genus of yeast-like fungi, species of which cause candidiasis (candidosis). *Candida albicans* is the most frequent aetiological agent of candidiasis but numerous other *Candida* species have now been implicated as pathogens in man, especially in compromised individuals. [L *candidus* white.]

candidiasis (kan·did·**i**·as·is). An acute or chronic, superficial or disseminated mycosis due to species of *Candida*, usually *Candida albicans.* Clinical forms are variable: mucous membranes—oral thrush, perlèche, vulvovaginitis; cutaneous—onychia, paronychia, intertrigo, generalized cutaneous candidiasis; bronchopulmonary; pulmonary; endocarditis. [*Candida*, Gk *-osis* condition.]

candidid (**kan**·did·id). An allergic skin manifestation in a subject infected cutaneously with *Candida.*

candidosis (kan·did·**o**·sis). Candidiasis. [*Candida*, Gk *-osis* condition.]

candiru (kan·de·**roo**). A small catfish, *Vandellia cirrhosa*, 6 cm long, 3-4 mm wide, native of parts of the Amazon. It penetrates the urethra of male bathers and, reaching the bladder, may cause death. [Port. from S. American Indian *canderu.*]

candle (**kan**·dl). A unit employed in the comparison of intensities of light. **Foot candle.** The amount of light received by a surface 1 ft^2 in area placed 1 ft from a standard candle. **International candle.** A photometric unit of luminous intensity decided on by international agreement in 1909; 1/10 the light of the standard pentane lamp. **Metre candle.** The intensity of illumination on a surface placed at right angles to the light falling on it from 1 international candle placed at 1 m distance. **Standard candle.** A candle burning at the rate of 120 grains of spermaceti per hour. [L *candela* light.]

canella (kan·**el**·ah). Canella bark (white or wild cinnamon bark), obtained from *Canella alba* Murray (family Canellaceae), indigenous to the West Indies and Florida. It contains volatile oil and a bitter principle. [dim. of L *canna* reed.]

caneotica (ka·ne·**ot**·ik·ah). A type of cutaneous leishmaniasis endemic in Crete. [*Canea*, in the island of Crete.]

canescent (kan·**es**·ent). Greyish; becoming grey or whitish. [L *canus* grey.]

caniculoplasty (kan·**ik**·ew·lo·**plas'**·te). An operation for the repair, enlargement or re-formation of the lacrimal canaliculus. [canaliculus, Gk *plassein* to mould.]

canine (**ka**·nine). 1. Pertaining to or of the nature of a dog. 2. The pointed tooth next to the incisors. *See* TOOTH. **Incisiform canines.** Canine teeth that are flattened, such as those of ruminants. [L *canis* dog.]

caniniform (ka·**nin**·e·form). Resembling or having the form of a typical canine tooth.

caninus (ka·**ni**·nus). The levator anguli oris muscle. [L canine.]

canities (kan·**ish**·e·eez). Greying or whitening of the hair. **Canities unguium.** White spots or streaks on the nails. [L.]

canker (**kang**·ker). 1. A corroding or sloughing ulcer. 2. Aphthous stomatitis. *See* STOMATITIS. [L *cancer* crab.]

Canna (**kan**·ah). A genus of plants of the family Cannaceae. The root of *Canna edulis* Edwards yields canna starch (Queensland arrowroot, tous-les-mois). [L a reed.]

cannabane (**kan**·ab·ane). Cannabene hydride, $C_{18}H_{22}$, a hydrocarbon obtained from Indian hemp, a variety of *Cannabis sativa.*

cannabene (**kan**·ab·een). $C_{18}H_{20}$, a hydrocarbon occurring in Indian hemp. [*Cannabis indica.*]

cannabine (**kan**·ab·een). An alkaloid from *Cannabis indica* (Indian hemp). It causes apparent stimulation of the motor areas and lower centres of the brain by depression of the higher centres. At one time it was used as a hypnotic in medicine.

cannabinine (kan·**ab**·in·een). A poisonous alkaloid found in the essential oil of Indian hemp. [*Cannabis indica.*]

cannabinol (kan·**ab**·in·ol). $C_{21}H_{30}O_2$. A red oil or resin from Indian hemp (*Cannabis indica*). It produces a state of euphoria, but has no rational use in medicine.

Cannabis BPC 1949 (**kan**·ab·is). Indian hemp, *Cannabis indica*, the dried flowering and fruiting tops of the female plants of *Cannabis sativa* Linn. (family Cannabinaceae). The plant is indigenous to central and western Asia and is cultivated in tropical India, Africa and North America. In temperate countries it does not produce the narcotic resin, but is grown specially for hemp fibre and hemp seed. Guaza and ganjah are names given to forms of the drug produced in India. Bhang, churrus and hashish are products of *Cannabis sativa* used by orientals for smoking and the preparation of electuaries. Dagga is the material used by addicts in South Africa, whilst marihuana is the Mexican name for the drug. Cannabis contains a soft resin (cannabinone), from which cannabinol has been isolated. The drug acts on the central nervous system, often producing pleasurable excitement, hallucinations, distortion of the sense of time and space, followed by lethargy and sleep. It has been used as a sedative in nervous disorders and spasmodic coughs, but is unreliable. [Gk *kannabis* hemp.]

cannabism (**kan**·ab·izm). Hashish intoxication. [*Cannabis indica.*]

cannabist (**kan**·ab·ist). One addicted to the taking of *Cannabis indica.*

cannibalism (**kan**·ib·al·izm). The practice of eating one's own kind. [Carib. *calina.*]

Cannizzaro, Stanislao (b. 1826). Rome chemist.

Cannizzaro's reaction. A reaction which is given by aromatic and certain aliphatic aldehydes when treated with dilute alkali. Two molecules of the aldehyde interact so that one is reduced to the alcohol and the other oxidized to the carboxylic acid: $2RCHO + H_2O \rightarrow RCH_2OH + RCOOH$. This reaction also occurs when aldehydes are brought into contact with a living tissue such as the liver, or with certain bacteria.

Cannon, Walter Bradford (b. 1871). Boston physiologist.

Cannon's ring. A ring of tonic contraction that may be felt in the right half of the transverse colon.

Cannon's theory. The emergency theory of the emotions which postulates that the characteristic arousal of the sympathetic nervous system rapidly mobilizes visceral and muscular energy to prepare the individual for fight or flight according to his conscious evaluation of the situation. The latter *Cannon–Bard* version stresses the role of the *hypothalamus* and the *limbic system* in activating both cortical and visceral processes. (*See also* JAMES-LANGE THEORY.)

cannon (kan·on). **Radium cannon.** A synonym for an applicator in teleradium therapy. [Fr. *canon*.]

cannula (**kan**·ew·lah). A glass or metal tube, or a blunt needle, used to effect a communication between a body cavity and the exterior. It may be inserted by open operation or by direct puncture, the cannula being then threaded for insertion over a sharp trocar. It is used *(a)* for the withdrawal of body fluids, e.g. blood, or urine, or cerebrospinal, ascitic, pleural or hydrocele fluid; *(b)* for the withdrawal of gas, e.g. air from a pneumothorax; *(c)* for the removal of a core of tissue for microscopic examination; *(d)* for the introduction of fluid, e.g. blood transfusion, or subcutaneous saline. **Aditus cannula.** A cannula for evacuation and irrigation of the middle ear from the mastoid antrum in mastoidectomy. **Ascites cannula.** A cannula for the withdrawal of fluid from the ascitic abdomen. **Blood-transfusion cannula.** A cannula for the introduction of blood into a vein. **Cyst cannula.** A cannula for the evacuation of an ovarian cyst too large to deliver through a laparotomy wound. **Epistaxis cannula.** A cannula for packing the posterior nares. **Evacuation cannula.** A cannula for flushing out material from a cavity, e.g. stone fragments after litholapaxy. **Exploring cannula.** One introduced in a solid organ to seek an abscess, or to locate pus or other fluid in a body cavity. **Infusion (intravenous) cannula.** One used to introduce saline or other fluids into a vein. **Irrigation cannula.** Perfusion cannula (see below). **Lacrimal cannula.** One for the irrigation of the lacrimal sac. **Laryngotomy cannula.** An intubation tube used after laryngotomy. **Perfusion cannula.** A double cannula used in the irrigation of a body cavity. **Sinus cannula.** A cannula for the evacuation and irrigation of frontal or sphenoidal sinus by way of the nasal cavity. **Tracheotomy cannula.** An intubation tube introduced after tracheotomy. **Transfusion cannula.** Blood-transfusion cannula (see above). **Venoclysis cannula.** A cannula for the introduction of saline or other fluid into a vein. **Ventricular cannula.** A cannula used through a trephine opening, or at operation, to evacuate fluid from the ventricle of the brain, or to introduce air for ventriculography. [L a small reed.]

See also: BAILEY (H.), BELLOCQ, CALVÉ, CANTLIE, COLT, HAHN, KIDD, SOUTHEY, TRENDELENBURG, WELLS (T. S.).

cannular (**kan**·ew·lar). Like a cannula in shape; tubular.

cannulate, cannulated (**kan**·ew·late, **kan**·ew·la·ted). Term descriptive of structures that have a passage. [L *cannula* a small reed.]

cannulation (kan·ew·**la**·shun). Cannulization.

cannulization (**kan**·ew·li·**za**′·shun). The insertion of a cannula.

Canny Ryall, Edward (b. 1865). London urologist.

Canny Ryall syringe. Urethral syringe. *See* SYRINGE.

Cantani test. A little-used serological test for syphilis.

Cantelli's sign. An unusual type of ocular palsy complicating diphtheria, and characterized by sluggish movements of the eyeballs and eyelids. As the head is raised the eyes are lowered, and vice versa.

canthal (**kan**·thal). Relating to a canthus of the eye.

cantharene (**kan**·thar·een). 1. Dihydro-orthoxylene, $C_6H_6(CH_3)_2$, a reduction product of *o*-xylene. 2. $C_{10}H_{12}O_3I_2$, a di-iodo derivative of cantharidin.

canthariasis (kan·thar·**i**·as·is). Any disease arising from the presence in the body of the larvae of beetles or other coleoptera. [Gk *kantharis* beetle.]

cantharidal (kan·**thar**·id·al). Containing or relating to cantharides.

cantharidate (kan·**thar**·id·ate). Any salt of cantharidic acid.

cantharidated (kan·**thar**·id·a·ted). Containing cantharides.

cantharides (kan·**thar**·id·eez). Dried Spanish flies *Lytta (Cantharis) vesicatoria;* the body of the fly contains a white crystalline substance, cantharidin, which is a vesicant. Cantharides is used as a counter-irritant in the form of a plaster, and is occasionally incorporated in small quantities in hair lotions to stimulate circulation in the scalp. When given by mouth it is excreted via the kidney unchanged, setting up irritation of the genito-urinary tract and acting as an aphrodisiac. Its use is liable to cause nephritis. [Gk *kantharis* beetle.]

cantharidic (kan·thar·**id**·ik). Relating to or obtained from cantharides.

cantharidin (kan·**thar**·id·in). Cantharidinum BPC 1949, $C_{10}H_{12}O_4$. The lactose of cantharidic acid and the active constituent of cantharides, the dried insects *Lytta (Cantharis) vesicatoria.* It is a white crystalline substance, very slightly soluble in water, with an irritant action on the skin and mucous membranes. After absorption, it is excreted by the kidneys, which may suffer damage, and the bladder and urethra may also be irritated causing strangury and priapism. It has been used as an aphrodisiac and was formerly employed as a counter-irritant.

cantharidism (kan·**thar**·id·izm). A toxic state caused by poisoning with cantharidin. **External cantharidism.** The condition resulting from absorption through the skin of toxins contained in the blister produced by local application of cantharides.

Cantharis BPC 1949 (**kan**·thar·is). Cantharides, Spanish fly, the dried beetle *Lytta (Cantharis) vesicatoria* Latr. (Order Coleoptera, family Meloidae). It contains cantharidin, a powerful rubefacient and vesicant. In medicine, cantharis has been largely replaced by cantharidin, which is used in plasters and liquors for its rubefacient properties. [Gk *kantharis* beetle.]

canthectomy (kan·**thek**·to·me). The removal by surgical methods of a canthus. [canthus, Gk *ektome* a cutting out.]

canthitis (kan·**thi**·tis). Inflammation affecting one canthus or several. [canthus, Gk *-itis* inflammation.]

cantholysis (kan·**thol**·is·is). The surgical procedure of cutting through one of the canthi or a palpebral ligament. [canthus, Gk *lysis* a loosing.]

canthomeatal (**kan**·tho·me·**a**′·tal). Pertaining to the canthus of the eye and the external auditory meatus.

canthoplastic (**kan**·tho·plas·tik). Referring to canthoplasty.

canthoplasty (**kan**·tho·plas·te). 1. Plastic surgery as applied to the palpebral fissure. 2. Incision of the lateral angle of the palpebral fissure in order to lengthen the latter. 3. Reparative surgery of a defective canthus. **Provisional canthoplasty.** In blepharospasm, the carrying out of canthotomy as a means of relief. [canthus, Gk *plassein* to mould.]

canthorrhaphy (kan·**thor**·af·e). The procedure of suturing any one or all of the canthi. [canthus, *raphe* suture.]

canthotomy (kan·**thot**·o·me). Division of the lateral canthus by surgical operation. [canthus, Gk *temnein* to cut.]

canthus (**kan**·thus). The part which forms the angle at each end of the palpebral fissure. **Inner canthus, Nasal canthus.** Forms the medial angle of the eye. **Outer canthus.** Forms the lateral angle of the eye. [Gk *kanthos* the corner of the eye.]

Cantlie, Sir James (b. 1851). London surgeon.

Cantlie's cannula. A slotted cannula designed for drainage of amoebic abscess of the liver, but now used in modified forms, with combinations of side-tubes, valves and taps, for many purposes, e.g. suprapubic cystostomy.

Cantor, Meyer O. (b. 1907). Detroit surgeon.

Cantor tube. A rubber tube with a leading mercury-laden bag to facilitate its passage; it is passed through the pharynx and guided into the small intestine in the relief of ileus, where there is no strangulation.

cantus galli (**kan**·tus **gal**·i). Laryngismus stridulus. [L *cantare* to sing, *gallus* cock.]

canula (**kan**·ew·lah). Cannula.

caoutchouc (**kowt**·chook). Indiarubber. The coagulated juice, or latex, of species of Euphorbiaceae grown in South America, India, Malaysia and elsewhere. It consists of a polymerized hydrocarbon, polyisoprene, $(C_5H_8)_n$, related to the terpenes, in a colloidal solution of protein, resins and mineral salts; it is soluble in chloroform and carbon disulphide, and combines with sulphur to form vulcanized rubber. [S. Amer. *cahuchu.*]

cap (kap). 1. A covering; any organ resembling a covering. 2. In dentistry, a covering for an exposed pulp. **Abduction cap.** An appliance made of leather or canvas to maintain the arm in abduction, in subacromial bursitis. **Cradle cap.** Common, harmless yellow crusting of the scalp in babies. **Duodenal cap.** The shadow cast by radio-opaque material in the first part of the duodenum. **Dutch cap.** A rubber diaphragm attached to a semirigid ring and fitting into the vagina, thereby preventing spermatozoa from reaching the cervical canal. **Enamel cap.** The thin layer of enamel laid down on the surface of dentine during tooth development. **Head cap.** The thin membrane enclosing the nucleus of the spermatozoon, subdivided into anterior and posterior head caps. **Knee cap.** The patella. **Metanephric cap.** Mesoderm of the nephrogenic cord of the embryo which surmounts the upper end of the ureteric bud and develops into the uriniferous tubules. **Metanephrogenic cap.** The mass of nephrogenic tissue which covers the expanded end of the ureteric rudiment in the embryo. **Nuclear cap.** Any crescentic mass of cytoplasm with specified staining properties which is applied to the surface of the nucleus. **Phrygian cap.** A band or constriction in the fundus of the gall bladder due to congenital septum, as seen by cholecystography. **Polar cap.** Specialized cytoplasm at opposite ends of the nucleus, from which the mitotic spindle is derived in some cells. **Pyloric cap.** Duodenal cap (see above). [AS *caeppe.*]

See also: DUMAS, STOPES.

capacitance (kap·**as**·it·ans). Electrostatic capacity. The quantity of electricity absorbed by a capacitor or other body in charging it to a certain potential; measured in farads or microfarads.

capacitator (kap·**as**·it·a·tor). A capacitor; an arrangement of conductors and dielectrics designed to store an electrostatic charge. [see foll.]

capacity (kap·**as**·it·e). 1. The ability to contain or absorb anything; the extent to which this may take place. 2. Volume. 3. Mental ability to learn and understand. 4. Physical ability to do work. **Buffer capacity.** *See* BUFFER. **Cranial capacity.** The volume contained within the cranial cavity; about 1450 ml in European males. **Fast vital capacity.** The rate at which after a maximum inspiration the air in the lungs can be expired. **Haemoglobin oxygen capacity.** A measure of the total amount of oxygen that a specimen of haemoglobin (or blood) can bind. One gramme of haemoglobin, when fully converted to oxyhaemoglobin, will bind 1.36 ml of O_2 at stp. **Heat capacity.** Thermal capacity (see below). **Loading capacity.** The maximum power (expressed in watts) that can be passed through an x-ray tube in a given time. **Oxygen capacity.** The amount of oxygen, expressed in ml per cent, absorbed, e.g. by blood, in the presence of an excess of oxygen; 16–24 ml is the oxygen capacity of blood. **Respiratory capacity.** Vital capacity (see below). **Testamentary capacity.** The capacity, expressed in law terms, to make a will, and depending on the physical and mental fitness of a person to understand the nature of such a document and its contents, and to sign or initial it in the presence of attesting witnesses. **Thermal capacity.** The amount of heat in joules (calories) required to raise the temperature of a body 1°C; the product of the mass of a body in kilograms (grams) and its specific heat. **Timed vital capacity.** The percentage of *predicted* vital capacity which can be expired forcefully in 1, 2 and 3 s after a maximal inspiration. The method differentiates between certain types of pulmonary disorder. **Total lung capacity.** The total maximal air content of the lungs; the vital capacity (see below) plus the residual air and the tidal air. **Vital capacity.** The maximal expiration preceded by a maximal inspiration. [L *capacitas.*]

capeline (kap·el·een). *See* BANDAGE. [Fr. hooded cape, or sunbonnet.]

Capgras, Jean Marie Joseph (b. 1873). French psychiatrist.

Capgras' syndrome. A rare psychiatric phenomenon wherein the patient believes that a person well known to him has been replaced by an identical double.

capiat (ka·pe·at). An instrument with which foreign objects can be removed from a body cavity, e.g. the uterus. [L let it take.]

capillarectasia (kap·**il**·ar·ek·**ta**'·ze·ah). Capillary dilatation. [capillary, *ektasis* a stretching.]

Capillaria (kap·**il**·a·re·ah). A genus of small round nematode worms of which *Capillaria aerophila*, normal to the lungs of cats and dogs, and *Capillaria hepatica*, normal to the liver of rats, have both been recorded in man. **Capillaria philippinensis.** A species, so far confined to the island of Luzon, Philippines, which parasitizes the gut of freshwater fish and shrimps. Heavy infection in man may cause a severe malabsorption syndrome. [L *capillaris* hair-like.]

capillariasis (kap·il·ar·i·as·is). Infection with the nematode *Capillaria.* **Intestinal capillariasis.** Infection of the small intestine with *Capillaria philippinensis.* It presents either symptomatically or as a gross maladsorption syndrome. Monkeys and gerbils can be infected experimentally by instillation of adult larvae or eggs of the nematode into the stomach. *Capillaria philippinensis* is a nematode recently recognized as a frequent human infection in Luzon, Philippines. The larvae may long remain dormant in the gut of certain freshwater fish and are transmitted to man when such fish are eaten raw. [L *capillaris* hair-like.]

Capillariidae (kap·il·a·re·e·dee). A family of nematodes; the genus *Capillaria* is of medical significance. [L *capillaris* hair-like.]

capillarimeter (kap·**il**·ar·**im**'·et·er). An instrument with which the diameter of a capillary vessel can be measured. [capillary, meter.]

capillariomotor (kap·**il**·ar·e·o·**mo**'·tor). A term descriptive of the functional activity of the capillary vessels. [capillary, L *motor* mover.]

capillaritis (kap·**il**·ar·**i**'·tis). A condition of inflammation affecting the capillary vessels. [capillary, Gk *-itis* inflammation.]

capillarity (kap·**il**·ar·it·e). 1. The state of being capillary or hair-like. 2. Capillary attraction; a surface tension effect, as exemplified by the elevation or depression of a liquid at the place at which it comes in contact with a solid, e.g. in capillary tubes. [L *capillaris* hair-like.]

capillaropathy (kap·**il**·ar·**op**'·ath·e). Any disease affecting the capillary vessels. [capillary, Gk *pathos* suffering.]

capillaroscopy (kap·**il**·ar·**os**'·ko·pe). Microscopical examination of the capillary vessels of the skin. [capillary, Gk *skopein* to watch.]

capillary (kap·**il**·ar·e). 1. Relating to a hair. 2. Hair-like. 3. Any one of the hair-like vessels comprising a network between the arterioles and the venules distributed through the body. **Arterial capillary.** A minute vessel which is the termination of an arteriole. **Erythrocytic capillaries, Erythropoietic capillaries.** Thin-walled sinusoids, lined by phagocytic cells, found in blood-forming tissues, e.g. the red bone marrow. **Fenestrated capillary.** A capillary whose endothelium contains small fenestrations. These are usually closed by a thin membrane but in some capillaries they may be true openings. **Lymph capillary.** One of the microscopic branches which constitute the beginnings of the lymph vessels originating in a lymph space. **Secretory capillary.** One of the tiny channels formed when the grooved surface of one gland cell is in apposition to that of another, e.g. bile capillaries of the liver. **Sinusoidal capillary.** A thin-walled vessel of irregular calibre lined by phagocytic cells (littoral histiocytes) and containing blood or lymph; they are present in bone marrow, the liver and lymph glands. **Venous capillary.** A capillary which terminates in a venule. **Capillary vessel.** *See* VESSEL. [L *capillaris* hair-like.]

See also: MEIGS (A. V.).

capilliculture (kap·il·e·kul·tcher). 1. The care of the hair. 2.

Systematic treatment of diseases of the hair or of baldness. [L *capillus* hair, culture.]

capillus (kap·il·us). 1. A hair, or any filament like a hair. 2. A hair's breadth. [L.]

capistration (kap·is·tra·shun). Phimosis; narrowing of the external urethral orifice and tightening of the prepuce, thus inhibiting retraction of the prepuce over the glans penis. A similar condition affects the clitoris. [L *capistrare* to halter.]

capitalis reflexa (kap·it·a·lis re·flex·ah). A recurrent bandage applied as a cap to an amputation stump by means of a single-headed roller bandage. [L of the head, turned back.]

capitate (kap·it·ate). Head-like in shape. [L *caput* head.]

capitate bone [os capitatum (NA)]. The largest of the carpal bones, placed in the distal row opposite the base of the 3rd metacarpal bone.

capitatum (kap·it·a·tum). The capitate bone of the carpus (os magnum). [L having a head.]

capitellum (kap·it·el·um). 1. Any knob-like bony process. 2. The capitulum of the humerus. 3. The bulb of a hair. [L little head.]

capitonnage (kap·it·on·ahzh). The closing of a cyst cavity by suture so that the opposing surfaces of the cavity are approximated. [Fr. padding.]

capitopedal (kap·it·o·ped′·al). 1. Relating to the head and the foot. 2. In biology, placed near or relating to the junction of head and foot. [L *caput* head, *pes* foot.]

capitular (kap·it·ew·lar). Relating to a capitulum.

capitulum [NA] (kap·it·ew·lum). A knob-like eminence or protuberance (the small head) at the end of a bone, associated with an articulation. **Capitulum of the humerus [capitulum humeri (NA)].** The lateral convex surface at the lower end of the humerus, articulating with the head of the radius. [L small head.]
See also: SANTORINI.

Caplan's syndrome. Rheumatoid arthritis associated with nodular fibrosis of the lungs, that has been described in miners; it is distinguishable from massive pulmonary fibrosis that occurs in complicated pneumoconiosis.

capnometry (kap·nom·et·re). The measurement of smoke density. [Gk *kapnos* smoke, meter.]

capnomore (kap·no·more). A rubber solvent obtained from tar oil. [Gk *kapnos* smoke, *moira* part.]

capnophilic (kap·no·fil·ik). Describing bacteria which are stimulated in their growth by carbon dioxide. [Gk *kapnos* smoke, *philein* to love.]

capotement (kap·ote·mahn). The splashing sound heard on auscultation of a dilated stomach. [Fr.]

capping (kap·ing). 1. The operation of placing a medicament in a protective cap over the exposed surface of the pulp of a tooth, in the hope that the pulp will lay down a barrier of secondary dentine and remain vital. 2. A medicament, often calcium hydroxide, which is placed over the exposed surface of the pulp of a tooth. [AS *caeppe.*]

Capps, Joseph Almarin (b. 1872). Chicago physician.
Capps' reflex. Fall of blood pressure, collapse, sweating and pallor, caused by irritation of the pleura; pleural shock.

caprate (kap·rate). A salt of capric acid.

Capreomycin (kap·re·o·mi′·sin). BP Commission approved name for an antibiotic produced by *Streptomyces capreolus.* **Capreomycin Sulphate BP 1973.** An antibiotic produced by the growth of *Streptomyces capreolus* and used in the treatment of infections with *Mycobacterium tuberculosis.* It is administered by intramuscular injection.

caprillic (kap·ril·ik). Goat-like. [L *caper* goat.]

capriloquism, capriloquium (kap·ril·o·kwizm, kap·ril·o·kwe·um). Aegophony; the bleating quality of voice heard on auscultation and characteristic of certain lung conditions, e.g. pleurisy with effusion. [L *caper* goat, *loqui* to speak.]

caprin (kap·rin). Name given to any of the 3 glyceryl caprates which occur in butter, particularly glyceryl tricaprate, $(C_9H_{19}COO)_3C_3H_5$, tricaprin.

caprinate (kap·rin·ate). A caprate

caprizant (kap·riz·ant). A term applied to an irregular leaping or bounding pulse. [L *caper* goat.]

caproate (kap·ro·ate). A salt of caproic acid.

caproin (kap·ro·in). Name given to any of the 3 glyceryl caproates occurring in butter, particularly glyceryl tricaproate, $(C_5H_{11}CO O)_3C_3H_5$, tricaproin.

caprone (kap·rone). Diamyl ketone, $CH_3(CH_2)_4CO(CH_2)_4CH_3$. A volatile oil obtained from butter.

Caproxamine (kap·rox·am·een). BP Commission approved name for 3′-amino-4′-methylhexanophenone-(2-aminoethyl)oxime; an antidepressant agent.

caproyl (kap·ro·il). The monovalent acyl radical $CH_3(CH_2)_4CO-$ from caproic acid.

caproylamine (kap·ro·il·am·een). $CH_3(CH_2)_5NH_2$, a ptomaine which arises during the decomposition of yeast, and fat oils becoming rancid.

capryl (kap·ril). The monovalent acyl radical $C_9H_{19}CO-$ from capric acid.

caprylate (kap·ril·ate). A salt of caprylic acid.

caprylin (kap·ril·in). Name given to any of the 3 glyceryl caprylates occurring in butter, particularly glyceryl tricaprylate, $(C_7H_{15}COO)_3C_3H_5$, tricaprylin.

capsaicin (kap·sa·is·in). $C_{18}H_{27}O_3N$, a crystalline substance obtained from *Capsicum minimum* and responsible for its characteristic pungency.

capsanthin (kap·san·thin). $C_{40}H_{58}O_3$, a carotenoid pigment which forms the colouring matter of capsicum.

capsanthinosis (kap·san·thin·o′·sis). Discoloration of the skin which results from the inclusion of an abnormal amount of paprika in the diet. [capsanthin, Gk *-osis* condition.]

capsicin (kap·sis·in). An oleoresin derived from capsicums. It is used as a counter-irritant or administered internally in dyspepsia.

capsicism (kap·sis·izm). Capsicum addiction.

capsicol (kap·sik·ol). The fixed oil yielded by species of *Capsicum.*

capsicum (kap·sik·um). Cayenne pepper, capsici fructus; consists of the dried ripe fruits of *Capsicum minimum* Roxb. (family Solanaceae). Three varieties of the drug, known commercially as *African chillies,* occur: Tanzania, Malawi and Sierre Leone. It contains the intensely pungent principle, capsaicin, a liquid alkaloid, a fixed oil and a red colouring matter. A tincture of the drug is given as a carminative in dyspepsia and flatulence. Externally, the drug is applied in the form of ointment, plaster, or medicated wool as a counter-irritant (BPC 1959). **Bombay and Natal capsicums.** Fruits derived from *Capsicum annuum* Linn.; they are larger and less pungent than the official capsicum. **Hungarian capsicums.** Paprika; the fruits of a mild variety of *Capsicum annuum* Linn., used as a condiment. [L *capsa* box.]

capsitis (kap·si·tis). An inflammatory condition affecting the capsule of the lens of the eye. [capsule, Gk *-itis* inflammation.]

capsotomy (kap·sot·o·me). Capsulotomy.

capsular (kap·sewl·ar). 1. Relating to a capsule. 2. Hollow and fibrous. [L *capsula* little box.]

capsulation (kap·sewl·a·shun). The enclosing of a drug in a capsule of gelatin or other soluble medium to enable it to be taken orally without taste.

capsule [capsula (NA)] (kap·sewl). 1. In anatomy, a sheath or envelope around an organ or structure. 2. Any structure or organ in the body resembling an envelope in form. 3. A case made of gelatin or starch used to dispense drugs which are nauseating or otherwise unpalatable. 4. The protective polysaccharide or protein covering of certain bacteria. 5. The metal envelope containing an expanding fluid which serves to control thermostatically the temperature within an incubator. **Adherent capsule.** A capsule of an organ such as the kidney which has become bound to the underlying surface by means of adhesions of scar tissue. **Adipose capsule.** Fatty capsule of the kidney (see below). **Anterior capsule.** The anterior part of the capsule of the lens (see below). **Articular capsule [capsula articularis (NA)].** This consists of 2 parts, an outer fibrous capsular ligament and an inner lining synovial layer. The capsular ligament forms an investing sleeve of white fibrous tissue typically attached near the perimeter of the articular surfaces and continuous with the periosteum of the bones forming the joint; one or more localized thickenings of the capsule form the ligaments, which may show circumscribed gaps through which protrusions of synovial membrane may occur to form bursae. The synovial layer consists of a thin stratum of vascular areolar tissue, on the free surface of which is an incomplete layer of mesothelial-like cells. It is attached to the edges of the articular surfaces and lines the inner surface of the capsular ligament and any intracapsular structure other than the articular surfaces. The more complex capsules of some of the larger joints are described separately below. **Articular capsule of the ankle joint.** A fibrous tissue sleeve surrounding the joint and attached to the edges of the articular surfaces. It is lax anteriorly and posteriorly. **Articular capsule of the elbow joint.** The investment of the elbow joint, the fibrous ligament of which is attached to the humerus near the capitular articular surface laterally and below the epicondyle medially. The synovial layer is attached to the perimeter of the articular surfaces of the humerus and ulna, and lines the internal surface of the fibrous ligament. **Articular capsule of the hip joint.** A strong investment for the joint, attached above to the margin of the acetabulum and below to the intertrochanteric line and the base of the femoral neck superiorly and inferiorly. It is loosely attached posteriorly to the middle of the neck. **Articular capsules of the interphalangeal joints.** Similar to those of the metatarsophalangeal joints (see below). **Articular capsule of the knee joint.** A thin cylindrical investment of fibrous tissue mostly obscured by overlying ligaments. There are deficiencies in front for the patella, and behind the medial condyle, for a bursa deep to the medial head of the gastrocnemius and semimembranosus, laterally for the tendon of the popliteus, and superiorly for the suprapatellar bursa. **Articular capsules of the metatarsophalangeal joints.** An investment for the joints, thickened laterally to form the collateral ligaments and inferiorly by the plantar ligament. The dorsal part is weak. **Articular capsule of the shoulder joint.** The lax capsular ligament attached to the periphery of the articular surfaces, except on the medial side of the humerus where it encroaches on the shaft. **Articular capsule of the talocalcanean joint.** A loose thin capsule attached around the articular margins. **Auditory capsule.** Periotic capsule (see below). **Brood capsule.** A chamber in which individuals are developed during asexual reproduction, particularly one of those on the inner surface of a hydatid cyst on which the scolices are formed. **Cell capsule.** A non-living cell wall outside the plasma membrane, such as the mucopolysaccharide capsule around developing cartilage cells. **Crystalline capsule.** The capsule of the lens (see below). **Enteric capsule.** Formalized capsule (see below) or capsule of other substance that resists the stomach acid. **External capsule [capsula externa (NA)].** A thin layer of white matter on the lateral aspect of the lentiform nucleus. **Fatty capsule of the kidney.** Renal fat; the fat-containing tissue in which the kidney lies comparatively loosely; it is enclosed in the perirenal fascia of Gerota. **Fibrous capsule of the kidney.** Renal capsule (see below). **Formalized capsule.** One which has been dipped into formaldehyde solution and dried. It passes through the acid stomach medium intact but is dissolved in the alkaline medium of the small intestine. **Gamma-ray capsule.** A small gamma-ray source container with sufficient wall thickness to reduce β-ray transmission to a negligible value. **Capsule of the glomerulus.** *See* GLOMERULUS, MALPIGHIAN. **Glutoid capsule.** Formalized capsule (see above). **Hepatobiliary capsule [capsula fibrosa perivascularis** (NA)]. The fibrous tissue around the lobules of the liver. **Internal capsule [capsula interna (NA)].** A broad band of fibres passing to and from the cerebral cortex, lying against the convex medial surface of the lentiform nucleus and therefore V-shaped when seen in horizontal sections of the brain. It has a lentiform part [pars sublentiformis capsulae internae (NA)] and a retrolentiform part [pars retrolentiformis capsulae internae (NA)]. **Joint capsule.** The fibrous capsule enclosing a joint. **Capsule of the lens [capsula lentis (NA)].** The transparent membrane round the lens of the eye. **Capsule of the lentiform nucleus.** A capsule which is divided into an external capsule or thin layer of fibres between the lentiform nucleus and the claustrum, and an internal capsule or thicker layer between the lentiform nucleus laterally and the caudate nucleus and thalamus medially. **Nasal capsule.** The cartilage formed round the developing olfactory organ and forming the ethmoid bone in the adult. **Otic capsule.** Periotic capsule (see below). **Perinephric capsule.** The fascia around the kidney. **Periotic capsule.** The otic or auditory capsule, a condensation of mesenchyme, later cartilaginous and bony, surrounding the otic vesicle. It develops into the petrous part of the temporal bone. **Posterior capsule.** The posterior part of the capsule of the lens (see above). **Capsule of the prostate.** An investment of fibrous tissue containing the prostatic plexus of veins. The posterior part differs from the remainder, being of tissue divided from the obliterated lower portion of the rectovesical pouch. The capsule is continuous anteriorly with the puboprostatic ligament and inferiorly with the fascia covering the deep perineal muscles. **Renal capsule [capsula fibrosa (NA)].** Fibrous capsule of the kidney; the connective-tissue capsule intimately attached to the kidney. **Capsule of the spleen.** The fibro-elastic coat of the spleen. **Suprarenal capsule.** Suprarenal gland. *See* GLAND. **Synovial capsule.** Articular capsule (see above). [L *capsula* little box.]

See also: BONNET, BOWMAN, GEROTA, GLISSON, MUELLER (J.), TENON, WRIGHT (A. E.).

capsulectomy (kap·sewl·**ek**·to·me). Surgical excision of a capsule, particularly the capsule of the lens of the eye, an articular capsule or the renal capsule. [capsule, Gk *ektome* a cutting out.]

capsulitis (kap·sewl·**i**·tis). An inflammatory condition affecting any capsule of the body. **Hepatic capsulitis.** Perihepatitis. **Capsulitis of the labyrinth.** Otosclerosis. [capsule, Gk *-itis* inflammation.]

capsulolenticular (kap·sewl·o·len·**tik**'·ew·lar). Relating to the lens of the eye and the capsule of the lens.

capsuloma (kap·sewl·o·mah). A tumour in the fibrous capsule of the kidney or one occurring in the subcapsular area. [capsule, Gk *-oma* tumour.]

capsuloplasty (kap·sewl·o·**plas**'·te). A plastic operation performed on an articular capsule. [capsule, Gk *plassein* to mould.]

capsulorrhaphy (kap·sewl·**or**·af·e). The suturing of a capsule, particularly an articular capsule to repair a laceration or to prevent dislocation. [capsule, Gk *rhaphe* suture.]

capsulotome (kap·sewl·o·tome). An instrument used for incising the lens capsule, usually some form of needle, e.g. Ziegler's or Bowman's. [capsule, Gk *temnein* to cut.]

capsulotomy (kap·sewl·**ot**·o·me). The operation of incising a capsule, particularly an articular capsule or that of the lens of the eye. **Renal capsulotomy.** The incising of the fibrous capsule of the kidney. [capsule, Gk *temnein* to cut.]

captation (kap·ta·shun). The earliest stage in the induction of hypnotism; term applied to the initial phase of trance. [L *captare* to catch.]

Captodiame (kap·to·**di**·am·e). BP Commission approved name for 4-butylthio-α-phenylbenzyl 2-dimethylamino-ethyl sulphide, a depressant of the central nervous system, and spasmolytic. It is used as a tranquillizer but it has little hypnotic action in normal dosage.

capture (kap·tcher). **Electron capture.** A nuclear transformation whereby a nucleus captures one of its orbital electrons. **Neutron capture.** Capture of a neutron by a nucleus, giving an isotope of 1 unit higher mass and the emission of a γ-ray by the excited nucleus. [L *captura* a catching.]

Capuron, Joseph (b. 1767). French physician.

Capuron's points, Capuron's cardinal points. Four fixed points of the pelvic inlet, the 2 iliopectineal points anteriorly and the 2 sacro-iliac points posteriorly.

caput [NA] (kap·ut) (pl. *capita*). A head, or part of a structure resembling a head; also sometimes applied to the origin of a muscle, e.g. caput breve, the short head of the biceps muscle. **Caput caudati.** The head, or expanded anterior part, of the caudate nucleus. **Caput distortum.** Torticollis. **Caput humeralis.** The head of the humerus which articulates with the scapula. **Caput natiforme.** Caput succedaneum (see below). **Caput obstipum.** Torticollis. **Caput planum.** Perthes' disease; osteochondritis of the hip. **Caput progeneum.** Abnormal forward projection of the mandible. **Caput succedaneum.** The swelling produced on the head of the fetus during labour, after the rupture of the membranes. The tissues of the scalp become oedematous from pressure, and present as a soft swelling at the most dependent part of the head. [L head.]

caraate (kar·ah·a·te). Pinta.

Carabelli, Georg C. (b. 1787). Vienna dentist.

Carabelli cusp, tubercle of Carabelli. A small tubercle of enamel often found on the antero-internal cusps of the second deciduous molar teeth or the first permanent molar teeth in the upper jaw.

caramel (**kar**·am·el). Saccharum ustum; burnt sugar; made by heating sucrose at 180–200°C until it oxidizes with the formation of some free carbon and has the appearance of a thick black mass, which is then diluted with water to a specific gravity of 1.4. It is used for colouring purposes, usually in the form of liquor sacchari usti, which consists of equal parts of caramel and chloroform water. [Sp. *caramelo.*]

caramelization (**kar**·am·el·i·**za**′·shun). The conversion of cane sugar into caramel by heating.

Caramiphen (kar·ah·**mif**·en). BP Commission approved name for 1-phenylcyclopentanecarboxylic acid 2-diethylaminoethyl ester, $C_{18}H_{27}NO_2$. A synthetic spasmolytic agent used in extrapyramidal motor disturbances, especially parkinsonism. The effects are mainly subjective; rigidity is alleviated but tremors are little affected. Side effects are common, including dyspnoea, blurred vision, vertigo, nausea and drowsiness, and the dose should be carefully built up. It is given as the hydrochloride (BP 1968).

carane (**kar**·ane). $C_{10}H_{18}$. A terpene hydrocarbon, isomeric with camphane, and consisting of a 6-membered carbon ring bridged in the *ortho* position. It occurs in essential oils, and is the parent of a family of terpenes.

carapace (**kar**·ah·pase). The body shell of crustaceans. [Sp. *carapacho.*]

Carassini's spool. A tube over which end-to-end intestinal anastomosis was once sometimes performed.

carate (kar·a·te). Pinta.

Caraway BP 1973 (**kar**·ah·wa). Carum; the dried ripe fruits of *Carum carvi* Linn., a biennial umbelliferous herb cultivated in Central and North European countries, particularly Holland. It is used as a carminative. [Ar. *karwiya.*]

Carbachol BP 1973 (**kar**·bak·ol). Carbamyl choline chloride, $[NH_2COOCH_2CH_2N(CH_3)_3]Cl$. A water-soluble crystalline substance with action similar to that of acetycholine but more resistant to cholinesterase and gastric juice, and, hence, more prolonged in effect and permitting oral administration. It is used in postoperative retention of urine, in hypertension and in glaucoma.

carbamate (kar·bam·ate). An ester or salt of carbamic acid; the esters are known as *urethanes,* and are important hypnotics.

Carbamazepine BP 1973 (kar·bam·**az**·ep·een). Dibenz[*b,f*]-azepine-5-carboxamide; it is used in the treatment of trigeminal neuralgia.

carbamic (kar·**bam**·ik). Name applied to compounds containing the divalent radical -NHCOO- which is derived from carbamic acid.

carbamide (**kar**·bam·ide). Urea, $CO(NH_2)_2$. A white crystalline substance, very soluble in water or alcohol; excreted in the urine of mammals, birds and certain reptiles, as the end-product of protein metabolism, being formed in the liver from the amino acids. The first organic compound to be synthesized in the laboratory, it condenses to biuret on heating and then cyanuric acid; combines with acids to form ureides, and with salts to give additive compounds.

carbamidine (kar·**bam**·id·een). Guanidine.

carbamine (**kar**·bam·een). Acetonitrile, methyl cyanide, CH_3CN. A colourless liquid with a pleasant odour found in coal tar and molasses; used in organic synthesis and the manufacture of perfumery.

carbaminohaemoglobin (kar·**bam**·in·o·he·mo·**glo**′·bin). A compound of haemoglobin and carbon dioxide present in the circulating blood. It is one of the forms in which CO_2 is transported, and is an unstable combination of the latter with an uncharged amino group of the haemoglobin.

Carbarsone BP 1958 (**kar**·bar·sone). Paracarbamidobenzene arsonic acid, $(OH)_2AsOC_6H_4NHCONH_2$. A pentavalent organic arsenical compound containing 28.5 per cent arsenic; used mainly in amoebic dysentery, the drug being active against vegetative forms and cysts in the alimentary tract. It has been found valueless in amoebic hepatitis. The drug is given by mouth and occasionally as a retention enema. It is relatively non-toxic, but mild skin rashes occasionally result from its administration

carbazide (**kar**·baz·ide). Name given to a number of compounds derived from urea and containing the group, -NHNHCONH NH-.

carbazotate (kar·baz·**o**·tate). A picrate; a salt of picric acid.

Carbenicillin (**kar**·ben·e·**sil**′·in). BP Commission approved name for 6-(α-carboxyphenylacetamido)penicillanic acid. **Carbenicillin Sodium BP 1973.** The disodium salt, an antibiotic.

Carbenoxolone (kar·ben·**ox**·o·lone). BP Commission approved name for 3β-(3-carboxypropionyloxy)-11-oxo-olean-12-en-30-oic acid; it is used in the treatment of peptic ulcer. **Carbenoxolone Sodium BP 1973.** Disodium enoxolone succinate, an anti-inflammatory agent used in the treatment of gastric ulcer. It is administered orally in tablets and variable results are reported. Side-effects may be serious, especially in patients with cardiac, renal or hepatic disease.

carbide (**kar**·bide). A binary compound of carbon and a metal or certain other elements; those derived from acetylene are known as *acetylides.* They vary in stability, from the explosive carbides of silver and copper to the extremely hard and abrasive carbides of silicon and boron. Those of the alkali metals and the metals of the alkali earths evolve acetylene with water; others give a mixture of acetylene, hydrogen, and methane.

Carbidopa (kar·be·**do**·pah). BP Commission approved name for L-2-(3,4,-dihydroxybenzyl)-2-hydrazinopropionic acid; a dopa-decarboxylase inhibitor.

Carbimazole BP 1973 (kar·**bim**·az·ole). 2-Carbethoxythio-1-methylglyoxaline,

$$C_2H_5OOCS\overline{C{=}NCH{=}CHN}(CH_3).$$

A drug used in the treatment of thyrotoxicosis. Also known as *CGI.*

carbimide (**kar**·bim·ide). Carbonylamine. 1. An isocyanate of the general formula O=C=NR, where R is a monovalent radical. 2. Isocyanic acid, HNCO.

carbinol (**kar**·bin·ol). 1. Methyl alcohol. 2. Designation of alcohols under a system of nomenclature whereby they are regarded as derivatives of methyl alcohol, with the hydrogens of the methyl group of the latter replaced by aliphatic or aromatic hydrocarbon groups.

Carbinoxamine (kar·bin·**ox**·am·een). BP Commission approved name for *p*-chloro-α-2-pyridylbenzyl-2-dimethylaminoethyl ether; an antihistaminic used in the treatment of hay fever and other allergic conditions.

Carbiphene (**kar**·be·feen). BP Commission approved name for α-ethoxy-*N*-methyl-*N*-[2-(*N*-methylphenethylamino)-ethyl]diphenylacetamide; an analgesic.

carbo (**kar**·bo). Charcoal. **Carbo activatus.** Activated charcoal, a form made by heating charcoal in steam or in an activating gas. This greatly increases its adsorptive powers, and renders it more efficient for the adsorption of toxic substances such as strychnine. **Carbo animalis.** Animal charcoal, made by burning bones and subsequently boiling with hydrochloric acid, then washing and drying. A 2 per cent aqueous suspension has been given intravenously, but there is risk of pulmonary embolism. **Carbo ligni.** Medicinal charcoal, a type of charcoal which occurs in stick and powdered form and is made by burning wood in the minimum of air. It is used mainly as an adsorbent in medicine, particularly in distension of the stomach, and for this purpose it is usually given in the form of a biscuit, or enclosed in a cachet. It also adsorbs toxins, and limits their absorption. It may be incorporated in linseed poultices and used externally as an application to ulcers. [L.]

Carbocloral (kar·bo·**klor**·al). BP Commission approved name for ethyl(2,2,2-trichloro-1-hydroxyethyl)carbamate; a hypnotic.

carbocyclic (kar·bo·**si**·klik). Alicyclic, isocyclic. Term applied to an organic compound having in its structure a closed ring consisting solely of carbon atoms. [carbon, Gk *kyklos* circle.]

carbodiimide (kar·bo·**di**·im·ide). Dicyclohexyl carbodiimide, $C_6H_{11}N{=}C{=}NC_6H_{11}$, a reagent widely employed in condensation reactions, i.e. nucleotide syntheses. It removes the elements of water from reactants, even in aqueous solution, with production of dicyclohexylurea.

carbogaseous (kar·bo·**ga**·se·us). Describing anything which is charged with carbon dioxide. [carbon, gas.]

carbohaemia (kar·bo·**he**·me·ah). 1. A condition in which there is not sufficient oxygenation of the blood. 2. A condition in which there is incomplete elimination of carbonic acid gas. [L *carbo* coal, Gk *haima* blood.]

carbohaemoglobin (kar·bo·he·mo·**glo**′·bin). A compound of haemoglobin and carbon dioxide. [L *carbo* coal, haemoglobin.]

carbohydrase (kar·bo·**hi**·draze). An enzyme which acts upon a carbohydrate, e.g. amylose, maltose, breaking them into simpler sugars. They belong to the class of enzymes called hydrolases, since they add H_2O to the substrate.

carbohydrate (kar·bo·**hi**·drate). Originally, organic compounds occurring in nature composed of 6 carbon atoms or multiples thereof, combined with hydrogen and oxygen in the proportions of water; the term is now extended to cover allied compounds, natural or synthetic, with other proportions of the 3 elements. They are classified as follows: 1. Monosaccharides, polyhydroxy ketones or aldehydes with a chain of 2–10 carbon atoms; they do not crystallize, are soluble in water and have a sweet taste: glucose is an example. 2. Compound saccharides, anhydrides of 2 or more molecules of monosaccharide; they crystallize, are soluble in water and are sweet: sucrose, $C_{12}H_{22}O_{11}$, is an example. 3. Polysaccharides, formed from monosaccharide units, have complex molecules which give colloidal solutions; they are not sweet: starch, $(C_6H_{10}O_5)_m$, is an example. 4. Hetero-saccharides, complex combinations of non-saccharides and sugar units: gums and pectins are in this class. 5. Glycosides, compounds of a saccharide with another substance, which occur in nature: the principles of vegetable drugs are of this type. **Reserve carbohydrate.** Carbohydrate such as starch or glycogen stored by a plant or animal as a reserve. [carbon, Gk *hydor* water.]

carbohydraturia (kar·bo·hi·drat·**ewr**′·e·ah). The presence of carbohydrate in the urine. The commonest forms are glycosuria, lactosuria and pentosuria.

carbohydrogenic (kar·bo·hi·dro·**jen**′·ik). Producing carbohydrate. [carbohydrate, Gk *genein* to produce.]

carbolate (**kar**·bol·ate). 1. To add phenol to a mixure. 2. A salt of carbolic acid; a phenate. [carbolic acid.]

carbolfuchsine (kar·bol·**fook**·seen). A staining solution containing basic fuchsine and phenol, being a mixture of a 10 per cent alcoholic solution of the former with a 5 per cent aqueous solution of the latter. It is used particularly in the well-known Ziehl-Neelsen method for tubercle bacilli, in which sections or smears are overstained in hot carbolfuchsine and then differentiated with 25 per cent sulphuric acid; the stain is removed from all but the acid-fast bacilli, which remain crimson. A weaker solution is used as a counterstain in Gram's method for classifying bacteria. [carbolic acid, fuchsine.]

carbolic (kar·**bol**·ik). Pertaining to carbolic acid or phenol. Originally, pertaining to coal tar. [L *carbo* coal.]

carbolism (**kar**·bol·izm). Phenol poisoning. [carbolic acid.]

carbolize (**kar**·bol·ize). 1. To wash or treat with phenol. 2. To mix with phenol. [see prec.]

carbolmarasmus (kar·bol·mar·**az**′·mus). Chronic phenol poisoning; the main symptoms are general wasting and sickness, vertigo, salivation, headache and nephritis. [carbolic acid, Gk *marasmos* decay.]

Carbolonium Bromide (kar·bol·o·ne·um **bro**·mide). BP Commission approved name for hexamethylenebis(carbamoylcholine bromide); a muscle relaxant.

carboluria (kar·bol·**ewr**·e·ah). The presence of phenol in urine, colouring it darkly, a sign of phenol poisoning. [carbolic acid, urine.]

carbolxylene, carbolxylol (kar·bol·**zi**·leen, kar·bol·**zi**·lol). A clearing agent used in microscopy, especially in the case of moist objects. It consists of pure phenol (1 part) and xylol (3 parts).

Carbomer (**kar**·bo·mer). BP Commission approved name for a polymer of acrylic acid cross-linked with allyl sucrose.

carbometer (kar·**bom**·et·er). A device with which the quantity of carbon dioxide in air can be measured. Cf. CARBONOMETER. [carbon, meter.]

carbomethane (kar·bo·**me**·thane). Ketene, $CH_2{=}CO$. A colourless gas derived from acetic anhydride and used as an acetylating agent.

carbometry (kar·**bom**·et·re). Carbonometry.

carbon (**kar**·bon). An element of atomic weight 12.011, atomic number 6 and chemical symbol C. It is a non-metal existing in several allotropic forms, and uncombined occurs naturally as graphite and diamonds. It is found very widely in combination, and is an essential component of all organic chemical compounds and so of all living matter. In medicine it is employed in the form of activated charcoal as an absorbent and deodorant. The stable isotope is ${}^{12}_{6}C$, occurring naturally to the extent of 98.9 per cent, the remaining 1.1 per cent consisting of the stable isotope ${}^{13}_{6}C$. There is also a radioactive isotope, ${}^{14}_{6}C$ that has a half-life of over 5000 years; it is a low-energy β-ray transmitter and has been much used as a tracer in metabolic studies. **Carbon dating.** A method of determining the age of an archaeological specimen of biological origin by measuring its content of the naturally-occurring radioactive isotope of carbon, ${}^{14}C$. This method cannot be applied to specimens of great age and is u··lly limited to those obtained from quarternary deposits. **Carbon dioxide.** CO_2, a gas which dissolves readily in water to form carbonic acid; it is one of the end-products of the tissue oxidation of carbohydrates and fats. It acts as a stimulus to the respiratory centre, and is administered for this purpose clinically (BP 1973) as a 5-7 per cent mixture with oxygen. Solid carbon dioxide (carbon dioxide snow) is used as a local application to destroy warts and naevi, which it does by virtue of its very low temperature. **Carbon disulphide.** CS_2, a clear, colourless, volatile, inflammable liquid, used in veterinary practice as a parasiticide, and an important industrial solvent. Poisoning by carbon disulphide is characterized by signs of damage to the central nervous system. **Carbon monoxide.** CO, a colourless gas, the chief constituent of coal gas. It combines more readily with haemoglobin than does oxygen to form carboxyhaemoglobin, which is a relatively stable compound; as a result the amount of haemoglobin available for oxygen transport is reduced. **Radioactive carbon.** One of a number of isotopes of carbon characterized by having an unstable nucleus and emitting ionizing radiation. Only one such isotope occurs naturally in the earth, ${}^{14}C$. **Carbon Tetrachloride BP 1953.** CCl_4, a clear, colourless, volatile liquid with characteristic odour and burning taste. It is employed as an anthelmintic, chiefly against tapeworms and hookworms. Toxic symptoms may be produced, chiefly headache, dizziness and sickness, and occasionally liver damage may result. Administration of the drug is generally preceded and followed by a saline purge. Its use as a cleaner and in fire extinguishers renders it an occupational hazard, since inhalation of the fumes leads to carbon tetrachloride poisoning, of which the chief symptom is acute nephritis. [L *carbo* coal.]

carbonaemia (kar·bon·e·me·ah). The presence of carbon dioxide in blood. [carbon, Gk *haima* blood.]

carbonate (**kar**·bon·ate). A salt of carbonic acid.

carbonated (**kar**·bon·a·ted). 1. Charged with carbon dioxide. 2. Rendered into a carbonate.

carbone (**kar**·bone). A carbuncle.

Carbonei Dioxidum (kar·**bon**·e·i di·**ox**·id·um). *European Pharmacopoeia* name for Carbon Dioxide BP 1973.

carboneum (kar·**bo**·ne·um). Latin for carbon in compounds; genitive *carbonei.*

carbonide (**kar**·bon·ide). A carbide.

carbonite (**kar**·bon·ite). 1. An oxalate. 2. A high-explosive mixture of nitroglycerin and sodium nitrate in a flour base [L *carbo* coal.]

carbonization (kar·bon·i·**za**′·shun). 1. The heating of organic substances in a closed space to form carbon. 2. The industrial process of coal distillation designed to produce coal gas, coke and by-products.

carbonize (**kar**·bon·ize). 1. To transform organic matter into charcoal. 2. To char. 3. To combine with carbon or to impregnate with carbon. [L *carbo* coal.]

carbonmonoxyhaemoglobin (**kar**·bon·mon·**ox**·e·he·mo·**glo**′·bin). *See* HAEMOGLOBIN.

carbonometer (kar·bon·**om**·et·er). A device with which the carbonic acid content of the blood can be measured. Cf. CARBOMETER. [carbon, meter.]

carbonometry (kar·bon·**om**·et·re). Estimation of the amount of carbonic acid gas exhaled with the breath, e.g. in the air of a room. [see prec.]

carbonous (**kar**·bon·us). Containing carbon.

carbonuria (kar·bon·**ewr**·e·ah). The presence of a carbon compound in urine. **Dysoxidative carbonuria.** Increase of amount of carbon compounds in urine as the result of too little oxygen circulating in the system.

carbonyl (**kar**·bon·il). The divalent radical CO=. **Carbonyl chloride.** Phosgene, $COCl_2$, a poisonous gas with a suffocating odour obtained by the oxidation of chloroform; used in organic synthesis and in chemical warfare. **Nickel carbonyl.** A gaseous industrial product arising in the hardening of steel and involving a risk of carcinoma of the nose, sinuses or bronchial tree.

carbonylamine (kar·bon·**il**·am·een). Carbimide. 1. An isocyanate of general formula O=C=NR. 2. Isocyanic acid, HNC=O.

carbonylhaemoglobin (**kar**·bon·il·he·mo·**glo**′·bin). Carboxyhaemoglobin.

Carborundum (kar·bor·**un**′·dum). Silicon carbide, SiC. An extremely hard abrasive, manufactured by heating carbon and silica together in an electric furnace. In dentistry, it is used as an abrasive for grinding and polishing. [Trade name.]

carbostyril (kar·bo·**stir**·il). $C_6H_4{=}NC(CH_2)_2OH$. 2-Hydroxyquinoline, the lactam of *o*-aminocinnamic acid; conjugated with glycuronic acid it is excreted in the urine.

carboxaemia (kar·box·e·me·ah). A condition in which the carbon dioxide content of the circulating blood is increased. [carbon, oxide, Gk *haima* blood.]

Carboxydomonas (kar·box·e·**do**·mo·nas). A genus of organisms (family Protobactereae) securing growth energy by oxidizing CO to CO_2. [carbon, oxide, Gk *monas* unit.]

carboxyhaemoglobin (kar·**box**·e·he·mo·**glo**′·bin). A compound of characteristic cherry-red colour formed by the contact of haemoglobin with carbon monoxide, for which it possesses 300 times greater affinity than for oxygen. Although more stable than oxyhaemoglobin, dissociation readily occurs in an atmosphere of pure oxygen or air. Its formation in the blood reduces the amount of oxygen that can be carried, and inhalation of carbon monoxide is therefore extremely dangerous. [carbon, oxide, haemoglobin.]

carboxyhaemoglobinaemia (kar·**box**·e·he·mo·glo·bin·**e**′·me·ah). The presence of carboxyhaemoglobin in the circulation which in sufficient saturation leads to tissue oxygen starvation (carbon monoxide poisoning). Death occurs at 60–80 per cent saturation, and prolonged coma may lead to bilateral softening of the globus pallidus. [carboxyhaemoglobin, Gk *haima* blood.]

carboxyl (kar·**box**·il). The monovalent group COOH- which confers acidic properties upon the majority of organic acids; the hydrogen atom is replaceable by elements and radicals to form salts and esters.

carboxylase (kar·**box**·il·aze). An enzyme catalysing a reaction involving CO_2 fixation. **Acetyl CoA carboxylase.** The first enzyme of fatty acid biosynthesis, it converts acetyl CoA to malonyl CoA. **Amino acid carboxylases.** Enzymes widely distributed in nature, in animal tissue and many bacteria, capable of decarboxylating specific amino acids, often with the production of toxic amines such as putrescine and cadaverine. **β-Carboxylase.** A widely occurring enzyme that reversibly catalyses the conversion of oxalo-acetic acid into pyruvic acid. **Propionyl CoA carboxylase.** An enzyme of propionate metabolism in liver catalysing the formation of methylmalonyl CoA. **Pyruvate carboxylase.** A regulatory enzyme important in fatty acid and carbohydrate synthesis, it catalyses the formation of oxaloacetate from pyruvate.

carboxymethylcellulose (kar·**box**·e·meth·il·**sel**′·ew·loze). An ion-exchanger, frequently used in protein purification. **Carboxymethylcellulose sodium.** A compound which forms colourless and tasteless mucilages that are neutral and inert.

Carboxymethylcysteine (kar·**box**·e·meth·il·**sis**′·te·een). BP Commission approved name for *S*-carboxymethylcysteine; a mucolytic agent.

carboxypeptidase (kar·**box**·e·**pep**′·tid·aze). A proteolytic enzyme from many sources including the pancreatic secretion; it cleaves carboxyl-terminal amino acids sequentially.

β-carboxypyridine (**be**·tah·kar·box·e·**pir**′·e·deen). Nicotinic acid. *See* ACID.

Carbromal BP 1973 (kar·**bro**·mal). Bromodiethylacetylurea, $NH_2CONHCOCBr(C_2H_5)_2$, a monoureide which has a mild sedative and hypnotic effect. It is less powerful than the barbiturates, but also less toxic.

carbuncle (**kar**·bung·kl). An infection of the skin and subcutaneous tissue by *Staphylococcus aureus* in which there is diffuse necrosis of the subcutaneous tissue as opposed to the localized necrotic core of the boil. It occurs particularly in dense integuments such as the back of the neck and the back, and is often associated with multiple openings in the skin through which pus discharges. **Renal carbuncle.** A low-grade inflammatory process in a part of the renal parenchyma usually arising as metastasis from infection elsewhere in the body, such as multiple boils. It may be controlled by appropriate antibiotics but, if not, forms a low-grade abscess which causes considerable destruction of kidney tissue, and may burst through the renal capsule to cause a perinephric abscess. [L *carbunculus* little coal.]

carbuncular (kar·**bung**·kewl·ar). Relating to, or having the characteristics of, a carbuncle.

carbunculosis (**kar**·bung·kewl·**o**′·sis). The condition characterized by the appearance in quick succession of several carbuncles. [carbuncle, Gk *-osis* condition.]

carbunculus (kar·**bung**·kewl·us). Carbuncle. [L little coal.]

Carbutamide (kar·**bew**·tam·ide). BP Commission approved name for *N*-butyl-*N*′-sulphanylurea. It proved of value in the treatment in relatively mild cases of diabetes, but was too toxic and has been largely superseded by tolbutamide, a drug with a very similar action but less toxic.

carbylamine (kar·bil·**am**·een). 1. An isocyanide; an isonitrile of general formula RN=C, where R is a monovalent radical. Colourless liquids with an alkaline reaction, poisonous and with an offensive smell. 2. Ethyl carbylamine, ethyl isocyanide, C_2H_5 N=C; it is liable to change tautomerically into the isomeric propionitrile, C_2H_5CN.

Carcassone, Maurice (fl. 1821). Montpelier surgeon.

Carcassone's ligament. The perineal membrane. *See* MEMBRANE.

carcinaemia (kar·sin·e·me·ah). The debilitated condition, dark complexion and emaciation that are typical of the sufferer from carcinoma; cancerous cachexia. [carcinoma, Gk *haima* blood.]

carcinectomy (kar·sin·**ek**·to·me). Surgical excision of carcinoma. [carcinoma, Gk *ektome* a cutting out.]

carcinelcosis (**kar**·sin·el·**ko**′·sis). An ulcerative state showing evidence of malignancy. [carcinoma, Gk *elkosis* ulceration.]

carcinogen (kar·**sin**·o·jen). Any substance which causes living tissues to become carcinomatous. [carcinoma, Gk *genein* to produce.]

carcinogenesis (**kar**·sin·o·**jen**′·es·is). The production of carcinoma in living tissues. [see prec.]

carcinogenic (**kar**·sin·o·**jen**′·ik). Giving rise to or producing carcinoma. [see foll.]

carcinogenicity (**kar**·sin·o·jen·**is**′·it·e). 1. The state that tends to produce carcinoma. 2. The power or ability to produce or give rise to carcinoma. [carcinoma. Gk *genein* to produce.]

carcinoid (**kar**·sin·oid). 1. Literally a tumour resembling a carcinoma histologically, but clinically benign. 2. A tumour derived from the argentaffin (Kulchitsky) cells of the appendix, intestines, stomach or bronchus. It runs a benign course in the appendix, but in other sites infiltrates and metastasizes, especially to the liver, though relatively slowly. **Carcinoid syndrome.** *See* SYNDROME. [carcinoma, Gk *eidos* form.]

carcinoidosis (**kar**·sin·oid·**o**′·sis). Carcinoid syndrome. *See* SYNDROME. [carcinoma, Gk *eidos* form, *-osis* condition.]

carcinology (kar·sin·**ol**·o·je). The science and study of carcinoma and its treatment. [carcinoma, Gk *logos* science.]

carcinolysin (kar·sin·**ol**·is·in). Any agent which destroys carcinoma cells. [see foll.]

carcinolysis (kar·sin·**ol**·is·is). The destruction of carcinomatous cells. [carcinoma, Gk *lysis* a loosing.]

carcinolytic (**kar**·sin·o·**lit**′·ik). Able to destroy carcinomatous cells. [see prec.]

carcinoma (kar·sin·o·mah). A malignant epithelial tumour which tends to spread locally, and generally throughout the body, destroying normal tissues as it progresses and eventually proving fatal. It is most common after middle age. **Acinic cell carcinoma.** Carcinoma of the salivary glands of intermediate malignancy composed of cells resembling acinar cells. **Acinous carcinoma.** Medullary carcinoma (see below). **Acute carcinoma.** A rapidly growing and highly malignant carcinoma. In the breast, the plugging of the lymphatic channels by permeating columns of carcinoma cells results in marked oedematous enlargement of the breast. **Adenocystic carcinoma.** Adenoid cystic carcinoma (see below). **Adenoid carcinoma, Adenomatous carcinoma.** Adenocarcinoma; a carcinoma with a strongly-marked glandular pattern. **Adenoid cystic carcinoma.** A relatively slowly growing tumour of the salivary glands, major and minor, the palate and paranasal sinuses, which shows a special tendency to infiltrate locally particularly along the sheaths of nerves, and because of this it is difficult to eradicate. **Adrenocortical carcinoma.** Carcinoma of the adrenal cortex. **Alveolar carcinoma.** A carcinoma in which the connective-tissue stroma clearly surrounds groups of carcinoma cells, imitating a glandular structure. **Anaplastic carcinoma.** A carcinoma composed of undifferentiated primitive cells. **Aniline carcinoma.** Carcinoma of the urinary bladder arising in workers in aniline dyes and dye-intermediates. **Argentaffin carcinoma.** Argentaffinoma. **Carcinoma asbolicum.** Chimney-sweeps' carcinoma (see below). **Atrophic scirrhus carcinoma.** A rare, very slowly growing carcinoma of the breast, often remaining localized to the breast for many years, in which carcinoma cells are scanty and the bulk of the tumour consists largely of reactive fibrous tissue. The breast may eventually be reduced to a small shrivelled remnant. **Basal-cell carcinoma, Basal-celled carcinoma, Carcinoma basocellulare.** A rodent ulcer. *See* ULCER. **Basisquamous carcinoma.** A tumour of the skin showing transition between basal and squamous carcinoma. There are 2 types: the intermediate form which is of low malignancy, differentiating towards hair follicle structure; and a mixed form of double origin with the squamous elements prone to metastasize. **Bronchogenic carcinoma.** Carcinoma orginating from a bronchus. **Chimney-sweeps' carcinoma.** Epithelioma of the scrotum occurring in chimney-sweeps, due to the irritant action of soot. **Chorionic carcinoma.** A carcinoma arising from retained chorionic elements within the uterus; a variety of malignant teratoma in males. **Chronic carcinoma.** Scirrhous carcinoma (see below). **Cloacogenic carcinoma.** An adenocarcinoma at the junction of the rectal and anal mucosae, possibly arising from epithelium or intramuscular glands which may be cloacal remnants. **Colloid carcinoma.** A carcinoma which secretes large amounts of mucus. **Comedo carcinoma.** One in which tiny yellowish or whitish greasy masses can be distinguished with the naked eye. **Cutaneous carcinoma, Carcinoma cutaneum.** A squamous-celled carcinoma of the skin. **Cylindrical carcinoma, Carcinoma cylindromatosum.** Adenocarcinoma; a variety of adenoid carcinoma in which the cancer cells have columnar shapes. **Duct carcinoma.** One which arises within the ducts of a gland, especially the ducts of the nipple. **Carcinoma durum.** Scirrhous carcinoma (see below). **Embryonal carcinoma.** A malignant teratoma. **Encephaloid carcinoma.** One which grows rapidly, is very soft and vascular, and resembles brain tissue on naked-eye examination. **Endo-epidermal carcinoma.** A precancerous condition; chronic superficial mucosal ulceration, lymphocytic inflammation with downgrowths into the epithelium. **Epidermoid carcinoma.** A squamous-celled carcinoma of the skin or some derivative of skin. **Epithelial carcinoma.** Epithelioma; a squamous-celled carcinoma. **Carcinoma epitheliale adenoides.** A basal-celled carcinoma in which a glandular pattern is prominent. **Carcinoma epitheliale adenoides cysticum.** A form of carcinoma epitheliale adenoides (see preceding) in which cystic spaces are prominent. **Fibromedullary carcinoma.** A carcinoma in which equal amounts of fibrous stroma and cells are present. **Fibrous carcinoma.** Scirrhous carcinoma (see below). **Gelatiniform carcinoma.** Colloid carcinoma (see above). **Carcinoma gigantocellulare.** One in which giant cells are numerous, as in some carcinomata of the liver. **Glandular carcinoma.** Adenoid carcinoma (see above). **Granulosa-cell carcinoma.** A tumour of the ovary which is associated with sex disturbances. **Hair-matrix carcinoma.** A basal-celled carcinoma arising from hair or hair rudiments. **Hyaline carcinoma.** Colloid carcinoma (see above). **Carcinoma in situ.** Malignant change in the character of epithelial cells without spread beyond the epithelium. **Inflammatory carcinoma.** Acute carcinoma associated with inflammatory changes from the reaction of normal tissues. In the breast it is often mistaken for an abscess. **Intraduct carcinoma.** Term applied to the phase in the development of carcinoma in glandular organs in which the cells fill the lumen of the ducts but have not yet penetrated the duct walls. Used particularly in relation to the breast. **Intra-epithelial carcinoma.** Carcinoma *in situ* in which there are atypical mitotic figures in individual cells of an abnormal (e.g. leucoplakic) epithelium. **Lenticular carcinoma.** A variety of scirrhous carcinoma (see below). **Lipomatous carcinoma.** One in which fat cells are numerous within the substance of the tumour. **Carcinoma mastitoides.** A medullary carcinoma (see following) which on section resembles a cow's udder. **Medullary carcinoma.** Carcinoma in which there is a high proportion of cells and a small amount of fibrous tissue, so that the tumour has a relatively soft consistency. **Melanoid carcinoma.** Cutaneous malignant melanoma. **Melanotic carcinoma.** A pigmented carcinoma, most often derived from skin, and very malignant. **Carcinoma molle.** Medullary carcinoma (see above). **Mucinous carcinoma.** A glandular cancer whose cells secrete mucin; a special instance is the Krukenberg tumour of the ovaries. **Carcinoma muciparum.** Colloid carcinoma (see above). **Carcinoma mucocellulare.** Mucinous carcinoma (see above). **Muco-epidermoid carcinoma.** A histological variety of carcinoma occurring in both major and minor salivary glands, but chiefly in the parotid. Usually of an intermediate degree of malignancy. To be distinguished from adenocarcinoma with mucoid degeneration. **Mucous carcinoma.** Colloid carcinoma (see above). **Carcinoma myxomatodes.** A variety of colloid carcinoma (see above). **Carcinoma nigrum.** Melanotic carcinoma (see above). **Oat cell carcinoma.** A histological type of poorly differentiated carcinoma of the bronchus. **Carcinoma ossificans, Osteoid carcinoma.**

Calcifying epithelioma; one containing much bone or calcified material. **Papillary carcinoma, Papilliferous carcinoma.** A cancer that protrudes from a surface in the form of a nipple-shaped projection. **Postcricoid carcinoma.** One often associated with iron-deficiency dysphagia. **Carcinoma psammosum.** One containing stratified, and often calcified, concretions. **Pultaceous carcinoma.** Colloid carcinoma (see above). **Reticulated carcinoma.** A carcinoma with a very prominent stroma. **Carcinoma sarcoma, Sarcomatous carcinoma.** An adenocarcinoma in which the stroma has undergone sarcomatous transformation. **Scirrhous carcinoma.** A carcinoma characterized clinically by a hard consistency and histologically by abundant fibrous tissue among the masses of carcinoma cells. The common type of carcinoma of the breast. **Carcinoma scroti, Carcinoma scroti asbolicum.** Chimney-sweeps' carcinoma (see above). **Seeding carcinoma.** A spreading carcinoma. **Carcinoma solanoid.** One which resembles a potato in section. **Carcinoma spongiosum.** One showing large and small cavities in its substance. **Squamous carcinoma, Squamous-cell carcinoma.** A carcinoma derived from the squamous epithelium of the skin, or closely related epithelium in other situations such as the oesophagus or neck of the uterus. **Tar carcinoma.** Carcinoma resulting from the application of tar or other substances. **Carcinoma telangiectaticum, Carcinoma telangiectodes.** A carcinoma which shows large blood vessels, or spaces filled with blood. **Thymic carcinoma.** Thymoma; cancer of the thymus gland. **Transitional-cell carcinoma.** Cancer derived from transitional-cell epithelium such as bladder epithelium. **Tuberous carcinoma.** Carcinoma in which, as a result of irregular contraction of bands of fibrous tissue, the surface has a nodular appearance. **Carcinoma ex ulcere.** A carcinoma arising in a chronic ulcer. **Carcinoma ventriculi.** Cancer of the stomach. **Villous carcinoma.** One showing numerous papillary processes, so that it resembles a papilloma. [Gk *karkinos* crab, *-oma* tumour.]

See also: ALIBERT, KRUKENBERG (G. P. H.).

carcinomatoid (kar·sin·o·mat·oid). Having resemblance to carcinoma. [carcinoma, Gk *eidos* form.]

carcinomatophobia (kar·sin·o·mat·o·**fo**′·be·ah). Unfounded or unreasonable fear or morbid conviction that carcinoma will develop, or that there is predisposition to carcinoma. [carcinoma, phobia.]

carcinomatosis (**kar**·sin·o·mat·**o**′·sis). 1. The pathological condition which gives rise to the development of carcinoma. 2. The condition in which carcinoma is widely distributed throughout the body and is developing in several places simultaneously. **Acute carcinomatosis.** A form which runs a rapidly fatal course. **Acute miliary carcinomatosis.** A form in which small carcinomatous nodules develop rapidly on the surface of, or within, an internal organ. **Miliary carcinomatosis.** A form in which there is development of secondary nodules that resemble miliary tubercles. **Carcinomatosis pleurae.** Secondary carcinoma of the pleura in which many nodules develop. **Pulmonary carcinomatosis.** Diffuse epithelial hyperplasia of the bronchic and alveolar cells of the lungs without metastasis. [carcinoma, Gk *-osis* condition.]

carcinomatous (kar·sin·**o**·mat·us). Relating to, or descriptive of, carcinoma.

carcinomectomy (**kar**·sin·o·**mek**′·to·me). Carcinectomy.

carcinomelcosis (**kar**·sin·o·mel·**ko**′·sis). Carcinelcosis.

carcinophilia (kar·sin·o·**fil**′·e·ah). A term referring to the medium on which carcinomatous cells freely flourish; applied to local as well as to general structures. [carcinoma, Gk *philein* to love.]

carcinophilic (**kar**·sin·o·**fil**′·ik). Suitable for the development of carcinomatous tissue. [see prec.]

carcinophobia (**kar**·sin·o·**fo**′·be·ah). Carcinomatophobia.

carcinosarcoma (**kar**·sin·o·sar·**ko**′·mah). A neoplasm in which the elements of both carcinoma and sarcoma are to be found. **Embryonal carcinosarcoma.** Wilms' tumour.

carcinosectomy (**kar**·sin·o·**sek**′·to·me). Carcinectomy.

carcinosis (kar·sin·**o**·sis). Carcinomatosis.

carcinostatic (**kar**·sin·o·**stat**′·ik). Checking the growth of a carcinoma. [carcinoma, Gk *statos* standing.]

carcinous (**kar**·sin·us). Carcinomatous.

carcinus (**kar**·sin·us). Carcinoma.

cardamom (**kar**·dam·om). The dried, nearly ripe fruit (Cardamom Fruit BP 1973) of *Elettaria cardamomum* Maton, var. *minuscula* Burkill. (family Zingiberaceae), cultivated in Sri Lanka and South India, and of which there are 4 commercial varieties: Mysore, Malabar, Mangalore and Aleppy. The seeds only are used, and should be stored in the capsules until required: they contain a volatile oil which has carminative properties. Cardamom is largely used as a flavouring agent. **Long wild native cardamoms.** The fruits of *Elettaria cardamomum* var. *major* Thwaites and the source of commercial cardamom oil, used in liqueurs. **Oil of cardamom.** An oil containing terpineol and cineole, distilled from the whole fruits. [Gk *kardamomon.*]

Cardarelli, Antonio (b. 1831). Naples physician.

Cardarelli's aphthae. Cachectic ulcers.

Cardarelli's sign. Lateral pulsation of the trachea in aneurysm or aneurysmal dilatation of the aortic arch; also attributed to Castellino. Cf. OLIVER'S SIGN.

Carden, Henry Douglas (d. 1872). Worcester surgeon.

Carden's amputation, or operation. Amputation of the femur just above its condyles, with the use of an anterior flap containing the patella.

cardia (**kar**·de·ah). 1. The cardiac (oesophageal) orifice of the stomach. 2. Sometimes misused as a synonym for fundus of the stomach. 3. The heart. [Gk *kardia* heart.]

cardiac (**kar**·de·ak). 1. Relating to the heart. 2. Situated near the heart. 3. An individual suffering from some form of heart affection. 4. Referable to the cardiac end of the stomach. 5. Name given to a drug which by its effect on heart muscle improves tone and restores power to the heart generally. **Black cardiac.** A bronchitic person, with a mild degree of cardiac insufficiency and severe cyanosis. **Cardiac notch.** *See* NOTCH OF THE LUNG, NOTCH OF THE STOMACH. **Cardiac plexus.** *See* PLEXUS. [see prec.]

cardiac veins. Veins draining the wall of the heart. **Anterior cardiac veins [venae cordis anteriores (NA)].** Small vessels from the front of the right ventricle, which open directly into the right atrium. **Great cardiac vein [vena cordis magna (NA)].** A tributary of the coronary sinus, draining mainly the front of the heart. **Middle cardiac vein [vena cordis media (NA)].** A tributary of the coronary sinus, draining the diaphragmatic surfaces of the ventricle. **Small cardiac vein [vena cordis parva (NA)].** A tributary of the coronary sinus; it lies in the posterior atrioventricular groove, and drains the adjacent parts of the right atrium and ventricle.

cardiacos negros (kar·de·**ah**·kos **ne**·gros). Ayerza's disease. [Sp. of the heart, black.]

cardiagra (**kar**·de·**ag**·rah). Pain in the heart due to gout. [Gk *kardia* heart, *agra* a catching.]

cardial (**kar**·de·al). Relating to the cardia.

cardialgia (kar·de·**al**·je·ah). 1. Cardiodynia. 2. Heartburn. **Cardialgia icterica.** Heartburn occurring with jaundice. **Cardialgia inflammatoria.** Gastritis. **Cardialgia sputatoria.** Heartburn. [Gk *kardia* heart, *algos* pain.]

cardialgic (kar·de·**al**·jik). Referring to, or affected by, cardialgia.

cardiameter (kar·de·**am**·et·er). An instrument with which the position of the cardia may be determined, the datum line being taken as the biting edge of the incisor teeth. [cardia, meter.]

cardiamorphia (**kar**·de·am·**or**′·fe·ah). Cardiac malformation or deformity. [Gk *kardia* heart, *a-*, *morphe* form.]

cardianastrophe (**kar**·de·an·**as**′·tro·fe). Cardio-anastrophe.

cardiant (**kar**·de·ant). Any heart stimulant. [Gk *kardia* heart.]

cardiasthenia (**kar**·de·as·**the**′·ne·ah). An obsolete term used to describe the symptom-complex due to a cardiac neurosis. *See* SYNDROME, EFFORT. [Gk *kardia* heart, *asthenia* lack of strength.]

cardiataxia (**kar**·de·at·**ax**′·e·ah). An obsolete term used to denote irregular action of the heart. *See* ARRYTHMIA, CARDIAC. [Gk *kardia* heart, *ataxia* incoordination.]

cardicentesis (kar·de·sen·**te**'·sis). Cardiocentesis.

cardiectasis (kar·de·**ek**·tas·is). Cardiac dilatation. [Gk *kardia* heart, *ektasis* a stretching.]

cardiectomized (kar·de·**ek**·to·mi·zd). 1. Having had the cardiac portion of the stomach removed by surgical means. 2. Having had the heart removed. [see foll.]

cardiectomy (kar·de·**ek**·to·me). 1. Surgical removal of the cardiac portion of the stomach. 2. Removal of the heart. [Gk *kardia* heart, *ektome*, a cutting out.]

Cardiette (kar·de·**et**). A particular type of small portable electrocardiograph. [trade name.]

cardinal (**kar**·din·al). Fundamental; of primary importance, on which other things hinge. [L *cardo* hinge.]

cardio-accelerator (**kar**·de·o·ak·**sel**'er·a·tor). Any agent which speeds up the rate of the heart's action. [Gk *kardia* heart, L *accelerare* to make swift.]

cardio-active (kar·de·o·**ak**'·tiv). Acting on the heart. [Gk *kardia* heart, L *agere* to act.]

cardio-amorphia (**kar**·de·o·am·**or**'·fe·ah). Malformation or deformity of the heart. [Gk *kardia* heart, *a-*, *morphe* form.]

cardio-anastrophe (**kar**·de·o·an·**as**'·tro·fe). A heart congenitally right-sided. [Gk *kardia* heart, *anastrophe* a turning back.]

cardio-angiography (**kar**·de·o·an·je·**og**'·raf·e). Angiocardiography.

cardio-angiology (**kar**·de·o·an·je·**ol**'·o·je). That branch of medicine which is concerned with the heart and the vascular system. [Gk *kardia* heart, angiology.]

cardio-aortic (**kar**·de·o·a·**aw**'·tik). Referring to the heart and the aorta. [Gk *kardia* heart, aorta.]

cardio-arterial (**kar**·de·o·ar·**teer**'·e·al). Relating to the heart and the arteries. [Gk *kardia* heart, artery.]

cardio-asthenia (**kar**·de·o·as·**the**'·ne·ah). Cardiovascular neurasthenia. [Gk *kardia* heart, asthenia.]

cardio-ataxia (**kar**·de·o·at·**ax**'·e·ah). Inco-ordination or irregularity of the heart's action. [Gk *kardia* heart, ataxia.]

cardio-atelia (kar·de·o·at·**e**'·le·ah). Atelocardia; an incompletely developed state of the heart. [Gk *kardia* heart, *ateleia* incompleteness.]

cardio-atrophia (**kar**·de·o·at·**ro**'·fe·ah). Cardiac atrophy. [Gk *kardia* heart, atrophy.]

cardio-augmentor (**kar**·de·o·awg·**men**'·tor). An agent which increases the force or the strength of the heartbeat. [Gk *kardia* heart, L *augmentare* to increase.]

cardiocairograph (**kar**·de·o·**ki**'·ro·graf). An apparatus which synchronizes the taking of x-ray pictures of the heart with any selected phase of the cardiac cycle. [Gk *kardia* heart, *kairos* time, *graphein* to record.]

cardiocele (**kar**·de·o·seel). A protrusion or hernia of the heart through a wound or fissure in the diaphragm. **Cardiocele abdominalis.** Hernia of the heart into the abdomen. [Gk *kardia* heart, *kele* hernia.]

cardiocentesis (**kar**·de·o·sen·**te**'·sis). Operative incision or puncture of the heart for the purpose of relieving engorgement. [Gk *kardia* heart, *kentesis* a pricking.]

cardiocinetic (**kar**·de·o·sin·**et**'·ik). Cardiokinetic.

cardiocirrhosis (**kar**·de·o·sir·**o**'·sis). Cardiac cirrhosis; existence together of cardiac disease and cirrhosis of the liver. [Gk *kardia* heart, *kirrhos* orange yellow.]

cardioclasia, cardioclasis (**kar**·de·o·**kla**'·ze·ah, kar·de·**ok**·las·is). Rupture of the heart. [Gk *kardia* heart, *klasis* a breaking.]

cardiodilator (**kar**·de·o·di·**la**'·tor). An instrument with which the cardiac portion of the stomach can be dilated in cases of stricture or cardiospasm. [cardia, L *dilatare* to widen.]

cardiodiosis (**kar**·de·o·di·**o**'·sis). The procedure of dilating the cardiac portion of the stomach. [cardia, Gk *dia*, *osmos* a thrusting.]

cardiodynamics (**kar**·de·o·di·**nam**'·ix). The science or the branch of medicine which treats of the work and power inherent in the action of the heart. [Gk *kardia* heart, *dynamis* force.]

cardiodynia (**kar**·de·o·**din**'·e·ah). A sharp sensation of pain in the region of the heart or in the organ itself. [Gk *kardia* heart, *odyne* pain.]

cardiogenesis (**kar**·de·o·**jen**'·es·is). The formation and development of the embryonic heart. [Gk *kardia* heart, *genein* to produce.]

cardiogenic (**kar**·de·o·**jen**'·ik). Produced by or having origin in the heart. [see prec.]

cardiogmus (kar·de·**og**·mus). 1. Cardiac aneurysm. *See* ANEURYSM. 2. Angina pectoris. 3. Cardialgia. **Cardiogmus strumosis.** Exophthalmic goitre. *See* GOITRE. [Gk *kardia* heart, *ogmos* furrow.]

cardiognost (**kar**·de·og·nost). A psychiatrist who has made a study of the characteristic quality of the several emotions and through his knowledge may be able to bring to the surface of the patient's mind those deep-seated emotional distortions and suppressions inimical to his well-being. [Gk *kardia* heart, *gnosis* knowledge.]

cardiogram (**kar**·de·o·gram). Electrocardiogram; the curve traced by the style of a cardiograph, or by the galvanometer mirror of an electrocardiograph. **Apex cardiogram.** The record of the movements of the apex of the heart as detected through the chest wall. **Oesophageal cardiogram.** An electrocardiogram obtained by placing an electrode in the oesophagus near the posterior surface of the heart. **Vector cardiogram.** Vectorcardiogram; a cardiogram showing the direction of spread of the electrical forces generated by contraction of the heart. [Gk *kardia* heart, *gramma* record.]

cardiograph (**kar**·de·o·graf). A device which records the force and character of the heart's motion. **Apex cardiograph.** The instrument used to record the movements of the apex of the heart as detected through the chest wall. [Gk *kardia* heart, *graphein* to record.]

cardiographer (kar·de·**og**·raf·er). A person who may be specially qualified by skill or experience to make observations and records by the cardiograph.

cardiographic (**kar**·de·o·**graf**'·ik). Referring or belonging to cardiography.

cardiography (kar·de·**og**·raf·e). The recording of the force and character of the heart's action. **Apex cardiography.** The recording of the movements of the apex of the heart as detected through the chest wall. **Ultrasound cardiography.** Echocardiography. [Gk *kardia* heart, *graphein* to record.]

cardiohepatic (**kar**·de·o·hep·**at**'·ik). Belonging to the heart and liver. [Gk *kardia* heart, *hepar* liver.]

cardiohepatomegaly (**kar**·de·o·**hep**·at·o·**meg**'·al·e). Hypertrophy of the heart and the liver. [Gk *kardia* heart, hepatomegaly.]

cardioid (**kar**·de·oid). Like a heart. [Gk *kardia* heart, *eidos* form.]

cardio-inhibitory (**kar**·de·o·in·**hib**'·it·or·e). Term applied to any agent that slows or inhibits the motions of the heart. [Gk *kardia* heart, L *inhibere* to restrain.]

cardiokinetic (**kar**·de·o·kin·**et**'·ik). 1. A remedy which stimulates the action of the heart. 2. Stimulating to the heart. [Gk *kardia* heart, *kinesis* movement.]

cardiokymography (**kar**·de·o·ki·**mog**'·raf·e). Kymography. [Gk *kardia* heart, kymography.]

cardiolipin (**kar**·de·o·**lip**'·in). A substance extracted from fresh beef hearts, consisting of phosphorylated polysaccharide esters of fatty acids. It is capable of acting as an artificial antigen in serum tests for syphilis when activated with lecithin or cholesterol. [Gk *kardia* heart, *lipos* fat.]

cardiolith (**kar**·de·o·lith). An area of calcareous degeneration or a concretion in the heart; cardiac calculus. [Gk *kardia* heart, *lithos* stone.]

cardiologist (kar·de·**ol**·o·jist). A heart specialist and consultant; one who has made a special study of cardiology.

cardiology (kar·de·**ol**·o·je). The science which is concerned with the heart and its functions. [Gk *kardia* heart, *logos* science.]

cardiolysin (kar·de·**ol**·is·in). A lysin which has an effect on the muscles of the heart. [Gk *kardia* heart, *lysis* a loosing.]

cardiolysis (kar·de·**ol**·is·is). 1. Destruction of the substance of the heart. 2. In adhesive mediastinopericarditis—a form of chronic adhesive pericarditis—the freeing of the heart and pericardium by removal of several ribs and costal cartilages and division of the adhesions to the sternal periosteum. [see prec.]

cardiomalacia (kar·de·o·mal·**a**′·she·ah). Degeneration and softening of the muscular walls of the heart. [Gk *kardia* heart, *malakia* softness.]

cardiomegalia, cardiomegaly (kar·de·o·meg·**a**′·le·ah, **kar**·de·o·**meg**′·al·e). Cardiac enlargement due either to hypertrophy or to dilatation of one or more of the chambers. **Cardiomegalia glycogenica.** Glycogen disease complicated by involvement of the heart. [Gk *kardia* heart, *megas* large.]

cardiomelanosis (kar·de·o·mel·an·**o**′·sis). Melanosis of the heart muscle. [Gk *kardia* heart, melanosis.]

cardiomentopexy (kar·de·o·**men**′·to·pex·e). The surgical treatment of diseases of the heart such as angina pectoris by making an incision in the diaphragm, drawing a part of the omentum through and suturing it to the heart so that a collateral circulation is established. [Gk *kardia* heart, omentopexy.]

cardiometer (kar·de·**om**·et·er). An instrument with which the force of the heart's action and the volume of the pulse can be measured. [Gk *kardia* heart, meter.]

cardiometry (kar·de·**om**·et·re). 1. Measurement of the force of the heart's action or of the volume of the pulse. 2. Estimation by means of palpation, percussion and auscultation of the diameter of the heart. [see prec.]

cardiomotility (kar·de·o·mo·**til**′·it·e). 1. The power of movement of the heart. 2. The sum of movements of the heart. [Gk *kardia* heart, L *movere* to move.]

cardiomyoliposis (kar·de·o·mi·o·lip·**o**′·sis). Fatty degeneration of the musculature of the heart. [Gk *kardia* heart, *mys* muscle, *lipos* fat.]

cardiomyopathy (kar·de·o·mi·**op**′·ath·e). Literally, disease of the heart muscle, but usually restricted to diffuse myocardial disease not resulting from coronary arterial disease, and sometimes only to disease of unknown aetiology. Various classifications have been proposed but none is universally accepted. **Alcoholic cardiomyopathy.** Myocardial disease believed to result from the ingestion of alcohol. **Congestive cardiomyopathy.** Diffuse myocardial disease presenting as cardiac enlargement and failure. **Constrictive cardiomyopathy.** Myocardial disease presenting with features indicating diastolic compliance of the ventricles, thereby imitating constrictive pericarditis. **Dystrophic cardiomyopathy.** Myocardial disease occurring as part of a skeletal muscular dystrophic syndrome. **Familial cardiomyopathy.** Myocardial disease occurring familially; the most common form is hypertrophic cardiomyopathy (see below) but glycogen storage disease and other more obscure forms of myocardial disease also occur. **Hypertrophic cardiomyopathy.** Myocardial disease characterized by great hypertrophy which is usually not evenly distributed, the ventricular septum most often being chiefly affected. The condition occurs both familially and sporadically but its exact nature is not known. It presents in a variety of clinical forms, a common one being obstruction to the outflow of the left ventricle (*hypertrophic obstructive cardiomyopathy* or *idiopathic hypertrophic subaortic stenosis*). **Inflammatory cardiomyopathy.** Myocardial disease characterized by an inflammatory reaction in the tissue, usually excluding rheumatic carditis. The aetiology is usually unknown but it can result from viral infection. **Jamaican cardiomyopathy.** A form of heart disease found in Jamaica which may present with atrioventricular valve incompetence stimulating ischaemic heart disease, features simulating constrictive pericarditis or as stenotic heart valve disease. It resembles endomyocardial fibrosis in some respects but differs from it in that the heart is generally larger in the Jamaican disease and mural thrombosis is less common. The aetiology is uncertain. **Non-coronary cardiomyopathy.** Myocardial disease resulting from some cause, known or unknown, other than coronary arterial disease. **Puerperal cardiomyopathy.** Myocardial disease with its onset shortly after childbirth; its existence as a true entity distinct from other forms of cardiomyopathy is disputed, but the aetiology in the described cases is unknown. **Restrictive cardiomyopathy.** Constrictive cardiomyopathy (see above). [Gk *kardia* heart, *mys* muscle, *pathos* disease.]

cardiomyopexy (kar·de·o·**mi**′·o·pex·e). An operation devised to improve the blood supply to the myocardium in coronary ischaemia (angina pectoris) by fixing the pectoral muscles directly to the heart. [Gk *kardia* heart, *mys* muscle, *pexis* a fixation.]

cardiomyotomy (kar·de·o·mi·**ot**′·o·me). Longitudinal division of the muscle of the lower end of the oesophagus down to, but not including, the mucous membrane, as in the Ramstedt operation for pyloric stenosis. The term is misleading and should be avoided. [cardiac sphincter, Gk *mys* muscle, *temnein* to cut.]

cardionecrosis (kar·de·o·nek·**ro**′·sis). Gangrene or necrosis affecting the tissues of the heart. [Gk *kardia* heart, necrosis.]

cardionecteur, cardionector (kar·de·o·**nek**′·ter, **kar**·de·o·**nek**′·tor). The structures which act as regulators of the heartbeat; the sinu-atrial node and the atrioventricular bundle (bundle of His). The first governs the atrial contraction and the second the ventricular contraction. [Gk *kardia* heart, L *nector* joiner.]

cardionephric (kar·de·o·**nef**′·rik). Referring to or involving the heart and the kidneys. [Gk *kardia* heart, *nephros* kidney.]

cardioneural (kar·de·o·**newr**′·ral). Relating to the heart and the nervous system. [Gk *kardia* heart, *neuron* nerve.]

cardioneurosis (kar·de·o·newr·**o**′·sis). Disturbance of normal activity of the heart, so that symptoms of palpitation, irregularity, shortness of breath, suffocation, flushing of the face and fear of death are produced. Other names: *pseudo-angina, cardiac neurasthenia.* [Gk *kardia* heart, neurosis.]

cardio-oesophageal (kar·de·o·e·sof·ah·**je**′·al). Relating to the cardia of the stomach and the oesophagus. [Gk *kardia* heart, *oisophagos* gullet.]

cardio-omentopexy (kar·de·o·o·**men**′·to·pex·e). Cardiomentopexy.

cardiopalmus (kar·de·o·**pal**′·mus). Palpitation of the heart. [Gk *kardia* heart, *palmos* palpitation.]

cardiopaludism (kar·de·o·**pal**′·ew·dizm). Heart disease resulting from invasion of that organ during an attack of malaria by *Plasmodium falciparum* so that there is internal sporulation and localized blocking of the capillaries. Degenerative myocardial changes mark the syndrome, which occasions breathlessness, congestive cardiac failure and cyanosis, and results occasionally in sudden death. The main signs are gallop rhythm, irregularity of pulse and dilatation of the right side of the heart. [Gk *kardia* heart, paludism.]

cardiopath (kar·de·o·path). A subject with heart disease. [Gk *kardia* heart, *pathos* disease.]

cardiopathia (kar·de·o·**path**·e·ah). Cardiopathy.

cardiopathic (kar·de·o·**path**′·ik). Referring to, or characterized by disease or disorder of the heart. [Gk *kardia* heart, *pathos* disease.]

cardiopathology (kar·de·o·path·**ol**′·o·je). Cardiology. [Gk *kardia* heart, pathology.]

cardiopathy (kar·de·**op**·ath·e). Collective term to include all diseases and disorders of the heart. **Arteriosclerotic cardiopathy.** Disease due to hardening of the arteries. **Fatty cardiopathy.** Disease due to fatty infiltration of the tissues of the heart. **Hypertensive cardiopathy.** Disease due to high arterial blood pressure. **Nephropathic cardiopathy.** Disease resulting from disorder of the kidneys. **Thyrotoxic cardiopathy.** Disease due to dysfunction of the thyroid gland. **Toxic cardiopathy.** Disease due to the action of toxins on the heart. **Valvular cardiopathy.** Disease resulting from affections of the valves of the heart. [Gk *kardia* heart, *pathos* disease.]

cardiopericardiopexy (kar·de·o·per·e·**kar**′·de·o·pex·e). One treatment of disease of the coronary arteries by establishing artificial (surgical) pericarditis; the pericardium and the heart become adherent and the cardiac muscle is thus supplied with an emergency vascular system. [Gk *kardia* heart, pericardium, Gk *pexis* fixation.]

cardiopericarditis (kar·de·o·**per**·e·kar·**di**′·tis). An inflammatory condition affecting both heart and pericardium. [Gk *kardia* heart, pericarditis.]

cardiophobia (**kar**·de·o·**fo**′·be·ah). Fear amounting to a phobia of falling a victim to heart disease. [Gk *kardia* heart, phobia.]

cardiophone (**kar**·de·o·fone). An instrument specially devised and used for the study of the sound made by the heart musculature at various stages of its activity. [Gk *kardia* heart, *phone* sound.]

cardiophrenia (**kar**·de·o·**fre**′·ne·ah). Cardiovascular neurasthenia. [Gk *kardia* heart, *phren* mind.]

cardioplasty (**kar**·de·o·**plas**′·te). The relief of achalasia of the cardia (stomach) by a plastic operative procedure. [Gk *kardia* heart, *plassein* to mould.]

cardioplegia (**kar**·de·o·**ple**′·je·ah). 1. Cardiac paralysis. 2. Direct injury to the heart as the result of trauma. [Gk *kardia* heart, *plege* stroke.]

cardiopneumatic (**kar**·de·o·new·**mat**′·ik). Referring to the heart and the respiration. [Gk *kardia* heart, *pneuma* breath.]

cardiopneumograph (**kar**·de·o·**new**′·mo·graf). An instrument which traces on a graph the movements of the heart and of respiration. [Gk *kardia* heart, pneumograph.]

cardiopneumonopexy (**kar**·de·o·**new**·mon·o·**pex**′·e). An operation aimed at improving the blood supply to the myocardium in the treatment of coronary ischaemia (angina pectoris) by bringing the heart into close proximity with the lung. [Gk *kardia* heart, *pneumon* lung, *pexis* a fixation.]

cardioptosia (**kar**·de·op·**to**′·se·ah). Cardioptosis.

cardioptosis (**kar**·de·op·**to**′·sis). A condition in which the heart is displaced downward. [Gk *kardia* heart, *ptosis* fall.]

cardiopulmonary, cardiopulmonic (**kar**·de·o·**pul**′·mon·ar·e, **kar**·de·o·pul·**mon**′·ik). Relating to the heart and lungs. [Gk *kardia* heart, pulmonary.]

cardiopuncture (**kar**·de·o·**pungk**′·tcher). 1. Cardiocentesis. 2. Any surgical or other puncture of the heart in a living subject. [Gk *kardia* heart, puncture.]

cardiopyloric (**kar**·de·o·pi·**lor**′·ik). Referring to both the cardiac and the pyloric portions of the stomach. [Gk *kardia* heart, pylorus.]

cardiorenal (**kar**·de·o·**re**′·nal). Relating to the heart and the kidneys. [Gk *kardia* heart, L *ren* kidney.]

cardiorespiratory (**kar**·de·o·res·**pir**′·at·or·e). Relating to the heart and the respiratory system. [Gk *kardia* heart, respiratory.]

cardiorrhaphy (kar·de·**or**·af·e). Surgical suture of the muscle of the heart. [Gk *kardia* heart, *rhaphe* suture.]

cardiorrheuma (**kar**·de·o·**roo**′·mah). Rheumatism affecting the heart. [Gk *kardia* heart, *rheuma* flux.]

cardiorrhexis (**kar**·de·o·**rex**′·is). Rupture of the heart. [Gk *kardia* heart, *rhexis* rupture.]

cardioschisis (kar·de·**os**·kis·is). A method of treatment of adhesive pericarditis which consists in the breaking-down of the adhesions between the heart and the wall of the thorax. [Gk *kardia* heart, *schisis* division.]

cardiosclerosis (**kar**·de·o·skler·o′·sis). The so-called fibroid heart; hardening of the cardiac tissues by development of fibroid elements. [Gk *kardia* heart, *skleros* hard.]

cardioscope (**kar**·de·o·skope). An instrument by means of which the interior of the heart may be examined. [Gk *kardia* heart, *skopein* to watch.]

cardiospasm (**kar**·de·o·spazm). Muscular spasm occurring at the lower end of the oesophagus. [Gk *kardia* heart, spasm.]

cardiosphygmogram (**kar**·de·o·**sfig**′·mo·gram). The record of movements of the heart made on paper by the style of a cardiosphygmograph. [see foll.]

cardiosphygmograph (**kar**·de·o·**sfig**′·mo·graf). An instrument which records on paper the movements of the heart simultaneously with those of the pulse of the radial artery. [Gk *kardia* heart, *sphygmos* pulse, *graphein* to record.]

cardiostenosis (**kar**·de·o·sten·**o**′·sis). Development of a constriction of the heart, especially of the infundibulum. [Gk *kardia* heart, *stenosis* a narrowing.]

cardiosurgery (**kar**·de·o·**ser**′·jer·e). Surgery of the heart. [Gk *kardia* heart, surgery.]

cardiosymphysis (**kar**·de·o·**sim**′·fis·is). Cardiac symphysis. *See* SYMPHYSIS.

cardiotachometer (**kar**·de·o·tak·**om**′·et·er). An instrument by which the total number of the heart beats can be counted over a long period of time during which the subject is allowed to be active. [Gk *kardia* heart, *tachos* speed, meter.]

cardiotherapy (**kar**·de·o·**ther**′·ap·e). Treatment of cardiac disease. [Gk *kardia* heart, therapy.]

cardiothyrotoxicosis (**kar**·de·o·**thi**·ro·tox·e·**ko**′·sis). Hypothyroidism complicated by severe heart disease or disorder. [Gk *kardia* heart, thyrotoxicosis.]

cardiotomy (kar·de·**ot**·o·me). 1. The making of an incision into the heart. 2. The division of the cardiac portion of the stomach in order to relieve stricture of the oesophagus. [Gk *kardia* heart, *temnein* to cut.]

cardiotonic (**kar**·de·o·**ton**′·ik). Having a stimulating effect on the heart; term applied to any substance or form of treatment with this action. [Gk *kardia* heart, *tonos* tone.]

cardiotopography (**kar**·de·o·to·**pog**′·raf·e). The topographical anatomy of the heart and the region around it. [Gk *kardia* heart, topography.]

cardiotopometry (**kar**·de·o·to·**pom**′·et·re). The measuring of the area of cardiac dullness. [Gk *kardia* heart, *topos* place, meter.]

cardiotoxic (**kar**·de·o·**tox**′·ik). Having a poisonous effect on the heart. [Gk *kardia* heart, *toxikon* poison.]

cardiovalvulotomy (**kar**·de·o·val·vew·**lot**′·o·me). More usually, valvulotomy; a method of treatment of stenosis of the heart valves (especially the mitral) by its blind rupture with finger dilatation, or by its division by a specially devised cutting instrument, a valvulotome. [Gk *kardia* heart, valve, Gk *temnein* to cut.]

cardiovascular (**kar**·de·o·**vas**′·kew·lar). Relating to the cardiovascular system. [Gk *kardia* heart, L *vasculum* little vessel.]

cardiovasology (**kar**·de·o·vas·**ol**′·o·je). Cardio-angiology. [Gk *kardia* heart, L *vas* vessel, Gk *logos* science.]

cardioversion (**kar**·de·o·**ver**′·shun). The process of converting the heart from an abnormal rhythm (most commonly atrial fibrillation) to normal sinus rhythm; defibrillation. [Gk *kardia* heart, L *vertere* to turn.]

cardioverter (**kar**·de·o·ver·ter). An instrument used to convert the heart from an abnormal rhythm (most commonly atrial fibrillation) to normal sinus rhythm; a d.c. current defibrillator. [Gk *kardia* heart, L *vertere* to turn.]

cardipericarditis (**kar**·de·per·e·kar·**di**′·tis). Cardiopericarditis.

carditis (kar·**di**·tis). A state of inflammation of any constituent of the heart, but generally involving any 2 of the following structures: endocardium, myocardium, pericardium. **Internal carditis.** Endocarditis. **Rheumatic carditis.** Carditis associated with acute rheumatism. [Gk *kardia* heart, *-itis* inflammation.]

See also: STERGES.

Carduus benedictus (**kar**·dew·us ben·e·**dik**·tus). Blessed thistle, the compositous herb *Cnicus benedictus* Linn. (*Carduus benedictus* Steud.), of Europe and North America. It has been used as a bitter tonic. [L.]

carene (**kar**·een). $C_{10}H_{16}$, a terpene hydrocarbon occurring in Indian turpentine.

Carfecillin (kar·fe·**sil**·in). BP Commission approved name for 6-(α-phenoxycarbonylphenylacetamido)-penicillanic acid; an antibiotic.

Cargile, Charles H. (b. 1853). American surgeon.

Cargile's membrane. Membrane composed of prepared ox peritoneum and used with the object of preventing peritoneal adhesions.

caribi (kar·**e**·be). Epidemic gangrenous proctitis, rectitis. [*Carib*, inhabitant of southern West Indian Islands.]

Carica (**kar**·ik·ah). 1. A genus of plants of the family Caricaceae. The juice of the unripe fruit of the tropical papaw, *Carica* *papaya* Linn., yields the proteolytic mixture of enzymes known as papain, which is sometimes used to assist protein digestion in dyspepsia. 2. The fig, the dried fruit of *Ficus carica* Linn. (family Moraceae). [L dried fig.]

caricin (kar·is·in). Papain BPC 1954; a proteolytic enzyme or mixture of enzymes obtained from the unripe fruit of *Carica papaya.* It is a white or light-brown powder, used as an aid to protein digestion when the natural ferments are deficient, as in pancreatic disease, and also in the manufacture of proteolysed liver preparations.

caricous (kar·ik·us). 1. Fig-shaped. 2. Resembling a fig in appearance; applied particularly to tumours. [L *carica* dried fig.]

caries (ka·reez). A gradual decay or death of bone as a result of chronic infection, usually tuberculous. The bone is gradually eroded by the infective granulation tissue. **Caries acuta.** Caries humida (see below). **Arrested caries.** Dental caries which produces collapse of the enamel on the occlusal surface of a tooth whereby the self-cleansing area which is produced presents conditions inhibitive to the progress of the carious process. It usually occurs in first permanent molar teeth, accompanied by staining. **Caries articulorum.** Caries affecting the articular end of a bone. **Backward caries.** Dental caries which, having penetrated the enamel along a narrow path as far as the dentine, spreads along the amelodentinal junction and invades the overlying enamel from its deep aspect; secondary enamel decay. **Central caries.** A central patch of necrotic bone. **Dental caries.** The process of invasion of the calcified tissues of a tooth by micro-organisms, producing softening and disintegration. **Dry caries.** Caries of the bone unaccompanied by pus formation. **Caries fungosa.** A form of tuberculosis of a bone. **Caries humida.** A moist type of dental caries which invades the tooth rapidly and usually produces exposure of the tooth pulp; caries acuta. **Necrotic caries.** A disease in which pieces of bone lie in a suppurating cavity. **Primary caries.** Dental caries which attacks either the pits and fissures, or the smooth surfaces of a tooth. **Caries sicca.** 1. Dry caries (see above). 2. A dry type of dental caries which, because of its slow progress, allows the tooth pulp to lay down a protective barrier of secondary dentine. **Spinal caries.** Tuberculous osteitis of the vertebrae and of the intervertebral cartilages. **Caries tuberculosa.** Caries due to tuberculosis of the bone. [L decay.]

See also: POTT.

carina (kar·i·nah). Any keel-like prominence or ridge. **Carina tracheae** [NA]. The triangular hook-shaped process which separates the two bronchi at the bifurcation of the trachea. [L keel.]

carinamide (kar·in·am·ide). Caronamide.

Carindacillin (kar·in·dah·sil·in). BP Commission approved name for 6-(α-indan-5-yloxycarbonylphenylacetamido)-penicillanic acid; an antibiotic.

cariosity (ka·re·os·it·e). The state of being carious. [L *caries* decay.]

carious (ka·re·us). Decaying; affected with caries.

Carisoprodol (kar·i·so·pro′·dol). BP Commission approved name for 2-carbamoylmethyl-2-*N*-isopropylcarbamoyloxy-methylpentane; a skeletal muscle relaxant.

Carlens, E. Scandinavian laryngologist.

Carlens' tube. A double-lumen tube, originally devised for differential bronchospirometry but also used in thoracic anaesthesia.

Carleton, Bukk G. (b. 1856). New York physician.

Carleton's spots. Localized areas of osteosclerosis occurring in chronic gonococcal infection.

carmalum (karm·al·um). A solution containing carminic acid (1 per cent solution) and potassium alum (10 per cent solution) used for bulk staining of embryos and for thick histological sections. It chiefly stains nuclear chromatin. Also called *Mayer's carmalum.*

Carman, Russell Daniel (b. 1875). American physician.

Carman's sign. Meniscus sign. *See* SIGN. The sign is attributed in the UK to *Kirklin* and not to *Carman.*

Carmichael, John P. (b. 1856). Milwaukee dentist.

Carmichael crown. A crown in which only the inner aspect of the natural crown of a tooth is artificially replaced; a three-quarter crown.

carminative (kar·min·at·iv). A drug which is used to facilitate the eructation of gas from the stomach. The active principle is usually a volatile oil, which has a pleasant flavour and serves the double purpose of relieving flatulence and rendering the medicine more palatable. Carminatives produce a mild irritation, promoting vascularity and relaxing the cardiac orifice of the stomach. The most important are: anethum (dill), which is a constituent of the familiar gripe mixture given to babies; peppermint oil, which contains menthol and stimulates the nerve-endings sensitive to cold; aniseed, reputed to have an expectorant action in addition to its carminative effect; caraway, cardamom seeds (usually used in the form of the tincture), cloves and ginger. [L *carminare* to cleanse.]

carmine (kar·mine). A natural colour derived from the cochineal insect, and the first stain to be used for microscopic work. It is combined with alum and the resulting co-ordination compound is a nuclear stain (BPC 1968). **Ammonia carmine.** A solution of carmine in ammonia used for bulk injection. **Borax carmine.** Borax and carmine used as a nuclear stain. **Indigo carmine.** *See* INDIGO. **Lithium carmine.** Orth's solution. **Magnesia carmine.** Used for bulk injection. **Carmine red.** $C_{11}H_{12}O_7$, a red stain derived from carmine. [Ar. *qirmize.*]

See also: GRENACHER.

carminophil (kar·min·o·fil). 1. Refers to a cell or tissue which easily takes the carmine stain. 2. Suitable for staining with carmine. [carmine, Gk *philein* to love.]

carnal knowledge (kar·nal nol·ij). Sexual connection or partial sexual connection with some degree of penetration. [L *caro* flesh, knowledge.]

carnallite (kar·nal·ite). The mineral potassium magnesium chloride, $KClMgCl_2{\cdot}6H_2O$, found in the Stassfurt salt deposits. [B. von *Carnall,* 19th century German mineralogist.]

carnauba (kar·naw·bah). The Brazilian palm, *Copernicia cerifera* Mart.; also its root, used medicinally in Brazil. **Carnauba wax.** The yellowish or greenish wax obtained from the surfaces of the leaves of this palm. It has a melting point of 83–86°C and is used in the manufacture of candles, varnishes and polishes. [Port. from S. Amer. Indian.]

carnaubanol (kar·naw·ban·ol). Carnaubyl alcohol, $CH_3(CH_2)_{23}OH$. A white solid occurring in lanolin and carnauba wax.

carneous (kar·ne·us). Fleshy; consisting of or like flesh. [L *carneus* of flesh.]

Carnett's sign. The abdomen is palpated whilst the patient contracts his anterior abdominal muscles; if tenderness is then present, it is produced by a lesion of the abdominal wall, but if palpated when the muscles are relaxed, tenderness may be due to a parietal or intra-abdominal lesion. If tenderness is present when the muscles are either relaxed or tense, it is due to a parietal lesion outside the abdominal cavity.

carniferrin (kar·nif·er·in). A compound of iron and phosphocarnic acid, of uncertain composition and formerly used as a tonic. [L *caro* flesh, *ferrum* iron.]

carnification (kar·nif·e·ka′·shun). The morbid process of turning to flesh or to a substance like flesh. It may occur in the tissues of some organs, e.g. the lung. [L *caro* flesh, *facere* to make.]

carnine (kar·neen). $C_7H_8N_4O_3{\cdot}H_2O$, a purine body found in meat extract. [L *caro* flesh.]

carnitine (kar·nit·een). $(CH_3)_3N^+(OH)CH_2CHOHCH_2COOH$, an intracellular metabolite involved in lipid metabolism and, in particular, in the transport of fatty acyl units across the mitochondrial membrane. **Acetyl carnitine.** Formed from acetyl CoA and carnitine by the action of carnitine acetyl transferase.

Carnivora (kar·niv·or·ah). An order of flesh-eating mammals. [L *caro* flesh, *vorare* to devour.]

carnivorous (kar·niv·or·us). Eating flesh habitually. [see prec.]

Carnochan, John Murray (b. 1817). New York surgeon.

Carnochan's operation. For the relief of trigeminal neuralgia:

removal of the semilunar ganglion and part of the trigeminal nerve by way of the maxillary antrum.

carnophobia (kar·no·fo·be·ah). Strong aversion to eating meat. [L *caro* flesh, phobia.]

carnosinaemia (kar·no·seen·e′·me·ah). A condition found rarely in mentally-defective epileptic children deficient in carnosinase which hydrolyses carnosine to histidine and β-alanine. [carnosine, Gk *haima* blood.]

carnosine (kar·no·seen). β-Alanylhistidine, an extractive of muscle of unknown significance. It is a dipeptide with formula $C_3N_2H_3CH_2CH(COOH)NHCOCH_2CH_2NH_2$.

carnosity (kar·nos·it·e). Any abnormal fleshy growth or excrescence. [L *carneus* of flesh.]

carnotite (kar·no·tite). A naturally occurring vanadate of uranium and potassium, and one of the principal ores from which radium is obtained.

Caro, Heinrich (b. 1834). German chemist.

Caro's acid. Peroxymonosulphuric acid. *See* ACID.

caroba (kar·o·bah). The leaves of *Jacaranda procera* Spreng. (family Bignoniaceae), used in Brazil as a cathartic and an alternative, and a popular remedy for venereal diseases.

caronamide (kar·on·am·ide). $C_6H_5CH_2SO_2NHC_6H_4COOH$, a compound formerly used to enhance the penicillin level in the blood by preventing tubular excretion, but now replaced by procaine penicillin.

carone (kar·one). $C_{10}H_{16}O$, a ketone of the carane group of bridged terpenes, found in peppermint oil; a colourless oil with a camphor smell.

Caronia, Giuseppe (b. 1884). Rome paediatrician.

Caronia's vaccine. An obsolete vaccine suggested for scarlet-fever prophylaxis.

carony bark (kar·o·nee bark). Angostura bark. [*Caroni*, Venezuelan river.]

carotenaemia (kar·ot·en·e′·me·ah). The condition in which there is carotene in the circulating blood; its presence may be shown by a yellow tinge of the skin resembling that present in jaundice. [L *carota* carrot, Gk *haima* blood.]

carotenase (kar·ot·en·aze). An enzyme which activates the splitting of the carotene molecule into vitamin A.

carotene (kar·ot·een). $C_{40}H_{56}$, a complex unsaturated hydrocarbon occurring as a pigment in carrots. It exists in 3 forms: α-carotene, an optically-active form; β-carotene, occurring also in palm kernel oil, red pepper and spinach; and γ-carotene, rarer in plants but present in certain bacteria. In the body they are to be found in the fat, serum and nerve tissue, and are converted by the liver into vitamin A. [L *carota* carrot.]

carotenodermia (kar·ot·en·o·der′·me·ah). Yellow coloration of the skin due to ingestion of carotene. [carotene, Gk *derma* skin.]

carotenoid (kar·ot·en·oid). 1. Having a yellow colour like that of carotene. 2. A name for a group of carotene-like plant pigments found in animal tissues. [L *carota* carrot, Gk *eidos* form.]

carotenosis (kar·ot·en·o′·sis). A pigmented condition of the skin due to the presence of carotene in the tissues. [L *carota* carrot, Gk *-osis* condition.]

carotic (kar·ot·ik). Referring or relating to a state of stupor; characterized by stupor. [Gk *karos* heavy sleep.]

caroticoclinoid (kar·ot·ik·o·kli′·noid). Relating to the internal carotid artery and the anterior clinoid process of the sphenoid bone.

caroticotympanic (kar·ot·ik·o·tim·pan′·ik). Referring to the carotid canal and the middle ear (tympanic cavity), or involving them.

caroticotympanic nerves [nervi caroticotympanici (NA)]. Twigs, superior and inferior, from the carotid sympathetic plexus to the tympanic plexus.

carotid (kar·ot·id). 1. The single arterial trunk in the lower part of the neck, the common carotid artery, which divides at the level of the upper border of the thyroid cartilage into the internal and external carotid arteries. 2. Relating to or situated near one of the carotid arteries. **Carotid groove.** *See* GROOVE. **Carotid plexus.** *See* PLEXUS. **Carotid sinus.** *See* SINUS. **Carotid siphon.** *See* SIPHON. **Carotid tubercle.** *See* TUBERCLE. [Gk *karos* heavy sleep.]

carotid arteries. Common carotid artery [arteria carotis communis (NA)]. The main artery of the neck, arising from the innominate artery on the right side and the arch of the aorta on the left. It divides at the level of the upper border of the thyroid cartilage into the internal and external carotid arteries. **External carotid artery [arteria carotis externa (NA)].** The smaller of the terminal divisions of the common carotid artery. It has multiple branches supplying the face and scalp, neck, mouth and contents, nose, submandibular and pterygoid regions, and terminates by dividing into the superficial temporal and maxillary arteries. **Internal carotid artery [arteria carotis interna (NA)].** The larger of the terminal divisions of the common carotid artery. It enters the skull through the carotid canal, runs through the cavernous sinus and, after giving off the ophthalmic artery, ends by dividing into the anterior and middle cerebral arteries. It supplies most of the cerebrum, the eyeball and its appendages, the forehead and nose, and the middle ear [ramus caroticotympanicus (NA)].

carotid nerves. External carotid nerves [nervi carotici externi (NA)]. Branches from the superior cervical sympathetic ganglion to the external carotid artery, where they form a plexus on the wall of the vessels. **Internal carotid nerve [nervus caroticus internus (NA)].** The sympathetic postganglionic fibres from the superior cervical ganglion which enter the skull with the internal carotid artery. It forms the internal carotid plexus in the carotid canal.

carotidynia (kar·ot·e·din′·e·ah). Carotodynia.

carotin (kar·ot·in). Carotene.

carotinaemia (kar·ot·in·e′·me·ah). Carotenaemia.

carotinase (kar·ot·in·aze). Carotenase.

carotinoid (kar·ot·in·oid). Carotenoid.

carotinosis cutis (kar·ot·in·o′·sis kew·tis). Aurantiasis cutis. [L *carota* carrot, Gk *-osis* condition, L *cutis* skin.]

carotodynia (kar·ot·o·din′·e·ah). Pain occurring in the maxillary region round the eyes and about the back of the neck, caused by pressure on the common carotid artery. [carotid, Gk *odyne* pain.]

carpagra (kar·pag·rah). A condition of painful spasm of the wrist, in which there is sudden seizure of the nature of acute cramp. [Gk *karpos* wrist, *agra* a catching.]

carpal (kar·pal). 1. Relating to or involving the carpus. 2. Relating to the wrist. [Gk *karpos* wrist.]

carpal bone [os carpi (NA)]. One of the wrist bones.

carpale (kar·pa·le) (pl. *carpalia*). Common term for any of the bones which constitute the carpus; a carpal bone. [Gk *karpos* wrist.]

carpectomy (kar·pek·to·me). Surgical removal of one or more of the carpal bones. [Gk *karpos* wrist, *ektome* a cutting out.]

carpel (kar·pel). In botany, that part of a flower which bears the ovules and the stigma. [Gk *karpos* fruit.]

Carperidine (kar·per·id·een). BP Commission approved name for ethyl-1-(2-carbamoylethyl)-4-phenylpiperidine-4-carboxylate; a cough suppressant.

Carphenazine (kar·fen·az·een). BP Commission approved name for 10-{3-[4-(2-hydroxyethyl)piperazin-1-yl]propyl}-2-propionylphenothiazine; a tranquillizer.

carphologia, carphology (kar·fol·o·je·ah, kar·fol·o·je). Floccilation; a sign typical of the typhoid state in which there is *inter alia* picking at the bedclothes. [Gk *karphos* chaff, *legein* to pick up.]

carpocarpal (kar·po·kar·pal). 1. Relating to 2 parts of the carpus. 2. Midcarpal; a term applied to the articulation between the 2 rows of carpal bones. [Gk *karpos* wrist.]

Carpoglyphus (kar·po·gli·fus). A genus of mites, including *Carpoglyphus lactis* (= *passularum*), which is restricted to dried fruits, and may cause grocers' itch. Mites of this genus have been found in sputum. [Gk *karpos* fruit, *glyphein* to carve.]

carpokyphosis (kar·po·ki·fo′·sis). Madelung's deformity. [Gk *karpos* wrist, kyphosis.]

carpometacarpal (kar·po·met·ah·kar′·pal). Relating to the carpus and the metacarpus, or involving them. **Carpometacarpal joint.** *See* JOINT.

carpopedal (kar·po·ped·al). Relating to the wrist and the foot, e.g. any of the structures of the carpus and tarsus or any of the fingers and toes. [Gk *karpos* wrist, L *pes* foot.]

carpophalangeal (kar·po·fal·an′·je·al). Relating to or involving the carpus and the phalanges.

carpoptosis (kar·po·to′·sis). Wrist drop. [Gk *karpos* wrist, *ptosis* fall.]

carpotroche braziliense (kar·po·tro·ke braz·il·e·en·se). An oil from Brazil used like chaulmoogra oil in leprosy.

Carpue, Joseph Constantine (b. 1746). London surgeon.

Carpue's operation. A rhinoplasty operation, sometimes called the Indian method.

carpus [NA] (kar·pus). 1. The wrist. 2. The structure composed of the 8 carpal bones taken together. **Carpus curvus.** Madelung's deformity. [Gk *karpos*.]

Carr, Francis Howard (b. 1874). London chemist.

Carr-Price test. For vitamin A: a transient blue colour is given by vitamin A when 0.2 ml of a chloroform solution containing the vitamin is mixed with 2 ml of chloroform saturated with antimony trichloride.

Carr-Price unit. A colour equal to 1 Lovibond blue unit given by 0.04 g of sample in 0.2 ml of solvent when mixed with 2 ml of antimony trichloride reagent shows unit vitamin A potency. The Carr-Price blue value may be converted to International Units per gram by multiplying by a factor which varies according to the material under examination, e.g. 32 for cod-liver oil, 23 for refined whale products.

carrageen, carragheen (kar·ag·een, kar·ag·heen). Chondrus BPC 1959, Irish moss: the dried red alga *Chondrus crispus* Stackh. (family Gigartinaceae), found mainly on the coasts of north-west Ireland, Brittany and Massachusetts. It is a brownish-purple substance (creamy-yellow when bleached), used as a demulcent, an emulsifying agent for cod-liver oil and a gum substitute, and in the preparation of nutrient jellies. [Irish *carraigeen* moss of the rock.]

carreau (kar·o). An enlarged and indurated condition of the abdomen as the result of disease of the walls and of the peritoneum. [Fr. hassock.]

Carrel, Alexis (b. 1873). New York surgeon.

Carrel flask. A flat, round, glass flask with a side arm, used for culturing cells. It has largely been superseded by Petri dishes.

Carrel method, or treatment. A method of treatment of wounds which was widely practised in World War I and which involved the free irrigation of wounds with hypochlorite solution introduced into their depths by a series of fine tubes (Carrel-Dakin tubes).

Carrel's mixture. A preparation consisting of soft paraffin, hard paraffin, beeswax, and castor oil, used for holding grafts in place on ulcerated surfaces.

Carrel tube, Carrel-Dakin tube. *See* CARREL METHOD.

Dakin-Carrel method. Carrel method (see above).

Carrel-Lindbergh perfusion apparatus. An apparatus for keeping alive intact organs, such as thyroid gland or kidney, after removal from the body.

carrier (kar·e·er). 1. An individual, without signs or symptoms, who carries the causal organisms of an infectious disease in some part of his body, either as the result of an attack of this disease or without having suffered from it, and who sheds the pathogens in his discharges, e.g. faeces, urine, throat, secretions. 2. A healthy person who similarly carries a hereditary disease trait. 3. A chemical substance used in conjunction with a toxoid or vaccine in order to improve its immunizing properties. 4. In biochemistry, any compound capable of undergoing reversible oxidation-reduction which acts as hydrogen carrier from enzyme dehydrogenase systems of tissue respiration to molecular oxygen. **Active carrier.** A carrier (main def. 1) excreting micro-organisms at the time of observation. **Chronic carrier.** A carrier (main def. 1) for a long period. **Closed carrier.** A non-infectious carrier. **Contact carrier.** A carrier (main def. 1) following recognizable contact with a known case. **Convalescent carrier.** A carrier (main def. 1) who has recently suffered from the disease himself, without being able to get rid of the micro-organisms. **Haemophilic carrier.** A female member of a haemophilic family who is herself not a bleeder, and who may be carrying the haemophilic trait in a gene contained in the X chromosome. Such a daughter of a haemophilic male can transmit the disease to half her sons and the recessive or hidden trait to half her daughters. **Healthy carrier.** A carrier (main def. 1) who has not contracted the disease himself; a symptomless carrier. **Incubation carrier.** A carrier (main def. 1) in the incubation period of a disease. **Intermittent carrier.** A periodic excretor of dangerous microbes who shows periods of apparently complete freedom from infection. **Intestinal carrier.** A carrier (main def. 1) excreting the infectious element in his faeces. **Precocious carrier.** An apparently healthy carrier (main def. 1) who subsequently develops the disease. **Temporary carrier.** A carrier (main def. 1) for a short period, possibly after recovery from a disease. Sometimes an intermittent carrier (see above). **Typhoid carrier.** A carrier (main def. 1) of typhoid bacilli, usually in the gall bladder and excreted in the faeces, or in the urinary tract and excreted in the urine. **Urinary carrier.** A carrier (main def. 1) excreting the infectious element in the urine. [OFr. *carier.*]

carrier-free (kar·e·er·fre′). A preparation of a radioisotope to which no carrier has been added and for which precautions have been taken to minimize contamination with other isotopes. [OFr. *carier,* AS *freo.*]

Carrión, Daniel Alcides (b. 1850). Peruvian medical student.

Carrión's disease. Oroya fever; a febrile disease that occurs in certain valleys in the western slopes of the Andes. It is caused by *Bartonella bacilliformis,* which is transmitted by sand flies to man. The disease is characterized by severe anaemia, and is often fatal. Those who recover may suffer at a later date from a granulomatous eruption known as *verruga peruana.*

carrot (kar·ot). The cultivated plant *Daucus carota* Linn. var. *sativa* DC (family Umbelliferae), grown as a table vegetable and cattle food. It is a source of carotene. **Wild carrot herb.** The aerial parts of *Daucus carota* Linn.; a diuretic, and a popular domestic remedy in affections of the bladder. [L *carota.*]

carrotene (kar·ot·een). Carotene.

Carsalam (kar·sal·am). BP Commission approved name for 1, 3-benzoxazine-2,4-dione; an analgesic.

Carswell, Sir Robert (b. 1793). London pathologist.

Carswell's grapes. A racemose arrangement of tuberculous infiltration around the bronchioles in pulmonary tuberculosis. Radiologically it resembles bunches of grapes.

Cartagena bark (kar·tah·hay·nah bark). Cinchona bark from Cartagena, Colombia, S. America. It is derived from *Cinchona lancifolia* Mutis.

Carter, Henry Vandyke (b. 1831). Indian Medical Service.

Carter's disease. Madura foot. *See* FOOT.

Carter, William Wesley (b. 1869). New York otologist.

Carter's operation. A cartilage rib graft for the correction of nasal deformity.

carthamus (kar·tham·us). Safflower, bastard saffron, American saffron; the flowers of *Carthamus tinctorius* Linn. (family Compositae), a plant indigenous to India. Like saffron it is used as a domestic remedy for infant disorders such as measles, and as a colouring agent. [Ar. *qartama* paint.]

Carticaine (kar·te·kane). BP Commission approved name for methyl 4-methyl-3-(2-propylaminopropionamido)thiophene-2-carboxylate; a local anaesthetic.

cartilage [cartilago (NA)] (kar·til·ij). A skeletal or connective tissue which is firm, flexible and slightly elastic, and which consists of specialized cells (chondrocytes) enclosed in a matrix of collagenous fibres and a chondromucoid. The latter gives the matrix a homogeneous glassy appearance *(hyaline cartilage).* When the matrix is permeated with large bundles of collagenous fibres, fibrocartilage, or white fibrocartilage, is formed; when elastic fibres are present, as in the cartilage of the auricle or pinna, the pharyngotympanic tube or the epiglottis, it is called yellow elastic fibrocartilage, or simply elastic cartilage. **Cartilages of the ala, small [cartilagines alares minores (NA)].** Small cartilaginous plates in the fibrous membrane that joins the back of the lower nasal cartilage to the frontal process of the maxilla. **Articular cartilage [cartilago articularis (NA)].** Cartilage covering the articulating surfaces of synovial joints; it is of the hyaline variety. **Arytenoid cartilage [cartilago arytenoidea (NA)].** A small paired pyramidal cartilage; the major part is hyaline in type; the apex [apex cartilaginis arytenoideae] is elastic fibrocartilage and is the highest point. The base [basis cartilaginis arytenoideae] has an articular facet [facies articularis (NA)] for articulation with the cricoid lamina. The anterolateral surface [facies anterolateralis (NA)] is the convex surface bearing the colliculus; the medial surface [facies medialis (NA)] is the narrow flat surface which bounds the rima glottidis laterally; and the posterior surface [facies posterior (NA)] is the triangular surface giving attachment to the transverse arytenoid cartilage. **Cartilage of the auricle [cartilago auriculae (NA)].** The framework of all but the lobe of the auricle, consisting of a single thin plate of elastic fibrocartilage continuous below and anteriorly with the cartilage of the external auditory meatus. That for the tragus is separated from the remainder by a cleft, the incisura terminalis of the auricle, which extends downwards almost to the meatal cartilage. Its irregular surface corresponds to the named grooves and eminences which form the landmarks of both surfaces of the auricle. **Bronchial cartilages.** Rings of hyaline cartilage in the walls of the main bronchi; also irregular plates of cartilage in the walls of the smaller bronchi. **Calcified cartilage.** Cartilage containing a deposit of calcium salts in its matrix; such deposition occurs in all cartilage about to be ossified or replaced by bone, though it may occur independently of bone replacement, e.g. in old age. **Cellular cartilage.** *See* EMBRYONIC CARTILAGE (below). **Central cartilage.** A term sometimes used for an orbital implant after enucleation of the eye. **Condylar cartilage.** The cartilage situated in the condyle of the mandible which, by progressive growth and conversion into bone, produces the downward and forward growth of the mandible. **Connecting cartilage.** Cartilage which may form a junction (primary synchondrosis) between 2 bones, usually temporary, e.g. in that between the basi-occipital bone and the body of the sphenoid in a child; such connecting cartilage is similar to epiphyseal cartilage. It is also known as *interosseous* or *synarthrodial cartilage.* **Corniculate cartilage [cartilago corniculata (NA)].** A small, conical, elastic fibrocartilage in the posterior margin of the aryepiglottic folds, immediately above the apex of the arytenoid cartilages. **Costal cartilage [cartilago costalis (NA)].** The bar of cartilage at the anterior end of each rib. **Cricoid cartilage [cartilago cricoidea (NA)].** An annular cartilage, shaped like a signet ring, made up of a narrow anterior arch and a wide quadrilateral lamina [lamina cartilaginis cricoideae] posteriorly. **Cuneiform cartilage [cartilago cuneiformis (NA)].** An elongated elastic fibrocartilage in the free edge of the aryepiglottic fold, above and anterior to the corniculate cartilage. **Diarthrodial cartilage.** Articular cartilage (see above). **Embryonic cartilage.** That containing many cells (*cellular cartilage*); much of the cartilage formed in the embryo is subsequently replaced by bone (*temporary cartilage, ossifying cartilage*), but some, such as the costal and laryngeal cartilages, and the cartilaginous rings of the trachea, remain as *permanent cartilage.* **Epiglottic cartilage [cartilago epiglottica (NA)].** The epiglottis. **Epiphyseal cartilage [cartilago epiphysialis (NA)].** That which persists between the epiphysis and shaft or main part of a developing bone, but which is eventually replaced by bone when growth is complete. **Cartilage of the external auditory meatus [cartilago meatus acustici (NA)].** The fibrocartilage of the external part of the meatus. **Fetal cartilage.** Embryonic cartilage (see above). **Growth cartilage.** Epiphyseal cartilage (see above). **Hyaline cartilage.** *See* MAIN DEF. (above). **Interosseous cartilage.** Connecting cartilage (see above). **Cartilages of the larynx [cartilagines laryngis].** The single thyroid and cricoid cartilages, the paired arytenoid, corniculate and cuneiform cartilages, and the epiglottis. **Loose cartilage.** A torn cartilage, usually one of the menisci in the knee joint. **Nasal cartilage, lower [crus laterale (NA)].** A thin cartilage situated below the upper cartilage and curling round the nostril to reach the lower part of the septum. It has an outer part and a septal process. **Nasal cartilage, upper [cartilago nasi lateralis (NA)].** A triangular cartilage attached to the nasal bone and the frontal process of the maxilla. **Cartilages of the nose [cartilagines nasi (NA)].** The group of hyaline cartilages in the anterior part of the lateral walls and septum of the external nose. **Ossifying cartilage.** *See* EMBRYONIC CARTILAGE (above). **Permanent cartilage.** *See* EMBRYONIC CARTILAGE (above). **Cartilage of the pharyngotympanic tube [cartilago tubae auditivae (NA)].** The cartilaginous basis of the inner two-thirds of the tube. It is shaped like an inverted gutter with a wide medial [lamina (cartilaginis) medialis (NA)] and narrow lateral [lamina (cartilaginis) lateralis] lamina. **Semilunar cartilage of the knee joint, lateral [meniscus lateralis (NA)].** A crescentic plate of fibrocartilage on the lateral part of the articular surface of the tibia, to which it is attached, and on which it is slightly mobile. **Semilunar cartilage of the knee joint, medial [meniscus medialis (NA)].** A crescentic plate of fibrocartilage on the periphery of the medial articular surface of the tibia, to which it is attached and on which it is slightly mobile. **Septal cartilage [cartilago septi nasi (NA)].** A flat quadrilateral plate of cartilage forming the skeleton of the lower anterior part of the nasal septum. It is attached posteriorly to the perpendicular plate of the ethmoid bone and vomer. **Sesamoid cartilage of the larynx [cartilago sesamoidea (NA)].** A nodule occasionally found on the external border of the arytenoid cartilage. **Sesamoid cartilages of the nose [cartilagines nasales accessoriae (NA)].** Small cartilages at the border of the lower nasal cartilages where they join the septum. **Subvomerine cartilage [cartilago vomeronasalis (NA)].** Strips of cartilage on the outer surface of the vomeronasal organ. **Synarthrodial cartilage.** Connecting cartilage (see above). **Tarsal cartilage.** The fibrocartilaginous plate within an eyelid. **Temporary cartilage.** *See* EMBRYONIC CARTILAGE (above). **Thyroid cartilage [cartilago thyroidea (NA)].** The largest cartilage of the larynx, consisting of 2 flat laminae (right and left [lamina dextra et sinistra (NA)], the anterior borders of which are fused inferiorly but separated above (the thyroid notch). The posterior borders are prolonged as slender superior [cornu superius (NA)] and inferior [cornu inferius (NA)] horns. **Tracheal cartilages [cartilagines tracheales (NA)].** 16–20 horseshoe-like hyaline cartilages extending the whole length of the trachea, the deficiency lying posteriorly. This is filled by a fibrous membrane containing many transversely-running muscle fibres (the trachealis muscle) and some longitudinal bundles. **Xiphoid cartilage.** The lowest piece of the sternum, so called because of its sword-like shape; the xiphoid process. [L *cartilago.*]

See also: EUSTACHIO, HUSCHKE, JACOBSON (L. L.), LUSCHKA, MECKEL, MEYER (E. V.) (MAYER), MORGAGNI, REICHERT (K. B.), SANTORINI, SEILER, WEITBRECHT, WRISBERG.

cartilagin (kar·til·aj·in). Chondrogen, a complex mixture of collagen and chondromucoid which forms the basis of the ground substance of cartilage.

cartilaginification (kar·til·aj·in·if·e·**ka'**·shun). Chondrification; changing into cartilage. [cartilage, L *facere* to make.]

cartilaginiform (kar·til·aj·**in'**·e·form). Cartilaginoid. [cartilage, form.]

cartilaginoid (kar·til·**aj**·in·oid). Like cartilage in structure and appearance. [cartilage, Gk *eidos* form.]

cartilaginous (kar·til·**aj**·in·us). 1. Composed of cartilage. 2. Resembling cartilage in firmness and toughness. 3. Gristly. **Cartilaginous joint.** *See* JOINT.

cartilago triticea [NA] (kar·til·a·go tri·**tis**·e·ah). A small cartilage often present in the lateral thyrohyoid ligament. [cartilage, L *triticeus* wheaten.]

cartilagotropic (**kar**·til·ag·o·**trop'**·ik). A term applied to any substance which is suitable for the growth of cartilage cells. [cartilage, Gk *tropos* a turning.]

carum (ka·rum). Carui fructus, Caraway BP 1958, caraway fruit, caraway seed: the dried ripe fruits of *Carum carvi* Linn., a biennial umbelliferous herb cultivated in Central and North European countries, particularly Holland. Its most important constituent is a volatile oil (Caraway Oil BPC 1959) containing 53-63 per cent of carvone. It has carminative properties and is used chiefly as Concentrated Caraway Water BPC 1959 for flatulence in infants. Large quantities are used as a culinary flavouring. [Gk *karon.*]

caruncle [caruncula (NA)] (kar·ung·kl). Any normal or abnormal fleshy excrescence, usually minute and often representing the healed remnants of a tag of torn flesh. **Lacrimal caruncle [caruncula lacrimalis (NA)].** The small reddish body situated in the medial angle of the eye. **Urethral caruncle.** A small fleshy growth which may develop from the mucous membrane at the urethral meatus of the female. It is painful and is prone to bleed. [see foll.]

See also: MORGAGNI.

caruncula [NA] (kar·ung·kew·lah). A small fleshy elevation. **Carunculae hymenales [NA], Carunculae myrtiformes.** Small protuberances round the vaginal orifice, remnants of the ruptured hymen. [L small piece of flesh.]

See also: SANTORINI.

caruncular (kar·ung·kew·lar). Like a caruncle or relating to a caruncle.

Carus, Karl Gustav (b. 1789). Dresden anatomist and gynaecologist.

circle, or curve of Carus. A curved line formed by joining the axes of a large number of planes in the pelvis and indicating the path travelled by the presenting part in delivery.

carus (ka·rus). 1. Deep lethargy. 2. Coma with insensibility. **Carus cataleptica, Carus ecstasis.** Catalepsy. **Carus lethargus.** Lethargy. [Gk *karos* heavy sleep.]

carvacrol (kar·vak·rol). Methylisopropylhydroxybenzene, $C_3H_7C_6H_3(CH_3)OH$. A colourless liquid, isomeric with thymol, and found with it in oil of thyme. It has weak antiseptic properties, and is also used in perfumery. **Carvacrol iodide.** $C_3H_7C_6H_2I(CH_3)OH$, an antiseptic used instead of iodoform as it is both colourless and odourless.

carvene (kar·veen). Hesperidene, D-limonene, $C_{10}H_{16}$. A terpene hydrocarbon which is the main constituent of oil of orange and lemon rind; also occurs in oils of lavender, bergamot and caraway. It is a colourless liquid with an odour of lemons, and is dextrorotatory.

carveol (kar·ve·ol). $C_{10}H_{16}O$, an alcohol occurring in the volatile oil of caraway.

carver (kar·ver). A sharp hand-instrument made in various forms for shaping and carving restorative materials in conservative dentistry. [AS *ceorfan.*]

carvol (kar·vol). Carvone.

carvone (kar·vone). $C_{10}H_{14}O$, a ketone of the terpene group, found in the volatile oils of caraway and cummin, also dill oil; a colourless liquid isomeric with carvacrol.

carvotanacetone (kar·vo·tan·as′·e·tone). Thujone, $C_{10}H_{16}O$. A ketone of the terpene series, found in thuja and sage oils.

Carwardine's saccharimeter. A simple apparatus for the determination of sugar in urine by the reduction of Fehling's solution.

cary-. For compounds beginning with **Cary-**, *see also* KARY-.

caryenchyma (kar·e·en·kim·ah). In cytology, an obsolete term for the nuclear sap. [Gk *karyon* nut, *en, chymos* juice.]

caryophyllin (kar·e·of·il·in). $(C_{10}H_{16}O)_3$, an odourless white ketonic substance of the terpene series, found in clove oil. [see foll.]

caryophyllum (kar·e·of·il·um). Clove BP 1953; the dried flower-buds of *Eugenia caryophyllus* (Spreng.) Sprague (family Myrtaceae), a tree indigenous to the Molucca Islands and cultivated in the islands of Zanzibar, Pemba and Penang. It contains 15-20 per cent of volatile oil, gallotannic acid and caryophyllin. It is used as an aromatic stimulant, carminative and flavouring agent. [Gk *karyon* nut, *phyllon* leaf.]

Casal, Gaspar (b. 1679). Spanish physician and author.

Casal's collar, or necklace. In pellagra, the erythematous pigmented area that appears on the neck.

casca bark (kas·kah bark). Sassy bark; the bark of *Erythrophloeum guineense* G. Don. (family Leguminosae), used at one time in Africa as an arrow poison. It contains the alkaloid erythrophloeine.

cascade (kas·kade). Term used to refer to enzyme systems, e.g. complement, kinins, clotting factors, characterized by a sequential reaction in which each enzyme activates the next one in the sequence.

cascara (kas·kar·ah). 1. A bark. 2. (BP 1973.) Cascara sagrada, the dried bark of *Rhamnus purshianus* DC. (family Rhamnaceae), which must be collected at least one year before being used; British Columbia, the Western States of the USA and Kenya are the main sources of supply. The constituents are incompletely known, but belong to the class of hydroxymethylanthraquinones (free and combined as glycosides). It is a most valuable mild purgative, usually administered in the form of liquid extract, or tablets prepared from the dry extract. **Cascara amarga.** Bitter bark, Honduras bark, the dried bark of *Sweetia panamensis* Bentham (family Simarubaceae). It contains the alkaloids sweetine and picramnine, and is a bitter tonic. **Cascara Sagrada BP 1953.** *See* MAIN DEF. 2 (above). [Sp. bark.]

Cascarilla BPC 1949 (kas·kar·il·ah). The dried bark of *Croton eluteria* Benn. (family Euphorbiaceae), a shrub indigenous to the Bahama Islands. It contains a volatile oil, a crystalline bitter principle (cascarillin) and alkaloids. It is an aromatic bitter, and is also used in fumigants. [Sp. dim. of *cascara* bark.]

cascarillin (kas·kar·il·in). $C_{12}H_{18}O_4$. A bitter substance from cascarilla bark.

case (kase). 1. Any particular instance of injury or disease. 2. A protective container. **Borderline case.** A case which has the characteristics of any two recognized diseases or conditions and does not typify either of them. **Brain case.** The upper parts of the skull which form a kind of box or case to enclose and protect the brain. **Custodial case.** Term used to describe a patient requiring care in an institution because of mental instability or criminal tendencies. **Case fatality rate.** *See* RATE. **Case history.** The past physical and psychical history of a patient with the history of his environment and family. **Coroners' cases.** Cases of death referred to the Coroner for enquiry and often post-mortem examination; usually sudden, unexplained, obscure or violent deaths, but also death from all unnatural causes, miscarriages of treatment, industrial and compensatable deaths, deaths of those in custody or prisons or for whom a certificate is either not forthcoming or unacceptable to the Registrar. **Missed case.** A case in which the symptoms and signs are so mild in degree or atypical of any particular disease that it remains unclassified clinically; a case in which evidences are undoubtedly present but in which the examining doctor has not noticed them. **Trial case.** In ophthalmology, the box or rack in which trial lenses are kept in a definite order. [L *casus* a happening.]

casease (ka·se·aze). A proteolytic enzyme formed by certain bacteria and capable of activating the solution of albumin and casein in milk and cheese. [L *caseus* cheese.]

caseate (ka·se·ate). 1. To become cheesy or undergo caseous degeneration. 2. Referring to lactates generally. [L *caseus* cheese.]

caseation, caseification (ka·se·a·shun, ka·se·if·e·ka′·shun). 1. In organic chemistry, the precipitation of casein while milk is undergoing the process of curdling. 2. A form of degeneration or necrosis in which structures or tissues are changed into a cheesy mass. [see prec.]

caseiform (ka·se·e·form). Resembling casein or cheese in appearance or structure. [L *caseus* cheese, form.]

casein (ka·se·in). A protein found in milk in the form of caseinogen. It contains phosphorus and sulphur and is a white powder, insoluble in water but soluble in alkalis. It is formed from caseinogen by the action of rennin in the presence of calcium. Casein is a "first-class" protein in that it contains all the amino acids considered essential in human and animal nutrition. Preparations of casein are used when the ability to digest natural protein food is impaired, and to supplement food intake in high-protein diets. **Glycerophosphated casein.** A preparation composed of 95 per cent of soluble casein and 2.5 per cent each of sodium and calcium glycerophosphates. **Casein hydrolysate.** A buff-coloured powder prepared by the enzyme hydrolysis of casein, and containing a mixture of amino acids, polypeptides and other breakdown products. It is used to maintain the amino acid intake in debilitated patients, or in whom protein digestion is impaired; it may be given by mouth or by intravenous drip in aqueous solution. **Soluble Casein BPC 1954.** Casein mixed with a small quantity of alkali, generally sodium carbonate; a white or yellowish-white powder with a characteristic taste and very soluble in water. It is the form in which casein is preferably administered as, being soluble, it is the more easily digested. [L *caseus* cheese.]

caseinate (ka·se·in·ate). A salt formed by solution of casein in a dilute alkali.

caseinogen (ka·se·**in**·o·jen). A phosphoprotein present in milk and convertible by the enzyme chymosin (rennin) into casein. (In the USA caseinogen is called *casein* and casein *paracasein.*) It is the substance which is precipitated when milk goes sour by the formation of lactic acid, and the precursor of the casein formed by rennin in the coagulation of milk. [casein, Gk *genein* to produce.]

caseogenous (ka·se·**oj**·en·us). Giving rise to caseation. [see prec.]

caseoiodine (ka·se·o·**i**'·o·deen). A compound formed by the union of casein with iodine, the iodine uniting with the tyrosine groups present in the protein. It has been used in the treatment of thyroid deficiency.

caseose (**ka**·se·oze). A peptone produced by the peptic digestion of casein. The hydrolysis of casein by pepsin in acid solution only proceeds as far as the proteose stage, and free amino acids are not produced.

caseoserum (ka·se·o·**seer**'·um). An antiserum against casein.

caseous (**ka**·se·us). Like or possessing the qualities of curd or cheese. [L *caseus* cheese.]

cashew nut (**kash**·oo nut). The fruit of *Anacardium occidentale* Linn. (family Anacardiaceae), a tree cultivated in the tropics. The fresh juice of the pericarp yields an acrid, vesicant oil used by the natives as an application for warts and corns; this oil also has anthelmintic properties. The roasted seed kernel is edible and nutritive. [Brazilian *acajiba.*]

Casilli's test. A micro-modification of the Kahn test for syphilis.

Casoni, Tomaso (b. 1880). Italian physician.

Casoni's test. An intracutaneous test for hydatid disease, of considerable practical value. With a tuberculin syringe 0.02 ml of filtered sterile hydatid fluid (or a diluted extract of scolices or of adult tapeworms) is injected into the skin: a positive result is indicated by the formation of a weal which increases to at least 1.0 cm in diameter and develops pseudopodia.

Caspar's ring opacity. A circular corneal opacity, generally the result of a contusion.

cassava (kas·**ah**·vah). 1. The Brazilian shrubs *Manihot utilissima* Pohl. (bitter cassava) and *Manihot aipi* Pohl. (sweet cassava); manioc. 2. The name given to the starchy substance obtained from the tubers of the manioc plant, and from which tapioca is prepared by purification. [Haitian *kasabi.*]

Casselberry, William Evans (b. 1859). Chicago laryngologist.

Casselberry's position. A position used after intubation, the patient lying prone so that he can swallow without the risk of fluid entering the intubation tube.

Casserio, Giulio (b. 1552). Padua anatomist.

Casserio's fontanelle. The posterolateral fontanelle. *See* FONTANELLE.

Casserio's ligament. The anterior ligament of the malleus; originally described by Casserio as the laxator tympani minor muscle.

Casserio's perforated muscle. The coracobrachialis muscle.

Casserio's perforating nerve. The musculocutaneous nerve of the arm.

cassette (kaz·**et**). 1. Reels of magnetic tape in a flat box used for recording speech or music. 2. A light-tight flat container used to hold an x-ray film in close contact with intensifying screens. [Fr. little box.]

Cassia (**kash**·e·ah). A genus of plants of the family Leguminosae, several species of which yield senna. *Cassia angustifolia* Vahl., cultivated in South India and known as Tinnevelly senna, and *Cassia acutifolia* Delile (Alexandrian senna) yield the official senna leaflets and pods. *Cassia auriculata* Linn. yields Palthé senna. *Cassia obovata* Colladon. yields dog senna. The wild plants of *Cassia angustifolia* growing in Arabia yield Bombay, Mecca and Arabian sennas. **Cassia bark.** Chinese cinnamon, the dried bark of *Cinnamomum cassia* Blume (family Lauraceae), cultivated in south-east China. It contains a volatile oil, mucilage, and tannin, and resembles cinnamon in properties but is less pleasantly aromatic. **Cassia buds.** The immature fruits of *Cinnamomum cassia;* they are used as a spice. **Cassia Fruit BPC 1959.** Cassia pod, purging cassia, the ripe fruits of *Cassia fistula* Linn., an Indian tree. They contain sugar and hydroxymethylanthraquinones, and are used for the preparation of cassia pulp, which is laxative and an ingredient of confection of senna. **Oil of cassia.** An oil distilled from the leaves and twigs of *Cinnamomum cassia* Blume; it is similar to cinnamon oil, but contains more cinnamic aldehyde and no eugenol. [Hebrew *qatsa* to peel off bark.]

cassiopeium (kas·e·**o**·pe·um). A name given to the rare-earth element now known as *lutetium.* [*Cassiopeia,* Ethiopian queen, and the name of a constellation.]

cast (kahst) 1. Any mass of pathological material thrown off from the surface of a cavity, or excreted in a body fluid such as urine. 2. In dentistry, the act of pouring or forcing a substance which subsequently sets or hardens into a pattern or mould. 3. Squint or strabismus. **Bacterial cast.** A cast of the renal tubules, found in the urine and composed of enormous numbers of bacteria. **Blood cast.** A cast composed of blood. **Coma cast.** A hyaline or granular renal cast thought by Kuelz to be diagnostic of impending diabetic coma; also called *Kuelz's cast* or *cylinder.* **Decidual cast.** The thick layer of mucous membrane which is cast off from the uterus after death of the ovum in certain cases of extra-uterine pregnancy. **Epithelial cast.** A cast composed of desquamated epithelium. **False cast.** Pseudocast; urinary sediment resembling a true cast. **Fatty cast.** A cast rich in fats or fat-containing cells. **Fibrinous cast.** A cast composed of fibrin. **Granular cast.** A cast composed of cells filled with protein and fatty granules. **Haemoglobin cast.** A cast composed of laked blood. **Hair casts.** Grey, keratin cylinders surrounding the hair shafts and resulting from prolonged traction on the hair during hairdressing procedures. **Hyaline cast.** A cast composed of cells showing hyaline degeneration. **Mucus cast.** A cast found in the faeces in cases of mucomembranous enteritis and mucous colitis. **Pus cast.** A cast composed of pus cells. **Renal cast.** A cast formed in the renal tubules and glomeruli as the result of disease. **Spiral cast.** A Curschmann's spiral. **Spurious cast.** False cast (see above). **Spurious tube cast.** A form of false cast. **Tube cast.** A cast formed in a renal tubule as the result of nephritis. **Tubular exudation cast.** A mucous mass discharged from the large gut in mucous colitis. **Urate cast.** A cast composed of urates. **Urinary cast.** A cast of a urinary tubule. **Waxy cast.** A cast composed of amyloid substance. [Old Norse *kasta.*]

See also: KUELZ.

Castaigne, Joseph (b. 1871). Paris physician.

Achard-Castaigne test. A test of renal function: a solution of methylene blue is injected intramuscularly and the time of appearance of the dye in the urine is noted. Normally, this occurs in about 30 min. This was one of the first substances used as a test of renal function by ingestion or injection. It has for long been superseded by other substances such as phenolsulphonephthalein (the phthalein test of Rowntree and Geraghty) or by indigo carmine.

Castanea (kas·ta·ne·ah). 1. A genus of trees which includes the chestnuts. 2. Chestnut leaves, the leaves of *Castanea vesca* Gaertn. (*Castanea vulgaris* Lam.). They have tonic and astringent properties, and are reputed to be of value in respiratory complaints. [Gk *kastanon* chestnut.]

Castañeda, M. Ruiz. Mexican virologist.

Castañeda's stain. For *Rickettsiae* and certain virus inclusion bodies: preparations are stained with 1 per cent alcoholic methylene blue 1:20 in formalized phosphate buffer at pH 7.5 for 3 min and counterstained with 0.2 per cent safranine in 0.1 per cent acetic acid. The *Rickettsiae* and inclusion bodies stain blue, tissue cells red.

Castañeda's vaccine. A typhus vaccine prepared from the lungs of infected mice.

Zinsser-Castañeda vaccine. A vaccine used in southern Mexico, consisting of four parts of murine rickettsiae and one part of epidemic rickettsiae (*Rickettsia prowazeki*).

Castañeda-negative, Castañeda-positive (kas·tan·ye·dah·**neg**'·a·tiv, kas·tan·ye·dah·**poz**'·it·iv). A classificatory term applied to inclusion bodies or viruses according to whether they do or do not stain blue with Castañeda's stain. [M. Ruiz *Castañeda.*]

Castellanella (kas·tel·an·**el**'·ah). A generic name sometimes used for *Trypanosoma;* it is not valid. [Aldo *Castellani.*]

Castellani, Aldo (b. 1877). Italian mycologist and physician in London, Rome and Lisbon.

Castellani's bronchitis, or disease. Haemorrhagic bronchitis due to spirochaetal infection.

Castellani's lotion. Castellani's paint (see below).

Castellani's mixture. A mixture consisting of tartar emetic, sodium salicylate, potassium iodide, sodium bicarbonate and water, used in the treatment of yaws. [Obsolete.]

Castellani's ointment. Unguentum resorcinolis et acidi salicylici.

Castellani's paint. The original formula is a saturated alcoholic solution of basic fuchsine 10 ml with 5 per cent aqueous carbolic acid solution 100 ml, which is filtered and boric acid 1 g added: after 2 h 5 ml of acetone is added, and 2 h later resorcin 10 g. It is kept in a dark-coloured bottle with glass stopper, and is used for the treatment of fungous infection of the skin, particularly epidermophytosis but has also been employed for intertrigo not necessarily due to this type of infection. Paint of Magenta BPC 1959 or paint of fuchsine which has very similar ingredients is the form in which this medicament is now used.

Castellani's pyosis. An ecthymatous eruption, usually affecting the legs.

Castellani's syndrome. Enlargement of the liver and spleen with arthritis.

Castellani's vaccine. A pentavalent or tetravalent vaccine containing typhoid and paratyphoid bacilli.

Castellani-Low sign. Fine tremor of the tongue in trypanosomiasis.

Castellanus castellanii (kas·tel·a·nus kas·tel·a·ne·i). *Shigella ceylonensis.*

Castellino, Pietro (b. 1864). Naples physician.

Castellino's sign. *See* CARDARELLI'S SIGN.

Castillon's powder. A mixture of powdered tragacanth, sage, salep, oyster shell and cochineal; it is boiled with milk and used in the treatment of diarrhoea and dysentery.

Castle, William Bosworth (b. 1897). Boston physician.

Castle's test. A clinicobiochemical test for the presence of haemopoietin (Castle's or intrinsic factor) in the gastric juice: gastric secretion aspirated (150 ml) from the patient is digested with 200 g of beef muscle or its muscle globulin at 37°C and pH 2.5–7.2 for about 2 h, and is then given daily by tube orally to a patient with uncomplicated pernicious anaemia not in remission. If the test gastric juice contains haemopoietin, then the patient with pernicious anaemia will show a clinical remission with a reticulocytosis; the gastric juice from a pernicious anaemia will not cause such a response.

castle (**kah**·sl). The arrangement of lead shielding around a Geiger counter to decrease the background count; descriptive of the usual cylindrical shape of the lead. [L *castellum.*]

castrate (**kas**·trate). 1. To remove the testes or the ovaries. 2. An individual who has undergone castration. [L *castrare* to geld.]

castration (kas·**tra**·shun). Orchidectomy. **Castration complex.** *See* COMPLEX. **Female castration.** Oöphorectomy. [see prec.]

castroid (**kas**·troid). Eunuchoid. [L *castrare* to geld.]

castrophrenia (kas·tro·**fre**·ne·ah). In schizophrenia, the idea held by a patient that his thoughts are being sucked out of his brain by some mechanism. It is so called by reason of the hypothesis that it is an expression of the castration complex. [L *castrare* to castrate, Gk *phren* mind.]

casualty (**kaz**·ew·al·te). 1. An accident, fatal or otherwise; the victim of such an accident. 2. An individual killed or wounded in war. **Casualty Department.** The name given to the emergency receiving room in many hospitals. [L *casus* a happening.]

casuistics (kaz·ew·**ist**·ix). The keeping of records of cases of injury or disease for the purpose of study. [L *casus* a happening.]

cata-. *See* KATA-.

catabasial (kat·ah·**ba**·ze·al). In craniology, indication that the basion is lower than the opisthion. [Gk *kata,* basion.]

catabasis (kat·**ab**·as·is). The stage of a disease at which it is abating. [Gk *kata, bainein* to go.]

catabatic (kat·ab·**at**·ik). Referring to the abatement of a disease. [see prec.]

catabiosis (**kat**·ah·bi·**o**'·sis). An activity in living tissue which causes the primary structure to influence contiguous structures to develop in harmony with it. [Gk *kata, bios* life.]

catabiotic (**kat**·ah·bi·**ot**'·ik). 1. Referring to catabiosis. 2. Functionally able to use up or dissipate, e.g., energy derived from food. 3. Descriptive of the functional activity of a cell. [see prec.]

catabolergy (kat·ab·**ol**·er·je). The energy used up by catabolic processes. [Gk *kata, ballein* to throw, *ergon* work.]

catabolic (kat·ab·**ol**·ik). Referring to catabolism.

catabolin (kat·**ab**·o·lin). Catabolite.

catabolism (kat·**ab**·ol·izm). The breaking-down of tissues so that the constituents of living matter are reduced to waste material and are eliminated from the body. Disintegration from a complex physiological state to one less complex. Metabolism in its destructive phase. Cf. ANABOLISM. [Gk *kata, ballein* to throw.]

catabolite (kat·**ab**·ol·ite). An end-product of a catabolic process.

catabythismomania (**kat**·ab·ith·is·mo·**ma**'·ne·ah). Suicidal mania which impels an individual to drown himself. [Gk *katabythismos* submergence, mania.]

catacausis (kat·ah·**kaw**·sis). Destruction of tissues, e.g. brought about by chemical changes; spontaneous combustion. [Gk *kata, kausis* a burning.]

cataclasis (kat·ah·**kla**·sis). 1. Catacleisis. 2. Fracture. [Gk *kata, klasis* a breaking.]

catacleisis (kat·ah·**kli**·sis). 1. Spasmodic closure of the eyelids. 2. Closure of the eyelids by adhesion. [Gk *kata, kleisis* a locking.]

cataclonus (kat·ah·**klo**·nus). Repetitive convulsive movements of muscle groups resulting from hysteria and not from organic disease. [Gk *kata, klonos* confused motion.]

cataclysm (**kat**·ah·klizm). 1. A sudden shock or upheaval. 2. An effusion. [Gk *kataklysmos* deluge.]

catacoustics (kat·ak·**oos**·tix). In physics, that branch of the science of acoustics which is concerned with echoes or reflected sounds. [Gk *kata, akouein* to hear.]

catacrotic (kat·ak·**rot**·ik). Referring to or characterized by catacrotism.

catacrotism (kat·**ak**·rot·izm). A particular abnormality in the beat of the pulse caused by secondary expansions of the artery. On the sphygmogram it is shown by the presence of one or more minor elevations on the descending curve. [Gk *kata, krotein* to strike.]

catadicrotic (kat·ah·di·**krot**′·ik). Referring to or characterized by catadicrotism.

catadicrotism (kat·ah·**dik**·rot·izm). Abnormality of the pulse consisting in double expansion of the artery and shown on the sphygmogram by a double interruption of the downward curve. [Gk *kata*, dicrotic.]

catadidymus (kat·ah·**did**·e·mus). A twin monster of which the upper part is fused and the lower part doubled. [Gk *kata*, *didymos* twin.]

catadioptric (kat·ah·di·**op**′·trik). In physics, referring to or produced by reflection and refraction of light. [Gk *kata*, *dioptra* levelling instrument.]

catagen (kat·ah·jen). The transitory degenerative phase of the cycle of hair growth, between anagen and telogen. It lasts for about 2 weeks and at any one time less than 1 per cent of scalp hairs are in catagen. It is the stage of hair detachment and shedding. [Gk *kata* down, *genesis* formation.]

catagenesis (kat·ah·**jen**·es·is). In biology, retrogressive evolution. [Gk *kata*, *genein* to produce.]

catagenetic (kat·ah·jen·**et**′·ik). Referring to or showing catagenesis.

catagmatic (kat·ag·**mat**·ik). 1. A remedy which promotes the consolidation of broken bones. 2. Having the quality of promoting union of broken bones. 3. Referring to a case of fracture. 4. Useful in cases of fracture. [Gk *katagma* fracture.]

catahaemoglobin (kat·ah·he·mo·**glo**′·bin). Parahaematin, a compound of haematin with denatured globin. [Gk *kata*, haemoglobin.]

catalase (**kat**·al·aze). A haem enzyme containing ferric ion, of molecular weight 250 000. It catalyses the decomposition of hydrogen peroxide into water and oxygen. It occurs in many tissues, especially liver, where it is located in the peroxisomes. **Milk catalase.** One of the enzymes occurring in small amounts in fresh milk. Bacterial contamination of the milk causes a rapid increase in the amount. [catalysis.]

catalepsy (kat·al·**ep**·se). A morbid condition in which there is sudden suspension of sensibility and voluntary movement, with waxy rigidity of the limbs and body, these maintaining any posture in which they are placed. The pulse and respiration rates are slow and the body is cold. The condition is of nervous origin and may be found in association with hypnosis, hysteria and epilepsy; the attack may last for any period between a few minutes and several days. **Local catalepsy.** Catalepsy in which a single group of muscles or one organ is affected. [Gk *kata*, *lambanein* to seize.]

cataleptic (kat·al·**ep**·tik). 1. Referring to or involving catalepsy. 2. An individual who is subject to catalepsy.

cataleptiform, cataleptoid (kat·al·**ep**·te·form, kat·al·**ep**·toid). Applied to a condition that has a resemblance to the state of catalepsy. [catalepsy, L *forme* form, Gk *eidos* form.]

catalogia (kat·al·o·je·ah). Verbigeration; in insanity, the persistent repetition of meaningless words and incoherent sentences. [Gk *katalegein* to count up.]

catalysation (kat·al·i·**za**′·shun). 1. In chemistry, the subjecting of any particular body to catalysis. 2. The process of becoming catalysed.

catalysator (**kat**·al·i·za′·tor). Catalyser.

catalyser (**kat**·al·i·zer). A substance which produces catalysis. **Negative catalyser.** A substance which retards the speed of a chemical reaction or a physical process. **Positive catalyser.** A substance which accelerates the speed of a chemical reaction. [Gk *katalein* to dissolve.]

catalysis (kat·**al**·is·is). The promotion or acceleration of a chemical reaction by the presence of a small amount of a substance, the substance itself appearing to be unchanged and unaffected by the reaction. **Contact catalysis.** The influencing of the speed of a chemical reaction by the power of absorption of surfaces in contact with one another. **Negative catalysis.** The retarding of a chemical reaction by a substance. **Positive catalysis.** The acceleration of a chemical reaction by the presence of a catalyser. [Gk *katalein* to dissolve.]

catalyst (**kat**·al·ist). Catalyser.

catalytic (kat·al·**it**·ik). 1. Referring to catalysis. 2. Causing catalysis, or involving it. 3. Having an alterative effect. 4. An alterative medicine.

catamenia (kat·ah·**me**·ne·ah). The menses, menstruation. [Gk *kata*, *men* month.]

catamenial (kat·ah·**me**·ne·al). Relating to menstruation or the menses. [see prec.]

catamenogenic (kat·ah·men·o·**jen**′·ik). Term applied to any substance or form of treatment that induces a menstrual flow. [catamenia, Gk *genein* to produce.]

catamnesis (kat·am·**ne**·sis). The subsequent case history of a patient from the time of his first examination. [Gk *kata*, *mnesis* memory.]

catamnestic (kat·am·**nes**·tik). Referring to catamnesis.

cataphasia, cataphasis (kat·ah·**fa**·ze·ah, kat·ah·**fa**·sis). A disorder of speech in which the same word or phrase is repeated involuntarily several times in succession. [Gk *kata*, *phanai* to speak.]

cataphonics (kat·ah·**fon**·ix). The study of reflected sound. [Gk *kata*, *phone* sound.]

cataphora (kat·**af**·or·ah). Somnolence; lethargy with periods of semicoma. [Gk *kataphora* lethargy.]

cataphoresis (kat·ah·for·**e**′·sis). 1. The movement of positively-charged colloid particles towards the cathode, occurring when colloid particles suspended in fluid come under the influence of an electric field. 2. The introduction into the tissues of substances carrying an electronegative charge by the passage of an electric current. 3. The "repletive" effect produced under the cathode, contrasted with the "depletive" effect occurring under the anode, a phenomenon made use of in electrotherapy. [Gk *kata*, *pherein* to bear.]

cataphoretic (kat·ah·for·**et**′·ik). Referring to cataphoresis or involving its employment.

cataphoria (kat·ah·**for**·e·ah). A tendency of the visual axes of both eyes to assume too low a plane. [Gk *kata*, *pherein* to bear.]

cataphoric (kat·ah·**for**·ik). Referring to cataphoria.

cataphrenia (kat·ah·**fre**·ne·ah). General mental weakness of the dementia type but having a tendency towards recovery of sanity. [Gk *kata*, *phren* mind.]

cataphylaxis (kat·ah·fil·**ax**′·is). 1. The concentration in the body of phylactic agents such as leucocytes and antibodies in the area in which there is infection. 2. The breaking-down of the natural defences of the body against infection. [Gk *kata*, phylaxis.]

cataplasia, cataplasis (kat·ah·**pla**·ze·ah, kat·ah·**pla**·sis). A form of atrophy in which the tissues degenerate to an earlier or embryonic stage of development. [Gk *kata*, *plassein* to mould.]

cataplasma, cataplasm (kat·ah·**plaz**·mah, **kat**·ah·plasm). A poultice often having kaolin and glycerine as a basis. **Cataplasma kaolini.** Kaolin Poultice BP 1958, a very effective poultice for application to local inflammations, being efficient in retaining heat and moisture. In addition to kaolin and glycerine, cataplasma kaolini contains thymol, methyl salicylate and oil of peppermint. These latter substances have some irritant effect and stimulate the blood flow through the affected part with, in addition, a slight antiseptic action. [Gk *kataplasma* poultice.]

cataplectic (kat·ah·**plek**·tik). 1. Referring to, involving or characterized by cataplexy. 2. Fulminant.

cataplexie du reveil (kat·ah·plex·e dew ra·va). Awakening and awareness of the psyche before the actual physical awakening with opening of the eyes. [Fr. cataplexy of awakening.]

cataplexis (kat·ah·**plex**·is). Cataplexy.

cataplexy (kat·ah·**plex**·e). 1. The sleep of hypnosis. 2. Sudden loss of muscular tone and weakness induced by strong emotion often associated with narcolepsy. 3. The extreme weakness induced by a sudden attack of disease. [Gk *kata*, *plexis* stroke.]

cataract (**kat**·ar·akt). Opacity in the crystalline lens of the eye which may be partial or complete. Since, with modern methods of examination, opacities can be found in almost all lenses, the word is, in practice, limited to those cases in which they are detected by ordinary clinical means. **Adherent cataract.** A cataract in which the affected lens is adherent to surrounding structures, the cornea, the iris or the anterior surface of the vitreous. **Adolescent cataract.** Cataract developing in adolescence. **Anterior polar cataract.** An opacity of the central portion of the anterior surface of the lens; usually the result of a perforating ulcer affecting the pupillary area of the cornea, but may be congenital due to contact of the lens and cornea in fetal life. **Arborescent cataract.** Coralliform cataract (see below). **Axial cataract.** A spindle-shaped opacity extending from the anterior to the posterior pole of the lens; congenital in origin. **Black cataract.** One in which the lens, at first yellow, from nuclear sclerosis, gradually becomes darker in colour. This may be due to oxidation of tyrosine or to deposition of melanin or lipofuscin. **Blue cataract.** A cataract characterized by a blue colour due to the optical effect of numerous small translucent opacities dispersing light irregularly, as in the sky. **Blue-dot cataract.** Numerous punctate opacities in the adult nucleus and cortex which disperse the light and appear blue. **Bottle-makers' cataract.** A variety of glass-blowers' cataract (see below). **Cachectic cataract.** A bilateral cortical cataract associated with acute toxic illness, or severe cachectic conditions. **Calcerous cataract.** Chalky deposits, usually in hypermature cataracts. **Capsular cataract.** An opacity due to thickening of the epithelial cells lining the capsule, usually due to disease of surrounding parts. **Capsulolenticular cataract.** A later stage of the preceding, where the opacity has spread into the substance of the lens. **Caseous cataract.** A late stage of cataract in which the substance of the lens has broken down into caseous material. **Central cataract.** A cataract involving the nucleus of the lens; it may be due to senile sclerosis or may be congenital. **Cerulean cataract.** Blue cataract (see above). **Cheesy cataract.** Caseous cataract (see above). **Cholesterin cataract.** One in which bright, sparkling crystals (cholesterin) are sometimes formed in advanced cases. **Choroidal cataract.** Cataract due to chronic, inflammatory or degenerative processes in the posterior segment of the eye, affecting first of all the posterior pole of the lens. **Complete cataract.** One in which all the layers of the lens are affected. **Complicated cataract.** A cataract due to other disease in the eye, usually inflammatory or degenerative, but also seen in glaucoma and in retinal detachment. **Concussion cataract.** Cataract due to a blow on the eye, causing a slight rupture of the capsule, followed by opacity of the lens fibres, which may become general or remain stationary for a long time. **Congenital cataract.** Cataract arising from faults in development of the lens. Numerous varieties have been described. **Congenital membranaceous cataract.** One associated usually with persistence of the central hyaloid artery and a gap in the posterior capsule through which fibrous tissue extends into the lens. **Contusion cataract.** Concussion cataract (see above). **Coralliform cataract.** Opacities with a tube-like appearance, radiating forward and outward from the centre of the lens and terminating in ampullae just short of the capsule. **Coronary cataract.** Numerous club-like opacities, radiating from the equator of the lens, and occupying the outer layers of the adult nucleus and inner layers of the cortex. It is non-progressive, often associated with small dots, rings and discs of opacity, and is present in 25 per cent of the population. **Cortical cataract.** Opacity affecting the cortex of the lens and not the nucleus. **Cuneiform cataract.** Spokes of opacity radiating from the periphery of the lens to its centre; the commonest form of senile cataract. **Cupuliform cataract.** Posterior saucer-shaped cataract (see below). **Dermatogenous cataract.** Bilateral cataract associated with the skin diseases neurodermatitis, sclerodermia and chronic eczema. **Diabetic cataract.** 1. Cataract of the ordinary senile form but tending to occur earlier and progress more rapidly. 2. True diabetic cataract with widespread subcapsular opacities rapidly progressive, usually in young patients. **Dilacerated cataract.** A cataract which is congenital or develops soon after birth; fine thin opacity like teased-out moss. **Dinitrophenol cataract.** Cataract occurring in susceptible persons who have taken this drug; it may not appear until some months after, and develops rapidly. **Dust-like cataract.** Perinuclear punctate cataract (see below). **Electric cataract.** Cataract resulting from the passage of an electric current through the body, as occurs when hit by lightning. **Embryonal nuclear cataract.** A central opacity situated in the embryonic nucleus of the crystalline lens of the eye. It has a familial tendency. Called also *cataracta centralis pulverulenta.* **Endocrine cataract.** Opacities in the crystalline lens often associated with endocrine disorders. It is characterized usually by punctate opacities in the cortex. **Fibroid cataract.** One due to maldevelopment of the lens and its replacement by fibrous tissue. **Floriform cataract.** A cataract with peculiar annular opacities in the adult nucleus and cortex. **Fluid cataract.** One in which the lens matter is of fluid consistency. **Fusiform cataract.** An opaque stripe passing from the anterior to the posterior pole of the lens, specified *axial,* or, if there are offshoots, *coralliform.* **Galactose cataract.** Cataract produced experimentally in animals by an excess of galactose in the diet. **Glass-blowers' cataract.** Cataract due to prolonged exposure to heat. It begins as a disc of opacity at the posterior pole. **Glaucomatous cataract.** 1. Cataract occurring in the course of glaucoma. 2. Cataract giving rise to glaucoma. **Green cataract.** A variant of blue cataract (see above). **Grey cataract.** An intermediate stage of senile cataract, before the opacity has become white. **Grumous cataract.** One in which the lens matter is of grumous consistency. **Gypseous cataract.** Calcification of the lens, usually taking place in the late stages of complicated cataract. **Hard cataract.** Cataract due to pathological intensification of the normal sclerosis of the lens, often becoming pigmented (black cataract). **Heat-ray cataract.** Glass-blowers' cataract (see above). **Heterochromic cataract.** Cataract occurring as a complication of heterochromic cyclitis. **Hyaloid cataract.** Opacity of the anterior part of the vitreous, noticeable after cataract extractions. **Hypermature cataract.** One in which the opaque lens loses water and becomes inspissated and shrunken. **Immature cataract.** An early stage of cataract in which only parts of the lens are opaque. **Incipient cataract.** The early stage of any form of cataract. **Infantile cataract.** Cataract developing in infancy, as opposed to congenital and senile forms, often hereditary. Some forms of lamellar cataract are infantile. **Intumescent cataract.** A late stage in the development of cataract, in which the lens swells. **Irradiation cataract.** Radiational cataract (see below). **Juvenile cataract.** Opacities occurring before the age of 40, also known as *presen le cataract;* often hereditary influence is found. **Lactose cataract.** Cataract occurring in experimental animals in whose diet lactose is from 50 to 70 per cent of the total carbohydrate. **Lamellar cataract.** Congenital cataract or occurring in early infancy: one or more lamellae of the lens are cloudy, surrounding the usually clear nucleus. Non-progressive. **Lenticular cataract.** Cataract involving the substance of the lens and not the capsule. **Mature cataract.** Cataract in which the lens is completely opaque and the opacity extends to the anterior capsule, as shown by the absence of iris shadow on lateral illumination. **Membranous cataract.** Deposits of lymph, fibrinous and plastic exudate following postoperative iridocyclitis. **Milk-dot cataract.** One in which the lens is studded with numerous white dots (punctate cataract) which have the bluish-white appearance of milk droplets. **Milky cataract.** Cataract in which some of the lens matter has liquefied to form a milky fluid. **Morgagnian cataract.** A long-standing cataract wherein the cortex of the lens has liquefied and the nucleus has sunk to the bottom of the capsule. **Nuclear cataract.** A senile cataract in which there is an increase in the density of the nucleus. **Perinuclear punctate cataract.** Thickening of the anterior and posterior parts of the adult nucleus associated with small dust-like opacities. A type of senile cortical cataract. **Polar cataract.** A cataract situated at the anterior or posterior pole of the lens. **Posterior saucer-shaped cataract (of Vogt).** Posterior corneal opacities which appear saucer-shaped on slit-lamp examination. A common type of senile cortical cataract more usually called *cupuliform cataract.* **Presenile cataract.** Juvenile cataract (see above). **Progressive cataract.** A cataract in development when opacities are increasing in size or number. **Punctate cataract, Punctiform cataract.** Punctate opacities situated in the cortex and nucleus, but mostly at the periphery, which are found on slit-lamp examination so frequently that they are considered physiological. These dots have a blue coloration (hence the usual name, *blue-dot cataract*) and never progress or interfere with vision. **Pupillary cataract.** Cataract occupying the pupillary area of the lens. **Pyramidal cataract.** Cataract due to adhesion between the anterior capsule of the lens and the back of the cornea, following a perforating ulcer of the latter. **Radiational cataract.** That due to inept radium or x-ray exposure. It has been proved that infra-red rays, x-rays and those emanating from radium will cause cataract, but there is doubt about visible light rays. **Reduplication cataract.** Similar opacities situated at different levels in the lens, often connected by a linear opacity. **Ripe cataract.** Mature cataract (see above). **Secondary cataract.** 1. Cataract secondary to other intra-ocular disease, e.g. iridocyclitis. 2. Remnants of lens matter and capsule left after extracapsular extraction. **Sedimentary cataract.** Morgagnian cataract (see above). **Senile cataract.** The commonest form of cataract, in which lens opacities develop with advancing age. There is great variation in their density and rate of growth. **Siliquose cataract.** A cataract exhibiting absorption of the lens substance and calcification of its capsule. **Snow-flake cataract.** True diabetic cataract (see above). **Soft cataract.** One in which the lens cortex becomes softened and opaque, the nucleus being relatively unaffected. **Spear-shaped cataract.** A congenital opacity, with a strong hereditary tendency, consisting of spiky processes radiating through the axial region of the crystalline lens, described by Vogt; it is very similar to coralliform cataract (see above). **Spindle cataract.** Cataract characterized by an opaque stripe passing from the front to the back of the lens, being wider in the nuclear region. **Spontaneous cataract.** Cataract arising without obvious cause. **Stationary cataract.** One in which the lens opacities remain unchanged, e.g. lamellar cataract (see above). **Stellate cataract.** A star-shaped opacity in the posterior subcapsular layers of the lens, usually traumatic. **Subcapsular cataract.** Opacity due to proliferation of the cells of the anterior capsule of the lens; it may be congenital or acquired, toxic or traumatic. It is sometimes applied to opacity affecting the superficial layers of the lens cortex. **Sunflower cataract.** A cataract formed in the anterior capsule of the lens of the eye and resembling a sunflower in shape; pathognomonic of chalcosis, a condition of the eye caused by the absorption of copper from a retained foreign body of this metal or one of its alloys. **Sutural cataract.** Opacity developing along the lines of junction of the lens fibres, most commonly Y- or ʎ-shaped. **Tetany cataract.** Opacities in the crystalline lens associated with either idiopathic tetany or tetany following thyroidectomy. The condition is characterized by small discrete opacities, which often form large flakes, and coloured crystals, all situated in the cortex, but having a clear zone just beneath the capsule. **Total cataract.** One in which the whole lens is opaque. **Toxic cataract.** Opacities in the crystalline lens associated with the administration of various substances, e.g. dinitrophenol, paradichlorobenzene and ergot (cataracta raphonica), and occasionally in acute toxic illness (cataracta cachectica). **Tremulous cataract.** A cataractous partially dislocated lens. **Ultra-violet cataract.** Ultra-violet rays cause slight degeneration of the lens fibres and subcapsular epithelium, and, although this may be a factor in cataract formation, authorities differ as to whether it can be the primary cause. **Unripe cataract.** One in which there is still some transparent lens substance. **Zonular cataract.** Lamellar cataract (see above). [Gk *katarrhaktes* a portcullis.]

See also: COPPOCK, VOGT (A.), VOSSIUS.

cataracta (kat·ar·akt·ah). Cataract. **Cataracta brunescens.** Black cataract. *See* CATARACT. **Cataracta cachectica.** *See* CATARACT, TOXIC. **Cataracta caerulea.** Punctiform cataract. *See* CATARACT. **Cataracta calcarea.** Gypseous cataract. *See* CATARACT. **Cataracta centralis pulverulenta.** Embryonal nuclear cataract. *See* CATARACT. **Cataracta dermatogenes.** Dermatogenous cataract. *See* CATARACT. **Cataracta neurodermatica.** Cataract arising in association with neurodermatitis. **Cataracta nigra.** Black cataract. *See* CATARACT. **Cataracta ossea.** The formation of bone in the lens occurring, very rarely, in the late stages of cataract when the capsule has ruptured or disintegrated. **Cataracta raphonica.** *See* CATARACT, TOXIC. **Cataracta syndermatotica.** Dermatogenous cataract. *See* CATARACT. [see prec.]

cataractopiesis (kat·ar·akt·o·pi·e′·sis). Couching; the operation, not now in use, of displacing the opaque lens of the eye in cataract by turning it down with a needle into the vitreous body, which eventually absorbed it. [Gk *katarassein* to dash down, *piesis* pressure.]

cataractous (kat·ar·akt·us). Affected with or having the characteristics of cataract.

cataria (kat·a·re·ah). Catnip, the herb *Nepeta cataria* Linn. (family Labiatae), which has been used for its carminative, diaphoretic and tonic properties. [L *catta*.]

catarrh (kat·ahr). The simplest form of inflammation of a mucous membrane, usually associated with an increase in the amount of the normal secretion of mucus. **Acute catarrh.** Acute catarrhal inflammation of a mucous surface. **Alveolar catarrh.** Exudate in the pulmonary alveoli; bronchopneumonia. **Atrophic catarrh.** Excessive dryness associated with the degeneration of mucus-secreting glands of the mucous membrane. **Autumnal catarrh.** Hay fever; allergic rhinitis due to the pollen of autumnal plants. **Bronchial catarrh.** Bronchitis. **Chronic catarrh.** A chronic form of catarrhal inflammation. **Dry catarrh.** Inflammation of a mucous surface, associated with thick viscid mucus, scanty in amount. **Endocervical catarrh.** Chronic cervicitis. **Epidemic catarrh.** Influenza. **Fruehjahr catarrh.** Vernal catarrh (see below). **Gastric catarrh.** Catarrhal gastritis. *See* GASTRITIS. **Haemorrhagic catarrh.** Bronchitis with blood-stained sputum. **Hypertrophic catarrh.** An inflammation of a mucous surface associated with hypertrophy of the mucous and submucous tissues. **Infectious catarrh.** Acute coryza; the common cold. **Intestinal catarrh.** Diarrhoea; enteritis. **Intoxication catarrh.** Catarrh produced by chemical or food poisoning. **Laryngeal catarrh.** Catarrhal inflammation of the larynx. **Lightning catarrh.** An acute vasomotor rhinitis, usually resulting from allergy. **Mycotic catarrh.** A catarrhal condition resulting from a fungus infection. **Nasal catarrh.** Rhinitis; an inflammation of the nasal passages. **Papillary catarrh.** Inflammation of the renal papillae. **Pharyngeal catarrh.** Catarrhal inflammation of the pharynx. **Pituitous catarrh.** Bronchorrhoea serosa. **Postnasal catarrh.** An inflammation of the postnasal space, most commonly secondary to nasal infection or infection of the air sinuses. **Pulmonary catarrh.** Bronchopneumonia. **Russian catarrh.** Influenza. **Spring catarrh.** Vernal catarrh (see below). **Suffocative catarrh.** Suffocative bronchitis; asthma. **Summer catarrh.** Hay fever. *See* FEVER. **Tracheal catarrh.** Tracheitis. **Vasomotor catarrh.** Allergic rhinorrhoea. **Vernal catarrh.** Vernal conjunctivitis; an interstitial form of conjunctivitis, manifested by flat-topped papules in the tarsal conjunctiva, sometimes by gelatinous swelling of the limbus, and of seasonal origin. The cause is thought to be allergic. **Vesical catarrh.** Catarrh of the bladder (see above). [Gk *kata, rhoia* flow.]

See also: BOSTOCK, LAËNNEC.

catarrhal (kat·ahr·al). Of the nature of, produced by or affected with catarrh.

Catarrhina (kat·ar·i·nah). A super-family of the primate sub-order Anthropoidea. It includes all Old World monkeys, all apes, and man. It is often divided into two as Cercopithecoidea and Hominoidea. [Gk *kata, rhis* nose.]

catastalsis (kat·as·tal·sis). During digestion, a downward moving wave of contraction which occurs in the alimentary tract, there not being any preceding wave of inhibition. Cf. ANASTALSIS; DIASTALSIS. [Gk *kata, stellein* to set.]

catastaltic (kat·as·tal·tik). 1. Referring to catastalsis. 2. Inhibitory. 3. Restraining evacuations because of astringent properties. 4. A medicinal agent (e.g. a sedative) which restrains or checks a process. 5. Moving from above downwards, e.g. a nerve impulse.

catastate (kat·as·tate). A result of catabolism. [Gk *katastatos* settled down.]

catastatic (kat·as·**tat**·ik). Relating to a catastate.

catastrophe (kat·**as**·tro·fe). **Otolithic catastrophe.** *See* SYNDROME, OTOLITH. [Gk *katastrophe* sudden turn.]

catatasis (kat·**at**·as·is). General term applied to the measures used in the reduction of a fracture or dislocation by extension. [Gk *katatasis* a stretching.]

catathermometer (kat·ah·ther·**mom**′·et·er). Katathermometer.

catathymia (kat·ah·**thi**·me·ah). The changes to which the psychic content is subjected by affective influences. [Gk *kata, thymos* mind.]

catathymic (kat·ah·**thi**·mik). Governed by the emotions, especially of reasoning, or an argument which superficially appears rational. [see prec.]

catatonia (kat·ah·**to**·ne·ah). 1. A state of increased tone in the muscles at rest, abolished during voluntary movement, and thereby to be distinguished from extrapyramidal rigidity. A special variety is waxy flexibility (flexibilitas cerea). 2. A clinical syndrome, falling within the schizophrenic group, characterized by periodic functional disturbance of muscular innervation of the type described, and also by sudden impulsive movements and attacks of excitement. [Gk *kata, tonos* tension.]

catatoniac (kat·ah·**to**·ne·ak). An individual suffering from catatonia.

catatonic (kat·ah·**ton**·ik). 1. Referring to or indicating a state of catatonia. 2. An individual suffering from catatonia.

catatony (kat·**at**·o·ne). Catatonia.

catatricrotic (kat·ah·tri·**krot**′·ik). Referring to or characterized by catatricrotism.

catatricrotism (kat·ah·**tri**·krot·izm). Abnormality of the pulse consisting in 3 secondary expansions of the artery and shown on the sphygmogram by minor elevations of the downward curve. [Gk *kata, treis* three, *krotein* to strike.]

catatropia (kat·ah·**tro**·pe·ah). Cataphoria. [Gk *kata, trepein* to turn.]

catechin (**kat**·e·kin). A substance present in catechu. Related compounds occur in tea, and catechin is regarded as the basis of many natural tannins.

catechol (**kat**·e·kol). 1. Pyrocatechin, 1=2-dihydroxybenzene, $C_6H_4(OH)_2$. A phenolic substance derived from phlobatannins and catechins, and occurring in wood tar and raw beet sugar. It is a colourless compound used as an antiseptic similar to resorcinol with which it is isomeric. 2. General name for members of a group of dihydroxy phenols derived from 1. above, including adrenaline and noradrenaline. **Catechol oxidase.** Polyphenoloxidase, an enzyme in bacteria, fungi and certain higher plants which specifically activates the oxidation of polyphenols but not of tyrosine.

catecholamines (kat·e·kol·**am**′·eenz). A general name for members of a group of dihydroxy phenols derived from catechol, including adrenaline and noradrenaline. *Catecholamine excretion* is increased in cases of phaeochromocytoma, neuroblastoma and sometimes other conditions in which adrenaline and noradrenaline are produced in excess; it is measured by estimating VMA excretion in urine.

catechu (**kat**·e·kew). Gambir, pale catechu. The dried aqueous extract of *Uncaria gambier,* a climbing shrub cultivated in the East Indies. It consists mainly of catechutannic acid, and a bitter substance, catechin. The tannic acid which the drug contains is released slowly when it is taken by mouth and produces an astringent effect which is useful in the treatment of diarrhoea (BPC 1968). **Black catechu, Catechu Nigrum BPC 1949.** Cutch, an extract of the heartwood of *Acacia catechu* similarly used as an astringent; also used in the tanning industry. [Malay *kachu.*]

catelectrotonus (kat·el·ek·tro·**to**′·nus). The increased irritability shown by a muscle or nerve when it is near the cathode. [Gk *kata,* electrotonus.]

catenating (**kat**·en·a·ting). 1. Referring to a disease which is linked with another. 2. Forming one of a connected series of symptoms. [L *catena* chain.]

catenoid, catenulate (**kat**·en·oid, kat·**en**·ew·late). Having resemblance to a chain. [L *catena* chain, Gk *eidos* form.]

caterpillars (**kat**·er·pil·arz). Name applied to the larvae of butterflies and moths; many are hairy and the hairs of some, particularly Arctiidae (tiger moths) and Saturniidae, can cause intense irritation and dermatitis when the larvae are handled. [L *catta pilosa* hairy cat.]

catfish (**kat**·fish). Siluridae. [L *catta,* AS *fisc.*]

catgut (**kat**·gut). Sterilized Surgical Catgut BP 1968, absorbable material for ligatures or sutures prepared from the submucous layer of the sheep's intestine, rendered aseptic by dry heat or chemical sterilization. **Carbolized catgut.** Catgut sterilized in phenol solution. **Chromic catgut, Chromicized catgut.** Catgut sterilized and rendered stronger and more durable by impregnation with chromium trioxide. **Formaldehyde catgut.** Catgut boiled in formaldehyde-alcohol solution. **I.K.I. catgut, Iodine catgut, Iodized catgut.** Catgut treated by immersion in iodine-potassium iodide solution. **Iodochromic catgut.** Catgut prepared by immersion in a solution of iodine, potassium iodide and potassium dichromate. **Silverized catgut.** Catgut impregnated with silver to increase its strength. [L *catta* gut.]

Catha (**kath**·ah). Arabian, African or Abyssinian tea; the dried leaves of *Catha edulis* Forsk. (family Celastraceae), a small tree of Abyssinia and Arabia. It is a stimulant narcotic, causing excitation of the central nervous system. The leaves are chewed by the Arabs as a stimulant. [Ar. *khat.*]

cathaeresis (kath·a·er·es·is). 1. Weakness or prostration caused by medication. 2. A caustic action of a mild kind. [Gk *kathairesis* a pulling down.]

catharsis (kath·**ar**·sis). 1. Natural or artificial purgation, e.g. of the bowels. 2. Purification, especially of the passions; in psychoanalysis, abreaction, one of the earliest conceptions of the mechanism of cure by the uncovering of unconscious memory or phantasy and the discharge of associated affect. The patient is induced to unburden himself of all the associations connected with the original trauma by re-experiencing and discharging the emotion formerly repressed. [Gk *katharsis* a cleansing.]

cathartate (kath·**ar**·tate). Name given to any salt or ester of cathartic acid.

cathartic (kath·**ar**·tik). 1. Having a purging action or relating to purgation. 2. The term is sometimes used loosely to describe any drug with a purgative action, but should be reserved for purgative drugs containing glycosidal resins, such as jalap, ipomoea, colocynth, podophyllum and scammony resin. The irritant aglycones contained in these drugs are liberated by the action of lipase and bile in the duodenum, causing violent irritation along the whole length of the intestine and increased peristalsis. [Gk *katharsis* a cleansing.]

cathartogenin (kath·ar·**toj**·en·in). An aglycone obtained by the hydrolysis of cathartic acid.

cathect (**kath**·ekt). Cathecticize.

cathectic (kath·**ek**·tik). Referring to cathexis.

cathecticize (kath·**ek**·tis·ize). To charge with mental energy and affect. [Gk *kathektikos* able to retain.]

cathelectrotonus (kath·el·ek·tro·**to**′·nus). Catelectrotonus.

Cathelin, Fernand (b. 1873). French urologist.

Cathelin's anaesthetic technique. Sacral anaesthesia.

Cathelin's segregator. An instrument, now obsolete, which was introduced into the bladder and had a partition device by which it was aimed to collect separately the urine passed into the bladder from each ureter.

Cathelineau's syndrome. Gilles de la Tourette's disease.

cathepsins (kath·**ep**·sinz). Enzymes; proteinases and peptidases of animal tissue. [Gk *kathepsis* a boiling down.]

cathepsis (kath·**ep**·sis). The process of protein synthesis or hydrolysis in living tissue, or autolysis in dead tissue. [Gk *kathepsis* a boiling down.]

catheter (**kath**·et·er). A tube for withdrawing fluid from a body cavity or for introducing fluid into a body cavity. **Balloon catheter.** A twin-lumen catheter through one lumen of which a balloon at the end of the catheter can be distended with air, water or a contrast medium. **Bicoudé catheter.** A catheter with a double angle close to its tip. **Cardiac catheter.** A tube of plastic material passed along a vein to the right auricle or one of the great central veins for collection of blood samples in measuring the cardiac output. **Coudé catheter.** A catheter with an angle near its tip for negotiating a urethra angled forward by an enlarged prostate. **Catheter à demeure.** A catheter left *in situ* for a period. **Elbowed catheter.** A catheter with an angle near the tip; coudé catheter (see above). **Eustachian catheter.** A catheter passed along the eustachian tube by which to distend the middle ear. **Female catheter.** A short silver or glass catheter for the female urethra. **Flexible catheter.** A catheter of malleable material such as rubber. **Gum-elastic catheter.** A flexible catheter of a plastic silk compound. **Indwelling catheter.** A catheter left in place for a period after its introduction. **Lobster-tail catheter.** A catheter jointed in 3 places near its tip. **Opaque catheter.** A catheter impregnated with lead for radioscopic visualization. **Phono catheter.** *See* PHONOCATHETER. **Prostatic catheter.** A long silver catheter with a wide curve. **Railway catheter.** A catheter threaded over a filiform guide passing through a urethral stricture. **Rat-tail catheter.** A catheter that runs to a fine point: used when the urethral opening is narrowed. **Red-rubber catheter.** A rubber catheter with an opening near its rounded tip used for the urethra or other hollow tube. **Self-retaining catheter.** A catheter fashioned to remain in place after its passage. **Sigmoid catheter.** An S-shaped catheter for the bladder in females. **Silver catheter.** A catheter of that metal for emptying of an obstructed bladder. **Soft catheter.** Red-rubber catheter (see above). **Two-way catheter.** A double-channelled catheter for irrigation. **Ureteric catheter.** A fine graduated gum-elastic catheter passed by way of a cystoscope into the ureter and up to the renal pelvis for the introduction of opaque fluid and radiological visualization of the kidney. **Ventricular catheter.** A catheter passed from the 4th ventricle along the aqueduct of the 3rd ventricle in operations for the relief of internal hydrocephalus. **Vertebrated catheter.** A flexible catheter of short-hinged segments. **Whistle-tip catheter.** A catheter with both a terminal and a lateral opening. **Winged catheter.** A self-retaining catheter with 2 lateral projections near its tip. [Gk *katheter* a thing lowered into.]

See also: BOZEMAN, DE PEZZER, FOLEY, FRITSCH, ITARD, MALECOT, SCHROETTER, SKENE.

catheterism (**kath**·et·er·izm). The condition of being habituated to the use of a catheter.

catheterization (**kath**·et·er·i·za'·shun). The passing of a catheter. **Cardiac catheterization.** The introduction of a flexible radio-opaque catheter by way of the median basilic or saphenous vein. A flow of saline and heparin in maintained through the catheter, which is passed under fluoroscopy into the superior vena cava, right atrium, right ventricle and pulmonary artery. It may also enter the inferior vena cava, the hepatic vein and, in the presence of abnormal openings, the other great vessels and cardiac chambers. Pressures may be recorded from the various cardiac chambers entered, and samples of blood withdrawn for determination of oxygen saturation. **Laryngeal catheterization.** Intubation. **Retro-urethral catheterization.** The passing of a catheter from the bladder end of the urethra. **Suprapubic catheterization.** The fixation of a catheter in the bladder by making a suprapubic opening surgically.

catheterize (**kath**·et·er·ize). To pass a catheter.

catheterostat (**kath**·et·er·o·stat). A container in which catheters may be sterilized and kept. [catheter, Gk *statos* standing.]

cathetometer (kath·et·**om**·et·er). 1. An instrument with which small differences in height, e.g. as between 2 columns of fluid or mercury, can be measured. It consists of a sliding telescopic levelling apparatus which can be moved up and down an upright standard on which fine gradations are marked. 2. A similar instrument with which other differences can be determined. In this case the telescope moves along a graduated bar. [Gk *kathetos* vertical height, meter.]

cathexis (kath·**ex**·is). That amount of energy, emotional or mental, which attaches to any object or idea. **Cathexis of the ego.** The psychic energy attached to objects or to mental processes. **Object cathexis.** The presence in someone of a cathexis towards a certain object. [Gk *kathexis* retention.]

cathisophobia (**kath**·is·o·**fo'**·be·ah). 1. A mental affection in which there is morbid fear of sitting still and consequently inability to do so. 2. A form of rhythmic chorea in which the subject is not able to remain seated for any length of time. [Gk *kathizein* to sit down, phobia.]

cathodal (kath·**o**·dal). Relating to a cathode.

cathode (**kath**·ode). The negative pole or electrode of an electric current, or of an electric battery, cell or other device. Cf. ANODE. **Cathode rays.** *See* RAY. [Gk *kata, hodos* way.]

cathodic (kath·**od**·ik). 1. Referring to a cathode. 2. Emanating from a cathode. 3. In physiology, indicating the efferent course of a nerve impulse.

catholysis (kath·**ol**·is·is). Electrolysis induced with the cathode needle.

catholyte (**kath**·ol·ite). In electrolysis, that portion of the electrolyte which is in immediate relationship to the cathode.

cation (**kat**·i·on). An ion which carries the positive charge in the direction of the current and delivers it at the cathode in electrolysis. Neutral molecules of electrolytes dissociate on solution into oppositely-charged ions: ions of metals and hydrogen carry positive charges and migrate towards the cathode; they are the cations, and are atoms which have lost one or more electrons, leaving the positively charged nuclei unneutralized. [Gk *kata*, ion.]

cationic (kat·i·**on**·ik). Of the nature of, or concerned with, a cation.

cationogen (kat·i·**on**·o·jen). Any substance which in solution produces cations. [cation, Gk *genein* to produce.]

catlin, catling (**kat**·lin, **kat**·ling). A sharp-pointed double-edged knife, long and straight, used in amputations. [dim. of AS *cat.*]

catmint, catnep, catnip (**kat**·mint, **kat**·nep, **kat**·nip). The herb *Nepeta cataria* Linn. (family Labiatae), which has been used for its carminative, diaphoretic and tonic properties. [AS *catminte.*]

catodont (**kat**·o·dont). An individual who has natural teeth only in the lower jaw. [Gk *kata, odous* tooth.]

catophoria (kat·o·**for**·e·ah). Cataphoria.

catoptric (kat·**op**·trik). 1. Referring to mirrors or reflected light. 2. Produced by or depending upon reflection. [Gk *katoptron* mirror.]

catoptrics (kat·**op**·trix). The branch of physics which is concerned with mirrors and reflected light. [see prec.]

catoptrophobia (kat·op·tro·**fo'**·be·ah). Unreasoning and excessive dread of mirrors. [Gk *katoptron* mirror, phobia.]

catoptroscope (kat·**op**·tro·skope). A device by means of which objects can be examined by reflected light. [Gk *katoptron* mirror, *skopein* to watch.]

catotropia (kat·o·**tro**·pe·ah). Cataphoria. [Gk *kato* downwards, *trepein* to turn.]

Cattaneo's sign. Red spots appearing over the spines of the dorsal vertebrae when strongly percussed indicate disease of the tracheobronchial lymph glands.

Cattell, Raymond Bernard (b. 1905). English psychologist.

Cattell culture-free test. A non-verbal intelligence test.

Catterall, Mary. British anaesthetist.

M.C. mask. An oronasal oxygen mask which prevents too high a blood oxygen tension being produced. Described in 1967.

cauda [NA] (**kaw**·dah). A tail or a tail-like appendage. **Cauda cerebelli.** The vermis of the cerebellum. **Cauda equina [NA].** A sheaf of roots (like a horse's tail) of the lumbar, sacral, and coccygeal nerves which runs down through the lower part of the spinal canal below the level of the 1st lumbar vertebra, where the spinal cord ends. **Cauda medullae.** A term for the spinal cord and the medulla oblongata taken as one structure. **Cauda muliebris.** The clitoris. **Cauda salax.** The penis. **Cauda striati.** The tail of the caudate nucleus. [L tail.]

caudal (**kaw**·dal). 1. Relating to or resembling a tail. 2. [Caudalis (NA).] Descriptive of a position towards the tail end of the long axis of the body. [see prec.]

caudate (kaw·date). 1. Having a tail-like appendage. 2. Tailed. **Caudate nucleus.** *See* NUCLEUS. **Caudate process of liver.** *See* PROCESS. [L *cauda* tail.]

caudation (kaw·**da**·shun). 1. The condition of having a tail-like appendage. 2. Elongation of the clitoris. [see prec.]

caudatolenticular (kaw·da·to·len·**tik**′·ew·lar). Relating to the caudate and the lentiform nuclei of the corpus striatum.

caudatum (kaw·**da**·tum). The caudate nucleus of the corpus striatum.

caudiduct (kaw·de·dukt). In anatomy, to carry backwards in the direction of the tail. [L *cauda* tail, *ducere* to lead.]

caul (kawl). 1. The greater sac of the peritoneum; the great omentum. 2. A part of the membranes enveloping the fetus which may cover the head and face and in labour be extruded in advance of them. **Pseudoperitoneal caul.** A pathological membranous structure formed about the colon. [ME *cawel* basket.]

Caulk, John Roberts (b. 1881). St. Louis urologist.

Caulk punch. A cautery punch for the removal of median bar prostatic enlargements. The tissue to be resected is rendered avascular by the diathermy current before resection.

caulophylline (kawl·o·fil·een). Methylcytisine, $C_{12}H_{16}ON_2$. An alkaloid obtained by precipitating the alcoholic tincture of caulophyllum or blue cohosh. It is a diuretic and emmenagogue.

caulophyllum (kawl·o·fil·um). Blue cohosh, papoose root; the rhizome and roots of *Caulophyllum thalictroides* (Linn.) Michx. (family Berberidaceae), of the USA and Canada. It contains saponins, an alkaloid and resin, and has been used as a diuretic, antispasmodic and emmenagogue. [Gk *kaulos* stalk, *phyllon* leaf.]

cauloplegia (kawl·o·**ple**·je·ah). Paralysis of the penis. [Gk *kaulos* stalk, *plege* stroke.]

caumaesthesia (kawm·es·**the**·ze·ah). A sensation of burning heat although the temperature of the patient and of the surrounding atmosphere is low. [Gk *kauma* heat, aesthesia.]

causalgia (kawz·**al**·je·ah). Burning pain, intense hypersensitivity and trophic changes in the cutaneous distribution of an injured peripheral nerve, especially the median and sciatic nerves. [Gk *kausis* a burning, *algos* pain.]

cause (kawz). Something that produces an effect; the condition from which something results. **Antecedent cause.** A predisposing factor. **Constitutional cause.** A cause that lies in the general condition of the body. **Determining cause.** The final factor which brings about an effect. **Efficient cause.** A cause which is sufficient in itself. **Endopathic cause.** A cause arising from some morbid condition within the body. **Essential cause.** A factor without which the effect could not be produced. **Exciting cause.** The final determining factor. **Exopathic cause, External cause.** A cause arising outside the body. **Immediate cause.** Exciting cause (see above). **Internal cause.** A cause arising from within the body. **Local cause.** A cause localized to a part of the body; not constitutional. **Predisponent cause, Predisposing cause.** Any condition that favours the essential or specific cause of a disease. **Primary cause.** The main or essential cause. **Proximate cause.** A cause immediately preceding an event. **Remote cause.** A cause that is not immediate in its effect but is predisposing. **Secondary cause.** One that aids the primary or essential cause. **Specific cause.** A factor that produces an effect specific to itself, e.g. the microbe of an infectious disease. **Ultimate cause.** The remote cause that initiated the train of events. [L *causa*.]

caustic (kaw·stik). 1. Exercising a corrosive or escharotic action. 2. Any substance which destroys tissue by chemical corrosion or burning. **Lunar caustic.** Toughened Silver Nitrate BP 1958. **Mitigated caustic.** Mitigated Silver Nitrate BPC 1959. *See* SILVER. **Perpetual caustic.** Fused silver nitrate. **Caustic potash.** Potassium Hydroxide BP 1958. **Caustic soda.** Sodium Hydroxide BP 1958. **Vienna caustic.** Vienna paste; potassium hydroxide and slaked lime made into a paste with alcohol and glycerin. **Zinc caustic.** Zinc chloride mixed with flour. [Gk *kaustikos* burning.]

See also: CHURCHILL, FILHOS, LANDOLFI, LUGOL, PLUNKET, ROUSSELOT.

causticity (kaws·**tis**·it·e). The quality or state of being caustic or corrosive.

causticize (kaws·tis·ize). 1. To make caustic. 2. To convert into a hydroxide by the use of lime.

cauter (kaw·ter). The metal instrument used for cauterization. [Gk *kauterion* branding iron.]

cauterant (kaw·ter·ant). 1. A caustic or cauterizing agent. 2. Cauterizing or caustic.

cauterization (kaw·ter·i·**za**′·shun). The process of burning a part with a cautery. **Cold cauterization.** Cauterization by the application of carbon dioxide snow. **Distant cauterization.** That carried out by keeping the hot iron at a distance from the part of the body surface to be cauterized. **Neapolitan cauterization.** Cauterization of deep tissues reached through an incision. **Objective cauterization.** Distant cauterization (see above). **Cauterization by points, Punctate cauterization.** Cauterization of deep tissues by means of a pointed iron. **Slow cauterization.** Cauterization in which a moxa is used. **Solar cauterization.** Burning by a lens focusing the rays of the sun. **Subcutaneous cauterization.** Cauterization of deep tissues by means of a cautery heat-insulated except at its tip, or by the subcutaneous injection of a caustic substance. **Sun cauterization.** Solar cauterization (see above). **Tubular cauterization.** The cauterizing of the walls of a cyst by means of an instrument connected to the negative pole of a battery.

cauterize (kaw·ter·ize). To cause local burning with a caustic agent or a cautery.

cautery (kaw·ter·e). 1. Cauterization. 2. A hot iron or other agent used in cauterization. **Actual cautery.** Red-hot or white-hot metal which produces its effect by heat as opposed to chemical action or diathermy. **Button cautery.** A handled hemisphere of iron applied momentarily at red heat to produce counter-irritation. **Dento-electric cautery.** An electric cautery used in dentistry. **Electric cautery, Galvanic cautery.** A wire cautery heated by galvanic current. **Gas cautery.** A gas flame adapted for burning tissues. **Steam cautery.** The treatment of benign uterine conditions, or the arrest of uterine haemorrhage, by the direct application of super-heated steam. [Gk *kauterion* branding-iron.]

See also: CORRIGAN, PAQUELIN, SOUTTAR.

cava (ka·vah). 1. A vena cava. 2. Any external hollow or cavity of the body. [L *cavum* cavity.]

caval (ka·val). 1. Relating to a vena cava. 2. Hollow. [see prec.]

Cavare's disease. Familial periodic paralysis. *See* PARALYSIS.

cavascope (kav·as·kope). An instrument with which the interior of a body cavity can be illuminated and examined. [L *cavum* cavity, Gk *skopein* to watch.]

cave (kave). *See* MECKEL, RETZIUS (A. A.). [L *cava* cavity.]

cavern (kav·ern). 1. A pathological cavity resulting from destruction of tissue, such as occurs in a tuberculous lung. 2. A hole in the optic disc which may be congenital, due to glaucoma, or of the Schnabel type. The word "cup" is more commonly used. [L *caverna* cavity.]

See also: SCHNABEL.

Cavernicola pilosa (kav·er·**nik**·o·lah pi·**lo**·sa). A reduviid bug which is a potential vector of American trypanosomiasis. [L *caverna* cavity, *colere* to inhabit, *pilosus* hairy.]

caverniloquy (kav·ern·**il**·o·kwe). The hollow low-pitched pectoriloquy which is a sign of the presence of a cavity in the chest. [cavern, L *loqui* to speak.]

cavernitis (kav·ern·**i**·tis). Inflammation of the corpus cavernosum of the penis or corpus cavernosum of the clitoris. **Fibrous cavernitis.** Peyronie's disease. [cavernosum, Gk *-itis* inflammation.]

cavernoma (kav·ern·**o**·mah). Cavernous angioma. *See* ANGIOMA. **Cavernoma lymphaticum.** Lymphangioma cavernosum. **Portal cavernoma.** A disorder of the portal venous system with dilated cavernous changes, probably developmental. [cavern, Gk *-oma* tumour.]

cavernoscope (kav·ern·o·skope). An instrument by means of which lung cavities can be examined. The instrument is pushed into the cavity by way of an intercostal space. [cavern, Gk *skopein* to watch.]

cavernoscopy (kav·ern·**os**·ko·pe). The use of a cavernoscope in examination of lung cavities.

cavernositis (kav·ern·o·**si′**·tis). Inflammation of the corpus cavernosum of the penis or corpus cavernosum of the clitoris. [cavernosum, Gk *-itis* inflammation.]

cavernostomy (kav·ern·**os**·to·me). The draining of an abscess of the lung through an incision. [cavern, Gk *stoma* mouth.]

cavernosum (kav·ern·o·sum). Corpus cavernosum. [L full of hollows.]

cavernotomy (kav·ern·**ot**·o·me). The cutting into and evacuation of the contents of a tuberculous pyocalyx. [cavern, Gk *temnein* to cut.]

cavernous (kav·ern·us). 1. Relating to or resembling a cavity. 2. Containing cavities. 3. Relating to the corpus cavernosa of the penis, or to the cavernous sinus in the base of the skull. **Cavernous plexus.** *See* PLEXUS. **Cavernous sinus.** *See* SINUS OF THE DURA MATER. [see prec.]

cavilla (kav·**il**·ah). The sphenoid bone. [L small cavity.]

cavitary (kav·it·ar·e). 1. Having or relating to a cavity or cavities. 2. In zoology, having an alimentary cavity or coelom.

cavitation (kav·it·a·shun). Bubbles or *cavitation voids* appearing in a liquid on application of high intensity alternating ultrasonic waves. [L *cavum* cavity.]

cavitis (ka·vi·tis). An inflamed condition of a vena cava. [vena cava, Gk *-itis* inflammation.]

cavity (kav·it·e). 1. A hole or space; in anatomy, often only a potential space [cavum (NA)]. 2. In dentistry, a decayed hollow in a tooth, or a prepared excavation. **Cavity of the abdomen [cavum abdominis (NA)].** The space bounded by the diaphragm above, by the muscular abdominal wall anteriorly and laterally, and by the vertebral column and associated muscles posteriorly. Below, it extends into the pelvis (pelvic cavity) which is closed by the pelvic diaphragm, made up chiefly of the levator ani muscles. **Amniotic cavity.** The fluid-filled cavity of the amniotic sac surrounding the developing embryo. **Arachnoid cavity.** The subarachnoid space. *See* SPACE. **Axial cavity.** A cavity in an axial surface of a tooth. **Body cavity.** The interior of the thorax and abdomen. **Buccal cavity.** 1. Vestibule of the mouth. 2. A cavity on the buccal aspect of a tooth. **Cerebral cavity.** The cavity of the skull which contains the brain, etc. **Coelomic cavity.** The coelom; the cavity formed in all vertebrates by the splitting of the mesoderm adjacent to the alimentary canal into somatic and splanchnic layers. In mammals the general coelomic cavity is always divided into 2 pleural cavities, a pericardial cavity, and a peritoneal cavity. **Complex cavity.** A cavity involving more than one surface of a tooth. **Cavity of the concha [cavum conchae (NA)].** The concave hollow of the auricle of the ear into which the external auditory meatus opens. **Cotyloid cavity.** The acetabulum. **Cranial cavity.** Cerebral cavity (see above). **Digital cavity.** The occipital horn of the lateral ventricle. **Epidural cavity.** The extradural space. *See* SPACE. **Epiploic cavity.** The lesser sac of the peritoneum. **Erosion cavity.** A cavity formed at the neck of the tooth as a result of erosion. **Fissure cavity.** A cavity commencing in a fissure on the surface of a tooth. **Gastrula cavity.** Archenteron. **Glenoid cavity [cavitas glenoidalis (NA)].** The shallow cavity on the scapula with which the head of the humerus articulates. **Infraglottic cavity [cavum infraglotticum (NA)].** The part of the laryngeal cavity below the rima glottidis. **Joint cavity [cavum articulare (NA)].** The potential cavity between the articulating surfaces of a synovial joint, enclosed by the synovial membrane and capsule. **Cavity of the larynx [cavum laryngis (NA)].** The interior of the larynx, communicating above with the pharynx and below with the cavity of the trachea. **Lymph cavity.** An imprecise term which may refer to the cisterna chyli or to the cavities of the larger lymph trunks. **Mastoid cavity.** The mastoid air cells. **Medullary cavity [cavum medullare (NA)].** The cylindrical cavity, filled with marrow, in the interior of a long bone. **Cavity of the mouth [cavum oris (NA)].** The cavity containing the teeth and part of the tongue. **Cavity of the mouth, proper [cavum oris proprium (NA)].** That part of the cavum oris bounded laterally by the teeth. **Nerve cavity.** Pulp cavity (see below). **Cavity of the nose [cavum nasi (NA)].** The cavity of the nose divided into halves by a sagittal septum. Each communicates through the anterior nares with the face, and through the posterior nares with the nasopharynx. They are bounded above by cribriform plates of the ethmoid, below by the hard palate and laterally by the paranasal air sinuses. **Occlusal cavity.** A cavity in the occlusal surface of a tooth. **Pelvic cavity, Cavity of the pelvis [cavum pelvis (NA)].** *See* CAVITY OF THE ABDOMEN (above). **Pericardial cavity [cavum pericardii (NA)].** The serous cavity between the visceral and parietal layers of the pericardium. Since the pericardium is filled by the heart, its cavity is potential only. **Cavity of the peritoneum [cavum peritonei (NA)].** The potential serous cavity between the layer of peritoneum covering the abdominal viscera and the parietal peritoneum covering the inside of the abdominal wall. **Cavity of the pharynx [cavum pharyngis (NA)].** The cavity comprising the nasopharynx, oral pharynx, and laryngeal pharynx. **Pit cavity.** A cavity commencing in a pit on the surface of a tooth. **Cavity of the pleura [cavum pleurae (NA)].** The potential serous cavity between the layer of pleura covering the lung and the parietal pleura on the inner aspect of the chest wall and upper surface of the diaphragm. **Pleuroperitoneal cavity.** The combined pleural and peritoneal cavities of the early embryo before their separation. **Proximal cavity.** A cavity in the proximal surface of a tooth. **Pulp cavity.** Cavity of a tooth (see below). **Segmentation cavity.** The cavity, or blastocoele, formed within the mass of dividing cells of the early developing ovum. **Cavity of the septum lucidum [cavum septi pellucidi (NA)].** The small cavity between the two leaves of the septum lucidum beneath the corpus callosum. **Serous cavity.** A space lined by serous mesothelium; the pleural, pericardial and peritoneal cavities, and the tunica vaginalis of the testis. **Somatic cavity.** The coelom; coelomic cavity (see above). **Splanchnic cavity, Subgerminal cavity.** The cavity which appears beneath the germinal disc during the early development of large-yolked eggs. **Cavity of the thorax [cavum thoracis (NA)].** The cavity enclosed by the ribs, sternum, thoracic part of the vertebral column and associated muscles, and by the diaphragm. **Cavity of a tooth [cavum dentis (NA)].** The physiological space in the centre of a tooth which contains the tooth pulp. **Tympanic cavity [cavum tympani (NA)].** The middle ear. *See* EAR. **Tympanic cavity, floor of the [paries jugularis (NA)].** The narrow inferior wall formed by a thin plate of bone which separates the cavity from the jugular fossa. **Tympanic cavity, roof of the [paries tegmentalis (NA)].** The superior wall formed of a thin plate of bone, the tegmen tympani, separating the epitympanic recess from the floor of the middle cranial fossa. **Tympanic cavity, anterior wall of the [paries caroticus (NA)].** A narrow wall merging above with the down-sloping anterior end of the roof. Its lower part is formed by a thin plate of bone separating the tympanum from the carotid canal. Between these there are the openings of 2 parallel canals; the smaller upper one lodges the tensor tympani muscles, the lower and larger is the bony pharyngotympanic tube. **Tympanic cavity, lateral wall of the [paries membranaceus (NA)].** A wall formed almost entirely by the tympanic membrane. **Tympanic cavity, medial wall of the [paries labyrinthicus (NA)].** This, which also forms the lateral wall of the labyrinth, is approximately rectangular. The first coil of the cochlea forms a large eminence on its anterior part, the promontory. Above and behind this an oval opening, the fenestra vestibuli, communicates with the bony vestibule and lodges the foot of the stapes. Behind and below, a round aperture, the fenestra cochlea, connects with the bony cochlea and is closed by the secondary tympanic membrane. Between the two is a depression, the sinus tympani. A thin shelf of bone terminating in a hook posteriorly, the processus cochleariformis, overhangs the fenestra vestibuli; the tendon of the tensor tympani muscle plays around it. **Tympanic**

cavity, posterior wall of the [paries mastoideus (NA)]. A thin narrow wall in the epitympanic portion of which is the opening of the aditus into the antrum. Below this is a conical projection, the pyramid, which has a hole at the summit transmitting the tendon of the stapedius muscle. Lateral to this is the opening of the posterior canaliculus for the chorda tympani nerve. **Cavity of the uterus [cavum uteri (NA)].** The cavity of the body of the uterus and the cervical canal; these are continuous at the internal os uteri. The former is a triangular-shaped cleft in the coronal plane, with its apex at the internal os and its base at the fundus. **Visceral cavity.** An imprecise term which might mean the cavity of a viscus (e.g. of the bladder or stomach), or refer to any of the serous cavities of the body (see above). **Yolk cavity.** Subgerminal cavity (see above). [L *cavum.*]

See also: BAER (K. E.), MECKEL, RETZIUS (A. A.), ROSENMUELLER.

cavogram (ka·vo·gram). An x-ray film obtained in the radiographical examination of the vena cava. [vena cava, Gk *gramma* record.]

cavography (ka·vog·raf·e). Radiographical examination of the vena cava after injection of an opaque contrast solution. [vena cava, Gk *graphein* to record.]

cavovalgus (ka·vo·val·gus). Talipes cavus with talipes valgus as a complication. [L *cavum* cavity, *valgu* bow-legged.]

cavum coronale [NA] (ka·vum kor·on·a·le). That part of the pulp cavity which lies immediately deep to the crown of a tooth. [L *cavum* cavity, *corona* crown.]

cavum trigeminale [NA] (ka·vum tri·jem·in·a′·le). A finger-like recess of the dura mater projecting from the posterior to the middle cranial fossa, and lodging parts of the roots and ganglion of the trigeminal nerve. [L *cavum* cavity, *trigeminus* triple.]

cavus (ka·vus). Talipes cavus. [L *cavum* cavity.]

Cazenave, Pierre Louis Alphée (b. 1795). Paris dermatologist.

Cazenave's disease. Pemphigus foliaceus.

c cell (see sel). The cells in the thyroid gland that secrete calcitonin.

ceasmic (se·az·mik). Marked by the persistence of embryonic fissures after birth. [Gk *keazein* to split.]

cebocephalia (se·bo·kef·a′·le·ah). A deformity of the fetal head, the features being monkey-like with eyes closely set and nose absent or rudimentary. [Gk *kebos* monkey, *kephale* head.]

cebocephalus (se·bo·kef·al·us). A fetus with a head like that of a monkey, closely-set eyes and rudimentary nose. [see prec.]

cebocephaly (se·bo·kef·al·e). Cebocephalia.

cec-. For words beginning with **Cec-**, *see* CAEC-.

cedar (se·dar). Strictly, trees belonging to the coniferous genus *Cedrus* Lawson., but in commerce the name is often applied to species of *Cedrela* or other genus. [Gk *kedros.*]

cedrene (sed·reen). $C_{15}H_{24}$, a liquid terpene hydrocarbon occurring in the oil of American red cedar, *Juniperius virginiana.*

cedron (se·dron). The seeds of *Simaba cedron* Planch. (family Simarubaceae), which have been used in malarial fevers; a febrifuge, bitter, and tonic.

Čejka, Johann Joseph (b. 1812). Prague physician.

Čejka's sign. Absence of change in the area of cardiac dullness on inspiration in cases of adherent pericardium. Normally the heart moves during respiration, and the area of dullness changes. The value of this sign is questionable, since on inspiration expansion of the lungs tends to cover the heart and decrease the area of dullness, irrespective of whether the heart lies fixed or mobile in the mediastinum.

ceke (the·ke). Elephantiasis of the scrotum. [Fiji word.]

cel-. For words beginning with **Cel-**, *see also* COEL-.

celandine (sel·an·dine). Chelidonium, greater celandine; the herb *Chelidonium majus* Linn. (family Papaveraceae) containing alkaloids, and with diuretic and cathartic properties. The fresh juice is a domestic application for warts. **Lesser celandine.** The herb *Ranunculus ficaria* Linn. (family Ranunculaceae), taken internally as an infusion, or used in the form of an ointment or suppository, for haemorrhoids. [Gk *chelidonion* swallow-wort.]

celation (sel·a·shun). Concealment of pregnancy or childbirth. [L *celare* to conceal.]

celectome (se·lek·tome). An instrument used for the removal of a piece of tissue from a tumour for microscopical and other examinations. [Gk *kele* hernia, *temnein* to cut.]

celery (sel·er·e). Apium, celery fruit, celery seed, apii fructus; the dried ripe fruits of cultivated plants of *Apium graveolens* Linn. [Gk *selinon* celery.]

cell (sel). 1. In biology, a unit from which living organisms and tissues are built. At some stage of its existence it is capable of reproduction by mitotic division. Each is a highly organized structure containing a nucleus (karyoplasm) surrounded by protoplasm (cytoplasm) and limited externally by a cell membrane. The cytoplasm contains organoids such as mitochondria and the reticular apparatus of Golgi, and in many cases such inclusions as secretory granules, pigment, fat droplets, glycogen, etc. In multicellular organisms, cells are differentiated in relation to different functions (e.g. secretory cells, nerve cells, germ cells, etc.). They are also classified according to their shape (e.g. columnar, cubical, squamous, etc.), or arrangement (e.g. stratified cells), or cytoplasmic inclusions (e.g. pigment cells, fat cells, etc.), or presence in a particular tissue (e.g. connective-tissue cells, cartilage cells), or from the possession of some special structural feature (e.g. ciliated cell, hair cell). 2. [Cellula (NA).] In anatomy, any small hollow space or cavity, such as an accessory nasal air sinus. 3. In electricity, a source of electrical energy depending upon chemical action and complete in itself. 4. In crystallography, an element of the structure of a crystal. **Acid cell.** A parietal cell of the gastric mucosa which secretes hydrochloric acid. **Acidophil cell, Acidophilic cell.** Any cell having an affinity for acid dyes such as eosin, or acid fuchsine. **Acoustic hair cells.** The neurosensory cells of the organ of Corti in the cochlea. **Adelomorphous cell.** Chief cell (see below). **Adipose cell.** Fat cell (see below). **Adventitial cell.** A type of phagocytic cell found in or around the wall of a blood or lymphatic vessel. **Albuminous cell.** Serous cell (see below). **Algoid cells.** Cells resembling algae, seen sometimes in the faeces when there is chronic diarrhoea. **Alpha cell.** One of the cell types of the anterior pituitary, pancreatic islets, or other glandular tissue possessing more than one cell type. It is usually applied to eosinophilic or acidophilic cells. **Alveolar cell.** A lining cell of lung alveolus. **Amacrine cell.** A type of retinal neurone found between the rods and cones on the one side and the ganglion cells on the other. No axon can be demonstrated. **Amoeboid cell.** A cell capable of active migration by the throwing out and retraction of pseudopodia, like an amoeba. **Ancestral cell.** A parent cell which by proliferation, and differentiation of some of the daughter cells, gives rise to adult fully functional cells. The earlier, more embryonic, less differentiated forerunner of a later, more mature cell. **Antipodal cell.** One of the lower 4 large blastomeres of an 8-cell segmenting ovum. **Apocrine cell.** A secretory cell in which the distal part of the cell is cast off with the secretory granules, as is the case in the sebaceous and mammary glands. **Apolar cell.** Any unpolarized cell, especially a nerve cell without processes. **Apoplectic cell.** A blood-filled cavity in the brain, resulting from cerebral haemorrhage or thrombosis. **Apud cells.** Endocrine cells which secrete polypeptide hormones. (The name is derived from *a*mine *p*recursor *u*ptake and *D*-carboxylation, including cells which secrete calcitonin, glucagon, insulin, gastrin, secretin and other hormones.) **Argentaffin cell.** A cell whose cytoplasm readily reduces silver salts, or which contains granules which do so, such as some of the epithelial cells of the intestinal crypts of Lieberkühn. **Argyrophil cell.** Any cell staining with reduced silver. **Arkyochrome cell.** A nerve cell in which the Nissl substance is arranged in the form of a network. **Auditory cell.** Acoustic hair cell (see above). **B cell.** Bone-marrow derived (or in birds, bursa-derived) lymphocyte mediating humoral immunity. **Balloon cells.** Cells described by Unna, and seen in herpes zoster. They are formed by a degenerative process affecting the rete mucosum; the affected cells become large and spheroidal and lose their fibrillary structure and intercellular processes. Their cytoplasm is transformed into a cloudy, homogeneous, eosinophilic mass. In the early forms, inclusion bodies are to be seen in the nuclei. **Banana cells.** The resistant ligneous cells developed in the banana fruit which, when found in the faeces of persons suffering from an intestinal disorder, have sometimes been mistaken for helminths or fungi. **Band cell.** A stage in the development of a granular leucocyte, in which the nucleus is unsegmented. **Barrier-layer photo cell.** A photovoltaic cell having a semitransparent metal layer sputtered on to a semiconductor, usually selenium, forming a "barrier layer" of high resistance between them. Photons absorbed in the semiconductor eject electrons into the metal film across the barrier layer, some of which return to the semiconductor by flowing through the external circuit connected between the electrodes. **Basal cell, Basilar cell.** A cell in the deepest or germinal layer of a stratified epithelium. **Basket cell.** 1. A degenerated leucocyte seen in blood smears, which has a basket-like form. 2. A large cell in the deep stratum of the molecular layer of the cerebellar cortex. **Basophilic cell.** A cell with an affinity for basophil stains, notably the basophilic leucocyte or mast cell, and the basophilic or stippled red cell. **Beaker cell.** Goblet cell (see below). **Beta cell.** One of the cell types in glands such as the anterior pituitary or the pancreatic islets, in which there is a mixture of cell types. Usually applied to the basophilic cells. **Bichromate cell.** A one-fluid cell containing a mixture of potassium bichromate and sulphuric acid in equal parts by weight, diluted with 7 parts of water by weight. The electrodes consist of a zinc plate between 2 carbon plates immersed in the electrolyte. It provides an e.m.f. of 2.1 V. **Binary nerve cell.** Bipolar nerve cell (see following). **Bipolar nerve cell.** A neurone with 2 processes. **Bladder cell.** A swollen epithelial cell found in the embryonic fingers and toes. **Blast cell.** A primitive cell of any group. **Bloated cell.** A swollen astrocyte, showing fatty degeneration. **Blood cell.** Any one of the many types of nucleated and non-nucleated cellular bodies that are found in the blood plasma, marrow and other body tissues: the main ones are the red cells (erythrocytes), white cells (leucocytes), platelets or thrombocytes, and the many early or primitive red cells (the several erythroblasts) and granular or non-granular white cells. **Bone cell.** The osteocyte; a flattened melon-seed-like cell with numerous spidery processes, characteristic of bony tissue. **Border cell.** The parietal cell of the gastric mucosa secreting hydrochloric acid. **Breviradiate cell.** A neuroglial cell with short processes. **Bristle cell.** A cell such as an auditory hair cell, or any of the hair cells of the maculae and cristae of the membranous labyrinth. **Bronchic cell.** A lung alveolus. **Brood cell.** A parent cell which gives rise to a cluster of daughter cells. **Brush cell.** A cell with a group of bristle-like processes at one extremity. **Burr cells.** Burr-shaped red blood corpuscles seen in the haemolytic-uraemia syndrome. **C cell.** An agranular cell-type from the islets of Langerhans. **Cadmium cell.** A standard cell having electrodes of mercury and cadmium amalgam in an electrolyte of cadmium sulphate, with mercurous sulphate as a depolarizer. It furnishes an e.m.f. of 1.108 V at 20°C. **Calciform cell.** Goblet cell (see below). **Calcigerous cell.** A cell which can cause the deposition of inorganic calcium in its immediate vicinity, e.g. an osteoblast. **Cameloid cell.** An ellipsoidal red blood cell (normal in the *Camelidae*). **Capsule cell.** One of the cells forming a capsule-like arrangement around the bodies of the ganglion cells in the spinal cord and sympathetic ganglia. **Carmine cell.** A phagocytic cell which will take up grains of carmine supravitally. **Cartilage cell.** The spherical cell typical of cartilaginous tissue. **Caryochrome cell.** Karyochrome cell (see below). **Castration cell.** A special pituitary cell which develops during gonadal insufficiency. **Caudate cell.** A neuroglial cell with the shape of a long-tailed comet. **Central cell.** Chief or peptic cell (see below). **Centro-acinar cell, Centro-acinous cell.** A cell of a pancreatic acinus at its junction with the duct. **Chalice cell.** Goblet cell (see below). **Chief cell.** 1. A pepsinogen-secreting cell of the gastric mucosa. 2. A chromophobe cell of the anterior pituitary. 3. A clear, non-secretory cell of the parathyroid. **Chromaffin cell.** A cell which stains brown with chrome salts, because of the presence of adrenaline or its derivatives, such as those of the adrenal medulla and the paraganglia. **Chromargentaffin cell.** Argentaffin cell (see above). **Chromatophore cell.** A pigment cell, or a cell which produces the precursor of a pigment. **Chromophil cell.** A cell of the anterior part of the pituitary gland, which has an affinity for acid or basic dyes. **Chromophobe cell.** A cell of the anterior pituitary which has little affinity for acid or basic dyes, and is thought to be a precursor of a chromophil cell. **Ciliated cell.** A cell which possesses hair-like actively motile processes at its free end. **Clear cells.** Water-clear cells; most common in parathyroid adenomas with functional activity, they are also found in the gut, the pancreas and the bile ducts. **Cleavage cell.** One of the cells of the segmenting ovum; a blastomere. **Clump cells.** Round pigmented cells without processes, found in the iris. **Cochlear cell.** Any cell of the spiral organ. **Columnar cell.** A type of epithelial cell in the shape of a hexagonal prism which appears approximately rectangular when sectioned along its long axis, the length being considerably greater than the width. **Cometal cell.** Caudate cell (see above). **Commissural cell.** A spinal neurone whose axon crosses to the opposite side in one of the commissures. **Compound granular cell.** A microglial cell distended with phagocytosed debris. **Cone cells.** Neurosensory cells of the retina, the receptive parts of which are cone-shaped. **Cone retinal cells.** Cells in the retina, most numerous in the central region, and associated with fine perception of contours and colour vision. **Connective-tissue cell.** Primarily a fibroblast, but the term may be applied to any of the cells found in connective tissue, e.g. macrophages, mast cells, lymphocytes, etc. **Constant cell.** A voltaic cell free from polarization, and therefore of constant voltage. **Contractile fibre cell.** An unstriped muscle cell. **Corneal cells.** Fibroblasts between the lamellae of the substantia propria of the cornea. **Counting cell.** A ruled glass slide of known depth for the enumeration of cells in blood and cerebrospinal or other fluids, e.g. Thoma-Zeiss counting cell. **Cover cell.** A cell whose apparent function is to protect an underlying cell. **Crescent cell.** A parietal serous cell of a mucous gland, lying between the principal mucous cells and the basement membrane where it is flattened in the form of a crescent. **Cribrose cell.** A cell whose walls show numerous perforations. **Cuboid cell, Cuboidal cell.** An epithelial cell whose height and breadth are of similar dimensions. **Cell culture.** Cells maintained *in vitro* by culture in artificial media usually containing salts, vitamins and serum. Monolayers or suspensions of cells so formed are used for investigations into the mechanisms of cell growth and division, and for the cultivation of, and research into, viruses. **Cylindrical cell.** Columnar cell (see above). **Cytochrome cell.** A neurone with a very small nucleus and inconspicuous cell body. **Daughter cell.** One of the cells resulting from division of a parent cell. **Decidual cell.** A large, clear, connective-tissue cell found in the uterine mucosa during pregnancy. **Delomorphous cell.** The parietal hydrochloric-acid-secreting cell of the gastric mucosa. **Delta cell.** One of the cell types of the islets of Langerhans. **Demilune cell.** Crescent cell (see above). **Dentin cell, Dentine cell.** Odontoblast. **Dichromate cell.** Bichromate cell (see above). **Dome cells.** The large cells of the outer layer of the fetal epidermis. **Dry cell.** A portable primary voltaic cell in which the electrolyte is in the form of a paste or is held in some absorbent material. Except for a small vent the cell is sealed. **Dust cell.** A phagocytic white cell containing dust or carbon particles, most commonly seen in the pulmonary alveoli and secretion. **Ectoplastic cell.** A cell which shows characteristic changes in the peripheral cytoplasm during its differentiation. **Egg cell.** The immature ovum. **Electrolytic cell.** A system consisting of electrodes and one or more electrolytes. **Elementary cell, Embryo cell, Embryonal cell, Embryonic cell.** An undifferentiated cell of the early embryo. **Embryoplastic cell.** One of the cells of the ovum which gives rise to the embryo proper, as distinct from the membranes. **Emigrated cell.** A leucocyte which has migrated from the blood stream by diapedesis through the capillary wall. **Enamel cell.** An ameloblast. **Encasing cell.** Cover cell (see above). **Endothelial** cell. One of the lining cells of a blood vessel or lymphatic. **Endothelioid cell.** A histiocyte or blood mononuclear leucocyte which has assumed the shape of an endothelial cell because of pressure from other cells. Endothelioid cells are characteristic of the tuberculous inflammatory lesion or "tubercle". **Enterochromaffin cell.** A type of cell with granular, argentophilic cytoplasm found among the ordinary epithelial cells of the intestinal and gastric glands. **Entoplastic cell.** A cell which differentiates by changes in the more central parts of its cytoplasm. **Eosinophil cell.** Any cell that takes eosin stain; an acidophil cell of the parathyroid gland, of no assigned function, but capable of secreting parathyroid hormone; of the anterior lobe of the pituitary; secretes growth hormone and prolactin. **Ependymal cell.** A ciliated columnar epithelial cell lining the ventricles of the brain and the central canal of the spinal cord. **Epidermic cell.** A cell from the epidermis of the skin. **Epithelial cell.** A cell belonging to the surface epithelium of the skin, alimentary, respiratory and genito-urinary passages, or their associated glands. **Epithelioid cell.** 1. A connective-tissue cell in the form of an epithelial cell. 2. Endothelial cell (see above). **Erythroid cell.** A cell of a red colour. **Ethmoid cell [cellula ethmoidalis (NA)].** One of the accessory nasal air sinuses in the lateral masses of the ethmoid bone, classified as anterior, middle and posterior. **Fat cell.** A connective-tissue cell loaded with neutral fat, in the form of either a single large cytoplasmic globule or a number of closely-packed globules. **Fatty granule cell.** A microglial cell filled with fatty debris. **Fibre cell.** A cell whose length is very much greater than its width. **Fibrillated cell.** A cell whose cytoplasm contains numerous fine fibrils. **Flagellate cell.** A motile unicellular organism equipped with one or more flagella. **Floor cells.** Cells found in the floor of the organ of Corti (spiral organ) in the ear. **Foam cells.** Vacuolated reticulo-endothelial cells filled with lipoids. **Follicle cell.** One of the cells forming the wall of a graafian follicle and surrounding the ovum before ovulation. **Follicular-lutein cell.** A cell of the ovarian corpus luteum, derived from a follicle cell. **Foot cells.** Basal supporting cells, such as those of Sertoli in the germinal epithelium. **Foreign-body giant cell.** A multinucleate giant cell that forms around foreign bodies such as ligatures, talc particles, cholesterol crystals, etc. **Formative cell.** An undifferentiated embryonic cell which gives rise to a specific tissue, organ or region of the later embryo. **Fusiform cell.** A spindle-shaped cell, such as a fibroblast. **Gametoid cells.** Cancer cells which resemble reproduction cells. **Ganglion cell.** 1. One of the neurone cell bodies of a spinal or sympathetic ganglion. 2. One of the large nerve cells from the inner layer of the retina. **Germ cell.** An ovum or spermatozoon, or one of their precursors. **Germinal cell.** 1. Germ cell (see preceding). 2. An ancestral or blast cell. 3. A cell from the inner layer of the early neural tube of the embryo from which the nerve cells are derived by proliferation and migration. **Ghost cell.** The last visible remnant of a degenerating cell. **Giant cell.** A very large cell, whether multinucleate or uninucleate. Examples are the osteoclast and megakaryocyte. **Giant pyramidal cell.** Betz cell; a giant pyramidal neurone of the motor cortex whose axons form part of the pyramidal tract subserving volitional movements. **Gitter cell.** Compound granular cell (see above). **Glandular fever cells.** Peculiar mononuclear cells, possibly of lymphatic origin, found in the peripheral blood of affected patients. **Glia cell.** Neuroglia cell (see below). **Glomus cell.** One of the epithelioid cells surrounding the coiled arteriovenous anastomosis of a glomus body in the fingers and toes. **Goblet cell.** A type of intestinal epithelial cell in which the distal cytoplasm is distended by a large globule of clear mucus which gives the cell the appearance of a goblet or chalice. **Granule cell.** A small nerve cell from the cerebellar or cerebral cortex. **Granulosa cell.** Follicle cell (see above). **Granulosa-lutein cell.** Follicular-lutein cell (see above). **Gravity cell.** A 2-fluid voltaic cell in which the lighter liquid floats on the heavier instead of being separated by a porous pot. **Guard cell.** A cell lining a stoma in a serous membrane. **Gustatory cell.** One of the cells of a taste bud. **Hair cell.** A type of epithelial cell from which projects one or more hair-like processes. **Heart cells, Heart-disease cells, Heart-failure cells, Heart-lesion cells.** Haematoidin-containing macrophages found in sputum in association with chronic bronchitis and cardiac disease. **Hecatomeral cell, Hecatomeric cell.** A nerve cell of the grey matter of the spinal cord whose axon branches to supply collaterals to the white matter of both sides. **Heckle cell.** A prickle cell. **Hela cells.** The cells composing the cultures of the first continuously cultured human cervical carcinoma. Often used in the culture of viruses. **Hepatic cell.** One of the epithelial cells of the liver acini. **Heteromeral cell, Heteromeric cell.** A nerve cell from the grey matter of the spinal cord whose axon passes to the opposite side. **Hilus cell.** A large epithelioid cell numbers of which are found in the hilus of the ovary and believed to have an endocrine function. **Histogenetic wandering cell.** A motile phagocytic cell derived from the connective tissues and capable of differentiating into one of the fixed connective-tissue cells. **Horizontal cell.** A type of nerve cell found in the retina, in which the processes run parallel to the surface. **Horn cell.** 1. A cornified and dead squamous cell from the outer layers of the epidermis. 2. A nerve cell from one of the horns of grey matter of the spinal cord. **Horny cell.** Horn cell (1st def.). **Hyperchromatic cell.** A cell whose nucleus stains intensely with basic dyes, due to the presence of large amounts of deoxyribonucleic acid. **Ichthyoid cell.** A megaloblast. **Imbricated cell.** One of a number of cells of an epithelium which overlap, like roofing tiles. **Indifferent cell.** An undifferentiated cell associated with a number of specifically differentiated cells. **Initial cell.** Germ cell (see above). **Interfollicular cell.** A cell apparently lying between adjacent follicles of the thyroid gland, but in reality an illusion due to the plane of sectioning. **Interstitial (Leydig) cell.** Stimulating hormone (CSH), the hormone produced in the cells lying in the interstices between the seminiferous tubules of the testes. **Islet cell.** One of the cells that compose the islets of Langerhans. **Juvenile cell.** A cell intermediate in development between a myelocyte and the youngest mature segmented polymorphonuclear leucocyte, having a nucleus which is sausage- or bean-shaped, with but little chromatin condensation of the nuclear protoplasm; metamyelocyte. **Juxtaglomerular cells.** The specialized cells of the juxtaglomerular apparatus of the kidney found in close association with the afferent glomerular arterioles. The cells contain granules and are probably the source of renin. **Karyochrome cell.** A nerve cell with a hyperchromatic nucleus and little perinuclear cytoplasm. **Kupffer cell.** Non-motile phagocytic macrophages lining the sinuses of the liver. **Lacis cell.** One of the non-granular cells of the juxtaglomerular apparatus. **Lacrimo-ethmoid cell.** An anterior ethmoidal air cell which is adjacent to the lacrimal bone. **L.E. cell.** A neutrophil that has phagocytosed the nucleus of another leucocyte already greatly altered following an interaction with the lupus erythematosus factor in the blood. **Lead-telluride photo cell.** A photoconductive cell used in the infra-red region up to a wavelength of 6 μm. **Lepra cell.** A mononuclear phagocyte (macrophage or histiocyte) full of *Mycobacterium leprae.* **Leucocytoid cell.** A blood mononuclear cell which is transformed into a fibroblast in scar tissue. **Littoral cell.** A phagocytic endothelial cell lining the lymph spaces of lymph nodes and the sinusoids of bone marrow, liver and spleen. **Liver cell.** The polygonal epithelial cell of which the bulk of the liver is constituted. **Locomotive cell.** Amoeboid cell (see above). **Longiradiate cell.** A neuroglial cell with long processes. **Lutein cell.** The polygonal epithelial cell of the corpus luteum of the ovary, which contains numerous fatty granules, often of a yellowish or orange colour. **Lymphadenoma cell.** The giant cell of Hodgkin's disease; also known as *Sternberg's giant cell.* **Lymphoid cell.** A cell, probably identical with a lymphocyte, found in large numbers in lymphoid organs such as the tonsils, adenoids, thymus, Peyer's patches, etc. **Lymphoid stem cell.** Lymphoblast. **Malpighian cell.** A cell of the deepest germinal layer of the epidermis. **Marginal cell.** Crescent cell (see above). **Marrow cell.** An immature red or white blood cell from the bone marrow. **Mast cell.** A type of connective-tissue cell containing numerous cytoplasmic granules which stain metachromatically with basic dyes. Found in mucous membrane of the small intestine, their function is uncertain, probably concerned with motility as well as secretion, and they are thought to manufacture heparin. **Mastoid air cells [cellulae mastoideae].** Air cells in the mastoid process of the temporal bone. **Medullary cell.** Marrow cell (see above). **Mesamoeboid cell.** The name given by Minot to the primitive blood cell formed in the embryo from the blood islands of the yolk sac. **Mesangial cell.** A cell lying in the intercapillary area in the central region of the renal glomerulus. Such cells are embedded in basement membrane-like material and display phagocytic properties. **Mesothelioma cells.** The flattened cells which line the serous cavities. They are the origin of the mesothelioma. **Microglia cell.** A small phagocytic neuroglial cell derived from the mesenchyme and belonging to the reticulo-endothelial system. **Migratory cell.** An amoeboid cell (see above). **Mitral cell.** A pyramidal nerve cell from the olfactory bulb which relays olfactory impulses brought in by the olfactory nerve. **Morula cell.** A cell shaped like a mulberry, seen, for example, in the perivascular infiltration in trypanosomiasis. **Mossy cell.** A type of neuroglial cell with numerous short branching processes. **Mother cell.** A cell which gives rise to a new generation of cells by repeated cell division. **Motor cell.** A cell from the ventral horn of grey matter of the spinal cord which sends its axon into the ventral root to supply muscle fibres. **Mucin cell, Muco-albuminous cell, Mucoserous cell, Mucous cell.** A cell containing mucinogen granules and which secretes mucin, as opposed to a serous cell. **Mucous neck cell.** A mucus-secreting cell from the neck region of a gastric gland. **Muscle cell.** An elongated contractile cell from either smooth, voluntary, striated, or cardiac muscle. **Myeloid cell.** Marrow cell (see above). **Myeloma cell.** The cell constituent of a myeloma. When well differentiated it closely resembles the plasma cell and manufactures various abnormal globulins. When less differentiated the resemblance to the plasma cell is not marked, although a percentage of the tumour cells still show the basophil staining of the mature cell. **Myo-epithelial cell.** An epithelial cell, usually lying around a glandular acinus, in which part of the cytoplasm has contractile properties, serving to empty the acinus of its secretion. **Myoid cell.** A striated-muscle-like cell from the thymus gland. **Naked cell.** A cell without a demonstrable cell membrane. **Nerve cell.** A cell specialized for the conduction of nervous impulses, typically in the form of a cell body containing the nucleus and Nissl granules, and several elongated processes, one of which, the axon or axis-cylinder, conveys nerve impulses away from the cell body, the others, the dendrites, serving to collect impulses and convey them towards the cell body. **Neuro-epithelial cell.** 1. A cell from a specialized sensory epithelium serving as an intermediary between the environment and the nerve-ending, such as the cells of a taste bud, or the hair cells of the cochlea. 2. A nerve cell whose body is in the form of an epithelial cell lining a sensory surface such as the olfactory epithelium of the nasal cavity. 3. A cell from the specialized ectoderm of the early embryo which becomes the neural tube. **Neuroglia cell.** A cell which subserves connective-tissue-like supporting functions within the central nervous system. Astrocytes and oligodendroglia are of ectodermal origin; microglia are of mesodermal origin. **Neuromuscular cell.** A cell from the ectoderm of lower invertebrates whose inner end is flattened and elongated as a contractile organ. **Neutrophil cell.** A blood leucocyte whose granules show no marked affinity for either acid or basic dyes. It is the commonest type of white blood cell. **Noble cell.** An old term for a fully differentiated adult type of cell. **Nuclear cell.** A nerve cell with short branching processes from the sensory cortex. **Nucleated cell.** A term applicable to all living cells. **Nurse cell, Nursing cell.** The Sertoli cell of the seminiferous tubule. **Oat-shaped cells.** Cells like oat grains, found in carcinoma of the lung. **Olfactory cell.** The specialized neuro-epithelial cell of the olfactory mucosa. **One-fluid cell.** A voltaic cell in which the 2 electrodes are immersed in the same electrolyte. **Osseous cell.** A bone corpuscle, or osteocyte. **Over-ripe cell.** A polymorphonuclear leucocyte. **Oxyntic cell.** A parietal, hydrochloric-acid-secreting cell from the gastric glands. **Oxyphil cell.** Acidophil cell (see above). **Palatine cell.** A posterior ethmoidal air cell which extends into the palatine bone. **Parafollicular cells.** Cells which lie between the follicles of the thyroid gland. They are believed to produce calcitonin. **Paraluteal cell, Paralutein cell.** A lutein cell from the corpus luteum, derived from the inner vascular layer of the graafian follicle. **Parent cell.** Mother cell (see above). **Parietal cell.** The hydrochloric-acid-secreting cell of the gastric glands. **Pavement cell.** A flattened squamous type of cell lining serous cavities. **Pediculated cell.** An astrocyte with a so-called sucker foot, attached to a capillary wall. **Peptic cell.** A chief, or pepsin-secreting, cell of the gastric mucosa. **Pericapillary cell.** A modified fibroblast from the delicate perithelium of connective tissue surrounding the capillary endothelium. **Pericellular cell.** A neuroglial cell from the capsule of a neurone cell body of a spinal ganglion. **Perichrome cell.** A nerve cell in which the Nissl substance lies peripherally against the cell membrane. **Peri-thelial cell.** Pericapillary cell (see above). **Perivascular cell.** A cell which is found immediately outside the basal lamina of the endothelial cells of capillaries and is itself enclosed in a basal lamina. **Persensitized cell.** Sensitized cell (see below). **Pessary cell.** A red blood cell in which the haemoglobin is seen only as a narrow band around the periphery of the cell. **Phagocytic cells.** Cells that pick up and absorb micro-organisms, cellular and other debris, and dead or obsolescent cells, and digest them. **Phalangeal cells.** Cells which support the hair cells of the spiral organ. **Pheochrome cell.** Chromaffin cell (see above). **Photo-conductive cell.** A photo-electric cell (see following) in which the decrease of electrical resistance of the detector with increase of intensity of light falling upon it is used to measure the intensity of the light. **Photo-electric cell.** A generic name used to describe any detector in which an electromotive force is produced, or a current varied in magnitude, by the action of visible light, or ultra-violet or infra-red radiation. **Photo-emissive cell.** A photo-electric cell (see preceding) in which electrons are ejected from the light-sensitive surface and pass *in vacuo* to a collecting electrode maintained at a positive potential to the emitting surface. **Photovoltaic cell.** A photo-electric cell in which an electromotive force is produced by the action of light falling upon the cell, the magnitude of which is a measure of the intensity of the incident radiation. **Physaliphorous cells.** Cells found in the chordoma which are intensely vacuolated by droplets of mucin. They are derived from the notochord. **Pigment cell.** Any cell containing pigmented granules as a normal constituent. **Pillar cells.** The cells which form the inner and outer pillars of the spiral organ. **Plasma cell.** Cell derived from the B-cell series (see above) which manufactures and secretes antibody. The cytoplasm is deeply basophilic and contains much rough endoplasmic reticulum. The nucleus is eccentric and its chromatin is arranged in a cartwheel distribution. **Pluricordonal cell.** A stellate type of neurone found in posterior horn cells of the embryonic spinal cord of the pigeon. **Pneumatic cell.** A cavity containing air, such as an accessory nasal air sinus. **Polar cell.** Polar body. *See* BODY. **Polychromatic cell, Polychromatophil cell.** An immature type of red blood cell possessing eosinophil and basophil granules. **Polyhedral cell.** A cell of polyhedral form with from 11 to 17 surface facets. **Polyplastic cell.** A cell which may assume several different forms. **Porous cell.** Porous pot; an unglazed earthenware pot serving as a diaphragm in a 2-fluid voltaic cell. **Pregnancy cell.** A modified chromophobe cell found in the anterior pituitary during pregnancy. **Prickle cell.** One of the cells from the inner layer of the epidermis which possesses numerous protoplasmic processes connecting it with neighbouring cells. **Primary cell.** 1. A voltaic cell in which chemical energy is converted into electrical energy. 2. An undifferentiated or embryonic cell. **Primary wandering cell.** The name given by Saxer to the primitive blood cell formed in the embryo from the blood islands of the yolk sac. **Primitive cell.** An undifferentiated or embryonic cell. **Primordial cell.** Elementary cell (see above). **Primordial germ cell.** One of a collection of cells that appear first in the wall of the yolk sac. They later migrate into the gonadal ridges of the embryo, where they ultimately give rise to all the germ cells. **Principal cell.** Chief cell (see above). **Protective cell.** A superficially placed cell overlying and protecting a deeper cell. **Psychic cell.** A cell from the grey matter of the cerebrum. **Pus cell.** A necrotic white cell. **Pyramidal cell.** A neurone whose cell body is pyramidal in shape, typically found in the grey matter of the cerebral cortex. **Pyrrole cell.** A phagocytic cell of the reticulo-endothelial system which takes up pyrrole dyes from the circulation. **RA cell.** Ragocyte. **Radium cell.** A radium container of very small size, so that a number may be used for filling radium tubes or needles to ensure an even, or planned uneven, distribution of the source. **Residential cell.** A fixed cell, as opposed to a wandering cell, especially in the cornea. **Resting cell.** A cell in an inactive, non-functional phase of its existence. **Resting wandering cell.** A temporarily non-motile macrophage. **Reticular cell.** A relatively undifferentiated stellate connective-tissue cell, found chiefly in the spleen, bone marrow, and lymph glands, and capable of differentiating into any of the connective-tissue cells or blood cells when suitably stimulated. **Reticulo-endothelial cell.** Any one of the phagocytic cells, reticular or endothelial, which comprise the reticulo-endothelial system, and characterized by its ability to store particulate dyes picked up from the circulation. **Reticulum cell.** Reticular cell (see above). **Rhagiocrine cell.** A histiocyte, or fixed connective-tissue macrophage. **Rod cell.** A light-sensitive cell from the outer layer of the retina, possessing an externally projecting rod-like process. **Round cell.** 1. Any cell with a spherical shape. 2. A lymphocyte. **Salivary cell.** A desquamated epithelial cell found in saliva. **Sarcogenic cell.** The embryonic cell which becomes a muscle fibre; myoblast. **Satellite cells.** Glial cells which accumulate around damaged ganglion cells. **Sauroid cell.** A nucleated red blood cell. **Scavenger cell.** A microglial cell of the central nervous system. **Secondary cell.** A voltaic cell which is reversible, and which after discharge can be brought back to its initial (charged) chemical condition by passing a current through it in the direction opposite to that of the discharge. **Segmentation cell.** A blastomere of the segmentary ovum. **Segmented cell.** A polymorphonuclear leucocyte with a segmented nucleus. **Selenium cell.** A light-sensitive cell in which the operative element is a photoconductive layer of selenium. **Seminal cell.** One of the desquamated epithelial cells found in seminal fluid. **Sensation cell.** A neurone of the sensory cortex of the brain. **Sensitized cells.** Usually sheep's red blood cells to which the specific haemolysin has been added, rendering them sensitive to the lytic action of complement. **Sensory cell.** A neurone whose processes are connected with a sense organ. **Sensory epithelial cell.** A modified epidermal or connective-tissue cell, adapted for the transmission of sensations to an associated nerve-ending. **Sentinel cell.** A type of epithelioid cell found in the wall of an afferent arteriole of a renal glomerulus. **Septal cell.** A flattened epithelial cell lining a lung alveolus. **Septate cell.** A cell whose cytoplasm is partially subdivided by a septum or deep indentation. **Serous cell.** A glandular cell which produces a clear, usually enzyme-containing secretion, found chiefly in the salivary-gland acini. **Serous fat cell.** A modified fat cell found in atrophic adipose tissue. **Shadow cell.** The faintly staining remnant of a degenerating cell, especially a spinal ganglion cell. **Sickle cell.** The characteristic crescentic or sickle-shaped red cell found in the hereditary form of anaemia which affects negroes and which is known as sickle-cell, drepanocytic, meniscocytic or African anaemia. **Signet cell.** A cell containing a central vacuole, usually filled by mucus which pushes and compresses the nucleus to the periphery. Usually seen in a mucus-secreting adenocarcinoma. **Silver cell.** Argentaffin cell (see above). **Simple cell.** One without a markedly differentiated cytoplasm or nucleus. **Sister cell.** One of the 2 daughter cells resulting from the division of a parent cell. **Skein cells.** Reticulocytes. **Skeletogenous cell.** An osteoblast or chondroblast. **Sleeping cell, Slumber cell.** An undifferentiated connective-tissue cell. **Smear cell, Smudge cell.** A degenerate and fragile lymphocyte found especially in lymphatic leukaemia, which breaks down when a blood film is made, and resembles a smear or a smudge. **Somatic cell.** A body cell, as opposed to a germ cell. **Somatochrome cell.** A neurone whose cell body contains a large amount of basophilic cytoplasm. **Sperm cell.** A spermatozoon, or one of its immature precursors. **Spermatogenic cell.** One of the precursors of a spermatozoon. **Spermatogonial cell.** The primordial male germ cell of the seminiferous tubules; spermatogonium. **Sphenoid cell.** The sphenoidal air sinus. **Spider cell.** A cell with many fine processes, such as an astrocyte or osteocyte. **Spindle cell.** A fusiform or spindle-shaped cell, such as a fibroblast. **Splanchnic cell.** A mesenchymal cell from the splanchnopleure surrounding the embryonic alimentary canal, as opposed to one from the body wall somatopleure. **Squamous cell.** A flattened plate-like cell with crenated outline, forming part of an endothelium, mesothelium, or epithelium. **Stab cell, Staff cell.** An abnormal mature polymorphonuclear leucocyte in which the usual process of segmentation of the nucleus has become arrested by toxic or other deleterious influences, so that the nucleus is narrow, ribbon-like, and often bent on itself to form curious shapes, whilst the nuclear material shows pyknosis and condensation. **Standard cell.** A cell prepared according to a given specification and employed to provide a standard of potential difference. **Star cells.** Large vacuolated cells in adamantinoma. **Stellate cell.** A star-shaped cell, such as a neuroglial cell or reticular cell. **Stellate cell of the liver.** Kupffer cell of the liver; one of the phagocytic epithelial cells lining the venous sinusoids of the liver. **Stem cell.** An ancestral cell which gives rise to generations of adult cells by cell division and differentiation. **Sterile cell.** One which is incapable of cell division. **Stichochrome cell.** A neurone whose Nissl substance is arranged in a stratified manner. **Stickle cell.** Prickle cell (see above). **Stipple cell.** A red cell which contains basophil-staining dots or granules or aggregations, all of which are known as stipples, which arise owing to deleterious action upon the reticular material in a young red cell from lead poisoning, as well as less constantly in severe anaemia, leukaemia and malaria. **Stroma cell.** One of the connective-tissue cells of an organ, as opposed to a glandular, epithelial, muscle, or other more highly differentiated cell; used especially in connection with the uterine mucosa and ovary. **Supporting cell.** A relatively undifferentiated cell whose function appears to be that of affording mechanical support and protection, and possibly also nutritive assistance, to other more highly differentiated cells in the vicinity. **Sustentacular cell.** 1. Supporting cell (see preceding). 2. Sertoli's cell. **Swarm cell.** A motile spore, e.g. of an alga. **Sympathetic cell.** A neurone of the sympathetic, as opposed to the somatic, nervous system. **Sympathicotrophic cell.** A large chromaffin cell from the hilum of the ovary. **Sympathochromaffin cell.** One of the embryonic cells of neural crest origin, from which the suprarenal medulla is developed. **Syncytial cell.** One of a number of cells which fuse to form a multinucleate syncytium. **T cell.** Thymus-derived lymphocyte, the cell responsible for cell-mediate immunity. **Tactile cell.** One of the cells composing a tactile sensory end-organ. **Tapetal cell, Tapetum cell.** One of the specialized pigment cells from the tapetum of the eye of carnivores and seals. **Target cell.** An abnormal red cell which, when stained, appears to have the haemoglobin arranged as a circular central disc and an external concentric ring, thus giving the appearance of a target. The cells are characteristic of Mediterranean anaemia, and are often numerous after splenectomy. **Tart cell.** A histiocyte-like cell found in the bone marrow in acute disseminated lupus and in that of severely ill persons with many other diseases. It has a secondary nucleus that stains somewhat differently from the primary nucleus. **Taste cell.** One of the cells comprising a taste bud. **Tautomeral cell.** A spinal nerve cell whose axon passes to the white matter of the same side. **Tegmental cell.** A cell from a delicate epithelium covering a thin membrane. **Tendon cells.** Fibroblasts between the bundles of collagenous fibres in a tendon. **Theca cell, Thecalutein cell.** A cell of the corpus luteum of the ovary, derived from the tunica interna of the graafian follicle. **Totipotential cell.** An embryonic type of cell which is totally undifferentiated, and can develop into any type of cell. **Touch cell.** Tactile cell (see above). **Transitional cell.** A monocyte which was thought by Ehrlich to be a transitional phase between the lymphocyte and the neutrophil granulocyte or polymorphonuclear leucocyte; it is formed from its precursor, the monoblast of the parathyroid gland. Derived from the chief cell and is the main source of parathyroid hormone. **Tropochrome cell.** A glandular cell containing both serous and mucous glands. **Tubal air cells [cellulae pneumaticae (NA)].** Air cells which extend from the middle ear into the petrous bone, close to the auditory tube. **Twin cell.** Sister cell (see above). **Two-fluid cell.** A voltaic cell in which the 2 electrodes are immersed in different electrolytes. **Tympanic air cells [cellulae tympanicae (NA)].** Air cells of the temporal bone related to the tympanic antrum. **Vacuolated cell.** A cell with clear rounded areas in its cytoplasm. **Vasofactive cell, Vasoformative cell.** An angioblast; the embryonic mesenchymal cell from which blood-vessel endothelium is derived. **Visual cell.** A rod or cone cell of the retina. **Voltaic cell.** A source of electricity produced by chemical action. **Wandering cell.** An amoeboid cell, especially a macrophage. **Water-clear cells.** Clear cells (see above). **Whip cell.** A motile cell with one or more flagella of the whip-lash type. **Wing cell.** A concavoconvex lentiform cell from the corneal epithelium. **Xanthoma cell.** Foam cell (see above). **Yolk cell.** 1. A cell-like globule of yolk. 2. An early entodermal cell of the embryo, filled with yolk granules. **Zinc-carbon cell.** A primary cell, either single or 2-fluid, with electrodes of zinc and carbon. **Zinc-copper cell.** A primary cell, either single or 2-fluid, with electrodes of zinc and copper. **Zymogenic cell.** An enzyme-secreting cell which exhibits a large number of rounded granules in the cytoplasm adjacent to the lumen during the resting stage. Such cells are found in the salivary glands, pancreas and crypts of Lieberkühn of the intestine. [L *cella* store-room.]

See also: ABBÉ, ALZHEIMER, ANITSCHKOW, ARMANNI, ASCHOFF, BEALE, BERGMANN (E.), BETZ, BEVAN-LEWIS, BIZZOZERO, BOETTCHER, BOLL, CALLEJA, CLARK (J. L.), CLARKE, CLAUDIUS, CORTI, COUNCILMAN, CROOKE, CUSTER, DANIELL, DAVIDOFF, DAVY (H.), DEITERS, DE LA RUE, DOGIEL, DRASCH, EBSTEIN, EDELMANN, FERRATA, FINKELDEY, FOA, FOULIS, FRIEDLAENDER, FULLER, GAUCHER, GEGENBAUR, GEHUCHTEN, GIANNUZZI, GIERKE (H. P.), GLEY, GOLGI, GOORMAGHTIGH, GRAWITZ, GRENET, GROVE, HEIDENHAIN, HENLE, HENSEN, HIS (W. SNR.), HODGKIN, HOFBAUER, HORTEGA, HUERTHLE, KULTCHITSKY, KUPFFER, KURLOV, LANGENDORFF, LANGERHANS, LANGHANS, LECLANCHÉ, LEYDEN, LEYDIG, LIPSCHUETZ, MARCHAND, MARIÉ DAVY, MARTINOTTI, MERKEL (F. S.), MEYNERT, MIKULICZ-RADECKI, MOSHER, NAGEOTTE, NEUMANN (E. F. C.), NIEMANN, NUSSBAUM, PAGET, PANETH, PELGER, PICK (L.), POGGENDORF, PURKINJE, RAMÓN Y CAJAL, RANVIER, REED, RIEDER, RINDFLEISCH, ROLANDO, ROLLET (A.), ROUGET, SAXER, SCHULTZE (M. J. S.), SCHWANN, SERTOLI, SÉZARY, SMEE, SNELL, SORBY, STERNBERG (K.), STILLING, THOMA, TOUTON, TUERK, UNNA, VIGNAL, VIMTRUP, VIRCHOW, WALDEYER-HARTZ, WARTHIN, WELSH, WESTON, ZANDER, ZEHBE, ZEISS.

cell islets (**sel**·i·letz). **Intra-alveolar cell islets.** The islets of Langerhans of the pancreas. [cell, OFr. *islette.*]

cella (**sel**·ah). 1. A cell. 2. A part of the lateral ventricle of the brain. **Cella lateralis.** The lateral ventricle of the brain. **Cella media.** The central part of the lateral ventricle of the brain. [L store-room.]

Cellacephate (sel·as·ef·ate). BP Commission approved name for a partial mixed acetate and hydrogen phthalate ester of cellulose; it is used as an enteric coating.

Cellia (**sel**·e·ah). A sub-genus of *Anopheles.*

celliferous (sel·**if**·er·us). Productive of or bearing cells. [cell, L *ferre* to bear.]

celliform (**sel**·e·form). Cell-like.

cellifugal (sel·**if**·ew·gal). Cellulifugal.

cellipetal (sel·**ip**·et·al). Cellulipetal.

cellobiase (sel·o·**bi**·aze). An enzyme found with cellulase, which breaks down the cellobiose produced by the latter from cellulose, and converts it into glucose.

cellobiose (sel·o·**bi**·oze). Cellose, $C_{12}H_{22}O_{11}$. A disaccharide entering into the structure of cellulose and obtained from it by hydrolysis. It is hydrolysed in turn by the enzyme cellobiase into glucose. A β-glucose glucoside, stereo-isomeric with maltose; less sweet and less soluble than the latter.

celloidin (sel·**oid**·in). A preparation of nitrocellulose dissolved in alcohol and ether, used as a histological embedding agent and in solution for the protection of wounds.

cellon (**sel**·on). Acetylene tetrachloride, tetrachlorethane, $CHCl_2$ $CHCl_2$. Formed by the combination of acetylene and chlorine, it is a liquid used as a solvent for fats, waxes, varnishes and sulphur; also as an insecticide against garden pests.

Cellophane (**sel**·o·fane). A thin, tough, transparent material, insoluble and non-inflammable, manufactured from viscose (the sodium salt of cellulose xanthate). It is used for wrapping purposes and bandages. [trade name.]

cellosan (**sel**·o·san). A hexosan formed from cellobiose.

cellose (**sel**·oze). Cellobiose.

cellula (**sel**·ew·lah). A small cell. [L little cell.]

cellular (**sel**·ew·lar). 1. Relating to a cell or cells. 2. Containing or consisting of cells.

cellularity (sel·ew·**lar**·it·e). The state of being made up of cells.

cellulase (**sel**·ew·laze). An enzyme secreted by soil organisms, wood-destroying fungi and certain marine worms, which converts the cellulose of wood and plants into the disaccharide cellobiose.

cellule (**sel**·ewl). A very small cell. [L *cellula.*]

See also: STOHR.

cellulicidal (sel·ew·le·**si**′·dal). Destructive to cells. [cellula, L *caedere* to kill.]

celluliferous (sel·ew·**lif**·er·us). In biology, term denoting the producing or the bearing of small cells. [cellula, L *ferre* to bear.]

cellulifugal (sel·ew·**lif**·ew·gal). 1. Moving in a direction away from a cell. The term is applied to those cells which are repelled by other cells, or to processes extending away from a cell body. 2. Relating to the carrying of impulses away from a nerve cell. [cellula, L *fugere* to flee.]

cellulin (**sel**·ew·lin). A substance of animal origin which is like cellulose.

cellulipetal (sel·ew·**lip**·et·al). 1. Moving in a direction towards a cell. The term is applied to those cells which are attracted to other cells or to processes which extend towards a cell body. 2. Relating to the carrying of impulses towards a nerve cell. [cellula, L *petere* to seek.]

cellulitis (sel·ew·**li**·tis). A diffuse inflammation of connective tissue, especially of subcutaneous tissue. **Dissecting cellulitis of the scalp.** Perifolliculitis capitis abscedens et suffodiens. **Ischiorectal cellulitis.** Cellulitis affecting the fatty tissue of the ischiorectal fossa. **Orbital cellulitis.** Inflammation affecting the cellular tissue within the orbit. **Pelvic cellulitis.** Inflammation affecting the connective tissue investing the uterus. **Phlegmonous cellulitis.** Diffuse phlegmon. *See* PHLEGMON. **Streptococcal cellulitis.** Cellulitis caused, as it usually is, by streptococci. [cellula, Gk *-itis* inflammation.]

cellulocutaneous (sel·ew·lo·kew·**ta**′·ne·us). Relating to, involving or composed of loose connective tissue and skin. [cellula, L *cutis* skin.]

cellulofibrous (sel·ew·lo·**fi**′·brus). Both cellular and fibrous.

celluloneuritis (sel·ew·lo·newr·**i**′·tis). Inflammation of nerve cells in acute conditions, e.g. anterior poliomyelitis, polyneuritis. **Acute anterior celluloneuritis.** Landry's paralysis, acute anterior poliomyelitis or polyneuritis, considered to be the one disease. [cellula, neuritis.]

cellulosa (sel·ew·**lo**·sah). A cellular layer or coat. **Cellulosa chorioideae.** The outer layer of the choroid. [cellula.]

cellulose (**sel**·ew·lose). A polysaccharide of between 100 and 200 glucose units, and with a molecular weight in the region of 30 000. It is the principal constituent of the plant cell-wall, either as such or as derivatives. When purified it is a tough white material, insoluble in water but soluble in various special reagents, e.g. Schweitzer's, and it is used in the manufacture of paper, artificial silk, plastics and explosives. It is ingested by herbivorous animals by means of specific bacteria of the digestive tract. **Methyl cellulose.** A "bulk preparation" used in cases of obesity to give a feeling of satiety and therefore prevent the patient from eating an excessive amount of food. **Microcrystalline Cellulose BPC 1968.** A partially depolymerized cellulose, prepared by acid hydrolysis of purified wood cellulose. In its various physical forms it has pharmaceutical applications in the preparation of tablets and as a suspending agent. **Oxidised Cellulose BP 1973.** An absorbable haemostatic prepared by oxidizing surgical gauze or cotton with nitrogen dioxide. Its main disadvantage is that it delays bone repair and inactivates penicillin, and that it cannot be sterilized by heat. [cellula.]

cellulosity (sel·ew·**los**·it·e). 1. The state of being composed of cells. 2. Cellulose substance.

cellulotoxic (sel·ew·lo·**tox**′·ik). Having a toxic effect on cells. [cellula, Gk *toxikon* poison.]

cellulous (**sel**·ew·lus). Consisting of cells or cellular in form.

celo-. For words beginning with **Celo-**, *see also* COELO- and KELO-.

celology (se·**lol**·o·je). The branch of surgery which is concerned with hernia. [Gk *kele* hernia, *logos* science.]

celosomia (se·lo·**so**·me·ah). Hernia of the viscera in the fetus. [Gk *kele* hernia, *soma* body.]

celotome (**se**·lo·tome). Kelotome; a surgical knife used in herniotomy. [Gk *kele* hernia, *temnein* to cut.]

celotomy (se·**lot**·o·me). Kelotomy; operative repair of a hernia. [see prec.]

Celsius, Anders (b. 1701). Swedish astronomer.

Celsius scale. A temperature scale in which there are 100 degrees between the melting point of ice (0°C) and the boiling point of water (100°C). Each degree Celsius is equal to a kelvin, but on the thermodynamic temperature scale zero kelvin (0 K) is absolute zero (−273.15°C).

Celsus, Aulus Aurelius Cornelius. 1st century A.D. Roman writer on medicine.

Celsus' papules. Acute papular eczema, or lichen agrius.

Celsus' quadrilateral. Redness, swelling, heat and pain: the 4 cardinal symptoms of inflammation.

Celsus' vitiligo. Alopecia.

Celsus-Knapp blepharoplasty. A sliding skin flap is pulled horizontally from the temporal area to fill lid defects, upper or lower. It is associated with 2 Burow's triangles at its base.

cement (se·**ment**). 1. Any substance which, mixed with water or other medium, sets to a hard mass. 2. A substance which sticks 2 articles together; in dentistry, a substance which attaches an artificial restoration to a tooth or denture. 3. An adhesive material used in filling a cavity in a tooth. 4. Cementum. **Acrylic cement.** Formed by mixing methylmethacrylate monomer and polymer in the presence of an activator and initiator. It is widely used in prosthetic replacement of bones and joints. **Oxyphosphate cement.** An adhesive cement, used to protect the vital tooth structures from the effects of a filling inserted in a cavity; also to retain in position a restoration to a tooth. **Silicate cement.** A translucent material used for filling a cavity in a tooth. [L *caementum* unhewn stone.]

cementicle (se·**ment**·ikl). A small discrete calcified body in the periodontal membrane surrounding the root of a tooth. [dim. of cementum.]

cementification (se·**ment**·if·ik·a′·shun). The formation of cementum on the root of a tooth. [cementum, L *facere* to make.]

cementin (se·**ment**·in). The cement substance which sometimes causes one cell to adhere to an adjacent one.

cementoblast (se·**ment**·o·blast). An osteoblast in the layer of bone-forming material which invests the root of a developing tooth. [cement, Gk *blastos* germ.]

cementoclasia (se·**ment**·o·kla′·ze·ah). The progressive resorption of the cementum on the root of a tooth. [cementum, Gk *klasis* a breaking.]

cementodentinary (se·**ment**·o·**den**′·tin·ar·e). Dentocemental.

cemento-exostosis (se·**ment**·o·ex·**os**′·to·sis). Hypercementosis; the formation by cementoblasts of the periodontal membrane of a mass of secondary cementum on the root of a tooth. It may involve all of the teeth in a patient suffering from Paget's disease. [cementum, exostosis.]

cementoma (se·**ment**·o·mah). A neoplasm the substance of which is similar to the cement of the teeth. [cement, Gk *-oma* tumour.]

cementome (se·**ment**·ome). An excessive irregular deposition of cementum around the apex of a tooth after it has been completely formed. [cement, Gk *-oma* tumour.]

cementoperiostitis (se·**ment**·o·per·e·os·**ti**′·tis). Pyorrhoea alveolaris. [cement, periostitis.]

cementosis (se·**ment**·o·sis). The formation and development of a cementoma. [cementum, Gk *-osis* condition.]

cementum (se·**ment**·um). The calcified tissue that immediately surrounds the dentine of the root of a tooth; cement, peridentine. There are 2 histological varieties, (*a*) primary cementum, and (*b*) secondary cementum. [L *caementum* unhewn stone.]

cen-. For words beginning **Cen-**, *see also* COEN-.

ceno-encephalocele (se·no·en·**kef**′·al·o·seel). Hernia of the brain through a fissure in the skull and without formation of a cyst. [Gk *kenos* empty, encephalocele.]

cenophobia (se·no·**fo**·be·ah). Kenophobia; morbid dread of large open spaces. [Gk *kenos* empty, phobia.]

cenosis (se·**no**·sis). 1. Inanition. 2. A morbid discharge. [Gk *kenos* empty.]

cenotic (se·**not**·ik). 1. Referring to cenosis. 2. Referring to a morbid discharge, or indicating its presence.

cenotoxin (se·no·**tox**·in). Kenotoxin; fatigue toxin. *See* TOXIN. [Gk *kenos* empty, *toxikon* poison.]

censor (**sen**·sor). **Freudian censor.** The psychic barrier which, according to Freud, does not allow certain unconscious wishes and thoughts to come to consciousness until they have been so disguised as to make their original form unrecognizable by the subject. [L *censere* to assess.]

centesimal (sen·**tes**·im·al). 1. In the proportion of 1 to 100. 2. Divided into hundredths, as on any scale. [L *centesimus* the hundredth.]

centesis (sen·**te**·sis). Tapping or puncture, e.g. of a tumour or cavity. [Gk *kentesis* a pricking.]

centibar (**sen**·te·bar). A unit of pressure, being a hundredth part of a bar and equal to 1000 pascal (1 kPa). [L *centum* hundred, bar.]

Centigrade (**sen**·te·grade). 1. Consisting of 100 divisions or grades. 2. Of a thermometer, as Celsius, having 100 degrees, with zero as the freezing point and 100 degrees as the boiling point of water. [L *centum* hundred, *gradus* step or degree.]

centigram (**sen**·te·gram). A weight equalling a hundredth part of a gram. [L *centum* hundred, Gk *gramma* small weight.]

centilitre (**sen**·te·le·ter). A measure of volume equalling a hundredth part of a litre. [L *centum* hundred, Gk *litra* pound.]

centimetre (**sen**·te·me·ter). A measure of length equal to a hundredth part of a metre. **Cubic centimetre.** A cube the edge of which is 1 centimetre long. 1 cubic centimetre is equivalent to 1 millilitre. [L *centum* hundred, Gk *metron* measure.]

centinem (**sen**·te·nem). Von Pirquet's term for a hundredth part of a nem, which is the unit of nutrition in his system of feeding. Cf. NEM. [L *centum* hundred, nem.]

centinormal (**sen**·te·norm·al). A term used to indicate that the strength of a solution used in volumetric analysis is a hundredth part of the standard or normal strength. [L *centum* hundred, *norma* rule.]

centipede (**sen**·te·peed). An arthropod with a flattened body and one pair of legs to each body segment. The larger species are tropical and their bites are painful but not dangerous, except through sepsis. Small forms are often found in the nasal cavities, which they enter during sleep. [L *centum* hundred, *pes* foot.]

centipoise (**sen**·te·poiz). A unit of viscosity, being a hundredth part of a poise and equal to a millipascal second (1 mPas). [L *centum* hundred, poise.]

centrad (**sen**·trad). A unit of angular measure, a hundredth part of a radian (about 0.57 degree). [L *centum* hundred, radian.]

centrage (sen·traje). The situation in which all the refracting surfaces of the eye are aligned. [centre.]

central (sen·tral). 1. Situated at, near or in the middle. 2. Relating to a, or the, centre; not peripheral. **Central lobule.** *See* LOBULE. **Central sulcus.** *See* SULCUS OF THE CEREBRUM, CENTRAL. [centre.]

central veins [venae centrales (NA)]. The main veins draining the liver lobules.

central vein of the suprarenal gland [vena centralis (NA)]. A vein lying near the centre of the medulla and formed by the union of tributaries which drain the sinusoids. It drains into the suprarenal vein.

centrality (sen·tral·it·e). The situation in which the origin of nervous phenomena is not in the peripheral nerves but in the central nervous system.

centraphose (sen·trah·foze). Any subjective sensation of darkness the origin of which is in the visual or optic centre. [centre, Gk *a, phos* light.]

centraxonial (sen·trax·o·ne·al). Having the axis in a median line. [centre, Gk *axon* axle.]

centre (sen·ter). 1. The mid-point of a line or surface; the central part of an organ or structure. 2. A restricted region in which a process begins, and from which it spreads, e.g. of ossification, or of chondrification. 3. An imprecise term used in neurology to denote a region or part of the nervous system the integrity of which is essential for the performance of a particular function. Often the centre does not correspond with any nucleus or part which can be defined in precise anatomical terms, its identification depending on observations that the function is activated or abolished by respective stimulation or destruction of the area. **Abdominal centre.** The part of the spinal cord, probably in the 10th thoracic segment, from which the abdominal cutaneous reflex is elicited. **Accelerating centre.** That part of the cardiac centre in the medulla oblongata which, when stimulated, causes acceleration of the heart rate via sympathetic nerve pathways. **Acoustic centre.** Auditory centre (see below). **Ankle clonus centre.** A region in the lumbosacral part of the spinal cord concerned with stretch reflexes from the tendo calcaneus (Achillis). **Anospinal centre.** The region of the lumbosacral spinal cord concerned with reflex contraction or relaxation of the sphincters of the anus. **Apneustic centre.** A centre which causes inhibition of respiration. **Arm centre.** The part of the motor area in the precentral gyrus from which movements of the upper limb can be elicited. **Articulate language centre.** Motor speech centre (see below). **Association centre.** An area of cerebral cortex which subserves no specific nervous function, but which is connected by association fibres with other areas. **Auditopsychic centre.** The cortex in the temporal lobe adjacent to the auditory area and thought to be concerned in building up complex auditory concepts such as words, sentences, music, etc., and the appreciation of their meaning. **Auditory centre.** The auditory cortex of the transverse temporal gyri. The term may also be applied to the inferior corpus quadrigeminum as an *auditory reflex centre,* or even to the cochlear nuclei of the hind-brain. **Automatic centre.** A centre concerned with automatic activity; one not under the control of the will and not solely concerned with reflex activity, although reflexes may influence its action, e.g. the respiratory centre. **Autonomic centre.** Any of the centres within the brain or spinal cord which regulate the activity of the autonomic nervous system via the sympathetic or parasympathetic nerves. **Brain centre.** Any area or group of cells in the brain with a special function. **Calorific centres.** Regions, probably in the hypothalamus, controlling body temperature. The corpus striatum has also been thought to control body temperature, but this is doubtful. **Cardiac centre.** The region of the hind-brain where stimulation causes acceleration (*cardio-accelerating centre*) or slowing (*cardio-inhibitory centre*) of the heart rate. Centres influencing the heart rate have also been identified in the hypothalamus. **Cardio-accelerating centre.** *See* CARDIAC CENTRE (preceding). **Cardio-inhibitory centre.** *See* CARDIAC CENTRE (above). **Cardiomotor centre.** An alternative name given to the atrioventricular node by Tawara, who considered that the cardiac contraction originated in this node instead of in the sinu-auricular node, as is now known. **Cardiovascular and circulatory centres.** Regions of the hind-brain, and possibly of the hypothalamus, concerned in the regulation of the heart rate and also of the degree of constriction or dilatation of the peripheral blood vessels. Terms such as *vascular centre, vasoconstrictor centre, vasodilator centre, vasomotor centre, vasotonic centre* are used in this connection. **Cheirokinaesthetic centre.** Probably the cortex in the lower part of the precentral gyrus, concerned with movements of the fingers, and the cortex immediately anterior to it, where the movements necessary for writing may be integrated. **Ciliospinal centre.** The pupillodilator centre in the 1st and 2nd thoracic segments of the spinal cord. **Colour centre.** The area of occipital cortex that is concerned with the perception of colour. **Convergence centre.** An area in the mid-brain situated centrally between the 3rd-nerve nuclei and responsible for convergence of the eyes. Also called *Perlia's nucleus.* **Convulsion centre.** A centre in the floor of the 4th ventricle, which, when stimulated, produces convulsions (it is doubtful whether this is an entity). **Co-ordination centre.** Any part of the nervous system concerned with co-ordination or integration of complex patterns of activity, e.g. the medulla oblongata for respiratory and cardiovascular reflexes. **Correlation centre.** Any part of the nervous system concerned, like the co-ordination centres, with complex patterns of activity; the term is more commonly used for the integration of afferent or sensory impulses than for motor patterns. **Cortical centre.** Any part of the cerebral cortex thought to be concerned with a particular activity or function; a *high-level centre,* as opposed to a *low-level* or spinal centre, or a *mid-level centre* in the brain stem. **Coughing centre.** The region of the hind-brain in which the activity of coughing is integrated; it is probably associated with the vagal nuclei. **Cremasteric centre.** A cutaneous reflex centre, probably in the 2nd lumbar segment, from which contraction of the cremaster muscle can be elicited. **Centre of curvature.** A term used in optics and ophthalmology as the centre of the sphere, a segment of which forms one of the surfaces of a lens or curved refracting surface such as the cornea. **Cutaneous reflex centre.** Any part of the nervous system (usually in the spinal cord) from which a particular movement can be elicited as a result of stimulating a particular area of the skin. **Defaecation centres.** Regions of the spinal cord which cause contraction of the pelvic colon and rectum, and relaxation of the anal sphincters. They probably lie in the 2nd, 3rd and 4th sacral segments from which the sacral parasympathetic nerves arise. **Deglutition centres.** Regions of the brain stem which control the movements of the jaws, tongue and pharynx; the motor nuclei of the 5th, 9th, 10th and 12th cranial nerves. **Diabetic centre.** Glycogenic centre (see below). **Ejaculation centre.** An area probably in the sacral and, possibly, lumbar segments of the spinal cord; it controls ejaculation and other genital functions. **Epigastric centre.** Abdominal centre (see above). **Erection centre.** A part of the genital centre located in the sacral and, possibly, lumbar segments of the spinal cord, concerned with the erection of the penis. **Eupraxic centre.** A cerebral centre concerned with the integration of muscular activity into willed purposive movements. **Excitomotor centre.** Motor centre, 1st def. (see below). **Expiratory centre.** *See* RESPIRATORY CENTRE (below). **Facial centre.** The region in the inferior part of the motor area of the precentral gyrus from which facial movements can be elicited. **Foot clonus centre.** Ankle clonus centre (see above). **Ganglionic centre.** Any one of the masses of grey matter in the basal ganglia (this term includes the thalamus and the corpus striatum, and many other basally situated centres). **Genital centre, Genitospinal centre.** A centre controlling genital function and including the ejaculation and erection centres (see above). **Germinal centre.** A primary follicle within lymphoid tissue undergoes a characteristic change in responding to antigen. The follicle enlarges and becomes filled with lymphoblasts and dendritic macrophages which are surrounded by a ring of small lymphocytes. This antigen-responding and antigen-localizing follicle is described as a germinal centre. **Glossokinaesthetic centre.** The centre concerned with movements of the tongue in articulation; it is situated in the posterior part of the 2nd frontal gyrus in the dominant hemisphere. **Gluteal centre.** The centre in the spinal cord which mediates the gluteal reflex; it is situated in the 4th lumbar segment. **Glycogenic centre.** A region in the floor of the lower part of the 4th ventricle where injury is associated with glycosuria. **Gustatory centre.** A centre concerned with taste, and thought to lie in the hypothalamus, but this is doubtful. **Health centre.** 1. An official or voluntary institution for organizing and co-ordinating various forms of health activities. 2. A system in the General Practitioner Services of the National Health Services based on premises technically equipped, staffed and maintained by the local health authorities at public cost. Health centres should afford facilities for the general medical and dental services, for many of the special clinic services of the local authorities, and sometimes also for outpost clinics of the hospital and specialist services. They should also serve as bases for various activities in health education. **Heat centre.** Calorific centre (see above). **Hypothalamic centres.** The nuclei of the hypothalamus, which are mainly concerned with regulation of autonomic activity; the anterior and middle nuclei are chiefly concerned with control of the parasympathetic system, the posterior nuclei with the sympathetic system. **Idea centre.** Name centre (see below). **Ideomotor centre.** Any one of the centres in the cerebral cortex which are concerned with ideomotor activities such as speech. **Independent centre.** Automatic centre (see above). **Inhibitory centres.** Regions the stimulation of which causes the cessation or inhibition of activity, e.g. the suppressor areas of the cerebral cortex. They may be defined according to position, e.g. cerebral, cerebellar, spinal, etc., or according to their particular function, e.g. cardio-inhibitory. **Inspiratory centre.** *See* RESPIRATORY CENTRE (below). **Kinaesthetic centres.** Regions for the appreciation of movements or position in parts of the body, lying in the post- and, possibly, also the pre-central gyrus. **Kinetic centre.** The centrosphere of a fertilized ovum. **Knee-jerk centre.** A centre for a stretch reflex of the quadriceps muscle in the 3rd and 4th lumbar segments of the spinal cord. **Language centre, Laryngeal cortical centre.** Motor speech centre (see below). **Mastication centre.** The part of the motor area in the precentral gyrus concerned with movements of the jaws; the term may also be applied to the motor nucleus of the trigeminal nerve. **Micturition centres.** Regions of the spinal cord causing contraction of the bladder and relaxation of the sphincters; like the defaecation centres, they are located in the 2nd, 3rd and 4th sacral segments. **Motor centre.** 1. Cortical; an area of cortex from which movement may be elicited by stimulation, notably the motor area of the precentral gyrus; excitomotor centre. 2. Bulbospinal: any of the motor nuclei of the brain stem, or of the anterior horn of the spinal cord. 3. Term which may be applied to any part of the nervous system from which a movement can be elicited or even modified by stimulation. **Motor speech centre.** A unilateral area in the posterior part of the inferior frontal gyrus on the side contralateral to that of the dominant hand associated with articulate speech; Brodmann's areas 44 and 45. **Musculotendinous centre.** Any centre in the spinal cord for a stretch reflex, e.g. knee jerk. **Name centre.** A cortical centre, mainly in the superior temporal gyrus, thought to be concerned with remembering names. **Nerve centre, Neural centre.** A mass of nerve cells performing some specific co-ordinating function. **Olfactory centre.** Any part of the brain in which olfactory-tract fibres end, e.g. the pyriform cortex of the uncus. **Oncology centre.** A group of facilities for basic research and prevention, diagnosis and treatment of cancer in one regional centre. **Optical centre.** In optics, applied to that point in a lens through which rays may pass without alteration in direction. Anatomically, the primary optical centres comprise the external geniculate bodies and the anterior corpora quadrigemina. **Ossification centre.** The region in which ossification begins in a tissue. Primary centres of ossification for the most part appear before birth, and from their extension the main part, shaft or body of the bone is formed. Epiphyses are ossified later from secondary centres of ossification. **Oval centre.** The centrum ovale; the outline of white matter of the cerebral hemispheres seen when the upper parts are removed by a horizontal cut just above the level of the corpus callosum. **Panting centre.** The region of the hypothalamus where stimulation causes increase in the rate of respiration. **Parenchymatous centre.** Any nerve centre, i.e. ganglion cells, found in the substance of a viscus. **Parturition centre.** A region in the lumbosacral part of the spinal cord where stimulation may cause contraction of the pregnant uterus. **Phonation centre.** Motor speech centre (see above). **Phrenic centre.** 1. The cells of origin for the motor fibres of the phrenic nerve in the 3rd, 4th and 5th cervical segments of the spinal cord. 2. The central tendon of the diaphragm. **Plantar reflex centre.** A centre probably situated in the 2nd sacral segment of the spinal cord; it is a cutaneous reflex centre. **Pneumotaxic centre.** Lumsden's centre; a centre partly responsible for the rhythmic character of respiration. **Polypnoeic centre.** Panting centre (see above). **Pontine centre for co-ordination of the movements.** Fuse's nucleus. **Psychocortical centre, Psychomotor centre.** That part of the cerebral cortex concerned with the production and control of voluntary movements. **Pteriotic centre.** A centre of ossification in the petrous part of the temporal bone. **Pupillary centre.** A term which can be applied to any part of the central nervous system where stimulation will give dilatation or constriction of the pupil, e.g. the 1st thoracic spinal segment (dilatation), the pretectal nucleus and, possibly, the superior corpora quadrigemina (constriction). **Pupillodilator centre.** *See* CILIOSPINAL CENTRE (above). **Radiotherapy centre.** A centre for the treatment of disease by radiotherapy and other means. **Receptive centre.** Peripheral or central nerve centres concerned with the reception of afferent impulses, some of which excite sensations; others do not reach consciousness but are concerned with reflex control of bodily activity. **Rectovesical centres.** The combined defaecation and micturition centres (see above). **Reflex centre.** Any part of the nervous system where the reception of afferent impulses is automatically followed by the emission of efferent impulses which in turn cause movement or other peripheral change. **Reserve centre.** Any nerve centre which is only brought into use under conditions of stress or excessive or abnormal activity. **Respiratory centres.** Regions of the medulla whose integrity and connections with the spinal cord and with peripheral nerves are essential for carrying out the activity of respiration. Sub-regions concerned with particular aspects of respiratory function have been identified, e.g. *inspiratory centre, expiratory centre* and an *apneustic centre* causing inhibition of respiration. A *pneumotaxic centre* is partly responsible for the rhythmic character of respiration. **Centre of rotation.** An imaginary point (it is actually a series of points) about which the eyeball rotates in its movements. **Salivary centre, Salivation centre.** Nerve cells in the floor of the 4th ventricle from which secretomotor fibres for the salivary glands are thought to arise. **Scapular centre.** The centre in the spinal cord which mediates the scapular reflex; it is situated in the 5th and 6th cervical segments of the cord. **Semi-ovale centre.** The centrum semi-ovale; the outline of the white matter of the one cerebral hemisphere seen when the upper part is removed by a horizontal cut just above the level of the corpus callosum. **Sensory centre.** Any part of the brain concerned with the conscious appreciation of sensation, e.g. the general sensory centre (the postcentral gyrus and adjacent parts of the parietal lobe), visual, auditory, olfactory centres. The term sensory should be restricted to centres of the forebrain, and probably to the cortex and thalamus, since there is no evidence that the reception of impulses in the spinal cord, brain stem or cerebellum can by itself cause sensation. **Smell centre.** Olfactory centre (see above). **Sneezing centre.** A region of the medulla oblongata, possibly part of or related to the respiratory centre (see above), from which sneezing is thought to be effected. **Somaesthetic centre.** The general sensory area of the postcentral gyrus. **Somatic centre.** A name given to the anterior lobe of the pituitary gland because of its property of controlling body growth. **Spasm centre.** Convulsion centre (see above). **Speech centre.** Motor speech centre (see above). **Sphenotic centre.** An undesirable term referring to the centre of ossification in the sphenoid bone which gives rise to the lingula. **Splenial centre.** An obsolete term for a centre of ossification in the mandible. **Spoken-word centre.** Motor speech centre (see above). **Sudorific centre.** That centre which controls diaphoresis, and which lies in the anterior hypothalamus. **Suprasegmental centre.** A cerebral centre which controls the inter-relationship of higher cerebral functions, or a centre in the brain which exerts a controlling influence over spinal-cord activity. **Swallowing centre.** Deglutition centre (see above). **Sweat centre.** Sudorific centre (see above). **Tactile centre.** A centre concerned with the appreciation of tactile impulses; it is situated in the sensory cortex, posterior to the central sulcus. **Taste centre.** Gustatory centre (see above). **Thermogenic centre, Thermo-inhibitory centre, Thermotaxic centre.** Centres concerned mainly with heat production, heat inhibition and heat conservation, respectively. **Thermolytic centre.** That centre controlling heat loss; it is associated with the sudorific centre in the anterior hypothalamus. **Trophic centre.** Any part of the nervous system whose activity is thought to be necessary for the nutrition of a peripheral structure or part of the body. **Vascular centre, Vasoconstrictor centre, Vasodilator centre, Vasomotor centre, Vasotonic centre.** *See* CARDIOVASCULAR AND CIRCULATORY CENTRES (above). **Vesical centre, Vesicospinal centre.** Micturition centre (see above). **Visual centre.** Generally, the visual area. The term may also be applied to the lateral geniculate body, or to the superior corpora quadrigemina. **Visuopsychic centre.** Visuopsychic area. *See* AREA. **Vomiting centre.** A part of the medulla oblongata, stimulation of which may cause vomiting; possibly the dorsal nucleus of the vagus. **Winking centre.** The centre in the pons near the facial-nerve nucleus, which is concerned with reflex winking. **Word centre, auditory.** A centre in the posterior part of the superior temporal convolution of the dominant hemisphere, concerned with the perception of spoken words. **Word centre, visual.** A centre in the dominant parietal lobe, concerned with the recognition and perception of written or printed words. **Written-word centre.** The visual word centre (see preceding). [Gk *kentron.*]

See also: BROCA, BUDGE, EXNER, FLECHSIG, HITZIG, KRONECKER, KUPRESSOFF, LUMSDEN, SETCHENOV, WERNICKE (K.).

centric (**sen**·trik). 1. Referring to a centre. 2. Central; neither peripheral nor acentric. 3. Referring to the centromere. 4. Of chromosomes or chromosome segments, having a centromere.

centricipital (sen·tre·**sip**·it·al). Relating to the centriciput; parietal.

centriciput (sen·**tris**·e·put). The central part of the head between the occiput and the sinciput. [centre, L *caput* head.]

centrifugal (sen·**trif**·ew·gal). 1. Efferent. 2. Proceeding away from a centre. 3. Tending to move outward from the cerebral cortex. [centre, L *fugere* to flee.]

centrifugalization, centrifugation (sen·**trif**·ew·gal·i·**za**′·shun, **sen**·trif·ew·**ga**′·shun). 1. A process by which a liquid is subjected to fast rotation so that one suspended component of a certain specific gravity is separated from other suspended components of different gravity. 2. A similar process for separating a liquid from a solid. **Density gradient centrifugation.** Centrifugation in a liquid whose density increases with distance from the rotor axis; it is used in immunochemistry for separating materials of different densities. [see foll.]

centrifuge (**sen**·tre·fewj). 1. A machine in which there is a rapidly rotating container for holding fluids or substances the components of which are to be separated. The centrifugal force throws the heavier components to the peripheral part of the container. 2. To subject to centrifugation. [centre, L *fugere* to flee.]

centring (**sen**·tring). 1. In optics, the adjustment of a lens so that its optic centre and the pupil of the eye are in the same axis. 2. In microscopy, the placing of an object so that its centre coincides with the optical axis of the instrument.

centriole (**sen**·tre·ole). One of a pair of short, hollow, cylindrical structures about 500 nm long which are found within the centrosome. They have a complex structure and, during mitosis, are involved in the formation of the spindle.

centripetal (sen·**trip**·et·al). 1. Afferent. 2. Tending to move towards the centre from the periphery. [centre, L *petere* to seek.]

centro-acinar (sen·tro·**as**·in·ar). In anatomy, denoting cubical cells which line the walls of the minute ducts of the pancreas at the points at which the ducts lead into the alveoli. [centre, L *acinus* grape.]

centrocinesia, centrocinesis (**sen**·tro·sin·e′·ze·ah, **sen**·tro·sin·e′·sis). Movement resulting from stimulation of the central nervous system. [centre, Gk *kinesis* movement.]

centrocinetic (**sen**·tro·sin·**et**′·ik). Referring to centrocinesia; excitomotor.

centrocyte (**sen**·tro·site). A certain type of cell containing groups of granules, some occurring singly and some in pairs, and which stain with haematoxylin. Centrocytes are found in the epidermis in measles, rubella, lichen planus and pityriasis rosea, and were described by Lipschuetz. [centre, Gk *kytos* cell.]

centrodesmose, centrodesmus (sen·tro·**des**·moze, sen·tro·**des**·mus). In mitosis, the achromatic fibril which connects the 2 centrosomes as they separate and gives rise to the achromatic spindle. [centre, Gk *desmos* band.]

centrodesome (sen·tro·**des**·ome). A thread connecting two nuclei in protozoa. [centre, Gk *desmos* band, *soma* body.]

centrodontous (sen·tro·**don**·tus). Having sharply pointed teeth. [Gk *kentron* sharp point, *odous* tooth.]

centrolecithal (sen·tro·**les**·ith·al). In embryology, denoting an ovum in which the yolk sac is centrally situated. [centre, Gk *lekithos* yolk.]

centromere (**sen**·tro·meer). 1. The region(s) of the chromosomes which become(s) associated with the spindle fibres at mitosis and meiosis. The position of the centromere (primary constriction) usually determines the shape of the chromosome. *See* ACROCENTRIC, TELOCENTRIC, METACENTRIC. 2. The neck of a spermatozoon (obsolete usage). **Centromere misdivision.** Transverse, instead of longitudinal, division of the centromere leading, usually, to the production of telocentric fragments of isochromosomes. [centre, Gk *meros* part.]

centromeric (sen·tro·**mer**·ik). Pertaining to the centromere.

centronervin (sen·tro·**ner**·vin). A substance present in the central nervous system that intensifies and modifies its activity.

centronucleus (sen·tro·**new**·kle·us). A nucleus that is made up of a single body composed of centrosome and spindle fibres, with the chromatin massed round it; a karyosome.

centro-osteosclerosis (sen·tro·**os**·te·o·skler·**o**′·sis). Osteosclerosis invading the medullary cavities of bones. [centre, osteosclerosis.]

centrophose (**sen**·tro·foze). Any subjective sensation of light the origin of which is in the visual or optic centre. [centre, Gk *phos* light.]

centroplasm (**sen**·tro·plazm). The protoplasm of the centrosome. [centre, Gk *plasma* something formed.]

centrosclerosis (**sen**·tro·skler·**o**′·sis). Centro-osteosclerosis.

centrosome (**sen**·tro·some). A cytoplasmic organelle present in most, but not all, animal cells, and usually close to the nucleus near the geometric centre of the cell. It appears as a spherical region of clear cytoplasm containing at its centre 2 minute centrioles which have a special affinity for Heidenhain's iron haematoxylin. During mitosis the centrosome divides into 2 parts which migrate to the opposite poles of the achromatic spindle. There each becomes surrounded by a wide clear zone known as the centrosphere, which in turn merges externally into the astrosphere. Little is known of the chemical composition or precise functional significance of these various structures. [centre, Gk *soma* body.]

centrosphere (**sen**·tro·sfeer). The cell centre; a clear area of the cytoplasm near the nucleus, containing the centrioles, and playing a vital part in cell division. [centre, sphere.]

centrostaltic (sen·tro·**stal**·tik). 1. Referring to a centre of movement. 2. Designating or referring to the action of nerve force in the spinal centre. [centre, Gk *stellein* to place.]

centrostigma (sen·tro·**stig**·mah). In morphology, a structure all the axes of which converge on a central point. [centre, Gk *stigma* point.]

centrotherapy (sen·tro·**ther**·ap·e). Treatment applied externally with the object of producing an effect on the nerve centres. [centre, therapy.]

centrum (**sen**·trum). 1. The centre or central part of an organ or region. 2. That part of the body of a vertebra which develops from the centre, or centres, of ossification for the body, i.e. excluding those parts which are developed from the bases of the neural arch. **Centrum medianum.** The central median nucleus of the thalamus; a nucleus situated in the posteromedial part of the thalamus and unconnected with the cerebral cortex. **Centrum ovale.** The oval area of white matter seen in the 2 central hemispheres taken together, when the brain is sliced horizontally at a level just above the corpus callosum. **Centrum semi-ovale.** The area of white matter seen in either of the cerebral hemispheres when the brain is sliced to expose the centrum ovale (see preceding). [L centre.]

See also: VIEUSSENS.

Centrurus exlicauda (sen·**troo**·rus ex·le·**kaw**·dah). A tropical poisonous scorpion, the bite of which may kill a child. [Gk *kentron* sting, *oura* tail.]

cephaeline (sef·a·el·een). $C_{28}H_{38}O_4N_2$, one of the chief alkaloids of ipecacuanha. It is a colourless substance with an irritant action on the gastric mucosa. As an amoebacide it is less powerful than emetine and is but little used in therapeutics. [see foll.]

Cephaelis (sef·a·el·is). A genus of tropical plants of the family Rubiaceae. *Cephaelis ipecacuanha* (Brot.) A. Rich, and *Cephaelis acuminata* Karsten yield the drug, ipecacuanha. [Gk *kephale* head, *eilein* to roll up.]

cephalaematocele (kef·al·e·mat·o·seel). Cephalhaematocele.

cephalaematoma (kef·al·e·mat·o′·mah). Cephalhaematoma.

cephalaemia (kef·al·e·me·ah). Congestion of the brain. [Gk *kephale* head, *haima* blood.]

cephalagra (kef·al·ag·rah). Severe pain in the head. [Gk *kephale* head, *agra* a catching.]

cephalalgia (kef·al·al·je·ah). Pain in the head. **Histamine cephalalgia.** Headache repeatedly affecting the region over the external carotid artery, combined with rhinorrhoea, lacrimation and local rise in temperature; the syndrome is caused by the liberation of histamine in the body or the administration of the substance. **Quadrantal cephalalgia.** A form of headache that affects only one quadrant of the head. [Gk *kephale* head, *algos* pain.]

cephalalgiagram (kef·al·al·je·ah·gram). A record of cerebrospinal fluid pressure which shows whether a particular variety of headache is the result of increased cerebrospinal pressure or of nervous or other origin. [Gk *kephale* head, *algos* pain, *gramma* record.]

cephalalgic (kef·al·al·jik). Referring to headache. [Gk *kephale* head, *algos* pain.]

cephalea (kef·al·e·ah). Cephalalgia. **Cephalea agitata, Cephalea attonita.** The violent headache which sometimes occurs in the early stages of infectious diseases, in association with intolerance of sound and light. [Gk *kephale* head.]

Cephalexin BP 1973 (kef·al·ex·in). 7-(D-aminophenylacetamido)-3-methyl-3-cephem-4-carboxylic acid; an antibiotic active in Gram-positive and Gram-negative infections. It is less potent than cephaloridine or cephalothin.

cephalhaematocele (kef·al·he·mat·o·seel). 1. A cephalhaematoma communicating with an intracranial venous sinus. 2. A blood-filled tumour occurring beneath the scalp and communicating through the bones of the skull with a dural sinus. [Gk *kephale* head, *haima* blood, *kele* hernia.]

See also: STROMEYER.

cephalhaematoma (kef·al·he·mat·o′·mah). 1. A haematoma occurring under the pericranium. 2. Caput succedaneum. **Cephalhaematoma deformans.** A calcified cephalhaematoma. [Gk *kephale* head, *haima* blood, *-oma* tumour.]

cephalhydrocele (kef·al·**hi**·dro·seel). In fracture of the skull, a collection of fluid beneath the epicranial aponeuroses. [Gk *kephale* head, *hydor* water, *kele* hernia.]

cephalic (kef·**al**·ik). 1. [Cranialis (NA).] Referring or relating to, situated near, or directed towards, the head. 2. A remedy for disorders of the head. [Gk *kephale* head.]

cephalic vein [vena cephalica (NA)]. The superficial vein of the pre-axial (radial) border of the upper limb. It commences at the dorsal venous arch, and ends by joining the axillary vein at the apex of the axilla. **Accessory cephalic vein [vena cephalica accessoria (NA)].** A vessel which arises from the ulnar side of the dorsal venous arch of the hand, and runs across the back of the forearm to join the cephalic vein. **Median cephalic vein [vena mediana cephalica (NA)].** *See* MEDIAN VEIN OF THE FOREARM (under FOREARM).

cephalin (kef·al·in). Any of a group of phospholipides which are glycerol esters of fatty acids and colamine phosphate, and occurring especially in brain, also present in nerve tissue and yolk of egg. They have the property of accelerating the coagulation of blood. [Gk *kephale* head.]

cephalitis (kef·al·i·tis). Encephalitis. **Cephalitis aegyptiaca.** A variety of encephalitis lethargica which occurs when the hot winds of early summer are prevalent in Egypt. **Cephalitis littriana.** Epiphysitis. **Cephalitis meningica.** Meningitis. **Cephalitis nervosa.** Whooping-cough. [Gk *kephale* head, *-itis* inflammation.]

cephalization (kef·al·i·za′·shun). In embryology, the localization of important organs and parts in or near the head end and the beginning of growth there. [Gk *kephale* head.]

cephalocathartic (kef·al·o·kath·ar′·tik). 1. Clearing or relieving the head, e.g. by inducing discharge of mucus from the nose and paranasal sinuses. 2. A remedy that clears the head or relieves disorders in it. [Gk *kephale* head, *katharsis* cleansing.]

cephalocaudal (kef·al·o·kaw′·dal). Cephalocercal. [Gk *kephale* head, L *cauda* tail.]

cephalocele (kef·al·o·seel). Protrusion of part of the brain through a cleft, congenital or traumatic, in the skull; cerebral hernia. [Gk *kephale* head, *kele* hernia.]

cephalocentesis (kef·al·o·sen·te′·sis). Puncture of the skull and brain, generally with a hollow needle, in order to drain off fluid or the contents of an abscess. [Gk *kephale* head, *kentesis* a pricking.]

cephalocercal (kef·al·o·ser′·kal). In anatomy, relating to the long axis of the body, i.e. head to tail. [Gk *kephale* head, *kerkos* tail.]

cephalochord (kef·al·o·kord). In embryology, that part of the notochord which extends into the region of the head. [Gk *kephale* head, *chorde* string.]

cephaloclast (kef·al·o·klast). Cephalotribe. [Gk *kephale* head, *klastos* broken.]

cephalocyst (kef·al·o·sist). A tapeworm. [Gk *kephale* head, *kystis* bag.]

cephalodymia (kef·al·o·di′·me·ah). In teratology, the merging or fusion of 2 fetal heads, so that a monster with a single head and/or one with 2 merged heads is produced. [Gk *kephale* head, *dymenai* to mingle.]

cephalodymus (kef·al·od·im·us). A twin monster with a single head, the latter as a product of fusion of 2 heads. [see prec.]

cephalodynia (kef·al·o·din′·e·ah). 1. Cephalalgia. 2. Pain referred from painful conditions in the neck, usually osteo-arthrosis and disc degenerative disease, into occiput and other parts of the head. [Gk *kephale* head, *odyne* pain.]

cephaloedema (kef·al·e·de′·mah). Oedema of the head; oedema of the brain. [Gk *kephale* head, *oidema* a swelling.]

cephalofacial (kef·al·o·fa′·shal). Having reference to the skull and the face. [Gk *kephale* head, L *facies* face.]

cephalogaster (kef·al·o·gas′·ter). 1. In embryology, that part of the alimentary canal nearest to the anterior pole. 2. The first part of the alimentary canal, as found in certain types of intestinal worm. [Gk *kephale* head, *gaster* stomach.]

cephalogenesis (**kef**·al·o·**jen**′·es·is). That branch of embryology which is concerned with the origins of the head. [Gk *kephale* head, *genein* to produce.]

Cephaloglycin (**kef**·al·o·**gli**′·sin). BP Commission approved name for 7-[D(−)-α-aminophenylacetamido]cephalosporanic acid; an antibiotic.

cephalograph (**kef**·al·o·graf). An instrument for registering the contours of the head so that the true plan and elevation may be drawn up. [Gk *kephale* head, *graphein* to record.]

cephalogyric (**kef**·al·o·**ji**′·rik). Referring to turning or circular movements of the head. [Gk *kephale* head, *gyros* turn.]

cephalohaematocele (**kef**·al·o·**he**′·mat·o·seel). Cephalhaematocele.

cephalohaematoma (**kef**·al·o·he·mat·**o**′·mah). Cephalhaematoma.

cephalohaemia (**kef**·al·o·**he**′·me·ah). Cephalaemia.

cephalohaemometer (**kef**·al·o·he·**mom**′·et·er). An instrument with which changes in pressure of the blood within the head may be estimated. [Gk *kephale* head, haemometer.]

cephalohydrocele (**kef**·al·o·**hi**′·dro·seel). Cephalhydrocele.

cephaloid (**kef**·al·oid). Shaped like the head, or resembling it. [Gk *kephale* head, *eidos* form.]

cephalology (kef·al·**ol**·o·je). The topographical appreciation of the cranium, with regard to measurements and landmarks. [Gk *kephale* head, *logos* science.]

cephaloma (kef·al·**o**·mah). Encephaloma; encephaloid carcinoma; soft cancer. [Gk *kephale* head, *-oma* tumour.]

cephalomelus (kef·al·**o**·mel·us). A monster from the head of which grows a supernumerary limb. [Gk *kephale* head, *melos* limb.]

cephalomenia (**kef**·al·o·**me**′·ne·ah). Vicarious menstruation in the form of a discharge of blood from the nose at the menstrual period. [Gk *kephale* head, *menes* menses.]

cephalomeningitis (**kef**·al·o·men·in·**ji**′·tis). Meningitis as affecting the meninges of the cerebral region. [Gk *kephale* head, meningitis.]

cephalometer (kef·al·**om**·et·er). Craniometer. [Gk *kephale* head, *metron* measure.]

cephalometry (kef·al·**om**·et·re). 1. Craniometry. 2. In dentistry, a dimensional appraisal of the craniofacial skeleton using standardized x-ray pictures which can be used in a serial study of growth and treatment changes. **Fetal cephalometry.** Measurement of the size of the fetal skull by radiographic or ultrasonic methods. **Radiographic cephalometry.** Measurement of the skull by radiographic methods. [see prec.]

cephalomotor (**kef**·al·o·**mo**′·tor). 1. Relating to movements of the head. 2. Term applied to muscles which move the head. [Gk *kephale* head, L *motor* mover.]

cephalone (**kef**·al·one). An idiot with a large head; the condition is usually associated with degeneration and hypertrophy of the brain sustance. [Gk *kephale* head.]

cephalonia (kef·al·**o**·ne·ah). The condition of having a large head and hypertrophy of the brain. [see prec.]

Cephalonium (kef·al·**o**·ne·um). BP Commission approved name for 3-(4-carbamoyl-1-pyridiniomethyl)-7-(2-thienylacetamido)-3-cephem-4-carboxylate; an antibiotic.

cephalont (**kef**·al·ont). A sporozoan immediately before production of spores. [Gk *kephale* head, *on* being.]

cephalo-orbital (**kef**·al·o·**or**′·bit·al). Referring to the skull and the orbits. [Gk *kephale* head, orbit.]

cephalo-orbitonasal (**kef**·al·o·**or**·bit·o·**na**′·zal). Referring to the skull, the orbits and the nose. [Gk *kephale* head, orbit, L *nasus* nose.]

cephalopagus, cephalopagy (kef·al·**op**·ag·us, kef·al·**op**·ah·je). Craniopagus; a twin monster the 2 heads of which are fused into one. **Cephalopagus parietalis.** United twins joined in the parietal region. [Gk *kephale* head, *pagos* joined.]

cephalopathy (kef·al·**op**·ath·e). General term to describe any disease of the head. [Gk *kephale* head, *pathos* suffering.]

cephalopelvic (**kef**·al·o·**pel**′·vik). Referring to the fetal head and the maternal pelvis. [Gk *kephale* head, pelvis.]

cephalopelvimetry (**kef**·al·o·pel·**vim**′·et·re). The radiological measurement of the fetal head when *in utero.* [Gk *kephale* head, L *pelvis* basin, Gk *metron* measure.]

cephalopharyngeus (**kef**·al·o·far·**in**′·je·us). An obsolete name for the superior constrictor muscle of the pharynx. [Gk *kephale* head, pharynx.]

cephaloplegia (**kef**·al·o·**ple**′·je·ah). Paralysis of the muscles of the head and face. [Gk *kephale* head, *plege* stroke.]

Cephaloram (kef·al·**or**·am). BP Commission approved name for 7-phenylacetamidocephalosporanic acid; an antibiotic.

Cephaloridine BP 1973 (kef·al·**or**·id·een). 7-(α-Thien-2-ylacetamido)-3-(pyrid-1-ylmethyl)-3-cephem-4-carboxylic acid betaine, an antibiotic with a broad spectrum of bactericidal activity against rapidly multiplying organisms.

cephalorrhachidian (**kef**·al·o·rak·**id**′·e·an). Relating to the head and the vertebral column. [Gk *kephale* head, *rhachis* spine.]

cephaloscopy (kef·al·**os**·ko·pe). Auscultation of the head. [Gk *kephale* head, *skopein* to watch.]

cephalosporin C (kef·al·o·**spor**·in **see**). Approved name for 7-(5-amino-5-carboxyvaleramido)cephalosporanic acid; an antibiotic.

cephalosporiosis (**kef**·al·o·spo·re·**o**′·sis). Infection due to the fungus *Cephalosporium;* not a generally accepted term, infections due to this species are usually grouped under the disease entity, e.g. mycetoma. [*Cephalosporium*, Gk *-osis* condition.]

Cephalosporium (**kef**·al·o·**spo**′·re·um). A genus of fungi, some of which are pathogenic for man, e.g. *Cephalosporium falciforme* and *C. recifei* have been isolated from maduromycetoma. **Cephalosporium granulomatis** Weidman and Kligman 1945. A species isolated from a case of mycetoma. [Gk *kephale* head, *sporos* seed.]

cephalostyle (**kef**·al·o·stile). The head end of the notochord. [Gk *kephale* head, *stylos* pillar.]

cephalotetanus (**kef**·al·o·**tet**′·an·us). Tetanus occurring as a complication of a head wound. [Gk *kephale* head, *tetanos* a stretching.]

Cephalothin (**kef**·al·o·thin). BP Commission approved name for 7-(2-thienylacetamido)cephalosporanic acid. **Cephalothin Sodium BP 1973.** The sodium salt, an antibiotic.

cephalothoracic (**kef**·al·o·thor·**as**′·ik). Referring to the head and the thorax. [Gk *kephale* head, thorax.]

cephalothoracopagus (**kef**·al·o·thor·ak·**op**′·ag·us). A twin monster the head and thorax of which are coalesced. [Gk *kephale* head, thorax, *pagos* joined.]

cephalotome (**kef**·al·o·tome). Craniotome; an instrument for use in operations on the cranium or in perforation and division of the fetal skull when delivery is otherwise impossible. [Gk *kephale* head, *temnein* to cut.]

cephalotomy (kef·al·**ot**·o·me). 1. Fetal craniotomy. 2. Dissection of the head. [see prec.]

cephalotractor (**kef**·al·o·**trak**′·tor). An obstetrical forceps. [Gk *kephale* head, L *trahere* to pull.]

cephalotribe (**kef**·al·o·tribe). An instrument like a strong-bladed forceps with a screw handle used to crush the head of the fetus in cases in which delivery otherwise is impossible. [Gk *kephale* head, *tribein* to crush.]

cephalotridymus (**kef**·al·o·**trid**′·im·us). A monster with 3 heads. [Gk *kephale* head, *tridymos* triple.]

cephalotripsy (**kef**·al·o·**trip**′·se). The operation of crushing the fetal head in a cephalotribe so that delivery may be accomplished. [Gk *kephale* head, *tribein* to crush.]

cephalotriptor (kef·al·o·**trip**′·tor). Cephalotribe.

cephalotropic (kef·al·o·**trop**′·ik). Having affinity for brain tissue. [Gk *kephale* head, *tropos* a turning.]

cephalotrypesis (kef·al·o·tri·**pe**′·sis). The operation of trephining the skull. [Gk *kephale* head, *trypesis* a boring.]

cephaloxia (kef·al·**ox**·e·ah). Torticollis. [Gk *kephale* head, *loxos* oblique.]

Cephamandole (kef·ah·**man**·dole). BP Commission approved name for 7-D-mandelamido-3-[(1-methyltetrazol-5-yl)thiomethyl]-3-cephem-4-carboxylic acid; an antibiotic agent.

Cephazolin (kef·a·zo·lin). BP Commission approved name for 3-[(5-methyl-1,3,4,-thiadiazol-2-yl)-thiomethyl]-7-(tetrazol-1-ylacetamido)-3-cephem-4-carboxylic acid; an antibiotic.

Cephoxazole (kef·**ox**·az·ole). BP Commission approved name for 7-(3-*o*-chlorophenyl-5-methylisoxazole-4-carboxamido)-cephalosporanic acid; an antibiotic.

Cephradine (**kef**·rah·deen). BP Commission approved name for 7-[D-2-amino-2-(1,4-cyclohexadien-1-yl)-acetamido]-3-methyl-3-cephem-4-carboxylic acid; an antibiotic.

ceptor (**sep**·tor). A general term covering any nerve-ending, either simple or specialized, which on receiving a stimulus passes it to the cell of which the ending is a part. **Chemical ceptor.** 1. A sensory nerve-ending specialized to respond to chemical stimuli, as in the carotid and aortic bodies. 2. In any living cell, that molecular configuration or side-chain which can react with certain extraneous chemical substances, thereby initiating changes in cellular activity. **Contact ceptor.** A ceptor which responds to direct physical stimuli. **Distance ceptor.** A ceptor which responds to stimuli at a distance; typically, auditory and optic sensory nerve-endings. **Nerve ceptor.** *See* MAIN DEFINITION (above). [L *capere* to take.]

cer-. For words beginning **Cer-**, *see also* KER-.

cera (**se**·rah). Wax. **Cera alba.** White Beeswax BP 1958; beeswax bleached by exposure to light and air. **Cera flava.** Yellow Beeswax BPC 1959, the ordinary beeswax obtained from the honeycomb. [L.]

ceraceous (ser·**a**·shus). Like wax in texture and appearance. [L *cera* wax.]

cerasine (**ser**·as·een). 1. A cerebroside in brain tissue; it is a galactolipin composed of galactose, sphingosine and lignoceric acid. 2. A red azo dye used as a biological stain. [Gk *kerasos* cherry tree.]

cerasus (**ser**·as·us). Red cherry, the fruit of *Prunus cerasus* Linn. var. *caproniana* DC. (family Rosaceae), cultivated in England, and used in the preparation of syrup of cherry and other fruit syrups. [Gk *kerasos.*]

cerate (**se**·rate). An external application containing wax which renders it plastic and less liable to melt than an ointment when spread. **Blistering cerate, Cantharides cerate.** Blistering plaster. *See* PLASTER. **Lead subacetate cerate.** A cerate composed of lead subacetate, lanolin, paraffin and camphor. **Rosin cerate.** A mixture of colophony, beeswax and lard. [L *cera* wax.]

See also: GALEN, GOULARD.

cerated (**se**·ra·ted). Covered or coated with wax. [L *cera* wax.]

ceratocricoid muscle [musculus ceratocricoideus (NA)] (**ser**·at·o·**kri**'·koid). A slip of the posterior crico-arytenoid muscle to the inferior horn of the thyroid cartilage. [Gk *keras* horn, cricoid.]

ceratoglossus (**ser**·at·o·**glos**'·us). A variable slip of muscle arising from the lesser cornu of the hyoid bone and inserted into the tongue with the hyoglossus. [Gk *keras* horn, *glossa* tongue.]

Ceratonia BPC 1949 (ser·at·o·**ne**·ah). Ceratoniae gummi, carob gum, the endosperms from the seeds of the locust bean, *Ceratonia siliqua* Linn. (family Leguminosae). It contains mannan, galactan, pentosans, proteins and cellulose, and produces a mucilage when boiled with water. It has uses similar to those of tragacanth, and is extensively employed in the food industry. [Gk *keratonia* carob.]

Ceratophyllidae (**ser**·at·o·**fil**'·id·e). A family of the insectan order Siphonaptera. The genera *Ceratophyllus, Oropsylla* and *Nosopsyllus* are of medical interest. [Gk *keras* horn, *phyllon* leaf, *eidos* form.]

Ceratophyllus (**ser**·at·o·**fil**'·us). Fleas of this genus are vectors of plague, potential vectors of tularaemia and arthropod hosts of *Hymenolepsis diminuta.* **Ceratophyllus fasciatus.** Nosopsyllus fasciatus. **Ceratophyllus montanus.** A vector of plague and a potential vector of tularaemia. **Ceratophyllus silantiewi.** A vector of plague. **Ceratophyllus telchinus.** A vector of plague. **Ceratophyllus tesquorum.** A vector of plague. [Gk *keras* horn, *phyllon* leaf.]

Ceratopogonidae (**ser**·at·o·po·**gon**'·id·e). A family of the dipteran sub-order Nematocera; biting midges. The genera *Culicoides* and *Forcipomyia* are of medical interest. [Gk *keras* horn, *pogon* beard, *eidos* form.]

ceratum (se·**ra**·tum). Cerate. [L.]

cercaria (ser·**ka**·re·ah). The somewhat tadpole-shaped final larval form of flukes. They develop from rediae within the secondary hosts and, after a short free-swimming life, encyst, developing into adults only if eaten by the primary hosts. Those of schistosomes bore actively into the primary host tissues. The name is used as a pseudogenus when the adult form is not recognized. [Gk *kerkos* tail.]

cercaricidal (**ser**·kar·e·**si**'·dal). Having a destructive effect on cercariae. [cercaria, L *caedere* to kill.]

cerclage (ser·**klahzh**). In oblique fracture or in fracture of a rounded surface, the binding together of the parts by encircling them with a metal ring or loop. [Fr. hooping.]

cercocystis (ser·ko·**sis**·tis). A larval tapeworm with a single invaginated scolex and a tail-like appendage to the bladder; characteristic of some *Hymenolepis* species. [Gk *kerkos* tail, *kystis* bladder.]

cercomonad (ser·ko·**mo**·nad). A general term for coprozoic flagellates found in faeces. [see foll.]

Cercomonas (ser·ko·**mo**·nas). A genus of coprozoic flagellates in human faeces but probably never parasitic. Numerous specific names have been given, but perhaps only *Cercomonas crassicauda* is correct. [Gk *kerkos* tail, *monas* unit.]

cercomoniasis (**ser**·ko·mo·**ni**'·as·is). The condition caused by infection with *Cercomonas.*

Cercopithecoidea (**ser**·ko·pith·e·**koid**'·e·ah). A super-family of the primate sub-order Anthropoidea. It includes all Old World monkeys. [Gk *kerkos* tail, *pithekos* ape, *eidos* form.]

Cercopithecus (ser·ko·**pith**·e·kus). A genus of monkeys; some are used in experimental malaria, and others are potential reservoirs of yellow fever in Africa. [Gk *kerkos* tail, *pithekos* ape.]

Cercospora (ser·ko·**spo**·rah). A fungus commonly parasitic on plants. One species, *Cercospora apii,* has been isolated from ulcerated, verrucous lesions in man. [Gk *kerkos* tail, *sporos* seed.]

cercosporamycosis (**ser**·ko·spo·rah·mi·**ko**'·sis). A single, well-documented case in an Indonesian boy. Extensive indurated, verrucous, ulcerated cutaneous and subcutaneous lesions were present on the face; dissemination occurred later to other areas; brown septate hyphae were found at all levels in skin and subcutaneous granulomas. [Gk *kerkos* tail, *sporos* seed, *mykes* fungus, *-osis* condition.]

cercus (**ser**·kus). A structure which is stiff and bristle-like. [Gk *kerkos* tail.]

cerea flexibilitas (se·re·ah flex·ib·**il**·it·as). In the insane, a condition of muscular tension which allows of the limbs being placed in any position or bent in any direction, the posture being retained until another is imposed. Generally referred to as *flexibilitas cerea.* [L wax-like flexibility.]

cerealose (**ser**·e·al·oze). A product of the enzyme hydrolysis of grain, consisting of maltose and glucose. [L *Ceres* goddess of agriculture.]

cerebellar (ser·e·**bel**·ar). Relating to the cerebellum, or involving it. **Cerebellar folium.** *See* FOLIUM. **Cerebellar notch.** *See* NOTCH.

cerebellar arteries. Anterior inferior cerebellar artery [arteria cerebelli inferior anterior (NA)]. A branch from the lower part of the basilar artery, supplying the anterior part of the inferior surface of the cerebellum. **Posterior inferior cerebellar artery [arteria cerebelli inferior posterior** (NA)]. *See* VERTEBRAL ARTERY. **Superior cerebellar artery [arteria cerebelli superior** (NA)]. A large artery from the upper part of the basilar artery. It winds round the cerebral peduncle just below the tentorium cerebelli to supply the upper surface of the cerebellum.

cerebellar veins. Inferior cerebellar veins [venae cerebelli inferiores (NA)]. Veins draining the inferior surface of the cerebellum into the adjacent occipital, sigmoid and petrosal sinuses. **Superior cerebellar veins [venae cerebelli superiores**

(NA)]. Veins draining the superior surface of the cerebellum into the adjacent straight, transverse and superior petrosal sinuses.

cerebellifugal (ser·e·bel·**if**′·ew·gal). Extending away from or tending to move away from the cerebellum. [cerebellum, L *fugere* to flee.]

cerebellipetal (ser·e·bel·**ip**′·et·al). Extending towards or tending to move towards the cerebellum. [cerebellum, L *petere* to seek.]

cerebellitis (ser·e·bel·**i**′·tis). A condition of inflammation of the cerebellum. [cerebellum, Gk *-itis* inflammation.]

cerebello-olivary (ser·e·**bel**·o·**ol**′·iv·ar·e). Relating to or connecting the cerebellum and the olive of the medulla oblongata.

cerebellopontile, cerebellopontine (ser·e·bel·o·**pon**′·tile, ser·e·bel·o·**pon**′·tine). Relating to the cerebellum and the pons.

cerebellorubral (ser·e·bel·o·**roo**′·bral). Relating to the cerebellum and the red nucleus of the tegmentum of the mid-brain, or involving them. [cerebellum, L *ruber* red.]

cerebellorubrospinal (ser·e·**bel**·o·roo·bro·**spi**′·nal). Relating to or involving the cerebellum, the red nucleus of the tegmentum of the mid-brain and the spinal cord. [cerebellum, L *ruber* red, spinal cord.]

cerebellospinal (ser·e·bel·o·**spi**′·nal). Relating to or affecting the cerebellum and the spinal cord.

cerebellum [NA] (ser·e·**bel**·um). The largest part of the hind-brain, a somewhat ovoid convoluted body lying behind the pons and the upper medulla in the posterior cranial fossa. It consists of a median vermis and lateral hemispheres both of which are divided by transverse grooves or sulci into *folia*. Superficially it is covered by a cortex of grey matter; more deeply are situated the cerebellar nuclei or independent centres of grey matter, and the white matter [corpus medullare (NA)]. It is connected to the brain stem on each side by 3 peduncles, which contain its afferent and efferent fibre tracts. Functionally, it is concerned with the co-ordination of muscle action in the performance of movement, or in the maintenance of equilibrium or posture. [L small brain.]

anterior lobe. The anterior part of the upper surface of the cerebellum, limited posteriorly by a deep fissure, the fissura prima.

lateral part. The part lateral to the vermis.

median part. That part of the vermis lying anterior to the fissura prima.

middle lobe. The major part of the cerebellum, lying between the anterior lobe and nodule (posterior or flocculonodular lobe).

lateral part. The part lateral to the inferior vermis.

median part. The part including the lobulus clivi.

posterior lobe. Term usually applied to the nodule plus the 2 flocculi; sometimes taken to include the middle lobe also, in which case the cerebellum is divided into anterior and posterior lobes only.

lateral part. The flocculus.

median part. The most anterior part of the inferior vermis; the nodule.

lower surface [facies inferior (NA)]. The surface formed by the middle lobe.

upper surface [facies superior (NA)]. The surface formed by the anterior and middle lobes.

cerebral (ser·e·bral). Relating to the cerebrum. **Cerebral sulcus.** *See* SULCUS.

cerebral arteries. Vessels supplying the cerebrum. **Anterior cerebral artery [arteria cerebri anterior (NA)].** The smaller of the 2 terminal branches of the internal carotid artery. It supplies central branches [rami centrales (NA)], piercing the anterior perforated substance, and cortical branches [rami corticales] supplying the medial surface of the cerebral hemisphere anterior to the parieto-occipital fissure and the upper part of the superolateral surface [rami frontales et parietales (NA)] and the orbital surface of the frontal lobe [rami orbitales (NA)]. **Middle cerebral artery [arteria cerebri media (NA)].** The larger of the 2 terminal branches of the internal carotid artery, running laterally in the lateral sulcus (sylvian fissure) to the surface of the insula. It supplies important central (medial and lateral striate) [rami striati (NA)] branches to the basal nuclei by perforating the anterior perforated substance [rami centrales (NA)], and cortical branches [rami corticales (NA)] to the greater part of the superolateral surfaces of the frontal [rami frontales, rami orbitales (NA)], parietal [rami parietales (NA)], and temporal [rami temporales (NA)] lobes. **Posterior cerebral artery [arteria cerebri posterior (NA)].** A terminal branch of the basilar artery, that supplies central branches [rami centrales (NA)] to the basal nuclei via the posterior perforated substance, choroid branches [rami choroidei posteriores (NA)] to the choroid plexuses of the 3rd and lateral ventricles, and cortical branches [rami corticales (NA)] to the occipital [rami occipitales (NA)] and part of the temporal lobes [rami temporales (NA)], and to the cuneus and precuneus [ramus parieto-occipitalis].

cerebral veins. Veins draining the cerebrum. **Anterior cerebral vein [vena cerebri anterior (NA)].** A tributary of the basal vein, accompanying the artery of the same name. **Deep middle cerebral vein [vena cerebri media profunda (NA)].** A tributary of the basal vein, draining the insula and floor of the lateral cerebral sulcus. **Great cerebral vein [vena cerebri magna (NA)].** A median vein, a tributary of the straight sinus, draining the choroid plexuses of the lateral and 3rd ventricles and adjacent structures in these regions. **Inferior cerebral veins [venae cerebri inferiores (NA)].** Veins draining the bases of the cerebral hemispheres, terminating according to the region drained in the superior sagittal, cavernous, superior petrosal, or transverse sinuses. **Internal cerebral veins [venae cerebri internae (NA)].** Bilateral tributaries of the great cerebral vein, formed by the union of the choroid vein draining the choroid plexus of the lateral ventricle of the brain, and the thalamostriate vein draining the adjacent parts of the thalamus and caudate nucleus. **Superficial middle cerebral vein [vena cerebri media superficialis (NA)].** A tributary of the cavernous sinus. It lies in the posterior ramus of the lateral sulcus, and drains the adjacent part of the cerebral hemisphere. **Superior cerebral veins [venae cerebri superiores (NA)].** Multiple tributaries of the superior sagittal sinus, draining much of the superolateral surface of the cerebral hemisphere and the adjacent part of the medial surfaces.

cerebralgia (ser·e·**bral**·je·ah). Any kind of pain occurring in the head. [cerebrum, Gk *algos* pain.]

cerebrasthenia (ser·e·bras·**the**′·ne·ah). The mental and physical weakness which is the result of a cerebral lesion. [cerebrum, asthenia.]

cerebration (ser·e·**bra**·shun). 1. The functional activity of the cerebrum. 2. Mental activity generally. **Unconscious cerebration.** Mental activity of which the subject is unaware.

cerebriform (ser·**eb**·re·form). Cerebroid. [cerebrum, form.]

cerebrifugal (ser·e·**brif**·ew·gal). Conveying impulses away from, or tending to move outwards from, the cerebral cortex. [cerebrum, L *fugere* to flee.]

cerebrin (ser·e·brin). A mixture of non-phosphorized nitrogenous substances obtained from brain tissue by alcoholic extraction; also a constituent of the medullary sheaths of nerves. [L *cerebrum* brain.]

cerebripetal (ser·e·**brip**·et·al). Conveying impulses towards the cerebral cortex. [cerebrum, L *petere* to seek.]

cerebritis (ser·e·**bri**·tis). Inflammation of the substance of the cerebrum. **Saturnine cerebritis.** Lead encephalopathy. *See* ENCEPHALOPATHY. [cerebrum, Gk *-itis* inflammation.]

cerebrocardiac (ser·e·bro·**kar**′·de·ak). Referring to the brain and the heart. [cerebrum, Gk *kardia* heart.]

cerebrogalactose (ser·e·bro·gal·**ak**′·toze). The monosaccharide, galactose, derived from a glycolipid (galactoside) on hydrolysis. So called from the occurrence of galactosides in brain tissue. [L *cerebrum* brain, galactose.]

cerebrogalactoside (ser·e·bro·gal·**ak**′·to·side). General name for a cerebroside, or lipid which contains no phosphorus, occurring in brain and nerve tissue and composed of galactose, a fatty acid and an organic base, sphingosine. Typical examples are phrenosin and kerasin.

cerebrohyphoid (ser·e·bro·**hi'**·foid). Having resemblance to brain tissue. [cerebrum, Gk *hyphe* tissue, *eidos* form.]

cerebroid (ser·e·broid). Resembling the brain or the brain substance. [cerebrum, Gk *eidos* form.]

cerebrol (ser·e·brol). An oil obtained from brain and nerve tissue; most probably a mixture of fats and sterols. [L *cerebrum* brain, *oleum* oil.]

cerebrolein (ser·e·**bro**·le·in). Cerebro-olein.

cerebrology (ser·e·**brol**·o·je). 1. The science of the brain and its functions. 2. The aggregate of knowledge regarding the brain. [cerebrum, Gk *logos* science.]

cerebromacular (ser·e·bro·**mak**·ew·lar). Referring to any condition affecting both the brain and the macula lutea, especially cerebral lipidosis. [cerebrum, macula.]

cerebromalacia (ser·e·bro·mal·**a'**·she·ah). Encephalomalacia; pathological softness of the brain. [cerebrum, Gk *malakia* softness.]

cerebromedullary (ser·e·bro·med·**ul'**·ar·e). Cerebrospinal. [cerebrum, L *medulla* marrow.]

cerebromeningeal (ser·e·bro·men·**in'**·je·al). Relating to the brain and its membranes, or affecting them. [cerebrum, Gk *menigx* membrane.]

cerebromeningitis (ser·e·bro·men·in·**ji'**·tis). A condition of inflammation of the brain and its membranes. [L *cerebrum* brain, meningitis.]

cerebrometer (ser·e·**brom**·et·er). An instrument with which the pulsations and movements of the brain can be measured. [cerebrum, meter.]

cerebro-ocular (ser·e·bro·**ok'**·ew·lar). Relating to or involving the brain and the eye. [cerebrum, L *oculus* eye.]

cerebro-olein (ser·e·bro·**o'**·le·in). An intermediate in the decomposition of brain tissue, consisting of lecithin mixed with aliphatic acids. [L *cerebrum* brain, *oleum* oil.]

cerebropathia, cerebropathy (ser·e·bro·**path'**·e·ah, ser·e·**brop**·ath·e). Any disease or disorder of the brain. **Psychic cerebropathy.** Mental disease caused by a lesion of the brain or spinal cord. **Cerebropathia psychica toxaemia.** Korsakoff's psychosis. [cerebrum, Gk *pathos* suffering.]

cerebrophysiology (ser·e·bro·fiz·e·**ol'**·o·je). The physiology of the brain. [L *cerebrum* brain, physiology.]

cerebropontile, cerebropontine (ser·e·bro·**pon'**·tile, ser·e·bro·**pon'**·tine). Relating to the cerebrum and the pons, or affecting them.

cerebrorrhachidian (ser·e·bro·rak·**id'**·e·an). Cerebrospinal. [cerebrum, Gk *rhachis* spine.]

cerebrosclerosis (ser·e·bro·skler·**o'**·sis). Hardening of the brain substance of the cerebral hemispheres. [cerebrum, Gk *skleros* hard.]

cerebroscope (ser·e·bro·skope). An ophthalmoscope used in the diagnosis of disease of the brain. [cerebrum, Gk *skopein* to watch.]

cerebroscopy (ser·e·**bros**·ko·pe). 1. Examination for disease of the brain by the use of a cerebroscope. 2. Examination of the brain *post mortem.*

cerebrose (ser·e·broze). Brain sugar, galactose. A monosaccharide occurring as a constituent of the cerebrosides or galactosides (now called *glycolipids*) in brain and nerve tissue. [L *cerebrum* brain.]

cerebroside (ser·e·bro·side). Galactoside; now called *glycolipid.* General term for compounds, obtained from brain and nerve tissue, which can be split into a carbohydrate (galactose), a fatty acid and an organic base, sphingosine. They are distinguished from lecithin and the other phospholipids by their containing no phosphorus. They include phrenosin, kerasin and nervone. [L *cerebrum* brain.]

cerebrosidosis (ser·e·bro·sid·**o'**·sis). A type of lipoidosis characterized by predominance of kerasin in the fatty tissues of the body, e.g. Gaucher's disease. [cerebroside, Gk *-osis* condition.]

cerebrosis (ser·e·**bro**·sis). Any disease of the cerebrum. [cerebrum, Gk *-osis* condition.]

cerebrospinal (ser·e·bro·**spi'**·nal). Relating to the brain and the spinal cord, or affecting them. **Cerebrospinal fluid.** *See* FLUID. **Cerebrospinal tract.** *See* TRACT. [see foll.]

cerebrospinant (ser·e·bro·**spi'**·nant). A drug or preparation which affects the brain or spinal cord. [cerebrum, spinal cord.]

cerebrostomy (ser·e·**bros**·to·me). Creation of a canal from the external surface of the head to the cerebrum. [cerebrum, Gk *stoma* mouth.]

cerebrotomy (ser·e·**brot**·o·me). 1. The anatomy of the brain. 2. Dissection of brain tissue. [cerebrum, Gk *temnein* to cut.]

cerebrotonia (ser·e·bro·**to'**·ne·ah). A variety of temperament described by Sheldon and characterized by hyperattentionality, or hyperconsciousness, and the inhibition of both viscerotonic and somatotonic expression. [cerebrum, Gk *tonos* tension.]

cerebrovascular (ser·e·bro·**vas'**·kew·lar). Relating or belonging to the arteries and veins of the brain, or affecting them. [cerebrum, L *vasculum* little vessel.]

cerebrum [NA] (ser·e·brum). The cerebral hemispheres and their commissure, the corpus callosum. [L brain.]

base of the cerebrum. The inferior surface.

frontal lobe [lobus frontalis (NA)]. The anterior portion of the cerebral hemisphere in front of the central sulcus and above the lateral sulcus.

inferior surface [facies inferior cerebri (NA)]. The surface which is in contact with the anterior and middle cranial fossae and with the tentorium cerebelli.

inferolateral border [margo inferior (inferolateralis) NA]. The border which lies between the superolateral and inferior (basal) surfaces.

inferomedial border [margo medialis (inferomedialis) NA]. The border which lies between the inferior (basal) surface and the medial surface.

occipital lobe [lobus occipitalis (NA)]. The portion of the cerebral hemisphere lying posterior to a line joining the pre-occipital notch to the parieto-occipital sulcus. It contains the calcarine cortex.

parietal lobe [lobus parietalis (NA)]. The lobe situated between the frontal, occipital and temporal lobes; its anterior part contains the sensory area.

superomedial border [margo superior (superomedialis) NA]. The border which lies between the medial surface and the superolateral surface.

temporal lobe [lobus temporalis (NA)]. That portion of the cerebral hemisphere below the lateral sulcus and anterior to the pre-occipital notch.

medial surface [facies medialis cerebri (NA)]. The flat surface of the hemisphere that faces the opposite cerebral hemisphere.

superolateral surface [facies superolateralis cerebri (NA)]. The dorsolateral convex surface.

Cerenkov, P. A. 20th century Russian physicist.

Cerenkov radiation. When a fast charged particle passes through a transparent material, it suffers a special kind of radiation loss of energy if its speed is greater than the velocity of light in the medium. This radiation loss is emitted partly as photons of visible light, which may be observed.

cereolus (se·re·o·lus) (pl. *cereoli*). A medicated bougie for insertion into the urethra. [L a wax taper.]

cereous (se·re·us). Waxy; made of wax. [L *cera* wax.]

ceresine (ser·e·seen). A hard paraffin wax used in the manufacture of candles and polishes, a bleached and purified form of the natural paraffin occurring in the Galicia and Baku oilfields. [L *cera* wax.]

cereus (ser·e·us). Night-blooming cereus, cactus grandiflorus, the fresh young shoots (usually preserved in alcohol) of *Cereus grandiflorus* Mill., a cactus indigenous to the West Indies. It is reputed to act as a heart stimulant and nerve tonic, but is of doubtful therapeutic value. [L waxen.]

cerevisia (ser·e·viz·e·ah). The Latin term for any malt liquor such as beer. In the plural (cerevisiae) it refers generally to many varieties of cultured yeast employed in brewing. **Cerevisiae fermentum.** Brewer's yeast, the cells and spores of varieties of

Saccharomyces cerevisiae. **Cerevisiae fermentum compressum.** Compressed yeast. **Cerevisiae fermentum siccatum.** Dried Yeast BPC 1959.

cerin (ser·in). 1. Cerotic acid. 2. A steroid substance found in cork.

cerite (se·rite). A mineral found chiefly in Scandinavia. It is a silicate of cerium and other rare-earth metals, and one of the principal sources of these elements. [see foll.]

cerium (se·re·um). An element of the rare earths, with atomic weight 140.12, atomic number 58 and chemical symbol Ce. It is a grey metal occurring in the cerite earths and monazite sands, and because of its high reactivity is used in pyrophoric alloys (lighter flints, tracer bullets and flash powders). The oxide is incorporated into gas-mantles. Compounds of cerium are poisonous but have been used medicinally in nervous disorders. **Cerium oxalate.** Cerous oxalate, $Ce_2(OOCCOO)_3 \cdot 9H_2O$, a pinkish compound usually with the oxalates of praseodymium, lanthanum and neodymium as impurities, has been employed in the treatment of the vomiting of pregnancy and various affections of the nervous system. **Cerium valerate.** Cerous valerate, Ce $(C_5H_9O_2)_3$, an insoluble compound used for the same purpose as the oxalate. [the planet *Ceres*.]

ceroma (se·ro·mah). A cystic tumour which has undergone waxy or fatty degeneration. [L *cera* wax, Gk *-oma* tumour.]

ceroplasty (se·ro·plas·te). The modelling of anatomical structures in wax. [L *cera* wax, Gk *plassein* to mould.]

cerosate (se·ro·sate). Any salt or ester of cerosic acid, e.g. cerosinyl cerosate, the wax of sugar cane.

cerosic (se·ro·sik). Pertaining to cerosin.

cerosin (se·ro·sin). A wax occurring in sugar cane.

cerotate (se·ro·tate). A salt of cerotic acid.

cerotin (se·ro·tin). Ceryl alcohol, $CH_3(CH_2)_{25}OH$. A colourless substance obtained from lanolin and Chinese wax.

cerous (se·rus). Denoting a compound of the rare-earth element cerium, in which the latter is trivalent.

certifiable (ser·te·fi·abl). Designating a patient with mental disease of such type that for his own protection and that of others he must be detained in a hospital. [L *certus* certain, *facere* to make.]

ceruloplasmin (se·roo·lo·plaz·min). A blue copper-containing alpha globulin found in blood plasma which is abnormally low in hepatolenticular degeneration (or Wilson's disease). [L *caelum* sky, Gk *plassein* to mould.]

cerumen (se·roo·men). Ear wax. **Inspissated cerumen.** Dried and powdered ear wax. [L *cera* wax.]

ceruminal (se·roo·min·al). Relating to ear wax. [see prec.]

ceruminoma (se·roo·min·o′·mah). A slowly growing adenocarcinoma of the external auditory meatus. [L *cera* wax, Gk *-oma* tumour.]

ceruminosis (se·roo·min·o′·sis). The secretion of ear wax abnormal in quantity or kind. [cerumen, Gk *-osis* condition.]

ceruminous (se·roo·min·us). Composed of ear wax. [cerumen.]

ceruse (se·rooz). White lead; the basic carbonate of lead, used in paint and at one time in cosmetics. **Antimony ceruse.** White antimonious oxide. [L *cerussa*.]

cervical (ser·vik·al). In anatomy, relating to the human neck, or to the cervix of an organ. **Cervical enlargement.** *See* ENLARGEMENT. **Cervical fascia.** *See* FASCIA. **Cervical lymph gland.** *See* GLAND. **Cervical plexus.** *See* PLEXUS. [L *cervix* neck.]

cervical arteries. **Ascending cervical artery [arteria cervicalis ascendens (NA)].** *See* THYROID ARTERY, INFERIOR. **Deep cervical artery [arteria cervicalis profunda (NA)].** A division of the costocervical trunk which ascends on the deep surface of the semispinalis capitis muscle, supplying a twig to the spinal canal, and ends by anastomosing with branches of the occipital and vertebral arteries. **Superficial cervical artery [arteria cervicalis superficialis (NA)].** The superficial branch of the transverse cervical artery when it occurs as a separate artery. The deep branch is then the descending scapular artery [arteria scapularis descendens dorsalis (NA)]. **Transverse cervical artery [arteria transversa colli (NA)].** A branch of the thyrocervical trunk running horizontally across the posterior triangle of the neck and dividing into superficial [ramus (arteria cervicalis) superficialis NA] and deep (ramus profundus (arteria scapularis descendens) NA] branches that anastomose, respectively, with branches from the occipital artery and with the scapular anastomosis.

cervical nerves [nervi cervicales (NA)]. Spinal nerves which arise from the cervical part of the spinal cord and emerge in relation to the cervical vertebrae. There are 8 pairs, the first [nervus suboccipitalis (NA)] emerging above the atlas and the last below the 7th cervical vertebra. The first 4 of the anterior primary rami [rami ventrales (NA)] form the cervical plexus and supply the head and neck; the remaining 4 supply the upper limb through the brachial plexus. The posterior primary rami [rami dorsales (NA)] supply muscular and cutaneous branches to the scalp and back of the neck [rami mediales, rami laterales (NA)], and the last 2 to the deep muscles of the back.

cervical veins. **Deep cervical vein [vena cervicalis profunda].** The venous drainage of the deep muscles at the back of the neck; it is a tributary of the vertebral vein. **Transverse cervical veins [venae transversae colli].** Tributaries of the external jugular vein.

cervicalis ascendens (ser·vik·a·lis as·en·denz). An obsolete term for the costocervicalis muscle. [L of the neck, ascending.]

cervicectomy (ser·vis·ek·to·me). Amputation of the neck of the uterus. [L *cervix* neck, Gk *ektome* a cutting out.]

cervicicardiac (ser·vis·e·kar′·de·ak). Relating to or serving the neck and the heart; the term is applied to certain branches of the vagus nerve. [L *cervix* neck, Gk *kardia* heart.]

cerviciplex (ser·vis·e·plex). The cervical plexus of the spinal nerves.

cervicispinal (ser·vis·e·spi′·nal). Referring to the neck and the spinal cord. [L *cervix* neck, spinal cord.]

cervicitis (ser·vis·i·tis). Inflammation of the cervix of the uterus. [cervix, Gk *-itis* inflammation.]

cervico-auricular (ser·vik·o·aw·rik′·ew·lar). Relating to the area of the cervical vertebrae and the auricle of the external ear.

cervico-axillary (ser·vik·o·ax·il′·ar·e). Relating to the neck and the axillae. [L *cervix* neck, axilla.]

cervicobasilar (ser·vik·o·ba′·sil·ar). Relating or belonging to the neck and the region of the basilar part of the skull. [L *cervix* neck, basilar.]

cervicobrachial (ser·vik·o·bra′·ke·al). Relating to the neck and the arm. [L *cervix* neck, Gk *brachion* arm.]

cervicobregmatic (ser·vik·o·breg·mat′·ik). Relating to the nape of the neck and the bregma. [L *cervix* neck, Gk *bregma* front of the head.]

cervicobuccal (ser·vik·o·buk′·al). Relating to the line angle formed by the cervical and buccal walls of a cavity prepared in a tooth.

cervicodorsal (ser·vik·o·dor′·sal). Relating to the neck and the back, or involving them. [L *cervix* neck, *dorsum* back.]

cervicodynia (ser·vik·o·din′·e·ah). Pain affecting the muscles of the back of the neck. [L *cervix* neck, Gk *odyne* pain.]

cervicofacial (ser·vik·o·fa′·shal). Relating or belonging to the neck and the face. [L *cervix* neck, *facies* face.]

cervicohumeral (ser·vik·o·hew′·mer·al). Relating to the neck and the upper arm, or affecting them. [L *cervix* neck, *humerus* shoulder.]

cervicolabial (ser·vik·o·la′·be·al). Appertaining to the cervical margin on the labial surface of a tooth.

cervicolingual (ser·vik·o·ling′·gwal). Pertaining to the cervical margin and the lingual surface of a tooth.

cervicomuscular (ser·vik·o·mus′·kew·lar). Having reference to the muscles of the neck, or involving them. [L *cervix* neck, muscle.]

cervico-occipital (ser·vik·o·ok·sip′·it·al). Belonging or in relation to the neck and the occiput. [L *cervix* neck, occiput.]

cervico-orbicular (ser·vik·o·or·bik′·ew·lar). Relating to the neck and the muscles of the orbit. [L *cervix* neck, orbit.]

cervicoplasty (ser·vik·o·plas′·te). Plastic surgery performed on the neck. [L *cervix* neck, Gk *plassein* to mould.]

cervicoscapular (ser·vik·o·skap'·ew·lar). In relation or belonging to the neck and the scapula. [L *cervix* neck, scapula.]

cervicothoracic (ser·vik·o·thor·as'·ik). Relating to the neck and the thorax, or affecting them. [L *cervix* neck, thorax.]

cervicovaginal (ser·vik·o·vaj·i'·nal). Relating to the cervix of the uterus and the vagina.

cervicovaginitis (ser·vik·o·vaj·in·i'·tis). Inflammation of the vagina and cervix uteri. [cervix, vagina, Gk *-itis* inflammation.]

cervicovesical (ser·vik·o·ves'·ik·al). Relating to the cervix of the uterus and the bladder. [cervix, L *vesica* bladder.]

cervimeter (ser·vim·et·er). An instrument with which the cervix of the uterus can be measured. [cervix, meter.]

cervisia (ser·viz·e·ah). Cerevisia.

cervix [NA] (ser·vix) (pl. *cervices*). A neck, or any part resembling a neck. **Cervix of an axon.** The constricted neck of an axon at the beginning of the myelin sheath. **Conical cervix.** A cervix uteri having a cone shape and usually smaller than normal; thus, conoid and conoidal. **Cervix cornu.** The neck of the posterior horn of grey matter in the spinal cord. **Cervix dentis.** The neck of a tooth; the constricted part between the crown and the root. **Cervix obstipa.** An obsolete term for congenital torticollis. **Tapiroid cervix.** A cervix uteri having an elongated anterior lip. **Cervix uteri.** Neck of the uterus. *See* UTERUS. [L neck.]

ceryl (se·ril). The monovalent radical, $CH_3(CH_2)_{25}$–, which occurs in ceryl alcohol. **Ceryl cerotate.** $CH_3(CH_2)_{25}COO(CH_2)_{25}CH_3$, the ester of ceryl alcohol and cerotic acid found in Chinese wax. **Ceryl palmitate.** $CH_3(CH_2)_{14}COO(CH_2)_{25}CH_3$, an ester of ceryl alcohol and palmitic acid found in Chinese wax. [L *cera* wax.]

Cesaris-Demel, Antonio (b. 1866). Milan pathologist.

Cesaris-Demel bodies. Degenerative granules sometimes seen in leucocytes in severe anaemia. Also known as *Bender's bodies.*

Cestan, Raymond (b. 1872). Toulouse neurologist.

Cestan's sign. In complete facial palsy of lower motor neurone type, an attempt to close both eyes slowly when the patient is looking forward will result in slight elevation of the affected upper eyelid, due to the action of the levator palpebrae superioris muscle.

Cestan's syndrome, Cestan-Chenais paralysis. Cestan-Chenais syndrome (see following).

Cestan-Chenais syndrome. A syndrome produced by a pontobulbar lesion, usually vascular, with ipsilateral palatal and laryngeal paralysis. Horner's syndrome and ataxia of the limbs, and contralateral hemiplegia and hemi-anaesthesia; due to involvement of the pyramidal tract, medial lemniscus, inferior cerebellar peduncle, nucleus ambiguus, and the ocular sympathetic pathway.

Dutemps and Cestan sign. Cestan's sign (see above).

Cestan-Raymond syndrome, Raymond-Cestan syndrome. Cestan-Chenais syndrome (see above).

Cestoda (ses·to·dah). The typical tapeworms, a sub-class of the Cestoidea, whose individuals have no intestine and are joined together to form a long "worm" of identical segments, with a "head" end usually bearing a spiny scolex. All have complex life histories and (except *Hymenolepis nana*) secondary hosts, but the adults are always intestinal parasites of vertebrates. The following genera are of medical interest, *Bertiella, Diphyllobothrium, Dipylidium, Echinococcus, Hymenolepis, Inermicapsifer, Multiceps, Raillietina, Taenia.* [see foll.]

cestode, cestoid (ses·tode, ses·toid). 1. Like a tapeworm, or having the characteristics of a tapeworm. 2. A tapeworm of the sub-class Cestoda. [Gk *kestos* girdle, *eidos* form.]

Cestoidea (ses·toid·e·ah). Platyhelminthes. A class of flatworms in which the intestine is absent; it includes the tapeworms in the sub-class Cestoda. [see prec.]

cetaceum (se·ta·se·um). Spermaceti BPC 1959, a common ingredient of toilet creams. It is a white, wax-like solid obtained from the sperm whale, and composed mainly of cetyl palmitate, $C_{15}H_{31}COOC_{16}H_{33}$. [Gk *ketos* whale.]

Cetalkonium Chloride (se·tal·ko·ne·um klor·ide). BP Commission approved name for benzylhexadecyldimethylammonium chloride; an anti-infective agent.

cetanol (se·tan·ol). Cetyl alcohol. *See* ALCOHOL.

cetin (se·tin). Cetyl palmitate, $CH_3(CH_2)_{14}COO(CH_2)_{15}CH_3$. A white crystalline substance occurring in spermaceti.

Cetomacrogol 1000 BP 1973 (se·to·mak·ro·gol). A mixture of ethers prepared by condensation of cetyl or cetostearyl alcohol with ethylene oxide under controlled conditions, having the general formula $CH_3(CH_2)_mO(CH_2OCH_2)_nCH_2OH$ in which m is 15 or 17 and n is 19-23. Soluble in water and in acetone, insoluble in light petroleum and liquid paraffin, and dispersible in vegetable oils, it is used in pharmacy as a non-ionic emulsifying agent, usually in combination with cetostearyl alcohol, and forms stable oil-in-water creams. It is also used as a solubilizing agent for the preparation of aqueous solutions of fat-soluble vitamins and volatile oils. BP Commission approved name.

Cetoxime (se·tox·eem). BP Commission approved name for *N*-benzylanilino-acetamidoxime; an antihistaminic used in the treatment of hay fever and other allergic conditions.

cetraria (se·tra·re·ah). Iceland moss, the dried foliaceous lichen, *Cetraria islandica* (Linn.) Ach. (family Parmeliaceae), collected mainly in Sweden and Central Europe. It contains the carbohydrate complexes lichenin and isolichenin, and a bitter principle. It has demulcent, nutritive and tonic properties. [L *caetra* a short shield.]

cetrarin (se·tra·rin). The name given to the bitter substance derived from the dried lichen *Cetraria islandica* (Iceland moss); it is probably a lichen acid of the orcin type.

Cetrimide BP 1973 (se·trim·ide). CTAB; a cationic detergent consisting of a mixture of alkylammonium bromides, principally cetyltrimethyl ammonium bromide, $C_{16}H_{33}N(CH_3)_3Br$. It is a synthetic quaternary ammonium compound, soluble in water to give a cationic surface-active agent having a strong surface tension-lowering property. It is both a detergent and bactericide, a 1 per cent solution having a high bactericidal action. It is specially active against Gram-positive organisms, less against Gram-negative: it will kill *Staphylococcus aureus, Streptococcus pyogenes, Bacterium coli* and *Pseudomonas pyocyanea.* A 1 per cent solution is also used for its powerful cleansing action. Clinical uses are many: it is valuable for cleaning dirty contaminated wounds, abrasions and burns, for skin disinfection, disinfecting surgical instruments and hospital vessels. It is also used in creams as an antiseptic application in the treatment of minor wounds and skin infections.

Cetrimidum (se·trim·i·dum). *European Pharmacopoeia* name for Cetrimide BP 1973.

Cetrimonium Chloride (se·trim·o·ne·um klor·ide). BP Commission approved name for hexadecyltrimethylammonium chloride, a cationic emulsifying agent with similar properties to those of cetrimide.

cetyl (se·til). The monovalent radical $CH_3(CH_2)_{15}$– occurring in cetyl alcohol. **Cetyl alcohol.** *See* ALCOHOL. **Cetyl palmitate.** Cetin. **Cetyl pyridinium bromide.** CPB, a cation-active detergent with bactericidal properties, used for sterilizing woollens. **Cetylpyridinium Chloride BP 1973.** $C_5H_5N(C_{16}H_{33})Cl$, a cationic detergent with antiseptic properties.

cevadilla (sev·ad·il·ah). Sabadilla, caustic barley, the ripe seeds of *Schoenocaulon officinale* A. Gray (family Liliaceae). It contains alkaloids, the most important being cevadine (crystalline veratrine) which is highly toxic and sternutatory. The mixture of alkaloids constitutes amorphous commercial veratrine. Cevadilla has been used as a parasiticide, particularly for pediculi capitis. [Sp. *cebeda* barley.]

cevadilline (sev·ad·il·een). Sabadilline, $C_{34}H_{53}O_8N$. An alkaloid obtained from cevadilla seeds, *Schoenocaulon officinale.*

cevadine (sev·ad·een). Veratrine, $C_{32}H_{49}O_9N$. A crystalline alkaloid found in cevadilla seeds.

cevine (sev·een). $C_{27}H_{43}O_8N$. An alkaloid derived from cevadine and found naturally in species of *Veratrum.*

chacaleh (chak·ah·la). Burning feet.

Chaddock, Charles Gilbert (b. 1861). St. Louis neurologist.

Chaddock reflex. 1. Extension and fanning of the fingers, with flexion of the wrist in a hemiplegic patient, caused by stimulation of the lower ulnar border of the affected forearm. 2. Chaddock's sign (see below).

Chaddock's sign. The production of an extensor-plantar response on scratching the skin in the region of the external malleolus in pyramidal-tract disease; also called the *external malleolar sign.*

chaerophobia (ke·ro·fo·be·ah). 1. A morbid fear of gaiety. 2. Excessive dislike or dread of being happy. [Gk *chairein* to rejoice, phobia.]

chaffbone (chaf·bone). The mandible. [etym. dub.]

Chagas, Carlos (b. 1879). Brazilian physician.

Chagas' disease. American trypanosomiasis; an acute febrile disease characterized in its early stages by local swellings, adenitis and anaemia, and in its later stages by cardiac, nervous and myxoedematous symptoms. Dilatation of hollow viscera is a common sequal; death from complete heart block in early adult life frequently occurs. It affects children mainly. It is caused by *Trypanosoma cruzi* and transmitted to man by reduviid bugs of the family Triatomidae, especially *Panstrongylus (Triatoma) megistus* and *Triatoma infestans.* The chief reservoir hosts are small mammals including the opossum and armadillo; certain domestic animals have been found infected, and probably also act as intermediaries.

Chagasia (chag·as·e·ah). A genus or sub-genus of anopheline mosquitoes which includes *Anopheles (Chagasia) fajardoi* from Brazil.

chagoma (chag·o·mah). The primary lesion of Chagas' disease. [Chagas' disease, Gk *-oma* tumour.]

chain (chane). 1. A connected series of events or objects. 2. A measure of length equalling 66 ft. 3. In bacteriology, cells joined end to end, a long chain consisting of 4 or more. 4. In chemistry, atoms linked by valency bonds. 5. A term used to define polypeptides in immunoglobulins. **Alpha chain.** The type of polypeptide chain that occurs in all normal human haemoglobins. **Alpha chain variant.** One of the class of abnormal human haemoglobins which contain an alternative amino acid, or other abnormality, in the alpha polypeptide chain. **Beta chain.** The class of polypeptide chains of human haemoglobin which, in association with alpha chains, produce the major adult haemoglobin species. **Beta chain variant.** One of the class of abnormal human haemoglobin which contains an alternative amino acid, or other abnormality, in the beta polypeptide chain. **Branched chain.** A chain of atoms branching to one side of a long chain, or from both sides simultaneously. **Carbon chain.** Carbon atoms connected by valency bonds. **Closed chain.** A chain of atoms joining ends by valency bonds to form a complete ring. **Delta chain.** The type of polypeptide chain that is characteristic of the minor adult human haemoglobin (haemoglobin A_2). **Delta chain variant.** One of the class of abnormal human haemoglobins which contain an alternative amino acid residue in the delta polypeptide chain. **Chain elongation.** The reactions by which amino acid residues are polymerized on the instructions specified by messenger RNA, once the initiating aminoacyl tRNA is in position on the mRNA on a functional ribosome. **Epsilon chain.** The type of polypeptide chain characteristic of human embryonal haemoglobins—that is, of haemoglobins Gower-1 and Gower-2. **Forked chain.** Two small chains branching from the last atom of a long chain. **Gamma chains.** The class of polypeptide chains which are characteristic of human fetal haemoglobin. **Gamma chain variant.** One of the class of abnormal human haemoglobins which contain an alternative amino acid, or other abnormality, in the gamma polypeptide chain. **Chain initiation.** The process by which the synthesis of polypeptide chains is started in living cells. **Lateral chain.** A small chain branching from an intermediate atom in a long chain. **Nascent chain.** Nascent polypeptide. *See* POLYPEPTIDE. **Open chain.** Atoms linked into a chain open at each end. **Ossicular chain.** The malleus, incus and stapes of the middle ear. **Periodic chain.** A diagrammatic arrangement of the chemical elements in order of their atomic weights. *See* TABLE, PERIODIC. **Radon-seed chain.** A length of joined radon seeds for implantation; an obsolete term. **Reaction chain.** A series of chemical reactions in which one reaction starts off the next, and so on. **Side chain.** A lateral chain. **Straight chain.** An open chain without lateral or forked chains. **Sympathetic chain.** Sympathetic trunk. *See* TRUNK. **Chain termination.** The process by which the synthesis of a polypeptide is completed and the polypeptide released from the ribosome on which it was synthesized. **Toxiphoric chain.** In the immunity theory, the chemical group which unites with any particular toxin. [L *catena.*]

chairamidine (cha·ram·id·een). $C_{22}H_{26}O_4N_2$, one of the less important alkaloids found in cinchona bark.

chairamine (cha·ram·een). $C_{22}H_{26}O_4N_2$, an alkaloid, isomeric with chairamidine, and occurring in the bark of *Reniyia purdieana.*

Chalara (kal·ar·ah). A genus belonging to the "miscellaneous" fungi imperfecti. The type species is *Chalara fusidoides* Corda. These are rare saprophytes which have not been studied from a morphological viewpoint. Only a single species has been reported pathogenic. **Chalara pyogenes** Roger, Sartory and Menard, 1914. A species found in subcutaneous gummatous nodules which yielded to treatment with potassium iodide. The fungus was pathogenic for guinea-pigs. [Gk *chalaros* supple.]

chalasia (kal·a·ze·ah). Cardio-oesophageal relaxation. *See* RELAXATION. [Gk *chaloun* to relax.]

chalaza (kal·az·ah). One of the 2 spirally-twisted cords which lie within the albumen at each end of a bird's egg. They are produced by the twisting of the egg in the oviduct, and serve to fix the yolk at the poles of the shell. [Gk hail.]

chalazia (kal·az·e·ah). 1. The hailstone sputum of bronchitis. 2. Plural of chalazion. 3. Congenital laxity of a muscle, e.g. the oesophagus. [Gk *chalazion* hailstone. Gk *chalasis* relaxation.]

chalazion (kal·az·e·on) (pl. *chalazia, chalazions*). Swelling and congestion of a tarsal gland of the eyelid, with retention of the secretion, the result being a hard tumour about the size of a pea on the eyelid, generally the upper eyelid. Sometimes referred to as *porosis palpebrae.* **Chalazion terreum.** A chalazion the contents of which have changed by a process of degeneration into calcium carbonate and cholesterin. [Gk *chalazion* hailstone.]

chalazodermia (kal·az·o·der′·me·ah). Dermatolysis. [Gk *chalazion* hailstone, *derma* skin.]

chalcitis (kal·si·tis). Chalkitis.

chalcone (kal·kone). 1. Any one of a series of unsaturated ketones obtained during the synthesis of flavones by the condensation of benzaldehyde with hydroxylated acetophenones; they are yellow substances of the general formula RCOCH=CHR′. 2. Benzylidene acetophenone, $C_6H_5CH{=}CHCOC_6H_5$. [Gk *chalkos* copper.]

chalcosis (kal·ko·sis). The condition in which deposits of copper are present in the tissues. **Chalcosis lentis.** Sunflower cataract. *See* CATARACT. **Ocular chalcosis.** Cataract. [Gk *chalkos* copper.]

chalicosis (kal·e·ko·sis). A form of pneumoconiosis brought on by inhalation of stone dust. [Gk *chalix* gravel, *-osis* condition.]

chalinoplasty (kal·in·o·plas′·te). 1. A plastic operation performed on the angle of the mouth for correction of defects. 2. The operation of constructing a new frenum for the tongue. [Gk *chalinos* bridle, *plassein* to mould.]

chalk (chawk). $CaCO_3$. An amorphous white form of calcium carbonate occurring naturally as the result of the deposition of the shells of microscopic marine foraminifera upon a sea bed. **Precipitated chalk.** Calcium carbonate. **Prepared Chalk BP 1973.** Creta praeparata, native chalk purified by grinding with water and freezing from the heavy siliceous materials by elutriation. It is used in indigestion powders and mixtures as an antacid. [L *calx.*]

chalkitis (kal·ki·tis). An ophthalmic disease of brass-workers, characterized by inflammation chiefly in the form of conjunctivitis caused by irritation of fine brass dust or by rubbing with the fingers. [Gk *chalkos* brass, *-itis* inflammation.]

chalone (**kal**·one). Colyone; an organic secretion which is carried in the blood stream to other organs on the function of which it has an inhibitory effect. [Gk *chaloun* to relax.]

chalonic (kal·**on**·ik). Colyonic.

chalybeate (kal·**ib**·e·ate). 1. A substance or mixture containing salts of iron. 2. A chalybeate medicine. [Gk *chalyps* steel.]

chamaecephalia, chamaecephaly (**kam**·e·kef·**a'**·le·ah, kam·e·**kef'**·al·e). The condition of having a flat receding skull, of a craniometrical index of not more than 70 degrees. [Gk *chamai* on the ground, *kephale* head.]

chamaecranious (kam·e·**kra**·ne·us). In craniometry, a skull low in proportion to its height, and having a length: height index of 70 degrees or less. [Gk *chamai* on the ground, *kranion* skull.]

Chamaelirium (kam·e·**lir**·e·um). A genus of plants of the family Liliaceae. The dried rhizome and roots of *Chamaelirium luteum* A. Gray (false unicorn root) is reputed to act as a uterine tonic and diuretic. [Gk *chamai* on the ground, *leirion* lily.]

chamaeprosopic (**kam**·e·pro·**so'**·pik). Brachyfacial. [see foll.]

chamaeprosopy (kam·e·**pro**·so·pe). The condition of being brachyfacial, i.e. having a short broad face. [Gk *chamai* on the ground, *prosopon* face.]

chamber (**chame**·ber). 1. An enclosed space. 2. A vessel, particularly one in which a process or investigation is being conducted. 3. In anatomy, a cavity, usually small (e.g. anterior chamber of the eye) or of medium size (e.g. chamber of the heart). **Air chamber.** A space on the centre of the fitting surface of an artificial upper denture which aids its retention by creating a partial vacuum. **Air-wall ionization chamber.** An ionization chamber used for the measurement of x- or γ-ray dose in which the atomic number of the material of the walls of the chamber has the same effective atomic number as that of air. **Anterior chamber of the eye [camera arterior bulbi (NA)].** The part of the aqueous chamber that lies anterior to the iris. **Aqueous chamber.** The space in the eyeball between the cornea and the anterior surface of the lens; it contains the aqueous humour. **Boyden chamber.** Apparatus used for measuring leucocyte chemotaxis. **Cavity ionization chamber.** An ionization chamber in which the gaseous volume in which the ions are collected is considered to be a cavity inside an extended medium. It is realized in practice by having the walls of the chamber of the same effective atomic number as the gas. **Cloud chamber.** A method of rendering visible the path of ionizing particles in a gas: a volume of gas in a cylinder which is saturated with water vapour is suddenly reduced in pressure, causing supersaturation of the vapour. Vapour condenses in droplets on the ions in the path of the particle, and this track is rendered visible for visual or photographic observation by orthogonal illumination. **Condenser ionization chamber.** An ionization chamber used for the measurement of x- or γ-ray dose which is charged and then removed from the potential source before use. After use the drop in potential V between the insulated electrode and the wall is measured. The total loss of charge Q of the electrode is equal to CV, where C is the electrical capacity of the chamber which acts as a condenser. The x-ray dose may be determined from Q and the geometry of the chamber. **Counting chamber.** A special heavy glass slide, having in its centre usually 2 accurately machine-ruled platforms separated from each other and from bars at each side by moats grooved in the slide so that when a special cover slip is put on top, thus resting on the lateral relatively "elevated" bars, it lies exactly 0.1 mm above the ruled central platforms. The platforms have exactly ruled areas divided into squares according to various haematologists' requirements, but the Neubauer ruling is the one usually employed. **Decompression chamber.** An air-tight chamber, able to withstand great changes in atmospheric pressure, the pressure within which can be reduced or increased. It is used in the treatment of caisson disease. Also patients subject to sinus or otitic barotrauma can be examined inside the chamber after sudden alterations in pressure, and patients suffering from acute barotraumatic lesions may have their symptoms relieved by being placed inside and decompressed to that pressure at which symptoms commenced; thereafter, they are slowly returned to normal barometric pressure. **Digestive chamber.** One of a number of fluid-filled cavities derived from the disintegration of the myelin sheath after section of the axon. **Extrapolation chamber.** An ionization chamber of adjustable volume which can be used for estimating the limiting value of the ionization current per unit volume as the volume decreases to vanishing point. **Free-air ionization chamber.** An ionization chamber so constructed that the irradiated volume of air is part of a larger air volume, and in which the walls of the chamber do not influence the ionization measured. **Chamber of the heart.** Any one of the atria or ventricles of the heart. **Hyperbaric chamber.** An airtight chamber containing air or oxygen under pressure; used in the treatment of vascular disease, certain infections and malignant disease. **Ionization chamber.** A container filled with air or some other gas with 2 or more electrodes (one of which is usually the wall). When ionizing radiation falls upon the chamber the gas is ionized and the amount of ionization produced is taken as a measure of the dose of radiation delivered. **Lethal chamber.** A chamber in which animals may be killed, usually by the introduction of coal gas. **Posterior chamber of the eye [camera posterior bulbi (NA)].** The part of the aqueous chamber which lies posterior to the iris. **Pulp chamber.** The cavity in the crown of a tooth containing the pulp (connective tissue, blood vessels, nerves, etc.). **Relief chamber.** The same as an air chamber (see above), to prevent pressure by an artificial denture on the tissues in the centre of the hard palate; used also to reduce the risk of fracture of an acrylic upper denture during mastication. **Resonance chamber.** Any air- or gas-containing space which behaves as a resonator. **Respiration chamber.** A special chamber in which the mechanism of respiration or the respiratory gas exchange may be studied. **Spark chamber.** A form of static imaging device for recording the distribution of a radionuclide within an organ or part of the body. **Thimble ionization chamber.** Originally an ionization chamber in the shape of a thimble; now applied to any ionization chamber of small volume. **Urogenital chamber.** The entodermal cloaca in the early embryo. **Vitreous chamber of the eye [camera vitrea bulbi (NA)].** The part of the cavity of the eyeball between the lens and the retina which contains the vitreous body. [Gk *kamara* anything with an arched cover.]

See also: HALDANE, NEUBAUER (O.), STORM VAN LEEUWEN, WILSON (C. T. R.).

Chamberlain, W. E. 20th century American radiologist.

Chamberlain's line. A radiographic line drawn from the posterior margin of the foramen magnum (opisthion) to the posterior border of the hard palate. It is used for assessing basilar impression.

Chamberland, Charles Edouard (b. 1851). Paris bacteriologist.

Chamberland filter. A bacterial filter made of unglazed porcelain.

Pasteur-Chamberland filter. A bacterial filter similar to the Coors or Kitasato filter.

Chamberlen forceps. The original obstetric forceps invented by either Peter Chamberlen, father, 1560–1631, or Peter Chamberlen, son, 1601–1683.

Chamomile (**kam**·o·mile). Roman chamomile, consisting of the dried flowerheads of the cultivated plants of *Anthemis nobilis* Linn. (family Compositae). It is used in the form of bitters to aid digestion (BPC 1954). **German chamomile.** The flowerheads of *Matricaria chamomilla* Linn. **Spanish chamomile.** Pellitory; the root of *Anthemis pyrethrum* (family Compositae), formerly used as a rubefacient and as a remedy for toothache. [Gk *chaimai* on the ground, *melon* apple.]

chamomilla (**kam**·o·mil·ah). Matricaria. [see prec.]

champacol (**cham**·pak·ol). $C_{15}H_{26}O$, a sesquiterpene obtained from guaiacum resin.

champagne (sham·**pane**). A wine made from grapes, especially those of the country in the vicinity of the Marne river in France;

it is effervescent and of many different qualities and strengths. Alcohol content varies from 5 to 13 per cent. In the past it was customary to recommend it as a stimulant and sedative (especially in seasickness) and as a tonic in convalescence. [*Champagne,* a district in France.]

Champetier de Ribes, Camille Louis Antoine (b. 1848). Paris obstetrician.

Champetier de Ribes' bag. A cone-shaped inflatable bag made of rubber or silk, used for dilating the neck of the uterus.

Championnière. *See* LUCAS-CHAMPIONNIÈRE.

Champy, Christian (b. 1885). Paris histologist.

Champy's fixing fluid. A solution of potassium bichromate, with chromic and osmic acids; it is especially suited to the preservation of mitotic figures within cells.

chancebone (**chans**·bone). The ischium. [OFr. *cheance,* bone.]

chancre (**shang**·ker). A venereal ulcer usually situated in the genital region at the point of infection, and a primary lesion of the disease. **Concealed chancre.** A chancre hidden within a tight prepuce. **Erosive chancre.** A non-indurated ulcerated chancre resembling an eroded papule. **Extragenital chancre.** A primary syphilitic lesion not occurring in the genital region, e.g. lip, finger, tongue. **Hard chancre.** Syphilitic chancre (see below). **Hunterian chancre.** The characteristic hard chancre of syphilis. **Mixed chancre.** A venereal sore from infection with both *Treponema pallidum* and *Haemophilus ducreyi.* **Non-infecting chancre.** Soft chancre (see below). **Parchment chancre.** A primary lesion of syphilis occurring as a dry sclerotic area of the skin with little induration and no ulceration. **Phagedenic chancre.** A chancre infected with pyogenic bacteria, leading to deep ulceration and local gangrene. **Recurrent chancre, Chancre redux.** A recurrence of a chancre on the site of a previous one. **Sclerotic chancre.** Parchment chancre (see above). **Simple chancre.** Soft chancre (see following). **Soft chancre.** Chancroid, soft sore; the local genital ulcer following infection with *Haemophilus ducreyi.* Inguinal buboes are a frequent accompaniment. **Sulcus chancre.** Hard chancre (see above). **Syphilitic chancre.** The primary lesion which develops at the site of inoculation with syphilis which is followed invariably by constitutional syphilis. The syphilitic sore does not develop into the classical hard (hunterian) chancre until a week or more has elapsed. At first the lesion is a small red papule which gradually hardens and erodes in the centre; later an ulcer forms, the margin and base of which become densely indurated. *Treponema pallidum* may be found by dark-ground microscopy in the secretion expressed from the lesion at any stage. Excision of a chancre does not prevent the onset of constitutional syphilis. **True chancre.** Hard chancre (see above). **Tuberculous chancre.** A primary tuberculous lesion in the skin or upper respiratory tract, presenting as a chronic inflammatory focus with regional lymphadenopathy which ultimately liquefies. [Fr. canker.]

See also: HUNTER (J.), RICORD.

chancriform (**shang**·kre·form). Like a chancre. [chancre, form.]

chancroid (**shang**·kroid). Soft chancre, soft sore, ulcus molle; a contagious venereal ulcer of the genitals due to infection with *Haemophilus ducreyi.* The lesion may be multiple from the outset, and extends locally, frequently causing a painful suppurating inguinal bubo. There is no constitutional disease, but after the first week the skin will react to an intradermal injection of a vaccine of *Haemophilus ducreyi.* A painful soft ulcer appears 3-5 days after infection and may extend rapidly and deeply but does not become hard. The surrounding tissues are inflamed and phagedena may ensue. *Haemophilus ducreyi* may be found in small numbers in scrapings from the edge of the ulcer, and auto-inoculation of skin in contact with the ulcer is not uncommon. It occurs chiefly in tropical and sub-tropical areas, and is infrequent in women. [chancre, Gk *eidos* form.]

chancroidal (shang·**kroid**·al). 1. Relating to chancroid. 2. Resembling chancroid.

chancrous (**shang**·krus). 1. Having chancres. 2. Having characteristics of chancre.

chandelier (shan·del·**eer**). **Favic chandeliers.** Antler-like hyphae, seen only in culture, and pathognomonic of *Trichophyton schoenleinii.* [L *candela* candle.]

change (**cha**·nj). An alteration or variation. **Change of life.** The menopause. **Change of note or sound.** An alteration of the percussion note with change of position or other cause. **Change of voice.** The loss of the treble quality of the voice and the assumption of the adult quality in adolescence; the alteration in timbre of the voice, resulting from a change from the chest register to the head register, or vice versa. **Conservative amino acid change.** A change in an amino acid at a given point in a polypeptide chain to one of very similar properties, during the course of evolution of the protein. **Radical amino acid change.** A change in an amino acid at a given point in a polypeptide chain to one of quite different properties during the course of evolution of the protein. **Secular change.** A change occurring over a period of time. [L *cambire* to change.]

See also: BIERMER, CROOKE, FRIEDREICH, GERHARDT (C. C. A. J.), HUTCHINSON, WINTRICH.

Chantemesse, André (b. 1851). Paris bacteriologist.

Chantemesse's reaction. A local allergic reaction of the eye following instillation into the conjunctival sac of typhoid bacterial protein. More injection of blood vessels, more itching and more lacrimation occur in patients suffering from typhoid fever than in normal subjects. The test is now obsolete.

Chantemesse's serum. An antityphoid serum prepared by immunizing horses with cultures and extracts of typhoid bacilli. Obsolete.

Chantemesse's vaccine. A specially prepared typhoid "toxin" or bacterial protein. Obsolete.

Chaoul, Henri (b. 1887). Berlin radiologist.

Chaoul applicator. An applicator for use with a Chaoul tube.

Chaoul therapy. Short-distance low-voltage (contact) x-ray therapy developed as an alternative to some surface and intracavity radium techniques by Zimmer, Schaefer and Witte, and later expanded for superficial therapy by Chaoul.

Chaoul tube. A transmission target x-ray tube for short-distance low-voltage x-ray treatment (*see* CHAOUL THERAPY). The x-rays passing through the anode are those used for treatment.

chap (chap). A cleft or crack in the skin; it occurs usually on the shins, the nipples, the backs of the hands and the lips. [ME *chappen* to crack.]

Chapman, John (b. 1822). English physician and publisher.

Chapman's bag. A long narrow bag, by which ice can be applied to the spine.

Chapman's agar. Salt agar. *See* AGAR.

chappa (**chap**·ah). A disease prevalent in Lagos and Southern Nigeria; the onset is accompanied by severe muscular and articular pains, going on to the development of multiple nodules ranging in size from a marble to a pigeon's egg. Over these, skin ulcers develop without abscess formation, and eventually the bones are involved. It is almost certainly a local manifestation of yaws. [W. Afr.]

chapped (chapt). Referring to a condition of the thinner epidermal layers of the skin in which there are areas of erosion and cracks, the cause being exposure to low atmospheric temperature. [ME *chappen* to crack.]

Chaput, Henri (b. 1857). French surgeon.

Chaput's method, or operation. A technique for the formation of an artificial anus.

character (**kar**·ak·ter). 1. The totality of the conscious life of the individual as expressed by patterns of thought and behaviour, determined by constitutional, developmental and environmental factors. 2. A feature, trait or characteristic of an organism, particularly the phenotypic expression in the individual of one of a pair of allelomorphic genes. **Acquired character.** One that is acquired during the lifetime of an individual in response to environmental influences. **Anal character.** The personality type which stems from the anal or excretory stage in mental development, characterized by orderliness, parsimoniousness and obstinacy. **Compound character.** One whose presence in the phenotype is dependent on the presence of more than one allelomorphic pair of genes. **Dominant character.** One which appears in the phenotype when only one of its controlling genes is present. In a cross between individuals, each of which is homozygous for one of an allelomorphic pair of genes, the dominant character will appear in all the F_1 generation and in three-quarters of the F_2. **IMViC character.** A mnemonic for the 4 important tests used to distinguish coliform organisms: indole production, methyl-red test, Voges–Proskauer reaction and the ability to utilize citrate as the sole source of carbon. Typical faecal coli are indole positive, methyl-red positive, and negative for the other 2 characters; the statement of inability to ferment citrate is only correct for true faecal strains. **Oral character.** The various personality types which stem from the oral or breast-sucking stage in mental development, either optimistic or pessimistic, hating or destructive, and sadistic. **Paranoid character.** The type of character distinguished by morbid suspicion. **Primary sex character.** One that is directly concerned with reproduction, gonads, accessory organs and copulatory apparatus. **Recessive character.** One which appears in the phenotype only when both its controlling genes are present. In a cross between individuals, each of which is homozygous for one of an allelomorphic pair of genes, the recessive character will not appear in the F_1 generation, but will appear in one-quarter of the F_2. **Secondary sex character.** One that differs in the two sexes and, though not directly concerned with insemination, may play a part in some other stage in the reproductive cycle. **Sex-limited character.** *See* SEX-LIMITED. **Sex-linked character.** *See* SEX-LINKED. **Unit character.** One known to be the phenotypic expression of a single pair of allelomorphic genes. [Gk *charassein* to engrave.]

characteristic (kar·ak·ter·is′·tik). Typical; a distinction. In mathematics, the whole number preceding the decimal (mantissa) in a logarithm. **Film characteristics.** Parameters defining the contrast and speed of a film which are obtained from the characteristic curve of the film; in this the optical density is plotted as ordinate against the logarithm of the exposure as abscissa. [see prec.]

charas (**kah**·ras). Churrus.

charbon (shar·**bon**). Anthrax. [Fr. coal.]

charcoal (**char**·kole). A fine black powder without taste or odour; an impure form of carbon prepared from a variety of animal, vegetable and mineral substances by incomplete combustion in the absence of air. The substances used in its preparation include coal, wood and bone. It is used in medicine in its activated form as an adsorbent of gases, as in intestinal flatulence, and of alkaloids and other drugs in cases of poisoning. It may also be used as an index of the rate of gastric emptying, or of the passage of food residue through the bowel. **Activated charcoal.** The form of charcoal chiefly used medicinally; the charcoal is rendered more active as an adsorbent, by heat or by chemical agents. **Animal charcoal.** Bone black, a form of charcoal prepared by the destructive distillation of bones and other animal tissues. **Medicinal Charcoal BPC 1968.** A purified form of activated charcoal. **Wood charcoal.** Charcoal made from wood by firing it in an enclosed space. [AS *cerr*, coal.]

Charcot, Jean Martin (b. 1825). Paris neurologist.

Charcot's artery. The largest lateral striate artery. It is from this vessel that cerebral haemorrhage frequently occurs.

Charcot's arthritis, arthropathy or arthrosis. Charcot's disease (see below).

Charcot's cirrhosis. Biliary cirrhosis. *See* CIRRHOSIS.

Charcot's sensory crossway. The retrolenticular part of the internal capsule.

Charcot's disease. Amyotrophic lateral sclerosis; a variety of motor neuron disease. *See* SCLEROSIS.

Charcot's disease, or joint. Neuropathic or neurogenic arthritis, tabetic arthropathy; a condition of osteoarthritis associated with gross disorganization of the affected joints, due to trophic disturbance resulting from associated disease of the central nervous system, generally tabes dorsalis, syringomyelia or leprosy. The larger weight-bearing joints, or the spine, are those commonly affected.

Charcot's fever. An intermittent biliary fever due to an impacted gallstone; also called *intermittent hepatic* (*or biliary*) *fever.*

Charcot's gait. The gait of Friedreich's ataxia, a combination of sensory and cerebellar ataxia.

Charcot's pain. An undesirable word for testicular neuralgia.

Charcot's sign. 1. In a facial palsy of lower motor neuron type the eyebrow on the affected side is raised; if contracture occurs it is lowered. 2. Charcot's syndrome (see following).

Charcot's syndrome. Intermittent claudication (cramp-like pains) usually in the calves of the legs, produced by effort and relieved by rest, due to ischaemia of muscle resulting from occlusive disease of the nutrient arteries.

Charcot's triad. Scanning speech, intention tremor and nystagmus; a triad of signs due to brain-stem involvement in disseminated sclerosis.

Charcot's laryngeal vertigo. Vertigo or even syncope after a paroxysm of coughing. *See* SYNDROME, COUGH.

Charcot's zone. Hysterogenic zone. *See* ZONE.

Erb–Charcot disease. Syphilitic spastic paraplegia.

Charcot–Guinon disease. Dementia complicating muscular dystrophy.

Charcot–Leyden crystals. Diamond-shaped crystals of undetermined composition occurring in the sputum in asthma. Similar crystals have been observed in the faeces in various pathological states, including amoebiasis, and in leukaemic spleens. It has been suggested that they consist of spermine phosphate, but this has not been confirmed.

Charcot–Marie symptom. Marie's sign.

Charcot–Marie–Tooth atrophy, disease or type. Peroneal muscular atrophy, a familial disease predominantly of the peripheral nerves characterized by weakness and wasting of the distal muscles of the lower and upper limbs, usually beginning in the peroneal group; pes cavus is common, and appreciation of vibration and position may be impaired in the lower limbs.

Charcot–Vigouroux sign. Diminished electrical resistance of the skin, said to be present in thyrotoxicosis.

charge (charj). **Space charge.** A region of space in which an electric charge of unchanging density distribution exists. The electron cloud which may surround the cathode of a thermionic valve is an example of a space charge. [L *carrus* cart.]

charlatan (**shar**·lat·an). A quack; one who claims medical skill that he does not possess; a fraudulent empiric. [Fr.]

charlatanism, charlatanry (**shar**·lat·an·izm, **shar**·lat·an·re). 1. The pretension to medical skill. 2. The practices of a charlatan. [see prec.]

Charles, Jacques Alexandre César (b. 1746). French physicist.

Charles' law. The volume of a given weight of gas at constant pressure is directly proportional to its absolute temperature. Thus, all gases expand by 1/273 of their volume at 0° C for every degree rise in temperature, provided the pressure remains the same.

Charles, Sir R. Haverlock. 20th century English surgeon.

Charles' operation (1912). Radical excision of hypertrophied skin and subcutaneous tissue of the leg in treatment of lymphoedema.

Charlouis, M. 19th century Dutch army surgeon in Java.

Charlouis' disease. Yaws.

Charlton, Willy (b. 1889). Berlin physician.

Schultz–Charlton phenomenon, reaction or test. A rash-extinction reaction or test, produced by injecting convalescent scarlet-fever serum or commercial streptococcus antitoxin intracutaneously into any area of bright red rash believed to be that of scarlet fever. Blanching at the site of injection indicates that the rash is that of scarlet fever.

Charnley, John. Orthopaedic surgeon from Lancashire.
Charnley's arthrodesis. A technique of compression arthrodesis applied to the hip, knee, shoulder, ankle and small joints of the toes.
Charnley low-friction arthroplasty. A prosthetic replacement of the hip using a plastic acetabulum and a stainless steel femoral head.

Charon (ka·ron). A genus of viruses of the yellow-fever group, causing diseases mainly characterized by acute non-contagious fever. Examples are *Charon ergatus* (yellow fever) and *Charon vallis* (Rift Valley fever). This nomenclature is of USA origin and is not widely accepted in the UK. [Gk *Charon* ferryman of the Styx.]

Charrière, Joseph François Bernard (b. 1803). Paris instrument maker.
Charrière's operation. An operation for lithotrity using a type of lithotrite incorporating a screw and clutch in the handle, by means of which the stone was crushed.
Charrière's scale. The French scale in general use for grading the size of urethral and ureteric catheters; a scale commonly used in Great Britain, the figures representing the measurement of the circumference in millimetres.

Charrin, Albert (b. 1857). Paris pathologist.
Charrin's disease. Infection by *Pseudomonas pyocyanea.*

chart (chart). A sheet of pasteboard or paper on which data relating to an illness or disease can be recorded in tabular or graphic form, e.g. urinary output, fluctuation in temperature or respiration. **Diplopia chart.** A record of the relative positions of the images seen by the two eyes in the various positions of gaze. This will indicate which is the paresed muscle. **Exposure chart.** 1. A set of exposure times and tube settings for radiography of different parts of the body for a given x-ray machine. 2. Similarly for photography of subjects, allowing for different lenses, film types, lighting conditions. [L *charta* paper.]
See also: GIBSON, HESS (W.R.), REUSS, SNELLEN.

charta (kar·tah). A piece of cartridge paper coated or impregnated with an active substance or preparation. **Charta oleata.** Paper rendered waterproof by treating it with a drying oil. **Charta potassii nitratis.** Paper impregnated with potassium nitrate solution. It is burnt and the smoke inhaled to relieve asthma; the process of burning converts some of the nitrate to nitrite which dilates the bronchi thereby affording relief. **Charta sinapis.** A plaster prepared from oil-free black mustard and rubber solution which is spread on paper; used as a counter-irritant and rubifacient. [L paper.]

Chase, Ira Carleston (b. 1868). Texas physician.
Chase's sign. Pain felt in the caecal region when the examiner's hand is passed quickly and deeply along the transverse colon from left to right while the descending colon is compressed with the other hand.
Sherman and Chase assay test. A test in which the aneurine hydrochloride content of a preparation was measured by noting its effect on the growth of rats kept on a diet deficient in aneurine. Now that crystalline preparations are available, the test is little used.

chasma (kaz·mah). 1. A yawn; yawning. 2. An opening or cleft. [Gk *chasma* wide opening.]

chasmatoplasson (kaz·mat·o·plas'·on). Plasson in its expanded form. Cf. PYKNOPLASSON. [Gk *chasma* wide opening, plasson.]

Chassaignac, Edouard Pierre Marie (b. 1804). Paris surgeon.
Chassaignac's bursa, or space. A fascial space between the pectoral fascia and the mammary gland.
Chassaignac's axillary muscle. An occasional bundle of muscle fibres from the lower border of the latissimus dorsi muscle which crosses the axillary floor to end in the pectoralis minor muscle or the deep fascia of the arm.
Chassaignac's tubercle. The carotid tubercle of the 6th cervical vertebra.

chaude-pisse (shode·pees). A sensation of scalding when urine is being passed: typical of the acute stage of gonorrhoea. [Fr. hot urine.]

chauffage (sho·fahzh). Treatment with a cautery at a low degree of heat. The iron is held about 6 mm away from the area to be treated and is moved backwards and forwards in front of it. [Fr. warming.]

Chauffard, Anatole-Marie-Emile (b. 1855). Paris physician.
Chauffard's point. A tender point beneath the right clavicle that may be present in disease of the gall bladder.
Chauffard's syndrome. Still-Chauffard syndrome (see below).
Minkowski-Chauffard syndrome, Chauffard-Minkowski syndrome. Acholuric familial jaundice. *See* JAUNDICE.
Still-Chauffard syndrome, Chauffard-Still syndrome. Rheumatoid arthritis with the onset in childhood; juvenile rheumatoid arthritis.

chauffie (cho·fe). Ancylostome dermatitis. *See* DERMATITIS. [A local name used in Grenada.]

chaulmoogra (chawl·moo·grah). A Burmese tree, *Taraktogenos kurzii* King (family Flacourtiaceae). **Chaulmoogra Oil BPC 1954.** The fixed oil expressed from the seeds of *Taraktogenos kurzii.* It consists mainly of the glycerides of chaulmoogric, hydnocarpic, palmitic and oleic acids. The oil, and its ethyl esters, were used in the treatment of leprosy, but have now been almost entirely superseded, first by hydnocarpus oil and then by the synthetic antileprotics. [Bengali *cal* rice, *mugra* plant.]

chaulmoograte (chawl·moo·grate). Any salt or ester of chaulmoogric acid.

chaulmugra (chawl·moo·grah). Chaulmoogra.

Chaussier, François (b. 1746). Paris and Dijon anatomist.
Chaussier's areola. In anthrax, the indurated ring surrounding the malignant pustule.
Chaussier's great muscular artery. The descending branch of the lateral circumflex femoral artery.
Chaussier's line. The median raphe of the corpus callosum.
Chaussier's sign. Epigastric pain as a premonitory sign of eclampsia.
Chaussier's tube. A trumpet-shaped tube used for the insufflation of the lungs.

Chavasse, Francis Bernard (b. 1889). Liverpool ophthalmologist.
Chavasse's hook. A curved hook with a sharp point, suitably mounted at right angles to the handle, resembling an aneurysm needle; for use in Chavasse's operation.
Chavasse's operation. For myectomy of the inferior oblique muscle: Chavasse's hook is passed through the conjunctiva beneath the globe and along the floor of the orbit, and hooks out the muscle, a piece of which is excised.

chavibetol (chav·e·be·tol). Allylguaiacol, $C_3H_5C_6H_3(OH)OCH_3$. A colourless liquid occurring in betel leaves; isomeric with eugenol.

chavicine (chav·e·seen). $C_{17}H_{19}O_3N$, an alkaloid present in pepper, and isomeric with piperine.

chavicol (chav·e·kol). *p*-Allylphenol, $C_3H_5C_6H_4OH$. An oil found in betel nuts, the dried seeds of *Areca catechu.* **Methyl chavicol.** $CH_3OC_6H_4C_3H_5$, occurs in oil of estragon (tarragon oil), and anise oil.

Cheadle, Walter Butler (b. 1835). British paediatrician.
Cheadle's disease. 1. Scurvy. 2. Rickets.

Cheatle, Sir George Lenthal (b. 1865). London surgeon.
Cheatle's forceps. A long forceps for the removal of basins and instruments from the steam sterilizer.

Chediak, Alejandro. 20th century Cuban physician.
Chediak-Higashi syndrome. A metabolic abnormality of circulating leucocytes which contain giant peroxidase granules in the cytoplasm. Granulocytopenia follows and the patients suffer recurrent infections, from which they die. Described by *Chediak* in Cuba and by *Higashi* in Japan.

cheek [bucca (mala) NA] (cheek). The wall of flesh which forms the side of the face. [AS *ceace.*]

cheek-bone (cheek·bone). The zygomatic bone. [AS *ceace,* bone.]

cheek-tooth (cheek·tooth). A molar tooth. *See* TOOTH. [AS *ceace,* tooth.]

cheese (cheez). The consolidated curd of milk, the curd having been separated from the whey by the action of a coagulating agent such as rennet. It is flavoured, coloured, compressed and allowed to ferment or ripen. [AS *cese.*]

cheese mite (**cheez** mite). *Tyroglyphus siro* of the order Acarina, the usual mite of cheese; also common on other stored products. It causes intestinal irritation if ingested in quantity, and dermatitis due to this species is common in vanilla workers. [AS *cese,* mite.]

cheese skipper (**cheez** skip·er). The larvae of the small fly *Piophila casei,* common in cheese and other high-protein foods. It may occur in intestinal myiasis, usually without symptoms. Though legless they can flick themselves several centimetres, whence the name. [AS *cese,* Scand. *skip.*]

Cheever's operation. Excision of the tonsil through an open operation through the neck for malignant disease.

cheilalgia (ki·**lal**·je·ah). Pain in the lips. [Gk *cheilos* lip, *algos* pain.]

cheilectomy (ki·**lek**·to·me). The surgical cutting away of irregular points round the cavity of a joint so that movement may be unimpeded. [Gk *cheilos* lip, *ektome* a cutting out.]

cheilectropion (ki·lek·**tro**·pe·on). Eversion of the lip. [Gk *cheilos* lip, *ektrepein* to turn away.]

cheilitis (ki·**li**·tis). Inflammation of the lips. This may occur alone or as part of a general stomatitis. It also occurs with herpes febrilis, erythema multiforme, eczema, psoriasis, urticaria, angioneurotic oedema, lupus, syphilis and anthrax. **Actinic cheilitis.** Cheilitis due to exposure to ultra-violet rays from the sun or from artifical sources. **Acute cheilitis.** Considerable swelling of the lip following injury or other affections such as a furuncle, herpes labialis or eczema. **Allergic cheilitis.** Cheilitis occurring in allergic subjects from contact with some substance to which they are sensitized. **Angular cheilitis.** Inflammation affecting the corners of the mouth which become cracked and sore. Seen in iron deficiency anaemia, uncontrolled diabetes and where inadequate labial support allows salivary leakage and maceration of the skin. Invariably secondarily infected with *Candida albicans.* Also due to *Staphylococcus aureus,* herpes or eczema and, rarely, riboflavine deficiency. **Exfoliative cheilitis.** Repeated and persistent exfoliation of the mucous membrane of the lips associated with seborrhoea. **Glandular cheilitis.** Chronic inflammation of the lower lip with swelling of the mucous glands; ulceration and small abscesses may form. **Granulomatous cheilitis.** A chronic inflammation of the lip with a sarcoid-type granuloma. **Impetiginous cheilitis.** A form occurring in children with impetigo contagiosa. **Lipstick cheilitis.** Erythematous scaly patches on the labial mucous membrane due to poisoning from ingredients of lipsticks. It may also affect the tip of the tongue. **Plasma-cell cheilitis.** A persistent non-indurated plaque on the lip with a plasma-cell infiltrate, of undetermined cause, comparable to plasma-cell balanitis. [Gk *cheilos* lip, *-itis* inflammation.]

cheilo-angioscope (ki·lo·**an**·je·o·skope). An instrument with which the blood may be observed in circulation in the vessels of the lips. [Gk *cheilos* lip, angioscope.]

cheilo-angioscopy (ki·lo·an·je·**os**'·ko·pe). The observation of the circulation in the lips by means of a cheilo-angioscope.

cheilocace (ki·**lok**·as·e). A reddish firm swelling of the lip seen in children with scrofula. [Gk *cheilos* lip, *kakos* bad.]

cheilocarcinoma (ki·lo·kar·sin·**o**'·mah). Carcinoma of the lip. [Gk *cheilos* lip, carcinoma.]

cheilognathopalatoschisis (ki·lo·**nath**·o·pal·at·**os**'·kis·is). The condition of having both hare-lip and cleft palate. [Gk *cheilos* lip, *gnathos* jaw, L *palatum* palate, Gk *schisis* division.]

cheilognathoprosoposchisis (ki·lo·**nath**·o·pro·so·**pos**'·kis·is). Persistence of the primary lateral facial cleft. [Gk *cheilos* lip, *gnathos* jaw, *prosopon* face, *schisis* division.]

cheilognathoschisis (ki·lo·nath·**os**'·kis·is). Hare-lip in which the cleft involves the jaw as well as the lip. [Gk *cheilos* lip, *gnathos* jaw, *schisis* division.]

cheilognathouranoschisis (ki·lo·**nath**·o·ewr·an·**os**'·kis·is). The condition of combined hare-lip and cleft palate. [Gk *cheilos* lip, *gnathos* jaw, *ouranos* roof of mouth, *schisis* division.]

cheilognathus (ki·lo·**nath**·us). Hare-lip. [Gk *cheilos* lip, *gnathos* jaw.]

cheilogramma (ki·lo·**gram**·ah). Jadelot's lines. [Gk *cheilos* lip, *gramma* a writing.]

cheiloncus (ki·**long**·kus). A tumour of the lip. [Gk *cheilos* lip, *ogkos* a swelling.]

cheilopalatognathus (ki·lo·**pal**·at·o·**nath**'·us). Combined cleft palate and fissure of the alveolar process of the maxilla. [Gk *cheilos* lip, L *palatum* palate, Gk *gnathos* jaw.]

cheilophagia (ki·lo·**fa**·je·ah). The habit of biting or chewing the lips. [Gk *cheilos* lip, *phagein* to eat.]

cheiloplastic (ki·lo·**plas**·tik). Relating or belonging to cheiloplasty.

cheiloplasty (ki·lo·**plas**·te). Plastic surgery for repair of defect or injury of the lip. [Gk *cheilos* lip, *plassein* to mould.]

cheilorrhaphy (ki·**lor**·af·e). The procedure of closing the lip or a wound of the lip with sutures. [Gk *cheilos* lip, *rhaphe* suture.]

cheiloschisis (ki·**los**·kis·is). Hare-lip. **Complicated cheiloschisis.** Hare-lip with fissure either of the palate or the alveolar arch. [Gk *cheilos* lip, *schisis* division.]

cheilosis (ki·**lo**·sis). A condition seen in cases of riboflavine deficiency; lesions appear at the angles of the mouth and on the lips. [Gk *cheilos* lip.]

cheilostomatoplasty (ki·lo·**sto**·mat·o·**plas**'·te). Plastic repair and restoration of the lips and shape of the mouth, e.g. subsequent to initial treatment for laceration or for removal of carcinoma. [Gk *cheilos* lip, *stoma* mouth, *plassein* to mould.]

cheilotomy (ki·**lot**·o·me). 1. The cutting away of a part of the lip. 2. Treatment of the end of bone for the removal of overgrowths which are hindering full movements at the joint concerned. [Gk *cheilos* lip, *temnein* to cut.]

cheimaphobia (ki·mah·**fo**·be·ah). Morbid fear of cold. [Gk *cheima* winter, *phobein* to fear.]

cheimetlon (ki·**met**·lon). An injury due to exposure to frost. **Mild cheimetlon.** Chilblain. **Severe cheimetlon.** Frostbite. [Gk *cheimetlon* chilblain.]

cheiragra (ki·**rag**·rah). Gout in the hand with or without tophi and twisting of the fingers. [Gk *cheir* hand, *agra* a catching.]

cheiralgia (ki·**ral**·je·ah). Cheiragra. **Cheiralgia paraesthetica.** Neuritis of the superficial branches of the radial nerve. [Gk *cheir* hand, *algos* pain.]

cheirapsia (ki·**rap**·se·ah). Massage or friction applied with the hand. [Gk *cheir* hand, *apsis* a touching.]

cheirarthritis (kire·ar·**thri**·tis). An inflammatory condition affecting the joints of hand and fingers. [Gk *cheir* hand, arthritis.]

cheirismus (ki·**riz**·mus). 1. Spasm of the hand. 2. A manipulative form of massage. [Gk *cheirismos* a handling.]

cheirocinaesthesia (ki·ro·sin·es·**the**'·ze·ah). Cheirokinaesthesia.

cheirocinaesthetic (ki·ro·sin·es·**thet**'·ik). Cheirokinaesthetic.

cheirognostic (ki·rog·**nos**·tik). 1. Indicating the ability to recognize the left and right hands, or to distinguish between the left side and the right. 2. Able to distinguish whether the right or the left side of the body is being touched. [Gk *cheir* hand, *gnostikos* knowing.]

cheirokinaesthesia (ki·ro·kin·es·**the**'·ze·ah). The power of being able to feel movements of the hand, e.g. during the process of writing. [Gk *cheir* hand, kinaesthesia.]

cheirokinaesthetic (ki·ro·kin·es·**thet**'·ik). Referring to the ability to feel movements of the hand. [see prec.]

cheirology (ki·**rol**·o·je). Dactylology; conversation by means of signs made with the fingers and hands. [Gk *cheir* hand, *logos* discourse.]

cheiromegaly (ki·ro·**meg**·al·e). A condition resembling acromegaly and marked by enlargement of the wrists, hands and ankles. [Gk *cheir* hand, *megas* large.]

cheirometer (ki·**rom**·et·er). In manual pelvimetry, an instrument devised by Oziander for measuring distances on index and middle fingers, and thus providing a basis for calculation of internal diameters of the pelvis. [Gk *cheir* hand, meter.]

cheiropelvimeter (**ki**·ro·pel·**vim**'·et·er). An instrument for measuring the hand, used in manual pelvimetry. [Gk *cheir* hand, L *pelvis* basin, meter.]

cheiroplasty (ki·ro·**plas**·te). The use of plastic surgery for repair or restoration of the hand. [Gk *cheir* hand, *plassein* to mould.]

cheiropompholyx (ki·ro·**pom**·fo·lix). An acute vesicular form of eczema affecting the hands and often the feet. Large vesicles filled with an inflammatory exudate appear, run together and form large blebs. [Gk *cheir* hand, *pompholyx* water-bubble.]

See also: DYSHIDROSIS.

cheiropractic, cheiropraxis (ki·ro·**prak**·tik, ki·ro·**prax**·is). A system of treatment inspired by the belief that in functional abnormality of the nervous system lies the origin of disease. Manipulation of the vertebral column and other structures of the body is carried out in an attempt to restore normal function. [Gk *cheir* hand, *praktikos* proficient.]

cheiropractor (**ki**·ro·prak·tor). A practitioner who treats certain diseases according to the system of cheiropraxis.

cheiroscope (**ki**·ro·skope). An instrument for correction of strabismus. It is based on the principle of stereoscopy, bringing the hand into play as an aid in the education of the eyes. [Gk *cheir* hand, *skopein* to watch.]

cheirospasm (**ki**·ro·spazm). A spasm, similar to that of writers' cramp, affecting the hand. [Gk *cheir* hand, spasm.]

cheken (**chek**·en). A Chilean shrub, *Myrtus cheken,* the bark of which is astringent. [Araucan *chequeñ.*]

chekenine (**chek**·en·een). $C_{13}H_{11}O_3$, a crystalline yellow alkaloid found in the leaves of cheken, *Myrtus cheken.*

chekenone (**chek**·en·one). $C_{40}H_{44}O_8$, a crystalline substance occurring in the leaves of cheken, *Myrtus cheken.*

chelate (**kel**·ate). 1. Term applied to organic complexes in which an atom of hydrogen or of a metal such as iron, nickel, cobalt, chromium or platinum, is held fast in a molecular ring-structure by residual valencies. 2. To enclose, as with a prehensile claw, another substance, rendering it inactive and thus non-toxic. **Chelate group.** A molecular group which is able to form a chelate ring. **Chelate ring.** A molecular ring-formation brought about by co-ordinate links with a central atom. [Gk *chele* claw.]

chelation (kel·**a**·shun). The ability of certain compounds to achieve a ring-structure by internal association through the residual valencies of certain atoms, usually oxygen, nitrogen or sulphur, which will form co-ordinate bonds with polyvalent metallic ions or with hydrogen. [see prec.]

chelerythrine (kel·er·ith·reen). $C_{21}H_{17}O_4N$, a red crystalline alkaloid obtained from the greater celandine, *Chelidonium majus,* closely resembling sanguinarine.

chelidonium (kel·e·**do**·ne·um). Greater celandine, the herb *Chelidonium majus* Linn. (family Papaveraceae), containing alkaloids with diuretic and cathartic properties. The fresh juice is a domestic application for warts. [Gk *chelidon* a swallow.]

cheloid, cheloma (**ke**·loid, ke·**lo**·mah). Keloid; a fibrous tumour developed in the substance of a scar. [Gk *kelis* scar, *eidos* form.]

chelonian (ke·**lo**·ne·an). Relating to the tortoise or the turtle. [Gk *chelone* tortoise.]

cheloplasty (**ke**·lo·plas·te). Keloplasty; plastic surgery performed for the purpose of altering or strengthening scar tissue. [Gk *kelis* scar, *plassein* to mould.]

chelotomy (ke·**lot**·o·me). Kelotomy; section of the constriction causing strangulated hernia and the resultant reduction of the latter. [Gk *kelis* scar, *temnein* to cut.]

Chelsea pensioner (**chel**·se **pen**·shun·er). Name given to an old-fashioned remedy for constipation, containing the mildly laxative principles guaiacum resin, rhubarb and sulphur, with potassium acid tartrate, nutmeg and honey. [*Chelsea* hospital for invalid soldiers, London.]

chemasthenia (kem·as·**the**·ne·ah). Inertia or weakness of the chemophysiological processes of the body. [chemical, asthenia.]

chemiatric (kem·e·**at**·rik). Iatrochemical; relating or belonging to iatrochemistry (chemiatry).

chemiatry (kem·e·**at**·re). Iatrochemistry; the system of treatment of which Paracelsus was the chief exponent, that life and health are founded on the proper chemical balance in, and action of the organs and fluids of, the body, and that disease should be treated chemically. [Gk *chemeia* alchemy, *iatreia* treatment.]

chemical (**kem**·ik·al). 1. Relating to chemistry. 2. Operated by the agency of a chemist. 3. A substance produced by a chemical process and therefore of known composition. [Gk *chemeia* alchemy.]

chemico-analytic (**kem**·ik·o·an·al·**it**'·ik). Referring to chemical analysis.

chemicobiological (**kem**·ik·o·bi·o·**loj**'·ik·al). Relating to the chemistry of living matter. [chemistry, biology.]

chemicocautery (**kem**·ik·o·**kaw**'·ter·e). Cauterization by means of the application of caustic chemicals.

chemicogenesis (**kem**·ik·o·**jen**'·es·is). Fertilization of an ovum by the action of a chemical agent. [chemical, Gk *genein* to produce.]

chemicophysical (**kem**·ik·o·**fiz**'·ik·al). 1. Relating to physical chemistry. 2. Relating to chemistry and physics.

chemicophysiological (**kem**·ik·o·fiz·e·o·**loj**'·ik·al). Referring to physiology and chemistry.

chemicovital (**kem**·ik·o·**vi**'·tal). Relating to the chemistry of life. [chemistry, L *vita* life.]

chemiluminescence (**kem**·e·loo·min·**es**'·ens). The production of light during a chemical reaction at low temperature, e.g. glow of phosphorus or freshly cut surfaces of sodium or potassium. Oxidation accompanies this type of luminescence. The production of light in animals is a special case of chemiluminescence due to oxidation of substances produced in the body cells.

cheminosis (kem·in·**o**·sis). Any disease resulting from the action of a chemical agent. [chemical, Gk *nosos* disease.]

chemiotaxis (**kem**·e·o·**tax**'·is). Chemotaxis.

chemiotherapy (**kem**·e·o·**ther**'·ap·e). Chemotherapy.

chemise (shem·**eez**). A surgical dressing consisting of a square piece of muslin or linen tied around a catheter passing out through its centre, the muslin holding in place a tampon packed round the catheter. The dressing is for use after operations such as perineal section. [Fr. shirt.]

chemism (**kem**·izm). 1. Chemical relationship, activity, property or force. 2. Iatrochemistry; the doctrine that the universe and its development are the results of chemical processes. [Gk *chemeia* alchemy.]

chemist (**kem**·ist). 1. Properly an individual skilled in chemistry or who studies the action of chemicals. 2. A pharmaceutical chemist. *See* PHARMACIST. **Dispensing chemist.** *See* PHARMACIST.

chemistry (**kem**·is·tre). The science which deals with the composition, structure and properties of the molecules of matter, and with the atoms which compose them. **Agricultural chemistry.** The chemistry of soils and fertilizers. **Analytical chemistry.** The application of chemical methods to the analysis of substances. **Applied chemistry.** The chemistry of industrial processes, or chemistry applied to the arts and manufactures and to the welfare of mankind. **Biological chemistry.** Biochemistry. **Colloidal chemistry.** The chemistry of substances in the colloidal state. **Dental chemistry.** The study of the chemical properties of materials used in dentistry. **Empirical chemistry.** Chemical knowledge gained as the result of haphazard experiment only; rule-of-thumb chemistry. **Fermentation chemistry.** The chemistry of enzymes and ferments. **Food chemistry.** Chemical knowledge applied to the manufacture of foodstuffs, and their analysis for purity and fitness for consumption. **Forensic chemistry.** Chemistry recruited for the elucidation of legal questions or the investigation of crime. **Industrial chemistry.** The industrial manufacture of chemical products. **Inorganic chemistry.** The branch of chemistry devoted to the study of non-living substances as distinct from the chemistry of carbon compounds; the chemistry of minerals and metals. **Medical chemistry.** Chemical science in the service of medicine for diagnostic and therapeutic purposes. **Metabolic chemistry.** Biochemistry. **Mineral chemistry.** Inorganic chemistry (see above). **Nuclear chemistry.** The chemistry of the nucleus of the atom. **Organic chemistry.** The branch of chemistry devoted to the study of carbon compounds, a large proportion of which occur in living things. **Pathological**

chemistry. The chemistry of abnormal tissue and the effects of disease. **Pharmaceutical chemistry.** The preparation, assay and dispensing of drugs. **Physical chemistry.** The branch of chemistry which studies the physical phenomena involved in chemical reactions and states. **Physiological chemistry.** The biochemistry of healthy plant or animal tissue. **Radiation chemistry.** The study of the chemical effects of radiation upon chemical compounds. The term is not synonymous with *Radiochemistry.* **Structural chemistry.** The study of the arrangement of atoms within the molecules of substances. **Synthetic chemistry.** The application of chemical methods to the building up of more complex compounds from simpler substances. **Theoretical chemistry.** The laws and theories that have been evolved from the study of chemical phenomena. **Therapeutical chemistry.** The knowledge of drugs especially with regard to their value in the cure of disease. **Toxicological chemistry.** That dealing with poisons. [Gk *chemeia* alchemy.]

chemo-antigen (kem·o·**an**·te·jen). A chemical compound which has the power of stimulating the production of antibody. [chemical, antigen.]

chemo-autotrophic (**kem**·o·awt·o·**trof**′·ik). Describing bacteria which are capable of deriving their metabolic energy from inorganic reactions. [chemical, Gk *autos* self, *trophe* nutrition.]

chemoceptors (kem·o·**sep**·torz). Chemoreceptors.

chemocoagulation (**kem**·o·**ko**·ag·ew·**la**′·shun). Of neoplasms, the state of being destroyed or of being formed into coagulations by the action of chemical agents applied to the area of the growth.

chemo-immunity (**kem**·o·im·**ewn**′·it·e). Immunochemistry; the branch of science which is concerned with substances that confer immunity and the reactions resulting from their injection into the blood. [chemical, immunity.]

chemo-immunology (**kem**·o·im·ewn·**ol**′·o·je). 1. The science of immunochemistry. 2. The study of the chemical processes and changes which occur while an organism is undergoing immunization.

chemokinesis (**kem**·o·kin·**e**′·sis). The increase that takes place in the activity of an organism as a result of the presence of a chemical agent. [chemical, Gk *kinesis* movement.]

chemoluminescence (**kem**·o·loo·min·**es**′·ens). Chemiluminescence.

chemolysis (kem·**ol**·is·is). The dissolution of organic matter due to the process of decay, the cause not being bacterial action but chemical reaction. [chemical, Gk *lysis* a loosing.]

chemomorphosis (kem·o·**mor**·fo·sis). Change of form resulting from chemical action. [chemical, metamorphosis.]

chemopallidectomy (**kem**·o·pal·id·**ek**′·to·me). The production of a lesion in the globus pallidus by the stereotactic injection of a chemical agent. [chemical, L *pallidus* pale, Gk *ektome* a cutting out.]

chemopallidothalamectomy (kem·o·**pal**·id·o·thal·am·**ek**′·to·me). The production of a lesion in the globus pallidus and the thalamus by the injection of a chemical agent. [chemical, L *pallidus* pale, Gk *thalamos* chamber, *ektome* a cutting out.]

chemopharmacodynamic (**kem**·o·**far**·mah·ko·di·**nam**′·ik). Referring to the relationship between chemical structure and pharmacological or biological action. [chemical, Gk *pharmakon* drug, *dynamis* force.]

chemophysiology (**kem**·o·fiz·e·**ol**′·o·je). Physiological chemistry. *See* CHEMISTRY.

chemoprophylaxis (**kem**·o·pro·fil·**ax**′·is). Prevention of disease by the administration or use of chemical agents. [chemical, prophylaxis.]

chemoreceptors (**kem**·o·re·**sep**′·torz). Cells sensitive to changes in $[H^+]$, PCO_2 or PO_2. Found in the carotid body and on the ventral surface of medulla. [chemical, L *recipere* to receive.]

chemoreflex (kem·o·**re**·flex). An alteration of function brought about by stimulation of a chemoreceptor in the carotid body, e.g. an increase in the respiratory rate during arterial hypoxaemia. [chemical, L *reflectere* to bend back.]

chemoresistance (**kem**·o·re·**zis**′·tans). The specific resistance set up in a cell to the chemical substances present.

chemosensitive (kem·o·**sen**·sit·iv). Responding to or affected by changes in chemical composition. [chemical, sensitive.]

chemoserotherapy (**kem**·o·seer·o·**ther**′·ap·e). Treatment consisting of administration of serum combined with chemotherapy.

chemosis (ke·**mo**·sis). Swelling around the cornea of the eye as the result of oedema of the conjunctiva. The condition is not necessarily inflammatory. [Gk *cheme* cockle, *-osis* condition.]

chemosmosis (kem·oz·**mo**·sis). Chemical reaction occurring through an intervening semipermeable membrane, e.g. in colloidal growth. [chemical, Gk *osmos* a thrusting.]

chemosmotic (kem·oz·**mot**·ik). Referring to chemosmosis.

chemostat (**kem**·o·stat). An apparatus whereby controlled multiplication of bacteria is maintained indefinitely by a continuous flow of culture medium having a limited concentration of a required nutrient. [chemical, *statos* standing.]

chemosuppression (**kem**·o·sup·**resh**′·un). The administration of a drug with the object of keeping an infection below the clinical level rather than of eradicating it altogether, e.g. the daily administration of mepacrine in a malarious country. [chemical, L *supprimere* to suppress.]

chemosurgery (kem·o·**ser**·jer·e). The combined use of surgery and caustic or cytotoxic substances to remove tumours of the skin. [chemical, Gk *cheirourgos* surgeon.]

chemosynthesis (kem·o·**sin**·thes·is). The utilization by certain organisms of the energy of chemical action for the purposes of growth, e.g. the oxidation of ammonia by nitrifying soil bacteria, or of hydrogen sulphide by the sulphur bacteria. Cf. PHOTOSYNTHESIS. [chemical, synthesis.]

chemotactic (kem·o·**tak**·tik). Referring to chemotaxis.

chemotaxis (kem·o·**tax**·is). Directional migration of cells in response to chemical substances. **Negative chemotaxis.** The moving away of certain living cells from other cells or substances which exert a chemical stimulus. **Positive chemotaxis.** The locomotion of cells towards other cells or substances which exert a chemical stimulus. [chemical, Gk *taxis* arrangement.]

chemothalamotomy (**kem**·o·thal·am·**ot**′·o·me). Chemopallidectomy. [chemical, thalamotomy.]

chemotherapeutical (**kem**·o·ther·ap·**ew**′·tik·al). Relating to chemotherapy.

chemotherapeutics (**kem**·o·ther·ap·**ew**′·tix). The science of chemotherapy.

chemotherapy (kem·o·**ther**·ap·e). The specific treatment with drugs of parasitic infections due to insects, worms, protozoa, spirochaetes, bacteria, fungi, rickettsiae and viruses. Though crude extracts of vegetable materials and other substances have been used in the treatment of disease for hundreds of years, e.g. cinchona bark in malaria and mercury in the treatment of syphilis, the first great advance in modern times was the discovery by Ehrlich of potent antispirochaetal drugs which could be given to man. He conceived the idea that drugs acted on the organisms and not the host because they had an affinity for specific cell receptors. Further progress in chemotherapy arose with developments in the dyestuff industry which resulted in new antimalarial drugs and the discovery of the first antibacterial drug, sulphanilamide, in 1935. This directed attention to the specific treatment of bacterial infections in man, until that time considered an impossibility. The third phase was opened in 1941 by the application of Fleming's discovery in 1929 of penicillin, a substance derived from moulds and antagonistic to the growth of a number of bacteria. Many modern drugs are the result of further investigation of moulds and soil bacteria. The modern conception of the mode of action of chemotherapeutic agents is that they compete with cell metabolites for enzyme systems essential to the metabolism of the cell, which is in fact the restatement of Ehrlich's original conception in terms of enzyme chemistry. Penicillin, streptomycin, chloramphenicol, aureomycin and other chemotherapeutic substances have to a great extent controlled the common infectious diseases. The improved substitutes for quinine have altered the picture of malaria; diethylcarbamazine that of filarial diseases; diamidines, kala-azar and trypanosome infections; and the sulphones, leprosy.

This does not mean that chemotherapy has conquered infectious disease. The treatment of virus diseases, for example, is just beginning and another great problem is the prevention of development of resistant strains of the parasites to the different chemotherapeutic agents. [chemical, Gk *therapeia* treatment.]

See also ANTIBIOTIC.

chemotic (ke·**mot**·ik). Referring to chemosis.

chemotransmitters (kem·o·**trans**·mitters). Chemical substances that are transmitted from one position to another—for example, from the hypothalamus to the anterior lobe of the pituitary by means of vessels—and produce a hormonal effect.

chemotrophy (kem·o·**tro**·fe). That type of bacterial nutrition in which chemical oxidation is the source of energy. [chemical, Gk *trophe* nutrition.]

chemotropism (kem·o·**tro**·pizm). Directional growth of an organism or movement of part of an organism in response to the presence of a chemical substance. [chemical, Gk *tropos* a turning.]

Chenais, Louis Jean (b. 1872). Paris physician.

Cestan-Chenais paralysis, or syndrome. A syndrome produced by a pontobulbar lesion, usually vascular, with ipsilateral palatal and laryngeal paralysis, Horner's syndrome and ataxia of the limbs, and contralateral hemiplegia and hemianaesthesia; due to involvement of the pyramidal tract, medial lemniscus, inferior cerebellar peduncle, nucleus ambiguus and the ocular sympathetic pathway.

chenocholic (ken·o·**ko**·lik). Relating to goose bile. [Gk *chen* goose, *chole* bile.]

Chenopodium (ken·o·**po**·de·um). American wormseed, the dried fruit of *Chenopodium ambrosioides* Linn. var. *anthelminticum* Gray (family Chenopodiaceae), a plant common in eastern USA. It contains a volatile oil which consists largely of ascaridole. The drug has anthelmintic properties, and is used for roundworms and hookworms (BPC 1949). **Chenopodium Oil BPC 1959.** The volatile oil steam-distilled from the fresh flowering and fruiting plants, excluding the roots, and containing not less than 65 per cent by weight of ascaridole. It is now practically the only form of the drug that is used. [Gk *chen* goose, *pous* foot.]

cheoplastic (ke·o·**plas**·tik). Relating to cheoplasty.

cheoplasty (ke·o·**plas**·te). The process of pouring molten metals or alloys into a preformed mould; in dentistry, the process of casting a metal tray in which an impression of the mouth is to be taken. [Gk *chein* to pour, *plassein* to mould.]

cherophobia (ker·o·**fo**·be·ah). A morbid fear of cheerfulness. [Gk *chairein* to rejoice, *phobein* to fear.]

cherry (**cher**·e). The fruit obtained from various species of *Prunus.* The cultivated red cherry is the fruit of *Prunus cerasus* Linn. var. *caproniana* DC. (family Rosaceae); cerasus. The black cherry is the fruit of *Prunus avium* Linn. **Cherry laurel, Cherry-laurel leaves.** Laurocerasus BPC 1949, the fresh leaves of the evergreen shrub *Prunus laurocerasus* Linn. **Wild Cherry Bark BPC 1968.** A bark derived from the American wild black cherry, *Prunus serotina* Ehrh., with mild sedative properties and used in cough mixtures; Virginian prune. [L *cerasus.*]

cherubism (**cher**·ub·izm). Familial disturbance in the growth and development of the jaws arising in childhood. The bone in the molar areas is replaced and expanded by multilocular masses of vascular fibrous tissue containing giant cells. The expanded face has been likened to that of a cherub.

Chervin, Claudius (b. 1824). French teacher.

Chervin's method, or treatment. A method of treating stuttering.

Cherwell, Lord. *See* LINDEMANN, FREDERICK ALEXANDER.

Cheselden, William (b. 1688). London surgeon.

Cheselden's operation. 1. For making an artificial pupil: iridotomy with a lance in a pulled-up iris. Of historical interest. 2. A form of perineal lithotomy.

chest (chest). The thorax. **Alar chest.** A chest with projecting (winged) scapulae owing to increased obliquity of the ribs and flatness of the chest. **Barrel chest.** A chest more rounded than normal with elevated ribs, a wide costal angle, prominent manubriosternal angle and generally some kyphosis. It is found with emphysema. **Blast chest.** A contused chest with intrapulmonary haemorrhages, the result of blast. **Cobblers' chest.** Pectus excavatum; a chest in which the lower part of the sternum is depressed and hollowed out like a funnel. **Emphysematous chest.** 1. Atrophic type, causing breathlessness, but no change in contour of the chest. 2. Hypertrophic type; barrel chest (see above). **Flail chest.** An injured chest with multiple fractures in which the loose portion behaves paradoxically, that is, it moves centrifugally on expiration. **Flat chest.** A long chest with reduced anteroposterior diameter. **Foveated chest.** Cobblers' chest (see above). **Frozen chest.** One in which there is a clotted haematoma: it is also caused by coagulated pus or fluid in tuberculous pleurisy or by an artificial pneumothorax effusion. **Funnel chest.** Cobblers' chest (see above). **Keeled chest.** A chest where the sternum projects sharply forward, resembling the keel of a boat. **Paralytic chest.** A long flat chest with increased obliquity of the ribs, a narrow costal angle and winged scapulae. **Pendel-luft chest.** A condition resulting from open pneumothorax in which the collapsed lung becomes partially inflated during expiration by air extruded from the opposite lung, resulting in a pendulum movement of the air. The heart and mediastinum also swing to and fro with each respiration. Cyanosis results from used air being sucked back into the functioning lung and from cardiac embarrassment due to displacement to and fro. **Phthinoid chest.** Paralytic chest (see above). **Pigeon chest.** Keeled chest (see above). **Postoperative chest.** A pathological condition, usually atelectasis, which may follow a surgical operation, especially one involving the anterior abdominal wall. **Rachitic chest.** A chest deformed by rickets, showing beading of the ribs, a transverse (Harrison's) furrow at the attachment of the diaphragm, and pigeon breast. **Stove-in chest.** A driving inwards of part of the chest wall as a result of a severe compression injury. **Tetrahedron chest.** A chest which appears to have 4 sides and on cross-section is more square than elliptical. [AS *cest* box.]

chétivism (**sha**·tiv·izm). A form of infantilism in which the somatic growth as a whole is arrested, there being no special emphasis on the retardation of any one part or organ. [Fr. *chétif* paltry.]

Cheyletiella (**sha**·let·e·**el**'·ah). A genus of Arachnida. *Cheyletiella parasitovorax*, an animal scabies affecting rabbits and sometimes conveyed by cats to man.

Cheyletus (ka·**le**·tus). A genus of mites, species of which have been found in sputum.

Cheyne, George (b. 1671). Scottish physician in Bath.

Cheyne's disease. Hypochondria.

Cheyne, John (b. 1777). Scottish physician in Dublin.

Cheyne's nystagmus, Cheyne-Stokes nystagmus. Nystagmus the eye movements of which resemble Cheyne-Stokes respiration in rhythm.

Cheyne-Stokes phenomenon, respiration or sign. Rhythmical waxing and waning of respiration, consisting of alternating periods of hyperpnoea (increased depth and rate of respiration), and apnoea (cessation of respiration). Respiration steadily increases in depth, then wanes, until finally it ceases entirely. After a few moments the cycle is repeated. During apnoea the pupils contract, and consciousness is often lost: during hyperpnoea the pupils dilate and consciousness is regained. Cheyne-Stokes respiration is due to an altered sensitivity of the respiratory centre, connected with reduced cerebral blood flow. It occurs in cerebral tumour, raised intracranial pressure, cerebral vascular accidents; in congestive cardiac failure (usually of the left ventricle); after narcotics such as morphine derivatives and barbiturates; and in uraemia. Occasionally it occurs in normal persons during sleep.

Cheyne-Stokes psychosis. A confusional state associated with Cheyne-Stokes respiration.

Cheyne, Sir William Watson (b. 1852). London surgeon.

Cheyne's operation. Repair of femoral hernia by use of a flap from the pectineus muscle.

Chiari, Hans (b. 1851). Prague and Strasbourg pathologist.

Chiari's disease. Arnold-Chiari disease (see below).

Chiari-Frommel syndrome. A condition of persistent lactation and amenorrhoea and failure to ovulate *post partum* due to continued secretion of prolactin with lack of FSH and LH production.

Chiari operation. An approach to the pituitary fossa through the orbito-ethmoidosphenoidal route.

Chiari's reticulum. An irregular muscular reticulum within the auricle of the right atrium.

Chiari's syndrome. Budd-Chiari syndrome (see below).

Arnold-Chiari deformity, disease, malformation or syndrome, Chiari-Arnold syndrome. Congenital elongation and caudal displacement of the brain stem and cerebellar tonsils, with herniation of the cerebellum and medulla through the foramen magnum; usually associated with meningocele or meningomyelocele and lumbosacral spina bifida. It commonly produces hydrocephalus.

Budd-Chiari disease, or syndrome. Thrombosis of the hepatic veins or of the inferior vena cava in its intrahepatic course, leading to enlargement of the liver, pain and ascites with portal hypertension.

Chiari, Karl. Viennese surgeon.

Chiari's operation. Osteotomy of the pelvis above a deficient acetabulum to obtain stability of a subluxing femoral head.

chiasm (ki·azm). Chiasma.

chiasma (ki·az·mah) (pl. chiasmata). 1. A decussation. 2. An X-shaped crossing. 3. The cross where individual chromosomes remain in contact during the late prophase (diplotene, diakinesis) and metaphase I of meiosis. Chiasmata are associated with exchange of genetic material due to crossing-over. **Optic chiasma [chiasma opticum (NA)].** The point in the hypothalamus at which the two optic nerves partially cross. It consists in a flat almost quadrilateral bundle of nerve fibres and is situated at the junction of the floor with the anterior wall of the 3rd ventricle. **Chiasma tendinum** [NA]. The point at which the tendons of the flexor digitorum profundus muscle pass through the openings in the tendons of the flexor digitorum sublimis muscle opposite the proximal phalanges of the fingers. [Gk *chiasma* two lines placed crosswise.]

See also: CAMPER.

chiasmal, chiasmatic (ki·az·mal, ki·az·mat·ik). 1. Relating to a chiasma. 2. Crosswise, as in a chiasma.

chiasmatypy (ki·az·mah·ti·pe). Term signifying crossing over, as of 2 nerves. [chiasma, Gk *typos* mark.]

chiastometer (ki·az·tom·et·er). An instrument with which can be measured any deviation of the optic axes from the normal state of parallelism. [chiasma, meter.]

Chiatopsylla (ki·at·op·sil·ah). A genus of rodent fleas some species of which transmit plague experimentally. **Chiatopsylla rossi.** A potential transmitter of plague.

Chibret's operation. For glaucoma: by corneal draining. [obsolete.]

chichism (che·kizm). A disease resembling pellagra and occurring in Central America.

chickenpox (chik·en·pox). Varicella; an acute, universally prevalent and highly infectious disease caused by a herpesvirus. It attacks mainly those in the middle years of childhood, causing a vesicular rash which passes through the stages of macule, papule, vesicle and pustule. Finally the lesions dry out and form crusts which separate without scarring. The spots develop in crops and the distribution is mainly on the face and trunk (centripetal distribution). In childhood there is relatively little constitutional upset and complications are rare. In adults, pneumonia may be a relatively common and serious complication. After recovery, the virus may lie dormant in sensory ganglia in the central nervous system and recrudesce many years later as herpes zoster (shingles). Bullous and haemorrhagic forms of the eruption occur rarely. The former may resemble pemphigus; the latter, in which a general bleeding tendency may be found, is a very serious complication and is particularly liable to occur in patients on cytotoxic drugs or steroids. [AS *cicen*, ME *pokkes*.]

chicle (chi·kl). Chicle gum, the gum of *Achras sapota*, a tree that grows in tropical America; it is used to make chewing-gum. [Mex. *tzictli*.]

chicory (chik·or·e). Succory, the root of *Cichorium intybus* Linn. (family Compositae), of Europe and Asia. It resembles dandelion root. Dried, roasted and ground, it is used as an addition to, or substitute for, coffee. [Gk *kichora*.]

Chiene, John (b. 1843). Edinburgh surgeon.

Chiene's incision. A gridiron incision continued medially to open the lateral part of the rectus sheath.

Chiene's lines. Arbitrary lines used to help in localizing cerebral centres.

Chiene's operation. Cuneiform osteotomy for correction of knock knee.

Chievitz, Johan Hendrik (b. 1850). Copenhagen anatomist.

Chievitz layer. An embryonic layer in the retina between the inner and outer neuroblastic layers. Also called *transitional fibre layer.*

Chievitz's organ. A small, transient, outgrowth of gland tissue from the postero-inferior portion of the developing parotid gland.

chigger (chig·er). American name for the larval stages of mites of the genus *Trombicula.* [Fr. *chique* from Carib name.]

chigoe (chig·o). South American name for the jigger or sand flea *Tunga penetrans* of the order Siphonaptera.

chikungunya (chik·un·gun·yah). An infective disease due to a group A arbovirus, with fever, joint pains (which may be excruciating) and a maculopapular rash. In Thailand it has been associated with a haemorrhagic fever. The insect vector is the mosquito, particularly *Aëdes* species. [Tanzanian dialect, that which bends.]

chil-. For words beginning with **Chil-**, *see also* CHEIL-.

chilblain (chil·blane). An inflammatory swelling due to exposure to cold which appears on hands or feet and may progress to ulceration. The lesion is painful and there are sensations of severe itching and burning; the desire to rub the affected part is so great that open sores may be caused. **Necrotized chilblain.** A severe chilblain with central necrotic ulceration. [AS *cele* cold, *bleyn* blister.]

child (chi·ld). A person under the age of 14. **Newborn child.** A child up to the age of 4 weeks—after which it is called an infant. [AS *cild*.]

childbed (chi·ld·bed). The puerperium; the puerperal state [AS *cild, bed*.]

childbirth (chi·ld·berth). Parturition. [AS *cild*, ME *bwith*.]

chile (chil·e). **Chile nitre, Chile saltpetre.** Caliche, crude sodium nitrate, $NaNO_3$, found in great deposits in Northern Chile; contains also sodium iodate, $NaIO_3$.

chill (chil). Convulsive shivering or shaking of the body with a sensation of cold and pallor of the skin as the result of exposure to wet or cold which causes involuntary contraction of the voluntary muscles. The condition usually is the precursor of an acute disorder or feverish illness, and is characteristic of the preliminary stages of malaria. **Brass chills, Brassfounders' chills, Braziers' chills.** Metal-fume fever. *See* FEVER. **Creeping chill.** A sensation of cold or chill unattended by any obvious shivering or chattering of the teeth. **Chills and fever.** A popular name for malaria. **Shaking chill.** A chill in which the shivering symptom is marked. **Spelter chills.** Metal-fume fever. *See* FEVER. **Urethral chill.** A sensation of cold or chill occurring after a catheter has been passed and sometimes attended by shivering. **Wind chill.** The extra cooling due to exposure to an air current, other factors being held constant. **Zinc chills.** Metal-fume fever caused by the inhalation of fumes from zinc. [AS *cele* cold.]

chillies (chil·eez). The commercial name applied to the fruit of *Capsicum minimum* Roxb. African chillies are varieties from Sierra Leone, Malawi and Tanzania; a less pungent, unofficial variety known as Japanese chillies is probably derived from *Capsicum frutescens* Linn. [Mex.]

Chilodon (ki·lo·don). A genus of ciliate protozoa. **Chilodon dentatus.** A coprozoic ciliate found in faeces, probably a contaminant. [Gk *cheilos* lip, *odous* tooth.]

Chilognatha (ki·lo·**nath**·ah). An order of Myriapoda including millipedes. Millipedes have 2 pairs of legs on each body segment, except the first few. They have been found in the alimentary canal and nasal passages but are purely adventitious. [Gk *cheilos* lip, *gnathos* jaw.]

chilomastigiasis (**ki**·lo·mas·tig·**i**'·as·is). Chilomastixiasis.

Chilomastix (ki·lo·**mas**·tix). A genus of Mastigophora. **Chilomastix mesnili.** A large flagellate common in the large intestine. It is world-wide but not pathogenic. [Gk *cheilos* lip, *mastix* whip.]

chilomastixiasis, chilomastosis (**ki**·lo·mas·tix·**i**'·as·is, **ki**·lo·mas·**to**'·sis). Infestation with the intestinal flagellate *Chilomastix mesnili.*

Chilopoda (ki·**lop**·o·dah). An order of Myriapoda, centipedes. Centipedes have one pair of legs to each body segment, and poison fangs on the head. The larger species are tropical and their bites though painful are not dangerous, except through sepsis. Small forms are often found in the nasal cavities, which they enter during sleep. [Gk *cheilos* lip, *pous* foot.]

chilopodiasis (**ki**·lo·po·**di**'·as·is). Invasion of a cavity of the body by one of the chilopoda or centipede family of insects. The cavity usually affected is the nasal.

chim-. For words beginning with **Chim-**, *see also* CHEIM-.

chimaera (ki·**me**·rah). An organism with cells derived from two or more distinct zygotes and, therefore, having different genomes. In contraposition to mosaic in which the cells with different genetic make-up derive from the same zygote. *Chimaera* and *mosaic* have sometimes been used as synonyms. [Gk *khimaros* goat.]

Chimani-Moos test. For simulated unilateral deafness: a tuning fork is held alternately at equal distances from each ear, and it is said to be heard better in the sounder ear. It is then placed on the vertex, and, with hesitation, the malingerer lateralizes the sound to the allegedly normal ear. On blockage of the meatus on this side, he will then state that the sound is no longer heard.

chimaphila (ki·**maf**·il·ah). Pipsissewa, the dried leaves of the evergreen plant *Chimaphila umbellata* (Linn.) Nutt. (family Pyrolaceae), containing a crystalline substance chimaphilin, arbutin, tannin, resin and gum. It is diuretic and astringent, and has been used in renal disease. [Gk *cheima* winter, *philein* to love.]

chimera (ki·**me**·rah). 1. A fire-spouting monster with a lion's head, a goat's body and a snake's tail. 2. Applied in botany to a plant that has tissues differing in genetic constitution, such as a graft hybrid. 3. Applied in zoology and then in medicine to binovular twins whose blood was originally of different groups but in whom there has been an interchange of blast cells *in utero* so that their bloods are of mixed groups, an anomaly that has persisted. [Gk *khimaros.*]

chimpanzee (chim·pan·**ze**). A man-like ape of tropical West and Central Africa, *Pan satyrus.* It is particularly useful in experimental work as it is affected by many diseases that are otherwise peculiar to man. [Angola name.]

chin [mentum] (chin). The triangular raised part of the outer surface of the mandible formed by the mental protuberance. **Chin cough.** *See* COUGH. **Double chin.** Buccula. **Galoche chin.** A thrusting prominent chin which is a congenital condition. **Chin jerk, Chin-jerk reflex.** *See* REFLEX. [AS *cin.*]

china (**ke**·nah). Quina, cinchona bark. [Peruv. *kina* bark.]

china-root (**chi**·nah·root). The name appears to have been applied to 3 different drugs: 1. The root of *Smilax china* Linn. (family Liliaceae), used locally in China, Japan and the East Indies, but almost obsolete in Europe. 2. Galanga, lesser galangal, the rhizome of *Alpinia officinarum* Hance (family Zingiberaceae), an aromatic carminative. 3. The dried rhizome of *Dioscorea villosa* Linn. (family Dioscoreaceae), of North America, which is diuretic. [China, root.]

chincumbi (chin·**kum**·be). Chiufa.

chineto (kin·**e**·to). Totaquine.

chinidine (**kin**·id·een). Quinidine.

chinine (**kin**·een). Quinine.

Chininii Chloridum. *European Pharmacopoeia* name for Quinine Hydrochloride BP 1973.

Chiniofon Sodium BP 1958 (**kin**·e·o·fon **so**·de·um). A bright yellow powder consisting of the sodium salt of 7-iodo-8-oxyquinoline-5-sulphonic acid with sodium bicarbonate. By virtue of its iodine content it kills amoebae in the intestinal tract whether they are in the motile or encysted form. It is given in acute or chronic intestinal amoebiasis, by mouth in tablet form during the day, and as a retention enema at night. Its action is, however, slower than that of emetine. It should not be used in patients intolerant of iodine or who have liver damage, and care should be taken in giving it in cases of thyroid disease.

chinkumbi (chin·**kum**·be). Chiufa.

chinoline (**kin**·o·leen). Quinoline.

chinone (**kin**·one). Quinone.

chinovin (**kin**·o·vin). Quinovin, a bitter glucoside present in cinchona bark.

chionablepsia (ki·on·a·**blep**'·se·ah). Snow blindness. *See* BLINDNESS. [Gk *chion* snow, ablepsia.]

Chionanthus (ki·o·**nan**·thus). A genus of trees of the family Oleaceae. The root bark of the American fringe tree, *Chionanthus virginicus* Linn., contains a glycoside chionanthin, and a saponin. It is a bitter tonic and diuretic. [Gk *chion* snow, *anthos* flower.]

chionophobia (ki·on·o·**fo**'·be·ah). Morbid fear of snow. [Gk *chion* snow, *phobein* to fear.]

chip-blower (**chip**·blo·er). Chip syringe. *See* SYRINGE. [dim. of *chop,* AS *blawan.]*

chir-. For words beginning with **Chir-**, *see also* CHEIR-.

Chirata BPC 1949 (ke·**ra**·tah). Indian gentian, the dried plant *Swertia chirata* Buch.-Ham. (family Gentianaceae), an annual herb of Northern India. It has bitter and tonic properties, and is used mainly in India. [Hind.]

chiratin (ki·**ra**·tin). $C_{26}H_{48}O_{15}$, a bitter substance from *Swertia chirata;* commonly used at one time as a tonic.

chiratta, chiretta (ke·**ra**·tah, ke·**ret**·ah). Chirata.

chirobrachialgia (**ki**·ro·bra·ke·**al**'·je·ah). Pain in the hand and arm. **Chirobrachialgia paraesthetica.** So called when paraesthesiae are also felt. [Gk *cheir* hand, *brachion* arm, *algos* pain.]

Chironomidae (ki·ro·**nom**·id·e). A family of non-biting midges. The biting midges Ceratopogonidae are sometimes included here. [Gk *cheironomos* one who gesticulates.]

chiropodist (ki·**rop**·o·dist). An expert in the treatment of minor diseases of the hands and feet and in the removal of bunions and corns. [Gk *cheir* hand, *pous* foot.]

chiropody (ki·**rop**·o·de). 1. The care of the feet and toenails, especially by a chiropodist. 2. The profession or business of a chiropodist.

chirurgia, chirurgery (ki·**rer**·je·ah, ki·**rer**·jer·e). Surgery. [Gk *cheir* hand, *ergon* work.]

chirurgic, chirurgical (ki·**rer**·jik, ki·**rer**·jik·al). Surgical. [see prec.]

chisel (**chiz**·el). A sharp cutting instrument of steel with a terminal blade bevelled at the cutting edge on one side only, for the division of a hard structure such as bone. [from L *caedere* to cut down.]

chitin (**ki**·tin). A complex polysaccharide composed of units of acetylglucosamine, $CH_3CONHC_6H_{11}O_5$, constituting the horny external skeleton of insecta and crustacea, and the supporting tissue of fungi. It is hard, insoluble and very stable, but is hydrolysed by concentrated hydrochloric acid into glucosamine and acetic acid: it corresponds to the cellulose of plants. [Gk *chiton* tunic.]

chitinization (ki·tin·i·**za**'·shun). 1. The process of becoming chitinous. 2. Transformation into chitin.

chitinous (ki·tin·us). 1. Of the nature of chitin. 2. Composed of chitin.

chitobiose (ki·to·bi·oze). A disaccharide composed of 2 units of glucosamine; obtainable from chitin.

chitoneure (ki·to·newr). A collective term for the sheaths of nerve fibres and other nerve structures such as the neurilemma and the perineurium. [Gk *chiton* tunic, *neuron* nerve.]

chitonitis (ki·ton·i·tis). A condition of inflammation of any investing membrane such as the peritoneum. [Gk *chiton* tunic, *-itis* inflammation.]

chitosamine (ki·to·zam·een). D-glucosamine, aminoglucose, $CH_2OH(CHOH)_3CH(NH_2)CHO$. An aminosaccharide obtained by the hydrolysis of chitin, and occurring widely in nature combined with protein as glycoproteins.

chitosan (ki·to·san). A polymer of acetylglucosamine, produced during the breaking down of chitin.

chitose (ki·toze). A monosaccharide obtained by reducing chitonic acid.

chitotriose (ki·to·tri·oze). A trisaccharide composed of 3 units of glucosamine; obtainable from chitin.

Chittenden, Russell Henry (b.1856). New Haven, Connecticut biochemist.

Chittenden's diet. A low diet containing 45–55 g of protein.

chittim bark (chit·im bark). Sacred bark, Cascara BP 1958, the dried bark of the California buckthorn, *Rhamnus Purshiana* DC. (family Rhamnaceae), occurring mostly in British Columbia, Western USA, and Kenya. It is a most valuable mild purgative, usually administered in the form of liquid extract, or tablets prepared from the dry extract.

Chitty's method of iodine therapy. A convenient way of giving iodine; 5 minims of liquor of iodine in half a tumblerful of milk thrice daily.

chiufa (ki·oo·fah). An acute inflammatory condition of the rectum, involving the vulva and vagina in the female, occurring in South America. Also described in Malawi.

Chlamydobacteriaceae (klam·id·o·bak·teer·e·a'·se·e). A family of non-pathogenic bacteria belonging to the order of Chlamydobacteriales, class Schizomycetes. Many species are sheathed and the elements show false branching. The sheaths usually contain iron. The organisms occur in water and soil. [Gk *chlamys* cloak, bacteria.]

Chlamydobacteriales (klam·id·o·bak·teer·e·a'·leez). An order of non-pathogenic bacteria, of the class Schizomycetes, found in water and soil. They grow as filamentous elements showing false branching; many species are sheathed and contain iron. [see prec.]

Chlamydophrys (klam·id·of·ris). A genus of Protozoa. **Chlamydophrys stercorea.** A shelled amoeba which occurs in stale faeces, but probably not in the intestine. [Gk *chlamys* cloak, *ophrys* brow.]

chlamydospore (klam·id·o·spor). The term for the converted terminal cells of pseudohyphae which become round, thick-walled, asexual resting spores. Amongst the truly filamentous fungi, cells of the mycelium may enlarge and form spores, which are also called chlamydospores. Those formed within the hypha are said to be intercalary; those at the end are called terminal; while those formed at the side of the hypha are termed lateral. Their function is to carry the fungus through unfavourable environmental conditions. [Gk *chlamys* cloak, *sporos* seed.]

chlamydozoa (klam·id·o·zo'·ah). Cloak animals, an old name for viruses or their intracellular inclusion bodies. [Gk *chlamys* cloak, *zoon* animal.]

chlamydozoan (klam·id·o·zo'·an). Any minute organism which belongs to the chlamydozoa.

chliasma (kli·az·mah). A poultice; a fomentation [Gk *chliainein* to make warm.]

chloasma (klo·az·mah). A general term for pigmentary discoloration of the skin occurring in spots or patches of yellow, brown or black. **Chloasma bronzinum.** A brown pigmented condition of the skin of the uncovered parts of the body, e.g. face and neck, resulting from long exposure to the rays of the tropical sun. **Chloasma cachecticorum.** Chloasma resulting from profound constitutional disorders such as malaria or syphilis. **Chloasma caloricum.** Chloasma resulting from constant exposure to heat or to the sun's rays. **Chloasma gravidarum.** The chloasma which is observable in women during pregnancy. **Chloasma hepaticum.** Chloasma occurring in conditions of dyspepsia. **Chloasma phthisicorum.** Chloasma occurring on the chest, forehead and cheeks of a tuberculous individual. **Symptomatic chloasma.** Chloasma regarded as a symptom of a disease such as tuberculosis or syphilis. **Chloasma toxicum.** Chloasma occurring during or after the local use of certain drugs. **Chloasma traumaticum.** The chloasma which results from friction or pressure on areas of the skin. **Chloasma uterinum.** Chloasma occurring in women during pregnancy or in diseases of the ovaries or uterus and affecting chiefly the face, the nipples and the median line of the abdomen. [Gk *chloazein* to be green.]

Chlophedianol (klo·fed·i·an·ol). BP Commission approved name for 1-*o*-chlorophenyl-3-dimethylamino-1-phenylpropan-1-ol; a cough suppressant.

chloracetone (klor·as·e·tone). Chloro-acetone, acetyl methyl chloride, $CH_2ClCOCH_3$. A colourless unstable liquid used as a war gas.

chloracetophenone (klor·as·et·o·fe'·none). Chloroacetophenone.

chloracetyl (klor·as·et·il). Chloro-acetyl. The monovalent radical CH_2ClCO-, occurring in chloracetic acid. **Chloracetyl chloride.** $CH_2ClCOCl$, a fuming colourless liquid.

chloracne (klor·ak·ne). A widespread acneiform eruption due to exposure to chlorinated naphthalenes, chlordiphenyls and chlordiphenyl oxides. It usually occurs in persons engaged in making insulating materials, or in electricians, by whom it is called *cable rash.* Heavily chlorinated hydrocarbons present in cutting oils may cause a similar condition in machinists and others exposed to the oils. [Gk *chloros* greenish, acne.]

chloraemia (klor·e·me·ah). 1. A condition in which the blood contains an excess of chlorides. 2. Chlorosis (green sickness). [Gk *chloros* greenish, *haima* blood.]

chloral (klor·al). Anhydrous chloral, CCl_3CHO. An oily liquid with a pungent odour, formed by the action of dry chlorine on ethyl alcohol. It is not itself used in medicine though its derivatives are valuable as hypnotics. **Chloral Betaine BP 1963.** Chloral hydrate-betaine adduct; a hypnotic and sedative. **Camphorated chloral.** A liquid composed of equal parts of camphor and chloral hydrate; used locally to relieve irritation of the skin. **Chloral formamide.** Chloralamide, $CCl_3CHOHNHCHO$, a colourless crystalline substance with a bitter taste. It has a sedative and hypnotic action resembling that of chloral hydrate, is less irritant to the stomach, but also less potent and more irregular in its action. **Chloral Hydrate BP 1973.** Trichlorethylidene glycol, $CCl_3CH(OH)_2$, a colourless crystalline substance with a pungent odour and bitter taste. It depresses the central nervous system, and is used as a hypnotic, its chief drawbacks being its taste and the fact that it may irritate the stomach and cause vomiting. In therapeutic doses it has a wide margin of safety and is a suitable hypnotic for children. When applied locally it has a mild irritant effect, followed by a slight degree of anaesthesia. **Syrup of Chloral BPC 1959.** A preparation consisting of chloral hydrate, water, and syrup; 1 ml contains 0.2 g of chloral hydrate. [Gk *chloros* greenish.]

chloralamide (klor·al·am·ide). $CCl_3CHOHNHCHO$, a colourless crystalline compound moderately soluble in water, and which decomposes on heating. It is sometimes used instead of chloral hydrate as a hypnotic: it decomposes in the body to chloral hydrate and ammonium formate producing hypnosis about one hour after ingestion.

chloralammonia (klor·al·am·o'·ne·ah). Chloralamide.

chloralcaffeine (klor·al·kaf·e·een). A granular white crystalline substance having analgesic and laxative properties when injected hypodermically. It is formed by mixing chloral hydrate and caffeine in alcoholic solution and evaporating. [Gk *chloros* greenish, caffeine.]

chloralformamid (klor·al·**form**·am·id). Chloralamide.

Chlorali (**klor**·al·i). **Chlorali Hydras.** *European Pharmacopoeia* name for Chloral Hydrate BP 1973.

chloralic (klor·**al**·ik). Pertaining to chloral.

chloralide (**klor**·al·ide). $C_4Cl_6H_2O_3$, an additive compound of chloral formed by heating it with trichloracetic acid.

chloralimide (klor·al·**im**·ide). $CCl_3CH{=}NH$, a compound used as a substitute for chloral but having no advantages over the latter as its action depends upon the liberation of chloral within the body.

chloralism (**klor**·al·izm). 1. The habitual taking of chloral 2. The poisonous effects that may arise from habitually taking chloral or from prolonged medical administration. The symptoms may be alimentary, nervous, cardiac and cutaneous (erythematous rashes and patches of oedema). Severe cases may simulate delirium tremens.

chloralization (**klor**·al·i·**za**′·shun). 1. Treatment with chloral or anaesthetization by the use of chloral. 2. Chloralism.

chloralize (**klor**·al·ize). To treat with or place under the influence of chloral.

chloralomania (**klor**·al·o·**ma**′·ne·ah). Psychotic addiction to the use of chloral as an intoxicant. [chloral, mania.]

chloralose (**klor**·al·oze). Glucochloral, $C_8H_{11}Cl_3O_6$. A colourless crystalline compound prepared from chloral and glucose. It has hypnotic properties, but is not used in therapeutics. Its chief use is as an anaesthetic in animal experiments, when its action in maintaining an elevated blood pressure is often an advantage.

chloralurethane (klor·al·**ewr**·e·thane). $CCl_3CH(OH)NHCOOC_2H_5$, a hypnotic sometimes used instead of chloral.

Chlorambucil BP 1973 (klor·**am**·bew·sil). γ-*p*-di-(2-Chloroethyl)-aminophenylbutyric acid, for oral administration in cases of lymphadenoma.

chloramine (klor·**am**·een). 1. The general name applied to any organic compound containing the group NCl. They are prepared by the action of a hypochlorite on an amine or imide, and have antiseptic properties. 2. (BP 1953), sodium *p*-toluene sulphonechloramide, $CH_3C_6H_4SO_2NClNa{\cdot}3H_2O$, a white crystalline powder with a slight odour of chlorine and a bitter taste. It decomposes slowly in air, becoming yellow, and has antiseptic properties due to the slow release of chlorine. It is inactivated by the presence of organic matter, but more slowly than the inorganic hypochlorites. It is soluble in water, the solution being almost neutral and non-irritant; a 2 per cent solution may be used as a local application or by irrigation, whilst a 0.5 per cent solution may be employed as a mouth-wash.

Chloramphenicol BP 1973 (klor·am·**fen**·ik·ol). D-*threo*-2-dichloroacetamido-1-(4-nitrophenyl)propane-1,3-diol, an antibiotic produced by the growth of *Streptomyces venezuelae* but now prepared synthetically. It has a wide spectrum of antibacterial activity, but side-effects are serious and include toxic depression of bone marrow. Its most important use is in the treatment of enteric fever. **Chloramphenicol Cinnamate BPC 1968.** The 3-cinnamic ester of chloramphenicol. **Chloramphenicol Palmitate BPC 1968.** The 3-palmitic ester of chloramphenicol. **Chloramphenicol Sodium Succinate BPC 1968.** The sodium salt of the 3-monosuccinic ester of chloramphenicol.

Chloramphenicolum (klor·am·fen·ik·**o**·lum). *European Pharmacopoeia* name for Chloramphenicol BP 1973.

chloramyl (**klor**·am·il). The monovalent radical $C_5H_{10}Cl$–, derived from the amyl group.

chloranaemia (klor·an·**e**·me·ah). A form of anaemia resembling chlorosis and occurring in cachectic conditions. **Achylic chloranaemia.** Chronic hypochromic anaemia. *See* ANAEMIA. **Idiopathic chloranaemia.** Idiopathic hypochromic anaemia. *See* ANAEMIA. [Gk *chloros* greenish, anaemia.]

chlorargentate (klor·**ar**·jen·tate). A double salt of the chlorides of silver and a metal or radical.

chlorarsenous (klor·**ar**·sen·us). Term applied to an arsenic compound which also contains chlorine.

chlorate (**klor**·ate). A salt of chloric acid. **Chlorate poisoning.** *See* POISONING.

chlorated (klor·**a**·ted). Treated with chlorine gas or chlorine water.

chlorazol (**klor**·az·ol). The name given to a family of synthetic azo dyes containing sulphonic acid groups and bearing chemical relationship to heparin. **Chlorazol fast pink.** A dye which has been used as anticoagulant in animal experiments. It is non-toxic and has few side effects, but cannot be used in man owing to its colouring propensities.

Chlorbetamide (klor·**bet**·am·ide). BP Commission approved name for dichloro-*N*-(2,4-dichlorobenzyl)-*N*-(2-hydroxyethyl)-acetamide; used in sulphonamide therapy.

chlorbromide (klor·**bro**·mide). Chlorobromide; name applied to any compound in which an organic radical is combined with both chlorine and bromine, e.g. trimethylene chlorbromide, $CH_2BrCH_2CH_2Cl$.

chlorbutanol (klor·**bew**·tan·ol). Chlorbutol BP 1973.

Chlorbutol BP 1973 (klor·**bew**·tol). Chlorobutanol, $CCl_3C(OH)(CH_3)_2$. A hypnotic which does not produce gastric irritation like chloral. It has some anaesthetic action on the gastric mucous membrane and has been used therefore to guard against travel sickness or seasickness. Also employed as a preservative in certain drug solutions.

chlorcamphor (klor·**kam**·for). 1. A substituted derivative of camphor produced by chlorination; it may be mono- or di-substituted, and one of several isomers in each case. 2. Camphorated chloral.

chlorcarvacrol (klor·**kar**·vak·rol). A chlorine derivative of carvacrol used as an antiseptic.

Chlorcyclizine (klor·**si**·kliz·een). BP Commission approved name for DL-1-(*p*-chlorobenzhydryl)-4-methylpiperazine, an antihistaminic drug. The official preparation is Chlorcyclizine Hydrochloride BP 1973.

Chlordantoin (klor·**dan**·to·in). BP Commission approved name for 5-(1-ethylpentyl)-3-(trichloromethylthio)hydantoin; an antifungal agent.

chlordiazepoxide (**klor**·di·az·ep·**ox**′·ide). Approved name for 7-chloro-2-methylamino-5-phenyl-3*H*-benzo-1,4-diazepine 4-oxide. **Chlordiazepoxide Hydrochloride BP 1973.** The hydrochloride of chlordiazepoxide, a drug with mild tranquillizing effects used in the treatment of neuroses characterized by anxiety and tension.

Chlorella (klor·el·ah). A genus of green (fresh-water) algae. [Gk *chloros* greenish.]

chlorephidrosis (**klor**·ef·id·**ro**′·sis). A condition in which the sweat has a greenish discoloration. [Gk *chloros* greenish, *ephidrosis* sweat.]

chlorethyl (klor·**eth**·il). Ethyl chloride, C_2H_5Cl. A highly volatile liquid packed in small glass cylinders for spraying on the tissues for its local anaesthetic effect due to rapid evaporation. Thawing may, however, be painful, and damage caused to the cells may delay healing. It is employed as a general anaesthetic, induction being quick, in very short operative procedures, but there is danger of laryngeal spasm, paralysis of the medullary centres, and, in the case of accidental overdose, primary cardiac failure.

chlorethylene (klor·**eth**·il·een). Chloroethylene.

chlorguanide hydrochloride (klor·**gwan**·ide hi·dro·**klor**·ide). Proguanil Hydrochloride BP 1958.

chlorhaematin (klor·**he**·mat·in). Haemin and haematin chloride.

Chlorhexadol (klor·**hex**·ad·ol). BP Commission approved name for 2-methyl-4-(2,2,2-trichloro-1-hydroxyethoxy)-pentan-2-ol; a hypnotic and sedative.

Chlorhexidine (klor·**hex**·id·een). BP Commission approved name for 1,6-di(4′-chlorophenyldiguanido)-hexane. **Chlorhexidine Acetate BPC 1968.** The diacetate of chlorhexidine, an antiseptic used in aqueous or alcoholic solution for disinfection of the hands and in the treatment of superficial wounds and burns. **Chlorhexidine Hydrochloride BP 1973.** The dihydrochloride of chlorhexidine; actions and uses are essentially those of the acetate (see above) but, as it is only sparingly soluble in water, the hydrochloride is used in dusting powders, ointments, creams and surgical dressings.

chlorhistechia (klor·his·**tek**·e·ah). Increased amount of chloride in the tissues. [chlorine, Gk *histos* tissue, *echein* to hold.]
chlorhydria (klor·**hi**·dre·ah). A condition in which there is too large a quantity of hydrochloric acid in the stomach.
chlorhydric (klor·**hi**·drik). Hydrochloric; pertaining to hydrogen chloride.
chlorhydrin (klor·**hi**·drin). Denoting a compound containing both hydroxyl and chloride radicals.
chlorhydroxyquinoline (**klor**·hi·drox·e·**kwin**′·o·leen). A common name for a large number of chemical isomers, the best-known of which is 7-chloro-8-hydroxyquinoline (7-chloro-oxine), a bacteriostatic. Its action, like that of oxine itself, depends on its ability to remove trace elements essential to bacteria.
chloric (**klor**·ik). 1. Relating to, or containing chlorine. 2. Term applied to compounds containing chlorine at the higher valencies. **Chloric ether.** 1. Ethyl chloride. 2. Spirit of chloroform.
chloridaemia (klor·id·**e**·me·ah). A condition in which chlorides are retained in the blood. [chloride, Gk *haima* blood.]
chloride (**klor**·ide). 1. A salt of hydrochloric acid. 2. A salt consisting of monovalent chlorine combined with an element or radical. **Acid chloride.** A derivative of an organic acid in which chlorine has replaced the hydroxyl of the acid COOH group. **Chloride ion.** The negative ion Cl^- produced by the dissociation of hydrochloric acid and chlorides. **Chloride of lime.** Chlorinated Lime BP 1958, bleaching powder, a mixture of basic calcium chloride, $CaCl_2Ca(OH)_2 \cdot H_2O$, and calcium hypochlorite, $Ca(OCl)_2$, used as a bleaching agent and disinfectant.
chloridimeter (klor·id·**im**·et·er). An apparatus with which the chlorides in fluids may be estimated. [chloride, meter.]
chloridimetry (klor·id·**im**·et·re). The estimation of the chloride content of a fluid. [see prec.]
chloridion (klor·id·i·on). Chloride ion.
chloridometer (klor·id·**om**·et·er). Chloridimeter.
chloriduria (klor·id·**ewr**·e·ah). A condition in which there is an excessive quantity of chlorides in the urine.
chlorimeter (klor·**im**·et·er). An apparatus for determining the quantity of free or available chlorine in compounds such as bleaching powder. [chlorine, meter.]
chlorimetry (klor·**im**·et·re). The quantitative determination of the free or available chlorine in bleaching powder and other compounds, by means of a chlorimeter.
chlorinated (**klor**·in·a·ted). Treated with or containing chlorine.
chlorination (klor·in·**a**·shun). Disinfection of water or sewage by treatment with free chlorine.
chlorine (**klor**·een). An element of the halogen family, with atomic weight 35.453, atomic number 17, and chemical symbol Cl. It is a greenish gas, heavier than air, with a characteristic pungent odour, occurring widely in nature in combined form, as a common salt in sea-water and rock salt, and as the chlorides of metals. It is a constituent of all plants and animals, mostly as the chlorine ion, and exerts a considerable influence in the processes of excretion, hydration, buffering and digestion. It is essential to the body, where it is present in the cells and extracellular fluid, in the blood, and in all secretions and excretions. The element is chemically highly reactive, especially when freshly released from one of its compounds, and many substances owe their antiseptic properties to the fact that when in contact with organic matter they release free chlorine which combines with the bacterial protein, thus killing the organism. The gas irritates mucous membranes and may cause conjunctivitis, bronchitis and bronchopneumonia, and gastritis; it has been used in chemical warfare as a choking gas. **Chlorine dioxide,** ClO_2, a poisonous yellow gas produced by the action of concentrated sulphuric or hydrochloric acid on potassium chlorate. It is one of the constituents of chlorine gargle. **Chlorine water.** A saturated solution of chlorine in water, used as an antiseptic, disinfectant and bleaching agent. [Gk *chloros* greenish.]
chlorinum (klor·i·num). Chlorine.
chloriodoform (klor·i·**o**·do·form). Dichloriodomethane, $CHCl_2I$. A yellow liquid used like iodoform.
Chlorisondamine Chloride (klor·i·**son**·dam·een **klor**·ide). BP Commission approved name for 4,5,6-tetra-chloro-2(2-dimethylaminoethyl)iso-indoline dimethochloride; a ganglion-blocking agent with gradual but prolonged action, for oral administration in cases of mild or moderate hypertension of whatever nature, but it should be used in small doses in renal disease.
chlorite (**klor**·ite). 1. A salt of chlorous acid. 2. Name given to a group of minerals.
Chlormadinone (klor·**mad**·in·one). BP Commission approved name for 6-chloro-17α-hydroxypregna-4,6-diene-3,20-dione. **Chlormadinone Acetate BP 1968.** 17α-Acetoxy-6-chloropregna-4,6-diene-3,20-dione, a progestational steroid.
Chlormerodrin (klor·**mer**·o·drin). BP Commission approved name for 3-chloromercuri-2-methoxy-propylurea, $HgClCH_2CH(OCH_3)CH_2NHCONH_2$. A compound administered orally for the treatment of oedema associated with congestive heart failure.
Chlormethiazole (klor·meth·i·az·ole). BP Commission approved name for 5-(2-chloroethyl)-4-methylthiazole; a hypnotic and sedative.
chlormethyl (klor·**meth**·il). Methylchloride.
Chlormezanone (klor·**mez**·an·one). BP Commission approved name for 2-(4-chlorophenyl)tetrahydro-3-methyl-1,3-thiazin-4-one 1,1-dioxide; it is used in the treatment of neuroses.
Chlormidazole (klor·**mid**·az·ole). BP Commission approved name for 1-(4-chlorobenzyl)-2-methylbenzimidazole; an antifungal agent.
chloro-acetone (klor·o·**as**·e·tone). 1. Chloracetone. 2. Methylchlorophenyl ketone, $CH_3COC_6H_4Cl$, a lacrimatory gas used in chemical warfare.
chloro-acetophenone (**klor**·o·as·et·o·**fe**′·none). Chloracetophenone, chlorophenylmethyl ketone, phenacyl chloride, $C_6H_5COCH_2Cl$. A crystalline substance with a lacrimatory vapour, used in chemical warfare as a tear gas (CAP).
chloro-acetyl (klor·o·**as**·et·il). Chloracetyl; the monovalent radical, CH_2ClCO–, occurring in chloracetic acid.
chloro-anaemia (**klor**·o·an·**e**′·me·ah). Chloranaemia.
chloroazodin (**klor**·o·az·**o**′·din). $NCl{=}C(NH_2)N{=}NC(NH_2){=}CNl$, a wound antiseptic having a prolonged action due to the slow liberation of chlorine. Its efficacy is not decreased by pus or serum, and it is active in very small concentration.
chlorobromhydrin (**klor**·o·brom·**hi**′·drin). 1. Denoting a compound which contains hydroxyl, chloride, and bromide radicals. 2. Allyl chlorobromhydrin, $CH_2ClCHOHCH_2Br$, a derivative of glycerol.
chlorobromide (klor·o·**bro**·mide). Chlorbromide.
chlorobutanol (klor·o·**bew**·tan·ol). Chlorbutol BP 1973.
Chlorocresol BP 1973 (klor·o·**kre**·sol). 6-Chloro-3-hydroxytoluene, $CH_3C_6H_3(OH)Cl$. A white crystalline compound which is not very soluble in water but more soluble in soap solution, in which form it is a constituent of certain germicidal preparations. It has a relatively low toxicity.
chloro-erythroblastoma (**klor**·o·er·**ith**·ro·blast·**o**′·mah). A neoplasm in which are included the elements of both chloroma and erythroblastoma.
chloroethylene (klor·o·**eth**·il·een). A term including the several chlorinated derivatives of ethylene. The only two of medical importance are trichloroethylene, $CHCl{=}CCl_2$, and tetrachloroethylene, $CCl_2{=}CCl_2$.
chloroform (**klor**·o·form). Trichloromethane, $CHCl_3$. A colourless volatile liquid with a characteristic odour and a burning, sweet taste, insoluble in water but mixing in all proportions with alcohol or ether. Its chief property, medically, is that of powerful depression of the central nervous system. It was first introduced as a general anaesthetic by Simpson, an Edinburgh obstetrician, in 1847, but is little used nowadays owing to its toxicity and the fact that better anaesthetics are available. Its dangers are cardiac irregularities, especially ventricular fibrillation, and toxic hepatitis (delayed chloroform poisoning); its advantages are smooth induction and good muscular relaxation. Applied to the skin it causes mild local irritation and redness, and it is sometimes incorporated in rubefacient liniments; internally it is

of value as a carminative. It is a useful general solvent, and is employed in histological work to clear tissues prior to embedding in paraffin wax. (BP 1973.) **Acetone chloroform.** Chlorbutol BP 1958, $CCl_3C(CH_3)_2OH$, a compound used as an anaesthetic for the gastric mucosa in seasickness and vomiting. **Chloroform of aconite.** An extract of aconite made by percolating the drug with chloroform and alcohol after moistening with ammonia. **Emulsion of Chloroform BP 1953.** A preparation containing 5 per cent of chloroform in water, emulsified with tragacanth; employed as a carminative. **Liniment of chloroform.** A rubefacient preparation composed of equal volumes of chloroform and liniment of camphor. **Chloroform Spirit BP 1973.** A carminative and flavouring agent consisting of 5 per cent chloroform in 90 per cent alcohol. **Chloroform Water BP 1973.** A solution of 0.25 per cent chloroform in water mainly employed as a flavouring agent. [chlorine, formyl.]

chloroformin (klor·o·**form**·in). A chloroform extract from tubercle bacilli with toxic properties, prepared by Auclaire in 1899; now only of historical interest.

chloroformism (**klor**·o·form·izm). 1. The habit of inhaling chloroform for its narcotic action and the morbid condition resulting from the practice. 2. The anaesthetizing effect of chloroform vapour.

chloroformization (**klor**·o·form·i·**za**'·shun). 1. Anaesthesia induced by administration of chloroform. 2. Chloroformism.

chloroleukaemia (**klor**·o·lew·**ke**'·me·**ah**). Chloroma. [Gk *chloros* greenish, leukaemia.]

chlorolymphoma (**klor**·o·lim·**fo**'·mah). 1. A variety of lymphoma. 2. Chloroma. [Gk *chloros* greenish, lymphoma.]

chlorolymphosarcoma (**klor**·o·lim·fo·sar·**ko**'·mah). Chloroma associated with an increase of lymphocytes in the blood. [chloroma, lymphosarcoma.]

chloroma (klor·o·mah). An atypical form of leukaemia in which tumours of a greenish colour form in the skull, the orbits, the long bones and abdomen, metastasizing by way of the lymph vessels. [Gk *chloros* greenish, *-oma* tumour.]

chloromethylchloroformate (klor·o·**meth**·il·klor·o·**for**'·mate). $CH_2ClCOOCl$, a lacrimatory liquid used in chemical warfare (palite).

chloromorphine (klor·o·**mor**·feen). An intermediate substance that may be formed during the conversion of morphine to apomorphine, and resembling diamorphine in its pharmacological actions. It may be present as a contaminant in commercial apomorphine.

chloromyeloma (**klor**·o·mi·el·**o**'·mah). Chloroma with which multiple growths in the bone marrow are associated. [Gk *chloros* greenish, myeloma.]

chloronaphthalene (klor·o·**naf**·thal·een). $C_{10}H_7Cl$, a compound occurring either as a colourless liquid (α-form) or in white laminae (β-form). Unprotected workers exposed to chloronaphthalene have sometimes developed hepatic necrosis.

chloropenia (klor·o·**pe**·ne·ah). A condition in which there is a deficiency of chlorine in the blood. [chlorine, Gk *penes* poor.]

chloropercha (klor·o·**per**·chah). A solution of gutta percha in chloroform, used as a filling material for the root canal of devitalized teeth.

chloropexia (klor·o·**pex**·e·ah). The process by which chlorine is fixed in the body tissues. [chlorine, Gk *pexis* fixation.]

chlorophane (**klor**·o·fane). A pigment of a greenish-yellow colour present in the retina. [Gk *chloros* greenish, *phainein* to show.]

chlorophenol (klor·o·**fe**·nol). 1. OHC_6H_4Cl, a mixture of the *ortho-* and *para-*isomers of monochlorphenol, obtained by the action of chlorine on phenol. The introduction of chlorine atoms into the molecule of phenol increases its germicidal power, but at the same time increases its toxicity and caustic properties. It is used only for sanitary purposes. 2. A term applied to any derivative of phenol containing chlorine. Such compounds have antiseptic properties which vary according to the number and position of the chlorine atoms substituted in the molecule. **Chlorophenol red.** Dichlorophenolsulphonephthalein, a compound used as an indicator, changing from yellow at pH 5.5 to red at pH 6.5. **Chlorophenol salicylate.** Chlorosalol.

chlorophenyl (klor·o·**fe**·nil). The radical C_6H_4Cl–, derived from chlorophenol.

chlorophyll (**klor**·o·fil). The green pigment of plants which absorbs solar energy and uses it to synthesize sugars from the carbon dioxide and water taken in by the plant. Chemically, it is related to the haemoglobin of blood except that the metal within the porphyrin ring is magnesium, in the case of chlorophyll, and the compound is esterified with methyl and phytyl alcohols. It occurs in plants in 2 forms, blue-green *chlorophyll a*, $C_{55}H_{72}Mg N_4O_5$, and an oxidized yellow-green *chlorophyll b*, $C_{55}H_{70}MgN_4 O_6$; the mechanism of photosynthesis depends, it is believed, on the interconvertibility of the two. **Crystalline chlorophyll.** The methylester or chlorophyllide produced by alcoholysis when green leaves are extracted with ethyl alcohol. **Water-soluble chlorophyll.** The mixture of water-soluble chlorophyllins produced by the alkaline hydrolysis of chlorophyll. [Gk *chloros* greenish, *phyllon* leaf.]

chlorophyllase (**klor**·o·fil·aze). An enzyme present in the leaves of plants, which brings about the alcoholysis of chlorophyll to give chlorophyllides, phytol and methyl alcohol.

chlorophyllide (**klor**·o·fil·ide). An alcoholic ester of chlorophyllin.

chlorophyllin (**klor**·o·fil·in). The tricarboxy acid of which chlorophyll is the methyl phytyl ester. It is a magnesium porphyran, and yields an aetioporphyrin almost identical with the protoporphyrin derived from haemoglobin.

chloropia (klor·o·pe·ah) Chloropsia.

chloropicrin (klor·o·**pik**·rin). Chlorpicrin, nitrochloroform, trichloronitromethane, CCl_3NO_2. A dense liquid with a suffocating lacrimatory vapour that also causes vomiting; used as a choking gas in chemical warfare.

Chloropidae (klor·**op**·id·e). A family of the dipteran suborder Cyclorrhapha. The genera *Hippelates* and *Siphunculina* are of medical interest. [Gk *chloros* greenish, *ops* eye.]

chloroplastin (klor·o·**plas**·tin). The name given to the protoplasm contained in grains of chlorophyll. [Gk *chloros* greenish, *plassein* to mould.]

chloroprivic (klor·o·**pri**·vik). 1. Deprived of chlorides, chlorine or hydrochloric acid. 2. Caused by loss of chlorides, chlorine or hydrochloric acid. [chlorine, L *privare* to deprive of.]

chloroprocaine hydrochloride (klor·o·**pro**·kane hi·dro·**klor**·ide). 2-Diethylaminoethyl-4-amino-2-chlorobenzoate hydrochloride, a local analgesic of the ester type, similar to procaine but less toxic and rather more potent.

chloropropane (klor·o·**pro**·pane). Propyl chloride, $CH_3CH_2CH_2 Cl$, or its isomer, isopropyl chloride, $CH_3CHClCH_3$, both of which have been used as anaesthetics.

chloropropene (klor·o·**pro**·peen). Propenyl chloride, $CH_3CH{=}CHCl$, or its isomer, isopropenyl chloride, $CH_2{=}CClCH_3$, both of which have been used as anaesthetics.

chloropsia (klor·**op**·se·ah). A form of disordered vision which makes all objects appear to be coloured green. [Gk *chloros* greenish, *opsis* sight.]

Chloropyrilene (klor·o·**pir**·il·een). BP Commission approved name for *N,N*-dimethyl-*N*-(2-pyridyl)-*N*-(5)-chloro-2-thienylethylenediamine hydrochloride. An antihistaminic used in allergic disorders such as hay fever, urticaria, allergic rhinitis, etc.

Chloroquine (**klor**·o·kween). BP Commission approved name for a synthetic antimalarial derived from 7-chloro-4-aminoquinoline. It is similar in action to mepacrine but even less toxic. It is the most efficient malarial schizonticide known. The two most commonly used salts are the phosphate (BP 1973) and the sulphate (BP 1973).

chloroquinone (klor·o·**kwin**·one). One of the several derivatives formed by the substitution of chlorine atoms in quinone.

chlorosalol (klor·o·**sal**·ol). Chlorophenol salicylate, $C_6H_4(OH) COOC_6H_4Cl$. A compound with mild antiseptic properties, used externally.

chlorosarcolymphadeny (klor·o·sar·ko·limf·**ad'**·en·e). Chlorolymphosarcoma. [Gk *chloros* greenish, *sarx* flesh, L *lympha* water, Gk *aden* gland.]

chlorosarcoma (**klor**·o·sar·**ko'**·mah). Chloroma. [Gk *kloros* greenish, *sarx* flesh, *-oma* tumour.]

chlorosarcomyeloma (klor·o·**sar**·ko·mi·el·**o'**·mah). Chloromyeloma containing elements of sarcoma. [Gk *chloros* greenish, *sarx* flesh, myeloma.]

chlorosis (klor·**o**·sis). Green sickness; an anaemic condition seen in young women and girls and thought to have been due to tight corsets, constipation, frequent pregnancies, poor hygiene and diet. It is rarely encountered now, and would appear to have been chronic hypochromic anaemia due to inadequate intake of iron, poor diet and living conditions, and excessive menstrual losses at a time of growth. **Achylic chlorosis.** Idiopathic hypochromic anaemia. *See* ANAEMIA. **Egyptian chlorosis.** Ancylostomiasis. **Chlorosis florida.** Idiopathic chronic hypochromic anaemia in which the complexion is florid. **Chlorosis gigantea.** Chlorosis occurring in a very obese patient. **Late chlorosis.** Chronic or idiopathic hypochromic anaemia. *See* ANAEMIA. **Chlorosis rubra.** Hypochromic anaemia in which the pallor of the skin is masked by dilatation of the peripheral blood vessels. **Chlorosis tarda.** Late chlorosis (see above). **Tropical chlorosis.** Ancylostomiasis. [Gk *chloros* greenish, *-osis* condition.]

Chlorothiazide BP 1973 (klor·o·**thi**·az·ide). 6-Chloro-7-sulphamoylbenzo-1,2,4-thiadiazine 1,1-dioxide, a powerful oral diuretic.

chlorothymol (klor·o·**thi**·mol). A potent bactericide, $C_{10}H_{13}OCl$. It is a white crystalline powder soluble in organic solvents but not in water. It is irritating to mucous membranes except in weak solutions.

chlorotic (klor·**ot**·ik). 1. Related to chlorosis. 2. An individual affected with chlorosis.

Chlorotrianisene BP 1973 (**klor**·o·tri·**an'**·is·een). 1-Chloro-1,2,2-tri(*p*-methoxyphenyl)ethylene, a synthetic oestrogen used in menopausal disorders and for the relief of symptoms in prostatic carcinoma.

chlorous (**klor**·us). Combined with chlorine. Usually it describes compounds of chlorine in which the proportion of the element is larger than that in chloric compounds.

chlorovinyldichloroarsine (klor·o·**vi**·nil·di·klor·o·**ar'**·seen). $AsCl_2CH{=}CHCl$. A vesicant liquid with a faint geranium odour. Lewisite, used in chemical warfare as a blister gas, is a mixture of this substance with dichlorovinylchloroarsine, $AsCl(CH{=}CHCl)_2$.

chloroxyl (klor·**ox**·il). Cinchophen hydrochloride (so-called), $C_{16}H_{12}ClNO_2$. A compound which, since it is insoluble in water, but soluble in ether and chloroform, is very unlikely to be a true hydrochloride. It has the same physiological properties as cinchophen itself.

Chloroxylenol BP 1958 (klor·o·**zi**·len·ol). Parachlorometaxylenol.

Chlorphenesin BP 1973 (klor·**fen**·es·in). 3-*p*-Chlorophenoxypropane-1,2-diol; a fungicide.

Chlorpheniramine (klor·fen·**ir**·am·een). The BP Commission approved name for 1-*p*-chlorophenyl-3-dimethyl-amino-1,2'-pyridyl propane, an antihistaminic drug with minimal side effects. **Chlorpheniramine Maleate.** The hydrogen maleate of the drug (BP 1973).

Chlorphenoctium Amsonate (klor·fen·**ok**·te·um **am**·son·ate). BP Commission approved name for 2,4-dichlorophenoxymethyldimethyloctylammonium 4,4'-diaminostilbene-2,2'-disulphonate; an antifungal agent.

chlorphenol (klor·**fe**·nol). Chlorophenol.

Chlorphenoxamine (klor·fen·**ox**·am·een). BP Commission approved name for 1-*p*-chlorophenyl-1-phenylethyl-2-dimethylaminoethyl ether; it is used in the treatment of parkinsonism.

Chlorphentermine (klor·**fen**·ter·meen). BP Commission approved name for 4-chloro-$\alpha\alpha$-dimethylphenethylamine; it is used in sedation and in the treatment of obesity.

chlorphenyl (klor·**fe**·nil). Chlorophenyl.

chlorpicrin (klor·**pik**·rin). Chloropicrin.

Chlorproguanil (klor·pro·**gwan**·il). BP Commission approved name for N^1-3,4-dichlorophenyl-N^5-isopropyldiguanide. **Chlorproguanil Hydrochloride BP 1973.** The hydrochloride of chlorproguanil, an antimalarial drug more potent than the parent substance proguanil, and used in the prevention and treatment of malaria.

Chlorpromazine (klor·**pro**·maz·een). BP Commission approved name for 3-chloro-10-(3'-dimethylamino-*n*-propyl)-phenothiazine. A sedative used in psychoses and psychoneuroses, as a premedicant, in anaesthesia to prevent vomiting, and in other forms of intractable vomiting, and in the induction of hypothermia. The official preparation is Chlorpromazine Hydrochloride BP 1973.

Chlorpropamide BP 1973 (klor·**pro**·pam·ide). *N-p*-chlorobenzenesulphonyl-*N*-propylurea; it is used in the treatment of diabetes.

chlorprophenpyridamine (klor·**pro**·fen·pir·**id'**·am·een). Chlorpheniramine.

Chlorprothixene (klor·pro·**thix**·een). BP Commission approved name for α-2-chloro-9-(3-dimethylaminopropylidene)-thiaxanthen; it is used in the treatment of psychoneuroses.

Chlorquinaldol (klor·**kwin**·al·dol). BP Commission approved name for 5,7-dichloro-8-hydroxy-2-methylquinoline; a fungicide.

chlorsalol (klor·**sal**·ol). Chlorosalol.

chlortetracycline (**klor**·tet·rah·**si'**·kleen). Aureomycin. **Chlortetracycline Hydrochloride BP 1973.** Aureomycin hydrochloride.

chlortetracyclini (**klor**·tet·rah·**si'**·klin·i). **Chlortetracyclini Hydrochloridum.** *European Pharmacopoeia* name for Chlortetracycline Hydrochloride BP 1973.

Chlorthalidone BP 1973 (klor·**thal**·id·one). 3-(4-chloro-3-sulphamoylphenyl)-3-hydroxy-iso-indolin-1-one; a diuretic. Its actions and uses are similar to those of chlorothiazide, but are more prolonged.

Chlorthenoxazin (klor·then·**ox**·az·in). BP Commission approved name for 2-(2-chloroethyl)-2,3-dihydro-4-oxobenz-1,3-oxazine; an anti-inflammatory and analgesic agent.

chlorum (**klor**·um). Chlorine.

chloruraemia (klor·ewr·**e**·me·ah). 1. A condition in which urinary chlorides are retained in the blood. 2. Chloridaemia. [chloride, urine, Gk *haima* blood.]

chloruria (klor·**ewr**·e·ah). A condition in which chlorides are present in urine.

chloryl (**klor**·il). Ethyl chloride.

Chlorzoxazone (klor·**zox**·az·one). BP Commission approved name for 5-chlorobenzoxazolin-2-one; a muscle relaxant.

Chmelia slovaca (**shme**·le·ah **slo**·vak·ah). A dematiaceous fungus isolated from verrucoid lesions of an external ear in a Czechoslovakian. Lesions were suggestive of chromomycosis, but tissue forms of the fungus were not typical.

choana (**ko**·an·ah). Any funnel-like opening or cavity. **Choana cerebri.** The infundibulum of the hypothalamus. **Choana narium.** The posterior aperture of the nose. [Gk *choane* funnel.]

choanal (**ko**·an·al). Relating to a choana.

choanoid (**ko**·an·oid). Infundibuliform. [choana, Gk *eidos* form.]

choc en dome (shok ahn **dome**). The expansile pulsation of the precordia associated with aortic regurgitation. [Fr. vault shock.]

choc en retour (shok ahn re·**toor**). 1. In internal ballottement, the impact of the descending fetus on the fingertip. 2. Infection believed to be communicated to the mother from a syphilitic fetus. [Fr. return shock.]

chocolate (**chok**·o·late). A confectionery product manufactured by grinding cocoa nibs with cocoa butter, cane sugar, and flavouring (plain or bitter chocolate). It sets into a hard dark-brown amorphous mass which has a high calorific value by virtue of its carbohydrate content (40–60 per cent) and fat (20–40 per cent). Powdered or condensed milk may be incorporated (milk chocolate), which increases its food value. [Mexican *chocolatl*.]

choke (choke). 1. Obstruction to breathing (and swallowing) by impaction of food, vomit or a foreign body in the throat or glottis; occurring frequently in inmates of mental institutions, or drunken or semiconscious persons. 2. To be unable to draw breath because of obstruction of the trachea or for other reasons. *See* CHOKING. **Cerebral choke.** Thoracic choke (see below). **Ophthalmovascular choke.** Obstruction of the circulation of the blood in the retina because the retinal vessels are pressing upon each other. **Thoracic choke.** Oesophageal obstruction in the thoracic region. **Water choke.** Spasm of the larynx due to the presence of fluid in it or between the vocal folds. [ME *choken.*]

choke-damp (**choke**·damp). An unbreathable atmosphere developing in a mine, shaft or well, and consisting of carbon dioxide and other asphyxiating gases. [ME *choken,* damp.]

chokes (choxe). A sensation of tightness of the chest, retrosternal pain and irritation in the throat; it is a symptom of decompression sickness. [ME *choken.*]

choking (**cho**·king). The feeling of strangulation resulting from the presence in any one of the upper respiratory tracts of a foreign body or morsel of food, or from inspiration of any unbreathable gas or vapour, so that passage of air to the lungs is partially or entirely prevented. [ME *choken.*]

cholaemia (ko·le·me·ah). A condition in which the circulating blood contains bile or bile constituents in abnormal amounts; it can be the result of liver insufficiency, but may have other causes. **Familial cholaemia.** Haemolytic jaundice of the newborn. *See* JAUNDICE. [Gk *chole* bile, *haima* blood.]

See also: GILBERT.

cholaemimetry (ko·le·**mim**·et·re). The process of estimating the quantity of bile constituents in the circulating blood. [Gk *chole* bile, *haima* blood, meter.]

cholagogia (ko·lag·**o**·je·ah). The flowing or expulsion of bile from the gall bladder. [Gk *chole* bile, *agagos* drawing forth.]

cholagogue (**ko**·lag·og). 1. A drug which promotes the flow of bile into the duodenum from the gall bladder and bile ducts. 2. Promoting the flow of bile. [Gk *chole* bile, *agogein* to draw forth.]

cholane (**ko**·lane). A saturated hydrocarbon with a 4-ring sterol structure, regarded as the parent of the bile acids. **Cholane ring.** Androstane ring, cyclopentenophenanthrene skeleton; three 6-membered rings in phenanthrene form fused with a 5-membered ring, and possessing a side-chain. This configuration is the basis of the sterols, steroids, sex hormones and bile acids; by fracture it gives rise to the carotenoids and cerebrosides.

cholangeitis (**ko**·lan·je·**i**′·tis). Cholangitis.

cholangia, cholangie (ko·**lan**·je·ah, ko·**lan**·je). A term generally applied to morbid processes of the bile passages that are not inflammatory. [Gk *chole* bile, *aggeion* small vessel.]

cholangiectasis (**ko**·lan·je·**ek**′·tas·is). Dilatation of biliary vessels. [Gk *chole* bile, angiectasis.]

cholangioduodenostomy (ko·**lan**·je·o·**dew**·o·de·**nos**′·to·me). The making of an anastomosis between the common bile duct or the hepatic ducts and the duodenum. [Gk *chole* bile, *aggeion* small vessel, duodenum, Gk *stoma* mouth.]

cholangio-enterostomy (ko·**lan**·je·o·en·ter·**os**′·to·me). The surgical procedure of making a communication between a bile duct and the intestine. [Gk *chole* bile, *aggeion* small vessel, enterostomy.]

cholangiogastrostomy (ko·**lan**·je·o·gas·**tros**′·to·me). The opening by surgical means of a communication between a bile duct and the stomach. [Gk *chole* bile, *aggeion* small vessel, gastrostomy.]

cholangiogram (ko·**lan**·je·o·gram). An x-ray picture of the gall bladder and the bile ducts. [Gk *chole* bile, *aggeion* small vessel, *gramma* a writing.]

cholangiography (**ko**·lan·je·**og**′·raf·e). The making of x-ray pictures of the gall bladder and bile ducts. **Operative cholangiography.** Radiographic demonstration of the biliary passages during the course of an operation by the direct injection of the radio-opaque medium into the gall bladder, cystic duct or common bile duct. **Transhepatic cholangiography.** Radiographic demonstration of the biliary passages either before operation by the introduction of a needle or cannula through the skin (*percutaneous transhepatic cholangiography*), or at operation by introduction of the needle or cannula directly into the liver. Used in cases of suspected obstructive jaundice as a diagnostic measure. [Gk *chole* bile, *aggeion* small vessel, *graphein* to record.]

cholangiohepatoma (ko·**lan**·je·o·hep·at·**o**′·mah). A tumour of the liver derived from the cells of the intrahepatic bile ducts. [Gk *chole* bile, *aggeion* vessel, *hepar* liver, *-oma* tumour.]

cholangiojejunostomy (ko·**lan**·je·o·jej·oon·**os**′·to·me). The operation of anastomosing the hepatic duct to the jejunum, employed especially in the relief of jaundice due to postoperative stricture of the common bile duct. [Gk *chole* bile, *aggeion* small vessel, jejunum, Gk *stoma* mouth.]

cholangiolitis (ko·**lan**·je·o·**li**′·tis). Inflammation of the intrahepatic bile ducts. It is associated with general inflammatory diseases of the liver such as infective hepatitis, cirrhosis and chronic venous congestion. [Gk *chole* bile, *aggeion* small vessel, *-itis* inflammation.]

cholangioma (**ko**·lan·je·**o**′·mah). Neoplasm originating in a bile duct. [Gk *chole* bile, *aggeion* small vessel, *-oma* tumour.]

cholangiostomy (**ko**·lan·je·**os**′·to·me). The surgical incision of a bile duct for the purpose of drainage. [Gk *chole* bile, *aggeion* small vessel, *stoma* mouth.]

cholangiotomy (ko·**lan**·je·**ot**′·o·me). Choledochotomy. [Gk *chole* bile, *aggeion* small vessel, *temnein* to cut.]

cholangitis (ko·lan·**ji**·tis). Inflammation of the biliary duct system, usually due to calculi; it may be *acute, chronic, recurrent* (Charcot's fever) or *suppurative* (may be due to parasitic infection). **Catarrhal cholangitis.** Infective hepatitis. **Cholangitis lenta.** A chronic inflammatory state of the bile ducts uncomplicated by the formation of biliary calculi. **Obliterative cholangitis.** Cholangitis resulting in occlusion of the bile ducts. **Sclerosing cholangitis.** *Primary*—progressive stenosis of extrahepatic bile ducts without stone or obvious cause. *Secondary*—sclerosis due to obstruction and causing thickening of bile ducts without narrowing of their lumen. [Gk *chole* bile, *aggeion* small vessel, *-itis* inflammation.]

cholanopoiesis (ko·**lan**·o·poi·**e**′·sis). The synthesis of cholic acid by the liver. [Gk *chole* bile, *poiesis* production.]

cholanopoietic (ko·**lan**·o·poi·**et**′·ik). Characterized by cholanopoiesis.

cholanthrene (ko·**lan**·threen). $C_{20}H_{14}$, a derivative of benzanthracene synthesized from desoxycholic acid. Under certain circumstances it has carcinogenic properties.

cholascos (ko·**las**·kos). Effusion of bile into the cavity of the peritoneum. [Gk *chole* bile, *askos* bag.]

cholate (**ko**·late). Any salt or ester of cholic acid.

cholebilirubin (**ko**·le·bil·e·**roo**′·bin). Direct bilirubin or the bilirubin of the bile, to distinguish it from the indirect bilirubin (haemobilirubin) of the reticulo-endothelial system which does not give an immediate colour reaction in van den Bergh's test. [Gk *chole* bile, bilirubin.]

Cholecalciferol (**ko**·le·kal·**sif**′·er·ol). BP Commission approved name for 9,10-secocholesta-5,7,10(19)-trien-3β-ol; it is used in the treatment of vitamin D deficiency. **Cholecalciferol D_3.** The active principal which is produced in the gut by the action of sunlight on 7-dehydrocholesterol in the skin.

cholechromeresis (**ko**·le·kro·mer·**e**′·sis). An increase in the excretion of bile pigments. [Gk *chole* bile, *chroma* colour, *eresis* removal.]

cholechromopoiesis (**ko**·le·kro·mo·poi·**e**′·sis). The synthesis of bile pigments in the liver. [Gk *chole* bile, *chroma* colour, *poiesis* production.]

cholecyanin (ko·le·**si**·an·in). Bilicyanin; a blue oxidation product of bilirubin formed in Gmelin's test, in which bilirubin is treated with fuming nitric acid. It is believed to be among the pigments which appear on the skin over a bruise. [Gk *chole* bile, *kyanos* blue.]

cholecyst (**ko**·le·sist). The gall bladder. [Gk *chole* bile, *kystis* bag.]

cholecystagogic (ko·le·sis·tag·**og**′·ik). Of the nature of, or pertaining to a cholecystagogue.

cholecystagogue (ko·le·**sis**·tag·og). A drug or action that promotes emptying of the gall bladder. [cholecyst, Gk *agogein* to draw forth.]

cholecystalgia (**ko**·le·sist·**al**′·je·ah). Biliary colic. *See* COLIC. [cholecyst, Gk *algos* pain.]

cholecystatony (**ko**·le·sist·**at**′·on·e). Atony of the gall bladder. [cholecyst, atony.]

cholecystectasia (**ko**·le·sist·ek·**ta**′·ze·ah). 1. Dilatation of the gall bladder. 2. A condition of distension of the gall bladder. [cholecyst, Gk *ektasis* a stretching.]

cholecystectomy (**ko**·le·sist·**ek**′·to·me). Excision of the gall bladder. [cholecyst, Gk *ektome* a cutting out.]

cholecystelectrocoagulectomy (**ko**·le·sist·el·**ek**·tro·ko·ag·ew·**lek**′·to·me). Cholecysto-electrocoagulectomy.

cholecystendysis (**ko**·le·sist·**en**′·dis·is). Cholecysto-endysis.

cholecystentero-anastomosis (**ko**·le·sist·**en**·ter·o·an·as·to·**mo**′·sis). Cholecysto-enterostomy. [cholecyst, Gk *enteron* bowel, anastomosis.]

cholecystenterorrhaphy (**ko**·le·sist·en·ter·**or**′·af·e). Cholecysto-enterorrhaphy.

cholecystenterostomy (**ko**·le·sist·en·ter·**os**′·to·me). Cholecysto-enterostomy.

cholecystgastrostomy (**ko**·le·sist·gas·**tros**′·to·me). Cholecysto-gastrostomy.

cholecystic (ko·le·**sist**·ik). Referring to the gall bladder. [see foll.]

cholecystis (ko·le·**sist**·is). The gall bladder. [Gk *chole* bile, *kystis* bag.]

cholecystitis (**ko**·le·sist·**i**′·tis). Inflammation of the gall bladder; it is most often due to obstruction of the cystic duct by a stone, or to bacterial infection, e.g. typhoid, and may be acute or chronic. **Emphysematous cholecystitis.** Infection of the gall bladder with the organisms of gas gangrene, and the consequent formation of gas bubbles in its wall. **Cholecystitis glandularis proliferans.** A condition in which there is a localized area of muscle hypertrophy in the gall-bladder wall containing epithelial-lined cystic spaces which may contain calculi (intramural). [cholecyst, Gk *-itis* inflammation.]

See also: EBERTH.

cholecystocolostomy (ko·le·**sist**·o·kol·**os**′·to·me). The establishment by operative means of a communication between the gall bladder and the colon. [cholecyst, colostomy.]

cholecystocolotomy (ko·le·**sist**·o·kol·**ot**′·o·me). Incision into the gall bladder and the colon. [cholecyst, colotomy.]

cholecystoduodenostomy (ko·le·**sist**·o·dew·o·de·**nos**′·to·me). The establishment by operative means of a communication between the gall bladder and the duodenum. [cholecyst, duodenostomy.]

cholecysto-electrocoagulectomy (ko·le·**sist**·o·el·**ek**·tro·ko·ag·ew·**lek**′·to·me). The operation of removing the gall bladder by the use of surgical diathermy. [cholecyst, electrocoagulectomy.]

cholecysto-endysis (ko·le·**sist**·o·**en**′·dis·is). A form of cholecystotomy in which the gall bladder is incised, the stone removed and the internal wound sutured and fastened to the abdominal incision, which is then closed. [cholecyst, Gk *endysis* an entering in.]

cholecysto-entero-anastomosis (ko·le·**sist**·o·en·ter·o·an·as·to·**mo**′·sis). Cholecysto-enterostomy. [cholecyst, Gk *enteron* intestine, anastomosis.]

cholecysto-enterorrhaphy (ko·le·**sist**·o·en·ter·**or**′·af·e). Surgical suture of the gall bladder to the intestinal wall. [cholecyst, enterorrhaphy.]

cholecysto-enterostomy (ko·le·**sist**·o·en·ter·**os**′·to·me). The surgical procedure of making a direct communication between the gall bladder and the intestine. [cholecyst, enterostomy.]

cholecysto-enterotomy (ko·le·**sist**·o·en·ter·**ot**′·o·me). Surgical incision of both the gall bladder and the intestine. [cholecyst, enterotomy.]

cholecystogastrostomy (ko·le·**sist**·o·gas·**tros**′·to·me). The operative establishment of a communication between the gall bladder and the stomach. [cholecyst, gastrostomy.]

cholecystogram (ko·le·**sist**·o·gram). An x-ray photograph of the gall bladder. [cholecyst, Gk *gramma* a writing.]

cholecystography (**ko**·le·sist·**og**′·raf·e). X-ray examination of the gall bladder. [cholecyst, Gk *graphein* to record.]

cholecysto-ileostomy (ko·le·**sist**·o·i·le·**os**′·to·me). The operative establishment of a communication between the gall bladder and the ileum. [cholecyst, ileostomy.]

cholecystojejunostomy (ko·le·**sist**·o·jej·oon·**os**′·to·me). The operative formation of a communication between the gall bladder and the jejunum. [cholecyst, jejunostomy.]

cholecystokinetic (ko·le·**sist**·o·kin·**et**′·ik). 1. An agent which stimulates the contractions of the gall bladder. 2. Having the property of exciting more vigorous contractions of the gall bladder. [cholecyst, Gk *kinesis* movement.]

cholecystokinin (**ko**·le·sist·o·**kin**′·in). A hormone formed by the duodenal mucosa in the presence of fat, acids, or egg-yolk, and which stimulates contraction of the gall bladder. [cholecyst, Gk *kinein* to move.]

cholecystokinin-pancreozymin (CCK) (**ko**·le·sist·o·**kin**′·in **pan**·kre·o·**zi**′·min). A gastric hormone in which the terminal pentapeptide is the same as that found in gastrin. Formerly believed to be 2 separate hormones, it is now thought that both actions are caused by the same hormone, secreted by cells in the mucosa of the upper small intestine, and causing contraction of the gall bladder and secretion of pancreatic juice rich in enzymes. [cholecyst, Gk *kinein* to move, pancreas, Gk *zyme* ferment.]

cholecystolithiasis (ko·le·**sist**·o·lith·**i**′·as·is). The condition in which there are gall-stones in the gall bladder. [cholecyst, Gk *lithos* stone.]

cholecystolithotripsy (**ko**·le·sist·o·**lith**′·o·trip·se). The operation of crushing gall-stones in the gall bladder with a lithotrite. [cholecyst, lithotripsy.]

cholecystomy (ko·le·**sist**·o·me). Cholecystotomy.

cholecystonephrostomy (ko·le·**sist**·o·nef·**ros**′·to·me). The surgical operation of making a communication between the gall bladder and the pelvis of the right ureter so that the bile is diverted from the intestines. [cholecyst, nephrostomy.]

cholecystopathy (**ko**·le·sist·**op**′·ath·e). Any disease affecting the gall bladder. [cholecyst, Gk *pathos* suffering.]

cholecystopexy (ko·le·**sist**·o·pex·e). The surgical procedure of stitching the gall bladder to the wall of the abdomen. [cholecyst, Gk *pexis* fixation.]

cholecystoptosis (**ko**·le·sist·op·**to**′·sis). Displacement of the gall bladder downwards. [cholecyst, Gk *ptosis* fall.]

cholecystorrhaphy (**ko**·le·sist·**or**′·af·e). The surgical process of stitching or suturing the gall bladder. [cholecyst, Gk *rhaphe* suture.]

cholecystostomy (**ko**·le·sist·**os**′·to·me). Incision into the gall bladder for the purpose of inserting a drainage tube. [cholecyst, Gk *stoma* mouth.]

cholecystotomy (**ko**·le·sist·**ot**′·o·me). The making of an incision into the gall bladder. [cholecyst, Gk *temnein* to cut.]

cholecystotyphoid (**ko**·le·sist·o·**ti**′·foid). Typhoid fever in association with acute cholecystitis.

choledochectasia (**ko**·le·dok·ek·**ta**′·ze·ah). Dilatation of the bile duct. [choledochus, Gk *ektasis* a stretching.]

choledochectomy (**ko**·le·dok·**ek**′·to·me). In carcinoma of the bile duct, the excising of the affected part of the duct. [choledochus, Gk *ektome* a cutting out.]

choledochendysis (**ko**·le·dok·**en**′·dis·is). Choledochotomy. [choledochus, Gk *endysis* an entering in.]

choledochitis (**ko**·le·dok·**i**′·tis). Inflammation of the bile duct. [choledochus, Gk *-itis* inflammation.]

choledochocholedochostomy (ko·le·**do**·ko·ko·le·do·**kos**′·to·me). Anastomosis of one portion of the common bile duct to another, e.g. after excision of a stricture of the duct. [choledochus, Gk *stoma* mouth.]

choledochodochorrhaphy (ko·le·**do**·ko·do·**kor**′·af·e). The suturing of the ends of the bile duct at any place at which it has been divided. [choledochus, Gk *rhaphe* suture.]

choledochoduodenostomy (ko·le·**do**·ko·**dew**·o·de·**nos**'·to·me). The operative establishment of a communication between the bile duct and the duodenum. [choledochus, duodenum, Gk *stoma* mouth.]

choledocho-enterostomy (ko·le·**do**·ko·**en**·ter·**os**'·to·me). The operative establishment of a communication between the bile duct and the intestine. [choledochus, Gk *enteron* bowel, *stoma* mouth.]

choledochogram (ko·le·**do**·ko·gram). An x-ray photograph of the bile duct. [choledochus, Gk *gramma* a writing.]

choledochohepatostomy (ko·le·**do**·ko·hep·at·**os**'·to·me). The operative measure of suturing the divided ends of the bile duct or the hepatic duct over the opening of the gall bladder. [choledochus, Gk *hepar* liver, *stoma* mouth.]

choledocho-ileostomy (ko·le·**do**·ko·i·le·**os**'·to·me). The operative establishment of a communication between the bile duct and the ileum. [choledochus, ileum, Gk *stoma* mouth.]

choledochojejunostomy (ko·le·**do**·ko·jej·oon·**os**'·to·me). The operative formation of a communication between the bile duct and the jejunum. [choledochus, jejunum, Gk *stoma* mouth.]

choledocholith (ko·le·**do**·ko·lith). A concretion or calculus in the bile duct. [choledochus, Gk *lithos* stone.]

choledocholithiasis (ko·le·**do**·ko·lith·**i**'·as·is). The condition in which a gall-stone or gall-stones are present in the bile duct. [see prec.]

choledocholithotomy (ko·le·**do**·ko·lith·**ot**'·om·e). The cutting open of the bile duct in order to remove calculi. **Transduodenal choledocholithotomy.** Operation for removal of a stone from the lower end of the common bile duct by first opening the second part of the duodenum and then exposing the duct by incising the medial wall above the ampulla of Vater. [choledocholith, Gk *temnein* to cut.]

choledocholithotripsy, choledocholithotrity (ko·le·**do**·ko·**lith**'·o·trip·se, ko·le·**do**·ko·lith·**ot**'·rit·e). The procedure of crushing a gall-stone within the bile duct by means of a lithotrite. [choledocholith, Gk *tribein* to crush.]

choledochoplasty (ko·le·**do**·ko·**plas**'·te). Any plastic operation on the bile duct, e.g. for biliary fistula. [choledochus, Gk *plassein* to mould.]

choledochorrhaphy (ko·le·do·**kor**'·af·e). The suturing of the edges of an incision made into the bile duct. [choledochus, Gk *rhaphe* suture.]

choledochoscope (ko·le·**do**·ko·skope). An instrument used for inspecting the interior of the common bile duct. [choledochus, Gk *skopein* to view.]

choledochoscopy (ko·le·do·**kos**'·ko·pe). Inspection of the common bile duct by means of a choledochoscope.

choledochostomy (ko·le·do·**kos**'·to·me). The operative establishment of an opening into the bile duct through the wall of the abdomen. [choledochus, Gk *stoma* mouth.]

choledochotomy (ko·le·do·**kot**'·o·me). Surgical incision into the bile duct. **Transduodenal choledochotomy.** The operation of opening into the lower end of the common bile duct from the lumen of the duodenum. [choledochus, Gk *temnein* to cut.]

choledochus (ko·**le**·do·kus). The bile duct. *See* DUCT. [Gk *chole* bile, *dochus* containing.]

choledocography (ko·le·do·**kog**'·raf·e). Radiography of the bile ducts, opacified by a contrast medium, which may be introduced either orally, intravenously or through a drainage tube after choledochostomy. [choledochus, Gk *graphein* to record.]

choledogastrostomy (ko·le·do·gas·**tros**'·to·me). The formation by surgical procedure of a communication between the bile duct and the stomach. [choledochus, Gk *gaster* stomach, *stoma* mouth.]

cholegenetic (ko·le·jen·**et**'·ik). Bile producing. [Gk *chole* bile, *genein* to produce.]

choleglobin (ko·le·**glo**·bin). Name given to a compound intermediate in the formation of bilirubin from haemoglobin by the coupled oxidation with free oxygen of haemoglobin or haemochromogen and oxidizable substances such as ascorbic acid or glutathione. [Gk *chole* bile, haemoglobin.]

cholehaemia (ko·le·**he**·me·ah). Cholaemia.

cholehaemothorax (ko·le·he·mo·**thore**'·ax). A condition in which blood and bile are present in the thorax. [Gk *chole* bile, *haima* blood, thorax.]

choleic (ko·**le**·ik). Derived from or referring to bile. [Gk *chole* bile.]

cholelith (ko·le·lith). A gall-stone. [Gk *chole* bile, *lithos* stone.]

cholelithiasis (ko·le·lith·**i**'·as·is). The condition in which there are gall-stones in the gall bladder or bile duct. [see prec.]

cholelithic (ko·le·**lith**·ik). 1. Caused by gall-stones. 2. Referring to gall-stones. [Gk *chole* bile, *lithos* stone.]

cholelithotomy (ko·le·lith·**ot**'·o·me). The operation of removing gall-stones through an incision into the gall bladder or bile duct. [cholelith, Gk *temnein* to cut.]

cholelithotripsy, cholelithotrity (ko·le·**lith**·o·trip·se, **ko**·le·lith·**ot**'·rit·e). The process of crushing gall-stones. [cholelith, Gk *tribein* to crush.]

cholemesis (ko·**lem**·es·is). The vomiting of bile. [Gk *chole* bile, *emesis* vomiting.]

cholepathia (ko·le·**path**·e·ah). 1. Any disease of a bile duct. 2. Irregularity in contractions of a bile duct. **Cholepathia spastica.** Spasm of a bile duct or bile ducts. [Gk *chole* bile, *pathos* suffering.]

choleperitoneum, choleperitonitis (ko·le·per·e·ton·**e**'·um, ko·le.per·e·ton·**i**'·tis). Occurrence of bile in the peritoneum as a result of rupture of the bile passages. [Gk *chole* bile, peritoneum.]

choleplania (ko·le·**pla**·ne·ah). Jaundice, the result of the presence of bile in the body protoplasm. [Gk *chole* bile, *plane* a wandering.]

cholepoiesis (ko·le·poi·**e**'·sis). The formation or secretion of bile. [Gk *chole* bile, *poiein* to make.]

cholepoietic (ko·le·poi·**et**'·ik). Secreting bile. [see prec.]

choleprasin (ko·le·**pra**·sin). Biliprasin; a light-green pigment which can be extracted from gall-stones. [Gk *chole* bile, *prasaios* leek-green.]

cholepyrrhin (ko·le·**pir**·in). 1. A mixture of bile pigments. 2. Bilirubin. [Gk *chole* bile, *pyrrhos* orange.]

cholera (**kol**·er·ah). Asiatic cholera, cholera orientalis, cholera morbus; a severe infectious epidemic disease due to *Vibrio cholerae,* characterized clinically by violent purgation, vomiting, and collapse. Epidemics occurring since 1964 have been due to the *Vibrio cholerae* biotype *El Tor,* which has almost universally replaced the classical strains of *Vibrio cholerae.* The average case exhibits 3 phases: evacuation, with painless passage of copious motions resembling rice water; the algid stage, with severe collapse; and the reaction stage. Dehydration and suppression of kidney function are prominent features. Treatment depends upon the replacement of water, sodium potassium and bicarbonate, at first by intravenous infusion, later by mouth, together with tetracycline, which is effective against the vibrio. Infected water supplies and flies are important factors in its spread, China and the Ganges Valley being the main endemic sites, and its spread usually follows the pilgrim routes. Preventive inoculation is efficacious in reducing both the mortality and incidence of the disease. **Algid cholera.** Cholera in which the second or collapse stage is severe. **Dry cholera.** Cholera sicca, cholera siderans; cholera in which the patient dies of acute toxaemia before diarrhoea and vomiting have had time to develop. **Cholera infantum.** Summer diarrhoea, acute gastroenteritis of children. It generally occurs in warm weather, is of bacterial or virus origin and is especially apt to occur in bottle-fed infants. It has no connection with true cholera. **Cholera nostras.** Diarrhoea and vomiting due to bacterial food poisoning, usually by organisms of the salmonella group. **Cholera sicca, Cholera siderans.** Dry cholera (see above). **Cholera typhoid.** Cholera in which the febrile reaction stage is prolonged with high continuous fever and great exhaustion. [Gk *chole* bile, *rhein* to flow.]

choleragenic (**kol**·er·ah·**jen**'·ik). Tending to produce or to spread cholera. [cholera, Gk *genein* to produce.]

choleraic (kol·er·**a**·ik). 1. Resembling cholera, or having the characteristics of cholera. 2. Referring to cholera.

choleraphage (kol·er·ah·faje). The bacteriophage of *Vibrio cholerae.*

choleresis (ko·ler·e·sis). The secretion of bile by the liver. [Gk *chole* bile, *eresis* removal.]

choleretic (ko·ler·et·ik). 1. An agent which actively aids the excretion of bile by the liver so that there is a greater flow of bile and greater excretion of biliary constituents. 2. Promoting the excretion of bile by the liver. [see prec.]

choleric (ko·ler·ik). 1. Having an abundance of bile. 2. Irascible in temper or easily excited to anger. [Gk *chole* bile.]

choleriform (kol·er·e·form). Choleroid. [cholera, form.]

cholerigenous (kol·er·ij·en·us). Giving rise to or causing cholera. [cholera, Gk *genein* to produce.]

cholerine (kol·er·een). One of the clinical types of cholera, characterized by sudden severe pain in the abdomen and the passing of many faeculent and rice-water motions. Recovery is rapid. This term is not in common use.

choleroid (kol·er·oid). Resembling cholera. [cholera, Gk *eidos* form.]

choleromania (kol·er·o·ma'·ne·ah). 1. A form of mania which may occur during the course of cholera. 2. Cholerophobia.

cholerophobia (kol·er·o·fo'·be·ah). A morbid dread of falling a victim to cholera. [cholera, phobia.]

cholerrhagia (ko·ler·a·je·ah). 1. Cholera. 2. A copious flow of bile. [Gk *chole* bile, *rhegnynein* to gush forth.]

cholestane (ko·les·tane). $C_{27}H_{48}$, a saturated cyclic hydrocarbon of sterol structure, derived from cholesterol by reduction.

cholestanol (ko·les·tan·ol). β-Cholestanol, $C_{27}H_{47}OH$. A reduction product of cholesterol; isomeric with coprosterol, or normal dihydrocholesterol, which occurs in the lipoids of the faeces.

cholestasia (ko·le·sta·se·ah). Cholestasis.

cholestasis (ko·le·sta·sis). Stasis of bile in the liver and biliary canaliculi. **Familial intrahepatic cholestasis.** A non-fatal disease of children, with steatorrhoea, hepatosplenomegaly and stunted growth. [Gk *chole* bile, *stasis* a standing still.]

cholestatic (ko·le·stat·ik). Referring to or resulting from cholestasis.

cholesteatoma (ko·le·ste·at·o'·mah). 1. A slow-growing intracranial tumour of uncertain origin and often symptomless. It has a glistening appearance and is made up of layers of flat polygonal cells composing a grey and greasy mass of which cholesterol is the basis; the strongly teratoid characteristics are shown in the presence of epithelial cells, hair and certain other constituents of skin. 2. A lesion of the membrane of the middle ear; the mucous membrane becomes tough and skin-like in character and sheds masses of dead epithelium in which cholesterol crystals and fat can be found. Formerly thought to be neoplastic; now regarded as the result of chronic otitis media. **Cholesteatoma verum tympani.** Congenital steatoma of the middle ear. [Gk *chole* bile, *stear* fat, *-oma* tumour.]

cholesteatomatous (ko·le·ste·at·o'·mat·us). 1. Relating to cholesteatoma. 2. Like cholesteatoma in nature, or having its characteristics.

cholesteatosis (ko·le·ste·at·o'·sis). A condition of steatosis arising from the presence of cholesterol esters in an organ or tissues; fatty degeneration. [Gk *chole* bile, *stear* fat, *-osis* condition.]

cholestene (ko·les·teen). $C_{27}H_{46}$, the unsaturated hydrocarbon from which cholesterol is derived.

cholestenone (ko·les·ten·one). $C_{27}H_{44}O$, a ketone obtained when cholesterol is dehydrogenated with copper oxide at 300°C. Reduction yields a saturated hydrocarbon, cholestane, $C_{27}H_{48}$.

cholesteraemia (ko·les·ter·e'·me·ah). Cholesterolaemia.

cholesterase (ko·les·ter·aze). An enzyme that brings about the hydrolysis of cholesterol.

cholesterilins (ko·les·ter·il'·inz). A series of hydrocarbons obtained by the action of sulphuric acid on cholesterol: they are believed to be allied to the terpenes.

cholesterin (ko·les·ter·in). Cholesterol.

cholesterinaemia (ko·les·ter·in·e'·me·ah). Cholesterolaemia.

cholesterinosis (ko·les·ter·in·o'·sis). Cholesterolosis.

cholesterinuria (ko·les·ter·in·ewr'·e·ah). Cholesteroluria.

cholesteroderma, cholesterodermia (ko·les·ter·o·der'·mah, ko·les·ter·o·der'·me·ah). Xanthoderma. [Gk *chole* bile, *stereos* solid, *derma* skin.]

cholesterohistechia (ko·les·ter·o·his·tek'·e·ah). Increase of cholesterol in the tissues. [cholesterol, Gk *histos* tissue, *echein* to hold.]

cholesterohydrothorax (ko·les·ter·o·hi·dro·thore'·ax). A condition in which effused fluid, containing cholesterol crystals, is present in the pleural cavity; a hydrothorax with a concentration of cholesterol.

cholesterol (ko·les·ter·ol). $C_{27}H_{45}OH$, an unsaturated secondary alcohol, one of the large groups of sterols containing the cholane ring. It is a waxy substance present in all cells and appears to be concerned in the biochemical reactions that take place at their surfaces. It occurs in bile, and occasionally forms gall-stones which may be dissolved in chloroform from which it crystallizes in characteristic plates. Its sterol structure relates it to the bile acids, the sex hormones and vitamin D. It takes part in the biosynthesis of steroid hormones and is present in large amounts in the zona fasiculata of the adrenal, where it is formed from acetate and converted into Δ^5-pregnenolone. **Blood cholesterol.** The level of cholesterol in blood, being fairly constant for each individual but showing comparatively wide variation between different individuals. The concentration lies normally between 4 and 6.5 mmol/l (150 and 250 mg per 100 ml) blood, but normal ranges of anything from 2.6 to 7.8 mmol/l (100 to 300 mg) or more have been reported. Greatest variation in disease occurs in the plasma cholesterol level; low concentrations may be found in hyperthyroidism and pernicious anaemia, and high concentrations in coronary arterial disease, lipaemia, nephrosis, hypothyroidism, biliary obstruction and untreated diabetes mellitus. About one-third of the cholesterol in blood is present in the free state, the remainder occurring as esters. [Gk *chole* bile, *stereos* solid.]

cholesterolaemia (ko·les·ter·ol·e'·me·ah). Hypercholesterolaemia; excess of cholesterol in the blood. [cholesterol, Gk *haima* blood.]

cholesterolopoiesis (ko·les·ter·ol·o·poi·e'·sis). Cholesterol synthesis. [cholesterol, Gk *poiesis* production.]

cholesterolosis (ko·les·ter·ol·o'·sis). A condition in which there is an abnormal deposit of cholesterol in the gall bladder as the result of hypercholesterolaemia. **Cholesterolosis cutis.** Xanthomatosis. [cholesterol, Gk *-osis* condition.]

cholesteroluria (ko·les·ter·ol·ewr'·e·ah). A condition in which there is cholesterol in the urine.

cholesterone (ko·les·ter·one). A ketone derived from cholesterol.

cholesterosis (ko·les·ter·o'·sis). Cholesterolosis.

cholesteryl (ko·les·ter·il). The monovalent radical $C_{27}H_{45}$– which occurs in cholesterol.

Cholestyramine (ko·le·sti·ram·een). BP Commission approved name for a styryl-divinylbenzene copolymer (about 2 per cent divinylbenzene) containing quaternary ammonium groups; a resin producing insoluble bile-acid complexes.

choletelin (ko·let·el·in). The end-product formed in Gmelin's reaction in which the bile pigment bilirubin is oxidized by fuming nitric acid. It is a reddish-yellow compound perhaps present when haemoglobin breaks down locally in bruises on the skin. [Gk *chole* bile, *telos* end.]

choletherapy (ko·le·ther·ap·e). The use of bile as a remedy. [Gk *chole* bile, therapy.]

choleuria (ko·le·ewr·e·ah). Choluria.

Cholewa, Erasmus Rudolph (b. 1845). German physician.

Itard-Cholewa sign. Anaesthesia of the tympanic membrane and external auditory meatus in otosclerosis.

choline (ko·leen). Bilineurine, ethylol trimethylammonium hydroxide, $OHCH_2CH_2N(CH_3)_3OH$. An amine base present in the blood, cerebrospinal fluid and urine, and which may be extracted from many of the body tissues, including skeletal and cardiac muscle. It may be formed from lecithin by putrefaction and so may be produced in the bowel. It is often classified as a member of the B complex of vitamins as it commonly occurs together with the other members of this group. Pharmacologically, it has a lipotropic action and disperses fat from the liver or prevents its accumulation in excess. In unphysiological concentrations, it has a stimulant action on intestinal and uterine muscle, and increases the tone of the detrusor urinae; such doses may also cause neuromuscular block. Its ester, acetylcholine, has an important function in the transmission of nerve impulses. Choline is used in therapeutics in the treatment of precirrhotic fatty infiltration of the liver. It has been used in the treatment of infective hepatitis but without conclusive benefit. **Choline acetylase.** The enzyme responsible for the formation of acetylcholine from acetyl CoA and choline. **Choline Salicylate.** BP Commission approved name for the choline salt of salicylic acid; it is used as an analgesic and antipyretic. **Choline Theophyllinate BP 1973.** The choline salt of theophylline, a preparation with the pharmacological actions of theophylline; it is given orally for its bronchodilator effect for the relief of mild asthma. [Gk *chole* bile.]

choline-acetylase (ko·leen·**as**′·et·il·aze). An enzyme concerned in the acetylation of choline, the energy for the endogenous process being provided by adenosine triphosphate.

cholinergic (ko·lin·**er**·jik). Relating to those nerve fibres that have actions similar to those caused by acetylcholine.

cholinesterase (ko·lin·**es**·ter·aze). An enzyme present in the blood and tissues at the endings of voluntary motor nerves and nerves of the parasympathetic division of the involuntary system, which inactivates by hydrolysis the acetylcholine produced there by nerve impulses, and prevents its accumulation.

cholithotomy (ko·lith·**ot**·o·me). Cholelithotomy.

chologenetic (ko·lo·jen·**et**′·ik). Cholegenetic.

chololith (**ko**·lo·lith). Cholelith.

chololithiasis (**ko**·lo·lith·**i**′·as·is). Cholelithiasis.

chololithic (ko·lo·**lith**·ik). Cholelithic.

cholopoiesis (**ko**·lo·poi·**e**′·sis). Cholepoiesis.

choloscopy (ko·**los**·ko·pe). 1. Testing of the function of the biliary system. 2. Examination of the biliary system. [Gk *chole* bile, *skopein* to watch.]

cholosis (ko·**lo**·sis). A disease associated with abnormality of bile secretion. [Gk *chole* bile, *-osis* condition.]

choluria (ko·**lewr**·e·ah). The presence of bile, bile salts or bile pigment in the urine. [Gk *chole* bile, urine.]

chondral (**kon**·dral). 1. In relation to cartilage, or involving it. 2. Cartilaginous. [Gk *chondros* cartilage.]

chondralgia (kon·**dral**·je·ah). A sensation of pain in or around a cartilage; chondrodynia. [Gk *chondros* cartilage, *algos* pain.]

chondralloplasia (**kon**·dral·o·**pla**′·ze·ah). Chondrodysplasia. [Gk *chondros* cartilage, *allos* other, *plassein* to form.]

chondrectomy (kon·**drek**·to·me). Operative removal of cartilage. [Gk *chondros* cartilage, *ektome* a cutting out.]

chondric (**kon**·drik). Chondral.

chondrification (**kon**·drif·ik·**a**′·shun). Conversion into or formation of cartilage. [Gk *chondros* cartilage, L *facere* to make.]

chondrify (**kon**·dre·fi). 1. To become cartilaginous. 2. To convert into cartilages. [see prec.]

chondrigen (**kon**·dre·jen). Chondrogen.

chondrin (**kon**·drin). A scleroprotein mixture which forms the chief constituent of cartilage matrix. It consists of a glycoprotein, chondromucoid, mixed with collagen. [Gk *chondros* cartilage.]

chondriome (**kon**·dre·ome). Mitochondria. [Gk *chondros* cartilage.]

chondriomite (**kon**·dre·o·mite). A filamentous chondriosome. [Gk *chondros* cartilage, *mitos* thread.]

chondriosome (**kon**·dre·o·some). Any one of the granular structures present in the cytoplasm of an animal cell. Cf. MITOCHONDRIA. [Gk *chondros* cartilage, *soma* body.]

chondriosphere (**kon**·dre·o·sfeer). A spherical chondriosome. [Gk *chondros* cartilage, *sphaira* ball.]

chondritis (kon·**dri**·tis). A condition of inflammation in cartilage. **Chondritis intervertebralis calcanea.** Intervertebral calcinosis. *See* CALCINOSIS. [Gk *chondros* cartilage, *-itis* inflammation.]

chondro-adenoma (**kon**·dro·ad·en·**o**′·mah). An adenoma in which there are cartilaginous elements. [Gk *chondros* cartilage, adenoma.]

chondro-albuminoid (**kon**·dro·al·**bew**′·min·oid). A protein occurring as a constituent of the organic matrix of cartilage. It is similar in properties to elastin. [Gk *chondros* cartilage, albuminoid.]

chondro-angioma (**kon**·dro·an·je·**o**′·mah). A neoplasm in which there are the elements of a chondroma and an angioma. [Gk *chondros* cartilage, angioma.]

chondro-arthritis (**kon**·dro·ar·**thri**′·tis). A condition of inflammation in the cartilage of joints. [Gk *chondros* cartilage, arthritis.]

chondroblast (**kon**·dro·blast). In the embryo, a cell of the primitive tissue from which cartilage develops. [Gk *chondros* cartilage, *blastos* germ.]

chondroblastoma (**kon**·dro·blas·**to**′·mah). A tumour with cells which characteristically become like cartilage cells and the sections of which resemble cartilaginous tissue; examples are chondroma and chondrosarcoma. [Gk *chondros* cartilage, *blastos* germ, *-oma* tumour.]

chondrocalcinosis (**kon**·dro·kal·sin·**o**′·sis). Calcification of joints. [Gk *chondros* cartilage, calcinosis.]

chondrocarcinoma (**kon**·dro·kar·sin·**o**′·mah). A carcinoma the framework of which contains cartilaginous elements. [Gk *chondros* cartilage, carcinoma.]

chondrocele (**kon**·dro·seel). A sarcocele in which is found material like cartilage. [Gk *chondros* cartilage, *kele* hernia.]

chondroclasis (kon·dro·**kla**·sis). Crushing of a cartilage. [Gk *chondros* cartilage, *klasis* a breaking.]

chondroclast (**kon**·dro·klast). Any giant cell of the kind that absorbs and removes cartilage. [see prec.]

chondroconia (kon·dro·**kon**·e·ah). Schridde's granules; granules which stain with acid fuchsine dyes, and which have been described in certain lymphocytes and plasma cells. [Gk *chondros* cartilage, *konis* dust.]

chondrocostal (kon·dro·**kos**·tal). In relation to the costal cartilages and the ribs, or involving them. [Gk *chondros* cartilage, L *costa* rib.]

chondrocranium (kon·dro·**kra**·ne·um). In the development of the skull in the embryo, the cartilaginous structure that is the forerunner of ossification. [Gk *chondros* cartilage, *kranion* skull.]

chondrocutaneous (**kon**·dro·kew·**ta**′·ne·us). Referring to cartilage and skin, e.g. a chondrocutaneous graft. [Gk *chondros* cartilage, L *cutis* skin.]

chondrocyte (**kon**·dro·site). A mature cartilage cell. **Isogenous chondrocyte.** One of a group of 2, 4, or 8 similar cells which have all been derived from the subdivision of a single precursor cell, and which lie close together within a common capsule of basophilic matrix. [Gk *chondros* cartilage, *kytos* cell.]

Chondrodendron (kon·dro·**den**·dron). A genus of South American plants of the family Menispermaceae. *Chondrodendron tomentosum*, Ruiz et Pav. (Pereira, Pereira Brava), yields the alkaloid, D-tubocurarine, which has the pharmacological activity of curare. [Gk *chondros* cartilage, *dendron* tree.]

chondrodermatitis (**kon**·dro·der·mat·**i**′·tis). Inflammation of a cartilage. **Chondrodermatitis nodularis chronica helicis.** The condition in which a nodular growth develops on the helix of the ear. [Gk *chondros* cartilage, dermatitis.]

chondrodynia (**kon**·dro·**din**·e·ah). Pain affecting a cartilage or the area around it. [Gk *chondros* cartilage, *odyne* pain.]

chondrodysplasia (**kon**·dro·dis·**pla**′·ze·ah). Dyschondroplasia. **Hereditary deforming chondrodysplasia.** Hereditary multiple ossifying ecchondromata. **Unilateral chondrodysplasia.** One of the 3 clinical conditions included under the term dyschondroplasia. The condition, the distribution of which is usually unilateral, occurs in children and may be familial. [Gk *chondros* cartilage, dysplasia.]

chondrodystrophia, chondrodystrophy (**kon**·dro·dis·**tro**′·fe·ah, kon·dro·**dis**·tro·fe). Anomalies of bone due to faulty growth of endochondral bone, apparently hereditary but not sex-linked.

Chondrodystrophia calcificans congenita. Stippled epiphyses and perhaps calcified costal cartilages and trachea, spots of calcification in the carpus and tarsus, and short limbs; it may cause asphyxiating thoracic dystrophy. Of variable inheritance. **Chondrodystrophia congenita punctata.** Dwarfism with underdeveloped long bones, cataracts and a red, scaly skin. **Chondrodystrophia fetalis.** Achondroplasia, a disturbance of endochondral bone formation which may originate at various periods of early intra-uterine life and results in a dwarf with short, bowed extremities and a depressed nose bridge; full growth of the trunk takes place however, and sex and mental development are normal. **Chondrodystrophia hyperplastica.** Multiple cartilaginous exostoses, a variety of chondrodystrophia in which cartilage forms large, nodular, poorly ossified projections at the ends of bones. **Chondrodystrophia hypoplastica.** A variety of chondrodystrophia in which the cartilage is under-developed and unable to proliferate. **Chondrodystrophia malacia.** Chondromalacia fetalis. [Gk *chondros* cartilage, dystrophy.]

chondro-ectodermal (**kon**·dro·ek·to·**der**′·mal). Describing those cartilaginous elements of the branchial skeleton which have apparently been derived from the neural crest of the head region, and hence are ectodermal in origin. **Chondro-ectodermal dysplasia** (Ellis van Creveld syndrome). Chondrodystrophy with ectodermal deformities such as polydactyly, short tibia, dysplasia of the teeth, sparse hair growth and congenital malformations of the heart and sweat glands. [Gk *chondros* cartilage, ectoderm.]

chondro-endothelioma (**kon**·dro·en·do·the·le·**o**′·mah). An endothelioma in which there are cartilaginous elements. [Gk *chondros* cartilage, endothelioma.]

chondro-epiphyseal (**kon**·dro·ep·e·**fiz**′·e·al). Relating to the epiphyseal cartilages. [Gk *chondros* cartilage, epiphysis.]

chondro-epiphysitis (**kon**·dro·ep·e·fiz·**i**′·tis). A condition of inflammation of the epiphyses and cartilaginous portions of bone. [Gk *chondros* cartilage, epiphysitis.]

chondrofibroma (**kon**·dro·fi·**bro**′·mah). A chondroma which contains fibrous elements. [Gk *chondros* cartilage, fibroma.]

chondrogen (**kon**·dro·jen). 1. Cartilagin, changed by boiling into chondrin. 2. A substance which, in embryonic and early life, is a component of the tissue of developing cartilage or of corneal tissue. [Gk *chondros* cartilage, *genein* to produce.]

chondrogenesis (kon·dro·**jen**·es·is). The process of forming cartilage. [see foll.]

chondrogenetic (**kon**·dro·jen·**et**′·ik). 1. Producing or forming cartilage. 2. Referring to chondrogenesis. [Gk *chondros* cartilage, *genein* to produce.]

chondrogenous (kon·**droj**·en·us). Giving rise to cartilage. [see prec.]

chondroglossus muscle [musculus chondroglossus NA] (kon·dro·**glos**·us). A slip of muscle, closely associated with the hyoglossus, arising from the lesser cornu of the hyoid and inserted into the tongue. [Gk *chondros* cartilage, *glossa* tongue.]

chondroglucose (**kon**·dro·**gloo**′·kose). A monosaccharide obtained by the hydrolytic splitting of chondrin.

chondroid (**kon**·droid). 1. Resembling cartilage in structure. 2. Amyloid. [Gk *chondros* cartilage, *eidos* form.]

chondroitic (kon·dro·**it**·ik). 1. Referring to cartilage. 2. Like cartilage. 3. Derived from cartilage. [Gk *chondros* cartilage.]

chondroitin sulphate (kon·**dro**·it·in **sul**·fate). A mucoid substance which may be obtained from cartilage. It is a polysaccharide, composed of glycuronic acid and chondrosamine units esterified with sulphuric acid. [Gk *chondros* cartilage.]

chondroituria (**kon**·dro·it·**ewr**′·e·ah). A condition in which there is chondroitic acid in the urine.

chondrolipoma (**kon**·dro·lip·o′·mah). A neoplasm in which there are elements of cartilaginous and fatty tissue. [Gk *chondros* cartilage, lipoma.]

chondrolysis (kon·**drol**·is·is). The destruction of cartilaginous tissue which takes place during the process of calcification. [Gk *chondros* cartilage, *lysis* a loosing.]

chondroma (kon·**dro**·mah) (pl. *chondromata*). A neoplasm composed of cartilaginous tissue. **External chondroma.** Perichondroma. **Multiple chondromata.** One of the 3 clinical conditions included under the heading dyschondroplasia; firm, rounded, elastic swellings appear in the fingers and toes in childhood and increase in size over a number of years; the condition is rare. **Chondroma sarcomatosum.** Chondrosarcoma. [Gk *chondros* cartilage, *-oma* tumour.]

chondromalacia (**kon**·dro·mal·**a**′·she·ah). A condition of abnormal softness of cartilage. **Chondromalacia auris.** Haematoma auris. **Chondromalacia fetalis.** A form of achondrodysplasia in which the limbs of the fetus, which is stillborn, are pliable and flabby because the epiphyseal cartilage is soft. **Chondromalacia patellae.** Focal degeneration of the articular cartilage of the patella. [Gk *chondros* cartilage, *malakia* softness.]

chondromatosis (**kon**·dro·mat·**o**′·sis). Multiple chondromata affecting the hands and feet. The disease, which is a form of dyschondroplasia, begins in childhood. Spontaneous fracture may occur and sarcoma may supervene. **Synovial chondromatosis.** A rare condition in which cartilage is formed in the synovial membranes of the joints, tendon sheaths or bursa, by metaplasia of the connective tissue beneath the surface of the membrane. Some metaplastic foci on the surface of the membrane may become sessile, and then pedunculated, and finally become detached, producing a number of loose bodies. [Gk *chondros* cartilage, *-oma* tumour, *-osis* condition.]

See also: REICHEL (F. P.).

chondromatous (kon·**dro**·mat·us). Having the characteristics of or relating to chondroma or cartilage.

chondromitome (kon·**dro**·mit·ome). Paranucleus. [Gk *chondros* cartilage, *mitos* thread.]

chondromucin, chondromucoid (kon·dro·**mew**·sin, kon·dro·**mew**·koid). The characteristic ground substance of cartilage, consisting of polymerized chondroitin sulphate bound to a protein. It is identified by its intense metachromatic reaction with certain basic dyes such as methylene blue or toluidine blue in very dilute solution. [Gk *chondros* cartilage, mucus.]

chondromyoma (**kon**·dro·mi·**o**′·mah). A mixed tumour combining the elements of chondroma and myoma.

chondromyxoma (**kon**·dro·mix·**o**′·mah). A mixed tumour combining the elements of chondroma and myxoma.

chondromyxosarcoma (**kon**·dro·mix·o·sar·**ko**′·mah). A mixed tumour in which there are elements of chondroma, myxoma and sarcoma.

chondro-osseous (kon·dro·**os**·e·us). Made up of cartilage and bone. [Gk *chondros* cartilage, *osteon* bone.]

chondro-osteoarthritis (**kon**·dro·os·te·o·ar·**thri**′·tis). Osteoarthritis involving also the cartilage of the joint. [Gk *chondros* cartilage, osteoarthritis.]

chondro-osteodystrophy (**kon**·dro·os·te·o·**dis**′·tro·fe). A rare deformity of the epiphyses leading to dwarfism with dorsolumbar kyphosis, pigeon-breast deformity and limitation of extension of the hips and knees. Brailsford–Morquio disease. [Gk *chondros* cartilage, osteodystrophy.]

chondro-osteoma (**kon**·dro·os·te·**o**′·mah). Exostosis multiplex cartilaginea. [Gk *chondros* cartilage, osteoma.]

chondropathology (**kon**·dro·path·**ol**′·o·je). The pathology of cartilage. [Gk *chondros* cartilage, pathology.]

chondropathy (kon·**drop**·ath·e). Any disease affecting cartilage. [Gk *chondros* cartilage, *pathos* suffering.]

chondropharyngeus (**kon**·dro·far·**in**′·je·us). The part of the middle constrictor muscle of the pharynx which arises from the lesser horn of the hyoid bone. [Gk *chondros* cartilage, pharynx.]

chondrophyma (kon·dro·**fi**·mah). 1. A tumour based on a cartilage. 2. Chondrophyte. 3. A tumour containing cartilaginous elements. [Gk *chondros* cartilage, *phyma* growth.]

chondrophyte (**kon**·dro·fite). A fungus-like growth springing from the articular cartilage of bone. [Gk *chondros* cartilage, *phyton* growth.]

chondroplast (**kon**·dro·plast). Chondroblast. [Gk *chondros* cartilage, *plassein* to form.]

chondroplastic (kon·dro·plas·tik). Referring to chondroplasty.

chondroplasty (kon·dro·plas·te). 1. The replacement of displaced or the repair of torn cartilage. 2. The act of performing plastic operations on cartilage. [Gk *chondros* cartilage, *plassein* to form.]

chondroporosis (kon·dro·po·ro'·sis). A porous condition of cartilage, to be noted normally during the period of ossification in the growing bone, and shown in thinning of cartilage and formation of spaces and sinuses. [Gk *chondros* cartilage, *poros* passage.]

chondroprotein (kon·dro·pro·te·in). A general term for the proteins of cartilage, of which chondromucoid is a typical example. [Gk *chondros* cartilage, protein.]

chondrosamine (kon·dro·sam·een). Aminogalactose, $CH_2OH(CHOH)_3CHNH_2CHO$. The prosthetic group of a glycoprotein present in cartilage.

chondrosarcoma (kon·dro·sar·ko'·mah). A sarcoma with incorporation of cartilaginous elements; growth is usually rapid. [Gk *chondros* cartilage, sarcoma.]

chondrosarcomatosis (kon·dro·sar·ko·mat·o'·sis). A condition in which multiple chondrosarcomata form. [chondrosarcoma, Gk *-osis* condition.]

chondrosarcomatous (kon·dro·sar·ko'·mat·us). Relating to or of the nature of chondrosarcoma.

chondroseptum (kon·dro·sep·tum). The part of the septum of the nose which is cartilaginous in type. [Gk *chondros* cartilage, L *septum* partition.]

chondrosidin (kon·dro·sid·in). A hyalin derived from chondrosin.

chondrosin (kon·dro·sin). $C_{12}H_{21}O_{11}N$, a substance produced during the hydrolysis of chondroitin sulphate, and which in turn hydrolyses to chondrosamine and glucuronic acid.

chondrosis (kon·dro·sis). 1. The forming of cartilage. 2. A neoplasm of cartilaginous type. [Gk *chondros* cartilage.]

chondroskeleton (kon·dro·skel·et·on). A cartilaginous skeleton. [Gk *chondros* cartilage, skeleton.]

chondrosome (kon·dro·some). The granular form of mitochondria. [Gk *chondros* cartilage, *soma* body.]

chondrosternal (kon·dro·ster·nal). Relating to costal cartilage and the sternum, or affecting them. [Gk *chondros* cartilage, *sternon* chest.]

chondrotome (kon·dro·tome). A strong scalpel-shaped knife for cutting cartilage. [Gk *chondros* cartilage, *temnein* to cut.]

chondrotomy (kon·drot·o·me). The dissection or cutting of cartilages. [see prec.]

chondroxiphoid (kon·dro·zif·oid). Relating to the xiphoid cartilage. [Gk *chondros* cartilage, *xiphos* sword, *eidos* form.]

Chondrus BPC 1959 (kon·drus). Carrageen, carragheen, Irish moss; the dried alga *Chondrus crispus* Stackh. (family Gigartinaceae), coming chiefly from the coasts of N.W. Ireland, Britanny and Massachusetts. It is a brownish-purple substance (creamy-yellow when bleached), consisting mainly of two substances corresponding to the formula $R(OSO_2O)_2Ca$, where R is a carbohydrate complex. It is used as a demulcent, as an emulgent for cod-liver oil and other oils, in the preparation of nutrient jellies and for various technical purposes as a gum substitute. [Gk *chondros* cartilage.]

chonechondrosternon (ko·ne·kon·dro·ster'·non). Funnel chest. *See* CHEST. [Gk *chone* funnel, chondrosternal.]

Chopart, François (b. 1743). Paris surgeon.

Chopart's amputation, or operation. Amputation through the midtarsal joint.

Chopart's joint. The transverse tarsal joint. *See* JOINT.

Chopra, Sir Ram Nath (b. 1882). Calcutta physician and pharmacologist.

Chopra's test. Antimony test. *See* TEST.

chorangioma (kor·an·je·o'·mah). Chorio-angioma.

chord (kord). Cord.

chorda (kord·ah). 1. Name applied to any cord-like structure, e.g. a tendon, or nerve filament. 2. The notochord. **Chorda anteriarum umbilicalium.** The obliterated umbilical artery. **Chorda dorsalis.** The notochord. **Chorda gubernaculum.** A fibromuscular band, found in the inguinal region of the embryo, which is connected to the lower pole of the testis or ovary and which gives rise to the lower parts of the gubernaculum testis and the round ligament of the uterus respectively. **Hippocratic chorda.** The tendo calcaneus. **Chorda magna.** An obsolete term for the tendo calcaneus. **Chorda Resorbilis Aseptica.** *European Pharmacopoeia* name for Sterilised Surgical Catgut BP 1973. **Chorda spermatica.** The spermatic cord. *See* CORD. **Chorda spinalis.** The spinal cord. *See* CORD. **Chordae tendineae [NA].** The fine fibrous ligaments by which the free margins and ventricular surfaces of the cusps of the mitral and tricuspid valves are attached to the papillary muscles and the ventricular walls of the heart. **Chorda tympani [NA].** A branch of the facial nerve which crosses the tympanic membrane and eventually supplies secretomotor fibres to the submandibular and sublingual glands, and special sensory (taste) fibres to the anterior two-thirds of the tongue. **Chorda umbilicalis.** The umbilical cord. *See* CORD. **Chorda vertebralis.** The notochord. **Chordae vocales.** The vocal folds of the larynx. [L, from Gk *chorde* string.]

chordal (kord·al). Relating to any cord or sinew, particularly the notochord.

chordamesoblast (kord·ah·mez·o·blast). The cells on the surface of the ovum before gastrulation which will later be invaginated at the blastopore or primitive streak to give rise to the chordamesoderm, from which the notochord and mesoderm of the embryo are differentiated. [Gk *chorde* string, *mesos* middle, *blastos* germ.]

chordamesoderm (kord·ah·mez·o·derm). The cells of the chordamesoblast after gastrulation but before they have clearly separated into notochord and mesoderm. [Gk *chorde* string, *mesos* middle, *derma* skin.]

Chordata (kord·a·tah). A phylum of the animal kingdom which contains all animals which have, at some stage in their life history, a dorsal notochord. All Craniata as well as such forms as Hemichorda (*Amphioxus*) and Urochorda (sea squirts) belong to it. [Gk *chorde* string.]

chordate (kord·ate). In zoology, having a notochord; a member of the phylum Chordata.

chordectomy (kord·ek·to·me). Cordectomy.

chordee (kord·a). A painful erection of the penis, which becomes bent laterally or downwards. The condition is a rare complication of gonorrhoea and is caused by inflammation in the corpus spongiosum or corpora cavernosa. [Fr *cordé* fastened with a cord.]

chorditis (kord·i·tis). A condition of inflammation of a vocal cord. **Chorditis cantorum.** Inflammation of the vocal cords of singers. **Chorditis fibrinosa.** Acute laryngitis with fibrinous deposits on the vocal cords, which in addition show erosion. **Chorditis nodosa, Chorditis tuberosa.** A condition affecting professional voice users, in which a small nodule may appear on one or both cords, usually at the junction of the anterior middle third of the cord. **Chorditis vocalis inferior.** Chronic laryngitis affecting mainly the undersurface of the vocal cords. [Gk *chorde* string, *-itis* inflammation.]

chordoblastoma (kord·o·blas·to'·mah). A neoplasm composed of cells which tend to acquire the characteristics of the cells of the notochord. [Gk *chorde* string, blastoma.]

chordocarcinoma (kord·o·kar·sin·o'·mah). Chordoma. [Gk *chorde* string, carcinoma.]

chordo-epithelioma (kord·o·ep·e·the·le·o'·mah). Chordoma. [Gk *chorde* string, epithelioma.]

chordoid (kord·oid). Having resemblance to the notochord. [Gk *chorde* string, *eidos* form.]

chordoma (kord·o·mah). 1. A neoplasm made up of notochordal tissue. 2. A small malignant neoplasm composed of notochordal tissue, which may occur at the union of the occipital with the sphenoid bone. 3. A term applied by Virchow to the upper portion of a persisting notochord. [Gk *chorde* string, *-oma* tumour.]

chordopexy (kord·o·pex·e). The operative treatment of laryngeal stenosis by displacement outwards of the vocal folds. [Gk *chorde* string, *pexis* fixation.]

chordotomy (kord·ot·o·me). Surgical division of any cord, e.g. an anterolateral column of the spinal cord for the relief of intractable pain. **Mesencephalic chordotomy.** Surgical division of nerve tracts in the mid-brain. [Gk *chorde* string, *temnein* to cut.]

chordurethritis (kord·ewr·e·thri'·tis). Chordee. [Gk *chorde* string, urethritis.]

chorea (ko·re·ah). Acute chorea; Sydenham's chorea. A disease chiefly affecting children and characterized by irregular involuntary movements of the limbs and face, commonest between the ages of 5 and 15 years and occurring in females more frequently than in males. It is often associated with signs of acute endocarditis and with symptoms or history of rheumatism. Some emotional instability may be exhibited, occasionally in very severe form as far as actual mania. Many so-called choreas are of hysterical or functional type (e.g. epidemic chorea, laryngeal chorea, chorea nutans), and do not come strictly under the definition; some are occupational neuroses (e.g. local chorea, chorea scriptorum), whilst others are of a different pathology altogether, such as paralysis agitans or hemiplegic (vascular) phenomena. **Chronic progressive hereditary chorea.** A rare condition seen in families, beginning after the age of 40. The symptoms are very similar to those of acute chorea but are accompanied by progressive mental degeneration. It is also called *Huntington's chorea* or simply *chronic chorea.* Sporadic cases with no familial association are also seen, the condition being then known as *chronic progressive non-hereditary chorea.* **Degenerative chorea.** Chronic progressive chorea (see preceding). **Chorea dimidiata.** Hemichorea. **Electrical chorea.** A variety of chorea minor in which the movements are very violent; an epidemic disease possibly related to encephalitis. Also called *Bergeron's disease, Dubini's disease.* **Epidemic chorea.** Choreomania. **Chorea festinans.** Paralysis agitans. **Chorea gravidarum.** Chorea seen in pregnancy. **Chorea gravis.** A severe form of chorea in which deglutition is difficult and the patient gets insufficient nourishment. His movements are ceaseless, so that he suffers from loss of rest and sleep. **Hemilateral chorea.** Hemichorea. **Hereditary chorea.** Chronic progressive hereditary chorea (see above). **Chorea insaniens.** Chorea associated with mental symptoms, and occasionally seen in pregnancy. **Laryngeal chorea.** Spasmodic involvement of the laryngeal muscles. **Limp chorea.** Limb paralysis sometimes seen in severe chorea. **Maniacal chorea.** Chorea insaniens (see above). **Chorea minor.** Symptoms of a mild degree in Sydenham's chorea. **Chorea mollis.** A condition of chorea in which paralytic symptoms occur; limp chorea (see above). **Chorea nocturna.** Choreic movements during sleep. **Chorea nutans.** Chorea with rhythmic nodding. **One-sided chorea.** Hemichorea. **Paralytic chorea.** Choreic hemiplegia; limp chorea (see above). **Posthemiplegic chorea.** Apoplectic chorea. **Procursive chorea.** Paralysis agitans. **Rhythmic chorea.** A form of chorea in which the movements are rhythmical and repeated; it is usually a hysterical condition. **Chorea scriptorum.** Writer's cramp. **Simple chorea.** Sydenham's chorea, ordinary acute chorea. [Gk *choreia* dance.]

See also: HUNTINGTON, SYDENHAM.

choreal, choreatic, choreic (ko·re·al, ko·re·at·ik, ko·re·ik). 1. Having relation or reference to chorea. 2. Of the nature of or having the characteristics of chorea. 3. Caused by chorea.

choreiform (ko·re·e·form). Similar in type to chorea. [chorea, form.]

choremania (ko·re·ma'·ne·ah). Choreomania.

choreo-athetoid (ko·re·o·ath'·et·oid). Relating to or resembling choreo-athetosis. [chorea, athetosis, Gk *eidos* form.]

choreo-athetosis (ko·re·o·ath·et·o'·sis). A nervous condition, the characteristic signs of which are choreic and athetoid movements.

choreoid (ko·re·oid). Choreiform. [chorea, Gk *eidos* form.]

choreomania (ko·re·o·ma'·ne·ah). Epidemic chorea; the hysterical dancing mania of the Middle Ages. [chorea, mania.]

choreophrasia (ko·re·o·fra'·ze·ah). A nervous condition characterized by the repetition of incomplete and meaningless phrases. [Gk *choreia* dance, *phrasein* to utter.]

chorial (ko·re·al). Chorionic.

chorio-adenoma (ko·re·o·ad·en·o'·mah). A tumour of the chorion, adenomatous in type and destructive to the placenta. It frequently becomes malignant, involving the uterine wall and spreading to the liver and lungs. A variety is sometimes found in males, arising from teratoma of the testicle.

chorio-allantois (ko·re·o·al·an'·to·is). Chorio-allantoic membrane; the outer embryonic membrane in a fertile egg immediately below the shell and shell membrane upon which some viruses can be grown.

chorio-angiofibroma (ko·re·o·an·je·o·fi·bro'·mah). Angiofibroma of the chorion.

chorio-angioma (ko·re·o·an·je·o'·mah). Angiomatous neoplasm of the chorion.

chorio-angiopagus (ko·re·o·an·je·op'·ag·us). Uniovular twins. **Chorio-angiopagus parasiticum.** Omphalosite. [chorion, Gk *aggeion* vessel, *pagos* fixed.]

chorioblastoma (ko·re·o·blas·to'·mah). Chorionepithelioma. [chorion, blastoma.]

chorioblastosis (ko·re·o·blas·to'·sis). 1. Hypertrophy of the chorion. 2. Any anomaly or overgrowth of the chorion and the underlying connective tissue. [chorion, Gk *blastos* germ.]

choriocapillaris (ko·re·o·kap·il·a'·ris). In the vascular coat of the eye, the choriocapillary lamina or inner vascular layer of the choroid. [Gk *chorion* a skin, L *capillus* hair.]

choriocarcinoma (ko·re·o·kar·sin·o'·mah). Chorionepithelioma. [chorion, carcinoma.]

choriocele (ko·re·o·seel). A choroidal herniation through the scleral envelope of the globe. [Gk *chorion* a skin, *kele* hernia.]

chorio-epithelioma (ko·re·o·ep·e·the·le·o'·mah). Chorionepithelioma. **Chorio-epithelioma malignum.** Syncytioma malignum.

choriogenesis (ko·re·o·jen'·es·is). Development of the chorion. [chorion, Gk *genein* to produce.]

chorioid (ko·re·oid). 1. Resembling the chorion. 2. Choroid. [Gk *chorion* a skin, *eidos* form.]

chorioidea (ko·re·oid·e·ah). Choroid.

chorioiditis (ko·re·oid·i'·tis). Choroiditis.

chorioidoretinitis (ko·re·oid·o·ret·in·i'·tis). Choroidoretinitis.

chorio-iritis (ko·re·o·i·ri'·tis). Inflammation of the choroid and iris. [choroid, iris, Gk *-itis* inflammation.]

chorioma (ko·re·o·mah). Chorionepithelioma.

choriomeningitis (ko·re·o·men·in·ji'·tis). Inflammation of the cerebral membranes with cellular infiltration of the meninges and infiltration of lymphocytes into the choroid plexuses. **Benign lymphatic choriomeningitis.** Armstrong's disease; generally a mild lymphocytic meningitis due to an arenovirus which normally infects mice and is rarely transmitted to man. Other forms of neurological or systemic disease may be seen. **Lymphocytic choriomeningitis.** A benign or inapparent virus infection of wild mice which may occasionally be transmitted to man, in whom it causes an acute febrile illness varying in severity from an influenza-like infection to an acute meningitis, rarely a meningo-encephalitis. The causative virus is an arenovirus. [Gk *chorion* a skin, meningitis.]

chorion (ko·re·on). The double-layered nutritive envelope which protects and covers the fertilized ovum, and within which the yolk sac lies. **Chorion frondosum.** The outer surface of the chorion, the villi of which are in contact with the decidua basalis; it constitutes the placental area. **Chorion laeve.** The smooth membranous surface which develops on that part in contact with the decidua capsularis when the villi have disappeared owing to lack of circulation as the amniotic cavity expands; it is not concerned in the formation of the placenta. **Shaggy chorion.** Chorion frondosum (see above). **Smooth chorion.** Chorion laeve (see above). [Gk a skin.]

chorionepithelioma (ko·re·on·ep·e·the·le·o'·mah). A neoplasm of the chorion which develops as a result of cystic degeneration and malignant epithelial proliferation of the chorionic villi. The condition is characterized by rapid increase in the size of the uterus, haemorrhage and the discharge of bloody clots containing whitish cysts. **Chorionepithelioma of the ovary.** *See* TERATOMA. [chorion, epithelioma.]

chorionic (ko·re·**on**·ik). Referring to the chorion.

chorionitis (**ko**·re·on·**i**'·tis). 1. A condition of inflammation of the corium, resulting in sclerodermia. 2. Placentitis. [Gk *chorion* a skin, *-itis* inflammation.]

chorioplacental (ko·re·o·plas·**en**'·tal). Relating to the chorion and the placenta.

chorioplaque (**ko**·re·o·plak). A multinuclear giant cell found in cellular infiltrations of the skin. [Gk *chorion* a skin, Fr. *plaque* slab.]

Chorioptes (ko·re·**op**'·teez). A genus of sarcoptid mites. *Chorioptes symbiotes* var. *bovis*, found on the legs of horses and cattle, has been recorded rarely from human heads. It causes few symptoms. [Gk *chorion* a skin, *optos* visible.]

chorioptosis (**ko**·re·op·**to**'·sis). Chorioptic sarcoptidosis; infestation with *Chorioptes. Chorioptes symbiotes* var. *bovis* has been found on human heads, but causes few symptoms. [*Chorioptes*, Gk *-osis* condition.]

chorioretinitis (ko·re·o·ret·in·**i**'·tis). Choroidoretinitis.

chorisis (**kor**·i·sis). In biology, the development of 2 or more members in place of the normal one. [Gk separation.]

chorista (kor·is·tah). A state of defective development characterized or resulting from separation or misplacement of the anlage. [Gk *choristos* separated.]

choristoblastoma (kor·is·to·blas·**to**'·mah). An autonomous neoplasm originating in a choristoma. [Gk *choristos* separated, blastoma.]

choristoma (kor·is·**to**·mah). A neoplasm developing as a result of aberrant anlage. [Gk *choristos* separated, *-oma* tumour.]

choroid [choroidea (NA)] (**kor**·oid). The main part of the vascular coat of the eye, lining the sclera and composed of 2 main layers, the suprachoroid lamina, and the choroid proper, the latter being further divisible into an outer layer of small vessels, and an inner capillary layer. **Choroid plexus.** *See* PLEXUS. [Gk *chorion* a skin, *eidos* form.]

choroid artery [arteria choroidea (NA)] . A branch of the internal carotid artery which runs backward between the uncus and optic tract to enter the inferior horn of the lateral ventricle. It supplies adjoining regions of the brain, including parts of the optic pathway before terminating in the choroid plexus of the lateral ventricle.

choroid vein [vena choroidea (NA)]. A vein draining the choroid plexus of the lateral ventricle of the brain.

choroidal (kor·**oid**·al). Having relation to the choroid.

choroidea (kor·**oid**·e·ah). Choroid.

choroidectomy (kor·oid·**ek**·to·me). Surgical removal of the choroid plexus in the lateral ventricle. [choroid, Gk *ektome* excision.]

choroideremia (**kor**·oid·er·**e**'·me·ah). Familial progressive choroidal atrophy, a sex-linked disorder fully developed in males but with minimal signs in females. Initially, there is night blindness and contracted fields. Central vision is not lost until middle age or later. [choroid, Gk *eremia* absence.]

choroiditis (kor·oid·i·tis). Inflammation of the choroid, but often applied to degenerative conditions. Since the retina is in close apposition, it is nearly always involved in the process, and it is customary therefore to use the term *choroidoretinitis;* if the inflammation spreads forward to involve the iris and ciliary body the condition is described as *uveitis.* The term *iridochoroiditis* is seen sometimes, but it is unlikely that the ciliary body should be unaffected. The classification of choroiditis is difficult because the reaction of the choroid to various noxa is often non-specific: where possible, the aetiological factor is used; in other cases the description is morphological, geographical, or eponymous bearing the name of the discoverer. **Anterior choroiditis.** Choroiditis occurring in the peripheral part of the fundus; usually syphilitic and often found in cases of interstitial keratitis. **Areolar choroiditis, Areolar central choroiditis.** A form, often binocular, which attacks the posterior pole of the fundus in the young. Foci are at first pigmented, closely set and coalescent, with the pigment gradually absorbed. It may be caused by infarction of the choriocapillaris. **Central choroiditis.** A generic term describing choroiditis affecting the posterior pole of the eye and often involving the macula. It is particularly applied to the form of choroiditis occurring in childhood with nystagmus and arrested mental development, or to choroiditis which is a complication of pregnancy toxaemia. **Diffuse choroiditis.** An exudative inflammation spreading over the choroid, caused usually by syphilis or tuberculosis but may also occur in acute illness, e.g. measles, as the result of focal infection or from no known cause; rare. **Disseminated choroiditis.** Numerous foci of inflammation scattered over the fundus and producing characteristic scars: the commonest cause is syphilis. **Exudative choroiditis.** A generic term applied to the various forms of choroiditis in which an exudate occurs. **Metastatic choroiditis.** Choroiditis due to metastatic bacterial emboli, e.g. syphilis, tuberculosis and pyaemia. **Myopic choroiditis.** A term applied to the degenerative changes consequent upon stretching of the choroid in progressive myopia. **Senile guttate choroiditis.** A term applied to localized thickening of Bruch's membrane in the region of the macula, producing so-called *colloid* or *drüsen bodies* often unassociated with defect of vision. **Serous choroiditis.** A term applied at one time to forms of non-purulent choroiditis in which there was no plastic exudate. **Suppurative choroiditis.** A suppurative process originating in the choroid or transferred to it from neighbouring structures. It may go on to panophthalmitis and shrinkage or loss of the eye. The infection may be endogenous or exogenous (traumatic). [choroid, Gk *-itis* inflammation.]

See also: DOYNE, FOERSTER (R.), HUTCHINSON, TAY.

choroidocyclitis (kor·**oid**·o·si·**kli**'·tis). A condition of inflammation of the choroid of the vascular coat and the ciliary processes of the eyeball. [choroid, cyclitis.]

choroido-iritis (kor·**oid**·o·i·**ri**'·tis). A condition of inflammation of the choroid of the vascular coat and of the iris. [choroid, iritis.]

choroidoretinitis (kor·**oid**·o·ret·in·**i**'·tis). A condition of inflammation of the choroid coat and the retina of the eye. [choroid, retinitis.]

See also: JENSEN (E. Z.).

chorology (ko·**rol**·o·je). The science which treats of the geographical distribution of organisms. [Gk *chora* land, *logos* science.]

choromania (kor·o·**ma**·ne·ah). A nervous condition marked by morbid desire to dance or make rhythmic movements. [Gk *choros* dance, mania.]

choronosologia (**ko**·ro·no·so·**lo**'·je·ah). 1. The science of the geographical distribution of the organisms of disease. 2. The science of the endemicity of disease. [Gk *chora* land, *nosos* disease, *logos* science.]

chortosterol (kor·to·**steer**·ol). A sterol found in grass. [Gk *chortos* grass, sterol.]

Christensen's culture medium. A medium prepared from peptone 1 g, sodium chloride 5 g, monopotassium phosphate 2 g, dextrose 1 g, phenol red 0.012 g, agar 20 g, distilled water 1 litre. To this is added 100 ml of a 20 per cent watery solution of urea.

Christian, Henry Asbury (b. 1876). Boston physician.

Christian syndrome, Christian-Schueller disease, Schueller-Christian disease. Hand-Schueller-Christian disease, or syndrome (see below).

Hand-Schueller-Christian disease, or syndrome. Xanthomatosis; a non-familial disturbance of lipoid (cholesterol) metabolism seen in young children, characterized by slight anaemia, defects in membranous bone, mainly skull, exophthalmos, diabetes insipidus, often with dwarfism, and a yellowish-brown colour (xanthomatosis) of the skin. Sometimes the liver, spleen and glands are enlarged to a moderate degree.

Letterer-Christian disease. The provisional name given to a group of diseases that includes Hand-Schueller-Christian, Letterer-Siwe, and Jaffe-Lichtenstein diseases. *Histiocytosis X* has also been suggested as a name.

Christian-Weber disease. Nodular, pyrexial, non-suppurative panniculitis.

Christiansen, Johanne Ostenfeld (b. 1882). Copenhagen physician.

Christiansen's method. A method of preparing the tubes of coagulated egg albumin used in Mett's method of determining peptic activity.

Christmas. The name of the patient whose case was the first recorded example of the disease named after him (see below).

Christmas disease. A hereditary bleeding disease affecting males and rarely females, and very closely resembling haemophilia in clinical and genetic features and in the reaction of the blood to the usual laboratory tests for haemophilia. It differs from haemophilia in that the blood contains the anti-haemophilic globulin in normal amounts but does not contain a serum factor (termed the Christmas factor) which is present in haemophilic blood.

Christmas factor, Christmas serum factor. A factor present in blood serum and necessary for normal blood thromboplastin formation. It is deficient or absent in Christmas disease. This Christmas factor is obtained readily from serum, and closely resembles Factor VII of Koller.

Christophers, Sir Samuel Rickard (b. 1873). British malariologist.

Christophers' dots, or spots. Coarse irregular markings in the cytoplasm of erythrocytes found only in association with heavy infections of the subtertian malaria parasite (*Plasmodium falciparum*). With Romanovsky stains they take on a reddish tinge. These markings are more frequently, but less justifiably, called *Maurer's dots* or *clefts*.

chromaesthesia (kro·mes·**the**·ze·ah). The perception of colours during the experience of sensations of taste, hearing, smell, or touch. [Gk *chroma* colour, aesthesia.]

chromaffin (kro·**maf**·in). A term applied to certain cells which take a strong stain of brownish yellow from chrome salts. The cells are present in certain glands and organs and in the nerves of the sympathetic system. [Gk *chroma* colour, L *affinis* having affinity for.]

chromaffinoblastoma (kro·**maf**·in·o·blas·**to**′·mah). A neoplasm the cells of which are early forms of chromaffin cells. [chromaffin, blastoma.]

chromaffinoma (kro·**maf**·in·**o**′·mah). A tumour the contents of which are chromaffin tissue. [chromaffin, Gk *-oma* tumour.]

chromaffinopathy (kro·**maf**·in·**op**′·ath·e). Any disease affecting the chromaffin system. [chromaffin, Gk *pathos* suffering.]

chromagogue (**kro**·mag·og). Having a tendency to eliminate pigments. [Gk *chroma* colour, *agogos* leading.]

chromaphil (**kro**·mah·fil). Chromatophil.

chromargentaffin (krome·ar·jen·**taf**′·in). A term applied to certain cells of the mucous coat of the alimentary canal which stain with chromium salts and can be impregnated with silver. [Gk *chroma* colour, argentaffin.]

chromate (**kro**·mate). 1. A salt of chromic acid. 2. In chemical practice, to treat a substance with a chromate or dichromate.

chromatelopsia (**kro**·mat·el·**op**′·se·ah). 1. The condition of being able to perceive colours only imperfectly. 2. Partial colour blindness. [Gk *chroma* colour, *ateles* incomplete, *opsis* sight.]

chromatic (kro·**mat**·ik). 1. Referring to colours. 2. Produced by colour or colours. 3. Taking the stain of dyes. 4. Chromatinic. [see foll.]

chromatid (**kro**·mat·id). The 2 halves into which a chromosome is longitudinally divided at mitosis and meiosis. These are held together at the centromere and part from each to become daughter chromosomes at anaphase of mitosis and anaphase II of meiosis. **Chromatid aberration.** *See* ABERRATION. **Chromatid break.** Breakage of only 1 of the chromatids of a chromosome. **Half chromatid.** One of the 2 strands forming a chromatid. **Sister chromatid.** One of the 2 chromatids formed by duplication of a chromosome. [Gk *chroma* colour.]

chromatin (**kro**·mat·in). *Formerly:* a substance distributed throughout the interphase nucleus and showing characteristic affinity for certain dyes. *Currently:* the component of the nucleus which contains the genetic material, i.e. the interphase form of the chromosomes. *See also* EUCHROMATIN, HETEROCHROMATIN. **Distributed chromatin.** Chromidia. **Chromatin dust.** *See* DUST. **Extranuclear chromatin.** Chromidia. **Chromatin mass.** An obvious mass of chromatin lying immediately beneath the nuclear membrane of the majority of cells in a *chromatin-positive* (female) individual. A *chromatin-negative* (male) individual has few, if any, cells with a chromatin mass. **Sex chromatin.** Term used to denote the chromocentre formed by the heterochromatic X chromosome (Barr body) in interphase cells of female mammals. Therefore, sex chromatin *positive* and *negative*, respectively, indicate cells and individuals showing or not showing Barr bodies. Recently, however, it has been suggested that *sex chromatin* should be used only as a collective term for X and Y chromatin. **X chromatin.** Barr body. **Y chromatin.** Y body. *See* BODY. [Gk *chroma* colour.] [see prec.]

chromatinic (kro·mat·**in**·ik). Referring to or composed of chromatin.

chromatinolysis (**kro**·mat·in·**ol**′·is·is). Chromatolysis.

chromatinorrhexis (**kor**·mat·in·o·**rex**′·is). The fragmentation or the splitting up of chromatin. [chromatin, Gk *rhexis* rupture.]

chromatism (**kro**·mat·izm). Abnormal pigmentation of a part. [Gk *chroma* colour.]

chromatize (**kro**·mat·ize). To subject to a chromium salt.

chromatoblast (**kro**·mat·o·blast). Chromatophore. [Gk *chroma* colour, *blastos* germ.]

chromatocinesis (**kro**·mat·o·sin·**e**′·sis). Chromatokinesis.

chromatodermatosis (**kro**·mat·o·der·mat·**o**′·sis). Any disease of the skin in which pigmentation is one of the main features. [Gk *chroma* colour, dermatosis.]

chromatodysopia (**kro**·mat·o·dis·**o**′·pe·ah). Almost complete colour blindness. [Gk *chroma* colour, dysopia.]

chromatogenous (kro·mat·**oj**·en·us). Productive of colouring matter or colour. [Gk *chroma* colour, *genein* to produce.]

chromatogram (**kro**·mat·o·gram). The zoned distribution, either in column or on paper, produced in chromatography.

chromatography (kro·mat·**og**·raf·e). A method of separating 2 or more chemical compounds in solution by taking advantage of the fact that they are removed from the solution at different rates when the latter is percolated down a column of a powdered adsorbent or passed across the surface of an absorbent paper. **Adsorption chromatography, Column chromatography.** The separation of the components of a mixture in solution by percolating the latter down a column of a powdered adsorbent such as chalk or alumina. Owing to differences in adsorptive affinity the components become distributed in zones at different levels in the column, where they can be identified either by their natural colours or by colours produced with appropriate reagents, or by their fluorescence in ultra-violet light. In this way plant pigments have been separated and vitamins isolated and purified. **Exclusion chromatography.** Gel filtration. *See* FILTRATION. **Filter-paper chromatography.** Paper chromatography (see below). **Gas chromatography.** A method of analysis by vaporization of volatile compounds through suitably packed columns, ending in a detector from which a recording is made; used extensively in forensic toxicology. **Ion-exchange chromatography.** The separation of the components of a mixture (usually metallic salts) in solution by percolating the latter through a long column of ion-exchange material. By subsequent elution with an acid the metal ions can be carried forward in bands which travel down the column and are re-adsorbed at lower levels to form distinctive zones. The method has been used for the isolation of metals of the rare earths and also to investigate the products of uranium fission. **Paper chromatography.** A laboratory method by which dissolved chemical and other substances can be identified by a chromatogram run out into paper and sprayed with colour reagent. Largely superseded by *thin layer chromatography* techniques, in which a silica gel spread on a glass plate develops the same differential spread of dissolved substances. **Partition chromatography.** The separation of the components of a mixture in solution into zones, either in a column of adsorbent material or on absorbent paper, which serve only to anchor a second solvent between which and the original solvent the components become distributed in accordance with their partition coefficients. The method has been used to separate protein hydrolysates (amino acids), and for the isolation of the anti-pernicious anaemia factor from liver extracts. **Thin layer chromatography.** A method of analysis by which dissolved chemical and drug substances can be identified by a chromatogram run out under electrical impulsion into a silica, or other 'thin layer', gel spread on a glass plate. [Gk *chroma* colour, *graphein* to record.]

chromatoid (kro·mat·oid). 1. Taking the stain of a dye deeply. 2. A chromatoid body. [Gk *chroma* colour, *eidos* form.]

chromatokinesis (kro·mat·o·kin·e'·sis). The movement of chromatin in taking up different forms of arrangement. [Gk *chroma* colour, *kinesis* movement.]

chromatology (kro·mat·ol'·o·je). The science of colour; investigation of colours by means of the spectroscope. [Gk *chroma* colour, *logos* science.]

chromatolysis, chromatolysm (kro·mat·ol·is·is, kro·mat·ol·izm). The breaking up and destruction by lysis of the chromatin. [Gk *chroma* colour, *lysis* a loosing.]

chromatolytic (kro·mat·o·lit'·ik). Referring to chromatolysis, or having relation to it.

chromatometer (kro·mat·om·et·er). 1. An instrument, bearing a scale of shades of colours, used in determining colour perception. 2. An apparatus with which the intensity of colour in a substance or liquid can be measured. [Gk *chroma* colour, meter.]

chromatometry (kro·mat·om·et·re). The measurement of colour perception. [see prec.]

chromatopathy (kro·mat·op·ath·e). Chromatodermatosis. [Gk *chroma* colour, *pathos* suffering.]

chromatopectic (kro·mat·o·pek·tik). Chromopexic.

chromatopexis (kro·mat·o·pex·is). Chromopexy.

chromatophagus (kro·mat·of·ag·us). A term applied to certain micro-organisms which destroy pigment or cause a loss of it. [Gk *chroma* colour, *phagein* to eat.]

chromatophil, chromatophile (kro·mat·o·fil, kro·mat·o·file). Any cell and substance which readily take up a dye. [Gk *chroma* colour, *philein* to love.]

chromatophilia (kro·mat·o·fil'·e·ah). The condition of being able to take stains readily. [see prec.]

chromatophilic, chromatophilous (kro·mat·o·fil'·ik, kro·mat·of·il·us). Chromatophil.

chromatophobia (kro·mat·o·fo'·be·ah). 1. A condition in which the patient shows morbid dislike of colours or of certain colours. 2. Of cells, taking stains badly. [Gk *chroma* colour, phobia.]

chromatophore (kro·mat·o·for). 1. Any pigment-bearing cell such as that found in the skin, or in the choroid coat of the eye. 2. In zoology, a coloured plastid found in some forms of protozoa. [Gk *chroma* colour, *pherein* to bear.]

chromatophoroma (kro·mat·o·for·o'·mah). A neoplasm composed of pigment-bearing cells of the skin or of the choroid coat of the eye. [chromatophore, Gk *-oma* tumour.]

chromatophoromatosis (kro·mat·o·for·o·mat·o'·sis). Melanomatosis. [chromatophoroma, Gk *-osis* condition.]

chromatophorotropic (kro·mat·o·for·o·tro'·pik). A term applied to the function of the middle part of the hypophysis cerebri which has a modifying effect on chromatophores. [chromatophore, Gk *trepein* to turn.]

chromatophorous (kro·mat·of·er·us). Bearing or containing pigment or pigment cells. [Gk chroma colour, *pherein* to bear.]

chromatoplasm (kro·mat·o·plazm). In biology, a general name for the pigment elements of cells. [Gk *chroma* colour, *plasma* something formed.]

chromatoplast (kro·mat·o·plast). Chromatophore. [Gk *chroma* colour, *plassein* to form.]

chromatopseudopsis (kro·mat·o·sewd·op'·sis). Colour blindness; a condition in which there is abnormal perception of colour. [Gk *chroma* colour, *pseudes* false, *opsis* sight.]

chromatopsia, chromatopsy (kro·mat·op·se·ah, kro·mat·op·se). 1. A condition in which coloured objects appear as unnaturally coloured, and colourless objects as coloured. 2. Partial colour blindness. 3. A state of disordered vision in which colours are seen subjectively as the result of ingestion of certain drugs or of disturbance of the optic centres, or after a cataract extraction. [Gk *chroma* colour, *opsis* sight.]

chromatoptometer (kro·mat·op·tom'·et·er). An instrument with which the degree of colour perception may be determined. [Gk *chroma* colour, optometer.]

chromatoptometry (kro·mat·op·tom'·et·re). Measurement of the degree of colour perception with a chromatoptometer.

chromatoscopy (kro·mat·os·ko·pe). 1. The testing of colour perception. 2. The testing of renal function by observation of the colour or urine passed after a dye has been administered either intravenously or by the mouth. **Gastric chromatoscopy.** Observation of the colour of the stomach contents in diagnosing the state of gastric function. [Gk *chroma* colour, *skopein* to view.]

chromatosis (kro·mat·o·sis). 1. Chromatodermatosis. 2. Pigmentation. [Gk *chroma* colour, *-osis* condition.]

chromatoskiameter (kro·mat·o·ski·am'·et·er). A particular apparatus for the testing of the sense of colour. The shadow of a pencil is cast on a white screen by the light from a lamp shining through differently coloured pieces of glass; a scale indicates when 2 or more shadows are equally clearly defined. [Gk *chroma* colour, *skia* shadow, *metron* measure.]

chromatosome (kro·mat·o·some). Chromosome. [obsolete term.]

chromatotaxis (kro·mat·o·tax'·is). In a cell nucleus, the influence exerted by certain substances which do not have an effect on the cell body but attract and destroy the chromatin. [Gk *chroma* colour, *taxis* arrangement.]

chromatotropism (kro·mat·o·trop'·izm). The state of turning towards a pigment or colour because of affinity for it. [Gk *chroma* colour, *trepein* to turn.]

chromaturia (kro·mat·ewr·e·ah). The condition in which urine of an abnormal colour is excreted. [Gk *chroma* colour, urine.]

chrome (krome). 1. A common name for chromium or its oxide. 2. Lead chromate. **Chrome alum.** Potassium or ammonium chromium sulphate. *See* ALUM. **Chrome green.** 1. Chromium sesquioxide, Cr_2O_3, a green powder used as a pigment. 2. A mixture of lead chromate and Prussian blue used in paint manufacture. **Chrome iron ore.** Chromite, ferrous chromite, Fe Cr_2O_4, the chief source of chromium, used also as a refractory for furnace linings. **Chrome red.** Basic lead chromate, formed by treating chrome yellow with lime. **Chrome yellow.** Lead chromate, $PbCrO_4$, an important pigment. [Gk *chroma* colour.]

chromhidrosis (krome·hid·ro·sis). The secretion of sweat coloured as the result of bacterial activity. [Gk *chroma* colour, *hidros* sweat.]

chromicize (kro·mis·ize). To mix or impregnate or treat with a chromium salt or compound.

chromidial (kro·mid·e·al). Composed of or relating to chromidia.

chromidiation (kro·mid·e·a'·shun). Chromidiosis.

chromidien (kro·mid·een). The extranuclear chromatin in an animal cell. [G.]

chromidiosis (kro·mid·e·o'·sis). The flow of chromatin and nuclear substance from the nucleus into the protoplasm of the cell body. [chromidium, Gk *-osis* condition.]

chromidium (kro·mid·e·um). (pl. *chromidia*). Any one of the granules of pigment which are present in the cell body outside the nucleus. [Gk *chroma* colour.]

chromidrosis (kro·mid·ro·sis). Chromhidrosis.

chromiole (kro·me·ole). Any one of the minute granules of chromatin contained within a chromosome.

chromism (kro·mizm). Coloration of unusual intensity. [Gk *chroma* colour.]

chromite (kro·mite). 1. Chrome ironstone, a naturally-occurring ferrous chromite, $FeCr_2O_4$, and the principal ore of chromium. 2. Any salt of the hypothetical chromous acid, $H_2Cr_2O_4$.

chromium (kro·me·um). An element of atomic weight 51.996, atomic number 24 and chemical symbol Cr. It is a hard crystalline bluish metal, malleable and with high melting point, resembling iron in properties and found with the latter in chrome ironstone (chromite) in Asia Minor, India, and Rhodesia. It is acid-resisting and is alloyed with nickel and iron in the manufacture of stainless steel and armour plating; also employed in chromium plating. All its compounds are characteristically coloured, and some are of value in therapeutics, but its medical importance lies in the risk of poisoning, either locally or from absorption, to which those engaged in industry are exposed. **Chromium potassium sulphate.** Chrome alum, $KCr(SO_4)_2 \cdot 12H_2O$, a violet-coloured crystalline compound, used in tanning, dyeing and photography. **Chromium sesquioxide.** Chromic oxide, Cr_2O_3, chrome green, an insoluble dark-green powder used in printing and glass making. **Chromium Trioxide BPC 1968.** Chromic acid anhydride, CrO_3, a dark-red crystalline compound or dark-brown mass. It is a strong oxidizing agent and a caustic employed as a local application to remove warts and superficial growths, or to stimulate healing in indolent ulcers. A dilute solution is used as a mouth-wash or gargle and as an astringent lotion. Used industrially in chromium plating, it may cause dermatitis with deep ulceration of the skin and nasal septum, and if absorbed may give rise to nephritis. [Gk *chroma* colour.]

chromo-aromatic (kro·mo·ar·o·**mat**′·ik). Descriptive of micro-organisms that are coloured and aromatic. [Gk *chroma* colour, *aroma* sweet smell.]

Chromobacteriae (kro·mo·bak·**teer**′·e·e). A division of the family Bacteriaceae that includes the genus *Chromobacterium.*

Chromobacterium (kro·mo·bak·**teer**′·e·um). Small non-sporing rods, usually motile organisms, and producing red, yellow or violet pigments. They are non-pathogenic and occur in soil and water. *Chromobacterium prodigiosum* produces a red or maroon pigment and a mawkish smell; a common contaminant of culture media. *Chromobacterium violaceum* produces a violet pigment. [Gk *chroma* colour, bacterium.]

chromoblast (kro·mo·blast). Chromatophore. [Gk *chroma* colour, *blastos* germ.]

chromoblastomycosis (kro·mo·blas·to·mi·**ko**′·sis). Chromomycosis; dermatitis verrucosa: a localized, chronic mycosis of skin and subcutaneous tissues characterized by verrucoid, ulcerated and crusted lesions, usually on exposed areas of the extremities. Infection is caused by dematiaceous fungi of the genus *Phialophora* and by *Cladosporium carrionii* which may be found on rotting wood. [chromoblast, Gk *mykes* fungus, *-osis* condition.]

chromocentre (kro·mo·**sen**·ter). The body formed in the interphase nucleus by densely packed chromosome material (chromatin). *See* HETEROCHROMATIN. [Gk *chroma* colour, *kentron* centre.]

chromocholoscopy (kro·mo·kol·**os**′·ko·pe). A method of investigation of the hepatic function by use of pigments, e.g. methylthionine chloride, the time and amount of the excretion of the latter being assessed. [Gk chroma colour, choloscopy.]

chromocrater (kro·mo·**kra**·ter). A bowl-shaped blood corpuscle. [Gk *chroma* colour, *krater* mixing vessel.]

chromocrinia (kro·mo·**krin**·e·ah). The secretion and excretion of colouring matter, e.g. in the sweat. [Gk *chroma* colour, *krinein* to separate.]

chromocystoscopy (kro·mo·sis·**tos**′·ko·pe). Cystoscopy after administration of a dye such as methylene blue so that renal function and the state of the orifices of the urinary system may be determined by the evidence of the passage and deposition of the dye. [Gk *chroma* colour, cystoscopy.]

chromocyte (kro·mo·site). Any cell or corpuscle bearing pigment, e.g. an erythrocyte. [Gk *chroma* colour, *kytos* cell.]

chromocytometer (kro·mo·si·**tom**′·et·er). Haemoglobinometer; an instrument with which the percentage of haemoglobin in the blood may be determined. [chromocyte, meter.]

chromocytometry (kro·mo·si·**tom**′·et·re). Haemoglobinometry; the determining of the percentage of haemoglobin in any specimen of blood. [see prec.]

chromodacryorrhoea (kro·mo·dak·re·o·**re**′·ah). The act of shedding tears in which there are elements of blood. [Gk *chroma* colour, *dakryon* tear, *rhoia* flow.]

chromodermatosis (kro·mo·der·mat·**o**′·sis). Chromatodermatosis.

chromodiagnosis (kro·mo·di·ag·**no**′·sis). Diagnosis which is based on change of colour in tests, e.g. diagnosis by examination through sheets of coloured gelatin or glass, diagnosis of haemorrhage in the central nervous system by the presence of a yellow discoloration (xanthochromia) in a specimen of cerebrospinal fluid, or diagnosis of urinary function by noting the rate at which a colouring substance, e.g. methylthionine chloride, is excreted, or by chromocystoscopy. [Gk *chroma* colour, diagnosis.]

chromogen (kro·mo·jen). Substances in biological liquids which by oxidation form coloured compounds, e.g. indigo. [Gk *chroma* colour, *genein* to produce.]

chromogene (kro·mo·jeen). Any parent-substance of a pigment-producing compound or dyestuff. [see prec.]

chromogenesis (kro·mo·**jen**·es·is). The production of colouring matter or pigment, e.g. by the action of bacteria. [Gk *chrome* colour, *genein* to produce.]

chromogenic (kro·mo·**jen**·ik). 1. Referring to a chromogen. 2. Producing colouring matter or a pigment. [see prec.]

chromo-isomerism (kro·mo·i·**so**′·mer·izm). Isomerism in which the isomers are differently coloured. [Gk *chroma* colour, isomer.]

chromoleucite (kro·mo·**lew**·site). Chromoplast. [Gk *chroma* colour, *leukos* white.]

chromolipoid (kro·mo·**lip**·oid). Lipochrome; any of the fat-soluble pigments of carotenoid type which occur naturally in oils and fats to which they give colour. [Gk *chroma* colour, lipoid.]

chromolume (kro·mo·lewm). An apparatus with which coloured rays of light can be produced for therapeutic purposes. **Electro-arc chromolume.** A device in which an arc light is used for solarization. [Gk *chroma* colour, L *lumen* light.]

chromolysis (kro·**mol**·is·is). Chromatolysis.

chromoma (kro·**mo**·mah). A malignant ulcerating neoplasm which is held to derive from chromatophore (melanophore) cells; a variety of malignant melanoma. [Gk *chroma* colour, *-oma* tumour.]

chromomere (kro·mo·meer). 1. Each of the serially aligned, dense, chromosomal segments visible in elongated chromosomes such as those of early prophase I of meiosis. 2. That part of a blood platelet which contains dark granules. [Gk *chroma* colour, *meros* part.]

chromometer (kro·**mom**·et·er). Colorimeter. [Gk *chroma* colour, meter.]

chromometry (kro·**mom**·et·re). Colorimetry. [see prec.]

chromomycosis (kro·mo·mi·**ko**′·sis). Chromoblastomycosis. [Gk *chroma* colour, mycosis.]

chromone (kro·mone). 1. A member of a group of yellow plant-pigments related to the flavones. 2. The heterocyclic compound, benzopyrone, $CO(C_6H_4)O(CH)_2$, and the parent of the group of pigments. [Gk *chroma* colour.]

chromoneme (kro·mo·neem). The smallest chromosomal strand visible with the light microscope. H. L. K. Whitehouse has recently proposed the use of this term for the DNA strand(s) containing the genetic information of bacteria and their viruses as well as for the DNA of plastids and mitochondria. [Gk *chroma* colour, *nema* thread.]

chromoparic, chromoparous (kro·mo·**par**·ik, kro·**mop**·ar·us). A term applied to chromogenic bacteria which colour their immediate environment. [Gk *chroma* colour, L *parere* to give birth.]

chromopathy (kro·**mop**·ath·e). Chromatodermatosis. [Gk *chroma* colour, *pathos* suffering.]

chromopexic (kro·mo·**pex**·ik). Of or pertaining to chromopexy.

chromopexy (kro·mo·pex·e). The fixation of pigment, e.g. of bile pigment, by the liver. [Gk *chroma* colour, *pexis* fixation.]

chromophage (kro·mo·faje). Pigmentophage; a phagocytic cell, and in particular of the hair, which destroys pigment. [Gk *chroma* colour, *phagein* to eat.]

chromophane (kro·mo·fane). 1. Any pigment of the retina. 2. The pigment of the inner retina of some animals. [Gk *chroma* colour, *phainein* to show.]

chromophil, chromophile, chromophilic, chromophilous (**kro**·mo·fil, **kro**·mo·file, kro·mo·**fil**·ik, kro·**mof**·il·us). Any histological element or a cell which readily takes stains. [Gk *chroma* colour, *philein* to love.]

chromophobe (**kro**·mo·fobe). A cell which takes stain either not at all or very lightly, e.g. any of the cells of the anterior lobe of the pituitary which take stain poorly because they contain few or no granules. [Gk *chroma* colour, *phobos* fear.]

chromophobia (kro·mo·**fo**·be·ah). Chromatophobia.

chromophobic (kro·mo·**fo**·bik). Referring to chromatophobia.

chromophore (**kro**·mo·for). A characteristic group such as -N=N- or $-NO_2$, which, introduced into an organic compound, affects its absorption spectrum and causes it to display colour. The compound is then known as a *chromogene*, and the further addition of strongly acid or basic groups such as COOH or NH_2 gives it full dyeing properties. [Gk *chroma* colour, *pherein* to carry.]

chromophoric, chromophorous (kro·mo·**for**·ik, kro·mo·**for**·-us). 1. Pertaining to a chromophore. 2. Applied to certain micro-organisms which are capable of producing pigment and imparting it to the surrounding medium. [see prec.]

chromophose (**kro**·mo·foze). A subjective sensation of there being a spot or patch of colour in the eye. [Gk *chroma* colour, *phos* light.]

chromophototherapy (**kro**·mo·fo·to·**ther**′·ap·e). The therapeutic use of coloured light. [Gk *chroma* colour, *phos* light, therapy.]

chromophytosis (**kro**·mo·fi·**to**′·sis). Pityriasis versicolor. [Gk *chroma* colour, *phyton* a growth.]

chromoplasm (**kro**·mo·plazm). In biology, the network of a cell nucleus which readily takes the stain of acid dyes. [Gk *chroma* colour, *plasma* something formed.]

chromoplast, chromoplastid, chromoplastidule (**kro**·mo·plast, kro·mo·**plas**·tid, kro·mo·**plas**·tid·ewl). In botany, any of the plastids which are the source of colour of most flowers and fruits. [Gk *chroma* colour, *plassein* to form.]

chromoprotein (kro·mo·**pro**·te·in). Any conjugated protein, in which a protein moiety is united with a chromogenic group, often a metallic porphyrin, giving the protein colour. The most important are haemoglobin, in which the basic protein, globin, is united to an iron-containing body, haem, and cytochrome, a haemochromogen in which the globin is de-natured. Chromoproteins occur in both animals and plants (phytochromes), and are intimately concerned in respiration. [Gk *chroma* colour, protein.]

chromopsia (kro·**mop**·se·ah). Chromatopsia.

chromoptometer (kro·mop·**tom**·et·er). Chromatoptometer.

chromoradiometer (**kro**·mo·ra·de·**om**′·et·er). A simple instrument for measuring x-rays, designed by Holzknecht (1902) based on the photochemical effect of the rays on a mixture of potassium chloride and sodium carbonate. Now obsolete. [Gk *chroma* colour, radiometer.]

chromoretinography (**kro**·mo·ret·in·**og**′·raf·e). Photography of the retina in colour. [Gk *chroma* colour, retinography.]

chromorhinorrhoea (**kro**·mo·ri·no·**re**′·ah). The discharge of pigmented fluid from the nose, as in cephalomenia. [Gk *chroma* colour, rhinorrhoea.]

chromosantonin (**kro**·mo·**san**′·ton·in). A yellow isomer of santonin produced by the effect of sunlight on the latter. [Gk *chroma* colour, santonin.]

chromoscopy (kro·**mos**·ko·pe). Chromatoscopy.

chromosochromic (**kro**·mo·so·**kro**′·mik). Describing any compound of chromium in which the element is both di- and tri-valent.

chromosomal (kro·mo·**so**·mal). Relating to a chromosome or chromosomes.

chromosome (**kro**·mo·some). Term proposed by Waldeyer (1888) for the individual thread-like structures in the cell nucleus. Chromosomes are formed by double helices of DNA complexed with basic proteins (usually histone) and containing also acidic proteins and RNA. They carry the genetic information of the cell in a linear array of functional units (genes) occupying specific positions called loci (singular *locus*). In 'resting' cells the chromosomes take the appearance of a network of threads packed more or less tightly (chromatin) and are not visible as separate entities. As the cells undergo division, the chromosomes contract and appear as separate rod-shaped bodies divided into halves (chromatids) held together at the centromere. At this stage the chromosomes can often be distinguished from each other by their length and position of the centromere and/or by a number of cytochemical properties. During the course of division (i.e. at anaphase of mitosis and anaphase II of meiosis) the chromatids come apart and migrate to opposite poles of the cell and they are then called *daughter chromosomes.* These, in turn, may reduplicate during the subsequent interphase to become double structures formed by two chromatids. Man has 23 pairs of chromosomes, i.e. 22 pairs of autosomes and 1 pair of sex chromosomes; this is a heteromorphic pair comprising a medium-size chromosome, the X, and a small chromosome, the Y. Normal females have 2 X chromosomes, while males have 1 X and a Y. Chromosomes belonging to the same pair usually carry the same loci and are called *homologous chromosomes* or *homologues.* At the first divisions of mitosis, homologues pair to form bivalents; then they usually exchange parts through crossing-over and appear held by chiasmata. Subsequently, they separate and segregate to opposite poles to form gametes containing 1 member of each pair. The X and Y chromosomes also segregate to produce a Y- and an X-bearing gamete; in man these are, respectively, the male and female determining gamete. **A chromosome.** A chromosome of the usual kind, in contraposition to B chromosome. **Accessory chromosome.** B chromosome (see below). **Chromosome arm.** One of the 2 parts into which a chromosome or chromatid (daughter chromosome) is divided by the centromere. Chromosomes with only 1 arm (telocentrics) are rare. The *chromosome-arm ratio* is the ratio of the longer to the shorter arm of a chromosome. **B chromosome.** One of a heterogeneous group of chromosomes which, in contrast to the A chromosomes, vary considerably in number in different cells, tissues, individuals or populations; they do not form chiasmata with any A chromosome and pair weakly with each other, show irregular segregation at meiosis and mitosis, are usually small and heterochromatic, and have only mild effects on the phenotype. **Chromosome break.** Discontinuity involving the whole cross-section of the chromosome, in contradistinction with chromatid break. **Christchurch chromosome.** A G group chromosome with extremely small short arm found in a family with high incidence of chronic lymphocytic leukaemia and believed at first to play a part in the aetiology of this condition. This has not been confirmed, and such chromosomes usually appear to be variants of little clinical significance. **Circular chromosome.** Ring chromosome (see below). **Chromosome complement.** The chromosomes with which a cell or an individual is endowed. **Derivative chromosome.** A structurally abnormal chromosome originated directly from the rearrangement of one or more chromosomes in the complement without any intervening process of meiotic crossing over. **Extra chromosome.** B chromosome (see above). **Giant chromosome.** A very large chromosome formed presumably by the lateral strands (polyteny). Chromosomes of this type are found in some tissues of a few organisms—for example, salivary glands of *Diptera.* **Chromosome imbalance.** The situation brought about by chromosome abnormalities and genome mutations which, by producing aneuploidy duplications and/or deficiencies, disturb the internal integration of the genotype essential for the normal development and function of the organisms. **Chromosome inheritance.** *See* INHERITANCE. **Chromosome lagging.** The failure to move or the slow movement of some chromosomes or pairing configuration at metaphase and/or anaphase of mitosis or meiosis, usually resulting in abnormal chromosome segregation. **Lampbrush chromosome.** A special conformation of the chromosome found during the diplotene stage in the primary oocyte of a variety of vertebrates and invertebrates, and in the spermatocytes of *Drosophila.* These chromosomes show a central axis from which a series of loops project in pairs. The loops show an axis, formed probably by one DNA double helix, and a matrix consisting of RNA and proteins. **Chromosome map.** Representation of a chromosome showing some of its genes arranged linearly according to their relative distances. The map is called *genetic* if it is constructed using recombination data so that the distances are expressed in crossing-over units, and *cytologic* if it is based on cytological data and the distances are measured in physical units. **Chromosome mapping.** The assignment of genes to chromosomes and the measurement of intergenic distances necessary for the construction of chromosome maps. **Marker chromosome.** A chromosome of distinct morphology present in only some members of a population of cells or individuals. **Mediocentral chromosome.** *See* METACENTRIC. **Chromosome modal number.** *See* NUMBER. **Nucleolar chromosome.** A chromosome carrying a nucleolar organizer region. **Chromosome pairing.** The intimate side-by-side association of homologous chromosome regions which usually occurs at meiosis (synapsis) or may occur in somatic cells (somatic pairing). Non-homologous chromosomes or chromosome regions may occasionally pair; this is called *non-specific pairing.* **Ph chromosome, Philadelphia chromosome.** A deleted chromosome of group G, presumably No. 22, which has lost from one-half to two-thirds of the long arm. This is usually found in the bone marrow cells of patients with chronic myeloid leukaemia. **Polytene chromosome.** Giant chromosome (see above). **Chromosome rearrangement.** Any chromosomal structural aberration; this may involve the loss, gain or change in position of chromosome material. **Recombinant chromosome.** A chromosome which has undergone genetic recombination or, in a more restricted sense, a structurally altered chromosome resulting from meiotic crossing-over within a rearranged chromosome segment in an individual heterozygous for a structural chromosomal change. **Chromosome restitution and reunion.** *See* REJOINING. **Ring chromosome.** A circular chromosome. In eukaryotes such a chromosome is always the result of rearrangements involving its distal segments. Ring chromosomes tend to be unstable in meiosis and mitosis, and show variation in size and number even within the same individual or cell population. **Chromosome set.** A minimum (monoploid) chromosome complement contributed by the gamete of a supposed ancestor. Diploid organisms have 2 chromosome sets in their somatic cells. **Sex chromosome.** A chromosome which is differentially represented in the male and female and is usually involved in the genotypic control of sex determination. *See* main definition (above) *and* DICENTRIC, DISJUNCTION, METACENTRIC, MONOCENTRIC, MUTATION, NON-DISJUNCTION, SUBACROCENTRIC, SUBMETACENTRIC, SUBTELOCENTRIC, TELOCENTRIC, TRICENTRIC. **Supernumerary chromosome.** B chromosome (see above). **Chromosome variant.** *See* VARIANT. **W chromosome.** The sex chromosome characteristic of females in species where these are heterogametic. **X chromosome.** The sex chromosome which is usually present in duplicate in females of species with heterogametic males. **Y chromosome.** The sex chromosome characteristic of males in species where they are heterogametic. **Z chromosome.** The sex chromosome normally disomic (present in duplicate) in the male of species with heterogametic females. [Gk *chroma* colour, *soma* body.]

chromospermism (kro·mo·**sperm**·izm). A condition of pigmentation of the semen. [Gk *chroma* colour, sperm.]

chromostroboscope (**kro**·mo·**stro**·bo·skope). A stroboscope in which the pictures are coloured. [Gk *chroma* colour, stroboscope.]

chromotherapy (kro·mo·**ther**·ap·e). Treatment of disease by application of rays from restricted areas of the spectrum—that is, by the use of light of specific colours. [Gk *chroma* colour, therapy.]

chromotoxic (kro·mo·**tox**·ik). 1. Caused by toxic action on haemoglobin. 2. Destructive of haemoglobin. [Gk *chroma* colour, *toxikon* poison.]

chromotrichia (kro·mo·**trik**·e·ah). Coloration of the hair. [Gk *chroma* colour, *thrix* hair.]

chromotrichomycosis (**kro**·mo·trik·o·mi·**ko**'·sis). Trichomycosis. [Gk *chroma* colour, trichomycosis.]

chromotropic (kro·mo·**trop**·ik). 1. Being drawn towards pigment or colour. 2. Having attraction for pigment or colour. [Gk *chroma* colour, *trepein* to turn.]

chromo-ureteroscopy, chromo-urinography (**kro**·mo·ewr·e·ter·**os**'·ko·pe, **kro**·mo·ewr·in·**og**'·raf·e). The endoscopic inspection of the ureteric orifice following the intravenous injection of a dye such as indigo carmine. The rapid excretion of indigo carmine by the kidneys leads to a coloured efflux of urine from the ureteric orifice. The method is used both to assist the cystoscopist in the identification of the ureteric opening and as a renal-function test by noting the time of the appearance of the dye following the intravenous injection. [Gk *chroma* colour, ureteroscopy, urinography.]

chronaxia, chronaxie (kron·**ax**·e·ah, kron·**ax**·e). A measurement of the excitability of nervous or muscular tissue; the shortest time that a current twice the strength of the rheo-base must be applied to stimulate a response. The more excitable a nerve or muscle, the shorter its chronaxia. [Gk *chronos* time, *axia* value.]

chronaximeter (kron·ax·**im**·et·er). A device with which chronaxia in nerve lesions can be measured.

chronaximetry (kron·ax·**im**·et·re). The process of measuring chronaxia.

chronaxy (kron·**ax**·e). Chronaxia.

chronic (**kron**·ik). Long continued; the opposite of acute. [Gk *chronos* time.]

chronicity (kron·**is**·it·e). The fact of being chronic.

chroniosepsis (kron·e·o·**sep**·sis). Chronic sepsis.

chronobiology (**kron**·o·bi·**ol**'·o·je). The science of the duration of life and the study of means of prolonging the span. [Gk *chronos* time, biology.]

chronognosis (kron·og·**no**·sis). Subjective perception of the passing of time. [Gk *chronos* time, *gnosis* knowledge.]

chronograph (**kron**·o·graf). An instrument with which short periods of time can be measured and recorded. It is used in experiments in psychophysics and physiology. [Gk *chronos* time, *graphein* to record.]

chronokymograph (kron·o·**ki**·mo·graf). An instrument with which alterations in pressure are measured against time. [Gk *chronos* time, kymograph.]

chronometry (kron·**om**·et·re). The measuring of time in periods or divisions. **Mental chronometry.** The study of mental processes in their relation to time and the measurement of their duration. [Gk *chronos* time, *metron* measure.]

chronomyometer (**kron**·o·mi·**om**'·et·er). An instrument for measuring chronaxia. [Gk *chronos* time, *mys* muscle, meter.]

chronophobia (kron·o·**fo**·be·ah). Pathological fear of time [Gk *chronos* time, phobia.]

chronophotograph (kron·o·**fo**·to·graf). Any one of a set of photographs taken of a moving object in order to record the successive phases of movement. [Gk *chronos* time, photograph.]

chronoscope (**kron**·o·skope). An instrument with which extremely short periods of time may be measured, as in the determination of reaction time in experiments or the velocity of a moving object. [Gk *chronos* time, *skopein* to watch.]

chronosphygmograph (kron·o·**sfig**·mo·graf). A sphygmograph which records the character of the pulse as well as its rhythm. [Gk *chronos* time, sphygmograph.]

chronotaraxis (**kron**·o·tar·**ax**'·is). Inability to orientate self correctly with regard to time. [Gk *chronos* time, *taraktos* disturbed.]

chronothermal (kron·o·**ther**·mal). 1. Relating to time and temperature, e.g. the periodicity of alterations in the temperature of the body. 2. Relating to the theory that in all diseases there are intermittent periods of alternating heat and chill. [Gk *chronos* time, *therme* heat.]

chronotropic (kron·o·**trop**·ik). 1. Referring to chronotropism. 2. A term applied to nerve fibres which modify the action of the heart; the vagus nerve retards and the nerves of the sympathetic system accelerate the rate of contraction. [Gk *chronos* time, *trepein* to turn.]

chronotropism (kron·**ot**·ro·pizm). Modification of the rapidity of a periodically-recurring phenomenon such as the heart beat. **Negative chronotropism.** Retardation of movement. **Positive chronotropism.** Acceleration of movement. [see prec.]

chrotoplast (**kro**·to·plast). An epithelial cell belonging to the skin. [Gk *chroa* skin, *plassein* to form.]

chrotopsia (kro·**top**·se·ah). Chromatopsia. [Gk *chroma* colour, *opsis* sight.]

chrysaniline (kris·**an**·il·een). Diaminophenylacridine, $C_{19}H_{15}N_3$. A yellow substance obtained from acridine; its nitrate is known as *phosphine*- or *leather-yellow.*

chrysarobin (kris·ah·**ro**·bin). An orange-yellow powder obtained from a deposit in cavities in the wood of *Vouacapoua araroba,* a tree of Brazil. The chief constituent of the powder is chrysophanolanthranol, which is irritant and fungicidal. It is insoluble in water and is usually incorporated in an ointment base when used to treat skin disorders. The official ointments containing about 4–6 per cent chrysarobin are effective against ringworm and psoriasis, though it may be necessary to use ointments of greater strength to get satisfactory results. [Gk *chrysos* gold, araroba.]

chrysene (**kri**·seen). Benzophenanthrene, $C_{18}H_{12}$. A hydrocarbon obtained in the distillation of coal tar, and from some natural fats and oils. It has no medical uses, but is carcinogenic.

chrysiasis (kris·**i**·as·is). Permanent pigmentation of the skin due to the parenteral administration of gold. The pigmentation is most noticeable on exposed areas and the discoloration varies from grey to lilac, mauve and prune. Also known as *chrysoderma.* [Gk *chrysos* gold.]

chrysitis (kris·**i**·tis). Litharge, the yellow monoxide of lead, PbO. [Gk *chrysos* gold.]

chrysocyanosis (**kris**·o·si·an·**o**′·sis). Chrysiasis. [Gk *chrysos* gold, *kyanos* blue, *-osis* condition.]

chrysoderma, chrysodermia (kris·o·**der**·mah, **kris**·o·**der**·me·ah). Chrysiasis. [Gk *chrysos* gold, *derma* skin.]

chrysoidine (kris·**oi**·deen). Diaminoazobenzene hydrochloride, $C_6H_5N{=}NC_6H_3(NH_2)_2HCl$. An orange-red dye used as a disinfectant and for the staining of bacteria.

Chrysomyia (kris·o·**mi**·e·ah). A genus of metallic blue-green blow-flies (Calliphoridae) of the Old World tropics. *Chrysomyia bezziana* normally oviposits in sores of living mammals, including man. The larvae feed on necrotic and living tissues and mature in about 10 days, when they fall out and pupate in the ground. Several other species may occasionally cause human myiasis, but they are normally saprophagous. [Gk *chrysos* gold, *myia* fly.]

chrysophanin (kris·**of**·an·in). $C_{20}H_{20}O_9$. The glucoside of chrysophanic acid, found in rhubarb.

chrysophanol (kris·o·**fan**·ol). Chrysophanic acid, 1,8-dihydroxy-3-methylanthraquinone, $C_6H_3(OH)(CO)_2C_6H_2(OH)CH_3$. An acidic substance obtained by the oxidation of chrysarobin; it occurs as glycosides in rhubarb, cascara bark and senna.

chrysophanolanthranol (**kris**·o·fan·ol·**an**′·thran·ol). One of the isomeric trihydroxy methyl anthracenes, and the chief constituent of chrysarobin.

chrysophyll (**kris**·o·fil). Xanthophyll; a dihydroxycarotene occurring as a yellow pigment in foliage. [Gk *chrysos* gold, *phyllon* leaf.]

Chrysops (**kri**·sops). A genus of horse-flies (Tabanidae), usually with metallic-coloured eyes. The females of all species feed on mammalian blood. Many feed readily on man and the after-effects of a bite are irritable and often painful. *Chrysops centurionis, C. Longicornis, C. silacea, C. dimidiata,* and *C. distinctipennis* are intermediate hosts of the nematode *Loa loa* in tropical Africa. *C. discalis,* the deer fly, transmits tularaemia in North America. [Gk *chrysos* gold, *ops* eye.]

chrysosis (kris·**o**·sis). Chrysiasis.

chrysotherapy (kris·o·**ther**·ap·e). The use of gold compounds in the treatment of disease. Gold was formerly used in tuberculosis, but is now seldom employed. The only condition for which gold is still used is rheumatoid arthritis, the preparation employed being gold sodium thiomalate. Associated with its use there is a definite risk of toxic effects, particularly on the bone marrow, the skin and the kidneys. [Gk *chrysos* gold, therapy.]

chthonophagia, chthonophagy (thon·o·**fa**·je·ah, thon·**of**·aj·e). Geophagia; the morbid habit or practice of eating clay and other earthy substances; it may be connected with malnutrition. [Gk *chthon* earth, *phagein* to eat.]

Churchill, Fleetwood (b. 1808). Dublin obstetrician.

Churchill's iodine caustic. A strong caustic solution of iodine in aqueous potassium iodide.

churganja (ker·**gan**·jah). Indian hemp. *See* GANJA. [Ind.]

churning (**chern**·ing). **Haustral churning.** The to-and-fro movements of the intestinal contents caused by the rhythmical contractions of the sacculations of the colon during the digestive process. [AS *cyrin.*]

churrus (**ker**·rus). Bhang, a product of *Cannabis sativa,* used for smoking and the preparation of electuaries. [Ind.]

Chvostek, Frantisek (b. 1835). Vienna surgeon.

Chvostek's sign, Chvostek-Weiss sign. In tetany, e.g. after total parathyroidectomy, tapping the 7th nerve results in twitching of the facial muscles.

Chvostek, Franz (b.1864). German surgeon.

Chvostek's anaemia. Anaemia associated with impaired pancreatic function.

chylaceous (ki·**la**·shus). Consisting of or having the properties of chyle.

chylaemia (ki·**le**·me·ah). A condition in which chyle is present in the peripheral circulation. [chyle, Gk *haima* blood.]

chylangioma (**ki**·lan·je·**o**′·mah). 1. Lymphangioma filled with a chylous fluid. 2. A condition in which there is dilatation of a lymph vessel due to retention of chyle. [chyle, angioma.]

chylaqueous (ki·**lak**·we·us). Like or composed of chyle and water. [chyle, L *aqua* water.]

chyle [chylus (NA)] (kile). The modified milk-white lymph contained in the lymph vessels of the small intestine after they have absorbed fat from foodstuffs; the emulsified fat gives the milky appearance. Chyle reaches the veins by way of the thoracic duct and the left subclavian vein. **Granular chyle.** The minute globules of fat in chyle. [Gk *chylos* juice.]

chylectasia (ki·lek·**ta**·ze·ah). A state of dilatation of a chyle-carrying vessel. [chyle, Gk *ektasis* a stretching.]

chylhidrosis, chylidrosis (kile·hid·**ro**·sis, ki·lid·**ro**·sis). Chylous sweating. [chyle, Gk *hidros* sweat.]

chylifacient (ki·le·**fa**·shent). Chyle-forming. [chyle, L *facere* to make.]

chylifaction (ki·le·**fak**·shun). The forming or producing of chyle. [see prec.]

chylifactive (ki·le·**fak**·tiv). Chylifacient.

chyliferous (ki·**lif**·er·us). Conveying, containing or forming chyle. [chyle, L *ferre* to bear.]

chylific (ki·**lif**·ik). Referring to chylification.

chylification (ki·lif·ik·**a**·shun). The process of forming chyle and its subsequent separation and absorption by the villi. [chyle, L *facere* to make.]

chylificatory (**ki**·lif·ik·**a**′·tor·e). Chylifacient.

chyliform (**ki**·le·form). Like or resembling chyle. [chyle, form.]

chylocele (**ki**·lo·seel). An effusion of chylous fluid into the tunica vaginalis testis. **Parasitic chylocele.** Dilatation of the lymph vessels of the scrotum such as may occur in filariasis; lymph scrotum. [chyle, Gk *kele* hernia.]

chylocyst (**ki**·lo·sist). The cisterna (receptaculum) chyli. [chyle, Gk *kystis* bag.]

chylocystic (ki·lo·**sis**·tik). Referring to the chylocyst or cisterna chyli.

chyloderma (ki·lo·**der**·mah). Lymph scrotum. *See* SCROTUM. [chyle, Gk *derma* skin.]

chylodochium (ki·lo·**do**·ke·um). The cisterna (receptaculum) chyli. [chyle, Gk *docheion* receptacle.]

chyloid (ki·loid). Chyliform. [chyle, Gk *eidos* form.]
chylology (ki·lol·o·je). The sum of knowledge concerning chyle and its function. [chyle, Gk *logos* science.]
chylomediastinum (ki·lo·me·de·as·ti′·num). Occurrence of chyle in the mediastinum.
chylomicrograph (ki·lo·mi·kro·graf). A graph showing the curve obtained from successive counts of chylomicrons.
chylomicrons (ki·lo·mi·kronz). Small, fat globules about 1 nm in diameter. They are formed of triglycerides complexed with lipoprotein, cholesterol ester and phospholipid. They enter the lymphatic system draining the intestine and are carried in the plasma to fat depots, where they are cleared from the plasma by the enzyme lipoprotein. [chyle, Gk *mikros* small.]
chylopericarditis (ki·lo·per·e·kar·di′·tis). A condition in which chyle is present in the serous pericardial sac as well as pericarditis.
chylopericardium (ki·lo·per·e·kar′·de·um). A condition in which there is a pericardial effusion containing chyle as a result of obstruction to the thoracic duct, usually by neoplasm.
chyloperitoneum (ki·lo·per·e·ton·e′·um). The condition in which there is an effusion of chyle into the peritoneal cavity.
chylophoric (ki·lo·for·ik). Chyliferous. [chyle, Gk *pherein* to bear.]
chylopleura (ki·lo·ploor·ah). The condition in which chyle is present in the cavity of the pleura.
chylopoiesis (ki·lo·poi·e′·sis). Chylifaction. [chyle, Gk *poiein* to make.]
chylopoietic (ki·lo·poi·et′·ik). 1. Referring to chylopoiesis. 2. Having a part in the making of chyle.
chyloptyalism (ki·lop·ti·al·izm). A condition in which the saliva is milky in appearance. [chyle, Gk *ptyalezein* to spit.]
chylorrhoea (ki·lo·re·ah). 1. A flow of chyle caused by rupture of the thoracic duct. 2. Excessive secretion of chyle. 3. Diarrhoea in which the faeces are of a milky colour as the result of rupture of the lymph vessels of the small intestine. [chyle, Gk *rhoia* flow.]
chylosis (ki·lo·sis). The process by which food is converted into chyle and that in turn taken up by the tissues. [chyle, Gk *-osis* condition.]
chylothorax (ki·lo·thor·ax). The condition in which there is an effusion of chyle into the thoracic cavity.
chylous (ki·lus). Relating to, resembling or mixed with chyle.
chyluria (ki·lewr·e·ah). The condition in which the urine is of a milky appearance because it contains chyle or lipoid matter. **Chyluria tropica.** Chyluria resulting from filariasis, the lymph vessels becoming obstructed by adult filaria.
chymase (ki·maze). A ferment produced in the gastric juice which accelerates the action of the pancreatic juice. [Gk *chymos* juice.]
chyme (kime). Food in a partly digested state and in the form of a thick greyish or brownish liquid passing from the stomach into the intestines for the completion of digestion. [Gk *chymos* juice.]
chymiferous (ki·mif·er·us). 1. Containing or carrying chyme. 2. Having the power to produce chyme. [chyme, L *ferre* to bear.)
chymification (ki·mif·e·ka′·shun). The process of conversion of food into chyme by the digestive action of the gastric juice. [chyme, L *facere* to make.]
chymopapain (ki·mo·pap·a′·in). An enzyme from papaya. [Gk *chymos* juice, papain.]
chymorrhoea (ki·mor·e·ah). An evacuation or flow of chyme. [chyme, Gk *rhoia* flow.]
chymosin (ki·mo·sin). The modern name for rennin, or chymase, the enzyme in gastric juice which converts the caseinogen of milk into insoluble casein in the presence of calcium ions (clotting). [Gk *chymos* juice.]
chymosinogen (ki·mo·sin·o·jen). The modern name for renninogen, the precursor of rennin (chymosin). [chymosin, Gk *genein* to produce.]
chymotrichy (ki·mot·rik·e). By derivation, wavy hair: not generally used in medical literature today. [Gk *kyma* a wave, *thrix* hair.]
chymotrypsin (ki·mo·trip·sin). An intestinal proteolytic enzyme. It is formed by the action of trypsin on the zymogen chymotrypsinogen. **Alpha chymotrypsin.** Employed in cataract extraction to digest the suspensory ligament of the lens. [Gk *chymos* juice, trypsin.]
chymotrypsinogen (ki·mo·trip·sin′·o·jen). The zymogen precursor of chymotrypsin. [Gk *chymos* juice, trypsin, Gk *genein* to produce.]
chymous (ki·mus). Relating to or composed of chyme.
Ciaccio, Carmelo (b.1877). Messina pathologist.
Ciaccio's methods. Various methods for staining lipoids involving fixation with potassium dichromate and staining with Sudan III.
Ciaccio, Giuseppe Vincenzo (b. 1824). Italian anatomist.
Ciaccio's glands. Accessory lacrimal glands. *See* GLAND.
Ciaglinski, Adam (fl. 1891). German anatomist.
Ciaglinski's tract. A tract of ascending fibres in the posterior grey commissure of the thoracic portion of the spinal cord.
Ciarrocchi, Gaetano (b. 1857). Rome dermatologist.
Ciarrocchi's disease. Symmetrical dermatitis of the third interdigital spaces of the hands.
cibarian (si·ba·re·an). Relating to food and the mouth parts, i.e. the organs of chewing and swallowing. [L *cibus* food.]
cibarious (si·ba·re·us). 1. Relating to food. 2. Edible or nutritious. [see prec.]
cibisotome (si·bis·o·tome). Cystitome; a fine scalpel used in cataract extraction for making an opening in the lens capsule. [Gk *kibisis* pouch, *temnein* to cut.]
cibophobia (si·bo·fo·be·ah). 1. Aversion to food. 2. An insane or morbid fear of eating. [L *cibus* food, phobia.]
cicatricial (sik·at·rish·al). Relating to or having the character of a scar. [L *cicatrix* scar.]
cicatricle (sik·at·rikl). The small disc present on the yolk of the fertilized egg of reptiles and birds from which the embryo develops. [see prec.]
cicatricose (sik·at·rik·oze). Bearing marks of scars or impressions like those of scars. [L *cicatrix* scar.]
cicatricotomy (sik·at·rik·ot′·o·me). 1. Removal of a scar by surgical means. 2. Incision into a scar. [cicatrix, Gk *temnein* to cut.]
cicatricula (sik·at·rik·ew·lah). A small scar. [L.]
cicatrisate (sik·at·ris·ate). Cicatricose.
cicatrisotomy (sik·at·ris·ot′·o·me). Cicatricotomy.
cicatrix (sik·at·rix) (pl. *cicatrices*). The fibrous scar resulting from the healing of a wound. **Exuberant cicatrix.** A scar with excessive fibrous proliferation. **Filtering cicatrix.** An incompletely healed wound of the eyeball, usually covered by conjunctiva, through which there is an escape of aqueous. This may be the result of trauma, or produced deliberately, as in glaucoma operations. **Hypertrophic cicatrix.** A scar with hypertrophied fibrous tissue. **Keloid cicatrix.** A new growth of fibrous tissue, distinguished from hypertrophy by its extension beyond the limits of the scar. **Manometric cicatrix.** A cicatrix or scar on the drum head, which tends to exaggerate the normal inward and outward movements of the drum head which follows variations of pressure on it. **Vibratory cicatrix.** A scar which shows pulsation. **Vicious cicatrix.** A scar that by its contraction causes serious deformity. [L scar.]
cicatrizant (sik·at·riz·ant). An agent which promotes the healing of a sore or wound by the formation of scar tissue. [see foll.]
cicatrization (sik·at·ri·za′·shun). The process or state of healing by formation of a scar. [L *cicatrix* scar.]
cicatrize (sik·at·rize). To heal in such a way as to leave a scar. [see prec.]
cicatrose (sik·at·roze). Cicatricose.
Cichorium (sik·or·e·um). A very small genus of the family Compositae. Two species are important as food plants, *Cichorium intybus* Linn. (chicory) and *Cichorium endivia* Linn. (endive). [Gk *kichorion.*]
Ciclopirox (si·klo·pi·rox). BP Commission approved name for 6-cyclohexyl-l-hydroxy-4-methyl-2-pyridone; a fungicide.
Cicloxolone (sik·lox·o·lone). BP Commission approved name for

3β-(*cis*-2-carboxycyclohexylcarbonyloxy)-11-oxo-olean-12-en-30-oic acid; it is used in the treatment of gastric ulcer.

Cicuta (sik·**ew**·tah). A small genus of plants of the family Umbelliferae. *Cicuta virosa* Linn. (cowbane, water hemlock) is the only British species; it is poisonous and is not used medicinally. [L hemlock.]

cicutine (**sik**·ew·teen). Coniine; a volatile, colourless liquid alkaloid obtained from *Cicuta virosa,* the water hemlock, probably identical with coniine. It depresses the central nervous system and has a paralytic effect on the nerve-endings in skeletal muscle.

cicutism (**sik**·ew·tism). Poisoning by water hemlock, *Cicuta virosa;* marked by dilatation of pupils, cyanosis of face, convulsions and coma.

cicutoxin (sik·ew·**tox**·in). A complex pyrone derivative from *Cicuta virosa,* the water hemlock. It is a stimulant to the central nervous system, resembling picrotoxin in its pharmacological actions. [*Cicuta,* toxin.]

ciguatera (sig·wah·**ta**·rah). A disease characterized by acute gastro-enteritis; it occurs in Central and South America, and is held to be caused by eating the poisonous fish *Sphyraena picuda.*

cilia (**sil**·e·ah). 1. The eyelashes. 2. Hair-like processes found on many cells, capable of lashing or vibratory movement which drives forward fluid or particles. 3. The prehensile and motile organs present in some micro-organisms. [L, eyelashes.]

ciliariscope (sil·e·**ar**·is·kope). A prism-like instrument with which the ciliary region of the eye can be examined. [cilium, Gk *skopein* to watch.]

ciliarotomy (**sil**·e·ar·**ot**′·o·me). The surgical procedure of dividing the ciliary zonule for the relief of glaucoma. [cilium, Gk *temnein* to cut.]

ciliary (**sil**·e·ar·e). 1. Relating to cilia. 2. Relating to the eyelids or the eyelashes. **Ciliary gland.** *See* GLAND. **Ciliary plexus.** *See* PLEXUS. **Ciliary ring.** *See* RING.

ciliary arteries. Anterior ciliary arteries [arteriae ciliares anteriores], Long posterior ciliary arteries [arteriae ciliares posteriores longae], Short posterior ciliary arteries [arteriae ciliares posteriores breves]. *See* OPHTHALMIC ARTERY.

ciliary muscle [musculus ciliaris (NA)]. An unstriped circular muscle in the ciliary body of the eye, consisting of circular fibres [fibrae circulares (NA)] (of Mueller) and meridional fibres [fibrae meridionales (NA)] (of Bruecke). It is the muscle of accommodation.

ciliary nerves. Long ciliary nerves [nervi ciliares longi (NA)]. Branches from the nasociliary nerve to the eye which do not traverse the ciliary ganglion. They contain sympathetic fibres for the dilator pupillae muscle. **Short ciliary nerves [nervi ciliares breves (NA)].** The branches of the ciliary ganglion to the eye, 6–10 in number. They contain parasympathetic and sensory fibres.

ciliary veins [venae ciliares (NA)]. Veins of the ciliary body arranged in 2 groups, anterior and posterior, the former draining the ciliary muscle and perforating the sclera near the cornea to join the veins of the recti muscles, the latter draining the ciliary processes into the choroidal veins.

Ciliata (sil·e·a·tah). A class of Protozoa whose individuals are covered with cilia which serve for locomotion and often to set up feeding currents. *Balantidium coli* is the only species of medical importance, causing balantidial dysentery in man. Species of *Balantiophorus, Lembus* and *Uronema* are coprozoic. [L *cilium* eyelash.]

ciliated (**sil**·e·a·ted). Having cilia.

ciliation (sil·e·a·shun). 1. A ciliate process. 2. The quality or state of being ciliated.

ciliectomy (sil·e·**ek**·to·me). 1. Surgical removal of a part of the ciliary body or ciliary muscle. 2. Surgical removal of part of the edge of the eyelid. [cilium, Gk *ektome* a cutting out.]

ciliogenesis (**sil**·e·o·**jen**′·es·is). The development or formation of cilia. [cilia, Gk *genein* to produce.]

ciliograde (**sil**·e·o·grade). Moving by means of cilia. [cilia, L *gradus* step.]

Ciliophora (sil·e·**of**·or·ah). A sub-phylum of the phylum Protozoa. The members are characterized by the presence of cilia in at least some stage of the life history. The class Ciliata is of medical interest. [L *cilium* eyelash, Gk *pherein* to bear.]

cilioretinal (**sil**·e·o·**ret**′·in·al). Relating to the retina and the ciliary body.

cilioscleral (**sil**·e·o·**skleer**′·al). Relating to the ciliary body and the sclera.

ciliospinal (**sil**·e·o·**spi**′·nal). Having relation to the ciliary body and the spinal cord.

ciliotomy (sil·e·**ot**·o·me). Operative division of the ciliary nerves. [cilium, Gk *temnein* to cut.]

cilium (**sil**·e·um). 1. The eyelid. 2. The outer margin of the eyelid. 3. An eyelash. 4. A hair-like process attached to a cell or a micro-organism. [L.]

cillosis (sil·**o**·sis). Spasmodic trembling of the upper eyelid. [cilium, Gk *-osis* condition.]

cillotic (sil·**ot**·ik). Referring to or affected with cillosis.

cimbia (**sim**·be·ah). A band of white fibres that extends across the anterior surface of the cerebral peduncle. [L girdle.]

cimbial (**sim**·be·al). Relating to cimbia.

Cimex (si·mex). A genus of wingless bugs whose members are blood suckers of birds and mammals. *Cimex lectularius,* the temperate bed bug, and *C. hemipterus* (=*rotundatus*), the tropical bed bug, are parasites of man and generally similar to each other in behaviour. In the former the prothorax is much wider than the head; in the latter but little wider. Adults are about 8 mm long, round bodied, much flattened, and brown; nymphs are whitish and less flattened. They live in wall and furniture cracks, emerging, usually at night, to feed. The life cycle can be completed in about 7 weeks, but under cold conditions and absence of food the individuals can live for very much longer. The bites give rise to painful irregular weals. Heavy infestations have a characteristic smell. Other species, whose normal hosts are pigeons and bats, occasionally bite man. No bug of this species has been incriminated as an important vector of any disease of man, but the above species and *C. bueti* and *C. hirundinis* have been shown to be potential vectors of American trypanosomiasis. [L bug.]

Cimicidae (si·**mis**·id·e). A family of the insectan order Hemiptera. The genera *Cimex, Haematosiphon* and *Oeciacus* are of medical interest. [L *cimex* bug, Gk *eidos* form.]

cimicifuga (sim·is·**if**·ew·gah). Black cohosh, black snake root, the dried rhizome and root of *Cimicifuga racemosa* Nutt. (family Ranunculaceae). It contains resin, isoferulic acid, and other acids and alcohols. It is a bitter and mild expectorant, and has also been used in the treatment of chorea, rheumatism and neuralgia. [L *cimex* bug, *fugare* to put to flight.]

cimicifugin (sim·is·**if**·ew·jin). A resinous substance derived from cimicifuga (black cohosh, black snake root); it is also known as *macrotin.* It has only slight pharmacological action apart from some depression of smooth muscle, but has been reported to be antispasmodic, expectorant and stomachic.

cimicosis (sim·ik·o·sis). An itching condition of the skin resulting from bites of the bed bug, *Cimex lectularius.* [*Cimex,* Gk *-osis* condition.]

cinaesthesia, cinaesthesis (sin·es·**the**·ze·ah, sin·es·**the**·sis). Kinaesthesia. 1. The sum of sensations by which weight, position and muscular motion are perceived. 2. The force which compels an individual to throw himself to the ground when looking down from a great height. [Gk *kinein* to move, aesthesia.]

cinanaesthesia (**sin**·an·es·**the**′·ze·ah). Derangement of deep sensibility causing inability to perceive the sensation of movement. [Gk *kinein* to move, anaesthesia.]

cinchamidine (sin·**kam**·id·een). Hydrocinchonidine, $C_{19}H_{24}ON_2$. An alkaloid from *Cinchona ledgeriana* which is isomeric with cinchotine.

cinching (**sin**·ching). The operative making of tucks (plicating) in a muscle of the orbit of the eye in order to shorten it. [L *cingere* to gird.]

cinchocaine (sin·ko·kane). $C_9H_5N(OC_4H_9)CONH(CH_2)_2N(C_2H_5)_2$, a local analgesic with action more prolonged than that of cocaine or procaine. It is used in the preparation of ointments or oily solutions (BPC 1968). **Cinchocaine Hydrochloride BP 1973.** The salt of the above used for procuring spinal, surface or infiltration anaesthesia.

cinchol (**sin**·kol). $C_{29}H_{50}O$, a sterol found in cinchona bark.

cinchona (sin·**ko**·nah). Peruvian bark, Jesuit bark; the bark of several species and hybrids of *Cinchona* (family Rubiaceae), trees indigenous to South America. Cinchona BPC 1963 is the dried bark of cultivated trees of *Cinchona calisaya* Wedd. (yellow bark), *C. ledgeriana* Moens (yellow bark), *C. officinalis* Linn. (pale bark), *C. robusta* Howard, and *C. succirubra* Pav. (red bark), or of hybrids of these. It is grown in India, Sri Lanka, Tanzania and particularly in Java (90 per cent of the world supply). It contains several alkaloids, the most important being quinine, quinidine, cinchonine and cinchonidine, combined with quinic and cinchotannic acids; a glycoside quinovin, and a phlobaphene, cinchona red, are also present. Cinchona preparations have bitter-tonic, stomachic and astringent properties. The bark is mainly used as a source of the alkaloids. *C. lancifolia* Mutis. yields Columbian and Carthagena barks. [Countess of *Chinchon,* d. 1641, was formerly erroneously credited with having introduced it into Europe.]

cinchonamine (sin·**kon**·am·een). $C_{19}H_{24}ON$, a cinchona alkaloid derived from Cuprea bark (*Remijia purdieana*), isomeric with cinchotine and cinchamidine. It is more toxic than quinine.

cinchonate (**sin**·kon·ate). Any salt or ester of cinchonic acid.

cinchonic (sin·**kon**·ik). Belonging or having reference to cinchona.

cinchonicine (sin·**kon**·is·een). Cinchotoxine, $C_{19}H_{23}ON_2$. An alkaloid from cinchona and cuprea barks. It is isomeric with cinchonine.

cinchonidine (sin·**kon**·id·een). $C_{19}H_{22}ON_2$, an alkaloid present in cinchona bark, laevorotatory and isomeric with cinchonine. Its pharmacological actions are similar to those of quinine, though it is less efficacious in the treatment of malaria; it is also more depressant to the heart and may cause convulsions. **Cinchonidine dihydrochloride.** $C_{19}H_{22}ON_2{\cdot}2HCl{\cdot}H_2O$, a crystalline compound which is very soluble in water and therefore suitable for injections. **Cinchonidine hydrochloride.** $C_{19}H_{22}ON_2HCl{\cdot}H_2O$, a salt less soluble in water but readily in chloroform. **Cinchonidine salicylate.** $C_{19}H_{22}ON_2C_6H_4(OH)COOH$, a compound used in oral administration of the drug. **Cinchonidine sulphate.** $(C_{19}H_{22}ON_2)_2H_2SO_4{\cdot}7H_2O$, a compound used similarly to the salicylate.

cinchonifine (sin·**kon**·if·een). Cinchotine.

cinchonine (**sin**·kon·een). $C_{19}H_{22}ON_2$, an alkaloid derived from cinchona bark, dextrorotatory and isomeric with cinchonidine. Pharmacologically its actions are similar to those of quinine, though in toxicity it is comparable with cinchonidine. **Cinchonine dihydrochloride.** Cinchonic acid hydrochloride, $C_{19}H_{22}ON_2{\cdot}2HCl$, a white crystalline powder soluble in water. **Cinchonine iodosulphate.** A brown substance which has been used for similar purposes to those of iodoform. **Cinchonine sulphate.** $(C_{19}H_{22}ON_2)_2H_2SO_4{\cdot}2H_2O$, a compound soluble in alcohol, used like quinine sulphate.

cinchonism (**sin**·kon·izm). A morbid condition produced by excessive or long-continued use of cinchona or any of the alkaloids of cinchona bark, also rarely after therapeutic dosage in the highly susceptible. Various toxic symptoms are produced, e.g. cerebral congestion, giddiness, tinnitus, rash, nausea, mental and cardiac disturbances, and circulatory or respiratory failure.

cinchonize (**sin**·kon·ize). To expose to the strong influence of cinchona or one of its alkaloids, particularly quinine.

cinchophen (**sin**·ko·fen). Phenylquinoline carboxylic acid, $C_6H_5C_9H_5NCOOH$. A synthetic compound with antipyretic properties similar to those of the salicylates but promoting a large excretion of uric acid by the kidneys, for which reason it has been used in the treatment of chronic gout. It has a toxic effect on the liver, however, producing hepatic necrosis. The drug (BP 1953) is always given by mouth, but may cause gastric irritation, which can be obviated by bicarbonate, which also renders the urine alkaline and prevents precipitation of urates. It is also known as *quinophan.* **Cinchophen hydrochloride.** A yellow crystalline insoluble powder formerly in use under the name chloroxyl.

cinchotannin (sin·ko·**tan**·in). Cinchotannic acid, $C_{14}H_{16}O_9$. A phlobatannin found in cinchona bark.

cinchotine (**sin**·ko·teen). Dihydrocinchonine, $C_{19}H_{24}ON_2$. An alkaloid from cinchona; also known as *hydrocinchonine.* It can be prepared by the oxidation of quinine.

cinchotoxine (sin·ko·**tox**·een). Cinchonicine.

cinclisis (sin·**kli**·sis). 1. Quick spasmodic movement affecting any part of the body. 2. Rapid breathing as in dyspnoea. 3. Rapid involuntary winking. [Gk *kigklisis* quick repeated motion.]

cine-angiocardiography (**sin**·e·**an**′·je·o·kar·de·**og**′·raf·e). Cinematographic angiocardiography. [Gk *kinesis* movement, angiocardiography.]

cine-angiography (**sin**·e·an·je·**og**′·raf·e). The technique of recording, by moving pictures, the intensified x-ray image of radio-opaque material injected into the circulation to show the chambers of the heart or the blood vessels. [Gk *kinema* motion, *aggeion* vessel, *graphein* to record.]

cinemadiagraphy (**sin**·e·mah·di·**ag**′·raf·e). Cinematography of the movement of the internal structures of the body. [Gk *kinema* motion, *dia, graphein* to record.]

cinemascopia, cinemascopy (**sin**·e·mas·**ko**′·pe·ah, sin·e·**mas**′·kop·e). Cinematoradiography. [Gk *kinema* motion, *skopein* to watch.]

cinematics (sin·e·**mat**·ix). Kinematics. The science of movements and motion in general, and body movements in particular. [Gk *kinema* motion.]

cinematization (**sin**·e·mat·i·**za**′·shun). Cineplastics.

cinematomicrography (**sin**·e·mat·o·mi·**krog**′·raf·e). The making and projection of photographic films of moving microscopic objects. [Gk *kinema* motion, micrography.]

cinematoradiography (sin·e·**mat**·o·ra·de·**og**′·raf·e). Cineradiography. [Gk *kinema* motion, radiography.]

cineole (**sin**·e·ole). 1. Any of the oxides or ethers of the menthane group of terpenes. 2. Eucalyptol, $C_{10}H_{18}O$, an oil contained in, and responsible for the characteristic odour of, eucalyptus oil; also in wormseed oil and cajuput oil. It is an irritant with some antiseptic action, and is generally preferred to the crude eucalyptus oil for inclusion in nasal drops. Most commonly used in inhalants and in toothpaste.

Cinepazet (si·ne·**pa**·zet). BP Commission approved name for ethyl-4-(3,4,5-trimethoxycinnamoyl)piperazin-l-ylacetate; it is used in the treatment of angina.

cineplastics, cineplasty (sin·e·**plas**·tix, sin·e·**plas**·te). Cineplastic amputation. *See* AMPUTATION. [Gk *kinein* to move, *plassein* to mould.]

cineraceous (sin·er·**a**·shus). Ash-grey. [L *cinereus* ashen coloured.]

cineradiography (**sin**·e·ra·de·**og**′·raf·e). The taking of x-ray moving pictures of bodily structures and organs for the purpose of diagnosis. [Gk *kinein* to move, radiography.]

cineradiology (**sin**·e·ra·de·**ol**′·o·je). The science of x-ray technique applied to moving x-ray pictures and organs for the purpose of diagnosis. [Gk *kinein* to move, radiology.]

cinerea (sin·**eer**·e·ah). The grey matter of the nervous tissue. [L *cinereus* ashen coloured.]

cinereal (sin·**eer**·e·al). Relating or belonging to the grey matter of the nervous tissue. [see prec.]

cineritious (sin·er·**ish**·us). Ash-grey. [L *cineritius* ashen grey.]

cineroentgenography (**sin**·e·runt·yen·**og**′·raf·e). Cineradiography. [Gk *kinein* to move, roentgenography.]

cinesalgia (sin·es·**al**·je·ah). Kinesalgia; pain caused by movement of the muscles. [Gk *kinesis* movement, *algos* pain.]

cinesia (sin·e·**ze**·ah). Any feeling of nausea, with or without vomiting, that is caused by motion, e.g. seasickness, car sickness. [Gk *kinesis* movement.]

cinesiatrics (sin·e·ze·**at**′·rix). Cinesitherapy. [Gk *kinesis* movement, *iatreia* treatment.]

cinesiology (sin·e·ze·**ol**'·o·je). That department of medical science which has reference to muscular movement, particularly in so far as its use in treatment is concerned. [Gk *kinesis* movement, *logos* science.]

cinesiotherapy (sin·e·ze·o·**ther**'·ap·e). Cinesitherapy.

cinesis (sin·e·sis). Kinesis.

cinesitherapy (sin·e·ze·**ther**'·ap·e). Treatment of disease by means of callisthenics or other types of active and passive movement. [Gk *kinesis* movement, therapy.]

cinetographic (sin·et·o·**graf**'·ik). Having reference to the graphical recording of movements. [Gk *kinesis* movement, *graphein* to record.]

cingule (sing·gewl). Cingulum.

cingulectomy (sing·gew·**lek**·to·me). The operation for removal, usually by suction-ablation, of parts of both cingulate gyri; used in treatment of certain mental disorders. [cingulum, Gk *ektome* excision.]

cingulum [NA] (sing·gew·lum). A long curved bundle of association fibres lying within the gyrus cinguli of the cerebral hemisphere. [L *cingulum* girdle.]

Ciniselli, Luigi (b.1803). Cremona surgeon.

Ciniselli's method. Electrocoagulation of aneurysm.

cinnabar (sin·ah·bar). A red mineral ore, mercuric sulphide HgS, found mostly in Spain and Tuscany; it is the chief source of mercury. [L *cinnabaris.*]

cinnaldehyde (sin·**al**·de·hide). An obsolete name for cinnamic aldehyde, derived from oil of cinnamon.

cinnamate (sin·am·ate). A salt of cinnamic acid.

cinnamein (sin·am·e·in). 1. A mixture of balsamic esters, principally benzyl benzoate and benzyl cinnamate, constituting 56–66 per cent of commercial balsam of Peru; used internally as an expectorant, externally as an antiseptic. 2. Benzyl cinnamate, $C_6H_5CH{=}CHCOOCH_2C_6H_5$, a colourless compound occurring in Peru and Tolu balsams, and used in perfumes.

cinnamene (sin·am·een). Styrene, phenyl ethylene, $C_6H_5CH{=}CH_2$. An unsaturated liquid hydrocarbon which occurs free in storax and in coal tar. It is prepared by heating cinnamic acid, and polymerises to a glassy substance, metastyrene, used in plastics manufacture.

cinnamol (sin·am·ol). Cinnamene.

Cinnamomum (sin·am·**o**·mum). 1. A genus of evergreen trees and shrubs of the family Lauraceae. 2. Cinnamon bark. *See* CINNAMON. **Cinnamomum burmanni.** The species which yields Java cinnamon. **Cinnamomum camphora.** A species the wood of which is the source of natural camphor. **Cinnamomum cassia.** The species which yields cassia bark; Chinese cinnamon. **Cinnamomum oliveri.** The species which furnishes oliver bark (black sassafras), used in Australia as a substitute for cinnamon. **Cinnamomum zeylanicum.** A species principally grown in Sri Lanka; it is the source of cinnamon bark; Ceylon cinnamon. [Gk *kinnamomon.*]

cinnamon (sin·am·on). The dried inner bark of *Cinnamomum zeylanicum*, a tree cultivated in Sri Lanka and elsewhere. It may be encountered as quills telescoped together or as a powder (BP 1973). The bark contains a volatile oil, Cinnamon Oil BP 1958, which is responsible for the characteristic aromatic odour and for the carminative action of preparations containing the drug. It is commonly used as a flavouring agent, particularly in preparations used to treat diarrhoea since the drug contains tannic acid which has a considerable astringent effect. **Chinese cinnamon.** Cassia bark. [see prec.]

cinnamylcocaine (sin·am·il·ko·**kane**'). Methylcinnamylecgonine, $C_{19}H_{23}O_4N$. An insoluble alkaloid isolated from Java coca leaves.

cinnamyl-eugenol (sin·am·il·**ew**'·jen·ol). Eugenol cinnamate, $C_6H_5CH{=}CHCOOC_6H_3(OCH_3)CH_2CH{=}CH_2$. A colourless compound with antiseptic properties similar to eugenol.

Cinnarizine (sin·**ar**·iz·een). BP Commission approved name for 1-*trans*-cinnamyl-4-diphenylmethylpiperazine; an antihistaminic drug.

cinology (sin·**ol**·o·je). Cinesiology.

cinometer (sin·**om**·et·er). Kinesimeter: 1. A device used to determine the degree of movement in a part. 2. A device for examination of the body surface in order to measure the degree of cutaneous sensibility. [Gk *kinein* to move, *metron* measure.]

cinoplasm (sin·o·plazm). Kinoplasm.

Cinoxacin (sin·**ox**·as·in). BP Commission approved name for 1-ethyl-4-oxo[1,3]dioxolo[4,5-*g*]cinnoline-3-carboxylic acid; an antibacterial agent.

Cinoxolone (sin·**ox**·o·lone). BP Commission approved name for cinnamyl 3β-acetoxy-11-oxo-olean-12-en-30-oate; it is used in the treatment of gastric ulcer.

cion (si·on). The uvula. [Gk *kion* pillar.]

cionectomy (si·on·**ek**·to·me). Uvulectomy. [Gk *kion* pillar, *ektome* a cutting out.]

cionitis (si·on·**i**·tis). Uvulitis. [Gk *kion* pillar, *-itis* inflammation.]

cionoptosis (si·on·op·**to**'·sis). Uvuloptosis. [Gk *kion* pillar, *ptosis* fall.]

cionorrhaphy (si·on·**or**·af·e). Palatoplasty. [Gk *kion* pillar, *rhaphe* suture.]

cionotome (si·on·o·tome). Uvulotome. [Gk *kion* pillar, *temnein* to cut.]

cionotomy (si·on·**ot**·o·me). Uvulotomy. [see prec.]

circadian (ser·**ka**·de·an). Diurnal; relating to a period of about 1 day, or 24 h. **Circadian rhythm.** The rhythm that varies at different intervals, such as daily, by which the activity of some process increases or decreases at certain different times. For instance, adrenocortical circadian rhythm is greatest in the early morning and falls during the day so that it is lowest at midnight. [L *circa* around or about, *dies* a day.]

circellus (ser·**sel**·us). A small circle. **Circellus venosus hypoglossi.** A network of veins which surrounds the hypoglossal nerve as it passes through the anterior condylar canal. [L.]

circinate (ser·sin·ate). Ring-shaped; having lesions that are circular or ring-shaped, e.g. in dermatological conditions. [L *circinare* to make round.]

circle (ser·kl). 1. A ring; a plane figure described by the end of a radius rotating about a centre. 2. In anatomy [circulus (NA)], any ring-shaped structure, usually one formed by blood vessels. **Circle absorber.** A canister of soda lime in an anaesthetic circuit which absorbs carbon dioxide. Unidirectional valves ensure circular motion of the gas mixture. **Arterial circle of the iris, greater [circulus arteriosus iridis major (NA)].** An arterial circle round the periphery of the iris. **Arterial circle of the iris, lesser [circulus arteriosus iridis minor (NA)].** An arterial circle round the pupillary margin. **Defensive circle.** The co-existence of 2 pathological conditions which antagonize each other, e.g. gout and tuberculosis. **Diffusion circle.** The blurred image produced on the retina when the eye is looking at, but not focused for, a point source of light. **Circle of dispersion, Circle of dissipation.** The minute disc-shaped image on the retina formed by the eye when it is focused on a point source of light. **Circles of the iris.** Arterial circles of the iris (see above). **Vascular circle of the optic nerve.** Circulus vasculosus of the optic nerve. **Vicious circle.** The term used when one disease or morbid condition causes another, which in turn aggravates the first, and so on, in a circle. [L *circulus.*]

See also: BERRY (G. A.), CARUS, HALLER, HOVIUS, HUGUIER, LEBER, MINSKY, ROBINSON (F. B.), WEBER (E. H.), WILLIS, ZINN.

circocele (ser·ko·seel). Varicocele. [Gk *kirsos* dilated vein, *kele* hernia.]

circuit (ser·kit). A single loop or complex network of electrical conductors through which current may flow. **Breathing circuits.** Different arrangements of breathing tubes used on anaesthetic machines. **Closed circuit.** A closed anaesthetic circuit to which oxygen is added and carbon dioxide absorbed by soda lime. **Constant potential circuit.** A circuit giving a constant direct potential from the alternating high voltage supplied from an x-ray transformer. **Extracorporeal circuits.** The technique of keeping the circulation of the blood going by the use of an artificial heart–lung machine, used in open operations on the heart. **Full-wave circuit.** A circuit for converting an alternating supply into a constant or pulsating direct potential in which both halves of the supply potential cycle are used. **Half-wave supply circuit.** The same as full-wave supply circuit (see above) except that only one half of the supply cycle is used. **Magnetic circuit.** A closed loop containing magnetic material which is mathematically analogous to an electric circuit, the intensity of magnetization taking the place of electric current. **Open circuit.** An anaesthetic circuit from which gases can escape through an expiratory valve. **Organic circuit.** Reflex arc. *See* ARC. **Printed circuit.** An electrical circuit formed as a unit by copper laminates on a phenol base. They may be deposited as a powder, photographed on a resist and etched, or deposited by electrodeposition. **Quenching circuits.** Electronic circuits designed to quench a Geiger discharge. **Reflex circuit.** Reflex arc. *See* ARC. **Scaling circuit.** An electronic circuit which divides the electrical pulses entering it by a constant number, and emits a pulse, for example, once every hundred entrant pulses. **Semi-closed (or semi-open) anaesthetic circuit.** A system in which the patient expires partly to the outside atmosphere and partly into a reservoir bag, depending on the flow of gases and the type of breathing. **Short circuit.** 1. A circuit in which one element possesses an unusually low resistance, allowing an abnormally high current flow. 2. The surgical establishment of a communication between a segment of the gastro-intestinal tract above an obstruction and a segment below it. **Circuit training.** Non-specific exercises carried out in sequence a set number of times. [L *circumire* to go round.]

See also: COCKROFT, GEIGER, GREINACHER, KOCH (R.), MARX, MUELLER (W.), NEHER-HARPER, VILLARD.

circulation (ser·kew·**la**·shun). Movements in a circular fashion or through a course which leads back to the starting point. **Allantoic circulation.** The circulation supplying blood in the fetus through the allantois and, later in development, through the umbilical vessels. **Assisted circulation.** The method of treating acute, severe circulatory insufficiency by some mechanical means such as an external pump or a pulsating balloon inserted into the aorta. **Blood circulation.** The movement of blood from the heart through the arteries, capillaries and veins back to the heart. **Capillary circulation.** The amount of blood circulating in the capillaries. **Chilblain circulation.** Acrocyanosis. **Chorionic circulation.** Umbilical circulation (see below). **Collateral circulation.** A compensatory circulation developed through enlargements of secondary channels following obstruction to a main blood vessel. **Coronary circulation.** The blood flow through the coronary vessels of the heart. **Cross circulation.** Perfusion of parts of the body of one animal by connecting its blood vessels to the circulation of a second animal. **Enterohepatic circulation.** Excretion in the bile of bile salts which are absorbed from the intestines, carried back to the liver, and re-excreted into the intestines from which they are again reabsorbed. **Extracorporeal circulation.** The circulation of blood outside the body through a heart-lung machine, artificial kidney, etc. **Fetal circulation.** The circulation of blood from the fetus to the mother's placenta and back to the fetus. **First circulation.** The primitive circulation of the embryo. **Greater circulation.** The general circulation of the body, excluding the circulation in the lungs. **Intervillous circulation.** That part of the maternal blood circulation in contact with the placental villi. **Lesser circulation.** The circulation of blood through the lungs for oxygenation and removal of carbon dioxide. **Lymph circulation, Lymphatic circulation.** The passage of lymph through lymphatic vessels, glands, and ducts. **Omphalomesenteric circulation.** Vitelline circulation (see below). **Placental circulation.** The circulation of maternal blood through the sinusoids of the placenta, and of the fetal blood via the fetal circulation (see above). **Portal circulation.** The passage of blood from the gastro-intestinal tract and spleen, through the portal vein and its tributaries, to the liver. **Pulmonary circulation.** Lesser circulation (see above). **Systemic circulation.** Greater circulation (see above). **Umbilical circulation.** The blood circulation between the fetus and placenta. **Vitelline circulation.** The circulation between the embryo and the yolk sac. [L *circulare* to go round.]

See also: BOSTON.

circulatory (ser·kew·**la**·tor·e). Relating to or concerned with circulation, e.g. of the blood.

circulus [NA] (**ser**·kew·lus). Circle, or ring. **Circulus arteriosus [circulus arteriosus cerebri (NA)].** The arterial anastomosis in the cisterna interpeduncularis at the base of the brain, formed by the anterior cerebral, anterior communicating, posterior cerebral and posterior communicating arteries. **Circulus arteriosus iridis.** The arterial circle of the iris, greater or lesser. **Circulus arbicularis vasculosus (NA).** An anastomotic ring formed by the blood vessels of the synovial membrane around the periphery of the articular cartilage of a synovial joint. **Circulus vasculosus of the optic nerve [circulus vasculosus nervi optici (NA)].** The vascular circle, circle of Haller (and of Zinn); small arteries in the sclerotic coat of the eye around the entrance of the optic nerve. **Circulus venosus.** The ring of veins around the base of the nipple. [L.]

circumagentes (ser·kum·aj·**en**'·teez). A term descriptive of muscles that cause a part to rotate, e.g. the oblique muscles of the orbit of the eye. [L *circum* around, *agere* to act.]

circumanal (ser·kum·**a**·nal). Perianal. **Circumanal gland.** *See* GLAND. [L *circum* around, anus.]

circumarticular (**ser**·kum·ar·**tik**'·ew·lar). Periarticular. [L *circum* around, *articulare* to divide into joints.]

circumaxillary (**ser**·kum·ax·**il**'·ar·e). Periaxillary. [L *circum* around, axilla.]

circumbuccal (ser·kum·**buk**·al). Around or surrounding the mouth. [L *circum* around, *bucca* cheek.]

circumbulbar (ser·kum·**bul**·bar). Peribulbar. [L *circum* around, bulb.]

circumcallosal (**ser**·kum·kal·**o**'·sal). Surrounding the corpus callosum, or passing around it. [L *circum* around, callosum.]

circumcision (ser·kum·**sizh**·un). The operation of removing the prepuce in the male or the labia minora in the female. **Circumcision of the cornea.** Peridectomy, 1st def. **Pharaonic circumcision.** Infibulation. [L *circum* around, *caedere* to cut.]

circumclusion (ser·kum·**kloo**·zhun). A form of acupressure. A wire is passed around the artery, attached to a pin inserted beneath the artery and made fast. [L *circumcludere* to enclose.]

circumcorneal (ser·kum·**kor**·ne·al). Surrounding the cornea. [L *circum* around, cornea.]

circumcrescent (ser·kum·**kres**·ent). In biology, growing over or around. [L *circum* around, *crescere* to grow.]

circumduction (ser·kum·**duk**·shun). The active or passive movement of a part in a circular manner. [L *circum* around, *ducere* to lead.]

circumference (ser·**kum**·fer·ens). Perimeter, periphery. **Articular circumference.** The circular plane surface of a joint. **Articular circumference of the head of the radius.** *See* RADIUS. **Articular circumference of the head of the ulna.** *See* ULNA. [L *circum* around, *ferre* to bear.]

circumferential (**ser**·kum·fer·**en**'·shal). 1. Encircling. 2. Relating to a circumference or perimeter. [see prec.]

circumflex (**ser**·kum·flex). Having a curve like a bow, or winding around another structure, e.g. shaft of a long bone. A term descriptive of a nerve and of some arteries and veins. [L *circum* around, *flectere* to bend.]

circumflex arteries. Lateral circumflex artery [arteria circumflexa femoris lateralis (NA)]. A branch of the profunda femoris or the femoral artery which winds around the lateral side of the upper thigh and supplies the muscles on this aspect of the thigh and in the gluteal region. Its ascending branch [ramus ascendens (NA)] supplies the hip joint; its transverse branch [ramus transversus (NA)] joins the crucial anastomosis; and its large descending branch [ramus descendens (NA)] accompanies the nerve to the vastus lateralis as far as the knee. **Medial circumflex artery [arteria circumflexa femoris medialis (NA)].** A branch of the profunda femoris artery which winds around the medial side of the upper thigh and supplies the muscles here and in the gluteal region [ramus profundus (NA)]. Its acetabular branch [ramus acetabularis (NA)] accompanies the acetabular branch of the obturator artery to the head of the femur; the transverse branch [ramus transversus (NA)] joins the cruciate anastomosis; and the ascending branch [ramus ascendens (NA)] accompanies the tendon of the obturator externus muscle into the trochanteric fossa.

circumflex humeral arteries (ser·kum·flex **hew**·mer·al). **Anterior circumflex humeral artery [arteria circumflexa humeri anterior (NA)].** A small branch from the third part of the axillary artery, running horizontally in front of the surgical neck of the humerus to anastomose with the posterior circumflex humeral artery. It sends a branch to the shoulder joint along the bicipital groove. **Posterior circumflex humeral artery [arteria circumflexa humeri posterior (NA)].** A large branch from the third part of the axillary artery, running backwards (with the circumflex nerve) through the quadrangular space and then winding laterally behind the surgical neck of the humerus. It supplies adjacent muscles, and anastomoses with the anterior circumflex, suprascapular and acromiothoracic arteries.

circumflex iliac arteries (ser·kum·flex **il**·e·ak). **Deep circumflex iliac artery [arteria circumflexa ilium profunda (NA)].** A branch of the external iliac artery supplying the muscles of the lower abdominal wall. **Deep circumflex iliac artery, ascending branch of the [ramus ascendens (NA)].** A constant branch of the deep circumflex iliac artery arising near the anterior superior iliac spine and supplying the lower abdominal muscles. **Superficial circumflex iliac artery [arteria circumflexa ilium superficialis (NA)].** A branch of the femoral artery to the skin and the superficial fascia and lymph glands in the fold of the groin.

circumflex iliac veins. Deep circumflex iliac vein [vena circumflexa ilium profunda (NA)]. A tributary of the external iliac vein, from the iliac fossa. **Superficial circumflex iliac vein [vena circumflexa ilium superficialis (NA)].** A tributary of the saphenous vein from the inguinal region.

circumflex nerve [nervus axillaris (NA)]. An important branch of the posterior cord of the brachial plexus (root value C5 and 6) which winds from the axilla to the posterior surface of the shoulder region to supply the deltoid muscle [ramus muscularis (NA)] and the skin over the muscle. It also supplies the shoulder joint and teres minor muscle.

circumflex scapular artery [arteria circumflexa scapulae] (ser·kum·flex **skap**·ew·lar). *See* SUBSCAPULAR ARTERY.

circumflex veins. Lateral circumflex veins [venae circumflexae femoris laterales (NA)]. Tributaries of the femoral vein, accompanying the correspondingly named arteries. **Medial circumflex veins [venae circumflexae femoris mediales (NA)].** Tributaries of the femoral vein, accompanying the correspondingly named arteries.

circumgemmal (ser·kum·**jem**·al). Perigemmal. [L *circum* around, *gemma* bud.]

circuminsular (ser·kum·**in**·sew·lar). Peri-insular. [L *circum* around, *insula* island.]

circumintestinal (ser·kum·in·**tes'**·tin·al). Around or surrounding the intestine. [L *circum* around, intestine.]

circumlental (ser·kum·**len**·tal). Perilenticular. [L *circum* around, lens.]

circumnuclear (ser·kum·**new**·kle·ar). Perinuclear. [L *circum* around, nucleus.]

circumocular (ser·kum·**ok**·ew·lar). Round the eye. [L *circum* around, *oculus* eye.]

circumolivary (ser·kum·**ol**·iv·ar·e). Around the olivary body. [L *circum* around, olivary.]

circumoral (ser·kum·**or**·al). Round the mouth. [L *circum* around, *os* mouth.]

circumorbital (ser·kum·**or**·bit·al). Round the orbit. [L *circum* around, orbit.]

circumpolarization (ser·kum·po·lar·i·**za'**·shun). The rotation of the plane of polarized light. [L *circum* around, polarize.]

circumrenal (ser·kum·**re**·nal). Perinephric. [L *circum* around, *ren* kidney.]

circumscribed, circumscriptus (ser·kum·skri·bd, ser·kum·**skrip**·tus). 1. Well defined. 2. Enclosed within narrow limits. [L *circum* around, *scribere* to draw.]

circumstantiality (ser·kum·stan·she·**al'**·it·e). In psychiatry, a conversation into which the patient introduces elaborate details not relevant to the subject. [L *circum* around, *stare* to stand.]

circumtonsillar (ser·kum·**ton**·sil·ar). Peritonsillar. [L *circum* around, tonsil.]

circumvallate (ser·kum·**val**·ate). Surrounded by an elevation, ridge or ditch. [L *circum* around, *vallare* to wall.]

circumvascular (ser·kum·**vas**·kew·lar). Perivascular. [L *circum* around, *vasculum* little vessel.]

circumvolute (ser·kum·**vol**·ewt). Enclosed in something which is wound round. [L *circum* around, *volvere* to roll.]

circumzygomatic (ser·kum·zi·go·**mat'**·ik). Around the zygoma. [L *circum* around, Gk *zygoma* bar.]

cirrhogenous (sir·**oj**·en·us). Productive of hardening or cirrhosis. [Gk *kirrhos* orange-yellow, *genein* to produce.]

cirrholysin (sir·**ol**·is·in). A compound of bismuth tri-iodide and thiosinamine (allyl sulphocarbamide). It was formerly employed for its reputed effect upon fibrous tissue and in the treatment of lupus, though its value has not been proved. [Gk *kirrhos* orange-yellow, *lysein* to dissolve.]

cirrhonosus (sir·**on**·o·sus). 1. A fetal disorder or disease marked macroscopically by yellow staining of the peritoneum and pleura. 2. An abnormally yellow tinge observed *post mortem* in the skin or any other tissue. [Gk *kirrhos* orange-yellow, *nosos* disease.]

cirrhosis (sir·o·sis). A term which is used in a general sense to mean progressive fibrous tissue overgrowth in an organ, and in a more special sense as synonymous with chronic, progressive, diffuse hepatitis associated with much liver tissue destruction and regeneration (cirrhosis hepatis). Both terms imply distortion, toughening and often atrophy of the affected organs. **Alcoholic cirrhosis.** Portal or Laënnec cirrhosis, an old term, implying alcohol as the cause of the cirrhosis, but now known to be incorrect. **Annular cirrhosis.** A form of cirrhosis of the liver in which bands of fibrous tissue completely surround the liver lobules. Although the term has no aetiological significance, it has value in indicating the advanced nature of the cirrhosis. **Atrophic cirrhosis.** Advanced portal cirrhosis associated with great shrinking of the liver. **Bacterial cirrhosis.** A form of cirrhosis caused by bacterial infection, especially streptococcal. **Biliary cirrhosis.** 1. *Primary* (Hanot's): Inflammation causing fibrosis with destruction of the bile ducts associated with deep jaundice, itching and high blood cholesterol level. 2. *Secondary* (obstructive): Obstruction due to stricture of the bile ducts after cholecystectomy, gall stones or tumour causing dilatation of large bile ducts and perforation of small ducts, with much cellular regeneration and fibrosis. **Biliary cirrhosis of children.** Cirrhosis in young children due to congenital anomalies of the bile ducts. **Calculus cirrhosis.** Biliary cirrhosis (see above), associated with gall-stones. **Capsular cirrhosis.** Chronic perihepatitis; capsular pseudo-cirrhosis. **Cardiac cirrhosis.** Fibrous tissue increase within the liver as the result of chronic cardiac failure; chronic myocarditis; fibrosis of the heart. **Cardiotuberculous cirrhosis.** Fibrosis of the liver associated with phthisis, and often alcoholism, in which the clinical features resemble those of cardiac failure. **Diffuse nodular cirrhosis.** Portal cirrhosis; cirrhosis of the liver (see below). **Fatty cirrhosis.** Cirrhosis which results from long-continued fatty infiltration of the liver the result of imperfect diet. **Hepatic cirrhosis.** Cirrhosis of the liver (see below). **Hypertrophic cirrhosis.** A form, or more correctly a stage, of cirrhosis in which the liver is greatly enlarged. **Infectious cirrhosis.** Cirrhosis resulting from infectious hepatitis. **Juvenile cirrhosis.** Portal cirrhosis found in young children, especially in India; occasionally biliary cirrhosis. **Cirrhosis of the kidney.** Chronic nephritis with replacement of much of the kidney by fibrous tissue. **Cirrhosis of the liver.** Cirrhosis hepatis, portal cirrhosis, fibrosis of the liver in which the fibrous tissue follows the course of the portal vein within the liver. **Cirrhosis of the lung.** A generalized form of fibrous tissue in one or both lungs, the result of pneumonia or certain dust diseases. **Lymphatic cirrhosis.** Cirrhosis associated with the deposits of lymphatic leukaemia in the liver. **Cirrhosis mammae.** Chronic interstitial mastitis. **Mixed cirrhosis.** A combination of unilobular and multilobular cirrhosis (see below). **Monolobular cirrhosis.** Cirrhosis of the kidney (see above). **Multilobular cirrhosis.** An artificial term for a type of cirrhosis in which prominent fibrous bands surround many lobules. **Muscular cirrhosis.** Atrophy and fibrous and fatty tissue replacement in a muscle; chronic myositis. **Obstructive cirrhosis.** Biliary cirrhosis (see above). **Periportal cirrhosis.** Cirrhosis of the liver (see above). **Pigmentary cirrhosis.** Cirrhosis of the liver with pigmentation of the skin, pancreas and some mucous membranes; haemochromatosis; bronzed diabetes. **Pipe-stem cirrhosis.** A variety of portal cirrhosis with unusually dense scars around the large portal veins. It is usually due to *Schistosoma mansoni.* **Portal cirrhosis.** Cirrhosis of the liver (see above). **Pulmonary cirrhosis.** Cirrhosis of the lung (see above). **Renal cirrhosis.** Cirrhosis of the kidney (see above). **Cirrhosis of the spleen.** Banti's disease. **Stasis cirrhosis.** Cardiac cirrhosis (see above). **Cirrhosis of the stomach.** Chronic interstitial gastritis. **Syphilitic cirrhosis.** Cirrhosis or fibrosis caused by syphilis. **Toxic cirrhosis.** Cirrhosis of the liver caused by chronic intoxication such as that of alcohol, solvents or phosphorus. **Tuberculous cirrhosis.** Cardiotuberculous cirrhosis (see above). **Turbinated cirrhosis.** Replacement of the erectile tissue of the turbinate bodies by fibrous tissue as the result of atrophic rhinitis. **Unilobular cirrhosis.** An artificial term for a type of cirrhosis in which the fibrous bands enclose single lobules. **Cirrhosis ventriculi.** Sclerosing fibrosis of the stomach. **Xanthomatous cirrhosis.** Cirrhosis associated with a heavy deposit of lipoid material within the liver cells. **Zooparasitic cirrhosis.** Cirrhosis which is the result of invasion by animal parasites and their deposited ova, e.g. in schistosomiasis. [Gk *kirrhos* orange-yellow, *-osis* condition.]

See also: BAUMGARTEN (W.), CHARCOT, CRUVEILHIER, GLISSON, HANOT, LAËNNEC, TODD (R. B.).

cirrhotic (sir·**ot**·ik). Affected with or characterized by the presence of cirrhosis.

cirsectomy (ser·**sek**·to·me). The surgical removal of a part of a varicose vein. [Gk *kirsos* dilated vein, *ektome* a cutting out.]

cirsenchysis (ser·**sen**·kis·is). A type of treatment of varicose veins which consists in the injecting of a sclerosing fluid into them. [Gk *kirsos* dilated vein, *enchysis* a pouring in.]

cirsocele (**ser**·so·seel). Varicocele. [Gk *kirsos* dilated vein, *kele* hernia.]

cirsodesis (ser·so·**de**·sis). The treatment of varicose veins by ligating them. [Gk *kirsos* dilated vein, *desis* ligation.]

cirsoid (**ser**·soid). Varicoid. [Gk *kirsos* dilated vein, *eidos* form.]

cirsomphalos (ser·**som**·fal·os). Varicomphalos. [Gk *kirsos* dilated vein, *omphalos* navel.]

cirsophthalmia (ser·sof·**thal**·me·ah). Varicula; a varicose condition of the veins supplying the conjunctiva. [Gk *kirsos* dilated vein, *ophthalmos* eye.]

cirsotome (**ser**·so·tome). A surgical knife used in varicotomy. [Gk *kirsos* dilated vein, *temnein* to cut.]

cirsotomy (ser·**sot**·o·me). Varicotomy. [see prec.]

cissa (**sis**·ah). Pica; an abnormal craving to eat substances not fit for food (e.g. wood, lead pencils, chalk), to which pregnant women are subject. The state may be found in patients with chlorosis and in certain types of hysteria and insanity. [Gk *kissa* craving for strange food.]

cissampeline (sis·**am**·pel·een). $C_{18}H_{21}O_3N$, an alkaloid from plants of the genus *Cissampelos* occurring in tropical Africa and South America. [Gk *kissos* ivy, *ampelos* vine.]

cisterna [NA] (sis·**ter**·nah). In an organism, a sac or space containing fluid. **Cerebellomedullary cisterna [cisterna cerebellomedullaris (NA)].** The dilatation of the subarachnoid space between the inferior surface of the cerebellum and the posterior surface of the medulla oblongata; it is this cistern which is tapped in the operation of cisternal puncture. **Chiasmatic cisterna [cisterna chiasmatis (NA)].** The subarachnoid space around the optic chiasma. **Cisterna chyli [NA].** The dilatation at the beginning of the thoracic duct into which the lumbar and intestinal lymph trunks open. **Cisterna corporis callosi.** The subarachnoid space above the corpus callosum where it contains the anterior cerebral arteries. **Interpeduncular cisterna [cisterna interpeduncularis (NA)].** The subarachnoid space between the 2 cerebral peduncles beneath the mid-brain and hypothalamus. **Cisterna of the lateral sulcus [cisterna fossae lateralis cerebri (NA)].** The dilatation of the subarachnoid space around the branches of the middle cerebral artery in the lateral sulcus (Sylvius' fissure) of the cerebrum. **Cisterna lateralis pontis.** A lateral extension of the cisterna pontis into the cerebellopontine angle. **Cisterna lumbaris.** The subarachnoid space around the cauda equina between the levels of the 1st lumbar and 2nd sacral vertebrae. **Cisterna magna.** Cerebellomedullary cisterna (see above). **Periotic cisterna.** The perilymphatic space in the vestibule of the inner ear. **Cisterna pontis.** The subarachnoid space anterior to the pons and containing the basilar artery. **Subarachnoid cisternae [cisternae subarachnoideales (NA)].** Any of the regions in which the subarachnoid space around the brain is enlarged, e.g. cerebellomedullary cisterna (see above) or cisterna magna, the space between the inferior surface of the cerebellum and the medulla. **Cisterna venae magnae cerebri.** The subarachnoid space around the great cerebral veins below and behind the splenium of the corpus callosum. [L a vessel.]

See also: PECQUET.

cisternal (sis·**ter**·nal). 1. Relating to a cisterna. 2. Relating to the cerebellomedullary cisterna.

cisternogram (sis·**tern**·o·gram). The result obtained from cisternography. [L *cisterna* a vessel, Gk *gramma* record.]

cisternography (sis·tern·**og**·raf·e). Contrast radiography of the intracranial cisterns. **Isotope cisternography.** External recording of the distribution of a radioactive nuclide or radiopharmaceutical in the cerebral cisterns and ventricles. [L *cisterna* a vessel, Gk *graphein* to record.]

cistron (**sis**·tron). A genetic unit of function; the sequence of DNA (or RNA in certain viruses) which contains the genetic information for a single polypeptide chain. The term is sometimes used as equivalent of *gene.* [L *cis* on this side, *trans* across.]

cisvestitism (sis·**vest**·it·izm). The practice of wearing clothes appropriate to one's own sex but to another calling or situation in life, e.g. in the case of a civilian who wears a service uniform. [L *cis* on this side of, *vestis* garment.]

Citellus (sit·**el**·us). A genus of ground squirrels in North America, numerous species of which have been found infected with sylvatic plague. *Citellus beecheyi, C. columbianus* and *C. richardsoni* are the most important in western USA; only *C. richardsoni* has been shown to be involved in Canada. *C. beecheyi* is also a carrier of tularaemia. *C. pygmaeus* is a species found in south-east USSR, an important reservoir of plague. [L squirrel.]

citral (**sit**·ral). $C_{10}H_{16}O$, an optically-inactive aldehyde present in lemon oil (Indian oil of verbena), lemon grass oil and other volatile oils. The natural product consists of a mixture of α-citral (geranial) and β-citral (neral); it is used in perfumery and to flavour food.

citrate (**sit**·rate). A salt of citric acid. **Citrate synthase, Citrate synthetase.** The mitochondrial enzyme responsible for the synthesis of citrate from acetyl CoA and oxaloacetate.

citrated (**sit**·ra·ted). Mixed with citric acid or a citrate. **Citrated ferrous chloride.** A buff powder composed of citric acid and ferrous chloride, $FeCl_2$, used for the administration of ferrous iron as it does not readily oxidize.

citric (**sit**·rik). An adjective sometimes applied to the various products of the citrus fruits, but more particularly to the acid which they contain. Citric acid is secreted by the prostate and is present in the semen. [Gk *kitron* citron.]

citrin (**sit**·rin). Vitamin P; a crystalline substance isolated from Hungarian red pepper. In combats the increased fragility and permeability of capillary walls that occurs in scurvy. The vitamin is also present in blackcurrant juice and in lemon juice. [see foll.]

citrine (sit·reen). Having a lemon colour. [Gk *kitron* citron.]

citrinin (sit·rin·in). An antibiotic produced by *Penicillium citrinium, Aspergillus terreus* and *A. candicus.* It is too toxic for chemotherapeutic use, but acts mainly on Gram-positive organisms. When ingested by laboratory animals, it results in renal damage.

Citromyces (sit·ro·mi·seez). An obsolete synonym for *Penicillium.* [citric acid, Gk *mykes* fungus.]

citron (sit·ron). 1. The orange-like tree, *Citrus medica,* of the family Rutaceae; the term is also applied to the fruit. 2. Shaped like a lemon; a term used in bacteriology. [Gk *kitron.*]

citronella (sit·ron·el·ah). Lemon grass, *Cymbopogon citratus,* an aromatic grass grown in Sri Lanka, yielding essential oils. **Citronella Oil BPC 1959.** A volatile oil from *Cymbopogon citratus,* containing geraniol and citronellal, and used as an insect repellent, in perfumes and as a flavouring agent. [dim. of citron.]

citronellal (sit·ron·el·al). $C_{10}H_{18}O$, the main component of citronella oil, also found in *Eucalyptus* species. It is a mixture of 2 isomers derived from the corresponding citronellols.

citronellol (sit·ron·el·ol). $C_{10}H_{20}O$, an unsaturated alcohol existing in 2 isomeric forms, and the main constituent of oil of rose and Spanish geranium oil.

citrophosphate (sit·ro·fos·fate). A compound of a citrate and a phosphate, especially the solution of dicalcium phosphate in ammonium citrate used in calcium deficiency diseases.

citropten (sit·rop·ten). Dimethoxycoumarin, $(CH_3O)_2C_6H_2O(CH{=}CH)CO$.

citrulline (sit·rul·een). α-Amino-δ-carbamidovaleric acid, $NH_2CONH(CH_2)_3CHNH_2COOH$. An amino acid which occurs free in watermelons (*Citrullus*), and also as a constituent of proteins. It is a monosubstituted urea, and is concerned in the ornithine cycle of urea formation. Mentally-defective epileptic babies with excessive citrulline in the blood have been described; the metabolic block lies between the conversion of citrulline and aspartic acid to arginosuccinic acid.

Citrullus (sit·rul·us). A genus of plants of the family Cucurbitaceae, consisting of 4 species indigenous to tropical Africa. **Citrullus colocynthis** (Linn.) Schrad. The species which yields colocynth. **Citrullus vulgaris** Schrad. A species widely cultivated for its edible fruit, the watermelon, and used medicinally in India. [O Fr. *citrulle* cucurbit.]

Citrus (sit·rus). A genus of evergreen trees and shrubs of the family Rutaceae, important for their fruits. **Citrus acida.** The source of lime (lime juice). **Citrus aurantium.** The orange tree; the variety *amara* yields the bitter or Seville orange, the variety *sinensis* the sweet orange. **Citrus bergamia.** The bergamot, a species cultivated for the essential oil from the peel of the fruit. **Citrus limonia.** The lemon tree. **Citrus medica.** The citron tree. [L citron.]

citta, cittosis (sit·ah, sit·o·sis). Cissa.

Civatte, Achille (b.1877). Paris physician.

Civatte's disease, or poikiloderma. Reticulated pigmented poikiloderma; erythroderma, pigmentation and atrophy affecting the face and neck, usually seen in women of middle age. Most observers consider it identical with Riehl's melanosis.

civet (siv·et). The secretion obtained from the perineal glands of the civet cat, *Viverra civetta,* of Africa, and other species of *Viverra.* It has a powerful odour, due to the unsaturated ketone, civetone, and is used in perfumery; it was formerly used in medicine as an antispasmodic and stimulant, like musk. [Ar. *zabbad.*]

Civiale, Jean (b.1792). Paris surgeon.

Civiale's operation. 1. So-called mediobilateral lithotomy. 2. Lithotrity practised by a perurethral instrument with expanding blades for grasping the stone.

Civinini, Filippo (b.1805). Pistoia anatomist.

Civinini's canal. The anterior canaliculus for the chorda tympani nerve. *See* CANALICULUS.

Civinini's ligament. The pterygospinous ligament. *See* LIGAMENT.

Civinini's process, or spine. A process on the lateral pterygoid plate of the sphenoid which is linked with the spinous process by a ligament (60–70 per cent) or a bar of bone (3 per cent).

cladiosis (klad·e·o·sis). A dermatomycosis caused by *Scopulariopsis blochii* (Matruchot) described by Bloch in a butcher; the fungus was isolated from chains of papuloverrucose lesions extending upwards from the hands to the upper arms. [Gk *klados* branch, *-osis* condition.]

Clado, Spiro (b.1856). Paris surgeon and gynaecologist.

Clado's anastomosis. An anastomosis between the appendicular and ovarian arteries in the infundibulopelvic ligament.

Clado's band. The infundibulopelvic ligament. *See* LIGAMENT.

Clado's ligament. An occasional fold of peritoneum joining the meso-appendix and the infundibulopelvic ligament.

Clado's point. A point of special tenderness observed in cases of appendicitis. It is situated at the point of intersection of the right semilunar line by a line drawn between the anterior superior iliac spines.

Cladonia (klad·o·ne·ah). A genus of lichens. **Cladonia rangiferina.** Reindeer moss, a species from Asia, Europe and North America; it is used as a food in famine seasons, and is locally distilled to give an alcoholic spirit. It was formerly used medicinally as a stomachic and pectoral. [Gk *klados* branch.]

cladosporiosis (klad·o·spo·re·o′·sis). A disease caused by species of *Cladosporium* having a predilection for tissues of the central nervous system, e.g. *Cladosporium trichoides,* brain abscesses commonly occurring. [cladosporium, Gk *-osis* condition.]

Cladosporium (klad·o·spo·re·um). A genus of fungi of which several species are pathogenic for man. **Cladosporium carrionii.** A causal organism of chromomycosis. **Cladosporium trichoides.** The causative agent of cladosporiosis. **Cladosporium werneckii.** An aetiologic agent of tinea nigra. [Gk *klados* branch, *sporos* seed.]

cladothricosis (klad·o·thrik·o′·sis). A disease caused by infection with cladothrix. [cladothrix, Gk *-osis* condition.]

Cladothrix (klad·o·thrix). The old name applied to species of *Actinomyces* and *Fusiformis.* [Gk *klados* branch, *thrix* hair.]

clairaudience (klare·awd·e·ens). 1. The ability to hear sounds which are too high-pitched normally to be heard. 2. An alleged faculty of being able subjectively to hear meaningful communications. [Fr. *clair* acute, L *audire* to hear.]

clairsentience (klare·sen·she·ens). An acute state of the sense in which phenomena are perceived which are normally not perceptible. [Fr. *clair* acute, L *sentire* to feel.]

clairvoyance (klare·voi·ans). An alleged faculty of being able subjectively to view scenes which convey information. The use has been extended to include more broadly an alleged faculty of being aware of events taking place at a distance, whether by visual imagery or not, and of a similar faculty of being aware of events which have taken place in the past but outside the experience of the possessor of the faculty, and also including precognition. [Fr. *clair* acute, *voyeur* an onlooker.]

Clamoxyquin (klam·ox·e·kwin). BP Commission approved name for 5-chloro-7-(3-diethylaminopropylaminomethyl)-8-hydroxyquinoline; it is used in the treatment of amoebiasis.

clamp (klamp). An instrument employed in surgical operations to clasp an organ or tissue with the intention of preventing escape of content, controlling haemorrhage, maintaining it in a desired position or steadying it against the application of force. **Anastomosis clamp.** A clamp used in anastomosis to appose 2 loops of gut, control bleeding from their walls and prevent escape of content. **Bone clamp, Bone-holding clamp.** A clamp used to maintain a bone in a required position, e.g. during plating of a fracture. **Bulldog clamp.** A short-bladed clamp applied to an artery or vein in vascular anastomosis. **Carotid clamp.** A screw clamp with rubber-covered blades applied to the common carotid artery to control bleeding in operations on the mouth and face. **Cholecystectomy clamp.** A clamp applied to the cystic duct in removal of the gall bladder. **Circumcision clamp.** A crushing clamp applied to the prepuce in circumcision. **Colectomy clamp.** A clamp used in the technique of aseptic colectomy. **Crushing clamp.** A heavy clamp applied to a hollow organ before division, to reduce the thickness of its wall and render its vessels less liable to bleed, or to control escape of content from a hollow organ in the process of removal. **Distraction clamp.** A bone clamp used to reduce fractures at open operation. **Fenestrated clamp.** A clamp with blades slotted to give a double grip. **Gastrectomy clamp.** A clamp, usually crushing, employed in excision of the stomach. **Gastro-enterostomy clamp.** A twin- or 3-bladed clamp to hold the jejunum to the stomach in gastro-enterostomy. **Haemostatic clamp.** Artery forceps. *See* FORCEPS. **Hysterectomy clamp.** A clamp used to control bleeding from the broad ligaments in hysterectomy. **Lever-compression clamp.** The common type of clamp, with fulcrum between blade and handle. **Light clamp.** A clamp exercising a gentle and temporary effect, as opposed to a crushing clamp. **Nasal-septum clamp.** A clamp for forcibly straightening the nasal septum. **Occlusion clamp.** A clamp intended to control bleeding and escape of content without damage to the wall. **Pedicle clamp.** A clamp applied to the vascular attachment of an organ before its removal. **Penile clamp.** A clamp applied to the penis, and released at intervals, for the control of certain types of urinary incontinence. **Pile clamp.** A clamp applied to the base of a mass of piles before its excision. **Rectal clamp.** A crushing clamp to control escape from the rectum during its excision. **Rubber-dam clamp.** In dentistry, an instrument which partially encircles the neck of a tooth and holds a rubber dam in position to maintain isolation of the tooth during operations of conservative dentistry. **Stomach clamp.** Gastrectomy clamp (see above). **Suturing clamp.** A crushing clamp bearing a device for the mechanical insertion of 2 rows of silver clips into the crushed tissue between its blades; an incision between the rows of sutures provides 2 closed ends. **Three-bladed clamp.** An anastomosis clamp which controls both hollow viscera and holds them in apposition. **Vaginal clamp.** A clamp applied across the vagina in hysterectomy. [AS *clam* to fasten together.]

See also: BLALOCK, BOEHLER, BRONNER, COPE (V. Z.), CRILE, DE MARTEL, DOYEN, FREIDRICH, GANT (S. G.), GOLDBLATT, GUSSENBAUER, LANE (W. A.), MICHEL, MIKULICZ-RADECKI, MILES, MOYNIHAN, PAYR, PETZ, POTT, PRINCE, PRINGLE (S. S.), RANKIN, SCHOEMAKER, SMITH (H), WILLETT.

clang (klang). The metallic quality of tone of the voice. **Clang association.** *See* ASSOCIATION. **Clang deafness.** *See* DEAFNESS. [L *clangere* to resound.]

clap (klap). A vulgar term for gonorrhoea. **Clap thread.** *See* THREAD. [etym. dub.]

Clapeyron, Benoit-Paul Emile (b.1799). French engineer.

Clapeyron's law. A principle in thermodynamics to the effect that any action tends to be counteracted by the forces it sets up.

clapotage, clapotement (klap·o·**tazh**, klap·oe·**mahn**). The plashing sound heard on succussion when liquid is present in the cavities of the body. [Fr. *clapoter* to plash.]

clappa (**klap**·ah). A term used in Cuba to denote a disease in which sporotrichosis occurs in leprotic tissue.

Clapton, Edward (b.1830). London physician and surgeon.

Clapton's line. Copper line; a green line at the bases of the teeth in copper poisoning.

clarificant (klar·**if**·ik·ant). Any agent used for clearing a solution. [L *clarus* clear, *facere* to make.]

clarification (**klar**·if·ik·**a**'·shun). The process by which a solution is rendered free from turbidity. [see prec.]

clarify (**klar**·if·i). To make a liquid or solution clear by freeing it of turbidity; hence *clarifying.* [L *clarus* clear, *facere* to make.]

Clark, Alonzo (b.1807). New York physician.

Alonzo Clark treatment. The administration of large doses of opium in cases of peritonitis to produce bowel rest.

Clark, Cecil.

Clark-Hadfield syndrome, Hadfield-Clark syndrome. Infantilism due to congenital insufficiency of the pancreas, probably identical with cystic fibrosis of the pancreas or fibrocystic disease of the pancreas.

Clark, Earl Perry (b.1892). American biochemist.

Clark-Collip method. For calcium in serum: mix in a centrifuge tube 2 ml serum, 2 ml water and 1 ml of 4 per cent ammonium oxalate. Stand at least 30 min, centrifuge, pour off supernatant and drain on filter paper. Wash the precipitate with 3 ml dilute ammonia, centrifuge, pour off supernatant and drain on filter paper. Dissolve the precipitate in 2 ml of hot 5 per cent sulphuric acid and titrate with N/100 potassium permanganate.

Clark, Josiah Latimer (b.1822). British engineer.

Clark cell. A standard voltaic cell having electrodes of mercury and zinc amalgam in an electrolyte of zinc sulphate, with mercurous sulphate as a depolarizer. It yields a constant e.m.f. of 1.433 V at 15°C, and was the first successful standard of electrical pressure.

Clark, Thomas (b.1801). British chemist.

Clark's scale. A scale of hardness of water, based on the number of grains of calcium carbonate per imperial gallon of the given water.

Clark's operation. Plastic operation for urethral fistula.

Clark's paralysis. Infantile cerebral paralysis.

Clark's rule. A rule for calculating dosage in children: adult dose multiplied by weight in pounds divided by 150.

clark (klark). **Clark I.** Diphenylchlorarsine, a highly toxic nose gas used in chemical warfare: DA. **Clark II.** Diphenylcyanarsine, a highly toxic nose gas used in chemical warfare: DC.

Clarke, Jacob Augustus Lockhart (b.1817). London neurologist.

Clarke's bundle. A bundle of nerve fibres in the spinal cord connecting the thoracic nucleus with the fasciculus cuneatus.

Clarke's cells, Stilling-Clarke cells. Large rounded or fusiform cells in the thoracic nucleus of the spinal cord.

Clarke's column, Stilling-Clarke column. The thoracic nucleus of the spinal cord. *See* NUCLEUS.

clasmacytosis (klas·mah·si·**to**'·sis). The fragmentation of clasmatocytes and resultant grouping of granules of debris. [clasmatocyte, Gk *-osis* condition.]

clasmatoblast (klaz·**mat**·o·blast). The precursor cell of the clasmatocyte, or tissue macrophage. [Gk *klasma* fragment, *blastos* germ.]

clasmatocyte (klaz·**mat**·o·site). One of the synonyms for the tissue macrophage or histiocyte, next to the fibroblast the commonest cell in loose connective tissue. It is a large cell, with simple reniform nucleus, and is actively phagocytic, especially towards cell debris; it is the resting wandering cell of the reticulo-endothelial system. [Gk *klasma* fragment, *kytos* cell.]

clasmatocytosis (klaz·**mat**·o·si·**to**'·sis). Clasmacytosis.

clasmatodendrosis (klaz·**mat**·o·den·**dro**'·sis). The process of breaking up of the branched processes of protoplasmic astrocytes. [Gk *klasma* fragment, *dendron* tree, *-osis* condition.]

clasmatosis (klaz·mat·**o**·sis). The process of breaking into fragments, such as occurs in cell changes. [Gk *klasma* fragment, *-osis* condition.]

clasp (klahsp). In surgery, any apparatus used for keeping tissues together, particularly bony structures. [AS *clapse* to slap.]

class (klahs). 1. In biology, a comprehensive group of animals or plants forming a category superior to that of an order. 2. A term used in statistics to denote a group of variables all members of which show either a defined or a particular value. **Frequency of class.** Frequency distribution. *See* DISTRIBUTION. [L *classis* collection.]

classification (**klas**·if·ik·**a**'·shun). The division, or the series resulting from such a division, of any group of individuals or class categories into a series of classes of increasing comprehensiveness. **Classification of burns.** *See* BURN. **Natural classification.** The division of living organisms into such a series. In the Kingdoms Animalium and Plantarum the divisions are based on the idea of degree of difference in the sum total of characters. In both Kingdoms the class category which is composed of individuals is by definition the Species. Species may be further subdivided into sub-species, varieties, forms or races. In the animal Kingdom the chief class categories are the Genus (composed of Species), Family, Order, Class, Phylum and Sub-kingdom. In the plant Kingdom they are Genus, Natural Order, Class, Division. The system also indicates the phylogenetic relationships of the evolutionary lines, though this is not inherent to it. All class category names are latinized, and international codes of procedure are in use. [L *classis* collection, *facere* to make.]

See also: ANGLE, ARNETH, BAZIN, BENNETT (N. G.), CALDWELL (W. E.), COOKE, DUKES (C. E.), DUPUYTREN, EDRIDGE-GREEN, GUEDEL, JAMES (S. P.), JANSKY, JENSEN (O.), KRAEPELIN, LANCEFIELD, LANDSTEINER, MOLOY, MOSS, PONDER, SCHILLING, WILKIE.

clastic (klas·tik). 1. Capable of being taken apart. 2. Showing a tendency to divide or break into parts. 3. Causing or undergoing division into parts. [Gk *klastos* broken.]

clastothrix (klas·to·thrix). Trichorrhexis nodosa. [Gk *klastos* broken, *thrix* hair.]

Clauberg, Karl Wilhelm (b.1893). Berlin bacteriologist.

Clauberg's test. A method of assay of progesterone in which the degree of endometrial development is assessed in immature rabbits previously treated with an oestrogen before giving the test or standard preparation.

Claude, Henri Charles Jules (b.1869). Paris psychiatrist.

Claude's hyperkinesis sign. Reflex contractions of paralysed or paretic muscles on painful stimulation.

Claude's syndrome. Paralysis of the 3rd cranial nerve with contralateral ataxia and tremor, due to a lesion in the tegmentum of the midbrain involving the red nucleus. More often referred to as the *syndrome of Benedikt.*

claudication (klawd·e·**ka**·shun). 1. Lameness. 2. Limping. 3. An obstruction. **Abdominal claudication.** Abdominal pain after eating, due to chronic midgut ischaemia. **Claudication of the cauda equina.** Pain produced in the back, buttocks and legs by compression of the lumbar and sacral nerves as they leave the spinal canal. A term not in common use. **Intermittent claudication.** A syndrome which is one of the earliest signs of partial impairment of the arterial flow. Severe pain in the legs, tension and weakness after the patient has been walking for a certain distance occur, and the symptoms increase as walking proceeds until further progress is impossible. After a short rest, during which the symptoms cease, walking becomes possible again. **Spontaneous claudication.** The lameness which is an early sign of coxarthrocace in children. **Venous claudication.** Intermittent claudication as the result of stasis due to venous congestion. [L *claudicatio.*]

claudicatory (klawd·e·**ka**·tor·e). Relating to claudication.

claudicometer (klawd·e·**kom**·et·er). An instrument for measuring the amount of work done by the muscles of an ischaemic limb before cramp develops in them. [claudication, meter.]

Claudius, Friedrich Matthias (b.1822). Marburg anatomist.

Claudius' cells. Polyhedral supporting cells in the outer part of the spiral organ of the cochlea.

Claudius' fossa. Ovarian fossa; a depression in the parietal peritoneum of the pelvis bounded in front by the obliterated umbilical artery and behind by the ureter and uterine vessels, and in which the ovary lies.

Clausen, Raymond John (b. 1890). London anaesthetist.

Clausen harness. A triradiate rubber strap for attachment to a hooked ring on the face-piece of an anaesthetic apparatus.

claustral (**klaw**·stral). 1. Relating to the claustrum. 2. Of the nature of a claustrum.

claustrophilia (klaw·stro·**fil**·e·ah). Morbid desire to shut doors and windows and to be closed within a confined space. [L *claustrum* barrier, Gk *philein* to love.]

claustrophobia (klaw·stro·**fo**·be·ah). Morbid dread of being within walls or in a house, or of being shut in a room or confined space; in some cases the fear of travelling in railway carriages is very great. Cf. AGORAPHOBIA. [L *claustrum* barrier, phobia.]

claustrum (**klaw**·strum). 1. [NA] A thin sheet of grey matter beneath the cortex of the insula separated from the lentiform nucleus by the fibres of the external capsule. It is a part of the basal ganglia of the cerebral hemispheres. 2. A term applied to an opening that can be closed to prevent entrance. **Claustrum oris.** The soft palate. **Claustrum virginale, Claustrum virginitatis.** The hymen. [L barrier.]

clausura (klaw·**sewr**·ah). Atresia. **Clausura tubalis.** Atresia tubalis. **Clausura uteri.** Atresia uteri. [L closure.]

clava (**kla**·vah). The gracile tubercle. *See* TUBERCLE. [L club.]

clavacin (**klav**·as·in). An antibiotic produced by *Aspergillus clavatus* on Czapek-Dox medium. It is active against Gram-positive and Gram-negative organisms as well as fungi, but is toxic to animals. It has been shown to be identical with the claviformin of *Penicillium claviforme* and the patulin of *P. patulum.*

claval (**kla**·val). Relating to the gracile tubercle (clava).

clavate (**kla**·vate). 1. Relating to the gracile tubercle (clava). 2. Club-shaped. [L *clava* club.]

clavatin (**klav**·a·tin). Clavacin.

clavatine (**klav**·at·een). $C_{16}H_{25}O_2N$, a laevorotatory alkaloid derived from *Lycopodium clavatum.* It is toxic to test-animals.

clavation (klav·a·shun). Gomphosis; a type of close articulation characterized by the fitting of a peg-like piece of bone into another; e.g. tooth and socket in jaw. [L *clavus* nail.]

Claviceps (**klav**·is·eps). A genus of fungi parasitic on wild and cultivated grasses and grain. About 20 species are known. **Claviceps purpurea.** A species parasitic on rye, and producing ergot. [L *clava* club, *caput* head.]

clavicepsin (klav·is·**ep**·sin). $C_{18}H_{34}O_{16}$, a glycoside of mannitol obtained from the ergot of *Claviceps purpurea.*

clavicle [clavicula (NA)] (**klav**·ikl). The long bone of the shoulder girdle shaped like the italic letter *f.* The acromial (lateral) end [extremitas acromialis (NA)] bears an articular facet for the medial side of the acromion [facies articularis acromialis (NA)], and the sternal (medial) end [extremitas sternalis (NA)] articulates with the clavicular notch of the manubrium sterni. [L *clavicula* little key.]

clavicotomy (klav·ik·**ot**·o·me). Surgical division of the clavicle. [clavicle, Gk *temnein* to cut.]

clavicular (klav·**ik**·ew·lar). Relating to the clavicle. **Clavicular notch.** *See* NOTCH.

claviculate (klav·**ik**·ew·late). 1. Having clavicles. 2. Ridged or wrinkled.

claviculectomy (klav·ik·ew·**lek**'·to·me). The operative removal of the clavicle. [clavicle, Gk *ektome* excision.]

claviculus (klav·**ik**·ew·lus). A perforating fibre of Sharpey. [L little nail.]

claviform (**kla**·ve·form). Clavate; club-shaped. [L *clava* club, form.]

claviformin (klav·e·**form**·in). An antibiotic produced by *Penicillium claviforme,* also by *Aspergillus giganteus* and a species of *Gymnoascus.* It is active against Gram-positive and Gram-negative organisms and also fungi, but is toxic to animals. It has been shown to be identical with clavacin and patulin.

clavipectoral (klav·e·**pek**·tor·al). Relating to the clavicle and the thorax. **Clavipectoral fascia.** *See* FASCIA. [clavicle, L *pectus* breast.]

clavitol (**klav**·it·ol). Gravitol, $N(C_2H_5)_2(CH_2)_2OC_6H_3(OCH_3)C_3H_5$. The diethylamino-ethyl ether of 2-methoxy-6-allylphenol, a complex synthetic compound which on injection into animals has ergot-like action, causing weak contraction of the uterus but also marked slowing of the heart.

clavus (**kla**·vus). 1. A corn. 2. A callous growth. **Clavus hystericus.** A painful sensation as if a nail were being driven into the head. It affects hysterical patients. **Clavus secalinus.** Ergot of rye. **Clavus syphiliticus.** A flat horny callosity on the foot or hand, held to be of syphilitic origin. [L nail.]

claw-foot (**klaw**·fut). A deformity of the foot caused by paralysis of the muscles. The heads of the metatarsal bones are depressed and there is extension of the first phalanges and flexion of the last. [AS *clawu,* foot.]

claw-hand (**klaw**·hand). A condition of hyperextension of the proximal phalanges of the fingers and flexion of the terminal 2 phalanges, associated with flattening of the hand. A paralytic condition associated with paralysis of the median and ulnar nerves. [AS *clawu,* hand.]

Claybrook, Edwin B. (b. 1871). American surgeon.

Claybrook's sign. Abnormal accentuation of the heart sounds and breath sounds heard on auscultation of the abdomen in cases of rupture of an abdominal viscus.

Claypole, Edith Jane. British physiologist and pathologist in the USA.

Gay and Claypole vaccine. A typhoid prophylactic prepared by sensitizing a typhoid vaccine with antityphoid serum, and then precipitating with alcohol and extracting with saline; it is now obsolete.

Clayton gas. Sulphur dioxide gas. The Clayton apparatus is specially constructed for generating sulphur dioxide, and is chiefly used to fumigate ships. The apparatus, named from the inventor, consists essentially of a chamber in which sulphur is burned and the gas thence passed into the compartment to be fumigated.

clean (kleen). In practical anatomy, to separate the vessels, nerves and other structures from the investing fat and connective tissue and to remove all such tissues from the field of dissection. [AS *claene.*]

cleansings (**klen**·zingz). The local discharges. [AS *claensian.*]

clear (kleer). 1. To clarify a solution or liquid. 2. To use a clearing agent on microscopical specimens in order to make them transparent. [L *clarus.*]

clearance (**kleer**·ans). The act of freeing from obstruction, or clearing. **Blood-urea clearance, Urea clearance.** The volume of blood which in the course of a minute is cleared of urea by the work of the kidneys. **Carbon clearance.** A test of mononuclear phagocyte function used in experimental animals. The ability of these cells, chiefly hepatic Kupffer cells, to clear injected carbon particles from the circulation is determined. [see foll.]

clearer (**kleer**·er). A clearing agent for use on microscopical specimens. [L *clarus* clear.]

cleavage (**kleev**·ij). 1. Segmentation, the furrowing of the cytoplasm which follows nuclear division. 2. The division of the fertilized egg (zygote) during the period preceding blastulation. **Holoblastic cleavage.** Total segmentation. **Cleavage nucleus.** *See* NUCLEUS. **Yolk cleavage.** Yolk segmentation. [AS *cleofan.*]

cleavers (**kleev**·erz). The herb *Galium aparine* Linn. (family Rubiaceae). It is an aperient, diuretic, tonic and alternative, used in the form of a liquid extract. [see prec.]

Clefamide (**klef**·am·ide). BP Commission approved name for α,α-dichloro-*N*-(2-hydroxyethyl)-*N*-[4-(4-nitrophenoxy)benzyl]-acetamide; it is used in the treatment of amoebiasis.

cleft (kleft). A fissure, notch, gap, depression, or incisura. **Alveolar cleft.** Cleft palate in which the failure of fusion extends forwards to involve the alveolus. **Anal cleft.** Gluteal cleft (see below). **Branchial cleft.** A linear superficial depression in the pharyngeal region of an early embryo opposite a branchial (pharyngeal) pouch. It is lined with ectoderm. **Cholesterol cleft.** A space in a histological section resulting from the loss of cholesterol crystals during preparation. **Coelomic cleft.** One of the spaces in the lateral plate mesoderm which presages the formation of the coelom in the embryo. **Facial cleft.** One of the gaps between the mandibular, maxillary and frontonasal processes in the early development of the facial region of the embryo. **Fetal cleft.** The ocular or choroidal cleft in the developing optic cup. **Genal cleft.** A congenital malformation, a persistence of the facial cleft involving the cheek. **Genital cleft.** The external depression over the cloacal membrane of the early embryo. **Gluteal cleft [crena ani (NA)].** The cleft between the nates. **Hyomandibular cleft.** The first branchial cleft, lying between the mandibular and hyoid arches of the early embryo. In fishes it becomes the spiracular opening; in higher vertebrates it forms the external auditory meatus. **Interdigital cleft.** One of the spaces between the fingers and toes. **Internatal cleft.** Natal cleft (see below). **Intratonsillar cleft [fossa supratonsillaris (NA)].** A cleft of variable size in the upper part of the tonsil. **Natal cleft.** The cleft between the nates or buttocks. **Postalveolar cleft.** Cleft palate behind an intact alveolus. **Pre-alveolar cleft.** Cleft of the soft tissues of the lip in front of the alveolus. **Pudendal cleft [rima pudendi (NA)].** The fissure between the labia majora, into which the urethra and vagina open. **Synaptic cleft.** The space, about 20 nm in width, between the cell membranes of 2 neurones at a synapse. **Visceral cleft.** Branchial cleft (see above). [ME *clift.*]

See also: LANTERMANN, LARREY, MAURER, SANTORINI, SCHMIDT (H. D.).

clegs (klegz). Biting flies of the family Tabanidae. [Old Norse *kleggi.*]

cleidagra (kli·**dag**·rah). Gouty pain affecting the clavicle. [Gk *kleis* key, *agra* a catching.]

cleidal (**kli**·dal). Clavicular. [Gk *kleis* key.]

cleidocostal (kli·do·**kos**·tal). Costoclavicular. [Gk *kleis* key, L *costa* rib.]

cleidocranial (kli·do·**kra**·ne·al). Belonging to the clavicle and the head, or involving them. [Gk *kleis* key, *kranion* skull.]

cleidocranialiasis (kli·do·**kra**·ne·al·**i**'·as·is). Cleidocranial dysostosis. *See* DYSOSTOSIS.

cleidohyoid (kli·do·**hi**·oid). Relating to the clavicle and the hyoid bone. [Gk *kleis* key, hyoid.]

cleidomastoid (kli·do·**mas**·toid). Relating to the clavicle and the mastoid process of the temporal bone. [Gk *kleis* key, mastoid.]

cleido-occipital (**kli**·do·ok·**sip**'·it·al). Relating to the clavicle and the occiput. [Gk *kleis* key, occiput.]

cleidorrhexis (kli·do·**rex**·is). The operation of fracturing the clavicles of the fetus in order to reduce the diameter of the shoulder girdle and so make delivery less difficult. [Gk *kleis* key, *rhexis* rupture.]

cleidoscapular (kli·do·**skap**·ew·lar). Relating to or affecting the clavicle and the scapula. [Gk *kleis* key, scapula.]

cleidosternal (kli·do·**ster**·nal). Sternoclavicular. [Gk *kleis* key, *sternon* chest.]

cleidotomy (kli·**dot**·o·me). The dividing by cutting of the clavicles of the fetus in order to reduce the diameter of the shoulder girdle and make delivery less difficult. [Gk *kleis* key, *temnein* to divide.]

cleidotripsy (kli·do·**trip**·se). The crushing of the clavicles of the fetus in order to reduce the diameter of the shoulder girdle and so make delivery less difficult. [Gk *kleis* key, *tribein* to crush.]

cleisagra (kli·**sag**·rah). Cleidagra.

cleithrophobia (kli·thro·**fo**·be·ah). Claustrophobia. [Gk *kleisis* closure, phobia.]

Cleland, John (b. 1835). Glasgow anatomist.

Cleland's skin ligaments. Cutaneophalangeal ligaments; a series of fascial slips connecting the skin of the finger to the underlying phalanges.

Clemastine (**klem**·as·teen). BP Commission approved name for (+)-2-[2-(4-chloro-α-methylbenzhydryloxy)ethyl]-1-methylpyrrolidine; an antihistamine.

clematine (**klem**·at·een). A poisonous alkaloid obtained from *Clematis flammula.* [Gk *klematis* branch.]

Clemizole (**klem**·iz·ole). BP Commission approved name for 1-*p*-chlorobenzyl-2-pyrrolidinomethylbenzimidazole; an antihistaminic drug.

Clerada apicicornis (**kler**·ah·dah a·pis·e·**kor**'·nis). A bug that is a potential vector of American trypanosomiasis.

Clérambault, Gatian de (b. 1872). Paris psychiatrist.

Clérambault-Kandinsky complex, or syndrome. In a psychotic state, the occurrence of paranoid ideas of reference or control.

Clérat, M. (fl. 1910). Paris physician.

Launois-Clérat syndrome. Acromegalic gigantism. [obsolete term.]

Cletoquine (klet·o·kween). BP Commission approved name for 7-chloro-4-[4-(2-hydroxyethylamino)-1-methylbutyl]aminoquinoline; an anti-inflammatory agent.

Clevedon positive-pressure respirator. An automatic portable respirator effecting pulmonary ventilation by intermittent positive pressure via a tracheotomy tube; used in respiratory failure with bulbar paralysis.

Clevenger, Shobal Vail (b. 1843). Chicago psychiatrist.

Clevenger's fissure. The inferior sulcus of the temporal lobe. *See* SULCUS.

click (klik). In cardiology, an abrupt sound occurring during the cardiac cycle observed on auscultation of the heart. **Ejection click.** An abrupt sound heard early in systole at the time of the commencement of the ejection of blood from the ventricles. It may arise from either aorta or pulmonary artery and is nearly always associated with dilatation of the relevant vessel, most commonly distal to stenosis of the corresponding valve. **Systolic click.** An abrupt sound heard in mid- or late systole commonly arising from the mitral valve apparatus and often followed by a late systolic murmur due to mitral regurgitation. [Fr. *cliquer.*]

clid-. For words beginning **Clid-**, *see* CLEID-.

Clidinium Bromide (kli·din·e·um bro·mide). BP Commission approved name for 3-benziloyloxy-1-methylquinuclidinium bromide; an anticholinergic.

climacophobia (kli·mak·o·fo'·be·ah). Pathological fear of climbing or of stairs. [Gk *klimakter* rung of a ladder, phobia.]

climacteric (kli·mak·ter·ik). Any critical period, but by common usage generally referring to the menopause; the word is also used adjectivally. **Male climacteric.** The subjective phenomena sometimes associated with the normal decline in sexual power in the male. [Gk *klimakter* rung of a ladder.]

climacterium (kli·mak·teer·e·um). The menopause. **Climacterium praecox.** Early menopause. [see prec.]

climatotherapeutics (kli·mat·o·ther·ap·ew'·tix). The science of climatotherapy; the practice of using it to cure disease.

climatotherapy (kli·mat·o·ther'·ap·e). Treatment of disease by sending a patient to a country or region the climate of which is different from that in which he is living or is more favourable to his particular condition. [Gk *klima* region, therapy.]

climax (kli·max). The stage of a disease during which it is most severe. [Gk *klimax* ladder.]

Clindamycin (klin·dah·mi·sin). BP Commission approved name for methyl 7-chloro-6,7,8-trideoxy-6-(*trans*-1-methyl-4-propyl-L-2-pyrrolidinecarboxamido)-1-thio-L-*threo*-α-D-galacto-octopyranoside; an antibiotic.

clinic (klin·ik). 1. Name given to a class of medical students which meets regularly in a ward or elsewhere and is conducted by a physician or surgeon; at this class instruction is given in the examination and treatment of patients. 2. In the out-patient department of a hospital, one of a number of special sections devoted to particular diseases, or groups of diseases, and under the leadership of a physician or surgeon. Patients who have been in hospital may attend clinics for after-treatment. 3. Any particular building or group of buildings set aside by medical authorities in which treatment is given to ambulant patients. [Gk *kline* bed.]

clinical (klin·ik·al). 1. Relating to a sickbed. 2. Having reference to a clinic or to treatment at a clinic. 3. Founded on observation and treatment of patients, not on the results of pathological or experimental work. [see prec.]

clinician, clinicist (klin·ish·an, klin·is·ist). An expert in clinical medicine or surgery.

clinicohaematological (klin·ik·o·he·mat·o·loj'·ik·al). Relating or pertaining to the correlation of the bed-side study of the patient and the investigation of his blood. [Gk *kline* bed, *haima* blood, *logos* science.]

clinicopathological (klin·ik·o·path·o·loj'·ik·al). Relating to the symptoms and pathology of disease. [see foll.]

clinicopathology (klin·ik·o·path·ol'·o·je). The study of the pathology of disease in relation to the clinical observations. Clinical pathology. [Gk *kline* bed, pathology.]

clinicoradiological, clinicoroentgenological (klin·ik·o·ra·de·o·loj'·ik·al, klin·ik·o·runt·yen·o·loj'·ik·al). Relating or pertaining to the correlation of the bed-side observation and radiological investigation of a patient or of patients generally. [Gk *kline* bed, radiology, roentgenology.]

clinocephalism (kli·no·kef·al·izm). Clinocephaly.

clinocephalus (kli·no·kef·al·us). A malformation of the head in which the vertex is flat or even hollow. [see foll.]

clinocephaly (kli·no·kef·al·e). The state of having a saddle-shaped or abnormally flat head, the result of premature closing of the sphenoparietal suture. [Gk *klinein* to bend, *kephale* head.]

clinocoris (kli·no·kor·is). *Cimex.* [Gk *kline* bed, *koris* bug.]

clinodactylism, clinodactyly (kli·no·dak·til·izm, kli·no·dak·til·e). A condition in which the fingers or toes are permanently deflected or abnormally curved. [Gk *klinein* to bend, *daktylos* finger.]

clinography (kli·nog·raf·e). A method by which various data are represented by charting and progressive plotting on curves; data such as pulse rate, temperature, urinary output, and so on, are thus recorded graphically. [Gk *kline* bed, *graphein* to record.]

clinoid (kli·noid). Like a bed. **Clinoid process of the sphenoid bone.** *See* PROCESS. [Gk *kline* bed, *eidos* form.]

clinology (kli·nol·o·je). 1. The science or study of retrograde changes in an animal organism after it has reached maturity, or in a group of organisms after the period of culmination is over. [Gk *klinein* to bend, *logos* science.] 2. The study of beds for the sick with regard to their suitability in various diseases and for certain individuals. [Gk *kline* bed, *logos* science.]

clinomania (kli·no·ma·ne·ah). A morbid or insane desire to remain lying down in bed or to lie flat. [Gk *kline* bed, mania.]

clinometer (kli·nom·et·er). An instrument designed by Stevens for measuring declinations of the retinal meridians. [Gk *klinein* to bend, *metron* measure.]

clinophilus (kli·nof·il·us). *Cimex.* [Gk *kline* bed, *philein* to love.]

clinoscope (kli·no·skope). Clinometer. [Gk *klinein* to bend, *skopein* to view.]

clinostatic (kli·no·stat·ik). 1. Referring to the recumbent position. 2. Occurring when the patient is in a recumbent position. [Gk *klinein* to recline, *stasis* a standing still.]

clinostatism (kli·no·stat·izm). The state of being in a recumbent positon. [see prec.]

clinotherapy (kli·no·ther·ap·e). Treatment by keeping the patient at rest in bed. [Gk *klinein* to recline, therapy.]

Clioquinol BP 1973 (kli·o·kwin·ol). 5-Chloro-8-hydroxy-7-iodoquinolone; iodochlorhydroxyquin. An antiseptic and amoebacide, used in the treatment of intestinal amoebiasis, especially when this is complicated by bacillary dysentery.

clip (klip). A device for holding tissues or materials together, or for controlling the rate of passage of a fluid in a tube. **Catheter clip.** A clip for preventing uncontrolled escape of urine from a bladder catheter. **Nasal clip.** A rubber-covered clip applied to the nose in certain forms of anaesthesia. **Silver clips.** Silver-wire clips used for ligating vessels in intracranial surgery. **Towel clip.** A forceps clip to fix towels to the edges of wounds, preventing the entrance of infection from adjacent skin. [AS *clyppan* to embrace.]

See also: CALLENDER, CUSHING (HARVEY W.), MICHEL.

cliseometer (kli·se·om·et·er). An instrument with which can be determined the degree of inclination of the axis of the pelvis with the vertebral column. [Gk *klisis* inclination, *metron* measure.]

clisis (kli·sis). In biology, the state of being sympathetic to or attracted by or having inclination towards. [Gk inclination.]

clithrophobia (kli·thro·fo·be·ah). Claustrophobia. [Gk *kleithria* door-bolt, phobia.]

clition (kli·te·on). In craniometry, the central point of the anterior border of the clivus. [Gk *klitys* slope.]

clitoral (klit·or·al). Pertaining to the clitoris. **Clitoral hypertrophy.** Enlargement of the clitoris.

clitoralgia (klit·or·**al**·je·ah). Pain referred to the clitoris. [clitoris, Gk *algos* pain.]

clitoridectomy (klit·or·id·**ek'**·to·me). Surgical removal of the clitoris. [clitoris, Gk *ektome* a cutting out.]

clitoriditis (klit·or·id·**i'**·tis). An inflammatory condition of the clitoris. [clitoris, Gk *-itis* inflammation.]

clitoridotomy (klit·or·id·**ot'**·o·me). Circumcision performed on the female. [clitoris, Gk *temnein* to cut.]

clitoris [NA] (**klit**·or·is). A small erectile organ in the female homologous to the penis in the male and situated at the anterior angle of the pudendum muliebre. It is partially hidden by the ends of the labia minora. [Gk *kleitoris.*]

Body [corpus clitoridis (NA)]. The portion of the organ distal to the body of the pubis and composed of the corpora cavernosa enveloped in a dense fibrous membrane.

clitoris, arteries of the. *See* PENIS, ARTERIES OF THE.

clitoris, nerves of the. *See* PENIS, NERVES OF THE.

clitoris, veins of the. *See* PENIS, VEINS OF THE. **Dorsal veins of the clitoris, deep [vena dorsalis clitoridis profunda (NA)].** Tributaries of the vesical plexus.

clitorism (**klit**·or·izm). Prolonged erection of the clitoris, a condition which may be attended with pain; it is analogous to priapism in the male. Tribadism.

clitoritis (klit·or·**i**·tis). Clitoriditis.

clitoromania (klit·or·o·**ma'**·ne·ah). Nymphomania. [clitoris, mania.]

clitorotomy (klit·or·**ot**·o·me). Clitoridotomy.

clitorrhagia (klit·or·**a**·je·ah). Haemorrhage from the clitoris. [clitoris, Gk *rhegnynein* to gush forth.]

clival (**kli**·val). Relating to the clivus.

clivis (**kli**·vis). The lobulus clivi. [L *declivis* sloping.]

clivus (**kli**·vus). A sloping surface, particularly of bone. **Clivus blumenbachii.** Clivus of the sphenoid bone (see below). **Clivus monticuli.** The lobulus clivi. **Clivus of the occipital bone [clivus (NA)].** The sloping upper surface of the occipital bone behind the body of the sphenoid. **Clivus of the sphenoid bone [clivus (NA)].** The sloping area behind the dorsum sellae of the sphenoid bone. [L slope.]

See also: BLUMENBACH.

cloaca (klo·**a**·kah). 1. The common urogenital and rectal chamber in the human embryo. In some vertebrates, the common chamber or cavity into which the ducts of the intestinal, urinary and reproductive systems open. 2. A passage in necrosed bone leading to a cavity containing a sequestrum. **Cloaca cloacae.** *Aerobacter cloacae.* **Congenital cloaca, Persistent cloaca.** Names applied to the malformation in which the opening of the rectum is into the genito-urinary tract, as a result of a failure of development of the urorectal septum or of trauma or disease. **Urogenital cloaca.** A malformation in which there is a common opening for the urethra and the vagina. **Ventral cloaca.** The ventral division of the embryonic cloaca. **Vesicorectovaginal cloaca.** Any malformation, natural or traumatic, in which the bladder, rectum and vagina have a common opening. [L sewer.]

cloacal (klo·**a**·kal). Having reference or relating to a cloaca.

Clobazam (**klo**·baz·am). BP Commission approved name for 7-chloro-1-methyl-5-phenyl-1,5-benzodiazepine-2,4-dione; a tranquillizer.

Clobetasol (klo·**be**·tah·sol). BP Commission approved name for 21-chloro-9α-fluoro-11β,17α-dihydroxy-16β-methylpregna-1,4-diene-3,20-dione; a corticosteroid.

Clobetasone (klo·**be**·tah·sone). BP Commission approved name for 21-chloro-9α-fluoro-17α-hydroxy-16β-methylpregna-1,4-diene-3,11,20-trione; a corticosteroid.

Clociguanil (klo·si·**gwan**·il). BP Commission approved name for 4,6-diamino-1-(3,4-dichlorobenzyloxy)-1,2-dihydro-2,2-dimethyl-1,3,5-triazine; an antimalarial agent.

Clofazimine (klo·**faz**·im·een). BP Commission approved name for 3-(4-chloroanilino)-10-(4-chlorophenyl)-2,10-dihydro-2-isopropyliminophenazine; it is used in the treatment of leprosy.

Clofibrate BP 1973 (klo·**fi**·brate). Ethyl-2-(4-chlorophenoxy)-2-methylpropionate; it is used to lower serum cholesterol and triglycerides in the treatment of hypercholesterolaemia.

Clofluperol (klo·**floo**·per·ol). BP Commission approved name for 4-(4-chloro-3-trifluoromethylphenyl)-1-[3-(4-fluorobenzoyl)propyl]piperidin-4-ol; a neuroleptic.

Clogestone (**klo**·jes·tone). BP Commission approved name for 6-chloro-3β,17-dihydroxypregna-4,6-diene-20-one; a progestational steroid.

Cloguanamile (klo·**gwan**·am·ile). BP Commission approved name for 1-amidino-3-(3-chloro-4-cyanophenyl)urea; an antimalarial agent.

Clomacran (**klo**·mah·kran). BP Commission approved name for *N,N*-dimethyl-3-(2-chloro-9,10-dihydroacridin-9-yl)propylamine; a tranquillizer.

Clomiphene (**klo**·me·feen). BP Commission approved name for 1-chloro-2-[4-(2-diethylaminoethoxy)phenyl]-1,2-diphenylethylene. **Clomiphene Citrate BP 1973.** The dihydrogen citrate of clomiphene, chemically related to chlorotrianisene. It is used in the treatment of anovulatory infertility and in various menstrual disorders.

Clomipramine (klo·**mip**·ram·een). BP Commission approved name for 3-chloro-5-(3-dimethylaminopropyl)-10,11-dihydrodibenz[*b,f*]azepine; an antidepressant.

Clomocycline (klo·mo·**si**·kleen). BP Commission approved name for N^2-(hydroxymethyl)chlorotetracycline; an antibiotic.

Clonazepam (klo·**na**·ze·pam). BP Commission approved name for 5-(2-chlorophenyl)-1,3-dihydro-7-nitro-2*H*-1,4-benzodiazepin-2-one; an anticonvulsant.

clone (klone). A population of cells or organisms derived from a single cell or organism through asexual reproduction (for example, mitosis). **Forbidden clone.** A hypothetical clone of antigenically competent tissue cells which, according to the clonal selection theory, have been suppressed in fetal life. [Gk *klon* cutting used for propagation.]

clonic (**klon**·ik). Referring or relating to clonus.

clonicity (klon·**is**·it·e). The state of being clonic; clonic quality.

clonicotonic (klon·ik·o·**ton'**·ik). Term applied to muscular spasms which are both clonic and tonic.

Clonidine (**klo**·nid·een). BP Commission approved name for 2-(2,6-dichloroanilino)-2-imidazoline; a hypotensive agent.

clonism, clonismus (**klon**·izm, klon·**iz**·mus). A continued state of clonic spasm; a succession of clonic spasms.

Clonitazene (klo·**ni**·taz·een). BP Commission approved name for 2-(4-chlorobenzyl)-1-(2-diethylaminoethyl)-5-nitrobenzimidazole; a narcotic analgesic agent.

clonogenic (klon·o·**jen**·ik). A cell able to produce a clone. [klone, Gk *genein* to produce.]

clonograph (**klon**·o·graf). An apparatus with which the movements occurring in clonic spasm may be recorded. [clonus, Gk *graphein* to record.]

clonorchiasis, clonorchiosis (klon·or·**ki**·as·is, **klon**·or·ke·**o'**·sis). A disease of the Far East characterized by infestation of the bile ducts with a trematode parasite (*Clonorchis sinensis*) of the family Opisthorchidae. It produces hepatomegaly, chronic cholangitis, biliary cirrhosis, cholangiocellular carcinoma (rarely), cachexia, dyspepsia, chronic jaundice and, occasionally, night blindness. [*Clonorchis*, Gk *-osis* condition.]

Clonorchis (klon·**or**·kis). A genus of trematode flukes. **Clonorchis sinensis.** A liver fluke of the Far East which is an important human parasite in regions where raw fresh-water fish are habitually eaten. The normal wild hosts of the adult fluke are a wide range of carnivores; intermediate hosts are snails of the genera *Bythinia, Melania* and *Parafossarulus,* and the cercariae encyst in the muscles of cyprinoid fish. Migration to the human liver takes place through the bile duct. It is very common in man where faeces are passed into fish ponds, the snail hosts feeding directly on the faeces. Individual infections have occurred throughout the world as the result of migration of people from endemic centres. [Gk *klon* branch, *orchis* testicle.]

clonospasm (**klon**·o·spazm). Clonic spasm. *See* SPASM.

clonothrix (klon·o·thrix). Filamentous organisms showing false branching. They live in waterworks and pipes and are frequently encrusted with iron and manganese deposits. They are non-pathogenic to man. [Gk *klon* branch, *thrix* hair.]

clonus (klo·nus). A sign of increased reflex activity as in upper motor neuron lesions, characterized by repetitive muscular contraction induced by stretch. **Ankle clonus.** A tendon reflex induced by extending the patient's leg and suddenly dorsiflexing the foot; continued pressure on the foot elicits a clonus at the ankle. **Anodal closure clonus.** ACCl, a rapid succession of contractions and relaxations which may occur in muscle under the anode when an electrical circuit is closed. **Anodal opening clonus.** AOCl, a rapid succession of contractions and relaxations which may occur in muscle under the anode when an electrical circuit is opened. **Cathodal closure clonus.** CCCl, clonus occurring in the muscles at the cathode when the electrical circuit is closed. **Cathodal opening clonus.** COCl, clonus occurring in the muscles at the cathode when the electrical circuit is opened. **Foot clonus.** Ankle clonus (see above). **Patellar clonus.** Clonus produced in the patella by taking it between the thumb and forefinger and forcibly pushing it down. **Toe clonus.** Clonus produced in the big toe by the sudden extension of the first phalanx. **Wrist clonus.** Clonus induced in the wrist by the forcible bending back of the hand. [Gk *klonos* tumult.]

Clopamide (klo·pam·ide). BP Commission approved name for 4-chloro-*N*-(2,6-dimethylpiperidino)-3-sulphamoylbenzamide; a diuretic.

Clopenthixol (klo·pen·thi·zol). BP Commission approved name for 1-[3-(2-chlorothiaxanthan-9-ylidene)propyl]-4-(2-hydroxyethyl)piperazine; a psychotropic agent.

Clopirac (klo·pir·ak). BP Commission approved name for 1-*p*-chlorophenyl-2,5-dimethylpyrrol-3-ylacetic acid; an anti-inflammatory agent.

Cloponone (klo·pon·one). BP Commission approved name for β,4-dichloro-α-dichloroacetamidopropiophenone; an antiseptic.

Cloquet, Hippolyte (b.1787). Paris anatomist and surgeon.

Cloquet's ganglion. A reputed ganglion on the long sphenopalatine nerve within the incisive canal; it is doubtful if such a ganglion exists.

Cloquet, Jules Germain (b.1790). Paris anatomist and surgeon.

Cloquet's canal. The hyaloid canal of the vitreous of the eye.

Cloquet's fascia. Loose areolar tissues within the femoral ring.

Cloquet's gland. The upper of the deep femoral lymph nodes which are usually 3 in number and lie between the femoral artery and vein.

Cloquet's hernia. A hernia which protrudes behind the posterior layer of the femoral sheath.

Cloquet's ligament. Vaginal ligament; the fibrous remnant of the obliterated processus vaginalis. It is found in the inguinal canal.

Cloquet's needle, or sign. An ordinary bright needle is inserted deeply into a muscle and left for 10 s. If life is still present the needle will be tarnished when withdrawn; obsolete.

Cloquet's septum. The femoral septum. *See* SEPTUM.

Cloquet's space. The zonular space between the suspensory ligament of the lens and the vitreous body.

Cloquinate (klo·kwin·ate). BP Commission approved name for chloroquine-di-(8-hydroxy-7-iodoquinoline-5-sulphonate); an amoebacide.

Clorexolone (klor·ex·o·lone). BP Commission approved name for 5-chloro-2-cyclohexyl-6-sulphamoylisoindolin-1-one; a diuretic.

Clorgyline (klor·ji·leen). BP Commission approved name for *N*-3-(2,4-dichlorophenoxy)propyl-*N*-methylprop-2-ynylamine; a monoamine oxidase inhibitor and antidepressant.

Clorindione (klor·in·di·one). BP Commission approved name for 2-(4-chlorophenyl)indane-1,3-dione; an anticoagulant.

Clorprenaline (klor·pren·al·een). BP Commission approved name for 1-(2-chlorophenyl)-2-isopropylaminoethanol; a sympathomimetic agent.

Clostebol Acetate (klo·ste·bol as·et·ate). BP Commission approved name for 17β-acetoxy-4-chloroandrost-4-en-3-one; an anabolic steroid.

clostridial (klos·trid·e·al). Relating to or caused by any bacterium of the genus *Clostridium.*

Clostridium (klos·trid·e·um). A genus of anaerobic or micro-aerophilic bacteria, which produce endospores that are usually wider than the bacillus, thus giving rise to the characteristic bulged or clostridial morphology. They are Gram-positive in young culture, though often become decolorized in older cultures or in pathological fluids. They act on both carbohydrates and proteins, and may be very active bio-chemically on one or the other (saccharolytic or proteolytic subdivision). Many species are pathogenic, and many form exotoxins. The primary invading organisms which give rise to gas gangrene are *Clostridium welchii, C. septicum* and *C. oedematiens.* Tetanus is produced by the powerful toxin which circulates when *C. tetani* multiplies in a local wound. Botulinus food poisoning (botulism) results from swallowing food containing preformed toxin produced by *C. botulinum.* All the above organisms, together with secondary invaders of gas-gangrene lesions such as *C. sporogenes* and *C. histolyticum,* as well as non-pathogenic organisms such as *C. butyricum,* are often present in soil, where they can survive for years as spores; any may occur in the intestinal tract of man or animals, and *C. welchii* are particularly numerous. The resistance of the spores of these organisms to heat makes them an important cause of spoilage in imperfectly canned food: acid conditions lessen this resistance. Their resistance to antiseptics raises difficulties, for example, in the sterilization of surgical catgut. Though the vegetative organisms are usually susceptible to sulphonamides and penicillin, these agents are of much greater prophylactic than therapeutic value in clostridial infections which are essentially toxic infections. Most strains of Clostridia are strictly anaerobic, and require special enriched media for cultivation (e.g. Robertson's cooked-meat media, liver-broth or thioglycollate media). The stricter anaerobes, such as *C. tetani,* require the McIntosh and Fildes anaerobic jar, or deep tubes of suitable solid media (nutrient "sloppy" agar). Separation of mixed cultures to obtain pure strains is, however, difficult and prolonged, and the isolation of the organisms from contaminated wounds does not necessarily establish the presence of bacterial infection or a diagnosis of gas gangrene, which latter must be made on clinical grounds, or on the evidence of bacterial multiplication by direct films or sections from the affected muscles. **Clostridium botulinum** (A, B, C, D, E types). Isolated from foodstuffs and associated with botulism in man (A, B, E) or with botulism-like diseases in animals (C, D and E). It is widely distributed in soil, and in the intestinal tracts of animals. Proteolytic, forming subterminal or free spores which are oval. Its toxins and antitoxins are specific. **Clostridium chauvoei.** A species causing blackleg in cattle and sheep, but non-pathogenic to man. It is mainly saccharolytic, and forms subterminal oval spores. Serologically it is homogeneous and has specific toxin and antitoxin: bears some relationship to *Clostridium septicum.* **Clostridium histolyticum.** A clostridium isolated from soil and the intestinal tract; a secondary invader in gas gangrene: toxin production and pathogenicity are variable. It is mainly proteolytic and oval subterminal spores are readily formed. **Clostridium novyi.** *C. oedematiens* (see following). **Clostridium oedematiens, Clostridium oedamatis.** An organism pathogenic for man, and many animals, forming large oval, subterminal or free spores and mainly saccharolytic. It is haemolytic, with specific homologous agglutinins and antitoxins. **Clostridium septicum.** *Vibrion septique* of Pasteur; a primary invader in gas gangrene in man, found in the soil. It has a specific exotoxin and antitoxin, and some strains show antigenic relationship to *C. chauvoei* (see above). It forms oval, subterminal or free spores, and is mainly saccharolytic. **Clostridium sordellii.** Pathogenic strains of *C. bifermentans* (see above). **Clostridium sporogenes.** A species isolated from soil and faeces; a secondary invader in gas gangrene, but not a pathogen. It has oval, subterminal, and many free spores, and is mainly proteolytic. **Clostridium tetani.** An organism isolated from cultivated soil, and the intestines of man and animals. It produces a powerful specific exotoxin, and is pathogenic to man, horses, mice, guinea-pigs and rabbits; birds are resistant. It is a very strict anaerobe with spherical, terminal spores giving a drumstick appearance. Not saccharolytic, but has a slight proteolytic action. There is a potent antitoxin of great value prophylactically and of some value therapeutically, and active immunization by tetanus toxoid is protective. **Clostridium tetanomorphum.** A non-pathogenic species resembling *C. tetani* morphologically, but actively saccharolytic. No toxin is produced. **Clostridium welchii** (A, B, C, D types). A primary invader in gas gangrene in man (type A), lamb dysentery (type B), "struck" enteritis (type C), and enterotoxaemia and pulpy kidney disease of sheep (type D). It is found in soil and the intestinal tracts of man and animals. Its spores are oval and subterminal, formed usually only under alkaline conditions. Capsules are formed in the animal body, and the organism is saccharolytic. [dim. of Gk *kloster* spindle.]

closure (klo·zyer). The act of closing or completing an electric circuit. [L *claudere* to shut.]

clot (klot). 1. A semi-solid mass produced by coagulation in blood, lymph, milk, etc.; a blood clot (see below). 2. To coagulate. **Agony clot.** The blood clot formed in the heart during the death agony. **Ante-mortem clot.** The blood clot formed in the heart before death. **Blood clot.** The solidified elastic mass of fibrin containing in its meshes red cells, white cells and platelets, produced when whole blood is allowed to coagulate or clot. **Chicken-fat clot.** A blood clot that has only a yellowish colour, resembling chicken fat, because clotting has taken place after the erythrocytes have sedimented. **Currant-jelly clot.** A reddish-coloured jelly-like blood clot due to the presence of haemoglobin from erythrocytes. **Distal clot.** The clot formed in a blood vessel on the distal side of a ligature. **External clot.** A clot formed outside a blood vessel. **Heart clot.** A blood clot formed within the cavities of the heart. **Internal clot.** A clot formed inside a blood vessel. **Laminated clot.** A blood clot formed in layers inside an aneurysm. **Marantic clot.** A clot due to enfeeblement and stagnation of the circulation. **Passive clot.** A blood clot formed in an aneurysm when the circulation through it is stopped. **Plastic clot.** A clot formed at the point of ligature of a blood vessel, causing permanent occlusion. **Post-mortem clot.** A blood clot formed within the heart after death. **Proximal clot.** A clot formed on the proximal side of a ligature. **Clot retraction.** *See* RETRACTION. **Stratified clot.** Laminated clot (see above). **White clot.** A decolorized blood clot. [AS *clott.*]

clotbur (klot·ber). The leaves of *Xanthium strumarium* (family Compositae), a domestic remedy for the bites of poisonous insects and venomous serpents; also an active styptic.

clotetasol (klo·tet·a·sole). A potent corticosteroid applied topically in main skin disorders. It may lead to signs of adrenocortical insufficiency which may persist for 3 or more months after treatment is discontinued.

Clothiapine (klo·thi·ap·een). BP Commission approved name for 2-chloro-11-(4-methylpiperazin-1-yl)dibenzo[*b,f*]-[1,4]thiazepine; a tranquillizer.

Clotrimazole (klo·tri·maz·ole). BP Commission approved name for 1-(α-2-chlorophenylbenzhydryl)imidazole; a broad spectrum fungistatic agent of the imidazole group, for topical application only.

clottage (klot·ij). The pathological or artificial blocking up of a duct or a canal by a clot of blood.

clouding (klowd·ing). **Clouding of consciousness.** A mental state in which the patient is not fully aware of his environment or is confused regarding it. [AS *clud.*]

Clough, Mildred Clark (b.1888). Baltimore physician.

Clough and Richter syndrome. An anaemia associated with marked auto-agglutination of erythrocytes usually indicative of myelomatosis.

Clove (klove). (BP 1953.) The dried flower buds of *Eugenia caryophyllata* (Spreng.) Sprague (family Myrtaceae); Caryophyllum. **Clove bark.** The aromatic bark of the tree *Dicypellium caryophyllatum.* **Clove Oil BP 1968.** *See* OIL. [L *clavus* nail.]

Clover, Joseph Thomas (b.1825). London anaesthetist.

Clover's apparatus. A portable regulating ether air inhaler, first described in 1877.

clownism (klown·izm). A hysterical state marked by the performance of absurd and awkward actions or by contortions of the body. [AS *clott* lump.]

Cloxacillin (klox·ah·sil'·in). BP Commission approved name for 6-[3-(2-chlorophenyl)-5-methylisoxazole-4-carboxamido]penicillanate. **Cloxacillin Sodium BP 1973.** The monohydrate of the sodium salt of cloxacillin; an antibiotic with an action similar to that of benzylpenicillin. It can be given by mouth as it is resistant to the action of the gastric juice.

Clozapine (klo·zap·een). BP Commission approved name for 8-chloro-11-(4-methylpiperazin-1-yl)-5*H*-dibenzo[*b,e*][1,4]diazepine; a sedative.

club (klub). A small protrusion of the nucleus of polymorphonuclear leucocytes which, unlike the drumstick, is not indicative of the cell X chromosome complement.

See also: LANDOLT.

club-foot (klub·fut). Talipes; congenitally distorted foot. **Heel club-foot.** Talipes calcaneus, deformed foot with the toes drawn up so that only the heel touches the ground. **Inward club-foot.** Talipes varus, deformed foot with the sole turned in so that the outer side of the foot touches the ground. **Outward club-foot.** Talipes valgus, deformed foot with the sole turned outwards so that the inner side of the foot touches the ground. [ME *clubbe,* foot.]

club-hand (klub·hand). A deformity of the hand which is analogous to talipes. [ME *clubbe,* hand.]

clubbing (klub·ing). Term applied to a condition which affects the fingers and toes in many diseases of widely different aetiology. The ends of the fingers and toes show a characteristic deformity which is most easily detected in the fingers. The soft tissues are enlarged but the most outstanding feature of clubbing is seen in the nails, which are curved both laterally and longitudinally, presenting a bulbous, shiny appearance which varies from a slight departure from normal, as in the early stages of infective endocarditis, to the gross changes described as *drumstick* or *parrot's beak* in septic pulmonary disease or some congenital cardiac diseases. Clubbing of the fingers is most commonly found in (1) diseases of the lung such as bronchiectasis, cancer, septic diseases of the lung and the pneumoconioses; (2) infective endocarditis and some other cardiac conditions; (3) steatorrhoea, ulcerative colitis, subphrenic abscess and polycythaemia. It is occasionally found as a familial condition unassociated with any of the conditions so far mentioned. Enlargement of the bones of the hands and feet, as well as enlargement of the soft tissues, is found in hypertrophic pulmonary arthropathy, which is occasionally associated with some of the conditions mentioned above. Some of the conditions mentioned as a cause of clubbing are associated with reduced oxygen tension in the blood. [ME *clubbe.*]

clucking hen (kluk·ing hen). A radiation detector which gave an audible "cluck" in a pair of earphones, the rate of clucking increasing with proximity of the detector to a γ-ray source. [obsolete] [AS *cloccian.*]

clump (klump). A mass of bacteria suspended in a fluid and in a quiescent state. [AS *clympre.*]

clumping (klump·ing). Agglutination; the aggregation of relatively large particles such as red cells or bacteria. Such clumping may occur as a physicochemical phenomenon, or as a result of specific antibody (agglutinin) action. It may be observed by the naked eye, by hand lens or under the microscope. The reaction forms the basis of identifying organisms by means of known agglutinins; it can also be used to detect agglutinins in the sera of patients using known suspensions of bacteria (Widal reaction). [see prec.]

clunis (**kloo**·nis) (pl. *clunes*). The buttock. [L.]

clupeine (**kloo**·pe·een). A strongly basic simple protein found associated with nucleic acid in herring sperms. It is similar in type to protamine, which is used in combination with insulin, and yields histidine as an amino derivative. [L *clupea* shad.]

Clupidae (**kloo**·pid·e). A genus of small fish that may be poisonous. [L *clupea* shad, Gk *eidos* form.]

Clurman, A. W. 19th-20th century New York bacteriologist.

Teague and Clurman agar. Brilliant-green eosin agar. *See* AGAR.

Clusia (**kloo**·se·ah). A genus of plants of the family Guttiferae; many species yield a gum resin known as West Indian balsam. **Clusia flava.** A West Indian species which affords a milky sap used as a substitute for copaiba. **Clusia hilanana.** A species of the West Indies and South America, yielding a gum which is used as a drastic and vulnerary; its fruit is edible, and its bark is employed as an astringent in diarrhoea. **Clusia insignis.** A Brazilian species which yields a milky sap used as a salve. **Clusia rosea.** A species from which is obtained a gum similar to gamboge. [L *clusus* closed.]

cluttering (**klut**·er·ing). A nervous, hurried way of speaking in which letters and syllables are dropped. [ME *clotter.*]

Clutton, Henry Hugh (b.1850). London surgeon.

Clutton's joint. Hydrarthrosis of the knee occurring in congenital syphilis.

clysis (**kli**·sis). The giving of a clyster, or cleansing by means of a clyster. [Gk *klysis.*]

clysma (**klis**·mah). A clyster. [Gk *klysma* a drenching.]

clyster (**klis**·ter). An injection *per rectum.* An enema. [Gk *klyster* wash-out.]

clysterize (**klis**·ter·ize). To treat by means of a clyster or an enema.

cnemis (**ne**·mis). 1. The lower leg or shin. 2. The tibia. [Gk *kneme* leg.]

cnemitis (ne·**mi**·tis). Inflammation of the tibia. [Gk *kneme* leg, *-itis* inflammation.]

cnemoscoliosis (**ne**·mo·sko·le·**o'**·sis). Bending of the leg in a lateral direction. [Gk *kneme* leg, scoliosis.]

cnicin (**ni**·sin). $C_{42}H_{56}O_2$, a crystalline compound, derived from various species of thistle, especially *Cnicus benedictus.* It is odourless and very bitter, and is reputed to possess emmenagogue and emetic properties.

Cnicus (**ni**·kus). A genus of plants of the family Compositae. **Cnicus benedictus.** The blessed thistle (*Carduus benedictus*), used as a tonic. [L thistle.]

cnidosis (ni·**do**·sis). Urticaria; nettle rash. [Gk *knide* nettle, *-osis* condition.]

coacervate (ko·**as**·er·vate). The aggregation of an emulsoid into droplets, either preparatory to becoming emulsified, or in the process of demulsification. [L *coacervatus* heaped-up.]

coadunation, coadunition (ko·ad·ew·**na'**·shun, **ko**·ad·ew·**nish'**·un). Junction or union of 2 or more dissimilar substances into one mass. [L *cum, ad, unus* one.]

coagglutination (**ko**·ag·loo·tin·a'·shun). A clumping of erythrocytes by mixtures of protein antigens and their antisera; the clumping occurs during the course of the interaction of the antigens and their antisera, but not under their separate influences. [L *cum,* agglutinate.]

coagulant (ko·**ag**·ew·lant). 1. Causing coagulation. 2. An agent that causes a coagulum to form. [L *coagulare* to curdle.]

coagulase (ko·**ag**·ew·laze). An enzyme produced by pathogenic strains of *Staphylococci.* It causes coagulation of plasma *in vitro* and *in vivo,* and partially explains the localization of staphylococcal lesions.

coagulate (ko·**ag**·ew·late). 1. To undergo the process of coagulation. 2. To cause to coagulate.

coagulation (ko·ag·ew·**la'**·shun). 1. The process of changing by chemical reaction from a fluid to a curdled or clotted state. 2. A coagulum. 3. The precipitation by means of heat, enzymes or chemical agents of colloids or proteins into a jelly-like soft mass. **Blood coagulation.** The process of clotting or coagulation of whole blood, the mechanism of which comprises a series of reactions involving calcium, thromboplastin (and platelets or damaged body tissues), prothrombin, fibrinogen and probably other factors. This can be prevented, delayed or accelerated by various chemical or physical factors. **Electric coagulation.** The process of breaking-down tissue and condensing it into a mass by applying to it a needle point or points charged with a bipolar current. **Laser coagulation.** Coagulation of tissue produced by laser energy, used in the treatment of retinal disease. **Light coagulation.** Coagulation of tissue produced by an intense beam of light, used in the treatment of retinal disease. **Massive coagulation.** A pathological condition of the spinal fluid in which it is transformed into almost completely solid curd, as occurs in cases of tumour or inflammation of the cord. **Coagulation necrosis.** *See* NECROSIS. **Coagulation time.** *See* TIME. [L *coagulare* to curdle.]

coagulative (ko·ag·ew·la·tiv). 1. Aiding the process of coagulation. 2. Associated with or characterized by the process of coagulation.

coagulin (ko·**ag**·ew·lin). Thromboplastin. [L *coagulare* to curdle.]

coagulometer (ko·**ag**·ew·**lom'**·et·er). An apparatus for ascertaining the rapidity of the process of coagulation of blood, or for determining its coagulability. [L *coagulare* to curdle, meter.]

coagulotomy (ko·**ag**·ew·**lot'**·o·me). Excision by the use of a strong electric current of low frequency (diathermic) so that bleeding is prevented by coagulation of the vessels in the raw surfaces. [L *coagulare* to curdle, Gk *temnein* to cut.]

coaguloviscosimeter (ko·ag·ew·lo·vis·ko·**sim'**·et·er). An apparatus with which the coagulation time of the blood can be determined. [L *coagulare* to curdle, *viscosus* gummy, meter.]

coagulum (ko·**ag**·ew·lum). 1. The coagulated mass of fibrin, serum and corpuscles into which blood changes when it is withdrawn from the body. 2. A curdled substance, as milk or insoluble albumin. [L.]

Coakley, Cornelius Godfrey (b.1862). New York otolaryngologist.

Coakley's operation. An operation with the approach to the frontal sinus through its anterior wall.

coalition (ko·al·**ish**·un). **Calcaneoscaphoid coalition.** A congenital abnormality in which the calcaneus and tarsal scaphoid are joined by a bar of bone. [L *coalescere* to grow together.]

coalitus (ko·**al**·it·us). 1. Coalescence. 2. Coalescent. **Coalitus artuum.** The coalescence of one part or limb with another, as fingers or toes. [L.]

coaptation (ko·ap·**ta**·shun). The fitting or the joining together of 2 surfaces, e.g. the lips of a wound or the ends of a broken bone. [L *coaptare* to fit together.]

coarctate (ko·**ark**·tate). 1. In biology, pressed or connected closely together. 2. Contracted or narrowed. [L *coarctare* to press together.]

coarctation (ko·ark·**ta**·shun). 1. A state of compression. 2. A condition of narrowing or of stricture. **Abdominal coarctation.** Coarctation of the abdominal aorta, a rare condition which is probably more often an acquired stenosis from arteritis rather than a developmental abnormality. **Aortic coarctation.** Coarctation or stenosis of the aorta; narrowing of the lumen of the aorta, which is due to congenital maldevelopment. The site is almost invariably at the isthmus and just above the ductus arteriosus. In the common "adult" type, the narrowing is localized, but in the "infantile" type it may be extensive and associated with complete interruption of the aorta or atresia of the ascending portion, combined with patency of the ductus arteriosus. Occasional cases of coarctation of the descending aorta and of the arch have been described. [see prec.]

coarctotomy (ko·ark·**tot**·o·me). Surgical division of a stricture. [L *coarctare* to press together, Gk *temnein* to cut.]

coarse (kors). 1. Not fine. 2. In microscopy, composed of large particles. [from the phrase *of course,* i.e. ordinary.]

coarticulation (**ko**·ar·tik·ew·**la'**·shun). Synarthrosis. [L *cum, articulare* to join.]

coat [tunica (NA)] (kote). In anatomy, a covering, often of fibrous tissue, which invests an organ or structure completely, or almost completely. **Adventitious coat [tunica adventitia].** The outer coat of a structure, derived from the surrounding connective tissue. **Buffy coat.** The greyish-white buffy coat, or layer, consisting mainly of the white blood corpuscles and platelets with varying amounts of erythrocytes, that lies on the surface of the main bulk of sedimented erythrocytes when blood plasma is allowed to stand; the quantity of this yellow layer depends on the speed of sedimentation and the total number of white blood corpuscles present. When removed it is sometimes known as *leucocytic cream*, and has been used therapeutically. The term is also applied to the buffy coat of similar composition plus fibrin that covers the surface of the blood clot when whole blood is allowed to stand and clot. It is also known as *crusta phlogistica* or *crusta inflammatoria*; *yellow layer*. **"Enseal" coat.** A proprietary coating for tablets; it resists acid but swells and bursts in the duodenum. **Fibrous coat [tunica fibrosa (NA)].** The fibrous tissue covering or lining an organ. **Internal elastic coat of an artery.** A layer of elastic tissue between the tunica intima and tunica media; the internal elastic lamina. **Middle coat of an artery.** The tunica media. **Mucous coat [tunica mucosa (NA)].** A rather vague term to denote the lining coat of hollow organs, tubes or cavities. The free surface is always moist and coated with a thin layer of mucus. **Muscular coat [tunica muscularis (NA)].** The muscular coat of tubes or hollow organs, usually composed of smooth or involuntary muscle. **Serous coat [tunica serosa (NA)].** The covering layer of organs or tubes that are related to a serous cavity, generally consisting of a thin stroma of connective tissue coated with a single layer of pavement epithelium, and moistened by a small amount of serous fluid to facilitate the gliding of these organs or tissues on one another and on adjacent structures. **Submucous coat [tela submucosa (NA)].** A lax areolar tissue layer underlying, and often facilitating the movement of, the mucous membranes on surrounding tissues. **Subserous coat [tela subserosa (NA)].** Loose areolar tissue underlying a serous coat and attaching it to the organ or tube covered. **Uveal coat.** The vascular tunic or uveal tract of the eyeball, consisting of the choroid, ciliary body, and iris. [OFr. *cote*.]

coating (ko·ting). A covering layer. **Enteric coating.** The coating given to a pill or tablet which will ensure that the ingredients will pass unchanged through the stomach into the intestines. **Coating of the tongue.** A condition of the tongue indicative of digestive disturbance; the surface is covered with a layer of viscous material. **Coating of pills.** Any substance (e.g. sugar) used to cover pills so that the ingredients cannot be tasted. [see prec.]

Coats, George (b.1876). London ophthalmologist.

Coats' disease, or retinopathy. Applied orginally to the development in the retina, usually of one eye only, of large yellowish-white masses deep to the vessels: the patients were healthy, young, and commonly males. It is realized now that it includes some 6 or more distinguishable retinal and choroidal conditions.

cobalt (ko·bawlt). An element of atomic weight 58.94, atomic number 27 and chemical symbol Co. It is a hard pinkish-white metal, slightly magnetic, and closely related to iron and nickel; used in alloys. Forms cobaltous salts C^{2+} which are pink or blue, and cobaltic Co^{3+} which enter into complex combinations. **Cobalt-60.** A radioactive isotope of cobalt used in radiotherapy. [G *Kobold* goblin found in mines.]

cobra (ko·brah). A poisonous snake of the Old World which can expand its neck region into a flattened hood. *Naia naia*, the Indian cobra, enters houses in search of rodent prey. *N. haie* is the commonest spitting cobra of Africa, whose venom is dangerous if it reaches the eyes or mucous membranes. *N. hannah*, the hamadryad or king cobra of India, may reach 4.5 m in length. The cape spitting cobra, Ringhalo *Sepedon haemachates*, occurs in South Africa. For other species *see* NAIA. [Port. from L *colubra* snake.]

cobraism (ko·brah·izm). The condition of being poisoned by cobra venom as the result of therapeutic administration.

cobralysin (ko·**bral**·is·in). The haemolytic substance derived from cobra venom. [cobra, Gk *lyein* to dissolve.]

coca (**ko**·kah). The dried leaves of *Erythroxylum coca* Lam. (Bolivian or Huanuco coca) and of *Erythroxylum truxillense* Rusby (Peruvian or Truxillo coca), of the family Erythroxylaceae. The shrubs are cultivated in Bolivia, Peru and Java, and the leaves contain important alkaloids, chiefly cocaine, cinnamylcocaine and α-truxilline, all derivatives of ecgonine. It is used by the people of Bolivia and Peru as a stimulant masticatory to allay hunger and fatigue, and is sometimes employed in medicine in the form of an elixir or liquid extract especially in convalescence. Its chief importance, however, is as a source of cocaine. [Sp.]

cocaethyline (ko·kah·**eth**·il·een). Homococaine, ethylbenzoylecgonine, $C_{18}H_{23}NO_4$. A synthetic alkaloid slightly soluble in water, and isomeric with methylcocaine. It is used as a local anaesthetic.

cocaine (ko·**kane**). Methylbenzoylecgonine, $C_{17}H_{21}O_4N$. An alkaloid obtained from coca, the dried leaves of *Erythroxylum coca* Lam. or of *Erythroxylum truxillense*. It is a colourless crystalline compound, only slightly soluble in water, insoluble in glycerine, but soluble in most other organic solvents. It is a very efficient surface anaesthetic, used for local anaesthesia of mucous surfaces and of the eye, but is seldom employed internally owing to its high toxicity and the danger of habit formation (BP 1973). First used as a local analgesic by Karl Koller of Vienna in 1884. **Cocaine Hydrochloride BP 1973.** $C_{17}H_{21}O_4NHCl$, a water-soluble salt of cocaine used for the administration of the latter in aqueous solution. **Lamellae of Cocaine BP 1953.** Lamellae each containing 1.3 mg of cocaine hydrochloride; used for ophthalmic purposes. **Cocaine muriate.** Cocaine hydrochloride (see above). **Cocaine nitrate.** $C_{17}H_{21}O_4NHNO_3$, a water-soluble salt of cocaine used in conjunction with silver nitrate to lessen the pain caused by the latter. **Cocaine salicylate.** $C_{17}H_{21}O_4NC_6H_4(OH)COOH$, a salt which is readily soluble in water and with good keeping properties. It has a similar action to cocaine hydrochloride. [coca.]

cocaini (ko·ka·ni). **Cocaini Hydrochloridum.** *European Pharmacopoeia* name for Cocaine Hydrochloride BP 1973.

cocainidine (ko·**ka**·nid·een). Methylcocaine, $C_{18}H_{23}NO_4$. An alkaloid base derived from commercial cocaine.

cocainine (ko·**ka**·neen). Truxilline.

cocainism (ko·**ka**·nizm). 1. The habitual use of cocaine in order to experience its intoxicating effects. 2. The diseased condition of mind and body which results from addiction to cocaine.

cocainist (ko·**ka**·nist). A cocaine addict.

cocainization (ko·**ka**·ni·**za**'·shun). The putting or the bringing of the system or an organ under the analgesic influence of cocaine. **Endomeningeal cocainization, Intraspinal cocainization.** Spinal cocainization (see following). **Spinal cocainization.** Making the abdomen and legs analgesic by injection of cocaine into the intradural or subarachnoid space by means of puncture at the space between the 3rd and 4th lumbar vertebrae. Sensibility to temperature and touch and muscular sensibility are not impaired. **Spinal-canal cocainization, Spinal subarachnoid cocainization, Subarachnoid cocainization.** Spinal cocainization (see preceding).

cocainize (ko·**ka**·nize). To put or bring under the analgesic influence of cocaine.

cocainomania (ko·**ka**·no·**ma**'·ne·ah). 1. Cocaine addiction. 2. Mental derangement resulting from cocaine addiction. [cocaine, mania.]

cocainomaniac (ko·**ka**·no·**ma**'·ne·ak). 1. A cocaine addict. 2. An individual who has become mentally deranged as the result of cocaine addiction. [see prec.]

cocamine (ko·kam·een). α-Truxilline, γ-isoatropylcocaine, $C_{38}H_{46}O_8N_2$. An alkaloid obtained from the leaves of Peruvian coca. It is an amorphous white base which hydrolyses into ecgonine.

co-carboxylase (ko·kar·**box**·il·aze). *See* THIAMINE PYROPHOSPHATE.

co-carcinogen (ko·kar·**sin**·o·jen). Anything that furthers the action of a carcinogenin producing a malignant tumour, such as a pre-existing chronic inflammation or the irritating effects of a chemical not itself a carcinogen. [L *cum*, carcinogen.]

co-carcinogenesis ((**ko**·kar·sin·o·**jen**′·es·is). The process by which a co-carcinogen acts.

Coccaceae (kok·**a**·se·e). A family of bacteria belonging to the order Eubacteriales. It comprises 3 tribes, Streptococceae, Neisserieae and Micrococcaceae; and 7 genera, *Micrococcus, Streptococcus, Neisseria, Leuconostoc, Rhodococcus, Sarcina* and *Staphylococcus*. The main characteristic of members of the family is that all cells are spherical, oval or kidney-shaped. Numerous species are pathogenic for man and animals, e.g. *Streptococcus pyogenes, Neisseria gonorrhoeae, Neisseria meningitidis, Micrococcus tetragenus* (*Gaffkya tetragena*), *Staphylococcus aureus* (*S. pyogenes*). [Gk *kokkos* berry.]

coccal (**kok**·al). Relating to or caused by a coccus or cocci.

coccerin (**kok**·se·rin). Cochineal wax, $C_{30}H_{60}(C_{31}H_{61}O_3)_2$. An ester of cocceryl alcohol and related acids which forms the coating of the body of the cochineal insect.

coccidia (kok·**sid**·e·ah). *See* COCCIDIUM.

coccidial (kok·**sid**·e·al). Relating to the coccidia, or belonging to them.

Coccidiida (kok·sid·**i**·id·ah). An order of sporozoa which includes the genus *Plasmodium*. [Gk *kokkos* berry, *eidos* form.]

coccidioidal (**kok**·sid·e·**oid**′·al). Relating to or caused by *Coccidioides*.

Coccidioides (**kok**·sid·e·**oid**′·eez). The dimorphic fungus *Coccidioides immitis* is the causal organism of coccidioidosis (coccidioidomycosis), a self-limiting respiratory infection that rarely develops a chronic granulomatous stage. The fungus is seen in pus, sputum or tissues as spherical thick-walled non-budding bodies, 5–50 μm in diameter, which develop into spherules containing numerous ellipsoid endospores disseminated by rupture of the wall of the spherule. Mycelium consisting of branching septate hyphae is common in cultures, but rare in the tissues. Also known as *Coccidioides esferiformis*. [Gk *kokkos* berry, *eidos* form.]

coccidioidin (**kok**·sid·e·**oid**′·in). An intradermal skin test antigen prepared from *Coccidioides immitis* and used in the diagnosis of coccidioidomycosis. [*Coccidioides*.]

coccidioidomycosis (**kok**·sid·e·**oid**·o·mi·**ko**′·sis). A mycotic infection caused by *Coccidioides immitis*. **Cutaneous coccidioidomycosis.** Primary skin lesions are rare; there must be no history of preceding respiratory infection and clear evidence of traumatic implantation with ulceration within 1–3 weeks of injury, together with regional lymphadenopathy. **Disseminated coccidioidomycosis.** A chronic, persisting, metastasizing infection involving skin, bones and viscera. **Primary coccidioidomycosis.** A mild self-limiting respiratory infection. [*Coccidioides*, Gk *mykes* fungus, *-osis*.]

coccidioidosis (kok·**sid**·e·oid·**o**′·sis). Coccidioidomycosis.

coccidiosis (**kok**·sid·e·**o**′·sis). A disorder due to the presence in the intestine of a coccidium, *Isospora hominis*, and characterized by copious discharge of watery mucoid stools. [coccidium, Gk *-osis* condition.]

Coccidium (kok·**sid**·e·um) (pl. *coccidia*). A name formerly given to a group of protozoa belonging to the order Sporozoa, parasitic in animals. They have a complex life cycle, resembling that of the malarial parasite. **Coccidium bigeminum.** *Isospora bigeminum*, a species parasitic in cats and dogs. **Coccidium cuniculi.** *Eimeria stiedae*, a species in rabbits and mice. **Coccidium hominis.** *Isospora hominis*, a species parasitic in man. **Coccidium oviforme.** *Coccidium cuniculi* (see above). [Gk *kokkos* berry.]

coccidynia (kok·sid·**in**·e·ah). Coccygodynia.

coccigenic (kok·se·**jen**·ik). Applied as a qualification of a disease, indicates that the aetiological factor is a micro-organism of the family Coccaceae. [coccus, Gk *genein* to produce.]

coccillana (kok·se·**ah**·nah). Cocillana.

coccinella (kok·sin·**el**·ah). Cochineal.

coccinellin (kok·sin·**el**·in). A little-used name for carminic acid, the colouring matter of cochineal.

coccobacillus (**kok**·o·bas·**il**′·us). A bacillus which is so short as to resemble a coccus.

coccobacteria (**kok**·o·bak·**teer**′·e·ah). 1. A general name for cocci of any kind. 2. *Serratia*. [Gk *kokkos* berry, *bakterion* rod.]

coccode (**kok**·ode). A granule which has the characteristics of a globe or a berry. [Gk *kokkos* berry, *eidos* form.]

coccogenous (kok·**oj**·en·us). Producing or yielding cocci. [Gk *kokkos* berry, *genein* to produce.]

coccoid (**kok**·oid). 1. Like a coccus. 2. Spherical. [Gk *kokkos* berry, *eidos* form.]

coccomelasma (**kok**·o·mel·**az**′·mah). A disorder of the skin characterized by the formation of pigmented granules. [Gk *kokkos* berry, *melas* black.]

cocculin (**kok**·ew·lin). $C_{19}H_{26}O_{10}$, a principle found in levant berries, the dried fruit, *Cocculus indicus*, of *Anamirta paniculata*. A tasteless crystalline narcotic.

Cocculus (**kok**·ew·lus). A genus of plants of the family Menispermaceae; many are medicinal, some actively poisonous. **Cocculus indicus.** The fruit of *Anamirta paniculata*, a climbing shrub indigenous to the Malay Archipelago and East India; it is collected when ripe and dried, and contains picrotoxin, a bitter poisonous substance, with a little cocculin (anamirtin). [L a little berry.]

coccus (**kok**·us). 1. Spherical or elliptical bacterial cells which may occur singly, in pairs, in clusters, or in chains; either Gram-positive, e.g. *Staphylococcus*, or Gram-negative, e.g. *Gonococcus*. 2. *Coccus cacti*. **Coccus cacti.** *See* COCHINEAL. [Gk *kokkos* berry.]

See also: TUNNICLIFF.

coccyalgia (kok·se·**al**·je·ah). Coccygodynia. [coccyx, Gk *algos* pain.]

coccycephalus (kok·se·**kef**·al·us). A monster the head of which is in the form of a beak-shaped process. [coccyx, Gk *kephale* head.]

coccydynia (kok·se·**din**·e·ah). Coccygodynia.

coccygalgia (kok·sig·**al**·je·ah). Coccygodynia. [coccyx, Gk *algos* pain.]

coccygeal (kok·**sij**·e·al). Belonging or relating to, or involving the coccyx. **Coccygeal plexus.** *See* PLEXUS. **Coccygeal whorl.** *See* WHORL.

coccygeal nerve [nervus coccygeus (NA)]. The last spinal segmental nerve emerging between the sacrum and coccyx and joining the coccygeal plexus. The anterior primary ramus [ramus ventralis (NA)] is small; the posterior [ramus dorsalis (NA)] unites with the posterior primary rami of the 4th and 5th sacral nerves.

coccygectomy (kok·sij·**ek**·to·me). Excision of the coccyx. [coccyx, Gk *ektome* a cutting out.]

coccygerector (kok·sij·e·**rek**·tor). The coccygeus muscle. [coccyx, L *erigere* to set up.]

coccygeus muscle [musculus coccygeus (NA)] (kok·**sij**·e·us). A small muscle which completes the muscular pelvic floor posteriorly; it is attached to the spine of the ischium and to the coccyx.

coccygodynia (**kok**·sig·o·**din**′·e·ah). Pain in the coccyx and the coccygeal region which may be referred. [coccyx, Gk *odyne* pain.]

coccygotomy (kok·sig·**ot**·o·me). 1. Coccygectomy. 2. The dissection and freeing of the coccyx from its attachments. [coccyx, Gk *temnein* to cut.]

coccyodynia (**kok**·se·o·**din**′·e·ah). Coccygodynia.

coccyx [os coccygis (NA)] (**kok**·six). The small triangular bone, directed downward and forward, with which the apex of the sacrum articulates. It is the lower end of the vertebral column. [Gk *kokkyx* cuckoo—from resemblance of the bone to a cuckoo's beak.]

Cochin-leg (**kot**·chin·leg). True elephantiasis (filarial elephantiasis); a pathological overgrowth of skin and subcutaneous tissues induced by reaction to a filarial infection.

Cochineal BP 1973 (kot·shin·**eel**). The dried bodies of the female insects of the species *Coccus cacti*. The red colouring matter which they contain is known as *carmine* and can be extracted with water or alcohol. It was formerly used to colour medicine, but as it is turned yellow by acids and purple by alkalis it has been replaced by synthetic dyes the colour of which is not so affected. Of certain value as an indicator for inorganic acids and alkalis (pH 6.0–7.0). [L *coccineus* scarlet.]

cochinilin (kot·shin·**il**·in). Carminic acid, $C_{22}H_{20}O_{13}$. An anthrapurpurin derived from cochineal and used as a stain in microscopy; also employed as a pH indicator (5.0–6.0).

cochlea [NA] (**kok**·le·ah). The conical spiral tube of the bony labyrinth of the internal ear containing the duct of the cochlea, the essential organ of hearing. The apex is directed forwards and laterally, and the base [basis cochleae (NA)] directed towards the bottom of the internal auditory meatus. [L snail shell.]

cochlear (**kok**·le·ar). 1. Relating or belonging to the cochlea. 2. Having reference to the cochlea. **Cochlear nucleus.** *See* NUCLEUS. **Cochlear recess of the vestibule.** *See* RECESS.

cochlear nerve [pars cochlearis (nervi octavi) (NA)]. One of the main divisions of the auditory nerve, the nerve of supply to the cochlea; the nerve of hearing. Its fibres arise in the cells of the spiral ganglion; the peripheral fibres end in relation to the hair cells of the organ of Corti, and the central fibres terminate in relation to the cochlear nuclei in the medulla oblongata.

cochleare (kok·le·a·re). A Latin word used in prescription writing, meaning a spoon. **Cochleare amplum.** A heaped spoonful. **Cochleare magnum.** A tablespoon. **Cochleare maximum, Cochleare medium.** A dessertspoon. **Cochleare minimum.** A teaspoon. **Cochleare modicum.** A dessertspoon. **Cochleare parvum.** A teaspoon. **Cochleare plenum.** A tablespoon.

Cochlearia (kok·le·a·re·ah). A genus of plants of the family Cruciferae. **Cochlearia armoracia.** The horseradish; the fresh root is collected from cultivated plants and contains the glycoside, sinigrin. It is used as a counter-irritant and vesicant. **Cochlearia officinalis.** Scurvy grass, used as an antiscorbutic and diuretic. [L *cochleare* spoon.]

cochleariform (kok·le·**ar**·e·form). 1. Spoon-shaped. 2. Shaped like a snail's shell. [L *cochlea* snail shell.]

cochleate (**kok**·le·ate). A term descriptive of one of the forms taken by bacterial cultures—that of a spiral coil. [L *cochlea* snail shell.]

cochleitis (kok·le·**i**·tis). Inflammation of the cochlea of the ear. [cochlea, Gk *-itis* inflammation.]

cochleovestibular (**kok**·le·o·ves·**tib**′·ew·lar). Relating to the cochlea and the vestibule of the ear.

Cochliomyia (**kok**·le·o·**mi**′·e·ah). A genus of metallic coloured blow flies (Calliphoridae) of the tropical and sub-tropical New World. **Cochliomyia hominivorax (americana).** A fly which oviposits normally in sores in living mammals, including man, particularly in the nose, and very occasionally in decaying organic matter. The larvae, called *screw-worms,* burrow in living tissue. **Cochliomyia macellaria.** A species normally saprophagous, which occasionally invades sores. **Cochliomyia megacephalia.** A species that may act as a mechanical vector of infection, as also may other species. [L *cochlea* snail shell, Gk *myia* fly.]

cochlitis (kok·**li**·tis). Cochleitis.

Cocillana BP 1968 (ko·se·**ah**·nah, ko·sil·**ah**·nah). Guapi bark; the bark of *Guarea rusbyi* from South America. It is stated to be equal to ipecacuanha in expectorant properties. It is also a tonic and laxative.

cocinin (**ko**·sin·in). A fatty substance, the main constituent of coconut oil. It is an ester of cocinic acid.

Cock, Edward (b.1805). London surgeon.

Cock's operation. External urethrotomy by perineal section without a guide.

Cock's peculiar tumour. A lesion simulating an epithelioma, formed by septic ulceration of a neglected sebaceous cyst on the scalp.

Cockayne, Edward Alfred (b.1880). London physician.

Cockayne's syndrome. Dwarfism, mental defect, impaired hearing, photosensitivity and retinal degeneration; autosomal recessive.

Cockett, Frank Bernard. London surgeon.

Cockett's operation. Ligature of the communicating veins of the leg in the treatment of varicose ulcer.

cockle (kokl). The corn cockle, *Agrostemma githago.* [AS *coccul.*]

cocklebur (**kokl**·ber). Agrimony, the plant *Agrimonia eupatoria.* [AS *coccul,* ME *burr.*]

cockroach (**kok**·roche). Members of the insect family Blattidae. Several species are cosmopolitan household pests: *Blatta orientalis,* the "black beetle", *Blatella germanica,* the steam fly or (USA) croton bug and *Periplaneta americana,* a large brown form, are the commonest. They may be important in bacterial dissemination and as intermediate hosts of several parasitic worms. [Sp. *cucaracha.*]

Cockroft, Sir John Douglas (b.1897). British physicist.

Cockroft-Walton circuit. A circuit used for the production of a direct high potential from an alternating supply by the addition of potentials developed across condensers in series with rectifiers.

cocktail (**kok**·tale). **Lytic cocktail.** A term coined in France in the early 1950s for the mixture of analgesic and phenothiazine derivatives used to potentiate anaesthesia. [etym. dub.]

cocoa (**ko**·ko). 1. The seeds of the tree *Theobroma cacao* grown in South and Central America, the West Indies and West Africa. 2. A food preparation made from the seeds of *Theobroma cacao* which are first fermented, then roasted (nibs), and ground to a fine powder, with the expression of a certain amount of the contained fat. It contains theobromine, which gives it a slight stimulant property, milder than that of tea or coffee, and is therefore of value in the diet of children and certain invalids. **Cocoa butter.** A fat consisting of the mixed glycerides of arachic, oleic, palmitic and stearic acids. It is used in the manufacture of chocolate and other confectionery, also in cosmetic and toilet preparations and as a basis for suppositories since it melts below body temperature. [Mexican *cacuatl.*]

co-conscious (ko·**kon**·shus). A psychological term describing something that can be remembered and brought into consciousness only when the conditions of consciousness itself are favourable. [L *cum,* consciousness.]

co-contraction (ko·kon·**trak**·shun). A muscular state in which antagonist muscles act in co-ordination for the purpose of holding a limb straight. [L *cum, contrahere* to draw together.]

coconut (**ko**·ko·nut). The nut of *Cocos nucifera,* a tropical palm yielding from its wood a sap known as *toddy* (palm wine). Of greater importance is the fruit or kernel—coconut—which is used in cooking. **Coconut oil.** An oil expressed from coconuts and used in the manufacture of candles, soap, margarine and certain toilet products; also applied to the skin as an embrocation. [Port. *coco* grimace.]

coction (**kok**·shun). 1. A name for digestion. 2. The process of boiling. [L *coquere* to cook.]

coctolabile (kok·to·**la**·bile). Referring to any substance which is altered in composition or even destroyed by heating to 100°C. [L *coquere* to cook, *labilis* liable to slip.]

coctostabile, coctostable (kok·to·**sta**·bile, kok·to·**sta**·bl). Describing anything which retains its properties even when raised to the boiling point of water (100°C). [L *coquere* to cook, *stabilis* stable.]

cod (kod). A salt-water fish *Gadus morrhua* (order Teleostei). **Cod-liver Oil BP 1958.** *See* OIL. [etym. dub.]

Codactide (ko·**dak**·tide). BP Commission approved name for D-Ser^{1}-Lys^{17,18}-$\beta^{1\text{-}18}$-corticotrophin amide; a corticotrophic peptide.

codamine (**ko**·dam·een). $C_{20}H_{25}O_4N$, a crystalline alkaloid obtained from opium. It is a benzyl isoquinoline derivative isomeric with laudanum.

code (kode). 1. A system of rules. 2. A set of groups of symbols with arbitrary meanings for the carriage of information in brief form. **Amino acid code.** Genetic code (see below). **Genetic code.** The information system in living cells that instructs the machinery for polypeptide synthesis to insert a particular amino acid in response to the nucleotide sequence of the genetic material. It comprises 64 nucleotide triplet sequences (called *codons*), of which 61 specify the 20 amino acids that occur in proteins and 3 (called *termination codons*) interrupt the further addition of any amino acid to a growing polypeptide chain. The code is degenerate, since most of the amino acids are coded for by more than 1 codon (thus, there are 6 different codons for each of the amino acids arginine, serine and leucine, but 1 each for tryptophan and methionine). It is universal, being of general application in viruses, bacteria, plants and animals. It is non-overlapping, since each nucleotide base is an integral part of only one codon and no other. **Triplet code.** The code of nucleic acid residues which is translated into amino acid sequences by the ribosomal apparatus. [L *caudex* book.]

co-dehydrogenase, co-dehydrase (ko·de·hi'·dro·jen·aze, ko·de·hi'·draze). Co-enzymes I and II, the prosthetic groups in certain pyridino-protein enzymes. They are derived from nicotinamide and act as hydrogen carriers in such systems as the oxidation of lactic acid, glucose and hexose monophosphate.

codeine (ko·de·een). Monomethylmorphine, $C_{18}H_{21}O_3N$. An alkaloid obtained from opium or prepared by the methylation of morphine. It is a white crystalline base, laevorotatory, moderately soluble in water (more so in alcohol or ether), which is used as a mild hypnotic since it causes less respiratory depression than morphine and is less constipating. It is of especial value in allaying irritating cough, and as an analgesic, usually with acetylsalicylic acid (BPC 1954). **Codeine hydriodide,** $C_{18}H_{21}O_3NHI{\cdot}2H_2O$. A salt similar in properties to the hydrobromide. **Codeine hydrobromide.** $C_{18}H_{21}O_3NHBr{\cdot}2H_2O$, a salt used for similar purposes to the phosphate: it has also been employed in the eye, like ethylmorphine. **Codeine hydrochloride.** $C_{18}H_{21}O_3NHCl{\cdot}2H_2O$, a salt similar in properties to the phosphate, and included in several Continental pharmacopoeias. **Codeine methyl bromide.** $C_{18}H_{21}O_3N(CH_3)Br$, eucodeine, a salt used as a sedative. **Codeine Phosphate BP 1973.** $C_{18}H_{21}O_3NH_3PO_4{\cdot}H_2O$, a granular crystalline white salt containing 69 per cent of the anhydrous alkaloid. It is soluble in water and is the compound most commonly used in the preparation of mixtures, linctuses and official tablets. **Codeine sulphate.** $(C_{18}H_{21}O_3N)_2H_2SO_4{\cdot}5H_2O$, a water-soluble salt. **Codeine valerianate.** $C_{18}H_{21}O_3NC_4H_9COOH$, a salt used as an antispasmodic and hypnotic. [Gk *kodeia* poppy-head.]

Codeinii Phosphas. *European Pharmacopoeia* name for Codeine Phosphate BP 1973.

codex (ko·dex). 1. A manuscript volume; especially an ancient classical text or an early Greek version of the Bible. 2. An authorized formulary. **British Pharmaceutical Codex.** BPC, a publication of the Pharmaceutical Society of Great Britain intended to be complementary to the *British Pharmacopoeia* and providing additional information about official and other medicinal substances, galenicals and compounded preparations. [L *caudex* book.]

Codivilla, Alessandro (b.1861). Italian surgeon.

Codivilla's extension. Extension of a limb by calipers or pins transfixing or fixed into the bone.

Codivilla's operation. An operation for non-union of a fracture with pseudarthrosis. The pseudarthrosis is surrounded by thin osteoperiosteal grafts.

Codman, Ernest Amory (b.1869). Boston surgeon.

Codman's bursa. The subacromial bursa. *See* BURSA.

Codman's bursitis. Subacromial bursitis. *See* BURSITIS.

Codman's bursal incision. An incision used for the removal of Codman's (subacromial) bursa and extending 5 cm (2 in) forward from the acromioclavicular joint.

Codman's sign. For rupture of the supraspinatus tendon: the arm can be passively abducted without pain but active abduction in the middle range of the movement is either impossible or painful.

Codman's triangle. A small deposit of subperiosteal bone at the periphery of a sarcoma of bone. In the x-rays this produces a triangular appearance on the surface of the bone at the edge of the tumour. The appearance is said to be characteristic of sarcoma of bone.

codol (ko·dol). Retinol, $C_{32}H_{16}$. A liquid hydrocarbon from the distillation of pitch or resin. It was formerly in use as a urinary antiseptic, and in the treatment of gonorrhoea.

codon (ko·don). The smallest unit of genetic information which specifies one amino acid residue in the synthesis of polypeptides in living cells; a nucleotide triplet on a DNA strand (or its complementary triplet on a strand of messenger RNA) which specifies a particular amino acid in cellular synthesis of proteins. **Imitation codon.** The codon on messenger RNA which signals the start for the translation of the information carried on the messenger into the amino acid sequence of a polypeptide chain in the process of polypeptide synthesis in living cells. **Synonym codon.** One of a group of codons which code for the same amino acid. **Termination codon.** One of 3 codons on mRNA which do not specify any of the amino acids involved in the protein synthesis in living cells. [code.]

coefficient (ko·e·fish·ent). 1. A factor; in mathematics, a multiplier of a function; in chemistry, the figure before the formula of a compound indicating the number of molecules of that compound taking part in a reaction. 2. Any measurement of a specific physical property of a substance, usually expressed as a ratio to a standard unit. **Absorption coefficient.** 1. A constant for radiation of a given wavelength the value of which depends on the atomic number of the material through which the radiation passes. When a beam of x-rays passes through an absorbing material its intensity is reduced according to the law, $I_x = I_o e^{-\tau x}$, where I_x is the intensity after passage through x centimetres of material, I_o is the initial intensity, and τ is the linear absorption coefficient per centimetre. 2. The intensity of a parallel beam of gamma radiation is reduced in passing through an absorber of thickness x, such that $\Delta I/I = \mu x$, where ΔI is the loss of intensity of a beam of intensity I, and μ is a constant, the linear absorption coefficient of the absorber. μ may be separated into components arising from the different methods of absorption of the incident radiation thus: $\mu = \mu_{\text{photoelectric}} + \mu_{\text{Compton scattering}} + \mu_{\text{pair production}} + \mu_{\text{nuclear absorption}}$, where the individual μs are the partial absorption coefficient of each individual process. 3. In the solution of gases in liquids, the volume of a particular gas (measured at 0°C and 101 kPa (760 mmHg) pressure) which will saturate a unit volume of solvent at a given temperature. **Biological coefficient.** The amount of energy used by the body at rest, compared with a normal body at rest. **Cubical coefficient.** *See* COEFFICIENT OF EXPANSION (below). **Coefficient of diffusion.**

$$k = -\frac{Q}{A}.\frac{dx}{dn}$$

where Q is the mass of a solute in grams carried across an area A cm² of a surface normal to the direction of a diffusion in one second, n is the concentration of the solute in g/ml at a point x cm distant from some arbitrary organ, and the ratio $-dn/dx$ is the gradient, or rate of decrease of concentration per cm in the direction of diffusion. **Distribution coefficient.** If a substance is soluble in 2 immiscible solvents, the constant ratio in which the substance distributes itself in equilibrium between the 2 solvents when the latter are shaken together. **Coefficient of electrical conductivity.** The amount of electricity in coulombs passing through a centimetre cube of a given substance when a potential difference of 1 V is applied to opposite faces of the cube. It is expressed in siemens (mhos). **Coefficient of expansion.** When the temperature of a given substance increases by 1°C, the amount by which unit length increases (linear coefficient), or the amount of increase of unit area (superficial coefficient), or the amount by which a unit volume increases (cubical coefficient). **Haemoglobin coefficient.** The amount of haemoglobin per 100 ml of blood, calculated at the rate of 14.8 g being equivalent to 100 per cent. **Internal conversion coefficient.** The ratio of the number of transitions in which internal conversion takes place to the remaining number of transitions between 2 given nuclear states. **Isometric coefficient of lactic acid.** The ratio of the total isometric tension a muscle can produce before fatigue to the milligrams of lactic acid it produces. **Linear coefficient.** *See* COEFFICIENT OF EXPANSION (above). **Olfactory coefficient.** A measurement of the strength of an odour, based on the number of cubic centimetres of air saturated with a given odour necessary for the recognition of the particular odour. **Coefficient of partage, Partition coefficient.** Distribution coefficient (see above). **Phenol coefficient.** A number which is intended to represent the ratio of bactericidal effectiveness of a substance compared to phenol as a standard. Also known as *Rideal-Walker coefficient.* **Red-blood-corpuscular coefficient.** The percentage of red corpuscles in the blood when the number enumerated is compared with the normal figure arbitrarily fixed at 5 000 000 per mm^3 being equal to 100 per cent. **Coefficient of refraction.** The ratio of refracted radiation energy to incident radiation energy. **Respiratory coefficient.** Respiratory quotient; the ratio of the volume of oxygen used and CO_2 produced by an organism or tissue. **Coefficient of solubility of a gas.** Absorption coefficient 3rd def. (see above). **Superficial coefficient.** *See* COEFFICIENT OF EXPANSION (above). **Temperature coefficient.** The ratio of the velocity of a chemical reaction at one temperature to the velocity at a higher temperature; the velocity is roughly doubled for every rise of 10°C. **Coefficient of thermal conductivity.** The amount of heat in joules (calories) passing through a metre (centimetre) cube of a given substance in 1 s when the temperature of opposite faces of the cube differs by 1°C. **Coefficient of variability.** In statistics, the standard deviation of a distribution expressed as a percentage of the mean of the distribution: it is equivalent to (standard deviation ÷ mean) × 100. In medical statistics, it adjusts the difficulties arising in the comparison of the variabilities of frequency distributions measured in different units. **Velocity coefficient.** In a chemical reaction, the time it takes for 1 g of a substance to be converted to end-products. **Viscosity coefficient.** The ratio of the shearing force per unit area, between 2 parallel layers of a liquid in motion, to the velocity gradient between the layers. It is usually symbolized by η. **Volume coefficient.** The normal corpuscular volume adjusted to a red-blood-corpuscular count of 5 000 000 per mm^3, which is 42 ml. [L *cum, efficere* to effect.]

See also: BUNSEN, RIDEAL, WALKER.

coelarium (se·la·re·um). The mesothelium (coelom epithelium). [Gk *koilos* hollow.]

coele (se·le). A ventricle of the brain. [see prec.]

co-electron (ko·el·**ek**·tron). The atomic core or atom of matter, consisting of the hydrogen nucleus with attached electron. [L *cum,* electron.]

Coelenterata (se·len·ter·a′·tah). A phylum of animals composed of only 2 cell layers and having a central cavity with 1 aperture. It contains, amongst others, jellyfish and sea anemones, which have numerous unicellular stinging organs capable of causing much pain and toxic rash. [see foll.]

coelenteron (se·**len**·ter·on). Archenteron; in zoology, the primitive cavity which forms at the conversion of an ovum into a gastrula, and from which the alimentary canal develops. [Gk *koilos* hollow, *enteron* intestine.]

coeliac (se·le·ak). Referring or relating to the abdomen. **Coeliac lymph gland.** *See* GLAND. **Coeliac plexus.** *See* PLEXUS. [Gk *koilos* hollow.]

coeliac artery [truncus celiacus (NA)]. A short thick trunk arising from the front of the abdominal aorta just below the aortic opening in the diaphragm. It divides into the left gastric, hepatic and splenic arteries.

coeliadelphus (se·le·ad·**el**′·fus). Coelio-adelphus.

coelialgia (se·le·**al**·je·ah). Abdominal pain; colic. [Gk *koilos* hollow, *algos* pain.]

coeliectasia (se·le·ek·**ta**′·ze·ah). A distended condition of the abdomen. [Gk *koilos* hollow, *ektasis* a stretching.]

coeliectomy (se·le·**ek**·to·me). 1. Removal by means of operation of any organ within the abdomen. 2. The relief of essential hypertension by surgical removal of the coeliac branches of the vagus nerve. [Gk *koilos* hollow, *ektome* a cutting out.]

coelitis (se·le·i·tis). Inflammation of the abdominal viscera. [Gk *koilos* hollow, *-itis* inflammation.]

coelio-adelphus (se·le·o·ad·**el**′·fus). A twin monstrosity the 2 bodies of which are united at the abdomen. [Gk *koilos* hollow, *adelphos* brother.]

coeliocele (se·le·o·seel). Abdominal hernia. *See* HERNIA. [Gk *koilos* hollow, *kele* hernia.]

coeliocentesis (se·le·o·sen·**te**′·sis). Surgical puncture of the abdomen. [Gk *koilos* hollow, *kentesis* a pricking.]

coeliocolpotomy (se·le·o·kol·**pot**′·o·me). Coeliotomy in which the vaginal route is taken. [Gk *koilos* hollow, colpotomy.]

coeliocyesis (se·le·o·si·**e**′·sis). Abdominal pregnancy. *See* PREGNANCY. [Gk *koilos* hollow, *kysis* pregnancy.]

coeliodynia (se·le·o·**din**′·e·ah). Coelialgia; abdominal pain; colic. [Gk *koilos* hollow, *odyne* pain.]

coelio-elytrotomy (se·le·o·el·it·**rot**′·o·me). Vaginal coeliotomy. *See* COELIOTOMY. [Gk *koilos* hollow, elytrotomy.]

coelio-enterotomy (se·le·o·en·ter·**ot**′·o·me). The operation of making an opening into the intestine through an incision in the abdominal wall. [Gk *koilos* hollow, enterotomy.]

coeliogastrotomy (se·le·o·gas·**trot**′·o·me]. Surgical incision of the stomach by means of abdominal section. [Gk *koilos* hollow, gastrotomy.]

coeliohysterectomy (se·le·o·his·ter·**ek**′·to·me). Caesarean section. *See* SECTION. [Gk *koilos* hollow, hysterectomy.]

coeliohystero-oöthecectomy (se·le·o·**his**·ter·o·o·o·the·**sek**′·to·me). Removal of the uterus and ovaries through an abdominal incision. [Gk *koilos* hollow, hystero-oöthecectomy.]

coeliohysterosalpingo-oöthecectomy (se·le·o·**his**·ter·o·**sal**·ping·go·o·o·the·**sek**′·to·me). Removal of the uterus, ovaries and uterine tubes through an abdominal incision. [Gk *koilos* hollow, hysterosalpingo-oöthecectomy.]

coeliohysterotomy (se·le·o·his·ter·**ot**′·o·me). 1. Caesarean section. *See* SECTION. 2. The operation of opening up the uterus through an abdominal incision. [Gk *koilos* hollow, hysterotomy.]

coeliolymph (se·le·o·limf). The cerebrospinal fluid. *See* FLUID. [Gk *koilos* hollow, L *lympha* water.]

coelioma (se·le·**o**·mah). An abdominal tumour. [Gk *koilos* hollow, *-oma* tumour.]

coeliomyalgia (se·le·o·mi·**al**′·je·ah). Pain affecting the muscles of the abdomen. [Gk *koilos* hollow, myalgia.]

coeliomyitis (se·le·o·mi·i′·tis). Coeliomyositis.

coeliomyodynia (se·le·o·mi·o·**din**′·e·ah). Coeliomyalgia. [Gk *koilos* hollow, myodynia.]

coeliomyomectomy, coeliomyomyotomy (se·le·o·mi·o·**mek**′·to·me, se·le·o·mi·o·mi·**ot**′·o·me). Removal of a uterine myoma through an abdominal incision. [Gk *koilos* hollow, myomectomy.]

coeliomyositis (se·le·o·mi·o·**si**′·tis). An inflamed condition of the abdominal muscles. [Gk *koilos* hollow, myositis.]

coelioncus (se·le·**ong**·kus). An abdominal tumour. [Gk *koilos* hollow, *ogkos* a swelling.]

coelioparacentesis (se·le·o·**par**·ah·sen·**te**′·sis). Abdominocentesis; puncture of the abdominal cavity, for diagnostic or therapeutic purposes. [Gk *koilos* hollow, paracentesis.]

coeliopathy (se·le·**op**·ath·e). Any disease of the abdomen. [Gk *koilos* hollow, *pathos* suffering.]

coeliophyma (se·le·o·**fi**′·mah). Coelioncus. [Gk *koilos* hollow, *phyma* a growth.]

coelioplegia (se·le·o·**ple**′·je·ah). An obsolete name for Asiatic cholera. [Gk *koilos* hollow, *plege* stroke.]

coeliopyosis (se·le·o·pi·**o**′·sis). A condition in which there is formation of pus in the abdominal cavity, as in purulent peritonitis. [Gk *koilos* hollow, pyosis.]

coeliorrhaphy (se·le·**or**·af·e). The suturing of a wound in the wall of the abdomen. [Gk *koilos* hollow, *rhaphe* suture.]

coeliosalpingectomy (**se**·le·o·sal·pin·**jek'**·to·me). The removal of a uterine tube through an abdominal incision. [Gk *koilos* hollow, salpingectomy.]

coeliosalpingo-oöthecectomy (se·le·o·**sal**·ping·go·**o**·o·the·**sek'**·to·me). Removal of the uterine tube and the ovary through an abdominal incision. [Gk *koilos* hollow, salpingo-oöthecectomy.]

coeliosalpingotomy (se·le·o·sal·ping·**got'**·o·me). Coeliosalpingectomy.

coelioschisis (se·le·**os**·kis·is). Congenital fissure of the abdominal wall, the cavity being open. [Gk *koilos* hollow, *schisis* a division.]

coelioscope (**se**·le·o·skope). An instrument with which a body cavity can be illuminated and examined. [see foll.]

coelioscopy (se·le·**os**·ko·pe). A method of examining the peritoneal cavity by inflating it with sterile air passed in through a hollow needle and inserting a cystoscope through a trocar into the space. [Gk *koilos* hollow, *skopein* to watch.]

coeliothelioma (**se**·le·o·the·le·**o'**·mah). Coelothelioma.

coeliotomy (se·le·**ot**·o·me). The operation of incising the abdomen. **Vaginal coeliotomy.** Incision of the vagina in order to gain access to the abdominal cavity. **Ventral coeliotomy.** Incision of the abdominal wall in order to gain access to the abdominal cavity. [Gk *koilos* hollow, *temnein* to cut.]

coelitis (se·**li**·tis). Any condition of inflammation affecting the abdomen. [Gk *koilos* hollow, *-itis* inflammation.]

coelom, coeloma (**se**·lom, se·**lo**·mah). The true body-cavity of the embryo. In mammals it divides into 2 main parts, the thorax and the abdomen. [Gk *koiloma* hollow.]

coelomic (se·**lo**·mik). Referring to the coelom.

coelonychia (se·lon·**ik**·e·ah). Koilonychia.

Coelopa (se·**lo**·pah). A genus of Diptera. The larvae feed on decayed seaweeds, and adults become a non-biting nuisance on beaches. There are records of outbreaks in dry-cleaning establishments in London. *Coelopa frigida* and *C. pilipes* are the important species.

coelophlebitis (**se**·lo·fle·**bi'**·tis). Inflammation of the vena cava. [Gk *koilos* hollow, *phlebe* vein, *-itis* inflammation.]

coeloschisis (se·**los**·kis·is). Coelioschisis.

coeloscope (**se**·lo·skope). Coelioscope.

coeloscopy (se·**los**·ko·pe). Coelioscopy.

coelosoma (se·lo·**so**·mah). A class of monster characterized by eventration through a body cleft, which may be extensive. In addition there is marked abnormality of the extremities, in the intestinal tract and the genito-urinary apparatus, often so great in degree that the whole trunk is involved. [Gk *koilos* hollow, *soma* body.]

coelothel (**se**·lo·thel). In embryology, the mesoderm which lines the coelom. [Gk *koilos* hollow, *thele* nipple.]

coelothelioma (**se**·lo·the·le·**o'**·mah). Mesothelioma; a tumour composed of mesothelial cells. [Gk *koilos* hollow, *thele* nipple, *-oma* tumour.]

coelothelium (se·lo·**the**·le·um). Mesothelium; the layer of flat multiform cells developed from the mesoderm which forms the internal covering of the coelum in the embryo. In adult life this layer makes up the squamous-celled stratum of the epithelium which lines the serous cavities of the body. [Gk *koilos* hollow, *thele* nipple.]

coelozoic (se·lo·**zo**·ik). Denoting extracellular parasitic protozoa which are present in the internal body cavities. [Gk *koilos* hollow, *zoon* animal.]

coenadelphus (se·nad·**el**·fus). 1. A twin monster of which both individuals are equally developed. 2. A twin monster the 2 parts of which have a common vital organ or organs. [Gk *koinos* common, *adelphos* brother.]

coenaesthesia (se·nes·**the**·ze·ah). The normal undifferentiated conscious state of awareness of being alive and of general organic sensation; vital sense. The state comprises the ordinary rise and fall of spirits, including normal mental function, within physiological limits. [Gk *koinos* common, aesthesia.]

coenaesthesic (se·nes·**the**·zik). Referring or belonging to coenaesthesia.

coenaesthesiopathy (**se**·nes·the·ze·**op'**·ath·e). Any disorder or disturbance of the state of coenaesthesia. [coenaesthesia, Gk *pathos* suffering.]

coenaesthetic (se·nes·**thet**·ik). Coenaesthesic.

coenaesthopathia (**se**·nes·tho·**path'**·e·ah). A state of morbid perversion of general consciousness. [Gk *koinos* common, aesthesia, Gk *pathos* suffering.]

coenobium (se·**no**·be·um). A cluster of independent cells or unicellular organisms held within a common envelope. [Gk *koinos* common, *bion* a living thing.]

coenocyte (**se**·no·site). 1. A multinucleate mass of protoplasm usually filamentous and without cell walls; syncytium. 2. The term applied to the multinucleated unicellular filaments of some algae. [Gk *koinos* common, *kytos* cell.]

coenotype (**se**·no·tipe). Prototype; the primary or original form from which all other types or forms have arisen. [Gk *koinos* common, type.]

coenurosis (se·newr·**o**·sis). Infection with so-called *Coenurus cerebralis*, the larva of the tapeworm *Multiceps multiceps*, rare in man but relatively common in sheep, in which the disease is known as "staggers". In man, the larvae may develop within the cerebral ventricles causing internal hydrocephalus. [*Coenurus*, Gk *-osis* condition.]

Coenurus (se·**newr**·us). A larval form of tapeworms in which there is more than one invaginated scolex and a large cyst: it is characteristic of the genus *Multiceps*. Coenuri of several species have occasionally been found in human muscle. **Coenurus cerebralis.** The larva of *Multiceps multiceps*, normal to sheep, which has been recorded from the human brain. [Gk *koinos* common, *oura* tail.]

co-enzyme (ko·**en**·zime). Properly the non-protein component which, with the apoenzyme, forms the active holoenzyme. Frequently covalently linked to the protein, it functions as a carrier from substrate to acceptor. **Coenzyme I.** Nicotinamide adenine dinucleotide. **Coenzyme II.** Nicotinamide adenine dinucleotide phosphate. **Coenzyme** A (CoA). An important metabolite, not a true coenzyme. It is involved in the citric acid cycle, fatty acid and amino acid metabolism, both free and combined as, for example, acetyl CoA. **Coenzyme F.** Tetrahydrofolic acid. *See* ACID. **Methylmalonyl coenzyme A.** An intermediate in the conversion of propionyl coenzyme A to succinyl coenzyme A. The metabolism of methylmalonyl CoA utilizes vitamin B_{12}. **Coenzyme Q.** An intermediate in the electron transport chain of mitochondria, its locus being between cytochromes b and c. Structurally similar to vitamin K, it is synthesized by condensation of isoprenoid units ultimately derived from acetyl CoA. **Co-enzyme R.** Biotin; vitamin H. [L *cum*, enzyme.]

coercible (ko·**er**·sibl). Describing any gas that may be liquefied by ordinary means. [see foll.]

coercive (ko·**er**·siv). Capable of being rendered magnetic and of thereafter resisting demagnetization. [L *coercere* to shut up.]

coetaneous (ko·e·**ta**·ne·us). 1. Belonging to the same period. 2. Of the same age. [L *cum*, *aetas* age.]

coeur en sabot (ker on sab·**o**). The name given to the shadow, shaped like a boot, which is observable in x-ray examination of the heart in the tetralogy of Fallot. [Fr.]

co-excitation (**ko**·ex·si·**ta'**·shun). Excitation occurring simultaneously with other phenomena. [L *cum*, excitation.]

co-ferment (ko·**fer**·ment). Any substance which acts as an auxiliary to an enzyme or ferment. Cf. CO-ENZYME. [L *cum*, ferment.]

Coffea (**kof**·e·ah). A genus of plants of the family Rubiaceae. The kernel of the dried ripe seeds of *Coffea arabica* Linn., *C. liberica* Bull. ex Hiern, *C. robusta* Linden, and other species, is used to make coffee, the seed coat being almost completely removed from the seed and the remainder roasted until it acquires a deep brown colour and characteristic odour. [see foll.]

coffee (kof·e). **Prepared Coffee BPC 1968.** The kernel of the dried ripe seed of various plants of the genus *Coffea,* roasted until deep brown in colour, a process which imparts flavour, and then ground. The infusion, taken as a beverage, contains caffeine (1 per cent), to which its stimulant effect is due. [Ar. *qahweh.*]

coffeinism (**kof**·e·in·izm). The state of morbid ill-health resulting from excessive coffee drinking.

Coffeinum (kof·**e**·in·um). *European Pharmacopoeia* name for Caffeine BP 1973. **Coffeinum Monohydricum.** *European Pharmacopoeia* name for Caffeine Hydrate BP 1973.

coffeol (**kof**·e·ol). Caffeol, $C_8H_{10}O_2$. An oil developed in coffee during the process of roasting and responsible for the characteristic odour.

Coffey, Robert Calvin (b.1869). Portland, Oregon, surgeon.

Coffey's operation. Transplantation of the ureters into the colon.

Coffey, Walter Bernard (b.1868). San Francisco surgeon.

Coffey–Humber treatment. The treatment of cancer by injections of an extract of the suprarenal cortex of sheep.

Cogan's disease. A non-syphilitic disease in young adults of rapid onset, characterized by labyrinthine involvement and interstitial keratitis. The onset is accompanied by tinnitus, vertigo and rapidly progressing deafness, which usually become complete and permanent. The speedy development of auditory impairment, the severity of the vertigo, the characteristic daily fluctuation in the ocular appearances, and the negative serological tests, distinguish this disease from the interstitial keratitis and perceptive deafness associated with congenital syphilis.

Coggins' stethoscope test. For simulated unilateral deafness: one ear-piece of a stethoscope is occluded with wax. Both ear-pieces are inserted into the patient's ears; the examiner stands behind the patient and speaks through the chest-piece. With the occluded ear-piece in his deaf ear, the patient should hear well. When this is reversed, if hearing still remains satisfactory, the patient is probably malingering.

cognac (**ko**·nyak). Brandy; the name usually applied to the wine produced in the Charente valley in France and particularly in Cognac. [Fr. *Cognac,* a town in France.]

cognition (kog·**nish**·un). A psychological term for that activity of the mind by which one "knows" things, i.e. the means by which one is aware of the processes of thinking and perceiving. The faculties of understanding and reasoning are included in the term. [L *cognoscere* to know.]

cognominal (kog·**nom**·in·al). Descriptive of a word derived from a surname, e.g. angstrom, curie, mackintosh. [L *cognomen* name.]

cohabitation (ko·hab·it·**a'**·shun). Living together as man and wife. [L *cum, habitare* to dwell.]

Cohen, Harold H. Chicago biochemist.

Falls, Freda and Cohen test. For pregnancy; an intradermal injection of colostrum is given and no reaction occurs if the patient is pregnant. Reactions were obtained in 96 per cent of non-pregnant patients. It requires further investigation before being accepted, as other workers have not reported such remarkable results.

cohesion (ko·**he**·zhun). 1. In physics, the attractive force which aggregates and holds together the molecules of a substance throughout the mass. 2. In botany, the union of similar parts. [L *cohaerere* to stick together.]

cohesive (ko·**he**·ziv). Sticking together or producing cohesion.

Cohnheim, Julius Friedrich (b.1839). German experimental pathologist.

Cohnheim's area, or field. An aggregation of myofibrils packed closely with little sarcoplasm intervening, seen in transverse sections of a striated muscle fibre.

Cohnheim's arteries. End-arteries to the basal ganglia of the cerebrum.

Cohnheim's frog. A frog in which physiological saline solution is substituted for blood.

Cohnheim rest, or tumour germs. Embryonal rest, epithelial rest, fetal rest; a minute collection of cells, embryonic or partly differentiated, which persists from the early stages of development of the human being throughout life in a dormant state, but sometimes assuming the features of growing tissue and even becoming malignant.

Cohnheim's theory. 1. Inflammatory processes are essentially associated with leucocyte emigration. 2. Tumours arise from embryonic rests in normal tissue.

Cohnistreptothrix israeli (ko·ne·**strep**·to·thrix iz·**ra**·li). *Actinomyces israeli,* which is probably identical with *A. bovis.*

cohobation (ko·ho·**ba**·shun). 1. Repeated distillation by pouring the liquor back upon the residue in the vessel in order to increase its purity. 2. A term signifying that the symptoms of a disease have returned. [L *cohobare* to redistil.]

cohort (**ko**·hort). A group of individuals, identified by a common characteristic (often year of birth), who are studied over a period of time. [L *cohortem* large group.]

cohosh (**ko**·hosh). Name given to several medicinal plants. **Black cohosh.** Cimicifuga. **Blue cohosh.** *Caulophyllum thalictroides.* **Red cohosh.** Baneberry. **White cohosh.** *Actea alba.* [Algonquin name.]

coil (koil). 1. An arrangement of wire, rope, tubing or spring, in spirals, loops or concentric circles. 2. A contraceptive device. A flexible loop introduced into the vagina. **Choke coil.** A coil of wire wound on a former, with or without an iron core, and introduced into a circuit to control an alternating or high-frequency electric current by its inductance. **Induction coil.** An electrical apparatus for producing high-voltage discharges, consisting of a coil of wire (primary) wound on a laminated iron core, upon which is wound in turn an independent coil of fine wire (secondary); rapid interruption of the current in the primary coil induces high-voltage current in the secondary. **Primary coil.** The primary winding of an induction coil. **Resistance coil.** A coil of standardized electrical resistance against which the resistance of a given object may be measured on a Wheatstone bridge. **Secondary coil.** The secondary winding of an induction coil. **Spark coil.** Induction coil (see above). [L *colligere* to bind.]

See also: LEITER, RUHMKORFF.

coilonychia (koi·lon·**ik**·e·ah). Koilonychia; a condition in which the edges of the nail at the sides are raised and there is a depression in the centre of the nail. [Gk *koilos* hollow, *onyx* nail.]

coin-catcher (**koin**·kach·er). An instrument with which a foreign body such as a coin can be seized and removed from the oesophagus. [Fr. *coin* wedge, OFr. *cachier.*]

co-indication (ko·in·de·ka'·shun). 1. One of several signs suggesting the same fact. 2. Confirmatory indication. [L *cum,* indication.]

Coiter, Volcher (b.1534). Bologna/Nuremberg anatomist.

Coiter's muscle. The corrugator muscle of the forehead formed by the medial part of the orbicularis oculi muscle.

coition (ko·**ish**·un). Coitus. [L *coire* to come together.]

coitophobia (**ko**·it·o·**fo'**·be·ah). Morbid dread of or aversion from coitus. [coitus, phobia.]

coitus (**ko**·it·us). Sexual union. **Coitus incompletus, Coitus interruptus.** Coitus in which the male organ is withdrawn from the vagina before ejaculation takes place. **Coitus reservatus.** Sexual intercourse in which the male withholds his orgasm until the female climax or as a means of contraception, or sometimes as a morbid condition associated with inability to ejaculate. **Coitus à la vache.** Coitus from behind with the female partner in the knee–chest position. [L *coire* to come together.]

coko (**ko**·ko). The Fijian name for framboesia or yaws.

cola seeds (**ko**·lah seedz). Kola BPC 1949.

colalgia (ko·**lal**·je·ah). Colic. [colon, Gk *algos* pain.]

colamine (**ko**·lam·een). $NH_2CH_2CH_2OH$, a compound related to the cholines and occurring in cephalin.

Colaspase (kol·**asp**·ase). BP Commission approved name for L-asparagine amidohydrolase obtained from cultures of *Escherichia coli.*

colatein (ko·lah·te·in). A phenolic derivative of kola nut, identified with D-catechol and L-epicatechol.

colation (ko·**la**·shun). The process or act of filtering or straining. [L *colare* to strain.]

colatorium (ko·lah·**to**·re·um). 1. In pharmacy, a sieve, strainer or colander. 2. The hypophysis cerebri. [L *colare* to strain.]

colature (**ko**·lah·tewr). In pharmacy, liquid which has been obtained by filtration or straining of a fluid. [see prec.]

colauxe (ko·**lawx**·e). Colectasia. [colon, Gk *auxe* increase.]

colchiceine (kol·chis·e·een). Acetyltrimethylcolchicinic acid, $C_{21}H_{23}O_6N$. An alkaloid derived from colchicine and less active than the latter.

Colchicine BP 1973 (**kol**·chis·een). $C_{22}H_{25}O_6N$, an alkaloid derived from the autumn crocus and other species of *Colchicum;* a pale-yellow crystalline substance with a bitter taste, soluble in water, alcohol or chloroform. It stimulates smooth muscle, especially that of the alimentary canal, but causing gastro-enteritis, sometimes of a severe nature. It has been found effective in the relief of pain in acute gout, for reasons which are not clear. The alkaloid is unique in its effect on mitosis: it inhibits the formation of the spindle and arrests division in the metaphase; the reversion of the nucleus to the resting state produces polyploidy. This phenomenon has been used in the breeding of giant plants and animals, but the arrest of cell division has proved non-specific for tumours and has no significant clinical applications as yet.

Colchicum (**kol**·chik·um, **kol**·kik·um). 1. A genus of plants of the family Liliaceae. 2. The dried corm of the meadow saffron, *Colchicum autumnale.* **Colchicum autumnale.** Meadow saffron; the corm (BP 1973) contains the alkaloid cochicine, and is used to relieve the pain and inflammation of acute gout. **Colchicum seed.** The dried ripe seed of *Colchicum autumnale;* it has a similar action to that of the corm. [Gk *kolchikon.*]

cold (**ko**·ld). 1. Deficient in heat; a person may be said to be cold when he is subject to an environmental temperature that is below comfort, so that the surface of the body is below 37°C (98.6°F) and the body mechanism for preserving body heat comes into action, viz. constriction of the peripheral arterioles and shivering. It may be fatal in small babies, rectal temperature falling below 32°C (90°F); rapid re-warming is dangerous. 2. A general term for coryza and other mild disorders of the respiratory system caused by a filtrable virus and often attributed to exposure of the individual to low temperature and damp. **Allergic cold.** The form of allergic paroxysmal rhinorrhoea known as hay fever. **Cold on the chest.** Acute tracheitis and/or bronchitis. **Common cold.** *See* MAIN DEF. 2 (above). **June cold.** Paroxysmal rhinorrhoea caused by allergy to the pollen of ripening grasses. **Rose cold.** Paroxysmal rhinorrhoea caused by allergy to rose pollen. **Cold sore.** *See* SORE. **Strangers' cold.** A term used in the Hebrides for a form of influenzal catarrh which is attributed by the islanders to infection brought in by visitors. [AS *kald.*]

Cole, Sydney William (b.1877). Cambridge biochemist.

Cole's test. For lactose in urine: shake 25 ml of urine with 1 g of activated charcoal, boil briefly, cool thoroughly and shake occasionally during 10 min. Filter, transfer the charcoal to a dish containing 10 ml of 10 per cent acetic acid. Heat to boiling, filter into a test-tube containing 0.1 g phenylhydrazine hydrochloride and 0.2 g sodium acetate. Heat the tube in boiling water for about 45 min, allow to cool slowly and examine for hedgehog crystals of lactosazone under the microscope.

Hopkins-Cole test. For tryptophan or proteins containing tryptophan: a glyoxylic acid reagent is prepared by adding 4 g of magnesium powder slowly to 100 ml of saturated oxalic-acid solution. When the reaction is complete, the solution is filtered and diluted to 400 ml with water. To 3 ml of test solution add 2 ml of reagent and layer with 3 ml of concentrated sulphuric acid. If tryptophan is present, a deep purple ring forms at the junction of the liquids.

Cole, Warren Henry. Chicago surgeon.

Graham-Cole test. Cholecystography.

colectasia (ko·lek·**ta**·ze·ah). Dilatation or distension of the colon. [colon, Gk *ektasis* a stretching.]

colectomy (ko·**lek**·to·me). Resection of the colon. **Complete colectomy, Total colectomy.** Surgical removal of the entire colon. [colon, Gk *ektome* a cutting out.]

coleitis (ko·le·**i**·tis). Vaginitis. [Gk *koleos* sheath, *-itis* inflammation.]

Coleman, Warren (b.1869). New York physician.

Coleman's diet. A high-calorie diet used in the treatment of a patient with typhoid fever.

coleocele (**ko**·le·o·seel). Colpocele; hernia into the vagina. [Gk *koleos* sheath, *kele* hernia.]

coleocystitis (**ko**·le·o·sis·**ti'**·tis). Colpocystitis. [Gk *koleos* sheath, cystitis.]

Coleoptera (ko·le·**op**·ter·ah). The beetles; an order of insects in which the front pair of wings is modified to form sclerotized covers over the hind pair. They are of medical importance as causative agents of canthariasis, and as producers of cantharidin or similar vesicants which may cause blisters on handling living insects. Of the former, the scarab genera *Caccobius* and *Onthophaga* are important, and of the latter, the genera *Lytta* and *Paederus.* Beetles which are intermediate hosts of human parasites comprise *Blaps, Calandra, Dermestes* and *Tenebrio.* [Gk *koleos* sheath, *pteron* wing.]

coleoptosis (**ko**·le·op·**to'**·sis). Coloptosis.

coleospastia (**ko**·le·o·**spas'**·te·ah). Colpospasm; vaginismus. [Gk *koleos* sheath, *spastia* spasm.]

coleotomy (ko·le·**ot**·o·me). Colpotomy. [Gk *koleos* sheath, *temnein* to cut.]

coles (**ko**·leez). The penis. **Coles femininus.** The clitoris. [L.]

Coleus aromaticus (**ko**·le·us ar·o·**mat**·ik·us). A common plant of Bengal, the juice from the leaves of which is reputed to control the diarrhoea in cholera and thereby to obviate intravenous saline therapy. [Gk *koleos* sheath, *aromatikos* fragrant.]

Coley, William Bradley (b.1862). New York surgeon.

Coley's fluid, or mixture. A preparation made by growing virulent streptococci in bouillon for 10 days; the culture is sterilized by heat, and mixed with a 10-day growth of *Chromobacterium (Bacillus) prodigiosum.* It is then incubated for a further 10 days, and again sterilized by heat. It can contain killed bacilli, or it can be filtered and contain only the toxin. It was a reputed cure for malignant disease, especially sarcomata, and was injected directly into the tumour if possible, otherwise intramuscularly.

Coley's toxin. The unfiltered culture of the streptococci and *Serratia marcescens* which has been used to treat inoperable neoplasms.

colibacillaemia (**ko**·li·bas·il·**e'**·me·ah). The condition in which *Bacterium (Bacillus) coli* is present in the blood. [colibacillus, Gk *haima* blood.]

colibacillary (ko·li·**bas**·il·ar·e). Relating to or caused by *Bacterium (Bacillus) coli.*

colibacillosis (**ko**·li·bas·il·**o'**·sis). The pathological condition resulting from infection by *Bacterium (Bacillus) coli.* [colibacillus, Gk *-osis* condition.]

colibacilluria (**ko**·li·bas·il·**ewr'**·e·ah). Infection of urine by the micro-organism *Bacterium (Bacillus) coli.*

colibacillus (**ko**·li·bas·**il'**·us). A term formerly used as a synonym for certain genera within the family Enterobacteriaceae, e.g. *Escherichia, Klebsiella.* [Gk *kolon* colon, L *bacillum* a small rod, staff or stick.]

colic (**kol**·ik). A severe spasmodic griping pain which increases in intensity to a climax then remits for a short period and returns with equal intensity. It differs from a severe continuous pain in which the intensity remains constant. **Appendicular colic.** A colicky pain arising in the appendix. **Biliary colic.** That due to the passage of a gall-stone in the bile duct. **Bilious colic.** Abdominal colic with vomiting of bile and the passage of bile in the stools. **Copper colic.** Colic occurring rarely among workers in copper and its compounds. **Crapulent colic, Crapulous colic.** That caused by the impaction of a bolus of food in the bowels. **Cystic colic.** Colicky pain produced in the bladder. **Devonshire colic.** Lead colic, from the lead pipes of cider presses. **Flatulent colic.** Pain due to flatulent distension of the bowels. **Gall-stone colic.** That due to the passage of a gall-stone. **Gastric colic.** Gastralgia. **Haemorrhoidal colic.** Spasmodic pain due to piles. **Hepatic colic.** Biliary colic (see above). **Herniary colic.** Pain due to a strangulated hernia. **Hill colic.** Hill diarrhoea. *See* DIARRHOEA. **Inflammatory colic.** The pain of gastro-enteritis. **Intestinal colic.** Spasmodic pain in intestinal disorders. **Lead colic.** The most frequent symptom in lead poisoning. **Meconial colic.** The colic of newborn infants; a term that is little used now. **Menstrual colic.** Abdominal pain occurring just before or during the menses; dysmenorrhoea. **Mucous colic.** The pain of mucomembranous colitis. **Nephritic colic.** That due to a renal calculus. **Painters' colic.** Lead colic (see above). **Pancreatic colic.** Pain produced by obstruction of the pancreatic duct. **Poitou colic.** Colica pictonum; lead colic (see above). **Pseudomembranous colic.** Mucous colic (see above). **Renal colic.** Pain produced by a renal calculus in the ureter. **Sabural colic.** The pain of enteritis. **Salivary colic.** Pain due to a salivary calculus. **Saturnine colic.** Lead colic (see above). **Stercoral colic.** That due to faecal impaction. **Tubal colic.** The severe pain caused by contraction of the fallopian tube in cases of tubal pregnancy. **Ureteral colic.** That due to the passage of a renal calculus in the ureter. **Uterine colic.** Pain of a spasmodic nature originating from the uterus, as in extrusion of a fibroid polyp or in spasmodic dysmenorrhoea. **Vermicular colic.** Appendicular colic (see above). **Verminous colic.** Intestinal pain caused by parasitic worms. **Wind colic.** Flatulent colic (see above). **Worm colic.** Verminous colic (see above). **Zinc colic.** Lead colic in zinc workers, due to lead as impurity in crude zinc. [Gk *kolikos* pain in the colon.]

colic arteries. Inferior left colic artery [arteria sigmoideae (NA)]. *See* MESENTERIC ARTERY, INFERIOR. **Middle colic artery [arteria colica media (NA)].** *See* MESENTERIC ARTERY, SUPERIOR. **Right colic artery [arteria colica dextra (NA)].** *See* MESENTERIC ARTERY, SUPERIOR. **Superior left colic artery [arteria colica sinistra (NA)].** *See* MESENTERIC ARTERY, INFERIOR.

colic veins. Inferior left colic veins [venae sigmoideae (NA)]. Tributaries of the inferior mesenteric vein, draining the pelvic colon. **Middle colic vein [vena colica media (NA)].** A tributary of the superior mesenteric vein. It accompanies the correspondingly named artery, and drains the transverse colon. **Right colic vein [vena colica dextra (NA)].** A tributary of the superior mesenteric vein from the ascending colon and hepatic flexure of the colon. **Superior left colic vein [vena colica sinistra (NA)].** A tributary of the inferior mesenteric vein, draining the left colic flexure (splenic flexure) and descending colon.

colica (kol·ik·ah). Colic. **Colica mucosa.** Mucous colitis. *See* COLITIS. **Colica passio.** Colic. **Colica pictonum.** Lead colic. *See* COLIC. **Colica scortorum.** The severe colicky pain accompanying inflammation of the uterine tubes. [L colic.]

colicin (ko·le·seen). A term first used for antibiotic-like substances produced by coliform bacilli and later applied to other genera within the family Enterobacteriaceae, e.g. *Shigella sonnei* (*see* BACTERIOCINE). [*Bacterium coli,* L *caedere* to kill.]

colicinogeny (ko·le·sin·**oj**′·en·e). The inheritable ability to produce colicin. [colicin, Gk *genein* to produce.]

colicodynia (ko·lik·o·**din**′·e·ah). Pain localized to the region of the colon. [colon, Gk *odyne* pain.]

colicolitis (ko·le·kol·i′·tis). Colitis as a result of infection by *Bacterium coli.*

colicoplegia (ko·lik·o·**ple**′·je·ah). Colic and paralysis resulting from poisoning by lead. [colic, Gk *plege* stroke.]

colicystitis (ko·le·sis·**ti**′·tis). Cystitis caused by coliform bacillus infection.

colicystopyelitis (ko·le·sis·to·pi·el·i′·tis). Inflammation of the urinary bladder and the ureteric (renal) pelvis resulting from coliform bacillus infection. [colicystitis, pyelitis.]

coliform (ko·le·form). 1. Having resemblance to *Bacterium coli.* 2. Cribriform. [*Bacterium coli,* form.]

coli-lisbonne (ko·li·liz·bon). A lysogenic strain of *Bacterium coli.*

colinearity (ko·lin·e·**ar**′·it·e). In molecular biology, connoting the fact that the sequence of nucleotide bases, in DNA or RNA polynucleotides, codes for, or is colinear with, the sequence of amino acids in derivative protein. [L *cum, linea* line.]

colinephritis (ko·le·nef·**ri**′·tis). Nephritis caused by coliform bacillus infection.

coliplication (ko·le·plik·**a**′·shun). Coloplication.

colipuncture (ko·le·pungk·tcher). Colocentesis. [colon, L *pungere* to prick.]

colipyelitis (ko·le·pi·el·**i**′·tis). Pyelitis resulting from infection by *Bacterium coli.*

colipyuria (ko·le·pi·**ewr**′·e·ah). A condition in which pus is present in the urine because of infection by *Bacterium coli.* [*Bacterium coli,* pyuria.]

colisepsis (ko·le·**sep**·sis). Infection by *Bacterium coli.* [*Bacterium coli,* sepsis.]

Colistin (ko·**lis**·tin). BP Commission approved name for a mixture of polypeptides produced by strains of *Bacillus polymyxa* var. *colistinus.* **Colistin Sulphate BP 1973.** The sulphate of colistin; an antibiotic with therapeutic applications similar to those of polymyxin B. **Colistin Sulphomethate Sodium BP 1973.** A compound derived from colistin sulphate with similar actions and uses, but it is suitable for intramuscular injection.

colitis (kol·i·tis). Inflammation of the colon. **Amoebic colitis.** Infection of the colon by the protozoon *Entamoeba histolytica;* amoebic dysentery. **Balantidial colitis.** Infection of the colon by the protozoon *Balantidium coli.* **Catarrhal colitis.** A catarrhal reaction of the colon resulting from over-use of purgatives and other medicaments or from other irritants, or from infections with pathogens, usually by extension from other parts of the intestinal tract. **Croupous colitis, Desquamative colitis, Diphtheroid colitis, Follicular colitis.** Terms used for the colitis that occurs as a secondary process in certain severe diseases, such as uraemia, cancer, etc. It begins as a follicular enteritis affecting the solitary glands, a diphtheroid membrane forms and there may be superficial or deep necrosis. It is part of a general enterocolitis. **Colitis gravis.** Ulcerative colitis (see below). **Ischaemic colitis.** Mesenteric artery occlusion causing ulceration of a part of the colon, usually at the splenic flexure, with symptoms of pain, obstruction and bleeding; it is often fatal. **Membranous colitis, Mucomembranous colitis, Myxomembranous colitis.** This condition is not usually recognized today; it is now considered to be a neuromuscular disorder of the colon, largely functional in origin, but aggravated by irritating purgatives and unsuitable food. **Mucous colitis.** Irritable bowel syndrome. *See* SYNDROME. **Colitis polyposa.** A sequel to inflammation of the mucous coat of the colon in which swelling of the mucosa goes on to the formation of innumerable polypi. It may follow ulcerative colitis. **Regional colitis.** Granulomatous inflammation of the colon, usually on the right side, as a manifestation of Crohn's disease. **Spastic colitis.** Irritable colon. *See* COLON. **Ulcerative colitis.** A severe ulcerative inflammation of the colon characterized by fever, anaemia and the passage of blood, mucus and pus from the bowels; there is often a psychosomatic basis. [colon, Gk *-itis* inflammation.]

colitoxaemia (ko·li·tox·**e**′·me·ah). Colibacillaemia. [*Bacterium coli,* toxaemia.]

colitoxicosis (ko·li·tox·e·**ko**′·sis). Colibacillosis. [*Bacterium coli,* toxicosis.]

colitoxin (ko·li·**tox**·in). The poisonous substance in *Bacterium coli* which is the cause of colibacillosis. [*Bacterium coli,* toxin.]

coliuria (ko·li·**ewr**·e·ah). Colibacilluria.

collacin (**kol**·as·in). Collastin.

collaemia (kol·e·me·ah). A condition in which the blood is glutinous or viscid as a result of the presence of colloid deposits or urates. [Gk *kolla* glue, *haima* blood.]

collagen (**kol**·aj·en). Name given to the class of scleroproteins occurring in bone and cartilage and forming the ground substance or white fibres of connective tissue. They are rich in glycine and proline and are hydrolysed into gelatin on boiling or treatment with acids. [Gk *kolla* glue, *genein* to produce.]

collagenase (kol·aj·en·aze). An enzyme that induces change in collagen substrate. This may precede ovulation and take place in the collagen of the follicular wall.

collagenic (kol·aj·en·ik). Producing or containing collagen.

collagenosis (kol·aj·en·o'·sis). A group of disorders in which there is a fibrinoid reaction of the collagen tissues producing various signs and symptoms of a so-called "rheumatic" nature. Included in the group are sclerodermia, dermatomyositis, disseminated lupus erythematosus and polyarteritis nodosa. It may be a manifestation of allergy in which the basic fault is damage to vascular endothelium and consequent increased permeability of the capillary walls. Most of the conditions in the group show some response to ACTH or cortisone therapy. [collagen, Gk *-osis* condition.]

collagenous (kol·aj·en·us). 1. Containing or resembling collagen or gelatin. 2. Associated with pathological changes in collagen.

collapse (kol·aps). 1. A breakdown in health; a state of extreme weakness with physical and mental depression. 2. The giving way of the structural framework of an organ; the reduction in size or the obliteration of the space within an air-containing organ. **Absorption collapse.** *See* COLLAPSE OF THE LUNG (below). **Circulatory collapse.** Shock; sudden circulatory failure. **Compression collapse.** *See* COLLAPSE OF THE LUNG (below). **Collapse of the lung.** A reduction in the amount of air in the lung and consequently of the volume of the lung. This may be caused by lessening of the intrapleural negative pressure and the elastic recoil of the lung (relaxation collapse), or to a positive intrapleural pressure caused by air or fluid in the pleural cavity (compression collapse). Obstruction of a bronchus followed by absorption of alveolar air causes absorption collapse. The collapse may affect a whole lung, a lobe, or lobules. **Massive collapse.** Due to obstruction of a large bronchus, causing collapse of a whole lung or of a whole lobe. It usually refers to the acute collapse such as may occur after an operation under general anaesthesia. **Neurocirculatory collapse.** A condition sometimes seen in decompression sickness and one which may develop hours after return to normal ambient pressure; it consists of shock, haemoconcentration and transient neurological disturbances. **Relaxation collapse.** *See* COLLAPSE OF THE LUNG (above). [L *collabi* to fall together.]

collapsotherapy (kol·aps·o·ther'·ap·e). Collapse therapy. *See* THERAPY.

collar (kol·ar). **Periosteal bone collar.** The thick and vascular periosteum that surrounds the diaphysis of young bones. **Venereal collar, Collar of Venus.** Melanoleucoderma colli. [L *collum* neck.]

See also: BIETT, CASAL, STOKES (SIR WILLIAM).

collar-bone (kol·ar·bone). The clavicle. [L *collum* neck, bone.]

collar-crown (kol·ar·krown). An artificial crown which is fitted to a tooth, and has a metal collar which surrounds the neck of the root of the tooth to provide additional strength.

collarette (kol·ar·et). 1. Casal's collar. 2. The circle formed behind the iris of the eye by the ciliary processes. [Fr. *collerette* collar.]

collastin (kol·as·tin). A degenerative product of collagen which stains with the acid dyes that are normally used to stain elastin.

collateral (kol·at·er·al). 1. Accessory or secondary. 2. Side by side or parallel in space. 3. A paraxon. **Collateral sulcus.** *See* SULCUS. **Collateral vessel.** *See* VESSEL. [L *cum, latus* side.]

collaurum (kol·aw·rum). Colloidal gold. *See* GOLD. [Gk *kolla* glue, L *aurum* gold.]

Colles, Abraham (b.1773). Dublin surgeon.

Colles' fascia. The membranous layer of the superficial fascia of the perineum forming the inferior boundary of Colles' space.

Colles' fracture. Fracture of the lower end of the radius with backward and radial displacement of the wrist and hand.

Colles' immunity. The immunity of a mother showing no signs of syphilis, to infection from her congenitally syphilitic child; *see* Colles' law (following).

Colles' law. The apparently healthy mother who gives birth to a syphilitic infant can suckle her child without developing signs of syphilis, whereas a healthy nurse, who suckles the infant, will often become infected. (These mothers invariably have a positive Wasserman test, and are considered to be cases of syphilis in its latent stage.)

Colles' ligament. The reflected part of the external oblique muscle.

Colles' space. The space between the perineal membrane above, and the membranous layer of superficial fascia below. It contains the root of the penis and its attendant muscles, the scrotal nerves and vessels, and the superficial transversus perinei muscle.

Collet, Frédéric-Justin (b.1870). Lyons otolaryngologist.

Collet's syndrome, Collet-Sicard syndrome. Paralysis of palatal, intrinsic laryngeal, pharyngeal, tongue, sternomastoid and trapezius muscles on one side, due to a lesion of the 9th, 10th, 11th and 12th cranial nerves.

colliculectomy (kol·ik·ew·lek'·to·me). Excision of the seminal colliculus. [colliculus, Gk *ektome* a cutting out.]

colliculitis (kol·ik·ew·li'·tis). Inflammation in the region of the seminal colliculus. [colliculus, Gk *-itis* inflammation.]

colliculus (kol·ik·ew·lus). 1. A small elevation. 2. One of the quadrigeminal bodies forming the tectum of the mid-brain. **Colliculus of the arytenoid cartilage [colliculus (NA)].** A small eminence at the superior end of the arcuate crest on the antero-lateral surface. **Facial colliculus [colliculus facialis (NA)].** An elongated swelling on the superior part of the floor of the 4th ventricle, produced in part by the ascending portion of the intramedullary root of the facial nerve. **Seminal colliculus [colliculus seminalis (NA)].** An elevation in the posterior wall of the prostatic part of the male urethra, the urethral crest; the orifices of the prostatic utricle and ejaculatory ducts are situated on it. **Colliculus urethralis.** The seminal colliculus (see preceding). [L little hill.]

collidine (kol·id·een). 1. One of the isomeric trimethylpyridines of formula $C_5H_2(CH_3)_3N$, found in bone oil; colourless liquids with a pungent odour. 2. Symmetrical collidine, γ-collidine, found in coal tar; it also occurs in decaying gelatin. **Acetaldehyde collidine.** Symmetrical collidine prepared from aldehyde ammonia. [Gk *kolla* glue.]

Collier, James Stansfield (b.1870). London neurologist.

tucked lid of Collier. The type of retraction of the upper eyelid sometimes seen in ophthalmoplegia resulting from a supranuclear lesion in the mid-brain.

Collier's tract. That part of the medial longitudinal bundle which lies in the tegmentum of the mid-brain.

collifixation (kol·e·fix·a'·shun). Collopexia. [L *collum* neck, fixation.]

colligative (kol·ig·a·tiv). Term applied to those physical properties such as freezing point, boiling point, vapour pressure or osmotic pressure, the value of which depend only on concentration of dissolved particles, ions and molecules, and not on their nature. [L *colligere* to bind.]

collimation (kol·im·a·shun). Strictly, to make parallel. In radiodiagnosis and radiotherapy, to limit a beam to the required size and thus protect the remainder of the patient from radiation; used in optics, etc. [see foll.]

collimator (kol·im·a·tor). 1. In isotope scanning, to restrict the beam of gamma rays to a predetermined area. That part of a spectrometer which converts the light rays diverging from the slit into a parallel pencil. It consists of a metal tube bearing at the end nearest the turntable an achromatic convex lens; at the far end is a vertical slit so adjusted as to lie in the focal plane of the lens. 2. In radiology, a device attached to the x-ray tube; the collimator is furnished with adjustable lead shutters and a light beam to define the size of the required x-ray beam. [L *collineare* to align.]

Collins, Edward Treacher (b.1862). British ophthalmologist. **Treacher Collins syndrome.** Mandibulofacial dysostosis; characterized by maldevelopment of the facial skeleton and associated with disturbances of the extremities such as radio-ulnar synostosis and oligodactylia.

Collinsonia (kol·in·so·ne·ah). 1. A genus of plants of the family Labiatae. 2. The rhizome of *Collinsonia canadensis.* **Collinsonia canadensis.** Stone root, knob root; a plant indigenous to Canada and the United States. It acts as an antispasmodic, and is used in gastric and intestinal flatulence, also in biliary colic. [Peter *Collinson,* 1694–1768, London botanist.]

Collip, James Bertram (b.1892). Montreal biochemist. **Clark-Collip method.** For calcium in serum: mix in a centrifuge tube 2 ml serum, 2 ml water and 1 ml of 4 per cent ammonium oxalate. Stand at least 30 min, centrifuge, pour off supernatant and drain on filter paper. Wash the precipitate with 3 ml dilute ammonia, centrifuge, pour off supernatant and drain on filter paper. Dissolve the precipitate in 2 ml of hot 5 per cent sulphuric acid and titrate with N/100 potassium permanganate.

colliquation (kol·e·**kwa**·shun). The degeneration of an organ or tissue with subsequent liquefaction. **Ballooning colliquation.** Liquefaction of the cell protoplasm leading to oedematous softening. **Reticulating colliquation.** Incomplete ballooning colliquation in which reticulations form in the cell protoplasm. [L *cum, liquare* to melt.]

colliquative (kol·ik·wat·iv). 1. Causing colliquation. 2. Descriptive of an excessive liquid discharge, e.g. colliquative diarrhoea. 3. Characterized by liquefying of the tissues.

colliquefaction (**kol**·ik·we·**fak**′·shun). Colliquation. [L *cum,* liquefaction.]

collision (kol·**izh**·un). 1. A state of being interlocked, as of twins. 2. In chemistry, the change in energy of a molecule produced by impact with another molecule. **Photo-electric collision.** Collision of a photon and an electron, with transfer of energy from the photon and ejection of the electron from the atom. **Scattering collision.** *See* COMPTON SCATTER. [L *cum laedere* to strike.]

Colliver's symptom. Muscular twitches and spasmodic movements in the preparalytic stage of poliomyelitis; they may be localized to the face and jaw or to the limbs, or may be generalized.

collocated (**kol**·o·ka·ted). Placed side by side; corresponding in regard to position, a term applied particularly to parts of the brain which are situated next to each other. [L *conlocare* to place together.]

collochemistry (kol·o·**kem**·is·tre). The chemistry of colloidal substances.

collodion, collodium (kol·**o**·de·on, kol·**o**·de·um). A solution of nitrocellulose in alcohol and ether (1:7), used in medicine to furnish a protective for the skin in the form of a film left on evaporation. Various medicated collodium preparations are made but they are not in common use, since usually the medicament is completely enclosed in the membrane formed when the application dries and is rendered thereby ineffective. **Collodium Acetonum BPC 1949.** Gun-cotton, clove oil and amyl acetate dissolved in a mixture of benzene and acetone; used as a wound dressing. **Blistering collodion, Collodium cantharidatum.** Collodion containing an acetone extract of cantharides; a vesicant. **Flexible Collodion BP 1973, Collodium flexile.** A solution of gun-cotton, colophony and castor oil in a mixture of alcohol and ether, used to provide a flexible film which does not shrink. **Haemostatic collodion.** Styptic collodion (see below). **Collodion of Salicylic Acid BPC 1959.** Collodion containing *Cannabis indica* (2 per cent) and salicylic acid (11 per cent); used for treating corns. **Collodium salicylicum compositum.** Collodium acetonum containing salicylic acid and cannabis; used for treating corns. **Simple Collodion BPC 1954, Collodium simplex.** Nitrocellulose (gun-cotton) dissolved in ether and alcohol. **Styptic collodion, Collodium stypticum.** Collodion containing tannic acid. [Gk *kolla* glue, *eidos* form.]

collogenesis (kol·o·**jen**·es·is). In biochemistry, a term indicating the supposed colloidal origin of life. [colloid, Gk *genein* to produce.]

colloid (**kol**·oid). A state of matter intermediate between true solution and suspension or emulsion. A colloidal solution or sol is now generally defined as one in which the dispersed particles have a diameter between 1 and 100 nanometres (nm), the colloid being termed the *disperse, internal* or *discontinuous phase,* and the medium the *dispersion medium,* or *external* or *continuous phase,* as distinct from solute and solvent. The chief characteristics of colloids are their surface properties and surface electrical charges, the optical Tyndall effect, Brownian movement and the fact that they may be separated mechanically from the dispersion medium by special methods such as ultracentrifugation. **Amyl colloid.** An anodyne collodion containing aconitine. **Bovine colloid.** Conglutinin; a substance in serum which causes a clumping of red blood cells when treated with a heated specific haemolytic serum plus fresh complement. **Emulsoid colloid.** The term emulsoid is generally applied to a liquid/liquid emulsion in which particles of the disperse phase are of colloid proportions. In some systems of colloid classification it also includes the hydrophilic colloids which behave in some respects as dispersed liquids. **"H" colloid.** A vasodilator of relatively low diffusibility released by tissue damage. **Hydrophilic colloid.** A substance which disperses in water to form a stable colloidal sol that is not coagulated by addition of small quantities of electrolytes. The stability of hydrophilic (water-loving) colloids is attributed to a protective sheath of water adsorbed on to the surface of the particles. They are also reversible colloids (see below). Examples are gelatin, starch and soaps. **Hydrophobic colloid.** A substance which forms a colloidal sol readily precipitated by addition of small amounts of electrolytes. This type of colloid includes the metals and metallic salts. **Irreversible colloid.** A colloid which will not reform a sol upon addition of the dispersion medium after separation from the medium by evaporation to dryness or other means of precipitation. **Lyophilic colloid.** A substance which forms a stable colloidal sol. The term is usually synonymous with hydrophilic colloid. **Lyophobic colloid.** A substance which forms a colloidal sol which is readily precipated. It is usually synonymous with hydrophobic colloid. **Protective colloid.** Any colloid of the hydrophilic type which when added to a sol of a hydrophobic colloid prevents the coagulating effect of small quantities of electrolytes. **Reversible colloid.** A colloid which will re-form a colloidal sol upon addition of dispersion medium after separation from the medium by evaporation to dryness or other means of precipitation. The term is practically synonymous with hydrophilic colloid. **Styptic colloid.** A styptic collodion containing tannic acid. **Suspension colloid.** Suspensoid; a term generally applied to the disperse phase of solid/liquid colloidal sols. It is restricted in some classifications, however, to be essentially synonymous with hydrophobic colloid. **Thyroid colloid.** The liquid contained in the lumen of the thyroid follicles of the thyroid gland, the chief constituent of which is thyroglobulin. [Gk *kolla* glue, *eidos* form.]

colloidal (kol·**oid**·al). Having the characters of a colloid. **Colloidal-S.** An iron preparation formerly given parenterally in various infections.

colloidin (kol·**oid**·in). $C_9H_{15}NO_6$, a substance formed during the colloid degeneration of epithelium.

colloidoclasia, colloidoclasis (**kol**·oid.o.**kla**′·ze·ah, **kol**·oid·o·**kla**′·sis). A disturbance of the equilibrium of colloids in the living body resulting in anaphylactic shock, such as may be produced by the introduction of unaltered colloids, e.g. proteins, into the blood stream. [colloid, Gk *klasis* a breaking up.]

colloidogen (kol·**oid**·o·jen). A hypothetical substance in the body held to be the agent which keeps the mineral elements in colloid solution. [colloid, Gk *genein* to produce.]

colloidopexic (kol·**oid**·o·**pex**′·ik). Referring to colloidopexy.

colloidopexy (kol·**oid**·o·**pex**′·e). In metabolism, the holding or fixing of colloids within the body, as by the action of the liver. [colloid, Gk *pexis* fixation.]

colloidoplasmatic (kol·**oid**·o·plaz·**mat**'·ik). Relating to colloids and plasma.
colloma (kol·**o**·ma). Colloid cancer; as a rule it implies that the degeneration of the tumour has reached a stage at which the contents are like glue. [Gk *kolla* glue, *-oma* tumour.]
collonema (kol·on·**e**·ma). 1. Myxosarcoma. 2. Myxoma. 3. A neoplasm arising from mucoid degeneration of a lipoma. [Gk *kolla* glue, *nema* tissue.]
collopexia (kol·o·**pex**·e·ah). Trachelopexy; the operation of cervical fixation of the uterus. [L *collum* neck, Gk *pexis* fixation.]
colloxylin (kol·**ox**·il·in). Pyroxylin, or nitrocellulose.
collunarium (kol·ew·**na**·re·um). A douche for the nose. [L *colluere* to rinse, *nares* nostril.]
collutorium, collutory (kol·ew·**to**·re·um, **kol**·ew·tor·e). A mouth-wash or gargle. **Collutorium acidi benzoici.** A mouth-wash containing benzoic acid, krameria, saccharin, alcohol and the oils of peppermint and cinnamon; it is astringent and antiseptic. **Collutorium acidi citrici.** A very dilute solution of formaldehyde flavoured with citric acid. **Collutorium arsenicale.** A mouth-wash composed of tincture of ipecacuanha, glycerin, hydrogen peroxide and liquor arsenicalis; it is used to treat Vincent's angina. **Collutorium formaldehydi.** Mouth-wash of Formaldehyde BPC 1959. **Collutorium hydrogeni peroxidi.** A diluted solution of hydrogen peroxide flavoured with peppermint and thymol and sweetened with saccharin. **Collutorium phenolis alkalinum.** Alkaline Mouth-wash of Phenol BPC 1959. **Collutorium sodii chloridi compositum.** Compound Mouth-wash of Sodium Chloride BPC 1959. **Collutorium zinci sulphatis et zinci chloridi.** Mouth-wash of Zinc Sulphate and Zinc Chloride BPC 1959. [L *colluere* to rinse.]
collyrium (kol·**ir**·e·um). An eye lotion. **Collyrium acidi borici.** A solution of boric acid in distilled water. **Collyrium hydrargyri perchloridi.** A weak solution of mercury perchloride in distilled water; sometimes combined with boric acid. **Collyrium Zinci Compositum BPC 1949.** An eye lotion similar to collyrium acidi borici but containing zinc sulphate and less boric acid. [Gk *kollyrion* eye salve.]
coloboma (kol·o·**bo**·mah) (pl. *colobomas* or *colobomata*). A gap in one of the structures of the eye, usually due to congenital malformation, but may be the result of trauma or of operation. **Atypical coloboma.** In the eye, a developmental defect of tissue situated other than below and slightly nasally and therefore not due to a faulty closure of the fetal cleft. **Bridge coloboma.** A coloboma which is not complete, in that there is a bridge of tissue uniting the 2 sides, leaving a gap above and below it; occurs in the iris. **Coloboma of the choroid.** A gap in the choroid and overlying retina due to defective closure of the fetal cleft, usually in the lower part of the fundus. A typical coloboma may occur in other parts, probably from intra-uterine inflammation. **Coloboma of the disc.** A condition in defective crescent of the optic disc in which there is partial failure in closure of the fetal cleft, with a wide exposure of sclerotic which is ectatic. **Facial coloboma.** Facial cleft. *See* CLEFT. **Coloboma iridis.** A gap in the iris continuous with the pupil and usually extending to the pupillary border; typically, it extends downwards or down and slightly inwards. It is often associated with coloboma of the choroid and is due to failure in closure of the fetal cleft. Atypical colobomata can occur in any situation. **Coloboma lentis.** A congenital abnormality, producing a notch usually in the inferior margin of the lens. **Macular coloboma.** A defect of the retina and choroid situated at the macula, originally considered to be an atypical colobomatous defect. Now, some cases are considered to be due to intra-uterine inflammatory changes or toxoplasmosis. **Coloboma of the optic nerve.** A developmental defect of the optic nerve head, the lesser degrees appearing as a hole or cup. **Coloboma palpebrae, Coloboma palpebrale, Coloboma palpebrarum.** A gap in the eyelid or eyelids. The congenital type usually affects the upper lid, to the inner side of the midline, and may be caused by amniotic bands or failure in closure of the fetal cleft. **Coloboma of the retina.** A developmental defect of the retina, associated with the choroid, situated below, due to faulty closure of the optic cup. **Coloboma of the vitreous.** A gap in the lower part of the vitreous, filled with connective tissue which projects into the eyeball. [Gk *koloboma* defect.]
See also: FUCHS (E.).
colocaecostomy (**ko**·lo·se·**kos**'·to·me). Caecocolostomy.
colocentesis (**ko**·lo·sen·**te**'·sis). The surgical puncturing of the colon in order to relieve distension. [colon, Gk *kentesis* a pricking.]
colocholecystostomy (**ko**·lo·ko·le·sis·**tos**'·to·me). Cholecystocolotomy.
colocleisis (ko·lo·**kli**·sis). Occlusion of the colon. [colon, Gk *kleisis* closure.]
coloclysis (ko·**lok**·lis·is). Colonic irrigation. [colon, Gk *klysis* a washing out.]
coloclyster (ko·lo·**klis**·ter). An enema given high up into the colon. [colon, Gk *klyster* wash-out.]
colocolic (ko·lo·**kol**·ik). Referring to 2 parts of the colon, e.g. colocolic fistula, a fistular opening between 2 loops of colon.
colocolostomy (**ko**·lo·kol·**os**'·to·me). The surgical establishment of a communication between 2 separate segments of the colon. [colon, colostomy.]
Colocynth BPC 1963 (**kol**·o·sinth). Colocynthidis pulpa; bitter apple; the dried pulp of the fruit *Citrullus colocynthis* (Linn.) Schrad. (family Cucurbitaceae), cultivated in Cyprus, Syria (Turkey colocynth), Sudan (Egyptian colocynth), Spain and Morocco. It is a powerful purgative, due to an amorphous alkaloid and resins. It is rarely prescribed alone, but usually with other ingredients which prevent griping. [Gk *kolokynthis.*]
colocynthein (kol·o·**sin**·the·in). $C_{40}H_{54}O_{13}$, a resinous product of the hydrolysis of colocynthin.
colocynthin (kol·o·**sin**·thin). $C_{56}H_{84}O_{23}$, a bitter purgative derived from colocynth, originally thought to be a glucoside, but now considered a combination of amorphous alkaloids.
colocystoplasty (**ko**·lo·sist·o·**plas**'·te). The employment of a segment of colon to form a urinary bladder. [colon, Gk *kystis* bag, *plassein* to mould.]
colodyspepsia (**ko**·lo·dis·**pep**'·se·ah). Dyspepsia caused by disturbance set up by conditions in the colon. [colon, dyspepsia.]
colo-enteritis (**ko**·lo·en·ter·**i**'·tis). Enterocolitis.
colofixation (**ko**·lo·fix·**a**'·shun). The surgical procedure of suspending or fixing the colon in cases of prolapse.
colohepatopexy (ko·lo·**hep**·at·o·pex·e). The surgical procedure of attaching the colon to the liver so as to provide protection against adhesions after operations on the gall bladder or removal of gall-stones. [colon, Gk *hepar* liver, *pexis* fixation.]
cololysis (ko·**lol**·is·is). The surgical freeing of the colon from adhesions. [colon, Gk *lysis* a loosing.]
colomba (kol·**om**·bah). Calumba.
colon [NA] (**ko**·lon). That part of the large intestine which extends from the ileocolic junction in the right iliac fossa to end in the pelvis by becoming the rectum in front of the 3rd sacral vertebra. It is characterized by sacculations, a division of the longitudinal muscle coat into 3 discrete bands (taeniae coli), appendices epiploicae and the absence of villi from the mucous membrane. It is divided into an *ascending colon* [colon ascendens (NA)] which passes upwards in a retroperitoneal position from the right iliac fossa to the hepatic flexure of the colon beneath the right lobe of the liver, a *transverse colon* [colon transversum (NA)] suspended by a transverse mesocolon which passes across the abdomen behind the great omentum to the splenic or left colic flexure where it joins the *descending colon* [colon descendens (NA)] which passes down on the left side, retroperitoneal in position, to the left iliac fossa, the part in this fossa being sometimes known as the *iliac colon* which is continued as the *pelvic* or *sigmoid colon* [colon sigmoideum (NA)]. This latter is suspended by a mesocolon from the pelvic brim and midline of the anterior aspect of the sacrum as far as the 3rd sacral vertebra where the pelvic colon becomes continuous with the rectum. **Coat of the colon, mucous [tunica mucosa NA)].** The inner coat of the colon; it is devoid of villi

and aggregated lymphatic nodules, but possesses tubular glands and presents a series of semicircular folds with intervening sacculi. **Coat of the colon, muscular [tunica muscularis (NA)].** The muscular coat of the large intestine comprising longitudinal and circular fibres. The longitudinal muscular fibres form 3 bands (taeniae coli) and the circular fibres an investment separated by connective tissue. **Coat of the colon, serous [tunica serosa (NA)].** The layer of visceral peritoneum partially or completely clothing the walls of the colon. **Coat of the colon, submucous [tela submucosa (NA)].** A layer of areolar tissue between the muscularis mucosae and the inner circular muscle coat of the colon. **Giant colon.** Megacolon; an abnormally large colon. **Irritable colon.** Disorder of intestinal mobility with variable diarrhoea or constipation, often following dysentery. **Lead-pipe colon.** A non-functioning hard tubular colon that may be seen in the late stages of ulcerative colitis. **Redundant colon.** One that is congenitally larger than normal, so that it is subject to excessive folding; said to lead to constipation. **Spastic colon.** Irritable bowel syndrome. *See* SYNDROME. **Thrift colon, Thrifty colon.** A colon with excessive absorption of water, so that the faeces become small and dry. [Gk *kolon.*]

colonalgia (ko·lon·**al**·je·ah). Colalgia; colic. [colon, Gk *algos* pain.]

colonic (ko·**lon**·ik). Having reference to the colon; applying to the colon.

colonitis (ko·lon·**i**·tis). Colitis.

colonization (**kol**·on·i·**za'**·shun). 1. The establishment of mental patients, or patients suffering from chronic infectious disease, in small communal groups instead of housing a large number under one roof. 2. Innidiation. [L *colonia* colony.]

Colonna, Paul Crenshaw (b.1892). Philadelphia orthopaedic surgeon.

Colonna's capsular arthroplasty. Used in reconstruction of the hip in congenital dislocation.

Colonna's reconstruction of the hip. An operation to restore stability after an ununited fracture of the neck of the femur (now obsolete).

colonometer (kol·on·**om**·et·er). An instrument with which the colonies of bacteria on a culture plate can be counted. [colony, Gk *metron* measure.]

colonopathy (ko·lon·**op**·ath·e). Any disorder or disease affecting the colon. [colon, Gk *pathos* suffering.]

colonopexy (**ko**·lon·o·**pex'**·e). Colopexy.

colonorrhagia (**ko**·lon·o·**ra'**·je·ah). Haemorrhage from the colon. [colon, Gk *rhegnynein* to gush forth.]

colonorrhoea (**ko**·lon·o·**re'**·ah). 1. Colitis. 2. Discharge of fluid from the colon. [colon, Gk *rhoia* flow.]

colonoscope (ko·**lon**·o·skope). A long speculum with which examination can be made of the colon. [colon, Gk *skopein* to watch.]

colonoscopy (ko·lon·**os**·ko·pe). Examination of the colon by means of a colonoscope.

colony (**kol**·on·e). A connected mass of bacterial growth originating from a single point. Material containing organisms, diluted if necessary, is distributed over the surface of a solid medium or through a liquid which is quickly set to a gel; when kept under suitable conditions, each cell, or small group of cells, multiplies and gives rise to a visible growth as a separate colony. **Bitten colony.** A bacterial colony with pieces apparently nibbled off the edges, the effect of bacteriophage. **Daughter colony.** A distinct colonial growth arising from a variant cell of the parent colony. **Disgonic colony, Dysgonic colony.** A difficult, sparse or thin colonial growth. **Eugonic colony.** An abundant, thick, luxuriant type of growth. **G colony, Gonidial colony.** Very small colonies, said to be produced by filtrable forms of organisms derived from parent colonies of normally non-filtrable organisms. **H colony.** [G *Hauch* film], a colony of motile, flagellated organisms spreading in a film over the medium. **Matt colony.** Rough colony (see below). **Nibbled colony.** Bitten colony (see above). **O colony.** [G *ohne Hauch* without film], the colony of a non-motile, non-flagellated variant of a normally motile organism, concentrated without a spreading film. **R colony, Rough colony.** A colony with an irregular surface; this often arises as a degenerate variant of an organism usually giving smooth colonies. **S colony.** Smooth colony (see below). **Satellite colony.** A colony that only grows in the neighbourhood of the growth of a colony of other organisms which produce growth factors in which the medium is deficient, e.g. *Haemophilus influenzae* growing near staphylococci on autoclaved nutrient agar. **Smooth colony.** A colony with a shiny surface. Degrees of degeneration are sometimes differentiated as M (mucoid)→MS (matt)→S(glossy) →R (rough), but the order is not always identical with the degree of roughness (e.g. matt streptococci→glossy streptococci). [L *colonia* colony.]

colopathy (ko·**lop**·ath·e). Colonopathy.

colopexia (ko·lo·**pex**·e·ah). Colopexy.

colopexostomy (**ko**·lo·pex·**os'**·to·me). Fixation of the ascending colon and caecum in a desired position by establishment of a temporary caecostomy or appendicostomy. [colon, Gk *pexis* fixation, *stoma* mouth.]

colopexy (ko·lo·**pex**·e). The surgical procedure of suturing the pelvic colon to the wall of the abdomen. [colon, Gk *pexis* fixation.]

colophene (**kol**·o·feen). $(C_{10}H_{16})_2$, a colourless hydrocarbon occurring in turpentine oil.

Colophony BP 1973 (kol·**of**·on·e). Rosin, resin. An oleoresin obtained from various species of pine. It is distilled to extract the turpentine; the glassy amber mass left, consisting mainly of abietic acid and resene, is used to a limited extent in pharmacy to prepare plasters and ointments, but is important in the manufacture of varnishes, soaps, waxes and linoleum. [*Colophon,* a city in Asia Minor.]

coloplication (**ko**·lo·pli·**ka'**·shun). In dilatation or distension of the colon, the operation of taking a fold or pleat in the colon. [colon, L *plica* fold.]

coloproctectomy (**ko**·lo·prok·**tek'**·to·me). Surgical removal of the colon and rectum, performed for ulcerative colitis. [colon, Gk *proktos* anus, *ektome* a cutting out.]

coloproctia (ko·lo·**prok**·she·ah). Colostomy. [colon, Gk *proktos* anus.]

coloproctitis (**ko**·lo·prok·**ti'**·tis). Proctocolitis.

coloproctostomy (**ko**·lo·prok·**tos'**·to·me). Colorectostomy. [colon, Gk *proktos* anus, *stoma* mouth.]

coloptosis (ko·lop·**to**·sis). Prolapse or downward displacement of the transverse colon. [colon, Gk *ptosis* fall.]

colopuncture (ko·lo·**pungk**·tcher). Colocentesis. [colon, L *pungere* to prick.]

colorectitis (**ko**·lo·rek·**ti'**·tis). Proctocolitis. [colon, L *rectum* straight (intestine), Gk *-itis* inflammation.]

colorectostomy (**ko**·lo·rek·**tos'**·to·me). The surgical establishment of a new communication between the colon and the rectum. [colon, L *rectum* straight (intestine), Gk *stoma* mouth.]

colorimeter (kol·or·**im**·et·er). An instrument with which the depth of colour in a substance or fluid can be measured, particularly in determining the proportion of haemoglobin in the blood.

See also: DUBOSCQ.

colorimetric (**kol**·or·im·**et'**·rik). Referring to the quantitative determination of depth of colour. [colour, meter.]

colorimetry (kol·or·**im**·et·re). Measuring the colour of a substance by means of a colorimeter.

colorrhaphy (ko·**lor**·af·e). Suture of the colon. [colon, Gk *rhaphe* suture.]

colorrhoea (ko·lor·**e**·ah). Colitis. [colon, Gk *rhoia* flow.]

colosigmoidostomy (**ko**·lo·sig·moid·**os'**·to·me). Surgical establishment of a communication between the descending colon and the pelvic colon. [colon, Gk *sigma* letter S, *stoma* mouth.]

colostomy (ko·**los**·to·me). A temporary or permanent artificial opening made through the abdominal wall into the colon. The site is usually indicated in its description, e.g. *iliac colostomy, left inguinal colostomy, lumbar colostomy, transverse colostomy.* **Defunctioning colostomy, Double-barrel colostomy.** Colostomy in which the colon is completely cut across and both ends brought out on to the abdominal wall so that no faeces passes beyond the colostomy. **Terminal colostomy.** Colostomy in which the proximal cut end of the colon is brought out on to the abdominal wall after the colon, distally, has been resected or closed. **Wet colostomy.** One through which the urine as well as the faeces drains and most often employed after the operation of pelvic evisceration. [colon, Gk *stoma* mouth.]

colostration (kol·os·**tra**·shun). A state of illness or disorder that may be present in newly-born infants as the result of sensitivity to colostrum in the mother's milk.

colostric (kol·**os**·trik). Referring to colostrum.

colostrorrhoea (kol·os·tro·**re**'·ah). 1. The profuse secretion of colostrum. 2. The spontaneous discharge of colostrum. [colostrum, Gk *rhoia* flow.]

colostrous (kol·**os**·trus). 1. Like colostrum. 2. Containing colostrum. 3. Colostric.

colostrum (kol·**os**·trum). The first milk secreted by the mammary gland; sometimes it may be found 48 h before the child is born. It is thin, white and opalescent, and contains a large amount of milk proteins. It has a laxative effect on the infant. **Colostrum gravidarum.** Colostrum secreted before childbirth. **Colostrum puerperarum.** Colostrum secreted after childbirth. [L.]

colotomy (ko·**lot**·o·me). The operation of opening the colon, usually performed through the abdominal wall. **Lumbar colotomy.** A colotomy through a lumbar incision. [colon, Gk *temnein* to cut.]

See also: LITTRÉ.

colotyphoid (ko·lo·**ti**·foid). Ulceration of the colon and lesions of the small intestine associated with typhoid fever.

colour (**kul**·or). An optical attribute of a substance due to its absorption of a portion of the spectrum and its reflection or transmission of the remainder. Colour has shade or hue, strength or purity, and brightness or intensity. **Colour analysis.** *See* ANALYSIS. **Basic colours.** As light—red, green and violet; as pigments—red, yellow and blue. **Binary colour.** One composed of 2 primary colours. **Colour blindness.** *See* BLINDNESS. **Complementary colours.** Two colours which, blended as light, produce white light: these differ from the so-called complementaries, or pigments which, when mixed together, form white. **Compound colour.** The colour produced by mixing 2 or more primary pigments. **Confusion colour.** A colour which, to a colour-blind person, appears identical with another colour. **Colour hearing.** *See* HEARING. **Impure colour.** A sensation produced by light containing more than one monochromatic component. **Incidental colour.** The colour that persists on the retina after the stimulating colour has been removed. **Colour index.** 1. The proportion of haemoglobin in each red blood corpuscle. 2. A numerical index of British dyestuffs. **Primary colours.** 1. The colours of the spectrum or rainbow, red, orange, yellow, green, blue, indigo and violet. 2. Basic colours (see above). **Pure colour.** The colour of a single wavelength of light. **Saturated colour.** A colour from which light of wavelengths above or below has been eliminated. **Secondary colour.** Compound colour (see above). [L *color.*]

colpalgia (kol·**pal**·je·ah). Colpodynia. [Gk *kolpos* vagina, *algos* pain.]

colpatresia (kol·pat·re·ze·ah). Occlusion or imperforation of the vagina. [Gk *kolpos* vagina, atresia.]

colpectasia, colpectasis (kol·pek·**ta**·ze·ah, kol·**pek**·tas·is). Dilatation or distension of the vagina. [Gk *kolpos* vagina, *ektasis* a stretching.]

colpectomy (kol·**pek**·to·me). Complete removal of the vagina by surgical means. [Gk *kolpos* vagina, *ektome* a cutting out.]

colpeurynter (kol·pewr·**in**·ter). An inflatable bag for use in dilating the vagina or the os uteri. [Gk *kolpos* vagina, *eurynein* to dilate.]

colpeurysis (kol·**pewr**·e·sis). Mechanical or operative dilatation of the vagina, particularly by use of a colpeurynter. [Gk *kolpos* vagina, *eurys* wide.]

colpismus (kol·**piz**·mus). Vaginismus. [Gk *kolpos* vagina.]

colpitic (kol·**pit**·ik). Referring to colpitis.

colpitis (kol·**pi**·tis). A condition of inflammation of the vagina. **Colpitis emphysematosa.** Colpitis in which small blebs develop on the mucous membrane. **Colpitis mycotica.** Colpitis caused by the presence of a mould. [Gk *kolpos* vagina, *-itis* inflammation.]

colpocele (**kol**·po·seel). 1. Colpoptosis. 2. Hernia into the vagina. [Gk *kolpos* vagina, *kele* hernia.]

colpocleisis (kol·po·**kli**·sis). Surgical obliteration of the lumen of the vagina. [Gk *kolpos* vagina, *kleisis* closure.]

colpocoeliotomy (**kol**·po·se·le·**ot**'·o·me). The method of incising the abdomen by the vaginal route. **Anterolateral colpocoeliotomy.** Anterolateral incision into the abdomen by the vaginal route, with division of the broad ligament of the uterus of one side. [Gk *kolpos* vagina, coeliotomy.]

colpocystic (kol·po·**sis**·tik). Referring to the vagina and the urinary bladder. [Gk *kolpos* vagina, *kystis* bag.]

colpocystitis (**kol**·po·sis·**ti**'·tis). A condition of inflammation involving the vagina and the urinary bladder. [Gk *kolpos* vagina, cystitis.]

colpocystocele (kol·po·**sis**·to·seel). Hernia of the urinary bladder associated with prolapse of the anterior wall of the vagina. [Gk *kolpos* vagina, *kystis* bag, *kele* hernia.]

colpocystoplasty (kol·po·**sis**·to·plas·te). Plastic surgery employed in repair of the vesicovaginal wall. [Gk *kolpos* vagina, *kysis* bag, *plassein* to mould.]

colpocystosyrinx (**kol**·po·sis·to·**sir**'·inx). Colpocystic fistula; vesicovaginal fistula. *See* FISTULA. [Gk *kolpos* vagina, *kystis* bag, *syrigx* pipe.]

colpocystotomy (**kol**·po·sis·**tot**'·o·me). Surgical incision into the urinary bladder through the wall of the vagina. [Gk *kolpos* vagina, *kystis* bag, *temnein* to cut.]

colpocysto-ureterocystotomy (kol·po·**sis**·to·ewr·e·ter·o·sis·**tot**'·o·me). Exposure of the orifices of the ureters in the bladder by incision of the vaginal and cystic walls. [Gk *kolpos* vagina, *kystis* bag, ureterocystotomy.]

colpodesmorrhaphy (kol·po·dez·**mor**'·af·e). The operation of suturing together the ruptured edges of the bulbospongiosus muscle of the perineum in the female. [Gk *kolpos* vagina, *desmos* band, *rhaphe* suture.]

colpodynia (kol·po·**din**·e·ah). Pain in the vagina. [Gk *kolpos* vagina, *odyne* pain.]

colpoedema (kol·pe·**de**·mah). Oedema affecting the vagina. [Gk *kolpos* vagina, *oidema* a swelling.]

colpohyperplasia (**kol**·po·hi·per·**pla**'·ze·ah). A condition of abnormal growth of the mucous membrane of the vagina. **Colpohyperplasia cystica.** The formation of gas-filled cysts in association with colpohyperplasia; the condition occurs during pregnancy. **Colpohyperplasia emphysematosa.** Colpohyperplasia as a result of bacillary infection, and occurring during pregnancy. [Gk *kolpos* vagina, hyperplasia.]

colpohysterectomy (**kol**·po·his·ter·**ek**'·to·me). Operative removal of the uterus by the vaginal route. [Gk *kolpos* vagina, hysterectomy.]

colpohysteropexy, colpohysterorrhaphy (**kol**·po·his·ter·o·**pex**'·e, **kol**·po·his·ter·**or**'·af·e). The operative fixation of the uterus through the vagina. [Gk *kolpos* vagina, hysteropexy, hysterorrhaphy.]

colpohysterotomy (**kol**·po·his·ter·**ot**'·o·me). Surgical incision of the uterus by the vaginal route. [Gk *kolpos* vagina, hysterotomy.]

colpolaparotomy (**kol**·po·lap·ar·**ot**'·o·me). Laparotomy via the vaginal route. [Gk *kolpos* vagina, laparotomy.]

colpomicroscope (kol·po·**mi**·kro·scope). A magnifying instrument for visualizing the cervix uteri in the living woman. It is mainly used to detect early malignant change and to identify sites for biopsy, with or without previous staining of the cervix. [Gk *kolpos* vagina, microscope.]

colpomycosis (**kol**·po·mi·**ko**'·sis). Colpitis mycotica; vaginal inflammation set up by a mould such as *Candida.* [Gk *kolpos* vagina, mycosis.]

colpomyomectomy, colpomyomotomy, colpomyotomy (**kol**·po·mi·o·**mek**'·to·me, **kol**·po·mi·o·**mot**'·o·me, **kol**·po·mi·**ot**'·o·me).

Removal of a myoma from the uterus by the vaginal route. [Gk *kolpos* vagina, myomectomy.]

colpoparovariocystectomy (kol·po·par·o·var·e·o·sis·tek'·to·me). Surgical removal of a cystic tumour of the epoöphoron by the vaginal route. [Gk *kolpos* vagina, *para*, ovary, cystectomy.]

colpopathy (kol·pop·ath·e). Any disease of the vagina. [Gk *kolpos* vagina, *pathos* suffering.]

colpoperineoplasty (kol·po·per·in·e·o·plas'·te). Plastic surgery used for repair or re-forming of the perineum and the vagina. [Gk *kolpos* vagina, perineoplasty.]

colpoperineorrhaphy (kol·po·per·in·e·or'·af·e). Repair of a perineal tear by plastic surgery and suturing of the torn edges. [Gk *kolpos* vagina, perineorrhaphy.]

colpopexy (kol·po·pex·e). Surgical fixation of the vagina to the abdominal wall in order to correct relaxation and prolapse. [Gk *kolpos* vagina, *pexis* fixation.]

colpoplasty (kol·po·plas·te). Any plastic surgical operation on the vagina. [Gk *kolpos* vagina, *plassein* to mould.]

colpopoiesis (kol·po·poi·e'·sis). The construction of an artificial vagina by plastic surgical procedures. [Gk *kolpos* vagina, *poiein* to make.]

colpopolypus (kol·po·pol·e·pus). Polypus of the vagina. [Gk *kolpos* vagina, polypus.]

colpoptosis (kol·pop·to·sis). Prolapse of the walls of the vagina. [Gk *kolpos* vagina, *ptosis* fall.]

colporectopexy (kol·po·rek·to·pex·e). The suturing of a prolapsed rectum to the walls of the vagina. [Gk *kolpos* vagina, rectopexy.]

colporrhagia (kol·po·ra·je·ah). Haemorrhage from the vagina. [Gk *kolpos* vagina, *rhegnynein* to gush forth.]

colporrhaphy (kol·por·af·e). 1. Repair of a vaginal tear by freshening and suturing the edges. 2. A plastic operation on the vaginal walls in order to narrow the lumen. [Gk *kolpos* vagina, *rhaphe* suture.]

colporrhexis (kol·po·rex·is). Laceration or rupture of the vaginal walls. [Gk *kolpos* vagina, *rhexis* rupture.]

colporrhoea (kol·po·re·ah). 1. Discharge of mucus from the vagina. 2. Leucorrhoea. [Gk *kolpos* vagina, *rhoia* flow.]

colposcope (kol·po·skope). An instrument with which the vagina and the neck of the uterus may be examined. [Gk *kolpos* vagina, *skopein* to watch.]

colposcopy (kol·pos·ko·pe). Examination of the vagina and the neck of the uterus by means of a colposcope.

colpospasm, colpospasmus (kol·po·spazm, kol·po·spaz·mus). Vaginismus. [Gk *kolpos* vagina, *spasmos* a drawing.]

colpostat (kol·po·stat). A device by means of which a therapeutic medium such as a radium applicator can be held in place in the vagina. [Gk *kolpos* vagina, *statos* a standing.]

colpostenosis (kol·po·sten·o'·sis). Constriction or narrowing of the vagina. [Gk *kolpos* vagina, stenosis.]

colpostenotomy (kol·po·sten·ot'·o·me). The surgical division of a vaginal stricture. [Gk *kolpos* vagina, stenosis, *temnein* to cut.]

colpotherm (kol·po·therm). An apparatus fitted with an electric element for the application of heat to the vagina and surrounding parts. [Gk *kolpos* vagina, *therme* heat.]

colpotomy (kol·pot·o·me). Any cutting operation in or surgical incision of the vagina. [Gk *kolpos* vagina, *temnein* to cut.]

colpo-ureterocystotomy (kol·po·ewr·e·ter·o·sis·tot'·o·me). Colpocysto-ureterocystotomy.

colpo-ureterotomy (kol·po·ewr·e·ter·ot'·o·me). The relief of ureteral stricture by surgical division by the vaginal route. [Gk *kolpos* vagina, ureterotomy.]

colpoxerosis (kol·po·zer·o'·sis). A condition of abnormal dryness of the vaginal canal and vulva. [Gk *kolpos* vagina, *xerosis* dryness.]

Colt, George Herbert (b.1878). Aberdeen and London surgeon.

Colt's cannula. A cannula for the introduction of coils of wire into the sac of an arterial aneurysm to produce a layered clot.

Colt's technique. The insertion of a long coiled wire into an aneurysmal sac to induce clotting.

Colt's wire. A spiral of wire inserted into an aneurysmal sac to encourage clotting and reduce the risk of rupture.

coltsfoot (koltz·fut). The plant *Tussilago farfara* Linn. (family Compositae); the dried leaves are used as a demulcent and relieve chronic and irritable cough. [AS *colt, fot.*]

Colubridae (kol·ew·brid·e). A family of snakes displaying large shield-like hard scales; it includes many harmless snakes, but also the poisonous coral snakes, cobras and kraits. [L *coluber* snake, Gk *eidos* form.]

Colubrinae (kol·ew·brin·e). A sub-family of snakes: there are several hundred species, mostly non-poisonous. [see prec.]

colubrine (kol·ew·breen). 1. $C_{22}H_{24}O_3N_2$, an alkaloid associated with strychnine and brucine in nux vomica seeds. It occurs in 2 isomeric forms, and takes its name from *Strychnos colubrina* of the East Indies. 2. Pertaining to snakes of the sub-family Colubrinae.

columbin (kol·um·bin). Calumbin.

columbium (kol·um·be·um). Name given to the rare metal related to tantalum and more usually known as *niobium*. [*Columbia*, USA]

columella (kol·um·el·ah). 1. A little column. 2. In mosses or moulds, the axis of the spore case around which the spores are set. **Columella cochleae.** The modiolus of the cochlea. **Columella fornicis.** The anterior column of the fornix of the rhinencephalon. **Columella nasi.** The terminal (fleshy) portion of the nasal septum. [L little column.]

column [columna (NA)] (kol·um). In anatomy, any elongated structure, often orientated vertically and sometimes supporting, or appearing to support, other structures; very commonly applied in the central nervous system to elongated systems of fibres or masses of grey matter. **Column of the abdominal ring.** Thickenings in the aponeurosis of the external oblique muscle which form the sides of the superficial inguinal ring. **Anal columns [columnae anales (NA)].** Vertical folds in the mucous membrane of the anal canal. **Anterolateral column.** The white matter of both the anterior and lateral columns of the spinal cord. **Branchial column.** The broken column of nuclei which innervate the musculature of the visceral arches; the motor nuclei of the trigeminal, facial, glossopharyngeal, vagus and spinal accessory nerves. **Direct cerebellar column.** The posterior spinocerebellar tract. *See* TRACT. **Enamel column.** Enamel prism. *See* PRISM. **Column of the external ring.** Column of the abdominal ring (see above). **Column of the fornix, anterior.** The anterior part of the fornix which descends behind the anterior commissure to the hypothalamus. **Column of the fornix, posterior [crus fornicis (NA)].** The part of the fornix towards the thalamus. **Fractionation column.** A glass or metal column employed in fractional distillation. **Fundamental column.** The intersegmental tracts, basis bundles or intersegmental fibres of the spinal cord. **Grey column, anterior [columna anterior (NA)].** The grey matter of the anterior horns in the spinal cord. **Grey column, lateral [columna lateralis (NA)].** The lateral horn of grey matter. **Grey column, posterior [columna posterior (NA)].** The posterior horns of grey matter in the spinal cord. **Positive column.** The glow extending from the positive electrode of a discharge tube. It is of uniform luminosity at pressures of about 1 mm, but when the pressure is reduced even more it generally breaks up into a series of bright and dark striae. **Postero-external column.** The fasciculus cuneatus. **Posteromedian column.** The fasciculus gracilis. **Rectal column.** Anal column (see above). **Renal columns [columnae renales (NA)].** Renal cortical tissue which extends between the pyramids of the kidney towards its hilum. **Respiratory column.** A term which has been applied, probably incorrectly, to the fasciculus solitarius. **Columns of rugae [columna rugarum (NA)].** The columns of rugae on the anterior [columna rugarum anterior (NA)] and posterior [columna rugarum posterior (NA)] walls of the vagina. **Somatic motor column.** The anterior horn of the spinal cord together with the somatic motor nuclei of the brain stem. **Somatic sensory column.** The posterior horn of the spinal cord together with the somatic sensory nuclei of the brain stem. **Spinal column.** Vertebral column (see below). **Columns of the spinal cord, grey [columnae griseae (NA)].** Columns of grey matter formed by the anterior, posterior or lateral horns of the spinal cord. **Columns of the spinal cord, white [funiculi medullae spinalis (NA)].** The bundles of nerve fibres arranged into anterior, lateral and posterior columns, surrounding the grey matter of the spinal cord. **Splanchnic column.** Nuclei in the brain stem which send fibres to the facial, vagus and glossopharyngeal nerves for the supply of smooth muscle and glands. **Vaginal columns.** Columns of rugae (see above). **Vertebral column [columna vertebralis (NA)].** The backbone, made up of the vertebrae and the intervertebral discs. **Vesicular column.** A column of nerve cells in the posterior horn of the spinal cord; Clarke's column. **Visceral motor column.** The lateral horn of grey matter of the spinal cord together with the splanchnic column of the brain stem. **Visceral sensory column.** Nerve cells in the central nervous system, thought to receive afferent connections from the viscera; their precise anatomical location is uncertain. **White column, anterior [funiculus anterior (NA)].** The white matter in the anterior part of the spinal cord between the anterior horns of grey matter. **White column, lateral [funiculus lateralis (NA)].** The white matter in the lateral part of the spinal cord between the posterior and anterior horns of grey matter and extending to the medulla oblongata. **White column, posterior [funiculus posterior (NA)].** The fibres between the posterior horn of grey matter in the spinal cord (the fasciculi cuneatus and gracilis). [L *columna* column.]

See also: BERTIN, BRUCE (A.), BURDACH, CLARKE, COTUGNO (COTUNNIUS), D'AZYR, FLECHSIG, GOLL, GOWERS, LISSAUER, MORGAGNI, ROLANDO, SERTOLI, SPITZKA (E. C.), STILLING, TUERCK.

columna [L.] (kol·um·nah). A column. **Columnae carneae.** The trabeculae carneae of the heart. **Columna extremitatis superioris.** The cell groups in the anterior horn of the cervical swelling of the spinal cord from which the muscles of the upper limb are innervated. [L column.]

columnar (kol·um·nar). Shaped like a column.

columnella (kol·um·nel·ah). Columella.

columning (kol·um·ing). A method of supporting a prolapsed uterus, or of preventing prolapse, by packing the vagina with tampons. [L *columna* column.]

columnization (kol·um·ni·za′·shun). The use of the method of columning in prolapse of the uterus.

colypeptic (ko·le·pep·tik). Preventing or retarding digestion. [Gk *kolyein* to hinder, *pepsis* digestion.]

colyphrenia (ko·le·fre·ne·ah). A state in which the workings of the mind and the process of thought are subjected to unusually strong inhibition. [Gk *kolyein* to hinder, *phren* mind.]

colyseptic (ko·le·sep·tik). Antiseptic. [Gk *kolyein* to hinder, *sepsis* decay.]

colytic (ko·lit·ik). 1. Inhibitory; the result of an obstruction. 2. Term applied to a temperament distinguished by the qualities of self-restraint and tranquillity of mind, combined with an inclination to play the passive parts of listener and spectator. [Gk *kolyein* to hinder.]

coma (ko·mah). The state of complete loss of consciousness from which the patient cannot be roused by any ordinary external stimulus; conjunctival and pupillary reflexes are absent and deep reflexes are usually abolished. It is due to serious disturbance of brain functions by trauma, vascular lesions, endogenous toxins or external poisons. **Alcoholic coma.** That due to alcoholic poisoning. **Apoplectic coma.** Coma caused by acute vascular lesions such as cerebral haemorrhage, thrombosis and embolism. **Diabetic coma.** That due to ketosis in hyperglycaemia. **Coma hepaticum.** Coma arising in hepatic insufficiency from acute yellow atrophy, or in the terminal stage of hepatic cirrhosis. It may be precipitated in persons with liver dysfunction by the administration of ammonia-containing cationic-exchange resins. **Hypoglycaemic coma.** Coma associated with a low level of the blood sugar. **Hypopituitary coma.** Coma that is liable to occur in any person with severe hypopituitarism. **Trance coma.** *See* TRANCE. **Uraemic coma.** Coma in renal failure. **Coma vigil.** A state of unconsciousness in which the patient lies with eyes wide open, a vacant gaze, lips parted, and the face pale and devoid of expression. There is incoherent muttering. It is most often seen in typhus but occurs also occasionally in typhoid fever. [Gk *koma* deep sleep.]

comatose (ko·mat·oze). Affected with coma; resembling coma.

combing (ko·ming). Hersage; in disease of any area served by a peripheral nerve, the operation of splitting the nerve sheath and so releasing the fibres, which are then teased out and left free. [ME *kemb.*]

combining power (kom·bi·ning pow·er). Valency. [LL *combinare*, power.]

combustion (kom·bust·yun). 1. Burning. 2. Oxidation of a substance with liberation of heat, sound or light, or all three together. **Slow combustion.** 1. Decay, as of the animal body. 2. The slow oxidation of a substance. **Spontaneous combustion.** Combustion of its own accord, without application of a flame. [L *comburere* to burn up.]

Comby, Jules (b. 1853). Paris paediatrician.

Comby's sign. Inflammation of the buccal mucous membrane, sometimes with white or yellowish patches adhering to cheeks and gums; used in the early diagnosis of measles, before the appearance of Koplik's spots.

Comby-Filatov treatment. The administration of arsenic in heavy dosage as treatment for chorea. Now obsolete.

comedo (kom·e·do) (pl. *comedones*). A plug of greasy matter commonly referred to as a *blackhead*, which blocks the superficial mouth of a sebaceous follicle; it is tipped by a blackened cap of dust and debris. Comedones are a sign of disorder of the sebaceous glands or of the development in them which takes place at puberty. They occur in the young chiefly, and are characteristic of acne vulgaris. The parasite *Demodex folliculorum* may be found in the comedones. [L *comedere* to eat up.]

comedocarcinoma (kom·e·do·kar·sin·o′·mah). Carcinoma of the breast in which the fine ducts are filled with firm masses of cancer cells which can be squeezed out by manual pressure. [comedo, carcinoma.]

comes (ko·meez). A vessel, such as an artery, which accompanies another vessel or a nerve trunk. [L companion.]

comfimeter (kum·fim·et·er). A device with which the cooling power of air at body temperature can be measured, so that a room can be kept at a comfortable warmth. [comfort, meter.]

comfrey (kum·fre). The plant *Symphytum officinale* Linn. (family Boraginaceae); the dried root and rhizome contain allantoin, and have been applied to wounds, sores and ulcers in the form of a decoction. [OFr. *confirie.*]

commasculation (kom·as·kew·la′·shun). Homosexuality among males. [L *cum, masculus* male.]

commensal (kom·en·sal). 1. An organism which, although not a parasite, lives in, on or with another and is nourished by the same food. Mutual benefit may result. 2. Having the character of a commensal. [L *cum, mensa* table.]

commensalism (kom·en·sal·izm). A state of symbiosis in which one of the associate organisms benefits and the other is unaffected for either better or worse. [see prec.]

comminuted (kom·in·ew·ted). Crushed or broken into many small pieces. The term is applied particularly to fracture of bone. [L *comminuire* to break into fragments.]

comminution (kom·in·ew·shun). 1. The fracture of a bone into a number of pieces. 2. The act of breaking into small pieces. 3. The condition of being broken into fragments. [see prec.]

Commiphora (kom·if·or·ah). A genus of shrubs and trees of the family Burseraceae. **Commiphora molmol.** A species which yields myrrh. **Commiphora opobalsamum.** A species which yields Mecca balsam (balm of Gilead). [Gk *kommi* gum, *pherein* to bear.]

commissural (kom·is·ewr·al). 1. Relating to a commissure. 2. Belonging to a commissure.

commissure [commissura (NA)] (kom·is·ewr). Any tissue joining 2 like masses of tissue or structures, usually, but not always, crossing the median sagittal plane of the body; most commonly in the central nervous system, where it is to be differentiated from a chiasma or decussation. **Anterior commissure [commissura anterior (NA)].** A bundle of fibres in the anterior wall of the 3rd ventricle of the forebrain, connecting the olfactory bulb and the cortex of the temporal lobes on one side with the same structures on the other. **Anterior commissure, olfactory part of the [pars anterior (NA)].** The majority of the fibres of the anterior commissure, which connect the olfactory bulbs, pyramids and pyriform areas of either side. **Anterior commissure, posterior part of the [pars posterior (NA)].** The remaining fibres of the anterior commissure. **Anterior grey commissure [commissura anterior grisea (NA)].** The grey matter in the spinal cord anterior to the central canal. **Anterior white commissure [commissura alba (NA)].** Fibres which cross in the spinal cord anterior to the central canal; many of these are decussating fibres passing to the spinothalamic tracts. **Commissure of the bulb.** The union anterior to the vagina of the 2 parts of the bulb of the vestibule. **Commissure of the cerebellum, dorsal.** Commissural fibres in the roof of the 4th ventricle in relation to which the body or corpus of the cerebellum develops. **Commissure of the cerebellum, lateral.** Fibres in the roof of the 4th ventricle connecting the vestibular nuclei of the 2 sides; the flocculonodular lobe of the cerebellum develops around it. **Commissure of the forebrain, dorsal.** In comparative anatomy, the hippocampal commissure (see below). **Fornix commissure.** Hippocampal commissure (see below). **Grey commissure.** Anterior and posterior grey commissures (see above and below). **Habenular commissure [commissura habenularum (NA)].** A commissure in the roof of the 3rd ventricle anterior to the stalk of the pineal body; it joins the habenular ganglia of the 2 sides, and contains fibres from the stria habenularis (stria medullaris or taenia thalami). **Hippocampal commissure [commissura fornicis (NA)].** Fibres from the fimbria and fornix which connect the hippocampal formations of the 2 sides and cross beneath the corpus callosum. **Commissures of the hypothalamus.** Postoptic commissures (see below). **Labial commissure [commissura labiorum (NA)].** The junction between the upper and lower lip at the angle of the mouth. **Commissura mollis.** A variable connection between the 2 thalami across the cavity of the 3rd ventricle; the connexus interthalamicus. It contains few commissural fibres in man. **Palpebral commissure, lateral [commissura palpebrarum lateralis (NA)].** The line of fusion of the 2 eyelids on the lateral side. **Palpebral commissure, medial [commissura palpebrarum medialis (NA)].** The line of fusion of the 2 eyelids on the medial side. **Posterior commissure [commissura posterior (NA)].** Fibres which cross in the roof of the aqueduct of the mid-brain anterior to the superior corpora quadrigemina. **Posterior grey commissure.** Grey matter in the spinal cord posterior to the central canal. **Postoptic commissure [commissurae supraopticae (NA)].** Commissural fibres above and behind the optic chiasma which connect the subthalamic regions, corpora striata, hypothalamic nuclei, and possibly the medial geniculate bodies of the 2 sides; 3 components are recognized, the commissures of Gudden, Meynert and Ganser. **Supraoptic commissure.** Postoptic commissure (see above). **Commissure of the vestibule.** A narrow band across the front of the vaginal orifice, uniting the 2 masses of erectile tissue on either side of it. **Commissure of the vulva, anterior [commissura labiorum anterior (NA)].** The junction between the labia majora anterior to the vulva. **Commissure of the vulva, posterior [commissura labiorum posterior (NA)].** The junction of the labia majora posterior to the vulva. [L *commissura* a join.]

See also: GANSER, GUDDEN, MEYNERT, WERNEKING.

commissurotomy (**kom**·is·ewr·**ot**'·o·me). Division of the angle of union of 2 margins, e.g. of the lips. **Mitral commissurotomy.** Division of the mitral valve (at the junction of its cusps) for the relief of mitral stenosis. [L *commissura* a join, Gk *temnein* to cut.]

commotio (kom·o·she·o). 1. A concussion or a violent shaking. 2. The shock resulting from concussion or being violently shaken up. **Commotio cerebri.** Concussion of the brain. **Commotio retinae.** Concussion of the retina. **Commotio spinalis.** 1. Concussion of the spine. 2. Railway spine. *See* SPINE. [L *commovere* to agitate.]

communicans (kom·**ew**·nik·anz). Term applied to a nerve, artery or other structure which forms a connection or communication between 2 similar structures, e.g. ramus communicans, the nerve joining a spinal nerve to the sympathetic chain of ganglia. [L communicating.]

communicating arteries of the brain (kom·**ew**·nik·a·ting). **Anterior communicating artery of the brain [arteria communicans anterior (NA)].** A short artery linking the 2 anterior cerebral arteries just anterior to the optic chiasma; it is part of the arterial circle of Willis. **Posterior communicating artery of the brain [arteria communicans posterior (NA)].** A vessel linking the internal carotid with the posterior cerebral artery; it is part of the arterial circle of Willis.

communis (kom·**ew**·nis). 1. Common; not specific. 2. Relating or belonging to more than one. 3. Not rare. [L.]

commutator (**kom**·ew·ta·tor). A device by means of which an electric current may be automatically interrupted or reversed. [L *commutare* to exchange.]

Comolli, Antonio (b. 1879). Italian pathologist.

Comolli's sign. A triangular swelling reproducing the shape of the scapula which is seen following fracture of this bone.

comose (**ko**·mose). 1. Having a heavy growth of hair. 2. In botany, bearing a tuft of soft hairs. [Gk *kome* hair.]

companion artery of the sciatic nerve [arteria comitans nervi ischiadici (NA)] (kom·**pan**·e·on). A branch of the inferior gluteal artery which accompanies the sciatic nerve, often considered as a remnant of the primitive axial artery of the lower limb.

comparascope (kom·**par**·ah·skope). An accessory instrument attached to a microscope so that 2 separate slides can be compared simultaneously. [L *comparare* to compare, Gk *skopein* to watch.]

comparator (kom·**par**·ah·tor). A form of colorimeter with which standard colour solutions can be compared. It may consist of a block of wood pierced by holes in which test-tubes containing the solutions are placed, and transected by other holes through which the colours can be inspected. [L *comparare* to compare.]

compatible (kom·**pat**·ible). Of drugs, not interfering chemically, physically or therapeutically the one with the other, and therefore suitable to be administered together. In blood transfusion, when the donor red cells do not carry antigens against which the recipient has the corresponding antibody. [see foll.]

compatibility (kom·pat·ib·**il**·it·e). A word used in dispensing to signify that when 2 or more drugs are compounded there will be no undesirable chemical reaction between them, nor will they have antagonistic therapeutic effects. Sometimes it is necessary to prescribe together 2 or more drugs which are physically incompatible, as, for example, when oils or resins are prescribed in an aqueous medium. In such a case the difficulty can be overcome by adding an innocuous gum to the mixture, thereby making an emulsion. [L *compatibilis* agreeing.]

compensation (kom·pen·**sa**·shun). 1. Making good the lack of something. 2. Making good a defect in constitution, function or structure. 3. Making good the failure of one part or organ by the assumption of its activities by another part or organ. 4. In psychology, the "buffer" mechanism in an individual which advances a valuable characteristic or trait in order to avert the shock that recognition of the opposite valueless trait would give to self-love, e.g. loving consideration (so-called) towards others covering the unamiable trait of possessiveness. **Broken compensation.** Weakness of heart action so that stagnation and congestion occurs because the blood is not driven at the requisite speed through the arteries. **Dosage compensation.** In genetics, any mechanism which secures the equality, or near equality, of the phenotypic effect of sex-linked genes acting on somatic traits and, thus, compensates for differences in gene dosage existing between the homo- and hetero-gametic sex. *See* LYON HYPOTHESIS. **Compensation neurosis.** *See* NEUROSIS. [L *compensare* to weigh together.]

compensator (**kom**·pen·sa·tor). A physical device to compensate for variation of surface contour and tissue density in external radiotherapy. [L *compensare* to weigh together.]

competence (**kom**·pet·ens). In bacterial transformation, the ability of recipient bacteria to take up donor DNA. Competence factor. *See* FACTOR. [L *competentia* capable.]

complaint (kom·**pla**·nt). A disease or ailment of the body. **Chief complaint.** The presenting symptom. **Summer complaint.** Cholera nostras. [LL *complangere* to beat the breast.]

complement (**kom**·ple·ment). 1. Alexin, cytase. An unstable substance present in normal serum or plasma, and destroyed by heating at 56°C for half an hour. It is necessary to complete the destructive action of antisera (bactericidal or bacteriolytic) on bacteria, or other cells (e.g. haemolysis of red blood cells which have been combined with their specific immune body; that is, sensitized cells). Complement is not increased by immunization, nor does it combine with or have any action on cells in the absence of immune bodies; it combines with most antigen-antitoxin complexes, but not with certain toxin-antitoxin compounds. 2. Those components present in normal serum which are removed by antigen-antibody complexes, a wider definition that includes substances which increase agglutination by antibodies. Some of the components of agglutinating complements are interchangeable with the components of lytic and bactericidal complements. **Complement deflection, Complement deviation.** 1. Incomplete fixation of complement; the immune body is present in great excess of the amount required to saturate the antigen and the complement therefore remains in solution, i.e. is deviated from the antigen-antibody complex. 2. The power with which a particular complement is fixed by antigen-antibody complexes (deviability of complement); this varies in different sera, e.g. from different species of animals. **Endocellular complement.** Endocomplement. **Complement fixation.** The removal of added complement from solution by antigen-antibody complexes, as when known specific antigens are used to detect antibodies in sera. Such solutions which have fixed complement will no longer lyse a second antigen-antibody system such as sensitized red cells. Examples are the detection of gonococcal antibodies, syphilitic antibodies, thyroid autoimmune antibodies in Hashimoto's disease and variola antibodies by gonococcal suspension, cardiolipin-lecithin-cholesterol suspensions and vaccinial lymph vaccine, respectively. Conversely, the reaction may be used with known antibodies to identify unknown antigens, e.g. sera of vaccinated rabbits to identify lymph from suspected smallpox cases. **Complement inhibition.** The non-specific inactivation of complement. Examples are inhibition by chylous sera, particulate antigens in the absence of antibodies and other absorbing suspensions. **Complement splitting.** The separation of complement into several distinct components by the precipitation of serum globulins, by treatment with carbon dioxide or with weak acids. The redissolved precipitate (middle piece) will combine with sensitized corpuscles, after which further combination with an unprecipitated component (end piece) will take place. A third component, stable at 55°C, and a fourth component, which is destroyed by ammonia, have also been differentiated. [L *complementum* anything which completes.]

complemental (kom·ple·**ment**·al). Relating to a complement; complementary.

complementary (kom·ple·**ment**·ar·e). 1. Serving to complete. 2. Accessory. 3. Term applied to anything (e.g. a drug) that makes good a deficiency or defect. [complement.]

complementation (**kom**·ple·ment·**a'**·shun). In genetics, the restoration of the non-mutant (wild) phenotype when 2 mutant chromosomes, or homologous parts of chromosomes, are present in the same cell. This indicates that the cell possesses a complete set of functional units (genes) and, therefore, that the mutations in the 2 chromosomes involve different genes. **Interallelic complementation, Intragenic complementation.** Complementation may sometimes be demonstrated in micro-organisms in which the 2 mutations involve the same function; in such cases the functional protein is usually composed of a number of identical polypeptide subunits which, if defective at different sites, may still compensate each other's defects in association. *See* CIS-TRANS TEST, COMPLEMENTATION TEST (under TEST). [complement.]

complementophil (kom·ple·**ment**·o·fil). Having the power of attracting complement; applied to groupings by which complement is attached to the antigen-antibody complex. [complement, Gk *philein* to love.]

complex (**kom**·plex). 1. A definite group of associated signs or symptoms due to a particular cause; a syndrome. 2. The wave complex of an electrocardiogram all of which relates to one event in the cardiac cycle, e.g. the QRS complex, due to ventricular excitation, or the QRST complex, which represents the whole of the ventricular activity in one cycle. 3. A group of repressed emotionally charged ideas with a common emotive tone which unconsciously determine a person's reaction to various situations, e.g. inferiority complex. **Aberrant complex.** Anomalous complex (see following). **Anomalous complex.** An atrial or ventricular complex which has an abnormal form; it is usually due to an impulse arising in an ectopic focus, or, in the case of an anomalous ventricular complex, to bundle-branch block. **Antigen antibody complex.** Immune complex. **Anxiety complex.** A complex in which expressed or repressed anxiety is a dominant feature. **Atrial complex.** The electrocardiographic waves which result from the electrical activity of the atria. The T wave represents the spread of the excitation wave over the atria; this is followed by the Ta wave due to repolarization, but this is small in amplitude and normally is buried in the succeeding ventricular (QRS) complex. **Auricular complex.** Atrial complex (see above). **Bios complex.** Bios I and bios II (*see* BIOS). **Cain complex.** Sib rivalry. **Castration complex.** The anxiety suffered by a male child that his father may deprive him of his genitalia (psychoanalysis). **Diana complex.** The group of masculine psychic tendencies in the female. **Electra complex.** The female counterpart of the Oedipus complex (see below). **Father complex.** 1. In a general sense, any abnormal emotional relationship to the father. 2. Oedipus complex (see below). **Immune complex.** Macromolecular complex of bound antigen and antibody molecules. **Immune complex disease.** Disease caused by the deposition of complement-fixing immune complexes *in vivo*, especially in capillaries, e.g. in the renal glomeruli. It causes an Arthus-type reaction and is believed to be responsible for the lesions of serum sickness and certain types of glomerulonephritis and possibly polyarteritis. **Inferiority complex.** A feeling of inferiority, or the attitude resulting from a repressed feeling of inferiority. **Initiation complex.** The complex which starts the process of polypeptide synthesis in living cells. It is formed by the binding together of messenger RNA, the first (or initiating) aminoacyl transfer RNA and a free 30*S* ribosomal subunit in the presence of 3 specific proteins called *initiation factors*. The formation of this complex requires energy, which is supplied by the hydrolysis of guanosine triphosphate. **Jocasta complex.** In psychoanalysis, the morbid attachment of a mother to her son. [*Jocasta*, mother of Oedipus.] **Junctional complex.** A collective name for the 3 specialized components of intercellular junctions—the zonula occludens, the zonula adherens and the macula adherens. **Lear complex.** Marked attachment of a father to his daughter. **Mother complex.** 1. In a general sense, any abnormal emotional relationship to the mother. 2. Oedipus complex (see following). **Oedipus complex.** The stage in infantile sexual development when there are sexual wishes in regard to the mother, and the father is perceived as an obstacle to them (psychoanalysis). **Ophthalmoganglionar complex.** Unilateral oedema of the eyelids and inflammation of the lacrimal gland in American trypanosomiasis (Chagas' disease). **Persecution complex.** A complex with ideas of persecution as the dominant motif. **Primary complex.** A primary lesion of syphilis, tuberculosis, leishmaniasis, deep fungal infection, or cowpox, in the skin. **QRS complex.** The deflections of the electrocardiogram which are produced by the electrical forces initiated by the spread of the excitation wave through the ventricular muscle during systole (ventricular depolarization). **QRST complex.** The ventricular complex of the electrocardiogram. It consists of the QRS complex (ventricular depolarization during systole), the S-T segment, the Q-T interval, the T wave and the U wave. The T and U waves represent ventricular repolarization during systole. **Sex complex.** 1. The correlation of the sexual functions with the endocrine glands and nervous system. 2. The psychological complex supposed to be based on repressed infantile sexuality. **Superiority complex.** A feeling of superiority, believed often due to a repressed feeling of inferiority. **Complex of symptoms.** A syndrome; a group of symptoms or signs which, associated together, form a clinical entity. **Synaptinemal complex.** A ribbon-like structure which is present in meiotic cells during the zygotene to diplotene state of prophase I and can be seen, under the electron microscope, to span the space between paired chromosomes. The synaptinemal complex is composed of proteins and consists of 3 longitudinal elements (that is, 2 electron-dense lateral bands flanking the chromosomal fibres and a central element of variable appearance) and transverse filaments. Its presence is associated with the occurrence of crossing-over and chiasmata and, therefore, is presumably instrumental in the process of genetic recombination. **Ventricular complex.** QRST complex (see above). [L *complexus* an embrace.]

See also: CLÉRAMBAULT, EISENMENGER, FRIEDMANN (M.), KANDINSKY, LUTEMBACHER.

complexion (kom·plek·shun). The texture and hue or colour of the skin, particularly of the face. [L *complexio* combination.]

complexus (kom·plex·us). The semispinalis capitis muscle. [L an embrace.]

compliance (kom·pli·ans). The property of alteration of the shape or size of a structure as the result of the application of a distorting force; i.e. reduced compliance means greater stiffness. It is measured in terms of the magnitude of the change in size or shape resulting from the application of a unit of distorting force. **Ventricular compliance.** The compliance of a cardiac ventricle in its resting state, which is a property of the thickness of the wall and the condition of the muscle; it determines the relationship between the filling of the ventricle and its diastolic pressure. [It. *complire* complete.]

complicated (kom·ple·ka·ted). Complex or involved; applied to a disease or injury with which another disease or injury has become associated so that the symptoms of the first are altered and the course changed. [L *complicare* to fold together.]

complication (kom·ple·ka·shun). 1. The co-existence in a patient of 2 or more separate diseases. 2. Any disease or condition that is co-existent with and modifies the course of the primary disease but need not be connected with it. [see prec.]

compligon (kom·ple·gon). Gonococcal culture filtrate.

component (kom·po·nent). Constituent part. **Active component.** Active current; that component of an alternating current which is in phase with the voltage. **Plasma thromboplastin component.** (P.T.C.). Christmas factor. **Somatic motor component.** Neurones conducting impulses to the voluntary musculature. **Somatic sensory component.** Neurones conducting impulses from the somatic sensory nerve-endings. **Splanchnic motor component.** Neurones conducting impulses to those organs containing involuntary muscle and that are supplied by the splanchnic nerves. **Splanchnic sensory component.** Neurones conducting afferent impulses from the area supplied by the splanchnic nerves. **Tagged components.** A compound or element in which some atoms are rendered physically observable by the substitution of a stable isotope of different mass or a radioactive isotope of the atom normally present. [L *componere* to put together.]

compos mentis (kom·pos men·tis). Of sound mind. [L.]

composition (kom·po·zish·un). 1. In chemistry, the respective proportions of the components forming a mixture, or of the elements forming a compound. 2. Compound powder of bayberry. 3. In dentistry, a hard material with a resin base which, becoming soft on heating, is used for taking impressions in the mouth. It is also used on a mould to hold a graft or epithelial inlay in position pending its attachment to the underlying tissues. **Atomic composition of tissue.** The overall proportions of the different elements in tissue. **Composition essence, Composition powder.** A preparation of bayberry, ginger, capsicum and clove, used as a remedy for colds. [L *componere* to put together.]

See also: STENT.

compound (kom·pownd). 1. To mix 2 or more substances together intimately, as with drugs. 2. Chemically, an individual, pure, homogeneous substance of constant composition, formed by the union of 2 or more atoms of different elements by valency bonds, which cannot be split up again except by reactions requiring energy. **Acyclic compound.** An organic compound consisting of atoms linked in an open chain. **Addition compound.** The combination of 2 simpler compounds into 1 more complex without the elimination of any part of the components. **Additive compound.** A new substance formed by the saturation of the double or triple bonds of an unsaturated compound. **Aliphatic compound.** A derivative of the acyclic fatty hydrocarbons. **Aromatic compound.** A derivative of benzene or quinone. **Asymmetric compound.** One displaying optical activity by reason of its containing an asymmetric carbon atom. **Azo compound.** One containing the group -N=N- between 2 alkyl radicals. **Benzene compound.** An aromatic compound derived from benzene. **Binary compound.** A compound composed of only 2 elements. **Carbamino compound.** Name given to any compound derived from urea (carbamide) and containing the group NH_2 CONH. **Carbon compound.** An organic compound (see below). **Closed-chain compound.** A compound containing a ring of atoms. **Coal-tar compound.** Usually an aromatic compound. **Condensation compound.** One formed by the union of 2 or more compounds, usually with the elimination of water. **Cyclic compound.** A closed-chain compound (see above). **Diazo compound.** One containing the group -N=N- between an aryl radical and an acid or OH group. **Endothermic compound.** One the formation of which is attended with the absorption of heat. **Exothermic compound.** One the formation of which is attended with the liberation of heat. **Fatty compound.** An aliphatic compound (see above). **Compound fracture.** *See* FRACTURE. **Heterocyclic compound.** One which contains a ring or rings which include other elements besides carbon. **Inorganic compound.** A compound of elements other than carbon except when the latter is in the form of a carbonate or carbide. **Isocyclic compound.** One containing a ring composed only of the same atoms. **Labelled compound.** Usually a compound in which one or more of the atoms of a proportion of the molecules is replaced by a radioactive isotope of the atom concerned. **Non-polar compound.** A non-electrolyte, one that does not dissociate ionically; most organic compounds. **Open-chain compound.** One the atoms of which are linked into a chain that does not join at the ends. **Organic compounds.** The compounds of carbon; those found in living tissues and processes. **Paraffin compound.** A derivative of the aliphatic hydrocarbons. **Quaternary compound.** A compound analogous to an ammonium compound except that all 4 hydrogen atoms are replaced by alkyl radicals. **Racemic compound.** An isomer of an optically-active compound which displays no optical rotation by reason of its being a mixture or loose molecular association in equal parts of the mutually compensating dextro- and laevorotatory isomers; it can be separated into the latter by physical or chemical methods. Usually denoted by the prefix *dl-* or *r-*, it derives its name from the racemic acid in grape juice. [Obsolete term.] **Ring compound.** One containing a closed chain of atoms. **Saturated compound.** One in which all valencies are fully absorbed. **Substitution compound.** A compound derived from another by the substitution of different elements or radicals in the first. **Symmetrical compound.** Any aromatic compound in which substituted groups are arranged round a benzene ring in a regular manner. **Tagged compounds.** Compounds to which isotopes and other substances have been attached in order to facilitate tracing them in the body. **Ternary compound.** A compound of 3 different elements.

Unsaturated compound. A compound containing double or triple bonds. [L *componere* to put together.]
See also: GRIGNARD.

compound 1080. Sodium fluoroacetate; a rodent poison.

compound B. Corticosterone.

compound E. Cortisone.
See also: KENDALL.

compound F. Hydrocortisone.
See also: KENDALL.

compounding (kom·**pownd**·ing). The art of the dispenser in mixing drugs to make a preparation which is both elegant and suitable for the purpose for which is is required. [L *componere* to put together.]

compress (**kom**·pres). A pad of damp, thickly-folded lint or linen, applied to an area for the relief of pain or the reduction of inflammation. A hot compress is known as a *fomentation.* **Electrothermic compress.** A pad consisting of material incorporating wires which is placed in contact with the body and heated by a strong electric current. [L *comprimere* to press together.]

compression (kom·**presh**·un). 1. The state of being compressed or of being pressed together into narrower compass. 2. The process of decreasing the volume and increasing the density of a body or a gas by means of force applied externally. **Compression arthrodesis.** *See* ARTHRODESIS. **Compression of the brain, Cerebral compression.** Increased intracranial pressure due to haemorrhage, inflammation, abscess, tumour or other cause. **Digital compression.** The arresting of haemorrhage by compressing a blood vessel with the fingers. **Instrumental compression.** Compression applied to a blood vessel by close application of an instrument or mechanical agent. **Compression plating.** The internal fixation of a fracture using a plate and a compressive device. **Compression treatment of fractures.** A method of acceleration of bony union by compressing together fractured surfaces with the aid of pins inserted into the bone and an external compression apparatus. Used also in arthrodesis. [see prec.]
See also: LERICHE.

compressor (kom·**pres**·or). 1. A surgical instrument for producing pressure on a part. 2. In anatomy, a muscle which compresses a tubular or saccular structure, orifice or gland; the term is seldom used now. **Aortic compressor.** An instrument for compressing the aorta through the abdominal wall. **Compressor bulbi proprius.** A part of the bulbospongiosus muscle. **Compressor labii.** A marginal bundle of fibres in the orbicularis oris muscle. **Compressor sacculi laryngis.** Fibres of the aryepiglottic and thyro-arytenoid muscles which compress the saccule of the larynx. **Compressor urethrae.** The sphincter of the membranous part of the urethra. [L *comprimere* to press together.]

compressor naris muscle (kom·**pres**·or **na**·ris musl). *See* NASAL MUSCLES, Pars transversa.

compressorium (kom·pres·**or**·e·um). A glass cell in which microscopic objects may be pressed under the cover glass, for examination. [L *comprimere* to press together.]

Compsomyia macellaria (komp·so·**mi**·e·ah mas·el·a·re·ah). *Cochliomyia macellaria.* [Gk *kompsos* elegant, *myia* fly, *makellon* slaughter house.]

Compton, Arthur Holly (b. 1892). American physicist.

Compton absorption. Absorption of electromagnetic radiation due to the Compton effect, in which a scattered photon of lower energy is emitted and an electron is given kinetic energy. The sum of the energies of the electron and scattered photon is equal to the energy of the incident photon.

Compton effect. When an x-ray quantum is scattered by a free electron, the wavelength of the scattered x-ray quantum is increased and the electron recoils. The principles of conservation of energy and of momentum are maintained in the process.

Compton scatter. Scatter of photons by the Compton effect with decrease of energy of the scattered photon, kinetic energy being given to the scattering electron.

compulsion (kum·**pul**·shun). In psychology, an irresistible urge, sometimes amounting to obsession, to perform a particular act which usually is carried out against the performer's will or better judgment. **Compulsion act.** Compulsive act. *See* ACT. **Compulsion neurosis.** *See* NEUROSIS. [L *compellere* to urge.]

compulsive (kum·**pul**·siv). Done under the stress of compulsion. **Compulsive act.** *See* ACT.

computer (kom·**pu**·ter). **Analogue computer.** A computer composed of circuits which can be made to form an analogue of the system to be studied, its parameters are continuously variable. **Digital computer.** A computer which handles data in digital form; it calculates using the binary scale.

conalbumin (kon·**al**·bew·min). A protein constituent of the white of eggs.

conamen (ko·**nam**·en). Attempted suicide. [L *conari* to attempt.]

conarial (ko·**na**·re·al). Relating to the pineal body (conarium).

conariohypophyseal (ko·**na**·re·o·hi·po·**fiz**'·e·al). Relating to the pineal body and the hypophysis cerebri. [conarium, hypophysis.]

conarium (ko·**na**·re·um). An obsolete name for the pineal body, originally conferred upon it because of its shape. [Gk *konarion* little cone.]

conation (ko·**na**·shun). In psychology: 1. The force which impels to exertion of any kind, or which directs it. 2. Any particular act of the impelling force. [L *conari* to attempt.]

conative (**kon**·at·iv). Relating to the striving force. [see prec.]

concameration (kon·kam·er·a'·shun). A system or arrangement of interconnecting cavities. [L *concamerare* to arch over.]

concassation (kon·kas·a·shun). 1. The comminution of fibres or roots of medicinal plants so that their active principles become separated. 2. The shaking up of medicines in a vessel or bottle. [L *concassare* to beat.]

concatenate (kon·**kat**·en·ate). Arranged in a connected series, row, or chain. [L *concatenare* to chain together.]

concatenation (kon·**kat**·en·**a**'·shun). 1. A series of structures arranged together in a row like the links of a chain, e.g. enlarged lymph glands. 2. The chain arrangement of cells that form a nerve or nerve tract. [see prec.]

Concato, Luigi Maria (b. 1825). Italian physician.

Concato's disease. Polyserositis.

Concato's pericarditis. Involvement of the pericardium with other serous cavities, probably from tuberculosis, resulting in chronic adhesive changes and producing constrictive pericarditis.

concave (**kon**·kave). 1. Hollowed. 2. Curved like the interior of an arched surface or line. [L *concavare* to make hollow.]

concavity (kon·**kav**·it·e). 1. A fossa. 2. The hollow space included by a concave line. 3. The inside of a curved organ or surface, or the hollow included in it. [see prec.]

concavoconcave (kon·**ka**·vo·**kon**'·kave). Concave on both sides.

concavoconvex (kon·**ka**·vo·**kon**'·vex). Having a concave and a convex surface, e.g. a lens.

concealment of birth (kon·**seel**·ment). The action of any person who after delivery of a child, whether it be alive or dead, endeavours to conceal the birth. The child must be properly concealed (i.e. hidden). [OFr. *conceler,* birth.]

conceive (kon·**seev**). To become pregnant. [L *concipere* to take in.]

concentrate (**kon**·sen·trate). 1. To focus, or direct to a common point. 2. To reduce the bulk and increase the strength of a solution, by evaporation of the solvent. 3. A strong solution provided for dilution before use. **Vitamin concentrate.** A medicinal preparation of vitamins. [L *cum, centrum* centre.]

concentration (kon·sen·**tra**·shun). 1. The state in which the attention is fixed upon and restricted to any particular matter. 2. The process of increasing the strength of a solution by evaporation of the solvent. 3. The increasing of the potency of a medicine by the elimination of inactive constituents. 4. The strength of a solution expressed as the number of gram-equivalents of the solute contained in a litre. **Hydrogen-ion concentration.** The number of grams of hydrogen ion present in a litre of solution: this is denoted by the symbol C_H; the logarithm of the reciprocal of the latter is the pH value of the solution. **Ionic concentration.** The number of gram-equivalents of an ion in a litre of solution. **Maximum permissible concentration.** The upper limit of concentration of radioactive material (usually in the air or in drinking water) such that, for continuous occupational exposure, the dose received by any body tissues cannot exceed the permissible dose. The limit depends upon a number of factors, such as the physical and chemical properties of the radioactive material, and the method of intake into the body. **Mean corpuscular haemoglobin concentration.** M.C.H.C., the mean haemoglobin concentration expressed as a percentage of the volume of a single red corpuscle; it is given by the formula:

$$\frac{\text{haemoglobin (grams per 100 ml blood)}}{\text{packed cell volume (\%)} \times 100}$$

The normal value is 33–38 per cent (mean 35 per cent). **Minimal alveolar concentration.** Of an anaesthetic vapour, the least possible alveolar concentration which will produce lack of reflex response to skin incision in 50 per cent of subjects tests. A concept propounded by G. Merkel and E. I. Eger in 1963. **Molecular concentration.** The concentration of a substance in solution expressed as the number of gram-molecular weights per unit volume of solution (litre). **Prothrombin concentration.** A measure of the amount of prothrombin in the blood plasma calculated from the plasma prothrombin time of the test sample and of a normal plasma. With the normal plasma prothrombin time adjusted to 12 s, the plasma prothrombin concentration is given by 302/(clotting time − 8.7). **Radioactive concentration.** The activity per unit quantity of any material containing a radionuclide. **Radio-isotope concentration.** The percentage content of a radio-isotope in solid or solution, expressed as mC/g or mC/cm^3. **Urea concentration.** A measurement of renal efficiency based upon the excretion of urea after a large dose of the latter has been given. [see prec.]

concentric (kon·**sen**·trik). Having a common centre. [L *cum, centrum* centre.]

concept (**kon**·sept). The image or notion which the mind forms of an action or a thing. [L *concipere* to take in.]

conception (kon·**sep**·shun). 1. The act of becoming pregnant. 2. The fertilization of the ovum by a spermatozoon and the beginning of the growth of the embryo. 3. Concept. **Imperative conception.** In psychiatry, a delusion of which the patient cannot rid himself although he knows it is not reasonable; it appears spontaneously and dominates his actions. [see prec.]

conceptive (kon·**sep**·tiv). Capable of conceiving. [see foll.]

conceptus (kon·**sep**·tus). The developing product of conception throughout the period of gestation. [L conception.]

concha (**kong**·kah) (pl. *conchae*). A shell; in anatomy, any structure thought to resemble a shell in form. **Concha of the auricle [concha auriculae (NA)].** The deep depression on the outer surface of the auricle, the lower part of which leads into the external auditory meatus. **Concha bullosa.** A distension of the turbinated bone, usually the middle, due to the formation of a cyst. **Nasal concha, highest [concha nasalis suprema (NA)].** A small supernumerary concha in the spheno-ethmoidal recess of the nose, above the superior nasal concha. **Nasal conchae, superior, middle, inferior [concha nasalis, superior, media, inferior (NA)].** Ridges of bone which project into the nasal cavity from its lateral wall and separate the superior, middle and inferior meatuses of the nose. **Concha santorini.** The highest nasal concha (see above). **Sphenoidal concha [concha sphenoidalis (NA)].** The thin papery bone which forms part of the anterior wall of the body of the sphenoid and partially encloses the sphenoidal air sinuses. [L.]

See also: SANTORINI.

conchiform (**kong**·ke·form). 1. Shell-shaped. 2. Having the form of one half of a bivalve shell. [Gk *kogche* shell, form.]

conchinine (**kon**·kin·een). Quinidine.

conchiolinosteomyelitis (**kong**·ke·o·lin·**os**·te·o·mi·el·**i**'·tis). A form of osteomyelitis which attacks pearl workers. [Gk *kogche* shell, osteomyelitis.]

conchitis (kong·**ki**·tis). A condition of inflammation of the concha of the ear, or of the nasal conchae. [concha, Gk *-itis* inflammation.]

conchoidal (kong·**koid**·al). 1. Like a shell. 2. Conchiform, 2nd def. [Gk *kogche* shell, *eidos* form.]

conchologist (kong·**kol**·o·jist). A specialist in conchology.

conchology (kong·**kol**·o·je). The science of shells: this includes the study of snails and shell-fish. [Gk *kogche* shell, *logos* science.]

conchoscope (**kong**·ko·skope). A speculum with attached mirror for inspection of the cavity of the nose (nasal conchae). [concha, Gk *skopein* to watch.]

conchotome (**kong**·ko·tome). A surgical knife used in removing part or the whole of the nasal conchae. [concha, Gk *temnein* to cut.]

conchotomy (kong·**kot**·o·me). The surgical removal of the nasal conchae. [see prec.]

conchyliologist (**kong**·ki·le·**ol**'·o·jist). Conchologist.

conchyliology (**kong**·ki·le·**ol**'·o·je). Conchology.

conclination (kon·klin·a·shun). Adtorsion; a condition in which both eyes turn inwards and their vertical meridians converge above instead of being parallel. [L *cum*, Gk *klinein* to incline.]

concoctio (kon·**kok**·she·o). The process of digestion. **Concoctio tarda.** Dyspepsia. [L *cum, coquere* to cook.]

concomitant (kon·**kom**·it·ant). Conjoined; accessory; accompanying. [L *cum, comitari* to accompany.]

conconscious (kon·**kon**·shus). In psychology, a term indicating that mental processes are going on in the mind of an individual of which he is not aware. [L *cum, scire* to know.]

concrement (**kon**·kre·ment). 1. A concretion. 2. A nodule or small mass which has become calcified. [L *cum, crescere* to increase.]

concrescence (kon·**kres**·ens). 1. The fusion of 2 parts which were originally separate. 2. The fusion together of the roots of the upper second and third molar teeth by seondary cementum; false or pathological germination. 3. Of protozoa, conjugation. [L *concrescere* to grow together.]

concrete (**kon**·kreet). Solid, formed into a hard mass. **Barium concrete.** Concrete containing a high proportion of barytes (barium sulphate). Used as a protective building material in the walls of x-ray rooms. [see prec.]

concretio cordis (kon·**kre**·she·o **kor**·dis). Chronic constrictive pericarditis. [L growing together of the heart.]

concretion (kon·**kre**·shun). 1. A calculus. 2. A hard or solid mass of foreign material present in a cavity of the body or within an organism. 3. The act or process of becoming solid or calcified. 4. An adhesion of 2 parts. **Alvine concretion.** A bezoar or a calculus present in the alimentary canal. **Arterial concretion.** A formation of chalky matter in one artery. **Calculus concretion.** Arthritic calculus. **Cutaneous concretion.** A concretion present in the tissues underlying the skin. **Intestinal concretion.** Enterolith. **Preputial concretion.** A concretion composed of smegma and urinary salts deposited beneath a tight foreskin. **Tophic concretion.** A tophus. **Umbilical concretion.** A concretion formed in the umbilical orifice by the gradual accumulation and drying of cornified epithelium. [L *concrescere* to grow together.]

concubitus (kon·**kew**·bit·us). Coitus. [L *cum, cumbere* to lie.]

concussion (kon·**kush**·un). 1. The sudden application of a violent force, or the results of that violence. 2. A state in which there is loss of consciousness, possibly only transient, which is usually followed by amnesia, resulting from a head injury. **Air concussion.** The effects of the blast of an explosion. **Concussion of the brain, Cerebral concussion.** Main def. 2 (see above). **Hydraulic abdominal concussion.** Abdominal injuries produced in a swimmer by underwater explosion. **Concussion of the labyrinth.** Damage to the labyrinth as a result of trauma. It may be from a blow, or from sudden overstimulation from a noise. **Pulmonary concussion.** Blast effect on the lungs. **Concussion of the retina.** When the front of the eye is struck, the retina being affected by contrecoup, usually at the posterior pole. The commonest reaction is the development of oedema, Berlin's oedema, or commotio retinae, which may subside completely or result in the formation of a "hole" at the macula with loss of central vision. **Concussion of the spine.** Temporary loss of function in the spinal cord due to spinal injury and associated with muscle paralysis and anaesthesia below the level of the injury. [L *concussio* a shaking together.]

concussor (kon·**kus**·er). An instrument which is used in massage and vibratory therapeutics for the purpose of applying light taps to the part under treatment. [see prec.]

condensability (kon·**den**·sab·**il**'·it·e). Degree to which matter is capable of being condensed. [L *condensare* to make thick.]

condensation (kon·den·**sa**·shun). 1. The act or process of becoming or being made more dense. 2. The process of reducing to another and denser form, as steam to water. 3. In psychoanalysis, a new mental image produced by a fusion of concepts, thoughts, or events, so that energy is spared. 4. In dentistry, the practice of making a filling in a tooth compact and therefore more resistant to the forces of mastication. [see prec.]

condensed (kon·**denst**). 1. Made more compact. 2. Reduced to a denser form, e.g. a gaseous to a liquid state. [see foll.]

condenser (kon·**den**·ser). 1. A device by means of which energy or matter may be condensed. 2. An optical arrangement of lenses and mirrors so that light may be concentrated on an object being examined under a microscope. 3. An apparatus with which gases or vapours may be cooled to a state of liquidity. 4. An apparatus consisting of a series of insulated conductors for the accumulation of electricity. **Cardioid condenser.** A device for use with the ultramicroscope so that light can be concentrated to give dark-field illumination. **Dark-ground condenser.** One that reflects the light in such a way that the objects in a microscope field are illuminated and stand out against a dark (unilluminated) background. **Paraboloid condenser.** A microscope condenser suited to dark-ground use. [L *condensare* to make thick.]

See also: ABBÉ.

conditioning (kon·**dish**·un·ing). 1. Improving a clinical condition by physical exercises. 2. In psychology, the acquisition of new stimulus-response connections. Includes *classical conditioning,* in which an indifferent stimulus, by being repeatedly associated with the specific stimulus exciting a response, leads eventually to that response, and *operant conditioning,* in which a naturally-occurring response is strengthened by positive reinforcement (reward) or weakened by negative reinforcement (punishment). [L *conditio* condition.]

condom (**kon**·dom, **kun**·dom). A sheath of thin rubber or similar material worn over the penis during coitus in order to contain the semen and prevent conception or infection. [*Condon,* London physician of the 18th century, the reputed inventor.]

conduct (kon·**dukt**). **Infamous conduct.** An older term used by the General Medical Council to describe conduct grossly unbecoming to a doctor's professional or moral code: adultery, advertisement, abuse of privileges, abortion practice of unlawful kind, association with unqualified persons, etc. [L *conducere* to conduct.]

conductance (kon·**duk**·tans). Conductivity. **Electrical conductance.** Electrical conductivity. *See* CONDUCTIVITY.

conductibility (kon·**duk**·tib·**il**'·it·e). 1. Conductivity. 2. Capability of being conducted, as nerve impulses. **Centrifugal conductibility.** The capability of carrying nervous impulses to the periphery from the centre. **Centripetal conductibility.** The capability of carrying nervous impulses to the centre from the periphery. [see foll.]

conduction (kon·**duk**·shun). The handing-on or transfer of a stimulus or wave motion; in medicine, the transmission through the tissues of heat, sound waves (e.g. those arising from the heart), or electrical currents (e.g. those passing along nerves). **Aberrant conduction.** Conduction of an impulse from the atria to the ventricles of the heart by any pathway or pathways other than the normal. It is recognized by the occurrence of abnormal QRS patterns in beats which are stimulated by conduction from preceding atrial activity. **Accelerated conduction.** *See* SYNDROME, ACCELERATED CONDUCTION. **Aerial conduction.** The conduction of sound waves from the outside air to the inner ear via the auditory meatus or middle ear, as distinct from bone conduction (see below). **Aerotympanal conduction.** Aerial conduction (see preceding). **Antidromic conduction.** Conduction of a nerve impulse in the reverse direction to the normal. **Atrioventricular conduction.** The conduction of the stimulating impulse from the atria of the heart to the ventricles, which is normally via the atrioventricular node and the His bundle system but may be via abnormal accessory pathways, as in the Wolff–Parkinson–White syndrome. **Avalanche conduction.** Conduction of a nerve impulse in which one neurone stimulates a number of others. **Bone conduction.** Conduction of sound waves to the inner ear through the bones of the skull. **Cardiac conduction.** The transmission through the heart of the nervous impulses that are responsible for the beating of the heart. **Concealed conduction.** The phenomenon of conduction of an impulse into some part of the heart which is not manifested by any electrocardiographic or mechanical activity. It cannot, by its nature, be demonstrated directly but may be deduced from evidence that the part of the heart concerned is subsequently refractory to stimulation. The phenomenon is usually observed in the branches of the His bundle system. **Cranial conduction.** Bone conduction (see above). **Decremental conduction.** Progressive slowing of conduction within the His bundle system with each successive beat until an impulse is blocked, after which conduction is restored to its initial velocity and the whole cycle is repeated: the mechanism of the *Wenckebach phenomenon.* **Delayed cardiac conduction.** Delay in the transmission of nervous impulses in the heart as a result of interference with the specialized conducting tissue. **Electric conduction.** The flow of an electric charge through a conducting medium between points of different potential. **Irreversibility of conduction.** The principle that the conduction of a nerve impulse can occur in only one direction in the pathway of a reflex. **Osteotympanic conduction.** Bone conduction (see above). **Reflex conduction.** The conduction of a nerve impulse from the afferent to the efferent side of a reflex arc. **Retrograde conduction.** The conduction of a stimulating impulse from the ventricles, usually arising from an ectopic force, backwards to the atria through either the normal His bundle system or through an accessory pathway, as found in the Wolff–Parkinson–White syndrome. **Saltatory conduction.** The mode of conduction of a nerve impulse along a myelinated nerve in which the action potential passes rapidly from node to node. **Supernormal conduction.** Conduction in the His bundle system occurring because of, and during, supernormal phase of recovery of the cells involved. **Synaptic conduction.** Conduction of a nerve impulse across a synapse. **Tissue conduction.** Allied to bone conduction, but sometimes used when the source of vibration is placed on a part of the body some distance from the ear. [L *conducere* to conduct.]

conductivity (kon·duk·**tiv**·it·e). The measure of the conduction of heat, light, sound, or electricity by a substance. **Electrical conductivity.** The amount of current that flows through a 1 m (1 cm) cube of a substance when a difference in potential of 1 V is applied between the faces: this unit is the siemens (mho), and the reciprocal of the unit of resistance, the ohm. **Thermal conductivity.** The number of joules (calories) that will pass through a 1 m (1 cm) cube of a substance in 1 s when there is a difference in temperature of 1°C between the faces. [see prec.]

conductor (kon·**duk**·tor). 1. A grooved sound for guiding the knife in surgery. 2. A part of the nervous system along which impulses pass. 3. An agent for the transmission of force-vibrations. 4. A substance through which electricity can pass. 5. The healthy and unaffected transmitter of a hereditary disease or condition, e.g. the daughter of a man suffering from psoriasis. **Sonorous conductor.** The nerve fibres of the corpus trapezoideum which run up to the lateral lemniscus in company with the auditory striae. [L *conducere* to conduct.]

See also: BERGMANN (G. H.).

conduit (**kon**·dit). An artificial channel; an aqueduct. **Colon conduit.** The use of an isolated loop of colon to which one, or both, ureters have been anastomosed, to drain urine to the skin surface. **Ileal conduit.** The use of an isolated loop of ileum to which one, or both, ureters have been anastomosed, to drain urine to the skin surface. [O.Fr.]

conduplicate (kon·**dew**·plik·ate). Folded back upon itself, so that one half of a surface lies along the surface of the other half. [L *cum, duplicare* to double.]

conduplicatio corporis (kon·**dew**·plik·**a**'·she·o **kor**·por·is). In transverse presentation, a doubled-up attitude of the fetus. [L doubling up of the body.]

condurango (kon·dew·**rang**·go). The bark obtained from the stem of the climbing plant *Marsdenia condurango* Nichols (family Asclepiadaceae), which contains a poisonous glycoside, or mixture of glycosides. It is used as a gastric sedative in the form of a liquid extract, and as a wine. [Sp.]

Condy, Henry Bollmann. 19th century British physician.

Condy's fluid. A disinfectant solution prepared from the permanganates of sodium and potassium.

condylar (kon·**di**·lar). Relating or belonging to a condyle, or involving it. **Condylar part of occipital bone.** *See* OCCIPITAL BONE. [Gk *kondylos* knuckle.]

condylarthrosis (kon·di·lar·**thro**'·sis). A condyloid articulation, e.g. that of the knee. [Gk *kondylos* knuckle, *arthron* joint.]

condyle (kon·dile). A rounded articular surface at the end of a bone, e.g. of the humerus. **External condyle.** Lateral condyle (see below). **Condyle of the humerus [condylus humeri (NA)].** The distal end of the bone. **Internal condyle.** Medial condyle (see below). **Lateral condyle [condylus lateralis (NA)].** 1. The prominent expansion of bone at the lower end of the femur on the lateral aspect. 2. The prominent mass of bone at the upper end of the tibia on the lateral aspect. **Condyle of the mandible.** The condyloid process of the mandible. *See* PROCESS. **Medial condyle [condylus medialis (NA)].** 1. The prominent expansion of bone at the lower end of the femur on the medial side. 2. The prominent mass of bone at the upper end of the tibia on the medial side. **Occipital condyle [condylus occipitalis (NA)].** An oval process situated inferiorly on the condylar part of the occipital bone and articulating with the atlas. [Gk *kondylos* knuckle.]

condylectomy (kon·di·**lek**·to·me). Amputation of a condyle. [condyle, Gk *ektome* a cutting out.]

condylicus (kon·**di**·lik·us). Condylar.

condylion (kon·**di**·le·on). The blunt point on the head of the condyloid process of the mandible which projects beyond the lateral surface of the other parts of the ramus.

condyloid (kon·**di**·loid). 1. Condylar. 2. Shaped like a knuckle or condyle. **Condyloid joint.** Ellipsoid joint. *See* JOINT. **Condyloid process of the mandible.** *See* PROCESS. [condyle, Gk *eidos* form.]

condyloma (kon·di·**lo**·mah) (pl. *condylomata*). A wart-like tumour formed by hypertrophy of the prickle-cell layer of the epidermis. **Condyloma acuminatum.** Fig wart; moist wart: pointed wart; venereal wart; verruca acuminata: a filiform or cauliflower-like soft, oedematous wart affecting the genitalia or nearby area. The lesion is a simple wart, modified by its situation; its association with venereal disease is fortuitous. **Flat condyloma, Condyloma latum.** A large moist, flat papule found commonly near the anus or on the vulva in secondary syphilis. The lesions are always multiple, and may occur also in the flexures and even between the toes. Condylomata may occur in children suffering from congenital syphilis who have passed the polymorphic eruption stage; they are rarely seen before the sixth month or after the sixth year. **Malignant condyloma.** A variety of giant condyloma acuminatum. **Condyloma neonatorum.** Condylomata at the angles of the mouth and in the flexures in congenital syphilis. **Pointed condyloma.** Condyloma acuminatum (see above). **Syphilitic condyloma, Condyloma syphiliticum.** Condyloma latum (see above). [Gk *kondyloma* knob.]

condylomatoid (kon·di·**lo**·mat·oid). Like a condyloma. [condyloma, Gk *eidos* form.]

condylomatosis (kon·di·lo·mat·**o**'·sis). The condition in which condylomata are present. [condyloma, Gk *-osis* condition.]

condylomatous (kon·di·**lo**·mat·us). 1. Characterized by the presence of condylomata. 2. Belonging to a condyloma.

condylosis (kon·di·**lo**·sis). A condition in which condylomata form. [condyloma, Gk *-osis* condition.]

condylotomy (kon·di·**lot**·o·me). A division or incision of a condyle. [condyle, Gk *temnein* to cut.]

condylus (kon·**di**·lus). Condyle. [L.]

cone (kone). 1. A solid geometrical figure with a circular base and a pointed apex. 2. A retinal cone (see below). **Adjusting cones.** Two hollow cones, employed in measuring the distance between the visual axes when they are parallel. **Antipodal cone.** That part of the aster opposite to the spindle of a dividing cell. **Attraction cone.** A conical projection from the surface of the ovum at the site of penetration of the spermatozoon. **Bifurcation cone.** A swelling on a dendrite at its bifurcation. **Cerebellar pressure cone.** Plugging of the cerebellar tonsils and medulla into the foramen magnum by pressure from above. **Ether cone.** An appliance for giving anaesthetic ether. **Fertilization cone.** Attraction cone (see above). **Fibrous cone.** The corona radiata of follicle cells around the mature ovum. **Graduated cone.** A cone-shaped body used for measuring the orifices of valves or the diameters of blood vessels at post-mortem examination. **Growth cone.** A swelling at the tip of a growing axon. **Implantation cone.** The swelling at the origin of an axon from a nerve-cell body. **Keratosic cone.** The horny elevations which sometimes occur on the palms of the hands and soles of the feet, in association with gonorrhoeal rheumatism. Also known as *keratoderma blennorrhagica,* or *keratosis blennorrhagica.* **Cone of light.** Those rays of light which pass through the pupil to form an image on the retina. *See also* OCULAR CONE (below). **Medullary cone.** The conus medullaris. **Ocular cone.** A cone of light (see above) whose base is taken as being on the cornea. In neither case are these strictly conical, because the direction of the rays is altered by the refraction of the lens. **Primitive cone.** A renal pyramid. **Radiographic cone.** A metallic cone (sizes variable) for attachment to a diagnostic x-ray tube to confine the x-ray beam. *See* COLLIMATOR. **Retinal cone.** The cone-shaped outer end of one of the 2 types of light-sensitive cell in the retina. **Sarcoplasmic cone.** One of the 2 clear areas of cytoplasm adjacent to the poles of the nucleus of a plain or cardiac muscle fibre. **Spermatic cone.** One of the conical masses composing the head of the epididymis; Haller's cone. **Tentorial pressure cone.** Plugging of the hippocampal gyrus, mid-brain, etc., into the tentorial hiatus by pressure from above. **Terminal cone.** The conus medullaris. **Theca interna cone.** A lunate wedge of theca interna cells covering the graafian follicle near the point where rupture will take place at ovulation. **Treatment cone.** Beam-therapy applicator. *See* APPLICATOR. **Twin cones.** Binucleated retinal cones formed by the fusion of adjacent cones. **Vascular cone.** Graduated cone (see above). **Visual cone.** Ocular cone (see above). [Gk *konos* cone.]

See also: HALLER, POLITZER, WILDE.

conessi bark (ko·**nes**·e bark). Kurchi; holarrhena: the dried bark from the stem and root of the small Indian tree, *Holarrhena antidysenterica* Wall. (family Apocynaceae). It contains the alkaloid conessine, and is used in India for the treatment of amoebic dysentery. [East Ind.]

conessine (ko·**nes**·een). An alkaloid, $C_{24}H_{40}N_2$, obtained from the dried bark of the small tree, *Holarrhena dysenterica* Wall. It is used in India in the indigenous systems of medicine and was tested very thoroughly by British and Indian pharmacologists with unimpressive results. Then it was again revived as a treatment of dysentery in the French tropical colonies and some good results were claimed. [see prec.]

confabulation (kon·**fab**·ew·**la**'·shun). The recital of experiences that have no foundation in fact and the glib untruthful answering of questions usually in compensation for a gap in memory. [L *cum, fabulari* to speak.]

confectio (kon·**fek**·she·o). Confection. [L.]

confection (kon·**fek**·shun). A sweet preparation containing drugs in the dry, raw state, or in the form of a soft extract, and mixed with sugar, honey or syrup. Such preparations have the consistency of a stiff paste. They are not commonly used in modern therapeutics. **Confection of rose.** A mixture of the pulp of the fruit of the dog rose, *Rosa canina,* and sugar. It is an old-fashioned pill excipient. **Confection of Senna BPC 1959.** A mixture of powdered senna, figs, tamarinds and prunes, all having a mild laxative action, with coriander, cassia and liquorice as flavouring agents, and sugar to sweeten the preparation. **Compound confection of senna.** A mixture of powdered jalap, senna and sulphur, with black treacle. It has a fairly potent laxative action. **Confection of sulphur.** A confection of precipitated sulphur and potassium acid tartrate, both with laxative action, glycerin, syrup and tincture of orange to flavour it, and gum tragacanth to stiffen the preparation. [L *conficere* to prepare.]

confertus (kon·fer·tus). Crowded, squeezed or crushed together, as in certain dermal lesions in which there is confluency and heaping up of crusts. [L *cum, ferre* to bring.]

configuration (kon·fig·ewr·a′·shun). 1. The general form and relative disposition of the parts of the body. 2. In chemistry, the spatial relationship of atoms in a molecule. 3. In gestaltism, interdependent parts organized into a whole, the whole being greater than the sum of the parts. **Chain configuration.** Open linear arrangement of chromosomes held together by chiasmata to form a multivalent in the first division of meiosis. *Chain of three, four, etc.*—chain configuration consisting of 3 chromosomes, 4 chromosomes, etc. **Ring configuration.** Closed linear arrangement of chromosomes taking part in the formation of a multivalent at the first meiotic division. [L *configurare* to form from or after something.]

confinement (kon·fine·ment). 1. The puerperal period. 2. Restriction to bed, room or house on account of illness. [Fr. *confiner* to restrain within limits.]

confirmatory (kon·ferm·at·or·e). Serving to confirm or corroborate. [L *confirmare* to make firm.]

conflict (kon·flikt). 1. In psychology, a state of mental hesitancy or inconsistency, in which the sufferer finds it impossible to do without any one form of satisfaction in order to achieve another. 2. Conflict between opposed and incompatible principles or impulses leading to repression and the development of psychoneurosis. **Intrapsychic conflict.** The presence of opposing forces in the mind usually relating to instinctive drives and controlling forces preventing their expression. [L *confligere* to strike together.]

confluence (kon·flew·ens). A running together. **Confluence of sinuses of the dura mater.** *See* SINUS. [see foll.]

confluent (kon·floo·ent). Coalescent or running together, as the pimples or pustules of an eruption, e.g. in confluent smallpox. [L *confluere* to flow together.]

confocal (kon·fo·kal). Having the same focus or foci. [L *cum, focus* hearth.]

conformation (kon·form·a·shun). The particular form, shape or structure of a molecule. [L *conformatio* shape.]

conformator (kon·form·a·tor). An apparatus with which the shape of anything can be determined, e.g. the outlines of the head in craniometry. [L framer.]

confrontation (kon·frun·ta·shun). *See* TEST, CONFRONTATION. [L *cum, frons* forehead.]

confusion (kon·few·zhun). The state of being muddled. [L *confundere* to mix up.]

confusional (kon·few·zhun·al). 1. Characterized by a state of confusion or bewilderment. 2. Having relation to a confused state.

congelation (kon·jel·a·shun). 1. Numbness as the result of exposure to intense cold. 2. The act or process of freezing. 3. Frostbite. 4. Coagulation. [L *cum, gelare* to freeze.]

congener (kon·je·ner). 1. An animal or vegetable organism belonging to the same species as another. 2. A congenerous muscle. 3. A drug belonging to the same group as, or having similar actions to, other drugs. [L of the same race.]

congenerous (kon·jen·er·us). 1. Kindred. 2. Allied as to cause or origin. 3. Having common function or action, as certain muscles. [see prec.]

congenital (kon·jen·it·al). 1. Constitutional or natural. 2. Existing before birth or at birth; dating from birth. [L *congenitus* born with.]

congested (kon·jes·ted). Referring to a part which contains an excessive accumulation of blood. [see foll.]

congestion (kon·jes·chun). Hyperaemia; an excessive accumulation of blood in an organ. **Active congestion, Fluxionary congestion.** An excess of blood in a part, caused by an increased flow or the dilatation of its blood vessels. **Functional congestion.** Active congestion determined by increased functional activity of a part. **Hypostatic congestion.** Congestion due to the action of gravity in a dependent part. **Neuroparalytic congestion.** Congestion due to vasomotor paralysis. **Neurotonic congestion.** Congestion due to vasomotor paralysis. **Passive congestion.** Congestion caused by increased venous pressure. **Physiological congestion.** Increased blood flow during functional activity of an organ. **Pleuropulmonary congestion, Pulmonary congestion.** Congestion of the lungs, either passive, as in heart failure, or active, as in inflammation. **Venous congestion.** Passive congestion due to increased venous pressure or obstruction. [L *congerere* to heap together.]

See also: POTAIN.

congestive (kon·jes·tiv). 1. Anything that causes a state of congestion. 2. Relating to, attended with, or causing congestion.

congius (kon·je·us). In pharmacy, a measure equal to about 4.5 litres (one gallon). [L a liquid measure.]

conglobate (kon·glo·bate). Formed or collected into a rounded mass, as in certain gland accumulations. [L *conglobare* to form into a ball.]

conglomerate (kon·glom·er·ate). 1. Made up of several parts gathered into a mass. 2. Closely crowded together and lacking order. [L *conglomerare* to wind into a ball.]

conglutinant (kon·gloo·tin·ant). 1. Causing to adhere together. 2. An agent which promotes healing together or union, as of the edges of a wound. [see foll.]

conglutinatio (kon·gloo·tin·a′·she·o). Conglutination. **Conglutinatio orificii externi.** Atresia of the external os of the cervix, usually limited to an agglutination of the mucous membrane. [L gluing together.]

conglutination (kon·gloo·tin·a′·shun). 1. The adhesion or sticking together of one object with another. 2. The sticking together or clumping of sensitized erythrocytes by certain constituents of normal serum and other substances such as bovine albumin and polymers such as dextran. Originally referred to the clumping of erythrocytes or bacteria with an antibody in the presence of complement and conglutinin present in serum. 3. Reaction produced by conglutinin. [see prec.]

conglutinin (kon·gloo·tin·in). Protein found in bovine serum which activates complement-containing immune complexes by reacting with activated complement component C3. Conglutinin is not an antibody. [L *conglutinare* to glue together.]

Congo Red BPC 1968 (kong·go red). Sodium diphenylbisazobisnaphthylamine sulphonate, $SO_3NaC_{10}H_5(NH_2)N_2C_6H_4C_6H_4N_2C_{10}H_5(NH_2)SO_3Na$. A benzidine dyestuff which is an indicator for mineral acids in the presence of organic acids (pH 3–5). It is used in the examination of gastric juice, becoming blue with free hydrochloric acid; also administered intravenously in the diagnosis of amyloid disease, the tissue being stained by the dye, and as a haemostatic in haemoptysis.

congressus (kong·gres·sus). Coitus. **Congressus interruptus.** Coitus interruptus. [L a friendly meeting.]

conhydrine (kon·hi·dreen). $C_8H_{17}ON$, a crystalline alkaloid derived from hemlock, *Conium maculatum* Linn. In action it resembles coniine but is less toxic.

coniasis (ko·ni·as·is). A condition in which there are dust-like particles in the bile duct or gall bladder. [Gk *konis* dust.]

coniceine (ko·nis·e·een). $C_8H_{15}N$, any one of a series of 6 alkaloids of the formula, prepared from conhydrine, or, in the case of γ-coniceine, obtained from *Conium maculatum* Linn. Whilst resembling coniine in pharmacological action, their toxicity is much greater.

conicine (ko·nis·een). An isomer of coniine.

conidial (ko·**nid**·e·al). 1. Belonging or relating to conidia. 2. Producing conidia. 3. Resembling conidia.

conidiophore (ko·**nid**·e·o·for). A special enlarged branch of mycelium in certain fungi. It produces the conidia. [conidium, Gk *phoros* bearer.]

conidiospore (ko·**nid**·e·o·spore). Conidium. [conidium, spore.]

conidium (ko·**nid**·e·um). (pl. *conidia*). In botany an asexual spore which develops and is set free by the dividing up of the summit of a conidiophore. [Gk *konidion* particle of dust.]

coniferin (kon·**if**·er·in). $C_6H_{11}OC_6H_3(OCH_3)CH{=}CHCH_2OH$, the natural glucoside of conifers; also found in asparagus. It is hydrolysed to coniferyl alcohol, and oxidized to vanillin.

coniine (**ko**·ne·een). α-Norpropylpiperidine, $C_5H_9NH(CH_2CH_2CH_3)$. A toxic alkaloid present in all parts of the hemlock plant, *Conium maculatum* Linn., and the first alkaloid to be prepared synthetically (Ladenburg, 1886). Its chief pharmacological action is on the motor nerves, where it causes paralysis of the peripheral endings; there is evidence that it also has effect upon the sensory nerves. It has been employed in spasmodic affectations such as whooping-cough and asthma, and also as an analgesic and sedative, but its use is dying out because of its toxic nature. Externally, it is sometimes incorporated in a soothing ointment. Death from the alkaloid is caused by asphyxia due to paralysis of the phrenic nerve-endings to the diaphragm. **Coniine hydrobromide.** $C_8H_{17}NHBr$, a soluble salt administered in cases of cardiac asthma. **Coniine hydrochloride.** $C_8H_{17}NHCl$, a soluble salt of coniine, formerly used for the same purposes as the hydrobromide.

coniism (ko·ni·izm). Poisoning by conium (hemlock).

coniocortex (**ko**·ne·o·**kor'**·tex). The granulous type of cortex of the sensory areas. [Gk *konis* dust, cortex.]

coniofibrosis (**ko**·ne·o·fi·**bro'**·sis). Pneumoconiosis produced by inorganic forms of dust which lead to pulmonary fibrosis, e.g. asbestosis, silicosis. [Gk *konis* dust, fibrosis.]

coniology (ko·ne·**ol**·o·je). The scientific study of atmospheric dust and its effects. [Gk *konis* dust, *logos* science.]

coniolymphstasis (**ko**·ne·o·**limf'**·stas·is). A type of pneumoconiosis caused by hard and gritty dusts which block up the lymph vessels, e.g. in anthracosis. [Gk *konis* dust, L *lympha* water, Gk *stasis* a standing still.]

coniometer (ko·ne·**om**·et·er). A device by means of which the amount of dust present in the atmosphere may be determined. [Gk *konis* dust, meter.]

coniophage (**ko**·ne·o·faje). A macrophage which absorbs particles of dust. [Gk *konis* dust, *phagein* to eat.]

conioscope (**ko**·ne·o·skope). Coniometer. [Gk *konis* dust, *skopein* to watch.]

coniosis (ko·ne·**o**·sis). The morbid condition which results from inhaling dust. [Gk *konis* dust, *-osis* condition.]

coniosporosis (**ko**·ne·o·spor·**o'**·sis). A hypersensitivity reaction after the inhalation of large numbers of spores of *Cryptostroma corticale* in workers stripping maple bark. [Gk *konis* dust, *sporos* seed.]

coniotomy (ko·ne·**ot**·o·me). In tracheotomy, making entry into the trachea through the cricovocal membrane. [Gk *konos* cone, *temnein* to cut.]

coniotoxicosis (**ko**·ne·o·tox·e·**ko'**·sis). Pneumoconiosis in which the dust invades the connective-tissue cells. [Gk *konis* dust, toxicosis.]

Conium (ko·**ni**·um). 1. A genus of plants of the family Umbelliferae. 2. Conium leaf, hemlock leaf, the fresh leafy tops of *Conium maculatum* Linn. **Conium maculatum.** The poison hemlock; it contains the alkaloids coniine, *N*-methylconiine and conhydrine. The extract is used in pills as a sedative and antispasmodic, and in ointments and suppositories in haemorrhoids. [Gk *koneion* hemlock.]

conization (ko·ni·**za**·shun). The excision of a cone-shaped piece of tissue, e.g. in partial cervicectomy. **Cervical conization.** The removal of a conical piece of tissue from the cervix uteri. **Cold conization.** The removal of a conical piece of tissue with a cold cutting instrument, in contradistinction to a diathermy knife.

conize (**ko**·nize). To remove a conical or wedge-shaped piece of tissue for histological examination.

conizer (**ko**·ni·zer). An appliance for carrying out conization.

conjugal (**kon**·joo·gal). 1. Affecting or relating to both partners in a marriage. 2. Relating to marriage or the marital relationship. [L *conjugere* to yoke together.]

conjugate (**kon**·joo·gate). 1. The conjugate diameter. *See* DIAMETER. 2. United in pairs or couples. **Anatomical conjugate.** True conjugate (see below). **Available conjugate.** Obstetric conjugate (see below). **External conjugate.** External conjugate diameter. *See* DIAMETER. **Internal conjugate.** Internal conjugate diameter. *See* DIAMETER. **Obstetric conjugate.** The distance between the upper posterior edge of the symphysis and the most projecting part of the vertebral column. **True conjugate [conjugatum (NA)].** In pelvimetry, the distance between the summit of the pubic symphysis and the most projecting part of the vertebral column. [see prec.]

conjugation (kon·joo·**ga**·shun). 1. In anatomy, 2 conjoined parts, e.g. a pair of cranial nerves. 2. The fusion of 2 organisms, involving union of nuclei or interchange of nuclear material. 3. The sexual fusion of 2 cells, involving partition of chromatins and division into 2 new cells. 4. In biochemistry, the combination of one compound (e.g. protein) with another compound to form a product of biological importance, as in detoxication. **Conjugation nucleus.** Cleavage nucleus. *See* NUCLEUS. [L *conjungere* to yoke together.]

conjunctiva [tunica conjunctiva (NA)] (kon·jungk·**ti**·vah). The mucous membrane lining the eyelids and forming a protective and nutritive covering for the anterior part of the eyeball. **Ocular part of the conjunctiva [tunica conjunctiva bulbi (NA)].** That portion which is reflected over the sclera and cornea. **Palpebral part of the conjunctiva [tunica conjunctiva palpebrarum (NA)].** That portion which lines the eyelids and which at the margin of the lids is continuous with the skin. **Tarsal conjunctiva.** Palpebral part of the conjunctiva (see above). [L *conjunctivus* connecting.]

conjunctival (kon·jungk·**ti**·val). Relating or belonging to the conjunctiva.

conjunctival arteries [arteriae conjunctivales anteriores et posteriores]. *See* OPHTHALMIC ARTERY.

conjunctival veins [venae conjunctivales (NA)]. Veins draining the tarsal and most of the bulbar conjunctiva and the palpebral veins. From the pericorneal region they drain into the muscular veins, forming a superficial conjunctival and a deep episcleral plexus.

conjunctiviplasty (kon·jungk·**ti**·ve·plast·e). Plastic repair of conjunctiva; keratoplasty. [conjunctiva, Gk *plassein* to mould.]

conjunctivitis (kon·**jungk**·tiv·**i'**·tis). Inflammation of the conjunctiva. Numerous varieties have been described which may be classified simply into *superficial* affecting principally the epithelium, and *interstitial* involving the deeper or connective-tissue layers of the conjunctiva in addition to the epithelial. **Acute epidemic mucopurulent conjunctivitis.** An acute, epidemic, mucopurulent, bilateral form, very contagious and therefore commonly seen in institutions. It is caused by the Koch–Weeks bacillus, and is also known as *Koch–Weeks conjunctivitis* or *pink eye.* **Allergic conjunctivitis.** An allergic reaction of the conjunctiva often associated with hay fever. **Angular conjunctivitis.** Conjunctivitis affecting principally the regions of the canthi and due to the bacillus of Morax and Axenfeld. **Catarrhal conjunctivitis.** The simple form may be due to various micro-organisms, though each does not always produce a specific picture, to irritation from mechanical stimuli (e.g. foreign bodies, inturned eyelashes), or to chemical and thermal causes, and ultra-violet light. It may occur in allergies, e.g. hay fever, or in association with numerous general diseases such as the exanthemata. **Caterpillar conjunctivitis.** That caused by transference of the hairs of certain caterpillars to the conjunctiva by means of the hands; it runs a short acute course. **Chronic catarrhal conjunctivitis.** Conjunctivitis that may result from simple catarrhal, angular, or mucopurulent forms. **Croupous conjunctivitis.** Pseudomembranous conjunctivitis (see below). **Eczematous conjunctivitis.** Phlyctenular conjunctivitis (see below). **Follicular conjunctivitis.** A form of conjunctivitis associated with hypertrophy of the conjunctival lymphatic follicles. **Glare conjunctivitis.** Conjunctivitis due to the effect of glare, e.g. sun or snow. **Gonococcal conjunctivitis.** That caused by *Neisseria gonorrhoeae;* it is a severe purulent conjunctivitis that may cause blindness, especially in infants. **Granular conjunctivitis.** Trachoma. **Hay-fever conjunctivitis.** Allergic conjunctivitis (see above). **Interstitial conjunctivitis.** *See* MAIN DEFINITION (above). **Conjunctivitis lymphatica.** Phlyctenular conjunctivitis (see below). **Membranous conjunctivitis.** A condition in which the surface of the conjunctiva is covered by a fibrinous membrane which may be of the croupous or diphtheritic variety, according to the severity of the reaction. It is caused typically by the diphtheria bacillus, but other organisms such as streptococci and pneumococci may be responsible. **Mucopurulent conjunctivitis.** So named because of its secretion, is frequently due to the Koch-Wells bacillus, and is called *pink eye.* It is highly infectious and is often associated with numerous small conjunctival haemorrhages. **Phlyctenular conjunctivitis.** An allergic form, commonly seen in children, and thought to be due to a sensitization of the conjunctiva to an endogenous protein, usually tuberculous. It is characterized by the formation of nodules astride the limbus which often ulcerate and invade the cornea. Also known as *eczematous conjunctivitis, scrofulous conjunctivitis* or *conjunctivitis lymphatica.* **Pseudomembranous conjunctivitis.** A form characterized by the formation of a pseudomembrane, formed by fibrinous exudate on the surface of, and not in, the conjunctival epithelium. It is a rare condition caused by many different organisms, e.g. haemolytic streptococcus and the Klebs-Loeffler bacillus. **Purulent conjunctivitis.** Conjunctivitis caused by virulent organisms, especially gonococci and some varieties of streptococci and pneumococci; ophthalmia neonatorum is usually purulent. **Scrofulous conjunctivitis.** Phlyctenular conjunctivitis (see above). **Superficial conjunctivitis.** *See* MAIN DEFINITION (above). **Swimming-bath conjunctivitis.** Enlargement of the conjunctival lymphatic follicles due to a filter-passing virus. **Syphilitic conjunctivitis.** Conjunctivitis occurring in a variety of forms, from a chancre through different manifestations of the secondary stage to gummata and congenital lesions. **Trachomatous conjunctivitis.** A chronic contagious disease affecting primarily the subepithelial tissues of the conjunctiva and cornea; in the latter it is associated with pannus. Healing takes place by cicatrization which entails much deformity of the lids and opacity of the cornea. The disease is probably due to a virus of the rickettsia type, and is almost universal in the countries to the south and east of the Mediterranean, but rare in Great Britain and the Scandinavian countries. **Tuberculous conjunctivitis.** A form which may be primary or associated with systemic tuberculosis. It appears as an ulcerated area on the palpebral conjunctiva with a variable amount of granulation. **Vernal conjunctivitis.** Spring catarrh, a form which tends to affect vagotonic persons, is possibly allergic in origin, and is of recurrent seasonal nature. It is characterized by the formation of flat-topped papules in the tarsal conjunctiva (palpebral type), or by the formation of fine nodular jelly-like excrescences round the limbus (ocular type). There is usually a milky discharge containing eosinophils. [conjunctiva, Gk *-itis* inflammation.]

See also: KOCH (R.), PARINAUD, WEEKS.

conjunctivodacryocystostomy (kon·jungk·**ti**·vo·**dak**·re·o·sis·**tos**'·to·me). An operation in which the lacrimal sac is sutured into the inner canthus of the eye, to overcome an obstructed lower canaliculus, causing epiphora. Also called *Stallard's operation.* [conjunctiva, Gk *dakryon* tear, *kystis* sac, *stoma* mouth.]

conjunctivoma (**kon**·jungk·tiv·**o**'·mah). A neoplasm developing on the eyelid and made up of tissue derived from the conjunctiva. [conjunctiva, Gk *-oma* tumour.]

conjunctivoplasty (kon·jungk·**ti**·vo·plas·te). Conjunctiviplasty.

Conn, W. J. Michigan physician.

Conn's syndrome. Primary hyperaldosteronism.

connatal, connate (kon·**a**·tal, **kon**·ate). Congenital; innate; occurring at the time of birth; produced together. [L *cum, nasci* to be born.]

connection (kon·**ek**·shun). **Intertendinous connection [connexus intertendineus (NA)].** Any of the bands connecting the tendons of the extensor digitorum muscles. [L *connexus* a joining.]

connective (kon·**ek**·tiv). 1. Binding. 2. Connecting. [L *cum, nectere* to bind.]

connectivum (kon·ek·**ti**·vum). Connective tissue. [L.]

connector (kon·**ek**·tor). A connector neurone. *See* NEURONE. [L *cum, nectere* to bind.]

Connell, Frank Gregory (b. 1875). Oshkosh, Wisconsin, surgeon.

Connell's suture. An inverted suture (interrupted or continuous) used in bowel anastomosis, the loop being always on the side of the mucosa; also called *loop-on-mucosa suture.*

Connell, Karl (b. 1878). New York physician.

Connell harness. A band passing behind the head and fixed to 2 hooks on the sides of the face-piece of an anaesthetic apparatus.

Connell meter. An apparatus for measuring gas flow, employing 2 small metal spheres enclosed in an inclined glass tube.

connexus interthalamicus [adhesio interthalamica (NA)] (kon·**ex**·us in·ter·thal·**am**·ik·us). The band of grey matter which crosses the cavity of the 3rd ventricle of the brain, joining the 2 thalami. [L *connexus* a joining, *inter,* thalamus.]

conoid (**ko**·noid). An imaginary three-dimensional figure enclosing rays of light after their passage through an astigmatic lens system. Successive sections show an ellipse, a straight line, a second ellipse, a circle, a third ellipse, and then a straight line whose long axes are perpendicular to that of the first and second ellipses. **Conoid part of the coracoclavicular ligament.** *See* LIGAMENT, CORACOCLAVICULAR. **Conoid tubercle.** *See* TUBERCLE. [cone, Gk *eidos* form.]

See also: STURM.

conoides (ko·**noid**·eez). The canine teeth. [Gk *konos* cone, *eidos* form.]

Conolly, John (b.1794). British alienist.

Conolly's system. A humanitarian system of treatment of the insane without the use of restraint.

conomyoidin (**ko**·no·mi·**oid**'·in). The contractile protoplasm in the retinal layer of rods and cones. It expands on exposure to light and contracts the cones, the reverse process occurring in darkness. [Gk *konos* cone, *mys* muscle, *eidos* form.]

conophthalmus (ko·nof·**thal**·mus). Staphyloma of the cornea. [Gk *konos* cone, *ophthalmos* eye.]

Conor, Alfred (b. 1870). French parasitologist.

Conor and Bruch disease. Fièvre boutonneuse; a tick-borne rickettsial fever caused by *Rickettsia conorii.*

conotruncal (ko·no·**trungk**·al). Pertaining to the conus (infundibulum) and the truncus arteriosus of the developing heart. [Gk *konos* cone, L *truncus* trunk.]

Conradi, Andrew Christian (b. 1809). Norwegian physician.

Conradi's line. A line drawn from the base of the xiphisternum to the cardiac apex which marks the normal upper limit of dullness due to the left lobe of the liver.

Conradi, Heinrich (b. 1876). Dresden bacteriologist.

Conradi-Drigalski agar, Drigalski-Conradi agar. A nutrient agar containing 1 per cent peptone, 1.9 per cent nutrose, 0.5 per cent calcium chloride, 1.5 per cent lactose, 0.001 per cent crystal violet and 15 per cent litmus solution.

consanguineous (kon·sang·**gwin**·e·us). Of the same blood; of the same parentage; descended from a common ancestor. [L *cum, sanguis* blood.]

consanguinity (kon·sang·**gwin**·it·e). The state of being related by blood, that is, being descended from a common ancestor. [see prec.]

consciousness (kon·shus·nes). 1. Mental experience; awareness; the response of the mind to stimuli received through the senses or to thought processes, varying from vague awareness to attention. 2. That part of mental experience which is the object of immediate attention, as distinguished from the subconscious and the unconscious. 3. A sense organ for the perception of psychic qualities. Disagreement arises among philosophical views on consciousness, ranging from denial of its existence or at least its importance, to the attribution of it to the simplest living things and even to the inorganic. **Collective consciousness.** The group mind; the devotion of the separate consciousnesses of the individuals composing a group towards some deliberately chosen end. **Colon consciousness.** Awareness of the activities of the colon, normally an unconscious process. **Double consciousness.** A psychopathic state in which a person has 2 distinct and unrelated mental lives, the experiences and emotions of one being forgotten whilst living the other. **Group consciousness.** Collective consciousness (see above). **Noetic consciousness.** Awareness of one's thoughts; cognition. **Objective consciousness.** The awareness of stimuli proceeding from external sources. **Subjective consciousness.** The awareness of stimuli arising in oneself and not perceptible by the consciousness of another. [L *conscire* to be aware of.]

consensual (kon·sen·sew·al). 1. A term descriptive of reflex excitement of one part as the result of stimulation of another, usually a conjugate part, e.g. the pupils of both eyes react alike although stimulation is applied to only one. 2. Involuntary movement accompanying voluntary movement. 3. In psychology, involuntary action combined with consciousness or sensation. [L *cum, sentire* to feel.]

consent (kon·sent). 1. Consent to medical or surgical treatment obtained by implication (*implied*), word of mouth (*verbal*) or, on paper, signed (*written*), necessary to avoid subsequent allegation of operative or other procedure without approval. 2. Implied or verbal consent to sexual intercourse, without which (except between married persons) the act is a criminal offence. [see prec.]

conservancy (kon·ser·van·se). Official care and supervision of matters relating to public health and its preservation. [L *conservare* to keep together.]

conservation (kon·ser·va·shun). 1. The guarding of the health and strength of a patient. 2. Of medicines and drugs, the keeping of them in an entire state and unaffected by injurious conditions. **Conservation of energy.** *See* ENERGY. [see prec.]

conservative (kon·ser·vat·iv). 1. Of treatment, of a type to restore function and preserve health; against heroic methods. 2. Preservative. [L *conservare* to keep together.]

consilia (kon·sil·e·ah) A special use of the word is its application to the letters describing the symptomatology of certain maladies and the therapy employed by physicians of the 15th, 16th and 17th centuries. [L consultations.]

consolidant (kon·sol·id·ant). 1. An agent which promotes healing. 2. Aiding the union or healing of parts and wounds. [L *consolidare* to make firm.]

consolidation (kon·sol·id·a′·shun). The process of being converted into a firm mass, as occurs in the lung when the alveoli fill with exudate in cases of pneumonia. [see prec.]

consolute (kon·sol·ewt). 1. A solution or liquid which can be merged in another solution or liquid. 2. Miscible in all proportions. [L *cum, solvere* to dissolve.]

consonation (kon·son·a·shun). The presence of pulmonary râles which on auscultation are heard in unison with another sound. [L *cum, sonare* to sound.]

conspersus (kon·sper·sus). A dusting-powder; usually a mixture of 2 or more substances in fine powder form, intended for external use. It should not be applied to broken skin surfaces. **Conspersus acidi borici et amyli.** Dusting-powder of boric acid and starch, a mixture of boric acid powder and starch used as an antiseptic to soothe and dry irritated and inflamed surfaces, mostly for infants. **Conspersus acidi salicylici compositus.** Compound dusting-powder of salicylic acid, a mixture of salicylic acid, boric acid and sterilized talc powder, used largely for the feet to allay sweating, keep the skin dry, and stop irritation. **Conspersus hydrargyri subchloridi compositus.** Compound dusting-powder of mercurous chloride, a mixture of powdered mercurous chloride, bismuth subgallate and sterilized talc, used as a germicide and astringent for dusting on sores, and as a protective. It should not be applied to extensive raw surfaces owing to its poisonous nature. **Conspersus talci borici.** Dusting-powder of boric talc, a mixture of powdered boric acid, starch and sterilized talc, used as an antiseptic for application to moist and inflamed surfaces. **Conspersus zinci oxidi et acidi borici.** Dusting-powder of zinc oxide and boric acid, a mixture of powdered boric acid and zinc oxide, applied as an astringent to the skin when inflamed, and to allay irritation in certain skin diseases. **Conspersus zinci oxidi et acidi salicylici.** Dusting-powder of zinc oxide and salicylic acid, a mixture of zinc oxide, salicylic acid and starch powder, used for application to the skin, particularly of the feet, to allay sweating and stop irritation. **Conspersus zinci oxidi et amyli.** Dusting-powder of zinc oxide and starch, a mixture of zinc oxide and starch powder, applied to the skin as a mildly astringent and soothing agent for inflamed surfaces, and in certain skin diseases. **Conspersus zinci oxidi et amyli compositus.** Compound dusting-powder of zinc oxide and starch, a mixture of zinc oxide, starch, boric acid and sterilized talc powder, used as a mildly astringent and soothing application on moist and inflamed surfaces. [L *cum, spargere* to sprinkle.]

constant (kon·stant). 1. Unchanging. 2. In mathematics, an invariable quantity. 3. In physics, a number expressing an attribute or relation that does not vary. **Absolute constant.** One that retains the same value in all circumstances. **Decay constant of radioactive substances.** In a radioactive substance the fraction of the atoms present which decay in a given time is constant. The fraction is numerically equal to the decay constant and its value depends upon the time chosen. This decay law leads to the relation $N = N_0e^{-\lambda t}$, where N is the number of atoms present after time t, N_0 the original number present and e the base of natural logarithms. The half-life of a radioactive substance = $0.69/\lambda$. **Derived constant.** A constant determined indirectly, as against an experimental constant. **Dielectric constant.** The measurement of the inductive capacity of a dielectric, ϵ, compared with air as unit. **Diffusion constant.** The characteristic factor of proportionality between the rate of diffusion of a substance in a given medium and the gradient of its concentration at the same point. **Dissociation constant.** The ratio of the product of the concentrations of ions of a substance in solution, to the concentration of the substance. **Equilibrium constant.** In the chemical theory of mass action the product of the concentrations of the products of a reaction divided by the product of the concentrations of the original substances entering into the reaction. **Experimental constant.** A physical constant arrived at by numerous independent experiments, and stated with its probable error. **Ionization constant.** Dissociation constant (see above). **Specific gamma ray constant.** Of a radioactive nuclide, the exposure dose rate produced by the gamma rays from a unit point source of that nuclide at unit distance. (Unit: roentgens per millicurie hour at 1 cm. Symbol: Γ.) **Statistical constant.** A statistical term used to express the value of a series of quantitative observations, e.g. arithmetical mean, standard error. [L *cum, stare* to stand.]

See also: AVOGADRO, FARADAY, LAPICQUE, MICHAELIS (L.), PLANCK, STEFAN.

constantan, constantin (kon·stan·tan, kon·stan·tin). An alloy of copper (60 per cent) and nickel (40 per cent) employed in thermocouples.

constellation (kon·stel·a·shun). A term used in psychiatry for a group of ideas associated with a central idea. It has come to mean in analysis a group of emotionally-coloured ideas, mostly repressed. [L *constellatio* a group of stars.]

constipated (kon·stip·a·ted). Costive; suffering from constipation.

constipation (kon·stip·a·shun). A condition in which the bowels are opened only infrequently and with difficulty, or in which the faeces are retained. **Atonic constipation.** That resulting from lack of tone of the intestine. **Gastrojejunal constipation.** Constipation as a condition secondary to disease of the alimentary canal. **Gerontal constipation.** That affecting elderly men with prostatic enlargement. **Proctogenous constipation.** The retention of the faeces in the rectum because of inefficiency of the defaecation reflex so that the sensation of fullness is lost. **Spastic constipation.** A form induced by neurasthenia, or by the effect of lead poisoning; there is constrictive spasm of part of the intestine. [L *constipare* to crowd together.]

constituents (kon·stit·ew·ents). A term used indiscriminately to describe the elements or substances which compose compounds and mixtures, but usually understood to refer to the elements or parts of a compound. [L *constituere* to set up.]

constitutio (kon·stit·ew·she·o). Constitution. **Constitutio lymphatica.** Lymphatic constitution. *See* CONSTITUTION. [see prec.]

constitution (kon·stit·ew·shun.) 1. The totality of the physical and mental qualities and functions determined by heredity and environment which determine the general bodily health, the reaction to adverse circumstances, the resistance to infection and the personality of an individual. 2. In chemistry, the way in which the atoms are linked together to form the molecule of a compound, as distinct from the composition of the latter. 3. In pharmacy, composition, e.g. of a preparation. **Allergic constitution.** One that shows a special tendency to react allergically. **Asthenic constitution.** One characterized by slender build, flattened long chest, and poor general physique and resistance to disease. **Epidemic constitution.** A metaphysical conception of the causation of epidemics propounded by Sydenham. An epidemic constitution was supposed to be a mysterious factor beyond and more powerful than ordinary atmospheric changes. It depended upon alterations in "the bowels of the earth" which gave rise to effluvia that polluted the atmosphere. The constitution determined the kind of fever prevalent at the time so that all would be alike in their symptoms. Since the constitution varied from year to year, so did the prevalent fevers; one year they were intermittent, another pestilential, and in yet others variolous, dysenteric or comatose according to the epidemic constitution dominant at the time. The conception is derived from Hippocrates and Galen, but, whereas they laid emphasis on the natural changes in atmosphere and climate to account for most fevers, Sydenham made it the central feature. The conception influenced medical theory and hindered epidemiological progress until the time of Pasteur and the germ theory. **Ideo-obsessional constitution.** A personality deviation characterized by excessive rigidity, with a tendency to repetitive and compulsive modes of thought and action. **Lymphatic constitution.** A slow, sluggish constitution associated with hyperplasia of the lymphatic system. **Neuropathic constitution.** A constitution which predisposes to nervous disorders. **Psychopathic constitution.** A personality deviation characterized by a tendency to psychopathy. **Vasoneurotic constitution.** One associated with irritability and instability of the vasomotor system. [L *constituere* to set up.]

constitutional (kon·stit·ew·shun·al). 1. Relating to the state of the constitution. 2. Inherent in the constitution of mind or body. 3. Relating to the bodily system as a whole.

constitutive (kon·stit·ew·tiv). Term applied to enzymes whose synthesis is not regulated but remains constant irrespective of growth conditions. [L *constituere* to set up.]

constrict (kon·strikt). 1. To bind closely together. 2. To contract. [L *constringere* to draw tight.]

constriction (kon·strik·shun). 1. Stenosis. 2. The contraction or the binding of a place or part. 3. A morbid subjective sensation as of being tightly squeezed or bound. **Nucleolar constriction.** A chromosomal secondary constriction associated with the nucleolus and presumably with the nucleolus organizer. **Primary constriction.** In cytogenetics, the centromere region of the chromosome. **Secondary constriction.** In cytogenetics, any chromosomal constriction in addition to the primary constriction **Pyloric constriction.** The narrow canal bounded by the pyloric sphincter. [see prec.]

constrictive (kon·strik·tiv). Pertaining to or characterized by constriction; causing constriction.

constrictor (kon·strik·tor). 1. Any muscle which causes contraction of a cavity or compresses an organ. (For named constrictor muscles see organ or structure concerned.) 2. Anything which squeezes or binds a part. 3. An instrument the use of which causes compression or tightening of a part. [see foll.]

constringent (kon·strin·jent). Astringent. [L *constringere* to draw tight.]

constructive (kon·struk·tiv). 1. Anabolic. 2. Belonging to a process of construction. [L *construere* to build up.]

consult (kon·sult). 1. To seek the opinion or advice of a physician, surgeon or other practitioner. 2. To confer with another practitioner over a case. [see foll.]

consultant (kon·sul·tant). 1. A physician or other practitioner called in by the physician in charge of a case to give advice about it. 2. A retired member of a hospital staff who can be called in for advice by the physician or surgeon in charge of a case. 3. A registered medical or dental practitioner who, by virtue of training and experience, has acquired specialist knowledge in some branch of medicine or dentistry which has been recognized by his colleagues in that on their recommendation he holds a hospital appointment within the National Health Service on the highest salary scale, or an honorary appointment of equivalent status. [L *consultare* to deliberate.]

consultation (kon·sul·ta·shun). Deliberation between 2 or more physicians or other practitioners over the diagnosis or treatment in any specified case. [see prec.]

consummate (kon·sum·ate). Of a marriage, to complete it by the act of coitus. [L *consummare* to accomplish.]

consummation (kon·sum·a·shun). The act of completing a marriage by coitus. [see prec.]

consumption (kon·sump·shun). Pulmonary tuberculosis; a condition in which the tissues of the body are progressively wasting away. **Buffers' consumption.** Silicosis. **Cell consumption.** Physiological degeneration of the blood cells. **Galloping consumption.** Acute miliary tuberculosis. *See* TUBERCULOSIS. **Luxus consumption.** The reserve of protein contained in the body beyond the amount required by metabolism. **Potters' consumption.** Silicosis. [L *consumere* to use up completely.]

consumptive (kon·sump·tiv). 1. An individual suffering from pulmonary tuberculosis. 2. Of the nature of pulmonary tuberculosis. [see prec.]

contact (kon·takt). 1. A touching; a connection. 2. The touching of 2 conductors to complete an electric circuit; the prepared spot, e.g. platinum point, where such a touching occurs. 3. An individual in close proximity to, but not necessarily touching, a source of infection, usually a person suffering from an infectious disease. 4. In dentistry, the touching of teeth. **Direct contact, Immediate contact.** A person who touches a diseased person, or is in his immediate vicinity; also the method of spreading disease by touching or by being in close contact with. **Indirect contact, Mediate contact.** A person infected by an intermediate person or object, without being in close proximity to the infecting case. Also the transference of disease by contaminated hands, food, toys, etc. **Contact point.** *See* POINT. **Proximal contact.** The touching of the distal surface of a tooth with the mesial surface of the adjacent tooth. **Contact therapy.** Low-voltage x-ray therapy in which the source of x-rays is brought close to the part to be treated (short target-skin distance). **Weak contact.** That form of contact in which a tooth barely touches the adjacent tooth. [L *contingere* to touch.]

contactant (kon·tak·tant). An allergen that produces the effects of hypersensitivity by contact with skin or mucous membrane. [see prec.]

contagion (kon·ta·jun). 1. Transmission of an infective disease by direct contact with a patient who has it, or by contact with a secretion of such a patient, or with some person or thing touched by him. 2. A contagious disease. 3. Any specific virus or germ which is the cause of a contagious disease. **Direct contagion, Immediate contagion.** Transmission of infective disease by direct contact. **Indirect contagion, Mediate contagion.** Transmission of infective disease by contact with a secretion of a patient who has it or with some person or thing touched by him. **Mental contagion.** The spread of hysterical symptoms from one person to another. **Psychic contagion.** Communication of a nervous disorder by the influence of the mind of an affected person on that of an unaffected person, e.g. by imitation. [L *contingere* to touch.]

contagiosity (kon·ta·je·**os**′·it·e). 1. The quality of being contagious. 2. The intensity of contagiousness of a disease.

contagious (kon·**ta**·jus). 1. Transmissible by contagion, a term used of certain infective diseases. 2. Relating to contagion.

contagium (kon·**ta**·je·um). An old term for the causal agent or microbe of any communicable disease. **Contagium animatum, Contagium vivum.** Obsolete terms for living agents, animal or vegetable, which might spread infection. [L *contingere* to touch.]

container (kon·**ta**·ner). **Gamma-ray source container.** A holder into which a gamma-ray source is sealed. **Radium container.** A holder into which a radium source is sealed. **Radon container.** A holder into which radon is sealed, usually a radon seed. [L *continere* to contain.]

contaminant (kon·**tam**·in·ant). An agent that causes contamination, e.g. a spore or mould which lodges by accident on a bacterial culture and grows on it. [L *contaminare* to bring in contact.]

contamination (kon·**tam**·in·a′·shun). 1. Pollution or soiling with infective material. 2. In Freudian psychology, a term for the running of one word into another. **Radioactive contamination.** Contamination of materials (animal, vegetable or mineral) with radioactive substances. In biological material the contamination may be superficial only (*external contamination*) or from metabolic uptake (*internal contamination*). **Verbal contamination.** The inordinate cropping up of a word or phrase, appropriately or not, in the speech or writing of an aphasiac. [see prec.]

contemplative (kon·**tem**·plat·iv). A sexual pervert who by an act of imagination can excite an orgasm. [L *contemplari* to contemplate.]

content (**kon**·tent). 1. Anything contained within something else. 2. In psychology, the symbolized form in which a dream appears to the consciousness of the dreamer. **Effective radium (radon) content.** The quantity of radium (radon) which, in the absence of wall absorption, produces the same effect as the given container of radium (radon). **Equivalent radium content.** The activity of a radium source determined by comparison of the γ-ray activity, with that of a standard. No correction is made for differences of screening which may exist between the unknown and the standard. **Latent content.** The part of a dream or thought which is hidden behind the symbol presented to consciousness and cannot be detected without specialized interpretation. **Manifest content.** The external form taken by a dream when remembered by the dreamer. **Oxygen content.** The amount of oxygen, expressed in ml per cent, at any one time, e.g. in blood, which is 15–23 ml in arterial and 10–18 ml in venous blood. **Radium content.** The actual radium content in mg of radium element. **Radon content.** The gaseous radium content of a vessel, expressed in millicuries. [L *continere* to contain.]

contiguity (kon·tig·**ew**·it·e). 1. Proximity or contact without continuity. 2. Intimate relation of one thing with another. 3. In psychology, proximity of impressions or ideas in time or place, as a principle of association of ideas. **Amputation in contiguity.** Amputation through a joint. **Solution of contiguity.** Dislocation of parts normally in contiguity. [L *contingere* to touch.]

contiguous (kon·**tig**·ew·us). 1. Applied to 2 or more parts in actual contact. 2. Adjacent without being in contact. [see prec.]

continence (**kon**·tin·ens). 1. Self-restraint or moderation in regard to sexual indulgence, particularly unlawful sexual indulgence. 2. Self-control. [L *continere* to contain.]

continued (kon·**tin**·ewd). Uninterruptedly persisting, without remission or intermission. [L *continuare* to join on.]

continuity (kon·tin·**ew**·it·e). The state of being continuous. **Amputation in continuity.** Amputation through a long bone between one joint and the next. **Continuity of germ plasma.** That property of the germ plasma which transmits in continuity from one generation to the next the substance of heredity. **Solution of continuity.** Separation of normally continuous bones or soft parts by fracture, laceration, incision or rupture. [see prec.]

contortion (kon·**tor**·shun). 1. A twisted state of the body or face. 2. A writhing of the body. [L *cum, torquere* to twist.]

contour (**kon**·toor). The normal outline of the body, or of one of its parts. **Dose contours.** In radiation therapy, the distribution of radiation dose within a three-dimensional body may be partially described by the dose distribution on certain plane surfaces which intersect the body. On these surfaces contour lines are drawn, on every point of which the radiation dose is constant. The number of dose contours drawn is arbitrary and depends upon the accuracy with which interpolation of the dose at a point not on a contour is required. **Isocount contours.** Lines joining points in space in the vicinity of a radioactive source at which equal count rates are obtained with a Geiger counter or other radiation detector. [L *cum, tornare* to turn.]

contoured (**kon**·toord). An irregular smoothly undulating surface. A term used in descriptive bacteriology to denote a bacterial colony the surface of which is in varied relief. [see prec.]

contouring (**kon**·toor·ing). The restoring to a part of its lost contour, e.g. by means of plastic surgery.

contra-. Latin prefix meaning *opposed.*

contra-angle (kon·trah·**ang**′·gl). A double angle in the length of a forceps or tube so arranged that the handles and the blades operate in the same vertical plane but lie in different horizontal planes. [L *contra,* angle.]

contra-aperture (**kon**·trah·**ap**′·er·tewr). A counter-opening made in an abcess so that the contents can flow away more easily. [L *contra,* aperture.]

contraception (kon·trah·**sep**·shun). The prevention of impregnation or conception. [L *contra, concipere* to take in.]

contraceptive (kon·trah·**sep**·tiv). 1. Any agent or measure used to prevent conception. 2. Descriptive of the agent or measure used. **Intra-uterine contraceptive.** A device variously shaped and made of plastics materials or non-irritant metal which is inserted into the uterus to prevent pregnancy or the implantation of the fertilized ovum. **Oral contraceptive.** A substance taken by mouth to prevent conception.

contract (kon·**trakt**). 1. To reduce or be reduced in size or length. 2. To draw together or to be drawn together. 3. To fall victim to a disease. [L *cum, trahere* to draw.]

contractile (kon·**trak**·tile). 1. Capable of shortening or of drawing together or being drawn together in response to application of stimuli. 2. Tending to draw together when stimulated. [see foll.]

contractility (kon·trak·**til**·it·e). The state of being able to draw together or shorten in response to appropriate stimuli. **Galvanic contractility.** Galvanocontractility. **Idiomuscular contractility.** That form of contractility peculiar to muscles which have undergone degeneration or have wasted. **Myocardial (ventricular) contractility.** The ill-defined concept of the variable vigour of contraction of the ventricle which is dependent upon the state of the myocardium and not related to heart rate, pre-load or after-load. **Neuromuscular contractility.** The physiological contractility of muscular tissue (under nervous control and direction) as distinct from pathological contractility. [L *cum, trahere* to draw.]

contractinogen (kon·trak·**tin**·o·jen). A blood fibrinogen fraction that is said to accelerate the erythrocyte sedimentation rate. [L *cum, trahere* to draw, fibrinogen.]

contractio praevia (kon·**trak**·she·o **pre**·ve·ah). The contraction of a lower segment of the uterus before the fetus passes through that segment. [L previous contraction.]

contraction (kon·**trak**·shun). The process of becoming smaller or shorter. **Anodal closure contraction.** ACC, the muscle contraction resulting from excitation with a constant current when the circuit is closed and the anode is the testing electrode. **Anodal opening contraction.** AOC, the muscle contraction resulting from excitation with a constant current when the circuit is opened and the anode is the testing electrode. **Auricular contraction.** *Normal:* contraction of the auricles as a result of stimulus from the sinu-auricular node. *Blocked:* a normal auricular contraction which is not followed by a ventricular contraction. *Blocked premature:* an auricular premature beat which is not followed by a ventricular contraction. **Cardiac contraction.** The shortening of the cardiac muscle fibres which results in reduction in size of the chambers of the heart and the expulsion from them of blood. **Carpopedal contraction.** Trousseau's sign; one of the manifestations of tetany, spontaneous or caused by pressure. There is painful spasm of the hands and feet, and the fingers and toes become fully extended but slightly flexed at the junctions of metacarpals with digits and metatarsals with toes. **Cathodal closure contraction.** CCC, the muscle contraction resulting from excitation with a constant current when the circuit is closed and the cathode is the testing electrode. **Cathodal opening contraction.** COC, the muscle contraction resulting from excitation with a constant current when the circuit is opened and the cathode is the testing electrode. **Cicatricial contraction.** Contraction due to shrinkage of the fibrous tissue of a scar. **Clonic contraction.** Alternating contraction and partial relaxation of muscle, or incomplete tetanus. **Closing contraction.** The muscle contraction occurring at the site of stimulation with either a constant or alternating current when the circuit is closed. **Ectopic contraction.** Premature contraction (see below). **Fibrillary contraction.** Spontaneous or induced contractions occurring successively in different bundles of the fibres of a diseased muscle. **Fixation contraction.** Reflex contraction of a muscle on maximum passive shortening; said to occur in paralysis agitans. Also called *Westphal's contraction.* **Front tap contraction.** Contraction of the gastrocnemius muscle on tapping the muscles of the front of the leg. **Galvanotonic contraction.** The continuous muscle contraction occurring near the cathode when a strong direct current is passed. **Hourglass contraction.** The contraction seen in the stomach from the shrinkage of the scar left by a healed gastric ulcer which may produce 2 chambers separated by a narrow channel. **Idiomuscular contraction.** The prolonged contracture occurring on direct stimulation of a wasted muscle. **Isometric contraction.** A contraction in which shortening of the muscle is almost entirely prevented by fixing it at both ends, so that tension changes alone may be measured. In cardiology, applied to that part of ventricular contraction which occurs whilst both the atrioventricular and semilunar valves are closed; the description, however, is only approximately true as there is a change in the shape of the ventricle and some shortening of muscle fibres must occur. **Isotonic contraction.** A muscle contraction during which shortening is permitted but tension is kept constant. **Isovolumic contraction.** In cardiology, that phase of ventricular contraction which occurs whilst both the atrioventricular and the semilunar valves are closed; although true in the sense that the volume of blood in the ventricle cannot change, the valve cusps may move before opening so that the volume contained by the muscular part of the chamber can alter. **Myoclonic contraction.** Abnormal spasmodic contractions of muscle. **Myotatic contraction.** Contraction induced by passive stretching of muscle, as by tapping of its tendon. **Opening contraction.** The muscle contraction occurring at the site of stimulation with either a constant or alternating current when the circuit is opened. **Palmar contraction.** A thickening of the palmar fascia causing slow-flexion deformity of the fingers and usually mainly affecting the ring- and little fingers. **Paradoxical contraction.** Contraction of muscle caused by passive reduction of its tension, as by approximating its ends. **Premature contraction.** A contraction arising from an ectopic focus in the auricle, nodal tissue or ventricle. **Rheumatic contraction.** A spasm of muscles, occurring especially in children and young adults in winter. Also called *rheumatic tetany* or *epidemic tetany.* **Tetanic contraction.** A state of apparently continuous contraction evoked in voluntary muscle by a rapid stream of nerve impulses. In uterine muscle, a continued and pathological contraction. **Tone contraction.** The normal state of slight tension occurring in muscles during waking hours, or tonus. **Tonic contraction.** A maintained contraction or spasm. **Ventricular contraction.** The contraction of the ventricular myocardium which initiates ventricular systole and which leads to the expulsion of blood. At the commencement of contraction the atrioventricular valve closes and the isometric or isovolumic phase of contraction occurs until the semilunar valve opens. Blood is then ejected rapidly at first and then more slowly, as contraction is completed, until the semilunar valve again closes. **Vermicular contraction.** Peristaltic contraction, e.g. of the intestines. [L *contractio* a drawing together.]

See also: BRAXTON HICKS, DUPUYTREN, GOWERS, WESTPHAL (A.K.O).

contracture (kon·**trak**·tewr). 1. A prolonged reversible contraction of skeletal muscle which may affect only a part, and in which no wave-like action potentials occur. Cf. TETANUS. 2. Deformity due to shortening of muscle, usually the result of fibrosis. **Fatigue contracture.** Myotatic contracture (see below.) **Functional contracture.** Deformity due to hysteria. **Hypertonic contracture.** In spastic paralysis, muscular contractions that are caused by repeated discharge of impulses; they do not occur during sleep. **Ischaemic contracture.** Contracture following ischaemia of muscle due to fibrous replacement. **Myostatic contracture.** Shortening of a muscle that is held in mechanical fixation. **Myotatic contracture.** Contractions that occur in a degenerated muscle when it is tapped or violently stretched. **Organic contracture.** Fixed deformity due to pathological change in the joints or muscles. **Postpoliomyelitic contracture.** Fixed deformity following poliomyelitis and due to disturbance of muscle balance. **Veratrine contracture.** The greatly prolonged contraction that occurs in skeletal muscle in the presence of veratrine. [L *contractura* a drawing together.]

See also: DUPUYTREN, VOLKMANN (R.).

contra-extension (kon·trah·ex·**ten**'·shun). Counter-extension. [L *contra,* extension.]

contrafissura, contrafissure (**kon**·trah·fis·**ewr**'·ah, **kon**·trah·**fish**'·er). Contrecoup. [L *contra, fissura* split.]

contra-incision (**kon**·trah·in·**sizh**'·un). Counter-opening made at or near the site of operation. [L *contra,* incision.]

contra-indicant (kon·trah·**in**·dik·ant). 1. A condition or symptom in a case which indicates that any particular method of treatment is prohibited by the special circumstances. 2. Serving to make the normal line of treatment inadvisable or improper. [L *contra, indicare* to make known.]

contra-indication (**kon**·trah·in·dik·**a**'·shun). The presence of a modifying condition or disease which renders it impossible or undesirable to treat the patient as in normal circumstances he would be treated, or to give him medicines that otherwise would be suitable. [see prec.]

contra-insular (kon·trah·**in**·sew·lar). Exerting an inhibiting effect on the secretory powers of the interalveolar cell-islets of the pancreas so that insulin is not produced. [L *contra, insula* island.]

contralateral (kon·trah·**lat**·er·al). Relating to the opposite side, e.g. when there is a sensation of pain or when paralysis occurs on the side opposite to that bearing the lesion. [L *contra, latus* side.]

contraparetic (**kon**·trah·par·**e**'·tik). Any preparation which is beneficial in cases of paresis. [L *contra,* Gk *paresis* relaxation.]

contraselection (**kon**·trah·sel·**ek**'·shun). In microbial genetics, the prevention of growth of certain genetic classes by the inclusion of inhibitors in, or the exclusion of growth factors from, the growth medium, e.g. drug-resistant mutants or recombinants are selected, and sensitive parental types contraselected, by adding the drug to the medium. [L *contra, seligere* to choose from among.]

contrast (**kon**·trahst). To show opposing qualities in anything, e.g. light and dark; such qualities themselves. **Contrast medium.** *See* MEDIUM. **Negative contrast.** Negative stain. *See* STAIN. **Radiographic contrast.** The difference in density between the various opacities in a radiograph. Factors which have the greatest bearing on contrast are the exposure, the wavelength of x-rays, the intensifying screens, and scattered radiation. **Contrast stain.** Counterstain or after-stain: in histology, a second stain, of contrasting colour, applied to a section of tissue after the primary stain, e.g. eosin (red) applied after haematoxylin (blue), whereby certain details in the section taking the one colour stand out clearly in contrast against details or background stained with the other. *See* STAIN. [L *contra, stare* to stand.]

contrastimulant (kon·trah·**stim**·ew·lant). An agent which is effective in counteracting response to a stimulant; one that has depressant effects. [L *contra, stimulare* to urge on.]

contrastimulism (kon·trah·**stim**·ew·lizm). The practice of using contrastimulant appliances or medicines.

contrastimulus (kon·trah·**stim**·ew·lus). Any influence which counteracts or obstructs the action of a stimulant or stimulus. [L *contra, stimulare* to urge on.]

contravolitional (kon·trah·vol·**ish**'·un·al). 1. Carried out by a person against his own will. 2. Carried out independently of the will; involuntary. [L *contra,* volition.]

contrayerva (kon·trah·**yer**·vah). The root of *Dorstenia contrayerva* Linn. (family Moraceae), a stimulant and diaphoretic. [Port.]

contrecoup (kontr·**koo**). An injury, usually to the brain, developing on the surface opposite to that part of the head injured; a feature of sudden acceleration or deceleration of the head, not of local penetrating injury. Also, although rarely, seen in the lung or the liver. [Fr. counterstroke.]

contrectation (kon·trek·**ta**·shun). 1. The impulse to touch with the hands or fondle a member of the opposite sex. 2. Sexual dalliance. [L *contrectare* to handle.]

control (kon·**trole**). An experiment or standard by which to check the validity of the deductions made from observation or other experiment. Proper controls vary according to the problem, and may be many or few persons, or animals, or experiments in which the only variable is the factor being studied. **Associative automatic control.** Nerve impulses arising in the corpus striatum and having a steadying effect on skeletal muscles, preventing tremor and excessive tonus. **Birth control.** The prevention or spacing of pregnancies by the use of contraceptives or by other methods. **Idiodynamic control.** Nerve impulses arising in the ventral horn cells upon which depend both function and normal nutritional state of skeletal muscle. **Reflex control.** Nerve impulses transmitted to any organ by a reflex arc, and by which activity is regulated. **Sex control.** The taking of measures to influence the sex of the offspring. **Synergic control.** Nerve impulses arising in the cerebellum, integrating the activity of skeletal muscles and so permitting the performance of skilled acts. **Tonic control.** Nerve impulses regulating the tone of skeletal muscles. **Vestibulo-equilibratory control.** Impulses arising in the sensory nerves of the labyrinths, and reflexly controlling posture. **Volitional control, Voluntary control.** Impulses arising in those areas of the cerebral cortex in which "will" is situated, and transmitted by the motor system to appropriate muscle groups. [Fr. *contrôle* check.]

controlled drugs. Drugs as defined in the Misuse of Drugs Act 1971.

controller (kon·**tro**·ler). An electrical arrangement which regulates the current to appliances. [see prec.]

contunding (kon·**tund**·ing). Producing a bruise. [L *contundere* to thump.]

contuse (kon·**tewz**). To bruise; to injure a part without breaking the skin. [L *contundere* to thump.]

contusion (kon·**tew**·zhun). A bruise; a superficial injury caused by a blow without breaking of the skin. [see prec.]

contusive (kon·**tew**·ziv). 1. Causing contusion. 2. Characterized by or belonging to contusion.

conular (**kon**·ew·lar). Conical.

conus (**ko**·nus) (pl. *coni*). 1. A cone; in anatomy, the term may be applied to any structure which is approximately conical in shape, though its use is becoming obsolete. 2. Applied loosely to the bulge which may develop at the posterior pole of a myopic eye. **Conus cordis.** Infundibulum of the heart. **Distraction conus.** A crescentic white conus associated with myopic crescent and produced when the optic nerve passes through the scleral canal in a markedly oblique direction. **Conus medullaris [NA].** The tapered conical end of the spinal cord, of which the filum terminale is a continuation. **Myopic conus.** Myopic crescent. *See* CRESCENT. **Conus retinalis.** The receptive ending of a cone cell in the retina. **Supertraction conus.** Displacement nasally of the pigment layer of the retina and of Bruch's membrane over the edge of the disc, which occurs usually in myopia and produces a grey or reddish-yellow conus. **Coni vasculosi.** The lobules of the head of the epididymis formed by the coiled parts of the efferent ducts of the testis. [Gk *konos* cone.]

convalescence (kon·val·**es**·ens). 1. The period of gradual recovery of health after illness. 2. The period of time between the termination of a disease and complete recovery of health. [L *convalescere* to grow strong.]

convalescent (kon·val·**es**·ent). 1. Applied to the stage of recovery from disease or debility. 2. Belonging to the recovery of health. 3. A patient during the period of convalescence. [see prec.]

convallamaretin (kon·val·am·**ar**'·et·in). An aglycone of uncertain constitution derived from convallamarin.

convallamarin (kon·val·**am**·ar·in). $C_{23}H_{44}O_{12}$, a crystalline glucoside found in the dried flowers of lily-of-the-valley, *Convallaria majalis* Linn. and of only slight cardiac activity. It hydrolyses to convallamaretin, glucose, and rhamnose. [*Convallaria,* L *amarus* bitter.]

convallaretin (kon·val·**ar**·e·tin). $C_{14}H_{26}O_3$, an aglycone yielded by the hydrolysis of convallarin.

Convallaria (kon·val·**a**·re·ah). 1. A genus of plants of the family Liliaceae. 2. Convallaria BPC 1949, convallaria flowers; the dried inflorescence of *Convallaria majalis* Linn. **Convallaria majalis.** Lily-of-the-valley; it is a cardiac stimulant and diuretic, similar to digitalis in action. [L *convallis* valley.]

convallarin (kon·**val**·ar·in). $C_{34}H_{26}O_{11}$, a crystalline glucoside derived from lily-of-the-valley, *Convallaria majalis* Linn. It is an insoluble compound which hydrolyses to convallaretin and glucose, acts like a saponin haemolytically on blood cells, and is used internally for its purgative effect.

convallatoxin (kon·val·ah·**tox**·in). $C_{29}H_{42}O_{10}$, the chief glycoside of the flowers, rhizome and root of lily-of-the valley, *Convallaria majalis* Linn. It consists of needle-like insoluble crystals and has a highly potent action upon the heart, resembling digitalis in effect. It yields on hydrolysis an aglycone identical with strophanthidin. [*Convallaria,* toxin.]

convection (kon·**vek**·shun). The process of transferring heat by the rise of heated liquids or gases and the fall of their colder parts; these in turn become heated and rise. [L *convehere* to bring together.]

convergence (kon·**ver**·jens). 1. The state of inclining towards a common focus or point. 2. A disjunctive movement of the eyes whereby the fixation axes, instead of remaining parallel, become inclined towards each other, so allowing a near object to be fixed and fusion maintained. 3. The meeting-point of 2 convergent lines. **Accommodative convergence.** Convergence induced by a stimulus to accommodate. **Convergence deficiency.** *See* DEFICIENCY. **Convergence excess.** *See* EXCESS. **Fusional convergence.** Convergence that can be produced in order to maintain binocular single vision without change in any other function. **Involuntary convergence.** Reflex convergence (see below). **Negative convergence.** Divergence or outward vergence of the eyes. **Positive convergence.** Inward vergence of the eyes. **Reflex convergence.** That taking place involuntarily as part of the near reflex. **Relative convergence.** The amplitude of convergence that can take place when the accommodation remains stationary. **Tonic convergence.** Convergence due to continuous basic muscle tone. **Voluntary convergence.** That initiated voluntarily. [L *convergere* to incline together.]

convergent (kon·**ver**·jent). Tending towards a common focus. [see prec.]

convergiometer (**kon**·ver·je·**om'**·et·er). An instrument for measuring the power of convergence of the visual axes. The best-known is the Livingston binocular gauge.

See also: LIVINGSTON.

conversion (kon·**ver**·shun). 1. During the progress of labour, manipulation of the body of the fetus or of a part of it for the purpose of placing it in a better position for expulsion. 2. In psychology, transformation of emotion into physical action. 3. In bacterial genetics, *lysogenic* or *phage* conversion means the acquisition of a new character or characters by bacteria following lysogenization with a temperate phage, the new character being determined by a phage gene, e.g. production of toxin by virulent *Corynebacterium diphtheriae* is determined by a specific prophage. **Internal conversion.** A transition between 2 energy states of a nucleus in which the energy difference is not emitted as a photon but is given to an orbital electron which is thereby ejected from the atom. Symbol IC. [L *cum, versari* to be turned.]

See also: MANTOUX.

converter (kon·**ver**·ter). A machine or appliance designed to change energy or material from one form into another, e.g. rotary converters to transform alternating current into direct, and the Bessemer converter used in steel manufacture. **Image converter.** A vacuum tube containing a photosensitive surface on which an optical image is projected. This image is scanned by an electron beam, variations in intensity of the image being converted to variations in potential of an electrical signal. [L *cum, vertere* to turn.]

convertin (kon·**ver**·tin). Stable component (Owren): a factor concerned in blood coagulation, according to Owren, formed by the action of calcium and thromboplastin on proconvertin. This stable component, together with calcium, produces a minimal conversion of prothrombin into thrombin insufficient to clot the blood but initiating a more active formation of thrombin via pro-accelerin (labile component), and accelerin (serum accelerator). [see prec.]

convex (**kon**·vex). Having a bulging or rounded outside surface. [L *convexus* vaulted.]

convexity (kon·**vex**·it·e). 1. The state of being convex. 2. The outer part of a curved surface, organ, or line.

convexoconcave (kon·**vex**·o·**kon'**·kave). Having one side convex and the other concave.

convexoconvex (kon·**vex**·o·**kon'**·vex). Having each of 2 sides or faces convex.

convolute (**kon**·vol·ewt). Rolled together, as one part upon another in a scroll. [L *convolvere* to roll together.]

convoluted (kon·vol·**ewt**·ed). 1. Coiled. 2. Folded and tortuous. [see prec.]

convolution (kon·vol·**ew**·shun). Gyrus; an elevation of the surface of the cerebral hemisphere, usually elongated in form, and bounded by irregular grooves or sulci. The formation of convolutions greatly increases the extent of the area of cerebral cortex contained in the cerebral cavity. **Uncinate convolution.** The hook of the hippocampal gyrus towards the end of the temporal lobe; the uncus. [L *convolvere* to roll together.]

See also: BROCA, DUVAL (M. M.), HESCHL, SCHWALBE.

convolutional, convolutionary (kon·vol·**ew**·shun·al, kon·vol·**ew**·shun·ar·e). Relating or belonging to a convolution.

convolvulin (kon·**vol**·vew·lin). Jalapin, $C_{31}H_{50}O_{16}$. A glucosidal resin obtained from jalap containing glucose and rhamnose units united to convolvulic, tiglic and other acids. It is probably the mildest of the resinous cathartics, but nevertheless produces a very fluid stool within 3-4 h. [see foll.]

Convolvulus (kon·**vol**·vew·lus). A genus of plants of the family Convolvulaceae. **Convolvulus scammonia.** A species which yields the gum resin scammony, a drastic purgative. [L bindweed.]

convulsant (kon·**vul**·sant). 1. Capable of producing convulsions. 2. Any drug which produces convulsions, either by stimulating muscle directly or by the stimulation of the central nervous system. Drugs acting in the latter way are more commonly known as analeptics. [L *convellere* to shake.]

convulsio cerealis (kon·**vul**·se·o seer·e·**a**·lis). The cramp-like muscular spasms which are a symptom of ergotism. [L cramp due to a cereal.]

convulsion (kon·**vul**·shun). A violent involuntary contraction, either prolonged or spasmodic, of the skeletal musculature. **Anaesthetic convulsion.** A convulsion associated with the inhalation of a volatile anaesthetic, usually to a patient with a high temperature or in a hot environment. It can also be caused by the injection of local analgesic agents. **Audiogenic convulsion.** Convulsion stimulated by sound. **Central convulsion.** A convulsion which has its origin in centrally situated nervous structures. **Choreic convulsion.** Any brief, localized, involuntary muscular contraction of the type seen in chorea. **Clonic convulsion.** A convulsion characterized by rhythmic alternate contraction and relaxation of muscle groups. **Co-ordinate convulsion.** A convulsion in which rhythmic movements occur which simulate natural willed activity. **Crowing convulsion.** Laryngismus stridulus. **Epileptiform convulsion.** Any convulsion in which consciousness is lost. **Essential convulsion.** One of central origin but of unknown cause; dependent upon functional and not organic changes in the central nervous system. **External convulsion.** Involuntary spasmodic muscular contraction, the visible element of a convulsion. **Hysterical convulsion.** Any episodic disturbance due to hysteria, which involves spasmodic muscular contractions. **Hysteroid convulsion.** An epileptic convulsion with hysterical features. **Infantile convulsion.** Involuntary muscular contractions due to many causes, characterized by sudden, generalized stiffness, the tonic stage, which may last for a few moments or several hours, and usually with unconsciousness, followed by the clonic stage where there are irregular movements of limbs, face and trunk, which precedes the return of consciousness. Its aetiology is diverse. There is a familial tendency with no epilepsy history; or it may be due to epilepsy, congenital malformation of the brain, cerebral trauma at birth or later, cerebral haemorrhage or cerebral infections. **Internal convulsion.** A slight spasmodic involuntary movement with no alteration in consciousness. **Jacksonian convulsion.** Those occurring in jacksonian epilepsy. **Local convulsion.** A convulsion in which the movements remain localized to one member or part of a member. **Mimetic convulsion, Mimic convulsion.** Habit spasm, or tic of facial muscles. **Oscillating convulsion, Oscillatory convulsion.** A convulsion in which there is successive, but not simultaneous, activation of separate muscle fasciculi. **Puerperal convulsion.** Any epileptiform fit occurring in the puerperium. It is usually eclamptic. **Salaam convulsion.** Spasmodic head nodding. **Spontaneous convulsion.** A convulsion occurring without apparent exciting cause. **Static convulsion.** Saltatory spasm. *See* SPASM. **Suffocative convulsion.** Convulsion due to disturbances of the blood chemistry affecting the brain centres, and associated with oxygen want. **Tetanic convulsion.** A generalized tonic muscular contraction without impairment of consciousness; or the violent prolonged muscular contraction typical of tetanus. **Tonic convulsion.** Prolonged, usually generalized, contraction of skeletal muscles. **Toxic convulsion.** A convulsion precipitated by the action of toxic substances, either endogenous or exogenous, upon the central nervous system. **Traumatic convulsion.** Convulsion due to head injury. **Uraemic convulsion.** One due to uraemia, or to the accumulation in the blood of non-protein nitrogenous substances. [L *convulsio* cramp.]

See also: JACKSON (J.H.).

convulsivant (kon·**vul**·siv·ant). A convulsant.

convulsive (kon·**vul**·siv). 1. Producing or attended with convulsion. 2. Affected or characterized by convulsion. 3. Of the nature of convulsion.

Cooke, William Edmond (b. 1881). Wigan pathologist.

Cooke's count, criterion, formula or index, Cooke and Ponder classification, formula or method. A simplification of Arneth's count or index in which the polymorphonuclear leucocytes are divided into 5 groups according to the number of their nuclear lobes united by fine filaments. The nucleus is considered to be undivided if parts of it are still united by even a small band of nuclear material.

Cooley, Thomas Benton (b. 1871). Detroit paediatrician.

Cooley's anaemia, or disease. A familial, haemolytic, erythroblastic anaemia which occurs usually in families of Mediterranean stock. It is seen in major and minor forms, may be overt or mild in adults but more marked in children, who often show developmental retardation, splenomegaly and skeletal changes, with a hypochromic microcytic anaemia and sometimes mongoloid facies; thalassaemia major.

Cooley's anaemia trait. Thalassaemia minor; a hereditary and familial condition affecting both sexes in patients of Mediterranean origin and related to thalassaemia major or Cooley's anaemia. In the trait, or thalassaemia minor, the heterozygous children are only mild cases, but the homozygous children have the severe, ultimately fatal, thalassaemia major.

Coolidge, William David (b. 1873). American physicist.

Coolidge tube. An evacuated tube containing a heated filament (the cathode) producing electrons, and a metal target (the anode), with a difference of potential between them which accelerates a stream of electrons from the cathode so that they strike the anode.

cooling (**kool**·ing). The process of reducing the body temperature.

Surface cooling. Cooling the body surface by, for example, ice bags in order to induce hypothermia. [AS *colian* cold or cool.]

Coombs, Carey F. (b. 1879). Bristol physician.

Carey Coombs murmur. A short, low-pitched murmur in early diastole occurring with mitral valvulitis in rheumatic carditis.

Coombs, Robin (b. 1921). Cambridge pathologist.

Coombs' test, indirect Coombs' test. An agglutination test used in haematology to detect the incomplete or "blocking" form of Rh antibody, necessary because most sera containing Rh antibody will not agglutinate Rh-positive cells suspended in saline. For testing, the donor's cells are incubated with the recipient's serum, then washed and tested against a potent antiglobulin rabbit serum (*Coombs' reagent*). The titre is the highest dilution of Coombs' reagent that will agglutinate Rh-positive cells sensitized with the incomplete Rh antibody in the recipient's serum.

Cooper, Sir Astley Paston (b. 1768). London surgeon and anatomist.

Cooper's disease. Cystic disease of the breasts.

Cooper's fascia. *See* COOPER'S SUSPENSORY LIGAMENT (below).

Cooper's hernia. A femoral hernia with spreading finger-like processes deep to the femoral vessels.

Cooper's ligament. The pectineal ligament. *See* LIGAMENT.

Cooper's ligament of the elbow. Transverse ligament of the elbow; a portion of the ulnar collateral ligament of the elbow joint which connects the medial sides of the coronoid and olecranon processes.

Cooper's suspensory ligament. Bands of fibrous tissue that anchor the breast to the overlying skin and to the underlying fascia on the pectoralis major muscle.

Cooper's operation. 1. Ligature of the external iliac artery by an incision above the inguinal ligament. 2. An incision of the drum head for acute suppurative otitis media.

Cooper, Georgia. New York bacteriologist.

Cooper's serum. A serum used for Type III pneumonia.

cooperativity (ko·**op**·er·at·**iv**'·it·e). The name given to the phenomenon of the interaction of binding sites and subunits within a protein molecule. *Positive cooperativity* occurs when binding of a ligand at one site increases the affinity of a second or further site for further ligands. [L *cum, operari* to work.]

Coopernail, George P. (b. 1876). New York surgeon.

Coopernail's sign. Ecchymosis in the perineum, a sign of fracture of the pelvis.

co-ordination (ko·**or**·din·**a**'·shun). The harmonious mutual adjustment of parts so that they combine to carry out a function, e.g. of several muscles or muscle groups in executing a complicated movement. [L *cum, ordinare* to arrange.]

Coors filter A cylindrical Chamberland filter; now obsolete.

co-ossification (**ko**·os·if·ik·**a**'·shun). 1. The growing together of bones or of parts of a bone. 2. The state of being grown together, as of bones. [L *cum*, ossification.]

co-ossify (ko·**os**·if·i). Of bones, to ankylose. [see prec.]

cooties (**koo**·teez). A slang term for the human louse *Pediculus humanus.* [Army slang from the Hindustani.]

Copaiba BPC 1949 (ko·**pi**·bah). The oleoresin obtained by incision from the trunk of *Copaifera landsdorfii* Desf. and other species of *Copaifera.* There are several commercial varieties named according to the parts from which they are exported, e.g. Bahia, Maracaibo, Maranham, Para. It contains a volatile oil, consisting mainly of sesquiterpenes, and resin in proportions which vary according to the variety. By virtue of its volatile oil it exerts a stimulant and antiseptic action on the genito-urinary tract and on the bronchioles; it is sometimes used in inflammatory conditions of the genito-urinary tract and in chronic bronchitis. [Port.]

copal (**ko**·pal). Gum animi, a hard resin obtained from the East African tree *Trachylobium hornemannianum.* It is used in varnishes and has been employed in plasters. [Mex. *copalli* incense.]

Cope, Edward Drinker (b. 1840). Philadelphia palaeontologist.

Cope's law. Less specialized organisms may give rise to a greater number of new types than more specialized ones.

Cope, Sir Vincent Zachary (b. 1881). London surgeon.

Cope's clamp. A lever-action instrument which applies, in one movement, 3 intestinal crushing clamps lying side by side. Removal of the middle one of them allows a clean division of the bowel. It is a modified form of de Martel's clamp.

Cope's point. The midpoint of the line from the umbilicus to the right anterior superior spine of the ilium; the point of maximum tenderness in appendicitis.

Cope's sign. The psoas test. *See* TEST.

Cope's test. For appendicitis: 1. Obturator test; 2. Psoas test. *See* TEST.

Copepoda (ko·pe·**po**·dah). A sub-class or order of the Crustacea. The genera *Cyclops* and *Diaptomus* are of medical interest. [Gk *kope* oar, *pous* foot.]

cophosis (ko·**fo**·sis). Deafness. [Gk *kophos* deaf.]

copiopia, copiopsia (ko·pe·o·pe·ah, ko·pe·**op**·se·ah). Eyestrain due to using the eyes too much or in unsuitable conditions. [Gk *kopos* fatigue, *opsis* sight.]

copodyskinesia (**ko**·po·dis·kin·**e**'·ze·ah). Any occupation neurosis due to the constant repetition of a particular action, e.g. writer's cramp. [Gk *kopos* fatigue, dyskinesia.]

copper (**kop**·er). An element of atomic weight 63.546, atomic number 29 and chemical symbol Cu (*cuprum*). It is a red metal, highly malleable and ductile, used as wire and sheet in the electrical industry, for boilers and utensils, and, in the form of alloys with zinc (brass) or tin (bronze), for various specific purposes. It occurs naturally free in Sweden and Canada, or in combination as ores, particularly in the Urals. It is present in small quantities in all body tissues, especially in the liver and spleen, and traces are in the red blood cells, minute amounts being necessary in the diet for normal red cell formation, though anaemia due to its dietary deficiency has not been shown to occur in man. Deficiency of copper in the food has, however, been associated with the incidence of swayback in lambs, a disease resembling disseminated sclerosis in some respects. The element occurs also biologically in the respiratory pigment of certain marine invertebrates, haemocyanin, in leguminous plants, and in turacin, the pigment of the feathers of the plantain-eater. Many compounds are used in medicine, the inorganic salts being of importance chiefly for their astringent and germicidal actions. The organic salts have been tried in rheumatoid arthritis, disseminated sclerosis, trigeminal neuralgia and other conditions, with doubtful benefit. **Copper acetate.** $(CH_3COO)_2Cu{\cdot}H_2O$, a soluble green compound used as a caustic. **Copper amalgam.** An alloy of copper and mercury used sometimes in children as a filling for carious teeth, its chief advantage being ease of insertion as it is slow to set firmly. It often causes staining and so is not used for permanent teeth. **Basic copper acetate.** Copper subacetate, verdigris, $(CH_3COO)_2CuCu(OH)_2{\cdot}5H_2O$, a greenish-blue powder used in veterinary practice. **Copper chloride.** Cupric chloride, $CuCl_2{\cdot}2H_2O$, a compound used like copper sulphate. **Copper citrate.** $C_6H_4O_7Cu_2{\cdot}2H_2O$, a compound used in ointment form in the treatment of trachoma. **Copper Sulphate BP 1958.** Cupric sulphate, blue vitriol, blue stone, $CuSO_4{\cdot}5H_2O$, a blue crystalline substance with strong astringent properties, occasionally used in solution as an emetic; more dilute solutions are used externally in various skin conditions. In solid form it is sometimes employed as a caustic. A constituent of Benedict's and Fehling's reagents. It is also employed to restrain the growth of algae in reservoirs, and to kill the snails which act as intermediate hosts to *Schistosoma*. [L *cuprum*.]

copper-nose (**kop**·er·noze). 1. Rosacea. 2. Rhinophyma. [copper, nose.]

copperas (**kop**·er·as). Ferrous sulphate. [copper, L *rosa* rose.]

copperhead (**kop**·er·hed). A poisonous snake of North America (*Agkistrodon mokasen*). [copper, head.]

Coppock. The family name of the patients who had a type of cataract named after them.

Coppock cataract. A disc of opacity, consisting of a single layer lying behind the nucleus and well in front of the posterior capsule.

copra (**kop**·rah). The dried and crushed white fleshy endosperm of the seed of the coconut, *Cocos nucifera* (family Palmae). From it is expressed coconut oil. [Hind.]

copracrasia (kop·rah·**kra**·se·ah). Inability to retain faeces. [Gk *kopros* dung, *a*, *kratos* power.]

copragogue (**kop**·rag·og). A cathartic. [Gk *kopros* dung, *agogos* leading.]

co-precipitation (ko·pre·sip·it·**a**'·shun). In radiochemistry, the precipitation of trace amounts of one chemical substance by causing a bulky precipitation of another (for example, ferric hydroxide). [L *cum*, precipitation.]

copremesis (kop·**rem**·es·is). Stercoraceous vomiting; a condition of emesis in which faecal matter is present in the vomited material. [Gk *kopros* dung, *emesis* vomiting.]

coprikin (**kop**·rik·in). A condition in which there is undigested animal matter in the faeces. [Gk *kopros* dung.]

coproctic (kop·**rok**·tik). Faecal. [Gk *kopros* dung.]

coprodaeum (kop·ro·**de**·um). That part of the large intestine, i.e. the rectum and a part of the colon, which is concerned actively with the expulsion of faeces. [Gk *koprus* dung, *hodos* way.]

coprolagnia (kop·ro·**lag**·ne·ah). A form of sexual perversion in which excitement is aroused by the thought or the sight of human faeces. [Gk *kopros* dung, *lagneia* lust.]

coprolalia (kop·ro·**lal**·e·ah). The involuntary utterance of disgusting or obscene words mainly concerning the excretions, a symptom encountered in some diseases and in certain states of insanity. [Gk *kopros* dung, *lalein* to babble like a child.]

coprolalomania (kop·ro·lal·o·**ma**'·ne·ah). The morbid tendency or desire to use disgusting and obscene language. [Gk *kopros* dung, *lalein* to babble like a child, mania.]

coprolith (**kop**·ro·lith). A hard mass of faeces in the bowel. [Gk *kopros* dung, *lithos* stone.]

coprology (kop·**rol**·o·je). The study of the faeces. [Gk *kopros* dung, *logos* science.]

coproma (kop·**ro**·mah). Stercoroma; an accumulation of hardened faeces which presents the appearance of a tumour in the rectum. [Gk *kopros* dung, *-oma* tumour.]

Copromonas (kop·ro·**mo**·nas). A genus of unicellular algae. **Copromonas subtilis.** A species sometimes found in stale faeces. [Gk *kopros* dung, *monas* unit.]

coprophagous (kop·**rof**·ag·us). Having the habit of eating faeces; this is the natural habit of some insects, e.g. beetles, but may be observed in certain psychoses. [see foll.]

coprophagus, coprophagy (kop·**rof**·ag·us, kop·**rof**·ah·je). 1. In zoology, the feeding on dung, as do certain beetles. 2. The habit of eating faeces, a symptom of certain forms of insanity. [Gk *kopros* dung, *phagein* to eat.]

coprophemia (kop·ro·**fe**·me·ah). Obscene speech. [Gk *kopros* dung, *phemis* speech.]

coprophil, coprophile (**kop**·ro·fil, kop·ro·**file**). Of bacteria and fungi, living in or on faecal matter. [Gk *kopros* dung, *philein* to love.]

coprophilia (kop·ro·**fil**·e·ah). A psychopathological condition in which there is shown attraction of a sexual kind to faeces and anything connected with them. [see prec.]

coprophilous (kop·**rof**·il·us). Coprophil.

coprophobia (kop·ro·**fo**·be·ah). A condition of abnormal loathing with regard to faeces and to movement of the bowels. [Gk *kopros* dung, phobia.]

coproplanesis (kop·ro·plan·**e**'·sis). The passing of faeces from the bowel through an abnormal opening, e.g. a fistula. [Gk *kopros* dung, *plane* a wandering.]

coproporphyria (kop·ro·por·**fi**'·re·ah). A metabolic disorder in which coproporphyrin is retained in the tissues. **Erythropoietic coproporphyria.** Light sensitivity with a high erythrocyte coproporphyrin concentration. **Hereditary coproporphyria.** A form of porphyria with abdominal pain, dark urine and neuropsychiatric symptoms. [Gk *kopros* dung, *porphyros* purple.]

coproporphyrin (kop·ro·**por**·fir·in). $C_{36}H_{38}N_4O_8$, a porphyrin pigment which is a by-product in normal haemopoiesis. It is excreted largely by the liver in bile, and thence in normal faeces and urine. Increased excretion occurs in porphyria and porphyrinuria, and has been reported in various other disorders. [Gk *kopros* dung, porphyrin.]

coproporphyrinuria (kop·ro·**por**·fir·in·**ewr**'·e·ah). Coproporphyrin occurring in urine.

coprostanol (kop·ro·**sta**·nol). Coprosterol.

coprostasia, coprostasis (kop·ro·**sta**·ze·ah, kop·**ros**·tas·is). 1. Chronic constipation. 2. Faecal impaction. [Gk *kopros* dung, *stasis* a standing still.]

coprosterin (kop·**ros**·ter·in). Coprosterol.

coprosterol (kop·ro·**steer**·ol). Normal dehydrocholesterol, $C_{27}H_{47}OH$. A fully saturated sterol formed in the intestine by the bacterial reduction of cholesterol, and excreted in the faeces. [Gk *kopros* dung, sterol.]

coprozoa (kop·ro·**zo**·ah). Coprozoic protozoa; protozoa that live in media rich in decomposing organic matter, e.g. sewage. [see foll.]

coprozoic (kop·ro·**zo**·ik). Found in faecal material, sewage, and any substance rich in decaying organic matter. [Gk *kopros* dung, *zoon* animal.]

Coptis (**kop**·tis). A genus of plants of the family Ranunculaceae. **Coptis trifolia.** Gold thread; the root is a bitter tonic. [Gk *koptein* to cut.]

coptosystole (kop·to·**sis**·to·le). The cutting off of a ventricular systole. [Gk *koptein* to cut, systole.]

copula (**kop**·ew·lah). 1. A yoke, bridge or connecting link. 2. The copula linguae (see below). 3. An obsolete term for amboceptor. **Copula linguae.** A transverse ridge in the floor of the primitive pharynx, connecting the 2 hyoid or second pharyngeal arches at an early stage in the development of the tongue. [L a band.]

copulation (kop·ew·**la**·shun). Coitus. [L *copulare* to couple.]

coquille (ko·**keel**). A lens or glass, generally smoked, of the shape of a watch-glass. [Fr shell.]

cor (kor). Heart. **Cor adiposum.** Fatty heart; a heart in which fatty degeneration or infiltration has occurred. The term is also used to denote an excessive accumulation of epicardial fat. **Cor biatriatum triloculare.** A congenital malformation due to failure of development of the ventricular septum; there are 2 atria and a single ventricle. **Cor biloculare.** A congenital malformation due to failure of development of atrial and ventricular septa; there is only 1 atrium and 1 ventricle. **Cor biventriculare triloculare.** A congenital malformation in which the atrial septum has failed to develop, resulting in a single atrium; there are 2 ventricles. **Cor bovinum.** Ox heart; a grossly enlarged heart resulting from great hypertrophy of the left ventricle, particularly seen in severe aortic valvular disease. **Cor dextrum.** The right side of the heart, i.e. the right atrium and ventricle. **Cor hirsutum.** Villous heart; a roughened, shaggy surface of the heart due to thick exudate in pericarditis. **Cor mobile.** Mobile heart; a heart which moves freely within the chest with respiration and changes in posture. **Cor pendulosum, Cor pendulum.** Drop heart; a long narrow heart shadow seen on radiography in persons of asthenic build and in asthmatic individuals with a low diaphragm. **Cor pulmonale.** Pulmonary heart disease; heart disease resulting from disease of the lungs or pulmonary circulation. It may be acute (pulmonary embolism) or chronic. The latter is divided into 2 types, anoxic (due to disease of the lung parenchyma, such as emphysema) and obstructive (due to narrowing of the pulmonary arterioles). **Cor sinistrum.** The left side of the heart, i.e. the left atrium and ventricle. **Cor taurianum.** Cor bovinum (see above). **Cor tometosum.** Cor hirsutum (see above). **Cor triatriatum.** A congenital malformation due to the development of an abnormal transverse septum which divides the left atrium into an upper and lower portion; there are thus 3 atria. **Cor venosum.** The right side of the heart, containing venous blood. **Cor villosum.** Cor hirsutum (see above). [L.]

coracidium (kor·as·**id**·e·um). Embryo of tapeworms of the order Pseudophyllidea, enclosed in a ciliated embryophore; that of *Diphyllobothrium latum.* [Gk *korakidion* hooklet.]

coraco-acromial (kor·ak·o·ak·ro′·me·al). Relating or belonging to the coracoid process and the acromion.

coracobrachialis (kor·ak·o·bra·ke·a′·lis). The coracobrachialis muscle. [coracoid, brachialis.]

coracobrachialis muscle [musculus coracobrachialis (NA)]. A muscle which lies on the medial side of the arm, and extends from the coracoid process to the middle of the humeral shaft.

coracoclavicular (kor·ak·o·klav·**ik**′·ew·lar). Relating or attached to the coracoid process and the clavicle.

coracohumeral (kor·ak·o·**hew**′·mer·al). Relating to or attached to the coracoid process and the humerus.

coracohyoid (kor·ak·o·**hi**′·oid). 1. Relating to the coracoid process and the hyoid bone. 2. Another name for the omohyoid muscle.

coracoid (kor·ak·oid). 1. The coracoid process. 2. Shaped like a crow's beak. **Coracoid process.** *See* PROCESS. [Gk *korax* crow, *eidos* form.]

coracoiditis (kor·ak·oid·i′·tis). A painful condition in the region of the scapula and of the coracoid process, with deltoid atrophy; attributed to injury of the coracoid process. [coracoid, Gk *-itis* inflammation.]

coracopectoralis (kor·ak·o·pek·tor·a′·lis). Another name for the pectoralis minor muscle. [coracoid, pectoral.]

coracoradialis (kor·ak·o·ra·de·a′·lis). The short head of the biceps muscle, arising from the apex of the coracoid process. [coracoid, radial.]

coraco-ulnaris (kor·ak·o·ul·**na**′·ris). Those fibres of the biceps muscle which are attached to the fascia of the forearm. [coracoid, ulna.]

coral (kor·al). The calcareous substance which is secreted by sea polyps and serves to form their skeleton. **Coral calculus.** *See* CALCULUS. [Gk *korallion.*]

coralliform (kor·al·e·form). 1. Resembling a coral in shape. 2. Having branches like a coral.

corallin (kor·al·in). Rosolic acid. *See* ACID. **Yellow corallin.** Sodium rosolate, a dye used as an indicator.

coralloid (kor·al·oid). Coralliform. [coral, Gk *eidos* form.]

Corallorhiza (kor·al·o·ri′·zah). A genus of plants of the family Orchidaceae. **Corallorhiza odontorhiza.** A species the root of which is an antipyretic and diaphoretic. [Gk *korallion* coral, *rhiza* root.]

corasthma (kor·**as**·mah). Hay fever; acute rhinitis with an allergic basis. [coryza, asthma.]

Corbus, Budd Clarke (b. 1876). Chicago urologist.

Corbus' disease. Gangrenous balanitis. *See* BALANITIS.

cord (kord). An elongated flexible structure with a circular, or approximately circular, cross-section. **Cord of the brachial plexus, lateral [fasciculus lateralis (NA)].** Part of the brachial plexus formed behind the clavicle by the union of the anterior divisions of the upper and middle trunks and hence carrying fibres from the 5th, 6th and 7th cervical roots. The branches mainly supply the flexor muscles of the arm and forearm and the skin on the flexor surface of the forearm and hand laterally. **Cord of the brachial plexus, medial [fasciculus medialis (NA)].** Part of the brachial plexus formed behind the clavicle by the anterior division of the lower trunk. It lies medial to the axillary artery and carries fibres from the 8th cervical and 1st thoracic roots. The branches mainly supply the flexor muscles of the forearm and small muscles of the hand and the skin on the flexor surface of the arm, forearm, and hand medially. **Cord of the brachial plexus, posterior [fasciculus posterior (NA)].** A segment of the brachial plexus, formed by the union of the posterior divisions of the three trunks and containing fibres from all the roots of the plexus. The branches of the posterior cord are, in the main, responsible for the supply of the dorsal or extensor skin and muscles of the arm, forearm and a large part of the hand. **Dental cord.** Dental lamina. *See* LAMINA. **Dorsal cord.** Notochord. **Enamel cord.** A cord of cells connecting the enamel organ with the dental lamina. **False cords [plicae vestibulares].** The vestibular folds, or false vocal cords; folds of mucous membrane which pass from the thyroid cartilage to the cuneiform cartilages above the vocal folds (true vocal cords). **Ganglionated cord.** The paravertebral chain of sympathetic ganglia. **Genital cord.** An elongated mass of mesodermal cells lying medial to the mesonephros of the embryo, from which the ovary or testis is derived. **Gubernacular cord.** "Gubernaculum". **Hepatic cord.** One of the columns of epithelial cells composing a liver lobule. **Lumbosacral cord.** The lumbosacral trunk, formed by the union of the anterior primary ramus of the 5th lumbar nerve with part of that of the 4th. **Medullary cord.** One of the epithelial strands found near the hilum of the fetal ovary, and thought to be homologous with the seminiferous tubules of the testis. **Nephrogenic cord.** In the early embryo, one of the paired cells running lengthwise in the posterior coelomic wall on either side of the gut mesentery from which the pro-, meso- and meta-nephros are derived. **Nerve cord.** A nerve trunk. **Oblique cord [chorda obliqua (NA)].** A fibrous band passing distally and laterally from the tuberosity of the ulna to the radius. **Sex cord, Sexual cord.** One of the strands of epithelial cells of the embryonic gonad from which the ovarian follicles and seminiferous tubules of the testis are derived. **Sonorous cords.** Vocal cords (see below). **Spermatic cord [funiculus spermaticus (NA)].** A cord-like structure formed by the vas deferens and the blood vessels, nerves and lymphatics of the testis, bound together by connective tissue. It extends from the upper pole of the testis to the deep inguinal ring. **Spinal cord [medulla spinalis (NA)].** The part of the central nervous system from the medulla oblongata to the filum terminale, lying within the vertebral canal. Named parts are cervical [pars cervicalis (NA)], thoracic [pars thoracica (NA)]. and lumbar [pars lumbalis (NA)]. **Splenic cord.** Billroth's cord; one of the anastomosing columns of reticular cells and erythrocytes composing the red pulp of the spleen. **Testicular cord.** Spermatic cord (see above). **Umbilical cord [funiculus umbilicalis (NA)].** The cord by which the fetus is attached to the placenta and containing 2 umbilical arteries and 1 umbilical vein. **Vocal cords [plicae vocales (NA)].** The vocal folds of the larynx; the true vocal cords, as distinct from the false cords (see above); folds of mucous membrane stretched between the thyroid and arytenoid cartilages and responsible for voice production. [Gk *chorde* string.]

See also: BERGMANN (G. H.), BILLROTH, BRAUN, FERREIN, HIPPOCRATES, PFLUEGER, WEITBRECHT, WILDE, WILLIS.

cordate (kord·ate). Heart-shaped. [L *cor* heart.]
cordectomy (kord·**ek**·to·me). Surgical removal of a vocal fold. [Gk *chorde* string, *ektome* a cutting out.]
Cordia (**kord**·e·ah). A genus of plants of the family Boraginaceae. **Cordia anbletti.** A species from Guyana; the leaves were used for tumours and skin diseases. **Cordia myxa.** A species from the East Indies and cultivated in Arabia and Egypt; the root was used as a purgative, the fruit for coughs and the powdered bark for ringworm. [Euricius *Cordius,* German botanist.]
cordial (**kord**·e·al). 1. An alcoholic liquor containing aromatic flavouring agents. Many so-called fruit cordials used as beverages contain virtually no alcohol. 2. A stimulant. [see foll.]
cordiale (kord·**e**·**a**·le). A cordial; it usually consists of a tincture flavoured and sweetened to make it more palatable. The various cordials which were once in common use are now obsolete. [L.]
See also: GODFREY.
Cordier's treatment. The injection of filtered air around the trunk of the sciatic nerve as treatment for sciatica. Now obsolete.
cordiform (**kord**·e·form). Cordate.
cordis (**kord**·is). Of the heart. **Accretio cordis.** External adhesive pericarditis. *See* PERICARDITIS. **Concretio cordis.** Internal adhesive pericarditis. *See* PERICARDITIS. [L.]
cordite (**kord**·ite). A smokeless, highly explosive substance, used in shells and cartridges. It is a gun-cotton dissolved in nitroglycerin, with castor oil or "Vaseline" as a moderant. Poisoning amongst cordite workers is a serious industrial risk. [cord, from its appearance.]
corditis (kord·**i**·tis). Inflammation of the spermatic cord. [cord, Gk *-itis* inflammation.]
cordoblastoma (**kord**·o·blas·**to**'·mah). Chordoblastoma.
cordocarcinoma (**kord**·o·kar·sin·**o**'·mah). Chordoma.
cordo-epithelioma (**kord**·o·**ep**·e·the·le·**o**'·mah). Chordoma.
cordoid (**kord**·oid). Chordoid.
cordoma (kord·**o**·mah). Chordoma.
Cordonnier's operation. Intraperitoneal transplantation of ureters.
cordopexy (**kord**·o·pex·e). Chordopexy.
cordotomy (kord·**ot**·o·me). Chordotomy.
Cordylobia (kor·dil·**o**·be·ah). A genus of blow-flies (Calliphoridae). **Cordylobia anthropophaga.** The tumbu fly of tropical Africa, a species which lives as a larva in the superficial tissues of rodents and frequently man. Single larvae cause boil-like swellings with a central respiratory aperture, but multiple infections may produce serious ulceration. The larval life is about 10 days. **Cordylobia rodhaini.** A species that may cause myiasis in man. [Gk *kordyle* club, lobe.]
core (kore). 1. The most vital part of anything. 2. The central part of anything. 3. The central mass of a carbuncle or boil. 4. The pupil of the eye. 5. The central iron former of an induction coil. **Atomic core.** Co-electron. [L *cor* heart.]
coreclisis (kor·e·**kli**·sis). Pathological occlusion or obliteration of the pupil of the eye. [Gk *kore* pupil, *kleiein* to shut up.]
corectasis (kor·**ek**·tas·is). Dilatation of the pupil of the eye, the result of disease. [Gk *kore* pupil, *ektasis* a stretching.]
corectome (kor·**ek**·tome). Iridectome; an instrument with a cutting edge used in excision of a portion of the iris. [Gk *kore* pupil, *temnein* to cut.]
corectomedialysis (kor·**ek**·to·me·di·**al**'·is·is). Iridectomesodialysis; the making of an artificial pupil by removal of the iris from the ciliary ligament. [Gk *kore* pupil, *ektemnein* to cut out, *dialyein* to set free.]
corectomy (kor·**ek**·to·me). Iridotomy; incision of the iris, with or without the formation of an artificial pupil. [Gk *kore* pupil, *ektemnein* to cut out.]
corectopia (kor·ek·**to**·pe·ah). The condition in which the pupil is abnormally situated. [Gk *kore* pupil, *ektopos* out of place.]
coredialysis (**kor**·e·di·**al**'·is·is). 1. The surgical procedure of cutting the ciliary body free from the ciliary border of the iris. 2. The surgical establishment of an artificial pupil at the ciliary border of the iris. [Gk *kore* pupil, dialysis.]
corediastasis (**kor**·e·di·**as**'·tas·is). Dilatation of the pupil of the eye. [Gk *kore* pupil, diastasis.]
corelysis (kor·**el**·is·is). 1. Operative destruction of the pupil of the eye. 2. The cutting through of adhesions between the capsule of the lens and the iris. [Gk *kore* pupil, *lysis* a loosing.]
coremium (kor·**em**·e·um). A sheaf of conidiophores or sometimes aerial hyphae bound together, usually erect and prominent on the surface of a fungus colony. [Gk *korema* sweepings.]
coremorphosis (kor·e·**mor**·fo·sis). The surgical establishment of an artificial pupil. [Gk *kore* pupil, *morphe* form, *-osis* condition.]
corenclisis (kor·en·**kli**·sis). Iridencleisis; a method of making an artificial pupil by using a small strip of iris tissue and fixing to the site of incision in the cornea. [Gk *kore* pupil, *egklein* to enclose.]
coreometer (kor·e·**om**·et·er). An instrument with which the width of the pupil of the eye may be measured. [Gk *kore* pupil, meter.]
coreometry (kor·e·**om**·et·re). The act of measuring the pupil of the eye. [see prec.]
coreoncion (kor·e·**on**·se·on). An iris forceps with a double hook. [Gk *kore* pupil, *ogkos* barb.]
coreoplasty (**kor**·e·o·**plas**'·te). 1. Plastic operation of any type performed on the pupil of the eye. 2. The establishment of an artificial pupil. 3. The correction by plastic means of a deformed pupil. [Gk *kore* pupil, *plassein* to mould.]
corepressor (ko·re·**pres**·or). The name given to the molecule which combines with repressor proteins to yield active repressor complexes which bind the operator regions of the DNA, and thus inhibit transcription. Thus, histidine is the corepressor involved in the inhibition of the synthesis of the enzymes of histidine biosynthesis. [L *cum, reprimere* to press back.]
corestenoma congenitum (**kor**·e·sten·**o**'·mah kon·**jen**·it·um). A congenital condition of partial occlusion of the pupil caused by outgrowths from the iris, these forming a grid-like mask over the pupil. [Gk *kore* pupil, *stenosis* a narrowing, L *congenitus* born with.]
coretomedialysis (kor·e·to·me·di·**al**'·is·is). The establishment of an artificial pupil by combined cutting and tearing of the iris. [Gk *kore* pupil, *temnein* to cut, *dialysis* division.]
coretomy (kor·**et**·o·me). 1. Iridotomy. 2. Any cutting operation performed on the iris of the eye. [Gk *kore* pupil, *temnein* to cut.]
Cori, Carl Ferdinand (b. 1896) and **Cori, Gerty Theresa** (b. 1896). American biochemists.
Cori cycle. Glucose-lactate cycle. *See* CYCLE.
Cori ester. Glucopyranose-1-monophosphate, $C_6H_{11}O_6PO(OH)_2$, formed from the glycogen of the liver and muscle with phosphate ions.
coriaceous (kor·e·**a**·shus). Of bacterial cultures, tough or leathery. [L *corium* leather.]
Coriander BP 1973 (kor·e·**an**·der). The dried ripe fruits of *Coriandrum sativum* Linn. (family Umbelliferae); it contains a volatile oil and is aromatic and carminative. By adding it to purgative medicines it prevents griping, e.g. Compound Rhubard Tincture BP 1958. [Gk *koriannon.*]
coriandrol (kor·e·**an**·drol). Linalool. [see prec.]
Coriaria (kor·e·**a**·re·ah). A genus of poisonous shrubs of the family Coriaraceae. **Coriaria myrtifolia.** A species used in dyeing and tanning; the leaves contain a glycoside which has tetanic properties like those of picrotoxin. **Coriaria sarmentosa.** A species the seed and shoots of which afford so-called toot poison; memory is said to be impaired after recovery from poisoning by this root. [L *corium* leather.]
coridine (**kor**·id·een). $C_{10}H_{15}N$, a substance related to pyridine, obtained when bones are distilled.
corium [dermis (NA)] (**ko**·re·um). The tough, flexible and highly elastic layer of vascular tissue lying immediately beneath the epidermis; also referred to as true skin or dermis. It contains the sebaceous and sweat glands and the hair follicles, and on its surface are vascular and sensitive papillae. **Corium phlogisticum.** Crusta phlogistica. [L leather.]
Corlett, William Thomas (b. 1854). Cleveland dermatologist.
Corlett's pyosis. Bullous staphyloderma. *See* STAPHYLODERMA.

Corley, Ralph Conner (b. 1901). American biochemist.
Corley and Denis method. A method for the estimation of calcium in tissues based on its precipitation as the oxalate.

corm (korm). A swollen underground plant stem holding reserves of plant food. [Gk *kormos* trunk.]

corn (korn). 1. A small, hard seed of a plant. [AS.] 2. Clavus; a small, circumscribed, painful, horny growth, formed in the skin over bony protuberances, on areas subjected intermittently to pressure. The toes are the sites of election. The lesion is a simple hyperkeratosis; in the centre a conical plug or core forms, which, by pressure on underlying sensory nerve-endings, causes a typical boring pain. **Hard corn.** A typical hard, dry corn. **Soft corn.** A corn which is macerated by sweat that is formed on the side of the toe. **Squirrel corn, Turkey corn.** *See* CORYDALIS. [L *cornu* horn.]

corn cockle (**korn** kokl). The plant *Agrostemma githago* the seeds of which cause githagism. [AS *corn, coccel* tares.]

corn smut (**korn** smut). A fungus, *Ustilago zeae.* [AS *corn,* ME *smut.*]

cornea [NA] (**kor**·ne·ah). The transparent anterior part of the fibrous coat of the eyeball, of which the posterior part is the sclera. It consists of a substantia propria, made up chiefly of collagenous fibres with a few cells (corneal corpuscles), and is avascular. It is covered anteriorly [facies anterior] by an anterior elastic lamina, outside which is the stratified corneal epithelium; posteriorly [facies posterior] is the posterior elastic lamina, and the endothelium of the anterior chamber of the eye. **Conical cornea.** Keratoconus. **Cornea farinata.** A degenerative change of the deeper layers of the cornea in old people; it is usually bilateral, and appears as numerous fine dust-like opacities. **Flat cornea.** Flattening of the cornea, occurring in shrinking atrophic eyeballs. **Cornea globata.** Megalocornea; a bilateral developmental abnormality in which the anterior segment of the eye is larger than normal. It differs from buphthalmos in the absence of raised intra-ocular pressure. **Cornea guttata.** A dystrophic condition of the corneal endothelium, visible in its early stages only with the slit lamp, and characterized by the formation of black spherules in the endothelial mosaic. It affects both eyes, and may go on to epithelial dystrophy (dystrophia epithelialis corneae). **Cornea opaca.** The sclerotic. **Cornea plana.** A congenital condition in which the cornea does not develop its normal amount of convexity. **Sugar-loaf cornea.** Keratoconus. [L *corneus* horny.]

corneal (**kor**·ne·al). Relating or belonging to the cornea.

Corneal Grafting Act 1952. *See* HUMAN TISSUE ACT 1961.

corneal splitter (**kor**·ne·al **split**·er). An instrument used in ophthalmic surgery for splitting the corneal lamella at the limbus.
See also: LAWFORD, TOOKE.

corneitis (kor·ne·**i**·tis). Inflammation of the cornea. [cornea, Gk *-itis* inflammation.]

Cornell, Ethel Letitia (b. 1892). New York psychologist.
Cornell index test. A questionary designed to pick out subjects with psychopathic personality or psychosomatic disorders.

corneoblepharon (kor·ne·o·**blef**'·ar·on). Adhesion between the surface of the eyelid and the cornea. [cornea, Gk *blepharon* eyelid.]

corneo-iritis (kor·ne·o·i·**ri**'·tis). Inflammation of the cornea and the iris. [cornea, iritis.]

corneosclera (kor·ne·o·**skleer**'·ah). The cornea and the sclera considered as a single organ, i.e. the fibrous coat of the eye.

corneosclerectomy (kor·ne·o·skler·**ek**'·to·me). An operation in which a portion of adjoining cornea and sclera is excised at the limbus, as in Elliot's corneoscleral trephining for glaucoma. [corneosclera, Gk *ektome* excision.]
See also: BERENS.

corneous (**kor**·ne·us). Hard; of a texture resembling that of horn. [L *cornu* horn.]

Corner, Edred Moss (b. 1873). London surgeon.
Corner's plug, or tampon. An omental plug used to close a perforated peptic ulcer.

Corner, George Washington (b. 1889). Rochester, N.Y., anatomist.
Corner–Allen test. A method of assaying progesterone based on the effects of progesterone on the uterus of the rabbit which has been mated and the ovaries removed 18 h later.
See also: MACPHAIL TEST.

Cornet, George (b. 1858). Berlin physician.
Cornet's forceps. A cross-action forceps for holding litmus paper in testing urine.

cornet (**kor**·net). 1. A small horn-shaped ear-trumpet which fits into the ear and is easily concealed by the hair; now little used. 2. A bony layer. **Sphenoid cornet.** One of the sphenoidal concha. [L *cornu* horn.]
See also: BERTIN.

corneum (**kor**·ne·um). The horny zone of the epidermis. [L.]

corniculate (kor·**nik**·ew·late). Having small horn-like processes or horns. **Corniculate cartilage.** *See* CARTILAGE. [L *corniculum* little horn.]

corniculum laryngis (kor·**nik**·ew·lum lar·**in**·jis). The corniculate cartilage. *See* CARTILAGE. [L little horn of the larynx.]

cornification (kor·nif·ik·a'·shun). 1. A callosity. 2. The process of being converted into horn or into horny tissue or substance such as the stratified squamous type of epithelium. 3. Cornification of the vaginal epithelium. Cornification index, the percentage of cornified cells (flattened, flaked superficial cells) found typically in high percentage at ovulation. [L *cornu* horn, *facere* to make.]

cornified (**kor**·nif·ide). Converted into horn or horny tissue. [see prec.]

Corning, James Leonard (b. 1855). New York neurologist.
Corning's anaesthesia. Anaesthesia by the application of cocaine to nerves.
Corning's puncture. Lumbar puncture; withdrawal of cerebrospinal fluid for diagnostic or therapeutic purposes through a needle introduced into the spinal subarachnoid space.

cornu [NA] (**kor**·new) (pl. *cornua*). A horn; in anatomy, a structure shaped like a horn. **Cornu ammonis.** The curved elongated projection of the hippocampal formation into the inferior horn of the lateral ventricle; the hippocampus, as opposed to the dentate gyrus and subiculum. **Coccygeal cornua [cornua coccygea** (NA)]. Bilateral projections from the back of the 1st coccygeal vertebra, representing the neural arch of that vertebra. **Cornu cutaneum.** An excrescence arising from the epidermis; it may develop from a wart, or be connected with a sebaceous cyst or a pilosebaceous follicle, and is formed by the hypertrophy of the prickle-cell and horny layers. At first the proliferation of the former is commensurate with the hyperkeratosis, but later the cornification preponderates; malignant degeneration may occur at the base. Such horns may be single or multiple, and vary greatly in length and diameter, though they are usually small. **Cornu descendens.** The descending, inferior or temporal horn of the lateral ventricle. **Cornu dorsale.** The dorsal, or posterior horn of grey matter in the spinal cord. **Ethmoid cornu.** The middle concha (obsolete). **Cornu of the falciform margin.** *See* MARGIN. **Cornu humanum.** Cornu cutaneum (see above). **Cornu laterale.** The lateral horn of grey matter in the thoracic and upper lumbar segments of the spinal cord. It contains the cell bodies of the preganglionic sympathetic neurones. **Cornu occipitale.** The posterior horn of the lateral ventricle. **Cornua ossis hyoidei.** The greater and lesser horns of the hyoid bone. **Pulp cornu.** That part of the tooth pulp that occupies a horn of the pulp chamber. **Sacral cornua [cornua sacralia** (NA)]. Projections from the posterior surface of the 5th sacral vertebra, representing its neural arch. **Cornua of the spinal cord.** The projections of grey matter into the white matter seen on the cut surface of a transverse section of the spinal cord, anterior (ventral), posterior (dorsal), and lateral. **Cornua of the uterus.** Straight or curved extensions from the lateral angles of the body of the uterus, resulting from an incomplete fusion of the bilateral paramesonephric ducts from which the uterus is developed. In most mammals, other than man, the uterus is normally bicornate. **Cornu ventrale.** The ventral, or anterior, horn of grey matter in the spinal cord. [L horn.]

cornual (**kor**·new·al). Relating to a cornu.

cornucommissural (**kor**·new·kom·**is**'·ewr·al). Relating to a cornu and a commissure.

Cornus (**kor**·nus). 1. A genus of plants of the family Cornaceae. 2. The root and bark of *Cornus florida* Linn. **Cornus circinata.** The round-leaved dogwood; it has properties similar to those of *C. florida.* **Cornus florida.** A species from Canada and the USA. The root bark is tonic and astringent and is used for intermittent fevers. [L dogwood tree.]

coroclisis (kor·o·**kli**·sis). Coreclisis.

corodiastasis (**kor**·o·di·**as**'·tas·is). Corediastasis.

corolla (ko·**rol**·ah). In botany, the inner perianth of the envelope of a flower, which is usually coloured, i.e. not green, and often scented to attract insects. It is constituted of a whorl of petals. [L little crown.]

corometer (kor·**om**·et·er). Coreometer.

corona [NA] (kor·o·nah). A crown; also used for a curved line, or circle. **Corona capitis.** The crown of the head. **Ciliary corona.** The ciliary crown; the anterior part of the ciliary body, as opposed to the posterior, or ciliary ring. **Corona glandis [NA].** The raised posterior margin of the glans penis. **Corona of a lymphatic nodule.** The peripheral zone of a lymphatic nodule, packed densely with small lymphocytes. **Corona radiata [NA].** 1. The fibres which radiate between the internal capsule and the cerebral cortex. 2. Follicular cells around a mature ovum, some of which may remain attached to the ovum for a period subsequent to ovulation. **Corona seborrhoeica.** An erythematous and scaling eruption associated with seborrhoeic dermatitis of the scalp, extending across the upper part of the forehead; the lower edge may be festooned. **Corona veneris.** A papular syphilitic eruption involving the upper margin of the forehead in a transverse band. [L crown.]

See also: BISCHOFF, ZINN.

coronal (kor·on·al). 1. Relating or belonging to the crown of the head. 2. Relating to any corona. **Coronal plane.** *See* PLANE. **Coronal suture.** *See* SUTURE. [see prec.]

coronale (kor·on·a·le). 1. The frontal bone. 2. In the coronal suture, the point at each end of the widest frontal diameter. [L *corona* crown.]

coronaria (kor·on·a·re·ah). A coronary artery. **Coronaria ventriculi.** An artery on the lesser curvature of the stomach formed by the joining of the gastric artery and the superior pyloric branch of the hepatic artery.

coronarism (**kor**·on·a·izm). A condition in which there is spastic contraction of the coronary arteries of the heart.

coronaritis (**kor**·on·ar·**i**'·tis). A state of inflammation of the coronary arteries of the heart. [coronary, Gk *-itis* inflammation.]

coronary (**kor**·on·ar·e). A term descriptive of certain anatomical structures which are in the form of a crown or circlet, e.g. coronary artery. **Coronary sinus.** *See* SINUS. **Coronary suture.** *See* SUTURE. [L *corona* crown.]

coronary arteries. Arteries supplying blood to the walls of the heart. **Left coronary artery [arteria coronaria sinistra (NA)].** An artery arising from the left posterior aortic sinus and running forward and to the left in the atrioventricular groove. After giving off an interventricular branch [ramus interventricularis anterior (NA)] along the anterior interventricular groove, it continues around the atrioventricular groove [ramus circumflexus (NA)] and ends by anastomosing with the right coronary artery. **Right coronary artery [arteria coronaria dextra (NA)].** An artery arising from the anterior aortic sinus and running to the right in the upper part, and to the left in the lower part, of the atrioventricular groove. It gives an interventricular branch [ramus interventricularis posterior (NA)] to the inferior interventricular groove, and ends by anastomosing with the left coronary artery.

coronavirus (**kor**'·o·nah·vi·rus). A group of viruses whose outer surface is studded with club-shaped projections giving a "setting-sun" appearance in the electron microscope. The particles are pleomorphic with an average size of about 100 nm. Members of the group include some of the causative agents of the common cold in man and other viruses causing a variety of diseases in animals. Similar agents have been found in stools by direct electron microscopy. They have been found in association with enteritis but their role in causation has to be confirmed. [L *corona* crown, *virus* poison.]

corone (kor·o·ne). The coronoid process of the mandible. *See* PROCESS.

coroner (**kor**·on·er). A judicial officer whose duty is to enquire into the manner of death of any person who is suspected of dying an unnatural death, or of one for which the cause is not evident, also of all persons dying in prison, and all deaths among persons certified as suffering from mental disease. Such deaths include those due to violence and industrial disease, and as a result of anaesthetics, and deaths among persons in receipt of disability pensions. He is appointed by the local authority and must be possessed of a legal or medical qualification and have practised for at least 5 years. **Coroners' cases.** *See* CASE. [L *corona* crown.]

Coronilla (kor·o·**nil**·ah). A genus of plants of the family Leguminosae. **Coronilla scorpiodes.** A species which contains a glycoside, coronillin; it is a cardiac tonic and diuretic. **Coronilla varia.** A diuretic and purgative species. [L *corona* crown.]

coronion (kor·o·ne·on). In craniometry, the tip of the coronoid process of the mandible; koronion. [Gk *korone* crow.]

coronium (kor·o·ne·um). An element believed to have been observed in the corona of the sun; it has not been found on the earth.

coronobasilar (**kor**·on·o·**ba**'·sil·ar). In head measurement, running from the coronal suture to the basilar portion of the skull.

coronofacial (**kor**·on·o·**fa**'·shal). In head measurement, having reference to the crown of the head and the face. [L *corona* crown, face.]

coronoid (**kor**·on·oid). 1. Like the beak of a crow in shape. [Gk *korone* crow, *eidos* form.] 2. Shaped like a crown or corona. **Coronoid process.** *See* PROCESS. [L *corona* crown, Gk *eidos* form.]

coroparelcysis (kor·o·par·**el**'·sis·is). The surgical readjustment of the pupil so that it is set over a transparent part of a partially opaque cornea. [Gk *kore* pupil, *parelkein* to draw aside.]

corophthisis (kor·o·**thi**·sis). Diminution in the size of the pupillary area of permanent kind as a result of general wasting of the eye. [Gk *kore* pupil, *phthein* to consume.]

coroscopy (kor·**os**·ko·pe). Retinoscopy; reflected shadow test of the retina by which the refraction potential of the eye may be assessed. [Gk *kore* pupil, *skopein* to watch.]

corotomy (kor·**ot**·o·me). Iridotomy. [Gk *kore* pupil, *temnein* to cut.]

corpora (**kor**·por·ah). *See* CORPUS.

corporal (**kor**·por·al). 1. Relating or belonging to the body. 2. Relating to a body. [L *corpus* body.]

corporeal (kor·**po**·re·al). 1. Consisting of matter or a material body—that is, physical, not mental. 2. Corporal. [L *corpus* body.]

corporic (kor·**po**·rik). Referring to the body of any organ. [see prec.]

corpse (korps). A dead human body. **Radioactive corpse.** Disposal is subject to a recommendation issued in 1957. Cremation is prohibited over the prescribed level set by the Ministry of Health Circular 95030/30/2. [see foll.]

corpulence, corpulency (**kor**·pew·lens, **kor**·pew·len·se). Obesity; bulkiness of body. [L *corpus* body.]

corpus [L.] (**kor**·pus) (pl. *corpora*). A body; the term may be used in anatomy for any large mass of tissue which can be delimited from its surroundings. **Corpus albicans [NA].** The scar tissue that replaces the corpus luteum (see below) at the beginning of the next menstrual cycle. It is seen as a depression on the ovary, with a yellow or yellowish-white hue. **Corpus alienum.** A foreign body. **Corpora amylacea.** Amyloid bodies. *See* BODY. **Corpora arantii.** Nodules of the aortic and pulmonary semilunar valves. **Corpora arenacea.** Brainsand granules, consisting mainly of the phosphates and carbonates of calcium and magnesium, which are found in the pineal body after the age of 7. **Corpora atretica.** Corpora albicans (see above). **Corpus bigeminum.** Either of the 2 superior quadrigeminal bodies; the term is commonly used only in connection with the brains of sub-mammalian vertebrates where the inferior quadrigeminal bodies are poorly developed and do not project on the surface. They are usually referred to as the optic lobes of the mid-brain. **Corpus callosum** [NA]. The large elongated commissure joining the cortex of one hemisphere with that of the other; it is found at the bottom of the fissure between the 2 hemispheres. **Corpora candicantia.** The mamillary bodies. *See* BODY. **Corpora cavernosa of the clitoris [corpus cavernosum clitoridis (dextrum et sinistrum)** NA]. Bodies of erectile tissue similar to but smaller than the corpora cavernosa penis (see following). **Corpora cavernosa penis** [NA]. The two columns of erectile tissue dorsal to the urethra and forming the main part of the body of the penis. **Corpus dentatum olivae.** The irregular layer of nerve cells forming the olivary nucleus; obsolete. **Corpus fibrosum.** The end result of a graafian follicle which has never reached maturity. **Corpus fimbriatum.** The fimbria. **Corpora flava.** Yellowish waxy bodies found in areas of degeneration of the central nervous system, possibly derived from nerve cells. **Corpus haemorrhagicum.** A blood clot formed in the cavity left by rupture of a graafian follicle; when the clot is old, it may be called a *corpus nigrum.* **Corpus highmori.** Mediastinum testis. **Corpus interpedunculare.** The interpenduncular nucleus. *See* NUCLEUS. **Corpora libera.** Loose bodies within a joint. **Corpus liberum pericardi.** A free mass lying in the pericardium; it is usually of fatty or fibro-fatty tissue, but may also be a foreign body or a neoplasm. **Corpora lutea** [NA]. Yellowish or orange bodies found in the ovary after rupture of graafian follicles and derived from the granulosa and theca cells. They secrete the hormone progesterone, which prepares the uterine mucosa for implantation of the fertilized ovum. **Corpora lutea atretica.** Corpora albicans (see above). **Corpus luysi.** The subthalamic nucleus. *See* NUCLEUS. **Corpora malpighiana.** Grey or whitish areas seen on the cut surface of the fresh spleen and forming the white pulp (diffuse and nodular lymphatic tissue) of the organ. **Corpus nigrum.** *See* CORPUS HAEMORRHAGICUM (above). **Corpora olivaria.** The oval projections on the ventral surface of the medulla, lateral to the pyramids and caused by the underlying olivary nuclei. **Corpus pampiniforme.** The epoöphoron, or peravarium. **Corpus papillare [stratum papillare** (NA)]. The superficial layer of the skin. **Corpus pontobulbare.** A rounded eminence on the lateral surface of the inferior cerebellar peduncle, close to the root of the 8th cranial nerve; it is formed by some outlying cells of the pontine nuclei. **Corpus pyramidale.** The pyramid on the ventral surface of the medulla. **Corpora quadrigemina.** Quadrigeminal bodies. *See* BODY. **Corpora santoriana.** The corniculate cartilages of the larynx. **Corpus spongiosum penis** [NA]. The erectile tissue surrounding the urethra, which is continuous with the bulb of the penis posteriorly and the glans penis anteriorly. **Corpus spongiosum urethrae.** Corpus spongiosum penis (see preceding). **Corpora striata** [NA]. The basal ganglia of the cerebral hemisphere, consisting chiefly of the caudate and lentiform nuclei. **Corpus subthalamicum.** The subthalamic nucleus. *See* NUCLEUS. **Corpus trapezoideum** [NA]. The trapezoid decussation found deep to the caudal part of the pons; it consists principally of fibres from the cochlear nuclei which, after crossing, form the lateral lemniscus. **Corpus trapezoideum, dorsal nucleus of the [nucleus dorsalis corporis trapezoidei** (NA)]. A nucleus in the reticular formation of the pons just dorsal to the lateral part of the trapezoid body, within which some of the fibres on the auditory pathway relay. **Corpus trapezoideum, ventral nucleus of the [nucleus ventralis corporis trapezoidei** (NA)]. A small nucleus ventral to the dorsal trapezoid nucleus. **Corpus triticeum.** A small cartilaginous nodule in the lateral thyrohyoid ligament. **Corpus wolffianum.** The wolffian body, or mesonephros. [L body.]

See also: ARANZIO, SANTORINI, SWAMMERDAM.

corpus cavernosography (**kor**·pus **kav**·ern·o·**sog**′·raf·e). The radiographical examination of a corpus cavernosum after instillation of a contrast medium [corpus cavernosum, Gk *graphein* to record.]

corpuscle [corpusculum (NA)] (**kor**·pusl). 1. Any small round body or mass. 2. In anatomy, a small discrete body, usually of microscopic dimensions; a term very commonly applied to the various forms of organized nerve-endings. **Amylaceous corpuscle, Amyloid corpuscle.** A small body resembling a starch grain. **Articular corpuscle [corpusculum articulare** (NA)]. An end-bulb found in the synovial membrane of the joints of the finger and certain other joints. **Basal corpuscle.** Basal granule; a small cytoplasmic granule at the base of a cilium. **Blood corpuscle.** Blood cell. *See* CELL. **Bone corpuscle.** An osteocyte or bone cell. **Bridge corpuscles.** Minute swellings which can be demonstrated on the fine protoplasmic bridges which join the cells of stratified epithelium (prickle cells). **Bulbous corpuscles [corpuscula bulboidea** (NA)]. Special nerve-endings found in the papillae of skin and the mucous membrane of the lip and tongue, consisting of a connective-tissue capsule within which the nerve fibre terminates as a plexus or bulb. They are believed to be receptive for cold. **Cancroid corpuscle.** A cell nest of epithelioma. **Cartilage corpuscle.** A cartilage cell or chondrocyte. **Cement corpuscle.** A cell in the cementum of a tooth, probably identical with an osteocyte. **Chorea corpuscles.** Round, laminated, strongly refractile bodies of hyaline structure found in perivascular sheaths in the corpus striatum in cases of chorea. **Chromophil corpuscle.** A Nissl granule of a nerve cell. **Colostrum corpuscle.** A large cellular body, not unlike a large leucocyte, found in colostrum; Donné's corpuscle. **Colourless corpuscles.** Leucocytes, or white blood corpuscles. **Compound granular corpuscles.** Microglia altered in appearance by the ingestion of lipoids set free as the result of damage to the brain. Also called *Gitterzellen* or *scavenger cells.* **Concentrated Human Red Blood Corpuscles BP 1968.** Whole Human Blood BP 1968 from which part of the plasma and anticoagulant solution have been removed. **Concentric corpuscle.** One of the small bodies found in the medulla of the thymus, formed of concentric layers of epithelial cells. **Corneal corpuscles.** Fibroblastic cells in the substantia propria of the cornea. **Dimpled corpuscle.** A target cell. *See* CELL. **End corpuscle [corpusculum nervosum terminale** (NA)]. Any encapsulated sensory end-organ. **Fusiform corpuscles.** Thrombocytes found in the blood of lower vertebrates, where no blood platelets are present. **Genital corpuscle [corpusculum genitale** (NA)]. An encapsulated sensory nerve-ending in the skin of the external genitalia and of the nipple. **Ghost corpuscle.** A red blood corpuscle (erythrocyte) containing such a small amount of haemoglobin pigment that it looks almost colourless. **Lamellated corpuscles [corpuscula lamellosa** (NA)]. Large encapsulated sensory nerve-endings found in the connective tissues in relation to the skin, muscles and peritoneum. The actual nerve-endings are surrounded by laminated cells. The corpuscles appear to respond to pressure stimuli. **Lymph corpuscle.** A leucocyte present in lymphatic fluids. **Lymphoid corpuscle.** An amoeboid cell resembling a leucocyte, seen in body tissues and lymph spaces. **Malpighian corpuscle.** 1. A lymphoid germinal centre in the spleen. 2. A glomerulus in the cortex of the kidney. **Marginal corpuscles.** Small, peripherally-situated granules seen occasionally in deeply stained red blood corpuscles in certain anaemias. **Meconium corpuscles.** Yellow granules in the epithelial cells of the small intestine in fetuses of 4 months or older. **Milk corpuscles.** Fine fat droplets that may be seen in milk "serum". **Molluscous corpuscle.** Molluscous body. *See* BODY. **Oval corpuscles [corpuscula tactus** (NA)]. Encapsulated sensory nerve-endings found in the dermal papillae of the skin of the palm, fingers, sole of the foot, and toes. They are thought to be receptors for the sensation of touch. **Pacchionian corpuscle.** Pacchionian body. *See* BODY. **Pacinian corpuscle.** Lamellated corpuscle (see above). **Pavement corpuscle.** 1. A squamous epithelial cell. 2. A blood leucocyte applied to the wall of a capillary prior to its emigration into an inflammatory focus. **Pessary corpuscle.** Pessary form. **Phantom corpuscle.** Ghost corpuscle (see above). **Polar corpuscle.** Polar body. *See* BODY. **Pus corpuscle.** Pus cell: a leucocyte especially of the polymorphonuclear type. **Red blood corpuscle.** Red blood cell; erythrocyte: a circular, biconcave, non-nucleated, haemoglobinated disc-like cell enclosed in an elastic membrane, of about 7.2 μm diameter. There are about five million in each mm³ of blood normally, but they show great variations in numbers, sizes and shapes, in different abnormal conditions of the blood. These cells stain red on account of the haemoglobin. **Renal corpuscle [corpusculum renis (NA)].** The part of the nephron formed by the glomerulus enclosed in Bowman's capsule. It is the filter of constituents from the plasma. Also known as *malpighian corpuscle.* **Reticulated corpuscle.** Reticulocyte. **Salivary corpuscle.** A round or oval cell several times larger than a leucocyte and containing granules of varying size, occurring in normal saliva. **Sensitized corpuscles.** Erythrocytes to which a specific amboceptor has been attached in order to facilitate lysis by complement, e.g. in complement-fixation tests. **Shadow corpuscle.** Ghost corpuscle (see above). **Splenic corpuscle.** Malpighian corpuscle; a lymphoid germinal centre in the spleen. **Tactile corpuscle.** Oval corpuscle (see above). **Target corpuscle.** Target cell. *See* CELL. **Taste corpuscle.** Taste bud. *See* BUD. **Tendon corpuscles.** Encapsulated sensory end-organs in tendon, resembling Pacini's or Golgi-Mazzoni corpuscles. **Terminal corpuscle.** End corpuscle (see above). **Third corpuscle.** A blood platelet. *See* PLATELET. **Thymus corpuscle.** Concentric corpuscle (see above). **Touch corpuscle.** Oval corpuscle (see above). **Typhic corpuscles.** Degenerate cells of lymph nodes in the intestine (Peyer's patches) in typhoid fever. **Washed corpuscles.** A red blood cell (erythrocyte) that has been separated by sedimentation or centrifugalization from its plasma, washed in a normal saline solution until free from plasma, and usually suspended in normal saline. **White blood corpuscle.** White blood cell; leucocyte: a circular, nucleated, non-haemoglobinated, disc-like cell enclosed in an elastic membrane. There are many types of normal and abnormal white cells, differing in size (7–22 μm), maturity, appearances of the nuclei and cytoplasm, staining reactions and numbers in the blood, marrow and other body tissues. The normal cells are the neutrophil, eosinophil and basophil polymorphonuclear cells, lymphocytes and monocytes, while there are many other cells (the precursors of these) not usually seen in normal blood, though present in the bone marrow. [L *corpusculum* little body.]

See also: BABÈS, BENNET, BIZZOZERO, BURCHARDT, DOGIEL, DONNÉ, DRYSDALE, ECKER, EICHHORST, ERNST, GIERKE (H. P.), GLUGE, GOLGI, GRANDRY, GUARNIERI, HALBERSTAEDTER, HASSALL, HAYEM, HERBST, KEY (E. A. H.), KRAUSE (W. J. F.), LANGERHANS, LAVERAN, LEBER, MALPIGHI, MAZZONI, MEISSNER, MERKEL (F. S.), MONTGOMERY, MORGAGNI, NORRIS, NUNN, PACCHIONI, PACINI, PATERSON (R.), PROWAZEK, PURKINJE, RAINEY, RETZIUS (M. G.), RUFFINI, SCHWALBE, TIMOFEEW, TOYNBEE, TRAUBE (L.), VATER, WAGNER (R.), WEBER (M. I.), WRISBERG, ZIMMERMANN (G. H. E.), ZIMMERMANN (K. W.).

corpuscular, corpusculous (kor·pus·kew·lar, kor·**pus**·kew·lus). Composed of, of the nature of, or belonging to corpuscles.

corpusculum [NA] (kor·**pus**·kew·lum). A small body, or corpuscle; use of the term in anatomy is becoming uncommon. **Corpusculum wrisbergii.** The cuneiform cartilage of the larynx. [L little body.]

See also: WRISBERG.

Corradi's operation. *See* MOORE-CORRADI.

correctant (kor·**ek**·tant). Corrigent.

correction (kor·**ek**·shun). 1. The remedying of error or defect, e.g. in muscles or retina. 2. The counteraction or modification of the injurious effect of one drug by combining with it another drug. [L *corrigere* to make straight.]

corrective (kor·**ek**·tiv). Corrigent.

correlated (**kor**·el·a·ted). 1. Mutually dependent. 2. Closely related. [see foll.]

correlation (kor·el·a·shun). 1. Reciprocal relationship, as of afferent impulses which according to Herrick are integrated in the sensory centres into appropriate responses. 2. Interdependence. In statistics, the variation of one variable with another; the degree of interdependence is denoted by the *coefficient of correlation,* or in the case of non-linear relationships by the *ratio of correlation,* and may permit the deduction of values of one variable from known values of the other. **Curvilinear correlation.** A correlation in which the regression equation is not expressed by a straight line. **Linear correlation.** A relationship between variables that can be shown graphically by a straight line. [L *cum, relatio* a bringing back.]

correspondence (kor·es·**pon**·dens). The relationship between corresponding points in the retinae of the 2 eyes: these may be defined as points the simultaneous stimulation of which gives rise to the sensation of a single object. **Abnormal retinal correspondence.** False associated fixation, false projection, secondary correspondence; the means whereby diplopia is avoided in concomitant squint and consists in the patient making the portion of retina on which the image of the squinting eye falls "correspond" with the fovea of the straight eye. There are two types: (*a*) *harmonious,* in which the angle of squint and the angle of anomaly are equal; (*b*) *unharmonious,* in which the angles are unequal. [L *cum, respondere* to answer.]

Corrigan, Sir Dominic John (b.1802). Dublin physician.

Corrigan's button, or button cautery. A metal hemisphere carried on a shaft and handle, heated red for momentary application on the skin to produce a form of counter-irritation.

Corrigan's disease. Aortic incompetence. *See* INCOMPETENCE.

Corrigan's line. Copper line; a green line at the bases of the teeth in copper poisoning. Also known as *Clapton's line.*

Corrigan's pulse, or sign. Visible abrupt distension and rapid collapse of the arterial pulse in the neck occurring with aortic regurgitation; it is the visible counterpart of the collapsing or water-hammer pulse. *Corrigan's sign* has also been applied to the tactile quality of this pulse and to the expansile pulsation of the abdominal aorta which occurs with an aneurysm of this vessel.

corrigent (**kor**·ij·ent). A corrective; a drug added to a preparation simply to correct any undesirable action of another constituent of the preparation. Alternatively it may be given separately to counteract an undesirable side-effect of a therapeutic agent: thus atropine may be incorporated in preparations containing strong purgatives, in order to relax the gut and prevent colicky pains which might otherwise be caused. [L *corrigere* to make straight.]

corrosion (kor·o·zhun). 1. Of tissue, the process of being impaired or worn away by a destructive agent. 2. Gradual disintegration. [see foll.]

corrosive (kor·o·siv). Any substance which causes the destruction and gradual erosion of tissue, as, for example, strong acids and alkalis. **Corrosive sublimate.** Mercuric chloride, $HgCl_2$, a compound which has a corrosive action by virtue of the fact that the precipitate of tissue proteins which it produces is soluble in an excess of salt solution; when applied to the abraded skin, it precipitates the proteins of the surface cells, the precipitate then dissolving in the surrounding plasma, and the process is repeated on the layer of cells below resulting in complete erosion of the tissue. [L *corrodere* to gnaw to pieces.]

corrugant (**kor**·ew·gant). The name applied to any drug, such as atropine, which checks secretion. [L *corrugare* to wrinkle.]

corrugator (**kor**·ew·ga·tor). 1. Anything which causes wrinkling, as those muscles which draw the skin together. 2. The small pyramidal muscle [musculus corrugator supercilii (NA)] which arises from the medial end of the superciliary arch. It is the "frowning" muscle of suffering and produces vertical wrinkles on the forehead. **Corrugator cutis ani.** A fine stratum of involuntary muscle that radiates from the anal orifice. [see prec.]

corset (**kor**·set). In surgery, a fitted covering, generally stiff, for the chest, the abdomen or the whole trunk, applied in cases of fracture, deformity, spinal defect or injury in order to give support and fix the position of the parts. [Fr. bodice.]

corsetage (**kor**·set·ij). A method of approximating the lips of an open wound. Strips of adhesive material to which hooks have been attached on the inner edges are fastened to the skin on each side of the operation area 48 h before the operation is performed. After operation, opposite hooks are drawn together by means of rubber bands passed over both, thus bringing in contact the edges of the wound. [see prec.]

cortex (**kor**·tex) (pl. *cortices*). 1. The bark of a tree or root. 2. The rind of a fruit. 3. In anatomy [NA], the outer or superficial part of an organ, when this can be distinguished from the inner medullary part. It is not applied to any capsule or sheath which is not an intrinsic part of the organ under consideration. **Adrenal cortex.** Cortex of the adrenal gland (see below). **Agranular cortex.** *See* CEREBRAL CORTEX (below). **Auditory cortex.** The auditory area in the cerebral cortex; Brodmann's areas 41 and 42. **Cortex aurantii.** The peel of the bitter orange. *Citrus aurantium* Linn. (family Rutaceae). **Calcarine cortex.** The cortex in and around the calcarine fissure of the cerebrum, commonly used as synonymous with *visual cortex, area striata,* or *Brodmann's area 17.* **Cerebellar cortex, Cortex of the cerebellum [cortex cerebelli (NA)].** The layer of grey matter on the surface of the cerebellum, consisting of an outer molecular layer [stratum moleculare (NA)], a layer of Purkinje cells [stratum gangliosum (NA)] and a layer of granule cells [stratum granulosum (NA)]; it is structurally uniform throughout its extent. **Cerebral cortex, Cortex of the cerebrum [cortex cerebri].** The layer of grey matter on the surface of the cerebral hemispheres, immediately superficial to the white matter. It consists of the cell bodies of neurones of many different types arranged in laminae of which 6 are usually recognized (*isocortex,* or *neocortex*): in other regions the laminated pattern is markedly different (*allocortex; archicortex; palaeocortex*). In addition to the broad distinction of iso- from allocortex, many subdivisions are recognized based on structural or physiological differences, e.g. *motor cortex, visual cortex, agranular cortex,* or are described by anatomical location, e.g. *prefrontal cortex, calcarine cortex,* etc. The network of fibres (axons and dendrites) with which the cells are surrounded is an equally important part of the cortical structure. **Cerebral cortex, parolfactory area of the [area subcallosa (NA)].** That part of the cerebral cortex on the medial side of the hemisphere immediately below the genu and rostrum of the corpus callosum; it contains also the septal nuclei. Its relation to olfaction is doubtful. **Cerebral cortex, striate area of the.** The visual cortex, adjacent to the calcarine sulcus, and characterized by the presence of the stria of Gennari; Brodmann's area 17. **Frontal premotor cortex.** Brodmann's area 6. **Cortex of the kidney [cortex renis (NA)].** That portion of the parenchyma of the kidney which lies immediately beneath the capsule; it dips down between the segments of the medulla in the corticomedullary zone. In it are situated the glomeruli and convoluted tubules. **Cortex of the kidney, convoluted part of the [pars convoluta (NA)].** The part of the cortex between the radiate parts. **Cortex of the kidney, radiate part of the [pars radiata (NA)].** The part in contact with the basal part of a renal pyramid. **Cortex of the lens [cortex lentis (NA)].** The soft outer part of the lens. **Cortex limonis.** The peel of the lemon, *Citrus limonia* Osbeck (family Rutaceae). **Cortex of a lymph gland [cortex (NA)].** Rounded masses of lymphoid tissue (lymphoid nodules) lying under the capsule, except at the hilum. **Motor cortex.** *See* CEREBRAL CORTEX (above). **Piriform cortex.** Piriform area. *See* AREA. **Postcentral cortex, Precentral cortex.** *See* AREA, POSTCENTRAL, PRECENTRAL. **Prefrontal cortex.** *See* CEREBRAL CORTEX (above). **Renal cortex.** Cortex of the kidney (see above). **Somatosensory cortex.** An ill-defined term used to denote the parietal region of the cerebral cortex; it includes the postcentral gyrus. **Visual cortex.** Calcarine cortex (see above). [L bark.]

Corti, Alfonso (b.1822). Italian anatomist.

arch of Corti. The arch formed by the inner and outer rods of Corti on the upper surface of the basilar membrane.

canal of Corti. Corti's tunnel (see below).

cell of Corti. Acoustic hair cell; a neurosensory cell of the organ of Corti in the cochlea.

Corti's fibres. Corti's rods; part of the spiral organ of the cochlea.

Corti's ganglion. The spiral ganglion of the cochlea. *See* GANGLION.

Corti's membrane. The tectorial membrane of the spiral organ of the cochlea. *See* MEMBRANE.

organ of Corti. The spiral organ. *See* ORGAN.

Corti's rods. Supporting cells of the tunnel of the organ of Corti.

Corti's tooth. Auditory tooth of Huschke. *See* HUSCHKE.

Corti's tunnel. The space between the inner and outer rods of Corti and the basilar membrane of the cochlea.

cortical (**kor**·tik·al). Relating or belonging to or composed of cortex, especially with reference to the cerebral or the suprarenal cortex. **Cortical dependency.** *See* DEPENDENCY. **Cortical substance.** *See* SUBSTANCE.

corticate (**kor**·tik·ate). Invested in cortex or any specially developed external substance.

cortices (**kor**·tis·eez). *See* CORTEX.

corticifugal (kor·tis·**if**·ew·gal). Corticofugal.

corticipetal (kor·tis·**ip**·et·al). Corticopetal.

cortico-adrenal (**kor**·tik·o·ad·**re**'·nal). Relating to the cortex of the adrenal gland.

cortico-afferent (**kor**·tik·o·**af**'·er·ent). Of certain nerve fibres, carrying impulses and impressions inward and upward to the cerebral cortex. [cortex, afferent.]

cortico-autonomic (**kor**·tik·o·aw·to·**nom**'·ik). Pertaining to the relationship of autonomic function with certain areas in the cerebral cortex.

corticobulbar (**kor**·tik·o·**bul**'·bar). Pertaining to the medulla oblongata and cerebral cortex. [cortex, bulb.]

corticocerebral (**kor**·tik·o·**ser**'·e·bral). Relating to the cerebral cortex.

corticodiencephalic (**kor**·tik·o·di·en·kef·**al**'·ik). Pertaining to the diencephalon and the cerebral cortex.

cortico-efferent (**kor**·tik·o·**ef**'·er·ent). Of certain nerve fibres, conducting impressions and impulses outward and downward from the cerebral cortex. [cortex, efferent.]

corticofugal (kor·tik·**of**·ew·gal). Proceeding away from the outer surface or cortex, as efferent nerve impulses. [L *cortex* bark, *fugere* to flee.]

corticoid (**kor**·tik·oid). Possessing, or exhibiting, an action similar to that of a steroid hormone of the adrenal gland. [adrenal cortex, Gk *eidos* form.]

corticomesencephalic (**kor**·tik·o·mez·en·kef·**al**'·ik). Pertaining to the mesencephalon and the cerebral cortex.

corticopeduncular (**kor**·tik·o·ped·**ung**'·kew·lar). Relating or belonging to the cerebral cortex and the peduncles of the brain.

corticopetal (kor·tik·**op**·et·al). Passing towards the outer surface or cortex, as afferent nerve impulses. [L *cortex* bark, *petere* to seek.]

corticopleuritis (**kor**·tik·o·ploor·**i**'·tis). A condition of inflammation of the visceral pleura. [L *cortex* bark, pleuritis.]

corticopontine (**kor**·tik·o·**pon**'·tine). In or associated with the tracts connecting the pons with the cerebral cortex.

corticopontocerebellar (**kor**·tik·o·pon·to·ser·e·**bel**'·ar). Pertaining to the nerve pathway that connects the cerebral cortex to the cerebellum via the pons.

corticospinal (**kor**·tik·o·**spi**'·nal). Relating or belonging to the cerebral cortex and the spinal cord.

corticosteroids (**kor**·tik·o·**steer**'·oids). Substances of steroid structure isolated from the adrenal cortex. They are classified according to the side chain at the carbon atom numbered 17 in the cyclopentenophenanthrene ring, and include cortisone and corticosterone.

corticosterone (**kor**·tik·o·**steer**'·one). A naturally-occurring glucocorticoid secreted by the adrenal gland. [adrenal cortex, Gk *stereos* solid.]

corticostriate (kor·tik·o·stri'·ate). Pertaining to nerve fibres connecting the cerebral cortex and corpus striatum.

corticothalamic (kor·tik·o·thal·am'·ik). In or associated with the tracts connecting the thalamus and cerebral cortex.

corticotrophic (kor·tik·o·tro'·fik). Term applied to any substance which nourishes and/or stimulates the cortex of the suprarenal gland. [cortex, Gk *trophe* nourishment.]

Corticotrophin BP 1973 (kor·tik·o·tro'·fin). Adrenocorticotrophic hormone (ACTH). Produced by the anterior pituitary gland, it causes release of corticosteroids from the adrenal gland. [adrenal cortex, Gk *trophe* nourishment.]

cortisol (kor·te·sol). Hydrocortisone; a naturally occurring glucocorticoid secreted by the adrenal gland in the greatest quantities. [adrenal cortex, solution.]

Cortisone (kor·tiz·one). An 11-keto breakdown product of cortisol, not secreted by the adrenal gland. Naturally-occurring cortisone produced in the liver does not normally enter the circulation as it is promptly broken down to form tetrahydrocortisone glucuronide. Synthetically-prepared cortisone has been used extensively in medical practice. Kendall's Compound E, 17(β)-[1-keto-2-hydroxy-ethyl]-Δ^4-androstene-3,11-dione-17(α)-ol. A secretion of the adrenal cortex having a predominantly glucocortical activity. Originally extracted from the glands of hogs, it has been synthesized from bile acids and from plant materials such as stigmasterol, from soya beans, sarmentogenin and certain genins from the Mexican yam, *Dioscorea mexicana*. It has been used with spectacular effects in certain cases of rheumatoid arthritis and rheumatic fever, and in others of the so-called collagen diseases, in which, however, the high dosage necessary carries with it the risk of dangerous side-effects. It is used in smaller and safer doses in the substitution therapy of Simmonds' disease and Addison's disease and after bilateral adrenalectomy. BP Commission approved name. **Cortisone Acetate BP 1973.** The acetate of cortisone, and the form in which the drug is usually administered.

cortisoni (kor·te·so·ni). **Cortisoni Acetas.** *European Pharmacopoeia* name for Cortisone Acetate BP 1973.

Cortodoxone (kor·to·dox·one). BP Commission approved name for 17,21-dihydroxypregn-4-ene-3,20-dione; a corticosteroid.

corundum (kor·un·dum). A native anhydrous aluminium oxide, Al_2O_3. It is a diamond-hard crystalline substance used as an abrasive for grinding and polishing (emery). Transparent forms of it, coloured with metallic oxides, constitute the gems ruby, sapphire and amethyst. It is used in the USA in dentistry as an abrasive. [Hind. *kwrand.*]

coruscation (kor·us·ka·shun). A condition in which there is a subjective sensation as of intermittent glittering or flashes of light before the eyes. [L *coruscare* to flash.]

Corvisart des Marets, Jean Nicolas (b.1755). French physician.

Corvisart's disease. Chronic hypertrophic myocarditis.

Corvisart's facies. Cardiac facies; the appearance of a person suffering from congestive cardiac failure, with low cardiac output, of long duration. The face is drawn, sunken and anxious, the skin pale, sallow and slightly cyanosed.

corybantism (kor·e·ban·tizm). A kind of maniacal frenzy or wild delirium in which the patient has tormenting hallucinations and convulsive jerkings and is unable to sleep. [Korybas, a priest of Cybele who accompanied the goddess with music and wild dancing on her travels.]

corydalis (kor·id·al·is). The dried tubers of the North American plants *Dicentra canadensis* Walp. (squirrel corn, turkey corn) and *Dicentra cucullaria* Bernh. (Dutchman's breeches), of the family Papaveraceae. The former contains the alkaloids protopine and corydine; the latter contains cryptopine and 2 other alkaloids. It is used in the form of a decoction as a tonic and diuretic. [Gk *korydallis* crested lark.]

coryl (kor·il). Name applied to one of many mixtures of ethyl and methyl chlorides used to produce local anaesthesia, cutaneous or buccal, by freezing.

Corynebacterium (kor·i·ne·bak·teer'·e·um). A genus of organisms showing specialized or differentiated forms consisting of short or long curved rods with swellings and irregular shapes (clubs, granules, bars, boat-shapes). They are Gram-positive, showing irregular staining with more specific stains, not acid-fast, and contain no sulphur, bacteriopurpurin or iron granules. Non-sporing, non-motile and usually strongly aerobic, they require complex proteins for growth. They never form gas in sugar media. The type species is *Corynebacterium diphtheriae* which produces a powerful toxin and is the cause of diphtheria. Non-pathogenic organisms of the group which resemble the diphtheria bacillus are often called *diphtheroids*. **Corynebacterium acnes.** A micro-aerophilic to anaerobic diphtheroid isolated from sebaceous glands, hair follicles and acne pustules; its growth is feeble on glucose agar at 37°C after 3–4 days. **Corynebacterium bovis.** A milk diphtheroid. **Corynebacterium diphtheriae gravis, intermedius, mitis.** Organisms isolated from cases, convalescents and carriers of diphtheria by means of swabs of the throat, nose, nasopharynx, larynx, vagina or wounds; originally described by Klebs from diphtheritic membranes of the throat and cultured by Loeffler on inspissated serum. They show much pleomorphism with arrangement in films in V- and Y-forms, and contain granules of volutin which are stained deeply by Neisser's stain; clubs or bars may be present. They can be cultured on coagulated serum in 12–24 h forming cream-coloured colonies; their growth in 24–48 h on media containing potassium tellurite with blood or serum enables the different types to be distinguished, and also suppresses competing organisms thus yielding a higher isolation. Glucose in serum water is fermented, but not saccharose. A single toxin neutralized by one antitoxin is produced by all types: a few strains otherwise indistinguishable fail to produce toxins, but all others on injection into guinea-pigs cause death in 2–4 days unless the animal is protected by antitoxin injection. Of the main epidemic types, *gravis* shows poor granules and barred staining, forms large grey convex or umbonate "daisy head" colonies on tellurite media and a coarse granular deposit in broth, ferments starch, and has the highest mortality and toxic complications; it forms only a slight membrane. *Intermedius* is predominantly of the barred form with granules, furnishes a small grey flat "frosted glass" colony on tellurite media and a fine granular deposit in broth, does not ferment starch, and approximates to *gravis* in mortality in epidemic times. *Mitis*, with clubs and granules, is characterized by a greyish-black smooth domed soft colony on tellurite media, turbidity in broth and no fermentation with starch, and is haemolytic; it forms a pronounced membrane and is of low mortality and toxicity. **Corynebacterium equi.** A cause of pneumonia in foals and chronic suppurations in other animals. **Corynebacterium minutissimum.** The causative organism of erythrasma, previously thought to be due to a *Nocardia* species. **Corynebacterium ovis.** The cause of pseudotuberculosis in sheep. **Corynebacterium pseudodiphtheriae.** *Corynebacterium hofmannii.* **Corynebacterium pyogenes.** A species associated with suppurative lesions in cattle, pigs, sheep, goats and rabbits. It ferments saccharose, and produces yellow pigment and a haemolysin. **Corynebacterium renale.** The cause of pyelonephritis in cattle. **Corynebacterium segmentosum.** A non-pathogenic saccharose-fermenting diphtheroid which produces yellow pigment. **Corynebacterium tenuis.** The causal organism of trichomycosis axillaris. **Corynebacterium typhi.** A species very similar to *Corynebacterium acnes* (see above). **Corynebacterium ulcerans.** A species associated with localized ulcerations of the throat; it resembles *C. ovis* (see above). **Corynebacterium ulcerogenes.** A non-pathogenic diphtheroid isolated from ulcers. **Corynebacterium vaginale.** A species causing a mild infective vaginitis in women, and possibly urethritis in men. One possible cause of non-specific genital infection. **Corynebacterium xerosis.** A saccharose-fermenting barred diphtheroid which produces granules. It is non-pathogenic and is common in nose, ear and eye swabs. [Gk *koryne* club, bacterium.]

coryza (kor·i·zah). Nasal catarrh. The common cold. **Acute infectious coryza.** The common cold due to filtrable virus. Other so-called colds are acute exacerbations of a persistent infection in the nasal sinuses, of bacterial origin. **Allergic coryza.** Paroxysmal rhinorrhoea occurring in allergic subjects who are sensitized to some air-borne substance, e.g. pollen as in hay fever, or to hairs, feathers and other animal emanations: house dust is a common cause. In some cases the sensitization is to bacteria infecting the upper respiratory passages. **Coryza caseosa.** Caseous rhinitis, a rare disease in which there is an accumulation of cheesy material with a very fetid odour. **Chronic coryza.** Chronic rhinitis; it may follow a series of colds; it is associated with chronic nasal obstruction or persistent infection of the accessory sinuses. **Coryza foetida.** Or atrophic rhinitis, a chronic condition characterized by atrophic changes in the mucous membrane of the nose and a mucropurulent secretion which dries into crusts with a foul odour (ozaena). [Gk *koryza* a running at the nose.]

cosensitize (ko·sen·sit·ize). To render the cells of the body sensitive to more than one infection. [L *cum, sentire* to feel.]

cosmesis (koz·me·sis). 1. The use of cosmetics. 2. The art of preserving or enhancing natural beauty; in therapeutics, treatment which concerns the appearance of the patient; and in surgery, the undertaking of an operation, plastic or otherwise, which will improve the appearance, or the avoidance of one which will have a disfiguring effect. [Gk *kosmesis* adornment.]

cosmetic (koz·met·ik). 1. Referring to cosmesis. 2. Denoting any procedure or application which will preserve or enhance natural beauty; beautifying. 3. Any application or preparation that helps to preserve the tissues and prevent deterioration of natural beauty. [see prec.]

cosmetology (koz·met·ol·o·je). The study of the appearance, including cleanliness and care of the body and the preservation of natural good looks. [cosmesis, Gk *logos* science.]

cosmic (koz·mik). Of the material universe; world-wide. **Cosmic rays.** *See* RAY. [Gk *kosmos* the universe.]

cosmonaut (koz·mo·nawt). Synonym for *astronaut* (q.v.) especially in the USSR where "cosmic" is synonymous with "space". [Gk *kosmos* the universe, *nautes* sailor.]

cosotoxin (ko·so·tox·in). Kosotoxin, $C_{26}H_{34}O_{10}$. A compound allied to filicic acid, and the chief constituent of cusso. It is used as an anthelmintic, particularly against tapeworms. Also known as *koussin* or *koussotoxin*. [cusso, toxin.]

costa (kos·tah). A rib. **Costa fluctuans.** Floating rib. *See* RIBS. **Costa fluctuans decima.** Loose attachment of the 10th rib. [L.]

costal (kos·tal). Relating to a rib or the ribs, or involving them. **Costal facet.** *See* FACET. **Costal groove.** *See* GROOVE. **Costal notch.** *See* NOTCH. **Costal process.** *See* PROCESS. [see prec.]

costalgia (kos·tal·je·ah). Pain occurring in the ribs, generally intercostal neuralgia. [L *costa* rib, Gk *algos* pain.]

costalis muscle [musculus iliocostalis thoracis (NA)] (kos·ta'·lis). A part of the iliocostocervicalis muscle.

costate (kos·tate). 1. Having ribs. 2. Having structural connections. [L *costa* rib.]

costatectomy, costectomy (kos·tat·ek·to·me, kos·tek·to·me). Surgical resection of a rib. [L *costa* rib, *ektome* a cutting out.]

Costen, James Bray (b.1895). American otolaryngologist.

Costen's syndrome. Neuralgia associated with overclosure of the temporomandibular joint in the edentulous individual. Earache, headache and dryness of the throat and tongue may occur. *See* Temporomandibular joint pain dysfunction SYNDROME.

costicartilage (kos·te·kar·til·ij). 1. Costal cartilage. *See* CARTILAGE. 2. A sternal rib in which ossification has not taken place. [L *costa* rib, cartilage.]

costicervical (kos·te·ser·vik·al). Costocervical.

costiferous (kos·tif·er·us). Bearing a rib, e.g. the dorsal vertebrae in man. [L *costa* rib, *ferre* to bear.]

costiform (kos·te·form). Shaped like a rib. [L *costa* rib, form.]

costispinal (kos·te·spi·nal). Relating to the ribs and the vertebral column. [L *costa* rib, spine.]

costive (kos·tiv). 1. Constipated. Indicating a condition in which condensed and hardened faecal matter is retained in the bowel. 2. Applied to drugs the action of which is to cause the above condition. [Fr. *costiver* to constipate.]

costiveness (kos·tiv·nes). The condition of being constipated. [see prec.]

costo-abdominal (kos·to·ab·dom'·in·al). In relation to the ribs and the abdomen. [L *costa* rib, abdomen.]

costocentral (kos·to·sen·tral). Relating to a rib and the body of a vertebra. [L *costa* rib, centre.]

costocervical (kos·to·ser·vik·al). Associated with a rib and the neck. **Costocervical trunk.** *See* TRUNK. [L *costa* rib, *cervix* neck.]

costocervicalis muscle [musculus iliocostalis cervicis (NA)] (kos·to·ser·vik·a'·lis). A part of the iliocostocervicalis muscle.

costochondral (kos·to·kon·dral). Relating to the ribs and their cartilages. [L *costa* rib, Gk *chondros* cartilage.]

costoclavicular (kos·to·klav·ik'·ew·lar). Relating to the ribs and the clavicle, or affecting them. [L *costa* rib, clavicle.]

costocolic (kos·to·kol·ik). Referring to the ribs and the colon. [L *costa* rib, colon.]

costocoracoid (kos·to·kor·ak·oid). Relating to or involving the ribs and the coracoid process of the scapula. [L *costa* rib, coracoid.]

costogenic (kos·to·jen·ik). Originating in a rib. [L *costa* rib, Gk *genein* to produce.]

costohumeral (kos·to·hew·mer·al). Relating to the ribs and the humerus. [L *costa* rib, humerus.]

costo-inferior (kos·to·in·feer'·e·or). Belonging to the lower ribs. [L *costa* rib, *inferior* lower.]

costophrenic (kos·to·fren·ik). Referring to the ribs and the diaphragm, e.g. the costal and the diaphragmatic pleurae. [L *costa* rib, Gk *phren* diaphragm.]

costopleural (kos·to·ploor·al). Relating to the ribs and the pleura. [L *costa* rib, pleura.]

costopneumopexy (kos·to·new·mo·pex·e). The surgical procedure of fixing the lung to a rib. [L *costa* rib, Gk *pneumon* lung, *pexis* fixation.]

costopulmonary (kos·to·pul·mon·ar·e). Relating to the rib and the lungs. [L *costa* rib, *pulmo* lung.]

costoscapular (kos·to·skap·ew·lar). Relating or belonging to or affecting the ribs and the scapula. [L *costa* rib, scapula.]

costoscapularis (kos·to·skap·ew·la'·ris). The serratus anterior muscle. [see prec.]

costosternal (kos·to·ster·nal). Relating or belonging to or involving a rib and the sternum. [L *costa* rib, sternum.]

costosternoplasty (kos·to·ster·no·plas·te). Surgical repair of funnel chest, a segment of rib being used to support the sternum. [L *costa* rib, sternum, *plassein* to mould.]

costosuperior (kos·to·sew·peer'·e·or). Relating or belonging to the upper ribs. [L *costa* rib, *superior* upper.]

costotome (kos·to·tome). An instrument in the form of a knife or a pair of strong shears with a hook instead of an underblade. It is used to resect or to cut through a rib or the costal cartilages. [L *costa* rib, Gk *temnein* to cut.]

costotomy (kos·tot·o·me). The surgical procedure of resecting or dividing a rib, particularly with the use of a costotome.

costotransverse (kos·to·trans·vers). Relating to or lying between the ribs and the transverse process of their articulating vertebrae. **Costotransverse joint.** *See* JOINT. **Costotransverse ligament.** *See* LIGAMENT. [L *costa* rib, transverse.]

costotransversectomy (kos·to·trans·ver·sek'·to·me). The surgical removal of part of a rib with the transverse process of the corresponding vertebra. [L *costa* rib, transverse, Gk *ektome* a cutting out.]

costovertebral (kos·to·ver·te·bral). Having reference or belonging to a rib and a vertebra, or ribs and vertebrae. [L *costa* rib, vertebra.]

costo-xiphoid (kos·to·zif·oid). Connecting or relating to the ribs and the xiphoid process of the sternum. [L *costa* rib, xiphoid.]

Cotard, Jules (b.1840). Paris neurologist.

Cotard's syndrome. Insanity of negation; a symptom of mental disorder in which the person denies many or all propositions.

cotarnine (ko·tar·neen). $C_{12}H_{15}O_4N$, an alkaloid obtained by the oxidation of narcotine and related to isoquinoline. It has been used for the control of uterine haemorrhage, but does not increase the coagulation time of the blood. **Cotarnine hydrochloride.** $C_{12}H_{13}O_3NHCl{\cdot}2H_2O$, a compound used in haemorrhages as a styptic. **Cotarnine phthalate.** $C_{12}H_{13}O_3NOOCC_6H_4COOH$, a yellow crystalline compound employed in uterine haemorrhage.

coto (ko·to). Paracoto; a bark obtained from the Bolivian tree *Ocotea pseudocoto* Rusby (family Lauraceae). It is used in the form of a tincture or liquid extract as an astringent in the treatment of diarrhoea. [Tupi (Brazil) name.]

cotoin (ko·to·in). Methoxy-2,6-dihydroxybenzophenone, $C_{14}H_{12}O_4$. A constituent of coto bark, with an irritant action on the skin and mucous membrane. **Cotoin formaldehyde.** Methylene dicotoin, $(C_{14}H_{11}O_4)_2CH_2$, a compound used as an astringent and antiseptic.

Co-trimoxazole (ko·tri·mox·az·ole). BP Commission approved name for compounded preparations of trimethoprim and sulphamethoxazole in the proportions of 1 part to 5 parts.

Cotte, Gaston (b.1879). Lyons surgeon.

Cotte's operation. Presacral neurectomy.

Cotting, Benjamin Eddy (b.1812). New York surgeon.

Cotting's operation. Removal of the edge of an ingrowing toenail with the adjacent nail fold.

cotton (kotn). The hairs or epidermal trichomes of the seeds of *Gossypium barbadense* and other species of *Gossypium.* **Absorbent cotton.** Absorbent Cotton Wool BPC 1959; a material prepared from cotton by removing the seeds and fatty matter and treating the hairs mechanically. It consists almost entirely of cellulose, and readily absorbs water. **Boric acid cotton.** Boric acid cotton wool; absorbent cotton impregnated with boric acid. **Capsicum cotton.** Capsicum Cotton Wool BPC 1959, absorbent cotton impregnated with capsicum and methyl salicylate. **Purified cotton.** Absorbent cotton (see above). **Salicylated cotton.** Absorbent cotton impregnated with salicylic acid. **Styptic cotton.** Absorbent cotton impregnated with styptic solution, and dried. **Cotton wool.** Absorbent cotton (see above). [Ar. *qutun.*]

cotton-mouth (kotn·mowth). A poisonous snake of swampy places in North America (*Agkistrodon piscivorus*). [cotton, mouth.]

cotton-rat (kotn·rat). A large rat of tropical North America (*Sigmodon hispidus*) used as a laboratory animal. [cotton, rat.]

cottonpox (kotn·pox). A name used in the USA for alastrim. [cotton, pox.]

Cotugno, Domenico (Dominicus Cotunnius) (b.1736). Naples anatomist.

aqueduct of Cotunnius, Cotunnius' canal. The aqueduct of the vestibule.

Cotunnius' columns. Columns in the osseous spiral lamina of the cochlea.

Cotugno's disease, Cotunnius' disease. Sciatic neuritis; inflammation of the sciatic nerve.

Cotunnius' nerve. The long sphenopalatine nerve.

Cotunnius' space. The interior of the membranous labyrinth.

co-twin (ko·twin). Either one of a pair of identical twins. [L *cum,* twin.]

cotyle (kot·il·e). Acetabulum. [Gk *kotyle* cup.]

cotyledon (kot·il·e·don). 1. The seed-leaf of the embryo of a plant. 2. One of the portions into which the human placenta may be divided, based on the natural cleavage lines present on the maternal surface of the organ. 3. One of the numerous independent rounded bodies composing the placenta of ungulates. 4. A genus of plants of the family Crassulaceae. [Gk *kotyledon* cup-shaped.]

cotyloid (kot·il·oid). 1. Acetabular; relating to the acetabulum. 2. Shaped like a cup. [Gk *kotyle* cup, *eidos* form.]

cotylopubic (kot·il·o·pew'·bik). Referring to the acetabulum and the pubis. [Gk *kotyle* cup, pubis.]

cotylosacral (kot·il·o·sa'·kral). Relating to the acetabulum and the sacrum. [Gk *kotyle* cup, sacrum.]

couch (kowch). **Contour couch.** A reclining seat which is accurately moulded to the astronaut's body to counteract excess gravitational force; the posture is semirecumbent. [Fr. *coucher* to lay down.]

couche (koosh). *See* SATTLER.

couching (kowch·ing). In cure of cataract, the operation of displacing the opaque lens of the eye by turning it down with a needle into the vitreous body, which eventually absorbs it. [Fr. *coucher* to lay down.]

cough (kof). A defensive reflex aimed at keeping the lower respiratory tract clear of foreign material. It is characterized by a sudden noisy expulsion of compressed air from the tracheo-bronchial tract through the glottis. The reflex is most often initiated by stimulation of vagus afferent nerve-endings in the laryngeal, tracheal and bronchial mucosa: other causes may be stimulation of afferent terminals in the pharyngeal, tonsillar or gastric mucosa, the parietal pleura and the external ear. The act of coughing consists of a deep inspiration followed immediately by closure of the glottis and a forcible expiratory effort so causing a considerable rise of pressure within the lungs; the glottis then suddenly opens and the compressed air with any foreign material in the air passages is forcibly and noisily expelled. **Barking cough.** A loud harsh, unproductive cough which may go on for months without disturbance of health; hysterical in origin and in some cases a form of respiratory tic. **Bovine cough.** A prolonged and wheezing cough associated with paralysis of the recurrent laryngeal nerve. **Brassy cough.** A high-pitched cough due to pressure on the trachea or irritation of the recurrent laryngeal nerve. **Chin cough.** A synonym for whooping-cough. **Croupy cough.** A harsh, hoarse cough occurring with partial obstruction of the larynx, as in diphtheritic laryngitis. **Dry cough.** An ineffective cough without production of sputum. **Emetic cough.** A cough ending in vomiting; it may occur in whooping-cough, chronic pharyngitis, especially in alcoholics and heavy smokers, and pulmonary tuberculosis. **Gander cough.** Brassy cough (see above). **Hacking cough.** A short weak cough frequently repeated, as in laryngeal irritation of the larynx from secretion trickling down from the nasopharynx. **Malt-house workers' cough.** A cough caused by moulds inhaled from the malt. **Miller's cough.** A cough due to the fungus *Aspergillus fumigatus* contaminating flour. **Moist cough.** A cough accompanied by the expectoration of sputum. **Paroxysmal cough.** Severe bouts of coughing occurring at intervals, as in whooping-cough, bronchiectasis and cavitation of the lung. **Privet cough.** One due to inhalation of the spores of privet, noted in China. **Productive cough.** One that effectively removes the secretion from the respiratory tract. **Tea-tasters' cough.** A cough due to inhalation of the fungus *Candida,* noted in tea workers in Sri Lanka. **Weavers' cough.** A condition similar to farmers' lung occurring in weavers handling damp mildewed cotton. **Whooping cough.** *See* WHOOPING-COUGH. [AS *cohhetan.*]

Coulomb, Charles Augustin de (b.1736). Paris physicist.

Coulomb's balance. A balance with which quantitative measurements of electric charges can be made by the use of a fine torsion fibre.

Coulomb's law. The force between 2 electric charges varies directly as the product of their charges and inversely as the square of the distance between them.

Coulomb scattering. The scattering of colliding charged elementary particles or atomic nuclei, brought about by the force between their electric charges. This force obeys Coulomb's law, depending on the inverse square of the distance.

coulomb (koo·lom). The unit of electrical quantity; the quantity of electricity transported in one second by a current of one ampere. [C. A. *de Coulomb.*]

01014700 01/09/77 (Vsn 00/00/00) Csys

coulometer (koo·**lom**·et·er). Voltameter. [coulomb, meter.]

coumarin (**koo**·mar·in).

$$C_6H_4\overline{(CH{=}CHCOO)},$$

the lactone of *o*-coumaric acid occurring in the common woodruff, in oil of lavender and in the Tonquin bean. It is a colourless compound, soluble in hot water, and with the smell of new-mown hay, on account of which it is used in perfumery; also employed as a flavouring in confectionery. Now manufactured synthetically from orthocresol. [*coumarou,* the local name for Tonquin beans grown in Guyana.]

Councilman, William Thomas (b.1854). Boston pathologist.

Councilman body. An eosinophilic mass of degenerated cytoplasm seen within liver cells in yellow fever and also in some other forms of acute hepatic necrosis.

Councilman cell. The characteristic cell in the liver in yellow fever. It is a parenchyma cell that has undergone an extreme degree of necrosis: it is round in outline, the nucleus has undergone chromatolysis and the chromatin is arranged marginally, and the cytoplasm contains hyaline eosinophil bodies, Councilman bodies (see above).

Councilman lesion. The characteristic histological lesion of yellow fever (see above two entries).

count (kownt). 1. A computation; a reckoning; the act of counting; the sum total. 2. To count, to make a count; to enumerate. *See also* COUNTING. **Background count.** A constant count rate present during the use of a radiation detector, such as a Geiger counter, which arises from cosmic rays, radioactive contamination or the presence of other sources. The count rate due to background must be subtracted from every reading to obtain the count rate due to the measured radiation. **Blood count.** The enumeration of the numbers of red and white cells per mm^3 of blood of an individual; in a broader sense the term may also include the differential white-cell count and haemoglobin value. **Differential blood count.** A count of the different types of normal and abnormal white blood cells per mm^3 of peripheral blood of an individual. **Direct platelet count.** A count of the total number of platelets per mm^3 of fresh blood, normally from 250 000 to 500 000. **Dust count.** The number of particles less than 10 μm in diameter per cubic metre (foot) of air present in a particular atmosphere, as enumerated by the "light field" method. The count is in use for the estimation of workers' risks from siliceous and other dusts. **Filament-non-filament count.** A method of enumerating the polymorphonuclear leucocytes according to the appearances of their nuclei: those cells in which 2 or more nuclear lobes are joined by a thin filament of chromatin are termed "filamented" cells, while those without filaments, although having segmented nuclei, are classed as "non-filamented" cells. **Indirect platelet count.** A relative count of the platelets in a fixed stained blood film compared with the number of red blood cells. **Reticulocyte count.** A count of the number of reticulocytes—that is, of red cells that show a fine network after they have been stained supravitally with cresyl blue. The result is expressed as a percentage of the total red cells. **Spurious count.** A count obtained when using a radiation detector which arises from a transient electrical pulse in some part of the apparatus and not from the arrival of radiation. **Staff count.** *See* SCHILLING'S BLOOD COUNT. [OFr. *conter.*]

See also: ADDIS, ARNETH, COOKE, SCHILLING, STOLL.

counter (**kown**·ter). 1. An instrument used for the purpose of counting anything. 2. A detector of radiation in which an electrical pulse of potential is given for each individual particle or quantum of radiation actuating the detector. 3. A term sometimes used for the electronic instrument which counts and registers pulses from a detector, as 2. Better terminology is "*scaler*" or "*scaling unit*". 4. A device used with a radiation detector to indicate the number of photons or particles detected. **Coincidence counter.** A radiation detector so arranged that it records only radiation the quanta of which arrive in simultaneous pairs. It is particularly applicable to the detection of annihilation radiation. **Crystal counter.** A counter in which the radiation is absorbed by a semiconductor such as a diamond, causing instantaneous changes of electrical resistance and hence potential pulses which may be counted. **Directional counter.** A counter in which the detection efficiency varies with the direction of incidence of the radiation relative to the axis of the counter. Usually the efficiency is a maximum in the direction of the long axis of the counter, due to increased intrinsic efficiency and to external lead shielding. **End-window counter.** A counter cylindrical in shape, with a window transparent to the particles detected at the end of the cylinder. The window is often aluminium, or for α-particles thin mica. **Counter for fast neutrons.** A device in which the passage of a fast neutron produces a detectable signal. The fast neutron communicates some kinetic energy to a charged recoil particle, e.g. a proton, which may produce ionization in a gas cavity leading to an electrical pulse which may be amplified, or which may produce in a suitable phosphor a scintillation which can be converted to an electrical pulse and amplified in a photomultiplier. Alternatively, the neutron may produce a detectable charged secondary particle by means of a nuclear disintegration, e.g. fission in uranium. **Gas counter.** A demountable counter such that a radioactive gas can be admitted into the sensitive volume of the counter. **Gaseous-flow counter.** A proportional counter for the determination of α or weak β activity, in which the source is placed inside the counter through which a stream of the counter gas is flowing. **Immersion counter.** A counter designed to be immersed in the liquid the activity of which is to be determined. **Jet dust counter.** A device for estimating the number of particles of dust in a measured sample of air. The sample is rendered moist and impelled at a high rate of speed through a narrow opening on to an upright plate, on which the particles collect. Afterwards, a microscopic count is made of them. *See also* DUST COUNT, IMPINGER, KONIMETER. **Liquid counter.** A cylindrical counter with an annular jacket in which the radioactive liquid is placed for assay. **Liquid-flow counter.** A liquid counter in which the radioactive liquid flows continuously through the annular jacket. **Liquid scintillation counter.** A counter where the sensitive volume is a liquid. **Neutron counter.** Any instrument which will detect the incidence of a neutron upon it and produce an electrical signal which may be counted electrically. The type of instrument used depends upon the energy of the incident neutron, and the intrinsic efficiency of neutron counters is low. **Non-self-quenching counter.** A device in which the electrical discharge initiated by the passage of an atomic particle continues indefinitely, and which must be stopped by external means, e.g. interruption of the voltage by an associated circuit. **Profile counter.** A radiation detector arranged to record at intervals along the axis of the body the radiation emanating from it. A graph of the results is plotted with distance along the body as abscissa and the radiation recorded at each cross-section of the body as ordinate. Such a graph is called a *radiation profile* for the body. **Proportional counter.** A Geiger counter in which the standing potential between the electrodes is reduced. The amplitude of the potential pulse produced by the passage of an ionizing particle is proportional to the number of ions initially formed by that particle in the gas; hence discrimination between α- and β-particles is possible, the more densely ionizing α-particle producing a larger pulse. **Scintillation counter.** A radiation detector whose sensitive volume emits flashes of light when ionizing radiation is absorbed within it. Scintillation counters are the most commonly used detectors of such radiation in medical applications. The sensitive volume is commonly a crystal, an organic liquid, or a plastic. **Self-quenching counter.** A device in which the electrical discharge initiated by the passage of an atomic particle ceases spontaneously after a short interval, e.g. a Geiger counter containing a mixture of argon and alcohol vapour. **Semiconductor counter.** A counter where the sensitive volume is a semiconductor. **Shadow shield counter.** A form of whole-body counter where the radiation detectors are heavily shielded from extraneous radiation so that they detect from points only within the radiation shadow so formed. The whole-body count is performed by slowly sliding the body on a stretcher through the shadow. A very small modification makes such an instrument perform also as a *profile counter.* **Counter for slow neutrons.** As for fast neutrons (see above), but in this case the charged secondary particle can only be obtained by a nuclear disintegration, e.g. of boron to give an α-particle. **Solid-state counter.** Semiconductor counter (see above). **Well counter.** A scintillation counter with a re-entrant hole in the sensitive volume. The radioactive sample in an appropriate container is placed in this hole. **Whole-body counter.** A counter which detects radiation from the whole body. [OFr. *conter.*]

See also: GEIGER, MUELLER (W.).

counteraction (kown·ter·**ak**·shun). Pharmacologically, the action of one drug in opposition to or antagonizing the action of another, of great importance in the prevention of undesirable side-reactions or as an antidote following overdosage with toxic drugs. The process may be physiological, as when adrenaline counteracts the effects of stimulation of the parasympathetic nervous system; pharmacological, as when the action is blocked by substrate competition at the receptors (e.g. antihistamine drugs) or by inactivation of enzyme systems (e.g. anticholinesterase drugs); or purely chemical neutralization, as in the counteraction of hyperchlorhydria by the administration of alkali. [L *contra,* action.]

counter-die (**kown**·ter·di). The "female" of a die, with which it is used, in conjunction, in the construction of the metallic bases for artificial dentures and crowns. [L *contra,* ME *de.*]

counter-extension (**kown**·ter·ex·**ten'**·shun). 1. Fixation of the upper part of a limb while traction is being applied to the lower part. 2. Counterbalance against extension of a limb, e.g. the raising of the foot of the bed so that the body is not pulled downwards by the weight attached to the leg. [L *contra,* extension.]

counter-fissure (kown·ter·**fish**·er). Contrecoup; an injury that is the result of a blow suffered on an opposite part or a part at a distance, e.g. a fracture appearing on the side of the skull opposite to that on which the blow fell. [L *contra,* fissure.]

counter-incision (**kown**·ter·in·**sizh'**·un). Counter-opening. [L *contra,* incision.]

counter-indication (**kown**·ter·in·dik·**a'**·shun). Contra-indication.

counter-investment (**kown**·ter·in·**vest'**·ment). Anticathexis. [L *contra,* investment.]

counter-irritant (kown·ter·**ir**·it·ant). 1. A substance which alleviates the pain arising from an internal organ, by irritating the sensory nerve-endings in that area of skin supplied by nerves which synapse at the same level in the spinal cord as the nerves from the internal organ concerned. Several theories have been advanced to explain this phenomenon, but the most likely is that which postulates that the impulses entering the cord from the stimulated nerve-endings in the skin send antidromic impulses down the nerves coming from the internal organ, and that these block the painful incoming stimuli. 2. Producing counter-irritation. [L *contra,* irritant.]

counter-irritation (**kown**·ter·ir·it·**a'**·shun). A superficial irritation artificially applied in order to disguise the effects of or relieve an irritation existing elsewhere, or to act beneficially on an abnormal process in an adjacent or deeper-lying part. [see prec.]

counter-opening (kown·ter·o·pen·ing). A second incision made opposite to a previous incision, e.g. in an abscess, so that drainage will be more satisfactory. [L *contra,* opening.]

counter-poison (kown·ter·**poi**·zn). A poison which acts as an antidote to another poison. [L *contra,* poison.]

counter-pressure (kown·ter·**presh**·er). A pressure or force acting in a direction contrary to that of another pressure or force. [L *contra,* pressure.]

counterpulsation (**kown**·ter·pul·**sa'**·shun). The techniques of applying a positive pressure to the arterial system in diastole and a reduction of pressure in systole, for the treatment of cardiogenic shock. [L *contra, pulsio* a beating.]

counterpulsator (**kown**·ter·pul·**sa'**·tor). An instrument used to provide counterpulsation. [L *contra, pulsio* a beating.]

counter-puncture (kown·ter·**pungk**·tcher). Counter-opening. [L *contra,* puncture.]

countershock (**kown**·ter·shok). An electric shock applied across the chest to restore normal ventricular function when life-threatening ventricular arrhythmias occur, i.e. a shock to counter the disturbance of ventricular action. [L *contra,* Fr. *choc.*]

counterstain (**kown**·ter·stane). In microscopical work, a stain applied so as to show up by contrast substances or structures already stained with another dye. [L *contra,* stain.]

counterstroke (**kown**·ter·stroke). Contrecoup; an injury that is the result of a blow, suffered on an opposite part or a part at a distance, e.g. a fracture appearing on the side of the skull opposite to that on which the blow fell. [L *contra,* stroke.]

counter-traction (kown·ter·**trak**·shun). A method of reducing fractures by applying traction from 2 opposite directions at the same time. [L *contra,* traction.]

counter-transference (kown·ter·**trans**·fer·ens). In psycho-analytical treatment, the development of an emotional (or transference) relationship on the part of the analyst towards his patient, which relationship accordingly ceases to be objective. Where this is positive, the analyst commonly over-values the patient, or attributes to him qualities he does not possess, but which are possessed by the analyst himself. [L *contra,* transference.]

counting (**kown**·ting). **Anti-coincidence counting.** The arrangement is similar to that for coincidence counting (see below), except that the circuit is arranged to work in the simplest case of 3 sources, A, B and C, to give a pulse if a pulse from C does not occur when pulses from A and B are coincident. **Coincidence counting.** Electrical pulses from 2 or more radiation detectors are applied to an electronic instrument which emits a pulse only when pulses from all the detectors arrive coincident in time within a certain instrumental limit. This limit is called the resolving time of the circuit. [OFr. *conter.*]

counting rate (**kown**·ting rate). The average number of pulses per unit time produced by ionizing radiation in counting equipment such as a Geiger–Mueller tube or a scintillation counter. **Background counting rate.** *See* COUNT, BACKGROUND. [OFr. *conter,* rate.]

coup (koo). A stroke. **Coup sur coup.** The administration of small doses of a drug given frequently in order to ensure that it will act continuously or that its effect will be complete or rapid. **Coup de fouet.** Sudden rupture of the plantaris muscle, an injury sustained by lawn-tennis players. **Coup de sang.** Cerebral congestion. **Coup de soleil.** Sunburn. [Fr. blow.]

couphonia (koo·**fo**·ne·ah). Auscultatory percussion; a method of percussion in which the resultant notes are observed and compared by means of the stethoscope. [Fr. *coup* blow, Gk *phone* voice.]

coupling (**kup**·ling). In cardiology, the frequent occurrence of 2 heart beats having the same relationship to each other, usually a normally conducted ventricular beat followed after a constant interval by a ventricular ectopic beat. [OFr. *copler* couple.]

courbometer (koor·**bom**·et·er). An apparatus designed to reproduce the characteristic sine curves of an alternating current. [Fr. *courbe* curve, meter.]

Courmont, Jules (b. 1865). French pathologist.

Arloing-Courmont test. An agglutination reaction similar to that of Widal's typhoid test, in which a dilute emulsified culture of *Mycobacterium tuberculosis* is mixed with a patient's serum and examined macroscopically and microscopically after incubation for a few hours. Clumping is said to indicate the presence of the specific antigen. Its reliability is questioned.

Cournand, André Frederic (b. 1895). New York physician.

Cournand catheter. A flexible, radio-opaque catheter with a single lumen and hole at the tip, used for venous catheterization of the heart.

Cournand needle. An indwelling arterial needle used for pressure recording or repetitive sampling of arterial blood.

courses (**kors**·ez). The menses, a term generally used by the laity. [L *cursus* running.]

Courtois sign. Unilateral hip and knee flexion on flexing the neck, described by Courtois in a comatose patient. The cerebral lesion responsible for the coma was discovered on the same side of the brain as the side on which the reflex occurred. (This reflex has not proved to be of any value in clinical neurology.)

Courvoisier, Ludwig (b. 1843). Basle surgeon.

Courvoisier's gall bladder. A chronically large gall bladder due to non-calculous obstruction of the cystic or common bile duct.

Courvoisier's incision. Kocher's incision.

Courvoisier's law, or sign. In a case of obstructive jaundice, if the gall bladder is palpable, the cause of the obstruction is unlikely to be gall-stones and is therefore, by exclusion, likely to be a malignant growth. It depends on the fact that obstruction of the common duct due to gall-stones is rarely complete and permanent.

Courvoisier-Terrier syndrome. Obstructive jaundice, distension of the gall bladder and clay-coloured faeces, indicating obstruction of the common bile duct, e.g. by a tumour of the ampulla of Vater.

cousso (**koo**·so). Cusso.

Coutard, Henri (b. 1876). Paris radiologist.

Coutard's method. A protracted-fractionated method of irradiation, based on experimental work by Regaud; a high dose is given at low dosage-rate in even daily fractions over a long time.

couvade (koo·**vahd**). A racial custom among many primitive peoples, and variously explained, according to which the father takes to bed when a child is born and remains there until the mother is up and about again. [Fr. *couver* to brood upon.]

Couvelaire, Alexandre (b. 1873). French obstetrician.

Couvelaire uterus. The condition of the uterine musculature in severe concealed accidental ante-partum haemorrhage.

couveuse (koo·**verz**). Incubator. [Fr. broody hen.]

Cova's point. The point at the apex of the lumbocostal angle which is tender to pressure in cases of pyelitis.

Covent Garden hummy (**kov**·ent **gar**·den **hum**·e). A bursa on the 7th cervical vertebra, in porters. [*Covent Garden* market, London.]

cover-glass (**kuv**·er·glahs). In microscopical or biological work, a thin glass scale or plate used to cover a specimen or a culture. [OFr. *cuvrir*, glass.]

covering (**kuv**·er·ing). Permitting medically unqualified persons the privileges of registered medical practitioners; conduct which, in a doctor, is liable to result in erasure of his name from the Register by the General Medical Council. [OFr. *cuvrir.*]

cow (cow). A small ion-exchange column on which is adsorbed a radionuclide which is the parent of the daughter nuclide of interest. By pouring a suitable liquid through the column a supply of the daughter nuclide is obtained. The process can be repeated at frequent intervals, the frequency being largely determined by the half-life of the daughter nuclide. This method of obtaining a daughter nuclide from its parent adsorbed on a column is called *milking.* [AS *cu.*]

Cowden. The family name of the propositus with the first recorded example of the disease described below.

Cowden's disease. Hypertrophy of the breasts, hypoplasia of the jaws, scrotal tongue, papillomatosis of the lips and mouth, multiple thyroid adenoma, scoliosis and pectus excavatum.

Cowell's operation. An iridotomy made with a lance in a contracted iris. Of historical interest as the first operation on the iris, 1798.

Cowgill's salt mixture. A mixture of sodium chloride, magnesium citrate, potassium and calcium hypophosphites, potassium chloride, ferric citrate and potassium iodide, used as an aperient and tonic.

cowhage (**kow**·ij). Cowitch, the hairs from the tropical plant *Mucana pruriens* DC. (family Leguminosae). Mixed with honey or treacle, it has been used as a vermifuge.

cowitch (**kow**·itch). Cowhage. [AS *cu*, itch.]

cowl (kowl). Caul. [AS *cugele.*]

Cowper, William (b. 1666). London surgeon.

Cowper's cyst, Cowperian cyst. A cyst of a bulbo-urethral gland.

Cowper's glands, Cowperian glands. The bulbo-urethral glands. *See* GLAND.

Cowperian (kow·**peer**·e·an). Associated with William Cowper.

cowperitis (kow·per·**i**·tis). A state of inflammation of the bulbo-urethral glands (Cowper's glands). [Cowper, Gk *-itis* inflammation.]

cowpox (**kow**·pox). A mild contagious virus disease affecting the teats and udders of cows. The virus can be transferred to the hands of milkers, causing a mild infection which can confer protection against the antigenically related smallpox virus. Jenner's observation of this fact led to his use of cowpox virus for vaccination. It is now a constituent of smallpox vaccine (*see* VACCINIA). [AS *cu*, ME *pokkes.*]

Cox, Harold Rae. Virologist, Montana and New York.

Cox vaccine. A typhus vaccine prepared from a yolk-sac culture of rickettsiae.

Cox, Wilhelm Hendrik (b. 1861). Dutch histologist.

Cox's modification of Golgi's corrosive sublimate method. Tissues are treated for some months in a mixture of potassium bichromate, mercuric chloride and potassium chromate, then the mercury precipitate is blackened with ammonia. Nerve cells and their processes and neuroglia are impregnated.

coxa (**cox**·ah). The hip joint. *See* JOINT. **Coxa adducta.** Adduction deformity of the hip. **Coxa flexa.** Flexion deformity of the hip. **Coxa magna.** A hip joint in which the head of the femur is abnormally large. **Coxa plana.** Perthes' disease; osteochondritis of the hip. **Coxa valga.** A deformity of the femoral neck in which the angle between the neck and the shaft is increased; the opposite of coxa vara. **Coxa vara.** A deformity of the femoral neck in which the angle between the shaft and the neck is decreased; the opposite of coxa valga. **Coxa vara luxans.** Coxa vara with dislocation of the head. [L.]

coxal (**kox**·al). Relating to the hip or the hip joint. [see prec.]

coxalgia (kox·**al**·je·ah). Pain in the hip joint. [coxa, Gk *algos* pain.]

coxalgic (kox·**al**·jik). Referring to coxalgia.

coxankylometer (**kox**·an·ki·**lom'**·et·er). An apparatus with which the degree of deformity in a diseased hip may be determined. [coxa, Gk *agkylos* bent, *metron* measure.]

coxarthria, coxarthritis (cox·**ar**·thre·ah, cox·ar·**thri**·tis). Coxitis. [coxa, Gk *arthron* joint, *-itis* inflammation.]

coxarthropathy (kox·ar·**throp**·ath·e). Any disease of the hip joint. [coxa, Gk *arthron* joint, *pathos* suffering.]

coxarthrosis (kox·ar·**thro**·sis). Degenerative arthritis of the hip joint. [coxa, arthrosis.]

Coxeter-Mushin apparatus. An apparatus for closed anaesthesia, working on the circle principle.

Coxiella (kox·e·**el**·ah). A microbial genus, closely related to *Rickettsia* but with certain distinguishing characters, including high resistance to heat and to disinfectants. **Coxiella burneti.** The causal organism of Q fever. [H.R. *Cox.*]

coxitis (kox·**i**·tis). Inflammation of the hip joint. **Coxitis cotyloidea.** Coxitis attacking mainly the acetabulum. **Coxitis fugax.** A temporary condition of mild inflammation of the hip joint. **Senile coxitis.** A form of rheumatoid arthritis of the hip joint which occurs in elderly people; there is stiffness, wasting and pain, without suppuration. [coxa, Gk *-itis* inflammation.]

coxodynia (kox·o·**din**·e·ah). Coxalgia. [coxa, Gk *odyne* pain.]

coxofemoral (kox·o·**fem**·or·al). Relating to the hip and the thigh. [coxa, femur.]

coxotomy (kox·**ot**·o·me). The surgical exploration of the hip joint. [coxa, Gk *temnein* to cut.]

coxotuberculosis (**kox**·o·tew·ber·kew·**lo'**·sis). Tuberculosis of the hip joint. [coxa, tuberculosis.]

co-zymase (ko·**zi**·maze). Coenzyme I, II; nicotinamide adenine dinucleotide and nicotinamide adenine dinucleotide phosphate.

crab, crab louse (krab, **krab**·lows). The sucking louse *Phthirus pubis*, a specific parasite of man, and confined to areas of coarse hair particularly in the pubic region, but also of the chest, axillae, and eyebrows and lashes. It causes irritation and purple patches at the hair bases, but is not apparently a disease vector. [AS *crabba*, louse.]

crachotement (krah·shote·**mahn**). A state caused by nervous reflex which may be the result of gynaecological operation. The patient has a strong desire to spit but is unable to do so, and there is often an accompanying tendency to syncope. [Fr. *crachoter* to spit often.]

crackle (krakl). **Egg shell crackle.** The sensation obtained in palpation of the superficial parts of a thin walled bone tumour, e.g. giant cell tumour around the knee. **Pleural crackle.** Bruit de cuir neuf heard in the early stages of acute dry pleurisy. [AS *cracian*.]

crackling (**krak**·ling). *See* DUPUYTREN. [see prec.]

cradle (kra·dl). A hooped framework of metal or wicker. **Bed cradle.** A cradle designed to support the weight of the bedclothes. **Electric cradle.** One for the application of radiant heat which is supplied by electric bulbs fixed inside it. **Fracture cradle.** One to which is suspended a splint for the support of a lower limb. **Ice cradle.** A cradle from which is suspended a metal tray for ice; used for the reduction of body temperature. **Radiant heat cradle.** Electric cradle (see above). [AS *cradel*.]

Crafoord, Clarence (b. 1899). Stockholm surgeon.

Crafoord's operation. Excision of a coarctation of the aorta with reconstitution by anastomosis. First performed in 1945.

Crafts, Leo Melville (b. 1863). Minneapolis neurologist.

Crafts' test. A clinical test for organic disease of the pyramidal tract: a stroke with a blunt point in an upward direction over the anterior surface of the ankle causes dorsiflexion of the great toe. This test or sign is simply the extensor plantar response of Babinski, evoked by stimulation of a skin area remote from the sole of the foot.

Craigia (**kra**·ge·ah). A supposed genus of intestinal flagellates. *Craigia hominis*, described as having amoeboid and flagellate stages, is probably a confusion of other forms. [Charles Franklin *Craig*, 1872–1950, US army surgeon and parasitologist.]

Craigie's tube. A test-tube containing semi-solid agar, inside which there is a smaller tube open at both ends, and with one end projecting above the agar; by inoculating within the inner tube and subculturing from outside it, organisms motile under the test conditions can be isolated. Its most common use is in the study of diphasic variation in the flagellar antigens of *Salmonellae* and in the identification of strains of this genus.

Cramer, Friedrich (b. 1847). Wiesbaden surgeon.

Cramer's splint. A malleable metal splint made of wires, in the shape of a ladder.

Cramer, William (b. 1878). London pathologist.

Cramer and Bannerman solution. A diluting fluid used in an indirect method for enumerating blood platelets; it consists of sodium citrate (0.2 g), sodium chloride (0.8 g), 1 per cent aqueous solution of brilliant cresyl blue (1 ml), formalin (2 ml) and distilled water to 100 ml.

cramp (kramp). Painful and involuntary contraction of muscles, leading to spasm of variable duration. It is associated with a rheumatic tendency and with exposure to cold. The condition may affect certain groups of muscles used in specific vocations, as in the case of ballet dancers, musicians (including violinists, piano players), seamstresses, tailors, telegraphers and writers and is commonly related to occupational neurosis; shaving cramp also occurs. **Heat cramp, Thermal cramp.** Cramp due to dehydration and salt-privation brought on by exposure to intense heat; it is accompanied by flushing, dilation of the pupils, vertigo and laboured breathing. [AS *crammian* to fill.]

Crampton, Charles Ward (b. 1877). New York physician.

Crampton's test. Of myocardial reserve: the pulse rate and blood pressure are measured in the recumbent position, and again after the subject suddenly assumes the erect position. Normally, increase in vascular tone in the splanchnic areas and lower half of the body prevents pooling of blood and maintains pulse rate and blood pressure in the standing position. A fall in blood pressure indicates inadequacy of this reflex mechanism, and may result in syncope (orthostatic hypotension). Individuals with sluggish or poor vascular control of the autonomic nervous system show a positive reaction to the test, which does not necessarily indicate organic cardiovascular disease.

Crampton, Sir Philip (b. 1777). Dublin surgeon.

Crampton's line. A line drawn from the tip of the last rib to nearly the crest of the ilium and then forward to a point just below and internal to the anterior superior iliac spine. It indicates the course of the common iliac artery.

Crampton's muscle. Meridional fibres of the ciliary muscle.

Crandon's scurvy. Experimental scurvy to show that wounds heal slowly and may break down in the absence of vitamin C in the diet.

cranial (kra·ne·al). Relating to the cranium.

cranial nerves [nervi craniales (NA)]. The nerves arising from the brain, 12 on each side, all traversing the cranium: *first*, olfactory; *second*, optic; *third*, oculomotor; *fourth*, trochlear; *fifth*, trigeminal; *sixth*, abducent; *seventh*, facial; *eighth*, auditory; *ninth*, glossopharyngeal; *tenth*, vagus; *eleventh*, accessory; *twelfth*, hypoglossal.

craniamphitomy (kra·ne·am·**fit**′·o·me). The circumferential division of the cranium in order to achieve wide decompression. [Gk *kranion* skull, *amphi*, *temnein* to cut.]

Craniata (kra·ne·a·tah). A division or sub-phylum of the phylum Chordata, which contains all those forms in which the brain is enclosed in a definite cranium. It includes all fish, amphibia, reptiles, birds and mammals. The more usual term is vertebrata. [Gk *kranion* skull.]

craniectomy (kra·ne·**ek**·to·me). The cutting away of a portion of the skull. **Linear craniectomy.** The cutting away of strips of the bones of the skull in order to relieve microcephaly. [Gk *kranion* skull, *ektome* a cutting out.]

craniencephalometer (kra·ne·en·kef·al·**om**′·et·er). A device by means of which the location of the gyri of the brain can be determined relative to the surface of the head. [Gk *kranion* skull, encephalometer.]

cranio-acromial (kra·ne·o·ak·**ro**′·me·al). Relating to the skull and the acromion. [Gk *kranion* skull, acromion.]

cranio-aural (kra·ne·o·aw′·ral). Relating to the skull and the ear, or involving them. [Gk *kranion* skull, L *auris* ear.]

craniobuccal (kra·ne·o·**buk**′·al). Relating to the head and the mouth. [Gk *kranion* skull, L *bucca* cheek.]

craniocaudal (kra·ne·o·**kaw**′·dal). Relating to the head and the tail as of an axis in embryology. [Gk *kranion* skull, L *cauda* tail.]

craniocele (kra·ne·o·seel). Encephalocele. [Gk *kranion* skull, *kele* hernia.]

craniocerebral (kra·ne·o·**ser**′·e·bral). Relating to the skull and the brain. [Gk *kranion* skull, cerebrum.]

craniocervical (kra·ne·o·**ser**′·vik·al). Relating to the skull and the neck. [Gk *kranion* skull, L *cervix* neck.]

cranioclasis, cranioclasm (kra·ne·**ok**·las·is, **kra**·ne·o·klazm). The crushing of the fetal skull with a cranioclast in order to make delivery possible. [Gk *kranion* skull, *klasis* a breaking.]

cranioclast (kra·ne·o·klast). A heavy instrument of the pincer type for use in cranioclasis. [see prec.]

cranioclasty (kra·ne·o·**klas**′·te). Cranioclasis.

craniocleidal (kra·ne·o·**kli**′·dal). Pertaining to the cranium and the clavicle. [Gk *kranion* skull, *kleis* key.]

craniocleidodysostosis (kra·ne·o·**kli**·do·dis·os·**to**′·sis). Cleidocranial dysostosis. *See* DYSOSTOSIS. [Gk *kranion* skull, *kleis* key, dysostosis.]

craniodidymus (kra·ne·o·**did**′·e·mus). Cephalopagus: craniopagus. [Gk *kranion* skull, *didymos* twin.]

craniofacial (kra·ne·o·**fa**′·shal). Relating to the skull and the face, or affecting both. [Gk *kranion* skull, L *facies* face.]

craniofenestria (kra·ne·o·fen·**es**′·tre·ah). Defective skull formation, with areas in the vault where no bone has formed. [Gk *kranion* skull, L *fenestra* window.]

craniognomy (kra·ne·**og**·no·me). The study of the shape and characteristics of the skull. [Gk *kranion* skull, *gnomen* understanding.]

craniograph (**kra**·ne·o·graf). An instrument with which drawings to scale can be made of the general outline of the skull and its diameters. [Gk *kranion* skull, *graphein* to record.]

craniography (kra·ne·**og**·raf·e). That branch of craniology which represents the skull and the bones of the face by means of drawings or photographs and descriptions of the relations of craniometric points and angles. [see prec.]

craniolacunia (**kra**·ne·o·lak·**ew**′·ne·ah). Defective skull formation, with depressed areas in the inner table of the vault. [Gk *kranion* skull, L *lacuna* hollow.]

craniology (kra·ne·**ol**·o·je). The study of skulls with regard to their shape, size and proportions, in particular for ethnical purposes. [Gk *kranion* skull, *logos* science.]

craniomalacia (**kra**·ne·o·mal·**a**′·she·ah). Craniotabes. [Gk *kranion* skull, *malakia* softness.]

craniomandibular (**kra**·ne·o·man·**dib**′·ew·lar). Relating to the skull and the mandible. [Gk *kranion* skull, mandible.]

craniomeningocele (**kra**·ne·o·men·**ing**′·go·seel). Hernia of the cerebral meninges through a defect in the skull. [Gk *kranion* skull, meningocele.]

craniometer (kra·ne·**om**·et·er). An instrument with which the diameters of the skull may be measured. [Gk *kranion* skull, meter.]

craniometric (**kra**·ne·o·**met**′·rik). Referring to craniometry.

craniometry (kra·ne·**om**·et·re). The measurement of skulls and their proportions and peculiarities. [Gk *kranion* skull, meter.]

craniopagus (kra·ne·**op**·ag·us). A twin monster the 2 heads of which are fused into one. **Craniopagus frontalis.** A double monster, twins attached in the frontal region. **Craniopagus occipitalis.** A double monster, twins attached in the occipital region. **Craniopagus parasiticus.** A craniopagus of which one fetus is small and rudimentary and is parasitic on the larger fetus. **Craniopagus parietalis.** A double monster, twins attached in the parietal region. [Gk *kranion* skull, *pagos* fixed.]

craniopathy (kra·ne·**op**·ath·e). Cephalopathy. **Metabolic craniopathy.** A condition in which headache, eye disorders and obesity are found in association with lesions of the skull. [Gk *kranion* skull, *pathos* suffering.]

craniopharyngeal (**kra**·ne·o·far·**in**′·je·al). Relating to the skull and the pharynx. [Gk *kranion* skull, pharynx.]

craniopharyngioma (**kra**·ne·o·far·**in**·je·**o**′·mah). A neoplasm originating in the remnants of the hypophyseal duct. These are chiefly suprasellar tumours occurring mainly in children and adolescents. [Gk *kranion* skull, pharynx, Gk *-oma* tumour.]

craniophore (**kra**·ne·o·for). An apparatus which holds the skull steady during craniometry. [Gk *kranion* skull, *phoros* bearer.]

cranioplasty (**kra**·ne·o·plas·te). 1. Surgical correction or restoration of defects of the skull. 2. Any plastic operation performed on the skull. [Gk *kranion* skull, *plassein* to mould.]

craniopuncture (kra·ne·o·**pungk**′·tcher). Exploratory puncture of the brain. [Gk *kranion* skull, puncture.]

craniorrhachischisis (**kra**·ne·o·rak·**is**′·kis·is). Congenital fissure of the skull and spinal column. [Gk *kranion* skull, *rhachis* spine, *schisis* division.]

craniosacral (kra·ne·o·**sa**′·kral). Relating to the skull and the sacrum. [Gk *kranion* skull, sacrum.]

cranioschisis (kra·ne·**os**·kis·is). Congenital fissure of the skull. [Gk *kranion* skull, *schisis* division.]

craniosclerosis (**kra**·ne·o·skler·**o**′·sis). A condition in which the bones of the skull become thickened, usually as a result of rickets. [Gk *kranion* skull, *skleros* hard.]

cranioscopy (kra·ne·**os**·ko·pe). Examination of the skull of a living individual for the purposes of diagnosis or in connection with phrenology or craniometry. [Gk *kranion* skull, *skopein* to watch.]

craniospinal (**kra**·ne·o·**spi**′·nal). Relating to the skull and the vertebral column. [Gk *kranion* skull, spine.]

craniostat (**kra**·ne·o·stat). An apparatus for taking standardized skull radiographs for comparative purposes. [Gk *kranion* skull, *statos* standing.]

craniostenosis (**kra**·ne·o·sten·**o**′·sis). Contraction of the skull as a result of obliteration of the cranial foramina and closure of the fissures. [Gk *kranion* skull, stenosis.]

craniostosis (kra·ne·**os**·to·sis). Congenital ossification of the skull with obliteration of the cranial sutures. [Gk *kranion* skull, *osteon* bone, *-osis* condition.]

craniosynostosis (**kra**·ne·o·sin·**os**′·to·sis). Premature closure of cranial sutures. [Gk *kranion* skull, *syn*, *osteon* bone, *-osis* condition.]

craniotabes (**kra**·ne·o·**ta**′·beez). A condition of the skull of an infant in which the bones in the occipital region become patchily thin and soft so that small depressions form in the bone substance. The cause may be syphilis, marasmus or rickets. [Gk *kranion* skull, L *tabes* a wasting.]

craniotabetic (**kra**·ne·o·tab·**et**′·ik). 1. Having reference to or belonging to craniotabes. 2. One suffering from craniotabes.

craniotome (**kra**·ne·o·tome). An instrument for use in operations on the cranium, or in perforation and division of the fetal skull when delivery is otherwise impossible. [Gk *kranion* skull, *temnein* to cut.]

craniotomy (kra·ne·**ot**·o·me). 1. Any operation on the skull. 2. The cutting away of a part of the skull. **Fetal craniotomy.** The breaking-up or division of the fetal skull, or the perforation and crushing of it with removal of the contents in order to make delivery possible. **Osteoplastic craniotomy.** The operation of opening the skull by raising a bone flap to which the muscles are left attached in order that the blood supply of the bone will be preserved. [see prec.]

craniotonoscopy (**kra**·ne·o·to·**nos**′·ko·pe). Auscultatory percussion of the skull used in combination with a special kind of pneumatoscope placed in the examiner's mouth, so that local thickening or thinning of the bony substance of the skull can be detected. [Gk *kranion* skull, *tonos* tone, *skopein* to watch.]

craniotopography (**kra**·ne·o·to·**pog**′·raf·e). The study of the skull with reference to the different portions of the brain beneath particular areas of the surface. [Gk *kranion* skull, topography.]

craniotractor (**kra**·ne·o·**trak**′·tor). A form of cranioclast which can be used as a tractor. [Gk *kranion* skull, L *trahere* to pull.]

craniotripsotome (**kra**·ne·o·**trip**′·so·tome). A special kind of cranioclast, described by G. Camagna (1891). [Gk *kranion* skull, *tripsis* a rubbing, *temnein* to cut.]

craniotrypesis (**kra**·ne·o·tri·**pe**′·sis). Trephination. [Gk *kranion* skull, *trypesis* a boring.]

craniotympanic (**kra**·ne·o·tim·**pan**′·ik). Referring to the skull and the middle ear (tympanum). [Gk *kranion* skull, *tympanon* drum.]

cranium [L.] (**kra**·ne·um). 1. The skull. 2. The part of the skull which encloses and protects the brain. **Cranium bifidum.** Congenital fissure of the skull. **Cranium cerebrale.** *See* MAIN DEF. 2 (above). **Visceral cranium, Cranium viscerale.** The bones of the face. [Gk *kranion.*]

crapulent, crapulous (**krap**·ew·lent, **krap**·ew·lus). Dissipated; characterized by or resulting from excess in eating or drinking. [L *crapulari* to intoxicate.]

crasis (**kra**·sis). The blending of various factors which together compose the individual constitution or temperament. **Blood crasis.** The state of the blood. **Parasitic crasis.** An enfeebled condition which is favourable to the harbouring of parasites in the body or is the result of being infested with parasites. **Verminous crasis.** A term formerly used to describe the disordered condition resulting from the presence of worms. [Obsolete term.] [Gk *krasis* a mingling.]

crassamentum (kras·ah·**ment**·um). 1. Blood clot. *See* CLOT. 2. Coagulum. 3. The sediment or the thick portion of a fluid. [L thickness.]

crataegin (krat·e·jin). A substance obtained from the fruit of the English hawthorn, *Crataegus oxyacantha*, and capable of causing a fall of blood pressure. If given intravenously, it has a depressant action on the respiratory centre and may cause auricular fibrillation and heart block.

Crataegus (krat·e·gus). A genus of trees and shrubs of the family Rosaceae. **Crataegus oxyacantha.** English hawthorn, haw; the fruits in the form of a liquid extract or tincture are used as a cardiac tonic. [Gk *krataigos* thorn.]

crater (kra·ter). 1. Niche. 2. The pit-like depression left when the slough of an ulcer has been cast out. 3. Outline of an active peptic ulcer as seen by x-ray examination. [Gk *krater* mixing-bowl for wine.]

crateriform (kra·ter·e·form). Hollow like a saucer, bowl or deep pit; said of bacterial colonies. [Gk *krater* mixing-bowl for wine, form.]

craunology (krawn·ol·o·je). Crenology.

craunotherapy (kraw·no·ther·ap·e). Crenotherapy.

craw-craw (kraw·kraw). The West African name applied to many itching eruptions, e.g. scabies and prurigo, but particularly to onchocerciasis.

crawling (krawl·ing). A form of paraesthesia in which there is a localized sensation as of ants crawling over the body. [Dan. *kravle* to scrabble with the hands.]

crayfish (kra·fish). A small fresh-water lobster. Several species, in the genera *Astacus* and *Cambarus*, are intermediate hosts of flukes of the genus *Paragonimus*. [ME *crevice*.]

cream (kreem). 1. The fatty layer which rises to the top when milk is left standing; it contains approximately 20 per cent of fat, with milk protein, lactose and salts. Better separation may be achieved with a centrifuge (up to 45 per cent fat), and such cream is used in making butter. 2. Name given to any semi-solid preparation in pharmacy, less viscous than an ointment and resembling the cream of milk in viscosity. **Aluminium hydroxide cream.** An aqueous suspension of colloidal aluminium hydroxide used in the treatment of peptic ulcer. **Aqueous Cream BP 1973.** Emulsifying ointment 300 g, water 699 g and chlorocresol 1 g. **Cold cream.** An unstable emulsion of water in an oil-beeswax medium; rubbing on to the skin breaks down the emulsion and the evaporation of the water droplets gives a sensation of coldness. **Leucocytic cream.** A buffy layer of concentrated whole blood corpuscles and platelets formed on the top of the red blood coil layer when blood plasma is allowed to sediment or is subjected to centrifugation; it has been used therapeutically and experimentally. **Cream of magnesia.** Magnesium Hydroxide Mixture BP 1973. **Marylebone cream.** A 50 per cent emulsion of arachis oil, containing vitamin D. **Purified cream of tartar.** Potassium Acid Tartrate BP 1958, COOH $(CHOH)_2COOK$, a white powder only slightly soluble in water, obtained from the crude tartar which separates out in wine-making. When administered, the tartrate ion is not easily absorbed from the gastro-intestinal tract; in consequence, some of it is retained in the bowel and with it sufficient water to render the solution isotonic. This increases the bulk of the faeces, stretching the muscular wall of the intestine and intensifying peristalsis. The stools are rendered fluid and purgation takes place 1½–2 h after the ingestion of the drug. It is also diuretic. [Gk *chrima* oil.]

creamometer (kre·mom·et·er). A device with which the quantity of fat in milk may be estimated. [cream, meter.]

crease (krees). A mark or line made by folding. **Gluteofemoral crease, Iliofemoral crease.** The fold of the buttock. **Simian crease.** A crease which goes across the palm of the hand and replaces the 2 transversal creases which are present in most normal individuals. [etym. dub.]

creasote (kre·as·ote). Creosote.

creat (kre·at). Kreat. The name given to *Andrographis paniculata* Nees. (family Acanthaceae). An infusion of the root is used in India as a bitter tonic and stimulant in diarrhoea and dysentery.

creatinaemia (kre·at·in·e′·me·ah). A condition in which there is an excessive amount of creatine in the blood. [creatine, Gk *haima* blood.]

creatinase (kre·at·in·aze). An enzyme which converts creatine into its anhydride, creatinine.

creatine (kre·at·een). $NH_2C(=NH)N(CH_3)CH_2COOH$, present in muscle as its phosphate ester. An end-product of nucleotide metabolism, it is excreted as *creatinine*. **Creatine phosphate.** A reservoir of high-energy phosphate in muscle, it serves to regenerate ATP from ADP in a reaction catalysed by creatine phosphokinase. **Creatine phosphokinase.** An enzyme of which the serum level rises when there is muscle damage, especially in pseudohypertrophic muscular dystrophy. **Creatine tolerance test.** *See* TEST. [Gk *kreas* flesh.]

creatininase (kre·at·in·in′·aze). An enzyme which hydrolyses creatinine into urea and sarcosine (*N*-methylglycine).

creatinine (kre·at·in·een). Methylglycocyamidine, $NH{=}C(NHCO)N(CH_3)CH_2$. The cyclic anhydride of creatine, which occurs in urine as the end-product of muscle metabolism. The amount excreted daily is constant for each individual, regardless of diet, depending entirely on the blood flow through the kidney.

creatininuria (kre·at·in·in·ewr′·e·ah). An excess of creatinine in the urine.

creatinuria (kre·at·in·ewr′·e·ah). A condition in which creatine is present in the urine.

creaton (kre·at·on). Oxalyl methyl guanidine, $NH{=}C(NHCO)N(CH_3)CO$. A derivative of creatine, which occurs in muscle.

creatorrhoea (kre·at·o·re′·ah). The presence in the stools of undigested muscle fibres, e.g. in certain diseases of the pancreas. [Gk *kreas* flesh, *rhoia* flow.]

creatotoxism, creatoxism (kre·at·o·tox′·izm, kre·at·ox·izm). A state of poisoning resulting from the eating of tainted or rotten meat. [Gk *kreas* flesh, *toxikon* poison.]

Credé, Karl Siegmund Franz (b.1819). Leipzig gynaecologist.

Credé's manoeuvre, or method. Expulsion of the retained placenta by pressure on the fundus uteri through the abdominal wall. The uterus is massaged until it contracts, and the attendant compresses the fundus between his fingers posteriorly and thumb anteriorly.

Credé's method. Of treatment of the eyes: the instillation of silver nitrate drops into the eyes of the newborn child to prevent gonococcal conjunctivitis.

creeps (creeps). An itchy sensation in the skin encountered in decompression sickness. [ME *créopan*.]

cremaster, artery to the, or to the round ligament of the uterus [arteria cremasterica et arteria ligamenti teretis uteri (NA)] (kre·mas·ter). A branch of the inferior epigastric artery which passes through the deep inguinal ring to the cremaster muscle, or in the female to the round ligament. [see foll.]

cremaster muscle [musculus cremaster (NA)]. A thin layer of muscle on the anterior and lateral aspects of the spermatic cord. *See* CREMASTER MUSCLE AND FASCIA. [Gk *kremastos* hanging.]

cremaster muscle and fascia [musculus cremaster et fascia cremasterica (NA)]. An investment for the spermatic cord and testis, derived from the internal oblique muscle of the abdomen and composed of connective tissue containing discrete strands of muscle. Its action is to elevate the testis and it can be caused to contract by stroking the skin on the inner side of the thigh (cremasteric reflex). [see prec.]

cremasteric (kre·mas·ter·ik). Referring to the cremaster muscle.

cremation (kre·ma·shun). Disposal of the bodies of the dead by burning. [L *cremare* to burn.]

crematorium, crematory (krem·at·or·e·um, krem·at·or·e). An establishment in which cremation is carried out by means of special furnaces.

cremnocele (krem·no·seel). Inguinolabial hernia; hernia into the labium majus. [Gk *kremnos* cliff, *kele* hernia.]

cremnophobia (krem·no·fo·be·ah). A morbid dread of precipices or steep places. [Gk *kremnos* cliff, phobia.]

cremor tartari (kre·mor tar·tar·i). Cream of tartar.

crena (kre·nah). 1. A cleft or notch. 2. One of the notches on the margins of the cranial sutures. **Crena chenium.** The natal cleft. **Crena cordis.** The atrioventricular groove of the heart. *See* GROOVE. [L.]

crenate, crenated (kre·nate, kre·na·ted). Having a scalloped or cog-wheel margin, e.g. erythrocytes when exposed to air. [L *crena* notch.]

crenation (kre·**na**·shun). 1. The notched or scalloped appearance of erythrocytes when they are exposed to unnatural conditions, e.g. strong saline solution. 2. The process of becoming crenated. 3. The state of being crenated. [see prec.]

crenocyte (**kre**·no·site). A crenated erythrocyte. [L *crena* notch, Gk *kytos* cell.]

crenocytosis (**kre**·no·si·**to**'·sis). A condition in which there are crenated erythrocytes in the blood. [crenocyte, Gk *-osis* condition.]

crenology (kren·**ol**·o·je). The science dealing with those mineral waters obtained from springs which are of therapeutic value. [Gk *krene* spring, *logos* science.]

crenotherapy (kren·o·**ther**·ap·e). The treatment of disease by mineral waters obtained from springs. [Gk *krene* spring, *therapeia* treatment.]

Crenothrix (**kren**·o·thrix). A genus of the family Crenothrichaceae. A filamentous organism found in stagnant water and reservoirs. It frequently fills pipes and causes nuisance, due to the formation of brownish masses incorporating a great deal of iron deposit. *Crenothrix polyspora* is the only recognized species. [Gk *krene* spring, *thrix* hair.]

crenulate (**kren**·ew·late). Minutely crenate. [L *crenula* little notch.]

crenulation (kren·ew·**la**·shun). Wavy edge; a term used to describe the waved appearance of the edges of erythrocytes parasitized by *Plasmodium ovale.* It is not necessarily present in all cases of such parasitism. [see prec.]

creolin (**kre**·o·lin). A soap solution of cresol or homologues of cresol, used as a disinfectant of the skin in 2 per cent concentration; also employed in ascarides infestations as a local application (alcoholic solution, 5-50 per cent). Strong solutions are effective in sanitary disinfection.

creophagism, creophagy (kre·**of**·ah·jizm, kre·**of**·ah·je). The habit of using the flesh of animals in the dietary. [Gk *kreas* flesh, *phagein* to eat.]

creosol (**kre**·o·sol). $CH_3OC_6H_4(OH)$, the monomethyl ether of guaiacol, and one of the major components of creosote.

creosote (**kre**·o·sote). A colourless or pale-yellow liquid of strong smoky odour and burning taste, obtained by fractional distillation of wood (generally beech) tar; a mixture of phenols, principally guaiacol and creosol. It resembles phenol in its properties, being antiseptic and deodorant, but is less toxic. It is used to deodorize the sputum in bronchiectasis, and may be inhaled from hot water or given internally in capsule form, as it is partly excreted by the bronchi. It has some local analgesic action and has been used to relieve toothache. In ointment form it is employed to treat certain parasitic skin diseases (BP 1953). Various derivatives have been tried at different times as substitutes; amongst these are creosote carbonate, calcium creosote and creosote phosphate. They are, however, little used now in medical treatment. **Inhalation of Creosote BPC 1954, Creosote vapour.** A mixture of creosote, light magnesium carbonate, and water, used as an inhalation in upper respiratory-tract infections. [Gk *kreas* flesh, *sozein* to preserve.]

creotoxin (kre·o·**tox**·in). Kreotoxin; any poisonous substance formed in meat by bacterial action. [Gk *kreas* flesh, *toxikon* poison.]

creotoxism (kre·o·**tox**·izm). Creotototoxism.

crepitant (**krep**·it·ant). Having or producing a rattling or crackling sound; having the character of crepitus. [L *crepitans* crackling.]

crepitation, crepitatio (krep·it·**a**·shun, krep·it·**a**·she·o). A crepitant râle; crepitus. [L *crepitare* to crackle.]

crepitus (**krep**·it·us). 1. The sound of 2 rough substances being rubbed together. 2. A crepitant râle. 3. The sound produced when pressure is applied to tissues filled with gas or air, e.g. in subcutaneous emphysema. **Articular crepitus.** Joint crepitus (see below). **Bony crepitus.** The grating noise produced by the rubbing or grinding together of the fractured ends of bones. **False crepitus.** Joint crepitus (see below). **Crepitus indux.** Râle indux. **Joint crepitus.** The grinding or grating sensation felt or sound heard when dry synovial surfaces of joints rub on one another. **Crepitus redux.** The coarse râles heard over an area of resolving pneumonia. **Silken crepitus.** A sensation in the hand when it is manipulating a joint affected with hydrarthrosis, as if 2 silk surfaces were being rubbed together between the fingers. [L a crackling.]

crepuscular (kre·**pus**·kew·lar). 1. Imperfectly clear. 2. Relating to a twilight state literally, but figuratively used in reference to bodily and mental states. [L *crepusculum* twilight.]

crescent (**kres**·ent). Anything shaped like a sickle, or new moon. **Epithelial crescent.** Proliferation of the epithelial lining of the glomeruli in subacute and chronic glomerulonephritis. **Grey crescent.** A grey pigmented area which appears in the pigmented ova of certain animals, e.g. the frog, subsequent to fertilization; its position has a definite relationship to the future craniocaudal and dorso-abdominal axes of the organism. **Malarial crescent.** The gametocyte or sexual form of the subtertian malaria parasite *Plasmodium falciparum;* it is crescentic in shape and both male and female stages are produced. **Myopic crescent.** A white crescent of exposed sclera, usually on the temporal side of the disc, and caused by myopic enlargement of the eyeball in its anteroposterior axis dragging on the retina and choroid on the temporal side of the disc. **Crescent sphere.** Malarial crescent (see above). **Crescent of the spinal cord.** The crescentic outline formed by the anterior and corresponding posterior horn of grey matter seen on the surface of a transverse section of the spinal cord. [L *crescere* to grow.]

See also: GIANNUZZI, HEIDENHAIN.

cresol (**kre**·sol). $CH_3C_6H_4OH$, a yellowish liquid consisting of a mixture of *ortho-*, *meta-* and *para-*cresols; with phenol it is the chief constituent of the crude carbolic acid obtained from coal tar and wood tar. It is a more potential bactericide than phenol and less toxic (BP 1973). In high concentrations it precipitates proteins and has a caustic action on the tissues. Applied to the skin it penetrates to the sensory nerve-endings and has a local anaesthetic effect. Systemically it stimulates and then depresses the central nervous system, and death occurs from paralysis of the respiratory centre. It is a powerful antipyretic, and in poisoning with cresol there is a marked fall in body temperature. Cresol is absorbed from all sites, and is either excreted in the urine conjugated with glycuronic or sulphuric acids or oxidized in the body to quinone and pyrocatechin; the urine often has a smoky appearance due to oxidation of the excretion products. When poisoning results from ingestion of cresol, corrosion of the mucous membranes of the intestinal tract takes place with considerable pain and vomiting; blood pressure is low, there is a cold sweat and much shock, whilst casts, albumin and free haemoglobin appear in the rather scanty urine. Treatment consists primarily in removing the compound from the gastro-intestinal tract by lavage with copious amounts of olive oil. **Cresol phthalein.** Cresolphthalein. **Cresol red.** Orthocresol sulphonephthalein, a compound used as a pH indicator (7.2-8.8). **Cresol and Soap Solution BP 1968.** *See* SOLUTION.

cresolphthalein (kre·sol·**thal**·een). A derivative of phenolphthalein used as an indicator.

cresomania (kre·so·**ma**·ne·ah). Croesomania.

cresorcin (kres·**or**·sin). Dimethylfluorescein, $C_{22}H_{16}O_5$. A yellow dye used as an indicator (pH 4-6).

cresorcinol (kres·**or**·sin·ol). Dihydroxytoluene, $CH_3C_6H_3(OH)_2$. An isomer of orcinol prepared from cresol.

cresotate (**kres**·o·tate). 1. A salt of cresotic acid. 2. A cresylate.

crest [crista (NA)] (krest). A narrow elongated elevation; a prominent superior border to a structure. The term is most commonly used in the description of bones, e.g. iliac crest, intertrochanteric crest, but sometimes for soft structures, e.g. urethral crest. **Ampullary crest [crista ampullaris (NA)].** The most prominent part of the septum transversum of the membranous ampulla. **Arcuate crest [crista arcuata (NA)].** A crest on the anterolateral surface of the arytenoid cartilage between the attachment of the vestibular ligament and those of the vocalis and crico-arytenoid muscles. **Basal crest.** The crista basilaris. **Conchal crest [crista conchalis (NA)].** A ridge on the medial aspect of the maxilla and palatine bone to which the inferior nasal concha is attached. **Ethmoidal crest of the maxilla [crista ethmoidalis (NA)].** A ridge in the medial aspect of the frontal process of the maxilla: posteriorly it articulates with the middle nasal concha; anteriorly it forms the agger nasi. **Ethmoidal crest of the palatine bone [crista ethmoidalis (NA)].** A ridge on the medial surface of the palatine bone which articulates with the middle nasal concha. **Crest of the fenestra cochleae [crista fenestrae cochleae (NA)].** The edge of the opening to which the annular ligament is attached. **Crest of the fibula, medial [crista medialis (NA)].** A ridge on the posterior surface of the fibula, separating the attachment of the tibialis posterior and flexor hallucis longus. **Frontal crest [crista frontalis (NA)].** A median sagittal projection from the frontal bone into the anterior cranial fossa. **Crest of the head of a rib [crista capitis costae (NA)].** The transverse ridge which separates the 2 facets on the head of a rib. **Iliac crest [crista iliaca (NA)].** The upper and outer border of the ilium. **Iliac crest, intermediate area of the [linea intermedia (NA)].** The roughened area between the inner and outer lips of the iliac crest. It gives attachment to the internal oblique muscle. **Infratemporal crest [crista infratemporalis (NA)].** A ridge on the greater wing of the sphenoid bone separating the temporal from the infratemporal surface. **Infundibuloventricular crest [crista supraventricularis (NA)].** A muscular ridge between the atrioventricular and pulmonary orifices of the right ventricle. **Intertrochanteric crest.** Trochanteric crest (see below). **Crest of the lacrimal bone [crista lacrimalis posterior (NA)].** A ridge on the lacrimal bone forming the posterior boundary of the fossa for the lacrimal sac. **Lacrimal crest of the maxilla [crista lacrimalis anterior (NA)].** The crest on the nose which forms the anterior boundary of the lacrimal fossa. **Medial crest of the shaft of the fibula [crista medialis (NA)].** *See* FIBULA, SHAFT. **Nasal crest of the maxilla [crista nasalis (NA)].** A ridge along the medial border of the palatal process articulating with the vomer. **Nasal crest of the palatine bone [crista nasalis (NA)].** A ridge along the medial border of the horizontal plate, articulating with the vomer. **Crest of the neck of a rib [crista colli costae (NA)].** The sharp upper border of a rib. **Neural crest.** The ridge of cells which proliferate from the lateral margin of the medullary plate in the early embryo; they form the nerve cells of sensory and autonomic ganglia as well as a number of other tissues. **Obturator crest [crista obturatoria (NA)].** The anterior border of the pectineal surface of the superior ramus of the pubis. **Occipital crest, external [crista occipitalis externa (var. protuberantia occipitalis externa) NA].** A ridge on the occipital bone to which the ligamentum nuchae is attached. **Occipital crest, internal [protuberantia occipitalis interna (var. crista occipitalis interna) (NA)].** A ridge on the occipital bone to which the falx cerebelli is attached. **Palatine crest [crista palatina (NA)].** A transverse bony ridge close to the posterior border of the hard palate. **Pubic crest [crista pubica (NA)].** The upper border of the body of the pubic bone. **Crest of the sphenoid [crista sphenoidalis].** An anterior projection from the body of the sphenoid which forms a small part of the septum of the nose. **Crest of the spine of the scapula.** The posterior subcutaneous border of the spine of the scapula. **Supinator crest [crista musculi supinatoris].** A lateral ridge near the upper end of the ulna, to which part of the supinator muscle is attached. **Supramastoid crest, Suprameatal crest.** A horizontal ridge on the squamous part of the temporal bone immediately above the mastoid process. **Temporal crest.** The ridge on the frontal, parietal and temporal bones. **Transverse crest [crista transversa].** A bony ridge at the bottom of the internal auditory meatus separating the facial and auditory nerves. **Crest of the trapezium [tuberculum ossis trapezii].** A ridge on the trapezium which forms one of the attachments of the flexor retinaculum. **Trochanteric crest [crista intertrochanterica].** A prominent ridge posteriorly at the junction of the neck and shaft of the femur, running from the greater to the lesser trochanter. **Urethral crest [crista urethralis].** In the male, an elevation in the posterior wall of the prostatic urethra on which the ejaculatory ducts open; in the female, a longitudinal fold of mucous membrane in the posterior wall of the urethra. **Vestibular crest [crista vestibuli].** A bony ridge in the vestibule of the inner ear between the utricle and the saccule. [L *crista* ridge.]

See also: KOELLIKER.

cresyl (kres·il). 1. The monovalent radical $(CH_3)C_6H_3OH$-, derived from the cresols, and giving rise to numerous isomeric compounds. 2. Cresol; cresylic acid. 3. Tolyl salicylate, $C_6H_4(OH)COOC_6H_4(CH_3)$, an antiseptic prepared from cresol. **Cresyl cinnamate.** $C_6H_5CH{=}CHCOOC_6H_4(CH_3)$, used in the treatment of tuberculous sores.

cresylate (kres·il·ate). 1. A salt of cresylic acid. 2. A compound formed by one of the isomeric cresols with a base, homologous with a phenate, and having the general formula $C_6H_4(CH_3)OR$.

cresylene (kres·il·een). Toluylene.

creta (kre·tah). Chalk. **Hydrargyrum cum creta.** Grey powder, consisting of 33 per cent of metallic mercury dispersed in chalk. The mercury is so finely divided in this preparation that an enormous surface is presented which results in some solution of the metal when it is taken internally. The very small amount of soluble mercury compounds formed irritate the gastro-intestinal mucosa and purgation takes place. **Creta praeparata.** Prepared Chalk BP 1958, naturally occurring calcium carbonate ground and purified. Given internally it reacts with the gastric acid to produce carbon dioxide and calcium chloride. In the alkaline duodenum, calcium carbonate is re-formed which covers and protects the mucous membrane and inhibits peristalsis. Thus in addition to acting as an antacid it causes some constipation, and is perhaps more frequently used to treat diarrhoea than hyperacidity. **Pulvis cretae aromaticus.** Aromatic powder of chalk, prepared chalk flavoured with powdered cinnamon, nutmeg, clove, cardamom and sugar. This preparation is used to treat diarrhoea, since, in addition to the constipating action of the chalk, the volatile oils contained in the flavouring agents cause relaxation of the intestinal musculature. **Pulvis cretae aromaticus cum opio.** Aromatic powder of chalk to which 2.5 per cent of opium is added. This preparation has an even greater constipating effect because the opium alkaloids check peristalsis more powerfully than chalk alone. **Pulvis cretae compositus.** A mixture of chalk, sugar and gum arabic. [L.]

cretaceous (kre·ta·shus). 1. Chalky. 2. A geological period, about 100 million years ago. [L *creta* chalk.]

cretin (kret·in). An individual affected with cretinism. [Fr.]

cretinism (kret·in·izm). A condition of congenital hypothyroidism, which may be endemic, sporadic or familial, and is often encountered in mountainous regions, particularly the Alpine valleys. Mental and physical development are arrested or retarded. The face is pasty and thick-skinned, the forehead wrinkled, the nose broad and the lips thick; the tongue lolls. The hair, eyebrows and eyelashes are scanty and dry. The term was originally, and is more properly, applied to the condition caused by congenital atrophy or absence of the thyroid gland, but now, with the prefix goitrous, it is applied to the condition of infantile myxoedema in which there is a congenital defect of enzyme action and a consequent failure of the conversion of iodine into thyroxine. [Fr. *crétin.*]

cretinoid (kret·in·oid). 1. Like the state of cretinism. 2. Resembling a cretin. [cretin, Gk *eidos* form.]

cretinous (kret·in·us). Pertaining to cretinism; having the characteristics of a cretin.

Creutzfeld, Hans Gerhard (b. 1885). Kiel neurologist.

Jakob-Creutzfeld disease. Spastic pseudosclerosis; a progressive disease of middle life, with dementia, peripheral muscular wasting, and degeneration of the pyramidal and extrapyramidal systems, giving spasticity and tremor or other involuntary movements.

crevice (krev·is). A cleft or fissure. **Gingival crevice.** The small fissure between the reflected gum and the neck of a tooth; the subgingival space. [ME *crevace.*]

crevicular (krev·**ik**·ew·lar). Relating to a crevice; especially the gingival crevice.

crib (krib). A shaped piece of metal attached to an artificial denture, or to any appliance worn in the mouth which aids retention by surrounding a natural tooth. [AS *cribb.*]

cribral (**krib**·ral). 1. Relating to the cribriform plate of the ethmoid bone. 2. Relating to any sieve-like structure. [L *cribrum* sieve.]

cribrate (**krib**·rate). Profusely pitted with depressions as is a sieve with holes. [see prec.]

cribration (krib·**ra**·shun). 1. The state of being marked with numerous punctures or depressions. 2. The process or act of passing drugs through a sieve in order to separate the coarser from the finer particles. [L *cribrum* sieve.]

cribriform, cribrose (**krib**·re·form, **krib**·roze). Containing many perforations or punctures, like a sieve. **Cribriform plate.** *See* PLATE. [L *cribrum* sieve, form.]

cribrum (**krib**·rum). The cribriform plate of the ethmoid bone. *See* PLATE. [L sieve.]

Cricetus (kri·**se**·tus). A genus of Old World rodents. **Cricetus auratus.** The golden hamster of Syria; a laboratory animal. **Cricetus cricetus.** The common hamster of Europe and Asia; a reservoir of plague in Russia. [Polish, *krecek.*]

Crichton Browne. *See* BROWNE, SIR JAMES CRICHTON.

Crick, Francis H. (b.1916). English molecular biologist. Nobel Prize winner 1962.

Crick's central dogma. The theory that the flow of information in living cells goes from nucleic acid (DNA via RNA) to protein but not vice versa.

Crick's wobble hypothesis. The hypothesis that the third nucleotide base in an anticodon triplet on a tRNA molecule can undergo slight fluctuations in its orientation (i.e. it can wobble) and in this way can form hydrogen bonds with more than one type of base in the corresponding position of a codon triplet on a messenger RNA.

Watson–Crick DNA double helix. The model of DNA structure in which the molecule is represented as consisting of 2 right-handed helical polynucleotide chains coiled around the same axis to form a double helix, the purine and pyrimidine bases of each strand being on the inside of the double helix and paired accordingly to the base-pairing rule such that adenine can only pair with thymine, and cytosine only with guanine.

Watson–Crick pair. The complementary nucleoside bases: adenine and guanine, cytosine and thymine or uracil.

Watson–Crick pairing. The formation of hydrogen bonds between complementary nucleoside base pairs.

crick (krik). Sudden painful muscular spasm affecting a region or set of muscles, e.g. the back of the neck. [onomat.]

crico-arytenoid (kri·ko·ar·e·**te**′·noid). Belonging to or extending between the cricoid and the arytenoid cartilages.

crico-arytenoid muscles. Lateral crico-arytenoid muscle [musculus crico-arytenoideus lateralis (NA)]. A small muscle passing upward and backward from the upper margin of the cricoid arch to the muscular process of the arytenoid cartilage. It closes the glottis by rotating the arytenoids medially. **Posterior crico-arytenoid muscle [musculus crico-arytenoideus posterior (NA)].** A triangular muscle arising from the back of the cricoid lamina and passing upward and laterally to be inserted into the muscular process of the arytenoid cartilage. It opens the glottis by rotating the arytenoids laterally.

cricoderma (kri·ko·**der**·mah). A dermatitis showing a dark central area of linear infiltration surrounded by a lighter similar ring. [Gk *krikos* ring, *derma* skin.]

cricohyoid (kri·ko·**hi**·oid). Relating to the cricoid cartilage and the hyoid bone.

cricoid (**kri**·koid). 1. Shaped like a ring. 2. The cricoid cartilage. *See* CARTILAGE. [Gk *krikos* ring, *eidos* form.]

cricoidectomy (kri·koid·**ek**·to·me). The operation of removing the cricoid cartilage. [cricoid, Gk *ektome* a cutting out.]

cricoidynia (kri·koid·**in**·e·ah). Pain affecting the cricoid cartilage. [cricoid, Gk *odyne* pain.]

cricopharyngeal (kri·ko·far·**in**′·je·al). Relating to the cricoid cartilage and the pharynx.

cricothyreotomy (kri·ko·thi·re·**ot**′·o·me). Surgical division of the cricoid and thyroid cartilages. [cricoid, thyroid, Gk *temnein* to cut.]

cricothyroid (kri·ko·**thi**·roid). Relating to or serving to connect the cricoid and thyroid cartilages. **Cricothyroid joint.** *See* JOINT. **Cricothyroid ligament.** *See* LIGAMENT.

cricothyroid muscle [musculus cricothyroideus (NA)]. The only extrinsic laryngeal muscle diverging from its origin on the anterolateral surface of the cricoid cartilage, to be inserted into the anterior margin of the inferior horn of the thyroid cartilage [pars obliqua (NA)] and the posterior part of the lower border of the lamina of the thyroid [pars recta (NA)]. Its function is to tense and elongate the vocal folds.

cricothyroidotomy (kri·ko·thi·roid·**ot**′·o·me). Cricothyreotomy.

cricothyrotomy (kri·ko·thi·**rot**′·o·me). Cricotomy with the additional cutting through of the cricovocal membrane. [cricoid, thyroid, Gk *temnein* to cut.]

cricotomy (kri·**kot**·o·me). The cutting through of the cricoid cartilage in laryngotomy. [cricoid, Gk *temnein* to cut.]

cricotracheal (kri·ko·trak·**e**′·al). Relating to the cricoid cartilage and the trachea.

cricotracheotomy (kri·ko·trak·e·**ot**′·o·me). Tracheotomy performed by incision through the cricoid cartilage.

cricovocal (kri·ko·**vo**·kal). [cricoid, L *vox* voice.]

Crigler, John Fielding Jnr. (b. 1919). American paediatrician.

Crigler–Najjar kernicterus. A form of kernicterus not associated with iso-immunization. It appears to be due to a congenital lack of enzymes responsible for the conversion of unconjugated bilirubin into its conjugated form.

Crigler–Najjar syndrome. Autosomal recessive hepatic deficiency of glucuronyl transferase activity with unconjugated hyperbilirubinaemic jaundice and kernicterus.

Crile, George Washington (b. 1864). Cleveland, Ohio, surgeon.

Crile's clamp. A light clamp the blades of which can be gradually tightened by a thumb-screw. It is used for trial occlusion of the internal or common carotid artery.

Crile forceps. An American artery forceps.

Crile's head-piece. A harness for applying weights for head traction in fractured spine.

Crile's operation. Block dissection of malignant neck glands.

criminal (**krim**·in·al). Involving crime or of the nature of crime. **Criminal responsibility.** Graded by the law defining the culpability of persons charged with criminal offences, particularly murder. Previously the assessment depended upon McNaghten rules but in current times the doctrine of diminished responsibility developed in the Homicide Act 1957 demanding proof of an abnormality of mind is more usually applied. Everyone is considered sane and responsible until the contrary is proved. [L *crimen* crime.]

criminaloid (**krim**·in·al·oid). In criminology, an individual with inborn criminal tendencies. [criminal, Gk *eidos* form.]

criminology (krim·in·**ol**·o·je). 1. The science and the study of crime as a social phenomenon and of criminals in their relation to society. 2. Crime and criminal studies from the psychological aspect. [L *crimen* crime, Gk *logos* science.]

criminosis (krim·in·**o**·sis). A form of neurosis in which the patient's behaviour shows criminal tendencies.

crina (**krin**·ah). Silkworm-gut; a thread extracted from killed silkworms. It has the same composition as silk but is of much wider gauge, and is used as a surgical suture for the same purposes as catgut.

crinis (**kri**·nis). Hair. **Crinis capitis.** The hair of the head. **Crinis pubis.** The pubic hair. [L.]

crinogenic (kri·no·**jen**·ik). 1. Increasing the function of a gland. 2. Causing secretion. [Gk *krinein* to separate, *genein* to produce.]

crinose (**kri**·noze). Hairy. [L *crinis* a hair.]

crinosin (**kri**·no·sin). A nitrogenized substance derived from brain tissue and crystallizing in filamentary form. [L *crinis* a hair.]

crisis (**kri**·sis). 1. The turning point in a disease, for better or for worse, e.g. a sudden drop in temperature associated with rapid improvement in other symptoms, as in the crisis of pneumonia. 2. A paroxysmal intensification of symptoms, including pain, usually associated with a disturbance of function of an organ that is the site of the pain. **Addisonian crisis, Adrenal crisis.** Acute failure of the adrenal glands, as occurs in Addison's disease, characterized by hypoglycaemia and sodium deficiency in varying proportions. **Anaphylactoid crisis.** Collapse which closely resembles an anaphylactic attack in its clinical features, but which is independent of a true hypersensitivity. It most frequently results from the parenteral administration of a foreign protein or colloid. **Asthmatic crisis.** Status asthmaticus. **Blood crisis.** A sudden appearance of large numbers of nucleated red blood cells (erythroblasts) in the circulating blood, as may occur in acute haemolytic anaemias. **Bronchial crisis.** An attack of dyspnoea due to tabes dorsalis, usually of laryngeal origin due to irritation of a larynx already the seat of an abductor palsy. **Cardiac crisis.** A severe attack of palpitation in a case of tabes dorsalis; it may be associated with other vasomotor phenomena and is then called a *vascular crisis.* **Cerebral crisis.** A sudden disturbance of cerbral activity, either generalized, causing loss of consciousness, or localized, causing, say, hemiplegia. **Cholinergic crisis.** An access of weakness and parasympathetic overactivity induced by overdosage with anticholinesterase drugs in myasthenia gravis. **Clitoris crisis.** An episode of sexual excitement in a tabetic female. **Coeliac crisis.** Sudden drop in weight, acidosis and dehydration or severe anorexia, produced during the course of the coeliac syndrome by dietetic mismanagement or intercurrent infection. It demands immediate control of the infection, eradication of any hidden septic focus, combined with reorganization of the diet to eliminate the acidosis and dehydration and to maintain the caloric and vitamin intake. **Colloidoclastic crisis.** Anaphylactoid crisis (see above). **Deglobulization crisis.** An acute and severe exacerbation of symptoms, anaemia, haemoglobinuria and reticulocytosis in haemolytic anaemias. **Enteralgic crisis.** A sharp attack of pain in the lower abdomen, and diarrhoea, in a case of tabes dorsalis. **Febrile crisis.** A sudden drop of temperature occurring in a fever. **Gastric crisis.** A paroxysm of intense upper abdominal pain, with intractable vomiting and retching, complicating tabes dorsalis. **Haematic crisis.** An acute and severe thrombocythaemia that may occur in certain conditions such as fevers, or after splenectomy. **Haemoclastic crisis, Haemolytic crisis.** Mass red-cell haemolysis. **Hepatic crisis.** A sudden attack of severe pain in the liver region. **Hypertensive crises.** Fits that occur during the course of Bright's disease. **Intestinal crisis.** Enteralgic crisis (see above). **Laryngeal crisis.** Episodic laryngeal spasm in tabes dorsalis, due to abductor palsy. **Mammary crisis.** Spasmodic galactorrhoea in tabes dorsalis. **Myelocytic crisis.** An acute and sudden appearance of immature myeloid leucocytes (usually myelocytes) in the circulating blood. **Nasal crisis.** Paroxysmal sneezing and rhinorrhoea, in tabes dorsalis. **Nefast crisis.** A sudden onset of severe symptoms occurring in experimental spirochaetal jaundice. **Nephralgic crisis, Nephritic crisis.** A painful paroxysm, resembling renal or ureteral colic, occurring in tabes dorsalis. **Nitritoid crisis.** A syncopal attack occurring during or immediately after the intravenous injection of arsphenamine, consisting of flushing of the face and conjunctivae, dyspnoea, cough, precordial pain and a feeling of distress. The pulse is rapid and feeble; the patient may become unconscious. The condition resembles amyl nitrite poisoning. **Ocular crisis.** Sudden intense pain, lacrimation and photophobia in the eyes. **Oculogyral crisis, Oculogyric crisis.** An attack lasting minutes or hours, in which involuntary deviation (usually upwards) and fixation of the eyeballs occurs; a feature of chronic encephalitis lethargica (postencephalitic parkinsonism). **Pharyngeal crisis.** Paroxysmal pharyngeal paraesthesiae with involuntary movements of deglutition, in a case of tabes dorsalis. **Rectal crisis.** Severe rectal pain and attendant constipation in tabes dorsalis. **Renal crisis.** Nephralgic crisis (see above). **Salivary crisis.** Paroxysmal sialorrhoea in tabes dorsalis. **Spastic vasoconstrictor crisis.** Sudden symptoms caused by vasoconstriction of the blood vessels of a limb or other part. **Tabetic crisis.** A paroxysm of pain in tabes dorsalis, with disturbance of function in the organ or organs to which the situation of the pain is automatically related. **Thoracic crisis.** An episode of chest pain like angina pectoris occurring in a tabetic subject, but associated with spasm of thoracic and upper limb musculature. **Thrombocytic crisis.** An acute and marked increase in blood platelets (thrombocythaemia) in the circulating blood; it may occur spontaneously or following splenectomy, or be associated with certain bone-marrow disturbances. **Thyroid crisis, Thyrotoxic crisis.** A sudden exacerbation of symptoms occurring in the course of exophthalmic goitre, characterized by tachycardia, hyperpyrexia, hyperhidrosis and extreme nervous excitability. **Vagal crisis.** *See* ATTACK, VAGAL. **Vascular crisis.** *See* CARDIAC CRISIS (above). **Vesical crisis.** Severe pain in the bladder, with dysuria, in tabes dorsalis. **Visceral crisis.** An attack of pain in any viscus, in tabes dorsalis. [Gk *krisis* turning point.]

See also: DIETL, LUNDVALL, PAL.

crispation (kris·**pa**·shun). 1. Crispatura. 2. An involuntary slight muscular quivering producing a sensation as of creeping of the skin. [L *crispare* to curl.]

crispatura (kris·pat·**ewr**·ah). A wrinkling or puckering. **Crispatura tendinum.** Dupuytren's contracture. [L.]

crista [NA] (**kris**·tah). 1. In anatomy, a crest. 2. (More usually cristae) the lamellae formed by the infolding of the inner mitochondrial membrane. **Crista basilaris [NA].** A periosteal thickening in the outer wall of the duct of the cochlea to which the basilar membrane is attached. **Crista dividens.** The curved free border of the septum secundum in the fetal heart which directs most of the blood from the inferior vena cava into the left atrium. **Crista galli [NA].** *The cock's comb,* a projection from the ethmoid in the midline of the anterior cranial fossa. Its anterior border carries small processes [alae cristae galli (NA)] which articulate with the frontal bone. **Crista quarta.** A ridge projecting into the posterior end of the lateral semicircular canal. **Crista supraventricularis.** A prominent muscular ridge which extends downwards and to the right from the posterior wall of the infundibulum of the right ventricle, separating the tricuspid from the pulmonary valve orifice, and which marks the lower limit of the bulbar part of the right ventricle. **Crista terminalis [NA].** A muscular ridge in the wall of the right atrium separating the atrium proper from the sinus venarum. [L ridge.]

cristal (**kris**·tal). Relating to a ridge or crest. [L *crista* ridge.]

cristate (**kris**·tate). Of bones or bony structures, ridged; of other organic structures, having a crest. [see prec.]

Critchett, George (b. 1817). London ophthalmologist.

Critchett's operation. 1. For squint: (*a*) advancement of muscle using Prince's forceps and suturing the muscle to the sclera just behind the limbus with silk sutures; (*b*) subconjunctival tenotomy. 2. Amputation of the anterior segment of the eye, used in cases of anterior staphyloma, leaving a movable bulb to which an artificial eye could be fitted. Historical.

criterion (kri·**teer**·e·on). *See* COOKE. [Gk *krites* judge.]

critical (**krit**·ikl). 1. Dangerous. 2. Belonging to or indicating a crisis. [Gk *krisis* turning point.]

crocidismus (kro·sid·**iz**·mus). Caphology. [Gk *krokydizein* to pick at.]

crocin (**kro**·sin). An impure colouring matter obtained from saffron (*Crocus sativus* Linn.).

croesomania (kre·so·**ma**·ne·ah). A hallucination of being in possession of great wealth. [*Croesus,* wealthy king of Lydia, mania.]

Crohn, Burrill Bernard (b. 1884). New York physician.

Crohn's disease. An inflammatory lesion of the intestines of unknown cause. Originally described in the ileum (regional ileitis) but now known to affect many other parts of the alimentary tract, especially the colon. Diseased areas are often separated by normal bowel.

Crooke, Arthur Carleton. Birmingham endocrinologist and pathologist.

Crooke's hyaline cells. Degenerated hyaline basophilic cells of the anterior pituitary gland (see below).

Crooke's changes. Hyaline degeneration of the basophilic cells of the anterior lobe of the pituitary gland, often accompanied by ballooning of their nuclei, swelling of the cells and loss of basophilic granules, associated with the clinical syndrome of Cushing's syndrome due to excess of cortisol.

Crookes, Sir William (b. 1832). English chemist and physicist.

Crooke's glass. A glass made in varying tints, which absorbs mainly the ultra-violet rays; used to avoid glare.

Crooke's lens. A spectacle lens tinted to absorb mostly the ultra-violet rays and prevent glare.

Crooke's radiometer. A special form of radiometer consisting of vanes, mounted on a central spindle in an exhausted tube, which rotate when a beam of light falls upon them.

Crooke's dark space. A dark space in a discharge tube, when the discharge is passing, between the cathode glow and the negative glow.

Crooke's tube. An evacuated glass vessel containing a gas at low pressure through which an electric discharge is passed.

Cropropamide (kro·**pro**·pam·ide). BP Commission approved name for *N,N*-dimethyl-2-(*N*-propylcrotonamido)butyramide; a respiratory stimulant.

Crosfill, J. W. L. Naval surgeon.

Crosfill's syndrome. Inherited dolichocolon and pseudodextrocardia with an allergic tendency.

Cross and Bevan reagent. A 33 per cent solution of zinc chloride in concentrated hydrochloric acid; it is a solvent for cellulose.

cross (kros). 1. Any structure that has the shape of a cross. 2. A crossbreed. **Occipital cross.** The cruciate arrangement of the dural venous sinuses at the internal occipital protuberance. **Silver cross.** Ranvier's cross; a cruciate figure seen at the nodes of Ranvier of a nerve fibre after silver impregnation. [L *crux* cross.]

See also: RANVIER.

cross-fire (**kros**·fire). A radiotherapy technique using multiple beams of radiation so directed that, entering the body through different regions, they cross in the depth at a place where it is intended to concentrate the amount of energy to be absorbed. A method of delivering a localized high dose of radiation beneath the body surface. [L *crux*, AS *fyr*.]

cross-foot (**kros**·fut). Talipes varus. [L *crux*, AS *fot*.]

cross-matching (**kros**·mach·ing). Direct matching of donor with recipient blood to prevent incompatible transfusion. *See* MATCHING.

cross-over (**kros**·o·ver). *See* CROSSING-OVER.

crossing-over (kros·ing·o·ver). The process of exchange between homologous chromatids taking place during prophase of the first meiotic division and resulting in the production of new combinations of linked genes. **Mitotic or somatic crossing-over.** Crossing-over taking place during mitosis in either somatic or germinal tissue. [L *crux*, AS *ofer*.]

cross-section (kros·**sek**·shun). Of a given nucleus or atom for a given radiation, that area perpendicular to the direction of the radiation which one has to attribute to the nucleus or atom to account geometrically for its interaction with the radiation. The *activation cross-section* usually refers to the formation of a particular radionuclide and, in computing it, one used either the total number of nuclei of the element being irradiated or that of the isotope that forms the nuclide in question. **Capture cross-section.** The cross-section for an interaction involving the capture of a particle by an atom or nucleus. **Differential cross-section.** The cross-section may be subdivided to express the probability of occurrence of the interaction when the paths of the product particles are required to lie within small angular ranges about specified directions. The ratio of the infinitesimal portion of the cross-section to the associated infinitesimal range of solid angle within which the path of one of the particles falls is called the *differential cross-section.* **Nuclear cross-section.** The cross-section for a specifically nuclear interaction. [L *crux*, *secare* to cut.]

cross-talk (**kros**·tawk). That part of a signal intended for one detector which is received in another, and vice versa. In nuclear medicine the term is used particularly when similar radiation detectors are sited over paired organs undergoing a dynamic study using a radioactive material *in vivo.* The cross-talk is the radiation received by the left detector from the right organ and by the right detector from the left organ of the pair. [L *crux* cross, ME *talken* talk.]

crossway (**kros**·wa). **Sensory crossway.** The posterior limb of the internal capsule of the brain. [L *crux*, AS *weg*.]

See also: CHARCOT.

crotalic (kro·**tal**·ik). Pertaining to the genus of snakes, *Crotalus.*

Crotalinae (kro·**tal**·in·e). A sub-family of the Viperidae, poisonous snakes of the New World including pit vipers and rattlesnakes. [Gk *krotalon* rattle.]

Crotalus (**krot**·al·us). A genus of New World crotaline snakes which contains the most important rattlesnakes. All species are highly poisonous. **Crotalus adamanteus.** The Florida diamondback of South-eastern USA. **Crotalus atrox.** The Texas rattlesnake; the Western diamondback. **Crotalus horridus.** The commonest rattlesnake in Eastern USA. **Crotalus oreganus.** The rattlesnake of the Pacific coast of USA. **Crotalus terrificus.** A large species, of tropical South America. **Crotalus viridis.** The prairie rattler of central USA. [Gk *krotalon* rattle.]

Crotamiton BP 1973 (kro·**tam**·it·on). Crotonyl-*N*-ethyl-*o*-toluidide. Used in the treatment of scabies and for the symptomatic relief of pruritus.

crotaphion (kro·**taf**·e·on). In craniometry, a point at the tip of the greater wing of the sphenoid bone. [Gk *krotaphos* temple (of head).]

crotchet (**krot**·shet). A hooked instrument used in extraction of the fetus after craniotomy. [Fr. *crochet* little hook.]

Crotethamide (cro·**teth**·am·ide). BP Commission approved name for 2-(*N*-ethylcrotonamido)-*N,N*-dimethylbutyramide; a respiratory stimulant.

crotin (**kro**·tin). A toxic substance in croton seeds.

Croton (**kro**·ton). A genus of plants of the family Euphorbiaceae. **Croton chloral hydrate.** Butylchloral hydrate. **Croton oil.** A fixed oil expressed from the seeds of *Croton tiglium* Linn. It is a violent cathartic even in minute doses: applied externally it is a vesicant and counter-irritant. [Gk *kroton* tick.]

crotonism (**kro**·ton·izm). A condition of gastro-enteritis with haemorrhage resulting from poisoning with croton oil.

crotonol (**kro**·ton·ol). Crotonolic acid, $C_8H_{13}COOH$. A vesicant cathartic found in croton oil.

crotoxin (kro·**tox**·in). A protein of the venom of the rattlesnake, e.g. *Crotalus terrificus.* [*Crotalus*, Gk *toxikon* poison.]

crounotherapy (kroo·no·**ther**·ap·e). Crenotherapy; the treatment of disease by mineral waters obtained from natural springs. [Gk *krounos* spring, *therapeia* treatment.]

croup (kroop). Any condition caused by respiratory obstruction, particularly acute inflammatory affections of the larynx and trachea in children, or reflex disturbances such as laryngismus stridulus and spasm of the glottis. The condition is characterized by a hoarse ringing cough and difficult breathing, and there may be local membranous deposit, frequently due to infection by viruses. **Artificial croup.** Traumatic membranous laryngitis. **Bronchial croup.** Croupous bronchitis. **Catarrhal croup.** An acute laryngitis with the characteristic croupy cough. **Diphtheritic croup.** Laryngeal diphtheria. *See diphtheria.* **False croup.** Laryngismus stridulus. **Fibrinous croup.** Membranous croup (see below). **Infectious croup.** An upper respiratory infection in which after a variable period hoarseness and stridor develop. One type is possibly due to a virus infection, a second to *Haemophilus influenzae* and a third to *Corynebacterium diphtheriae.* **Intestinal croup.** Colitis. **Membranous croup,**

Pseudomembranous croup. Acute laryngitis with formation of membrane and a croupy cough. **Spasmodic croup.** Laryngismus stridulus. **True croup.** Membranous croup (see above). **Uterine croup.** Exudative inflammation of the mucous membrane lining the uterus. [Scot. to croak.]

croupine (kroop·een). Laryngismus stridulus. [see prec.]

croupous (kroop·us). 1. Relating to croup. 2. Like croup.

croupy (kroop·e). 1. Like croup. 2. Affected with croup.

Crouzon, Octave (b. 1874). Paris neurologist.

Crouzon's disease. Ocular hypertelorism; hereditary craniofacial dysostosis; a familial disease with malformation of the skull, exophthalmos, optic atrophy, and divergent squint.

Crowe, Henry Warren (b. 1879). London physician.

Crowe's vaccine. A mixed vaccine for use in rheumatism.

Crowe, Samuel James (b. 1883). Baltimore physician.

Crowe's sign. Engorgement of the retinal veins on compression of the opposite jugular vein in cases of cavernous sinus thrombosis.

crown (krown). 1. [Corona (NA)] Any ring-like structure with a crenated edge, resembling a regal crown. 2. [Vertex (NA)] Of the head, the highest part of the cranium. 3. A restoration used in conservative dentistry which is fixed on the root of a tooth to replace a natural crown which has been lost by caries or fracture or which is unsightly; an artificial crown. **Anatomical crown.** That part of the tooth which is covered by enamel. **Ciliary crown [corona ciliaris (NA)].** The anterior part of the ciliary body, as opposed to the posterior, or ciliary ring. **Clinical crown [corona clinica (NA)].** The portion of a tooth which projects into the mouth cavity. It does not necessarily coincide with the anatomical crown. **Collar crown.** An artificial crown which encircles the neck of the root of a natural tooth. **Dowel crown.** A type of artificial porcelain crown used in dentistry, which has a channel running part of the way from the base to the biting edge to provide for its attachment. **Jacket crown.** An artificial crown which fits over the natural crown of a tooth from which the enamel has been removed, and which reproduces the natural appearance of the tooth. **Post crown.** An artificial crown which is fixed to the root of a tooth by means of a post which extends into the root canal. **Radiating crown.** Bischoff's crown; the corona radiata of the granulosa cells around the ovum. **Three-quarter crown.** A crown in which only the inner aspect of the natural crown of a tooth is artificially replaced; Carmichael crown. **Crown of a tooth [corona dentis].** *See* TOOTH. [L *corona.*]

See also: BISCHOFF, CARMICHAEL.

crowning (krown·ing). The stage in childbirth when the scalp of the fetus becomes visible, and with successive uterine pains distends the vulva more and more. [see prec.]

crownwork (krown·werk). In dentistry, the science and practice of making an artificial crown to replace part of a tooth when it is missing; also applied to the artificial crown itself. [crown, AS *weorc.*]

Cruchet, Jean René (b. 1875). Bordeaux surgeon.

Cruchet's disease. Epidemic encephalitis lethargica; also called *von Economo's disease.*

crucial (kroo·shal). 1. Shaped like a cross, e.g. an incision. 2. Decisive. 3. Very critical or severe. [L *crux* cross.]

cruciate (kroo·shate). 1. Shaped like a cross, e.g. certain ligaments. 2. Crossed. [see prec.]

crucible (kroo·sibl). A conical vessel used in chemistry, with a rounded or truncated base and made of a refractory substance. It is used for the melting or calcining of materials such as metals which require to be exposed to strong heat. [LL *crucibulum* hanging lamp.]

See also: GOOCH (F. A.).

cruciform (kro·se·form). Cross-shaped. [L *crux* cross, form.]

crude (krood). 1. Undigested. 2. Unrefined or raw, as chemicals or drugs. [L *crudus* raw.]

cruels (kroo·elz). Scrofula. [Fr. *écrouelles.*]

Cruise, Sir Richard Robert (b. 1877?). London ophthalmologist.

Cruise's operation. For chronic glaucoma: a corneoscleral wedge-shaped trap-door is made, hinged at the limbus under a conjunctival flap; no iridectomy. Regular massage is necessary until a filtering cicatrix is formed.

cruor (kroo·or). Coagulated blood containing erythrocytes. [L blood.]

crura (kroo·rah). *See* CRUS.

cruraeus (kroo·re·us). The vastus intermedius muscle, arising from the femur and inserted through the common tendon of the quadriceps into the patella. [L *crus* leg.]

crural (kroo·ral). 1. Relating or belonging to any of the crura, especially the crura cerebri. 2. Relating or belonging to the thigh or leg. [L *crus* leg.]

cruritis (kroo·ri·tis). Phlegmasia alba dolens. [L *crus* leg, Gk *-itis* inflammation.]

crurogenital (kroo·ro·jen·it·al). Relating to the thigh and the genital organs. [L *crus* leg, genitalia.]

crus [NA] (kroos) (pl. *crura*). A leg; in anatomy, an elongated process or part of a structure more or less comparable to a leg. **Ampullary crura [crura ossea ampullaria (NA)].** The parts of the semicircular canals immediately adjacent to the utricle. **Crura of the antihelix [crura anthelicis (NA)].** The 2 ridges into which the antihelix divides superiorly; they enclose the triangular fossa. **Crus of the atrioventricular bundle [crus (dextrum et sinistrum) (NA)].** The main bundle of Purkinje fibres which leaves the atrioventricular node and passes through the trigonum fibrosum dextrum to divide at the upper edge of the muscular part of the interventricular septum into left and right branches. **Crus cerebelli.** A peduncle of the cerebellum. **Crus of the cerebrum [crus cerebri (NA)].** The ventral part of the cerebral peduncles; the large band of white fibres running on either side of the midline on the ventral surface of the mid-brain from the pons to the cerebral hemisphere. **Crus of the clitoris [crus clitoridis (NA)].** The part of the corpus cavernosum of the clitoris attached to the ischiopubic ramus. **Crus commune [crus osseum commune (NA)].** A single channel formed by the union of the posteromedial end of the superior with the upper end of the posterior semicircular canal. **Crura of the diaphragm, right and left [crus dextrum, crus sinistrum (NA)].** Musculotendinous origins of the diaphragm, the right crus from the sides of the bodies of the first 3 lumbar vertebrae, passing upwards and to the left in front of the left crus and splitting to enclose the oesophageal opening, the left crus arising from the upper 2 lumbar vertebrae. **Crus helicis [NA].** The anterior end of the helix of the external ear. **Inferior crus.** *See* CRUS OF THE INGUINAL RING. **Crus of the inguinal ring.** Two, superior and inferior [crus mediale, crus laterale (NA)], forming the corresponding margins of the superficial inguinal ring. **Crura of the internal capsule, anterior and posterior [crus anterius capsulae internae, crus posterius capsulae internae (NA)].** The anterior and posterior limbs of the internal capsule. **Crura membranacea [NA].** The limbs of a semicircular canal which attach it to the utricle. **Crus membranaceum ampullare [NA].** The limb of a semicircular canal bearing the ampulla. **Crus membranaceum commune [NA].** The common stem of the superior and posterior semicircular ducts. **Crus membranaceum simplex [NA].** The limb of a lateral semicircular canal not bearing the ampulla. **Crus olfactorium.** The olfactory peduncle. *See* PEDUNCLE. **Crus of the penis [crus penis (NA)].** The part of the corpus cavernosum of the penis which is attached to the ischiopubic ramus. **Crus osseum simplex [NA].** The crus of a semicircular canal that joins the utricle independently. **Superior crus.** *See* CRUS OF THE INGUINAL RING (above). [L a leg.]

crush (krush). To squeeze or press violently. **Phrenic crush.** Phreniclasia. **Crush syndrome.** *See* SYNDROME. [OFr. *cruisir.*]

crust (krust). 1. Any outer covering or layer. 2. A hardening mass of dried secretions, pus, or blood occurring superficially on the body. **Buffy crust.** Crusta phlogistica. **Bullock's-liver crust.** The red-brown scab which forms on a scorbutic ulcer. **Limpet-shell crust.** The blackish scab which forms over the lesions in syphilitic rupia. [see foll.]

crusta (krus·tah). 1. A crust. 2. The basis pedunculi of the cerebral peduncles of the mid-brain. **Crusta adamantina dentium.**

The enamel of the teeth. **Crusta inflammatoria.** *See* COAT, BUFFY. **Crusta lamellosa.** Psoriasis. **Crusta osteoides, Crusta petrosa.** The cement covering the root of teeth. **Crusta phlogistica.** *See* COAT, BUFFY. **Crusta radicis.** Crusta osteoides (see above). [L.]

Crustacea (krus·ta·she·ah). A class of Arthropoda characterized by their complex biramous appendages and absence of true head. They are (except for woodlice) aquatic and the following genera are of importance as intermediate hosts of parasitic worms: *Astacus, Cambarus, Cyclops, Eriocheir, Potamon.* [L *crusta* crust.]

crustal (krus·tal). Relating to a crust or crusta.

crutch (kruch). A long stick or staff fitted with a padded concave cross-piece into which the armpit fits so that the weight of the body rests on the staff. **Axillary crutch.** The usual form of crutch with which the weight is taken in the axilla. **Elbow crutch.** A form of crutch that obviates the pressure exerted by the ordinary crutch in the axilla. It does not provide the same degree of support as an axillary crutch (see above). It usually consists of a single shaft from which the grip projects at a right angle at a suitable height; at the upper end there is a padded U shaped projection which fits around the arm and adds stability. **Hand crutch.** A form of crutch with a pair of which the patient can support his whole weight on his hands. It usually consists of 2 shafts joined at the bottom, where they fit into a ferrule, and separated at the top by a cylindrical or fusiform grip: there is usually a cross-bar in the middle to add stability. **Perineal crutch.** A device used to support the leg of a patient in the lithotomy position and so made that the angle of the height at which the limb is held can be altered as is necessary. [AS *cryce.*]

Crutchfield, W. Gayle (b. 1900). Richmond, Virginia, surgeon.

Crutchfield tongs. An appliance inserted into the skull for applying skeletal traction to the cervical spine.

Cruveilhier, Jean (b. 1791). Paris pathologist and anatomist.

Cruveilhier's atrophy, or disease. Progressive muscular atrophy. *See* ATROPHY.

Cruveilhier's fascia. The superficial fascia of the perineum. *See* FASCIA OF THE ABDOMINAL WALL, SUPERFICIAL.

Cruveilhier's joint. The median atlanto-axial joint. *See* JOINT, ATLANTO-AXIAL.

Cruveilhier's nerve and plexus. 1. The branch from the inferior cervical ganglion to the plexus surrounding the vertebral artery, together with that plexus. 2. A plexus formed by small branches of the posterior primary rami of the first 3 cervical nerves.

Cruveilhier's paralysis. The progressive muscular atrophy type of motor neuron disease. Also called *Aran–Duchenne disease.*

Cruveilhier's plexus. Plexiform aneurysm; an angioma or a congenital abnormality composed of varicose vessels.

Cruveilhier's sign. If a swelling in the groin is felt whilst the patient coughs, a tremor as though a jet of water was entering the swelling occurs with a varicose saphenous vein.

Cruveilhier's valve. The lacrimal fold. *See* FOLD.

Cruveilhier-Baumgarten cirrhosis, or syndrome. Thrombosis of the portal vein, often within its hepatic course, with cirrhosis of the liver, portal hypertension, and splenomegaly; it occurs in young children.

crux (krux) (pl. *cruces*). A cross. **Hair cruces [cruces pilorum (NA)].** Hair distributed in the form of a cross. **Crux of the heart.** On the external surface of the heart, that point at which the atrioventricular groove crosses the interventricular groove, or the corresponding structural portion of the heart. [L cross.]

Cruz, Osvaldo Gonçalves (b. 1872). Rio de Janeiro bacteriologist.

Cruz trypanosomiasis. Chagas' disease caused by *Trypanosoma cruzi.*

cry (kri). 1. The sudden vehement utterance of a loud inarticulate vocal sound. 2. To utter such a sound. 3. To weep. **Arthritic cry, Articular cry.** Night cry (see below). **Cerebral cry.** A sudden shrill cry, often repeated, by young infants with cerebral irritation. **Epileptic cry.** The loud outcry often made by an epileptic as he falls to the ground at the beginning of an attack. **Hydro-encephalic cry, Hydrocephalic cry.** The involuntary loud cry uttered at night by a child with tuberculous meningitis or acute acquired hydrocephalus. **Joint cry, Night cry.** A loud scream uttered by a child during sleep at night. It may be a symptom of the beginning of some form of tuberculous arthritis or other disease of the joints. **Starting cry.** A spontaneous cry made at night by children suffering from tuberculosis of the hip joint. *See also:* REFLEX, CRY. [OFr. *crier.*]

See also: DOUGLAS (J.).

cryaesthesia (kri·es·**the**·ze·ah). The state of being extremely sensitive to cold. [Gk *kryos* cold, aesthesia.]

cryalgesia (kri·al·**je**·ze·ah). Pain caused by application of cold. [Gk *kryos* cold, *algos* pain.]

cryanaesthesia (kri·an·es·**the'**·ze·ah). Loss of the perception of cold by the skin. [Gk *kryos* cold, anaesthesia.]

crymo-anaesthesia (kri·mo·an·es·**the'**·ze·ah). Anaesthesia by refrigeration. [Gk *krymos* frost, anaesthesia.]

crymodynia (kri·mo·**din**·e·ah). 1. Cryalgesia. 2. Pain of rheumatic type caused by damp or cold weather. [Gk *krymos* frost, *odyne* pain.]

crymophilia (kri·mo·**fil**·e·ah). Cryophilia. [Gk *krymos* frost, *philein* to love.]

crymophilic (kri·mo·**fil**·ik). Cryophilic. [see prec.]

crymophylactic (kri·mo·fil·**ak'**·tik). Cryophilactic. [Gk *krymos* frost, *phylax* guard.]

crymotherapeutics (kri·mo·ther·ap·**ew'**·tix). Cryotherapeutics. [Gk *krymos* frost, therapeutics.]

crymotherapy (kri·mo·**ther**·ap·e). The use of extreme cold as a local therapeutic measure. [Gk *krymos* frost, therapy.]

cryo-aerotherapy (kri·o·a·er·o·**ther'**·ap·e). The therapeutic use of cold air. [Gk *kryos* cold, aerotherapy.]

cryochem (kri·o·kem). A desiccation procedure in which rapid freezing constitutes a stage. [Gk *kryos* cold, *chymos* juice.]

cryo-extraction (kri·o·ex·**trak'**·shun). Removal of a lens by a probe which produces an adherent ice-ball within its substance. [Gk *kryos* cold, L *ex, trahere* to draw.]

cryo-extractor (kri·o·ex·**trak'**·tor). A probe with the tip cooled to −80°C, employed for the removal of a cataractous lens. [Gk *kryos* cold, L *ex, trahere* to draw.]

cryofibrinogenaemia (kri·o·fi·brin·o·jen·**e'**·me·ah). A blood protein resembling fibrinogen which precipitates from plasma on cooling, causing purpura and necroses. [Gk *kryos* cold, fibrinogen, Gk *haima* blood.]

cryogen (kri·o·jen). A freezing mixture; any substance used to produce very low temperatures, e.g. carbon dioxide snow. [Gk *kryos* cold, *genein* to produce.]

cryogenic (kri·o·**jen**·ik). 1. Producing low temperatures. 2. Referring to the production of low temperatures. [see prec.]

cryoglobulin (kri·o·**glob**·ew·lin). A specific form of serum globulin that separates out on cooling. [Gk *kryos* cold, globulin.]

cryoglobulinaemia (kri·o·**glob**·ew·lin·**e'**·me·ah). The presence of the abnormal globulin, cryoglobulin, in the blood; it is usually found in association with certain rare forms of reticulosis resembling or related to leukaemia and myelomatosis. [cryoglobulin, Gk *haima* blood.]

cryohydrate (kri·o·**hi**·drate). Eutectic mixture; the name applied to what was formerly considered a compound of any soluble salt and ice, which separates out in crystals at the lowest temperature attainable when a solution is cooled below the freezing point of water. [Gk *kryos* cold, hydrate.]

cryolite (kri·o·lite). A naturally-occurring sodium aluminium-fluoride, Na_3AlF_6, used in the manufacture of aluminium.

cryometer (kri·**om**·et·er). A thermometer used in measuring very low temperatures. [Gk *kryos* cold, meter.]

cryopallidectomy (kri·o·pal·id·**ek'**·to·me). Cryosurgical destruction of part of the thalamus in the treatment of Parkinson's disease. [Gk *kryos* cold, L *pallidus* pale, Gk *ektome* a cutting out.]

cryopathy (kri·**op**·ath·e). Any deleterious effect on tissues due to a cold, or disease caused by cold. [Gk *kryos* cold, *pathos* suffering.]

cryophilia (kri·o·**fil**·e·ah). In bacteriology, the state of thriving best at low temperatures. [Gk *kryos* cold, *philein* to love.]

cryophilic (kri·o·**fil**·ik). In bacteriology, describing bacteria which thrive best at low temperatures. [see prec.]

cryophylactic (kri·o·fil·**ak**′·tik). Term applied to bacteria which show resistance to low temperatures and which are not destroyed at freezing point. [Gk *kryos* cold, *phylax* guard.]

cryoscope (**kri**·o·skope). A device used in chemical and physiological research with which the freezing point of a liquid can be determined. [Gk *kryos* cold, *skopein* to watch.]

cryoscopic, cryoscopical (kri·o·**skop**·ik, kri·o·**skop**·ikl). Referring to cryoscopy.

cryoscopy (kri·**os**·ko·pe). The determination of the freezing point of a fluid (in medicine, urine, blood, and so on) as compared with that of distilled water. There is depression of the freezing point as the content of solids increases. [Gk *kryos* cold, *skopein* to watch.]

cryostat (**kri**·o·stat). An apparatus for controlling temperatures at very low levels. [Gk *kryos* icy, *statos* a standing.]

cryosurgery (kri·o·**ser**·jer·e). Surgical procedures in which tissue is destroyed by freezing. [Gk *kryos* cold, surgery.]

cryotherapeutics (kri·o·ther·ap·**ew**′·tix). The science of the use of cold as a therapeutic measure. [see foll.]

cryotherapy (kri·o·**ther**·ap·e). Use of cold or freezing as a therapeutic measure, e.g. carbon dioxide snow for the removal of angiomas, xanthelasmas and warts. [Gk *kryos* cold, therapy.]

cryotolerant (kri·o·**tol**·er·ant). Able to bear abnormally low temperatures. [Gk *kryos* cold, L *tolerare* to bear.]

crypt (kript). A small blind pocket or recess, usually microscopic in size. **Anal crypt.** Anal sinus, one of the small pockets formed by crescentic folds of mucous membrane joining the lower ends of the anal columns. **Dental crypt.** Crypt of a tooth (see below). **Crypt of the iris.** A small irregular pit on the anterior surface of the iris, chiefly near the ciliary and pupillary borders. **Crypt of the tongue.** A small tubular invagination of the stratified epithelium of the surface into the lymphoid tissue of the lingual tonsil. **Crypts of the tonsils [cryptae tonsillares (NA)].** Small tubular invaginations of the stratified epithelium of the surface into the lymphoid tissue of the palatine and nasopharyngeal tonsils. **Crypt of a tooth.** Sometimes applied to the cavity in which a tooth develops before eruption; dental crypt. [Gk *kryptos* hidden.]

See also: LIEBERKÜHN, MORGAGNI.

cryptaesthesia (kript·es·**the**·ze·ah). Extrasensory perception. *See* PERCEPTION. [Gk *kryptos* hidden, aesthesia.]

cryptamnesia, cryptanamnesia (kript·am·**ne**′·ze·ah, **kript**·an·am·**ne**′·ze·ah). Cryptomnesia. [Gk *kryptos* hidden, *amnesia* forgetfulness, *anamnesis* a calling to mind.]

cryptectomy (kript·**ek**·to·me). The operation of obliterating or excising a tonsillar pit or other crypt. [crypt, Gk *ektome* a cutting out.]

cryptic (**kript**·ik). 1. Concealed. 2. Adapted to conceal. 3. Larval. [Gk *kryptos* hidden.]

cryptitis (kript·**i**·is). A state of inflammation of a crypt. **Urethral cryptitis.** Inflammation of the mucous follicles of the external orifice of the female urethra. [crypt, Gk *-itis* inflammation.]

cryptocephalus (kript·o·**kef**·alus). A monster the head of which is imperfectly developed and almost concealed. [Gk *kryptos* hidden, *kephale* head.]

cryptococcosis (**kript**·o·kok·**o**′·sis). An acute, subacute or chronic pulmonary, systemic or meningeal mycosis due to *Cryptococcus neoformans.* The pulmonary form is presumably transitory, mild and unrecognized. Cutaneous, skeletal and visceral lesions may occur during dissemination of the disease, but involvement of the central nervous system with meningitis is the most familiar form of the mycosis. [*Cryptococcus,* Gk *-osis* condition.]

Cryptococcus (kript·o·**kok**·us). A yeast-like fungus reported to have a Basidiomycete state. It is a spherical fungus which reproduces by budding and only rarely produces filamentous forms. *Cryptococcus neoformans* is pathogenic for man and other animals showing a marked preference for the central nervous system, but it may also involve skin, lungs and viscera. **Cryptococcus capsulatus.** The name suggested by Castellani and Chalmers (1919) for *Histoplasma capsulatum,* but not generally accepted.

cryptocrystalline (kript·o·**kris**·tal·een). Microcrystalline. [Gk *kryptos* hidden, *krystallos* rock-crystal.]

cryptocystis (krip·to·**sis**·tis). A larval form in the tapeworms in which the cyst is not enlarged: characteristic of *Dipylidium caninum.* [Gk *kryptos* hidden, *kystis* bladder.]

cryptodidymus (krip·to·**did**·im·us). A double monster of which one fetus is concealed within and is parasitic upon the other. [Gk *kryptos* hidden, *didymos* twin.]

crypto-empyema (**krip**·to·em·pi·e′·mah). An empyema the presence of which cannot be detected by means of puncture. [Gk *kryptos* hidden, empyema.]

cryptogam (**krip**·to·gam). In botany, a general term for plants in which the reproductive parts are not clearly demarcated as flowers, particularly algae, fungi, mosses and ferns. [Gk *kryptos* hidden, *gamos* marriage.]

cryptogenetic, cryptogenic (**krip**·to·jen·**et**′·ik, krip·to·**jen**·ik). 1. Of diseases, of unknown, indeterminate, or obscure origin. 2. Living as a parasite within another living organism and always having done so. [Gk *kryptos* hidden, *genein* to produce.]

cryptoglioma (**krip**·to·gli·**o**′·mah). That stage in development of glioma of the retina at which the growth is concealed because cyclitis has caused the eyeball to shrink. [Gk *kryptos* hidden, glioma.]

cryptoleukaemia (**krip**·to·lew·**ke**′·me·ah). Any hyperplastic condition of the blood in which abnormal cells are not to be found in the blood stream. [Gk *kryptos* hidden, leukaemia.]

cryptolith (**krip**·to·lith). A calculus contained in a crypt. [crypt, Gk *lithos* stone.]

cryptolithiasis (**krip**·to·lith·**i**′·as·is). The calcification of tumours of the skin and underlying tissues. [see prec.]

cryptomenorrhoea (**krip**·to·men·or·**e**′·ah). Retention of the menstrual flow due to congenital or acquired genital-canal stenosis. [Gk *kryptos* hidden, menorrhoea.]

cryptomere (**krip**·to·meer). A sac-like or cystic condition of a part. [Gk *kryptos* hidden, *meros* part.]

cryptomerorrhachischisis (**krip**·to·me·ro·rak·**is**′·kis·is). Spina bifida occulta. [Gk *kryptos* hidden, *meros* part, *rhachis* spine, *schisis* division.]

cryptomnesia (krip·tom·ne·ze·ah). Subconscious memory; memory in which the thing remembered appears to be a new experience and not something experienced before. [Gk *kryptos* hidden, *amnesia* forgetfulness.]

cryptoneurous (krip·to·**newr**·us). Descriptive of an organism that has not any recognizable or defined nervous system. [Gk *kryptos* hidden, *neuron* nerve.]

cryptophthalmia (krip·tof·**thal**·me·ah). Congenital adhesion of the eyelids so that the eyeballs cannot be seen. [Gk *kryptos* hidden, *ophthalmos* eye.]

cryptophthalmos (krip·tof·**thal**·mos). 1. An individual affected with cryptophthalmia. 2. Cryptophthalmia.

cryptopine (**krip**·to·peen). $C_{21}H_{23}O_5N$, an alkaloid found in opium and species of *Dicentra.* It resembles papaverine in its general effects. [Gk *kryptos* hidden, opium.]

cryptoplasmic (krip·to·**plaz**·mik). A term applied to an infection the causative organism of which has been able to conceal itself. [Gk *kryptos* hidden, *plasma* something formed.]

cryptopodia (krip·to·**po**·de·ah). A condition in which the lower part of the leg and the dorsum of the foot are so much swollen that the shape of the entire foot is lost, the sole remaining visible as a kind of pad. [Gk *kryptos* hidden, *pous* foot.]

cryptoporous (krip·**top**·or·us). Having hidden imperceptible pores. [Gk *kryptos* hidden, *poros* passage.]

cryptopsoriasis (**krip**·to·so·**ri**·as·is). Hidden, latent psoriasis. [Gk *kryptos* hidden, *psoriasis* itch.]

cryptopsychism (krip·to·si·kizm). The science of phenomena beyond the domain of ordinary or physiological psychology and having relation to telepathic or clairvoyant processes, for example. [Gk *kryptos* hidden, *psyche* mind.]

cryptopyic (krip·to·**pi**·ik). Referring to or marked by concealed suppuration. [Gk *kryptos* hidden, *pyon* pus.]

cryptoradiometer (**krip**·to·ra·de·**om**′·et·er). An instrument with which the power of penetration of x-rays can be measured. [Gk *kryptos* hidden, radiometer.]

cryptorchid (kript·**or**·kid). An individual in whom the testicles have not descended into the scrotum, but are retained in either the abdomen or the inguinal canal. [Gk *kryptos* hidden, *orchis* testis.]

cryptorchidism (kript·**or**·kid·izm). A failure of development resulting in the testes being retained in the inguinal canal or the abdomen. [Gk *kryptos* hidden, *orchis* testis.]

cryptorchism (kript·**or**·kizm). Cryptorchidism.

cryptorrhoea (krip·to·**re**·ah). Excessive secretion from an endocrine gland. [Gk *kryptos* hidden, *rhoia* flow.]

cryptorrhoeic, cryptorrhoetic (krip·to·**re**·ik, krip·to·**ret**·ik). 1. Referring to the normal internal secretions. 2. Referring to cryptorrhoea. [see prec.]

cryptoscope (**krip**·to·skope). Fluoroscope. [Gk *kryptos* hidden, *skopein* to watch.]

See also: SATVIONI.

cryptoscopy (krip·**tos**·ko·pe). Fluoroscopy. [see prec.]

cryptosterol (krip·to·**steer**·ol). A cholesterol which is found in cryptogams.

cryptotoxic (krip·to·**tox**·ik). Term applied to solutions which in the normal state are non-toxic but in which toxic properties may develop should there be disturbance of the colloidal balance. The term indicates that such a solution has hidden toxic properties. [Gk *kryptos* hidden, *toxikon* poison.]

cryptotrichotillomania (**krip**·to·trik·o·til·o·**ma**′·ne·ah). A psychopathy in which hairs are plucked and eaten. *kryptos* hidden, *thrix* hair, *tillein* to pull, *mania* madness.]

cryptoxanthin (krip·to·**zan**·thin). Kryptoxanthin, $C_{40}H_{55}OH$. A carotenoid (hydroxy-β-carotene) and a precursor of vitamin A in the body. It is found in species of *Physalis.* [Gk *kryptos* hidden, *xanthos* yellow.]

cryptozoite (krip·to·**zo**·ite). A phase of the malarial parasites' development in the human liver which has been demonstrated comparatively recently. It is believed to account for the incubation period and for the well-known relapses of the disease. Both pre-erythrocytic and exo-erythrocytic phases are recognized, although the latter does not occur in the case of *Plasmodium falciparum.* [Gk *kryptos* hidden, *zoon* animal.]

cryptozygous (krip·to·**zi**·gus). Having a narrow face and wide skull so that when the head is looked at from above, the zygomatic arches are not visible. [Gk *kryptos* hidden, *zygoma* cheekbone.]

crystal (**kris**·tal). A solid particle the external form of which shows plane faces intersecting at definite angles to give a characteristic symmetry. Crystal form arises from a systematic lattice arrangement of the atoms or molecules of which the solid is composed. **Cockle-burr crystals.** Brown ammonium-urate crystals occurring in alkaline urine. **Coffin-lid crystal.** A form of triple-phosphate crystal occurring in some urinary deposits. **Dumb-bell crystal.** A form of calcium oxalate crystal occurring in some urinary deposits. **Ear crystals.** Minute hexagonal particles of crystalline calcium carbonate, suspended in the gelatinous substance covering the hair cells of the maculae of the saccule and utricle, and less marked in man than in some lower animals. Small vacuoles have been found in their centre. Occasionally they are seen in small numbers in the cristae acusticae of the ampullae. Also known as *otoliths, ear stones* or *otoconia.* **Envelope crystal.** A form of calcium oxalate crystal occurring in some urinary deposits. **Haemin crystals.** Yellow to chocolate-brown rhomboid microcrystals of haematin chloride formed by the action of hot glacial acetic acid upon dried blood in the presence of sodium chloride and separating upon cooling. The reaction is used to detect blood stains. **Knife-rest crystal.** A form of triple-phosphate crystal occurring in some urinary deposits. **Rock crystal.** A colourless, glassy variety of quartz. **Triple-phosphate crystals.** Crystals that occur normally in alkaline urine. They are composed of the phosphates of calcium, magnesium and the ammonium radical. [Gk *krystallos* rock-crystal.]

See also: CHARCOT, FLORENCE, LEYDEN, TEICHMANN-STAWIARSKI, VIRCHOW.

crystalbumin (kris·**tal**·bew·min). Usually referred to as *γ-crystallin,* a protein extracted from the lens of the eye and representing its total albuminous content. [crystalline lens, albumin.]

crystalfibrin (kris·tal·**fi**·brin). A form of fibrin said to be extracted from the crystalline lens by the action of hydrochloric acid.

crystallin (**kris**·tal·in). The name given to 2 globulins, α- and β-crystallin, occurring in the lens of the eye. They differ in their sulphur content and in certain precipitation reactions. [crystalline lens.]

crystalline (**kris**·tal·een). 1. Transparent and clear like a crystal. 2. Belonging to crystals. 3. Having the characteristics of a crystal.

crystallitis (kris·tal·**i**·tis). Phacitis; an inflamed condition of the lens of the eye. [crystalline lens, Gk *-itis* inflammation.]

crystallization (**kris**·tal·i·**za**′·shun). The formation of crystals either by the concentration of a solution until the solute is deposited in this way, or by the cooling of a liquid or gas into the solid phase. **Alcohol of crystallization.** The molecular combination of alcohol with a compound to form crystals. **Fractional crystallization.** The purification of a compound by successive crystallizations from solution. **Water of crystallization.** The water retained in molecular association by a compound crystallizing from an aqueous solution.

crystallize (**kris**·tal·ize). To convert, or to become converted, to a crystalline form.

crystallography (kris·tal·**og**·raf·e). The study of crystals, and their classification according to geometrical forms. **X-ray crystallography.** A technique for studying the diffraction patterns of crystals and crystal complexes produced by x-rays; the contour maps of electron density determined for the crystal unit cell can then, by extensive computation, be converted into a molecular structure. [crystal, Gk *logos* science.]

crystalloid (**kris**·tal·oid). 1. Having the properties of a crystal. 2. Formerly applied to a substance which dissolved to give a true solution, and crystallized, as against a colloid. The term is now held to denote a solute the particles of which are less than 1 μm in diameter. [crystal, Gk *eidos* form.]

crystalloiditis (**kris**·tal·oid·**i**′·tis). Crystallitis.

crystallomagnetism (**kris**·tal·o·**mag**′·net·izm). The behaviour of crystals in a magnetic field; the tendency of certain crystals such as magnetite and pyrrhotite to orientate themselves with respect to the earth's magnetic field.

crystallometry (kris·tal·**om**·et·re). The measurement of the angles of the faces and edges of crystals; also the measurement of their physical attributes, such as optical properties. [crystal, meter.]

crystallophobia (**kris**·tal·o·**fo**′·be·ah). The condition of being morbidly afraid of glass and objects made of glass. [crystal, phobia.]

crystallose (**kris**·tal·oze). A sweetening agent; sodium saccharate.

crystallurhidrosis (**kris**·tal·ewr·**hid**′·ro·sis). A condition in which the sweat contains urinary salts which on excretion crystallize on the skin. [crystal, urhidrosis.]

crystalluria (kris·tal·**ewr**·e·ah). The condition in which crystals are present in the urine and cause renal irritation, e.g. certain crystals of the sulphonamide group.

crystalluridrosis (**kris**·tal·ewr·id·**ro**′·sis). Crystallurhidrosis.

Csillag's disease. Dermatitis lichenoides chronica atrophicans.

Ctenocephalides (**te**·no·kef·**al**′·id·eez). A genus of fleas of which *Ctenocephalides canis* of the dog and *C. felis* of the cat have a cosmopolitan distribution with their domestic hosts. In temperate countries they are common in summer, and in civilized areas are to be found more often on man, whom they bite freely, than is *Pulex irritans. Ctenocephalides canis* is intermediate host to the tapeworms *Hymenolepis diminuta* and *Dipylidium caninum*, and both species may be secondarily involved in plague transmission. [Gk *kteis* comb, *kephale* head.]

ctenocephalus (te·no·**kef**·al·us). Ctenocephalides.

Ctenodactylus (te·no·**dak**·til·us). A genus of North African rodents, *Ctenodactylus gundi*. *See* GONDI. [Gk *kteis* comb, *daktylos* finger.]

Ctenophthalmus (te·nof·**thal**·mus). Fleas of this genus are vectors of plague. [Gk *kteis* comb, *ophthalmos* eye.]

Ctenus (**te**·nus). A genus of spiders of which *Ctenus nigriventer* of Brazil bites with dangerous and sometimes fatal results. [Gk *kteis* comb.]

ctetology (te·**tol**·o·je). The branch of biology which is concerned with the acquired characters of an organism. [Gk *ktetos* that may be acquired, *logos* science.]

ctetosome (**te**·to·some). An accessory chromosome. [Gk *ktetos* that may be acquired, *soma* body.]

cube root (kewb **root**). Lonchocarpus. [Gk *kybos*, root.]

cubeb (**kew**·beb). Cubebae fructus, tailed pepper; the dried unripe fruits of *Piper cubeba* Linn. (family Piperaceae), used as a stimulating and antiseptic expectorant in the form of lozenges or as a tincture of liquid extract (BPC 1954). It contains 10–18 per cent of oil, mainly terpenes, and about 3 per cent of amorphous resin. **Cubeb camphor.** A camphor-like substance obtained from oil of cubeb. **Oil of cubeb.** A pale greenish-yellow oil with the smell of camphor. **Oleoresin of cubeb.** A substance obtained from cubeb by extraction with ether. [Ar. *kabāba.*]

cubebein, cubebin (kew·beb·**e**·in, kew·**beb**·in). $C_{20}H_{20}O_6$, a crystalline resinous compound derived from the volatile oil of cubeb.

cubebism (kew·**beb**·izm). Poisoning due to cubebs (*Piper cubeba*). Severe gastro-enteritis is a characteristic symptom.

cubital (**kew**·bit·al). Relating to the forearm or the ulna. [L *cubitum* elbow.]

cubital vein, median [vena mediana cubiti (NA)]. The vein connecting the cephalic and basilic veins across the anterior surface of the elbow.

cubitale (kew·**bit**·a·le). The cuneiform bone of the carpus. [L *cubitum* elbow.]

cubitalis (kew·bit·**a**·lis). Any one of the ulnar muscles. [see prec.]

cubitocarpal (**kew**·bit·o·**kar**′·pal). Relating to the radius and the carpus. [cubitus, carpus.]

cubitoradial (**kew**·bit·o·**ra**′·de·al). Relating to the ulna and the radius. [cubitus, radius.]

cubitus (**kew**·bit·us). 1. The forearm. 2. The elbow. **Cubitus valgus.** A deformity of the forearm in which there is a marked angle between the upper and lower arm at the elbow which is seen when the arm is held down by the side of the body. A characteristic feature of Turner's syndrome. **Cubitus varus.** Gunstock deformity. *See* DEFORMITY. [L *cubitum* elbow.]

cuboid (**kew**·boid). 1. The cuboid bone. 2. Cube-like in shape. [Gk *kybos* cube, *eidos* form.]

cuboid bone [os cuboideum (NA)]. An irregular cuboidal bone on the lateral side of the foot, articulating with the anterior surface of the calcaneum and carrying the lateral 2 metatarsal bones.

cuboidal (kew·**boid**·al). Relating or belonging to the cuboid bone.

cuboideonavicular (kew·**boid**·e·o·nav·**ik**′·ew·lar). Cubonavicular.

cuboides (kew·**boid**·eez). The cuboid bone.

cubonavicular (**kew**·bo·nav·**ik**′·ew·lar). Pertaining to the cuboid and navicular bones.

Cucurbita (kew·**ker**·bit·ah). 1. A genus of plants, including the pumpkin. 2. Melon pumpkin seed; the fresh seeds of *Cucurbita maxima* Duchesne (family Cucurbitaceae), used as a taenicide. No substance of physiological activity has, however, been isolated. [L gourd.]

cucurbitula (kew·ker·**bit**·ew·lah). A small cupping glass. **Cucurbitula cruenta.** Wet cup, i.e. a cupping glass applied for the purpose of draining blood after scarification. **Cucurbitula sicca.** Dry cup, i.e. a cupping glass applied without scarification. [L little gourd.]

cucurbocitrin (**kew**·ker·bo·**sit**′·rin). A glucoside found in the seeds of the watermelon, *Cucurbita citrullus*, and used in the treatment of hypertension since it causes dilatation of the capillaries. Also known as *citrin* (not to be confused with citrin, vitamin P).

cudbear (**kud**·bare). Persio. [after *Cuthbert* Gordon.]

cuff (kuf). The inflatable balloon on an endotracheal or endobrachial tube. **Musculotendinous cuff.** The combined insertion of the supraspinatus, infraspinatus and teres minor muscles to the humerus. [etym. dub.]

cuffing (**kuf**·ing). The pathological process by which tiny blood vessels are ringed round by collections of inflammatory cells, as in syphilis. [etym. dub.]

cuirass (kwer·**as**). An unyielding bandage closely fitting over the chest. **Cuirass cancer.** Cancer en cuirass. **Cuirass respirator.** *See* RESPIRATOR. **Tabetic cuirass.** The area of diminished sensibility to touch which sometimes encircles the chest in cases of tabes dorsalis. [Fr. *cuirasse* breastplate.]

culdocentesis (**kul**·do·sen·**te**′·sis). Introduction of a needle into the recto-uterine pouch through the posterior fornix in order to aspirate pus or other intraperitoneal exudates. [cul-de-sac (recto-uterine pouch), Gk *kentesis* a pricking.]

culdoscope (**kul**·do·skope). An instrument with a light attachment which is inserted through the posterior fornix of the vagina enabling inspection of the pelvis to be carried out. [cul-de-sac, Gk *skopein* to view.]

culdoscopy (kul·**dos**·ko·pe). Inspection of the pelvis by means of a culdoscope passed through the posterior fornix of the vagina.

culdotomy (kul·**dot**·o·me). Surgical incision of the pouch of Douglas to allow inspection or palpation of the pelvic viscera. [cul-de-sac (recto-uterine pouch), Gk *temnein* to cut.]

Culex (**kew**·lex). A genus of mosquitoes, many species of which bite man. **Culex alis.** A potential vector of filariasis. **Culex annulirostris.** A potential vector of filariasis. **Culex apicalis.** A potential vector of tularaemia. **Culex coronator.** A vector of St. Louis encephalitis. **Culex erythrothorax.** A potential vector of filariasis. **Culex fatigans** (= *quinquefasciatus* in American literature.) The chief intermediate host of *Wuchereria bancrofti* in tropical and sub-tropical zones; it is also a vector of St. Louis encephalitis and a potential vector of yellow fever. **Culex fuscocephalus.** A potential vector of filariasis. **Culex habilitator.** A potential vector of filariasis. **Culex nigripalpus.** A potential vector of yellow fever. **Culex pipiens.** A vector of St. Louis, equine, autumn and Japanese encephalitis, and a potential vector of filariasis. **Culex quinquefasciatus.** *Culex fatigans* (see above). **Culex stigmatosoma.** A vector of equine encephalitis. **Culex tarsalis.** A species considered a possible vector of encephalitis, both St. Louis and equine; a potential vector of filariasis. **Culex thalassius.** A vector of yellow fever. **Culex tritaeniorrhynchus.** A vector of autumn encephalitis and of Japanese encephalitis. **Culex vagans.** A potential vector of filariasis. **Culex vishnui.** A potential vector of filariasis. **Culex whitmorei.** A potential vector of filariasis. [L *culex* gnat.]

culicicide (kew·**lis**·is·ide). Culicide.

Culicidae (kew·**lis**·id·e). A family of flies of the order Diptera, which contains the true mosquitoes in the sub-family Culicinae. [L *culex* gnat.]

culicidal (kew·lis·**i**·dal). Destructive to mosquitoes or gnats. [see foll.]

culicide (**kew**·lis·ide). Any agent with which mosquitoes or gnats can be destroyed. [L *culex* gnat, *caedere* to kill.]

culicifuge (kew·**lis**·e·fewj). Any preparation applied to the skin for the purpose of keeping mosquitoes and gnats away. [L *culex* gnat, *fugare* to drive away.]

Culicinae (kew·**lis**·in·e). A sub-family of the mosquitoes of which the tribes Anophelini and Culicini are of medical importance. [L *culex* gnat.]

Culicini (kew·**lis**·in·i). A tribe of mosquitoes of which the genera *Aëdes* and *Culex* are of medical importance. [see prec.]

Culicoides (kew·lik·**oid**·eez). A genus of biting midges of the family Ceratopogonidae. The adults are very small greyish flies and the larvae mostly aquatic. Many species cause intense irritation by their bites, and because of their abundance can render large areas of land almost uninhabitable in the summer months. *Culicoides austeni* and *C. grahami* are intermediate hosts of the filaria *Acanthocheilonema* species in tropical Africa and America, whilst *Culicoides furens* is intermediate host of the filaria *Mansonella ozzardi* in the West Indies. *Culicoides trichopis* is another species that transmits *Acanthocheilonema* species. [L *culex* gnat, Gk *eidos* form.]

Culiseta (kew·le·se·tah). A genus of mosquitoes that are vectors of St. Louis encephalitis and of equine encephalitis; the species implicated are *Culiseta incidens* and *C. inornata*. [L *culex* gnat.]

Cullen, Glenn Ernest (b. 1890). American biochemist.

Van Slyke and Cullen method. For urea in blood: blood is treated with urease and the mixture is made alkaline with potassium carbonate, and aerated. The ammonia is absorbed in standard acid and the excess of acid titrated with standard alkali.

Cullen, Thomas Stephen (b. 1868). Baltimore gynaecologist.

Cullen's sign. The bluish discoloration sometimes seen in the region of the umbilicus in cases of intraperitoneal bleeding, especially ruptured ectopic gestation.

culmen (kul·men) (pl. *culmina*). The lobulus culminus. [L ridge.]

culminal (kul·min·al). Relating to the lobulus culminus. [see prec.]

cult (kult). Therapeutic principles, usually of an unorthodox kind and based on theories which are unproved or discredited. [L *cultus* care.]

cultivation (kul·tiv·a·shun). The artificial multiplication of pathogenic bacteria *in vitro* by providing the necessary food in the form of media, together with the appropriate gaseous and heat requirements. The gaseous environment may be aerobic or anaerobic, or a mixture of air or oxygen with carbon dioxide. Growth on solid media generally takes the form of colonies. [LL *cultivare* to cultivate.]

cultural (kul·tcher·al). Relating or belonging to a culture.

culture (kul·tcher). 1. The technique of growing and maintaining cells, tissues and organs under artificial conditions. Such techniques are named according to the physical character of the media employed (e.g. agar, broth, clot, liquid, solid, etc.), or to the type of container used (e.g. flask, plate, slide, etc.), or according to the method of inoculation (e.g. stab, smear, streak, etc.) or by the type of material cultured. 2. A crop of cells produced by one of the preceding methods. They are usually designated by their physical or biological characteristics (e.g. pure, stock, virulent, attenuated, giant) or according to the nutrient medium used (e.g. blood agar, tetrathionate broth). The terms *positive* and *negative culture* are used to denote growth or absence of growth, respectively. 3. An inoculated medium. **Blood (lymphocyte) culture.** The culture of peripheral lymphocytes which are stimulated into division by phytohaemagglutinin or other substances. **Lysogenic culture.** A culture of bacteria which is carrying a bacteriophage active against the cells of heterologous clones, but not against the carrier cells. **Monolayer culture.** *See* MONOLAYER. **Primary culture.** A culture which is started directly from cells, tissues or organs of an individual and has not yet been subcultured. **Stab culture.** A culture made by dipping a needle into the inoculum and then thrusting it into a transparent solid medium (gelatin or agar); the nature of the growth at different depths and of the degree of liquefaction can be judged after incubation. **Suspension culture.** A culture system where cells are grown in suspension in the medium rather than attached to a surface. **Thrust culture.** Stab culture (see above). **Tissue, or organ, culture.** The maintenance or growth *in vitro* of tissues, organ primordia, or the whole or parts of an organ, in conditions which allow differentiation and preservation of structure and/or function. [L *colere* to cultivate.]

culture medium (kul·tcher me·de·um). A preparation used to grow crops of micro-organisms; it may be in either liquid or solid form. Nutrient media may contain the materials necessary for the growth of a specific micro-organism, either natural (e.g. peptone, meat infusion) or synthetic. *Selective media* are designed to favour the growth of one genus of micro-organism and inhibit or discourage the growth of others, and are exemplified by the tellurite media for diphtheria bacilli, and the desoxycholate-citrate media for *Salmonella* or *Shigella*. *Enrichment media*, as liquids allow the desired organism to grow faster than its competitors, e.g. the selenite and tetrathionate broth media used to isolate intestinal pathogenic bacteria. The term also refers to the nutrient medium used to maintain animal cells in culture. *See also:* AGAR, BOUILLON, BROTH, MILK, SLOPE. **Aesculin culture medium.** A blood-agar crystal-violet plate containing aesculin, used in the diagnosis of bovine mastitis. **Agar culture medium.** A solution of agar in a basal medium, forming a gel which, with 0.1 per cent agar is sloppy, with 1-2 per cent agar, soft, and with 2.5-5 per cent agar, firm. The best agars dissolve at 90-100°C, and only solidify on cooling below 45°C. **Ascitic-fluid culture medium.** A peptone medium to which ascitic fluid has been added; it is used for the culture of *Neisseria*. **Bile-salt culture medium.** Nutrient broth containing bile salts, for the isolation of members of the family *Enterobacteriaceae*. **Bismuth culture medium.** Wilson and Blair bismuth sulphite agar; a complex selective and differential medium for the isolation of typhoid or paratyphoid organisms from sewage or faeces. **Brilliant-green-eosin culture medium.** An inhibitory selective medium used to isolate *Salmonellae* from faeces. **Citrate culture medium.** Koser's medium; a synthetic medium which contains citrate as the sole source of carbon. It is used in the examination of water to differentiate soil coliforms which can grow in it from faecal coliforms which cannot. **Coagulated-blood-serum culture medium.** Koch's coagulated blood serum; serum coagulated at 75°C and intermittently sterilized. **Cooked-meat culture medium.** A medium prepared from 500 g minced fresh meat cooked in 500 ml N/20 sodium hydroxide. The meat is added to tubes of 1 per cent peptone infusion broth in proportion of 3 parts of broth to 1 of cooked meat. **Gelatin culture medium.** A variety of media used to test for the proteolytic powers of organisms. There are numerous such media in which gelatin is incorporated; these are variously named, either according to the other, or another, ingredient, e.g. agar, dextrose, fish, lactose, litmus, meat extract, potato, etc., as agar gelatin culture medium, etc., or with the name of the first introducer. **Litmus-milk culture medium.** A medium used in the identification of *Clostridium* and other organisms. **N.N.N. culture medium.** Novy-Nicolle-McNeal culture medium, a medium for the cultivation of *Leishmania*. It is essentially a normal-saline agar (2 per cent) medium to which freshly drawn rabbit's blood is added while it is still warm; the percentage of blood and the addition of other ingredients are varied by different workers. **PABA culture medium.** A medium containing *p*-aminobenzoic acid. **Penicillinase culture medium.** A medium containing penicillinase, to hydrolyse any penicillin contained in the inoculum. **Peptone-water culture medium.** A liquid medium containing 1 per cent peptone and 0.5 per cent sodium chloride. **Selenite culture medium.** Sodium selenite and peptone in a phosphate buffer. It is an enrichment medium used for the isolation of *Salmonellae*. There are three formulae: F. for faeces, M. for milk and S. for sewage. *Selenite F. culture medium* is a medium prepared from sodium acid selenite 4 g, peptone 5 g, lactose 4 g, disodium hydrogen phosphate 9.5 g, sodium dihydrogen phosphate 0.5 g, and distilled water to 1 litre. The *M.* and *S.* media slightly vary from this in composition. **Serum-dextrose culture medium.** 1 per cent dextrose dissolved in a mixture of 1 part serum and 3 parts distilled water. Phenol red is usually added as an indicator. **Serum-water culture medium.** 1 part of serum mixed with 3 parts of distilled water. **Tellurite culture medium.** A medium containing potassium tellurite for the isolation of the diphtheria bacillus. **Tetrathionate culture medium.** An enrichment selective medium for the isolation of *Salmonellae* and *Shigellae* from faeces. **Thioglycollate culture medium.** Brewer's medium; a medium prepared from nutrient broth to which is added pork-infusion solids 1 per cent, peptone 1 per cent, sodium chloride 0.5 per cent, sodium thioglycollate 0.1 per cent, agar 0.05 per cent, dextrose 1 per cent and methylene blue 0.0002 per cent. **Tissue culture medium.** A solution of physiological salts, vitamins and serum used to grow and maintain cells in culture. **Trypsin-digest-agar culture medium.** A solid medium prepared by adding agar to tryptic digest broth. [L *colere* to cultivate, medium.]

See also: ABE, ANDERSON, ARONSON, BASS, BOECK (W. C.), BORDET, BREWER (J. H.), BROWNING, CHRISTENSEN, CZAPEK-DOX, DORSET, DUBOS, FILDES, FLETCHER, GASPERINI, GENGOU, HOYLE, KIRSCHNER, KORTHOF, KOSER, LEIFSON, LOEWENSTEIN, MCLEOD, MCNEAL, NICOLLE, NOGUCHI, NOVY, PETRAGNANI, PETROFF, ROBERTSON, SABOURAUD, SCHUEFFNER, SENEKJIE, SMITH (E. F.).

Culver's physic, Culver's root. Leptandra.

cum. The Latin for with. In the forms *co-*, *col-*, *com-*, *con-*, *cor-*, a prefix meaning *together with.*

cumarin (kew·mar·in). Coumarin.

Cumbo's sign. In a radiograph, a crescentic translucent area enclosed between 2 opaque convexities, due to air intrusion outside a hydatid cyst of the lung.

cumenyl (kew·men·il). Cumyl. The monovalent radical $(CH_3)_2CH$ C_6H_4–, occurring in derivatives of cumene.

cumenylamine (kew·men·il·am·een). Cumidine.

Cumetharol (kew·meth·ar·ol). BP Commission approved name for 4,4′-dihydroxy-3,3-(2-methoxyethylidene)dicoumarin; an anticoagulant.

cumidine (kew·mid·een). Aminocumene, cumenylamine, $(CH_3)_2CHC_6H_4NH_2$. A colourless liquid prepared from the volatile oils of cumin and caraway.

cumin (kew·min). Cuminum, 2nd def.

Cuminum (kew·mi·num). 1. A genus of plants of the family Umbelliferae. 2. The ripe fruit of *Cuminum cyminum* Linn. It contains an aromatic volatile oil and is used as a carminative, mainly in spices and in veterinary preparations. [Ar. *kammun.*]

cumulative (kew·mew·lat·iv). 1. Increasing by successive additions. 2. Adding to. [L *cumulare* to heap up.]

cumulus (kew·mew·lus). A collection or heap. **Ovarian cumulus, Cumulus ovaricus [cumulus oöphorus (NA)].** In the vesicular ovarian (graafian) follicles of the human ovary, the inner of the two strata into which the investing follicular cells are split by the liquor folliculi. [L heap.]

cumyl (kew·mil). Cumenyl.

cundurango (kun·dew·rang·go). Condurango.

cuneate, cuneiform (kew·ne·ate, kew·ne·e·form). Wedge-shaped. **Cuneate tubercle.** *See* TUBERCLE. **Cuneiform tubercle.** *See* TUBERCLE. [cuneus, form.]

cuneiform bones. Three wedge-shaped tarsal bones. **Intermediate cuneiform bone [os cuneiforme intermedium (NA)].** The smallest of the 3 wedge-shaped tarsal bones, lying between the navicular and the metatarsal of the second toe. **Lateral cuneiform bone [os cuneiforme laterale (NA)].** A wedge-shaped tarsal bone situated between the navicular and the metatarsal of the third toe. **Medial cuneiform bone [os cuneiforme mediale (NA)].** The largest of 3 wedge-shaped tarsal bones, lying between the navicular and the metatarsal of the great toe. **Cuneiform osteotomy.** *See* OSTEOTOMY.

cuneocuboid (kew·ne·o·kew′·boid). Belonging to the cuneiform and the cuboid bones, or affecting them.

cuneohysterectomy (kew·ne·o·his·ter·ek′·to·me). As a means of correcting anteflexion of the uterus, the operation of cutting out a wedge of uterine tissue. [L *cuneus* wedge, Gk *hystera* womb, *ektome* a cutting out.]

cuneonavicular (kew·ne·o·nav·ik′·ew·lar). Relating or belonging to the cuneiform and the navicular (scaphoid) bones of the tarsus.

cuneoscaphoid (kew·ne·o·skaf′·oid). Relating to the triquetral (cuneiform) and the scaphoid bones of the carpus.

cuneus [NA] (kew·ne·us). On the medial surface of the cerebral hemisphere, a wedge-shaped area lying between the parieto-occipital and the postcalcarine sulci. [L wedge.]

cunicular (kew·nik·ew·lar). Furrowed; descriptive of the burrow in the skin made by the itch mite. [see foll.]

cuniculus (kew·nik·ew·lus). The burrow made in the skin by the itch mite. [L underground passage.]

cunnilinction (kun·e·lingk·shun). Licking of the vulva. [L *cunnus* vulva, *linguere* to lick.]

cunnilinguist (kun·e·ling·gwist). A person who applies friction to the vulva with the tongue. [L *cunnus* vulva, *lingua* tongue.]

cunnus (kun·us). The vulva. [L.]

cup (kup). 1. A cup-shaped hollow space. 2. A cupping glass; a cup-shaped vessel in which a partial vacuum is produced so that, when applied to the skin over a part, a swelling with hyperaemia forms. 3. The act of using a cupping glass. 4. A drinking vessel. **Antimonial cup.** An antimony vessel used in olden times to render the contents emetic. **Atrophic cup.** A depression of the optic disc, usually shallower than the glaucomatous type, due to atrophy of the optic nerve. **Bitter cup.** A quassia-wood vessel intended to render the contents bitter. **Dry cup.** Cupping in which no external bleeding occurs. **Favus cup.** The sulphur-coloured, cup-shaped mass of adherent fungus characteristic of favus. Single "cups" are seldom seen; usually there are many of them. **Glaucomatous cup.** A cup-shaped depression of the optic disc, often with overhanging edges, occurring in association with ocular hypertension. **Impression cup.** A container which holds the material with which an impression of the teeth or jaws is taken. **Ocular cup, Ophthalmic cup.** Optic cup (see following). **Optic cup [caliculus ophthalmicus (NA)].** The double-layered cup-shaped structure attached to the brain by means of a hollow optic stalk which develops into the retina and inner layers of the ciliary body and iris. It is formed by the invagination of the outer wall of the optic vesicle; later, nerve cells develop in its invaginated layer and some of these send their axons back along the optic stalk to form the optic nerve. **Physiological cup.** The normally depressed area at the head of the optic nerve, as seen at the back of the eye by means of an ophthalmoscope. **Retinal cup.** An obsolete term applied to cupping of the disc, whether glaucomatous or not. **Suction cup.** A cupping glass (see main def. 2 above). **Wet cup.** Cupping in which the skin is scarified or incised, so allowing blood to escape. [L *cupa* cask.]

See also: BIER, HEATLEY, MONTGOMERY.

cupola (kew·po·lah). 1. The top of one of the solitary glands (lymphatic nodules) of the small intestine. 2. [Cupola cochleae (NA)]. The dome-shaped apex of the cochlea. [L little vault.]

cupping (kup·ing). 1. The process of formation of a hollow depression like a cup. 2. The practice of using or the act of applying a cupping glass. **Dry cupping.** Cupping without scarification. **Wet cupping.** Cupping after scarification, so that the blood comes into the cup.

cupraemia (kew·pre·me·ah). A condition in which copper is present in the blood. [L *cuprum* copper, Gk *haima* blood.]

cuprammonia (kew·pram·o·ne·ah). A deep-blue solution formed by dissolving cupric hydroxide in ammonia, containing the cuprammonium ion, $Cu(NH_3)_4^{2+}$. This solution dissolves cellulose, and has been used in the manufacture of artificial silk (Schweitzer's reagent.]

cuprammonic (kew·pram·o·nik). Containing cuprammonia or the cuprammonium ion.

cuprammonium (kew·pram·o·ne·um). The complex ion $Cu(NH_3)_4^{2+}$, produced by the solution of a cupric salt in an excess of ammonia. **Cuprammonium reagent.** Schweitzer's reagent. *See* CUPRAMMONIA.

cuprea bark (kew·pre·ah bark). The bark of species of *Remijia.* It contains the alkaloid cupreine and other allied alkaloids, and has been employed as a substitute for cinchona. [L *cuprum* copper.]

cupreine (kew·pre·een). The name given to the molecule obtained by converting the methoxy group of quinine into a hydroxyl group; alternatively cupreine may be regarded as hydroxy-cinchonidine.

cuprene (kew·preen). A yellow solid hydrocarbon of indefinite formula formed by the polymerization of acetylene in the presence of fine copper.

cuprescent (kew·pres·ent). Like copper in appearance. [L *cuprum* copper.]

cupressin (kew·**pres**·in). An oil obtained from cypress trees, formerly used in the treatment of whooping-cough.

cupric (**kew**·prik). Term applied to a compound of divalent copper. Most cupric salts are blue, and many are used as pigments. **Cupric citrate.** Copper citrate. **Cupric sulphate.** Copper sulphate, blue vitriol, $CuSO_4·5H_2O$. [L *cuprum* copper.]

cuprichloramine (kew·pre·**klor**·am·een). A compound of cuprammonia and chlorine, used in the treatment of reservoirs for the destruction of algae.

cuprosopotassic (kew·**pro**·so·pot·**as'**·ik). Describing a double salt of monovalent copper and potassium.

cuprosulphate (kew·pro·**sul**·fate). A double sulphate of copper and another metal.

cuprotartrate (kew·pro·**tar**·trate). A tartrate of copper combined with that of another metal, as in the case of Fehling's solution which is formed by adding caustic soda to a solution of copper sulphate in sodium potassium tartrate (Rochelle salt).

cuprous (**kew**·prus). Term denoting compounds of monovalent copper. They are less stable than cupric compounds, breaking up readily into the latter and metallic copper: used in organic synthesis for the preparation of halides from diazonium compounds. [L *cuprum* copper.]

cuproxoline (kew·**prox**·o·leen). Cupric bis-[8-hydroxy-quinoline di-(diethyl-ammonium sulphate)], $C_{34}H_{56}N_6O_{14}S_4Cu$. It occurs as green platelets, soluble in water and has been recommended for rheumatoid arthritis, chronic gout and psoriatic arthritis.

cuprum (**kew**·prum). Copper. [L.]

cupula (**kew**·pew·lah). **Cupula of the ampullary crest [cupula (NA)].** A gelatinous mass forming a cap over the cristae in the ampullae of the semicircular canals of the ear. **Cupula pleurae.** The cervical pleura. **Cupula radii.** The shallow hollow on the upper surface of the head of the radius for articulation with the capitulum of the humerus. [L a cup.]

cupular, cupulate (**kew**·pew·lar, **kew**·pew·late). Cup-shaped. [see prec.]

cupulogram (**kew**·pew·lo·gram). A logarithmic record of vestibular function obtained from the performance of cupulometry. The durations of the after-sensation of rotation and of the after-nystagmus are plotted against the measured rotational impulses of different strengths applied to induce these phenomena. A cupulogram is valuable in cases of labyrinthine disorder, and since the given stimulus is known, regulable, and innocuous, it can be used in the examination of very ill patients. Patients are examined in a rotating chair. Noise, draughts, light and other disturbing stimuli are reduced to a minimum by the test being conducted in a sound-damped chamber and the chair being surrounded by dark curtains. A subthreshold acceleration is applied to the chair until a certain, consistent, angular velocity is achieved. When all reactions have ceased, the chair is rapidly stopped and the duration of the after-nystagmus and after-sensation recorded. Rotational stimuli from 0.75 degree per second up to 90 degrees per second are applied; the smallest stimulus capable of producing a reaction is also recorded. Tests are performed after clockwise and anti-clockwise rotation. In normal individuals, the cupulogram is in the form of a straight line. [cupulometry, Gk *gramma* a record.]

cupulometry (kew·pew·**lom**·et·re). A method of investigating vestibular function which examines one pair of semicircular canals at a time, and employs a rotation test using small regulable stimuli. The results are recorded in the form of a cupulogram. [L *cupula* little cup, Gk *metron* measure.]

curage (kewr·**ahzh**). 1. Curettage. 2. The cleansing of a morbid surface, e.g. of an ulcer. 3. A term for the clearing of the cavity of the uterus by the use of a finger. 4. The cleansing of the eye. [Fr. a cleansing.]

curare (kew·**rah**·re). A substance obtained from the root-bark of certain poisonous plants, the most important of which is *Strychnos toxifera.* It was used by the natives of South America and elsewhere to poison the tips of their arrows, but is now of considerable importance medically as a paralysant. It contains the alkaloid curarine amongst others, and the constitution of any particular sample depends upon its source of origin, indicated by the type of packing in which it has been exported (tube, pot, gourd or calabash). Extensively used in anaesthesia as tubocurarine chloride obtained from the plant *Chondrodendron tomentosa* and first employed in modern anaesthesia by Harold R. Griffith of Montreal in 1942. It has no action when taken orally, but intravenous injection produces muscular paralysis by its effect on the motor nerve-endings in striped muscle. The paralysis follows a definite order commencing with the extrinsic ocular muscles and ending with the diaphragm, when death results from respiratory failure. Curare is rapidly destroyed in the tissues, however, and if respiration can be maintained recovery takes place in the reverse order. Its action can usually be reversed by anticholinergic drugs, e.g. neostigmine. It is a non-depolarizing, anti-depolarizing or competitive myoneural blocking agent. It has no action upon the brain. [South American Indian *ourari* or *woorari.*]

curarine (kew·**rah**·reen). $C_{19}H_{26}ON_2$, an alkaloid obtained from gourd curare, with a paralysant effect upon striped muscle. It is also known as *calabashcurarine* to distinguish it from the other curarines, e.g. tubocurarine, the composition and pharmacological effects of which differ.

curarization (**kew**·rah·ri·za'·shun). The subjecting of an individual, animal or tissue to the influence of curare, or of its essential alkaloid, curarine. Muscular paralysis due to failure of conduction at the myoneural junction results. The term is also (incorrectly) used, by analogy, for similar failure of neuromuscular conduction due to different causes, such as the action of drugs other than curarine. **Neostigmine-resistant curarization.** An abnormal state in a patient in which a reasonable dose of non-depolarizing muscle relaxant is not reversed by neostigmine.

curarize (**kew**·rah·rize). To bring any animal (including a human being) under the influence of curare.

curcin (**ker**·sin). A toxic substance resembling ricin. It is found in purging nut, *Jatropha curcas.*

Curcuma BPC 1949 (**ker**·kew·mah). Turmeric; the dried rhizome of *Curcuma domestica.* A bright orange-yellow powder used in curry; the tincture is sometimes used as a colouring agent. [Ar. *kurkum* saffron.]

curcumin (**ker**·kew·min). $C_{21}H_{20}O_6$, a yellow pigment obtained from turmeric, the dried rhizome of *Curcuma domestica.* It is used as a colouring matter for foodstuffs, a vegetable dye, and as an indicator, changing from yellow to brown round pH 8. Employed medicinally by intravenous injection to promote the flow of bile.

curd (kerd). The coagulum of clotted milk produced by the action of rennin upon caseinogen in the presence of calcium salts, as distinguished from the fluid part or whey. [ME.]

cure (kewr). 1. A particular method of treatment designed to restore health. 2. To restore health. **Faith cure.** A cure by means of implicit and unquestioning acceptance of its certainty. certainty. **Hunger cure.** The treatment of disease by starvation. **Milk cure.** Treatment by the administration of a purely milk diet. **Mind cure.** A cure by psychological means. **Spontaneous cure.** Recovery that occurs in the natural course of the disease, with or without treatment; in the former case the implication is that the treatment had little to do with the cure. Or the sudden, unexpected remission in a chronic disease without any obvious explanation. **Thirst cure.** Treatment of disease by limiting the intake of fluids. [L *cura* care.]

curettage (kewr·**et**·ij). 1. The operation of removing neoplasms and other growths or foreign bodies from the skin or from the wall of a cavity. 2. Treatment with a curette, especially of the uterine cavity. [see foll.]

curette (kewr·**et**). A scraper in spoon or scoop shape with which neoplasms and other growths or foreign bodies may be removed from the wall of a cavity. It may have either a cutting or a blunt edge. **Suction curette.** An instrument which, having scraped a piece of tissue from the wall of an organ, picks it up by suction. [Fr. scoop.]

See also: HARTMANN (A.), SHARMAN, YANKAUER.

curettement, curetting (kewr·et·ment, kewr·et·ing). Curettage.

Curie, Marie Sklodowska (b. 1867). Paris scientist and discoverer of radium.

Curie's therapy. Treatment with any radioactive element.

Curie, Pierre (b. 1859). Paris scientist.

Curie's law. In paramagnetic substances, the magnetic susceptibility varies inversely as the absolute temperature.

Curie's therapy. Treatment with any radioactive element.

curie (kewr·e). The unit of radioactivity. One curie is 3.7×10^{10} nuclear transformations per second. Symbol Ci. **Curie hour.** The amount of emanation produced by 1 g of radium in 1 h. [Named after Marie and Pierre *Curie*.]

curiegram (kewr·e·gram). A photographic print produced by the action of radium emanation. [Curie, Gk *gramma* a record.]

curietherapy (kewr·e·ther·ap·e). Term formerly used for radium therapy but now applied to any interstitial radiotherapy. [Marie and Pierre *Curie*, therapy.]

curine (kewr·een). Bebeerine, $C_{36}H_{38}O_6N_2$. An alkaloid from bebeera bark; it is used as the sulphate, a commercial form soluble in water. As it is an aromatic bitter it is sometimes employed as a stomachic.

curium (kewr·e·um). A transuranic element of atomic number 96 and chemical symbol Cm. It was synthesized in 1945 by bombarding plutonium with α-particles in the cyclotron, and has a half-life of 150 days. [Marie and Pierre *Curie*.]

curled (kerld). A term used in descriptive bacteriology to designate the parallel chains in wavy bands seen at the edge of anthrax and similar colonies. [ME *croll*.]

Curling, Thomas Blizard (b. 1811). London surgeon.

Curling's ulcer. Acute duodenal ulcer found as an infrequent but dangerous complication of extensive burns.

current (kur·ent). 1. Anything in the act of flowing. 2. The flow of electricity or electrons along a conducting material. **Abnerval current.** An electrical current passing from a nerve to a muscle. **Abterminal current.** That electrical current passing from the tendinous end towards the body of a muscle. **Action current.** The current occurring when a cell, or any part of it, becomes active. **Adterminal current.** That electrical current passing from the body of a muscle towards its insertion. **After current.** That current occurring in muscle or nerve after the original stimulus has been withdrawn, and indicating the level of excitability of the nerve. **Alternating current.** A.C., an electric current which continually reverses its direction in a regular periodic manner, flowing first in one direction round the circuit and then in the other. **Anelectrotonic current.** That current produced near the anode on passage of a constant current through a nerve, and resulting in a diminution of excitability of the nerve. **Anionic current.** That part of the current passing through a discharge tube, carried by the positive ions. **Ascending current.** That current passing along a motor nerve when the anode, or positive electrode, is nearer the muscle than the cathode, or negative electrode. **Axial current.** The central portion of the flowing blood mass in the vessels. **Battery current.** Electric current flowing in a circuit containing a primary or a secondary cell. **Blaze current.** That current occurring in tissues as the result of mechanical stimulation. **Branch curent.** Electric current flowing in a branch circuit. **Catelectrotonic current.** Katelectrotonic current (see below). **Cathodic current.** That part of the current passing through a discharge tube, carried by the cathode or negative particles. **Centrifugal current.** Descending current (see below). **Centripetal current.** Ascending current (see above). **Combined current.** Summation of currents from branch circuits arriving at a point in a system. **Compensating current.** That current which balances the electric current in a muscle. **Conduction current.** The flow of an electric charge through a conducting medium, the current being the rate of transfer of charge. **Constant current.** Electric current showing no fluctuation. **Continuous current.** An uninterrupted flow of electricity which may be constant or variable. **Damped current.** *See* OSCILLATING CURRENT (below). **Demarcation current.** That current which flows from the normal depolarized surface of a muscle towards the polarized area at the site of an injury; current of injury. **Derived current.** Induced current (see below). **Descending current.** That current passing along a motor nerve when the cathode, or negative electrode, is nearer the muscle than the anode, or positive electrode. **Direct current.** D.C., an electric current flowing in one direction only, and non-pulsating. **Direct vacuum-tube current.** The current passing from the positive to the negative electrode through a discharge tube. **Electric current.** The flow of electricity through a conductor caused by the difference of potential between the ends of the conductor. The current in amperes flowing between the 2 points of a conductor is equal to the difference of potential in volts divided by the resistance in ohms between the 2 points. **Electrostatic current.** Direct current produced from an electrostatic machine. **Electrotonic current.** That current induced in the sheath of a nerve by another current passing along the axon. **Electrovital current.** An old expression referring to certain currents supposed to exist in animal bodies. **Eye current.** The electrical changes occurring in the optic nerve as a result of the stimulation of the retina by light. **Faradic current.** An interrupted current derived from an induction coil, usually from the secondary winding though occasionally from the primary, used in treatment of diseases by stimulation of muscles and nerves. **Galvanic current.** A steady direct current possessing constant polarity, supplied by a battery of voltaic cells or an electrostatic machine, or it may be rectified current from an alternator. **High-frequency current.** An alternating current more than 1000 Hz (cycles per second) when the current is confined mainly to the surface of the conducting wire. **High-potential current, High-tension current.** A current having high electromotive force, such as that obtained from the secondary winding of an induction coil. **Induced current.** The current produced in a circuit (the secondary) caused by the change in magnetic flux through the circuit due to the variation in the current flowing in the circuit or in a neighbouring independent circuit (the primary). **Inducing current.** The current in the primary circuit which gives rise to the current in the secondary circuit. **Induction current, Inductive current.** Current produced by change of magnetic flux through a circuit. **Current of injury.** Demarcation current (see above). **Interaxonal current.** The current produced in one set of nerve fibres by the action potentials occurring in a nearby group. **Interrupted current.** A current flowing in a circuit which is frequently opened and closed. **Inverse current.** Current flowing through a discharge tube in the wrong direction when the alternating current is not properly rectified. **Ionization current.** Current arising from the movement of ions in an electric field. **Katelectrotonic current.** That current produced near the cathode on passage of a constant current through a nerve, and resulting in an increase of excitability of the nerve. Also called *catelectrotonic current.* **Labile current.** That current applied with one or both electrodes moving over the surface. **Low-frequency current.** An alternating current which does not change rapidly in direction, e.g. a current executing 50-120 Hz (cycles per second). **Monophasic action current.** An action current in which the change of potential is in one direction only. It is seen when one lead is taken from a part of the nerve that has been injured, so that this part becomes permanently negative, and the change accompanying excitation is absent at that point. **Nerve action current.** Action current (see above). **Oscillating current.** An alternating current of constant or of gradually decreasing amplitude; it is called *undamped current* when the amplitude is constant, and *damped current* when the amplitude gradually decreases. **Primary current.** Current flowing in the primary circuit of an induction coil or closed-core transformer. **Pulsating current.** A regularly interrupted current whose pulses are of constant size. **Reversed current.** Current flowing in a direction opposite to the normal flow of current. **Saturation current.** That value of the current between 2 electrodes which remains constant if the potential between the electrodes is increased. For example, in an ionization chamber saturation current is obtained when the potential is raised so that collection of ions in the electrodes is equal to the rate of production of ions in the chamber. **Secondary current.** Current flowing in the secondary circuit of an induction coil or a closed-core transformer. **Sine-wave current.** An alternating current the wave shape of which has the regular sine form; a sinusoidal current. **Sinusoidal current.** An alternating current, consecutive values of which fall on a regular sine-wave curve, showing that the values of the current alternate regularly between maxima and minima. **Spark-gap current.** Static current (see below). **Stable current.** That current applied with both electrodes in fixed positions. **Static current.** Electric current obtained from an electrostatic machine. **Static-induced current.** An electrostatic current passed through a patient. **Static-wave current.** That current occurring in a patient raised to a high potential by means of an electrostatic machine, when suddenly discharged. **Surgical current.** Diathermy current passed through a special knife in order to produce a bloodless dissection. **Swelling current.** Electric current varying in strength. **Undamped current.** *See* OSCILLATING CURRENT (above). **Uniform current.** A current of constant magnitude. **Voltaic current.** Electric current resulting from chemical action. [L *currere* to run.]

See also: D'ARSONVAL, DE WATTEVILLE, LEDUC, OUDIN, TESLA.

Curry, Rodney Campbell. British surgeon.

Curry's test. A test for function of the parotid gland by measuring the amount of parotid saliva secreted in 5 min following intravenous injection of 5 mg of pilocarpine.

Curschmann, Hans (b. 1875). Rostock physician.

Curschmann's solution. A solution of camphor in ether and olive oil, administered by injection.

Curschmann, Heinrich (b. 1846). Leipzig physician.

Curschmann's disease. Perihepatitis with thickened capsule.

Curschmann's sign, or spirals. Spiral bodies found in the sputum of patients with bronchitic asthma.

curtometer (ker·tom·et·er). Cyrtometer.

curvature (ker·vat·ewr). A normal or abnormal bending or curving of a line from a rectilinear direction, as in kyphosis. **Angular curvature.** Pott's curvature. **Anterior curvature.** Kyphosis. **Backward curvature.** Lordosis. **Compensatory curvature.** In spinal curvature the secondary bend with which the vertebral column seeks to maintain its normal upright position. **Gingival curvature.** The inward curve of the gum at its attachment to the neck of a tooth. **Greater curvature [curvatura ventriculi major (NA)].** The convex line of the stomach which extends from the cardiac notch, in a backward and upward arch and then downward, to the pylorus. **Lateral curvature.** Scoliosis. **Lesser curvature [curvatura ventriculi minor (NA)].** The concave line of the stomach which extends between the cardiac and pyloric orifices and forms the posterior or right border, ending at the pylorus. **Spinal curvature.** Any bending or abnormal curve of the vertebral column. [L *curvatura* bend.]

See also: POTT.

curve (kerv). 1. A curvature; a line or plane with a deviation from the straight, and not angular in form. 2. A graph, usually curved, showing the relation between two dependent variables. **Base curve.** A term used in optics: in meniscus, periscopic or toric lenses (e.g. those with a concave surface towards the eye), the flatter of the 2 curved surfaces. This usually remains constant and the other curve is varied to attain the required refractive power. **Buccal curve.** The curve formed by the buccal surfaces of the premolar and molar teeth. **Camel curve.** A temperature chart recording 2 periods of elevation separated by an interval of normal or low temperature. **Dental curve.** The curve of the teeth in the dental arch. **Distribution curve.** Frequency curve (see below). **DNA melting curve.** A graph relating the absorbance at 260 nm of a sample of DNA versus temperature. **Frequency curve.** In statistical methods, the curve obtained by plotting graphically the number of times a certain value of a variable (e.g. height, age, test scores, etc.) occurs in a given sample, against the particular value of the variable. The probability of a value occurring within a given range may be estimated by comparison of the area under the curve, between the limits, with the total area. **Gaussian curve.** Normal curve of distribution (see below). **Growth curve.** A graphic representation of the numbers of bacteria present in a culture medium at varying intervals after inoculation, the culture medium being kept at a constant temperature. The number of bacteria present is usually expressed as the logarithm. **Haemoglobin oxygen-dissociation curve.** A graph relating oxygen content of a specimen of haemoglobin (expressed as oxygen saturation %) to the partial pressure of oxygen. The P_{50} value is derived from it. A 'shift to the left' in the curve implies greater oxygen affinity and lower ability to release oxygen than normal; a 'shift to the right' in the curve implies lower oxygen affinity and greater ability to release oxygen than normal. **Indicator dilution curve.** A graph of the variation of the dilution of an indicator with respect to time, obtained when using an indicator dilution method to investigate flow in a circulating system. **Isodose curves.** Dose contours; lines joining points receiving the same radiation dose. **Labial curve.** The curve formed by the labial surfaces of the incisor and canine teeth. **Logistic curve.** A name given to a group of curves used in biometrics defined by the equation

$$y = \frac{a}{b + c^x}$$

where a, b, c are constants and x is the independent variable. This group of curves is derived from the exponential type of curve, being in a way the reciprocal of the exponential group. The shape of the curve depends on the value of c. If c is less than 1, the curve rises from its initial value of

$$\frac{a}{b + 1}$$

when $x = 0$ and approaches the asymptotic value a/b its approach being steep or gradual, depending on the actual value of c. If c is extremely small, the rise to the asymptote is very rapid; if c is not very small (but still less than 1), the curve has the shape of an elongated S. If c is greater than 1, the curve falls from its initial value of

$$\frac{a}{b + 1}$$

when $x = 0$ and approaches its asymptotic value 0. If c is extremely large, the fall to the asymptote is very rapid. If c is not very large (but still larger than 1) the fall to the asymptote is slow, and the curve has the shape of a downward S. **Luetic curve.** *See* LANGE'S COLLOIDAL GOLD TEST. **Meningitic curve.** *See* LANGE'S COLLOIDAL GOLD TEST. **Muscle curve.** A record showing the tension changes occurring in muscle during contraction. **Normal curve of distribution.** In statistical methods, a symmetrical inverted bell-like curve obtained by plotting a frequency distribution; it is the form of frequency curve most encountered in biology and genetics. **Oxygen dissociation curve.** A graph, first worked out by Barcroft and Poulton in 1913, showing the relationship between the partial pressure of oxygen in the blood and the percentage saturation of haemoglobin. **Paretic curve.** *See* LANGE'S COLLOIDAL GOLD TEST. **Pressure curve.** The graphic representation of changes in the pressure within a contracting organ. A simple pressure curve consists of an upstroke produced by the increasing pressure, a rounded summit or plateau, and a downstroke inscribed as the pressure falls to the original level. **Probability curve.** Frequency curve (see above). **Pulse curve.** A sphygmogram. **Radioactive decay curve.** The graph representing the rate of fall of activity of a radioactive isotope by disintegration. **Saddleback temperature curve.** A temperature curve (see below) that shows 2 peaks during the course of the disease, e.g. in dengue. **Solubility curve.** *See* SOLUBILITY. **Staircase curve.** Staircase phenomenon. *See* PHENOMENON. **Strength-duration curve.** The curve produced by plotting the strength of current which, applied to the motor point of a muscle, is just sufficient to cause a twitch against the duration of the current. When muscle is denervated, the strength of current required with brief shocks is much increased. **Temperature curve.** A graph showing the variations in a patient's temperature as recorded at regular intervals. **Tension curve.** A curvature in the trabeculae of cancellous bone, thought to be related to tension stresses. **Time-concentration curve.** *See* RADIOCARDIOGRAPHY. [L *curvare* to bend.]

See also: BRAGG, CARUS, DAMOISEAU, DONDERS, ELLIS (C.), GARLAND, HARRISON (E.), HERING (K. E. K.), MONSON, POISSON (S. D.), PRICE-JONES, SPEE, TRAUBE (L.), WUNDERLICH.

Cusco, Edouard Gabriel (b. 1819). Paris surgeon.

Cusco's speculum. An adjustable bivalve speculum.

Cushing, Harvey Williams (b. 1869). Boston neurosurgeon.

Cushing's basophilism. Cushing's syndrome (see below).

Cushing's silver clip. An angled clip of malleable metal applied to a vessel, usually of the brain, and squeezed tight over it to prevent haemorrhage.

Cushing's law. Increase in the intracranial tension raises the blood pressure to a level slightly greater than the pressure exerted upon the medulla.

Cushing's operation. 1. For trigeminal neuralgia: exposure of the gasserian ganglion by the temporal approach. 2. Hypophysectomy; the nasal septum is approached and removed, through a sublabial incision, and by this route the sphenoidal sinus is approached and subsequently the pituitary fossa.

Cushing's phenomenon. Arterial hypertension due to increased intracranial pressure.

Cushing's syndrome. A disease characterized by obesity of the trunk, purple striae atrophicae on the abdomen and flanks, hypertension, polycythaemia, osteoporosis and glycosuria in either sex and by hypertrichosis, excessive bruising and amenorrhoea in women. In an individual patient, some of these characteristics may be absent. It is caused by overproduction of glucocorticoids by the adrenal cortex due either to primary disease of the adrenal glands (e.g. tumour) or to excessive stimulation by the basophil cells of the anterior pituitary gland produced by increased output of corticotrophin-releasing hormone (CRH) by the hypothalamus or by a basophil tumour of the pituitary. It may also be caused by corticotrophin or corticosteroid secretion occurring elsewhere than in the pituitary or adrenal gland—for example, in a bronchial carcinoma.

Cushing's thermic reaction. Injection of a small quantity of an extract of the anterior lobe of the pituitary of an ox subcutaneously produces a rise of temperature of 1 or 2 degrees in cases of hypopituitarism. Obsolete as a test.

Cushing's ulcer. Acute gastric ulcer associated with injury to the central nervous system or neurosurgery.

Cushing, Hayward Warren (b. 1854). Boston surgeon.

Cushing's suture. A continuous invaginating intestinal suture of the mattress type.

cushion (kushn). In anatomy, any structure resembling a pad or cushion. **Endocardial cushion.** One of the masses of mesenchymal cells lying between the muscular and endothelial walls of the embryonic heart which forms the basis of a valve cusp. **Cushion of the epiglottis.** Epiglottic tubercle. *See* TUBERCLE. **Eustachian cushion.** The tubal elevation behind the pharyngeal orifice in the cartilaginous part of the pharyngotympanic (eustachean) tube. **Polar cushion of the glomerulus.** The locally thickened wall of an afferent arteriole to a renal glomerulus; the juxtaglomerular apparatus. **Sucking cushion.** A pad filled with lobules of fat which lies over the buccinator muscle in young babies. [O Fr. *coissin.*]

cusp (kusp). 1. A pointed projection. 2. [Cuspis (coronae) dentis (NA).] One of the small prominences on the crown of a tooth which assists in the mastication of food. Adjacent cusps are separated from one another by a depression or fissure. 3. One of the triangular segments of the valves of the heart. *See* VALVE, ATRIOVENTRICULAR. **Canine cusp.** The labial cusp on the crown of a premolar tooth. **Distal cusp.** A cusp situated on the posterior part of the occlusal surface of a tooth. **Mesial cusp.** A cusp situated on the anterior part of the occlusal surface of a tooth. [L *cuspis* point.]

See also: CARABELLI, MOON (H.), PASSAVANT.

cusparia (kus·pa·re·ah). The bark of *Cusparia angostura.* This contains a bitter substance, angosturin, and several bitter alkaloids. It is used medically as an aromatic bitter tonic in the form of an infusion, and is one of the constituents of angostura bitters. [S. American *cuspare.*]

cuspidate (kus·pid·ate). 1. Of a tooth, indicating that it bears a cusp or cusps. 2. Ending in a sharp hard point. [L *cuspidare* to make pointed.]

Cusso BPC 1949 (kus·o). The dried panicles of the fertilized pistillate flowers of *Brayera anthelmintica* Kunth (family Rosaceae), a tree indigenous to North-eastern Africa and cultivated in Ethiopia. It contains the active principle kosotoxin, and the inactive substances protokosin and kosidin. It is employed as an anthelmintic, especially against tapeworm, in the form of an infusion, which should be preceded by a dose of sodium bicarbonate and a saline purge; a further purge after administration is not always necessary. Also known as *cousso* and *kousso.* [Ethiopian name.]

Custer cells. Elongated reticulo-endothelial cells found in lymph nodes in certain reticulo-endothelial diseases.

cutaneomucosal (kew·**ta**·ne·o·mew·**ko**′·sal). Mucocutaneous.

cutaneous (kew·**ta**·ne·us). Affecting or associated with the skin; superficial. **Cutaneous nerve.** *See* ARM, FOREARM, THIGH. [L *cutis* skin.]

cutaneous nerve, perforating. A branch of the anterior primary rami of the 2nd and 3rd sacral nerves. It perforates the sacrotuberous ligament and supplies the skin over the lower and medial part of the buttock.

cutch (kuch). Black catechu. *See* CATECHU. [Malay *kachu.*]

cuticle (kew·tikl). 1. The epidermis. 2. An external membranous skin overlapping the free surface of epithelial cells. 3. In a special sense, the epidermis that is spread over the base of the nails from the surrounding skin. **Enamel cuticle.** Cuticle of a tooth (see below). **Keratose cuticle.** The vascular lamina (outer layer) of the choroid. *See* CHOROID. **Prism cuticle.** The organic tissue surrounding each enamel prism in a tooth. **Cuticle of a root sheath.** The delicate skin of the inner root-sheath of a hair which lies next to the hair itself. **Cuticle of a tooth [cuticula dentis (NA)].** The distinct thin horny membrane, consisting of 2 layers, which covers the crown of a young tooth. [L *cuticula* little skin.]

See also: NASMYTH.

cuticolour (kew·te·kul·or). Flesh colour or skin colour. The term is applied to medicaments used in affections of the skin so that their presence will be as little noticeable as is possible and that they may mask the external appearance of the condition. [L *cutis* skin, colour.]

cuticula (kew·**tik**·ew·lah). The cuticle. **Cuticula pili.** Cuticle of a root sheath. [L little skin.]

cuticular (kew·**tik**·ew·lar). Pertaining to the cuticle.

cuticularization (kew·**tik**·ew·lar·i·**za**′·shun). The forming of a skin over a wound or abrasion during the process of healing. [L *cuticula* little skin.]

cutification (kew·tif·ik·**a**′·shun). 1. The forming of skin. 2. Cuticularization. [L *cutis* skin, *facere* to make.]

cutin (kew·tin). 1. A waxy substance which, combined with cellulose, forms the cuticle of plants; also known as *suberin.* 2. A preparation of the muscular layers of the gut of cattle, used as a substitute for catgut. [L *cutis* skin.]

cutinization (kew·tin·i·**za**′·shun). The plastic operation of lining a cavity with skin, e.g. in the case of a bony fistula. [L *cutis* skin.]

cutireaction (kew·te·re·**ak**′·shun). Cutaneous reaction. *See* REACTION.

cutis (kew·tis). 1. A skin. 2. A bark, rind, peel or outermost coat. 3. In anatomy, the skin; the flexible continuous covering of the body, comprising the epidermis, cutis vera and hypoderm, with the vascular, glandular, nervous and other tissues contained therein. The skin is the largest organ of the body, and if taken to include only that portion of the hypoderm which ensheaths its deepest appendages, then its weight is about 3-4 kg, or 6 per cent of the body weight. The average thickness of human skin is 0.22 cm. **Cutis anserina.** Goose flesh; the appearance of the skin caused by contraction of the arrectores pilorum muscles. It may be provoked by cold or by emotions such as fear. **Aurantiasis cutis.** A golden-yellow discoloration of the skin caused by the ingestion of colouring matter in the food, e.g. in fruit and vegetables. It is of no clinical significance, and is curable by abstention. **Cutis elastica, Cutis hyperelastica.** Elastic skin, india-rubber skin, dermatorrhexis; a localized or generalized, usually hereditary, cutaneous abnormality in which the skin is smooth, soft, slightly thinned, very supple and elastic, so that when a fold is pulled out from the body and then released it may return to its original place with an audible snap. Whilst the elasticity may be general, it is usually most noticeable on the face and near the large joints. The condition is often associated with fragility of the skin and blood vessels, overextensibility of the joints, pseudotumours (red or blue in colour and resembling haemangiomata) which follow injuries, and subcutaneous nodules which may be formed of fatty or fibrous tissue. It is this combination of signs and symptoms that is known as *Ehlers-Danlos syndrome.* **Cutis laxa.** Chalazodermia, dermatolysis, lax skin, pachydermatocele. Two conditions have been described under this name: a variety of neurofibromatosis in which large pendulous tumours arise, and a congenital abnormal laxation of the skin. The clinical appearance of most cases is of thickened, often pigmented, skin, so loosely attached to underlying structures that it hangs in baggy folds. Atrophy of the abnormal skin may occur producing a condition that has been named *lipoatrophia circumscripta.* The sites of election are the face, neck, shoulders and thighs. **Cutis marmorata.** Marbled skin; a bluish-red network formed by congested blood vessels, generally seen on the forearms and legs, which may be intensified by cold or friction. The condition is believed particularly to occur in tuberculous persons with a chilblain circulation. **Cutis pendula.** Cutis laxa (see above). **Cutis rhomboidalis frontalis.** Excessive furrowing of the forehead, as seen in porphyria variegata. **Cutis rhomboidalis nuchae.** An atrophic condition of the skin of the nape, usually seen in men who have spent much of their lives exposed to the elements (e.g. gardeners, fishermen). The skin is thickened, may be wrinkled and slightly pigmented, and its surface is cross-hatched by a pattern of deep lines. **Cutis unctuosa.** A shiny, greasy skin, the condition being due to seborrhoea, i.e. over-activity of the sebaceous glands, of the face (faciei) and the nose (nasi). **Cutis vera.** Corium, dermis, true skin; the dense, fibrous layer of the skin which lies immediately under the epidermis, chiefly composed of white fibrous tissue and a variable amount of yellow elastic tissue, in the interstices of which are migratory and fixed cells. The average thickness of the human corium has been estimated as 2 mm. It is described as having an upper papillary layer and a reticular layer; the papillae are conical projections into the epidermis arranged on ridges of varying height, more or less parallel to each other. Blood vessels, nerves, lymphatics, nerve corpuscles, hair, sweat and sebaceous glands, muscles and fat cells are to be found in the true skin. **Cutis verticis gyrata.** MacLeod described this condition as "a peculiar affection of the scalp, in which it is unusually lax, easily movable, having the appearance, especially about the vertex, of being too big for the cranium, so that it forms irregular gyri and furrows like those of the cerebrum". Usually the condition is most marked at the vertex. There are various theories concerning the aetiology. Fischer considers that local causes such as naevi, fibromata or inflammatory changes may be responsible, but also it may be produced by systemic disorders such as acromegaly, myxoedema, cretinism or leukaemia. One variety may be due to anomalous congential development. [L skin.]

cutisector (kew·te·sek·tor). 1. An instrument for the removal of small sections or cylinders of skin from a living subject for examination under a microscope. 2. An instrument with which pieces of skin of varying thickness can be cut away for the purpose of grafting them at another place. [L *cutis* skin, *secare* to cut.]

cutitis (kew·ti·tis). Dermatitis; an inflamed condition of the skin. [L *cutis, Gk -itis* inflammation.]

cutization (kew·ti·za·shun). The process by which exposed mucous membrane acquires the characters of corium. [L *cutis.*]

Cutler, H. H. American biochemist.

Cutler, Power and Wilder test. A chemical test for Addison's disease which depended upon the induction of an exacerbation of the disease by the withholding of salt. It is now obsolete because of its danger.

Cutler, Norman Leon (b. 1901). Wilmington, Delaware, surgeon.

Cutler's operation. The insertion of an implant into Tenon's capsule following enucleation. This is stitched to the muscles and later the artificial eye is fitted into the centre of the implant giving good movement. It is usually extruded in time.

Cutler's solution. A paint of phenol, iodine, and chloral hydrate, used for alopecia.

Cuvier, Georges Léopold Chrétien Frédéric Dagobert. Baron (b. 1769). Paris anatomist and naturalist.

canal of Cuvier. The sinus venosus.

duct of Cuvier. One of the paired common cardinal veins of the embryo, opening into the sinus venosus. In man, the right one becomes the terminal portion of the superior vena cava, the left one the oblique vein of the left atrium.

Cuvier's sinus. The common cardinal vein of the embryo.

cyanacetic acid hydrazine (si·an·as·e′·tik as·id **hi**·draz·een). $CNCH_2CONHNH_2$, a compound recently tested as a substitute for isoniazid in the treatment of tuberculous patients unable to tolerate the latter compound. Radiological improvement was noted in half the cases under test, but no important change in physical signs or symptoms. In some cases the drug had to be discontinued because of severe side-effects. CAH.

cyanacetyl (si·an·**as**·et·il). Acetyl isocyanide, CH_3CONC.

cyanaemia (si·an·e·me·ah). A bluish colour of the blood owing to insufficient aeration, e.g. in cyanosis. [Gk *kyanos* blue, *haima* blood.]

cyanalcohol (si·an·**al**·ko·hol). Cyanhydrin; a compound prepared from an aldehyde and hydrocyanic acid, containing the hydroxyl OH and cyano CN radicals united to the same carbon atom, as in ethylidene cyanhydrin, $CH_3CH(OH)CN=$, useful in organic synthesis as a means of lengthening a chain of carbon atoms.

cyanaldehyde (si·an·**al**·de·hide). $CNCH_2CHO$, a substance derived from acetaldehyde by substitution.

cyanamide (si·**an**·am·ide). Cyanogen amide, $CNNH_2$. A colourless hygroscopic solid, the anhydride of urea, prepared from cyanogen chloride and ammonia: it polymerizes readily to dicyandiamide on heating. **Calcium cyanamide.** A fertilizer manufactured by passing air over heated calcium carbide.

cyanate (si·an·ate). A salt of cyanic acid.

cyanephidrosis (si·an·ef·id·**ro**′·sis). The excretion of sweat of a bluish tint. [Gk *kyanos* blue, ephidrosis.]

cyanhaematin (si·an·**he**·mat·in). A compound formed between potassium cyanide and haematin.

cyanhaemoglobin (**si**·an·he·mo·**glo**′·bin). A compound believed in the past to be formed in hydrocyanic acid poisoning, but giving no characteristic spectrum. The bright-red colour alleged to be due to this compound in the blood is actually due to the action of hydrocyanic acid on the tissue oxidases which prevents the utilization of oxygen: the colour is attributed to oxyhaemoglobin.

cyanhidrosis (si·an·hid·**ro**′·sis). Cyanephidrosis.

cyanhydrin (si·an·**hi**·drin). Cyanalcohol.

cyanide (**si**·an·ide). A salt of hydrocyanic acid containing the monovalent group -CN combined with a metal or radical. **Phenyl cyanide.** Benzonitrile. **Cyanide poisoning.** *See* POISONING. **Cyanide process.** In mining, the process of dissolving gold from its crushed ore with potassium cyanide solution. **Vinyl cyanide.** Acrylonitrile. [Gk *kyanos* blue.]

cyanidin (si·**an**·id·in). Pentahydroxy flavylium chloride, $C_{15}H_{11}O_6Cl$. The chloride of a hydroxylated base, the glycosides of which constitute the colouring matters of chrysanthemums, cranberries, the leaves of the copper-beech, and, as a diglucoside, of blue cornflowers.

cyanidrosis (si·an·id·**ro**′·sis). Cyanephidrosis.

cyanin (**si**·an·in). 1. A member of a family of anthocyanins which form the blue colouring matter of cornflowers, violas, violets, and irises. 2. The diglucoside of cyanidin, $C_{27}H_{30}O_{16}$, which occurs in red rose petals, and, as a potassium salt, forms the blue pigment of cornflowers. It is a useful indicator for acids, varying from red at pH 3 to blue at pH 11.

cyanine (si·an·een). Quinoline blue, $C_{29}H_{35}N_2I$. A dye used in the sensitization of photographic plates. **Cyanine dyes.** A family of blue dyes containing pairs of quinoline rings in their structure, which are of special importance in photography as colour sensitizers for panchromatic plates; used in medicine as antiseptics.

cyanmethaemoglobin (si·an·met·he·mo·glo′·bin). Cyanhaemoglobin.

cyanochroia (si·an·o·kroi′·ah). Cyanosis. [Gk *kyanos* blue, *chroia* skin.]

Cyanocobalamin BP 1973 (si·an·o·ko·bal′·am·in). α-(5,6-Dimethylbenzamidazol-2-yl)cobamide cyanide, a cobalt-containing substance which "may be produced in suitable media by the growth of certain micro-organisms or obtained from liver" (*BP*). Its actions and uses are essentially those of hydroxocobalamin but it is more rapidly excreted and has other minor disadvantages therapeutically. **Cyanocobalamin (^{57}Co) and (^{58}Co) BP 1973.** Cyanocobalamin labelled with radioactive cobalt (^{57}Co) and (^{58}Co); these preparations are used "to measure the absorption of orally administered cyanocobalamin in the investigation of megaloblastic anaemias" (BPC 1968).

Cyanocobalaminum (si·an·o·ko·bal·am′·in·um). *European Pharmacopoeia* name for Cyanocobalamin BP 1973.

cyanoderma (si·an·o·der′·mah). Cyanosis. [Gk *kyanos* blue, *derma* skin.]

cyanoform (si·an·o·form). Tricyanomethane, $CH(CN)_3$. A crystalline compound prepared from chloroform by the substitution of cyanogen radicals for chlorine atoms with alcoholic potassium cyanide.

cyanogen (si·an·o·jen). Oxalonitrile, ethane dinitrile, dicyanogen, CNCN. An extremely poisonous colourless gas with an odour of bitter almonds, occurring in coal gas and blast-furnace gases, being stable at high temperatures. It polymerizes to a brown substance, paracyanogen $(CN)_x$. **Cyanogen bromide.** CNBr, a crystalline compound used in chemical warfare because of its lacrimatory properties. **Cyanogen chloride.** CNCl, a colourless gas, poisonous and lacrimatory, used for the fumigation of ships' holds and warehouses. [see foll.]

cyanogenesis (si·an·o·jen′·es·is). The production or yielding of cyanogen or hydrocyanic acid. [Gk *kyanos* blue, *genein* to produce.]

cyanogenetic (si·an·o·jen·et′·ik). Producing or yielding cyanogen or hydrocyanic acid. [see prec.]

cyanomycosis (si·an·o·mi·ko′·sis). A condition giving rise to blue pus, due to infection with *Pseudomonas aeruginosa (pyocyanea).* The organism is resistant to penicillin, but may be sensitive to streptomycin, or to chloramphenicol. It is often a troublesome invader in ear or wound infections. [Gk *kyanos* blue, *mykes* fungus, *-osis* condition.]

cyanopathy (si·an·op·ath·e). Cyanosis. [Gk *kyanos* blue, *pathos* suffering.]

cyanophil (si·an·o·fil). Capable of being stained by blue dyes; e.g. a cell nucleus which readily takes a blue stain. [Gk *kyanos* blue, *philein* to love.]

cyanophilous (si·an·of·il·us). Taking blue dye stains readily. [see prec.]

cyanophoric (si·an·o·for′·ik). Term denoting those natural glycosides which produce hydrocyanic acid when hydrolysed. [cyanogen, Gk *pherein* to carry.]

cyanophose (si·an·o·foze). A blue phose. [Gk *kyanos* blue, *phos* light.]

cyanophyceae (si·an·o·fi′·se·e). An order of blue-green algae, some forms of which may obstruct water purification by their over-growth. [Gk *kyanos* blue, *phykos* seaweed.]

cyanopia, cyanopsia (si·an·o·pe·ah, si·an·op·se·ah). A condition in which everything looked at appears to be tinted with a blue colour. [Gk *kyanos* blue, *ops* eye.]

cyanosis (si·an·o·sis). A blue appearance of the skin and mucous membranes, which may be general but is most prominent in the extremities, hands and feet, and in superficial highly vascular parts such as the lips, cheeks and ears. It is due to deficient oxygenation of the blood in the minute blood vessels, and depends upon the absolute amount of reduced haemoglobin present. **Central cyanosis.** Cyanosis which originates in the "centre", in that the arterial blood is not normally oxygenated. It occurs as a result of the shunting of venous blood past the pulmonary bed, as in cyanotic congenital heart disease, or with impaired oxygenation of blood flowing through the pulmonary bed. **Congenital cyanosis.** Cyanosis present at birth; it is usually due to congenital heart disease or atelectasis of the lungs. **Delayed cyanosis.** Tardive cyanosis (see below). **Differential cyanosis.** The uncommon occurrence of differing degrees of cyanosis in the upper and lower parts of the body. It is seen with persistent ductus arteriosus when there is pulmonary hypertension so that venous blood is shunted into the arch of the aorta and flows principally to the lower part of the body. **Enterogenous cyanosis.** Cyanosis associated with the presence of methaemoglobin or sulphmethaemoglobin in the red cells, both of which may be formed from substances absorbed in the intestine. Methaemoglobinaemia may occur as a congenital disorder, but is most often due to certain poisons, e.g. sulphonamides, chlorates, and certain coal-tar derivatives, e.g. acetanilide, sulphonal, phenacetin, trional and after some local analgesic agents, e.g. prilocaine. Sulphaemoglobinaemia may be caused by drugs or by a reducing agent, possibly of bacterial origin, permitting the formation of sulphaemoglobin with minute traces of sulphuretted hydrogen. **Heliotrope cyanosis.** A peculiarly pale cyanosis seen in influenza with severe respiratory complications. **Peripheral cyanosis.** Cyanosis which originates in the "periphery", in that the arterial blood is normally oxygenated but the tissue extraction of oxygen is excessive so that the amount of reduced haemoglobin in the venules which contribute to the visible colour of the part is sufficient to give rise to the cyanotic appearance. It occurs as a result of peripheral vasoconstriction or gross reduction in cardiac output. **Tardive cyanosis.** Cyanosis occurring in congenital interauricular septal defect only after cardiac failure. [Gk *kyanos* blue, *-osis* condition.]

Cyanthomastix (si·an·tho·mas′·tix). A genus of protozoa now known as *Chilomastix.* **Cyanthomastix hominis.** *Chilomastix mesnili.*

cyanurea (si·an·ewr·e′·ah). $NH_2CONHCN$, a compound formed from urea by cyanogen halides.

cyanuria (si·an·ewr·e·ah). A condition in which the urine is of a blue colour. [Gk *kyanos* blue, urine.]

cyanuric (si·an·ewr·ik). 1. Containing cyanurea. 2. Referring to cyanuria. **Cyanuric chloride.** Trichlorocyanogen, $(C_3Cl_3)N_3$. Crystals formed by the polymerization of cyanogen chloride.

cyasma (si·az·mah). The freckling of the skin which may be present during pregnancy. [Gk *kyein* to be pregnant.]

cyathus (si·ath·us). 1. The funnel-shaped recess in the infundibulum of the hypothalamus of the cerebrum. 2. In botany, a cup-shaped organ or cavity. 3. A glass or cup. [Gk *kyathos* cup.]

cybernetics (si·ber·net·ix). The study of similarities in performance and behaviour of machines and living individuals, and of the underlying electrical and mechanical processes which determine them. [Gk *kybernetes* steersman.]

Cyclandelate (si·klan·del·ate). BP Commission approved name for 3,3,5-trimethylcyclohexyl mandelate; it is used in the treatment of vascular disorders.

Cyclarbamate (si·klar·bam·ate). BP Commission approved name for 1,1-di(phenylcarbamoyloxymethyl)cyclopentane; a muscle relaxant and tranquillizer.

cyclarthrodial (si·klar·thro·de·al). Belonging or related to a pivot joint. [Gk *kyklos* circle, *arthron* joint.]

cyclarthrosis (si·klar·thro·sis). A pivot joint. *See* JOINT. [see prec.]

Cyclaster scarlatinalis (sik·las·ter skar·lat·in·a′·lis). A protozoon claimed to have been observed in the epithelial cells of the skin in scarlet fever, and formerly believed by some to be the cause of the infection. This view of the aetiology was given up many years ago from lack of supporting evidence. [Gk *kyklos* circle, *aster* star, scarlatina.]

Cyclasterion scarlatinale (sik·las·**teer**·e·on **skar**·lat·in·**a**'·le). *Cyclaster scarlatinalis.*

cyclatron (**si**·klat·ron). Cyclotron.

cycle (**si**·kl). A complete series of events which recurs at intervals. **Anovulatory cycle.** A sexual cycle without extrusion of an ovum. **Biliary cycle.** The passage into the bile of absorbed biliary constituents, notably of bile salts, demonstrated by Schiff about 1870. **Cardiac cycle.** The changes which occur in the heart during each beat, consisting of auricular systole and diastole, and ventricular systole and diastole. They may be divided into mechanical events (pressure changes) and electrical events (electrocardiographic changes). The length of the cycle varies inversely with the heart rate. *Pressure changes:* 1. Auricles. The pressure changes in the right auricle are transmitted to the jugular veins and can be measured from a tracing of the jugular venous pulse. Auricular contraction (systole) causes a positive (*a*) wave, which is succeeded by a negative wave (*x*). The tricuspid valve is open during auricular systole (so that blood enters the ventricle), and closes at the commencement of a second positive wave (*c*), the summit of which coincides with the opening of the semilunar valves. A second negative wave (x^1) follows the (*c*) wave, and is succeeded by a gradual positive wave (*v*) due to the inflow of blood from the great veins during auricular diastole. Finally, a third negative wave (*y*) occurs as blood flows from auricle to ventricle after opening of the tricuspid valve. The duration of auricular systole is 0.1 s and of diastole 0.7 s, when the heart is beating at 70 per minute. 2. Ventricles. Ventricular contraction (systole) is divided into 3 phases, isometric-contraction phase, maximal-ejection phase and reduced-ejection phase. The first phase lasts until the opening of the aortic and mitral valves and is then succeeded by the maximal-ejection and reduced-ejection phases, respectively, during which time blood is being forced into the aorta and the pulmonary artery. Ventricular relaxation (diastole) follows the reduced-ejection phase, and commences with the protodiastolic phase, which lasts until the aortic and pulmonary valves close, and is followed by the isometric-relaxation phase until the opening of the atrio-ventricular valves initiates the phase of rapid filling. The duration of ventricular systole is 0.3 s and of diastole 0.5 s, at a heart rate of 70 a minute. *Electrical changes:* these are recorded by the electrocardiograph, and consist of auricular depolarization and repolarization during auricular systole (P wave, and auricular T wave, respectively), and ventricular depolarization and repolarization during ventricular systole (QRS complex and T wave, respectively). The electrical events of the cardiac cycle slightly precede the mechanical events. **Cardiovascular cycle.** The circulation of the blood through the heart, arteries, capillaries and veins, back to the heart. **Cell cycle.** The life cycle of a cell. In proliferating somatic cells this consists of division (mitosis) and interphase. The latter usually consists of the G_1, S and G_2 periods; G_1 is the interval between mitosis and the beginning of DNA replication, S is the period of DNA synthesis, and G_2 is the interval between the end of S and mitosis. **Citric acid cycle.** The cycle of reactions whereby the intermediate products of carbohydrate, fats and amino acid metabolism are converted to CO_2 and water in the mitochondrion. **Cytoplasmic cycle.** The cycle of development of a parasite within the cytoplasm of a cell. **Endogenous cycle.** The cycle of development within the definite host. **Exogenous cycle.** The cycle of development of a parasite outside the host, e.g. of *Strongyloides stercoralis* in the soil. **Genesial cycle.** The reproductive period of a woman's life. **Glucose lactate cycle.** An intermediate cycle of carbohydrate metabolism stimulated by exercise, in which muscle glycogen→blood lactate→liver glycogen→blood glucose→muscle glycogen. **Growth cycle.** The time taken or the processes involved in the replication of micro-organisms, including bacteria and viruses. **Human cycle.** The cycle of development within the human host, e.g. of *Strongyloides stercoralis.* **Intranuclear cycle.** The cycle of development within a nucleus, e.g. of certain rickettsiae. **Life cycle.** Of arthropods, the series of stages from any one stage in one generation to the same stage in the next. **Lytic cycle.** The sequence of events that leads to bursting of a sensitive bacterial cell following infection by bacteriophage. **Menstrual cycle.** A term used to describe the cyclical changes that occur in the female reproductive organs. **Mosquito cycle.** The phase of development of the malaria parasite in the gut wall (stomach) of the appropriate species of *Anopheles* mosquito. The oöcyst produced by the penetration of the oökinete develops just beneath the epithelium; inside the oöcysts sporozoites are produced. **Oestrous cycle.** The periodic changes that take place under the influence of the sex hormones. **Oögenetic cycle.** Ovarian cycle (see following). **Ovarian cycle.** The cyclic changes that take place in the ovary during reproductive life. **Pulse cycle.** The period between the beginning of one pulse wave and the beginning of the next. **Restored cycle.** After a "returning cycle" (see following), or completed premature ventricular contraction, there is a compensatory pause, during which the refractory period of the ventricle wears off. The next normal ventricular beat is known as the "restored cycle". **Returning cycle.** A term based on the "re-entry" theory of causation of coupled premature ventricular contractions, in which the original impulse from the auriculoventricular node, having produced a normal ventricular beat, is thought to cause a second premature response by re-entering the ventricle. Such a premature contraction may be known as a "returning cycle". **Schizogenic cycle, Schizogenous cycle.** The asexual cycle in sporozoa. **Sex cycle, Sexual cycle.** 1. Menstrual cycle (see above). 2. In animals, that part of the reproductive cycle in which sexual forms must be present for reproduction to occur. **Sporogenic cycle, Sporogenous cycle.** The sexual cycle in sporozoa. **Tricarboxylic acid cycle.** Citric acid cycle (see above). [Gk *kyklos* circle.]

See also: CORI, KREBS (H. A.), ROSS (R.), SCHIFF (H.).

cyclectomy (si·**klek**·to·me). 1. Surgical removal of a part of the ciliary body or ciliary muscle. 2. Surgical removal of part of the edge of the eyelid. [Gk *kyklos* circle, *ektome* a cutting out.]

cyclencephalus (si·klen·**kef**·al·us). A monster in which the 2 cerebral hemispheres are fused into one. [Gk *kyklos* circle, *egkephalos* brain.]

cyclic (**si**·klik). 1. Having the characteristics of a cycle. 2. Describing phenomena occurring in series at different periods of time; a term used by Hirsch and others for the exacerbations of epidemic diseases, e.g. influenza, over long periods of time. Also used, rarely, for certain diseases which run a characteristic course, e.g. lobar pneumonia. 3. In chemistry, describing a compound which has in its structure a closed ring of atoms. [Gk *kyklikos* circular.]

cyclic AMP (**si**·klik amp). (3′,5′-Adenosine monophosphate.) It is formed by the actions of the enzyme adenyl cyclase present in cell membranes on ATP (adenosine triphosphate) in the cytoplasm. AMP may be activated by certain compounds and homones affecting the cell. For instance, catecholamines cause glycolysis in hepatic cells and lipolysis in fat cells. Adenyl cyclase may also be inhibited by prostaglandins, for instance.

cyclicotomy (si·klik·**ot**·o·me). A surgical measure for relieving tension in glaucoma, consisting in the dividing of the ciliary body. [Gk *kyklos* circle, *temnein* to cut.]

cyclite (**si**·klite). Benzyl bromide, $C_6H_5CH_2Br$. A colourless liquid with a lacrimatory vapour; used in chemical warfare as a tear-gas.

cyclitis (si·**kli**·tis). Inflammation of the ciliary body. **Heterochromic cyclitis.** A chronic intractable form of cyclitis affecting one eye and resulting in depigmentation of the iris so that the two eyes appear to differ in colour. Secondary cataract is a frequent complication. **Plastic cyclitis.** Cyclitis associated with a copious fibrinous exudate into the posterior chamber which forms a dense membrane behind the lens; this becomes organized into fibrous tissue and by contraction leads to shrinkage of the eyeball. **Purulent cyclitis.** A severe form of cyclitis, associated with exudation of pus, some of which accumulates at the bottom of the anterior chamber (hypopyon). **Serous cyclitis.** A mild form of cyclitis with deepening of the anterior chamber, precipitation of dots on the back of the cornea (keratitic precipitates) and turbidity of the aqueous. [Gk *kyklos* circle, *-itis* inflammation.]

Cyclizine (si·kliz·een). BP Commission approved name for 1-methyl-4-α-phenylbenzylpiperazine. It is used in pregnancy, postanaesthetic, and in travel sickness. **Cyclizine Hydrochloride BP 1973.** 1-diphenylethyl-4-methyl-piperazine monohydrochloride, a white, almost odourless crystalline powder with a bitter taste. An antihistamine compound used in the prevention and relief of motion sickness.

cyclo-anaemization (si·klo·an·e·mi·**za**·shun). Operation for glaucoma to reduce the blood supply to the ciliary body; diathermy over the long ciliary arteries combined with temporary tenotomy of rectus muscles of the orbit. [Gk *kyklos* circle, *a*, *haima* blood.]

cyclobarbital (si·klo·**bar**·bit·al). Cyclobarbitone BP 1958.

cyclobarbitalum (si·klo·bar·bit·**a'**·lum). **Cyclobarbitalum Calcicum.** *European Pharmacopoeia* name for Cyclobarbitone Calcium BP 1973.

Cyclobarbitone BP 1958 (si·klo·**bar**·bit·one). 5-Ethyl-5-Δ'-cyclohexenyl barbituric acid, $CO(NHCO)_2C(C_2H_5)(C_6H_9)$. A short-acting comparatively mild barbiturate used for insomnia due to anxiety or nervous unrest. **Cyclobarbitone Calcium BP 1973.** The calcium derivative of cyclobarbitone, a white, almost odourless powder with a bitter taste; it is administered orally in the treatment of insomnia.

cyclocephalus (si·klo·**kef**·al·us). 1. A monster in which the organs of vision are rudimentary and fused in the median line and the olfactory organs are defective or absent. 2. A cyclops. [Gk *kyklos* circle, *kephale* head.]

cycloceratitis (si·klo·ser·at·**i'**·tis). Cyclokeratitis.

cyclochoroiditis (si·klo·kor·oid·**i'**·tis). Inflammation of the ciliary body and of the choroid of the vascular coat of the eye. [Gk *kyklos* circle, choroid, Gk *-itis* inflammation.]

Cyclocoumarol (si·klo·**koo**·mar·ol). BP Commission approved name for 5',6'-dihydro-6'-methoxy-6'-methyl-4'-phenylpyrano-(3',2',3,4) coumarin, an anti-coagulant, three or four times as potent as dicoumarol, the therapeutic level of which can be reached within 72 h. The maintenance dosage can be reduced to alternate days, and over-action controlled by vitamin K.

cyclocryotherapy (si·klo·kri·o·**ther'**·ap·e). Cryotherapy over the ciliary body to reduce the secretion of aqueous. [Gk *kyklos* circle, *kryos* cold, *therapeia* treatment.]

cyclodialysis (si·klo·di·**al'**·is·is). In glaucoma, the operation of establishing a communication between the anterior chamber of the eye and the perichoroidal space in order to lessen tension. The operation is a relatively slight one and can be employed when more serious ones are contra-indicated. [Gk *kyklos* circle, *dialysis* a dissolution.]

cyclodiathermy (si·klo·**di**·ah·ther·me). Diathermy used for the purpose of destroying the ciliary body of the eye. [Gk *kyklos* circle, diathermy.]

cyclodiplopia (si·klo·dip·**lo'**·pe·ah). Torsional diplopia. *See* DIPLOPIA. [Gk *kyklos* circle, diplopia.]

cycloduction (si·klo·**duk**·shun). The range of rotation of one eye around an anteroposterior axis, through which binocular single vision can be maintained. It is measured on a synoptophore or similar instrument by rotating one of the fusional slides. [Gk *kyklos* circle, L *ducere* to draw.]

Cyclofenil (si·klo·**fe**·nil). BP Commission approved name for 4,4'-diacetoxybenzhydrylidenecyclohexane; it is used in the treatment of infertility.

cyclogeny (si·**kloj**·en·e). The life cycle of a micro-organism. [Gk *kyklos* circle, *genein* to produce.]

cyclogram (si·klo·gram). 1. A chart of the field of vision made by means of a cycloscope. 2. An endocrinogram. [Gk *kyklos* circle, *gramma* a writing.]

cyclohexane (si·klo·**hex**·ane). Hexahydrobenzene, hexamethylene, $CH_2{=}(CH_2CH_2)_2{=}CH_2$. A colourless fragrant liquid hydrocarbon resembling a paraffin in properties, found in petroleum from the Caucasus and Galicia. It is prepared synthetically by passing benzene and hydrogen over a hot nickel catalyser.

cyclohexanol (si·klo·**hex**·an·ol). Hydroxycyclohexane, hexahydrophenol, $CH_2{=}(CH_2CH_2){=}CHOH$. A crystallizable liquid prepared from phenol by catalytic reduction with hydrogen; a commercial solvent for waxes, gums, rubber and nitrocellulose; also an emulsifier.

cycloheximide (si·klo·**hex**·im·ide). An inhibitor of eukaryotic cytoplasmic protein synthesis. It acts at the level of translation.

cycloid (si·kloid). 1. A descriptive term applied to individuals who are round-faced, jolly and rubicund, apparently without a care in the world. 2. A term applied to individuals who tend towards the manic-depressive type of insanity. [Gk *kyklos* circle, *eidos* form.]

cyclokeratitis (si·klo·ker·at·**i'**·tis). A state of inflammation of the cornea and the ciliary body. [Gk *kyklos* circle, keratitis.]

cyclol (si·klol). A unit in protein structure based upon the diketopiperazine ring (cyclopeptide), in which 6 amino acid residues are joined by cyclol bonds, =NC(OH)=, into a "cyclol 6". A number of these form a closed cage which is considered the globular molecule of such proteins as insulin, pepsin, lactoglobulin and haemoglobin.

cyclomastopathy (si·klo·mas·**top'**·ath·e). A general name for a group of lesions of the breast which are marked by excessive growth of connective tissue with or without epithelial proliferation. [Gk *kyklos* circle, mastopathy.]

Cyclomethycaine (si·klo·**meth**·e·kane). BP Commission approved name for 3-(2-methylpiperidino)propyl-*p*-cyclo-hexyloxybenzoate, a local anaesthetic used in creams, etc., for sunburn and other superficial dermatological lesions. **Cyclomethycaine Sulphate BP 1973.** The hydrogen sulphate of cyclomethycaine, a white, odourless crystalline powder with a bitter taste followed by a sensation of numbness. A local anaesthetic, it is used for abrasions and some types of skin lesions, painful conditions arising in the mucous membrane of the rectum and vagina, and before cystoscopy, except in cases of injury.

cyclonopathy (si·klon·**op**·ath·e). A condition in which the individual is made uneasy and uncomfortable by the approach of inclement weather. [cyclone, Gk *pathos* suffering.]

cycloparaffin (si·klo·**par**·af·in). Any one of a series of saturated aliphatic compounds composed of methylene groups, CH_2, linked in a ring, e.g. cyclopropane,

$$\overline{CH_2CH_2CH_2}.$$

cycloparesis (si·klo·par·e·sis). Weakness of a ciliary muscle of the eye. [Gk *kyklos* circle, paresis.]

cyclopean (si·**klo**·pe·an). Of, or pertaining to a cyclops.

cyclopentamine (si·klo·**pen**·tam·een). BP Commission approved name for 1-cyclopentenyl-2-methylamino propane, $C_5H_9CH_2CH(CH_3)NHCH_3$. A sympathomimetic amine used as a local vasoconstrictor to maintain blood pressure in operations.

cyclopentane (si·klo·**pen**·tane). Pentamethylene, $CH_2{=}(CH_2)_3{=}CH_2$. A cycloparaffin homologous with cyclohexane, and found with it in certain petroleums; a liquid which can be prepared synthetically from calcium adipate.

cyclopentenobenzanthracene (si·klo·pen·ten·o·ben·**zan'**·thrah·seen). 5,6-Cyclopenteno-1,2-benzanthrene, $C_{21}H_{17}$. An oestrogenic and potentially carcinogenic compound prepared in the investigations which led to the discovery of stilboestrol.

cyclopentenoperhydrophenanthrene (si·klo·**pen**·ten·o·per·hi·dro·fen·**an'**·threen). Perhydro-1,2-cyclopentenophenanthrene. A compound constituted of a phenanthrene ring-system with a 5-membered ring fused to it at the 1,2-position. It is this structure that forms the characteristic unit of the steroids.

cyclopentenophenanthrene (si·klo·**pen**·ten·o·fen·**an'**·threen). A chemical group or skeleton composed of three 6-membered carbon rings united to one 5-membered carbon ring, the former being in the phenanthrene configuration. It is the basic structure of the sterols and steroids, which include compounds of such biological importance as cholesterol, the sex hormones, provitamins D, the bile acids, the hormones of the adrenal cortex, the saponins and heart poisons, and certain carcinogenic hydrocarbons.

Cyclopenthiazide BP 1973 (si·klo·pen·**thi**′·az·ide). 1,2,4-Benzothiadiazine-7-sulphonamide 1,1-dioxide, a non-mercurial diuretic with actions and uses similar to those of chlorothiazide.

Cyclopentolate (si·klo·**pen**·to·late). BP Commission approved name for 2-dimethylamino-ethyl α-1-hydroxocyclopentyl-α-phenylacetate. **Cyclopentolate Hydrochloride BP 1973.** The hydrochloride of cyclopentolate; a mydriatic and cycloplegic drug used in ophthalmology for diagnostic and therapeutic purposes.

cyclopeptide (si·klo·**pep**·tide). A ring compound with the diketopiperazine structure, formed by the union of the respective amino and carboxyl groups of 2 amino acids. It is considered that the linkage of such rings by cyclol bonds builds up the molecules of globular proteins.

cyclophoria (si·klo·**for**·e·ah). A latent tendency for the eye to rotate on an anteroposterior axis. When the eye is covered, the 6 to 12 o'clock meridian of the cornea may lean outwards (excyclophoria) or inwards (incyclophoria). **Accommodative cyclophoria.** A condition of cyclophoria which occurs only on looking at near objects and is probably associated more with convergence than with accommodation. [Gk *kyklos* circle, *pherein* to bear.]

cyclophorometer (si·klo·for·**om**′·et·er). An instrument with which the degree of cyclophoria can be measured. [cyclophoria, meter.]

Cyclophosphamide BP 1973 (si·klo·**fos**·fam·ide). 2-[Di-(2-chloro-ethyl)amino]-1-oxa-3-aza-2-phosphacyclohexane 2-oxide; an alkylating drug used in the treatment of malignant tumours.

cyclophrenia (si·klo·**fre**·ne·ah). Circular insanity; manic-depressive psychosis. *See* PSYCHOSIS. [Gk *kyklos* circle, *phren* mind.]

Cyclophyllidea (si·klo·fil·**id**′·e·ah). An order of the cestode subclass Cestoda. Members of the families Anoplocephalidae, Davaineidae, Dipylidiidae, Hymenolepididae, Mesocestoididae, Taeniidae are of medical interest. [Gk *kyklos* circle, *phyllon* leaf.]

cyclopia (si·**klo**·pe·ah). The state of being a cyclops. **Cyclopia synophthalmus.** Synophthalmus.

cycloplegia (si·klo·**ple**·je·ah). Paralysis of a ciliary muscle of the eye, leading to loss of accommodation. [Gk *kyklos* circle, *plege* stroke.]

cycloplegic (si·klo·**ple**·jik). 1. Appertaining to cycloplegia. 2. Any drug such as atropine which causes temporary cycloplegia.

Cyclopropane BP 1973 (si·klo·**pro**·pane). Trimethylene,

$$\overline{CH_2CH_2CH_2}.$$

A colourless gas which is a potent anaesthetic even when mixed with large quantities of oxygen. It is non-irritating to the air passages, but produces cardiac irregularities, whilst its wide range of inflammability and explosibility necessitates its being given in a closed system.

cyclops (si·klops). 1. Synophthalmus; a fetal monster with both eyes fused into one medially. 2. A genus of small fresh-water Copepoda. Numerous species are intermediate hosts to tapeworms of the genus *Diphyllobothrium* including *Sparganum,* and to the guinea-worms *Dracunculus medinensis* and *D. insignis.* [*Cyclops* the one-eyed giant of Greek mythology.]

Cycloquanil Embonate (si·klo·**kwan**·il **em**·bon·ate). BP Commission approved name for 4,6-diamino-1-(4-chlorophenyl)-1,2-dihydro-2,2-dimethyl-1,3,5-triazine compound (2:1) with 4,4′-methylenedi-(3-hydroxy-2-naphthoic acid); an antimalarial.

Cyclorrhapha (si·klo·**ra**·fah). A sub-order of the insectan order Diptera. It contains those flies which have 3 segmented antennae and a coarctate pupa. The families Gastrophilidae, Glossinidae, Hippoboscidae, Muscidae, Oestridae, Oscinidae, Phoridae, Stratiomyidae and Syrphidae are of medical interest. [Gk *kyklos* circle, *rhaphe* suture.]

cycloscope (si·klo·skope). Any apparatus designed for measuring the field of vision. [Gk *kyklos* circle, *skopein* to view.]

cyclose (si·**kloze**). Designation of a member of a family of cyclo-sugars which are hydroxy derivatives of cyclohexane; the quercitol of acorns, and inositol from heart muscle are examples.

Cycloserine BP 1973 (si·klo·**seer**·ine). An antibiotic obtained from species of *Streptomyces.* It is active against tuberculosis and is well absorbed when given orally, but it has toxic side-reactions.

cyclosis (si·**klo**·sis). Cytoplasmic streaming movements, chiefly in plant cells. [Gk *kyklos* circle.]

cyclospasm (si·klo·spazm). Spasm of accommodation. [Gk *kyklos* circle, spasm.]

cyclostage (si·klo·staje). The stage in the life cycle of a micro-organism during which development takes place. [Gk *kyklos* circle, stage.]

cyclostat (si·klo·stat). A glass cylinder in which an experimental animal can be rotated. [Gk *kyklos* circle, *statos* standing.]

Cyclothiazide (si·klo·**thi**·az·ide). BP Commission approved name for 3-(bicyclo[2,2,1]hept-5-en-2-yl)-6-chloro-3,4-dihydro-1,2,4-benzothiadiazine-7-sulphonamide 1,1-dioxide; a diuretic.

cyclothyme (si·klo·thime). In psychiatry, a character trend, possibly amounting to mental disorder, in which occur the fundamental psychological symptoms of manic-depressive psychosis in the form of personality traits. [Gk *kyklos* circle, *thymos* mind.]

cyclothymia (si·klo·**thi**·me·ah). Circular insanity; manic-depressive insanity of mild type. [Gk *kyklos* circle, *thymos* mind.]

cyclothymiac (si·klo·**thi**·me·ak). An individual suffering from circular insanity. [see prec.]

cyclothymic (si·klo·**thi**·mik). Referring or belonging to the state of cyclothymia; affected with cyclothymia.

cyclothymosis (si·klo·thi·**mo**′·sis). Any mental disease belonging to the circular insanity group. [Gk *kyklos* circle, *thymos* mind.]

cyclotol (si·klo·tol). A cyclic alcohol such as inositol.

cyclotome (si·klo·tome). A surgical knife used for incising or dividing the ciliary muscle, and for other operations on the eye. [Gk *kyklos* circle, *temnein* to cut.]

cyclotomy (si·**klot**·o·me). Incision of the ciliary body. [Gk *kyklos* circle, *temnein* to cut.]

cyclotron (si·klo·tron). An electromagnetic machine designed to accelerate charged atomic particles to velocities corresponding to several million electronvolts, by causing them to spiral between the poles of a gigantic magnet from one hollow semicircular electrode to another and back again, receiving meanwhile the high-voltage impulse of a high-frequency oscillator. Used in the production of radioactive isotopes, and for generating a stream of neutrons in the treatment of cancer. [Gk *kyklos* circle, electron.]

cyclotropia (si·klo·**tro**·pe·ah). A condition of permanent cyclophoria: in excyclotropia, the 6 to 12 o'clock meridian of the cornea leans outwards; in incyclotropia, the meridian is inclined in the opposite direction. [Gk *kyklos* circle *trepein* to turn.]

cyclotus (si·**klo**·tus). A monster in which the ears are fused beneath the skull. [Gk *kyklos* circle, *ous* ear.]

Cycrimine (si·**krim**·een). BP Commission approved name for 1-cyclopentyl-1-phenyl-3-piperidinopropan-1-ol; it is used in the treatment of Parkinson's syndrome.

Cydonia BPC 1949 (si·**do**·ne·ah). Cydoniae semen; quince; quince seeds: the seeds of the quince tree *Cydonia oblongata* Mill. (family Rosaceae), cultivated in temperate Europe and South Africa. They contain about 20 per cent of mucilage and are used as a demulcent, also, in the form of a mucilage, as a suspending agent for toilet preparations. [Gk *kydonion.*]

cydonin (si·**do**·nin). $C_{18}H_{28}O_{14}$, the mucilaginous substance in quince seeds used as an emulsifying agent in the manufacture of toilet preparations and hair creams.

cyema (si·e·mah). The fetus *in utero* from the moment of fertilization of the ovum until birth has taken place. [Gk *kyema* fetus.]

cyematocardia (si·e·mat·o·**kar**′·de·ah). Rhythm of the heart beat as heard in the fetus. [Gk *kyema* fetus, *kardia* heart.]

cyemology (si·e·**mol**·o·je). Embryology. [Gk *kyema* fetus, *logos* science.]

cyesiognosis (si·e·se·og·**no'**·sis). Diagnosis of pregnancy. [Gk *kyesis* pregnancy, *gnosis* knowledge.]

cyesiology (si·e·se·**ol'**·o·je). That branch of medical science which is concerned with pregnancy. [Gk *kyesis* pregnancy, *logos* science.]

cyesis (si·e·sis). Pregnancy. [Gk *kyesis*.]

cyesoedema (si·e·se·**de'**·mah). The appearance of bloating or slight local oedema that is to be noted in some women during pregnancy: the face particularly is affected. [Gk *kyesis* pregnancy, oedema.]

cyestein, cyesthein (si·**es**·te·in, si·**es**·the·in). A thin scum which sometimes forms on urine which has been allowed to stand for some hours. It was formerly regarded as a sign of pregnancy. [Gk *kyesis* pregnancy, *esthes* garment.]

cyetic (si·e·tik). Having reference to or occurring during pregnancy. [Gk *kyesis* pregnancy.]

cylicotomy (sil·ik·**ot**·o·me). An obsolete operation for glaucoma, consisting of division of the ciliary body. [ciliary body, Gk *temnein* to cut.]

cylinder (**sil**·in·der). 1. A solid body having a rectangular or square longitudinal section and a circular transverse section. 2. A cylindrical lens. *See* LENS. 3. Any object, e.g. a cast, roughly cylindrical in shape. **Cross cylinder, Crossed cylinders.** An instrument used for determining the amount and axis of astigmatism, consisting of cylinders of equal strength placed at right angles to each other. **Gas cylinder.** A metal container holding a gas or mixture of gases under pressure, e.g. oxygen, nitrous oxide, carbon dioxide. **Terminal cylinder.** Organ of Ruffini; a cylindrical brush-like structure composed of the terminal branches of a sensory nerve fibre in the skin. **Urinary cylinder.** Urinary cast. *See* CAST. [Gk *kylindros*.]

See also: KUELZ, RUFFINI.

cylindrarthrosis (sil·in·drar·**thro'**·sis). A joint the articular surfaces of which are approximately cylindrical. [cylinder, Gk *arthron* joint.]

cylindraxile (sil·in·**drax**·ile). An axon. [cylinder, axle.]

cylindrical, cylindriform (sil·**in**·drik·al, sil·**in**·dre·form). Shaped like or having the properties of a cylinder.

cylindro-adenoma (**sil**·in·dro·ad·en·**o'**·mah). A neoplasm composed of the degenerated cells of an adenoma and containing collections of hyaline matter in the form of cylinders.

cylindrocellular (**sil**·in·dro·**sel'**·ew·lar). Relating to, containing, or composed of cylindrical cells.

cylindrodendrite (**sil**·in·dro·**den'**·drite). Paraxon; a collateral branch of the axon of a nerve cell which is given off at a right angle. [cylinder, Gk *dendron* tree.]

cylindroid (**sil**·in·droid). A body of cylindrical shape but with elliptical ends. The term is applied to the false cast found occasionally in urine deposits, distinguished from true casts by its extremities, which are usually tapering, its variations in width along its length, and sometimes by the presence of twists and bends. [Gk *kylindros* cylinder, *eidos* form.]

cylindroma (sil·in·**dro**·mah). A perithelioma or endothelioma with a hyaline supporting stroma. **Dermal cylindroma.** A tumour of sweat gland origin usually on the scalp and consisting of multiple nodules. [Gk *kylindros* cylinder, *-oma* tumour.]

cylindrosarcoma (**sil**·in·dro·sar·**ko'**·mah). A sarcoma in which there is hyaline degeneration, as in a cylindroma.

cylindruria (sil·in·**drewr**·e·ah). The presence of cylindroids or hyaline tube casts in the urine.

cyllosis (sil·o·sis). 1. Club-foot. 2. Any deformity of the leg or foot. [Gk *kyllos* lame.]

cyllosoma, cyllosomus (sil·o·**so**·mah, sil·o·**so**·mus). A variety of monster of the class Coelosoma, characterized by lateral eventration chiefly of the lower part of the abdomen and underdevelopment of the leg on the same side. In some cases the leg is entirely absent. [Gk *kyllos* lame, *soma* body.]

cymarin (**si**·mar·in). $C_{30}H_{44}O_9$, a glycoside obtained by the partial hydrolysis of K-strophanthin-β from the seeds of *Strophanthus kombé*. It is itself hydrolysed to strophanthidin and the sugar, cymarose.

cymarose (**si**·mar·oze). Methyl-digitoxose. $CH_3(CHOH)_2C(CH_3)OHCH_2CHO$. A desoxyhexose which occurs as a sugar unit in cardiac glycosides of *Strophanthus* and *Apocynum* species.

cymba conchae [NA] (**sim**·bah **kon**·ke). The upper smaller part of the concha of the auricle. [Gk *kymbe* boat, concha.]

cymbiform (**sim**·be·form). A biological term meaning boat-shaped. [Gk *kymbe* boat, form.]

cymbocephalia (**sim**·bo·kef·**a'**·le·ah). The condition of having a skull hollowed out in boat or bowl shape. [Gk *kymbe* boat, *kephale* head.]

cymbocephalic, cymbocephalous (**sim**·bo·kef·**al'**·ik, sim·bo·**kef**·al·us). Having a boat-shaped or bowl-shaped skull, depressed in the middle of the upper surface. [see prec.]

cymbocephaly (sim·bo·**kef**·al·e). Cymbocephalia.

cymene (**si**·meen). Isopropyl *p*-methylbenzene, $CH_3C_6H_4CH(CH_3)_2$. A liquid hydrocarbon with a pleasant odour, found in the oils of caraway, eucalyptus, cumin and thyme; it can be prepared from camphor and turpentine. It is closely related to the terpenes.

cymenyl (**si**·men·il). The monovalent radical $CH_3C_6H_3CH(CH_3)_2$–, derived from cymene, which enters into combination to form phenols and sulphonic acids.

cymograph (**si**·mo·graf). Kymograph.

cymol (**si**·mol). Cymene alcohol, $CH_3C_6H_3(OH)CH_2(CH_3)_2$. A methyl isopropyl phenol isomeric with thymol and carvacrol.

cymyl (**si**·mil). Cymenyl.

cynanche (si·**nang**·ke). Any severe affection of tonsils, throat or windpipe, with inflammation and swelling, difficulty of breathing and swallowing, and a sensation as of threatening suffocation. The term is not now in general use. **Cynanche dysarthritica.** A sore-throat which accompanies an attack of arthritis, and may go on to abscess formation. **Cynanche maligna.** A form of acute septic pharyngitis with gangrene of the throat: the exciting cause is usually streptococcal. **Cynanche sublingualis.** An acute inflammation of the submaxillary connective tissue. **Cynanche suffocativa.** Any acute affection of the throat which causes croup. **Cynanche tonsillaris.** Peritonsillar abscess. *See* ABSCESS. [Gk *kyon* dog, *agchein* to choke.]

cynanthropia, cynanthropy (si·nan·**thro**·pe·ah, si·**nan**·thro·pe). A form of delusional insanity in which the patient believes himself to be changed into a dog and imitates a dog's voice and behaviour. [Gk *kynos* dog, *anthropos* man.]

cynic (**sin**·ik). 1. Having the characteristics or qualities of a snarling dog. 2. Having the grinning expression produced by risus sardonicus. [Gk *kynos* dog.]

Cynictis penicillinata (sin·**ik**·tis pen·is·**il**·in·**a'**·tah). The meercat. It may transmit rabies. [Gk *kynos* dog, *iktis* weasel, L *penicillus* paint-brush.]

cynocephalic, cynocephalous (si·no·kef·**al'**·ik, si·no·**kef**·al·us). Having the head or face shaped like that of a dog. [see foll].

cynocephalus (si·no·**kef**·al·us). 1. A baboon that can be infected with *Trypanosoma gambiense*. 2. A monster fetus with a head resembling that of a dog. [Gk *kynos* dog, *kephale* head.]

cynodont (si·no·dont). A canine tooth. *See* TOOTH. [Gk *kynos* dog, *odous* tooth.]

cynolyssa (si·no·**lis**·ah). Rabies. [Gk *kynos* dog, *lyssa* frenzy.]

Cynomolgus (si·no·**mol**·gus). A genus of monkey of which some species are susceptible to yaws and others harbour a plasmodium. [Gk *kynos* dog, *molgos* skin.]

Cynomyia (si·no·**mi**·e·ah). A genus of blow flies (Calliphoridae) of the American continent. The several species usually lay on decaying flesh, but larvae have been recorded from wounds. [Gk *kynos* dog, *myia* a fly.]

Cynomys (si·no·mis). A genus of rodents, the prairie dogs, several species of which have been responsible for outbreaks of sylvatic plague in Western USA. [Gk *kynos* dog, *mys* mouse.]

cynophobia (si·no·**fo**·be·ah). 1. Morbid dread of dogs. 2. Pseudorabies. [Gk *kynos* dog, phobia.]

cynorexia (si·no·**rex**·e·ah). Bulimia; perpetual and voracious appetite for food in large quantities, as a result of increased hunger sense, to a morbid degree [Gk *kynos* dog, *orexis* appetite.]

cyogenic (si·o·**jen**·ik). Giving rise to a state of pregnancy. [Gk *kyos* fetus, *genein* to produce.]

Cyon, Elie de (b. 1843). St. Petersburg (Leningrad) physiologist.

Cyon's experiment. The demonstration of the stronger contraction of a muscle obtained by stimulation of its intact anterior nerve root than that of the peripheral end of the cut motor nerve.

Cyon's nerve. A cervical cardiac branch of the vagus nerve described as arising from the superior laryngeal nerve.

cyophoria (si·o·**for**·e·ah). The state of pregnancy. [Gk *kyos* fetus, *pherein* to bear.]

cyophoric (si·o·**for**·ik). Having reference to pregnancy or child-bearing. [see prec.]

cyotrophy (si·**ot**·rof·e). Fetal nutrition; a term which covers all aspects of supply and use of nourishment of the unborn child. [Gk *kyos* fetus, *trophe* nutrition.]

Cypenamine (si·**pen**·am·een). BP Commission approved name for 2-phenylcyclopentylamine; an antidepressant.

cyphoscoliosis (**si**·fo·sko·le·**o**'·sis). Kyphoscoliosis.

cyphosis (si·**fo**·sis). Kyphosis.

cyphotic (si·**fot**·ik). Kyphotic.

Cyprenorphine (si·pren·**or**·feen). BP Commission approved name for *N*-cyclopropylmethyl-19-methylnorovinol; a narcotic antagonist.

cyprian (**sip**·re·an). 1. A term applied to any substance containing copper. [Island of *Cyprus*, early source of copper.] 2. A courtesan. Aphrodite. [Gk *Kypris* Aphrodite.]

cypridology (sip·rid·**ol**·o·je). Venereology. [Gk *Kypris* Aphrodite, *logos* science.]

cypridopathy (sip·rid·**op**·ath·e). Any venereal disease. [Gk *Kypris* Aphrodite, *pathos* suffering.]

cypridophobia (**sip**·rid·o·**fo**'·be·ah). 1. Morbid fear of coitus. 2. Excessive and morbid fear of contracting venereal disease. 3. An erroneous morbid belief on the part of an individual that he is suffering from some venereal disease. [Gk *Kypris* Aphrodite, phobia.]

cypriphobia (sip·re·**fo**·be·ah). Cypridophobia, 1st def.

Cyproheptadine (si·pro·**hep**·tad·een). BP Commission approved name for 4-(1,2:5,6-dibenzocycloheptatrienylidene)-1-methylpiperidine. **Cyproheptadine Hydrochloride BP 1973.** The hydrochloride sesquihydrate; an antihistamine.

Cyproterone (si·**pro**·ter·one). BP Commission approved name for 6-chloro-17α-hydroxy-1α,2α-methylenepregna-4,6-diene-3,20-dione; a steroid with anti-androgenic properties which inactivates epididymal function, thus destroying sperm mobility and lability in small doses though not affecting other accessory genital glands, spermatogenesis and libido. In large doses it is used in the management of aberrant and increased male libido.

Cyriax, James Henry. London physician.

Cyriax's syndrome. Pain in the chest due to "slipping" or overlapping ribs.

cyrtocephalus (ser·to·**kef**·al·us). An individual with an abnormally short head. [Gk *kyrtos* curved, *kephale* head.]

cyrtocoryphus (ser·to·**kor**·e·fus). In craniometry, a term descriptive of a skull the parietal angle of which is between 122 and 132 degrees (Lissauer). [Gk *kyrtos* curved, *koryphe* crown of head.]

cyrtograph (**ser**·to·graf). A cyrtometer which records the movements of the chest wall in respiration. [Gk *kyrtos* curved, *graphein* to record.]

cyrtoid (**ser**·toid). Curved like a hump. [Gk *kyrtos* curved, *eidos* form.]

cyrtometer (ser·**tom**·et·er). An instrument for measuring the curves of the body and its curved surfaces, especially the chest. The procedure is known as *cyrtometry.* [Gk *kyrtos* curved, meter.]

cyrtometopus (**ser**·to·met·**o**'·pus). In craniometry, a term descriptive of a skull of which the angle formed by the lines extending from the nasion to the metopion and from the metopion to the bregma is between 120 and 135.5 degrees. [Gk *kyrtos* curved, *metopon* forehead.]

cyrtometry (ser·**tom**·et·re). The measurement of the curvature of surfaces, e.g. of the chest, by the use of the cyrtometer.

cyrtosis (ser·**to**·sis). 1. Curvature of the bones. 2. Kyphosis. [Gk *kyrtos* bent.]

cyrturanus (ser·tew·**ra**·nus). In craniometry, a term descriptive of a skull of which the angle of the hard palate is between 132 and 147.5 degrees (Lissauer). [Gk *kyrtos* curved, *ouranos* roof of mouth.]

cyst (sist). 1. A cavity lined by a well-defined epithelium, fibrous tissue, or degenerating, inflamed or neoplastic tissue. 2. A parasitic cyst; a stage, usually the resting stage, in the life cycle of a protozoal or helminthic parasite, which may occur within or outside the body of a host. **Air cyst.** A gas-containing cavity within the lungs or the intestinal wall. **Allantoic cyst.** A dilated portion of the persistent allantois. **Alveolodental cyst.** A cyst arising within the alveolus and derived from an embryonic tooth remnant. **Amoebic cyst.** 1. *General:* the cystic stage of an amoeba. 2. *Special:* the cystic, infective stage of *Entamoeba histolytica.* **Aneurysmal bone cyst.** A vascular bone cyst usually eccentrically placed. **Cyst of the anterior lingual glands.** Cyst of the glands of Blandin and Nuhn, rare cyst resulting from obstruction to the duct of one of the anterior lingual glands situated beneath the anterior part of the tongue. **Apoplectic cyst.** A cavity arising within a cerebral haemorrhage as the result of absorption of part of the blood clot. **Arachnoid cyst.** A cyst due to adhesions obstructing the pia-arachnoid space. **Atheromatous cyst.** A variety of sebaceous cyst. **Bile cyst.** A dilatation of a large bile duct as the result of congenital malformation or an infection. **Blood cyst.** A cavity arising from softening and absorption of a blood clot. **Blue-dome cyst.** A cystic dilatation of a mammary duct into which bleeding has occurred. **Bone cyst.** Osteitis fibrosa cystica. **Branchial cyst, Branchial-cleft cyst, Branchiogenetic cyst, Branchiogenous cyst.** A cyst derived from a branchial remnant in the neck. **Cyst of the broad ligament.** A cyst arising from the peritoneum, or an embryonic remnant with the broad ligament of the uterus. **Bursal cyst.** A distended bursa. **Butter cyst.** Softening of fat necrosis. **Cervical cyst.** Nabothian cyst (see below). **Chocolate cyst.** A cyst occurring in endometriosis. **Choledochus cyst.** Cystic dilatation of the common bile duct. **Chyle cyst.** A cystic dilatation of chyle-containing lymphatics within the mesentery. **Ciliated epithelial cyst.** A cyst arising from ciliated epithelium, such as that in a bronchus. **Coli cyst.** The cystic stage of *Entamoeba coli.* **Colloid cyst.** 1. A follicle of the thyroid gland greatly distended with colloid secretion. 2. A cyst of the 3rd ventricle leading to hydrocephalus; derived from paraphysis. **Compound cyst.** Multilocular cyst (see below). **Conjunctival cyst.** A cyst formed by obstruction of a conjunctival gland, or downgrowth or implantation of the epithelium. **Coronodental cyst.** Alveolodental cyst (see above). **Corpus-luteum cyst.** Excessive distension of a corpus luteum by its contents. **Cowperian cyst.** A cyst of a bulbo-urethral gland. **Craniobuccal cyst.** A cyst arising from Rathke's pouch. **Cutaneous cyst, Cuticular cyst.** A cyst arising from skin or its derivatives, such as the sebaceous glands. **Daughter cyst.** A first derivative of a hydatid cyst. **Degeneration cyst.** A cavity formed within normal or neoplastic tissue through softening and degeneration. **Dental cyst.** 1. Any alveolodental cyst (see above). 2. A cyst occurring in the alveolus of the jaw, formed by the proliferation and breaking down of the debris of Malassez in the periodontal membrane of an infected dead tooth; a periodontal cyst. **Dentigerous cyst.** 1. A cyst arising from some pathological change in the root of the tooth. 2. A cyst occurring in the alveolus of the jaw that contains part of an unerupted tooth, usually in the crown. **Dermoid cyst.** A cyst resulting from profound embryonic disturbance, usually in the skin or deep midline structures. **Development cyst.** A cyst of the dermoid or epidermal type. **Dilatation cyst, Distension cyst.** A cyst caused by dilatation of a duct of a gland or of the gland cavity. **Echinococcus cyst.** Hydatid cyst (see below). **Endometrial cyst.** A neoplastic cyst of the endometrium, as in endometriosis; the term is also applied to a cyst arising from distension of endometrial glands. **Endothelial cyst.** A microscopic cyst arising from the lining cells of serous membranes such as the pericardium or pleura. **Enteric cyst.** A cyst arising in the wall of the small intestine. **Ependymal cyst.** A cyst arising within a ventricle of the brain because of ependymal adhesions or abnormalities. **Epidermal cyst, Epidermoid cyst.** A cyst lined by epidermis resulting either *congenitally*, from sequestration of epidermis during the course of development, e.g. at the outer angle of the orbit, or *acquired* from downward growth of the skin surface along a sinus leading to a granulation-tissue-lined cavity. **Epithelial cyst.** A general term for cysts arising from and lined by epithelium of any kind. **Eruption cyst.** A cyst which forms in the soft tissues overlying an erupting tooth. **False cyst.** A cyst produced by softening and absorption within a pathological tissue, as opposed to a cyst lined by epithelium. **Fissural intra-alveolar cyst.** Globulomaxillary cyst (see below). **Flagellate cyst.** The cystic stage of an intestinal flagellate. **Follicular cyst.** An ovarian cyst derived from graafian follicles. **Gartnerian cyst.** A cystic dilatation of Gartner's duct. **Gas cyst.** Air cyst (see above). **Giardia cyst.** The cystic stage of the intestinal flagellate, *Giardia intestinalis.* **Globulomaxillary cyst.** A cyst produced by the proliferation and degeneration of epithelial cells included at the junction of the globular and maxillary processes. It lies in the alveolus between the roots of the lateral incisor and the canine teeth. **Granddaughter cyst.** The offspring of daughter hydatid cysts. **Haemorrhagic cyst.** Blood cyst (see above). **Histolytica cyst.** The cystic, infective stage of *Entamoeba histolytica.* **Hydatid cyst.** The encysted stage in the tissues, usually in the liver, of man (and also of sheep and cattle) of the tapeworm, *Echinococcus granulosus* (see DISEASE, HYDATID). **Hypophyseal cyst.** Rathke's cyst. **"I" cyst.** Iodamoeba cyst. **Implantation cyst.** Epidermal cyst (see above). **Incisive-canal cyst.** Nasopalatine cyst (see below). **Inclusion cyst.** Epidermal cyst (see above). **Intra-epithelial cyst.** A cavity formed by displacement of epithelium by fluid. **Intra-ligamentous cyst.** A bursal or fascial cyst. **Involution cyst.** Cystic distension of milk ducts after lactation has ceased, or after hormonal stimulation of the breast. **Iodamoeba cyst, Iodine cyst.** The cystic stage of the intestinal parasite, *Iodamoeba bütschlii,* which contains a prominent iodine-staining vacuole. **Lacteal cyst.** Chyle cyst (see above). **Lamblia cyst.** The cystic stage of the intestinal flagellate, *Giardia intestinalis* (previously called *Lamblia intestinalis).* **Lutein cyst.** Corpus-luteum cyst (see above). **Median-maxillary cyst.** A cyst arising in the midline of the maxilla. **Meibomian cyst.** A cystic distension of a meibomian gland due to obstruction of its duct. **Milk cyst.** A cyst resulting from obstruction of the lactiferous sinus or of a milk duct. **Morgagnian cyst.** A cyst of the hydatid of Morgagni attached to the testis. **Mother cyst.** Hydatid cyst (see above). **Mucoid cyst, Mucous cyst.** A cyst formed either by the distension of a mucous gland with mucus or, more commonly, by the extravasation of mucus into the interstitial tissues and the formation of an adventitious fibrous tissue wall. **Multilocular cyst.** A general term applied to any cyst with multiple compartments. **Myxoid cyst.** A cyst containing mucoid material due to degeneration of the connective tissue, usually near a finger joint, particularly the distal one. **Nabothian cyst.** A mucous cyst of the cervix of the uterus. **Naevoid cyst.** A vascular cyst. **Nasolabial cyst.** A cyst formed external to the bone by the sequestration and proliferation of epithelium at the junction of the globular, lateral nasal, and maxillary processes; naso-extra-alveolar cyst. **Nasopalatine cyst.** A rounded or heart-shaped cyst resulting from the proliferation and breaking down of epithelium contained in the incisive canal in the midline of the maxilla. **Necrotic cyst.** A cavity formed in the midst of dead tissue through absorption of the softened central tissue. **Neural cyst.** A congenital cyst of the neural canal. **Odontogenic cyst.** A cyst derived from epithelial remnants of the tooth-forming structures; the types are primoidral cyst, eruption cyst, dental cyst, and dentigerous cyst. **Oil cyst.** Butter cyst (see above). **Oöphoritic cyst.** Ovarian cyst (see following). **Ovarian cyst.** Cystic enlargement of the ovary. This may be a true tumour or due to disordered function. **Pancreatic cyst.** A cyst arising within or in close proximity to the pancreas. **Paradental cyst.** A form of alveolodental cyst (see above). **Paranephric cyst.** A cyst caused by inflammation of the tissues close to the kidneys. **Paraphysial cyst.** A cavity arising within the paraphysis of long bones: a form of osteitis fibrosa cystica. **Parasitic cyst.** A cyst which is either a stage in the life history of a parasite, or the result of parasitic activity in a tissue. **Parent cyst.** Hydatid cyst (see above). **Paröophoritic cyst.** A congenital cyst occurring in close proximity to the ovary. **Pearl cyst.** A solid, or cystic, greyish-white tumour found in the iris or angle of the anterior chamber of the eye. It always follows perforating injury, and is a form of implantation cyst, being made up of epithelial cells, often found around an implanted eyelash. **Periodontal cyst.** A variety of alveolodental cyst. **Periosteal cyst.** A cyst of the normal or inflamed periosteum. **Piliferous cyst, Pilocystic cyst, Pilonidal cyst, Pilous cyst.** 1. A cyst containing hairs. In the sacrococcygeal region it is not a true cyst but an infective granuloma around hairs acting as foreign bodies. 2. A dermoid cyst, e.g. a teratomatous cyst of the ovary in which the hairs are derived from the skin of the teratomatous element. **Primordial cyst.** A cyst found in the alveolus usually in the mandibular third molar region, formed by degeneration of the cells of the enamel organ prior to tooth formation. **Proliferous cyst, Proligerous cyst.** A cyst produced by proliferation of the lining cells of a duct, as in the breast. **Pyelogenic renal cyst.** A renal cyst in open communication with the renal pelvis, so as to resemble a calyceal diverticulum. The aetiology of the cyst is unknown, but it occurs in the absence of any inflammatory or ulcerative lesion. **Radicular cyst, Radiculodental cyst.** Root cyst (see below). **Renal cyst.** A cyst resulting from distension of the renal tubules. **Residual cyst.** A dental cyst which has continued to grow after the tooth on which it formed has been extracted. **Retention cyst.** A general term applied to all cysts formed by the abnormal retention of glandular secretions. **Retinal cyst.** Retinoschisis. **Root cyst.** A cyst attached to the root of a tooth. **Sanguineous cyst.** Blood cyst (see above). **Sebaceous cyst.** A cyst derived from a sebaceous gland through obstruction of its duct. **Secretory cyst.** Retention cyst (see above). **Seminal cyst.** A retention cyst involving seminal ducts in the testis or epididymis. **Sequestration cyst.** An epidermoid or dermoid cyst. **Serous cyst.** A cystic derivative of a serous membrane such as the pleura or pericardium. **Softening cyst.** Necrotic cyst (see above). **Solitary cyst of bone.** A simple cyst lined by a fibrous membrane and filled with fluid occurring in the metaphysis of long bones, usually in children. **Spring-water cyst.** A cyst of the mediastinum which contains a clear water-like fluid. **Steatoid cyst.** A cyst filled with sebaceous matter and cell debris which usually becomes pustular later, as in acne vulgaris. **Sterile cyst.** A cyst which is not infected. **Sublingual cyst.** A ranula. **Subsellar cyst.** A pituitary or pituitary-derivative cyst, situated in the region of the sella turcica. **Subsynovial cyst.** A cyst arising beneath the synovial membrane of a joint, usually from the escape of synovial fluid. **Suprasellar syst.** Craniopharyngioma. **Synovial cyst.** A localized collection of synovial fluid within an inflamed joint; a herniation of synovial membrane. **Tarsal cyst.** 1. A cyst of a tarsal bone. 2. A meibomian cyst (see above). **Thecal cyst, Thecalutein cyst.** A variety of ovarian cyst. **Thyroglossal cyst.** A cyst arising from the thyroglossal duct in the neck. **Thyrolingual cyst.** A cyst arising from the terminal portion of the thyroglossal duct in the tongue. **Traumatic bone cyst.** Blood cyst (see above). **True cyst.** A cyst lined with epithelium. **Tubo-ovarian cyst.** A cyst formed by adhesion of the fimbriated end of a tube and the ovary. **Umbilical cyst.** A congenital cyst arising from some component of the umbilicus. **Unicameral bone cyst.** A single cyst, usually situated towards one end of a long bone. **Unilocular cyst.** A cyst composed of a single compartment. **Urachal cyst.** A cyst derived from the urachus. **Urinary cyst.** Renal cyst (see above). **Vitelline macular cyst.** A form of congenital macular degeneration which has the ophthalmoscopic appearance of an egg yolk. **Vitello-intestinal cyst.** A congenital cyst derived from remnants of the yolk sac. **Wolffian cyst.** A cyst of the wolffian duct. [Gk *kytis* bag.]

See also: BAKER, BLANDIN, BLESSIG, COWPER, GARTNER, KOBELT, MEIBOM, MORGAGNI, NABOTH, NUHN, RATHKE, SAMPSON.

cyst-passer (**sist**·pah·ser). One who passes cysts. Many persons harbour *Entamoeba histolytica* but may suffer no pathological lesions; such persons pass cysts in their faeces which are probably a source of infection to others.

cystadenocarcinoma (sist·**ad**·en·o·kar·sin·**o'**·mah). A cancer of glandular origin which forms many cysts as it grows; cystic adenocarcinoma.

cystadenoma (**sist**·ad·en·**o'**·mah). Any adenoma in which fluid has accumulated in the spaces to form cysts. **Cystadenoma adamantinum.** Adamantinoma. **Apocrine cystadenoma.** A skin tumour, usually near the outer canthus of the eye, produced by adenomatous cystic proliferation of apocrine glands. **Giant cystadenoma.** An innocent, rapidly growing tumour of the breast which may attain a large size and cause pressure necrosis of the overlying skin. **Papillary cystadenoma lymphomatosum.** Adenolymphoma; a rare innocent tumour of salivary gland or its embryonic precursor. **Cystadenoma partim simplex partim papilliferum.** An adenoma composed of cysts and tiny projections from the cyst walls, with serous fluid. **Proliferous cystadenoma.** Giant cystadenoma (see above). **Pseudomucinous cystadenoma.** A cystadenoma in which the spaces contain mostly mucin. **Serous cystadenoma.** Adenoma of the ovary which forms many cysts containing serous fluid.

cystadenosarcoma (**sist**·ad·en·o·sar·**ko'**·mah). A cystadenoma in which there are sarcomatous elements.

cystalgia (sist·**al**·je·ah) Pain in the urinary bladder. [Gk *kystis* bag, *algos* pain.]

cystanastrophe (sist·an·**as**·tro·fe). Inversion of the urinary bladder. [Gk *kystis* bag, *anastrophe* a turning back.]

cystathioninaemia (sist·ah·**thi**·o·neen·**e'**·me·ah). A condition occurring with cystathioninuria in some persons; it is inherited in autosomal recessive fashion but its clinical significance is uncertain. [cystathionine, Gk *haima* blood.]

cystathionine (sist·ah·**thi**·o·neen). A sulphur-containing amino acid formed by the condensation of homocysteine and serine. It is formed in the body as an intermediate compound in the conversion of methionine to cysteine.

cystathioninuria (sist·ah·**thi**·o·neen·**ewr**·e·ah). Urinary excretion of cystathionine, an inherited condition found in patients with neural or hepatic diseases. [cystathionine, Gk *ouron* urine.]

cystatrophia (sist·at·**ro**·fe·ah). Atrophy of the urinary bladder. [Gk *kystis* bag, atrophy.]

cystauchenitis (**sist**·aw·ken·**i'**·tis). A condition of inflammation of the neck of the urinary bladder. [Gk *kystis* bag, *auchen* neck, *-itis* inflammation.]

cystauchenotomy (**sist**·aw·ken·**ot'**·o·me). Surgical incision into the neck of the urinary bladder; cystotrachelotomy [Gk *kystis* bag, *auchen* neck, *temnein* to cut.]

cystauxe (sist·**aux**·e). Enlargement or thickening of the urinary bladder. [Gk *kystis* bag, *auxe* increase.]

cystectasia, cystectasy (sist·ek·**ta**·ze·ah, sist·**ek**·tas·e). 1. Surgical dilatation of the neck of the urinary bladder, with or without stretching of the prostatic part of the urethra or slitting of the membranous part of the urethra. The procedure was undertaken for the extraction of stone, but is now obsolete. 2. Dilatation of the urinary bladder; it may be carried out under anaesthesia in the treatment of interstitial cystitis. [Gk *kystis* bladder, *ektasis* extension.]

cystectomy (sist·**ek**·to·me). Removal in part (*partial cystectomy*) or whole (*total cystectomy*) of the urinary bladder. [Gk *kystis* bag, *ektome* a cutting out.]

cysteine (**sis**·te·een). $SHCH_2CH(NH_2)COOH$, one of 2 important and closely related amino acids derived from propionic acid, the other being cystine. Two molecules of cysteine are produced by the reduction of 1 molecule of cystine. It is a constituent of many proteins, and forms a valuable source of sulphur in the metabolism. **Methyl Cysteine.** BP Commission approved name for methyl-α-amino-β-mercaptopropionate; a nasal decongestant.

cystelcosis (sist·el·**ko**·sis) Ulceration of the urinary bladder. [Gk *kystis* bag, *elkosis* ulceration.]

cystencephalus (sist·en·**kef**·al·us). A monster with internal hydrocephaly so that the skull is almost entirely filled by a sac distended with fluid. [Gk *kystis* bag, *egkephalos* brain.]

cystendesis (sist·en·**de**·sis). The suturing of a wound in the urinary bladder or gall bladder. [Gk *kystis* bag, *endesis* a binding together.]

cysterethism (sist·**er**·e·thizm). Irritability of the urinary bladder. [Gk *kystis* bag, *erethismos* irritation.]

cysthypersarcosis (**sist**·hi·per·sar·**ko'**·sis). Abnormal thickening of the muscular walls of the urinary bladder. [Gk *kystis* bag, hypersarcosis.]

cystic (**sist**·ik). 1. Referring to a cyst. 2. Referring to the urinary bladder or the gall bladder, or affecting either. 3. Giving the physical signs of elasticity and fluctuation. [Gk *kystis* bag.]

cystic artery [arteria cystica (NA)]. An artery from the right branch of the hepatic artery to the surface of the gall bladder.

cystic vein [vena cystica (NA)]. A tributary of the right branch of the portal vein, draining the gall bladder.

cysticercoid (sis·te·**ser**·koid). A larval form of tapeworms in which most of the body remains solid, the scolex being contained in a small bladder; characteristic of *Dipylidium, Hymenolepis* and other genera with invertebrate intermediate hosts. [cysticercus, Gk *eidos* form.]

cysticercosis (**sis**·te·ser·**ko'**·sis). Infestation with cysticercus. [cysticercus, Gk *-osis* condition.]

cysticercus (sis·te·**ser**·kus). A larval form of tapeworms in which there is only a single invaginated scolex and a large cyst. It is characteristic of the genus *Taenia.* Cysticercus cellulosae, the larva of *Taenia solium,* is the cause of measly pork. Cysticercus bovis, that of *Taenia saginata,* occurs in measly beef. The former also occurs in the tissues of man and causes symptoms appropriate to its location, e.g. in the brain it causes epileptic seizures. [Gk *kystis* bag, *kerkos* tail.]

cysticolithectomy (**sist**·e·ko·lith·**ek'**·to·me). The removal of gall-stones through an incision made in the cystic duct. [Gk *kystis* bag, *lithos* stone, *ektome* a cutting out.]

cysticolithotripsy (**sist**·e·ko·**lith'**·o·trip·se). The procedure of crushing a gall-stone in the cystic duct. [Gk *kystis* bag, *lithos* stone, *tribein* to crush.]

cysticorrhaphy (sist·e·**kor**·af·e). The suturing of the cystic duct. [Gk *kystis* bag, *rhaphe* suture.]

cysticotomy (sist·e·**kot**·o·me). The making of an incision into the cystic duct. [Gk *kystis* bag, *temnein* to cut.]

cystidocoeliotomy (**sist**·e·do·se·le·**ot'**·o·me). Cystidolaparotomy. [Gk *kystis* bag, coeliotomy.]

cystidolaparotomy (**sist**·e·do·lap·ar·**ot'**·o·me). Incision of the urinary bladder by way of the abdominal wall. [Gk *kystis* bag, laparotomy.]

cystidomyeloma (**sist**·e·do·mi·el·**o'**·mah). Medullary carcinoma of the urinary bladder. [Gk *kystis* bag, myeloma.]

cystidotrachelotomy (**sist**·e·do·trak·el·**ot'**·o·me). Incision into the neck of the urinary bladder; cystotrachelotomy. [Gk *kystis* bag, *trachelos* neck, *temnein* to cut.]

cystifellotomy (**sist**·e·fel·**ot'**·o·me). Cholecystotomy; the making of an incision into the gall bladder. [Gk *kystis* bag, L *fel* bile, Gk *temnein* to cut.]

cystiferous (sist·**if**·er·us). Cystigerous. [Gk *kystis* bag, L *ferre* to bear.]

cystiform (**sist**·e·form). 1. Looking like or shaped like a cyst or bladder. 2. Encysted. [Gk *kystis* bag, form.]

cystigerous (sist·**ij**·er·us). Containing or bearing a cyst or cysts. [Gk *kystis* bag, L *gerere* to bear.]

cystinaemia (sist·in·e·me·ah). The condition in which the peripheral blood contains cystine. [cystine, Gk *haima* blood.]

cystine (sis·teen). β-Dicysteine, $HOOCCH(NH_2)CH_2SSCH_2CH(NH_2)COOH$. An important amino acid occurring in the diet and one of the principal sources of sulphur for the metabolism. It takes part in the formation of the keratin of hair, and of the crystalline lens. When reduced, it yields 2 molecules of cysteine. In a rare inborn error of metabolism it is excreted in the urine, a condition known as *cystinuria.*

cystinosis (sist·in·o·sis). Cystine deposition in tissues, with amino-aciduria, hypophosphataemia and acidosis, resembling Fanconi's disease. [cystine, Gk *-osis* condition.]

cystinuria (sist·in·**ewr**·e·ah). A metabolic disorder in which cystine appears in the urine.

cystinuric (sist·in·**ewr**·ik). 1. Belonging or referring to the condition of cystinuria. 2. A person affected with cystinuria.

cystipherous (sist·**if**·er·us). Cystigerous. [Gk *kystis* bag, *pherein* to bear.]

cystirrhagia (sist·e·ra·je·ah). Cystorrhagia.

cystirrhoea (sist·e·**re**·ah). Cystorrhoea.

cystis (**sist**·is). 1. A cyst. 2. A bladder. [Gk *kystis* bag.]

cystistaxis (sist·is·**tax**·is). The oozing of blood into the urinary bladder from its mucous membrane. [Gk *kystis* bag, *staxis* a dropping.]

cystitis (sist·**i**·tis). Inflammation of the urinary bladder following injury or due to organismal infection, a foreign body (e.g. stone or indwelling catheter), or a chemical irritant. **Acute catarrhal cystitis.** The common form of cystitis characterized by frequent and painful micturition with pyuria, and often haematuria. **Allergic cystitis.** An abacterial inflammation of the bladder, of obscure aetiology. It has been suggested that the causal organism may be a virus. **Chemical cystitis.** Inflammation of the bladder as a result of instillations of a chemical irritant. **Chronic cystitis.** That which occurs when the source of the infection persists, or a cause of chronic irritation remains. The symptoms vary in severity. **Cystitis colli.** Inflammation of the neck of the urinary bladder. **Cystitis cystica.** A low form of chronic inflammation of the urinary bladder associated with the inclusion of numerous cell follicles in the submucosa of the trigone. Central cellular degeneration or the secretion of mucus leads to the translucent appearance of the cysts. **Encrusted cystitis.** A chronic inflammation of the urinary bladder associated with phosphatic deposit on the catarrhal mucous membrane. The urine is alkaline with an ammoniacal odour. **Exfoliative cystitis.** A severe form of cystitis occurring in the debilitated, and associated with the sloughing of the mucous membrane of the bladder. There is marked prostration. **Cystitis follicularis.** A chronic inflammation of the urinary bladder with hyperplasia of the submucous lymphatic follicles. **Cystitis glandularis.** A granular type of chronic inflammatory lesion of the bladder epithelium, which undergoes metaplasia with central cavitation, or, alternatively, the crypts of secreting glands become occluded and the mucinous secretion is retained. The terms *cystitis cystica* and *cystitis follicularis* are sometimes used for the same condition. **Interstitial cystitis.** Cystitis occurring on the roof of the bladder as a stellate fissured ulcer which readily bleeds when the bladder wall is stretched. There is reduction in the bladder capacity, and considerable suprapubic pain and urgency prior to voiding. **Pseudomembranous cystitis.** A condition in which a false membrane may form either from inspissated debris or in association with necrotic mucous membrane following irradiation therapy or cystodiathermy in the treatment of bladder tumours. [Gk *kystis* bag, *-itis* inflammation.]

cystitome (**sist**·e·tome). A surgical knife used in opening the capsule of the lens of the eye. [Gk *kystis* bag, *temnein* to cut.]

cystitomy (sist·**it**·o·me). Capsulotomy; the operation of incising a capsule, particularly that of the lens of the eye. [see prec.]

cysto-adenoma (**sist**·o·ad·en·**o**′·mah). Cystadenoma.

cysto-adenosarcoma (**sist**·o·ad·en·o·sar·**ko**′·mah). Cystadenosarcoma.

cystobubonocele (**sist**·o·bew·**bon**′·o·seel). Protrusion of the urinary bladder into an inguinal hernia. [Gk *kystis* bag, *boubon* groin, *kele* hernia.]

cystocarcinoma (**sist**·o·kar·sin·**o**′·mah). The presence of cysts in association with carcinoma.

cystocele (**sist**·o·seel). Hernia of the urinary bladder. [Gk *kystis* bag, *kele* hernia.]

cystochondroma (**sist**·o·kon·**dro**′·mah). A tumour in which there are elements of cystoma and chondroma.

cystochromoscopy (**sist**·o·kro·**mos**′·ko·pe). Chromocystoscopy; cystoscopy after administration of a dye such as methylene blue so that renal function and the state of the orifices of the urinary system may be determined by the evidence of the passage of the dye. [Gk *kystis* bag, *chroma* colour, *skopein* to watch.]

cystocolostomy (**sist**·o·kol·**os**′·to·me). The surgical operation of establishing permanent communication between the urinary bladder and the colon, so that urine is passed *per rectum.* [Gk *kystis* bag, colostomy.]

cystodiaphanoscopy (**sist**·o·di·ah·fan·**os**′·ko·pe). The examination of the contents of the abdomen by means of a diaphanoscope. [Gk *kystis* bag, diaphanoscopy.]

cystodiathermy (**sist**·o·di·ah·**ther**′·me). Removal of bladder tumours by means of the diathermy knife. [Gk *kystis* bag, diathermy.]

cystodynia (sist·o·**din**·e·ah). Cystalgia. [Gk *kystis* bag, *odyne* pain.]

cysto-elytroplasty (**sist**·o·el·it·ro·**plas**′·te). Plastic operation for the repair of vesicovaginal fistula or vaginal injury involving the bladder. [Gk *kystis* bag, elytroplasty.]

cysto-enterocele (sist·o·**en**·ter·o·seel). Hernia of part of the urinary bladder and intestine. [Gk *kystis* bag, *enteron* bowel, *kele* hernia.]

cysto-enterostomy (**sist**·o·en·ter·**os**′·to·me). The making of an anastomosis between a cyst and the intestine; performed as treatment of pseudocysts of the pancreas. [Gk *kystis* bag, *enteron* bowel, *stoma* mouth.]

cysto-epiplocele (**sist**·o·ep·**ip**′·lo·seel). Hernia of part of the urinary bladder and the omentum. [Gk *kystis* bag, *epiploon* omentum, *kele* hernia.]

cysto-epithelioma (**sist**·o·ep·e·the·le·**o**′·mah). An epithelioma containing fluid-filled cysts.

cystofibroma (**sist**·o·fi·**bro**′·mah). A fibroma with formation of cysts within it.

cystogastrostomy (**sist**·o·gas·**tros**′·to·me). The making of an anastomosis between a cyst and the stomach; performed as treatment of pseudocysts of the pancreas. [Gk *kystis* bag, *gaster* stomach, *stoma* mouth.]

cystogenia, cystogenesis (sist·o·**je**·ne·ah, sist·o·**jen**·es·is). The process of forming or developing cysts. [Gk *kystis* bag, *genesis* origin.]

cystogram (**sist**·o·gram). A skiagram of the urinary bladder. [Gk *kystis* bag, *gramma* a record.]

cystography (sist·**og**·raf·e). Radiographical examination of the bladder by the introduction, either through a cystoscope or urethral catheter, of a radio-opaque substance, usually sodium iodide. [Gk *kystis* bladder, *graphein* to record.]

cystoid (**sist**·oid). 1. Like a bladder or cyst. 2. A cyst-like pulpy tumour lacking a capsule or other containing membrane. 3. Made up of a number of cysts. 4. Pseudocyst. [Gk *kystis* bag, *eidos* form.]

cystolith (**sist**·o·lith). Vesical calculus. *See* CALCULUS. [Gk *kystis* bag, *lithos* stone.]

cystolithectomy (**sist**·o·lith·**ek**′·to·me). The operation of opening the urinary bladder in order to remove vesical calculus. [cystolith, Gk *ektome* a cutting out.]

cystolithiasis (**sist**·o·lith·**i**′·as·is). The presence of a calculus in the urinary bladder and the general condition associated with stones in the bladder. [Gk *kystis* bag, *lithos* stone.]

cystolithic (sist·o·**lith**·ik). Referring to vesical calculus. [see prec.]

cystolithotomy (**sist**·o·lith·**ot**′·o·me). Cystolithectomy.

cystoma (sist·o·mah). A neoplasm containing cysts, particularly with regard to the ovary. **Cystoma glandulare proliferum.** Proliferating cystoma (see below). **Mesonephric cystoma.** A cyst of the wolffian body. **Myxoid cystoma.** A proliferating ovarian cyst the inner surface of which behaves as a mucous membrane. **Parovarian cystoma.** A cyst of the parovarium; paroöphoritic cyst. **Proliferating cystoma, Cystoma proliferum papillare.** A form of cyst often found in the ovary or pancreas and of glandular origin; papillomatous growths or follicles line the inner surface of the cyst. **Cystoma serosum simplex.** A simple ovarian cyst containing serous fluid. **Simple cystoma.** A sac which contains liquid or a semisolid. **Tubo-ovarian cystoma.** A cyst derived from the oviducts and ovary. [Gk *kystis* cyst, *-oma* tumour.]

cystomatitis (sist·o·mat·i′·tis). A condition of inflammation affecting a cyst or cysts within a cystoma. [cystoma, Gk *-itis* inflammation.]

cystomatous (sist·o·mat·us). Pertaining to a cystoma.

cystomerocele (sist·o·me·ro·seel). Hernia of the urinary bladder through the femoral ring. [Gk *kystis* bag, *meros* thigh, *kele* hernia.]

cystometer (sist·om·et·er). An instrument used to measure the pressure within the urinary bladder and variations in its content. [Gk *kystis* bag, meter.]

See also: WELLS (C.A.).

cystometrogram (sist·o·met·ro·gram). A graphic record of the pressure within the urinary bladder. [cystometer, Gk *gramma* record.]

cystometrography (sist·o·met·rog′·raf·e). The making of a traced record of urinary-bladder capacity and pressure by means of a cystometer. [cystometer, Gk *graphein* to record.]

cystometry (sist·om·et·re). The study of urinary-bladder pressure and capacity by the use of a cystometer and examination of the records it traces.

cystomorphous (sist·o·mor·fus). Bladder-like or cyst-like in shape. [Gk *kystis* bag, *morphe* shape.]

cystomyoma (sist·o·mi·o′·mah). A myoma in which pseudocysts of necrotic or vascular origin have formed.

cystomyxo-adenoma (sist·o·mix·o·ad·en·o′·mah). A combined form of myxoma and adenoma with cyst-like formation.

cystomyxoma (sist·o·mix·o′·mah). Myxoma with formation of cysts.

cystonephrosis (sist·o·nef·ro′·sis). Cystic enlargement or dilatation of the kidney. [Gk *kystis* bag, *nephros* kidney.]

cystoneuralgia (sist·o·newr·al′·je·ah). Neuralgic pain in the urinary bladder. [Gk *kystis* bag, *neuron* nerve, *algos* pain.]

cystoparalysis (sist·o·par·al′·is·is). Paralysis affecting the urinary bladder. [Gk *kystis* bag, paralysis.]

cystopexia, cystopexy (sist·o·pex·e·ah, sist·o·pex·e). Surgical fixation of the urinary bladder to the wall of the abdomen as a measure for the cure of cystocele. [Gk *kystis* bag, *pexis* fixation.]

cystophorous (sist·of·or·us). Cystigerous; containing or bearing a cyst or cysts. [Gk *kystis* bag, *pherein* to carry.]

cystophotography (sist·o·fo·tog′·raf·e). Photography of the inside of the urinary bladder, used in diagnosis. [Gk *kystis* bag, photography.]

cystophthisis (sist·o·thi·sis). Tuberculosis of the urinary bladder. [Gk *kystis* bag, *phthiein* to consume.]

cystoplasty (sist·o·plas·te). Any plastic operation for repair or reconstruction of the urinary bladder. [Gk *kystis* bag, *plassein* to mould.]

cystoplegia (sist·o·ple·je·ah). Cystoparalysis. [Gk *kystis* bag, *plege* stroke.]

cystoproctostomy (sist·o·prok·tos′·to·me). The surgical establishment of a communication between the urinary bladder and the rectum. [Gk *kystis* bag, *proktos* anus, *stoma* mouth.]

cystoptosis (sist·op·to·sis). Prolapse into the urethra of a portion of the mucous coat of the urinary bladder. [Gk *kystis* bag, *ptosis* fall.]

cystopyelitis (sist·o·pi·el·i′·tis). The presence of pyelitis as a complication of cystitis.

cystopyelography (sist·o·pi·el·og′·raf·e). X-ray photography of the urinary bladder and the ureteric pelvis. [Gk kystis bag, *pyelos* pelvis, *graphein* to record.]

cystopyelonephritis (sist·o·pi·el·o·nef·ri′·tis). Inflammation of the urinary bladder, the renal pelvis and the renal parenchyma. The infection may be descending when it is haematogenous, or ascending in the presence of urinary obstruction. [Gk *kystis* bag, *pyelos* pelvis, *nephros* kidney, *-itis* inflammation.]

cystoradiography (sist·o·ra·de·og′·raf·e). X-ray photography of the urinary bladder. [Gk *kystis* bag, radiography.]

cystorectostomy (sist·o·rek·tos′·to·me). Cystoproctostomy. [Gk *kystis* bag, rectum, Gk *stoma* mouth.]

cystorrhagia (sist·o·ra·je·ah). Haemorrhage from the urinary bladder. [Gk *kystis* bag, *rhegnynein* to gush forth.]

cystorrhaphy (sist·or·af·e). The surgical suturing of a wound in the urinary bladder. [Gk *kystis* bag, *rhaphe* suture.]

cystorrhexis (sist·o·rex·is). Rupture of the urinary bladder. [Gk *kystis* bag, *rhexis* rupture.]

cystorrhoea (sist·o·re·ah). 1. Catarrh of the bladder. 2. Bleeding from the inner bladder wall. 3. Polyuria. [Gk *kystis* bag, *rhoia* flow.]

cystosarcoma (sist·o·sar·ko′·mah). Sarcoma in which cysts have formed. **Cystosarcoma phyllodes, Cystosarcoma phylloides.** Adenofibrosarcoma of the breast or of the uterus; the latter is especially found in children.

cystoschisis (sist·os·kis·is). Congenital fissure of the urinary bladder, a condition resulting from imperfect development of the organ. [Gk *kystis* bag, *schisis* division.]

cystoscirrhus (sist·o·skir·us). Scirrhus of the urinary bladder. [Gk *kystis* bag, *skirrhos* hard.]

cystosclerosis (sist·o·skler·o′·sis). Of cysts, a condition in which they have become hardened or fibrotic. [Gk *kystis* bag, *skleros* hard.]

cystoscope (sist·o·skope). A tubular instrument fitted with an electric-light bulb with which the inside of the urinary bladder may be examined. [Gk *kystis* bag, *skopein* to watch.]

See also: KIDD, MCCARTHY (J.F.).

cystoscopic (sist·o·skop·ik). Referring to cystoscopy.

cystoscopy (sist·os·ko·pe). The examining of the interior of the urinary bladder with a cystoscope. **Air cystoscopy.** Cystoscopy with the bladder full of air. **Water cystoscopy.** Cystoscopy with the bladder full of water.

cystose (sist·oze). 1. Cystomorphous. 2. Cystigerous. [Gk *kystis* bag.]

cystospasm (sist·o·spazm). Spasmodic contraction of the bladder. [Gk *kystis* bag, spasm.]

cystospermitis (sist·o·sper·mi′·tis). Inflammation of a seminal vesicle. [Gk *kystis* bag, *sperma* seed, *-itis* inflammation.]

cystostaxis (sist·o·stax·is). Cystistaxis.

cystosteatoma (sist·o·ste·at·o′·mah). Sebaceous cyst. *See* CYST. [Gk *kystis* bag, *stear* fat, *-oma* tumour.]

cystostomy (sist·os·to·me). The surgical establishment of a permanent or semipermanent opening into the urinary bladder. [Gk *kystis* bag, stoma mouth.]

cystotome (sist·o·tome). 1. An instrument with which incision may be made into the urinary bladder. 2. Cystitome. [Gk *kystis* bag, *temnein* to cut.]

cystotomy (sist·ot·o·me). Surgical incision into the urinary bladder. **Perineal cystotomy.** Cystotomy by the perineal route. **Suprapubic cystotomy.** Incision into the urinary bladder at a point immediately above the pubic symphysis. [see prec.]

cystotrachelotomy (sist·o·trak·el·ot′·o·me). Surgical incision into the neck of the urinary bladder. [Gk *kystis* bag, *trachelos* neck, *temnein* to cut.]

cysto-ureteritis (sist·o·ewr·e·ter·i′·tis). A condition of inflammation of the urinary bladder and the ureters. [Gk *kystis* bag, ureteritis.]

cysto-ureterogram (sis·to·ewr·e′·ter·o·gram). A skiagram of the urinary bladder and the ureters. [Gk *kystis* bag, ureter, Gk *gramma* record.]

cysto-ureteropyelitis (sist·o·ewr·e·ter·o·pi·el·i′·tis). Cysto-ureteropyelonephritis.

cysto-ureteropyelonephritis (sist·o·ewr·e·ter·o·pi·el·o·nef·ri′·tis).

A condition of inflammation of the urinary bladder, the ureters and their pelves. [Gk *kystis* bag, ureteropyelonephritis.]

cysto-urethritis (sist·o·ewr·eth·ri′·tis). A condition of inflammation of the urinary bladder and the urethra. [Gk *kystis* bag, urethritis.]

cysto-urethrocele (sist·o·ewr·e′·thro·seel). Prolapse of the anterior vaginal wall and bladder neck. [Gk *kystis* bladder, urethra, Gk *kele* hernia.]

cysto-urethrogram (sist·o·ewr·e′·thro·gram). A radiograph of the urinary bladder and urethra, made after intraluminal injection of a contrast medium. [Gk *kystis* bladder, urethra, Gk *gramma* record.]

cysto-urethrography (sist·o·ewr·e·throg′·raf·e). Radiography of the urinary bladder and urethra, made after intraluminal injection of a contrast medium. [Gk *kystis* bladder, urethra, Gk *graphein* to record.]

cysto-urethroscope (sist·o·ewr·e′·thro·skope). A tubular instrument with which the interior of the bladder and the posterior part of the urethra can be examined. [Gk *kystis* bag, urethra, Gk *skopein* to watch.]

cysto-urethroscopy (sist·o·ewr·e·thros′·ko·pe). Cystoscopy and urethroscopy carried out through the same instrument if a direct-vision system is used, or with a panendoscope with an oblique-lens system.

cystous (sist·us). Cystose.

cytaemia (si·te·me·ah). The condition in which extraneous cells are present in the blood. [Gk *kytos* cell, *haima* blood.]

cytagenin (si·taj·en·in). The name given to an unidentified substance in the blood said to have anti-anaemic properties.

cytamoeba (si·tam·e·bah). An amoeba present within a cell. [Gk *kytos* cell, amoeba.]

Cytarabine (si·tar·ab·een). BP Commission approved name for 1-β-D-arabinofuranosylcytosine; an antiviral agent.

cytase (si·taze). 1. Name given by Metchnikoff to complement. 2. An enzyme occurring in the seeds of various plants and having the power of rendering soluble the material of the cell wall. [Gk *kytos* cell.]

cytaster (si·tas·ter). Aster; in mitosis, the star shape taken by the arrangement of chromosomes around the equator of the cell. [Gk *kytos* cell, *aster* star.]

cyte (site). A cell; the word is rarely used by itself, but frequently as a suffix. [Gk *kytos* cell.]

cythaemolysis (si·the·mol·is·is). Haemocytolysis; destruction of blood corpuscles by dissolution. [Gk *kytos* cell, *haima* blood, *lysis* a loosing.]

cythaemolytic (si·the·mo·lit′·ik). Referring to haemocytolysis. [see prec.]

cytherean (sith·er·e·an). Venereal. **Cytherean shield.** A condom. [Gk *Kythereia* Aphrodite.]

cytheromania (sith·er·o·ma′·ne·ah). Nymphomania. [Gk *Kythereia* Aphrodite, mania.]

cytidine (si·tid·een). The nucleoside composed of cytosine and D-ribose. A component of both RNA and DNA. **Cytidine triphosphate.** The immediate precursor of cytidine residues in nucleic acids. It is involved in phospholipid synthesis through the formation of cytidine diphosphate, choline, etc.

cytisine (sit·is·een). $C_{11}H_{14}ON_2$, an alkaloid present in laburnum, *Cytisus laburnum*. It causes ganglionic block, like nicotine.

cytisism (sit·is·izm). Poisoning from eating seeds of the laburnum tree, *Cytisus laburnum*.

Cytisus (sit·is·us). A genus of plants of the family Leguminosae. **Cytisus laburnum.** The laburnum tree. **Cytisus scoparius.** A shrub indigenous to temperate Europe; the tops are used in medicine as Scoparium BPC 1949. [Gk *kytisos* a kind of clover.]

cyto-architecture (si·to·ar·ke·tek·tcher). The constructive arrangement of cells in a tissue or an organ. [Gk *kytos* cell, L *architectura* architecture.]

cytobiology (si·to·bi·ol′·o·je). The study of biology in its relation to cells. [Gk *kytos* cell, biology.]

cytobiotaxis (si·to·bi·o·tax′·is). Cytoclesis. [Gk *kytos* cell, *bios* life, *taxis* arrangement.]

cytoblast (si·to·blast). 1. A blastocyte. 2. A cell nucleus. 3. Micelle, 1st def. [Gk *kytos* cell, *blastos* germ.]

cytoblastema (si·to·blas·te′·mah). Cytoplasm (obsolete). [Gk *kytos* cell, *blastema* bud.]

cytocentrum (si·to·sen·trum). Centrosome. [Gk *kytos* cell, centre.]

cytocerastic (si·to·ser·as′·tik). Cytokerastic.

cytochemism (si·to·kem·izm). The chemical activity of living cells, e.g. their reaction to chemical agents. [Gk *kytos* cell, chemical.]

cytochemistry (si·to·kem·is·tre). That branch of biological chemistry which is concerned with the chemical activities of living cells. [Gk *kytos* cell, chemistry.]

cytochromatin (si·to·kro·mat·in). The basophilic granular material of the cytoplasm of some cells, especially the Nissl substance of a nerve cell, which resembles in some of its staining reactions the chromatin of the nucleus. [Gk *kystos* cell, chromatin.]

cytochrome (si·to·krome). One of a group of proteins involved in electron transport systems. All contain haem groups and iron, and alternate between the ferrous and ferric states. *Cytochromes a, b and c* are involved in the mitochondrial oxidative system which is coupled to ATP synthesis. *Cytochrome oxidase* is the terminal acceptor of the mitochondrial oxidative system which is reoxidized by oxygen. *Cytochromes b_5 and P450* are associated with extramitochondrial electron transport in the liver, involved with "mixed function oxidation" reactions and in drug detoxication. [Gk *kytos* cell, *chroma* colour.]

cytochylema (si·to·ki·le′·mah). Hyaloplasm. [Gk *kytos* cell, *chylos* juice.]

cytocidal (si·to·si·dal). Descriptive of any agent that causes the death of cells. [Gk *kytos* cell, L *caedere* to kill.]

cytocide (si·to·side). Any agent that causes the death of cells. [see prec.]

cytocinesis (si·to·sin·e′·sis). Cytokinesis.

cytoclasis (si·tok·las·is). 1. The destruction or fragmentation of living cells. 2. Cell necrosis. [Gk *kytos* cell, *klasis* a breaking.]

cytoclastic (si·to·klas·tik). Breaking up or destroying cells. [see prec.]

cytoclesis (si·to·kle·sis). The influence exerted on some living cells by other cells. [Gk *kytos* cell, *klesis* a calling for.]

cytocyst (si·to·sist). A host cell so distended by multiplying protozoal parasites, e.g. merozoites of malaria, that a mere cyst-like cell outline remains. [Gk *kytos* cell, *kystis* bag.]

cytode (si·tode). 1. A non-nucleated cell, e.g. an erythrocyte. 2. A mass of protoplasm. [Gk *kytos* cell, *eidos* form.]

cytodendrite (si·to·den·drite). Any dendrite given off directly from the body of a nerve cell and carrying impulses towards the cell body. Cf. AXODENDRITE. [Gk *kytos* cell, *dendron* tree.]

cytodesma (si·to·dez·mah). A name for the intercellular substance which holds animal cells together. [Gk *kytos* cell, *desmos* band.]

cytodiaeresis (si·to·di·er′·es·is). Mitosis. [Gk *kytos* cell, *diairesis* separation.]

cytodiagnosis (si·to·di·ag·no′·sis). The study of cells contained in an exudate or transudate in order to determine the nature of any pathological process. It is used in gynaecology (*cervical cytodiagnosis*) and in thoracic medicine (*bronchial cytodiagnosis*), also in bullous skin diseases and in vesicular virus conditions. **Exfoliative cytodiagnosis.** Diagnosis of the presence and nature of tumours from the microscopical character of cells shed or removed from their surface. [Gk *kytos* cell, diagnosis.]

cytodistal (si·to·dis·tal). 1. Of the axons of nerve cells, indicating the extremity away from the cell body. 2. Descriptive of a neoplasm formed at a distance from its cells of origin. [Gk *kytos* cell, distal.]

cytoflavin (si·to·fla·vin). Warburg's yellow respiratory enzyme; a compound of riboflavine and phosphoric acid which is a component of many dehydrogenase systems and is thus essential to normal oxidative processes in the body. [Gk *kytos* cell, flavin.]

cytogenesis (si·to·jen·es·is). Cell formation and development. [Gk *kystos* cell, genesis.]

cytogenetic (si·to·jen·**et**′·ik). 1. Referring to cytogenetics. 2. Referring or belonging to cytogenesis; having reference to cell formation or development. [Gk *kytos* cell, genesis.]

cytogenetics (**si**·to·jen·**et**′·ix). The branch of genetics concerned with the structure and function of the cell, especially the chromosomes. [see prec.]

TABLE OF SYMBOLS COMMONLY USED IN CYTOGENETICS

Symbol	Meaning
→	from—to.
+, −	signs used after a chromosome or a structural designation (for example, arm, satellite, and so on) to indicate in the first instance the presence in excess or the absence of the chromosome, and in the second instance a plus or minus change in the size of the relevant structure. For greater clarity, it has now been suggested that these signs should be placed in front of the chromosome designation and after the structural symbols to which they refer.
/	diagonal used to separate the cell lines contributing to the formation of a mosaic or chimera.
:	indicating a break not followed by reunion as in terminal deletions.
: :	indicating a break followed by reunion.
?	the question mark in front of a chromosome or structural designation indicates doubt about their identification.
1–22	the number assigned to the 22 pairs of autosomes.
A, B, C, D, E, F, G	the 7 groups of human chromosomes—they are used as a chromosome designation when this has been assigned to a group but has not been further identified.
ace	acentric.
cen	centromere.
del	deletion.
der	derivative chromosome.
dic	dicentric.
dup	duplication.
end	endoreduplication.
h	secondary constriction or region staining negatively (weakly) with ordinary stains (for example, orcein).
i	isochromosome.
ins	insertion.
inv	inversion.
inv ins	insertion where the inserted segment is inverted.
mar	marker chromosome.
mat	maternal origin.
p	short arm of a chromosome.
pat	paternal origin.
q	long arm of a chromosome.
r	ring chromosome.
rec	recombinant chromosome.
rep	reciprocal translocation.
rob	Robertsonian translocation.
s	satellite.
t	translocation.
tan	tandem translocation.
ter	terminal part of a chromosome arm (for example, p ter and q ter are the terminal part of the short and long arms, respectively).
tri	tricentric.
X, Y	the sex chromosomes.

Using the symbols listed above, shorthand descriptions of karyotypes can be made as follows: The total chromosome number is indicated first, followed by a comma and then by the description of the sex chromosome complement. The autosomes, which are shown only when involved in abnormalities, are separated from the sex chromosomes and from each other by commas. Rearranged chromosomes should be shown in parentheses preceded by the symbols which specify the type of rearrangement. Chromosomes that arise from the same rearrangement are shown in the same parenthesis and are separated by semicolons. Recently new staining techniques have revealed distinctive banding patterns along the human chromosomes. These bands allow the description of chromosome abnormalities in greater detail, but have made nomenclature and symbolism more complex.

cytogenic (si·to·**jen**·ik). Producing cells. [Gk *kytos* cell, *genein* to produce.]

cytogenics (si·to·**jen**·ix). Cytogenetics.

cytogenous (si·**toj**·en·us). Cytogenic.

cytogeny (si·**toj**·en·e). Cytogenesis.

cytoglobin, cytoglobulin (si·to·**glo**·bin, si·to·**glob**·ew·lin). A protein substance derived from leucocytes and from lymph glands. [Gk *kytos* cell, globin.]

cytoglycopenia (si·to·gli·ko·**pe**′·ne·ah). A condition in which the blood cells are deficient in glucose. [Gk *kytos* cell, *glykys* sweet, *penes* poor.]

cytogony (si·**tog**·on·e). The process of reproduction by cytogenesis. [Gk *kytos* cell, *gone* seed.]

cytohistogenesis (**si**·to·his·to·**jen**′·es·is). The structural development of a cell. [Gk *kytos* cell, histogenesis.]

cytohistology (**si**·to·his·**tol**′·o·je). Histology with special reference to the individual cells. [Gk *kytos* cell, histology.]

cytohormone (si·to·**hor**·mone). A cell hormone. [Gk *kytos* cell, hormone.]

cytohyaloplasm (si·to·**hi**·al·o·plazm). Cytoreticulum. [Gk *kytos* cell, hyaloplasm.]

cytohydrolyst (si·to·**hi**·dro·list). An enzyme which destroys the wall of a cell by hydrolytic action. [Gk *kytos* cell, hydrolyst.]

cytoid (**si**·toid). Having resemblance to a cell. [Gk *kytos* cell, *eidos* form.]

cyto-inhibition (**si**·to·in·hib·**ish**′·un). The action of phagocytic cells in protecting ingested bacteria or viruses from chemotherapeutic agents. It is displayed in the inhibitory action of pus for chemotherapeutic agents, such as the sulphonamides. [Gk *kytos* cell, L *inhibere* to restrain.]

cytokerastic (**si**·to·ker·**as**′·tik). Referring to cells which have developed into a higher order. [Gk *kytos* cell, *kerastos* mingled.]

cytokinesis (**si**·to·kin·**e**′·sis). The changes that take place in the cytoplasm of a cell during cell division. [Gk *kytos* cell, kinesis.]

cytolergy (si·tol·**er**·je). Cell activity. [Gk *kytos* cell, *ergon* work.]

cytologic, cytological (si·to·**loj**·ik, si·to·**loj**·ik·al). Referring to cytology.

cytologist (si·**tol**·o·jist). An expert in cytology.

cytology (si·**tol**·o·je). The science of the form and functions of cells, i.e. their anatomy, physiology, pathology and chemistry. **Exfoliative cytology.** The microscopic study of cells shed from various sites into the body fluids and cavities, and used to detect cancer or cellular changes which may be forerunners to malignant disease. In the female genital tract it is used also for assessing sex hormone status. [Gk *kytos* cell, *logos* science.]

cytolymph (si·to·limf). Hyaloplasm. [Gk *kytos* cell, *lympha* water.]

cytolysate (si·tol·is·ate). The clear fluid resulting from the lysis of cells. **Blood cytolysate.** The fluid resulting from the lysis of washed erythrocytes. [Gk *kytos* cell, *lyein* to loosen.]

cytolysin (si·tol·is·in). An antibody or substance produced in the body and able to dissolve partially or completely an animal cell; certain cytolysins are specialized. [see prec.]

cytolysis (si·tol·is·is). The destruction by disintegration or dissolution of living cells. **Immune cytolysis.** Lysis of cells, other than red blood cells, by antibody in the presence of complement. [Gk *kytos* cell, *lysis* a loosing.]

cytolyst (si·to·list). Cytolysin.

cytolytic (si·to·lit·ik). Referring or belonging to, or causing cytolysis.

cytoma (si·to·mah). A cell tumour, e.g. sarcoma, in which the arrangement of cells is atypical. [Gk *kytos* cell, *-oma* tumour.]

cytomachia (si·to·mak·e·ah). The struggle between the protective cells of the body and invading bacteria when the cells organize to resist infection and are active in producing dissolution of the invaders. [Gk *kytos* cell, *mache* battle.]

cytomegalovirus (si·to·meg′·al·o·vi·rus). Salivary gland virus. A herpesvirus with particular affinity for the salivary glands, giving rise to infections known as cytomegalic inclusion disease, visceral disease, inclusion body disease, etc., as well as neonatal or congenital infections. The virus is widely distributed, about 50 per cent of the population having antibody to it, but overt infection is rare. Clinical infection may follow depression of normal defences and may be found particularly in patients who have had organ transplants. The disease then presents as a serious, or fatal, pneumonia or as an atypical mononucleosis. Congenital or neonatal infections cause hepatosplenomegaly, jaundice, blood dyscrasias and microcephaly. Salivary gland viruses of other species are not related and all cytomegaloviruses are very species-specific. [Gk *kytos* cell, *megas* large, L *virus* poison.]

cytomegaly (si·to·meg·alli). Enlargement of the cell. [Gk *kytos* cell, *megas* great.]

cytometaplasia (si·to·met·ah·pla′·ze·ah). Change in the form or activity of a cell. [Gk *kytos* cell, metaplasia.]

cytometer (si·tom·et·er). An apparatus accessory to a microscope with which cells can be measured and/or counted. **Eyepiece cytometer.** An eyepiece micrometer; a round piece of glass with a scale etched on it, that is put into the eyepiece of a microscope. **Stage cytometer.** A cytometer that is used on the stage of a microscope, e.g. a haemocytometer. [Gk *kytos* cell, meter.]

cytometry (si·tom·et·re). The counting and measuring of blood cells. [see prec.]

cytomicrosome (si·to·mi·kro·some). *See* MICROSOME. [Gk *kytos* cell, microsome.]

cytomitoma, cytomitome (si·to·mi·to′·mah, si·tom·it·ome). Cytoreticulum. [Gk *kytos* cell, *mitos* thread.]

cytomorphology (si·to·mor·fol′·o·je). The morphology of the cells of the body. [Gk *kytos* cell, morphology.]

cytomorphosis (si·to·mor·fo·sis). The structural alterations and other changes undergone by a cell during the course of its life. [Gk *kytos* cell, *morphosis* a shaping.]

cytomycosis (si·to·mi·ko′·sis). A fungal infection of particular cells. **Reticulo-endothelial cytomycosis.** Histoplasmosis. [Gk *kytos* cell, mycosis.]

cyton, cytone (si·ton, si·tone). The body of a nerve cell as distinct from its processes. [Gk *kytos* cell.]

cytopathic (si·to·path·ik). The power of an agent, particularly of a virus, to injure a living cell. [Gk *kytos* cell, *pathos* suffering.]

cytopathology (si·to·path·ol′·o·je). Cellular pathology. *See* PATHOLOGY. [Gk *kytos* cell, pathology.]

cytopathy (si·top·ath·e). Any disease of the living cell. [Gk *kytos* cell, *pathos* suffering.]

cytopenia (si·to·pe·ne·ah). Poverty of cellular elements in the blood or other tissues. [Gk *kytos* cell, *penes* poor.]

Cytophaga (si·tof·ag·ah). A genus of cellulose-destroying organisms which break down vegetable tissue. [Gk *kytos* cell, *phagein* to eat.]

cytophagocytosis (si·to·fag·o·si·to′·sis). The destruction by absorption of some cells by other cells. [Gk *kytos* cell, *phagein* to eat, *-osis* condition.]

cytophagus (si·tof·ag·us). Belonging to or having the nature of a phagocyte; devouring or destructive to cells. [see prec.]

cytophagy (si·tof·aj·e). Cytophagocytosis.

cytophil, cytophile, cytophilic (si·to·fil, si·to·file, si·to·fil·ik). Having affinity for cells, or attracted by cells. Cf. AMBOCEPTOR. [Gk *kytos* cell, *philein* to love.]

cytophylactic (si·to·fil·ak′·tik). Referring to cytophylaxis. [see foll.]

cytophylaxis (si·to·fil·ax′·is). 1. The process of increasing the activity of leucocytes in defence of the body against infection. 2. The protecting of cells from infection and other lytic agents. [Gk *kytos* cell, *phylaxis* guarding.]

cytophyletic (si·to·fil·et′·ik). Referring or belonging to the genealogy or line of development of cells. [Gk *kytos* cell, *phyle* tribe.]

cytophysics (si·to·fiz·ix). That branch of physics which is concerned with cell activity. [Gk *kytos* cell, physics.]

cytophysiology (si·to·fiz·e·ol′·o·je). That branch of physiology which is concerned with the living cell. [Gk *kytos* cell, physiology.]

cytopigment (si·to·pig·ment). Pigment present in a cell. [Gk *kytos* cell, pigment.]

cytoplasm, cytoplasma (si·to·plazm, si·to·plaz·mah). The contents of the cell invested by the cell membrane, excluding the nucleus. [Gk *kytos* cell, *plasma* something formed.]

cytoplasmic (si·to·plaz·mik). Referring or belonging to, or contained in the cytoplasm.

cytoplastin (si·to·plas·tin). The hyaloplasm of the cell body. [Gk *kytos* cell, *plastos* formed.]

cytopoiesis (si·to·poi·e′·sis). The process of cell development. [Gk *kytos* cell, *poiesis* production.]

cytoproximal (si·to·prox·im·al). Of the axons of nerve cells, indicating the end nearest to the cell of origin. [Gk *kytos* cell, L *proximus* next.]

cytoreticulum (si·to·ret·ik′·ew·lum). The delicate honeycomb-like structure which is part of the cell body. [Gk *kytos* cell, L *reticulum* network.]

Cytoryctes (si·tor·ik·teez). The name given by Guarnieri (1892) to bodies found in the cytoplasm of epithelial cells of the skin in smallpox and vaccinia lesions, and called by him *Cytoryctes variolae* and *Cytoryctes vacciniae* in the mistaken belief that they were protozoal in nature. It is now accepted that these inclusion bodies consist of a collection of virus elementary bodies contained in a matrix. Similar bodies have also been described in cell cytoplasm in rabies, molluscum contagiosum, trachoma, scarlet fever and many animal diseases caused by viruses. The name is now only of historic interest. [Gk *kytos* cell, *oryktes* digger.]

cytoryctology (si·to·rik·tol′·o·je). The study of *Cytoryctes* and similar organisms. The term is now obsolete. [*Cytoryctes*, Gk *logos* science.]

cytoscopy (si·tos·ko·pe). Cytodiagnosis. [Gk *kytos* cell, *skopein* to watch.]

cytosiderin (si·to·sid·er·in). An intracellular iron-containing pigment derived from the breakdown of the haemoglobin of erythrocytes. [Gk *kytos* cell, *sideros* iron.]

cytosine (si·to·seen). Oxyaminopyrimidine, $C_4H_5ON_3$. A pyrimidine base which, with phosphoric acid and D-ribose or D-2-deoxyribose, forms nucleotide units in the nucleic acids; an end-product of the digestion of nucleoprotein.

cytoskeleton (si·to·**skel**·et·on). The structural framework of a cell. [Gk *kytos* cell, skeleton.]
cytosol (**si**·to·sol). The name given to the non-particle-containing "soluble" fraction of cellular material; often used interchangeably with *cytoplasm.* [Gk *kytos* cell, L *solutus* dissolved.]
cytosome (**si**·to·some). The body of a living cell with the exclusion of its nucleus. [Gk *kytos* cell, *soma* body.]
cytospongium (si·to·**spun**·je·um). Cytoreticulum. [Gk *kytos* cell, *spoggia* sponge.]
cytostasis (si·**tos**·tas·is). The blocking of the capillaries by the leucocytes, which marks the early stage of inflammation. [Gk *kytos* cell, *stasis* a standing still.]
cytosteatonecrosis (si·to·ste·at·o·nek·**ro**'·sis). Adiponecrosis subcutanea neonatorum. [Gk *kytos* cell, *steas* fat, necrosis.]
cytostome (**si**·to·stome). The mouth opening of some one-celled animals, e.g. certain protozoa. [Gk *kytos* cell, *stoma* mouth.]
cytostromatic (si·to·stro·**mat**'·ik). Referring to the cell stroma. [Gk *kytos* cell, *stroma* a covering.]
cytotactic (si·to·**tak**·tik). Referring or belonging to cytotaxis.
cytotaxia (si·to·**tax**·e·ah). Cytotaxis.
cytotaxis (si·to·**tax**·is). 1. The influence which directs living cells into any particular arrangement or order. 2. The function in the living cell which governs the direction of its movement. **Negative cytotaxis.** A form of cytotaxis which causes some living cells to be repelled by others. **Positive cytotaxis.** A form of cytotaxis which causes isolated living cells to select and be attracted to one another. [Gk *kytos* cell, *taxis* arrangement.]
cytotherapy (si·to·**ther**·ap·e). 1. Organotherapy; the use in treatment of the organs of animals (e.g. liver) or of preparations made from them (e.g. desiccated hog's stomach). 2. The use of cytolytic or cytotoxic serums in treatment of disease. [Gk *kytos* cell, therapy.]
cytothesis (si·to·**the**·sis). The reparative or restorative process by which an injured cell returns to a condition of health. [Gk *kytos* cell, *thesis* a placing.]
cytotoxic (si·to·**tox**·ik). Referring to a cytotoxin.
cytotoxicosis (si·to·tox·ik·**o**'·sis). The condition produced by the effect of a cytotoxin. [cytotoxin, Gk *-osis* condition.]
cytotoxigen (si·to·**tox**'·igen). A substance or particle which activates cytotoxins, e.g. immune complexes which cause release of chemotactic factors from complement.
cytotoxin (si·to·**tox**·in). A chemotactic factor which directly attracts leucocytes. Cf. HAEMATOTOXIN, HEPATOTOXIN, LEUCOTOXIN, NEPHROTOXIN, SPERMATOTOXIN. [Gk *kytos* cell, *toxikon* poison.]
cytotrochin (si·to·**trok**·in). The substance in a toxin which bears the active poisonous element to the cell. [Gk *kytos* cell, *trochia* track.]
cytotropal (si·to·**tro**·pal). Cytotropic.
cytotrophoblast (si·to·**tro**·fo·blast). The inner cellular layer of the wall of the blastocyst. [Gk *kytos* cell, trophoblast.]
cytotrophoblastic (si·to·tro·fo·**blas**'·tik). The inner cellular layer (Langhans' cells) surrounding fertilized ovum gives rise to outer non-cellular nucleated layer, thus forming trophoblastic covering. [see prec.]
cytotrophy (si·to·**tro**·fe). The process of growth and nourishment of living cells. [Gk *kytos* cell, *trophe* nutrition.]
cytotropic (si·to·**trop**·ik). Attracted to or having affinity for cells. [Gk *kytos* cell, *trepein* to turn.]
cytotropism (si·to·**tro**·pizm). The attraction inherent in certain living cells of the body for particular chemicals, drugs, bacteria, or viruses. [see prec.]
cytozoic (si·to·**zo**·ik). Descriptive of parasites which are attached to cells or live within them. [see foll.]
cytozoon (si·to·**zo**·on). A parasite such as a protozoon which lives within the cells of the body. [Gk *kytos* cell, *zoon* animal.]
cyttarrhagia (sit·ah·**ra**·je·ah). Haemorrhage from the socket of a tooth. [Gk *kyttaros* socket, *rhegnynein* to gush forth.]
cytula (**sit**·ew·lah). In biology: the parent cell or the ferilized egg cell of an organism. [dim. of Gk *kytos* cell.]
cytuloplasm (**sit**·ew·lo·plazm). In biology, the mingled protoplasm of ovum and spermatids in a cytula. [cytule, Gk *plasma* something formed.]
cyturia (si·**tewr**·e·ah). The presence of any kind of cell in the urine. [Gk *kytos* cell, urine.]
Czapek-Dox culture medium, or solution. A synthetic medium used for the culture of fungi.
Czermak, Johann Nepomuk (b. 1828). Graz and Leipzig physiologist.
  Czermak's line. One of the microscopic lines formed in dentine by rows of interglobular spaces.
  Czermak's spaces. The interglobular spaces of the dentine.
Czermak, W. Prague ophthalmologist.
  Czermak's operation. For cataract: extraction of the lens through a section in the lower half of the limbus cut with scissors, the whole operation being performed subconjunctivally. Of historical interest.
Czerny, Adalbert (b. 1863). Berlin paediatrician.
  Czerny's anaemia. A deficiency anaemia seen in infants on defective or inadequate diets.
Czerny, Vincenz (b. 1842). Heidelberg surgeon.
  Czerny's operation. Ligation and excision of the sac of an inguinal hernia.
  Czerny's suture, Czerny–Lembert suture. A haemostatic 2-layer intestinal suture consisting of a mucosal in addition to a Lembert (seromuscular) suture.
Cziky's sign. A sign of hypotonia, which may occur in tabes dorsalis, cerebellar disease, or myatonia congenita: if the patient sits with the legs apart and knees extended, hypotonia is present if the spine of the 7th cervical vertebra can be brought below the level of the greater trochanter of the femur.
Czocor, Johann (fl. 1880). Vienna physician.
  Czocor's cochineal solution. A combination of alum and cochineal used as a nuclear stain.

D

Daae, Anders (b. 1838). Norwegian physician.

Daae's disease, Daae-Finsen disease. Epidemic pleurodynia.

daboia, daboya (**dab**·oi·ah). 1. The Indian name for Russell's viper *(Vipera russelli)*, a large and very poisonous snake of India, Burma and Thailand. 2. The venom of Russell's viper used as a coagulant in haemophilia. [Hind. *dabna* to lurk.]

Da Costa, Jacob Mendes (b. 1833). Philadelphia physician.

Da Costa's disease, or syndrome. Neurocirculatory asthenia, soldier's heart, effort syndrome and disordered action of the heart.

Mendes da Costa's syndrome. Erythrokeratoderma variabilis.

d'Acosta, José (b. 1539). Jesuit missionary.

d'Acosta's disease. Anoxia.

dacro-. *See* DACRYO-.

dacrocystitis (**dak**·ro·sis·**ti**′·tis). Dacryocystitis.

dacroma (dak·**ro**·mah). Dacryoma.

dacryadenalgia (**dak**·re·ad·en·**al**′·je·ah). Dacryo-adenalgia.

dacryadenitis (**dak**·re·ad·en·**i**′·tis). Dacryo-adenitis.

dacryadenoscirrhus (**dak**·re·ad·en·o·**sir**′·us). Dacryo-adenoscirrhus.

dacryagogatresia (**dak**·re·ag·o·gat·**re**′·ze·ah). Dacryo-agogatresia.

dacryagogue (dak·**re**·ag·og). 1. An agent that induces a flow of tears. 2. Acting as a channel for the flow of tears. 3. Causing an outpouring of tears. [Gk *dakryon* tear, *agogos* leading.]

dacrycystalgia (**dak**·re·sis·**tal**′·je·ah). Dacryocystalgia.

dacrycystitis (**dak**·re·sis·**ti**′·tis). Dacryocystitis.

dacryelcosis (**dak**·re·el·**ko**′·sis). Dacryohelcosis.

dacryo-adenalgia (**dak**·re·o·ad·en·**al**′·je·ah). Pain in the lacrimal gland. [Gk *dakryon* tear, adenalgia.]

dacryo-adenectomy (**dak**·re·o·ad·en·**ek**′·to·me). Surgical removal of the lacrimal gland. [Gk *dakryon* tear, adenectomy.]

dacryo-adenitis (**dak**·re·o·ad·en·**i**′·tis). Inflammation of the lacrimal gland. [Gk *dakryon* tear, adenitis.]

dacryo-adenoscirrhus (**dak**·re·o·ad·en·o·**sir**′·us). Scirrhus affecting the lacrimal gland. [Gk *dakryon* tear, *aden* gland, *skirrhos* hard.]

dacryo-agogatresia (**dak**·re·o·ag·o·gat·**re**′·ze·ah). A condition of imperforation or closure of the duct of the lacrimal gland. [Gk *dakryon* tear, *agogos* leading, atresia.]

dacryoblennorrhoea (**dak**·re·o·blen·o·**re**′·ah). Chronic discharge of mucus from the duct of the lacrimal gland, with inflammation. [Gk *dakryon* tear, *blennos* mucus, *rhoia* flow.]

dacryocanaliculitis (**dak**·re·o·**kan**·al·ik·ew·**li**′·tis). Inflammation of the lacrimal sac and canaliculi. [Gk *dakryon* tear, *L canaliculus* small channel, Gk *-itis* inflammation.]

dacryocele (**dak**·re·o·seel). Dacryocystocele.

dacryocyst (**dak**·re·o·sist). The lacrimal sac. [Gk *dakryon* tear, *kystis* bag.]

dacryocystalgia (**dak**·re·o·sis·**tal**′·je·ah). A sensation of pain in the lacrimal sac. [dacryocyst, Gk *algos* pain.]

dacryocystectasia (**dak**·re·o·sis·tek·**ta**′·ze·ah). Dilatation of the lacrimal sac. [dacryocyst, Gk *ektasis* a stretching.]

dacryocystectomy (**dak**·re·o·sis·**tek**′·to·me). Surgical removal of the wall of the lacrimal sac. [dacryocyst, Gk *ektome* a cutting out.]

dacryocystitis (**dak**·re·o·sis·**ti**′·tis). Inflammation of the wall of the lacrimal sac. It may be acute, associated with pain and redness, or chronic, in which the sac contains mucopus but signs of inflammation are absent. **Dacryocystitis blennorrhoeica.** A form of dacryocystitis associated with conjunctivitis. **Dacryocystitis phlegmonosa.** A condition of inflammation of the tissues of the lacrimal sac and of the soft area immediately surrounding it. **Syphilitic dacryocystitis.** An infection of the lacrimal sac due to syphilis, usually found in the tertiary stage either as a secondary infection to a periostitis of the nearby bones, or as a gumma of the sac itself. **Trachomatous dacryocystitis.** A trachomatous infection of the lacrimal sac caused by spread down the canaliculus from the affected conjunctiva. This is rare, and most cases of dacryocystitis associated with trachoma are due to secondary infection. **Tuberculous dacryocystitis.** An infection of the lacrimal sac due to the tubercle bacillus. It is common in children, especially girls, and can be primary, or secondary to infection of the nose, conjunctiva, skin or bone. [dacryocyst, Gk *-itis* inflammation.]

dacryocystitome (**dak**·re·o·sis′·te·tome). A surgical instrument for cutting strictures of the lacrimal apparatus or for incising the lacrimal sac. [dacryocyst, Gk *temnein* to cut.]

dacryocystoblennorrhoea (**dak**·re·o·sis·to·blen·o·**re**′·ah). Chronic inflammation and catarrh of the lacrimal sac, with decomposition of the tears. The condition is caused by a narrowing of the nasolacrimal duct. [dacryocyst, blennorrhoea.]

dacryocystocele (**dak**·re·o·**sis**′·to·seel). Dilatation of the lacrimal sac by mucus or mucopus. [dacryocyst, Gk *kele* hernia.]

dacryocystogram (**dak**·re·o·**sis**′·to·gram). The radiograph made during dacryocystography. [dacryocyst, Gk *gramma* record.]

dacryocystography (**dak**·re·o·sis·**tog**′·raf·e). The technique of radiographic visualization of the lacrimal duct after the injection of a radio-opaque contrast medium into the lumen. [dacryocyst, Gk *graphein* to record.]

dacryocystoptosis (**dak**·re·o·sis·top·**to**′·sis). Downward displacement or prolapse of the lacrimal sac. [dacryocyst, Gk *ptosis* fall.]

dacryocystorrhinostenosis (**dak**·re·o·**sis**·to·ri·no·sten·**o**′·sis). A narrowing of the nasolacrimal duct. [dacryocyst, Gk *rhis* nose, stenosis.]

dacryocystorrhinostomy (**dak**·re·o·**sis**·to·ri·**nos**′·to·me). An operation to effect an anastomosis, by way of the lacrimal bone, between the lacrimal sac and the middle meatus of the nose. [dacryocyst, Gk *rhis* nose, *stoma* mouth.]

dacryocystorrhinotomy (**dak**·re·o·**sis**·to·ri·**not**′·o·me). Dacryorrhinocystotomy.

dacryocystostenosis (**dak**·re·o·**sis**·to·sten·**o**′·sis). Stricture or narrowing of the lacrimal sac. [dacryocyst, stenosis.]

dacryocystostomy (**dak**·re·o·sis·**tos**′·to·me). The incision of the lacrimal sac to establish drainage. [dacryocyst, Gk *stoma* mouth.]

dacryocystosyringotomy (**dak**·re·o·**sis**·to·sir·ing·**got**′·o·me). Surgical incision of the lacrimal sac and its duct. [dacryocyst, Gk *syrigx* pipe, *temnein* to cut.]

dacryocystotome (**dak**·re·o·**sis**′·to·tome). Dacryocystitome.

dacryocystotomy (**dak**·re·o·sis·**tot**′·o·me). Surgical piercing or opening of the lacrimal sac. [dacryocyst, Gk *temnein* to cut.]

dacryogenic (**dak**·re·o·**jen**′·ik). Causing tears to flow. [Gk *dakryon* tear, *genein* to produce.]

dacryohaemorrhoea (**dak**·re·o·hem·o·**re**′·ah). 1. A flow of blood-stained tears. 2. A flow of blood from the duct of the lacrimal gland. [Gk *dakryon* tear, *haima* blood, *rhoia* flow.]

dacryohelcosis (**dak**·re·o·hel·**ko**′·sis). Ulceration of the lacrimal sac or its duct. [Gk *dakryon* tear, *helkosis* ulceration.]

dacryoid (**dak**·re·oid). Resembling a tear or tears. [Gk *dakryon* tear, *eidos* form.]

dacryolin (**dak**·re·o·lin). A name which has been applied to the soluble protein present in tears. [Gk *dakryon* tear.]

dacryolith (**dak**·re·o·lith). A calculus found in the lacrimal apparatus. [Gk *dakryon* tear, *lithos* stone.]
dacryolithiasis (**dak**·re·o·lith·**i**′·as·is). The condition in which stones are present in the lacrimal apparatus. [see prec.]
dacryoma (dak·re·**o**·mah). 1. A tear-filled cyst caused by obstruction of a duct of the lacrimal gland. 2. Stoppage of one of the puncta lacrimalia so that the tears overflow. [Gk *dakryon* tear, *-oma* tumour.]
dacryon (**dak**·re·on). 1. A tear. 2. In craniometry, the point at which the anterosuperior angle of the lacrimal bone unites with the frontal bone and the frontal process of the maxilla. [Gk *dakryon* tear.]
dacryops (**dak**·re·ops). 1. A cystic dilatation caused by fluid retained in the duct of the lacrimal gland. 2. A chronic condition of excess of tears in the eye. [Gk *dakryon* tear, *ops* eye.]
dacryopyorrhoea (**dak**·re·o·pi·o·**re**′·ah). A flow of tears mingled with pus. [Gk *dakryon* tear, *pyon* pus, *rhoia* flow.]
dacryopyosis (**dak**·re·o·pi·**o**′·sis). Suppuration affecting the lacrimal apparatus. [Gk *dakryon* tear, *pyon* pus, *-osis* condition.]
dacryorrhinocystotomy (**dak**·re·o·ri·no·sis·**tot**′·o·me). The surgical procedure of probing through the lacrimal sac into the cavity of the nose. [Gk *dakryon* tear, *rhis* nose, *kystis* bag, *temnein* to cut.]
dacryorrhoea (**dak**·re·o·**re**′·ah). An excessive flow of tears. [Gk *dakryon* tear, *rhoia* flow.]
dacryosinusitis (**dak**·re·o·si·nus·**i**′·tis). Inflammation of the lacrimal ducts and ethmoidal sinuses. [Gk *dakryon* tear, sinus, Gk *-itis* inflammation.]
dacryosolen (**dak**·re·o·**so**′·len). 1. A lacrimal canaliculus. 2. Duct of the lacrimal gland. [Gk *dakryon* tear, *solen* pipe.]
dacryosolenitis (**dak**·re·o·so·len·**i**′·tis). Inflammation affecting the duct of the lacrimal gland or the nasolacrimal duct. [dacryosolen, Gk *-itis* inflammation.]
dacryostenosis (**dak**·re·o·sten·**o**′·sis). Narrowing or stricture of the duct of the lacrimal gland. [Gk *dakryon* tear, stenosis.]
dacryosyrinx (**dak**·re·o·**sir**′·ingx). 1. A lacrimal fistula. 2. An instrument for syringing out the duct of the lacrimal gland. [Gk *dakryon* tear, *syrigx* pipe.]
dactyl (**dak**·til). A digit of the hand or foot. [Gk *daktylos* finger.]
dactylar (**dak**·til·ar). Dactylic.
dactylate (**dak**·til·ate). Having digit-like processes. [see foll.]
dactylic (dak·**til**·ik). Belonging to a finger or a toe. [Gk *daktylos* finger.]
dactyliferous (dak·til·**if**·er·us). Dactylate. [Gk *daktylos* finger, L *ferre* to carry.]
dactylion (dak·**til**·e·on). Syndactylism: a condition in which the fingers are wholly or partly united; webbed fingers, often congenital. [Gk *daktylos* finger.]
dactylitis (dak·til·**i**·tis). Inflammation of one or more fingers or toes. **Dactylitis strumosa.** Dactylitis tuberculosa (see below). **Dactylitis syphilitica.** An inflammatory affection of the fingers and toes which occurs in tertiary syphilis; the spongy substance of the bones and the subcutaneous connective tissue are infiltrated by a gummatous substance, and severe deformity results. **Dactylitis tuberculosa.** Inflammation of the fingers or toes which is tuberculous in character. [Gk *daktylos* finger, *-itis* inflammation.]
dactylium (dak·**til**·e·um). Dactylion.
dactylocampsodynia (**dak**·til·o·kamp·so·**din**′·e·ah). Painful contraction of one or more fingers or toes. [Gk *daktylos* finger, *kampsis* a curving, *odyne* pain.]
dactyloedema (**dak**·til·e·**de**′·mah). Oedema affecting the fingers or the toes. [Gk *daktylos* finger, *oidema* a swelling.]
dactylogram (dak·**til**·o·gram). A fingerprint made for the purpose of individual identification. [Gk *daktylos* finger, *gramma* record.]
dactylography (dak·til·**og**·raf·e). The study of fingerprints. [Gk *daktylos* finger, *graphein* to write.]
dactylogryposis (**dak**·til·o·grip·**o**′·sis). Permanent contraction of the fingers or toes. [Gk *daktylos* finger, *gryposis* curve.]
dactyloid (**dak**·til·oid). Resembling a finger. [Gk *daktylos* finger, *eidos* form.]
dactylology (dak·til·**ol**·o·je). The practice of carrying on conversation by means of signs made with the fingers and hands. [Gk *daktylos* finger, *logos* discourse.]
dactylolysis (dak·til·**ol**·is·is). The spontaneous dropping off of fingers and toes such as occurs in leprosy or ainhum. [Gk *daktylos* finger, *lysis* a loosing.]
dactylomegaly (**dak**·til·o·**meg**′·al·e). A condition in which one or more fingers are abnormally large. [Gk *daktylos* finger, *megas* large.]
dactylophasia (**dak**·til·o·**fa**′·ze·ah). Dactylology. [Gk *daktylos* finger, *phanai* to speak.]
dactyloscopy (dak·til·**os**·ko·pe). Examination of fingerprints in order to establish identity. [Gk *daktylos* finger, *skopein* to watch.]
dactylose (**dak**·til·oze). 1. Having finger-like processes. 2. Bearing five appendages or rays. [Gk *daktylos* finger.]
dactylospasm (**dak**·til·o·spazm). Spasmodic contraction of a finger or toe. [Gk *daktylos* finger, spasm.]
dactylosymphysis (**dak**·til·o·**sim**′·fis·is). Syndactylism; a condition, often congenital, in which the fingers have grown together or are united by webs. [Gk *daktylos* finger, *syn* together, *phyein* to grow.]
dactylous (**dak**·til·us). Dactylose.
dactylus (**dak**·til·us). A finger or a toe. [Gk *daktylos.*]
Dacuronium Bromide (dak·ewr·o·ne·um **bro**·mide). BP Commission approved name for 3α-acetoxy-2β,16β-dipiperidino-5α-androstan-17β-ol dimethobromide; a neuromuscular blocking agent.
dadyl (**da**·dil). A camphene isomer obtained when bornyl chloride is treated with lime.
dagga (**dag**·ah). An African name for a preparation of Indian hemp.
dahlia (**da**·le·ah). A plant of the family Compositae, much esteemed in the garden for its flowers, the bulbs of which contain inulin and a purple dye. **Dahlia B.** A dye related to methyl violet, being a mixture of methyl rosaniline chlorides, and used as an antiseptic. **Dahlia paper.** A paper impregnated with the purple dye of dahlia species and used as an indicator (acids, red; alkalis, green). **Dahlia violet.** A methylated ethyl violet with bactericidal properties. [A. *Dahl*, 18th century Swedish botanist.]
dahlin (**dah**·lin). Inulin. [see prec.]
dahllite (**dahl**·ite). A double salt of calcium carbonate and phosphate having the approximate composition $CaCO_3.2Ca_3,(PO_4)_2$, which mainly constitutes the inorganic matter of bone and teeth.
daisy (**da**·ze). Term applied to the rosette form assumed by mature schizonts of *Plasmodium malariae*, the causal agent of quartan malaria. [AS *daeges eage* day's-eye.]
Dakin, Henry Drysdale (b. 1880). New York biochemist.

Dakin's antiseptic, or solution. A solution of sodium hypochlorite and boric acid which has proved of value in the continuous irrigation of wounds.

Carrel–Dakin tube, Dakin–Carrel method. *See* CARREL METHOD.

Dakin and West liver fraction. An extract of liver containing the haemopoietic factor and used in the treatment of pernicious anaemia.

Dakinization (da·kin·i·**za**′·shun). The treating of a patient with Dakin's solution. [Henry Drysdale *Dakin.*]
dakryon (**dak**·re·on). Dacryon.
dakryops (**dak**·re·ops). Dacryops.
Dale, Sir Henry Hallett (b. 1875). London physiologist.

Dale phenomenon, or reaction. Schultz-Dale reaction (see below).

Schultz-Dale reaction, or test. Smooth muscle taken from an animal that has been made anaphylactic shows a powerful contraction in the presence of minute amounts of the same antigen: the smooth muscle is capable of being desensitized. Schultz used intestinal muscle, and Dale uterine muscle from virgin guinea-pigs.

Dalen, Johan Albin (b. 1866). Swedish ophthalmologist.

Dalen's spots. Small white spots seen on the retina in the early stages of sympathetic ophthalmitis, due to changes in the pigment epithelium.

Dalen–Fuchs nodules. Nodules formed in the pigment epithelium of the iris and choroid in sympathetic ophthalmitis. The cells of the epithelium swell up and proliferate, and are finally invaded by lymphocytes and epithelioid cells, so forming nodules.

Dalldorf, Gilbert Julius (b. 1900). New York pathologist.

Dalldorf's test. A biological test for capillary fragility: a suction cup is applied to the arm for a measured period. The number of petechiae found in the cupped area is counted.

Dalrymple, John (b. 1803). London ophthalmic surgeon.

Dalrymple's disease. Inflammation of the cornea and ciliary body.

Dalrymple's sign. Wideness of the palpebral fissure, as often seen in exophthalmic goitre. (Obsolete name.)

Dalton, John (b. 1766). English chemist.

Dalton's law. Henry's law.

Dalton–Henry law. In the case of a mixture of gases in equilibrium with a liquid, the amount of any one particular gas dissolved is directly proportional to its partial pressure.

dalton (**dawl**·ton). An obsolete unit of atomic mass; 1/16 of the mass of the oxygen atom. [John *Dalton.*]

Daltonism (**dawl**·ton·izm). Blindness to colour. [John *Dalton.*]

dam (dam). In dentistry, a thin sheet of rubber which is placed around a tooth and held in position by a metal clamp or a silk ligature to isolate it from saliva during conservative work; also referred to as a *rubber-dam.* [AS.]

damar, damaria (**dam**·ar, dam·a·re·ah). Dammar.

damiana (dam·e·a·nah). Turnera; the dried leaves of the herb *Turnera diffusa* Willd. var. *aphrodisiaca* Urb., and probably of other species of *Turnera* found in Texas and Mexico. It contains a mildly irritant volatile oil which is excreted in the urine and may be responsible for the reputed aphrodisiac properties of the drug. It is also a mild purgative. [Sp.]

dammar (**dam**·ar). A gummy exudate from certain East Indian plants of the family Dipterocarpaceae. Dissolved in chloroform, it is used in microscopy. [Hind. resin.]

dammaran (**dam**·ar·an). A neutral resin occurring as a constituent of dammar.

dammarin (**dam**·ar·in). An acid resin, one of the constituents of dammar.

Damoiseau, Louis Hyacinthe Céleste (b. 1815). Paris physician.

Damoiseau's curve, line or sign, Ellis–Damoiseau curve, line or sign. The S-shaped curve that on percussion marks the upper limit of dullness caused by a pleural effusion. Also known as *Ellis's curve.*

damp (damp). 1. Moisture in the air, or impregnating a surface. 2. The foul air in a mine. **After damp.** *See* AFTER-DAMP. **Black damp, Choke damp.** A mixture of carbon dioxide and nitrogen accumulating in mine workings and rendering the atmosphere unbreathable. **Cold damp.** A humid atmosphere containing much carbon dioxide. **Fire damp.** *See* FIREDAMP. **Stink damp.** Sulphuretted hydrogen. **White damp.** Carbon monoxide. [AS.]

damper (**dam**·per). 1. Any device intended to check oscillation or reduce vibration. 2. A device incorporated in a galvanometer to reduce the amplitude of swing. 3. A metal plate in a flue which controls the draught. [AS.]

damping (**dam**·ping). The gradual reduction of the amplitude of vibrations or wave motion. **Damping period.** The time during which an electron in an excited atom emits radiation and falls back into its original state. [AS.]

Dana, Charles Loomis (b. 1852). New York neurologist.

Dana's operation. Posterior rhizotomy.

Putnam–Dana symptom complex. Putnam–Dana syndrome (see below).

Dana–Putnam syndrome, Putnam–Dana syndrome. Sclerosis of the lateral columns of the spinal cord, with variable dorsal column involvement. The description can be applied to many cases of disseminated sclerosis, and it is doubtful if the syndrome is a separate entity.

Danazol (**dan**·az·ol). BP Commission approved name for 17α-pregna-2,4-dien-20-yno[2,3-*d*]isoxazol-17-ol; an anterior pituitary suppressant.

Dance, Jean Baptiste Hippolyte (b. 1797). Paris physician.

Dance's sign. A depression in the right iliac fossa is felt in cases of intussusception.

dance (dahns). **Dance of the arteries.** Very strongly marked arterial pulsation such as occurs in cases of aortic incompetence. **Hilar dance, Hilus dance.** Pulsation of large pulmonary arteries seen during cardioscopy in Eisenmenger's syndrome and patent ductus arteriosus. [ME.]

Dancel, Jean François (b. 1804). French physician.

Dancel's treatment. The treatment of obesity by drastic restriction of fluid intake.

dandelion (**dan**·de·li·on). The plant *Taraxacum officinale,* family Compositae. The fresh or dried root constitutes the drug taraxacum, which is used as a tonic and bitter, also as a mild laxative. [Fr. *dent de lion* lion's tooth.]

dandruff (**dan**·druf). 1. The bran-like scales occurring on the scalp in seborrhoeic dermatitis. 2. Scaling of the scalp which as a rule is not associated with any inflammatory condition, but due to the ordinary scaling of the epidermis. [dial. E. *dander* scurf.]

Dandy, Walter Edward (b. 1886). Baltimore neurosurgeon.

Dandy's operation. Section of the preganglionic trigeminal root by the posterior fossa approach; also intracranial section of the 9th nerve for glossopharyngeal neuralgia.

dandy (**dan**·de). A litter for carrying the wounded; it consists of a cloth hammock suspended from a bamboo pole. [Hind. *dandi.*]

Dane particles (**dayn** par·tiklz). Particles about 42 nm in diameter found in the serum of patients with serum hepatitis. By electron microscopy they are seen in association with particles of hepatitis B antigen and may be mature virus particles. They are named after their discoverer, Dr David S. Dane, a London virologist.

dangerous drugs (**dane**·jer·us **drugz**). *See* MISUSE OF DRUGS ACT 1971.

Daniell, John Frederick (b. 1790). London physicist and chemist.

Daniell cell. A two-fold primary voltaic cell consisting usually of a copper can holding a saturated solution of copper sulphate in which is immersed a porous pot containing dilute sulphuric acid and a zinc rod or plate. It furnishes an e.m.f. of 1.07 V.

Daniell's hygrometer. An instrument consisting of two connected bulbs containing ether, the vapour of which is cooled by external evaporation until the dew point is reached as shown by an enclosed thermometer.

daniell (**dan**·e·el). An obsolete unit of electromotive force, originally based on the voltage of the Daniell cell; 1.07 V. [John Frederick *Daniell.*]

Danielssen, Daniel Cornelius (b. 1815). Bergen, Norway, physician.

Danielssen's disease. Leprosy.

Danlos, Henri Alexandre (b. 1844). Paris dermatologist.

Danlos' syndrome. *See* EHLERS-DANLOS DISEASE.

Ehlers–Danlos disease, or syndrome. Cutis hyperelastica; dermatorrhexis: increased elasticity of the skin with increased laxity of the joints, fragility of the skin, pseudotumours resembling haemangiomata and reduction of subcutaneous fat; occasionally subcutaneous nodules are present.

Danthron BP 1973 (**dan**·thron). 1,8-Dihydroxyanthraquinone; an anthraquinone purgative.

Dantrolene (dan·tro·**leen**). BP Commission approved name for 1-(5-*p*-nitrophenylfurfurylideneamino)imidazoline-2,4-dione; a skeletal muscle relaxant.

Danysz, Jean (b. 1860). Polish pathologist in Paris.

bacillus of Danysz. *Salmonella enteritidis.*

Danysz's effect, or phenomenon. The decrease in neutralizing power of an antitoxin when the toxin is added to it in portions instead of all at once.

Danysz's vaccine. A vaccine made from a mixed culture of all the organisms growing in the bowel. It is believed to have an anti-anaphylactic effect in certain allergic states.

Danysz virus. A culture of *Salmonella enteritidis* or allied organism, used for rat extermination.

Daphne (daf·ne). A genus of trees and shrubs of the family Thymelaeaceae. The dried barks of *Daphne mezereum* Linn., *D. laureola* Linn. and *D. gnidium* Linn. yield the drug mezereum. [Gk laurel.]

daphnism (daf·nizm). Gastro-enteritis with haemorrhage and later on delirium and collapse as the result of poisoning by a species of *Daphne* or an allied shrub. [see prec.]

Dapsone BP 1973 (dap·sone). 4,4′-Diaminodiphenyl-sulphone, $(NH_2)C_6H_4SO_2C_6H_4(NH_2)$, a drug used in the treatment of leprosy. It has a bacteriostatic action, and is thought to act by preventing the use by bacteria of certain metabolites essential to their normal development. Also called *DADPS.*

Darányi, Julius von (b. 1888). Budapest bacteriologist.

Darányi test. A flocculation test for tuberculosis in which the patient's serum is mixed with an alcohol and sodium chloride solution, and incubated for 20 min at 60°C. Readings as to flocculation are taken at intervals of 30 min–24 h; the flocculation is said to occur with increasing rapidity according to the activity of the disease. It is unreliable.

d'Arcet's metal. An alloy of lead, bismuth and tin used in dentistry.

Dare, Arthur (b. 1868). Philadelphia physician.

Dare's method. For the direct estimation of the haemoglobin content of undiluted capillary blood: a drop of blood is placed between two glass plates into a stratum of exact thickness, illuminated and compared with a movable glass colour scale.

Reiker–Dare haemoglobinometer. An instrument in which a film of undiluted blood of uniform depth is compared with a standardized red glass plate of graduated intensity, as a means of estimating the haemoglobin content.

Darier, Ferdinand Jean (b. 1856). Paris dermatologist.

Darier's disease. Keratosis follicularis.

Darier's erythema. Erythema annulare centrifugum.

Darier's pityriasis simplex. Pityriasis alba.

Darier–Roussy sarcoid. Subcutaneous lesions similar to those of erythema induratum, but not necessarily confined to the lower limbs, probably of tuberculous origin.

Darkshevich, Liverij Osipovich (b. 1858). Moscow neurologist.

Darkshevich fibres. A bundle of nerve fibres connecting the optic tract and the habenular nucleus.

Darkshevich's ganglion, or nucleus. A nucleus of large cells just lateral to the upper end of the aqueduct of the mid-brain sending efferents to the medial longitudinal bundle and the posterior commissure.

Darling, Samuel Taylor (b. 1872). Ancon, Panama, physician.

Darling's disease. Histoplasmosis.

darmous (dar·moos). A North African name for fluorine poisoning. [Ar.]

Darnall, Carl Rogers (b. 1867). USA Army surgeon.

Darnall filter. A filter of Canton flannel used to purify drinking water; it is becoming obsolete.

darrengardera (dar·en·gar·der·ah). A trypanosome infection of horses.

Darrow, Daniel Cady (b. 1895). New Haven, Connecticut, paediatrician.

Darrow's solution. A solution of potassium chloride, sodium chloride and sodium lactate, used for gastro-enteritis in children.

d'Arsonval, Jacques Arsène (b. 1851). Paris physicist and physiologist.

d'Arsonval current. A high-frequency alternating current used to stimulate metabolism.

d'Arsonval galvanometer. Mirror galvanometer; a galvanometer in which a mirror attached to the magnet reflects a beam of light on to a graduated scale.

d'Arsonvalism, d'Arsonvalization (dar·son·val·izm, dar·son·val·i·za′·shun). Treatment by means of a high-frequency alternating current; d'Arsonval's original high-frequency apparatus was the forerunner of the diathermy apparatus of today. It produced intermittent trains of heavily damped oscillations of high voltage but low amperage, the current having very little heating effect on the bodily tissues. [Jacques Arsène *d'Arsonval.*]

dartoic (dar·to·ik). Dartoid.

dartoid (dar·toid). 1. Like or consisting of the dartos muscle. 2. Having contractions of the slow involuntary kind like those of the dartos muscle. [Gk *dartos* flayed, *eidos* form.]

dartos (dar·tos). The dartos muscle. **Dartos muliebris.** A structure similar to the dartos muscle and present beneath the skin of the labia majora. [Gk flayed.]

dartos muscle [tunica dartos (NA)]. A subcutaneous layer of smooth muscle fibres enclosing the scrotum.

dartre (dar·ter). Herpetiform disease of the skin; the term is used without any specific meaning. [Fr. tetter.]

dartrous (dar·trus). Herpetic. [see prec.]

Darwin, Charles Robert (b. 1809). English naturalist.

Darwin's auricle. The apex of the auricle.

Darwin's ear. An exaggeration of Darwin's tubercle.

Darwin's theory. *See* DARWINISM.

Darwin's tubercle. The tubercle of the helix of the auricle.

Darwinism (dar·win·izm). The theory of natural selection propounded by Darwin that those varieties of offspring survive which are best adapted to their environment. [Charles Robert *Darwin.*]

dasetherapy (das·e·ther·ap·e). The treatment of disease by requiring the patient to live in a region where pines and balsams grow. [Gk *dasos* forest, therapy.]

Dastre, Jules Albert François (b. 1844). Paris physiologist.

Dastre–Morat law. Constriction of the blood vessels of the skin is usually associated with dilatation of the splanchnic blood vessels, and vice versa.

dasymeter (da·sim·et·er). A hollow sphere of thin glass the weight of which is determined in various gases, thus affording a comparison of their densities. [Gk *dasys* density, meter.]

Dasypus (das·e·pus). A genus of armadillos, some species of which are reservoirs of *Trypanosoma cruzi.* [Gk rabbit.]

data (dar·tah). **Dental data.** 1. The charted details of teeth present, filled, repaired or missing from the jaws. 2. Data of wear and tear in erupted teeth providing information on the age (Gustafson formulae or data).

Dattner, Bernhard (b. 1887). Austrian neurologist in New York.

Dattner needle. A needle for the aspiration of cerebrospinal fluid, consisting of an outer needle of moderate bore containing a fine inner needle which is protruded to perforate the spinal dura mater.

Datura (dat·ewr·ah). A genus of plants of the family Solanaceae. **Datura leaf.** The dried leaves and flowering tops of *Datura metel* Linn. and *D. innoxia* Miller. It contains hyoscine, with only traces of hyoscyamine and atropine, and is used as a source of the former. It is employed in India for the same purpose as belladonna and stramonium. **Datura seed.** The dried seeds of *D. metel* Linn., used in India similarly to stramonium seed. [Sanskrit *dhattūra.*]

daturine (dat·ewr·een). An alkaloid present in stramonium, the leaves and flowering tops of *Datura stramonium* Linn.; most probably hyoscyamine, or a mixture of the latter with atropine. [Sanskrit *dhattura* datura.]

daturism (dat·ewr·izm). The morbid condition resulting from poisoning with stramonium. [see prec.]

Daubenton, Louis Jean Marie (b. 1716). Paris physician and naturalist.

Daubenton's angle. The occipital angle, between the plane in which the foramen magnum lies and a plane including the posterior border of the foramen magnum and the infra-orbital margins.

Daubenton's line. A line joining the infra-orbital margin and the posterior border of the foramen magnum.

Daubenton's plane. A plane passing through the infra-orbital margins and the opisthion.

dauciform (**daw**·se·form). Like a carrot. [Gk *daukon* carrot, form.]

daucine (**daw**·seen). $C_{11}H_{18}N_2$, an alkaloid related to pyrrolidine and found in the leaves of the wild carrot, *Daucus carota;* it has a diuretic action. [Gk *daukon* carrot.]

daucoid (**daw**·koid). Dauciform. [Gk *daukon* carrot, *eidos* form.]

daunorubicin (daw·no·**roo**·bis·in). An antibiotic produced by two strains of *Streptomyces coeruloerubidus.* It is effective against Gram-positive organisms but rarely used to combat infections because of its harmful effect on bone marrow; occasionally given to combat acute leukaemia.

Davaine, Casimir Joseph (b. 1812). Paris pathologist and parasitologist.

Davaine's bacillus. A bacillus described by Davaine in 1863, presumably *Bacillus anthracis,* causing septicaemia in sheep.

Davainea (da·va·ne·ah). A genus of tapeworms which at one time included *Raillietina.* [Casimir Joseph *Davaine.*]

Davaineidae (da·va·ne·i'·de). A family of the cestode order Cyclophyllidea. The genus *Raillietina* is of medical interest. [Casimir Joseph *Davaine.*]

Davat's operation. Cure of varicocele by compressing the veins by acufilopressure.

David, Walter (b. 1890). Berlin physician.

David's disease. A form of purpura seen in women and characterized by severe purpura or haemorrhages from the mucous membranes, with normal blood-platelet counts in the early stages but with the development of thrombocytopenia later.

Davidoff, M. (d. 1904). Munich and St. Petersburg physician.

Davidoff's cell. An eosinophil granular epithelial cell from the intestinal crypts of Lieberkühn, probably secreting digestive enzymes; Paneth's cell.

Davidsohn, Hermann (b. 1842). Berlin physician.

Davidsohn's reflex, or sign. Loss of the light reflex on the side of a diseased antrum when a light is placed in the mouth.

Daviel, Jacques (b. 1693). Paris ophthalmic surgeon.

Daviel's operation. For cataract: the first operation performed in which the lens was removed from the eye, 1752. An incision below with the keratome is enlarged with a knife and scissors. Of historical interest.

Daviel's scoop, or spoon. A narrow, spoon-like instrument used in expressing the lens in extracapsular cataract extraction; first used by Daviel in the original cataract extraction.

Davies-Colley, John Neville Colley (b. 1842). London surgeon.

Davies-Colley operation. Removal of a bone wedge from the foot to correct talipes.

Davis, John Staige (b. 1872). Baltimore surgeon.

Davis graft. Pinch graft; small circular deep grafts a few millimetres in diameter sliced off so that the centre is of whole skin, the periphery of epidermis only.

Davis' sign. Emptiness and paleness of the arteries after death.

Davy, Sir Humphry (b. 1778). British chemist.

Marié-Davy cell. A two-fluid cell the two electrodes of which are zinc and carbon immersed, respectively, in zinc sulphate and mercuric sulphate, the latter acting as a depolarizer. It yields an e.m.f. of 1.4 V.

Davy, Richard (b. 1838). London surgeon.

Davy's lever. A wooden appliance at one time used to compress the iliac artery by insertion into the rectum.

Dawbarn, Robert Hugh Mackay (b. 1860). American surgeon.

Dawbarn's sign. In acute subacromial bursitis, pain is produced by pressure on the bursa with the arm to the side, but disappears when the arm is abducted.

Day, Richard Lawrence (b. 1905). American paediatrician.

Riley-Day syndrome. Familial dysautonomia. *See* DYSAUTONOMIA.

d'Azyr, Felix Vicq (b. 1748). Paris physician and anatomist.

Vicq d'Azyr's band, or stripe. Band of Gennari; a white band which is characteristic of the visual area of the cerebral cortex. It is continuous with the outer line of Baillarger and is more usually known as *Gennari's band, layer, line, stria or stripe.* The cortical area concerned is often called the *striate area.*

Bundle, column or tract of Vicq d'Azyr. The mamillothalamic tract.

Vicq d'Azyr's foramen. The depression at the lower border of the pons which coincides with the termination of the anterior median fissure of the medulla oblongata.

Vicq d'Azyr's operation. Laryngotomy.

de-. Prefix, from the Latin *de,* meaning *away, from.*

deacetylation (de·as·et·il·a'·shun). The process of removing an acetyl group from a compound. [L *de,* acetyl.]

deacidification (de·as·id·if·e·**ka**'·shun). The correcting of acidity by neutralization or removal of an acid. [L *de,* acid, L *facere* to make.]

deactivation (de·ak·tiv·**a**'·shun). 1. In chemistry, the process of causing inactivity or of becoming inactive. 2. Loss of radioactivity of a substance. [L *de,* activation.]

deadly nightshade (**ded**·le **nite**·shade). The plant *Atropa belladonna* Linn. (family Solanaceae). It contains the alkaloids hyoscyamine and atropine, and is the source of belladonna. [AS *déad, nihtscada.*]

deaf (def). Partially or wholly deprived of the sense of hearing. [AS *déaf.*]

deaf-mute (def·**mewt**). An individual who is deaf and dumb. [AS *déaf,* L *mutus.*]

deaf-mutism (def·**mewt**·izm). The state of being both deaf and dumb; the mutism being the result of the inability to hear. The causative deafness may be present at birth, in which case it is known as *congenital deaf-mutism,* or it may be first established during the speech-learning age, when it gives rise to an acquired form of deaf-mutism. **Congenital deaf-mutism.** Deaf-mutism as a result of congenital deafness. **Hysterical deaf-mutism.** A form occurring suddenly as the result of hysteria. **Symptomatic deaf-mutism.** Deaf-mutism indicative of either congenital anatomical abnormalities or infections, such as syphilis or meningitis acquired during fetal development or in early life. [see prec.]

deafferentate (de·af·er·en·tate). To cut the afferent-nerve supply. [L *de,* afferent nerve.]

deafferentation (de·af·er·en·ta'·shun). The cutting of the afferent-nerve supply. [see prec.]

deafness (**def**·nes). The inability to appreciate the stimuli resulting from sound waves, as a result of lack of development or disease of the auditory mechanism. **Bass deafness.** Impairment of hearing for low-frequency sounds. **Blast deafness.** Deafness due to the traumatic effect of an explosion at close quarters. **Boilermakers' deafness.** A form of deafness resulting from degeneration of the cochlea as a result of prolonged overstimulation by noise. It is common among boilermakers and riveters. **Central deafness.** Deafness due to a lesion in the auditory pathway, as opposed to deafness resulting from injury to the cochlea or the auditory nerve. **Cerebral deafness.** That due to damage of the higher auditory centres and cerebellum. As hearing has a bilateral cerebral representation, complete cerebral deafness is rare, since destruction of the higher auditory centres on both sides is unusual. **Ceruminous deafness.** That due to complete blockage of the outer ear passage by a plug of wax. **Clang deafness.** Inability to appreciate small variations in tone. **Conduction deafness.** Deafness resulting from disordered function of the sound-conducting mechanism, which includes the ear-drum and ossicular chain. **Cortical deafness.** A term used to imply deafness of a hysterical nature; it is seen in cases of shell shock and battle fatigue. **Functional deafness.** Deafness resulting from a functional disorder and not from organic disease. **Gun deafness.** Deafness occurring in naval and army gunners and ordnance officers as the result of frequent exposure to the noise of gunfire. **Hysterical deafness.** Deafness consequent on a functional or hysterical disorder of the auditory mechanism without actual organic disease. **Labyrinthine deafness.** That resulting from disease of the internal ear or labyrinth; it is another form of perceptive deafness (see below). **Middle-ear deafness.** Deafness resulting from middle-ear disease. **Music deafness.** Another form of tone deafness (see below). **Nerve deafness.** Deafness due to damage or disease of the auditory nerve. The term is sometimes used to cover all types of deafness produced by damage to the sound-perceiving mechanism. **Nervous deafness.** A functional disorder which arises in an individual who, as a result of mental excitement or confusion, fails to appreciate sounds. **Organic deafness.** That associated with disease of the auditory mechanism; the opposite of hysterical deafness (see above). **Paradoxical deafness.** The ability to hear speech better in noisy surroundings; Willis' paracousis. **Perceptive deafness.** Deafness due to damage of any part of the sound-perceiving mechanism, that is, any part of the mechanism including the cochlea, the auditory nerve and its central connections. **Pocket-handkerchief deafness.** A form of deafness which results from over-stretching of the tympanic membrane due to air under pressure being forced up the eustachian tubes during vigorous and injudicious blowing of the nose. **Psychic deafness.** Deafness resulting from a disturbed mental state. **Psychogenic deafness.** A hysterical deafness seen commonly as a war neurosis and in battle fatigue; not to be confused with malingering. **Sensory deafness.** Psychic deafness (see above). **Speech deafness.** Deafness in which simple sounds can be heard and appreciated, but not the complex sound patterns of speech which the auditory mechanism is unable to analyse and appreciate. **Tone deafness.** An inability to appreciate the pitch or changing pitch of a note. **Toxic deafness.** Deafness due to an adverse effect of poisons on the ear, particularly on the nerve of hearing. Certain drugs, such as quinine and salicylates, and tobacco may be responsible. **Transmission deafness.** Conduction deafness (see above). **Vascular deafness.** Deafness due to disorder of the blood supply to the inner ear. **Word deafness.** Auditory imperception. Failure to appreciate the words which go to make up speech; it is due to damage of the auditory word centres following on destruction of the left first temporal gyrus. [AS *déaf.*]

dealbation (de·al·**ba**·shun). Bleaching, or blanching. [L *de, albare* to whiten.]

dealcoholization (**de**·al·ko·hol·i·za′·shun). 1. The process of removing alcohol from a liquid. 2. In histology, the freeing of a specimen from the alcohol in which it has previously been immersed. [L *de,* alcohol.]

deallergization (**de**·al·er·jiz·**a**′·shun). The process of counteracting to various degrees the sensitivity of an individual to any particular substance or drug. [L *de,* allergy.]

deamidase (de·**am**·id·aze). Deaminase.

deamidation (de·**am**·id·**a**′·shun). Deamination.

deamidization (de·**am**·id·i·za′·shun). 1. Deamination. 2. The replacement of the NH_2 group in an amide by another radical.

deamidize (de·**am**·id·ize). Deaminize.

deaminase (de·**am**·in·aze). One of a class of enzymes responsible for deamination. **α-Deaminase.** Amino-acid oxidase, an enzyme which is found in the liver and kidney; it oxidizes α-amino acids to keto acids. **Adenosine deaminase.** An enzyme which catalyses the conversion of adenosine to hypoxanthine and ammonia. **Adenylic deaminase.** An enzyme which catalyses the conversion of adenylic acid to inosinic acid and ammonia. **Cysteine desulphurase deaminase.** An enzyme which degrades cysteine to pyruvate. **Cytidine deaminase.** An enzyme which catalyses the conversion of cytidine to uridine and ammonia. **Guanosine deaminase.** An enzyme which catalyses the conversion of guanosine to xanthosine and ammonia. **Guanylic-acid deaminase.** An enzyme which catalyses the conversion of guanylic acid to xanthylic acid and ammonia. **Serine deaminase.** An enzyme which degrades serine to pyruvate. **Threonine deaminase.** An enzyme which degrades threonine to 2-oxobutyrate.

deamination, deaminization (de·**am**·in·**a**′·shun, de·**am**·in·i·**za**′·shun). The process of removing amino groups or imino linkages from amino acids and related nitrogenous compounds by hydrolysis, oxidation or reduction, thereby liberating ammonia and producing the corresponding alcohol or fatty acid. [L *de,* amine.]

deaminize (de·**am**·in·ize). To perform the process of deamination.

deammoniated (de·am·**o**·ne·a·ted). Freed from ammonia. [L *de,* ammonia.]

deanaesthesiant (**de**·an·es·**the**′·ze·ant). Any agent or means by which a patient can be roused from the stuporous influence of an anaesthetic. [L *de,* anaesthesia.]

Deanol (**de**·an·ol). BP Commission approved name for 2-dimethylamino-ethanol; it is used in the treatment of psychoneuroses.

deaquation (de·ak·**wa**·shun). The process of dehydrating a substance; that is, of removing moisture or water. [L *de, aqua* water.]

Dearborn test. An intelligence test consisting of a variety of non-verbal tasks.

dearterialization (**de**·ar·teer·e·al·i·**za**′·shun). The process of converting arterial into venous blood. Cf. ATMOSPHERIZATION. [L *de,* artery.]

dearticulation (**de**·ar·tik·ew·**la**′·shun). 1. Dislocation of a joint. 2. Diarthrosis. [L *de,* articulation.]

death (deth). The final cessation of life; the cessation of all vital functions in a living organism. **Apparent death.** The condition in which the vital functions are so feebly maintained as to be scarcely apparent. **Black death.** Purpuric plague. **Cot death.** A perplexing form of death in which infants, often in their first year, are found dead in cots or beds, sometimes face down. The pathology is obscure, though there is a seasonal incidence in late winter. Little, or nothing, emerges from post-mortem examination or laboratory investigation. **Death certification.** The certification of all deaths on the standard death (or stillbirth) certificate, or notified to the Coroner. **Intra-uterine death.** Death of a fetus while still in the uterus. **Limes death.** The smallest amount of a bacterial toxin which, when mixed with one unit of the homologous antitoxin and injected into a susceptible animal of standard weight, will kill that animal in 96 h on the average. **Local death.** Death of a part of the body only; necrosis. **Molar death.** Death of the whole mass of a part of the body. **Molecular death.** Death of the tissues; this may occur later than somatic death, so that, for instance, electrical stimuli may cause some response. **Moment of death.** The *final* moment of spontaneous cessation of heart beat and respiration. **Muscular death.** The condition of the muscles when they fail to react to any stimulus. **Neonatal death.** The death of an infant under one month of age. **Red death.** A salmon-pink colour assumed by muscles in a limb affected by gas gangrene. **Reports of death to Coroner.** Cases of sudden, unexpected death, or deaths from unknown cause; cases not seen within 14 days, deaths from violence or miscarriages of treatment or drug use; suspicious maternal and infant deaths; deaths in places of lawful confinement, e.g. prison. *See also* COT DEATH (above). **Serum death.** Death due to anaphylaxis following the injection of serum into a heterologous animal. **Signs of death.** Such signs as cessation of respiration and circulation, the non-response to mechanical stimuli, the fall of body temperature, hypostasis, rigor mortis, etc. **Somatic death.** Death of the whole body. **Thymineless death.** The death of bacteria which is observed to follow deprivation of thymine, which is an essential component of DNA. **Thymus death.** Sudden death occurring in persons with status lymphaticus, a condition of hyperplasia of the lymphatic system with enlarged thymus gland. [AS *déath.*]

death adder (**deth ad**·er). An Australasian poisonous snake of the genus *Acanthophis.* The tip of the tail is flattened and bears a spine. [AS *déath, nàedre* serpent.]

death certificate (**deth** ser·**tif**·ik·ate). A certificate issued on a prescribed form and signed by a registered medical practitioner, stating to the best of his knowledge and belief the cause of death, with other relevant particulars of the person whom he has attended in the last illness. The certificate may be posted *or* handed to the "qualified informant" by the practitioner to the Registrar of Births and Deaths for the district. A Coroner, or High Court Judge acting as such, may also issue a Death Certificate for authority to dispose of a dead body. *See also:* STILLBIRTH. **Standard death certificate.** A form of death certificate recommended by the United States Bureau of the Census and in general use throughout the United States of America.

Deaver, John Blair (b. 1855). Philadelphia surgeon.

Deaver's incision. Incision for removal of the appendix through the sheath of the right rectus abdominis muscle with medial retraction of the muscle.

Deaver's windows. Translucent, fat-free areas of the mesentery in the small intestine, framed by the arterial arcades.

Debaryomyces neoformans (de·**bar**·e·o·**mi'**·seez ne·o·**for**·manz). An obsolete synonym for *Cryptococcus neoformans.*

debilitant (de·**bil**·it·ant). 1. A sedative. 2. Causing debility or weakness. [L *debilis* weak.]

debility (de·**bil**·it·e). 1. Weakness or languor the result of loss of general tone in the tissues, especially the muscles. 2. The state of being feeble or without strength. **Nervous debility.** Neurasthenia. [see prec.]

deblocking (**de**·blok·ing). The technique whereby an anomic aphasiac is assisted in his search for an elusive word by showing it to him in print along with a series of other and inappropriate terms.

débouchement (de·boosh·**mahn**). 1. The orifice of one passage in a canal or passage of another. 2. The point at which one canal or passage opens into another. 3. Emptying or opening into another passage or canal. [Fr. outlet.]

Débove, Maurice Georges (b. 1845). Paris pathologist.

Débove's disease. Splenomegaly.

Débove's layer, or membrane. The basement membrane of the respiratory and intestinal epithelia.

Débove's treatment. Forced feeding for the treatment of tuberculosis.

Débove's tube. A tube for washing out the stomach.

Debré, Robert (b. 1882). Paris paediatrician and bacteriologist.

Debré's phenomenon. The local prevention of the development of the rash of measles by injecting measles convalescent serum or gamma globulin. It is rarely applicable in practice, since the serum must be injected from one to two days before the general rash appears.

Debré-De Toni-Fanconi syndrome. *See* FANCONI'S DISEASE.

débridement (de·breed·**mahn**). 1. Literally, to make an incision to relieve tension. 2. Excision from a wound of dead tissue or tissue the blood supply of which has been so seriously interfered with that it is likely to die, in order to remove a pabulum on which organisms can grow. **Chemical débridement.** Removal of dead tissue from a wound by chemical, usually enzymatic, action. **Larval débridement.** Removal of dead tissue from a wound by digestion by maggots. [Fr. an incision.]

debris (**da**·bree). 1. An accumulation of fragments of broken-down or necrosed organic tissue. 2. In dentistry, foreign matter lying on the surface of a tooth or in a cavity prepared in a tooth. **Epithelial debris.** Malassez' debris; the unatrophied remains of the epithelial sheath of Hertwig found in the periodontal membrane which may contribute to the formation of cysts associated with a tooth. **Word debris.** The indistinct and incoherent fragmentary attempts at speech made by an individual affected with aphasia. [Fr. remains.]

Debrisoquine (deb·ri·so·kween). BP Commission approved name for 2-amidino-1,2,3,4-tetrahydroisoquinoline; a hypotensive agent.

decagram (**dek**·ah·gram). Ten grams. [Gk *deka* ten, gram.]

decalcification (de·kal·sif·e·**ka'**·shun). Freeing from calcareous matter or lime salts. [L *de,* calcification.]

decalcify (de·**kal**·sif·i). To remove lime salts or calcareous matter from bone or tissue. [see prec.]

decalitre (**dek**·ah·le·ter). Ten litres. [Gk *deka* ten, litre.]

decalvant (de·**kal**·vant). 1. Having the property of destroying or removing hair. 2. An agent which destroys or removes hair. [L *decalvare* to make bald.]

decamethonium (dek·ah·meth·**o'**·ne·um). An organic radical derived by substitution from ammonium. It is the decamethylene member of a series of polymethylene bis(trimethylammonium) radicals of general formula $(CH_3)_3N^+(CH_2)_nN^+(CH_3)_3$ known as *methonium bases, n* in this case being 10. The simple salts (e.g. the iodide) are muscle relaxants behaving superficially like curare, but differing fundamentally in mode of action in that they block transmission at the neuromuscular junction by depolarization of the motor end-plate. The block is not diminished by neostigmine, but is antagonized by D-tubocurarine, the action of which in itself antagonizes neostigmine. **Decamethonium bromide.** $(CH_3)_3NBr(CH_2)_{10}NBr(CH_3)_3$, a compound similar to the iodide and with the same pharmacological action. **Decamethonium Iodide BPC 1959.** C10, decamethylene bis(trimethylammonium iodide), $(CH_3)_3NI(CH_2)_{10}NI(CH_3)_3$; a synthetic depolarizing muscle relaxant used by anaesthetists. It is particularly free from side-effects such as the paralysis of the ganglia seen with curare, and histamine release. Its duration with therapeutic doses is of the order of 20–30 min. Neostigmine is not an effective antidote, and thus the period of action cannot be shortened. Furthermore, in sensitive individuals the duration may be excessively prolonged, and the lack of a suitable antidote is a definite disadvantage. While the drug is claimed to have a sparing effect on the respiratory muscles, artifical respiration is often necessary. [Gk *deka* ten, methonium.]

decametre (**dek**·ah·me·ter). Ten metres. [Gk *deka* ten, metre.]

decane (**dek**·ane). $C_{10}H_{22}$. A saturated liquid hydrocarbon, the tenth in the methane series, which occurs in petroleum. [Gk *deka* ten.]

decanem (**dek**·ah·nem). Equivalent to 10 nems (= units of nutrition in von Pirquet's system). [Gk *deka* ten, nem.]

decannulation (de·kan·ew·**la'**·shun). The act of removing a cannula or tube, particularly after tracheotomy. [L *de,* cannula.]

decanormal (dek·ah·**nor**·mal). In volumetric analysis, a standard solution ten times normal strength; denoted by 10N. [Gk *deka* ten, normal.]

decantation (de·kan·**ta**·shun). The separation of a liquid or solid sediment by pouring off the overlying layer of clear liquid. [L *de,* Gk *kanthos* lip of a vessel.]

decapeptide (dek·a·**pep**·tide). A protein molecule consisting of 10 amino acids linked in a chain by peptide bonds. [Gk *deka* ten, peptide.]

decapitation (de·kap·it·**a'**·shun). The act of cutting off the head, e.g. of a bone; particularly, removal of the fetal head when delivery otherwise is not possible. [L *de, caput* head.]

decapitator (de·**kap**·it·a·tor). An instrument with which the head of a fetus may be removed in order to make delivery possible. [see prec.]

Decapoda (dek·ah·**po**·dah). 1. An order of the class Crustacea; crabs, lobsters, etc. The genera *Astacus, Cambarus, Eriocheir* and *Potamon* are of medical interest. 2. A sub-order of the molluscan class Cephalopoda, which contains all cuttle-fish and squids. [Gk *deka* ten, *pous* foot.]

decapsulation (de·kap·sew·**la'**·shun). 1. Surgical removal of a capsule or sheath. 2. Surgical removal of the capsule of the kidney. **Renal decapsulation.** The sloughing off of the capsule of the kidney in Bright's disease. [L *de, capsula* little box.]

decarbonated (de·**kar**·bon·a'·ted). Having had carbon or carbon dioxide removed. [L *de,* carbon.]

decarbonation (de·kar·bon·a'·shun). The process of removing carbon dioxide from a compound or from a solution. [L *de,* carbon.]

decarbonization (de·**kar**·bon·i·**za'**·shun). 1. The act of removing carbon from a substance. 2. The act of saturating the lungs with oxygen in order to remove carbon dioxide from the blood. [see prec.]

decarboxylase (de·kar·**box**·il·aze). An enzyme catalysing a reaction involving the release of carbon dioxide. **Amino-acid decarboxylases.** Enzymes which convert amino acids into the corresponding amines. **Pyruvate decarboxylase.** A microbial enzyme catalysing the conversion of pyruvate into acetaldehyde. [L *de,* carboxyl group.]

decarboxylation (de·kar·**box**·il·**a'**·shun). 1. Decarboxylization. 2. The process taking place during the bacterial decomposition of proteins by certain enzymes whereby amino acids are converted into amines with the liberation of carbon dioxide. [L *de,* carboxyl group.]

decarboxylization (de·kar·**box**·il·i·**za'**·shun). The process in which certain enzymes attack the carboxyl radical of organic acids, liberating carbon dioxide and producing aldehydes or lower acids. [see prec.]

decay (de·**ka**). 1. The gradual mental and physical deterioration which accompanies the decline of life; senility. 2. To waste away. 3. The gradual chemical decomposition of dead organic matter when exposed to the effects of atmospheric oxygen. 4. The process of disintegration of radioactive substances. **Alpha decay.** The mode of radioactive decay (disintegration) in which the atomic nucleus emits an alpha particle. **Anile decay.** Old age in women. **Beta decay.** The mode of radioactive decay (disintegration) in which the atomic nucleus emits a beta particle. **Radioactive decay.** The process of disintegration in which a radioactive isotope of an element transforms into another isotope of the same element, or into another element. The isotope resulting from the disintegration may itself be radioactive or may be stable. Radioactive decay follows an exponential law $R_t = R_0e^{-\lambda t}$ where R_0 and R_t are the radioactivity at zero time and time *t*, respectively, and λ is the decay constant for the radionuclide of interest. [L *de, cadere* to fall.]

deceleration (**de**·sel·er·**a'**·shun). Decrease of speed, as in the heart rate. [L *de, accelerare* to hasten.]

decentration (de·sen·**tra**·shun). 1. The state of being or becoming decentred. 2. The process of removing from a centre. [L *de, centrum* centre.]

decentred (de·**sen**·terd). 1. Situated or placed eccentrically or out of the common centre. 2. In optics, indicating that the visual axis of a lens does not coincide with the axis of the lens. [see prec.]

decerating, deceration (de·ser·a·ting, de·ser·**a**·shun). In histology, the freeing of a section from paraffin wax in preparation for the microscope. [L *de, cera* wax.]

decerebellation (de·**ser**·e·bel·**a'**·shun). Removal of the cerebellum. [L *de,* cerebellum.]

decerebrate (de·**ser**·e·brate). 1. To remove the brain or, in physiology, to cut the brain stem above the level of the red nucleus. 2. One that has been subjected to decerebration. [L *de,* cerebrum.]

decerebration (de·ser·e·**bra'**·shun). The process of removing the brain, or cutting the brain stem above the level of the red nucleus. [see prec.]

decerebrize (de·**ser**·e·brize). To decerebrate.

dechloridation, dechlorination (**de**·klor·id·**a'**·shun, **de**·klor·in·**a'**·shun). The process of reducing the quantity of sodium chloride in the body by the use of a salt-free diet. [L *de,* chloride, chlorine.]

dechlorurant (de·**klor**·ewr·ant). Any agent which induces dechloruration.

dechloruration (**de**·klor·ewr·**a'**·shun). The decreasing of the quantity of chlorides excreted in the urine by use of a salt-free diet. [L *de,* chloride, urine.]

decholesterolization (de·kol·es·ter·ol·i·**za'**·shun). Reduction of cholesterol in the blood. [L *de,* cholesterol.]

decibel (**des**·e·bel). One-tenth of a bel; the unit used for measurement of the intensity of sound in a logarithmic scale based on the reference level of 20 μPa. Used particularly in recording the degree of deafness and the sound level of noise. [L *decimus* tenth, bel.]

decidua [membrana decidua] (de·**sid**·ew·ah). The name applied to the mucous membrane lining the uterus after fertilization has taken place; it becomes thickened and vascular whilst the interglandular tissue is congested with decidual cells. **Decidua basalis [NA].** The area of endometrium to which the ovum is attached, and into which the synctium grows; formerly known as the *decidua serotina.* **Decidua capsularis [NA].** Formerly *decidua reflexa,* the decidua that covers the ovum after fertilization and which stretches as the ovum grows. **Catamenial decidua.** A term not in common use today denoting the decidua-like reaction that occurs in the endometrium after ovulation has taken place; also called *decidua menstrualis.* **Decidua graviditatis.** The decidua of pregnancy. **Decidua parietalis [NA].** The decidua that is not in contact with the ovum; the true decidua or decidua vera. **Decidua vera.** The decidua that is neither basalis nor capsularis; the true decidua lining the rest of the uterus. [L *decidere* to fall off.]

decidual (de·**sid**·ew·al). Relating to the decidua.

decidualitis (de·**sid**·ew·al·**i'**·tis). A condition in which, as the result of bacterial infection, inflammatory changes occur in the decidua. [decidua, Gk *-itis* inflammation.]

deciduation (de·**sid**·ew·**a'**·shun). The shedding of the decidua during the menstrual periods. [L *decidere,* to fall off.]

deciduitis (de·**sid**·ew·**i'**·tis). Decidual endometritis. [decidua, Gk *-itis* inflammation.]

deciduoma (de·**sid**·ew·**o'**·mah). A neoplasm developed within the uterus and containing decidual cells; it is held by some to arise from retained fragments of the decidua after abortion. **Deciduoma malignum.** Chorionepithelioma. [decidua, Gk *-oma* tumour.]

See also: LOEB.

deciduomatosis (de·**sid**·ew·o·mat·**o'**·sis). A condition of the non-gravid uterus in which decidual tissue forms irregularly and in excessive quantity. [deciduoma, Gk *-osis* condition.]

deciduosarcoma (de·**sid**·ew·o·sar·**ko'**·mah). Chorionepithelioma. [decidua, sarcoma.]

deciduous (de·**sid**·ew·us). 1. Shed at maturity. 2. Impermanent. **Deciduous teeth.** The first set of temporary teeth which erupt during the first and second years of life. [L *decidere* to fall off.]

decigram (**des**·e·gram). The tenth part of a gram; 100 mg. [L *decimus* tenth, gram.]

decilitre (**des**·e·le·ter). The tenth part of a litre; 100 ml. [L *decimus* tenth, litre.]

decimetre (**des**·e·me·ter). One-tenth of a metre; 10 cm. [L *decimus* tenth, metre.]

decimolar (des·e·**mo**·lar). Of a solution, the tenth part of the molecular weight of a substance dissolved in 1 litre of solvent, usually distilled water. [L *decimus* tenth, molecule.]

decinem (**des**·e·nem). One-tenth of a nem, the unit proposed by von Pirquet in his system of nutritive values. [L *decimus* tenth, nem.]

decinormal (des·e·**nor**·mal). In volumetric analysis, a standard solution one-tenth of normal strength; denoted by N/10. [L *decimus* tenth, normal.]

decipara (des·**ip**·ah·rah). A woman who is bearing her tenth child or has borne 10 children. [L *decem* ten, *parere* to give birth.]

decitellization (**de**·si·til·i·**za'**·shun). The extermination of ground squirrels which are plague carriers in the USA. [L *de, citellus* ground squirrel.]

declination (dek·lin·a·shun). Cyclophoria. **Magnetic declination.** The angle by which a magnetic needle at any place deviates from the true north. [L *declinare* to slope away.]

declinator (**dek**·lin·a·tor). An instrument with which parts can be retracted and held out of the way during an operation. [see prec.]

decline (de·**kline**). 1. Decay. 2. Diminution. 3. Any wasting or chronic progressive disease. 4. Pulmonary tuberculosis. 5. That stage of a paroxysm, disorder or disease when the symptoms begin to abate. [L *declinare* to slope away.]

declive (de·**klive**). 1. The lobulus clivi. 2. The lowest part, e.g. of a wound. [L *de, clivus* hill.]

declivis cerebelli (de·**kli**·vis ser·e·**bel**·i). The lobulus clivi. [L hill of the little brain.]

decoction (de·**kok**·shun). An extract of the water-soluble substances in a drug made by boiling it for 10 min in distilled water. Decoctions are best prepared fresh, but concentrated decoctions are made usually to be diluted 1 to 7. Alcohol must be added to concentrated decotions to a strength of at least 20 per cent in order to preserve them. [L *de, coquere* to boil.]

decoctum (de·**kok**·tum). A decoction. **Decoctum acaciae corticis.** A 6 per cent decoction of the bark of *Acacia arabica* or *A. decurrens* used as an astringent and in gargles. **Decoctum Aloes Compositum BPC 1949.** A decoction containing 1 per cent aloes with myrrh, potassium carbonate, liquorice and compound tincture of cardamom; a cathartic. **Decoctum Cinchonae Concentratum BPC 1949.** A decoction of cinchona bark concentrated to 1 in 7. [L.]

decollation (de·**kol**·a·shun). Decapitation. [L *de, collum* neck.]

decollator (de·**kol**·at·or). Decapitator. [see prec.]

décollement (de·kol·**mahn**). The separation by surgical means of two structures which normally or pathologically are adherent. [Fr. detachment.]

decolorant (de·**kul**·or·ant). An agent that absorbs or destroys a colour. [see foll.]

decoloration (de·kul·or·a′·shun). Loss or removal of colour by bleaching. [L *de*, colour.]

decolorize (de·**kul**·or·ize). To bleach, whiten or destroy or remove a colour by means of an agent. [see prec.]

decombustion (de·kom·**bust**·yun). The process of removing oxygen from a substance, as when heated strongly with charcoal. [L *de, combuere* to burn up.]

decompensation (de·kom·pen·**sa**′·shun). Failure of compensation; any condition in which an organ, that has hitherto been meeting the normal demands of the body despite some defect or any additional demands, fails to meet these demands. **Cardiac decompensation.** Heart failure; inability of the heart to fulfil adequately the demands made upon it. In clinical practice, the term is often used to describe congestive cardiac failure. **Hepatic decompensation.** The failure of a damaged liver to meet minimum functional requirements. [L *de*, compensation.]

decompose (de·kom·**poze**). 1. To rot or putrefy after death; a consequence of the disintegration of tissues from the action of enzymes and bacteria. 2. To break up a compound into its constituents. 3. To analyse, split up or break down a substance. 4. To disintegrate. [L *de, componere* to put together.]

decomposition (de·kom·po·**zish**′·un). 1. A state of being decomposed. 2. The process of decomposing. **Double decomposition.** Metathesis, 2nd def. **Decomposition of movement.** A condition met with in disease of the cerebellum in which muscular movement lacks smoothness, any movement of a limb appearing as a series of separate mechanical motions. **Single decomposition.** Analysis. [see prec.]

decompression (de·kom·**presh**·un). Removal or relief of pressure. The term is applied in particular to the gradual or "stage" decompression of caisson workers and divers to prevent "bends" from the formation of bubbles of nitrogen gas in the blood and tissues, for which recompression may be necessary. **Cardiac decompression.** Removal of a large pericardial effusion (pericardial aspiration), a haematoma (pericardiotomy) or a constriction of the pericardial sac (pericardiolysis), relieving compression of the heart and permitting adequate filling in diastole. **Cerebral decompression.** Removal of a portion of the skull, with or without the dura mater, to relieve intracranial tension. **Explosive decompression.** A rapid reduction of ambient pressure occurring in one-tenth of a second or less. **Decompression of the heart.** Cardiac decompression (see above). **Nerve decompression.** Splitting of the fibrous or bony containment of a swollen nerve. **Decompression of the pericardium.** Cardiac decompression (see above). **Decompression sickness.** *See* SICKNESS. **Decompression of the spinal cord.** Laminectomy or similar operation to remove pressure on the cord. [L *de, comprimere* to press together.]

decongestive (de·kon·**jes**·tiv). 1. An agent for the relief or reduction of congestion. 2. Having the property of reducing or relieving congestion. [L *de, congerere* to heap up.]

decontamination (de·kon·tam·in·**a**′·shun). The freeing of an individual, any object or the environment from an injurious agent such as a poison or radioactive material. [L *de, contaminare* to bring in contact.]

decortication (de·kor·tik·**a**′·shun). 1. Decapsulation. 2. The stripping-off of parts of the cortical substance of the brain. 3. Removal of the cortex of any organ or structure. 4. In pharmacy, the divesting of a seed, plant or root of its external layer, e.g. shell or hull. **Arterial decortication.** Periarterial sympathectomy. *See* SYMPATHECTOMY. **Decortication of a lung, Pulmonary decortication.** Pleurectomy. **Renal decortication.** Surgical removal of the cortex of the kidney. [L *de, cortex* rind.]

decrement (**dek**·re·ment). 1. Stadium decrementi; the stage in the course of a pyretic disease during which the temperature falls. 2. A decreasing. [L *de, crescere* to grow.]

decrepitate (de·**krep**·it·ate). 1. To crackle as salt does when exposed to strong heat. 2. To expose a moist substance to strong heat. [L *decrepitare* to crackle.]

decrepitation (de·krep·it·**a**′·shun). 1. The property of crystals, e.g. salt, to explode with a crackle when they are exposed to strong heat. 2. Crepitation. [see prec.]

decrepitude (de·**krep**·it·ewd). The state of general feebleness and decline of old age; senility. [L *de, crepare* to creak.]

decrudescence (de·kroo·**des**·ens). A lessening in the severity of symptoms of a disease. [L *de, crudescere* to become bad.]

decrustation (de·krus·**ta**·shun). Removal of a crust by artificial means or its detachment as the process of healing goes on. [L *de*, crust.]

decubation (de·kew·**ba**·shun). The last stage of an infectious disease; it extends from the disappearance of the specific symptoms to the time when the patient is completely recovered. [L *decumbere* to lie down.]

decubitus (de·**kew**·bit·us). The posture assumed by a patient lying in bed over a long period. **Decubitus sore or ulcer, Chronic decubitus, Decubitus chronicus.** *See* ULCER. [L *decumbere* to lie down.]

See also: ANDRAL.

decurrent (de·**kur**·ent). Moving or extending downwards from above. [L *de, currere* to run.]

decurtate (de·**ker**·tate). Curtailed or shortened. [L *decurtare* to cut short.]

decurtation (de·ker·**ta**·shun). 1. The cutting-off of a part. 2. The shortening of a structure. 3. The shortening of the normal duration of a condition. [see prec.]

decussate (de·**kus**·ate). 1. To intersect or cross. 2. Crossing, as the arms of an X. [L *decussare* to cross like an X.]

decussation [decussatio (NA)] (de·kus·a·shun). A crossing, generally used of fibres in the central nervous system which cross in their passage from a region on one side to a different region on the opposite side. Also known as a *chiasma.* **Decussation of the brachium conjunctivum.** Decussation of the superior cerebellar peduncles (see below). **Dorsal tegmental decussation.** Fountain decussation (see below). **Fillet decussation.** Sensory decussation (see below). **Fountain decussation.** The decussation of the tectospinal tracts in the mid-brain; the dorsal tegmental decussation. **Decussation of the lemniscus.** Sensory decussation (see below). **Motor decussation.** Decussation of the pyramids (see below). **Optic decussation.** Optic chiasma. *See* CHIASMA. **Decussation of the pons.** The transverse fibres of the pons which arise from cells in the pontine nuclei on one side and pass across to the middle cerebellar peduncle of the other. **Decussation of the pyramids [decussatio pyramidum (NA)].** The crossing of the fibres of the cortico-spinal motor tract which occurs on the ventral side of the lower part of the medulla oblongata. **Decussation of rubrospinal tracts.** A decussation of fibres in the tegmentum between the two red nuclei and ventral to the tectospinal decussation. **Sensory decussation [decussatio lemniscorum sensoria (NA)].** The crossing of the fibres of the medial lemniscus which occurs in the medulla oblongata; these fibres arise from cells in the cuneate and gracile nuclei and pass to the thalamus. **Decussation of the superior cerebellar peduncles [decussatio pedunculorum cerebellarium superiorum (NA)].** The crossing of fibres from the dentate nuclei to the red nucleus and thalamus which occurs in the tegmentum of the mid-brain. **Decussation of the tectospinal tracts.** The decussation below the central grey matter of fibres arising in the superior corpora quadrigemina. **Decussation of the tegmentum [decussatio tegmenti (NA)].** A term which can be applied to any fibres crossing the midline in the tegmentum of the mid-brain, e.g. the dorsal or ventral tegmental decussations or the decussation of the brachium conjunctivum. **Trapezoid decussation.** The decussating fibres from the ventral cochlear nucleus. **Trochlear decussation, Decussation of the trochlear nerves [decussatio nervorum trochlearium (NA)].** The crossing of the fibres of the trochlear nerve which occurs in the superior medullary velum. **Ventral tegmental decussation.** The crossing of the rubrospinal tracts in the tegmentum of the mid-brain; also known as *Forel's decussation.* [see prec.]

See also: FOREL, HELD, MEYNERT.

decussorium (de·kus·or·e·um). An instrument used in trephining to keep the dura mater depressed. [L.]

dedentition (de·den·**tish**·un). Shedding of teeth; loss of teeth, particularly as a result of disease of the supporting alveolar bone. [L *de, dens* tooth.]

dedifferentiation (**de**·dif·er·en·she·**a**'·shun). Differentiation of a tissue to a more primitive structure, the successive stages being gone through in reverse order to that of development. [L *de*, differentiation.]

dedolation (de·do·**la**·shun). 1. The removal of a shaving of skin by an oblique slicing cut. 2. A subjective sensation of bruising in the arms and legs. [L *dedolare* to hew away.]

dee (de). The name given to a cyclotron electrode which is a shallow metal box shaped like a letter D. Accelerated particles travel in spiral orbits inside two dees arranged thus: ᗡD

de-electronation (**de**·el·ek·tron·**a**'·shun). A term used in the electrochemical theory of oxidation-reduction, to denote oxidation itself, or the loss by an element of a negatively charged electron. [L *de*, electron.]

deep [profundus (NA)] (deep). Below the surface. [AS *diop.*]

Deetjen, Hermann (b. 1867). Kiel and Berlin physician.

Deetjen's body. Blood platelet. *See* PLATELET.

defaecalgesiophobia (de·fe·kal·**je**·se·o·**fo**'·be·ah). Dread of evacuating the bowels on account of attendant pain. [defaecation, Gk *algos* pain, phobia.]

defaecation (de·fe·**ka**·shun). Evacuation of the bowels. **Chemical defaecation.** Freeing a solution of adulterating matter by means of an added reagent which separates off impurities. **Fragmentary defaecation.** Slight evacuation of the bowels occurring at intervals of a few hours. [L *defaecare* to remove dregs.]

defatigation (**de**·fat·ig·**a**'·shun). Over-fatigue of the nervous or muscular system to a dangerous extreme. [L *defatigatio* weariness.]

defatted (de·**fat**·ed). Freed from or deprived of fat. [L *de*, fat.]

defect (de·**fekt**). 1. Deficiency; absence or loss of something necessary for wholeness. 2. Lack of a physical or mental quality. 3. Failure in ordinary function. 4. Lack of a part or organ. **Afferent pupil defect.** Gunn's pupillary sign. **Aortopulmonary septal defect.** A developmental abnormality in which there is incomplete separation of the primitive truncus into the aorta and pulmonary artery so that a communication exists between them where they lie side by side at their origin. **Atrial septal defect.** A developmental abnormality in which the septum separating the right and left atria of the heart is incomplete. There are various forms distinguished by their anatomy or embryology. The *ostium primum type* arises from persistence of the primitive ostium primum and is often associated with endocardial cushion defects. The *ostium secundum type* arises from persistence of the ostium secundum. The *sinus venosus type* occurs high in the atrial septum involving the lower part of the superior vena cava and is usually associated with some anomalous drainage of pulmonary veins distally into the vena cava or the right atrium. **Congenital ectodermal defect.** Hereditary ectodermal dysplasia. **Endocardial cushion defect.** A developmental abnormality of the heart arising from failure of the complete normal development of the structures which should arise from the endocardial cushions; the principal forms are the ostium primum type of atrial septal defect usually with defects in tricuspid or mitral valve cusps and various degrees of common atrioventricular canal. **Filling defect.** 1. A defect, detected radiologically by use of contrast medium, in the wall or lumen of a hollow organ, due to the presence of some space-occupying body, either innocent or malignant. 2. In dentistry, a fault or a leak in a filling due to its imperfect contact with the walls of the cavity in which it has been inserted. **Retention defect.** A defect in that process of learning which is involved in the preservation of registered material. **Ventricular septal defect.** A developmental abnormality in which the septum separating the right and left ventricles of the heart is incomplete. There are various forms distinguished by their position in the septum, and the names are self-explanatory: *defect of the membranous septum, low muscular defect, supracristal defect, infracristal defect. [L defectus* a failing.]

defective (de·**fek**·tiv). 1. Imperfect. 2. One suffering from a severe subnormality within the meaning of the Mental Health Act 1959. [see prec.]

defectiveness (de·**fek**·tiv·nes). **Mental defectiveness.** Mental deficiency. *See* DEFICIENCY. [L *defectus* a failing.]

defemination, defeminization (**de**·fem·in·**a**'·shun, de·**fem**·in·i·**za**'·shun). 1. Weakness or loss of female secondary characters with increase of male characters; the condition may be the result of oöphorectomy. 2. Perversion in a woman of the female sexual impulse into that of the male. [L *de, femina* woman.]

defence (de·**fens**). 1. Resistance against an attack of disease. 2. Behaviour of an individual with the object of protecting himself from harm or injury. **Muscular defence.** Rigidity and tension in muscles associated with local inflammation or pain. **Perceptual defence.** Selective perception which excludes stimuli with unpleasant associations. [L *defendere* to repel.]

Defer's method. The treatment of hydrocele by evacuation and cauterization of the sac with silver nitrate. This method is out-of-date, and has been superseded by the injection of quinine hydrochloride and urethane after evacuation.

deferens (**def**·er·enz). The vas deferens. [L carrying away.]

deferent (**def**·er·ent). 1. Relating to the vas deferens. 2. Efferent; carrying away from a centre. [see prec.]

deferentectomy (**def**·er·ent·**ek**·to·me). Vasectomy. [vas deferens, Gk *ektome* a cutting out.]

deferentiovesical (def·er·**en**·she·o·**ves**'·ikl). Relating or belonging to the vas deferens and the urinary bladder. [vas deferens, L *vesica* bladder.]

deferentitis (**def**·er·en·**ti**'·tis). Vasitis; an inflammatory condition of the vas deferens. [vas deferens, Gk *-itis* inflammation.]

defervescence (de·fer·**ves**·ens). The period of subsidence of fever. [L *defervescere* to grow cool.]

defervescent (de·fer·**ves**·ent). 1. Any agent or remedy which reduces a febrile condition. 2. Causing or relating to defervescence. [see prec.]

defibrillation (**de**·fib·ril·**a**'·shun). 1. Blunt dissection of tissue fibres. 2. A method of brain dissection used to demonstrate the natural lines of cleavage, the cerebral tissues being pulled gently apart. 3. In cardiology, the process of abolishing atrial or ventricular fibrillation to allow the resumption of normal rhythm, achieved by the passage of electric currents through the heart. [L *de, fibrilla* little thread.]

defibrillator (de·**fib**·ril·a·tor). An instrument used to achieve defibrillation of the atria or ventricles of the heart. **Alternating current (a.c.) defibrillator.** A defibrillator which delivers a shock of alternating current, derived from the electrical mains through a transformer. **Direct current (d.c.) defibrillator.** A defibrillator which delivers a predominantly monophasic electrical discharge, derived from a precharged capacitance. [L *de*, *fibrilla* little thread.]

defibrinate (de·**fi**·brin·ate). To remove the fibrin and, in the case of fresh blood, thereby to stop clotting. [L *de*, fibrin.]

defibrination (**de**·fi·brin·**a′**·shun). The removal of fibrin from a body fluid such as blood after it has been drawn so that it will not clot or thicken. [see prec.]

deficiency (de·**fish**·en·se). 1. A lack of anything; the amount by which anything falls short. 2. In cytogenetics, this term was used originally to indicate the loss from the complement of a terminal acentric chromosome segment. Now it is often used as a near synonym of *deletion* or, in general, to indicate the loss of genetic information ensuing from chromosome structural changes. **Acid maltase deficiency.** An inborn error of metabolism causing glycogen storage in skeletal and heart muscle. Pompe's disease. **Convergence deficiency.** A weakness of the convergence power; a common cause of eye strain. **Disaccharidase deficiency.** This may be *primary*, a combined deficiency of ability to digest sucrase and isomaltose, or *secondary* to other conditions, especially gastro-enteritis or gluten enteropathy. Lactose and/or sucrose deficiency are more common than maltose or isomaltose deficiency. All cause diarrhoea and often severe subnutrition, but in secondary cases there is a strong tendency to recover if the offending sugar is removed from the diet. **Enzyme deficiencies.** A group of digestive disorders due to lack of enzymes, often congenital, causing gastro-intestinal symptoms, especially vomiting and diarrhoea. Most of these are rare congenital abnormalities of infants or children. **Hereditary disaccharidase deficiency.** Lack of enzymes (lactase, invertase, isomaltase) which may cause diarrhoea with acid stools; often called *intestinal carbohydrate dyspepsia.* **Lactase deficiency.** A congenital or acquired disorder commonly present amongst Negroes, Chinese and Cypriots; it causes diarrhoea and abdominal distension, especially after drinking milk or milk products. **Lecithin-cholesterol acyl transferase deficiency.** A syndrome in which cholesterol is not esterified. There is increased free cholesterol and hyperlipaemia, corneal opacity and normochromic anaemia. **Lipocaic deficiency.** Decreased function of the parenchyma of the pancreas. **Mental deficiency.** 1. A state of incomplete mental development which renders the subject incapable of independent social adaptation (Wood Report). 2. Obsolete term now reclassified into four specific forms of "mental disorders" under the Mental Health Act 1959. **Phosphofructokinase deficiency.** Deficiency of this enzyme in muscle with weakness, cramp and myoglobinuria. Probably autosomal recessive. **Phosphoglucomutase deficiency.** Deficiency of this enzyme in muscle with weakness and cramp. **PTA deficiency.** Deficiency of factor XI; haemophilia C. A mild bleeding disease treatable by normal serum or plasma. **Sulphite oxidase deficiency.** Decreased sulphate excretion in urine with increased sulphite, thiosulphate and *S*-sulpho-L-cysteine; there may be neurological disease. **Taste deficiency.** Absence of sense of taste, or inability to taste certain substances. [L *de*, *facere* to make.]

deficit (**def**·is·it). A deficiency. **Alkali deficit.** *See* ACIDOSIS. **Base deficit.** Base concentration per litre of blood measured by alkali titration at pH 7.4. **Oxygen deficit.** Anoxia: anoxaemia. **Pulse deficit.** The difference between the rate of the pulse and that of the heart. [see prec.]

definition (def·in·**ish**·un). 1. The precise determination of the limits of anything, e.g. a disease process. 2. In optics, the power of a lens to give precision of detail and distinctness of outline of an object. 3. The sharpness of the edges of the various shadows in a radiograph or on a fluorescent screen. Maximum sharpness is produced by many technical factors, the more important of which are a small tube focus, immobility of the object, long focus-film distance and short object-film distance. 4. The clarity of the object or objects viewed under a microscope. 5. In medical literature, a concise description of the important points in a disease. [L *definire* to limit.]

deflagration (de·flag·**ra**·shun). Combustion accompanied by a self-propagating flame. [L *de*, *flagrare* to burn.]

deflagrator (de·flag·**rate**·or). An apparatus designed to burn substances in a strongly oxidizing atmosphere. [L *de*, *flagrare* to burn.]

deflection (de·**flek**·shun). Deflexion.

deflexion (de·**flek**·shun). 1. Turning from a straight course. 2. Downward deviation. 3. The action of moving to one side. 4. In optics, the bending of rays of light at the surface of an opaque body. Cf. REFLECTION. 5. In psycho-analysis, an unconscious diverting of ideas from conscious attention. **Deflexion of the complement.** Deviation of the complement. **Intrinsicoid deflexion.** *See* R WAVE (under WAVE). **QRS deflexion.** The portion of the electrocardiogram which represents depolarization of the ventricular muscle, consisting of an initial negative Q wave, succeeded by a positive R wave, and after that a negative S wave. The Q wave indicates initial depolarization of the upper part of the interventricular septum, the R wave depolarization of the base of the septum and the myocardium of the right and left ventricles, and the S wave depolarization of the basal portion of the ventricles. [L *deflectere* to bend aside.]

deflocculator (de·**flok**·ew·la·tor). A surface-active agent which reduces the formation of loose aggregates in colloidal solutions. Deflocculators have importance in industry in conjunction with detergents and wetting agents. [L *de*, *floccus* wool.]

defloration (de·flor·**a**·shun). The act of rupturing the hymen. [L *deflorare* to deflower.]

deflorescence (de·flor·**es**·ens). The fading of the exanthema in diseases such as scarlet fever. [L *deflorescere* to fade.]

defluvium (de·**floo**·ve·um). A falling out. **Defluvium capillorum.** Alopecia. **Defluvium unguinum.** Loss of the nails. [L.]

defluxio (de·**flux**·e·o). A sudden loss, as of hair or eyelashes. **Defluxio capillorum.** Alopecia. **Defluxio ciliorum.** A sudden falling out of the eyelashes such as may occur in alopecia. [L *defluere* to fall out.]

defluxion (de·**fluk**·shun). 1. A sudden copious loss or discharge, as of fluid in catarrh. 2. A sudden loss as of hair or eyelashes. 3. A sudden flow of blood to a part. [see prec.]

deform (de·**form**). To cause deviation from the normal form or shape. [see foll.]

deformation (de·for·**ma**·shun). 1. Deformity; any aberration from the normal in shape. 2. The process of becoming deformed or disfigured. [L *de*, *formare* to shape.]

See also: SPRENGEL.

deformity (de·**for**·mit·e). Distortion of any part of the body. **Boutonnière deformity.** A flexion deformity of the proximal interphalangeal joint of a finger due to damage to the middle strand of the extensor tendon. **Dinner-fork deformity.** Deformity of the wrist, typical of Colles' fracture. **Funnel-neck deformity of the bladder.** *See* SCHRAMM'S PHENOMENON. **Gunstock deformity.** Reversal of the normal angle between the arm and forearm, the result of fracture at the elbow. **Hottentot deformity.** Steatopyga. **Mushroom deformity.** A radiological feature of psoriatic arthropathy in which the tapered distal end of one phalanx is impacted into the proximal end of the next. **Parrot-beak deformity.** A self-explanatory description given to a form of lupus vulgaris involving the nose. **Pencil and cup deformity.** Mushroom deformity (see above). **Seal-fin deformity.** The position of ulnar deviation which the fingers tend to assume in sufferers with chronic rheumatoid arthritis. **Simian deformity.** Any condition in which the tip and the anterior part of the nasal septum have been eroded so that the openings of the nares face forwards, as in most species of apes. **Swan-neck deformity.** Characteristic deformity of the finger in rheumatoid arthritis with hyperextension at the proximal interphalangeal joint and flexion at the terminal interphalangeal joint. [L *deformis* misshapen.]

See also: ÅKERLUND, ARNOLD (J.), CHIARI, MADELUNG, SPRENGEL.

defunctionalization (de·**fungk**·shun·al·i·**za′**·shun). 1. The process of depriving of function. 2. Loss of function. [L *de*, function.]

defundation, defundectomy (de·fun·**da**·shun, de·fun·**dek**·to·me). Surgical removal of the fundus of the uterus together with the uterine tubes. [L *de, fundus* bottom, Gk *ektome* a cutting out.]

defurfuration (de·**fer**·fer·**a'**·shun). The forming of branny scales on the skin and the shedding of them. [L *de, furfur* bran.]

defuselation (de·**few**·zel·**a'**·shun). In the manufacture of spirits, the removal of fusel oil from raw alcohol. [L *de*, fusel oil.]

defusion (de·**few**·zhun). In psycho-analysis, the mental process in which the two primal instincts, sexual (life) instinct and death instinct, previously blended, are separated. [L *de, fundere* to pour.]

deganglionate (de·**gang**·gle·on·ate). To take away ganglia. [L *de*, ganglion.]

degeneracy (de·**jen**·er·as·e). 1. Reversion to a lower type. 2. A condition in which physical and mental powers decline. 3. In criminology, "moral" deterioration. 4. Degeneracy of the genetic code. Implies that two or more codons (sequences of three nucleotides) may specify a single amino acid. **Inferior degeneracy.** Degeneracy in which there is physical deformity or mental deterioration. **Superior degeneracy.** Reversion to a lower type in association with intellectual brilliance. [L *degenerare* to deviate from kind.]

degenerate (de·**jen**·er·ate). 1. Of a condition, to grow worse. 2. To revert to a lower type. 3. An individual with congenital characteristics of a type lower than the normal of his kind. 4. In criminology, an individual lacking in physical, mental, or moral qualities who has a tendency to commit crime or has perverted instincts. [see prec.]

degeneratio (de·**jen**·er·**a'**·she·o). Degeneration. **Degeneratio micans.** The glassy translucent matter formed by degenerating neuroglia cells. [see foll.]

degeneration (de·**jen**·er·**a'**·shun). 1. A breaking-down of an organized structure into one less organized in form or function. 2. Mental or moral deterioration. **Abiotrophic degeneration.** Primary degeneration or trophic failure; degeneration owing to loss of vitality. **Adipose degeneration.** The deposition of fat within cells in abnormal amounts; the invasion of organs with fatty tissue. **Albuminoid degeneration, Albuminous degeneration.** Cloudy-swelling degeneration (see below). **Amyloid degeneration.** A condition in which extracellular deposits of amyloid occur in the spleen, liver, kidney, heart muscle, and elsewhere; the finer connective-tissue elements swell and become translucent and homogenous. It is usually preceded by long-standing tuberculosis, but may follow other chronic diseases. Owing to interference with the circulation of the part, cells may atrophy. Later, much of the specialized structure of an organ may disappear. **Anaemic degeneration.** Polychromatophilia. **Angiolithic degeneration.** Calcareous degeneration of blood vessels; a form of arteriosclerosis. **Ascending degeneration.** The centripetal advance of wallerian degeneration in nerve fibres from the periphery to the spinal cord and the brain. **Atheromatous degeneration.** Degeneration of the coats of an artery due to atheroma (atherosclerosis), affecting mainly the larger vessels. It begins as a proliferation of the subintimal connective tissue which becomes infiltrated with lipides (cholesterol), calcium is deposited and an atheromatous nodule forms. The intima proliferates and becomes hyalinized, whilst fragments of the nodule may be washed away in the blood stream, leaving an atheromatous ulcer. **Axonal degeneration.** That degeneration occurring in a nerve fibre following injury or section. Peripherally, the myelin sheath breaks up, the cells of the neurolemma proliferate, and most specialized nerve-endings alter but do not completely disappear. Centrally, some degree of degeneration occurs, but unless the injury is very close to the cell body it is usually not complete, so that regeneration may ultimately occur. **Bacony degeneration.** Amyloid degeneration (see above). **Balloon degeneration.** A pathological change, noted by Unna, which occurs in the prickle cells of the epidermis in zoster. These cells swell, become spheroid and lose their filaments of attachment to other cells, whilst their protoplasm becomes opaque, fibrinous and vacuolated; the nuclei increase in number and inclusion bodies may be seen in many of them. **Basic degeneration, Basophilic degeneration.** The appearance of basophil-staining granules (i.e. punctate basophilia) in red blood corpuscles that are degenerating through exposure to toxic substances such as lead, malarial and other cachexial conditions, and diseases such as leukaemia and severe anaemias. **Calcareous degeneration.** Calcification; deposition of calcium and other mineral salts at the site of fatty degeneration or necrosis in tissues, especially in the walls of arteries. **Caseous degeneration.** Caseation; a form of fatty degeneration leading to necrosis in the cells which accumulate around the tubercle bacillus when it lodges in a susceptible tissue. **Cellulose degeneration.** Amyloid degeneration (see above). **Cerebromacular degeneration.** A group of heredofamilial disorders characterized by visual loss and progressive spastic paralysis, resulting from the abnormal storage of lipoid in the central nervous system. The infantile form, Tay-Sachs' disease or amaurotic family idiocy, gives rise to progressive paralysis, dementia, blindness, convulsions and death within 2 years. On ophthalmoscopy, a cherry-red spot may be seen at the macula. The late infantile form is called *Bielschowsky-Jansky disease*, the juvenile *Spielmeyer-Vogt disease*, and the late juvenile *Kufs' disease*. **Cheesy degeneration.** Caseous degeneration (see above). **Chitinous degeneration.** Amyloid degeneration (see above). **Cloudy-swelling degeneration.** The commonest and possibly the mildest deterioration of cells, usually produced by a soluble toxic substance circulating in the blood, especially a bacterial toxin. The organs are swollen, pale and cloudy, the individual cells are swollen and often irregular in outline; their protoplasm contains granules which consist partly of protein. The liver, kidney and heart muscle may all be affected. Typically seen in acute infectious fevers, and in other infections and toxaemias. **Cobblestone degeneration of the retina.** A benign peripheral retinal degeneration. **Colloid degeneration.** Formation of a glue-like deposit within cells, especially in the pituitary and thyroid glands, and the kidney; often used as synonym for *mucoid degeneration*. **Combined degeneration.** Degeneration of the posterior and lateral columns of the spinal cord giving rise to paraesthesia, sensory ataxia and sometimes spastic paraplegia; in its subacute form it occurs as a manifestation or complication of pernicious anaemia, and responds to specific treatment. Similar cord changes may rarely occur in other nutritional disorders. Also referred to as *ataxic paraplegia, combined sclerosis*, or *SCD*. **Comma degeneration.** Degeneration of the nerve fibres of the comma tract of Schultze. **Congenital macular degeneration.** Various types of congenital degeneration have been described, affecting the macular region of the retina in each eye and unassociated with degenerative changes in the central nervous system. They tend to occur at times of physiological stress and the following varieties are described: infantile, juvenile, adolescent, presenile and senile. Many names are associated with these, e.g. Jonathan Hutchinson, Warren Tay, Rayner Batten, Best, Stargardt, Behr, Vossius and others. **Cystic adventitial degeneration.** A rare lesion of the popliteal artery in which a mucinous cyst, which may compress the artery, forms in the adventitia. **Cystic degeneration.** Degeneration leading to cyst formation. **Cystoid degeneration.** Cysts commonly forming in the peripheral retina with advancing age (Blessig). They may also be associated with advanced vascular disease, or follow trauma (usually the cyst is at the macula), infective and oedematous conditions, retinal detachment, glaucoma and choroidal tumours. **Descending degeneration.** The centrifugal spread of wallerian degeneration along nerve fibres. **Disciform degeneration of the macula.** Macular degeneration which appears disc-shaped. It usually begins as a detachment of the pigment epithelium, and central vision is permanently affected. **Earthy degeneration.** Calcareous degeneration (see above). **Elastoid degeneration.** Hyaline change of the elastic fibres in the wall of an artery, especially during involution of an organ such as the breast or uterus. **Endoglobular degeneration.** Degenerating macrocytes (megalocytes) which may show irregularly-shaped areas in the cell apparently devoid of pigment and resembling vacuoles. **Familial colloid degeneration.** *See* DOYNE'S FAMILIAL HONEYCOMBED CHOROIDITIS. **Fascicular degeneration.** The type of degeneration of voluntary muscles seen in disease of anterior-horn cells or motor neurones. **Fatty degeneration.** Adipose degeneration (see above). **Fibrinoid degeneration, Fibrinous degeneration.** Swelling and tinctorial change in fibrous tissue whereby it comes to resemble fibrin; common in rheumatic infections. **Fibroid degeneration.** A change into fibrous tissue. **Fibrous degeneration.** Increase in the fibrous tissue of an organ as the result of chronic inflammation. **Fibrous degeneration of the heart.** Cardiac fibrosis; replacement of cardiac muscle by fibrous tissue as a result of ischaemia or inflammatory conditions, or in association with rare cardiopathies such as haemochromatosis. **Gelatiniform degeneration.** Colloid degeneration (see above). **Glassy degeneration.** Amyloid degeneration (see above). **Glistening degeneration.** The appearance of glistening collections of tissue during glial degeneration. **Glycogenic degeneration.** The deposition of large amounts of glycogen within cells, especially in the liver and kidneys. **Granular degeneration.** Basophilic degeneration (see above). **Granulovascular degeneration.** A form of degeneration in which vacuoles containing condensed granules of protoplasm develop within ganglion cells. **Grey degeneration.** Demyelination of the white matter of the spinal cord, resulting in a greyish coloration. **Haematohyaloid degeneration.** A hyaline degeneration of thrombi containing red blood cells and/or platelets. **Haemoglobinaemic degeneration.** A degeneration leading to the concentration of the cellular haemoglobin in the middle of the red blood corpuscle. **Hepatolenticular degeneration.** Wilson's disease; a progressive disease, often familial, beginning in the first or second decade, and characterized by tremor, muscular rigidity, involuntary movements of many types, loss of control of emotional reactions and evidence of hepatic dysfunction. Kayser-Fleischer pericorneal pigment rings may be seen. Symptoms are due to an inborn error of metabolism leading to accumulation of toxic concentrations of copper. Also referred to as the *pseudosclerosis of Westphal* and *progressive lenticular degeneration*. **Hyaline degeneration.** Formation of a glassy material in the connective tissue of blood vessels and in old scars, which resembles amyloid in all but certain of its staining reactions. **Hyaloid degeneration.** Amyloid degeneration (see above). **Hydrocarbonaceous degeneration.** Paschutin's degeneration; glycogenic degeneration in diabetes mellitus. **Hydropic degeneration.** Intracellular oedema. **Keratoid degeneration.** Increase of keratin in the skin or a derivative of skin. **Lardaceous degeneration.** Amyloid degeneration (see above). **Lattice degeneration of the cornea.** Haab's degeneration. **Lattice degeneration of the retina.** A peripheral degeneration which may lead to retinal holes and detachment. **Lenticular degeneration.** A term covering a number of progressive disorders due to degeneration of the lenticular nucleus, including acquired bilateral athetosis, spasmodic torticollis, dystonia musculorum deformans or torsion spasm, and Wilson's disease. *See* HEPATOLENTICULAR DEGENERATION, above. **Lipoidal degeneration.** Deposition of fat-like substances within cells; a variety of adipose degeneration (see above). **Mineral degeneration.** Calcification. **Mucinoid degeneration.** A form of mucoid degeneration, especially in the ovaries. **Mucoid degeneration, Mucous degeneration.** The deposition of mucus in the connective tissue of an organ or within epithelial cells of certain sites, especially the alimentary canal, uterus and some cancers. **Myelinic degeneration.** Formation of myelins or lipoid substances in degenerating nerve fibres and within the epithelial cells of the renal tubules. **Myxomatous degeneration.** Mucoid degeneration (see above). **Neurosomatic degeneration.** The end-result of repeated or continuous epileptic convulsions, consisting of dementia, parkinsonism and widespread muscular contractures. **Pallidal degeneration.** Damage of the globus pallidus of the lentiform nucleus of the brain. **Parenchymatous degeneration.** Degeneration of the parenchyma cells, of the nature of cloudy-swelling degeneration (see above) is usually implied. **Parenchymatous degeneration of the kidney.** Cloudy swelling and fatty degeneration of the tubule epithelium of the kidney as the result of nephritis or a poor blood supply. **Pigmental degeneration, Pigmentous degeneration.** Pigmentation of the muscles or of organs such as the liver in old age. **Polychromatophilic degeneration.** Polychromatophilia. **Polypoid degeneration.** Polyposis. **Primary calcareous degeneration of the cornea.** Dystrophia calcarea corneae, a rare condition in which calcium salts are deposited beneath the corneal epithelium in otherwise healthy eyes. **Primary fatty degeneration of the cornea.** Dystrophia adiposa corneae. **Primary progressive cerebellar degeneration.** A familial form of progressive cerebellar disease beginning in middle age, characterized clinically by the slow development and progression of ataxia and nystagmus, and pathologically by degeneration of the inferior olivary nucleus and cerebellar cortex (Holmes). **Progressive lenticular degeneration.** Wilson's disease; hepatolenticular degeneration (see above). **Putrid degeneration.** Hospital gangrene. **Red degeneration.** A condition occurring in a uterine fibroid, usually during pregnancy, in which a red staining of the fibroid is found on section. **Reticular degeneration.** Haab's degeneration. **Rim degeneration.** Degeneration of the periphery of the spinal cord. **Sclerotic degeneration.** Fibroid degeneration (see above); fibrosis. **Secondary degeneration.** Wallerian degeneration. **Senile degeneration.** Atrophy of old age. **Spongy degeneration of white matter.** Familial fatal demyelination with spongy zone in deep layers of the cerebral cortex. **Tapetoretinal degeneration.** A group of hereditary degenerations of the retina and choroid. Leber believed that the initial disturbance was in the tapetum nigrum or pigment epithelium. **Theroid degeneration.** A state in which an insane person has beast-like qualities. **Trabecular degeneration.** Hypertrophy of the elastic and connective tissue surrounding the bronchi and their cartilages. **Traumatic degeneration.** Degenerative changes induced in cells by trauma. **Turbid-swelling degeneration.** Cloudy-swelling degeneration (see above). **Vacuolar degeneration.** A form of hydropic degeneration (see above). **Wallerian degeneration.** Fatty degeneration in nerve fibres following their transection or rupture. **Waxy degeneration.** Amyloid degeneration (see above); Zenker's degeneration. [L *degenerare* to deviate from kind.]

See also: ABERCROMBIE, ARMANNI, BIBER, DIMMER, EHRLICH, GOMBAULT, GRAWITZ, HAAB, HOLMES (G. M.), MARAGLIANO, MOENCKEBERG, NISSL, PASCHUTIN, QUAIN, TUERCK, VIRCHOW, WALLER, ZENKER (F. A.).

degenerative (de·jen·er·a·tiv). Relating or belonging to degeneration. [see prec.]

degenerescence (de·jen·er·**es′**·ens). An initial state of degeneration. [degeneration, L *crescere* to grow.]

degenitalization (de·jen·it·al·i·**za′**·shun). In psycho-analysis, the mental process in which the sexual instincts are expressed to a non-sexual end. [L *de*, genital.]

Degkwitz, Rudolf (b. 1889). Hamburg paediatrician.

Degkwitz's serum. An anti-measles serum prepared by immunizing sheep, and used for prophylaxis. (Obsolete term.)

degloving (de·**gluv**·ing). The tearing off, by injury, of the skin of the forearm and hand or the leg and foot in a manner comparable to that of taking off a glove. [L *de*, AS *glof*.]

deglutible (de·**gloo**·tibl). Suitable for being swallowed. [L *deglutire* to swallow down.]

deglutitio impedita (de·gloo·**tish**·e·o im·ped·i·tah). Dysphagia. [L a swallowing obstructed.]

deglutition (de·gloo·**tish**·un). The process or the act of swallowing, e.g. food. [L *deglutire* to swallow down.]

deglutitive, deglutitory (de·**gloo**·tit·iv, de·**gloo**·tit·or·e). Relating or belonging to deglutition. [see prec.]

degradation (deg·rad·**a**·shun). 1. Physical or histological degeneration. 2. The changing of a chemical compound into one less complex, or containing fewer carbon atoms. [L *de*, *gradus* step.]

degranulation (de·gran·ew·**la′**·shun). The process undergone by certain granular cells in losing their granules. [L *de*, granule.]

degrease (de·**grees**). To remove grease or fatty matter from a structure; especially applied in the case of osteological specimens; hence *degreasing.* [L *de,* grease.]

degree (de·**gre**). 1. A station in a qualitative series. 2. A unit of angular measurement. 3. One of the divisions or intervals marked on any scale for the measurement of temperature. 4. An academic rank conferred on attainment of a relevant stage of proficiency. 5. A stage in amount or intensity. [Fr. *degré.*]

degrowth (de·**gro**·th). Decrease in the mass of an organic body after it has gone through a period of growth. [L *de,* growth.]

degustation (de·gus·**ta**·shun). 1. The sense of taste. 2. The function or act of tasting. [L *degustare* to taste.]

dehaem (de·**heem**). To remove the haem portion from a haemoprotein. [L *de,* Gk *haima* blood.]

dehaematize (de·**he**·mat·ize). To deprive a part of the body of blood by application of pressure, or by the process of bleeding. [L *de,* Gk *haima* blood.]

dehaemoglobinize (de·he·mo·**glo'**·bin·ize). To remove the haemoglobin from erythrocytes. [L *de,* haemoglobin.]

dehepatized (de·**hep**·at·i·zd). Having had the liver removed, applied to experimental animals. [L *de,* Gk *hepar* liver.]

dehiscence (de·**his**·ens). Gaping. **Wound dehiscence.** Complete breakdown and falling apart of an operation wound. [L *dehiscere* to gape.]

dehumanization (de·**hew**·man·i·**za'**·shun). The process of losing those qualities which characterize the human species, e.g. pity, tenderness, which is to be found in profound psychotic states. [L *de, humanitas* human nature.]

dehydrase (de·**hi**·draze). A dehydrogenase.

dehydrate (de·**hi**·drate). To render free from water or watery elements. [L *de,* Gk *hydor* water.]

dehydration (de·hi·**dra**·shun). 1. The restriction of water in the dietary. 2. The removal of water from the body or its tissues. 3. A state in which there is less than the normal volume of water present in the tissue or organism. Dehydration may relate to the extracellular fluid or, if more severe, to the cells also. 4. In chemistry, rendering free from water. [see prec.]

dehydro-androsterone (de·**hi**·dro·an·dro·**steer'**·one). $C_{19}H_{28}O_2$, a substance of predominantly androgenic activity which occurs in the urine of men and of women with adrenal tumours. Its systemic name is Δ^5-androstene-3(β)-ol-17-one.

dehydrobilirubin (de·**hi**·dro·bil·e·**roo'**·bin). Biliverdin.

dehydrocholate (de·hi·dro·**ko'**·late). Any salt or ester of dehydrocholic acid.

dehydrocholesterol (de·hi·dro·ko·**les'**·ter·ol). Cholestadien-3-ol, $C_{27}H_{47}OH$. The precursor of vitamin D_3, into which it is converted by ultraviolet irradiation. The product thus formed is identical with the principal form of vitamin D found in cod-liver oil and other liver oils.

dehydrocorticosterone (de·**hi**·dro·kor·tik·o·**steer'**·one). $C_{21}H_{28}O_4$, a substance which occurs in the adrenals and has a glucocorticoid activity; known also as *Kendall's compound A.* Its systemic chemical name is 17(β)-[1-keto-2-hydroxyethyl]-Δ^4-androstene-3,11-dione.

Dehydroemetine (de·**hi**·dro·**em**·et·een). BP Commission approved name for 3-ethyl-1,6,7,11b-tetrahydro-9,10-dimethoxy-2-(1,2,3,4-tetrahydro-6,7-dimethoxy-1-isoquinolylmethyl)-4*H*-benzo[*a*]quinolizine; it is used in the treatment of amoebiasis.

dehydroepiandrosterone (DHA) (de·**hi**·dro·epi·an·dro·**steer**·-one). An androgenic steroid normally found in the adrenal cortex only and present in excess in cases of adrenal hyperplasia and carcinoma.

dehydrogenase (de·**hi**·**droj**·en·aze). An enzyme catalysing an oxidoreduction reaction of the general form RH_2 + oxidized co-enzyme $\rightleftharpoons$ R + reduced co-enzyme. The co-enzyme is NAD^+, $NADP^+$, FMN or FAD. Alcohol, glycerol 3-phosphate, glyceraldehyde 3-phosphate, β-hydroxybutyrate, β-hydroxyacyl CoA, lactate, malate and 3-phosphoglycerate dehydrogenases all require NAD^+; glucose 6-phosphate and 6-phosphogluconate dehydrogenases require $NADP^+$; glutamate and isocitrate dehydrogenases use either NAD^+ or $NADP^+$; fatty acyl CoA and succinate dehydrogenases are flavin-linked; oxoglutarate and pyruvate dehydrogenases are high molecular weight enzyme complexes whose turnover involves both NAD^+ and flavin. **Acetaldehyde dehydrogenase.** An enzyme that activates the conversion of acetaldehyde into acetic acid. **Aerobic dehydrogenase.** One which activates the oxygen of the air as an acceptor and forms hydrogen peroxide in the system. **Alcohol dehydrogenase.** Found in the liver in conjunction with co-enzyme I, it activates the oxidation of primary and secondary alcohols into aldehydes and ketones. **Anaerobic dehydrogenase.** One that activates an oxidation without the assistance of molecular oxygen, by the removal of hydrogen. **Aspartic dehydrogenase.** An enzyme of muscle and liver which activates the transamination of aspartic acid in the building up of amino acids within the body. **3-Beta-dehydrogenase.** Found in the microsomal fraction of the adreno-cortical cells. An enzyme that plays a part in the biosynthesis of adrenocortical hormones. **Beta-hydroxybutyric dehydrogenase.** The enzyme occurring in liver and muscle which, in the presence of co-enzyme I, activates the oxidation of β-hydroxybutyric acid into aceto-acetic acid. **Citric dehydrogenase.** Found in liver, muscle and vegetables; activates the conversion of citric acid into acetone dicarboxylic acid. **Co-enzyme dehydrogenase.** Diaphorase, an enzyme which activates the oxidation of a reduced co-enzyme. **18-Dehydrogenase.** The enzyme which, together with 18-hydroxylase, converts corticosterone to aldosterone. **Glucose dehydrogenase.** In liver, activates the oxidation of glucose into gluconic acid. **Glucose-6-phosphate dehydrogenase.** An enzyme which catalyses the reaction glucose-6-phosphate $\rightleftharpoons$ phosphogluconate. Its determination in red blood cells is of significance in certain types of drug-induced haemolytic anaemia. **Glutamic-acid dehydrogenase.** An enzyme which with either co-enzyme I or II, activates the oxidation of L-glutamic acid into α-ketoglutaric acid. **Glycerophosphate dehydrogenase.** In yeast and tissues, with adenosine triphosphate as co-enzyme, it takes part in glycolysis, forming glyceraldehyde phosphate. **Hexosediphosphate dehydrogenase.** In muscle and liver, it activates fructose diphosphate in the conversion of glycogen to lactic acid. **Hexosemonophosphate dehydrogenase.** An enzyme in erythrocytes and in yeast. In the presence of co-enzyme II it specifically activates the oxidation of glucose-6-monophosphate to 6-phosphogluconic acid. **Isocitrate dehydrogenase.** An enzyme which catalyses the oxidative decarboxylation of isocitrate with production of 2-oxoglutarate and CO_2. It is involved in the citric-acid cycle. Two mitochondrial enzymes, one of which utilizes NAD^+, the other $NADP^+$. The enzyme in the cytoplasm is specific for $NADP^+$. **Lactic dehydrogenase.** In muscle, brain and yeast, it activates the oxidation of lactic acid into pyruvic acid. **Malic dehydrogenase.** An enzyme which, in the presence of co-enzyme I, activates the conversion of malic acid into oxalo-acetic acid. **Oxoglutarate dehydrogenase.** A multi-enzyme complex which acts on oxyglutarate with the production of succinyl CoA and NADH. **Pyruvate dehydrogenase.** An enzyme complex which catalyses the conversion of pyruvate to acetyl co-enzyme A and which is essential to the oxidation of glucose and to the biosynthesis of fatty acids from glucose. The enzyme requires thiamine pyrophosphate and lipoate as co-enzymes. **Pyruvic dehydrogenase.** An enzyme which activates the oxidation of pyruvic acid in the citric acid cycle. **Succinate dehydrogenase.** The flavoprotein-linked dehydrogenase which catalyses the formate of fumarate from succinate. **Triosephosphate dehydrogenase.** An enzyme in yeast and muscle which, in the presence of co-enzyme I, has a selective action on L-3-phosphoglyceraldehyde; it takes part in muscle metabolism and yeast fermentation. **Xanthine dehydrogenase.** In the liver, it activates the oxidation of xanthine into uric acid in the purine metabolism.

See also: ROBISON.

dehydrogenate (de·**hi**·dro·jen·ate). Dehydrogenize.

dehydrogenation (de·**hi**·dro·jen·**a'**·shun). The process of oxidation by the removal of hydrogen atoms, such as occurs in living tissues through the intermediary of dehydrogenases. [L *de*, hydrogen.]

dehydrogenize (de·hi·dro·jen·ize). In chemistry, to remove hydrogen from organic compounds. [see prec.]

dehydro-iso-androsterone (de·hi·dro·i·so·and·dro·steer′·one). Dehydro-androsterone.

dehydromorphine (de·hi·dro·mor·feen). $C_{34}H_{36}O_6N_2.3H_2O$, pseudomorphine or oxydimorphine, an alkaloid found in opium. It is formed by the elimination of two atoms of hydrogen from two molecules of morphine.

dehypnotization (de·hip·no·ti·za′·shun). The process or act of arousing an individual from a state of hypnosis. [L *de*, hypnosis.]

dehypnotize (de·hip·no·tize). To arouse an individual from a state of hypnosis. [see prec.]

de-inebriating (de·in·e·bre·a·ting). The application of any measure that counteracts the intoxication produced by alcohol. [L *de*, *inebriare* to make drunk.]

de-insectization (de·in·sek·ti·za′·shun). Disinsectization.

de-intoxication (de·in·tox·ik·a′·shun). The process of nullifying the effects of toxins. [L *de*, *in-*, Gk *toxikon* poison.]

deiteral (di·ter·al). Relating to Deiters' nucleus (lateral vestibular nucleus). [Otto Friedrich Karl *Deiters*.]

Deiters, Otto Friedrich Karl (b. 1834). Bonn histologist.

Deiters' cell. 1. One of the supporting cells of the organ of Corti. 2. A neuroglial cell.

Deiters' formation. Formatio reticularis.

Deiters' nucleus. The lateral vestibular nucleus.

Deiters' phalanges. Processes from supporting cells of the spiral organ connecting them to the reticular membrane.

Deiters' process. An axis-cylinder.

Deiters' tract. The vestibulospinal tract.

déjà vécu (da·zhah va·koo). Descriptive of the sensation that an apparently new experience has been previously encountered. [Fr. already lived.]

déjà vu (da·zhah voo). Applied to the impression that something seen for the first time has been seen before. Normal persons are occasionally subject to the delusion, but it occurs most frequently in some types of mental disorder. [Fr. already seen.]

dejecta (de·jek·tah). Faeces; a general term for excrements. [L *dejicere* to throw down.]

dejection (de·jek·shun). 1. A mood or state of melancholy and depression. 2. Excrement. 3. The discharge of excrement. **Alvine dejections.** The faeces. [see prec.]

Déjérine, Joseph Jules (b. 1849). Paris neurologist.

Déjérine's disease. Déjérine–Sottas atrophy (see below).

Déjérine's sign. Aggravation of the pain of nerve-root irritation by coughing, sneezing or straining at stool.

Déjérine's syndrome. 1. Bulbar syndrome. 2. Sensory impairment of cortical type; there is loss of tactile discrimination, stereognosis, judgement of intensity of stimulation, appreciation of position and other highly integrated sensory functions. 3. Loss of appreciation of deep pressure sensation, with retention of tactile discrimination, as occurs in tabes dorsalis.

Déjérine type. The amyotrophic lateral sclerosis form of motor neurone disease.

Déjérine–Landouzy atrophy, myopathy or type, Landouzy–Déjérine atrophy, dystrophy, myopathy or type. Facioscapulohumeral muscular dystrophy; a heredofamilial form, probably an incomplete mendelian dominant. It is a slowly progressive disease, producing weakness and wasting of the facial and shoulder-girdle muscles and later affecting the pelvic girdle. A characteristic smooth facies with pouting lips develops, lumbar lordosis is accentuated and there is a waddling gait.

Déjérine–Lichtheim phenomenon. A phenomenon sometimes seen in expressive aphasia: a patient unable to speak may be able, by a show of fingers, to indicate the number of syllables in a word.

syndrome of Déjérine–Roussy, Roussy–Déjérine syndrome. Thalamic syndrome. *See* SYNDROME.

Déjérine–Sottas atrophy, disease or neuropathy, Sottas–Déjérine atrophy, disease or neuropathy. Progressive hypertrophic interstitial neuritis of infants.

Dejerine, Auguste (b. 1859). Paris neurologist.

Dejerine–Klumpke's paralysis or syndrome. A birth-palsy involving the 7th and 8th cervical and 1st dorsal nerves, usually with a Horner's syndrome, ptosis and miosis due to sympathetic nervous involvement.

Dejust's test. A chemical test for carbon monoxide: air suspected of containing carbon monoxide is passed through a test-tube of ammoniated silver solution; if CO is present it causes a deposit of metallic silver in the test-tube and the solution turns black or dark brown.

dekatron (dek·ah·tron). A cold-cathode-glow discharge tube in which the cathode glow may exist on any of 10 wire cathodes arranged in a circular pattern inside the glass envelope of the valve. The cathode glow may be transferred between adjacent cathodes by application of a potential pulse, 10 pulses causing 1 complete rotation of the glow round the valve. An arrangement of such valves in series may be used for counting electrical pulses. [Gk *deka* ten, electron.]

De La Camp's sign. Dullness over and to each side of the 5th and 6th dorsal vertebrae, due to an enlargement of bronchial glands.

delacerate (de·las·er·ate). To lacerate severely or tear to strips. [L *de*, *lacerare* to tear.]

delactation (de·lak·ta·shun). 1. The cessation of lactation. 2. The process of weaning. [L *de*, *lactare* to give milk.]

Delafield, Francis (b. 1841). New York pathologist.

Delafield's haematoxylin. *See* HAEMATOXYLIN.

delamination (de·lam·in·a′·shun). 1. The process of forming and separating into layers. 2. In embryology, the formation of the bilaminar or trilaminar blastoderm by the migration of individual cells from a wide area of the original single-layered blastoderm, instead of by a localized mass invagination. [L *de*, *lamina* thin plate.]

De Lange, Cornelia Catharina (b. 1871). Dutch paediatrician.

De Lange sign. Persistent extension or scissoring of the legs in the neonatal period.

De Lange syndrome. Congenital muscular hypertrophy with mental deficiency and rigidity, low hairline on neck, long upper lip with central "beak", low-set ears and many other anomalies of bodily development.

De Lapersonne, F. (fl. 1903). Paris ophthalmologist.

De Lapersonne's operation. For ptosis: tucking of the tendon of the levator palpebrae superioris muscle, approached from the skin surface of the lid.

De La Rue, Warren (b. 1815). British astronomer and chemist.

De La Rue cell. A two-fluid voltaic cell with zinc and silver electrodes, the zinc being immersed in zinc-chloride solution and the silver embedded in a stick of fused silver chloride. It furnishes an e.m.f. of 1.42 V.

delay (de·la). In a conditioned reflex, the short period that elapses between the application of the conditioned stimulus (e.g. ringing a bell) and the presentation of the unconditioned stimulus (food). **Duodenal delay.** Prolongation of the emptying time of the duodenum due either to local disorder or to reflex inhibition from stimulation of the peritoneum somewhere along the alimentary canal. **Synaptic delay.** The retardation of a nerve impulse at the synapse between neurones. [Fr. *délai*.]

Delbet, Paul (b. 1866). Paris surgeon.

Delbet's sign. In aneurysm of the main artery, adequate nutrition of a limb distal to the aneurysm indicates that the collateral circulation may be sufficient, even though the distal pulses are absent.

Delbet, Pierre Louis Ernest (b. 1861). Paris surgeon.

Albee–Delbet operation. An operation for fractured femoral neck; the fracture is fixed to a bone graft driven up a hole drilled in the neck of the femur.

De Lee, Joseph Bolivar (b. 1869). Chicago obstetrician.

De Lee's manoeuvre. A method of changing a face or brow

presentation into a vertex, by flexion of the fetal head. It is carried out by combined internal and external manipulation.

deletion (de·le·shun). In cytogenetics, a chromosomal structural change resulting in loss from the complement of part of its genetic material. It has been used sometimes in contradistinction to *deficiency* to indicate the loss of an acentric intercalary chromosome segment. **Terminal deletion.** A deletion involving one end of a chromosome. [L *deletionum* destruction.]

deligation (de·lig·a·shun). Ligation. [L *de, ligare* to bind.]

De Lima's operation. Transantral ethmoidectomy with preservation of the mucosa of the lateral nasal wall.

delimitation (de·lim·it·a'·shun). 1. Determination of the extent of a pathological process or the limits of a diseased tissue in the body. 2. Prevention of the spread of disease in a community. 3. The process of ascertaining the boundaries of the various organs, regions and areas of the body. [L *de, limes* boundary.]

delineascope (de·lin·e·ah·skope). A form of projection apparatus bearing a slide carrier, a reflector of silvered glass and a special bulb filled with nitrogen. [L *de, linea* line, Gk *skopein* to watch.]

delinquency (de·ling·kwen·se). Criminal or antisocial conduct, especially in a juvenile. It usually implies a psychotherapeutic, rather than judicial, attitude to the offender. [L *delinquere* to fail.]

See also: CHILDREN AND YOUNG PERSONS ACT.

deliquescence (del·e·kwes·ens). In chemistry, the process of gradual liquefaction by the absorption of water from the atmosphere. [L *deliquescere* to dissolve.]

deliquescent (del·e·kwes·ent). Term applied to a substance which becomes damp when exposed to the air, and eventually dissolves completely in the condensed water. [see prec.]

deliquiation (del·ik·we·a'·shun). Deliquescence. [L *deliquare* to clarify.]

deliquium (del·ik·we·um). 1. Syncope. 2. Failure or weakness of vitality of body or mind. 3. Melancholy or lowness of spirits. **Deliquium animi.** Fainting or syncope. [L failure.]

deliriant (de·lir·e·ant). 1. Delirifacient. 2. An individual affected with delirium. [L *delirare* to rave.]

delirifacient (de·lir·e·fa'·shent). 1. A drug such as belladonna which can cause delirium. 2. Able to cause delirium. [L *delirare* to rave, *facere* to make.]

delirious (de·lir·e·us). Wandering in mind; affected with delirium.

delirium (de·lir·e·um). A symptom of disordered functions of the higher portions of the central nervous system, exhibited in various ways by hallucination, illusions, disorientation, excitement and restlessness. It is associated with many different states such as fever, toxic conditions, head injuries, senility and inanition, and ranges in degree from acute maniacal types to quiet low muttering, depending upon the underlying factors. **Active delirium.** Delirium with excitement. **Acute delirium.** Very severe delirium with gross excitement. **Afebrile delirium.** Delirium not attended by fever, often associated with inanition. **Delirium alcoholicum.** Delirium tremens; that due to acute or chronic alcoholism. **Asthenic delirium.** Delirium that occurs with long wasting diseases, with or without fever. **Emergence delirium.** An acutely disturbed state sometimes seen during emergence from anaesthesia, especially cyclopropane. **Exhaustion delirium.** Afebrile delirium (see above). **Febrile delirium.** That seen in many acute fevers. **Grave delirium.** Active delirium (see above). **Hysterical delirium.** Delirium due to the psychological mechanisms of hysteria. **Inanition delirium.** Asthenic delirium (see above). **Lingual delirium.** Delirium in which meaningless words and sentences are uttered. **Low delirium.** Delirium with slow mental processes and confusion. **Macroptic delirium.** Delirium with delusions of great size of the body or its members. **Microptic delirium.** Delirium with delusions of smallness of the body. **Delirium mussitans.** Low muttering delirium. **Oneiric delirium.** Delirium associated with dreams. **Delirium of persecution.** Delirium with delusions of persecution. **Quiet delirium.** Low delirium (see above). **Specific febrile delirium.** Acute and active delirium (see above). **Toxic delirium.** Delirium caused by poisons. **Traumatic delirium.** Delirium associated with injury. **Delirium tremens.** Delirium alcoholicum (see above). [L *delirare* to rave.]

delitescence (del·it·es·ens). 1. The incubation period of an infection. 2. The latent period in cases of poisoning before the symptoms appear. 3. The sudden subsidence of symptoms of disease. 4. The disappearance of the signs of the presence of a tumour or lesion. [L *delitescere* to lie hid.]

deliver (de·liv·er). 1. To aid the natural process of giving birth. 2. To remove or extract from an enclosed space, e.g. the lens of the eye in cataract, or a tumour from its capsule. [L *de, liberare* to free.]

delivery (de·liv·er·e). 1. The act of being delivered of the products of conception, e.g. by normal birth. 2. The removal or expulsion of a structure such as the placenta after childbirth or the lens of the eye in cataract. **Abdominal delivery.** Caesarean section. *See* SECTION. **Immature delivery.** Expulsion of a viable fetus before the seventh month. **Post-mortem delivery.** Caesarean section performed in order to save the child after the death of the mother. **Premature delivery.** The giving birth to a living child before full term and after the beginning of the seventh month of pregnancy. [see prec.]

delle (del·e). The lighter central portion of a stained erythrocyte.

dellen (del·en). A transient shallow depression in the surface of the cornea, usually secondary to an adjacent swelling of the limbal tissue or to contact lens wear. [D *del* small hollow.]

Delmadinone (del·mad·in·one). BP Commission approved name for 6-chloro-17α-hydroxypregna-1,4,6-triene-3,20-dione; a progestational steroid.

Delmege's sign. Flattening of the deltoid muscle on the side of a tuberculous lung.

delomorphic, delomorphous (del·o·mor·fik, del·o·mor·fus). Having definite form within clear limits. [Gk *delos* manifest, *morphe* form.]

Délorme, Edmond (b. 1847). Paris surgeon.

Délorme's operation. Excision of thickened pericardium in chronic pericarditis.

delouse (de·lows). To free from infestation with lice. There is a school of thought that prefers the verb *to louse* in this connection. [L *de*, louse.]

Delpech, Jacques Mathieu (b. 1777). Montpellier orthopaedic surgeon.

Delpech's abscess. An abscess which rapidly produces severe constitutional disturbance, but is accompanied by only slight fever.

Delphinium (del·fin·e·um). A genus of plants of the family Ranunculaceae, including the larkspurs. **Delphinium staphisagria.** A species grown in southern Europe; the seed constitutes the drug staphisagria. [Gk *delphinion* larkspur.]

delphos, delphys (del·fos, del·fis). The womb. [Gk *delphys*.]

delta (del·tah). 1. Δ or δ, the fourth letter of the Greek alphabet. 2. Any space having the shape of a triangle, or capital Greek Δ. **Delta cell.** *See* CELL. **Delta chain.** *See* CHAIN. **Delta fornicis.** The triangular space made by the curving upward and towards each other of the two posterior columns of the fornix on the posterior aspect of the splenium. **Delta granule.** *See* GRANULE. **Delta mesoscapulae.** The smooth triangular area into which the crest of the spine of the scapula expands at its medial end. **Delta position.** In an organic compound comprising a straight chain of carbon atoms, the fourth carbon atom from that to which the characteristic group is attached. **Delta rhythm.** *See* RHYTHM. **Delta wave.** *See* WAVE. [Gk letter Δ corresponding to D.]

See also: GALTON.

deltoid (del·toid). 1. Triangular in shape or outline. 2. The deltoid muscle. [delta, Gk *eidos* form.]

deltoid muscle [musculus deltoideus]. The large muscle covering the shoulder region and running from the scapula and clavicle to the middle of the shaft of the humerus. It is the main abductor of the humerus.

deltoiditis (del·toid·i·tis). A condition of inflammation affecting the deltoid muscle. [deltoid, *-itis* inflammation.]

delusion (de·**loo**·zhun, de·**lew**·zhun). A false belief, not susceptible to argument or reason, and determined, pathologically, by some form of mental disorder: the belief of a primitive people in sorcery, therefore, is not covered by this definition. The mental disorder need not be of any organic nature caused by a structural lesion, or even be one of the functional psychoses such as schizophrenia. In a close family circle, a delusion may be passed from one member of the family to another by a process of psychological contagion and still, even in the secondary case, be regarded as a delusion. There is an element of circularity in the definitions of delusion and mental disorder, as the existence of a delusion presupposes a mental disorder, and mental disorder is itself defined as a condition in which abnormal mental phenomena may be shown, e.g. delusions. **Autochthonous delusion.** The primary or core element in a schizophrenic delusional system from which secondary elaborations are comprehensibly derived. **Depressive delusion.** A delusion whose content can be explained by a prevailing mood of depresion, e.g. that the subject is infected by syphilis, that he has so infected his family, or that he is a wicked man and will go to hell. **Expansive delusion.** Delusion of grandeur (see following). **Delusion of grandeur.** A delusion exalting the personality of the subject, e.g. that he is a millionaire, that he is of royal blood, or a new Messiah. **Large delusion.** Delusion of grandeur (see above). **Delusion of negation.** Nihilistic delusion (see following). **Nihilistic delusion.** A delusion, usually depressive, involving loss, destruction or absence of a normal possession of the individual, e.g. that bowel function has completely ceased, or that wife and children have been destroyed. **Delusion of parasitosis.** A delusion of the skin being infested with insects. Fragments of epidermal horn, sebum or extraneous matter are often presented by the patient to substantiate the belief. **Delusion of persecution.** A delusion involving the hostility of the environment, taking such forms as that the subject is being followed or watched, or that his mind is being interfered with by telepathy. **Delusion of reference.** A delusional belief that occurrences, which the normal individual would suppose to have no connection with him, involve the subject, have some special meaning for him, or refer to him in some way, e.g. that paragraphs in the newspaper refer to him though without mentioning his name, or that strangers in the street are talking about him. Such delusions nearly always have a persecutory quality. **Somatic delusion.** A delusional belief involving one of the organs of the body, e.g. that the stomach has a hole in it so that the food taken drops to the bottom of the abdominal cavity, or that the genitalia are changing their form into those of the opposite sex. **Systematized delusions.** Delusions which are logically interrelated: once a single delusional premise is granted, the remaining delusions appear as natural consequences. Systematized delusions are usually of slow growth in a well-preserved and integrated, even though disordered, personality. **Unsystematized delusion.** A delusion that bears no logical relation to another delusion, and may even be mutually contradictory. [L *deludere* to deceive.]

delusional (de·**loo**·zhun·al). 1. Characterized by delusions. 2. Relating to or of the nature of a delusion. [see prec.]

demagnetization (de·**mag**·net·i·**za**′·shun). Any method by which an object is freed from or deprived of its magnetic properties. [L *de*, magnetism.]

demagnetize (de·**mag**·net·ize). To free from or deprive any object of its magnetic properties. [see prec.]

demarcation (de·mar·**ka**·shun). 1. The act of setting or settling a limit. 2. The determination of boundaries. **Surface demarcation.** A term used in recording the mechanical effects of electric current on muscle and denoting the line marking the end of paralysed and the beginning of functioning muscle. [L *de*, *marcare* to mark.]

Demarquay, Jean Nicolas (b. 1811). Paris surgeon.

Demarquay's sign. Fixation of the trachea on phonation or on deglutition, due to peritracheal adhesions; found in syphilis.

De Martel's clamp. A three-bladed crushing clamp used in colon resection.

demasculinization (de·**mas**·kew·lin·i·**za**′·shun). Loss of normal male characteristics from any cause. [L *de*, *masculus* male.]

Dematiaceae (de·mat·i·**a**′·se·e). A family of fungi characterized by dark-coloured hyphae. A number of species are plant pathogens and some genera have been implicated in disease in man, e.g. *Phialophora, Cladosporium.* [Gk *demation* little bundle.]

dematiaceous (de·mat·i·**a**′·se·us). Pertaining to the *Dematiaceae.*

Dematium (de·**ma**·she·um). A genus of chromogenic fungi. **Dematium werneckii.** An obsolete synonym for *Cladosporium werneckii,* the causative organism of tinea nigra. [Gk *demation* little bundle.]

Demecarium Bromide (de·mek·a·re·um **bro**·mide). BP Commission approved name for decamethylenebis(*m*-dimethylaminophenyl *N*-methylcarbamate) dimethobromide; it is used in the treatment of glaucoma.

demeclocycline (de·**mek**·lo·**si**′·kleen). 7-Chloro-4-dimethylamino-1,4,4α,5,5α,6,11,12α-octahydro-3,6,10,12,12α-pentahydroxy-1,11-dioxonaphthacene-2-carboxyamide. **Demeclocycline Hydrochloride BP 1973.** The hydrochloride of the base; a yellow, odourless, amphoteric crystalline powder with a bitter taste. An antibiotic produced by a strain of *Streptomyces aureofaciens.*

demeclocyclini (de·**mek**·lo·**si**′·klin·i). Demeclocycline. **Demeclocyclini Hydrochloridum.** *European Pharmacopoeia* name for Demeclocycline Hydrochloride BP 1973.

Demecolcine (de·mek·**ol**·seen). BP Commission approved name for methyldeacetylcolchicine. A colchicine derivative with one-thirtieth the toxicity of the parent drug. It is used in myeloid leukaemia but contra-indicated in lymphatic leukaemia.

demedication (de·med·ik·**a**′·shun). The process of removing drugs from the system. **Catalytic demedication, Cataphoretic demedication, Electrophoretic demedication.** Demedication by the use of electrophoresis. [L *de*, medicament.]

dement (de·**ment**). A person who has dementia, especially to contrast this psychotic state with that of amentia. [L *de*, *mens* mind.]

demented (de·**men**·ted). Suffering from dementia.

dementia (de·**men**·she·ah). A form of mental disorder in which the cognitive and intellectual functions of the mind are prominently or predominantly affected; invariably a symptom of organic cerebral disease and, as a rule, impairment of memory is one of the earliest signs. Dementia necessarily implies some degree of permanent change: totally recoverable confusional states, in which also cognitive changes are prominent, are thus excluded. **Alcoholic dementia.** The dementia resulting from chronic alcoholism. **Apoplectic dementia.** Dementia following cerebral haemorrhage. **Circular dementia.** Dementia in which phases of excitement and depression follow in regular succession. **Epileptic dementia.** Dementia which may ensue in some cases of epilepsy, usually after years of incompletely controlled epileptic fits. Some of its main features are shown in slowness and circumstantiality of utterance, narrowing of the span of attention and interest, a clinging to detail, and impoverished grasp of the abstract and the essential. **Dementia myoclonica.** A term applied to the mental disorder of paramyoclonus multiplex. **Dementia paralytica.** General paralysis of the insane; a specific disease of the brain and meninges found in late states of syphilis, and caused by *Treponema pallidum.* If allowed to progress untreated, dementia, paralysis and death ensue, but if found in the earliest stages, it may be so successfully treated as to obviate any intellectual impairment, or dementia in the true sense. **Dementia paranoides.** An old term of psychiatric classification intended to distinguish a distinct clinical syndrome, largely co-extensive with the paranoid form of schizophrenia but involving severe deterioration of personality. **Paretic dementia.** Dementia paralytica (see above). **Dementia praecoccissima.** A disease of unknown aetiology, but often attributed to an exceptionally early and malignant form of schizophrenia, which may affect a child after some years of apparently normal mental and physical growth and development, progressively impairing intelligence and personality. **Dementia praecox.** Kraepelin's formulation of the severer and more typical forms of schizophrenia, in which marked destruction of the personality occurs. There is no dementia in the true sense, unless some form of organic cerebral disease is superimposed. **Dementia presenilis.** Dementia supervening in years too early for a senile dementia to be spoken of (any age from the thirties to the sixties). The condition is usually idiopathic and hereditary, but may sometimes be caused by organic disease such as cerebral arteriopathy. The clinically most distinct forms of presenile dementia are Huntington's chorea, Pick's disease and Alzheimer's disease. **Primary dementia.** An obsolete term for dementia praecox, emphasizing the distinction from secondary dementia. **Dementia pugilistica.** A condition tending to supervene in boxers in the later stages of their careers, attributed to repeated minor cerebral contusions, and showing itself in impairment of memory and power of concentration, and in temperamental changes. In boxing circles the affected subject is spoken of as "punch drunk". **Secondary dementia.** An organically determined deteriorative process affecting especially memory and cognition, which supervenes in the later stages of many psychoses, e.g. epilepsy, manic-depressive psychoses. **Semantic dementia.** A term invented by Cleckley to explain the abnormal psychological signs shown by psychopaths of the improvident, unreliable, impulsive type, such as spongers and confidence tricksters. It was suggested that such persons were unable to appreciate semantically the concepts of truth, honour or justice. **Senile dementia.** The dementia which eventually affects all aged people, provided they live long enough: the pathological picture is distinctive, and shows such features as senile plaques. **Tabetic dementia.** The dementia sometimes found in cases of tabes dorsalis. **Terminal dementia.** A dementia, supervening in the latest stages of many psychoses and organic diseases of the brain, which may herald a fatal termination. **Toxic dementia.** Dementia caused by a toxic process, e.g. alcoholism, plumbism. **Traumatic dementia.** Dementia after an accident that causes damage to the brain. [L *de, mens* mind.]

See also: ALZHEIMER, PICK (A.).

demethylation (de·**meth**·il·**a**'·shun). The process of removing methyl groups from a compound. [L *de*, methyl group.]

Demianoff's sign. Lasègue's sign.

demibain (**dem**·e·bane). A sitz bath. [Fr. half-bath.]

demic (**dem**·ik). Pertaining to the living body of man. [Gk *demos* people.]

demifacet (dem·e·**fas**·et). One half of an articulation surface which is shaped to articulate with 2 bones. [L *dimidius* half, Fr. *facette* little face.]

demigauntlet (dem·e·**gawnt**·let). A bandage for the fingers and the hand. [L *dimidius* half, Fr. *gant* glove.]

demilune (**dem**·e·lewn). A crescent-shaped cell, especially a serous cell at the periphery of an alveolus of mucous cells from a salivary gland. [L *dimidius* half, *luna* moon.]

See also: ADAMKIEWICZ, GIANNUZZI, HEIDENHAIN.

demimineralization (**dem**·e·min·er·al·i·**za**'·shun). Excessive loss of the mineral salts from the blood and tissues as occurs in certain diseases. [L *dimidius* half, mineral.]

demimonstrosity (**dem**·e·mon·**stros**'·it·e). 1. A monstrosity in which the malformation is not so extreme as to prevent the continuance of life. 2. A malformation which does not inhibit the functioning of the affected part. [L *dimidius* half, *monstrum* portent.]

demipenniform (dem·e·**pen**·e·form). Applied to organs or structures which are wing-shaped on 1 of 2 sides or with 1 of 2 edges winged. [L *dimidius* half, *penna* wing, form.]

demodectic (de·mo·**dek**·tik). Caused by or relating to the mite, *Demodex*.

Demodex (**de**·mo·dex). A genus of mites of which *Demodex folliculorum hominis*, the sebaceous mite, is a parasite of man. The adults are vermiform, less than 1 mm long and with 8 short legs anteriorly. They live in sebaceous glands and hair follicles, causing blackheads, and possibly but more rarely a chronic dermatitis; said to be common and world-wide but rarely observed, though a closely allied species occurs in cats and dogs. [Gk *demos* tallow, *dex* woodworm.]

Demodicidae (de·mo·**dis**·id·e). A family of the acarine superfamily Demodicoidea. The genus *Demodex* is of medical interest. [Gk *demos* tallow, *dex* woodworm, *eidos* form.]

demodicosis (**dem**·o·de·**ko**'·sis). Infestation with *Demodex folliculorum hominis*, causing scaling, follicular papulopustules and, sometimes, blepharitis. It may be a feature of rosacea. [Gk *demos* tallow, *dex* woodworm, *-osis* condition.]

demography (de·**mog**·raf·e). The social science of people considered collectively: race, occupation, habitation, physical, moral and intellectual conditions, and vital statistics. **Dynamic demography.** The collective study of conditions within a particular community with reference to vital statistics considered over the period of the duration of the community. **Static demography.** The collective study of the anatomy of a community, e.g. numbers, sex, age, social position, occupation, environment. [Gk *demos* the people, *graphein* to record.]

Demoivre, Abraham (b. 1667). London mathematician.

Demoivre's formula. A formula used by Demoivre to determine the expectation of life, which he stated as equal to two-thirds of the difference between the age of the individual and the figure 80.

demoniac (de·**mo**·ne·ak). An individual suffering from frenzy. [Gk *daimon* demon.]

demonolatry (de·mon·**ol**·at·re). Spirit worship. [Gk *daimon* demon, *latreia* service.]

demonology (de·mon·**ol**·o·je). The branch of learning dealing with demons or beliefs about demons, especially an early branch of learning which taught that a mentally disordered individual was possessed of a demon and that the only effective treatment was exorcism. [Gk *daimon* demon, *logos* science.]

demonomania (de·mon·o·**ma**'·ne·ah). The insane belief by any individual that an evil spirit or spirits are in possession of him. [Gk *daimon* demon, *mania* madness.]

demonomaniac (**de**·mon·o·**ma**'·ne·ak). An individual suffering from demonomania.

demonomy (de·**mon**·o·me). The laws or science of human activities considered as a whole. [Gk *demos* the people, *nomos* law.]

demonopathy (de·mon·**op**·ath·e). Demonomania. [Gk *daimon* demon, *pathos* suffering.]

demonophobia (**de**·mon·o·**fo**'·be·ah). Fear of the devil or of evil spirits. [Gk *daimon* demon, *phobia* fear.]

De Morgan, Campbell Greig (b. 1811). London physician.

De Morgan's spot, Campbell de Morgan's spot. A small red vascular haemangioma, resembling naevus araneus, but without the typical adjacent capillary dilatation, usually noted on the trunk. There are frequently several of the spots to be seen. Originally believed to be evidence of internal cancer, the spots are now usually regarded as late-developing naevi, or are formed by vascular dilatation due to localized degeneration of supporting connective tissue, having no pathological significance, and being almost within the limits of normal change in middle-aged and elderly persons.

demorphinization (**de**·mor·fin·i·**za**'·shun). Gradual withdrawal of morphine in treatment of cases of addiction. [L *de*, morphine.]

Demours, Pierre (b. 1702). Paris ophthalmic surgeon.

Demours' membrane. The posterior elastic lamina of the cornea.

demucosation (**de**·mew·ko·**sa**'·shun). The cutting away of the mucosa of any part. [L *de*, mucosa.]

demulcent (de·**mul**·sent). A substance which protects the mucous membranes and allays irritation. Demulcents consist of colloidal solutions of gums or proteins which become adsorbed on to the surface of the mucous membrane and form a protective coat. Tragacanth and acacia gums, milk and solutions of gelatin are examples. [L *demulcere* to smooth down.]

de Mussy. *See* GUÉNEAU DE MUSSY.

demutization (de·**mew**·ti·**za**'·shun). The process of overcoming dumbness by teaching deaf-mutes to copy the movements of the lips made in pronouncing words and thus to make sounds approximately correct, or by teaching them dactylology. [L *de*, *mutus* dumb.]

demyelinate (de·mi·el·in·ate). To take away or destroy the myelin of nerve tissue. [L *de*, Gk *myelos* marrow.]

demyelination, demyelinization (de·mi·el·in·a′·shun, de·mi·el·in·i·za′·shun). The removal and destruction of the myelin of nerve tissue. **Disseminated demyelinization.** Disseminated sclerosis. *See* SCLEROSIS. [L *de*, myelin.]

demyelinize (de·mi·el·in·ize). Demyelinate.

denarcotize (de·nar·kot·ize). 1. To remove narcotine from an opiate. 2. To deprive of narcotic properties. [L *de*, narcotic.]

denatality (de·na·tal·it·e). A falling in the birth rate in a community. [L *de*, *natus* birth.]

Denatonium Benzoate (de·na·to·ne·um ben·zo·ate). BP Commission approved name for benzyldiethyl-(2,6-xylylcarbamoylmethyl)ammonium benzoate; an alcohol denaturant.

denaturant (de·na·tewr·ant). A substance that causes denaturation. [L *de*, *natura* nature.]

denaturation (de·na·tewr·a′·shun). 1. The rendering of a substance such as salt or alcohol unfit for food, although still fit for other purposes, by adding a harmful or inert substance. 2. The alteration of an organic biological substance by subjecting it to the action of heat or chemicals or by adding another substance to it. **Protein denaturation.** A change in the nature of proteins induced by the action of heat, of strong acids and of alcohol, by which they are rendered insoluble in water or in neutral salt solutions. It is regarded as being a structural rather than a chemical change. [see prec.]

denatured (de·na·tewrd). Of a substance: 1. Rendered unfit for food. 2. Altered from its normal character. [L *de*, *natura* nature.]

denaturization (de·na·tewr·i·za′·shun). Denaturation.

Dendraspis (den·dras·pis). A genus of snakes of which *Dendraspis angusticeps*, the common mamba, is the most important species. [Gk *dendron* tree, *aspis* asp.]

dendraxon (den·drax·on). A type of axon which is shorter than normal, and which therefore tends to branch very soon after leaving the nerve cell; it may or may not be covered with a sheath. [Gk *dendron* tree, *axon* axle.]

dendric (den·drik). Dendritic.

dendriceptor (den·dre·sep·tor). A point at the end of a minute terminal twig of a dendrite which picks up the stimuli or impulses originating in or imparted by other neurones. [Gk *dendron* tree, L *recipere* to receive.]

dendriform (den·dre·form). Branched. [Gk *dendron* tree, form.]

dendrite (den·drite). The protoplasmic process of a nerve cell which, freely branching, conveys nerve impulses to the cell and communicates physiologically with dendrites of other nerve cells. [Gk *dendron* tree.]

dendritic (den·drit·ik). 1. Relating to a dendrite or having dendrites. 2. Having branches like a tree. [see prec.]

dendroid (den·droid). Having branches like a tree. [Gk *dendron* tree, *eidos* form.]

dendron (den·dron). Dendrite.

dendrophagocytosis (den·dro·fag·o·si·to′·sis). The process by which microglial cells absorb the debris of degenerating astrocytes. [Gk *dendron* tree, *phagein* to eat, *kytos* cell, *-osis* condition.]

dendrophilia (den·dro·fil·e·ah). Love of trees; abnormal or obsessional love of trees. [Gk *dendron* tree, *philein* to love.]

denematize (de·nem·at·ize). To disinfest an individual of nematode worms. [L *de*, nematode.]

denervate (de·ner·vate). To cut off or interfere with the nerve supply to a part, by blocking it with a drug, by division or excision, or by a disease process. [L *de*, nerve.]

dengue (deng·ge). Break-bone fever; an endemic and epidemic fever occurring in the tropics and sub-tropics, mainly in sea-coast towns. It is caused by a group B arbovirus, transmitted mostly by *Aëdes aegypti* mosquitoes, and there are four serotypes. The seven-day fever remits temporarily about the third to fifth day; a secondary rise of temperature then occurs giving the characteristic saddle-back chart. A measles-like rash appears about the fifth day. Pains in the muscles, joints and back are severe, and the pulse is slow throughout. Mortality is negligible, but debility may be severe and prolonged. [Sp.]

denidation (de·ni·da·shun). The disintegration and stripping off of epithelial elements from the superficial mucous membrane of the uterus, a process believed to take place during menstruation. [L *de*, *nidus* nest.]

Denig, Rudolf Carl Robert (b. 1867). New York ophthalmologist.

Denig's operation. The use of mucous-membrane grafts to cover denuded areas of conjunctiva. Also in trachomatous pannus, removal of adjacent conjunctiva and replacement with mucous membrane.

Denigès, Georges (b. 1859). Bordeaux biochemist.

Denigès' reagent. For acetone: add 20 ml of concentrated sulphuric acid to 100 ml of water and dissolve 5 g of mercuric oxide in the hot solution.

Denigès' test. For acetone: to 2 ml of solution add 2 ml of Denigès' reagent and place in boiling water. A heavy white precipitate is produced in a few minutes.

denigration (de·ni·gra·shun). 1. The process of becoming black. 2. The act of blackening. [L *denigrare* to blacken.]

Denis, Prosper Sylvain (b. 1799). French biochemist.

Denis' plasmin. Tryptase, fibrinolysin; a proteolytic enzyme present in and carried by the globulin fraction of normal blood plasma. It is concerned in the mechanism of fibrinolysis, whereby fibrin is aseptically dissolved.

Denis, Willey Glover (b. 1879). American biochemist.

Denis' method. For magnesium in serum: precipitate the calcium as oxalate by the Clark-Collip method. To the filtrate add ammonium phosphate solution and ammonia. After standing overnight, centrifuge, and wash the precipitate with dilute ammonia. Determine the magnesium ammonium phosphate by the method for phosphate of Fiske and Subbarow.

Benedict and Denis method. This is essentially Benedict's method for total sulphur in urine, except that 25 ml urine is mixed with 5 ml of a reagent made up from copper nitrate 25 g, sodium chloride 25 g, ammonium nitrate 10g, water to 1 litre.

Corley and Denis method. A method for the estimation of calcium in tissues based on its precipitation as the oxalate.

Folin and Denis method. A method for determining the total nitrogen of urine by direct nesslerization of the diluted digest obtained by the micro-Kjeldahl procedure.

Denis Browne. *See* BROWNE, DENIS.

denitration (de·ni·tra·shun). 1. The extraction of nitrates from a medium such as the soil. 2. The removal of nitrogroups, NO_2, from a compound. [L *de*, nitrate.]

denitrification (de·ni·trif·ik·a′·shun). The taking away of nitrogen from a compound or medium. [L *de*, nitrogen, L *facere* to make.]

denitrifier (de·ni·trif·i·er). Any substance or agent, particularly a micro-organism, which is able to remove nitrogen from a medium such as soil. [L *de*, nitrogen.]

denitrify (de·ni·trif·i). To take away nitrogen or nitrates from a substance as do certain micro-organisms which reduce nitrogen compounds down to ammonia or even free nitrogen. [see prec.]

denitrogenation (de·ni·tro·jen·a′·shun). The displacement of nitrogen dissolved in plasma by pure oxygen, a technique sometimes employed by anaesthetists. [L *de*, Gk *nitron* soda, *genein* to produce.]

Denker, Alfred (b. 1863). German otorhinolaryngologist.

Denker's operation. A radical operation for the treatment of suppuration of the maxillary air sinuses.

Denonvilliers, Charles Pierre (b. 1808). Paris anatomist and surgeon.

Denonvilliers' fascia. The fascia between the rectum behind and the prostate in front.

Denonvilliers' operation. Plastic correction of a nostril deformity by a skin flap from the side of the nose.

dens (denz) (pl. *dentes*). Tooth. **Dens of the axis vertebra.** The odontoid process of the axis. **Dens in dente.** A geminated composite odontome, arising as a result of invagination of the epithelium of the enamel organ into the coronal aspect of the dentine germ during development. **Dens serotinus [NA].** The third molar, or wisdom tooth. [L tooth.]

densimeter (den·sim·et·er). Hydrometer. [L *densus* thick, meter.]

densimetric (den·sim·et·rik). Referring to the use of a densimeter (hydrometer).

densitometer (den·sit·om·et·er). 1. A hydrometer for measuring the action of added bacteriophage or antiseptic on the growth of bacteria. 2. A device for measuring the dose of radiation delivered, by means of the degree of blackening of x-ray or photographic film. [L *densus* thick, meter.]

densitometry (den·sit·om·et·re). The science of determining the amount of radiation. [L *densus* thick, meter.]

density (den·sit·e). 1. Thickness, compactness. 2. The concentration of matter, as in outer space. 3. The mass of a unit volume of a substance. **Current density.** The amount of electricity passing through unit area. **Electric density.** Surface density of an electric charge, the charge per unit of surface; volume density of an electric charge is the charge per unit volume. **Mosquito density.** An estimate of the number of insects per volume, area, person, house or similar unit. **Optical density.** The ratio of light transmitted by a translucent or transparent substance. **Parasite density.** The average number of parasites per chosen unit. **Photographic density.** The comparative thickness of a photographic image on a negative. **Relative density.** The weight of a certain volume of a substance compared with the weight of the same volume of a standard such as water or hydrogen. **Vapour density.** The weight of a volume of gas or vapour compared with the weight of the same volume of hydrogen, both measured at stp. [L *densus* thick.]

densography (dens·og·raf·e). The comparative measurement of the varying densities of the image on an x-ray plate by the use of a photo-electric cell. [density, Gk *graphein* to record.]

dental (den·tal). 1. Relating to the teeth or a tooth. 2. In phonetics, formed or sounded by contact of the tip of the tongue and the teeth, e.g. the letter *t*. **Dental arch.** *See* ARCH. **Dental foramen.** *See* FORAMEN. **Dental papilla.** *See* PAPILLA. [L *dens* tooth.]

dental arteries. Arteries entering the pulps and supplying the teeth. **Anterior superior dental arteries [arteriae alveolares superiores anteriores].** *See* MAXILLARY ARTERY. **Inferior dental artery [arteria alveolaris inferior].** The sole artery to the lower teeth, from the maxillary artery. **Posterior superior dental arteries [arteriae alveolares superiores posteriores].** *See* MAXILLARY ARTERY.

dental nerves. Nerves carrying pain sensations from the teeth. **Anterior superior dental nerve [rami alveolares superiores anteriores (NA)].** The branch of the infra-orbital nerve to the incisor and canine teeth. It also supplies the side wall and floor of the nasal cavity. **Inferior dental nerve [nervus alveolaris inferior (NA)].** One of the main branches of the mandibular nerve, supplying the teeth of the lower jaw [rami dentales inferiores (NA)] and the gum over the lower jaw [rami gingivales inferiores (NA)], the motor nerve to the mylohyoid muscle [nervus mylohyoideus (NA)], and, by its terminal branch, the skin of the chin [rami mentales] and lower lip [rami labiales inferiores (NA)]. **Middle superior dental nerve [ramus alveolaris superior medius (NA)].** The branch of the infra-orbital nerve to the premolar teeth. **Posterior superior dental nerves [rami alveolares superiores posteriores (NA)].** Branches of the maxillary nerve, usually 2 in number, which run on the back of the maxilla and then in the bone to the upper molar teeth. They also give twigs to the mucous membrane of the maxillary sinus and the upper gums.

dental veins. **Inferior dental vein.** A vein following the artery of the same name, draining the lower jaw and teeth into the pterygoid plexus. **Superior dental veins.** Tributaries of the infra-orbital vein or pterygoid plexus direct.

dentalgia (den·tal·je·ah). Tooth-ache. [L *dens* tooth, Gk *algos* pain.]

dentaphone (den·tah·fone). A piece of metal worn between the teeth to assist the hearing. Of historical interest only. [L *dens* tooth, Gk *phone* sound.]

dentata (den·ta·tah). The 2nd cervical vertebra. [L *dens* tooth.]

dentate (den·tate). Having tooth-like projections or a sharp serrated edge. **Dentate nucleus.** *See* NUCLEUS. [see prec.]

dentation (den·ta·shun). 1. The state of being dentate. 2. A sharp tooth-like projection, e.g. on a leaf margin. [L *dens* tooth.]

dentatum (den·ta·tum). The dentate nucleus of the cerebellum. [see prec.]

dentelation (den·tel·a·shun). The condition of having tooth-like processes. [L *dens* tooth.]

dentia (den·she·ah). The process of teething. **Dentia praecox.** The condition in which there are erupted teeth at birth, or shortly afterwards. **Dentia tarda.** A condition of delayed eruption of the teeth. [L early teething.]

dentiaskiascope (den·te·ah·ski′·as·kope). A dental x-ray apparatus. (Obsolete term.) [L *dens* tooth, skiascope.]

dentibuccal (den·te·buk·al). Relating to the teeth and the cheek. [L *dens* tooth, *bucca* cheek.]

denticle (den·tikl). 1. A small projecting point or tooth-like process. 2. A pulp stone or nodule. 3. A small tooth. **Adherent denticle.** A pulp stone fixed to the dentine wall of the pulp chamber. **False denticle.** An amorphous deposition of calcium salts with an irregular outline in the tooth pulp. **Free denticle.** A pulp stone lying free in the substance of the tooth pulp. **Interstitial denticle.** An irregular nodule sunk into the dentine of a tooth. **True denticle.** A pulp stone with an irregular system of tubes. [L *denticulus* little tooth.]

denticulate (den·tik·ew·late). 1. Having very small tooth-like projections. 2. Having diminutive teeth. **Denticulate suture.** *See* SUTURE. [see prec.]

denticule (den·tik·ewl). A sharp projection of bone. [L *denticulus* little tooth.]

denticulus (den·tik·ew·lus). Denticle; a small tooth. [L.]

dentification (den·tif·ik·a′·shun). 1. The process of forming dentine. 2. The formation of calcified masses within a soft-tissue tumour. [L *dens* tooth, *facere* to make.]

dentiform (den·te·form). Tooth-shaped. [L *dens* tooth, form.]

dentifrice (den·te·fris). Any liquid, paste or powder used for cleansing the teeth. [L *dens* tooth, *fricare* to rub.]

dentigerous (den·tij·er·us). 1. Containing teeth. 2. Bearing tooth-like structures or teeth. [L *dens* tooth, *gerere* to bear.]

dentilabial (den·te·la·be·al). Relating to the teeth and lips. [L *dens* tooth, *labium* lip.]

dentilave (den·te·lave). An antiseptic wash for the teeth or mouth. [L *dens* tooth, *lavare* to wash.]

dentilingual (den·te·ling·gwal). Relating to the teeth and the tongue. [L *dens* tooth, *lingua* tongue.]

dentimeter (den·tim·et·er). An instrument for measuring the size of a tooth. [L *dens* tooth, meter.]

dentinal (den·tin·al). Composed of or relating to dentine.

dentinalgia (den·tin·al·je·ah). Pain felt in the dentine. [dentine, Gk *algos* pain.]

dentine [dentinum (NA)] (den·teen). A calcified tissue containing about 25 per cent of organic matter, surrounding the pulp of a tooth, and covered with enamel in the crown and cementum in the root. It is permeated by a system of tubes running outwards, each containing a protoplasmic prolongation of the odontoblast cells of the pulp, tissue fluid and possibly nerve fibres. It normally contains some interglobular spaces and is attacked by caries when the protective enamel has been lost. **Adventitious dentine.** Secondary dentine (see below). **Circumpulpar dentine.** That part in which the fibres forming the dentine matrix are running in a radial direction; it lies nearest to the pulp chamber. **Hereditary opalescent dentine.** Dentinogenesis imperfecta. **Hypoplastic dentine.** Poorly calcified dentine associated with deficiency diseases during calcification. It contains many interglobular spaces and is therefore rapidly affected by caries.

Mantle dentine. That part in which the fibres forming the dentine matrix are running parallel to the surface of the tooth; the outer part of the dentine. **Primary dentine.** That part of the dentine which is laid down during the physiological development of the tooth. **Secondary dentine.** A protective barrier of dentine laid down by the cells of the pulp as a result of stimulation due to attrition, abrasion and erosion, and the approach of caries. [L *dens* tooth.]

dentinification (den·tin·if·ik·a′·shun). The formation of dentine by the odontoblasts. [dentine, L *facere* to make.]

dentinoblast (den·tin·o·blast). Odontoblast. [dentine, Gk *blastos* germ.]

dentinogenesis (den·tin·o·jen′·es·is). The formation and development of the dentine by the odontoblasts. **Dentinogenesis imperfecta.** A brown discoloration of the teeth that is caused by a hereditary defect in calcification of the dentine. [dentine, Gk *genesis* origin.]

dentinoid (den·tin·oid). 1. Structurally resembling or similar to dentine. 2. The matrix upon which calcium salts are deposited to form dentine. [dentine, *Gk eidos* form.]

dentinoma (den·tin·o·mah). An odontoma composed mainly of an irregular mass of dentine. [dentine, Gk *-oma* tumour.]

dentinosteoid (den·tin·os·te·oid). Odontoma containing bone material. [dentine, Gk *osteon* bone, *eidos* form.]

dentiparous (den·tip·ar·us). Belonging to the production of teeth. [L *dens* tooth, *parere* to give birth.]

dentiphone (den·te·fone). Dentaphone.

dentist (den·tist). A practitioner of dentistry. [L *dens* tooth.]

dentistry (den·tis·tre). That part of the science and practice of medicine and surgery which concerns the oral cavity, the teeth, the bone of the jaws and the overlying soft tissues, together with the diagnosis and treatment of diseases thereof. **Ceramic dentistry.** The practice and art of using porcelain in conservative and prosthetic dentistry; dental ceramics. **Conservative dentistry.** That part of the practice of dentistry which involves the restoration of teeth by fillings. **Forensic dentistry.** The knowledge of the law as it affects dental practitioners, and of the legal obligations of such practitioners towards their patients; dental jurisprudence. **Preventive dentistry.** The science and practice of the prevention of diseases of the teeth and associated parts. **Prosthetic dentistry.** That part of the practice of dentistry which involves the replacement of missing teeth by artificial bridges and dentures. [see prec.]

dentition (den·tish·un). 1. The process of teething. 2. The number, arrangement and shape of teeth characteristic of a particular species or genus. 3. The teeth as arranged in the mouth. **Deciduous dentition.** The 20 deciduous teeth that are replaced by the permanent teeth at the age of 12 years. **Permanent dentition.** The 32 teeth that commence to erupt at the age of 6 years, and should remain in position during the rest of life. **Primary dentition.** Deciduous dentition (see above). **Secondary dentition.** Permanent dentition (see above). [L *dentia* early teething.]

dento-alveolar (den·to·al·ve′·o·lar). Relating to the alveolus of a tooth. [L *dens* tooth, alveolus.]

dento-alveolitis (den·to·al·ve·o·li′·tis). Pyorrhoea alveolaris. [L *dens* tooth, alveolus, Gk *-itis* inflammation.]

dentocemental (den·to·se·men′·tal). Appertaining to the dentine and cementum of a tooth, as the dentocemental junction. [L *dens* tooth, *caementum* rubble.]

dentofacial (den·to·fa·shal). Relating to the dental arches and their effects upon facial contour. [L *dens* tooth, face.]

dentoid (den·toid). 1. Dentiform. 2. Odontoid. [L *dens* tooth, Gk *eidos* form.]

dentolegal (den·to·le·gal). Appertaining to the legal aspects of the practice of dentistry.

dentolingual (den·to·ling·gwal). Belonging to the teeth and the lingual nerve or the tongue. [L *dens* tooth, *lingua* tongue.]

dentoliva (den·to·li·vah). The olivary nucleus of the medulla oblongata. [L *dens* tooth, *oliva* olive.]

dentology (den·tol·o·je). Odontology. [L *dens* tooth, Gk *logos* science.]

dentoma (den·to·mah). An odontoma made up of dentine. [L *dens* tooth, Gk *-oma* tumour.]

dentomechanical (den·to·mek·an′·ik·al). Relating or belonging to the science of dental mechanics. [L *dens* tooth, Gk *mechane* machine.]

dentomental (den·to·men·tal). Relating to the teeth and the chin. [L *dens* tooth, *mentum* chin.]

dentonasal (den·to·na·zal). Relating to the teeth and the nose. [L *dens* tooth, nose.]

dentonomy (den·ton·om·e). Classification of teeth. [L *dens* tooth, Gk *nomos* law.]

dentosurgical (den·to·ser·jik·al). Relating to or used in surgical dentistry.

dentural (den·tewr·al). Belonging to a denture.

denture (den·tewr). A set of teeth, either natural or artificial. **Artificial denture.** An appliance constructed of metal, vulcanite or acrylic resin, which supports one or more artificial teeth to replace missing natural teeth. **Denture fixative.** A powder composed mainly of gum tragacanth, which is applied to the fitting surface of an artificial denture to improve its adhesion to the soft tissues of the mouth. **Full denture.** A denture which replaces all the natural teeth in either upper or lower jaw. **Immediate denture.** An artificial denture, either full or partial, which is inserted in the mouth immediately after the extraction of natural teeth, in order that appearance, facial contour and mastication can be maintained. **Partial denture.** A denture which replaces less than the full complement of natural teeth in either jaw. **Permanent denture.** An artificial denture which is inserted in the mouth after all alveolar resorption occurring as a result of the extraction of the natural teeth has taken place. [L *dens* tooth.]

Denucé, Jean Louis Paul (b. 1824). Bordeaux surgeon.

Denucé's ligament. The quadrate ligament of the superior radio-ulnar joint.

denucleated (de·new·kle·a·ted). Having had the nucleus removed. [L *de*, nucleus.]

denudation (de·new·da·shun). 1. The act or process of stripping bare. 2. The state of being deprived of a protecting layer or covering, e.g. a body surface of its epithelium. [L *denudare* to make bare.]

denude (de·newd). To strip off a protective covering or to make bare. [see prec.]

denutrition (de·new·trish·un). A condition of degeneration and atrophy of tissues as the result of failure or withdrawal of nutrition. [L *de*, nutrition.]

deobstruent (de·ob·stroo·ent). 1. Having the property of getting rid of matter causing any blockage, e.g. of the bowel. 2. Any drug or preparation that acts in bringing about a clearance. [L *de*, *obstruere* to obstruct.]

deodorant (de·o·der·ant). An agent that corrects, masks or removes unpleasant odours. [L *de*, odour.]

deodoriferant (de·o·der·if″·er·ant). 1. Deodorant. 2. Capable of masking unpleasant odours. [L *de*, odour, *ferre* to carry.]

deodorize (de·o·der·ize). To free from odour, particularly unpleasant odour. [L *de*, odour.]

deodorizer (de·o·der·i·zer). A deodorant.

deolepsy (de·o·lep·se). A form of psycholepsy in which the patient is convinced that he has a god within him, and has divine powers and reactions. [L *deus* god, Gk *lambanein* to seize.]

deontology (de·on·tol·o·je). Medical ethics. [Gk *deon* obligation, *logos* science.]

deoppilant (de·op·il·ant). Aperient. [L *de*, *oppilare* to ram down.]

deoppilation (de·op·il·a′·shun). The removing of an obstruction, as of the bowels. [see prec.]

deoppilative (de·op·il·a·tiv). Deoppilant.

deorality (de·or·al·it·e). In psycho-analysis, the state in which an instinct or activity connected with the oral region is expressed in another way. [L *de*, *os* mouth.]

deorsum (de·or·sum). Downward. **Deorsum vergens.** Turning downwards. [L.]

deorsumduction (de·or·sum·**duk**'·shun). The action of turning downwards; of the eyes, rotation of the eyeball downwards on its transverse axis. [L *deorsum* downward, *ducere* to lead.]

deorsumvergence (de·**or**·sum·**ver**'·jens). Deorsumduction. [L *deorsum* downward, *vergere* to bend.]

deorsumversion (de·**or**·sum·**ver**'·shun). 1. Deorsumduction. 2. The turning downwards of both eyes simultaneously. [L *deorsum* downward, *vertere* to incline.]

deossification (de·**os**·if·ik·**a**'·shun). The removal or loss of the mineral constituents of bone. [L *de*, ossification.]

deoxidation (de·ox·e·**da**'·shun). In chemistry, the removal of oxygen from a compound. [L *de*, oxygen.]

deoxidize (de·**ox**·id·ize). 1. To remove oxygen from its chemical combination. 2. To deprive of chemically-combined oxygen. [see prec.]

deoxycorticosterone (de·ox·e·**kor**·tik·o·**steer**'·one). Deoxycortone. **Deoxycorticosterone trimethylacetate.** Deoxycortone Pivalate BPC 1968.

11-deoxycortisol (de·ox·e·**kor**·ti·**sole**). A compound formed in the biosynthesis of cortisol in the adrenal gland by adding oxygen at the 11-position; 21-hydroxylase converts hydroxyprogesterone to cortisol via deoxycortisol; 21-hydroxylase deficiency is consequently the commonest cause of congenital adrenal hyperplasia.

deoxycortone (de·ox·e·**kor**·tone). $C_{21}H_{30}O_3$, a steroid compound, Δ^4-pregnene-21-ol-3,20-dione, isolated from the cortex of the suprarenal gland and now prepared synthetically. It is chiefly concerned with the regulation of the salt and water metabolism, and therefore does not give complete replacement therapy in adrenal insufficiency since it has little effect on the regulation of the carbohydrate metabolism. It is usually employed as the acetate or propionic ester. **Deoxycortone Acetate BP 1973.** DOCA; the acetate of deoxycortone. Has been available for over 30 years and at one time was the only corticostoid therapy available and, together with salt, was used in the treatment of Addison's disease; for prolonged action deoxycortone pivalate is given by intramuscular injection and is effective for 2 or 3 weeks. **Deoxycortone Acetate Implants BP 1973.** Sterile cylinders prepared by fusion or heavy compression of deoxycortone acetate. **Deoxycortone Acetate Injection BP 1973.** A sterile solution of deoxycortone acetate in ethyl oleate or a suitable fixed oil. **Deoxycortone Pivalate BPC 1968.** 21-Pivaloyloxypregn-4-ene-3,20-dione. The pivalate has the same actions, uses and side-effects as the acetate; it is only slightly soluble in water and, after intramuscular injection, its action lasts from 2 to 3 weeks. **Deoxycortone Trimethylacetate BP 1963.** 21-Pivaloyl oxypregn-4-ene-3,20-dione. A white, odourless crystalline powder, almost insoluble in water, slightly soluble in fixed oils and soluble in alcohol. It is administered in the form of intramuscular injection in the treatment of Addison's disease. It remains effective for 3–4 weeks.

deoxyephedrine (de·ox·e·**ef**'·ed·reen). Methylamphetamine.

deoxygenate (de·**ox**·e·jen·ate). To remove oxygen. [L *de*, oxygen.]

deoxygenation (de·ox·e·jen·**a**'·shun). Deoxidation.

2-deoxyglucose. *See* GLUCOSE.

deoxyhaemoglobin (de·ox·e·he·mo·**glo**'·bin). *See* HAEMOGLOBIN.

deoxyribonuclease (de·**ox**·e·ri·bo·**new**'·kle·aze). A class of endonucleases which are specific for the hydrolysis of deoxyribonucleic acids. [deoxyribose, nuclease.]

deoxyribonucleoprotein (de·ox·e·**ri**·bo·new·kle·o·**pro**'·te·in). A class of conjugated proteins that contain deoxyribonucleic acid. The protein factor is generally very basic, and is usually a histone or a protamine. [DNA, Gk *proteois* of first rank.]

deoxyribonucleotide (de·**ox**·e·ri·bo·**new**'·kle·o·tide). A class of nucleotide in which the pentose is 2-deoxy-D-ribose. [deoxyribose, nucleotide.]

deoxyribose (de·**ox**·e·**ri**'·boze). The sugar moiety in DNA and its precursors. The term *desoxyribose* is used in the USA.

deozonize (de·o·zo·nize). To deprive of ozone. [L *de*, ozone.]

Depage, Antoine (b. 1862). Brussels surgeon.

Depage's position. The prone position with the pelvis elevated so that the body with the legs forms an inverted V.

depancreatize (de·**pan**·kre·at·ize). To excise the pancreas. [L *de*, pancreas.]

Depaul, Jean Anne Henri (b. 1811). Paris surgeon.

Depaul's tube. A tube for the insufflation of the lungs.

depauperate (de·**paw**·per·ate). In mycology, a relative deficiency in the special reproductive structures or spore forms which is reflected in lack (or absence) of distinctive morphological characters. [L *de*, *pauperare* to impoverish.]

dependence (de·**pen**·dens). In a drug addict, that state of body and mind which is conditioned by ingestion of a certain quantity of the drug or an increasing quantity of it. Any decrease in dose gives rise to abstinence symptoms. [L *de*, *pendere* to hand.]

dependency (de·**pen**·den·se). The state of being dependent. **Cortical dependency.** That portion of the brain supplementary to the cerebral cortex. [see prec.]

depepsinized (de·**pep**·sin·izd). Describing gastric juice that has been inactivated by removal of the pepsin. [L *de*, pepsin.]

depersonalization (de·**per**·son·al·i·**za**'·shun). A state in which the subject feels that he is unreal. [L *de*, *persona* mask.]

de Pezzer, Michael Benvenuto (b. 1853). French surgeon.

de Pezzer catheter. A self-retaining catheter with a bulbous tip.

dephlogisticate (de·flo·**jis**·tik·ate). To subdue or remove inflammation in a part. [L *de*, Gk *phlegein* to burn.]

depigmentation (de·pig·men·**ta**'·shun). The removal or destruction of natural pigment from a tissue by either physiological or chemical means. [L *de*, *pigmentum* paint.]

depilate (**dep**·il·ate). To strip or remove the hairs from a part. [L *depilare* to deprive of hair.]

depilation (dep·il·**a**·shun). Epilation. The act of removing hair; loss of hair. [see prec.]

depilatory (dep·**il**·at·or·e). Capable of removing hair; a term applied to any substance, such as barium sulphide, which removes the hair by external application, or thallium acetate, which, administered internally, produces a falling-out of the hair by its effect on the sympathetic innervation. [L *depilare* to deprive of hair.]

See also: ATKINSON.

depilous (**dep**·il·us). Hairless. [see prec.]

depletion (de·**ple**·shun). 1. The removal of solids or fluids from the system, as by blood-letting or purgation. 2. Exhaustion of strength as the result of haemorrhage or excessive discharge of fluid from the system. **Plasma depletion.** The operation of withdrawing a copious amount of blood, centrifuging it in order to separate the corpuscles, substituting Locke's solution for the plasma, and returning this and the corpuscles into the blood vascular system (Abel). [L *deplere* to empty.]

depletive (de·**ple**·tiv). 1. An agent that depletes. 2. Depletory. [L *deplere* to empty.]

depletory (de·**ple**·tor·e). Serving to deplete; causing depletion. [see prec.]

deplumation (de·ploo·**ma**·shun). Loss of the eyelashes as the result of disease, local or general. [L *deplumare* to strip of feathers.]

depolarization (de·**po**·lar·i·**za**'·shun). 1. The prevention, reduction or elimination of polarization. As applied to the motor end-plate, acetylcholine (or a synthetic depolarizing muscle relaxant) combines with anionic sites on the end-plate plasma membrane, alters its permeability, permits free entry of sodium ions and results in depolarization. 2. Electrically, the removal of the layer of gas which polarizes the positive plate in a voltaic cell. 3. The neutralizing effect of introducing a depolarizer into a polariscope. 4. The electrical events that occur when an impulse travels down a nerve axon or from one heart cell to another. It results from a sudden change in the conductivity of the cell membrane with the consequent movement of ions into and out of the cell. **Cellular depolarization.** The process of extinction of the resting polarized state of muscle and nerve cells when they are activated. There is a rapid flux of ions across the cell membrane and the resting positive charge on the external surface of the cell, as compared with the interior of the cell, is abolished; simultaneously, in the case of muscle cells, the contraction process is initiated. The electrical fields created by the depolarization and repolarization processes are the basis of electrocardiography, electromyography and electro-encephalography. [L *de*, Gk *polos* pivot.]

depolarize (de·**po**·lar·ize). 1. To remove or prevent polarization. 2. To deprive of polarity. [L *de*, Gk *polos* pivot.]

depolarizer (de·**po**·lar·i·zer). 1. An optical arrangement for reconverting polarized light into ordinary light. 2. The chemical oxidizing agent surrounding the positive plate in a voltaic cell to prevent the formation of the layer of hydrogen gas which would polarize the cell. [see prec.]

deportation (de·port·**a**·shun). A process in the development of the embryo that causes the chorionic villi to atrophy and disappear from the fetal placenta (Veit). [L *deportare* to carry away.]

deposit (de·**poz**·it). 1. A precipitate. 2. Dregs. 3. A collection of extraneous inorganic particles present in a viscus or cavity, or in the tissues. 4. The material, calcareous or otherwise, which sticks fast to the surface of a tooth. **Active deposit.** The mixture of radioactive substances which are formed in the decay of a radioactive gas, e.g. radon, and which deposit on nearby solid surfaces. **Brick-dust deposit.** A rust-coloured sediment of urates observed in urine. [L *deponere* to lay down.]

deposition (de·po·**zish**·un). Medicolegally, written records of evidence given orally in a court of justice. They must be read by or to a witness before he signs them. [see prec.]

depositive (de·**poz**·it·iv). Descriptive of the papular condition of the skin that is caused by exudation of inflammatory lymph into the derma. [L *deponere* to lay down.]

depot (**dep**·o). A place where things are deposited and stored. **Drug depot.** A quantity—usually several times more than the individual pharmacopoeial dose—of a drug in a form in which it is only slowly absorbable, either in a solid or a fluid but concentrated form, often dissolved in oil, placed in or injected into the tissues. From this depot the drug is slowly absorbed and thus exerts a continuous and prolonged effect. [Fr. *dépôt.*]

depravation (de·prav·**a**·shun). 1. Change for the worse. 2. Morbid perversion or deterioration occurring in physiological functions or in the tissues or secretions. [L *depravare* to corrupt.]

depraved (de·**pra**·vd). 1. Characterized by degeneration. 2. Deteriorated. 3. Perverted or corrupt. [see prec.]

deprementia (de·pre·**men**·she·ah). A psychosis the result of autotoxaemia and characterized by amnesia, melancholy and depression of spirits. [L *deprimere* to press down, *mens* mind.]

depressan (de·**pres**·an). Name given to a urinary extract containing a mixture of non-specific substances, most likely depressor amines, which on intravenous injection lowers the blood pressure of an anaesthetized rabbit. [L *deprimere* to press down.]

depressant (de·**pres**·ant). 1. Having the ability to lessen the general activity of the body, reduce the degree of function or lower the general vital response. 2. Any drug, agent or causal factor that diminishes normal tone or functional activity. Gastric depressants include the barbiturates, bismuth salts, chloral, opium and the bicarbonates of potassium and sodium. Among depressants affecting the central nervous system are: alcohol; the anaesthetics, such as ether, chloroform and cyclopropane; the barbiturates; opium and its derivatives; synthetic analgesics, such as methadone; sedatives, including chloral, the bromides, hyoscine, etc. Respiratory depressants include most drugs depressing the central nervous system, particularly alcohol, anaesthetics, barbiturates, opium and its derivatives. [see prec.]

depressed (de·**prest**). 1. Forced down below the level of surrounding parts, e.g. a fracture. 2. Below the normal level of function. 3. Lowered in vitality. 4. Dejected in spirits. [L *deprimere* to press down.]

depressing (de·**pres**·ing). In ophthalmology, couching, especially with reference to the now obsolete operation for cataract. [see prec.]

depression (de·**presh**·un). 1. In anatomy, any circumscribed part of the surface of an organ or structure which is lower than the general level of the surface. 2. Any displacement to form a hollow. 3. The reduction of function by a drug or other agent. 4. In psychiatry, the affective attitude of unhappiness and hopelessness. **Adolescent depression.** Depression occurring in adolescence. **Agitated depression.** Depression accompanied by restlessness. **Anaclitic depression.** A syndrome shown by infants as a result of prolonged separation from the mother or mother substitute. **Anxious agitated depression.** Depression accompanied by anxiety and restlessness. **Auricular depression.** A term referring to the pressure phases of the right auricle of the heart: the positive wave of auricular systole seen in the jugular venous pulse is succeeded by a negative wave (depression) during auricular diastole. It is also known as the "*x-descent*" *wave.* **Averse depression, Aversion depression.** A depression characterized by evidence of aversion to the facts of the illness and to the medical care which it necessitates. **Depression of cataract.** Reclination or couching; an operation for cataract in which the opaque lens is dislocated downwards and backwards into the vitreous, by means of an instrument introduced through the cornea. It was much used in ancient times, but now very rarely because of its liability to be followed by secondary glaucoma and blindness. **Involutional depression.** Either of two forms of depression occurring in the involutional period of life, the first characterized by depression with agitation, the second by depression with hypochondriacal delusions. **Otic depression.** The depression in the embryo that eventually develops into the ear. **Pacchionian depressions.** Small depressions on the inner surface of the parietal bones, adjacent to the sagittal suture, found in the elderly; they lodge the pacchionian (arachnoid) granulations. **Postdormitial depression.** Momentary mental depression after sleep. **Pterygoid depression.** A depression on the anteriomedial surface of the neck of the mandible where the lateral pterygoid muscle is attached. **Radial depression.** The radial fossa on the anterior surface of the lower end of the humerus. **Reactive depression.** A depression in which a predominant causative factor is an environmental stress. **Retarded depression.** Depression accompanied by the slowing of both mental and physical processes. **Supratrochlear depression.** The coronoid fossa on the anterior surface of the lower end of the humerus. **Systolic depression.** Systolic retraction; recession of the sternum or ribs overlying the heart during systole, due to adherence of the pericardium to the chest wall. **Ventricular depression.** A term referring to the jugular venous pulse curve and denoting the portions of the curve between ventricular and auricular systole. [L *deprimere* to press down.]

See also: PACCHIONI, TROELTSCH.

depressive (de·**pres**·iv). Causing depression, or tending to depress. [see prec.]

depressomotor (de·**pres**·o·**mo**'·tor). 1. Diminishing or lowering the capacity for movement. 2. An agent, such as a bromide, that retards or lessens the activity of the motor centres. [L *deprimere* to press down, motor.]

depressor (de·**pres**·or). 1. A nerve or muscle which lessens or inhibits the activity of an organ or depresses or draws down a part. 2. A surgical appliance or instrument which holds down or draws out of the way any part during an examination or operation. 3. An agent which restrains or lessens physiological function, e.g. blood pressure. **Tongue depressor.** An apparatus for holding the tongue down against the floor of the mouth. [L *deprimere* to press down.]

See also: SIMS.

depressor anguli oris muscle [musculus depressor anguli oris (NA)] (de·**pres**·or ang·gew·li **or**·is musl). A muscle attached below to the oblique line on the mandible and above to the angle of the mouth. Its fibres blend with the superficial layer of the orbicularis oris muscle.

depressor labii inferioris muscle [musculus depressor labii inferioris (NA)] (de·**pres**·or **la**·be·i in·feer·e·**or**·is musl). A muscle attached below to the mandible from the symphysis to below the mental foramen, and above to the skin of the lower lip.

depressor septi muscle [musculus depressor septi (NA)] (de·**pres**·or **sep**·ti musl). A facial muscle attached to the incisive fossa of the maxilla and to the posterior part of the ala and adjacent part of the nasal septum.

depressor supercilii muscle [musculus depressor supercilii (NA)] (de·**pres**·or sew·per·**sil**·e·i musl). That part of the orbital portion of the orbicularis oculi muscle whose fasciculi interweave with the fibres of the frontalis and corrugator supercilii muscles and also insert into the skin and subcutaneous tissue of the eyebrow.

deprival, deprivation, deprivement (de·**pri**·val, dep·riv·**a**·shun, de·**prive**·ment). A condition of lack or loss of parts or powers, or of being in want of anything necessary for normal health. **Sensory deprivation.** Reduced cues about the environment; a condition in which exteroceptive sensory input (touch, temperature, noise, smell, kinaesthesia, etc.) is reduced to a minimal steady state.

Deprodone (**dep**·ro·done). BP Commission approved name for 11β,17β-dihydroxypregna-1,4-diene-3,20-dione; a corticosteroid.

depside (**dep**·side). A class of substances which occur in nature as gallotannins. They are formed by the linking of two or more hydroxy aromatic acids into chains, and are known accordingly as di-, tri- and tetradepsides.

depth (depth). Deepness; profundity. The measurement from a surface downwards, as with a liquid, or horizontally from front to back, as in penetration. **Focal depth, Depth of focus.** The distance through which an object can be moved and still give a clear image through an optical system. It depends on the size of the aperture of the system. [AS *diop.*]

Deptropine (**dep**·**tro**·peen). BP Commission approved name for 3-(1,2:4,5-dibenzocycloheptadien-3-yloxy)tropane; a bronchodilator.

depula (**dep**·ew·lah). In embryology, that transitional stage of development of the ovum in which it is changing from a blastula to a gastrula. [Gk *depas* goblet.]

depulization (de·pew·li·**za**′·shun). The act or process of freeing dwellings from plague-carrying fleas; a term used by anti-plague workers. [L *de, pulex* flea.]

depurant (**dep**·ewr·ant). 1. Any agent or drug which promotes the elimination of waste material from the system. 2. Eliminating waste material. [L *depurare* to purify.]

depurated (**dep**·ewr·a·ted). Freed from impurities. [see prec.]

depuration (dep·ewr·**a**·shun). The act or process of cleansing or purifying from waste products. [L *depurare* to purify.]

depurative (dep·**ewr**·at·iv). 1. Tending to cleanse or purify. 2. An agent that purifies the blood. [see prec.]

depurator (**dep**·ewr·a·tor). 1. A depurant. 2. An apparatus by means of which the excretory powers of the skin are stimulated. [L *depurare* to purify.]

Deputy Director of Medical Services. DDMS; the representative of the Director of Medical Services at the headquarters of an army or of a corps. USA equivalent, *Army* or *Corps Surgeon.*

Depuy splint. A splint for fractures of the clavicle.

Dequalinium Acetate BP 1973 (de·kwol·**in**·e·um **as**·et·ate). Decamethylenedi-(4-aminoquinaldinium acetate), a white, odourless, slightly hygroscopic powder with a bitter taste. It is an antiseptic active against a wide range of micro-organisms and several species of fungi.

Dequalinium Chloride BP 1973 (de·kwol·**in**·e·um **klor**·ide). A quaternary ammonium-type antiseptic compound, decamethyl enedi-(4-aminoquinaldinium chloride). Its activity is against a wide range of micro-organisms, except spores. It is administered as a mouth-wash or lozenges.

de Quervain's thyroiditis (de·ker·vans thi·roid·**i**·tis). Associated with pain and fever, the gland is infiltrated with fibrosis, round cells, polymorphs and giant cells.

deradelphus (der·ad·**el**·fus). A twin monster with single head, fused neck and thorax, 3 or 4 arms, and 4 legs. [Gk *dere* neck, *adelphos* brother.]

deradenitis (der·ad·en·**i**′·tis). Inflammation of the lymph glands of the neck. [Gk *dere* neck, *aden* gland, *-itis* inflammation.]

deradenoncus (der·ad·en·**ong**′·kus). A tumour or swelling of a lymph gland of the neck. [Gk *dere* neck, *aden* gland, *ogkos* a swelling.]

deranencephalia (der·an·en·kef·a′·le·ah). A condition of fetal monstrosity in which the head, brain and upper portion of the spinal cord are defective or lacking, but the neck is present. [Gk *dere* neck, *a, egkephalos* brain.]

derangement (de·**ra**·nj·ment). 1. Disturbance of the proper or regular order and arrangement of a system. 2. Irregularity of, or in, a part or organ. 3. Mental disturbance or intellectual confusion. 4. Insanity. [Fr. *dérangement* act of disturbing.]

See also: HEY (W.).

Dercum, Francis Xavier (b. 1856). Philadelphia neurologist.

Dercum's disease. Adiposis dolorosa.

derealization (de·re·al·i·**za**′·shun). Loss of the sense of reality, when external objects and events seem unfamiliar and unreal. [L *de,* realization.]

dereism (**de**·re·izm). In psychiatry, thinking controlled and directed not by logic and reality but by the wishes, conscious and unconscious, of the subject. [L *de, res* thing.]

derencephalocele (der·en·**kef**·al·o·seel). Partial extrusion of the brain substance through a fissure in one or more of the cervical vertebrae. [Gk *dere* neck, *egkephalos* brain, *kele* hernia.]

derencephalous (der·en·**kef**·al·us). Having the characteristics of a derencephalus.

derencephalus (der·en·**kef**·al·us). A single monster with open skull, rudimentary skull bones, and bifid cervical vertebrae within which the very small brain is enclosed. [Gk *dere* neck, *egkephalos* brain.]

derencephaly (der·en·**kef**·al·e). A double monster having 1 head. [see prec.]

derepression (de·re·**presh**·un). The switching-on of transcription of a structural gene by removal of a repressor molecule from an operator gene; the process involves binding of a small molecular weight molecule, called an *inducer,* to the repressor protein. [L *de, reprimere* to press back.]

deric (**der**·ik). Referring to the ectoderm. Cf. ENTERIC. [Gk *deros* skin.]

derism (**de**·rizm). Dereism.

derivation (der·iv·**a**·shun). 1. A drawing of body fluids or blood to one area (by blistering or cupping, for example) in order to relieve congestion in another. 2. The transference of a disease from one part to another. 3. The process by which the blood was thought to be sucked through the heart. 4. A lead in electrocardiography. 5. The synthesis of an organic compound from another closely related to it. 6. The structural relationship between a parent compound and its derivative. [L *derivatio* a drawing off.]

derivative (der·**iv**·at·iv). 1. Anything produced by derivation. 2. Any substance stained by another substance. 3. A compound formed by chemical means from a parent compound. 4. A compound closely related structurally to another compound, but not necessarily prepared from it. [see prec.]

derm, derma (derm, **der**·mah). The corium. [Gk *derma* skin.]

dermabrasion (der·mab·**ra**·zhun). A procedure of surgical skin planing, usually performed with a rapidly-rotating burr. The skin is frozen by a jet of dichlortetrafluorethane, thus rendering the area to be treated anaesthetic, firm and bloodless. The technique is used for removing superficial benign lesions and tattoo marks, also for rendering pitted scars of acne vulgaris less conspicuous. [Gk *derma* skin, L *abrasio* a scraping.]

Dermacentor (der·mah·**sen**·tor). A genus of ticks, holarctic in distribution, with many species. The larvae and nymphs are usually parasites of rodents and rabbits, but the adults prefer larger hosts, including man; they are thus very suitable vectors of rodent diseases. The bites easily become infected, and those of mature females may cause tick paralysis. The following species are of medical importance: *Dermacentor andersoni* of Western USA is the most important vector of Rocky Mountain spotted fever and also conveys tularaemia, equine encephalitis, Colorado tick fever and Q fever, and is a cause of tick paralysis; *D. nuttalli, D. variabilis* of Central and Eastern USA, and *D. occidentalis* of the West Coast are less well known vectors of spotted fever; *D. parumapterus,* a species which may also be involved as a vector of spotted fever. *D. silvarum* is also a potential vector of tularaemia. [Gk *derma* skin, *kentein* to pierce.]

Dermacentroxenus rickettsii (der·mah·sen·**trox**′·en·us rik·**et**·se·i). The causal agent of Rocky Mountain spotted fever; rickettsia bodies found in the stomach of the arthropod host *Dermacentor.* The name was originally proposed by Wolbach, but it is now called *Rickettsia rickettsii.* [*Dermacentor,* Gk *xenos* host.]

dermadrome (**der**·mah·drome). The cutaneous manifestation of an internal disorder; "the skin part of a syndrome" (Wiener, 1947). [Gk *derma* skin, syndrome.]

dermagraph (**der**·mah·graf). 1. Dermatograph. 2. An instrument with which hyperalgesic areas of the body can be localized. [Gk *derma* skin, *graphein* to write.]

dermagraphy (der·**mag**·raf·e). 1. An anatomical description of the skin. 2. Dermatographia. [see prec.]

dermahaemia (der·mah·**he**·me·ah). Hyperaemia of the skin. [Gk *derma* skin, *haima* blood.]

dermal (**der**·mal). Relating or belonging to the skin, particularly the corium. [Gk *derma* skin.]

dermalaxia (der·mal·**ax**·e·ah). Pathological relaxation or softening of the skin. [Gk *derma* skin, *malaxis* a softening.]

dermalgia (der·**mal**·je·ah). Dermatalgia.

dermametropathism (**der**·mah·met·**rop**′·ath·izm). A method of diagnosing skin disease by noting the intensity and nature of the markings made when an instrument with a blunt point is pressed on or drawn across the skin. [Gk *derma* skin, *metron* measure, *pathos* suffering.]

dermamyiasis (**der**·mah·mi·**i**′·as·is). Myiasis of the skin. **Dermamyiasis linearis migrans oestrosa.** The term suggested by Kumberg for the disorder named *creeping eruption* (Lee), *larva migrans* (Crocker) or *hyponomoderma* (Kaposi), which is characterized by narrow, slightly elevated, red, linear lesions which may be straight, curved, festooned or looped, produced by the burrowing of larvae, particularly those of *Ancylostoma, Gastrophilus* (botfly), *Hypoderma* (warble fly) and *Gnathostoma.* [Gk *derma* skin, myiasis.]

dermanaplasty, dermanoplasty (der·**man**·ah·plas·te, der·**man**·o·plas·te). Dermatoplasty.

Dermanyssus (der·man·**is**·us). A genus of mites of which *Dermanyssus gallinae* is an important parasite of domestic birds and occurs frequently on men associated with them. It may give rise to poultrymen's itch, a violent rash, particularly on hands and forearms. Other species normal to birds and mammals have been found on man. **Dermanyssus avium.** A mite which infests poultry, pigeons, starlings, cage-birds, sparrows and other species. On man, the mite may cause papular urticaria or a rash resembling scabies. [Gk *derma* skin, *nyssein* to prick.]

dermapostasis (der·map·**os**·tas·is). Any disease of the skin with formation of abscesses or hard spots. [Gk *derma* skin, *apostasis* defection.]

Dermaptera (der·**map**·ter·ah). An order of insects, the earwigs, characterized by the pair of forceps posteriorly and the fan-like hind wings which fold under the small forewings. The genera *Forficula* and *Anisolabis* are of medical interest. [Gk *derma* skin, *pteron* wing.]

dermaskeleton (der·mah·**skel**·et·on). Exoskeleton; applied, in man, to the very rudimentary superficial coverings of the body, i.e. the nails and the teeth. [Gk *derma* skin, *skeletos* dried up.]

dermatalgia (der·mat·**al**·je·ah). A local sensation of pain in the skin; it is based on nervous disease or may be of reflex origin. There is no organic structural lesion, and usually there is paraesthesia. [Gk *derma* skin, *algos* pain.]

dermataneuria (**der**·mat·an·**ewr**′·e·ah). Anaesthesia of the skin because of derangement of its nerve supply. [Gk *derma* skin, *a, neuron* nerve.]

dermatatrophia (**der**·mat·at·**ro**′·fe·ah). A condition of thinning or atrophy of the skin. [Gk *derma* skin, *a, trophe* nutrition.]

dermatauxe (der·mat·**awx**·e). Hypertrophy of the skin. [Gk *derma* skin, *auxe* increase.]

dermatergosis (**der**·mat·er·**go**′·sis). Any occupational disease of the skin. [Gk *derma* skin, *ergon* work, *-osis* condition.]

dermathaemia (der·mat·**he**·me·ah). Hyperaemia of the skin. [Gk *derma* skin, *haima* blood.]

dermatic (der·**mat**·ik). 1. Dermal. 2. Any remedy for skin disease. [Gk *derma* skin.]

dermatitis (der·mat·i·tis) (pl. *dermatitides*). Inflammation of the skin. **Acid dermatitis.** That due to contact with strong or weak acids; in the latter case repeated contact first causes sensitization to subsequent contacts. **Acriflavine dermatitis.** Dermatitis medicamentosa (see below) due to acriflavine. **Dermatitis actinica.** Cutaneous inflammation due to the sun's rays, ultra-violet rays, x-rays or the radiations from radioactive substances. **Acute infectious bullous dermatitis.** Pemphigus acutus. **Dermatitis aestivalis.** Heat rash: prickly heat. **Alkali dermatitis.** A condition analogous to acid dermatitis. **Allergic dermatitis.** An eruption due to an altered state of reactivity of the skin to allergens or haptens. **Dermatitis ambustionis.** That due to a burn. **Ammoniacal dermatitis.** A form of napkin dermatitis in which faecal organisms form ammonia from urea in the urine. **Ancylostome dermatitis.** Ground itch from hookworm infection. **Arsenical dermatitis.** Eczematous eruptions and ulceration occurring from exposure to solutions, powders or pigments containing arsenic; acute or chronic eruptions caused by the ingestion or injection of drugs containing arsenic. **Arsphenamine dermatitis.** Arsenical dermatitis (see above). **Dermatitis artefacta.** Self-inflicted traumatic dermatitis. **Asteatotic dermatitis.** Dermatitis with dry, cracked skin affecting mostly the limbs of elderly persons particularly in the winter. Xerodermatous individuals may also suffer, particularly after excessive soaping of the skin. **Atopic dermatitis.** Atopic eczema. **Dermatitis atrophicans diffusa.** Diffuse idiopathic atrophy of the skin. **Dermatitis atrophicans lipoidis diabetica.** Necrobiosis lipoidica diabeticorum (Urbach). **Dermatitis atrophicans maculosa.** Idiopathic cutaneous atrophy affecting small areas. **Dermatitis atrophicans pustulosa.** A follicular pustular condition of the legs and sometimes of the thighs and forearms occurring in Africans and Asians. Atrophic scars result. **Dermatitis atrophicans reticularis.** Poikiloderma vascularis atrophicans. **Autophytic dermatitis.** Self-inflicted dermatitis. **Bakers' dermatitis.** 1. An allergic dermatitis. 2. Bakers' itch. **Berlock dermatitis, Berloque dermatitis.** Dermatitis due to the photosensitizing action of oil of bergamot or other essential oils used in perfumery. **Bhilwanol dermatitis.** Marking-nut dermatitis (see below). **Bismuth dermatitis.** A rare condition due to bismuth injections. **Dermatitis blastomycetica.** Cutaneous blastomycosis. **Blister-beetle dermatitis.** Seasonal bullous dermatitis (see below). **Brucella dermatitis.** Dermatitis caused by *Brucella abortus.* **Dermatitis bullosa striata pratensis.** A patterned bullous dermatitis due to exposure of the skin to certain meadow plants and grasses. **Dermatitis calorica.** Dermatitis of various grades due to heat or cold. **Cane dermatitis.** An occupational dermatitis among cane cutters. **Carpenters' dermatitis.** A dermatitis that is a recognized occupational risk in carpenters. Certain woods themselves may cause sensitization and eventually dermatitis, but in addition carpenters come in contact with irritating substances such as glues, resins and lacquers. **Caterpillar dermatitis.** Urticarial lesions following direct contact with certain caterpillars, or with shed caterpillar hairs. **Cement dermatitis.** Dermatitis caused by contact with cement. It may be either of the primary irritant variety or due to allergic hypersensitivity to the chromate content of the cement. **Cercarial dermatitis.** Schistosome dermatitis (see below). **Chromium dermatitis.** Dermatitis caused by contact with chromium-plated objects or with chromium salts which may be present in cement, diesel-oil engines and leather objects. **Chronic superficial dermatitis.** A chronic eczematous condition resembling parapsoriasis en plaques but not proceeding to a reticulosis. **Dermatitis chronica atrophicans.** Idiopathic atrophy of the skin. **Chrysanthemum dermatitis.** Dermatitis venenata (see below) due to contact with chrysanthemums. **Clothing dermatitis.** Dermatitis caused by dyes, formalin, chromates or other chemicals in clothing. **Dermatitis colonica.** A chronic eruption characterized by the appearance of oval scaling lesions on the thighs, arms and lower abdomen, attributed to abnormality of the intestinal flora. **Colostomy dermatitis.** Inflammation of the skin around a colostomy. **Dermatitis congelationis.** Cutaneous inflammation due to cold; chilblains, frostbite, immersion foot and trench foot are included in this category. **Contact dermatitis.** Cutaneous inflammation caused by exposure to deleterious agents. **Contagious pustular dermatitis.** Orf; normally a disease of sheep, it may occasionally infect those who come in contact with an infected animal. In man, it causes single lesions on the hand or, occasionally, on the face, which resolve spontaneously, though slowly. The disease is caused by a pox virus which is a member of the paravaccinia group. **Dermatitis contusiformis.** Erythema nodosum. **Cosmetic dermatitis.** Dermatitis due to sensitization to some constituent of a cosmetic. **Cotton-seed dermatitis.** An occupational dermatitis caused by contact with cotton seed. **Dhobie-mark dermatitis.** Marking-nut dermatitis (see below). **Diaper dermatitis.** Napkin-area dermatitis (see below). **Dress-shield dermatitis.** Dermatitis of the axillary folds caused by sensitization, usually to rubber, in shields designed to protect clothing from sweat. **Dermatitis dysmenorrhoeica.** A dermatitis described by R. Matzenauer and R. Polland (1912), characterized by the appearance in dysmenorrhoeic women at the menstrual periods, and at no other time, of an eruption (usually symmetrical) on the face, trunk or limbs, which is usually vesicular but which may be solely erythematous or urticarial. **Eczematoid dermatitis.** Dermatitis infectiosa eczematoides (see below). **Endogenous dermatitis.** Inflammatory disease of the skin of internal origin, e.g. endogenous eczema. **Dermatitis exfoliativa, Exfoliative dermatitis.** A confusing descriptive term limited in its application to a variety of maladies of differing aetiology, and usually, but not invariably, connoting generalized redness of the skin with scaling of the upper layer of the epidermis, but without vesiculation or oozing. Primary exfoliative dermatitis is synonymous with pityriasis rubra; secondary exfoliative dermatitis may develop as a sequel to eczema, dermatitis venenata, pityriasis rubra pilaris and seborrhoeic dermatitis, or as a result of the injudicious use of local applications of, for example, dithranol or chrysarobin, or following the administration of arsenic and arsenical preparations, gold salts, mepacrine and certain other drugs. The erythrodermias noted in some cases of Hodgkin's disease and in the premycotic stage of mycosis fungoides constitute a form of exfoliative dermatitis. **Dermatitis exfoliativa epidemica.** Savill's disease, a disease of obscure aetiology with a mortality of from 5 to 13 per cent. A moist and a dry form have been recorded, the latter regarded as indistinguishable from pityriasis rubra. **Dermatitis exfoliativa infantum, Dermatitis exfoliativa neonatorum.** Ritter's disease, a malady of very young infants which commences in a localized area, often on the face, and spreads to involve the whole body surface; vesicles and bullae are noted. It is caused by staphylococcal infection. **Dermatitis exfoliatrice** (Brocq). Exfoliative dermatitis (see above). **Exudative discoid and lichenoid chronic dermatitis.** Exudative discoid and lichenoid chronic dermatosis. **Dermatitis factitia.** Dermatitis artefacta (see above). **Flexural dermatitis.** Inflammation of the skin covering the flexor surfaces of joints. **Friction dermatitis.** Traumatic dermatitis due to friction. **Fruit dermatitis.** An allergic dermatitis from handling fruit. **Fungoid dermatitis.** Dermatitis of fungous origin. **Fusospirillary dermatitis.** Dermatitis caused by Vincent's fusiform bacillus and spirochaete. **Dermatitis gangraenosa.** Gangrene of the skin. **Dermatitis gangraenosa infantum.** Multiple disseminated gangrene of the skin in infants; pemphigus gangraenosa; rupia escharotica; gangrenous infantile ecthyma. The malady may develop as a complication of, or as a sequel to, an acute specific fever, e.g. varicella (varicella gangraenosa), rubeola or scarlatina, or may occur independently. It is a severe ecthymatous process associated with the formation of areas of gangrene. **Genitocrural dermatitis.** Dermatitis of the genitocrural folds caused by bacterial, candidal and fungal infections, psoriasis or contact sensitivity. **Dermatitis glandularis erythematosa.** Lupus erythematosus. **Glue dermatitis.** An occupational disease in wood workers. **Gluteal dermatitis.** Napkin-area dermatitis (see below). **Gold dermatitis.** A condition due to gold infections: it responds to treatment by BAL. **Grain dermatitis.** Grain itch; a dermatitis caused by a mite that lives in straw. **Hairnet dermatitis.** Dermatitis around the nape of the neck caused by a dye in a hairnet. **Harara dermatitis.** A form of heat rash common in Anatolia, Syria and Palestine. **Harvest-mite dermatitis.** Dermatitis due to *Trombicula* mites of various species. **Hatband dermatitis.** Dermatitis in the hatband area caused by leather, plastics, formaldehyde or antiseptics. **Heat dermatitis.** An ill-defined term, including prickly heat. **Dermatitis herpetiformis.** Duhring's disease, a malady in which the eruption can take several forms, the most characteristic of which is the occurrence of intensely itching vesicles, usually grouped, symmetrically distributed and developing in crops; their sites eventually are marked by pigmentation of varying degree. Papular, pustular and bulbous lesions may occur, and the malady is very chronic and usually afebrile. The cause is unknown, and it may occur at all ages, but mostly in adult life. **Dermatitis hiemalis.** A recurrent eruption noted during the winter in the Great Lake region of North America. **Hypostatic dermatitis.** Stasis dermatitis (see below). **Ileostomy dermatitis.** Maceration, redness and erosions around an ileostomy cap, caused by alkaline proteolytic intestinal juice. **Industrial dermatitis.** A skin eruption caused by exposure at work to deleterious agents. **Dermatitis infectiosa eczematoides, Infectious eczematoid dermatitis.** A scaling or oozing eruption due to bacterial infection (usually staphylococcal), in which the process is continued by sensitization as well as by infection. **Infective dermatitis.** Inflammation in skin flexures and follicles caused by bacteria (staphylococci, streptococci, *Pseudomonas pyocyanea* and other organisms), also *Candida albicans.* **Insect dermatitis.** That produced by contact with insects of a wide variety. **Juvenile papular dermatitis.** A diffuse or discrete lichenoid papular eruption of children, probably caused by trauma, e.g. builders' sand. **Dermatitis lichenoides chronica atrophicans.** Lichen sclerosus et atrophicus. **Light-sensitization dermatitis.** Dermatitis in a person who is naturally, or who has become, hypersensitive to light. **Malignant papillary dermatitis.** Paget's disease of the nipple. **Marine dermatitis.** Seabathers' dermatitis caused by contact with corals, jellyfish, the Portuguese man-of-war and other marine animals and plants, including sensitization to *Alcyonidium gelatinosum,* a marine animal resembling seaweed, which is the cause of "Dogger Bank Itch". **Marking-nut dermatitis.** Local irritation caused by bhilawanol oil, used by the washermen in India (dhobie) to mark clothes. **Match-box dermatitis.** Dermatitis due to contact with irritant chemicals on the striking surface of a match box. **Meadow dermatitis.** Phytophoto dermatitis with streaky bullae produced by contact with certain plant juices which cause light sensitivity. **Dermatitis medicamentosa.** A drug eruption; any eruption due to ingestion, injection or absorption of a medicinal substance, as distinct from contact dermatitis caused by medicinal agents. **Mercury dermatitis.** Dermatitis medicamentosa (see above) due to mercury. **Metabolic dermatitis.** A rare condition associated with thyroid deficiency; it may occur in ichthyotic subjects. **Dermatitis micropapulosa erythematosa hyperhidrotica nasi.** Granulosis rubra nasi. **Mite dermatitis.** Scrub itch. *See* ITCH. **Moth dermatitis.** Dermatitis produced by contact with the hairs of the wings of moths of several species, and also by the hairs of the larvae of certain other species. **Dermatitis multiformis.** Dermatitis herpetiformis (see above). **Mycotic dermatitis.** That caused by a fungus infection. **Napkin-area dermatitis.** Dermatitis resulting from the irritation of contact with a wet urine-soaked napkin. **Necklace dermatitis.** Dermatitis caused by nickel-plated clasps, lacquered pearls or exotic woods in necklaces. **Nickel dermatitis.** A condition that occurs in almost everybody who is constantly in contact with nickel salts. **Dermatitis nodosa.** Onchocerciasis. **Dermatitis nodosa rubra.** A persistent nodular eruption of uncertain cause. **Dermatitis nodularis necrotica.** An eruption affecting the extremities, resembling papulonecrotic tuberculide and in many instances identical with it; a few cases have been associated with bacterial endocarditis. **Non-sensitization dermatitis.** Dermatitis in which the cutaneous reaction is not caused by or associated with allergic or anaphylactic phenomena. **Occupational dermatitis.** A skin eruption due to one or more hazards of the individual's occupation. **Oil dermatitis.** Dermatitis caused by exposure to oil. **Onchocercal dermatitis.** Pruritis, with or without urticaria, caused by *Onchocerca volvulus.* **Onion-mite dermatitis.** Insect dermatitis (see above). **Dermatitis palmaris et plantaris.** Pompholyx or sweat desquamation of the hands and feet, secondary to tinea pedis. **Dermatitis papillaris capillitii.** Folliculitis keloidalis, a chronic irritating eruption commencing as a folliculitis and passing through a stage of papulation to the formation of keloidal plaques. The nape of the neck is the site of election. **Dermatitis papulosa nigra.** A papular eruption peculiar to members of the negro races. **Dermatitis papulosa somaliensis.** A papular or nodular eruption affecting particularly the anterior surfaces of the legs. **Paraphenylenediamine dermatitis.** Dermatitis caused by sensitization to paraphenylenediamine or to one of its oxidation products. This dermatitis, which can be very acute, occasionally occurs among those who have their hair dyed with a certain range of dyes which contain this chemical, and can develop after wearing furs which have been similarly treated. **Parasitic dermatitis.** Dermatitis caused by infestation with parasites. **Penicillin dermatitis.** Dermatitis medicamentosa (see above) due to penicillin. **Perfume dermatitis.** Dermatitis due to contact with essential oils in perfume. **Perianal dermatitis.** Inflammation of the skin around the anus caused by oxyuriases, fungal infections, contact irritants or sensitizers, haemorrhoids, proctitis or local skin disease. **Perioral dermatitis.** A papular eruption around the mouth, mostly of women, sometimes of undetermined cause and sometimes as a manifestation of rosacea. **Peripheral-nerve dermatitis.** Eczematoid dermatitis, sometimes associated with trophic ulceration, following trauma or section of the peripheral nerves. **Photocontact dermatitis.** Dermatitis of areas of skin exposed to sunlight and due to photo-allergic or phototoxic actions of substances which have come into contact with the skin. **Phytophoto dermatitis.** Cutaneous inflammation due to photosensitization after exposure to certain plants or to vegetable extracts. **Pigmented purpuric lichenoid dermatitis.** A chronic, usually symmetrical, eruption occurring most commonly on the legs, but sometimes affecting the upper limbs or trunk, and characterized by small, slightly raised papules which, pink at first, become purpuric, telangiectatic or pigmented. **Dermatitis pigmentée en forme de coulée.** Berlock dermatitis (see above). **Plant dermatitis.** Dermatitis due to contact with many species of flowers or other plants. **Plurifactor dermatitis.** Dermatitis the cause of which is not only some precipitating factor, but a predisposing factor that may be, for example, previous sensitization or a hereditary tendency. **Poison-ivy dermatitis.** Dermatitis resulting from contact with *Rhus toxicodendron.* **Dermatitis polymorphes douloureuses.** Dermatitis herpetiformis (see above). **Dermatitis pratensis.** A tropical malady of uncertain cause. The primary lesion is a papule which spreads and ulcerates. **Pre-cancerous dermatitis.** Bowen's disease. **Primary irritant dermatitis.** Dermatitis caused by primary irritants, that is substances which can cause cell damage even on only one contact in most individuals provided the contact is long enough and of sufficient concentration or temperature. A primary toxic reaction results in the skin. **Primrose dermatitis, Primula dermatitis.** Dermatitis due to contact with primrose or primula in sensitive persons. **Dermatitis psoriasiformis nodularis.** A guttate variety of parapsoriasis; *parapsoriasis en gouttes* (Brocq). **Pyococcal dermatitis.** Pyogenic dermatitis (see below). **Pyocyaneus dermatitis.** Ulceration or gangrene due to *Pseudomonas pyocyanea:* some forms of ecthyma gangraenosum may be included in this category. **Pyogenic dermatitis.** Dermatitis caused by pyogenic organisms. **Rat-mite dermatitis.** Weals, papules or vesicles caused by the blood-sucking rat-mite *Liponyssus bacoti.* **Recurrent herpetiform dermatitis repens.** Familial benign chronic pemphigus. **Dermatitis repens.** A chronic inflammatory eruption which usually develops on a finger and spreads relentlessly, the affection being characterized by an area of red, denuded, slightly oozing epithelium, bordered by an irregular collar of epidermis raised by clear or turbid fluid. It is probably the same as acrodermatitis perstans. **Rhus dermatitis.** Poison-ivy dermatitis (see above). **Ring dermatitis.** Dermatitis caused by substances accumulated beneath a ring or by the ring itself. **Roentgen-ray dermatitis.** X-ray dermatitis (see below). **Rubber dermatitis.** An industrial dermatitis due to contact with rubber during manufacture or to contact with rubber in a garment or utensil. **Satinwood dermatitis.** Occupational dermatitis among wood workers. **Dermatitis scarlatiniformis recidivans.** Scarlatiniform erythema. **Schistosomal dermatitis.** A dermatitis that may be caused by the species that normally infect man but also by several species of animal and bird schistosome, e.g. *Trichobilharzia szidati* of ducks. Carp breeders in Germany are affected by this species. **Schistosome dermatitis.** Swimmers' itch, cercarial dermatitis; a pruriginous dermatitis caused by penetration of the skin by cercariae. **Seasonal bullous dermatitis.** An eruption caused by Meloidae (blister beetles), attributed to cantharidin. **Seaweed dermatitis.** Dogger Bank itch, a dermatitis caused by sensitization to *Alcyonidium gelatinosum,* a marine animal resembling seaweed. **Dermatitis seborrhoeica, Seborrhoeic dermatitis.** An inflammatory disease of the skin beginning usually upon the scalp and characterized by scaliness, redness and fatty hypersecretion, with a tendency to downward extension (Schamberg). An adequate and comprehensive definition of the eruptions classified under this name is wanting. The malady may be acute, subacute or chronic, varying widely in intensity and appearance, and tending chiefly to affect certain sites of election but also spreading from these. The eruption ranges from localized, scarcely erythematous, furfuraceous patches, to severe erythematous oozing widespread lesions, and from intertrigos of varying severity to petaloid chronic localized yellowish-pink lesions with greasy scales; seborrhoeic folliculitis is also recognized. The affected individuals manifest a diathesis which has been named the *seborrhoeic state.* **Sensitization dermatitis.** Dermatitis, usually of an eczematous type, caused by an allergic reaction in the skin. **Shoe dermatitis.** Dermatitis caused by some constituent of footwear. **Silk-winders' dermatitis.** An occupational dermatitis occurring amongst workers in silk factories. **Dermatitis simplex.** Erythema. **Dermatitis skiagraphica.** X-ray dermatitis (see below). **Dermatitis solaris.** Sunburn. **Stasis dermatitis.** Dermatitis due to obstruction of the blood in any part; hypostatic dermatitis. **Straw-mat dermatitis.** Grain itch; a dermatitis caused by a mite that lives in straw. **Sulphonamide dermatitis.** Dermatitis, often widespread, not infrequently associated with hypersensitivity to light, following the application of sulphonamides to the skin or mucosae, or after the ingestion of one of this group of drugs. **Sulphur dermatitis.** Cutaneous inflammation following the application of sulphur to the skin. **Swimmers' dermatitis.** Schistosome dermatitis (see above). **Tar-workers' dermatitis.** An occupational dermatitis due to sensitization through repeated contact with tar. **Tetryl dermatitis.** An occupational dermatitis. **Dermatitis traumatica, Traumatic dermatitis.** Cutaneous inflammation caused by injury. The term is not used in regard to anaphylactic, allergic or toxic eruptions. **Trichloroethylene dermatitis.** Dermatitis, usually of an allergic type, following exposure to trichloroethylene. The liquid is much used as a degreasing agent. Possibly the vapour rising from tanks containing this substance can also produce dermatitis. **Tyrothricin dermatitis.** Allergic dermatitis attributed to exposure to tyrothricin. **Uncinarial dermatitis.** Ground itch, mazamorra; an eruption usually affecting the feet, caused by the larvae of *Ancylostoma duodenale* or of *Nectar americanus.* **Universal dermatitis** (of children at the breast). Erythroderma desquamativa; exfoliative dermatitis of infants (dermatitis exfoliativa infantum; see above), associated with intestinal disturbances and not infrequently proceeding to a fatal conclusion. **Dermatitis urticariodes parasitica.** Grain itch, straw itch and similar eruptions caused by *Pediculoides ventricosus.* **Vacciniformis infantum dermatitis.** More correctly, *dermatitis vacciniformis infantum;* an ulcerating streptococcal infection of the skin of infants and young children. The buttocks and the genitals are the sites of election; the lesions commence as tiny erythematous macules which are soon covered by small umbilicating vesicles filled with serum that rapidly becomes purulent. They often resemble closely the lesions of varicella. **Vanilla dermatitis.** Dermatitis from contact with vanilla beans. **Varicose dermatitis.** Stasis dermatitis (see above). **Dermatitis vegetans.** *Pyodermite végétante* (Hallopeau); a rare eruption characterized in the early stages by pustule formation and crusting, and later by the formation of vegetations. The groins, genitalia, axillae and scalp are the commonest sites, but the lips and mucosae of the mouth may be involved, in which case the pustules may be followed by ulcers. The name has been also applied to some cutaneous lesions of blastomycosis. **Dermatitis veldtis.** Veldt sore. **Dermatitis venenata.** Contact dermatitis, the onset of which is usually acute. The affected area may be oedematous as well as erythematous, and bullae together with vesicles may be numerous. **Dermatitis vernalis aurium.** Juvenile spring eruption; a papular or vesicular eruption on the helices of the ears, occurring in spring, in boys more than girls. **Dermatitis verrucosa, Dermatitis verrucosa blastomycotica, Dermatitis verrucosa chromomycotica.** Chromoblastomycosis. **Vesicular dermatitis in industrial workers.** Dermatitis due to the rat mite *Bdellonyssus bacoti.* **Weeping dermatitis.** A dermatitis in which there is a profuse serous exudate. **X-ray dermatitis.** Cutaneous inflammation due to x-rays. [Gk *derma* skin, *-itis* inflammation.]

See also: JACQUET, SCHAMBERG.

dermato-arthritis (der·mat·o·ar·**thri**′·tis). **Lipoid dermato-arthritis.** Reticulohistiocytic xanthomatous giant-cell granulomata on the skin, mucous membranes and synovial membranes. The prognosis is good but deforming arthritis may occur. [Gk *derma* skin, arthritis.]

dermato-autoplasty (der·mat·o·**aw**′·to·plas·te). The grafting of skin taken from another part of the patient's body and applied to the part under treatment. [Gk *derma* skin, *autos* self, *plassein* to mould.]

Dermatobia (der·mat·o·be·ah). A genus of botflies of the family Oestridae. *Dermatobia hominis* (*cyaniventris*) is an important parasite in the skin of man and animals in tropical America. The eggs are laid on mosquitoes, usually *Psorophora* species, and other blood-sucking arthropods. The larvae hatch while the carrier feeds, and bore into intact skin, living to maturity in boil-like swellings with a central aperture. Pupation takes place in the soil. [Gk *derma* skin, *bios* life.]

dermatobiasis (der·mat·o·**bi**′·as·is). Infection from *Dermatobia* present in the body.

dermatocele (der·mat·o·seel). Dermatolysis. **Dermatocele lipomatosa.** Pedunculated lipoma with cystic degeneration. [Gk *derma* skin, *kele* hernia.]

dermatocelidosis (der·mat·o·sel·id·**o**′·sis). Dermatokelidosis.

dermatocellulitis (der·mat·o·sel·ew·**li**′·tis). A condition of inflammation of the skin and the subcutaneous connective tissue. [Gk *derma* skin, cellulitis.]

dermatochalasis (der·mat·o·kal·**a**′·sis). Abnormal looseness of skin. [Gk *derma* skin, *chalasis* a slackening.]

dermatoconiosis (der·mat·o·kon·e·**o**′·sis). Any disease of the skin caused by dust irritation, particularly in occupations such as stone-cutting. [Gk *derma* skin, *konis* dust, *-osis* condition.]

dermatoconjunctivitis (der·mat·o·kon·jungk·tiv·**i**′·tis). An inflamed condition of the skin around the eyes and of the conjunctiva. [Gk *derma* skin, conjunctivitis.]

dermatocyst (der·mat·o·sist). A cystic tumour of the skin. [Gk *derma* skin, cyst.]

dermatocystoma (der·mat·o·sis·**to**′·mah). A cystic new growth of the skin. [Gk *derma* skin, *kystis* bladder, *-oma* tumour.]

dermatodynia (der·mat·o·**din**′·e·ah). Dermatalgia. [Gk *derma* skin, *odyne* pain.]

dermatodyschroia (der·mat·o·dis·**kro**′·e·ah). A state of abnormal pigmentation of the skin. [Gk *derma* skin, *dys-*, *chroia* skin.]

dermatodysplasia verruciformis (der·mat·o·dis·**pla**′·ze·ah ver·oo·se·**for**′·mis). A condition in which warts occur all over the body. [Gk *derma* skin, dysplasia, L *verruca* wart, form.]

dermatofibroma (der·mat·o·fi·**bro**′·mah). A fibrous tumour of the skin. **Dermatofibroma lenticulare, Dermatofibroma verum histiocytoma.** Nodular subepidermal fibrosis. [Gk *derma* skin, fibroma.]

dermatofibrosarcoma (der·mat·o·fi·bro·sar·**ko**′·mah). A fibrosarcoma of the skin. **Dermatofibrosarcoma protuberans.** A locally malignant tumour consisting of one or more dermal nodules, usually on the trunk. [Gk *derma* skin, fibrosarcoma.]

dermatofibrosis lenticularis disseminata (der·mat·o·fi·**bro**′·sis **len**·tik·ew·**la**′·ris **dis**·em·in·**a**′·tah). Nodular subepidermal fibrosis. The lesions, which are almost asymptomatic, are firm, reddish nodules; their surface may be raised above or depressed below the level of the surrounding skin. The cause is uncertain. [Gk *derma* skin, fibrosis, L *lens* lentil, *disseminare* to sow.]

dermatogen (der·**mat**·o·jen). An antigen which acts particularly in diseases of the skin. [Gk *derma* skin, antigen.]

dermatogenic, dermatogenous (der·mat·o·**jen**′·ik, der·mat·**oj**·en·us). 1. Producing skin. 2. Producing or causing a skin disease. [Gk *derma* skin, *genein* to produce.]

dermatoglyphics (der·mat·o·**glif**′·ix). The line and ridge patterns of the skin and, in particular, those of the fingers and palms of the hands and the toes and soles of the feet. [Gk *derma* skin, *glyphe* a carving.]

dermatograph (der·**mat**·o·graf). An instrument with which the anatomical landmarks of the body can be marked on the skin. [Gk *derma* skin, *graphein* to write.]

dermatographia (der·mat·o·**graf**′·e·ah). A state in which writing on the skin with a blunt instrument causes the skin development of a red weal; it is present in certain allergic conditions. Also called *factitious urticaria.* **Dermatographia alba.** The white line appearing on the skin in the adrenaline test. **Black dermatographia.** The dark-coloured mark appearing on the skin when it is stroked with a soft metal. [see prec.]

dermatographic (der·mat·o·**graf**′·ik). Marked by or referring to dermatographia (factitious urticaria).

dermatographism (der·mat·o·**graf**′·izm). Dermatographia (factitious urticaria).

dermatography (der·mat·**og**·raf·e). 1. An anatomical description of the skin. 2. Dermatographia. [Gk *derma* skin, *graphein* to write.]

dermatoheteroplasty (der·mat·o·**het**′·er·o·plas·te). The operation of grafting on skin taken from another individual. [Gk *derma* skin, *heteros* another, *plassein* to mould.]

dermatoid (der·mat·oid). Dermoid; skin-like. [Gk *derma* skin, *eidos* form.]

dermatokelidosis (der·mat·o·kel·id·**o**′·sis). A freckled or spotted state of the skin. [Gk *derma* skin, *kelis* stain, *-osis* condition.]

dermatokeras (der·mat·o·**ker**′·as). Cornu cutaneum. [Gk *derma* skin, *keras* horn.]

dermatokoniosis (der·mat·o·kon·e·**o**′·sis). Dermatoconiosis.

dermatologist (der·mat·**ol**·o·jist). A specialist in diseases of the skin. [Gk *derma* skin, *logos* science.]

dermatology (der·mat·**ol**·o·je). That branch of medicine which is concerned with the skin and diseases affecting the skin. [see prec.]

dermatolysis (der·mat·**ol**·is·is). A condition in which there are soft fibromata of the skin and mucous membranes, these forming large, misshapen and pendulous masses, which may be pedunculated. **Dermatolysis palpebrarum.** Blepharochalasis. [Gk *derma* skin, *lysis* a loosing.]

dermatoma (der·mat·o·mah). 1. A skin tumour. 2. A local

circumscribed patch of hypertrophy or thickness of the skin. [Gk *derma* skin, *-oma* tumour.]

dermatomalacia (der·mat·o·mal·a′·she·ah). Abnormal softening of the skin due to pathological conditions. [Gk *derma* skin, *malakia* softness.]

dermatome (der·mat·ome). 1. An instrument for cutting split-skin transplants. 2. The lateral part of an embryonic somite. 3. An area of skin sending afferent nerve fibres to a single posterior spinal nerve root. 4. The area of skin supplied by a spinal nerve. **Electric dermatome.** A graduated instrument working on a similar principle to that of a barber's hair clippers by which, through the rapid alternating action of a moving blade, split-skin grafts of varying thickness can be cut. **Onion-peel dermatomes.** The segments of pain and temperature sensation in the face, which are arranged in concentric laminae centering upon the mouth, the more peripheral segments being represented more caudally in the trigeminal nucleus. [Gk *derma* skin, *temnein* to cut.]

dermatomelasma (der·mat·o·mel·az′·mah). Addison's disease. [Gk *derma* skin, *melas* black.]

dermatomere (der·mat·o·meer). Mesodermic somite. [Gk *derma* skin, *meros* part.]

dermatomic (der·mat·om·ik). Referring or belonging to one of the skin segments of the embryo. [Gk *derma* skin, *temnein* to cut.]

dermatomucosomyositis (der·mat·o·mew·ko·so·mi·o·si′·tis). An inflamed condition of the skin, of the mucosa of the nose, mouth and throat, and of the muscles. [Gk *derma* skin, mucus, myositis.]

dermatomycid (der·mat·o·mi′·sid). Dermatophytid. [Gk *derma* skin, *mykes* fungus.]

dermatomycin (der·mat·o·mi′·sin). Trichophytin, one of a number of antigenic preparations derived from dermatophytes and used for the diagnosis of fungal infections of the skin. [Gk *derma* skin, *mykes* fungus.]

dermatomycosis (der·mat·o·mi·ko′·sis). A term often employed as a synonym for dermatophytosis, but more correctly used as a generic term for all cutaneous infections, whether superficial or deep, due to fungi. **Dermatomycosis favosa.** An infection of the glabrous skin due to favus. **Dermatomycosis furfuracea.** Pityriasis versicolor. [Gk *derma* skin, *mykes* fungus, *-osis* condition.]

dermatomyiasis (der·mat·o·mi·i′·as·is). Any skin disease caused by flies or maggots. [Gk *derma* skin, *myia* fly.]

dermatomyoma (der·mat·o·mi·o′·mah). A myomatous tumour of, or in, the skin; usually multiple. [Gk *derma* skin, myoma.]

dermatomyositis (der·mat·o·mi·o·si′·tis). One of the group of collagen disorders characterized by polymyositis in association with an erythematous or violaceous rash affecting any part of the body. There may be oedema of the skin and subcutaneous calcification. There is an association with malignant disease. [Gk *derma* skin, myositis.]

dermatoneurology (der·mat·o·newr·ol′·o·je). A subdivision of medicine in which dermatologists and neurologists have a combined interest. [Gk *derma* skin, neurology.]

dermatoneurosis (der·mat·o·newr·o′·sis). Neurodermatosis.

dermatonosus (der·mat·o·no′·sus). Dermatopathy. **Neuropathic dermatonosus.** Neurodermatosis. [Gk *derma* skin, *nosos* disease.]

dermato-ophthalmitis (der·mat·o·of·thal·mi′·tis). An inflamed condition of the skin and of all the structures of the eye. [Gk *derma* skin, ophthalmitis.]

dermatopathia (der·mat·o·path′·e·ah). Dermatopathy.

dermatopathic (derm·at·o·path′·ik). Referring to disease of the skin. [Gk *derma* skin, *pathos* suffering.]

dermatopathology (der·mat·o·path·ol′·o·je). The pathology of the skin. [Gk *derma* skin, pathology.]

dermatopathophobia (der·mat·o·path·o·fo′·be·ah). Morbid dread of contracting skin diseases and excessive preoccupation with anything to do with the skin and its condition. [Gk *derma* skin, pathophobia.]

dermatopathy (der·mat·op′·ath·e). Any disease or disorder of the skin. [Gk *derma* skin, *pathos* suffering.]

Dermatophagoides (der·mat·o·fag·oi′·deez). A genus of sarcoptiform mites. *Dermatophagoides culinae* or *pteronyssinus* has recently been shown to be associated with house-dust allergy. The mite is present in bedding and antigenic extracts from it have been shown to give immediate hypersensitivity reactions in susceptible persons. *D. saitoi* has been recorded from Japan in sputum, *D. scheremetewskyi* recorded rarely in foot and scalp dermatitis, perhaps secondary, and *D. takeuichii* recorded from Japan in urine. [Gk *derma* skin, *phagein* to eat, *eidos* form.]

dermatophiliasis (der·mat·o·fil·i′·as·is). Infestation with *Tunga (Dermatophilus) penetrans.*

Dermatophilus (der·mat·of·il·us). A genus of Actinomycetaceae of importance in veterinary medicine. **Dermatophilus congolensis.** The cause of streptotrichosis and mycotic dermatitis in animals; occasional infections occur in man. [Gk *derma* skin, *philein* to love.]

dermatophobe (der·mat·o·fobe). An individual suffering from dermatophobia. [Gk *derma* skin, phobia.]

dermatophobia (der·mat·o·fo′·be·ah). Morbid and excessive dread of contracting skin disease or of injuring the skin. [see prec.]

dermatophone (der·mat·o·fone). A particular kind of stethoscope through which the sounds of the blood coursing through the skin can be heard. [Gk *derma* skin, *phone* sound.]

dermatophylaxis (der·mat·o·fil·ax′·is). Any method of protecting the skin against infection. [Gk *derma* skin, *phylax* guard.]

dermatophyte (der·mat·o·fite). A member of a closely-related group of fungi which cause specific infections of man and animals by invading only the superficial keratinized areas of the body (skin, hair and nails). Three genera are recognized—*Microsporum, Trichophyton* and *Epidermophyton.* Commonly occurring species are *Microsporum audouinii, M. canis, M. gypseum, Trichophyton mentagrophytes, T. rubrum, T. sulphureum, T. schoenleinii, T. verrucosum* and *Epidermophyton floccosum.* [Gk *derma* skin, *phyton* plant.]

dermatophytid (der·mat·of·it·id). A secondary reaction due to hypersensitivity in a patient affected with dermatophytosis. [Gk *derma* skin, *phyton* plant.]

dermatophytosis (der·mat·o·fi·to′·sis). A superficial fungus infection of keratinized tissues (i.e. hair, skin, nails) by the dermatophyte fungi. Agents of tinea nigra, tinea versicolor and cutaneous candidiasis are excluded. **Dermatophytosis interdigitale.** Athlete's foot. [Gk *derma* skin, *phyton* plant, *-osis* condition.]

dermatoplasia (der·mat·o·pla′·ze·ah). The power possessed by the skin to make good injury inflicted on it. [Gk *derma* skin, *plassein* to form.]

dermatoplastic (der·mat·o·plas′·tik). Referring to skin grafting or to plastic surgery of the skin. [Gk *derma* skin, *plassein* to form.]

dermatoplasty (der·mat·o·plas·te). Any reparative operation on the skin; the plastic replacement of skin by the use of grafts or flaps. [see prec.]

dermatopolyneuritis (der·mat·o·pol·e·newr·i′·tis). Acrodynia; an acute epidemic disease of infants and young children, in which there is an itching rash variable in character, photophobia, anorexia, swelling of the hands and feet, disturbance of sensation, and change in disposition and in the spinal cord and nerve roots. [Gk *derma* skin, polyneuritis.]

dermatorrhagia (der·mat·o·ra′·je·ah). 1. Haemorrhage from the skin. 2. Haemathidrosis. [Gk *derma* skin, *rhegnynai* to burst forth.]

dermatorrhexis (der·mat·o·rex′·is). The condition known as elastic skin or cutis hyperelastica; Ehlers–Danlos syndrome. [Gk *derma* skin, *rhexis* a breaking.]

dermatorrhoea (der·mat·o·re′·ah). Hyperhidrosis. [Gk *derma* skin, *rhoia* flow.]

dermatosclerosis (der·mat·o·skler·o′·sis). Sclerodermia; a cutaneous disease characterized by the formation of rigid, indurated and thickened pigmented patches. Degenerative changes occur in the fibrous-tissue bundles in the dermis and subcutaneous tissue, fibrous tissues replacing the fat in the latter. [Gk *derma* skin, sclerosis.]

dermatoscopy (der·mat·**os**·ko·pe). Examination of the skin, particularly of the superficial capillaries, with a microscope and lens of high power. [Gk *derma* skin, *skopein* to watch.]

dermatosiophobe (der·mat·**o**·se·o·fobe). Dermatophobe.

dermatosiophobia (der·mat·**o**·se·o·**fo**'·be·ah). Dermatophobia.

dermatosis (der·mat·**o**·sis) (pl. *dermatoses*). Commonly, but incorrectly, used as a synonym for dermatitis. More accurately, a pathological state of the skin in which inflammation is not necessarily of most importance. **Acarine dermatosis.** That due to a mite. **Acute febrile neutrophilic dermatosis.** A febrile illness with an eruption of raised painful plaques in which there is an infiltrate of polymorphonuclear neutrophils. It may be a severe atypical form of erythema multiforme. **Angioneurotic dermatosis.** A vasomotor disturbance. **Chronic haemosideric dermatosis.** A condition in which haemosiderin occurs in the skin; included under this heading are Schamberg's disease, pigmented purpuric lichenoid dermatitis and stasis dermatitis. **Exudative discoid and lichenoid chronic dermatosis.** An eruption of unknown cause particularly affecting Jewish men of middle age. **Gonorrhoeal dermatosis.** Cutaneous manifestation of gonorrhoeal infection, including erythema, urticarial and erythema-nodosum-like lesions, haemorrhagic and bullous eruptions, and keratosis blenorrhagica. **Hysteric dermatosis.** 1. A self-inflicted eruption. 2. An eruption in a hysterical subject caused by subconscious psychological mechanisms. **Industrial dermatosis.** Occupational dermatitis. **Lichenoid dermatosis.** A condition suggestive of lichen planus. **Menopausal dermatosis.** Any skin condition alleged to be caused by endocrine changes of the climacteric. Most such conditions are more accurately linked with ageing. **Menstrual dermatosis.** Dermatosis associated with the menstrual period. **Metabolic dermatosis.** Any of a wide group of disorders caused by metabolic disturbances, but otherwise unrelated: thus diabetic xanthoma and phrynoderma are both examples. **Dermatosis nigro-annulata.** An eruption characterized by black annular chronic lesions, and of uncertain aetiology. **Dermatosis papulosa nigra.** A papular eruption of the face in negroes; probably an epithelial naevus. **Dermatosis pigmentaria.** Berlock dermatitis. **Dermatoses pigmentée peribuccale** (Brocq). Symmetrical peribuccal brown or brownish-red pigmentation occurring in young girls or women. **Precancerous dermatosis.** Any pathological change of the skin to which carcinomatous degeneration is the sequel, e.g. keratoma senilis. The lesions, which may be multiple, are brown, crusted, superficial plaques of various sizes. Bowen's precancerous dermatosis (Bowen's disease) is now considered a squamous-cell epithelioma from the outset. **Progressive pigmented purpuric dermatosis.** Schamberg's disease. **Stasis dermatosis.** That due to blood and lymph stasis. **Streptococcal dermatosis.** Any eruption due to streptococcal infection of the skin. **Subcorneal pustular dermatosis.** A chronic, benign, relapsing, pustular eruption with subcorneal bullae containing polymorphonuclear leucocytes. [Gk *derma* skin, *-osis* condition.]

See also: BOWEN, KAPOSI, SCHAMBERG.

dermatospasm (der·mat·o·spazm). Cutis anserina (goose flesh). [Gk *derma* skin, spasm.]

dermatostomatitis pluriorificialis (der·mat·o·sto·mat·**i**'·tis ploor·e·**or**·if·ish·e·**a**'·lis). Ectodermatosis erosiva pluriorificialis: eruptive fever with stomatitis and ophthalmia; probably a variety of erythema multiforme. [Gk *derma* skin, stomatitis, L *plus* more, *orificium* mouth.]

dermatosyphilis (der·mat·o·**sif**'·il·is). The signs of syphilis which are observable on the skin. [Gk *derma* skin, syphilis.]

dermatotherapy (der·mat·o·**ther**'·ap·e). The treatment of affections and diseases of the skin. [Gk *derma* skin, therapy.]

dermatothlasia (der·mat·o·**thla**'·ze·ah). A morbid and uncontrollable or spasmodic impulsion to bruise, pinch or rub selected areas of the skin (Fournier). [Gk *derma* skin, *thlasis* a bruising.]

dermatotome (der·mat·o·tome). 1. A skin segment of the fetus. 2. Surgical knife or other instrument used for cutting skin grafts. [Gk *derma* skin, *temnein* to cut.]

dermatotomy (der·mat·**ot**·o·me). 1. Dissection of the skin. 2. Anatomy of the skin. [see prec.]

dermatotropic (der·mat·o·**trop**'·ik). 1. Acting especially on the skin. 2. Having particular affinity for the skin and mucosa. [Gk *derma* skin, *trepein* to turn.]

dermatoxerasia (der·mat·o·zer·**a**'·se·ah). Xerodermia.

dermatozoiasis (der·mat·o·zo·**i**'·as·is). Dermatozoonosus.

dermatozoon (der·mat·o·**zo**'·on). Any animal parasite of the skin. [Gk *derma* skin, *zoon* animal.]

dermatozoonosus (der·mat·o·zo·on·**o**'·sus). Any disease of the skin caused by the presence of animal parasites, e.g. *Sarcoptes scabiei.* [Gk *derma* skin, *zoon* animal, *nosos* disease.]

dermatrophia, dermatrophy (der·mat·**ro**·fe·ah, der·**mat**·ro·fe). Thinning or atrophy of the skin. [Gk *derma* skin, *atrophia* unnourished.]

dermectasia (der·mek·**ta**·ze·ah). Dermatolysis. [Gk *derma* skin, *ektasis* a stretching.]

dermepenthesis (der·mep·**en**·the·sis). Dermatoplasty. [Gk *derma* skin, *epenthesis* insertion.]

dermhelminthiasis (derm·hel·min·**thi**'·as·is). An affection of the skin caused by the presence of a parasitic worm. [Gk *derma* skin, helminthiasis.]

dermic (der·mik). Belonging or relating to the skin or the dermis in particular. [Gk *derma* skin.]

dermis (der·mis). 1. The skin. 2. The corium [NA (Dermis)]. [Gk.]

dermite livedoide (der·meet le·va·do·eed). The blockage of an artery by bismuth that has been administered for therapeutic purposes. Severe cases are described as being of the Nicolau type, whilst benign cases are referred to as of the Freudenthal type. [Fr. livid dermatitis.]

dermites infantiles simples (der·meet ahn·fan·**teel sahm**·pl). Erythematous, erythematovesicular or papular-erosive lesions occurring as manifestations of the dermatitis of Jacquet. [Fr. simple infantile dermatitis.]

dermitis (der·**mi**·tis). Dermatitis.

dermo-actinomycosis (der·mo·ak·tin·o·mi·**ko**'·sis). Actinomycosis of the skin; granulomatous infection of the skin due to the presence of *Actinomyces;* the neck and scalp are the parts most affected. The disease occurs in association with actinomycosis in deeper structures. [Gk *derma* skin, actinomycosis.]

dermo-anergy (der·mo·**an**·er·je). A condition in which the skin does not react to the injection of an antigen. [Gk *derma* skin, anergy.]

dermoblast (der·mo·blast). In embryology, the somatic layer of the mesoderm (mesodermic somites) which develops into the corium. [Gk *derma* skin, *blastos* germ.]

dermocyma, dermocymus (der·mo·**si**·mah, der·mo·**si**·mus). Fetus in fetu, a monster fetus containing another small fetus within it. [Gk *derma* skin, *kyma* fetus.]

dermo-epidermal (der·mo·ep·e·**der**'·mal). Applied to skin grafts which take in the superficial and deep layers of the skin. [Gk *derma* skin, epidermis.]

dermoglyphics (der·mo·**glif**·ix). Dermatoglyphics.

dermograph (der·mo·graf). Dermatograph.

dermographia (der·mo·**graf**·e·ah). Dermatographia.

dermographic (der·mo·**graf**·ik). Dermatographic.

dermographism, dermography (der·mo·**graf**·izm, der·**mog**·raf·e). Dermatographia.

dermohaemia (der·mo·**he**·me·ah). Dermathaemia.

dermoid (der·moid). 1. A teratomatous cyst in which skin elements are prominent, the contained fluid being opaque from shed epithelium and sebaceous material, and hairs usually being present. 2. A cyst or sinus lined by skin. 3. Like skin. **Dermoid of the spine.** A tumour of the spinal cord derived from dermoid tissue and usually situated in the lumbar area. **Epibulbar dermoid.** A dermoid on the eyeball, as in oculo-auriculovertebral dysplasia. **Implantation dermoid.** A cyst in which the skin lining is derived from skin accidentally implanted deeply by puncture of the overlying skin. It is rare but commonest on the hands. **Inclusion dermoid, Sequestration dermoid.** A cyst formed by sequestration of skin during the course of development. It occurs at the site of developmental infoldings, e.g. in the middle line of the back, at the external angle of the orbit. **Tubular dermoid.** A cyst formed by the persistence of developmental tube-like structures, e.g. the thyroglossal duct. Not strictly a dermoid. [Gk *derma* skin, *eidos* form.]

dermoidectomy (der·moid·**ek**·to·me). The surgical removal of a dermoid cyst. [dermoid, Gk *ektome* a cutting out.]

dermolabial (der·mo·**la**·be·al). Relating to the skin and the lips. [Gk *derma* skin, L *labium* lip.]

dermolipoma (der·mo·lip·**o**′·mah). Lipoma of the skin. [Gk *derma* skin, lipoma.]

dermolysis (der·**mol**·is·is). Dermatolysis.

dermometer (der·**mom**·et·er). An instrument used in dermometry.

dermometry (der·**mom**·et·re). The measurement of the resistance of the skin to the passage of a direct electrical current; the resistance increases with increased vascularity, and vice versa. If a sensory loss is present and accompanied by loss of vascular control, then areas of abnormal skin resistance correspond to areas of sensory loss. [Gk *derma* skin, meter.]

dermomuscular (der·mo·**mus**·kew·lar). In embryology, those tissues which have relation to the muscles and the skin. [Gk *derma* skin, muscle.]

dermomycosis (der·mo·mi·**ko**′·sis). Dermatophytosis. [Gk *derma* skin, mycosis.]

dermonecrotic (der·mo·nek·**rot**′·ik). Causing necrosis of the skin, or of certain elements of the skin. [Gk *derma* skin, necrosis.]

dermoneurosis (der·mo·newr·**o**′·sis). Neurodermatitis. [Gk *derma* skin, neurosis.]

dermonosology (der·mo·no·**sol**′·o·je). The science of the classification of diseases of the skin. [Gk *derma* skin, nosology.]

dermopathic (der·mo·**path**·ik). Dermatopathic.

dermopathy (der·**mop**·ath·e). Dermatopathy.

dermophlebitis (der·mo·fleb·**i**′·tis). An inflamed condition of the superficial veins and the surrounding skin. [Gk *derma* skin, phlebitis.]

dermophobe (**der**·mo·fobe). Dermatophobe.

dermophylaxis (der·mo·fil·**ax**′·is). Dermatophylaxis.

dermophyma venereum (der·mo·**fi**·mah ven·**eer**·e·um). A soft lump or tumour of syphilitic origin, found usually in the rectum or superficially on the genitals. [Gk *derma* skin, *phyma* growth, L *venereus* of Venus.]

dermophyte (**der**·mo·fite). Dermatophyte.

dermoplasty (**der**·mo·plas·te). Dermatoplasty.

dermoreaction (der·mo·re·**ak**′·shun). Cutaneous reaction. *See* REACTION. [Gk *derma* skin, reaction.]

dermorrhagia (der·mo·**ra**·je·ah). Dermatorrhagia: 1. Haemorrhage from the skin. 2. Haemathidrosis. [Gk *derma* skin, *rhegnynai* to burst forth.]

dermoskeleton (der·mo·**skel**·e·ton). Exoskeleton; in man, the rudimentary skeletal coverings of the body consisting of the nails and the teeth. [Gk *derma* skin, skeleton.]

dermostenosis (der·mo·sten·**o**′·sis). 1. Shrinkage of the skin due to disease. 2. A tightening of the skin caused by the presence of a swelling underneath it, or as in sclerodermia. [Gk *derma* skin, stenosis.]

dermostosis (der·**mos**·to·sis). Ossification of the corium. [Gk *derma* skin, ostosis.]

dermosynovitis (der·mo·si·no·**vi**′·tis). An inflamed condition of the skin over an inflamed subcutaneous bursa or tendon sheath. **Dermosynovitis plantaris ulcerosa.** Severe perforating ulcer of the sole of the foot as the result of inflammation of the bursa underlying a callus. [Gk *derma* skin, synovitis.]

dermosyphilography (der·mo·sif·il·**og**′·raf·e). That department of medicine which is concerned with the skin as affected by syphilis. [Gk *derma* skin, syphilography.]

dermosyphilopathy (der·mo·sif·il·**op**′·ath·e). Any skin disease of which syphilis is the cause. [Gk *derma* skin, syphilopathy.]

dermotactile (der·mo·**tak**·tile). The sensibility to touch of the skin. [Gk *derma* skin, tactile.]

dermotherapy (der·mo·**ther**·ap·e). Dermatotherapy.

dermotomy (der·**mot**·o·me). Dermatotomy.

dermotropic (der·mo·**trop**·ik). Dermatotropic.

dermovaccine (der·mo·**vak**·seen). A strain of vaccine virus maintained by passage through the skin and obtained by scraping the skin lesions. [Gk *derma* skin, vaccine.]

dermovascular (der·mo·**vas**·kew·lar). Relating to the blood vessels of the skin. [Gk *derma* skin, vascular.]

dermovirus (der·mo·**vi**·rus). Dermovaccine. [Gk *derma* skin, virus.]

derodidymus, derodymus (de·ro·**did**·im·us, de·**rod**·im·us). A monster with 2 necks and heads but only 1 body. [Gk *dere* neck, *didymos* twin.]

derrid (**der**·id). A resin from *Derris elliptica.* It is a toxic substance used as an arrow poison.

Derris BPC 1949 (**der**·is). The powdered dried rhizome of *Derris elliptica.* It contains resins and a crystalline substance, rotenone, all of which are toxic to insects. It is used as a horticultural and agricultural insecticide. [Gk fur.]

desacetylmethylcolchicine (dez·**as**·et·il·**meth**·il·**kol**′·chis·een). Demecolcine, an alkaloid obtained from the roots of *Colchicum autumnale* and used in the treatment of myelogenous leukaemia.

desalination (de·sal·in·**a**′·shun). The process of removing salts from a substance. [L *de, sal* salt.]

De Salle, Eusèbe François (b. 1796). Marseilles physician.

De Salle's line. A furrow running from the side of the nose round the angle of the mouth.

desamidization (dez·**am**·id·i·**za**′·shun). Deamination; the removal of amino or imino groups from amino acids and related compounds, with the production of ammonia and the corresponding alcohol or fatty acid.

desanimania (dez·an·e·**ma**′·ne·ah). Amentia. [L *de, animus* mind, mania.]

desaturation (de·sat·ewr·**a**′·shun). The formation of an unsaturated compound from one already saturated. [L *de,* saturation.]

Desault, Pierre Joseph (b. 1744). Paris surgeon.

Desault's bandage. A roller bandage for the support of a fractured clavicle.

Desault's ligature. Ligature of the femoral artery for popliteal aneurysm.

Desault's operation. For stricture of the nasolacrimal duct: by cauterizing threads passed through the duct; obsolete.

Descartes, René (b. 1596). French anatomist, mathematician, philosopher and scientist.

Descarte's law. *See* SNELL'S LAW.

Descemet, Jean (b. 1732). Paris surgeon and anatomist.

Descemet's membrane. One of the deep layers of the cornea of the eye, lying between the substantia propria externally and the endothelium internally.

descemetitis (des·e·met·**i**′·tis). A form of deep keratitis. [Jean *Descemet,* Gk *-itis* inflammation.]

descemetocele (des·e·**met**·o·seel). Hernia of Descemet's membrane. [Jean *Descemet,* Gk *kele* hernia.]

descendens cervicalis nerve. A nerve formed from a branch of the 2nd cervical nerve and one from the 3rd.

descendens hypoglossi nerve. The descending branch of the hypoglossal nerve.

descending (de·**sen**·ding). Directed or extending downward. [L *descendere* to descend.]

descensus (de·**sen**·sus). Descent. **Descensus uteri.** Prolapse of the uterus. **Descensus ventriculix.** Gastroptosis. [L.]

descent (de·**sent**). Motion downward. **Descent of the testis [descensus testis (NA)].** The passage of the testis from the intracoelomic site of its formation down the posterior abdominal wall, through the inguinal canal, and into the scrotum. **Theory of descent.** The theory that higher organisms evolve from lower earlier forms of the same organism, and therefore "descend" from them. The theory is in contradistinction from that of special creation. [L *descendere* to descend.]

Deschamps, Joseph François Louis (b. 1740). French surgeon.

Deschamps' needle. A special needle used in the ligature of deep-seated arteries.

desensitization (de·**sen**·sit·i·**za**'·shun). Hypersensitization. A procedure used in patients with immediate hypersensitivity to a specific antigen. The patient is given a graded series of doses of the antigen to stimulate IgG antibody production. On later contact, the IgG antibody should react with the antigen, thus preventing it from reacting with cell-bound IgE. **Desensitization block.** *See* BLOCK. [L *de, sentire* to feel.]

desensitize (de·**sen**·sit·ize). 1. In general, to remove or reduce sensitivity or to deprive of sensation. 2. To paralyse a sensory nerve by blocking its pathway or by cutting it across. 3. To reduce susceptibility to infection or to the action of a foreign protein. 4. Removal of the antibody from sensitized cells to prevent allergy or anaphylaxis. [see prec.]

Deserpidine (de·**ser**·pid·een). BP Commission approved name for 11-demethoxyreserpine, a tranquillizing drug used in the treatment of psychotic disorders.

desexualization (de·**sex**·ew·al·i·**za**'·shun). In psychoanalysis, the mental mechanism postulated by theory in which libido is directed to other than sexual aims, and in this process of sublimation is desexualized. [L *de*, sex.]

desexualize (de·**sex**·ew·al·ize). To castrate. [see prec.]

Desferrioxamine (**des**·fer·e·**ox**'·am·een). BP Commission approved name for 30-amino-3,14,25-trihydroxy-3,9,14,20,25-pentaazatriacontane-2-10,13,21,24-pentaone. **Desferrioxamine Mesylate BP 1973.** The methanesulphonate, a chelating agent.

deshydraemia (des·hi·**dre**·me·ah). A condition in which the watery element of the blood is reduced. [L *de*, Gk *hydor* water, *haima* blood.]

desiccant (**des**·ik·ant). Drying, or a drying agent. [L *desiccare* to dry up.]

desiccate (**des**·ik·ate). To deprive of moisture. [see prec.]

desiccation (des·ik·**a**·shun). 1. The process of rendering dry. Many species of microbes are preserved by rapid and complete removal of moisture, preferably while frozen in glass ampules which are sealed in a high vacuum after removal of air; the ampules can then be stored at room temperature in the dark. *See* LYOPHILIZATION. 2. The act of drying up. **Electric desiccation.** The destruction of new growths and the treatment of other diseases by the electric cautery or the diathermy current, which dry up the tissues. [L *desiccare* to dry up.]

desiccative (**des**·ik·a·tiv). Causing or promoting desiccation. Any agent which dries up secretions. [see prec.]

desiccator (**des**·ik·a·tor). A glass vessel containing a desiccant, and used to keep substances dry. **Vacuum desiccator.** One which can be pumped free of air and moisture after the substance to be kept dry has been placed inside. [L *desiccare* to dry up.]

17-desinolase (**dez**·in·o·**lase**). Enzyme concerned with conversion of 17α-hydroxy-progesterone to androstenedione.

Desipramine (des·**ip**·ram·een). BP Commission approved name for 10,11-dihydro-5-(3-methylaminopropyl)dibenz[*b,f*]-azepine; a central nervous system stimulant.

Desipramine Hydrochloride BP 1973 (dez·**ip**·ram·een hi·dro·**klor**·ide). The hydrochloride of 10,11-dihydro-5-(3-methylaminopropyl)dibenz[*b,f*]azepine. The actions and uses are similar to those of imipramine, but its effects develop in 3 or 4 days after starting treatment.

Desjardin, Abel. 19th-20th century Paris surgeon.

Desjardin's forceps. A forceps for removing stones from the common bile duct.

Desjardin's point. A point on the abdominal wall which lies over the head of the pancreas. It lies on an imaginary line from the umbilicus to the anterior axillary fold and is placed 5-7 cm from the former.

Desjardin's gall-stone probe. A flexible-spring metal probe with a bulbous leading end, used to detect stones in the bile ducts.

Deslanoside BP 1973 (des·**lan**·o·side). Deacetyl-lantoside C, a cardiac glycoside with actions and uses similar to those of lantoside C. It is given intravenously for rapid digitalization of patients with pulmonary oedema due to heart failure.

desloughing (de·**sluf**·ing). The removal of slough from a wound or infected lesion. [L *de*, ME *sluh* a husk.]

desmalgia (dez·**mal**·je·ah). Pain in a ligament. [Gk *desmos* band, *algos* pain.]

Desmarres, Louis Auguste (b. 1810). Paris ophthalmologist.

Desmarres' operation. For pterygium: the pterygium is dissected off from the corneal end right back to its root; the inferior conjunctival flap is then mobilized, and the head of the pterygium sutured as far down as possible underneath it.

Desmarres' retractor. A curved, shallow, metal retractor designed for placing in the conjunctival fornix, when retracting the lid or lids to examine the eye.

Guérin and Desmarres operation. For corectopia (obsolete term).

desmectasia, desmectasis (dez·mek·**ta**·ze·ah, dez·**mek**·tas·is). A stretched condition of a ligament. [Gk *desmos* band, *ektasis* a stretching.]

desmepithelium (dez·mep·e·**the**'·le·um). 1. The epithelial parts of the mesoderm. 2. The lining epithelium of the blood vascular system and the serous cavities of the body. [Gk *desmos* band, epithelium.]

desmiognathus (**dez**·me·o·**nath**'·us). A monster with a supplementary head attached to the lower jaw by muscular tissue or a ligamentary structure. [Gk *desmos* band, *gnathos* jaw.]

desmitis (dez·**mi**·tis). An inflamed condition of a ligament. [Gk *desmos* band, *-itis* inflammation.]

desmocranium (dez·mo·**kra**·ne·um). The membranous precursor of the bony and cartilaginous skull, formed of condensed mesenchyme and fine connective-tissue fibres. [Gk *desmos* band, *kranion* skull.]

desmocyte (**dez**·mo·site). A fibroblast, one of the varieties of cell composing areolar tissue. [Gk *desmos* band, *kytos* cell.]

desmocytoma (**dez**·mo·si·**to**'·mah). Sarcoma. [Gk *desmos* band, cytoma.]

Desmodillus (dez·mo·**dil**·us). A genus of small rodents. **Desmodillus auricularis.** A gerbille, a reservoir of plague.

Desmodus (dez·**mo**·dus). A genus of bats. **Desmodus rotundus.** A vampire bat, vector of rabies usually manifested as an acute ascending myelitis. **Desmodus rufus.** The common vampire bat of the neotropics. [Gk *desmos* band, *odous* tooth.]

desmodynia (dez·mo·**din**·e·ah). Desmalgia. [Gk *desmos* band, *odyne* pain.]

desmogenous (dez·**moj**·en·us). Formed of, originating in or pertaining to connective tissue or ligaments. [Gk *desmos* band, *genein* to produce.]

desmography (dez·**mog**·raf·e). The study and description of the ligaments. [Gk *desmos* band, *graphein* to write.]

desmoid (**dez**·moid). 1. Fibroma or a hard, fibrous tumour. 2. Resembling a ligament or a tendon in appearance. [Gk *desmos* band, *eidos* form.]

desmolase (**dez**·mol·aze). Lyase. A class of enzyme which disrupts the linkage between carbon atoms and brings about the cleavage of organic substances in such vital processes as respiration and glycolysis. [Gk *desmos* band.]

desmology (dez·**mol**·o·je). 1. That branch of anatomy which is concerned with the ligaments. 2. The art of applying bandages. [Gk *desmos* band, *logos* science.]

desmoma (dez·**mo**·mah). Fibroma. [Gk *desmos* band, *-oma* tumour.]

desmon, desmone (**dez**·mon, **dez**·mone). Amboceptor. [Gk *desmos* band.]

desmoneoplasm (dez·mo·**ne**·o·plazm). A tumour consisting of connective-tissue elements. [Gk *desmos* band, neoplasm.]

desmopathology (**dez**·mo·path·**ol**'·o·je). Pathology in its relation to ligaments. [Gk *desmos* band, pathology.]

desmopathy (dez·**mop**·ath·e). Any disease affecting the ligaments. [Gk *desmos* band, *pathos* suffering.]

desmopexia (dez·mo·**pex**·e·ah). Correction of uterine displacement by suturing the round ligaments to the wall of the vagina or of the abdomen. [Gk *desmos* band, *pexis* fixation.]

desmoplasia (dez·mo·**pla**·ze·ah). An abnormal tendency of part of the body to form fibrous adhesions or bands. [Gk *desmos* band, *plassein* to form.]

desmoplastic (dez·mo·**plas**·tik). Stimulating or initiating the development of cellular connective tissue or adhesions. [see prec.]

Desmopressin (des·mo·**pres**·in). BP Commission approved name for 1-deamino-8-D-arginine-vasopressin; it is used in the treatment of diabetes insipidus.

desmopyknosis (**dez**·mo·pik·**no'**·sis). The shortening of the round ligaments of the uterus by removing a patch of epithelium from the anterior wall of the vagina and suturing the ligaments to the wall at that place (Dudley). [Gk *desmos* band, *pyknosis* a packing close.]

desmorrhexis (dez·mo·**rex**·is). Rupture of a ligament or ligaments. [Gk *desmos* band, *rhexis* rupture.]

desmosis (dez·**mo**·sis). Any disease of connective tissue. [Gk *desmos* band, *-osis* condition.]

desmosome (**dez**·mo·some). Macula adherens, a component of the junctional complex between two cells. [Gk *desmos* band, *soma* body.]

desmotomy (dez·**mot**·o·me). Surgical division or dissection of a ligament. [Gk *desmos* band, *temnein* to cut.]

desmotropism (dez·**mot**·tro·pizm). A dynamic tautomerism in which one form of a substance may change into the other and back again, or exist with it in equilibrium, according to the conditions. [Gk *desmos* band, *tropos* a turning.]

desmotroposantonin (**dez**·mo·tro·po·**san'**·ton·in). $C_{15}H_{18}O_3$, a tautomeric isomer of santonin.

desmurgia, desmurgy (dez·**mer**·je·ah, dez·**mer**·je). The science of applying ligatures or bandages to a part. [Gk *desmos* band, *ergein* to do.]

desoleolecithin (des·o·le·o·**les'**·ith·in). Lysolecithin: a haemolytic substance produced by removal of the unsaturated fatty acid of lecithin when lecithinase A of cobra venom acts on lecithin in blood. It is antagonized by cholesterol, forming a non-haemolytic compound. [L *de, oleum,* oil, lecithin.]

desolution (de·sol·**ew**·shun). The reduction in solubility, and eventual throwing out of solution, of a solute. [L *de, solvere* to dissolve.]

Desomorphine (des·o·**mor**·feen). BP Commission approved name for dihydrodeoxymorphine, a modified morphine having similar properties to morphine itself.

Desonide (**dez**·on·ide). BP Commission approved name for 11β,21-dihydroxy-16α,17α-isopropylidenedioxypregna-1,4-diene-3,20-dione; an anti-inflammatory agent.

desoxy-. For words beginning **desoxy-**, *see also* DEOXY-.

desoxycholaneresis (dez·**ox**·e·ko·lan·er·**e'**·sis). Increase of desoxycholic acid in the bile. [L *de,* Gk *oxys* sharp, *chole* bile, *a, eresis* removal.]

desoxycorticosterone (dez·ox·e·**kor**·tik·o·**steer'**·one). Deoxycorticosterone, deoxycortone.

desoxycortone (dez·**ox**·e·**kor'**·tone). Deoxycortone.

Desoxycortoni (des·**ox**·e·kor·**to**·ni). **Desoxycortoni Acetas.** *European Pharmacopoeia* name for Deoxycortone Acetate BP 1973.

desoxyhexose (dez·ox·e·**hex**·oze). A hexose sugar containing one or more oxygen atoms fewer than the normal hexose, $C_6H_{12}O_6$. Thus digitoxose, $CHOCH_2(CHOH)_3CH_3$, is 2,6-desoxyallose, and rhamnose, $CHO(CHOH)_4CH_3$, is 6-desoxymannose.

Desoxymethasone (dez·**ox**·e·**meth'**·az·one). BP Commission approved name for 9α-fluoro-11β,21-dihydroxy-16α-methylpregna-1,4-diene-3,20-dione; a topical corticosteroid.

desoxymorphine (dez·ox·e·**mor**·feen). Dihydrodesoxymorphine, $C_{17}H_{19}O_2N$. A derivative of morphine synthesized by Small and Mosettig. It is more potent but also more toxic than morphine. It is much less constipating than morphine but has only a short period of action.

desoxyribose (dez·ox·e·**ri**·boze). *See* DEOXYRIBOSE.

desoxy-sugar (dez·ox·e·**shug**·ar). Name applied to a monosaccharide which has lost an oxygen atom. [L *de,* Gk *oxys* sharp, Arab. *sukkar.*]

despeciation (de·spe·se·**a'**·shun). Loss of or deviation from the normal physical characteristic of species. [L *de,* species.]

despecification (de·spes·**if**·ik·a·shun). Removal with pepsin of the Fc fragment of IgG antibody molecules used in passive immunization, e.g. diphtheria or tetanus antitoxins. This reduces the antigenicity of the protein and thus reduces the incidence of hypersensitivity reactions in subjects receiving it.

D'Espine, Jean Henri Adolphe (b. 1844). French physician.

D'Espine's sign. Pectoriloquy is heard lower than the normal limit on auscultation over the vertebral spines in enlargement of the bronchial glands.

despumation (des·pew·**ma**·shun). 1. The rising of scum and impurities to the surface of a liquid. 2. The clarifying of a liquid by removal of scum and impurities. [L *de, spuma* froth.]

desquamatio neonatorum (des·kwam·a·she·o **ne**·o·nat·**o'**·rum). The peeling off of the epidermis of newborn infants during the first few days after birth. [L a scaling off of the newborn.]

desquamation (des·kwam·**a**·shun). 1. The casting off of the epidermis in shreds or scales. 2. The peeling off of epithelial elements from structures such as the mucosa. **Furfuraceous desquamation.** The shredding of the epidermis in branny scales. **Lamellar desquamation of the newborn.** This may be a benign, transitory, or a persistent genetically-determined phenomenon; in the latter, the skin is covered with a shiny, red, cracked, collodion-like film which peels off, leaving ichthyosiform erythroderma or lamellar ichthyosis. **Membranous desquamation.** Desquamation in large sheets. **Siliquose desquamation.** The shedding of the epithelial covering of a part in an unbroken husk-like form. [L *desquamare* to scale off.]

desquamative (des·**kwam**·at·iv). Marked by desquamation.

desquamatory (des·**kwam**·at·or·e). Attended by or associated with desquamation.

Desse's spaces. Spaces between the sinusoids of the liver and the liver cells, containing tissue fluids and lymphatics.

dessertspoonful (dez·**ert**·spoon·ful). A domestic measure roughly equivalent to one centilitre.

Dessy, G.

Dessy's vaccine. A variety of typhoid vaccine prepared from numerous strains of typhoid bacilli grown on alkaline-agar medium.

desternalization (de·**ster**·nal·i·**za'**·shun). Separation from the sternum; refers to the costal cartilages. [L *de,* Gk *sternon* chest.]

desthiobiotin (dez·**thi**·o·**bi'**·o·tin). A competitive analogue of ascorbic acid: biotin in which two hydrogen atoms have replaced the sulphur atom.

destrudo (de·**stroo**·do). In psycho-analysis, the psychic energy associated with the death instinct. Cf. LIBIDO. [L *destruere* to destroy, libido.]

desudation (de·sew·**da**·shun). Sweating, particularly of a profuse or morbid nature, with sometimes a later eruption of pimples, giving the clinical picture of sudamina or sweat rash. [L *de, sudare* to sweat.]

desudatory (de·**sew**·dat·or·e). Applied to any kind of bath of heat intended to induce sweating. [see prec.]

desumvergence (de·sum·**ver**·jens). Deorsumduction. [L *desursum* from above, *vergere* to incline.]

Desvoidea (des·**voi**·de·ah). *Armigeres.*

desynapsis (**de**·sin·**ap'**·sis). The falling apart, prior to metaphase I of meiosis, of homologues which appeared to be normally paired at pachytene. [L *de,* Gk *synaptein* to join.]

detachment (de·**tach**·ment). **Detachment of the retina.** A condition where the retina, in part or whole, becomes separated from the choroid. The line of cleavage is inter-retinal, between the pigment layer and the layer of rods and cones. [Fr. *détachement.*]

De Takats, Geza (b. 1892). Chicago surgeon.

De Takats' test. A test based on the increase in clotting times following a standardized dose of heparin. Coagulation times are determined before, and 10, 20, 30 and 40 min after the intravenous injection of 10 mg heparin. Absence of increase in clotting time occurs immediately after surgical operations, and in vascular thrombosis and embolism. The test has been used to predict an increased general tendency to thrombosis.

detector (de·**tek**·tor). Anything which discovers and reveals the presence of another thing. **Lie detector.** An apparatus recording blood pressure, pulse and respiration rate in individuals under police questioning or medical analysis, designed to indicate tension in the telling of lies. **Semiconductor detector.** A radiation detector which depends upon the property of semiconduction. **Sterility detector.** A method employed to test the efficiency of sterilization by autoclaving. It may consist in chemical test papers, or ampoules containing liquid, or in the introduction into the autoclave of a package containing spores of known heat resistance; subsequent failure to grow living organisms from these indicates efficient sterilization. [L.]

detelectasis (de·tel·**ek**·tas·is). Collapse due to lack of normal inflating contents. [L *de*, Gk *telos* end, *ektasis* a stretching.]

detergent (de·**ter**·jent). A cleansing agent. Commonly applied to a surface-active agent in solution which influences surface tension ionically. [L *detergere* to wipe off.]

deterioration (de·**teer**·e·or·a′·shun). The act or process of becoming worse. **Emotional deterioration.** A psychical state in which the emotions are dulled and do not respond to ordinary stimuli. **Mental deterioration.** A condition in which the personality has become perverted or debased and the mental calibre has decreased. [L *deteriorare* to worsen.]

deteriorative (de·**teer**·e·or·a′·tiv). Descriptive of a psychosis marked by steady impairment of mental function and degrading change, or loss, of personality. [see prec.]

determinant (de·**ter**·min·ant). The determining cause. **Antigenic determinant.** The small site on the antigen to which antibody is specifically able to become attached by its combining site. A single antigenic molecule may carry several different antigenic determinants. Haptens attached to it will form new determinants. [L *determinare* to limit.]

determination (de·**ter**·min·a′·shun). The imposition of a limit; the measurement or establishment of a value. **Embryonic determination.** The point at which embryonic tissue undergoes specific development to become specialized tissue. **Phototurbidometric determination.** Determining the degree of turbidity by photo-electric methods. **Sex determination.** 1. The shift of the developmental programme of an individual towards femaleness or maleness. 2. The procedure for determining the sex of an organism. 3. In its forensic aspects, now resting more upon cellular sex identification than upon physical characteristics. Cell chromosome and Barr body identification effected in mucous membrane epithelium now regarded as a sounder guide in the problems of inter-sex. In the dead, organ or skeletal differences, hair changes and cell sexing where tissues are fresh enough is decisive. [L *determinare* to limit.]

determiner (de·**ter**·min·er). Biophore. [see prec.]

determinism (de·**ter**·min·izm). The doctrine that every occurrence is necessarily determined by a cause. **Psychic determinism.** The doctrine that human thought and action are not free, but necessarily determined by causes and motives. [L *determinare* to limit.]

detersive (de·**ter**·siv). Detergent.

dethyroidism (de·**thi**·roid·izm). The condition or complex of symptoms which occurs after the thyroid gland has been removed. Cf. ATHYREOSIS. [L *de*, thyroid.]

dethyroidized (de·**thi**·roid·i·zd). Having had the thyroid gland excised. [see prec.]

De Toni, Giovanni (b. 1895). Modena paediatrician.

Debré–De Toni–Fanconi syndrome. *See* FANCONI'S DISEASE.

detorsion (de·**tor**·shun). 1. A defect in a normal process of twisting during development. 2. The correction of any bodily deformity or curvature. 3. Distorsion. [L *detorquere* to turn about.]

detoxicate (de·**tox**·e·kate). 1. To make harmless a poisonous substance, or to lessen the virulence of a harmful organism. 2. To overcome the effects of having been poisoned. [L *de*, Gk *toxikon* poison.]

detoxication (de·tox·e·**ka**′·shun). 1. Rendering harmless a poisonous substance or a pathogenic organism. 2. Recovery from the effects of poisoning. **Metabolic detoxication.** The metabolic process which lessens the toxicity of an ingested substance. [see prec.]

detoxification (de·tox·if·e·**ka**′·shun). The capacity to destroy or reduce the poisonous attributes of a substance. [L *de*, Gk *toxikon* poison, L *facere* to make.]

detoxify (de·**tox**·e·fi). Detoxicate.

detrital (de·**tri**·tal). Composed of or pertaining to detritus.

detrition (de·**trish**·un). A process of wearing away through use or by friction. [see foll.]

detritus (de·**tri**·tus). 1. The product of disintegration. 2. The calcareous substance which adheres to the teeth or the fragments of disintegrating tooth substance. [L a rubbing away.]

detruncation (de·trung·**ka**·shun). 1. Decapitation; this refers chiefly to the fetus. 2. Shortening by cutting off. [L *detruncare* to cut off.]

detrusion (de·**troo**·zhun). 1. An outward and downward thrust. 2. Expulsion or ejection. [L *detrudere* to thrust away.]

detrusor urinae (de·**troo**·zor **ewr**·in·e). The muscular coat of the bladder, consisting of 2 layers of longitudinal fibres and 1 layer of circular fibres. [L thruster of urine.]

detubation (de·tew·**ba**·shun). The extraction or removal of a tube. [L *de*, tube.]

detuberculization (de·tew·**ber**·kew·li·**za**′·shun). Any process, natural or artificial, intended to rid a person or a community of tuberculous infection. [L *de*, tubercle.]

detumescence (de·tewm·**es**·ens). 1. The diminution or subsidence of any swelling. 2. The ejaculation of seminal fluid (Ellis). [L *de*, *tumere* to swell.]

deutencephalon (dew·ten·**kef**·al·on). Diencephalon. [Gk *deuteros* second, *egkephalos* brain.]

deuteranomalopia (**dew**·ter·an·om·al·**o**′·pe·ah). Deuteranomaly. [Gk *deuteros* second, *anomalos* irregular, *ops* sight.]

deuteranomaly (**dew**·ter·an·**om**′·al·e). A form of partial colour blindness classified as anomalous trichromatic; all 3 primary colours, red, green and blue, are appreciated, but the green portion of the spectrum only is imperfectly perceived. [Gk *deuteros* second, *anomalos* irregular.]

deuteranope (**dew**·ter·an·ope). An individual affected with deuteranopia; a green-blind person. [Gk *deuteros* second, anopia.]

deuteranopia, deuteranopsia (**dew**·ter·an·**o**′·pe·ah, **dew**·ter·an·**ops**′·e·ah). A form of partial colour blindness of the dichromatic type, in which only 2 of the 3 primary colours, red and blue, are appreciated; the green portion of the spectrum is not perceived. Also called *green blindness.* [Gk *deuteros* second, *a*, *opsis* vision.]

deuterion (dew·**teer**·e·on). A deuteron.

deuteripara (dew·ter·**ip**·ar·ah). Secundipara; a woman who has had or is in the process of giving birth to her second child. [Gk *deuteros* second, L *parere* to give birth.]

deuterium (dew·**teer**·e·um). This is heavy hydrogen, ^{2}H, a non-radioactive isotope of hydrogen which has a nucleus consisting of a proton and a neutron. **Deuterium oxide.** Heavy water, D_2O, a colourless liquid with chemical properties very similar to water, but inimical to growth in concentration. It occurs in rain and natural waters (about 1 part in 9000): used as a labelled atom in the study of metabolism. [Gk *deuteros* second.]

deutero-albumose (**dew**·ter·o·al·**bew**·mose). Deuteroproteose.

deutero-anopia (**dew**·ter·o·an·**o**′·pe·ah). Deuteranopia.

deuterofat (**dew**·ter·o·fat). Any fat in which the hydrogen is in the form of the isotope, deuterium.

deuterogenic (**dew**·ter·o·**jen**′·ik). Secondary in origin. [Gk *deuteros* second, *genein* to produce.]

deuterohaemin (**dew**·ter·o·**he**′·min). $C_{30}H_{28}O_4N_4FeCl$, a derivative of haemin formed during the synthesis of haematoporphyrin.

deuterohydrogen (dew·ter·o·hi′·dro·jen). Deuterium. [Gk *deuteros* second, hydrogen.]
deuterology (dew·ter·ol·o·je). The biology of the placenta. [Gk *deuteros* second (substance), *logos* science.]
deuteromycetes (dew·ter·o·mi·se′·teez). Fungi imperfecti. [Gk *deuteros* second, *mykes* fungus.]
deuteron (dew·ter·on). The nucleus of the atom of deuterium, or heavy hydrogen. It has a mass of 2, and unit charge: employed as an atomic projectile in the cyclotron for the production of radioactive isotopes. [Gk *deuteros* second.]
deuteropathic (dew·ter·o·path′·ik). Referring to a disease associated with or secondary to another. [Gk *deuteros* second, *pathos* suffering.]
deuteropathy (dew·ter·op·ath·e). A disease secondary to another disease. [see prec.]
deuteroplasm (dew·ter·o·plazm). Deutoplasm.
deuteroporphyrin (dew·ter·o·por′·fir·in). A porphyrin, $C_{30}H_{30}N_4O_4$, occurring in faeces and derived from the breakdown of haemoglobin or myoglobin. Its constitution differs from that of protoporphyrin by having 2 hydrogen atoms in place of 2 vinyl groups.
deuteroproteose (dew·ter·o·pro′·te·oze). A secondary proteose, soluble in water, formed by the hydrolytic rupture of the protein molecule, and precipitated by strong salt solutions. [Gk *deuteros* second, proteose.]
deuterostoma (dew·ter·o·sto′·mah). A secondary blastopore. [Gk *deuteros* second, *stoma* mouth.]
deuterotocia, deuterotoky (dew·ter·o·to′·se·ah, dewt·er·ot·o·ke). Parthenogenesis in which the offspring are of both sexes. [Gk *deuteros* second, *tokos* birth.]
deutiodide (dew·ti·o·dide). Deutoiodide.
deutipara (dew·tip·ar·ah). Secundipara. [Gk *deuteros* second, L *parere* to give birth.]
deutobromide (dew·to·bro·mide). The analogue of a deutochloride, containing twice the bromine of the lowest bromide of a series of bromides. [Gk *deuteros* second, bromide.]
deutochloride (dew·to·klor·ide). Of the several chlorides of a metal or radical, the term applied to that which contains twice the chlorine of the lowest member of the series. [Gk *deuteros* second, chloride.]
deutohydrogen (dew·to·hi·dro·jen). Deuterium. [Gk *deuteros* second, hydrogen.]
deutoiodide (dew·to·i·o·dide). The iodide, analogous with a deutochloride, which contains twice the iodine of the lowest member of a series of iodides. [Gk *deuteros* second, iodide.]
deuton (dew·ton). A deuteron.
deutonephron (dew·to·nef·ron). The mesonephros (wolffian body), the second of the three sets of excretory organs which appear in the embryo during the course of development of the urogenital organs. [Gk *deuteros* second, *nephros* kidney.]
deutoplasm (dew·to·plazm). The nutritive yolk; the reserve food material present in the ovum, composed mainly of fatty matter and lecithin. In the mammal it serves the embryo in the early stages only. [Gk *deuteros* second, protoplasm.]
deutoplasmolysis (dew·to·plaz·mol′·is·is). Disintegration or destruction of deutoplasm. [deutoplasm, Gk *lysis* a loosening.]
deutosclerous (dew·to·skler·us). Indicating a hard spot or patch formed as the result of an independent morbid condition. [Gk *deuteros* second, sclerous.]
Deutschlaender, Karl Ernst Wilhelm (b. 1872). Hamburg surgeon.
Deutschlaender's disease. March foot. *See* FOOT.
Deutschmann's theory. A theory that the involvement of the sympathizing eye in sympathetic ophthalmia is caused by a spread of infection via the lymphatic channels of the optic nerves and chiasma. Hence the name *migratory ophthalmia.*
devalgate (de·val·gate). Bow-legged. [L *de, valgus* bow leg.]
devaporation (de·vap·or·a′·shun). The condensation of vapour. [L *de, vaporare* to steam.]
devasation (de·vas·a·shun). Destruction of the blood vessels of an organ or tissue. **Senile cortical devasation.** Insanity due to arteriosclerosis of the blood vessels of the cerebral pallium (cortex). [L *de, vas* vessel.]
devascularization (de·vas·kew·lar·i·za′·shun). 1. The drawing away of blood from a part. 2. Lessening or stopping the blood supply of any part of the body by blocking the nutrient vessels. [L *de,* vascular.]
development (de·vel·op·ment). The series of changes by means of which the individual embryo becomes a mature organism. **Psychosexual development.** The unfolding of the personality of an individual as he passes from babyhood through adolescence to adult life. [Fr. *développer.*]
developmental (de·vel·op·men′·tal). 1. Evolutionary. 2. Characterized by or belonging to the process of development. [see prec.]
Deventer, Hendrik van (b. 1651). Dutch obstetrician.
Deventer's oblique diameter. The oblique diameter of the pelvic inlet.
Devergie, Marie Guillaume Alphonse (b. 1798). Paris physician.
Devergie's attitude. The posture of a corpse, marked by flexion of the knees, elbows and fingers, and the extension of the ankles.
Devergie's disease. Pityriasis rubra pilaris.
Puits de Devergie. Minute perforations with serous crusts remaining after eczematous vesicles have ruptured.
deviation (de·ve·a·shun). 1. A variation from the normal, or from some given standard. 2. In ophthalmology, inco-ordination of the eyes. 3. In statistics, the difference of any member of a series of values from the mean value. **Animal deviation.** A term employed by medical entomologists to describe a habit of *Anopheles maculipennis* and its geobiotypes in feeding on animal blood in preference to that of humans; anthropophilism. **Average deviation.** Mean deviation (see below). **Axis deviation.** Deviation of the mean electrical axis of the heart in the frontal plane from the usual limits of $-10°$ and $+100°$. **Deviation of complement.** Also known as the *Neisser-Wechsberg phenomenon,* and differing from fixation of complement. When more specific amboceptor is added to a mixture of antigen and complement than can be absorbed by the antigen, the excess amboceptor may combine with the complement. This prevents the complement from acting on the antigen-amboceptor complex. **Conjugate deviation.** In ophthalmology, applied to movements of the two eyes in which their visual axes remain parallel. **Immune deviation.** Selective alteration of the immune response to an antigen caused by prior contact with the same antigen. **Latent deviation.** Heterophoria. **Deviation to the left.** Shift to the left. **Left axis deviation.** Deviation of the mean electrical axis of the heart in the frontal plane to the left (less than $-10°$) occurring when the heart lies in a horizontal position and the cardiac apex is disposed upwards and to the left. The sum of the QRS deflexions is positive in lead I of the electrocardiogram and negative in lead III. It may be due to extracardiac factors which affect the position of the heart, or because of hypertrophy of the left ventricle when the increased muscle mass displaces the apex upwards and to the left. **Manifest deviation.** The amount in degrees by which the visual axis of one eye deviates from that of its fellow in cases of squint, when both eyes are open. **Mean deviation.** Average deviation; in statistics, the arithmetical average of the differences between each observation made in a series and the mean of the series irrespective of the sign denoting the differences. **Minimum deviation.** The deviation of a ray of light when it passes symmetrically through a prism. **Primary deviation.** Applied to cases of uniocular paralytic squint to describe the deviation of the affected eye when the unaffected one looks at an object. **Deviation to the right.** Shift to the right. **Right axis deviation.** Deviation of the mean electrical axis of the heart in the frontal plane to the right (more than $+100°$) occurring when the heart is vertical and the apex directed downwards and to the right. The sum of the QRS deflexions is negative in lead I and positive in lead III. It may be due to extracardiac factors or to hypertrophy of the right ventricle. **Secondary deviation.** The deviation of the sound eye when the

fellow eye with a paretic muscle or muscles takes up fixation. It is commonly greater than the primary deviation (see above). **Skew deviation.** Vertical divergence of the eyes due to a brain-stem lesion. It may or may not be concomitant and can sometimes be differentiated from a partial muscle palsy only by the presence of other brain-stem signs. **Standard deviation.** In statistics, a measure of dispersion of scatter which takes into account the deviation of every value of a variable such as height, age or test score, from the mean value of the sample under consideration. Mathematically it is the square root of the average of the squares of the amounts by which each value differs from the average, and is denoted by the Greek letter σ, or SD. **Strabismic deviation.** The angle of squint. **Deviation of teeth.** The condition of lying in an abnormal position in the dental arch. [L *deviare* to turn aside.]

See also: HERING (K. E. K.), HILLEBRAND.

Devic's disease. Neuromyelitis optica.

device (de·vise). **Rotating devices.** Appliances for correcting the rotation of a tooth and bringing it into its normal position. [OFr. *devise.*]

See also: DUKE-ELDER.

deviometer (de·ve·**om**·et·er). An instrument for measuring the angle of squint; a type of strabismometer. [deviation, meter.]

devisceration (de·vis·er·a·shun). Evisceration. [L *de, viscus* any large internal organ.]

devitalization (de·vi·tal·i·za′·shun). The deprivation of life or vitalizing properties. [L *de, vita* life.]

devitalize (de·vi·tal·ize). To deprive of vitalizing properties or of life. [see prec.]

devitrifaction, devitrification (de·vit·re·**fak**′·shun, de·**vit**·rif·e·**ka**′·-shun). The process by which transparency disappears because of crystallization, e.g. glass becomes opaque when acted on by certain chemicals or age. [L *de, vitrum* glass, *facere* to make.]

devolution (de·vol·**ew**·shun). 1. Degeneration. 2. Catabolism. 3. Involution. [L *de, volvere* to roll.]

devorative (de·**vor**·at·iv). A medicinal substance which is to be swallowed without being first chewed. [L *devorare* to swallow up.]

De Vries, Hugo (b. 1848). Amsterdam botanist.

De Vries' theory. The theory that evolution has occurred by a series of saltations rather than by continuous small changes.

Dew, Sir Harold Robert (b. 1891). Sydney, New South Wales, surgeon.

Dew's sign. With a subdiaphragmatic hydatid abscess the area of resonance moves caudally when the patient is in the knee-elbow position.

Dewar, Sir James (b. 1842). British chemist.

Dewar flask. A double-walled vacuum flask used in work with liquid air.

dewatering (de·**waw**·ter·ing). The process in the purification of sewage, of removing a portion of the water contained in the sludge by draining, pressing, centrifuging or other natural or mechanical processes. [L *de*, water.]

De Watteville current. A combination of galvanic and faradic currents.

Dewees, William Potts (b. 1768). American obstetrician.

Dewees' sign. Expectoration of tough, whitish mucus as a sign of pregnancy. The sputum was said to resemble a silver coin.

De Wesselow, Owen Lambert Vaughan Simpkinson (b. 1883). British pathologist.

Maclean-De Wesselow test. Urea concentration test. *See* TEST.

Dexamethasone BP 1973 (dex·ah·**meth**·az·one). 9α-Fluoro-16α-methylprednisolone; it is used in corticosteroid therapy. **Dexamethasone Acetate BP 1963.** 21-Acetoxy-9α-fluoro-11β, 17α-dihydroxy-16α-methylpregna-1,4-diene-3,20-dione; a white, odourless powder used in corticosteroid therapy.

Dexamphetamine (dex·am·**fet**·am·een). BP Commission approved name for D-amphetamine, $C_6H_5CH_2CH(CH_3)NH_2$. A compound whose action and toxic effects are similar to those of amphetamine, which it has largely replaced in the treatment of obesity. **Dexamphetamine Sulphate BP 1958.** The dextroisomer of amphetamine sulphate $[C_6H_5CH_2CH(NH_2)CH_3]_2H_2SO_4$. In the treatment of obesity, it is preferred to the racemic form.

Dexetimide (dex·**et**·im·ide). BP Commission approved name for (+)-3-(1-benzyl-4-piperidyl)-3-phenylpiperidine-2,6-dione; it is used in the treatment of Parkinson's syndrome.

dexiocardia (dex·e·o·**kar**′·de·ah). Dextrocardia. [Gk *dexios* on the right hand, *kardia* heart.]

dexiotropic (dex·e·o·**trop**′·ik). Dextrotropic. [Gk *dexios* on the right hand, *trepein* to turn.]

Dexpanthenol (dex·**pan**·then·ol). BP Commission approved name for (+)-2,4,-dihydroxy-*N*-(3-hydroxypropyl)-3,3-dimethylbutyramide; it is used in the treatment of paralytic ileus and post-operative distension.

Dexpropanolol (dex·pro·**pan**·o·lol). BP Commission approved name for (+)-1-isopropylamino-3-(1-naphthyloxy)propan-2-ol; it is used in the treatment of arrhythmia.

dexter (**dex**·ter). Pertaining to the right-hand side. [L on the right side.]

dextral (**dex**·tral). 1. Relating or belonging to the right as opposed to the left. 2. An individual who shows a preference for using the right hand and any other right-sided part of the body (e.g. eye, foot, and so on). [see prec.]

dextrality (dex·**tral**·it·e). Right-handedness; having more efficiency on the right than on the left side, or being different on the right side. [L *dexter* on the right side.]

Dextran (**dex**·tran). BP Commission approved name for polyanhydroglucose. A gummy substance produced by the action of certain bacteria on polysaccharides. A solution of dextran is employed extensively for transfusion, and is also used in perfusion experiments in animals. The official *British Pharmacopoeia* preparations are dextran 40, 70, and 110 injections, where the numerals refer to the average size of the molecules contained in the solution.

dextransucrase (dex·tran·**sew**·kraze). A ferment which converts the sucrose of molasses and beet-juice into dextran.

dextrase (**dex**·traze). An enzyme concerned with the formation of lactic acid from dextrose (glucose).

dextren (**dex**·tren). Relating inherently to the right side. [L *dexter* on the right side.]

Dextriferron (dex·tri·**fer**·on). BP Commission approved name for a colloidal solution of ferric hydroxide in complex with partially hydrolysed dextrin; it is used in the treatment of iron-deficiency anaemia.

dextrin (**dex**·trin). Starch gum, British gum, $(C_6H_{10}O_5)_n$. A hexosan, or polymer of glucose, obtained by the hydrolysis of starch, being an intermediate during the conversion of the latter into monosaccharides. It is a tasteless, colourless, gummy substance, soluble in water and dextrorotatory; used as a mucilage. The industrial product obtained by heating potato starch dry, or *in vacuo* with citric acid, contains amylodextrin, erythrodextrin and achro-odextrin, all of which are highly dextrorotatory. **Animal dextrin, Liver dextrin.** Glycogen.

dextrinase (**dex**·trin·aze). An enzyme found in starch, which synthesizes dextrinose (isomaltose) from the products of maltase fermentation.

dextrinate, dextrinize (**dex**·trin·ate, **dex**·trin·ize). 1. To impregnate with dextrin. 2. To convert into dextrin.

dextrinose (**dex**·trin·oze). Isomaltose, $C_{12}H_{22}O_{11}$. A glucose-β-glucoside, synthesized by the action of enzymes or hydrochloric acid on molecules of glucose which occurs naturally in beer and honey. It is dextrorotatory and nonfermentable.

dextrinuria (dex·trin·**ewr**·e·ah). The presence of dextrin in the urine.

dextro- (**dex**·tro). 1. A prefix to the name of an organic substance indicating that it is dextrorotatory. In modern nomenclature, D- is not an abbreviation for "dextro" and therefore does not necessarily mean that the substance is dextrorotatory; it is purely a configuration symbol. Optical activity is indicated by a plus or minus sign following the prefix, e.g. D(+)-glucose. 2. Prefix, from the Latin *dexter*, meaning *right.* [L *dexter* on the right side.]

dextro-amphetamine (dex·tro·am·**fet**′·am·een). Dexamphetamine.

dextro-aural (dex·tro·**awr**·al). Having better hearing on the right side than on the left. [L *dexter* on the right side, *auris* ear.]

dextrocardia (dex·tro·**kar**·de·ah). A developmental abnormality in which the apex of the heart is directed towards the right. If this occurs as part of total situs inversus, the heart may be functionally normal but its anatomy is a mirror image of the normal. **Isolated dextrocardia.** Dextrocardia occurring with normal visceral situs; the heart is always anatomically abnormal. [L *dexter* on the right side, Gk *kardia* heart.]

dextrocardiogram (dex·tro·**kar**·de·o·gram). The complex derived from a unipolar electrode facing the right ventricle, consisting of a small R wave and a large S wave. Cf. LAEVOCARDIOGRAM. [L *dexter* on the right side, electrocardiogram.]

dextrocerebral (dex·tro·**ser**·e·bral). 1. Indicating that the right cerebral hemisphere is functioning more actively than is the left. 2. Situated in the right cerebral hemisphere. [L *dexter* on the right side, cerebrum.]

dextroclination (dex·tro·klin·**a**′·shun). Dextrotorsion. [L *dexter* on the right side, Gk *klinein* to bend.]

dextrocompound (dex·tro·**kom**·pownd). A compound that is dextrorotatory in solution. [L *dexter* on the right side, compound.]

dextrocycloduction (dex·tro·si·klo·**duk**′·shun). Dextrotorsion. [L *dexter* on the right side, Gk *kylos* circle, L *ducere* to draw.]

dextroduction (dex·tro·**duk**·shun). Movement of the visual axis of either eye towards the right. [L *dexter* on the right side, *ducere* to draw.]

dextrogastria (dex·tro·**gas**·tre·ah). The condition in which the stomach is displaced to the right, usually in association with dextrocardia. [L *dexter* on the right side, Gk *gaster* stomach.]

dextroglucose (dex·tro·**gloo**·koze). Dextrose.

dextrogram (**dex**·tro·gram). Dextrocardiogram.

dextrogyral, dextrogyrate (dex·tro·**ji**·ral, dex·tro·**ji**·rate). Dextrorotatory. [see foll.]

dextrogyration (**dex**·tro·ji·**ra**′·shun). Dextrorotation. [L *dexter* on the right side, *gyrare* to turn round.]

dextrogyre (**dex**·tro·jire). Dextrorotatory. [see prec.]

dextromanual (dex·tro·**man**·ew·al). Right-handed. [L *dexter* on the right side, *manus* hand.]

dextromenthol (**dex**·tro·**men**·thol). D-Menthol, $C_{10}H_{19}OH$. A dextrorotatory form of menthol which does not occur naturally but is produced by the reduction of the corresponding menthone.

Dextromethorphan (dex·tro·meth·**or**′·fan). BP Commission approved name for D-3-methoxy-*N*-methylmorphinan, the methyl ether of levorphanol (3-hydroxy-*N*-methylmorphinan). It is claimed to be free from undesirable effects such as addiction and central depression; a useful cough suppressant. **Dextromethorphan Hydrobromide BP 1973.** The hydrobromide monohydrate; a drug credited with a selective depressant action on the cough centre. No harmful effects have been reported and it is non-addictive.

Dextromoramide (dex·tro·**mor**·am·ide). BP Commission approved name for (+)-1-(β-methyl-γ-morpholino-αα-dephenylbutyryl)-pyrrolidine. **Dextromoramide Tartrate BP 1973.** The hydrogen tartrate, a potent narcotic analgesic given either by mouth or injection and used for the relief of severe pain, with side-effects similar to those of methadone hydrochloride; a drug of addiction.

dextro-ocular (dex·tro·**ok**·ew·lar). Right-eyed, i.e. using the right eye more than the left. [L *dexter* on the right side, *oculus* eye.]

dextro-ocularity (**dex**·tro·ok·ew·**lar**′·it·e). The condition in which the right eye is stronger than the left and therefore is used more than the left, particularly in work with a microscope. [see prec.]

dextropedal (dex·**trop**·ed·al). Right-footed; using the right foot in preference to the left. [L *dexter* on the right side, *pes* foot.]

dextropedality (**dex**·tro·ped·**al**′·it·e). Being right-footed. [see prec.]

dextrophobia (dex·tro·**fo**·be·ah). A morbid fear of any object at the right hand or on the right side. [L *dexter* on the right side, Gk *phobos* fear.]

dextrophoria (dex·tro·**for**·e·ah). The condition in which the visual lines tend towards the right. [L *dexter* on the right side, Gk *pherein* to carry.]

dextroposition (**dex**·tro·poz·**ish**′·un). A term sometimes applied to the heart when the apex appears to be directed to the right. [L *dexter* on the right side, L *positio* position.]

Dextropropoxyphene (**dex**·tro·pro·**pox**′·e·feen). BP Commission approved name for (+)-α-4-dimethylamino-3-methyl-1,2-diphenyl-2-propionyloxybutane; an analgesic. **Dextropropoxyphene Hydrochloride BP 1973.** The hydrochloride; its potency is comparable with that of codeine but, although it may cause nausea and drowsiness, constipation does not occur. **Dextropropoxyphene Napsylate BP 1973.** The monohydrate of the naphthalene-2-sulphonate; this preparation is less bitter and less irritating to the gastric mucosa.

dextrorotation (**dex**·tro·ro·**ta**′·shun). A turning or twisting to the right, as in movements of the eye or of the plane of polarization of light. **Cardiac dextrorotation.** Dextrocardia supposedly due to rotation to the right about the long axis of the body of an otherwise normally developed heart. [L *dexter* on the right side, *rotare* to swing around.]

dextrorotatory (**dex**·tro·ro·**ta**′·tor·e). Turning towards the right hand, particularly the plane of polarization of luminous rays. [see prec.]

Dextrorphan (**dex**·tror·fan). BP Commission approved name for (+)-3-hydroxy-*N*-methylmorphinan; a narcotic analgesic.

dextrosamine (dex·**tro**·sam·een). Glucosamine, $CH_2OH(CHOH)_3CH(NH_2)CHO$. An aminosaccharide obtained by the hydrolysis of chitin, and occurring widely in nature in the prosthetic group of glycoproteins. [dextrose, amine.]

dextrosazone (dex·**tro**·sa·zone). Glucosazone, $CH_2OH(CHOH)_3CN(NHC_6H_5)CH{=}NNHC_6H_5$. A reaction product of glucose with an excess of phenylhydrazine: only slightly soluble in water, its crystals are characteristic in shape and serve to identify glucose. This same osazone, however, is formed by fructose and mannose.

Dextrose BP 1973 (**dex**·troze). Dextrose monohydrate; glucose; grape sugar; $C_6H_{12}O_6{\cdot}H_2O$. The principal hexose, occurring widely in fruit and plants, honey and the blood and tissue of animals; the product of carbohydrate digestion, appearing free in diabetic urine. A white crystalline substance, very soluble in water, giving a solution that is sweet, dextrorotatory and readily fermentable, and which reduces alkaline cupric reagents such as Fehling's solution. *Anhydrous Dextrose BP 1973* and *Dextrose Monohydrate for Parenteral Use BP 1973* conform to the requirements of the *European Pharmacopoeia* for *Dextrosum Anhydricum ad Usum Parenterale* and *Dextrosum Monohydricum ad Usum Parenterale,* respectively.

dextrosinistral (dex·tro·**sin**·is·tral). 1. Extending in a right and left direction. 2. Extending from the right to the left. 3. Applied to an individual who is naturally left-handed but has been trained to use the right hand when there is a choice. [L *dexter* on the right side, *sinister* left.]

dextrosum (dex·**tro**·sum). Dextrose. **Dextrosum Anhydricum ad Usum Parenterale.** *European Pharmacopoeia* name for Anhydrous Dextrose BP 1973. **Dextrosum Monohydricum ad Usum Parenterale.** *European Pharmacopoeia* name for Dextrose Monohydrate for Parenteral Use BP 1973.

dextrosuria (dex·tro·**zewr**·e·ah). The presence of dextrose in the urine.

Dextrothyroxine (**dex**·tro·thi·**rox**′·een). BP Commission approved name for D-α-amino-β-[4-(4-hydroxy-3,5-di-iodophenoxy)-3,5-di-iodophenyl]propionic acid; it is used in the treatment of hypercholesterolaemia.

dextrotorsion (dex·tro·**tor**·shun). A disjunctive movement of the two eyes together form extorsion of the right eye, intorsion of the left eye. [L *dexter* on the right side, *torquere* to turn about.]

dextrotropic, dextrotropous (dex·tro·**trop**·ik, dex·tro·**tro**·pus). 1. Tending or turning towards the right. 2. Twisting in a right-hand spiral. [L *dexter* on the right side, Gk *trepein* to turn.]

dextroversion (dex·tro·ver·zhun). 1. Turning towards the right. 2. Of the eye, a movement towards the right. **Cardiac dextroversion.** Cardiac dextrorotation. *See* DEXTROROTATION. [L *dexter* on the right side, *vertere* to turn.]

dextroverted (dex·tro·ver·ted). Turned to the right or towards the right. [see prec.]

dezymotize (de·zi·mo·tize). 1. To destroy ferments or enzymes. 2. To disinfect. [L *de*, Gk *zyme* ferment.]

d'Herelle, Felix (b. 1873). France and USA bacteriologist.

d'Herelle's phenomenon, Twort-d'Herelle phenomenon. The lysis of a bacterial culture by bacteriophage: it is transmissible and specific.

dhooley (doo·le). A simple kind of litter with a cover used in India as an army ambulance. [Hind. *doli* to swing.]

di- . 1. Prefix, from the Latin *dis*, meaning *apart, separation, the opposite of.* 2. Prefix, from the Greek *dis*, meaning *twice, twofold, double.*

dia- . Prefix, from the Greek *dia*, meaning *through, across, between, apart.*

diabetes (di·ah·be·teez). 1. Without qualification the word is usually taken to mean *diabetes mellitus* (see below). 2. Any one of a group of diseases in which there is polyuria and/or an error of metabolism, especially of carbohydrate metabolism. **Acromegalic diabetes.** Hyperglycaemia associated with acromegaly; it occurs in about 17 per cent of persons with the latter condition. **Alimentary diabetes.** Diabetes assumed to be due to an excessive intake and absorption of sugar. **Alloxan diabetes.** A diabetes-like condition that follows the injection of alloxan, an oxidation product of uric acid. **Artificial diabetes.** Experimental glycosuria such as that produced by puncture of the 4th ventricle. **Bronzed diabetes.** Haemochromatosis; a rare chronic disease in which haemosiderin is deposited in the liver, pancreas, skin and other organs. It is characterized by cirrhosis of the liver, glycosuria and a bronzed pigmentation of the skin. **Cerebral diabetes.** Glycosuria caused by disease or injury to the brain. **Experimental diabetes.** That produced in animals by artificial methods. **Fat diabetes.** Diabetes mellitus associated with obesity. **Gouty diabetes.** Glycosuria in a gouty person. **Diabetes innocens.** Renal glycosuria. **Diabetes insipidus.** A disease characterized by polydipsia and polyuria, the urine having a very low specific gravity and a low salt content. It is caused by any lesion that destroys parts of the tracks of nerve fibres which run from the supraoptic and paraventricular nuclei to the posterior lobe of the pituitary gland, or the adjacent part of the hypothalamus or the hypophysis cerebri or, in some familial cases, to renal tubular lack of response to antidiuretic hormone. **Lipo-atrophic diabetes.** Lipo-atrophy associated with diabetes. **Lipogenous diabetes.** Diabetes mellitus associated with obesity. **Diabetes mellitus.** A disease, of which there are several forms, characterized by a high-fasting blood sugar, an exaggerated rise in the blood sugar after the ingestion of glucose and a failure of the blood sugar to return in a normal time to normal values. In the *juvenile form,* the clinical characteristics are hyperglycaemia, glycosuria, polydipsia, polyuria, wasting and ketosis, culminating in coma and death. In the *senile form,* wasting does not occur, obesity is common, ketosis is absent or mild and coma is rare, death occurring by reason of late complications. The late complications in both types are arterial changes, glomerular nephrosis, retinitis and cataract. The pancreas, anterior pituitary gland, adrenal cortex and liver may each be concerned in its aetiology. **Pancreatic diabetes.** Diabetes mellitus caused by deficiency of insulin from a defect of the islet cells of the pancreas. **Phloridzin diabetes.** Glycosuria due to the action of phloridzin on the renal tubules which lose their power to reabsorb glucose from the urine. **Piqûre diabetes, Puncture diabetes.** Glycosuria in experimental animals caused by puncture of the floor of the 4th ventricle. **Renal diabetes.** Glycosuria due to a low renal threshold so that small amounts of glucose can be excreted in the urine although the blood sugar may be low. **Skin diabetes.** Urbach and Lentz (1945) suggested that there is in the skin an intermediary carbohydrate metabolism independent of the general carbohydrate metabolism of the body. They used the term "independent cutaneous glycohistechia" to designate a rise in the skin-sugar level, not accompanied or preceded by a rise in the blood-sugar level and not related to diabetes mellitus. They suggested that this condition occurred in certain resistant cases of furunculosis, sweat-gland abscesses, eczema and pruritus, and that the term "skin diabetes" should serve as a designation for the syndrome of therapy-resistant skin disease, high-fasting skin-sugar level associated with a normal blood-sugar curve, and great improvement of the lesions associated with a reduction of the high skin-sugar level when the patient is given a low carbohydrate diet, sometimes combined with injections of insulin. These views are not universally accepted. **Temporary diabetes.** Transient glycosuria occurring in healthy persons as a result of excitement. **Diabetes tenuifluus.** A condition due to an excessive secretion of the posterior pituitary antidiuretic hormone which results in oliguria, with retention of fluid in the tissues and an increase in perspiration. **True diabetes.** That due to a deficiency of insulin. [Gk *diabainein* to pass through.]

diabetic (di·ah·be·tik, di·ah·bet·ik). Suffering from or relating to diabetes.

diabetid (di·ah·be·tid). A skin eruption occurring as a symptom of diabetes.

diabetogenic, diabetogenous (di·ah·be·to·jen'·ik, di·ah·be·toj'·en·us). 1. Causing diabetes. 2. Caused by diabetes. [diabetes, Gk *genein* to produce.]

diabetometer (di·ah·be·tom'·et·er). A type of polariscope used for ascertaining the presence of sugar and the amount of it in urine passed by patients with diabetes. [diabetes, Gk *metron* measure.]

diabetophobia (di·ah·be·to·fo'·be·ah). The morbid dread of falling a victim to diabetes. [diabetes, Gk *phobos* fear.]

diabetotherapy (di·ah·be·to·ther'·ap·e). The treatment of diabetes.

diabolepsy (di·ab·o·lep·se). A form of psycholepsy in which the patient thinks he is in communication with evil spirits or is possessed by a devil. [Gk *diabolos* devil, *lambanein* to seize.]

diabrosis (di·ab·ro·sis). Ulcerative perforation of the walls of a vessel or organ, the result of constant corrosion or of erosion. [Gk ulceration.]

diabrotic (di·ab·rot·ik). Corrosive, erosive or ulcerative. [see prec.]

diacaustic (di·ah·kaw·stik). 1. Strongly caustic. 2. An instrument with a double convex lens for cauterizing a surface by means of refracted rays. [Gk *dia*, *kausis* a burning.]

diacele (di·ah·seel). Diacoele.

diacetaemia (di·as·et·e'·me·ah). Acidosis induced by the presence of diacetic acid in the blood. [diacetic acid, Gk *haima* blood.]

Diacetamate (di·as·et·am·ate). BP Commission approved name for 4-acetamidophenyl acetate; an analgesic.

diacetanilide (di·as·et·an'·il·ide). $C_6H_5N(COCH_3)_2$, the diacetyl derivative of acetanilide; it has similar properties to acetanilide but is more potent.

diacetate (di·as·et·ate). A salt of diacetic acid.

diaceticaciduria (di·as·e·tik·as·id·ewr'·e·ah). Ketonuria. [diacetic acid, urine.]

diacetin (di·as·et·in). Glyceryl acetate, $(CH_3COOCH_2)_2CHOH$. An acetic ester of glycerol; a colourless liquid soluble in water.

diacetonuria, diaceturia (di·as·et·on·ewr'·re·ah, di·as·et·ewr'·e·ah). Ketonuria. [diacetic acid, urine.]

diacetyl (di·as·et·il). α-Diketobutane, $CH_3COCOCH_3$. A yellowish-green liquid with a pungent odour which occurs naturally in butter, where it is formed by lactic-acid bacteria, and to which butter largely owes its flavour. It is used as a reagent for arginine and creatine. **Diacetyl monoxime.** $CH_3COC(NOH)CH_3$, a compound used in testing for the amino acid, citrulline (diacetyl test). **Diacetyl peroxide.** $CH_3COOOCOCH_3$, a compound used as an antiseptic.

diacetylaminoazotoluene (di·as·et·il·am·in·o·az·o·tol'·ew·een). Dimazon, $CH_3C_6H_4N{=}NC_6H_3(CH_3)N(OCCH_3)_2$. An acetylation product of ammoazotoluene. It has the properties of stimulating the growth of epithelial cells as does scarlet red, and may be applied as an ointment to promote epithelial growth in such surgical conditions as chronic ulcers and bedsores.

diacetylmorphine (di·**as**·et·il·**mor'**·feen). Diamorphine, heroin, $C_{21}H_{23}O_5N$. A synthetic derivative of morphine produced by acetylation of both OH groups. It resembles morphine in its general effects but has stronger excitatory actions, and is a more powerful and quicker-acting analgesic, but at the same time is more toxic, especially on the respiratory centre. Though it depresses the cough centre, the drug offers no real advantage over morphine in this respect, apart from a reduced incidence of nausea and vomiting. In view of its severe addictive properties, the use of this drug is sometimes opposed. It causes intense euphoria together with excitation, and addiction once produced is most difficult to treat successfully. It is usually administered in the form of the hydrochloride.

Diacetylnalorphine (di·**as**·et·il·**nal'**·or·feen). BP Commission approved name for diacetyl-*N*-allylnormorphine. It bears the analogous relationship to nalorphine that diamorphine bears to morphine, i.e. it is much more potent. It is used to counteract poisoning by diamorphine and in the treatment of addiction.

diachesis (di·ak·e·sis). A state of mental confusion. [Gk *dia, chein* to pour.]

diachorema (**di**·ak·o·**re'**·mah). Faeces. [Gk excrement.]

diachoresis (**di**·ak·o·**re'**·sis). The passing of faeces. [Gk excretion.]

diachylon (di·**ak**·il·on). Plaster mass of lead. Emplastrum plumbi in massa; a crude oleate of lead prepared from lead monoxide and olive oil, used in lumbago and as a protective. **Compound diachylon.** Galbanum plaster, prepared from lead oleate, galbanum, turpentine and Burgundy pitch. **Diachylon ointment.** Hebra's ointment, a plaster composed of lead oleate and phenol, used for its astringent action in eczema. **Yellow diachylon.** Compound diachylon (see above). [Gk *diachylos* juicy.]

diacid (di·**as**·id). Term applied to a base with 2 available hydroxyl groups, or capable of neutralizing 1 molecule of a dibasic acid. [Gk *di-*, acid.]

diaclasia, diaclasis (di·ak·**la**·ze·ah, di·**ak**·la·sis). 1. A fracture which has been produced with intention, as in the correction of a deformity. 2. Refraction. [Gk *dia, klasis* a breaking.]

diaclast (**di**·ak·last). An instrument used in craniectomy for crushing or perforating the skull of the fetus. [see prec.]

diacoele, diacoelia (**di**·ah·seel, di·ah·**se**·le·ah). The 3rd ventricle. [Gk *dia, koilos* hollow.]

diacope (di·**ak**·op·e). 1. A longitudinal fracture or cut. 2. A deep incision, particularly of any part of the skull or head. [Gk *dia, koptein* to cut.]

diacoustics (di·ak·**oos**·tix). That branch of physics concerned with refraction of sound and the different media causing it. [Gk *dia, akouein* to hear.]

diacrinous (di·**ak**·rin·us). Excreting outwardly or directly, or via a duct. [Gk *dia, krinein* to separate.]

diacrisis (di·**ak**·ris·is). 1. A morbid alteration in a secretion. 2. A critical discharge occurring in a disease. 3. Diagnosis. **Follicular diacrisis.** Morbid alteration of follicular secretion. [Gk *dia, krinein* to separate.]

diacritic, diacritical (di·ak·**rit**·ik, di·ak·**rit**·ik·al). Diagnostic. [see prec.]

diactinic (di·ak·**tin**·ik). Capable of transmitting the actinic rays of light. [Gk *dia*, actinic.]

diactinism (di·**ak**·tin·izm). The power of transmitting the actinic rays of light. [Gk *dia*, actinism.]

diad (**di**·ad). A divalent element or radical. [Gk *di-*.]

diaderm (**di**·ah·derm). In embryology, the name applied to the blastoderm when the two plates representing ectoderm and entoderm are at the stage before active cell growth from the sides of the primitive streak separates these layers. [Gk *dia, derma* covering.]

diadermic (di·ah·**der**·mik). 1. Referring to the diaderm. 2. A term applied to medication by inunction. [see prec.]

diadexis (di·ah·**dex**·is). Metastasis of a disease with accompanying change in its characteristics. [Gk metastasis.]

diadochocinesia (**di**·ad·o·ko·sin·**e'**·ze·ah). Diadochokinesia.

diadochocinetic (**di**·ad·o·ko·sin·**et'**·ik). Diadochokinetic.

diadochokinesia, diadochokinesis (**di**·ad·o·ko·kin·**e'**·ze·ah, **di**·ad·o·ko·kin·**e'**·sis). The normal power of the muscles to move a limb alternately into opposite positions, e.g. flexion and extension. [Gk *diadochos* successor, kinesis.]

diadochokinetic (**di**·ad·o·ko·kin·**et'**·ik). Referring to diadochokinesis.

diaeresis (di·**er**·es·is). The separation of two parts which normally are in continuity by operation or trauma. [Gk *diairesis* separation.]

diagnose (**di**·ag·noze). 1. To recognize the presence of a disease by examination and assessment of the symptoms and signs. 2. To identify or determine the nature of a disease. [Gk *dia, gnosis* knowledge.]

diagnosis (di·ag·**no**·sis). 1. The term which denotes the disease from which a person suffers, e.g. pulmonary tuberculosis, measles, cerebral thrombosis; such labels are useful for certificates, vital statistics and hospital records. 2. The art of applying scientific methods to the elucidation of the problems presented by a sick patient. This implies the collection and critical evaluation of all the evidence obtainable from every possible source and by the use of any method necessary. From the facts so obtained, combined with a knowledge of basic principles, a concept is formed of the aetiology, pathological lesions and disordered functions which constitute the patient's disease. This may enable the disease to be placed in a certain recognized category but, of far greater importance, it also provides a sure basis for the treatment and prognosis of the individual patient. **Aetiological diagnosis.** Diagnosis based on aetiology; in the case of an infective disease, the recognition of the causal micro-organism, its source, mode of infection and the factors, extrinsic and intrinsic, which determine the patient's susceptibility. **Anatomical diagnosis.** Determination of the organ or region of the body concerned in a pathological process. **Biological diagnosis.** The use of animals for certain diagnostic tests, e.g. the Ascheim–Zondek test. **Clinical diagnosis.** Diagnosis by bedside methods without the aid of laboratory tests. **Cytohistological diagnosis, Cytological diagnosis.** That based on the presence of exfoliated specific cells in the exudates. **Differential diagnosis.** The recognition of a particular condition from amongst others which closely resemble it in certain respects. **Niveau diagnosis.** The determination of the level of a lesion, such as a tumour, in the spinal cord. **Regional diagnosis.** Anatomical diagnosis (see above). **Serum diagnosis.** The use of specific sera to identify a micro-organism. **Therapeutic diagnosis.** The immediate favourable response to a specific drug in a doubtful condition, e.g. to sodium salicylate in a doubtful case of acute rheumatism, or to antimalarial drugs in a doubtful fever. **Topographical diagnosis.** Anatomical diagnosis (see above). [Gk *dia, gnosis* knowledge.]

diagnostic (di·ag·**nos**·tik). 1. Indicating or determining the nature of a disease. 2. Aiding in or belonging to diagnosis. [see prec.]

diagnosticate (di·ag·**nos**·tik·ate). To diagnose.

diagnostician (**di**·ag·nos·**tish'**·un). 1. A person skilled in diagnosis. 2. The person who has made the diagnosis in a specific case.

diagnostics (di·ag·**nos**·tix). The science of diagnosis considered as a branch of medicine.

diagnostitial (**di**·ag·nos·**tish'**·al). Indicating any procedure undertaken for the purpose of diagnosis or as an aid to diagnosis.

diagometer (di·ag·**om**·et·er). An obsolete instrument used to compare the electrical conductivities of substances. [Gk *diagein* to transmit, meter.]

diagraph (**di**·ah·graf). A drawing instrument with which the outlines of an area or part, e.g. cranium, can be recorded. [Gk *dia, graphein* to record.]

diahydric (di·ah·**hi**·drik). A sound that has been transmitted through fluid or water, e.g. a percussion note. [Gk *dia, hydor* water.]

diakinesis (**di**·ah·kin·**e'**·sis). The final stage in prophase of meiosis, during which the paired homologous chromosomes shorten and thicken and take on the tetrad form. [Gk *dia, kinesis* motion.]

dial (di·al). **Astigmatic dial.** Black radiating lines on a white background at intervals of 10° for either 180° or 360° used for a subjective test for assessing the axis and degree of astigmatism. The patient views at 6 m, and is asked which line (or lines) is clearest and blackest. This indicates the axis of the astigmatism. [L *dialis* daily.]

dialectrolysis (di·al·ek·**trol**'·is·is). Term denoting electrolytic treatment with therapeutic ions; also known as *iontophoresis.* [Gk *dia,* electrolysis.]

dialectrothermy (di·al·ek·tro·**ther**'·me). Short-wave diathermy. *See* DIATHERMY.

Dialister (di·al·is·ter). A genus of organisms of the tribe Haemophileae in the family Parvobacteriaceae; minute rod-shaped cells, which are anaerobic and parasitic. The type species is *Dialister pneumosintes,* which is found in the nasopharyngeal washings of man, but seems to have no pathogenic properties.

diallyl (di·al·il). 1. Denoting an organic compound which contains two allyl, $CH_2{=}CHCH_2$-, groups. 2. Hexadienol, $CH_2{=}CHCH_2CH_2CH{=}CH_2$, a hydrocarbon of the acetylene series; a colourless liquid with a garlic odour. **Diallyl sulphide.** Allyl sulphide, $(CH_2{=}CHCH_2)S$, a yellowish liquid occurring in garlic; used orally in the treatment of phthisis and bronchitis, and externally in lupus and tuberculous abscesses.

diallylmalonylurea (di·**al**·il·mal·on·il·ewr·**e**'·ah). Allobarbitone.

diallylnortoxiferine (di·al·il·nor·tox·**if**'·er·een). A muscle relaxant, an alkaloid of calabashcurarine.

dialurate (di·al·**ewr**·ate). A salt formed by dialuric acid.

dialysable (di·al·i·zabl). Able to pass through a natural or artificial membrane. [Gk *dia, lysis* a loosing.]

dialysance (di·**al**·is·ans). The minute rate of net exchange of a substance between blood and bath fluid per unit blood-bath concentration gradient; a parameter in artificial kidney kinetics (non-filtration) functionally equivalent to the clearance of the natural kidney. [Gk *dia, lysis* a loosing.]

dialysate (di·**al**·is·ate). In dialysis, the crystalloid filtrate which has passed through a membrane.

dialyse (di·al·ize). To separate from a solution by dialysis.

dialyser (di·al·i·zer). 1. The apparatus used in dialysis. 2. A semipermeable membrane for use in dialysis.

dialysis (di·**al**·is·is). The process of separating the soluble crystalloid substances from the colloids in a mixture by means of a dialyser. **Peritoneal dialysis.** Dialysis in which the peritoneum is used as a dialysing membrane. Dialysing fluid is introduced via a catheter into the peritoneal cavity, where it remains for 1h, and is then drained. This cycle is repeated hourly until blood chemistry is satisfactory. **Dialysis retinae.** A tear occurring in the retina at the ora serrata; a frequent cause of retinal detachment. [Gk *dia, lysis* a loosing.]

dialytic (di·al·**it**·ik). 1. Pertaining to dialysis. 2. Evolutionary. 3. A remedy that induces relaxation. [see prec.]

diamagnetic (di·ah·mag·**net**'·ik). 1. Repelled by a magnet. 2. Tending to take a position at right angles to the lines of force in a magnetic field. [Gk *dia,* magnet.]

Diamanus (di·**am**·an·us). A genus of fleas of which *Diamanus montanus* is the commonest. It occurs on *Citellus beecheyi* and other ground squirrels in Western USA and is a vector of sylvatic plague.

diameter (di·**am**·et·er). 1. The chord passing through the centre of a circle, and hence applied to any line joining opposite points of a circular, or roughly circular, structure. 2. In anatomy, a straight line across any more or less circular structure or space and passing through its centre. The term is used most frequently to specify certain dimensions of the female pelvis. **Anteroposterior diameter.** 1. Of the brim of the pelvis: the line from the lumbosacral angle to the symphysis pubis. 2. Of the pelvic outlet: the line from the tip of the coccyx to the lower border of the symphysis pubis. **Auricular diameter.** In craniometry, the distance between the mid-points of the external auditory meati. **Bi-acromial diameter.** The transverse distance between the acromia. **Bi-ischial diameter.** The line joining the ischial tuberosities; the transverse diameter of the pelvic outlet. **Bimastoid diameter.** The transverse distance between the mastoid processes. **Biparietal diameter.** The transverse distance between the two parietal eminences. **Bispinous diameter.** The transverse distance between the ischial spines. **Bitemporal diameter.** The distance between the most distant parts of the coronal suture. **Bitrochanteric diameter.** The distance between the uppermost points of the greater trochanters. **Bituberous diameter.** A measurement used in radiological pelvimetry—the distance between the ischial tuberosities. **Buccolingual diameter.** The diameter of the crown of a tooth from the buccal to the lingual surface. **Cervicobregmatic diameter.** Submentobregmatic diameter (see below). **Coccygeopubic diameter.** Anteroposterior diameter of the pelvic outlet (see above). **Conjugate diameter.** Anteroposterior diameter of the inlet of the pelvis (see above). **Dental diameter.** The diameter of the crown of a tooth, either in a buccolingual or in a mesiodistal direction. **Diagonal conjugate diameter.** In obstetrics, the distance between the outer border of the symphysis pubis and the sacral promontory. **External conjugate diameter.** The line from the depression above the spine of the 1st sacral vertebra on the surface of the body to the upper border of the symphysis pubis; Baudelocque's diameter. **Fronto-occipital diameter.** A line from the depression at the root of the nose to the most projecting point on the occiput. **Intercristal diameter.** The greatest transverse distance between corresponding points on the crests of the right and left iliac bone. **Internal conjugate diameter.** The true conjugate diameter; the term is, however, not in general use today. **Interspinous diameter.** The distance between the outer edges of the anterior superior iliac spines. **Intertuberal diameter.** The distance between the ischial tuberosities. **Mean corpuscular diameter, MCD.** The mean diameter of erythrocytes obtained by direct measurement of from 200 to 500 according to techniques such as that of Price-Jones; the normal range is from 6.7 to 7.7 μm (mean 7.2 μm) according to Price-Jones. **Mentovertical diameter.** The distance between the point of the chin and the most distant point on the vertex. **Oblique diameter of the pelvic inlet [diameter obliqua (NA)].** The distance from the sacro-iliac joint to the iliopubic (iliopectineal) eminence. **Occipitofrontal diameter.** Fronto-occipital diameter (see above). **Parietal diameter.** Biparietal diameter (see above). **Posterior sagittal diameter.** The distance from the mid-point of a line joining the ischial tuberosities to the last sacral vertebra. **Pubotuberous diameter.** The vertical distance between the superior pubic ramus and the point of the tuberosity of the ischium. **Submentobregmatic diameter.** The line from the junction of the chin and neck in front to the middle of the anterior fontanelle. **Suboccipitobregmatic diameter.** The line from the junction of the head and neck behind to the middle of the anterior fontanelle. **Suboccipitofrontal diameter.** The line from the junction of the head and neck behind to the prominence of the forehead. **Suprasubparietal diameter.** The transverse distance between a point just above one parietal eminence and a point just below the other parietal eminence. **Trachelobregmatic diameter.** Submentobregmatic diameter (see above). **Transverse diameter of the pelvic inlet [diameter transversa (NA)].** The greatest transverse distance between corresponding joints on the brim of the pelvis, at right angles to the true conjugate. **Transverse diameter of the pelvic outlet.** Bi-ischial diameter (see above). **True conjugate diameter.** The distance between the sacral promontory and the middle of the inner aspect of the symphysis pubis. **Vertical diameter of the fetal head.** That extending from the highest point of the head to the anterior margin of the foramen magnum. **Zygomatic diameter.** The width of the skull at the level of the zygomatic arches. [Gk *diametros* measuring across.]

See also: BAUDELOCQUE, DEVENTER.

diamide (di·**am**·ide). 1. General term denoting an organic compound which contains two amido, $-CONH_2$, radicals. 2. Oxamide, $NH_2COCONH_2$, the amide of oxalic acid; an insoluble white crystalline substance. 3. Also applied, incorrectly, to a diamine and to hydrazine.

diamidine (di·am·id·een). General term for an organic compound which contains two amidine, NH=C(NH_2)-, groups: examples are propamidine and stilbamidine.

diamine (di·am·een). 1. General term denoting a compound which contains two amino, NH_2, groups. 2. Hydrazine, diamide, NH_2NH_2, a colourless liquid of value in organic synthesis, and the parent of a number of important derivatives. **Diamine oxidase.** Histamine oxidase, an enzyme which oxidizes diamines.

diamino-acridine (di·am·in·o·ak′·rid·een). Proflavine, $NH_2C_6H_2=(CHN)=C_6H_3NH_2$. A compound which is an effective germicide against Gram-positive micro-organisms in alkaline media, and at one time used as a trypanocide. It is excreted unchanged in the urine and acts as an effective urinary antiseptic. A 0.1 per cent solution is employed as a germicide for mucous membranes and for washing out wounds; also incorporated as an oleate in ointments and emulsions for application to open wounds. It has a weaker antiseptic action than acriflavine, but is more rapid and less toxic.

diaminodihydroxyarsenobenzene (di·am·in·o·di·hi·drox·e·ar·sen·o·ben′·zeen). Arsphenamine base, 3,3′-diamino-4,4′-dihydroxyarsenobenzene, $NH_2C_6H_3(OH)As{=}AsC_6H_3(OH)NH_2$. An amorphous yellow powder, the hydrochloride of which is soluble in water and was used formerly in the treatment of syphilis. It has now been largely replaced by penicillin.

diaminodiphosphatide (di·am·in·o·di·fos′·fat·ide). A member of a group of phospholipides which contain 2 phosphate groups and 2 basic nitrogenous groups.

diaminomonophosphatide (di·am·in·o·mon·o·fos′·fat·ide). A member of a group of phospholipides which contain 1 phosphate group and 2 basic nitrogenous groups.

2,4-diaminopyrimidines (di·am·in·o·pir·im′·id·eenz). A series of compounds to which the antimalarial, pyrimethamine, belongs.

diaminuria (di·am·in·ewr′·e·ah). The presence of diamine compounds in the urine.

Diamocaine (di·am·o·kane). BP Commission approved name for 1-(2-anilinoethyl)-4-(2-diethylaminoethoxy)-4-phenylpiperidine; a local anaesthetic.

Diamond, Joseph Solomon (b. 1881). New York physician.

Wallace and Diamond method. For urobilinogen in urine: urine is diluted stepwise until the red colour obtained with Ehrlich's reagent is just discernible, the result being expressed as the limiting dilution.

Diamond, Louis K. 20th century American physician.

Blackfan–Diamond syndrome. Congenital anaemia due to lack of red blood corpuscle precursors.

diamorphine (di·ah·mor·feen). Diacetylmorphine. **Diamorphine Hydrochloride BP 1973.** A crystalline compound more soluble than heroin and used hypodermically.

diamorphosis (di·ah·mor·fo′·sis). The condition of growing normally into shape. [Gk *dia*, morphosis.]

diamotosis (di·ah·mo·to′·sis). Packing of a wound or a lesion such as an abscess with lint. [Gk *dia*, *motos* lint.]

Diampromide (di·am·pro·mide). BP Commission approved name for *N*-[2-(*N*-methylphenethylamino)propyl]-propionanilide; an analgesic.

Diamthazole (di·am·thaz·ole). BP Commission approved name for 6,2′-diethylamino-ethoxy-2-dimethylaminobenzo-thiazole; a fungicide.

diamylene (di·am·il·een). $CH_2{=}CH(CH_3)_7CH_3$, an unsaturated liquid hydrocarbon of the olefine series.

diamylose (di·am·il·oze). Bisamylose, $C_{12}H_{20}O_{10}$. The anhydride of maltose, consisting of 2 α-glucopyranose rings, and considered the fundamental unit in the molecular structure of starch.

diandry (di·an·dre). The presence in the product of gametic fusion of 2 male nuclei and 1 female nucleus. [Gk *di-*, *aner* man.]

dianoetic (di·an·e·tik). Descriptive of intellectual function, particularly discursive reasoning. [Gk *dia*, *nous* mind.]

dianthin (di·an·thin). Erythrosin. **Dianthin B.** Sodium tetraiodofluorescein, a dyestuff used as an indicator for pH, changing at 2.0 from magenta to orange. **Dianthin G.** Potassium di-iodofluorescein.

diapason (di·ah·pa·zon). 1. A tuning-fork used in the diagnosis of ear affections and diseases to determine the degree of deafness present. 2. Generally, a harmonious combination of notes in music or a fixed standard of musical pitch; a burst of harmony. [Gk *dia*, *pason* (*chordon*) all (strings).]

diapedesis (di·ah·ped·e′·sis). The insinuation of intact cells (e.g. leucocytes) through a capillary wall. [Gk *dia*, *pedesis* an oozing.]

diapedetic (di·ah·ped·et′·ik). Referring to diapedesis.

diaphane (di·ah·fane). 1. The condensation of cell protoplasm which forms the transparent plasma membrane surrounding a cell. 2. The electric light used in a diaphanoscope. [Gk *diaphanes* shining through.]

diaphaneity (di·ah·fan·e′·it·e). The quality or state of being transparent. [see prec.]

diaphanometer (di·ah·fan·om′·et·er). An instrument with which, by means of transmitted light, the transparency of liquids or air can be measured. [Gk *diaphanes* shining through, *metron* measure.]

diaphanometry (di·ah·fan·om′·et·re). The measurement of transparency of a fluid or of air. [see prec.]

diaphanoscope (di·ah·fan·o·skope). An instrument with which a body cavity can be lighted up, its interior examined and its limits defined. [Gk *diaphanes* shining through, *skopein* to watch.]

diaphanoscopy (di·ah·fan·os′·ko·pe). Examination of a body cavity with a diaphanoscope.

diaphanous (di·af·an·us). Transparent or translucent. [Gk *diaphanes* shining through.]

diaphemetry (di·ah·fe·met′·re). The measurement of the degree of subjective tactile sensibility. [Gk *dia*, *haphe* touch, *metron* measure.]

diaphorase (di·af·or·aze). The flavoprotein which catalyses the reoxidation of NADH by the mitochondrial electron transport chain.

diaphoresis (di·ah·for·e′·sis). Sweating, particularly profuse perceptible sweating artificially induced. [Gk *dia*, *pherein* to carry.]

diaphoretic (di·ah·for·et′·ik). 1. Sudorific; producing sweat. 2. A drug which induces perspiration; also known as a *sudorific.* The chief drugs administered internally for this purpose are pilocarpine, ipecacuanha, and ipecacuanha with opium (Dover's powder). Pilocarpine stimulates the sweat glands directly; ipecacuanha, which is not effective, acts by causing vasodilatation; opium itself does not induce sweating but appears to augment the action of ipecacuanha. Diaphoresis may also be promoted by application of moist heat to the skin (Turkish baths). The salicylates and other antipyretics cause perspiration, chiefly during fevers. Other substances which are used include aconite, alcohol, ammonium acetate, ammonium chloride, antimony and potassium tartrate, camphor, physostigmine, potassium citrate and spirit of nitrous ether. [see prec.]

diaphotoscope (di·ah·fo·to·skope). A particular kind of endoscope. [Gk *dia*, *phos* light, *skopein* to watch.]

diaphragm (di·ah·fram). 1. A disc placed in an optical system to cut off a portion of a beam of light passing through the system. 2. A septum, such as that used in dialysis. 3. In anatomy [diaphragma (NA)], a thin layer of tissue stretched across an opening; in particular, the musculotendinous sheet which separates the abdominal from the thoracic cavity; the thoraco-abdominal diaphragm. **Central-stop diaphragm.** A diaphragm to cut off the central portion of a beam of light traversing an optical system. **Condensing diaphragm.** An iris diaphragm situated below the stage of a microscope for varying the amount of illumination, and so altering its character by reducing the size of the cone of emergent light. **Contraceptive diaphragm.** A rubber cap that fits over the cervix uteri. **Graduating diaphragm.** A graduated plate dropped into an eye-piece between the lenses, with which the sizes of particles or their number per unit area can be measured under the microscope. **Iris diaphragm.** An adjustable circular hole in the centre of an opaque circular disc to cut off the marginal portion of a beam of light traversing an optical system. **Diaphragm opening.** The aperture of an opaque diaphragm. **Opening in the diaphragm, aortic [hiatus aorticus (NA)].** A tendinous aperture between the medial borders of the crura in front of the body of the 12th thoracic vertebra. **Opening in the diaphragm, oesophageal [hiatus esophageus (NA)].** An opening in the musculature of the right crus opposite the 10th thoracic vertebra. **Opening in the diaphragm, vena-caval [foramen venae cavae (NA)].** A tendinous aperture in the posterior border of the central tendon at the junction of the right and central leaf. **Part of the diaphragm, costal [pars costalis (NA)].** That part arising from the lower 6 ribs and costal cartilages. **Part of the diaphragm, sternal [pars sternalis (NA)].** That part arising from the back of the xiphisternum. **Part of the diaphragm, vertebral [pars lumbalis (NA)].** That portion which arises from the lumbar vertebrae via the crura and from the arcuate ligaments. **Pelvic diaphragm [diaphragma pelvis (NA)].** The muscular partition between the pelvic cavity and the peritoneum which is formed by the levatores ani and the coccygei muscles. **Perineal diaphragm.** Urogenital diaphragm (see below). **Thoraco-abdominal diaphragm.** The diaphragm. *See* MAIN DEF. 3 (above). **Urogenital diaphragm [diaphragma urogenitale (NA)].** A double fibrous layer enclosing the sphincter urethrae and the deep transverse muscle of the perineum, and stretching across the subpubic arch. [Gk *diaphragma* partition.]

See also: BUCKY, POTTER (H. E.).

diaphragma (di·ah·**frag**·mah). Diaphragm. **Diaphragma oris.** The floor of the mouth, formed by the 2 mylohyoid muscles. **Diaphragma sellae (NA).** A circular fold of dura mater which forms the roof over the pituitary fossa of the sphenoid bone; it is pierced centrally by the stalk of the pituitary body. [Gk partition.]

diaphragmalgia, diaphragmatalgia (di·ah·frag·**mal**'·je·ah, di·ah·-frag·mat·**al**'·je·ah). A sensation of pain in the diaphragm. [diaphragm, Gk *algos* pain.]

diaphragmatic (di·ah·frag·**mat**'·ik). Pertaining to a diaphragm.

diaphragmatitis (di·ah·frag·mat·**i**'·tis). Inflammation of the diaphragm. [diaphragm, Gk *-itis* inflammation.]

diaphragmatocele (di·ah·frag·**mat**'·o·seel). Diaphragmatic hernia. *See* HERNIA. [diaphragm, Gk *kele* hernia.]

diaphragmitis (di·ah·frag·**mi**'·tis). Diaphragmatitis.

diaphragmodynia (di·ah·frag·mo·**din**'·e·ah). Diaphragmalgia. [diaphragm, Gk *odyne* pain.]

diaphylactic (di·ah·fil·**ak**'·tik). Prophylactic. [Gk *diaphylaktikos* preserving.]

diaphyseal (di·ah·**fiz**·e·al). Belonging to or affecting the shaft of a long bone. [diaphysis.]

diaphysectomy (di·ah·fiz·**ek**'·to·me). Surgical removal of the shaft of a long bone. [diaphysis, Gk *ektome* a cutting out.]

diaphysis [NA] (di·**af**·is·is). The shaft of a long bone. [Gk *dia*, *phyein* to grow.]

diaphysitis (di·af·iz·**i**'·tis). Inflammation of the shaft of a long bone. [diaphysis, Gk *-itis* inflammation.]

diapiresis (di·ah·pi·**re**'·sis). Diapedesis. [Gk *diapeirein* to push through.]

diaplacental (di·ah·plas·**en**'·tal). By way of the placenta. [Gk *dia*, placenta.]

diaplasis (di·**ap**·las·is). Reduction of a dislocation or fracture. [Gk a putting into shape.]

diaplastic (di·ah·**plas**·tik). Referring to diaplasis.

diaplex (di·ah·plex). The choroid plexus of the 3rd ventricle. [Gk *dia*, plexus.]

diaplexal (di·ah·**plex**·al). Relating to the diaplex.

diaplexus (di·ah·**plex**·us). Diaplex.

diapnoe (di·**ap**·no·e). Slight invisible sweating; insensible perspiration. [Gk *diapnon* exhalation.]

diapnoic (di·ap·**no**·ik). Inducing or pertaining to mild sweating. [see prec.]

diapophysis (di·ah·**pof**·is·is). The articular portion, on the superior aspect, of a vertebral transverse process. [Gk *dia*, apophysis.]

Diaptomus (di·**ap**·to·mus). A genus of copepods of which several species act as intermediate hosts to *Diphyllobothrium latum.*

diapyema (di·ah·pi·**e**'·mah) (pl. *diapyemata*). Abscess. [Gk *dia*, *pyon* pus, *haima* blood.]

diapyesis (di·ah·pi·**e**'·sis). Pyosis. [Gk *dia*, *pyon* pus.]

diapyetic (di·ah·pi·**et**'·ik). Producing or causing suppuration. [see prec.]

diarrhoea (di·ar·e·ah). The frequent passage of unformed liquid stools. **Acute diarrhoea.** Diarrhoea of sudden onset. **Diarrhoea alba.** Hill diarrhoea (see below). **Cachectic diarrhoea.** A terminal event in severe cachectic diseases. **Catarrhal diarrhoea.** Diarrhoea due to enteritis. **Choleraic diarrhoea.** Diarrhoea due to cholera, or severe acute diarrhoea with very frequent passage of watery cholera-like stools. **Chronic diarrhoea.** Persistent diarrhoea. **Climatic diarrhoea.** Diarrhoea due to exposure to cold. **Cochin-China diarrhoea.** Hill diarrhoea (see below). **Colliquative diarrhoea.** Profuse watery diarrhoea leading to dehydration. **Critical diarrhoea.** Diarrhoea occurring at the crisis of an acute disease. **Dysenteric diarrhoea.** Diarrhoea with blood and mucus in the stools. **Epidemic diarrhoea of infants.** Summer diarrhoea of children; an infectious disease. **Epidemic diarrhoea of the newborn.** A term used to describe a severe gastro-enteritis of any type occurring in epidemic form in the newborn. **Fatty diarrhoea.** Diarrhoea with undigested fat in the stools. **Fermentative diarrhoea.** Diarrhoea associated with organisms causing fermentation of carbohydrates. **Flagellate diarrhoea.** Diarrhoea associated with the presence of flagellate organisms, e.g. *Giardia intestinalis,* in the stools. **Gastrogenous diarrhoea.** Diarrhoea of gastric origin, due to deficiency or absence of hydrochloric acid in the gastric juice. **Hill diarrhoea.** An outmoded concept of an acute sprue-like diarrhoea that attacks newcomers, especially Europeans, at high altitudes in the Himalayas, no longer considered a specific disease. **Infantile diarrhoea.** Epidemic diarrhoea of infants (see above). **Inflammatory diarrhoea.** Catarrhal diarrhoea (see above). **Irritative diarrhoea.** That due to mechanical or chemical irritants in the food. **Lienteric diarrhoea.** Diarrhoea occurring immediately after meals. **Membranous diarrhoea.** Mucomembranous colitis. **Mucous diarrhoea.** Diarrhoea with excess of mucus in the stools. **Neonatal diarrhoea.** Diarrhoea in the newborn. **Nervous diarrhoea.** Diarrhoea due to excessive peristalsis from emotional disturbance. **Diarrhoea pancreatica, Pancreatogenous diarrhoea.** Diarrhoea from failure of pancreatic digestion. **Paradoxical diarrhoea.** The passage of fluid mucoid stool occurring with constipation and due to the irritation of hard faecal masses. **Parasitic diarrhoea.** Diarrhoea due to the irritation of intestinal parasites. **Parenteral diarrhoea.** Diarrhoea of which the cause lies outside the bowel. **Postprandial diarrhoea.** Lienteric diarrhoea (see above). **Putrefactive diarrhoea.** Offensive alkaline stools from excessive putrefaction. **Soapy diarrhoea.** Diarrhoea in which the stools contain fatty acids and soaps from deficient absorption, but with normal pancreatic digestion. **Summer diarrhoea.** Epidemic diarrhoea of infants (see above). **Toxic diarrhoea.** Diarrhoea caused by the ingestion of toxic material in the food. **Traveller's diarrhoea.** An acute gastro-enteritis due to bacterial infection acquired on journeys or in foreign countries due to contaminated food, often by an *Escherichia coli.* **Trench diarrhoea.** Diarrhoea due to infections under the conditions of trench warfare. **Tropical diarrhoea.** Hill diarrhoea (see above). **Tuberculous diarrhoea.** Diarrhoea due to tuberculous ulceration of the bowel. **Uraemic diarrhoea.** Diarrhoea occurring in advanced chronic nephritis. **Verminous diarrhoea.** That due to parasitic worms. **Virus diarrhoea.** Diarrhoea due to a filtrable virus. **Watery diarrhoea.** Excessively liquid stools. **Zymotic diarrhoea.** Hill diarrhoea (see above). [Gk *dia*, *rhein* to flow.]

See also: REIMANN.

diarrhoeal (di·ar·e·al). Belonging, simulating or characterized by the presence of diarrhoea.

diarthric (di·**ar**·thrik). Relating to 2 joints. [Gk *di-*, *arthron* joint.]

diarthrodial (di·ar·**thro**·de·al). Relating to or of the nature of a diarthrosis. [diarthrosis, Gk *eidos* like.]

diarthrosis (di·ar·**thro**·sis). A type of articulation which permits of movement in any direction, the opposing bones being held in apposition. **Diarthrosis ambigua.** Amphiarthrosis. **Diarthrosis obliqua.** A variable articulation which may occur between the spines of adjacent lumbar vertebrae. **Diarthrosis obliqua accessoria.** A double articulation sometimes occurring between the spines of adjacent thoracic or lumbar vertebrae near the roots of the articular processes. **Planiform diarthrosis.** Arthrodia. **Diarthrosis rotatoria, Rotatory diarthrosis, Synarthrodial diarthrosis, Trochoid diarthrosis, Diarthrosis trochoides.** Pivot joint. *See* JOINT. [Gk articulation.]

diarticular (di·ar·**tik**·ew·lar). Biarticular. [Gk *di-*, L *articulare* to divide into joints.]

diaschisis (di·**as**·kis·is). A loss of functional activity due to damage or disease interrupting the passage of stimuli along neurons. [Gk *dia, schizein* to split.]

diascope (**di**·as·kope). 1. A flat glass plate through which, when it is pressed against the skin, superficial lesions and changes in the tissues can be clearly observed. 2. Diaphanoscope. [Gk *dia, skopein* to watch.]

diascopic (di·as·**kop**·ik). Referring to a diascope, or to anything seen by means of a diascope.

diascopy (di·**as**·ko·pe). 1. Examination of the skin through a diascope. 2. Diaphanoscopy.

diasostic (di·as·**os**·tik). 1. Hygienic. 2. The guarding of health. 3. Diateretic. [Gk *diasozein* to preserve.]

diastalsis (di·as·**tal**·sis). Movement in the small intestine which consists in a wave of inhibition followed by a downward moving wave of contraction (Cannon). Cf. ANASTALSIS, CATASTALSIS. [Gk *dia, stellein* to set.]

diastaltic (di·as·**tal**·tik). Referring to reflex action effected by way of the spinal cord. [see prec.]

diastasaemia (**di**·as·ta·**se**′·me·ah). The separation from each other of the constituents of the erythrocytes, resulting in various degrees of anasarca. [Gk *diastasis* separation, *haima* blood.]

diastase (**di**·as·taze). Amylase; any of a class of enzymes occurring widely in animal and plant tissues which break down starch and glycogen to give dextrins and maltose. In animals the richest source is the pancreas, whilst the chief vegetable source is malt. Diastase occurs normally to a slight extent in blood and urine, but becomes greatly increased in acute pancreatitis. **Salivary diastase.** Ptyalin. **Urinary diastase.** Diastase excreted in the urine. The amount is normally quite small, but is greatly increased in acute pancreatitis. *See* WOHLGEMUTH'S TEST. [Gk *diastasis* separation.]

diastasic (di·as·**ta**·sik). 1. Referring to diastase. 2. Diastatic.

diastasimetry (**di**·**as**·ta·**zim**′·et·re). Determination of the power of starch-digesting extracts to convert starch into sugar. [diastase, Gk *metron* measure.]

diastasis (di·**as**·tas·is). 1. Forcible simple separation of parts that normally are joined. 2. Dislocation of 2 bones between which a synovial joint does not exist. **Diastasis cordis.** The latter part of diastole in the cardiac cycle when there is a period of apparent rest, the blood entering the ventricle only slowly under pressure from the veins. **Iris diastasis.** A colobomatous defect of the peripheral part of the iris, leaving the pupillary margin intact; rarely multiple iridodiastasis. **Diastasis recti abdominis.** A condition in which there is an abnormal gap between the rectus abdominis muscles, as may occur after abdominal operations or during pregnancy. [Gk separation.]

diastasum (di·as·ta·sum). Diastase.

diastasuria (**di**·**as**·ta·**sewr**′·e·ah). The presence of diastase in the urine.

diastatic (di·as·**tat**·ik). 1. Referring to diastasis. 2. Referring to diastase. 3. Converting starch into sugar. [Gk *diastasis* separation.]

diastem, diastema (**di**·as·tem, di·as·**te**·mah). 1. A pronounced gap between the lateral incisor and canine teeth of the upper jaw in some animals, into which an enlarged lower canine bites. 2. The equatorial plate of modified cytoplasm along which a cell divides in mitosis. 3. In dentistry, a space between 2 teeth not produced by loss of the tooth or teeth normally lying between them. [Gk *diastema* interval.]

diastematocrania (di·as·te·mat·o·**kra**′·ne·ah). A congenital fissure along the median line of the skull. [diastema, Gk *kranion* skull.]

diastematomyelia (di·as·**te**·mat·o·mi·**e**′·le·ah). Congenital splitting of a part of the spinal cord or of its entire length. [diastema, Gk *myelos* marrow.]

diastematopyelia (di·as·**te**·mat·o·pi·**e**′·le·ah). A congenital fissure which runs along the median line of the pelvis. [diastema, Gk *pyelos* trough.]

diaster (di·**as**·ter). Amphiaster. [Gk *di-, aster* star.]

diastole (di·**as**·to·le). The period of the cardiac cycle from the closure of the aortic and pulmonary valves to the beginning of the next ventricular contraction. The period when the heart fills with blood and dilates. **Arterial diastole.** The dilatation of an artery after the ventricular systole. **Atrial diastole.** That period of time other than when the atrium is contracting. **Auricular diastole.** Atrial distole (see above). **Cardiac diastole.** The phase of relaxation and expansion after a cardiac contraction. **Reflex diastole.** The change from red to white of the line marked on the skin when a blunt point is drawn firmly across it. **Ventricular diastole.** Diastole of the ventricles of the heart. [Gk *dia, stellein* to set.]

diastolic (di·as·**tol**·ik). Referring or belonging to diastole.

diastolization (di·**as**·tol·i·**za**′·shun). 1. Dilatation. 2. The dilatation of the nasal passages and massage of the mucous membrane as a method of treatment of hypertrophic rhinitis. The instrument used is a hollow rubber bougie, the inflation and deflation of which is controlled by pressure on a rubber bulb. [Gk *dia, stellein* to set.]

diastomyelia (di·**as**·to·mi·**e**′·le·ah). Diastematomyelia.

diataxia (di·at·**ax**·e·ah). Ataxia affecting both sides of the body. **Cerebral diataxia, Diataxia cerebralis infantilis.** Cerebral birth palsy in which there is bilateral paralysis of ataxic type. [Gk *di-*, ataxia.]

diatela, diatele (di·at·e·lah, **di**·at·eel). The roof of the 3rd ventricle of the forebrain. [Gk *dia*, L *tela* web.]

diateretic (**di**·at·er·**et**′·ik). Referring to the practical application of hygienic science. [Gk *diaterein* to watch closely.]

diathermacy (di·ah·**ther**·mas·e). The quality or condition of being able to absorb heat rays. [Gk *diathermasia* a warming through.]

diathermanous (di·ah·**ther**·man·us). Allowing the passage of heat rays. [Gk *diathermainein* to warm through.]

diathermia (di·ah·**ther**·me·ah). Diathermy.

diathermic (di·ah·**ther**·mik). Referring to diathermy.

diathermocoagulation (di·ah·**ther**·mo·ko·ag·ew·**la**′·shun). Surgical diathermy. [diathermy, L *coagulare* to curdle.]

diathermometer (**di**·ah·ther·**mom**′·et·er). An instrument for measuring the thermal conductivity of a substance. [Gk *dia*, thermometer.]

diathermy (di·ah·**ther**·me). A method of providing "deep" heat by high-frequency electrical currents (ultra-short-wave or short-wave), electromagnetic waves (microwaves) or very-high-frequency vibrations (ultrasonics or ultrasound). **Conventional diathermy.** The generation of heat in the body tissues as the result of the passage of an oscillating electric current of frequency from 500 000 to 1 500 000 Hz, and wavelengths between 100 and 600 m. **Long-wave diathermy.** Medical diathermy employing high-frequency currents of wavelengths between 100 and 300 m. **Medical diathermy.** The use of a high-frequency current to generate heat in the tissues sufficient to warm but not damage them. **Microwave diathermy.** Medical diathermy employing high-frequency currents of wavelengths from 10 cm to 1 m. **Short-wave diathermy.** Medical diathermy employing high-frequency currents of wavelengths between 3 and 30 m. **Surgical diathermy.** The passage of a high-frequency electric current by knife or button electrode to generate heat in the tissues for the destruction of pathological tissue, the coagulation of bleeding vessels or the bloodless division of tissues. **Ultra-short-wave diathermy.** Medical diathermy employing high-frequency currents of wavelengths less than 10 m. **Ultrasonic diathermy.** A mechanical form of treatment using the propagation and absorption of very-high-frequency vibrations. [Gk *dia, therme* heat.]

diathesis (di·ath·es·is). The inborn constitutional make-up of an individual that predisposes him to a certain disease or group of diseases; the genetical factors which determine the way the tissues of the body react to certain noxious stimuli of exogenous or endogenous origin. It is not a sharply defined condition because, like stature, it is determined by a number of genes, i.e. a polygenic system, in constrast to well-defined familial diseases such as haemophilia and night blindness which are due to a single dominant or recessive gene. **Allergic diathesis.** A tendency to suffer from urticaria, eczema, prurigo, asthma and other disorders of allergic origin. **Contractional diathesis.** A tendency to develop contractures: often hysterical. **Exudative diathesis.** Allergic diathesis (see above). **Furuncular diathesis.** Chronic furunculosis. **Gouty diathesis.** A predisposition to suffer from an excess of uric acid in the blood, due to a fault of the purine metabolism. **Hereditary haemorrhagic diathesis.** Hémogénie diathéseque, a familial non-thrombocytopenic haemorrhagic condition transmitted to either sex, characterized by bleeding from the nose and mucous membranes, prolonged bleeding time, but normal coagulation time, clot retraction and platelet count. Tourniquet (Hess) test may be positive. There are two groups, thrombo-asthenia (Glanzmann), and constitutional thrombopathy (von Willebrand) or pseudohaemophilia in which the bleeding tendency is inherited in both sexes as a dominant sex-linked character. **Hypersthenic gastric diathesis.** A diathesis associated with hyperchlorhydria and usually a short, high, rapidly-emptying stomach. It predisposes to peptic ulcers. **Hyposthenic gastric diathesis.** One associated with hypochlorhydria and achlorhydria, and with a long, low, slowly-emptying stomach. It predisposes to cholecystitis, intestinal infections and anaemia. **Neuropathic diathesis.** A tendency to respond to mental stress by the production of an abnormal mental reaction, i.e a neurosis. **Oxalic diathesis.** A tendency to develop oxaluria. **Psychopathic diathesis.** The predisposition to develop mental disease; the particular type of mental disease is also determined by the diathesis, e.g. manic-depressive diathesis, schizophrenic diathesis. **Scrofulous diathesis.** Tuberculous diathesis (see below). **Thrombo-asthenic diathesis.** Hereditary haemorrhagic diathesis (see above). **Tuberculous diathesis.** A tendency to develop tuberculous disease. **Uric-acid diathesis.** Gouty diathesis (see above). **Varicose diathesis.** A tendency to develop varicose veins. [Gk arrangement.]

diathetic (di·ath·et·ik). Referring or belonging to a diathesis.

diatom (di·at·om). Any microscopical unicellular seaweed or freshwater alga, the cell wall of which is siliceous and persists as a skeleton after the animal's death. Each individual cell is composed of 2 halves or valves. [Gk *diatomos* cut in two.]

diatomaceous (di·at·om·a'·shus). Composed of the shells of diatoms. **Diatomaceous earth.** Kieselguhr, a porous form of silica found in deposits in Germany and Scotland, and composed of the fossilized shells of diatoms; was used in the manufacture of dynamite and as a polishing powder. [see prec.]

Diatomea (di·at·o·me'·ah). A class of unicellular algae with silica walls; diatoms. [Gk *diatomos* cut in two.]

diatomic (di·at·om·ik). 1. Describing a molecule in which there are 2 atoms only. 2. Applied to an acid that has 2 replaceable hydrogen atoms, or to an alcohol or base that has 2 replaceable hydroxyl groups. [Gk *di-*, atom.]

Diatomite BPC 1949 (di·at·om·ite). Purified kieselguhr. A white or faintly buff powder, light and bulky, used as a filtering medium and as a dusting absorbent.

diatoric (di·at·or·ik). A type of artificial tooth with a channel running in an anteroposterior direction to provide attachment for the material forming the base of an artificial denture. [Gk *diatoros* pierced.]

diauchenos (di·awk·en·os). A monster with 2 heads and necks. [Gk *di-*, *auchen* neck.]

diaxon, diaxone (di·ax·on). A nerve cell with 2 axons. [Gk *di-*, axon.]

diazene (di·az·een). A diazo compound; one of a group of organic compounds containing the radical -N=N-.

Diazepam BP 1973 (di·az·e·pam). A tranquillizer or sedative of the benzodiazepine group which can be given intravenously or by mouth. It can be used for the induction of anaesthesia.

diazine (di·az·een). 1. A general term for a member of a series of heterocyclic compounds containing a 6-membered ring, comprising 2 nitrogen and 4 carbon atoms. 2. Any ring compound containing 2 nitrogen atoms in its structure.

diazo (di·az·o). A distinctive prefix denoting that the compound to which it is applied contains the group -N=N-. **Diazo compound.** *See* COMPOUND. **Diazo reaction.** *See* REACTION.
See also: EHRLICH.

diazobenzene (di·az·o·ben'·zeen). The monovalent radical, $C_6H_5N{=}N$-, occurring in many diazo compounds.

diazoma (di·az·o·mah). The diaphragm. [Gk.]

diazone (di·ah·zone). One of the markings seen in a section of enamel due to groups of enamel prisms being cut transversely. [Gk *dia*, *zone* belt.]

diazotization (di·az·o·ti·za'·shun). In chemical synthesis, the process of converting amino NH_2 groups into diazo N_2 groups, by treating a primary amine with nitrous acid.

diazotize (di·az·o·tize). To bring about diazotization.

Diazoxide (di·az·ox·ide). BP Commission approved name for 7-chloro-3-methyl-1,2,4-benzothiadiazine 1,1-dioxide; a hypotensive.

dibasic (di·ba·sik). 1. Bibasic. Term applied to an acid that has 2 atoms of hydrogen replaceable by a metal or radical. *See* BASICITY. 2. Of an alcohol, one containing 2 hydroxyl groups. [Gk *di-*, basic.]

dibenzanthracene (di·benz·an·thras·een). $C_{22}H_{14}$, a polycyclic hydrocarbon derived from coal tar. It gives rise to epithelial tumours and sometimes sarcomas when injected into susceptible animals such as the rat and mouse.

Dibenzepin (di·benz·e·pin). BP Commission approved name for 4-(2-dimethylaminoethyl)-1,4-dihydro-1-methyl-2,3:6,7-dibenzo-1,4-diazepin-5-one; an antidepressant.

dibenzyl (di·ben·zil). 1. A prefix denoting a compound that contains 2 benzyl, $C_6H_5CH_2$-, groups. 2. $C_6H_5CH_2CH_2C_6H_5$, a crystalline hydrocarbon prepared by condensation from benzyl chloride.

dibenzylamine (di·ben·zil·am·een). $C_6H_5CH_2NHCH_2C_6H_5$, a colourless oily liquid.

dibenzyl-β-chloroethylamine (di·ben·zil·be·tah·klor·o·eth·il·am'·een). *N,N*-dibenzyl-beta-chloroethylamine, $(C_6H_5CH_2)_2NCH_2CH_2Cl$. A compound related chemically to the nitrogen-mustard compounds, which opposes the stimulatory actions of adrenaline and noradrenaline, and hence reverses the rise in blood pressure produced by the adrenaline. It is effective against injected and circulating adrenaline and, in larger doses, against adrenergic nerve stimulation; it does not block the cardiac effects of adrenaline. Side-effects include stimulation of the central nervous system and orthostatic hypotension. It may be used as a diagnostic in phaeochromocytoma, and is of value in moderately advanced hypertension (not in essential). Since it increases peripheral blood flow, it may prove helpful in frostbite and Raynaud's disease.

dibenzyline (di·ben·zil·een). A synthetic adrenergic blocking agent.

diblastic (di·blas·tik). Of twofold origin. [Gk *di-*, *blastos* germ.]

diblastula (di·blas·tew·lah). A blastula in which entodermal and ectodermal areas are present. [Gk *di-*, blastula.]

diborated (di·bor·a·ted). Applied to a compound which has in its composition 2 boric-acid radicals. [Gk *di-*, boric acid.]

dibothriocephaliasis (di·both·re·o·kef·al·i'·as·is). Diphyllobothriasis. [Gk *di-*, *bothrion* pit, *kephale* head.]

Dibothriocephalus (di·both·re·o·kef'·al·us). *Diphyllobothrium*, a genus of tapeworms. [see prec.]

dibromated (di·bro·ma·ted). Applied to a compound which has 2 bromine atoms in its structure. [Gk *di-*, bromine.]

dibromethane (di·brom·e·thane). Dibromoethane, ethylene dibromide, $BrCH_2CH_2Br$. A colourless liquid similar in properties to chloroform and prepared from glycol.

dibromethylene (di·brom·eth·il·een). $C_2H_2Cl_2$, an additive compound derived from acetylene. It is a non-steriod oestrogen.

dibromide (di·bro·mide). A salt of hydrobromic acid which contains 2 bromine atoms.

dibromoethane (di·bro·mo·e′·thane). Dibromethane.

dibromoketone (di·bro·mo·ke′·tone). Methyl dibromoethyl ketone, $CH_3COCHBrCH_2Br$. A poisonous vapour used in chemical warfare.

Dibromopropamidine Isethionate BP 1973 (di·bro·mo·pro·pam′·id·een i·zeth·i·on·ate). $[NH_2C(=NH)C_6H_3BrO]_2(CH_2)_3 2C_2H_5{=}HSO_4$, a compound used for the prophylaxis of skin infections. It is almost as active against Gram-positive organisms as penicillin.

dibucaine hydrochloride (di·bew·kane hi·dro·klor·ide). Cinchocaine Hydrochloride BP 1958.

Dibupyrone (di·bew·pi·rone). BP Commission approved name for sodium 2,3-dimethyl-1-phenyl-5-pyrazolon-4-yl-*N*-isobutylaminomethanesulphonate; an analgesic.

dibutyl (di·bew·til). 1. Applied to a compound containing two butyl, $CH_3CH_2CH_2CH_2$–, groups. 2. Octane, C_8H_{18}, a hydrocarbon, eighth of the methane series, which occurs in petroleum. **Dibutyl Phthalate BP 1963.** $C_4H_9OOCC_6H_4COOC_4H_9$, the dibutyl ester of phthalic acid. It is slightly less effective than dimethyl phthalate as a general insect repellent, but is more specific in its action against trombidiid mites and is therefore more useful in the prevention of scrub typhus.

dibutyrin (di·bew·tir·in). Glycerol dibutyrate, $(CH_3CH_2CH_2COO)_2C_3H_5OH$. An oily liquid formed by the pancreatic digestion of butyrin.

dicacodyl (di·kak·o·dil). Cacodyl, tetramethyldiarsine, $(CH_3)_2As As(CH_3)_2$. A colourless liquid, insoluble in water, formed from cacodyl chloride. Its vapour has a disgusting odour that causes vomiting, is exceedingly poisonous and is liable to ignite spontaneously.

dicalcic (di·kal·sik). Applied to a compound which contains 2 atoms of calcium. **Dicalcic orthophosphate.** Dicalcium phosphate. [Gk *di-*, calcium.]

dicalcium phosphate (di·kal·se·um fos·fate). Dicalcic orthophosphate, dibasic calcium phosphate, calcium hydrogen phosphate, $CaHPO_4{\cdot}2H_2O$. An insoluble crystalline substance precipitated from acid solutions of a calcium salt by sodium phosphate, and appearing in the urine in phosphaturia. It is of value in calcium therapy.

dicamphendion (di·kam·fen·de·on). $(C_{10}H_{14}O)_2$, a yellow crystalline substance formed by the condensation of 2 molecules of bromocamphor with metallic sodium.

dicamphor (di·kam·for). $(C_{10}H_{15}O)_2$, colourless crystals formed at the same time as dicamphendion in the condensation of bromocamphor molecules with metallic sodium.

dicarbonate (di·kar·bon·ate). A term rarely used, bicarbonate being the more customary.

dicarboxylic (di·kar·box·il′·ik). With 2 carboxyl groups.

dicelous (di·se·lus). Dicoelous.

Dicentra (di·sen·trah). A genus of North American plants of the family Fumariaceae. **Dicentra canadensis.** Squirrel corn, Turkey corn; a species containing the alkaloid protopine. **Dicentra cucullaria.** Dutchman's breeches; a species containing, among other alkaloids, cryptopine. With the former species it is used in the form of a decoction as a tonic and diuretic (corydalis). [Gk *dikentros* with 2 points.]

dicentric (di·sen·trik). Of chromosomes or chromatids, with 2 centromeres. [Gk *di-*, L *centrum* centre.]

dicentrine (di·sen·treen). $C_{20}H_{21}O_4N$, an alkaloid isolated from *Dicentra pusilla* (family Fumariaceae). It has a paralysing effect on the respiratory centre.

dicephalism (di·kef·al·izm). The condition of being two-headed. [Gk *di-*, *kephale* head.]

dicephalous (di·kef·al·us). Two-headed. [see prec.]

dicephalus (di·kef·al·us). A two-headed monster. [Gk *di-*, *kephale* head.]

dicephaly (di·kef·al·e). Dicephalism.

dichastasis (di·kas·tas·is). Biological spontaneous subdivision. [Gk division.]

dicheirus, dichirus (di·ki·rus). A congenital abnormality; duplication of the hand. [Gk *di-*, *cheir* hand.]

Dichloralphenazone BP 1973 (di·klor·al·fen′·az·one). A complex of chloral hydrate and phenazone; a hypnotic and sedative.

dichloramine (di·klor·am·een). Dichloramine-T, toluene-*p*-sulphondichloramide, $CH_3C_6H_4SO_2NCl_2$. An organic compound containing loosely-linked chlorine. It differs from chloramine-T in having 2 chlorine atoms attached to the nitrogen atom, and in being soluble in oil and organic solvents but not in water. It is a powerful germicide owing to the release of active chlorine and is employed most usually dissolved in chlorinated paraffin. This solution, which is stable for a few days, produces a sustained antiseptic action. For application to wounds a 5 per cent solution is employed and for mucous mebranes 1–2 per cent. It may become irritating owing to the formation of hydrochloric acid, and both the drug and its solution should be protected from sunlight.

dichlorbenzene, dichlorbenzol (di·klor·ben·zeen, di·klor·ben·zol). Paradichlorobenzene, $C_6H_4Cl_2$. A white compound used as an insecticide, and especially valuable for killing moths, the vapour being toxic to insects, larvae and eggs. It is poisonous to humans.

dichlordioxydiamido-arsenobenzol (di·klor·di·ox·e·di·am·id·o-ar·sen·o·ben′·zol). Arsphenamine hydrochloride.

dichlorethyl sulphide (di·klor·eth·il sul·fide). Dichorodiethyl sulphide.

dichlorethylarsine (di·klor·eth·il·ar′·seen). Ethyldichlorarsine, $C_2H_5AsCl_2$. A liquid used in chemical warfare as a nose gas under the name *dick.* It is an irritant to the nasal mucous membranes and to the lungs, producing an asthmatic condition; also a powerful vesicant.

dichlorhydrin (di·klor·hi·drin). α-Dichlorhydrin, $(CH_2Cl)_2CHOH$. A colourless ether-like liquid which dissolves resins, and is used in the manufacture of varnishes and lacquers.

dichloride (di·klor·ide). A salt of hydrochloric acid which contains 2 atoms of chlorine.

dichlormethane (di·klor·me·thane). Dichloromethane, methylene chloride, CH_2Cl_2. A heavy volatile liquid closely resembling chloroform, from which it can be prepared.

dichlorocresol (di·klor·o·kre′·sol). An antiseptic of the chlorinated phenol type having a wider range of activity than chloroxylenol.

dichlorodiethyl sulphide (di·klor·o·di·eth′·il sul·fide). $\beta\beta$-Dichlorethyl sulphide, mustard gas, yperite, $(CH_2ClCH_2)_2S$. Prepared industrially from ethylene and sulphur chloride, an oily vesicant liquid used in chemical warfare as a blister gas.

Dichlorodifluoromethane BPC 1968 (di·klor·o·di·floo·or·o·me′·thane). Emperical formula CCl_2F_2, a refrigerant and an aerosol propellant, gaseous at ordinary temperatures but liquefied by compression and supplied in suitable metal containers. It is usually mixed with other compounds of the same type, such as dichlorotetrafluoroethane, as vehicles for analgesic or anaesthetic sprays.

dichlorodiphenyltrichloro-ethane (di·klor·o·di·fe·nil·tri·klor·o·e′·thane). Dicophane BP 1958.

dichlorodivinylchloroarsine (di·klor·o·di·vi·nil·klor·o·ar′·seen). Di-β-chlorovinylchloroarsine, $AsCl(CH{=}CHCl)_2$. A vesicant liquid; mixed with chlorovinyldichloroarsine it forms *lewisite*, a blister gas used in chemical warfare.

dichlorohydroxymethylquinoline (di·klor·o·hi·drox·e·meth·il·kwin′·o·leen). 5,7-Dichloro-8-hydroxy-2-methylquinoline. A synthetic bacteriostatic related to oxine (8-hydroxyquinoline). It is used in ointment form for bacterial and mycotic skin infections.

dichloromethane (di·klor·o·me′·thane). Dichlormethane.

dichloromethyl ether (di·klor·o·meth·il e·ther). $(CH_2Cl)_2O$. A colourless liquid used in chemical warfare as a blister gas.

Dichlorophen BP 1973 (di·klor·o·fen). di-(5-Chloro-2-hydroxyphenyl)methane, an anthelminthic used especially against the human tapeworm, *Taenia saginata.*

Dichlorophenarsine (di·**klor**·o·fen·**ar**′·seen). BP Commission approved name for 3-amino-4-hydroxyphenyldichloroarsine, $NH_2C_6H_3(OH)AsCl_2$. A base, the hydrochloride of which in alkaline buffer solution is used intravenously in the treatment of syphilis.

dichlorophenol-indophenol sodium (di·klor·o·**fe**·nol·in·do·**fe**′·nol **so**·de·um). Sodium 2,6-dichlorophenol indophenol, $O{=}C_6H_2Cl_2NC_6H_4ONa$. A compound used in standard solution for the volumetric titration of solutions of ascorbic acid, e.g. in the estimation of the excretion of the latter in urine.

Dichlorotetrafluoroethane BPC 1968 (di·**klor**·o·tet·rah·**floo**·or·o·**e**′·thane). Empirical formula $C_2Cl_2F_4$. *See* DICHLORODIFLUOROMETHANE. Dichlorotetrafluoroethane is added to dichlorodifluoromethane to modify the action as a propellant.

dichlorovinylchloroarsine (di·**klor**·o·vi·nil·klor·o·**ar**′·seen). Dichlorodivinylchloroarsine.

Dichloroxylenol (**di**·klor·o·**zi**′·len·ol). BP Commission approved name for 2,4-dichloro-3,5-xylenol, a bacteriostatic closely related to parachlorometaxylenol, but more effective, especially against *Staphylococcus aureus.*

Dichlorphenamide BP 1973 (di·klor·**fen**·am·ide). 4,5-Dichlorobenzene-1,3-disulphonamide; a carbonic anhydrase inhibitor used as a diuretic and to lower the intra-ocular pressure.

dichogeny (di·**koj**·en·e). Change in development of tissues which is brought about by alteration in the conditions affecting them. [Gk *dicha* in two, *genein* to produce.]

dichotomy (di·**kot**·om·e). 1. Bifurcation, particularly repeated bifurcation, e.g. as of a vein. 2. A cutting in two. 3. Division of the fee paid to a consultant or surgeon with the general practitioner who has brought him into the case; the procedure is entirely unethical and is not practised in Great Britain. **Anterior dichotomy, Cephalic dichotomy.** Describing a double monster which is united as far up as the arms. **Posterior dichotomy.** Describing a double monster which is united above the legs. [Gk *dicha* in two, *temnein* to cut.]

dichroa febrifuga (di·**kro**·ah feb·rif·**ew**·gah). A root with reputed antimalarial properties, used in Chinese indigenous medicine. [Gk *di-*, *chroa* colour, L *febris* fever, *fugare* drive away.]

dichroic (di·**kro**·ik). Pertaining to dichroism.

dichroism (**di**·kro·izm). A phenomenon displayed by certain crystals, which are different in colour when they are viewed by reflected and by transmitted light. Similarly, the colour may vary with the axis along which the light is transmitted. [Gk *di-*, *chroa* colour.]

dichromasia, dichromasy (di·kro·**ma**·ze·ah di·**kro**·mas·e). The ability to see only 2 of the 3 primary colours, red, blue and green. [Gk *di-*, *chroma* colour.]

dichromat (**di**·kro·mat). An individual affected with dichromasia.

dichromate (di·**kro**·mate). A salt of the hypothetical dichromic acid which provides the orange dichromate ion, $Cr_2O_7{}^{2-}$.

dichromatic (di·kro·**mat**·ik). 1. Having or showing 2 colours. 2. Referring to dichromasia. [Gk *di-*, *chroma* colour.]

dichromatism (di·**kro**·mat·izm). A state of being dichromatic.

dichromatopsia (di·kro·mat·**op**′·se·ah). The state of vision of a dichromat, i.e. of a patient who can see only 2 out of the 3 primary colours. There are thus 3 varieties, red blindness, green blindness or blue blindness. [Gk *di-*, *chroma* colour, *opsis* vision.]

dichromic (di·**kro**·mik). 1. Having 2 colours. 2. Possessing 2 atoms of chromium. [Gk *di-*, *chroma* colour, chromium.]

dichromism (di·**kro**·mizm). 1. Dichroism. 2. Dichromatopsia. [Gk *di-*, *chroma* colour.]

Dichromium Trioxide (di·**kro**·me·um tri·**ox**·ide). BP Commission approved name for chromium sesquioxide; a diagnostic aid.

dichromophil, dichromophile (di·**kro**·mo·fil di·**kro**·mo·file). Term used of a tissue that takes an acid dye at one part and a basic dye at another. [Gk *di-*, chromophil.]

dichromophilism (di·kro·**mof**·il·izm). The power to take 2 stains, e.g. acid and basic. [see prec.]

dicinchonicine, dicinchonine (di·sin·**kon**·is·een, di·**sin**·kon·een). $C_{38}H_{44}O_2N_4$, a minor alkaloid of the cinchona group, obtained from the species *Cinchona rosulenta* and *C. succirubra.*

Dick, George Frederick (b. 1881) **and Gladys Rowena Henry Dick** (b. 1881). Chicago physicians.

Dick reaction, or test. A biological skin test for immunity to scarlet fever, analogous to the Schick test in diphtheria: a suitable amount of scarlet-fever toxin is injected intradermally into the forearm (heated toxin is often also injected as a control). A local reaction to the toxin is regarded as positive (=susceptible).

Dick's serum. Dochez' serum; scarlet-fever antitoxin; haemolytic streptococcus antitoxin; antitoxin prepared by immunizing horses against scarlet-fever toxin. It alleviates toxic symptoms, and is therefore useful in treatment.

Dick toxin. The toxic substance produced in cultures of haemolytic streptococci isolated from cases of scarlet fever. It is used in the Dick test for demonstrating susceptibility to scarlet fever; in appropriate doses it immunizes against scarlet fever and converts a positive Dick test into a negative one. Antitoxic serum produced against this toxin gives good results in the treatment of scarlet fever and also gives a positive Schultz-Charlton reaction.

dick (dik). Ethyldichlorarsine; a nose gas used in chemical warfare.

Dickey, Clifford Allen (b. 1901). San Francisco ophthalmologist.

Dickey's operation. For ptosis: a modification of Motais' operation; a fascial sling is passed under the tendon of the superior rectus muscle and anchored to the tarsal plate.

Dickey, John Stuart (b. 1882). Belfast anatomist.

Dickey's fibres, or suspensory ligament. Fibres of the scalenus anterior muscle that end at the suprapleural membrane (Sibson's fascia).

dicliditis (dik·lid·i·tis). Valvulitis. [Gk *diklides* valve, *-itis* inflammation.]

diclidostosis (**dik**·lid·os·**to**′·sis). Ossification of the valves of the veins. [Gk *diklides* valve, *osteon* bone, *-osis* condition.]

diclidotomy (dik·lid·**ot**·o·me). 1. Valvulotomy. 2. The cutting of a horizontal fold of the rectum. [Gk *diklides* valve, *temnein* to cut.]

Diclofenac (di·**klo**·fen·ak). BP Commission approved name for [2-(2,6-dichloroanilino)phenyl]acetic acid; an anti-inflammatory agent.

dicoelous (di·**se**·lus). Having 2 cavities. [Gk *di-*, *koilos* hollow.]

Dicophane BP 1973 (**di**·ko·fane). Dichlorodiphenyltrichloroethane; DDT, 1,1,1-trichloro-2,2-bis(*p*-chlorophenyl)ethane, $(C_6H_4Cl)_2{=}CHCCl_3$. A powerful insecticide. It was introduced into general use during World War II and revolutionized the preventive treatment of malaria, typhus, relapsing fever, sandfly fever and many insect-transmitted diseases; it also proved valuable in preventing house-fly-spread diseases, e.g. cholera, typhoid and dysentery. It is almost universally known as DDT.

dicoria (di·**kor**·e·ah). Diplocoria; double pupil. [Gk *di-*, *kore* pupil.]

dicoumarin (di·**koo**·mar·in). Dicoumarol BPC 1954.

Dicoumarol BPC 1954 (di·**koo**·mar·ol). Dicoumarin, 3,3′-methylene-bis-(4-hydroxycoumarin), $C_9H_4O(OH)CH_2O_2C_9H_4O(OH)$. A white crystalline compound originally isolated from "spoiled" sweet clover hay following the investigation of haemorrhagic diseases in cattle; now prepared synthetically and used as an anticoagulant. Unlike heparin it is active by mouth and it is usually administered orally, but can also be injected. It acts by depressing the prothrombin level in the blood, apparently through affecting its production by the liver. It also reduces adhesiveness of the platelets and prolongs clot-retraction time. The onset is much slower than with heparin and once established is much more prolonged. Its action is, however, extremely variable, not only from patient to patient, but also from day to day in the same patient. Daily determinations of the blood prothrombin level are therefore necessary. A further disadvantage is the difficulty in counteracting the effects of overdosage with dicoumarol: it is essential to transfuse relatively large quantities of fresh blood without delay to provide prothrombin, followed by an injection of menaphthone (water-soluble vitamin K) intravenously to counteract the effects of the drug on the liver. Now largely replaced by ethyl biscoumacetate and phenindione.

dicranous (di·**kra**·nus). Dicephalous. [Gk *di-*, *kranion* skull.]

dicrocoeliasis (**dik**·ro·se·**li**'·as·is). Infection with dicrocoelium. [Gk *dikroos* forked, *koilia* bowel.]

Dicrocoeliidae (**dik**·ro·**se**'·li·id·e). A family of the trematode sub-order Distomata or Fasciolidea. The genera *Dicrocoelium* and *Eurytrema* are of medical interest. [Gk *dikroos* forked, *koilia* bowel, *eidos* form.]

Dicrocoelium (dik·ro·**se**·le·um). A genus of small elongate flukes. *Dicrocoelium dendriticum (lanceolatum),* normal to sheep, is a not uncommon liver parasite of man in Europe and Asia. Intermediate hosts are land snails, e.g. species of *Helicella.* [Gk *dikroos* forked, *koilia* bowel.]

dicrotic (di·**krot**·ik). 1. Pertaining to dicrotism. 2. Referring to the second dilatation of the artery in a dicrotic pulse. [Gk *dikrotos* twofold beating.]

dicrotism (**di**·krot·izm). A condition of the pulse in low arterial tension: there are 2 beats or waves to each beat of the heart. [see prec.]

dictamnine (dik·**tam**·neen). $C_{12}H_9O_2N$, an alkaloid of the quinoline group obtained from white dittany root, *Dictamnus albus* Linn., *Skimmia repens* and other plants.

dictyitis (dik·te·**i**·tis). Retinitis. [Gk *diktyon* net, *-itis* inflammation.]

dictyocyte (**dik**·te·o·site). A cell that forms reticulin. [Gk *diktyon* net, *kytos* cell.]

dictyokinesis (**dik**·te·o·kin·**e**'·sis). In mitosis, the division and the distribution of the dictyosomes to the 2 daughter cells. [Gk *diktyon* net, *kinesis* movement.]

dictyoma (dik·te·**o**·mah). A tumour of the ciliary epithelium which represents the embryonic retina. [Gk *diktyon* net, *-oma* tumour.]

dictyosome (**dik**·te·o·some). Golgiosome; a cytoplasmic body, having similar staining reactions to the Golgi apparatus, and thought to represent a dispersed element of the latter. The Golgi apparatus of vertebrates may disperse in various physiological and pathological conditions; in invertebrates the dispersed condition is apparently normal. [Gk *diktyon* net, *soma* body.]

dictyotene (**dik**·te·o·teen). Arrested prophase I of mammalian female meiosis lasting, usually, from fetal or early postnatal life to just before ovulation. It occurs during diplotene when the chromosomes, instead of contracting and entering diakinesis, become progressively longer and thinner and the nucleus assumes again an interphase appearance. [Gk *diktyon* net, *tainia* ribbon.]

dicyanate (di·si·an·ate). Bicyanate.

Dicyclomine (di·**si**·klo·meen). BP Commission approved name for 2-diethylamino-ethyl dicyclohexyl-1-carboxylate, a spasmolytic of atropine type used in the treatment of gastric and duodenal ulcers, and spasm of biliary and urinary tracts. **Dicyclomine Hydrochloride BP 1973.** The hydrochloride of dicyclomine; a synthetic preparation with weak atropine-like effects and used mainly in gastro-intestinal disorders for its anticholinergic actions.

dicysteine (di·**sis**·te·een). L-Cystine, diamino-β-thiopropionic acid, $S_2(CH_2CH(NH_2)COOH)_2$. An α-amino acid which occurs in the keratin of human hair and of wool, and in albumin and casein. It is the principal source of sulphur for the organism, and is excreted in the urine in the abnormal condition known as *cystinuria.*

dicytosis (di·si·**to**·sis). The relative percentages of polymorphonuclear and of mononuclear cells in the blood in a comparative analysis of the leucocyte content. [Gk *di-*, cytosis.]

didactylism (di·**dak**·til·izm). The congenital condition of having only 2 fingers on a hand or 2 toes on a foot. [Gk *di-*, *daktylos* finger.]

Diday, Charles Joseph Paul Edouard (b. 1812). Lyons syphilologist.

Diday's law. When congenital syphilitic infection continues to occur throughout a family of children, it shows a tendency to decrease in severity in each successive child until it finally comes to an end.

didelphic (di·**del**·fik). Possession of a double uterus. [Gk *di-*, *delphys* womb.]

Didelphis, Didelphys (di·**del**·fis). A genus of marsupials; the opossum: a reservoir of *Trypanosoma cruzi* in South America and also of Q fever. [see prec.]

didermoma (di·der·**mo**·mah). Bidermoma; a teratoid growth involving 2 germ layers. [Gk *di-*, *derma* skin, *-oma* tumour.]

diduction (di·**duk**·shun). Withdrawal or separation of a part, or abduction of 2 parts. [L *diducere* to draw apart.]

diductor (di·**duk**·tor). A muscle the action of which produces diduction, e.g. an abductor muscle. [see prec.]

didymalgia (did·im·**al**·je·ah). Orchiodynia; testicular pain. [Gk *didymos* twin (testis), *algos* pain.]

didymitis (did·im·**i**·tis). Orchitis. [Gk *didymos* twin (testis), *-itis* inflammation.]

didymium (did·**im**·e·um). Originally considered a single element, a mixture of the rare-earth metals, neodymium and praseodymium, found in cerite. **Didymium salicylate.** A non-irritant and desiccant substance used as a dusting powder in various skin diseases. [Gk *didymos* twin, from the absorption bands in its spectrum.]

didymodynia (**did**·im·o·**din**'·e·ah). Orchiodynia. [Gk *didymos* twin (testis), *odyne* pain.]

didymous (**did**·im·us). Twofold or twin. [Gk *didymos* twin.]

didymus (**did**·im·us). 1. One of twins. 2. A twin monster. 3. A testis. [see prec.]

die (di). In dentistry, a model of the mouth cast in metal (used in conjunction with a counter-die) upon which the metallic base of a restoration for the mouth is accurately swaged into shape. **Amalgam die.** A model of a tooth which has been prepared for the reception of an inlay or crown. [L *datum* given.]

diechoscope (di·**ek**·o·skope). A type of stethoscope with which 2 different sounds in 2 different parts of the body can be heard at the same time. [Gk *di-*, *echos* sound, *skopein* to examine.]

Dieffenbach, Johann Friedrich (b. 1792). Berlin surgeon.

Dieffenbach's amputation. A form of disarticulation of the hip. An elastic tourniquet is applied, a circular flap cut through the thigh, and the vessels are secured: the tourniquet is then removed and a lateral vertical incision made downwards over the greater trochanter to meet the circular incision; the disarticulation is then completed.

Dieffenbach's operation. 1. Dieffenbach's amputation (see preceding). 2. Blepharoplasty, for the lower lid: a triangle of skin is removed with the base at the lid margin and the apex downwards. A parallelogram lateral to this triangle is marked out, being left attached only below; this is then swung medially to fill the original triangle. 3. For squint: the first operation performed for convergent squint, by division of the belly of the internal rectus muscle. Of historical interest.

diego. *See* Blood GROUP.

Dieldrin (di·**el**·drin). BP Commission approved name for a product containing 85 per cent of 1,2,3,4,10,10-hexachloro-6,7-epoxy-1,4,4a,5,6,7,8,8a-octahydro-*exo*-1,4-*endo*-5,8-dimethanonaphthalene; it is used in the treatment of arthropod infestation.

dielectric (di·el·**ek**·trik). A non-conducting medium capable of transmitting an electrostatic charge by induction. **Dielectric constant.** *See* CONSTANT. [Gk *dia*, electric.]

Diels, Otto (b. 1876). German chemist.

Diels' hydrocarbon. Methyl cyclopentenophenanthrene, $C_{18}H_{16}$, the parent of the sterols.

diembryony (di·**em**·bre·on·e). The development of 2 embryos in a single ovum. [Gk *di-*, embryo.]

diencephalic (**di**·en·kef·**al**'·ik). Pertaining to the diencephalon.

diencephalohypophyseal (di·en·**kef**·al·o·hi·**pof**'·iz·e·al). Pertaining to the diencephalon and the hypophysis cerebri.

diencephalon [NA] (di·en·**kef**·al·on). The central part of the forebrain, consisting of paired masses of nervous tissue surrounding the 3rd ventricle. It is subdivided into the *epithalamus,* with which is associated the pineal body and the choroid plexus of the 3rd ventricle, the *hypothalamus,* with which is associated the pituitary body, the *thalamus* proper, and the *subthalamus,* which is wedged in between the thalamus and hypothalamus posteriorly. [Gk *dia, egkephalos* brain.]

Dienoestrol BP 1973 (di·en·e·strol). 3,4-Bis(*p*-hydroxyphenyl)-2,4-hexadiene, $C_6H_4(OH)C(=CHCH_3)C(=CHCH_3)C_6H_4(OH)$. A synthetic oestrogen related to stilboestrol and hexoestrol, but much less toxic than the former. It is seldom now used in the treatment of ovarian hypofunction, and for temporary symptomatic relief of cancer of the prostate.

Dientamoeba (di·ent·am·e′·bah). A genus of amoebae. *Dientamoeba fragilis* occurs in the colon. It is very small (approximately 10 μm), and world-wide though usually rare; as normally encountered, it has 2 nuclei. It does not invade tissues and is probably harmless, though intestinal disorders have been attributed to it. [Gk *di-, endon* within, *amoibe* change.]

diet (di·et). The normal or specially prescribed daily intake of food and drink. The more important components of a complete diet include proteins, fats, carbohydrates, vitamins, mineral salts and water. The principal function of the protein of the diet is to build new body protein and to replace its waste. The protein requirement is assessed as about 70 g per day for an average-sized man: this, however, depends on the supply of essential amino acids of which the protein is composed, and a relative deficiency of one or more amino acids in one protein may be made up by the supplementary action of another protein which contains them. The essential amino acids required by animals (and probably by man) are 10 in number, namely, tryptophan, lysine, methionine, phenylalanine, histidine, leucine, isoleucine, valine, threonine and arginine. In general, animal proteins are more complete in their amino-acid make-up than some vegetable proteins. The rôle of carbohydrate in nutrition is essentially as a source of calories (body heat). Fats are also a source of calories. The heat available from the three main components of foods are as follows: carbohydrate, 17.2 kJ (4.1 calories, large, or kilogram-calories) per gram; fat, 39.6 kJ (9.45 calories) per gram; protein, 23.7 kJ (5.65 calories) per gram. The requirement for an average man doing moderate muscular work is reckoned to be about 12.56 MJ (3000 calories) per day, the factors determining it including physical activity, size of subject, sex, age and superficial area of body. The more important vitamins needed in the diet include vitamin A, vitamin B_1, nicotinamide, riboflavine, and vitamins C and D; lack of any of these may give rise to the corresponding vitamin-deficiency disease. The estimated daily requirements for an adult are as follows: vitamin A, 3000 international units; vitamin B_1, 300 I.U.; vitamin C, 30 mg; riboflavine, 1.8 mg; nicotinamide, 12 mg; and, for an infant, vitamin D, 400 I.U. The essential mineral and "trace" elements in foods include sodium, chlorine, potassium, sulphur, calcium, phosphorus, magnesium, iron, iodine, copper, cobalt, manganese, zinc. Those most liable to be deficient include iron, calcium and (in goitrous areas) iodine. The daily requirement of calcium is of the order of 1 gram per day, and of iodine 0.1 milligram per day. Foodstuffs of importance in the diet as source of proteins include meat, fish, dairy products; of fats, margarine, butter, dairy products, fatty meats and cooking oils; of carbohydrates, cereals, potatoes, sugar; of calcium, milk and cheese; of vitamin A, margarine, milk, butter, green vegetables, carrots; of vitamin B_1, wheatmeal bread, potatoes; of vitamin C, citrus fruits, cabbage and greenstuffs, potatoes; of vitamin D, fish-liver oils, egg yolk, margarine; of nicotinamide, wheatmeal bread and various protein-rich foods. In the planning of diets of infants and children, important points are: the use of milk as a basis, and supplementation with vitamin D (e.g. as concentrates, or preparations of fish-liver oils), vitamin C (e.g. as orange or blackcurrant juice, or ascorbic acid) and iron. For adults, the "normal middle-class" diet is likely to be adequate provided it is reasonably varied and contains a small helping of protein food daily (fish, meat, milk, cheese, eggs), fresh fruit, vegetables or salad (for vitamin C) and wheatmeal bread (white bread being low in B vitamins). In regions where dietary deficiency disease is endemic, appropriate measures need to be taken, e.g. substitution of parboiled rice for milled white rice (or addition of vitamin B_1 in other ways) to combat beriberi, the supplementation of maize diets with other foodstuffs to prevent pellagra, and the use of vitamin C concentrates in some far-northern areas. **Balanced diet.** One which contains all the dietary ingredients, including the vitamins, in the ideal proportions. **Colitis diet.** A diet relatively free from residue and low in fat; all vegetables are puréed and eggs added in the later stages. **Diabetic diet.** A diet which is carefully assessed according to its ingredients, in which sugar and carbohydrates generally are relatively low. **Gluten-free diet.** A diet from which all wheat and rye flour has been excluded; used in cases of coeliac disease and idiopathic steatorrhoea. **High-calorie diet.** One containing more calories than the subject would normally require; e.g. for an average man doing sedentary work, 12.56 MJ (3000 calories) would normally be sufficient, and 16.75 MJ (4000 calories) would be a high-calorie diet. **High-protein diet.** One containing more than the normal 100 g (for an average man) of protein. **Ketogenic diet.** One containing relatively and actually an excess of fats, which are reduced to ketones: not now popular, but once used in the treatment of epilepsy and of urinary *Bacterium coli* infections. **Line-ration diet.** A dietetic scheme that simplifies the dieting of diabetics in relation to the insulin that they are receiving. **Low-calorie diet.** One containing less calories than the subject would normally require. **Low-fat diet.** One low in fat, i.e. with 50 g or less. **Nephritic diet.** A high-protein diet, 120 g or more. **Purine-free diet.** A diet in which meat, red or white, and fish are avoided and the proteins and calories made up by milk and cheese. **Reducing diet.** A low-calorie diet planned to reduce the weight of an obese subject. **Salt-free diet.** A diet containing the minimum amount of sodium chloride, less than 1.0 g. **Sprue diet.** A high-protein, low-fat and low-carbohydrate diet with the proportion P:F:C = 1:0.3:1.3 instead of 1:1:5. [Gk *diaita* a way of living.]

See also: CHITTENDEN, COLEMAN, HAY (W.H.), KARELL, LENHARTZ, MEULENGRACHT, SIPPY, WITTS.

dietary (di·et·ar·e). The whole system of food intake based on the requirements of the body and the distribution of this throughout the day; applied to the individual, a group of individuals or a whole population. [see prec.]

dietetic (di·et·et·ik). Referring to diet or to a dietary.

dietetics (di·et·et·ix). The science of relating diet or food to health and disease and sytematically regulating it accordingly. [Gk *diaita* a way of living.]

Diethadione (di·eth·ad·i′·one). BP Commission approved name for 5,5-diethyloxazine-2,4-dione; an analeptic.

Diethanolamine Fusidate BPC 1968 (di·eth·an·ol′·am·een few·sid·ate). The diethanolamine salt of fusidic acid, an antibiotic having an antibacterial action against Gram-positive organisms, including penicillin-resistant strains of *Staphylococcus aureus,* and also against some Gram-negative organisms.

Diethazine Hydrochloride BP 1973 (di·eth·az·een hi·dro·klor′·ide). *N*-2-diethylaminoethylphenothiazine hydrochloride, $(C_{12}H_8NS)CH_2CH_2N(C_2H_5)_2HCl$. A synthetic drug widely used in Parkinson's syndrome; it possesses both sympathicolytic and parasympathomimetic action.

diethoxin (di·eth·ox·in). $C_2H_5OC_6H_4COO(CH_2)_2N(C_2H_5)_2$, a local anaesthetic similar to procaine.

diethyl (di·eth·il). An organic prefix signifying the presence in a compound of 2 ethyl radicals. **Diethyl acetal.** Acetal, $C_2H_4(OC_2H_5)_2$, a volatile liquid obtained by the condensation of acetaldehyde and ethyl alcohol, and used in medicine as a hypnotic. **Diethyl glycocoll guaiacol.** $(C_2H_5)_2NCH_2COOC_6H_4OCH_3$, a compound the hydrochloride of which is employed as an antiseptic, and in the treatment of the common threadworm. **Diethyl Phthalate BPC 1968.** Ethyl *o*-benzenedicarboxylate; a solvent and plasticizer for cellulose acetate, nitrocellulose and rubber.

diethylamine (di·eth·il·**am**′·een). $(C_2H_5)_2NH$, a secondary amine which arises during the bacterial decomposition of fish. It is a colourless liquid, prepared from ethyl bromide and ammonia.

Diethylcarbamazine Citrate BP 1973 (di·**eth**·il·kar·**bam**′·az·een **sit**·rate). 1-Diethylcarbamyl-4-methylpiperazine dihydrogen citrate, $C_{16}H_{29}O_8N_2$. A synthetic drug with a specific action in several filarial infections, especially useful in bancroftian filariasis and in loiasis: it kills the microfilaria rapidly and thereby prevents the spread of the infection to others, but it also sterilizes and often kills the adult worm, so that there is no relapse of microfilaraemia. Its administration is sometimes associated with headaches, drowsiness and vomiting, and with allergic reactions of various kinds, but these are thought to be caused by the dead filariae; these reactions can be controlled by antihistamine drugs.

diethylenediamine (di·**eth**·il·een·**di**′·am·een). Hexahydropyrazine, piperazine, $NH=(CH_2CH_2)_2=NH$. A white crystalline substance, soluble in water or alcohol. It is used in medicine to dissolve uric acid in the treatment of gout, rheumatism and urinary calculi.

diethylether (di·**eth**·il·**e**′·ther). Ethyl ether, sulphuric ether, $(C_2H_5)_2O$. A colourless liquid with a distinctive odour; volatilizes readily and is very inflammable. Prepared by the action of sulphuric acid on ethyl alcohol, it is used as a solvent for fats, resins, iodine and certain alkaloids; in medicine, it is valuable as an anaesthetic, internally as a stimulant and carminative, and for its solvent action on gallstones, also externally as an antiseptic.

diethylketone (di·**eth**·il·**ke**′·tone). Pentanone $(C_2H_5)_2CO$. A colourless volatile liquid, soluble in water or alcohol; used in medicine as a hypnotic.

diethylmalonylurea (di·**eth**·il·mal·o·nil·ewr·**e**′·ah). Barbitone, diethylbarbituric acid, $(C_2H_5)_2C=(CONH)_2=CO$. A compound with a strong hypnotic action.

Diethylpropion (di·**eth**·il·**pro**′·pe·on). BP Commission approved name for α-diethylaminopropiophenone; an appetite suppressant used in the treatment of obesity.

diethylstilboestrol (di·eth·il·**stil**·be·strol). Stilboestrol BP 1958, $HOC_6H_4C(C_2H_5)=C(C_2H_5)C_6H_4OH$, a synthetic chemical compound occurring as colourless crystals or as a crystalline powder, and with oestrogenic properties. It is effective by mouth as well as by injection, though oral administration may cause nausea and vomiting. The chief clinical indications are the menopausal syndrome, natural hormone deficiency as in ovarian agenesis, to inhibit lactation, and in certain forms of malignant disease, particularly prostatic carcinoma. **Diethylstilboestrol dipropionate.** The dipropionic ester of stilboestrol. It has the same therapeutic properties as the parent compound, but is more suitable for injections in an oily solution in cases where the oral use of the latter causes nausea and vomiting.

Diethylthiambutene (di·**eth**·il·thi·am·**bew**′·teen). BP Commission approved name for 3-diethylamino-1,1-di-2′-thienylbut-1-ene, an analgesic for subcutaneous administration to dogs and other small animals.

Diethyltoluamide (di·**eth**·il·**tol**′·ew·am·ide). BP Commission approved name for *N,N*-diethyl-*m*-toluamide; an insect repellent.

dietician, dietitian, dietist (di·et·**ish**·an, **di**·et·ist). A specialist in dietary; an officer appointed in a hospital or institution to plan and supervise dietaries with the approval of the medical staff. [Gk *diaita* a way of living.]

Dietl, Joseph (b. 1804). Cracow physician.

Dietl's crisis. Severe symptoms due to kinking and partial obstruction of the ureter, occurring with floating kidney.

dietotherapy (**di**·et·o·**ther**′·ap·e). The application of the principles of dietetics in treatment. [diet, therapy.]

dietotoxic (**di**·et·o·**tox**′·ik). Having a harmful effect when used in certain food combinations. [see foll.]

dietotoxicity (**di**·et·o·tox·**is**′·it·e). The quality inherent in some food substances which causes them to become poisonous when not counterbalanced by other food substances in the diet. [diet, Gk *toxikon* poison.]

Dieudonné, Adolf (b. 1864). Munich hygienist.

Dieudonné's medium, or agar. A medium consisting of defibrinated ox blood steamed with caustic soda, aged 10 days, and added (3 parts) to 3 per cent nutrient agar (7 parts). It is used for the culture of *Vibrio cholerae.*

Dieulafoy, Georges (b. 1839). Paris physician.

Dieulafoy's aspirator. A graduated syringe, fitted with a two-way device, which enables fluid to be withdrawn from a cavity through one channel, and expelled from the syringe by another.

Dieulafoy's disease, or erosion. Ulceration of the gastric mucous membrane, occurring in pneumonia.

Difetarsone (di·fet·**ar**·sone). BP Commission approved name for *N,N*′-ethylene-1,2-diarsanilic acid; an arsenical.

difference (**dif**·er·ens). **Optical-path difference.** The difference between the optical length of a pair of rays of light passing from an object point through an optical system to an image point. [L *differentia.]*

differential (dif·er·**en**·shal). Relating to, constituting or creating a difference. [see prec.]

differentiation (**dif**·er·en·she·a′·shun). 1. Specialization. The acquisition of a distinct or separate character. 2. The ascertaining of the specific difference between one disease and another or between one thing and another. **Correlative differentiation.** Differentiation caused by the mutual effect and modification of parts of an organism. **Sex differentiation.** The process which leads to the development in an individual of the sex organs and of the characteristics proper of males and females. [L *differentia* difference.]

diffluence (**dif**·loo·ens). 1. Fluidity. 2. The process of liquefying. 3. The state of being almost fluid. [L *diffluere* to flow off.]

diffluent (**dif**·loo·ent). 1. Deliquescent. 2. Dissolving or flowing away readily. [see prec.]

diffraction (dif·**rak**·shun). A phenomenon peculiar to wave-motion, whereby a wave is deflected at a sharp edge. With parallel light waves a series of interference fringes may be set up. **Electron diffraction.** A beam of electrons of homogenous velocity possesses a wave character, the wavelength of the beam being $\lambda = hmv$, where h is Planck's constant, m the electron mass and v its velocity. Diffraction phenomena analogous to those obtained with light may be obtained with the beam in quantitative agreement with the postulation of a wavelength as given above. **Diffraction grating.** A glass or metal plate, the surface of which is cut with very close parallel lines to produce spectra by diffraction. **X-ray diffraction.** X-rays passed through crystals are diffracted by the regular arrangement in space of their atoms, ions or molecules, just as light rays are diffracted by closely-ruled lines on glass. Each crystalline chemical or element produces its characteristic diffraction pattern. An unknown material may be identified by matching its diffraction pattern against standard patterns of known pure materials. [L *dis-*, *frangere* to break.]

diffractometer (dif·rak·**tom**·et·er). An instrument for measuring the intensities and diffraction angles of beams of radiation or particles. **Neutron diffractometer.** An instrument for measuring the intensities and diffraction angles of neutron beams coherently scattered by a specimen the atoms of which are arranged in a regular structure. **X-ray diffractometer.** An instrument used for measuring the intensities and diffraction angles of x-ray beams coherently scattered by a specimen the atoms of which are arranged in a regular structure.

diffusate (**dif**·ew·zate). In dialysis, the liquid which passes through the semipermeable membrane; the dialysate. [L *diffundere* to pour out.]

diffuse (dif·**ewz**). 1. Widespread, dispersed or copious. 2. To extend or spread widely; to spread into another substance, e.g. through a membrane. [L *diffundere* to pour out.]

diffusibility (dif·**ewz**·ib·**il**′·it·e). The ability to diffuse possessed by a gas, liquid, and to a small extent, by a solid. **Diffusibility of gases.** The property, due to the kinetic energy of their molecules, whereby 2 or more gases will expand to occupy completely any volume, and each exert its own pressure independent of the others. [L *diffundere* to pour out.]

diffusible (dif·**ewz**·ibl). 1. Capable of diffusing or of being diffused. 2. Acting rapidly but temporarily, e.g. as a stimulant, affecting or invading all parts of the body or organism quickly. [see prec.]

diffusiometer (dif·**ewz**·e·**om**'·et·er). An apparatus with which the diffusibility or rate of diffusion of a gas can be estimated. [diffusion, Gk *metron* measure.]

diffusion (dif·**ew**·zhun). The random movement of particles, ions or molecules resulting from their thermal energy (Brownian movement). This may occur in gaseous, liquid or solid states and has the effect of producing a uniform concentration of the substance. **Diffusion analysis.** *See* ANALYSIS. **Anodal diffusion.** Cataphoresis, the diffusion of charged particles from an anode placed in a medium. **Diffusion circle.** *See* CIRCLE. **Free diffusion.** Diffusion of one substance through another, freely, without any intervening membrane. **Diffusion hypoxia.** *See* HYPOXIA. **Impeded diffusion.** Diffusion that is restrained by an interposed membrane or porous partition. **Diffusion length.** *See* LENGTH. **Diffusion oxygenation.** *See* OXYGENATION. **Diffusion vacuole.** *See* VACUOLE. [L *diffundere* to pour out.]

Diflucortolone (di·floo·**kor**·to·lone). BP Commission approved name for 6α,9-difluoro-11β,21-dihydroxy-16α-methylpregna-1,4-diene-3,20-dione; a glucocorticoid.

Diflumidone (di·**floo**·mid·one). BP Commission approved name for 3'-benzoyldifluoromethanesulphonanilide; an anti-inflammatory agent.

difluordiphenyl, difluorodiphenyl, difluorphenyl (di·**floo**·or·di·**fe**'·nil, di·**floo**·or·o·di·**fe**'·nil, di·**floo**·or·**fe**'·nil). $C_6H_4FC_6H_4F$, a derivative of diphenyl used as an antiseptic.

digametic (di·gam·**et**·ik). Capable of producing 2 types of gametes, in particular, male- and female-determining gametes. [Gk *di-*, gamete.]

digastric (di·**gas**·trik). 1. Pertaining to the digastric muscle. 2. Having 2 stomachs or muscle bellies. [Gk *di-*, *gaster* stomach.]

digastric muscle [musculus digastricus]. A muscle consisting of 2 bellies; the posterior [venter posterior (NA)] attached to the mastoid notch of the temporal bone, and the anterior [venter anterior (NA)] beside the symphysis of the lower jaw. The intermediate tendon pierces the stylohyoid muscle and is bound to the hyoid bone by a loop of fascia. This muscle forms the inferior boundary of the digastric triangle. [see prec.]

digastricus (di·**gas**·trik·us). The digastric muscle.

Digenea (di·**je**·ne·ah). A sub-class of the platyhelminth class Trematoda; characterized by an alternation of generation in the life cycle. All flukes of medical interest are members of it. [Gk *di-*, *genein* to produce.]

digenesis (di·**jen**·es·is). Alternation of generation. Reproduction by successive sexual and asexual methods, as in the life cycle of the malaria parasite. [Gk *di-*, genesis.]

digenetic (di·jen·**et**·ik). 1. Characterized by digenesis. 2. Referring to the Digenetica, one of the primary orders of trematode worms to which the liver fluke belongs, or requiring, as do these worms, more than 1 host during the course of life. [see prec.]

digenism (**di**·jen·izm). 1. Digenesis. 2. The combined or concurrent action of 2 causes. [Gk *di-*, *genein* to produce.]

digerent (**dij**·er·ent). 1. Digestant. 2. An agent used to expedite pus formation and discharge in wounds. [L *digerere* to digest.]

digest (di·**jest**). 1. To convert food in the alimentary tract into simpler chemical compounds so that it can be absorbed and assimilated. 2. In pharmacy, to soften by exposure to moisture. 3. In chemistry, to disintegrate substances by subjecting them to the action of heat and strong agents. [see prec.]

digestant (di·**jes**·tant). Promoting or aiding digestion.

digester (di·**jes**·ter). 1. An autoclave. 2. A large strong iron vessel or kettle with a fitted lid and a safety valve, in which substances can be softened, decomposed and cooked, usually in liquid, at high temperature and pressure. 3. Any apparatus in which substances can be warmed or heated for the purpose of extracting a soluble ingredient. [L *digerere* to digest.]

digestion (di·**jes**·chun). 1. The process whereby food is broken down to smaller units ready for absorption in the gastro-intestinal tract. 2. In chemistry, the process of heating substances for long periods with chemical reagents, sometimes under pressure as well, in order to soften them or decompose them entirely. **Artificial digestion.** Solubilization of foodstuffs by artificial means, or by enzyme action outside the body. **Gastric digestion.** Digestion by gastric juice, normally in the stomach. **Gastro-intestinal digestion.** Digestion in the stomach followed by that in the intestine. **Intestinal digestion.** Digestion in the intestinal lumen. **Intracellular digestion.** Digestion within a cell. **Pancreatic digestion.** Digestion by the action of pancreatic juice. **Parenteral digestion.** Digestion occurring outside the alimentary canal. **Peptic digestion.** Digestion by pepsin, normally in the stomach. **Salivary digestion.** Digestion of starch by the amylase of saliva. **Sludge digestion.** The process in sewage purification by which the suspended or floating particles of sewage (sludge) in septic tanks and contact beds are acted on chemically and by bacteria. The process comprises firstly hydrolysis, a splitting up of the complex organic molecules of the sludge by the introduction of hydrogen and hydroxyl (OH) derived from water; substances such as CO_2, amino acids and substituted ammonias are formed, no free oxygen is needed, and this stage is usually performed anaerobically: and secondly, oxidation of the amino bodies into nitrites and nitrates through the agency of nitrifying bacteria. The purified sewage liquor is drained off from the bottom of the contact bed and constitutes the "bacterial effluent". **Tryptic digestion.** Digestion of protein by trypsin, or, loosely, by pancreatic juice. [L *digerere* to separate.]

digestive (di·**jes**·tiv). 1. A substance or drug which promotes or aids the digestion of food. 2. Pertaining to digestion.

Dighton, Charles Allen Adair (b. 1885). Liverpool otologist.

Adair-Dighton syndrome. Osteogenesis imperfecta; also known as *Eddowes' syndrome, Lobstein's syndrome.*

digit (dij·it). 1. A finger or toe. 2. A single figure. **Accessory digits.** Additional digits occurring as a congenital abnormality either on the hands or feet. **Binary digit.** A digit in a scale of 2; used in computers. **Supernumerary digits.** Accessory digits (see above). **Webbed digits.** A congenital abnormality in which the digits are connected together by a flap of skin. [L *digitus* finger.]

digital (**dij**·it·al). 1. Referring to or associated with a finger. 2. Bearing the characteristics of a finger imprint. 3. Of data, when they are recorded by discrete signals or marks. **Digital markings.** A neuroradiological term describing the appearance of the inner wall of the skull vault, sometimes called *beaten silver* appearance; seen almost entirely in children and sometimes indicating raised intracranial pressure. The markings are an imprint of the cerebral convolutions. [see prec.]

digital arteries. Arteries of the digits. **Dorsal digital arteries [arteriae digitales dorsales (NA)].** Branches of the dorsal metacarpal or metatarsal arteries to the sides of the fingers or toes. **Palmar digital arteries.** *See* PALMAR ARCH, SUPERFICIAL (under ARCH). **Plantar digital arteries [arteriae digitales plantares communes, arteriae digitales plantares propriae (NA)].** Branches of the plantar metatarsal arteries, or of the plantar arch or lateral plantar artery, to the sides of the toes.

digital nerves. Nerves of the digits. **Dorsal digital nerves of the foot [nervi digitales dorsales pedis (NA)].** 1. Nerves from the medial branch of the musculocutaneous nerve which supply the medial side of the great toe and the adjacent sides of the 2nd and 3rd toes. 2. Nerves from the lateral branch of the musculocutaneous nerve which supply the contiguous sides of the 3rd, 4th and 5th toes. **Dorsal digital nerves of the hand [nervi digitales dorsales (NA)].** 1. Of the ulnar nerve: 2 nerves arising from the dorsal branch of the ulnar nerve. One runs on the medial side of the little finger and the second on the contiguous side of the little and ring fingers. They supply the backs of the fingers as far as the distal interphalangeal joint; occasionally a third nerve supplies the contiguous sides of the middle and ring fingers. 2. Of the radial nerve: 5 nerves arising from the termination of the radial nerve. The first 3 supply the lateral and medial sides of the thumb and the lateral side of the index finger.

The remaining 2 supply the contiguous sides of the index, middle and ring fingers; the fifth is occasionally replaced by a branch from the ulnar nerve. They supply the backs of the fingers as far as the distal interphalangeal joint. **Palmar digital nerves, common [nervi digitales palmares communes (NA)].** 1. Of the median nerve: 2 nerves arising from the medial branch of the median nerve and running to the clefts between the index, middle and ring fingers. 2. Of the ulnar nerve: a nerve arising from the superficial branch of the ulnar nerve and running to the cleft between the ring and little fingers. **Palmar digital nerves, proper [nervi digitales palmares proprii (NA)].** 1. Of the median nerve: the nerves which supply and run at the sides of the lateral three and a half digits. Those for the thumb and lateral side of the index finger arise directly from the median nerve (lateral branch); the remainder arise from the common palmar digital branches of the nerve (medial branch). 2. Of the ulnar nerve: the nerves which supply and run at the sides of the medial one and a half fingers. That for the medial side of the little finger arises directly from the superficial branch of the ulnar nerve; the remaining 2 arise from the common palmar digital branch of that nerve. **Plantar digital nerves, common [nervi digitales plantares communes (NA)].** 1. Of the medial plantar nerve: 3 branches of the medial plantar nerve which run to the clefts between the great, 2nd, 3rd and 4th toes, and give rise to the proper plantar digital nerves. 2. Of the lateral plantar nerve: a branch of the lateral plantar nerve which runs to the cleft between the 4th and 5th toes, and gives rise to the proper digital branches. **Plantar digital nerves, proper [nervi digitales plantares proprii (NA)].** 1. Of the medial plantar nerve: nerves which supply and run at the sides of the medial three and a half toes. That for the medial side of the great toe arises directly from the medial plantar nerve and supplies the flexor hallucis brevis muscle. The remainder arise from the common digital plantar nerves of the medial plantar nerve. 2. Of the lateral plantar nerve: the nerves which supply and run along the side of the lateral one and a half toes. That for the lateral side of the little toe arises direct from the lateral plantar nerve and also supplies the flexor digiti minimi brevis muscle and the 2 interossei muscles of the fourth space. The remaining 2 arise from the common plantar digital nerve of the lateral plantar nerve.

digital veins. Veins of the digits. **Palmar digital veins [venae digitales palmares (NA)].** Veins on either side of the digits, and on the palmar surfaces, draining into the dorsal venous network. **Plantar digital veins [venae digitales plantares (NA)].** The veins draining the plantar surfaces of the toes into the plantar metatarsal veins.

digitalein (dij·it·a·le·in). A term applied loosely to a mixture of soluble glycosides obtained from digitalis leaves and present in commercial digitalis.

digitaligenin (dij·it·al·ij'·en·in). $C_{23}H_{30}O_3$, an aglucone found combined with digitalose in the glycoside, digitalin.

digitalin (dij·it·a·lin). Digitalinum purum germanicum; amorphous digitalin. A standardized preparation of glycosides made from the seeds of *Digitalis purpurea* Linn.; it is adjusted by comparison with International digitalis powder to an activity of 100 units per gram. It is a yellowish-white powder with a bitter taste, and is used for the same conditions as digitalis (BPC 1954). The name has also been applied to the glycoside forming the chief constituent of the above preparation, and to several other digitalis preparations, thus causing confusion. **Crystallized digitalin.** Digitoxin BPC 1959; a preparation from Digitalis Leaf, chiefly composed of the crystalline glycoside, digitoxin, with traces of other glycosides. It is a white powder with a very bitter taste, the most potent glycoside obtained from digitalis, and perhaps less prone to cause nausea than other digitalis preparations. It is employed clinically in the same condition as digitalis. **French digitalin.** An amorphous preparation of digitalis; it is insoluble in water, and of uncertain composition. **German digitalin.** An amorphous preparation principally digitonin, obtained from the seeds of digitalis; it is soluble in water.

See also: HOMOLLE, KILIANI, NATIVELLE.

digitalis (dij·it·a·lis). The dried leaf of *Digitalis purpurea,* the purple foxglove. It contains the active glycosides digitoxin, gitoxin and gitalin, the aglucone in each case being steroid in structure with its pharmacological action dependent on its linkage with the sugar. It has a slowing effect upon the heart by stimulation of the vagal centre in the medulla and sensitization of the heart to vagal action; it also slows conduction in the auriculoventricular bundle, thus preventing irregularities of the ventricular rhythm in cases of auricular flutter. Its most important use is in the treatment of congestive heart failure, where it reduces the size and rate of the heart, lowers the blood pressure and improves the oxygenation of the blood which has deteriorated through indifferent pulmonary circulation: increased flow through the kidneys produces diuresis and relieves the oedema accompanying the condition. Its action is cumulative, as the heart muscle removes the drug from circulation and retains it for long periods; treatment therefore consists of a large dose initially, followed by smaller daily maintenance doses. In some patients it may stimulate the vomiting centre and cause emesis. The commercial drug is a yellowish powder with a very bitter taste: it must be assayed biologically to ensure standardization. It is employed in the form of tablets or as a tincture. Toxic doses produce excessive slowing of the heart, the vagal action being augmented by reduced conduction of the impulses and lessening of the number emitted by the pacemaker. **Austrian digitalis.** Woolly foxglove leaf. **Digitalis dispert.** An aqueous solution of the soluble constituents of digitalis leaves. **Digitalis folium.** The first or second year leaves of *Digitalis purpurea;* dried and powdered they are used in the preparation of tablets and the tincture. **Infusum digitalis recens.** An infusion standardized to 0.05 units of activity per millilitre. **International digitalis standard.** A standard preparation of a mixture of dried, powdered, digitalis leaves, obtained from *Digitalis purpurea,* which has been established by the World Health Organization as the standard for use in the biological assay of digitalis preparations. **International digitalis unit.** A unit based on the specific activity contained in such an amount of the standard preparation (see above) as the World Health Organization and the Medical Research Council may from time to time indicate. **Digitalis Lanata Leaf BPC 1968.** Austrian foxglove, woolly foxglove; a species indigenous to Austria and the Balkans, but cultivated in Britain. It contains the glycoside digoxin, in addition to gitoxin and digitoxin, and is used as a source of it. **Digitalis Leaf BP 1973.** Digitalis folium (see above). **Prepared Digitalis BP 1973, Powdered digitalis, Digitalis pulverata.** Digitalis leaves powdered and standardized to 10 points of activity per gram. **Digitalis purpurea.** The common foxglove; a biennial plant common in Europe. It contains the cardiac glycosides digitoxin, gitoxin and gitalin, of which digitoxin is separated commercially. **Tincture of Digitalis BP 1953.** Made by percolating the leaves or powder with alcohol and standardized to 1 unit of activity per millilitre. [L of the fingers.]

digitalism, digitalismus (dij·it·al·izm, dij·it·al·iz'·mus). The symptoms of poisoning produced by digitalis.

digitalization (dij·it·al·i·za'·shun). The process of administering digitalis to a patient until the desired physiological effects are produced.

digitaloid (dij·it·al·oid). Resembling or related to digitalis. [digitalis, Gk *eidos* form.]

digitalose (dij·it·al·oze). $CH_3(CHOH)_3CH(OCH_3)CHO$, a methylpentose produced by the hydrolysis of digitalin in which, with glucose, it forms a unit combined with digitaligenin. It is isomeric with cymarose.

digitanide (dij·it·an·ide). The name given to complex glycosides, A, B and C, which are actually present in *Digitalis* species, and which are the precursors of the glycosides, digitoxin, gitoxin, digoxin and digitalin, produced by hydrolysis in the presence of specific enzymes. They are compounds of steroid genins, a digitose, glucose and acetic acid.

digitate (dij·it·ate). 1. Having fingers or processes resembling fingers. 2. Having faintly-marked depressions as though fingers had been pressed on the part. [L *digitatus* having fingers.]

digitation (dij·it·a·shun). 1. A process resembling a finger; the term is used particularly of a muscle. 2. A method of amputation by which the stump is divided into a fork-like process so that it can be used to grip objects. [see prec.]

digitiform (dij·it·e·form). Shaped like a finger. [L *digitus* finger, form.]

digitigrade (dij·it·e·grade). Walking on the toes. [L *digitus finger (toe), gradus* step.]

digitizer (dij·it·i·zer). Apparatus which will receive data and record them in digital form. [L *digitus* finger.]

digitofibular (dij·it·o·fib'·ew·lar). Pertaining to the fibular aspect of the toes. [L *digitus* finger (toe), fibular.]

digitometatarsal (dij·it·o·met·ah·tar'·sal). Pertaining to the toes and the metatarsus. [L *digitus* finger (toe), metatarsus.]

digitonin (dij·it·o·nin). $C_{56}H_{92}O_{29}$, a saponin found in the seeds of *Digitalis purpurea* Linn. It forms insoluble compounds with cholesterol and ergosterol, and is employed in the estimation of the latter (digitonin reaction).

digitoplantar (dij·it·o·plan'·tar). Pertaining to the toes and the sole of the foot. [L *digitus* finger (toe), *planta* sole.]

digitoradial (dij·it·o·ra'·de·al). Pertaining to the radial aspect of the fingers. [L *digitus* finger, radius.]

digitose (dij·it·oze). The general name for the methylpentoses, digitoxose and digitalose, which constitute units in the digitalis glycosides.

digitotibial (dij·it·o·tib'·e·al). Pertaining to the tibial aspect of the toes. [L *digitus* finger (toe), tibia.]

digito-ulnar (dij·it·o·ul'·nar). Pertaining to the ulnar aspect of the fingers. [L *digitus* finger, ulna.]

digitoxigenin (dij·it·ox·ij'·en·in). $C_{23}H_{34}O_4$, an aglucone occurring in the leaves of *Digitalis purpurea* Linn. combined with digitoxose as the glycoside, digitoxin.

Digitoxin BP 1973 (dij·it·ox·in). Crystallized digitalin; $C_{41}H_{64}O_{13}$. The most important of the three cardiotoxic glycosides found in the leaves of *Digitalis purpurea.* It is composed of digitoxigenin united to digitoxose.

digitoxinum. (dij·it·ox·in·um). *European Pharmacopoeia* name for Digitoxin BP 1973.

digitoxose (dij·it·ox·oze). $CH_3(CHOH)_3CH_2CHO$, a desoxy-methylpentose obtained by the hydrolysis of digitoxin, digoxin and gitoxin, the glycosides of *Digitalis* species. It exerts a considerable influence on the cardiotoxic action of the aglucones with which it is associated in the natural glycosides.

digitus (dij·it·us). A finger or a toe. **Digitus auricularis.** Little finger. **Digitus clavatus.** Clubbed finger. **Digitus demonstrativus.** Index finger. **Digitus hippocraticus.** Hippocratic finger. **Digitus medicus.** Ring finger. **Digitus mortuus.** Acro-asphyxia. **Digitus recellens.** Trigger finger. **Digitus valgus.** Displacement or permanent deviation of a finger or fingers to the ulnar side. **Digitus varus.** Displacement or permanent deviation of a finger or fingers to the radial side. [L.]

diglossia, diglossus (di·glos·e·ah, di·glos·us). Bifid tongue. *See* TONGUE. [GK *di-, glossa* tongue.]

diglutathione (di·gloo·tah·thi'·one). The double sulphide of glutathione formed by the elimination of hydrogen between the sulphydryl groups of 2 molecules of glutathione. This process of oxidation is reversible and is believed to play a part in tissue respiration, the glutathione of the tissues acting as an oxygen carrier. It would appear that traces of copper are essential for the process.

diglyceride (di·glis·er·ide). An ester of glycerol in which the hydrogen of 2 of the hydroxyl groups is replaced by an acyl radical.

diglycol (di·gli·kol). Name applied to any compound which contains two alcoholic groups, CH_2OH. **Diglycol stearate.** A base used for making tar ointment.

dignathus (di·na·thus). A monster with a double lower jaw. [Gk *di-, gnathos* jaw.]

digoxigenin (dij·ox·ij·en·in). $C_{23}H_{34}O_5$, an aglucone which, combined with digitoxose, occurs as the glycoside, digoxin, in the leaves of *Digitalis lanata* Ehrh.

Digoxin BP 1958 (dij·ox·in). $C_{41}H_{64}O_{14}$, a crystalline glycoside obtained from the leaves of *Digitalis lanata* Ehrh., the woolly foxglove. It is administered orally for the same purposes as digitalis, and is the most widely employed single cardiac glycoside, having displaced mixtures such as digitalin, etc. It is more rapidly excreted than the other cardiac drugs, and is hence less cumulative.

digoxinum (dij·ox·in·um). *European Pharmacopoeia* name for Digoxin BP 1973.

Di Guglielmo, Giovanni (b. 1886). Pavia and Naples haematologist.

Di Guglielmo's anaemia, or disease. Acute erythraemic myelosis; acute erythraemia; immature-cell erythraemia: a very rare, fatal, acute anaemic condition resembling acute leukaemia, having a severe erythroblastic bone marrow with large numbers of immature red cells and variable numbers of early immature white cells in the peripheral blood.

digyny (di·ji·ne). The presence in the product of gamete fusion of 2 female nuclei and 1 male nucleus. [Gk *di-, gyne* woman.]

diheterozygote (di·het·er·o·zi'·gote). In genetics, an individual heterozygous for 2 characters. [Gk *di-*, heterozygote.]

dihexose (di·hex·oze). Name applied to a disaccharide like sucrose, because it is composed of 2 hexose molecules. [Gk *di-*, hexose.]

dihexoside (di·hex·o·side). Dihexose.

dihybrid (di·hi·brid). The offspring of a cross in which the parents differ in 2 characters. [Gk *di-*, hybrid.]

Dihydrallazine (di·hi·dral·az·een). BP Commission approved name for 1,4-dihydrazinophthalazine, a blood-pressure depressant.

dihydrate (di·hi·drate). 1. A general term for compounds which possess 2 hydroxyl, OH, groups. 2. A compound which has crystallized with 2 molecules of water. [Gk *di-, hydor* water.]

dihydrated (di·hi·dra·ted). Combined with 2 molecules of water of crystallization. [see prec.]

dihydric (di·hi·drik). Term applied to an alcohol that contains 2 hydroxyl, OH, groups.

dihydride (di·hi·dride). A substance formed by the combination of 2 atoms of hydrogen with 1 atom of an element, or with a divalent radical.

dihydrocholesterol (di·hi·dro·kol·es'·ter·ol). $C_{27}H_{47}OH$. 1. A reduction product of cholesterol found with it in animal tissues. 2. Normal dihydrocholesterol, coprosterol, a natural sterol occurring in the intestine and found in the fatty matter of faeces.

dihydrocodeine (di·hi·dro·ko'·de·een). **Dihydrocodeine Acid Tartrate BPC 1968, Dihydrocodeine Tartrate BP 1973.** The hydrogen tartrate of the 3-methyl ester of 7,8-dihydromorphine. An analgesic with potency and side-effects nearer to those of morphine than of codeine; also used as a cough suppressant.

dihydrocodeinone (di·hi·dro·ko'·de·in·one). A synthetic alkaloid of the morphine group, used orally in the form of the acid tartrate for its action on the cough centre in coughs and respiratory affections. The hydrochloride is sometimes employed subcutaneously.

dihydrodiethylstilboestrol (di·hi·dro·di·eth·il·stil·be'·strol). Hexoestrol, $OHC_6H_4CH(C_2H_5)CH(C_2H_5)C_6H_4OH$. A synthetic non-steroid oestrogen derived from 4,4-dihydroxystilbene, with an activity equal to that of oestradiol, but more soluble in water and capable of being given orally. It is less toxic than diethylstilboestrol, and may be used for the same conditions as those for which the natural oestrogens are prescribed. *See* HEXOESTROL.

dihydro-equilenin (di·hi·dro·ek·wil'·en·in). $C_{18}H_{20}O_2$, a naturally-occurring steroid oestrogen.

dihydro-ergocornine (di·hi·dro·er·go·kor'·neen). One of the alkaloid constituents of ergotoxine. It is adrenalytic and sympatheticolytic, and has been used therapeutically for lowering blood pressure.

dihydro-erythroidine (di·hi·dro·er·ith·**roi**'·deen). A hydrogenated derivative of β-erythroidine, an alkaloid obtained from species of *Eythrina.* It has a curare-like effect on motor nerve-endings and is used in surgery, as its action is more prolonged and more intense than the parent alkaloid.

dihydromorphinone (di·hi·dro·**mor**·fe·none). $C_{17}H_{19}O_3N$, an analgesic about 5 times as active as morphine, but weaker in hypnotic action. It is employed in the form of the hydrochloride.

dihydroresorcin, dihydroresorcinol (di·**hi**·dro·res·**or**'·sin, di·**hi**·-dro·res·**or**'·sin·ol). $C_6H_6(OH)_2$, a compound formed by the reduction of resorcinol with sodium amalgam. It has antibacterial properties.

dihydrostreptomycin (di·**hi**·dro·strep·to·**mi**'·sin). $C_{21}H_{41}O_{12}N_7$, a streptomycin derivative, more stable than the latter. **Dihydrostreptomycin Sulphate BP 1958.** $(C_{21}H_{41}O_{12}N_7)_2{\cdot}3H_2SO_4$, a white solid, soluble in water, insoluble in alcohol, prepared by the hydrogenation of streptomycin and conversion to the sulphate.

Dihydrotachysterol BP 1968 (di·**hi**·dro·tak·e·**steer**'·ol). 9,10-Secoergosta-5,7,22-trien-3β-ol, a synthetic compound with actions resembling those of calciferol and vitamin D_3.

dihydrotestosterone (di·**hi**·dro·tes·to·**steer**·one). An androgen with biological properties formed from its inactive precursor testosterone within androgen-responsive target cells by means of an intranuclear enzyme, 5α-reductase.

dihydrotheelin (di·**hi**·dro·**the**'·lin). Oestradiol.

dihydroxyacetone (di·**hi**·drox·e·**as**'·et·one). The simplest keto-sugar. Not a normal metabolite but is utilized by the liver in a reaction catalysed by triokinase and yielding dihydroxyacetone phosphate. **Dihydroxyacetone phosphate.** $CH_2OHCOCH_2OPO_3H_2$, an intermediate in glycolysis and gluconeogenesis.

dihydroxyanthranol (di·hi·drox·e·**an**'·thran·ol). Dithranol BP 1958.

dihydroxyanthraquinone (di·hi·**drox**·e·an·thrah·**kwin**'·one). A purgative of anthraquinone type; used mainly in veterinary medicine.

dihydroxybenzene (di·hi·drox·e·**ben**'·zeen). Dioxybenzene, $C_6H_4(OH)_2$. The general term for the isomeric dihydric phenols, catechol, resorcinol and quinol, having the hydroxyl groups in the *ortho-*, *meta-* and *para-*positions, respectively.

1,25-dihydroxycholecholesterol. *See* VITAMIN D.

dihydroxydiethylstilbene (di·hi·**drox**·e·di·eth·il·**stil**'·been). Diethylstilboestrol.

dihydroxyoestrin (di·hi·drox·e·**e**'·strin). Oestradiol BPC 1959. **Dihydroxyoestrin monobenzoate.** Oestradiol Benzoate BP 1958.

dihydroxyphenylalanine (di·hi·**drox**·e·fe·nil·**al**'·an·een). DOPA; an amino acid formed by tyrosine oxidation in animal tissues. A precursor of the catecholamines and of melanin.

dihydroxyphenylethylmethylamine (di·hi·**drox**·e·fe·nil·eth·il·-meth·il·**am**'·een). $C_6H_3(OH)_2CH_2CH_2NH_2$. Dopamine, a catecholamine which is the precursor of noradrenalin and adrenaline.

dihydroxyphthalophenone (di·hi·**drox**·e·thal·o·**fe**'·none). Phenolphthalein, $C_6H_4(COO){=}C(C_6H_4OH)_2$. A crystalline white compound prepared from phenol and phthalic anhydride. It dissolves in dilute alkalis with a red coloration: used as an indicator (pH 8–10), and in medicine as a mild purgative.

dihydroxypropyl bismuthate (di·hi·drox·e·**pro**'·pil **biz**·muth·ate). $C_3H_5(OH)_2BiO_3$, an anti-treponema drug, used in the oral treatment of yaws and syphilis.

dihydroxytheelin (di·hi·**drox**·e·**the**'·lin). Oestradiol.

dihypercytosis (di·**hi**·per·si·**to**'·sis). Hyperleucocytosis in which there is relative increase in neutrophil cells. [Gk *di-*, hypercytosis.]

dihysteria (di·his·**teer**·e·ah). The abnormal state of having a double uterus. [Gk *di-*, *hystera* womb.]

di-iodide (di·i·o·dide). A salt of hydriodic acid which contains 2 atoms of iodine. [see foll.]

di-iodo- (di·i·o·do). A prefix signifying that an organic compound contains 2 iodine atoms. [Gk *di-*, iodine.]

di-iodofluorescein (di·i·o·do·floo·or·**es**'·e·in). An iodine derivative of fluorescein, used as a dye. Di-iodofluorescein in which radioactive iodine, ^{131}I, is substituted for some stable iodine atoms has been used for the attempted localization of brain tumours, since this dye is selectively taken up by the tumour. The position of the tumour is assessed by measurement of the external γ-ray field around the head arising from the ^{131}I. Considerable technical difficulties attend this method, and it is unsuitable for posterior-fossa tumours.

di-iodoform (di·i·o·do·form). Ethylene periodide, ethylene tetra-iodide, C_2I_4. A yellow odourless compound used as a substitute for iodoform.

di-iodohydroxypropane (di·i·**o**·do·hi·drox·e·**pro**'·pane). $C_3H_5I_2(OH)$, an oily preparation containing 80 per cent iodine; used for external application.

Di-iodohydroxyquinoline BP 1973 (di·i·o·do·hi·drox·e·**kwin**'·o·-leen). $C_9H_4I_2(OH)N$, a non-toxic amoebacidal drug given by mouth.

di-iodomethane (di·i·o·do·**me**'·thane). Methylene iodide, CH_2I_2. A yellow liquid employed in the density determination of substances that would dissolve if water were used.

di-iodothyronine (di·i·o·do·**thi**'·ron·een). An iodine-containing compound found in the thyroid gland. It has a very weak thyroxine-like activity.

di-iodotyrosine (di·i·o·do·**ti**'·ro·seen). Iodogogoric acid, $OHC_6H_2I_2CH_2CH(NH_2)COOH$, an iodine-containing amino acid found in the thyroid gland and believed to be an intermediary in the synthesis of thyroxine. It has been used in the treatment of hyperthyroidism but its effects are no different from those of inorganic iodine compounds.

di-isopropylfluorophosphonate (di·i·so·**pro**·pil·floo·or·o·**fos**'·fon·-ate). DFP; dyflos, $(CH_3)_2CHOFPOOCH(CH_3)_2$. A powerful miotic which relieves tension in glaucoma when other drugs fail. It is also used in myasthenia gravis. It is a dangerous drug that should be handled with caution; in large therapeutic doses it may cause bronchial constriction, muscular fibrillation, salivation, diarrhoea, and even cardiospasm. Atropine sulphate counteracts the effect.

dikaryon (di·**kar**·e·on). A cell, spore or mycelium containing 2 nuclei. [Gk *di-*, *karyon* nut.]

dikephobia (di·ke·**fo**·be·ah). A morbid fear of justice. [Gk *dike* right, *phobos* fear.]

diketocamphane (di·**ke**·to·**kam**'·fane). Camphorquinone.

diketone (di·**ke**·tone). An organic compound which has in its structure 2 carbonyl, CO, groups.

diketopiperazine (di·ke·to·pip·**er**'·az·een). Glycine anhydride, $(NHCH_2CO)_2$. A crystalline compound which is obtained, together with certain of its substitution products, in small amounts on hydrolysis of proteins. According to the cyclol theory, the diketopiperazine ring structure forms an integral part of protein molecules.

dikwakwadi (dik·wak·**wah**·de). Witkop; a non-contagious infection of the scalp resembling favus, which affects South African natives suffering from syphilis and is characterized by the presence of crusts which run together so that the head appears to be covered with a white skull-cap. [S. African Bantu name.]

dilaceration (di·las·er·**a**'·shun). 1. The act of tearing apart; term used particularly of the tearing in half of a cataract after an incision has been made in it. 2. The condition of a tooth a portion of which, during development, has been displaced and has continued to develop in its new environment, so that the fully formed tooth is bent in its long axis. [L *dilacerare* to tear apart.]

dilapidation (dil·**ap**·id·**a**'·shun). Deterioration or disintegration. [L *dilapidare* to scatter like stones.]

dilatation (di·lat·a·shun). The enlargement or increase in volume of a hollow organ, cavity or tube. **Congenital idiopathic dilatation of the colon.** Hirschsprung's disease; megacolon. **Digital dilatation.** The stretching of an orifice by the fingers.

Gastric dilatation. Enlargement of the cavity of the stomach, from either muscular atony or obstruction of the pyloric orifice. **Dilatation of the heart.** Enlargement of the heart resulting from stretching of the muscular walls due to weakening of the myocardium; it is a manifestation of cardiac failure. **Hydrostatic dilatation.** Dilatation due to fluid pressure. **Prognathic dilatation.** Dilatation of the pyloric end of the stomach causing a protrusion seen on x-ray examination. **Dilatation of the stomach.** Gastric dilatation (see above). [L *dilatare* to widen.]

dilate (di·late). 1. To enlarge or extend in size and bulk. 2. To stretch apart. [see prec.]

dilation (di·la·shun). Dilatation or distension.

dilator (di·la·tor). An instrument for the enlargement of a body opening, or tube, by stretching. **Anal dilator.** An instrument for stretching the anal orifice. **Hydrostatic dilator.** An oesophageal dilator, the essential part of which is a rubber and linen bag which is dilated by means of a syringe that injects water. **Laryngeal dilator.** An instrument with 2 or more blades for stretching the larynx in cases of laryngeal stricture. **Oesophageal dilator.** A bougie or hydrostatic apparatus for widening a narrowed oesophagus. **Tracheal dilator.** An instrument for enlarging a tracheotomy wound to admit the passage of a tracheotomy tube. **Dilator tubae.** A few fibres of the tensor palati muscle which are attached to the cartilage of the auditory (eustachian) tube and which dilate the latter slightly during swallowing. **Vaginal dilator.** A glass or plastics cylinder used to enlarge the vaginal orifice. [L *dilatare* to widen.]

See also: ARNOTT (N.), BARNES, BOSSI, HEGAR, NETTLESHIP.

dilator muscle of the pupil [musculus dilatator pupillae (NA)]. Radiating smooth muscle fibres of the iris, innervated by sympathetic nerves.

dilator naris muscle. *See* NASAL MUSCLE, pars alaris.

dildo, dildoe (dil·do). An artificial penis. [Jamaican word from *dildo*, West Indian cactus with columnar joints.]

Dilepididae (di·lep·id′·id·e). A family of the cestode order Cyclophyllidea. The genus *Dipylidium* is sometimes included in it. [Gk *di-*, *lepis* scale, *eidos* form.]

Dill BPC 1954 (dil). Anethum, dill fruit; the dried fruits of the annual umbelliferous herb *Anethum graveolens* Linn. cultivated in Western Europe. [AS *dili.*]

dilo (di·lo). Caulophyllum, blue cohosh, papoose or squaw root; the rhizome and roots of *Caulophyllum thalictroides* (Linn.) Michx. (family Berberidaceae), grown in the USA and used as an emmenagogue and diuretic.

Diloxanide (di·lox·an·ide). BP Commission approved name for dichloroacet-4-hydroxy-*N*-methylanilide, used in the treatment of amoebic dysentery. **Diloxanide Furoate BP 1973.** 4-(*N*-methyldichloroacetoamido)phenyl 2-furoate, a white, odourless, tasteless crystalline powder. An anti-amoebic agent used, sometimes in conjunction with other drugs, in the treatment of various types of amoebiasis.

diluent (dil·ew·ent). 1. Diluting. 2. A weak drink. 3. An agent for effecting dilution of any of the body fluids. 4. An inert liquid or solid used to increase the bulk of another substance or solution. [L *diluere* to wash away.]

dilupine (di·loo·peen). $C_{16}H_{26}O_2N_2$, a minor alkaloid of *Lupinus* species.

dilute (di·lewt). 1. To make weaker or more liquid by admixture, e.g. of water, to increase bulk. 2. Term qualifying solutions which have been so diluted. [L *diluere* to wash away.]

dilution (di·lew·shun). 1. The process or act of reducing the strength of a solution or mixture. 2. Any substance which has been subjected to a dilution process. **Dye dilution.** Indicator dilution using a substance identifiable by its colour. **Indicator dilution.** A method for examining the flow in a circulating system (e.g. the circulation of the blood) which involves the introduction of a known amount of an indicator, which can be detected downstream, into the circulation and monitoring its passage downstream. The time pattern of the degree of dilution of the indicator provides information about the flow in the system. **Isotope dilution.** A method for determination of the content, C_A, of substance A in a mixture. To the mixture is added a known amount X of the substance A, specially produced so that one of the constituent atoms of its molecule has for a particular isotope an increased relative abundance, B, from that in the substance A which is to be analysed. The final increased isotopic abundance B' in the mixture is measured, so that

$$C_A = \left(\frac{B}{B'} - 1\right)X$$

Thermal dilution. Dilution using fluid that is warmer or cooler than the natural fluid, detectable by a change of temperature. [see prec.]

dimargarin (di·mar·gar·in). A glyceride consisting of 2 molecules of margaric acid and 1 molecule of glycerol.

Dimastigamoeba (di·mas·tig·am·e′·bah). A genus of amoebae of which *Dimastigamoeba gruberi* is frequent in stale faeces. Individuals exist in either amoeboid or flagellate forms, the latter having 2 flagella. [Gk *di*, *mastix* whip, amoeba.]

dimazon (di·ma·zon). Diacetylaminoazotoluene.

Dimefline (di·mef·leen). BP Commission approved name for 8-dimethylaminomethyl-7-methoxy-3-methylflavone; a respiratory stimulant.

Dimenhydrinate BP 1973 (di·men·hi·drin·ate). 2-(Benzohydryloxy)-*N*,*N*-dimethylethylamine 8-chlorotheophyllinate. An antihistamine drug, but its main uses are against motion sickness, radiation sickness and the vomiting of pregnancy.

Dimenoxadole (di·men·ox·ad·ole). BP Commission approved name for 2-dimethylaminoethyl-2-ethoxy-2,2-diphenylacetate; a narcotic analgesic.

Dimepheptanol (di·mep·hep·tan·ol). BP Commission approved name for 6-dimethyl-amino-4,4-diphenylheptan-3-ol, a central analgesic and narcotic. It has properties similar to those of morphine.

Dimepregnen (di·me·preg·nen). BP Commission approved name for 3β-hydroxy-6α,16α-dimethylpregn-4-en-20-one; an anti-oestrogen.

Dimepropion (di·mep·ro·pe·on). BP Commission approved name for α-dimethylaminopropiophenone; an anorexigenic agent.

Dimercaprol BP 1973 (di·mer·kap·rol). British Anti-Lewisite, BAL, 2,3-dimercaptopropanol, $CH_2(SH)CH(SH)CH_2OH$. A compound developed during World War II as an antidote for vesicants containing arsenic, e.g. lewisite; the thiol SH groups react with the arsenic and thus protect the essential SH groups of the cell protoplasm. Damage to the skin can be prevented by the application either before or within 2 h of contamination. It is also an effective antidote in poisoning by antimony, bismuth, mercury, gold, chromium and nickel, but is relatively useless in lead poisoning. It is particularly valuable against the haemorrhagic encephalitis or exfoliative dermatitis due to organic arsenicals employed in the treatment of syphilis, being usually injected intramuscularly in peanut oil.

Dimercaprolum (di·mer·kap·rol·um). *European Pharmacopoeia* name for Dimercaprol BP 1973.

dimerous (dim·er·us). Consisting of 2 parts; bipartite. [Gk *di-*, *meros* part.]

dimers (di·merz). Compounds comprising 2 molecules. [Gk *di-*, *meros* part.]

Dimesone (di·mes·one). BP Commission approved name for 9α-fluoro-11β,21-dihydroxy-16α,17-dimethylpregna-1,4-diene-3,20-dione; an anti-inflammatory steroid.

dimetallic (di·met·al·ik). Of molecules, containing 2 atoms of a metallic element. [Gk *di-*, metal.]

Dimethicone (di·meth·e·kone). BP Commission approved name for a silicone with water-repellent and skin-adherent properties. It is employed in industrial barrier creams as a skin protective agent, and in creams, ointments and lotions as a prophylactic against bedsores and the traumatic effect of ammonia in urine on dermal contact.

Dimethindene (di·meth·in·deen). BP Commission approved name for 2-{1-[2-(2-dimethylaminoethyl)inden-3-yl}ethyl]-pyridine; an antihistamine.

Dimethisoquin (di·meth·i·so·kwin). BP Commission approved name for 3-butyl-1-(2-dimethylamino-ethoxy)isoquinoline; an antipruritic.

Dimethisterone BP 1973 (di·meth·is·ter·one). 6α-21-Dimethylethisterone; an orally active progestational agent with no androgenic, oestrogenic or anabolic activity. It is used in the treatment of amenorrhoea and threatened abortion.

Dimethothiazine (di·meth·o·thi·az·een). BP Commission approved name for 10-(2-dimethylaminopropyl)-2-dimethylsulphamoyl-phenothiazine; it is used in the treatment of migraine.

Dimethoxanate (di·meth·ox·an·ate). BP Commission approved name for 2-(2-dimethylaminoethoxy)ethyl phenothiazine-10-carboxylate; a cough suppressant.

dimethyl- (di·meth·il). In organic chemistry, a prefix signifying the presence in a compound of 2 methyl, CH_3, groups. **Dimethyl Phthalate BP 1968.** $C_6H_4(COOCH_3)_2$, a colourless or slightly yellow liquid which is an insect repellent, being effective against fleas, mosquitoes, mites, ticks and midges. It may be applied to the skin or clothing and is non-irritant to the normal skin but may affect the conjunctiva and mucous membranes. It is sometimes dispensed as a cream which should contain not less than 35 per cent dimethyl phthalate. **Dimethyl sulphate.** $(CH_3O)_2SO_2$, a very poisonous liquid formed from sulphur trioxide and methyl ether; used in organic synthesis to introduce the methyl group, and in chemical warfare as a poison gas. **Dimethyl sulphoxide.** BP Commission approved name for methyl sulphoxide; a topical anti-inflammatory agent. **Dimethyl yellow.** Dimethylamino-azobenzene.

dimethylacetal (di·meth·il·as′·et·al). $CH_3CH(OCH_3)_2$, a compound which is anaesthetic in action, but too toxic for general use in medicine.

dimethylamine (di·meth·il·am′·een). $(CH_3)_2NH$, a secondary amine which occurs in guano, and in decomposing nitrogenous matter, especially fish. It is a heavy soluble vapour with an ammoniacal smell, and is used in dealing with weevil infestation.

dimethylamino-antipyrine (di·meth·il·am′·in·o·an·te·pi′·reen). Amidopyrine BPC 1954.

dimethylamino-azobenzene (di·meth·il·am·in·o·az·o·ben′·zeen). Dimethyl yellow, $C_6H_5N{=}NC_6H_4N(CH_3)_2$. A dye used as an indicator, with a pH range of 2.8 (red) to 4.0 (yellow). It is also the indicator used in Toepfer's test for free hydrochloric acid in gastric juice.

dimethylaminobenzaldehyde (di·meth·il·am·in·o·ben·zal′·de·hide). $(CH_3)_2NC_6H_4CHO$, a yellowish-white crystalline powder, a solution of which in absolute alcohol and hydrochloric acid is used as a test for indole production by bacteria (Ehrlich's rosindole reagent). A solution in 20 per cent hydrochloric acid is used to test for excess urobilinogen in urine.

dimethylarsine (di·meth·il·ar′·seen). 1. $(CH_3)_2AsH$, a colourless liquid related to cacodyl. 2. The cacodyl radical, $(CH_3)_2As$-, which enters into combinations like an alkali metal.

dimethylated (di·meth·il·a·ted). Term, applied to a compound which has had 2 methyl groups introduced into its molecule.

dimethylbenzene (di·meth·il·ben′·zeen). Xylene, xylol, $C_6H_4(CH_3)_2$. A homologue of benzene which occurs in 3 colourless aromatic liquids, used as solvents in microscopy, and for sterilizing catgut.

dimethylcarbinol (di·meth·il·kar′·bin·ol). Isopropyl alcohol, secondary propyl alcohol, $(CH_3)_2CH(OH)$. A liquid occurring in fusel oil and also as a petroleum by-product. Used as a solvent, denaturant and surgical antiseptic, and in the manufacture of perfumes.

dimethyldicocoammonium chloride (di·meth·il·di·ko·ko·am·o′·ne·um klor·ide). A quaternary ammonium salt with very efficient non-wetting anticoagulant properties, used to coat needles and syringes for drawing blood to prevent the surface influence on clotting of the blood.

dimethyldiphenylene disulphide (di·meth·il·di·fe′·nil·een di·sul′·fide). Mesulphen.

dimethylethylcarbinol (di·meth·il·eth·il·kar′·bin·ol). Amylene hydrate, amylene alcohol, $(CH_3)_2C(C_2H_5)(OH)$. A colourless volatile liquid with hypnotic properties. It is used as a solvent for bromethol, whose action it enhances.

dimethylethylpyrrole (di·meth·il·eth·il·pir′·ole). $C_8H_{13}N$; 2 compounds of this composition, haemopyrrole, 2,3-dimethyl-4-ethyl-pyrrole, and kryptopyrrole, 2,4-dimethyl-3-ethyl-pyrrole, have been isolated as ultimate fission products of haemin, chlorophyll and bilirubin.

dimethylketone (di·meth·il·ke′·tone). Acetone.

dimethylmercaptopropanol (di·meth·il·mer·kap·to·pro′·pan·ol). Dimercaprol.

dimethylmorphine (di·meth·il·mor′·feen). Thebaine, $C_{19}H_{21}NO_3$. A phenanthrene alkaloid in opium which is much less narcotic than morphine. Chemically its structure is the same as morphine except that both hydroxy groups have methyl radicals inserted. Toxic doses can cause strychnine-like convulsions and paralysis of peripheral motor nerves, particularly in animals which are susceptible to the stimulating effects of morphine and its derivatives. It is not used medicinally as such, except as it occurs in opium and its preparations.

dimethylparaphenylenediamine (di·meth·il·par·ah·fe·nil·een·di′·am·een). A compound used in bacteriology as a substrate for an oxidase possessed by members of the genus *Neisseria.* When a solution of the compound is poured on to a plate on which neisseriae are growing, the colonies develop a purple colour within a second or two. The test is used to detect gonococcal colonies in mixed cultures.

dimethylphenanthrene (di·meth·il·fen·an′·threen). $(CH_3)_2C_{14}H_8$, a carcinogenic and oestrogenic hydrocarbon derivable from coal tar.

dimethylphosphine (di·meth·il·fos′·feen). $(CH_3)_2PH$, a colourless liquid, insoluble in water and easily oxidized. It has been used against infusoria.

dimethylsulphanilamidoisoxazole (di·meth·il·sul·fan·il·am·id·o·i·zox′·az·ole). A sulphonamide drug that is used against urinary infections.

Dimethylthiambutene (di·meth·il·thi·am′·bew·teen). BP Commission approved name for 3-dimethylamino-1,1-di-2′-thienyl-but-1-ene, the dimethyl analogue of diethylthiambutene; its properties are closely similar.

dimethylthianthrene (di·meth·il·thi·an′·threen). Mesulphen.

Dimethyltubocurarine (di·meth·il·tew·bo·kew·rah′·reen). BP Commission approved name for the dimethyl ether of D-tubocurarine iodide. It is a muscle relaxant resembling the parent compound in properties.

dimethylxanthine (di·meth·il·zan′·theen). $C_7H_8O_2N_4$, a substituted purine which occurs in 3 isomeric forms: theophylline (1,3), theobromine (3,7) and paraxanthine (1,7).

dimetria (di·met·re·ah). The anatomical state in which there is a double uterus. [Gk *di-*, *metra* womb.]

Dimitri, Vicente. 20th century Buenos Aires neurologist.

Dimitri's disease, Weber-Dimitri disease. Sturge-Kalischer-Weber disease.

Dimitry, Theodore John (b. 1879). New Orleans ophthalmologist.

Mules-Dimitry operation. Evisceration followed by insertion of a glass, gold or bone ball into the sclerotic, the sclera and conjunctiva being stitched over it.

Dimmer, Friedrich (b. 1855). Vienna ophthalmologist.

Dimmer's keratitis. An infiltration of the superficial part of the cornea in the form of discs, occurring in young land workers and usually unilateral.

Dimmer's operation. For ectropion: the lower lid is split through the grey line along the lid margin, and a triangle of conjunctiva and tarsal plate is removed from the centre of the lower lid, with its base at the lid margin. A slightly larger triangle of skin, base up, is removed lateral to the outer canthus. The edges of the 2 triangles are sutured, the skin being slid laterally.

Biber-Haab-Dimmer degeneration. A familial type of dystrophy or degeneration of the corneal epithelium, beginning about puberty and characterized by the formation of fine lattice-like superficial lines.

dimorphic (di·**mor**·fik). Marked by dimorphism; existing as 2 distinct forms. [Gk *di-*, *morphe* form.]

dimorphism (di·**mor**·fizm). 1. In genetics, the occurrence in the population of 2 forms with different genotypes and/or chromosome complement. 2. In biology, a difference in outward appearance or structure occurring between 2 individuals of the same species. **Physical dimorphism.** In chemistry, crystallization of certain substances in 2 different forms. **Sexual dimorphism.** The condition present in the early embryo of having properties of both sexes. [see prec.]

dimorphobiotic (di·**mor**·fo·bi·**ot**'·ik). An organism the life cycle of which shows alternation of generations and parasitic and non-parasitic phases. [Gk *di-*, *morphe* form, *bios* life.]

dimorphous (di·**mor**·fus). Dimorphic.

dimple (dimpl). 1. A slight natural indentation or depression on the surface of a part of the body. 2. A slight indentation resulting from contracting scar tissue or from trauma. **Hilum dimple.** The appearance of a dimple beside the sternum in the 2nd intercostal space when the breath is held at the end of an inspiration, caused by enlarged mediastinal lymph glands. **Postnatal dimple.** Coccygeal sinus. *See* SINUS. [ME *dympull.*]

See also: FUCHS (E.).

dineric (di·**ner**·ik). 1. Relating to the phenomena peculiar to the interfacial area between 2 liquids. 2. Describing the whirling motion of the interface of liquids. [Gk *dinos* a whirling.]

dineuric (di·**newr**·ik). A nerve cell which has 2 axons. [Gk *di-*, *neuron* nerve.]

dinic (**di**·nik). An agent which relieves vertigo or dizziness. [Gk *dinos* a whirling.]

dinical (**di**·nikl). Relating to, belonging to, or relieving dizziness or vertigo. [see prec.]

dinitrate (di·**ni**·trate). A compound which contains 2 nitrate, NO_2, groups.

dinitrated (di·**ni**·tra·ted). Having had 2 nitro, NO_2, groups introduced into its molecule.

dinitrocellulose (di·**ni**·tro·**sel**'·ew·loze). $C_6H_8O_5(NO_2)_2$, a nitrated cellulose obtained by the action of nitric and sulphuric acids on defatted cotton wool; mixed with the tetranitrate formed in the process it constitutes pyroxylin, used as a basis of collodion.

dinitrocresol (di·**ni**·tro·**kre**'·sol). Dinitro-orthocresol, $CH_3C_6H_2(OH)(NO_2)_2$. An orange dye formed by the nitration of cresol and known commercially as *saffron substitute.* It increases the oxidative metabolism in relation to fat and is used like dinitrophenol in the treatment of obesity, but is more potent and correspondingly more toxic. The toxic symptoms produced are skin eruptions, neuritis, damage to the liver and kidneys, and, less commonly, cataract. It does not cause ketosis or acidosis. It is now employed as a crop spray, and has caused poisoning in farm workers.

dinitro-orthocresol (di·**ni**·tro·or·tho·**kre**'·sol). Dinitrocresol.

dinitrophenol (di·ni·tro·**fe**·nol). $C_6H_3(OH)(NO_2)_2$, a compound formed by the catalytic nitration of benzene with nitric oxides, yielding the 2,4 isomer. It brings about an increase in the metabolism when injected, raises the temperature considerably and has been used in obesity; its toxicity renders such use inadvisable. An uncoupler of oxidative phosphorylation.

dinomania (di·no·**ma**·ne·ah). Choromania; epidemic chorea; dancing mania. [Gk *dinos* a whirling, mania.]

dinophobia (di·no·**fo**·be·ah). Unreasoning or morbid fear of becoming dizzy. [Gk *dinos* a whirling, phobia.]

Dinoprost (**di**·no·prost). BP Commission approved name for 7-[3α,5α-dihydroxy-2β-(3-*S*-hydroxy-*trans*-oct-1-enyl)cyclopent-1]-yl-*cis*-hept-5-enoic acid; a smooth muscle activator.

Dinoprostone (di·no·**pros**·tone). BP Commission approved name for 7-[3α-hydroxy-2β-(3-*S*-hydroxy-*trans*-oct-1-enyl)-5-oxocyclopent-1-yl]-*cis*-hept-5-enoic acid; a smooth muscle activator used in gynaecology and obstetrics.

Dinopsyllus lypusus (di·**nop**·sil·us **lip**·us·us). A wild-rodent flea which transmits plague. [Gk *deinos* terrible, *psylla* flea.]

dinormocytosis (**di**·nor·mo·si·**to**'·sis). Isonormocytosis; normal condition of the leucocytes in the blood. [Gk *di-*, normocytosis.]

dinucleotide (di·**new**·kle·o·tide). In the splitting up of a nucleic acid, the intermediary association of 2 mononucleotides which, on further hydrolysis, break down into the latter completely. **Nicotinamide-adenine dinucleotide** (NAD). New nomenclature for diphosphopyridine nucleotide (co-enzyme I). In reactions it is written NAD^+. **Nicotinamide-adenine dinucleotide phosphate** (NADP). New nomenclature for triphosphopyridine nucleotide (co-enzyme II).

dinus (**di**·nus). 1. Dizziness. 2. Vertigo. [Gk *dinos* a whirling.]

Dioctophyme (di·**ok**·to·**fi**·me). A genus of round nematode worms containing *Dioctophyme renale (gigas),* the giant cosmopolitan nematode of dogs. Up to 40 cm long and blood red, it occurs in the kidney, which it hollows out, and in the coelom. A very few cases have been reported from man. [Gk *di-*, *okto* eight, *phyme* nodule.]

Dioctophymeata (di·**ok**·to·fi·me·**a**'·tah). A sub-order of the nematode order Enoplata. The family Dioctophymeidae is of medical interest. [see prec.]

Dioctophymeidae (di·**ok**·to·fi·**me**'·id·e). A family of the nematode sub-order or order Dioctophymeata. The genus *Dioctophyme* is of medical interest. [Gk *di-*, *okto* eight, *phyme* nodule, *eidos* form.]

Dioctyl Sodium Sulphosuccinate (di·**ok**·til **so**·de·um sul·fo·**suk**'·sin·ate). BP Commission approved name for di-(2-ethylhexyl) sodium succinate; a non-laxative faecal softener.

diode (**di**·ode). 1. A two-electrode electronic valve, usually a rectifier. 2. A semiconductor device with two terminals, analogous in use to the valve diode. [Gk *di-*, *hodos* way.]

Diodon (**di**·o·don). A genus of spiny fish of tropical seas, the porcupine fish. Their flesh is poisonous. [Gk *di-*, *odous* tooth.]

diodone (**di**·o·done). An intravenous contrast medium for visualizing the urinary tract radiologically (Diodone Injection BP 1968). It is formed from 3,5-di-iodo-4-pyridone-*N*-acetic acid and diethanolamine by loose combination.

dioecious (di·e·shus). Animals and plants which are sexually distinct, individuals being of one or the other sex. [Gk *di-*, *oikos* house.]

dioesophagus (di·e·**sof**·ag·us). A partial or complete congenital reduplication of the oesophagus. [Gk *di-*, oesophagus.]

dioestrous (di·**es**·trus). Referring to a dioestrum.

dioestrum (di·**es**·trum). In a female animal, an abnormally short period of rest between 2 periods of heat. [Gk *dia*, *oistros* mad desire.]

dioestrus (di·**es**·trus). A period of sexual inactivity in female lower animals during gestation and lactation. [see prec.]

diogenism (di·**oj**·en·izm). The leading of a simpler and more natural life without the restraining influences of civilization; or the efforts to lead such a life. [*Diogenes*, the Greek philosopher who is said to have lived in a barrel to show his contempt for the effete state of civilization then obtaining.]

diolefine (di·**ol**·ef·een). An aliphatic hydrocarbon possessing 2 double bonds.

dionism (**di**·o·nizm). Heterosexuality. [*Dione*, Greek goddess, the mother of Aphrodite.]

diophthalmus (di·of·**thal**·mus). Diprosopus; a monster with two faces and heads or with any part of the face duplicated. [Gk *di-*, *ophthalmos* eye.]

diopsimeter (di·op·**sim**·et·er). An instrument with which the field of vision can be explored and its limits determined. [Gk *dia*, *opsis* view, meter.]

dioptometer (di·op·**tom**·et·er). Optometer; an instrument with which the strength and distance of distinct vision may be estimated and the state of refraction of the eye determined. [see foll.]

dioptometry (di·op·**tom**·et·re). The measuring of the accommodative and refractive power of the eye. [dioptre, meter.]

dioptoscopy (di·op·**tos**·ko·pe). The measuring of the refractive power of the eye by means of an ophthalmoscope. [dioptre, Gk *skopein* to watch.]

dioptre (di·**op**·ter). The unit of refractive power of a lens, the number of dioptres being the reciprocal of the focal length measured in metres. **Dioptres of accommodation.** A measurement of the amplitude of accommodation of the eye measured in dioptres, i.e. the change in spherical refraction on focusing. **Prism dioptre.** *See* PRISM. [Gk *dioptra* levelling instrument.]

dioptric (di·**op**·trik). Referring to transmitted and refracted light or to refraction. [see prec.]

dioptrics (di·**op**·trix). That branch of optics which is concerned with the refraction of light, particularly by the transparent medium of the eye. [Gk *dioptra* levelling instrument.]

dioptrometer (di·op·**trom**·et·er). Dioptometer.

dioptrometry (di·op·**trom**·et·re). Dioptometry.

dioptroscopy (di·op·**tros**·ko·pe). Dioptoscopy.

dioptry (di·**op**·tre). Dioptre.

Diorchitrema (**di**·or·ke·**tre'**·mah). A genus of Trematoda. *Diorchitrema pseudocirratum*, and perhaps other species, normal to dogs and cats, which have occurred in the intestine and elsewhere in man, in the tropical Far East, e.g. in Manila. It is probably not pathogenic. [Gk *dia, orchis* testis, *trema* hole.]

diorthosis (di·or·**tho**·sis). Surgical repair of an injured or deformed limb. [Gk a making straight.]

diose (**di**·oze). Glycollic aldehyde, CH_2OHCHO. The simplest of the monosaccharides, formed from the tartaric acid in ripening grapes.

diosmic (di·**oz**·mik). A compound which contains 2 atoms of tetravalent osmium.

diosmin (di·**oz**·min). $C_{34}H_{44}O_{21}$, a glycoside occurring in buchu leaves, *Barosma betulina* (Thunb.) Bartl. (family Rutaceae) and in other plants. It consists of rhamnose and glucose units combined with diosmetin, a methoxyflavone. [Gk *dios* divine, *osme* smell.]

diosmosis (di·oz·**mo**·sis). Osmosis; the passage of water through a semipermeable membrane from a weak solution into a stronger, until both solutions are equalized in strength. [Gk *dia, osmos* thrust.]

diosmotic (di·oz·**mot**·ik). Relating to diosmosis.

diosphenol (di·os·**fe**·nol). Buchu camphor, barosma camphor, $C_{10}H_{16}O_2$. An unsaturated phenolic ketone extracted from the volatile oil of *Barosma betulina* (Thunb.) Bartl. (buchu oil).

diostosis (di·os·**to**·sis). Displacement of a bone. [Gk *dia, osteon* bone.]

diotic (di·**o**·tik). Pertaining to both ears. [Gk *di-, ous* ear.]

Dioxamate (di·**ox**·am·ate). BP Commission approved name for 4-carbamoyloxymethyl-2-methyl-2-nonyl-1,3-dioxolan; it is used in the treatment of Parkinson's syndrome.

dioxane (di·**ox**·ane). Diethylene dioxide, $(CH_2CH_2)_2O_2$. A colourless liquid miscible with water and many organic solvents. It is employed as a dehydrating agent in the process of paraffin embedding in histological technique, and as an industrial solvent for cellulose acetate. This substance has toxic effects on the liver and kidneys.

Dioxaphetyl Butyrate (di·ox·ah·**fe**·til **bew**·tir·ate). BP Commission approved name for ethyl-4-morpholino-2,2-diphenylbutyrate; a narcotic analgesic.

dioxide (di·**ox**·ide). An oxide which contains 2 atoms of oxygen.

dioxyanthranol (di·**ox**·e·**an'**·thran·ol). Dithranol BP 1958.

dioxybenzene (di·ox·e·**ben'**·zeen). Dihydroxybenzene, $C_6H_4(OH)_2$. The general term for the isomeric dihydric phenols, catechol, resorcinol and quinol, having the hydroxyl groups in the *ortho-, meta-*, and *para*-positions, respectively.

dioxydiamino-arsenobenzol (di·**ox**·e·di·am·in·o·**ar**·sen·o·**ben'**·zol). Arsphenamine.

dioxyfluoran (di·**ox**·e·**floo'**·or·an). Fluorescein.

dioxyphenylalanine (di·**ox**·e·fe·nil·**al'**·an·een). Dihydroxyphenylalanine.

dip (dip). 1. The angle of inclination of a vertically suspended magnetized needle along the earth's lines of force. This varies with the latitude, being least at the equator and greatest at the magnetic poles. 2. In the otological sense, a trough or depression in the auditory curve resulting from a loss of hearing at a particular pitch. In the range of human hearing the most frequent loss is at from 4000 to 4096 double vibrations per second. **Dip circle.** The arrangement of magnetized needle and a circular scale graduated in degrees, both in a vertical plane, for the direct reading of dip. [ME *dippen.*]

Dipenine Bromide (di·**pen**·een **bro**·mide). BP Commission approved name for 2-dicyclopentylacetoxyethyltriethylammonium bromide; an antispasmodic.

dipentene (di·**pen**·tene). $C_{10}H_{16}$, a terpene hydrocarbon found in Swedish and Russian turpentine, and in the oils of cinea, cubeb and citronella. It is an inactive isomer of limonene, and is formed by the polymerization of isoprene when rubber is distilled.

dipeptidase (di·**pep**·tid·aze). An enzyme present in the pancreas and intestine, also in yeast and micro-organisms: highly specific for the splitting of dipeptides.

dipeptide (di·**pep**·tide). A simple compound formed by the union of 2 amino acids, the link being between the carboxyl of one and the amino group of the other, thus: $NH_2CH(R^1)CO\text{-}NHCH(R^2)COOH$, R^1 and R^2 being alkyl radicals.

Diperodon (di·**per**·o·don). BP Commission approved name for 1,2-di(phenylcarbamoyloxy)-3-piperidinopropane. **Diperodon hydrochloride.** A local anaesthetic; it is the diphenylurethane derivative of piperidinopropanediol.

Dipetalonema (di·**pet**·al·o·**ne'**·mah). *Acanthocheilonema.*

dipetalonemiasis (di·**pet**·al·o·ne·**mi'**·as·is). Infection with *Dipetalonema perstans (Acanthocheilonema perstans).*

diphalia (di·**fal**·e·ah). Possessing a double penis. [Gk *di-, phallos* penis.]

diphallus (di·**fal**·us). An individual with a double penis. [see prec.]

diphasic (di·**fa**·zik). Occurring in 2 stages or phases. [Gk *di-*, phase].

Diphemanil Methylsulphate (di·fem·**an**·il meth·il·**sul**·fate). BP Commission approved name for 4-diphenylmethylene-1,1-dimethylpiperidinium methylsulphate, a cholinergic blocking-agent with atropine-like action on the gastrointestinal tract. It is used in the treatment of bronchial asthma, duodenal ulcer and hyperhidrosis.

Diphenadione (**di**·fen·ah·**di'**·one). BP Commission approved name for 2-diphenylacetylindane-1,3-dione; an anticoagulant.

Diphenan BP 1953 (di·**fe**·nan). *p*-Benzylphenylcarbamate, $C_6H_5CH_2C_6H_4COONH_2$. An anthelmintic, used especially against threadworm *(Enterobius vermicularis)* infections.

Diphenhydramine Hydrochloride BP 1973 (di·fen·**hi**·dram·een hi·dro·**klor**·ide). $(C_6H_5)_2CHOCH_2CH_2N(CH_3)_2HCl$, one of the most widely used antihistaminic drugs. Its action is rapid, but of short duration. Diphenhydramine is the BP Commission approved name.

Diphenidol (di·**fen**·e·dol). BP Commission approved name for 1,1-diphenyl-4-piperidinobutan-1-ol; an anti-emetic.

Diphenoxylate (di·fen·**ox**·il·ate). BP Commission approved name for ethyl-1(3-cyano-3,3-diphenylpropyl)-4-phenylpiperidine-4-carboxylate. **Diphenoxylate Hydrochloride BP 1973.** The hydrochloride, used in the treatment of diarrhoea.

diphenoxypropane (**di**·fen·ox·e·**pro'**·pane). Propamidine.

diphenyl (di·**fe**·nil). 1. The monovalent radical, $C_6H_5C_6H_4$-, derived from phenylbenzene. 2. Denoting that the molecule of a compound contains 2 phenyl, C_6H_5, groups. 3. The hydrocarbon, phenylbenzene, $C_6H_5C_6H_5$, a colourless crystalline solid which occurs in coal tar, and is the parent of many important derivatives.

diphenylamine (di·**fe**·nil·**am'**·een). Phenylaniline, $NH(C_6H_5)_2$. A colourless compound prepared from aniline, and of importance in the manufacture of dyestuffs. A solution in sulphuric acid affords a very delicate test for nitric acid, with which it becomes intensely blue; it is also used as an indicator in the volumetric analysis of ferrous salts.

diphenylaminearsine chloride (di·**fe**·nil·am·een·**ar'**·seen **klor**·ide). Diphenylaminechlorarsine.

diphenylaminechlorarsine, diphenylaminechloroarsine (di·**fe**·nil·am·een·klor·**ar'**·seen, di·**fe**·nil·am·een·klor·o·**ar'**·seen). Diphenylaminearsine chloride, $NH(C_6H_4)_2AsCl$. A yellow substance used in chemical warfare, under the names *adamsite* and *DM*, because of the irritating effect of its vapour upon the nasal mucous membrane.

diphenylamino-azobenzene (di·fe·nil·am·in·o·az·o·ben′·zeen). $C_6H_5N{=}NC_6H_4N(C_6H_5)_2$, an azo-dye, used as an indicator (pH 1-2).

diphenylchlorarsine, diphenylchloroarsine (di·fe·nil·klor·ar′·seen, di·fe·nil·klor·o·ar′·seen). $(C_6H_5)_2AsCl$, a nose gas used in chemical warfare under the names *Clark I, sneezing gas* and *DA*.

diphenylcyanarsine, diphenylcyanoarsine (di·fe·nil·si·an·ar′·seen, di·fe·nil·si·an·o·ar′·seen). $(C_6H_5)_2AsCN$, a highly toxic nose gas used in chemical warfare under the names *Clark II* and *DC*.

diphenylhydantoin (di·fe·nil·hi·dan·to′·in). $(C_6H_5)_2C{=}(CONHC{=}N)OH$, a derivative of hydantoin. **Diphenylhydantoin sodium.** Phenytoin Sodium BP 1958, $(C_6H_5)_2C{=}(CONHC{=}N)ONa$, a white, odourless powder, moderately hydroscopic, and absorbing carbon dioxide when exposed to the air. It is freely soluble in water. It has a strong anticonvulsant action on the motor cortex, and very little hypnotic effect; it is thus a valuable drug in the treatment of epilepsy, chiefly effective in major and psychomotor attacks, but with no effect in minor epilepsy. Toxic effects are not infrequent and include gastrointestinal disturbances, skin rashes, hyperplasia of the gums, and a variety of neurological symptoms such as ataxia, tremors, diplopia and mental disturbances.

Diphenylpyraline (di·fi·nil·pi′·ral·een). BP Commission approved name for diphenylmethyl 1-methyl-4-piperidyl ether, an antihistamine compound of the substituted piperidine series.

diphonia (di·fo·ne·ah). The production of 2 simultaneous tones during vocal utterance. [Gk *di-*, *phone* sound.]

diphosgene (di·foz·jeen). Trichloromethylchloroformate, $ClCO{-}OCCl_3$. A choking gas with a severely irritant effect on the lungs, used in chemical warfare under the names *perstoff* and *superpalite*.

diphosphopyridine nucleotide (di·fos·fo·pir′·id·een new·kle·o·tide). Nicotinamide adenine dinucleotide.

diphtheria (dif·theer·e·ah). A specific infectious disease caused by virulent strains of a bacillus, *Corynebacterium diphtheriae* or Klebs-Loeffler bacillus, which gains a lodgement and usually forms a fibrinous exudate on the throat or elsewhere in the upper respiratory tract. Much less frequently, other mucous membranes or the skin may be invaded by the microbes. In addition to the local symptoms, generalized constitutional symptoms and toxaemia result from diffusion of a powerful exotoxin produced by the bacilli at the site of exudate. Disturbances in the circulatory system (myocardial damage) and nervous system (postdiphtheritic paralyses) are liable to occur, and are of toxic origin. **Aural diphtheria.** A condition in which virulent or non-virulent diphtheria bacilli are present more or less saprophytically in aural discharges. The extension of actual membrane from the nasopharynx to the middle ear is rare. **Circumscribed diphtheria.** A variety, not clearly or usefully defined, in which a circumscribed slough appears on one tonsil, or possibly elsewhere. **Conjunctival diphtheria.** Diphtheritic infection of the conjunctiva. **Cutaneous diphtheria.** Diphtheria of the skin, an acute form occurring in association with throat lesions. A chronic variety which is common in hot climates may be superimposed on other skin lesions or infections, and may be associated with paralyses. **False diphtheria.** A disease somewhat resembling diphtheria, but not due to diphtheria bacillus. **Faucial diphtheria.** Diphtheritic infection of the fauces. **Gangrenous diphtheria.** A rare and severe form of diphtheria with gangrene of the skin or mucous membrane. **Diphtheria gravis.** Diphtheria caused by *Corynebacterium diphtheriae* var. *gravis,* one of the three types of true diphtheria bacilli, the others being *intermedius* and *mitis.* The differentiation is made principally by the behaviour of the bacteria to starch, and by the appearance of the colony on tellurite media. The percentage of cases which develop severe or fatal attacks is slightly higher with *gravis* strains than with *intermedius* and very much higher than with *mitis.* It is not synonymous with malignant diphtheria. **Haemorrhagic diphtheria.** Malignant diphtheria (see below). **Laryngeal diphtheria.** Diphtheria with spread of the membrane to the larynx. In children there may be croup, characterized by cough, hoarseness and respiratory stridor. In adults laryngeal infection is rare, and may be overlooked; the larynx is wider and croup is absent. At all ages extension of the membrane down the trachea may lead to pulmonary complications and a high mortality. **Latent diphtheria.** Infection due to the diphtheria bacillus, but without obvious membrane formation. **Malignant diphtheria.** A severe or hypertoxic variety, characterized by rapid extension of the membrane and restlessness, followed by prostration, drowsiness, pallor and other manifestations of a depressant toxaemia (typhoid symptoms). Haemorrhages into the local lesion and the skin are common, and this form is often fatal. Even in patients who eventually recover, prolonged rest in bed is essential, so as to modify or prevent myocardial or nervous sequelae. **Nasal diphtheria.** Anterior nasal diphtheria, a relatively mild form in which the membrane is limited to the mucosa of the anterior nares, leading to nasal discharge that is frequently blood-stained. When the postnasal mucosa is involved, it is usually the result of spread of membrane from the fauces (*pharyngonasal* or *nasopharyngeal diphtheria*). This is a much more serious condition than anterior nasal diphtheria. **Non-membranous diphtheria.** A condition in which the diphtheria bacillus is present, but without giving rise to the ordinary symptoms of diphtheria. The immune state of the patient is the usual explanation for such an atypical infection, or for the complete absence of signs of infection (carrier state). **Pharyngeal diphtheria.** Sometimes regarded as synonymous with faucial diphtheria. A preferable classification is that *faucial* is synonymous with *tonsillar,* the membrane being confined to the area between the pillar of the fauces and therefore mainly on the tonsils (the term *faucial-tonsillar* has also been used for this type). When the membrane extends beyond the faucial pillars, the term *faucial-pharyngeal* or more simply *pharyngeal* diphtheria is applied, generally a more severe condition than the tonsillar (or faucial) type. **Postscarlatinal diphtheria.** Scarlatinal diphtheria (see below). **Preputial diphtheria.** Diphtheritic infection of the prepuce. **Scarlatinal diphtheria.** Diphtheria superimposed on scarlet fever; usually of the mild nasal type, with blood-stained discharge and sores around the nose and lips. **Septic diphtheria.** Diphtheria rendered serious by concomitant infection with streptococci and other pyogenic bacteria. **Surgical diphtheria.** Secondary diphtheritic infection of surgical wounds, e.g. the umbilical stump, or the penis following circumcision. **Umbilical diphtheria.** Diphtheritic infection of the umbilical cord in infants. **Vaginal diphtheria.** Diphtheritic infection of the vagina. **Vulval diphtheria.** Diphtheritic infection of the vulva. **Wound diphtheria.** Extra-respiratory diphtheria, in which the infection has usually been conveyed from the nose or the throat to wounds, sores or abrasions. There may be much crusting, although typical membrane formation may have been prevented by surgical dressings. [Gk leather skin or membrane.]

See also: BRETONNEAU.

diphtherial (dif·theer·e·al). Pertaining to or characterized by the presence of diphtheria.

diphtheriaphor (dif·theer·e·ah·for). A carrier of the diphtheria bacillus, *Corynebacterium diphtheriae* (Klebs-Loeffler bacillus). [diphtheria, Gk *phoros* bearer.]

diphtheric (dif·ther·ik). Diphtheritic.

diphtherin (dif·ther·in). A diphtheria antigen used in serum tests.

diphtheriolysin (dif·ther·e·ol′·is·in). A lysin with special affinity for the diphtheria bacillus, *Corynebacterium diphtheriae.* [diphtheria, Gk *lysis* a loosing.]

diphtheritic (dif·ther·it·ik). 1. Pertaining to diphtheria. 2. With characteristics resembling those of diphtheria, particularly the forming of a false membrane.

diphtheritis (dif·ther·i·tis). Diphtheria. [diphtheria, Gk *-itis* inflammation.]

diphtheroid (**dif**·ther·oid). 1. Pseudodiphtheria bacilli, non-virulent organisms identical in appearance with *Corynebacterium diphtheriae* (Klebs–Loeffler bacillus) found sometimes in the throat, more often in the nose and ear. 2. Any disease with membranous formation resembling diphtheria. [diphtheria, Gk *eidos* form.]

diphtherotoxin (**dif**·ther·o·**tox**'·in). Diphtheria toxin; toxin obtained from culture of *Corynebacterium diphtheriae* (Klebs-Loeffler bacillus). [diphtheria, Gk *toxikon* poison.]

diphthongia (dif·**thon**·je·ah). Diphonia; the production of 2 simultaneous tones during vocal utterance. [Gk *di-*, *phthoggos* voice.]

diphyllobothriasis (di·fil·o·both·**ri**'·as·is). Infection with a tapeworm belonging to the genus *Diphyllobothrium.* It is generally due to the eating of raw or partially cooked infected fish. [Gk *di-*, *phyllon* leaf, *bothrion* pit.]

Diphyllobothriidae (**di**·fil·o·both·**ri**'·id·e). A family of the cestode order Pseudophyllidea. The genera *Diphyllobothrium, Diplogonoporus* and *Sparganum* are of medical interest. [Gk *di-*, *phyllon* leaf, *bothrion* pit, *eidos* form.]

Diphyllobothrium (di·**fil**·**o**·**both**'·re·um). A genus of tapeworms. There has been much confusion about the specification but there are probably 2 important groups each containing several closely related forms. **Diphyllobothrium cordatum.** A species normal to seals, which has been recorded from man once. **Diphyllobothrium erinacei, Diphyllobothrium mansoni.** Under these names are included forms, of the subgenus *Spirometra,* whose plerocercoids occur in human subcutaneous tissues, particularly round the eyes. Such infections, in the Far East, are said to be caused by the local practice of placing opened frogs on wounds and bad eyes. Normal hosts of adults are small carnivores, and there is one record from man in China. *Sparganum proliferum* is a name given to plerocercoids which multiply by budding, perhaps as response to abnormal hosts. **Diphyllobothrium houghtonium.** A fish tapeworm that rarely infects man. **Diphyllobothrium latum.** The giant fish tapeworm of Europe and North America which grows to 10m. It is common in man where fresh-water fishing is an important industry. The coracidia larvae are eaten by copepods (*Diaptomus* and *Cyclops*) and form onchospheres and later procercoids. If the copepods are eaten by fish, they form large plerocercoids or *Sparganum* larvae in the muscles. These will develop to adults only if eaten by suitable mammal hosts (mostly carnivora and seals); if eaten by other fish, they can reinvade the muscles several times. **Diphyllobothrium mansoni.** *See* DIPHYLLOBOTHRIUM ERINACEI (above). **Diphyllobothrium minus.** Of Lake Baikal, a closely-related form with similar life history to *Diphyllobothrium latum.* Infection in man gives similar symptoms to *Taenia,* but also, in a minority of cases, causes severe anaemia. **Diphyllobothrium parvum.** A species once found in a Syrian immigrant. [Gk *di-*, *phyllon* leaf, *bothrion* pit.]

diphyodont (**dif**·e·o·dont). An animal, e.g. man, having 2 successive sets of teeth, deciduous and permanent. [G *di-*, *phyein* to grow, *odous* tooth.]

Dipipanone (di·**pip**·an·one). BP Commission approved name for 4,4-diphenyl-6-piperidinoheptan-3-one. The piperidine analogue of methadone and having very similar analgesic actions to it. **Dipipanone Hydrochloride BP 1973.** 4,4-Diphenyl-6-piperidinoheptan-3-one hydrochloride monohydrate, a white, almost odourless crystalline powder with a bitter taste followed by a sensation of numbness and burning. It has a strong analgesic, sedative and hypnotic action, and can be used to combat the symptoms produced by the withdrawal of morphine or pethidine.

Diplacanthus (dip·lah·**kan**·thus). A genus of tapeworms now included in *Hymenolepsis.*

diplacusis (dip·lah·**koo**·sis). A condition in which there is difference of perception of sound by the two ears, either in pitch or in time. **Diplacusis binauralis dysharmonica.** The condition in which a tone is heard as higher in pitch by one ear than it is by the other, the opposite ear being closed. **Diplacusis binauralis echoica.** The condition in which in the affected ear there is a weak echo of the tone heard. **Diplacusis monauralis, Diplacusis uni-auralis.** The condition in which, while one ear is closed, a single tone is heard as 2 sounds by the other ear. [Gk *diploos* double, *akouein* to hear.]

diplasmatic (di·plaz·**mat**·ik). Descriptive of cells which contain other matter as well as protoplasm. [see foll.]

diplastic (di·**plas**·tik). Term used of cells constituted of 2 substances. [Gk *di-*, *plasma* something formed.]

diplegia (di·**ple**·je·ah). Paralysis of similar parts on both sides of the body. **Atonic-astatic diplegia.** Diplegia in which there is reduction in muscle tone instead of excessive tension. **Cerebral diplegia.** A congenital bilateral disturbance of mobility, affecting the lower more severely than the upper limbs, with spastic paralysis as the main feature. Cerebellar ataxia, mental retardation and epilepsy may also occur. **Facial diplegia.** Bilateral facial paralysis. **Infantile diplegia.** Birth palsy. *See* PALSY. **Masticatory diplegia.** Paralysis of all the muscles of mastication. **Spastic diplegia.** Congenital spastic paraplegia. [Gk *di-*, *plege* stroke.]

diplegic (di·**ple**·jik). 1. Characterized by diplegia. 2. Referring to diplegia.

diplo-albuminuria (**dip**·lo·al·bew·min·**ewr**'·e·ah). A condition in which there is co-existence or alternation of pathological (nephritic) and physiological (non-nephritic) albuminuria. [Gk *diploos* double, albuminuria.]

diplobacillary (**dip**·lo·bas·**il**'·ar·e). Caused by or referring to a diplobacillus.

diplobacillus (**dip**·lo·bas·**il**'·us). A micro-organism in which bacilli occur in pairs, e.g. *Moraxella.* [Gk *diploos* double, bacillus.]

See also: MORAX.

diploblastic (dip·lo·**blas**·tik). Formed of 2 germinal layers. [Gk *diploos* double, *blastos* germ.]

diplocardia (dip·lo·**kar**·de·ah). A condition in which a fissure slightly separates the two lateral halves of the heart. [Gk *diploos* double, *kardia* heart.]

diplocephalus (dip·lo·**kef**·al·us). A monster with 2 heads on a single body. [Gk *diploos* double, *kephale* head.]

diplocephaly (dip·lo·**kef**·al·e). The condition of there being 2 heads on a single body. [see prec.]

diplochromosome (dip·lo·**kro**·mo·some). A chromosome which has reduplicated twice without separation into daughter chromosomes (endoreduplication) and is therefore formed by 4 chromatids. [Gk *diploos* double, *chroma* colour, *soma* body.]

diplococcaemia (**dip**·lo·kox·e'·me·ah). The condition in which diplococci are present in the blood. [diplococcus, Gk *haima* blood.]

diplococcal (dip·lo·**kok**·al). 1. Relating to a diplococcus. 2. Caused by diplococci.

diplococcoid (dip·lo·**kok**·oid). Resembling a diplococcus. [diplococcus, Gk *eidos* form.]

diplococcus (dip·lo·**kok**·us). A term used to describe bacteria of the family Coccaceae, occurring as pairs of cocci. It was based on microscopic morphology alone, and used for both Gram-positive and Gram-negative cocci. In the light of the most recent classification of the Coccaceae it is no longer in use in medical bacteriology except for a few species which do not fall naturally into recognized genera. The names in current use, of the more important diplococci found as parasites or saprophytes in man, are listed. **Diplococcus catarrhalis.** *Neisseria catarrhalis.* **Diplococcus crassus.** An organism of doubtful position, but apparently related to the meningococcus. **Diplococcus gonorrhoeae.** *Neisseria gonorrhoeae.* **Diplococcus intracellularis, Diplococcus intracellularis meningitidis.** *Neisseria meningitidis.* **Diplococcus of pertussis.** *Haemophilus pertussis.* **Diplococcus pneumoniae.** *Streptococcus pneumoniae.* **Diplococcus rheumaticus, Diplococcus scarlatinae.** *Streptococcus pyogenes.* [Gk *diploos* double, *kokkos* berry.]

See also: AXENFELD, MORAX, WEICHSELBAUM.

diplocoria (dip·lo·**kor**·e·ah). A condition of the eye in which there is a double pupil. [Gk *diploos* double, *kore* pupil.]

Diplodia (dip·lo·de·ah). A genus of fungi which may attack maize. It was formerly regarded as a possible causative agent in the production of pellagra.

diploë [NA] (dip·lo·e). The spongy substance filled with red bone marrow which lies between the outer and the inner tables of the skull. [Gk fold.]

diplogen (dip·lo·jen). One of the names proposed for the isotope of hydrogen, now generally known as *deuterium.*

diplogenesis (dip·lo·jen·es·is). 1. The development of a twin or double monstrosity or of one having some parts doubled. 2. The process of formation of congenital tumours by the inclusion of embryonic remains (Pignè). [Gk *diploos* double, genesis.]

Diplogonoporus (dip·lo·gon·op′·or·us). A genus of Cestoda. **Diplogonoporus grandis.** A species which is normally a parasite of whales, rarely of man, in Japan. [Gk *diploos* double, *gone* seed, *poros* pore.]

diplogram (dip·lo·gram). A skiagram consisting of 2 exposures. [Gk *diploos* double, *gramma* a writing.]

diploic (dip·lo·ik). Relating or belonging to the diploë.

diploic veins [venae diploicae NA]. Veins of the diploë, classified according to their main sites of drainage into frontal [vena diploica frontalis (NA)], anterior and posterior parietal [venae diploicae temporales, anterior et posterior (NA)] and occipital [vena diploica occipitalis (NA)].

diploid (dip·loid). Term indicating that the chromosome complement of a cell or organism is formed by 2 homologous chromosome sets so that each chromosome—except the sex chromosomes of the heterogametic sex—is represented twice. [Gk *diploos* double, *eidos* form.]

diplokaryon (dip·lo·kar·e·on). A nucleus in which there is twice the diploid number of chromosomes, that is, tetraploid. [Gk *diploos* double, *karyon* nut.]

diplomellituria (dip·lo·mel·it·ewr′·e·ah). The condition in which there is co-existent or alternating diabetic and non-diabetic glycosuria. [Gk *diploos* double, mellituria.]

diplomeric (dip·lo·mer·ik). In embryology, term applied to muscles derived from 2 myotomes. [Gk *diploos* double, *meros* part.]

diplomyelia (dip·lo·mi·e′·le·ah). Apparent duplication of the spinal cord because of the presence of a longitudinal fissure within it. [Gk *diploos* double, *myelos* marrow.]

diplon (dip·lon). Obsolete term for the deuteron. [Gk *diploos* double.]

diplonema (dip·lo·ne·mah). A term for the chromosome thread at the diplotene stage of meiosis. [Gk *diploos* double, *nema* thread.]

diploneural (dip·lo·newr·al). Applied to structures, including muscles, which have a double nerve supply. [Gk *diploos* double, *neuron* nerve.]

diplopagus (dip·lop·ag·us). Conjoined twins who have some vital organ in common. [Gk *diploos* double, *pagos* anything fixed.]

diplophase (dip·lo·faze). That stage in life cycles in which the chromosomes are in a diploid condition. [diploid, phase.]

diplophonia (dip·lo·fo·ne·ah). The production of double vocal sounds that sometimes occurs in disease of the larynx; diphonia. [Gk *diploos* double, *phone* sound.]

diplopia (dip·lo·pe·ah). Double vision; the appearance of single objects as double. **Artificial diplopia.** That produced by artificial means, e.g. by placing a prism in front of one eye or by altering the visual axis of one eye by pressure with the finger. **Binocular diplopia.** A form due to stimulation of non-corresponding points in the two retinae. **Congruous diplopia.** Diplopia when, in pathological binocular diplopia, the distance between the two images measured in degrees of arc is equal to the angle of deviation of the visual axes, the usual form. **Crossed diplopia.** Diplopia when, in the lateral form of binocular diplopia, the false image is situated, as regards the true image, on the opposite side to the deviated eye. Found in divergent squints. **Fore and aft diplopia.** Diplopia when the two images appear to be one in front of the other. **Heteronymous diplopia.** Crossed diplopia (see above). **Homonymous diplopia.** Diplopia when, in the lateral form of binocular diplopia, the false image is situated, as regards the true image, on the same side as the deviated eye. Found in convergent squints. **Horizontal diplopia.** Diplopia when the two images are displaced laterally or side by side. **Incongruous diplopia.** Diplopia when, in pathological binocular diplopia, the distance between the two images measured in degrees of arc does not equal the deviation of the visual axes. This is the uncommon form and is due to abnormal retinal correspondence. **Lateral diplopia.** Horizontal diplopia (see above). **Pathological diplopia.** Diplopia that may be due to: (*a*) weakness or over-action of one or more of the extra-ocular muscles resulting in inability to fix both eyes simultaneously on the same object (in cases of long standing, such as convergent squint, it may be overcome by suppression of the image in the deviating eye); (*b*) displacement of the image on the retina of the one eye by optical means, such as occurs in the correction of high degrees of anisometropia; or (*c*) by inequality in size of the retinal images (aniseikonia), such as occurs after extraction of uni-ocular cataract. **Physiological diplopia.** The basis of stereoscopy, consisting in the doubling of all objects which are not on the horopter of that which is being observed. For objects nearer, the diplopia is crossed, i.e. the right image belongs to the left eye and the left image to the right eye; for those beyond, the diplopia is uncrossed or homonymous. **Torsional diplopia.** Diplopia when there is tilting of one or both of the images. Cyclodiplopia. **Uncrossed diplopia.** Homonymous diplopia (see above). **Uni-ocular diplopia.** Diplopia due to some disturbance in the refracting media of the eye which may cause the production of 2 images (sometimes more than 2, *polyopia*) of the object regarded. The commonest cause is early cataract: others are partial dislocation of the lens so that its equator lies across the pupil, high uncorrected error of refraction (usually astigmatism) and deformities of the cornea such as occur from cicatrization after chemical burns. If this occurs in both eyes, it is called *bilateral uni-ocular diplopia* or *amphodiplopia.* **Vertical diplopia.** Diplopia when 2 images are displaced vertically, one above the other. [Gk *diploos* double, *opsis* vision.]

diplopic (dip·lo·pik). 1. Affected with diplopia. 2. Relating or referring to diplopia.

diplopiometer (dip·lo·pe·om′·et·er). An instrument with which the presence of diplopia can be detected and its degree estimated.

Diplopoda (dip·lo·po·dah). Millipedes which have 2 pairs of legs on each body segment, except the first few. They have been recorded from the alimentary canal and nasal passages, but are purely adventitious. [Gk *diploos* double, *pous* foot.]

Diploscapter (dip·lo·skap·ter). A genus of threadworms of which *Diploscapter coronata,* normally free-living, has been recorded from the stomach in cases of acid deficiency. [Gk *diploos* double, *skapter* digger.]

diploscope (dip·lo·skope). An instrument with which binocular vision can be studied and anomalies investigated. [Gk *diploos* double, *skopein* to watch.]

diplosomatia (dip·lo·so·ma′·she·ah). A condition in which twins, which appear to be complete and independent each of the other, are joined together at one or more parts of their bodies. [see foll.]

diplosome (dip·lo·some). 1. A paired sex chromosome. 2. A double centrosome. [Gk *diploos* double, *soma* body.]

diplosomia (dip·lo·so·me·ah). Diplosomatia.

diplotene (dip·lo·teen). The stage of the first meiotic prophase during which the chromatids of homologous pairs begin to separate and appear to be held together by chiasmata. [Gk *diploos* double, *tainia* ribbon.]

diploteratology (dip·lo·ter·at·ol′·o·je). That branch of teratology which is concerned with joined twins. [Gk *diploos* double, teratology.]

Dipodipus sagitta (di·pod·ip·us saj·it·ah). A gerbille, incriminated as a reservoir of plague in south-east Russia.

dipolar (di·po·lar). Bipolar. [see foll.]

dipole (di·pole). A combination of 2 equal and opposite electric charges or magnetic poles separated by a finite distance. **Electric dipole.** Two equal and opposite electric charges, separated by a finite distance. Many important biological phenomena depend on the presence of dipolar ions, e.g. in the case of proteins and amino acids, and the phenomena of detergency are due to the electric dipoles of large molecules. **Magnetic dipole.** Two opposite magnetic poles separated by a finite distance. The moment is the product of either pole (or in the case of an electric dipole, either charge) and the finite distance; it equals the couple necessary to keep the dipole at right angles to a magnetic (or electric) field of unit intensity. [Gk *di-*, pole.]

Dippel, Johann Konrad (b. 1673). German physician and alchemist.

Dippel's animal oil. An oil obtained by the destructive distillation of bones and other animal matter. It contains pyridine, and is not used in medical practice.

dipping (**dip**·ing). Palpation of a solid organ in the abdomen, e.g. the liver, by sudden downward pressure of the fingers with the hand flat on the surface of the body. By this movement any intervening matter is displaced. [AS *dyppan.*]

dippoldism (**dip**·ol·dizm). Flogging of children to satisfy emotional or sexual abnormality in the adult. [*Dippold,* the name of a German schoolmaster.]

Diprenorphine (di·pren·**or**·feen). BP Commission approved name for *N*-cyclopropylmethyl-7,8-dihydro-7α-(1-hydroxy-1-methylethyl)-O^6-methyl-6,14-*endo*ethanonormorphine; a narcotic antagonist.

Diprophylline (di·**pro**·fil·een). BP Commission approved name for 7-(2,3-dihydroxypropyl)theophylline; it is used in the treatment of angina pectoris and bronchospasm.

diprosopus (di·pro·**so**·pus). A monster with 2 faces and heads, or with any part of the face duplicated. **Diprosopus tetra-ophthalmus.** A monster with a fused double face, a central double eye and 2 lateral eyes. [Gk *diprosopos* two-faced.]

dipsesis (dip·**se**·sis). Extreme thirst; craving for abnormal kinds of drink. [Gk *dipsa* thirst.]

dipsetic (dip·**set**·ik). 1. Tending to produce thirst. 2. Attended by thirst. 3. Referring to dipsesis. [see prec.]

dipsomania (dip·so·**ma**·ne·ah). Imperative morbid craving, which may be recurrent, particularly for alcoholic spirits and indulgence in these to excess. [Gk *dipsa* thirst, mania.]

dipsomaniac (dip·so·**ma**·ne·ak). An individual who is affected with dipsomania.

dipsopathy (dip·**sop**·ath·e). 1. Dipsotherapy. 2. The abnormal nervous condition of which dipsomania is a characteristic symptom. [Gk *dipsa* thirst, *pathos* suffering.]

dipsorexia (dip·so·**rex**·e·ah). The early stage of alcoholism when the craving for drink is established but organic lesions have not appeared. [Gk *dipsa* thirst, *orexis* appetite.]

dipsosis (dip·**so**·sis). Dipsesis. [Gk *dipsa* thirst, *-osis* condition.]

dipsotherapy (dip·so·**ther**·ap·e). Thirst cure; treatment of disease by limiting the intake of fluids. [Gk *dipsa* thirst, therapy.]

Diptera (**dip**·ter·ah). An order of insects containing the two-winged flies, which are characterized by having only the anterior pair of wings well developed, the hind pair being represented by small stalked knobs, the halteres. The larvae are always legless, and in many the head is reduced or absent: where this is so they are called *maggots.* In the lower form the pupa is free, but in the higher it is enclosed in the last larval skin, the puparium. The lower forms (Nematocera) usually have elongate antennae and abdomens, but in the higher (Brachycera) they are short. Numerous genera, particularly in the following families, contain species of medical importance: Psychodidae (moth flies), Culicidae (mosquitoes), Ceratopogonidae (midges), Simuliidae (buffalo gnats), Tabanidae (clegs), Muscidae (house flies, etc.), Calliphoridae (bluebottles, etc.) and Oestridae (botflies). [Gk *dipteros* two-winged.]

Dipterocarpus (**dip**·ter·o·**kar**′·pus). A genus of trees found in Southern Asia and yielding gurjun balsam. **Dipterocarpus turbinatus.** The principal source of gurjun balsam. [Gk *dipteros* two-winged, *karpos* fruit.]

dipterous (**dip**·ter·us). 1. Belonging to the Diptera. 2. Having 2 wings, as flies and other insects of the order Diptera. 3. In botany, having 2 wing-like processes or wings. [Gk *dipteros* two-winged.]

dipygus (di·**pi**·gus). A monster with a fused double lower part of the spinal column and pelvis and with double genitalia and lower limbs. **Dipygus parasiticus.** Gastrothoracopagus dipygus. [Gk *di-*, *pyge* rump.]

Dipylidiidae (**di**·pil·id·**i**′·id·e). A family of the cestode order Cyclophyllidea; sometimes treated as a subfamily Dipylidiinae of the family Dilepididae. The genus *Dipylidium* is of medical interest. [Gk *dipylos* having two entrances, *eidos* form.]

Dipylidium (di·pil·**id**·e·um). A genus of tapeworms of which *Dipylidium caninum* is normal to the dog. Many human cases are recorded, particularly in children. Intermediate hosts to the cysticercoids are fleas (*Ctenocephalides* species and *Pulex irritans*), and the dog louse (*Trichodectes canis*). [Gk *dipylos* having two entrances.]

Dipyridamole (di·pi·**rid**·am·ole). BP Commission approved name for 2,6-di-[di-(2-hydroxyethyl)amino]-4,8-dipiperidinopyrimido-(5,4-*d*)pyrimidine; a coronary vasodilator.

Dipyrone (di·**pi**·rone). BP Commission approved name for sodium 2,3-dimethyl-1-phenyl-5-pyrazolon-4-yl-*N*-methylaminomethanesulphonate; an analgesic.

Dirck's fibril. A radial elastic fibre in the media of a blood vessel.

direction (di·**rek**·shun). **Beam direction.** Methods of defining the path taken by the beam in a patient during radiotherapy. [see foll.]

director (de·**rek**·tor). Any device or object that guides. **Beam director.** Any device which indicates the path of a beam of radiation in the body. **Grooved director.** A surgical instrument consisting of a sound or probe with which a knife, sliding in a groove within, can be guided to the site of operation (as in the slitting of a sinus) and its motion limited as desired. [L *dirigere* to direct.]

See also: HEY GROVES.

Director of Medical Services. DMS; the head of the army medical services in the field. USA equivalent, *Theater Surgeon.*

directoscope (di·**rek**·to·skope). An instrument with which the larynx can be directly examined. [L *dirigere* to direct, Gk *skopein* to watch.]

dirhinic (di·**ri**·nik). Referring to both halves of the nasal cavity. [Gk *di-*, *rhis* nose.]

dirhinus, dirhynus (di·**ri**·nus). Duplication of the nose. [see prec.]

dirigation (dir·ig·**a**·shun). Voluntary control of an involuntary or instinctive bodily function such as digestion or temperature by concentrating the attention on the function or organ involved. [L *dirigere* to direct.]

dirigomotor (**dir**·ig·o·**mo**′·tor). Producing or directing muscular motion. [L *dirigere* to direct, motor.]

Dirofilaria (**di**·ro·fil·**a**′·re·ah). A genus of Filaria. **Dirofilaria immitis.** Heartworm, a species which occurs in the dog and other animals; an antigen prepared from this is used in the diagnosis of filarial diseases. **Dirofilaria lobuisianensis.** A rare accidental parasite of doubtful pathogenicity. **Dirofilaria repens.** A rare parasite in man. [L *dirus* dread, filaria.]

dis- . 1. Prefix, from the Latin *dis,* meaning *apart, separation, the opposite of.* 2. Prefix, from the Greek *dis,* meaning *twice, twofold, double.*

disable (dis·a·bl). In law, to disable is to do something that creates a permanent disability and not merely a temporary injury. [L *dis-*, able.]

disaccharidase (di·**sak**·ar·id·aze). A general term for the class of enzymes which break down disaccharides into monosaccharides.

disaccharide (di·**sak**·ar·ide). 1. The general term for a carbohydrate formed by the union of any 2 monosaccharide molecules. 2. Most usually applied to the dihexosides, which include sucrose, lactose and maltose, and have the formula $C_{12}H_{22}O_{11}$. **Reducing disaccharide.** A disaccharide that reduces Fehling's solution.

disaccharose (di·**sak**·ar·oze). Disaccharide.

disacidify (dis·as·**id**·e·fi). To neutralize or remove the acid present in a mixture. [L *dis-*, acidify.]

disaesthesia (dis·es·**the**·ze·ah). A sensation of unease or discomfort. [L *dis-*, aesthesia.]

disaggregation (dis·ag·re·**ga**′·shun). A disconnection of an idea or group of ideas whereby it is relatively isolated from other mental contents. [L *dis, ad, gregare* to collect into a flock.]

disallergization (dis·al·er·ji·**za**′·shun). The rendering neutral of allergic activity or the destroying of it. [L *dis-*, allergy.]

disamidize (dis·**am**·id·ize). Deaminize. [L *dis-*, amide.]

disarticulation (dis·ar·tik·ew·**la**′·shun). Separation or amputation at a joint, without cutting through bone. [L *dis-*, articulation.]

disassimilation (dis·as·im·il·**a**′·shun). 1. Retrograde metabolism. 2. The oxidation of assimilated material and consequent liberation of active energy and waste products. [L *dis-*, assimilation.]

disassociation (dis·as·o·se·**a**′·shun). The splitting on heating of a compound with associated molecules, e.g. water $(H_2O)_3$, into single molecules (steam, H_2O) which re-associate on cooling. [L *dis-*, association.]

disc (disk). 1. A flat, circular, coin-shaped structure. 2. In anatomy, a rounded plate-like structure; the term is commonly used for plates of fibrocartilage separating the articulating surfaces of bone. 3. Colloquially, the optic disc, or the field visible with the retinoscope. **A disc.** The dark anisotropic band of a striated muscle fibre. **Accessory disc.** A thin dark line across a striated muscle fibre, occasionally present between Krause's membrane and the main dark band. **Anangioid disc.** An optic disc in which no blood vessels can be seen. **Anisotropic disc, Anisotropous disc.** A disc (see above). **Articular disc [discus articularis (NA)].** A disc of fibrocartilage between the articular surfaces of a synovial joint. **Articular disc of the acromioclavicular joint [discus articularis (NA)].** The occasional wedge-shaped fibrocartilage occupying the upper part of the acromioclavicular joint. **Articular disc of the inferior radio-ulnar joint [discus articularis (NA)].** The triangular fibrocartilage attached by its apex to the base of the ulnar styloid process and by its base to the medial edge of the inferior end of the radius. **Articular disc of the mandibular joint [discus articularis (NA)].** *See* MANDIBULAR JOINT (under JOINT). **Articular disc of the sternoclavicular joint [discus articularis (NA)].** The flat, circular, biconcave disc attached especially to the upper posterior border of the articular surface of the clavicle and to the first costal cartilage near its junction with the sternum. **Bilaminar embryonic disc.** The two-layered (ectomesoderm and entoderm) stage in the early developing embryo. **Blastodermic disc.** 1. The flat plate of embryonic cells lying on the surface of the yolk of large-yolked eggs. 2. The embryonic disc formed of apposed layers of ectodermal and entodermal cells between the amniotic and yolk-sac cavities of mammalian ova; it develops into the embryo proper, as opposed to the fetal membranes. **Blood disc.** A blood platelet. **Carborundum disc.** A dental disc charged with carborundum. **Cervical disc.** An intervertebral disc in the cervical region. **Choked disc.** A swollen optic disc due either to oedema (also called *papilloedema*), or to inflammation of the nerve head (also called *optic neuritis*). **Cloth discs.** Circular pieces of cloth used for polishing. **Cupped disc.** Excavation of the optic disc, either physiological, glaucomatous, or following atrophy of the optic nerve. **Cutting disc.** A disc charged with an abrasive material, which is used for cutting a tooth. **Cuttle-fish disc.** A dental disc charged with powdered cuttle-fish bone. **Dental disc.** A thin circular piece of cardboard or metal covered with abrasive powder which is rotated rapidly to grind a tooth or polish a filling in a tooth. **Diamond disc.** A dental disc charged with small fragments of diamond, or with diamond dust. **Emery disc.** A dental disc charged with emery powder. **Epiphyseal disc.** The plate of cartilage (growth cartilage) which separates an epiphysis from the shaft or body of an immature bone. **Equatorial disc.** The disc-like mass of chromosomes at the equator of a dividing cell in metaphase. **Gelatin disc.** Lamella; a medicament incorporated in a disc of gelatin base, for application to the eye. The base dissolves and the medicament is absorbed. **Germinal disc.** Blastodermic disc; the flat plate of embryonic cells lying on the surface of the yolk of large-yolked eggs. **Hair disc.** A slightly raised minute area of skin adjacent to the emergence of the shaft of a hair; it is richly innervated, and may represent a rudimentary sense organ. **Herniated disc.** Prolapsed disc (see below). **I disc.** The isotropic or isotropous disc of a striated muscle fibre. **Interarticular disc.** A plate of fibrocartilage separating the articulating surfaces of bones. **Intercalated discs.** Transverse lines seen in cardiac muscle fibres which are formed by the closely applied cell membranes of adjacent muscle cells. **Intermediate disc.** Krause's membrane; the dark band hemisecting the light isotropic band of a striated muscle fibre and separating adjacent sarcomeres. **Interpubic disc [discus interpubicus (NA)].** A lamina of fibrocartilage covered on each surface by a thin layer of hyaline cartilage uniting the two pubic bones. **Intervertebral disc [discus intervertebralis (NA)].** The fibrocartilaginous tissue between the bodies of successive vertebrae. Peripherally the fibrous tissue is most in evidence, forming an annulus fibrosus; centrally the tissue is soft and jelly-like, the nucleus pulposus. **Isotropic disc, Isotropous disc.** One of the pale bands between adjacent dark bands of a striated muscle fibre. **J disc.** I disc (see above). **Light disc.** I disc (see above). **Lumbosacral disc.** The intervertebral disc between the 5th lumbar vertebra and the sacrum. **M disc.** M line. **Micrometer disc.** A small round disc with a number of equally-spaced lines engraved on it at right angles to the diameter; this is fitted into the ocular of a microscope, calibrated against an object of known size, and subsequently used for measuring objects under the microscope (eyepiece micrometer). **Nuclear disc.** Equatorial disc (see above). **Optic disc [disci nervi optici (NA)].** The round light disc which can be seen in the retina, 3 mm on the nasal side of the macula lutea. It is formed by the optic nerve as it pierces the 3 main layers of the eyeball. **Ovigerous disc.** The cumulus oöphoron or discus proligerus of granulosa cells around the ovum in a graafian follicle. **Polishing disc.** A dental disc charged with a polishing rather than an abrasive material. **Prolapsed disc.** Posterior displacement of part of an intervertebral disc, causing symptoms of pressure on the nerve roots or the cord. **Proligerous disc.** Ovigerous disc (see above). **Q disc.** One of the dark anisotropic bands of a striated muscle fibre. **Sandpaper disc.** A dental disc charged with finely crushed silica. **Sarcous disc.** The dark anisotropic disc of a striated muscle fibre. **Scleral disc.** The disc removed from the sclera in a trephine operation. **Slipped disc.** Prolapsed disc (see above). **Stenopaeic disc.** An opaque, flat, circular disc with a narrow slit, used for testing irregular astigmatism. **Discs of striated muscle fibres.** The transverse striations seen in voluntary or skeletal muscle. Two principle types alternate, a dark anisotropic A disc and a light isotropic I disc; a dark band, the Z disc, can be seen in the middle of the I disc, and a light band, Hensen's disc, in the middle of the A disc. Hensen's disc is further subdivided by a dark, very thin M disc. The appearance of the discs is probably due to the regular arrangement of regions of different chemical and physical constitution along the course of the myofibrils. **Tactile disc.** A disc-like expansion on an intra-epithelial nerve-ending in contact with a specialized epithelial cell; Merkel's corpuscle. **Theminal disc.** Intermediate disc (see above). **Transverse disc.** A disc (see above). **Vitelline disc.** Ovigerous disc (see above). **Z disc.** Z line. [Gk *diskos* quoit.]

See also: AMICI, BARDEEN, BECQUEREL, BLAKE, BOWMAN, ENGELMANN, HENSEN, MERKEL (F. S.), NEWTON (I.), PLACIDO, RANVIER, REKOSS, SCHIEFFERDECKER.

discharge (dis·**charj**). 1. To emit, expel, unload or release anything. 2. An emission. 3. The draining away of the normal or pathological contents of a cavity. 4. A pathological secretion. 5. The sudden release or escape of energy, usually electrical or chemical. 6. The relinquishment by a conductor of an electrostatic charge to other conductors of lower potential. **Alvine discharge.** Faeces. **Brush discharge.** A characteristic brush-like manifestation appearing at the pointed pole of an induction coil or high-frequency generator, caused by the ionization of the surrounding air. **Conductive discharge.** An electrical discharge effected through a conductor or series of conductors. **Convective discharge.** An electrical discharge brought about by the convection stream of ions in the surrounding medium. **Delta discharge.** Abnormal slow activity in the 1-4 Hz range of the electroencephalogram, indicative of structural or functional nerve-cell damage. **Diencephalic autonomic discharge.** A discharge of nerve cells in the diencephalon, leading to autonomic effects. **Disruptive discharge.** A noisy and instantaneous discharge in spark form, resulting from the sudden breakdown of the dielectric in the neighbourhood of the poles. **Nervous discharge, Neural discharge.** The disseminated impulses which result from the stimulation of a nerve centre. **Systolic discharge.** Stroke volume. *See* VOLUME. [OFr. *deschargier.*]

discharger (dis·**charj**·er). An extendible conductor with insulated handles, used to discharge electrostatic machines and condensers. [see prec.]

dischromatopsy (dis·**kro**·mat·**op**′·se). Dyschromatopsia: partial colour blindness; a condition in which there is difficulty in distinguishing colours. [L *dis-*, chromatopsia.]

disciform (**dis**·e·form). Disc-shaped. [disc, form.]

discission (dis·**ish**·un). 1. A cutting through or incision of a part, as a cataract. 2. The operation of removing a soft cataract by needling the capsule so as to break up the substance of the lens and allow its absorption. 3. Ransohoff's operation. **Discission of cataract.** Division of the lens capsule, used in 2 conditions: (*a*) the capsule is divided in cases of cataract, under the age of 25, to allow the aqueous to dissolve the lens; (*b*) after extracapsular extraction of cataract, an opaque membrane, composed of capsule and lens remnants, may form in the pupil and require division. **Discission of the cervix uteri.** The relief of stricture of the neck of the uterus by making incisions on the sides of it. **Discission of the pleura.** Ransohoff's operation. **Posterior discission.** The incising of the capsule of a cataract from behind. [L *discindere* to cut apart.]

discitis (disk·i·tis). 1. Inflammation of any disc. 2. Meniscitis. [disc, Gk *-itis* inflammation.]

disclination (dis·klin·a·shun). Abtorsion. [L *dis-*, *clinare* to bend.]

discoblastic (dis·ko·**blas**·tik). Undergoing or showing disc-like segmentations of the egg yolk. [disc, Gk *blastos* germ.]

discogenetic, discogenic (**dis**·ko·jen·**et**′·ik, dis·ko·**jen**·ik). Referring to or caused by displacement of an intervertebral disc. [disc, Gk *genein* to produce.]

discography (dis·**kog**·raf·e). Demonstration of a disc of a joint by the injection of a radio-opaque medium. [disc, Gk *graphein* to record.]

discoid, discoidal (**dis**·koid, dis·**koid**·al). 1. Disc-shaped. 2. A medicated tablet in the shape of a disc. 3. A disc-shaped excavator for dental work. [disc, Gk *eidos* form.]

discolorations (**dis**·kol·or·**a**′·shunz). Chloasma; a general term for pigmentary discolorations of the skin occurring in spots or patches of yellow, brown or black. [L *dis-*, coloration.]

Discombe, George. 20th century London pathologist.

Discombe's diluting fluid, or solution. A diluting fluid for use in the enumeration of eosinophils, containing aqueous eosin γ (1.0 per cent) 5 vols, acetone 5 vols, distilled water 100 vols.

discophorous (dis·**kof**·or·us). Bearing a disc or disc-like structure or organ. [disc, Gk *pherein* to bear.]

discoplacenta (**dis**·ko·plas·**en**′·tah). A disc-shaped placenta.

discoplasm (**dis**·ko·plazm). The plasma of the erythrocytes. [disc, plasma.]

discoria (dis·**kor**·e·ah). Dyscoria.

discrete (dis·**kreet**). 1. Composed of distinct parts. 2. Not confluent. 3. Marked by lesions that are separated and do not become incorporated in one another. [L *discretus* separated.]

discrimination (dis·krim·in·**a**′·shun). The act or faculty of distinguishing or differentiating. **One-point discrimination.** The faculty of localizing a single point of pressure or contact. **Tactile discrimination.** The faculty of being able to discriminate accurately by means of touch. **Tonal discrimination.** The faculty of distinguishing tone values. **Two-point discrimination.** The faculty of differentiating pressure or touch at 2 points; in the normal person this faculty is dependent on these points being a short distance apart, and the acuity of the faculty is in inverse ratio to the minimum distance apart at which these 2 points can be differentiated. [L *discrimen* division.]

discriminator (dis·**krim**·in·a·tor). **Pulse amplitude discriminator.** An electrical circuit to which are applied potential pulses of different amplitudes, and which transmits only those equal to or greater than a fixed reference value. The reference value or "discriminator level" may be varied by a control. [see prec.]

discus (**dis**·kus). A disc. **Discus intervertebralis.** Intervertebral disc. **Discus oöphorus.** The cumulus oöphorus. **Discus opticus.** The optic disc. **Discus proligerus.** The cumulus oöphorus. [L quoit.]

discussive, discutient (dis·**kus**·iv, dis·**kew**·shent). 1. Able to disperse morbid matter or effect resolution; dispersing. 2. An agent which effects the disappearance of inflammatory exudates or the dispersal of swellings and tumours. [L *discutere* to strike asunder.]

disdiaclast (dis·**di**·ah·klast). Any one of the particles making up the doubly-refracting discs of contractile muscle fibres. [Gk *dis*, *diaklan* to break in two.]

disease (diz·**eez**). In general, a departure from the normal state of health. More specifically, a disease is the sum total of the reactions, physical and mental, made by a person to a noxious agent entering his body from without or arising within (such as a micro-organism or a poison), an injury, a congenital or hereditary defect, a metabolic disorder, a food deficiency or a degenerative process. These cause pathological changes in organs or tissues which are revealed by characteristic signs and symptoms. Since a particular agent tends to produce a pathological and clinical picture peculiar to itself, although modified by individual variations in different patients, a mental concept of the average reactions or a composite picture can be formed which, for the convenience of description, is called a particular disease or clinical entity. But a disease has no separate existence apart from a patient, and the only entity is the patient. **āaā disease.** Ancylostomiasis. **Accumulation disease.** A metabolic disorder in which some product is abnormally stored in reticulo-endothelial cells, e.g. lipoidosis. **Acute disease.** A disease arising quickly, and having a short course. **Acute respiratory disease.** An acute epidemic pharyngitis, due to an adenovirus. **Acute specific disease.** An acute disease due to a microbic infection. **Disease of adaptation** (Selye). Any disease resulting from distortion of the basic pattern of the glucocorticoid and mineral corticoid hormones produced by the adrenal cortex in the general adaptation syndrome (*see* SYNDROME). Typical diseases are Addison's, Cushing's and Simmonds', but the syndrome is concerned in many others which may seem unrelated, e.g. allergic states, nephrosclerosis, hypertension, ulcerative colitis and peptic ulcer, in which stress appears to play a part. **Akamushi disease.** Tsutsugamushi disease (see below). **Akureyri disease.** (Syn. Iceland disease.) Benign myalgic encephalitis. *See* ENCEPHALITIS. **Alkali disease.** 1. Tularaemia; so called because it was first observed in Tulare County in eastern California, which borders on the alkali desert areas of Nevada. 2. Selenium poisoning in animals. **Alligator-skin disease.** Ichthyosis. **Allogeneic disease.** Transplantation disease (see below). **Alpha-chain disease.** A disorder occurring in children, with diarrhoea, weight loss and finger clubbing, due to abnormal synthesis of an immunoglobulin peptide. **Altitude disease.** Mountain sickness; anoxia due to the low oxygen pressure at great heights. **Amyloid disease.** Waxy or lardaceous disease; a condition in which amyloid material is deposited in certain tissues. **Andes disease.** Erythemic symptoms seen in people crossing the Andes; Monge's disease. **Angiospasmodic disease.** A disorder in which spasm of various blood vessels occurs. **Anserine disease.** Wasting of the extremities. **Aortic valvular disease.** Disease of the aortic valve which may produce obstruction (stenosis), incompetence (regurgitation), or a combination of both. It may be congenital or acquired, and in the latter case is usually due to rheumatic fever or syphilis. **Arc-welders' disease.** Siderosis. **Association disease.** Epilepsy with myoclonus. **Attic disease.** Disease of the attic or epitympanic recess, usually of a suppurative type; it may be acute or chronic. **Australian X disease.** Australian X encephalitis. *See* ENCEPHALITIS. **Autochthonous disease.** A disease that is endemic within the country in which it is encountered. **Autogenous disease.** Any disease produced by internal causes. **Aviators' disease.** Anoxaemia due to the low oxygen pressure at great altitudes. **Barbed-wire disease.** Any mental disorder attributable to the psychological effects of being a prisoner of war. **Barcoo disease.** Barcoo rot; a characteristic shallow chronic septic sore that occurs in the sandy desert of the Barcoo River area of West Australia, probably identical with desert or veldt sore. **Barometer-makers' disease.** A form of mercurial poisoning from the handling of mercury. **Big spleen disease.** A syndrome described in Africa and New Guinea associated with endemic malaria and believed to be due to an abnormal cellular immune reaction to this infection. In addition to hyperplasia of the lymphoid tissues in the spleen, the hepatic sinusoids are densely infiltrated with lymphocytes. Hypersplenism accompanies the condition. **Bleeders' disease.** Haemophilia. **Blue disease.** 1. Rocky Mountain spotted fever. 2. Congenital heart disease. **Borna disease.** An infectious meningo-encephalomyelitis of horses (and occasionally of cattle and sheep), due to a virus. **Bornholm disease.** A painful inflammation of muscles, frequently the intercostal muscles, due to group B Coxsackie viruses. Named after the Danish island of Bornholm, where there was an extensive outbreak in 1930, it has now been observed in many parts of the world. Also called *epidemic pleurodynia, epidemic myalgia,* and *devil's grip.* **Brassfounders' disease, Braziers' disease.** That due to inhalation of zinc dust. Also called *brassfounders' ague* and *metal-fume fever.* **Bridegrooms' disease.** Thrombosis of the pampiniform plexus. **Bronzed disease.** Addison's disease. **Bush disease.** Tauranga; a cattle disease in New Zealand. **Caisson disease.** Conditions ensuing upon too rapid release of pressure in those returning from pressurized work under water, or in other caissons, to normal atmospheric conditions; it is marked by muscle and joint pains (bends), headaches, confusion and twitchings. **California disease.** Coccidioidal granuloma *(Coccidioides immitis).* **Caloric disease.** Disease due to exposure to high temperature. **Carapata disease.** African relapsing fever due to *Borrelia duttoni.* **Carcinoid heart disease.** Endocardial fibrosis leading to tricuspid regurgitation, pulmonary stenosis and right heart failure, developing secondary to carcinoid (argentaffin) tumours secreting vaso-active substances. **Cat-scratch disease.** Systemic symptoms of infection with regional lymph node enlargement sometimes related to a cat's scratch. It is benign but there may be encephalomyelitis. Possibly rickettsial. **Central core disease.** A genetically determined benign disease of muscle causing weakness and hypotonia; on section many muscle fibres contain a core with distinct staining properties. **Chicago disease.** Blastomycosis. **Chignon disease.** Beigel's disease. **Cholesterin disease, Cholesterol disease.** A condition in which cholesterol is deposited in the tissues. **Chronic disease.** A disease having a long course. **Chronic granulomatous disease.** Recurrent and chronic infections in patients whose polymorphonuclear leucocytes can phagocytose but not kill bacteria. It occurs mainly in males. **Chronic rheumatic diseases.** A generic term for the collagen group of diseases, including many forms of arthritis and such entities as systemic lupus erythematosus, sclerodermia, dermatomyositis, polyarteritis nodosa, polymyalgia rheumatica. **Chylopoietic disease.** Digestive disturbance due to malabsorption by the lacteals. **Climatic disease.** Disease due to climatic changes, or to adverse climatic conditions; a vague term best avoided. **Coal-miners' disease.** Silicosis. **Coeliac disease.** A type of malabsorption syndrome due to congenital or acquired sensitivity to gluten, a protein derived from wheat or rye flour. It is associated with villous atrophy in the duodenum and jejunum, leading to malabsorption of all food elements, especially fats, minerals and vitamins. The symptoms abate when a gluten-free diet is imposed. Although spontaneous remissions may occur, the defect is usually carried on into adult life. The common symptoms are primarily digestive, such as anorexia, passage of large, fatty stools and diarrhoea, followed later by growth anomalies. The common signs are associated with the digestive disorder, such as enlarged abdomen due to hypotonia and intestinal flatus, varying loss of subcutaneous fat particularly in the gluteal regions, undersize and underweight. Associated signs, mainly due to the failure of normal fat and vitamin absorption, are those of skeletal rickets, hypochromic and less commonly hyperchromic anaemia, periodic oedema, etc. The stools are usually bulky, offensive and glistening with fatty-acid crystals. They contain a greatly increased total quantity of fat, which is normally balanced between split and unsplit factors, together with an increase of starch granules. Also known as *Gee's, Gee-Herter, Gee-Herter-Heubner, Herter* or *Herter-Heubner disease.* **Coko disease.** A Fijian name for yaws. **Collagen diseases.** *See* CONNECTIVE-TISSUE DISEASE (below). **Combined-system disease.** Subacute combined degeneration of the cord. **Communicable disease.** A disease communicable from one human being to another, or from an animal to a human being, by direct contact or through a vector. **Complicating disease.** A disease occurring as a complication of a primary disease. **Compressed-air disease.** Caisson disease (see above). **Congenital disease.** A disease present at birth. **Connective-tissue disease.** A group of diseases of varied aetiology, all involving derangement of connective tissue; the skin, muscles, joints and blood vessels are particularly affected. The group contains such disorders as disseminated lupus erythematosus, polyarteritis nodosa, dermatomyositis, scleroderma, rheumatoid arthritis and polymyalgia rheumatica. They are also called *collagen diseases.* **Constitutional disease.** A disease due to general causes arising from the constitution of a patient. **Contagious disease.** A disease communicated by direct contact or by infected secretions. (The distinction between infectious, communicable and contagious diseases has now become artificial, the term used depending on individual or national preference.) **Creeping disease.** Larva migrans. **Cyclic disease.** A disease which recurs in cycles. **Cystic disease of the breast.** Fibrosis and cyst formation of the breasts. **Cysticercus disease.** Disease due to the cysticercus stage of *Taenia solium.* **Cytomegalic inclusion body disease.** A disease usually contracted *in utero* while the mother is apparently healthy, due to cytomegalovirus. Manifestations include haemorrhage, thrombocytopenia, anaemia, hepatomegaly, splenomegaly and calcification around the cerebral ventricles. **Deer-fly disease.** Tularaemia. **Deficiency disease.** Any disease due to the lack of vitamins or other essential food elements. **Demyelinating disease.** A term applicable to many diseases of the central nervous system in which destruction of nerve myelin sheaths occurs. **Deprivation disease.** Any disease due to starvation. **Diffuse disease.** A disease in which several tracts of the spinal cord are involved. **Divers' disease.** Caisson disease (see above). **Dog's disease.** A name that has been used for both sandfly fever and dengue. **Drug disease.** Drug addiction. **Dust disease.** Pneumoconiosis. **Dynamic disease.** Functional disease (see below). **Elevator disease.** Pneumoconiosis occurring in grain-elevator workers. **Endemic disease.** *See* ENDEMIC. **English disease.** Rickets. **Epidemic disease.** *See* EPIDEMIC. **Epidemic haemorrhagic disease.** Songo fever, Korin fever, Kokka disease, Nodoko disease; a haemorrhagic disease, noted in Korea, characterized by petechial rash, haemoptysis, haematemesis, haematuria or melaena, albuminuria and pyrexia, which may last about 7 days, usually clearing up in about 14 days, but a low-grade form may last several weeks. It is thought to be a virus disease, transmitted by mites, and shows about 10 per cent mortality. **Familial disease.** A disease that occurs in more than one member of the same family. Such a disease may be hereditary, but the implication is rather that it is environmental. **Fat-deficiency disease.** A disease due to deficiency of the fat-soluble vitamins A and D. **Fatigue disease.** The physical and/or mental symptoms due to physical or mental exertion. **Fellmongers' disease.** Anthrax: the infection is transmitted from the hides of infected animals while the hides are being handled.

Fetal haemolytic (erythroblastic) disease. Erythroblastosis fetalis. **Fibrocystic disease of bone.** Osteitis fibrosa cystica. **Fibrocystic disease of the pancreas.** A disease better described as *mucoviscidosis.* It occurs in infants and may present as meconium ileus, as recurrent pulmonary infection or, later, as a pancreatic deficiency. The sodium and chloride concentration is increased in the sweat. **Fifth disease.** Cheinesse's (1905) name for erythema infectiosum (Stricker, 1899) or megalerythema epidemicus (Plachte, 1904), an epidemic disease resembling rubella. **Fifth venereal disease.** Granuloma inguinale. **File-cutters' disease.** Lead poisoning due to inhalation of fumes from molten lead used in the process. **First disease.** Measles. **Fish-handlers' disease.** Erythema serpens (erysipeloid). **Fish-skin disease.** Ichthyosis. **Fish-slime disease.** Septic poisoning from a prick by a spine of a fish. **Fish-tapeworm disease.** A pernicious anaemia-like disease that is associated with infection by the fish tapeworm *Diphyllobothrium latum;* however, only a relatively small percentage of persons so infected suffer from the disease. Morbidity probably depends on the location of the worm or worms: when they are in the upper part of the small intestine, they take up the vitamin B_{12} before it has been absorbed. **Flax-dressers' disease.** A fibroid pneumonic condition due to inhalation of fine particles of flax by those employed in dressing flax. **Fleshworm disease.** Trichiniasis. **Flint disease.** Silicosis. **Focal disease.** A disease localized in a definite focus such as the tonsils or a dental abscess. **Foot and mouth disease.** A virus disease of farm animals which may infect man, causing malaise, headache, fever, soreness and vesiculation of the mouth, palms and soles, sometimes with ulceration. Resolution occurs within a week. **Fourth disease.** A disease once believed to be intermediate between scarlet fever, measles and rubella, but regarded no longer as a separate entity. **Fourth venereal disease.** Specific and ulcerative gangrenous balanoposthitis; other diseases have also been called by this name. **Frien disease.** A dermatitis occurring among wood choppers. **Functional disease.** A disease with no perceptible organic lesion. **Gannister disease.** Silicosis in workers in gannister, or coal-miners. Gannister is a hard, close-grained siliceous stone which frequently forms the stratum beneath a coal-seam. **Genetotrophic disease.** A conditioned nutritional disease. **Glassblowers' disease.** Inflation by air of Stensen's duct, forming a tumour of the parotid gland. Some tumours contain a mixture of air, saliva and pus; in rare cases there are gaseous crepitant tumours of the gland substance. It occurs in glass-blowers, and in musicians playing on wind instruments. **Glycogen disease, Glycogen-storage disease.** A disease in which there is an abnormal deposit of glycogen in the tissues, especially in the liver. *Type I:* von Gierke's disease, hepatorenal deficiency of glucose-6-phosphatase. *Type II:* Pompe's disease, cardiac deficiency of alpha-1,4-glucosidase. *Type III:* Forbes' disease, liver and muscle deficiency of 2 de-branching enzymes in various combinations; limit dextrinosis. *Type IV:* Andersen's disease. *Type V:* McArdle's syndrome, muscle deficiency of phosphorylase. *Type VI:* Hers' disease, deficient liver phosphorylase. **Grinders' disease.** Silicosis. **Guinea-worm disease.** Dracontiasis; an infection by the nematode worm, *Dracunculus medinensis.* This worm is ingested in water in its larval stage and reaches the soft tissues where it develops into a worm that may grow to 1.2 m in length and causes a severe local reaction. The infection is endemic in certain localities in Asia, including India, and in Africa. **Habit disease.** Drug addiction. **Haemolytic disease of the newborn.** Anaemia caused by the presence of incompatible maternal antibodies in the fetal circulation. **Haemopoietic disease.** A disease affecting the haemopoietic or blood-forming system. **Haemorrhagic disease of the newborn.** A disease associated with bleeding manifestations such as haemophilia, purpura, melaena neonatorum, prothrombin deficiency. **Haff disease.** A disease that was reported among fisherfolk in the Königsberg Haff. The symptoms were muscular pain and cramps, extreme generalized muscular weakness, and myohaemoglobinaemia and myohaemoglobinuria. It is thought to have been caused by arsenic in the waters of the Haff that was introduced in the waste products from cellulose factories. **Hand and foot disease.** A trophoneurosis causing ulceration of the hands and feet. **Hand-foot-and-mouth disease.** A painful ulcerative stomatitis of tongue, gingival and buccal mucosae, anterior fauces and soft palate, associated with intravesicular eruption on hands and feet; incubation period is from 3 to 5 days, duration 1 week. It is attributed to several types of Coxsackie A virus. **Hard-metal disease.** A pneumoconiosis caused by industrial exposure to tungsten carbide, silicon carbide or cobalt dust. **Heart disease.** Disease of the heart. *See* HEART. **Heart-water disease.** Haemoglobinuria of sheep. **Hepatolenticular disease.** Hepatolenticular degeneration; Kinnier Wilson's disease. **Hereditary disease.** Any disease of genetic origin. **Heredoconstitutional disease.** A non-progressive inherited constitutional disease. **Heredodegenerative disease.** Any one of the hereditary degenerative disorders of the nervous system. **Heterotoxic disease.** One due to toxins foreign to the body. **Holla disease.** An endemic haemolytic jaundice with recurrent attacks of anaemic crises, named after the town of Holla. **Hookworm disease.** Ancylostomiasis. **Hunger disease.** Excessive hunger with abnormal eating. It may be a neurosis or due to hyperinsulinism or other causes. **Hyaline membrane disease.** *See* PULMONARY HYALINE MEMBRANE DISEASE (below). **Hydatid disease.** A disease occurring in sheep, cattle and pigs, as well as man. It is caused by the larval stage of *Echinococcus granulosus,* a small tapeworm that occurs in the intestine of dogs, from which man and other animals become infected. The cyst develops slowly to a large size in the liver or other organs and produces pathological changes mainly by pressure. The cycle of transmission is completed when the dog eats the hydatid-infected organs, usually of sheep. **Hydrocephaloid disease.** Appearances resembling those of hydrocephalus, but with depression of fontanelles, occurring in dehydrated or wasted infants. **Iceland disease.** Benign myalgic encephalitis. *See* ENCEPHALITIS. **I-cell disease.** A form of mucopolysaccharidosis resembling gargoylism but with unusual inclusions in cultured fibroblasts. **Idiopathic disease.** Any disease which occurs without obvious cause. **Immunity deficiency disease.** Disease due to inability to resist infection; causes are impaired cell function, impaired haemoglobin function, or cellular and immunoglobulin deficiency. **Inclusion-body disease.** Infection due to cytomegalovirus. **Infectious disease.** Communicable disease (see above). **Inhalation disease.** Any disease due to inhalation of noxious material, including infectious micro-organisms. **Inherited disease.** Any disease of genetic origin. **Insufficiency disease.** A deficiency disease (see above). **Intercurrent disease.** A disease running concurrently with another. **Interstitial disease.** A disease of the connective tissue. **Jeep disease.** Pilonidal sinus of the coccygeal region. **Jeune disease.** Respiratory failure in infancy due to thoracic osseous disease. **Jumping disease.** Choromania; leaping, jumping movements of hysterical origin, similar to saltatory spasm. **Kabure disease.** A name given to the local irritation and urticarial rash that follows the entry of cercaria into the skin. **Katayama disease.** The invasion stage of human oriental schistosomiasis. It is characterized by fever, urticaria and eosinophilia. **Kedani disease.** Tsutsugamushi disease (see below). **Knife-grinders' disease.** Formerly regarded as chronic bronchitis occurring in knife-grinders through inhalation of steel dust, it is now usually held to be a form of silicosis, often associated with pulmonary tuberculosis. **Kokka disease.** Epidemic haemorrhagic disease (see above). **Kyasanur Forest disease.** An acute illness of haemorrhagic type due to a virus transmitted by the bite of larval ticks of the family Haemaphysalis. The disease occurs in forested areas of northern Mysore in India. It has a reservoir in small mammals and in monkeys. **Lardaceous disease.** Amyloid disease (see above). **Local disease.** A disease confined to one part of the body. **Madura disease.** Mycetoma. **Malignant disease.** Cancer. **Maple-syrup urine disease.** An autosomal recessive condition in which urine smells like maple syrup, with increased valine, leucine and isoleucine in blood and urine; there is physical and mental deterioration. **Marble-bone disease.** A dystrophy of bone associated with apparent increased density and obliteration of the distinction between cortex and medulla. **Marburg virus disease.** A severe and sometimes fatal febrile illness with a rash and haemorrhages, due to a virus transmitted from African green monkeys. **Masai disease.** A disease of East Africa marked by fever, vomiting and abdominal tenderness. It is thought to be filarial. **Mast-cell disease.** Urticaria pigmentosa. **Mastoid disease.** An inflammatory disease of the mastoid antrum or air cells. **Mediterranean disease.** Thalassaemia. **Medullary cystic disease.** Term comprising medullary sponge kidney with small cavities in renal medulla (good prognosis), medullary cystic disease with cortical fibrosis (causing renal failure) and nephronophthisis (presenting with anaemia and later renal failure). **Meleda disease.** Mal de Meleda. **Mental disese.** Any disease with predominantly mental symptomatology, whether of mental or physical causation. **Miana disease, Mianeh disease.** Tick-borne relapsing fever of Iran due to infection by *Borrelia persica* or *Borrelia sogdiana.* **Miasmatic disease.** Malaria. **Microdrepanocytic disease.** A type of chronic haemolytic anaemia due to the doubly heterozygous inheritance of the genes for sickle cell or S haemoglobin and that for thalassaemia. The spleen is usually much enlarged, whereas in sickle-cell anaemia it is usually totally infarcted. **Milk-borne disease.** Disease in which the infection is conveyed by milk. **Minamata disease.** A chronic neurological disease occurring near Minamata Bay in Japan, characterized by peripheral neuropathy, ataxia and blindness, and attributed to mercury poisoning from contaminated fish. **Mitral disease.** Disease of the mitral valve, nearly always due to the effects of rheumatic fever (rheumatic endocarditis) which may be increased by superadded bacterial infection. Distortion of the valve cusps interferes with valve function and causes obstruction to the orifice (stenosis) or ineffective closure of the valve, leading to regurgitation of blood through it during ventricular systole (incompetence). Very rarely it may be congenital (Duroziez's disease), consisting of stenosis, or failure of development of the valve (atresia). **Mljet disease.** Mal de Meleda. **Molecular disease.** An inherited disease which arises from the production inside the body of a molecule that is structurally and functionally different from that produced in normal persons. Examples include sickle-cell anaemia and the inborn errors of metabolism. **Motor neuron disease.** A progressive disease of middle life, predominant in males, and characterized by degeneration of anterior-horn cells, motor cranial nerve nuclei and the pyramidal tracts. It may be seen in three clinically distinct forms: progressive muscular atrophy, progressive bulbar palsy and amyotrophic lateral sclerosis. **Mountain disease.** Mountain sickness; anoxaemia of altitude. **Mucous disease of the bowel.** Mucous colitis. **Mule-spinners' disease.** A disease of workers in cotton mills. The lubricating oil used for the spinning mules caused chronic irritation of the skin with perifolliculitis and warts which became malignant. The common form was cancer of the scrotum. **Multiglandular disease.** Disease due to combined disorder of several endocrine glands. **Myocardial disease.** Disease of the muscle of the heart. **Nanukayami disease.** A form of spirochaetal jaundice. **Nervous disease.** Any functional disorder or organic disease of the nervous system. **Newcastle disease.** (*a*) Dysentery caused by *Shigella flexneri* var. *newcastle;* (*b*) a highly infectious virus disease of fowls, involving the central nervous, respiratory and gastro-intestinal systems. **Nodoko disease.** Epidemic haemorrhagic disease (see above). **Nutritional disease.** Any disease due to nutritional deficiency. **Occupational disease.** An organic or functional disease associated with the occupation of the individual affected. Examples are: *organic,* silicosis; *functional,* writers' cramp, an occupational neurosis. **Organic disease.** Any disease with pathological lesions. **Pandemic disease.** Any widespread epidemic disease. **Parenchymatous disease.** One affecting the cellular structure of an organ. **Parodontal disease.** Disease of the gingival margin which may spread to the periodontal membrane and alveolar bone. **Paroxysmal disease.** One occurring in sudden short attacks repeated at intervals. **Periodical disease.** A disease recurring at regular intervals. **Periodontal disease.** Parodontal disease (see above). **Perna disease.** *See* PERNA. **Pink disease.** A disease of children with pink, cold, sweating hands and feet, tachycardia, hypotonia and lassitude. It is due to hypersensitivity to mercury which may be given in teething powders, worm cakes, etc. Also known as *acrodynia, Feer's disease, Swift's disease.* **Pinta disease.** Pinta. **Pneumatic-hammer disease.** Loriga's disease; traumatic vasospastic disease of the hands; dead fingers, white fingers: an affection of the hands seen in pneumatic-hammer operatives, especially stone-cutters. The occupation impedes the local circulation, as shown by numbness and pallor of the fingers. **Pock diseases.** Smallpox, chickenpox and alastrim. **Pollen disease.** Hay fever. *See* FEVER. **Polycystic disease.** A congenital error of development resulting in the massive formation of cysts; it occurs most often in the kidneys and is then bilateral. A similar condition may occur in the liver and more rarely in the lungs, ovaries, uterus, pancreas and spleen. Severe polycystic disease of the kidneys causes death, either before or just after birth: those who survive may be free from symptoms for many years and die in middle age from uraemia or cerebral haemorrhage. Such kidneys may give rise to large palpable renal tumours. **Porcupine disease.** Ichthyosis hystrix gravior. **Prescribed disease.** One of certain occupational diseases "prescribed" by the Minister of National Insurance in regulations under the National Insurance (Industrial Injuries) Acts, for which benefit is available, e.g. lead poisoning, anthrax, pneumoconiosis. **Protozoal disease.** Any disease caused by protozoa. **Psychosomatic disease.** A disease characterized by one or more of the following: a disease in which it is necessary to study the mental processes of the patient in order to reach its full understanding; a specific premorbid personality structure; exacerbation or amelioration of the disease in response to specific or non-specific psychological factors; a disturbance of somatic function resulting from psychological factors; a disturbance of somatic structure resulting from psychological factors. **Pulmonary heart disease.** Cor pulmonale; heart disease resulting from disease of the lungs or pulmonary circulation. It may be acute (pulmonary embolism) or chronic. The latter is subdivided into anoxic and obstructive types: the anoxic type is due to lung disease which interferes with oxygenation (emphysema, bronchitis, bronchiectasis, pulmonary fibrosis); the obstructive type results from obstructive changes in the pulmonary vessels which increase pulmonary vascular resistance and embarrass the right ventricle (repeated pulmonary emboli, pulmonary endarteritis, periarteritis, idiopathic pulmonary hypertension). **Pulmonary hyaline-membrane disease.** Perinatal distress syndrome; the commonest pulmonary lesion found at post-mortem examination in premature babies, weighing less than 2500 g, who die during the first week of life. It is also found in full-term babies of diabetic mothers and in babies born by caesarean section who die from respiratory distress. The whole of the lungs are affected simultaneously and show a deep red-purple coloration, with infiltration of eosinophilic deposits in alveoli, respiratory ducts and bronchioles. Peripheral alveoli collapse and interstitial emphysema occurs; capillaries are intensely engorged and some oedema may result; cellular response by mononucleate and multinucleate phagocytes, without inflammatory cells, is typical. Resolution begins after 1 or 2 days. Hyaline membrane has disappeared by 7–8 days after birth. Aetiology is still indefinite; prevention depends upon prevention of prematurity; treatment is non-specific but must consist of vigorous efforts to prevent secondary infection, together with maintaining an airway. **Pulseless disease.** Takayusu disease; lack of peripheral pulses caused by diffuse arteritis with obstruction. Renal and cerebral vessels may be affected also. **Rag-pickers' disease, Rag-sorter's disease.** 1. A synonym for anthrax, occurring in the cutaneous form as *malignant pustule,* or in the pulmonary form as *woolsorters' disease.* It arises from infected animal products such as wool, hair, etc. 2. A distinct disease due to *Proteus hominis capsulatus* of Bordoni-Uffreduzzi. **Ray-fungus disease.** Actinomycosis. **Respiratory disease.** Disease of the lungs or upper respiratory tract. **Rheumatic heart disease.** Endocarditis, myocarditis or pericarditis due to rheumatic fever. **Rice disease.** Beriberi. **Royal Free disease.** An epidemic disease of unknown cause affecting young adults in institutions and characterized by muscular pain and weakness, sensory symptoms and depression, but with few physical signs. *Benign myalgic encephalomyelitis.* (Royal Free Hospital, London.) **Runt disease.** An often fatal condition characterized by failure to thrive, wasting and a liability to infections occurring in animals that have been grafted with tissue from a donor of another strain and due to a graft versus host reaction. **Sandworm disease.** Larva migrans. **San Joaquin Valley disease.** Coccidioidomycosis. **Sartian disease.** Dermatosis affecting the face; endemic in Asiatic Russia. **Scythian disease.** Atrophy of the male external genitalia. **Second disease.** Scarlatina. **Senecio disease.** Cirrhosis of the liver caused by *Senecio* poisoning. **Septic disease.** Any disease caused by pyogenic organisms. **Serum disease.** Allergic phenomena after injection of serum. **Seven-day disease.** Seven-day fever; relapsing fever. Also used for a disease similar to dengue, but due to *Leptospira hebdomadis.* **Sexually-transmitted diseases.** Diseases usually transmitted by some form of sexual contact. As well as the venereal diseases (syphilis, gonorrhoea, chancroid), included are lymphopathia venereum, granuloma inguinale, non-specific genital infections, trichomoniasis, candidiasis, genital scabies, pediculosis pubis, genital herpes, warts and molluscum contagiosum. **Shimamushi disease.** Mite-borne typhus or scrub typhus of the Far East. **Shipyard disease.** Shipyard eye. **Shuttlemakers' disease.** An affection, whose chief symptoms are fainting attacks, headache, dyspnoea and nausea, caused by inhaling the toxic dust of certain woods used in making shuttles. **Silk-stocking disease.** Erythrocyanosis crurum puellarum frigidum. **Simian B disease.** Severe myelitis caused by a *Herpesvirus* transmitted to man by the bite of an infected monkey. **Sirkari disease.** An old name for kala-azar in Assam. **Sixth disease.** Exanthema subitum. **Sixth venereal disease.** Lymphopathia venereum. **Specific disease.** 1. Disease due to any specific micro-organism. 2. A euphemism for syphilis. **Sponge-divers' disease, Sponge-gatherers' disease.** A disease of sponge-divers due to the poisonous secretion of a species of *Actinia* present in sea-water. The secretion on the skin causes an itching swelling, then a papule and finally a deep black ulcer, accompanied by shivering, pain, and pyrexia. Also called *Skevas-Zerfus disease.* **Sporadic disease.** A scattered disease, occurring as a case (or group of cases) here and there; not epidemic. **Storage disease.** A disease in which a metabolic product is stored in abnormal amount in the tissues. **Straw-mattress disease.** Acrodermatitis urticarioides. **Structural disease.** A disease in which there is damage to tissues. **Stuttgart disease.** Leptospiral infection in dogs. **Subacute disease.** A disease of longer course, and less intense, than an acute disease. **Subchronic disease.** A disease intermediate between a subacute and chronic one. **Suffocation disease.** A disease due to destruction of the myenteric plexus in the muscular coats of the oesophagus, stomach, duodenum, colon and ureter in Chagas' disease. Migration of trypanosomes into these organs leads to rupture of the pseudocysts and to granulomatous inflammation in the muscular layer, and by lymphatic spread to destruction of the nerve plexuses, resulting in inco-ordination of the peristaltic movements and achalasia of the cardiac sphincter. **Swineherds' disease.** An acute non-fatal disease affecting pigkeepers and pork dealers. It is due to a virus transmitted from swine to man by the hog louse. It first causes intestinal disorder, followed by a remission period and then by meningeal symptoms. Also called *Bouchet's disease.* **System disease.** A disease confined to one system of the body; in a nervous disease, one in which a particular tract in the brain or cord is affected; uncommon usage in Great Britain. **Systemic disease.** A generalized disease, one affecting the whole body (system) as opposed to a localized disease. (This meaning is almost directly opposed to that of a system disease, a term apparently used in the USA.) **Tangier disease.** Familial lipoprotein deficiency with low blood cholesterol and large, orange or grey tonsils. **Tanners' disease.** Anthrax. **Tarabagan disease.** Bubonic plague. **Tea-tasters' disease.** A bronchopulmonary disease due to infection with a fungus of the genus *Candida.* **Tete disease.** Tick-borne relapsing fever, in Central Africa. **Third disease.** Rubella. **Tokelau disease.** Tinea imbricata; a superficial ringworm infection due to *Trichophyton concentricum* characterized by the formation of concentric scaling areas which may cover the entire surface of the skin in native populations in the tropics, especially in the South Pacific Islands, Southern China, Sri Lanka, South Africa, and South and Central America. **Topical disease.** A purely local disease. **Traumatic vasospastic disease of the hands.** Pneumatic-hammer disease (see above). **Tricuspid disease.** Disease of the tricuspid valve, usually the result of rheumatic fever (rheumatic endocarditis). Distortion of the valve cusps interferes with function, causing obstruction to the flow of blood (stenosis) or regurgitation of blood back through the valve during ventricular systole (incompetence); frequently both occur together. Less commonly it is due to congenital maldevelopment (tricuspid atresia, Ebstein's syndrome). Dilatation of the tricuspid valve, causing incompetence, occurs not infrequently in conditions which are associated with hypertrophy, dilatation and failure of the right ventricle (pulmonary stenosis, pulmonary hypertension, mitral stenosis with pulmonary hypertension, etc.). **Trinidad disease.** Paralyssa. **Tropical disease.** An ill-defined term, but it may be taken to mean those diseases (*a*) that occur exclusively, or almost exclusively, in hot countries, (*b*) that are more prevalent in hot countries and (*c*) that assume greater significance in hot countries. They are, in fact, mainly the diseases of hygienically backward peoples, many of which were at one time prevalent throughout the world. **Tsetse-fly disease.** Trypanosomiasis. **Tsutsugamushi disease.** Mite typhus or scrub typhus due to bites of the larval trombidia (microtrombidia), *Trombicula akamushi* or *Trombicula deliensis.* The causal organism is *Rickettsia tsutsugamushi (orientalis).* **Tunnel disease.** Ancylostomiasis. **Vagabonds' disease, Vagrants' disease.** Chronic pediculosis vestimentorum with harsh, dry, scratched, crusted skin. **Valvular disease.** Any disease affecting the valves of the heart. **Vanishing-bone disease.** Massive osteolysis. **Venereal diseases.** Diseases transmitted by venery. In the UK they are defined legally, by an Act of Parliament in 1917, as syphilis, gonorrhoea and chancroid. In the USA the legal definition also includes lymphogranuloma venereum and granuloma inguinale. **Veno-occlusive disease of the West Indies.** A disease resembling the Budd–Chiari syndrome, frequently encountered in West Indian children. Gross hepatomegaly with ascites and portal hypertension develop as a result of occlusive phlebitis of the sub-lobular and central veins. Cirrhosis of Laennec type is a late result. It is attributed to the consumption of "bush teas" or infusions of so-called medicinal herbs, especially when these contain *Crotolaria* and *Senecio* (ragwort) leaves. **Virus disease.** A disease caused by infection with a virus. **Waxy disease.** Amyloid disease (see above). **White-spot disease.** 1. Morphoea guttata. 2. Lichen sclerosus et atrophicus. **Winter vomiting disease.** Epidemic vomiting syndrome. *See* SYNDROME. **Woolsorters' disease.** Respiratory or gastro-intestinal anthrax due to the inhalation or swallowing of wollen particles, conveying anthrax spores or bacilli, by persons handling wool. **X disease.** A state of ill-health associated with various functional disturbances of digestion, respiration, and circulation described by Mackenzie. **Zymotic disease.** Any epidemic infectious disease. [L *dis-*, Fr. *aise* ease.]

See also: ABRAMI, ADAMS (R.), ADDISON (T.), ALBARRAN, ALBERS-SCHOENBERG, ALBRIGHT, ALIBERT, ALMEIDA, ALZHEIMER, ANDERS, APERT, APPELBAUM, ARAN, ARMSTRONG (C.), ARNOLD (J.), AUFRECHT, AUJESZKY, AYALA, AYERZA, BAELZ, BAERENSPRUNG, BAKER, BALLET, BALLINGALL, BALÓ, BAMBERGER (E.), BAMBERGER (H.), BANG (B. L. F.), BANNISTER, BANTI, BARLOW, BARRAQUER (J. A.), BARTHÉLEMY, BASEDOW, BATEMAN, BATTEN, BAYLE, BAZIN, BEARD, BEAUVAIS, BECHTEREW, BEGBIE, BEHÇET, BEHR, BEIGEL, BENSON, BERCHILLET-JOURDAIN, BERGERON, BERLIN, BERNHARDT (M.), BESNIER, BEST (F.), BEURMANN, BEVAN-LEWIS, BIEDL, BIELSCHOWSKY, BIERMER, BIETT, BIGNAMI, BILLROTH, BIRD (G.), BLOCQ, BOECK (C. P. M.), BONFIL, BOSTOCK, BOUCHARD, BOUCHET, BOUILLAUD, BOURNEVILLE, BOUVERET, BOWEN, BRAILSFORD, BREDA, BRETONNEAU, BRIGHT, BRILL, BRIN-

TON, BRION, BRISSAUD, BROCQ, BRODIE (B. C.), BROOKE, BROWN (C. L.), BROWN-SÉQUARD, BRUCK-LANGE, BRUGSCH (K. L. T.), BUCHMAN, BUDD, BUEDINGER, BUERGER, BUHL, BURNS (B. H.), BURY, BUSCHKE, BUSQUET, BUSSE, CALVÉ, CARRIÓN, CARTER (H. V.), CASTELLANI, CAVARE, CAZENAVE, CHAGAS, CHARCOT, CHARLOUIS, CHARRIN, CHEYNE (G.), CHIARI, CHRISTIAN, CHRISTMAS, CIARROCCHI, CIVATTE, COATS, COGAN, CONCATO, CONOR, COOLEY, COOPER (A. P.), CORBUS, CORRIGAN, COTUGNO (COTUNNIUS), CREUTZFELDT, CROHN, CROUZON, CRUCHET, CRUVEILHIER, CSILLAG, CURSCHMANN (HEINRICH), CUSHING (HARVEY W.), CZERNY, DAAE, DA COSTA, D'ACOSTA, DALRYMPLE, DANIELSSEN, DANLOS, DARIER, DARLING, DAVID, DÉBOVE, DÉJÉRINE, DERCUM, DEUTSCHLAENDER, DEVERGIE, DEVIC, DIEULAFOY, DI GUGLIELMO, DIMITRI, DOEHLE, DOLAGE, DRESBACH, DRESSLER, DUBINI, DUCHENNE, DUHRING, DUKES (C.), DURAND (J.), DURAND (P.), DUROZIEZ, DUTTON, DZIERZYNSKY, EALES, EBERTH, EBSTEIN, ECONOMO, EDSALL, EHLERS, EICHHORST, EICHSTEDT, ENGMAN, ERB, ERICHSEN, EULENBURG, FAHR, FALLOT, FANCONI, FAUCHARD, FAVRE, FEDE, FEIL, FELIX, FENWICK (S.), FERNEL, FIEDLER, FILATOV, FINSEN (J. C.), FLAJANI, FLATAU, FOERSTER (R.), FORDYCE, FOTHERGILL (J.), FOURNIER, FOX (G. H.), FRANCIS, FRANKL-HOCHWART, FREIBERG, FRIEDLAENDER, FRIEDMANN (M.), FRIEDREICH, FUERSTNER, GAISBOECK, GARBE, GARRÉ, GAUCHER, GEE, GENSOUL, GERHARDT (C. C. A. J.), GERLIER, GIBERT, GIERKE (E.), GILCHRIST, GILFORD, GILLES DE LA TOURETTE, GIOVANNINI, GLANZMANN, GLÉNARD, GOLDFLAM, GOLDSCHEIDER, GOUGEROT, GOURAUD, GOWERS, GRAEFE, GRAVES, GREENFIELD, GREENHOW, GREPPI, GRIESINGER, GROSS (S. D.), GRUBY, GUINON, GULL, HABERMANN, HAILEY (H. E.), HAILEY (W. H.), HALL (M.), HALLERVORDEN, HALLOPEAU, HAMMAN, HAMMOND, HAND, HANOT, HANSEN, HARLEY, HASHIMOTO, HASS, HAYEM, HEBERDEN, HEBRA, HEERFORDT, HEINE (J.), HELLER (A. L. G.), HENDERSON (M. S.), HENOCH, HERTER, HERXHEIMER, HEUBNER, HILDENBRAND, HIPPEL, HIRSCHFELD (F.), HIRSCHSPRUNG, HIS (W. JNR.), HODARA, HODGKIN, HODGSON, HOFFMAN (J.), HOPF, HUCHARD, HUNT (J. R.), HUNTINGTON, HUPPERT, HURLER, HUTCHINSON, HUTINEL, HYDE, INMAN, ISAMBERT, JACQUET, JADASSOHN, JAFFE, JAKOB, JAKSCH, JANET, JANSKY, JENSEN (E. Z.), JOHNE, JOHNSON, JONES (H. T.), JUENGLING, KAHLBAUM, KAHLER, KALISCHER, KAPOSI, KAYSER (B.), KAYSER (H.), KIENBOECK, KIMMELSTIEL, KLEBS, KLEMPERER, KOEBNER, KOEHLER, KORSAKOFF, KOZHEVNIKOFF, KRABBE, KRAEPELIN, KRISHABER, KUEMMELL, KUFS, KUNDRAT, KUSSMAUL, LAËNNEC, LAEWEN, LAIN, LAMBRINUDI, LANCEREAUX, LANDOUZY, LANDRY, LASÈGUE, LEBER, LEDERER, LEGG, LEICHTENSTERN, LEINER, LELOIR, LETTERER, LÉVI, LÉVY, LEWANDOWSKY, LEYDEN, LIBMAN, LICHTENSTEIN, LICHTHEIM, LINDAU, LITTLE (W. J.), LORAIN, LORIGA, LUCAS-CHAMPIONNIÈRE, LUDLOFF, LUTEMBACHER, LUTZ (H. C.), MACKENZIE (J.), MAGITOT, MAIER, MAJOCCHI, MALASSEZ, MANSON, MARCHIAFAVA, MARFAN, MARIE, MATHIEU, MAUCLAIRE, MAURIAC, MAXCY, MAYOU, MEDIN, MEIGE, MÉNIÈRE, MERZBACHER, MEYER (H. W.), MIBELLI, MICHELI, MIKULICZ-RADECKI, MILKMAN, MILLAR, MILLS, MILROY, MILTON, MINOR, MINOT, MITCHELL, MOEBIUS, MOELLER (J. O. L.), MONGE, MORAND, MOREL, MORGAGNI, MORQUIO, MORTIMER, MORTON (T. G.), MORVAN, MOUCHET, MOZER, MUCHA, MUENCHMEYER, MUNK, MURRI, MYÀ, NEFTEL, NETTLESHIP, NEUMANN (I.), NICOLAS, NIEMANN, NORDAU, OGUCHI, OHARA, OLDBERG, OLLIER, OPITZ, OPPENHEIM (H.), OPPENHEIM (M.), OSGOOD (R. B.), OSLER, OTTO (A. W.), OWREN, PAGE, PAGET, PALTAUF, PANNER, PARIS, PARKINSON (J.), PARROT, PARRY, PAVY, PAXTON, PAYR, PEL, PELIZAEUS, PELLEGRINI, PERTHES, PETIT (J. L.), PEYRONIE, PFEIFFER (E.), PICK (A.), PICK (F.), PICK (F. J.), PICK (L.), PINKUS, PLUMMER, POLLITZER, PONCET, POSADA, POTAIN, POTT, POULET, PRINGLE (J. J.), PURTSCHER, QUERVAIN, QUINCKE, QUINQUAUD, RAUZIER, RAYER, RAYNAUD, RECKLINGHAUSEN, RECLUS, REED, REFSUM, REICHMANN, REITER, RENDU, RIEDEL, RIETTI, RIGA, RIGGS, RITTER (G.), RIVALTA (S.), ROBINSON (A. R.), ROBLES, ROGER (H. L.), ROKITANSKY, ROMBERG, ROSENBACH (A. J. F.), ROSSBACH, ROTH (M.), ROTH (V. K.), ROUSSY, ROWLAND, RUNEBERG, RUYSCH, SACHS (B.), SACKS, ST. AGATHA, ST. AIGNAN, ST. ANTHONY, ST. APPOLONIA, ST. AVERTIN, ST. AVIDUS, ST. BLASIUS, ST. DYMPHNA, ST. ERASMUS, ST. FIACRE, ST. FRANCIS, ST. GERVASIUS, ST. GETE, ST. GILES, ST. HUBERT, ST. MAIN, ST. MATHURIN, ST. MODESTUS, ST. ROCH, ST. VALENTINE, ST. VITUS, ST. ZACHARY, SANDER, SANDERS, SAUNDERS (E. W.), SAVILL, SCHAMBERG, SCHAUMANN, SCHENCK, SCHEUERMANN, SCHILDER, SCHIMMELBUSCH, SCHLATTER, SCHMORL, SCHOENLEIN, SCHOLZ, SCHOTTMUELLER, SCHRIDDE, SCHUELLER (A.), SCHULTZ, SECRÉTAN, SENEAR, SEVER, SIMMONDS, SIMONS (A.), SINDING-LARSEN, SIWE, SJÖGREN, SKEVAS-ZERFUS, SMITH (E.), SMITH (T.), SOTTAS, SPATZ, SPIELMEYER, STANTON, STARGARDT, STEINERT, STERNBERG (K.), STEVENS (A. M.), STICKER, STIEDA (A.), STILL, STILLER, STOCK, STOKES (WILLIAM), STOKVIS, STRACHAN, STRUEMPELL, STURGE, SUDECK, SULZBERGER, SUTTON (H. G.), SUTTON (R. L.), SYMMERS, TAENZER, TAKAYASU, TALMA, TAY, TAYLOR (R. W.), THAYSEN, THEILER, THOMSEN, THOMSON (M. S.), TILLAUX, TOMMASELLI, TOOTH, TROUSSEAU, UNDERWOOD, UNNA, UNVERRICHT, URBACH, USHER, VALSUANI, VAN BUREN, VAN NECK, VAQUEZ, VINCENT, VIRCHOW, VOGT (C.), VOGT (O.), VOLHARD (F.), VOLTOLINI, WAGNER (E. L.), WALDENSTRÖM (J. H.), WARDROP, WARTENBERG, WASSILIEFF, WEBER (F. P.), WEIL (A.), WEINGARTNER, WEPFER, WERDNIG, WERLHOF, WERNER (H.), WERNICKE (K.), WERNICKE (R. J.), WESTBERG, WESTPHAL (C. F. O.), WHIPPLE (G. H.), WHITE (J. C.), WHITEHEAD (W.), WHYTT, WIDAL, WIETHE, WILKINSON, WILLAN, WILLEBRAND, WILLIS (T.), WILSON (C.), WILSON (S. A. KINNIER), WILSON, (W. J. E.), WINCKEL, WINDSCHEID, WINKLER (M.), WOILLEZ, ZAGARI, ZIEHEN.

disengagement (dis·en·**gaje**·ment). 1. The process or act of setting free. 2. During labour, the emergence of the head from the vaginal canal. 3. The emergence of an impacted tumour. [Fr. *désengager*.]

disequilibrium (dis·e·kwel·**ib'**·re·um). 1. Absence or loss of equilibrium in any sense. 2. Unstable mental balance. 3. Absence or lack of normal adjustment between the intellectual and the moral faculties. [L *dis-*, equilibrium.]

disfigure (dis·**fig**·ewr). In law, to disfigure is to do some external injury which may detract from an individual's personal appearance. [L *dis, fingere* to fashion.]

disgerminoma (dis·jer·min·**o'**·mah). A malignant tumour of the testicle or ovary originating in cells which have remained undifferentiated to either the male or female type. [L *dis, germen* germ, Gk *-oma* tumour.]

disgregation (dis·gre·**ga**·shun). Dispersion into individual units. [L *disgregare* to separate.]

dish (dish). An open, shallow receptacle used in laboratory work. **Culture dish.** A saucer-like receptacle on which bacteria are cultured. [AS *disc.*]

See also: PETRI.

disimmune (dis·im·**ewn**). Referring to an organism, e.g. human being, which has been deprived of its immunity. [L *dis-*, immune.]

disimmunity (dis·im·**ewn**·it·e). The state of having lost or been deprived of immunity, and the resultant condition. [see prec.]

disimmunize (dis·**im**·ewn·ize). To bring about the loss of immunity in an organism. [L *dis-*, immune.]

disimpaction (dis·im·**pak**·shun). The reduction of an impacted fracture. [L *dis-*, *impingere* to strike against.]

disinfect (dis·in·**fekt**). 1. To render innocuous. 2. To destroy or free from pathogenic organisms. [L *dis-*, *inficere* to corrupt.]

disinfectant (dis·in·**fek**·tant). 1. Having a lethal effect upon germs. 2. A germicide; any substance which kills bacteria and their spores. The term is generally restricted to substances which are too toxic to be applied directly to the tissues, but which can be used for decontaminating drains and faecal matter, and for the sterilizing of instruments and apparatus. They include oxidizing and reducing agents, halogens and halogen compounds, metallic salts, phenols, cresols and certain dyes. **Coal-tar disinfectant.** Creosote, or other disinfectant, derived from coal tar. **Complete disinfectant.** A disinfectant which is effective not only against vegetative bacteria but also against bacterial spores. **Incomplete disinfectant.** One that has no action on the spores of bacteria but only on the vegetative forms. [see prec.]

disinfection (dis·in·**fek**·shun). The process or act of disinfecting; the freeing of any person or object from harmful germs. **Aerial**

disinfection. Disinfection of the air, e.g. in an operating theatre or ward: various methods of filtration, chemical sprays and ultraviolet-light applications are used. **Concurrent disinfection.** Disinfection carried out continuously during the whole course of a disease by the immediate disposal and destruction of discharges and infectious matter and the cleansing of infected objects and linen. **Terminal disinfection.** The disinfecting of the room and the destruction or cleansing of infectious materials at the end of the infective stage of a disease. [L *dis-*, *inficere* to corrupt.]

disinfector (dis·in·**fek**·tor). An apparatus with which disinfectants can be applied and in this way the disinfection of buildings and objects be achieved. [see prec.]

See also: THRESH.

disinfestation (**dis**·in·fes·**ta**'·shun). Freeing a person or place from infestation, e.g. by ectoparasites, noxious rodents or other vermin. [L *dis-*, *infestare* to attack.]

disinhibition (**dis**·in·hib·**ish**'·un). The countering and removal of the mechanism of inhibition. [L *dis-*, *inhibere* to restrain.]

disinomenine (di·sin·**om**·en·een). $(C_{19}H_{22}O_4N)_2 2CH_3OH$, an alkaloid occurring in *Sinomenium acutum*, a Japanese plant of the family Menispermaceae; also formed by the gentle oxidation of sinomenine. It is a convulsive poison.

disinsect (dis·in·**sekt**). To free from any kind of insect or vermin. [L *dis-*, insect.]

disinsection, disinsectization (dis·in·**sek**·shun, **dis**·in·sek·tiz·**a**'·shun). The removal of insects from a person or object. [see prec.]

disinsector (dis·in·**sek**·tor). An apparatus with which individuals or clothes can be freed from insects or vermin. [L *dis-*, insect.]

disinsertion (dis·in·**ser**·shun). 1. Rupture of a tendon at the point of insertion into a bone. 2. Retinodialysis. [L *dis-*, *inserere* to connect in.]

disintegrate (dis·**in**·teg·rate). 1. Of a substance, to break up or become decomposed. 2. To be converted from a higher to a lower state of organization. [L *dis-*, *integrare* to make whole.]

disintegration (**dis**·in·teg·**ra**'·shun). 1. The act or process of breaking up or decomposing. 2. Decay. 3. Catabolism. **Disintegration of bacteria.** To obtain cell-free extracts or toxins. Methods vary from mechanical use of pestle and mortar with a suitable abrasive, shaking at high speed with glass beads, extrusion through small orifices by high pressure, and alternate freezing and thawing, to the use of sonic and ultrasonic waves. **Radioactive disintegration.** The emission of an alpha or beta particle by a radioactive element which is thereby transformed into another element. [see prec.]

disintoxication (**dis**·in·tox·ik·**a**'·shun). 1. Detoxication. 2. Any treatment given to a drug addict for the purpose of freeing him from craving. [L *dis-*, *in*, Gk *toxikon* poison.]

disinvagination (**dis**·in·vaj·in·**a**'·shun). The relieving or reduction of an invagination. [L *dis-*, *in*, *vagina* sheath.]

disjoint (dis·**joint**). 1. To separate the joints of any structure. 2. To put out of joint. 3. To separate parts united by joints. [L *disjungere* to disjoint.]

disjugate (**dis**·joo·gate). 1. Unequally paired. 2. In certain cases the opposite of conjugate. [L *dis-*, *jugum* yoke.]

disjunction (dis·**jungk**·shun). The separation of chromosomes at anaphase of the first meiotic division or of daughter chromosomes (chromatids) at anaphase of mitosis and second meiotic division. [L *disjungere* to disjoint.]

disjunctive (dis·**jungk**·tiv). In ophthalmology, referring to movements of the two eyes together when the fixation axes do not remain parallel, e.g. divergence, convergence and supravergence. [L *disjungere* to disjoint.]

disk (disk). *See* DISC.

dislocation (dis·lo·**ka**·shun). 1. Displacement of one part upon another; usually confined to the abnormal displacement of one bone upon another at a joint. 2. In cytogenetics, chromosome structural change due to loss or displacement of chromosome material. **Central dislocation.** Dislocation of the head of the femur through the acetabulum. **Closed dislocation.** A dislocation in which there is no wound involving the joint. **Complete dislocation.** A dislocation in which the constituent articular surfaces of the joint are entirely separated. **Complicated dislocation.** A dislocation associated with damage to other important structures. **Compound dislocation.** A dislocation with an associated wound communicating with the joint. **Congenital dislocation.** A dislocation present at birth. **Fracture dislocation.** Dislocation associated with fracture of bony components of joints. **Dislocation of the globe.** Displacement of the eyeball forwards so that the lids close behind it; also called *luxation of the globe.* **Habitual dislocation.** A dislocation which repeatedly recurs after reduction. **Incomplete dislocation.** Subluxation; partial abnormal separation of the articular surface of a joint. **Infra-acromialis dislocation.** Dislocation of the shoulder where the head of the humerus lies below the acromion process. **Infraglenoid dislocation.** Dislocation of the shoulder where the head of the humerus lies below the glenoid fossa. **Intra-uterine dislocation.** A dislocation which occurs *in utero.* **Dislocation of the lens.** Displacement of the crystalline lens of the eye from its normal position. **Obturator dislocation.** Dislocation of the hip, the head of the femur lying in the obturator foramen. **Old dislocation.** A dislocation which has been present for some time. **Paralytic dislocation.** Dislocation resuling from paralysis and wasting of the supporting muscles. **Partial dislocation.** Incomplete dislocation (see above). **Pathological dislocation.** Dislocation due to disease of the joint or of its constituent bones. **Perineal dislocation.** Dislocation of the hip with the head of the femur displaced into the perineum. **Pubic dislocation.** Dislocation of the hip anteriorly, with the head of the femur lying on the pubic bone. **Recent dislocation.** A dislocation seen shortly after the causative injury. **Recurrent dislocation.** Habitual dislocation (see above). **Relapsing dislocation.** Habitual dislocation (see above). **Sciatic dislocation.** Dislocation of the hip, the head of the femur lying in the sciatic notch. **Simple dislocation.** Closed dislocation (see above). **Subastragalar dislocation.** Dislocation of the calcaneum upon the astragalus. **Subclavicular dislocation.** Dislocation of the shoulder where the head of the humerus lies immediately below the clavicle. **Subcoracoid dislocation.** Dislocation of the shoulder, with the head of the humerus lying below the coracoid process. **Subglenoid dislocation.** Anterior dislocation of the shoulder where the head of the humerus lies below the glenoid fossa of the scapula. **Subpubic dislocation.** Anterior dislocation of the hip where the femoral head lies immediately below the pubis. **Subspinous dislocation.** Backward dislocation of the shoulder where the head of the humerus lies in the subspinous fossa of the scapula. **Subtalar dislocation.** Dislocation of the subtalar joint. **Traumatic dislocation.** Dislocation due to injury. [L *dis-*, *locare* to place.]

See also: KOCHER.

dismemberment (dis·**mem**·ber·ment). Amputation of a limb or limbs or of a part of a limb. [L *dis-*, *membrum* limb.]

dismutation (dis·mew·**ta**·shun). A chemical reaction involving 2 molecules of the same substance, one of which is oxidized at the expense of reduction of the second, producing 2 new compounds, one an oxidized derivative of the original substance, the other a reduced derivative. The phenomenon is a familiar one among the aldehydes (Cannizzaro reaction), benzaldehyde yielding on treatment with caustic potash equimolecular amounts of benzyl alcohol and benzoic acid. [Gk *dis-*, L *mutare* to change.]

disocclude (dis·ok·**lood**). In dentistry, to put out of occlusion. [L *dis-*, *occludere* to shut.]

disodic (di·**so**·dik). Term applied to a compound that contains 2 sodium atoms in its molecule. [Gk *dis-*, sodium.]

disodium (di·**so**·de·um). A compound which contains 2 atoms of sodium. **Disodium Edetate BP 1973.** Disodium dihydrogen ethylenediamine-*N,N,N′,N′*-tetra-acetate dihydrate; a chelating substance which has a strong affinity for divalent and trivalent metals. It is of particular value in the management of hypercalcaemia. **Disodium ethylenediaminotetra-acetate dihydrate.** An anticoagulant substance, with non-wettable characteristics, that does not adversely affect the activity of the platelets when used for transfusing platelet-rich plasma suspensions. **Disodium hydrogen citrate.** Sodium Acid Citrate BP 1958. **Disodium hydrogen phosphate.** Sodium Phosphate BP 1958. **Disodium phenylphosphate.** $Na_2(C_6H_5)PO_4$, a compound that is used in the King and Armstrong method for the estimation of alkaline phosphates. [see prec.]

disoma (di·so·mah). A monster with a double trunk. [Gk *dis-*, *soma* body.]

disomic (di·so·mik). Of cells or individuals, with a member of their chromosome complement represented twice. In contradistinction with monosomic, trisomic, tetrasomic, etc. [Gk *dis-*, *soma* body.]

disomus (di·so·mus) (pl. *disomi*). Disoma.

Disopyramide (di·so·pi·ram·ide). BP Commission approved name for 4-di-isopropylamino-2-phenyl-2-(2-pyridyl)butyramide; an anti-arrhythmic agent.

disorder (dis·or·der). Any indisposition or infirmity of the body. **Acting-out disorder.** A term for neurotic delinquency in which children act out unconscious impulses without understanding why, e.g. stealing because of rejection by parents. **Mental disorder.** Defined by the Mental Health Act 1959 as mental illness, arrested or incomplete development of mind, psychopathic disorder and any other disorder or disability of mind. **Nutritional disorder, Vegetative disorder.** Any disorder affecting growth, particularly of a kind to inhibit growth. [L *dis-*, *ordo* rank.]

disorganization (dis·or·gan·i·za′·shun). 1. The destroying of the organic structure of the body. 2. Complete degenerative change in a tissue or organ so that character and function are lost. [L *dis-*, Gk *organon* organ.]

disorientation (dis·or·e·en·ta′·shun). Uncertainty about one's bearings. Lack of orientating cues in fog or darkness or conflict of orientating information. **Spatial disorientation.** Uncertainty about one's position and velocity in space. In aviation, orientation is relative to the earth's surface; space travellers orientate with respect to their vehicle and to their target. [L *dis-*, *oriens* east.]

disoxidation (dis·ox·e·da′·shun). Deoxidation.

dispar (dis·par). Unequal. [L.]

disparasitize (dis·par·ah·sit·ize). To free from infestation with parasites. [L *dis-*, parasite.]

disparate (dis·par·ate). 1. Essentially different or distinct in character. 2. Not corresponding. 3. Unequally paired. [L *dispar* unlike.]

disparity (dis·par·it·e). Unequalness; incongruity. A word applied particularly to non-corresponding points in the retinae, simultaneous stimulation of which gives rise to diplopia or, if the points are nearly corresponding and in the horizontal meridian, to stereoscopic vision. If the object whose image stimulates disparate points is inside the horopter, there is crossed disparity, the right image being seen by the left eye and vice versa; if the object is beyond the horopter, there is uncrossed disparity, the right image being seen by the right eye and the left image by the left eye. **Fixation disparity.** Disparity occurring during binocular single vision when the fixation point stimulates non-corresponding retinal elements within Panum's area. [see prec.]

dispense (dis·pens). 1. To issue medicines, as from a dispensary. 2. To compound a drug or mixture of drugs in such a manner that the product will have the pharmacological action required by the prescriber. The considerations which govern dispensing are: the route by which the medicament is to be administered, its chemical nature and the compatibility between the drugs of which it is compounded. [L *dis-*, *pensare* to weigh.]

disperme (di·sper·me). Dispermy.

dispermine (di·sper·meen). Piperazine, diethylenediamine, $NH(CH_2)_4NH$. A colourless crystalline cyclic compound which is readily soluble in water, forming a solution which is itself a uric-acid solvent. It has been used in the treatment of gout, rheumatism and uric-acid gravel.

dispermy (di·sper·me). The entry of 2 spermatozoa into a single ovum. [Gk *dis-*, *sperma* seed.]

disperse (dis·pers). 1. To disseminate or scatter the finely-divided particles of a substance. 2. The extension of the term to mean the dispersed particles themselves, as in the colloidal state. **Disperse medium.** In a colloidal solution, the continuous external phase, or solvent. **Disperse particles.** The particles suspended in the disperse medium, or the internal phase of a colloidal system. **Disperse phase.** The discontinuous or internal phase of a colloidal solution; the disperse particles. **Disperse system.** A colloidal system. [L *dis-*, *spargere* to scatter.]

dispersible (dis·per·sibl). 1. Of a kind that can be dispersed, such as a tumour. 2. Capable of being dispersed, such as colloid particles. [see prec.]

dispersidology (dis·per·sid·ol′·o·je). Colloid chemistry; the chemistry of the colloid state. [L *dis-*, *spargere* to scatter, Gk *eidos* form, *logos* science.]

dispersion (dis·per·shun). 1. The scattering or dissemination of the finely-divided particles of a substance. 2. The permeation of one substance through the bulk of another. 3. The colloidal solution. 4. In optics, the phenomenon of white light being split into its coloured constituents, as in a rainbow or spectroscope. **Chromatic dispersion.** The separation of white light into its constituent colours by passage through a prism. **Coarse dispersion.** A suspension of large particles in a liquid. **Colloidal dispersion.** A colloidal solution. **Insect dispersion.** The distance from their breeding place that insects appear, as the result of either their own efforts (*active dispersion*) or having been transported there (*passive dispersion*). **Dispersion of light.** The production of the spectral colours of a complex light by refraction or diffraction. **Molecular dispersion.** A true solution. [L *dis-*, *spargere* to scatter.]

dispersity (dis·per·sit·e). The amount of dispersion in a colloidal solution, dependent on the size of the disperse particles. [see prec.]

dispersoid (dis·per·soid). A substance in such a finely-divided state that it gives a colloidal solution. [L *dis-*, *spargere* to scatter, Gk *eidos* form.]

dispersonalization (dis·per·son·al·i·za′·shun). The loss of sense of personal integrity in which feelings, emotions and physical bodily sensations are unfamiliar and unreal. [L *dis-*, *persona* mask.]

Dispholidus typus (dis·fol·id·us ti·pus). The boomslang: a poisonous snake of South Africa.

dispira, dispirem, dispireme (di·spi·rah, di·spi·rem, di·spi·reem). Terms applied to the early prophase chromosomes which, in mitosis, appear to be in the form of a continuous coiled double thread. It is now known that this appearance is illusory and that the chromosomes are discrete at all stages. [Gk *dis-*, *speirema* coil.]

displacement (dis·plase·ment). 1. Alteration or removal from the normal position or place. 2. In dentistry, the malposition of a tooth whose axis lies parallel to the position it should normally occupy. 3. In psychiatry, the transfer of affect from one object or end to another. **Backward displacement, Dorsal displacement of arm.** Nuchal displacement of arm (see below). **Fetal displacement.** An unusual position of the fetus. **Fish-hook displacement.** A common x-ray appearance of the stomach in which the lesser curvature turns upward at an acute angle in the pyloric part of the stomach. **Nuchal displacement of arm.** A term used to describe an extended arm in a breech presentation when the hand and forearm are behind the neck or head. **Uterine displacement.** Any variation of uterine position from the normal. [Fr. *déplacement*.]

disporous (di·spo·rus). In biology, two-spored. [Gk *dis-*, spore.]

disposition (dis·po·zish·un). 1. An inherent physical or mental tendency, e.g. to become affected by certain diseases. 2. Temperament. [L *disponere* to dispose.]

disproportion (dis·pro·por·shun). The state of being out of proportion; the absence of normal proportion between 2 factors. **Cephalopelvic disproportion.** The absence of the correct proportion between the pelvic opening and the head of the fetus, the latter being abnormally large or the former abnormally small. [L *dis-*, proportion.]

dissect (dis·**ekt**). 1. In anatomy, to separate or cut the tissues apart carefully so that the structure and relations of a part may be studied. 2. In surgery, to cut or tear the connective tissue so as to separate structures according to their natural limits instead of making a wide cut or incision. [L *dissecare* to cut apart.]

dissection (dis·**ek**·shun). 1. The separating or dividing of animal structures for the purpose of anatomical study or in surgical procedures. 2. The result of this procedure. [see prec.]

dissector (dis·**ek**·tor). 1. One who carries out dissection. 2. A special instrument used in surgery and for the dissection of anatomical structures. 3. Name commonly given to a manual of anatomy containing instructions for carrying out dissections. [L *dissecare* to cut apart.]

See also: LANG.

disseminated (dis·**em**·in·a·ted). Dispersed or spread throughout an organ, a tissue or the whole body. [L *dis-*, *seminare* to sow.]

dissemination (dis·**em**·in·**a**′·shun). The act or process of disseminating or the state of being disseminated. [see prec.]

dissepiment (dis·**ep**·e·ment). 1. Partition. 2. A separating septum or tissue. [L *dis-*, *saepire* to hedge in.]

dissimilate (dis·**im**·il·ate). To subject to disassimilation.

dissimilation (dis·**im**·il·**a**′·shun). Disassimilation; catabolism.

dissociable (dis·**so**·she·abl). 1. Lending itself readily to separation into component parts. 2. In psychology, capable of being separated from associations. [L *dis-*, *sociare* to unite.]

dissociant (dis·**so**·she·ant). A variant differing sharply from the normal form, appearing in a pure culture of a micro-organism, for example in an old culture in a fluid medium. [see prec.]

dissociated (dis·o·she·**a**′·ted). In psychology, separated from normal consciousness. [L *dis-*, *sociare* to unite.]

dissociation (dis·o·she·**a**′·shun). 1. Separation, either of parts or of function. 2. In chemistry, the splitting of a molecule of a compound into other molecules or into ions, under certain conditions, in a process which is temporary, usually incomplete, and reversible. 3. Term applied in cardiology to heart block, when the atria and ventricles beat independently. 4. The process whereby a part of the patient's consciousness becomes separated from the main stream and operates independently without contact with the main stream. It is the characteristic mechanism underlying hysterical symptom formation. **Albuminocytological dissociation.** Increase in the level of cerebrospinal fluid protein with no increase in the cell count, as in the *Guillain–Barré syndrome.* **Atrioventricular (auricoventricular) dissociation.** Loss of the normal co-ordination of the atrial and ventricular contractions; it occurs as a result of atrioventricular block, but the term is often restricted to situations where such block is not complete but the ventricles beat at normal or faster than normal rates independent of impulses conducted from the atria. **Auriculoventricular dissociation.** A disturbance of the normal co-ordination of impulses between auricles and ventricles, due either to auriculoventricular heart block or to ventricular escape. **Dissociation of bacteria.** The occurrence in a pure culture of bacteria, derived from a single cell, of individuals which differ markedly from the parent organism, e.g. the appearance of rough mutants in cultures of a pure strain. **Electrolytic dissociation.** Ionic dissociation (see below). **Interference dissociation, Dissociation by interference.** When a nodal rhythm occurs at a fast rate, the sinu-atrial node may activate the auricles at a slower rate. This produces atrioventricular dissociation. Although retrograde conduction is thus blocked, antegrade conduction can occur, and, if an atrial impulse reaches the ventricle when the latter is not refractory, a premature ventricular beat may result. **Ionic dissociation.** The splitting of a molecule of a substance in solution into ions with opposite electric charges; ionization. **Isorhythmic atrioventricular dissociation.** Atrioventricular dissociation (see above) but with the atria and ventricles beating at the same rate; this is the phenomena of *accrochage.* **Microbic dissociation.** Dissociation of bacteria (see above). **Peripheral dissociation.** Sensory loss in the periphery, as occurs in the hands and feet in polyneuritis; an unsatisfactory term. **Syringomyelic dissociation.** The dissociated anaesthesia of syringomyelia, consisting of loss or impairment of pain and temperature sense with retention of touch perception, tactile discrimination, and muscle and joint sense. It is due to interruption of fibres subserving pain as they cross in the anterior grey commissure of the spinal cord. **Tabetic dissociation.** Loss of appreciation of pain on deep pressure and of vibration and position sense, as occurs in tabes dorsalis. **Thermal dissociation.** The splitting of a molecule of a substance on heating into other molecules which recombine on cooling, e.g. ammonium chloride dissociates on heating into ammonia and hydrochloric acid. [see prec.]

dissolecule (dis·**ol**·e·kewl). The particular state of dissociation of the molecule of a substance when in solution and at the temperature of the latter. It is the molecular weight of this that is determined by the boiling-point method.

dissolution (dis·ol·**ew**·shun). 1. Death. 2. Liquefaction of organic tissues. 3. Disintegration of mental powers. 4. Solution. 5. In chemistry, the separation of a compound into its simpler constituents. [L *dissolvere* to loose.]

dissolve (diz·**olv**). 1. To bring about the dispersion of the molecules of a substance invisibly throughout the bulk of a liquid. 2. To enter into the state of solution. [see prec.]

dissolvent (diz·**ol**·vent). 1. The continuous phase of a solution, or the medium in which the solute is dissolved. 2. Having the power to dissolve. 3. A therapeutic administered with the intention of dissolving and removing calculi. [L *dissolvere* to loose.]

dissonance (**dis**·on·ans). 1. The unpleasant sound produced by discords. 2. The interference between the waves of sounds of different pitch which produces a rhythmic beat. [L *dis-*, *sonare* to sound.]

distal [distalis (NA)] (**dis**·tal). 1. Farthest from the median line. 2. Farthest from a central point. 3. Farthest from the trunk, e.g. a segment of a limb. 4. Remote from the point of attachment or origin. 5. Peripheral. 6. In opposition to proximal. [L *distare* to be distant.]

distalia (dis·**ta**·le·ah). The bones composing the distal row of the carpus or tarsus. [see prec.]

distance (**dis**·tans). The intervals between 2 objects. **Focal distance.** The distance of the focal point from the centre of a lens or spherical mirror. **Focus-film distance.** The distance between the source of x-rays and the radiographic film. It is an important factor influencing definition and sharpness. Other factors being equal, the greater the distance the sharper the radiographic image. **Focus-skin distance.** The distance between the focal spot on the target of an x-ray tube and the skin of the patient at the centre of the irradiated field. **Hearing distance.** The distance at which certain (unspecified) sounds can be heard. **Infinite distance.** In ophthalmology, 6 m or more, because the rays of light from an object seen at this distance or over are almost parallel. **Interpediculate distance.** The distance between the inner aspects of the right and left pedicles of each vertebra, as seen in an anteroposterior radiograph. The distance may be increased in expanding vertebral lesions. **Interpupillary distance.** The distance between the pupils of the two eyes. It is important for correct centring of spectacle lenses. **Object-film distance.** The distance between the object and the film in radiography. The closer the object the sharper is the definition. A magnified, but less sharp image results from a long object-film distance. **Pupillary distance.** Interpupillary distance (see above). **Short target-skin distance.** The distance between the source of x-rays (x-ray tube target) and the area of skin under treatment. Short distances are generally understood to be distances less than 15 cm. In the case of special so-called contact tubes this distance may be as short as 2 cm. **Source-skin distance.** Distance between gamma ray source and skin surface of the patient in the central axis of the field. **Source-tumour distance.** Distance between the gamma ray source and the centre of the tumour volume in the central axis of the field. **Working distance.** The distance between the foremost lens of a microscopic objective and the object examined, when the latter is in focus. [L *distantia* distance.]

distemper (dis·**tem**·per). Indisposition or disorder of body or mind: a morbid systemic state; a condition of malaise. The term is generally applied to animals. **Canine distemper.** A virus infection in dogs. [L *dis-*, *temperare* to regulate.]

distension (dis·**ten**·shun). 1. The act of distending or dilating. 2. The state of being enlarged, dilated or distended. [L *distendere* to stretch.]

distichia, distichiasis (dis·**tik**·e·ah, dis·tik·**i**·as·is). A condition in which there is an anterior and a posterior row of eyelashes on one lid, the posterior and sometimes also the anterior turning inwards against the eyeball. [Gk *dis-*, *stichos* row.]

Distigmine Bromide (di·**stig**·meen **bro**·mide). BP Commission approved name for *N,N′*-hexamethylenedi-[1-methyl-3-(methylcarbamoyloxy)pyridinium bromide]; an anticholinesterase.

distil (dis·**til**). To separate a volatile liquid from admixture with another and less volatile liquid or from dissolved impurities by boiling in a special apparatus and collecting the condensed vapour. [L *distillare* to drop down.]

distillate (**dis**·til·ate). The product of distillation. [see prec.]

distillation (dis·til·**a**·shun). The process of distilling. **Cold distillation.** Distillation at ordinary temperatures under reduced pressure. **Destructive distillation.** Distillation at relatively high temperature which splits up the original substance into simpler products which can be condensed. **Dry distillation.** Distillation of dry solids. **Fractional distillation.** The separation of the components of a liquid mixture by taking advantage of their different boiling-points and collecting them as distillates at the appropriate temperatures. **Molecular distillation.** The condensation of molecules escaping from the surface of a liquid. [L *distillare* to drop down.]

distinctometer (dis·tingk·**tom**·et·er). A form of palpatorium with which the boundaries of the abdominal organs can be identified and the amount of pressure exerted on them by the apparatus measured. [L *distinguere* to mark off, meter.]

distinctor (dis·**tingk**·tor). Palpatorium: an instrument used in abdominal palpation for the purpose of detecting tender areas during examination with a fluoroscope. [L *distinguere* to mark off.]

distobuccal (dis·to·**buk**·al). Relating to the distal and buccal surfaces of the teeth.

distobucco-occlusal (dis·to·**buk**·o·ok·**loo**′·zal). Relating to the distal, buccal and occlusal surfaces of bicuspid or molar teeth, particularly the angle formed by the meeting of these surfaces.

distobuccopulpal (**dis**·to·buk·o·**pul**′·pal). Relating to the distal, buccal and pulpal walls of the cavity of a tooth.

distoceptor (**dis**·to·sep·tor). A distance receptor. *See* RECEPTOR.

distocervical (dis·to·**ser**·vik·al). Relating to the distal and cervical walls of the cavity of a tooth.

distocia (dis·**to**·she·ah). The giving birth to a second child. [Gk *dis-*, *tokos* birth.]

distoclusal (dist·ok·**loo**·zal). Disto-occlusal.

distoclusion (dist·ok·**loo**·zhun). Disto-occlusion.

distokia (dis·**to**·ke·ah). Distocia.

distolabial (dis·to·**la**·be·al). Relating to that part of a tooth bounded by its distal and labial surfaces.

distolingual (dis·to·**ling**·gwal). Relating to the distal and lingual surfaces of a tooth.

distolinguocclusal (**dis**·to·ling·gwok·**loo**′·zal). The junction between the distal, lingual and occlusal surfaces of the crown of a tooth.

distoma (**dis**·to·mah). The old generic name for many flukes which are now correctly placed in separate genera. The liver fluke, *Distoma hepatica*, for example, has become *Fasciola hepatica*. [Gk *di-*, *stoma* mouth.]

distomata (dis·**to**·mah·tah). A sub-order of the trematode order Prostomata. The families Dicrocoeliidae, Echinostomatidae, Fasciolidae, Heterophyidae, Isoparorchidae, Opisthorchidae and Troglotrematidae are of medical interest. [see prec.]

distomatosis, distomia (**dis**·to·mat·**o**′·sis, dis·**to**·me·ah). 1. The congenital state of having 2 mouths. 2. Distomiasis. [Gk *di-*, *stoma* mouth, *-osis* condition.]

distomiasis (dis·to·**mi**·as·is). Any infection by trematodes or flukes: the term is now obsolete since the worms formerly in the genus *Distoma* are now correctly placed in other genera. The term still survives in medical textbooks, with many qualifying adjectives. **Haemic distomiasis.** Schistosomiasis. **Hepatic distomiasis.** Infection by *Fasciola hepatica*, *Clonorchis sinensis*, and other trematodes. **Intestinal distomiasis.** Infection by *Fasciolopsis buskii* and other trematodes. **Pulmonary distomiasis.** Caused by one fluke only, *Paragonimus westermani*. [Gk *di-*, *stoma* mouth.]

distomum (**dis**·to·mum). Distoma.

distomus (dis·**to**·mus). Double-mouthed monster. [Gk *di-*, *stoma* mouth.]

disto-occlusal (**dis**·to·ok·**loo**′·zal). Relating to the distal and occlusal surfaces of a tooth.

disto-occlusion (**dis**·to·ok·**loo**′·zhun). A condition in which the lower teeth meet the upper teeth in a position behind that which they should normally occupy. [distal, L *occludere* to shut.]

distoplacement (dis·to·**plase**·ment). In dentistry, the displacement of a tooth in a distal direction.

distortion (dis·**tor**·shun). 1. A twisting or bending out of normal shape or position; a deformity. 2. In ophthalmology, irregular alteration in the shape of objects seen due to astigmatism of the cornea or crystalline lens, or to changes in the retina. 3. In psycho-analysis, the change undergone by an unconscious idea in passing the censor to emerge in the conscious mind. [L *distorquere* to twist.]

distortor oris (dis·**tor**·tor **or**·is). The zygomaticus minor muscle. [L distorter of mouth.]

distractibility (dis·**trak**·tib·**il**′·it·e). A state of mental confusion in which the attention cannot remain concentrated on any one thing but is easily made to waver from one thing to another. [L *distrahere* to draw asunder.]

distraction (dis·**trak**·shun). 1. Dislocation in which there is separation of the bones of a joint without displacement or rupture of ligaments. 2. A method of treating disease or fracture of a joint by applying extension and counter-extension so as to draw and hold apart the bones of the joint. 3. Separation of bone fragments in a fracture of a long bone, usually resulting from excessive traction. 4. Agitation of the mind so that the attention turns aside from the central theme or most important aspect of an experience to settle on a trivial aspect, or misses the main theme altogether by being divided up among all the aspects. 5. Directing attention away from a disease or disability. [see prec.]

distribution (dis·trib·**ew**·shun). 1. The branching of an artery or nerve on its way to the different organs and tissues it supplies. 2. The area supplied by the branches of an artery or nerve and the arrangement of the branches within it. 3. Presence or arrangement in different parts of the body, as of hair, fat, etc. **Adjacent distribution.** Of those orientation and distributions of the chromosomes, forming a ring or chain at the first meiotic division of translocation heterozygotes, which lead to migration of adjacent chromosomes to the same pole. Two types may be distinguished: *adjacent 1* where the adjacent chromosomes which migrate together have non-homologous centromeres, and *adjacent 2* where these chromosomes have homologous centromeres. **Alternate distribution.** Referring to the orientation and distribution of the chromosomes forming a ring or chain configuration at the first meiotic division of translocation heterozygotes which leads to the migration of alternate chromosomes to the same pole. **Frequency distribution.** A table or histogram showing the numbers, or proportions, of individuals occurring in each of a series of defined classes. [L *distribuere* to allot.]

See also: FERMI (E.).

districhiasis (dis·trik·**i**·as·is). The condition in which 2 hairs grow from the same follicle. [Gk *dis-*, *thrix* hair.]

distrix (**dis**·trix). An affection in which the hairs split at the ends. [see prec.]

disturbance (dis·**ter**·bans). Interruption of continuity. **Time-zone disturbance.** Flights parallel to the equator (travelling "with the sun or against it") lengthen or shorten the day or night of the journey, depending on the number of time zones crossed; this may distort passengers' sleep and circadian rhythms, causing temporary malaise. [ME *destorben.*]

disubstituted (di·**sub**·stit·ew·ted). Term denoting a compound formed by the replacement of 2 of the atoms or radicals of another compound by different atoms or radicals. [Gk *di-*, L *substituere* to substitute.]

Disulfiram (di·**sul**·fir·am). BP Commission approved name for tetraethylthiuram disulphide, used in the treatment of alcoholism. Administration of the drug causes no untoward symptoms unless alcohol is subsequently taken, when extreme nausea, vomiting and collapse occur. Such substances should only be used under the strictest medical supervision, as death has been known to result from the treatment.

Disulphamide (di·**sulf**·am·ide). BP Commission approved name for 5-chloro-2,4-disulphamoyltoluene; a diuretic.

disulphanilamide (di·sul·fan·**il**'·am·ide). Sulphanilyl sulphanilamide, $NH_2C_6H_4SO_2NHC_6H_4SO_2NH_2$. A bactericidal compound.

disulphate (di·**sul**·fate). 1. Bisulphate. One of a series of acid sulphates of general formula $MHSO_4$, where M is a monovalent metal. 2. Also applied to a pyrosulphate of general formula $M_2S_2O_7$.

disulphide (di·**sul**·fide). 1. Bisulphide. A binary compound of 2 atoms of sulphur combined with 1 atom of another element. 2. Any organic compound containing 2 linked atoms of sulphur. -S=S-.

disulpho- (di·**sul**·fo). A prefix indicating the presence in an organic compound of 2 sulphur atoms.

disvitaminosis (**dis**·vi·tam·in·**o**'·sis). Avitaminosis. [L *dis-*, vitaminosis.]

disvolution (dis·vol·**ew**·shun). 1. Degeneration. 2. Catabolism. 3. Involution. [L *dis-*, *volvere* to roll.]

dita bark (**de**·tah bark). Alstonia, Australian fever bark; the dried bark of *Alstonia solidans* and of *Alstonia constricta* (family Apocynaceae). It contains the alkaloids echitenine, echitamine, alstonine, porphyrine, etc., and is used in the Far East in the treatment of diarrhoea and as a tonic in cases of malaria.

Dithiazanine (di·thi·**az**·an·een). BP Commission approved name for 3,3'-diethylthiadicarbocyanine; an anthelminthic.

dithio- (di·**thi**·o). 1. A prefix denoting the presence in a compound of 2 sulphur atoms, usually linked together. 2. Name given to the linkage -S=S- [Gk *di-*, *theion* brimstone.]

Dithranol BP 1973 (**dith**·ran·ol). Dioxyanthranol, 1,8-dihydroxyanthranol, $C_{14}H_{10}O_3$. A synthetic substance like chrysarobin in action used for the treatment of fungal infections of the skin, e.g. ringworm, usually in the form of an ointment.

ditokus (**dit**·o·kus). Biological term meaning giving birth to twins or laying 2 eggs at one time. [Gk *di-*, *tokos* birth.]

Ditophal BP 1963 (**di**·to·fal). Diethyl dithiolisophthalate; it is used in the treatment of leprosy.

Dittel, Leopold von (b. 1815). Vienna surgeon.

Dittel's operation. An operation for transvesical enucleation of the lateral lobes of an enlarged prostate (1885).

Dittrich, Franz (b. 1815). Prague physician.

Dittrich's plugs. Small yellow bodies composed of compact secretion, with a very offensive smell in the sputum, in suppurative bronchitis.

Dittrich's stenosis. Stenosis of the conus arteriosus or primitive outflow tract of the heart in early fetal life. Failure of the conus to develop correctly after it has become differentiated into the outflow tract or infundibulum of the right ventricle results in infundibular pulmonary stenosis, sometimes with involvement of the pulmonary valve.

Buhl-Dittrich law. The presence of acute miliary tuberculosis always has as an antecedent a caseous focus somewhere in the body.

diurate (di·**ewr**·ate). Biurate. An acid urate; a salt of uric acid in which one of the replaceable hydrogen atoms has been exchanged for a metallic atom or basic group.

diureide (di·**ewr**·e·ide). Any one of a class of cyclic ureides formed from 2 molecules of urea, e.g. uric acid. They contain 2 -CONHCO- groups.

diuresis (di·ewr·**e**·sis). The excretion of urine; usually denoting an excessive quantity. **Alcohol diuresis.** Diuresis resulting from inhibition of release of antidiuretic hormone from the posterior pituitary gland. **Osmotic diuresis.** Diuresis due to a high concentration of osmotically-active substances in the renal tubules preventing reabsorption of water. **Tubular diuresis.** Diuresis caused by the presence in the renal tubules of dissolved substances exerting an osmotic pressure which counterbalances forces tending to reabsorption, so that the water is retained in the tubules. [Gk *dia*, *ourein* to urinate.]

diuretic (di·ewr·**et**·ik). 1. Producing an increase in the amount of urine. 2. Any substance which increases the volume of the urine. The effect may be achieved by increasing the flow of blood through the kidneys, by stimulating more glomeruli to action, by inhibiting reabsorption in the tubules or by augmenting the concentration of non-threshold substances in the blood. **Acidifying diuretic.** A drug which promotes an increased formation of urine by producing a degree of acidosis. The kidney excretes the excess acid together with some fixed base and extra water. Ammonium chloride is an example. **Alkaline diuretic.** Any salt of potassium, such as the acetate, bicarbonate or citrate; the potassium ion is not retained by the kidney and these salts cause diuresis whilst rendering the urine alkaline. **Cardiac diuretic.** Any of the digitalis glycosides used to treat congestive heart failure and improve the circulation; they increase the blood flow through the kidney. **Mercury diuretic.** Any compound of mercury that is irritant to the kidney, and to the tubules, thereby inhibiting reabsorption. The organic compounds are less likely to cause nephritis than the inorganic; they are given either intramuscularly or intravenously. The treatment of oedema due to renal disease with mercury diuretics is not to be recommended, as they may increase the damage to the kidney. **Osmotic diuretic.** A drug which increases the amount of urine formed by virtue of being itself excreted in the urine and by its osmotic action diminishing tabular reabsorption of water. Urea is an example. **Purine diuretic.** The purines, caffeine, theophylline and theobromine; theophylline is the one most used, having a more powerful diuretic effect than theobromine and less influence on the central nervous system than caffeine. **Saline diuretic.** Any neutral salt that has a low renal threshold and therefore acts as a diuretic; given by mouth in weak solution the volume of liquid may be greater than the diuresis produced, whilst if the concentration is increased, it may cause vomiting. **Volatile-oil diuretic.** A volatile oil or oleoresin used at one time to produce diuresis by reason of its irritant action on the tubules; it thus inhibited reabsorption. Volatile oils also have an antiseptic action in the urinary tract. [see prec.]

diuria (di·ewr·e·ah). Frequency of micturition during the daytime. [L *dies* day, urine.]

diurnal (di·**er**·nal). 1. Occurring during the day. 2. Recurring every day. [L *diurnalis* of a day.]

divagation (di·vag·a·shun). Incoherence of mind or speech. [L *divagari* to wander about.]

divalent (di·va·lent). Bivalent. [Gk *di-*, L *valentia* strength.]

divaricatio palpebrarum (di·var·e·ka'·she·o pal·pe·**bra**·rum). Ectropion. [L stretching of the eyelids.]

divarication (di·var·e·**ka**'·shun). 1. Separation or stretching. 2. Diastasis. [L *divaricare* to stretch apart.]

divaricator (di·**var**·ik·a·tor). A splint for reducing and maintaining reduction of a congenital dislocation of the hip. [see prec.]

divergence (di·**ver**·jens). 1. Separation, and progression in different directions. 2. In ophthalmology, binocular abduction of the eyes from the midline. It is said to be comitant when the angle between the visual axes does not change with alteration in direction of gaze, and non-comitant, usually due to paralysis or paresis of one or more extra-ocular muscles, when the angle varies with alteration in direction of gaze. [L *di-*, *vergere* to incline.]

divergent (di·ver·jent). 1. Radiating. 2. Tending to move apart. 3. Differing from type. [see prec.]

diverticular (di·ver·tik·ew·lar). 1. Resembling a diverticulum. 2. Relating or belonging to a diverticulum.

diverticularization (di·ver·tik·ew·lar·i·za′·shun). The forming of sacs or diverticula while development is in progress.

diverticulectomy (di·ver·tik·ew·lek′·to·me). Surgical removal of a diverticulum. [diverticulum, Gk *ektome* a cutting out.]

diverticuleve (di·ver·tik·ew·leev). A surgical instrument with which a diverticulum of the bladder can be raised up so that the underlying portion of the bladder wall may be divided off. [diverticulum, L *levare* to lift.]

diverticulitis (di·ver·tik·ew·li′·tis). A condition of inflammation of a diverticulum or diverticula in the colon which may lead to colic and constipation, and eventually to intestinal obstruction or to abscess and fistula formation. [diverticulum, Gk *-itis* inflammation.]

See also: MECKEL.

diverticulogram (di·ver·tik·ew·lo·gram). A skiagram of a diverticulum. [diverticulum, Gk *gramma* a writing.]

diverticulopexy (di·ver·tik·ew·lo·pex′·e). A method of surgical treatment of pharyngeal pouch (pharyngeal diverticulum) by fixing it upside down in the neck. [diverticulum, Gk *pexis* a fixation.]

diverticulosis (di·ver·tik·ew·lo′·sis). The presence of diverticula in the colon, without complicating inflammation or any symptoms. Their presence can usually be detected by x-ray examination after an opaque meal, and the condition is a relatively common one. Only about 15 per cent of subjects with diverticulosis eventually develop diverticulitis. [diverticulum, Gk *-osis* condition.]

diverticulum (di·ver·tik·ew·lum). A pouch or cul-de-sac of a hollow organ. **Allanto-enteric diverticulum.** An entodermal outgrowth from the yolk sac into the mesenchyme of the body stalk which represents the allantois in the human embryo. **Diverticula of the ampulla of the ductus deferens [diverticula ampullae (NA)].** Outpockets between the folds of mucous membrane in the ampulla of the ductus deferens. **Bladder diverticulum.** Vesical diverticulum (see below). **Calyceal diverticulum.** Pyelogenic renal cyst. **Cervical diverticulum.** Diverticulum in the neck, derived from the cervical pouch. **Congenital diverticulum.** Diverticulum at birth, usually of the oesophagus or intestine. **Epiphrenic diverticulum.** Pulsion diverticulum of the oesophagus at the lower end of the oesophagus associated with achalasia cardia. **False diverticulum.** A protrusion of mucous membrane through a defect in the muscular coat of a hollow organ. **Ganglion diverticulum.** Hernial protrusion of synovial membrane. **Gastric diverticulum.** A small pouch of the stomach, usually near the pyloric end, sometimes found in connection with a peptic ulcer. **Hepatic diverticulum.** An entodermal outgrowth from the junction of the foregut and mid-gut of the embryo which gives rise to the epithelial elements of the liver and biliary passages. **Diverticulum ilei verum.** Meckel's diverticulum: a small pouch, comparable in size with the vermiform appendix, which projects from the ileum about 1 m from the ileocolic junction in about 2 per cent of people; it is a persistent part of the embryonic connection between the gut and the yolk sac (vitellointestinal duct). **Intestinal diverticulum.** A diverticulum of the intestine. **Laryngeal diverticulum.** An extension of the laryngeal ventricle; it is known in its gross form as a laryngocele. **Oesophageal diverticulum.** A local sacculation (pouch) in some part of the oesophagus, caused by a developmental defect, by traction on the wall from without or pressure from within (pulsion diverticulum). When due to traction, it is found anteriorly in the middle third, and is caused by adhesions between tuberculous glands at the bifurcation of the trachea and the oesophageal wall. **Pancreatic diverticulum.** One of 2 entodermal outgrowths from the junction of the foregut and mid-gut of the embryo which give rise to the glandular and epithelial elements of the pancreas. **Pharyngeal diverticulum** Pulsion diverticulum (see below) of the pharynx. **Pineal diverticulum.** The outgrowth from the caudal part of the roof of the 3rd ventricle of the embryo from which the pineal gland is developed. **Pituitary diverticulum.** Term which may be applied to the outgrowth from the floor of the 3rd ventricle of the brain which forms the posterior lobe of the pituitary, or to the ectodermal pouch (Rathke's pouch) from which the anterior lobe, pars intermedia hypophyseos, and the pars tuberalis hypophyseos are formed. **Pulsion diverticulum.** A diverticulum produced by an outward bulging of a hollow organ in response to an increase of pressure in it. **Diverticulum of the small intestine.** A diverticulum most commonly in the duodenum (usually single) and jejunum (often multiple); it may cause malabsorption symptoms. **Synovial diverticulum.** A protrusion of the synovial membrane of a joint or tendon sheath through its fibrous covering. **Thyroid diverticulum.** An entodermal outgrowth from the floor of the embryonic pharynx in the midline at the level of the first branchial arch: it gives rise to the thyroglossal duct and part, if not all, of the glandular elements of the adult thyroid gland. **Traction diverticulum.** A bulge and diverticulum produced in a hollow organ by the pull of an adhesion outside it. **True diverticulum.** A diverticulum whose wall includes all layers of the wall of the hollow organ through which it arises. **Ureteral diverticulum.** A congenital anomaly which occurs as a sharply demarcated extra-ureteral sac that communicates with the lumen of the ureter. **Vesical diverticulum.** A pouch lined with mucous membrane that protrudes through the muscular coat of the bladder. It is a disease of old age. [L *diverticulare* to turn aside.]

See also: EUSTACHIO, HAUDEK, HEISTER, KIRCHNER, MECKEL, NUCK, PERTIK, ROKITANSKY, VATER, ZENKER (F. A.).

divicine (di·vi·seen). $C_4H_6N_4O_2$, a toxic pyrimidine base; it has been recovered from the vetch, *Vicia sativa*, a contaminant of the crops of *Lathyrus sativa*, and thought possibly to be an aetiological factor in lathyrism.

divinyl (di·vi·nil). Denoting a compound which contains 2 vinyl $-CH{=}CH_2$, groups. **Divinyl ether.** Vinyl Ether BP 1958, $(CH_2{=}CH)_2O$. A highly inflammable liquid used as an inhalation anaesthetic for short-term anaesthesia. It is more potent than ether, with a smoother and more rapid induction, and can be given by the open-drop method or by gas and air machine. It is liable to cause hepatic injury, but is not as toxic as chloroform. Especially valuable for short operations or prior to the administration of ethyl ether.

division (div·izh·un). 1. The separation of anything into a number of parts; in mathematics the several parts are equal. 2. A limiting boundary or partition. 3. In the classification of plants, a group of classes, equivalent to the phylum in animals. **Cell division.** The division of a cell into 2 daughter cells, characterized by peculiar changes in the nucleus and cytoplasm of which rounding of the cell, loss of the nuclear membrane, disappearance of the nucleolus, appearance of the achromatic spindle, visualization and movement of the chromosomes, and constriction of the cell at its middle are outstanding events. *See* AMITOSIS, MEIOSIS, MITOSIS. **Equational division, Equatorial division.** Cell division (see preceding) in which individual chromosomes divide longitudinally and are distributed to identically constituted daughter nuclei. In meiosis, i.e. the maturation divisions of the germ cell, equational division follows reduction division. **Heterotypical cell division.** The first or reduction division of meiosis. **Reduction division.** Cell division in which homologous chromosomes pair and later separate, so that daughter cells have only one-half the normal number of chromosomes. This type of division occurs in the maturation of the germ cells. [L *dividere* to divide.]

divulse (di·**vuls**). To rend or pluck away with force. [L *divellere* to rend.]

divulsion (di·**vul**·shun). The act of rending or forcibly pulling asunder. [see prec.]

divulsor (di·**vul**·sor). An instrument with which forcible dilatation of a canal or cavity can be performed. [L *divellere* to rend.]

dizygotic (di·zi·**got**·ik). 1. Referring to a double birth, 2 cells having been fertilized, and therefore 2 zygotes produced. 2. Fraternal. [Gk *di-*, *zygotos* yolked together.]

dizziness (**diz**·e·nes). Colloquially used to describe any sensation of imbalance or of a lack of stable relationship with the immediate environment. [ME *dusi* foolish.]

djenkol (**jen**·kol). Jenkol: a poisoning caused by the eating of a bean *Pithecolobium lobatum.* Sharp crystals of jenkolic acid are precipitated in the kidney, and cause a train of urinary symptoms often ending in anuria. [Indonesian name.]

Dobell, Horace Benge (b. 1828). London physician.

Dobell's solution. A solution of borax, sodium bicarbonate, phenol and glycerin in water, used as an antiseptic.

Dobie, William Murray (b. 1828). Chester physician.

Dobie's globule, or line. Krause's line.

Dobie's layer. Krause's membrane.

Dobutamine (do·**bewt**·am·een). BP Commission approved name for (±)-4-[2-(3-*p*-hydroxyphenyl-1-methylpropylamino)ethyl]-pyrocatechol; a cardiac stimulant.

Dochez, Alphonse Raymond (b. 1882). New York bacteriologist.

Dochez' serum. Dick's serum; scarlet-fever antitoxin; haemolytic streptococcus antitoxin: antitoxin prepared by immunizing horses against scarlet-fever toxin. It alleviates toxic symptoms, and is therefore useful in treatment.

Dochez-Avery reaction. Typing of the causal pneumococcus by precipitin test on the patient's urine, using the type-specific antisera.

dochogram (**do**·ko·gram). Contrast radiography of a duct. [Gk *dochos* containing, *gramma* record.]

docimasia (dos·e·**ma**·ze·ah). 1. An analysis or assay. 2. An examination. 3. An official test. **Auricular docimasia.** Wreden's sign. **Hepatic docimasia.** The process of examining the liver for signs of the presence of glycogen or glucose. **Pulmonary docimasia.** The examination of the lungs of a dead infant in order to ascertain whether or not it was alive when born. [Gk *dok mazein* to assay.]

docimastic (dos·e·**mas**·tik). 1. Referring to docimasia. 2. Using tests or assays. 3. Proving by experiment or test. [see prec.]

doctor (**dok**·ter). 1. A person of learning, or a teacher. 2. The recipient of the highest degree in a faculty of a university. 3. The holder of the degree of doctor of medicine (MD or DM) from a university, but also used generally to describe any qualified medical practitioner. 4. A magician or medicine man of a savage tribe. 5. To apply remedies; the treatment of patients by a physician. 6. Colloquially, to tamper with or falsify. [L teacher.]

doctrine (**dok**·trin). A system of principles. [L *docere* to teach.]

See also: ARRHENIUS, MALTHUS, RASORI.

Dodds, Sir Edward Charles (b. 1900). London biochemist.

Dodds' nipples. The black pigmentation of the nipples which results from the administration of stilboestrol but no other oestrogen.

dodecadactylitis (do·dek·ah·dak·til·i′·tis). Duodenitis. [Gk *dodeka* twelve, *daktylos* finger (with regard to length of the duodenum), *-itis* inflammation.]

dodecadactylon (do·dek·ah·**dak**′·til·on). The duodenum. [see prec.]

Dodecyl Gallate BP 1973 (do·**dek**·il **gal**·ate). Dodecyl 3,4,5-trihydroxybenzoate; an anti-oxidant used for preserving oils and fats.

Dodicin (**do**·di·sin). BP Commission approved name for 3,6,9-triazadocosanoic acid; a surface-active agent.

Doederlein, Albert Siegmund Gustav (b. 1860). Leipzig and Munich gynaecologist.

Doederlein's bacillus. The predominant organism in the healthy vagina during the reproductive period.

Doehle, Karl Gottfried Paul (b. 1855). Kiel pathologist.

Doehle bodies. Precipitated nucleoprotein inclusions in neutrophil leucocytes, found in severe infections and in the May-Hegglin anomaly.

Doehle disease, Heller-Doehle aortitis, or disease. Syphilitic aortitis.

Doellinger, Johann Ignaz Josef (b. 1770). Würzburg and Munich physiologist.

Doellinger's tendinous ring. A thickening of the posterior elastic lamina of the cornea.

Doerfler-Stewart test. In cases of simulated deafness: the patient's hearing for speech is tested in a background of masking noise. In malingerers, the adopted subjective reference level is disturbed, and on repeat testing their responses are found to be variable.

Doering, Hans (b. 1871). German physician.

Neisser-Doering phenomenon. A phenomenon noted when an antihaemolytic substance is present in the blood capable of preventing the normal haemolysis of the red blood corpuscles.

Dofamium Chloride (do·**fam**·e·um **klor**·ide). BP Commission approved name for 2-(*N*-dodecanoyl-*N*-methylamino)ethyldimethyl-(phenylcarbamoylmethyl)ammonium chloride; an antiseptic.

dog rose (dog roze). *Rosa canina* Linn. (family Rosaceae) the fruits of which, and of other British species of wild rose, constitute Rose Fruit BPC 1954 (hips). The latter is used as a natural source of vitamin C in the form of a syrup standardized to contain 2 mg ascorbic acid per ml. **Dog rose fruits.** Rose Fruit BPC 1954. [OFr. *docga* dog, L *rosa* rose.]

Dogiel, Jan (b. 1830). St. Petersburg and Kasan anatomist and physiologist.

Dogiel's cell. Either of 2 types of nerve cell found in autonomic ganglia, particularly in the wall of the intestinal canal. One type represents a parasympathetic postganglionic neuron, the other an associational neurone synapsing with a number of cells of the first type.

Dogiel's corpuscle, end-bulb, or nerve-ending. A type of bulbous sensory end-organ present in the oronasal mucous membrane and the skin of the genitalia.

dogma (**dog**·mah). A doctrinal system laid down by authority. In molecular biology, the **Central dogma,** laid down by F. H. C. Crick, states that genetic information flows from nucleic acids to protein but never in the reverse direction. [Gk a thinking.]

dogmatists (**dog**·mat·ists). The first of the schools of medicine which came into being after the time of Hippocrates; they introduced speculative theory which soon became crystallized in formal doctrine. Aetiology, hygiene, physiology, symptomatology and therapeutics comprised the entire medical science of the Dogmatists. [Gk *dogma* a thinking.]

dogwood (**dog**·wud) The flowering dogwood, *Cornus florida.* **Jamaica dogwood.** Piscidia: the root bark of *Piscidia erythrina* Linn. (family Leguminosae) used in the form of a liquid extract as an analgesic and sedative. [OFr. *docga* dog, AS *wudu.*]

Doisy, Edward Adelbert (b. 1893). St. Louis biochemist (Nobel prizewinner, 1943).

Allen-Doisy test. A test for estimating the oestrogenic content of a body fluid by determining its effect on the vaginal epithelium after injection into mice.

Thayer-Doisy unit. Mouse unit. *See* UNIT.

dolabrate, dolabriform (do·**lab**·rate, do·**lab**·re·form). Shaped like an axe or hatchet. [Gk *dolabra* hatchet (from the shape of the folds), form.]

Dolage's disease. Dystrophia myotonica.

Dolbeau, Henri Ferdinand (b. 1830). Paris surgeon.

Dolbeau's operation. An operation for lithotomy in which a median incision was made in the urethra, the stone being crushed in the bladder with a lithotrite, followed by evacuation of debris.

dolichocephalia (**dol**·ik·o·kef·**a'**·le·ah). Dolichocephalism.

dolichocephalic (**dol**·ik·o·kef·**al'**·ik). In craniometry, having the transverse diameter of the head less than 75 per cent of the anteroposterior diameter, i.e. a cephalic index below 75. [see foll.]

dolichocephalism (**dol**·ik·o·**kef'**·al·izm). The state of having a relatively long skull. [Gk *dolichos* long, *kephale* head.]

dolichocephalous (**dol**·ik·o·**kef'**·al·us). Dolichocephalic.

dolichocephalus (**dol**·ik·o·**kef'**·al·us). A skull with a relatively long cephalic diameter. **Dolichocephalus simplex.** Dolichocephalus occurring as the result of synostosis of the sagittal suture. [Gk *dolichos* long, *kephale* head.]

dolichocephaly (**dol**·ik·o·**kef'**·al·e). Dolichocephalism.

dolichochamaecephalus (**dol**·ik·o·kam·e·**kef'**·al·us). A skull formation which is chamaecephalic as well as dolicephalic, or an individual having such a skull. [Gk *dolichos* long, *chamai* low, *kephale* head.]

dolichochamaecranial (**dol**·ik·o·kam·e·**kra'**·ne·al). With a long flat skull. [Gk *dolichos* long, *chamai* low, *kranion* skull.]

dolichocnemic (**dol**·ik·o·**ne'**·mik). Indicating that the length of the leg below the knee is almost equal to the length of the thigh. [Gk *dolichos* long, *kneme* leg.]

dolichocolon (**dol**·ik·o·**ko'**·lon). An abnormally long colon of normal diameter. [Gk *dolichos* long, colon.]

dolichocranial (**dol**·ik·o·**kra'**·ne·al). Dolichocephalic. [Gk *dolichos* long, *kranion* skull.]

dolichoderus (**dol**·e·ko·**de'**·rus). An individual who has a long neck. [Gk *dolichos* long, *dere* neck.]

dolichoeuromesocephalus (**dol**·ik·o·**ewr**·o·me·zo·**kef'**·al·us). An individual with a long skull broad in the temporal region. [Gk *dolichos* long, *eurys* wide, *mesos* middle, *kephale* head.]

dolichoeuro-opisthocephalus (**dol**·ik·o·**ewr**·o·o·pis·tho·**kef'**·al·us). An individual with a long skull broad in the occipital region. [Gk *dolichos* long, *eurys* wide, *opisthe* behind, *kephale* head.]

dolichoeuroprocephalus (**dol**·ik·o·**ewr**·o·pro·**kef'**·al·us). An individual with a long head broad in the frontal region. [Gk *dolichos* long, *eurys* wide, *pro* before, *kephale* head.]

dolichofacial (**dol**·ik·o·**fa'**·she·al). Having a relatively or abnormally long face. [Gk *dolichos* long, L *facies* face.]

dolichogastry (**dol**·ik·o·**gas'**·tre). Gastroptosis; the centre of the stomach is lengthened by stretching. [Gk *dolichos* long, *gaster* stomach.]

dolichohieric (**dol**·ik·o·hi·**er'**·ik). Referring to or having a relatively long sacrum. [Gk *dolichos* long, *hieron* sacrum.]

dolichokerkic (**dol**·ik·o·**ker'**·kik). Referring to a scapula of which the angle formed by the crest of the scapular spine and the vertebral border is over 80°. [Gk *dolichos* long, *kerkis* shuttle.]

dolichoknemic (**dol**·ik·o·**ne'**·mik). Dolichocnemic.

dolicholeptocephalus (**dol**·ik·o·lep·to·**kef'**·al·us). An individual with a skull that is abnormal in length, height and narrowness. [Gk *dolichos* long, *leptos* thin, *kephale* head.]

dolichomorphic (**dol**·ik·o·**mor'**·fik). Referring to a slight and long type of bodily build. [Gk *dolichos* long, *morphe* shape.]

dolichopellic, dolichopelvic (**dol**·ik·o·**pel'**·ik, **dol**·ik·o·**pel'**·vik). Referring to a person whose pelvis is of abnormal length. [Gk *dolichos* long, *pellis* bowl, pelvis.]

dolichoplatycephalus (**dol**·ik·o·plat·e·**kef'**·al·us). An individual with a long and flat skull. [Gk *dolichos* long, platycephaly.]

dolichoprosopic (**dol**·ik·o·pro·**so'**·pik). Dolichofacial. [Gk *dolichos* long, *prosopon* face.]

dolichorrhine (**dol**·ik·or·ine). Long-nosed. [Gk *dolichos* long, *rhis* nose.]

Dolichos (**dol**·ik·os). A genus of tropical plants of the pea family, characterized by stinging hairs on their seed pods. **Dolichos bifloris.** In blood group serology a source of anti-$A_1(\alpha_1)$ antibody. **Dolichos pruriens, Dolichos pubes.** Mucuna. [Gk long.]

dolichosigmoid (**dol**·ik·o·**sig'**·moid). An abnormally long loop of the pelvic colon. [Gk *dolichos* long, *sigma* Gk letter s.]

dolichostenomelia (**dol**·ik·o·sten·o·**me'**·le·ah). Arachnodactyly. [Gk *dolichos* long, *stenos* narrow, *melos* limb.]

dolichouranic, dolichuranic (**dol**·ik·o·ewr·**an'**·ik, **do**·lik·ewr·**an'**·ik). Referring to a long alveolar arch of the maxilla. [Gk *dolichos* long, *ouranos* palate.]

Dollo, Louis (b. 1857). Brussels zoologist.

Dollo's law. Organs or structures once lost during evolution cannot be regained.

dolor (**do**·lor) (pl. *dolores*). Physical pain; mental anguish; painful heat. Cf. ARDOR, CALOR, FERVOR. **Dolor capitis.** Pain in the head, particularly that caused by changes in bones or scalp. **Dolores vagi.** Wandering pains. [L pain.]

dolorific (do·lor·**if**·ik). Causing physical pain or mental anguish. [L *dolor* pain, *facere* to make.]

dolorimeter (do·lor·**im**·et·er). A device for the measurement of pain. [see foll.]

dolorimetry (do·lor·**im**·et·re). The measuring of pain. [L *dolor* pain, Gk *metron* measure.]

dolorogenic (**do**·lor·o·**jen'**·ik). Producing pain, e.g. certain kinds of stimulation. [L *dolor* pain, Gk *genein* to produce.]

dolorosus (do·lor·o·sus). Term indicating that pain is the outstanding symptom and its intensity is such that the pain is almost unbearable. [L *dolor* pain.]

domatophobia (**do**·mat·o·**fo'**·be·ah). Pathological fear of being inside a house. [L *domus* house, phobia.]

dominance (**dom**·in·ans). The property of a character or gene being dominant. **Cerebral dominance, Hemispherical dominance.** The normal state in which the function of speech, for example, is located in one cerebral hemisphere (the left in right-handed subjects): this is then referred to as the dominant hemisphere. **Ocular dominance.** The condition in which one eye is relied on, and used more than its fellow; almost universally present to a greater or lesser degree. **One-sided dominance.** One-handedness; this can usually be correlated with cerebral dominance (see above). [L *dominari* to rule.]

dominant (**dom**·in·ant). In genetics, a gene which will produce the same effects when it is present in hetero- or homozygote. In the heterozygous condition the potential effects of the other allelomorph are entirely absent, such a gene being known as a recessive. [L *dominans* ruling.]

Dominici, Henri (b. 1867). Paris radiologist and haematologist.

Dominici's tube. A silver radium container to filter α and β rays so as to make use of γ rays only.

Domiphen Bromide BP 1973 (**dom**·if·en **bro**·mide). Dodecyldimethyl-2-phenoxyethylammonium bromide, an antiseptic employed, usually in the form of tablets, for sore throat and oral infections.

Donahue's syndrome. *See* LEPRECHAUNISM.

Donald, Archibald (b. 1860). Manchester gynaecologist.

Donald's operation. The original Manchester operation for repair of uterovaginal prolapse. Donald first performed the operation in 1888 and combined amputation of the cervix with anterior and posterior colporrhaphy.

Donaldson, Robert (b. 1877). London pathologist.

Donaldson's stain. A stain for protozoal cysts, especially amoebae, in faeces: a saturated solution of iodine in 5 per cent potassium iodide to which is added an equal amount of saturated solution of eosin in normal saline. The cysts take the iodine stain and stand out against a pink background. The chief limitation of the method is that it does not stain the chromidial bars in the *Entamoeba histolytica* cysts.

Donaldson's broach. In dentistry, a barbed broach; a broach with fine barbs, used for removing the contents of a root canal.

Donath, Julius (b. 1870). Vienna physician.

Donath phenomenon, Donath-Landsteiner phenomenon. When blood taken from a patient with paroxysmal haemoglobinuria is cooled to 5°C, a cold haemolysin in the plasma combines with the red blood cells; when the temperature is allowed to rise, the sensitized red cells are then haemolysed by the complement normally present in the blood.

donatism (don·at·izm). A form of hypnotic trance in which imitation plays a predominant part. It is named after Donato, the stage name of Alfred d'Hont, 1845-1900, a Belgian hypnotist.

donator (do·na·tor). A compound which parts with a portion of itself to another compound in a reaction. **Hydrogen donator.** In a reaction, the compound which gives hydrogen to the acceptor. **Oxygen donator.** A substance which gives up oxygen to an acceptor in an oxidizing reaction. [L *donare* to give.]

donda ndugu (don·da ndoo·goo). A disease often encountered in the coastal regions of East Africa. It attacks the legs particularly, which become inflamed and oedematous, the affected skin later sloughing off. The causal organism abounds in stagnant water. [African name.]

Donders, Frans Cornelis (b. 1818). Utrecht physician and ophthalmologist.

Donders' curve. A curve showing the gradual diminution of accommodation with age.

Donders' law. Every oblique position of the eyeball is associated with a constant amount of torsional movement. For any determinate position of the line of fixation of the eyes with respect to the head, there corresponds a definite and invariable angle of torsion, independent of the volition of the observer and independent of the manner in which the line of fixation has been brought into the position in question.

Donders' hair optometer. An instrument for measuring the near point of accommodation: a number of fine hairs on a white background are brought up to the eye until they blur and cannot be differentiated.

Donders' pressure. An increase of intratracheal pressure as recorded by a manometer when the chest of a dead body is opened. It is due to collapse of the lungs.

Donnan, Frederick George (b. 1870). English physical chemist.

Donnan effect or equilibrium. The effect occurring when there is an ion on one side of a membrane which cannot diffuse through the membrane. If there are 3 different ions, one of which is non-diffusable, the product of the concentrations of the diffusable ions on one side of the membrane will equal that on the other side. However, the sum on one side of the membrane of all types of anion is not equal to the sum of the cations on either side of the membrane, resulting in an electrical potential difference between the two sides.

Donné, Alfred (b. 1801). Paris physician.

Donné's body, or corpuscle. A colostrum corpuscle.

donor (do·nor). Anyone who voluntarily gives blood or parts of tissues for use in treatment of, or grafting on, another individual. **General donor.** Universal donor (see below). **Skin donor.** An individual from whom skin is taken for grafting on another individual. **Universal donor.** Term sometimes applied to blood donors belonging to group O because they have neither A nor B antigens on their red cells; they are ABO compatible with everyone. As recipients, only group O blood is compatible. [L *donare* to give.]

Donovan, Charles (b. 1863). Scottish physician formerly in the Indian Medical Service.

Donovan's body. An organism, probably a bacterium, found in large numbers in pathognomonic cells in ulcerating granuloma of the pudenda; granuloma venereum.

Leishman-Donovan body. The round or resting stage of the protozoon *Leishmania donovani*, the causal organism of kala-azar; this is the stage in which the parasites occur in the tissues of the vertebrate host. The term is also, not inappropriately, applied to the similar stage of other species of *Leishmania* which is morphologically identical, e.g. that of *Leishmania tropica*.

Donovan, Michael (b. 1760). Dublin apothecary.

Donovan's solution. An aqueous solution of the iodides of mercury and arsenic, used in venereal diseases.

donovania granulomatis (don·o·van·e·ah gran·ew·lo·mat·is). The name suggested by Goodpasture and his colleagues for the Donovan body, the causal organism of granuloma venereum.

dopa (do·pah). Dioxyphenylalanine.

Dopamine (do·pam·een). BP Commission approved name for 2-(3,4-dihydroxyphenyl)ethylamine; a sympathomimetic drug acting as a neurotransmitter and secreted by neurons situated in the ventral hypothalamus, amongst other places, and passing along axons to the medial eminence from which it releases into the hypophyseal portal system factors which have either an inhibitory or releasing effect. One of the dopamine agonists is bromocriptine.

dopa-oxidase (do·pah·ox·id·ase). An enzyme found in certain epithelial cells which activates the conversion of dopa (dioxyphenylalanine) into the pigment melanin. It is thought that lack of this enzyme is a contributing cause of albinism.

dopase (do·paze). Dopa-oxidase.

Doppler, Christian Johann (b. 1803). Austrian physicist and mathematician.

Doppler's effect, phenomenon or principle. The apparent frequency of a source of sound varies with the motion of the source, observer, and medium through which the sound is propagated. The variation is given by

$$n = n_s\left(\frac{V + w + v_o}{V + w - v_s}\right)$$

where w is the velocity of the medium in the direction of the motion of energy, v_o the velocity of the observer towards the source, v_s the velocity of the source towards the observer, V the velocity of energy in the medium and n_s the real frequency of the source.

Doppler principle flowmeter. An instrument designed to measure the velocity of blood-flow, using the Doppler principle, by directing a beam of ultrasound along the line of flow and detecting the change in frequency of the sound waves reflected from the moving red blood cells.

Doppler, Karl (b. 1887). Vienna surgeon.

Doppler's operation. Bisection of, or injection of phenol into the tissues around, the sympathetic nerve leading to the gonads with the object of increasing hormone production and producing sexual rejuvenation. Also called *sympathicodiaphtheresis*.

Dopter, Charles Henri Alfred (b. 1873). Paris physician.

Dopter's serum. A serum against the parameningococcus.

doraphobia (do·rah·fo·be·ah). A morbid fear of animal skin or fur or of touching it. [Gk *dora* hide, *phobein* to fear.]

Dorello, Primo (b. 1872). Perugia anatomist.

Dorello's canal. An occasional bony canal at the apex of the petrous part of the temporal bone, transmitting the abducent nerve.

Dorendorf, Hans (b. 1866). Berlin surgeon.

Dorendorf's sign. A pulsatile swelling in the supraclavicular fossa in cases of aneurysm of the arch of the aorta. Swelling and pulsation in the right supraclavicular fossa may denote an aneurysm of the innominate artery.

dormancy (dor·man·se). 1. The state of being dormant or in abeyance. 2. In bacteriology, that quality of some bacteria which consists in their remaining quiescent for a time before they start to multiply. [L *dormire* to sleep.]

dormoron (dor·mor·on). A lethargic mentally stupid individual whose general state is trance-like. [L *dormire* to sleep, Gk *moros* stupid.]

Dorner's method. For the demonstration of bacterial spores in wet unfixed mounts: the spores are stained red by basic fuchsine, and the unstained bacterial bodies are outlined against the dark background of nigrosin.

doromania (dor·o·ma·ne·ah). Pathological tendency to give presents. [Gk *doron* gift, mania.]

dorsal [dorsalis (NA)] (dor·sal). 1. Relating to the back. 2. Relating to a dorsum. 3. Situated on or near the back of a part or organ. [L *dorsalis* of the back.]

dorsales linguae veins [venae dorsales linguae (NA)] (dor·sa·leez ling·gwe). Veins draining the dorsum of the tongue; they are tributaries of the lingual vein which accompanies the lingual artery.

dorsalgia (dor·sal·je·ah). Pain in the back. [L *dorsum* back, Gk *algos* pain.]

dorsalis (dor·sa·lis). Dorsal; term descriptive of blood vessels, or nerves or muscles situated in or supplying the back or dorsum of a part or organ. [L of the back.]

dorsalis nasi artery [arteria dorsalis nasi (NA)] (dor·sa·lis na·zi). *See* OPHTHALMIC ARTERY.

dorsalis pedis artery [arteria dorsalis pedis (NA)] (dor·sa·lis **ped**·is). A continuation of the anterior tibial artery along the dorsum of the foot, ending by passing through the first intermetatarsal space to the sole to anastomose with the lateral plantar artery [ramus plantaris profundus (NA)].

Dorset, Marion (b. 1872). Washington bacteriologist.

Dorset's egg culture medium. A medium used for the stock culture of the tubercle bacillus and for the maintenance of stock cultures of other organisms: it is prepared from new-laid hen eggs and water, solidified by heat in the inspissator at 75°C.

dorsicolumn (dor·se·**kol**·um). The posterior white column of the spinal cord. [L *dorsum* back, column.]

dorsicommissure (dor·se·**kom**·is·ewr). The posterior grey commissure of the spinal cord (Wilder). [L *dorsum* back, commissure.]

dorsicornu (dor·se·**kor**·new). The posterior grey horn of the spinal cord. [L *dorsum* back, cornu.]

dorsicumbent (dor·se·**kum**·bent). Supine. [L *dorsum* back, *cumbere* to lie.]

dorsiduct (**dor**·se·dukt). To draw or turn backwards or towards the back. [L *dorsum* back, *ducere* to draw.]

dorsiflexion (dor·se·**flek**·shun). Backward flexion of the fingers or toes. [L *dorsum* back, flexion.]

dorsimesal (dor·se·**me**·zal). Situated along or on the median longitudinal line of the back. [L *dorsum* back, Gk *mesos* middle.]

dorsimeson (dor·se·**me**·zon). The median longitudinal line of the back. [see prec.]

dorsispinal (dor·se·**spi**·nal). Relating to the back and the vertebral column. [L *dorsum* back, spine.]

dorsiventral (dor·se·**ven**·tral). Dorso-abdominal. [L *dorsum* back, *venter* belly.]

dorso-abdominal (**dor**·so·ab·**dom**'·in·al). 1. Extending from the back to the abdomen. 2. Relating to the dorsal and abdominal regions. [L *dorsum* back, abdomen.]

dorso-anterior (**dor**·so·an·**teer**'·e·or). A term applied to the position of the fetus *in utero* when its back is towards the anterior wall of the mother's abdomen. [L *dorsum* back, anterior.]

dorsocervical (dor·so·**ser**·vik·al). Referring to the back and the neck. [L *dorsum* back, *cervix* neck.]

dorsocostal (dor·so·**kos**·tal). Referring to the back and the ribs. [L *dorsum* back, *costa* rib.]

dorsodynia (dor·so·**din**·e·ah). Dorsalgia; pain in the dorsal region of the back. [L *dorsum* back, Gk *odyne* pain.]

dorso-epitrochlearis muscle (**dor**·so·ep·e·trok·le·**ar**'·is musl). An occasional muscular slip running from the lower border of the tendon of the latissimus dorsi muscle to the long head of the triceps. It is constant in many animals. [L *dorsum* back, epitrochlea.]

dorso-intercostal (**dor**·so·in·ter·**kos**'·tal). Referring to the intercostal regions of the back. [L *dorsum* back, intercostal.]

dorso-interosseal, dorso-interosseous (**dor**·so·in·ter·**os**'·e·al, **dor**·so·in·ter·**os**'·e·us). 1. Situated on the back of the hand and between the metacarpal bones. 2. Situated on the dorsum of the foot and between the metatarsal bones. [L *dorsum* back, *inter*, *os* bone.]

dorsolateral (dor·so·**lat**·er·al). Relating to the dorsal aspect and either of the two sides. [L *dorsum* back, *latus* side.]

dorsolumbar (dor·so·**lum**·bar). Relating or belonging to the back and the lumbar region. [L *dorsum* back, *lumbus* loin.]

dorsomedian, dorsomesal (dor·so·**me**·de·an, dor·so·**me**·zal). Belonging to the median longitudinal line of the back. [L *dorsum* back, median.]

dorsonasal (dor·so·**na**·zal). Relating to the posterior part of the nose. [L *dorsum* back, nose.]

dorsonuchal (dor·so·**new**·kal). Relating to the back and the nape of the neck. [L *dorsum* back, Ar. *nukha* spinal cord.]

dorso-occipital (dor·so·ok·**sip**'·it·al). Relating to the back and the back of the head. [L *dorsum* back, occiput.]

dorsoposterior (**dor**·so·pos·**teer**'·e·or). A term applied to the position of the fetus *in utero* when its back is towards the mother's back. [L *dorsum* back, posterior.]

dorsoradial (dor·so·**ra**·de·al). Relating to or situated on the radial border and back of the forearm, hand or finger. [L *dorsum* back, radius.]

dorsosacral (dor·so·**sa**·kral). Referring to the back and the sacrum. [L *dorsum* back, sacrum.]

dorsoscapular (dor·so·**skap**·ew·lar). Relating or belonging to the dorsal surface of the scapula. [L *dorsum* back, scapula.]

dorsothoracic (**dor**·so·thor·**as**'·ik). Referring to the back and the thorax. [L *dorsum* back, thorax.]

dorso-ulnar (dor·so·**ul**·nar). Referring to the ulnar border and the back of the forearm, hand or finger. [L *dorsum* back, ulna.]

dorsoventral (dor·so·**ven**·tral). Dorso-abdominal. [L *dorsum* back, *venter* belly.]

dorsum [NA] (**dor**·sum). 1. The back. 2. Any part corresponding in position to the back, e.g. of the hand. **Dorsum of the foot [dorsum pedis (NA)].** The upper part of the foot. **Dorsum of the hand [dorsum manus (NA)].** The back of the hand. **Dorsum ilii.** The external part of the ilium. **Dorsum of the nose.** *See* NOSE. **Dorsum of the penis [dorsum penis (NA)].** *See* PENIS. **Dorsum sellae [NA].** The plate of bone which extends upward and forward behind the hypophyseal fossa of the sphenoid bone. **Dorsum of the tongue.** *See* TONGUE. [L back.]

Dorylaimata (dor·e·la·**ma**·tah). A sub-order of the nematode order Enoplata. The family Trichuridae is of medical interest.

dosage (**do**·sij). The gradation and regulation of doses. **Dosage compensation.** *See* COMPENSATION. **Electrical dosage.** The dosage applied to any form of electric current used therapeutically. **Dosage meter.** Dosemeter. [Gk *dosis* a giving.]

dose (dose). 1. The quantity of medicament to be administered to a patient, as directed by the physician. 2. In radiotherapy, a measure of the quantity of radiation energy absorbed at a point in tissue or other material. **Absorbed dose.** Of any ionizing radiation: the amount of energy imparted to matter by ionizing particles per unit mass of irradiated material at the place of interest. Expressed ideally in rads, but for x- and γ-rays of quantum energy up to 3 MeV, the roentgen (r) may be used. **Air dose.** A misnomer for the intensity of a beam of radiation. The intensity of radiation measured in air at the point of interest, in the absence of patient (or phantom) or other object, thus excluding secondary radiation, apart from that arising from the air or associated with the source. **Amitogenic dose.** The dose required to arrest mitosis. **Booster dose.** An interim dose; a smaller dose than the standard dose of a vaccine, that is given after a relatively short interval in order to increase the immunity before it has fallen below the safe level. **Cancericidal dose.** The dose which produces permanent tumour regression *in vivo.* **Cumulative dose.** A concept of dose modifed by time, which makes an allowance for loss of effect between exposures. **Daily dose.** Total dose during a 24 h period, whether administered all at once or at definite intervals. **Depth dose.** The dose at a point at a given depth in the tissues. **Epilation dose.** The dose required to produce a temporary loss of hair. **Erythema dose.** A dose of ionizing radiation, ultraviolet light or sunlight therapy that is just sufficient to produce a mild and short-lived reddening of the exposed part of the skin. **Exit dose.** The dose to the tissues at the point of exit of the central ray of a beam of radiation. **Free air dose.** Air dose (see above). **Integral absorbed dose.** The integration of the energy absorbed through a given region of interest. The unit is the gram-rad or gram-roentgen. (1 gram-rad = 10 μJ.) **Intoxicating dose.** The dose of an antigen required to produce the allergic response. **L₊dose.** Limes tod dose, the smallest amount of diphtheria toxin injected subcutaneously which, when mixed with one unit of antitoxin, will kill a 250-gram guinea-pig within 4 days. **L_f dose.** The amount of diphtheria toxin which will produce the maximum flocculation when mixed with 1 unit of antitoxin. **L_h dose.** The immunological symbol for limes (or limit) of reaction, used in haemolytic tests: the test dose of a toxin equivalent to 1 unit (or other fixed amount) of antitoxin, at a point where the haemolysis of red blood corpuscles is at a definite standard. **L_o dose.** Limes nul dose, the largest amount of diphtheria toxin which, when mixed with 1 unit of diphtheria antitoxin and injected subcutaneously into a 250-gram guinea-pig, will produce no reaction. **L_r dose.** The smallest quantity of diphtheria toxin which, when mixed with 1 unit of antitoxin and injected intracutaneously into a guinea-pig, causes a small characteristic reaction at the site of the injection. **Lethal dose.** The dose of a poisonous substance required to kill the animal to which it is administered. **Limes nul dose.** L_o dose (see above). **Limes tod dose.** L_+dose (see above). **Maintenance dose.** The dose (e.g. of insulin) required to maintain the physiological status quo. **Maximum dose.** The largest safe dose; an elastic figure, but most pharmacopoeias lay down quantities as suggested maxima. **Mean effective dose.** Median effective dose (see below). **Mean lethal dose.** Median lethal dose (see below). **Median effective dose.** ED_{50}, the dose calculated to produce a particular effect in 50 per cent of the test objectives. It is usually determined by injecting the drug at ascending dose levels into groups of animals and calculated statistically from the percentage in each group showing the effect. **Median lethal dose.** LD_{50}, a dose relative to the weight of the animal of a drug or other toxic substance that will kill 50 per cent of the animals to which it is administered. **Median paralysing dose.** A dose causing paralysis in 50 per cent of animals inoculated. **Minimal dose.** The smallest dose of a drug or other substance that may possibly produce the desired effect; such a dose may be too small to produce the effect in the individual concerned. **Minimal erythema dose.** MED, one of a number of expressions proposed for the measurement of dose of radiation in biological terms (also TED, threshold erythema dose, and SED, skin erythema dose), variously defined in terms of the conditions required to produce a visible erythema in a given proportion of persons exposed. **Minimum haemolytic dose.** MHD, the smallest amount of reagent which gives complete lysis of a specified quantity of red blood corpuscles. **Minimum haemolytic dose of amboceptor.** Haemolysin, haemolytic amboceptor, immune body, haemolytic unit, amboceptor unit: the smallest amount of amboceptor which gives complete lysis of a specified quantity of red blood corpuscles in the presence of an excess of complement in a recognized haemolytic titration. **Minimum haemolytic dose of complement.** The smallest amount of complement which gives complete lysis of a specified quantity of red blood corpuscles (previously sensitized by an excess of amboceptor) in a titration by a recognized method. **Minimum haemolytic dose of haemolysin.** Minimum haemolytic dose of amboceptor (see above). **Minimum infective dose.** The smallest dose that will cause an infection. **Minimum lethal dose.** MLD, the smallest dose relative to the weight that will kill an experimental animal. It is a less satisfactory measurement of toxicity than the LD_{50} (median lethal dose, above), as it does not take account of the variability in the resistance of the animals concerned. **Optimum dose.** The dose which has been found by experiment to be the best for a particular patient; it is of great importance in replacement therapy (e.g. insulin, in diabetes). **Percentage depth dose.** The dose at a point at a given depth, expressed as a percentage of the maximum dose on the surface, usually at the centre of the field of irradiation. **Permissible dose.** In radiology, the dose of ionizing radiation that, in the light of present knowledge, is not expected to cause appreciable bodily injury to a person at any time during his lifetime. ("Appreciable bodily injury" means any bodily injury or effect that the person involved would regard as objectionable and/or that competent medical authorities would regard as being deleterious to the health and well-being of the individual.) **Permissible weekly dose.** Dose of ionizing radiation accumulated in 1 week of such magnitude that, in the light of present knowledge, exposure at this weekly rate for an indefinite period of time is not expected to cause appreciable bodily injury to a person at any time during his lifetime. (One week, as used here, means any 7 consecutive days, not a calendar week.) **Reacting dose.** The second dose of a substance used to produce an anaphylactic or allergic response in an animal which has received a sensitizing dose (see following). **Sensitizing dose.** The first dose of a substance used to produce an anaphylactic or allergic response. **Skin dose.** The dose to a point on the skin, usually the centre of a field of irradiation. **Skin erythema dose.** SED, one of a number of expressions proposed for the measurement of dose of radiation in biological terms, defined by the conditions required to produce a visible erythema in a given proportion of persons exposed. **Skin test dose.** The dose of a drug introduced into the skin to produce a reaction. **Threshold erythema dose.** *See* MINIMAL ERYTHEMA DOSE (above). **Tissue dose.** Absorbed dose when the irradiated medium is tissue. **Tissue tolerance dose.** The maximum dose the normal tissues will tolerate without necrosis. **Total field dose.** The total dose to the tissues at the central point of a field of radiation during a course of treatment. **Total skin dose.** The dose at one specified skin point from all fields during a course of treatment. Loosely used to denote the sum of the total field doses. **Tumour dose.** The dose at a point in a tumour; usually expressed as a maximum and a minimum tumour dose. **Tumour lethal dose.** Cancericidal dose (see above). [Gk *dosis*, a giving.]

dose contours (dose **kon**·toorz). Isodose curves; lines joining points receiving the same radiation dose.

dose finder (dose **fi**·nder). An instrument for finding the dose at any point from a number of treatment fields using isodose curves.

dosemeter, dosimeter (**dose**·me·ter, do·**sim**·et·er). An instrument for measuring radiation dose. **Integrating dosemeter.** An instrument for measuring the total sum dose of radiation received over a period of time. **Thermoluminescent dosemeter.** A radiation dosemeter depending on thermoluminescence. [dose, Gk *metron* measure.]

dosimetric (do·sim·**et**·rik). Referring or belonging to dosimetry.

dosimetry (do·**sim**·et·re). 1. The system of accurate measurement and determination of medicinal doses. It is based upon many factors, including age (e.g. children require smaller doses than adults), sex, physical condition, idiosyncrasies, tolerance, cumulative and synergistic effects of the drug, and the pathological conditions involved. 2. The measurement of radiation dose. [dose, Gk *metron* measure.]

dot (dot). A small round spot or speck. [AS *dott* head of boil.]

See also: CHRISTOPHERS, GUNN, MAURER, SCHUEFFNER, STEPHENS, TRANTAS, WORTH.

dothienesia (**do**·the·en·e′·ze·ah). Furunculosis. [Gk *dothien* boil.]

Dothiepin (do·**thi**·ep·in). BP Commission approved name for 11-(3-dimethylaminopropylidene)-6*H*-dibenz[*b,e*]thiepin; an antidepressant.

Dott, Norman McOmish (b. 1897). Edinburgh neurosurgeon.

Dott's gag. A self-retaining adjustable mouth gag with tongue-piece adaptable to intratracheal or intrapharyngeal anaesthesia.

double blind (dubl **bli**·nd). An experimental design often applied in clinical drug trials, in which neither the experimenter nor the patients know which patients are in the experimental and which are in the control groups until the trial has been completed. [L *duplus* double, AS *blind*.]

doublet (**dub**·let). A birefracting quartz prism, invented by Wollaston and used in the keratometer to double the images of the mires. [L *duplus* double.]

douche (doosh). A stream of liquid applied at moderate pressure, localized by means of a tube, and directed into a body cavity through a natural orifice, or on to a body surface. **Air douche.** A current of air blown into a cavity. It is used to re-open the eustachian tube by means of a eustachian catheter, Politzer's bag or auto-inflation. **Aix douche.** A douche that is an important part of the Aix spa therapy. **Alternating douche.** A douche in which hot and cold liquids are used alternately. Also known as a *Scotch douche.* **Hot-air douche.** A device for directing a stream of hot air on to the body surface for the purpose of inducing a therapeutic hyperaemia. **Scotch douche.** Alternating douche (see above). **Vichy douche.** A douche of warm water directed on to a part of the body whilst massage is in progress. [Fr.]

Doughty, Andrew. Contemporary British anaesthetist.

Doughty gag. A mouth gag used for tonsillectomy under orotracheal anaesthesia.

Douglas, Beverly (b. 1891). Nashville surgeon.

Douglas' graft. A graft cut by an elaborate dermatome apparatus.

Douglas, Claude Gordon (b. 1882). English physiologist.

Douglas bag. A large gas-tight bag used for the collection of expired air when its analysis is required for the estimation of oxygen consumption.

Douglas, James (b. 1675). Scottish anatomist and surgeon in London.

Douglas' abscess. An abscess in the recto-uterine pouch.

Douglas' cry. A long, sharp cry uttered by a patient undergoing laparotomy when the recto-uterine pouch is mopped out.

Douglas' semilunar fold, or line. The arcuate line of the rectus sheath; a horizontal curved ridge in the posterior wall of the rectus sheath made by the lower margin of the fused aponeuroses of the internal oblique and transversus abdominis muscles. It is usually about half-way between the umbilicus and the symphysis pubis.

Douglas' ligaments. The recto-uterine peritoneal folds.

Douglas' pouch. The recto-uterine pouch.

Douglas' septum. The urorectal septum; the dividing septum of the primitive cloaca.

Douglas' space. Douglas' pouch (see above).

Douglas, Stewart Ranken (b. 1871). London pathologist.

Douglas' tellurite-copper sulphate agar (Allison and Ayling's modification). A medium composed of trypsinized serum with copper sulphate, or potassium tellurite, agar. It is a slow-growing medium for diphtheria.

douglascele (dug·las·seel). A hernia through the recto-uterine (Douglas') pouch. [Douglas' pouch, Gk *kele* hernia.]

douglasitis (dug·las·i·tis). A condition of inflammation of the recto-uterine pouch. [Douglas' pouch, Gk *-itis* inflammation.]

dourine (doo·reen). A contagious disease of cattle caused by *Trypanosoma equiperdum.* [Ar. *darin* filthy.]

Dover, Thomas (b. 1660). Sea-captain and Bristol physician.

Dover's powder. Ipecacuanha and Opium Powder BP 1958, a mixture of powdered ipecacuanha, opium and lactose, standardized to contain 1 per cent of morphine. It is used as a diaphoretic and anodyne for acute catarrh and coryza.

dowel (dow·el). A metal pin fixed in the root of a natural tooth to provide attachment for an artificial crown. [ME plug.]

Dowieism (dow·e·izm). A form of faith cure practised by the Dowieites, a religious sect of America. [John Alexander *Dowie,* founder of the sect, 19th-20th century.]

down [lanugo (NA)] (down). The coating of fine hairs on the skin of the newly-born infant. [Gk *dayne,* first covering of young birds.]

Down, John Langdon (b. 1828). London physician.

Down's syndrome. Mongolism; associated with an error in chromosomal separation during the formation of the germ cells. Most frequently seen in the offspring of elderly mothers. There is, however, a rare genetic form. Congenital heart disease is a common occurrence.

Downey, Hal (b. 1877). Minneapolis haematologist.

Downey's types. The mononuclear white cells encountered in normal and disease states differentiated into a number of groups to which Downey gave numbers. More recently these have been studied further and differentiated more clearly, and Downey's groupings have been largely abandoned. The term Downey Type II is still sometimes used for what is now usually called a glandular-fever cell.

Downie's flocculation test. A test for smallpox.

Downie's test. A test for syphilis.

dowser (dow·ser). One who claims to be able to detect hidden materials, e.g. metals in the ground, underground water. Usually such a person has recourse to a simple device such as a pendulum or a springy twig, the movement of which supposedly indicates the presence of the material sought.

Doxapram (dox·ah·pram). BP Commission approved name for 1-ethyl-4-(2-morpholinoethyl)-3,3-diphenyl-2-pyrrolidone. **Doxapram hydrochloride.** A respiratory stimulant acting on the respiratory centre, after the manner of nikethamide.

Doxepin (dox·ep·in). BP Commission approved name for 11-(3-dimethylaminopropylidene)-6*H*-dibenzo[*b,e*]oxepin (a 1 in 5 mixture of *cis* and *trans*); an antidepressant.

Doxorubicin (dox·o·roo·be·sin). BP Commission approved name for 14-hydroxydaunorubicin; an antibiotic produced by *Streptomyces peuceticus* var. *caesius.*

Doxybetasol (dox·e·be·tah·sol). BP Commission approved name for 9α-fluoro-11β,17α-dihydroxy-16β-methylpregna-1,4-diene-3,20-dione; a corticosteroid.

Doxycycline (dox·e·si·kleen). BP Commission approved name for 6-deoxy-5-hydroxytetracycline. **Doxycycline Hydrochloride BP 1973.** The hydrochloride of 4-dimethylamino-1,4,4a,5,5a,6,11,12,12a-octahydro-3,5,10,12,12a-pentahydroxy-6α-methyl-1,11-dioxonapthacene-2-carboxyamide, an antimicrobial substance obtained from oxytetracycline and methacycline.

Doxylamine (dox·il·am·een). BP Commission approved name for 2-(α-2-dimethylaminoethoxy-α-methylbenzyl)pyridine, $(C_6H_5)(C_5H_4N)(CH_3)COCH_2CH_2N(CH_3)_2$. An antihistaminic of the benadryl series.

Doyen, Eugène Louis (b. 1859). Paris surgeon.

Doyen's clamp. A light metal clamp, straight or curved, to control the escape of content and bleeding from the intestine during excision or anastomosis.

Doyen gag. A type of incisor gag.

Doyen's operation. An operation of eversion of the sac, for the relief of hydrocele.

Doyère, Louis (b. 1811). Paris physiologist.

Doyère's eminence, or hillock. A papilla on a muscle fibre at the point of entry of the motor nerve fibre. It is possibly an artefact.

Doyne, Robert Walter (b. 1857). Oxford ophthalmologist.

Doyne's familial honeycombed choroiditis. A hyaline degeneration of Bruch's membrane causing irregular thickening and the appearance of light-coloured patches of colloid material in the vicinity of the disc and macula, arranged in a ring. Onset between 12 and 19 years, and probably due to a hereditary degeneration of the pigment epithelium that attacks both eyes.

drachm (dram). A unit of weight (apothecaries), equivalent to 3.888 g (60 grains). It is symbolized in prescriptions by ʒ. **Fluid drachm.** A unit of liquid measure equal to 3.696 millilitres (one-eighth of a fluid ounce; 60 minims). On prescription it is represented by the symbol ʒ. [Gk *drachme,* a weight of about the same value.]

dracontiasis (drak·on·ti·as·is). Guinea-worm disease; infestation by *Dracunculus medinensis,* the result of drinking water containing *Cyclops* or water fleas carrying the larval stages of the worms. The female, when gravid, migrates to subcutaneous regions liable to be often wetted, thus usually to the feet and legs. When the skin is moist, the female secretes a blister-forming enzyme, the resulting lesion bursts under osmosis and the vulval orifice protrudes to discharge a milky fluid containing innumerable larvae. Secondary infection in the track of the worm leads to cellulitis, periarticular fibrosis and arthritis. [Gk *drakontion* little dragon.]

dracuncular (drak·ung·kew·lar). Belonging to or caused by *Dracunculus.*

Dracunculoidea (drak·ung·kew·**loi**'·de·ah). A superfamily of the nematode sub-order Camallanata. The family Dracunculidae is of medical interest. [Gk *drakontion* little dragon, *eidos* form.]

dracunculosis (drak·**ung**·kew·**lo**'·sis). Dracontiasis.

Dracunculus (drak·**ung**·kew·lus). A genus of round worms which includes *Dracunculus (Filaria) medinensis*, the guinea-worm, a parasite of man of serious import in the tropical Old World, particularly in the more arid regions where water is obtained from step wells. The worm may calcify in the soft tissues and may mimic a urinary calculus. In America a similar worm found in animals and rarely in man has been called *Dracunculus insignis*. Female guinea-worms, about 10 cm long, form boil-like swellings in the subcutaneous tissues, particularly of the feet and legs. The males are small and seldom observed. The larvae are shed in batches at separate contacts with water: intermediate hosts are copepods (*Cyclops* species). [L from Gk *drakontion* little dragon.]

Dragendorff, Johann George Noel (b. 1836). German physician and pharmacist.

Dragendorff's reagent. For alkaloids: a suspension of bismuth subnitrate in potassium iodide solution, acidified with hydrochloric acid.

Dragstedt, Lester Reynold (b. 1893). Chicago surgeon.

Dragstedt's operation. Vagotomy.

drain (drane). An appliance that affords and maintains a communication between a body cavity and the exterior, or a channel of exit for discharge from a wound. **Capillary drain.** A wick of worsted or similar absorbent material which drains by capillary attraction. **Cigarette drain.** A drain of gauze surrounded by waterproof material, rubber or gutta percha. **Intercostal drain.** A rubber tube inserted between the ribs to drain the pleural cavity. **Quarantine drain.** A drain left in the peritoneal cavity after operation. **Redon drain.** A small-bore tube attached to a suction bottle used to prevent the accumulation of wound haematoma. **Stab-wound drain.** A drain inserted through a puncture incision separate from the operation. **Suction drain.** Redon drain (see above). **Sump drain.** A drain inserted into a collection of fluid, consisting of an outer tube of large diameter and an inner smaller tube which lies free in the outer tube and to which suction or gravity is applied. **T-tube drain.** A rubber tube with a terminal crosspiece of the same material for drainage or repair of the common bile duct. **Tube drain.** A tube of glass, metal, or rubber plastic material for employment as a drain. [AS *draehen* a tear drop.]

See also: KEITH (T.), MIKULICZ-RADECKI, MOSHER, PENROSE, WYLIE.

drainage (dra·nij). In medicine, the withdrawal of fluids or pus from body cavities, abscesses or wounds, either actively, or passively by means of tubes, wicks, etc., left *in situ*. **Basal drainage.** Drainage of the cisterna magna of the subarachnoid space at the base of the brain. **Capillary drainage.** Drainage by fine strands of catgut or thread along which blood escapes to the exterior by capillary attraction. **Closed drainage.** Drainage of a wound or cavity in which the entry of air is obviated. **Negative-pressure drainage.** Suction drainage (see below). **Partial anomalous pulmonary venous drainage.** The connection, directly or indirectly, of one or more, but not all, of the pulmonary veins to the right atrium instead of the left. **Postural drainage.** Encouragement of drainage of secretions from various parts of the lungs by alteration of the patient's posture and thus enlisting the aid of gravity. **Suction drainage.** Drainage by a tube subjected to negative pressure at the opposite end. **Through drainage.** Drainage by establishing through an inflamed area a track or canal with 2 openings in which a drainage tube or drainage material lies. **Tidal drainage.** Drainage of the urinary bladder by a gravity apparatus which alternately fills the cavity by the introduction of a known quantity of fluid under gravity, and empties it by suction. **Total anomalous pulmonary venous drainage.** The connection of the whole of the pulmonary venous drainage, directly or indirectly, to the right atrium; an associated atrial septal defect is obligatory for the maintenance of the circulation. There are 2 main varieties, the *supradiaphragmatic* and the *infradiaphragmatic*, distinguished by whether the venous channel is entirely above or partially below the diaphragm; the latter is more serious because of the pulmonary congestion consequent upon the compression of the venous channel by the intra-abdominal pressure. **Underwater seal drainage.** A closed system of drainage by means of a tube leading from the chest to a bottle containing water, under the surface of which the tube dips. Air, blood and fluid can then be removed from the pleural space and lung expansion maintained after lung surgery. [see prec.]

See also: MONALDI, WANGENSTEEN.

dram (dram). Alternative spelling of drachm.

dramatism (**dram**·at·izm). The pompous morbidly dramatic manner of speaking and acting which is characteristic of certain forms of insanity. [Gk *drama* deed.]

dramatization (**dram**·at·i·**za**'·shun). Conversion into theatrical form of behaviour. [see prec.]

drape (drape). To cover with a cloth. **Surgical drapes.** The arrangement of sterile surgical cloths around the area of an operation. [ME *drap* cloth.]

Draper's law. In photochemical actions, only light which is actually absorbed is capable of producing chemical effect.

drapetomania (**drap**·et·o·**ma**'·ne·ah). Insane or uncontrollable impulsion to wander away from home. [Gk *drapetes* a runaway, mania.]

Drasch, Otto (b. 1849). Graz histologist.

Drasch's cells. Cuneiform cells in the tracheal mucous membrane, now known to be mucous cells in a resting condition.

drastic (**dras**·tik). 1. Any agent which gives rise to a major physiological response. 2. Term applied to a purgative of violent action. [Gk *drastikos* effective.]

draught (draft). Haustus: a quantity of medicament in a fluid form intended to be taken at a single dose. **Black draught.** Compound Mixture of Senna BPC 1959. [AS *dragan* to draw.]

draw-shave (**draw**·shave). In surgery, a long-handled knife so shaped that it can remove thin slices of tissue from within a cavity as the blade is drawn towards the operator. [AS *dragan* to draw, *scafan* shave.]

dream (dreem). 1. The life of the mind during sleep; a series of fragmentary or distorted images, thoughts or emotions occurring during sleep. 2. To be conscious of images, ideas or events during sleep. 3. Mental experience during sleep, commonly regarded as symbolizing wish-fulfilment or the solution of a mental conflict. **Clairvoyant dream.** A vivid, clearly defined and coherent dream in which what purports to be a real event or experience is presented to the mind of the sleeper. **Day dream.** An unreal reverie in day-time. **Veridical dream.** A dream in which the sleeper sees the images of events unknown to him and coinciding with the real events themselves. **Wet dream.** A dream associated with the ejaculation of semen during sleep. **Dream work.** The metamorphosis of latent dream content into manifest dream content. [ME.]

dream-pain (**dreem**·pane). Hypnalgia. [ME *dream*, L *poena* penalty.]

Drepanidotaenia (drep·**an**·id·o·**te**'·ne·ah). A genus of tapeworms related to *Hymenolepis*. *Drepanidotaenia lanceolata*, infecting ducks and geese, has been recorded once from a child in Europe. [Gk *drepane* sickle, L *taenia* ribbon.]

drepanocytaemia (**drep**·an·o·si·**te**'·me·ah). Sickle-cell anaemia. *See* ANAEMIA. [drepanocyte, Gk *haima* blood.]

drepanocyte (**drep**·an·o·site). An erythrocyte which has assumed a crescentic shape (sickle cell). [Gk *drepane* sickle, *kytos* cell.]

drepanocytic (**drep**·an·o·**si**'·tik). 1. Referring to a sickle-shaped cell. 2. Having sickle-shaped cells. [see prec.]

drepanocytosis (**drep**·an·o·si·**to**'·sis). Sickle-cell anaemia or the sickle-cell trait. [Gk *drepane* sickle, *kytos* cell, *-osis* condition.]

Dresbach, Melvin (b. 1874). Philadelphia physiologist.

Dresbach's anaemia, disease or syndrome. Sickel-cell anaemia.

dressing (**dres**·ing). 1. A covering which is applied to a wound for protection and to promote healing. 2. A medicament applied to a surface, usually to the skin. **Air dressing.** Treatment by exposure. **Antiseptic dressing.** Gauze or lint which is impregnated with an antiseptic. **Cross dressing.** Transvestitism. **Dry dressing.** An application of dry gauze or lint. **Fixed dressing.** A dressing which is designed to adhere to the affected part, thus providing local immobilization. **Occlusive dressing.** A dressing, usually adhesive, applied to exclude air, and consequently all bacteria, from a wound. **Pressure dressing.** A dressing exerting pressure on a wound, usually by adhesive strapping, with the object of preventing oozing. Used particularly to prevent free skin grafts being floated off from the area being grafted. [OFr. *dresser* to arrange.]

See also: SCOTT.

Dressler's disease. Recurrent haemoglobinuria.

Dreyer, Georges (b. 1873). Oxford pathologist.

Dreyer's test. A form of Widal's agglutination reaction for the diagnosis of typhoid and paratyphoid fever; formolized cultures of known and constant agglutinability were used, and were mixed with the serum dilutions; all measurements were made by a drop method. This test is obsolete in its original form, but modifications are in use.

drift (drift). In immunology, the successive emergence of new antigenic variants of a virus which replace the pre-existing antigenic determinants, as in influenza virus A. [AS *drifan* to drive.]

drifting (**drif**·ting). The horizontal movement of natural teeth in the jaws when they have lost the support of the adjacent teeth with which they are normally in contact. [AS *drifan* to drive.]

Drigalski, Karl Wilhelm von (b. 1871). Berlin bateriologist.

Conradi-Drigalski agar, Drigalski-Conradi agar. A nutrient agar containing 1 per cent peptone, 1.9 per cent nutrose, 0.5 per cent calcium chloride, 1.5 per cent lactose, 0.001 per cent crystal violet and 15 per cent litmus solution.

drill (dril). An instrument used in conservative dentistry for deep penetration of tooth structure, as in opening infected pulp canals; a somewhat similar instrument is used in bone surgery. [D *drillen* to bore.]

drilling (**dril**·ing). In dentistry, the operation of using a drill. **Metaphyseal drilling.** The operation of making drill holes in the metaphysis of a bone to increase the blood supply. [see prec.]

Drinker, Philip (b. 1893). Boston public health engineer.

Drinker respirator. An apparatus for performing artificial respiration for long periods of paralysis of the respiratory muscles. It is popularly known as the *iron lung.*

Drinker-Collins resuscitation. Resuscitation by the use of the Drinker respirator.

drip (drip). Continuous administration of fluid into the body by allowing it to flow from a container into a tube connected either to a needle or cannula for parenteral use, or to a stomach or rectal tube. Parenteral drips may be subcutaneous, intravenous or (less often) intramuscular. **Intravenous drip.** Administration of a solution (e.g. saline or glucose) by a drip method into a vein. **Nasal drip.** A method of feeding individuals who are incapable of taking food in the normal way, fluids being introduced through a soft rubber catheter inserted into the nostril. The external end of the catheter is fixed to the skin, usually behind the ear, with adhesive plaster: the internal end of the tube reaches as far as the postnasal space. The fluids used should be at body temperature and sterile in case of inhalation into the bronchial tree. The method has been discontinued with infants and small children because of the danger of inhalation and of infection of the ears through the eustachian tube. **Postnasal drip.** Postnasal discharge; a term used more commonly in the USA than in the UK. [AS *dryppan.*]

See also: MURPHY (J. B.).

drip-chamber (**drip**·chame·ber). A glass container from which fluid runs into a vein and into which more fluid drips visibly from a container held above it. Part of a drip-set. [AS *dryppan,* Gk *kamara* anything with an arched cover.]

drip-set (**drip**·set). A system of sterile tubes consisting of a drip-chamber and tubing inserted above into a bottle of intravenous fluid, and below attached to a needle in a vein. [AS *dryppen,* L *secta* faction.]

drive (drive). The impelling force of an instinctive impulse. **Kinetic drive.** Overstimulation of the kinetic system. **Meiotic drive.** Any process taking place during meiosis and resulting in the non-random assortment of chromosomes into cells forming functional gametes. [AS *drifon.*]

drivel (drivl). The flowing of saliva from the mouth, such as occurs in infancy, senility and imbecility. [ME *drivelen* to slaver.]

dromograph (**dro**·mo·graf). An instrument with which can be recorded the velocity of the blood circulation. [Gk *dromos* course, *graphein* to record.]

dromomania (dro·mo·**ma**·ne·ah). 1. An obsession for roaming or wandering. 2. Drapetomania. [Gk *dromos* course, mania.]

dromophobia (dro·mo·**fo**·be·ah). Pathological fear of running. [Gk *dromos* course, phobia.]

dromotropic (dro·mo·**trop**·ik). A term applied to a set of fibres said to be present in the cardiac nerves and to affect the speed of induction and transmission of the contractile wave (T. W. Engelmann). [Gk *dromos* course, *trepein* to turn.]

dromotropism (dro·**mot**·rop·izm). Alteration of the normal conducting power of a nerve. **Negative dromotropism.** Decrease in nerve conductivity. **Positive dromotropism.** Increase in nerve conductivity. [see prec.]

drop (drop). 1. The largest quantity of a liquid which can form on the end of a rod or tube. Drops vary in size, according to the diameter of the rod or tube, the temperature and the viscosity of the liquid. 2. A troche. 3. The falling of a hand or foot, or any part, such as occurs in paralysis. **Ankle drop.** Inability to dorsiflex the foot due to paralysis of the leg muscles. **Balm drop.** Compound Benzoin Tincture BP 1958. **Dutch drop.** Balsam of sulphur, i.e. sulphur boiled in olive oil. **Enamel drop.** Enamel pearl. *See* PEARL. **Foot drop.** Paralysis of dorsiflexion of the foot. **Hanging drop.** A drop of fluid culture medium on the undersurface of a microscopical coverslip or slide, that maintains its position by surface tension. Air pressure is obviated, and the specimen can be examined in this condition under the microscope. **Hot drop.** A tincture containing capsicum and myrrh. **Knock-out drops.** A solution of chloral hydrate used as a narcotic. **Drop serene.** Gutta serena; amaurosis due to glaucoma, so called as it is painless and no opacity is seen in the pupil; in contradistinction to gutta opaca; obsolete but of historical interest. **Steel drops.** Steel tincture; a solution containing 15 per cent w/v of ferric chloride and from 22 to 24 per cent v/v of ethyl alcohol. It is a powerful styptic and astringent. **Stomach drop.** A carminative tincture containing gentian. **Thick drop.** Thick smear; a blood film made specially thick for examination for scanty or sparsely occurring malaria parasites, cells (eosinophil and basophil leucocytes), polychromasia, punctate basophilia and chromatic material. **Wrist drop.** Paralysis of extension of the wrist. [AS *dropa.*]

dropacism (**drop**·as·izm). Depilation by means of pitch plaster. [Gk *dropax* plaster.]

Droperidol (dro·**per**·id·ol). BP Commission approved name for 1-{1-[3-(4-fluorobenzoyl)propyl]-1,2,3,6-tetrahydro-4-pyridyl}-benzimidazolone; a neuroleptic, sedative and tranquillizer.

droplet (**drop**·let). A very small drop. **Flügges droplets.** Name given to the spray of droplets emitted by the mouth in loud or forcible speaking which may spread infection among listeners. [AS *dropa.*]

dropped (dropt). In a state of ptosis. [see prec.]

dropper (**drop**·er). A teat pipette or stoppered bottle so designed as to permit dispensing of a liquid drop by drop. [AS *dropa.*]

Dropropizine (dro·**pro**·pe·zeen). BP Commission approved name for 1-(2,3-dihydroxypropyl)-4-phenylpiperazine; a cough suppressant.

dropsical (**drop**·sik·al). Relating or belonging to dropsy; suffering from dropsy. [Gk *hydrops* dropsy.]

dropsy (**drop**·se). The abnormal collection of serous fluid in tissue spaces or serous cavities. **Abdominal dropsy.** Ascites. **Acute**

dropsy. Dropsy of sudden onset. **Dropsy of the amnion.** Hydramnion. **Articular dropsy.** Serous effusion into a joint. **Dropsy of the belly.** Ascites. **Dropsy of the brain.** Hydrocephalus. **Cachectic dropsy.** Dropsy occurring in cachectic conditions due to enfeebled circulation. **Cardiac dropsy.** Cardiac oedema. **Dropsy of the chest.** Hydrothorax; fluid in the pleural cavities. **Cutaneous dropsy.** Subcutaneous oedema. **Encysted dropsy.** Accumulation of fluid in an enclosed space. **Epidemic dropsy.** A condition somewhat resembling cardiac beriberi, but without paralysis or anaesthesia. The onset is sudden, accompanied by fever with aching of the body. An exanthem, erythematous on the face, rubeolar on the trunk and limbs, is frequently seen, as are also nodular eruptions. A not uncommon complication is acute glaucoma. It is especially prevalent in rice-eating populations, and is apparently caused by eating mustard oil containing argemone oil, the latter coming from *Argemone mexicana* (Mexican or prickly poppy), a contaminant of the mustard crop. **False dropsy.** Subcutaneous swellings giving the appearance of oedema, but caused by myxoedematous material or fat. **Famine dropsy.** Nutritional oedema. **Dropsy of the gall bladder.** Distension of the gall bladder with fluid secretion. **General dropsy.** Anasarca: general oedema of subcutaneous tissues and serous cavities. **Dropsy of the head.** Hydrocephalus. **Hepatic dropsy.** Oedema in cirrhosis of the liver. **Lymphatic dropsy.** That due to obstruction of lymph vessels. **Mechanical dropsy.** Oedema due to mechanical constriction of veins, e.g. by a ligature. **Nutritional dropsy.** Oedema due to lowered concentration of plasma protein, as in famine, cachectic states, marasmus, etc. **Passive dropsy.** That due to passive venous congestion. **Dropsy of the pericardium.** Hydropericardium; the accumulation of transudate in the pericardial sac (pericardial effusion). It occurs as part of a generalized oedematous state (anasarca). **Peritoneal dropsy.** Accumulation of fluid in the peritoneal cavity. **Renal dropsy.** Oedema caused by nephritis. **Symptomatic dropsy.** Oedema occurring as a result of some general disease. **Tubal dropsy.** Hydrosalpinx. **Uterine dropsy.** Hydrometra. **War dropsy.** Famine oedema; nutritional dropsy (see above). **Wet dropsy.** A term employed to describe extensive "soft" oedema, as in oedematous beriberi. [see prec.]

Drosophila (dro·**sof**·il·ah). A genus of small brachyceran flies. Several species, called *bar flies*, are seasonally abundant in bars and restaurants. They are a rare cause of myiasis in man. **Drosophila melanogaster.** The fruit fly or banana fly, a species which has been used in genetical research by reason of its prolificness, easy culture and the fact that it has 4 pairs of chromosomes only, all readily recognizable. [Gk *drosos* dew, *philein* to love.]

Drostanolone (dro·**stan**·o·lone). BP Commission approved name for 17β-hydroxy-2α-methyl-5α-androstan-3-one; an anabolic steroid.

Drotebanol (dro·**teb**·an·ol). BP Commission approved name for 3,4-dimethoxy-17-methylmorphinan-6β,14-diol; an analgesic and antitussive agent.

Droxypropine (drox·e·**pro**·peen). BP Commission approved name for 1-[2-(2-hydroxyethoxy)ethyl]-4-phenyl-4-propionylpiperidine; a cough suppressant.

drug (drug). 1. Any chemical substance, synthetic or extracted from plant or animal tissue and of known or unknown composition, which is used as a medicament to prevent or cure disease. 2. To administer medicine for the prevention or cure of disease. 3. To administer a narcotic. **Antagonistic drug.** One that counteracts the effect of another drug. **Crude drug.** An unrefined drug containing impurities derived from its source. **Dangerous drugs.** Pharmaceutical preparations designated as "Dangerous Drugs" by the older Dangerous Drugs Acts 1925–1968, now obsolete in England. Also known as "hard" drugs: preparations of opium, morphine, heroin and synthetic substitutes for these, such as pethidine, methadone, physeptone, and cocaine preparations. **Ganglioplegic drug.** A drug which temporarily blocks transmission through ganglia of the autonomic nervous system; blockage may be predominantly in sympathetic ganglia or in parasympathetic ganglia. **Habit-forming drug.** One that leads to addiction, e.g. opium. **Neuroplegic drugs.** *See* NEUROPLEGIC. **Noxious drug.** In law, a drug taken or administered for an unlawful purpose, e.g. to procure abortion. **Psychotropic drug.** A drug which exerts a powerful action on the higher parts of the central nervous system and on mental state and behaviour. [Fr. *drogue.*]

drug-fast (**drug**·fahst). A term describing micro-organisms which are resistant to the action of any drug or medicament.

drum (drum). The ear-drum; the tympanic membrane. **Drum belly.** Tympanites. **Drum head.** The tympanic membrane. **Drum membrane.** The tympanic membrane. [D *trom.*]

Drummond, Sir David (b. 1852). Durham surgeon.

Drummond-Morison operation. An operation for the relief of ascites in which the surfaces of the liver, spleen and parietal peritoneum are roughened to encourage adhesions, the omentum being also roughened and sutured to the abdominal wall.

Drummond, Sir Jack Cecil (b. 1891). London biochemist.

Rosenheim and Drummond method. For total and ethereal sulphates in urine: inorganic sulphates are precipitated with benzidine, and the benzidine sulphate titrated with standard alkali. Total sulphates are determined similarly after hydrolysis with hydrochloric acid.

Rosenheim-Drummond test. A colour test used for detecting vitamin A in cod-liver oil. It is based on the violet colour which is formed when 1 drop of concentrated sulphuric acid is added to 1 or 2 drops of cod-liver oil previously dissolved in anhydrous fat solvent.

drumstick (**drum**·stik). The drumstick-like appendage visible in the nuclei of a small proportion of polymorphonuclear leucocytes from individuals with at least 2 X chromosomes. Typical drumsticks have a near-spherical body of 1.5 μm diameter attached to the nucleus by a thread-like stalk; they must be distinguished from smaller appendages, either sessile or with a wide stalk, which are called *clubs* and are not an expression of the sex chromosome complement of the cells. **Drumstick bacillus.** *See* BACILLUS. [D *trom*, AS *sticca.*]

Drury, Phoebe E. 20th century Boston biochemist.

Stoddard and Drury method. For total fatty acids in blood: whole blood, plasma or serum is extracted with hot alcohol-ether. The filtered extract is boiled with alkali to saponify the free and combined fatty acids; the fatty acids are then separated, washed, dissolved in alcohol and titrated with standard alkali using phenol blue as indicator.

drüsen (**dree**·zen). 1. Small hyaline excrescences occurring in the optic disc or Bruch's membrane. 2. Clusters of granules that appear in the suppurative lesions of actinomycosis. [G *Drüse* gland.]

dry (dri). With the minimum of moisture. [AS *dryge.*]

Dryopteris filix-mas (dri·**op**·ter·is fil·ix·**mas**). The source of male fern. *See* FERN. [Gk *drys* oak, *pteris* fern, L *filix* fern, *mas* male.]

Drysdale, Thomas Murray (b. 1831). Philadelphia gynaecologist.

Drysdale's corpuscles. Tiny transparent cells found in the fluid of ovarian cysts.

D-stoff (**de**·shtof). Phosgene; a colourless gas with suffocating odour, used in chemical warfare as a choking gas. [G *Stoff* substance.]

dualism (**dew**·al·izm). 1. The doctrine that man is composed of 2 principles, mind and matter, which are independent of one another. 2. The polyphyletic theory that blood cells have a double origin. 3. The belief that psychic phenomena have no fundamental connection with those of the physical world. 4. The theory that molecules of all chemical compounds are electrically dipolar, one part negative, the other positive. [L *dualis* double.]

dualistic (dew·al·**is**·tik). Consisting of 2 members or parts. [see prec.]

Duane, Alexander (b. 1858). New York ophthalmologist.

Duane's syndrome. Retraction syndrome.

dubhium (doob·e·um). Symbol Db, a reputed element, later found to be identical with ytterbium.

dubi (doo·be). A name for yaws, used in Ghana.

Dubin, Isadore Nathan (b. 1913). American pathologist.

Dubin-Johnson syndrome. Chronic jaundice due to difficulty in getting conjugated bilirubin out of the hepatic cell, which contains dark pigment granules.

Dubini, Angelo (b. 1813). Milan physician.

Dubini's disease. Electrical chorea; also called *Bergeron's disease.*

dubo (dew·bo). Double strength milk or other nourishment (von Pirquet). [L *lac duplex bovinum* double cow's milk.]

Du Bois, Eugene Floyd (b. 1882). New York physiologist.

Aub-DuBois standards. Tables of calories per square metre of body surface per hour, for different ages.

Dubois, Paul (b. 1795). Paris obstetrician.

Dubois' abscess. An abscess of the thymus gland considered by Dubois to be associated with congenital syphilis; a questionable entity.

Dubois, Paul Charles (b. 1848). Berne psychiatrist.

Dubois' method, or treatment. The treatment of mental disorder by the inculcation of a loftier set of ideals.

Duboisia (dew·boi·se·ah). A genus of tropical plants of the Far East (family Solanaceae). *Duboisia myoporoides,* the corkwood elm of Australia, and other species, yield hyoscyamine and hyoscine.

duboisine (dew·boi·seen). Name given to an alkaloidal substance obtained from *Duboisia myoporoides* (family Solanaceae) and considered by some to be mainly hyoscyamine. It is used in solution (0.2–0.5 per cent) as a mydriatic.

Dubois-Reymond, Emil Heinrich (b. 1818). Berlin physiologist.

Dubois-Reymond's inductorium. A special form of induction coil in which the primary circuit remains unbroken.

Dubois-Reymond key. An electrical appliance consisting of 4 terminals arranged in connected pairs, and between them a movable switch of highly conducting material. When the switch forms a bridge between the 2 pairs, i.e. is closed, then part of the circuit is shorted.

Dubois-Reymond law. Variation in current density, and not its absolute value at any given moment, is the effective stimulus to muscle or nerve.

Dubos, René Jules (b. 1901). New York bacteriologist.

Dubos culture medium. A medium for the culture of mycobacteria, giving diffuse instead of granular growth: prepared from potassium dihydrogen phosphate, disodium hydrogen phosphate, sodium citrate, magnesium sulphate, Tween 80 and casein hydrolysate, to which is added sterile bovine albumin.

Duboscq, Jules (b. 1817). French optician.

Duboscq colorimeter. An instrument designed by Duboscq for the determination of small quantities of substances in solutions such as serum and fractions by direct comparison of colours, developed by appropriate reagents, against a standard.

Dubreuilh, William (b. 1857). French dermatologist.

Dubreuilh's elastoma. Diffuse, thickened plaques on the face or neck, resulting from prolonged exposure to sunlight.

Dubreuilh's precancerous circumscribed melanosis. Lentigo maligna; xeroderma pigmentosum.

Duchenne, Guillaume Benjamin Amand (b. 1806). Paris neurologist.

Duchenne's attitude. Dropping of the shoulder with clockwise rotation of the scapula, due to trapezius paralysis.

Duchenne's disease. 1. Tabes dorsalis. 2. Progressive bulbar palsy type of motor neuron disease.

Duchenne dystrophy. Progressive hypertrophic muscular dystrophy.

Duchenne's paralysis. Progressive bulbar paralysis.

Duchenne's sign. Recession of the epigastrium resulting from paralysis of the diaphragm, and said also to occur in hydropericardium.

Duchenne's syndrome. Labioglossopharyngeal paralysis, as seen in the progressive bulbar palsy type of motor neuron disease.

Duchenne's trocar. A trocar and cannula designed to core or punch out fragments of buried tissue, usually tumour, for microscopical examination.

Aran-Duchenne atrophy, disease or type. Progressive spinal muscular atrophy; motor neuron disease of the progressive muscular atrophy type.

Duchenne-Erb palsy, or syndrome, Erb-Duchenne palsy, or paralysis. Erb's palsy or paralysis.

Duchenne-Griesinger disease. Pseudohypertrophic muscular dystrophy.

duckering (duk·er·ing). A method by which hair and wool can be disinfected in order to destroy any anthrax bacilli present. [G. F. *Duckering.*]

Duckworth, Sir Dyce (b. 1840). London physician.

Duckworth's phenomenon, or sign. In fatal conditions in which the intracranial pressure is increased, the heart may continue to beat for some hours after respiration has ceased.

Ducrey, Augosto (b. 1860). Rome dermatologist.

Ducrey's bacillus. *Haemophilus ducreyi.*

duct [ductus (NA)] (dukt). A channel for conducting fluid. **Aberrant duct.** A duct which is not normally present, or which takes an abnormal course. **Alveolar ducts [ductuli alveolares (NA)].** Branched tubes, the walls of which contain muscle fibres, leading from the terminal (respiratory) bronchioles. **Archinephric duct.** An old term for the wolffian or mesonephric duct of the embryo. **Arterial duct.** Ductus arteriosus. **Bile duct [ductus choledochus (NA)].** An important duct, about 8 cm long, formed by the union of the common hepatic and cystic ducts (see below); it lies at first in the free border of the lesser omentum, then behind the first part of the duodenum and the pancreas, which it grooves. It is usually joined by the pancreatic duct just before opening into the second part of the duodenum. **Cloacal duct.** A temporary communication between the urogenital sinus and the rectum before their complete separation by the downgrowth of the cloacal septum. **Duct of the cochlea [ductus cochlearis (NA)].** A spiral tube within the bony canal of the cochlea, consisting in man of 2¾ turns. Its roof [paries vestibularis ductus cochlearis (membrana vestibularis) NA] is formed by the vestibular membrane, its floor [paries tympanicus ductus cochlearis (membrana spiralis) NA] by the basilar membrane or lamina and the outer part of the osseous spiral lamina, and its lateral wall [paries externus ductus cochlearis (NA)] by the vascular, modified periosteum lining the bony canal. **Craniopharyngeal duct.** A remnant of the stalk of Rathke's pouch forming a temporary communication between the stomatodeum and the anterior lobe of the pituitary in the early embryo. **Cystic duct [ductus cysticus (NA)].** The duct of the gall bladder, usually about 4 cm long, joining the common hepatic duct to form the common bile duct. **Ejaculatory duct [ductus ejaculatorius (NA)].** A slender tube, about 3 cm long, formed just outside the prostate by the union of the vas deferens and the duct of the seminal vesicle. It traverses the prostate to open in the posterior wall of the prostatic urethra. **Endolymphatic duct of the membranous labyrinth [ductus endolymphaticus [aqueductus vestibuli (NA)].** A blind membranous tube connected to the saccule and the utriculosaccular duct. It passes into the aqueduct of the vestibule and ends under the dura mater on the posterior surface of the petrous temporal bone as the dilated endolymphatic sac. **Duct of the epoöphoron [ductus epoöphori longitudinalis (NA)].** The caudal part of the mesonephric duct which, normally degenerating, may persist in the female. **Excretory duct.** A duct which is conductive only. **Frontonasal duct.** A fine duct in the lateral wall of the nasal cavity. It proceeds from the ethmoid bone to the frontal sinus. **Hepatic duct, common [ductus hepaticus communis (NA)].** A duct, 2.5 cm long, formed at the right end of the portal hepatic ducts. It unites with the cystic duct to form the common bile duct. **Hepatic duct, left [ductus hepaticus sinister (NA)].** The main duct draining bile from the left, quadrate and most of the caudate lobes. It is formed by the junction of medial [ramus medialis (NA)] and a lateral [ramus lateralis (NA)] duct, the latter draining the left lobe. **Hepatic duct, right [ductus hepaticus dexter (NA)].** The main duct draining bile from the right lobe, except for the quadrate and part of the caudate lobes. It is formed by the junction of anterior and posterior ducts **[rami anterior et posterior** (NA)] which drain anterior and posterior segments separated by an oblique plane. **Hypophyseal duct.** Craniopharyngeal duct (see above). **Incisive duct [ductus incisivus (NA)].** A rudimentary fold of mucous membrane into the incisive canal of the maxilla. **Interlobular ducts [ductuli interlobulares (NA)].** Tributaries of the hepatic ducts, running between the liver lobules with the interlobular veins. **Lactiferous ducts [ductus lactiferi (NA)].** The main ducts of the mammary gland, which number from 15 to 30, and open on to the nipple. **Longitudinal duct of the epoöphoron.** *See* DUCT OF EPOÖPHORON (above). **Lymphatic duct, right [ductus lymphaticus (thoracicus) dexter (NA)].** A short trunk, about 1 cm long, entering the junction of the right subclavian and internal jugular veins. It receives the right jugular, right subclavian and right bronchomediastinal trunk. Not uncommonly absent. **Mesonephric duct [ductus mesonephricus (NA)].** The Wolffian duct, a paired embryological tube; it forms part of the bladder and urethra, and the ureter grows from its lower end in both sexes. In the male it forms the vas deferens and the duct of the epididymis; in the female it mainly disappears. *See* EPOÖPHORON. **Mullerian duct.** Paramesonephric duct (see below). **Nasolacrimal duct [ductus nasolacrimalis (NA)].** A canal 2 cm long, draining tears from the lacrimal sac into the inferior meatus of the nose. It has an imperfect valvular fold just above its opening. **Omphalomesenteric duct.** The connecting stalk between the mid-gut and the yolk sac of the embryo; part of it may persist as a Meckel's diverticulum. **Pancreatic duct [ductus pancreaticus (NA)].** A duct running through the gland from left to right, receiving on either side of the lobular ducts. It lies nearer the posterior surface, and at the neck turns downwards and posteriorly to join the bile duct in its left side. The two pass obliquely through the duodenal wall and unite in its substance. **Pancreatic duct, accessory [ductus pancreaticus accessorius (NA)].** A commonly-occurring structure which drains the lower part of the head of the pancreas, and running upwards ventral to the main duct, with which it communicates, empties into the duodenum about 2 cm proximal to the ampulla. **Paramesonephric duct [ductus paramesonephricus (NA)].** The female sex duct of the embryo which becomes the uterine tube, uterus and vagina. Its homologue in the male atrophies, one remnant being found near the upper pole of the testis and one in the prostate. **Para-urethral ducts [ductus para-urethrales (NA)].** Ducts of small glands lying on each side of the urethra; they open on the lateral margins of the external urethral orifice. **Parotid duct [ductus parotideus (NA)].** The duct of the parotid gland, which runs over the cheek to open into the vestibule of the mouth opposite the second upper molar tooth. **Pronephric duct.** The duct of the pronephros or primitive kidney of the embryo. **Prostatic duct [ductulus prostaticus (NA)].** One of 12-20 small ducts draining the gland which open on the posterior wall of the prostatic urethra on either side of the urethral crest. **Salivary ducts.** The ducts that convey saliva to the mouth, the parotid, the submandibular, the submaxillary in man, and the corresponding ducts in animals and insects. **Segmental duct.** One of the paired pronephric or mesonephric ducts of the embryo, draining the segmental excretory tubules of the pronephros or mesonephros into the cloaca. **Semicircular ducts [ductus semicirculares (NA)].** Membranous tubes within the osseous semicircular canals. The medial end of the superior duct [ductus semicircularis anterior (NA)] and the upper end of the posterior duct [ductus semicircularis posterior (NA)] join and open into the utricle by a common opening; the other ends of these ducts and both ends of the lateral duct [ductus semicircularis lateralis (NA)] open independently. **Duct of a seminal vesicle [ductus excretorius (NA)].** The short, narrow, inferior portion which joins the vas deferens to form the ejaculatory duct (see above). **Sublingual ducts [ductus sublingualis major et ductus sublinguales minores (NA)].** Ducts of the sublingual gland, some of which open into the submandibular duct or directly into the floor of the mouth [ductus minores (NA)] and some of which unite to form a larger duct [ductus major (NA)]. **Submandibular duct [ductus submandibularis (NA)].** The sole duct of the gland of the same name. It opens into the mouth on the sublingual papilla. **Duct of a sweat gland [ductus sudoriferus (NA)].** The more or less straight superficial part of the gland, leading to the surface of the skin. **Thoracic duct [ductus thoracicus (NA)].** The larger of 2 terminal valved lymph vessels. It arises from the cisterna chyli in the upper abdomen, passes through the thorax on the vertebral column and empties into the junction of the left internal jugular and subclavian veins. It commonly receives all lymph except from the right arm and right half of the head and thorax. **Thyroglossal duct [ductus thyroglossus (NA)].** The embryonic connection of the thyroid gland with the floor of the mouth. It is not present in the adult, but when remnants persist they may give rise to a thyroglossal cyst or fistula. **Thyrolingual duct.** Thyroglossal duct (see preceding). **Umbilical duct.** Omphalomesenteric duct (see above). **Urogenital duct.** One of the muellerian or mesonephric ducts of the embryo. **Utriculosaccular duct [ductus utriculosaccularis (NA)].** A fine canal joining the utricle to the endolymphatic duct just behind its connection with the saccule. **Vitelline duct.** Omphalomesenteric duct (see above). **Vitello-intestinal duct.** The duct connecting the yolk sac with the intestine in the embryo. **Wolffian duct.** Mesonephric duct (see above). [L *ducere* to lead.]

See also: ARANZIO, BARTHOLIN (C.), BELLINI, BERNARD (C.), BLASIUS (G.), BOCHDALEK, BOTALLO, CUVIER, GARTNER, HALLER, HENSEN, HOFFMANN (M.), LEYDEN, MUELLER (J.), PECQUET, RATHKE, REICHEL (F. P.), RIVINUS, SANTORINI, SCHUELLER (K. H. A. L. M.), SKENE, STENSEN, WALTHER, WHARTON, WIRSUNG, WOLFF (K. F.).

ductile (**duk**·tile). Of metals, capable of being permanently drawn out into the thinness of wire. [see prec.]

duction (**duk**·shun). In opthalmology, the movement of an eye either laterally—abduction and adduction, vertically—supraduction and infraduction, or rotatory (around the anteroposterior axis)—cycloduction. **Binocular duction.** Fusion duction power; the range of disjunctive movements (adduction, abduction, vertical or rotatory movements in the opposite directions) which can be made on a synoptophore or similar instrument while maintaining binocular single vision. [see foll.]

ductless (**dukt**·les). Without an excretory duct, e.g. the ductless or endocrine glands. [L *ducere* to lead.]

ductule [ductulus (NA)] (**duk**·tewl). 1. Any very small duct. 2. The terminal portion of a duct nearest the alveolus of a gland. **Bile ductules [ductuli biliferi (NA)].** The excretory channels running between adjacent hepatic cell columns. **Efferent ductules [ductuli efferentes testis (NA)].** The excretory ducts in which the straight seminiferous tubules of the testis terminate. [L *ductulus* little duct.]

ductulus [NA] (**duk**·tew·lus). A small duct. **Ductulus aberrans, superior [ductulus aberrans superior (NA)].** The first epigenital tubule, persisting as an isolated remnant in the epididymis of the adult. **Ductuli aberrantes [NA].** From 12 to 20 tubules linking the rete testis to the lobules of the epididymis. [L.]

ductus [NA] (**duk**·tus). Duct. **Ductus aberrans.** Aberrant duct. **Ductus arteriosus** [NA]. A channel connecting the left pulmonary artery to the terminal part of the aortic arch in the fetus. It is normally occluded soon after birth but sometimes remains patent and requires surgical treatment. **Ductus auditorius.** Duct of the cochlea. **Ductus caroticus.** The portion of the embryonic dorsal aorta which lies between the third and fourth aortic arches and which normally disappears. **Ductus cuvieri.** Cuvier's duct. **Ductus deferens.** Vas deferens. **Patent ductus arteriosus, Persistent ductus arteriosus.** Persistence of the normal fetal patency of the ductus arteriosus beyond the first few weeks of life; it is associated with a shunt of blood from the aorta to the pulmonary artery, unless there is severe pulmonary hypertension, with the production of a characteristic continuous murmur.

Ductus reuniens [NA]. A membranous tube connecting the saccule to the commencement of the cochlear duct. **Ductus venosus** [NA]. The embryonic venous channel which joins the portal sinus to the inferior vena cava and transmits between one-third and two-thirds of the placental blood directly to the heart. It becomes occluded immediately after birth.

Duddell, Benedict (fl. 1729). English ophthalmologist.

Duddell's membrane. The posterior elastic lamina of the cornea.

Dudley, Emilius Clark (b. 1850). Chicago gynaecologist.

Dudley's operation. 1. Posterior incision of the cervix for dysmenorrhoea and sterility; obsolete. 2. A modification of Gilliam's operation for retrodisplacement of the uterus.

Duehrssen, Jacobus Alfred (b. 1862). Berlin gynaecologist.

Duehrssen's operation. 1. A type of vaginal caesarean section. 2. A vaginal fixation of the uterus for the treatment of prolapse; obsolete.

Duffy. *See* Blood GROUP.

Dugas, Louis Alexander (b. 1806). Augusta surgeon.

Dugas' test. In dislocation of the shoulder the hand cannot be placed on the opposite clavicle with the elbow touching the side.

Duguet, Jean Baptiste Nicolas (b. 1837). Paris physician.

Duguet's siphon. A trocar with a rubber tube, for aspirating a cavity by siphonage.

ulceration of Duguet. Ulceration of the fauces, observed in typhoid fever.

Duhot, Robert (b. 1867). Brussels urologist and dermatologist.

Duhot's line. A line joining the anterior superior iliac spine with the sacrococcygeal joint.

Duhring, Louis Adolphus (b. 1845). Philadelphia dermatologist and financial benefactor of dermatology.

Duhring's disease, Duhring–Brocq disease. Dermatitis herpetiformis.

Duhring's pruritus. Pruritus hiemalis; a malady of northern climates: the itching occurs only during cold weather when the patient undresses. The legs are usually affected, but other areas may be involved.

duipara (dew·**ip**·ah·rah). Secundipara. [L *duo* two, *parere* to give birth.]

Duke, William Waddell (b. 1883). Kansas City pathologist.

Duke's method. A method for the estimation of bleeding time by observing the time taken for bleeding to cease from a single needle puncture wound in the lobe of the ear when the drop of blood is removed every 30 s with blotting paper. Normal 2–5 min.

Duke-Elder, Sir William Stewart (b. 1898). London ophthalmologist.

Duke-Elder device. *See* STENOPEIC.

Duke-Elder lamp. A lamp fitted with quartz lenses for irradiation of the eye with ultraviolet light.

Dukes, Clement (b. 1845). Rugby physician.

Dukes' disease, Filatov–Dukes disease. Fourth disease; formerly believed to be intermediate between scarlet fever, measles and rubella, but regarded no longer as a separate entity.

Dukes, Cuthbert Esquire (b. 1890). London pathologist.

Dukes' classification. A classification of rectal carcinoma.

dulcin, dulcine (**dul**·sin, **dul**·seen). Sucrol, phenetidinurea, $C_2H_5OC_6H_4NHCONH_2$. A compound used as a sweetening agent; it is moderately soluble in water, and about 200 times as sweet as sugar. [L *dulcis* sweet.]

dulcite, dulcitol, dulcose (**dul**·site, **dul**·sit·ol, **dul**·koze). $CH_2OH(CHOH)_4CH_2OH$, a hexahydric crystalline alcohol, isomeric with mannitol, but optically inactive. It occurs in species of *Euonymus,* and is used as a sweetening agent. [see prec.]

dull (dul). Not clear or sharp (e.g. of mind, pain, sound and, particularly, of percussion sound). Muffled. [ME *dul.*]

dullness (**dul**·nes). Lessened resonance of percussion sound; the sound obtained when percussion is made over a nonvibratory solid part. **Postcardial dullness.** The dullness of sound evident when percussion is made on the back over the heart. **Shifting dullness.** Dullness on percussion over the abdominal cavity which persists but shifts in level as the patient is rolled from one side to the other. The sound is a sign of the presence of free fluid in the cavity. **Tympanic dullness.** Resonance of a dull and poor quality. **Wooden dullness.** Resonance as if percussion were being made on wood. [see prec.]

See also: GROCCO.

Dulong, Pierre Louis (b. 1785). French physicist and chemist.

Dulong and Petit law. The atomic heats (i.e. atomic weight multiplied by specific heat) of almost all solid elements are constant. Exceptions are elements of low atomic weight and high melting point.

Dumas cap. An occlusive cap, used for contraceptive purposes.

dumb (dum). Deprived of the faculty of speech. [AS.]

dumb-bell (**dum**·bel). *See* SCHAFER.

dumbness (**dum**·ness). Mutism; a state of inability to speak. [AS.]

dummy (**dum**·e). In dentistry, a dummy tooth; one which replaces a natural tooth. [AS *dumb.*]

dumping (**dum**·ping). The rapid emptying of a vessel. **Jejunal dumping.** A condition which may appear after gastrojejunostomy; the contents of the stomach pass rapidly into the jejunum. [ME *dumpen* to throw down.]

Dunbar, William Phillips (b. 1863). American physician in Hamburg.

Dunbar's serum. A serum prepared against pollen for treatment of hay fever.

Duncan, Charles Henry (b. 1880). New York physician.

Duncan's method. Autotherapy.

Duncan, James Matthews (b. 1826). Edinburgh and London obstetrician.

Duncan's folds. The peritoneal folds associated with the uterus.

Duncan's position. A low insertion of the placenta, causing it to be delivered maternal surface first.

Duncan's ventricle. The cavum septi pellucidi; the 5th ventricle.

Dungern, Emil Adolf Wilhelm Joseph, Baron von (b. 1867). Ludwigshafen physician.

von Dungern's test. *See* TEST FOR CANCER.

Dunham, Edward Kellogg (b. 1860). New York bacteriologist and pathologist.

Dunham's clearing agent. A mixture of 4 parts white oil of thyme and 1 part clove oil, used in histology to soften and clear celloidin sections.

Dunham's peptone, or solution. A 1 per cent solution of peptone in 0.5 per cent saline, used in the indole test for *Bacterium coli.*

Dunham, Henry Kennon (b. 1872). Cincinnati physician.

Dunham's fans. Pyramidal or triangular areas of increased density seen in the chest radiograph of a silicotic patient. They are formed by the lung tissue as a reaction to a foreign body, i.e. silica. In the dust removed from a segment of silicotic lung, the silica is found in its unchanged state.

Dunhill, Sir Thomas Peel (b. 1876). London surgeon.

Dunhill's forceps, an English artery forceps for use in thyroid operations.

Dunn, Naughton (b. 1884). Birmingham orthopaedist.

Dunn's arthrodesis, or operation. Fusion of the midtarsal and subastragaloid joints, with backward displacement of the foot relative to the astragalus, in poliomyelitis.

Dunn syringe. A type of hypodermic syringe used for extensive tissue infiltration; the barrel is re-filled from a reservoir of solution as the piston is pulled back, without the necessity of removing the needle from the site of injection or of separating the syringe from the needle.

Du Noüy, Pierre Lecomte (b. 1883). Paris physicist.

Du Noüy balance. A balance in which the unknown force produces torsion in a stretched wire. This may be calibrated with respect to angular deflexion, or the instrument used in a null method, by application of a known restoring couple.

Du Noüy phenomenon. The demonstration that the surface tension of blood serum is only temporarily reduced for a short time by the addition of sodium oleate.

duodenal (dew·o·**de**·nal). Relating or belonging to the duodenum. **Duodenal papilla.** *See* PAPILLA. **Duodenal recess.** *See* RECESS.

duodenectomy (**dew**·o·de·**nek**'·to·me). Partial or total excision of the duodenum. [duodenum, Gk *ektome* a cutting out.]

duodenitis (**dew**·o·de·**ni**'·tis). A condition of inflammation of the duodenum. [duodenum, Gk *-itis* inflammation.]

duodenocholangeitis, duodenocholangitis (dew·o·**de**·no·ko·lan·je·**i**'·tis, du·o·**de**·no·ko·lan·**ji**'·tis). A condition of inflammation of the duodenum and the bile duct. [duodenum, cholangitis.]

duodenocholecystostomy (dew·o·**de**·no·ko·**le**·sis·**tos**'·to·me). The surgical establishment of a communication between the duodenum and the gall bladder. [duodenum, cholecystostomy.]

duodenocholedochotomy (dew·o·**de**·no·ko·le·do·**kot**'·o·me). Surgical incision first of the duodenum and secondly of the bile duct.

duodenocolic (dew·o·**de**·no·**kol**'·ik). Relating to the duodenum and colon.

duodenocystostomy (dew·o·**de**·no·sis·**tos**'·to·me). Surgical establishment of a communication between the duodenum and the urinary bladder. [duodenum, cystostomy.]

duodeno-enterostomy (dew·o·de·no·en·ter·**os**'·to·me). Surgical establishment of a communication between the duodenum and a lower portion of the small intestine. [duodenum, enterostomy.]

duodenogram (dew·o·**de**·no·gram). A radiograph of the duodenum. [duodenum, Gk *gramma* a writing.]

duodenohepatic (dew·o·**de**·no·hep·**at**'·ik). Referring to the duodenum and the liver. [duodenum, Gk *hepar* liver.]

duodeno-ileostomy (dew·o·**de**·no·i·le·**os**'·to·me). The surgical establishment of a communication between the duodenum and the ileum. [duodenum, ileostomy.]

duodenojejunal (dew·o·**de**·no·jej·**oon**'·al). Relating or belonging to the duodenum and the jejunum.

duodenojejunostomy (dew·o·**de**·no·jej·oon·**os**'·to·me). The surgical establishment of a communication between the duodenum and the jejunum. [duodenum, jejunostomy.]

duodenopancreatectomy (dew·o·**de**·no·**pan**·kre·at·**ek**'·to·me). Pancreatoduodenectomy.

duodenorenal (dew·o·**de**·no·**re**'·nal). Referring to the duodenum and the kidney. [duodenum, L *ren* kidney.]

duodenorrhaphy (**dew**·o·de·**nor**'·af·e). The surgical suturing of the duodenum. [duodenum, Gk *rhaphe* suture.]

duodenoscopy (**dew**·o·de·**nos**'·ko·pe). Inspection of the duodenum with an endoscope. [duodenum, Gk *skopein* to watch.]

duodenostomy (**dew**·o·de·**nos**'·to·me). The surgical establishment of a permanent artificial opening (duodenal fistula) in the duodenum through the wall of the abdomen. [duodenum, Gk *stoma* mouth.]

duodenotomy (**dew**·o·de·**not**'·o·me). The operation of cutting into the duodenum. [duodenum, Gk *temnein* to cut.]

duodenum [NA] (dew·o·**de**·num). Name applied to the first 20-25 cm (8-10 in) of the small intestine extending from the pylorus to the beginning of the jejunum. It consists of a first [pars superior (NA)], second [pars descendens], third [pars horizon alis inferior (NA)] and fourth [pars ascendens (NA)] part and forms a loop round the head of the pancreas. In man it is retroperitoneal except at its beginning. [L *duodeni* twelve each, being in length the width of twelve fingers.]

duodenum, suspensory muscle of the [musculus suspensorius duodeni (NA)]. A muscle band, partly striped and partly unstriped, attaching the terminal part of the duodenum and the duodenojejunal flexure to the right crus of the diaphragm.

duoparental (**dew**·o·par·**en**'·tal). Derived from 2 sex elements or from 2 parents. [L *duo* two, *parere* to give birth.]

duovirus (**dew**·o·vi·rus). *See* ROTAVIRUS.

Duplay, Emmanuel Simon (b. 1836). Paris surgeon.

Duplay's bursitis. Subacromial bursitis.

Duplay's operations. Operations for plastic reconstruction of the urethra in epispadias and hypospadias.

Duplay's syndrome. Limited abduction and rotation of the area due to fibrositis at the shoulder; frozen shoulder.

duplication (dew·plik·**a**·shun). The result of a chromosome structural change causing doubling of part of the genome. [L *duplicare* to double.]

duplicature (**dew**·plik·at·ewr). A fold, as of a membrane upon itself. [L *duplicare* to double.]

duplicitas (dew·**plis**·it·as). Congenital malformation caused by the doubling at one or the other pole. **Duplicitas anterior.** A monster with double head and upper parts of the body. **Duplicitas asymmetros.** Conjoined twins of which one is parasitic on the other. **Duplicitas posterior.** A monster the pelvic region of which and the dependent parts are doubled. **Duplicitas symmetros.** Conjoined twins of equal development. [L doubleness.]

dupp (dup). In auscultation, the term expressive of the second sound heard at the apex of the heart. It is higher in pitch and shorter than the first sound, lubb. [onomat.]

Dupré (fl. 1699). Paris surgeon.

Dupré's muscle. Articularis genu muscle.

Dupré, Ernest Pierre (b. 1862). Paris physician.

Dupré's syndrome. Meningismus.

Dupuy-Dutemps, Louis (b. 1871). Paris ophthalmologist.

Dupuy-Dutemps operation. 1. Blepharoplasty. 2. For blocked nasopharyngeal duct: resection of the bone medial to the lacrimal sac, with incision of the underlying nasal mucosa into 2 flaps which are sutured to the 2 edges of a vertical incision into the sac.

Dupuy-Dutemps phenomenon. In paralysis of the 7th cranial nerve, on attempted closure of the lids when the patient is looking downwards, the upper lid on the paralysed side elevates.

Dutemps and Cestan sign. Cestan's sign.

Dupuytren, Guillaume, Baron (b. 1777). Paris surgeon.

Dupuytren's canals. Venous spaces in the diploë of the cranial bones.

Dupuytren's classification of burns. 1st degree, reddening of the skin; 2nd degree, blistering of skin; 3rd degree, partial skin destruction; 4th degree, total skin destruction; 5th degree, charring of muscle; 6th degree, charring of bone.

Dupuytren's contraction, or contracture. Palmar contraction; a thickening of the palmar fascia causing slow flexion deformity of the fingers and usually mainly affecting the ring and little fingers. It may sometimes be associated with alcoholic cirrhosis.

Dupuytren's false contraction. A condition simulating Dupuytren's contraction, due to sepsis in the palm.

Dupuytren's egg-shell crackling. The crackling that is felt when a medullary sarcoma of bone is palpated.

Dupuytren's fascia. The palmar fascia.

Dupuytren's finger. Dupuytren's contraction (see above).

Dupuytren's fracture. A fracture dislocation of the ankle in which the astragalus is displaced upward between the tibia and fibula.

Dupuytren's hydrocele. Bilocular hydrocele of the tunica vaginalis testis.

Dupuytren's operation. Removal of the arm at the shoulder joint.

Dupuytren's paste. A caustic made of arsenic trioxide, gum and calomel.

Dupuytren's phlegmon. Cellulitis in the anterior triangle of the neck.

Dupuytren's powder. A caustic powder consisting of arsenic trioxide and calomel; it is not in general use now.

Dupuytren's sign. Telescoping of the femur in congenital dislocation of the hip.

Dupuytren's tourniquet. A metal compressor for the abdominal aorta.

dura (dewr·ah). The dura mater.

dura mater [dura mater encephali (NA)] (dew·rah ma·ter). The outermost meninx of the brain, thick, dense, and inelastic. It lines the interior of the skull and is two-layered, meningeal and endosteal. **Spinal dura mater [dura mater spinalis (NA)].** The meninx surrounding the spinal cord like a kind of loose sheath; it represents the meningeal layer of the dura mater of the brain. [L hard mother.]

dural (dewr·al). Relating to the dura mater.

duralumin (dewr·al·ew·min). A hard, strong and resistant alloy of aluminium and copper from which surgical appliances are made. [L *durus* hard, aluminium.]

duramatral (dewr·ah·ma·tral). Relating to the dura mater.

Duran-Reynals, Francisco (b. 1899). Yale bacteriologist.

Duran-Reynals factor. Spreading factor. *See* FACTOR.

Durand, Joseph (b. 1876). Lyons physician.

Durand-Nicolas-Favre disease. Lymphopathia venereum.

Durand, P. (b. 1895). French physician in Tunis.

Durand's disease. *See* DURAND'S VIRUS (below).

Durand's virus. A virus, from 36 to 57 nm in size, isolated during yellow-fever investigations in Tunis in 1940. Its significance is under investigation.

Laigret-Durand vaccine. A living vaccine, dried, suspended in egg yolk and in olive oil. One two-hundredth part of the brain of an infected rat is injected against endemic typhus in Tunisia.

durango (dew·rang·go). *Centrurus exlicauda*, a scorpion found in Mexico.

duraplasty (dewr·ah·plas·te). Any reconstructive operation on the dura mater, e.g. grafting. [dura mater, Gk *plassein* to mould.]

durene (dewr·een). Symmetrical tetramethylbenzene, $C_6H_2(CH_3)_4$. A colourless solid hydrocarbon occurring in coal tar, or prepared from toluene.

Duret, Henri (b. 1849). Paris and Lille neurosurgeon.

Duret's nuclear arteries. The ganglionic branches of the posterior cerebral artery.

Duret's lesion. Bleeding in the mid-brain and 4th ventricle following closed head injury.

Duret's rivers. Subarachnoid spaces leading into the subarachnoid cisternae.

Durham, Arthur Edward (b. 1834). London surgeon.

Durham's trocar. Piloting trocar; a handled trocar for the insertion of a jointed Durham's tracheotomy tube.

Durham's tube. A jointed (lobster-tailed) tracheotomy tube.

Durham, Herbert Edward (b. 1866). English bacteriologist.

Durham's peptone water. Peptone-water culture medium.

Durham's tube. A narrow-gauged tube which is placed with the opening downwards in a test-tube containing coloured fermentable sugar solutions; any gas that is formed fills this tube and displaces the coloured sugar solution. It is used to study gas production by the organisms inoculated.

duritis (dewr·i·tis). Pachymeningitis; an inflamed condition of the dura mater. [dura mater, Gk *-itis* inflammation.]

duro-arachnitis (dewr·o·ar·ak·ni'·tis). An inflamed condition of the dura mater and the arachnoid mater. [dura mater, arachnoid, Gk *-itis* inflammation.]

durosarcoma (dewr·o·sar·ko'·mah). Meningioma. [dura mater, sarcoma.]

Duroziez, Paul Louis (b. 1826). Paris physician.

Duroziez's disease. Congenital mitral stenosis.

Duroziez's murmur, or sign. Traube's phenomenon; in conditions associated with high arterial pulse pressure (aortic incompetence), a systolic murmur is heard over the femoral or other large artery when the vessel is compressed. If compression just distal to the stethoscope is increased to a critical level, a diastolic murmur is also heard.

Dusart, Lucien O. (fl. 1850-1890). Paris pharmacist.

Dusart's syrup. A syrup very similar to syrup of calcium lactophosphate; a tonic.

Dusseau's injector. A trocar and cannula for injection of cylindrical hormone pellets.

dust (dust). Fine powder or dry particles light enough to be raised and conveyed by the wind. **Blood dust.** Haemoconia. **Chromatin dust.** Tiny red granules that may be present at the periphery of stained erythrocytes. **Ear dust.** Otoconia. **Luminous dust.** *See* ENTOPIC PHENOMENON (under PHENOMENON). [AS.]

See also: MUELLER (J.).

dusting-powder (dust·ing·pow·der). 1. A name most commonly applied to preparations having talc, kaolin and zinc oxide as a basis, and used for application to the body after bathing. 2. Any medicament applied to the skin or mucous membranes in a finely powdered form. [AS *dust*, powder.]

Dutton, Joseph Everett (b. 1877). Liverpool pathologist.

Dutton's disease. An obsolete term applied to both trypanosomiasis and relapsing fever.

Duval, Charles Warren (b. 1876). New Orleans pathologist.

Duval's bacillus. *Shigella sonnei.*

Duval, Mathias Marie (b. 1844). Paris anatomist.

Duval's plaited or tufted convolution. The dentate gyrus.

Duval's nucleus. An islet of multipolar nerve cells in the reticular formation of the medulla oblongata.

Duval, Pierre (b. 1874). Paris surgeon.

Duval's forceps. A lung-holding forceps.

Duval's operation. Exposure of the heart by removal of costal cartilage.

Duval-Barasty operation. Splitting of the sternum and incision of the diaphragm to explore the pericardium.

Duverney, Joseph Guichard (b. 1648). Paris anatomist.

Duverney's fissure, or incisura. A fissure in the cartilage of the external ear at the base of the tragus.

Duverney's foramen. The opening into the lesser sac of the peritoneum.

Duverney's glands. The greater vestibular glands.

Duverney's muscle. The portion of the orbicularis oculi muscle arising from the fascia covering the lacrimal sac.

dwarf (dwawf). A person of deficient stature. There may be no other abnormal features, or the less than normal growth may be associated with infantilism or deformities. **Achondroplastic dwarf.** A congenital dwarf with a normal trunk and large head, but with short limbs due to a disturbance of bone formation. **Asexual dwarf.** A dwarf with failure of sexual development. **Ateleiotic dwarf.** A dwarf of normal intelligence, and physically proportionate, but in miniature, with childish features and exhibiting primary hereditary infantilism. **Chondrodystrophic dwarf.** Achondroplastic dwarf (see above). **Deformed dwarf.** A dwarf with deformities due to rickets or other causes. **Hypophyseal dwarf.** Pituitary dwarf (see below). **Infantile dwarf.** A dwarf with marked retardation of physical, mental and sexual development. **Micromelic dwarf.** Achondroplastic dwarf (see above). **Normal dwarf.** A dwarf of retarded stature, but without other defects. **Ovarian dwarf.** A small under-developed female without ovaries. **Phocomelic dwarf.** Achondroplastic dwarf (see above). **Physiological dwarf.** Normal dwarf (see above). **Pituitary dwarf.** A dwarf of the Lévi-Lorain type, due to hypopituitarism. **Primordial dwarf.** Normal dwarf (see above). **Pure dwarf.** A dwarf of short stature but normal proportions. **Rachitic dwarf.** A dwarf due to severe and prolonged rickets. **Renal dwarf.** A dwarf due to renal infantilism with rickets secondary to chronic interstitial nephritis. **Sexual dwarf.** A dwarf with normal development of the sexual organs. **True dwarf.** A normally developed but small individual. [AS *dweorge.*]

See also: BRISSAUD, PALTAUF.

dwarfism (dwawf·izm). 1. The condition of sub-normal height below 1.25 m (about 50 in). 2. A term including various conditions of which lack of height is only one feature. **Amsterdam dwarfism.** De Lange syndrome. **Camptomelic dwarfism.** Congenital dwarfism with bent limb bones, especially the tibia. **Diatrophic dwarfism.** Short limbs usually associated with talipes; later kyphoscoliosis and dislocation of hip or knee may develop, followed by ossification in the external ear. **Metatropic dwarfism.** Short limbs, normal face and severe early kyphoscoliosis. **Polydystrophic dwarfism** (of Maroteaux and Lamy). A syndrome characterized by coarse features, lumbar kyphosis and genu valgum. Chondroitin sulphate is excreted in the urine. **Senile (pituitary) dwarfism.** Progeria. [see prec.]

See also: LÉVI, LORAIN, PALTAUF.

dwi-manganese (dwi·mang·an·eez). Name given by Mendeléeff to the element predicted in the Periodic Table by the vacant space two below that occupied by manganese. It was subsequently isolated and named *rhenium*. [Sanskrit *dwi* two, manganese.]

dyad (di·ad). 1. A bivalent radical or element. 2. One of the groups of 2 chromosomes formed by the division of a tetrad. 3. In morphology, a secondary unit composed of an aggregate of monads. 4. A pair or couple. 5. Consisting of 2. [Gk *dyas* the number 2.]

dyaster (di·as·ter). Amphiaster; in karyokinesis, 2 asters joined by a spindle. [Gk *dyas* the number 2, *aster* star.]

Dydrogesterone BP 1973 (di·dro·jes·ter·one). 9β,10α-pregna-4,6-diene-3,20-dione; a synthetic oral progestogen which reproduces the normal physiological changes of the endometrium when suitably primed. It seldom prevents ovulation when given in the first half of the menstrual cycle, though usually prevents dysmenorrhoea from taking place in the cycle in which it is given.

dye (di). 1. Dyestuff; any substance, usually in solution, which can be applied to a material in such a way as to colour it, the colour not subsequently washing out or fading. Originally organic colouring matters obtained from natural sources, nowadays dyes are synthesized artificially for particular requirements. Synthetic dyes are used extensively: (*a*) in histology and cytology, which studies are dependent on dyes for differential staining of tissues; (*b*) in bacteriology, for staining of bacteria; (*c*) in dermatology both for diagnosis and surface therapy; and (*d*) in parasitology, for diagnosis and chemotherapy—nearly all modern antimalarials developed from the observation that methylene blue would cure malaria. Also to a less extent in many other branches of medicine; in ophthalmology, for example, dyes are used to stain and thereby visualize corneal ulcers. 2. To colour a material by means of a dyestuff. Cf. STAIN. **Acid dye.** A dye, usually of silk or wool, taken up from an acid dye-bath. **Acridine dye.** Any dye containing the acridine ring; they are yellow or orange basic dyes and include acriflavine and mepacrine. **Azo dye.** Any dyestuff derived from or related to azobenzene; they include methyl orange and Biebrich scarlet. **Basic dye.** A dye, usually of silk or wool, basic in nature and taken up from an alkaline dye-bath. **Diazo dye.** Any dyestuff derived from diazobenzene. **Direct dye.** Substantive dye (see below). **Disazo dye.** Any dyestuff containing 2 azo groups. **Monoazo dye.** Any dyestuff containing only 1 azo group. **Mordant dye.** Any dyestuff which requires that the material be first impregnated with a mordant, the dye then combining with the latter to form a fast *lake*. **Rosaniline dye.** Triphenylmethane dye (see below). **Substantive dye.** Any dye which can be applied to cotton or artificial silk without a mordant. **Triphenylmethane dye.** Any dye derived from or related to triphenylmethane; they include fuchsine, methyl violet and crystal violet. **Triple dye.** A dye containing 1 per cent each of gentian violet, brilliant green and acriflavine. **Vat dye.** Any dye such as indigo which develops its colour on the material by oxidation of the leuco compound with which it has been previously impregnated. **Vital dye.** One used for staining tissues *in situ* during life. [AS *deag.*]

See also: BONNEY.

dyestuff (di·stuf). Any substance capable of colouring another by virtue of chemical or physical combination with the substance coloured. It is usually taken to mean a textile dye. **Indifferent dyestuff.** A dye showing very little selectivity in its staining. **Neutral dyestuff.** A dye that is neither an acid nor a base. [AS *deag*, OFr. *estoffe*.]

Dyflos (di·flos). BP Commission approved name for di-isopropyl phosphorofluoridate; it is used in the treatment of glaucoma.

dying declaration (di·ing dek·lar·a·shun). A statement made by a dying person in connection with a charge which might relate to his own death. At the time the dying person must know that he is dying and believe that he has no hope of living.

dynactinometer (di·nak·tin·om'·et·er). An instrument for measuring the value of photogenic rays. [Gk *dynamis* force, *aktis* ray, meter].

dynameter (di·nam·et·er). Dynamometer.

dynamic (di·nam·ik). Active; pertaining to force in action, as opposed to static. [Gk *dynamis* force.]

dynamics (di·nam·ix). A branch of physics dealing with force and motion. **Vital dynamics.** That concerned with the inherent power and motion of a living organism. [see prec.]

dynamimeter (di·nam·im·et·er). Dynamometer.

dynamo (di·nam·o). A machine for producing electrical energy from mechanical energy. [Gk *dynamis* force.]

dynamogenesis (di·nam·o·jen'·es·is). The production of development of force or energy, muscular, nervous or mental, as a result of associated sensory excitation. [Gk *dynamis* force, *genein* to produce.]

dynamogenic (di·nam·o·jen'·ik). 1. Referring to dynamogenesis or the development of power. 2. Generating or producing force or power, particularly muscular or nervous. 3. Aiding or favourable to the development of power or force. [see prec.]

dynamogeny (di·nam·oj·en·e). Dynamogenesis.

dynamograph (di·nam·o·graf). A dynamometer fitted with a device for the automatic graphic registration of muscular power. [Gk *dynamis* force, *graphein* to record.]

dynamography (di·nam·og·raf·e). 1. The graphic registering of muscular strength by means of a dynamograph. 2. Mechanics. [see prec.]

dynamometer (di·nam·om·et·er). An instrument with which the power of contraction of the muscles can be measured. **Optical dynamometer.** One with which the magnifying power of a lens can be estimated. **Squeeze dynamometer.** A dynamometer with which the strength of the hand grip can be determined. [Gk *dynamis* force, meter.]

dynamometry (di·nam·om·et·re). The use of a dynamometer measuring force. **Vital dynamometry.** The estimation of the force or power inherent in any particular individual. [see prec.]

dynamoneure (di·nam·o·newr). A spinal motor neurone. [Gk *dynamis* force, neurone.]

dynamopathic (di·nam·o·path'·ik). 1. Functional. 2. Having an effect on function. [Gk *dynamis* force, *pathos* suffering.]

dynamophany (di·nam·of·an·e). The release of psychic energy. [Gk *dynamis* power, *phainein* to show.]

dynamophore (di·nam·o·for). Any substance from which the body can derive energy, e.g. food. [Gk *dynamis* force, *pherein* to bear.]

dynamoscope (di·nam·o·skope). A special kind of stethoscope with which the contractions of muscles can be heard. [Gk *dynamis* force, *skopein* to watch.]

dynamoscopy (di·nam·os·ko·pe). 1. Auscultation of muscular contraction with a dynamoscope. 2. The observation of renal function by means of ureteral catheterization. [see prec.]

dynatherm (di·nah·therm). A diathermy apparatus. [Gk *dynamis* force, *therme* heat.]

dyne (dine). A unit of force equal to 10 μN. The force which will accelerate a mass of one gram, one centimetre per second. The megadyne is a million dynes. [Gk *dynamis* force.]

dys-. Greek prefix meaning *bad, difficult.*

dysacousia, dysacousis (dis·ak·oo·se·ah, dis·ak·oo·sis). Difficulty of hearing. [Gk *dys-*, *akouein* to hear.]

dysacousma (dis·ak·oos·mah). A condition in which a sensation of discomfort or pain is experienced when hearing even moderately loud sounds or noises. [see prec.]

dysacusia (dis·ak·ew·ze·ah). Dysacousia.

dysadaptation (dis·ad·ap·ta'·shun). A condition of the eye in which the iris and the retina are unable to accommodate properly to variations in the intensity of light. [Gk *dys-*, adaptation.]

dysadrenia (dis·ad·re·ne·ah). A condition of disordered renal function. [Gk *dys-*, L *ad*, *ren* kidney.]

dysaemia (dis·e·me·ah). Any disease or deteriorated condition of the blood. [Gk *dys-*, *haima* blood.]

dysaesthesia (dis·es·the·ze·ah). 1. Impairment, not to the point of anaesthesia, of any of the senses, particularly the sense of touch. 2. A condition in which pain is attached to any sensation not normally painful, e.g. persistent painfulness of a part that has been lightly touched. 3. An unpleasant sensation, either spontaneous or produced by normally innocuous stimulation. **Auditory dysaesthesia.** Dysacousma. [Gk *dys-*, aesthesis.]

dysaesthetic (dis·es·thet·ik). Referring to or characterized by the presence of dysaesthesia.

dysallilognathia (dis·al·il·og·nath'·e·ah). A condition in which there is disharmony between the size of the upper and lower jaws. [Gk *dys-*, *allos* other, *gnathos* jaw.]

dysanagnosia (dis·an·ag·no'·ze·ah). A variety of dyslexia in which there is inability to recognize certain words. [Gk *dys-*, *anagnosis* reading.]

dysantigraphia (dis·an·te·graf'·e·ah). A form of agraphia, due to a nerve lesion, in which there is inability to copy written or printed matter. [Gk *dys-*, *antigraphein* to write back.]

dysaphe, dysaphia (dis·af·e, dis·af·e·ah). A condition in which there is morbid or disordered sense of touch. [Gk *dys-*, *haphe* touch.]

dysaptation (dis·ap·ta·shun). Dysadaptation.

dysarteriotony (dis·ar·teer·e·ot'·on·e). A state of abnormal blood pressure, i.e. either too high or too low. [Gk *dys-*, *arteria* artery, *tonos* tone.]

dysarthria (dis·ar·thre·ah). Difficulty of articulating words caused by disease of the central nervous system. **Dysarthria literalis.** Stammering. **Dysarthria syllabaris spasmodica.** Stuttering. [Gk *dys-*, *arthroun* to articulate.]

dysarthric (dis·ar·thrik). Referring to or characterized by dysarthria.

dysarthrosis (dis·ar·thro·sis). 1. Any pathological condition of a joint caused by disease, dislocation or deformity, and diminishing the power of movement. 2. Dysarthria. 3. A false joint. [Gk *dys-*, arthrosis.]

dysautonomia (dis·awt·o·no·me·ah). **Familial dysautonomia.** A congenital disorder transmitted by autosomal recessive inheritance. It comprises hyperhidrosis, hypertension, indifference to pain, epilepsy and dysphagia, and death occurs in childhood. (syn. *Riley-Day syndrome.*)

dysbarism (dis·bar·izm). An inclusive term for the effects of a pressure differential between the ambient pressure and the pressure of the dissolved and free gases in living matter. The effects will depend upon whether the external pressure is greater *(hyperbarism)* or less *(hypobarism)* than the internal pressure and upon the speed of development, as in explosive decompression. [Gk *dys-*, *baros* weight.]

dysbasia (dis·ba·se·ah). Any kind of difficulty in walking and particularly that caused by a nerve lesion. **Dysbasia angiosclerotica.** Claudication due to arteriosclerosis of the legs and the resultant pain on walking. **Dysbasia angiospastica, Dysbasia intermittens angiosclerotica.** Intermittent claudication. **Dysbasia lordotica progressiva.** Dystonia musculorum deformans. **Dysbasia neurasthenica intermittens.** Claudication of neurasthenic origin. [Gk *dys-*, *basis* a stepping.]

dysbiotrophy (dis·bi·ot·ro·fe). **Renal dysbiotrophy.** A form of chronic nephritis which occurs without a past history of acute nephritis or other known cause. It may be a cause of uraemia in infants, or renal infantilism and rickets, or high blood pressure in older children. It is assumed to be due to a congenital tissue inferiority of the kidneys. [Gk *dys-*, *bios* life, *trophe* nourishment.]

dysbolism (dis·bol·izm). Disordered metabolism, not necessarily morbid in nature. [Gk *dys-*, metabolism.]

dysboulia (dis·boo·le·ah). 1. Perversion of will. 2. Weakening or impairment of will power. [Gk *dys-*, *boule* will.]

dysboulic (dis·boo·lik). Referring to dysboulia.

dysbulia (dis·bew·le·ah). Dysboulia.

dyscalculia (dis·kal·kew·le'·ah). Difficulty in dealing with numbers. [Gk *dys-*, L *calculare* calculus.]

dyscatabrosis (dis·kat·ah·bro'·sis). Dysphagia. [Gk *dys-*, *katabrosis* a swallowing down.]

dyscataposia (dis·kat·ah·po'·ze·ah). Dysphagia. [Gk *dys-*, *kata*, *posis* a drinking.]

dyscheiria (dis·ki·re·ah). A derangement of sensibility which makes it impossible for a patient to tell on which side of the body he has been touched although sensation apparently is not lost. [Gk *dys-*, *cheir* hand.]

dyschesia, dyschezia (dis·ke·ze·ah). Difficulty or pain in passing faeces. [Gk *dys-*, *chezein* to go to stool.]

dyschiasia, dyschiasis (dis·ki·a·ze·ah, dis·ki·as·is). A condition in which there is disorder of sense localization. [Gk *dys-*, *chi* letter X.]

dyschiria (dis·ki·re·ah). Dyscheiria.

dyschizia (dis·kiz·e·ah). Dyschesia.

dyscholia (dis·ko·le·ah). A disordered or morbid condition of the bile. [Gk *dys-*, *chole* bile.]

dyschondroplasia (dis·kon·dro·pla'·ze·ah). A term for a group of 3 clinical conditions which have in common perverted growth or arrest of growth in the normal endochondral ossification of the long bones. [Gk *dys-*, *chondros* cartilage, *plasis* a forming.]

dyschondrosteosis (dis·kon·dro·ste·o'·sis). Shortened, often curved, distal bones of the extremities. An autosomal dominant condition with Madelung's deformity is called *Léri–Weill's syndrome.* [Gk *dys-*, *chondros* cartilage, *osteon* bone, *-osis* condition.]

dyschroa, dyscroia (dis·kro·ah, dis·kroi·ah). Discoloration of the skin. [Gk *dys-*, *chroma* colour, *chroia* skin.]

dyschromasia (dis·kro·ma·ze·ah). 1. Dyschromatopsia. 2. Dyschromia. [Gk *dys-*, *chroma* colour.]

dyschromatodermia (dis·kro·mat·o·der'·me·ah). Dyschroa. [Gk *dys-*, *chroma* colour, *derma* skin.]

dyschromatope (dis·kro·mat·ope). A person who is affected with dyschromatopsia.

dyschromatopsia (dis·kro·mat·op'·se·ah). Partial colour blindness; a condition in which there is difficulty in distinguishing colours. [Gk *dys-*, *chroma* colour, *opsis* sight.]

dyschromia (dis·kro·me·ah). 1. Any abnormal pigmentation of the skin. 2. Any disease or disorder which affects the pigment cells of the epidermis. [Gk *dys-*, *chroma* colour.]

dyschromodermia (dis·kro·mo·der'·me·ah). Dyschromatodermia.

dyschronism (dis·kron·izm). 1. Separation as to time. 2. Disorder of relation in time. [Gk *dys-*, *chronos* time.]

dyschronous (dis·kron·us). Separate as to time; not synchronous. [see prec.]

dyschylia (dis·ki·le·ah). A disordered condition of the chyle. [Gk *dys-*, *chylos* juice.]

dyscinesia (dis·sin·e·ze·ah). Dyskinesia.

dyscoimesis (dis·koi·me·sis). Dyskoimesis.

dyscoria (dis·kor·e·ah). 1. A condition in which the pupil of the eye is faulty in shape. 2. A state of abnormal reaction of the pupils of the eyes. [Gk *dys-*, *kore* pupil.]

dyscrasia (dis·kra·ze·ah). An old term meaning an abnormal mixture of the 4 humours. Its meaning today is little different from that of disease, but it has a more limited use; it is applied somewhat arbitrarily to developmental and metabolic (in the widest sense) disorders, and it usually excludes infective diseases. **Blood dyscrasia.** A developmental disorder of the blood. **Lymphatic dyscrasia.** A disease of the formative elements of the lymph glands, e.g. Hodgkin's disease, status lymphaticus. [Gk *dys-*, *krasis* a mingling.]

dyscrasic, dyscratic (dis·kra·zik, dis·krat·ik). Relating to a dyscrasia.

dyscrinism (dis·krin·izm). The condition or state which results from alteration or perversion of any glandular secretion, particularly of the endocrine glands. [Gk *dys-*, *krinein* to secrete.]

dysdiadochocinesia, dysdiadochokinesia, dysdiadochokinesis (dis·di·ad·o·ko·sin·e'·ze·ah, dis·di·ad·o·ko·kin·e'·ze·ah, dis·di·ad·o·ko·kin·e'·sis). The slow, clumsy and irregular performance of alternating movements of a limb that characterizes the presence of a lesion of the cerebellum. [Gk *dys-*, diadochokinesis.]

dysdiaemorrhysis (**dis·di·em·or′·is·is**). Sluggishness of the capillary circulation. [Gk *dys-*, *dia*, *haima* blood, *rhysis* a flowing.]

dysdipsia (dis·**dip**·se·ah). The condition of experiencing difficulty in drinking. [Gk *dys-*, *dipsa* thirst.]

dysecoia (dis·e·**koi**·ah). Dysacousia. [Gk *dysekoia* deafness.]

dysembryoma (**dis**·em·bre·**o′**·mah). A tumour originating in embryonic sex cells which have followed an unnatural line of development. [Gk *dys-*, embryoma.]

dysembryoplasia (dis·**em**·bre·o·**pla′**·ze·ah). Malformation occurring prenatally. [Gk *dys-*, embryo, Gk *plassein* to form.]

dysemesia, dysemesis (dis·em·**e**·ze·ah, dis·**em**·es·is). Vomiting associated with retching; painful vomiting. [Gk *dys-*, *emesis* vomiting.]

dysendocrinia (**dis**·en·do·**krin′**·e·ah). Disordered or deficient function of the endocrine glands and the state of illhealth resulting from it. [Gk *dys-*, endocrine.]

dysendocriniasis (dis·**en**·do·krin·**i′**·as·is). A condition in which there is disorder of any of the internal secretory glands or secretions. [see prec.]

dysendocrinism (dis·**en**·do·krin·izm). Dysendocrinia.

dysendocrinosis (dis·**en**·do·krin·**o′**·sis). Dysendocriniasis.

dyseneia (dis·en·**e**·ah). Articulatory defects arising from defects of hearing. [Gk *dysenios* refractory.]

dysenteria (dis·en·**teer**·e·ah). Dysentery. **Dysenteria splenica.** Melaena. [Gk *dys-*, *enteron* intestine.]

dysenteric (dis·en·**ter**·ik). Referring or relating to dysentery.

dysenteriform, dysenterioid (dis·en·**ter**·e·form, dis·en·**ter**·e·oid). Resembling dysentery. [dysentery, Gk *eidos* form.]

dysentery (**dis**·en·ter·e). Inflammation of the colonic mucosa resulting in the passage of blood and mucus with tormina and tenesmus. **Amoebic dysentery.** Infection of the large intestine with *Entamoeba histolytica,* a protozoon which invades the intestinal mucosa and forms ulcers. This pathological condition produces diarrhoea with blood and mucus in the stools. As a rule it is accompanied by considerable abdominal pain, with flatulence, borborygmi and other intestinal disturbances. When the ulceration is prominent in the rectum, tenesmus may occur. Amoebic dysentery exists in two forms: *acute,* with acute symptoms as above, and *chronic,* with alternating diarrhoea and constipation; the latter form may eventually resolve itself into the carrier state where cystic forms of the amoeba are present in great numbers in the stools, a condition often unassociated with symptoms of any kind. The disease can be treated by drugs such as emetine and its compounds, various quinoxyl compounds, arsenicals, e.g. carbarsone, and recently the antibiotics aureomycin and oxytetracycline have been shown to have curative value in association with emetine. Metronidazole is largely effective as a single agent in both intestinal and hepatic amoebiasis. **Asylum dysentery.** Bacillary dysentery (see following). **Bacillary dysentery.** An acute form of dysentery generally occurring in epidemics during the late summer. It is due to various forms of dysentery bacilli *(Shigella)* which attack the mucous membrane of the large intestine, causing necrosis. The symptoms are more acute than those of ameobic dysentery and include acute diarrhoea with blood and mucus in the stools, great abdominal pain, and fever. It may become chronic and last for years. Complications are characteristic and due to absorption of dysenteric toxins; the most striking are iritis and arthritis. Since the introduction of sulphonamides it is seldom any longer a fatal disease: most efficacious are sulphaguanidine and sulphasuxidine. Oral tetracycline and streptomycin plus sulphonamides are very effective. Bacillary dysentery, especially *Shigella shigae* infection, is apt to assume a severe form in small children. **Balantidial dysentery.** Dysentery and diarrhoea associated with the presence of a large ciliate protozoon, *Balantidium coli,* in the faeces. The symptoms resemble those of amoebic dysentery but the balantidia may invade the lymphatic glands. The treatment of balantidiasis by drugs is not satisfactory. **Bilharzial dysentery.** The term applied to the dysenteric syndrome as it occurs in patients infected with *Schistosoma (Bilharzia)* of the 3 species, especially *mansoni.* The eggs of the parasite are found in the faeces as well as in the intestinal lesions. Treatment is efficacious, antimony compounds, especially in the form of sodium antimonyl tartrate, being given intravenously; recently lucanthone hydrochloride by mouth has been attended with a certain degree of success. Niridazole is a highly effective oral drug, but should not be used in the presence of a damaged liver. **Catarrhal dysentery.** A mild form of dysentery mainly characterized by the appearance of mucus in the stools. It is usually associated with mild infections of the dysentery bacilli. The term has, however, dropped out of usage. **Ciliary dysentery, Ciliate dysentery.** Balantidial dysentery (see above). **Flagellate dysentery.** A term somewhat loosely applied to a chronic diarrhoea associated with flagellate intestinal protozoa such as *Trichomonas hominis, Chilomastix mesnili* and *Giardia intestinalis.* The two former are regarded mainly as commensals and not of primary pathological importance; the last-named lives in the small intestine to the mucous surface of which it adheres by means of a sucking disc, giving rise when in large numbers to a lienteric diarrhoea. It occurs most commonly in children and is apt to spread in an epidemic wave. The parasites can be seen both in the adult and cystic stages in the faeces. Mepacrine is a specific. **Fulminant dysentery.** A severe form of dysentery, usually bacillary, which may end fatally. **Japanese dysentery.** The term applied to *Shigella shigae* infections, especially in children in Japan (ekiri). **Malarial dysentery.** The dysenteric syndrome often accompanying severe subtertian malaria *(Plasmodium falciparum).* It is caused by massive multiplication of the trophozoites of this organism in the intestinal capillaries. **Protozoal dysentery.** That due to protozoa, including amoebic dysentery (see above), and giardial dysentery (*see* FLAGELLATE DYSENTERY above). **Schistosomal dysentery.** Bilharzial dysentery (see above). **Scorbutic dysentery.** The dysenteric syndrome occurring in association with scurvy. It may represent a sign of the malady or be the result of superinfection with dysentery bacilli. **Viral dysentery.** Caused by a virus, usually acute watery diarrhoea. [Gk *dys-*, *enteron* intestine.]

See also: FLEXNER, SHIGA, SONNE.

dysepulotic (**dis**·ep·ew·**lot′**·ik). Slowly forming an imperfect cicatrix. [Gk *dys-*, *epoulousthai* to scar over.]

dyserethism (dis·**er**·eth·izm). A condition in which there is only slow response to stimulation. [Gk *dys-*, *erethizein* to irritate.]

dysergasia (dis·er·**ga**·ze·ah). A state of mind characterized by hallucinations, delirium and other phases of disorientation, based on cerebral instability; in mild cases neurasthenic reactions are the main signs (Meyer). [Gk *dys-*, *ergon* work.]

dysergastic (dis·er·**gas**·tik). Referring to dysergasia.

dysergasy (dis·er·**ga**·ze). Dysergasia.

dysergia (dis·**er**·je·ah). A condition in which there is inharmonious action between the muscles which effect any particular voluntary movement. The cause is irregularity of the efferent nerve impulses. [Gk *dys-*, *ergon* work.]

dysfunction (dis·**fungk**·shun). A state of abnormal, incomplete or impaired function of an organ. **Papillary muscle dysfunction.** Weakness of contraction of a papillary muscle, usually the posterior one of the mitral valve, which may occur with myocardial ischaemia or after infarction, leading to regurgitation through the valve. [Gk *dys-*, function.]

dysgalactia (dis·gal·**ak**·te·ah). A state of disordered or impaired secretion of milk, or entire stoppage of it. [Gk *dys-*, *gala* milk.]

dysgammaglobulinaemia (**dis**·gam·ah·**glob**·ewl·in·**e′**·me·ah). Deficient quantity or function of one or two of the main types of serum immunoglobulins. [Gk *dys-*, gamma, globulin, Gk *haima* blood.]

dysgenesis (dis·**jen**·es·is). 1. Impairment or loss of the power to procreate. 2. A condition in which the offspring of a crossbreed are fertile when bred with either of the parent races but sterile when bred among themselves. 3. Lack of proper development. **Gonadal dysgenesis.** Incomplete, defective formation of the gonads. *Mixed gonadal dysgenesis* is a form of intersexuality where one gonad is represented by a streak of connective tissue and the other by an ill-formed testis; this is often associated with 45,X/46,XY mixoploidy. *Pure gonadal dysgenesis* is a condition characterized by female appearance, primary amenorrhoea, lack of development of secondary sex characteristics, infantile female internal genitalia (uterus and tubes), lack of gonads but with normal height and none of the somatic malformations of Turner's syndrome; this is usually associated with a normal male or a normal female karyotype and, more rarely, with mixoploidy and/or structural aberrations of the sex chromosomes. **Ovarian dysgenesis.** Incomplete, defective formation of the ovaries. It is often found in individuals with anomalies of the sex chromosomes. Two syndromes can be distinguished: ovarian dysgenesis with short stature and webbing of the neck or Turner's syndrome, and ovarian dysgenesis with short stature but without webbing of the neck. Individuals with the latter syndrome lack the somatic anomalies of the former and are more often mixoploid (45,X/46,XX) or heterozygous for a structural abnormality of the X chromosome than monosomic for the X chromosome (45,X). [Gk *dys-*, *genein* to produce.]

dysgenetic (dis·jen·**et**·ik). Showing the property of disorderly growth. [Gk *dys-*, *genein* to produce.]

dysgenic (dis·**jen**·ik). 1. Referring to dysgenesis. 2. Term applied to factors which have a detrimental effect on the mental and physical qualities of the race. [see prec.]

dysgenics (dis·**jen**·ix). The science which deals with the effects of marriage between individuals of bad or defective heredity. [Gk *dys-*, *genein* to produce.]

dysgenitalism (dis·**jen**·it·al·izm). Any condition which results from defect or abnormality of the organs of generation, e.g. eunuchism. [Gk *dys-*, genitalia.]

dysgenopathy (dis·jen·**op**·ath·e). Any defect, disorder or impairment of physical development. [Gk *dys-*, *genein* to produce, *pathos* suffering.]

dysgerminoma (dis·jer·min·**o**'·mah). Disgerminoma; a malignant tumour of the testicle or ovary originating in cells which have remained undifferentiated to either the male or the female type. [Gk *dys-*, L *germen* germ, Gk *-oma* tumour.]

dysgeusia (dis·**gew**·ze·ah). Abnormality, impairment or perversion of the sense of taste. [Gk *dys-*, *geusis* taste.]

dysglandular (dis·**glan**·dew·lar). Relating to or caused by any abnormality or disorder in the action and functioning of a gland, particularly to deficiency or excess in the internal secretions of a gland or glands. [Gk *dys-*, gland.]

dysglycaemia (dis·gli·**se**·me·ah). Any abnormality of blood-sugar metabolism. [Gk *dys-*, *glykys* sweet, *haima* blood.]

dysgnosia (dis·**no**·ze·ah). 1. A state of disordered function of the intellect. 2. Any intellectual anomaly. [Gk *dys-*, gnosia.]

dysgonesis (dis·go·**ne**·sis). A state of disordered function of the organs of generation. [Gk *dys-*, *gone* seed.]

dysgonic (dis·**gon**·ik). Term applied to bacterial cultures which grow only sparsely on culture material. [see prec.]

dysgrammatism (dis·**gram**·at·izm). A state of difficulty in the proper use of words, caused by disease of the cerebrum. [Gk *dys-*, *gramma* letter.]

dysgraphia (dis·**graf**·e·ah). 1. Writers' cramp. 2. Difficulty in writing due to the existence of a brain lesion. The condition is not as severe as that of agraphia. [Gk *dys-*, *graphein* to write.]

dyshaematopoiesis (dis·**he**·mat·o·poi·**e**'·sis). Imperfection or defect in the blood-forming mechanism. [Gk *dys-*, haematopoiesis.]

dyshaphia (dis·**haf**·e·ah). A condition in which there is morbid or disordered sense of touch. [Gk *dys-*, *haphe* touch.]

dyshepatia (dis·hep·a·she·ah). Abnormal or incomplete functioning of the liver. **Lipogenic dyshepatia.** Disorder of the liver in children caused by excess of fat in their diet. [Gk *dys-*, *hepar* liver.]

dyshidrosis (dis·**hid**·ro·sis). 1. A disturbance of the sweating mechanism. 2. Pompholyx; cheiropompholyx: an acute or subacute vesicular or bullous eruption, symmetrical in distribution, affecting the hands and/or feet, representative of a definite type of cutaneous reaction, and characterized by numerous itching vesicles arising on skin which is not erythematous. Bullae may be formed during the course of the eruption. Whimster (1950) has suggested that true dyshidrosis may arise in conditions of excessive heat, or as a complication of an acute fever, whilst the term pompholyx (Hutchinson) should be reserved for a similar but eczematous type of reaction due to other causes such as emotion, fungous infections or, rarely, to drugs or exogenous allergens. **Trichophytic dyshidrosis.** Pompholyx arising during the course of a *Trichophyton* infection. [Gk *dys-*, *hidrosis* a sweating.]

dyshydrosis (dis·hi·**dro**·sis). Dyshidrosis.

dyshypophysia, dyshypophysism (dis·**hi**·po·**fiz**'·e·ah, dis·hi·**pof**'·is·izm). Dyspituitarism. [Gk *dys-*, hypophysis.]

dysidrosis (dis·**id**·ro·sis). Dyshidrosis.

dysimmunity (dis·im·**ew**·nit·e). Wrongly directed or irregular immunity. [Gk *dys-*, immunity.]

dysinsulinism, dysinsulinosis (dis·**in**·sew·lin·izm, dis·**in**·sew·lin·**o**'·sis). A condition in which disordered activity of the interalveolar cell-islets (islets of Langerhans) of the pancreas causes excess or deficiency in the secretion of insulin. [Gk *dys-*, insulin, Gk *-osis* condition.]

dyskeratosis (dis·ker·at·**o**'·sis). 1. Abnormal cornification of the cells of the epidermis. 2. Premature or embryonic keratinization of epidermal cells. The abnormality may be of the benign type, as seen in Darier's disease, or malignant, in which there is individual cell keratinization, as in Bowen's disease and squamous-cell carcinoma. **Dyskeratosis congenita.** A rare congenital anomaly in which may be noted areas of depigmented atrophic skin, areas of reticular, bluish-grey pigmentation, chronic atrophic acrodermatitis of the hands and feet, dystrophy or absence of the nails, absence of hair on some areas, and leucoplakia of the tongue and buccal mucosa. **Hereditary benign intra-epithelial dyskeratosis.** A genetically-determined dyskeratosis of the oral and ocular epithelium. [Gk *dys-*, *keras* horn, *-osis* condition.]

dyskesis (**dis**·ke·sis). The premature termination of pregnancy from any cause. [Gk *dys-*, *kesis* pregnancy.]

dyskinesia (dis·kin·e·ze·ah). 1. Impairment of voluntary motion, causing movements that are incomplete or only partial. 2. Involuntary movement (incorrect usage). **Dyskinesia algera.** A hysterical condition in which active movements cause pain but gentle movements can be performed. **Biliary dyskinesia.** Functional spasm affecting the ampullary fibres (sphincter of Oddi) in the terminal part of the bile duct. **Dyskinesia intermittens.** Intermittent limping caused by faulty circulation inducing disability. **Occupational dyskinesia.** Occupational neurosis. **Uterine dyskinesia.** A sensation of pain in the uterus on movement, the result of a displacement. [Gk *dys-*, *kinesis* movement.]

dyskinetic (dis·kin·**et**·ik). Referring to dyskinesia.

dyskoimesis (dis·koi·**me**·sis). A condition in which there is difficulty in getting to sleep. [Gk *dys-*, *koimesis* sleeping.]

dyslalia (dis·**lal**·e·ah). Difficulty in utterance or speaking caused by abnormality in the tongue or other external organs of speech (Kussmaul). [Gk *dys-*, *lalein* to babble like a child.]

dyslexia (dis·**lex**·e·ah). Difficulty in reading (innate or acquired); more precisely, difficulty in dealing with words. As a part of a learning disorder, two varieties are recognized: (1) primary or developmental (specific) dyslexia, and (2) secondary, as when resulting from minimal brain damage. The accepted definition of developmental dyslexia promulgated by The World Federation of Neurology (1968) is: "A disorder manifested by difficulty in learning to read despite conventional instruction, adequate intelligence and socio-cultural opportunity. It is dependent upon fundamental cognitive disabilities which are frequently of constitutional origin." Acquired dyslexia is part of an aphasia due to a brain-lesion occurring in a literate adult. [Gk *dys-*, *lexis* word.]

dyslochia (dis·**lo**·ke·ah). An abnormal condition of the lochia, e.g.

the cessation of the lochial discharge before the normal time. [Gk *dys-*, lochia.]

dyslogia (dis·**lo**·je·ah). 1. Impairment of the faculty or power of reasoning. 2. Inability to express ideas in words. [Gk *dys-*, *logos* discourse.]

dyslysin (dis·**li**·sin). $C_{24}H_{36}O_3$, a substance which appears in the decomposition of the bile acids; it is an anhydride of cholic acid. [Gk *dys-*, *lysis* a loosing.]

dysmasesia, dysmasesis (dis·mas·e·se·ah, dis·mas·e·sis). Difficulty in mastication. [Gk *dys-*, *masesis* a chewing.]

dysmegalopsia (dis·meg·al·**op**'·se·ah). Dysmetropsia. [Gk *dys-*, *megas* large, *opsis* appearance.]

dysmenorrhoea (dis·men·o·**re**'·ah). Pain occurring in the back and lower abdomen at or about the time of the menses. **Acquired dysmenorrhoea.** *See* SECONDARY DYSMENORRHOEA (below). **Congenital dysmenorrhoea.** Spasmodic dysmenorrhoea (see below). **Congestive dysmenorrhoea.** A condition of secondary dysmenorrhoea caused by pelvic congestion arising out of any disease which produces an increased blood supply to the pelvis. **Essential dysmenorrhoea.** Spasmodic dysmenorrhoea (see below). **Functional dysmenorrhoea.** Pain beginning with or exacerbated by mental anxiety or disturbance; psychogenic dysmenorrhoea. **Inflammatory dysmenorrhoea.** *See* SECONDARY DYSMENORRHOEA (below). **Dysmenorrhoea intermenstrualis.** Mittelschmertz: pain occurring at the time of ovulation. **Mechanical dysmenorrhoea.** Obstructive dysmenorrhoea (see below). **Membranous dysmenorrhoea.** An uncommon form of spasmodic dysmenorrhoea which is accompanied by the passing of a cast of the uterine cavity. **Obstructive dysmenorrhoea.** Dysmenorrhoea caused by the impeding of the passage of the products of menstruation. It may be real, as with a congenitally occluded cervix horn or of a bicornate uterus, or relative, when the calibre of the genital passage is normal but the products do not appear to be able to pass through easily: also known as *mechanical dysmenorrhoea.* **Ovarian dysmenorrhoea.** Usually applied to congestive pain in the premenstruum. **Primary dysmenorrhoea.** That occurring within a year or two of puberty in patients where there is no obvious pathological cause. **Psychogenic dysmenorrhoea.** Functional dysmenorrhoea (see above). **Secondary dysmenorrhoea.** Dysmenorrhoea occurring when there has been little or no pain until some disease has occurred in the pelvis; it is commonly associated with pelvic inflammation, endometritis and fibroids. *Inflammatory* and *acquired dysmenorrhoea* are secondary conditions of this nature. **Spasmodic dysmenorrhoea.** Pain occurring just before or at the commencement of the menstrual flow, increasing for about 8 h and then subsiding. It is not usually associated with any gross pelvic pathological condition but is said to be due to or associated with a pinhole os, under-development of the uterus, defective polarity of the latter, or small clots being extruded through the os; for this reason it is sometimes known as *congenital dysmenorrhoea.* [Gk *dys-*, *men* month, *rhein* to flow.]

dysmerogenesis (dis·mer·o·**jen**'·es·is). Division into dissimilar parts. [Gk *dys-*, *meros* part, *genein* to produce.]

dysmetria (dis·**met**·re·ah). 1. A form of dysergia in which there is inability to measure correctly the distance involved in any muscular act, e.g. in stretching the arm out to pick up an object the hand will overshoot the mark. 2. Disturbance of the power to arrest muscular movement at the point desired. [Gk *dys-*, *metron* measure.]

dysmetropsia (dis·met·**rop**·se·ah). Inability to judge correctly by sight the size or the measure of an object. [Gk *dys-*, *metron* measure, *opsis* sight.]

dysmimia (dis·**mim**·e·ah). Defect in ability to use gestures or signs to express thoughts; lack of the power to mimic. [Gk *dys-*, *mimeisthai* to mimic.]

dysmnesia (dis·**ne**·ze·ah). Impaired or naturally poor memory. [Gk *dys-*, *mnesis* memory.]

dysmnesic (dis·**ne**·zik). Referring to dysmnesia, i.e. masked by poor, impaired or disordered memory.

dysmorphia (dis·**mor**·fe·ah). Ill shape; deformity. [Gk *dys-*, *morphe* form.]

dysmorphism (dis·**mor**·fizm). 1. Allomorphism. 2. The quality of being able to take a different form in different environments, e.g. a fungus may grow in saprophytic conditions in a way quite different from that in parasitic conditions. [see prec.]

dysmorphophobia (dis·**mor**·fo·**fo**'·be·ah). Insane fear of becoming deformed. [Gk *dys-*, *morphe* form, *phobos* fear.]

dysmorphopsia (dis·mor·**fop**·se·ah). The distortion of objects in the visual image. [Gk *dys-*, *morphe* shape, *opsis* vision.]

dysmorphosis (dis·mor·**fo**·sis). Malformation. [Gk *dys-*, *morphe* form, *-osis* condition.]

dysmyotonia (dis·mi·o·**to**'·ne·ah). 1. An abnormal state of tonicity of muscles. 2. Atony. [Gk *dys-*, myotonia.]

dysneuria (dis·**newr**·e·ah). Impairment of nerve function. [Gk *dys-*, *neuron* nerve.]

dysnomia (dis·**no**·me·ah). Partial nominal aphasia. [Gk *dys-*, *onoma* name.]

dysoaemia (dis·o·e·me·ah). Dysaemia.

dysodontiasis (dis·o·don·**ti**'·as·is). Difficult, delayed or irregular eruption of the teeth. [Gk *dys-*, *odous* tooth.]

dysodynia (dis·o·**din**·e·ah). Labour pains which are not of any effect in furthering the progress of the fetus. [Gk *dys-*, *odyne* pain.]

dysontogenesis (dis·on·to·**jen**'·es·is). Faulty development of any individual organism. [Gk *dys-*, ontogenesis.]

dysontogenetic (dis·on·to·jen·**et**'·ik). Referring to dysontogenesis; caused by faulty development during the embryonic stage. [see prec.]

dysopia, dysopsia (dis·o·pe·ah, dis·**op**·se·ah). Impaired or defective vision. **Dysopia algera.** Impaired vision caused by headache and pain in the eyes when the sight is fixed on any object. [Gk *dys-*, *opsis* sight.]

dysorexia (dis·or·**ex**·e·ah). Loss, perversion or impairment of appetite. [Gk *dys-*, *orexis* appetite.]

dysorganoplasia (dis·**or**·gan·o·**pla**'·ze·ah). Faulty formation or irregular development of an organ. [Gk *dys-*, organ, Gk *plasis* a forming.]

dysosmia (dis·**oz**·me·ah). Defective or impaired sense of smell. [Gk *dys-*, *-osme* odour.]

dysosteogenesis (dis·os·te·o·**jen**'·es·is). Dysostosis. [Gk *dys-*, osteogenesis.]

dysostosis (dis·os·**to**·sis). 1. Defective formation of bone. 2. Defective ossification from fetal cartilage. **Cleidocranial dysostosis.** A rare congenital condition characterized by defective ossification of the cranial vault giving rise to many wormian bones, bossing of the frontal bones, a diminutive maxilla, failure to shed the deciduous dentition with unerupted permanent successors, i.e. pseudo-anodontia, partial or complete absence of the clavicles and varying defects of the pelvis and lower limbs. **Hereditary craniofacial dysostosis.** Ocular hypertelorism. **Dysostosis hypophysaria.** Craniohypophyseal xanthoma. **Mandibulofacial dysostosis, Treacher–Collins syndrome.** An autosomal condition giving rise to many bilateral malformations of the facial structures; these include antimongoloid palpebral fissures due to deficient or absent malar bones, colobomas of the outer third of the lower eyelids and absent cilia medially, and deformities of the external and middle ears. The mandible is usually small. **Metaphyseal dysostosis.** A condition in children in which bones show radiological appearance of rickets but there are no chemical changes in the blood. **Dysostosis multiplex.** Type I mucopolysaccharidosis, gargoylism. **Orodigitofacial dysostosis.** Abnormal oral frenula that cleft the tongue, jaws and lip, digital malformations, dystopia canthorum, hypoplasia of the skull base, mental retardation and trembling. The condition is probably x-linked dominant, limited to females and lethal in males. [Gk *dys-*, ostosis.]

dysovarism (dis·**o**·var·izm). Imperfect or impaired internal secretion of the ovary. [Gk *dys-*, ovary.]

dysoxidative (dis·**ox**·e·**da**'·tiv). Lacking in oxygen. [Gk *dys-*, oxygen.]

dysoxidizable (dis·ox·e·di'·zabl). Difficult to oxidize. [see prec.]

dyspancreatism (dis·pan·kre·at·izm). Disorder or impairment of the functional activity of the pancreas. [Gk *dys-*, pancreas.]

dysparathyroidism (dis·par·ah·thi'·roid·izm). Impairment or irregularity in the functioning of the parathyroid glands. [Gk *dys-*, parathyroid.]

dyspareunia (dis·par·ew·ne·ah). Difficulty or pain in coitus. **Climacteric dyspareunia.** Painful or difficult coitus occurring after the menopause. **Psychological dyspareunia.** Dyspareunia without any apparent somatic cause. [Gk *dys-*, pareunia.]

dyspepsia (dis·pep·se·ah). Difficulty in digestion; a term usually applied to functional derangements of digestion due to nervous or reflex causes without demonstrable pathological changes in the stomach. They are characterized by symptoms such as vague abdominal discomfort or a feeling of fullness after food, flatulence, heartburn, nausea or vomiting; these occur irregularly and the clinical picture presents little constancy. The appetite is poor, and food fads are common, whilst physical and radiological examinations do not show any abnormality. The symptoms are brought on or increased by emotional disturbances, and are generally absent on holidays. **Habit dyspepsia.** Dyspepsia due to faulty habits such as irregular meals, bolting of food, imperfect mastication or violent exercise after meals. **Intestinal carbohydrate dyspepsia.** Hereditary disaccharidase deficiency. *See* DEFICIENCY. **Reflex dyspepsia.** Gastric symptoms of an irregular nature occurring in association with chronic cholecystitis, chronic appendicitis or colitis. [Gk *dys-*, *peptein* to digest.]

dyspepsodynia (dis·pep·so·din'·e·ah). Gastralgia. [Gk *dys-*, *pepsis* digestion, *odyne* pain.]

dyspeptic (dis·pep·tik). Having dyspepsia, related or belonging to dyspepsia. [Gk *dys-*, *pepsis* digestion.]

dysperistalsis (dis·per·is·tal'·sis). Abnormal or atypical peristalsis. [Gk *dys-*, peristalsis.]

dysphagia, dysphagy (dis·fa·je·ah, dis·fa·je). Difficulty in swallowing. Interference with the act of swallowing may be due to many causes and occurs at several sites. The first or voluntary stage of swallowing, by which food is propelled from the mouth to the pharynx, may be impeded by painful affections of the throat and larynx and by paralysis of the buccal muscles concerned due to faucial diphtheria, bulbar paralysis or myasthenia gravis. The second stage, in which the sensory nerves of the pharynx are stimulated and reflexly set up the complex co-ordinated involuntary movements by which food passes into the oesophagus, is impeded in Plummer–Vinson syndrome; this syndrome is the result of iron deficiency which causes atrophy of the pharyngeal mucosa and a loss of sensibility, and involves the pharyngo-oesophageal sphincter. Another cause at this site is a pharyngeal pouch. In the oesophagus, obstruction may be caused by external pressure from an aneurysm or mediastinal tumour, or by disease of the oesophagus itself such as oesophagitis, peptic ulcer, fibrous stricture and, most often, cancer. At the lower end the cardiac opening may fail to relax (achalasia of the cardia). **Hysterical dysphagia.** A form of dysphagia caused by paralysis or inco-ordination of the voluntary muscles concerned in the first and second stages of swallowing. **Syncopal dysphagia.** Syncope occurring on swallowing. There are two main varieties: in one, temporary heart block is induced by swallowing, usually in patients with oesophageal stricture or diverticula; in the other, sinus arrest or slowing occurs in patients with glossopharyngeal neuralgia. **Tropical dysphagia.** A disease of Brazil in which attacks of dysphagia are severe and recurrent. [Gk *dys-*, *phagein* to eat.]

dysphasia (dis·fa·ze·ah). Difficulty in speaking, with inability to co-ordinate words and arrange them in correct order. The condition is due to a lesion in the central nervous system; the mind may be very little affected. [Gk *dys-*, *phasis* a speaking.]

dysphasiac (dis·fa·ze·ak). A person suffering from dysphasia.

dysphasic (dis·fa·zik). Affected with dysphasia.

dysphemia (dis·fe·me·ah). Disordered utterance, such as stuttering, of psychoneurotic origin. [Gk *dys-*, *pheme* speech.]

dysphonia (dis·fo·ne·ah). 1. Difficulty or pain in speaking. 2. Hoarseness. 3. Impairment of the voice. **Dysphonia clericorum.** Pharyngitis due to much use of the voice and giving rise to hoarseness and pain on speaking; clergyman's sore throat. **Dysphonia plicae ventricularis.** Disturbed phonation due to movements of the ventricular bands instead of the true vocal cords, producing a deep, rough voice, often double in nature. **Dysphonia puberum.** The breaking of the voice in boys at puberty. **Dysphonia spastica.** Phonatory spasm. [Gk *dys-*, *phone* voice.]

dysphoria (dis·for·e·ah). 1. The condition of being ill at ease. 2. Bodily discomfort. 3. Fidgetiness. 4. Morbid restlessness. [Gk *dys-*, *pherein* to bear.]

dysphotia (dis·fo·she·ah). Myopia. [Gk *dys-*, *phos* light.]

dysphrasia (dis·fra·ze·ah). Dysphasia. [Gk *dys-*, *phrasis* speech.]

dysphrenia (dis·fre·ne·ah). Any mental disorder not caused by organic brain disease. **Dysphrenia hemicranica.** Psychiatric symptoms associated with an attack of migraine. [Gk *dys-*, *phren* mind.]

dyspinealism (dis·pin·e·al·izm). The condition resulting from deficiency of secretion of the pineal body. [Gk *dys-*, pineal body.]

dyspituitarism (dis·pit·ew·it·ar·izm). The morbid condition caused by irregular activity, disease or destruction of the hypophysis cerebri (pituitary body). [Gk *dys-*, pituitary body.]

dysplasia (dis·pla·ze·ah). Abnormal development of tissue. **Anhidrotic ectodermal dysplasia.** A genetically determined syndrome of partial or complete absence of sweat glands and other epidermal appendages, with hypodontia or anadontia. **Dysplasia of the brain.** Any defect of brain development, often associated with failure of the skull to fuse in the midline. Many degrees of the defect are seen, from cranium bifidum to anencephalia. **Chondro-ectodermal dysplasia.** Dyschondroplasia, ectodermal dysplasia, polydactylism and congenital heart disease. **Cleidocranial dysplasia.** A congenital abnormality characterized by defects in the vault of the skull and absence of part or the whole of the clavicles. **Congenital anhidrotic ectodermal dysplasia.** A syndrome combining deficiency in teeth, fine scanty hair, chronic rhinitis, and deficiency of sweat and sometimes lacrimal glands. **Cretinoid dysplasia.** The abnormality of development characteristic of cretinism. **Encephalo-ophthalmic dysplasia.** Severe malformations of the eyes, with dysplasia of the retina and rosette formation, associated with cerebral dysplasia. **Dysplasia epiphysealis multiplex.** A developmental disorder of the epiphyses which interferes with bony development and results in dwarfism. **Dysplasia epiphysealis punctata.** An abnormality of the epiphyses in which the epiphyseal bone shows a curious slipped appearance in x-rays. **Hereditary ectodermal dysplasia.** A condition characterized by defective dermal structures in teeth, hair and skin, lack of sweat glands, intolerance of heat, inflammation of the larynx and nasal part of the pharynx, and impaired mentality. **Hidrotic ectodermal dysplasia.** Hypotrichosis, hyperpigmentation, dystrophic nails with hyperkeratosis of palms and soles. Various types have been distinguished: *Basan's*, with fragile nails and smooth palms; *Clouston's*, with thick palms and soles, enamel hypoplasia and curly hair; *Feinmesser's*, with rudimentary nails and deafness; *Marshall's*, with cataract and deafness, pili torti and deafness; *Robinson's*, with peg-shaped teeth and deafness. **Macular dysplasia.** Macular coloboma. **Metaphyseal dysplasia.** An abnormality of development of the bone of the metaphysis. **Monostotic fibrous dysplasia.** Fibrous dysplasia occurring in one bone only. **Nuclear dysplasia.** Maldevelopment of cerebral nuclei, particularly those of cranial nerves. **Oculo-auriculo-vertebral dysplasia** (syn. Goldenhar's syndrome). A syndrome consisting of epibulbar dermoids and/or lipodermoids, auricular appendages and pretragal sinuses, micrognathia, vertebral anomalies and mental defect. **Oculodentodigital dysplasia.** A condition characterized by a thin nose with hypoplastic alae and narrow nostrils, microphthalmos and lesions of the iris, syndactyly and camptodactyly of the 4th and 5th fingers, anomalies of the middle digits of the 5th fingers and toes, and dental enamel hypoplasia. **Osteo-onycho dysplasia.** A hereditary disease characterized by hypoplasia of the radial heads and patellae, prominent iliac bones and medial femoral condyles, and dystrophic fingernails. **Polyostotic fibrous dysplasia.** Albright's disease; osteitis fibrosa cystica or disseminata; osteodystrophia fibrosa: fibrous dysplasia of more than one bone; if with brown patches and precocious puberty it is known as the *McCune-Albright syndrome.* **Renal dysplasia.** Congenital malformation of the kidney with faulty development of the nephron. **Dysplasia spondylepiphysaria congenita.** An autosomal dominant dysplasia mainly affecting the spine and hips, which may be confused with eccentrochondrodysplasia. **Spondylo-epiphyseal dysplasia.** Chondrodystrophy resembling achondroplasia but not present at birth; the head is not affected. [Gk *dys-*, *plasis* a forming.]

dysplasmatic, dysplastic (dis·plaz·**mat**·ik, dis·**plas**·tik). 1. Characterized by dysplasia. 2. Of a physical build not conforming to any one of the 3 main classes: asthenic, athletic, pyknic. 3. Cacoplastic; of a low or imperfect grade of organization. [see prec.]

dyspnoea (disp·**ne**·ah). The subjective feeling of discomfort or distress which occurs when the need for increased pulmonary ventilation has reached the point of obtruding unpleasantly into consciousness. Breathing is normally performed unconsciously; it begins to enter consciousness when ventilation is doubled, and causes discomfort when increased fourfold. This occurs physiologically in normal subjects during severe exertion, and varies in degree with the vital capacity, mechanical efficiency (training) and the efficiency of oxygen exchange in the lungs. Pathologically it occurs in many conditions and from several causes, such as increased matabolism, anoxaemia, disturbed acid-base ratio, reduced vital capacity, and all diseases of the lungs which impede the oxygenation of the blood. **Cardiac dyspnoea.** Dyspnoea secondary to heart disease and nearly always the result of pulmonary venous congestion; less commonly it is related to the biochemical consequences of low arterial oxygen saturation in patients with cyanotic heart disease. When it is due to left heart failure, it is usually at first noticed only on effort, but later may occur at rest, particularly at night. **Expiratory dyspnoea.** That occurring in spasm of the bronchioles, as in asthma. **Inspiratory dyspnoea.** Dyspnoea due to obstruction of the larynx, trachea or larger bronchi, necessitating prolonged deep inspirations in the attempt to overcome the obstruction. **Paroxysmal cardiac dyspnoea.** Episodic dyspnoea occurring at rest and frequently during the night (paroxysmal nocturnal dyspnoea), secondary to left heart failure. **Paroxysmal nocturnal dyspnoea.** Paroxysmal cardiac dyspnoea occurring at night. **Renal dyspnoea.** Dyspnoea in renal failure due to reduction of the alkali reserve of the blood. [Gk *dys-*, *pnoia* breath.]

dyspnoeic (disp·**ne**·ik). Having, referring to or caused by dyspnoea.

dyspnoeoneurosis (disp·**ne**·o·newr·**o**'·sis). Shortness of breath due to nerve disease or a neurosis. [dyspnoea, neurosis.]

dyspoietic (dis·poi·**et**·ik). Term applied to anything, e.g. a structure, showing faulty development. [Gk *dys-*, *poien* to make.]

dyspragia (dis·**pra**·je·ah). Painful carrying out of a function. **Dyspragia intermittens angiosclerotica intestinalis.** Painful intestinal spasm caused by disordered blood supply to the intestines. [Gk *dys-*, *pragos* act.]

dyspraxia (dis·**prax**·e·ah). Impairment of the ability to perform co-ordinated movements. **Articulatory dyspraxia.** Varying degrees of failure to perform the movements required to reproduce speech sounds accurately. [Gk *dys-*, *prassein* to do.]

dysprosium (dis·**pro**·se·um). An element of the rare-earth series, with atomic weight 162.50, atomic number 66 and chemical symbol Dy. It is found in certain rare minerals such as samarskite and gadolinite.

dysproteose (dis·**pro**·te·oze). A product of protein cleavage, derived by the hydration of heteroproteose.

dysraphia (dis·**raf**·e·ah). Status dysraphicus, a developmental defect in which there is non-closure or partial and defective closure of the primary neural tube. [Gk *dys-*, *rhaphe* seam.]

dysraphism (dis·raf·izm). Malformation arising from the abnormal splitting of the notochord. **Spinal dysraphism.** Any failure of fusion in the midline in the spinal region. [see prec.]

dysrhythmia (dis·**rith**·me·ah). 1. Defect or disturbance of rhythm. 2. Irregularity or abnormality of rhythm in speaking. **Cortical dysrhythmia.** Abnormal electrical potentials arising within the cerebral cortex, as distinct from those which arise in deeper structures but which may be conducted to the cortex. **Electro-encephalographic dysrhythmia.** Irregularity or disturbance of rhythm shown in an electro-encephalogram. **Paroxysmal cerebral dysrhythmia.** Epilepsy. **Dysrhythmia pneumophrasia.** Dysrhythmia in speaking due to taking breath at wrong times and so breaking up the natural groupings of words. **Dysrhythmia prosoda.** Dysrhythmia in speaking due to the placing of stress on the wrong words. **Dysrhythmia tonia.** Dysrhythmia in speaking due to defective inflection of voice. [Gk *dys-*, rhythm.]

dyssebacea (dis·se·**ba**·se·ah). A disorder of the sebaceous glands of the skin, especially that due to riboflavine deficiency. [Gk *dys-*, sebum.]

dyssomnia (dis·**som**·ne·ah). Disordered sleep. [Gk *dys-*, L *somnus* sleep.]

dysspermia (dis·**sper**·me·ah). 1. Imperfection of the semen. 2. Impairment of the discharge or deposition of seminal fluid; bradyspermatism. 3. A condition in which ejaculation of seminal fluid causes discomfort or pain in the male. [Gk *dys-*, sperm.]

dysstasia (dis·**sta**·ze·ah). A condition in which there is difficulty in standing. [Gk *dys-*, *stasis* a standing still.]

dysstatic (dis·**stat**·tik). Referring to dysstasia.

dyssymbolia, dyssymboly (dis·sim·**bo**·le·ah, dis·**sim**·bo·le). Inability to form mental concepts and resultant inability to clothe thoughts intelligently in words. [Gk *dys-*, symbol.]

dyssynergia (dis·sin·**er**·je·ah). Ataxia. **Dyssynergia cerebellaris myoclonica.** Cerebellar dyssynergia in association with myoclonus and epilepsy. **Dyssynergia cerebellaris progressiva.** Disordered cerebellar function with resultant disturbance of muscle tone and co-ordination and the occurrence of generalized tremor. [Gk *dys-*, synergy.]

dyssynergy (dis·**sin**·er·je). In cardiology, an impairment of the normal co-ordinated contraction of the ventricular myocardium, especially of the left ventricle and as a result of abnormal conduction of the stimulating impulse or of local impaired contraction secondary to ischaemia. [Gk *dys-*, *syn* together, *ergein* to work.]

dyssystole (dis·**sis**·to·le). Hyposystole. [Gk *dys-*, systole.]

dystasia (dis·**ta**·ze·ah). Dysstasia.

dystaxia (dis·**tax**·e·ah). Partial ataxia. **Dystaxia agitans.** A condition of tremor resembling that of paralysis agitans and caused by irritation of the spinal cord. Paralysis is not present. [Gk *dys-*, *taxis* order.]

dystectia (dis·**tek**·she·ah). A condition in which the neural tube is not perfectly closed, giving rise to various malformations, e.g. meningocele and spina bifida. [Gk *dys-*, L *tectum* roof.]

dysteleology (dis·te·le·**ol**'·o·je). 1. A term for that branch of biology which is concerned with rudimentary and apparently useless organs, such as the vermiform appendix. 2. In biology, lack of purposefulness. [Gk *dys-*, *teles* perfect, *logos* science.]

dysthanasia (dis·than·a·ze·ah). A lingering and painful death. [Gk *dys-*, *thanatos* death.]

dysthesia (dis·**the**·ze·ah). 1. A condition of ill-health or of illness. The term is applied particularly to such a condition when caused by a non-febrile vascular disorder. 2. The impatience, fretfulness or bad temper engendered by illness. [Gk *dys-*, *thesis* a placing.]

dysthetic (dis·**thet**·ik). 1. Referring to dysthesia. 2. Cachectic.

dysthymia (dis·**thi**·me·ah). 1. The condition which is the result of faulty secretion of the thymus gland in early years. 2. War neurosis. 3. Morbid melancholy or mental depression. 4. Any anomaly of mind or mentation. **Dysthymia algetica.** A morbid mental state resulting from irritation of the peripheral nerves. **Dysthymia neuralgica.** A morbid mental state due to trigeminal or other form of neuralgia. [Gk *dys-*, thymus.]

dysthymiac (dis·thi·me·ak). Anyone suffering from dysthymia.

dysthyreosis (dis·thi·re·o′·sis). Imperfect functioning of the thyroid gland. [Gk *dys-*, thyroid, Gk *-osis* condition.]

dysthyroidea, dysthyroidism (dis·thi·roid·e·ah, dis·thi·roid·izm). Imperfect development of the thyroid gland leading to abnormality of function. [Gk *dys-*, thyroid.]

dystimbria (dis·tim·bre·ah). Defect of resonance or imperfect quality of the tones of the voice. [Gk *dys-*, timbre.]

dystocia (dis·to·se·ah). Abnormal or pathological labour. **Cervical dystocia.** A term used to indicate slow or difficult dilation of the cervix in labour, usually without pathological cause. It is a form of maternal dystocia (see below), and the term is sometimes applied loosely to cases in which there is some organic disease in the cervix. **Constriction-ring dystocia.** Difficult labour due to a constriction ring. **Dystocia dystrophia.** Dystocia dystrophia syndrome. *See* SYNDROME. **Fetal dystocia.** Difficult labour attributable to fetal causes such as hydrocephaly, monstrosity or complex presentation. **Maternal dystocia.** Difficult labour due to maternal causes such as contracted pelvis or uterine inertia, as distinguished from fetal dystocia (see preceding). **Placental dystocia.** Difficulty in delivering the placenta, as with contraction ring or placenta accreta. [Gk *dys-*, *tokos* birth.]

dystonia (dis·to·ne·ah). Lack of tonicity of any tissue; a state of disordered tonicity. **Dystonia lenticularis.** Dystonia caused by a lesion of the lentiform nucleus. **Dystonia musculorum deformans.** A rare disease of adolescence causing grave incapacity and deformity from involuntary muscular contraction, particularly involving the trunk. **Torsion dystonia.** Dystonia musculorum deformans (see preceding). [Gk *dys-*, tone.]

dystonic (dis·ton·ik). Referring to or characterized by dystonia.

dystopia (dis·to·pe·ah). Malposition or displacement of any organ; allotopia; heterotopia. **Dystopia canthorum.** Lateral displacement of the inner canthi. [Gk *dys-*, *topos* place.]

dystopic (dis·top·ik). Referring to dystopia, i.e. misplaced.

dystrophia, dystrophy (dis·tro·fe·ah, dis·tro·fe). A disorder, usually congenital, of the structure and functions of an organ or tissue, such as muscles or bones, due to perverted nutrition. **Dystrophia adiposa corneae.** Primary fatty degeneration of the cornea. **Adiposogenital dystrophy, Dystrophia adiposogenitalis.** 1. A condition in which obesity is present with under-development of the genital organs. 2. Froehlich's syndrome, in which obesity and genital under-development are due to a chromophobe adenoma of the pituitary gland. **Albipunctate dystrophy.** A familial condition where there are innumerable small discrete white dots in the fundus of the eye. In the progressive form there may be night blindness and contracted fields. The stationary form is known as *fundus albipunctatus.* **Dystrophia brevicollis.** Dwarfism associated with shortness of the neck. **Dystrophia bullosa.** A rare, genetically-determined syndrome of bullae, loss of hair, reticulate pigmentation and macular atrophy with mental retardation, occurring only in boys. **Dystrophia calcarea corneae.** A primary deposition of calcium salts in the cornea. The condition is extremely rare, and is also called *primary calcareous degeneration of the cornea.* **Corneal dystrophy.** Bilateral hereditary degenerations of the cornea, stationary or slowly progressive. **Dystrophia endothelialis corneae.** Cornea guttata; degeneration of the endothelium. **Dystrophia epithelialis corneae.** Grey opacities in the endothelium of the cornea: also called *Fuchs' dystrophy.* **Facioscapulohumeral dystrophy.** A comparatively benign form of muscular dystrophy, transmitted by dominant inheritance, in which facial muscles are always involved: *Landouzy-Déjérine dystrophy.* **Familial corneal dystrophy.** A hereditary degenerative disease of the subepithelial layers of the cornea, with deposits of hyaline material, bilateral and starting at puberty. *See* NODULAR- and RETICULAR- TYPES OF CORNEAL DYSTROPHY (below). **Familial hyperplastic periosteal dystrophy.** A hereditary abnormality in which there is hypertrophy of subperiosteal bone. **Granular corneal dystrophy.** Nodular-type corneal dystrophy (see below). **Hypophyseal dystrophy.** Nutritional disorder of the pituitary gland (obsolete term). **Dystrophia hypophyseopriva chronica.** Chronic nutritional disorder of the body due to removal or destruction of the pituitary gland; the term is obsolete, hypopituitarism or Simmonds' disease having taken its place. **Juvenile progressive muscular dystrophy.** Any form of muscular dystrophy with onset in adolescence. **Lamellar dystrophy of nail.** Splitting of the free border of a finger nail into layers, usually due to chemical injury. **Lattice dystrophy of the cornea.** A dominant condition characterized by fine lines in the anterior layers of the stroma. **Limb girdle muscular dystrophy.** A form of muscular dystrophy with variable inheritance, affecting mainly proximal muscles. **Macular corneal dystrophy.** Nodular-type corneal dystrophy (see below). **Marginal dystrophy of the cornea.** Marginal degeneration of the cornea; a rare disease starting as an opacity, similar to arcus senilis, but continuing to guttering of the peripheral parts of the cornea, and finally ectasia. **Dystrophia mediana canaliformis.** A rare disorder of the nails, especially of the thumbs, characterized by longitudinal grooves. **Dystrophia mesodermatis congenita.** Marfan's syndrome or arachnodactyly; subluxation of the crystalline lens of the eye associated with elongation of the long bones of the hands and feet. **Dystrophia myotonica.** A heredofamilial disease, probably an incomplete mendelian dominant, characterized by myotonia, peripheral myopathy (muscular wasting), weakness of sternomastoids, frontal baldness, ptosis and sometimes myopathy of ocular muscles, myopathic facies, cataracts, genital atrophy, sometimes mental impairment and evidence of cardiac insufficiency, and often characteristic radiological changes in the skull. Also called *myotonia atrophica.* **Nodular-type corneal dystrophy** (described by Groenouw). Milk-white subepithelial spots; familial. **Ocular muscular dystrophy.** Dystrophy predominantly of ocular muscles. **Oculocerebrorenal dystrophy.** A disease of male children, with hypotonia, loss of reflexes, mental deterioration, glaucoma, cataracts, and excretion of organic and amino acids in urine; Lowe's syndrome. **Papillary and pigmentary dystrophy.** Acanthosis nigricans. **Dystrophia periostalis hyperplastica familiaris.** A familial condition in which oxycephaly is associated with thickness and shortness of the long bones of the limbs. **Progressive muscular dystrophy.** Progressive weakness and wasting of muscles owing to myopathic degeneration, affecting particularly muscles of the shoulder and pelvic girdles, but sometimes facial and ocular muscles or distal limb muscles; this term covers all the forms of muscular dystrophy. **Pseudohypertrophic dystrophy, Pseudohypertrophic muscular dystrophy.** Dystrophy beginning in early childhood, transmitted by sex-linked recessive inheritance and characterized by severe weakness of predominantly proximal muscles. Pseudohypertrophy (the enlargement of weak muscles) is common. The prognosis is bad. **Reflex sympathetic dystrophy.** Reflex changes, often consisting of pallor, sweating and oedema, in the skin overlying the site of an injury such as a fracture or a sprain. **Reticular-type corneal dystrophy** (described by Biber, Haab and Dimmer). Lattice-like subepithelial lines; familial. **Thoracic asphyxiant dystrophy.** Jeune's disease; dysplasia of ribs causing respiratory failure. There is also shortening of other long bones. **Dystrophia unguis mediana canaliformis.** A longitudinally guttered nail dystrophy, usually of the thumb nail and caused by repeated trauma to the nail matrix from a habit of manipulating the centre of the nail fold, usually with the middle finger. **Dystrophia unguium.** An abnormality of the nails closely resembling pachyonychia congenita, which may occur with dyskeratosis congenita and leucokeratosis oris. **Dystrophia urica corneae.** Deposits of urea and sodium-urate crystals in the corneal stroma. The urea output is normal, and the condition is not found in gouty patients. It is extremely rare. [Gk *dys-*, *trophe* nourishment.]

See also: BIEDL, DÉJÉRINE, ERB, FUCHS (E.), GOWERS, LANDOUZY, LAURENCE, LEYDEN, MOEBIUS, MOON (R. C.), SALZMAN.

dystrophic (dis·tro·fik). Referring to dystrophia.

dystrophoneurosis (dis·tro·fo·newr·o′·sis). 1. Any nervous disease or disorder caused by poor nutrition or undernourishment. 2. The disturbance of nutritive processes which results from disorders of the nervous system. [Gk *dys-*, *trophe* nourishment, neurosis.]

dystrophy (dis·tro·fe). *See* DYSTROPHIA.

dystropic (dis·tro·pik). Referring to abnormal concentration of intellectual interest either on other people or on oneself. [Gk *dys-*, *trope* turn.]

dystropy (dis·tro·pe). Abnormality of behaviour. [see prec.]

dystrypsia (dis·trip·se·ah). Any dyspepsia caused by impaired secretion of pancreatic juice. [Gk *dys-*, trypsin.]

dysuria (dis·ewr·e·ah). A condition in which the passing of urine is painful or difficult. **Psychic dysuria.** Inability to pass urine when other persons are present. **Spastic dysuria.** Difficulty in voiding urine caused by spasm of the urinary bladder. [Gk *dys-*, *ouron* urine.]

dysuriac (dis·ewr·e·ak). Anyone affected with dysuria.

dysuric (dis·ewr·ik). Referring to or suffering from dysuria.

dysury (dis·ewr·e). Dysuria.

dysvitaminosis (dis·vi·tam·in·o'·sis). Any deficiency disorder or disease caused by lack of vitamins in the diet. [Gk *dys-*, vitamin.]

Dzierzynsky's disease. Familial hyperplastic periosteal dystrophy.

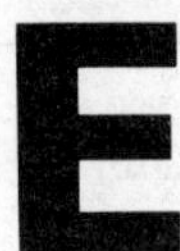

e-. Prefix, from the Latin *e*, meaning *from, out of, without.*

Ea (a·ah). A god of Babylonian legend, begotten by Anu (the sky). He was god of the earth and of the waters under the earth, and also of the healing art. His son was the national hero, Marduk, or Ashur, in the Assyrian version of the legend. Ea is invoked in Assyrian medical recipes and charms written on tablets.

Eagle, Harry (b. 1905). American cell biologist.

Eagle's medium. A balanced salt solution containing amino acids, glucose and some vitamins. It is widely used as the basis for a medium in which cells can be cultured *in vitro.*

Eales, Henry (b. 1852). Birmingham ophthalmic surgeon.

Eales' disease. Recurrent intra-ocular haemorrhages in young adults, principally male.

ear [auris (NA)] (eer). The organ of hearing. *See* ORGAN. **Acute ear.** An acute inflammation of the ear; a generic term used colloquially, and almost amounting to a slang expression. **Aviator's ear.** Traumatic inflammation of the ear due to changes in atmospheric pressure. **Aztec ear.** A congenital deformity of the ear associated with absence of the lobule; also associated with microcephalic idiocy. **Bat ears.** Prominent ears due either to excessive development or to defects in the antihelix. **Beach ear.** An external otitis resulting from bathing. **Boxers' ear.** Aural haematoma. **Cagot ear.** A deformity of the ear found in cretins. **Cat's ear.** Falling over of the auricle, making the ear appear to be folded on itself. **Cauliflower ear.** A distorted, fibrosed, thickened ear resulting from repeated trauma, as in boxing, causing perichondritis. **Diabetic ear.** Mastoiditis sometimes found in a diabetic patient. **Divers' ear.** An acute and painful condition, affecting the middle ear and causing temporary deafness, to which divers making sudden descents to great depths are subject. Trauma is brought about by an increase in pressure external to the tympanic membrane, combined with an inability to ventilate the middle ear by means of the eustachian tube. The tympanic membrane becomes indrawn and congested, and may rupture. Haemorrhages may occur and effusions into the middle-ear cavity take place. Treatment consists of re-ascent, auto-ventilation and the use of nasal decongestives; occasionally myringotomy is indicated. **External ear [auris externa (NA)].** The external part of the ear consisting of an expanded external portion, the auricle, and a tubular portion, the external auditory meatus, leading to the tympanum. **Faun ear.** A congenital anomaly of the auricle in which there is failure in the development of the helix. Imperfect folding of this structure produces a prominent Darwin's tubercle projecting upwards and backwards, which can be corrected by plastic surgery. Also known as *prick ear.* **Hong Kong ear.** Singapore ear (see below). **Hot-weather ear.** A loose term for external otitis found in hot climates; it is usually a mycotic infection, but may be due to mite infestation. **Insane ear.** Haematoma of the ear which is found in the insane and sometimes in congenital idiots. **Internal ear [auris interna (NA)].** A series of membranous sacs and ducts concerned with the sensations of hearing and balance, contained within the petrous part of the temporal bone. **Lop ear.** A deformity of the pinna which makes the ears project unduly from the side of the head. **Middle ear [auris media (NA)].** A slit-like cavity in the petrous part of the temporal bone, interposed between the external auditory meatus and the inner ear, and containing a chain of 3 ossicles which transmit sound waves from the former to the latter. Anteriorly it communicates with the nasopharynx via the pharyngotympanic tube, and posteriorly with the antrum via the aditus. **Oxygen ear.** After an oxygen-enriched atmosphere has been breathed, the excess oxygen remaining in the middle ear may be absorbed, causing barotitis. **Panama ear.** Otomycosis. **Prick ear.** Faun ear (see above). **Rabbit's ears.** Dilatation of the cisterna corporis callosi seen at air encephalography; it is usually an indication of a mass in the posterior cranial fossa. **Scroll ear.** A rolling over of the pinna, resembling a scroll. **Singapore ear.** Otomycosis which is relatively common in all the humid tropical countries. **Summer ear.** Otitis externa. **Surfers' ear.** Otomycosis. **Tank ear.** Otomycosis from bathing. **Tropical ear.** Hot-weather ear and Singapore ear (see above). [AS *eare.*]

See also: BLAINVILLE, DARWIN, MOREL, STAHL (F. K.), WILDERMUTH.

ear-drops (eer·drops). Auristillae; solutions of medicaments in oil or water for instillation into the external auditory meatus. [AS *eare, dropa.*]

ear-drum (eer·drum). The tympanic membrane, or tympanum. [AS *eare,* drum.]

ear-plug (eer·plug). A device, usually of plastics or rubber for permanent use, or of cotton wool for temporary use, which when placed in the ear deadens sound and protects the drum from the ill-effect of loud noises or from rapid changes of atmospheric pressure. [AS *eare, plugge.*]

earache (eer·ake). Otalgia; any pain in the ear, especially that associated with otitis media. [AS *eare, acan.*]

earth (erth). 1. The soil. 2. Name given by the alchemists to any non-metallic substance that withstood fire, e.g. alkaline earths (lime and magnesia); the term has continued into modern usage, e.g. rare earths. 3. An easily powdered mineral undergoing no other preparation than washing and drying, e.g. fuller's earth. **Alkaline earths.** The general name applied to magnesia, lime, strontia and baryta; it thus designates the metals of Group IIa of the Periodic Table (beryllium, magnesium, calcium, strontium, barium and radium). **Diatomaceous earth.** Infusorial earth (see below). **Fuller's Earth BPC 1959.** A natural clay-like mineral, mainly the hydrated silicate of aluminium with iron, magnesium and calcium silicates admixed. It is used as an absorbent for decolorizing oils and fats, as a filler for textiles (hence the name) and in cosmetic powders. **Infusorial earth.** Kieselguhr, a siliceous material composed of the fossilized shells of diatoms, found in deposits in Germany and Scotland, and used as an absorbent, filtering agent, and as a constituent of dynamite. **Purified siliceous earth.** Diatomite BPC 1949. **Rare earths.** A group of metallic oxides occurring in monazite and other rare minerals and affording cerium, lanthanum and other metals rare but of growing importance. **Siliceous earth.** Infusorial earth (see above). [AS *earthe.*]

Easton, John Alexander (b. 1807). Glasgow physician.

Easton's syrup. A syrup containing the phosphates of ferrous iron, quinine and strychnine, with glycerin. It was at one time the most popular tonic, but is now becoming replaced by tablets of ferrous sulphate.

Eaton, M. L. 20th century American physician.

Eaton-Lambert syndrome. Myasthenia occasionally accompanying bronchial carcinoma.

eau (o). Water. **Eau d'Alibour.** An astringent lotion containing copper and zinc sulphates, tincture of saffron and camphor. **Eau de Cologne.** A toilet water containing orange, lemon, bergamot, rosemary and orange-flower oils dissolved in 90 per cent alcohol. [Fr.]

ebb (eb). 1. The gradual decline of the opsonic index when the positive phase is over. 2. Any gradual decline or subsidence, e.g. of infection. [AS *ebba* flowing back.]

Eberstaller, Oscar. 19th-20th century Graz anatomist.

Eberstaller's sulcus. An occasional sulcus in the inferior parietal lobule.

Eberth, Karl Joseph (b. 1835). Halle pathologist.

Eberth's cholecystitis. That due to the presence of *Salmonella typhi* (*Eberthella typhosa*).

Eberth's disease. Typhoid fever. *See* FEVER.

Eberth's line. The intercalated disc of cardiac muscle fibres.

Eberthella (e·bert·el·ah). A genus of bacteria which has now been merged with the tribe Salmonellae (family Enterobacteriaceae). The only organism of significance as a human pathogen in the former genus *Eberthella* was the typhoid bacillus, now known as *Salmonella typhi,* an actively motile, Gram-negative, rod-shaped organism, the cause of typhoid fever in man and found in the human intestine. [Karl Joseph *Eberth.*]

Ebner, Victor (b. 1842). Graz and Vienna histologist.

Ebner's fibril. A collagen fibril of the dentine or cement of a tooth.

Ebner's glands. Serous glands of the tongue.

Ebner's liquid. A microscopical reagent for decalcification, consisting of hydrochloric acid in a saturated solution of common salt.

Ebner's reticulum. A cellular network in the convoluted seminiferous tubules.

ebonite (eb·on·ite). Hard black vulcanized rubber. [Gk *ebeninos,* ebon.]

ebrietas (e·bri·et·as). Drunkenness; refers especially to the toxic state resulting from acute or chronic alcoholic poisoning. [L drunkenness.]

ebriety (e·bri·et·e). Inebriety. [ebrietas.]

Ebstein, Wilhelm (b. 1836). Gottingen physician.

Ebstein's angle. The angle between the right border of cardiac dullness and the upper limit of hepatic dullness, in the anterior part of the 5th right intercostal space; the cardiohepatic angle.

Ebstein's anomaly of the tricuspid valve. A rare congenital abnormality of the heart in which the tricuspid valve is malformed and displaced into the cavity of the right ventricle, so that the right side of the heart consists of an atrio-ventricular chamber and a distal right ventricular chamber more or less effectively separated, depending upon the severity of the malformations of the valve. A defect of the atrial septum is commonly associated and, when present, almost always allows a shunt from right to left, producing cyanosis.

Ebstein's diet, method or treatment. The treatment of obesity by exclusion of carbohydrates from the diet whilst permitting proteins and fats.

Ebstein's disease. Ebstein's anomaly of the tricuspid valve (see above).

Ebstein's sign. Dullness to percussion in the 5th intercostal space to the right of the sternum, due to obtuseness of the cardiohepatic angle, in cases of pericardial effusion.

Armanni-Ebstein cells. Terminal convoluted renal cells filled with glycogen in diabetes mellitus.

Pel-Ebstein disease, or syndrome. Lymphadenoma with periodical pyrexia resembling undulant fever.

Pel-Ebstein fever. The characteristic undulant fever of Hodgkin's disease: a remittent pyrexia that occurs daily and reaches its highest point (40°C, 104°F or so) after about 5 days, then gradually subsides, to recur after a period of about 10 days.

ebullism (e·bul·izm). The formation of bubbles of gas in biological fluids owing to reduction of ambient pressure; the term is usually confined to the boiling of body liquids at low ambient pressure. [L *ebullire* to bubble up.]

ebullition (e·bul·ish·un). 1. Boiling; the rapid vaporization of a liquid, with turbulence and the formation of bubbles. 2. Effervescence. [L *ebullire* to bubble up.]

ebur dentis (e·ber **den**·tis). Dentine. [L ivory of tooth.]

eburnated (e·ber·**na**'·ted). 1. Dense and hard, like ivory. 2. In dentistry, descriptive of dentine the tubules of which have been filled up and obliterated by calcareous material. [see foll.]

eburnation (e·ber·**na**·shun). 1. A degenerated condition of bone or cartilage in which it is converted into a dense hard mass like ivory, as in osteosclerosis. 2. Increased density of bone as the result of inflammation. 3. Of a tumour, infiltration of calcareous material. 4. In dentistry, the condition of dentine which when exposed becomes hard and polished, and may be any colour from yellow to black. [L *ebur* ivory.]

eburneous (e·**ber**·ne·us). Like ivory, particularly in regard to colour. [see prec.]

écarteur (a·kar·**ter**). Retractor. [Fr.]

ecaudate (e·**kaw**·date). Without any tail or tail-like appendage. [L *e, cauda* tail.]

Ecballium (ek·**bal**·e·um). A genus of plants of the family Cucurbitaceae. **Ecballium elaterium.** The species which affords elaterium, a drastic hydragogue cathartic. [Gk *ekballein* to throw out.]

ecbolic (ek·**bol**·ik). 1. Oxytocic; producing contraction of the uterus and hence promoting parturition or abortion. 2. An oxytocic drug; a drug which hastens parturition. Cathartics and certain volatile oils act reflexly through irritation of the large intestine, but the chief ecbolics used are ergot, extract of pituitary and quinine, which act directly upon the uterine muscle, especially during parturition. [Gk *ekballein* to throw out.]

ecboline (**ek**·bol·een). The name given to one of the first alkaloidal substances prepared from ergot, and most probably an impure ergotoxine. [see prec.]

ecbolium (ek·**bo**·le·um). Any ecbolic or abortifacient drug. Quinine, ergot and lead salts are such, but their use is attended with serious dangers. [Gk *ekballein* to throw out.]

eccentric (ek·**sen**·trik). 1. Deviating or proceeding from a centre; occurring or situated away from a centre. 2. Departing from the usual course or practice. 3. Of conduct or behaviour, odd and unconventional but without necessarily any insane tendencies. 4. Anomalous. [Gk *ek,* centre.]

eccentricity (ek·sen·**tris**·it·e). 1. An aberration. 2. Oddness of behaviour or conduct without insanity. [see prec.]

eccentrochondrodysplasia, eccentro-osteochondrodysplasia (ek·**sen**·tro·kon·dro·dis·**pla**'·ze·ah, ek·**sen**·tro·**os**·te·o·kon·dro·dis·**pla**'·ze·ah). A familial form of dyschondroplasia in which, instead of a single centre of ossification there are multiple discrete centres. The effect on the bodily framework is to cause twisting of bones and various deformities. [eccentric, Gk *osteon* bone, chondrodysplasia.]

eccentropiesis (ek·**sen**·tro·pi·e'·sis). The exerting of pressure from within outwards. [eccentric, Gk *piesis* pressure.]

eccephalosis (ek·kef·al·o'·sis). Removal of the fetal head in order to assist delivery of the fetus. [Gk *ek, kephale* head, *-osis* condition.]

ecchondroma (ek·on·**dro**·mah) (pl. *ecchondromata*). An innocent cartilaginous tumour which grows from the surface of normal cartilage or bone. [Gk *ek, chondros* cartilage, *oma* tumour.]

ecchondromatosis (ek·on·dro·mat·o'·sis). Multiple chondromata. [ecchondroma, Gk *-osis* condition.]

ecchondrosis (ek·on·**dro**·sis). The state in which ecchondromata are present. **Ecchondrosis ossificans.** Diaphyseal aclasis. *See* ACLASIS. [see prec.]

ecchondrotome (ek·**on**·dro·tome). A surgical instrument for the removal of eccondromata. [ecchondroma, Gk *temnein* to cut.]

ecchordosis physaliphora (ek·kor·**do**·sis fiz·al·e·**for**·ah). A pathological condition in which the vertebral column or the base of the skull, or both, show a number of soft swellings of notochordal origin, composed of swollen, mucin-filled physaliphorous cells and a mucinous intercellular matrix. [Gk *ek, chorde* cord, *-osis* condition, *physallis* bubble, *pherein* to bear.]

ecchymoma (ek·e·**mo**·mah). A small haematoma arising on the site of a bruise. [ecchymosis, Gk *-oma* tumour.]

ecchymosis (ek·e·**mo**·sis) (pl. *ecchymoses*). 1. A swollen livid or blue-black spot on the skin caused by effusion of blood into the areolar tissue as the result of a contusion. 2. An extravasation of blood. **Cadaveric ecchymoses.** Post-mortem stains. **H-shaped ecchymosis.** That seen in rupture of the tendo calcaneus. [Gk *ek*, *chymos* juice.]

See also: BAYARD.

ecchymotic (ek·e·**mot**·ik). Referring or belonging to an ecchymosis.

eccrine (ek·rine). Excretory. [Gk *ekkrinein* to secrete.]

eccrinology (ek·rin·**ol**·o·je). That branch of medical science which is concerned with secretions and excretions. [Gk *ekkrinein* to secrete, *logos* science.]

eccrisiology (ek·ris·e·**ol**'·o·je). Eccrinology. [eccrisis, Gk *logos* science.]

eccrisis (ek·ris·is). 1. Excretion or expulsion of waste products. 2. Excrement. [Gk *ek*, *krisis* separation.]

eccyclomastoma, eccyclomastopathy (ek·si·klo·mas·**to**'·mah, ek·si·klo·mas·**top**'·ath·e). A tumour of the breast consisting of an isolated mass of epithelial proliferation or connective-tissue overgrowth such as is found in cyclomastopathy. [Gk *ek*, *kyklos* circle, *mastos* breast, *-oma* tumour, *pathos* disease.]

eccyesis (ek·si·e·sis). Ectopic pregnancy. *See* PREGNANCY. [Gk *ek*, *kyesis* pregnancy.]

ecdemic (ek·**dem**·ik). Applied to a disease which is neither endemic nor epidemic but is brought into a region from another distant region. [Gk *ekdemos* away from home.]

ecdemomania (ek·**dem**·o·**ma**'·ne·ah). The impulsion to wander away from home which is characteristic of certain forms of insanity. [Gk *ekdemos* away from home, mania.]

ecderon (**ek**·der·on). 1. The ectoderm. 2. The outer layer of mucous membrane. 3. The epidermis. [Gk *ek*, *deros* skin.]

ecdysis (ek·di·sis). 1. Desquamation. 2. The shedding of the outer covering in the metamorphosis of certain arthropods, snakes, etc. [Gk *ekdysis* a stripping off.]

ecdysone (ek·di·sone). The insect moulting hormone. [Gk *ekdysis* a stripping off.]

ecgonine (ek·gon·een). Tropine carboxylic acid, $C_8H_3N(OH)COOH$. A crystalline substance prepared from the crude alkaloids of coca leaves, or by the hydrolysis of cocaine. It occurs in 4 isomeric forms: the ordinary form is laevorotatory, and cocaine is its methyl-benzoyl derivative.

echeosis (ek·e·o·sis). A neurosis caused by noise. [Gk *eche* noise, neurosis.]

echidnase (ek·**id**·naze). A poisonous ferment principle of snake venom causing swelling and inflammation. [Gk *echidna* viper.]

Echidnophaga (ek·id·**nof**·ag·ah). A genus of fleas of which *Echidnophaga gallinacea*, the tropical hen flea, often attacks man. The female is "sticktight", that is remaining with the mouth parts inserted for long periods, and partially burrowing in habits; the male is free-living. [Gk *echidna*, viper, *phagein* to eat.]

echidnotoxin (ek·id·no·**tox**'·in). A poisonous substance identified in the venom of vipers. [Gk *echidna* viper, *toxikon* poison.]

echidnovaccine (ek·id·no·**vak**'·seen). A vaccine prepared from viper venom heated at 68°C, the neurotoxin present being more heat-stable than the other irritant toxins of the venom. Immunization of horses with this vaccine produces an antivenom effective against snake bite; e.g. that derived from the horned viper of Africa, *Cerastea cornutus*, is of value against the bite of the British adder. [Gk *echidna* viper, vaccine.]

echinate (ek·in·ate). Echinulate.

echinenone (ek·**in**·en·one). One of the active carotenoid pigments which is a provitamin, being converted into vitamin A in the animal body. It is isolated from the sex glands of the sea-urchin (Echinoidea). [Gk *echinos* sea-urchin.]

Echinochasmus (ek·in·o·**kaz**·mus). A genus of intestinal flukes. *Echinochasmus perfoliatus* in Europe and *Echinochasmus japonicus* in Japan, both normal to cats and dogs, have been recorded from man. *Echinochasmus paraulum* is a common pigeon parasite also recorded in man. Primary intermediate hosts are freshwater snails; secondary are fish. [Gk *echinos* hedgehog, *chasmos* open mouth.]

echinococciasis, echinococcosis (ek·i·no·kok·**i**'·as·is, ek·i·no·kok·**o**'·sis). Infestation with the tapeworm, *Echinococcus granulosus*, i.e. hydatid disease. [*Echinococcus*, Gk *-osis* condition.]

echinococcotomy (ek·i·no·kok·**ot**'·o·me). The evacuation or cutting out of an echinococcus (hydatid) cyst. [echinococcus, Gk *temnein* to cut.]

Echinococcus (ek·i·no·**kok**'·us). A genus of tapeworms. *Echinococcus granulosus* is, in its larval stage, a dangerous if uncommon parasite of man. The adult, less than 1 cm long, is found in dogs and wild carnivores; the larva, hydatid cyst, normally in domestic herbivores, usually in the liver. Hydatids may grow to enormous size, containing several gallons of fluid. Normally the cyst is simple, having within it numerous daughter cysts filled with brood chambers in which are developing scolices. Mature scolices are liberated into the cavity of the cyst as hydatid sand. Occasionally multilocular cysts are formed with numerous smaller cysts around a central core; these smaller cysts may break away and form new multilocular cysts in other places. They are sometimes distinguished as *Echinococcus multilocularis*, but this is not a valid species. [Gk *echinos* hedgehog, *kokkos* berry.]

echinoderm (ek·i·no·derm). A member of the division of marine animals, echinodermata. [Gk *echinos* hedgehog, *derma* skin.]

echinodermous (ek·i·no·**der**'·mus). Having a spine-bearing skin. [see prec.]

echino-ophthalmia (ek·i·no·of·**thal**'·me·ah). An inflamed condition of the eyelids causing the eyelashes to project. [Gk *echinos* hedgehog, ophthalmia.]

echinosis (ek·in·o·sis). A condition in which the erythrocytes have lost their smooth outline and become crenated like the shell of a sea-urchin. [Gk *echinos* hedgehog, *-osis* condition.]

Echinostoma (ek·in·os·to·mah). A genus of flukes with an anterior collar of spines. **Echinostoma iliocanum, E. jassyense.** Species which occasionally cause diarrhoea in man. **Echinostoma macrorchis.** A specis which occasionally causes diarrhoea in man. **Echinostoma revolutum.** A species normal to aquatic birds, has been reported from human intestine in Europe, Asia and Mexico; its secondary hosts are freshwater snails. [Gk *echinos* hedgehog, *stoma* mouth.]

Echinostomatidae, echinostomidae (ek·in·**os**·to·**mat**'·id·e, ek·in·os·**to**·mid·e). A family of the trematode sub-order Distomata. The genera *Echinochasmus*, *Echinostoma* and *Paryphostomum* are of medical interest. [Gk *echinos* hedgehog, *stoma* mouth, *eidos* form.]

echinulate (ek·**in**·ew·late). 1. Having pointed processes or spines. 2. In bacteriology, describing a colony which grows out laterally in spines from a stab inoculation. [Gk *echinos* hedgehog.]

Echis (ek·is). A genus of vipers occurring in Africa and India. **Echis carinatus.** A viper (subfamily Viperinae) locally known as the *phoorsa*. It is very small but highly poisonous. [Gk viper.]

echma (**ek**·mah). A stoppage. [Gk.]

echmasis (**ek**·mas·is). 1. Echma. 2. An obstructive disease.

echo (ek·o). A reverberation which may be heard in auscultation of the chest. **Amphoric echo.** A term used when the hollow sound heard on auscultation of the chest while the patient is speaking is appreciably delayed. The sound is resonant as if the voice were speaking into the neck of a bottle. **Metallic echo.** In pneumopericardium and pneumothorax, the abnormal ringing sound which may be heard when the beat of the heart is listened to. **Echo sign.** *See* SIGN. **Echo speech.** *See* SPEECH. [Gk sound.]

echo-acousia (ek·o·ak·**oo**'·se·ah). A subjective disturbance of hearing in which there appears to be a repetition of a sound heard. [echo, Gk *akouein* to hear.]

echocardiography (ek·o·kar·de·**og**'·raf·e). The graphical representation of the movements of the structures of the heart obtained by detecting the echoes from these structures using pulses of ultrasound. [Gk *echo* sound, *kardia* heart, *graphein* to record.]

echo-encephalography (ek·o·en·kef·al·**og**'·raf·e). The recording of ultrasonic echoes from the brain, particularly to diagnose displacement of the midline structures. [echo, encephalography.]

echogram (ek·o·gram). The recording of ultrasonic waves from an organ, e.g. gravid uterus, heart, brain, abdominal organs. [echo, Gk *gramma* record.]

echographia (ek·o·graf·e·ah). 1. A type of agraphia in which the patient can write what is dictated to him or can copy anything written, but cannot himself give expression to his thoughts in writing. 2. In aphasia: (*a*) the patient, in writing, rewrites much of what he has already written; (*b*) questions given to the patient are copied in writing by him without any comprehension of their meaning. [echo, Gk *graphein* to write.]

echokinesis (ek·o·kin·e′·sis). Automatic purposeless mimicry of a gesture made by another person, such as occurs in latah. [echo, Gk *kinesis* movement.]

echolalia (ek·o·la·le·ah). Involuntary repetition of a word or sentence just spoken by another person. [echo, Gk *lalein* to babble like a child.]

echolalus (ek·o·la·lus). An individual who, under hypnosis, repeats words spoken to him without comprehending their meaning. [see prec.]

echomatism (ek·o·mat·izm). In hypnosis, the automatic mimicry of any act when the hand is pressed on the crown of the subject's head. [echo, Gk *matizein* to strive to do.]

echomimia (ek·o·mim·e·ah). Echopathy. [echo, Gk *mimesis* imitation.]

echomotism (ek·o·mo·tizm). Echomatism.

echopathy (ek·op·ath·e). A morbid condition in which the patient automatically repeats words he hears and imitates actions he sees. [echo, Gk *pathos* suffering.]

echophony (ek·of·on·e). In auscultation of the chest, an immediate echo of a voice sound. [echo, Gk *phone* voice.]

echophotony (ek·o·fot·on·e). The mental association of tones in sound with particular colours. [echo, Gk *phos* light, *tonos* tone.]

echophrasia (ek·o·fra·ze·ah). Echolalia. [echo, Gk *phrasein* to utter.]

echopraxia, echopraxis, echopraxy (ek·o·prax·e·ah, ek·o·prax·is, ek·o·prax·e). 1. Echomatism. 2. The patient imitates the gestures or movements of the examiner, rather than performing an act to command. [echo, Gk *praxis* a doing.]

echovirus (ek·o·vi·rus). A group of viruses forming a subgenus of the picornaviruses and distinguished from polioviruses and Coxsackie A and B viruses by their failure to grow in suckling mice. The name is an acronym from enteric, cytopathic, human, orphan viruses. They are human viruses isolated from the gut, causing cytopathic effects in cell culture and originally thought, incorrectly, not to be associated with disease. There are 32 serotypes by neutralization and complement fixation. Two other former echoviruses have been re-allocated to other groups: Echo 10 is classed as a reovirus and Echo 28 is classed as a rhinovirus. Some echovirus serotypes are associated with respiratory infections, particularly in children, and types 4, 6 and 9 have been recovered from cases of aseptic meningitis.

Eck, Nicolai Vladimirovich (b. 1847). Russian physiologist.

Eck's fistula. A communication between the portal vein and the inferior vena cava.

Eck's fistula in reverse. A surgical communication designed to return the blood from the lower part of the body through the portal vein and liver when the inferior vena cava is blocked.

Ecker, Alexander (b. 1816). Freiburg anatomist.

Ecker's corpuscle. A blood platelet.

Ecker's fissure. Ecker's sulcus (see below).

Ecker's gyrus. Gyrus descendens.

Ecker's plug. York plug. *See* PLUG.

Ecker's sulcus. The transverse sulcus of the occipital lobe.

eclabium (ek·la·be·um). Eversion of the lip or lips. [Gk *ek*, L *labium* lip.]

eclampsia (ek·lamp·se·ah). An attack of convulsions; the word is now almost entirely confined to that associated with pregnancy. An acute toxaemia of pregnancy in pregnant (antepartum), parturient (intrapartum), or puerperal (postpartum) women, the essential feature being convulsions accompanied by high blood pressure, albuminuria and oedema of varying degree. Its onset is heralded by severe headache, dizziness, visual disturbances, epigastric pain and vomiting, and preliminary twitchings and mental confusion usually precede the convulsion, which passes through a tonic state of rigidity to a clonic contraction and relaxation of the muscles with noisy breathing and cyanosis; a coma ensues which may last any time, the patient remembering nothing of the event after regaining consciousness. **Eclampsia nutans.** Nodding spasm. *See* SPASM. **Eclampsia rotans.** Gyrospasm. [Gk *ek*, *lampein* to flash.]

eclampsism (ek·lamp·sizm). Puerperal eclampsia without convulsions, but with typical toxaemia.

eclamptic (ek·lamp·tik). Referring to or of the nature of eclampsia.

eclamptogenetic, eclamptogenic, eclamptogenous (ek·lamp·to·jen·et′·ik, ek·lamp·to·jen′·ik, ek·lamp·toj·en·us). Convulsive. [eclampsia, Gk *genein* to produce.]

eclectic (ek·lek·tik). 1. Referring to eclecticism. 2. A physician who follows a selective method of treatment. [see foll.]

eclecticism (ek·lek·tis·izm). 1. The choosing, from various systems of medicine by a special medical cult, of the most valued remedies to form a system of therapeutics in which the importance of indigenous plant remedies was emphasized. 2. The advocacy of this system. [Gk *eklektikos* selecting.]

eclimia (ek·lim·e·ah). Bulimia. [Gk *ek*, *limos* hunger.]

eclipsis (ek·lip·sis). 1. Temporary loss of consciousness. 2. Catalepsy. [Gk *ekleipsis* a failing.]

eclosion (ek·lo·zhun). An entomological term indicating the hatching of the larva from the ova or the imago from the pupa. [L *e*, *clausus* shut.]

eclysis (ek·lis·is). 1. Slight syncope; a tendency to syncope. 2. A loosening, as of the bowels. [Gk *eklysis* release.]

ecmetropia (ek·met·ro·pe·ah). Ametropia. [Gk *ek*, *metron* measure, *opsis* sight.]

ecmnesia (ek·ne·ze·ah). A form of amnesia in which there is total, but as a rule temporary, forgetfulness of recent events, the memory of more distant ones remaining unimpaired. [Gk *ek*, *mnesis* memory.]

ecnoea (ek·ne·ah). Insanity. [Gk *ek*, *nous* mind.]

eco-. For words beginning with **Eco-**, *see also* OECO-.

ecochleation (e·kok·le·a′·shun). 1. Enucleation. 2. Surgical removal of the cochlea. [L *e*, cochlea.]

ecology (e·kol·o·je). The branch of biology which deals with the mutual relations between an organism and its environment. **Human ecology.** The relationship between man and his environment.

Economo, Konstantin von (b. 1876). Vienna neurologist.

von Economo's disease or encephalitis. Epidemic encephalitis lethargica; less commonly called *Cruchet's disease.*

economy (e·kon·o·me). 1. The principles of the arrangement or working of anything. 2. The system according to which the processes of assimilation and excretion are carried on in an organism. **Animal economy.** The body of an animal considered as an organized whole; an old term for physiology. [Gk *oikos* house, *nomos* law.]

écorché (a·kor·sha). An anatomical figure or manikin deprived of its skin so that the muscular system is exposed. [Fr. *écorcher* to flay.]

ecostate (e·kos·tate). Ribless. [L *e*, *costa* rib.]

Ecothiopate Iodide BP 1973 (ek·o·thio·pate i·o·dide). *S*-2-dimethylaminoethyl diethyl phosphorothioate methiodide, an anticholinesterase used topically in the treatment of glaucoma.

ecphoria, ecphory (ek·for·e·ah, ek·for·e). Activation of a memory trace (engram) by an appropriate stimulus. [Gk *ek*, *pherein* to bear.]

ecphronia (ek·fro·ne·ah). Insanity. [Gk *ek*, *phren* mind.]

ecphyadectomy (ek·fi·ad·ek′·to·me). Appendicectomy. [ecphyas, Gk *ektome* a cutting out.]

ecphyaditis (ek·fi·ad·i′·tis). Appendicitis. [ecphyas, Gk *itis* inflammation.]

ecphyas (ek·fi·as). The vermiform appendix. [Gk *ekphyas* appendix.]

ecphylactic (ek·fi·**lak**·tik). Referring to, characterized by or belonging to ecphylaxis.

ecphylaxis (ek·fi·**lax**·is). A condition in which the phylactic agents or antibodies in the blood or tissues have lost their potency. [Gk *ek, phylaxis* a guarding.]

ecphyma (ek·**fi**·mah). A protuberance on the skin; an outgrowth, as a wart. **Ecphyma globulus.** A contagious skin disease formerly endemic in Ireland in which tubercles form on the skin and progress to soft raspberry-like tumours. It has a resemblance to yaws. [Gk *ek, phyma* a growth.]

écrasement (a·krahz·**mahn**). An operation carried out with an écraseur. [Fr. a crushing.]

écraseur (a·krahz·er. A surgical instrument consisting of a mechanically operated wire loop, cord or steel chain which, looped round a part, divides it by a slow process of bruising. **Galvanic écraseur.** A type through which a current can be passed while it is being used so that the wire becomes red hot. [Fr. a crusher.]

ecrodactylia (ek·ro·dak·**til**'·e·ah). The spontaneous separation of fingers or toes that occurs in, for example, ainhum. [Gk *ekrein* to flow forth, *daktylos* finger.]

ecstaltic (ek·**stal**·tik). A term applied to nerve impulses which are sent out from cell stations in the spinal cord or from other nerve centres. [Gk *ek, stellein* to set.]

ecstasy (**ek**·stas·e). A term used in psychiatry and in theology to denote a state of "merging" whereby the subject becomes identified with external reality which itself is endowed with a feeling of complete personal significance. Syn. cosmic consciousness. William James spoke of its four factors of transiency, passivity, ineffability and noëtic quality. [Gk *ekstasis* derangement.]

ecstatic (ek·**stat**·ik). Marked by ecstasy; belonging to ecstasy.

ecstrophy (**ek**·stro·fe). Exstrophy; congenital eversion of a hollow organ, e.g. the bladder. [Gk *ekstrophe* a turning out.]

ectacolia (ek·tah·**ko**·le·ah). Dilatation of the colon. [Gk *ektakos* capable of being stretched, colon.]

ectal (**ek**·tal). 1. Outer. 2. Superficial. 3. In comparison of position, placed farther from hypothetical centre than is the object compared. [Gk *ektos* outside.]

ectasia, ectasis (ek·**ta**·ze·ah, **ek**·tas·is). Natural or artificial dilatation of a canal or hollow organ. **Alveolar ectasia.** Distension of the alveoli of the lungs, i.e. emphysema of the lungs. **Corneal ectasia.** Bulging and thinning of the cornea due to either disease of the cornea or raised intra-ocular pressure. Also called *staphyloma of the cornea.* **Diffuse arterial ectasia.** Cirsoid aneurysm. **Hypostatic ectasia.** Dilatation of a blood vessel, particularly a vein, in a dependent portion of the body, as a varicose vein. **Ectasia iridis.** Displacement of the iris so that the pupil of the eye is diminished. **Papillary ectasia.** A raised red spot on the skin caused by circumscribed dilatation of the capillary vessels. **Peripapillary ectasia.** A congenital condition in which the coats of the eye directly surrounding the optic disc are thinned and form a deep cup as seen from the inside, the optic disc lying at the bottom of the cup. **Peripheral corneal ectasia.** Marginal corneal dystrophy. **Scleral ectasia.** Bulging and thinning of the sclera due to either disease or raised intra-ocular pressure. It can be total, as in buphthalmia, or partial as in staphyloma. **Senile ectasia.** Tufts of dilated capillaries or veins immediately under the epidermis that cause discoloured patches in the skin of old people. **Ectasia ventriculi.** Dilatation of the stomach. **Ectasia ventriculi paradoxa.** Bilocular stomach. *See* STOMACH. [Gk *ektasis* a stretching.]

ectatic (ek·**tat**·ik). 1. Dilated or stretched. 2. Referring to or characterized by ectasis. [see prec.]

ectental (ek·**ten**·tal). In biology, relating to both the ectoderm and the entoderm, as ectental line. [Gk *ektos* outside, *entos* within.]

ectethmoid (ek·**teth**·moid). Describing either of the 2 labyrinths of the ethmoid bone. [Gk *ektos* outside, ethmoid bone.]

ecthyma (ek·**thi**·mah). A deep or dermic type of impetigo. The initial lesion is either a vesicopustule or a small bulla having an erythematous areola. This spreads peripherally, a crust forms, and under it an indolent ulcer will be found. The lesions are discrete and usually develop on the lower limbs; they are bacterial in origin, inoculable and auto-inoculable, and the majority of patients are debilitated. **Ecthyma contagiosum.** Orf; sheep-pox: a zoonosis caused by a filtrable virus contracted from sheep suffering from contagious pustular dermatitis. The initial lesion is an indurated painless papule which later becomes umbilicated and resembles a large red molluscum-contagiosum lesion. **Ecthyma gangraenosum.** Pyoderma gangraenosum: furunculous lesions which rapidly break down so that ulcers are formed; areas of necrosis and gangrene are then noted. Almost invariably the malady is associated with ulcerative colitis. **Gangrenous infantile ecthyma.** Dermatitis gangraenosum. **Ecthyma terebrans infantum, Ecthyma térébrant.** Dermatitis gangraenosa infantum. [Gk *ek, thyein* to rush.]

ecthymatiform, ecthymiform (ek·thi·**mat**·e·form, ek·**thi**·me·form). Having resemblance to ecthyma. [ecthyma, form.]

ecthyreosis (**ek**·thi·re·**o**'·sis). A condition resulting from absence, or complete removal, of the thyroid gland. [Gk *ek*, thyroid.]

ectillotic (ek·til·**ot**·ik). A depilatory. The chief ectillotics are the sulphides of calcium and barium; they act by dissolving the keratin of the hair, and are applied to the skin in the form of a paste with water, allowed to remain for 5 min and then washed off, when the hair usually comes away. If left on too long, irritation of the skin may occur. Thallium acetate used internally and externally in ringworm of the scalp, often with toxic effects, like x-ray epilation is now superseded by the antibiotic griseofulvin in the therapy of ringworm infections. [Gk *ek, tillein* to pluck.]

ecto-antigen (ek·to·**an**·te·jen). An antigen which diffuses from the living cell or is produced by the cells in the external medium, e.g. exotoxins of diphtheria and tetanus organisms. [Gk *ektos* outside, antigen.]

ectobatic (ek·to·**bat**·ik). Centrifugal or efferent. [Gk *ektos* outside, *bainein* to go.]

ectoblast (**ek**·to·blast). 1. The wall of a cell. 2. Ectoderm. 3. Any outer membrane. [Gk *ektos* outside, *blastos* germ.]

ectocardia (ek·to·**kar**·de·ah). Any congenital misplacement of the heart. **Ectocardia abdominalis.** A congenital malformation in which the heart is situated within a sac in the lower part of the thorax or entirely within the abdominal cavity. **Ectocardia cephalica, Ectocardia cervicalis.** Misplacement of the heart to the base of the neck. **Ectocardia extrathoracica.** A malformation in which the heart is situated outside the thoracic cavity. **Ectocardia intrathoracica.** A malformation in which the heart lies within the thorax. **Ectocardia pectoralis.** Misplacement of the heart to the front of the chest. [Gk *ektos* outside, *kardia* heart.]

ectochoroidea (**ek**·to·kor·**oid**'·e·ah). The suprachoroid lamina of the vascular coat of the eye. [Gk *ektos* outside, choroid.]

ectocinerea (**ek**·to·sin·**e**'·re·ah). The grey matter of the cortex of the brain. [Gk *ektos* outside, cinerea.]

ectocinereal (**ek**·to·sin·**e**'·re·al). Relating to the cortical grey matter of the cerebrum. [see prec.]

ectocolon (ek·to·**ko**·lon). Dilatation of the colon. [Gk *ektasis* a stretching, colon.]

ectocolostomy (**ek**·to·kol·**os**'·to·me). The surgical establishment of an opening into the colon through the wall of the abdomen. [Gk *ektos* outside, colostomy.]

ectocondylar (**ek**·to·kon·**di**'·lar). Relating to the lateral condyle of a bone. [see foll.]

ectocondyle (ek·to·**kon**·dile). The lateral condyle of a bone. [Gk *ektos* outside, condyle.]

ectocondyloid (**ek**·to·kon·**di**'·loid). Ectocondylar.

ectocornea (ek·to·**kor**·ne·ah). The corneal epithelium or outermost layer of the cornea. [Gk *ektos* outside, cornea.]

ectocranial (ek·to·**kra**·ne·al). Relating or belonging to the exterior of the skull. [Gk *ektos* outside, cranium.]

ectocuneiform (ek·to·kew·**ne**′·e·form). The lateral cuneiform bone. [Gk *ektos* outside, cuneiform bone.]

ectocyst (**ek**·to·sist). The outer layer of a dermoid or hydatid cyst. [Gk *ektos* outside, cyst.]

ectocytic (ek·to·**si**·tik). Outside the cell wall; not part of its organization. [Gk *ektos* outside, *kytos* cell.]

ectodactylism (ek·to·**dak**·til·izm). The condition of lacking one or more fingers or toes. [Gk *ektos* outside, *dactylos* finger.]

ectoderm (**ek**·to·derm). The outer germinal layer of the early embryo which gives rise to the epidermis and its derivatives (e.g. sweat glands, hair follicles, mammary glands), the lining of the mouth and nose, the central and peripheral nervous systems, and the lens of the eye. **Amniotic ectoderm.** The epithelial layer of the amnion. **Basal ectoderm.** The inner layer of the multilayered fetal epidermis which becomes the germinal or malpighian layer of the skin. **Blastodermic ectoderm.** The outer epithelial layer of the primitive blastoderm before gastrulation. **Chorionic ectoderm.** The epithelial layer of the chorion which covers both the chorionic membrane and the chorionic villi of the placenta. **Epidermal ectoderm.** Ectoderm which gives rise to the epidermis of the skin. **Neural ectoderm.** That part of the primitive ectoderm which invaginates to become the neural tube and neural crest. **Primitive ectoderm.** The undifferentiated outer epithelial layer of the early embryo. **Two-layered ectoderm.** The embryonic epidermis, consisting of a basal layer and an outer layer or periderm. [Gk *ektos* outside, *derma* skin.]

ectodermal (ek·to·**der**·mal). 1. Relating or belonging to the ectoderm. 2. Originating in the ectoderm.

ectodermatosis (ek·to·der·mat·**o**′·sis). Any disorder arising from congenital maldevelopment of ectodermal organs, e.g. skin, nervous system. **Ectodermatosis erosiva pluriorificialis.** A form of erythema multiforme in which the mucous membrane of, for example, the anus, penis, mouth, show eroding lesions. [ectoderm, Gk *-osis* condition.]

ectodermic (ek·to·**der**·mik). Ectodermal.

ectodermoidal (ek·to·der·**moid**′·al). Resembling or having the characteristics of ectoderm. [ectoderm, Gk *eidos* form.]

ectodermosis (ek·to·der·**mo**′·sis). Ectodermatosis.

ecto-enzyme (ek·to·**en**·zime). An extracellular enzyme, excreted into the surrounding tissue or medium. Cf. ENDOENZYME. [Gk *ektos* outside, enzyme.]

ecto-ethmoid (ek·to·**eth**·moid). Ectethmoid.

ectogenic, ectogenous (ek·to·**jen**·ik, ek·**toj**·en·us). 1. Originating outside the organism, e.g. bacteria of an infectious disease. 2. Able to develop or grow outside the body, e.g. a parasite or bacterium. [Gk *ektos* outside, *genein* to produce.]

ectoglia (ek·**tog**·le·ah). In embryology, the thin non-nucleated superficial layer of cells laid down when the neural tube begins to form. [Gk *ektos* outside, neuroglia.]

ectoglobular (ek·to·**glob**·ew·lar). Not formed within a globular body, particularly a blood corpuscle. [Gk *ektos* outside, globe.]

ectogluteus (ek·to·**gloo**·te·us). The gluteus maximus muscle. [Gk *ektos* outside, gluteus.]

ectogony (ek·**tog**·in·e). The effect exerted on the maternal system by the developing embryo. [Gk *ektos* outside, *gone* seed.]

ectokelostomy (ek·to·ke·**los**′·to·me). The operation of draining the infected sac of an inguinal hernia through the wall of the abdomen as preparation for radical treatment. [Gk *ektos* outside, *kele* hernia, *stoma* mouth.]

ectolecithal (ek·to·**les**·ith·al). In embryology, having the yolk material concentrated at the periphery of the ovum. [Gk *ektos* outside, *lekithos* yolk.]

ectolysis (ek·**tol**·is·is). Lysis of the plasma membrane. [ectoplasm, lysis.]

ectomeninx (ek·to·**men**·ingx). The layer of condensed mesenchyme surrounding the developing central nervous system, from which the dura mater and part of the skull are developed. [Gk *ektos* outside, *meninx* membrane.]

ctomere (**ek**·to·meer). Any one of the blastomeres which take part in forming the ectoderm. [Gk *ektos* outside, *meros* part.]

ectomesoblast (ek·to·**mez**·o·blast). In embryology, the layer of undifferentiated matter, including cells from which ectoblastic and mesoblastic tissue will be formed. [Gk *ektos* outside, mesoblast.]

ectomesoderm (ek·to·**mez**·o·derm). Mesoderm derived from the upper layer of a bilaminar embryonic disk. [Gk *ektos* outside, mesoderm.]

ectomorphy (ek·to·**mor**·fe). The type of build of the body in which the predominating tissues are those derived from the ectoderm. [Gk *ektos* outside, *morphe* form.]

ectomy (**ek**·to·me). Amputation or excision of a part or organ. **Subtotal ectomy.** The surgical removal of a portion of a part or organ. [Gk *ektome* a cutting out.]

ectonuclear (ek·to·**new**·kle·ar). Relating to the part of a cell outside the nucleus. [Gk *ektos* outside, nucleus.]

ecto-organism (ek·to·**or**·gan·izm). An organism, such as an ectoparasite, which exists externally to another organism. [Gk *ektos* outside, organism.]

ectopagus (ek·**top**·ag·us). A twin monster joined at the side along the entire extent of the thorax. [Gk *ektos* outside, *pagos* fixture.]

ectoparasite (ek·to·**par**·ah·site). A parasite which spends all or some part of its life on the outside of the body of its hosts. Lice and itch mites are permanent ectoparasites of man; fleas are partial ectoparasites. [Gk *ektos* outside, parasite.]

ectopectoralis (**ek**·to·pek·tor·**a**′·lis). The pectoralis major muscle. [Gk *ektos* outside, L *pectus* breast.]

ectoperitoneal (**ek**·to·per·e·ton·**e**′·al). Relating to the abdominal surface or the external surface of the peritoneum. [Gk *ektos* outside, peritoneum.]

ectoperitonitis (**ek**·to·per·e·ton·**i**′·tis). Inflammation of the abdominal surface or the external surface of the peritoneum. [Gk *ektos* outside, peritonitis.]

ectophylaxination (**ek**·to·fil·ax·in·**a**′·shun). Immunization by transference of a prophylactic substance from one animal to another. [Gk *ektos* outside, prophylaxis.]

ectophyte (**ek**·to·fite). A vegetable ectoparasite; a vegetable growth parasitic on the skin. [Gk *ektos* outside, *phyton* plant.]

ectopia (ek·**to**·pe·ah). A morbid congenital malposition or traumatic displacement of an organ or part. **Ectopia ani.** Prolapse of the anus. **Ectopia bulbi.** Ectopia oculi (see below). **Ectopia cordis.** Congenital displacement of the heart outside the cavity of the thorax. **Ectopia lentis.** Displacement, congenital or traumatic, of the lens of the eye. **Ectopia oculi.** Malposition of the eyeball within the orbit. **Ectopia pupillae congenita.** Corectopia. **Ectopia renis.** Floating kidney. *See* KIDNEY. **Ectopia testis.** Abnormal position or dislocation of the testis. **Ectopia vesicae.** A condition of the bladder in which it is turned inside out (extrophia). **Visceral ectopia.** Congenital umbilical hernia. [Gk *ek*, *topos* place.]

ectopic (ek·**top**·ik). 1. Referring to, characterized by, or belonging to ectopia. 2. An organ or substance not in its proper position, or of a pregnancy, (ectopic gestation) occurring elsewhere than in the cavity of the uterus. 3. In cardiology, indicating a heart beat resulting from an impulse generated somewhere in the heart other than the sinu-atrial node and, more particularly, in an unidentifiable focus in the atrial or ventricular myocardium.

ectopism (**ek**·to·pizm). Anatopism. [Gk *ek*, *topos* place.]

ectoplasm (**ek**·to·plazm). The compact outer hyaline layer surrounding the protoplasm of a cell (plasma membrane); it is formed by condensation of the protoplasm. [Gk *ektos* outside, plasma.]

ectoplasmatic (**ek**·to·plaz·**mat**′·ik). 1. Referring or belonging to ectoplasm. 2. Situated away from the cell protoplasm.

ectoplast (**ek**·to·plast). Ectoplasm.

ectoplastic (ek·to·**plas**·tik). 1. Formed at the periphery. 2. Occurring or forming upon the surface or in the ectoplasm; a term applied to cells. [Gk *ektos* outside, plasma.]

ectopocystis (**ek**·to·po·**sis**′·tis). A condition in which the bladder is displaced. [Gk *ek*, *topos* place, *kystis* bag.]

ectopotomy (ek·to·**pot**·o·me). In cases of ectopic pregnancy,

abdominal section in order to remove the fetus or the contents of the gestation sac. [Gk *ek, topos* place, *temnein* to cut.]
ectopterygoid (ek·to·**ter**·e·goid). The lateral pterygoid muscle of the head. [Gk *ektos* outside, pterygoid muscle.]
ectopy (**ek**·to·pe). Ectopia.
ectoretina (ek·to·**ret**·in·ah). The stratum opticum (outermost layer) of the retina. [Gk *ektos* outside, retina.]
ectorhinal (ek·to·**ri**·nal). Outside the nose. [Gk *ektos* outside, *rhis* nose.]
ectosarc (**ek**·to·sark). The ectoplasm (outer membrane) of a unicellular organism such as an amoeba. [Gk *ektos* outside, *sarx* flesh.]
ectoscopy (ek·**tos**·ko·pe). 1. The general assessment of position and outline of the lungs and other internal organs by means of visual inspection. 2. The diagnosis of disease of an internal organ by watching movement of the thorax or abdominal walls while the patient is uttering vocal sounds. [Gk *ektos* outside, *skopein* to watch.]
ectosite (**ek**·to·site). Ectoparasite.
ectoskeletal (ek·to·**skel**·et·al). Relating to the ectoskeleton.
ectoskeleton (ek·to·**skel**·et·on). Exoskeleton. [Gk *ektos* outside, skeleton.]
ectosphenoid (ek·to·**sfe**·noid). The lateral cuneiform bone of the foot, sometimes referred to as the ectocuneiform bone. [Gk *ektos* outside, sphenoid.]
ectosphere (**ek**·to·sfeer). The outer zone of a centrosome. [Gk *ektos* outside, sphere.]
ectosteal (ek·**tos**·te·al). 1. Relating or belonging to ectostosis. 2. Situated on the outside of a bone. [Gk *ektos* outside, *osteon* bone.]
ectostosis (ek·tos·**to**·sis). Ossification beginning under the perichondrium and gradually surrounding or replacing cartilage. [Gk *ektos* outside, *osteon* bone, *-osis* condition.]
ectosuggestion (ek·to·suj·**es**′·chun). Suggestion coming from the environment or from someone other than the subject: the opposite of autosuggestion. [Gk *ektos* outside, suggestion.]
ectothrix (**ek**·to·thrix). General term for fungi producing arthrospores on the surface of the hair shaft. [Gk *ektos* outside, *thrix* hair.]
ectotoxaemia (ek·to·tox·e′·me·ah). Toxaemia the source or cause of which is outside the body. [Gk *ektos* outside, toxaemia.]
ectotoxin (ek·to·**tox**·in). Exotoxin. [Gk *ektos* outside, toxin.]
ectotriceps (ek·to·**tri**·seps). The lateral head of the triceps brachii muscle. [Gk *ektos* outside, triceps muscle.]
Ectotrichophyton (ek·to·trik·o·fi·ton). Archaic name for the genus *Trichophyton*, one of the dermatophytic fungi. [Gk *ektos* outside, *thrix* hair, *phyton* plant.]
ectotrochanter (ek·to·tro·**kan**′·ter). The greater trochanter. [Gk *ektos* outside, trochanter.]
ectozoon (ek·to·**zo**·on) (pl. *ectozoa*). A name for external animal parasites in general. [Gk *ektos* outside, *zoon* animal.]
ectrodactylia, ectrodactylism, ectrodactyly (ek·tro·dak·**til**′·e·ah, ek·tro·**dak**·til·izm, ek·tro·**dak**·til·e). Congenital absence of one or more fingers or toes. [Gk *ektrosis* miscarriage, *daktylos* finger.]
ectrogenic (ek·tro·**jen**·ik). Referring to, characterized by or caused by ectrogeny.
ectrogeny (ek·**troj**·en·e). Congenital absence or defect of a part of the body. [Gk *ektrosis* miscarriage, *genein* to produce.]
ectromelia (ek·tro·**me**·le·ah). Congenital lack of one or more limbs. **Infectious ectromelia.** Mouse pox; a virus disease of mice caused by a poxvirus. The extremities become gangrenous and are sloughed in the classical form of the disease. It may also present mainly as a visceral disease (pneumonia or hepatitis) or remain latent in laboratory mouse stocks. [Gk *ektrosis* miscarriage, *melos* limb.]
ectromelic (ek·tro·**me**·lik). 1. Referring to ectromelia. 2. Referring to an ectromelus.
ectromelus (ek·**trom**·el·us). A monster without limbs or with defective ones. [Gk *ektrosis* miscarriage, *melos* limb.]
ectromely (ek·**trom**·el·e). Ectromelia.
ectropia (ek·tro·pe·ah). Exstrophy. **Intestinal ectropia.** Adenoma of the umbilicus. [Gk *ek, trope* turn.]
ectropic (ek·**trop**·ik). 1. Everted. 2. Inside out. 3. Referring to an exstrophy. [see prec.]
ectropion, ectropium (ek·**tro**·pe·on, ek·**tro**·pe·um). Eversion, usually of the eyelids, especially of the lower. **Cervical ectropion.** Eversion of the external os uteri, exposing the endocervix. **Cicatricial ectropion.** Ectropion due to contraction of scar tissue in the lids. **Flaccid ectropion.** Drooping of the lower lid with eversion. **Ectropion luxurians.** Ectropion sarcomatosum (see below). **Mechanical ectropion.** Eversion of the eyelid due to extreme proptosis or thickening of the conjunctiva such as occurs after severe conjunctivitis. **Paralytic ectropion.** Ectropion due to paralysis of the orbicularis oculi muscle, affecting only the lower lid. **Ectropion sarcomatosum.** Ectropion arising out of luxuriant overgrowth of the exposed palpebral conjunctiva which has a fleshy appearance. **Senile ectropion.** That due to senile relaxation of the palpebral portion of the orbicularis ocul muscle. **Ectropion spasticum.** Ectropion due to spasm of the lid when they are well supported by the globe; it occurs mos commonly in phlyctenular disease. **Ectropion uveae.** Tha affecting the iris and consisting in a portion of the posterio pigment layer growing or being drawn round the pupil margin s as to appear in front. It is commonly seen in absolute glaucoma and may occur as a late result of severe iritis. A congenital form consists in a circular mass of dark colour projecting round th margin of the pupil to reach the front surface of the iris. It occur in horses. [Gk *ek, trepein* to turn.]
ectropodism (ek·**trop**·od·izm). The congenital condition of bein without a toe or toes. [Gk *ektrosis* miscarriage, *pous* foot.]
ectrosyndactyly (ek·tro·sin·**dak**′·til·e). A congenital condition i which one or more of the fingers are lacking and the others ar fused into one. [Gk *ektrosis* miscarriage, syndactyly.]
Ectylurea (ek·til·**ewr**·e·ah). BP Commission approved name fo α-ethylcrotonylurea; a sedative.
ectype (**ek**·tipe). Mental or physical constitution outstanding c unusual in type. [Gk *ek, typos* mark.]
ectypia (ek·**tip**·e·ah). Any deviation from type. [see prec.]
eczema (**ek**·ze·mah). A non-contagious inflammatory disease the skin with much itching and burning. It may be acut subacute or chronic, and takes the form of erythema at th outset, with papules, vesicles or pustules that may develop in scales and crusts. It may occur at any age, and may be caused b a variety of internal and external factors. By some the name applied only to cases of *sensitization dermatitis.* **Allergic eczem** Eczema caused by endogenous or exogenous allergens or b haptens. **Asteatotic eczema.** Dry, fissured eczema, most marke on the limbs, occurring in the winter, particularly in the elder or in xerodermatous individuals. **Atopic eczema.** Atopic dermat tis; eczema occurring as a part of the symptom complex of th atopic state. **Bakers' eczema.** Bakers' dermatitis. *See* DERMAT TIS. **Bleachers' eczema.** Contact dermatitis occurring in perso engaged in a bleaching process, particularly in one of the texti industries. The agents which may be responsible include caust soda, sodium carbonate, chlorine, hypochlorites and oxa acid. **Eczema circumscriptum.** A chronic papulo-erythemato and slightly scaling eruption, chiefly affecting the lower le **Eczéma craquelé.** A form of eczema in which shallow cracks fissures form in the epidermis: these extend only to the rete. some places the superficial layers of the epidermis are detach at the edges of the cracks and may be everted, but the th cuticular scales are quite adherent except at their borders. T pattern resembles cracked china. **Eczema crustosum.** Eczen with yellowish crusts. **Discoid eczema.** Nummular eczema (s below). **Endogenous eczema.** Eczema due to some system condition. **Eczema erythematosum** (archaic). 1. A sca erythematous eruption often associated with oedema. 2. Inte trigo. **Eczema exfoliativum.** An eczematous eruption characte ized by exfoliation; exfoliative dermatitis. *See* DERMATI **Eczema fissum.** 1. Fissured eczema; the fissures tend most eas

to develop on the face when that area is affected by a squamous or scaling dermatitis, or on the hands when affected by a thickened, hyperkeratotic dermatitis. 2. Chapped hands. **Fissured eczema.** 1. Eczema fissum (see above). 2. Eczéma craquelé (see above). **Follicular eczema, Eczema folliculorum.** A papulovesicular eruption in which the lesions arise in the neighbourhood of the follicles. **Gravitational eczema.** Hypostatic eczema (see below). **Eczema herpeticum.** Kaposi's varicelliform eruption. **Eczema herpetiforme.** A name for the eruption now called *Kaposi's varicelliform eruption.* **Herpetoid eczema.** Nummular eczema (see below). **Eczema hiemalis.** Asteatotic eczema (see above). **Hyperkeratotic eczema of the palms.** A chronic, fissured, hyperkeratotic condition of the palms of elderly men, sometimes a variant of lichen simplex. **Hypostatic eczema.** Chronic eczema of the legs arising from impaired venous return and sometimes complicated by infection or by sensitization to topical applications. **Eczema hypertrophicum.** Mycosis fungoides. **Infantile eczema.** Eczema of infants, whether atopic or allergic; some authors loosely include seborrhoeic eruptions in infants in this category. **Eczema intertrigo.** Erythema intertrigo; intertrigo. **Eczema madidans.** *See* ECZEMA RUBRUM (below). **Eczema marginatum.** Tinea cruris. Hebra gave this name (not recognizing the cause of the malady) to "a peculiar form of eczema, distinguished from all others by its constant localization on the inner surface of the thighs, the pubes and the buttocks. By its centrifugal progress and simultaneous involution at the centre, by its well-defined raised border, and by its almost exclusive occurrence in the male sex, and especially in shoemakers". **Nummular eczema, Eczema nummulare.** A form of eczema in which the lesions occur in small round or oval areas, and consist of groups of papules or vesicles. **Occupational eczema.** Sensitization dermatitis caused by exposure to deleterious agents during the course of the patient's employment. **Eczema papillomatosum.** Papilliferous excrescences arising on a pseudo-eczematous surface and associated with a foul-smelling discharge; the condition may arise from secondary infection of an eczema, but often the eruption is not a manifestation of the latter. **Eczema papulosum.** Eczema characterized by the formation of minute red papules. **Phlyctenular eczema.** A vesicular eruption of the thenar eminences and wrists. **Eczema pustulosum.** Eczema characterized by the formation of pustules. **Eczema rhagadiforme.** Eczema fissum (see above). **Eczema rubrum.** A stage of eczema characterized by redness, swelling, infiltration and moisture. The outer layers of the epidermis are lost, and crusting is noted. If the lesions are red and oozing, the condition is named *eczema madidans.* **Eczema sclerosum.** The most chronic and least inflammatory of eczematous eruptions, characterized by thickening and infiltration; usually seen on the hands, ankles or soles. **Eczema seborrhoeicum.** A form of seborrhoeic dermatitis. **Eczema siccum.** Dry, scaly eczema. **Eczema solare.** Light-sensitization dermatitis. *See* DERMATITIS. **Eczema tyloticum.** That usually seen on limited areas on the hands; the term refers to the carapace of horny tissue which occasionally forms during the healing stage of a vesicular eczema. The condition was thought to resemble tylosis. **Eczema unguinum.** Changes in the nails secondary to eczema of the peri-ungual areas. **Eczema vaccinatum.** Kaposi's varicelliform eruption, or eruptions confused with this malady. **Varicose eczema, Eczema varicosum.** Hypostatic eczema (see above). **Eczema verrucosum.** Crowded wart-like excrescences on a bluish-red area, usually situated near the ankle. **Vesicular eczema, Eczema vesiculosum, Weeping eczema.** A form of eczema characterized by a fluid exudate. [Gk *ekzein* to boil over.]

See also: BROCQ, HEBRA.

eczematid (ek·zem·at·id). A loose term for an allergic sequel to an eczematous condition. [see prec.]

eczematization (ek·zem·at·i·za′·shun). 1. Eczema occurring secondarily to an already existing dermatitis. 2. Persistent eczematous lesions of the skin caused by trauma from continued scratching. [Gk *ekzein* to boil over.]

eczematoid (ek·zem·at·oid). Having the characters of eczema. [eczema, Gk *eidos* form.]

eczematosis (ek·zem·at·o′·sis). 1. An extensive attack of eczema. 2. Any skin disease eczematous in character. [eczema, Gk *-osis* condition.]

eczematous (ek·zem·at·us). Affected with or resembling eczema.

eczemogenous (ek·zem·oj·en·us). Giving rise to eczema. [eczema, Gk *genein* to produce.]

Eddowes, Alfred (b. 1850). London physician.

Eddowes's syndrome. Osteogenesis imperfecta.

Eddyism (ed·e·izm). Christian Science. [Mary Baker Glover *Eddy*, 1821–1910, American founder of the sect.]

ede-. For words beginning with **Ede-**, *see also* OEDE-.

Edebohls, George Michael (b. 1853). New York surgeon.

Edebohls' incision, or operation. Nephropexy by means of mattress sutures through the true capsule of the kidney after decapsulation, through a vertical lumbar incision (Edebohls' incision) along the outer border of the sacrospinalis muscle.

Edebohls' position. The dorsosacral position; the patient lies on his back with the legs flexed at the knees, and the thighs flexed on to the abdomen with the legs abducted.

Edelmann, Adolf (b. 1885). Vienna physician.

Edelmann's anaemia. Anaemia of chronic infections.

Edelmann's cell. One of the small motile particles of plasma thought to represent a fourth type of corpuscle in addition to the red blood cell, white blood cell and platelet.

edema (e·de·mah). *See* OEDEMA.

edentate (e·den·tate). 1. An edentulous person. 2. A mammal which normally has no teeth. [L *e, dens* tooth.]

edentia (e·den·she·ah). Absence of teeth. [see prec.]

edentulous (e·den·tew·lus). Toothless (having lost the teeth). [L *e, dens* tooth.]

edestin (ed·es·tin). A crystallizable globulin obtained from hemp seed and certain other seeds such as the castor-oil bean. It contains all the essential amino acids, and will support growth in a diet free from other proteins. It has been used as substrate in determining peptic activity. [Gk *edestos* edible.]

edge (ej). **Incisive edge [margo incisalis (NA)].** The cutting edge of a tooth.

edge-strength (ej·strength). A term used to express the property of resistance to distortion and fracture of a dental filling material.

Edinger, Ludwig (b. 1855). Frankfurt neurologist.

Edinger's bundle. Fibres in the middle part of the medial lemniscus.

Edinger's law. Neurons respond by increased growth to maintained and slowly increasing stimulation, but undergo atrophy in response to excessive and intermittent stimulation.

Edinger's nucleus, Edinger–Westphal nucleus. A nucleus ventrolateral to the upper end of the aqueduct of the midbrain giving origin to oculomotor nerve fibres to the sphincter of the pupil and ciliary muscles.

Edison, Thomas Alva (b. 1847). American inventor.

Edison effect. The emission of charged particles from a hot filament *in vacuo*; thermionic effect.

Edogestrone (e·do·jes·trone). BP Commission approved name for 17-acetoxy-3,3-ethylenedioxy-6-methylpregn-5-en-20-one; a progestational steroid.

Edridge-Green, Frederick William (b. 1863). London ophthalmologist.

Edridge-Green classification. A classification of colour blindness based on the division of the spectrum into 6 colours, namely, red, orange, yellow, green, blue and violet.

Edridge-Green lamp, or lantern. A special lantern designed to test colour vision, used by the Board of Trade.

Edridge-Green lantern test. A test for colour vision designed for testing transport and shipping personnel: an Edridge-Green lantern is viewed from 6 m (20 ft) in a subdued light and the aperture, colour and intensity of the light from the lantern can be varied to simulate lights seen under all conditions.

Edrophonium Chloride BP 1973 (ed·ro·**fo**·ne·um **klor**·ide). Ethyl-*m*-hydroxyphenyldimethylammonium chloride, an anticholinesterase drug with a relatively short action. It is also sometimes used intravenously as a diagnostic test for myasthenia gravis.

Edsall, David Linn (b. 1869). Boston physician.

Edsall's disease. Heat cramp.

educt (e·dukt). 1. An extract. 2. Any chemical substance obtained from another in which it was present in the same form. Cf. PRODUCT. [L *e*, *ducere* to draw.]

edulcorant (e·dul·kor·ant). 1. Tending to correct acidity or acridity. 2. Sweetening, or tending to sweeten. 3. An agent which has the effect of rendering the body fluids less acid. [see foll.]

edulcorate (e·**dul**·kor·ate). 1. To free from acidity or acridity; to render sweet. 2. In chemistry, to purify. [L *edulcorare* to sweeten out.]

edulcoration (e·**dul**·kor·a'·shun). 1. The making of a substance sweet by the addition of sweetening agents. 2. The removal of acid or bitter-tasting constituents. [see prec.]

Edwards, John Hilton. 20th century British geneticist.

Edwards' syndrome. Deformed ears, micrognathia, prominent occiput, abnormal posture of fingers. Due to trisomy 17-18. It is usually fatal.

eelworm (eel·werm). One of many small species of nematodes which are free-living or plant-parasitic. **Vinegar eelworm.** *Anguillula* (= *Turbatrix*) *aceti*, which develops in vinegar. [AS *ael*, *wyrm*.]

effect (ef·**ekt**). 1. The result of an action or condition; a consequence. 2. The term has come to be applied to certain physical or chemical phenomena produced under specific conditions and usually of important theoretical significance. **Additive effect.** The combined effect of drugs used in combination, which given separately produce similar actions, but used together have an enhanced effect. **Ageing effect.** Of radiation, a chronic effect of the absorption by a living organism of ionizing radiation. The evidence for this effect in man is equivocal. **Clasp-knife effect.** Sudden flexion of a limb following an initial and abnormal resistance. **Contrary effect.** Aggravation of an infection following a small dose of a chemotherapeutic drug. **Coriolis effect.** An illusion of movement and a sense of vertigo caused by moving the head in a direction different from the axis of movement of the body. **Cumulative effect.** Actions of a drug produced after a number of doses have been given without producing such an effect. It may be due to delayed excretion or destruction of the drug, and may represent a form of toxic effect, seen in the case of digitalis and some hypnotic drugs. Applied also to the long-term deleterious effect of repeated doses of ionizing radiation. **Cupola effect.** A radiological sign in intussusception. It consists of a concave outline in the head of a barium enema at the upper level of the intussusceptum within the intussuscipiens. **Cytopathic effect, Cytopathogenic effect.** Localized or generalized degeneration of a cell sheet in culture, due to the presence of a virus or some other agent. Localized areas of degeneration are called *plaques*, the number of which is proportional to the amount of virus present. **Electrotonic effect.** The altered state of excitability of a nerve or muscle due to electrotonus. **Inverse photo-electric effect.** The emission of x-rays from a surface when bombarded by a beam of electrons. **Inverse piezo-electric effect.** The contraction or expansion which takes place when 2 opposite faces of a quartz crystal are subjected to a difference of electric potential. **Isotope effect.** Differences that may be detectable in the chemical or physical behaviour of 2 isotopes of the same element, or of their compounds. **Photechic effect.** The effect which certain substances have on the emulsion of a photographic plate when in close proximity to it, and detected when the plate is developed in the ordinary way. **Photo-electric effect.** Phenomena which occur when photons are absorbed, resulting in the ejection of electrons. Such phenomena include photoconductivity, photo-emissivity, etc. **Piezo-electric effect.** The production of a difference of potential between opposite faces of certain crystals (e.g. quartz, tourmaline) when subjected to differences of pressure, compressional or tensional. **Pressure effect.** The change that occurs in tissues subjected to pressure. **Skin effect.** The effect observed with alternating current when the current density is greater at the surface than at the centre of a conductor. With very high frequencies the current is practically confined to the surface. **Thermionic effect.** The emission of electrons by hot incandescent bodies. **Thermoelectric effect.** The electromotive force produced on account of a difference of temperature between 2 junctions of dissimilar materials in the same circuit. **Wall effect.** The effect on the ionization current of the variation of thickness and material of which the wall of a cavity ionization chamber is made. [L *effectus*.]

See also: BOHR, COMPTON, DANSYZ, DOPPLER (C. J.), EDISON, FERMI (E.), HALLWACH, JOULE, ORBELI, PASTEUR, PELTIER, RAMAN, RUSSELL (W. J.). SCHOTTKY, SEEBECK, SORET, STAUB, THOMSON (W. (LORD KELVIN)), TRAUGOTT, TYNDALL, VOLTA, ZEEMAN.

effectiveness. Relative biological effectiveness. The inverse ratio of the doses of 2 kinds of radiation that produce the same biological effect. [L *effectus*.]

effector (ef·**ek**·tor). 1. One of the specialized nerve-endings in the skeletal muscles through which impulses are passed to set in motion muscle contraction and gland secretion. 2. A molecule whose action is to stimulate or inhibit a process, usually an enzymatic reaction. **Allosteric effector.** A compound which, when bound to an allosteric site of an allosteric enzyme, modifies the catalytic activity. The effector may exert a positive effect (increasing catalytic activity) or a negative one (decreasing catalytic activity). **Somatic effector.** One of the specialized nerve-endings in striped skeletal muscle. **Visceral effector.** One of the specialized nerve-endings in smooth muscle. [L *efficere* to accomplish.]

effeminacy (ef·**em**·in·as·e). Feminism; the condition in males in which physical and mental characteristics correspond to those of the female sex, with or without arrested development of the male generative organs. [see foll.]

effemination, effeminization (ef·**em**·in·a'·shun, ef·**em**·in·i·**za**'·shun). In a man, the state or condition of being womanly in character and disposition. [L *effeminare* to make womanish.]

efferent (ef·er·ent). 1. Term applied to those blood vessels and other structures which convey or discharge outwards or away from a part. 2. A nerve which carries impulses away from the nerve centre to the organs. 3. Carrying impulses out from a nerve centre. Cf. AFFERENT. [L *effere* to bear out.]

effervesce (ef·er·**ves**'). To produce small bubbles or foam on the escape of gas from a fluid. [see foll.]

effervescence (ef·er·**ves**·ens). 1. The action of effervescing. 2. The onset of the symptoms of an infectious disease. [L *effervescere* to foam up.]

effervescent (ef·er·**ves**·ent). 1. Bubbling. 2. Giving off gas bubbles as in an aerated drink such as soda water. [see prec.]

efficiency (e·**fish**·en·se). The amount of achievement compared with the effort expended. **Electrical efficiency.** The ratio between current and the energy expended to produce it. **Geometrical efficiency of counters.** The solid angle subtended by a Geiger counter at the source divided by 4π, giving the fraction of the particles emitted by the source which enter the counter. **Intrinsic counter efficiency.** The percentage of particles or quanta arriving at a counter which cause an actuation of the latter. **Mechanical efficiency.** The ratio of energy produced by a machine to energy supplied in the same period. **Visual efficiency.** *See* VISUAL. [L *efficere* to accomplish.]

effluerage (ef·loor·**ahzh**). The gentle stroking movement in massage. [Fr. skimming.]

efflorescence (ef·lor·es·ens). 1. An eruption such as that which occurs in measles. 2. Any redness or lesion of the skin. 3. In chemistry, the property of a crystalline substance to become dry and crumble when exposed to the air, e.g. washing soda. [L *efflorescere* to bloom.]

efflorescent (ef·lor·es·ent). In chemistry, tending to become powdery on account of loss of water of crystallization. [see prec.]

effluent (ef·lew·ent). 1. Flowing out. 2. An outflow, as of a stream. 3. Term applied to any fluid discharged from sewage works, or to untreated fluid collected from sewage dumps, which may pollute streams. [see foll.]

effluvium (ef·lew·ve·um). 1. A flowing out. 2. A malodorous exhalation, particularly one liable to cause harm to animals, including human beings. **Effluvium capillorum.** Falling out of hair. **Telluric effluvium.** Miasmatic exhalation. [see prec.]

effraction (ef·rak·shun). Outburst or solution of continuity as the result of degeneration and weakening of tissues involved. [L *effrangere* to break up.]

effracture (ef·rak·tewr). Depressed fracture of the skull. [see prec.]

effumability (ef·ewm·ab·il′·it·e). The property of dissolving easily and rapidly into fumes (volatilization). [L *e, fumus* smoke.]

effuse (ef·ewz). Spread over the surface in a thin veil; particularly applied to bacterial cultures, e.g. the growth of *Clostridium tetani* or *Proteus* on solid media. [see foll.]

effusion (ef·ew·zhun). 1. Escape of fluid, e.g. blood, on account of rupture of or exudation through the walls of a vessel. 2. A fluid discharge. 3. In chemistry, the escape of gas under pressure through a small opening. **Haemorrhagic effusion.** One in which blood is present in the fluid. **Joint effusion.** A collection of fluid within a joint due to arthritis, infection or trauma. **Pericardial effusion.** Any effusion into the pericardium. **Pleural effusion.** Fluid present in the pleural sac. **Purulent effusion.** An effusion in which pus is present in the fluid. **Serous effusion.** An effusion of a serous nature. **Synovial effusion.** An effusion within a synovial joint. [L *effundere* to pour out.]

egersis (e·ger·sis). Excessive wakefulness. [Gk a waking.]

egesta (e·jes·tah). Any waste material thrown off from the body; excrement. [L *egerere* to discharge.]

egg (eg). The reproductive cell derived from the ovary of the female which is capable, after fertilization, of developing into a new individual. **Egg flip.** A draught of brandy, egg yolk, sugar and cinnamon water. **Embryonated egg.** One containing a mature or near-mature embryo. **Holoblastic egg.** Usually a small-yolked egg in which the entire cell undergoes subdivision during segmentation. **Meroblastic egg.** One in which only the cytoplasm at one pole of the egg cell undergoes subdivision during segmentation. Meroblastic eggs are usually large-yolked. [AS *aeg.*]

Eggers, George William Nordholtz (b. 1896). American orthopaedic surgeon.

Eggers' operation. An orthopaedic procedure to lengthen the hamstring muscles contracted owing to spasticity.

Eggleston, Cary (b. 1884). New York physician.

Eggleston's method. The administration of digitalis in large doses at frequent intervals in severe cases of heart failure when rapid digitalization is necessary. A single large dose is given, followed by smaller doses at intervals of from 4 to 6 h until the patient is digitalized, after which the treatment is continued with a maintenance dose. Since digitalis is irregularly absorbed, digitoxin is to be preferred.

eglandular, eglandulous (e·glan·dew·lar, e·glan·dew·lus). Devoid of glands. [L e, gland.]

Eglis' glands. Small mucous glands in the pelvis of the ureter.

ego (e·go, eg·o). 1. The living conscious subject or being. 2. In psychology, the self of an individual in its aspect either of conscious contrast to the self of other individuals or of a unity of clear and co-ordinated states of consciousness. [Gk I.]

egocentric (eg·o·sen·trik). Applied to a person who is entirely self-centred and whose ideas are concentrated on his or her own being. [ego, centre.]

egodystonic (eg·o·dis·ton′·ik). Incompatible with an individual's image of himself. [ego, Gk *dys-, tonos* tone.]

egomania (eg·o·ma·ne·ah). Self-esteem carried almost to the point of insanity. [ego, mania.]

egophony (e·gof·on·e). *See* AEGOPHONY.

egosyntonic (eg·o·sin·ton′·ik). Harmonizing with the ego and its unconscious ideals. [ego, Gk *syn, tonos* tone.]

egotropic (eg·o·trop·ik). 1. Self-centred. 2. Introspective [ego, Gk *trope* turn.]

Ehlers, Edvard (b. 1863). German dermatologist.

Ehlers-Danlos disease, or syndrome. Cutis hyperelastica; dermatorrhexis: increased elasticity of the skin with increased laxity of the joints, fragility of the skin, psuedotumours resembling haemangiomata and reduction of subcutaneous fat; occasionally subcutaneous nodules are present.

Ehrenritter, Johann (d. 1790). Vienna anatomist.

Ehrenritter's ganglion. The superior ganglion of the glossopharyngeal nerve.

Ehrlich, Paul (b. 1854). Frankfurt bacteriologist and pathologist.

Ehrlich's anaemia. Aplastic anaemia. *See* ANAEMIA.

Ehrlich's haemoglobinaemic bodies. Small rounded eosinophilic granules appearing in erythrocytes haemolysing after severe sepsis.

Ehrlich's acid haemotoxylin. *See* HAEMATOXYLIN.

Ehrlich's megaloblast. A primitive nucleated red cell which Ehrlich described as a pathological type of erythroblast seen only in pernicious anaemia in relapse and perhaps in early embryonic blood, but not in normal marrow and taking no part in normal adult erythropiesis; the cell is larger (19–27 μm) than the normoblast (12–19 μm) and the nuclear chromatin has a finer and more delicate structure, whilst there is relatively more cytoplasm; it passes through stages in its development similar to those undergone by the normoblast.

Ehrlich's postulate. Ehrlich's side-chain theory (see below).

Ehrlich's diazo reaction. The production of a pink or red coloration when diazobenzenesulphonic acid and ammonia are added to urine. A positive reaction occurs in febrile disorders, especially in measles, and typhoid fever, in which conditions it has a certain diagnostic value; in tuberculosis a positive result is reputed to have prognostic significance.

Ehrlich's reagent. For rosindole reaction: *p*-dimethylaminobenzaldehyde, 4 g, absolute alcohol, 380 ml, concentrated hydrochloric acid, 80 ml.

Ehrlich's diazo reagent. For the diazo reaction in urine: (*a*) Dissolve 5 g of sodium nitrite in 1 litre of distilled water. (*b*) Dissolve 5 g of sulphanilic acid in 50 ml of hydrochloric acid and 1 litre of water. For use, mix 1 of (*a*) with 50 or 100 of (*b*).

Ehrlich's triacid stain. For dried-blood films. This stain, containing acid fuchsine, orange G and methyl green, is that with which Ehrlich originally identified acidophil, neutrophil and basophil granules within the granular leucocytes.

Ehrlich's test. 1. Diazo reaction (see above). 2. For urobilinogen: mix 1 part of urine with 1 part of Ehrlich's *p*-dimethylaminobenzaldehyde reagent (see above). A red colour is produced if urobilinogen is present. 3. For indole and skatole: to 10 ml of test solution add 1 ml of 5 per cent alcoholic solution of *p*-dimethylaminobenzaldehyde and 1 ml of concentrated hydrochloric acid. Indole produces a red colour and skatole a blue colour.

Ehrlich's side-chain theory. A theory attempting to account for the phenomena of antigen-antibody reactions and the production of antibodies. It postulates receptor side-chains in the molecules of the host's cells, which react specifically with antigens and, as they are blocked by this reaction, are replaced by similar side-chains. This process is carried to excess, and redundant side-chains are then cast off to circulate in the blood plasma as antibody molecules. A precursor of modern theories of antibody production and now superseded by them.

Armanni-Ehrlich degeneration. Hyaline change in the epithelial cells of Henle's loops in the diabetic kidney.

Ehrlich-Biondi-Heidenhain triple stain. A mixture of acid fuchsine, orange G and methyl green, used for staining blood films.

Ehrlich-Hata treatment. Arsphenamine therapy for syphilis.

Heinz-Ehrlich bodies. Round refractile eosinophilic particles seen in mature red blood corpuscles usually in haemolytic anaemia, but not in reticulocytes; these are produced both *in vivo* and *in vitro* by the action of substances such as phenylhydrazine that are able to transform haemoglobin into verdoglobin. They are said to be denatured globin united with a green haem (verdoglobin) and fixed to the stroma of surface membrane by a layer of altered lipoid and stromal protein.

Ehrlich-Westphal method. Tissues are fixed in weak alcohol and stained in a mixture of alum carmine and dahlia, with glycerin, alcohol and acetic acid added. The granules of mast cells are stained violet against a red background.

Eichhorst, Hermann (b. 1849). Zürich physician.

Eichhorst's corpuscle. A type of microcyte seen in the blood of patients with pernicious anaemia.

Eichhorst's disease, or neuritis. Adventitial neuritis; a form of neuritis in which the pathological changes involve not only nerve sheaths but also interstitial tissue of the muscles supplied.

Eichhorst's type. Progressive muscular atrophy (motor neuron disease) affecting particularly the femoral and tibial muscles.

Eichstedt, Karl Ferdinand (b. 1816). Griefswald physician.

Eichstedt's disease. Pityriasis versicolor.

Eicken, Karl von (b. 1873). Giessen and Berlin otolaryngologist.

von Eicken's method. A method of examination of the larynx and hypopharynx with the head in extreme extension, by means of a specially designed oesophageal spatula.

eidetic (i·**det**·ik). 1. Referring to the power of exact visual reproduction of anything previously seen or imagined. 2. An individual who is able to call up at will a clear picture of any object or event he has seen or imagined. [Gk *eidos* form.]

eidoptometry (i·dop·**tom**·et·re). The measuring of the power of perception as applied to form. [Gk *eidos* form, *optikos* of sight, meter.]

eigon, eigone (i·gon, i·gone). General name given to a group of compounds of albumin with iodine or bromine. Pharmacologically they behave like iodides or bromides.

Eijkman, Christiaan (b. 1858). Dutch physiologist.

Eijkman's test. A method used for identifying faecal *Escherichia coli* in water supplies; it depends on the ability of *E. coli* to grow at a temperature of 44°C which non-faecal coliform bacilli fail to do.

eikonometer (i·kon·**om**·et·er). An instrument for measuring the size of the images of the two eyes in cases of aniseikonia. Also called *aniseikometer.* [Gk *eikon* image, *metron* measure.]

eiloid (i·loid). Resembling a roll or a coil in appearance. [Gk *eilein* to twist, *eidos* form.]

Eimer, Theodor (b. 1843). German zoologist.

Eimer's body, or organ. A sensory nerve-ending said to be present in the skin of the snout of *Talpa europea.*

Eimeria (i·me·re·ah). A genus of coccidial parasites. They are normally parasites of animals and fish, but the oöcysts are occasionally found in human faeces and rarely elsewhere and may be mistaken for those of *Isospora*; however, the oöcyst of the former contains 4 sporocysts with 2 sporozoites in each, whereas that of the latter contains 2 sporocysts with 4 sporozoites in each. **Eimeria gubleri.** A species which has been found in the liver. **Eimeria hominis.** A species which has been found in the purulent discharge from an empyema. **Eimeria stiedae.** A species found in rabbits and mice. **Eimeria wenyoni.** A species occasionally found in the faeces in man, possibly identical with *Eimeria cluperarum*, a parasite of herrings and other fish. [Theodor *Eimer.*]

Einhorn, Max (b. 1862). New York physician.

Einhorn's method. Chemical tests for the digestion of proteins, carbohydrates and fats by analysis of the duodenal contents.

Einhorn's saccharimeter. An apparatus for the measurement of sugar concentration in urine by fermentation. It consists of a graduated tube closed at the top and connected at the base by a U-tube to a reservoir. The amount of sugar in the urine is indicated by the volume of gas which has collected in the tube after fermentation with yeast.

Einhorn spring test. A method of localizing the sites of minimal persistent gastro-intestinal bleeding proximal to the ligament of Treitz. Umbilical tape is inserted overnight and its visual inspection after withdrawal supplemented by chemical testing for occult blood. The segment passing into the duodenum is bile-stained.

Einstein, Albert (b. 1879). German and USA physicist.

Einstein's viscosity formula. A theoretical formula for the viscosity of a suspension of rigid spheres in a viscous liquid. It states that $\eta_s = \eta(1 + 2.5\phi)$, where η_s is the viscosity of the suspension, η is the viscosity of the medium and ϕ the aggregate volume of spheres in unit volume of the suspension.

einsteinium (ine·sti·ne·um). A transuranic element first reported in 1954 as having been produced by the bombardment of uranium-238 with nitrogen nuclei. It has an atomic number 99, and symbol Es. It is short-lived and changes into berkelium. [Albert *Einstein.*]

Einthoven, Willem (b. 1860). Leyden physiologist.

Einthoven's formula, or hypothesis. The assumption that the heart lies in the centre of an equilateral triangle in the frontal plane of the body, defined by the right shoulder (R. arm), left shoulder (L. arm) and symphysis pubis (L. leg). The potential differences in electrocardiographic lead II (R. arm-L. leg) are equal to the sum of the potential differences of leads I (R. arm–L. arm) and III (L. arm–L. leg). The algebraic sum of the potentials at the 3 points of the triangle is always zero.

Einthoven galvanometer. String galvanometer, thread galvanometer; a very sensitive galvanometer consisting of a fine platinum or silvered quartz thread held taut in a powerful magnetic field. Minute currents in the thread cause movements which can be observed with the aid of a microscope.

Einthoven's triangle. A hypothetical equilateral triangle in the frontal plane of the body. *See* EINTHOVEN'S FORMULA (above).

eis-. Prefix from the Greek *eis*, meaning *into.*

eisanthema (i·zan·them·ah). Enanthema. [Gk *eis, anthema* blossoming.]

Eisenlohr, Carl (b. 1847). Hamburg physician.

Eisenlohr's syndrome. Bulbar paralysis with weakness and numbness of the limbs.

Eisenmenger, Victor (fl. 1897). German physician.

Eisenmenger complex, or syndrome. A type of congenital heart disease in which there is a defect of the ventricular septum associated with dextroposition of the aortic root which overrides the septum, and a dilated pulmonary artery.

Eisenmenger reaction. A term sometimes applied to the development of pulmonary hypertension in patients with any form of congenital communication between the two sides of the heart. The condition was not described by Eisenmenger but derives from the similarity of patients with this condition to those with *Eisenmenger's syndrome.*

eisodic (i·so·dik). Esodic.

eisophoria (i·so·**for**·e·ah). Esophoria.

Eitelberg, Abraham (b. 1847). Vienna otologist.

Eitelberg's test. To differentiate labyrinthine and middle-ear disease: a tuning fork is kept in repeated vibration at the meatus for 20 min. For lesions of the perceptive mechanism auditory fatigue is said to occur more rapidly than in a normal ear, and the length of time during which the tuning fork is perceived becomes less and less.

ejaculatio (e·jak·ew·la′·she·o). Ejaculation. **Ejaculatio deficiens.** Deficient ejaculation. **Ejaculatio praecox.** Premature ejaculation. **Ejaculatio retardata.** Delayed ejaculation. [L *ejaculari* to throw out.]

ejaculation (e·jak·ew·la′·shun). The emission of the seminal fluid. **Premature ejaculation.** Emission of the seminal fluid at the beginning of the sexual act. [see prec.]

ejaculatory (e·jak·ew·la′·tor·e). 1. Relating to an ejaculation. 2. Serving to ejaculate.

ejecta (e·jek·tah). Material thrown out; excreta. [L *ejicere* to cast out.]

ejection (e·jek·shun). 1. Violent excretion. 2. The casting-out of waste products. 3. Any waste product cast out. **Ventricular ejection.** The forceful expulsion of blood from the cardiac ventricles into the great arteries. The term is also used more particularly to refer to the exact pattern or time course of the expulsion of the blood in relation to the analysis of ventricular function. [see prec.]

ek-. Prefix, from the Greek *ek*, meaning *out.*

eka- (e·kah). A prefix denoting predicted element occupying place in periodic system directly beneath specified element. [Sanskrit *eka* one.]

eka-caesium (e·kah·**se**·se·um). Now Francium. [Sanskrit *eka* one, caesium.]

eka-iodine (e·kah·i·o·deen). Now Astatine. [Sanskrit *eka* one, iodine.]

eka-manganese (e·kah·**mang**·gan·eez). Now Technetium. [Sanskrit *eka* one, manganese.]

eka-tantalum (e·kah·**tan**·tal·um). Now Protactinium. [Sanskrit *eka* one, tantalum.]

Ekbom, Karl-Axel. Swedish neurologist.

Ekbom's syndrome. A condition without physical signs and of unknown cause in which there is severe discomfort in the legs, only relieved by movement; restless legs.

Ekehorn, Jol. Gustav (b. 1875). Swedish surgeon.

Ekehorn's operation. Correction of rectal prolapse by subcutaneous ligature around the anus.

ekiri (e·ki·ri). A form of infantile diarrhoea endemic in Japan. Its course is acute and fatal. [Japanese name.]

ekphorize (**ek**·for·ize). To bring a latent memory picture up into consciousness. [Gk *ek, pherein* to carry.]

elaboration (e·**lab**·or·a′·shun). In physiology, the natural process by which basic food material is converted into an assimilable or useful form. **Secondary elaboration.** In dream analysis, the reducing of the inconsistent and bizarre dream content to an orderly arrangement. [L *elaborare* to work out.]

elacin (**el**·as·in). Elastic tissue that has degenerated, as seen in the wrinkled skin of aged persons. [Gk *elaunein* to drive.]

elaeoma (el·e·o·mah). A swelling in the tissues due to the injection of oil. [Gk *elaion* oil, *-oma* tumour.]

elaeometer (el·e·**om**·et·er). A type of hydrometer used for the determination of the specific gravity of an oil, and for estimating its purity. [Gk *elaion* oil, meter.]

elaeomyenchysis (el·e·o·mi·**en**′·kis·is). The process of injecting oil into the muscles for the relief of local clonic spasm or other therapeutic purpose. [Gk *elaion* oil, *mys* muscle, *egchysis* a pouring in.]

elaeopathia, elaeopathy (el·e·o·**path**·e·ah, el·e·**op**·ath·e). Fatty infiltration of the subcutaneous tissue, especially around the joints of the legs, causing oedema-like swellings. It was described as occurring after contusions and dislocations sustained in warfare and attributed to the irritation of an oily substance on the tissues. **Pathomimic elaeopathia.** Swellings simulating disease, produced by the subcutaneous injection of liquid paraffin. [Gk *elaion* oil, *pathos* disease.]

elaeoplast (el·e·o·plast). A foreign-body giant cell containing drops of oil which appears in areas of fat necrosis or effusions of oil resulting from trauma. [Gk *elaion* oil, *plassein* to form.]

elaeoptene (el·e·**op**·teen). That part of an essential oil that is liquid and volatile. Cf. STEAROPTENE. [Gk *elaion* oil, *ptenos* volatile.]

elaeosaccharum (el·e·o·**sak**′·ar·um). An essential oil to which sugar has been added. [Gk *elaion* oil, *sakcharon* sugar.]

elaidin (el·a·id·in). Glycerol tri-elaidate, $(C_{17}H_{33}CO)_3C_3H_5$. A solid fat, isomeric with olein, and derived from castor and other oils. [Gk *elaion* oil.]

elain (e·la·in). Elaeoptene.

elaioma (el·a·o·mah). Elaeoma.

elaiometer (el·a·**om**·et·er). Elaeometer.

elaiopathia, elaiopathy (el·a·o·**path**·e·ah, el·a·**op**·ath·e). Elaeopathia.

elaioplast (el·a·o·plast). Elaeoplast.

Elapinae (e·**lap**·in·e). A subfamily of snakes, most of which are highly poisonous; it includes the cobra, *Naia naia.* [Gk *elops* snake.]

Elaps (e·laps). A genus of poisonous American snakes including the harlequin and coral snakes. The many species are usually banded black and red. [see prec.]

elastance (e·**las**·tans). The reciprocal of compliance; a measure of the increase in airway pressure for a given increase in volume of gas or air. [elastic.]

elastase (e·**las**·taze). An enzyme which, when activated by trypsin, cleaves bonds adjacent to neutral amino acids in elastin. [Gk *elaunein* to drive, *aze* enzyme.]

elastic (e·**las**·tik). Able to recover size and shape after being compressed, stretched, bent or otherwise distorted. [Gk *elaunein* to drive.]

elastica (e·**las**·tik·ah). 1. The tunica media of a blood vessel. 2. Caoutchouc. [see prec.]

elasticity (e·las·**tis**·it·e). The quality of being elastic. [Gk *elaunein* to drive.]

elastin (e·**las**·tin). A protein of the scleroprotein class occurring in the yellow elastic fibres of connective tissue, cartilage, ligaments and walls of arteries. Elastins, in contrast to collagens and keratins, are easily hydrolysed by pepsin and trypsin, yielding hydrolysates, comparatively rich in glycine and leucine. [see prec.]

elastinase (e·**las**·tin·aze). A ferment or enzyme which has a dissolving effect on elastic tissue.

elastogel (e·**las**·to·jel). A gel which has strongly-marked elastic properties.

elastoid (e·**las**·toid). A substance found in the uterine blood vessels after delivery, and formed by hyaline degeneration of the elastic layer of the intima of the vessels. [elastic, Gk *eidos* form.]

elastoma (e·las·**to**·mah). Any tumour of the skin in which elastic tissue predominates; pseudoxanthoma elasticum. **Juvenile elastoma.** A congenital hyperplastic condition of the elastic tissue of the corium. **Perforating elastoma.** A defect of elastic tissue with down-growths of the overlying epidermis which engulf the elastic tissue, forming linear, arciform or annular horny-plugged papules, usually on the neck, sometimes on the cheeks, arms or thighs. [elastic, Gk *-oma* tumour.]

elastometer (e·las·**tom**·et·er). A device with which the elasticity of any particular body or of the animal tissues can be ascertained and the degree of oedema present determined.

elastometry (e·las·**tom**·et·re). The process of measuring the elasticity of any body or tissue.

elastopathy (e·las·**top**·ath·e). A condition in which there is a deficiency of elastic tissue. [elastic, Gk *pathos* disease.]

elastorrhexis (e·**las**·to·rex′·is). Rupture of elastic tissue. [elastic, Gk *rhexis* a breaking.]

elastosis (e·las·**to**·sis). Any disorder of elastic fibres. **Elastosis atrophicans.** Pseudoxanthoma elasticum. **Diffuse elastosis.** A form of solar elastotic degeneration (Dubreuilh). **Elastosis dystrophica.** A syndrome in which there is a degeneration in the elastic tissues, of the skin, of the systemic arteries and of Bruch's membrane in the retina. **Elastosis senilis.** The cutaneous degeneration of old age; usually most marked on the backs of hands, around genitalia and anus, and on the lower limbs. **Solar elastosis.** Elastic degeneration of areas of skin repeatedly and excessively exposed to sunlight. [elastic, Gk *-osis* condition.]

elaterin (e·**lat**·er·in). The name given to a mixture of principles, alcohols, fatty acids and resin extracted with alcohol from elaterium. It contains roughly 70 per cent of alpha elaterin. **Alpha elaterin.** $C_{20}H_{28}O_3$, a physiologically inactive laevorotatory compound occurring in commercial elaterin and in colocynth. **Beta elaterin.** A purgative dextrorotatory isomer accompanying alpha elaterin in elaterium, [Gk *elaterios* driving.]

elaterium (e·lat·e·re·um). The dried sediment from the juice of the squirting cucumber, *Ecballium elaterium* (family Cucurbitaceae). It contains elaterin, which causes it to be a powerful hydragogue cathartic. [see prec.]

elaterometer (e·**lat**·er·**om**′·et·er). An instrument used for the purpose of measuring elasticity in gases. [Gk *elater* driver, meter.]

elation (e·la·shun). 1. A condition of strong emotional stimulation which has an accelerating effect on the physical and mental processes. 2. In psychiatry, an intensified feeling of gaiety or excitement, or the exaggerated expression of such feeling. [L *elatus* raised.]

Elaut, L. Ghent pathologist.

Elaut's triangle. A triangle bounded by the lumbosacral joint and the common iliac vessels.

elbow [cubitus (NA)] (el·bo). The joint between the arm and the forearm. **Beat elbow.** A cutaneous cellulitis occurring as a result of devitalization of the tissues and probably associated infection from pressure, friction or repeated trauma over the olecranon process. **Elbow crutch.** *See* CRUTCH. **Golfers' elbow.** Medial humeral epicondylitis; pain and stiffness of the joint with generalized tenderness of the whole forearm, especially over the medial epicondyle. It responds to local anaesthesia, rest and physiotherapy. **Elbow joint.** *See* JOINT. **Miners' elbow.** Olecranon bursitis. **Pulled elbow.** Partial dislocation of the head of the radius. **Tennis elbow.** Painful condition of the elbow due to a tender spot over the external epicondyle of the humerus in the origin of the extensor muscles of the hand. [AS *elboga.*]

elder (el·der). The tree *Sambucus nigra* Linn. (family Caprifoliaceae), common in Britain, the remainder of Europe, Western Asia and West Africa. The dried corollas and stamens of the flowers constitute sambucus. **Elder leaves.** The fresh leaves of *Sambucus nigra* Linn. One part digested with 3 parts of linseed oil forms green oil of elder, used as an external emollient application. [AS *ellaern.*]

elecampane (el·e·kam·pane). Inula: the dried rhizome and roots of *Inula helenium* Linn. (family Compositae). The leaves of elecampane are used as an adulterant of digitalis. [L *inula* elecampane, *campus* field.]

elective (e·lek·tiv). 1. Selective. 2. Term descriptive of treatment or procedure decided upon by doctor or patient that is of advantage to the particular patient under treatment but not fundamental in the therapy of the case. 3. Tending to act on or combine with one particular substance rather than another. [L *eligere* to choose out.]

electrician (el·ek·trish·an). 1. One who manipulates electrical appliances and apparatus. 2. One who is versed in the science of electricity. **Medical electrician.** A practitioner or technician who uses electricity as a therapeutic measure. [see foll.]

electricity (el·ek·tris·it·e). 1. The branch of science which deals with electrical phenomena. 2. A manifestation of energy associated with electrons and protons at rest (static), or in motion (dynamic); it is said to be negative or positive according to the particles concerned. **Animal electricity.** Electric potentials created in animal tissue, as in the transmission of nerve impulses or the contraction of heart muscle. **Chemical electricity.** Electricity produced by chemical action. **Current electricity.** Electrons in motion along a conductor. **Dynamic electricity.** Electricity in motion; current electricity: it is characterized by accompanying magnetic effects. **Faradic electricity.** Induced electricity (see below). **Franklinic electricity.** Static electricity (see below). **Frictional electricity.** Electricity produced in certain non-conductors such as glass by rubbing them with dry materials. **Galvanic electricity.** Electric current generated by a galvanic cell. **Induced electricity.** Electricity produced by induction, as in the secondary winding of an induction coil. **Negative electricity.** Electricity resulting from the presence of surplus electrons. **Positive electricity.** Electricity resulting from a surplus of protons or a deficiency of electrons. **Resinous electricity.** Electricity produced by the act of rubbing resin. **Static electricity.** The accumulation of a charge of electricity on a non-conductor which may produce a spark when brought near to an object at a lower electrical potential. **Thermo-electricity.** Electricity produced by the effect of heat, as in thermocouples; also the electrical production of heat. **Vitreous electricity.** Electricity produced by the act of rubbing glass. **Voltaic electricity.** Electric current generated by a voltaic cell. [Gk *elektron* amber.]

electrify (el·ek·tre·fi). To charge with electricity. [electricity, L *facere* to make.]

electro-affinity (el·ek·tro·af·in′·it·e). A measure of the degree to which ions are capable of retaining their charge. [electron, L *affinis* related.]

electro-anaesthesia (el·ek·tro·an·es·the′·ze·ah). 1. Local anaesthesia induced by application of an electric current to the surface of the skin to which an anaesthetizing substance has been applied. 2. Insensibility of the skin to the stimulus of an electric current.

electro-analysis (el·ek·tro·an·al′·is·is). Analysis of chemical substances using electrical methods, as by electrolytic deposition, or the determination of end-point in titrations by measurement of electrode potential.

electro-anastomosis (el·ek·tro·an·as·to·mo′·sis). Intestinal anastomosis performed by means of electrocautery.

electro-appendicectomy (el·ek·tro·ap·en·dis·ek′·to·me). Appendicectomy performed by electrocautery.

electrobasograph (el·ek·tro·ba′·so·graf). An electric apparatus with which a record of a patient's gait can be obtained and the extent to which weight is borne by each limb ascertained. [electricity, Gk *basis* a stepping, *graphein* to record.]

electrobiology (el·ek·tro·bi·ol′·o·je). 1. The branch of biology that is concerned with the electrical activities of living organisms. 2. An obsolete term for hypnotism or mesmerism.

electrobioscopy (el·ek·tro·bi·os′·ko·pe). The examination of the body by means of an electric current in order to determine whether or not life is present. [electricity, bioscopy.]

electrocapillarity (el·ek·tro·kap·il·ar′·it·e). Electrocapillary action. *See* ACTION.

electrocardiogram (el·ek·tro·kar′·de·o·gram). A record of the electrical potentials generated by the activation process of the muscle of the heart. These potentials produce an electrical field within the tissues of the body, resulting in the development of potential differences between various parts of the body surface; the presence of these differences is detected and recorded by electrodes placed on the limbs or the trunk and connected to a suitable detecting and recording instrument (an electrocardiograph). Abbreviation ECG or ecg. **Bipolar electrocardiogram.** An electrocardiogram showing the difference between the potentials developed at 2 electrical sites on the body; for example, between 2 limbs. **Scalar electrocardiogram.** The conventional representation of an electrocardiographic lead as a change of voltage magnitude with time; the term is used in distinction from the *vector cardiogram.* **Unipolar electrocardiogram.** An electrocardiogram ostensibly showing the potentials developed at one electrode site, the second electrode or combination of electrodes reputedly being maintained at zero potential. [electricity, Gk *kardia* heart, *gramma* record.]

electrocardiograph (el·ek·tro·kar′·de·o·graf). An apparatus used for recording electrocardiograms.

electrocardiography (el·ek·tro·kar·de·og′·raf·e). The method of recording the electrocardiogram. **Precordial electrocardiography.** Electrocardiography employing electrodes applied to the precordium; originally performed using a bipolar system with a second electrode on the limb, yielding records designated CR, CL or CF, with the second electrode on the right arm, left arm or a leg (foot), respectively, but now, by international convention, almost exclusively using a unipolar system employing the 3 standard limb electrodes joined together to yield record labelled V, with numbers added to identify the position of the precordial electrode. [electricity, Gk *kardia* heart, *graphein* to write.]

electrocardiophonogram (el·ek·tro·kar·de·o·fo′·no·gram). The record made by an electrocardiophonograph; a phonocardiogram.

electrocardiophonograph (el·ek·tro·kar·de·o·fo′·no·graf). Phonocardiograph; an electrical apparatus which records graphically the sounds and murmurs produced by the beating of the heart. [electricity, Gk *kardia* heart, *phone* voice, *graphein* to record.]

electrocardiophonography (el·ek·tro·kar·de·o·fo·nog′·raf·e). The recording of heart sounds electrically. [see prec.]

electrocardioscopy (el·**ek**·tro·kar·de·**os**′·ko·pe). A method of studying the movements of the heart and the shape of the heart and great vessels, by means of x-rays. [electricity, Gk *kardia* heart, *skopein* to watch.]

electrocatalysis (el·**ek**·tro·kat·**al**′·is·is). Chemical decomposition of the tissues as the result of the application of electric currents to the body. [electricity, Gk *katalein* to dissolve.]

electrocautery (el·**ek**·tro·**kaw**′·ter·e). An instrument for the controlled destruction of tissue by heat. An electric current is passed through a loop, button or bayonet-shaped blade of platinum which is thereby rendered red or white hot and applied to the tissue under treatment. [electricity, Gk *kausis* a burning.]

electrochemistry (el·**ek**·tro·**kem**′·is·tre). The study of electrical phenomena accompanying chemical action, and chemical processes brought about by electrical means.

electrochemy (el·**ek**·tro·kem·e). The production of chemical effects in the tissues for therapeutic purposes by the application of an electric current. The main methods employed are electrolysis, iontophoresis and cataphoresis.

electrocholecystectomy (el·**ek**·tro·**ko**·le·sis·**tek**′·to·me). Surgical removal of the gall bladder by electrical cauterization. [electricity, cholecystectomy.]

electrocholecystocausis (el·**ek**·tro·**ko**·le·sis·to·**kaw**′·sis). Electrical cauterization of the gall bladder. [electricity, cholecyst, Gk *kausis* a burning.]

electrocision (el·**ek**·tro·**sizh**′·un). Surgical removal of malignant tumours by endothermy knife. [electricity, L *caedere* to cut.]

electrocoagulation (el·**ek**·tro·ko·ag·ew·**la**′·shun). The control of haemorrhage from vessels divided in the course of a surgical operation, by the application to their open bleeding ends, directly or by way of the forceps occluding them, of a high-frequency current. The term is also applied to the actual destruction of abnormal tissues, warts and hair follicles (*see also* ELECTROLYSIS). [electricity, coagulation.]

electrocoma (el·**ek**·tro·**ko**′·mah). Coma produced in electroshock therapy.

electroconductivity (el·**ek**·tro·kon·duk·**tiv**′·it·e). The quality or power of conducting, receiving or transmitting electricity.

electrocontractility (el·**ek**·tro·kon·trak·**til**′·it·e). The quality of being able to contract when electrically stimulated; a term applied to muscular tissue.

electrocorticogram (el·**ek**·tro·**kor**′·tik·o·gram). An electrocorticographic reading.

electrocorticography (el·**ek**·tro·kor·tik·**og**′·raf·e). The recording of electrical potentials by means of electrodes placed directly on the cerebral cortex. [electricity, cortex, Gk *graphein* to write.]

electrocryptectomy (el·**ek**·tro·krip·**tek**′·to·me). Obliteration and cicatrization of unhealthy tonsillar crypts by means of surgical diathermy. [electricity, cryptectomy.]

electrocution (el·**ek**·tro·**kew**′·shun). 1. Death of an individual brought about by contact with a strong electric current. [electric execution.]

electrocystoscope (el·**ek**·tro·**sis**′·to·skope). A cystoscope fitted with a minute high-powered lamp which lights when it is connected to a battery. [electricity, cystoscope.]

electrode (el·**ek**·trode). 1. The conductor by means of which current enters or leaves an electrolytic cell or a vacuum tube; the positive electrode is referred to as the *anode*, the negative electrode as the *cathode*. 2. In medicine, the medium for transmitting electrical energy from a conductor to the patient. 3. Either of the ends of a spark gap or electric arc. **Active electrode.** 1. The electrode applied to the point of election in electrotherapy. 2. In the precipitation of solid or liquid particles held in suspension in a gas by means of a unidirectional electric field between electrodes, the *insulated* or *discharge electrode* distinguished from the *passive* or *collecting electrode*, which is earthed and upon which the precipitated particles collect, this being usually the anode. **Brush electrodes.** Contacts in the form of wire brushes used in some electrostatic machines. **Calomel electrode.** A standard electrode developing a constant potential, used in determining hydrogen-ion concentration: it consists of mercury in a solution of potassium chloride and saturated with mercurous chloride (calomel). **Collecting electrode.** *See* ACTIVE ELECTRODE (above). **Colon electrode.** An electrode which can be applied *per rectum.* **Deglutible electrode.** An electrode which can be swallowed. **Discharge electrode.** *See* ACTIVE ELECTRODE (above). **Dispersing electrode.** Silent electrode (see below). **Exciting electrode.** Therapeutic electrode (see below). **Hydrogen electrode.** An arrangement consisting of a base coated with spongy platinum, palladium or other suitable material and saturated with hydrogen, in a solution containing hydrogen ions; it is used in connection with the determination of hydrogen-ion concentration. **Impregnated electrode.** Therapeutic electrode (see below). **Indifferent electrode.** An inactive electrode. **Insulated electrode.** *See* ACTIVE ELECTRODE (above). **Irreversible electrode.** A single-electrode system in which a considerable change in the potential of the electrode occurs when the current passing slightly increases or decreases. **Localizing electrode.** Therapeutic electrode (see below). **Multiple-point electrode, Multiterminal electrode.** An electrode to which several connections can be made. **Negative electrode.** Cathode. **Oxygen electrode.** A device for measuring the oxygen tension in small samples of blood. It consists of a silver anode and a platinum cathode in an electrolyte solution. (Described by Clark in 1956.) **Passive electrode.** *See* ACTIVE ELECTRODE (above). **Point electrode.** A pointed piece of metal, as in a point/point or point/plane spark gap, usually mounted in an ebonite handle. **Positive electrode.** Anode. **Prescription electrode.** Therapeutic electrode (see below). **Press-stud electrode.** A form of electrode to which the connecting lead is attached by means of a metal device similar to the press-stud often used as a fastener for clothing. **Reversible electrode.** A single-electrode system in which a small or negligible change in the potential of the electrode occurs when the current passing slightly increases or decreases. **Silent electrode.** An inactive electrode. **Spark-ball electrode.** 1. A metal sphere fixed at the end of a metal rod mounted in an insulating handle. 2. One of the electrodes of a sphere spark gap. **Therapeutic electrode.** An electrode for introduction of drugs into the skin by ionization. Also known as *exciting, impregnated, localizing* or *prescription electrode.* [electricity, Gk *hodos* way.]

electrodermatome (el·**ek**·tro·**der**′·mat·ome). An electrical form of razor for the cutting of skin grafts. [electricity, Gk *derma* skin, *temnein* to cut.]

electrodesiccation (el·ek·tro·des·ik·a′·shun). Tissue destruction produced by the local application of a high-frequency, high-voltage, low-amperage current by means of a metal-needle electrode. Destruction is caused by dehydration and charring, and there is little tissue coagulation. Also known as *fulguration.* [electricity, L *desiccare* to dry up.]

electrodiagnosis (el·**ek**·tro·di·ag·**no**′·sis). Diagnosis of disease, or the determination of the nature of a disease, by observing the changes in those tissues of the body which react to electrical stimulation. Usually confined to the responses of peripheral nerves and skeletal muscles to varying forms of electrical stimulation.

electrodialysis (el·**ek**·tro·di·**al**′·is·is). Accelerated dialysis of electrolytes from admixture with colloids by placing electrodes outside the solution; the ions are attracted through the membrane to anode and cathode, respectively.

electrodiaphake (el·**ek**·tro·**di**′·ah·fake). A two-pronged probe which adheres to a lens when an electric current is passed from one prong to the other; used in cataract extraction. [electricity, Gk *dia, phakos* lens.]

electrodiaphane (el·**ek**·tro·**di**′·af·ane). Diaphanoscope; an illuminating instrument with which a body cavity can be lighted up, its interior examined and its limits defined. [electricity, diaphanoscope.]

electrodiaphany (el·**ek**·tro·di·**af**′·an·e). Diaphanoscopy; examination of a body cavity with a diaphanoscope. [see prec.]

electrodynamometer (el·**ek**·tro·di·nam·**om**′·et·er). An instrument with which the intensity of faradic and alternating currents can be measured. [electricity, dynamo, meter.]

electro-encephalogram (el·**ek**·tro·en·**kef**'·al·o·gram). The graphic record made during the course of electro-encephalography. Various wave frequencies and forms have been recognized and assigned names: alpha (α) waves (8–13 Hz) emerge mainly in the occipital region with eyes closed and the patient physically and mentally relaxed; beta (β) (15–30 Hz) are seen frontally, sometimes prominent in certain toxic or degenerative encephalopathies; delta (δ) ($\frac{1}{2}$–3 Hz) slow high voltage, generalized in profound coma, or localized at the site of regional brain damage; theta (θ) (4–7 Hz) bitemporally in certain forms of epilepsy or psychopathic states and in some midline deep lesions; kappa (κ) (not well-established) mainly frontal and when mental activity occurs; lambda (λ), low-voltage occipital waves apparently associated with visual activity; wave-and-spike (dome-and-spike) activity, paroxysms of 3 Hz wave-forms considered to be diagnostic of petit mal. Abbreviation e.e.g. [electricity, Gk *egkephalos* brain, *gramma* record.]

electro-encephalograph (el·**ek**·tro·en·**kef**'·al·o·graf). An instrument for recording the brain's electrical activity ("brain waves") made with electrodes on the intact scalp. It is used in the diagnosis of epilepsy where certain patterns of wave forms commonly occur, and also sometimes to indicate the site of a local brain lesion (tumour, etc.) by the localized change in wave pattern. [electricity, Gk *egkephalos* brain, *graphein* to record.]

electro-encephalography (el·**ek**·tro·en·**kef**·al·**og**'·raf·e). The use of the electro-encephalograph in registering the electric current set up in the cerebral cortex by the action of the brain.

electro-endosmosis (el·**ek**·tro·en·**doz**'·mo·sis). An osmotic effect achieved by a difference of electric potential between the liquids on opposite sides of a semipermeable membrane. [electron, Gk *endon* within, osmosis.]

electro-enterostomy (el·**ek**·tro·en·ter·**os**'·to·me). Enterostomy carried out by electrosurgical methods.

electrofit (el·**ek**·tro·fit). A fit, or convulsions, due to an electrotherapeutic shock.

electrofluoroscopy (el·**ek**·tro·floo·or·**os**'·ko·pe). The use of a fluoroscope in electrocardiography.

electrogastro-enterostomy (el·**ek**·tro·**gas**·tro·en·ter·**os**'·to·me). Gastro-enterostomy carried out by electrosurgical methods.

electrogastrogram (el·**ek**·tro·**gas**'·tro·gram). A record of the electrical changes occurring in the muscles of the stomach during their contraction. Leads may be taken from inside the stomach, or through the anterior abdominal wall in very thin persons. The exact significance of the curves obtained is not yet well established. [electricity, Gk *gaster* stomach, *gramma* record.]

electrogenesis (el·**ek**·tro·**jen**'·es·is). 1. The results produced by the application of electricity. 2. Generating electricity. [electricity, Gk *genein* to produce.]

electrogram (el·**ek**·tro·gram). Electrograph.

electrograph (el·**ek**·tro·graf). 1. A skiagraph. 2. The record in the form of a graph of the electric current set up by the contracting of any muscular organ, e.g. the heart. [electricity, Gk *graphein* to write.]

electrography (el·ek·**trog**·raf·e). 1. The procedure of recording by means of an electrograph. 2. Electrology.

electrohaemostasis (el·**ek**·tro·he·**mos**'·tas·is). The arrest of haemorrhage by electrocauterization so that the tissues are shrivelled and the vessels closed. [electricity, Gk *haima* blood, *stasis* a standing still.]

electrohysterography (el·**ek**·tro·his·ter·**og**'·raf·e). The recording of electrical activity in uterine muscle. [electricity, Gk *hystero* womb, *graphein* to record.]

electro-ionic (el·**ek**·tro·i·**on**'·ik). Referring to iontophoresis, i.e. that method of treatment in which ions of different kinds are driven from solutions of salts into the skin by means of an electric current.

electrokinetic (el·**ek**·tro·kin·**et**'·ik). 1. Referring to electrokinetics. 2. Referring to movement produced by an electric current.

electrokinetics (el·**ek**·tro·kin·**et**'·ix). 1. That branch of electrical science which is concerned with electricity in motion as distinguished from electricity at rest. 2. The application of direct current for therapeutic purposes. [electricity, Gk *kinesis* movement.]

electrokymogram (el·**ek**·tro·**ki**'·mo·gram). A graphic paper record of the motion of the heart border made with an electrokymograph.

electrokymograph (el·**ek**·tro·**ki**'·mo·graf). A device for recording motion of the heart border: the screen image of the heart border falls on the aperture of a pick-up device which converts the varying areas of light and shade into an electric current. This operates the string of an electrocardiograph, which records on paper the position of the heart border in respect to time. A synchronous tracing of the carotid pulse is used to correlate movements of various points on the heart border during the examination. [electricity, Gk *kyma* wave, *graphein* to record.]

electrokymography (el·**ek**·tro·ki·**mog**'·raf·e). A method of recording the motion of the heart border with an electrokymograph.

electrolithotrity (el·**ek**·tro·**lith**'·o·trit·e). Destruction of bladder stone with an electrode attached to an electrodynamic instrument called *URAT 1*. [electricity, lithotrity.]

electrology (el·ek·**trol**·o·je). The science of electricity, its phenomena and properties. [electricity, Gk *logos* science.]

electrolysis (el·ek·**trol**·is·is). 1. The destruction of body tissues resulting from application of an electric current. It produces focal inflammation reaction in the skin and is often used for epilation and removal of telangiectases. 2. The decomposing of any chemical compound by passing an electric current through it. **Cupric electrolysis.** Electrolysis applied to a diseased part of the body through chemically pure copper so that microbes are killed by the copper oxychloride generated. [electricity, Gk *lysis* a loosing.]

electrolyte (el·**ek**·tro·lite). 1. The liquid constituent of an electric cell. 2. A compound which, in solution, dissociates into electrically-charged particles (ions) which will conduct electricity. 3. The ionized salts in the blood. [electricity, Gk *lytos* soluble.]

electrolytic (el·**ek**·tro·**lit**'·ik). Referring to electrolysis.

electrolyzer (el·**ek**·tro·**li**'·zer). An electrolytic apparatus by means of which a urethral stricture or a fibroma can be treated.

electromagnet (el·**ek**·tro·**mag**'·net). A piece of soft iron to which magnetic properties can be imparted when an electric current is passed through a coil of insulated wire surrounding it. The iron loses these properties when the current is shut off.

electromagnetics (el·**ek**·tro·mag·**net**'·ix). The branch of science which is concerned with the relations between electricity and magnetism.

electromagnetism (el·**ek**·tro·**mag**'·net·izm). Magnetism developed by means of an electric current.

electromanometer (el·**ek**·tro·man·**om**'·et·er) An instrument for the measurement of pressure or pressure changes, in which an electrical signal is produced proportional to the magnitude of the measured quantity. [electricity, Gk *manos* rare, *metron* measure.]

electromassage (el·**ek**·tro·mas·**ahzh**'). A method of combining electrical treatment with massage by the use of massage apparatus charged with electricity.

electromedication (el·**ek**·tro·med·ik·**a**'·shun). The use of an electric current to drive certain chemical remedies into the tissues. [electricity, medication.]

electrometer (el·ek·**trom**·et·er). An instrument used to measure electrical potential. **Capillary electrometer.** A fine capillary tube containing dilute sulphuric acid in contact with the surface of a mercury thread; minute differences of potential between the two can be measured by movement of the mercury due to alteration of surface tension (Lippmann). **Gold-leaf electrometer.** A gold-leaf electroscope fitted with a quadrant scale for quantitative comparison of radioactive substances. **Quadrant electrometer.** A magnetic needle suspended horizontally within a coil; deflexion of the needle measures the electric current passing through the coil. **String electrometer.** An electrometer in which the moving element in a conducting fibre, measured on an eyepiece graticule, indicates the potential applied to the electrometer. **Vacuum-tube electrometer.** An electrometer in which the unknown electric potential is applied to one of the grids of a thermionic valve, and so changes the current flowing to the other electrodes of the valve by a determinable amount. **Vibrating-reed electrometer.** An electrometer in which the unknown electric potential is applied to a metallic strip or reed vibrating at a constant frequency and maintained thus electromagnetically. The movements of the reed cause oscillations of the potential of a fixed metal plate, called the anvil, which is close to the reed. These regular oscillations of potential are amplified by a conventional a.c. amplifier which provides an output signal that is a measure of the unknown potential applied to the reed. This is the most sensitive form of electrometer.

See also: LINDEMANN (F. A.).

electrometrogram (el·**ek**·tro·**met′**·ro·gram). An electrical apparatus which records uterine contractions. [electricity, Gk *metra* womb, *gramma* a writing.]

electromotive (el·**ek**·tro·**mo′**·tiv). 1. Producing mechanical motion by electricity. 2. Relating to electrical action. 3. Producing electricity. 4. Relating to the passing of electricity in a circuit.

electromyogram (el·**ek**·tro·**mi′**·o·gram). The graphic record after amplification of muscle-action potentials. [electricity, Gk *mys* muscle, *gramma* record.]

electromyography (el·**ek**·tro·mi·**og′**·raf·e). The process of recording, after suitable amplification, of muscle-action potentials and the clinical interpretation of the results obtained. [electricity, Gk *mys* muscle, *graphein* to record.]

electron (el·**ek**·tron). 1. Obsolete name of an alloy of magnesium (90 per cent) and aluminium, with traces of zinc and other metals for strength. 2. The negatively-charged particle (charge $e = -1.60 \times 10^{-19}$ C, mass $m = 9.11 \times 10^{-28}$g) which forms a constituent of all atoms, its positively charged counterpart of equal mass and charge being called the *positron.* However, the term electron is often used to include both negative electrons (negatrons) and positive electrons (positrons). **Auger electrons.** Those electrons emitted from an atom owing to the filling of a vacancy in an inner electron shell. **Emission electron.** An electron emitted in radioactivity. **Free electron.** An electron by virtue of which a metal is able to conduct electricity. **Heavy electron.** A heavy particle present in cosmic rays. **Electron microscope.** *See* MICROSCOPE. **Orbital electron.** One of the constituent electrons of the atom bound in a definite energy state, and visualized according to the original Bohr concept as circulating round the nucleus in a definite orbit like a planet round the sun. **Electron pair.** A positive and negative electron produced together by the interaction of a high-energy photon with matter. **Secondary electron.** A free electron which has been removed from its normal orbit by the absorption of energy from any type of ionizing radiation. **Subvalency electron.** An electron of an inner and complete shell, as distinguished from a valency electron of the outermost shell. **Electron theory.** *See* THEORY. **Electron therapy.** *See* THERAPY. **Thermionic electron.** An electron produced by the action of heat on a substance. **Valency electron.** An electron on the surface of the atom which effects chemical combination either by passing to another atom or by forming a common bond between the two. [Gk *elektron* amber.]

electronarcosis (el·**ek**·tro·nar·**ko′**·sis). A state of narcosis resulting from the use of electricity; the electrodes which discharge the current are placed on the patient's temples.

electronation (el·**ek**·tron·**a′**·shun). In oxidation-reduction theory, the supply of one or more electrons to an element which constitutes reduction.

electronecrosis (el·**ek**·tro·nek·**ro′**·sis). 1. Electrocution. 2. Local necrosis of an organ or tissue due to the action of an electric current.

electronegative (el·**ek**·tro·**neg′**·at·iv). 1. Having a negative charge of electricity. 2. In electrolysis, appearing at the positive pole.

electroneurolysis (el·**ek**·tro·newr·**ol′**·is·is). The destruction of nerve tissue brought about by use of an electric needle. [electricity, Gk *neuron* nerve, *lysis* a loosing.]

electronic (el·ek·**tron**·ik). Relating to electrons, or operated by electrons.

electronics (el·ek·**tron**·ix). The electrical technology of apparatus generally containing semiconductors or thermionic valves, apparatus often small and not containing moving parts, as distinct from *electrical engineering,* dealing with electric motors, etc. [Gk *elektron* amber.]

electronization (el·**ek**·tron·i·**za′**·shun). Irradiation used for the purpose of bringing diseased cells back to a healthy state by restoring their electrical equilibrium. [see prec.]

electronograph (el·ek·**tron**·o·graf). The picture produced by an electron microscope. [electron, Gk *graphein* to record.]

electronystagmogram (el·**ek**·tro·nis·**tag′**·mo·gram). A graphic record obtained by electronystagmography. [electron, nystagmus, Gk *graphein* to record.]

electronystagmography (el·**ek**·ro·nis·tag·**mog′**·raf·e). A method of recording the eye movements in spontaneous or induced nystagmus using the electrical potential of the moving eyeball to activate a galvanometer. [electron, nystagmus, Gk *graphein* to record.]

electro-oculogram (el·**ek**·tro·**ok′**·ew·lo·gram). A recording of changes in electrical potential around the eye, induced by eye movements; used in the study of eye movements and retinal function. [electricity, L *oculus* eye, Gk *gramma* record.]

electro-optics (el·**ek**·tro·**op′**·tix). The branch of physics which deals with optical phenomena produced by electromagnetic and electrostatic fields.

electro-osmophoresis (el·**ek**·tro·**oz**·mo·for·**e′**·sis). **Immune electro-osmophoresis.** Counter-current electrophoresis; a method of detecting antigens by causing them to migrate in an agar or agarose gel towards the anode by electrophoresis, whereas antibody moves in the reverse direction towards the antigen by endosmosis. The effect is to cause precipitation where the antigen meets antibody with a considerable increase in sensitivity over the otherwise very similar immuno-diffusion. The technique is widely used in the detection of Australia (serum hepatitis) antigen. [electron, Gk *osmos* impulse, *pherein* to bear.]

electro-osmosis (el·**ek**·tro·oz·**mo′**·sis). 1. An osmotic effect produced by a difference of electric potential between the liquids on opposite sides of a semipermeable membrane. 2. Cataphoresis.

electropathology (el·**ek**·tro·path·**ol′**·o·je). The study of the morbid condition of a part as shown by its response to electrical stimulation. [electricity, pathology.]

electrophobia (el·**ek**·tro·**fo′**·be·ah). Excessive fear of electricity and of anything electrical. [electricity, Gk *phobia* fear.]

electrophonoide (el·**ek**·tro·**fo′**·noid). An instrument designed by Zünd-Burguet which is capable of producing a wide range of sounds and harmonics equalling the whole range of the human voice. These sounds are produced by mechanical larynges set in vibration electrically. The purpose of the instrument is to produce a physiological stimulation of the ear and lead to re-education of the dormant auditory function. It is used in the treatment of deafness. [electricity, Gk *phone* voice, *eidos* form.]

electrophore (el·**ek**·tro·for). Electrophorus.

electrophoresis (el·**ek**·tro·for·**e′**·sis). The motion of charged colloidal particles towards electrodes placed in the solution. **Counter-current electrophoresis.** Immune electro-osmophoresis. *See* ELECTRO-OSMOPHORESIS. **High-voltage electrophoresis.** A modification of electrophoresis in which a voltage of 1000–5000 V is used. **Microscopic electrophoresis.** Modification of the method of electrophoresis for the study of particles of a size visible by microscopy or ultramicroscopy. **Moving-boundary electrophoresis.** Modification of the method of electrophoresis for the study of dissolved substances. It is of particular use for studying solutions of mixtures of biological substances. **Paper electrophoresis.** A method of chromatography for detecting abnormal haemoglobins. **Zone electrophoresis.** A modification of the method of electrophoresis so that the electrical field is produced on some solid support. Thus: filter, starch gel, agar gel, starch block, polyacrylamide gel electrophoresis. [electron, Gk *pherein* to bear.]

electrophoretic (el·**ek**·tro·for·**et**′·ik). Referring to electrophoresis. **Electrophoretic migration.** Electrophoretic mobility. *See* MOBILITY. **Electrophoretic mobility.** *See* MOBILITY.

electrophorus (el·ek·**trof**·or·us). A simple device for producing an electrostatic charge. A flat disc of resin or other dielectric is charged initially, and induced charges taken from it repeatedly by a brass disc of the same size fitted with an insulated handle. [electricity, Gk *pherein* to bear.]

electrophototherapy (el·**ek**·tro·fo·to·**ther**′·ap·e). Therapeutic use of rays from an electric light. [electricity, Gk *phos* light, therapy.]

electrophysiology (el·**ek**·tro·fiz·e·**ol**′·o·je). That branch of science which is concerned with healthy bodily processes and their relation to electrical phenomena. [electricity, physiology.]

electropism (el·**ek**·tro·pizm). Electrotropism.

electroplexy (el·**ek**·tro·**plex**′·e). 1. The production of a major epileptic convulsion by the use of an electrical stimulus, e.g. the discharge of a condenser transmitted through poles placed on the patient's forehead. 2. The method of treating patients by means of electrically-induced convulsions. [electricity, Gk *plege* stroke.]

electropneumatotherapy (el·**ek**·tro·new·mat·o·**ther**′·ap·e). The treatment of functional vocal fatigue by passing an electric current into the larynx whilst the vocal cords are in action. [electricity, Gk *pneuma* air, therapy.]

electropneumograph (el·**ek**·tro·**new**′·mo·graf). An electrical apparatus with which the movements of respiration can be recorded. [electricity, pneumograph.]

electropoion (el·**ek**·tro·**poi**′·on). Acidulated potassium dichromate used as an electrolyte in the biochromate cell. [electricity, Gk *poiein* to make.]

electropositive (el·**ek**·tro·**poz**′·it·iv). 1. Pertaining to positive electricity or a positive electrode (anode). 2. Describing anything bearing a positive charge, e.g. positive ion.

electropuncture (el·**ek**·tro·**pungk**′·tcher). The passing of an electric current into tissue or tumour through needles used as electrodes. [electricity, puncture.]

electropyrexia (el·**ek**·tro·pi·**rex**′·e·ah). The artificial raising of the body temperature to fever height by passing electric currents into the tissues by means of a special apparatus (pyrexia or fever therapy). [electricity, pyrexia.]

electroradiology (el·**ek**·tro·ra·de·**ol**′·o·je). The study of the diagnostic and therapeutic use of x-rays and electricity. [electricity, radiology.]

electroradiometer (el·**ek**·tro·ra·de·**om**′·et·er). A modified form of electroscope used in the differential measurement of radiant energy. [electricity, radiometer.]

electroresection (el·**ek**·tro·re·**sek**′·shun). The excision of a part by use of an electric cautery or similar instrument. [electricity, L *resecare* to cut off.]

electroretinogram (el·**ek**·tro·**ret**′·in·o·gram). A tracing that records the electrical variations that take place in the retina on exposure to light. [electricity, retina, Gk *gramma* record.]

electrosalivogram (el·**ek**·tro·sal·**i**′·vo·gram). A record of the electrical changes occurring in the salivary glands during their activity. The significance of the records has not been assessed as yet. [electricity, salivary glands, Gk *gramma* record.]

electroscission (el·**ek**·tro·**sizh**′·un). The use of an electric cautery or knife in cutting into or through tissue. [electricity, L *scindere* to cut.]

electroscope (el·**ek**·tro·skope). An instrument for demonstrating the presence of an electrostatic charge. **Gold-leaf electroscope.** A pair of gold leaves suspended from a rod, which take an induced charge and repel one another when an electrified body is brought near them. [electricity, Gk *skopein* to watch.]

electrosensibility (el·**ek**·tro·sen·sib·**il**′·it·e). The sensitiveness and response of a sensory nerve to electrical stimulation.

electroshock (el·**ek**·tro·**shok**′). A form of therapy used in psychiatry, where an electric current is passed through the brain. [electricity, Fr. *choc.*]

electrosol (el·**ek**·tro·sol). A colloidal solution of a metal formed by passing an arc between wires of the metal immersed in iced distilled water. [electricity, sol.]

electrosome (el·**ek**·tro·some). A chondriosome that is a centre of chemical activity. [electron, Gk *soma* body.]

electrospectrogram (el·**ek**·tro·**spek**′·tro·gram). The graph or tracing produced in electrospectrography. [electricity, L *spectrum* image, Gk *gramma* record.]

electrospectrography (el·**ek**·tro·**spek**·**trog**′·raf·e). The analysis of the complex wave-form of an electro-encephalogram, and the recording of the constituent wave systems. [electricity, L *spectrum* image, Gk *graphein* to record.]

electrospinogram (el·**ek**·tro·**spi**′·no·gram). The record of the action potential of the spinal cord. [electricity, spinal cord, Gk *gramma* record.]

electrostatic (el·**ek**·tro·**stat**′·ik). Relating to static electricity, or electrons in a state of rest. **Electrostatic generator.** A machine for producing static electricity by friction or influence. [electricity, Gk *stasis* a standing still.]

electrostatics (el·**ek**·tro·**stat**′·ix). The branch of physics which deals with the phenomena of static electricity. [see prec.]

electrostenolysis (el·**ek**·tro·sten·**ol**′·is·is). 1. The electrodeposition of a metal within the interstices of a porous material. 2. The electronic interchange that takes place at a porous membrane when there is a wide difference in potential between electrodes placed on opposite sides, reproducing oxidative and reductive changes. [electricity, Gk *stenos* narrow, *lysis* a loosing.]

electrostethograph (el·**ek**·tro·**steth**′·o·graf). An electrical apparatus which amplifies and records respiratory and cardiac sounds of the chest. [electricity, Gk *stethos* test, *graphein* to record.]

electrostethophone (el·**ek**·tro·**steth**′·o·fone). An electrically-amplified stethoscope. [electricity, stethoscope, Gk *phone* voice.]

electrosurgery (el·**ek**·tro·**ser**′·jer·e). The use of electricity for surgical purposes, e.g. by means of the electric knife or by surgical diathermy.

electrosynthesis (el·**ek**·tro·**sin**′·thes·is). In chemistry, synthesis or the forming of a compound brought about by electrical action.

electrotaxis (el·**ek**·tro·**tax**′·is). The movement of protoplasm or small organisms under the stimulus of an electric current. **Negative electrotaxis.** That in which the living cell or organism is attracted towards the anode and repelled from the cathode. **Positive electrotaxis.** That in which the living cell or organism is attracted towards the cathode and repelled from the anode. [electricity, Gk *taxis* arrangement.]

electrothanasia (el·**ek**·tro·than·**a**′·ze·ah). Electrocution, other than judicial execution. [electricity, Gk *thanatos* death.]

electrotherapeutics (el·**ek**·tro·ther·ap·**ew**′·tix). The science of electrotherapy.

electrotherapeutist (el·**ek**·tro·ther·ap·**ew**′·tist). Electrotherapist.

electrotherapist (el·**ek**·tro·**ther**′·ap·ist). A medical practitioner or a technician who uses electricity, particularly, in the treatment of disease. [see foll.]

electrotherapy (el·**ek**·tro·**ther**′·ap·e). Treatment based on the application of low-frequency (faradic) and direct (galvanic) currents, used to produce contractions of weak innervated muscles (faradic) or contractions of denervated muscles (galvanic). Also the effects of these agents on the relief of pain, especially that caused by injury or neuritis. [electricity, therapy.]

electrotherm (el·**ek**·tro·therm). An apparatus with which electricity can be applied superficially, and by the heat generated cause relief of pain. [electricity, Gk *therme* heat.]

electrothermal (el·**ek**·tro·**ther**′·mal). Relating to both heat and electricity. [see prec.]

electrothermotherapy (el·**ek**·tro·ther·mo·**ther**′·ap·e). A method of treatment in which heat is produced in the body in response to electrical stimulation. [electricity, Gk *therme* heat, therapy.]

electrotome (el·**ek**·tro·tome). 1. A needle or wire loop carrying a high-frequency current and used for the incision or resection of living tissues. The high-frequency currents are designed for two purposes, cutting and electrocoagulation. 2. A device, which may act automatically, attached to an electrical apparatus for breaking the circuit. **Prostatic electrotome.** An endoscopic instrument consisting of a cystoscope through which passes a wire loop carrying a diathermy current. It is used for resection of the prostate, especially when the latter is the site of malignant disease. [electricity, Gk *temnein* to cut.]

See also: MCCARTHY (J. F.).

electrotomy (el·ek·trot·o·me). An electrosurgical method of excision utilizing a high-frequency, high-voltage and low-amperage current. The cutting electrode is a wire loop which engages the part to be excised. [see prec.]

electrotonic (el·**ek**·tro·**ton**′·ik). Referring to electrotonus.

electrotonus (el·**ek**·tro·**to**′·nus). 1. The stimulated condition of a nerve or muscle whilst an electric current is passing through it. 2. The modified excitability and conductivity of a muscle or nerve produced by the passage of an electric current. [electricity, Gk *tonos* tension.]

electrotrephine (el·**ek**·tro·tref·**ine**′). A trephine electrically operated.

electrotropism (el·**ek**·tro·**trop**′·izm). The power of attraction or repulsion associated with certain electric currents when applied to an organism. [electricity, tropism.]

electrovagogram (el·**ek**·tro·**va**′·go·gram). An unsatisfactory general term applied to recordings of the electrical changes occurring in the vagus nerve which depend on the passage of a large number of both motor and sensory impulses. [electricity, vagus, Gk *gramma* record.]

electrovalence, electrovalency (el·**ek**·tro·**va**′·lens, el·**ek**·tro·**va**′·len·se). An ionic linkage between atoms or radicals in a compound by mutual donation or receipt of electrons to give each participator a completed electron shell. [electron, valency.]

electrovection (el·**ek**·tro·**vek**′·shun). 1. The passing of medicaments into the system by means of an electric current. 2. Cataphoresis. [electricity, L *vehere* to carry.]

electuary (e·**lek**·tew·ar·e). A confection; a drug compounded into a sweet paste with honey or sugar. **Electuary of senna.** Confection of senna. [Gk *ekleikton* that which is licked away.]

eleidin (el·e·id·in). A substance of protein nature formed by solution of the keratohyalin of the stratum granulosum of the skin during formation of the stratum lucidum. [Gk *elaia* olive tree.]

element (el·e·ment). 1. Any of the simplest components into which a thing may be analysed; any of the ultimate parts of which anything is built up. 2. Matter consisting of atoms having the same atomic number. **Alkaline element.** Name given to any member of the first group of the Periodic Table, i.e. the alkali metals. **Amphoteric element.** Any element, such as zinc, the oxide of which dissolved in water acts both as an acid and a base. **Anatomical element.** Any primary component of histological structure, such as a cell, fibre, nucleus, mitochondria, etc. **Appendicular element.** A part of the cartilaginous skull derived from the pharyngeal arches. **Biological element.** Any element concerned with plant or animal life. **Electronegative element.** Any element, for the most part the non-metals, which takes up electrons and forms negative ions. **Electropositive element.** Any element, for the most part hydrogen and the metals, which gives up electrons and forms positive ions. **Galvanic element.** Either of the elements forming with an electrolyte (or electrolytes) an electric cell. **Labile element.** The cell of a tissue which retains the ability to divide. **Morphological element.** Anatomical element (see above). **Radioactive element.** Radio-element; an element that exhibits radioactivity, either natural or artificially induced. **Rare-earth element.** Any of the rare elements comprising a series of 14 in the Periodic Table; they include cerium and gadolinium and resemble aluminium in chemical properties. **Sarcous element.** Any of the hypothetical primary granular elements composing a muscle fibre. **Stable element.** The cell of a tissue which does not divide, in contrast to a labile element (see above). **Tissue element.** One of the primary components, e.g. cells or fibres, of which a tissue is composed. **Trace element.** Name applied to any element, such as cobalt or copper, observed as a microconstituent of plant or animal tissue and of beneficial, harmful or even doubtful significance. **Tracer element.** Any isotope that can be detected by radioactivity or other means, and is used for this reason to investigate the rôle played by the particular element (e.g. phosphorus, iodine) in biological processes. **Transition element.** Name given to members of 3 series of elements in the Periodic Table, each displaying similarity horizontally and mostly several valencies. **Transuranic element, Transuranium element.** Any of the artificial elements formed by nuclear reaction and included in the Periodic Table beyond uranium; they include neptunium and plutonium. [L *elementum.*]

See also: BOWMAN.

elementary (el·e·**ment**·ar·e). 1. Fundamental or simple. 2. Relating or belonging to an element. 3. Having the characters of an element. 4. Uncompounded or consisting of a single element.

eleo-. For words beginning **Eleo-**, *see* ELAEO-.

elephantiasic (el·ef·an·ti·**as**′·ik). Referring to, associated with or suffering from elephantiasis.

elephantiasis (el·ef·an·**ti**′·as·is). Gross lymphatic oedema of the limbs or areas of the trunk or head, leading to hypertrophy of the connective tissues and thickening and overgrowth of the malpighian layer of the skin. The overall appearance roughly, in the case of the legs, resembles the forelegs of an elephant. **Elephantiasis anaesthetica.** Elephantiasis graecorum (see below). **Elephantiasis arabum.** Filarial elephantiasis. (see below). **Elephantiasis asturiensis.** Pellagra. **Congenital elephantiasis.** A term formerly applied to elephantiasis nostras (see below). **Filarial elephantiasis.** Formerly known as *elephantiasis arabum*, is caused primarily by mechanical blockage of the main lymphatic channels and glands of the leg, arm, breast or scrotum by adult *Wuchereria bancrofti* (*Filaria bancrofti*). The presence of these worms, when alive, and when dead and cretified, gives rise to chronic, progressive lymph stasis. During this process most, if not all, adult worms are killed and the embryos, or microfilariae, disappear from the circulation. **Elephantiasis gingivae.** Hypertrophy of the gums without any associated disease; macrogingivae. **Elephantiasis graecorum.** A term formerly applied to the chronic oedema of the skin and subjacent tissues in tuberculoid leprosy. **Elephantiasis neuromatosa.** Pachydermatocele; a plexiform neuroma attaining large dimensions and producing a condition resembling elephantiasis. **Elephantiasis nostras.** 1. Milroy's disease, which presents from the clinical aspect a similar condition and is due to congenital stenosis of the main lymphatic trunks. 2. Elephantiasis caused by recurrent streptococcal infections. **Elephantiasis oculi.** Chronic inflammation and thickening of the eyelids. **Elephantiasis scroti.** Filarial elephantiasis of the scrotum; it may also occur in other forms of lymphatic obstruction. **Streptococcal elephantiasis.** Elephantiasis due to streptococcal infection of the lymphatics which causes blocking and subsequent stasis of lymph. **Surgical elephantiasis.** Elephantiasis resulting from surgical procedures that have interfered with the lymphatic drainage of a limb. **Elephantiasis telangiectodes.** A term applied to a limited area of skin affected by elephantiasis. [Gk *elephas* elephant.]

elephantoid (el·ef·an·toid). 1. Elephant-like. 2. Resembling elephantiasis. [elephantiasis, Gk *eidos* form.]

elevation (el·e·va·shun). An eminence. **Dicrotic elevation.** In dicrotism, the secondary rise in the wave shown in the sphygmogram. **Tactile elevation [torulus tactilis (NA)].** Any one of the tiny raised areas on the palms and soles at which many sensory nerve-endings are clustered together; lamellated (Pacini's) corpuscle. **Tubal elevation [torus tubarius (NA)].** A prominence behind the pharyngeal opening of the pharyngotympanic tube, produced by the cartilage of the tube covered by mucous membrane. [see foll.]

elevator (el·e·va·tor). 1. A levator muscle. 2. An instrument with which a depressed portion of a bone can be lifted. 3. An instrument used for removing teeth or the roots of teeth: there are many shapes and sizes. **Apical elevator.** An instrument used for the removal of the apex of a tooth which has fractured during the process of extraction. **Curved elevator.** An instrument used mainly for the removal of roots which have been retained in the jaw. **Periosteum elevator.** Am instrument for stripping the periosteum from a bone. **Straight elevator.** An instrument used mainly for the removal of third molar teeth. [L *elevare* to raise.] *See also:* WINTER.

Elford membrane. Gradocol membrane. *See* MEMBRANE.

eliminant (e·lim·in·ant). An agent which promotes or increases excretion of waste products. [see foll.]

elimination (e·lim·in·a'·shun). The process or act of excreting or discharging waste products. [L *eliminare* to expel.]

elinin (el·in·in). A lipoprotein fraction separated from erythrocytes that contains the A, B and Rh agglutinogens.

Eliocharis (el·e·ok·ar·is). A genus of flowering plants. Cercariae of *Fasciolopsis buski* often encyst on the nuts of *Eliocharis tuberosa*, the water chestnut, which are eaten by man, thus causing infection.

elixir (el·ix·er). A liquid containing active drugs, to which syrup, glycerin or alcohol have been added to mask the unpleasant taste. **Elixir anisi.** A carminative mixture composed of the oils of aniseed, fennel and bitter almonds in alcohol, with syrup and water. **Elixir Bromoformi BPC 1949.** An elixir of bromoform flavoured with glycerin, tincture of orange and compound tincture of cardamoms; it is used as a sedative. **Elixir of Caffeine Iodide BPC 1959.** An elixir with a diuretic action, composed of caffeine and sodium iodide flavoured with liquid extract of liquorice, decoction of coffee and sweetened with chloroform. **Cascara Elixir BP 1958.** Made by percolating cascara, liquorice and light magnesium oxide with boiling water, evaporating, and flavouring with glycerin and a volatile oil, usually coriander oil, which is most effective in masking the bitterness of cascara. It is used as a purgative, and is very effective in children. **Elixir of Diamorphine and Terpin BPC 1959.** A mixture containing diamorphine hydrochloride, terpin hydrate, alcohol, glycerin and wild cherry syrup; it is used in the treatment of coughs. **Elixir of Nux Vomica BPC 1959.** A mixture of nux vomica tincture, compound cardamom tincture, syrup and chloroform water. **Elixir of Phenobarbitone BPC 1959.** A mixture of phenobarbitone, alcohol, compound tartrazine solution, glycerin and compound orange spirit; it is used as a sedative in nervous and anxiety states. **Elixir saccharini.** A 5 per cent solution of saccharin in bicarbonate to which alcohol has been added as a preservative; used as a sweetening agent in mixtures. **Elixir Valerianae et Chloralis Composition BPC 1949.** An elixir containing potassium bromide, chloral hydrate and liquid extract of valerian, flavoured with oils of orange, lemon, coriander and aniseed, in syrup, alcohol and water; it is used as a sedative in hysteria. [Ar. *el-iksir* philosopher's stone.]

Ellermann, Wilhelm (b. 1871). Copenhagen pathologist.

Ellermann and Erlandsen test. Injections of tuberculin of various dilutions made to determine the highest dilution that will produce a local reaction. Reaction to 1 in 10 000 or more is said to indicate active disease. It is not specific.

Elliot, George Thompson (b. 1851). New York dermatologist.

Elliot's sign. The induration to be noted at the peripheries of certain syphilitic lesions of the skin.

Elliot, John Wheelock (b. 1852). Boston surgeon.

Elliot's position. A position on the operating table in which access to the gall bladder and bile ducts is facilitated by arching the back over a support, the patient being supine.

Elliot, Robert Henry (b. 1864). Ophthalmologist and Lt-Col, Indian Medical Service.

Elliot's operation. For chronic glaucoma: corneoscleral trephining at the limbus under a conjunctival flap with a peripheral iridectomy.

Elliot's trephine. The manual trephine devised by Elliot for his corneoscleral trephining operation.

Elliot Smith. *See* SMITH, SIR GRAFTON ELLIOT.

Elliott, Charles Robert (b. 1879). New York gynaecologist.

Elliott treatment. The treatment of pelvic inflammatory disease by passing heated water through a rubber bag inserted into the vagina.

Elliott, Thomas Renton (b. 1877). London physician.

Elliott's law. The activity of adrenaline is due to its action on structures innervated by the sympathetic nervous system.

ellipsis (el·ip·sis). In psychological medicine, the omission by a patient of meaningful ideas or words while he is undergoing psycho-analysis. [Gk *elleipsis* omission.]

elliptocytary (el·ip·to·si'·tar·e). Characterized by the presence of numerous oval or elliptical erythrocytes in the blood. [Gk *elleipsis* ellipse, *kytos* cell.]

elliptocyte (el·ip·to·site). An oval or elliptical erythrocyte. [see prec.]

elliptocytosis (el·ip·to·si·to'·sis). A condition in which there are numerous oval or elliptical erythrocytes in the blood. [elliptocyte, Gk *-osis* condition.]

elliptocytotic (el·ip·to·si·tot'·ik). Elliptocytary.

Ellis, Sir Arthur William Mickle (b. 1883). London physician.

Swift-Ellis treatment. Autoserosalvarsan treatment.

Ellis, Calvin (b. 1826). Boston physician.

Ellis's curve, line or sign, Ellis-Damoiseau curve, line or sign, Ellis-Garland curve, line or sign. The S-shaped line that on percussion marks the upper limit of dullness caused by a pleural effusion.

Ellis, George Viner (b. 1812). London anatomist and physician.

Ellis' muscle. The corrugator cutis ani muscle.

Ellis, Richard White Bernard (b. 1902). Edinburgh paediatrician.

Ellis-van Creveld syndrome. Chondro-ectodermal dysplasia; a syndrome of bilateral manual polydactylism, chondrodysplasia of the long bones resulting in acromelic dwarfism, hidrotic ectodermal dysplasia affecting the nails and hair, and congenital malformations of the heart. *See* CHONDRO-ECTODERMAL DYSPLASIA.

Ellison, Edwin H. (b. 1918). American physician.

Zollinger-Ellison syndrome. Intractable peptic ulceration and gastric hyperacidity associated with islet-cell adenomata of the pancreas. In 50 per cent of cases a low-grade malignancy occurs.

elm (elm). A tree of the genus *Ulmus* (family Ulmaceae). **Corkwood elm.** The tree *Ulmus fulva.* The corkwood elm of Australia is *Duboisia myoporoides.* **Slippery elm, Slippery elm bark.** The dried bark of a small American tree *Ulmus fulva* (family Ulmaceae). It contains mucilage and a little tannin and is used internally as a demulcent; mixed with hot water it is employed as a poultice. The bark, broken into strips, is used by abortionists as tent-like insertions into the cervix of the uterus for the purpose of terminating a pregnancy. [AS.]

elodes (e·lo·deez). Malaria. **Elodes icteroides.** Yellow fever. [Gk *swampy.]*

elongatio (e·long·ga·she·o). Elongation. **Elongatio colli.** A pathological state of the neck of the uterus in which it is enlarged and lengthened. [L a prolonging.]

elongation (e·long·ga·shun). 1. The state of being lengthened or extended. 2. The process of lengthening. **Chain elongation.** *See* CHAIN. [see prec.]

Elsberg, Charles Albert (b. 1871). New York surgeon.

Elsberg's procedure. Two-stage removal of intramedullary spinal tumours.

Elsberg's test. Of olfactory function: a series of quantitative tests of olfactory function, the tests involving the injection of air containing volatile substances into the nasal cavities during a period of voluntary apnoea. From a series of observations, the minimum identifiable odour (MIO) can be determined as well as the duration of fatigue of olfactory sensation. Elsberg has suggested that variations in these values are of use in the differentiation between intracerebral and extracerebral tumours in the region of the frontal lobe.

Elschnig, Anton (b. 1863). German ophthalmologist.

Elschnig's bodies, or pearls. Clumps of transparent vesicles formed by the proliferation of subcapsular epithelium from the remnants of lens capsule following extracapsular cataract extraction.

Elschnig's spots. Spots of black pigment associated with a red or yellow halo, seen in the fundus in malignant hypertension.

eluate (el·ew·ate). That which is washed out by elution.

eluent (el·ew·ent). The solvent used in elution.

elute (el·ewt). To perform the process of elution.

elution (el·ew·shun). The process of separating the constituents of a mixture of powdered substances by washing with a selective solvent. If the eluates are subsequently reabsorbed in suitable media, complete separation may be achieved, as in chromatography. [L *e*, *luere* to wash.]

elutriation (el·ew·tre·a′·shun). A mechanical process of separating solids of different densities by crushing them to a fine powder which is then agitated in a suitable liquid: the lighter particles float to the top, the heavier sink. [L *elutriare* to wash out.]

Ely, Leonard Wheeler (b. 1868). San Francisco orthopaedic surgeon.

Ely's test. For contracture of the lateral fascia of the thigh: with the patient prone, flexion of the leg at the knee will cause abduction at the hip and lifting of the buttocks.

Ely's operation. For chronic suppurative otitis media; skin grafts are applied to the middle-ear cavity in cases with gross destruction of the tympanic membrane.

elytritis (el·it·ri·tis). A condition of inflammation of the vagina. [Gk *elytron* sheath, *-itis* inflammation.]

elytrocele (el·it·ro·seel). 1. Colpoptosis. 2. Hernia into the vagina. [Gk *elytron* sheath, *kele* hernia.]

elytroceliotomy (el·it·ro·se·le·ot′·o·me). Repair of an enterocele. [Gk *elytron* sheath *kele* hernia, *temnein* to cut.]

elytroclasia (el·it·ro·kla′·ze·ah). Rupture of the vagina. [Gk *elytron* sheath, *klasis* a breaking.]

elytrocleisis (el·it·ro·kli′·sis). Surgical obliteration of the lumen of the vagina. [Gk *elytron* sheath, *kleisis* closure.]

elytronitis (el·it·ron·i′·tis). 1. Capsulitis. 2. Colpitis; vaginitis. [Gk *elytron* sheath, *-itis* inflammation.]

elytroplastic (el·it·ro·plas′·tik). Referring to elytroplasty.

elytroplasty (el·it·ro·plas·te). Any plastic surgical operation on the vagina. [Gk *elytron* sheath, *plassein* to mould.]

elytropneumatosis (el·it·ro·new·mat·o′·sis). The accumulation of air in the vagina. [Gk *elytron* sheath, pneumatosis.]

elytropolypus (el·it·ro·pol′·e·pus). A polypus in the vagina. [Gk *elytron* sheath, polypus.]

elytroptosis (el·it·rop·to′·sis). Prolapse of the vagina. [Gk *elytron* sheath, *ptosis* fall.]

elytrorrhaphy (el·it·ror·af·e). Colporrhaphy. [Gk *elytron* sheath, *rhaphe* suture.]

elytrorrhoea (el·it·ro·re′·ah). Colporrhoea. [Gk *elytron* sheath, *rhoia* flow.]

elytrostenosis (el·it·ro·sten·o′·sis). Colpostenosis. [Gk elytron sheath, stenosis.]

elytrotome (el·it·ro·tome). A type of knife used in elytrotomy.

elytrotomy (el·it·rot·o·me). Colpotomy; any cutting operation in or surgical incision of the vagina. [Gk *elytron* sheath, *temnein* to cut.]

Elzholz, Adolf (b. 1863). Vienna neurologist.

Elzholz's bodies. Droplets of disintegrating myelin seen during nerve degeneration.

Elzholz's mixture. A solution of eosin in glycerin and water, used for the estimation of leucocytes.

emaciated (e·ma·se·a·ted). In a state of emaciation.

emaciation (e·ma·se·a′·shun). The state of extreme leanness; extreme loss of the subcutaneous fat. [L *emaciare* to become lean.]

emaculation (e·mak·ew·la′·shun). The process of removing spots, freckles and other blemishes from the skin, particularly that of the face. [L *e*, *macula* spot.]

emailloblast (em·a·lo·blast). Ameloblast. [Fr. *émail* enamel, Gk *blastos* germ.]

eman (e·man). An obsolete unit expressing the amount of (radon) present in a given volume of gas or liquid.

emanation (em·an·a·shun). 1. That which issues or proceeds from any source. 2. A radioactive gas occurring in each of the 3 radioactive series (radium, thorium and actinium), chemically similar to the inert gases. All 3 have nuclei bearing the same charge; they obey the ordinary gas laws, diffuse at a rate corresponding to their high atomic weights and condense at about −150°C. They are important because they yield active deposits in a pure state and in extremely thin layers. **Actinium emanation.** Actinon; Ac.Em or $_{86}Rn^{219}$, a gaseous element derived from actinium X. It has a half-life period of 3.92 s, and emits an α-particle, becoming actinium A. **Radium emanation.** $_{86}Rn^{222}$, radon, formerly known as *niton*; a gaseous element which is the direct product of the disintegration of radium; it has a half-life period of 3.8 days, and emits an α-particle, becoming radium A. **Thorium emanation.** Th.Em or $_{86}Rn^{220}$, thoron, a gaseous element formed by thorium X; it has a half-value period of 54.5 s, and emits an α-particle, becoming thorium A. [L *emanare* to flow forth.]

emanator (em·an·a·tor). An instrument which gives off radioactive emanations and at the same time applies them to the body. [Obsolete term.] [see prec.]

emanatorium (em·an·at·or′·e·um). An institute or room for the treatment of patients by emanation therapy. [Obsolete term.]

emancipation (e·man·sip·a′·shun). The acquisition of developmental independence by a region of the embryo previously subjected to external organizing influences. [L *emancipare* to set free.]

emanotherapy (em·an·o·ther′·ap·e). Treatment of disease with radon or other radioactive emanation. [Obsolete term.] [emanation, therapy.]

emansio mensium (e·man·se·o men·se·um). 1. Total failure of the menses to become established as a function. 2. Tardiness in first appearance of the menses. [L absence of the menses.]

emasculation (e·mas·kew·la′·shun). 1. Removal of all the male external genital organs. 2. Castration. [L *emasculare* to make impotent.]

Embadomonas (em·bad·o·mo·nas). A genus of small intestinal flagellates. *Embadomonas intestinalis* is a rare but geographically widely distributed species found in man; *Embadomonas sinensis* from China is doubtfully distinct. [Gk *embadon* surface, *monas* unit.]

embalm (em·balm). To preserve a dead body from decay by treating it with special antiseptic preparations. [ME *embaumen.*]

embalmment (em·bahm·ment). 1. The act of embalming. 2. The application to a wound of antiseptic ointment as an emergency measure, to prevent its infection until definitive treatment can be undertaken.

Embden ester. Glucopyranose 6-monophosphate, $C_6H_{11}O_5PO(OH)_2$, a constituent of Robison ester in muscle.

embed (em·bed). In histology, to fix tissue in a solid material such as paraffin wax so that it can be cut into thin sections. [Gk *en*, AS *bed.*]

embelate (em·bel·ate). A salt of embelic acid.

Embelia (em·be·le·ah). 1. A genus of plants of the family Myrsinaceae. 2. The dried fruits of *Embelia ribes* Burm. f. and *Embelia robusta* Roxb., used in India and the East as a taenicide, but of doubtful value. It contains the benzoquinone derivative, embelic acid.

embolaemia (em·bo·le·me·ah). A condition in which emboli are present in the blood. [embolus, Gk *haima* blood.]

embolalia (em·bo·la·le·ah). Embololalia.

embole (em·bo·le). 1. Reduction of a dislocated limb. 2. Embolism. [Gk, a thrusting in.]

embolectomy (em·bo·lek·to·me). Removal of an embolus by operation. [embolus, Gk *ektome* a cutting out.]

embolia (em·bo·le·ah). Embole.

embolic (em·bol·ik). Referring or belonging to an embolus or to embolism.

emboliform (em·bol·e·form). 1. Emboloid. 2. Wedge-shaped. [embolus, form].

embolism (em·bol·izm). The sudden blocking of a blood vessel, usually an artery, by fragments of a blood clot, or by clumps of bacteria or other foreign bodies introduced into the circulation.

Air embolism. Interference with the flow of blood by bubbles of air. **Amniotic embolism.** Embolism from amniotic fluid entering the maternal circulation during childbirth. **Bacillary embolism.** Obstruction caused by clumps of bacteria in septicaemia. **Bland embolism.** An embolism which produces no serious signs or symptoms. **Bone-marrow embolism.** Obstruction of a blood vessel due to particles of bone marrow entering the circulation after a fracture. **Capillary embolism.** A small embolus lodging in a capillary vessel. **Cerebral embolism.** Embolism of one of the arteries supplying the brain. **Coronary embolism.** Embolism of the coronary arteries of the heart. **Crossed embolism.** Paradoxical embolism (see below). **Fat embolism.** An embolism caused by globules of fat, usually following a fracture. **Haematogenous embolism.** An embolism due to a blood clot. **Infective embolism.** One attributable to clumps of bacteria, or from an infected blood clot, and giving rise to a metastatic abscess. **Lymphogenous embolism.** An embolism reaching the circulation from the lymphatic system. **Miliary embolism.** Multiple small emboli. **Multiple embolism.** Numerous emboli occurring at the same time or successively. **Oil embolism.** Embolism due to oil droplets, often the result of accidental injection of a medicinal oil into the circulation. **Paradoxical embolism.** Embolism caused by an embolus reaching the heart through the systemic veins but reaching the systemic arterial circulation because of a right-to-left shunt as, for example, in *Fallot's tetralogy.* **Peripheral artery embolism.** Embolism of an artery in a limb. **Pulmonary embolism.** Embolism of the pulmonary artery; if large may cause sudden death. **Pyaemic embolism.** An infective embolus producing an abscess. **Retinal embolism.** Embolism of the central artery of the retina, resulting in loss of vision in the affected eye. **Retrograde embolism.** An obstruction in a vein due to an embolus carried in a direction opposite to that of the circulation. **Spinal embolism.** An embolism of the spinal arteries. **Splenic embolism.** Embolism of the splenic artery which causes sudden pain and enlargement of the spleen. **Trichinous embolism.** Embolism attributable to *Trichinella* (*Trichina*) *spiralis.* **Venous embolism.** Embolism originating in a vein. [Gk *embolos* plug.]

embolization (**em**·bol·i·**za**′·shun). A neologism for *embolism.* [Gk *embolos* plug.]

emboloid (**em**·bol·oid). Having resemblance to an embolus. [embolus, Gk *eidos* form.]

embololalia (**em**·bol·o·**la**′·le·ah). A speech disorder in which irrelevant words are interpolated in a spoken sentence. [Gk *embolos* something thrust in, *lalein* to babble like a child.]

embolomycotic (**em**·bol·o·mi·**kot**′·ik). Referring to or caused by an infective embolus. [embolus, Gk *mykes* fungus.]

embolophrasia (**em**·bol·o·**fra**′·ze·ah). Embololalia. [Gk *embolos* something thrust in, *phrasein* to utter.]

embolus (**em**·bol·us). A foreign body, such as a blood clot, a mass of fat, tumour cells or a bubble of air, impacted within a blood vessel during life. **Air embolus.** A bubble of air impacted within a blood vessel as the result of trauma, decompression or infection with gas-forming bacteria. **Cancer embolus.** An embolus of cancer cells formed by the spread of a tumour into a blood vessel. **Cellular embolus.** An embolus composed of detached normal cells, such as liver cells, bone marrow cells or placental cells. **Foam embolus.** Air embolus (see above). **Gas embolus.** That caused by nitrogen gas being given off from the blood when a person is released too rapidly from a high-pressure atmosphere. **Obturating embolus.** An embolus producing obstruction of the vessel in which it is impacted. **Paradoxical embolus.** An embolus which appears to have spread in a direction contrary to that determined by the normal laws of blood flow. **Riding embolus, Saddle embolus, Straddling embolus.** An embolus which is balanced across, or straddles, a dividing blood vessel. **Tumour embolus.** Cancer embolus (see above). [Gk *embolos* plug.]

emboly (**em**·bo·le). In embryology, the process by which the hollow blastule becomes invaginated to form the gastrula. [Gk *embole* a thrusting in.]

Embramine (em·bram·een). BP Commission approved name for *N* - 2 - (4 - bromo - α - methylbenzhydryloxy)ethyldimethylamine; an antihistamine.

embrasure (em·**bra**·zher, em·**bra**·zhewr). The space formed by the contour and position of adjacent teeth. **Buccal embrasure.** In molar and premolar teeth, the embrasure opening out towards the cheeks. **Labial embrasure.** In incisor and canine teeth, the embrasure opening towards the lips. **Lingual embrasure.** An embrasure on the lingual sides of the teeth. **Occlusal embrasure.** The space bounded by the marginal ridge on the distal aspect of one tooth and that on the mesial aspect of the adjacent tooth and the contact points. [Fr. *ébraser* to make on opening.]

embrocation (em·bro·**ka**·shun). A liniment; a preparation designed to be applied to the intact skin. It usually contains a rubefacient drug which, irritating the sensory nerve-endings, causes vasodilatation by a local axon reflex; used to increase the blood flow to any particular part of the body surface, or as a counter-irritant. Embrocations are applied with friction which enhances this rubefacient effect, and nearly all contain oily substances, most frequently as emulsions. The most common rubefacients employed are turpentine and methyl salicylate; other substances sometimes incorporated are acetic acid, ammonia, capsicum and aconite. The emulsifying agent in oil-containing embrocations is usually soap. [Gk *en, brechein* to wet a surface.]

embryectomy (em·bre·**ek**·to·me). In ectopic pregnancy, the surgical removal of the embryo. [embryo, Gk *ektome* a cutting out.]

embryo (**em**·bre·o). 1. In botany, a young plant in process of development from an ovum, usually contained within a seed. 2. In zoology, an animal at some stage of its development from a fertilized ovum up to the point of birth or hatching. In man the term is usually restricted to the first 8 weeks of intrauterine life, the term *fetus* being employed after that. [Gk *en, bryein* to grow.]

See also: HERTIG, ROCK.

embryoblast (**em**·bre·o·blast). That portion of the developing ovum from which the embryo develops, in contrast with those parts from which the fetal membranes are formed. [embryo, Gk *blastos* germ.]

embryocardia (**em**·bre·o·**kar**′·de·ah). Disturbance of the rhythm of the heart beat, which may be present in cases of dilatation of the heart. The sounds resemble those of the fetal heart, the first and second sounds being alike in quality with a shortening of the long pause. **Jugular embryocardia.** Auricular flutter. *See* FLUTTER. [embryo, Gk *kardia* heart.]

embryochemical (**em**·bre·o·**kem**′·ik·al). Pertaining to the chemical changes taking place in the developing embryo.

embryoctony (em·bre·**ok**·ton·e). The destruction of the embryo or the fetus, as in induced abortion. [embryo, Gk *kteinein* to kill.]

embryogenesis (**em**·bre·o·**jen**′·es·is). Embryogeny.

embryogenetic, embryogenic (**em**·bre·o·jen·**et**′·ik, **em**·bre·o·**jen**′·ik). Referring or belonging to embryogeny.

embryogeny (em·bre·**oj**·en·e). 1. The formation and course of development of the embryo. 2. That branch of biology which is concerned with the development of the fertilized ovum. [embryo, Gk *genein* to produce.]

embryograph (**em**·bre·o·graf). A microscope with camera-lucida attachment which is used in drawing outlines of the embryo. [embryo, Gk *graphein* to draw.]

embryoid (**em**·bre·oid). Embryoniform. [embryo, Gk *eidos* form.]

embryoism (**em**·bre·o·izm). Embryonism.

embryolemma (**em**·bre·o·**lem**′·ah). The fetal membranes, such as the allantois and the amnion. [embryo, Gk *lemma* husk.]

embryologic, embryological (**em**·bre·o·**loj**′·ik, **em**·bre·o·**loj**′·ik·al). Relating or belonging to embryology.

embryologist (em·bre·**ol**·o·jist). One who makes a special study of embryology.

embryology (em·bre·**ol**·o·je). That branch of biological science which is concerned with the origin and development of the embryo from the ovum to the stage of extra-uterine life.

Experimental embryology. The study of the developing egg or embryo under artificial conditions. [embryo, Gk *logos* science.]

embryoma (em·bre·o·mah). 1. A neoplasm originating in embryonal elements or a blighted ovum. 2. A dermoid cyst of the ovary or testis, held by some to be a rudimentary embryo. [embryo, Gk *-oma* tumour.]

embryomorphous (em·bre·o·**mor'**·fus). 1. Concerning the formation and structure of an embryo. 2. Descriptive of abnormal rudimentary structures or embryonal rests in the body; they may be fragments of a blighted ovum. [embryo, Gk *morphe* form.]

embryon (em·bre·on). Embryo. [Gk.]

embryonal, embryonary (em·bre·on·al, em·bre·on·ar·e). Belonging to the embryo.

embryonate (em·bre·on·ate). 1. Fertilized. 2. Having an embryo. 3. Embryoniform.

embryonic (em·bre·**on**·ik). 1. Referring or belonging to an embryo. 2. Rudimentary or incipient.

embryoniform (em·bre·**on**·e·form). Resembling an embryo in form.

embryonin (em·bre·o·nin). A nucleoprotein present in embryo extracts which stimulates cell growth in tissue culture.

embryonism (em·bre·on·izm). The state of being an embryo.

embryonization (em·bre·on·i·**za'**·shun). Reversion of a cell or tissue to an embryonic form.

embryonoid (em·bre·on·oid). Embryoniform. [embryo, Gk *eidos* form.]

embryopathology (em·bre·o·path·**ol'**·o·je). That branch of pathology which is concerned with defective or abnormal development of the embryo.

embryophore (em·bre·o·for). A membrane which surrounds the developing oncosphere in tapeworm eggs. It is ciliated in *Diphyllobothrium* and its allies, and the whole, known as a *coracidium*, has a short free-swimming life. [embryo, Gk *pherein* to bear.]

embryoplastic (em·bre·o·**plas'**·tik). Descriptive of cells which participate in or belong to the forming and developing of an embryo. [embryo, Gk *plassein* to form.]

embryoscope (em·bre·o·skope). An instrument with which the embryo in a shell egg may be studied at different stages of development. [embryo, Gk *skopein* to watch.]

embryospastic (em·bre·o·**spas'**·tik). Referring to instrumental extraction of the fetus. [embryo, Gk *span* to draw.]

embryotocia (em·bre·o·**to'**·se·ah). Abortion. [embryo, Gk *tokos* birth.]

embryotome (em·bre·o·tome). Any cutting instrument used in embryotomy.

embryotomy (em·bre·**ot**·o·me). 1. The dismemberment and mutilation of the fetus so that it can be removed from the uterus when delivery by natural means is not possible. 2. Dissection of an embryo or fetus. [embryo, Gk *temnein* to cut.]

embryotoxon (em·bre·o·**tox'**·on). A congenital condition of the eye in which the margin of the cornea is opaque. The condition resembles that of arcus senilis, and is sometimes referred to as *arcus juvenilis.* **Anterior embryotoxon.** A benign ring-shaped opacity of the peripheral cornea present at, or shortly after, birth. Also called *arcus juvenilis.* **Posterior embryotoxon.** An accentuation of Schwalbe's line. [embryo, Gk *toxon* bow.]

embryotrophe (em·bre·o·trofe). The maternal glandular secretions, extravasated blood, etc., which provide nourishment for the early embryo. [embryo, Gk *trophe* nourishment.]

embryotrophy (em·bre·**ot**·ro·fe). Fetal nutrition. [see prec.]

embryulcia (em·bre·**ul**·se·ah). 1. Extraction of the embryo or fetus from the uterus by mechanical means. 2. Embryotomy. [embryo, Gk *elkein* to draw.]

embryulcus (em·bre·**ul**·kus). Obstetric forceps blunt and shaped like a hook, used in extraction of the dead fetus from the uterus. [see prec.]

Embutramide (em·**bew**·tram·ide). BP Commission approved name for *N*- [2 - ethyl - 2 - (3 - methoxyphenyl)butyl] - 4 - hydroxybutyramide; a narcotic analgesic.

emedullate (e·med·**ul**·ate). To extract the marrow or the pith from anything. [L *e*, *medulla* marrow.]

Emepronium Bromide (e·mep·**ro**·ne·um **bro**·mide). BP Commission approved name for ethyldimethyl - 1 - methyl - 3,3 - diphenylpropylammonium bromide; an anticholinergic.

emesia (em·e·ze·ah). Emesis. **Emesia gravidarum.** The vomiting that occurs in pregnancy.

emesis (**em**·es·is). 1. Vomiting. 2. An isolated act of vomiting, occurring as a single incident, or as one of a series of emetic incidents. [Gk vomiting.]

emetamine (em·**et**·am·een). $C_{29}H_{36}O_4N_2$, an alkaloid present in ipecacuanha root. It differs from emetine in possessing 4 hydrogen atoms fewer, corresponding to the presence of 2 additional double bonds, and has very little therapeutic value.

emetatrophia (em·et·at·**ro'**·fe·ah). Emaciation or atrophy as the result of vomiting which has gone on for a considerable period. [emesis, atrophy.]

emetic (em·**et**·ik). 1. Pertaining to emesis. 2. Causing vomiting. 3. Any substance that causes vomiting. **Central emetic.** An emetic that acts directly on the vomiting centre, e.g. apomorphine. **Peripheral emetic, Reflex emetic.** An emetic acting reflexly by irritation of the sensory vagal fibres in the mucous membrane of the stomach, e.g. tartar emetic, mustard, common salt, alum and the sulphates of copper or zinc. **Tartar emetic.** Antimony Potassium Tartrate BP 1958, $C_4H_4O_6(SbO)K$, a compound used as an expectorant by mouth, but in larger doses as an emetic; it is given by injection in the treatment of leishmania infections. [Gk *emesis* vomiting.]

emetine (em·et·een). Methylcephaeline, $C_{28}H_{37}(CH_3)N_2O_4$. An alkaloid present in ipecacuanha, and prepared from this, or synthetically. It has an irritant action on mucous membranes, and may cause vomiting when taken by mouth. Its chief medical use is in the treatment of amoebiasis, and occasionally in schistosomiasis. It is used either as the hydrochloride or as a complex iodide with bismuth. **Emetine and Bismuth Iodide BP 1973.** $C_{29}H_{40}N_2O_42HIBiI_3H_2O$, a complex iodide of emetine and bismuth, prepared from emetine hydrochloride. It is a reddish-orange powder with a very bitter taste, insoluble in water and alcohol. It is used in the treatment of amoebic dysentery, in both the acute and chronic state, and of carriers, but is not of value in other forms of amoebiasis. It is given by mouth, preferably in gelatin capsules, and not as compressed tablets. It may cause nausea, vomiting and diarrhoea. **Emetine Hydrochloride BP 1973.** $C_{29}H_{40}N_2O_4HCl7H_2O$, the hydrochloride of emetine; a colourless crystalline powder, without odour but with a bitter taste. It is soluble in water, giving a neutral or faintly acid solution, has an irritant action on mucous membranes and may cause vomiting if given orally. It is not used as an emetic. Its chief medical use is in the treatment of amoebiasis, especially in the acute stage of intestinal infections or in visceral infections, chiefly hepatic, as amoebic liver abscess. It is of no value in the chronic stage of amoebic dysentery or in the carrier state. It is administered by subcutaneous or intramuscular injection. It may have a toxic effect on the myocardium, producing arrhythmias. **Emetine periodide.** $C_{29}H_{40}N_2O_4I_6$, a substitute for emetine and bismuth iodide; although it is less toxic, it is also less effective.

emetism (em·et·izm). A condition of poisoning resulting from excessive ingestion of ipecacuanha, generally in one dose, but occasionally in several doses, the cumulative effect of which may be that of a single overdose. [emetine.]

emetocatharsis (em·et·o·kath·**ar'**·sis). 1. The condition in which vomiting and purging occur simultaneously. 2. Vomiting and purging effected by the same agent. [emesis, catharsis.]

emetocathartic (em·et·o·kath·**ar'**·tik). 1. An agent that produces vomiting and purgation at the same time. 2. Causing simultaneous vomiting and purging. [see prec.]

emetomorphine (em·et·o·**mor'**·feen). Apomorphine.

emetophobia (em·et·o·**fo'**·be·ah). Morbid fear of emetics or dread of vomiting. [emesis, phobia.]

emiction (e·**mik**·shun). Micturition. [L *e*, *mingere* to pass urine.]

emictory (e·mik·tor·e). 1. Diuretic. 2. A diuretic agent. [see prec.]

emigration (em·e·gra·shun). The passage of leucocytes through the walls of blood vessels into areolar or other surrounding tissue. [L *emigrare* to move out.]

eminence [eminentia (NA)] (em·in·ens). A prominence; usually applied to a rounded area raised slightly above the level of the surface on which it is situated. **Arcuate eminence [eminentia arcuata (NA)].** The raised area on the superior surface of the petrous part of the temporal bone under which lies the superior semicircular canal. **Collateral eminence [eminentia collateralis (NA)].** A raised part of the floor of the inferior horn of the lateral ventricle of the brain in the anterior part of the collateral trigone, just lateral to the hippocampus. **Eminence of the concha [eminentia conchae (NA)].** An elevation on the cranial surface of the auricular cartilage, corresponding to the conchal depression on the lateral surface. **Frontal eminence [tuber frontale (NA)].** The most prominent part of the frontal bone of the skull on each side. **Hypothenar eminence [hypothenar].** The eminence on the medial border of the palm. **Iliopubic eminence [eminentia iliopubica (NA)].** A raised area on the inner surface of the innominate bone, approximately marking the site of junction of its iliac and pubic parts, and situated just above the brim of the true pelvis (iliopectineal line). **Intercondylar eminence [eminentia intercondylaris (NA)].** The tibial spine; a pointed elevation on the upper surface of the tibia between the two articular surfaces for the femoral condyles. **Parietal eminence [tuber parietale (NA)].** The most prominent part of the parietal bone of the skull on each side. **Eminence of the scaphoid fossa [eminentia scaphae (NA)].** An elevation on the cranial surface of the auricular cartilage, corresponding to the scaphoid fossa. **Thenar eminence [thenar (NA)].** The eminence on the palm at the base of the thumb. **Eminence of the triangular fossa [eminentia fossae triangularis (NA)].** A rounded elevation on the cranial surface of the auricular cartilage, corresponding to the triangular fossa. **Vagal eminence.** The eminence in the floor of the 4th ventricle formed by the dorsal nucleus of the vagus nerve. [L *eminentia* a projection.]

See also: DOYÈRE, MUELLER (J.).

eminentia [NA] (em·in·en·she·ah). An eminence. **Eminentia abducentis.** The facial colliculus. **Eminentia acoustica.** A raised area near the lateral angle of the floor of the 4th ventricle, crossed superficially by the auditory striae. **Eminentia annularis.** The pons of the brain. **Eminentia articularis [tuberculum articulare (NA)].** That part of the inferior surface of the temporal bone lying just in front of the articular fossa of the head of the mandible. **Eminentia carpi radialis, Eminentia carpi ulnaris.** Eminences of the radial and ulnar sides of the front of the wrist, caused by the scaphoid and pisiform bones, respectively (obsolete terms). **Eminentiae cruciatae [eminentiae cruciformes (NA)].** The raised lines radiating from the internal occipital protuberance, superiorly, inferiorly and laterally, which divide the inner surface of the occiput into 4 areas, forming a superior cerebral and an inferior cerebellar fossa on each side (obsolete terms). **Eminentia facialis.** The facial colliculus. **Eminentia gracilis.** The gracile tubercle. *See* TUBERCLE. **Eminentia hypoglossi.** The raised area in the posterior part of the floor of the 4th ventricle, between the midline and the vagal trigone on each side, overlying the nucleus of the hypoglossal nerve. **Eminentia medialis [NA].** An elongated elevation in the anterior part of the floor of the 4th ventricle beside the midline; the posterior part forms the facial colliculus. **Eminentia restiformis.** The region of the medulla oblongata on its dorsilateral surface, raised up by the inferior cerebellar peduncles, **Eminentia trigemini.** The area on the lateral surface of the medulla oblongata, raised up by the descending root and nucleus of the trigeminal nerve. [L.]

emissary (em·is·ar·e). 1. An efferent duct. 2. An outlet for fluid. 3. Providing an outlet. [L *emittere* to send out.]

emissary veins [venae emissariae (NA)]. Veins connecting the venous sinuses inside the skull with the veins of the scalp. These are usually named according to their position: parietal [vena emissaria parietalis (NA)], mastoid [vena emissaria mastoidea (NA)], posterior condylar [vena emissaria condylaris (NA)], occipital [vena emissaria occipitalis (NA)], anterior condylar [plexus venosus canalis hypoglossi (NA)], foramen ovale [plexus venosus foraminis ovalis (NA)] and carotid-canal emissary veins [plexus venosus caroticus internus (NA)].

emission (e·mish·un). A discharge. **Beta emission.** A loose term that should be avoided, meaning either the emission of beta-particles or the beta-particle emitted. **Field emission.** The emission of electrons from a material by application of an electric field to the surface of the material. **Nocturnal emission.** Involuntary seminal discharge occurring during sleep. **Seminary emission.** Emission of semen. **Thermionic emission.** Ions and electrons emitted from a heated body. [L *emittere* to send out.]

emmenagogic (em·en·ag·og·ik). 1. Belonging to the menstrual process. 2. Promoting menstruation. [see foll.]

emmenagogue (em·en·ag·og). 1. A drug or other agent that promotes or assists the menstrual flow as distinct from an ecbolic. 2. Inducing menstruation. **Direct emmenagogue.** An agent that directly affects the organs of reproduction, e.g. ergot. **Indirect emmenagogue.** An agent that breaks down an inhibitory condition. [Gk *emmena* menses, *agogos* leading.]

emmenia (em·e·ne·ah). The menses. [Gk *emmena* menses.]

emmenic (em·en·ik). Referring to the menses. [see prec.]

emmenin (em·en·in). A crude extract of the human placenta, having oestrogenic activity due to the presence of oestriol sodium glucuronate. [Gk *emmena* menses.]

emmeniopathy (em·en·e·op′·ath·e). A comprehensive term including all defects and abnormalities of menstruation. [Gk *emmena* menses, *pathos* disease.]

emmenology (em·en·ol·o·je). That branch of medical science which is concerned with menstruation, its physiology and pathology. [Gk *emmena* menses, *logos* science.]

Emmet, Thomas Addis (b. 1828). New York gynaecologist.

Emmet's needle. A strong curved handled needle.

Emmet's operation. 1. A method of repairing a lacerated perineum. 2. Trachelorrhaphy, or suture of the edges of a lacerated cervix uteri. 3. Artificially-formed vesicovaginal fistula to secure drainage of the bladder in cystitis.

emmetrope (em·et·rope). Anyone with normal visual accommodation and refraction. [see foll.]

emmetropia (em·et·ro·pe·ah). The condition of perfect vision, or the condition of normal refraction and accommodation of the eye. [Gk *emmetros* proportioned, *opsis* vision.]

emmetropic (em·et·rop·ik). Referring to emmetropia; characterized by emmetropia.

Emmonsia (em·on·se·ah). A commonly occurring fungus in the soil. *Emmonsia crescens* and *E. parva* species cause adiaspiromycosis in man and in small rodents. Inhaled aleuriospores increase in diameter from 2–4 μm to 200–700 μm. Germination, reproduction and dissemination of the enlarged spore does not occur, but displaced pulmonary tissue impairs lung function. Granulomatous tissue forms in some cases. There is generally little host reaction in animals.

Emmonsiella (em·on·se·el′·ah). A genus of soil fungi. *Emmonsiella capsulata* (Kwong-Chung), the perfect (sexual) stage of *Histoplasma capsulatum*, the causative organism of histoplasmosis.

emodin (em·o·din). Any one of a class of anthraquinone derivatives found in aloe, cascara, rhubarb and senna, either free or combined as a glycoside. They are mild laxatives, acting only on the large intestine and causing an increase in propulsive movement probably due to an irritant effect; the purgation is slow because of the time required to reach the large intestine and the liberation there by hydrolysis of the active principle from the glycosides. They are used in the treatment of simple constipation, and are liable to impart a colour to the urine. **Aloe emodin.** $C_6H_3(OH)(CO)_2C_6H_2(OH)CH_2OH$, an emodin derived from aloin, and also occurring in rhubarb and senna. **Frangula emodin.** $C_6H_2(OH)_2(CO)_2C_6H_2(OH)CH_3$, an emodin from species of rhubarb and also contained in cascara. [*Emodi*, a species of Rheum.]

emollient (e·**mol**·e·ent). Any substance that softens the skin and renders it more pliant. These are for the most part oils, ointments with a paraffin basis or creams, which are emulsions of fat, paraffin or oil with water; sometimes insoluble substances such as French chalk are used for the purpose, but are generally less efficient. [L *emollire* to soften.]

emotiometabolic (e·**mo**·she·o·met·ah·**bol'**·ik). Referring to or inducing metabolic change as a result of emotion.

emotiomotor (e·**mo**·she·o·**mo'**·tor). Inducing activity consequent upon emotion. [emotion, motor.]

emotiomuscular (e·**mo**·she·o·**mus'**·kew·lar). Relating to muscular activity as the result of emotion.

emotion (e.**mo**·shun). Aroused state involving intense feeling, autonomic activation and related behavour (see CANNON THEORY and JAMES-LANGE THEORY). [L *emovere* to disturb.]

emotional (e·**mo**·shun·al). Relating or belonging to emotion or the emotions.

emotiovascular (e·**mo**·she·o·**vas'**·kew·lar). Relating to or producing some vascular change, e.g. blushing, as a result of emotion.

emotive (e·**mo**·tiv). Causing, expressing or having the characteristics of emotion.

emotivity (e·mo·**tiv**·it·e). 1. Emotional capacity. 2. Sensitivity of response to emotional stimulus.

empathic (em·**path**·ik). Referring to or marked by empathy.

empathize (**em**·path·ize). 1. To enter into the feelings or to take the place emotionally of another, 2. To ascribe one's own feelings to another. [see foll.]

empathy (**em**·path·e). 1. The condition of entering into the emotional state of another, or the feeling on the part of one person that he is emotionally in the place of another. 2. The ascription of human qualities to any object and the feeling on the part of an individual that he is in that object and is a part of it. [Gk *en*, *pathos* feeling.]

emperipolesis (**em**·peri·**polee**·sis). Penetration of lymphocytes into cells of other types.

emphatics (**em**·fa·tiks). Expressive features, emotional overtones. pauses, and non-verbal utterances which may accompany spoken speech. [Gk *emphasis* a declaration of speech.]

emphlysis (**em**·flis·is). Any exanthematous or vesicular eruption, such as pemphigus. [Gk *en*, *phlysis* eruption.]

emphractic (em·**frak**·tik). 1. Referring to emphraxis. 2. Closing or obstructing the ducts of the skin. 3. An agent that clogs or closes the ducts of the skin.

emphraxis (em·**frax**·is). 1. An obstruction, particularly with regard to the glandular ducts of the skin. 2. Infarction. impaction or congestion. [Gk, a blocking up.]

emphyma (em·**fi**·mah) (pl. *emphymata*). A tumour. [Gk *en*, *phyma* a growth.]

emphysatherapy (**em**·fiz·ah·**ther'**·ap·e). In therapeutics, the injection of gas into a body cavity or organ in order to dilate it or otherwise to alter the physical condition. [Gk *emphysan* to inflate, therapy.]

emphysema (em·fi·**se**·mah). A condition in which the alveoli of the lungs are dilated. **Acute vesicular emphysema.** The result of severe inspiratory efforts in patients with partially obstructed bronchi. It occurs in suffocation, acute bronchopneumonia, whooping cough and sometimes asthma. **Bullous emphysema.** An area of vesicular emphysema within the lung substance and separated from the pleura by lung parenchyma. It is due to bronchial obstruction with a check-valve action, commonly caused by chronic pulmonary tuberculosis, pneumoconiosis, chronic bronchitis and asthma. Giant bullae are usually unilateral and occasionally result from bronchial carcinoma. The check-valve action can be caused either by the growth itself or by pressure of enlarged glands. In such cases emphysema tends to be of segmental or zonal type, and may be associated with areas of collapse. **Chronic atrophic emphysema.** A form occurring with old age as part of the general atrophy. The alveolar walls are thinned and may give way so that adjacent alveoli coalesce, and the lungs are small and shrivelled (*small-lunged emphysema*). **Chronic hypertrophic emphysema.** Large-lunged emphysema. The term *hypertrophic* is a misnomer, as there is actually *atrophy* of the alveolar walls and the increase in volume is due to over-distension. Rupture of the walls may cause bullae, especially at the least supported sites such as the apices and margins. It is due to inspiratory stress associated with partial bronchial obstruction and is the type seen with chronic bronchitis. **Compensatory emphysema.** Expansion of healthy parts of the lung when other portions are collapsed, destroyed or filled with exudate. It is a physiological reaction to increase the functioning respiratory surface and to fill up the space caused by mediastinal shift. It may be temporary, as in temporary collapse, pneumothorax or pneumonia, or permanent, as with fibrosis, thoracoplasty or lobectomy. It may affect only part of a lung, or the whole of a lung when the other lung is out of action. **Interstitial emphysema.** A state in which air has escaped into the interstitial tissues of the lung from penetrating wounds or alveoli ruptured from violent respiratory efforts, as in the paroxysms of whooping cough. It is an occasional complication of labour. The air may enter the mediastinum and track into the subcutaneous tissues of the neck or chest wall, causing surgical emphysema. **Large-lunged emphysema.** Chronic hypertrophic emphysema (see above). **Small-lunged emphysema.** *See* CHRONIC ATROPHIC EMPHYSEMA (above). **Surgical emphysema.** A condition in which air is present in the subcutaneous tissues either from injury to, or operation on, the lungs or air passages, or occasionally from suction of air into a wound direct from the exterior. **Tissue emphysema.** Air in the tissues. **Traumatic emphysema.** Surgical emphysema (see above). [Gk *en*, *physema* a blowing.]

emphysematous (em·fi·**se**·mat·us). 1. Of the type of or belonging to emphysema. 2. Affected with emphysema.

empiric (em·**pir**·ik). 1. Founded on experience. 2. Anyone, e.g. a medical practitioner, who relies solely or chiefly on practical experience and observation, 3. A quack or charlatan. [Gk *empeirikos* experimental.]

empirical (em·**pir**·ik·al). Based on experience and observation, without regard to science or knowledge of principles. [see prec.]

empiricism (em·**pir**·is·izm). 1. The practice of medicine founded on experience and observation, 2. Quackery. [Gk *empeirikos* experimental.]

Empirics (em·**pir**·ix). A school of Medicine (about 280 BC) founded by Philenos of Cos and Serapion of Alexandria. The Empirics held that the original causes of disease were insoluble, and therefore devoted their attention to the immediate causes of maladies and the treatment of symptoms. Clinical observation and experience guided them in therapeutics. **Tripod of the Empirics.** The 3 rules upon which the system of the Empirics was based: (*a*) the observation of symptoms; (*b*) the learning and experience of contemporary and past physicians; (*c*) the formation of an opinion as to the nature and treatment of new diseases from those relating to analogous diseases. [see prec.]

emplastic (em·**plas**·tik). 1. Adhesive and suitable to be applied as a plaster. 2. The plaster as such. 3. Having a constipating effect. 4. A drug which has a constipating effect. [Gk *emplastikos* clogging.]

emplastration (em·plas·**tra**·shun). The applying of a salve or plaster. [see foll.]

emplastrum (em·**plas**·trum). A plaster; once a common form of medication, now rarely used. It consists of an active substance mixed with an adhesive base and spread on paper or other material cut to the shape of the surface to which it is to be applied. Blistering agents and counter-irritants were commonly incorporated with soap or resin, heated and applied in this way. **Emplastrum belladonnae.** An emplastrum containing 0·25 per cent of belladonna-root alkaloids in resin. **Emplastrum cantharidini.** Cantharidin, acetone, castor oil, beeswax and lanolin. **Emplastrum colophonii.** Resin plaster containing colophony, lead oleate and hard soap. **Emplastrum plumbi.**

Diachylon plaster; crude oleate of lead, which is itself adhesive. **Emplastrum sinapis.** A plaster composed of oil-free black mustard mixed with rubber solution. [Gk *emplastron.*]

empodistic (em·po·**dis**·tik). 1. Preventing or checking. 2. A prophylactic or preventive agent. [Gk *empodizein* to hinder.]

emprosthotonos, emprosthotonus (em·pros·**thot**·on·os, em·pros·**thot**·on·us). A spasmodic contraction associated with tetanus in which the head and feet are brought forwards so that the back is tensely curved with concavity forward. [Gk *emprosthen* forward, *tenein* to stretch.]

emprosthozygosis (em·**pros**·tho·zi·**go**'·sis). The condition of a twin monster in which there is anterior fusion. [Gk *emprosthen* forward, *zygosis* a joining.]

emptysis (**emp**·tis·is). 1. Expectoration. 2. Haemoptysis. [Gk, a spitting.]

empyema (em·pi·e·mah). A collection of pus in a cavity, particularly in the pleural cavity. **Empyema articuli.** Distension of the synovial membrane of a joint with pus. **Empyema benignum.** Pleural empyema without fever or other marked disturbance of health. **Empyema of the chest.** Pus in the pleural cavity. **Diaphragmatic empyema.** An empyema encysted between the pleura and the diaphragm: the physical signs are often obscure. **Empyema of the gall bladder.** Acute cholecystitis with distension of the gall bladder with pus. **Interlobar empyema.** A collection of pus between the lobes of a lung. **Latent empyema.** An empyema whose presence is unsuspected owing to the absence of symptoms. **Loculated empyema.** An empyema which is localized by pleural adhesions. **Mastoid empyema.** An abscess of the mastoid antrum and air cells. **Metapneumonic empyema.** One which is a sequel to lobar pneumonia and occurs when the infection has passed the crisis and the lung is resolving, **Empyema necessitatis.** The condition in which pus from the pleural cavity has tracked through an intercostal space and formed a subcutaneous swelling, **Empyema of the pericardium.** Purulent pericarditis. **Pneumococcal empyema.** An empyema caused by a pneumococcal infection. **Pulsating empyema.** An empyema necessitatis (see above) which transmits the cardiac pulsations and simulates an aneurysm. **Putrid empyema.** An empyema with foul-smelling pus. **Streptococcal empyema.** One caused by a streptococcal infection, **Synpneumonic empyema,** One that occurs during the active stage of a bronchopneumonia when widespread inflammation of the lung and severe toxaemia may be present. It is characteristic of a streptococcal infection. **Thoracic empyema.** A collection of pus in the pleural cavity. **Tuberculous empyema.** An empyema caused by a tuberculous infection. [Gk *en, pyon* pus.]

empyematic, empyematous, empyemic (em·pi·e·**mat**'·ik, em·pi·e·mat·us, em·pi·e·mik). Of the nature of or like empyema.

empyesis (em·pi·e·sis). 1. Any pustular eruption, such as smallpox. 2. Any disease in which there is an eruption of pustules which gradually fill with purulent fluid. 3. Hypopyon. [Gk *en, pyon* pus.]

empyocele (em·**pi**·o·seel). A suppurating scrotal hydrocele. [Gk *en, pyon* pus, *kele* hernia.]

empyomphalus (em·pi·**om**·fal·us). A circumscribed collection of pus at the umbilicus. [Gk *en, pyon* pus, *omphalos* navel.]

empyreuma (em·pi·**roo**·mah). The peculiar odour given off by animal or vegetable matter undergoing destructive distillation by being burned in a closed vessel. [Gk *empyreuein* to set on fire.]

empyreumatic (**em**·pi·roo·**mat**'·ik). Obtained from an organic substance by subjecting it to strong heat. [see prec.]

Emsher tank. A form of digestion tank for the treatment of sewage.

emulgent (e·**mul**·jent). 1. Literally, straining or filtering off; hence, an expression applied to the renal arteries or veins. 2. An emulsifying agent (see EMULSIFICATION) such as mucilages, soaps, etc., used to form emulsions. [L *emulgere* to milk out.]

emulsification (e·**mul**·sif·ik·**a**'·shun). The dispersion of 2 immiscible liquids one within the other, most commonly an oil and water. It is achieved by the aid of an emulsifying agent which acts by reducing the surface tension at the interface between the liquids; such agents may be gums (e.g. acacia, tragacanth), egg yolk (lecithin), soluble casein, malt extract, or the saponins and soaps. Bile plays an important part in the emulsification of fats in digestion. [emulsion, L *facere* to make.]

emulsifier (e·**mul**·sif·i·er). An emulsifying agent, such as egg yolk or gum arabic, used to produce an emulsion of a fixed oil.

emulsify (e·**mul**·sif·i). To form an emulsion with, or to convert into an emulsion. [emulsion, L *facere* to make.]

emulsin (e·**mul**·sin). Almond emulsion; a mixture of enzymes (prunase, amygdalase, oxynitrilase, principally), found in almonds and responsible for the hydrolysis of the respective glucosides present.

emulsion, emulsio (e·**mul**·shun, e·**mul**·se·o). A preparation of 2 immiscible liquids, usually oil and water, in which fine droplets of one (disperse phase) are dispersed throughout the body of the other (continuous phase). This effect is achieved by means of an emulsifying agent which also maintains the emulsion when formed; the latter may be diluted with the liquid of the continuous phase, but more of the disperse-phase liquid cannot be added without interfering with the stability. Commercially, such emulsions are prepared by forcing the liquids together with the emulsifier through a fine aperture to which a shearing action is imparted; they are used in creams and liniments. In pharmacy an emulsion is often made to disguise the taste of an oil, by dispersing the latter in another liquid which can itself be flavoured. **Emulsio acriflavinae.** A water-in-oil emulsion of liquid paraffin and water, containing 1 part per 1000 of acriflavine. **Benzyl benzoate emulsion.** An emulsion of benzyl benzoate and water used in the treatment of scabies. **Emulsion of Chloroform BPC 1959.** A 1 in 20 emulsion of chloroform in water made with the aid of tincture of quillaia and gum tragacanth; it is used to facilitate the making of chloroform water in dispensing. **Chylomicron emulsion.** An emulsion of minute fat particles, such as that which reaches the blood during fat metabolism. **Emulsion of Cod-liver Oil BPC 1959.** An emulsion of cod-liver oil with the latter in the disperse phase to disguise its taste. **Liquid Paraffin Emulsion BP 1958.** A palatable form of liquid paraffin for laxative purposes, containing 50 per cent v/v of liquid paraffin dispersed in an aqueous continuous phase by means of acacia and tragacanth gums, and flavoured with vanilla. Its action is often augmented by the addition of phenolphthalein, magnesia, cascara extract, etc. **Emulsion of Liquid Paraffin with Cascara BPC 1959.** A mixture of liquid paraffin emulsion and cascara elixir. **Emulsion of Liquid Paraffin and Magnesium Hydroxide BPC 1959.** An emulsion of liquid paraffin, also containing magnesium hydroxide and agar; it is used as a laxative. **Emulsion of Liquid Paraffin and Phenolphthalein BPC 1959.** Liquid paraffin emulsion with the addition of phenolphthalein (0·34 per cent). **Emulsion of Peppermint BPC 1959.** A 1 in 10 emulsion of oil of peppermint and water, made with the aid of tincture of quillaia. **Photographic emulsion.** The thin layer of gelatin containing light-sensitive silver salts that covers photographic plates or transparent plastic films. [L *emulgere* to milk out.]

emulsive (e·**mul**·siv). 1. Producing emulsion. 2. Transformable into an emulsion. 3. Producing a fixed oil when subjected to pressure.

emulsoid (e·**mul**·soid). 1. Emulsion. 2. An emulsion colloid. [emulsion, Gk *eidos* form.]

emulsum (e·**mul**·sum). Emulsion. [L.]

emunctory (e·**mungk**·tor·e). 1. Any organ of the body the function of which is to carry off waste, e.g. kidneys, skin; an excretory duct or organ. 2. Purifying. [L *emungere* to cleanse.]

Emylcamate (e·mil·**kam**·ate). BP Commission approved name for 1 - ethyl - 1 - methylpropyl carbamate; it is used in the treatment of neuroses.

en-. A prefix, from the Greek preposition *en,* meaning *in, into.*

enadelphia (en·ad·el·fe·ah). The type of monstrosity known as fetal inclusion, in which one twin encloses the other. [Gk *en, adelphos* brother.]

enamel [enamelum (NA)] (en·**am**·el). A very hard whitish substance, composed mainly of calcium carbonate and calcium phosphate, which covers the dentine of the anatomical crown of a tooth. **Curled enamel.** Enamel in which the bundles of prisms take a wavy course. **Dwarfed enamel.** Enamel which is thinner than normal. **Gnarled enamel.** Enamel in which the bundles of prisms run in very tortuous directions. **Mottled enamel.** Enamel which presents patches of white or brownish pigmentation owing to the child drinking water containing more than one per million of fluorine during the process of enamel calcification (endemic fluorosis). **Nanoid enamel.** Dwarfed enamel (see above). **Straight enamel.** Enamel in which the bundles of prisms take a fairly straight course. [OFr. *esmail.*]

enameloblast (en·**am**·el·o·blast). Ameloblast. [enamel, Gk *blastos* seed.]

enameloblastoma (en·**am**·el·o·blas·**to**′·mah). Adamantinoma. [enamel, Gk *blastos* seed, *-oma* tumour.]

enameloma (en·**am**·el·o′·mah). Enamel pearl; a small, smooth nodule of enamel just below the cemento-enamel junction of a tooth. [enamel, Gk *-oma* tumour.]

enanthem (en·**an**·them). Enanthema.

enanthema (en·**an**·them·ah). The rash or eruption produced by the action of an organism or its toxins on the small blood vessels of mucous membranes; e.g. in the mouth, where it may be of considerable diagnostic value. [Gk *en, anthema* blossoming.]

enanthematous (en·an·**them**·at·us). Relating or belonging to, or of the nature of, an enanthema.

enanthesis (em·an·**the**·sis). The process that causes the appearance of an enanthema. [Gk *en, anthesis* bloom.]

enanthrope (en·**an**·thrope). 1. An auto-infection. 2. Any disease originating within the body. [Gk *en, anthropos* man.]

enantiobiosis (en·**an**·te·o·bi·o′·sis). The condition in which organisms living in the same medium are antagonistic to and restrict each other's development. [Gk *enantios* opposite, *bios* life.]

enantiolalia (en·**an**·te·o·**la**′·le·ah). Speaking in opposites. [Gk *enantios* opposite, *lalia* talk.]

enantiomorph (en·**an**·te·o·morf). A term denoting either of the dextrorotatory or laevorotatory forms of an optically-active substance. [Gk *enantios* opposite, *morphe* form.]

enantiomorphic, enantomorphous (en·**an**·te·o·**mor**′·fik, en·**an**·te·o·**mor**′·fus). 1. Of similar but reversed or contrasted form, e.g. the two hands and the two feet. 2. In crystallography, said of a crystal which is similar to another and corresponds with it as the mirrored image does with the object mirrored. [Gk *enantios* opposite, *morphe* form.]

enantiopathia, enantiopathy (en·**an**·te·o·**path**′·e·ah, en·**an**·te·**op**′·ath·e). 1. A state of mutual antagonism between 2 diseases. 2. A disease antagonistic to another disease. Cf. ALLOPATHY, HOMOEOPATHY. [Gk *enantios* opposite, *pathos* disease.]

enarkyochrome (en·**ar**·ke·o·krome). Any arkyochrome, the network of which is single. [Gk *en*, arkyochrome.]

enarthritis (en·ar·**thri**·tis). Inflammation of a ball-and-socket (enarthrodial) joint. [Gk *en, arthron* joint, *-itis* inflammation.]

enarthrodial (en·ar·**thro**·de·al). Relating or belonging to a ball-and-socket joint (enarthrosis).

enarthrosis (en·ar·**thro**·sis). A ball-and-socket joint, e.g. the hip joint. [Gk *en, arthron* joint, *-osis* condition.]

enarthrum (en·**ar**·thrum). A foreign body inside a joint. [Gk *en, arthron* joint.]

Enbucrilate (en·**bew**·kril·ate). BP Commission approved name for butyl 2-cyanoacrylate; a surgical tissue adhesive.

encanthis (en·**kan**·this). A localized enlargement and inflammation of the caruncle and semilunar fold of the conjunctiva, which may go on to the formation of a small abscess. [Gk *en, kanthos* angle of the eye.]

encapsulated (en·**kap**·sew·la·ted). Enclosed in a sheath or capsule. [see foll.]

encapsulation (en·**kap**·sew·**la**′·shun). 1. Physiological enclosure in a capsule or sheath composed of a substance foreign to the protoplasm of the part. 2. The process of enclosing in a capsule or membrane. [Gk *en*, capsule.]

encarditis (en·kar·**di**·tis). Endocarditis.

encephalaemia (en·**kef**·al·**e**′·me·ah). Congestion of the brain. [encephalon, Gk *haima* blood.]

encephalalgia (en·**kef**·al·**al**′·je·ah). Any pain affecting the inside of the head; headache. **Encephalalgia hydropica.** Hydrocephalus. [encephalon, Gk *algos* pain.]

encephalasthenia (en·**kef**·al·as·**the**′·ne·ah). Defective brain power or lack of brain power. [encephalon, asthenia.]

encephalatrophy (en·**kef**·al·**at**′·ro·fe). Atrophy of the brain. [encephalon, atrophy.]

encephalauxe (en·**kef**·al·**awx**′·e). Hypertrophy of the brain. [encephalon, Gk *auxe* increase.]

encephalic (en·kef·**al**·ik). 1. Referring or belonging to the brain or the encephalon, 2. Situated within the skull.

encephalitic (en·**kef**·al·**it**′·ik). Referring or belonging to encephalitis.

encephalitis (en·**kef**·al·**i**′·tis) (pl. *encephalitides*). Inflammation of the brain. **Acute disseminated encephalitis.** Post-infection encephalitis, encephalomyelitis; inflammation of the brain and spinal cord, developing spontaneously, or arising during convalescence from an infection, or following vaccination against smallpox or rabies. **Acute superior encephalitis.** Wernicke's encephalopathy. **Australian X encephalitis.** An acute encephalomyelitis with a high mortality rate which occurred in epidemic form in Australia in 1917-1918; a transmissible virus has been demonstrated and is related to that of louping-ill. **Autumn encephalitis.** Japanese encephalitis (see below). **Benign myalgic encephalitis.** A benign but often relapsing epidemic disease of unknown cause. **Buffalo encephalitis.** Virus encephalitis of the Asiatic water buffalo. **California encephalitis.** A generally benign meningo-encephalitis caused by arboviruses of the California group, which forms part of the Bunyamwera supergroup. Despite its name, the disease is not confined to California, having also been found elsewhere in both North and South America, as well as in Africa and in Europe. **Central European tick-borne encephalitis.** A viral encephalitis due to a group B arbovirus. **Chronic progressive subcortical encephalitis.** Degeneration of subcortical white matter owing to atherosclerotic changes which are severe in subcortical vessels, the cortical vasculature escaping; an encephalopathy rather than an encephalitis, it affects particularly the temporal and occipital lobes. The clinical features are those of organic dementia, often with progressive visual impairment. Also called *Binswanger's encephalitis.* **Cortical encephalitis, Encephalitis corticalis.** Chronic encephalitis, or encephalopathy, in which pathological changes are most advanced in the cerebral cortex. **Epidemic encephalitis, Encephalitis epidemica.** Terms including all types of encephalitis due to arbovirus infections and occurring in epidemics. **Equine encephalitis.** A viral encephalitis of horses due to group A arboviruses and transmissible to man by mosquitoes. Eastern, Western and Venezuelan forms are described and are due to different viruses. **Forest spring encephalitis.** A virus encephalitis occurring in spring and early summer in eastern Russia, and carried by a wood tick, *Ixodes persulcatus.* **Fox encephalitis.** A virus disease of foxes associated with intranuclear cell inclusions. **Haemorrhagic encephalitis.** Any encephalitis in which foci of haemorrhage occur. **Haemorrhagic arsphenamine encephalitis.** A severe and acute encephalopathy occurring as a sensitivity reaction to arsphenamine, **Encephalitis haemorrhagica superior.** A haemorrhagic form of encephalopathy occurring in alcoholism and other conditions where the intake of vitamin B_1 may be deficient. Pathological changes are most evident in the mid-brain and produce confusion, nystagmus and ocular palsy; also called *Wernicke's encephalopathy.* **Herpes simplex encephalitis, Herpetic encephalitis.** A necrotizing encephalitis following infection with herpes simplex virus. A rare, but serious, complication with a high case-mortality. **Encephalitis hyperplastica.** Acute non-suppurative encephalitis, a term originally applied by Hayem, but not applicable in the light of modern pathological evidence. **Ilhéus encephalitis.** A type produced experimentally in animals following inoculation with a virus, isolated from mosquitoes at Ilhéus (Brazil). **Inclusion body encephalitis.** A fatal, subacute disease of children or adolescents characterized by progressive dementia, myoclonus and rigidity. Neuronal inclusion bodies are found. The disease is probably caused by the measles virus. Characteristic electroencephalographic changes occur as well as an abnormality in the Lange curve in the cerebrospinal fluid. *Subacute sclerosing panencephalitis. Dawson-type encephalitis.* **Infantile encephalitis,** A term covering the encephalopathies of infancy, sometimes complicating the exanthemata, and sometimes of no apparent cause. They often give rise to cerebral palsies, e.g. hemiplegia; now believed to be probably of allergic origin. **Influenzal encephalitis.** Haemorrhagic encephalitis or encephalopathy occurring in epidemic influenza; some such cases were probably encephalitis lethargica (see below). **Japanese B encephalitis.** An endemic and occasionally epidemic benign encephalitis due to a group B arbovirus, characterized by fever, stiff neck, confusion, tremor, nausea and vomiting. **Lead encephalitis.** An encephalopathy due to lead intoxication; convulsions occur and cerebral oedema is found in the occasional fatal cases. **Encephalitis lethargica, Lethargic encephalitis.** An epidemic virus encephalitis giving rise to lethargy, reversal of the sleep rhythm and disturbances of ocular accommodation. Pathologically, inflammation is most severe in the substantia nigra and mid-brain. If the disease becomes chronic, a parkinsonian syndrome results. Also called *sleepy sickness, Economo's disease, type-A encephalitis.* **Murray Valley encephalitis.** An acute arthropod-transmitted encephalomyelitis due to a group B arbovirus occurring in Australia and closely related to that of Japanese B encephalitis. It mostly attacks children and has a high case-mortality. **Encephalitis neonatorum.** Encephalitis or encephalopathy in the first 4 weeks of life. **Otitic encephalitis.** Inflammation of the brain occurring during the course of middle-ear or mastoid disease. It occurs most commonly in the form of an abscess, either in the temporosphenoidal lobe or in the cerebellum. **Encephalitis periaxalis, Encephalitis periaxalis diffusa.** A cerebral demyelinating disease of infancy, beginning in the occipital lobes, and giving rise to progressive blindness, deafness, dementia and paralysis; Schilder's disease. **Encephalitis periaxalis scleroticans.** Disseminated sclerosis. **Postexanthematous encephalitis.** Encephalitis following one of the acute exanthematous fevers, especially measles. The causal relationship is uncertain. **Postinfection encephalitis.** An acute encephalitis or encephalopathy following a variety of infective diseases; now believed to be allergic in origin. **Postvaccinal encephalitis.** Acute encephalitis or encephalopathy following vaccination. **Purulent encephalitis, Pyogenic encephalitis.** Encephalitis due to pyogenic bacteria; it may be diffuse in pyaemia, but if localized, a brain abscess is produced. **Russian epidemic encephalitis, Russian Far-East encephalitis, Russian spring encephalitis, Russian spring-summer encephalitis, Russian tick-borne encephalitis.** An endemic encephalitis due to a tick-borne group B arbovirus. The virus is closely related to those of Central European tick-borne encephalitis, louping-ill and Kyasanur Forest disease. **St Louis encephalitis.** A benign encephalitis due to a group B arbovirus. The virus is closely related to that of Japanese B encephalitis but causes a less severe illness. **Semliki forest encephalitis.** A type produced experimentally in animals inoculated with a virus, isolated from mosquitoes caught in Uganda. **Serous encephalitis.** Brown–Symmers disease; a rapidly fatal encephalitis of children below the age of 7 years. **Encephalitis siderans.** Encephalitis lethargica of fulminating, apoplectiform onset; rapidly fatal. **Subacute inclusion encephalitis.** An encephalitis of children, usually fatal. Perivascular infiltration with inflammatory cells and gliosis widespread in the grey matter of the cerebral cortex, basal ganglia and brain stem. Inclusion bodies are present in nerve cells and less commonly in neuroglia; cell degeneration and inflammation affect the white matter. Symptoms are those of a progressive encephalitis ending in stupor, complete dementia and quadriplegia. A variation of the condition described by van Bogaert (1945) as "subacute sclerosing leuco-encephalitis". **Encephalitis subcorticalis chronica.** Chronic progressive subcortical encephalitis (see above). **Suppurative encephalitis.** Purulent encephalitis (see above). **Torula encephalitis** (now known as cryptococcal encephalitis). Encephalitis resulting from infection with *Cryptococcus neoformans (Torula histolytica).* **Toxoplasma encephalitis, Toxoplasmic encephalitis.** Toxoplasmosis. **Track encephalitis.** Encephalitis in which the inflammatory process follows the track of the trigeminal nerve. **Trichinosis encephalitis.** Encephalitis resulting from the presence of the larval form of the worm *Trichinella spiralis* in the brain. **Type-A encephalitis.** Encephalitis lethargica (see above). **Type-B encephalitis.** Japanese encephalitis (see above). **Type-C encephalitis.** St. Louis encephalitis (see above). **Vaccinal encephalitis.** Postvaccinal encephalitis (see above). **Venezuelan equine encephalitis.** A form of epidemic encephalitis mainly confined to South America. Also called *type-A encephalitis.* **Vernal encephalitis.** Forest spring encephalitis (see above). **West Nile encephalitis.** A type produced experimentally in animals inoculated with the West Nile virus, related to St. Louis and Japanese B viruses. It may give rise to human disease ranging from a mild, short-term fever to acute and sometimes fatal encephalitis. Isolated from a woman with mild fever; it does not cause human encephalitis. **X encephalitis.** A form of encephalitis in New South Wales. [Gk *enkephalos* brain, *-itis* inflammation.]

See also: BINSWANGER, ECONOMO, SCHILDER.

encephalitogenic (en·kef·al·it·o·**jen**′·ik). Producing or causing encephalitis. [encephalitis, Gk *genein* to produce.]

encephalitozoon (en·kef·al·it·o·**zo**′·on). A sporulating protozoon, described by Levaditi, Nicolau and Schoen (1924) and Doerr and Zdansky (1924), and claimed to be the cause of spontaneous encephalomyelitis in rabbits. It gives rise to difficulties in the experimental-animal investigation of virus diseases in man. **Encephalitozoon cuniculi.** A sporozoon causing meningoencephalitis in rabbits. **Encephalitozoon hominis.** A sporozoon believed by some to be a cause of encephalitis in man. There has possibly been some confusion in the past between this organism and *Toxoplasma.* [Gk *enkephalos* brain, *zoon* animal.]

encephalization (en·kef·al·i·**za**′·shun). In embryology, the developing process by which the head takes shape. [encephalon.]

encephalo-arteriography (en·kef·al·o·ar·teer·e·**og**′·raf·e). Examination of the supply of blood to the brain by combined encephalography and arteriography.

encephalocele (en·**kef**·al·o·seel). Hernial protrusion of the brain or part of it through a congenital or traumatic fissure in the skull. [encephalon, Gk *kele* hernia.]

encephalocoele (en·kef·al·o·**se**′·le). 1. The entire cavity enclosed by the skull. 2. The cerebral ventricles as a whole. [encephalon, Gk *koilia* cavity.]

encephalocystocele (en·kef·al·o·**sist**′·o·seel). Hydrencephalocele; a hernia of the brain, the latter filled with cerebrospinal fluid communicating with the ventricles. [encephalon, Gk *kystis* bag, *kele* hernia.]

encephalodialysis (en·kef·al·o·di·**al**′·is·is). Softening of the brain. [encephalon, Gk *dialysis* dissolution.]

encephalodynia (en·kef·al·o·**din**′·e·ah). Encephalalgia. [encephalon, Gk *odyne* pain.]

encephalodysplasia (en·kef·al·o·dis·**pla**′·ze·ah). An abnormality of the brain; usually applied to congenital abnormalities. [encephalon, dysplasia.]

encephaloedema (en·kef·al·e·**de**′·mah). Oedema of the brain. [encephalon, oedema.]

encephalogram (en·**kef**·al·o·gram). Any x-ray film obtained in the radiological examination of the ventricles and subarachnoid space of the brain, by the use of air as a contrast medium. The air is introduced by lumbar or cisternal puncture. [encephalon, Gk *gramma* record.]

encephalograph (en·**kef**·al·o·graf). An instrument for recording the electrical activity of the brain. Small changes in electrical potential are measured by a sensitive galvanometer and amplifying device connected with electrodes placed on the scalp. [encephalon, Gk *graphein* to write.]

encephalography (en·kef·al·**og**′·raf·e). Radiological examination of the ventricles, cisterns and subarachnoid spaces of the brain by the introduction of a contrast substance, usually a gas, through a lumbar or cisternal injection. **Gamma encephalography.** The use of radio-isotopes emitting gamma-rays in the detection of intracranial abnormalities. **Isotope encephalography.** The study of the cerebrospinal fluid pathways within the cranium by the injection at lumbar puncture of a radioactive isotope in the form of albumin labelled with ^{131}I. [encephalon, radiography.]

encephalohepatitis (en·**kef**·al·o·hep·at·**i**′·tis). Vomiting followed by delirium, convulsions, coma and usually death. There is cerebral oedema and fatty degeneration of the liver. [encephalon, hepatitis.]

encephaloid (en·**kef**·al·oid). 1. Encephaloid carcinoma. *See* CARCINOMA. 2. Encephalocele. 3. Resembling brain substance or the brain. [encephalon, Gk *eidos* form.]

encephalolith (en·**kef**·al·o·lith). A cerebral calculus. [encephalon, Gk *lithos* stone.]

encephaloma (en·**kef**·al·**o**′·mah). 1. Encephaloid carcinoma. *See* CARCINOMA. 2. Encephalocele. 3. Brain tumour. [encephalon, Gk *-oma* tumour.]

encephalomalacia (en·**kef**·al·o·mal·**a**′·she·ah). Softening of the brain. [encephalon, malacia.]

encephalomeningitis (en·**kef**·al·o·men·in·**ji**′·tis). Inflammation of the brain and the meninges. [encephalitis, meningitis.]

encephalomeningocele (en·**kef**·al·o·men·**ing**′·go·seel). Hernia of the substance of the brain within its membranes through a fissure in the skull. [encephalon, meningocele.]

encephalomeningopathy (en·**kef**·al·o·men·ing·**gop**′·ath·e). Any disease that implicates the brain and the meninges. [encephalon, meninges, Gk *pathos* disease.]

encephalomere (en·**kef**·al·o·meer). In embryology, any one of the serial segments which compose the primitive brain. [encephalon, Gk *meros* part.]

encephalometer (en·**kef**·al·**om**′·et·er). An instrument for measuring the skull and determining the position of the cortical centres and regions of the brain. [encephalon, meter.]

encephalomyelic (en·**kef**·al·o·mi·**el**′·ik). Cerebrospinal. [encephalon, Gk *myelos* marrow.]

encephalomyelitis (en·**kef**·al·o·mi·el·**i**′·tis). A group of conditions caused by various forms of virus which attack the nervous system in particular. In some the effects are restricted to the nervous system by damage to the cells of the brain or spinal cord, and these viruses are described as strictly neurotropic; in other conditions the effects of infection are seen also in epithelial and vascular structures, the viruses being pantropic. There is a close relation between some animal virus diseases and human pathology (e.g. rabies, louping-ill of sheep). Instances of infection among workers in certain animal diseases are well established. **Acute disseminated encephalomyelitis.** Postinfection encephalitis, affection of the brain and spinal cord following acute infectious disease, or vaccination. **Allergic encephalomyelitis.** Encephalomyelitis resulting from the allergic response to an antigen introduced in the body, e.g. postvaccinal encephalomyelitis. **Benign myalgic encephalomyelitis.** *Royal Free disease*; an epidemic disease of unknown cause affecting young adults in institutions and characterized by muscular pain and weakness, sensory symptoms and depression, but with few physical signs. **Equine encephalomyelitis.** Epidemic infection of horses by a virus carried by mosquitoes and sometimes communicated to man. **Granulomatous encephalomyelitis.** A disease attributed to *Encephalitozoon* in which there is granulomatous affection and necrosis of the cerebral and spinal ventricles. **Mengo encephalomyelitis.** A human form due to a virus first isolated from animals in the Mengo District of Uganda. The virus was later shown to be identical with the Columbia SK and MM viruses. **Toxoplasmic encephalomyelitis.** Affection of the brain and spinal cord by *Toxoplasma* species. **Vaccinial encephalomyelitis.** Encephalomyelitis following anti-smallpox vaccination. **Virus encephalomyelitis.** An inflammation of the brain and spinal cord due to a virus; also used as a synonym for the various forms of equine encephalitis. [encephalon, Gk *myelos* marrow, *-itis* inflammation.]

encephalomyeloneuropathy (en·**kef**·al·o·**mi**·el·o·newr·**op**′·ath·e). Any disease implicating the brain, the spinal cord and the nerves. [encephalon, Gk *myelos* marrow, *neuron* nerve, *pathos* disease.]

encephalomyelopathy (en·**kef**·al·o·mi·el·**op**′·ath·e). Any disease of both the brain and the spinal cord. [encephalon, Gk *myelos* marrow, *pathos* disease.]

encephalomyeloradiculitis (en·**kef**·al·o·**mi**·el·o·rad·ik·ew·**li**′·tis). An inflamed condition of the brain, the spinal cord and the roots of the spinal nerves. [encephalitis, myeloradiculitis.]

encephalomyeloradiculoneuritis (en·**kef**·al·o·**mi**·el·o·rad·**ik**·ew·lo·newr·**i**′·tis). Guillain-Barré syndrome. [encephalitis, myeloradiculitis, neuritis.]

encephalomyeloradiculopathy (en·**kef**·al·o·**mi**·el·o·rad·ik·ew·**lop**′·ath·e). Any disease which implicates the spinal cord and nerve roots and the brain. [encephalon, myeloradiculopathy.]

encephalon (en·**kef**·al·on). The brain, i.e. the cerebrum, cerebellum, pons and medulla oblongata; a comprehensive term for the contents of the cranium. **Epichordal encephalon.** In embryology, the part of the brain that is developed behind the notochord. [Gk *enkephalos.*]

encephalonarcosis (en·**kef**·al·o·nar·**ko**′·sis). A state of coma or stupor resulting from disease of the brain. [encephalon, narcosis.]

encephaloncus (en·**kef**·al·**ong**′·kus). Cerebral neoplasm. [encephalon, Gk *ogkos* a swelling.]

encephalopathic (en·**kef**·al·o·**path**′·ik). Referring to any disease of the brain. [see foll.]

encephalopathy (en·**kef**·al·**op**′·ath·e). Cerebral disease due to various causes, vascular or degenerative, or to local disease in the cerebrum. **Demyelinating encephalopathy.** Any one of a large group of conditions in which there is progressive demyelination in the white matter of the brain. These disorders are often hereditary or familial and may be referred to as *cerebral sclerosis.* The term includes Schilder's disease, Pelizaeus-Merzbacher's disease, Krabbe's disease, Balo's disease, Scholz's disease and others. **Hepatic encephalopathy.** Cerebral symptoms due to hepatic failure, notably tremor and dementia leading to coma. **Hypertensive encephalopathy.** Acute transient local neurological signs and disturbance of consciousness associated with a great rise in blood pressure in hypertensive subjects. **Isoniazid encephalopathy.** Confusion, coma and convulsions caused by isoniazid intoxication. **Infantile subacute necrotizing encephalopathy.** Patchy necrosis of grey matter; onset in infancy usually proceeds to death after weeks or years. Probably autosomal recessive. **Lead encephalopathy.** Changes in the structure and function of the brain in consequence of chronic lead (or tetra-ethyl lead) poisoning; delirium convulsions, or mania. **Progressive subcortical encephalopathy.** Encephalopathy with symptoms relating to local subcortical lesions. **Saturnine encephalopathy.** Lead encephalopathy (see above). **Subacute necrotizing encephalopathy.** A rare disease of infants transmitted by autosomal recessive inheritance, characterized by progressive paralysis, optic atrophy and fits. There is widespread cellular necrosis in the brain. **Subacute spongiform encephalopathy.** A sporadic disease of adults characterized by progressive dementia, myoclonus and rigidity, and death at 6 months from the onset. Spongiform degeneration is present in the brain; *Jakob-Creutzfeldt disease.* **Traumatic encephalopathy.** Encephalopathy resulting from trauma, e.g. concussion. [encephalon, Gk *pathos* disease.]

See also: WERNICKE (K.).

encephalophyma (en·**kef**·al·o·**fi**′·mah). Cerebral neoplasm. [encephalon, Gk *phyma* a growth.]

encephalopsy (en·**kef**·al·**op**′·se). Colour association; the appearance of certain colours calls to the patient's mind in each case various numerals or words, or sensations of smell or taste. [encephalon, Gk *opsis* vision.]

encephalopsychosis (en·**kef**·al·o·si·**ko**′·sis). Any disease of the mind resulting from a focal lesion of the brain. [encephalon, psychosis.]

encephalopuncture (en·**kef**·al·o·**pungk**′·tcher). Puncture of the brain substance. [encephalon, puncture.]

encephalopyosis (en·**kef**·al·o·pi·**o**′·sis). Abscess or purulent inflammation of the brain. [encephalon, pyosis.]

encephalorrhachidian (en·**kef**·al·o·rak·**id**′·e·an). Cerebrospinal. [encephalon, Gk *rhachis* spine.]

encephalorrhagia (en·**kef**·al·o·**ra**′·je·ah). Apoplexy; haemorrhage from the capillaries of the brain. [encephalon, Gk *rhegnynai* to burst forth.]

encephalosclerosis (en·**kef**·al·o·skler·**o**′·sis). Hardening of the brain substance. [encephalon, sclerosis.]

encephaloscope (en·**kef**·al·o·skope). A form of speculum fitted with a removable disc, with which an abscess or other cavity in the brain can be examined through an opening in the skull. [encephalon, Gk *skopein* to watch.]

encephaloscopy (en·**kef**·al·**os**′·ko·pe). Direct inspection of the brain or of an abscess or other cavity of the brain by means of an encephaloscope.

encephalosepsis (en·**kef**·al·o·**sep**′·sis). Septic inflammation of the brain. [encephalon, sepsis.]

encephalosis (en·**kef**·al·**o**′·sis). 1. Any organic disease of the brain. 2. Degenerative disease of the brain as distinct from inflammatory disease. [encephalon, Gk *-osis* condition.]

encephalospinal (en·**kef**·al·o·**spi**′·nal). Relating to the brain and the vertebral column. [encephalon, spine.]

encephalothlipsis (en·**kef**·al·o·**thlip**′·sis). Pressure on the brain. [encephalon, Gk *thlipsis* pressure.]

encephalotome (en·**kef**·al·o·tome). An instrument used in dissection of the brain. [see foll.]

encephalotomy (en·**kef**·al·**ot**′·o·me). 1. Fetal craniotomy. 2. Anatomy or dissection of the brain, [encephalon, Gk *temnein* to cut.]

encheiresis (en·ki·**re**·sis). Any procedure in which the hands are used, e.g. the introduction of a sound or bougie. [Gk *en, cheir* hand.]

enchondral (en·**kon**·dral). Endochondral.

enchondroma (en·kon·**dro**·mah). A cartilaginous tumour forming in the interior of a bone. *See also* ECCHONDROMA. **Multiple congenital enchondroma.** Dyschondroplasia. **Enchondroma petrificum.** Osteochondroma. [Gk *en, chondros* cartilage, *-oma* tumour.]

enchondromatosis (en·**kon**·dro·mat·**o**′·sis). Dyschondroplasia. [enchondroma, Gk *-osis* condition.]

enchondromatous (en·kon·**dro**·mat·us). Relating or belonging to enchondroma.

enchondrosarcoma (en·**kon**·dro·sar·**ko**′·mah). Sarcomatous change in an enchondroma. [enchondroma, sarcoma.]

enchondrosis (en·kon·**dro**·sis). The process of development of an enchondroma. [Gk *en, chondros* cartilage.]

enchylema (en·ki·**le**·mah). The more fluid material which fills the cytoreticulum of the cell body. [Gk *en, chylos* juice.]

enchyma (en·**ki**·mah). A fluid elaborated from the chyme and serving to form and repair cells and other tissues. [Gk *egchyma* infusion.]

enclave (en·klave). 1. Any detached mass of tissue enclosed within tissue of a different kind or within another organ; the occurrence of some foreign element in particular protoplasmic arrangement, e.g. an isolated portion of gland tissue separated from the main gland and enclosed in muscular tissue. 2. An exclave in its relation to the surrounding part. [Fr. something enclosed.]

enclavement (en·**klave**·ment). 1. Retention due to a constriction. 2. Impaction of the fetal head in the pelvic outlet. [see prec.]

enclitic (en·**klit**·ik). In obstetrics, referring to the planes of the fetal head presenting obliquely to those of the maternal pelvis. [Gk *egklinein* to incline.]

encoelialgia (en·se·le·**al**′·je·ah). Pain in one of the viscera. [Gk *en, koilia* belly, *algos* pain.]

encoelitis (en·se·**li**·tis). An inflamed condition of any of the abdominal viscera. [Gk *en, koilia* belly, *-itis* inflammation.]

encolpism (en·**kol**·pizm). Treatment by giving injections into the vagina or by placing medicated pessaries within the vaginal cavity. [Gk *en, kolpos* vagina.]

encolpismus (en·kol·**piz**·mus). A medicated pessary for introduction into the vagina. [see prec.]

encolpitis (en·kol·**pi**·tis). Endocolpitis.

encopresis (en·kop·**re**·sis). Involuntary passing or incontinence of faeces. [Gk *en, kopros* dung, *eresis* removal.]

encranial (en·**kra**·ne·al). Intracranial. [Gk *en, kranion* skull.]

encyesis (en·si·e·sis). Normally-sited pregnancy. [Gk *en, kyesis* pregnancy.]

encyopyelitis (en·si·o·pi·el·**i**′·tis). Inflammation of the kidney occurring in pregnancy. [Gk *en, kyos* fetus, pyelitis.]

encyst (en·**sist**). To become enclosed in a resistant capsule; to become a cyst. [Gk *en, kystis* bag.]

encystation (en·sis·**ta**·shun). Development by an organism into an encysted state, one in which it is surrounded by a resistant outer envelope, the cyst. [see prec.]

encystment (en·**sist**·ment). 1. The state of being encysted. 2. The process of forming and becoming enclosed in a capsule.

end-artery (**end**·ar·ter·e). An artery which does not have any anastomosis with its neighbours. [AS *ende*, artery.]

end-body (**end**·bod·e). A component of complement. [AS *ende, bodig.*]

end-brain (**end**·brane). The telencephalon. [AS *ende, bragen.*]

end-brush (**end**·brush). The synaptic terminal portion of the axis cylinder of a nerve cell; it may have a brush-like end. [AS *ende*, ME *brusshe.*]

end-bud, end-bulb (**end**·bud, **end**·bulb). One of the minute oval or cylindrical bodies in which the axon of a sensory nerve cell ends. They are present in certain parts of the skin and mucous membranes. [AS *ende*, Gk *bolbos* onion.]

See also: DOGIEL, KRAUSE (W. J. F.).

end-fibril (end·**fi**·bril). One of the fine terminal branches of an axon, acting as a sensory receptor. [AS *ende*, fibril.]

end-flake (**end**·flake). End-plate.

end-lobe (**end**·lobe). The occipital lobe of the cerebral hemisphere. [AS *ende*, Gk *lobos* lobe.]

end-nucleus (end·**new**·kle·us). Nucleus of termination; a localized mass of grey matter in which a fibre tract of the brain or spinal cord ends. [AS *ende*, nucleus.]

end-organ (**end**·or·gan). Any nerve ending in which the terminal nerve filaments are encapsulated. **Neuromuscular end-organ.** A muscle spindle; an encapsulated group of 4 thin striated muscle fibres abundantly innervated with both motor and sensory nerve-endings, found in most skeletal muscles, and responsive to stretch stimuli. [AS *ende*, organ.]

See also: RUFFINI.

end-piece (**end**·pees). 1. A component of complement produced in complement splitting. 2. The terminal part of the tail of a spermatozoon; it is sheathless and consists only of axial filament. [AS *ende*, ME *pece.*]

end-plate (**end**·plate). The localized flat, round or oval expansions in which motor axons terminate in the skeletal muscles. [AS *ende*, ME *plat.*]

endadelphos, endadelphus (end·ad·**el**·fos, end·ad·**el**·fus). A double monster of which one twin is a parasite enclosed in a cyst upon the other, or is contained within the body of the other. [Gk *endon* within, *adelphos* brother.]

Endamoeba (end·am·e·bah). *See* ENTAMOEBA. *Endamoeba* is used for *Entamoeba* almost exclusively in American medical literature. [Gk *endon* within, amoeba.]

endamoebiasis (**end**·am·e·**bi**′·as·is). Entamoebiasis. [endamoeba.]

endangeitis (**end**·an·je·**i**′·tis). Intimitis. [Gk *endon* within, *aggeion* vessel, *-itis* inflammation.]

endangiitis (**end**·an·je·**i**′·tis). Intimitis. [see prec.]

endangium (end·**an**·je·um). Endo-angium.

endanthem (end·**an**·them). Any eruption appearing on a mucous surface. [Gk *endon* within, *anthein* to bloom.]

endaortic (end·a·or·tik). Endo-aortic.
endaortitis (end·a·or·ti′·tis). Endo-aortitis.
endarterectomy (end·ar·ter·ek′·to·me). Endarteriectomy.
endarterial (end·ar·teer·e·al). 1. Relating to the tunica intima of an artery. 2. Within an artery. [Gk *endon* within, artery.]
endarteriectomy (end·ar·teer·e·ek′·to·me). The operation of the removal of the intimal lining of an artery. **Disobliterative endarteriectomy.** The operation of coring out the innermost (intimal) coat or lining of a localized segment of an artery occluded by disease, together with the organized clot that blocks it, the outer coat being left to act as a new channel. **Gas endarteriectomy.** The technique for detaching the endarterium by means of the injection of gas (carbon dioxide) between it and the media of the vessel wall. [Gk *endon* within, artery, *ektome* a cutting out.]
endarteritis (end·ar·ter·i′·tis). An inflamed condition of the tunica intima of an artery. **Endarteritis deformans.** Chronic endarteritis with accompanying fatty degeneration of arterial tissue and calcareous deposits. **Embolic endarteritis.** Reactive changes in the intima of an artery which has become obstructed by an embolus; recanalization of the obstructing mass may occur and endothelium grow over the embolus. If the embolus is infected, the organisms may produce an infective endarteritis and may invade the other coats, causing weakening of the arterial wall with the production of an aneurysm. **Non-infective endarteritis.** Degeneration and/or proliferation of the intima of an artery which is not due to a specific infection. It may occur in hypertensive arteriosclerosis, endarteritis obliterans (see below), thrombo-angiitis obliterans, polyarteritis nodosa, giant-cell arteritis and atherosclerosis obliterans. **Endarteritis obliterans, Obliterating endarteritis.** A normal reaction of an artery or arteriole to a reduction in the functional demands made upon it, or to an external irritant. It consists of concentric thickening of the intima, without degenerative change, and gradual reduction and final obliteration of the lumen of the vessel. It occurs in the neighbourhood of ulcerating lesions to prevent haemorrhage (e.g. in gastric ulcer), and in chronic irritative or infective lesions (syphilitic or tuberculous). **Endarteritis proliferans.** Chronic endarteritis with accompanying marked increase of fibrous tissue in the tunica intima of the aorta. **Syphilitic endarteritis.** Proliferative endarteritis with the formation of granulation tissue and, later, fibrous tissue, extending in from the adventitia, or part of a panarteritis. Capillaries grow in the intima from the vasa vasorum to maintain the nutrition of the newly-formed connective tissue. In small vessels, complete obliteration of the lumen may occur. **Tuberculous endarteritis.** Endarteritis in tuberculosis, mainly of the simple obliterative type (endarteritis obliterans; see above). Tubercles are usually found in the adventitia, but caseation may weaken the vessel wall and lead to aneurysm formation. [Gk *endon* within, artery, Gk *-itis* inflammation.]
See also: HEUBNER.
endarterium (end·ar·teer·e·um). The tunica intima of an artery. [Gk *endon* within, artery.]
endaxoneuron (end·ax·o·newr′·one). A neuron of the central nervous system, the axon of which remains within the confines of the spinal cord and does not have a synapsis outside it. [Gk *endon* within, axoneuron.]
endchondral (end·kon·dral). Endochondral.
endeictic (en·dike·tik). 1. Indicative. 2. Symptomatic. [Gk *endeixis* a pointing out.]
endeixis (en·dixe·is). A sign or symptom. [Gk a pointing out.]
endemia (en·de·me·ah). Any endemic disease.
endemic (en·dem·ik). As an adjective qualifying disease or infection indicating that it is one that is caused by factors constantly present in the affected community, in contrast to *epidemic*, in which such causes are "not generally present". However, an endemic disease may become epidemic when some additional newly introduced factor upsets the equilibrium. It is usually confined to infections transmitted directly or indirectly from man to man, and not from animal to animal (enzootic) from which man is infected sporadically as in so-miscalled endemic typhus, a name that is now being replaced by murine typhus or flea-borne typhus. [Gk *endemos* native.]
endemiology (en·dem·e·ol′·o·je). That branch of medical science which is concerned with endemic diseases. [endemic, Gk *logos* science.]
endemism (en·dem·izm). The state or quality of being endemic.
endemo-epidemic (en·dem·o·ep·e·dem′·ik). Applied to a disease which is endemic by nature but on occasion becomes epidemic.
endemy (en·dem·e). Endemia.
endepidermis (end·ep·e·der′·mis). The deeper stratum (germinative zone) of the epidermis. [Gk *endon* within, epidermis.]
endergic (end·er·jik). Denoting a chemical action or change which involves an absorption of energy. [Gk *endon within, ergein* to work.]
endermatic, endermic (en·der·mat·ik, en·der·mik). Descriptive of remedies applied to the surface of the skin, through which they are absorbed into the body. The surface skin may be either sound or denuded of the epidermis by a blister. [Gk *en, derma* skin.]
endermically (en·der·mik·al·e). Indicating that application of a remedy is made directly to the skin. [see prec.]
endermism (en·der·mizm). The practice of administering medicaments and remedies endermically.
endermosis (en·der·mo·sis). 1. Endermism; administration of medicaments by inunction. 2. Any eruptive or herpetic disease or affection of mucous membranes. [Gk *en, derma* skin, *-osis* condition.]
enderon (en·der·on). The corium. [Gk *endon* within, *derma* skin.]
end-feet (end·feet). Terminal boutons. [AS *ende, fot.*]
Endo, Shigeru (b. 1869). Tokyo bacteriologist.
Endo's agar. An agar preparation used for the isolation of non-lactose-fermenting bacteria. It is prepared from peptone 10 g, agar 15 g, alcoholic basic fuchsine 0.3 g, lactose 10 g, potassium phosphate 3.5 g, sodium sulphite 0.25 g and distilled water to 1 litre.
endo-abdominal (en·do·ab·dom′·in·al). Within the abdomen. [Gk *endon* within, abdomen.]
endo-aneurysmorrhaphy (en·do·an·ewr·iz·mor′·af·e). An operation for the radical cure of aneurysm; the aneurysmal sac is opened, the contents are evacuated and the internal openings closed by continuous sutures (Matas' operation). [Gk *endon* within, aneurysmorrhaphy.]
endo-angiitis (en·do·an·je·i′·tis). Intimitis. [Gk *endon* within, *aggeion* vessel, *-itis* inflammation.]
endo-angium (en·do·an·je·um). The tunica intima of a blood vessel. [Gk *endon* within, *aggeion* vessel.]
endo-antitoxin (en·do·an·te·tox′·in). Intracellular antitoxin. [Gk *endon* within, antitoxin.]
endo-aortic (en·do·a·or′·tik). Within the aorta. [Gk *endon* within, aorta.]
endo-aortitis (en·do·a·or·ti′·tis). An inflammatory condition of the tunica intima of the aorta. [Gk *endon* within, aorta, Gk *-itis* inflammation.]
endo-appendicitis (en·do·ap·en·dis·i′·tis). The catarrhal form of acute appendicitis affecting only the mucosa. [Gk *endon* within, appendicitis.]
endo-arterial (en·do·ar·teer′·e·al). Endarterial.
endo-arteritis (en·do·ar·ter·i′·tis). Endarteritis.
endo-arterium (en·do·ar·teer′·e·um). Endarterium.
endobacillary (en·do·bas·il·ar·e). Contained in a bacillus. [Gk *endon* within, bacillus.]
endobiotic (en·do·bi·ot′·ik). Referring to a parasite living within the host. [Gk *endon* within, *bios* life.]
endoblast (en·do·blast). 1. Entoderm. 2. The nucleus of a cell. [Gk *endon* within, *blastos* germ.]
endoblastic (en·do·blas·tik). 1. Referring to the endoblast (entoderm). 2. Referring to a cell nucleus.
endobronchitis (en·do·brong·ki′·tis). Catarrhal bronchitis of the smaller bronchi; the result of inflammation of the bronchial mucosa. [Gk *endon* within, bronchitis.]

endocardiac, endocardial (en·do·**kar**·de·ak, en·do·**kar**·de·al). 1. Pertaining to the endocardium. 2. Within the heart. [Gk *endon* within, *kardia* heart.]

endocarditic (**en**·do·kar·**dit**'·ik). Referring to endocarditis.

endocarditis (**en**·do·kar·**di**'·tis). Inflammation of the endocardium, the lining membrane of the heart, caused either by microbial infection (bacterial endocarditis) or by a generalized inflammatory disorder such as rheumatic fever or a collagen-vascular disease (Libman-Sacks endocarditis). The damage ensuing to the heart valves may be responsible for stenosis or incompetence of the valves. **Acute endocarditis.** Endocarditis which is usually the result of rheumatic infection (*rheumatic endocarditis*) or bacterial infection (*bacterial endocarditis*) of the heart valves. **Bacterial endocarditis.** Infection of the heart valves by bacteria, usually after they have been previously damaged by rheumatic or congenital disease, causing fever, sweating, emboli and signs of septicaemia. Subacute bacterial endocarditis (*endocarditis lenta*) is commonly caused by infection with *Streptococcus viridans* (*viridans endocarditis*); it produces vegetations on the heart valves which may be polypoid or cause ulceration and perforation of the valve cusps (*ulcerative endocarditis*), and which may extend over to the chordae tendineae of the mitral valve or to the walls of the heart chambers (*mural endocarditis*). Acute bacterial endocarditis attacks normal valves, and is caused by the pyogenic bacteria (*pneumococcal, gonococcal, haemolytic streptococcal endocarditis*). **Calcific endocarditis.** Calcification, with consequent rigidity, of the heart valves which may occur as a late consequence of previous rheumatic damage or of congenital abnormality. **Chronic endocarditis.** Endocarditis which is either the late result of acute endocarditis (see above), or due to syphilis or atheroma. It affects usually the valves (*valvular endocarditis*), making them stenotic or incompetent. **Fetal endocarditis.** *In utero* infection of the heart valves. **Gonococcal endocarditis.** *See* BACTERIAL ENDOCARDITIS (above). **Haemolytic streptococcal endocarditis.** *See* BACTERIAL ENDOCARDITIS (above). **Infective endocarditis.** Bacterial endocarditis (see above). **Endocarditis lenta.** *See* BACTERIAL ENDOCARDITIS (above). **Malignant endocarditis.** Bacterial endocarditis (see above). **Mural endocarditis.** *See* BACTERIAL ENDOCARDITIS (above). **Mycotic endocarditis.** Infection of the heart valves by fungi, usually yeasts, in tissues previously damaged or in patients with lowered immune responses, or in drug addicts. **Non-bacterial thrombotic endocarditis.** The formation of fibrinous vegetations on the heart valves in the terminal stages of many cachectic illnesses. **Pneumococcal endocarditis.** *See* BACTERIAL ENDOCARDITIS (above). **Rheumatic endocarditis.** *See* ACUTE ENDOCARDITIS (above). **Sclerotic endocarditis.** Calcific endocarditis (see above). **Septic endocarditis.** Bacterial endocarditis (see above). **Subacute bacterial endocarditis.** *See* BACTERIAL ENDOCARDITIS (above). **Syphilitic endocarditis.** Thickening, stretching and weakening of the cusps of the aortic valves due to extension of syphilitic infection from the aorta, producing aortic valvular incompetence. **Tuberculous endocarditis.** Tuberculosis of a heart valve, very rarely affecting the endocardium of the heart wall. **Ulcerative endocarditis.** *See* BACTERIAL ENDOCARDITIS (above). **Valvular endocarditis.** *See* CHRONIC ENDOCARDITIS (above). **Verrucose endocarditis.** Warty vegetations on the heart valves. **Viridans endocarditis.** *See* BACTERIAL ENDOCARDITIS (above). [Gk *endon* within, *kardia* heart, *-itis* inflammation.]

See also: LIBMAN, SACKS.

endocardium [NA] (en·do·**kar**·de·um). The smooth thin endothelial membrane which lines the chambers of the heart and is continuous with the endothelium of the large blood vessels. [Gk *endon* within, *kardia* heart.]

endocellular (en·do·**sel**·ew·lar). Intracellular; within a cell. [Gk *endon* within, cell.]

endocervical (en·do·**ser**·vik·al). Within the neck of the uterus (cervix uteri). [Gk *endon* within, L *cervix* neck.]

endocervicitis (**en**·do·ser·vis·**i**'·tis). An inflamed condition of the lining membrane of the neck of the uterus; endotrachelitis. [Gk *endon* within, cervicitis.]

endocervix (en·do·**ser**·vix). The endometrium of the cervix uteri. [Gk *endon* within, L *cervix* neck.]

endochondral (en·do·**kon**·dral). Within the substance of a cartilage. [Gk *endon* within, *chondros* cartilage.]

endochorion (en·do·**kor**·e·on). In embryology, the layer of primary mesenchyme which forms the inner part of the chorion. [Gk *endon* within, chorion.]

endochrome (**en**·do·krome). The colouring matter within a cell. [Gk *endon* within, *chroma* colour.]

endochylema (**en**·do·ki·**le**'·mah). The more fluid material which fills the cytoreticulum of the cell body. [Gk *endon* within, *chylos* juice.]

endocoeliac (en·do·**se**·le·ak). 1. Within a ventricle or other cavity of the brain. 2. Within one of the cavities of the body. [Gk *endon* within, *koilia* cavity.]

endocolitis (**en**·do·kol·**i**'·tis). Catarrhal colitis. *See* COLITIS. [Gk *endon* within, colitis.]

endocolpitis (**en**·do·kol·**pi**'·tis). Inflammation of the mucous membrane of the vagina. [Gk *endon* within, colpitis.]

endocomplement (en·do·**kom**·ple·ment). Complement present in the erythrocytes, and not in the plasma. [Gk *endon* within, complement.]

endocorpuscular (**en**·do·kor·**pus**'·kew·lar). Within a corpuscle. [Gk *endon* within, corpuscle.]

endocranial (en·do·**kra**·ne·al). 1. Intracranial. 2. Relating to the dura mater of the brain. [see foll.]

endocranium (en·do·**kra**·ne·um). 1. The cerebral dura mater. 2. The inner surface of the cranium. [Gk *endon* within, cranium.]

endocrine (**en**·do·krine). 1. Of or pertaining to internal secretions; of a gland, secreting directly into the blood stream, not into a duct; of a secretion, secreted by an endocrine gland; of a disease, due to an abnormality of an endocrine gland. 2. An internal secretion. [Gk *endon* within, *krinein* to secrete.]

endocrinologist (**en**·do·krin·**ol**'·o·jist). 1. A physician who makes a special study and undertakes treatment of disease originating in the endocrine glands and their dysfunction. 2. Any other scientist who studies the physiological and pathological relations of the endocrine glands. [see foll.]

endocrinology (**en**·do·krin·**ol**'·o·je). The science of the endocrine glands and their secretions. [endocrine, Gk *logos* science.]

endocrinopathic (**en**·do·krin·o·**path**'·ik). Referring to or affected with an endocrinopathy.

endocrinopathy (**en**·do·krin·**op**'·ath·e). Any disease or disorder caused by abnormality of quantity or quality of secretion from any of the endocrine glands, or by an abnormal condition of the glands themselves. [endocrine, Gk *pathos* disease.]

endocyclic (en·do·**si**·klik). An unsaturated cyclic compound in which the double bond occurs within the ring structure. [Gk *endon* within, cyclic.]

endocyma (en·do·**si**·mah). A double monstrosity the autosite of which encloses the parasite. [Gk *endon* within, *kyma* anything swollen.]

endocyst (**en**·do·sist). The inner layer of a cyst wall. [Gk *endon* within, cyst.]

endocystitis (**en**·do·sis·**ti**'·tis). An inflamed condition of the mucous membrane lining the bladder. [Gk *endon* within, *kystis* bag, *-itis* inflammation.]

endocyte (**en**·do·site). Anything contained within a cell which does not belong to the cell itself. [Gk *endon* within, *kytos* cell.]

endoderm (**en**·do·derm). Entoderm. [Gk *endon* within, *derma* skin.]

endodermal (en·do·**der**·mal). Entodermal. [see prec.]

endodermoreaction (en·do·**der**·mo·re·**ak**'·shun). The reaction due to specific hypersensitivity which follows the intradermal injection of tuberculin (or other analogous preparation) and manifests itself as a flare reaction of the skin round the area of injection in persons who are suffering from or have previously been in contact with the specific infection or agent concerned. Cf. ALLERGY. [Gk *endon* within, *derma* skin, reaction.]

endodontia (en·do·**don**·she·ah). The science and practice of root-canal therapy in a tooth from which the vital pulp tissue has been removed. [Gk *endon* within, *odous* tooth.]

endo-ectothrix (en·do·**ek**·to·thrix). Term applied to any fungus growing on and in the hair: a type of growth of *Trichophyton* (large-spore ringworm). [Gk *endon* within, *ektos* outside, *thrix* hair.]

endo-enteritis (en·do·en·ter·**i**′·tis). Inflammation of the mucous coat of the intestine. [Gk *endon* within, *enteron* bowel, *-itis* inflammation.]

endo-enzyme (en·do·**en**·zime). An enzyme which is not passed out into the surrounding tissues but is retained in the elaborating cell. Cf. ECTO-ENZYME. [Gk *endon* within, enzyme.]

endo-erepsin (en·do·er·**ep**′·sin). Erepsin to be found within the cell. [Gk *endon* within, erepsin.]

endofaradism (en·do·**far**·ad·izm). The use of faradic (low frequency) electricity on the interior of a body cavity or hollow organ. [Gk *endon* within, faradism.]

endogalvanism (en·do·**gal**·van·izm). The use of galvanic (direct) electricity in the interior of a body cavity or in a hollow viscus. [Gk *endon* within, galvanism.]

endogamy (en·**dog**·am·e). 1. Marriage within a social or religious group. 2. Inbreeding, characterized by the fact that both parents have the same chromosomal make-up. [Gk *endon* within, *gamos* marriage.]

endogastrectomy (en·do·gas·**trek**′·to·me). The entire removal of the mucous coat of the stomach. [Gk *endon* within, *gaster* stomach, *ektome* a cutting out.]

endogastric (en·do·**gas**·trik). Within the stomach. [Gk *endon* within, *gaster* stomach.]

endogastritis (en·do·gas·**tri**′·tis). An inflamed condition of the mucous coat of the stomach. [Gk *endon* within, gastritis.]

endogenesis (en·do·**jen**·es·is). 1. A growing or developing from within. 2. The forming of new cells inside the parent cell. [Gk *endon* within, genesis.]

endogenote (en·do·jen·ote). In partially diploid bacteria, produced by infection with an F-prime factor or a localized transducing phage, the term refers to the homologue located in the resident bacterial chromosome. [Gk *endon* within, *genein* to produce.]

endogenous (en·**doj**·en·us). Having origin within the organism. [Gk *endon* within, *genein* to produce.]

endognathion (en·do·**na**·the·on). The inner segment of the inter-maxillary bone. [Gk *endon* within, *gnathos* jaw.]

endogonidium (en·do·go·**nid**′·e·um). Gonidium. [Gk *endon* within, gonidium.]

endoherniotomy (en·do·her·ne·**ot**′·o·me). An operation for hernia in which the sac is opened and the contents dealt with, after which the openings of the sac are sutured. [Gk *endon* within, herniotomy.]

endo-intoxication (en·do·in·tox·ik·**a**′·shun). A condition of poisoning resulting from the presence of a toxin formed within the organism. [Gk *endon* within, intoxication.]

endolabyrinthitis (en·do·lab·ir·in·**thi**′·tis). An inflamed condition of the membranous labyrinth of the ear. [Gk *endon* within, labyrinthitis.]

endolaryngeal (en·do·lar·**in**′·je·al). Within the larynx. [Gk *endon* within, larynx.]

endolarynx (en·do·**lar**·ingx). The cavity or interior of the larynx. [Gk *endon* within, larynx.]

endolemma (en·do·**lem**·ah). Neurolemma. [Gk *endon* within, *lemma* sheath.]

Endolimax (en·do·**li**·max). A genus of amoebae of which *Endolimax nana* is a harmless commensal in the large intestine. Trophozoites are about 10 μm in diameter; they are sluggish and feed on bacteria and general detritus. The cysts have 4 nuclei, but are much smaller than those of *Entamoeba histolytica.* It is world-wide in distribution. [Gk *endon* within, *limax* slug.]

endolumbar (en·do·**lum**·bar). Within the lumbar enlargement of the spinal cord. [Gk *endon* within, lumbar.]

endolymph [endolympha (NA)] (en·do·limf). The fluid which fills the membranous labyrinth of the ear. [Gk *endon* within, lymph.]

endolymphangial (en·do·lim·**fan**′·je·al). Situated inside or pertaining to the inside of a lymph vessel. [Gk *endon* within, lymphangial.]

endolymphatic, endolymphic (en·do·lim·**fat**′·ik, en·do·**lim**·fik). Referring or belonging to or containing endolymph. [Gk *endon* within, lymphatic.]

endolysin (en·do·**li**·sin, en·**dol**·is·in). A substance present in cells which has a specific destructive action against bacteria. **Leucocytic endolysin.** Leukin. [Gk *endon* within, lysin.]

endolysis (en·do·**li**·sis, en·**dol**·is·is). The breaking-up or dissolution of the protoplasm of a cell (cytoplasm). [Gk *endon* within, lysis.]

endomastoiditis (en·do·mas·toid·**i**′·tis). Inflammation affecting the tympanic cavity and the mastoid air-cells of the temporal bone. [Gk *endon* within, mastoiditis.]

endomeninx (en·do·**men**·ingx). The loose inner layer of mesenchyme, probably of neural-crest origin, which immediately surrounds the developing central nervous system and from which the pia-arachnoid is differentiated. [Gk *endon* within, *menigx* membrane.]

endomesoderm (en·do·**mes**·o·derm). Mesoderm derived from the lower layer of a bilaminar embryonic disc. [Gk *endon* within, mesoderm.]

endometrectomy (en·do·me·**trek**′·to·me). Complete removal of the mucous coat of the uterus. [Gk *endon* within, metrectomy.]

endometrial (en·do·**me**·tre·al). 1. Pertaining to or composed of endometrium. 2. Within the uterus. [Gk *endon* within, *metra* womb.]

endometrioid (en·do·**me**·tre·oid). Having the characters of the endometrium. [endometrium, Gk *eidos* form.]

endometrioma (en·do·me·tre·**o**′·mah). A mass of endometrial tissue, apart from and having no relationship to the uterine cavity. [endometrium, Gk *-oma* tumour.]

endometriosis (en·do·me·tre·**o**′·sis). The presence of endometrial tissue in abnormal situations in the body. **External endometriosis.** The ectopic occurrence of endometrial tissue in the ovary or intestine or superficially on the uterus or elsewhere outside the uterus or tubes. **Internal endometriosis.** The ectopic occurrence of endometrial tissue in a uterine tube or in the wall of the uterus. **Endometriosis vesicae.** The presence of endometrial tissue in or on the urinary bladder. [endometrium, Gk *-osis* condition.]

endometritis (en·do·me·**tri**′·tis). An inflammation of the inner mucous membrane of the uterus. **Acute endometritis.** An inflammatory condition of the endometrium, usually associated with infection of the myometrium, uterine tubes or other pelvic tissues. It occurs in puerperal and post-abortal uterine infection and in cases of acute salpingitis; it may result from curettage without full aseptic precautions or from radium insertion. **Chronic endometritis.** A sequel to acute endometritis, and often due to a chronic salpingitis or to post-partum or post-abortal uterine infection; it is less commonly associated with an infected polyp, a Graefenberg ring or intra-uterine radiation. After the menopause, it is referred to as *senile endometritis* and is then often associated with pyometra. A characteristic feature is plasma-cell infiltration of the endometrium. **Puerperal endometritis.** Acute endometritis (see above). **Senile endometritis.** *See* CHRONIC ENDOMETRITIS (above). **Tuberculous endometritis.** Infection of the endometrium by tubercle bacilli, usually secondary to a tuberculous salpingitis, but often an isolated condition. [endometrium, Gk *-itis* inflammation.]

endometrium (en·do·**me**·tre·um). The mucous membrane which lines the uterus. It is subdivided into a pars functionalis, which is shed during menstruation, and a pars basalis, which is not shed but remains in contact with the myometrium and provides a basis for the regeneration of the endometrium after each menstrual period. **Swiss-cheese endometrium.** Hyperplasia of the endometrium producing a pitting effect like Swiss Gruyère cheese. [Gk *endon* within, *metra* womb.]

endometrorrhagia (en·do·me·tro·**ra**'·je·ah). Metrorrhagia. [endometrium, *rhegnynai* to burst forth.]

endometry (en·**dom**·et·re). Measurement of the capacity of a cavity or organ of the body. [Gk *endon* within, *metron* measure.]

endomitosis (en·do·mi·**to**'·sis). Duplication of the chromosomes without segregation of daughter chromosomes and formation of daughter nuclei. This results in doubling of the cell ploidy. **Masked endomitosis.** Endoreduplication. [Gk *endon* within, *mitos* thread.]

endomorphic (en·do·**mor**·fik). Marked by or referring to endomorphy.

endomorphy (en·do·mor·fe). The type of bodily structure characterized by the presence of tissues derived from the entoderm. [entoderm, Gk *morphe* form.]

endomycopsis (en·do·mi·**kop**'·sis). A genus showing abundant development of true mycelium with blastospores; in addition, budding cells of various shape and, in most species, pseudomycelium. Arthrospores may occur. [Gk *endon* within, *mykes* fungus.]

endomyocarditis (en·do·mi·o·kar·**di**'·tis). A condition of inflammation of the lining membrane of the heart (endocardium) and of the muscular fibres (myocardium). [endocardium, myocardium, Gk *-itis* inflammation.]

endomysial (en·do·**mis**·e·al). Pertaining to or having the characteristics of endomysium.

endomysium (en·do·**mis**·e·um). The prolongations of connective tissue which hold together the striped muscular fibres within the connective-tissue sheath (perimysium) of a fasciculus. [Gk *endon* within, *mys* muscle.]

endonasal (en·do·**na**·zal). Within the nose. [Gk *endon* within, nose.]

endonephritis (en·do·nef·**ri**'·tis). Pyelitis. [Gk *endon* within, nephritis.]

endoneural (en·do·**newr**·al). Within a nerve. [Gk *endon* within, *neuron* nerve.]

endoneurial (en·do·**newr**·e·al). Pertaining to the endoneurium.

endoneuritis (en·do·newr·**i**'·tis). An inflamed condition of the endoneurium. [endoneurium, Gk *-itis* inflammation.]

endoneurium (en·do·**newr**·e·um). In a nerve trunk, the sheath of fine connective tissue which invests each medullated nerve fibre outside the neurolemma. [Gk *endon* within, *neuron* nerve.]

endoneurolysis (en·do·newr·**ol**'·is·is). Hersage. [Gk *endon* within, *neuron* nerve, *lysis* a loosing.]

endonuclear (en·do·**new**·kle·ar). Within the nucleus of an animal cell. [Gk *endon* within, nucleus.]

endonuclease (en·do·**new**·kle·aze). A class of hydrolytic enzymes which attack the linkages away from the ends of polynucleotides; an example is pancreatic nuclease. [Gk *endon* within, nuclease.]

endonucleolus (en·do·new·**kle**'·o·lus). A minute spot in the centre of a nucleolus which does not take any stain. [Gk *endon* within, nucleolus.]

endo-ocular (en·do·**ok**·ew·lar). Intra-ocular. [Gk *endon* within, L *oculus* eye.]

endo-oesophagitis (en·do·e·sof·ah·**ji**'·tis). An inflamed condition of the mucous coat of the oesophagus. [Gk *endon* within, oesophagitis.]

endo-oxidase (en·do·**ox**·id·aze). An intracellular oxidase. [Gk *endon* within, oxidase.]

endoparasite (en·do·**par**·ah·site). A parasite that spends all or some of its life within the body of the host; mostly protozoa and worms, but also some arthropods, including mites. [Gk *endon* within, parasite.]

endoparasitic (en·do·par·ah·**sit**'·ik). Pertaining to or having the characteristics of an endoparasite.

endopathy (en·**dop**·ath·e). Any disease originating within the organism. [Gk *endon* within, *pathos* disease.]

endopelvic (en·do·**pel**·vik). Within the pelvis. [Gk *endon* within, pelvis.]

endopeptidase (en·do·**pep**·tid·aze). A proteinase, or proteolytic enzyme acting on the middle linkages of peptides; examples are pepsin and trypsin. [Gk *endon* within, peptidase.]

endoperiarteritis (en·do·**per**·e·ar·ter·**i**'·tis). Endarteritis and periarteritis occurring simultaneously.

endopericardial (en·do·per·e·**kar**'·de·al). Pertaining to both the endocardium and the pericardium.

endopericarditis (en·do·per·e·kar·**di**'·tis). Endocarditis and pericarditis occurring simultaneously.

endoperimyocarditis (en·do·per·e·**mi**'·o·kar·**di**'·tis). An inflamed condition occurring simultaneously in the endocardium, the pericardium and the myocardium. [endocardium, pericardium, myocardium, Gk *-itis* inflammation.]

endoperineuritis (en·do·per·e·newr·**i**'·tis). An inflamed condition affecting both the endoneurium and the perineurium. [endoneurium, perineurium, Gk *-itis* inflammation.]

endoperitoneal (en·do·per·e·ton·**e**'·al). Inside the peritoneal cavity. [Gk *endon* within, peritoneum.]

endoperitonitis (en·do·per·e·ton·**i**'·tis). Peritonitis. [Gk *endon* within, peritonitis.]

endophasia (en·do·**fa**·ze·ah). The forming of a word or words with the lips without utterance of sound. [Gk *endon* within, *phasis* a speaking.]

endophasy (en·do·fa·zy). Inner speech. [Gk *endo* within, *phasis* speech.]

endophlebectomy (en·do·fleb·**ek**'·to·me). Removal of a thrombus from a vein. [Gk *endon* within, *phleps* vein, *ektome* a cutting out.]

endophlebitis (en·do·fleb·**i**'·tis). An inflamed condition of the tunica intima of a vein. **Endophlebitis hepatica obliterans.** Obliterative thrombophlebitis of hepatic veins. **Proliferative endophlebitis.** Intimal proliferation that may result in the blocking of a vein. [Gk *endon* within, phlebitis.]

endophthalmitis (end·of·thal·**mi**'·tis). A generic term signifying suppurative inflammation of the interior of the eyeball. Three varieties are recognized: (*a*) in which the exudate remains in the vitreous (abscess of the vitreous); (*b*) in which the inflammation extends to the anterior chamber or begins in this region (purulent iritis); and (*c*) where the whole of the interior of the eye is affected (panophthalmitis). **Phaco-anaphylactic endophthalmitis.** A generalized inflammation of the uveal tract produced by the liberation of lens proteins in persons who are hypersensitive to this substance. It occurs most commonly when one eye has already been operated upon for cataract, and almost certainly requires the intervention of some microorganism, usually a staphylococcus, for its production. [Gk *endon* within, *ophthalmos* eye, *-itis* inflammation.]

endophyte (en·do·fite). A plant which grows within a vegetable or animal organism and which may be parasitic in it. [Gk *endon* within, *phyton* plant.]

endoplasm (en·do·plazm). The inner layer of the cytoplasm. [Gk *endon* within, plasma.]

endoplast (en·do·plast). The nucleus of an animal cell, e.g. a protozoon. [Gk *endon* within, *plassein* to form.]

endoplastic (en·do·**plas**·tik). Possessing internal formative power. [see prec.]

Endopterygota (end·op·ter·e·go'·tah). A sub-class of the arthropod class Insecta; characterized by the presence of a pupal stage in the life history. Members of the orders Coleoptera, Diptera, Hymenoptera and Siphonaptera are of medical interest. [Gk *endon* within, *pteryx* wing.]

endoradiography (en·do·ra·de·**og**'·raf·e). X-ray examination of organs and cavities within the body after radio-opaque substances have been administered. [Gk *endon* within, radiography.]

endoreduplication (en·do·re·dew·plik·**a**'·shun). Chromosome duplication without nuclear division. It has also been called *masked endomitosis* because it occurs in the absence of morphological events comparable to those of normal mitoses. If endoreduplication is followed by a normal nuclear division, the chromosomes appear in close association with their duplicates (diplochromosomes). Successive endoreduplication may lead to a high degree of polyploidy. [Gk *endon* within, L *re-*, *duplicare* to double.]

endorrhachis (en·do·**ra**·kis). The dura mater of the spinal cord. [Gk *endon* within, *rhachis* spine.]

endorrhinitis (**en**·do·ri·**ni**'·tis). 1. An inflamed condition of the mucous membrane of the nasal cavity. 2. Coryza. [Gk *endon* within, rhinitis.]

endosalpingitis (**en**·do·sal·pin·**ji**'·tis). Inflammation of the mucous coat of the uterine tube. [Gk *endon* within, salpingitis.]

endosalpingoma (**en**·do·sal·ping·**go**'·mah). Adenomyoma of the uterine tube. [Gk *endon* within, *salpigz* trumpet, *-oma* tumour.]

endosalpingosis (**en**·do·sal·ping·**go**'·sis). Adenomyosis affecting the uterine tube. [Gk *endon* within, *salpigx* trumpet, *-osis* condition.]

endosarc (**en**·do·sark). The fluid-like constituent of the cytoreticulum of the cell body. [Gk *endon* within, *sarx* flesh.]

endoscope (**en**·do·skope). An instrument with which the interior of a hollow organ can be examined. [Gk *endon* within, *skopein* to watch.]

endoscopy (en·**dos**·ko·pe). The examination of hollow organs of the body by means of an endoscope. **Pleural endoscopy.** Direct examination of the cavity of the pleura with an endoscope.

endosecretory (**en**·do·se·**kre**'·tor·e). Pertaining to the internal secretions. [Gk *endon* within, secretion.]

endosepsis (en·do·**sep**·sis). Autosepticaemia; septicaemia which originates from an infection within the body. [Gk *endon* within, sepsis.]

endosite (**en**·do·site). Endoparasite. [Gk *endon* within, parasite.]

endoskeleton (en·do·**skel**·e·ton). The internal supporting framework of an animal, as distinct from the exoskeleton. [Gk *endon* within, skeleton.]

endosmic (end·**oz**·mik). Referring or belonging to endosmosis.

endosmometer (end·oz·**mom**·et·er). An instrument which shows the rate at which endosmosis is taking place. [endosmosis, meter.]

endosmosis (end·oz·**mo**·sis). The passage of water molecules through a semipermeable membrane into a solution contained therein. [Gk *endon* within, *osmos* drive.]

endosmotic (end·oz·**mot**·ik). Endosmic.

endosoma (en·do·**so**·mah). The matter contained in the envelope of an erythrocyte. [Gk *endon* within, *soma* body.]

endosperm (**en**·do·sperm). The protein, or nutritive element, contained in seed plants, and concerned with the nourishment of the embryo. [Gk *endon* within, sperm.]

endospore (**en**·do·spore). A spore developed endogenously within a closed receptacle. It may be formed asexually in large numbers by successive nuclear divisions, as in the sporangiospores of *Mucor*, or sexually in number up to 4 and multiples of 4, as in the *Ascomycetes*. [see foll.]

endosporium (en·do·**spo**·re·um). The inner sheath, e.g. of a pollen grain, of the envelope of a spore. [Gk *endon* within, spore.]

endosteal (end·**os**·te·al). Relating to the endosteum.

endosteitis (**end**·os·te·i'·tis). An inflamed condition of the endosteum. [endosteum, Gk *-itis* inflammation.]

endosteoma (**end**·os·te·**o**'·mah). 1. A neoplasm within the medullary cavity of a bone. 2. A bony tumour within a bone. [Gk *endon* within, *osteon* bone, *-oma* tumour.]

endosteum (end·**os**·te·um). The membrane of highly vascular areolar tissue which lines the medullary cavity of the long bones. [Gk *endon* within, *osteon* bone.]

endostitis (end·os·**ti**·tis). Endosteitis.

endostoma (end·os·**to**·mah. Endosteoma.

endostosis (end·os·**to**·sis) (pl. *endostoses*). Ossification originating in the substance of a cartilage. [Gk *endon* within, *osteon* bone.]

endotendineum (en·do·ten·**din**'·e·um). The areolar connective tissue within a tendon, between the bundles of tendon fibres. [Gk *endon* within, tendon.]

endotenon (en·do·**ten**·on). The pliant connective-tissue framework which contains and separates the bundles of fibrils making up the structure of a tendon. [Gk *endon* within, *tenon* tendon.]

endothelial (en·do·**the**·le·al). Relating to or composed of endothelium.

endotheliitis (**en**·do·the·le·**i**'·tis). An inflamed condition of the endothelium. [endothelium, Gk *-itis* inflammation.]

endothelio-angiitis (en·do·**the**·le·o·an·je·**i**'·tis). An inflammatory process involving the inner lining (endothelium) and walls of blood vessels in many organs. It is common to a number of vascular diseases. [endothelium, angiitis.]

endothelioblastoma (en·do·**the**·le·o·blas·**to**'·mah). A rare malignant tumour arising from primitive endothelial cells of blood or lymphatic vessels or from the endothelium which lines serous membranes; in its structure and behaviour it mimics a sarcoma or a carcinoma. Most of these tumours are anaplastic secondary carcinomas, often arising from the adrenals or from developing nerve cells. [endothelium, blastoma.]

endotheliocyte (en·do·**the**·le·o·site). An endothelial phagocytic cell; a large mononuclear cell wandering freely in the blood and body tissues as a scavenger cell, and said to arise from the blood-vessel endothelium, or represent migrated reticulo-endothelia. It is closely related to the monocyte. [endothelium, Gk *kytos* cell.]

endothelioid (en·do·**the**·le·oid). Having resemblance to endothelium. [endothelium, Gk *eidos* form.]

endothelioinoma (en·do·**the**·le·o·in·**o**'·mah). A malignant fibrous neoplasm of the endothelium (inoma). [endothelium, Gk *is* fibre, *-oma* tumour.]

endothelioleiomyoma (en·do·**the**·le·o·li·o·mi·**o**'·mah). Myosarcoma; a sarcoma containing non-striated muscular tissue. [endothelium, leiomyoma.]

endotheliolysin (**en**·do·the·le·**ol**'·is·in). An antibody which causes endothelial tissue to dissolve or disintegrate. [endothelium, lysin.]

endotheliolytic (en·do·**the**·le·o·**lit**'·ik). Able to cause dissolution or disintegration of endothelial tissue. [see prec.]

endothelioma (**en**·do·the·le·**o**'·mah). A malignant tumour originating in the endothelium (haemangio-endothelioma, lymphangio-endothelioma), which often resembles a sarcoma and at times a carcinoma. **Endothelioma capitis.** A multiple endothelioma of large size occurring on the scalp. **Endothelioma cutis.** Endothelioma occurring on the skin in the form of violet-coloured papules. **Dural endothelioma.** A fibroblastoma or neurofibroma originating in the endothelial cells of the subdural space or the arachnoid mater. [Gk *endon* within, *thele* nipple, *-oma* tumour.]

endotheliomatosis (en·do·**the**·le·o·mat·**o**'·sis). A condition in which multiple endotheliomata are diffusely spread throughout a tissue. [endothelioma, Gk *-osis* condition.]

endotheliomyoma (en·do·**the**·le·o·mi·**o**'·mah). A myoma or myomatous tumour derived from endothelium or having endothelial elements.

endotheliomyxoma (en·do·**the**·le·o·mix·**o**'·mah). A myxoma or myxomatous tumour derived from endothelium or having endothelial elements.

endotheliorhabdomyoma (en·do·**the**·le·o·rab·do·mi·**o**'·mah). A rhabdomyoma derived from endothelium and malignant in character.

endotheliotoxin (**en**·do·the·le·o·**tox**'·in). A toxin acting on the endothelium of blood vessels and producing haemorrhage.

endothelium [NA] (en·do·**the**·le·um). The lining cell of various body cavities and of the blood-vascular system. It is composed of flat nucleated cells of different shapes. **Endothelium of the anterior chamber [endothelium camerae anterioris (NA)].** The layer of flattened cells on the anterior face of the iris. **Subepithelial endothelium.** Débove's membrane. **Vascular endothelium.** The cells lining the chambers of the heart and the blood and lymph vessels. [Gk *endon* within, *thele* nipple.]

endothermal, endothermic (en·do·**ther**·mal, en·do·**ther**·mik). 1. Referring to the production of heat within an organism. 2. Characterized by the storing up of potential energy or heat. 3. Absorbing heat. 4. In chemistry, denoting compounds which absorb heat during their formation. 5. Pertaining to an endotherm or to endothermy. [Gk *endon* within, *therme* heat.]

endothermy (en·do·ther·me). Diathermy; causing mild heat to penetrate and raise the temperature of bodily tissues by applying a high-frequency current. [see prec.]

endothoracic (en·do·thor·as′·ik). Within the thorax. [Gk *endon* within, thorax.]

endothrix (en·do·thrix). General term applied to fungi living and producing arthrospores inside the hair shaft. [Gk *endon* within, *thrix* hair.]

endothyropexy (en·do·thi·ro·pex·e). In surgery, the separation of the thyroid gland from the trachea, displacing it forwards and to one side and fastening it in a space between the sternomastoid muscle and the skin. [Gk *endon* within, thyroid, Gk *pexis* fixation.]

endotin (en·do·tin). The name given to a preparation of old tuberculin which has been treated with various organic solvents.

endotome (en·do·tome). Strong decapitation shears used by obstetrical surgeons for beheading the fetus. [Gk *endon* within, *temnein* to cut.]

endotoscope (end·o·to·skope). An endoscope with which the ear can be examined. [Gk *endon* within, otoscope.]

endotoxic (en·do·tox·ik). Of or pertaining to an endotoxin.

endotoxicosis (en·do·tox·ik·o′·sis). A condition of poisoning arising from the presence of an endotoxin. [endotoxin, Gk *-osis* condition.]

endotoxin (en·do·tox·in). Toxin that is released only after death of the bacterial cell. Nowadays the term is a synonym for the lipopolysaccharides (O antigen) of Gram-negative bacteria. [Gk *endon* within, *toxikon* poison.]

endotoxoid (en·do·tox·oid). A toxoid formed from an endotoxin. [endotoxin, Gk *eidos* form.]

endotracheitis (en·do·trak·e·i′·tis). An inflamed condition of the mucous coat of the trachea. [Gk *endon* within, tracheitis.]

endotrachelic (en·do·trak·el′·ik). Endocervical. [Gk *endon* within, *trachelos* neck.]

endotrachelitis (en·do·trak·el·i′·tis). Endocervicitis. [Gk *endon* within, *trachelos* neck, *-itis* inflammation.]

endo-urethral (en·do·ewr·e′·thral). Intra-urethral. [Gk *endon* within, urethra.]

endo-uterine (en·do·ew·ter·ine). Intra-uterine. [Gk *endon* within, uterus.]

endovaccination (en·do·vak·sin·a′·shun). Oral administration of a vaccine. [Gk *endon* within, vaccination.]

endovascular (en·do·vas·kew·lar). Intravascular. [Gk *endon* within, vascular.]

endovasculitis (en·do·vas·kew·li′·tis). Intimitis. [Gk *endon* within, vasculitis.]

endovenitis (en·do·ven·i′·tis). A condition of inflammation inside a vein, particularly when caused for therapeutic purposes. [Gk *endon* within, L *vena* vein, Gk *-itis* condition.]

endovenous (en·do·ve·nus). Intravenous. [Gk *endon* within, L *vena* vein.]

end-plate (end·plate). The motor end-plate, an area consisting of the terminal membrane of the nerve axon, the post-junctional membrane of the muscle and the subneural space between the two. The myoneural junction. [AS *ende*, ME *plat*.]

endyma (en·dim·ah). Ependyma.

enelectrolysis (en·el·ek·trol′·is·is). The removal of superfluous hair by killing the root with an electric needle inserted into the funnel-shaped opening of the hair follicle after the hair has been pulled out. [Gk *en*, electrolysis.]

enema (en·em·ah) (pl. *enemas* or *enemata*). An injection of fluid into the rectum for cleansing, healing, sedative, diagnostic or nutritive purposes. **Alum enema.** An astringent enema of powdered alum dissolved in warm water. **Anaesthetic enema.** A rectal injection of a prescribed drug given to produce anaesthesia. **Anthelminthic enema.** An enema given to expel or kill intestinal worms. **Antiketosis enema.** Sodium bicarbonate in warm water. **Asafoetida enema.** Asafoetida added to starch mucilage as a carminative. **Astringent enema.** An enema given to control bleeding or diarrhoea by constriction of the blood vessels in the bowel wall; it may be composed of alum solution, boracic-acid solution or tannic-acid solution. **Barium enema.** A rectal injection of barium sulphate which, being opaque to x-rays, is used for purposes of diagnosis. **Blind enema.** An erroneous term referring to the passing of a flatus tube, by which no fluid is introduced. **Carminative enema.** An enema given to expel flatus from the bowel. **Castor-oil enema.** A purgative enema of castor oil mixed with olive oil. **Coffee enema.** 0.25 litre of strong coffee injected slowly and retained for purposes of stimulation. **Contrast enema.** An enema of radio-opaque material for radiography. **Double-contrast enema.** An enema of radio-opaque material, followed by evacuation and injection of air; radiography then shows the mucosal pattern. **Drop enema.** *See* DRIP. **Evacuant enema.** Purgative enema (see below). **Glycerin enema, Enema Glycerini BPC 1949.** An evacuant enema consisting of 2-8 drachms (3-14) g of warm glycerin, which is injected into the rectum by means of a vulcanite syringe. **High enema.** An enema which is injected into the colon by means of a long catheter, usually for purposes of irrigation. **Hypertonic saline enema.** 1. Two teaspoonfuls of common salt to 0.5 litre (1 pint) of warm water, used as an anthelmintic. 2. 0.1 litre of hypertonic magnesium-salt solution (25-50 per cent) injected slowly and retained for as long as possible, to relieve intracranial pressure. **Normal-saline enema.** From 0.25 to 0.5 litre (0.5 to 1 pint) of normal saline injected slowly and retained in order to combat shock or replace fluids lost; it may also be given quickly for irrigation. **Nutrient enema.** An enema which was formerly given in an attempt to introduce nutriment *per rectum*: it is now obsolete except for saline and glucose. **Olive-oil enema.** 0.2 litre of warm olive oil injected and retained for 2 h to soften impacted faeces prior to irrigation with soap and water. **Opaque enema.** Barium enema (see above). **Ox-bile enema.** A carminative enema composed of 0.6-1.3 g of ox bile in 0.25 litre of soap solution. **Purgative enema.** An enema producing purgation. **Quassia-chip enema, Enema Quassiae BPC 1949.** An infusion of 0.1 litre of a 1 per cent solution of quassia chips, given as an anthelmintic. **Sedative enema.** 1. For general sedation, paraldehyde, bromethol, bromide and chloral, sometimes given as a retention enema. 2. For local sedation in diarrhoea, starch mucilage or opium in starch is used. **Simple enema.** From 0.5 to 1.0 litres of warm water. The term is sometimes used for a soap-and-water enema. **Enema of Soap BPC 1959, Soap-and-water enema.** An evacuant enema composed of 28 g (1 oz) of soft soap dissolved in boiling water, and made up to 1 litre (2 pints) at a temperature of 38°C (100°F). **Starch enema.** A sedative enema composed of starch mucilage (1 tablespoonful of starch mixed to a smooth paste with cold water and thickened with boiling water). **Starch-and-opium enema.** Starch mucilage to which is added 30 minims of tincture of opium. **Stimulative enema.** An enema given in shock or dehydration, usually composed of normal saline, or saline with glucose, or coffee. **Treacle enema.** 0.1 litre (4 oz) of warm black treacle in 0.25 litre (0.5 pint) of water, given as a carminative. **Enema of Turpentine BPC 1959.** An evacuant and carminative enema, composed of 14-28 g (0.5-1.0 oz) of turpentine, 56 g (2 oz) of olive oil, and 0.5-1.0 litre (1-2 pints) of soap solution. **Veripaque enema.** An evacuant enema of dihydroxyphenyl isatin on an inert base used in the preparation of the bowel for barium enema examination. [Gk clyster.]

energetics (en·er·jet·ix). The science or the study of the laws governing manifestations of energy. [Gk *energein* to be in activity.]

energid (en·er·jid). 1. The part of the nucleus of an animal cell which carries the active formative properties. 2. The nucleus of an animal cell and the cytoplasm surrounding it and lying within its sphere of influence (Sachs). [Gk *energein* to be in activity.]

energometer (en·er·gom·et·er). An apparatus for measuring the forces and volume of the pulse wave. [energy, meter.]

energy (en·er·je). 1. The capacity to work or bring about physical changes; it exists in many forms which are interconvertible. 2. Defined in mechanics as $\frac{1}{2}mv^2$, where m is the mass and v the velocity of a body. **Binding energy.** The mass of an atomic nucleus is less than the sum of the masses of the constituent protons and neutrons. This mass defect may be equated to energy, and considered to be the binding energy of the nuclear particles, i.e. the energy that would theoretically be required to break the nucleus into its component particles. **Biologically-equivalent energy.** The quantity (expressed in rads) of x-ray energy absorbed in tissue which produces the same biological effect as the quantity (in rads) of absorbed energy of the radiation under consideration. **Biotic energy.** The energy of living things. **Chemical energy.** The energy that takes part in chemical actions. **Conservation of energy.** The idea that it is impossible to create or destroy energy; only transformations from one form to another may be effected, and that without gain or loss. **Coulomb energy.** The potential energy possessed by an electric charge in a region of space containing other charges, the energy existing because of the force between charges. **Dynamic energy.** Kinetic energy (see below). **Free energy.** The energy of a system available for performance of external work. **Kinetic energy.** The energy possessed by a body in virtue of its motion: a force capable of moving a body upon impact (or, if not, converted into heat and sound). A force of mass *m* and speed (velocity) *v* has a kinetic energy of $\frac{1}{2}mv^2$. **Latent energy.** Potential energy (see below). **Nuclear energy.** That released when the atom is split. **Potential energy.** The undiscernible energy contained in a body, due to its position in space, internal structure or stresses imposed upon it. **Quantum energy.** The energy contained in a quantum of radiation and proportional to the frequency of the radiation waves. (The energy *E* of a quantum of radiation of frequency *v* is *hv*, where *h* is Planck's constant.) **Radiant energy.** Energy transmitted by electromagnetic radiation. **Surface energy.** Energy associated with forces of tension in a surface, e.g. of a drop of liquid. [Gk *energeia.*]

enervate (**en**·er·vate). To deprive of nervous strength or force. [L *enervare* to cause to weaken.]

enervation (en·er·**va**·shun). 1. Neurasthenia. 2. General languor. 3. Nerve resection. [see prec.]

enflagellation (en·**flaj**·el·a·shun). 1. The development and formation of flagella. 2. Flagellation. [Gk *en*, flagella.]

enflurane (en·**floo**·rane). 2 - Chloro - 1,1,2 - trifluoroethyl difluoromethyl ether; a nonflammable volatile anaesthetic introduced in 1968 by A. B. Dobkin, an American anaesthesiologist.

engagement (en·**gaje**·ment). In obstetrics, the entrance of the presenting part of the fetus into the inlet of the pelvis as labour begins. [Fr.]

engastrius (en·**gas**·tre·us). A double monster of which the parasite is contained either partly or wholly within the abdomen of the autosite. [Gk *en, gaster* belly.]

Engel, P. 20th century German pathologist.

Engel's alkalimetry. The volumetric estimation of blood alkalinity by titration with a standard solution of tartaric acid.

Engelmann, Theodor Wilhelm (b. 1843). Utrecht and Berlin physiologist.

Engelmann's disc. The isotropic I or J disc of a striated muscle fibre; also known as *Hensen's disc.*

engine (**en**·jin). A mechanical device used for generating power. **Dental engine.** An instrument, activated by either an electric motor or a foot treadle, which induces rotary movement in the chuck of an attached handpiece, which in turn produces rotation at speed of cutting instruments such as burrs and drills. [L *ingenium* contrivance.]

englobe (en·**globe**). To absorb, applied in the case of phagocytic cells which ingest bacteria or foreign bodies by flowing round and completely enclosing them. [Gk *en*, L *globus* globe.]

Engman, Martin Feeney (b. 1868). New York and St Louis dermatologist.

Engman's disease. Chronic infectious eczematoid dermatitis.

engomphosis (en·gom·**fo**·sis). Gomphosis. [Gk *en, gomphos* bolt.]

engorged (en·**gorjd**). Filled to excess and distended with fluid, especially blood; in a state of congestion. [Fr. *engorger* to stop up.]

engorgement (en·**gorj**·ment). 1. Excessive filling or fullness of a vessel or vessels with blood. 2. Hyperaemia, or congestion of a part. [Fr. a stopping up.]

engram (**en**·gram). A memory picture, or trace; in particular its postulated physical substratum. [Gk *en, gramma* mark.]

engraphia (en·**graf**·e·ah). The process of implanting engrams. [Gk *en, graphein* to record.]

enhancement (en·hahns·ment). Improvement of radiation effect on tissues by agents such as oxygen and other chemical substances. **Oxygen enhancement ratio.** *See* RATIO. [O Fr. *enhaucer.*]

enissophobia (en·is·o·**fo**′·be·ah). Fear of reproach. [Gk *enissein* to reproach, phobia.]

enkatarrhaphy (en·kat·ar·af·e). The burying of a structure by the suture over it of adjacent tissues. [Gk *enkatarrhaptein* to sew in.]

enlargement (en·**larj**·ment). The swelling of an organ or part. **Cervical enlargment of the spinal cord [intumescentia cervicalis (NA)].** The swelling of the spinal cord, extending from the 3rd cervical to the 2nd thoracic vertebrae, to which the large nerves of the upper limbs are attached. **Lumbar enlargement of the spinal cord [intumescentia lumbalis (NA)].** The swelling of the spinal cord extending from the 12th thoracic vertebral level above, and tapering below at the junction of the 1st and 2nd lumbar vertebrae into the conus medullaris. It corresponds to the attachments of the nerves of the lower limbs. [OFr. *enlarger.*]

enmorphic (en·**mor**·fik). Normolineal. [Gk *en, morphe* form.]

ennui (on·**we**). Boredom. [Fr.]

enol (**e**·nol). The form into which a ketone may pass tautomerically by the oscillation of a hydrogen atom, the characteristic keto arrangement, $-CH_2C{=}O-$, becoming the alcoholic (enolic) $-CH{=}C(OH)-$, the two forms existing in equilibrium.

enolase (**e**·nol·aze). An enzyme of muscle which catalyses the production of phosphopyruvic acid from 2-phosphoglyceric acid in the cycle of muscle contraction.

enophthalmia, enophthalmos, enophthalmus (en·of·**thal**·me·ah, en·of·**thal**·mos, en·of·**thal**·mus). Recession of the eyeball into the cavity of the orbit. [Gk *en, ophthalmos* eye.]

Enoplata (e·no·**pla**·tah). An order of the Nematoda which includes worms of the genera *Trichinella, Trichuris* and *Capillaria.* [Gk *enoplos* armed.]

enorchia (en·**or**·ke·ah). Cryptorchism; a failure of development resulting in the testes being retained in the inguinal canal or the abdomen. [Gk *en, orchis* testis.]

enorganic (en·or·**gan**·ik). Innately characteristic of or arising within an organism. [Gk *en*, organism.]

enosimania (en·o·se·ma′·ne·ah). An irrational and extreme state of terror in association with insanity. [Gk *enosis* a trembling, mania.]

enostosis (en·os·**to**·sis). A bony growth arising inside the skull or within the medullary cavity of a bone. [Gk *en, osteon* bone.]

enoxidase (en·**ox**·id·aze). Oenoxidase.

Enoxolone (en·**ox**·o·lone). BP Commission approved name for 3β - hydroxy - 11 - oxo - olean - 12 - en - 30 - oic acid; it is used in the treatment of skin diseases.

Enpiprazole (en·**pip**·raz·ole). BP Commission approved name for 1 - (2 - chlorophenyl) - 4 - [2 - (1 - methylpyrazol - 4 - yl)ethyl]piperazine; a psychotropic drug.

enriched (en·**richd**). Containing a proportion of a specified isotope larger than that found in the naturally-occurring chemical element. [Gk *en*, AS *rice* rich.]

Enroth's sign. Swelling and oedema of the eyelids, especially the upper, in thyrotoxic exophthalmos.

ens morbi (enz **mor**·bi). The pathological basis or essence of a disease, as distinct from its cause. [L *ens* abstract being, *morbus* disease.]

ensheathed (en·**sheethd**). Encysted.

ensiform (**en**·se·form). Sword-shaped. [L *ensis* sword, form.]

ensisternal (en·se·**ster**·nal). Relating to the xiphoid process of the sternum. [see foll.]

ensisternum (en·se·**ster**·num). The xiphoid process of the sternum. [L *ensis* sword, sternum.]

ensomphalus (en·**som**·fal·us). A twin monster of which each individual is able to function almost by itself, but is joined to the other by bands in the abdomen or side. [Gk *en, soma* body, *omphalos* navel.]

enstrophe (**en**·stro·fe). 1. Inversion of a part. 2. Entropion. [Gk *en, strophe* twist.]

entaconid (en·tah·**ko**·nid). In the tritubercular theory of evolution, the name given to the postero-internal cusp of the lower permanent molar tooth. [Gk *entos* within, *konos* cone.]

entacoustic (ent·ak·**oos**·tik). 1. Pertaining to the ear in its capacity as the organ of hearing. 2. Of sounds, a hallucination of noises occurring in or immediately around the ear. [Gk *entos* within, *akouein* to hear.]

ental (**en**·tal). Central; inner. [Gk *entos* within.]

entallantoic (**ent**·al·an·**to**′·ik). Within the allantois. [Gk *entos* within, allantois.]

entamniotic (**ent**·am·ne·**ot**′·ik). In embryology, within the amnion. [Gk *entos* within, amnion.]

Entamoeba (ent·am·**e**·bah). A genus of amoebae of great medical importance. **Entamoeba coli.** A harmless commensal, exceedingly common throughout the world. Trophozoites are the same size as or larger than *Entamoeba histolytica*; the ectoplasm layer is much thinner, the pseudopodia more numerous, but movement is sluggish. The food is general detritus and very seldom erythrocytes. Cysts contain 8 nuclei. **Entamoeba dispar.** A smaller and less malign form than *Entamoeba histolytica* sometimes considered as a separate species. **Entamoeba gingivalis.** Confined to the mouth, and known only as trophozoites which are resistant to temperature changes. It is capable of histolysis; the causal agent of gingivitis and intimately associated with pyorrhoea though not certainly its prime cause. It occurs also in tonsils. **Entamoeba hartmanni.** A smaller form of *Entamoeba histolytica* recognized by many European workers; considered to be a commensal or at least a lumen-inhabiting parasite. **Entamoeba histolytica.** The causal agent of amoebic dysentery. The trophozoites are normally from 20 to 30 μm in diameter, with clear ectoplasm making one-third and granular endoplasm two-thirds; the living nucleus is hard to observe. Active forms produce a single ectoplasmic pseudopodium and move rapidly. Cysts contain 4 nuclei. Trophozoites inhabit the large intestine and form pockets in the mucosa and, more rarely, in muscle layers. Cysts are passed in faeces and remain viable up to several weeks under cold, damp conditions; they are killed rapidly on desiccation or on heating above 50°C (120°F). Trophozoites feed on cell contents and on erythrocytes. Secondary infections of the liver, and less often of lungs, brain and skin, occur. Though particularly associated with the tropics, the species occurs throughout the world especially in all backward areas. **Entamoeba hystolitica hartmanni.** *Entamoeba hartmanni* (see above). [Gk *entos* within, amoeba.]

entamoebiasis (**ent**·am·e·**bi**′·as·is). Infection with a parasite of the genus *Entamoeba.*

Entamoebidae (ent·am·**e**·bid·e). A family of the class Rhizopoda, order Amoebida. The species are all parasitic, those of medical interest being included in the genera *Dientamoeba, Endolimax, Entamoeba* and *Iodamoeba.* [Gk *entos* within, amoeba, Gk *eidos* form.]

entasia, entasis (en·**ta**·ze·ah, **en**·tas·is). 1. Tonic spasm. 2. Any disease in which tonic spasms occur. [Gk a straining.]

entatic (en·**tat**·ik). 1. Referring to entasia. 2. Causing spasm or strain. 3. Aphrodisiac. [see prec.]

entecephalic (**en**·te·kef·**al**′·ik). Of sensations, those arising internally within the brain. [Gk *entos* within, *kephale* head.]

entelechy (en·**tel**·ek·e). 1. A completion or realization; the full realization or expression of some vital function or principle. 2. In philosophical biology, a hypothetical vital principle which properly directs and controls living organisms. [Gk *entelecheia* completion.]

entepicondyle (**ent**·ep·e·**kon**′·dile). The medial epicondyle of the humerus. [Gk *entos* within, epicondyle.]

enteraden (en·**ter**·ad·en). Any gland of the alimentary canal. [Gk *enteron* bowel, *aden* gland.]

enteradenitis (**en**·ter·ad·en·**i**′·tis). Inflammation of the glands of the alimentary canal. [enteraden, Gk *-itis* inflammation.]

enteraemia (en·ter·**e**·me·ah). Congestion of the intestines. [Gk *enteron* bowel, *haima* blood.]

enteral (**en**·ter·al). 1. Within the intestines. 2. By the intestinal route. [Gk *enteron* bowel.]

enteralgia (en·ter·**al**·je·ah). Colic, or other pain in any part of the intestinal tract. [Gk *enteron* bowel, *algos* pain.]

enterectasis (en·ter·**ek**·tas·is). Distension or dilatation of any part of the intestine. [Gk *enteron* bowel, *ektasis* a stretching.]

enterectomy (en·ter·**ek**·to·me). Surgical excision of a part of the intestine. [Gk *enteron* bowel, *ektome* a cutting out.]

enterelcosis (**en**·ter·el·**ko**′·sis). An ulcerated condition of the intestine. [Gk *enteron* bowel, *elkosis* ulceration.]

enterepiplocele (**en**·ter·ep·**ip**′·lo·seel). Entero-epiplocele.

enteric (en·**ter**·ik). Relating to the intestine. **Enteric coating.** Coating given to a pill or tablet which will ensure that the ingredients will pass unchanged through the stomach into the intestines. [Gk *enteron* bowel.]

entericoid (en·**ter**·ik·oid). Resembling typhoid fever. [typhoid (enteric) fever, Gk *eidos* form.]

enteritic (en·ter·**it**·ik). Pertaining to enteritis.

enteritis (en·ter·**i**·tis). Inflammation of the mucous membrane of the intestines. The term is usually restricted to that of the small intestine, although the stomach and colon may be involved in the same process, producing a gastro-enteritis or enterocolitis. **Acute enteritis.** Enteritis usually due to bacterial food poisoning, especially with organisms of the *Salmonella* group and staphylococci. It may accompany acute infections such as influenza and septicaemia, or be caused by chemical poisons. Epidemic diarrhoea of children is a distinct form of enteritis. **Allergic enteritis.** Swelling of the mucous membrane, and diarrhoea, caused by ingestion of some substance to which an allergic patient is sensitized. **Chronic enteritis.** A form which may be a sequel to acute enteritis or secondary to gastric disease. It may be produced by errors of diet and the use of strong purgatives. **Ischaemic enteritis.** Occlusion of mesenteric arteries causing pain (*abdominal angina*) after eating, obstructive symptoms and sometimes stricture. **Mucomembranous enteritis.** A disease characterized by spasticity of the bowel, constipation and the passage of strips of mucus which may be casts of the bowel. The colon is more involved than the small intestine (mucomembranous colitis). It is a psychosomatic disorder in which there is overaction of the parasympathetic. **Enteritis necroticans.** Haemorrhagic necrosis of the small intestine due to infection with *Clostridium welchii.* **Post-irradiation enteritis.** Persistent diarrhoea following x-ray treatment. **Regional enteritis.** Regional ileitis; Crohn's disease: a condition in which the mucous membrane is inflamed and ulcerated, and all the coats become swollen and rigid. The inflammation is followed by fibrosis and the lumen is narrowed, whilst neighbouring parts of the bowel may become adherent and fistulae form. The terminal part of the ileum is first involved, and the disease may then spread to the caecum and other parts of the small intestine and colon. **Staphylococcal enteritis.** Severe diarrhoea which may follow antibiotic treatment, especially after surgical operations on the stomach or alimentary tract. **Viral enteritis.** Diarrhoea mainly of infants and children, due to enteroviruses (*Coxsackie virus* or *Echovirus*). [Gk *enteron* bowel, *-itis* inflammation.]

entero-anastomosis (**en**·ter·o·an·as·to·**mo**′·sis). Surgical anastomosis between 2 segments of intestine. [Gk *enteron* bowel, anastomosis.]

entero-antigen (**en**·ter·o·**an**′·te·jen). An antigen having origin in the intestine. [Gk *enteron* bowel, antigen.]

entero-apocleisis (**en**·ter·o·ap·o·**kli**′·sis). Isolating a portion of the intestine by surgical means. [Gk *enteron* bowel, *apokleisis* a shutting out.]

Enterobacteriaceae (**en**·ter·o·bak·teer·e·a′·se·e). A family of Gram-negative bacterial rods, either motile with peritrichous flagella, or non-motile. They are non-sporing, grow well in ordinary media and on bile-salt media (e.g. McConkey's medium), all ferment glucose with or without gas-formation and all reduce nitrates to nitrites. Some genera are intestinal pathogens and most of them do not ferment lactose, e.g. *Salmonella, Shigella*; some are potentially pathogenic, e.g. *Escherichia, Klebsiella, Proteus*, and some are saprophytic and found in soil or water. [Gk *enteron* bowel, *bakterion* small staff.]

enterobacteriotherapy (en·ter·o·bak·teer·e·o·**ther**′·ap·e). The therapeutic use of vaccines made from intestinal bacteria. [Gk *enteron* bowel, bacteriotherapy.]

enterobiasis (en·ter·o·**bi**′·as·is). Infestation with *Enterobius vermicularis*.

enterobiliary (en·ter·o·**bil**′·e·ar·e). Forming a connection between the intestine and the bile ducts. [Gk *enteron* bowel, bile.]

Enterobius (en·ter·o·be·us). A genus of roundworms of which *Enterobius vermicularis*, the threadworm, pinworm or seatworm, is probably the commonest internal parasite of white man, and the causal agent of oxyuriasis. Adults (females 1.5 cm, males 0.5 cm) live in the caecum and colon. The females migrate to lay eggs perianally, or may disintegrate after passing through the anus; eggs are therefore infrequent in faeces, but may be widely disseminated in dust. [Gk *enteron* bowel, *bios* life.]

enterocele (en·ter·o·seel). Any intestinal hernia. In obstetrics, hernia of the posterior vaginal wall. [Gk *enteron* bowel, *kele* hernia.]

enterocentesis (en·ter·o·sen·**te**′·sis). Surgical puncture of the intestine with a hollow needle to withdraw distending fluid or gas. [Gk *enteron* bowel, centesis.]

enterochirurgia (en·ter·o·ki·**rer**′·je·ah). Surgery of the intestines. [Gk *enteron* bowel, *cheirourgia* surgery.]

enterocholecystostomy (en·ter·o·**ko**·le·sis·**tos**′·to·me). Surgical anastomosis between the gall bladder and the intestine. [Gk *enteron* bowel, cholecystostomy.]

enterocholecystotomy (en·ter·o·**ko**·le·sis·**tot**′·o·me). Surgical incision of both the gall bladder and the intestine. [Gk *enteron* bowel, cholecystotomy.]

enterocinesia (en·ter·o·sin·**e**′·ze·ah). Peristalsis. [Gk *enteron* bowel, *kinesis* movement.]

enterocinetic (en·ter·o·sin·**et**′·ik). Peristaltic. [see prec.]

enterocleisis (en·ter·o·**kli**′·sis). Occlusion of the intestine, or surgical closure of a wound in the intestine. **Omental enterocleisis.** Closure of a wound or perforation of the intestine by fastening down a portion of omentum over it. [Gk *enteron* bowel, *kleisis* closure.]

enteroclysis (en·ter·**ok**·lis·is). 1. The injection into the rectum of a large quantity of fluid so that it reaches the small intestine (high enema). 2. The injection of a nutrient fluid into the rectum. [Gk *enteron* bowel, *klysis* a washing out.]

enteroclysm (en·ter·o·klizm). 1. Enteroclysis. 2. A syringe, used for enteroclysis.

enterococcus (en·ter·o·**kok**′·us). The characteristic streptococci of the human intestine, which grow on media containing 10 per cent bile; they usually withstand 60°C for 30 min, ferment mannitol and tend to be diplococcal. Species of Lancefield group D streptococci often alluded to as enterococci are: *Streptococcus bovis, S. durans, S. faecalis, S. liquefaciens* and *S. zymogenes*. [Gk *enteron* bowel, coccus.]

enterocoele (en·ter·o·**se**′·le). The cavity of the abdomen. [Gk *enteron* bowel, *koilia* cavity.]

enterocolectomy (en·ter·o·ko·**lek**′·to·me). Excision of the terminal ileum, the caecum and the ascending colon. [Gk *enteron* bowel, colon, Gk *ektome* a cutting out.]

enterocolitis (en·ter·o·kol·**i**′·tis). An inflamed condition of the small intestine and the colon. **Granulomatous enterocolitis.** Regional ileitis. *See* ILEITIS. **Pseudomembranous enterocolitis.** An as yet imperfectly understood but not infrequently fatal syndrome characterized clinically by the passage of frequent watery motions suggestive of cholera; there results severe shock from the loss of fluid, which may amount to 1000 ml/h, and sometimes septicaemia. Aetiologically, it has been associated with both *Staphylococcus pyogenes* and *Clostridium welchii*. The former infection has followed the administration of broad-spectrum antibiotic, e.g. oxytetracycline, which leaves an undesirable bacterial vacuum in the bowel. [Gk *enteron* bowel, colitis.]

enterocolostomy (en·ter·o·ko·**los**′·to·me). Surgical anastomosis between the small intestine and the colon. [Gk *enteron* bowel, colostomy.]

enterocrinin (en·ter·**ok**·rin·in). A hormone derived from the mucosa of the small intestine of certain animals which is held to be specific in stimulating and controlling the glands of the small intestine of man. [Gk *enteron* bowel, *krinein* to secrete.]

enterocyanosis (en·ter·o·si·an·**o**′·sis). Enterogenous cyanosis: cyanosis associated with the presence of methaemoglobin or sulphmethaemoglobin in the red cells both of which may be formed from substances absorbed in the intestine. Methaemoglobinaemia may occur as a congenital disorder, but it is most often due to certain poisons, e.g. sulphonamides, chlorates and certain coal-tar derivatives, e.g. acetanilide, sulphonal, phenacetin, etc. Sulphaemoglobinaemia may be caused by drugs or by a reducing agent, possibly of bacterial origin, permitting the formation of sulphaemoglobin with minute traces of sulphuretted hydrogen. [Gk *enteron* bowel, *kyanos* blue.]

enterocyst (en·ter·o·sist). A benign cyst of the wall of the intestine, arising from the extraperitoneal tissue. [Gk *enteron* bowel, cyst.]

enterocystocele (en·ter·o·**sist**′·o·seel). Hernia of the walls of both the intestine and the urinary bladder. [Gk *enteron* bowel, cystocele.]

enterocystoma (en·ter·o·sist·**o**′·mah). A congenital cystic tumour formed by irregular development of the intestine owing to persistence of a part of the vitelline duct. [Gk *enteron* bowel, cystoma.]

enterodialysis (en·ter·o·di·**al**′·is·is). The complete traumatic severing of the intestine. [Gk *enteron* bowel, *dia, lysis* a loosing.]

enterodynia (en·ter·o·**din**′·e·ah). Enteralgia. [Gk *enteron* bowel, *odyne* pain.]

entero-enterostomy (en·ter·o·en·ter·**os**′·to·me). Surgical anastomosis between 2 separate parts of the intestine. [Gk *enteron* bowel, *stoma* mouth.]

entero-epiplocele (en·ter·o·ep·**ip**′·lo·seel). A hernia containing small intestine and omentum. [Gk *enteron* bowel, epiplocele.]

enterogastritis (en·ter·o·gas·**tri**′·tis). Inflammation of the small intestine and the stomach. [Gk *enteron* bowel, gastritis.]

enterogastrocele (en·ter·o·**gas**′·tro·seel). Abdominal hernia in which loops of the walls of the stomach and intestine are involved. [Gk *enteron* bowel, *gaster* stomach, *kele* hernia.]

enterogastrone (en·ter·o·**gas**′·trone). A peptide secreted by the intestinal mucosa in response to the presence of acid in the stomach. It inhibits gastric acid secretion and motility. Uncertainty has existed as to its distinction from secretin and cholecystokinin-pancreozymin. [Gk *enteron* bowel, *gaster* stomach.]

enterogenetic, enterogenous (en·ter·o·jen·**et**′·ik, en·ter·**oj**·en·us). Of intestinal origin. [Gk *enteron* bowel, *genein* to produce.]

enteroglucagon (en·ter·o·**glu**·ca·gon). Gut glucagon, glucagon-like immunoreactivity GLIY.

enterogram (en·ter·o·gram). The tracing made by an enterograph.

enterograph (en·ter·o·graf). A type of myograph with which movements of the intestine can be recorded and measured. [Gk *enteron* bowel, *graphein* to record.]

enterography (en·ter·**og**·raf·e). The tracing of intestinal movements by the enterograph. [see prec.]

enterohaemorrhage (en·ter·o·**hem**′·or·ij). Haemorrhage from the intestines. [Gk *enteron* bowel, haemorrhage.]

enterohepatitis (en·ter·o·hep·at·**i**′·tis). Inflammation of the liver combined with intestinal inflammation. [Gk *enteron* bowel, hepatitis.]

enterohepatocele (en·ter·o·**hep**′·at·o·seel). In infants, umbilical hernia involving the liver and portions of the intestine. [Gk *enteron* bowel, *hepar* liver, *kele* hernia.]

enterohepatopexy (en·ter·o·**hep**'·at·o·pex·e). The operation of anchoring the small intestine to the liver. [Gk *enteron* bowel, *hepar* liver, *pexis* fixation.]

enterohydrocele (en·ter·o·**hi**'·dro·seel). Hydrocele existing in conjunction with hernia. [Gk *enteron* bowel, hydrocele.]

enteroidea (en·ter·**oid**·e·ah). The group of fevers caused by infection with intestinal bacteria, e.g. typhoid fever, paratyphoid fever. [Gk *enteron* bowel, *eidos* form.]

entero-intestinal (en·ter·o·in·**tes**'·tin·al). Relating or belonging to 2 different parts of the intestine. [Gk *enteron* bowel, intestine.]

entero-intoxication (en·ter·o·in·tox·ik·**a**'·shun). Autointoxication of intestinal origin. [Gk *enteron* bowel, intoxication.]

enterokinase (en·ter·o·**kin**'·aze). An intestinal proteolytic enzyme that catalyses the conversion of trypsinogen to trypsin. [Gk *enteron* bowel, *kinesis* movement, *aze* enzyme.]

enterokinesia (en·ter·o·kin·**e**'·se·ah). Peristalsis. [Gk *enteron* bowel, *kinesis* movement.]

enterokinetic (en·ter·o·kin·**et**'·ik). Peristaltic. [see prec.]

enterokleisis (en·ter·o·**kli**'·sis). Enterocleisis. [Gk *enteron* bowel, *kleisis* closure.]

enterolith (**en**·ter·o·lith). Any calculus or concretion formed or present in the intestine. The nucleus may be a hard foreign body such as the stone of a fruit. [Gk *enteron* bowel, *lithos* stone.]

enterolithiasis (en·ter·o·lith·**i**'·as·is). The formation of calculi or concretions in the intestine, or their presence there. [see prec.]

enterology (en·ter·**ol**·o·je). The science of the abdominal viscera. [Gk *enteron* bowel, *logos* science.]

enterolysis (en·ter·**ol**·is·is). The surgical procedure of freeing the intestine from adhesions. [Gk *enteron* bowel, *lysis* a loosing.]

enteromalacia (en·ter·o·mal·**a**'·she·ah). Morbid softening of the intestinal walls. [Gk *enteron* bowel, malacia.]

enteromegalia, enteromegaly (en·ter·o·meg·**a**'·le·ah, en·ter·o·**meg**'·al·e). An unusually large size of the intestine. [Gk *enteron* bowel, *megas* large.]

enteromenia (en·ter·o·**me**'·ne·ah). Flow of the menses by way of the bowel; a type of vicarious menstruation. [Gk *enteron* bowel, *menes* menses.]

enteromere (**en**·ter·o·meer). In embryology, one of the blocks of paraxial mesoderm from which the alimentary canal arises. [Gk *enteron* bowel, *meros* part.]

enteromerocele (en·ter·o·**meer**'·o·seel). A femoral hernia containing a loop of intestine. [Gk *enteron* bowel, merocele.]

enteromesenteric (en·ter·o·mez·en·**ter**'·ik). Referring to the intestine and the mesentery. [Gk *enteron* bowel, mesentery.]

enterometer (en·ter·**om**·et·er). An instrument used in surgery for measuring the lumen of the small intestine. [Gk *enteron* bowel, meter.]

Enteromonas (en·ter·o·**mo**·nas). A genus of flagellates of which *Enteromonas hominis* (*intestinalis*), a small form with 4 flagella, is a rare and harmless inhabitant of the intestine. [Gk *enteron* intestine, *monas* unit.]

enteromphalus (en·ter·**om**·fal·us). Hernia of the intestine through the umbilicus. [Gk *enteron* bowel, omphalus.]

enteromycodermitis (en·ter·o·**mi**·ko·der·**mi**'·tis). Inflammation of the mucous coat of the intestine. [Gk *enteron* bowel, mycodermitis.]

enteromycosis (en·ter·o·mi·**ko**'·sis). Intestinal disease of fungal origin. [Gk *enteron* bowel, mycosis.]

enteromyiasis (en·ter·o·mi·**i**'·as·is). Intestinal disease caused by the presence in the intestine of the larvae of flies. [Gk *enteron* bowel, *myia* fly.]

enteron (**en**·ter·on). The intestine. [Gk bowel.]

enteroncus (en·ter·**ong**·kus). A neoplasm of the intestine. [Gk *enteron* bowel, *ogkos* a swelling.]

enteroneuritis (en·ter·o·newr·**i**'·tis). Inflammation of the nerves supplying the intestine. [Gk *enteron* bowel, neuritis.]

enteronitis (en·ter·on·**i**'·tis). Enteritis; inflammation of the small intestine. **Polytropous enteronitis.** Acute infective gastroenteritis marked by the sudden onset of nausea or vomiting, with dull headache, abdominal distress and diarrhoea. [Gk *enteron* bowel, *-itis* inflammation.]

enteroparalysis (en·ter·o·par·**al**'·is·is). Paralysis involving the intestines. [Gk *enteron* bowel, paralysis.]

enteroparesis (en·ter·o·par·**e**'·sis). Diminished or arrested peristalsis leading to flaccidity and dilatation of the walls of the intestine. [Gk *enteron* bowel, *paresis* relaxation.]

enteropathy (en·ter·**op**·ath·e). Any intestinal disease. **Protein-losing enteropathies.** Disorders in which loss of protein occurs through the gastro-intestinal tract and may lead to general oedema; a characteristic feature of giant hypertrophic gastritis. Syn. Menetrier's disease (*see* GASTRITIS). [Gk *enteron* bowel, *pathos* disease.]

enteropeptidase (en·ter·o·**pep**'·tid·aze). Enterokinase. [Gk *enteron* bowel, *peptein* to digest, *aze* enzyme.]

enteropexia, enteropexy (en·ter·o·**pex**'·e·ah, **en**·ter·o·pex·e). The surgical procedure of fixing a segment of the intestine to the wall of the abdomen to relieve visceroptosis. [Gk *enteron* bowel, *pexis* fixation.]

enterophthisis (en·ter·o·**thi**'·sis). Tuberculosis of the intestines. [Gk *enteron* bowel, phthisis.]

enteroplasty (**en**·ter·o·plas·te). Plastic surgery of the intestine, sometimes used in closing a perforation or relieving a constriction. [Gk *enteron* bowel, *plassein* to mould.]

enteroplegia (en·ter·o·**ple**'·je·ah). Enteroparalysis. [Gk *enteron* bowel, *plege* stroke.]

enteroproctia (en·ter·o·**prok**'·she·ah). The condition of having an artificial anus, an opening into the bowel for the discharge of faeces. [Gk *enteron* bowel, *proktos* anus.]

enteroptosia (en·ter·op·**to**'·se·ah). Enteroptosis.

enteroptosis (en·ter·op·**to**'·sis). Downward, with sometimes forward, displacement of intestine within the cavity of the abdomen. It may occur with the falling of the other viscera in splanchnoptosis. [Gk *enteron* bowel, *ptosis* fall.]

enteroptotic (en·ter·op·**tot**'·ik). Referring or belonging to or suffering from enteroptosis.

enterorenal (en·ter·o·**re**'·nal). Relating to both the intestine and the kidney. [Gk *enteron* bowel, L *ren* kidney.]

enterorrhagia (en·ter·o·**ra**'·je·ah). Intestinal haemorrhage. [Gk *enteron* bowel, *rhegnynai* to burst forth.]

enterorrhaphy (en·ter·**or**·af·e). The surgical procedure of suturing a perforation or a wound of the intestine. **Circular enterorrhaphy.** In cases of complete division of the intestine, the invagination of one cut end in the other and suturing the two together. [Gk *enteron* bowel, *rhaphe* seam.]

enterorrhexis (en·ter·o·**rex**'·is). Rupture of the bowel. [Gk *enteron* bowel, *rhexis* rupture.]

enterorrhoea (en·ter·o·**re**'·ah). Diarrhoea. [Gk *enteron* bowel, *rhoia* flow.]

enterosarcocele (en·ter·o·**sar**'·ko·seel). Intestinal hernia in conjunction with sarcocele. [Gk *enteron* bowel, sarcocele.]

enterosarcoma (en·ter·o·sar·**ko**'·mah). Sarcoma involving the intestine. [Gk *enteron* bowel, sarcoma.]

enteroscope (**en**·ter·o·skope). In surgery, a form of speculum fitted with a small electric light used for examination of the interior of the intestine. [Gk *enteron* bowel, *skopein* to watch.]

enterosepsis (en·ter·o·**sep**'·sis). Decomposition of the contents of the intestine, with resultant sepsis. [Gk *enteron* bowel, sepsis.]

enterosite (**en**·ter·o·site). Any parasite which infests the intestines. [Gk *enteron* bowel, parasite.]

enterospasm (**en**·ter·o·spazm). Irregular painful spasm of the intestine, the result of increased peristalsis; spasmodic colic. [Gk *enteron* bowel, spasm.]

enterostasis (en·ter·o·**sta**'·sis). Intestinal stasis; a condition in which the passage of food along the intestine is abnormally delayed or stopped. [Gk *enteron* bowel, stasis.]

enterostaxis (en·ter·o·**stax**'·is). The oozing of blood from the mucous coat of the intestine. [Gk *enteron* bowel, *staxis* a dropping.]

enterostenosis (en·ter·o·sten·**o**'·sis). Narrowing of the lumen of the intestine. [Gk *enteron* bowel, stenosis.]

enterostomy (en·ter·**os**·to·me). The establishment, usually by the operative insertion of a tube, of an external opening in the small intestine to drain the distended bowel above an obstruction, or for the purpose of artificial feeding in a patient with an obstruction in the upper part of the digestive tract. **Gun-barrel enterostomy.** Enterostomy in which both ends of the gut are patent at the opening in the abdominal wall. [Gk *enteron* bowel, *stoma* mouth.]

enteroteratoma (en·ter·o·ter·at·**o**′·mah). A teratoma arising from the alimentary canal or its derivatives. [Gk *enteron* bowel, teratoma.]

enterotome (**en**·ter·o·tome). An instrument, such as a knife or pair of scissors, specially devised for incising and slitting open the intestine, particularly in the formation of an artificial anus. [see foll.]

See also: MIKULICZ-RADECKI.

enterotomy (en·ter·**ot**·o·me). 1. Incision, division or dissection of the intestine. 2. The anatomy of the intestine. [Gk *enteron* bowel, *temnein* to cut.]

enterotoxaemia (en·ter·o·tox·**e**′·me·ah). The presence in the circulating blood of toxins absorbed from the intestinal canal. [Gk *enteron* bowel, toxaemia.]

enterotoxication (en·ter·o·tox·ik·**a**′·shun). Enterointoxication.

enterotoxin (en·ter·o·**tox**′·in). A bacterial exotoxin which acts on the tissues of the intestine. Enterotoxins produced by different species of bacteria probably act differently on the bowel mucosa, e.g. large amounts of preformed staphylococcal enterotoxin, when ingested in contaminated food, cause a sharp attack of vomiting and diarrhoea of short duration; the enterotoxin of *Vibrio cholerae* is produced *in situ* and causes intense and continuous purgation resulting in severe dehydration and hypovolaemic shock. [Gk *enteron* bowel, *toxikon* poison.]

enterotoxism (en·ter·o·**tox**′·izm). 1. Enterosepsis. 2. Enterointoxication. [Gk *enteron* bowel, *toxikon* poison.]

enterotribe (**en**·ter·o·tribe). Enterotome. [Gk *enteron* bowel, *tribein* to rub.]

See also: MIKULICZ-RADECKI.

enterotropic (en·ter·o·**trop**′·ik). 1. Attacking the intestines. 2. Attracted by or having affinity for the intestines. [Gk *enteron* bowel, *tropos* a turning.]

enterovaccine (en·ter·o·**vak**′·seen). An oral vaccine prepared from members of the family Enterobacteriaceae.

enterovirus (en·ter·o·**vi**′·rus). A genus of RNA-containing viruses which preferentially inhabit the intestinal tract of vertebrates. They are comparatively resistant to low pH, which allows them to reach the gut through the stomach. They are among the smallest animal viruses and are spherical with a diameter of 25 nm. The genus includes polioviruses, Coxsackie viruses and echo-viruses among viruses infecting man, together with a number of species found in other vertebrates. [Gk *enteron* bowel, L *virus* poison.]

enterozoic (en·ter·o·**zo**′·ik). Referring to animal parasites which live in or infest the intestines. [see foll.]

enterozoon (en·ter·o·**zo**′·on). An animal parasite living in or infesting the intestine. [Gk *enteron* bowel, *zoon* animal.]

enteruria (en·ter·**ewr**·e·ah). The presence of urine in the intestine. [Gk *enteron* bowel, urine.]

enthelminth (ent·**hel**·minth). A worm parasitic in human intestines. [Gk *entos* within, *helmins* worm.]

entheomania (en·the·o·**ma**′·ne·ah). Religious mania; in most cases the affected person is convinced that he is especially inspired for his work. [Gk *entheos* inspired, mania.]

enthesis (en·**the**·sis). The use of non-vital material, e.g. metal or plastics, in making good deficiency or correcting deformity of the tissues or bony structure of the body. [Gk *en, tithenal* to set.]

enthetic (en·**the**·tik). 1. Referring to enthesis. 2. Exogenous.

enthlasis (en·thlas·is). Depressed fracture of the skull with comminution. [Gk *en, thlan* to dent.]

entiris (ent·**i**·ris). The posterior surface of the pigmented layer of the iris. [Gk *entos* within, iris.]

entity (**en**·tit·e). 1. Independent existence. 2. Personality. 3. That which in itself is a complete whole. [L *ens* abstract being or thing.]

entoblast (**en**·to·blast). 1. Entoderm. 2. The nucleolus of an animal cell. [Gk *entos* within, *blastos* germ.]

entoccipital (ent·ok·**sip**·it·al). Ento-occipital.

entocele (**en**·to·seel). Any hernia which occurs internally and does not affect the bodily contour and/or one containing an intestinal loop. [Gk *entos* within, *kele* hernia.]

entochondrostosis (en·to·kon·dros·**to**′·sis). The development of bone within cartilage. [Gk *entos* within, *chondros* cartilage, ostosis.]

entochorioidea, entochoroidea (en·to·kor·e·**oid**′·e·ah, en·to·kor·**oid**′·e·ah). The choriocapillary lamina of the choroid of the eye. [Gk *entos* within, *chorioeides* skin-like.]

entocinerea (en·to·sin·**e**′·re·ah). Term applied to grey matter which is not of cortical situation but which lies on the walls of cerebral and spinal spaces or cavities. [Gk *entos* within, L *cinereus* ashen-coloured.]

entocnemial (en·to·**ne**·me·al). On the medial side of the tibia. [Gk *entos* within, *kneme* leg.]

entocoeliac (en·to·**se**·le·ak). Endocoeliac. [Gk *entos* within, *koilia* cavity.]

entocondylar (en·to·kon·**di**′·lar). Relating to a medial condyle. [see foll.]

entocondyle (en·to·**kon**·dile). Any medial condyle of a long bone. [Gk *entos* within, condyle.]

entocornea (en·to·**kor**·ne·ah). The posterior elastic lamina of the cornea, or the anterior layer of Descemet's membrane. [Gk *entos* within, cornea.]

entocranial (en·to·**kra**·ne·al). Endocranial. [Gk *entos* within, *kranion* skull.]

entocuneiform (en·to·**kew**·ne·e·form). The medial cuneiform bone of the foot. [Gk *entos* within, cuneiform.]

entocyte (**en**·to·site). That which is contained within an animal cell and inherent in it. [Gk *entos* within, *kytos* cell.]

entoderm (**en**·to·derm). The inner of the 3 germ layers of the embryo. It gives rise to the epithelial lining of the respiratory system with the exception of that of the nose; to almost the whole of the alimentary canal and the glands opening into it; to some of the ductless glands; to the prostate gland and the urinary bladder and the adjoining segment of the urethra. **Primitive entoderm.** Hypoblast. **Yolk-sac entoderm.** The layer of entodermal cells lining the yolk sac and continuous with the entoderm of the embryonic gut at the umbilicus. [Gk *entos* within, *derma* skin.]

entodermal (en·to·**der**·mal). Pertaining to, derived from or originating in the entoderm.

entogastric (en·to·**gas**·trik). Endogastric. [Gk *entos* within, *gaster* stomach.]

entogenous (en·**toj**·en·us). Endogenous. [Gk *entos* within, genesis.]

entoglossal (en·to·**glos**·al). Within the tongue. [Gk *entos* within, *glossa* tongue.]

entohyal (en·to·**hi**·al). Relating to the medial aspect of the hyoid bone. [Gk *entos* within, *hyoid* bone.]

entomarginal (en·to·**mar**·jin·al). Situated medially and close to the margin. [Gk *entos* within, margin.]

entome (**en**·tome). A surgical knife used for the relief of stricture of the urethra. [Gk *en, temnein* to cut.]

entomiasis (en·to·**mi**·as·is). Any disordered or diseased condition the result of insect infestation. [Gk *entomon* insect.]

entomology (en·to·**mol**·o·je). The department of zoology which is concerned with insects. [Gk *entomon* insect, *logos* science.]

entomophobia (en·to·mo·**fo**′·be·ah). Pathological fear of insects. [Gk *entomon* insect, phobia.]

Entomophthora (en·to·**mof**·thor·ah). A cosmopolitan fungus often parasitic on insects, e.g. *Entomophthora muscae* on house flies. One species, *Entomophthora coronata,* is a causative organism of phytomycosis in man and animals, especially horses. It has a predilection for the nasal and paranasal sinuses and subcutaneous tissues of the face. Tissue form is characterized by the presence of wide, irregular, branched, sparingly septate hyphae.

Entomophthorales (en·to·mof·thor·**a**′·leez). An order of fungi, most members of which are parasitic on insects or protozoa and nematodes. Some genera are parasitic for man and animals, causing phycomycosis (e.g. *Basidiobolus, Entomophthora* and *Hyphomyces*).

entonox (en·to·nox). An apparatus for the administration of premixed nitrous oxide and oxygen in equal proportions, i.e. a 50:50 mixture.

ento-occipital (en·to·ok·**sip**'·it·al). Situated between the occipital gyrus of the cerebral hemisphere and the median plane of the skull. [Gk *entos* within, occiput.]

entoparasite (en·to·**par**·ah·site). Endoparasite. [Gk *entos* within, parasite.]

entophthalmia (ent·of·**thal**·me·ah). Endophthalmitis. [Gk *entos* within, ophthalmitis.]

entophyte (en·to·**fite**'). Endophyte. [Gk *entos* within, *phyton* plant.]

entopic (en·**top**·ik). In the normal place. [Gk *en, topos* place.]

entoplasm (en·to·plazm). Endoplasm [see foll.]

entoplastic (en·to·**plas**·tik). Endoplastic. [Gk *entos* within, *plassein* to form.]

entopterygoid (en·to·**ter**·e·goid). 1. The pterygoid process of the sphenoid bone. 2. The medial pterygoid muscle. 3. Situated medially and shaped like a wing. [Gk *entos* within, *pteryx* wing, *eidos* form.]

entoptic (ent·**op**·tik). Referring to the internal parts of the eye, to objects situated or visual phenomena originating within the eye. [Gk *entos* within, *optikos* of sight.]

entoptoscope (ent·**op**·to·skope). An instrument with which the interior of the eye can be examined. [Gk *entos* within, *ops* eye, *skopein* to watch.]

entoptoscopic (ent·**op**·to·**skop**'·ik). Referring to entoptoscopy.

entoptoscopy (ent·op·**tos**·ko·pe). Examination of the interior of the eye. [Gk *entos* within, *ops* eye, *skopein* to watch.]

entoretina (en·to·**ret**·in·ah). The inner nervous stratum of the retina. It consists of 5 layers held together by an internal limiting membrane. [Gk *entos* within, retina.]

entorganism (ent·**or**·gan·izm). Endoparasite. [Gk *entos* within, organism.]

entorrhagia (en·to·**ra**·je·ah). Internal haemorrhage. [Gk *entos* within, *rhegnynai* to burst forth.]

entosarc (en·to·**sark**'). 1. Endosarc. 2. The cytoplasm of a protozoon. [Gk *entos* within, *sarx* flesh.]

entosteosis (ent·**os**·te·**o**'·sis). Enostosis.

entosthoblast (en·**tos**·tho·blast). 1. The nucleolus of an animal cell. 2. A granular body present in a nucleolus, sometimes referred to as the nucleolar nucleus. [Gk *entosthe* from within, *blastos* germ.]

entostosis (ent·os·**to**·sis.) Enostosis.

entotic (en·**tot**·ik). 1. Originating or situated within the ear. 2. Referring or belonging to the interior of the ear. [Gk *entos* within, *ous* ear.]

entotrochanter (en·to·tro·**kan**'·ter). The lesser trochanter of the femur. [Gk *entos* within, trochanter.]

entotympanic (en·to·tim·**pan**'·ik). Within the middle ear. [Gk *entos* within, tympanum.]

entozoal (en·to·**zo**·al). Dependent on or arising from entozoa.

entozoon (en·to·**zo**·on) (pl. *entozoa*). An animal parasite living within the body of another animal. [Gk *entos* within, *zoon* animal.]

entrance-pupil (en'·trans·**pew**·pil). The image formed in an optical system which subtends the smallest angle at the object.

entripsis (en·**trip**·sis). Inunction. [Gk *en, tripsis* a rubbing.]

entropia (en·**tro**·pe·ah). Any condition in which there is a turning inwards of the tissues. [Gk *en, tropos* a turning.]

entropion (en·**tro**·pe·on). Inversion of the edges of the eyelids which may affect either or both, with resultant irritation of the eye by the lashes and the epithelial surfaces of the lid rubbing against it. **Bulbar entropion.** A falling-in of the lids when the eyeball is shrunken or absent. **Cicatricial entropion.** Entropion due to cicatricial contraction of the palpebral conjunctiva produced by trauma (burns), blepharitis or chronic conjunctivitis, especially trachoma. **Contraction entropion.** Cicatricial entropion (see preceding). **Muscular entropion.** A form which may be present at birth from overdevelopment of the orbicularis oculi muscle and is the basis of the spasmodic type (see below). **Organic entropion.** Entropion caused by failure of development of the conjunctiva. **Senile entropion.** Entropion affecting the lower lid in old people, with redundant lid skin and loss of orbital fat. There is probably also an element of orbicularis spasm. **Spasmodic entropion.** A form which occurs as a result of conjunctivitis, keratitis or foreign bodies, and may develop from bandaging the eye. It is produced by spasm of the orbicularis oculi muscle. **Spastic entropion.** That due to spastic contraction of the marginal fibres of the orbicularis oculi muscle and affecting usually the lower lid. **Superciliary entropion.** The curving of the hair of the eyebrows towards the conjunctiva. **Uveal entropion.** Inversion of the pupillary margin, usually the result of an iritis with exudate; rarely congenital. [Gk *en, tropos* a turning.]

entropionize (en·**tro**·pe·on·ize). 1. To cause to turn inwards. 2. To put into a state of entropion. [see prec.]

entropium (en·**tro**·pe·um). Entropion.

entropy (**en**·tro·pe). That part of the internal energy of a body or substance which is not available for mechanical work but is used internally. [Gk *en, tropos* a turning.]

enucleate (e·**new**·kle·ate). 1. To shell-out whole. 2. To deprive a cell of its nucleus. [L *e*, nucleus.]

enucleation (e·**new**·kle·**a**'·shun). 1. The removal of an organ from its capsule or a tumour from its covering cleanly and in its entirety, as a nut from the shell. 2. The operation of removing the eyeball. [see prec.]

enula (**en**·ew·lah). The medial aspect of the gums. [Gk *en, oula* gums.]

enuresis (en·ewr·e·sis). Involuntary voiding of urine. **Nocturnal enuresis.** Enuresis occurring during sleep at night. [Gk *enourein* to urinate.]

envelope (**en**·vel·ope). 1. A wrapper or covering. 2. A capsule. 3. A lipoprotein membrane, derived from host-cell membrane during virus release, which surrounds the nucleocapsid of some viruses. **Nuclear envelope.** The double membrane surrounding the nucleus. [Fr. *enveloppe.*]

See also: BUNYAN, STANNARD.

envenomation (en·**ven**·om·**a**'·shun). The therapeutic administration of snake poison. [Gk *en*, venom.]

enzootic (en·zo·**ot**·ik). Term descriptive of disease affecting animals and corresponding to endemic disease in man. [Gk *en, zoon* animal.]

enzooty (en·**zo**·ot·e). An enzootic disease.

enzygotic (en·zi·**got**·ik). Arising from a single fertilized ovum, as a pair of identical twins. [Gk *e, zygotos* yoked together.]

enzymatic (en·zi·**mat**·ik). Referring to an enzyme.

enzyme (**en**·zime). A protein substance which will catalyse a biochemical reaction. It may act independently of the living cell by which it is secreted, but is an essential constituent of it. In addition to the general properties of catalysts, the enzyme possesses certain characteristics of its own: it is a colloid, highly specific in its action, heat-labile, sensitive to pH and to particular substances which may act as activators, co-enzymes or toxins. The enzyme is classified according to the type of reaction it catalyses, and is commonly named by adding the suffix *-ase* to the particular substrate upon which it acts. The most important groups of enzymes are the *lyases,* which bring about hydrolysis, the *oxidoreductases,* which are concerned in biological oxidation, and the *desmolases,* which catalyse the breaking-up or formation of carbon chains. Each main group is divided into various sub-groups which particularize the reactions still further, and of these the following are of chief importance: *carbohydrases, esterases* and *proteases,* which catalyse the decomposition of carbohydrates, esters (including fats) and proteins, respectively, and belong to the hydrolase group, and *dehydrogenases, oxidases* and *catalases,* which are concerned chiefly in the oxidative processes of cell respiration and belong to the oxidoreductase group. **Allosteric enzyme.** A class of enzymes, the activity of which can be modified by the binding of one (or more) allosteric effector to a site which is not the active site. **Amylolytic enzyme.** Any enzyme which depolymerizes starch or glycogen, yielding intermediate dextrins and, ultimately, maltose. **Autolytic enzyme.** Any enzyme which promotes autolysis of the cell by which it is secreted. Such an enzyme is normally stimulated by increase in acidity and by lack of available oxygen, and is usually of the cathepsin type. **Cardiac enzymes.** Various enzymes derived from cardiac muscle which are present in increased amounts or following damage to myocardial fibres, as in myocardial infarction; the estimation of these enzymes can provide evidence concerning the possibility of recent myocardial infarction. **Catheptic enzyme.** An enzyme of the cathepsin type: an intracellular enzyme which catalyses hydrolytic protein degradation, occurring in animal tissues and responsible for autolysis. It may be activated by cyanide and by thiol compounds such as reduced glutathione and hydrogen sulphide. **Citrate cleavage enzyme.** ATP citrate lyase, the cytoplasmic enzyme responsible for the ATP-dependent cleavage of citrate with generation of oxalo-acetate and acetyl CoA for fatty-acid synthesis. **Condensing enzyme.** Citrate synthase. **Diastatic enzyme.** Amylolytic enzyme (see above). **Digestive enzyme.** Any enzyme of the alimentary tract responsible for hydrolysis of the protein, carbohydrate and fat of food preparatory to absorption. **Ferroporphyrin protein enzyme.** Any of a group of enzymes which have ferroporphyrin compounds as their prosthetic groups. They have an intermediate action in the oxidation of most metabolites in animal tissues, acting as oxygen carriers. **Glycolytic enzyme.** One which catalyses the oxidation of sugar in body tissues. **Hydrolytic enzyme.** One of the hydrolase group (see main def. above). **Inducible enzyme.** An enzyme, the concentration of which in a living cell is greatly increased in the presence of an inducer. **Joining enzyme.** A class of enzymes that can join the ends of 2 DNA chains, or join the 2 ends of a single DNA chain to form a circular molecule. **Lab enzyme.** *See* LAB. **Lipolytic enzyme.** An esterase which catalyses the hydrolysis of fat into fatty acid and glycerol. **Mucolytic enzyme.** Any of the enzymes which split mucoproteins. They are termed *mucinases*, and examples are lysozyme and hyaluronidase. **Proteoclastic enzyme, Proteolytic enzyme.** Any enzyme which catalyses the hydrolytic degradation of proteins. **Receptor-destroying enzyme.** Any enzyme found in a bacteria-free filtrate of a broth culture of cholera vibrios. It splits off from the surface of red blood cells the carbohydrate receptors by which viruses attach to the cells. Similar enzymes are found in cobra venom and as the neuraminidase on the surface of influenza and para-influenza viruses. **Repair enzyme.** A class of enzymes that have been postulated to be involved in the repair of DNA strands in which breaks have been produced by heat, folding or bending, or in which thymine dimers formed by covalent bonding between adjacent bases have been induced by ultraviolet radiation. DNA ligase and DNA polymerase I are thought to function as repair enzymes. **Repressible enzyme.** An enzyme, synthesis of which in a living cell can be decreased or completely prevented by the presence of a particular compound. **Respiratory enzyme.** Any enzyme of certain classes of enzymes, such as oxidase or dehydrogenase, which is concerned with the oxidative processes of tissue respiration. It usually acts as in conjunction with another substance known as the respiratory carrier. **Steatolytic enzyme.** Lipolytic enzyme (see above). **Uricolytic enzyme.** Uricase; an enzyme present in the liver of most mammals and the kidney of some, which oxidizes uric acid to allantoin and carbon dioxide. **Viral enzyme.** A virus-specific enzyme which is either part of the virus structure or induced in the host cell as part of the virus-replication process. [Gk *en, zyme* ferment.]

See also: SCHARDINGER, WARBURG (O. H.).

enzymic (en·zi·mik). 1. Having the characteristics of an enzyme. 2. Enzymatic.

enzymology (en·zi·**mol**·o·je). That branch of science which is concerned with enzymes and their action. [enzyme, Gk *logos* science.]

enzymolysis (en·zi·**mol**·is·is). The chemical change or disintegration produced by the action of an enzyme. [enzyme, Gk *lysis* a loosing.]

enzymosis (en·zi·**mo**·sis). Enzymolysis, with special reference to fermentation.

enzymuria (en·zime·**ewr**·e·ah). The presence of enzymes in the urine.

eocyte (**e**·o·site). A wandering cell, e.g. a leucocyte which has emigrated from a blood vessel. [L *eo* I go, Gk *kytos* cell.]

eocytosis (e·o·si·**to**'·sis). Leucocytosis. [see prec.]

eonism (**e**·o·nizm). A type of sexual abnormality in which there is a desire to adopt the dress of the opposite sex. Transvestism. [Chevalier *d'Eon*, French diplomat.]

eopsia (e·**op**·se·ah). Orthropsia. [L *e*, Gk *opsis* vision.]

eosin (e·o·sin). 1. One of a series of fluorane derivatives used as cytoplasmic stains in histology and haematology. 2. Eosin BPC 1959, the sodium (or potassium) salt of tetrabromofluorescein, used as a dye for silk and wool; also as an adsorption indicator. **Soluble eosin.** The sodium salt of eosin. **Eosin W, Eosin WS, Water-soluble eosin, Eosin Y, Yellow eosin.** Tetrabromofluorescein; a yellowish water-soluble dye of great importance as a cytoplasmic stain. Colour index 768. [Gk *eos* dawn.]

eosinoblast (e·o·**sin**·o·blast). A myeloblast which later becomes an eosinophil leucocyte. [eosin, Gk *blastos* germ.]

eosinocyte (e·o·**sin**·o·site). An eosinophil leucocyte. *See* LEUCOCYTE. [eosin, Gk *kytos* cell.]

eosinopenia (e·o·sin·o·**pe**'·ne·ah). An abnormally small number of eosinophil leucocytes in the blood; hypo-eosinophilia. **Hormonal eosinopenia.** Eosinopenia following the administration of certain adrenocorticotrophic steroids or agents stimulating the secretion of these. It is usually associated with lymphopenia. [eosin, Gk *penes* poor.]

eosinophil (e·o·**sin**·o·fil). 1. An eosinophil leucocyte. *See* LEUCOCYTE. 2. Any histological element or cell which readily takes the stain of eosin such as the eosinophil cells of the anterior pituitary which secrete growth hormones and prolactin. [eosin, Gk *philein* to love.]

eosinophile (e·o·**sin**·o·file). Readily taking an eosin stain. [see prec.]

eosinophilia (e·o·sin·o·**fil**'·e·ah). 1. The condition in which there is abnormal increase in the number of eosinophil leucocytes in the blood; it may be a relatively benign eosinophilic leucocytosis of idiopathic aetiology, a secondary to an allergic condition in the patient, a concomitant of parasitic infestation, skin lesions, acute infections or Hodgkin's disease, or a more serious but rare acute or chronic eosinophilic leukaemia of unknown cause. 2. A reaction of certain cells, tissues, bacteria and micro-organisms that leads to their taking up the stain of eosin. **Tropical eosinophilia.** An ill-defined clinical entity, occurring in association with asthma, bronchitis, pyrexia and sometimes splenomegaly; it is observed in the seaboard areas of India and Sri Lanka, and other tropical countries. It has been suggested that it is due to mites infesting the bronchi and bronchioles, but this is improbable. It usually responds to arsphenamine. Loeffler's syndrome is a similar condition without splenomegaly, occurring in the dry climate of the Middle East and Europe. [eosin, Gk *philein* to love.]

See also: LOEFFLER (W.).

eosinophilic, eosinophilous (e·o·sin·o·**fil**'·ik, e·o·sin·**of**'·il·us). Eosinophile.

eosinotactic (e·o·sin·o·**tak**'·tik). Exerting attraction or repulsion on eosinophil leucocytes or other cells. [eosinophil, Gk *taxis* arrangement.]

eosolate (e·o·so·late). One of the soluble disinfectants formed by treating the fatty esters of the cresols with alkalis.

eosophobia (e·o·so·**fo**'·be·ah). Pathological fear of the dawn. [Gk *eos* dawn, phobia.]

epacme (ep·**ak**·me). Of a disease, the period of increasing symptoms. [Gk *epi, akme* point.]

epactal (ep·**ak**·tal). 1. Supernumerary. 2. Interposed; applied to a sutural (wormian) bone of the skull. [Gk *epaktos* brought in.]
eparsalgia (ep·ar·**sal**·je·ah). Any pain or disorder caused by the unaccustomed use or overstrain of a muscle, joint or organ. [Gk *epairein* to lift, *algos* pain.]
eparterial (ep·ar·**teer**·e·al). Situated on or over an artery. [Gk *epi*, artery.]
epauxesiectomy (ep·awx·e·ze·**ek**'·to·me). Surgical excision of a neoplasm. [Gk *epauxesis* increase, *ektome* a cutting out.]
epaxial (ep·**ax**·e·al). Situated above or behind an axis, or extending over it. [Gk *epi*, axis.]
Epeira diadema (ep·e·i·rah di·ad·e·mah). The "cross spider"; a poisonous spider whose venom contains a powerful haemolysin. [Gk *epeiryein* to pull to, *diadema* crown.]
epencephalon (ep·en·**kef**·al·on). Rhombencephalon; the hind-brain. [Gk *epi*, *egkephalos* brain.]
ependopathy (ep·en·**dop**·ath·e). Ependymopathy.
ependyma [NA] (ep·**en**·dim·ah). The layer of ciliated epithelium which lines the central canal of the spinal cord and the ventricles of the brain. [Gk *ependyma* an upper garment.]
ependymal (ep·**en**·dim·al). 1. Relating or belonging to the ependyma. 2. Composed of ependymal tissue.
ependymitis (ep·en·dim·**i**'·tis). An inflamed condition of the ependyma. [ependyma, Gk *-itis* inflammation.]
ependymoblastoma (ep·**en**·dim·o·blas·**to**'·mah). A tumour composed of embryonic ependymal cells. [ependyma, blastoma.]
ependymocyte (ep·**en**·dim·o·site). Ependymoblast. [ependyma, Gk *kytos* cell.]
ependymocytoma (ep·**en**·dim·o·si·**to**'·mah). Ependymoma.
ependymoma (ep·**en**·dim·**o**'·mah). A tumour arising from the lining cells of the ventricular system of the brain, seen most commonly in young people. Histologically, ependymomas vary in their structure, from easily identifiable ependymal cells lining canals and forming rosettes around blood vessels to undifferentiated sarcomatous types (ependymoblastoma). *Myxopapillary ependymomas* are seen most commonly in the region of the filum terminale; the papillary processes are embedded in mucus derived from degeneration of the fibrous tissue stroma. [ependyma, Gk *-oma* tumour.]
ependymopathy (ep·**en**·dim·**op**'·ath·e). Any disease of the ependyma. [ependyma, Gk pathos disease.]
ephebic (ef·**e**·bik). Puberal, adolescent. [Gk *ephebos* an adolescent.]
ephebogenesis (**ef**·e·bo·**jen**'·es·is). The process of bodily change which occurs during puberty. [Gk *ephebos* an adolescent, genesis.]
ephebogenic (**ef**·e·bo·**jen**'·ik). 1. Relating to ephebogenesis. 2. Caused by the changes taking place during the phase of puberty.
ephebology (ef·e·**bol**·o·je). That branch of medical science which is concerned with puberty and adolescence and the changes caused by them. [Gk *ephebos* an adolescent, *logos* science.]
Ephedra (**ef**·ed·rah). 1. A genus of plants of the family Ephedraceae. 2. Ephedra BPC 1954, the dried stem of the Chinese herbs *Ephedra sinica* Stapf. and *Ephedra equisetina* Bunge, known as *ma-huang*, and of the Indian species *Ephedra gerardiana* Wall. It contains the alkaloids ephedrine and pseudoephedrine, which are responsible for its action as a vasoconstrictor and cardiac stimulant. It is administered as a liquid extract. [Gk *epi*, *hedra* seat.]
ephedrine (**ef**·ed·reen). Phenylmethylamino propanol, $C_6H_5CH(OH)CH(CH_3)NHCH_3$. An alkaloid obtained from certain species of *Ephedra*, or prepared synthetically. It is a colourless crystalline substance, odourless, but a slight aromatic odour may develop on storage. In its pharmacological activity it resembles adrenaline in many respects: it stimulates the myocardium, and raises the blood pressure by causing peripheral vasoconstriction, but there is no vasodilator effect as with adrenaline. It relaxes bronchial muscle, decreases intestinal motility, relaxes the bladder detrusor muscle and closes the sphincter. It also raises the blood-sugar level, may contract the uterus and dilates the pupil. In general, its actions are less intense but more prolonged than those of adrenaline. Unlike the latter, it is effective when taken by mouth. Also unlike adrenaline, it has a potent stimulant effect on the cerebrum and the medullary centres. It has a wide range of clinical usefulness, the main indications being as follows: it is given, orally as a rule, in asthma, laryngospasm in children, nocturnal enuresis, narcolepsy, myasthenia gravis, urticaria and allied allergic disorders; by intramuscular injection to restore or maintain the blood pressure during spinal analgesia; and used locally in dilute solution as a mydriatic, and as a decongestive in upper respiratory-tract infections (BP 1958). **Anhydrous ephedrine.** A very deliquescent, almost colourless substance, soluble in water, alcohol and oils. It is prepared from ephedrine by vacuum distillation, and its pharmacological actions are the same. **Ephedrine Hydrochloride BP 1973.** $C_{10}H_{15}ONHCl$, a colourless crystalline substance with a bitter taste. It is soluble in water, the solution being neutral to litmus. Its actions are those of ephedrine, which is commonly prescribed in this form. **Ephedrine Sulphate BPC 1954.** $(C_{10}H_{15}ON)_2H_2SO_4$, a colourless crystalline substance. Its actions and uses are similar to those of ephedrine hydrochloride.
ephelis (ef·**e**·lis) (pl. *ephelides*). A freckle.
ephemera (ef·**em**·er·ah). A fever of short duration, and usually of unknown aetiology. The term is of historical value only, having been applied at various times to fevers which have proved to be Malta fever, yellow fever, malaria, etc. [Gk *epi*, *hemera* day.]
ephialtes (ef·e·**al**·teez). Nightmare. [Gk *Ephialtes*, mythological demon believed to cause nightmare.]
ephidrosis (ef·e·**dro**·sis). Hyperhidrosis. **Ephidrosis cruenta.** The excretion of sweat mixed with blood. [Gk excessive sweating.]
ephippium (ep·**hip**·e·um). The sella turcica. [Gk *epi*, *hippos* horse.]
epi-. A prefix, from the Greek *epi*, meaning *upon, above, beside, among, on the outside, in addition.*
epi-allopregnanolone (**ep**·e·al·o·preg·**na**'·no·lone). A steroid hormone present in the urine of pregnant women. Its systematic name is 17(β)-[1-keto-ethyl]-androstane-3(α)-ol.
epiblast (**ep**·e·blast). Ectoderm. [Gk *epi*, *blastos* germ.]
epiblastic (ep·e·**blas**·tik). Ectodermal. [see prec.]
epiblepharon (ep·e·**blef**·ar·on). An abnormality of the lower eyelid consisting of a fold of skin stretching the length of the margin so that the eyelashes are pressed against the eyeball. [Gk *epi*, *blepharon* eyelid.]
epibole, epiboly (ep·**ib**·o·le). 1. In embryology, the overgrowth of one set of cells by another and more rapidly-dividing set. 2. The cellular movement accompanying gastrulation in Amphibia whereby the ectodermal cells of the animal hemisphere of the blastula grow over the entodermal cells of the vegetative hemisphere. [Gk cover.]
epibulbar (ep·e·**bul**·bar). 1. Situated on the eyeball. 2. Situated on any bulb-like part. [Gk *epi*, bulb.]
epicanthus (ep·e·**kan**·thus). A fold of skin of the upper eyelid prolonged over the medial angle (inner or nasal canthus) of the eye. [Gk *epi*, *kanthos* lip of a vessel.]
epicarcinogen (**ep**·e·kar·**sin**'·o·jen). A substance that augments the carcinogenic action of another substance. [Gk *epi*, carcinoma, Gk *genein* to produce.]
epicardia (ep·e·**kar**·de·ah). That part of the oesophagus which lies between the cardiac orifice of the stomach and the oesophageal opening of the diaphragm. [Gk *epi*, *kardia* heart.]
epicardial (ep·e·**kar**·de·al). 1. Relating to the epicardia. 2. Relating to the epicardium.
epicardiectomy (**ep**·e·kar·de·**ek**'·to·me). The operation of excising the pericardium. [Gk *epi*, *kardia* heart, *ektome* a cutting out.]
epicardiolysis (**ep**·e·kar·de·**ol**'·is·is). The operation of stripping the visceral pericardium from the heart muscle. [Gk *epi*, *kardia* heart, *lysis* a loosing.]
epicardium (ep·e·**kar**·de·um). The visceral layer of the pericardium; it covers the heart and parts of the great vessels. [Gk *epi*, *kardia* heart.]
epicauma (ep·e·**kaw**·mah). An ulcer or burn on the eyeball. [Gk *epi*, *kauma* burn.]

Epicauta (ep·e·**kaw**·tah). A genus of beetles of the family Canthariidae. The numerous species (mostly American) produce irritant, often vesicant, substances. [Gk *epikautos* burnt at the end.]

epicentral (ep·e·**sen**·tral). Arising from or attached to the centrum of a vertebra. [Gk *epi*, centre.]

epicerebral (ep·e·ser·e·bral). Situated over or on the brain. [Gk *epi*, cerebrum.]

epichitosamine (ep·e·ki·**to**'·zam·een). An isomer of chitosamine derived from mannose.

epichlorhydrin, epichlorohydrin (ep·e·klor·**hi**'·drin, ep·e·klor·o·**hi**'·drin). The internal anhydride of α-monochlorhydrin; a colourless liquid with a chloroform odour, used to dissolve resins.

epichordal (ep·e·**kor**·dal). Situated on or above the notochord. The term is applied particularly to structures which develop on the dorsal side of the notochord. [Gk *epi*, chorda.]

epichorial (ep·e·**kor**·e·al). 1. Situated on the chorion. 2. Relating to the epichorion. [see foll.]

epichorion (ep·e·**kor**·e·on). In embryology, the decidua capsularis, that portion of the decidua which covers the ovum. [Gk *epi*, chorion.]

Epicillin (ep·e·**sil**·in). BP Commission approved name for 6 - (D - α - aminocyclohexa - 1,4 - dien - 1 - ylacetamido)penicillanic acid; an antibiotic agent.

epicoeloma (ep·e·se·**lo**'·mah). In embryology, that part of the coelom which is in closest relation to the notochord. [Gk *epi*, coelom.]

epicolic (ep·e·**kol**·ik). Situated on or over the colon. The term is applied to the part of the abdomen adjacent to the colon. [Gk *epi*, colon.]

epicomus (ep·e·**ko**·mus). A double monster the parasite of which is united with the autosite at the top of the head. [Gk *epi*, *kome* hair.]

epicondylalgia (ep·e·kon·di·**lal**'·je·ah). Muscular pain around the elbow as the result of overstrain of the forearm. **Epicondylalgia externa.** Tennis elbow, *See* ELBOW. [epicondyle, Gk *algos* pain.]

epicondylar (ep·e·**kon**·dil·ar). Belonging or relating to an epicondyle.

epicondyle (ep·e·**kon**·dile). Any eminence on a long bone on or above the condyle. **Lateral epicondyle [epicondylus lateralis (NA)].** 1. The most prominent point on the lateral aspect of the lateral condyle of the femur. 2. The slight eminence on the lateral part of the condyle of the humerus. **Medial epicondyle [epicondylus medialis (NA)].** 1. The most prominent point on the medial surface of the medial condyle of the femur. 2. The conspicuous blunt eminence on the medial side of the lower end of the humerus. [Gk *epi*, condyle.]

epicondylian, epicondylic (ep·e·kon·**dil**'·e·an, ep·e·kon·**dil**'·ik). Epicondylar.

epicondylitis (ep·e·kon·dil·**i**'·tis). Inflammation of the epicondyle of the humerus or of the area immediately surrounding it. **External humeral epicondylitis, Radiohumeral epicondylitis.** Tennis elbow. *See* ELBOW. **Medial humeral epicondylitis.** Pain and stiffness of the elbow joint with generalized tenderness of the forearm, commonly referred to as *golfer's elbow.* [epicondyle, Gk *-itis* inflammation.]

epiconus (ep·e·**ko**·nus). Term applied to the part of the lumbar enlargement of the spinal cord immediately above the point at which the conus medullaris begins. [Gk *epi*, conus medullaris.]

epicoracoid (ep·e·**kor**·ak·oid). Situated above or on the coracoid process of the scapula. [Gk *epi*, coracoid process.]

epicorneascleritis (ep·e·kor·ne·ah·skler·**i**'·tis). Chronic inflammation of the cornea and sclera. [Gk *epi*, cornea, scleritis.]

epicostal (ep·e·**kos**·tal). Situated on or above a rib. [Gk *epi*, L *costa* rib.]

epicranial (ep·e·**kra**·ne·al). Relating to the epicranium.

epicranium (ep·e·**kra**·ne·um). The 5 layers of the scalp regarded as a whole. [Gk *epi*, *kranion* skull.]

epicranius muscle [musculus epicranius (NA)] (ep·e·**kra**·ne·us musl). A broad flat muscle lying under the skin of the scalp, consisting of 2 bellies joined in the centre by a flat tendon (the epicranial aponeurosis). The posterior belly arises from the occipital bone and is inserted into the aponeurosis; the anterior belly arises from the aponeurosis and is inserted into the skin in the supra-orbital region, blending with the orbicularis oculi muscle. [Gk *epi*, *kranion* skull.]

epicrisis (ep·e·**kri**·sis). 1. A secondary crisis occurring in the course of a disease. 2. The discussion or analysis of a case of disease after it is closed. [Gk *epi*, *krisis* decision.]

epicritic (ep·e·**krit**·ik). 1. Referring to an epicrisis. 2. Term applied to the system of sensory nerve fibres supplying the skin which enables the finer degrees of sensation (epicritic sensibility), such as those of temperature and touch, to be distinguished. [see prec.]

epicrusis (ep·e·**kroo**·sis). Massage by beating or striking. [Gk *epi*, *krousis* a striking.]

epicyesis (ep·e·si·**e**'·sis). Superfetation; a second impregnation occurring in an already pregnant uterus. [Gk *epi*, cyesis.]

epicystitis (ep·e·sist·**i**'·tis). An inflamed condition of the cellular tissues overlying the urinary bladder. [Gk *epi*, *kytis* bag, *-itis* inflammation.]

epicystotomy (ep·e·sist·**ot**'·o·me). Surgical incision above the pubic symphysis into the urinary bladder for the removal of stone. [Gk *epi*, *kystis* bag, *temnein* to cut.]

epicyte (**ep**·e·site). 1. An epithelial cell. 2. The plasma membrane investing an animal cell or a protozoon. [Gk *epi*, *kytos* cell.]

epicytoma (ep·e·si·**to**'·mah). A malignant epithelial tumour. [Gk *epi*, *kytos* cell, *-oma* tumour.]

epidemic (ep·e·**dem**·ik). 1. A period of increased prevalence of a particular disease in a population. 2. Adjectivally: "prevalent among a people or a community at a special time and produced by some special causes not generally present in the affected community" (*Syd. Soc. Lex.*), as opposed to "endemic", in which the "special cause" is constantly present. Within the above limitations, the word was usually confined to infections transmitted from man to man directly or through the agency of insects, in contradistinction to an epizootic (when applied to a disease of man), in which the infection is transmitted from animal to animal and only incidentally to man. The term is now also used to describe an increase in the prevalence of non-infectious diseases. [Gk *epi*, *demos* the people.]

epidemicity (ep·e·dem·**is**'·it·e). Being epidemic, or prevailing in epidemic form.

epidemiological (ep·e·**dem**·e·o·**loj**'·ik·al). Relating to epidemiology.

epidemiologist (ep·e·dem·e·**ol**'·o·jist). One who specializes in the study of epidemiology.

epidemiology (ep·e·dem·e·**ol**'·o·je). The study of disease, and disease attributes, in defined populations. It concerns the distribution and aetiology of disease. In the 19th century it was mainly concerned with infectious diseases such as typhoid and cholera. Now the techniques of studying disease in defined populations are widely used in non-communicable disease. Epidemiology is the scientific basis for public health and especially preventive medicine. [Gk *epi*, *demos* the people, *logos* science.]

epiderm (**ep**·e·derm). Epidermis.

epiderma (ep·e·**der**·mah). 1. Epidermis. 2. Anything abnormal growing out from the epidermis.

epidermal (ep·e·**der**·mal). Pertaining to the epidermis.

epidermatic (ep·e·der·**mat**'·ik). Referring to the epidermis.

epidermatoid (ep·e·**der**·mat·oid). Epidermoid.

epidermatomycosis (ep·e·**der**·mat·o·mi·**ko**'·sis). Dermatomycosis. [epidermis, mycosis.]

epidermatoplasty (ep·e·**der**·mat·o·plas·te). 1. Any plastic repair of tissue or replacement of skin. 2. Skin grafting in which the grafts are taken from the epidermis and the superficial layer of the corium; the Reverdin or Thiersch method of skin grafting. [epidermis, Gk *plassein* to mould.]

epidermatous (ep·e·**der**·mat·us). Epidermatic.

epidermic (ep·e·der·mik). Epidermatic.

epidermicula (ep·e·der·**mik**'·ew·lah). A very thin covering membrane such as the cuticle of the shaft of a hair. [epidermis.]

epidermidalization (ep·e·der·mid·al·i·**za**'·shun). The production by mucous cells (columnar cells) of stratified epithelium, forming a tissue of epidermal rather than of mucous type.

epidermidolysis (ep·e·der·mid·**ol**'·is·is). Epidermolysis.

epidermidosis (ep·e·der·mid·**o**'·sis). 1. A group of skin diseases which principally affect the epidermis. 2. Any irregular epithelial growth. [epidermis, Gk *-osis* condition.]

epidermis [NA] (ep·e·**der**·mis). The outer protective layer of the skin, composed of stratified pavement epithelium of ectodermal origin, fused to the underlying dermis of the skin. From within outwards, the following layers are described: stratum germinativum, or germinal layer; stratum spinosum, or prickle-cell layer, sometimes called the stratum mucosum; stratum granulosum, containing granules of keratohyalin; stratum lucidum; and stratum corneum. The 2 last-named layers are composed of dead cells. [Gk *epi, derma* skin.]

epidermitis (ep·e·der·**mi**'·tis). A condition of inflammation of the epidermis. [epidermis, Gk *-itis* inflammation.]

epidermization (ep·e·der·mi·**za**'·shun). 1. The formation of epidermis. 2. Skin grafting in which the epidermis is used.

epidermodysplasia verruciformis (ep·e·**der**·mo·dis·**pla**'·ze·ah ver·oo·se·**for**·mis). Generalized verrucosis. [epidermis, dysplasia, L *verruca* wart, *forma* form.]

epidermoid (ep·e·**der**·moid). 1. Belonging to or resembling epidermis. 2. A neoplasm, particularly of the brain or meninges, in which epidermic cells are included. [epidermis, Gk *eidos* form.]

epidermolysis (ep·e·der·**mol**·is·is). Loosening of the epidermis, usually with the development of blisters. **Epidermolysis bullosa.** Acantholysis bullosa, congenital pemphigus; an inherited affection of the skin in which vesicles or bullae arise after mild degrees of injury. The disorder does not cause systemic disturbance, and treatment is unavailing. **Epidermolysis bullosa dystrophica.** Epidermolysis in which the cleavage is lower and usually takes place at the junction of the epidermis and corium, so that not only do the lesions cause scarring but also epidermal cysts may ensue from the residual remains of rete pegs in the floors of the bullae. **Epidermolysis bullosa polydysplastica.** A severe form of epidermolysis bullosa with large, flaccid, sometimes haemorrhagic bullae, leaving atrophic scars and milia. Scar tissue may cause pseudo-webbing of the fingers or toes. Squamous epithelioma may supervene. The mucous membranes are also affected. **Epidermolysis bullosa simplex.** A form in which the bullae arise as a result of cleavage between the epidermal cells and heal without scarring. **Epidermolysis bullosa vegetans.** Epidermolysis bullosa polydysplastica with persistent vegetating masses from secondary infection. **Epidermolysis necroticans combustiformis.** Toxic epidermal necrolysis. *See* NECROLYSIS. [epidermis, Gk *lysis* a loosing.]

epidermoma (ep·e·der·**mo**'·mah). An irregular outgrowth of the skin, such as a wart. [epidermis, Gk *-oma* tumour.]

epidermomycosis (ep·e·**der**·mo·mi·**ko**'·sis). Dermatophytosis: any skin disease which is caused by a fungus. [epidermis, mycosis.]

epidermophyte (ep·e·**der**·mo·fite). A fungus of the genus *Epidermophyton.*

epidermophytid (ep·e·der·**mof**'·it·id). A skin eruption due to hypersensitivity of an individual to infection by the fungus *Epidermophyton.*

epidermophytin (ep·e·der·**mof**'·it·in). A product of *Epidermophyton* cultures producing a hypersensitivity (analogous to tuberculin); used in the treatment of epidermophytosis.

Epidermophyton (ep·e·der·**mof**'·it·on). A genus of dermatophytes, infecting skin and nails but not hair, and causing ringworm; examples are infection of the axillae or groin (dhobie itch) and athletes' foot. A monospecific genus *Epidermophyton floccosum.* [epidermis, Gk *phyton* plant.]

epidermophytosis (ep·e·**der**·mo·fi·**to**'·sis). Infection of the skin by *Epidermophyton.* The term is often incorrectly used as a synonym for dermatophytosis, but denotes a fungous infection of the skin without invasion of hair follicles, and the malady has certain sites of election. **Epidermophytosis axillaris.** Tinea axillaris. **Epidermophytosis cruris.** Tinea cruris. **Epidermophytosis interdigitalis.** Ringworm of the toes. [epidermophyte, Gk *-osis* condition.]

epidermosis (ep·e·der·**mo**'·sis). 1. A group of skin diseases which principally affect the epidermis. 2. Any irregular epithelial growth. [epidermis, Gk *-osis* condition.]

epidermotropic (ep·e·der·mo·**trop**'·ik). Being particularly attracted to epidermal tissues. [epidermis, Gk *trepein* to turn.]

epidiascope (ep·e·**di**·ah·skope). An optical apparatus similar to a projection lantern, in which solid objects, diagrams or photographs are illuminated strongly and their image focused on a screen for demonstration purposes. [Gk *epi, diaskopein* to look through.]

epididymal (ep·e·**did**·im·al). Relating or belonging to the epididymis.

epididymectomy (ep·e·did·im·**ek**'·to·me). Removal of the epididymis by surgical means. [epididymis, Gk *ektome* a cutting out.]

epididymis [NA] (ep·e·**did**·im·is). An elongated mass attached to the upper part of the testis, the main portion of which [corpus epididymidis (NA)] is composed of the first part of the efferent duct of the testis. There is an enlarged upper part [caput epididymidis (NA)] and a lower pointed end [cauda epididymidis (NA)]. [Gk *epi, didymos* twin (testis).]

epididymitis (ep·e·did·im·**i**'·tis). An inflamed condition of the epididymis. [epididymis, Gk *-itis* inflammation.]

epididymodeferentectomy (ep·e·**did**·im·o·def·er·en·**tek**'·to·me). Surgical removal of the epididymis and the vas deferens. [epididymis, deferentectomy.]

epididymodeferential (ep·e·**did**·im·o·def·er·**en**'·shal). Relating to the epididymis and the vas deferens. [epididymis, vas deferens.]

epididymo-orchitis (ep·e·**did**·im·o·or·**ki**'·tis). A condition of inflammation involving both the epididymis and the testis. [epididymitis, orchitis.]

epididymotomy (ep·e·did·im·**ot**'·o·me). Surgical incision into the epididymis, carried out usually for the relief of tension and pain. [epididymis, Gk *temnein* to cut.]

epididymovasectomy (ep·e·**did**·im·o·vas·**ek**'·to·me). Surgical removal of the epididymis and the major part of the vas deferens. [epididymis, vasectomy.]

epididymovasostomy (ep·e·**did**·im·o·vas·**os**'·to·me). Surgical anastomosis between the epididymis and the vas deferens. [epididymis, vasostomy.]

epidural (ep·e·**dewr**·al). Situated on the outside of or over the dura mater. [Gk *epi,* dura mater.]

epifascial (ep·e·**fash**·e·al). 1. On the fascia of a muscle or external to it. 2. As qualifying certain antisyphilitic injections (mercury, arsenic) which are made into the fascia lata and not into the fibres of the underlying muscle. [Gk *epi,* fascia.]

epifolliculitis (ep·e·fol·ik·ew·**li**'·tis). Inflammation of the hair follicles of the scalp. [Gk *epi,* folliculitis.]

epigamous (ep·e·**gam**·us). Denoting the theory that the sex of an individual is determined not at the time of fertilization of the ovum, but by external factors influencing the development of the embryo. [Gk *epi, gamos* marriage.]

epigaster (ep·e·**gas**·ter). The hind-gut; the embryonic basis of the colon. [Gk *epi, gaster* belly.]

epigastralgia (ep·e·gas·**tral**'·je·ah). Pain in the epigastrium. [epigastrium, Gk *algos* pain.]

epigastric (ep·e·**gas**·trik). Referring to the epigastrium.

epigastric arteries. Inferior epigastric artery [arteria epigastrica inferior (NA)]. A branch of the external iliac artery ascending on the deep surface of the lower part of the anterior abdominal wall, which it supplies. **Inferior epigastric artery, obturator branch of the [ramus obturatorius (NA)].** The anastomotic branch to the obturator artery. **Inferior epigastric artery, pubic branch of the [ramus pubicus (NA)].** A branch of the inferior epigastric artery which ramifies on the back of the pubis. It anastomoses with the pubic branch of the obturator artery, and is sometimes enlarged to become the abnormal obturator artery. **Superficial epigastric artery [arteria epigastrica superficialis (NA)].** A branch of the femoral artery to the skin and superficial fascia of the lower part of the anterior abdominal wall. **Superior epigastric artery [arteria epigastrica superior (NA)].** A terminal branch of the internal mammary artery lying in the sheath of the rectus abdominis muscle, at first behind and then within the muscle. It anastomoses with the inferior epigastric artery.

epigastric veins. Inferior epigastric vein [vena epigastrica inferior (NA)]. A tributary of the external iliac vein, from the lower abdominal wall. **Superficial epigastric vein [vena epigastrica superficialis (NA)].** A tributary of the saphenous vein from the superficial tissues of the lower part of the anterior abdominal wall. **Superior epigastric veins [venae epigastricae superiores (NA)].** Veins accompanying the artery of the same name and draining the upper part of the rectus abdominis muscle and overlying subcutaneous tissue [venae subcutaneae abdominis (NA)] into the internal mammary vein.

epigastrium (ep·e·**gas**·tre·um). The epigastric region of the abdomen. [Gk *epi, gaster* stomach.]

epigastrius (ep·e·**gas**·tre·us). A double monster, the small and incomplete parasite of which, in the form of a tumour, is attached to the epigastrium of the autosite. [see prec.]

epigastrocele (ep·e·**gas**·tro·seel). A hernia situated in the epigastric region of the abdomen. [epigastrium, Gk *kele* hernia.]

epigastrorrhaphy (**ep**·e·gas·**tror**′·af·e). Placing skin sutures in an epigastric wound and so closing the primary incision. [epigastrium, Gk *rhaphe* seam.]

epigenesis (ep·e·**jen**·es·is). 1. The occurrence of secondary or accessory symptoms which are not antagonistic to the primary symptoms. 2. The theory, now universally accepted in its strict form, that organ systems develop anew in the embryo, and are not preformed as such. [Gk *epi, genein* to produce.]

epigenetic (**ep**·e·jen·**et**′·ik). Referring or belonging to epigenesis.

epiglottectomy (**ep**·e·glot·**ek**′·to·me). Surgical removal of the epiglottis. [epiglottis, Gk *ektome* a cutting out.]

epiglottic, epiglottidean (ep·e·**glot**·ik, **ep**·e·glot·**id**′·e·an). Referring to or connected with the epiglottis.

epiglottidectomy (**ep**·e·glot·id·**ek**′·to·me). Epiglottectomy.

epiglottiditis (**ep**·e·glot·id·**i**′·tis). Inflammation of the epiglottis. [epiglottis, Gk *-itis* inflammation.]

epiglottis [NA] (ep·e·**glot**·is). A thin plate of fibrocartilage lying at the root of the tongue and in front of the entrance to the larynx. Its function is to fold back over the aperture of the larynx during the act of swallowing so that food or fluid does not pass into the larynx, trachea or bronchi. **Turban epiglottis.** Oedema of the epiglottis and aryepiglottic folds, producing the appearance of the folds of a turban. [Gk *epi, glossa* tongue.]

epiglottitis (**ep**·e·glot·**i**′·tis). Epiglottiditis.

epiglotto-hyoidean (ep·e·**glot**·o·hi·**oid**′·e·an). Applicable to both the epiglottis and the hyoid bone.

epignathous (ep·**ig**·nath·us). Having the characteristics of an epignathus.

epignathus (ep·**ig**·nath·us). A double monster of which the rudimentary acardiac parasite is attached to the maxilla of the autosite. [Gk *epi, gnathos* jaw.]

epigonal (ep·e·**go**·nal). Situated on or over a gonad or rudimentary germ gland. [Gk *epi, gone* seed.]

epiguanine (ep·e·**gwan**·een). $C_6H_7N_5O$, a purine base occurring in urine, principally in leukaemia.

epihyoid (ep·e·**hi**·oid). Situated on or over the hyoid bone. Sometimes denoting certain accessories of the thyroid gland which are situated above the geniohyoid muscle. [Gk *epi,* hyoid bone.]

epilamellar (**ep**·e·lam·**el**′·ar). On the outside of or above a basement membrane. [Gk *epi,* lamella.]

epilation (ep·il·**a**·shun). The removal of hair by the destruction of hair follicles to prevent further growth. [L *e, pilus* hair.]

epilatory (e·**pil**·at·or·e). Depilatory. [see prec.]

epilemma (ep·e·**lem**·ah). The neurolemma of fine terminal nerve fibrils. [Gk *epi, lemma* sheath.]

epilemmal (ep·e·**lem**·al). Relating to an epilemma.

epilepidoma (**ep**·e·lep·id·**o**′·mah). A tumour composed of hyperplastic tissue derived from the ectoderm (epiblast). [Gk *epi,* lepidoma.]

epilepsia (ep·il·**ep**·se·ah). Epilepsy. **Epilepsia cursiva.** Cursive epilepsy. **Epilepsia larvata.** Latent epilepsy. **Epilepsia major.** Major epilepsy. **Epilepsia media.** Latent epilepsy. **Epilepsia minor.** Minor epilepsy. **Epilepsia partialis continua.** Continuous partial epilepsy. **Epilepsia procursiva.** Cursive epilepsy. **Epilepsia retinae.** Retinal epilepsy. **Epilepsia rotatoria.** Turning movements of the body in epileptic convulsion. *See* EPILEPSY. [Gk seizure.]

epilepsy (ep·il·**ep**·se). An affection of the nervous system characterized by recurrent paroxysmal symptoms, the epileptic fit, resulting from excessive or disordered discharge of cerebral neurons. **Abdominal epilepsy.** Recurrent abdominal pain in children considered to be epileptic in origin. **Accelerative epilepsy.** Cursive epilepsy (see below). **Adversive epilepsy.** Epileptic fits beginning with turning of the head and eyes to the side away from the responsible cerebral lesion. **Affect epilepsy.** A psychosomatic state resulting from the stimulus of strong emotion, characterized by loss of colour, trembling of the limbs and hands, and sometimes leading to loss of consciousness. **Akinetic epilepsy.** Epilepsy characterized by falling without convulsion or loss of consciousness. **Centrencephalic epilepsy.** Epilepsy thought by Penfield to arise from disordered function of central cerebral structures, without anatomical lesions; idiopathic epilepsy. **Cerebellar epilepsy.** Attacks of generalized tonic spasm due to decerebrate rigidity in advanced cases of cerebellar tumour. **Continuous epilepsy.** A rare type showing major attacks and, at intervals, clonic movements. **Continuous partial epilepsy.** Long-continued epileptic clonic jerking confined to one limb or group of muscles; *Kozhevnikoff's epilepsy.* **Cortical epilepsy.** Epilepsy arising from a focus in the cerebral cortex. **Cryptogenic epilepsy.** Epilepsy of unknown cause. **Cursive epilepsy.** Epilepsy with preliminary symptoms of forward running before falling. **Diencephalic epilepsy.** Epilepsy arising from the upper brain stem and characterized by symptoms of overactivity of the autonomic nervous system. **Diurnal epilepsy.** That characterized by attacks during the daytime. **Essential epilepsy.** Any type of epilepsy not due to any obvious organic cerebral or metabolic cause. Syn: *idiopathic, true, or genuine epilepsy.* **Flicker-sensitive epilepsy.** Epileptic fits provoked by flickering lights; photogenic epilepsy. **Focal epilepsy.** Epilepsy arising from a localized area of the brain, usually in the cerebral cortex. Syn: partial epilepsy. **Frontal adversive area epilepsy.** A type of partial epilepsy in which the responsible lesion or site of neuronal discharge lies in the frontal adversive area. **Gelastic epilepsy.** Gelolepsy. **Generalized epilepsy.** Epilepsy characterized by seizures which are generalized from the start. **Genuine epilepsy.** Essential or idiopathic epilepsy. **Grand-mal epilepsy.** Major epilepsy (see below). **Idiopathic epilepsy.** 1. Epilepsy beginning in childhood or adolescence, not due to structural lesions of the brain and characterized either by grand mal without focal features, or by petit mal, or by both these forms of it; centrencephalic epilepsy. 2. Epilepsy of unknown cause; cryptogenic epilepsy. **Infantile epilepsy.** Seizures occurring in the newborn before the age of about 3 years, the upper age limit being somewhat indefinite. **Inhibitory epilepsy.** Epileptic fits characterized by loss of muscle power and tone, without convulsion. **Insular epilepsy.** A partial epileptic episode in which the neuronal discharge and lesion provoking the seizures is located in the insular area. The symptomatology is complex and consists mainly in manifestations of gustatory type and of autonomic phenomena. **Jacksonian epilepsy.** Epilepsy beginning unilaterally with clonic jerking or abnormal sensations confined to a portion of a limb or of the face, but often spreading to other structures on the same side or becoming generalized, when consciousness may be lost. Focal motor, focal sensory epilepsy. **Laryngeal epilepsy.** Laryngeal syncope. *See* SYNCOPE. **Latent epilepsy.** Epilepsy in which the unconscious stage is very brief and the movements, though automatic, appear to be voluntary. **Major epilepsy.** A form of epileptic fit in which consciousness is lost and there is generalized tonic muscular contraction followed by clonic jerking in which the tongue may be bitten. Urinary incontinence is common. After the convulsion, coma persists for a variable period. *Grand-mal epilepsy.* **Matutinal epilepsy.** Epilepsy in which the seizures occur mainly or exclusively in the morning. **Menstrual epilepsy.** Epilepsy in which the seizures occur mainly around the time of menstrual periods. **Metabolic epilepsy.** Epilepsy resulting from a metabolic disorder. **Migrainous epilepsy.** A rare form of epilepsy in which seizures alternate with typical attacks of migraine. **Masked epilepsy.** Latent epilepsy (see above). **Minor epilepsy.** Epilepsy in which the convulsive element is less marked than in major epilepsy. **Movement epilepsy.** A variety of seizure triggered off by a sudden movement. **Musicogenic epilepsy.** Epileptic fits provoked by music. **Myoclonic epilepsy.** 1. Violent jerking of one or both arms, usually in the early morning, affecting some patients with petit mal. 2. A genetically determined disease, with onset in childhood or adolescence, in which major epilepsy and myoclonus are associated with progressive dementia, ataxia and sometimes blindness, leading to death after a few years. **Nocturnal epilepsy.** Epilepsy in which the attacks occur predominantly during sleep. **Partial epilepsy.** Jacksonian epilepsy (see above). **Partial continuous epilepsy.** Continuous partial epilepsy (see above). **Petit-mal epilepsy.** A form of epilepsy characterized by abrupt loss of consciousness without falling or incontinence, and lasting for a few seconds. Convulsive movements are absent or confined to slight twitching. The onset is in childhood. **Photic epilepsy.** Photogenic epilepsy (see below). **Photogenic epilepsy.** Epilepsy induced by flickering light. **Post-traumatic epilepsy.** Epilepsy caused by head injury. **Procursive epilepsy.** Cursive epilepsy (see above). **Psychomotor epilepsy.** A form of epileptic fit characterized by clouding of consciousness and co-ordinated but inappropriate movements, often accompanied by a hallucinatory experience. **Reading epilepsy.** A form of seizure provoked by the act of silent reading. It may depend upon photic stimulation due to the jerky movement of the eyes when scanning a text, or it may be the effect of the emotional or intellectual aspects of the reading-matter. **Reflex epilepsy.** Epilepsy induced by specific external stimuli. **Renal epilepsy.** Seizures secondary to the metabolic disturbances of chronic renal insufficiency not necessarily uraemic in nature. **Retinal epilepsy.** Attacks of loss of vision due to transient retinal ischaemia (obsolete term). **Retrocursive epilepsy.** That in which an attack begins with backward movements. **Saturnine epilepsy.** Epileptic attacks as a symptom of lead encephalopathy. **Senile epilepsy.** Epilepsy developing in old age. **Sensory epilepsy.** Epilepsy characterized by paroxysmal abnormal sensations, usually somatic. **Serial epilepsy.** Frequent epileptic fits but with recovery of consciousness between fits. **Somatosensory epilepsy.** A partial epileptic attack manifested principally by subjective hallucinatory sensations resulting from neuronal discharge in the specific somatosensory cortex or its vicinity. **Startle epilepsy.** Seizures provoked by a brief, unexpected stimulus. The stimulus is usually auditory, less often tactile in nature. **Somnambulistic epilepsy.** Epilepsy associated with automatism. **Symptomatic epilepsy.** Epilepsy as the result of some known or presumed disease or focal lesion. **Tap epilepsy.** A rare type of epilepsy where attacks are provoked by unexpected contacts. **Tardive epilepsy.** Tardy epilepsy, epilepsy of late onset. **Television epilepsy.** Epileptic fits provoked by the flicker of the television tube. **Temporal-lobe epilepsy.** Epilepsy due to abnormal discharges from the temporal lobe. The fits vary from gland-mal to psychomotor epilepsy with formed auditory or visual hallucinations. **Tonic epilepsy.** Epileptic fits characterized by tonic muscle contraction only. **Traumatic epilepsy.** Post-traumatic epilepsy (see above). **Uncinate epilepsy.** A type of temporal epilepsy in which the neuronal discharge, or the provocative lesion, is located in the anteromesial part of the temporal lobe more particularly in the uncus. It is often preceded by an aura of smell. **Vasomotor epilepsy.** Epilepsy with extreme contractions of the arteries. **Versive epilepsy.** Epileptic fits beginning with turning of the eyes, head or trunk. **Vestibulogenic epilepsy.** Epilepsy provoked by disease of the vestibular apparatus. **Visual reflex epilepsy.** Epilepsy provoked by visual stimuli. [Gk *epilepsia* seizure.]

See also: BRAVAIS, JACKSON (J. H.), KOZHEVNIKOFF.

epileptic (ep·il·**ep**·tik). 1. Pertaining to or marked by epilepsy. 2. One who is liable to periodic attacks of epilepsy.

epileptiform (ep·il·**ep**·te·form). Resembling epilepsy. [epilepsy, form.]

epileptogenic, epileptogenous (ep·il·**ep**·to·**jen**′·ik, **ep**·il·ep·**toj**′·en·us). Causing epileptic attacks. **Epileptogenic focus.** A focal brain-lesion, whatever its nature, around which perexcitable neurons are prone to manifest localized epileptic discharges. [epilepsy, Gk *genein* to produce.]

epileptoid (ep·il·**ep**·toid). Having resemblance to epilepsy. [epilepsy, Gk *eidos* form.]

epileptosis (ep·il·ep·**to**′·sis). Any mental disorder which belongs to the epileptic group. [epilepsy, Gk *-osis* condition.]

epiloia (ep·il·**oi**·ah). A rare, and usually congenital, condition of mental deficiency with associated tumours of the kidney and heart, adenoma sebaceum and tuberous sclerosis of the brain. Epileptic attacks often occur. *See* TUBEROSE, TUBEROUS SCLEROSIS.

epilose (ep·il·oze). Bald; without hair. [L *e*, *pilus* hair.]

epilymph (ep·e·limf). Perilymph; the fluid, identical in substance with the cerebrospinal fluid, which fills the bony labyrinth and separates it from the membranous labyrinth of the ear. [Gk *epi*, lymph.]

epimandibular (ep·e·man·**dib**′·ew·lar). On or above the mandible. [Gk *epi*, mandible.]

epimenorrhagia (ep·e·men·o·**ra**′·je·ah). Excessively profuse menstruation occurring at abnormally short intervals, a condition often present at the menopause. [Gk *epi*, menorrhagia.]

epimenorrhoea (ep·e·men·o·**re**′·ah). Menstruation occurring at abnormally short intervals. [Gk *epi*, menorrhoea.]

epimer (**ep**·e·mer). One of a pair of isomeric substances which differ only in the positioning of H- and OH- attached to an asymmetric carbon atom. [see foll.]

epimere (**ep**·e·meer). In embryology, the dorsal muscle-forming mass of tissue derived from the myotome of a mesodermal somite. [Gk *epi*, *meros* part.]

epimerization (ep·e·mer·i·**za**′·shun). In organic chemistry, the formation of isomers (epimers) by the change-over in position of an H- and OH- about an asymmetric carbon atom, e.g. in carbohydrates. [Gk *epi*, *meros* part.]

epimorphosis (ep·e·mor·**fo**′·sis). Repair of the injured tissues of an organism and regeneration of any destroyed portion by proliferation of cells. [Gk *epi*, *morphe* form.]

epimyocardium (ep·e·mi·o·**kar**′·de·um). Incompletely differentiated tissue in the embryo which develops into the epicardium and myocardium. [Gk *epi*, *mys* muscle, *kardia* heart.]

Epimys (**ep**·e·mis). *Rattus*; a very large genus of rodents, the rats. [Gk *epi*, *mys* mouse.]

epimysium (ep·e·**mis**·e·um). The connective tissue which surrounds and holds together the bundles of fibres in striped muscle. [Gk *epi*, *mys* muscle.]

epinephral (ep·e·**nef**·ral). Suprarenal. [Gk *epi*, *nephros* kidney.]

epinephrectomy (ep·e·nef·**rek**′·to·me). Surgical excision of the suprarenal glands. [Gk *epi*, *nephros* kidney, *ektome* a cutting out.]

epinephrinaemia (ep·e·nef·rin·**e**′·me·ah). An excess of epinephrine in the blood. [epinephrine, Gk *haima* blood.]

epinephrine (ep·e·**nef**·reen). Adrenaline BP 1958. [Gk *epi*, *nephros* kidney.]

epinephritis (ep·e·nef·**ri**′·tis). Inflammation of a suprarenal gland; hypernephritis. [Gk *epi*, *nephros* kidney, *-itis* inflammation.]

epinephroma (ep·e·nef·**ro**′·mah). Hypernephroma. [Gk *epi*, *nephros* kidney, *-oma* tumour.]

epinephros (ep·e·**nef**·ros). The suprarenal gland. *See* GLAND. [Gk *epi*, *nephros* kidney.]

epineural (ep·e·**newr**·al). 1. In embryology, arising from or attached to the neural arch of a vertebra. 2. Situated on the neural arch of a vertebra, e.g. a process. [Gk *epi, neuron* nerve.]

epineurial (ep·e·**newr**·e·al). Relating or belonging to the epineurium.

epineurium (ep·e·**newr**·e·um). The sheath of connective tissue which binds together the bundles of fibres composing a nerve trunk. [Gk *epi, neuron* nerve.]

epinosic (ep·e·**no**·sik). Referring to a compensatory benefit obtained after or in the course of an illness. [see foll.]

epinosis (ep·e·no·sis). A state of imaginary illness or of disordered mentality complicating a primary illness. [Gk *epi, nosos* disease.]

Epioestriol (ep·e·e·stre·ol). BP Commission approved name for oestra-1,3,5(10)-triene-3,16β,17β-triol; a derivative of oestratriol employed in the form of a cream to reduce excessive sebaceous gland activity which often gives rise to acne vulgaris. It can be used in the male because it has no other oestrogenic effects.

epionychium (**ep**·e·on·**ik'**·e·um). Eponychium.

epiorchium (ep·e·**or**·ke·um). The visceral layer of the tunica vaginalis testis. [Gk *epi, orchis* testis.]

epiotic (ep·e·**ot**·ik). 1. In man, that part of the temporal bone which is the centre of ossification for the mastoid portion. 2. On the temporal bone, just above the ear. 3. On the cartilage of the ear. [Gk *epi, ous* ear.]

epiparonychia (**ep**·e·par·on·**ik'**·e·ah). Simultaneous eponychia and paronychia.

epipastic (ep·e·**pas**·tik). A dusting-powder. [Gk *epipassein* to sprinkle over.]

epipharyngitis (**ep**·e·far·in·**ji'**·tis). Inflammation of the nasal part of the pharynx. [epipharynx, Gk *-itis* inflammation.]

epipharynx (ep·e·**far**·ingx). The nasal part of the pharynx. [Gk *epi*, pharynx.]

epiphenomenon (**ep**·e·fen·**om'**·en·on). A symptom or sequel of a disease that is not invariably present or necessarily associated with the disease; an unusual occurrence in the course of a disease. [Gk *epi*, phenomenon.]

epiphora (e·**pif**·or·ah). Continuous accumulation and overflow of tears, the result of excessive secretion or obstruction of the lacrimal passages. [Gk downflow.]

epiphrenal (ep·e·**fre**·nal). Above the diaphragm. [Gk *epi, phren* diaphragm.]

epiphylactic (**ep**·e·fil·**ak'**·tik). Pertaining to or characterized by epiphylaxis.

epiphylaxis (**ep**·e·fil·**ax'**·is). Therapeutic reinforcement (generally by vaccine or similar therapy) of the natural defences of the body against infection. [Gk *epi*, phylaxis.]

epiphyseal (ep·e·**fiz**·e·al). Pertaining to or having the characteristics of an epiphysis. **Epiphyseal dysplasia multiplex.** Occurring mainly in the second decade. The epiphyses of the long bones are stippled or fragmented, as seen also in infantile hypothyroidism. **Epiphyseal stapling.** Epiphysiodesis.

epiphyseitis (ep·e·fiz·e·**i'**·tis). Epiphysitis.

epiphyseodesis (ep·e·**fiz**·e·o·**de'**·sis). Epiphysiodesis.

epiphyseolysis (**ep**·e·fiz·e·**ol'**·is·is). Separation or loosening of an epiphysis from the shaft of the bone. [epiphysis, Gk *lysis* a loosing.]

epiphyseopathy (**ep**·e·fiz·e·**op'**·ath·e). 1. Any disorder of an epiphysis. 2. Any disorder of the pineal body (epiphysis cerebri). [epiphysis, Gk *pathos* disease.]

epiphysial (ep·e·**fiz**·e·al). Epiphyseal.

epiphysiodesis (ep·e·**fiz**·e·o·**de'**·sis). An operation to obliterate an epiphysis. [epiphysis, Gk *desis* a binding.]

epiphysioid (ep·e·**fiz**·e·oid). Applied to carpal and tarsal bones that develop from centres of ossification in the same way as do epiphyses. [epiphysis, Gk *eidos* form.]

epiphysiolysis (**ep**·e·fiz·e·**ol'**·is·is). Epiphyseolysis.

epiphysiopathy (**ep**·e·fiz·e·**op'**·ath·e). Epiphyseopathy.

epiphysis [NA] (ep·**if**·is·is). A secondary bone-forming centre attached to a bone and separated from it by cartilage. After a certain number of years, different for each epiphysis, it becomes ossified and takes its place as an integral part of the main bone. **Epiphysis cerebri.** The pineal body of the thalamencephalon. **Stippled epiphysis.** An abnormality of epiphyseal bone in which there is a peculiar mottled appearance in x-rays. [Gk *epi, phyein* to grow.]

epiphysitis (**ep**·e·fiz·**i'**·tis). A condition of inflammation of an epiphysis. **Epiphysitis juvenilis.** Osteochondrosis of the navicular bone. **Vertebral epiphysitis.** Osteochondrosis of the vertebrae. [epiphysis, Gk *-itis* inflammation.]

epiphyte (**ep**·e·fite). 1. A vegetable parasite growing on the surface of the body, e.g. a fungus. 2. A vegetable organism growing on another plant or a tree, but not as a parasite; e.g. moss. [Gk *epi, phyton* plant.]

epiphytic (ep·e·**fi**·tik). Pertaining to or caused by an epiphyte.

epipial (ep·e·**pi**·al). On the pia mater of the brain or spinal cord. [Gk *epi*, pia mater.]

epiplasm (**ep**·e·plazm). That portion of the cytoplasm of an ascus in the Ascomycetes which is not used up in the production of ascospores. [Gk *epi*, plasm.]

epipleural (ep·e·**ploor**·al). 1. On a rib or on the area of the ribs. 2. On the side of the thorax. [Gk *epi, pleura* rib.]

epiplexus (ep·e·**plex**·us). The choroid plexus of the 4th ventricle. [Gk *epi, plexein* to interlace.]

epiplocele (ep·**ip**·lo·seel). A hernia containing a portion of omentum. [Gk *epiploon* caul, *kele* hernia.]

epiplo-ectomy (**ep**·ip·lo·**ek'**·to·me). Omentectomy. [Gk *epiploon* caul, *ektome* a cutting out.]

epiplo-enterocele (**ep**·ip·lo·**en'**·ter·o·seel). A hernia in which there is a loop of intestine and a certain amount of omentum. [Gk *epiploon* caul, enterocele.]

epiploic (ep·ip·**lo**·ik). Relating or belonging to the omentum. [Gk *epiploon* caul.]

epiplo-ischiocele (**ep**·ip·lo·**is'**·ke·o·seel). Hernia of the omentum through the greater sciatic notch. [Gk *epiploon* caul, ischiocele.]

epiploitis (**ep**·ip·lo·**i'**·tis). Omentitis. [Gk *epiploon* caul, *-itis* inflammation.]

epiplomerocele (**ep**·ip·lo·**me'**·ro·seel). A femoral hernia that contains a portion of omentum. [Gk *epiploon* caul, merocele.]

epiplomphalocele (ep·ip·**lom**·fal·o·seel). Umbilical hernia containing a part of the omentum. [Gk *epiploon* caul, omphalocele.]

epiploon (ep·ip·**lo**·on). The omentum. [Gk caul.]

epiplopexy (**ep**·ip·lo·**pex'**·e). Omentopexy. [Gk *epiploon* caul, *pexis* fixation.]

epiploplasty (**ep**·ip·lo·plas·te). In plastic surgery of the abdomen, the covering of raw surfaces with pieces taken from the omentum. [Gk *epiploon* caul, *plassein* to mould.]

epiplorrhaphy (ep·ip·**lor**·af·e). Omentorrhaphy. [Gk *epiploon* caul, *rhaphe* seam.]

epiplosarcomphalocele (**ep**·ip·lo·sar·kom·**fal'**·o·seel). A hernial protrusion of omentum, usually umbilical, the skin over which is ulcerated so that the swelling fungates as a raw mass. [Gk *epiploon* caul, *sarx* flesh, *omphalos* navel, *kele* hernia.]

epiploscheocele (ep·ip·**los**·ke·o·seel). A scrotal hernia the main content of which is a portion of omentum. [Gk *epiploon* caul, oscheocele.]

epipteric (ep·ip·**ter**·ik). Above or near the pterion. [Gk *epi*, pterion.]

epipygus (ep·e·**pi**·gus). Pygomelus. [Gk *epi, pyge* buttocks.]

epirotulian (**ep**·e·ro·**tew'**·le·an). On the patella. [Gk *epi*, L *rotula* little wheel.]

episarcidium (**ep**·e·sar·**sid'**·e·um). Anasarca. [Gk *epi, sarx* flesh.]

episclera (ep·e·**skle**·rah). The free connective tissue between the sclera and the conjunctiva. [Gk *epi*, sclera.]

episcleral (ep·e·**skleer**·al). 1. Referring to the episclera. 2. On the sclera of the eye.

episcleral arteries [arteriae episclerales (NA)]. *See* OPHTHALMIC ARTERY.

episcleral veins [venae episclerales (NA)]. Veins of the deep part of the pericorneal conjunctiva.

episcleritis, episclerotitis (**ep**·e·skler·**i'**·tis, **ep**·e·skler·ot·**i'**·tis). 1. An inflamed condition of the outer surface of the sclera. 2. An inflamed condition of the tissues lying immediately over the sclera. **Episcleritis periodica fugax.** Hyperaemia of the sclera and the conjunctiva overlying it. The condition develops suddenly, is transient and is liable to recur. [Gk *epi*, sclera, *-itis* inflammation.]

episiocele (ep·is·e·o·seel). Hernia occurring in the vulvar region. [Gk *episeion* pudenda, *kela* hernia.]

episioclisia (ep·is·e·o·kli′·ze·ah). Surgical occlusion of the vulva. [Gk *episeion* pudenda, *kleiein* to shut up.]

episio-elytrorrhaphy (ep·is·e·o·el·it·ror′·af·e). The suturing of a longitudinal fold in the vagina so that it and the vulva are narrowed to give support to a prolapsed uterus; in most cases there is rupture of the perineum as the initial lesion. [Gk *episeion* pudenda, elytrorrhaphy.]

episiohaematoma (ep·is·e·o·he·mat·o′·mah). A haematoma or haematocele of the vulva or pudenda. [Gk *episeion* pudenda, haematoma.]

episioitis (ep·is·e·o·i′·tis). An inflamed condition of the pudenda. [Gk *episeion* pudenda, *-itis* inflammation.]

episioperineoplasty (ep·is·e·o·per·in·e′·o·plas·te). A plastic operation for repair of the perineum and the vulva. [Gk *episeion* pudenda, perineum, *plassein* to mould.]

episioperineorrhaphy (ep·is·e·o·per·in·e·or′·af·e). The suturing of a lacerated perineum and vulva to give support to a prolapsed uterus. [Gk *episeion* pudenda, perineorrhaphy.]

episioplasty (ep·is·e·o·plas·te). 1. Plastic repair of the vulva. 2. Any plastic operation carried out in the pudendal region. [Gk *episeion* pudenda, *plassein* to mould.]

episiorrhagia (ep·is·e·o·ra′·je·ah). Vulvar haemorrhage. [Gk *episeion* pudenda, *rhegnynai* to burst forth.]

episiorrhaphy (ep·is·e·or′·af·e). The suturing of lacerations of the labia majora or the pudenda. [Gk *episeion* pudenda, *rhaphe* suture.]

episiostenosis (ep·is·e·o·sten·o′·sis). Narrowing or contraction of the pudendal cleft. [Gk *episeion* pudenda, *stenosis* a narrowing.]

episiotomy (ep·is·e·ot′·o·me). Lateral incision of the orifice of the vagina to prevent teating of the perineum during child-birth. [Gk *episeion* pudenda, *temnein* to cut.]

episode (ep·is·ode). A separate or unusual incident occurring in the normal course of events. **Psycholeptic episode.** In psychological medicine, a strongly-marked psychic experience which obtains and retains a hold on the patient's mind to the extent that he believes it to be responsible for his disordered condition and cannot free himself from its influence. [Gk *epeisodion* a coming in besides.]

episome (ep·e·some). A genetic element of bacteria, additional to the normal genome, which can replicate either autonomously or as part of the bacterial chromosome, e.g. the sex factor F, and the DNA of certain temperate bacteriophages. *See* PLASMID, of which it is a category. [Gk *epi*, *soma* body.]

epispadia (ep·e·spa·de·ah). Epispadias.

epispadias (ep·e·spa·de·as). A congenital deformity in which the urethra opens on the dorsum of the glans penis or the penis. **Female epispadias.** The condition in which the upper wall of the female urethra is cleft. [Gk *epi*, *spadon* a rent.]

epispastic (ep·e·spas·tik). 1. Inducing a serous discharge or a blister. 2. A blistering agent. [Gk *epi*, *spastikos* drawing in.]

epispinal (ep·e·spi·nal). 1. Situated on the vertebral column. 2. Situated on a spine or any structure like a spine. [Gk *epi*, spine.]

episplenitis (ep·e·splen·i′·tis). A condition of inflammation of the tunica albuginea of the spleen. [Gk *epi*, spleen, *-itis* inflammation.]

epistasis (ep·is·tas·is). 1. The suppression of a secretion or discharge. 2. A film or pellicle which forms on the surface of urine after it has been left standing for a time. [Gk a stopping, scum.]

epistatic (ep·is·tat·ik). In mendelian heredity, a term applied to characters which override the appearance of other characters determined by genes at other loci. [Gk *epistatos* standing over.]

epistaxis (ep·e·stax·is). Bleeding from the nose. It may be due to a local disease of the nasal passages, or sometimes occurs as a manifestation of a general disease, as in the early stages of acute fevers and in some of the blood diseases, and also in high blood pressure from any cause. [Gk a dropping.]

See also: GULL.

episternal (ep·e·ster·nal). 1. Relating to the episternum. 2. Situated on or over the sternum.

episternum (ep·e·ster·num). The manubrium sterni. [Gk *epi*, sternum.]

episthotonos, episthotonus (ep·is·thot·on·os, ep·is·thot·on·us). Emprosthotonos. [Gk *epi*, *tenein* to stretch.]

episylvian (ep·e·sil·ve·an). Situated above the lateral sulcus of the cerebral hemisphere (Sylvius' fissure). [Gk *epi*, Sylvius' fissure.]

epitarsus (ep·e·tar·sus). A congenital abnormality of the conjunctiva; a fold of it extends from the fornix to a point near the margin of the lid. [Gk *epi*, tarsus.]

epitela (ep·e·te·lah). The transparent white substance of which the superior medullary velum of the 4th ventricle is composed (Vieussens' valve). [Gk *epi*, L *tela* web.]

epitendineum (ep·e·ten·din′·e·um). The white fibrous tissue which surrounds a tendon. [Gk *epi*, tendon.]

epithalamic (ep·e·thal·am′·ik). 1. Referring to the epithalamus. 2. Applied to any structure which is situated on the thalamus.

epithalamus [NA] (ep·e·thal·am·us). That portion of the thalamencephalon made up of the pineal body, the habenula, the habenular commissure and the trigonum habenulae. [Gk *epi*, thalamus.]

epithalaxia (ep·e·thal·ax′·e·ah). The scaling off of epithelium or of epithelial cells, particularly of the mucous coat of the intestine. [epithelium, Gk *allaxis* a shedding.]

epithelia (ep·e·the·le·ah). 1. Plural of epithelium. 2. Cells forming epithelium.

epithelial (ep·e·the·le·al). Pertaining to or composed of epithelium.

epithelioblastoma (ep·e·the·le·o·blas·to′·mah). Tumours composed of primitive epithelial cells. [epithelium, blastoma.]

epithelioceptor (ep·e·the·le·o·sep′·tor). That specialized constituent of a gland cell to which the stimulus from the terminal expansion of a nerve fibril is applied. [epithelium, L *recipere* to receive.]

epitheliochorial (ep·e·the·le·o·kor′·e·al). Describing the form of placentation in which there is apposition but no fusion of fetal membranes to the uterine mucosa. [epithelium, chorium.]

epitheliofibril (ep·e·the·le·o·fi′·bril). Any one of the fibrils present in the protoplasm of certain epithelial cells, and often passing from one cell to another in protoplasmic bridges.

epitheliogenetic (ep·e·the·le·o·jen·et′·ik). Originating in or caused by abnormal multiplication of epithelial cells. [epithelium, Gk *genein* to produce.]

epitheliogenic (ep·e·the·le·o·jen′·ik). Productive of epithelium. [see prec.]

epithelioglandular (ep·e·the·le·o·glan′·dew·lar). Belonging to glandular epithelium.

epithelioid (ep·e·the·le·oid). Having resemblance to epithelium. [epithelium, Gk *eidos* form.]

epitheliolysis (ep·e·the·le·ol′·is·is). The destruction of epithelial cells caused by lysins. [see foll.]

epitheliolytic (ep·e·the·le·o·lit′·ik). Referring to epitheliolysis; able to destroy, or causing destruction of epithelial cells. [epithelium, Gk *lysis* a loosing.]

epithelioma (ep·e·the·le·o′·mah) (pl. *epitheliomata*). A carcinoma arising from squamous or transitional epithelium or their derivatives, such as that found in the skin, oesophagus and external genital organs, or from areas of metaplasia in regions normally lined by simple forms of epithelium, such as stomach, neck of the uterus or bronchus. **Epithelioma adamantinum.** Adamantinoma. **Epithelioma adenoides cysticum.** A rodent ulcer in which a glandular pattern is pronounced. **Basal-cell epithelioma.** Basal-cell carcinoma; a general term for locally malignant epithelial tumours arising, in the case of skin, from the basal cells of the epidermis, and including the rodent ulcer. **Benign calcifying epithelioma** (of Malherbe). Found on the neck and arms and situated deep in the dermis. It often calcifies or ossifies. The squamous cells gradually lose their ability to stain, and appear as ghost cells which may eventually calcify. **Epithelioma caniculatum.** A plantar epithelioma with multiple sinuses and an offensive greasy discharge. **Chorionic epithelioma.** Chorionic carcinoma, chorio-epithelioma; a very malignant carcinoma arising from the chorionic villi in the uterus and, rarely, in a teratoma of mediastinum or testis. **Columnar epithelioma, Cylindrical epithelioma.** A carcinoma derived from columnar epithelium, as in the bowel or body of the uterus; adenocarcinoma. **Familial self-healing squamous epitheliomata.** Multiple tumours on the face, resembling kerato-acanthoma, which are shed spontaneously leaving depressed scars. The inheritance is autosomal dominant. **Intra-epidermal epithelioma.** A spread of cancer cells between the epidermal cells of the skin, as in Paget's disease of the nipple. **Epithelioma molluscum.** A term sometimes used for an epithelioma which imitates closely molluscum contagiosum; found on the face, it is always benign and is often self-healing. **Multiple benign cystic epithelioma.** Epithelioma adenoides cysticum (see above). **Epithelioma myxomatoides psammosum.** A cancer which shows much mucoid degeneration and calcification; common in the ovary or uterus. **Squamous-cell epithelioma.** Squamous-cell carcinoma. *See* CARCINOMA. **Tubular epithelioma.** Columnar epithelioma (see above). [epithelium, Gk *-oma* tumour.]

epitheliomatosis (ep·e·**the**·le·o·mat·**o′**·sis). The condition in which epitheliomata are present, or tend to develop. [epithelioma, Gk *-osis* condition.]

epitheliomatous (**ep**·e·the·le·**o′**·mat·us). Pertaining to or having the characteristics of an epithelioma.

epitheliosis (**ep**·e·the·le·**o′**·sis). 1. Term used by Axenfeld to describe the active proliferating changes of the epithelium of the conjunctiva in trachoma. 2. Any viral infection with a special affinity for epithelium, e.g. smallpox and vaccinia. 3. Precancerous intraductal proliferation of duct epithelium of the breast. Found in Paget's disease of the breast and in 20 per cent of all breast cancers (Cheatle). **Epitheliosis desquamativa conjunctivae.** A condition resembling trachoma, reported from the Samoan islands. [epithelium, Gk *-osis* condition.]

epithelite (ep·e·**the**·lite). A name sometimes given to the stage of radiation reaction characterized by moist desquamation of the skin, or membrane formation on a mucous membrane. [epithelium.]

epithelitis (**ep**·e·the·**li′**·tis). Inflammation and overgrowth of the mucosal epithelium, e.g. as a result of an x-ray or radium burn. [epithelium, Gk *-itis* inflammation.]

epithelium [NA] (ep·e·**the**·le·um) (pl. *epithelia*). 1. A closely-packed sheet of cells arranged in one or more layers, the component cells of which usually adhere to each other along their edges and surfaces. It covers the external surface of the entire body and lines all hollow structures within the body with the exception of blood vessels and lymphatics, whose lining is properly called an *endothelium,* and serous cavities, whose lining is a *mesothelium.* Epithelia are mostly of ectodermal or entodermal origin, but those of the genito-urinary system arise from the mesoderm. They are classified primarily into *simple* or one-layered, and *stratified* or multilayered. Simple epithelia include *squamous, cuboidal, columnar* and *ciliated columnar* types, all of whose constituent cells touch underlying connective-tissue cells. Stratified epithelia comprise *stratified squamous, stratified columnar* and *stratified columnar ciliated* varieties, only some of whose constituent cells touch underlying connective tissue. *Pseudostratified* and *pseudostratified ciliated* epithelia appear superficially to be multilayered, but in fact all the cells reach the underlying connective tissue. 2. The pigment epithelium of the retina. 3. The outer layer of the retina. **Ciliated epithelium.** Epithelial cells with fine hair-like strands on their free borders. Their movement can pass particles upward in the respiratory tract and thus act protectively. In the fallopian tubes they aid propulsion of the ovum towards the uterus. **Epithelium of the cornea [epithelium anterius corneae (NA)].** A layer of stratified epithelium covering the front of the cornea and continuous on all sides with the epithelium of the conjunctiva. **Germinal epithelium.** 1. The layer of epithelial cells covering the free surface of the ovary at all stages of development, as well as in the adult. 2. The layer of epithelial cells covering the developing testis of the early embryo. **Glandular epithelium.** Epithelium containing many glandular cells. **Heterotopic epithelium.** Epithelium characteristic of one organ present in another organ, e.g. intestinal epithelium in the stomach. **Epithelium of the lens [epithelium lentis (NA)].** Transparent columnar cells covering the front of the lens. **Mucous epithelium.** 1. A layer of epithelial cells among which numerous goblet cells are to be found; each goblet cell is a mucus-secreting gland. 2. The rete mucosum, or deeper proliferating layer, of a stratified squamous epithelium. **Nerve epithelium.** Sensory epithelium (see below). **Pavement epithelium.** A sheet of flattened scale-like cells adhering edge-to-edge. **Protective epithelium.** Epithelium with a protective function, e.g. the skin. **Respiratory epithelium.** That which lines the respiratory tract. **Epithelium of the semicircular duct [epithelium ductus semicircularis (NA)].** The epithelial lining of the semicircular canal; it is for the most part composed of a single layer of polygonal cells, but it is thickened and specialized at the ampullary crest. **Sense epithelium, Sensory epithelium.** That related to the special sense organs. **Squamous epithelium.** Pavement epithelium (see above). **Subcapsular epithelium.** Epithelium on the posterior surface of the anterior capsule of the lens. **Tegumentary epithelium.** Epidermis. **Transitional epithelium.** The term used to describe the stratified columnar epithelium of the urinary passages. [Gk *epi, thele* nipple.]

epithelization (**ep**·e·the·li·**za′**·shun). The process of being converted into epithelium.

epithesis (ep·**ith**·es·is). 1. The correcting of a deformity of a limb or other structure by surgical means. 2. A mechanical appliance such as a splint for the correction of deformity. [Gk a putting on.]

Epithiazide (ep·e·**thi**·az·ide). BP Commission approved name for 6 - chloro - 3,4 - dihydro - 3 - (2,2,2 - trifluoroethylthiomethyl) - benzo - 1,2,4 - thiadiazine - 7 - sulphonamide 1,1 - dioxide; it is used in the treatment of hypertension.

epitonic (ep·e·**ton**·ik). 1. Overstrained or overstretched. 2. Unnaturally tense. 3. Characterized by great tension or unusual tightness. [see foll.]

epitonos, epitonus (ep·e·to·nos, ep·**e**·**to**·nus). 1. The state of being abnormally tense. 2. Descriptive of something stretched or exhibiting extreme tension between one point and another. [Gk *epi, tonos* tone.]

epitope (ep·e·tope). Antigenic determinant of known structure.

epitrichial (ep·e·**trik**·e·al). Having relation to the epitrichium.

epitrichium (ep·e·**trik**·e·um). 1. The outer layer or periderm of flattened cells of the embryonic epidermis. 2. The layer of epidermal cells covering the unerupted hair shaft. [Gk *epi, trichion* small hair.]

epitrochanteric (**ep**·e·tro·kan·**ter′**·ik). Situated on or above the trochanters. [Gk *epi,* trochanter.]

epitrochlea (ep·e·**trok**·le·ah). The medial (inner) epicondyle of the humerus. [Gk *epi,* trochlea.]

epitrochlear (ep·e·**trok**·le·ar). Relating to the epitrochlea; applied to the superficial group of the flexor muscles of the forearm which are attached to the epitrochlea.

epitrochleo-anconeus muscle (ep·e·**trok**·le·o·an·**ko′**·ne·us musl). An occasional muscle of the elbow, from the humerus to the olecranon process.

epituberculosis (**ep**·e·tew·ber·kew·**lo′**·sis). 1. A condition of hyperaemia and inflammation infiltrating round about a tuberculous focus; epituberculous infiltration. 2. A benign condition of consolidation which may affect the whole lobe of a lung of a tuberculous infant. Recovery is the rule. 3. Paratuberculosis. [Gk *epi,* tuberculosis.]

epiturbinate (ep·e·**ter**·bin·ate). The soft tissues which cover the nasal conchae. [Gk *epi,* L *turbo* spinning top.]

epitympanic (**ep**·e·tim·**pan′**·ik). In the upper part of, or above, the middle ear (tympanum). [Gk *epi,* tympanum.]

epitympanitis (ep·e·tim·pan·i'·tis). Inflammation of the middle ear involving the region of the attic or epitympanum. [epitympanum, Gk *-itis* inflammation.]

epitympanum (ep·e·tim·pan·um). The epitympanic recess; the attic: that part of the middle ear which is above the level of the tympanic membrane, and which contains part of the malleus and most of the incus. [Gk *epi*, tympanum.]

epitype (ep·e·type). Generic term for a family of related epitopes.

epityphlitis (ep·e·tif·li'·tis). 1. Appendicitis. 2. Paratyphlitis; inflammation affecting the connective tissue near the caecum. [epityphlon, Gk *-itis* inflammation.]

epityphlon (ep·e·tif·lon). The vermiform appendix. *See* APPENDIX. [Gk *epi, typhlon* caecum.]

epivertebral (ep·e·ver·te·bral). Situated on or over a vertebra. [Gk *epi*, vertebra.]

epizoic (ep·e·zo·ik). 1. Pertaining to epizoa. 2. Growing parasitically on living animals. 3. Epizootic. [epizoon.]

epizoicide (ep·e·zo·is·ide). Any preparation or other agent destructive of epizoa. [epizoon, L *caedere* to kill.]

epizoon (ep·e·zo·on) (pl. *epizoa*). An external animal parasite. [Gk *epi, zoon* animal.]

epizoonosis (ep·e·zo·on·o'·sis). An affection of the skin due to the presence of external animal parasites. [epizoon, Gk *nosos* disease.]

epizootic (ep·e·zo·ot'·ik). 1. An outbreak of disease affecting a large number of animals within a short time. 2. Relating to such a disease. [Gk *epi, zoon* animal.]

epizootiology (ep·e·zo·ot·e·ol'·o·je). The science and study of epizootic disease. [epizoon, Gk *logos* science.]

épluchage (a·ploosh·ahzh). Cutting away from an infected wound all the bruised and morbid tissues. Cf. DÉBRIDEMENT. [Fr. paring.]

epoikic (ep·oi·kik). Applied to diseases which occur within a limited locality or in a particular household. [Gk *epi, oikos* house.]

eponychia (ep·on·ik·e·ah). A blister affecting the eponychium.

eponychium [NA] (ep·on·ik·e·um). 1. The thin narrow cuticular fold of skin that overlaps the proximal part of the lunula of a nail. 2. The area of sensitive flesh (quick) below the nail. 3. In embryology, the horny layer of epidermis which is built up from the epitrichium to form the fetal nail. [Gk *epi, onyx* nail.]

eponym (ep·on·im). In medicine, a disease, procedure or anatomical structure of any kind that bears a person's name, generally that of the one who discovered or first described it, e.g. Hodgkin's disease, Syme's operation, duct of Cuvier. [Gk *eponymos* named after.]

eponymous (ep·on·e·mus). 1. Referring to or of the nature of an eponym. 2. Named after a particular person.

epoöphorectomy (ep·o·of·or·ek'·to·me). The removal by surgical means of the epoöphoron. [epoöphoron, Gk *ektome* a cutting out.]

epoöphoron [NA] (ep·o·of·or·on). A rudimentary structure situated between the ovary and the uterine tube. It consists of several short tubules, all that remains of the mesonephros; the parovarium. [Gk *epi, oöphoron* ovary.]

epostoma (ep·os·to·mah). Any projecting bony outgrowth; an exostosis. [Gk *epi, osteon* bone, *-oma* tumour.]

epsilon (ep·sil·on). The fifth letter of the Greek alphabet ε. ϵ_H. The type of human embryonal haemoglobin which contains only the epsilon type of polypeptide chains; haemoglobin Gower-1. **Epsilon chain.** *See* CHAIN.

Epstein, Albert Arthur (b. 1880). New York physician.

Epstein's nephrosis. Nephrosis considered due to a metabolic dyscrasia in which the plasma protein has undergone a change in composition and is got rid of by the kidneys which play a secondary part.

Epstein's syndrome. The nephrotic syndrome.

Epstein, Alois (b. 1849). Prague paediatrician.

Epstein's pearls, or sign. Tiny, whitish-yellow raised masses seen on the hard palate in newborn babies.

Epstein's symptom. The imperfect movement of the upper lid on looking downwards, which occurs in certain types of neuropathic children; probably of the same aetiology as von Graefe's sign in dysthyroidism.

Epstein, Michael Anthony. Bristol pathologist.

Epstein-Barr virus, EB virus. A herpes virus, antigenetically distinct from other members of the group, which is the cause of infectious mononucleosis (glandular fever). It is also found in about 5 per cent of cells cultured from the tumours of Burkitt's lymphoma. Antibody to the virus is widely distributed in man and its exact role in disease, other than in glandular fever, has yet to be determined.

epulis (ep·ew·lis). A small hard fibrous or sarcomatous tumour commonly affecting the gum or alveolar process of the jaw and generally having its origin in the periosteum. **Epulis fibromatosa.** Fibroma arising from the alveolar periosteum. **Epulis fissurata.** Hypertrophy of the gums, taking a bifid form. **Epulis gigantocellularis.** Giant-cell tumour of the alveolar process. **Epulis granulomatosa.** Local overgrowth of gum epithelium due to irritation. **Malignant epulis, Myeloid epulis.** A giant-cell sarcoma affecting the jaw. [Gk *epi, oulon* gum.]

epulo-erectile (ep·ew·lo·e·rek'·tile). Erectile and resembling an epulis.

epulofibroma (ep·ew·lo·fi·bro'·mah). A fibrous epulis. [epulis, fibroma.]

epuloid (ep·ew·loid). Having resemblance to an epulis. [epulis, Gk *eidos* form.]

epulosis (ep·ew·lo·sis). 1. The process of healing by cicatrization. 2. A cicatrix or scar. [Gk *epi, oule* scar, *-osis* condition.]

epulotic (ep·ew·lot·ik). 1. Referring to epulosis. 2. Cicatrizing. 3. An agent which promotes the healing over or the forming of skin or a cicatrix on a sore or wound. [see prec.]

equalization (e·kwal·i·za'·shun). The action of making equal. **Pressure equalization.** A term applied to the equalization of the pressure in the external and middle ears after they have been altered by changes in the barometric pressure, such as occur in rapid descents in aircraft. Equalization is brought about by auto-inflation, eustachian catheterization or paracentesis auris, or by the use of a decompression chamber. [L *aequare* to make equal.]

equate (e·kwate). 1. To render things equal. 2. To express in the form of an equation. 3. The faculty of the eye to combine 2 colours, obtaining the impression of a third, a fact which is taken advantage of in colour-printing. [L *aequare* to make equal.]

equation (e·kwa·shun). 1. The expression in symbols of an equivalence or equality. 2. The mathematical representation of a scientific law. 3. The statement of a chemical or physical change, showing on one side the new condition, on the other the condition prior to the change. **Chemical equation.** A system of formula whereby the participants in a chemical reaction are equated on the left with their products on the right. **Personal equation.** The factor of error which must be taken into consideration in scientific observations, due to the psychological and physical peculiarities of the observer. [see prec.]

See also: GIBBS, HASSELBALSH, HENDERSON.

equator (e·kwa·tor). A line circumscribed round a sphere midway between its poles, dividing it into 2 equal halves. **Equator of the eyeball [equator (NA)].** An imaginary line encircling the eyeball midway between the two poles of the eyeball. **Equator of the lens [equator lentis (NA)].** The marginal circumference of the lens. [L *aequare* to make equal.]

equilenin (ek·wil·en·in). $C_{18}H_{18}O_2$, an oestrogenic follicular hormone of steroid structure, isolated from the urine of pregnant mares, but not existing in that of pregnant women. Its systematic name is $\Delta^{1,3,5:10,6,8}$-estrapentaene-3-ol-17-one. [L *equus* horse.]

equilibration (e·kwil·ib·ra'·shun). 1. The state of being balanced or in equilibrium. 2. The maintaining of equipoise. 3. Restoration to the normal state of balance or equilibrium.

equilibrium (e·kwil·ib·re·um). A state of rest or balance, the result of an equality of opposing processes or forces. **Acid-base equilibrium.** Acid-base balance. **Body equilibrium.** A state of the body in which it remains at rest. **Carbon equilibrium.** Equality of intake and output of carbon. **Equilibrium in chemical systems.** The state in which the speed of a chemical reaction is equal to the speed of the reverse reaction, i.e. there is no net change in the concentrations of the various reactants. **Dynamic equilibrium.** An equilibrium of forces. **Homeostatic equilibrium.** The factor ensuring the constancy in the physiological state of the body. **Membrane equilibrium.** A state of thermodynamic equilibrium at membrane surfaces. **Metabolic equilibrium.** An even balance between intake of food on the one hand, and the utilization and excretion of waste products on the other. **Mobile equilibrium.** Dynamic equilibrium (see above). **Nitrogen equilibrium, Nitrogenous equilibrium.** A condition in which the daily intake of nitrogen in the food is equal to the daily loss of nitrogen by the excreta. **Nutritive equilibrium.** A steady state of nutrition in which the losses and gains of the body as regards its various constituents are equal. **Protein equilibrium.** Nitrogen equilibrium (see above). **Radioactive equilibrium.** A situation (not a true equilibrium) in which a particular atom is being produced by the radioactive breakdown of a precursor while it is itself breaking down, the two breakdowns matching so that the overall concentration of the atom in question remains constant. **Water equilibrium.** A state of the body in which water gains and losses are equal, so that the body weight is constant. [L *aequilibrium.*]

See also: DONNAN.

equilin (ek·wil·in). $C_{18}H_{20}O_2$, a follicular hormone with oestrogenic activity isolated from the urine of pregnant mares but not from that of pregnant women. Its systematic name is $\Delta^{1,3,5:10,7}$-estratetraene-3-ol-17-one. [L *equus* horse.]

equimolar (e·kwe·**mo**·lar). Said of solutions, when they contain the same number of mols of solute per given volume. [L *aequus* equal, mol.]

equimolecular (e·kwe·mol·**ek**'·ew·lar). 1. Denoting gases or solutions which contain the same number of molecules. 2. Term applied to a mixture of substances in the proportion of their molecular weights. [L *aequus* equal, molecule.]

equinia (e·**kwi**·ne·ah). Glanders. **Equinia mitis.** A mild form of glanders sometimes seen in man and contracted from horses. [L *equinus* pertaining to a horse.]

equinocavus (e·**kwi**·no·**ka**'·vus). A condition of combined talipes cavus and talipes equinus.

equinovarus (e·**kwi**·no·**va**'·rus). A condition of combined talipes equinus and talipes varus.

equinus (e·**kwi**·nus). Talipes equinus. **Equinus dorsalis.** A condition in which, as a result of extreme flexion of the toes, walking takes place on the dorsal surfaces. **Equinus plantaris.** Talipes equinus characterized by extension of the toes at the metatarsophalangeal joint or throughout their whole length. [L *equinus,* pertaining to a horse.]

equipotential (e·kwe·po·**ten**'·shal). 1. Denoting bodies that have the same electric potential. 2. Term applied to surfaces or lines of force which have the same electric potential. [L *aequus* equal, potential.]

equivalence, equivalency (e·**kwiv**·al·ens, e·**kwiv**·al·ens·e). 1. The state of being equivalent. 2. Valency; the number of atoms of hydrogen that an element or radical will combine with or displace. 3. In immunology, combination of antigen and antibody in proportions such that all available combining sites and determinants are combined with one another. [L *aequus* equal, *valere* to be strong.]

equivalent (e·**kwiv**·al·ent). 1. Equal in value. 2. In chemistry, that weight of an element or radical which combines with, displaces, or is in any way equivalent to, a standard unit. **Dose equivalent.** The product of absorbed dose, quality factor, and any other necessary modifying factor, at the point of interest. It is the absorbed dose of radiation of standard quality, uniformly delivered, which would give rise to the same biological effect as does the absorbed dose of the particular radiation of interest. Symbol *H.* **Endosmotic equivalent.** The number representing the amount of water passing through a membrane by endosmosis in the same time that a unit quantity of another substance will pass through the membrane in the opposite direction by exosmosis. **Epileptic equivalent.** Psychomotor epilepsy; paroxysmal behaviour disturbances or automatic acts, now recognized to be due to epileptic discharges arising in the temporal lobes. It used to be thought that they occurred in place of grand-mal attacks, and so seizures of this type were called epileptic equivalents. **Glucose equivalent.** The amount of glucose which is oxidized by the aid of 1 unit of insulin, as estimated by the lowering of the blood sugar of a standard rabbit in standard time. **Gram-equivalent.** The equivalent of an element or compound expressed in grams. **Lead equivalent.** That thickness of lead which would have the same radiation-absorption characteristic for the radiation of interest as has the material in question. **Psychical equivalent.** An attack of psychomotor epilepsy characterized by alteration in mentality or behaviour with no motor accompaniment. **Roentgen equivalent.** *See* ROENTGEN-EQUIVALENT. **Starch equivalent.** A number relating the amount of oxygen required for complete combustion of a given weight of fat to that required for complete combustion of the same weight of starch, approximately 2.4. **Thermometric equivalent.** The temperature on scale A equivalent to a value T° on scale B, where A and B are any two scales of temperature. **Toxic equivalent.** The amount of toxin necessary to kill an animal, expressed in terms of the amount required to kill a standard animal. Thus the intravenous minimal lethal dose of diphtheria toxin for mice is 60 times the guinea-pig subcutaneous minimum lethal dose. **Water equivalent.** The product of the mass of a calorimeter and its specific heat, i.e. the mass of water that would require the same amount of heat as the calorimeter to raise its temperature 1°C. [L *aequus* equal, *valere* to be strong.]

See also: JOULE.

equivocal (e·**kwiv**·o·kal). Applied to statements or symptoms which are of misleading or doubtful significance. [L *aequus* equal, *vocare* to call.]

eradication (e·**rad**·ik·a'·shun). The process of completely destroying; entire removal; extirpation. [L *eradicare* to take out by the root.]

erasion (e·**ra**·zhun). The scraping away of diseased tissue, particularly bone tissue. **Erasion of a joint.** Arthrectomy. [L *eradere* to scrape out.]

Eratyrus (er·at·i·rus). A genus of reduviid bugs, incriminated in the transmission of American trypanosomiasis (Chagas' disease). **Eratyrus cuspidatus.** A potential vector of Chagas' disease.

Erb, Wilhelm Heinrich (b. 1840). Heidelberg neurologist.

Erb's disease, dystrophy or syndrome. Juvenile (scapulohumeral) progressive muscular dystrophy; a slowly progressive form (usually beginning between the ages of 15 and 25) producing weakness and atrophy, often asymmetrical, first in the shoulder-girdle muscles, later in the pelvic girdle.

Erb's palsy, or paralysis. The upper plexus type of birth injury to the brachial plexus; a traction injury of the 5th and perhaps the 6th cervical root. There is paralysis of the deltoid, brachialis, biceps and brachioradialis muscles, giving inability to abduct the arm or to flex or supinate the forearm.

Erb's paraplegia. Spastic paraplegia due to spinal neurosyphilis.

Erb's phenomenon, or sign. In tetany, the reversal of the usual response to an anodal current; the anodal-opening current is more effective than the anodal-closing current, also the motor nerves respond to a weaker cathodal stimulation than in the normal person.

Erb's point. Surface marking of the upper trunk of the brachial plexus, 2 fingers' breadth above the clavicle and 1 finger's breadth lateral to the posterior border of the sternocleidomastoid muscle; frequently misused to refer to the upper trunk itself. Stimulation at this point causes contraction of the deltoid, biceps and other arm muscles.

Erb's myotonic reaction. In myotonia congenita or Thomsen's disease, a prolonged contraction with slow relaxation when a muscle is stimulated electrically with a galvanic or faradic current, just as occurs in a patient with this condition when he attempts to contract his own muscles.

Erb's sclerosis. A condition at one time thought to be a primary lateral sclerosis of the spinal cord, but now generally considered to be due to syphilitic meningomyelitis; the name is thus inappropriate.

Erb's wave. The wave-like contractions in a muscle that are produced by a strong constant current; they are probably fibrillary movements in a muscle damaged by the strong current.

Erb–Charcot disease. Syphilitic spastic paraplegia.

Erb–Duchenne palsy, or paralysis, Duchenne–Erb palsy, paralysis or syndrome. Erb's palsy, or paralysis (see above).

Erb–Goldflam disease, or syndrome, Goldflam–Erb disease. Myasthenia gravis.

Erb–Landouzy disease. Progressive muscular dystrophy.

Erb–Westphal sign, Westphal–Erb sign. Loss of the patellar reflex; as first described, this applies particularly to cases of tabes dorsalis.

Erb–Zimmerlin type. The Erb (juvenile, scapulohumeral) type of muscular dystrophy.

Erben, Siegmund (b. 1863). Vienna neurologist.

Erben's phenomenon, reflex or sign. Bradycardia when the head and trunk are bent forwards; said to be due to vagal hyperexcitability.

erbium (er·be·um). The rare-earth element of atomic weight 167.26, atomic number 68 and chemical symbol Er. A trivalent metal forming pink salts. [Ytt*erby* in Sweden.]

erect (e·**rekt**). 1. Upright. 2. Standing rigidly up or out from the body through engorgement of tissues. [L *erigere* to erect.]

erectile (e·**rek**·tile). Capable of erecting or of being erected.

erection (e·**rek**·shun). The state of a part which has become erect and rigid through engorgement of tissues.

erector (e·**rek**·tor). 1. An erector muscle. 2. Nervi erigentes. 3. In physics, a prism in the eyepiece of an optical instrument which causes the image to appear in an upright instead of an inverted position. [L *erigere* to erect.]

eredosome (e·**red**·o·some). The haemoglobin in the stromal network of the red blood cell.

eremacausis (er·e·mah·**kaw**′·sis). The slow oxidation and gradual decay that takes place when organic matter is exposed to the action of moisture and air. [Gk *erema* by degrees, *kausis* a burning.]

eremiophobia (er·e·me·o·**fo**′·be·ah). Morbid fear of absence of noise or of stillness. [Gk *eremia* stillness, phobia.]

eremophobia (er·e·mo·**fo**′·be·ah). Excessive or morbid fear of being away from the society of other people. [Gk *eremos* solitary, phobia.]

erepsin (er·**ep**·sin). A mixture of enzymes, chiefly polypeptidases, present in the intestinal mucosa and capable of converting polypeptides into amino acids.

ereptase (er·**ep**·taze). Erepsin.

ereptic (er·**ep**·tik). Containing or having relation to erepsin.

erethetical (er·e·**thet**·ik·al). Erethismic.

erethism (**er**·e·thizm). 1. A state of excessive nervous irritability. 2. The quality of reacting strongly and rapidly to stimulation; the opposite of apathism. **Erethism mercurialis.** Severe mental symptoms occurring in chronic mercurial poisoning. There is excessive irritability and sensitiveness, the patient is easily upset, dislikes being watched at work, loses his temper and self-control; depression, loss of memory and insomnia may follow. Hallucinations, delusions and mania may occur rarely. **Sexual erethism.** Excessive response to sexual stimuli. [Gk *erethismos* irritation.]

erethismic (er·e·**thiz**·mik). Referring to erethism.

erethisophrenia (er·e·thiz·o·**fre**′·ne·ah). A condition in which there is excessive mental excitability and irritability. [Gk *erethizein* to irritate, *phren* mind.]

erethistic (er·e·**this**·tik). 1. Affected with erethism. 2. Provoking irritability, or exacerbating an irritation already present.

erethitic (er·e·**thit**·ik). A term for the kind of temperament which keeps the individual in a state of constant and extreme stimulation and activity of emotions, mind and body (Hunt). [Gk *erethizein* to irritate.]

erg (erg). The unit of work or energy in the CGS system equal to 10^{-7} joules; defined as the work done by a force of one dyne moving over one centimetre, or the energy required to move one gram one centimetre against a force of one dyne. [Gk *ergon* work.]

ergamine (er·gam·een). The name originally applied to histamine isolated from ergot.

ergasia (er·**ga**·ze·ah). 1. A substance supposed to be responsible for enhancing the activity of the animal cell. 2. A term for integrated psychobiological function of any kind (Meyer). [Gk work.]

ergasiatrics, ergasiatry (er·ga·se·**at**′·rix, er·gas·i·at·re). A term for psychiatry (Meyer). [Gk *ergasia* work, *iatrikos* healing.]

ergasidermatosis (er·**ga**·se·der·mat·**o**′·sis). Any industrial dermatitis. [Gk *ergasia* work, dermatosis.]

ergasiology (er·ga·se·**ol**′·o·je). Objective psychobiology, the science concerned with the functioning of personality. [Gk *ergasia* work, *logos* science.]

ergasiomania (er·ga·se·o·**ma**′·ne·ah). Frenzied desire to be always at work on something, irrespective of the kind of work. [Gk *ergasia* work, mania.]

ergasiophobia (er·ga·se·o·**fo**′·be·ah). Extreme fear or dislike of doing work of any kind. [Gk *ergasia* work, phobia.]

ergasthenia (er·gas·**the**·ne·ah). Any symptom, debility or weakness caused by overwork. [Gk *ergasia* work, asthenia.]

ergastic (er·**gas**·tik). 1. Referring to ergasia, or showing its characteristics. 2. Applied to the non-active material produced or stored in an animal cell, e.g. fat, which is potentially energetic.

ergastoplasm (er·**gas**·to·plazm). That region of the protoplasm of certain cells, e.g. the exocrine cells of the pancreas, which shows a high affinity for basic dyes such as pyronine and methylene blue, owing to the presence of nucleoproteins in high concentration. Is synonymous with *granular endoplasmic reticulum.* [Gk *ergaster* workman, plasm.]

ergine (**er**·geen). 1. General term for catalytic hormones and enzymes. 2. $C_{16}H_{17}N_3O$, an ergot alkaloid, the amine of lysergic acid; it has a slight pressor action, the iso- form being more active and resembling ergometrine.

ergo-aesthesiograph (er·go·es·**the**′·ze·o·graf). An instrument which records muscular ability to counterbalance variable resistances and therefore shows the muscular aptitude. It is of use particularly in judging the fitness in this respect of candidates for training in aviation. [Gk *ergon* work, *aisthesis* feeling, *graphein* to record.]

ergobasine (er·go·**ba**·seen). Name applied to an alkaloid of ergot subsequently identified with ergometrine.

Ergocalciferolum. *European Pharmacopoeia* name for Calciferol BP 1973.

ergoclavine (er·go·**klav**·een). An equimolecular mixture of 2 less-important alkaloids of ergot, ergosine and ergosinine.

ergocristine (er·go·**kris**·teen). $C_{35}H_{39}N_5O_5$, an ergot alkaloid isomeric with ergotinine.

ergocristinine (er·go·**kris**·tin·een). $C_{35}H_{39}N_5O_5$, an ergot alkaloid, the isomer of ergocristine, and obtained from the latter by boiling.

ergodermatosis (er·go·der·mat·**o**′·sis). Occupational dermatitis. [Gk *ergein* to work, dermatosis.]

ergodynamograph (er·go·di·**nam**′·o·graf). An instrument which records the force of muscular contractions and the value of the work that is accomplished by them. [Gk *ergon* work, *dynamis* force, *graphein* to record.]

ergogenesis, ergogeny (er·go·**jen**·es·is, er·**goj**·en·e). A biological term for the potential and kinetic energy involved in the processes of adaptation carried out by animal organisms. [Gk *ergon* work, *genein* to produce.]

ergogram (**er**·go·gram). The tracing recorded by an ergograph. [Gk *ergon* work, *gramma* writing.]

ergograph (**er**·go·graf). An instrument which measures and records the amount of movement or the extent of work done by a single contracting muscle or set of muscles, the amount it is capable of doing, the value of the exertion, the rate of fatigue, and so on. [Gk *ergon* work, *graphein* to record.]

ergographic (er·go·**graf**·ik). Referring or belonging to an ergograph and to the record obtained by its use.

ergomania (er·go·**ma**·ne·ah). Ergasiomania. [Gk *ergon* work, mania.]

ergometer (er·**gom**·et·er). Dynamometer. [Gk *ergon* work, meter.]

ergometrine (er·go·**met**·reen). $C_{19}H_{23}O_2N_3$, a crystallizable alkaloid obtained from ergot, and the one to which ergot owes the property of producing strong rhythmic contractions of the uterus. It is a derivative of lysergic acid, more soluble in water than ergotoxine, and more effective and prompt than the other ergot alkaloids by reason of its rapid absorption. In therapeutic doses it evokes immediate rapid contractions of the uterus followed by a period of rhythmic contractions interspaced with relaxation. Its duration of action is shorter than that of ergotoxine, and it differs from the latter and from ergotamine in not causing adrenaline reversal and in having an excitatory rather than a blocking effect on the sympathetic nervous system. Furthermore, it is relatively much less toxic, rarely causes gangrene, has little influence on blood pressure and is free from unpleasant constitutional results. It is usually administered, by mouth or injection, in the form of the maleate. Also known as *ergonovine.* **Ergometrine Maleate BP 1973.** $C_{19}H_{23}O_2N_3C_4H_4O_4$, the acid maleate, used where ergot is indicated for oxytocic activity. It has little effect on the central nervous system, though it is sometimes used orally for migraine.

Ergometrinii Maleas. *European Pharmacopoeia* name for Ergometrine Maleate BP 1973.

ergomonamine (er·go·**mon**·am·een). $C_{19}H_{19}O_4N$, a crystalline alkaloid isolated from ergot; it does not give the indole colour reaction like the other ergot alkaloids.

ergonomics (er·go·**nom**·ix). 1. That branch of medicine which is concerned with human energy. 2. The study of human factors in work machine control and equipment design. [Gk *ergon* work, *nomos* law.]

ergonovine (er·go·**no**·veen). Ergometrine.

ergophobia (er·go·**fo**·be·ah). Ergasiophobia. [Gk *ergon* work, phobia.]

ergophore (**er**·go·for). Toxophore. [Gk *ergon* work, *pherein* to carry.]

ergosine (**er**·go·seen). $C_{30}H_{37}O_5N_5$, an ergot alkaloid with action similar to that of ergotoxine.

ergosinine (**er**·go·sin·een). $C_{30}H_{37}O_5N_5$, an ergot alkaloid isomeric with ergosine, which it forms on boiling with alcoholic potash.

ergostanol (er·**gos**·tan·ol). $C_{28}H_{50}O$, a steroid which occurs in ergot and yeast.

ergostat (**er**·go·stat). 1. An apparatus for the therapeutic exercise of muscles. 2. An apparatus by means of which the strength of muscles can be estimated. [Gk *ergon* work, *statikos* standing still.]

ergosterol (er·**gos**·ter·ol). $C_{28}H_{43}OH$, a phytosterol present in plants, yeast, ergot and certain higher fungi, which on irradiation with ultraviolet rays is converted into vitamin D_2 or calciferol. Ergosterol is used on a large scale commercially in the preparation of calciferol concentrates employed in antirachitic therapy.

ergostetrine (er·go·**stet**·reen). Ergometrine.

Ergot (**er**·got). The dried sclerotium of *Claviceps purpurea* Tulasne, a fungus which attacks the ovary of rye, *Secale cereale* Linn., breaking down the rye proteins. It contains a number of active principles, the most important being the alkaloids, ergotoxine, ergotamine and ergometrine, the last-mentioned being the one mainly responsible for the characteristic action of ergot upon the pregnant uterus, where it increases both the strength of the contractions and the tone of the muscle. Fluid extracts injected intravenously cause a rise in blood pressure due to contraction of the arterioles, and the drug has a haemostatic value, especially as a prophylactic against post-partum haemorrhage (BPC 1968). Prolonged administration may lead to ergotism, with gangrene of the extremities and disturbances of the central nervous system leading to convulsions. **Prepared Ergot BPC 1968.** Powdered ergot that has been defatted with light petroleum and adjusted to contain 0.2 per cent of total alkaloids. It is being replaced by the pure alkaloidal salts, e.g. ergotoxine ethanesulphonate, ergometrine maleate. [Fr. *argot*, a disease of cereals.]

See also: MORAND.

ergotamine (er·**got**·am·een). An alkaloid obtained from certain species of ergot. **Ergotamine Tartrate BP 1973.** The tartrate of ergotamine used almost exclusively in the treatment of migraine.

Ergotaminii Tartras. *European Pharmacopoeia* name for Ergotamine Tartrate BP 1973.

ergotaminine (er·got·**am**·in·een). $C_{33}H_{35}N_5O_5$, an alkaloid of ergot, isomeric with ergotamine, but physiologically inactive.

ergotherapy (er·go·**ther**·ap·e). The use of bodily exercise in treatment of disease. [Gk *ergon* work, therapy.]

ergothioneine (er·go·thi·**on′**·e·een). Thiolhistidine betaine, thioneine, erythrothioneine, $SHC_3H_2N_2CH_2CHCOON(CH_3)_2$. A cyclic base derived from histidine, which occurs in ergot and has also been observed in blood corpuscles.

ergothionone (er·go·**thi**·o·none). An inert base obtained from ergot.

ergotin (**er**·got·in). An aqueous extract of ergot.

ergotine (**er**·got·een). A solid preparation of ergot obtained by precipitating the aqueous extract with alcohol and evaporating the filtrate.

See also: BONJEAN.

ergotinine (er·**got**·in·een). $C_{35}H_{39}O_5N_5$, the first alkaloid isolated from ergot (Tanret 1875). It is a pharmacologically inactive compound. **Ergotinine series.** A series of dextrorotatory ergot alkaloids all with weak physiological activity, as distinct from the more potent members of the ergotoxine series.

ergotism (**er**·got·izm). A chronic disease resulting from wrong or excessive use of medicinal preparations made from ergot, or from eating meal made from rye affected with ergot. There are 2 known types of ergotism, as follows: (*a*) a form in which there is dry gangrene of fingers, toes, lobes of ear or tip of nose, with agonizing pain in the affected part (St. Anthony's fire) and later anaesthesia of the part, which turns livid and then black; (*b*) a form in which there is numbness and muscular twitching; fits, deafness and stupidity may occur, ending in dementia.

ergotized (**er**·got·i·zd). 1. Under the toxic influence of ergot. 2. Under the therapeutic influence of ergot.

ergotocine (er·go·**to**·seen). Name given by independent investigators to an alkaloid of ergot eventually proved identical with ergometrine.

ergotoxine (er·go·**tox**·een). Hydro-ergotinine, $C_{35}H_{41}O_6N_5$. A pharmacologically active alkaloid from ergot. Its most important action is upon smooth muscle, especially that of the uterus, small doses causing marked contraction, larger doses tending to produce spasm. Though it will stimulate an immature uterus, the gravid uterus is more sensitive, and the action is fairly specific. Large doses cause constriction of the smaller blood vessels and bradycardia; the capillary endothelium is damaged and gangrene may result. The drug paralyses the vasoconstrictor response to injected adrenaline, and a fall of blood pressure occurs with the latter instead of a rise. **Ergotoxine ethanesulphonate.** $C_{35}H_{41}O_6N_5C_2H_5SO_3H$, colourless crystals containing about 83 per cent ergotoxine; soluble in alcohol, and may be given orally, subcutaneously or intramuscularly. **Ergotoxine phosphate.** $C_{35}H_{41}O_6N_5H_3PO_4{\cdot}H_2O$, colourless crystals which darken on exposure to light; soluble in boiling alcohol but only sparingly in water. **Ergotoxine series.** The series of physiologically active laevorotatory ergot alkaloids which include ergotoxine and ergotamine.

ergotropic (er·go·**trop**·ik). Relating or belonging to ergotropy.

ergotropy (er·**got**·ro·pe). The injection of non-specific animal or vegetable proteins or the giving of medicinal baths or other treatment in order to energize the plasma and tissues of the body so that its power of resistance to pathogenic agents in general is increased. [Gk *ergon* work, *tropos* a turning.]

Erhard's test. For simulated unilateral deafness: a loudly ticking watch is approximated to the deaf ear, the meatus on the sound side being blocked. At a distance of about 1 m the tick should be heard in the good ear; denial of any sound is presumptive evidence of malingering.

Erichsen, Sir John Eric (b. 1818). London surgeon.

Erichsen's disease, or spine. Railway spine; post-traumatic neurosis following railway accidents, with symptoms suggesting a spinal origin but without pathological changes; also called *Page's disease.*

erigens (**er**·e·jenz). Causing erection, as applied to certain nerves. [L *erigere* to erect.]

Eriocheir (**er**·e·o·kire). A genus of fresh-water crabs, mitten crabs. *Eriocheir japonicus* and *E. sinensis,* from Japan and China, respectively, are secondary intermediate hosts of the lung fluke *Paragonimus westermani.* [Gk *erion* wool, *cheir* hand.]

eriodictin (er·e·o·**dik'**·tin). Eriodictyol.

eriodictyol (**er**·e·o·**dik'**·te·ol). 1. The flavone derivative $C_{15}H_{12}O_6$ found in *Eriodictyon californicum.* 2. Citrin, vitamin P, $C_{28}H_{38}O_{17}$. A vegetable colouring matter which occurs in lemon juice, orange peel and paprika, and is considered essential in the diet to give strength to capillary walls; it prevents the haemorrhages of scurvy. It is a flavone glucoside.

Eriodictyon (e·re·o·**dik'**·te·on). A genus of plants of the family Hydrophyllaceae. The dried leaves of *Eriodictyon californicum* (Hook. and Arn.) Greene, an evergreen shrub of California, are used as a bitter tonic, and as an expectorant in the form of a liquid extract. [Gk *erion* wool, *diktyon* net.]

eriometer (er·e·**om**·et·er). An instrument that takes advantage of the diffraction of light as a means of measurement. It can be used for determining the mean diameter of red cells by passing a beam of white light through a very thin film of blood which diffracts the light, producing concentric spectral rings: these can be so adjusted on a screen that measurement of the radius of the yellow circle enables the mean cell diameter to be calculated. [Gk *erion* wool, meter.]

eriometry (er·e·**om**·et·re). The measuring of minute particles or dried erythrocytes by means of an eriometer.

erisiphac, erisiphake (er·is·e·fak, er·is·e·fake). An instrument bearing a small cup at its tip and connected with a vacuum pump. It is used for the intracapsular extraction of cataract by suction. [Gk *eresis* removal, *phakos* lens.]

Eristalis (er·**is**·tal·is). A genus of hover flies. The larvae of several species, called *rat-tailed maggots,* particularly *Eristalis tenax,* have been found occasionally in intestinal myiasis. [L a precious stone.]

Erlandsen, Alfred (b. 1878). Copenhagen hygienist.

Ellermann and Erlandsen test. Injections of tuberculin of various dilutions made to determine the highest dilution which will produce a local reaction. Reaction to 1 in 10 000 or more is said to indicate active disease. It is not specific.

Erlenmeyer, Friedrich Albrecht (b. 1849). Bendorf neurologist.

Erlenmeyer's mixture. A mixture of the bromides of sodium, potassium and ammonium, used as a sedative.

Erlicki's fluid. A fixative for histological purposes, containing potassium bichromate and copper sulphate.

Ernst, Paul (b. 1859). German pathologist.

Babes-Ernst body, corpuscle, or granule. Metachromatic granule (*see* GRANULE) seen in *Corynebacterium diphtheriae.*

erodent (e·**ro**·dent). 1. Causing erosion. 2. Caustic. 3. A caustic or corrosive drug. [L *erodere* to eat out.]

erogenous (er·**oj**·en·us). Erotogenic.

eromania (er·o·**ma**·ne·ah). Erotomania.

erose (e·**rose**). 1. Uneven or irregular in outline, as if partly worn away. 2. In botany, having an irregularly notched border, as a leaf. [L *erodere* to eat out.]

erosion (e·**ro**·zhun). 1. Any superficial destructive process; a wearing away of a tissue. 2. In dentistry, the loss of the hard tissues at the neck of a tooth, due to causes other than abrasion. **Aphthous erosion.** Superficial ulceration of the oral mucous membrane in infants. **Cervical erosion.** A reddened, slightly raised area of columnar epithelium around the external os. It is velvety on palpation and usually does not bleed easily except during pregnancy. **Interdigital blastomycetic erosion.** Red, eroded finger webs, usually between the third and fourth fingers, due to infection with *Candida albicans.* It particularly occurs with diabetes mellitus and obesity or with rheumatoid arthritis. **Papillary erosion.** An erosion in which the downgrowth of the glandular epithelium has been more prolific, and the erosion appears more exuberant. [L *erodere* to eat out.]

See also: DIEULAFOY.

erosive (e·**ro**·siv). 1. Corrosive. 2. Erodent, 3. Marked by erosion.

erotic (er·**ot**·ik). Referring or belonging to sexual love or to lust; lustful; amatory. **Anal erotic.** An adult in whom the anal eroticism of childhood has persisted and who continues to show the characteristic traits of abnormal orderliness and neatness, and great economy and obstinacy. [Gk *eros* love.]

eroticism (er·**ot**·is·izm). 1. The character of being erotic. 2. The state of having morbid sexual desires or instincts. 3. A tendency towards erotomania. 4. The displaying of erotic characteristics. **Anal eroticism.** The derivation of sexual pleasure from the passages of faeces through the anus. **Muscle eroticism.** A state of sexual desire induced or stimulated by muscular exercise. **Stuff eroticism.** Hephephilia.

eroticomania (er·ot·ik·o·**ma'**·ne·ah). Erotomania.

erotism (er·**ot**·izm). Eroticism.

erotogenesis (er·ot·o·**jen'**·es·is). The initiation of erotic feelings. [see foll.]

erotogenic (er·**ot**·o·**jen'**·ik). Producing erotic sensations, sexual excitement or lustful desire. [Gk *eros* love, *genein* to produce.]

erotology (er·ot·**ol**·o·je). The study or description of love or love-making. [Gk *eros* love, *logos* science.]

erotomania (er·**ot**·o·**ma'**·ne·ah). 1. Excessive sexual passion. 2. A state of exaggerated reaction to sexual stimulation; a mental disorder caused or marked by feelings of extreme affection for or by erotic behaviour towards individuals of the opposite sex. [Gk *eros* love, mania.]

erotomaniac (er·**ot**·o·**ma'**·ne·ak). An individual suffering from erotomania.

erotopath (er·**ot**·o·path). An individual with abnormal or perverted sexual instincts and impulses. [Gk *eros* love, *pathos* disease.]

erotopathy (er·ot·**op**·ath·e). The condition of having abnormal or perverted sexual impulses or instincts. [see prec.]

erotophobia (er·**ot**·o·**fo'**·be·ah). A state of morbid aversion to sexual feelings and their physical expression. [Gk *eros* love, phobia.]

erotopsychic (er·**ot**·o·**si'**·kik). Referring to or characterized by erotopathy. [Gk *eros* love, *psyche* mind.]

erotosexual (er·**ot**·o·**sex'**·ew·al). Belonging to sexual love, or having the characteristics of it. [Gk *eros* love, sex.]

errhine (**er**·ine). 1. Any drug which has the effect of a nasal irritant, so that an increased discharge is produced. 2. Causing increased nasal discharge. [Gk *en, rhis* nose.]

Erro (**er**·o). A genus of viruses including those that cause the encephalitides. This nomenclature is American in origin and not widely accepted in the UK. **Erro equinus.** The virus of equine encephalomyelitis. [L wanderer.]

error (**er**·or). **Inborn error of metabolism.** *See* METABOLISM. **Probable error.** A measure of the distribution of the random errors in making an experimental observation. The probable error has a magnitude such that in making an observation there is a 50 per cent chance that the error of a single observation is greater than or less than the probable error. For a gaussian distribution the probable error is 0.67 of the standard deviation. **Random error.** Random variation. *See* VARIATION. **Standard error.** In statistics, the standard deviation of the errors between a series of estimated values and the series of true values. [L a wandering.]

erubescence (**er**·oo·**bes**·ens). A flushing or reddening of the skin of any surface. [L *erubescere* to grow red.]

eructation (e·ruk·**ta**·shun). A violent uprise of wind from the stomach; the act of belching wind. **Nervous eructation.** A gastric neurosis in which air is belched up after it has been swallowed. [L *eructare* to belch.]

erugation (e·roo·ga·shun). Removing or freeing from wrinkles. [L *e, ruga* wrinkle.]

erugatory (e·roo·gat·or·e). Applied to a medicament which tends to remove wrinkles. [see prec.]

eruption (e·rup·shun). 1. A breaking-out of any kind, so as to become visible, e.g. a tooth. 2. A rash on the skin. **Bullous eruption.** An eruption in which bullae predominate, e.g. pemphigus and erythema bullosum. **Corymbose eruption.** A syphilitic eruption. **Creeping eruption.** A linear eruption produced by the larvae of various parasites, especially *Gastrophilus.* **Crustaceous eruption.** An eruption in which the lesions are crusted. **Drug eruption.** A rash caused by the ingestion of a drug. **Erythematous eruption.** A red rash. **Feigned eruption.** Dermatitis artefacta. **Fixed eruption.** A form of drug rash (see above) in which erythematous plaques, often followed by hyperpigmentation, occur on the same sites whenever a dose of the drug is taken. **Iodine eruption.** An eruption caused by the ingestion of iodine. **Juvenile spring eruption.** A papulovesicular eruption on the helices and sometimes on the hands, mostly of boys, occurring in the spring. **Lichenoid eruption.** An eruption resembling lichen planus and caused by drugs or by exposure to colour developers. **Macular eruption.** A rash made up of macules. **Medicinal eruption.** Drug eruption (see above). **Monomorphic eruption.** An eruption in which all the lesions are of the same kind. **Morbilliform eruption.** A rash resembling measles. **Papular eruption.** A rash made up of papules. **Petechial eruption.** An eruption consisting chiefly of petechiae. **Polymorphic eruption.** An eruption consisting of different kinds of lesions. **Pustular eruption.** A rash in which pustules predominate. **Recurrent summer eruption.** Hydroa aestivale. **Ringed eruption.** Granuloma annulare. **Sandworm eruption.** An eruption occurring in Natal and Zululand, caused by creeping larvae. **Scaly eruption.** Squamous eruption (see below). **Scarlatiniform eruption.** An eruption resembling scarlet fever. **Scratch eruption.** A localized area of thickening and loss of elasticity of the skin resulting from repeated scratching or other forms of friction. **Serum eruption.** An eruption, often accompanied by fever, occurring between 1 and 30 (usually from 6 to 10) days after the administration of serum; commonly urticarial, polymorphic, scarlatiniform or morbilliform. **Simulated eruption.** Dermatitis artefacta. **Squamous eruption.** A scaly rash. **Summer eruption.** Miliaria. **Eruption of a tooth.** The complex process by which a tooth which is formed within the bone of the jaw moves in a vertical direction until the physiological crown is uncovered and is in occlusion with the corresponding tooth or teeth in the opposite jaw. **Tubercular eruption.** An eruption in which the individual lesions are nodules. **Vaccinal eruption.** Various eruptions following vaccination, the commonest being roseola vaccinia. [L *eruptio* a bursting forth.]

See also: KAPOSI.

eruptive (e·rup·tiv). 1. Producing or belonging to efflorescence or eruption. 2. Attended by or characterized by the presence of an eruption. 3. Favourable to the appearance of a rash or eruption.

Erwinia (er·win·e·ah). A genus of plant pathogens of the family Bacteriaceae. [*Erwin* F. Smith, 1854–1927, American bacteriologist.]

erysipelas (er·e·sip·el·as). An acute inflammation of the skin and subcutaneous tissues caused by *Streptococcus pyogenes* and giving rise to an acute feverish illness. **Ambulant erysipelas.** Erysipelas spreading rapidly at one border, the older part clearing at the same time. **Black erysipelas.** Severe erysipelas in which part of the lesion becomes dark purple. **Erysipelas bullosum.** Erysipelas with the formation of bullae on the lesions. **Coast erysipelas.** The nodular skin eruption in onchocerciasis. **Erysipelas diffusum.** Erysipelas in which the lesion lacks its usual sharp edge. **Erysipelas erraticum.** Erysipelas migrans (see below). **Facial erysipelas.** Erysipelas affecting the face. **Gangrenous erysipelas.** Erysipelas complicated by local gangrene. **Erysipelas glabrum.** Erysipelas in which the skin is smooth and shiny. **Idiopathic erysipelas.** Spontaneous erysipelas (see below). **Internal erysipelas.** Erysipelas of the vagina. **Lombardy erysipelas.** Pellagra. **Medical erysipelas.** Spontaneous erysipelas (see below). **Erysipelas migrans.** Erysipelas which clears rapidly from one site, reappearing elsewhere, and continuing to wander for some weeks. **Erysipelas perstans faciei.** 1. Recurrent erysipelatous eruption of the face. 2. Acute disseminated lupus erythematosus with erysipelatous appearance of the face. **Phlegmonous erysipelas.** Erysipelas complicated by subcutaneous suppuration. **Phlyctenular erysipelas.** Erysipelas vesiculosum (see below). **Erysipelas pustulosum.** Erysipelas vesiculosum (see below) in which the vesicles have become purulent. **Recurrent erysipelas.** Mild erysipelas or erysipelas-like eruption which recurs. **Relapsing erysipelas.** Chronic erysipelatous disease characterized by rashes. **Serpiginous erysipelas.** Erysipelas which spreads in different directions, giving a serpiginous appearance. **Spontaneous erysipelas.** Erysipelas which does not follow trauma or surgery. **Surgical erysipelas.** Erysipelas following a surgical operation. **Swine erysipelas.** An acute septicaemia of pigs caused by *Erysipelothrix rhusiopathiae.* **Traumatic erysipelas.** Erysipelas following trauma. **Erysipelas verrucosum.** Erysipelas in which the affected area has a warty surface. **Erysipelas vesiculosum.** Erysipelas in which vesicles appear on the plaque. **Wandering erysipelas.** Erysipelas migrans (see above). **White erysipelas.** Erysipelas with extreme degree of oedema, giving a pale-rose colour. **Zoonotic erysipelas.** Erysipeloid (Morrant Baker). **Erysipelas zoster.** Zoster. [Gk *erythos* red, *pella* skin.]

erysipelatous (er·e·sip·el'·at·us). 1. Pertaining to erysipelas. 2. Resembling erysipelas or having some of its characteristics. 3. Suffering from erysipelas.

Erysipelococcus (er·e·sip·el·o·kok'·us). *Streptococcus pyogenes.* It was first described by Fehleisen (1883) under the name *Erysipelkokken* as the causal agent of erysipelas. [erysipelas, Gk *kokkos* berry.]

erysipeloid (er·e·sip·el·oid). Non-contagious human infection with the bacillus of swine erysipelas, *Erysipelothrix rhusiopathiae,* appearing as an infective dermatitis at the site of a cut or abrasion of the skin of the forearm or hand. The cause is as a rule the handling of infected fish, carcases or cadavers, and the condition may become generalized and septic. Also called *fish-handlers' disease.* [erysipelas, Gk *eidos* form.]

See also: ROSENBACH (A. J. F.).

Erysipelothrix (er·e·sip·el·o·thrix). A Gram-positive rod-shaped organism, the type species of which, *Erysipelothrix rhusiopathiae,* causes swine erysipelas. Infection in man occurs in epidemic and sporadic forms, and it is encountered usually in those who handle meat, fish, game or cheese. The cutaneous form of the disease is known as *erysipeloid* (Rosenbach's). **Erysipelothrix monocytogenes.** A rod-shaped branching filamentous bacillus that causes a monocytosis in rabbits. Septicaemia, meningitis, bacterial endocarditis and other infections have been reported in man. [erysipelas, Gk *thrix* hair.]

erythema (er·e·the·mah). Redness of the skin due to hyperaemia. **Erythema ab igne.** Erythema in a reticular pattern due to exposure to heat. It is usually seen on the anteriolateral surface of the lower legs of women. **Erythema annulare.** A form of erythema multiforme in which the lesions are circular with a pale centre and a raised erythematous margin. **Erythema annulare centrifugum.** A form in which the primary lesions are red papules or small plaques which spread peripherally whilst the skin in the centres becomes a normal colour: relatively large circular lesions are thus produced. The trunk and the proximal parts of the limbs are the sites of election. The malady often persists for months; the aetiology is uncertain and treatment unsatisfactory. **Erythema arthriticum epidemicum.** Epidemic arthritic erythema (see below). **Erythema atrophicans.** Lupus erythematosus; a non-commital name suggested by Morris, which has now been discarded. **Erythema brucellum.** Erythema in sensitized persons dealing with cows suffering from contagious abortion. **Erythema bullosum.** Erythema multiforme (see below) with bullous lesions. **Erythema bullosum vegetans.** Pemphigus vegetans. **Erythema caloricum.** Transitory erythema produced by heat or cold. **Erythema chronicum migrans.** A slowly extending ringed eruption of uncertain aetiology. **Circinate syphilitic erythema.** Tertiary circinate erythema (see below). **Erythema circinatum.** Erythema annulare (see above). **Erythema dyschromicum perstans.** Ash-grey areas of skin with a red infiltrated margin, of undetermined cause but resembling late pinta. **Erythema elevatum diutinum.** A chronic painless nodular eruption believed to be a form of granuloma annulare. **Epidemic arthritic erythema.** Haverhill fever; an acute febrile infection characterized by constitutional symptoms, a skin eruption and arthritis, caused by *Actinomyces muris (Streptobacillus moniliformis).* Sporadic cases may be due to rat bites (*Actinomyces muris* is a saprophyte of the nasopharynx of rats) and epidemics due to a milk-borne infection. The eruption is rubelliform or morbilliform and not infrequently becomes haemorrhagic. In severe cases petechiae may be noted on the feet. **Erythema epidemicum.** Acrodynia. **Erythema exudativum multiforme.** Erythema multiforme (see below). **Erythema figuratum.** A form of erythema annulare (see above) in which the lesions coalesce to form gyrate figures. **Erythema figuratum perstans.** A rare chronic eruption characterized by persistent erythematous patches, which assume annular, marginate or gyrate forms. **Erythema fugax.** Transitory cutaneous erythema occurring in limited areas and probably a form of urticaria, although itching is usually not a symptom. **Erythema gangraenosum.** Dermatitis artefacta with escharotic or gangrenous lesions. **Erythema gyratum persistens.** Erythema figuratum perstans (see above). **Erythema gyratum repens.** A condition in which regular waves of erythema spread over the skin and produce an appearance like the graining of wood. It is associated with a malignant focus, usually in the breast or lung, and is reversible if the focus is eiliminated. **Erythema hydroa.** *See* ERYTHEMA IRIS (below). **Erythema hyperaemicum.** Localized or diffuse cutaneous hyperaemia. **Erythema induratum.** Bazin's disease; tuberculosis indurativa subcutanea: a chronic recurring malady almost invariably in young girls or women, characterized by the formation of subcutaneous nodules which undergo necrosis and cause ulceration. The lower legs are the sites of election. There is a tendency nowadays to use the term for tuberculous cases and to differentiate other cases into their proper denominations, e.g. sarcoid, nodular vasculitis. **Erythema infantum.** Diaper rash. *See* RASH. **Erythema infectiosum, Infectious erythema.** An epidemic disease occurring in children and resembling rubella, with an incubation period of from 6 to 14 days: fifth disease. **Erythema intertrigo.** Intertrigo. **Erythema iris.** Herpes iris: a variety of erythema multiforme (see below). The lesions commence as red macules or papules which heal in the centre and spread peripherally, being limited by raised red circular borders. New central papules appear which develop similarly, and typical patterns are formed consisting of 2 or more concentric circles surrounding a central red papule. Occasionally the rings become vesicular and the central papule is replaced by a vesicle, in which case the terms *herpes iris* (Willan) or *erythema hydroa* (Besnier) are applicable. **Erythema laeve.** The shiny redness of the skin seen in some cases of oedema of the extremities. **Erythema marginatum.** A form of erythema multiforme in which the erythematous patches fade in the centre, leaving raised marginal bands. **Erythema migrans.** Erysipeloid. **Erythema multiforme.** An acute inflammatory disease characterized by red or purplish-red variously-sized patches of erythema, sometimes with vesicles and bullae; the lesions, which are numerous, may be scattered or grouped. The eruption is usually accompanied by constitutional disturbances. **Erythema neonatorum.** A common, benign, blotchy, macular erythema of unknown cause, usually occurring 1-2 days after birth, sometimes with wealing, and clearing spontaneously within 2 days. **Ninth-day erythema.** Milian's ninth-day erythema: a morbilliform or scarlatiniform eruption associated with fever and other constitutional symptoms, lasting only for a few days, occurring about the ninth day after the administration of a drug, particularly arsphenamine. The eruption is probably a biotropic phenomenon. **Erythema nodosum.** An acute inflammatory disease of the skin, characterized by the formation of oval or round, tender, red swellings; the sites of election are the anterior surfaces of the lower legs. The malady is usually associated with fever and pains in the joints. It is often associated with an underlying infective or inflammatory disease such as sarcoidosis or pulmonary tuberculosis. **Erythema nodosum leprosum.** Histologically, not a true erythema nodosum, the outstanding feature being oedema. Clinically, there are crops of red nodules or plaques; there may also be fever, iridocyclitis, oedema of the glottis, epistaxis, swollen joints, painful swollen nerves, bone pains, lymphadentitis and orchitis. **Erythema nuchae.** The common telangiectatic naevus at the nape of the neck. **Palmar erythema.** A condition, sometimes accompanied by stellate haemangiomata, possibly due to increased circulating oestrogens. It may occur in pregnancy, liver disease, rheumatoid arthritis, or in apparent normal health as a dominant hereditary trait. **Erythema papulatum vel papulosum.** A variety of erythema multiforme (see above) characterized by papular lesions. **Erythema papulosum rheumaticum.** Erythema multiforme (see above). **Erythema paratrimmea.** Congested redness of the skin due to pressure, particularly preceding a bedsore. **Erythema pernio.** A chilblain. **Erythema perstans.** A group of eruptions resembling variations of erythema multiforme in which the eruption is a recurring erythema. Ormsby and Montgomery (1948) include erythema annulare centrifugum, erythema chronicum migrans, erythema figuratum perstans and erythema simplex gyratum under this heading. **Erythema punctatum.** Erythema scarlatiniforme (see below). **Erythema scarlatiniforme.** A generalized eruption, mimicking scarlatina but with fewer constitutional symptoms, not associated with strawberry tongue, and terminating with desquamation. A subacute as well as an acute variety of the eruption is recognized. The eruption may be caused by idiosyncrasy to drugs or food, or may be a symptom of toxaemia. **Erythema serpens.** Rosenbach's disease; the name given by Morrant Baker in 1873 to the condition later described by Rosenbach (1877) as erysipeloid. It has been described in fish-handlers, and has been called *fish-handlers' disease*; but it occurs in other persons, and is caused by *Erysipelothrix rhusiopathiae.* **Erythema simplex.** Erythema hyperaemicum (see above). **Erythema simplex gyratum.** Possibly a variety of urticarial erythema in which circinate and gyrate lesions appear, usually on the breast, neck or extremities, and last a few days, when new lesions appear. **Erythema solare.** Sunburn. **Erythema subitum.** Roseola infantum. **Symmetric erythema of the soles.** Symmetric lividity of the soles (Pernet); "scalded feet": a form of acute hyperhidrosis, affecting the soles and margins of the feet, associated with erythema of the areas of pressure and of the lateral and posterior margins of the feet. **Symptomatic erythema.** Erythema that is symptomatic of physical or mental disorder, embarrassment or shame. **Tertiary circinate erythema.** Circinate syphilitic erythema; circular patches or narrow rings, red or reddish-yellow in colour, and without infiltration, due to tertiary syphilis. **Toxic erythema.** A loose term applied to erythematous eruptions of undetermined cause in which a chemical agent, virus, mycoplasma or bacterial infection is suspected. **Traumatic erythema, Erythema traumaticum.** Erythema caused by injury; the source of the injury may be physical or chemical, but sensitization plays no part in the development of the erythema. **Erythema tuberculatum** vel **tuberculosum.** A variety of erythema multiforme (see above) in which the lesions are nodular. **Erythema urticans.** A variety of urticaria. **Erythema urticatum.** An itching form of erythema multiforme (see above). **Variolous erythema.** Generalized or localized erythema occurring as a prodromal sign of smallpox. **Erythema venenatum.** Cutaneous redness caused by contact with an irritant substance. **Erythema vesiculosum.** A rare variety of erythema multiforme (see above) in which vesicles form on the surface of the lesions. [Gk *redness.*]

See also: HEBRA, JACQUET, MILIAN.

erythematoid (er·e·**the**·mat·oid). Resembling erythema. [erythema, Gk *eidos* form.]

erythematous (er·e·the·mat·us). Marked by, relating to or having the characteristics of erythema.

erythemogenic (er·e·the·mo·jen′·ik). Causing or producing erythema. [erythema, Gk *genein* to produce.]

erythemoid (er·e·the·moid). Erythematoid.

erythra (er·ith·rah). 1. A skin eruption. 2. The menses. [Gk *erythros* red.]

erythraematoid (er·ith·re·mat·oid). Like erythraemia in appearance. [erythraemia, Gk *eidos* form.]

erythraemia (er·ith·re·me·ah). Polycythaemia vera. [Gk *erythros* red, *haima* blood.]

erythraemoid (er·ith·re·moid). Erythraematoid.

erythralgia (er·ith·ral·je·ah). Erythromelalgia.

erythrasma (er·ith·raz·mah). An infection of the horny layer of the epidermis in a body flexure due to a diphtheroid *Corynebacterium minutisssimum.* Affected areas are pink to brown irregular patches with fine creasing and they show a coral-pink fluorescence under Wood's rays. [Gk *erythros* red.]

See also: BAERENSPRUNG.

erythrene (er·ith·reen). CH_2=CHCH=CH_2, a colourless gas used as an anaesthetic, and also, by polymerization, to manufacture synthetic rubber.

erythrism (er·ith·rizm). 1. The condition of having a fresh rosy complexion, perhaps freckled, with red hair and beard. Among the pure-bred dark-haired races such as the Jews, the condition is or may be due to some functional derangement (Broca). 2. In biology, a condition of excessive redness of hair or plumage without reference to season, age or sex. [Gk *erythros* red.]

erythristic (er·ith·ris·tik). Pertaining to or characterized by the presence of erythrism.

erythrite, erythritol (er·ith·rite, er·ith·rit·ol). Erythrol.

erythrityl (er·ith·rit·il). The tetravalent organic radical C_4H_6, derived from the tetrahydric alcohol, erythrol, **Diluted erythrityl tetranitrate, Erythrityl tetranitrate (50 per cent).** $CH_2NO_3(CHNO_3)_2CH_2NO_2$, a drug which has pharmacological properties similar to those of the nitrites, but slower in action and longer in duration owing to gradual liberation of nitro groups. It causes vasodilatation by direct action on the smooth-muscle coat of the arterioles; its relief in angina pectoris is due to coronary vasodilatation.

Erythrobacillus (er·ith·ro·bas·il′·us). The name given to a group of micro-organisms producing red or pink pigment, and now classified as *Chromabacterium* (Topley and Wilson) or *Serratia* (Bergey). [Gk *erythros* red, bacillus.]

erythroblast (er·ith·ro·blast). A general term that includes all the differentiated nucleated red blood cells, namely, the proerythroblasts, normoblasts and megaloblasts. These are the intermediate cells between the haemocytoblasts and the non-nucleated red blood cells; they are not found in normal circulating blood after about the third month of intra-uterine development. **Primary erythroblast.** An early form of erythroblast; a nucleated precursor of the red blood cell containing much polychromatophilic cytoplasm and coarse nuclear chromatin. It closely resembles Ehrlich's megaloblast, and is seen in primitive marrow, also sometimes in fetal blood, but is gradually replaced by the ordinary erythroblasts at a later stage. [Gk *erythros* red, *blastos* germ.]

erythroblastaemia (er·ith·ro·blas·te′·me·ah). An abnormal condition of the blood in which erythroblasts are present, occurring, for example, in erythroblastosis fetalis. [erythroblast, Gk *haima* blood.]

erythroblastic (er·ith·ro·blas′·tik). Relating or belonging to erythroblasts.

erythroblastoma (er·ith·ro·blas·to′·mah). A tumour the component cells of which resemble erythroblasts; a variety of myeloma. [erythroblast, Gk *-oma* tumour.]

erythroblastomatosis (er·ith·ro·blas·to·mat·o′·sis). A condition in which erythroblastomata develop, or which is favourable to their development. [erythroblastoma, Gk *-osis* condition.]

erythroblastosis (er·ith·ro·blas·to′·sis). The occurrence in the circulating blood of erythroblasts (nucleated red blood corpuscles), usually associated with various severe haemolytic anaemias, and especially with the haemolytic or erythroblastic anaemias of fetal life, the newborn and children. **Erythroblastosis fetalis.** A severe haemolytic anaemia with large numbers of erythroblasts in the blood of the fetus, hepatomegaly and diffuse cirrhosis, splenomegaly, very active marrow and a large oedematous placenta. Early intra-uterine death produces a macerated fetus, or there may be an oedematous fetus either dead, or dying a few hours after birth (hydrops fetalis). In less severe cases the infant may live a few days or even longer but die with jaundice and liver failure; in such an event there may be bile staining of the basal nuclei of the brain (kernicterus). The survivors may have extrapyramidal nervous symptoms. This haemolytic condition is due to iso-immunization of the mother by a red cell antigen present in the fetus which she lacks, to produce antibody against the fetal red cells. This occurs most commonly in the case of the Rhesus blood group system when an Rh-negative mother pregnant with an Rh-positive fetus produces anti-D (Rh_0) antibody. In the absence of prior transfusions with Rh-positive blood, such a mother is unlikely to produce antibodies during the first pregnancy with an Rh-positive fetus. The passage of antibody across the placenta results in haemolysis of the fetal red cells. Immunization of Rh-negative women by the fetal red cells that enter the circulation at parturition can be prevented by the injection of potent anti-D gamma globulin just after delivery. Haemolytic disease of the newborn due to materno-fetal incompatibilities of other antigens, e.g. A, can occur rarely. **Erythroblastosis neonatorum.** A haemolytic disease of the newborn; icterus gravis neonatorum; congenital anaemia of the newborn: a type of severe jaundice, with or without a severe erythroblastic or a macrocytic anaemia, occurring in newborn babies. Its aetiology is the same as that of erythroblastosis fetalis (see preceding). [erythroblast, Gk *-osis* condition.]

erythrocatalysis (er·ith·ro·kat·al′·is·is). The destruction of large numbers of erythrocytes by phagocytosis. [erythrocyte, catalysis.]

erythrochloropia, erythrochloropsia (er·ith·ro·klor·o′·pe·ah, er·ith·ro·klor·op′·se·ah). A form of partial colour-blindness in which only the colours red and green can be clearly recognized. [Gk *erythros* red, *chloros* green, *opsis* sight.]

erythrochromia (er·ith·ro·kro′·me·ah). Stained or coloured red; of the spinal fluid, indicating the presence of blood. [Gk *erythros* red, *chroma* colour.]

erythroclasis (er·ith·rok·las·is). Of erythrocytes, the splitting up into fragments. [erythrocyte, Gk *klasis* a breaking.]

erythroclastic (er·ith·ro·klas′·tik). Referring to erythroclasis.

erythroconte (er·ith·ro·kont). One of the fine rod-like bodies staining faintly azurophilic that are occasionally seen in the stippled erythrocytes in certain anaemic conditions such as pernicious anaemia. [Gk *erythros* red, *kontos* pole.]

erythrocyanosis (er·ith·ro·si·an·o′·sis). A condition of the legs, occurring chiefly in young women, in which there is swelling and blueness and often chilblains. The cause is vascular spasm due to inadequate protection in cold weather. The full name of the condition is *erythrocyanosis crurum puellarum frigidum*; it is also known as *erythrocyanosis puellaris* and *erythrocyanosis supramalleolaris.* [Gk *erythros* red, *kyanos* blue.]

erythrocyte (er·ith·ro·site). A mature, non-nucleated, red blood cell; in man it is a circular biconcave disc with a complex histological structure and physiochemical constitution, behaving as though it were enclosed in a flexible semipermeable membrane. Its main function is to transport oxygen in combination with the pigment haemoglobin contained in the cell, and to remove the carbon dioxide. It is orthochromatic but younger cells may be polychromatic. Normally it has a mean diameter of 7.25 μm (6.7–7.7) and volume 86 μm^3 (78–94), and the blood contains 4 200 000–6 400 000 (average 5 500 000; females 4 800 000) per mm^3. They vary in size, shape and quality according to disease and other factors; thus, anisocytosis refers to abnormal variations in size, and of these the *macrocyte* (*megalocyte*) is greater than 9 μm in diameter, while the *microcyte* has a diameter less than 6 μm. *Leptocytes* are abnormally thin bowl-shaped red cells which are seen in thalassaemia; these cells stain so that the haemoglobin appears to be concentrated in the centre and around the periphery of the cell, producing the appearance of a target, and so characterizes the *target cell. Ovalocytes* (*oval cells*) may be seen in the familiar condition of ovalocytosis (elliptocytosis). Poikilocytosis occurs especially in pernicious anaemia, the red cells showing very great changes in shape, many being pear-shaped. The *sickle-shaped cells* (*meniscocytes*) are seen in the haemolytic disease, sicklaemia. The *siderocyte* is a red cell containing granules that stain blue with Prussian Blue; they are much increased in toxic and haemolytic conditions. A more or less spherical or biconvex red cell (*spherocyte*) is usually seen in chronic haemolytic anaemias. Of alterations in the cellular haemoglobin content (normal values: 14.8 g/100 ml blood; mean corpuscular haemoglobin 29 ± 2γγ; mean corpuscular haemoglobin concentration 34 ± 2 per cent), increased haemoglobin is noted in hyperchromic anaemias, diminution in hypochromic conditions. *Punctate basophilic* or *stippled cells* are characterized by the presence of basophil-staining granules in the cytoplasm, whilst *reticulocytes* are red cells with reticulated or basket-like chromatin network stained by "vital" stains. Other bodies may be seen, in special conditions, in the red cells, such as Cabot's rings, Auer's, Howell-Jolly, Heinz, Pappenheimer's bodies and Schueffner's dots. **Basophilic erythrocyte.** *See* BASOPHILIA. **Crenated erythrocyte.** One with a crinkled outline; this is caused by withdrawal of fluid from within the cell, e.g. by suspension in hypertonic saline. **Dichromatic erythrocyte.** One still retaining some basophilic staining; not yet quite mature. **Polychromatic erythrocyte.** An erythrocyte that stains irregularly and takes both acid and basic staining. [Gk *erythros* red, *kytos* cell.]

erythrocythaemia (er·ith·ro·si·**the**′·me·ah). Polycythaemia vera. [Gk *erythros* red, *kytos* cell, *haima* blood.]

erythrocytic (er·ith·ro·**sit**′·ik). Having relation to erythrocytes.

erythrocytoblast (er·ith·ro·**si**′·to·blast). Erythroblast: in the development of the vascular system, an erythrocyte at the first stage of its development from the primitive cell before it reaches the normoblastic stage. [erythrocyte, Gk *blastos* germ.]

erythrocytolysin (er·ith·ro·si·**tol**′·is·in). Haemolysin. [erythrocyte, lysin.]

erythrocytolysis (er·ith·ro·si·**tol**′·is·is). Plasmolysis of the erythrocytes; reduction of corpuscular volume because of the escape of soluble substances. **Erythrocytolysis megalosplenica.** Polycythaemia vera. [erythrocyte, lysis.]

erythrocytometer (er·ith·ro·si·**tom**′·et·er). 1. An apparatus used for counting erythrocytes. It consists of a graduated glass capillary tube with a bulb-like expansion near the upper end containing a cube-shaped glass bead which acts as a stirrer. 2. An apparatus with which the diameter of erythrocytes can be measured. [erythrocyte, meter.]

erythrocytometry (er·ith·ro·si·**tom**′·et·re). 1. The counting of erythrocytes. 2. The measuring of the diameter of erythrocytes. [see prec.]

erythrocyto-opsonin (er·ith·ro·si·to·**op**′·son·in). Haemopsonin. [erythrocyte, opsonin.]

erythrocytopenia (er·ith·ro·si·to·**pe**′·ne·ah). Erythropenia.

erythrocytopoiesis (er·ith·ro·si·to·poi·**e**′·sis). Erythropoiesis.

erythrocytorrhexis (er·ith·ro·si·to·**rex**′·is). Plasmorrhexis of erythrocytes, i.e. their rupture with resultant loss of cytoplasm. [erythrocyte, Gk *rhexis* rupture.]

erythrocytoschisis (er·ith·ro·si·**tos**′·kis·is). Plasmoschisis of erythrocytes; the splitting up of the corpuscles and resulting formation of disk-like plaques resembling blood platelets. [erythrocyte, Gk *schisis* a splitting.]

erythrocytosis (er·ith·ro·si·**to**′·sis). A condition in which the red blood cells and haemoglobin are transiently or permanently increased above normal values due to certain stimuli; it is seen in newborn infants, congenital or acquired heart disease, chronic pulmonary disease, Cushing's disease, Ayerza's syndrome, individuals living at high altitudes, and following poisoning by phosphorus and many metallic salts or benzene derivatives. Also called *polycythaemia*; the latter name is preferred where the cause is unknown. [erythrocyte, Gk *-osis* condition.]

erythrocytotropic (er·ith·ro·si·to·**trop**′·ik). Denoting that a substance has an abnormally great attraction for erythrocytes or a particular selective affinity for them. [erythrocyte, Gk *tropos* a turning.]

erythrocyturia (er·ith·ro·si·**tewr**′·e·ah). Haematuria. [erythrocyte, urine.]

erythrodegenerative (er·ith·ro·de·**jen**′·er·a·tiv). Characterized by or relating to deterioration of erythrocytes as the result of disease. [erythrocyte, L *generare* to beget.]

erythroderma (er·ith·ro·**der**′·mah). Universal, or almost universal, erythema, with scaling and infiltration in the skin. **Atopic erythroderma.** Widespread cutaneous erythema, perhaps with exudation and scaling, occurring as a manifestation of atopy. It is usually, but not invariably, a manifestation of one form of infantile eczema. **Erythroderma desquamativa.** Chronic exfoliative dermatitis of children, with seborrhoeic dermatitis of the scalp. *See* DERMATITIS. **Exfoliative erythroderma.** Pityriasis rubra. **Erythroderma ichthyosiforme congenitum.** Erythroderma beginning in infancy, with features resembling ichthyosis and marked involvement of the flexures. **Leukaemic erythroderma.** Erythroderma complicating lymphatic leukaemia. **Lymphoblastic erythroderma.** Very chronic erythroderma, with lymphocytosis and lymph-node enlargement. **Malignant erythroderma.** Erythroderma as a manifestation of mycosis fungoides, Hodgkin's disease or some related disorder. **Primary erythroderma.** Erythroderma arising *de novo* without known cause. **Erythroderma psoriaticum.** Erythroderma following psoriasis. **Resistant maculopapular scaly erythroderma.** Parapsoriasis en plaques. **Secondary erythroderma.** Erythroderma caused by a drug, or following some other dermatosis. **Stocking erythroderma.** Eczema madidans. [Gk *erythros* red, *derma* skin.]

erythrodermatitis (er·ith·ro·der·mat·**i**′·tis). An inflamed condition of the skin marked by abnormal redness. [Gk *erythros* red, dermatitis.]

erythrodextrin (er·ith·ro·**dex**′·trin). A class of dextrin which is soluble in 55 per cent alcohol and gives a red colour with iodine. It is produced during enzymatic digestion of starch intermediate to the end-product, maltose. [Gk *erythros* red, dextrin.]

erythrodontia (er·ith·ro·**don**′·she·ah). Reddish-brown staining of teeth. [Gk *erythros* red, *odous* tooth.]

erythroedema polyneuropathy (er·ith·re·**de**′·mah pol·e·newr·**op**′·ath·e). Acrodynia. [Gk *erythros* red, *oidema* a swelling, polyneuropathy.]

erythrogenesis (er·ith·thro·**jen**′·es·is). The process of formation of erythrocytes. [erythrocyte, Gk *genein* to produce.]

erythrogenetic, erythrogenic (er·ith·ro·jen·**et**′·ik, er·ith·ro·**jen**′·ik). 1. Relating to the formation or production of erythrocytes. 2. Giving rise to a sensation that the colour red is present. 3. Causing the occurrence of a rash. [see prec.]

erythroglucin (er·ith·ro·**gloo**′·sin). Erythrol.

erythrogone, erythrogonium (er·ith·ro·gone, er·ith·ro·**go**′·ne·um). A pro-erythroblast. [erythrocyte, Gk *gone* seed.]

erythroid (er·ith·roid). Red or reddish in colour. [Gk *erythros* red, *eidos* form.]

erythroidine (er·ith·**ro**·id·een). $C_{16}H_{19}O_3N$, an alkaloid obtained from plants of the *Erythrina* species. It is a base with a curare-like action.

erythrol (er·ith·rol). Erythrityl alcohol, butane tetrol, $CH_2OH(CHOH)_2CH_2OH$. A tetrahydric alcohol occurring in certain lichens and algae as an ester of orsellinic acid; it can be oxidized to erythrose. **Erythrol tetranitrate.** Erythrityl tetranitrate.

erythrolein (er·ith·**ro**·le·in). A red substance obtained from species of lichen; it is a constituent of commercial litmus.

erythroleucoblastosis (er·ith·ro·lew·ko·blas·**to**′·sis). Haemolytic disease of the newborn. [Gk *erythros* red, *leukos* white, *blastos* germ.]

erythroleucothrombocythaemia (er·ith·ro·lew·ko·**throm**·bo·si·**the**′·me·ah). Leuco-erythroblastic anaemia; erythroleukaemia;

Di Guglielmo's anaemia or disease. [Gk *erythros* red, *leukos* white, thrombocyte, *haima* blood.]

erythroleukaemia (er·ith·ro·lew·ke′·me·ah). 1. A type of anaemia in which the blood contains an abnormally large number of imperfectly developed leucocytes and erythrocytes. 2. The apparent simultaneous occurrence of erythraemia and leukaemia in the same subject. [Gk *erythros* red, *leukos* white, *haima* blood.]

erythrolitmin (er·ith·ro·lit′·min). $C_{26}H_{23}O_{13}$, a red colouring matter which is contained in commercial litmus. [Gk *erythros* red, litmus.]

erythrolysin (er·ith·rol·is·in). Haemolysin. [erythrocyte, lysin.]

erythrolysis (er·ith·rol·is·is). Erythrocytolysis.

erythromania (er·ith·ro·ma′·ne·ah). A condition in which there is an uncontrollable propensity to blush. [Gk *erythros* red, mania.]

erythromelalgia (er·ith·ro·mel·al′·je·ah). A painful condition involving the extremities, with marked cutaneous vasodilatation, usually bilateral, more commonly affecting the feet than the hands. It is characterized by redness and mottling of the skin, raised skin temperature and burning pain. It may occur with polycythaemia, gout, neurological disease, heavy metal poisoning or idiopathically. **Erythromelalgia of the head.** Histamine headache; pain in the temple and one eye, also affecting the face and neck, due to carotid vascular dilatation produced by circulating histamine. [Gk *erythros* red, *melos* limb, *algos* pain.]

erythromelia (er·ith·ro·me′·le·ah). A condition in which areas of progressive centrifugal redness of the skin over the extensor muscles of arms and legs occurs. The condition is painless and there is no swelling. [Gk *erythros* red, *melos* limb.]

erythrometer (er·ith·rom·et·er). 1. An apparatus in the form of a colour scale with which degrees of redness can be determined and measured. 2. Erythrocytometer. [Gk *erythros* red, meter.]

erythrometry (er·ith·rom·et·re). 1. The measuring of the degree of redness with an erythrometer. 2. Erythrocytometry. [see prec.]

Erythromycin BP 1973 (er·ith·ro·mi′·sin). An antibiotic produced by the growth of *Streptomyces erythreus.* It has a range of action similar to that of penicillin but is also effective against penicillin-resistant staphylococci and *Haemophilus* species. It is mainly used in the treatment of patients who are sensitive to penicillin. Preparations of erythromycin include Erythromycin Estolate BP 1973, Erythromycin Ethyl Carbonate BPC 1968 and Erythromycin Stearate BP 1973.

Erythromycinum (er·ith·ro·mi′·sin·um). *European Pharmacopoeia* name for Erythromycin BP 1973.

erythron (er·ith·ron). A comprehensive term used to describe as one functioning organ or tissue the red cells and their precursors in the peripheral blood and the bone marrow. [Gk *erythros* red.]

erythroneocytosis (er·ith·ro·ne·o·si·to′·sis). A condition in which regenerative forms of erythrocytes are found in the general circulation. [erythrocyte, Gk *neos* new, *kytos* cell.]

erythronoclastic (er·ith·ron·o·klas′·tik). Destructive of erythron. [erythron, Gk *klasis* a breaking.]

erythroparasite (er·ith·ro·par′·ah·site). A micro-organism parasitic on erythrocytes.

erythropathy (er·ith·rop·ath·e). Any disordered condition of the erythrocytes. [erythrocyte, Gk *pathos* disease.]

erythropenia (er·ith·ro·pe′·ne·ah). A state in which there are too few erythrocytes in the blood. [erythrocyte, Gk *penes* poor.]

erythrophage (er·ith·ro·faje). Any phagocytic cell which ingests blood corpuscles or blood pigment. [Gk *erythros* red, *phagein* to eat.]

erythrophagia (er·ith·ro·fa′·je·ah). The process of ingestion of erythrocytes or blood pigment by phagocytic cells. [see prec.]

erythrophagocytosis (er·ith·ro·fag·o·si·to′·sis). The condition in which there is ingestion of erythrocytes by phagocytes. [erythrocyte, phagocytosis.]

erythrophagous (er·ith·rof·ag·us). Denoting the destructive action which certain phagocytes have on erythrocytes and blood pigment. [Gk *erythros* red, *phagein* to eat.]

erythrophil (er·ith·ro·fil). Any histological element or cell which readily stains with red dye; that part of the nucleus of a cell, animal or vegetable, which takes the stain of red dye (Auerbach). [Gk *erythros* red, *philein* to love.]

erythrophilous (er·ith·rof·il·us). Rapidly or easily taking a red stain. [see prec.]

erythrophloeine (er·ith·ro·fle′·een). $C_{28}H_{43}O_7N$, an alkaloid derived from *Erythrophloeum guineense.*

Erythrophloeum (er·ith·ro·fle′·um). 1. A genus of plants of the family Leguminosae. 2. Casca bark, sassy bark, ordeal bark; the bark of *Erythrophloeum guineense* G. Don, containing a poisonous alkaloid, erythrophloeine. It has been used as an anaesthetic in dentistry. [Gk *erythros* red, *phloios* bark.]

erythrophobia (er·ith·ro·fo′·be·ah). 1. Intolerance of red colours, a condition which sometimes occurs after extraction of cataract. 2. Excessive dislike of and aversion to the colour red. 3. Morbid fear of blushing. 4. A type of neurosis in which the sufferer blushes without any, or with only the slightest, reason. [Gk *erythros* red, phobia.]

erythrophoric (er·ith·ro·for′·ik). 1. Bearing red or of red coloration. 2. Containing red. [Gk *erythros* red, *pherein* to carry.]

erythrophose (er·ith·ro·foze). Any subjective sensation of red colour or light present in the line of vision; a red phose. [Gk *erythros* red, phose.]

erythropia (er·ith·ro·pe·ah). Erythropsia.

erythroplakia (er·ith·ro·pla′·ke·ah). Erythroplasia. Erythroplakia would appear to be the better word etymologically, but is not in general use. [Gk *erythros* red, *plax* a plain.]

erythroplasia (er·ith·ro·pla′·ze·ah). A condition in which painless red patches form on areas covered by pavement epithelium. They are precancerous lesions. [Gk *erythros* red, *plasis* a forming.]

See also: QUEYRAT.

erythroplastid (er·ith·ro·plas′·tid). A normal non-nucleated erythrocyte of man and some mammals. [Gk *plassein* to mould.]

erythropoiesis (er·ith·ro·poi·e′·sis). The formation of erythrocytes by the red marrow. **Capillary erythropoiesis.** Blood-cell formation within the erythropoietic capillaries. [erythrocyte, Gk *poiein* to make.]

erythropoietic (er·ith·ro·poi·et′·ik). Having relation or belonging to erythropoiesis; forming erythrocytes.

erythroprosopalgia (er·ith·ro·pro·so·pal′·je·ah). A neuropathy similar to erythromelalgia; it is characterized by a red colour of the face and also by neuralgic pain in the face. [Gk *erythros* red, *prosopon* face, *algos* pain.]

erythropsia (er·ith·rop·se·ah). A condition of vision in which all objects appear to be tinged with red. It is often present after removal of the lens. [Gk *erythros* red, *ops* eye.]

erythropsin (er·ith·rop·sin). Rhodopsin: a purple colouring material of the retina which becomes bleached, opaque and clouded on exposure to light. [see prec.]

erythrorrhexis (er·ith·ro·rex′·is). Erythrocytorrhexis.

erythrose (er·ith·roze). $CH_2OH(CHOH)_2CHO$, a tetrose monosaccharide formed by the oxidation of erythrol. **Erythrose 4-phosphate.** An intermediate of the pentose phosphate pathway.

erythrosedimentation (er·ith·ro·sed·e·men·ta′·shun). Erythrocyte sedimentation.

erythrosin (er·ith·ro·sin). 1. $C_{13}H_{18}O_6N_2$, a red substance formed from tyrosine with nitric acid. 2. $C_{20}H_8O_5I_4$, a yellowish-red fluorescent dyestuff. **Erythrosin B.** Bluish erythrosin, sodium tetraiodofluorescein, $C_{20}H_6O_5I_4Na_2$, a dyestuff used as an indicator (pH 2; orange in acids, magenta in alkalis). **Erythrosin BB.** Phloxine, potassium tetrachlorotetrabromofluorescein, $C_{20}H_2O_5Cl_4Br_4K_2$. **Bluish erythrosin.** Erythrosin B (see above). **Erythrosin G.** Potassium di-iodofluorescein, $C_{20}H_8O_5I_2K_2$. **Yellowish erythrosin.** Sodium di-iodofluorescein. $C_{20}H_8O_5I_2Na_2$. [Gk *erythros* red.]

erythrosinophil, erythrosinophile (er·ith·ro·sin′·o·fil, er·ith·ro·sin′·o·file). Readily taking the stain of erythrosin. [erythrosin, Gk *philein* to love.]

erythrosis (er·ith·ro·sis). 1. The florid complexion due to arterial plethora. 2. An abnormal tendency to blush. 3. A condition in which there is cyanotic or red discoloration of the skin and mucosa such as is present in polycythaemia. 4. Hyperplasia of the tissues from which erythrocytes are formed. [Gk *erythros* red.]

erythrothioneine (er·ith·ro·thi·on′·e·een). Ergothioneine, thiolhistidine betaine, thioneine, $HSC_3H_2N_2CH_2CHCOON(CH_3)_3$. A cyclic base derived from histidine and observed in blood corpuscles. It also occurs in ergot.

erythrothrombomonoblastosis (er·ith·ro·throm·bo·mon·o·blas·to′·sis). A severe fatal disease of the haemopoietic system, resembling acute leukaemia, in which the peripheral blood shows thrombocytopenia, erythroblastaemia and monocytosis; splenomegaly is frequently found.

erythrotoxin (er·ith·ro·tox′·in). Any poisonous substance which affects the erythrocytes. [erythrocyte, toxin.]

erythroxylin (er·ith·rox·il·in). 1. Cocaine, the alkaloid of *Erythroxylum* species. 2. An alcoholic extract of *Erythroxylum coca*, formerly used as a tonic.

erythroxylon (er·ith·rox·il·on). *Erythroxylum.*

Erythroxylum (er·ith·rox·il·um). A genus of plants of the family Erythroxylaceae, occurring in South America, Sri Lanka and the East Indies. The dried leaves of *Erythroxylum coca* Lam. (Bolivian or Huanuco leaf) or of *E. truxillense* Rusby (Peruvian or Truxillo leaf) are used as a source of cocaine. [Gk *erythros* red, *xylon* wood.]

erythrulose (er·ith·roo·loze). $CH_2OHCOCHOHCH_2OH$, a ketotetrose isomeric with erythrose, and obtained by the oxidation of erythrol.

erythruria (er·ithr·ewr·e·ah). The condition in which urine of a red colour is passed. [Gk *erythros* red, urine.]

Esbach, Georges Hubert (b. 1843). Paris physician.

Esbach's apparatus. A simple apparatus for the estimation of protein in urine by Esbach's method.

Esbach's method. For protein in urine: urine is placed in Esbach's tube to a mark U, and Esbach's reagent is added to another mark R. The tube is stoppered, inverted several times to mix the contents and allowed to stand for 24 h. The precipitated protein settles to the bottom of the tube and the amount, in gram per litre, is given by the graduation corresponding to the surface level of the precipitate.

Esbach's reagent. For protein in urine: dissolve 1 g of picric acid and 2 g of citric acid in 100 ml of water.

Esbach's tube. A graduated tube used in Esbach's method.

escape (es·kape). Release of the heart from an inhibitory influence. **Atrioventricular escape, Auriculoventricular escape.** Ventricular escape (see below). **Nodal escape.** Ventricular escape (see below). **Vagal escape.** In cardiac standstill as a result of excessive vagal stimulation: release of the heart from inhibition and recommencement of beating may occur, even though the stimulation be continued. **Ventricular escape.** When the rate of discharge of impulses from the sinu-atrial node (pacemaker) falls below the natural rate of impulse formation of the atrioventricular node, escape of the latter and the temporary taking-over of the function of pacemaker. It may occur during sinus arrhythmia after a long pause between sinus beats, and is often associated with excessive vagal tone (vagal escape, see above). [OFr. *escaper.*]

eschar (es·kar). The slough or dry scab, e.g. that forms on an area of skin that has been burned. **Neuropathic eschar.** A decubitus ulcer (bedsore) that develops in those with disease of the spinal cord. [Gk *eschara* scab.]

escharosis (es·kar·o·sis). 1. Any process that results in the formation of an eschar. 2. Caustic or corrosive action. [Gk *eschara* scab, *-osis* condition.]

escharotic (es·kar·ot·ik). 1. Tending or serving to form an eschar. 2. Caustic. 3. A corrosive or caustic agent the effect of which is to produce a slough. [see prec.]

Escherich, Theodor (b. 1857). Munich paediatrician.

Escherich's reflex, or sign. Pouting of the lips as a result of stimulation of the labial mucosa by tapping the lip.

Escherich's syndrome, or symptom complex. *Bacterium coli* infection in infants.

Escherich's test. A modification of the tuberculin reaction in which dilutions of tuberculin are given at intervals in increasing strength in order to produce local, general or focal reactions. The last-named is accompanied by an increase of symptoms with alteration in the physical signs over the site of the suspected lesion, such as râles or altered breath sounds. General reaction includes malaise and pyrexia with local tenderness and swelling at the site of injection. Focal reactions are not without danger of reactivation of a quiescent lesion, and the method is not now used.

Eschericheae (esh·er·ik·e·e). A tribe of Enterobacteriaceae which contains *Aerobacter, Escherichia* and *Klebsiella.* They are Gram-negative aerobic and facultative anaerobic rods, growing in the presence of bile. They have marked fermentative characters and normally inhabit the intestines of man and animals, though in the tissues they may cause pyogenic infections. [Theodor *Escherich.*]

Escherichia (esh·er·ik·e·ah). A genus of the family Enterobacteriaceae found in the faeces of man and animals; it is sometimes pathogenic to man, causing such infections as gastroenteritis, pyelitis and cystitis. **Escherichia coli.** Gram-negative motile rods, fermenting lactose and glucose usually with gas-formation; it is divisible into many serotypes, some of which are associated with acute gastro-enteritis in infants. [Theodor *Escherich.*]

eschomelia (es·ko·me·le·ah). A monster with a defective limb. [Gk *eschatos* worst, *melos* limb.]

escorcin (es·kor·sin). $C_9H_8O_4$, a derivative of esculin; a brownish powder used to stain and thereby identify corneal defects.

esculent (es·kew·lent). Suitable to be used as food by man; edible. [L *esca* food.]

esculin (es·kew·lin). Aesculin.

eseptate (e·sep·tate). Not provided with a septum or septa. [L *e, saeptum* partition.]

eseramine (es·er·am·een). $C_{16}H_{25}N_4O_3$, an alkaloid found in Calabar beans, *Physostigma venenosum* Balf.; it has little known physiological action. [see foll.]

eserine (es·er·een). Physostigmine, $C_{15}H_{21}N_3O_2$. An alkaloid obtained from Calabar beans, the dried seeds of *Physostigma venenosum.* It inhibits the action of cholinesterase, the enzyme which destroys the acetylcholine liberated at parasympathetic nerve-endings, and potentiates all the muscarinic effects of acetylcholine, though its influence on the nicotinic properties is more complex. It increases the cholinergic response at neuromuscular junctions in skeletal muscle so that close arterial injection of acetylcholine to such a junction, which would normally produce a single twitch of the muscle, causes a tetanic response after eserine. Similarly, if the muscle has been curarized, eserine will tend to restore conduction. In sympathetic ganglia eserine potentiates inhibitor effects rather than excitor. It is sometimes used to reduce intra-ocular pressure by instilling a few drops of solution into the eye; the pupil is constricted, thus opening the canal of Schlemm in the filtration angle of the eye. It is also used in a similar way to reverse the effects of homatropine when the latter has been administered for diagnostic purposes. Together with posterior pituitary extract it has been employed to restore intestinal tone after operations, but is less effective than carbachol in this respect. Because of its action at neuromuscular junctions in skeletal muscle it has also been tried in myasthenia gravis, though neostigmine has proved more effective in doses that do not produce circulatory disturbance. **Eserine salicylate.** Physostigmine Salicylate BP 1958. **Eserine sulphate.** $(C_{15}H_{21}N_3O_2)_2H_2SO_4$, a deliquescent salt soluble in water or alcohol. [*esere*, the West African name for the Calabar bean.]

eseroline (es·er·o·leen). $C_{13}H_{18}ON_2$, an alkaloid derived from Calabar beans and formed by alkalis from physostigmine; it has no miotic properties. [see prec.]

Esmarch, Johann Friedrich August von (b. 1823). Kiel surgeon.

Esmarch's bandage, or tourniquet. A broad, flat, rubber bandage applied to the proximal part of a limb which has been emptied of blood by the application of an elastic bandage distoproximally.

Esmarch's mask. An anaesthetic mask not now used.

Esmarch's operation. Osteotomy of the mandible for temporomandibular ankylosis.

Esmarch's paste. A caustic of morphine, arsenic, calomel and acacia.

eso-. For words beginning with **Eso-**, *see also* OESO-.

esocataphoria (e·so·kat·ah·**for**′·e·ah). In ophthalmology, a condition in which there is an inward and downward direction of the visual axis. [Gk *eso* inward, cataphoria.]

esocolitis (e·so·kol·**i**′·tis). 1. An inflamed condition of the mucous coat of the colon. 2. Dysentery. [Gk *eso* inward, colitis.]

esodeviation (e·so·de·ve·**a**′·shun). 1. In ophthalmology, esophoria. 2. A turning inwards. [Gk *eso* inward, deviation.]

esodic (e·**so**·dik). 1. Afferent. 2. Centripetal. [Gk *eso* inward, *odos* way.]

eso-ethmoiditis (e·so·eth·moid·**i**′·tis). A condition of inflammation within the ethmoidal sinuses. [Gk *eso* inward, ethmoiditis.]

esogastritis (e·so·gas·**tri**′·tis). An inflamed condition of the mucous coat of the stomach. [Gk *eso* inward, gastritis.]

esogenetic (e·so·jen·**et**′·ik). Produced from within the organism. [Gk *eso* inward, *genein* to produce.]

esohyperphoria (e·so·hi·per·**for**′·e·ah). Hyperesophoria: the tendency on the part of an eye to deviate upwards and inwards because of muscular insufficiency; a type of heterophoria. [Gk *eso* inward, hyperphoria.]

esophagus (e·**sof**·ag·us). *See* OESOPHAGUS.

esophoria (e·so·**for**·e·ah). Latent convergent strabismus; a condition in which the visual axes of the two eyes show more than a normal tendency to converge. This tendency is controlled by corrective fusion movements of the eyes, and it is only when the stimulus to fusion is removed, e.g. by covering one eye, that the visual axis of this eye will deviate inwards, only to recover again when the eye is uncovered. Cf. HETEROPHORIA. [Gk *eso* inward, *pherein* to bear.]

esophoric (e·so·**for**·ik). Pertaining to or marked by esophoria.

esophylactic (e·so·fil·**ak**′·tik). Referring to esophylaxis, indicating that the body is protected from within against attacks of disease.

esophylaxis (e·so·fil·**ax**′·is). Defence and protection against attacks of disease effected by the biological action of the body cells and fluids. Cf. EXOPHYLAXIS. [Gk *eso* inward, phylaxis.]

esosphenoiditis (e·so·sfe·noid·**i**′·tis). Osteomyelitis of the sphenoid bone. [Gk *eso* inward, sphenoid bone, Gk *-itis* inflammation.]

esoteric (e·so·**ter**·ik). 1. In physiology, indicating origin within the organism. 2. Confidential or secret. [Gk *esoteros* inner.]

esotoxin (e·so·**tox**·in). Any poisonous substance the production of which occurs within the body. [Gk *eso* inward, toxin.]

esotropia (e·so·**tro**·pe·ah). Manifest convergent strabismus; when the fixation axis of one or other eye becomes deviated inwards, so that it does not pass through the fixation object, corresponding retinal points are not stimulated and single binocular vision does not take place. [Gk *eso* inward, *trope* a turning.]

esotropic (e·so·**trop**·ik). Pertaining to or marked by the presence of esotropia.

espnoeic, espnoic (esp·**ne**·ik, esp·**no**·ik). 1. Relating to the therapeutic use of gases or vapours injected into the body. 2. Inspiratory. [Gk *es* into, *pnoe* a blowing.]

espundia (es·**pun**·de·ah). Mucocutaneous leishmaniasis; espundia is the name given to the form of mucocutaneous leishmaniasis that occurs in the hot humid forest areas of the plains of tropical America. Nasopharyngeal ulceration is a common sequel and occurs metastatically. Cf. UTA. [Sp.]

esquillectomy (es·kwil·**ek**·to·me). The operative removal of fragments of bone in cases of comminuted fracture. [Fr. *esquille* bone splinter, Gk *ektome* a cutting out.]

essence (es·ens). A volatile oil or concentrated tincture, e.g. essence of lemon (lemon oil), essence of ginger (concentrated tincture of ginger). **Essence of bergamot.** Oleum Bergamottae BPC 1949. **Essence of ginger.** Strong Ginger Tincture BP 1958. **Essence of peppermint.** Peppermint Spirit BP 1958. [L *essentia* quality.]

See also: RUBINI.

essential (es·**en**·shal). 1. The necessary condition or part of a thing, without which it could not exist. 2. Self-existent; without obvious cause; idiopathic. [L *essentia* quality.]

Esser, Johannes Fredericus Samuel (b. 1878). Dutch plastic surgeon.

Esser graft. A buried graft of skin.

ester (es·ter). 1. A compound ether; an ethereal salt; an alkyl salt formed by the combination of an organic acid and an alcohol. When no specific alcohol is mentioned, the ethyl ester is implied. 2. The term is also extended to include combinations of alcohols with inorganic acids, and of organic acids with metals. **Acid ester.** An ester in which there are still carboxyl groups available for further combination. **Basic ester.** An ester in which there are still hydroxyl groups available for further combination. **Internal ester.** A combination between the OH and COOH groups within the molecule of a hydroxy acid; a lactone. **Mixed ester.** An ester containing 2 different alkyl radicals. [coined word from Gk *aither* air, G *Saüre* acid.]

See also: CORI, EMBDEN, HARDEN-YOUNG, NEUBERG, ROBISON.

esterapenia (es·ter·a·**pe**′·ne·ah). A deficiency of blood cholinesterase. [esterase, Gk *penes* poor.]

esterase (**es**·ter·aze). A class of enzyme which hydrolyses carboxylic or other esters with the production of the constituent acid and alcohol or base. Included in this class are the lipases and phosphatases. **Acetylcholine esterase.** Cholinesterase; the enzyme which acts upon acetylcholine at the nerve-endings to produce choline and acetic acid. Its action is inhibited by eserine and physostigmine.

esterification (es·**ter**·if·ik·**a**′·shun). The combining of an organic acid with an alcohol to form an ester; the action may be accelerated by the use of catalysts, or by dehydrating agents to remove the water as it is formed. [ester, L *facere* to make.]

esterize (**es**·ter·ize). 1. To convert into an ester. 2. To undergo conversion into an ester.

Estes, William Lawrence (b. 1885). American surgeon.

Estes' operation. The implantation of the ovary (with its vascular connections intact) into the uterine wall so that its surface is exposed to the uterine cavity. It is used in the hope of restoring fertility when both fallopian tubes have been removed.

esth-. For words beginning with **Esth-**, *see also* AESTH-.

esthiomene (es·the·**om**·en·e). 1. Elephantiasis of the vulva resulting from lymphatic obstruction in lymphopathia venereum. 2. Lupus vulgaris. [Gk *esthiomenos* eating.]

esthiomenous (es·the·**om**·en·us). 1. Destructive and corrosive of the substance of the tissues, e.g. ulcus tropicum. 2. Of the nature of or pertaining to esthiomene. [see prec.]

estimation (es·tim·**a**·shun). An approximate value, or the arrival at such; often used for a more accurate determination. **Ventricular estimation.** The measurement of the capacity of the cerebral ventricles by the amount of fluid withdrawn at ventricular tap. [L *aestimare* to value.]

See also: FANTUS.

estivation (es·tiv·**a**·shun). Aestivation. [L *aestivare* to pass the summer.]

Estlander, Jakob August (b. 1831). Helsinki surgeon.

Estlander's operation. The resection of ribs over an empyema cavity so that the chest wall collapses.

estr-. For words beginning with **Estr-**, *see* OESTR-.

estrus (e·strus). *See* OESTRUS.

esuritis (es·ewr·**i**·tis). Gastric ulceration resulting from starvation or continued hunger. [L *esuries* hunger, Gk *-itis* inflammation.]

Etafedrine (e·tah·**fed**·reen). BP Commission approved name for 2

- (ethylmethylamino) - 1 - phenylpropan - 1 - ol; a bronchodilator.

Etamiphylline (et·am·i·fil·een). BP Commission approved name for 7 - (2 - diethylaminoethyl)theophylline; a smooth-muscle relaxant.

état (a·tah). A condition, or state. **État criblé.** 1. Multiple irregular perforations in the swollen Peyer's patches of the intestine in typhoid fever. 2. Generalized dilatation of perivascular lymphatic spaces in the brain, usually due to senility. **État lacunaire.** The pathological end-result of multiple small cerebral infarcts. **État mammelonné.** A form of chronic gastritis in which the mucous membrane has a rough, wrinkled, mammelated appearance. **État marbré.** Global shrinkage of basal ganglia, due to loss of nerve cells in the lenticular nucleus and globus pallidus, and their replacement by nests or whorls of myelinated fibrils, giving a "marbled" appearance. Possibly due to asphyxia neonatorum, it may produce choreo-athetosis and spasticity. Also called *status marmoratus*, or *Vogt's disease.* **État vermoulu.** The irregular "worm-eaten" state of the cerebral cortex which may result from advanced atherosclerosis. [Fr.]

Etenzamide (et·en·zam·ide). BP Commission approved name for 2 - ethoxybenzamide; an analgesic.

ethal (e·thal). Cetyl alcohol. *See* ALCOHOL.

Ethambutol (eth·am·bew·tol). BP Commission approved name for (+) - *NN'* - di - (1 - hydroxymethylpropyl)ethylenediamine. **Ethambutol Hydrochloride BP 1973.** The dihydrochloride of ethambutol, used in the treatment of *Mycobacterium tuberculosis* infections.

Ethamivan (eth·am·e·van). BP Commission approved name for *NN* - diethylvanillamide; a respiratory stimulant and analeptic with effects similar to those of nikethamide.

Ethamsylate (eth·am·si·late). BP Commission approved name for diethylammonium 2,5 - dihydroxybenzenesulphonate; a haemostatic.

ethane (e·thane). Methyl methane dimethyl, ethyl hydride, C_2H_6. A saturated gaseous hydrocarbon, the second in the methane or paraffin series; it occurs in the gas of petroleum wells.

ethanediamine (e·thane·di·am·een). Ethylenediamine, diaminoethane, $NH_2CH_2CH_2NH_2$. A liquid of ammoniacal odour used in organic synthesis, and in 30 per cent solution employed pharmaceutically as a solvent for theophylline. Its dihydrochloride decomposes in the body in the same way as ammonium chloride, and has been used internally, in the form of keratin-coated tablets, to acidify the urine.

ethanol (eth·an·ol). Ethyl alcohol. *See* ALCOHOL.

Ethanolamine (eth·an·ol·am·een). Monoethanolamine, $NH_2CH_2CH_2OH$. A water-soluble amino-alcohol which, esterified with oleic acid, is used as a sclerosing agent for varicose veins (BP 1958). **Ethanolamine oleate.** A compound employed in sterile solution with benzyl alcohol as a sclerosing agent for the treatment of varicose veins. (Ethanolamine Oleate Injection BP 1958.)

ethanolysis (eth·an·ol·is·is). Alcoholysis brought about by ethyl alcohol.

ethaverine hydrochloride (eth·av·er·een hi·dro·klor·ide). The tetraethyl analogue of papaverine hydrochloride. A coronary vasodilator with a more prolonged action than that of papaverine itself, it is used in the treatment of smooth-muscle spasm.

Ethchlorvynol BP 1973 (eth·klor·vi·nol). 1 - Chloro - 3 - ethylpent - 1 - en - 4yn - 3 - ol, a hypnotic, producing sleep lasting from 4 to 6 h. It is administered in capsules.

Ethebenecid (eth·e·ben·e·sid). BP Commission approved name for *p* - diethylsulphamoylbenzoic acid; it is used in the treatment of gout.

ethene (eth·een). Ethylene. **Ethene chloride.** Ethylene dichloride.

ethenoid (eth·en·oid). Denoting a compound which contains the ethene linkage, $-CH_2CH_2-$. [ethene, Gk *eidos* form.]

ethenol (eth·en·ol). Vinyl alcohol. *See* ALCOHOL.

etheogenesis (e·the·o·jen'·es·is). In protozoa, non-sexual reproduction by the male gamete. [Gk *etheos* bachelor, *genein* to produce.]

ether (e·ther). 1. The name given to any organic compound in which two radicals are linked through an oxygen atom; they have the general formula R-O-R', and are prepared by the elimination of a molecule of water from 2 molecules of the alcohol or alcohols. Also known as *alkyl oxides.* 2. Commonly applied to ethyl ether (see below). 3. The medium formerly postulated as filling all space, and in which electromagnetic waves were formerly thought to be transmitted; now regarded as unnecessary for modern theory. **Acetic ether.** A name given loosely to ethyl acetate, which is not a true ether. **Anaesthetic Ether BP 1973.** Purified ether used in anaesthesia; a colourless liquid obtained from ethyl alcohol and sulphuric acid, and freed from acetone, acetaldehyde, methyl alcohol or peroxides. It is used less than formerly but is still perhaps the safest anaesthetic for the production of surgical anaesthesia. There is a wide margin of safety with it between surgical anaesthesia and medullary depression, it is relatively non-toxic to the heart and does not affect the liver; on the other hand, it is inflammable and explosive, has a long induction period and causes considerable irritation resulting in excessive secretion of mucus, which can, however, be reduced by premedication with hyoscine or atropine. It stimulates the sympathetic centres and causes a rise in blood pressure, heart rate and blood sugar; it may give rise to ketosis and albuminuria, but the effect is transitory and not serious. **Chloric ether.** Chloroform Spirit BP 1958, a mixture of chloroform and alcohol. **Complex ether.** Mixed ether (see below). **Compound ether.** An ester. **Ether cone.** An appliance for the administration of ether in anaesthesia practice. **Dibromethyl ether.** $BrCH_2OCH_2Br$, a poison gas used in warfare. **Diethyl ether.** Ethyl ether (see below). **Dimethyl ether.** $(CH_3)_2O$, a gas, used in refrigeration, and also tried as a general anaesthetic but abandoned, as it caused cyanosis and lung congestion. **Divinyl ether.** $(CH_2{=}CH)_2O$, a colourless liquid, highly inflammable and explosive. It is a good general anaesthetic producing deep surgical anaesthesia, but the margin between that and depression of the respiratory centre is small. It does not affect uterine muscle and can therefore be used in labour where deep anaesthesia is required; also of value in short operations. It is liable to decompose into formic acid and formaldehyde. **Ethyl ether.** $(C_2H_5)_2O$, sulphuric ether; a colourless, volatile, highly-inflammable liquid with a characteristic odour and sweet taste, prepared by the action of sulphuric acid on ethyl alcohol. It is slightly soluble in water, and miscible with alcohol, chloroform or fixed oils; used as a solvent and in anaesthesia (*anaesthetic ether*; see above). **Formic ether.** Name applied to ethyl formate, wrongly, as it is not an ether. **Hydrobromic ether.** Ethyl bromide. **Methyl ether.** Dimethyl ether (see above). **Mixed ether.** An ether in which the two alkyl groups linked to the oxygen atom are not identical. **Nitrous ether.** A name applied to ethyl nitrite, wrongly, since it is not an ether. **Oenanthic ether, Pelargonic ether.** $C_6H_{13}OC_2H_5$, Cognac oil, a liquid used as a flavouring. **Petroleum ether.** 1. A light paraffin containing principally pentane, used in vaporizing preparations. 2. Petroleum benzine, a light fraction from petroleum distillation, used as a solvent. **Phenylmethyl ether.** Anisole. **Simple ether.** An ether in which the two alkyl groups linked to the oxygen atom are identical. **Solvent Ether BP 1973.** Ethyl ether used as a solvent for oils and resins, and also for cleaning the skin. **Sulphur ether.** An alkyl sulphide, analogous to an ether but in which the oxygen atom has been replaced by sulphur. **Sulphuric ether.** Ethyl ether (see above). **Vinyl Ether BP 1958.** *See* VINYL. **Xylostyptic ether.** Styptic collodion. [Gk *aither* air.]

ethereal (e·the·re·al). 1. Made, prepared with or containing ether. 2. Resembling ether, i.e. extremely volatile. 3. Characterized by extreme delicacy, as a structure. 4. Evanescent. 5. Belonging to the ether or to the upper air. [Gk *aither* air.]

etheride (e·ther·ide). An acid halide; an organic acid in which the OH group of the carboxyl has been replaced by a halogen atom.

etherification (e·ther·if·ik·a'·shun). 1. Esterification. 2. The process of converting an alcohol into an ether. [ether, L *facere* to make.]

etherify (e·ther·if·i). 1. To perform the process of etherification. 2. To add ether to a mixture. 3. To extract a constituent selectively by adding ether in which it is more readily soluble.

Etherington-Wilson, William (b. 1894). Torquay surgeon.
Etherington-Wilson technique. Time-diffusion technique; a form of spinal analgesia in which the upward level of the anaesthesia is controlled by sitting the patient upright for a measured number of seconds after the intrathecal injection of a hypobaric solution of an analgesic drug, usually cinchocaine.

etherism (e·ther·izm). 1. The physiological condition caused by administration of ether or by the excessive use of ether. 2. Etheromania.

etherization (e·ther·i·za'·shun). 1. The process of inducing anaesthesia by giving ether. 2. The condition produced by inhalation of ether.

etherize (e·ther·ize). 1. To anaesthetize with ether. 2. To convert into ether.

etheromania (e·ther·o·ma'·ne·ah). Addiction to ether, because of its stimulant properties. [ether, mania.]

etherometer (e·ther·om·et·er). An apparatus by means of which the mechanical administration of ether for the production of anaesthesia can be controlled and measured.

etheryl (e·ther·il). Ethylene.

Ethiazide (eth·i·az·ide). BP Commission approved name for 6 - chloro - 3 - ethyl - 3,4 - dihydro - 1,2,4 - thiadiazine - 7 - sulphonamide 1,1 - dioxide; it is used in the treatment of hypertension.

ethics (eth·ix). The science of moral conduct. **Medical ethics.** The moral rules and principles which govern a member of the medical profession in the exercise of his profession. [Gk *ethikos* character.]

ethidene (eth·id·een). The divalent radical $CH_3CH=$, derived from ethane; ethylidene. **Ethidine chloride.** Ethylidene chloride, 1,1-dichloroethane, CH_3CHCl_2, a compound formed during the preparation of chloral and used as an anaesthetic. **Ethidene diamine.** $CH_3CH(NH_2)_2$, a toxic compound arising during the decomposition of fish.

Ethinamate (eth·in·am·ate). BP Commission approved name for 1-ethynylcyclohexyl carbamate, an open-chain ureide; it is a mild sedative and hypnotic.

ethine (eth·een). Acetylene.

ethinyl (eth·in·il). Acetenyl; the monovalent organic radical, $HC\equiv C-$, derived from acetylene.

ethinylandrostenediol (eth·in·il·an·dro·steen'·di·ol). $C_{19}H_{29}O_2C\equiv CH$, a synthetic derivative of androstenediol with sex-hormone activity, which can be given orally since the ethinyl radical protects the molecule in the stomach and intestine.

Ethinyloestradiol BP 1973 (eth·in·il·e·strad·i'·ol). 17(β)-Ethinyl-$\Delta^{1,3,5:10}$-oestratriene-3,17(α)-diol, $C_{20}H_{24}O_2$. An artificial oestrogen highly active when administered orally.

ethinyltestosterone (eth·in·il·tes·tos'·ter·one). Ethisterone BP 1958.

Ethionamide BP 1973 (eth·i·on·am·ide). 2 - Ethylisonicotinthio - amide; it is used in the treatment of tuberculosis. Its action resembles that of sodium aminosalicylate.

ethionine (eth·i·o·neen). The ethyl analogue of methionine. An inhibitor of protein synthesis, it acts on the translational step. This and mestranol are the two alternative components of the combined contraceptive pill and are given in 0.05 mg doses.

ethiopification (e·the·op·if·e·ka'·shun). Aethiopification. [Gk *Aithiops* Negro, L *facere* to make.]

Ethisterone BP 1973 (eth·is·ter·one). Anhydrohydroxyprogesterone, ethinyltestosterone, pregneninolone. 17(β) - ethinyl - Δ^4 - androstene - 3 - one - 17(α) - ol, $C_{21}H_{28}O_2$. A synthetic preparation not found in the animal body, with pharmacological action similar to that of progesterone, though weaker; unlike the latter it is almost as active by mouth as when injected.

ethmocarditis (eth·mo·kar·di'·tis). A chronic condition of inflammation and proliferation of the cardiac connective tissue. [Gk *ethmos* sieve, carditis.]

ethmocephalus (eth·mo·kef·al·us). A variety of single monster in which the head is imperfect; there is a rudimentary proboscis-like nose, turning upward, with one or two nostrils and eyes united together to some degree. [Gk *ethmos* sieve, *kephale* head.]

ethmocranial (eth·mo·kra·ne·al). Concerning the ethmoid bone and the skull. [ethmoid, Gk *kranion* skull.]

ethmofrontal (eth·mo·frun·tal). Ethmoidofrontal.

ethmoid (eth·moid). 1. The ethmoid bone. 2. Ethmoidal. 3. Having a number of small openings or apertures; pierced like a sieve. [Gk *ethmos* sieve, *eidos* form.]

ethmoid bone [os ethmoidale]. An unpaired cranial bone lying in front of the sphenoid bone and composed of a perpendicular plate, forming the upper part of the nasal septum, and a lateral mass on either side filled with air cells and lying between the nose and the orbit. These masses are connected to the perpendicular plate by a cribriform plate forming part of the roof of the nasal cavity and separating it from the anterior cranial fossa.

ethmoidal (eth·moid·al). 1. Relating or belonging to the ethmoid bone. 2. In the region of the ethmoid bone.

ethmoidal arteries. Anterior ethmoidal artery [arteria ethmoidalis anterior], Posterior ethmoidal artery [arteria ethmoidalis posterior]. *See* OPHTHALMIC ARTERY.

ethmoidal nerves. Anterior ethmoidal nerve [nervus ethmoidalis anterior (NA)]. The continuation of the nasociliary nerve to the mucous membrane and skin of the nose. **Anterior ethmoidal nerve, external nasal branch of the [ramus nasalis externus (NA)].** The branch of the anterior ethmoidal nerve to the skin of the nose. **Anterior ethmoidal nerve, internal nasal branches of the [rami nasales interni].** The main branches of the anterior ethmoidal nerve to the mucous membrane of the nose lateral and medial [rami nasales laterales et mediales (NA)]. **Posterior ethmoidal nerve [nervus ethmoidalis posterior (NA)].** A branch of the nasociliary nerve to the ethmoidal and sphenoidal sinuses.

ethmoidal veins [venae ethmoidales (NA)]. Two vessels, anterior and posterior, draining, respectively, the nose and the ethmoidal sinuses into the ophthalmic vein.

ethmoidectomy (eth·moid·ek·to·me). Surgical excision of a portion of the ethmoid bone or of the ethmoidal sinuses. **Transantral ethmoidectomy.** Ethmoidectomy through the antrum. **Transmaxillary ethmoidectomy.** Removal of cells in the ethmoidal labyrinth by means of an approach through the canine fossa and maxillary sinus. [ethmoid, Gk *ektome* a cutting out.]

ethmoiditis (eth·moid·i·tis). Inflammation affecting the ethmoid bone or the ethmoidal sinuses. [ethmoid, Gk *-itis* inflammation.]

ethmoidofrontal (eth·moid·o·frun'·tal). Having relation or belonging to the ethmoid bone and the frontal bone.

ethmoidolacrimal (eth·moid·o·lak'·rim·al). Having relation or belonging to the ethmoid bone and the lacrimal bone.

ethmoidomaxillary (eth·moid·o·max·il'·ar·e). Relating or belonging to the ethmoid bone and the maxilla.

ethmoidonasal (eth·moid·o·na'·zal). Relating or belonging to the ethmoid bone and the nasal bone.

ethmoidopalatal (eth·moid·o·pal'·at·al). Relating or belonging to the ethmoid bone and the bones of the palate.

ethmoidopalatine (eth·moid·o·pal'·at·ine). Relating or belonging to the ethmoid bone and the palatine bone, or any of the structures in the region of the palatine bone.

ethmoidosphenoid (eth·moid·o·sfe'·noid). Relating or belonging to the ethmoid bone and the sphenoid bone.

ethmoidotomy (eth·moid·ot·o·me). Surgical incision into one of the ethmoidal sinuses. [ethmoid, Gk *temnein* to cut.]

ethmoidovomerine (eth·moid·o·vo'·mer·een). Belonging to the ethmoid bone and the vomer, or in relation to them.

ethmolacrimal (eth·mo·lak·rim·al). Ethmoidolacrimal.

ethmomaxillary (eth·mo·max·il'·ar·e). Ethmoidomaxillary.

ethmonasal (eth·mo·na·zal). Ethmoidonasal.

ethmopalatal (eth·mo·pal·at·al). Ethmoidopalatal.

ethmopalatine (eth·mo·pal·at·ine). Ethmoidopalatine.

ethmosphenoid (eth·mo·sfe·noid). Ethmoidosphenoid.

ethmoturbinal (eth·mo·ter·bin·al). Relating or belonging to the superior and middle nasal conchae (turbinate bones). [ethmoid, turbinate.]

ethmovomerine (eth·mo·vo·mer·een). Ethmoidovomerine.

ethmyphitis (eth·me·fi·tis). Cellulitis. [Gk *ethmos* sieve, *hyphe* tissue, *-itis* inflammation.]

ethnics (eth·nix). Ethnology.

ethnography (eth·nog·raf·e). That branch of anthropology which is concerned with the history of races and nations. [Gk *ethnos* nation, *graphein* to record.]

ethnology (eth·nol·o·je). The comparative study and analytical classification of peoples and races, including origin, distribution, relations and peculiarities. [Gk *ethnos* nation, *logos* science.]

ethnopsychology (eth·no·si·kol'·o·je). The study of the psychology of races, especially of primitive and uncivilized races. [Gk *ethnos* race, psychology.]

ethocaine (eth·o·kane). Procaine.

Ethoglucid (eth·o·gloo·sid). BP Commission approved name for triethyleneglycol diglycidyl ether; a cytotoxic agent.

Ethoheptazine (eth·o·hep·taz·een). BP Commission approved name for ethyl (±) - 1 - methyl - 4 - phenylazacycloheptane - 4 - carboxylate; an analgesic.

ethology (e·thol·o·je). The study of animal behaviour. [Gk *ethos* character, *logos* science.]

Ethomoxane (eth·o·mox·ane). BP Commission approved name for 2 - butylaminomethyl - 8 - ethoxy - 1,4 - benzodioxan; an adrenaline antagonist.

Ethopropazine (eth·o·pro·paz·een). BP Commission approved name for *N* - (2 - diethylamino - *n* - propyl) - phenothiazine. An autonomic blocking agent that also has a spasmolytic action; it is used in extrapyramidal parkinsonism and in nervous syndromes originating in the corpus striatum. The official preparation is Ethopropazine Hydrochloride BP 1973.

Ethosalamide (eth·o·sal·am·ide). BP Commission approved name for salicylamide - 2 -ethoxyethyl ether; an analgesic.

Ethosuximide BP 1973 (eth·o·sux·im·ide). α - Ethyl - α - methylsuccinimide; an anticonvulsant.

Ethotoin BP 1973 (eth·o·to·in). 3 - Ethyl - 5 - phenylhydantoin; it is used in the treatment of epilepsy.

ethoxide (eth·ox·ide). An ethylate; a compound of ethyl alcohol and a metal, the latter taking the place of the hydroxyl hydrogen.

ethoxy (eth·ox·e). The monovalent organic radical, C_2H_5O-, which is obtained from ethyl alcohol.

ethrisin (eth·ris·in). Acetysalicylamide.

Ethybenztropine (eth·e·benz·tro·peen). BP Commission approved name for 3 - benzhydryloxy - 8 - ethylnortropane; an anticholinergic.

ethydene (eth·id·een). Ethidene.

ethyl (eth·il). The monovalent aliphatic organic radical C_2H_5-, derived from the hydrocarbon, ethane. **Ethyl acetate.** Acetic ether, $CH_3COOC_2H_5$, the ethyl ester of acetic acid; a colourless liquid used principally as a solvent. **Ethyl alcohol.** *See* ALCOHOL. **Ethyl aminobenzoate.** Benzocaine BP 1958. **Ethyl Biscoumacetate BP 1958.** Bis - 3,3' - (4 - oxycoumarinyl) - ethyl acetate, $C_{22}H_{16}O_8$, an anticoagulant of the dicoumarin series. It has replaced the parent compound, dicoumarin, in therapy because it is more rapidly absorbed and excreted and thus allows the prothrombin level to return to normal more rapidly after withdrawal of the drug. **Ethyl bromide.** C_2H_5Br, a heavy liquid used as an anaesthetic. **Ethyl butyl barbiturate.** Butobarbitone, $C_2H_5(C_4H_9)C(CONH)_2CO$, a long-acting hypnotic producing immediate and heavy sleep. **Ethyl butyrate.** $C_3H_7COOC_2H_5$, a liquid with the odour of pineapple when diluted; used as a flavouring. **Ethyl carbamate.** Urethane BP 1958, $NH_2COOC_2H_7$, colourless crystals, soluble in water; used as a hypnotic combined with quinine it has been employed as a sclerosing agent in the treatment of varicose veins. **Ethyl carbinol.** Propyl alcohol. **Ethyl cellulose.** An ether of cellulose obtained by the action of ethyl chloride, and used in plastics manufacture. **Ethyl Chloride BP 1973.** C_2H_5Cl, a gas at ordinary temperatures, but liquefied under pressure. It evaporates quickly when sprayed on the skin, producing local anaesthesia; it also acts as a general anaesthetic, having a quick induction period, but is suitable only for short operations. **Ethyl Dibunate.** BP Commission approved name for ethyl 2,7 - di - *tert* - butylnaphthalenesulphonate; a cough suppressant. **Ethyl di-iodosalicylate.** $C_6H_2(OH)I_2COOC_2H_5$, a compound which is colourless and soluble in alcohol; used in place of iodoform. **Ethyl formate.** $HCOOC_2H_5$, a liquid used as a flavouring (rum). **Ethyl hydrocupreine.** $C_{19}H_{24}ON_2OC_2H_5$, a white crystalline powder, soluble in water, and used in eye affections, and as a prophylactic when the cornea has been lacerated; it produces some anaesthesia. **Ethyl iodide.** C_2H_5I, hydriodic ether; a colourless liquid used in the treatment of bronchitis. **Ethyl nitrite.** C_2H_5ONO, a compound which, dissolved in alcohol (Spirit of Nitrous Ether BPC 1959), has been used in angina pectoris with limited effect; occasionally used also as a diaphoretic. **Ethyl Oleate BP 1973.** $C_{20}H_{38}O_2$, a pale-yellow oil with an offensive odour, prepared by the esterification of oleic acid with ethyl alcohol. **Ethyl orange.** An azo dye used as an indicator. **Ethyl oxide.** Ethyl ether. **Ethyl pelargonate.** $C_8H_{17}COOC_2H_5$, a liquid used as a flavouring (wine). **Ethyl pyrophosphate.** BP Commission approved name for tetraethyl pyrophosphate, TEPP; a compound used in myasthenia gravis and postoperative paralytic ileus: it inhibits the action of cholinesterase. Its action is less than that of neostigmine, but it is longer-lasting. **Ethyl salicylate.** $C_6H_4(OH)COOC_2H_5$, a liquid used like oil of wintergreen. **Ethyl sulphide.** Ethyl thio-ether, $(C_2H_5)_2S$, an offensive-smelling liquid used in organic synthesis. [ether, Gk *hyle* stuff.]

ethylate (eth·il·ate). An ethoxide.

ethylation (eth·il·a·shun). The introduction of an ethyl C_2H_5 group into a compound.

ethylbenzoylecgonine (eth·il·ben·zo·il·ek'·go·neen). Cocaethyline.

ethylbromacetate, ethylbromoacetate (eth·il·brom·as'·et·ate, eth·il·bro·mo·as'·et·ate). $CH_2BrCOOC_2H_5$, a colourless liquid, the vapour of which is lacrimatory; used as a tear gas in chemical warfare.

ethylchloralurethane (eth·il·klor·al·ewr'·e·thane). $CCl_3CH(OC_2H_5)NHCOOC_2H_5$, a hypnotic similar in action to chloral hydrate and related chemically to it.

ethylchlorosulphonate (eth·il·klor·o·sul'·fon·ate). $C_2H_5SO_3Cl$, a substance used in chemical warfare to produce smoke screens, and as a tear gas.

ethyldichlorarsine, ethyldichloroarsine (eth·il·di·klor·ar'·seen, eth·il·di·klor·o·ar'·seen). $C_2H_5AsCl_2$, a liquid used in chemical warfare as a nose gas under the name *Dick.* It is vesicant and highly irritant to the lungs, producing asthma.

ethylene (eth·il·een). Ethene, olefiant gas, $CH_2{=}CH_2$. A colourless gas that burns with a luminous flame, occurring in the natural gas from petroleum wells, in illuminating gas and in the gases formed by the cracking of oils. It is employed as a general anaesthetic for its rapid action and freedom from undue toxicity, but it is not very powerful, often causes vomiting, and the fact that mixtures with air or oxygen are explosive prevents its use with cautery or in diathermy. **Ethylene bichloride, Ethylene dichloride.** CH_2ClCH_2Cl, a heavy colourless oil formed by the action of chlorine on ethylene. It has been used to some extent as a general anaesthetic, its effect resembling that of chloroform, but prolonged use is said to damage the cornea. **Ethylene glycol.** CH_2OHCH_2OH, a compound not itself used in medicine, but the ethers of which are powerful bacteriostatics, particularly phenoxyethanol, the monophenyl ether, $CH_2OHCH_2OC_6H_5$. **Ethylene oxide.** C_2H_4O, a gas used to sterilize equipment. **Ethylene periodide.** $CI_2{=}CI_2$, a yellow odourless crystalline substance, insoluble in water or alcohol, but soluble in most organic solvents and used as a substitute for iodoform; also known as *di-iodoform.*

ethylenediamine (eth·il·een·di'·am·een). Ethanediamine, $NH_2CH_2CH_2NH_2$. A liquid with an ammoniacal odour, used in organic synthesis, and as a 30 per cent solution as a solvent for theophylline. The dihydrochloride decomposes in the body in the same way as ammonium chloride and has been used in the form of keratin-coated tablets to acidify the urine. Ethylenediamine Hydrate BP 1973 is the official preparation.

ethylene-ethenyldiamine (eth·il·een·eth·en·il·**di**'·am·een). Lysidine, methylglyoxalidine. A condensation product of ethylene and ethylidene diamine which is supposed to have a powerful solvent action on uric acid and is therefore used in the treatment of gout. It is soluble in water or alcohol, but is incompatible with acids and alkaloids.

ethylhydrocupreine (eth·il·hi·dro·**kew**'·pre·een). $C_{21}H_{28}O_2N_2$, a derivative of quinine, formerly used for pneumonia but now replaced by the more efficient and less toxic sulphonamide drugs. **Ethylhydrocupreine hydrochloride.** $C_{21}H_{28}O_2N_2HCl$, a compound not employed internally as it is too toxic, but in solutions used locally for eye affections. Only the free base is suitable for internal use.

ethylic (eth·**il**·ik). Relating to the ethyl radical or containing it.

ethylidene (eth·**il**·id·een). Ethidene. The divalent radical $CH_3CH=$ derived from ethane. **Ethylidene diamine.** Ethidene diamine.

ethyliodoacetate (eth·il·i·o·do·**as**'·et·ate). $CH_2ICOOC_2H_5$. A heavy liquid used in chemical warfare as a tear gas under the name KSK.

ethylism (eth·il·izm). A condition of intoxication or poisoning by ethyl alcohol.

Ethylmethylthiambutene (eth·il·**meth**·il·thi·**am**'·bew·teen). BP Commission approved name for 3 - ethylmethylamino - 1,1 - di - α - thienyl - 1 - butene, an analgesic-hypnotic drug used in veterinary practice. It has properties similar to those of morphine.

ethylmorphine (eth·il·**mor**·feen). $C_{19}H_{23}O_3N$, a homologue of morphine obtained by ethylation. **Ethylmorphine Hydrochloride BPC 1968.** $C_{19}H_{23}O_3NHCl·2H_2O$, a compound resembling codeine in pharmacological action and used mainly for coughs, also as a sedative and narcotic; it is less powerful than heroin but much safer.

ethylnoradrenaline hydrochloride (eth·il·nor·ad·**ren**'·al·een hi·dro·**klor**·ide). A sympatheticomimetic amine closely related to adrenaline and recommended as a bronchial antispasmodic.

ethylnorepinephrine hydrochloride (eth·il·nor·ep·e·**nef**'·reen hi·dro·**klor**·ide). Ethylnoradrenaline hydrochloride.

Ethyloestrenol (eth·il·e·stren·ol). BP Commission approved name for 17α - ethyloestr - 4 - en - 17β - ol; an anabolic agent which has nitrogen- and calcium-retaining properties. It is a 17α-alkylated preparation and these may have cholestatic effects and cause jaundice. This preparation is usually given in doses too small to produce this effect.

ethylol (eth·il·ol). 1. Ethyl chloride. 2. The monovalent organic radical CH_2OHCH_2–.

Ethynodiol (eth·in·o·di·ol). BP Commission approved name for 19 - nor - 17α - pregn - 4 - en - 20 - yne - 3β,17 - diol. **Ethynodiol Diacetate BP 1973.** 3β,17β - Diacetoxy - 19 - nor - 17α - pregn - 4 - en - 20 - yne; a derivative of the synthetic progestogen 19 - nor - testosterone, which with oestradiol is used as an oral contraceptive.

ethynyl (eth·in·il). The monovalent organic radical, HC≡C–, derived from acetylene.

Etidocaine (et·i·do·kane). BP Commission approved name for (±) - 2 - (*N* - ethylpropylamino)butyro - 2′,6′xylidide; a local anaesthetic agent.

Etifoxine (e·te·**fox**·een). BP Commission approved name for 6 - chloro - 2 - ethylamino - 4 - methyl - 4 - phenyl - 4*H* - 3,1 - benzoxazine; a tranquillizer.

etio-. For words beginning with **Etio-**, *see also* AETIO-.

etiocholanolone (e·te·o·ko·**lan**'·o·lone). Etiocholan - 3(α) - ol - 17 - one, $C_{19}H_{30}O_2$. One of the 17-ketosteroids excreted in human urine. It is a metabolic reduction product of testosterone.

etiolation (e·te·o·la'·shun). Pallor or paleness of the skin due to lack of light, a condition seen in patients whom illness has kept indoors for a long time. [Fr. *étioler* to whiten by excluding the sun's rays.]

etiology (e·te·**ol**·o·je). *See* AETIOLOGY.

etiquette (et·e·ket). The conventional rules of behaviour. **Professional etiquette.** The code of ethical conduct observed by a medical practitioner in relation to his patients and his professional brethren. It is based upon the hippocratic oath. [Fr. label.]

Etonitazene (e·to·**ni**·taz·een). BP Commission approved name for 1 - (2 - diethylaminoethyl) - 2 - (4 - ethoxybenzyl) - 5 - nitrobenzimidazole; a narcotic analgesic.

Etorphine (et·**or**·feen). BP Commission approved name for 7,8 - dihydro - 7α - [1(*R*) - hydroxy - 1 - methylbutyl] - O^6 - methyl - 6,14 - *endo*ethenomorphine; a narcotic analgesic.

Etoxeridine (et·ox·**er**·id·een). BP Commission approved name for ethyl 1 - [2 - (2 - hydroxyethoxy)ethyl] - 4 - phenylpiperidine - 4 - carboxylate; a narcotic analgesic.

etrohysterectomy (e·tro·his·ter·**ek**'·to·me). Hysterectomy performed through an incision made in the hypogastric region of the abdomen. [Gk *etron* hypogastrium, hysterectomy.]

etrotomy (e·**trot**·o·me). Abdominal incision. [Gk *etron* hypogastrium, *temnein* to cut.]

Etryptamine (e·**trip**·tam·een). BP Commission approved name for α - ethyltryptamine; it is used in the treatment of neuroses.

eu-. A prefix, from the Greek *eu*, meaning *good, well.*

euaesthesia (ew·es·**the**·ze·ah). Normal vigour and a normal condition of the senses; the sense of general physical and mental well-being. [Gk *eu*, aesthesia.]

euangiotic (ew·an·je·**ot**'·ik). Applied to a part which has a good supply of blood vessels. [Gk *eu*, *aggeion* vessel.]

Eubacteriales (ew·bak·teer·e·**a**'·leez). The name given, in the botanical classification of micro-organisms, to one of the orders of the class Schizomycetes. The order with its various families, genera and species includes most of the micro-organisms pathogenic to man and animals. [Gk *eu*, bacteria.]

eubiotics (ew·bi·**ot**·ix). The science of healthy and hygienic living. [Gk *eu*, *bios* life.]

eubolism (ew·bol·izm). The state in which body metabolism is proceeding normally. [Gk *eu*, metabolism.]

eucaine (ew·ka·een). Commonly applied to β-eucaine, one of the earliest synthetic substitutes for cocaine, prepared from acetone. **Alpha eucaine.** $N(CH_3)[C(CH_3)_2CH_2]_2C(COOCH_3)COOC_6H_5$, a derivative of piperidine γ-carboxylic acid which is less toxic than cocaine, but with irritant disadvantages. **Beta eucaine.** Benzamine, trimethylbenzoyloxypiperidine, $NH[C(CH_3)_2CH_2(CHCH_3CH_2)]CHCOOC_6H_5$, a compound used in the form of the hydrochloride or the lactate as a local analgesic. **Eucaine hydrochloride.** Benzamine Hydrochloride BPC 1954. **Eucaine lactate.** Benzamine lactate.

Eucalyptol BP 1958 (ew·kal·**ip**·tol). $C_{10}H_{18}O$, the anhydride of menthan - 1,8 - diol; it may be obtained from oil of eucalyptus, which is distilled from the leaves of various species of eucalyptus plants. A colourless liquid with an aromatic odour resembling camphor, employed in the symptomatic treatment of upper respiratory infections, either incorporated in tablets or pastilles, or inhaled with steam, or as a spray. Used also as an antiseptic in toothpaste, and in temporary dental fillings, combined with zinc oxide.

Eucalyptus (ew·kal·**ip**·tus). A genus of trees and shrubs of the family Myrtaceae; the dried leaves of the Australian tree *Eucalyptus globulus* Labill. are a source of eucalyptus oil. A tincture of the leaves has been used in the treatment of asthma and chronic bronchitis. **Eucalyptus Oil BP 1968.** *See* OIL. [Gk *eu*, *kalyptos* covered.]

eucanthus (ew·**kan**·thus). Any enlargement of the lacrimal caruncle at the medial (inner) angle of the eye. [Gk *eu*, canthus.]

eucapnia (ew·**kap**·ne·ah). The presence of a normal quantity of carbon dioxide in the blood. [Gk *eu*, *kapnos* vapour.]

eucaryote (ew·**kar**·e·ote). Eukaryote.

Eucatropine (ew·**kat**·ro·peen). BP Commission approved name for 4 - mandeloyloxy - 1,2,2,6 - tetramethylpiperidine, a mandelic ester of α-eucaine used as a mydriatic in aqueous solution instead of atropine, being more transient or with little effect as far as accommodation is concerned. **Eucatropine hydrochloride.** The salt most frequently used as a mydriatic in 10 per cent solution.

euchlorhydria (ew·klor·**hi**·dre·ah). The presence of a normal quantity of free hydrochloric acid in the gastric juice. [Gk *eu, chloros* green, *hydor* water.]

euchlorine (ew·**klor**·een). A solution of chlorine and chlorine dioxide in water, prepared by treating potassium chlorate with concentrated hydrochloric acid and dissolving the gases liberated. It is also known as *chlorine gargle.*

eucholia (ew·**ko**·le·ah). A condition in which the bile is normal in quantity and quality. [Gk *eu, chole* bile.]

euchromatic (ew·kro·**mat**·ik). Of chromosomes or chromosome regions, showing the properties characteristic of euchromatin. [Gk *eu, chroma* colour.]

euchromatin (ew·**kro**·mat·in). The chromatin of the chromosome regions which show a normal pattern of coiling and stainability, in contradistinction to heterochromatin. Euchromatin replicates earlier and has a greater influence on the phenotype than heterochromatin. [Gk *eu, chroma* colour.]

euchromatinization (ew·kro·mat·in·i·**za**′·shun). The process by which heterochromatic chromosome regions assume a euchromatic behaviour. [Gk *eu,* chroma *colour.*]

euchromatization (ew·kro·mat·i·**za**′·shun). Euchromatinization.

euchromatopsia, euchromatopsy (ew·**kro**·mat·**op**′·se·ah, ew·**kro**·mat·**op**′·se). The condition of being able correctly to recognize colours; normal colour vision. [Gk *eu, chroma* colour, *opsis* vision.]

euchromosome (ew·**kro**·mo·some). Autosome; any ordinary paired chromosome. [Gk *eu,* chromosome.]

euchylia (ew·**ki**·le·ah). The condition in which the chyle is normal in quantity and quality. [Gk *eu, chylos* juice.]

eucinesia (ew·sin·e·se·ah). Eukinesia.

eucodeine (ew·**ko**·de·een). Codeine methyl bromide, $C_{18}H_{21}O_3N(BrCH_3)$. A derivative of codeine used as a sedative.

eucolloid (ew·**kol**·oid). A colloid which, by reason of its large-chain molecules and cross-linkages between side-chains, is insoluble. [Gk *eu,* colloid.]

eucrasia (ew·**kra**·se·ah). 1. Physical well-being; normal health. 2. Lessened susceptibility to disease. 3. Diminished sensitivity to the action of certain foods or drugs. [Gk *eu, krasis* a mingling.]

eudiaphoresis (ew·**di**·ah·for·**e**′·sis). Normal free healthy excretion of sweat, giving a feeling of relief and comfort. [Gk *eu,* diaphoresis.]

eudiometer (ew·de·**om**·et·er). A vertical stout glass tube, straight or U-shaped, with platinum electrodes sealed into the upper closed end; it is used to fire mixtures of gases by an electric spark in gas analysis. [Gk *eudios* clear air, meter.]

eudiometry (ew·de·**om**·et·re). Gasometric analysis. *See* ANALYSIS. [see prec.]

euergasia (ew·er·ga·ze·ah). Balanced psychobiological functioning. [Gk *eu, ergein* to work.]

euflavine (ew·**fla**·veen). Neutral acriflavine, neutral flavine: a mixture of acriflavine (2,8 - diamino - 10 - methyl - acridinium chloride) with 2,8 - diaminoacridine monohydrochloride, prepared by neutralizing acriflavine with sodium carbonate and precipitating with sodium chloride. It is being displaced as an antiseptic by the more homogeneous Proflavine Hemisulphate BP 1958.

eugenesis (ew·**jen**·es·is). In biology, fertility, particularly between hybrids. [Gk *eu, genein* to produce.]

eugenetics (ew·jen·**et**·ix). Eugenics.

Eugenia (ew·**je**·ne·ah). A genus of plants of the family Myrtaceae. **Eugenia caryophyllatus.** An evergreen tree which is the source of cloves. [Named after Prince Eugène of Savoy.]

eugenic (ew·**jen**·ik). Referring or belonging to eugenics.

eugenics (ew·**jen**·ix). The science of the improvement of the human stock. Concerned with improvement in living conditions and in mental and moral environment for the benefit of coming generations, it includes sexual selection and improved co-operation and social relations between the sexes. [Gk *eugeneia* nobility of birth.]

eugenin (ew·jen·in). $C_{10}H_{12}O_2$, a terpene isomeric with eugenol and chavibetol; obtained from clove oil and other essential oils.

eugenism (ew·jen·izm). The sum total of good hereditary and environmental conditions which make possible a life of health and happiness (Galton). [eugenics.]

eugenist (ew·jen·ist). One who has made a study of the science of eugenics and is an authority.

Eugenol BP 1973 (ew·jen·ol). 4 - Allyl - 2 - methoxyphenol, $CH_2CHCH_2C_6H_3OHOCH_3$. A phenolic compound occurring in clove oil (85 to 90 per cent) and oil of cinnamon leaf. It is a colourless or straw-coloured liquid with the odour and taste of cloves, and is used in dentistry as an antiseptic and mild analgesic; as it hardens when mixed with zinc oxide, it is of value as a temporary dental filling.

eugenothenics (ew·**jen**·o·**then**′·ix). The science concerned with racial improvement by means of sexual selection and controlled environment. [Gk *eugeneia* nobility of birth, *euthenia* well-being.]

Euglena (ew·**gle**·nah). A genus of fresh-water flagellate protistan organisms usually classified with the unicellular algae, but often having no chlorophyll. **Euglena gracilis.** A species used in the biological assay of vitamin B_{12}. [Gk *eu, glene* socket.]

euglobulin (ew·**glob**·ew·lin). The name given to that fraction of serum globulin which is precipitated by dialysis of serum against distilled water. The name implies that this fraction is a typical globulin by reason of its insolubility in water. [Gk *eu,* globulin.]

eugnosia (ew·**no**·se·ah). The normal state in which an individual is perfectly aware of the form of his body image and of the significance of all forms of sensory stimuli. [Gk *eu, gnosis* knowledge.]

eugonic (ew·**gon**·ik). Denoting a bacterial culture of luxuriant growth. [Gk *eu, gone* seed.]

eukaryon (ew·**kar**·e·on). The nucleus of a eukaryote. [Gk *eu, karyon* nut.]

eukaryote (ew·**kar**·e·ote). An organism with cells containing a membrane-surrounded nucleus. The cells are larger and more complex than prokaryotic cells and contain other membranous organelles (such as mitochondria, Golgi bodies, endoplasmic reticulum and, in photosynthetic cells, chloroplasts). Such cells are characteristic of animals, plants, protozoa, fungi and some algae. [Gk *eu, karyon* nut.]

eukaryotic (ew·kar·e·**ot**′·ik). Appertaining to cells of higher organisms which are characterized by complex chromosome structure, a nuclear membrane and division by mitosis and meiosis. [Gk *eu, karyon* nut.]

eukeratin (ew·**ker**·at·in). The normal or true keratin of epidermal derivatives such as hair and nails. [Gk *eu,* keratin.]

eukinesia (ew·kin·e·se·ah). The normal perception of muscular movements. [Gk *eu, kinesis* movement.]

Eulenburg, Albert (b. 1840). Berlin neurologist.

Eulenburg's disease. Paramyotonia congenita.

eulexine (ew·**lex**·een). Cytisine, $C_{11}H_{14}ON_2$. A purgative emetic alkaloid obtained from the seed of *Cytisus laburnum.* It is very toxic, resembling nicotine in its pharmacological action.

eumelanin (ew·**mel**·an·in). A brown-black hair pigment derived from tyrosine. [Gk *eu,* melanin.]

eumenorrhoea (ew·men·o·**re**′·ah). A state in which the menstrual function is normal. [Gk *eu,* menorrhoea.]

eumetria (ew·**me**·tre·ah). 1. That amount of muscular effort necessary for achieving any particular result. 2. A condition of normalcy of nerve impulses. [Gk goodness of measure.]

eumorphics (ew·**mor**·fix). That branch of orthopaedics which is concerned with the restoration of a structure to its normal shape or form. [Gk *eu, morphe* form.]

eumorphism (ew·**mor**·fizm). The retention or preservation of the normal form of a cell despite pathological changes occurring in it. [see prec.]

Eumyces, Eumycetes (ew·**mi**·seez, ew·mi·se·teez). True fungi, i.e. neither *Myxomycota* nor *Bacteria.* [Gk *eu, mykes* fungus.]

eunoia (ew·**noi**·ah). The condition in which there is normal liveliness of mind and power of will. [Gk *eu, nous* mind.]

eunuch (ew·nuk). A male from whom the testes and/or penis have been removed or who has been mutilated so that he is impotent. **Fertile eunuch,** *see* FERTILE. [Gk *eune* couch, *echein* to guard.]

eunuchism (ew·nuk·izm). The condition of being a eunuch. **Pituitary eunuchism.** Impotence resulting from disease or dysfunction of the hypophysis cerebri (pituitary gland).

eunuchoid (ew·nuk·oid). 1. Resembling or having the characteristics of a eunuch, i.e. lack of masculinity of appearance. 2. Term applied to a male in whom the testes have not developed or atrophied and who therefore has the appearance of a eunuch, and a light, high falsetto voice. **Eunuchoid gigantism.** A condition in which the man is tall because, owing to the lack of testosterone, the epiphyses of the long bones have not united and the legs (and arms) are unduly long. [eunuch, Gk *eidos* form.]

eunuchoidism (ew·nuk·oid·izm). A condition of eunuchism in which the external genital organs or the testes are complete but the internal secretion is lacking, so that sexual power is impaired and there is a eunuchoid appearance.

euonymin (ew·**on**·im·in). The dried alcoholic extract of euonymus bark (*Euonymus atropurpureus*) mixed with calcium phosphate; it is a mild cathartic.

Euonymus (ew·**on**·im·us). 1. A genus of trees and shrubs of the family Celastraceae. 2. Euonymus BPC 1954. Wahoo bark; the dried root bark of *Euonymus atropurpureus* Jacq. (spindle-tree). It is a mild cathartic administered in the form of an extract, tincture or elixir, and as tablets, in conjunction with other cathartics. [Gk *eu*, *onoma* name.]

euosmia (ew·**oz**·me·ah). 1. The state of having normal keenness of the sense of smell. 2. Term for an odour that is agreeable or pleasant. [Gk *eu*, *osme* odour.]

eupad (**ew**·pad). A mixture of equal parts of dry chlorinated lime and boric-acid powder; when required for use, 28 g (1 oz) is mixed into a paste with water and made up to 1 litre (1 quart), shaken, allowed to stand, and finally filtered. The solution, known as *eusol*, is employed as an antiseptic. The powder itself is used sometimes for application to wounds.

eupancreatism (ew·**pan**·kre·at·izm). The condition in which there is normal activity of the pancreatic function. [Gk *eu*, pancreas.]

eupareunia (ew·par·**ewn**·e·ah). Sexual suitability existing between any particular pair of persons of opposite sexes; sexual compatibility. [Gk *eu*, pareunia.]

Euparyphium (ew·par·**if**·e·um). A genus of small intestinal flukes. *Echinostoma* is the generic name now more frequently used. **Euparyphium ilocanum.** A species whose normal hosts are rats; common in man in Java and the Philippines. The intermediate host is the fresh-water snail *Gyraulus prashadi*, and encystment takes place in other snails, particularly *Pila luzonica*. **Euparyphium jassyense.** A species recorded from man, once, in Europe. **Euparyphium malayanum.** A species occurring in man in Malaysia and South China. Intermediate snail hosts have not yet been identified. [Gk *eu*, *paryphe* border.]

eupathia (ew·**path**·e·ah). The mental state of content or happiness. [Gk *eu*, *pathos* feeling.]

Eupatorium (ew·pat·**or**·e·um). A genus of plants of the family Compositae. The leaves of *Eupatorium rebaudinianum*, contain the saponins, eupatorin and rebaudin, each several hundred times as sweet as sugar. [Gk *eupatorion* agrimony.]

eupepsia, eupepsy (ew·**pep**·se·ah, ew·**pep**·se). The condition in which the power and function of the digestion are good; in particular, the condition in which the gastric juice contains that quantity of pepsin required for normal digestive function. [Gk *eu*, *pepsis* digestion.]

eupeptic (ew·**pep**·tik). 1. Indicating that the digestion is good. 2. Applied to substances that are easily digested or that aid the process of digestion. 3. Belonging to the state of eupepsia. [see prec.]

euperistalsis (ew·per·is·**tal'**·sis). Normal healthy and painless peristaltic movement. [Gk *eu*, peristalsis.]

euphagia (ew·**fa**·je·ah). The proper mastication of food so that the digestive processes are not impaired or obstructed. [Gk *eu*, *phagein* to eat.]

euphonia (ew·**fo**·ne·ah). The normal condition of the voice, i.e. clear, of good tone and pleasing to the ear. [Gk *eu*, *phone* voice.]

Euphorbia (ew·**for**·be·ah). 1. A genus of plants of the family Euphorbiaceae, including the spurges. 2. Euphorbia BPC 1954. Euphorbia herb, euphorbia pilulifera, Australian shakeweed, cat's hair; a tropical herb, *Euphorbia hirta* Linn., used in the form of a liquid extract or tincture in the treatment of asthma and bronchitis. [Gk *euphorbion* spurge.]

euphorbism (ew·**for**·bizm). The condition of being poisoned by any of the euphorbia: the characteristic signs are asphyxia and severe inflammation of the alimentary canal.

euphoria (ew·**for**·e·ah). The bodily sense of well-being and comfort. Often used to denote an exaggerated sense of well-being. [Gk a bearing well.]

euphoric (ew·**for**·ik). Referring or belonging to or characterized by a state of euphoria.

euphoristic (ew·for·**is**·tik). Term applied to anything which produces a state of euphoria or causes its occurrence.

Euphractus (ew·**frak**·tus). A genus of armadillo, some species of which are reservoirs of *Trypanosoma cruzi*. [Gk *euphraktos* well protected.]

euplastic (ew·**plas**·tik). 1. Adapted to the formation of, or capable of being transformed into, healthy tissue. 2. Applied to a wound, indicating that it heals readily and well. 3. Having the capacity of readily becoming organized. [Gk *eu*, *plassein* to form.]

euploid (**ew**·ploid). In genetics, denoting a chromosome complement, a cell or an organism with 1 complete chromosome set or multiples thereof (monoploid, diploid, polyploid). [Gk *eu*, *-ploos* folds (multiple).]

euploidy (ew·**ploi**·de). The condition of a cell or organism with a euploid chromosome complement. [Gk *eu*, *-ploos* folds (multiple).]

eupnoea (ewp·**ne**·ah). Normal respiration, easy and free; the opposite of dyspnoea. [Gk *eu*, *pnein* to breathe.]

eupraxia (ew·**prax**·e·ah). A condition in which there is normal ability to perform co-ordinated movements. [Gk *eu*, *praxis* a doing.]

eupraxic (ew·**prax**·ik). 1. Having relation to eupraxia. 2. Belonging to or having a part in proper functional activity.

eupyknotic (ew·pik·**not**·ik). Euchromatic. [Gk *eu*, *pyknos* thick.]

eurodontia (ewr·o·**don**·she·ah). Dental caries. *See* CARIES. [Gk *euros* mould, *odous* tooth.]

europium (ewr·**o**·pe·um). A rare-earth element, of atomic weight 151.96, atomic number 63, and chemical symbol Eu. A trivalent metal forming pink compounds; it occurs in cerium minerals. [*Europe*.]

Eurotiaceae (**ewr**·o·te·**a'**·se·e). A family of fungi which includes the genus *Allescheria*. [Gk *euros* mould.]

Eurotium (ewr·**o**·she·um). A genus of fungi; the perfect states of the *Aspergilli*, some members being pathogenic for man and animals. [Gk *euros* mould.]

eurycephalic, eurycephalous (ewr·e·kef·**al'**·ik, ewr·e·**kef**·al·us). Characterized by having a wide head or skull. [Gk *euyrs* wide, *kephale* head.]

eurycranial (ewr·e·**kra**·ne·al). Eurycephalic. [Gk *eurys* wide, *kranion* skull.]

eurygnathic (ewr·ig·**nath**·ik). Having a broad or large jaw. [Gk *eurys* wide, *gnathos* jaw.]

eurygnathism (ewr·**ig**·nath·izm). The condition of having large or broad jaws. [see prec.]

euryon (**ewr**·e·on). In craniometry, the point at each end of a line drawn through the greatest transverse diameter of a skull. [Gk *eurys* wide.]

euryopia, euryopsia (ewr·e·o·pe·ah, ewr·e·**op**·se·ah). The condition in which the eyes are abnormally widely opened. [Gk *eurys* wide, *ops* eye.]

euryphotic (ewr·e·**fo**·tik). Term denoting ability to see in widely varying intensities of light. [Gk *eurys* wide, *phos* light.]

euryprosopic (ewr·e·pro·**so'**·pik). With a wide face, i.e. facial index between 80 and 85. [Gk *eurys* wide, *prosopon* face.]

eurysma (ewr·iz·mah). 1. Dilatation. 2. Any structure that has been dilated. [Gk *eurynein* to dilate.]

eurysomatic (ewr·e·so·mat′·ik). Short and thick-set in body. [Gk *eurys* wide, *soma* body.]

eurythermal (ewr·e·ther·mal). Able to bear a wide range of temperature. [Gk *eurys* wide, *therme* heat.]

eurythermic (ewr·e·ther·mik). Applied to bacteria which can exist and grow in widely differing temperatures. [see prec.]

Eurytrema (ewr·e·tre·mah). A genus of small liver flukes, *Eurytrema pancreaticum*, normal to cattle; it is occasionally recorded from man in China and Indo-China. [Gk *eurys* wide, *trema* hole.]

euscope (ew·skope). A device used with a microscope for projecting the image on a screen mounted in a darkened room to facilitate observation. [Gk *eu*, *skopein* to view.]

euscopy (ew·sko·pe). Examination by means of a euscope.

Euscorpius (ew·skor·pe·us). A genus of scorpions. *Euscorpius flavicaudis* of southern France and *E. italicus* of the eastern Mediterranean are small forms with but slightly toxic sting. [Gk *eu*, *skorpios* scorpion.]

Eusimulium (ew·sim·ew·le·um). A genus of small black flies of which several species have been incriminated as the vectors of the filarial worm, *Onchocerca volvulus*, the cause of onchocerciasis. [Gk *eu*, L *simulare* to make like.]

eusitia (ew·sit·e·ah). The normal condition of the appetite. [Gk *eu*, *sitos* food.]

eusol (ew·sol). A useful antiseptic solution made by dissolving a mixture of equal parts chlorinated lime and boric acid (eupad) in water, at the rate of 28 g (1 oz) of mixture per litre (quart) and filtering. [*E*dinburgh *U*niversity *s*olution *o*f *l*ime.]

eusplanchnia (ew·splangk·ne·ah). The condition in which the internal organs are normal. [Gk *eu*, *splagchnon* entrail.]

eusplenia (ew·sple·ne·ah). The condition in which the spleen is functioning normally. [Gk *eu*, spleen.]

Eustace Smith *See* SMITH, EUSTACE.

Eustachio, Bartolomeo (b. 1520). Rome anatomist.

Eustachian canal. The canal of the pharyngotympanic tube.

Eustachian cartilage. The cartilaginous part of the pharyngotympanic tube.

Eustachian diverticulum. An abnormal invagination of the lower part of the pharyngotympanic tube.

Eustachian tube. The pharyngotympanic tube. *See* TUBE.

Eustachian valve. The valve of the inferior vena cava.

eustachitis (ew·sta·ki·tis). An inflamed condition of the pharyngotympanic (eustachian) tube. [eustachium, Gk *-itis* inflammation.]

eustachium (ew·sta·ke·um). The pharyngotympanic (eustachian) tube. [Bartolomeo *Eustachio*.]

eusthenia (ew·sthe·ne·ah). The condition in which bodily strength and activity are normal. [Gk *eu*, sthenia.]

Eustoma rotundatum (ew·sto·mah ro·tun·da·tum). Dutch herring worm; an intestinal worm of herrings carried or distributed by seagulls. If dead herrings are not quickly frozen the worm leaves the gut and enters muscles. Raw or poorly cooked herrings, when eaten, liberate worms which enter mucosa of the small intestine of man and sensitize it. Ingestion of further worms subsequently leads to an intense allergic oedema, with eosinophilic granulomata. Symptoms then closely simulate regional ileitis (Crohn's disease), with eosinophilia.

Eustrongylus (ew·stron·jil·us). *Dioctophyme*. [Gk *eu*, *strongylos* rounded.]

eusystole (ew·sis·to·le). In the cardiac cycle of the heart, systole that is normal in time and force. [Gk *eu*, systole.]

eusystolic (ew·sis·tol·ik). Referring to or characterized by normal cardiac systole. [see prec.]

Eutamias (ew·tam·e·as). A genus of rodents, the chipmunks. The species may act as reservoirs of sylvatic plague in Western Canada and the USA. [Gk *eu*, *tamias* storer.]

eutaxia (ew·tax·e·ah). A state of good order and normal condition of the body. [Gk *eu*, *taxis* arrangement.]

eutectic (ew·tek·tik). 1. Term applied to a mixture that melts and resolidifies without the separation of its constituents. 2. Having the lowest possible melting point or freezing point. [Gk *eu*, *tekein* to melt.]

eutelegenesis (ew·tel·e·jen′·es·is). Artificial insemination practised, especially in animal breeding, on eugenic principles. [Gk *eu*, *teleos* end, *genein* to produce.]

eutexia (ew·tex·e·ah). The state of being eutectic, the condition of a mixture of such proportions that the result has a lower melting point than any other mixture of the same substances.

euthanasia (ew·than·a·ze·ah). 1. The process of dying easily, quietly and painlessly. 2. The act or practice of procuring, as an act of mercy, the easy and painless death of a patient who has an incurable and intractably painful and distressing disease. [Gk *eu*, *thanatos* death.]

euthenic (ew·then·ik). 1. Referring to euthenics. 2. Term applied to any measure that aims at providing a good regulated environment so that thereby the race may be improved.

euthenics (ew·then·ix). The science of the improvement of human stock through good environment. [Gk *eu*, *tithenai* to place.]

eutherapeutic (ew·ther·ap·ew′·tik). Applied to any substance that has good healing or curative properties. [Gk *eu*, therapy.]

Eutheria (ew·the·re·ah). A sub-class of the class Mammalia which contains all mammals except marsupials and monotremata. [Gk *eu*, *therion* wild animal.]

euthermic (ew·ther·mik). Promoting or conducive to warmth. [Gk *eu*, *therme* heat.]

euthesia (ew·the·ze·ah). The state of being in good health or of having a good bodily constitution. [Gk *eu*, *thesis* a placing.]

euthymia (ew·thi·me·ah). Peace of mind. [Gk *eu*, *thymos* mind.]

euthymism (ew·thi·mizm). A condition in which the thymus gland is healthily active and normal. [Gk *eu*, thymus gland.]

euthyroidism (ew·thi·roid·izm). The condition in which there is normal healthy function of the thyroid gland. [Gk *eu*, thyroid gland.]

eutocia (ew·to·se·ah). Natural and normal labour leading to easy delivery. [Gk *eu*, *tokos* childbirth.]

eutopic (ew·to·pik). Normally placed, in contrast to ectopic. [Gk *eu*, *topos* place.]

Eutriatoma (ew·tri·at·o·mah). A genus of reduviid bugs; potential vectors of Chagas' disease. [Gk *eu*, *Triatoma*.]

eutrichosis (ew·trik·o·sis). Normal development and growth of the hair. [Gk *eu*, *thrix* hair, *-osis* condition.]

Eutrombicula (ew·trom·bik·ew·lah). A genus of mites. The larva of *Eutrombicula alfreddugési* is the most important chigger, or bête rouge, of North and Central America. [Gk *eu*, *Trombicula*.]

eutrophia (ew·tro·fe·ah). The state of being well nourished and of normal growth. [Gk *eu*, *trophe* nutrition.]

eutrophic (ew·trof·ik). 1. Referring to or promoting eutrophia. 2. Any drug or other agent which promotes nutrition or the general health of the individual.

euxanthone (ew·zan·thone). $O(C_8H_3OH)_2CO$, a yellow crystalline derivative of xanthone, extracted from puree, Indian yellow, a pigment made in India from cows' urine. [Gk *eu*, *xanthos* yellow.]

evacuant (e·vak·ew·ant). 1. A purgative. 2. Any medicine or agent which causes an organ to discharge its contents, e.g. an emetic. [see foll.]

evacuation (e·vak·ew·a′·shun). 1. Discharge of faeces from the bowel. 2. An emptying of waste solid or fluid material from an organ by natural or artificial means, through either the natural passages of the body or an artificial opening. 3. The diminishing of the body fluids, e.g. by venesection. 4. That which is discharged from the body, e.g. faeces. 5. Withdrawal or removal of patients from hospital. [L *evacuare* to empty.]

evacuator (e·vak·ew·a·tor). 1. An instrument with which the emptying of a cavity, e.g. the urinary bladder, is effected, or for the removal of impacted faeces from the bowel. 2. An instrument with which small particles may be removed from a cavity, e.g. fragments of calculus from the urinary bladder. 3. An agent which causes evacuation. [see prec.]

evagination (e·vaj·in·a'·shun). 1. Eversion of an inner surface. 2. Protrusion of an organ or part from its covering membrane or sheath. **Optic evagination.** In embryology, the process that causes the appearance of a hollow diverticulum (the rudiment of the optic cup) on the lateral aspect of the forebrain. [L *e*, *vagina* sheath.]

Evans, Herbert (b. 1882). American anatomist.

Evans' blue. A non-toxic blue tetrazo dye suitable for intravenous injection for the purpose of determining blood and plasma volumes. *See* AZOVAN BLUE (under BLUE).

Evans'-blue method. A dye method for the estimation of the blood volume.

evaporation (e·vap·or·a'·shun). 1. The changing of a liquid or solid into vapour. 2. The removal of a volatile solvent by heating a solution. [L *e*, *vaporare* to steam.]

Eve, Frank Cecil (b. 1871). Hull physician.

Eve's method. *See* ARTIFICIAL RESPIRATION (under RESPIRATION).

evectics (e·vek·tix). 1. Methodical acquirement of bodily vigour and good bodily habits. 2. A term formerly used for hygiene. [L *evehere* to lift up.]

evenomation (e·ven·om·a'·shun). The process of neutralizing the effects of poisoning by venom. [L *e*, venom.]

eventration (e·ven·tra·shun). 1. Protrusion of the intestines through the abdominal walls. 2. Evisceration. **Diaphragmatic eventration, Eventration of the diaphragm.** Congenital left-sided maldevelopment of the diaphragm so that it lies high in the thoracic cavity (Petit's disease). [L *e*, *venter* belly.]

Everbusch, Oskar (b. 1853). Munich and Erlangen ophthalmologist.

Everbusch's operation. For ptosis: a resection and advancement of the levator palpebrae superioris muscle and resection of a small amount of the tarsal plate. The levator is sutured to the anterior surface of the tarsal plate below the cut edge. Approach is from the skin surface of the lid.

Everitt's salt. Potassium ferricyanide.

eversion (e·ver·shun). 1. The state of turning or of being turned inside out. 2. The state of being turned outwards. **Eversion of the eyelid.** Ectropion; the act of turning an eyelid outward and rolling it back so as to expose the conjunctiva or the sulcus sclerae. **Eversion of the foot.** The act of turning the whole foot so that the plantar surface faces laterally. [see foll.]

evert (e·vert). 1. To turn outward, as of the feet. 2. To turn inside out, as the eyelid. [L *e*, *vertere* to turn.]

evidence (ev·id·ens). **Direct evidence.** Evidence of fact by an eye-witness. **Documentary evidence.** Evidence in the form of written report or statement, or a printed document, or photostat or photograph, as distinct from the spoken word. **Oral evidence.** Statement made in court by witnesses in person after swearing to tell the truth on oath or by affirmation. **Written evidence.** Affidavits, deeds, records, i.e. statements made on oath. [L *evidens* clear.]

eviration (e·vi·ra·shun). 1. Loss of sexual power in the male. 2. A type of paranoia in which the patient is under the deep delusion that he is a woman and, losing the masculine characteristics, permanently assumes the feminine. 3. Loss or absence of masculine characteristics leading to the acquirement of feminine characteristics. 4. Emasculation. [L *e*, *vir* man.]

eviscerate (e·vis·er·ate). To remove the abdominal viscera. [see foll.]

evisceration (e·vis·er·a'·shun). 1. Removal of the abdominal viscera; eventration. 2. Removal of the contents of an organ or part. **Evisceration of the eye.** Removal of the contents of the eyeball with the exception of the sclera. **Obstetrical evisceration.** Removal of the contents of the thoracic and abdominal cavity of the fetus for the purpose of making delivery possible. **Evisceration of the orbit.** Surgical removal of the entire contents of the orbit and its periosteum. [L *e*, viscera.]

evisceroneurotomy (e·vis·er·o·newr·ot'·o·me). Division of the optic nerve combined with evisceration of the eye. [evisceration, neurotomy.]

e-viton (e·vi·ton). A unit of erythemal flux used in the USA in computing the output of sources of ultraviolet rays.

evocator (ev·ok·a·tor). Any chemical substance, naturally produced *in situ* or artificially introduced as an implant, which is capable of stimulating the differentiation of an organized tissue from the undifferentiated cells of a developing organism. **Primary evocator.** The substance produced by the dorsal lip of the blastopore during amphibian gastrulation and responsible for the evocation or induction of the neural tube. [L *evocare* to call out.]

evolution (e·vol·ew·shun). 1. Change in the characters of organisms which takes place over a series of generations. Evolutionary theory postulates that all living organisms are derived by such a process, the changes being, in general, irreversible and showing a trend from a more generalized organization towards a more specialized one. The theory, though associated with the name of Charles Darwin, is much older. Darwin contributed substantial evidence in support of it, and suggested a mechanism by which it might come about, i.e. survival of the fittest in the struggle for existence by means of natural selection. 2. The concept of the origin of organisms from earlier and unlike organisms, as opposed to their origin by special creation. **Adaptive evolution.** That which proceeds only by a selection of genotypes that are best fitted to the environment. **Convergent evolution.** That by which similar structures or functions are evolved in lines that are not closely related. **Determinate evolution.** Orthogenic evolution (see below). **Emergent evolution.** That by the production of new organ systems that could not be predicted from those of ancestors. **Organic evolution.** *See* MAIN DEFINITION 2 (above). **Orthogenic evolution.** That which proceeds in a definite direction without relation to the influences of the external environment. **Parallel evolution.** That by which similar structures or functions are evolved in lines that are closely related, as a result of their similarity of genetic make-up. **Spontaneous evolution.** In obstetrics, spontaneous delivery in which the shoulder or arm presents and is driven down into the pelvis, becoming fixed underneath the symphysis pubis. The trunk, breech and limbs are then delivered, and finally the head and other shoulder. [L *evolvere* to unroll.]

evolutive (e·vol·ew·tiv). 1. Belonging to evolution. 2. Tending to promote development. 3. Term denoting defective mentality caused by slowing down of the developmental processes.

evulsion (e·vul·shun). 1. Tearing out by force, as of a nerve or neoplasm. 2. Avulsion. [L *e*, *vellere* to pluck.]

Ewald, Carl Anton (b. 1845). Berlin physician.

Ewald's test-meal. A meal consisting of 56 g (2 oz) of toast without butter and 0.25 litre (0.5 pint) of tea without milk, employed to test the secretory function of the stomach.

Ewart, William (b. 1848). London physician.

Ewart's sign. The area of dullness to percussion near the inferior angle of the left scapula found in cases of pericardial effusion and thought to be due to collapse of the base of the left lung by pressure from the distended pericardial sac, but more likely the result of an associated pleural effusion.

Ewing, James (b. 1866). New York pathologist.

Ewing's postulates. A series of conditions proposed by Ewing to give proof that a tumour developing after injury had grown as a consequence of trauma: 1. Previous normality in the area. 2. Adequate and proven trauma. 3. An appropriate interval of time. 4. Tumour at the site of injury. 5. Histological confirmation.

Ewing's sarcoma, or tumour. A radiosensitive endothelioma of the bone marrow of long bones. Histologically, it can be difficult to distinguish from secondary deposits of neuroblastoma.

Ewing's operation. For entropion: a horizontal incision is made through the conjunctiva and tarsal plate in the whole length of the lid. Mattress sutures are passed from the upper conjunctival edge, through the substance of the lid, to be tied just above the lash margin, so everting the lid margin.

Ewing's sign. Tenderness of the medial part of the floor of the frontal air sinus elicited by digital compression, and suggestive of sinus infection.

ex-. 1. Prefix, from the Latin *ex*, meaning *from, out of, without.* 2. Prefix, from the Greek *ex*, meaning *out.*

exacerbation (ex·as·er·ba'·shun). Increase in severity of a disease or in violence of symptoms. [L *exacerbare* to irritate intensely.]

exaemia (ex·e·me·ah). A condition in which a considerable quantity of blood is temporarily removed from general circulation, as in shock when blood accumulates in the abdomen, or when a limb is ligatured. [Gk *ex, haima* blood.]

exaltation (ex·awl·ta·shun). 1. Abnormal intensification of organic or functional power. 2. Abnormal increase in mental activity. 3. In psychological medicine, exaggerated sense of personal well-being and power, with spiritual ecstasy and delusions of grandeur. [L *exaltare* to raise high.]

examination (ex·am·in·a'·shun). Critical investigation and inspection for diagnostic purposes.

exangeia, exangia (ex·an·je·ah). A state of dilatation of a blood vessel. [Gk *ex, aggeion* vessel.]

exanimation (ex·an·im·a'·shun). 1. A state of unconsciousness or coma. 2. A state of fainting. 3. Death. [L *ex, animus* soul.]

exanthem (ex·an·them). The rash or eruption produced by the action of an organism or its toxins on the small blood vessels of the skin. **Boston exanthem.** A febrile illness with a macular exanthem and, sometimes, an oral enanthema, caused by *Echovirus 16.* [Gk *ex, anthema* blossoming.]

exanthema (ex·an·the·mah) (pl. *exanthemata*). One of a group of infectious diseases in which a specific rash is an important clinical feature and may assist diagnosis. **Exanthema subitum.** Pseudorubella: an eruptive disease resembling rubella in its rash, the enlargement of glands of the neck, and fever, but differing from it in its age incidence, which is exclusively from 6 months to 2 years. The rash fades in 2 or 3 days, and there are no sequelae. Leucopenia with marked relative lymphocytosis may help in diagnosis. [see prec.]

exanthematous (ex·an·them·at·us). 1. Belonging or relating to or having the characteristics of an exanthem. 2. Showing the character of an eruptive disease.

exanthesis (ex·an·the·sis). Any eruption of the skin; an exanthem. **Exanthesis rosalia arthrodynia.** Dengue. [Gk a blossoming.]

exanthrope (ex·an·thrope). Any source outside the human body that gives rise to disease. [Gk *ex, anthropos* man.]

exanthropia (ex·an·thro·pe·ah). Morbid aversion to and avoidance of human society. [see prec.]

exanthropic (ex·an·throp·ik). 1. Referring to an exanthrope or exanthropia. 2. Originating outside of or not existing within the human body.

exarteritis (ex·ar·ter·i'·tis). A condition of inflammation of the tunica adventitia of an artery. [Gk *ex*, artery, Gk *-itis* inflammation.]

exarthrima (ex·ar·thrim·ah). Dislocation of a joint. [Gk *ex, arthron* joint.]

exarticulation (ex·ar·tik·ew·la'·shun). 1. Dislocation. 2. Amputation of a limb through a joint. 3. Excision of a part of a joint. [L *ex, articulatio* joint.]

excalation (ex·kal·a·shun). The exclusion or suppresion of one or more parts or members of a series, as a digit or a vertebra. [L *ex, calare* to call.]

excavation (ex·kav·a·shun). The process of scooping out. **Dental excavation.** The process of removing caries from a cavity in a tooth by means of an excavator. **Excavation of the optic disc.** Pallor and hollowing-out of the nerve head; also called *cupping.* It may be *physiological,* confined to the centre of the disc; *glaucomatous,* extending to the edge of the disc and often deep with overhanging edges; *postatrophic,* shallow and saucer-like; or *cavernous,* very deep and thought to be arteriosclerotic in nature, as it is not associated with raised tension. **Excavation of the disc of the optic nerve [excavatio disci (NA)].** The depression at the entry of the optic nerve into the retina; sometimes also termed the *physiological cup.* [L *ex, cavus* hollow.]

See also: SCHNABEL.

excavator (ex·kav·a·tor). 1. A large sharp spoon or scoop used to clear a cavity of morbid tissue. 2. In dentistry, an instrument used to clear out a tooth cavity preparatory to the insertion of a filling. **Spoon excavator.** A spoon-shaped dental excavator. [see prec.]

excentric (ek·sen·trik). 1. Eccentric. 2. Away from the centre or the median line. 3. Efferent. [L *ex,* centre.]

excerebration (ek·ser·e·bra'·shun). 1. In obstetrics, removal of the fetal brain in the operation of embryotomy. 2. Removal of the brain in dissection. [L *ex,* cerebrum.]

excess (ek·ses). Departure from normal. **Base excess.** Base concentration per litre of blood measured by acid titration to pH 7.4. **Convergence excess.** A form of muscle imbalance in which there is a tendency to converge, which is more marked for near vision than for distance. [L *excedere* to go out.]

exchange (ex·cha·nj). In cytogenetics, denoting chromosome mutations due to exchange of segments between chromatids of the same chromosome (*intrachange*) or between different chromosomes (*interchange*). [L *ex-, cambire* to change.]

excipient (ek·sip·e·ent). A binding agent enabling powdered drugs to be made into pills. Among the liquid excipients are syrup of glucose, mucilage of acacia and simple sugar; among the solids are gum acacia, liquorice, powdered soap and a mixture of gum acacia and tragacanth. Excipients must not have therapeutic action of their own, nor should they be of such a nature as to render the resultant pill insoluble. Colour must also be taken into account, and a white excipient used with white ingredients of a pill. [L *excipere* to take up.]

excise (ek·size). 1. To hollow out. 2. To amputate. 3. To cut away as diseased matter from healthy matter. [L *ex, caedere* to cut.]

excision (ek·sizh·un). The act or operation of excising or amputating a part. **Excision of a wound, Wound excision.** Débridement. [see prec.]

See also: LOCKHART-MUMMERY.

excitability (ek·si·tab·il'·it·e). 1. Irritability. 2. A property of living organisms causing them to respond quickly to the action of stimulants or a stimulus. [L *excitare* to rouse.]

excitable (ek·si·tabl). 1. Responding rapidly to stimulus. 2. Capable of being stimulated or excited. [see prec.]

excitant (ek·si·tant). 1. Tending to stimulate. 2. Any agent that stimulates or augments organic activity. 3. Any agent or remedy that stimulates mental function or the vital functions. [see foll.]

excitation (ek·si·ta·shun). 1. A state of being mentally or nervously excited. 2. The condition of being stimulated. 3. The act of increasing the rapidity or the intensity of a process. 4. In physics, the addition of energy to a system, transforming it from its ground state to an excited state. **Anomalous atrioventricular excitation.** Pre-excitation. Wolff–Parkinson–White syndrome. **Direct excitation.** Muscular stimulation brought about by placing an electrode on the muscle itself. **Indirect excitation.** The act of stimulating a muscle by stimulating its nerve. [L *excitare* to rouse.]

excitatory (ek·si·ta·tor·e). 1. Tending or serving to excite or stimulate. 2. Tending to induce disassimilation. [see prec.]

excitement (ek·site·ment). The second stage of anaesthesia. [L *excitare* to rouse.]

excito-anabolic (ek·si·to·an·ab·ol'·ik). Stimulating the process of anabolism. [excitation, anabolism.]

excitocatabolic (ek·si·to·kat·ab·ol'·ik). Stimulating the process of catabolism. [excitation, catabolism.]

excitoglandular (ek·si·to·glan'·dew·lar). Stimulating activity of a gland. [excitation, gland.]

excitometabolic (ek·si·to·met·ab·ol'·ik). Stimulating the activity of the metabolic process; giving rise to changes in metabolism. [excitation, metabolism.]

excitomotor, excitomotory (ek·si·to·mo'·tor, ek·si·to·mo'·tor·e). 1. Producing or increasing rapidity of movement. 2. Promoting motor function. 3. Any agent, e.g. a drug, that excites or induces functional or nervous activity or movement. [excitation, motor.]

excitomuscular (ek·si·to·mus′·kew·lar). Causing or increasing muscular activity. [excitation, muscle.]

excitonutrient (ek·si·to·new′·tre·ent). Inducing or stimulating nutritive activities. [excitation, nutrient.]

excitor (ek·si·tor). Any agent, nervous or chemical, that induces activity in an organ. [L *excitare* to rouse.]

excitosecretory (ek·si·to·se·kre′·tor·e). 1. Stimulating to increased secretion. 2. Term applied to anything that excites secretion. [excitation, secretion.]

excitovascular (ek·si·to·vas′·kew·lar). 1. Increasing circulatory activity. 2. Inducing vascular changes leading to increased activity of the part supplied by the vessels, e.g. engorgement, blushing. [excitation, L *vasculum* little vessel.]

exclave (ex·klave). A detached outlying portion of a gland or other organ, e.g. pancreas, thyroid gland; an accessory gland. [L *ex, clavis* key (signifying closed in).]

exclusion (ex·kloo·zhun). 1. The act of disconnecting or shutting out from the main part. 2. The act of ejecting or expelling, e.g. a fetus. 3. In operative surgery, the separation of a part of an organ from the main portion without removing it from the body. [L *excludere* to shut out.]

excochleation (ex·kok·le·a′·shun). The scraping out of the contents of a cavity; curettage. [L *ex, cochlea* spoon.]

excoriation (ex·kor·e·a′·shun). 1. The breaking and wearing away of the superficial protective surface, as of the skin by galling or scratching. 2. The raw surface left as the result of abrasion or scraping, as on a mucous membrane. **Neurotic excoriations.** Oval areas of skin gouged out with a finger nail, usually on the extensor aspects of a limb or on a face (acné excorié), occurring in some individuals with personality disorders. [L *excoriare* to flay.]

excortication (ex·kor·tik·a′·shun). Decortication. [L *ex, cortex* rind.]

excrement (ex·kre·ment). 1. Faeces. 2. Any waste matter discharged from the body. [L *excrementum.*]

excrementitious (ex·kre·men·tish′·us). Belonging to or having the characteristics of excrement.

excrescence (ex·kres·ens). 1. Natural or normal outgrowth from the surface, e.g. hair. 2. Morbid or unnatural outgrowth or appendage, e.g. a wart. **Cauliflower excrescence.** 1. An epithelioma of the neck of the uterus. 2. A tumour having an uneven surface similar to that of a cauliflower, caused by the occurrence close together of numbers of filiform warts. 3. Condyloma acuminatum. **Fungating excrescence, Fungous excrescence.** A fungous granulome occurring on the umbilicus after the cord has been separated. [L *ex, crescere* to grow.]

See also: LAMBL.

excrescent (ex·kres·ent). Resembling or having the character of an excrescence.

excreta (ex·kre·tah). 1. Any waste matter eliminated from the body. 2. Faeces. [see foll.]

excrete (ex·krete). To eliminate or discharge waste or harmful material from the body. [L *excernere* to sift out.]

excretion (ex·kre·shun). 1. The act or process of eliminating normal waste material from the body; the excretory function. 2. The waste or harmful matter discharged from the body. [see prec.]

excretory (ex·kre·tor·e). 1. Belonging to excretion. 2. Assisting or of use in excretion.

excursion (ex·ker·shun). 1. Departure or deviation from a direct or normal course. 2. The distance travelled by the eyes from a central position. **Respiratory excursion.** The extent of movement of the chest during 1 complete respiration. [L *ex, currere* to run.]

excurvation, excurvature (ex·ker·va·shun, ex·ker·vat·ewr). 1. Outward curvature from a central part. 2. Abnormal structure of the upper eyelid in which the tarsus of the upper eyelid turns outwards. [L *ex*, curve.]

excyclophoria (ex·si·klo·for′·e·ah). A condition in which the vertical meridians of the eyes are parallel when both are open, but the upper end of either tends to deviate outwards on covering. [Gk *ex, kyklos* circle, *pherein* to bear.]

excyclotropia (ex·si·klo·tro′·pe·ah). A condition in which the vertical meridians of the two eyes are divergent when traced from below upwards. [Gk *ex, kyklos* circle, *trepein* to turn.]

excyclovergence (ex·si·klo·ver′·jens). Disjunctive reciprocal motion of the eyes in which the upper poles of the cornea are rotated outwards; abtorsion. [L *ex*, Gk *kyklos* circle, L *vergere* to bend.]

excystation (ex·sis·ta·shun). Escape from a cyst; particularly of parasitic protozoa with a resistant cyst stage. [L *ex*, cyst.]

exencephalia (ex·en·kef·a′·le·ah). In teratology, the condition in which a defect in the skull exposes the whole or a part of the brain, which is imperfect. [Gk *ex, egkephalos* brain.]

exencephalocele (ex·en·kef·al·o·seel). Cerebral hernia. [Gk *ex, egkephalos* brain, *kele* hernia.]

exencephalous (ex·en·kef·al·us). 1. Relating to exencephalia or an exencephalus. 2. Marked by the condition of exencephalia.

exencephalus (ex·en·kef·al·us). A class of monster in which the skull is so malformed that at least a part of the imperfect brain lies outside the calvaria. [Gk *ex, egkephalos* brain.]

exencephaly (ex·en·kef·al·e). Exencephalia.

exenterate (ex·en·ter·ate). Eviscerate. [Gk *ex, enteron* bowel.]

exenteration (ex·en·ter·a′·shun). Evisceration. **Pelvic exenteration.** Surgical removal of all the pelvic organs in the treatment of advanced cancer.[see prec.]

exenteritis (ex·en·ter·i′·tis). A condition of inflammation of the visceral peritoneum. [Gk *ex*, enteritis.]

exercise (ex·er·size). Physical or mental exertion. **Active exercise.** Exercise voluntarily undertaken by the patient. **Active resistive exercise.** Voluntary movements performed against resistance provided either by mechanical means or by another person. **Exercise bone.** *See* BONE. **Corrective exercise.** The use of voluntary movements to correct minor deformities or to restore or maintain normal function. **Free exercise.** Voluntary movements in which there is no external aid and no resistance other than by gravity. **Muscle-setting exercise.** The repetitive contraction and relaxation of muscles which does not produce movement at the appropriate point. **Passive exercise.** Exercise of the muscles by mechanical or electrical means without involving the will of the patient. **Postural exercise.** Exercise to improve posture and thereby correct minor deformities. **Provocative exercises.** Exercises designed to test out the efficiency of part of the body. **Static exercise.** Muscle-setting exercise (see above). **Therapeutic exercise.** Any exercise that is designed to correct deformity or improve health. **Underwater exercise.** Remedial exercise carried out in a pool or special bath such as a Hubbard tank. [L *exercere* to keep at work.]

See also: BUERGER, FRENKEL (H. S.), TOGNA.

exeresis (ex·er·e·sis). Surgical removal or excision of a part, organ or structure. [Gk *ex, eresis* removal.]

exergic (ex·er·jik). Applied to a chemical action that is accompanied by the liberation of energy. [Gk *ex, ergein* to work.]

exesion (ex·e·shun). The slow destruction of superficial tissue and bone such as occurs through some corrosive agency or in ulceration. [L *exedere* to eat out.]

exfetation (ex·fe·ta·shun). Ectopic pregnancy. *See* PREGNANCY. [L *ex*, foetus.]

exflagellation (ex·flaj·el·a′·shun). The development of microgametes (flagellates) from a microgametocyte of a malarial parasite. This occurs after malarial blood is withdrawn from the human body, and takes place normally in the stomach of a mosquito after feeding on human infected blood. [L *ex*, flagellum.]

exfoliatio (ex·fo·le·a′·she·o). Exfoliation. **Exfoliatio areata linguae, Exfoliatio linguae.** Geographical tongue; term descriptive of an eczematous itching condition affecting the tongue in which circinate patches of desquamation spread and fuse together while healing occurs in the central areas. The tongue may become covered with such patches defined by sinuous lines like boundary markings on a map. [L *ex, folium* leaf.]

exfoliation (ex·fo·le·a′·shun). 1. A sequestrum. 2. The splitting off or coming away from the surface in thin scales or pieces, such as occurs in certain forms of desquamation. [see prec.]

exfoliative (ex·**fo**·le·a·tiv). Marked by desquamation or exfoliation.

exhalant (ex·**ha**·lant). 1. Having the quality of exhaling or emitting. 2. That which is exhaled. 3. Any organ of exhalation. [see foll.]

exhalation (ex·hal·**a**·shun). 1. The act of giving off in the form of steam or vapour. 2. Expiration, as of breath. 3. Any emanation or effluvium; the waste products of the body which are given off as vapour by the skin and lungs. **Miasmatic exhalation.** The supposedly noxious effluvium that arises from marshy land and was supposed to be the cause of febrile disease, especially malaria. [L *exhalare* to breathe out.]

exhale (ex·**hale**). To give off in the form of a vapour; to breath out. [see prec.]

exhaustibility (eg·**zawst**·ib·**il**'·it·e). **Faradic exhaustibility.** The decrease of excitability of a muscle after long repeated stimulation with low frequency current. [see foll.]

exhaustion (eg·**zawst**·chun). 1. The loss of mental and/or physical power due to fatigue or illness. 2. The state of a drug after all the therapeutically valuable ingredients have been removed. **Anhidrotic exhaustion.** Anhidrosis. **Cold exhaustion.** Failure to compensate for lowered environmental temperature; the symptoms are drowsiness and fatigue, and finally loss of consciousness. **Heat exhaustion.** Caused fundamentally by subjection to excessive heat, in a hot climate, or in other conditions: the determining causes are numerous and include excessive clothing and excessive exercise, but 3 pathogenic forms stand out clearly; (*a*) heat exhaustion due to salt deficiency, (*b*) heat exhaustion due to water deficiency and (*c*) anhidrotic heat exhaustion due to failure of the sweating mechanism. This may be acute or chronic; in the chronic form there may be acute exacerbations. The symptoms are vague discomfort, anorexia, irritability, tiredness, faintness and dizziness; there is often some cyanosis and then fever. This may lead to sudden collapse with a thready or no pulse, or to hyperpyrexia; or these 2 conditions may alternate, especially if treatment is too vigorous. The onset may, however, be sudden and may be accompanied by maniacal behaviour. **Nervous exhaustion.** A psychoneurosis attributed to a hypothetical exhaustion of nervous tissue. [L *exhaurire* to drain out.]

exhibit (eg·**zib**·it). To administer or give a drug or remedy. [L *exhibere* to offer.]

exhibition (ex·ib·**ish**·un). 1. The administering of a drug or remedy. 2. In medical jurisprudence, the exposure to public view of the genitalia. [see prec.]

exhibitionism (ex·ib·**ish**·un·izm). 1. A form of sexual behaviour consisting in the exposure to view of the body or any part of it, especially the genitalia, for the purpose (which may not be conscious) of gratifying sexual impulses. 2. The state in which an individual uses any means to attract attention to himself. [L *exhibere* to offer.]

exhibitionist (ex·ib·**ish**·un·ist). A person who practises exhibitionism.

exhilarant (eg·**zil**·ar·ant). 1. Stimulating to the mind. 2. Causing cheerfulness. 3. Anything which enlivens or cheers. [L *exhilarare* to gladden.]

exhumation (ex·hewm·**a**'·shun). The removal of a dead body from its place of burial; disinterment. [L *ex, humus* the ground.]

exinanition (ex·in·an·**ish**'·un). Enfeebling and extreme exhaustion. [L *exinanire* to empty completely.]

exitus (ex·it·us). 1. Exit or outlet. 2. A term for death. **Exitus pelvis.** The pelvic outlet. [L. exit.]

Exner, Siegmund (b. 1846). Vienna physiologist.

Exner's centre, or plexus. An interlacing plexus of nerve fibres near the surface of the cerebral cortex and said by Exner to be due to the junction of sensory and motor fibres. [Obsolete term.]

Exner's method. The demonstration of myelin sheaths by means of 1 per cent osmic acid.

Exner's nerve. A slender branch from the pharyngeal plexus to the cricothyroid muscle, believed to contain fibres from the superior laryngeal branch of the vagus nerve.

Call–Exner bodies. 1. Round dark masses among the follicular cells of a low-developing ovarian follicle; probably centres of secretion of follicular fluid. 2. Ova-like cells, the result of hydropic degeneration, around which other cells are arranged in rosettes in granulosa-cell tumours of the ovary.

exo-. Prefix, from the Greek *exo*, meaning *outside*.

exo-antigen (ex·o·**an**·te·jen). Ecto-antigen; an antigen which diffuses from the living cell or is produced by the cells in the external medium, e.g. exotoxins of diphtheria and tetanus organisms. [Gk *exo*, antigen.]

exobiology (ex·o·bi·**ol**·o·je). The study of the effects of extraterrestrial environments on living matter and the search for extraterrestrial life. [Gk *exo*, biology.]

exocardia (ex·o·**kar**·de·ah). 1. Congenital displacement of the heart. 2. An abnormal position of the heart within the thoracic cavity. [Gk *exo, kardia* heart.]

exocardiac, exocardial (ex·o·**kar**·de·ak, ex·o·**kar**·de·al). 1. Having relation to exocardia. 2. Situated outside the heart. 3. Developing or arising outside the heart.

exoccipital (ex·ok·**sip**·it·al). Situated at the side of the foramen magnum of the occipital bone. **Exoccipital bone.** One of a pair of bones bounding the foramen magnum laterally and forming part of the occipital region in lower vertebrates. It is present as a separate ossifying centre in higher vertebrates which fuses with the basi-occipital and supra-occipital centres to form the single occipital bone. [Gk *exo*, occiput.]

exochorion (ex·o·**kor**·e·on). In embryology, that part (the external layer) of the chorion which derives from the primitive ectoderm. [Gk *exo*, chorion.]

exocoelom (ex·o·**se**·lom). The fluid-filled cavity of the extra-embryonic mesoderm surrounding the yolk sac, amniotic sac and allantois, and bounded externally by the chorion. In the early embryo it is continuous through the umbilical orifice with the peritoneal cavity. [Gk *exo*, coelom.]

exocolitis (ex·o·kol·**i**'·tis). A condition of inflammation of the peritoneal coat of the colon. [Gk *exo*, colitis.]

exocranium (ex·o·**kra**·ne·um). The outer surface of the bones of the skull; the pericranium. [Gk *exo, kranion* skull.]

exocrin, exocrine (ex·o·krin, ex·o·krine). 1. Secreting externally; diacrinous. 2. The external secretion of a gland. [Gk *exo, krinein* to separate.]

exocrinous (ex·**ok**·rin·us). Belonging to any external glandular secretion. [Gk *exo, krinein* to secrete.]

exocyclic (ex·o·**si**·klik). An unsaturated cyclic compound in which the double bond occurs in the side chain. [Gk *exo*, cyclic.]

exocystis (ex·o·**sist**·is). A prolapsed condition of the urinary bladder. [Gk *exo, kystis* bag.]

exodeviation (ex·o·de·ve·**a**'·shun). Deviation of one eye outwards. It occurs typically in cases of uni-ocular defect, or loss of sight in one eye. [Gk *exo*, deviation.]

exodic (ex·**od**·ik). 1. Efferent. 2. Centrifugal. [Gk *ex, odos* way.]

exodontia, exodontics (ex·o·**don**·she·ah, ex·o·**don**·tix). 1. Extraction of teeth. 2. Forward protrusion of the teeth. [Gk *ex, odous* tooth.]

exo-enzyme (ex·o·**en**·zime). An enzyme secreted by a cell into the medium surrounding it; an extracellular enzyme. Included in this class are the bacterial enzymes that are capable of attacking large molecules to which the bacterial cell wall is impermeable. [Gk *exo*, enzyme.]

exo-erythrocyte (ex·o·er·**ith**'·ro·site). A malarial parasite in any tissue phase, including the pre-erythrocytic phase. [Gk *exo*, erythrocyte.]

exo-erythrocytic (ex·o·er·ith·ro·**sit**'·ik). External to erythrocytes; applied to malarial parasites in a tissue phase. [see prec.]

exogamy (ex·**og**·am·e). In protozoa, fertilization by union of gametes derived from different individuals. [Gk *exo, gamos* marriage.]

exogastric (ex·o·**gas**·trik). Having relation to the serous coat of the stomach. [Gk *exo, gaster* stomach.]

exogastritis (ex·o·gas·**tri**'·tis). Inflammation of the serous coat of the stomach; perigastritis. [Gk *exo*, gastritis.]

exogenetic (ex·o·jen·**et'**·ik). Exopathic, 2nd def. [see foll.]

exogenic, exogenous (ex·o·**jen**·ik, ex·**oj**·en·us). 1. Developing outside the body. 2. Belonging to aetiological factors outside the organism. 3. Growing from or by addition to the outside or outer surface, as bone. 4. In botany, belonging to the exogenae. [Gk *exo, genein* to produce.]

exogenote (ex·o·**jen**·ote). In partially diploid bacteria, produced by infection with an F-prime factor or a localized transducing phage; the term refers to the homologue located in the immigrant factor or phage DNA. [Gk *exo, genein* to produce.]

exognathia (ex·og·**nath**·e·ah). Prognathism. [see foll.]

exognathion (ex·og·**nath**·e·on). The alveolar process of the maxilla. [Gk *exo, gnathos* jaw.]

exognosis (ex·og·**no**·sis). Diagnosis by exclusion. [Gk *exo, gnosis* knowledge.]

exohysteropexy (ex·o·**his**·ter·o·pex·e). The operation of fastening the fundus of a prolapsed uterus into the abdominal wall outside the peritoneum under the fascia. [Gk *exo*, hysteropexy.]

exolinguistics (ex·o·**lin**·gew·is·tix). Metalinguistics. [Gk *exo*, L. *lingua* tongue.]

exometra (ex·o·**me**·trah). 1. A state of inversion of the uterus. 2. Prolapse of the uterus. [Gk *exo, metra* womb.]

exometritis (ex·o·met·**ri'**·tis). A condition of inflammation of the peritoneal surface of the uterus; perimetritis. [Gk *exo, metra* womb, *-itis* inflammation.]

exomphalia (ex·om·**fal**·e·ah). A condition in which there is protrusion of the navel. [Gk *ex, omphalos* navel.]

exomphalocele (ex·**om**·fal·o·seel). Umbilical hernia. [Gk *ex, omphalos* navel, *kele* hernia.]

exomphalos (ex·**om**·fal·os). 1. A condition in which a portion of the abdominal viscera protrudes into the umbilical cord. 2. Umbilical hernia. [Gk *ex, omphalos* navel.]

exomysium (ex·o·**mis**·e·um). Perimysium; the connective-tissue sheath investing each bundle of muscular fibres. [Gk *exo, mys* muscle.]

exonuclease (ex·o·**new**·kle·aze). A class of hydrolytic enzymes which only attack the terminal linkages of polynucleotides; examples are snake-venom nuclease and spleen nuclease. [Gk *exo*, nuclease.]

exopathic (ex·o·**path**·ik). 1. Referring to an exopathy. 2. Belonging to aetiological factors outside the organism.

exopathy (ex·**op**·ath·e). Any disease produced by a cause external to the organism or outside the body. [Gk *exo, pathos* disease.]

exopeptidase (ex·o·**pep**·tid·aze). A class of proteolytic enzymes which will only attack the terminal linkages of the protein molecule; previously known as *peptidase* or *ereptase.* Erepsin of the intestinal mucosa is an example. [Gk *exo*, peptide.]

exopexy (**ex**·o·pex·e). The surgical fixation outside a body cavity of any organ normally lying within that cavity. [Gk *exo, pexis* fixation.]

exophasy (ex·o·**fa**·see). Vocal, audible language. [Gk *exo, phasis* speech.]

exophoria (ex·o·**for**·e·ah). A tendency of one or both eyes to divergent strabismus; a type of heterophoria. [Gk *exo, pherein* to bear.]

exophoric (ex·o·**for**·ik). Referring or having relation to exophoria.

exophthalmia (ex·of·**thal**·me·ah). Exophthalmos.

exophthalmic (ex·of·**thal**·mik). 1. Referring or belonging to exophthalmos. 2. Marked by a state of exophthalmos.

exophthalmometer (ex·**of**·thal·**mom'**·et·er). An instrument with which the degree of protrusion of the eyes can be ascertained. [exophthalmos, meter.]

exophthalmos, exophthalmus (ex·of·**thal**·mos, ex·of·**thal**·mus). Prominence or protrusion of the eyeball, due to disease, to such an extent that the eyelids will not cover it, **Endocrine exophthalmos.** Exophthalmos associated with pituitary or thyroid abnormality. **Malignant exophthalmos, Pituitary-diencephalic exophthalmos, Progressive exophthalmos.** Thyrotropic exophthalmos (see below). **Exophthalmos-producing substance (EPS).** Active in fish, but its relation to Graves' disease is doubtful. **Pulsating exophthalmos.** Arteriovenous aneurysm of the orbit. **Thyrotoxic exophthalmos.** Real or apparent exophthalmos, and usually of moderate degree, associated with other marked signs of thyrotoxicosis. **Thyrotropic exophthalmos.** Progressive exophthalmos, with external ophthalmoplegia, associated with either slight signs of thyrotoxicosis or normal or subnormal thyroid activity, frequently following thyroidectomy. It is also known as *exophthalmic ophthalmoplegia.* [Gk *ex, ophthalmos* eye.]

exophylactic (**ex**·o·fil·**ak'**·tik). Relating or belonging to exophylaxis.

exophylaxis (**ex**·o·fil·**ax'**·is). Defence of the body against disease from without, such as that provided by the protective properties of the skin. Cf. ESOPHYLAXIS. [Gk *exo*, phylaxis.]

exoplasm (**ex**·o·plazm). Ectoplasm. [Gk *exo*, plasma.]

exopneumopexy (ex·o·**new**·mo·pex·e). The operation of bringing the lung outside the chest cavity and fixing it there, a procedure undertaken as a temporary measure in certain chest lesions. [Gk *exo*, pneumopexy.]

Exopterygota (**ex**·op·ter·e·**go'**·tah). A sub-class of the arthropod class Insecta; characterized by the absence of a pupal stage in the life history. The orders Anoplura, Dermaptera, Hemiptera and Orthoptera are of medical interest. [Gk *exo, pteryx* wing.]

exorbitism (ex·**or**·bit·izm). Exophthalmos. [Gk *ex*, orbit.]

exormia (ex·**or**·me·ah). Any skin disease of papular character. [Gk *exormaein* to rush forth.]

exosepsis (ex·o·**sep**·sis). Septic poisoning or a condition of sepsis due to some infection external to the body or organism. [Gk *exo*, sepsis.]

exoserosis (**ex**·o·se·**ro'**·sis). An exudation or oozing of serum such as occurs in oedema and in certain diseases of the skin. [Gk *exo*, serum, Gk *-osis* condition.]

exoskeleton (ex·o·**skel**·et·on). The Greek derivation of the word "skeleton" indicates that the thickened and hardened tissue of which it is composed dries up and remains after the rest of the body has disappeared. In many of the lower (invertebrate) animals the skeleton is on the surface, and is therefore known as the *exoskeleton*; it acts as a protective as well as a supporting framework. In contrast, higher (vertebrate) animals have an internal or *endoskeleton.* With but little justification, epidermal appendages such as nails, hair and hooves have been regarded as being exoskeletal. [Gk *exo*, skeleton.]

exosmosis (ex·oz·**mo**·sis). The passage of fluids through a membrane (osmosis) from within outwards, as through the walls of a blood vessel or a diaphragm. [Gk *ex*, osmosis.]

exosmotic (ex·oz·**mot**·ik). 1. Referring or belonging to exosmosis. 2. Characterized by exosmosis.

exosomaesthesia (**ex'**·o·som·es·**the**·ze·ah). A sensory illusion sometimes encountered in patients with parietal lobe lesions, whereby a tactile stimulus is located to some point outside the body.

exosplenopexia, exosplenopexy (ex·o·sple·no·**pex'**·e·ah, ex·o·**sple**·no·pex·e). The operation of attaching the tunica albuginea of the spleen within the wound in the abdominal wall or to the outside of the body. It is performed as an alternative to splenectomy. [Gk *exo*, splenopexy.]

exospore (ex·o·spor). The outer layer of a spore wall. [Gk *exo, sporos* seed.]

exosporium (ex·o·**spor**·e·um). In botany, the coating or outer layer of the spore wall. [Gk *exo*, spore.]

exostosectomy (ex·**os**·to·**sek'**·to·me). Surgical removal of an exostosis. [exostosis, Gk *ektome* a cutting out.]

exostosis (ex·os·**to**·sis). 1. Any outgrowth of bone from the surface of a bone. 2. The formation by cementoblasts of the periodontal membrane of a mass of secondary cementum on the root of a tooth; it may involve all teeth in a patient suffering from Paget's disease; hypercementosis. **Exostosis bursata.** A cartilaginous exostosis arising near to a joint and possessing a synovial covering which is derived from and may communicate with the joint. **Cartilage capped exostosis, Exostosis cartilaginea.** An exostosis rich in cartilage arising at the ends of long bones. **Ivory exostosis.** A flat, smooth, ivory-like bony protuberance from the skull or from the shaft of a long bone. **Multiple exostosis, Exostosis multiplex.** A mixed cartilage and bony tumour which arises from many long bones, especially at or near the epiphyseal cartilages. **Exostosis multiplex cartilaginea.** Multiple cartilaginous tumours arising close to the epiphyses of long bones of young people or children. [Gk *ex*, *osteon* bone.]

exostotic (ex·os·**tot**·ik). 1. Referring or belonging to an exostosis. 2. Having the character of an exostosis.

exoteric (ex·o·**ter**·ik). 1. Exopathic; belonging to aetiological factors outside the organism. 2. Ectodermal. [Gk *exoterikos* external.]

exothelioma (ex·o·the·le·**o'**·mah). Meningioma. [Gk *exo*, *thele* nipple, *-oma* tumour.]

exothermal, exothermic (ex·o·**ther**·mal, ex·o·**ther**·mik). 1. Relating to the surface heat of the body. 2. In chemistry; (*a*) formed with or characterized by the evolution or liberation or escape of heat; (*b*) indicating a substance from which heat is liberated during its formation. [Gk *exo*, *therme* heat.]

exothymopexy (ex·o·**thi**·mo·pex·e). The operation of removing the thymus gland entire from its position and fixing it to the superior aspect of the sternum. [Gk *exo*, thymus gland, Gk *pexis* fixation.]

exothyreopexy, exothyroidopexy, exothyropexy (ex·o·**thi**·re·-o·pex·e, ex·o·**thi**·roi·do·pex·e, ex·o·**thi**·ro·pex·e). The operation of making a median incision over an enlarged thyroid gland, enucleating it and fixing it outside the incision so that atrophy is induced. [Gk *exo*, thyroid gland, Gk *pexis* fixation.]

exotic (eg·**zot**·ik). Of a disease, foreign to any particular country. [Gk *exotikos* foreign.]

exotospore (ex·**o**·to·spor). Malarial sporozoite. [Obsolete term.] [Gk *exo*, *sporos* seed.]

exotoxic (ex·o·**tox**·ik). 1. Referring or belonging to an exotoxin. 2. Originating in an exotoxin, or produced by it.

exotoxin (ex·o·**tox**·in). Extracellular toxin which is secreted by multiplying bacterial cells and diffuses through the body to cause tissue damage in sites removed from the focus of bacterial growth; examples are diphtheria and tetanus toxins and the toxins of *Clostridia* that cause gas gangrene. [Gk *exo*, *toxikon* poison.]

exotropia (ex·o·**tro**·pe·ah). Divergent strabismus. [Gk *exo*, *tropos* a turning.]

expansion (ex·**pan**·shun). The state of being spread out. **Expansion of the arch.** The act of increasing the size of the dental arch by means of an orthodontic appliance. [see foll.]

expansive (ex·**pan**·siv). 1. Spread out, as a structure. 2. Extending widely; comprehensive. 3. Unrestrained. [L *expandere* to spread out.]

expansiveness (ex·**pan**·siv·nes). Extrovertal behaviour. [see prec.]

expectant (ex·**pek**·tant). Waiting and watching for; term applied to treatment limited to the relief of symptoms only, until such time as symptoms appear that indicate some more definite action, e.g. an operation. [L *ex*, *spectare* to look.]

expectation (ex·pek·**ta**·shun). The awaiting of a favourable or unfavourable event in an illness, e.g. the crisis in lobar pneumonia. **Expectation of life.** The average number of years lived beyond any specified age by the survivors of a group at that age when exposed subsequently to some selected mortality rate. This is the *complete expectation of life*, and is not, by definition, the most probable lifetime of any individual. *Curtate expectation of life*, a value rarely used, gives the average number of whole years lived after attaining any given age, as distinct from the complete expectation, which takes into account the fraction lived in the year of death. [see prec.]

expectorant (ex·**pek**·tor·ant). 1. Aiding the secretion of the mucous membrane of the air passages and the removal of fluid by spitting. 2. Any of the drugs which aid the removal of bronchial secretions. They act chiefly by increasing the secretion, thus rendering it less viscous; such action may be reflex, central or peripheral. Small doses of emetics such as ipecacuanha, ammonium chloride, squill and senega act reflexly by irritating the mucous membrane of the stomach; apomorphine in small doses acts centrally, while muscarine-like drugs, especially pilocarpine, stimulate the secretory glands directly. Iodides, accumulating in the cells of the glands, induce a secretion of a thin watery fluid, and most volatile oils, which are excreted to some extent in the lungs, produce a slight local irritation that increases the bronchial secretion. [see foll.]

expectorate (ex·**pek**·tor·ate). To eject matter from the respiratory tract via the mouth. [Gk *ex*, *pectus* breast.]

expectoration (ex·**pek**·tor·a'·shun). 1. The ejection of mucus and fluids from the lungs and trachea by coughing. 2. Sputum. **Prune-juice expectoration.** A type of sputum observed in old persons suffering from a severe type of pneumonia and in patients with carcinoma or gangrene of the lung, the ejected material being darkly coloured with altered blood. **Rusty expectoration.** Rusty sputum. *See* SPUTUM. [see prec.]

expellent (ex·**pel**·ent). A drug employed for expelling worms from the alimentary canal. [L *expellere* to drive out.]

experiment (ex·**per**·e·ment). A scientific procedure in the form of a practical test under conditions previously determined by the operator, either to elicit some fact not already known or to demonstrate some known princple. **Check experiment.** An experiment designed to give a clear-cut and final answer to the problem being investigated. **Control experiment.** An experiment performed collaterally with another but from which the factor under investigation has been omitted. **Heat-puncture experiment.** Injury to the corpus striatum which results in a rise in body temperature. [L *experimentum.*]

See also: CYON, GOLTZ, KUESS, MARIOTTE, MUELLER (J.), NUSSBAUM, O'BEIRNE, SCHEINER, STENSEN, TOYNBEE, VALSALVA.

expert (**ex**·pert). A specialist. **Medical expert.** In medical jurisprudence, a person who by reason of his experience and knowledge is entitled to give an opinion upon facts that he has ascertained himself or from evidence he has heard. He is not, however, in a position to express any opinion which would normally be for the decision of the jury. **Medicolegal expert.** A medically- or scientifically-qualified person with special experience in the field, usually of crime and investigation, performing autopsy or laboratory examinations or giving evidence as an accredited expert. **Qualified expert.** In radiology, a person having the knowledge and training needed to measure ionizing radiations and to advise regarding radiation hazard. His qualification should be certified by a national committee. [L *experiri* to try.]

expiration (ex·pir·**a**·shun). The phase of respiration when the gases are expelled from the lungs; exhalation. [L *expirare* to breathe out.]

expiratory (ex·**pir**·at·or·e). 1. Employed in the expiration of air from the lungs, applied to muscles. 2. Belonging or relating to expiration.

expire (ex·**pire**). 1. To breathe out; exhale. 2. To die. [L *expirare* to breathe out.]

expirium (ex·**pi**·re·um). The air expired from the lungs. [see prec.]

expiscation (ex·pis·**ka**·shun). The laborious and prolonged investigation of symptoms for the purposes of diagnosis. [L *expiscari* to fish out.]

explant (ex·**plant**). 1. To remove a piece of tissue and transplant it to another animal or, as in tissue culture, into a culture medium. 2. The fragment of tissue so transplanted or subcultured. [L *ex*, *plantare* to set in the ground.]

explode (ex·**plode**). 1. To induce sudden and violent chemical decomposition. 2. To decompose suddenly and radically. 3. To break out suddenly, as an epidemic. [L *ex*, *plaudere* to clap.]

exploration (ex·plor·**a**·shun). 1. Physical examination by touch or with an instrument in order to aid diagnosis. 2. An exploratory operation. **Hydrostatic exploration.** The diagnosis of disease of the abdomen by palpating the abdomen while the subject is lying covered with water in a bath. [L *explorare* to search out.]

exploratory (ex·**plor**·at·or·e). 1. Searching. 2. Connected with or belonging to exploration, applied to an operation. [see prec.]

explorer (ex·**plor**·er). Any instrument used in investigation for diagnostic purposes. [L *explorare* to search out.]

explosion (ex·**plo**·zhun). 1. The sudden and violent appearance of a symptom. 2. Sudden and violent functioning. 3. The discharge of a nerve cell. 4. A sudden and violently expressive outburst of emotion. 5. In chemistry, violent and noisy expansion after the sudden production of great pressure. [L *ex, plaudere* to clap.]

explosive (ex·**plo**·siv). 1. Capable of or tending towards explosion. 2. Marked by explosion. 3. Of disease, characterized by suddenness and violence of outbreak.

exponent (ex·**po**·nent). In mathematics, the superior index placed to the right and above a term, indicating the power to which it is to be raised, as the *x* in e^x. **Hydrogen exponent.** pH, the negative value of the power to which the base 10 has to be raised to equal the concentration in grams per litre of hydrogen ions in a solution. [L *exponere* to lay out.]

exponential (ex·pon·**en**·shal). In mathematics, e^x; the value of e, the base of the natural logarithms, raised to the power of the exponent *x*. [see prec.]

exposure (ex·**po**·zewr). 1. Displaying or laying bare, as in exhibitionism. 2. The state of being without shelter or protection, e.g. from weather or an attack of disease. 3. In medical physics, the total quantity of ionizing radiation to which an object, body or part of a body is exposed, in contrast to the quantity of energy absorbed from that radiation. The unit of exposure is the roentgen. **Exposure of person.** Medicolegally, the exposure of genitalia in a public place where members of the opposite sex may be present. **Surgical exposure.** Term used to describe the technique of a surgical approach to an organ. [L *exponere* to lay out.]

expression (ex·**presh**·un). 1. The act of pressing out, or that which is pressed out in the process. In pharmacy, a method by which juices, fixed oils or volatile oils are extracted from drugs by pressure; in obstetrics, delivery of the fetus by applied pressure. 2. The external manifestation (in the face, voice, etc.) of an emotion or mental state; the facies. **Expression of the fetus.** Assistance to the delivery of the fetus by pushing on the fundus or sides of the uterus. **Hippocratic expression.** The hippocratic facies in which the skin is pale or livid, the nose pinched, the cheeks drawn in, the eyes dull and sunken, the temples hollow, the lower jaw dropped and the mouth open. It is an indication of impending death. **Expression of the placenta.** Delivery of the placenta by pushing on the fundus of the uterus. **Rectal expression.** Delivery of the fetal head by pressure in the region of the anus. [L *expressio.*]

See also: KRISTELLER.

expressivity (ex·pres·**iv**·it·e). The extent to which a gene or set of genes is manifest in the characteristic or characteristics which it or they govern. [L *exprimere* to press out.]

expulsion (ex·**pul**·shun). The act or process of expelling or driving out. **Spontaneous expulsion.** The unaided expelling of the fetus or placenta by the natural forces. [L *expellere* to drive out.]

expulsive (ex·**pul**·siv). 1. Term denoting expelling or forcing out. 2. Having the power or serving to expel or drive out. The term is used in connection with the passage of urine and faeces, and the expulsion of the fetus or placenta in childbirth. [see prec.]

exsanguinate (ex·**sang**·gwin·ate). 1. To drain away or deprive of blood. 2. Exsanguine. [L *ex, sanguis* blood.]

exsanguination (ex·sang·gwin·**a′**·shun). 1. The act or process of rendering bloodless. 2. The draining away or expulsion of blood from a part. [see foll.]

exsanguine (ex·**sang**·gwin). Of a particular part, devoid of blood; anaemic. [L *ex, sanguis* blood.]

exsanguinity (ex·sang·**gwin′**·it·e). 1. A state of bloodlessness. 2. A state of abnormal pallor. 3. Anaemia. [see prec.]

exsanguinotransfusion (ex·**sang**·gwin·o·trans·**few′**·zhun). An exchange transfusion or replacement transfusion; a technique, usually employed for the treatment of erythroblastosis fetalis, in which the child's blood is removed while fresh donor blood is being given simultaneously. [exsanguination, transfusion.]

exsect (ek·**sekt**). To cut out a part of an organ or structure; to excise. [L *ex, secare* to cut.]

exsection (ek·**sek**·shun). Excision. [see prec.]

exsector (ek·**sek**·tor). A surgical instrument used in excision. [L *ex, secare* to cut.]

exsiccant (ek·**sik**·ant). 1. Term applied to any agent that has a drying effect. 2. An agent which causes moisture to evaporate or dry up; a dusting powder. [see foll.]

exsiccate (**ek**·sik·ate). 1. To exhaust moisture from, or to dry or drain completely. 2. In chemistry, to evaporate the water of crystallization from a crystalline substance. [L *exsiccare* to dry up.]

exsiccation (ek·sik·**a**·shun). 1. The process of causing to dry up. 2. The act of drying or draining thoroughly. 3. In chemistry, the process of causing the water of crystallization to evaporate from a crystalline substance. [see prec.]

exsiccator (**ek**·sik·a·tor). An apparatus in which substances can be exsiccated.

exsiccosis (ek·sik·**o**·sis). The physical condition of dryness of the tissues; dehydration. [L *exsiccare* to dry up, Gk *-osis* condition.]

exsomatized (ek·**so**·mat·i·zd). Removed or taken out of the body. [Gk *ex, soma* body.]

exstrophy (**ex**·tro·fe). Congenital eversion of a hollow organ. **Exstrophy of the bladder.** Extroversion of the bladder. [Gk *ex, strophe* a twist.]

exsufflation (ex·suf·**la**·shun). The forced expulsion of the breath from the lungs. [L *ex, sufflare* to blow.]

exta (**ex**·tah). The viscera; particularly the thoracic viscera. [L entrails.]

extasis (**ex**·tas·is). Ecstasy.

extension (ex·**ten**·shun). 1. A straightening out, e.g. of a flexed limb. 2. The action whereby the ends of a part are distracted; traction. 3. The spatial attribute in perception. **Nail extension.** Traction on a distal fragment of fractured bone into which is inserted a nail or pin (Steinmann's nail) to facilitate this. **Extension per saltam.** The spread of disease by the formation of metastases. **Skeletal extension.** Nail extension (see above). [L *extendere* to stretch out.]

See also: BUCK, CODIVILLA, STEINMANN.

extensity (ex·**ten**·sit·e). The spatial attribute in sensation. [see prec.]

extensor (ex·**ten**·sor). An extensor muscle. [L *extendere* to stretch out.]

extensor carpi radialis brevis muscle [musculus extensor carpi radialis brevis (NA)] (ex·**ten**·sor **kar**·pi ra·de·**a**·lis **brev**·is). A muscle which lies deep to the extensor carpi radialis longus muscle and extends from the lateral epicondyle to the base of the 3rd metacarpal bone.

extensor carpi radialis longus muscle [musculus extensor carpi radialis longus (NA)] (ex·**ten**·sor **kar**·pi ra·de·**a**·lis **long**·gus). A muscle on the radial side of the forearm, alongside the brachioradialis muscle. It extends from the lower shaft of the humerus to the base of the 2nd metacarpal bone.

extensor carpi ulnaris muscle [musculus extensor carpi ulnaris (NA)] (ex·**ten**·sor **kar**·pi ul·**na**·ris). A muscle placed on the ulnar side of the forearm and extending from the lateral epicondyle and the posterior border of the ulna to the base of the 5th metacarpal bone. It has 2 heads, the humeral [caput humerale (NA)], the part of the muscle arising from the tendon attached to the external epicondyle (the common extensor tendon), and the ulnar [caput ulnare (NA)], the part of the muscle that arises by an aponeurotic sheet from the posterior (subcutaneous) border of the ulnar.

extensor digiti minimi muscle [musculus extensor digiti minimi (NA)] (ex·**ten**·sor **dij**·it·i **min**·im·i). An extensor muscle of the 5th digit arising from the lateral epicondyle. It is inserted with the corresponding tendon of the extensor digitorum muscle.

extensor digitorum muscle [musculus extensor digitorum (NA)] (ex·**ten**·sor dij·it·**or**·um). The principal extensor muscle of the medial 4 digits. It extends from the lateral epicondyle to the bases of the middle and distal phalanges. Its tendons receive accessions from the lumbrical and interosseous muscles.

extensor digitorum brevis muscle [musculus extensor digitorum brevis (NA)] (ex·**ten**·sor dij·it·**or**·um **brev**·is). Any of the short extensor muscles of the toes arising from the dorsum of the tarsus and dividing into the tendons to the medial 4 toes. That to the big toe goes to the dorsum of the first phalanx; in the other toes they join the long extensor tendons.

extensor digitorum longus muscle [musculus extensor digitorum longus (NA)] (ex·**ten**·sor dij·it·**or**·um **long**·gus). An extensor muscle of the ankle and toes. Arising in the upper two-thirds of the leg, it is inserted by slips into the middle and distal phalanges of the lateral 4 toes.

extensor hallucis brevis muscle [musculus extensor hallucis brevis (NA)] (ex·**ten**·sor **hal**·oo·sis **brev**·is). A portion of the extensor digitorum brevis muscle which is sometimes separated from the remainder and is inserted into the dorsum of the first phalanx of the big toe.

extensor hallucis longus muscle [musculus extensor hallucis longus (NA)] (ex·**ten**·sor **hal**·oo·sis **long**·gus). A muscle which arises from the middle of the fibula and adjacent fascia and is inserted into the distal phalanx of the big toe. It is an extensor muscle of this toe and of the ankle.

extensor indicis muscle [musculus extensor indicis (NA)] (ex·**ten**·sor **in**·dis·is). A muscle that extends from the lower part of the shaft of the ulna and the interosseous membrane to join the tendon of the extensor digitorum muscle to the index finger.

extensor pollicis brevis muscle [musculus extensor pollicis brevis (NA)] (ex·**ten**·sor **pol**·is·is **brev**·is). The extensor muscle of the first phalanx of the thumb, arising from the radius and the interosseous membrane and inserted into the base of that phalanx.

extensor pollicis longus muscle [musculus extensor pollicis longus (NA)] (ex·**ten**·sor **pol**·is·is **long**·gus). The extensor muscle of the distal phalanx of the thumb, arising from the shaft of the ulna and interosseous membrane and inserted into the base of that phalanx.

extenuation (ex·ten·ew·**a'**·shun). 1. The act of making thin. 2. Thinness. 3. Weakness or delicacy. [L *extenuare* to make thin.]

exterior (ex·**teer**·e·or). 1. Outward, or external. 2. Of position, near or on the outside of the body or of a part of the body. [L outer.]

exterioration, exteriorization (ex·**teer**·e·or·**a'**·shun, ex·**teer**·e·or·i·**za'**·shun). 1. The surgical fixation of an internal organ, usually diseased, outside the surface of the body by way of an operation wound, for purposes of drainage or subsequent removal. 2. In psychology, the process of objectivating interests or affects. [see foll.]

exteriorize (ex·**teer**·e·or·ize). 1. To fix outside the body. 2. Psychologically, to objectivate interests or affects. [L *exterior* outer.]

external [externus (NA)] (ex·**ter**·nal). 1. Exterior, or on the outside. 2. Relating to the outside, as of a body, 3. Acting from without. 4. Situated on the side distant from the median line of the body; obsolete usage, lateral preferred. [L *externus* outward.]

externalia (ex·ter·**na**·le·ah). The external genitalia.

externalize (ex·**ter**·nal·ize). In psychology, to embody in outward form. Thus, an idea in the mind may be transformed into hallucination, e.g. voices, apparitions. [L *externus* outward.]

exteroceptive (ex·ter·o·**sep'**·tiv). Having the function of an exteroceptor, as applied to the surface of the body which receives stimuli from outside.

exteroceptor (ex·ter·o·**sep'**·tor). A sensory receptor, such as a visual receptor, which is affected by stimuli arising outside the body, as contrasted with a *proprioceptor* such as a muscle sensory receptor, which is affected by stimuli arising within the body itself. [L *exterus* outside, *recipere* to receive.]

exterofection (ex·ter·o·**fek'**·shun). The condition of responsiveness to environment which is brought about in the body by the activities of the central nervous system. [L *exterus* outside, *facere* to do.]

exterofective (ex·ter·o·**fek'**·tiv). Term applied to the central nervous system indicating that response to external stimulation originates in it (W. B. Cannon). [see prec.]

extima (**ex**·tim·ah). The tunica adventitia of an artery or vein. [L *extimus* outermost (coat).]

extinction (ex·**tingk**·shun). 1. The state of being completely destroyed or lost, e.g. the sense of hearing. 2. Partial abeyance or loss, as of the voice. [L *extinguere* to quench.]

extirpation (ex·ter·**pa**·shun). Total eradication; removal of an entire pathological structure, organ or part. [L *extirpare* to root out.]

Exton, William G. (b. 1876). American physician.

Exton's reagent. For protein in urine: dissolve 200 g of crystalline sodium sulphate in 800 ml of water, cool to 35°C and add 50 g of sulphosalicylic acid. When dissolved dilute to 1 litre with water.

extorsion (ex·**tor**·shun). Rotation of the vertical meridian of the cornea outwards, effected by the inferior oblique muscle when the eye is abducted and by the inferior rectus muscle when it is adducted. [L *ex, torquere* to twist.]

extra-. Prefix, from the Latin *extra*, meaning *outside of, beyond the scope of*. Not to be confused with the English adverb *extra*.

extra-amniotic (ex·trah·am·ne·**ot'**·ik). Indicating a structure lying outside the amnion, between it and the chorion. [L *extra*, amnion.]

extra-anthropic (ex·trah·an·**throp'**·ik). Exanthropic: 1. Having the character of an exanthrope. 2. Originating outside of or not existing within the human body. [L *extra*, Gk *anthropos* man.]

extra-articular (ex·trah·ar·**tik'**·ew·lar). 1. Occurring on the outside of a joint. 2. In the region of a joint but not involving the structures of the joint. 3. Systemic features of an arthritis (e.g. rheumatoid) involving tissues other than the joints. [L *extra*, articulation.]

extrabronchial (ex·trah·**brong**·ke·al). 1. Situated or occurring outside the bronchi. 2. Existing independently of the bronchi. [L *extra*, bronchus.]

extrabuccal (ex·trah·**buk**·al). On the outside of the mouth; outside the buccal cavity. [L *extra, bucca* cheek.]

extrabulbar (ex·trah·**bul**·bar). On the outside of or at a distance from any bulb, e.g. the medulla oblongata. [L *extra*, bulb.]

extracapsular (ex·trah·**kap**·sew·lar). Situated on the outside of the capsule of a joint, or occurring outside it. [L *extra*, capsule.]

extracardial (ex·trah·**kar**·de·al). Situated or occurring outside the heart. [L *extra*, Gk *kardia* heart.]

extracarpal (ex·trah·**kar**·pal). 1. Beyond the region of the carpus or wrist. 2. Unrelated to the carpus. [L *extra*, carpus.]

extracellular (ex·trah·**sel**·ew·lar). Outside the cell. [L *extra, cella* store-room.]

extracerebral (ex·trah·**ser**·e·bral). Within the cranium but outside the brain. [L *extra, cerebrum* brain.]

extracorporeal (ex·trah·kor·**po'**·re·al). 1. Without relation to the body or to any anatomical body. 2. Descriptive of those stages in the life cycle of a parasite which are not passed within the body of the host. 3. Extracorporeal circuits; the technique of keeping the circulation of the blood going by the use of an artificial heart–lung machine. It is used in open operations on the heart. [L *extra*, corpus.]

extracorpuscular (ex·trah·kor·**pus'**·kew·lar). Outside the corpuscles, particularly those of the blood. [L *extra*, corpuscle.]

extracostal (ex·trah·**kos**·tal). 1. Situated on the outside of a rib. 2. External to the ribs. [L *extra, costa* rib.]

extracranial (ex·trah·**kra**·ne·al). Outside the skull or on the outside of it. [L *extra*, Gk *kranion* skull.]

extract (**ex**·trakt). A preparation of a plant or animal substance, containing the therapeutically-active principles of the original but none of the cellular material. It is made with a suitable solvent and is known accordingly as an aqueous, alcoholic or acetic extract. The term may sometimes be wrongly applied, as in Goulard's extract, which is a mere solution of lead subacetate. There are 3 main classes of extract, dry, soft and liquid or fluid, according to the consistency of the product (see below). Most extracts of necessity contain extraneous material and are therefore only suitable for oral administration; those sufficiently free, e.g. from protein, to render them fit for parenteral administration are usually referred to as *injections.* The following official extracts are listed in the BP 1973: Belladonna Dry Extract, Cascara Dry Extract, Cascara Liquid Extract, Colchicum Liquid Extract, Ipecacuanha Liquid Extract, Liquorice Liquid Extract, Male Fern Dry Extract, Nux Vomica Liquid Extract. **Adrenal-cortex extract.** An extract of the suprarenal glands specially prepared for injection; it contains corticosterone, dehydrocorticosterone, deoxycorticosterone and other steroids, and is used in the treatment of Addison's disease. **Beef extract.** An extract containing the proteins of beef in a concentrated form; there are many proprietary brands. **Compound extract.** One containing the ingredients of 2 or more drugs. **Dry extract.** An extract prepared either by maceration, in which the drug in a suitable state of division is immersed in the solvent or menstruum for a definite time and the liquid filtered, or by percolation, in which the solvent is poured over the powdered drug packed into a glass solumn, the solution passing out through the bottom. In either case the liquid obtained is evaporated to dryness, if necessary, as with drugs containing ingredients unstable to heat, *in vacuo.* Sometimes the dried residue is mixed with an inert substance to adjust it to a required strength, the diluent being usually lactose or calcium phosphate. Dry extracts are used in making pills, being more concentrated than the powdered drug itself. **Infundibular extract.** Extract of pituitary (see below). **Liquid extract.** An extract prepared from the liquid obtained by maceration or percolation as in dry extract (see above), evaporated to a definite volume so that 28 ml (1 fl. oz) of the product contains the same quantity of active ingredient as 28 g (1 oz) by weight of the powdered dry drug. **Extract of liver.** An aqueous extract of liver, containing the specific antiperniciousanaemia principle and adjusted in strength so that 56 ml (2 fl. oz) is equivalent to 0.45 kg (1 lb) of fresh mammalian liver. It is administered orally, but is now being replaced by purer preparations suitable for injection, which possess the advantage that the effect of each dose lasts several days, whereas the oral extract has to be given more frequently. **Extract of malt.** An aqueous extract of malt or germinating barley evaporated *in vacuo* to the consistency of toffee. It contains maltose, dextrin and other carbohydrates, and is of value as a food. It is usually given mixed with cod-liver oil, to the presence of which its beneficial effects are almost entirely due. **Parathyroid extract.** An aqueous extract of the parathyroid glands, used to control the calcium content of the blood, and therefore administered to relieve tetany due to insufficient blood calcium. **Extract of pituitary.** An extract of the posterior lobe of the pituitary. It is used in midwifery to contract the uterus, as an antidiuretic and in postoperative ileus. **Placental extract.** Immune globulin, an extract of human placenta containing globulins and used to immunize children against measles. **Protein extract.** The extract of the protein of a substance to which sensitivity is suspected; the extract may be used for both diagnosis and treatment. **Rice-polishings extract.** The soluble extract of the pericarp, aleurone layer and germ of rice, which is removed when rice is milled or "polished", that is, made white and glistening; these contain vitamins, especially B_1. **Soft extract.** The liquid obtained in the dry-extract processes, evaporated to the consistency of a soft mass only; such extracts are awkward to handle and are passing out of use. **Thymus extract.** An aqueous acid extract of the thymus glands from 2-6 week-old calves, said to increase the growth, development, and fertility of rats. **Thyroid extract.** Thyroid BP 1958, dry thyroid; the thyroid glands of oxen, sheep or pigs, after removal of connective tissue, drying, powdering and defatting by means of light petroleum. The product is diluted with lactose to contain 0.09-0.11 per cent of iodine. [L *ex, trahere* to draw.]

See also: GOULARD, HANSON, LIEBIG.

extraction (ex·**trak**·shun). 1. The act or process of drawing out, as of a tooth. 2. The process of making an extract, e.g. by separating the active constituents of drugs. **Breech extraction.** A breech delivery that requires interference. **Extracapsular extraction.** Removal of the lens leaving part of the capsule in place. **Extraction of cataract.** The operation of removing a cataract from the eye. **Flap extraction.** Surgical removal of cataract through a semicircular incision of the cornea so that the latter may be folded back like a flap. **Intra-capsular extraction.** Removal of the whole lens with its capsule. [L *ex, trahere* to draw.]

extractive (ex·**trak**·tiv). That constituent of a mixture or of an organized tissue which may be extracted with a specific solvent such as water, ether or alcohol. [see prec.]

extractor (ex·**trak**·tor). An instrument, e.g. forceps, for the extraction of foreign bodies or sequestra, or with which to draw or pull out any natural part, such as a tooth. **Vacuum extractor.** A suction instrument used to aid delivery of the fetus (perfected by Malmstrom in 1957). A metal cup, provided in 3 sizes, is attached to tubing which contains a metal chain ending in a traction handle. The tubing passes through the handle and extends to enter a vacuum container fitted with a screw release valve and a pressure gauge. A short piece of tubing leaves the container to attach to a pump. The cup is applied to the scalp. It is used as an alternative to obstetrical forceps during the first or second stages of labour. [L *ex, trahere* to draw.]

extractum (ex·**trak**·tum). Extract. All official preparations are now under *extract*: prior to the BP 1953 they were under *extractum.* The following Extracta which appeared in the BP 1948 are now omitted: Extractum Colchici Siccum, Extractum Colocynthidis Compositum, Extractum Ergotae Liquidum, Extractum Fellis Bovini, Extractum Glycyrrhizae, Extractum Hepatis Liquidum, Extractum Krameriae Siccum, Extractum Senegae Liquidum. [L.]

extracurrent (ex·trah·**kur**·ent). Term applied to an electrically induced current; a current outside the primary current. [L *extra,* current.]

extracystic (ex·trah·**sis**·tik). 1. On the outside of, or situated beyond, the bladder or gall bladder. 2. Outside a cyst, or on the outside of it. 3. Unrelated to any bladder or cystic tumour. [L *extra,* Gk *kystis* bag.]

extradural (ex·trah·**dewr**·al). Situated on the outside of or lying outside the dura mater. [L *extra,* dura mater.]

extra-embryonic (ex·trah·em·bre·**on'**·ik). Term applied to those structures of the fertilized ovum which do not enter into the formation of the embryo proper but are situated outside it, e.g. the amnion. [L *extra,* embryo.]

extra-epiphyseal (ex·trah·ep·e·**fiz'**·e·al). 1. Not connected with or related to an epiphysis. 2. At a distance from an epiphysis. [L *extra,* epiphysis.]

extra-epithelial (ex·trah·ep·e·**the'**·le·al). Outside or on the outside of the epithelium. [L *extra,* epithelium.]

extra-expiratory (ex·trah·ex·**pir'**·at·or·e). Having relation to acts of forced expiration; beyond the normal range of breathing. [L *extra,* expiration.]

extragenital (ex·trah·**jen**·it·al). Unrelated to the genital organs; indicating a chancre that is not situated on the external genitalia. [L *extra,* genitalia.]

extrahepatic (ex·trah·hep·**at'**·ik). 1. Not connected with the liver. 2. On the outside surface of the liver. or outside the organ altogether. [L *extra,* Gk *hepar* liver.]

extraligamentous (ex·trah·lig·am·**en'**·tus). 1. Not connected with a ligament. 2. Occurring outside, or on the outer aspect of, a ligament. [L *extra,* ligament.]

extralobular (ex·trah·**lob**·ew·lar). Situated or occurring on the outside of or lying outside a lobe. [L *extra,* lobe.]

extramalleolus (ex·trah·mal·**e'**·o·lus). The lateral malleolus of the ankle joint. [L *extra,* malleolus.]

extramarginal (ex·trah·**mar**·jin·al). Beyond the limits of consciousness. [L *extra,* margin.]

extramastoiditis (ex·trah·mas·toid·**i'**·tis). An inflamed condition of those tissues contiguous to but lying outside the mastoid process and in association with inflammation of the outer surface of the process. [L *extra*, mastoiditis.]

extramedullary (ex·trah·med·**ul**'·ar·e). Outside a medulla or marrow, particularly the medulla oblongata, the spinal cord or the bone marrow. [L *extra*, *medulla* marrow.]

extrameningeal (ex·trah·men·**in**'·je·al). Occurring outside, or on the outside of, the meninges. [L *extra*, meninges.]

extramural (ex·trah·**mewr**·al). 1. Outside the wall of a part. 2. Studies or instruction conducted outside a school or university. [L *extra*, *murus* wall.]

extraneous (ex·**tra**·ne·us). 1. Foreign; of outside origin. 2. Originating, coming from or existing outside the organism. 3. Not essential. [L *extraneus* strange.]

extranuclear (ex·trah·**new**·kle·ar). Outside, or on the outside of, a nucleus. [L *extra*, nucleus.]

extra-ocular (ex·trah·**ok**·ew·lar). 1. On the outside of, or outside, the eyeball. 2. In biology, term applied to the antennae that are not placed near the eyes of the insect. [L *extra*, *oculus* eye.]

extra-oesophageal (ex·trah·e·sof·ah·**je**'·al). Outside the oesophagus but in close proximity to it. [L *extra*, oesophagus.]

extraparenchymal (ex·trah·par·**en**'·kim·al). 1. Unrelated to the parenchyma of an organ. 2. Originating or formed outside, or on the outside of, the parenchyma. [L *extra*, parenchyma.]

extrapelvic (ex·trah·**pel**·vik). 1. Not connected with or related to the pelvis. 2. In a situation outside the pelvis or occurring outside it. [L *extra*, pelvis.]

extrapericardial (ex·trah·per·e·**kar**'·de·al). Outside the pericardium. [L *extra*, pericardium.]

extraperineal (ex·trah·per·in·**e**'·al). Not connected with, or away from, the perineum. [L *extra*, perineum.]

extraperiosteal (ex·trah·per·e·**os**'·te·al). 1. Outside the periosteum. 2. Not connected with, independent of or unrelated to the periosteum. [L *extra*, periosteum.]

extraperitoneal (ex·trah·per·e·ton·**e**'·al). External to the peritoneal cavity. [L *extra*, peritoneum.]

extrapial (ex·trah·**pi**·al). External to the pia mater. [L *extra*, pia mater.]

extraplacental (ex·trah·plas·**en**'·tal). Unrelated to, or independent of, the placenta. [L *extra*, placenta.]

extraplantar (ex·trah·**plan**·tar). Occurring on the outside of the sole of the foot. [L *extra*, *planta* sole.]

extrapleural (ex·trah·**ploor**·al). Outside the cavity of the pleura. [L *extra*, pleura.]

extraprostatic (ex·trah·pros·**tat**'·ik). 1. Situated outside, or on the outside of, the prostate. 2. Independent of, or not connected with, the prostate. [L *extra*, prostate.]

extraprostatitis (ex·trah·pros·tat·**i**'·tis). An inflamed condition of the tissues in the neighbourhood of the prostate gland. [L *extra*, prostatitis.]

extrapulmonary (ex·trah·**pul**·mon·ar·e). 1. Outside the lungs. 2. Not having any connection with or relation to the lungs. [L *extra*, *pulmo* lung.]

extrapyramidal (ex·trah·pir·**am**'·id·al). Outside the cerebrospinal (pyramidal) tracts. [L *extra*, pyramid.]

extraradical (ex·trah·**rad**·ik·al). Term applied to any reaction or substitution which does not involve the characteristic radicals of a compound. [L *extra*, radical.]

extrarectus (ex·trah·**rek**·tus). The lateral rectus muscle of the orbit. [L *extra*, *rectus* straight.]

extrarenal (ex·trah·**re**·nal). On the outside surface of, or external to, the kidney. [L *extra*, *ren* kidney.]

extraserous (ex·trah·**seer**·us). Outside a serous cavity. [L *extra*, serum.]

extrasomatic (ex·trah·so·**mat**'·ik). 1. Outside the body. 2. Unrelated to, or not connected with, the body. [L *extra*, Gk *soma* body.]

extrasystole (ex·trah·**sis**·to·le). A premature contraction of the heart due to impulses which are abnormal either in their site of origin or in their timing in relation to the existing cardiac rhythm, or in both these respects; such beats may interfere with, or replace, the existing rhythm and are usually coupled to a preceding beat. The terms *premature beat* and *ectopic beat* are often used synonymously, but some extrasystoles are not premature and they can arise in the sinus node. Extrasystoles are most commonly ventricular in origin, **Atrial extrasystole.** An extrasystole arising from a focus in the atria. **Atrioventricular nodal extrasystole.** An extrasystole arising in the atrioventricular node. **Frustrate extrasystole.** An extrasystole occurring so soon after the previous beat that the resulting ventricular contraction fails to open the semilunar valves. **Infranodal extrasystole.** An extrasystole having its focus of origin below the atrioventricular node. **Interpolated (ventricular) extrasystole.** An extrasystole which occurs sufficiently early after one beat so as not to inhibit the normal succeeding beat; it must also fail to be conducted to the sinus node so as not to interfere with its normal cycle. **Multifocal extrasystoles.** Extrasystoles observed in one subject arising from more than one focus during any one period of observation. **Nodal extrasystole.** An extrasystole having its origin in the atrioventricular node. **Nomotropic extrasystole.** An extrasystole arising from a focus in or near to the sinus node. **R on T extrasystole.** An early extrasystole occurring so that the electrocardiographic **R** wave of the extrasystole falls within the T wave of the preceding beat; this occurrence has a greater likelihood of initiating ventricular fibrillation than an extrasystole occurring later. **Reciprocal extrasystole.** Reciprocal beat. *See* BEAT. **Retrograde extrasystole.** Conduction of an impulse arising from a ventricular focus retrogradely to the atria. **Return extrasystole.** Reciprocal beat. *See* BEAT. **Ventricular extrasystole.** An extrasystole arising from a focus in the ventricles. [L *extra*, Gk *systole* contraction.]

extrathoracic (ex·trah·thor·**as**'·ik). Outside the cavity of the thorax. [L *extra*, thorax.]

extratracheal (ex·trah·trak·**e**'·al). Situated or occurring outside the trachea. [L *extra*, trachea.]

extratubal (ex·trah·**tew**·bal). Situated outside any tube, with special reference to the pharyngotympanic or the uterine tube. [L *extra*, tube.]

extratympanic (ex·trah·tim·**pan**'·ik). Outside the middle ear (tympanum). [L *extra*, tympanum.]

extra-uterine (ex·trah·**ew**·ter·ine). Originating, occurring or situated outside the uterus, as of pregnancy. [L *extra*, uterus.]

extravaginal (ex·trah·**vaj**·in·al). 1. Outside the vagina. 2. Outside any sheath-like structure. [L *extra*, vagina.]

extravasate (ex·**trav**·as·ate). To flow or pass out from the proper channel. [L *extra*, *vas* vessel.]

extravasation (ex·**trav**·as·**a**'·shun). 1. The process of exuding from a containing vessel into the tissues, e.g. blood, serum, lymph or urine. 2. Substance or fluid present in the tissues and having escaped or exuded from its containing vessel; an exudate. 3. The act of forcing a fluid out of, or allowing it to escape from, its proper duct or vessel. **Punctiform extravasation.** An extravasation which covers the affected tissue with minute spots of blood. [L *extra*, *vas* vessel.]

extravascular (ex·trah·**vas**·kew·lar). Occurring outside or situated outside any vessel or vessels. [L *extra*, *vasculum* small vessel.]

extraventricular (ex·trah·ven·**trik**'·ew·lar). Occurring or situated outside any ventricle, particularly a ventricle of the heart. [L *extra*, ventricle.]

extraversion (ex·trah·**ver**·shun). Extroversion. [L *extra*, *vertere* to turn.]

extravert (ex·trah·vert). Extrovert.

extremital (ex·**trem**·it·al). 1. Relating or belonging to an extremity. 2. Situated at an extremity. 3. Distal.

extremity (ex·**trem**·it·e). 1. An arm or a leg. 2. A hand or a foot. 3. [Extremitas (NA)] The distal end or part of an organ or structure. **Lower extremity.** The hip, thigh, leg, ankle and foot regarded as one structure; the pelvic limb. **Upper extremity.** The shoulder, arm, forearm, wrist and hand regarded as one structure; the thoracic limb. [L, *extremitas*.]

extrinsic (ex·**trin**·sik). 1. External; originating outside any particular structure or organism. 2. Denoting parts of an organ or structure which are not wholly contained within it but stretch to it from another organ or structure, e.g. certain muscles. 3. Non-essential. [L *extrinsecus* on the outside.]

extrophia, extrophy (ex·tro·fe·ah, ex·tro·fe). A congenital condition in which there is malformation of an internal organ. **Extrophy of the bladder.** Ectopia vesicae. [Gk *ex, trophe* nutrition.]

extrospection (ex·tro·spek·shun). The outward expression of the mental condition of mysophobia, i.e. the continual inspection by the patient of his own skin to make certain that it is clean and uncontaminated. [L *extra, spectare* to look.]

extroversion (ex·tro·ver·shun). 1. Congenital eversion of a hollow organ. 2. In psychology, the turning of an individual's attention and interest outward to other people and things and away from himself. **Extroversion of the bladder.** Congenital malformation associated with absence of the anterior bladder wall and the lower part of the abdominal wall, and eversion of the posterior bladder wall, which is seen as a moist mucous surface from which there is a discharge of urine. The 2 ureter openings are visible on the everted posterior bladder wall. Cf. INTROVERSION. [L *extra, vertere* to turn.]

extrovert (ex·tro·vert). One whose interest and attention is centred on other people and external objects. [see prec.]

extrude (ex·trood). To thrust out, e.g. from alignment or from a surface. [L *extrudere* to push out.]

extrusion (ex·troo·zhun). The pushing out; as in dentistry, pushing of a tooth from its normal alignment. [see prec.]

extubate (ex·tew·bate). To remove a tube, particularly from the larynx after intubation. [L *ex, tuba* tube.]

extubation (ex·tew·ba·shun). The process or the act of removing a tube, particularly from the larynx after intubation. [see prec.]

extuberance (ex·tew·ber·ans). Protuberance; a swelling. [L *ex, tuber* tumour.]

extumescence (ex·tew·mes·ens). A swelling or rising; a projection. [L *ex, tumescere* to swell.]

exuberant (eg·zew·ber·ant). 1. Copious or superabundant production or supply. 2. Marked by excessive proliferation. [L *exuberare* to be very fertile.]

exudate (ex·ew·date). 1. An exuded substance. 2. A fluid extravasated into a cavity or the tissues. 3. Any additional substance deposited on or in the tissues as the result of a vital process or a condition of disease. **Fibrinous exudate.** A coagulation of fluid in the spaces or cavity into which it has seeped. **Serofibrinous exudate.** Serous fluid containing small coagulated flakes of fibrous matter. **Serous exudate.** An exudate composed chiefly of serum. [L *exudare* to sweat out.]

exudation (ex·ew·da·shun). 1. The discharge of moisture, serum or pus. 2. The deposition of an additional substance in or on the tissues as the result of a vital process or the action of a disease. [see prec.]

exudative (ex·ew·dat·iv). Marked by, belonging to or having the character of an exudation.

exulcerans (ex·ul·ser·anz). Ulcerating. [L making sore.]

exulceratio simplex (ex·ul·ser·a'·she·o sim·plex). Superficial gastric ulcer. [L simple ulceration.]

exulceration (ex·ul·ser·a'·shun). 1. Ulceration. 2. A sore. [L *exulcerare* to make sore.]

exumbilication (ex·um·bil·ik·a'·shun). 1. Umbilical hernia. *See* HERNIA. 2. Noticeable protrusion of the navel. [L *ex*, umbilication.]

exutory (ex·ew·tor·e). 1. Drawing, as of the blood, to the surface of the body or the promoting of suppuration of an abscess. 2. A substance or remedy that effects this. [L *exuere* to strip off.]

exuviae (ex·ew·ve·e). Any slough or material cast-off, particularly epidermis. [L what is stripped off.]

exuviation (ex·ew·ve·a'·shun). The casting-off of an epidermal part. [see prec.]

eye [oculus (NA)] (i). The visual organ. Almost spherical, it consists of 3 layers: a tough fibrous outer coat, the sclera, becoming clear in front to form the cornea; a vascular and pigmented middle layer, the choroid; and an inner and perceptive layer, the retina. The cornea, aqueous, lens and vitreous act as a refractive unit that forms an image on the retina. **Amblyopic eye.** An eye with subnormal vision, to account for which no disease can be seen; amblyopia occurs in squinting eye through lack of use, in hysteria, and in tobacco and other poisonings. **Angle of the eye, lateral [angulus oculi lateralis (NA)].** The lateral extremity of the palpebral fissure. **Angle of the eye, medial [angulus oculi medialis (NA)].** The medial extremity of the palpebral fissure. **Aphacic eye.** An eye in which the crystalline lens is absent. The term can be used for an eye in which the crystalline lens is not in the pupillary area and therefore cannot act as a refractive unit. **Arc eye.** Conjunctivitis and superficial punctate corneal ulceration found in oxyacetylene welders. **Artificial eye.** A glass or plastics shell, coloured to resemble a normal eye, which fits into the conjunctival sac following enucleation, or occasionally over a shrunken eye. **Bi-uniac eye.** Binoculus. **Black eye.** Bruising, by a blow, of the soft tissues around the eye against the bony rim of the orbit. **Cat's eye.** A human eye with complete congenital coloboma of the iris, resembling the slit-like pupil of the cat. **Cinema eye.** Conjunctivitis formerly found in film actors following exposure to arc lamps (Klieg lights); also called Klieg eye. It is caused by the ultraviolet rays. **Coat of the eye, fibrous [tunica fibrosa bulbi (NA)].** The sclera and the cornea. **Coat of the eye, nervous [tunica interna bulbi (NA)].** The inner coat of the eye comprising the retina. **Coat of the eye, vascular [tunica vasculosa bulbi (NA)].** The choroid, ciliary body and iris. **Cross eye.** Also called *squint*; deviation from the normal of the visual axis of one or other eye, so that single binocular vision cannot take place. **Cyclopean eye.** A single eye situated in the centre of the forehead; an extremely rare congenital abnormality. **Cystic eye.** A congenital deformity in which the eyeball is replaced by a cyst. This is caused by the failure of the primary optic vesicle to involute and thus a cyst is formed. **Dark-adapted eye.** An eye which has been protected from daylight, especially the lower end of the spectrum, to allow regeneration of the visual purple and other changes to take place. Also called *scotopic eye.* **Exciting eye.** Term used in sympathetic ophthalmia, denoting the injured eye which is primarily affected. **Fixing eye.** Term used in squint to denote the eye the visual axis of which passes through the object fixed. **Gas eye.** An affection of the eye prevalent among workers with natural gas. **Hare eye.** A condition in which the eye does not close during sleep. Also called *lagophthalmia.* **Hop eye.** Acute conjunctivitis found in hop-pickers, caused by irritation from the spinal hairs of the hop plant. **Hot eye.** Congestion of the conjunctiva, combined with a hot gritty feeling, associated with gout (described by Jonathan Hutchinson). **Klieg eye.** Cinema eye (see above). **Lazy eye.** An eye with poor vision due to lack of use; amblyopic eye. **Light-adapted eye.** An eye which has been in the bright light long enough for various chemical and physiological changes to have taken place. Also called *photopic eye.* **Nairobi eye.** A term that has been applied to a severe ocular lesion caused by the secretions of certain vesicating or blistering beetles, *Paederus,* that are common in Nairobi. Vesicating beetles of this and other allied genera occur in many other tropical areas, causing both skin and ocular lesions that are given both local and other names, e.g. *spider lick.* **Ox eye.** The unusually large eye found in infantile glaucoma. **Photopic eye.** Light-adapted eye (see above). **Pink eye.** Epidemic acute conjunctivitis common in institutions, due to the Koch–Weeks bacillus. **Reduced eye.** An eye where the optical systems are reduced diagrammatically to a single refracting unit; first described by Donders. **Schematic eye.** One in which the optical systems are reduced diagrammatically to 2 refractive units; first described by Listing. **Scotopic eye.** Dark-adapted eye (see above). **Shipyard eye.** Epidemic keratoconjunctivitis. An infection due to an adenovirus (type 8) spread by contaminated fluids applied to injured eyes, usually in busy eye casualty stations such as those in shipyards. **Squinting eye.** Denoting the eye the visual axis of which deviates from the normal, in contradistinction to fixing eye (above). **Sympathetic eye, Sympathizing eye.** Term used in sympathetic ophthalmia to denote the uninjured eye which becomes secondarily affected. **Watery eye.** Epiphora. [AS *éage.*]

See also: GULLSTRAND.

eye-cup (i·kup). 1. The optic cup. 2. A small vessel of glass or porcelain for use in bathing the eye, curved to fit the orbit. [AS *éage, cuppe.*]

eye fly (i fli). Any fly, of several genera, which habitually settles on the mucosal margins of the eyelids. *Hippelates pusio, H. flavipes* and others in the genus are serious nuisances in southern USA and Central America, and are associated with the spread of conjunctivitis and yaws. *Siphunculina (=Microneureum) funicola* plays a similar rôle in India and the East Indies. [AS *éage, flyge.*]

eye ground (i grownd). That part of the fundus of the eye that can be examined with the ophthalmoscope. [AS *éage, grund.*]

eye-minded (i·mind·ed). Term applied to a person whose thoughts and memories are mainly composed of visual images. [AS *éage,* ME *mynd.*]

eye-shield (i·sheeld). A covering for the eye, of various design, worn as a protection from glare or injury. [AS *éage, sceld.*]

eye spot (i spot). 1. In embryology, the rudiment of the eye, i.e. the hollow diverticulum which appears on each lateral aspect of the forebrain. 2. A chromatophore or coloured spot in a unicellular organism. [AS *éage,* ME *spot.*]

eye stone (i stone). A lid of a small smooth marine shell or a similar object inserted beneath the eyelid in order to facilitate removal of foreign bodies from the eye. [AS *éage, stan.*]

eye wash (i wash). A collyrium. [AS *éage, wascan.*]

eyeball [bulbus oculi (NA)] (i·bawl). The globular organ of sight, excluding the accessory structures such as eyelids and muscles. [AS *éage,* ME *bal.*]

eyebrow [supercilium (NA)] (i·brow). The raised arch of skin above each orbit together with the short thick hairs growing on it. [AS *éage, bru.*]

eyeglass (i·glahs). 1. A single lens for wear in one eye; a monocle. 2. A small glass vessel for use in bathing the eye, curved to fit the orbit. **Eyeglasses.** A form of spectacles without sidepieces, held in place by a bridge fitted with a spring; generally referred to as *pince-nez.* [AS *éage, glaes.*]

eyelash [cilium (NA)] (i·lash). One of the hairs growing from the free edges of the eyelid. [AS *éage,* ME *lasche.*]

eyelids [palpebrae (NA)] (i·lidz). Thin movable folds, upper [palpebra superior (NA)] and lower [palpebra inferior (NA)], in front of the eyeball, closing in sleep or to protect it from injury. **Borders of the eyelids, anterior [limbi palpebrales anteriores (NA)].** The curved anterior borders of the lid margins. **Borders of the eyelids, posterior [limbi palpebrales posteriores].** The sharp, almost angular, posterior borders of the lid margins. **Fused eyelid.** The failure of the eyelids of the fetus or newborn child to separate: normally, *in utero,* fusion occurs about the ninth week and persists until the seventh month. **Surface of the eyelid, anterior [facies anterior palpebrarum (NA)].** The surface covered by skin. **Surface of the eyelid, posterior [facies posterior palpebrarum (NA)].** The surface covered by the conjunctiva. [AS *éage, hlid.*]

eyepiece (i·pees). An ocular; in an optical instrument such as a microscope or telescope, the magnifying system of lenses through which the eye views the image formed by the objective. **Huyghenian eyepiece.** Huyghenian ocular. *See* OCULAR. **Eyepiece micrometer.** *See* MICROMETER. [AS *éage,* OFr. *pece.*]

eyestrain (i·strane). The tired condition of the eye resulting from uncorrected defective focusing; asthenopia. [AS *éage,* L *stringere* to draw tight.]

eyewater (i·waw·ter). 1. Tears. 2. A collyrium. [AS *éage, waeter.*]

Eysson, Henrique (b. 1620). Gröningen anatomist.

Eysson's bones. The mental ossicle.

F

fabella (fab·el·ah). A seed-like sesamoid of fibrocartilage or bone which is sometimes contained in the tendon of the lateral head of the gastrocnemius muscle. [L little bean.]

Faber, Knud Helge (b. 1862). Copenhagen physician.

Faber's anaemia, or syndrome. An idiopathic hypochromic microcytic anaemia with achlorhydria.

fabism (fa·bizm). Favism: 1. An acute haemolytic anaemia with abdominal pain, vomiting and diarrhoea brought on by the eating of certain kinds of bean, including the Italian lentil, *Vicia fava.* It is always associated with a deficiency of the enzyme glucose-6-dehydrogenase within the erythrocytes. 2. A disorder resembling hay fever caused by inhalation of the pollen of certain kinds of bean. [L *faba* bean.]

Fabricius ab Aquapendente, Hieronymus (b. 1533). Padua anatomist.

Fabricius' bursa. A mass of lymphoid tissue found in birds just above the cloaca. Its removal in the newly-hatched chick destroys the animal's ability to produce a normal antibody response.

Fabricius' ship. An allegorical description of the outlines of the frontal, sphenoid and occipital bones.

Fabricus–Moller urine test. For amylase in urine: dilute 1 ml of urine with 29 ml distilled water. Dissolve 0.1 g of soluble starch in 100 ml of buffer, pH 6.7, and add 0.45 g of sodium chloride. Place 2 ml of starch solution in each of 6 tubes and add 6 drops of diluted urine to the first, 5 to the second, and so on, to 1 drop in the sixth tube. Incubate the tubes at 40°C for 30 min, cool and test for starch with iodine solution. Increased amylase is indicated by complete digestion of starch in more than the first 3 tubes.

Fabry, J. (b. 1860). German dermatologist.

Fabry's disease. Angiokeratoma corporis diffusum; a familial inborn error of lipid metabolism which results in lipid deposition in many tissues, including blood vessels, heart muscle, kidney, cornea and nervous tissue. It results in a complex range of symptoms and signs, and death usually occurs in middle age from renal or heart failure.

face [facies (NA)] (fase). The front of the head, including the forehead and chin but excluding the ears. **Adenoid face.** Adenoid facies. *See* FACIES. **Bird face.** A malformation in which the forehead is prominent and the midface recessed. The upper lip is lengthened and the chin projects. **Bony face [facies].** The facial skeleton. **Bovine face.** Bovina. **Brandy face.** Rosacea. **Cow face.** Facies bovina. **Dish face, Dished face.** Bird face (see above). **Frog face.** The face in hereditary craniofacial dysostosis, in which there is a broad nasal bridge, a beaked nose, and a prognathous lower jaw, together with ocular manifestations such as exophthalmos, divergent squint, and optic atrophy. Mental impairment is usual. **Hippocratic face.** Facies hippocratica. **Hippopotamus face.** The peculiar facial appearance produced by chronic general hypertrophy of the gums. **Mask-like face.** An immobile expressionless face. The palpebral fissures are wider than normal, the eyes are staring, and blinking is infrequent. The mouth is slightly open and saliva may run from it. It is characteristic of the parkinsonian syndrome. **Moon-shaped face.** The appearance of the face, round and highly coloured, characteristically seen in Cushing's disease and occasionally in patients treated with too much cortisone or corticotrophin. **Myasthenic face.** Myasthenic facies. *See* FACIES. **Stove-in face.** Appearance caused by part of the face having been driven inwards as a result of a severe compression injury. **Tabetic face.** Tabetic facies. *See* FACIES. [L *facies* face.]

face-bow (fase·bo). An instrument used in prosthetic dentistry to ensure that artificial dentures, as far as possible, function anatomically in the same manner as the natural teeth which they replace. [face, AS *boga.*]

facet [facies (NA)] (fas·et). A smooth flat or nearly flat surface of a bone or other hard structure. **Articular facet, acromial [facies articularis acromialis (NA)].** *See* CLAVICLE. **Articular facet of the acromion [facies articularis acromii (NA)].** *See* ACROMION. **Articular facet of the arytenoid cartilage [facies articularis (NA)].** A facet on the under-surface for articulation with the posterior lamina of the cricoid cartilage. **Articular facet of the atlas, inferior [fovea articularis inferior (NA)].** The laterally-placed surface under the atlas for articulation with the axis vertebra. **Articular facet of the atlas, superior [fovea articularis superior (NA)].** The joint surface on the lateral mass of the atlas for articulation with the occipital bone of the skull. **Articular facet of the lateral malleolus [facies articularis malleoli (NA)].** A large articular facet on the medial surface of the lateral malleolus, for the lateral side of the talus. **Articular facet, sternal [facies articularis sternalis (NA)].** The surface on the medial end of the clavicle that articulates with the manubrium sterni. **Facet for the arytenoid cartilage [facies articularis arytenoidea (NA)].** A small articular surface on the upper lateral corners of the cricoid lamina. **Calcanean facet of the talus, anterior [facies articularis calcanea anterior (NA)].** A facet on the inferior surface of the neck, sometimes fused with the middle facet. **Calcanean facet of the talus, middle [facies articularis calcanea media (NA)].** A facet lying posteromedial to, and sometimes fused with, the anterior facet on the inferior surface of the neck. **Calcanean facet of the talus, posterior [facies articularis calcanea posterior (NA)].** A large, obliquely-placed facet on the inferior aspect of the body. **Costal facet of a thoracic vertebra [fovea costalis transversalis (NA)].** The articular facet on the front of the transverse process of a thoracic vertebra, for the tubercle of the rib. **Costal facet of a thoracic vertebra, inferior [fovea costalis inferior (NA)].** The lower articular surface on the body of a thoracic vertebra, for the head of a rib. **Costal facet of a thoracic vertebra, superior [fovea costalis superior (NA)].** The upper articular surface on the body of a thoracic vertebra, for the head of a rib. **Facet for the cuboid [facies articularis cuboidea (NA)].** A facet occupying the anterior surface of the calcaneum. **Malleolar facet [facies articularis malleolaris (NA)].** A comma-shaped articular surface on the medial malleolus of the tibia articulating with the medial side of the body of the talus. **Malleolar facet of the lateral surface of the talus [facies malleolaris lateralis (NA)].** A large triangular facet for the lateral malleolus. **Malleolar facet of the medial surface of the talus [facies malleolaris medialis (NA)].** A sickle-shaped facet, broad in front and pointed behind, for articulation with the medial malleolus. **Navicular facet of the talus [facies articularis navicularis (NA)].** The large articular facet on the head. **Facet for the odontoid process [fovea dentis (NA)].** An oral facet on the posterior surface of the anterior arch of the atlas, for articulation with the odontoid process of the axis. **Facets of the odontoid process [facies articularis anterior et posterior (NA)].** The articular areas on the odontoid process, a constant one in front for the anterior arch of the atlas (anterior articular facet) and an occasional one on the posterior surface caused by the transverse ligament (posterior articular facet).

Squatting facet. A plane area on the anterior part of the lower extremity of the tibia and on a corresponding area on the anterior surface of the talus found in many Oriental races. **Facet for the talus, anterior [facies articularis talaris anterior (NA)].** A facet, sometimes continuous with the middle facet, on the anterior end of the superior surface of the calcaneum. **Facet for the talus, middle [facies articularis talaris media (NA)].** A facet on the superior surface of the sustentaculum tali, sometimes continuous with the anterior facet. **Facet for the talus, posterior [facies articularis talaris posterior (NA)].** The large facet on the superior surface, about its middle. **Facet for the thyroid cartilage [facies articularis thyroidea (NA)].** The facet at the junction of the arch and lamina of the cricoid cartilage, for articulation with the inferior horn of the thyroid cartilage. [Fr. *facette* little face.]

See also: LENOIR.

facetectomy (fas·et·ek·to·me). Surgical excision of the articular facet of a vertebra. [facet, Gk *ektome* a cutting out.]

facette (fas·et). Facet.

facial (fa·she·al, fa·shal). 1. Belonging to the face. 2. Belonging to a facet or the surface of anything. 3. In dentistry, denoting the collective outer surfaces of the teeth.

facial artery [arteria facialis (NA)]. One of the largest branches of the external carotid artery. It hooks around the lower border of the mandible anterior to the masseter muscle, where it can be palpated to run tortuously as far as the medial angle of the eye. It supplies the submandibular salivary gland [rami glandulares (NA)], the tonsil, the submental region, the tongue, the lips [arteria labialis superior et inferior (NA)], the soft palate, and the pharyngotympanic tube. **Transverse facial artery [arteria transversa faciei (NA)].** *See* TEMPORAL ARTERY, SUPERFICIAL.

facial bones [ossa faciei (NA)]. The bones of the face, including the maxilla, mandible and palatine and zygomatic bones.

facial nerve [nervus facialis (NA)]. The 7th cranial nerve. It is mixed motor and sensory, arising from motor nuclei in the pons and medulla oblongata and a sensory ganglion in the petrous temporal bone, supplying motor fibres to the muscles of facial expression, and sensory fibres to the mucous membrane of the palate and possibly the nose, taste fibres to the tongue and mouth, also secretomotor fibres to the submandibular and sublingual salivary glands. *See* CHORDA TYMPANI.

buccal branches [rami buccales (NA)]. Motor branches to supply the muscles of the face associated with the nose and upper lip.

cervical branch [ramus colli (NA)]. A motor branch in the parotid gland and descending to the neck to supply the platysma.

communicating branch with the glossopharyngeal nerve [ramus communicans cum nervo glossopharyngeo (NA)]. A twig of communication with the glossopharyngeal nerve arising from the facial nerve as it leaves the stylomastoid foramen.

communicating branch with the tympanic plexus [ramus communicans cum plexu tympanico (NA)]. A small branch arising from the facial ganglion and believed to convey parasympathetic fibres to the tympanic plexus through which they pass to join the lesser superficial petrosal nerve.

digastric branch [ramus digastricus (NA)]. An extracranial branch.

mandibular branch [ramus marginalis mandibulae (NA)]. A motor branch to the muscles of the lower lip and chin.

stylohyoid branch [ramus stylohyoideus (NA)]. An extracranial branch.

temporal branches [rami temporales (NA)]. Motor branches to supply the orbicularis oculi and the frontal belly of the occipitofrontalis muscles.

zygomatic branches [rami zygomatic (NA)]. A motor branch to the lower part of the orbicularis oculi muscle.

nucleus [nucleus nervi facialis (NA)]. A nucleus lying deeply within the reticular formation at the lower part of the pons; the source of impulses to the muscles of expression.

roots. Medial (motor) and lateral (sensory) [nervus intermedius (NA)] roots appearing in the interval between the olive and the inferior cerebellar peduncle, at the lower border of the pons.

facial veins. Main veins draining the face, communicating with the neck veins and the venous sinuses of the dura mater. **Anterior facial vein.** The main vein of the anterior part of the face, commencing at the inner canthus and terminating at the upper part of the neck in the common facial vein. **Common facial vein [vena facialis (NA)].** The large vein formed in the neck by the union of the anterior facial vein and the anterior division of the posterior facial vein; it is a tributary of the internal jugular vein. **Deep facial vein [vena faciei profunda (NA)].** A large communication between the anterior facial vein and the pterygoid (venous) plexus. **Posterior facial vein [vena retromandibularis (NA)].** A vein draining the scalp and posterior part of the face. It is formed by the union of the superficial temporal and maxillary veins, and ends below by dividing into two branches, one to join the common facial, and the other to the external jugular veins. **Transverse facial vein [vena transversa faciei (NA)].** A vessel draining the side of the face into the posterior facial vein.

facies (fa·se·eez, fa·she·eez). 1. The facial expression or appearance. 2. [NA] A surface. **Facies abdominalis.** A dull, pinched, sunken appearance of the face, seen in severe abdominal infections such as peritonitis, typhoid fever, etc. **Adenoid facies.** A facial expression characterized predominantly by the wide-open mouth and general vacant expression which is associated with mouth breathing; it is secondary to nasal obstruction, and commonly in nasal obstruction resulting from adenoid hypertrophy. **Facies antonina.** A facial expression often seen in advanced leprosy. Paralysis of the orbicularis oculi muscle, with eversion of the lids and corneal opacities give a peculiar staring appearance. The lacrimal secretion may be diminished, or tears may run down the cheek from eversion of the punctum lacrimale. The 5th and 7th nerves may be paralysed and there may be nodulation of the skin of the face. **Aortic facies.** Facial pallor without anaemia, associated with chronic aortic-valve incompetence. **Facies bovina.** Cow face; the facial appearance in hypertelorism, in which the eyes are widely separated owing to an unusual breadth of the nasal bridge. The nose is retroussé, the forehead bulging, and an external squint may be present. **Cardiac facies.** The appearance of a person suffering from congestive cardiac failure, with low cardiac output, of long duration. The face is drawn, sunken and anxious, the skin pale, sallow and slightly cyanosed. **Facies dolorosa.** A drawn appearance of the face expressive of pain. **Facies hepatica.** A drawn face with sunken cheeks and eyes, and a sallow complexion with dilated capillaries and spider angiomata. **Facies hippocratica.** A pale or livid face with dull sunken eyes, pinched nose, hollow cheeks and temples, open mouth and dropped lower jaw. It is indicative of impending dissolution. **Facies leontina.** The lionlike countenance in nodular leprosy. **Mitral facies.** The flushed, slightly cyanotic cheeks of patients with mitral stenosis. **Mongoloid facies.** The face of a mongolian idiot. It is characterized by narrow tilted eye slits with epicanthic folds; the bridge of the nose is somewhat depressed and the nostrils forward looking; the cheeks are red and may be cyanosed; the pinnae of the ears overhang at the upper angle; the tongue is fissured and protruded and the teeth are irregular; the hair is coarse, straight and scanty; there is increased interzygomatic breadth, and the skull is brachycephalic with a vertical occipital region. **Myasthenic facies.** A face in which there is symmetrical or asymmetrical ptosis, most marked on looking upwards, and without the usual compensatory wrinkling of the forehead; the external ocular muscles are affected, causing strabismus. The muscles of the face are weak and the smile has a peculiar snarling appearance. It occurs in myasthenia gravis. **Myopathic facies.** A dull and expressionless face, the nasolabial fold being absent, the lips separated and the lower lip projecting. In smiling the mouth forms a straight line and the power of whistling is lost. **Facies ovarica, Facies ovarina.** The drawn and pinched face seen in women with an ovarian tumour. **Facies scaphoidea.** A face produced by a congenital malformation in which the skull is elongated and narrow and has a median ridge or keel running anteroposteriorly. **Tabetic facies.** A face showing a partial bilateral ptosis with wrinkling of the forehead owing to compensatory contraction of the frontalis muscle. It occurs in late stages of tabes. **Typhoid facies, Facies typhosa.** The characteristic facial expression often seen in the second week of enteric fever. There is a slight, hectic-looking flush, lustrous conjunctivae, heavy and possibly sunken eyes, languor and apathy. In the third week the flush may become more marked and generally diffused. [L face.]

See also: CORVISART DES MARETS, HALL (M.), PARKINSON (JAMES), WELLS (T. S.).

facilitation (fas·il·it·a'·shun). 1. The easy rendering or the promotion of the performance of function. 2. The reinforcement of a reflex or other nervous activity by the arrival at the reflex centre of nervous impulses having their origin elsewhere. **Proprioceptive neuromuscular facilitation (P.N.F.).** A special technique of resisted exercises used in rehabilitation. Cf. LAW OF FACILITATION. [L *facilitas* easiness.]

See also: KABAT, WEDENSKY.

facing (fa·sing). A piece of porcelain or acrylic resin fixed to a supporting metal backing on a crown, bridge or denture; used to replace a natural tooth and resembling it in appearance and shape. [L *facies* face.]

faciobrachial (fa·she·o·bra'·ke·al). Relating or belonging to, or affecting the face and the arm; a term used to denote a form of juvenile muscular dystrophy. [face, L *brachium* arm.]

faciocephalalgia (fa·she·o·kef·al·al'·je·ah). Neuralgic pain in the head, face and neck. [face, Gk *kephale* head, *algos* pain.]

faciocervical (fa·she·o·ser'·vik·al). Relating or belonging to, or affecting the face and the neck. [face, cervix.]

faciolingual (fa·she·o·ling'·gwal). Relating or belonging to, or affecting the face and the tongue. [face, L *lingua* tongue.]

faciomaxillary (fa·she·o·max·il·ar·e). Relating or belonging to, or affecting the face and the jaws. [face, L *maxilla* jaw.]

facioplasty (fa·she·o·plas·te). Any plastic operation on the face. [face, Gk *plassein* to mould.]

facioplegia (fa·she·o·ple'·je·ah). Facial paralysis; Bell's palsy. [face, Gk *plege* stroke.]

facioscapulohumeral (fa·she·o·skap·ew·lo·hew'·mer·al). Relating or belonging to, or affecting the face, scapula and arm; denoting a form of muscular dystrophy or infantile progressive muscular atrophy. [face, scapula, humerus.]

factitious (fak·tish·us). Produced artificially or unintentionally, or by unusual or abnormal causes; not natural. [L *facticius* artificial.]

factor (fak·tor). 1. In mathematics, a number by which another number is exactly divisible. 2. One of a number of elements contributing to a whole result or one which effects a specific result. 3. A gene; hereditary factor. **Accessory factor, Accessory food factor.** The term originally applied to a vitamin. **Animal protein factor,** APF. A factor occurring in liver, meat, fish and milk. It is an essential growth factor for many species of birds and animals, but is replaceable by vitamin B_{12}. **Anti-acrodynia factor.** Adermin; vitamin B_6; pyridoxine. **Anti-anaemia factor.** Intrinsic factor (see below) and vitamin B_{12}. **Anti-black-tongue factor.** Nicotinic acid. **Anticanitic factor, Antichromotrichia factor.** Pantothenic acid. **Antidermatitis factor.** Adermin; vitamin B_6; pyridoxine. **Anti-egg-white factor.** Biotin. **Anti-grey-hair factor.** *p*-Aminobenzoic acid which in rats cures a greyness of hair caused by their food. **Antihaemorrhagic factor.** Vitamin K. **Anti-insulin factor.** Glycotropic factor (see below). **Antineuritic factor.** Vitamin B_1. **Antinuclear factor.** An antibody to nuclear components characteristically present in disseminated lupus erythematosus but also present in weak dilution in other collagen disorders. **Antipellagra factor.** Nicotinic acid. **Anti-pernicious-anaemia (liver) factor.** An active principle, present in normal livers, that will produce remissions in pernicious anaemia. It is possibly cyanocobalamin (vitamin B_{12}) or a very closely-related substance. **Antirachitic factor.** Vitamin D. **Anti-Rh factor.** Anti-Rh agglutinin. *See* AGGLUTININ. **Antiscorbutic factor.** Vitamin C. **Antisterility factor.** Vitamin E. **Antixerophthalmia factor.** Vitamin A. **Antixerotic factor.** Vitamin A. **Backscatter factor.** The ratio between the dose at a point in an irradiated body to the dose which would be measured at the same point in relation to the source of radiation in the absence of the body. The ratio is greater than unity, due to the contribution of radiation scattered back to the point in question from within the body. This factor depends on the size of the field irradiated, the quality of the radiation and the composition of the material irradiated. **Be blood factor.** A "private" blood factor or antigen (Be or Berrens) reported by Davidson and others (1953), and producing a Be immune iso-antibody in a woman transfused with blood from her husband (having the Be antigen) after a first pregnancy. Also known as *Be agglutinogen.* **Cabbage factor.** A substance occurring in cabbage-fed animals which apparently inhibits the oxidation of ascorbic acid to the active dehydro-ascorbic acid: it is thought that this factor is in turn antagonized by ACTH, whereby the formation of dehydro-ascorbic acid is facilitated. **Chemotactic factor.** Any chemical substance which induces cells to move towards or away from it. **Chromotrichia factor.** Aminobenzoic acid. *See* ACID. **Citrovorum factor.** Folic acid. **Co-enzyme factor.** Diaphorase. **Competence factor.** A substance produced by competent bacteria which can render non-competent cells competent. **Diabetogenic factor.** A factor present in anterior-lobe pituitary extracts which lowers carbohydrate tolerance and induces glycosuria. **Elongation factor.** One of a group of three proteins essential for the reactions by which amino-acid residues are added to a growing polypeptide chain in living cells. **Eluate factor.** Pyridoxine. **Erythrocyte maturation factor.** Intrinsic factor (see below). **Excess factor.** A form of electro-encephalographic abnormality, formerly thought to be characteristic of schizophrenia. **Extrinsic factor.** A substance present in many foodstuffs, including meat, that is said to react with the intrinsic factor (see below) in the stomach to produce or liberate the anti-pernicious-anaemia (liver) factor (see above). Inadequate amounts may be ingested in starvation or incorrect dieting, so that a macrocytic anaemia resembling pernicious anaemia may be produced, but it is cured by proper diet or by giving the extrinsic factor. The extrinsic factor appears to be closely identified with vitamin B_{12} or cyanocobalamin. **F factor.** An episome which confers fertility, i.e. the ability to conjugate and transfer genetic material to other bacteria which lack the factor, on *Escherichia coli* and certain other coliform bacilli. **F-prime factor.** An F factor which has incorporated a piece of bacterial chromosome into its structure. **Fy factor.** Duffy factor. *See* AGGLUTINOGEN. **G factor.** A protein, isolated from bacterial sources, which is responsible for translocation with concomitant hydrolysis of GTP. **Galactopoietic factor.** Prolactin. **Hr factor.** Hr agglutinogen. *See* AGGLUTINOGEN. **Hypothalamic releasing factors.** A group of oligopeptides secreted into the hypothalamic portal system. They are specific releasing factors for the several hormones of the anterior pituitary. The structures of a number have been elucidated and total syntheses achieved. **Initiation factors.** F_1, F_2 and F_3, three protein factors required for the initiation of protein synthesis in micro-organisms. **Intrinsic factor.** Castle's anti-pernicious-anaemia stomach principle or substance, and identical with Wilkinson's haemopoietin, which is a constituent of normal gastric juice and reacts with the extrinsic factor (see above) in the food to form the anti-pernicious-anaemia (liver) principle or factor (see above) essential for the normal formation of the normoblast from the pro-erythroblast in the marrow. It is an enzyme of unknown constitution, distinct from pepsin, rennin and lipase, and readily destroyed at temperatures above 40°C. **Ketogenic factor.** A factor present in extracts of the anterior lobe of the pituitary which is said to induce formation of β-hydroxybutyric acid and thus stimulate ketosis. **K-k factor.** Kell-Cellano factor. *See* AGGLUTINOGEN. **Labile factor.** Factor V (see below). **Lactobacillus casei factor.** Folic acid. **Lactobacillus lactis dorner factor.** Vitamin B_{12}.

Lactogenic factor. Prolactin. **Le factor.** Lewis factor. *See* AGGLUTINOGEN. **Liver factor.** Anti-pernicious-anaemia (liver) factor (see above). **Liver filtrate factor.** Pantothenic acid. **Lu factor.** Lutheran factor. *See* AGGLUTINOGEN. **Lysogenic factor.** Bacteriophage. **Maturation factor.** 1. Any chemical substance which induces cellular differentiation and maturation. 2. The substance produced by the interaction of the intrinsic and extrinsic factors (see above) which promotes the maturation of erythrocytes in the bone marrow. **Multiple factor.** In inheritance, two or more factors which combine to produce a character. **Norite eluate factor.** Folic acid; a factor shown by Snell and Petersen to be necessary for the growth of *Lactobacillus casei.* **P.A. factor.** The factor that protects against pernicious anaemia. **Pellagra-preventing factor, P-P factor.** Nicotinic acid. **Plasma labile factor.** A factor in normal plasma, other than prothrombin, thromboplastin and calcium, that is essential for the formation of thrombin. **Plasma prothrombin conversion factor.** Plasma labile factor (see preceding). **Quality factor.** The factor by which an absorbed dose of radiation of a particular quality must be multiplied in order to derive the corresponding absorbed dose of radiation of standard quality which would entail as great a biological effect. For radiation likely to be used in nuclear medicine, the quality factor is 1. Symbol Q. **R factor.** A sex factor which carries drug resistance determinants. **Reflux factor.** When the tube is set up for the determination of the erythrocyte sedimentation rate by the Westergren method, there is a reflux of the adherent plasma and cells in the tube above the zero mark down on to the blood meniscus, and this reflux factor may affect the sedimentation rate of oxalated blood. **Releasing factor.** A chemical substance produced in the hypothalamus and transported by the hypophyseal portal system to the anterior lobe of the pituitary, which it stimulates to produce a trophic hormone. **Resistance transfer factor.** A sex factor carrying determinants of bacterial resistance to chemotherapeutic agents, responsible for transmissible drug resistance among bacteria. **Restropic factor.** A substance in the blood that is said to stimulate the reticulo-endothelial system. **Rh factor, Rhesus factor.** Rh agglutinogen. *See* AGGLUTINOGEN. **Sex factor.** A general term to connote fertility factors. **Rheumatoid factors.** Antigamma globulin antibodies found in the sera of most patients with rheumatoid arthritis, and of some patients with lupus erythematosus, Sjögren's syndrome, scleroderma, sarcoidosis, liver disease, syphilis and other chronic infections. They are detectable by the Rose-Waaler test. **Rho factor.** A soluble protein isolated from bacteria that causes synthesis of RNA by the enzyme RNA polymerase to stop at certain nucleotide sequences on a DNA template. It is not part of the polymerase molecule. **Risk factor.** A factor which if present increases the risk of the subsequent development of some diseases; most frequently used in the context of coronary artery disease in which hyperlipidaemia, obesity, hypertension and the habit of smoking are, for example, recognized as risk factors. **Sigma factor.** A component of the nucleotide of RNA polymerase which is required for the initiation of RNA synthesis on a DNA template. **Spreading factor.** Hyaluronidase; an enzyme with mucolytic properties, produced by highly-invasive strains of staphylococci and streptococci, and acting as a spreading factor in tissues by depolymerizing and hydrolysing hyaluronic acid. It is present in extracts of testicular tissue and is used therapeutically to extend the range of spread of injected fluids. **T factor.** A protein factor which catalyses the GTP-dependent binding of aminoacyl transfer RNAs to the ribosome in micro-organisms. **Termination factor.** One of a group of three proteins involved in the release of the completed polypeptide chain from its combination to tRNA at the completion of biosynthesis of a polypeptide chain; they are called R_1, R_2 and S. **Transfer factor.** Sex factor (see above). **Factor V, V factor** (Owren). Labile factor, Ac-globulin, thrombogen; a constituent of normal blood plasma that is essential for the formation of thrombin from prothrombin. It is unstable, being oxidized during storage, but is not affected by vitamin K deficiency or anti-coagulant therapy with dicoumarol and similar substances. It is regarded as a plasma prothrombin conversion factor in the formation of thrombin. **Factor VII.** A factor in the blood serum, according to Koller and others, that is necessary for the action of brain thromboplastin; it closely resembles, but may not be quite identical with, the Christmas factor. **X factor.** 1. In bacteriology, an essential factor in the aerobic growth of *Haemophilus influenzae,* probably haemin. 2. Biotin. **Yeast eluate factor.** Pyridoxine. **Yeast filtrate factor.** Pantothenic acid. [L a maker.]

See also: BITTNER, CASTLE, CHRISTMAS, DURAN-REYNALS, KOLLER, MENKIN, SIMON (C. E.), WARBURG (O. H.).

facultative (**fak**·ul·ta·tiv). 1. Having the capacity or power to perform an action but not being obliged to do so; potential. 2. Optional. 3. Voluntary. 4. In biology, having the power to live under different conditions, as a plant that may exist either parasitically or non-parasitically, or as a micro-organism aerobically or anaerobically. [L *facultas* capability.]

faculty (**fak**·ul·te). 1. Any function or power present in a normal person. 2. Capacity to perform any natural function. 3. Mental or other capability in some particular direction. 4. Any normal power or capacity of the mind, e.g. the will. 5. The members of a profession or calling, as a medical faculty. 6. A department of university teaching. **Affective faculties.** The emotions, qualities and tendencies peculiar to man. **Fusion faculty.** The power to blend the two images seen by the two eyes into one complete image. [see prec.]

faecal (**fe**·kal). Relating to, containing or having the character of faeces.

faecalith (**fe**·kal·ith). Coprolith. [faeces, Gk *lithos* stone.]

faecaloid (**fe**·kal·oid). 1. Faecal. 2. Resembling faeces or faecal matter. [faeces, Gk *eidos* form.]

faecaloma (fe·kal·**o**·mah). Stercoroma. [faeces, Gk *-oma* tumour.]

faecaluria (fe·kal·**ewr**·e·ah). A condition in which faeces or faecal matter is present in the urine.

faeceometer (fe·se·**om**·et·er). An apparatus with which the amount of faeces passed and the rate of discharge can be measured.

faeces (**fe**·seez). The undigested residue of food and other forms of waste matter and alimentary refuse discharged from the bowel during defaecation; excrement. [L dregs.]

faecula (**fe**·kew·lah). 1. Sediment obtained by infusion. 2. Starch. 3. The starchy constituents of a seed. [L lees.]

faeculent (**fe**·kew·lent). 1. Of a faecal nature. 2. Containing sediment or dregs. [L *faeculentus* dreggy.]

faex (feex). Yeast. **Faex medicinalis sicca.** Dried Yeast BPC 1959 in the form of tablets, employed in all deficiency diseases which are due to lack of B-group vitamins. [L lees.]

Faget, Jean Charles (b. 1818). New Orleans physician.

Faget's law, or sign. In yellow fever, a rise in temperature without a corresponding increase in pulse rate or a fall in pulse rate with a maintained fever.

fagine (**fa**·jeen). 1. An alkaloid of uncertain composition occurring in the nuts of the beech, *Fagus sylvatica.* 2. Choline, $OHC_2H_4N(CH_3)_3OH$, a base occurring in lecithin and of great physiological importance.

fagopyrism (fag·o·**pi**·rizm). Poisoning resulting from the eating of buckwheat. It is an allergic condition and is marked by nausea and vomiting, urticaria and irritation of nasal and conjunctival mucous membranes. [L *fagus* beech, Gk *pyros* wheat.]

Fahr, Karl Theodor (b. 1877). Hamburg pathologist.

Fahr-Volhard disease, Volhard-Fahr disease. Malignant hypertension.

Fåhraeus, Robin Sanno (b. 1888). Uppsala pathologist.

Fåhraeus phenomenon. When fresh citrated whole blood is placed in a vertical glass column, the blood corpuscles settle or sediment at a rate (erythrocyte sedimentation rate) depending on various factors and especially on the particular pathological or physiological state of the patient.

Fahrenheit, Daniel Gabriel (b. 1686). German physicist.

Fahrenheit scale. The scale of the Fahrenheit thermometer on which 32°F corresponds to the freezing point of water (0°C) and 212°F to the boiling point (100°C), under standard atmospheric pressure.

Fahrenheit thermometer. A thermometer calibrated by the Fahrenheit scale.

failure (fa·lewr). A term applied with reference to bodily organs, systems or processes when their function fails to fulfil demands made on them, e.g. *hepatic failure, renal failure.* **Congestive cardiac failure.** *See* HEART FAILURE. **Metabolic failure.** A complete or partial failure in metabolism on the part of a group of cells, of an organ, of a group of organs, or of the whole organism. [L *fallere* to deceive.]

faint (fa·nt). 1. Syncope. 2. As an adjective, denoting a weak and languid condition, with threatened syncope. 3. As a verb, to suffer from syncope. **Ear faint.** A form of syncope occurring in persons suffering from disease of the ear. [O Fr. *faindre* to feign.]

Fairley, Sir Neil Hamilton (b. 1891). London physician.

Fairley's fixation test. A complement-fixation test for schistosomiasis with an antigen made from infected snails.

Fajans, Kazimierz (b. 1887). Polish chemist.

Fajans' law. In the transmutation of the radioactive elements, emission of an α-particle involves the movement of the new element to a position in the Periodic Table two places lower than the parent element; emission of a β-ray (electron) on the other hand places the new element one position higher, with a corresponding increase in valency.

Fajersztajn, J. 19th-20th century Austrian neurologist.

Fajersztajn's crossed sciatic sign. In sciatica the hip joint can be flexed when the knee is bent, but if the knee is extended this movement is painful; further, straight-leg raising on the unaffected side may cause pain on the affected side.

falcadina (fal·kah·**de**·nah). A disease occurring on the peninsula of Istria, Italy, marked by the development of papillomata.

falcate (**fal**·kate). Falciform.

falces (**fal**·seez). *See* FALX.

falcial (**fal**·shal). 1. Sickle-shaped. 2. Relating or belonging to a falx, e.g. falx cerebri. [L *falx* sickle.]

falciform (**fal**·se·form). 1. Crescentic. 2. Shaped like a sickle. [L *falx* sickle, form.]

falcula (**fal**·kew·lah). The falx cerebelli. [L small sickle.]

falcular (**fal**·kew·lar). 1. Falciform. 2. Belonging to the falx cerebelli.

fallacia (fal·a·se·ah). A hallucination; any erroneous idea of the insane. **Fallacia auditoria.** An auditory illusion. **Fallacia optica.** An optical illusion. [L *fallere* to deceive.]

fallectomy (fal·**ek**·to·me). Salpingectomy. [fallopian (uterine) tube, Gk *ektome* a cutting out.]

falling sickness. (fal·lin **sik**·nes). Epilepsy. [Obsolete term.]

Fallopio (Fallopius), Gabriele (b. 1523). Padua anatomist.

aqueduct of Fallopius. The facial canal in the petrous part of the temporal bone; obsolete.

Fallopius' canal. The canal for the facial nerve.

hiatus fallopii. The hiatus for the greater superficial petrosal nerve.

fallopian muscle. The pyramidalis muscle.

fallopian tube. The uterine tube.

fallopian valve. The ileocolic valve.

fallostomy (fal·**os**·to·me). Salpingostomy. [fallopian (uterine) tube, Gk *stoma* mouth.]

Fallot, Etienne-Louis Arthur (b. 1850). Marseilles physician.

Fallot's disease, tetrad of Fallot, tetralogy of Fallot. A form of congenital heart disease consisting of a defect of the ventricular septum, dextroposition of the aorta, which overrides the septum, and pulmonary-artery stenosis; the fourth component of the tetrad is right ventricular hypertrophy which is the result of the pulmonary-artery stenosis.

Fallot's pentalogy. A term sometimes used to describe the combination of atrial septal defect and Fallot's tetralogy.

trilogy of Fallot. Pulmonary stenosis with atrial septal defect and large right ventricle.

fallotomy (fal·**ot**·o·me). Salpingotomy. [fallopian (uterine) tube, Gk *temnein* to cut.]

Falls, Frederick Howard (b. 1885). Chicago gynaecologist.

Falls, Freda, and Cohen test. For pregnancy: an intradermal injection of colostrum is given and no reaction occurs if the patient is pregnant.

Falret, Jean Pierre (b. 1794). Paris psychiatrist.

Falret's type. Manic-depressive psychosis. *See* PSYCHOSIS.

falx [NA] (falx) (pl. *falces*). Name applied to any structure comparable to a sickle in shape; most commonly to folds of membrane or fascia. **Falx cerebelli [NA].** A small sickle-shaped fold of dura mater which projects into the posterior cerebellar notch from the occipital bone. **Falx cerebri [NA].** The sickle-shaped fold of dura mater which lies in the great longitudinal fissure between the two cerebral hemispheres. [L a sickle.]

familial (fam·**il**·e·al). Characteristic of some or all of the members of a family, e.g. a familial disease.

family (**fam**·il·e). 1. A group of living individuals consisting of parents and their offspring, with others connected by affinity or blood. 2. A group of individuals, living and dead, of common ancestry. 3. In taxonomy, the main category between the order and the genus. Most families contain a group of related genera, but some may contain only a single genus. Family names of animal groups terminate in *-idae*, those of plant groups usually in *-eae*. [L *familia* household.]

Famprofazone (fam·**pro**·faz·one). BP Commission approved name for 4 - isopropyl - 2 - methyl - 3 - [*N* - methyl - *N* - (α-methyl - phenethyl)aminomethyl] - 1 - phenyl - 5 - pyrazolone; an analgesic and antipyretic.

fan (fan). *See* DUNHAM (H. K.).

fanapepea (fan·ah·**pe**·pe·ah). *chilomastix.*

fanaticism (fan·**at**·is·izm). A condition of mental imbalance characterized by unreasoning zeal or excessive enthusiasm for, or extravagant notions connected with, any subject, particularly religion. The condition may be a warning of the approach of mental disease, or the result of insanity. [L *fanaticus* inspired by divinity.]

Fanconi, Guido (b. 1892). Zürich paediatrician.

Fanconi's anaemia. Familial, usually fatal, anaemia of the aplastic or hypoplastic type with certain endocrine changes, developing mostly in the first decade of life. A high frequency of spontaneous chromosome breakages and rearrangement has been reported in this condition.

Fanconi's disease, or syndrome, Debré-De Toni-Fanconi syndrome. Amino-aciduria in association with renal rickets; an inherited disorder, due either to functional deficiency of proximal renal tubules or to biochemical disturbances of the deamination process. Symptoms are polyuria, and failure of growth, with changes in the bones similar to those in rickets. Signs are albuminuria and glycosuria in an alkaline urine, increase of amino-acid excretion with low serum inorganic phosphorus and normal alkaline phosphatase. Liver function is gradually affected. Treatment is dietetic only, with the hope of controlling the cellular changes: an alkaline diet with high vitamin D intake may lessen the symptoms, and protein intake should be low. No curative measures are known, however, and patients usually die before the age of ten.

Fanconi's familial nephronophthisis. Medullary cystic disease of the kidney with uraemia, probably genetic and usually fatal during childhood.

fango (**fang**·go). Mud obtained from the thermal springs at Battaglia, Italy, and used in the treatment of rheumatic and gouty conditions. [It. mud.]

fangotherapy (fang·go·**ther**·ap·e). Treatment of rheumatic and other similar affections by the application of packs of fango or other mud or by immersion in mud baths. [fango, therapy.]

Fannia (**fan**·e·ah). A genus of small house flies. The larvae of the lesser house fly (*Fannia canicularis*) and the latrine fly (*F. scalaris*) develop in manure or stored protein food, and have caused intestinal myiasis after ingestion of eggs, and, rarely, urinary myiasis. Other species are very occasionally involved. [Gk *phanos* conspicuous.]

fantast (**fan**·tast). A person who indulges in day dreams and wish-fulfilling fantasies to an abnormal degree. [Gk *phantasia* appearance.]

fantasy (**fan**·tas·e). A quality of the imagination, leading to the development of thought or imagery from conventional paths into ones lacking one or more of the prerequisites of reality; concretely, a mental picture or invented story having a dream-like quality. The term has no precise usage in medicine. [Gk *phantasia* appearance.]

Fanthridone (**fan**·thrid·one). BP Commission approved name for 5-(3-dimethylaminopropyl)phenanthridone; an antidepressant.

Fantus, Bernard (b. 1874). Chicago physician.

Fantus antidote. Against poisoning with mercury: intravenous injections of sulphurated-lime solution.

Fantus' estimation. A rapid method of estimating the chloride content of urine. To 10 drops of urine delivered into a small tube from a teat pipette is added 1 drop of 10 per cent potassium chromate. Silver nitrate solution (2.9 w/v) is then added drop by drop from the same pipette, after rinsing it with water, until a brick-red colour is produced. Each drop is equivalent to 1 g of chloride per litre of urine.

Farabeuf, Louis Hubert (b. 1841). Paris surgeon.

Farabeuf's amputation, or operation. Amputation of the leg at the site of election, a large flap being formed on the outer side.

Farabeuf's saw. An adjustable saw.

Farabeuf's triangle. A triangle in the neck formed by the hypoglossal nerve, the internal jugular vein and the common facial vein.

farad (**far**·ad). The unit of capacitance; defined as the capacitance of a body the potential of which is raised 1 volt by a charge of 1 coulomb. [Michael *Faraday.*]

faradaic (fa·**ad**·a·ik). Faradic.

Faraday, Michael (b. 1791). English scientist.

Faraday's constant. The amount of electricity necessary to liberate 1 gramme-equivalent of a substance in electrolysis: 96 494 coulombs.

Faraday's laws. Relating to electrolysis: (*a*) the chemical action of an electric current is directly proportional to the quantity of electricity which passes; (*b*) the weights of different substances deposited by a given quantity of electricity are proportional to their chemical equivalents.

Faraday dark space. The dark space in a discharge tube between the negative glow and the positive column.

faradic (far·**ad**·ik). Referring to faradism or belonging to it.

faradimeter (far·ad·**im**·et·er). An instrument with which the strength of faradic currents can be measured.

faradipuncture (**far**·ad·e·**pungk**'·tcher). The insertion of needle electrodes into the tissues in order to allow a faradic current to pass through. [faradism, puncture.]

faradism (**far**·ad·izm). 1. The phenomenon of the induced or faradic electric current. 2. Electricity produced through induction by a rapidly interrupted or alternating current. 3. Faradization. **Surging faradism.** An induced current that increases and decreases gradually and rhythmically. [Michael *Faraday.*]

faradization (**far**·ad·i·**za**'·shun). The therapeutic use of the faradic (induced) current for the purpose of stimulating nerves or muscles. It is customary to surge the current, thereby producing rhythmical contraction and relaxation of muscles. **Galvanic faradization.** The therapeutic application of the constant (galvanic) current combined with the surged (faradic) current. **General faradization.** The therapeutic application of the surged faradic current to the main muscle groups of the arms, legs and trunk. It is sometimes employed in the treatment of obesity. [see prec.]

faradize (**far**·ad·ize). 1. To apply stimulation by means of a faradic current. 2. To place under the influence of an induced electric current.

faradocontractility (**far**·ad·o·kon·trak·**til**'·it·e). The state of contractility of muscles while they are being stimulated by a faradic current.

faradomuscular (**far**·ad·o·**mus**'·kew·lar). Resulting from the direct application of a faradic current to a muscle.

faradonervous (**far**·ad·o·**ner**'·vus). Resulting from faradization of a nerve trunk.

faradopalpation (**far**·ad·o·pal·**pa**'·shun). The use of the faradic current for the localization of trigger spots in painful myofascial conditions. [faradism, palpation.]

faradopuncture (**far**·ad·o·**pungk**'·tcher). Faradipuncture.

faradotherapy (**far**·ad·o·**ther**'·ap·e). Treatment by means of faradization. [faradism, therapy.]

Farber, Sidney (b. 1903). American pathologist.

Farber's disease. Disseminated lipogranulosis; originally thought to be a disorder of lipid metabolism, now known to be a disorder of mucopolysaccharides. Characterized by nodular periarticular swellings, ankylosis, joint contractures and mental retardation in infants; they often have hoarse voices and are liable to recurrent infections.

farcinoma (far·sin·**o**·mah). 1. A granulomatous tumour such as occurs in glanders. 2. A farcy bud. [farcy, Gk *-oma* tumour.]

farctus (**fark**·tus). 1. An obstruction. 2. An infarction. [L *farcire* to stuff.]

farcy (**far**·se). The form of glanders which attacks the subcutaneous tissues following accidental inoculation of the skin. It gives rise to a spreading lymphangitis with subcutaneous nodules (farcy buds) which soften and form abscesses. It may be *acute* and usually fatal with the general picture of pyaemia, or *chronic* with the formation of a local granulomatous condition that breaks down to an irregular ulcer which spreads superficially and deeply and may persist for many months. **Button farcy.** A form of glanders in which tubercular nodules occur in the limbs and trunk. [L *farcire* to stuff.]

farfara (**far**·far·ah). **Farfarae flores.** Coltsfoot flower; the dried flowers of *Tussilago farfara* Linn. (family Compositae) used in the form of a liquid extract or as a syrup to relieve chronic irritable cough. **Farfarae folia.** Coltsfoot leaf, the leaves of *Tussilago farfara* Linn. after having been dried. It is a demulcent, used to relieve coughs. [L *farfarus* coltsfoot.]

farina (far·**i**·nah). The starchy flour or meal of wheat, barley, rye, maize and other cereal grains. **Farina avena.** Oatmeal. **Farina tritici.** Wheatmeal. [L meal.]

farinaceous (far·in·**a**·shus). 1. Starchy or containing starch. 2. Consisting of or made with flour or meal. 3. Yielding or having the character of farina. [see prec.]

farinometer (far·in·**om**·et·er). An instrument for determining the percentage of gluten in flour, or for measuring the viscosity of dough in order to evaluate any particular flour. [farina, meter.]

Farmer, Chester Jefferson (b. 1886). Chicago chemist.

Folin and Farmer method. A micro-Kjeldahl method of determining the total nitrogen in urine, the ammonia being separated by aeration and then nesslerized.

Farr, William (b. 1807). English medical statistician.

Farr's law. "Subsidence is a property of all zymotic diseases." This can be demonstrated graphically: in an epidemic outbreak the curve of incidence at first has a rapid ascent; then it rises more slowly to its maximum, after which the curve descends more rapidly than it ascended.

Farrant method. A histological mounting medium containing glycerin, gum arabic and arsenious acid. It is used after fat stains, as neither the fat nor the stain is extracted by it.

Farre, Arthur (b. 1811). London obstetrician.

Farre's white line, Farre–Waldeyer line. The boundary between the germinal epithelium of the ovary and the peritoneum of the ovarian mesentery.

Farre, John Richard (b. 1775). London physician.

Farre's tubercle. A secondary malignant growth in the liver.

fascia [NA] (**fash**·e·ah) (pl. *fasciae*). A layer or sheet of connective tissue separating or enclosing groups of muscles or other organs; the connective-tissue sheath of an organ. **Fascia of the abdominal wall, superficial.** Thick subcutaneous fascia continuous below with that of the perineum (superficial fascia of the perineum) and differentiated into a superficial fatty layer (Camper's fascia) and a deep membranous layer (Scarpa's fascia). **Anal fascia [fascia diaphragmatis pelvis inferior (NA)].** The thin fascia on the inferior surface of the levator ani muscle. **Antebrachial fascia [fascia antebrachii (NA)].** The deep fascia of the forearm. **Aponeurotic fascia.** A thickened fascia which gives attachment to a muscle. **Axillary fascia [fascia axillaris (NA)].** The thickened part of the pectoral fascia which forms the floor of the axillary space. **Bicipital fascia.** The bicipital aponeurosis, a broad aponeurosis passing from the tendon of the biceps muscle downwards and medially across the brachial artery to the deep fascia of the forearm. **Brachial fascia [fascia brachii (NA)].** The deep fascia of the arm, mostly transverse fibres, thin over the biceps brachii muscle but thicker over the triceps brachii muscle and the epicondyles of the humerus. **Buccopharyngeal fascia [fascia buccopharyngea (NA)].** A thin fascia covering the constrictor muscles and extending forwards over the buccinator muscle. **Fascia bulbi.** Tenon's fascia. **Cervical fascia, deep [fascia cervicalis (NA)].** The deep fascia of the neck, consisting of an enveloping layer [lamina superficialis (NA)], a pretracheal layer and a prevertebral layer. **Cervical fascia, superficial.** The superficial fascia of the neck. **Fascia cinerea.** A raised band of grey matter passing round the splenium of the corpus callosum and continuous with the indusium griseum above and with the dentate gyrus below. **Clavipectoral fascia [fascia clavipectoralis (NA)].** Costocoracoid membrane; the fascia beneath the pectoralis major muscle, lying between the clavicle and subclavius above and the pectoralis minor muscle below. **Fascia of the clitoris [fascia clitoridis (NA)].** A fibrous sheath continuous with the deeper membranous layer of the superficial fascia in adjacent regions; it invests the organ. **Coraclavicular fascia.** Clavipectoral fascia (see above). **Cremasteric fascia [fascia cremasterica (NA)].** *See* CREMASTER MUSCLE AND FASCIA. **Cribriform fascia [fascia cribrosa (NA)].** A deep layer of the superficial fascia of the thigh, covering the fossa ovalis and perforated by the long saphenous vein and other small blood vessels and lymphatics. **Crural fascia [fascia cruris (NA)].** The deep fascia of the leg. **Deep fascia.** The connective-tissue sheath which encloses all regions of the body and lies immediately beneath the superficial fascia and the skin. **Fascia dentata, Dentate fascia.** The dentate gyrus. **Dorsal fascia of the foot [fascia dorsalis pedis (NA)].** The deep fascia of the dorsum of the foot. **Dorsal fascia of the hand [fascia dorsalis manus (NA)].** The deep fascia of the back of the hand. **Endothoracic fascia [fascia endothoracica (NA)].** A fascial sheet which separates the parietal pleura from the chest wall and diaphragm (phrenicopleural fascia) and a thickened portion superiorly which attaches to the medial border of the first rib (suprapleural membrane) and meets the apex of the lung. **Extrapleural fascia.** Endothoracic fascia (see above). **Fibro-areolar fascia.** Superficial fascia (see below). **Fascia iliaca [NA].** The fascia covering the psoas and iliacus muscles. **Iliopectineal fascia.** The fascia passing from the inguinal ligament to the hip bone, and separating the femoral vessels from the psoas major, iliacus and the femoral nerve. **Infundibuliform fascia.** Spermatic fascia, internal (see below). **Intercolumnar fascia.** Curved tendinous fibres in the aponeurosis of the external oblique muscle, stretching between the two crura of the subcutaneous inguinal ring. **Ischiorectal fascia.** The fascia covering the perineal side of the levator ani muscle. **Lacrimal fascia.** Fascia forming the roof of the fossa for the lacrimal gland. **Fascia lata [NA].** The deep fascia of the thigh. **Fascia lata, saphenous opening of the [hiatus saphenus (NA)].** The aperture in the fascia lata through which the great saphenous vein passes to join the femoral vein. **Lumbar fascia [fascia thoracolumbalis (NA)].** The fascia covering the sacrospinalis muscle; above it is continuous with the deep fascia of the neck, and below it gives off two deep layers, one anterior to the sacrospinalis muscle, the other anterior to the quadratus lumborum muscle. **Masseteric fascia [fascia masseterica (NA)].** Part of the parotid fascia (see below). **Fascia nuchae [NA].** Fascia covering the back of the neck and overlying the cervical part of the sacrospinalis muscle. **Obturator fascia [fascia obturatoria (NA)].** That part of the parietal pelvic fascia which covers the obturator internus muscle. **Fasciae of the orbit, muscular [fasciae musculares (NA)].** The tubular prolongations of the fascial sheath of the eyeball which cover the orbital muscles. They blend with the perimysium on the rectus muscles and are continued on the inferior oblique muscle to the floor of the orbit and on the superior oblique muscle to its pulley. **Orbital fasciae [fasciae orbitales (NA)].** The periosteal lining of the orbit which is loosely attached to the bones. **Palmar fascia.** An aponeurosis which forms the deep fascia of the palm and receives the insertion of the palmaris longus muscle; the palmar aponeurosis. **Palpebral fascia.** The orbital septum; a thin membrane attached to the periosteal margins of the orbit and to the tarsal plates. **Parotid fascia [fascia parotidea (NA)].** A part of the deep cervical fascia that ensheaths the parotid gland. **Pectoral fascia [fascia pectoralis (NA)].** A fascia on the anterior wall of the thorax, covering the pectoralis major muscle. **Pelvic fascia [fascia pelvis (NA)].** The fascial sheath of the pelvic muscles and viscera. **Pelvic fascia, parietal [fascia pelvis parietalis (NA)].** The fascia lining the pelvic walls above the level of origin of the levator ani muscle and over the piriformis muscle. **Pelvic fascia, visceral [fascia pelvis visceralis (NA)].** The fascia covering the upper surface of the levator ani muscle and continued from it around the pelvic viscera. **Fascia of the penis, deep [fascia penis profunda (NA)].** The membranous layer continuous with the deep layer of the superficial fascia of the abdominal wall (Scarpa) and the fascia covering the scrotum and urogenital triangle of the perineum (Colles). **Fascia of the penis, superficial [fascia penis superficialis (NA)].** The loose areolar tissue, almost devoid of fat, continuous with the fatty layer of the superficial fascia of the abdominal wall (Camper). **Perineal fascia, Fascia of the perineum, superficial [fascia superficialis perinei (NA)].** Layers of fascia of the perineum (*see* FASCIA OF ABDOMINAL WALL, SUPERFICIAL, above). **Pharyngobasilar fascia [fascia pharyngobasilaris (NA)].** Connective tissue between the mucous and muscular layers of the pharyngeal wall. **Phrenicopleural fascia [fascia phrenicopleuralis (NA)].** *See* ENDOTHORACIC FASCIA (above). **Plantar fascia.** Plantar aponeurosis, a strong aponeurosis in the sole of the foot, stretching from the calcaneum to the toes; it is divided into central, medial and lateral parts. **Pretracheal fascia [lamina pretrachealis (NA)].** A part of the deep cervical fascia anterior to the trachea and forming a sheath for the thyroid gland. **Prevertebral fascia [lamina prevertebralis (NA)].** Fascia in front of the prevertebral muscles in the neck. **Prostatic fascia.** Sheath of the prostate. **Rectovesical fascia [fascia diaphragmatis pelvis superior (NA)].** A fascia between the rectum and the bladder that ensheaths the seminal vesicles and ductus deferentes. **Renal fascia.** A sheath formed from the retroperitoneal connective tissue which encloses the kidney and perirenal fat. **Scalene fascia.** The part of the prevertebral fascia of the neck which extends laterally in front of the scalenus muscles. **Spermatic fascia, external [fascia spermatica externa (NA)].** An investment for the spermatic cord and testis, derived from the aponeurosis of the external oblique muscle of the abdomen. **Spermatic fascia, internal [fascia spermatica interna (NA)].** A funnel-shaped fascia extending round the spermatic cord and derived from the transversalis fascia. **Subperitoneal fascia [fascia subperitonealis (NA)].** The loose areolar tissue outside the parietal peritoneum. **Superficial fascia.** The fascia found immediately beneath the skin and containing a variable quantity of fat. **Temporal fascia [fascia temporalis (NA)].** A strong aponeurosis covering the temporalis muscle, attached above to the superior temporal line, and below by two laminae [lamina superficialis, lamina profunda (NA)] to the zygomatic arch. **Thyrolaryngeal fascia.** The fascial sheath of the thyroid gland. **Transversalis fascia [fascia transversalis (NA)].** The fascia on the posterior surface of the anterior abdominal wall, superficial to the peritoneum. **Fasciae of the urogenital diaphragm, inferior and superior.** *See* PERINEAL MEMBRANE (under MEMBRANE). [L band.]

See also: ABERNETHY, BUCK, CAMPER, CLOQUET (J. G.), COLLES, COOPER (A. P.), CRUVEILHIER, DENONVILLIERS, DUPUYTREN, GEROTA, GODMAN, HESSELBACH, PORTER, RICHET, SCARPA, SIBSON, TENON, THOMSON (A.), TOLDT, TREITZ, TYRRELL, ZUCKERKANDL.

fasciagram (fash·e·ah·gram). An x-ray photograph of fascia. [fascia, Gk *gramma* writing.]

fasciagraphy (fash·e·ag·raf·e). The injection of air into fascia and subsequent x-ray photography. [fascia, Gk *graphein* to record.]

fascial (fash·e·al). Relating or belonging to, or having the character of, any fascia.

fasciaplasty (fash·e·ah·plas·te). Any plastic operation on fascia.

fasciation (fash·e·a·shun). The art of binding up or bandaging. [L *fascia* band.]

fascicle (fas·ikl). Fasciculus.

fascicular, fasciculate, fasciculated (fas·ik·ew·lar, fas·ik·ew·late, fas·ik·ew·la·ted). 1. Relating or belonging to a fasciculus. 2. Arranged in clusters or bundles.

fasciculation (fas·ik·ew·la'·shun). 1. The process of formation of fasciculi. 2. Arrangement in the form of clusters or bundles. 3. Spontaneous contraction of bundles of muscle fibres visible through the skin. 4. Fibrillary twitching of voluntary muscles seen, for example, after the injection of a depolarizing myoneural blocking agent.

fasciculus [NA] (fas·ik·ew·lus) (pl. *fasciculi*). A bundle or collection of fibres, all with the same orientation; the term is applied most commonly to nerve fibres but also to the more distal branches of the His-Purkinje conducting system of the heart. **Fasciculus acousticus.** The auditory striae in the floor of the 4th ventricle. **Atrioventricular fasciculus [fasciculus atrioventricularis (NA)].** The atrioventricular bundle. *See* BUNDLE. **Central tegmental fasciculus [tractus tegmentalis centralis (NA)].** Fibres in the tegmentum of the mid-brain and pons which descend to terminate in the olivary nucleus; some of these are considered to arise from the thalamus (thalamo-olivary fasciculus, see below). **Fasciculus cerebrospinalis.** Fibres from the precentral gyrus of the cerebral cortex which form the pyramids in the medulla oblongata and end in the spinal cord; the pyramidal tract. *See* TRACT. **Fasciculus circumolivaris pyramidalis.** Afferent fibres to the corpus pontobulbare which sweep dorsally from the region of the pyramid round the caudal end of the olivary eminence. **Corticothalamic fasciculi [fasciculi corticothalamici (NA)].** Bundles of fibres connecting the cerebral cortex to the thalamus. They include descending fibres from the frontal lobe. **Crossed pyramidal fasciculus.** Lateral cerebrospinal tract. *See* TRACT. **Fasciculus cuneatus [NA].** Fibres which ascend in the lateral part of the posterior columns of the spinal cord; they arise from cells in the spinal ganglia from the level of the 6th thoracic nerve upwards, pass up in the medulla oblongata [fasciculus cuneatus (NA)], and end in the nucleus cuneatus. **Direct pyramidal fasciculus.** Anterior cerebrospinal tract. *See* TRACT. **Dorsolateral fasciculus [fasciculus dorsolateralis (NA)].** Ascending and descending branches of posterior spinal nerve root fibres which lie between the posterior horn of grey matter and the surface of the spinal cord; Lissauer's tract. **Fastigiobulbar fasciculus.** Uncinate fasciculus, def. 2 (see below). **Fundamental fasciculus.** Anterior intersegmental tract. *See* TRACT. **Fasciculus gracilis [NA].** Fibres which ascend in the medial part of the posterior columns of the spinal cord; they arise from cells in the spinal ganglia from the level of the 7th thoracic segment downwards, pass up in the medulla oblongata, and end in the nucleus gracilis. **Fasciculus interfascicularis [fasciculus semilunaris (interfascicularis) (NA)].** Descending branches from fibres in the posterior columns of the spinal cord which run between the cuneate and gracile fasciculi: the comma tract of Schultze. **Longitudinal fasciculi, dorsal, inferior, medial, posterior, superior.** *See* LONGITUDINAL BUNDLE (under BUNDLE). **Maculary fasciculus.** Those fibres in the optic nerve and tract which originate from the macula in the retina. **Fasciculus marginalis ventralis.** Superficial fibres in the anterior columns of the spinal cord. **Fasciculus occipitofrontalis.** A long association tract linking the cortex of the frontal, parietal, occipital and temporal lobes of the cerebrum. It lies on a deeper plane than the superior longitudinal fasciculus. **Fasciculus precommissuralis.** Fibres of various origins which pass through the septum in front of the anterior commissure and the lamina terminalis. **Fasciculus retroflexus [NA].** A bundle of fibres passing from the habenular nucleus to the interpeduncular nucleus in the mid-brain; Meynert's bundle. **Rubroreticular fasciculus [fasciculus rubroreticulares (NA)].** Fibres from the red nucleus to the reticular formation in the brain stem and spinal cord. **Septomarginal fasciculus.** Descending branches from the fibres in the posterior columns of the spinal cord which lie close to the posterior median septum. **Fasciculus solitarius, Solitary fasciculus.** Root fibres of the 7th, 9th and 10th cranial nerves which descend along the nucleus solitarius in which they end. **Fasciculus subcallosus [NA].** A bundle of fibres beneath the corpus callosum, running along the upper border of the head and body of the caudate nucleus; they probably arise in the cerebral cortex and end in the corpus striatum. **Fasciculus sulcomarginalis.** Fibres adjacent to the anteromedian fissure of the spinal cord. **Fasciculus teres.** A longitudinal elevation in the floor of the 4th ventricle next to the median sulcus; its caudal part forms the trigonum hypoglossi. **Thalamocortical fasciculi [fasciculi thalamocorticales (NA)].** Bundles of fibres connecting the thalamus to the cerebral cortex. They include sensory fibres going to the postcentral gyrus. **Thalamo-olivary fasciculus.** Fibres of the central tegmental fasciculus (see above), thought to arise from the thalamus, and ending in the olivary nucleus. **Triangular fasciculus [fasciculus triangularis (NA)].** An intersegmental tract in the spinal cord. **Uncinate fasciculus.** 1. Association fibres from the cortex on the orbital surface of the frontal lobes of the cerebrum to the cortex of the anterior part of the temporal lobe. 2. The fastigiobulbar fasciculus; efferent fibres of the fastigial nuclei of the cerebellum to nuclei in the medulla, chiefly the vestibular nuclei; some fibres may reach the spinal cord. **Fasciculus ventrolateralis superficialis.** Anterior spinocerebellar tract. *See* TRACT. [L little bundle.]

See also: ARNOLD (F.), BURDACH, FLECHSIG, FOVILLE, GOLL, GOWERS, LISSAUER, MEYNERT, MONAKOW, ROLANDO, SCHULTZE (M. J. S.), SMITH (G. E.), TARIN, TUERCK.

fasciectomy (fash·e·ek·to·me). Surgical removal of fascia, especially by the method of stripping (Kondoleon operation). [fascia, Gk *ektome* a cutting out.]

fasciitis (fas·e·i·tis). Inflammation of any layer of fascia. **Plantar fasciitis.** Pain under the heel on walking, sometimes due to trauma or associated with ankylosing spondylitis, Reiter's disease and calcaneal spurs. **Pseudosarcomatous fasciitis.** A tumour, usually subcutaneous and perhaps inflammatory, recurring in children. [fascia, Gk *-itis* inflammation.]

fascination (fas·in·a·shun). A form of induced hypnotic sleep in which the subject is in a state of trance rather deeper than somnambulism and not as deep as catalepsy. [L *fascinare* to cast a spell over.]

fasciodesis (fash·e·o·de'·sis). The operation of attaching a fascia to another fascia or to a tendon. [fascia, Gk *desis* a binding together.]

Fasciola (fas·e·o·lah). A genus of liver flukes. **Fasciola gigantea.** A species of the Old World tropics which has occurred occasionally in man. **Fasciola hepatica.** The liver fluke, normally a sheep parasite but occurring occasionally in man. Secondary hosts are water snails, particularly *Lymnaea truncatula,* and the cercariae encyst on plants. Human infection occurs through eating such plants raw, particularly watercress (*Nasturtium officinale*). [L a little band.]

fasciola (fas·e·o·lah). The dentate gyrus of the rhinencephalon. **Fasciola cinerea.** The splenial gyrus, an extension of the dentate gyrus. [see prec.]

fasciolar (fas·e·o·lar). Relating or belonging to the fasciola (dentate gyrus and splenial gyrus).

fascioliasis (fas·e·o·li'·as·is). A condition in which there is infection with parasitic flukes of the family Fasciolidae, e.g. the common liver fluke, *Fasciola hepatica.*

Fasciolidae (fa·se·o·lid·e). A family of the trematode order Distomata or Fascioloidea. The general *Fasciolopsis* and *Fasciola* are of medical interest. [L *fasciola* a little band, Gk *eidos* form.]

fasciolopsiasis (fas·e·o·lop·si′·as·is). A condition of infection with the giant parasitic fluke, *Fasciolopsis buski*, as a result of eating the corms of certain water plants. [see foll.]

Fasciolopsis (fas·e·o·lop′·sis). A genus of intestinal flukes. **Fasciolopsis buski.** An important human parasite in India, Eastern China and much of the tropical Far East. The adults live in the small intestine, causing acute diarrhoea as well as toxic symptoms. Eggs passed in the faeces hatch in water, and the secondary hosts are water snails, particularly species of *Segmentina*. The cercariae encyst on water plants. This fluke is particularly associated with the cultivation of water nuts of the genus *Trapa*, known as caltrop and ling, and of *Eliocharis*; such nuts are often eaten raw and peeled with the teeth. Pigs are also true hosts and act as reservoirs. [L *fasciola* a little band, Gk *opsis* appearance.]

fascioplasty (fash·e·o·plas·te). Fasciaplasty.

fasciorrhaphy (fash·e·or·af·e). Aponeurorrhaphy; the suturing together of cut or torn aponeuroses or fasciae. [fascia, Gk *rhaphe* suture.]

fasciotomy (fash·e·ot·o·me). Surgical division of fascia. [fascia, Gk *temnein* to cut.]

fascitis (fash·i·tis). Fasciitis. **Pseudosarcomatous fascitis.** Fascitis with superficial resemblance to sarcoma. [fascia, Gk *-itis* inflammation.]

fast (fahst). 1. To eat only specified food, or to go without any food at all for a certain length of time. [AS *faestan* to observe.] 2. Of bacteria, denoting resistance to destruction or to staining. 3. Of dyes, durable in colour. [AS *faest* firm.]

fastidium (fas·tid·e·um). Disgust for food, or loathing for food and drink. [L loathing.]

fastigatum (fas·tig·a·tum). The nucleus fastigii, one of the four paired centres of grey matter embedded in the white matter of the cerebellum. [L *fastigatus* narrowing at the top.]

fastigium (fas·tij·e·um). The period in a fever when the temperature is at its height. [L ridge.]

fastness (fahst·nes). Denoting the degree to which a tissue or organism is capable of resisting the action of destructive agents, e.g. the resistance of stained bacteria to decolorization by acid (acid-fastness), or the resistance of a micro-organism to streptomycin (streptomycin-fastness). [AS *faest* firm.]

fat (fat). 1. Stout, corpulent; greasy. 2. Any member of a class of natural organic substances which act as structural and storage materials in plants and animals. They are mixtures of glycerol esters of the general formula $(CH_2COOR')(CHCOOR'')(CH_2COOR''')$ where R′, R″ and R‴ may be the same or different fatty-acid residues. They are insoluble in water, but soluble in ether, burn readily and are hydrolysed to glycerol and the fatty acids. Fats differ from oils only in being solid at 20°C. **Bound fat.** The lipoidal contents of a cell which are not stained with ordinary fat stains. **Brown fat.** The peculiar fatty deposits found between the shoulder blades in many mammals, particularly those which hibernate. **Butter fat.** Milk fat (see below). **Chyle fat.** A highly emulsified form of fat present in the milky fluid (chyle) of the lymphatics of the intestine. **Corpse fat.** Adipocere; a waxy substance which forms in the flesh of corpses exposed to water in the absence of air. **Depot fat.** Excess fat stored in large amounts in certain anatomical areas, e.g. the omentum and abdominal wall; in fat starvation these depots are drawn upon. **Grave fat.** Corpse fat (see above). **Hydrous Wool Fat BP 1958.** Wool fat to which purified water has been added. **Masked fat.** Bound fat (see above). **Fat mass.** Lean body mass, q.v.+triglyceride. **Milk fat.** The emulsified fat present to the extent of about 3 to 5 per cent in mammalian milk. It is distinguished from the other natural fats by its high proportion of esters of the lower fatty acids, particularly butyric acid. It is also referred to as *butter fat*. **Fat-mobilising substance.** It is claimed that restriction of calories and carbohydrates leads to the appearance of a fat-mobilising substance in the urine. **Molecular fat.** Intracellular fat in a highly emulsified state. **Moruloid fat.** The fat of the cells of the interscapular gland, so designated because of the mulberry-like appearance of the closely-packed fat globules in each cell. **Mulberry fat.** Moruloid fat (see preceding). **Neutral fat.** Fat entirely unsplit, i.e. containing no free fatty acid. **Orbital fat.** The fat body of the orbit, a mass of soft fat within the orbit. **Renal fat [capsula adiposa (NA)].** The firm fat enclosing the kidney and passing through the hilum into the renal sinus. **Saturated fat.** A fatty acid, the carbon chain of which is connected by single bonds exclusively; called saturated because it is not capable of absorbing any more hydrogen. **Split fat.** Fat which has been hydrolysed to yield free fatty acids and glycerol. If the hydrolysis occurs in alkaline media, soaps are formed by combination of the fatty acids with alkali. **Unsaturated fat.** A fatty acid, the carbon chain of which possesses one or more double or triple bonds; called unsaturated because it is capable of absorbing additional hydrogen. **Unsplit fat.** Fat which has not been hydrolysed. This term is of especial significance with respect to the fat in faeces in which a high proportion of unsplit fat usually indicates pancreatic or biliary dysfunction. **Wool Fat BP 1958.** Anhydrous lanolin; adeps lanae; a fat-like substance obtained from sheep's wool, consisting essentially of cholesterol and its esters. It is used in pharmacy as a basis of various ointments and creams. [AS *faett.*]

fat-ball (fat·bawl). A localized collection of fatty tissue. [AS *faett*, ME *bal.*]

See also: BICHAT.

fat-pad (fat·pad). A mass of adipose tissue; the sucking pad; the buccal pad of fat. **Synovial fat-pad.** A localized pad of fat in the synovial membrane of joints. [AS *faett, paeth.*]

See also: BICHAT.

fat-soluble (fat·sol·ewbl). Soluble in fat: a term used especially with reference to the vitamins A and D. [AS *faett*, soluble.]

fatal (fa·tal). Inevitable; causing death. [L *fatalis* preordained.]

fatigability (fat·e·gah·bil′·it·e). 1. A condition in which the subject becomes easily tired or exhausted. 2. The tendency to tire quickly. 3. A condition of loss of power that affects cells or organs which have passed through a period of excessive activity. [fatigue, L *habilis* apt.]

fatigue (fat·eeg). The feeling of weariness of mind and body following exertion, associated with a desire for rest and a disinclination or inability to make further effort; it ranges from slight lassitude to exhaustion. In muscular fatigue the muscles feel stiff and heavy from the accumulation of exuded fluid; physicochemical changes set up afferent impulses which cause a feeling of aching discomfort, and the brain is affected by slight anoxia and an increased hydrogen-ion concentration from the accumulation of lactic acid in the blood. Psychical factors play an important part, as fatigue occurs less readily when exercise is taken congenially in pleasant surroundings, and more readily under conditions of boredom. The insane maniacal patient is relatively unfatigable and undertakes activities which would soon tire a normal person. Posturing muscles are also relatively unfatigable. Pathologically, fatigue is the predominant symptom of myasthenia gravis and the threshold of fatigue is lowered in most conditions of ill-health. Extreme degrees of fatigue were experienced in World War II caused by great mental and physical stress combined with a loss of sleep and rest and sometimes extremes of heat or cold. They were given names such as *battle fatigue, convoy fatigue, pilot fatigue* or *operational fatigue.* **Stance fatigue.** Fatigue produced by standing for a long period in one position. [L *fatigare* to tire.]

fatty (fat·e). 1. Containing fat or bearing a heavy deposit of fat. 2. Derived from fat. 3. Having the qualities of fat. [AS *faett.*]

fauces [NA] (faw·seez). The constricted opening between the mouth and the oral part of the pharynx. [L throat.]

Fauchard, Pierre (c. 1678–1761). Paris dentist.

Fauchard's disease. Chronic suppurative periodontitis; pyorrhoea.

faucial (faw·shal). Pertaining to the fauces.

fauna (faw·nah) (pl. *faunae*). The aggregate of animals in any given geographical locality, region or area, or of any given geological period. [L *Faunus*, deity of fields and herds.]

Faust, Ernest Carroll. 20th century New Orleans parasitologist.
Faust's zinc-sulphate centrifugal floatation method. A floatation method for protozoal cysts and metazoal ova; a modification of Willis' method.

Fauvel, Sulpice Antoine (b. 1813). French physician and hygienist.
Fauvel's granule. Peribronchitic abscess. *See* ABSCESS.

favaginous (fa·vaj·in·us). 1. Having a resemblance to favus. 2. Formed like or having resemblance to a honeycomb. [L *favus* honeycomb.]

faveolar (fa·ve·o·lar). Relating or belonging to a faveolus.

faveolate (fa·ve·o·late). 1. Pitted, or having cavities or cells like those of a honeycomb. 2. Alveolate. [see foll.]

faveolus (fa·ve·o·lus). 1. A small depression, pit or cell, like that of a honeycomb. 2. An alveolus. [L small honeycomb cell.]

favid, favide (fa·vid). A widespread eruption occurring in connection with favus, usually of the scalp, closely resembling other dermatophytids and with an analogous aetiology, possibly of an allergic nature.

faviform (fa·ve·form). Resembling a honeycomb in appearance and structure, as a type of ulcer or ulcerated surface. [favus, form.]

favism (fa·vizm). 1. An acute haemolytic anaemia, associated with a deficiency of red blood cell glucose 6-phosphate dehydrogenase, associated chemically with abdominal pain, vomiting and diarrhoea brought on by the eating of certain kinds of bean (e.g. vetch), including the Italian lentil, *Vicia fava*. 2. A disorder resembling hay fever, caused by inhalation of the pollen of certain kinds of bean. Also called *fabism*. [It. *fava* bean.]

favoso-areolate (fa·vo·so·ar·e'·o·late). So pitted as to resemble the surface of a honeycomb. [favus, areola.]

Favre, Maurice (b. 1876). Lyons dermatologist.
Favre disease, Durand-Nicolas-Favre disease. Lymphopathia venereum.

favus (fa·vus). A chronic infection of the skin and hair or the nails with *Trichophyton schoenleinii*; less frequently *T. violaceum* are the causal fungi. Usually the scalp is affected, occasionally the glabrous skin or the nails, and the malady is characterized by the formation of yellow cup-shaped crusts called scutula, and a mouse-like odour. The dermis is involved and eventually there is cutaneous atrophy, or scar formation with baldness. On the glabrous skin scutula are usually noted, but a vesicular eruption is seen on rare occasions (favus herpeticus). Favus of the nails does not differ in appearance from tinea unguium. Animal favus may be transmitted to man, e.g. *Trichophyton quinckeanum* (mouse favus) or *T. gallinae* (fowl favus); the latter species only rarely causes ringworm infection in man. [L honeycomb.]

Fazadinium Bromide (fa·zah·din·e·um bro·mide). BP Commission approved name for 1,1'-azobis(3-methyl-2-phenylimidazo[1,2-α]pyridinium bromide); a neuromuscular blocking agent.

Fazio-Londe atrophy, or type. The Werdnig-Hoffmann paralysis affecting particularly the bulbar and facial muscles: it is usually familial.

fear (feer). 1. A phobia. 2. Painful apprehension or alarm. 3. A state of dread or alarm. [ME *fer* danger.]

feature (fe·tewr). 1. Any individual characteristic of the face, such as the nose. 2. Any marked characteristic, e.g. symptom, sign or complication of a case. 3. Any noticeable peculiarity of mind or body. [L *factura* a making.]

febricant (feb·rik·ant). Febrifacient.

febricide (feb·ris·ide). Febrifuge. [L *febris* fever, *caedere* to kill.]

febricity (feb·ris·it·e). 1. The state of being feverish. 2. The quality of being feverish; febrility. [L *febricitare* to have a fever.]

febricula (feb·rik·ew·lah). A slight fever characterized by a rise of temperature rarely above 37.5°C (100°F) and lasting but a short time and indefinite in origin. [L little fever.]

febriculose (feb·rik·ew·loze). Feverish to only a slight degree. [see foll.]

febriculosity (feb·rik·ew·los'·it·e). Slight feverishness. [L *febricula* little fever.]

febrifacient (feb·re·fa·shent). 1. Febrific. 2. An agent which produces a state of feverishness. [L *febris* fever, *facere* to make.]

febriferous (feb·rif·er·us). 1. Febrific. 2. Carrying fever. [L *febris* fever, *ferre* to bear.]

febrific (feb·rif·ik). Causing or producing fever. [L *febris* fever, *facere* to make.]

febrifugal (feb·rif·ew·gal). Mitigating or dispelling fever; antifebrile; antipyretic. [see foll.]

febrifuge (feb·rif·ewj). 1. Any remedy or drug which mitigates or removes fever. 2. Preventing fever. [L *febris* fever, *fugere* to flee.]

febrile (feb·rile, fe·brile). Feverish; having the character of or belonging to a fever; characterized by the presence of fever. **Febrile convulsions.** Convulsions occurring during episodes of fever most often seen in infancy. [see foll.]

febrility (feb·ril·it·e). 1. Feverishness. 2. The quality of being feverish; febricity. [L *febris* fever.]

febriphobia (feb·re·fo·be·ah). 1. Abnormal dread of having a high temperature; pyrexiophobia. 2. The condition of anxiety induced in a patient whose temperature is high. [L *febris* fever, phobia.]

febris (feb·ris, fe·bris). Fever. **Febris acuta.** Acute fever. **Febris bullosa.**Impetigo neonatorum. **Febris castrensis.** Camp fever; typhus fever. *See* FEVER. **Febris castrensis epidemica.** Typhus fever. *See* FEVER. **Febris catarrhalis.** Influenza; herpetic fever. *See* FEVER. **Febris comatosa.** A term used by Sydenham in the 17th century; possibly encephalitis lethargica. **Febris dysenterica.** Bacillary dysentery. *See* DYSENTERY. **Febris enterica.** Typhoid fever. *See* FEVER. **Febris entericoides.** Entericoid fever. *See* FEVER. **Febris famelica.** Famine fever. *See* FEVER. **Febris flava.** Yellow fever. *See* FEVER. **Febris innominata.** Fever of unknown origin. **Febris melitensis.** Malta fever. *See* FEVER. **Febris nervosa.** Fever due to nervous causes. **Febris pallida.** A form of acute infective endocarditis. **Febris petechialis.** Typhus fever or cerebrospinal fever. *See* FEVER. **Febris quintana.** Trench fever. *See* FEVER. **Febris recurrens.** Relapsing fever. *See* FEVER. **Febris remittens.** Remittent fever. *See* FEVER. **Febris rubra.** Scarlatina. **Febris sudoralis.** Sweat fever; miliaria. **Febris tritaea.** Tertian fever. *See* MALARIA. **Febris undulans.** Undulant fever; brucellosis. **Febris uveoparotidea.** The uveoparotid syndrome in which enlargement of the parotid glands and inflammation of the uveal tract are associated with an intermittent pyrexia. Swelling of other salivary glands, the lacrimal glands, lymph glands and spleen, together with peripheral neuritis, may be present. It is a manifestation of sarcoidosis. **Febris variolosa.** Smallpox. **Febris wolhynica.** Trench fever. *See* FEVER. [L.]

Fechner, Gustav Theodor (b. 1801). German philosopher and physicist.
Fechner's law. Sensation varies as the logarithm of the stimulus (i.e. it increases in arithmetical progression as the stimulus increases in geometrical progression).
Weber-Fechner law. Psychophysical law. *See* LAW.

fecundate (fek·un·date). In biology, to impregnate or to fertilize. [L *fecundare* to make fruitful.]

fecundation (fek·un·da·shun). 1. The state of being impregnated or fertilized. 2. The act of impregnating or fertilizing. **Artificial fecundation.** Artificial impregnation, i.e. that caused by instrumental injection of seminal fluid into the uterus. [see prec.]

fecundity (fek·un·dit·e). 1. The power or quality of being able to produce offspring. 2. Fertility. [L *fecunditas* fruitfulness.]

Fede, Francesco (b. 1832). Naples paediatrician.
Fede's disease. Sublingual fibroma.
Fede-Riga disease, Riga-Fede disease. Traumatic ulceration, with induration, of the frenulum of the tongue, caused by trauma from the lower incisor teeth during the process of suckling, and occurring therefore only during the suckling period after the eruption of the lower incisors.

Federici, Cesare (b. 1832). Palermo physician.
Federici's sign. Audibility of the heart sounds on auscultation of the abdomen in cases of intestinal perforation with gas in the peritoneal cavity.

feeblemindedness (fe·bl·mine′·ded·nes). A state of arrested or incomplete development of mind which includes subnormality of intelligence. This is one of the four specific forms of mental disorder under the Mental Health Act 1959. [L *flebilis* lamentable, ME *mynd.*]

feedback (feed·bak). A process whereby a part of the output of a system is returned to the input. The feedback may be negative or positive, dependent upon whether the phase of the feedback signal is out of phase or in phase with the input signal. Negative feedback tends to result in a stable output, whereas positive feedback may cause instability or oscillations. In biological systems, feedback plays an important role in stabilizing certain variables such as blood pressure; the feedback comes from the operation of the reflex mechanism associated with pressure control, e.g. carotid-body baroreceptors. **Feedback inhibition.** *See* INHIBITION. **Feedback mechanisms.** In endocrinology chiefly applied to the trophic hormones of the anterior pituitary, the secretion of which are stimulated by deficiency in the circulation of the hormones of their target glands acting directly on the anterior pituitary or through the hypothalamic releasing hormones which stimulate the appropriate pituitary hormone. Increased concentration of the target organ hormone diminishes the feedback of the trophic hormone—negative feedback. Positive feedback is due to increased amounts of the target gland hormone stimulating the secretion of the hormone of the controlling gland as may occur in the secretion of gonadotrophius. [AS *faedan, baec.*]

feeder (fe·der). A device used to administer food by force to those persons who refuse to take food. [see foll.]

feeding (fe·ding). The act of giving or taking food; the insertion into the mouth, mastication and swallowing, of nutritive material. **Artificial feeding.** 1. The introduction of food into the body by any means other than by the mouth, e.g. intravenous and rectal injections of water, salt, glucose or protein hydrolysates. 2. The general term used for the nourishment of an infant when the mother's breast milk is not available. **Feeding centre.** A nucleus laterally placed in the hypothalamus. If damaged the animal (or person) develops anorexia. **Extrabuccal feeding.** Giving food by a path other than the mouth, e.g. by the rectum. **Forced feeding, Forcible feeding.** Giving food to a resistant person, e.g. by intranasal or gastric tube. **Parenteral feeding.** Feeding by a route other than the intestinal canal, e.g. intravenously. **Feeding by the rectum.** The insertion of nutritive materials into the rectum. **Sham feeding.** An experimental method in which food is taken into the mouth, masticated and swallowed, but is prevented, by an oesophageal fistula or other method, from entering the stomach. [AS *faedan.*]

See also: FINKELSTEIN.

feeling (fe·ling). 1. The mental experience resulting from stimulation of the sensory nerves. 2. A mental state with an emotional tone; affect. **Ambivalent feeling.** One of a pair of mutually contradictory emotional states experienced at the same time, e.g. like and dislike, suspicion and trust, wishing to do something and also wishing not to do it. **Compulsive feeling.** The feeling that something has to be done, even though the subject is aware on the rational level that the act is unnecessary. **Déjà vu feeling.** The conviction that something one is looking at, presumably for the first time, has been seen before; a quasi-emotional experience the factual basis of which may be denied by reason and memory. [AS *felan.*]

Feer, Emil (b. 1864). Swiss paediatrician.

Feer's disease. Pink disease. *See* DISEASE.

fefe (fe·fe). Elephantiasis. [Samoan name.]

Fegan, William George. 20th century Dublin surgeon.

Fegan's method of treating varicose veins. A combination of sclerosing injections into the veins and prolonged compression of the veins by a special method of bandaging.

Fehling, Hermann Christian von (b. 1812). Stuttgart chemist.

Fehling's reagent, or solution. *Solution 1.* Crystalline copper sulphate, 34.64 g, concentrated sulphuric acid 0.5 ml, distilled water to 500 ml. *Solution 2.* 176 g of Rochelle salt are dissolved in 400 ml of water and 77 g of potassium hydroxide added. When dissolved the solution is cooled and made up to 500 ml with water. For use mix equal volumes of Solutions 1 and 2.

Fehling's test, for reducing sugar in urine. Boil a little of the urine with Fehling's reagent. A red precipitate of cuprous oxide appears if glucose or other reducing sugar is present.

Feil, André (b. 1884). Paris neurologist.

Feil-Klippel syndrome, Klippel-Feil disease, or syndrome. Shortness of the neck and limitation of neck movements due to congenital fusion of the cervical vertebrae; the growth of hair on the back of the neck reaches an abnormally low level.

Feitis' flecked spleen. A spleen mottled with small necrotic areas which are the result of ischaemia from arteriosclerosis.

fel (fel). Bile; most commonly ox-bile, the form employed medicinally. It is concentrated and the protein matter removed by the addition of alcohol and filtration; it contains salts of the bile acids (glycocholic and taurocholic acids), and is administered orally to promote peristalsis, and also as an enema to remove impacted faeces. [L.]

Feleki, Hugo von (b. 1861). Budapest urologist.

Feleki's instrument. An apparatus used in massage of the prostate gland.

Felix, Arthur (b. 1887). London bacteriologist.

Felix Vi serum. An antityphoid serum containing antibodies to the Vi and O antigens of the typhoid bacillus.

Felix-Weil reaction. A diagnostic test for typhus with a specific strain of *Proteus* (X19) which is agglutinated by sera of typhus patients.

Weil-Felix test. An agglutination test, originally for typhus fever but now extended to some other rickettsial infections, in which the patient's serum is reacted with suspensions of proteus strains (OX19, OXa, OXk) containing a heterophile antigen.

Felix's disease. Osteochondrosis of the epiphysis of the femoral trochanter.

Fell, George Edward (b. 1850). Buffalo physician.

Fell's apparatus, Fell-O'Dwyer apparatus. An apparatus for performing artificial respiration and preventing collapse of the lung in operation on the chest.

fellatio (fel·a·she·o). The act of introducing the penis into the mouth of the other partner. [L.]

fellator (fel·at·or). A male who is the passive partner in fellatorism. [L.]

fellatorism (fel·at·or·izm). Fellatio.

fellatrice (fel·at·rees). A female who is the passive partner in fellatorism. [see prec.]

fellifluous (fel·if·loo·us). Term indicating that bile is in ample supply. [fel, L *fluere* to flow.]

felo-de-se (fel·o·de·se′) (pl. *felos-de-se, felones-de-se*). In law: felonious, i.e. criminal, self-killing. The term is now obsolete. [LL crime against self.]

felon (fel·on). Whitlow; a suppurative infection of a finger, usually of the terminal phalanx. **Bone felon.** Infection of the terminal phalanx of the finger with erosion and inflammation of the bone. **Subcutaneous felon.** Suppurative inflammation of the pulp of the terminal phalanx of a finger. **Subcuticular felon, Subepithelial felon, Superficial felon.** A pustule arising between the epidermis and corium. **Thecal felon.** Suppurative inflammation of a finger involving the tendon sheath. [L *fel* bile.]

Felsen, Joseph (b. 1892). New York pathologist.

Felsen treatment. The use of rectal injections of oxygen in the treatment of ulcerative colitis or dysentery.

felspar (fel·spar). A mineral composed of the silicates of potassium and aluminium. [G *Feld* field, *Spath* spar.]

felt treatment. The subcutaneous injection of successive doses of 2 mg, 2.6 mg, and 3 mg of atropine at 48-hour intervals, as treatment of sciatica. Now obsolete.

Felton, Lloyd Derr (b. 1885). American physician.

Felton's serum. A concentrated antipneumococcal serum.

Felton's unit. A unit of antipneumococcal serum.

Felty, Augustus Roi (b. 1895). Hartford, Connecticut, physician. **Felty's syndrome.** Splenomegaly and lymphadenopathy in association with rheumatoid arthritis in adults. As a result of the hypersplenism there is neutropenia and often anaemia and thrombocytopenia.

Felypressin (fe·li·**pres**·in). BP Commission approved name for 2-phenylalanine-8-lysinevasopressin; a vasoconstrictor sometimes used with local analgesic drugs instead of adrenaline.

female (**fe**·male). 1. A human being or animal of the sex which conceives and gives birth. 2. Belonging or relating to or characteristic of woman. 3. In botany, any plant organ which after fecundation produces fruit. 4. Of an instrument, a hollow part into which a complementary (male) part fits. **XO female.** A female with only one sex chromosome (the X). In man, such individuals usually have Turner's syndrome and, more rarely, ovarian dysgenesis without webbing of the neck. **XXX female.** A female with a diploid complement of autosomes but trisomic for the X chromosome. In man, females of this chromosome constitution have been called *triple X, superfemale* or *metafemale.* The phenotype is variable. Some are essentially normal and fertile, but others show secondary amenorrhoea and some impairment of mental and psychological development. **XXXX** and **XXXXX female.** A female tetrasomic and pentasomic for the X chromosome. In man, such individuals have a more abnormal phenotype and particularly greater mental retardation than XXX females. [L *femella* little woman.]

femineity (fem·in·e·it·e). Femininity.

feminilism (fem·in·il·izm). Feminism.

femininity (fem·in·**in**·it·e). 1. The normal nature or quality of the female sex. 2. Womanhood; womanliness. [L *femina* woman.]

feminism (**fem**·in·izm). 1. Advocacy of women's rights on the grounds of equality of the sexes. 2. The condition in males in which physical and mental characteristics correspond to those of the female sex with or without arrested development of the male generative organs. **Mammary feminism.** Gynaecomastia. [see prec.]

feminity (fem·**in**·it·e). Femininity.

feminization (**fem**·in·i·za′·shun). In a male, the process of developing female qualities and characteristics. *See* TESTICULAR FEMINIZATION. [L *femina* woman.]

femoral (**fem**·or·al). Relating or belonging to the femur or the thigh. **Femoral ring.** *See* RING. **Femoral surface.** *See* ISCHIUM. **Femoral triangle.** *See* TRIANGLE.

femoral artery [arteria femoralis (NA)]. The main artery to the lower limb, a continuation of the external iliac artery in the thigh. Its branches are the superficial gastric artery, the superficial circumflex iliac artery, the superficial external pudendal artery, the deep external pudendal artery, muscular branches to the sartorius, vastus medialis and adductor muscles, and the profunda femoris artery. It ends by passing into the popliteal fossa where it becomes the popliteal artery.

femoral nerve [nervus femoralis (NA)]. The largest branch of the lumbar plexus (root value L2,3,4) supplying the extensor muscles [rami musculares (NA)] and skin on the front and medial sides of the thigh, and the skin on the medial side of the leg and foot through its saphenous branch.

femoral vein [vena femoralis (NA)]. The main vein of the lower limb. It is an upward continuation in the thigh of the popliteal vein.

femoro-articular (**fem**·or·o·ar·**tik**′·ew·lar). Referring to the part of bone which articulates with, or the process of articulating with, the femur.

femorocele (**fem**·or·o·seel). Femoral hernia. *See* HERNIA. [femur, Gk *kele* hernia.]

femoro-iliac (**fem**·or·o·**il**′·e·ak). Relating or belonging to the femur and the ilium.

femoropretibial (**fem**·or·o·pre·**tib**′·e·al). Relating to the thigh and the front of the leg. [femur, L *pre* tibia.]

femorotibial (**fem**·or·o·**tib**′·e·al). Belonging or relating to the femur and the tibia.

femto-. A prefix indicating that the quantity which follows is to be multiplied by 10^{-15}; thus, a femtogram (1 fg) = 10^{-15} g.

femur [NA] (**fe**·mur). 1. The thigh bone, or long bone of the thigh. 2. The thigh. **Head of the femur [caput femoris (NA)].** The hemispherical upper end of the femur articulating with the acetabulum; it is smooth except for a central pit [fovea capitis femoris] for the ligamentum teres. **Neck of the femur [collum femoris (NA)].** The portion of the femur connecting the head with the shaft, set at an angle to the shaft of about 130° in the adult, and lying partly within the capsule of the hip joint. Developmentally it is an upward extension of the shaft. **Pilastered femur.** A thigh bone on which the linea aspera is of unusual height. **Shaft of the femur [corpus femoris (NA)].** The main part of the thigh bone, supporting the upper and lower end. In its middle part it is triangular in cross-section with the ridge of the linea aspera posteriorly separating the medial and lateral surfaces which are in turn separated from the anterior surface by ill-defined medial and lateral borders. These surfaces give origin to the vastus muscles. At its upper and lower ends the shaft expands to produce an additional posterior surface in the position of the linea aspera. The posterior surface at the upper end bears the gluteal tuberosity on its lateral edge, while the posterior surface of the lower third forms part of the floor of the popliteal fossa and is called the popliteal surface. **Shaft of the femur, popliteal surface of the [facies poplitea (NA)].** A triangular, flattened area on the posterior surface of the lower end of the shaft of the femur, forming the floor of the popliteal fossa. **Surface of the femur, patellar [facies patellaris (NA)].** A concave area on the anterior surface of the condyles of the femur articulating with the patella. [L thigh.]

Fencamfamin (fen·**kam**·fam·in). BP Commission approved name for *N*-ethyl-3-phenylbicyclo[2,2,1]hept-2-ylamine; a central nervous system stimulant and appetite suppressant.

fence (fens). In erysipelas, a band of cross-scarification made on the skin to which a germicide is applied in order to limit the area and prevent the spread of the infection. [abbr, form of *defence.*]

fenchone (**fen**·chone). $C_{10}H_{16}O$, a ketonic camphane which is a constituent of fennel oil; it is isomeric with common camphor.

Fenclofenac (fen·**klo**·fen·ak). BP Commission approved name for 2-(2,4-dichlorophenoxy)phenylacetic acid; an anti-inflammatory agent.

fenestra (fen·**es**·trah). A surgical or anatomical opening in the wall of a cavity or hollow organ; a slit in the blade of a forceps. **Fenestra cochleae [NA].** An opening on the inner wall of the tympanic cavity covered by the secondary tympanic membrane. It leads to the cochlea. **Fenestra nov-ovalis.** The new oval window made through the vestibular dome in the Lempert fenestration operation for otosclerosis. **Fenestra ovalis.** Fenestra vestibuli (see below). **Fenestra rotunda.** Fenestra cochleae (see above). **Fenestra vestibuli [NA].** An opening on the inner wall of the tympanic cavity, covered by the foot of the stapes. It leads to the vestibule. [L window.]

fenestral, fenestrate, fenestrated (fen·**es**·tral, fen·**es**·trate, fen·es·tra·ted). 1. Having numerous small openings or apertures, as a membrane. 2. Reticular. [see prec.]

fenestration (fen·es·**tra**·shun). 1. The condition or state of having openings or perforations. 2. The act of perforating surgically. 3. The act of making openings, generally referred to as windows, in the dressing over a wound so that the progress of healing may be observed. [L *fenestra* window.]

Fenethylline (fen·eth·il·een). BP Commission approved name for 7-[2-(α-methylphenethylamino)ethyl]-theophylline; a cerebral stimulant.

Fenfluramine (fen·**floo**·ram·een). BP Commission approved name for 2-ethylamino-1-(3-trifluoromethylphenyl)propane, **Fenfluramine Hydrochloride BP 1973.** The hydrochloride of fenfluramine, a sympathomimetic agent but free from stimulant effect on the central nervous system. It is used to reduce appetite in treatment of obesity.

Fenimide (**fen**·im·ide). BP Commission approved name for 3-ethyl-2-methyl-2-phenylsuccinimide; a tranquillizer.

Fenisorex (fen·i·so·rex). BP Commission approved name for (±)-cis-7-fluoro-1-phenylisochroman-3-ylmethylamine; it is used in the treatment of anorexia.

Fenmetramide (fen·**met**·ram·ide). BP Commission approved name for 5-methyl-6-phenyl-3-morpholinone; an antidepressant.

Fennel BPC 1968 (**fen**·el). The dried fruit of the umbelliferous plant *Foeniculum vulgare* Mill., cultivated in Southern France, Saxony and Russia. It contains a volatile oil of aromatic odour and taste, mainly pinene, limonene, fenchone and anethole, and is used as a carminative. [L *foeniculum.*]

Fenoprofen (fe·no·**pro**·fen). BP Commission approved name for 2-(3-phenoxyphenyl)propionic acid; an anti-inflammatory and analgesic agent.

Fenpipramide (fen·**pip**·ram·ide). BP Commission approved name for 2,2-diphenyl-4-piperidinobutyramide; a spasmolytic.

Fenpiprane (fen·**pip**·rane). BP Commission approved name for 1-(3,3-diphenylpropyl)piperidine; a spasmolytic.

Fentanyl (fen·tan·il). BP Commission approved name for 1-phenethyl-4-(*N*-propionylanilino)piperidine; a narcotic analgesic. **Fentanyl citrate.** A potent narcotic analgesic with an effect similar to that of morphine but of shorter duration. Used with droperidol in neurolept analgesia to produce a state of calmness and indifference to reality.

Fenticlor (**fen**·te·klor). BP Commission approved name for di-(5-chloro-2-hydroxyphenyl) sulphide; an antiseptic and fungicide.

Fenton, William Hugh (b. 1854). London gynaecologist.

Fenton's operation. A plastic operation for enlarging the vaginal introitus.

Fenwick, Edwin Hurry (b. 1856). London urologist.

Fenwick's solitary ulcer. Ulcer of the bladder trigone.

Fenwick, Samuel (b. 1821). London physician.

Fenwick's disease. Primary atrophy of the stomach.

Feprazone (fe·praz·one). BP Commission approved name for 4-(3-methylbut-2-enyl)-1,2-diphenylpyrazolidine-3,5-dione; an analgesic and inflammatory agent.

Féréol, Louis Henri Félix (b. 1825). Paris physician.

Féréol's nodes. Subcutaneous nodes which may occur in the course of acute rheumatism.

Féréol-Graux type of ocular palsy. Paralysis of the internal rectus muscle of one side and of the external rectus muscle of the other.

Ferguson gag. A type of molar gag.

Fergusson, Sir William (b. 1808). London surgeon.

Fergusson's operation. Excision of the maxilla.

Fergusson's speculum. A tubular metal speculum used to visualize the cervix and vaginal walls.

ferment (**fer**·ment). 1. To undergo fermentation. 2. A biological catalyst that brings about fermentative changes. Though the term is often used synonymously with enzyme, it is usually held to mean those micro-organisms formerly known as *organized ferments* which work only in association with the living cells that produce them. Cf. ENZYME. **Amyloclastic ferment, Amylolytic ferment.** A diastatic ferment which splits starch into sugar. **Animal ferment.** A ferment produced in animal tissue. **Autolytic ferment.** A ferment which, upon the death of the tissue, proceeds to decompose it. **Chemical ferment.** A so-called *unorganized ferment,* or extracellular enzyme which will act apart from the cell. **Coagulating ferment.** A ferment that assists the curdling of milk or the clotting of blood. **Conform ferment.** An autolytic ferment that digests the bacteria which secrete it. **Curdling ferment.** The milk-clotting ferment, rennin. **Defensive ferment.** One of the ferments which act in the defensive mechanism of immunity. **Diastatic ferment.** A ferment that hydrolyses starch into sugars. **Digestive ferment.** One of the several ferments concerned in food digestion. **Fibrin ferment.** The ferment, thrombin, in blood which coagulates the fibrinogen in clotting. **Glycoclastic ferment, Glycolytic ferment.** 1. A ferment in the blood and tissues which breaks down complex sugars into simpler ones and even to lactic acid. 2. A liver ferment that hydrolyses starch. **Heteroform ferment.** A ferment that digests bacteria other than those which produce it. **Hydrolytic ferment.** A ferment that acts by the hydrolysis of its substrate. **Inversive ferment, Inverting ferment.** A ferment that splits sugar into glucose and fructose. **Lab ferment.** Rennin. **Lactic ferment.** A ferment produced by bacteria infecting milk which converts lactose into lactic acid thereby causing souring. **Leucocytic ferment.** A ferment with cytolytic properties secreted by leucocytes. **Lipolytic ferment.** A fat-splitting ferment which converts fats into fatty acids and glycerol. **Living ferment.** Term formerly applied to an organized ferment (see below). **Metallic ferment.** A colloidal metal used as a catalyst. **Milk-curdling ferment.** The ferment, Rennin, which coagulates casein and thereby clots milk. **Myosin ferment.** A ferment which clots muscle plasma by converting myogen into insoluble myosin. **Organized ferment.** Original name for the microorganisms which act only in association with living cells and are responsible for natural fermentations. **Oxidation ferment, Oxidizing ferment.** A ferment in tissue respiration which activates oxidation by functioning as an oxygen-carrier. **Protective ferment.** A ferment with cytolytic properties that is secreted into the blood to protect the body against invading organisms. **Proteoclastic ferment, Proteolytic ferment.** A protein-splitting ferment which attacks the peptide linkages of proteins, converting them into peptones and albumoses. **Soluble ferment.** Unorganized ferment (see below). **Steatolytic ferment.** Lipolytic ferment (see above). **Unorganized ferment.** Original name for an enzyme or chemical ferment which can be extracted from the living cell and will continue to act independently. **Urea ferment.** A ferment which activates the alkaline fermentation of urine, forming ammonia and carbon dioxide from urea. [L *fermentum* yeast.]

See also: WARBURG (O. H.).

fermentable (fer·**ment**·abl). Susceptible to fermentation.

fermentaemia (fer·ment·e·me·ah). The presence of a ferment in the circulating blood. [ferment, Gk *haima* blood.]

fermental (fer·**men**·tal). 1. Relating or belonging to or originating in a ferment. 2. Capable of producing fermentation.

fermentation (fer·men·**ta**·shun). 1. The conversion of sugars by yeast into ethyl alcohol during the manufacture of beer and wine, with the frothing liberation of carbon dioxide gas. 2. The slow non-putrefactive decomposition of complex organic substances into simpler forms through the intermediary of biological catalysts which themselves undergo no change. **Acetic fermentation.** The formation of vinegar (acetic acid) from a weak solution of ethyl alcohol by the action of *Acetobacter aceti* and similar organisms. **Alcoholic fermentation.** The formation of ethyl alcohol from natural sugars by species of *Saccharomyces* (yeasts). **Ammoniacal fermentation.** The conversion of the urea of urine into ammonia and carbon dioxide by *Micrococcus ureae.* **Amylic fermentation.** The production of amyl alcohol from natural sugars during alcoholic fermentation. **Amylolytic fermentation.** The conversion of starch into dextrins by the ptyalin of saliva. **Butyl alcohol fermentation.** The formation of butyl alcohol and acetone from maize starch by *Clostridium acetobutyricum.* **Butyric fermentation.** The formation of butyric acid from sugar and starch by anaerobic organisms of the type *Clostridium butyricum* contained in sour milk. **Caseous fermentation.** In cheese-making, the action of rennet to clot the milk by coagulating the casein. **Cellulose fermentation.** The fermentation of cellulose into acetic and butyric acids by the heat-resistant organisms of stable manure. **Dextran fermentation.** The formation of dextran from the glucose in beet syrup or wine by the action of certain cocci. **Diastatic fermentation.** The conversion of starch into dextrins and maltose by ptyalin or amylases. **Frog-spawn fermentation.** Dextran fermentation, from the ropy appearance of the intermediate substrate. **Intestinal fermentation.** The result of defective starch digestion, characterized by distended abdomen and loose stools. **Lactic fermentation, Lactic-acid fermentation.** The conversion of the lactose of milk into lactic acid by the lactic bacilli, causing the milk to become sour. **Propionic fermentation.** The conversion of sugar into propionic acid by the action of *Bacillus cavicidus.*

Saccharobutyric fermentation. The production of butyric acid from carbohydrates by *Clostridium welchii* in the intestine. **Stormy fermentation.** The rapid and frothy fermentation of milk by *Clostridium welchii.* **Viscous fermentation.** The formation of ropy or glutinous substances in substrates such as milk or wine by certain organisms. [L *fermentare* to cause to rise.]

fermentoid (fer·men·toid). A ferment which has been subjected to alteration so that the active properties are lost. [ferment, Gk *eidos* form.]

fermentum (fer·men·tum). Yeast. [L.]

Fermi, Claudio (b. 1862). Rome physician.

Fermi's treatment. A method of inoculation against rabies by serovaccination, i.e. the subcutaneous injection of mixtures of a vaccine of phenolized virus, and a serum prepared by the immunization of horses with the vaccine.

Fermi, Enrico (b. 1901). Italian physicist.

Fermi distribution of beta-particle energy. A theory which predicts the shape of the spectrum of number versus beta-particle energy, and gives a relationship between disintegration energy and half-life of the beta emitter.

Fermi effect. The formation of radioactive elements by neutron bombardment, discovered by Fermi in 1934; a process due to (n, γ) reaction.

fermium (fer·me·um). A transuranic element reported in 1954 by the University of California and the Argonne National Laboratory. It was produced in the reactor from plutonium by the absorption of 15 neutrons. It has an atomic number of 100, and has been given the symbol Fm. Its half-life is 3 hours, and it decays by the emission of alpha particles. [Enrico *Fermi.*]

fern (fern). The general name for Pteridophyta of the order Filicales. **Lady fern.** Filix femina, *Athyrium filix-foemina* (Linn.) Roth. **Male Fern BP 1973.** Filix mas; the dried rhizome and frond bases of the plant *Dryopteris filix-mas* (L.) Schott, used in the treatment of tapeworm. **Shield fern.** *Dryopteris spinulosa* (Müll.) Watt. **Fern test,** "ferning". A sample of vaginal or cervical secretion spread on a slide is dried by mild heat and produces crystallization in a fern pattern at the time of ovulation or when there is an excess of oestrogen. [AS *fearn.*]

Fernel, Jean François (b. 1497). Paris physician.

Fernel's disease. Aortic aneurysm.

Ferrata, Adolfo (b. 1880). Pavia physician.

Ferrata's cell. The hypothetical stem cell of all blood cells.

ferrated (fer·a·ted). 1. Charged with or containing iron. 2. Combined with iron. [L *ferrum* iron.]

Ferrein, Antoine (b. 1693). Paris surgeon and anatomist.

Ferrein's canal. A canal believed to be formed by the margins of the eyelids during sleep to carry the tears to the puncta lacrimalia.

Ferrein's cords. The vocal cords.

Ferrein's foramen. A foramen in the petrous part of the temporal bone which transmits the greater superficial petrosal nerve.

medullary rays or pyramids of Ferrein. An extension of the renal pyramid into the cortex of the kidney.

Ferrein's tubules. Those parts of the convoluted tubules that are included in the medullary rays of Ferrein.

Ferrein's vasa aberrantia. Intrahepatic bile canaliculi not continuous with the biliary tract.

ferri-albuminic (fer·e·al·bew′·min·ik). A compound of iron with egg albumin, used in the treatment of anaemia. [L *ferrum* iron, albumin.]

ferric (fer·ik). 1. Containing iron. 2. Term applied to any compound of iron in which the metal is trivalent. *See* IRON. **Ferric Ammonium Citrate BP 1973.** A preparation in scale form used widely in the treatment of anaemia. **Ferric ammonium sulphate.** Ammonioferric alum, iron alum, $NH_4Fe(SO_4)_2 \cdot 12H_2O$; a violet crystalline compound used as an astringent and styptic. **Ferric chloride,** $FeCl_3 \cdot 6H_2O$. The salt of choice when it is desired to administer iron in solution. Such solutions are also used as styptics, whilst a solution in glycerin is employed as a throat paint. **Ferric Glycerophosphate BPC 1963.** Iron glycerophosphate, a preparation made from ferric hydroxide and glycerophosphoric acid, used for its reputed tonic properties. **Ferric hydroxide.** A hydrated form of iron oxide, $Fe_2O_3 \cdot 3H_2O$, easily obtained as a gel by the action of alkalis on solutions of ferric salts. Mixed with a suspension of magnesium oxide it is an antidote for arsenical poisoning. **Ferric Hypophosphite BPC 1963.** Iron hypophosphite, a compound reputed to have tonic properties. **Red ferric oxide.** Rouge, Armenian bole, Fe_2O_3; an impure form of iron oxide used as a pigment, also as a polishing powder. **Ferric subsulphate.** Monsel's salt, $Fe_4O(SO_4)_5$; solutions are used for haemostatic purposes. **Ferric valerate, Ferric valerianate.** A salt, insoluble in water, which has been used in anaemia. [L *ferrum* iron.]

ferricyanide (fer·e·si·an·ide). Any salt of the hypothetical ferrocyanic acid, $H_3Fe(CN)_6$.

ferricyanogen (fer·e·si·an′·o·jen). Name given to the trivalent ferricyanide ion $Fe(CN)_6^{3-}$ which produces the blue pigment, Turnbull's blue.

Ferrier, P. 20th century French physician.

Ferrier's treatment. A treatment of pulmonary tuberculosis by the administration of calcium salts in an endeavour to promote calcification.

ferrihaemoglobin (fer·e·he·mo·glo′·bin). Haemoglobin in which the iron atoms are in the ferric state. [L *ferrum* iron, haemoglobin.]

Ferris Smith. *See* SMITH, FERRIS.

ferrisalipyrine (fer·e·sal·e·pi′·reen). A brown compound of iron and phenazone salicylate.

ferritin (fer·it·in). An iron-protein complex which plays a part in absorption, transport and storage of iron. [L *ferrum* iron.]

ferro-alumen (fer·o·al·ew′·men). Ferric ammonium sulphate, iron alum, $(NH_4)Fe(SO_4)_2 \cdot 12H_2O$. Pale-violet crystals used as a standard reagent and as an indicator in the volumetric analysis of silver. Employed medicinally as an astringent and styptic.

ferrocyanic (fer·o·si·an′·ik). Denoting a compound which contains the tetravalent radical ≡Fe(CN)₆.

ferrocyanide (fer·o·si·an·ide). Any salt of the hypothetical ferrocyanic acid, $H_4Fe(CN)_6$.

ferrocyanogen (fer·o·si·an′·o·jen). Name given to the tetravalent ferrocyanide ion $Fe(CN)_6^{4-}$ which forms the several Prussian blues.

ferrocyanuret (fer·o·si·an·ewr′·et). Ferrocyanide.

ferroferric (fer·o·fer·ik). Ferrosoferric.

ferrohaemoglobin (fer·o·he·mo·glo′·bin). Haemoglobin in which the iron atoms are in the ferrous state. [L *ferrum* iron, haemoglobin.]

ferroheme (fer·o·heem). Haematin or haem. [L *ferrum* iron, haem.]

ferromagnetic (fer·o·mag·net′·ik). Having magnetic properties similar to iron. [L *ferrum* iron, magnet.]

ferrometer (fer·om·et·er). An instrument for ascertaining the proportion of iron in the circulating blood. [L *ferrum* iron, meter.]

ferropectic (fer·o·pek·tik). Having the ability to hold iron in combination. [see foll.]

ferropexy (fer·o·pex·e). The retention of iron in a combined form. [L *ferrum* iron, Gk *pexis* fixation.]

ferroporphyrin (fer·o·por·fir·in). A combination of iron and a porphyrin. [L *ferrum* iron, porphyrin.]

ferroprotein (fer·o·pro·te·in). An enzyme in which the prosthetic group, a ferroporphyrin, is combined with a specific protein. Such enzymes act as hydrogen carriers in tissue respiration. [L *ferrum* iron, protein.]

Ferrosi Sulfas (fer·o·si sul·fas). *European Pharmacopoeia* name for Ferrous Sulphate BP 1973.

ferrosilicon (fer·o·sil·ik·on). A steel alloy containing 2 per cent silicon which gives it added strength and hardness. [L *ferrum* iron, silicon.]

ferrosin (fer·o·sin). A red pigment made from ferric oxide with lime and albumin.

ferrosoferric (fer·o·so·**fer**′·ik). Denoting a compound of iron in which both ferrous and ferric atoms are present; it may be regarded as derived from ferrosoferric oxide, Fe_3O_4.

ferrosoferrous (fer·o·so·**fer**′·us). A term not in frequent use, denoting a substance composed of two ferrous salts.

ferrotherapy (fer·o·**ther**·ap·e). Treatment by administration of iron and iron compounds or chalybeates. [L *ferrum* iron, therapy.]

ferrous (**fer**·us). 1. Containing iron, or of the nature of iron, e.g. minerals. 2. Denoting a compound of iron in which the element is in its reduced state, i.e. has a valency of two. *See* IRON. With albumin, ferrous salts form compounds that are soluble, non-irritant and non-corrosive; they are therefore of value in iron-deficiency diseases. **Ferrous bromide,** $FeBr_2 \cdot 6H_2O$. A red crystalline soluble compound. **Ferrous carbonate,** $FeCO_3$. An insoluble compound which is converted to some extent into ferrous chloride in the stomach; it is a constituent of Blaud's pill. **Ferrous chloride,** $FeCl_2 \cdot 4H_2O$. A soluble green compound. **Citrated ferrous chloride.** A scale preparation obtained by evaporating a solution of ferrous chloride containing citric acid. It is a stable form of ferrous iron, used as a tonic, usually in enteric-coated tablets as it tends to cause nausea otherwise. **Dried Ferrous Sulphate BP 1973.** Ferrous sulphate (see below) that has been deprived of water of crystallization by drying at 40°C. It is rapidly replacing more complex iron preparations, e.g. Easton's syrup; on account of its astringency it is almost always administered in tablet form. **Ferrous Fumarate BP 1973,** $C_4H_2FeO_4$. A preparation of iron used in the prevention and treatment of iron-deficiency anaemias; it is dispensed in tablets. **Ferrous Gluconate BP 1973,** $C_{12}H_{22}O_{14}Fe2H_2O$. An iron preparation used in the treatment of anaemia. **Ferrous iodide,** $FeI_2 \cdot 5H_2O$. A deliquescent green compound incorporated in tonic syrups. **Ferrous lactate,** $(CH_3CHOHCOO)_2Fe$. A compound composed of pale-green scales, employed in anaemia. **Ferrous phosphate.** Iron Phosphate BPC 1968. **Ferrous Succinate BP 1973.** A basic salt which may be prepared by the interaction of sodium succinate and ferrous sulphate in boiling aqueous solution; it is dispensed in capsules. **Ferrous Sulphate BP 1958,** $FeSO_4 \cdot 7H_2O$. Green vitriol, and the anhydrous $FeSO_4$; the most commonly used form of iron in medicine. It is employed as a tonic. [L *ferrum* iron.]

ferruginated (fer·**oo**·jin·a·ted). 1. Having the qualities and activities of iron. 2. Ferruginous. [see foll.]

ferruginous (fer·**oo**·jin·us). 1. Charged with or containing iron. 2. Having the colour and appearance of iron rust. [L *ferrugo* iron rust.]

ferrule (**fer**·ool, **fer**·ul). A metallic ring applied around the circumference of a tooth to which an artificial crown is being fitted, in order to provide additional strength and retention. [L *ferrum* iron.]

ferrum (**fer**·um). Iron; genitive *ferri.* **Ferrum Redactum BPC 1949, Ferrum reductum.** Quevenne's iron, reduced iron, obtained by passing hydrogen over heated ferric oxide; contains not less than 80 per cent of metallic iron mixed with ferrosoferric oxide, Fe_3O_4. [L.]

Ferry, Newell Simmons (b. 1876). Detroit physician.

Ferry's serum. 1. An antistreptococcal serum prepared for use in measles (obsolete). 2. An antitoxic serum prepared in horses in the belief that meningococci produce a soluble toxin. Formerly used in the treatment of cerebrospinal meningitis.

Ferry's toxin. 1. A toxin from meningococci studied by Ferry. 2. A toxin from an organism isolated from the blood in measles, but not accepted as causal.

fertile (**fer**·tile). 1. Capable of conceiving and giving birth. 2. Of ova, capable of developing and growing into a new individual. **Fertile eunuch.** Owing to ICSH deficiency the patient is eunuchoid and impotent. Treatment with testosterone or HCG will render him potent and therefore capable of inducing conception. [L *fertilis.*]

fertilization (**fer**·til·i·**za**′·shun). 1. Impregnation. 2. The process of making fertile. 3. In biology, the union of the male germ cell with the female germ cell; the process which is essential to the development of the fertilized ovum. **Cross fertilization.** The fusion of male and female gametes from different individuals. **Double fertilization.** In plants (angiosperms), the fusion of a male gamete to the egg occurring while another male and female gamete fuse to produce the nutritive tissue for the embryo (endosperm). In animals the entry of two sperms into one egg cell. **Self fertilization.** The fusion of male and female gametes from the same individual. [see prec.]

Ferula (**fer**·ew·lah). A genus of plants of the order Umbelliferae. Asafoetida is obtained from the species *Ferula foetida* Regel and *F. rubricaulis* Boiss., grown in Persia and Afghanistan. *Ferula communis* Linn. and *F. marmarica* Aschers and Taub. are the sources of Moroccan and Cyrenian ammoniacum, *F. galbaniflua* of galbanum and *F. sumbul* Hook f. of sumbul. [L fennel-giant.]

fervescence (fer·**ves**·ens). 1. Increase in the bodily temperature. 2. Heightening in the degree of fever present. [L *fervescere* to become boiling hot.]

fervor (**fer**·vor). Glowing (fever) heat. Cf. ARDOR, CALOR, DOLOR. [L excessive heat.]

fester (**fes**·ter). 1. To become superficially inflamed and discharge pus. 2. To grow virulent. 3. A pustule or small suppurating sore or ulcer. [L *fistula* a kind of ulcer.]

festinant (**fes**·tin·ant). Hastening or accelerating in movement; term applied to the gait in certain nervous diseases, especially paralysis agitans. [see foll.]

festination (fes·tin·**a**·shun). The involuntary acceleration in the rate of walking observed in certain nervous diseases such as paralysis agitans. It is an involuntary attempt to overtake the displaced centre of gravity. [L *festinare* to hasten.]

festoon (fes·**toon**). Term applied to the curving shape of the gum as it rounds the neck of the teeth. [Fr. *feston* garland.]

fetal (**fe**·tal). 1. Relating or belonging to a fetus. 2. In the condition or at the stage of a fetus.

fetalism (**fe**·tal·izm). The persistence in the body throughout life of certain fetal structures or characteristics.

fetalometry (fe·tal·**om**·et·re). 1. The act of measuring the fetus *in utero.* 2. Fetography. [fetus, meter.]

fetation (fe·**ta**·shun). 1. The state of pregnancy. 2. The process of development of the fetus *in utero.*

fetichism (**fet**·ish·izm). Fetishism.

fetichist (**fet**·ish·ist). Fetishist.

feticide (**fe**·tis·ide). 1. Abortion with intention. 2. The act of intentionally destroying the fetus *in utero.* [fetus, L *caedere* to kill.]

feticulture (**fe**·te·kul·tcher). The application of the laws of hygiene in pregnancy, with special reference to the developing fetus. [fetus, culture.]

fetid (**fe**·tid). Having a foul or offensive odour. [L *fetere* to stink.]

fetish (**fet**·ish). 1. Any object the thought or sight of which arouses lustful feelings. 2. Any natural or artificial material object regarded with awe as possessing magical powers. In some types of insanity any object may be regarded as a fetish. [Fr. *fétiche* sorcery.]

fetishism (**fet**·ish·izm). 1. A form of sexual perversion in which lustful feelings are aroused by the contemplation of such objects as an article of clothing belonging to a member of the opposite sex, or a lock of hair. 2. The attaching of abnormal or morbid interest to and feelings of veneration for any object which has belonged to someone dead or far away. [see prec.]

fetishist (**fet**·ish·ist). Anyone who indulges in fetishism in either of its forms.

fetography (fe·**tog**·raf·e). The photographing, by means of x-rays, of the fetus *in utero*; embryography. [fetus, Gk *graphein* to record.]

fetometry (fe·**tom**·et·re). 1. Fetalometry. 2. Measure of the intra-uterine fetus, particularly the head, by radiology. **X-ray fetometry.** The measurement, by means of x-rays, of the head of the fetus *in utero.*

fetoplacental (fe·to·plas·**en**′·tal). Relating or belonging to the fetus and the placenta.

fetor (fe·tor). A foul odour or stench. **Fetor hepaticus.** The distinctive odour of the breath noticeable in persons with disease of the gall bladder. **Fetor narium.** Ozaena. **Fetor ex ore, Fetor oris.** Foul breath; halitosis. [L stench.]

Fetoxylate (fe·tox·il·ate). BP Commission approved name for 2 - phenoxyethyl 1 - (3 - cyano - 3,3 - diphenylpropyl) - 4 - phenylpiperidine - 4 - carboxylate; it is used in the treatment of diarrhoea.

fetus (fe·tus). The later stage in the development of the embryo of a viviparous animal. In man the term is applied to the embryo from the end of the eighth week up to birth. **Fetus acardiacus, Fetus amorphus.** A condition which occurs in one of uni-ovular twins: part of the fetus becomes an amorphous mass. The upper or lower part of the fetus may be affected. **Fetus compressus.** In twin pregnancy, one fetus which dies and becomes flattened out between the membranes of the living child and the uterine wall. **Fetus in fetu.** A fetus which has within it parts of another fetus. **Harlequin fetus.** One which is affected with ichthyosis congenita. **Papyraceous fetus.** Fetus compressus (see above). **Parasitic fetus.** Another fetus or part of a fetus attached to an otherwise normal fetus. **Fetus sanguinolentis.** A macerated fetus. **Sirenoform fetus.** A fetus with fused lower limbs and feet. [L *fētus.*]

Feulgen, Robert (b. 1884). Giessen biochemist.

Feulgen reaction, staining method, or test. A specific histochemical staining technique for the demonstration of deoxyribonucleic acid within the cell nucleus and its differentiation from ribonucleic acid. After preliminary hydrolysis with MHCl at from 50° to 60°C for from 3 to 40 minutes, according to the method of fixation, sections are placed in Schiff's reagent (basic fuchsine decolorized with sulphurous acid) whereupon a magenta colour develops gradually in the nuclear chromatin. Such a result is said to be *Feulgen-positive*; a negative result, showing the absence of deoxyribose, is *Feulgen-negative.*

fever (fe·ver). 1. A rise above the normal body temperature due to disordered temperature regulation and disturbance of the balance between heat production and heat loss. 2. The whole of the complex reactions of the body to an infection or other fever-producing agent. These include, besides a raised temperature, a subjective feeling of heat and discomfort, a flushed skin or a rash, increased pulse and respiration rates, nervous restlessness and insomnia, a scanty high-coloured urine, furred tongue, constipation, etc. 3. An acute infectious disease, e.g. typhoid fever, scarlet fever, smallpox, etc. **Abortus fever.** Brucellosis due to infection with *Brucella abortus*; it usually takes a more chronic form than Malta fever (see below). **Absorption fever.** A fever occurring just after delivery, supposedly due to tissue damage. **Acclimation fever.** Fever occurring on changing residence to a hot climate. This may be due to a disturbance of heat regulation, or to mild infections. **Acute haemorrhagic fever.** Epidemic haemorrhagic disease. *See* DISEASE. **Aden fever.** A short febrile attack, very like sandfly fever (see below), that occurs at certain times of the year in Aden, usually after the wind has been blowing from the Somali coast opposite; it is almost certainly a fever of the sandfly-dengue group, probably transmitted by vectors blown across the Straits. **Adynamic fever.** A low type of fever occurring in asthenic patients. **Aestivo-autumnal fever.** Malignant tertian malaria. *See* MALARIA. **African Coast fever.** Rhodesian fever (see below): piroplasmosis of cattle. **African haemoglobinuric fever.** Blackwater fever (see below). **African tick fever.** Relapsing fever due to *Borrelia duttoni* and conveyed by the tick *Ornithodorus moubata.* **Algid pernicious fever.** An old term applied to a choleraic form of malignant malaria. **Alimentary fever.** Fever due to gastro-intestinal disorders. **Andaman fever.** A term that has been applied to leptospirosis that is caused by a strain of *Leptospira icterohaemorrhagiae*, a leptospire first isolated in the Andaman Islands. **Aphthous fever.** Foot and mouth disease. *See* DISEASE. **Argentinian haemorrhagic fever.** A virus disease characterized by generalized lymphadenopathy and haemorrhagic necrosis. It is caused by an arenovirus. **Artificial fever.** Therapeutic fever (see below). **Aseptic fever.** Fever occurring in the absence of infection, e.g. by the breakdown of proteins. **Assam fever.** Kala-azar. **Asthenic fever.** Fever occurring in asthenic patients who make little response to infection, as shown by collapse, feeble pulse and respiration, and a low type of fever. **Auric fever.** That due to injections of gold. **Australian Q fever.** Q fever (see below). **Autumnal fever.** Nanukayami; an autumnal disease in Japan resembling Weil's disease. **Barbeiro fever.** South American trypanosomiasis. *See* TRYPANOSOMIASIS. **Bed fever.** A raised temperature which persists whilst the patient remains in bed, but disappears when he gets up. **Bilious fever.** Fever with bilious vomiting; also a form of remittent malarial fever. *See* MALARIA. **Bilious remittent fever.** An old term applied to malignant tertian malaria with jaundice. **Black fever.** Kala-azar. **Blackwater fever.** A haemoglobinuric or malignant malaria; a single massive haemoclastic crisis in which more than half the circulating erythrocytes are haemolysed intravenously, or repeated smaller crises occur. The disease is very frequently fatal. It occurs mainly among foreigners in malarial countries, who have previously had attacks of malignant tertian malaria that have been inadequately treated by quinine: quinine often precipitates an attack. The disease is now almost unknown where the new synthetic antimalarial drugs are used. **Blister fever.** Pemphigus acutus. **Blue fever.** Rocky Mountain spotted fever (see below). **Bouquet fever.** Dengue. **Boutonneuse fever.** Mediterranean tick fever caused by *Rickettsia conorii* carried by a dog tick, *Rhipicephalus sanguineus.* **Brain fever.** Usually applied to meningitis, but has also been used by laymen in cases of encephalitis and the typhoid state. **Brazilian fever.** São Paulo fever. **Break-bone fever.** Dengue. **Brisbane fever.** Q fever (see below). **Bulam fever, Bulama fever.** Probably Pym's fever. **Bullis fever.** A febrile disease first encountered in Bullis Camp, Texas, which was apparently transmitted by the tick *Amblyomma americanum* (lone-star tick). The fever is of abrupt onset and lasts for from 3 to 13 days and the symptoms are similar to those of dengue. A virus has been isolated, but some observers have suspected a rickettsia. **Bullous fever.** The fever accompanying pemphigus. **Burdwan fever.** A severe outbreak of fever which, in the middle of the 19th century, caused many deaths, and which at the time was thought to be a severe form of malaria, but some years later was recognized, retrospectively, as almost certainly kala-azar. The name is now seldom used, and in any case has no special significance today. It was named after a town and district in Bengal. **Bushy Creek fever.** Fort Bragg fever (see below). **Bwambi fever.** A mild yellow-fever-like disease caused by a virus. **Cachectic fever, Cachexial fever.** A vague term applied to a febrile disease with splenomegaly, e.g. kala-azar. **Camp fever.** Typhus fever (see below). **Canicola fever.** Leptospirosis due to *Leptospira canicola.* **Carapata fever.** Tick-borne relapsing fever. *See* RELAPSING FEVER (below). **Carbohydrate fever.** Pyrexia attributed to intestinal carbohydrate dyspepsia. **Cat-bite fever, Cat-scratch fever.** A virus disease conveyed by a cat bite or scratch. **Catarrhal fever.** Influenza: herpetic fever (see below). **Catheter fever.** Pyrexia following catheterization. **Cavité fever.** A dengue-like fever prevalent in Cavité in Manila Bay (the naval station in the Philippines). **Cerebrospinal fever.** Cerebrospinal meningitis. *See* MENINGITIS. **Cesspool fever.** Typhoid fever (see below). **Chagres fever.** A name given by the inhabitants of Panama to a severe fever with a high mortality, usually malignant malaria, that is prevalent in the area of the Chagres river. **Channel fever.** Sea-sickness experienced when a ship enters the Channel or a land-locked sea after an ocean voyage. **Childbed fever.** Puerperal fever (see below). **Climatic fever.** 1. An old name that covered the fever in many tropical infections. 2. A low fever for which no specific cause can be discovered, occurring in hot climates and probably due to the direct effects of a hot climate. **Coastal fever.** Scrub typhus in Queensland. **Colombian tick fever.** A severe form of tick typhus; Tobia fever. **Colombo fever.** Paratyphoid fever (see below). **Colorada tick fever.** A dengue-like disease caused by a virus. **Congolese red fever.** A typhus-like fever occurring in the Congo (Zaire), but probably not a single clinical entity. **Continued fever, Continuous fever.** A fever which does not show remissions. **Cotton-mill fever.** Byssinosis. **Cretan fever, Cyprus fever.** Undulant fever (see below). **Dandy fever.** Dengue. **Death fever.** Visceral leishmaniasis. *See* LEISHMANIASIS. **Deer-fly fever.** Tularaemia. **Dehydration fever.** Pyrexia common in infants, due to lack of fluids. **Dengue fever.** Break-bone fever; a virus disease conveyed by the mosquito *Aëdes aegypti*, and characterized by a 5- to 7-day pyrexia with a saddle-back course, a measly rash and severe pains in the back and limbs. **Desert fever.** Coccidioidomycosis. **Digestive fever.** A slight rise of temperature during digestion of a meal. **Drug fever.** Fever resulting from the administration of a drug, e.g. some sulphonamides may cause fever in certain individuals. **Dum Dum fever.** Kala-azar. There was a British military cantonment at Dum Dum near Calcutta, India. It was in postmortem material from a soldier who had contracted the disease there that Sir William Leishman found the causal parasite of kala-azar, now placed in the genus *Leishmania*. The name is now seldom used. **Dust fever.** Undulant fever (see below). **East Coast fever.** Rhodesian fever (see below). **Elephantoid fever.** Filariasis. **Enteric fever.** Typhoid or paratyphoid fever. It has not the same specific meaning in the USA; there, it refers to any intestinal febrile disease. **Entericoid fever.** Parenteric fever; any fever resembling typhoid or paratyphoid clinically, but due to a different organism. **Ephemeral fever.** A rise of temperature lasting only a short time, such as a few hours or a day. **Epidemic haemorrhagic fever.** Epidemic haemorrhagic disease. *See* DISEASE. **Eruptive fever.** 1. One accompanied by a rash. 2. Boutonneuse fever (see above). **Essential fever.** Pyrexia of unknown origin. **Exanthematous fever.** Eruptive fever (see above). **Familial Mediterranean fever.** A genetically determined illness found in Sephardic Jews, Armenians and Arabs. It gives rise to intermittent pyrexial bouts accompanied by acute abdominal or pleuritic pain. Joint lesions suggestive of acute rheumatoid arthritis, also splenomegaly, may develop. The onset is usually between 10 and 20 years and the disease is usually complicated by renal amyloidosis, causing a fatal nephrotic syndrome. Amyloidosis may be the sole manifestation, while some sufferers never develop this complication. There is no effective treatment, though indomethacin has been recommended. **Famine fever.** Typhus and relapsing fevers (see below). **Fatigue fever.** One occurring after violent exercise. **Fermentation fever.** Fever due to absorption of products of alimentary fermentation. **Field fever.** A form of spirochaetosis occurring in field workers, especially in warm weather after flooding. **Five-day fever.** Term applied to trench fever (see below), and from time to time to other fevers of 5 days' duration. **Flood fever.** Tsutsugamushi fever (see below). **Food fever.** Pyrexia attributed to digestive disturbances. **Fort Bragg fever.** A dengue-like fever but caused by *Leptospira autumnalis* and characterized by a rash on the anterior aspect of the legs; also called *pretibial fever*; Bushy Creek fever. **Foundryman's fever.** Metal-fume fever (see below). **Fracture fever.** Fever occurring after fracture of a bone. **Gaol fever.** Typhus fever (see below). **Gastric fever.** Typhoid fever (see below). **Gibraltar fever.** Undulant fever (see below). **Glandular fever.** Infectious mononucleosis. *See* MONONUCLEOSIS. **Goat fever, Goat's-milk fever.** Malta fever (see below). **Guaitâra fever.** Oroya fever (see below). **Haemoglobinuric fever.** Blackwater fever (see above). **Haemorrhagic fever.** A widespread capillaritis due to some arboviruses of which the best known is yellow fever. As well as pyrexia, there is a haemorrhagic tendency to liver damage impairing clotting mechanisms. Haemorrhagic episodes are associated with the following arbovirus diseases: Chikungunya, Crimean haemorrhagic fever, dengue, Omsk haemorrhagic fever and yellow fever. **Harvest fever.** A fever affecting harvest workers; a vague term, probably leptospirosis in many instances. **Haverhill fever.** A disease due to *Actinomyces muris*, characterized by febrile illness, morbilliform rash and non-suppurative flitting arthritis. Diagnosis is based on blood cultures or agglutination tests. **Hay fever.** An acute affection of the mucous membranes of the upper respiratory tract, also involving the eyes and extending to the bronchial passages, causing asthma. It is due to an allergic reaction with some protein substance (pollen) to which the individual is sensitive. Its onset is usually seasonal, depending on the time of year when particular grasses and plants are about. The attacks may, however, be non-seasonal, being precipitated in such cases by some allergen other than plant pollens. The chief symptoms are coryza, sneezing and irritation of the nasal and upper respiratory mucous membranes, thought to be due to the liberation of histamine. Antihistamine drugs are effective in treatment. **Hectic fever.** A remittent or intermittent fever with severe chills and sweats. **Hepatic fever.** Infective hepatitis. *See* HEPATITIS. **Herpetic fever.** A common cold complicated by facial herpes infection. **Hyperpyrexial fever.** Fever in which the temperature exceeds 40.5°C (105°F). **Hysterical fever.** Fever arising as a hysterical symptom. **Icterohaemorrhagic fever.** Leptospiral jaundice. *See* JAUNDICE. **Inanition fever.** A fever due to lack of fluids in infants, but usually secondary to other diseases. **Intermenstrual fever.** A rise of temperature midway between the menstrual periods. **Intermittent fever.** Fever in which the temperature falls to, or below, normal between paroxysms. **Intermittent hepatic fever.** A fever due to cholecystitis associated with intermittent impaction of a gall-stone in the common bile duct; Charcot's fever. **Island fever.** Tsutsugamushi fever (see below). **Izumi fever.** A febrile disease of Japan of uncertain aetiology associated with a rash (scarlatiniform-morbilliform). It is a relapsing type of fever of rapid onset, sometimes diphasic lasting up to 21 days. **Jail fever.** Typhus fever (see below). **Japanese flood fever, Japanese river fever.** Tsutsugamushi fever (see below). **Jungle fever.** Malaria. **Jungle yellow fever.** Yellow fever (see below) in forests where *Aëdes aegypti* is not found and where monkeys form the reservoir of infections and *Haemagogus* and other jungle mosquitoes are the vectors. **Korin fever.** Epidemic haemorrhagic disease. *See* DISEASE. **Kriim fever.** An endemic infectious disease of Iceland and the Faroe Islands. **Land fever.** Channel fever (see above). **Lassa fever.** An acute febrile illness with a high mortality rate occurring in West Africa, reported first from Lassa, a village in Northern Nigeria. The causal agent is a small spherical virus allied to the viruses which cause South American haemorrhagic fevers. While the disease is transmitted naturally, probably by an arthropod vector from an unknown animal reservoir, direct contact is the only proved mode of transmission. The disease has a high infectivity. It is manifested by fever, oral ulceration, albuminuria and a haemorrhagic capillaritis causing multiple organ damage. There is no specific treatment. **Lechuguilla fever.** Swelled head; a disorder of sheep and goats in Texas caused by eating the toxic plant, *Agave lechuguilla*. **Lemming fever.** An infectious disease in Norway attributed to contamination of water by lemmings. **Lent fever.** Typhoid fever (see below). **Leprotic fever.** The febrile stage of leprosy; reaction fever in leprosy. **Lone-star fever.** Bullis fever (see above). **Low fever.** Asthenic fever (see above). **Lung fever.** Pneumonia. **Macular fever.** Typhus fever (see below). **Malarial fever.** Malaria. **Malignant fever.** Epidemic typhus fever (see TYPHUS); a very severe and fatal form of a specific infectious fever. **Malta fever.** Undulant fever due to infection with *Brucella melitensis*. **Marsh fever.** Old name for malaria. **Mediterranean fever.** Malta fever (see above). **Mediterranean fever, familial.** A periodic syndrome with recurrent fever and pain in the abdomen, chest and joints, found mainly in Sephardic Jews; in some cases amyloidosis develops, with nephrotic syndrome. Autosomal recessive transmission. **Mediterranean tick fever.** Boutonneuse fever (see above). **Melanuric fever.** Blackwater fever (see above). **Metabolic fever.** The complex response of the body to changes in metabolism. One of these responses is a rise in temperature, due to a disordered condition of the heat-regulating mechanism. In addition, dehydration, disturbed electrolyte balance in the blood and changes in the pulse/respiration ratio may occur. **Metal-fume fever.** Brassfounders' disease, ague or chills; spelter-workers' ague, shakes or chills. Zinc heated to a temperature near its boiling point, as in the smelting of zinc ores, casting of brass, galvanizing and oxyacetylene welding or cutting of galvanized iron, gives off particles of freshly sublimed zinc oxide which, when inhaled, destroy cells in the lung alveoli; the resulting proteins are absorbed and, after a latent period, cause a train of malaria-like symptoms: malaise, nausea, shivering, fever, muscular pains, sweating and prostration, and a leucocytosis. Recovery is usually complete in about 24 hours. The maximum allowable concentration of zinc oxide fume is 15 mg/m^3 of air. Metal-fume fever is also caused by the fume of other metals besides zinc. **Miliary fever.** Miliaria. **Milk fever.** 1. Sometimes used to denote puerperal fever (see below). 2. A fever due to inflammation of the breasts or their engorgement. 3. A disease of milking cows, associated with cerebral anaemia and paralysis. **Miniature scarlet fever.** Generalized rash with malaise and vomiting. It is observed very rarely during immunization with scarlet-fever prophylactic, and is due to the limit of tolerance to the toxin contained in the prophylactic being exceeded. **Mite fever.** Tsutsugamushi fever (see below). **Monday fever.** Byssinosis. **Mossman fever.** A fever prevalent among the cutters of sugar cane; it was probably a rickettsial infection of the scrub typhus variety. **Mud fever.** Leptospirosis. **Muma fever.** Tropical pyomyositis. *See* PYOMYOSITIS. **Naples sandfly fever.** Sandfly fever due to the Naples serotype. **Neapolitan fever.** Malta fever (see above). **Neurogenic fever.** Fever of nervous origin, all other causal factors being excluded. **Nightsoil fever.** Typhoid fever (obsolete). **Nine-mile fever.** Q fever (see below). **Nodal fever, Nodular fever.** Erythema nodosum. **Oroya fever.** The acute febrile stage of Carrion's disease caused by *Bartonella bacilliformis* and transmitted by sandflies. **Pahvant Valley fever.** Tularaemia. **Paludal fever.** Malaria. **Pappataci fever.** Sandfly fever (see below). **Papular fever.** Erythema multiforme. **Paramalta fever, Paramelitensis fever.** Terms sometimes applied to any febrile disease similar to Malta fever, but in the absence of *Brucella melitensis*; abortus fever caused by *B. abortus.* **Paratyphoid fever.** A disease resembling typhoid fever and included with it under the term *typhoid fevers.* Paratyphoid A, B and C infections are described, and are due respectively to *Salmonella paratyphi A, B* and *C.* The symptoms are sometimes milder than those of typhoid. **Para-undulant fever.** Paramalta fever (see above). **Parenteric fever.** Entericoid fever (see above). **Parrot fever.** Psittacosis. **Peach fever.** Respiratory catarrh, conjunctivitis, and dermatitis, occasionally attacking salesmen and other persons handling peaches. **Periodic fever.** Familial Mediterranean fever (see above). **Petechial fever.** Acute meningococcal meningitis; epidemic cerebrospinal meningitis. *See* MENINGITIS. **Pharyngoconjunctival fever.** An acute febrile illness that occurs epidemically, usually among schoolchildren. It is characterized by pharyngitis, rhinitis, conjunctivitis and enlarged cervical lymph glands, and is caused by *Adenovirus* of several types. **Phlebotomus fever.** Sandfly fever (see below). **Pinta fever.** A name used for a tick typhus of the Rocky Mountain fever type that occurs in South America; it is in no way associated with the disease pinta that also occurs there. **Pneumonic fever.** Acute pneumonia. **Polyleptic fever.** Relapsing fever (see below). **Polymer-fume fever.** A fever, similar to metal-fume fever, caused by the fumes from certain polymers when they are subjected to high temperatures in the manufacture of plastics. **Porcelain fever.** Urticaria. **Post-typhoid fever.** Rises of temperature interrupting the convalescent stage of typhoid fever (see below), and distinct from relapse. **Pretibial fever.** Fort Bragg fever (see above). **Prison fever.** Epidemic typhus. *See* TYPHUS. **Protein fever.** Fever produced by the parenteral injection of a protein. **Puerperal fever.** A fever in the puerperium. **Puerperal scarlet fever.** A rash resembling scarlet fever (*see* SCARLATINA) which may occur in streptococcal puerperal sepsis. **Pulmonary fever.** Pneumonia. **Purulent fever.** Pyaemia. **Pythogenic fever.** Typhoid fever (see below). **Q fever.** A world-wide rickettsial infection originally discovered in Australia caused by *Coxiella burnetii* and characterized by fever, pneumonia, muscle pains and headache. The disease is acquired from cattle or by drinking infected milk. **Quartan fever.** Infection with *Plasmodium malariae,* causing a rise of temperature at intervals of 3 days. **Queensland fever, Queensland coastal fever.** A rickettsia fever of the scrub-typhus group. *See* TYPHUS. **Quinine fever.** Pyrexia and a skin eruption attacking persons employed in the preparation of quinine. **Quintan fever, Quintana fever.** Trench fever (see below). **Quotidian fever.** An intermittent fever with daily paroxysms. **Rabbit fever.** Tularaemia, deer-fly fever, Pahvant Valley fever; a plague-like infectious disease of small rodents. It is caused by *Brucella tularensis* which is conveyed by blood-sucking flies and ticks. It was first discovered in ground squirrels in California and is transmissible to man. Many cases have been recorded in North America, Norway, Russia and Japan. It produces an indolent primary lesion in the form of a necrotic papule, followed by a persistent enlargement of the lymph glands of the affected area. These may suppurate and break down with considerable fever and constitutional disturbance. In some cases there is fever and much malaise without a local lesion. The disease is not usually fatal but causes a long disability. **Rat-bite fever.** A febrile disease due to *Spirillum minus* or to *Actinomyces muris*; transmitted by the bite of a rat. **Recurrent fever.** Relapsing fever (see below). **Red fever.** 1. Dengue. 2. Swine erysipelas. **Redwater fever.** Texas fever in cattle (see below). **Relapsing fever.** A group of spirochaetal diseases conveyed by ticks and lice; they are characterized by spells of pyrexia with apyrexial intervals. **Remittent fever.** Fever in which there is a considerable swing in the daily temperature chart but in which the normal line is never reached. **Rheumatic fever.** Acute rheumatism. **Rhodesian fever.** East Coast fever: African Coast fever: a disease of cattle caused by *Theileria parva* and transmitted by the bite of a tick. **Rice-field fever.** Leptospirosis. **Rift Valley fever.** Epizootic virus hepatitis, due to an arbovirus, which may be transmitted to man by direct infection. **Rock fever.** Malta fever (see above). **Rocky Mountain spotted fever.** A tick-borne infection of man occurring in North and South America, caused by *Rickettsia rickettsii* and transmitted by *Dermacentor andersoni* and other ticks. **Roman fever.** Malaria. **Russian intermittent fever.** Probably the same as trench fever (see below). **Russian spring-summer fever.** Russian epidemic encephalitis. *See* ENCEPHALITIS. **Sakushu fever.** A 7-day epidemic fever of Japan. **Salmonella fever.** A typhoid-like fever caused by a member of the genus *Salmonella* (it now includes the typhoid and paratyphoid bacteria, as well as organisms associated with food poisoning). **Sandfly fever.** A 3-day fever caused by a virus conveyed by the sandfly *Phlebotomus papatasii.* **San Joaquin Valley fever.** Coccidioidomycosis. **São Paulo fever.** São Paulo typhus. *See* TYPHUS. **Scarlet fever.** Scarlatina. **Sellar fever.** A name given to a dengue-like disease in Northern India. **Septic fever.** Fever due to septic infection. **Seven-day fever.** Dengue fever (see above). **Shin-bone fever.** Trench fever (see below). **Ship fever.** Typhus fever (see below). **Shoddy fever.** A disease in shoddy workers, of which the main symptoms are pyrexia, cough and difficult breathing, caused by inhaling dust of old wool obtained from woven fabrics (shoddy) which is made fit for remanufacture. **Sicilian sandfly fever.** Sandfly fever due to the Sicilian serotype. **Simple continued fever.** A non-remittent continuous fever. **Songo fever.** Epidemic haemorrhagic disease. *See* DISEASE. **South African tick-typhus fever.** A tick typhus transmitted by *Haemaphysalis* ticks. **Spirillum fever.** Relapsing fever (see above). **Splenic fever.** Anthrax in animals. **Spotted fever.** 1. Rocky Mountain spotted fever and other rickettsial fevers. 2. Epidemic cerebrospinal (meningococcal) meningitis. *See* MENINGITIS. **Sthenic fever.** Higher fever with hot dry skin, full strong pulse and often active delirium. **Stiffneck fever.** Epidemic cerebrospinal meningitis. *See* MENINGITIS. **Sulphonamide fever.** Continuous administration of a sulphonamide drug may cause a rise of temperature to 38.5°C (101°F) or so, after 4–8 days; this rise may be confused with that caused by the infection for which the drug was given. Usually sulphonamides cause a drop of temperature within 3 days, so that fever occurring later without accompanying signs of renewed infection should be regarded as due to the drug; administration should at once be stopped or serious toxic symptoms may occur. The drug fever usually falls within 48 hours and later toxic symptoms are unlikely. **Sumatran mite fever.** Tsutsugamushi fever (see below). **Sun fever.** Dengue. **Suppurative fever.** Fever occurring in suppurative processes. **Surgical fever.** Fever occurring after operations in pre-antiseptic days. **Swamp fever.** Weil's disease. **Sweat fever.** Miliaria. **Swine fever.** An epizootic virus fever among pigs, associated with loss of appetite, diarrhoea, emaciation and ecchymosis; swine cholera. **Symptomatic fever.** Fever from a non-specific cause. **Syphilitic fever.** Pyrexia caused by syphilis. **Fever of tension.** Fever caused by stitch abscesses. **Tertian fever.** Malarial fever with paroxysms at intervals of 48 hours. **Tetanoid fever.** Acute cerebrospinal meningitis. *See* MENINGITIS. **Texas fever.** An enzootic cattle disease caused by *Babesia* and transmitted by ticks. **Therapeutic fever.** Treatment of disease by the induction of fever, usually by the inoculation of malaria, by the injection of a pyrogenic substance, or by applying external heat. **Thermic fever.** Heat stroke. **Thirst fever.** The feverish state which results from the removal of water from the body in the absence of adequate replacement. Sweating, vomiting, diarrhoea and starvation will cause this disturbed physical state. **Three-day fever.** Sandfly fever (see above). **Threshing fever.** Inflammation of the respiratory tract by dust produced during threshing. **Thyroid fever.** Fever due to a thyrotoxic crisis. **Tick fever.** Relapsing fever; the term is also used for tick typhus. **Tick-bite fever.** Boutonneuse fever (see above). **Tobia fever.** Colombian tick fever, a severe form of typhus. **Traumatic fever.** One following injury. **Trench fever.** An acute, non-fatal, louseborne infection first recognized on many fronts in World War I, and probably caused by a species of *Rickettsia, R. quintana.* The illness resembles mild typhus fever and lasts several days. It did not reappear in World War II to any extent. **Trent Valley fever.** A benign encephalitis associated with a mumps epidemic, but sporadic cases have also appeared. The disease runs a mild febrile course and lasts about 6 days. **Tropical fever.** Malaria. **Trypanosome fever.** Trypanosomiasis. **Tsutsugamushi fever.** Japanese river fever. Asiatic or scrub typhus; caused by *Rickettsia orientalis* and transmitted by *Trombicula akamushi* and other mites. The lesion resembles those seen in house-borne typhus. **Typhoid fever.** The most important member of the enteric group of fevers which also includes the paratyphoids. It is due to the typhoid bacillus or *Salmonella typhi,* which is ingested in contaminated water, milk or foodstuffs. Numerous epidemics have been traced to carriers. The incubation period is usually 12–14 days, the onset of the typical case being insidious, with lassitude, headache, vague pains, constipation *or* diarrhoea and nose-bleeding. The temperature rises progressively and may reach 40°C (104°F) after 1 week. After being maintained at this level for 1-2 weeks, it falls by lysis. At the height of the illness, there may be prostration, muttering delirium, dry tongue, foul mouth and diarrhoea with typical "pea-soup" stools. Rose-coloured spots appear in crops from about the seventh day onwards. The third week is the most critical period, because of exhaustion and dangerous complications including intestinal perforation and haemorrhage. In unfavourable cases, the toxaemia may produce the typhoid state, i.e. extreme prostration, with ashen face, muttering delirium, subsultus tendinum and incontinence of urine and faeces. In uncomplicated cases, the patient improves rapidly during the fourth week. Relapses are fairly common. Aids to diagnosis include blood culture, agglutination and isolation of the bacillus from the stools. Treatment involves good nursing and chloramphenicol which often acts like a specific. Typhoid or TAB vaccine is used in prophylaxis. **Typhoid fever, abenteric.** Typhoid fever in which the intestines are apparently not affected. **Typhoid fever, abortive.** A variety of typhoid fever in which symptoms develop abruptly, but the duration of the disease is cut short. **Typhoid fever, afebrile.** Typhoid fever with the usual symptoms, often quite severe, but with very little or no fever (never above 38°C (100°F). **Typhoid fever, ambulatory.** Typhoid fever so mild that the patient is not confined to bed. **Typhoid fever, apyretic, apyrexial.** Typhoid fever, afebrile (see above). **Typhoid fever, bilious.** A term dating back to the 18th century when fevers were imperfectly differentiated. It seems to have been applied to forms of malaria and relapsing fever but was regarded by some as a transition form between these and typhoid fever. Probably cases of typhus fever, yellow fever or Weil's disease were included. **Typhoid fever, haemorrhagic.** A fatal toxic type with bleeding from mucous membranes and into the skin. **Typhoid fever, Manchurian.** A form of typhus seen in the Russo-Japanese War. **Typhoid fever, provocation.** Typhoid fever brought on, instead of being prevented, by the injection of typhoid vaccine during the incubation period of the disease. **Typhoid fever, subcontinuous.** A typhoid-like fever showing intermittent quiescent phases, occasionally seen in subtertian malaria. **Typhoid fever, sudoral.** Typhoid fever with pronounced sweating and prostration. **Typhoid fever, walking.** Typhoid fever, ambulatory (see above). **Typhomalarial fever.** Malignant malaria with prolonged pyrexia. **Typhus fever.** One of a group of febrile diseases caused by a variety of species of *Rickettsia* and transmitted by a variety of arthropods: the fevers vary in their clinical form and in their severity. *See also* TYPHUS. **Undulant fever.** Brucellosis; Malta and abortus fevers, a disease caused by infection with any of the *Brucella* organisms. It is usually transmitted from animal (cattle, goats) to man, either by close contact or from the ingestion of milk from the infected animal; it is characterized by remittent febrile attacks accompanied by headache, muscular pains and lassitude. **Urban fever.** A vague term, but used to indicate the urban form of tropical typhus usually flea-borne. *See* TYPHUS. **Urethral fever, Urinary fever.** Pyrexia after catheterization. **Uveoparotid fever.** Intermittent pyrexia accompanying enlargement of the salivary glands and inflammation of the uveal tract; a form of sarcoidosis. **Vaccinal fever.** Fever following vaccination. **Valley fever.** Coccidioidomycosis. **Vesicular fever.** Impetigo neonatorum. **Volhynia fever.** Trench fever (see above). **Worm fever.** The rise of temperature due to the presence of worms living a parasitic existence in the body. **West Nile fever.** A mild fever with a rubelliform rash due to a group B arbovirus, similar antigenically to the Japanese B, Murray Valley and St Louis encephalitis viruses. The natural hosts are probably birds with occasional spread to man, in whom the virus causes either a subclinical infection or a mild dengue-like illness. **Wound fever.** Traumatic fever (see above). **Yangtze Valley fever.** Schistosomiasis; infection with *Schistosoma japonicum.* **Yellow fever.** A mosquito-borne infection due to a group B arbovirus. It is characterized by pyrexia, jaundice and a haemorrhagic tendency. It occurs in Africa and Central America in two forms, *sylvan* or *jungle,* where man is rarely involved, and *urban* where man is an important host. **Zinc-fume fever.** Metal-fume fever (see above). [L *febris.*]

See also: CHARCOT, EBSTEIN, HERXHEIMER, JACCOUD, PEL, PFEIFFER (E.), PYM.

feveret (fe·ver·et). 1. Ephemeral fever; febricula. 2. Influenza.

feverish (fe·ver·ish). 1. Suffering from a slight degree of fever. 2. Term applied to any symptom characteristic of or condition characterized by fever. 3. Applied to a locality, term denoting that fever is prevalent.

fexism (fex·izm). A form of cretinism met with in Styria, Austria. [G *Bergfex* alpinist.]

fibraemia (fi·bre·me·ah). 1. A condition in which formed fibrin is present in the blood, the cause of embolism or thrombosis. 2. Inosaemia. [fibrin, Gk *haima* blood.]

fibration (fi·bra·shun). 1. The process of formation of fibres. 2. The system of arrangement of fibres in a structure.

fibre [fibra (NA)] (fi·ber). A long thread composing certain plant and animal tissues. **A fibres.** That group of nerve fibres having the greatest diameter and most rapid rate of impulse propagation, up to 120 m/s. **Accelerator fibres.** Those nerve fibres of the sympathetic nervous system that transmit impulses causing acceleration of the rate of the heart beat and an increase in its force. **Accessory fibre.** A fibre of the zonule of Zinn which does not attach to the lens capsule. **Adrenergic fibre.** Any nerve fibre that liberates an adrenaline-like substance at its termination, i.e.

most postganglionic sympathetic nerve fibres, and probably a number of fibres in the central nervous system also. **Alpha fibre.** The most rapidly conducting member of the A group of nerve fibres (see above); it is myelinated and may be somatic motor or proprioceptive sensory. **Amianthoid fibre.** A peculiar type of fibre seen in degenerating cartilage, resembling an asbestos filament. **Arcuate fibres, anterior external [fibrae arcuatae externae ventrales (NA)].** Fibres said to arise in the lateral part of the nucleus cuneatus, passing ventrally through the medulla to emerge at the anterior median fissure, then sweeping laterally over the surface of the olive to enter the inferior cerebellar peduncle; probably a pathway to the cerebellum for proprioceptive impulses from the upper limb. **Arcuate fibres, internal [fibrae arcuatae internae (NA)].** Fibres arising in the gracile and cuneate nuclei, curving forwards and medially round the central grey matter of the medulla to decussate with those of the upper side, then turning upwards as the medial lemniscus; the main pathway for proprioceptive impulses to the thalamus. **Arcuate fibres, posterior external [fibrae arcuatae externae dorsales (NA)].** Fibres running laterally from the lateral part of the nucleus cuneatus into the interior cerebellar peduncle, carrying proprioceptive impulses from the upper limb. **Argentaffine fibre, Argentophil fibre.** Argyrophil fibre (see foll.). **Argyrophil fibre.** A connective-tissue fibre with a special affinity for silver salts, such as a fine collagen or reticular fibre (see below). **Asbestos fibre.** Amianthoid fibre (see above). **Association fibres [fibrae arcuatae cerebri (NA)].** Fibres connecting ipsilateral gyri. **Augmentor fibres.** Accelerator fibres (see above). **Auxiliary fibre.** Accessory fibre (see above). **Axial fibre.** 1. Axis-cylinder of neurone. 2. Central filament of the tail of spermatozoon. **B fibre.** A myelinated autonomic nerve fibre, with propagation rate from 11 to 17 m/s. **Beta fibre.** A moderately rapidly conducting member of the A group of nerve fibres (see above); it is myelinated, and may be somatic motor, somatic sensory, perhaps from skin, or visceral afferent. **Bone fibre.** A stout collagen fibre running through bone and connected with a tendon or fascia outside the bone. **Bulbospiral fibre.** One of a group of heart-muscle fibres which run a spiral course through the auricles and ventricles. **C fibre.** A fine non-myelinated nerve fibre with propagation rate of about 0.7 m/s. It is generally autonomic, but may also be somatic sensory, carrying pain impulses. **Cerebropontine fibres.** Axons of the primary neurons in the cerebro-ponto-cerebellar tracts, arising in the frontal, temporal and occipital lobes, and terminating in the nuclei pontis. **Cerebrospinal fibres [fibrae corticospinales (NA)].** Fibres from cells in the motor and premotor areas of the cerebral cortex which terminate directly or through an internuncial neuron around the anterior horn cells in the spinal medulla. **Chief fibre.** One of the principal radial fibres of the zonule of Zinn which attaches to the lens capsule. **Cholinergic fibre.** Any nerve fibre that liberates acetylcholine at its termination, i.e. somatic motor nerves, postganglionic parasympathetic, all preganglionic fibres and probably some fibres of the central nervous system. **Chromatic fibre.** The spireme of early mitosis, incorrectly supposed to be a continuous tangled thread composed of all the chromosomes joined end to end. It is now known that the chromosomes are always discrete bodies and that the spireme, in the sense of a continuous thread, does not exist. **Chromosomal fibre.** One of the spindle fibres which is apparently attached to a chromosome in mitosis and appears to draw it towards the aster. **Ciliopostero-capsular fibre.** One of the principal fibres of the zonule of Zinn which passes to the back of the lens capsule. **Climbing fibre of the cerebellum.** The type of afferent fibre which traverses the white matter of the cerebellum via the middle cerebellar peduncle and synapses with dendrites of the Purkinje cells in the cerebellar cortex. **Collagenous fibre.** A basic constituent of the extracellular matrix of connective tissues and forming the chief component of fascias, tendons, ligaments, etc. and an essential in bone and cartilage. It is a white and inelastic fibre, composed of bundles of ultramicroscopic protein filaments, and gives rise to gelatin on boiling. **Collateral fibre.** A side branch from an axis-cylinder, chiefly found in the central nervous system. **Continuous fibre.** One of the spindle fibres in mitosis which pass without interruption from one aster to the other, in contradistinction to the chromosomal fibres (see above). **Corticonuclear fibres [fibrae corticonucleares (NA)].** Fibres from cells in the motor and premotor areas of the cerebral cortex which descend with the cerebrospinal fibres (see above) and terminate around the cells of origin of the efferent (motor) nuclei of the cranial nerves. **Corticoreticular fibres [fibrae corticoreticulares (NA)].** Scattered projection fibres which pass from the cerebral cortex to the reticular formation in the mid-brain, pons and medulla. **Corticostriate fibre.** Any one of the fibres, forming part of the extrapyramidal motor system, which transmit nervous impulses from the premotor area to the corpus striatum. **Corticothalamic fibre.** A fibre which transmits efferent impulses from the cerebral cortex to the thalamus; these fibres are believed to exert control over the thalamic reaction to sensory stimuli. **Dark fibre.** A muscle fibre rich in sarcoplasm, with a dark appearance. **Dendritic fibre.** A fibre which branches in tree-like fashion. **Depressor fibres.** Afferent nerve fibres arising in the heart and great vessels which on stimulation cause inhibition of the vasoconstrictor, and stimulation of the cardio-inhibitory centre, thus resulting in a fall in arterial pressure. **Elastic fibre.** One of the basic constituents of loose connective tissue, elastic cartilage and the dermis of the skin. It is yellowish and highly refractile, runs singly and is branched. **Fibroglia fibre.** One of the fine fuchsinophil fibrils present in the cytoplasm of fibroblasts. **Frontopontine fibres.** Fibres which have their cells of origin in the frontal cortex and terminations around the cells of the nuclei pontis; the upper part of the frontoponto-cerebellar pathway. **Gamma fibre.** The slowest conducting member of the A group of nerve fibres (see above); it is myelinated and may be afferent or efferent. **Geminal fibre.** Name used to describe certain fibres of the pyramidal tract in the spinal cord. Individual fibres are thought to split into two parts, one of which continues on the same side whilst the other crosses to the opposite side. **Grey fibre.** An unmyelinated axon. **Half-spindle fibre.** Chromosomal fibre (see above). **Impulse-conducting fibre.** Better known as *Purkinje fibre*; a primitive or modified muscle fibre lying under the endocardium and conducting the contractile impulse to the heart muscle. **Interciliary fibre.** A fibre of the zonule of Zinn which connects adjacent ciliary processes. **Intercrural fibres of the inguinal canal [fibrae intercrurales (NA)].** Curved fibres in the aponeurosis of the external oblique muscle, just above the apex of the external inguinal ring. **Interzonal fibre.** The central fibre of the spindle in mitosis. **Intrafusal fibre.** One of the fine muscle fibres composing a muscle spindle. **Involuntary-muscle fibre.** A non-striated plain-muscle fibre whose actions are not normally under the control of the will. **Itinerant fibres.** Fibres connecting the cerebral cortex with the lower parts of the brain and the spinal cord; projection fibres. **Lattice fibre.** Argyrophil or reticular fibre (see below). **Fibres of the lens [fibrae lentis (NA)].** Elongated ribbon-like fibres arranged in laminae within the lens. **Light fibre.** A type of striated muscle fibre which has a low content of myohaemoglobin and is therefore relatively transparent. **Main fibre.** Chief fibre (see above). **Mantle fibre.** Chromosomal fibre (see above). **Medullated fibre.** A nerve fibre provided with a myelin sheath. **Moss fibres.** Nerve fibres of the cerebellar cortex which have their origin outside the cerebellum and end in the granular layer. **Muscle fibre.** The unit constituent of muscle, whether voluntary, cardiac or plain. **Myelinated fibre.** Medullated fibre (see above). **Nerve fibre.** The long process of a neuron, usually the axon, but a fused dendrite and axon in the case of the primary sensory neurone. **Non-medullated fibre.** A nerve fibre devoid of a myelin sheath. **Osteo-collagenous fibre.** One of the collagen fibres of bone matrix. **Perforating fibre.** A connective-tissue fibre which passes from the exterior into the cortex of a bone; Sharpey's fibre. **Periventricular fibres [fibrae periventriculares (NA)].** Fine non-medullated fibres which occur dorsally from the posterior hypothalamic region to the tegmentum of the mid-brain; they are believed to be splanchnic motor in nature. **Fibres of the pons, transverse [fibrae pontis transversae (NA)].** Fibres originating in the nuclei pontis and passing into the cerebellum via its middle peduncles; the terminal portion of the corticoponto-cerebellar pathway. **Precollagenous fibre.** Argyrophil or reticular fibre (see below). **Preganglionic fibre.** An axon of the autonomic nervous system which passes from the bulb or spinal cord to a peripheral ganglion. **Pressor fibre.** Any nerve fibre, afferent or efferent, that on stimulation causes a contraction of the arterioles and a rise in arterial pressure. **Principal fibre.** Chief fibre (see above). **Projection fibres.** Itinerant fibres (see above). **Pyramidal fibres.** The corticospinal fibres which decussate in the midline of the lower part of the medulla oblongata and enter the lateral corticospinal tract. **Reticular fibre.** One of the very fine argyrophil fibres (see above) of young connective tissue and of the supporting tissue of lymphoid and myeloid tissue. **Rivet fibre.** One of the processes of the basal end of an epithelial cell which helps to anchor it to the underlying connective tissue. **Secretomotor fibre, Secretory fibre.** An axon of the autonomic nervous system which ends in a gland and causes it to secrete. **Spindle fibre.** One of the elements composing the achromatic spindle visible during cell division. **Spiral fibre.** Bulbospiral fibre (see above). **T fibre.** A collateral coming off at right angles from the parent axon. **Thalamocortical fibres.** Fibres passing from the thalamus to the cerebral cortex. **Traction fibre.** Chromosomal fibre (see above). **Ultraterminal fibre.** A fine branch arising from the terminal ramification of a motor nerve at the muscle end-plate. **Varicose fibre.** An axon with a beaded appearance, either as a normal condition or as a result of degenerative changes. **Vasoconstrictor fibre.** A nerve fibre, usually sympathetic, which when stimulated causes constriction of the arterioles and capillaries to which it is supplied. Presumably this is effected by release of adrenaline at the nerve-endings. **Vasodilator fibre.** A nerve fibre, often parasympathetic, but sometimes sympathetic, which when stimulated causes dilatation of the arterioles and possibly of the capillaries to which it is supplied. This is probably effected by release of acetylcholine at the nerve-endings. **White fibre.** Collagenous fibre (see above). **Yellow fibre.** Elastic fibre (see above). **Zonular fibres of the ciliary zonule [fibrae zonulares (NA)].** The fibres passing from the ciliary body to the lens, collected mainly into posterior layers enclosing a canal, triangular in cross-section. [L *fibra*.]

See also: BEALE, BERGMANN (E.), BERNHEIMER, BOGROW, BURDACH, CORTI, DARKSHEVICH, DICKEY (J. S.), GERDY, GOTTSTEIN, GRATIOLET, HELIE, HENLE, HERXHEIMER, KORFF, MEYNERT, MUELLER (H.), MUMMERY, NÉLATION, PRUSSAK, PURKINJE, REISSNER, REMAK (R.), RETZIUS (A. A.), RITTER (J. W.), SAPPEY, SCHROEDER VAN DER KOLK, SHARPEY, STILLING, TOMES (J.), WEISMANN, WEITBRECHT, WERNICKE (K.).

fibriform (fi·bre·form). Like a fibre in shape. [fibre, form.]

fibril, fibrilla (fi·bril, fi·bril·ah). A fine fibre. **Achromatic fibril.** One of the constituent fibres of the mitotic spindle. **Chromatic fibril.** A prophase chromosome. **Collagen fibril.** One of the very fine fibres which compose a collagen fibre proper. **Dentinal fibril.** One of the collagenous fibrils composing the matrix of dentine, not to be confused with the dentinal fibre, which is a process of an odontoblast. **Fibroglia fibril.** One of the fine fibrils in the cytoplasm of a connective-tissue cell. **Muscle fibril, Muscular fibril.** One of the fine fibrils running longitudinally in a muscle fibre. **Nerve fibril.** A neurofibril; one of the numerous filaments observed in the cytoplasm of nerve cells after certain types of fixation. **Nuclear fibril.** Chromatic fibril (see above). [L *fibrilla* small fibre.]

See also: DIRCK, EBNER, GOLGI, TOMES (J.).

fibrillar, fibrillary (fi·bril·ar, fi·bril·ar·e). Relating or belonging to one or more fibrils, or affecting them.

fibrillated (fi·bril·a·ted). 1. Fibrous in structure. 2. Composed of fibrils. 3. Fringed.

fibrillation (fi·bril·a·shun). 1. The condition of being fibrillar or fibrillated. 2. Spontaneous contraction of individual muscle fibres; a sign of denervation. **Atrial fibrillation.** A common disorder of cardiac rhythm in which the atria undergo a continuous process of inco-ordinate multifocal activity. The process, once initiated, is usually self-sustaining. The mechanism of the fibrillation process is uncertain but is possibly the development of multiple irregular re-entry circuits within the atrial myocardium. The atrioventricular node is bombarded by very frequent impulses, some of which are irregularly transmitted to the ventricles resulting in an irregular pulse, usually at a fast rate in the untreated patient. It is most common in patients with mitral valve disease but it also occurs in many other forms of heart disease and may occur paroxysmally with hyperthyroidism. **Auricular fibrillation.** Atrial fibrillation (see above). **Flutter fibrillation.** A type of atrial fibrillation where the irregular contractions of the atrium resemble those seen in atrial flutter. **Ventricular fibrillation.** The condition in which continuing inco-ordinate multifocal activity of the ventricles takes the place of regular co-ordinated contractions. It results in circulatory arrest and thereby is a common immediate cause of death. It is most frequently the consequence of myocardial hypoxia. [L *fibrilla* small fibre.]

fibrilloblast (fi·**bril**·o·blast). Odontoblast. [fibril, Gk *blastos* germ.]

fibrillolysis (fi·bril·**ol**·is·is). The process of destruction of fibrils by breaking up, dissolution or other means. [fibril, lysis.]

fibrillolytic (fi·bril·o·**lit'**·ik). Having the power to dissolve or otherwise destroy fibrils. [see prec.]

fibrin (**fi**·brin). An insoluble protein formed from the soluble protein of blood-plasma fibrinogen by the action of the enzyme, thrombin. The formation of fibrin is the fundamental process of the clotting of blood. **Canalized fibrin.** A stratified deposit of a fibrin-like material upon and within degenerate placental villi. **Myosin fibrin.** The insoluble form of myosin formed in salt solution or in water on standing. **Stroma fibrin.** Fibrin obtained from lysed erythrocytes. [L *fibra* fibre.]

fibrinaemia (fi·brin·**e**·me·ah). Fibraemia.

fibrination (fi·brin·**a**·shun). The process of acquiring an excess of fibrin or the condition of having it.

fibrinocellular (**fi**·brin·o·**sel'**·ew·lar). Composed of fibrin and cells, as certain exudates.

fibrinogen (fi·**brin**·o·jen). A soluble protein of the globulin class which occurs in blood plasma and is converted into an insoluble protein, fibrin, in the clotting process. **Dried Human Fibrinogen BP 1973.** A dried preparation of the soluble protein of liquid blood plasma, which is formed into fibrin by the addition of human thrombin. [fibrin, Gk *genein* to produce.]

fibrinogenaemia (fi·**brin**·o·jen·e'·me·ah). Excessive blood fibrinogen. [fibrinogen, Gk *haima* blood.]

fibrinogenase (fi·brin·**oj**·en·aze). An enzyme which hydrolyses fibrinogen.

fibrinogenic (**fi**·brin·o·**jen'**·ik). 1. Referring to fibrinogen. 2. Fibrinogenous.

fibrinogenopenia (fi·**brin**·o·jen·o·**pe'**·ne·ah). A condition in which the blood contains an abnormally small quantity of fibrinogen. [fibrinogen, Gk *penes* poor.]

fibrinogenous (fi·brin·**oj**·en·us). 1. Able to form fibrin. 2. Having the characteristics of or having properties similar to those of fibrinogen. [fibrin, Gk *genein* to produce.]

fibrinoglobulin (**fi**·brin·o·**glob'**·ew·lin). A fibrin globulin combination.

fibrinoid (**fi**·brin·oid). A material having many of the staining properties of fibrin, found in degenerate parts of the placenta, especially in the chorionic and decidual plates. It is probably derived from the maternal blood. **Canalized fibrinoid.** Stratified fibrinoid found in the placenta in the latter half of pregnancy, the spaces between individual strata appearing as canals in histological sections. [fibrin, Gk *eidos* form.]

fibrinolysin (fi·brin·**ol**·is·in). An enzyme formed after death and rendering fluid the blood clot formed in the body either within the blood vessels or in the tissues. [L *fibra* fibre, Gk *lysein* to loosen.]

fibrinolysis (fi·brin·**ol**·is·is). The partial decomposition or dissolution of fibrin by the action of fibrinolysin.

fibrinolytic (fi·brin·o·**lit'**·ik). Able to dissolve or split up fibrin. [fibrin, lysis.]

fibrinopenia (**fi**·brin·o·**pe'**·ne·ah). Fibrinogenopenia. **Hereditary fibrinopenia.** A familial hereditary condition in which there is a deficiency of fibrinogen in the blood, and consequently a deficiency of fibrin formation leading to impaired blood clotting. [fibrin, Gk *penes* poor.]

fibrinoplastic (**fi**·brin·o·**plas'**·tik). Resembling fibrinoplastin.

fibrinoplastin (**fi**·brin·o·**plas'**·tin). A globulin present in blood serum, cells, lymph and other body tissues. [fibrin, plastin.]

See also: SCHMIDT (A.).

fibrinopurulent (fi·brin·o·**pewr'**·ew·lent). Composed of fibrin which contains pus.

fibrinorrhoea plastica (fi·brin·o·**re'**·ah **plas**·tik·ah). Membranous dysmenorrhoea. *See* DYSMENORRHOEA. [fibrin, Gk *rhoia* flow, *plastikos* a forming.]

fibrinoscopy (fi·brin·**os**·ko·pe). Diagnosis of the presence of disease or of micro-organisms by dissolving in a pepsin digestive mixture the fibrinous elements in any of the body fluids. [fibrin, Gk *skopein* to watch.]

fibrinose (**fi**·brin·oze). An albuminose derivative of fibrin.

fibrinosis (fi·brin·o·sis). A diseased condition in which there is an excessive quantity of fibrin in the circulating blood. [fibrin, Gk *-osis* condition.]

fibrinous (**fi**·brin·us). Having the properties of or containing fibrin.

fibrinuria (fi·brin·**ewr**·e·ah). The presence of fibrin in the urine.

fibro-adenia (**fi**·bro·ad·**e'**·ne·ah). Fibrous degeneration of a gland or of gland tissue, as in splenic anaemia; e.g. in Banti's disease, increase in the stroma of the lymphatic nodules of the spleen and reduction in the number of lymphocytes. [fibre, Gk *aden* gland.]

fibro-adenoma (**fi**·bro·ad·en·**o'**·mah). An adenoma in which there is dense formation of fibrous tissue. **Intracanalicular fibro-adenoma.** A fibro-adenoma of the breast in which the fibrous tissue encroaches on the glandular adenomatous portions, converting it into slit-like structures. **Pericanalicular fibro-adenoma.** A fibro-adenoma of the breast in which the fibrous tissue forms concentric rings around the glandular portion, without distorting the lumina.

fibro-adenosis (**fi**·bro·ad·en·**o'**·sis). A common paraphysiological condition of the breast in which there is a diffuse non-neoplastic proliferation of fibrous and epithelial elements. A histological change and usually not detectable clinically since it is symptomless and gives no physical signs. [fibro-adenoma, Gk *-osis* condition.]

fibro-adipose (fi·bro·**ad**·ip·oze). Containing or relating to tissues which are both fibrous and fatty. [fibre, adipose.]

fibro-angioma (**fi**·bro·an·je·**o'**·mah). An angioma in which a considerable quantity of fibrous tissue is present.

fibro-areolar (**fi**·bro·ar·**e'**·o·lar). Indicating connective tissues which are fibrous as well as areolar.

fibroblast (**fi**·bro·blast). The common connective-tissue cell; flat and irregular in outline with a large oval nucleus and a granular, lightly-staining cytoplasm. [fibre, Gk *blastos* germ.]

fibroblastic (fi·bro·**blas**·tik). 1. Relating to or belonging to fibroblasts. 2. Fibroplastic.

fibroblastoma (fi·bro·blas·**to'**·mah). A tumour having its origin in the cells of connective tissues, e.g. fibroma. **Arachnoid fibroblastoma.** Meningioma. **Perineural fibroblastoma.** A fibroma arising in the connective sheath or perineurium of a nerve. [fibre, blastoma.]

fibrobronchitis (**fi**·bro·brong·**ki'**·tis). Fibrinous bronchitis, in which the sputum contains fibrinous casts.

fibrocalcareous (**fi**·bro·kal·**ka'**·re·us). Indicating a fibroma or a fibrous tumour in which calcareous degeneration has taken place.

fibrocarcinoma (fi·bro·kar·sin·**o'**·mah). Carcinoma in which there is a considerable amount of fibrous tissue.

fibrocartilage [fibrocartilago (NA)] (fi·bro·**kar**·til·ij). A firm but resilient tissue composed of bundles of white fibrous tissue interspersed with islands of cartilage cells surrounded by relatively sparse cartilage matrix. **Interarticular fibrocartilage [meniscus articularis (NA)].** A disc-like structure interposed between the articulating surfaces of certain joints. **Intervertebral fibrocartilage.** The intervertebral disc between the bodies of adjacent vertebrae. **Semilunar fibrocartilage.** One of the interarticular fibrocartilages (menisci) of the knee joint.

fibrocartilaginous (**fi**·bro·kar·til·**aj'**·in·us). 1. Relating to fibrocartilage. 2. Containing or made up of fibrocartilage.

fibrocaseose (fi·bro·**ka**·se·oze). Describing matter that is cheesy or curd-like as well as fibrous. [fibre, L *caseus* cheese.]

fibrocellular (fi·bro·**sel**·ew·lar). Having both fibrous and cellular elements.

fibrochondritis (**fi**·bro·kon·**dri'**·tis). An inflamed condition of fibrocartilage. [fibre, chondritis.]

fibrochondroma (**fi**·bro·kon·**dro'**·mah). A combined fibroma and chondroma, i.e. a tumour composed of mixed fibrous and cartilaginous tissue.

fibrocyst (**fi**·bro·sist). A cystic fibroma.

fibrocystic (fi·bro·**sist**·ik). 1. Referring to a cystic fibroma. 2. Fibrous primarily and subsequently affected with cystic degeneration.

fibrocystoid (fi·bro·**sist**·oid). Like a cystic fibroma in pattern. [fibrocyst, Gk *eidos* form.]

fibrocystoma (**fi**·bro·sist·**o'**·mah). A neoplasm in which there are fibromatous and cystomatous elements; a fibrocystic tumour.

fibrocyte (**fi**·bro·site). Fibroblast. [fibre, Gk *kytos* cell.]

fibrocytogenesis (**fi**·bro·si·to·**jen'**·es·is). The formation and development of fibrils of connective tissue. [fibrocyte, Gk *genein* to produce.]

fibrodysplasia (**fi**·bro·**dis**·pla·ze·ah). **Fibrodysplasia ossificans progressiva.** Myositis ossificans progressiva. [fibre, dysplasia.]

fibro-elastic (**fi**·bro·e·**las'**·tik). Term applied to a tumour that is composed of both fibrous tissue and elastic tissue.

fibro-elastosis (**fi**·bro·e·las·**to'**·sis). Proliferation of fibrous and elastic tissue. **Endocardial fibro-elastosis.** A developmental fibrosis accompanied by proliferation of elastic fibres under the endocardium of the ventricles of the heart, and revealing itself by disordered heart action in infancy or sudden death in the first or second decade. [fibre, elastic, Gk *-osis* condition.]

fibro-enchondroma (**fi**·bro·en·kon·**dro'**·mah). An enchondroma with fibromatous elements.

fibrofibrous (fi·bro·**fi**·brus). Connecting or joining one fibre with another, or one bundle of fibres with another.

fibroglia (fi·**brog**·le·ah). The supporting tissue of fibroblasts corresponding to the neuroglia of neuroblasts; inoglia. [fibre, Gk *glia* glue.]

fibroglioma (**fi**·bro·gli·**o'**·mah). A tumour of which the elements are those of both glioma and fibroma.

fibrogranuloma (**fi**·bro·gran·ew·**lo'**·mah). A fibrosing granuloma.

fibrohaemorrhagic (**fi**·bro·hem·or·**aj'**·ik). Characterized by or referring to haemorrhage and the formation of fibrin.

fibroid (**fi**·broid). 1. Resembling fibrous tissue or a fibrous structure. 2. A fibroma, myoma, fibromyoma or leiomyofibroma especially of the uterus. [fibre, Gk *eidos* form.]

See also: PAGET.

fibroidectomy (fi·broid·**ek**·to·me). Surgical removal of a fibrous tumour, more especially of a fibromyoma from the uterus or its accessory structures. [fibroid, Gk *ektome* a cutting out.]

fibrolaminar (fi·bro·**lam**·in·ar). Relating to a layer of fibrous tissue. [fibre, lamina.]

fibroleiomyoma (**fi**·bro·li·o·mi·**o'**·mah). Leiomyofibroma.

fibrolipoma (**fi**·bro·lip·**o'**·mah). A fibrous neoplasm containing fatty elements. [fibre, lipoma.]

fibrolipomatous (**fi**·bro·lip·**o'**·mat·us). Belonging or relating to fibrolipoma, or having the characteristics of a fibrolipoma.

fibrolymphangioblastoma (**fi**·bro·lim·**fan**·je·o·bas·**to'**·mah). Fibrosing lymphangioma; a cellular lymphangioma in which much fibrous tissue develops, often with replacement of the tumour by scar tissue. [fibre, lymphangioma, blastoma.]

fibroma (fi·**bro**·mah) (pl. *fibromata*). An innocent tumour composed chiefly of connective tissue. **Ameloblastic fibroma.**

An odontome consisting of a circumscribed mass of fibromyxomatous tissue containing islands of ameloblastic epithelium. **Aponeurotic fibroma.** Juvenile palmoplantar fibromatosis. **Fibroma cavernosum.** A fibroma rich in blood vessels or lymphatics, with a honeycomb appearance. **Fibroma of the choroid.** Fibrosis choroideae corrugans. **Concentric fibroma.** A leiomyofibroma encircling the uterine cavity. **Fibroma cutis.** A fibroma of the skin. **Cystic fibroma.** A fibroma rich in lymphatics, some of which have fused to form cysts, or are undergoing central softening to form cysts. **Fibroma durum.** A fibroma composed of dense mature fibrous tissue, which grows very slowly. **Fibroma ematodes cysticum.** A cystic fibrous polyp of the nose. **Fibroma fungoides.** A fibroma of exuberant growth projecting from a surface or into a cavity. **Hard fibroma.** Fibroma durum (see above). **Intracanalicular fibroma.** A fibroadenoma of the breast in which fibrous tissue obliterates the lumen of the ducts or distorts them into narrow slits. **Fibroma lipoidicum, Fibroma lipomatodes.** Xanthoma tuberosum. **Fibroma molle.** A fibroma composed of loose oedematous newly-formed fibrous tissue, which grows fairly rapidly. **Fibroma molluscum.** A benign neurofibroma. **Fibroma mucinosum.** Myxofibroma, a fibroma very rich in mucoid material. **Multiple fibroma.** Neurofibromatosis. **Fibroma myxomatodes.** A complex benign tumour of mucoid and fibrous tissue. **Non-osteogenic fibroma (of bone).** A fibromatous deposit in bone usually seen as an eccentrically-placed cystic lesion. **Odontogenic fibroma.** A rare soft tumour occurring around the root of a tooth, composed mainly of fibroblasts derived from the tooth follicle. **Papillary fibroma.** A stalked fibroma which projects from a surface or into a cavity. **Parasitic fibroma.** Originally a subserous, pedunculated leiomyofibroma which becomes separated from the uterus and attached to other abdominal organs from which it obtains its blood supply. **Fibroma pendulum.** A pedunculated fibroma. **Perineural fibroma.** Neurofibroma. **Periungual fibroma.** Smooth, firm excrescences protruding from the nail fold in tuberous sclerosis. **Fibroma sarcomatosum.** A sarcoma arising in a fibroma. **Sclerotic fibroma.** Fibroma durum (see above). **Fibroma simplex.** Histiocytoma. **Soft fibroma.** Fibroma molle (see above). **Submucous fibroma.** A fibroma arising in the submucous coat of the stomach or intestine. **Subperitoneal fibroma.** A fibroma arising in the subserous tissue of the peritoneum. **Telangiectatic fibroma.** A fibroma in which blood vessels, especially veins, are prominent and dilated. **Fibroma thecocellulare xanthomatodes.** A theca-cell tumour of the ovary. **Fibroma xanthoma.** Xanthoma tuberosum. [L *fibra* fibre, Gk *-oma* tumour.]

fibromatogenic (fi·**bro**·mat·o·**jen′**·ik). Causing the formation of or producing fibromata. [fibroma, Gk *genein* to produce.]

fibromatoid (fi·**bro**·mat·oid). 1. Resembling a fibroma. 2. Descriptive of a neoplasm composed mainly of fibrous tissue, either without a capsule at all or with only a part of one. [fibroma, Gk *eidos* form.]

fibromatosis (fi·bro·mat·**o′**·sis). A diffuse or nodular, cellular and collagenous proliferation found in the palmar fascia, the plantar fascia and in the limb. The proliferating fibrous tissue is non-encapsulated and may be difficult to distinguish from a fibrosarcoma. **Congenital generalized fibromatosis.** Fibroblastic nodules occurring in the subcutis, myocardium, lungs, liver and intestines. **Gingival fibromatosis.** A genetically-determined condition, with hypertrichosis. **Fibromatosis osteoplastica osseum.** Leontiasis ossea. **Palmoplantar fibromatosis.** A unilateral condition occurring in children sometimes malignant and necessitating wide excision. **Plantar fibromatosis.** Dupuytren's contraction. **Pseudosarcomatous subcutaneous fibromatosis.** Nodular fasciitis. *See* FASCIITIS. **Radiation fibromatosis.** A diffuse fibrous proliferation following x-irradiation, resembling fibrosarcoma from which it has to be differentiated clinically and histologically. **Fibromatosis ventriculi.** Cirrhosis ventriculi; linitis plastica. [fibroma, Gk *-osis* condition.]

fibromatous (fi·**bro**·mat·us). Relating or belonging to, or having the character of fibroma.

fibromectomy (fi·bro·**mek**·to·me). Surgical removal of a fibroma, particularly of a fibromyoma from the uterus or its surrounding structures. [fibroma, Gk *ektome* a cutting out.]

fibromembranous (fi·bro·**mem**·bran·us). Term applied to any membranous structure of which fibrous tissue forms a large part.

fibromucous (fi·bro·**mew**·kus). Descriptive of a growth the component parts of which are fibrous and mucosal.

fibromuscular (fi·bro·**mus**·kew·lar). Relating to or consisting of both fibrous and muscular tissues.

fibromyectomy (fi·bro·mi·**ek′**·to·me). Fibromyomectomy.

fibromyitis (fi·bro·mi·**i′**·tis). A condition of inflammation of a muscle resulting in its fibrous degeneration; fibromyositis. [fibre, Gk *mys* muscle, *-itis* inflammation.]

fibromyoma (fi·bro·mi·**o′**·mah). A neoplasm made up of fibrous and muscular tissue. [fibre, myoma.]

fibromyomectomy, fibromyomotomy (fi·bro·mi·o·**mek′**·to·me, fi·bro·mi·o·**mot′**·o·me). Surgical removal of a fibromyoma. [fibromyoma, Gk *ektome* a cutting out.]

fibromyositis (fi·bro·mi·o·**si′**·tis). An inflamed condition of muscular tissue. **Nodular fibromyositis.** Inflammation of muscular tissue in which there is characteristic development of nodules. [fibre, myositis.]

fibromyotomy (fi·bro·mi·**ot′**·o·me). Fibromyomectomy.

fibromyxolipoma (fi·bro·mix·o·lip·**o′**·mah). A mixed tumour composed of fat, fibrous and mucoid tissue. It is commonly found in the skin and fatty subcutaneous tissue. [fibre, Gk *myxa* mucus, lipoma.]

fibromyxoma (fi·bro·mix·**o′**·mah). A tumour which is a combined fibroma and myxoma.

fibromyxosarcoma (fi·bro·mix·o·sar·**ko′**·mah). 1. A myxosarcoma containing fibrous tissue. 2. A sarcoma which has become fasciculated and undergone myxoid degeneration.

fibroneuroma (fi·bro·newr·**o′**·mah). A tumour in which fibrous tissue is combined with nerve cells and fibres. [fibre, neuroma.]

fibroneurosarcoma (fi·bro·newr·o·sar·**ko′**·mah). Fibrosing neuroblastoma; a cellular and more rapidly growing variety of neurofibroma. [fibre, neurosarcoma.]

fibronuclear, fibronucleated (fi·bro·**new**·kle·ar, fi·bro·**new**·kle·a·ted). Relating to or descriptive of tissue composed of nucleated fibres.

fibro-osteoma (fi·bro·os·te·**o′**·mah). Osteofibroma; a tumour made up of bony and fibrous tissue. [fibre, osteoma.]

fibropapilloma (fi·bro·pap·il·**o′**·mah). A papilloma in which there is a considerable quantity of fibrous tissue; it is found occasionally in the urinary bladder.

fibropericarditis (fi·bro·per·e·kar·**di′**·tis). Fibrinous pericarditis, a type of pericarditis in which there are fibrous adhesions.

fibroplasia (fi·bro·**pla**·ze·ah). The forming of fibrous tissue such as occurs, for instance, in wound healing. **Retrolental fibroplasia.** Fibrosis of the retina, perhaps with detachment, and structure anterior to it, occurring in premature babies who have been given too much oxygen. [fibre, Gk *plassein* to form.]

fibroplastic (fi·bro·**plas**·tik). Producing or giving rise to fibres or fibrous tissue. [see prec.]

fibroplastin (fi·bro·**plas**·tin). Fibrinoplastin.

fibroplate (fi·bro·plate). An interarticular disc of fibrocartilage. [fibre, plate.]

fibropolypus (fi·bro·**pol**·e·pus). A polypus composed mainly of fibrous tissue.

fibropsammoma (fi·bro·sam·**o′**·mah). A new growth in which fibromatous and psammomatous elements are mixed.

fibropurulent (fi·bro·**pewr**·ew·lent). Applied to a discharge consisting of pus in which flakes of fibrin are present. [fibrin, L *purulentus* purulent.]

fibroreticulate (fi·bro·ret·**ik′**·ew·late). Relating to or characterized by a network of fibrous tissue. [fibre, L *reticula* little net.]

fibrosarcoma (fi·bro·sar·**ko′**·mah). A fibrous tumour in which there are a considerable number of imperfectly differentiated elements and cells of fibrous and sarcomatous nature. **Mucocellular fibrosarcoma, Fibrosarcoma ovarii mucocellulare carcinomatodes.** Krukenberg's tumour.

fibrose (fi·broze). 1. Fibrous. 2. To produce or form fibrous tissue.

fibroserous (fi·bro·seer·us). Denoting a membrane, such as the pericardium, which is composed of fibrous tissue with a serous lining.

fibrosis (fi·bro·sis). Sclerosis; cirrhosis: the development of fibrous tissue in a part or an organ. **Arteriocapillary fibrosis.** Chronic inflammation of the endothelium of small arterioles and capillaries, causing fibrosis and narrowing of the lumen, and finally occlusion by thrombosis (endarteritis obliterans). It occurs especially in syphilitic and tuberculous lesions. **Cardiac fibrosis.** Myocardial fibrosis (see below). **Fibrosis chorioideae corrugans.** The formation of a thick layer of fibrous tissue in the suprachoroid lamina following an attack of choroiditis; on contraction this throws the choroid into folds. It is also called *fibroma of the choroid.* **Condensation fibrosis.** The showing-up of fibrous tissue in an organ through disappearance of the parenchyma, and resulting in a false impression of proliferative fibrosis (see below). **Cystic fibrosis.** Fibrocystic disease of the pancreas. *See* DISEASE. **Endocardial fibrosis.** Thickening of the myocardium by fibrous tissue. **Endomyocardial fibrosis (EMF).** A condition described mainly from Africa, commonest in the second and third decades. Fibrosis of subendocardial myocardium is accompanied by gross thickening of the endocardium. Starting at the apex of either ventricle, it slowly eliminates the ventricular cavity and often causes shortening of the papillary muscles of the tricuspid or mitral valves and terminates in obstructive cardiac failure. The aetiology remains uncertain. **Hepatolienal fibrosis, Hepatosplenic fibrosis.** Displacement of the parenchyma cells of the liver and spleen by fibrous tissue. **Myocardial fibrosis.** Fibrosis of the myocardium, either as a result of previous acute inflammation, or as a result of ischaemia due to disease of the coronary arteries or prolonged severe anaemia. It may also occur in certain cardiopathies, or as a result of prolonged congestive heart failure. **Neoplastic fibrosis.** The fibrosis which develops as a response to the growth of tumour cells in a part. **Nodular subepidermal fibrosis.** Dermatofibroma verum histiocytoma; fibroma durum; fibroma simplex (Unna); noduli cutanei (Arning and Lewandowsky); dermatofibroma lenticulare (Schreus); fibroma en pastille (Civatte); histiocytoma (Woringer); sclerosing haemangioma (Gross and Wolbach): a cutaneous affection usually characterized by the formation of a single nodule, although multiple discrete and scattered lesions may be noted. Probably arising at the site of trauma or inflammation, a typical nodule is formed of spindle cells, fibroblasts and strands of collagen, occupying the upper two-thirds of the cutis and adherent to the overlying epidermis, but not invading the subcutaneous tissue and not attached to the deep fascia. When first noted the lesion may be a few millimetres in diameter, but may increase in size to one or more centimetres; occasionally it is pedunculated. The colour varies from the normal flesh tint to yellow, brown, red or bluish-black, and the overlying epidermis may appear atrophic and scaly, or smooth and round. The surface may be flat or conical. **Oral submucous fibrosis.** The formation of inelastic fibrous bands in the oral submucosa, leading to progressive extra-articular ankylosis of the mandible. Found principally in India and attributed to chewing the betel quid (*Pan supari*) or eating chillies. **Panmural fibrosis.** Fibrous-tissue replacement of the components of a complex structure, such as the pancarditis of rheumatism. **Postfibrinous fibrosis.** Replacement of fibrinous adhesions by fibrous tissue during healing, as in adhesion formation in pleurisy. **Proliferative fibrosis.** New formation of fibrous tissue in an organ through proliferation of connective-tissue cells. **Pulmonary fibrosis.** Fibrosis of the lungs, occurring as a sequel to any inflammatory or irritative process, such as the bronchopneumonias, chronic tuberculosis, the pneumoconioses. Localized fibrosis occurs with abscesses, bronchiectasis, infarction and similar conditions of local damage. **Renal fibrosis.** Increase of the interstitial tissue of the kidneys which occurs as a sequel to nephritis, diffuse hyperplastic sclerosis or senile atherosclerosis. **Replacement fibrosis.** Replacement of the specialized parenchyma of an organ by fibrous tissue. **Retroperitoneal idiopathic fibrosis.** Fibrosis of unknown origin causing compression of great vessels and, sometimes, renal obstruction. **Fibrosis uteri.** A condition of the uterus in which there is an undue proportion of fibrous tissue. [fibre, Gk *-osis* condition.]

fibrositis (fi·bro·si·tis). A form of non-articular rheumatism in which there are inflammatory changes in the fibrous tissues, causing pain and difficulty in movement. The subcutaneous tissue and fat, the muscle sheaths, the fibrous portions of joints, and the perineurium are the structures principally involved. **Subcutaneous fibrositis.** An inflamed condition of the thin fascia immediately underlying the skin. [fibre, Gk *-itis* inflammation.]

fibrotic (fi·brot·ik). Relating or belonging to fibrosis, or characterized by the presence of fibrosis.

fibrotuberculoma (fi·bro·tew·ber·kew·lo′·mah). A fibrosing tuberculoma. **Laryngeal fibrotuberculoma.** A fibrosing tuberculoma of the larynx.

fibrotuberculosis (fi·bro·tew·ber·kew·lo′·sis). Fibroid tuberculosis, one of the clinically distinguishable forms of pulmonary tuberculosis; fibroid phthisis.

fibrous (fi·brus). Composed of or characterized by the presence of fibres; like or of the nature of fibre.

fibroxanthoma (fi·bro·zan·tho′·mah). Fibroma lipomatodes; a brownish-yellow tumour composed of cells rich in lipoid globules. It is common in the eyelids, but also occurs in multiple form in other regions; one form is frequent in diabetes mellitus. [fibroma, xanthoma.]

fibula [NA] (fib·ew·lah). The slender lateral bone of the leg, the homologue of the ulna in the arm. [L clasp.]

head [caput fibulae (NA)]. The proximal extremity of the fibula. It bears a facet [facies articularis capitis fibulae (NA)] for articulation with the tibia.

shaft [corpus fibulae (NA)]. The main part of the bone supporting the upper and lower end. It is slender and appears twisted. It has three borders, anterior [margo anterior (NA)], posterior [margo posterior (NA)] and interosseous [margo interossea (NA)], and three surfaces, posterior, anterior and lateral. The interosseous border is adjacent to the tibia and gives attachment to the interosseous membrane. A sharp ridge, the medial crest [crista medialis (NA)], branches off from the lowest third of the medial side of the posterior border and extends upwards the length of the shaft. The anterior border ends below at the apex of a relatively smooth, subcutaneous triangular area.

anterior surface [facies medialis (NA)]. That which affords origin to the extensor muscles of the toes and the peroneous tertius muscle.

lateral surface [facies lateralis (NA)]. That which affords origin to the peroneus longus and brevis muscles.

posterior surface [facies posterior (NA)]. That which gives origin to the soleus muscle above and flexor hallucis longus muscle below.

fibula, nutrient artery to the. A branch of the peroneal artery to the fibula.

fibular [fibularis (NA)] (fib·ew·lar). 1. Relating or belonging to the fibula. 2. Relating or belonging to the lateral side of the leg. **Fibular notch.** *See* NOTCH.

fibulation (fib·ew·la·shun). Infibulation.

fibulocalcaneal (fib·ew·lo·kal·ka′·ne·al). Of or pertaining to the fibula and calcaneum.

ficaria (fik·a·re·ah). Pilewort, lesser celandine; the fresh herb *Ranunculus ficaria* Linn. (family Ranunculaceae), a common British perennial plant used in the form of an ointment or as suppositories in the treatment of haemorrhoids. [L *ficus* fig.]

Fich's axes. Axes of the eyeball: X, the horizontal or frontal axis; Y, the sagittal axis; Z, the vertical axis.

Fichera, Gaetano (b. 1880). Italian pathologist.

Fichera's treatment. The use of hypodermic injections of autolysed human fetal tissue in cancer.

ficiform (fi·se·form). Shaped like a fig. [L *ficus* fig, form.]

ficin (fi·sin). The sap of the fig tree. It is used as an anthelminthic, as it contains an enzyme which digests the parasites; especially effective in cases of infection by *Trichuris*. Used in blood group serology to treat red cells after which they can be agglutinated in saline suspensions by blocking antibodies. [L *ficus* fig.]

Fick, Adolf Eugen (b. 1829). German physiologist.

Fick's principle. The amount of a substance (or indicator) taken up or given off by an organ (or by the whole body) per unit of time equals the difference between the arterial and venous concentration of the substance multiplied by the blood flow. (Fick originally applied it to the O_2 consumption and the A-V O_2 content difference, as a means of measuring cardiac output. However, all indicator dilution methods for measuring the cardiac output are based on the same principle.)

Fick's law of diffusion. The rate at which the molecules of a solute diffuse through a liquid solvent is proportional to the concentration of the former.

Ficker, Martin (b. 1868). Berlin bacteriologist.

Ficker's reaction. An obsolete name for the agglutination of typhoid bacilli by the patient's serum in typhoid fever.

Fickling, Benjamin. 20th century London oral surgeon.

Fickling's "inkwell" repair of oro-antral fistulae. The fistulous tract is incised free from the oral mucosa and inverted into the antrum with a purse-string suture; a buccal flap is then extended over this area for complete closure.

ficosis (fi·ko·sis). Coccogenic sycosis barbae. [L *ficus* fig, Gk *-osis* condition.]

Ficus (fi·kus). 1. A genus of trees, including the fig tree. 2. Fig BPC 1959. [L fig.]

fidicinales (fid·is·in·a′·leez). The lumbrical muscles of the fingers. [L *fides* a lute, referring to the muscles used in playing it or other stringed instruments.]

fiebre (fe·eb·re). Fever. **Fiebre amarilla.** Yellow fever. *See* FEVER. [Sp.]

Fiedler, Carl Ludwig Alfred (b. 1835). Dresden physician.

Fiedler's disease. Leptospiral jaundice. *See* JAUNDICE.

Fiedler's myocarditis. Acute isolated myocarditis, an acute or subacute interstitial myocarditis characterized by widespread infiltration of the interstitial tissue with leucocytes, particularly mononuclear cells, and degenerative changes in the muscle fibres. It is of unknown aetiology.

field (feeld). 1. A limited area. 2. In embryology, the territory of influence of an organizer. 3. In electricity and magnetism, the region round a charged body or magnet in which a force would be exerted upon another charged body or magnet. 4. In ophthalmology, the field of vision. **Absolute field.** That defined region of the cerebral cortex, injury to which causes paralysis or spasticity of its related muscles. **Absolute field of vision.** That which is obtained when the eye is fixed and the face turned so as to exclude the limiting effects of the nose and orbital margins. **Adversive field.** Any area of the cerebral cortex which, when stimulated, evokes rotatory movements of parts of the body towards the opposite side. **Binocular field.** The field of vision when both eyes are open. **Centrocaecal area of field.** A central portion of the field which includes the fixation point and the physiological blind spot. **Field of consciousness.** The object or objects to which mental attention is directed at any one time. **Cribriform field of vision.** A field of vision with holes in it, i.e. discrete areas of blindness or scotomata. **Dark field.** The dark background used in the compound microscope and in the ultramicroscope to observe minute particles by scattered light; in the latter, particles having diameter of 10 nm can be observed in this way. **Deaf field.** One of the points near the external auditory meatus where the vibrating tuning fork cannot be heard by air conduction. **Electric field.** The field existing in a region of space in which a force is exerted on an electric charge placed in that region. **Electromagnetic field.** A region in space in which a force is exerted on an isolated magnetic pole placed in that region. **Electrostatic field.** Electric field (see above). **Exhaustion field, Fatigue field.** Oscillating field (see below). **Field of fixation.** An area whose boundary represents the limits of movement of the eye. **Flicker field of vision.** The field of vision as outlined by a flickering light. **Frontal adversive field.** That part of the frontal cortex (Brodmann's area 8) which, when stimulated, causes rotation of eyes, head and trunk towards the opposite side. **Gourd-shaped field.** A form of defect met with in chiasmal lesions, in which the outline is shaped like a gourd. **Magnetic field.** The region around a magnet throughout which its influence can be detected. **Maximum field.** Absolute field of vision (see above). **Field of a microscope.** The field of view of a microscope; the area of surface that can be seen at one time by a microscope. **Myelinogenetic field.** A region of nerve or tract where myelination of fibres is occurring more or less simultaneously throughout. **Occipital eye field.** An area of cerebral cortex, situated laterally in the occipital regions, stimulation of which causes conjugate deviation of the eyes to the opposite side. **Oscillating field.** Defects occurring in functional conditions, the size of the field varying from time to time. **Overshot field of vision.** A rare form of hemianopia in which the dividing line between the blind and seeing halves is several degrees to one side of the vertical meridian. **Parietal adversive field.** An adversive field situated in the parietal cortex. **Primary nail field.** *See* NAIL. **Relative field.** The field of vision obtained when the head is not moved. **Spiral field.** A type of field of vision obtained in functional cases, wherein it becomes progressively smaller as the examination is continued. **Field strength.** The value of an electrostatic or magnetic field, defined from the force on unit charge or pole respectively placed in that field. **Surplus field of vision.** That portion of the seeing area in partial hemianopia which encroaches on the blind area. **Tactile field.** That area of the body within which discrimination of a double stimulus is not possible. **Tubular field.** Sometimes applied to concentric contraction, but should be reserved for those cases in which the field, say at 1 m, has the same area as at $\frac{1}{3}$ m, whereas it ought to be 9 times bigger. Both these conditions are functional in origin. **Uncinate field.** Gourd-shaped field (see above). **Unpaired portion of field.** That part of the temporal field of one eye which is not overlapped by the nasal field of the other. **Field of vision.** That portion of space in which objects are visible at the same time without movement of the eye. [AS *feld*.]

See also: COHNHEIM, FLECHSIG, FOREL, KROENIG, WERNICKE (K.).

Fielding, George Hunsley (b. 1801). Tonbridge ophthalmologist.

Fielding's membrane. The tapetum of the choroid.

fièvre (fe·a·vr). Fever. **Fièvre boutonneuse.** Boutonneuse fever; Mediterranean tick fever. *See* FEVER. [Fr.]

Fig BPC 1968 (fig). Ficus; the dried fruit of the fig tree, *Ficus carica* Linn. (family Moraceae). It contains about 50 per cent of sugar (glucose) and small quantities of organic acids; used as a mild laxative. [L *ficus* fig.]

fig wart (fig wort). Condyloma acuminatum. [L *ficus* fig, AS *wearte*.]

figurate (fig·ewr·ate). Applied to skin eruptions or lesions which assume a distinct and fixed shape or arrangement. [see foll.]

figure (fig·er). Form; outline. **Achromatic figure, Achromatin figure.** The achromatic spindle. *See* SPINDLE. **Bistellate figure.** The amphiaster of dividing cells. **Chromatic figure, Chromatin figure.** The chromosome pattern in cell division. **Fortification figure.** One feature of the aura of migraine, characterized by bright jagged lines, often in the form of battlements, usually limited to half the visual field. Commonly called *fortification spectrum*. **Nuclear figure.** Chromatic figure (see above). [L *figura* form.]

See also: PURKINJE, STIFEL, ZOELLNER.

filaceous (fi·la·shus). Filamentous. [L *filum* thread.]

filament (fil·am·ent). A thin thread-like structure. **Axial filament.** The central filament of the tail of a spermatozoon. **Bacterial filament.** An elongated, unsegmented, thread-like form of bacteria, of uniform diameter. **Linin filament.** A thread-like precipitate of chromatin in fixed nuclei. **Spermatic filament.**

Axial filament (see above). **Terminal filament.** The end portion of the tail of a spermatozoon. [L *filamentum*.]

See also: AMMON.

filamentation (fil·am·en·ta'·shun). The formation of long thread-like forms by micro-organisms. Many of these, notably *Haemophilus pertussis, H. influenzae* and *Salmonella typhi*, normally exist as short rods, but show greatly increased numbers of filamentous forms after prolonged subculture in artificial media or when growing in unfavourable environments, as for example in immune serum or in low concentrations of antibiotics. [see prec.]

filamentous (fil·am·en·tus). 1. Threadlike. 2. Fibrillar. 3. In bacterial culture, denoting a colony composed of long irregularly-disposed and interwoven threads. 4. Capable of being drawn out into thread-like structures, as mucus is. 5. Containing a thread-like or stringy substance. [L *filamentum* thread.]

filar (fi·lar). Filamentous.

Filaria (fil·a·re·ah). A genus of nematode worms parasitic in the subcutaneous tissues and the lymphatics. **Filaria bancrofti.** Now known as *Wuchereria bancrofti*, a thread-like white worm found in the lymphatic vessels and glands. It has a wide tropical distribution, also reaching south Spain and the USA. The male is coiled; the female has a tapering anterior end with a rounded swelling. The embryos (microfilariae, formerly known as *Filaria sanguinis hominis*) exhibit a nocturnal periodicity, being present in the peripheral blood during the night but scanty or absent during the day, in most endemic areas; in others they are diurnal. Development takes place in the night-biting *Culex fatigans* and *C. pipiens*, and in various species of *Anopheles*. It is the cause of lymphangitis, filarial abscess and a number of other conditions, the highest expression of which is elephantiasis. **Filaria (Wuchereria) bancrofti var. pacifica.** A non-periodic form of *Wuchereria bancrofti* developing in *Aedes scutellaris pseudo-scutellaris* found in the Philippines and the Pacific Islands. **Filaria (Wuchereria) vauceli.** A variety of *Wuchereria bancrofti* confined to the west coast of Africa and Madagascar. **Filaria conjunctivae.** A filaria worm reported from cystic tumours of the eyelid and from the eyeball in Italy, Sicily and India. **Filaria demarquayi.** *Filaria (Mansonella) ozzardi* (see below). **Filaria (Dirofilaria) immitis.** The heartworm of the dog, found throughout the tropics. **Filaria loa.** *Loa loa*, the eye-worm of West Africa, the cause of allergic transient swellings known as Calabar swellings. The adults inhabit the connective tissues and migrate, appearing beneath the skin and under the ocula conjunctiva. The microfilariae resemble those of *Filaria bancrofti*, but have a diurnal periodicity and development takes place in the day-biting mangrove flies *Chrysops silacea* and *C. dimidiata*. **Filaria (Dirofilaria) magalhaesi.** Discovered in the left ventricle of the heart of a child in Brazil, is considered identical with *Filaria* (*Dirofilaria*) *immitis* of the dog. **Filaria (Wuchereria) malayi.** Found in South-east Asia, resembles *Filaria* (*Wuchereria*) *bancrofti*, except that the embryos differ in morphology and develop in the mosquito *Mansonioides*. **Filaria (Dracunculus) medinensis.** The guinea-worm of India, Africa and South America. The female may reach 0.6 m (2 ft) in length and lies in the connective tissues. The embryos formed in a blister on the skin are released into water, develop in a species of *Cyclops* and are swallowed in larval state by man. It is the cause of serious inflammatory affections of the legs, arms and other tissues. **Filaria (Mansonella) ozzardi.** Identical with *Filaria demarquayi*, is found in the West Indies, Guyana and South America. Its embryo develops in the midge *Culicoides furens* and appears non-periodically in the blood. **Filaria palpebralis.** *Filaria conjunctivae* (see above). **Filaria (Acanthocheilonema) perstans.** Found throughout central Africa and in the West Indies and South America, it has a small unsheathed non-periodic embryo which develops in species of *Culicoides*; it does not cause clinical symptoms. **Filaria (Wuchereria) philippinensis.** A variety of *Filaria* (*Wuchereria*) *bancrofti*, found in the Philippines and the Pacific islands; it is non-periodic and develops in *Aëdes scutellaris*. **Filaria (Dirofilaria) recondita.** A filarial worm found in the dog in China. **Filaria (Dipetalonema) streptocerca.** Found only in central Africa and probably a parasite of the chimpanzee, resembles *Filaria* (*Acanthocheilonema*) *perstans* in its adult form; the microfilariae are found in the corium of the skin and are distinguished by their "walking-stick handle" tail extremity. **Filaria taniguchii.** A species found in the groin gland of a Japanese. **Filaria (Onchocerca) volvulus.** Found in Africa and central America, it occurs in nodules on the body. The microfilariae formed in the fluid of the cyst, migrate into the eye and invade the cornea, causing filarial blindness; they develop in the buffalo gnat *Simulium damnosum*. [L *filum* thread.]

filariae (fil·a·re·e). A general term, not used taxonomically, for nematode worms of the super-family or sub-order Filarioidea. Worms of the genera *Acanthocheilonema, Loa, Onchocerca* and *Wuchereria* are included. [L *filum* thread.]

filarial (fil·a·re·al). Relating or belonging to, or caused by filariae.

filariasis (fil·ar·i·as·is). In man infection by worms of the super-family Filarioidea. Species are: *Wuchereria bancrofti*, transmitted by *Culex* and other mosquitoes, causing Bancroft's filariasis, a condition characterized clinically in its early stages by lymphangitis, lymphadenitis and occasional short bouts of fever, and in its later stages by elephantiasis, lymph varicocele and other effects of lymphatic obstruction; *W. malayi*, transmitted by *Taeniorhynchus* (*Mansonioides*) mosquitoes, causing Brug's filariasis, a condition similar to that caused by *W. bancrofti*; and *Mansonella ozzardi*, transmitted by *Culicoides furens*, causing Ozzard's filariasis which has no recognizable symptoms. Infections with *Acanthocheilonema perstans, Loa loa*, and *Onchocerca volvulus* satisfy the above definition, but are usually referred to as acanthocheilonemiasis, loiasis or loasis, and onchocerciasis, respectively.

See also: BANCROFT, BRUG, OZZARD.

Filariata (fil·a·re·a'·tah). Spirurata; a sub-order or order of the nematode order or sub-class Spirurida. The super-families or sub-orders Filarioidea and Spiruroidea are of medical interest. [L *filum* thread.]

filaricidal (fil·ar·is·i'·dal). Fatal to or destructive of filaria or filariidae. [see foll.]

filaricide (fil·ar·is·ide). Any agent (e.g. a drug) that kills or destroys filaria or filariidae. [*Filaria*, L *caedere* to kill.]

filariform (fil·ar·e·form). Having resemblance to filariae. [*Filaria*, form.]

Filarioidea (fil·a·re·oi'·de·ah). Filariae; a super-family of the nematode sub-order Spirurata, or a sub-order of the order Filariata. The families Filariidae and Philometridae are of medical interest. [L *filum* thread, Gk *eidos* form.]

Filatov, Nil Feodorowich (b. 1847). Moscow paediatrician.

Filatov's disease, Filatov-Dukes' disease. Dukes' disease; fourth disease.

Filatov's spots. Koplik's spots.

Filatov treatment, Comby-Filatov treatment. The administration of arsenic in heavy dosage as treatment for chorea. Now obsolete.

Fildes, Sir Paul Gordon (b. 1882). London bacteriologist.

Fildes' culture medium. A peptic digest blood medium for the growth of *Haemophilus influenzae* and other organisms.

McIntosh and Fildes jar or method. A method used to obtain oxygen-free conditions for the growth of anaerobic bacteria.

Filhos' caustic. A mixture of caustic potash and quicklime.

filicin (fil·is·in). The mixture of ether-soluble acidic substances occurring in the male fern, *Aspidium filix-mas*.

filicism (fil·is·izm). A condition of poisoning resulting from the excessive use of filicin, the active principle of male fern.

filiform (fil·e·form). Shaped like a filament or thread. In bacteriology, referring to stab or stroke cultures, a uniform growth confined to the line of the inoculation. **Filiform papilla.** *See* PAPILLA. [L *filum* thread, form.]

filings (fi·lingz). Metal debris produced by a coarse file. [AS *feol*.]

filioma (fil·e·o·mah). Fibroma durum. [L *filum* thread, Gk *-oma* tumour.]

Filipovitch, Casimir. 19th–20th century Polish physician.
Filipovitch's sign, or phenomenon. Palmoplantar phenomenon. *See* PHENOMENON.

filipuncture (fil·e·pungk·tcher). The surgical treatment of an aneurysm by puncturing the sac with a fine wire or thread or hair in order to induce coagulation. [L *filum* thread, puncture.]

filix (fi·lix) (pl. *filices*). Fern. **Filix femina.** Lady fern, *Athyrium filix-foemina* (Linn.) Roth. **Filix mas.** Male Fern BP 1958. [L.]

fillet (fil·et). A loop of thread or tape for suspending or retracting a tissue during operation. **Spinal fillet.** The spinal lemniscus. *See* LEMNISCUS. [L *filum* thread.]

filling (fil·ing). 1. The operation of inserting a filling material in a cavity prepared in a tooth. 2. The material used in the operation of filling a cavity prepared in a tooth, usually gold, amalgam, silicate cement or methyl methacrylate. **Combination filling, Composite filling.** A filling made of two materials placed one on top of the other. **Compound filling.** A filling in a compound cavity, i.e. a cavity involving two or more surfaces of the tooth. **Contour filling.** A filling which restores the original contour of the tooth. **Non-leaking filling.** A filling whose perfect contact with the walls of the cavity in which it has been inserted prevents the penetration of moisture and micro-organisms. **Permanent filling.** Any filling which it is proposed to leave in a cavity permanently. **Root-canal filling.** A filling inserted in the root canal of a tooth after the pulp has been removed. **Submarine filling.** An amalgam filling which contains a high percentage of copper, and sets when submerged by saliva. **Temporary filling.** A filling, usually of temporary cement or gutta percha, which is intended to remain in place only for a short time. [AS *fyllan.*]

film (film). 1. A membrane or pellicle. 2. A strip of thin transparent material coated with a light-sensitive emulsion for photographic purposes, or the negative therefrom. **Fixed blood film.** A small drop of fresh blood spread on a slide or cover slip, dried rapidly in air and fixed when the alcoholic staining solution is added; it is used for the examination and the counting of the cells present. **Nylon film.** A substance used for surgical dressings; it has the advantage of protecting from superinfection but at the same time allowing inspection and the passage of water vapour. **Stripping film.** A type of photographic emulsion frequently used in autoradiography which can be stripped off the supporting glass plate and laid directly on the specimen; improved resolution is thereby obtained. [AS *filmen* membrane.]

film-badge (film·baj). A small piece of photographic film in a suitable holder worn on the person, from which exposure to ionizing radiation may be assessed by a measurement of the blackening after development. [AS *filmen* membrane, ME *badge.*]

filoma (fil·o·mah). Filioma.

filopodium (fi·lo·po·de·um) (pl. *filopodia*). A fine, slender, thread-like pseudopodium. [L *filum* thread, Gk *pous* foot.]

filopressure (fi·lo·presh·er). The temporary compression of a blood vessel by ligating it with a thread or other fine ligature; the thread is removed when the blood has ceased to escape. [L *filum* thread, pressure.]

filovaricosis (fi·lo·var·ik·o'·sis). A condition in which there are unnatural swellings along the course of the axon of a nerve fibre. [L *filum* thread, varicose.]

filter (fil·ter). 1. A device consisting of a membrane or other substance (e.g. filter paper) arranged to prevent the passage through it of some of the components of a mixture. 2. Material (e.g. aluminium, copper) placed in the path of a heterogeneous beam of x-rays to reduce selectively the intensity of certain wavelength components. 3. In sound, any device to reduce or eliminate undesired frequencies. 4. In photography, a transparent coloured disc superimposed upon the lens to reduce selectively the intensity of certain colours. **Collodion filter.** Gradocol filter (see below). **Compensation filter.** *See* COMPENSATOR. **Composite filter.** A filter of two or more materials usually so arranged that the second material filters secondary radiation produced in the first, and so on. **Flattening filter.** A filter for flattening radiation beam isodoses. **Gradocol filter.** Gradocol membrane, a filter made from an acetone solution of collodion by controlled evaporation The pore size can be varied from 3 μm to 10 μm. **Intermittent sand filter.** A filter composed of sand in a sewage disposal system. The sewage is allowed to flow through the sand filter for a limited time, and is then drained off and exposed to the oxidizing action of the air. **Mechanical filter.** A filter of sand or other porous material used for the removal of gross particles. **Membrane filter.** A filter made from cellulose acetate with a narrow range of porosities. Such filters are available in various grades and the finer grades can be used to sterilize fluids by removing organisms of virus size and upwards. **Multivee air filter.** A form of air filter used in surgical dressing-rooms. **Percolating filter.** Porous filter-beds in a sewage disposal system. The sewage percolates slowly through the beds to drains beneath, and in so doing its organic matter becomes oxidized and purified. **Pollen filter.** A device for removing pollen from the air. **Primary filter.** The material (usually heavy metal) used to absorb the primary β-rays and softer γ-rays from radioactive sources. **Roughing filter.** A filter composed of coarse particles (coke fragments) used in water purification. It is placed before sand filters in order to remove the grosser suspended material from sewage water, which otherwise might clog the sand filters. **Scrubbing filter.** Roughing filter (see above). **Secondary filter.** The material (usually light metal or rubber) used to absorb secondary radiation produced in a primary filter (see above) round radioactive sources. **Sintered-glass filter.** A bacterial filter of porous glass of known pore size. **Slow sand filter.** A filter constructed of gravel and sand used in water purification. The water percolates slowly and is purified partly by mechanical filtration, but mainly by the vital layer of zoogloea in the upper 1 cm of the filter which consists of microorganisms. **Sprinkling filter.** A percolating filter-bed to which a well-digested effluent is distributed evenly over the whole of its surface by a mechanical sprinkler. A biologically-active film forms on the surface of the coke or other material of the filter. **Trickling filter.** Percolating filter (see above). **Ultraviolet filter.** One which allows ultraviolet rays to pass, but cuts out longer rays. **Wedge filter.** A wedge-shaped filter for altering isodose contours of a radiation beam. [Fr. *filtre.*]

See also: BERKEFELD, CHAMBERLAND, COORS, DARNALL, GOOCH (F. A.), JENKINS, KITASATO, MANDLER, PASTEUR, REICHEL (J.), SEITZ, THORAEUS.

filter-passer (fil·ter·pah·ser). Any micro-organism which can pass through a filter (e.g. of porcelain or diatomaceous earth) that does not allow passage to bacteria or microscopic protozoa; a non-filtrable virus.

filterable, filtrable (fil·trah·bl). Capable of passing through a porous filter such as those made of diatomaceous earth or porcelain.

filtrate (fil·trate). That which passes through a filter. **Bacterial filtrate.** The filtrate obtained when a fluid culture of bacteria is passed through a bacteria-proof filter. Such filtrates may contain toxin and other metabolic products, bacteriophage and L forms of bacteria. **Glomerular filtrate.** The fluid filtered off in the glomeruli from the blood plasma during its flow through the kidneys. It is similar in composition to plasma but contains no protein. About 99 per cent of the glomerula filtrate is reabsorbed in the renal tubules, the remaining 1 per cent being excreted as urine. The normal rate of glomerular filtration is of the order of 120 ml/min, but is markedly decreased in kidney disease.

filtration (fil·tra·shun). 1. The removal of particles of a precipitate from a liquid by draining away the latter through a porous material which retains the solid. 2. In x-ray work, the absorption of the soft rays by an interposed aluminium plate which allows the harder rays to pass through. **Centrifugal filtration.** The separation of a liquid from solid particles by centrifugal force in a rotating filter. **Gel filtration.** The fractionation of substances in solution by their ability to penetrate or to be excluded from a porous gel or molecular sieve. The fractionation depends on the molecular sizes of the solutes. **Inherent filtration.** The filtration of a beam of x-rays by the parts of the tube and tube shield through which it passes. **Pressure filtration.** Forced filtration by the application of air pressure. **Vacuum filtration.** Accelerated filtration achieved by suction. [filter.]

filtratometer (fil·trah·**tom**·et·er). An instrument with which the filtrates obtained from various samples of gastric contents may be measured.

filtros (**fil**·tros). Porous or vitrified fine concrete plates or tiles employed as diffusers for delivering air in minute bubbles in the activated sludge process of sewage purification. [American term.]

filum [NA] (**fi**·lum). A thread-like structure. **Filum of the spinal dura mater [filum durae matris spinalis (NA)].** The lowest end of the dura mater where it blends into the filum terminale. **Filum terminale [NA].** The continuation of the spinal cord, consisting mainly of pia mater, below the 2nd lumbar vertebra. It lies on the lower part of the spinal canal, eventually becoming attached to the periosteum of the coccyx. [L thread.]

fimbria (**fim**·bre·ah) (pl. *fimbriae*). Very fine filamentous appendages attached to the cell wall of both motile and non-motile genera in the family Enterobacteriaceae; they are far more numerous and much shorter and finer than flagella, and probably act as organs of adhesion to tissue cells. The alternative term *pilus* (pl. *pili*) is commonly used in American literature. **Bacterial fimbriae.** Pili; filamentous protein appendages commonly found on Gram-negative coliform bacilli. **Fimbria of the hippocampus [fimbria hippocampi (NA)].** A bundle of nerve fibres which forms a fringe along the concave border of the hippocampus; the fibres begin in the hippocampus, pass through the fimbria into the fornix and on to the mamillary body of the hypothalamus where they end. **Ovarian fimbria [fimbria ovarica (NA)].** A thread-like process from the margin of the pelvic opening of the uterine tube and attached to the tubal extremity of the ovary. **Sex fimbria.** A special type of fimbria determined by a sex factor and essential for fertility. **Fimbria of the uterine tube [fimbria tubae (NA)].** Thread-like processes from the margin of the pelvic opening of the uterine tube, each lined by mucous membrane similar to that lining the tube. One of these fimbriae is attached to the ovary as the ovarian fimbria (see above). [L a fringe.]

fimbrial (**fim**·bre·al). Relating or belonging to a fimbria or characterized by the presence of fimbriae.

fimbriate, fimbriated (**fim**·bre·ate, **fim**·bre·a·ted). Fringed; having an extremity or border bearing fringe-like processes or hairs. [L *fimbria* a fringe.]

frimbriation (fim·bre·a′·shun). Crenulation; a condition sometimes found in malaria: in thin blood smears the red cells are seen to have slightly crenated (wavy) margins. [see prec.]

fimbriocele (**fim**·bre·o·seel). A hernia of the fimbriae of the uterine tube, or a hernia that contains such fimbriae. [fimbria, Gk *kele* hernia.]

fin (fin). **Nasal fin.** In embryology, a vertical epithelial plate which separates the maxillary process from the frontonasal process below the nasal sac.

finder (**fi**·nder). A squared slide attached to a microscope which is an aid to the picking up of any particular object in the field of vision. [AS *findan.*]

finding (**fi**·nding). 1. An observation made on a particular case of illness or disease. 2. Any condition discovered during the course of a disease. 3. Conclusion arrived at as a result of examination. [see prec.]

fine (fine). Not coarse; thin or attenuated. [Fr. *fin.*]

finger [digitus manus (NA)] (**fing**·ger). Any one of the digits of the hand. Named surfaces are the dorsal [facies dorsalis (NA)], palmar [facies palmaris (NA)], lateral (radial) [facies lateralis (radialis) NA], and medial (ulnar) [facies medialis (ulnaris) NA]. **Clubbed fingers.** Enlargement of the terminal phalanges of the fingers with increased size and curvature of the nails, giving a parrot-beak appearance, or in severe cases drum-stick fingers. The condition is sometimes familial, but is most often associated with chronic suppurative diseases of the lungs, congenital heart disease, infective endocarditis and other diseases in which there is increased vascularity of the finger tips. **Dead fingers.** A white, cold, numb condition of the fingers brought on by exposure to cold. **Drum-stick fingers.** Severe clubbing of the fingers. *See* CLUBBED FINGER (above). **Fifth finger [digitus minimus (digitus V) NA].** The little finger. **First finger [pollex (digitus I) NA].** The thumb. **Fourth finger [digitus anularis (digitus IV) NA].** The ring finger. **Giant fingers.** Macrodactyly; hypertrophy of all the tissues of the fingers. **Hippocratic finger.** Clubbed finger (see above). **Index finger [index (digitus II) NA].** The finger next to the thumb; also called *second finger* or *forefinger.* **Insane finger.** Paronychia as found, but not specifically, in insane persons. **Little finger.** Fifth finger (see above). **Madonna fingers.** Thin delicate fingers occurring in pituitary infantilism. **Mallet finger.** Avulsion of the extensor tendon, producing a flexion deformity of the terminal phalanx of the finger. **Middle finger.** Third finger (see below). **Ring finger.** Fourth finger (see above). **Seal finger.** Erysipeloid. **Second finger.** Index finger (see above). **Snapping finger.** Trigger finger (see below). **Spider fingers.** Arachnodactyly; a congenital condition in which the fingers and toes are long and slender with unduly mobile joints. **Spring finger.** Snapping finger (see above). **Third finger [digitus medius (digitus III) (NA)].** The middle finger. **Trigger finger.** The temporary fixation of the finger in flexion, due to a narrowing of the fibrous flexor tendon sheath and a secondary thickening of the tendon, which on active or passive extension of the finger is overcome with a sudden jerk. **Tulip fingers.** Dermatitis venenata of the fingers due to handling tulips. **Washerman's fingers, Washerwoman's fingers.** Shrivelled fingers, as after immersion in water for a long time; a similar condition is caused in the dehydrated state, as for example in cholera. **Waxy finger.** Dead finger (see above). **Webbed finger.** Syndactylism; a condition in which some or all of the fingers are congenitally joined by skin and fibrous tissue. **White fingers.** A circulatory disease occurring in users of the pneumatic hammer. [AS.]

See also: DUPUYTREN.

finger-stall (**fing**·ger·stawl). A rubber or leather cap for the protection of the fingers. [AS *finger, steall.*]

fingerprint (**fing**·ger·print). 1. The pattern left on a surface by contact of the pad of a finger or thumb; a whorl or loop or compound pattern of the fine ridges marking the skin and capable of delineation to such a degree as to identify the finger making it. No two identical prints occur, unless from the same finger, even in twins. 2. The pattern of spots obtained by resolving a partial digest of a macromolecule (e.g. a protein or a nucleic acid) on a sheet of filter paper (or other solid support) by high-voltage electrophoresis in one direction and chromatography in a direction at right-angles to the first. **Latent prints.** Requiring treatment by dusting or chemical development to become visible. [AS *finger*, ME *prent.*]

Finkeldey, Wilhelm. 20th century Augsburg pathologist.

Warthin-Finkeldey giant cell. A multinucleated giant cell identified in the lymphatic tissue of tonsils, appendix and elsewhere, and formerly believed to be pathognomonic of early measles. The claim is unconfirmed; giant cells are not seen in autopsies of fatal cases.

Finkelstein, Heinrich (b. 1865). Berlin paediatrician.

Finkelstein's albumin milk, or feeding. A specially prepared milk, rich in casein and fat, for use in diabetes and cases requiring high-protein diets, e.g. nephrosis, nutritional oedema.

Finney, John Miller Turpin (b. 1863). Baltimore surgeon.

Finney's operation. A form of pyloroplasty.

Finochietto, Enrique (b. 1881). Buenos Aires surgeon.

Finochietto's tourniquet. A metal tourniquet controlled by a screw, applied around the head just above the ears and eyebrows to control haemorrhage from the scalp.

Finsen, Jon Constant (b. 1826). Icelandic physician.

Daae-Finsen disease. Epidemic pleurodynia.

Finsen, Niels Ryberg (b. 1860). Copenhagen physician.

Finsen apparatus, or lamp. A source of ultraviolet-light radiation designed for the local treatment of lupus. It consists of a carbon-arc lamp of high amperage. By means of a system of filters and quartz lenses radiation, rich in ultraviolet rays, is concentrated on to a small area of the skin. The lamp is water cooled.

Finsen bath. The irradiation of the body with light from electric arcs.

Finsen light. Irradiation with Finsen apparatus.

Finsen ray. Light emitted from a Finsen lamp, rich in violet and ultraviolet rays.

Finsen treatment. The treatment of lupus vulgaris by local ultraviolet irradiation with the Finsen lamp; this is now seldom employed since as good an effect can be obtained by calciferol.

Finsen-Lomholt lamp. A lamp that emits ultraviolet rays of wavelength mainly from 330 to 360 nm; the light rays are all filtered out and the heat rays absorbed. The ultraviolet rays constitute 75 per cent of the total, and the irradiation time is only one-third of that required with the Finsen lamp; obsolescent.

Finsen-Lomholt treatment. Treatment of lupus vulgaris by filtered ultraviolet rays emanating from a Finsen-Lomholt lamp.

Finsen-Reyn lamp. A modification of the Finsen lamp.

Finsterer, Hans (b. 1877). Vienna surgeon.

Finsterer gastrectomy. A Pólya-type operation in which the upper part of the opening in the gastric remnant is closed and the jejunum is united by anastomosis to the lower part of that opening, but is stitched also to the closed upper part of the transected stomach.

Finzi, Neville Samuel (b. 1881). London radiotherapist.

Finzi-Harmer operation. Treatment of vocal-cord cancer by means of radium needles. The needles are placed in a window in the thyroid ala formed by a partial removal of a quadrilateral area of cartilage.

fire (fire). Fever. **Fire measles.** Rubella. **St. Anthony's fire.** 1. Erysipelas. 2. Ergotism. 3. Hospital gangrene. 4. Anthrax. **St. Francis' fire, Wild fire.** 1. Erysipelas. 2. Impetigo contagiosa bullosa. 3. An endemic bullous disease of Brazil. [AS *fyr.*]

firedamp (**fire**·damp). A gas which occurs sometimes in sealed pockets in coal-mines where it has been formed by the decomposition of organic matter. It is a mixture of methane (not less than 60 per cent) and nitrogen. Special precautions are necessary, as it is liable to explode when mixed with air. [AS *fyr, damp.*]

first aid (**ferst** ade). Immediate treatment given on the spot in cases of accidental or other injuries, usually by experienced but not necessarily medically-qualified persons, before more expert medical or surgical attention can be obtained; in more serious accidents it includes life-saving measures such as the control of haemorrhage and the facilitating of transport. [AS *fyrst,* O Fr. *aider.*]

first intention (ferst in·**ten**·shun). That form of wound healing which occurs under aseptic conditions, the wound healing by granulation and, later, fibrous tissue with an epithelial covering, without any period of suppuration. [AS *fyrst,* ME *entent.*]

Fischer, E. 19th century Munich histologist.

Fischer's tufts. A basket-like expansion of nerve fibrils between touch corpuscles.

Fischer, Hans (b. 1881). Munich physician and biochemist.

Neubauer and Fischer test. *See* TEST FOR CANCER.

Fischer, Louis (b. 1864). New York paediatrician.

Fischer's murmur. A systolic murmur arising from the temporal region or anterior fontanelle in rickets.

Fischer, Martin Henry (b. 1879). Cincinnati physiologist.

Fischer's treatment. A solution of sodium chloride 14 g and sodium carbonate 10 g in 1000 ml of water, given rectally or intravenously for anuria in nephritis or eclampsia.

Fischer apparatus. An apparatus specifically designed for the analysis of producer gas, water gas and similar gaseous mixtures.

fish berry (**fish** ber·e). Levant berry, cocculus indicus, the fruit of *Anamirta paniculata* Colebr., used in the treatment of pediculi. [AS *fisc, bere.*]

Fisher, Sir Ronald Aylmer (b. 1890). Cambridge geneticist.

Fisher and Race notation. *See* NOTATION.

Fisher, Theodore (b. 1863). London physician.

Fisher's sign. A presystolic murmur said to occur in cases of adherent pericardium. There is no evidence that adherent pericardium produces such a murmur, and if found in association with rheumatic adherent pericardium, it is then likely to be due to mitral stenosis. Also called *Eustace Smith's sign.*

fishing (**fish**·ing). In bacterial technique, the picking off from a culture medium of a colony of bacteria for subculture and further investigation. [AS *fisc.*]

Fiske, Cyrus Hartwell (b. 1890). Boston biochemist.

Fiske's method. For total fixed base in urine: urine is boiled with dilute sulphuric acid and nitric acid to convert the bases to sulphates. Water is added, the reaction adjusted to just acid to methyl orange, and the phosphates precipitated with ferric chloride solution. The filtrate is evaporated and ignited. Sulphates in the residue are determined with benzidine and expressed as milli-equivalents of total fixed base per litre.

Fiske and Subbarow method. 1. For phosphate in urine: 0.5 ml urine is diluted to 5 ml with water, 0.7 ml of 60 per cent perchloric acid, 0.7 ml of 5 per cent aqueous ammonium molybdate and 0.5 ml of aminonaphtholsulphonic-acid reagent (0.2 g, 1,2,4-aminonaphtholsulphonic acid; 12 g sodium metabisulphite; 2.4 g, crystalline sodium sulphite; water to 100 ml) are added. The solution is diluted to 10 ml and the colour compared with standards after 10 min. 2. For inorganic phosphate in blood: 2 ml blood, serum or plasma are added to 8 ml 10 per cent trichloro-acetic acid. The mixture is shaken, filtered and 5 ml of filtrate treated as for urine.

fissible (**fis**·ibl). Fissile.

fissile (**fis**·ile). Able to split; to undergo fission. [L *fissilis* easily split.]

fission (**fish**·un). 1. A form of asexual reproduction in which there is spontaneous division of the body into two equal parts, each of which develops into a complete organism, as in the case of bacteria. 2. Of a cell or cell nucleus, the splitting into two equal parts. 3. A nuclear reaction in which a heavy nucleus splits into two approximately equal parts. **Atomic fission.** *See* MAIN DEF. 3 (above). **Binary fission.** Division into two equal parts; in the case of many protozoa the nucleus first divides and then the cytoplasm separates into two identical parts. **Bud fission.** In certain protozoa, reproduction by the budding-off of a portion of protoplasm. **Cellular fission.** *See* MAIN DEF. 2. (above). **Fission fragments,** The primary atomic particles formed with high kinetic energy at the moment of fission of a nucleus. Any one nucleus gives rise to one pair of fragments, but there are many possible pairs which occur with characteristic frequencies. **Multiple fission.** Division into many parts by a process of repeated division of the nucleus first, then later of the cytoplasm. **Nuclear fission.** 1. *See* MAIN DEF. 2 (above). 2. Atomic fission; *see* MAIN DEF. 3 (above). **Fission products.** The various nuclear species produced through fission of an atomic nucleus, i.e. the original fission fragments together with all the radioactive daughter products. [L *fissio* a splitting.]

fissionable (**fish**·un·abl). Fissile.

fissipara (fis·**ip**·ar·ah). Organisms which reproduce by division. [see foll.]

fissiparism, fissiparity (fis·**ip**·ar·izm, fis·ip·**ar**·it·e). In biology, reproduction by fission. [L *fissio* a splitting, *parere* to give birth.]

fissiparous (fis·**ip**·ar·us). Reproducing by division, as in many protozoa. [see prec.]

fissura (fish·**ewr**·ah). Fissure. **Fissura antitragohelicina [NA].** A slit-like fissure, open downwards, separating the tail of the helix from the antihelix. **Fissura prima [NA].** A deep V-shaped fissure crossing the whole width of the upper surface of the cerebellum. **Fissura secunda [NA].** The fissure which develops transversely across the inferior vermis, separating the pyramid from the uvula. [L.]

fissural (fish·ewr·al). Relating or belonging to a fissure.

fissuration (fish·ewr·a·shun). 1. Term applied to the pattern in which the natural fissures in certain structures (e.g. the brain) are arranged. 2. Fission.

fissure [fissura (NA)] (fish·ewr). 1. A groove, cleft or furrow; a sulcus; a natural one due to infolding during development, e.g. between the cerebral convolutions, or a pathological one, e.g. the partial fracture of a bone. *See also:* SULCUS. 2. In dentistry, a shallow groove or depression in the enamel on the surface of a tooth which forms a line of demarcation between the cusps and commonly forms the site of the commencement of dental caries. **Anal fissure.** A painful ulcer of the anal skin. **Ape fissure.** A deep vertical groove in the lateral aspect of the cerebral hemisphere ending superiorly in the parieto-occipital fissure. It is present in all higher primates except adult Man. **Avulsion fissure.** A separation of the tubercle of the tibia from the shaft by a sudden violent traction on the achilles tendon, **Branchial fissure.** The ectodermal cleft overlying a pharyngeal pouch in the early embryo. **Fissures of the cerebellum [fissurae cerebelli (NA)].** Curved furrows running across the surfaces of the cerebellum. **Fissure of the cerebrum, longitudinal [fissura longitudinalis cerebri (NA)].** The interval between the medial surfaces of the cerebral hemispheres. **Fissure of the cerebrum, transverse [fissura transversa cerebri (NA)].** The interval between the splenium of the corpus callosum and the roof of the 3rd ventricle and thalami. **Choroid fissure [fissura choroidea (NA)].** 1. The site of invagination of the choroid plexus of a cerebral hemisphere. 2. Choroidal fissure; the invagination on the under side of the optic cup and stalk of the developing eye. **Enamel fissure.** *See* MAIN DEF. 2 (above). **Floccular fissure.** Post-nodular fissure (see below). **Fetal fissure.** Choroid fissure (see above). **Genal fissure.** Genal cleft. *See* CLEFT. **Genitovesical fissure.** A groove between the bladder and genital cord (future uterus) which becomes the uterovesical fossa of the pelvic cavity. **Horizontal fissure [fissura horizontalis cerebelli (NA)].** The fissure which divides the superior and inferior surfaces of the ansiform lobule. **Interarytenoid fissure.** The groove between the arytenoid swellings of the embryonic larynx. **Fissure for the ligamentum teres [fissura ligamenti teretis (NA)].** A groove passing forward from the left end of the porta hepatis to the lower border of the liver. **Fissure for the ligamentum venosum [fissura ligamenti venosi (NA)].** A deep fissure on the posterior surface of the liver, running vertically to meet the left extremity of the porta hepatis. The lesser omentum is attached here; the ligamentum venosum lies in the floor of the fissure. **Lip fissure.** Hare-lip. **Fissure of the lung, oblique [fissura obliqua (NA)].** A fissure extending downward and forward from the level of the 3rd thoracic vertebra behind to the level of the 6th costal cartilage in front; it corresponds approximately to the medial border of the scapula when the arm is abducted. **Mandibular fissure.** The groove between the approaching mandibular arches of the developing face. **Oral fissure [rima oris (NA)].** The cleft between the upper and lower lips, leading into the cavity of the mouth. **Orbital fissure, inferior [fissura orbitalis inferior (NA)].** The interval between the floor and the lateral wall of the orbit opening posteriorly into the pterygopalatine fossa. **Orbital fissure, superior [fissura orbitalis superior (NA)].** The interval between the lateral wall and roof of the orbit, transmitting vessels and nerves. **Palpebral fissure [rima palpebrarum (NA)].** The gap between the eyelids when the eyes are open. **Parafloccular fissure.** A fissure of the cerebellum. **Parieto-occipital fissure.** Parieto-occipital sulcus. *See* SULCUS. **petro-occipital fissure [fissura petro-occipitalis (NA)].** A fissure extending backward from the foramen lacerum between the basi-occipital bone and the posterior and inner border of the petrous portion of the temporal bone. **Petrosquamous fissure [fissura petrosquamosa (NA)].** The anterior of two fissures into which the squamotympanic fissure divides medially. **Petrotympanic fissure.** A part of the squamotympanic fissure through which the chorda tympani passes. **Postcentral fissure.** 1. A fissure on the lateral surface of the cerebrum behind and parallel to the central sulcus. 2. The posterior of two fissures that run across the anterior lobe of the cerebellum. **Postlingual fissure.** The anterior of two fissures that run across the anterior lobe of the cerebellum. **Postlunate fissure.** A Y-shaped fissure crossing the upper surface of the middle lobe of the cerebellum. **Postnodular fissure [fissura posterolateralis (NA)].** The fissure separating the nodule from the remainder of the inferior vermis, frequently called the prepyramidal fissure on morphological grounds. **Postpyramidal fissure.** The deep fissure separating the lobulus tuberis from the pyramid. **Preculminative fissure.** Postcentral fissure (see above). **Prepyramidal fissure.** Postnodular fissure (see above). **Pterygoid fissure.** A gap between the anterior borders of the pterygoid plates below which lodges the tubercle of the palatine bone. **Pterygomaxillary fissure [fissura pterygomaxillaris (NA)].** A triangular interval formed by the divergence of the maxilla from the pterygoid process of the sphenoid bone. **Retrotonsillar fissure.** The fissure separating the tonsil from the inferior surface of the ansiform lobule. **Fissure of the right lung, horizontal [fissura horizontalis (pulmonis dextri) (NA)].** A transverse cleft beginning in the oblique fissure at the midaxillary line and running forward to cut the anterior border of the lung at the level of the 4th costal cartilage. **Rolandic fissure.** The central sulcus of the cerebrum. *See* SULCUS. **Spheno-occipital fissure.** The line of junction between the basilar parts of the occipital and sphenoid bones. A plate of cartilage occupies the interval until approximately the twenty-fifth year. **Sphenopetrosal fissure [fissura sphenopetrosa (NA)].** A fissure between the posterior edge of the great wing of the sphenoid bone and the petrous portion of the temporal bone, **Fissure of the spinal cord, anterior median [fissura mediana anterior (NA)].** A deep midline fissure extending the whole length of the front of the spinal cord, **Squamotympanic fissure [fissura petrotympanica (NA)].** A fissure lying in, and medial to, the mandibular fossa. At its inner end it is divided into petrosquamous and petrotympanic fissures by the edge of the tegmen tympani. **Tympanomastoid fissure [fissura tympanomastoidea (NA)].** A fissure between the tympanic plate and the mastoid, transmitting the auricular branch of the vagus. **Tympanosquamous fissure [fissura tympanosquamosa (NA)].** The fissure between the upper border of the tympanic plate and the posterior border of the articular surface of the squamous part of the temporal bone. **Urogenital fissure.** The narrow elongated opening of the urogenital sinus to the exterior of the embryo, which persists as the deeper part of the vulval cleft in the female, but which is closed in the male during the later development of the penile urethra. **Zygal fissure.** A transverse cerebral sulcus at right-angles to and uniting two parallel sulci to form an H, as in the case of the orbital sulcus. [L *fissura* cleft.]

See also: AMMON, BICHAT, BROCA, BURDACH, CLEVENGER, DUVERNEY, ECKER, HENLE, MONRO (II), PANSCH, ROLANDO, SANTORINI, SCHWALBE, SYLVIUS, WERNICKE (K.).

fist (fist). 1. The clenched hand. 2. The fungus, *Lycoperdon bovista.* [AS *fyst.*]

fistula (fis·tew·lah). An unnatural communication between an organ and the body surface, or between one organ and another. **Abdominal fistula.** A communication between a hollow abdominal organ and the surface of the body. **Aerial fistula.** An open communication between the larynx or trachea and the skin surface of the neck, or between a bronchus and the skin surface of the chest. **Anal fistula, Fistula in ano.** An open channel from the anus or rectum to the skin near the anus; loosely, any deep track in the region of the anus. **Angular fistula.** A congenital fistula at the angle of the mouth. **Anoperineal fistula.** A fistula from the rectum to the perineum. **Anovaginal fistula.** A fistula between the anal canal and the vagina. **Arteriovenous fistula.** A direct communication between an artery and a vein. **Fistula auris congenita.** A developmental pit sometimes seen in the front of the helix; ear pit. **Biliary fistula.** An opening discharging bile on the skin surface from the gall bladder, bile duct or liver. **Fistula bimucosa.** A fistula between two hollow organs or between two segments of the same hollow organ as when a track passes from the rectum into surrounding tissue and returns to open into the rectum at another place. **Blind fistula.** *External:* a deep channel which opens on the surface, and which does not communicate with a hollow organ. *Internal:* a track leading from the interior of a hollow organ into the tissues around it but without an opening to the exterior. **Bone fistula.** A patent track from the surface down to the bone marrow, which is maintained by suppuration in the latter. **Branchial fistula.** An abnormal communication between the pharynx and the exterior of the neck, resulting from an error in development of the branchial region. **Bronchial fistula.** An abnormal track between a bronchus and either the pleural cavity or the body surface. **Bronchobiliary fistula.** A communication between the bronchus and a bile duct whereby bile enters the air passages. **Bronchomediastinal fistula.** A fistula leading from a bronchus into the mediastinum, e.g. from the bronchial stump following a lung resection. **Bronchopleural fistula.** Communication between a bronchus and either the pleural cavity or the skin. **Carotico-cavernous fistula.** A fistula between the internal carotid artery and the cavernous sinus, usually the result of head injury. A pulsating exophthalmos with a bruit is the usual clinical concomitant. **Cervical fistula.** 1. An aerial fistula in the neck. 2. A fistula of the cervix uteri. **Cholecystoduodenal fistula.** A fistula between the gall bladder and the duodenum. **Cholecystogastric fistula.** A patent opening between the gall bladder and stomach resulting from a stone in the former ulcerating through both walls. **Cholecysto-intestinal fistula.** A patent opening between the gall bladder and intestine, which may have originated from a gall-stone or from an intestinal ulcer. **Chylous fistula.** A fistula in the neck or mediastinum which has resulted from an operation involving damage to the thoracic duct. **Coccygeal fistula.** A congenital pit over the coccyx; an opening near the coccyx communicating with a dermoid cyst. **Fistula colli congenita.** A congenital fistula in the neck communicating with the pharynx. **Colonic fistula.** Any fistula opening from the colon. **Colpocystic fistula.** Vesico-vaginal fistula (see below). **Complete fistula.** A fistula that opens both on the skin and into a hollow organ. **Fistula corneae.** An open track through the cornea. **Coronary-cameral fistula.** A vascular malformation supplied by a coronary artery and draining into a cardiac chamber, most commonly the right atrium or right ventricle. **Cysticocolic fistula.** A communication between the bladder and the colon. **Enterocutaneous fistula.** A communication between the small intestine and the external surface of the body. **Enterovaginal fistula.** A communication between the small intestine and the vagina. **Enterovesical fistula.** A communication between the small intestine and the bladder. **External fistula.** Any fistula that opens on the surface; usually a blind fistula. **Extrasphincteric fistula.** A rectal fistula that opens on the surface by passing outside the ring of the anal sphincter. **Faecal fistula.** A track from the bowel to the exterior. **Folliculovestibular fistula.** A track leading to a focus of inflammation in the region of the female urethra. **Gastric fistula.** A direct communication between the stomach and the exterior of the abdomen. **Gastrocolic fistula.** A communication between the stomach and the colon. **Gastrocutaneous fistula.** A communication between the stomach and the external surface of the abdomen. **Gastroduodenal fistula.** An unnatural communication between the stomach and the duodenum. **Gastro-intestinal fistula.** A communication between the stomach and the intestine. **Gastrojejunocolic fistula.** A fistula between the stomach, the jejunum and the colon, occurring as a complication of an anastomotic (jejunal, stomal) ulcer, usually following gastrojejunostomy. It leads to rapid emaciation. **Genito-urinary fistula.** A communication between the urinary tract and the exterior, through which urine is discharged at an unnatural site. **Hepatic fistula.** A fistula draining bile from the liver to the exterior. **Hepatopleural fistula.** A fistula between the liver and the pleural cavity. **Hepatopulmonary fistula.** A fistula leading from the liver, through the diaphragm, to the lung, e.g. as a complication of liver or subphrenic abscess. **Horseshoe fistula.** A canal-like inflammatory track around the rectum, opening on the exterior at one or more points and sometimes into the rectum as well. **Ileorectal fistula.** A patent opening between the ileum or rectum, resulting from an ulcer in either viscus first causing adhesions and eventually penetration. **Ileo-umbilical fistula.** A fistula between the ileum and the surface of the umbilicus. **Incomplete fistula.** Blind fistula (see above). **Internal fistula.** An abnormal communication between two hollow internal organs. **Intestinal fistula.** A track from the intestine to the exterior of the abdomen. **Lacrimal fistula.** A fistula leading from the surface into any part of the lacrimal passages, usually the lacrimal sac. **Laryngostomic fistula.** A surgical opening made through the neck into the larynx. **Lymphatic fistula, Fistula lymphatica.** A wound discharging lymph from a lymphatic channel to the exterior. **Mamillary fistula.** A fistula connected with a major mammary duct and presenting at the margin of the areola. It is associated with change in character of epithelium of the affected duct, and often presents as recurrent subareolar abscess. **Mammary fistula.** A leaking of milk which may occur if the lactating breast is incised. **Mediastinobronchial fistula.** Bronchomediastinal fistula (see above). **Oesophagobronchial fistula.** A fistula leading from the oesophagus to a bronchus: a complication of cancer or tuberculosis in either of them. **Oesophagocutaneous fistula.** A fistula leading from the oesophagus to the skin, e.g. following an operation on the cervical oesophagus. **Oesophagotracheal fistula.** A fistulous communication between the oesophagus and the trachea, commonly due to a cancer of the oesophagus or to a congenital opening, **Oroantral fistula.** A pathological communication between the mouth and the maxillary sinus. **Fistula of the pancreas.** A fistulous opening from the pancreas to the surface after an operation involving the pancreas. The erosion of tissue that results in a severe case may eventually prove fatal. **Parietal fistula.** A fistula through the abdominal wall or chest wall. **Parotid fistula.** A fistula from the parotid gland or duct to the surface. **Perineovaginal fistula.** An abnormal opening from the vagina to the exterior. **Perirectal fistula.** Anal fistula (see above). **Pharyngeal fistula.** An unnatural opening of the pharynx on the surface of the neck. **Pilonidal fistula.** A blind track containing hair, usually near the coccyx. **Pleurobronchial fistula.** Bronchopleural fistula (see above). **Pleurocutaneous fistula.** A patent opening from the pleural cavity through the skin, following an operation. **Pleuropulmonary fistula.** A breach in the pulmonary layer of the pleural membrane allowing alveolar air to escape into the pleural space. It is usually due to tuberculosis of the underlying lung but it may occur as a spontaneous rupture in apparently healthy subjects, leading to a pneumothorax. Collapse of the lung then often leads to healing and re-expansion; if this does not occur, intrapleural insufflations may be given to produce non-bacterial inflammation of the pleura to promote closure and the formation of adhesions which prevent occurrence. **Pre-auricular fistula.** A congenital deformity consisting of a short blind canal anterior to the tragus and lined with squamous epithelium which is liable to become infected and discharge. **Pulmonary fistula.** A track leading from the lung to the skin surface. **Rectal fistula.** A fistula from the rectum to the surface. **Rectolabial fistula.** A track leading from the surface of the labium majus to the rectum. **Rectovaginal fistula.** A communication between the rectum and the vagina. **Rectovesical fistula.** A communication between the rectum and the bladder. **Rectovulvar fistula.** An opening from the rectum to the vulva. **Sacrococcygeal fistula.** Pilonidal fistula (see above). **Salivary fistula.** An abnormal opening on the skin of the face discharging saliva from a salivary gland or duct. **Scrotal fistula.** A fistulous opening between the testes or epididymis and the skin surface of the scrotum. **Sigmoidovesical fistula.** A vesico-enteric fistula involving the sigmoid flexure of the colon. **Spermatic fistula.** A communication, discharging semen, from the epididymis or vas deferens to the exterior. **Stercoral fistula.** Faecal fistula (see above). **Submental fistula.** A salivary fistula opening below the chin. **Sylvian fissure.** The lateral sulcus of the cerebral hemisphere. **Thoracic fistula.** Fistula of the chest. **Thyroglossal fistula.** A fistula situated in the midline of the neck just above the thyroid isthmus and due to persistence of the embryonic thyroglossal duct. **Tracheal fistula.** An abnormal opening into the trachea. **Tracheo-oesophageal fistula.** A fistula between the trachea and the oesophagus. **Umbilical fistula.** A fistulous opening at the umbilicus from the bowel, due to congenital remnants. **Urachal fistula.** Persistence of the urachus, discharging urine from the bladder to the umbilicus. **Ureteral fistula.** A patent opening from the ureter to the surface. **Ureterocervical fistula.** A patent opening between the ureter and the cervix uteri. **Ureterorectal fistula.** A patent opening between the ureter and the rectum. **Ureterovaginal fistula.** A patent opening between the ureter and the vagina. **Urethral fistula.** A fistula from the urethra to the surface. **Urethrorectal fistula.** A patent opening between the urethra and the rectum. **Urethrovaginal fistula.** A patent opening between the urethra and the vagina. **Urinary fistula.** Any abnormal opening into the urinary passages, discharging urine. **Urogenital fistula.** Genito-urinary fistula (see above). **Uterorectal fistula.** A patent opening between the uterus and the rectum. **Uterovaginal fistula.** A patent opening between the uterus and the vagina. **Uterovesical fistula.** A patent opening between the uterus and the bladder. **Vaginocutaneous fistula.** An abnormal patent opening between the vagina and the surface of the perineum as a result of an obstetric tear in this region. **Vesical fistula.** An opening into the bladder. **Vesicocervical fistula.** A fistula between the bladder and the cervix uteri. **Vesicocolonic fistula.** A vesico-enteric fistula involving the colon. **Vesicocutaneous fistula.** A fistula between the bladder and the skin. **Vesico-enteric fistula, Vesico-intestinal fistula.** A communication between the bladder and intestines. **Vesicorectal fistula.** A patent opening between the bladder and any part of the rectum. **Vesico-uterine fistula.** A communication between the bladder and the uterus. **Vesicovaginal fistula.** A communication between the bladder and the vagina. [L pipe.]

See also: BOLLMAN, ECK, MANN (F. C.), THIRY, VELLA.

fistular, fistulate (**fis**·tew·lar, **fis**·tew·late). Relating or belonging to or having the character of a fistula.

fistulation (fis·tew·**la**·shun). Fistulization.

fistulatome (**fis**·tew·lat·ome). A knife used in incising a fistula; a syringotome. [fistula, Gk *temnein* to cut.]

fistulatomy (fis·tew·**lat**·o·me). The surgical incision of a fistula; syringotomy. [see prec.]

fistulectomy (fis·tew·**lek**·to·me). The surgical removal of a fistula; syringectomy. [fistula, Gk *ektome* a cutting out.]

fistulization (**fis**·tew·li·**za'**·shun). 1. The process of formation of a fistula. 2. The surgical incision of an organ, e.g. the urinary bladder, and the establishment in it of artificial drainage. **Fistulization of the eyeball.** Surgical incision of the sclera and establishment of artificial drainage.

fistulo-enterostomy (**fis**·tew·lo·en·ter·**os'**·to·me). The surgical formation of a new permanent canal along which the bile can pass into the small intestine, with closure of an external biliary fistula. [fistula, enterostomy.]

fistulous (**fis**·tew·lus). Affected with or having the form or characters of fistula.

fit (fit). A colloquial term applied to many forms of sudden disorder of function, especially of consciousness, e.g. fainting fit (syncope), apoplectic fit (stroke). Medically now almost always confined to the paroxysmal symptoms of the various forms of epilepsy. **Auditory fit.** Epileptic fit consisting of auditory hallucinations. **Epileptiform fit.** A term loosely applied to a major epileptic fit from any cause in a patient who does not have chronic epilepsy, e.g. fits in uraemia. **Focal fit.** Epileptic fit with evidence of origin in a localized area of the brain, usually the cerebral cortex. **Hysterical fit.** Symptoms in hysteria mimicking epilepsy; usually bizarre muscular contractions, violent movements and apparent disturbance of consciousness. **Jacksonian fit.** A motor or sensory fit beginning unilaterally. **Olfactory fit.** Epileptic fit characterized by hallucinations of smell, due to a lesion of the uncinate gyrus. **Psychomotor fit.** An epileptic fit characterized by co-ordinated but inappropriate movements and clouding of consciousness. **Sensory fits.** Sensory hallucinations of a great variety that may originate in any part of the body. **Visual fits.** Complex visual hallucinations or simple visual phenomena, e.g. flashes of light, or fits of a negative nature (dimness of vision or temporary complete loss of vision). [AS *fitt.*]

Fitz, Reginald (b. 1885). Boston physician.

Van Slyke and Fitz method, for alkali reserve. Urine is collected for 24 h, the volume is measured and the ammonia and titratable acidity determined as ml 0.1 M per litre of urine. The sum of the latter figures multiplied by the 24-h volume in litres gives the rate of excretion per 24 h, *D.* The plasma carbon dioxide capacity = 80-5 D/W, where W is the body weight of the patient.

Fitz, Reginald Heber (b. 1843). Boston surgeon.

Fitz's law, or syndrome. Acute pancreatic necrosis should be suspected when an apparently healthy person is afflicted with a sudden violent pain in the upper abdomen, shortly followed by vomiting and collapse, and within a few hours by abdominal distension, rigidity and a slight rise of temperature.

Fitzmaurice-Kelly, M. World War I surgeon.

Fitzmaurice-Kelly amputation. Disarticulation of the hip using a large posterior flap.

fix (fix). 1. To make stable or to fasten. 2. In ophthalmology, so to turn the eye that the image in the field of vision falls on the fovea centralis. 3. In biology, to establish permanently, by means of selective breeding, any characteristic or peculiarity in animal or plant. 4. In chemistry, to render solid or non-volatile or to induce solidification. 5. In histology, to treat tissue rapidly with a fixative so that it hardens and the elements remain permanently in the same relation that they had when they were part of a living organism. [see foll.]

fixation (fix·**a**·shun). 1. The act of holding or fastening parts in a fixed position. 2. Loss of mobility at a joint; immobilization of a fracture or diseased joint by open operation. 3. In photography, the rendering of an emulsion on a plate, film or paper, insensitive to the further action of light by dissolving out (e.g. with "hypo") the unaffected silver salts. 4. The condition when a mental presentation of an instinctual component is denied entry into consciousness, and persists unaltered in the unconscious mind with the instinct attached to it (psycho-analysis). **Alexin fixation.** Fixation of the complement (see below). **Binocular fixation.** Directing both eyes at an object so that its image falls on the fovea. **Fixation of the complement.** That which occurs when an antigen is allowed to react or combine with its specific antibody in the presence of complement. **Eccentric fixation.** A monocular condition in which fixation is with a point on the retina other than the fovea. *See* MACULA. **External skeleton fixation.** The holding together of the fragments of a broken bone by means of a device applied externally. **Freudian fixation.** *See* MAIN DEF. 4 (above). **Internal fixation.** The holding together of fragments of broken bone by wire, screws, etc. applied directly to the bony fragments. **Nitrogen fixation.** The conversion of free atmospheric nitrogen into nitrogenous compounds (e.g. ammonia, nitric acid) which can be used as fertilizers. This may be achieved by the direct union of nitrogen and oxygen in an electric arc, by the combination of nitrogen and hydrogen to form ammonia in the presence of a catalyst, or by the formation of nitrides, cyanamides, cyanides, etc. Certain bacteria such as *Azotobacter*, occurring in the soil, are capable of fixing atmospheric nitrogen. **Parent fixation.** An undue emotional attachment to, and dependence upon, a parent. [L *figere* to fasten.]

fixative (fix·at·iv). 1. Any agent employed to prepare biological specimens for staining and microscopical examination. 2. In histology, a chemical or physical agent employed to preserve and harden tissues prior to section, by denaturing, precipitating and rendering insoluble the proteins. **Dental fixative.** A preparation containing gum tragacanth used for retaining a loose artificial denture in position in the mouth. **"Susa" fixative.** *See* "SUSA" FIXATIVE. [L *figere* to fasten.]

fixator (fix·a·tor). Amboceptor. [see prec.]

fixing fluid (fix·ing floo·id). A solution used to harden and preserve the shape of the cells in tissue intended for microscopical sections. [L *figere* to fasten, *fluere* to flow.]

See also: CHAMPY, HELLY, REGAUD.

fixity (fix·it·e). In early labour, the stage at which the head of the fetus becomes engaged in the pelvis. [L *figere* to fasten.]

flaccid (flak·sid). 1. Flabby and soft; boneless. 2. Relaxed. [L *flaccus* flabby.]

Flack, Martin William (b. 1882). London physiologist.

Flack's node, Node of Keith and Flack. The sinu-atrial node.

Flack test, for respiratory efficiency. The subject takes a full inspiration and then expires as long as he can into a mercury manometer at a pressure of 5.3 kPa (40 mm Hg).

flag (flag). The common name for monocotyledonous plants with sword-shaped leaves. **Blue flag.** *Iris versicolar* Linn.; the dried rhizome and root is used as a cathartic. **Sweet flag.** Calamus; the dried rhizome of *Acorus calamus* Linn. used as a stomachic. [ME *flagge.*]

flagella (flaj·el·ah). *See* FLAGELLUM.

flagellar (flaj·el·ah). Of or pertaining to a flagellum.

Flagellata (flaj·el·a·tah). A synonym of Mastigophora, a class of protozoa. [L *flagellum* whip.]

flagellate (flaj·el·ate). 1. Shaped like a flagellum or whip. 2. Bearing whip-like processes, as do certain protozoa. [see prec.]

flagellation (flaj·el·a·shun). 1. A form of massage in which there is quick tapping of the fingers on the part under treatment, or application of light blows or strokes; an electrical appliance can be used instead of the fingers. 2. Exflagellation. 3. A form of sexual perversion or eroticism in which lustful feelings are aroused and satisfied by self-whipping or whipping another person. [L *flagellare* to scourge.]

flagelliform (flaj·el·e·form). 1. Shaped like a flagellum. 2. Long, slender, flexible and tapering like a whip-lash. [L *flagellum* whip, form.]

flagellin (flaj·el·in). The monometric protein resembling myosin which polymerizes to form bacterial flagella. [L *flagellum* whip.]

flagellosis (flaj·el·o·sis). Intestinal infection with *Giardia intestinalis* or some other form of flagellate protozoon. [Flagellata, Gk *-osis* condition.]

flagellospore (flaj·el·o·spore). A spore bearing a flagellum or flagella; a zoospore.

flagellula (flaj·el·ew·lah). Flagellospore.

flagellum (flaj·el·um) (pl. *flagella*). An elongate motile process of a cell or of a protistan individual, used for producing currents in fluid media and thence for locomotion. The tail portion of the spermatozoon which provides it with its motility. It is characteristic of the Mastigophora. [L whip.]

Flagg, Paluel J. 20th century American anaesthetist.

Flagg's can. A simple metallic can adapted so that a patient can inhale from it a volatile anaesthetic vapour in air.

flail (flale). The free-swinging state of an extremity when not under muscular control. **Flail joint.** *See* JOINT. [ME *fleyl* whip.]

Flajani, Giuseppe (b. 1741). Rome surgeon.

Flajani's disease. Exophthalmic goitre.

Flajani's operation. Iridodialysis, by an obsolete method.

flame (flame). A zone of active chemical reaction, usually oxidation, in gases and vapours, accompanied by heat and often light. **Capillary flame.** Capillary telangiectases that are occasionally seen in the face of a newly-born infant. **Manometric flame.** A flame of gas which is made to pulsate as a result of transmitted vibrations of a column of air or other gaseous material. It is used in the study of sound waves. **Flame picture.** The pattern made by the flame of the flame manometer. [L *flamma.*]

flank [latus (NA)] (flangk). That part of the body bounded above by the lowest rib, and below by the ilium. **Flank bone.** The ilium. [Fr. *flanc.*]

flannel (flan·el). **Vegetable flannel.** A kind of woven material made in Germany from the fibre of *Pinus sylvestris* and used by patients with rheumatism, for which it is held to be of benefit. **Welsh flannel.** A term for a particular kind of loosely-woven material made from the wool of Welsh sheep and used for the same purpose as vegetable flannel (see prec.). The wool in Welsh flannel has a high fatty content. [Welsh *gwlan* wool.]

flap (flap). A layer of skin or other tissue separated by dissection from deeper structures, either to afford surgical exposure to these deeper parts or to be used to cover some other area which has lost its integument as a result of surgery, accident or disease. **Amputation flap.** The skin flap raised, usually from the limb just below the level of bone division, to serve in covering the end of the amputation stump. **Artery flap.** A skin flap raised so that the blood vessels supplying it remain undamaged in its hinge. **Bipedicled flap.** A skin flap which remains attached at both extremities. **Bone flap.** A segment of bone, usually of skull, raised on a hinge of periosteum or other membrane. **Bridge flap.** Bipedicled flap (see above). **Cellulocutaneous flap.** A flap composed both of skin and of subcutaneous tissue. **Cineplastic flap.** A skin flap in which tendon is incorporated after amputation for manipulation of a mechanical prosthesis. **Circular flap.** A tube of soft tissues raised like a sleeve before bone division to be used to cover an amputation stump. **Compound flap.** A flap of skin together with other tissue. **Cross arm flap.** A pedicled flap formed from the skin of one arm and transferred to fill a skin defect on the other arm. **Cross finger flap.** A pedicled flap formed from the skin of one finger and transferred to fill a skin defect on the other finger. **Cross leg flap.** A pedicled flap formed from the skin of one leg and transferred to fill a skin defect on the other leg. **Delayed flap.** A flap which, after being cut, is temporarily resutured at its site of origin. **Filleted finger flap.** Removal of all tissues except skin from a severely injured finger and using it as a pedicle graft to fill a defect elsewhere in the hand. **Island flap.** A skin flap whose circumference is separated from deeper tissues but whose central attachment remains. **Jump flap.** A skin flap moved from one position to another by successive division and re-attachment of its ends. **Mediastinal flap.** Lateral movement of the mediastinum during breathing with an open pneumothorax, which interferes with both circulation and respiration and can be controlled by intermittent positive pressure respiration. **Muscle flap.** A flap of muscle used to fill up a cavity, e.g. an empyema cavity. **Musculocutaneous flap.** A flap of skin, subcutaneous tissue and muscle. **Osteoplastic flap.** 1. A hinged flap of skin and bone used to cover an amputation stump. 2. A portion of skull elevated on a hinge of pericranium in craniotomy. **Oval flap.** An amputation flap obtained by oblique incision. **Pedicle flap.** A flap fashioned as a tube by suture of its edges, one end remaining attached and the other being transplanted to a new position. **Pocket flap.** A skin flap raised by an incision at one of its edges only so that material to be covered—for example a skinless hand—may be inserted underneath. **Rectangular flap.** A skin flap with three straight sides, the fourth remaining attached. **Skin flap.** A flap of skin only. **Sliding flap.** A skin flap moved horizontally to cover an adjacent raw area. **Swinging flap.** A flap swinging on its pedicle to cover an adjacent raw area. **Tubed flap.** A skin flap attached at one or both ends and fashioned into a tube by suture of its edges so that the epidermis faces outwards. **Tunnel flap.** A skin flap attached at one or both ends and fashioned into a tube by suture of its edges so that the epidermis faces inwards. **V-Y flap.** An angled flap whose apex is advanced to cover a raw area. **Waltzing flap.** A skin flap moved to its new position by division and re-attachment of its ends alternately. **Z flap.** Two angular flaps, produced by a Z-shaped incision, whose bases can be distracted from each other, their apices being sutured to each other. [ME *flappe.*]

flare (flare). 1. The sudden development of a lesion in tissue which previously has appeared to be healthy, e.g. in pulmonary tuberculosis. 2. The zone of hyperaemia surrounding the area of local reaction to injury. **Aqueous flare.** Tyndall phenomenon in the anterior chamber of the eye. [etym. dub.]

Flarer, Francesco (b. 1791). Italian ophthalmologist.

Flarer's operation, for trichiasis. Removal of the line of the cilia. Not often used.

flash (flash). Flashes; an American version of the British expression "hot flushes".

flask (flask). 1. A narrow-necked glass vessel, often with round bottom, used in chemistry for boiling liquids. 2. A metal container in which artificial dentures are processed. **Culture flask.** A flask used to contain fluid media for the growth of bacteriological or other cultures. **Florence flask.** A round-bottomed glass flask employed in chemical distillation. **Volumetric flask.** A pear-shaped glass flask with a long thin neck; the latter bears a single graduation. Filling the flask to this graduation measures accurately a stated volume of liquid. [L *vasculum* small vessel.]

See also: BAILEY, DEWAR.

flasking (**flask**·ing). The shutting of a dental plate into a moulding flask during the process of vulcanization.

flat (flat). 1. Having an even surface in one plane. 2. Of the voice or a percussion note, dull, monotonous, without resonance and low in pitch. 3. Of pitch of sound, below the normal. **Optical flat.** A surface, usually on quartz, that has been ground so flat that differences from a true plane surface are small in comparison with the wavelength of light. [AS *flet* floor.]

flat foot (**flat** fut). Pronated foot, pes valgus; a condition of the foot in which the inner longitudinal arch is lowered or is absent. **Spastic flat foot.** Flattening of the longitudinal arch of the foot, associated with eversion of the heel and spasm of the peroneal muscles. [flat, AS *fot*.]

Flatau, Edward (b. 1896). Warsaw neurologist.

Flatau's law. The longer the nerve fibres of the spinal cord, the nearer they are to the surface of the cord.

Flatau-Schilder disease. Progressive subcortical encephalopathy or encephalitis periaxialis diffusa; usually called *Schilder's disease.*

flatness (**flat**·nes). 1. The condition of being flat. 2. The peculiar dull sound elicited by percussion over an abnormally solid part, or over an organ in which there is not any air, or over a large collection of fluid in a tissue.

flatulence (**flat**·ew·lens). The presence of an excessive amount of gas in the stomach and alimentary canal, leading to distension of the organs; tympanites. [flatus.]

flatulent (**flat**·ew·lent). 1. Characterized by flatus. 2. Suffering from flatulence or flatus. 3. Of an organ, distended by gas generated within it; tympanitic.

flatus (**fla**·tus). 1. Gas or air present in the alimentary canal or the stomach. 2. The act of expelling air from the lungs. 3. The air expelled from the lungs in expiration. 4. Air or gas expelled through the anus. 5. Air or gas expelled from the stomach in eructation. **Flatus vaginalis.** Loud expulsion of gas from the vagina. [L a blowing.]

flatworm (**flat**·werm). A member of the phylum Platyhelminthes. [flat, AS *wyrm*.]

flavedo (flav·**e**·do). 1. A jaundiced or yellowish colour of the skin. 2. Sallowness. [L yellowness.]

flavescens, flavescent (flav·**es**·ens, flav·**es**·ent). 1. Turning yellow. 2. Yellowish. [L *flavescere* to turn yellow.]

flavicid (**flav**·is·id). Dimethyl - 3 - dimethyl - amino - 6 - amino - 10 - methyl acridinum chloride, $(CH_3)_2NC_7H_5{=}CHN(CH_3)Cl{=}C_7H_5NH_2$. A brown dye, soluble in water, and used as an antiseptic.

flavicidin, flavicin (flav·**is**·id·in, **flav**·is·in). An antibiotic obtained from the mould *Aspergillus flavus.* It consists mainly of penicillin F.

flavin (**fla**·vin, **flav**·in). 1. Iso-alloxazine, $C_{10}H_6N_4O_2$; a heterocyclic ketone. 2. General name for the lyochromes, nitrogenous water-soluble yellow pigments with a greenish-yellow fluorescence in neutral solutions: they are derived from iso-alloxazine and related closely to riboflavine or vitamin B_2. They occur with phosphate and protein in the biological oxidation-reduction systems of plants and animals, [L *flavus* yellow.]

flavine (**fla**·veen, **flav**·een). The generic term for members of the group of bacteriostatics derived from acridine which includes acriflavine, proflavine and aminacrine; the name is often applied loosely to the individual compounds. [L *flavus* yellow.]

Flavivirus (**fla**·ve·vi·rus). The official generic name for the Group B arboviruses. Members of the genus include many of the arboviruses causing severe disease in man such as dengue and the encephalitides due to Japanese B, Murray Valley, St. Louis and equine viruses. The type species is yellow fever virus, hence the name, and members possess a similar haemagglutinating antigen.

Flavobacterium (**fla**·vo·bak·**teer**'·e·um). A genus of non-pathogenic bacteria (family Achromobacteriaceae) which form a yellow pigment on culture media. They are of medium size, are usually Gram-negative, sometimes motile, and are found in water and soil. [L *flavus* yellow, bacterium.]

flavone (**fla**·vone). 1. Phenylbenzopyrone, phenylchromone, anthoxanthin, $\overline{C_6H_4COCHCO}C_6H_5$. A colourless substance, the parent of numerous vegetable colouring matters. 2. General term for a group of polyhydroxy and methoxy derivatives of flavone which occur in the form of glycosides as the orange and yellow pigments of certain flowers and fruits: some, like citrin from lemon peel, have a capillary-strengthening property (vitamin P).

flavonoid (**fla**·vo·noid). 1. Related to, or of the nature of flavone. 2. Resembling, or belonging to the group of anti-haemorrhagic so-called vitamin-P substances. [flavone, Gk *eidos* form.]

flavonol (**fla**·vo·nol). 1. $\overline{C_6H_4COC(OH)CO}C_6H_5$, a hydroxy derivative of flavone. 2. General term for a group of vegetable dyes derived from 1.

flavoprotein (fla·vo·**pro**·te·in). A protein containing a flavin prosthetic group, usually FMN or FAD.

flavopurpurin (fla·vo·**per**·pewr·in). Alizarin X, trihydroxyanthraquinone, $C_6H_3(OH)(CO)_2C_6H_2(OH)_2$. A yellow substance used as a dyestuff. [L *flavus* yellow, *purpura* purple.]

flavour (**fla**·vor). 1. That quality in a substance which affects the sense of taste with or without involving the sense of smell. 2. Any therapeutically inert substance gratifying to the palate which is added to a food or a medicinal prescription in order to mask the disagreeable taste of other ingredients or give taste to an insipid mixture. [prob. O Fr. *flaur* odour.]

flavoxanthin (fla·vo·**zan**·thin). $C_{40}H_{56}O_3$, a yellow vegetable colouring matter of carotenoid structure occurring in the flowers of species of *Ranunculaceae.*

Flavoxate (fla·**vox**·ate). BP Commission approved name for 2 - piperidinoethyl 3 - methylflavone - 8 - carboxylate; an antispasmodic.

flavus (**fla**·vus). Yellow. [L.]

flax (flax). A European annual plant, *Linum usitatissimum* Linn. (family Linaceae). The dried ripe seed constitutes linseed; linen is manufactured from the xylem fibres of the stem. [AS *fleax*.]

flaxseed (**flax**·seed). Linseed BPC 1954; the dried ripe seeds of *Linum usitatissimum* Linn. (family Linaceae). [AS *fleax, saed.*]

flay (fla). To strip off the skin. [ME *flean* to tear.]

Flazalone (**flaz**·al·one). BP Commission approved name for 3 - (4 - fluorobenzoyl) - 4 - (4 - fluorophenyl) - 1 - methylpiperidin - 4 - ol; an anti-inflammatory agent.

flea (fle) 1. A member of the insect order Siphonaptera (= Aphaniptera), characterized by lateral flattening, absence of wings, piercing and sucking mouth parts, and jumping hind legs. All adult fleas are parasites of mammals and birds; the larvae live in host nests. 2. In combinations, the term is used of many small arthropods with jumping powers, e.g. water flea. **Asiatic rat flea.** *Xenopsylla.* **Cat flea.** *Ctenocephalides felis.* **Chigger flea.** *Tunga.* **Common flea.** *Pulex irritans.* **Dog flea.** *Ctenocephalides canis.* **Hen flea.** *Ceratophyllus.* **Human flea.** *Pulex irritans.* **Jigger flea.** *Tunga.* **Rat flea.** *Nosopsyllus.* **Sand flea.** *Tunga.* **Sticktight flea.** One whose adult female remains attached to the host in one place for long periods, e.g. *Tunga, Echidnophaga.* **Tropical hen flea.** *Echidnophaga gallinacea.* **Tropical rat flea.** *Xenopsylla.* **Water flea.** Crustaceans of the order Cladocera; *Daphnia.* [AS.]

fleam (fleem). 1. An instrument for letting blood or lancing the gums. 2. A lancet used for bleeding horses. [Gk *phlebe* vein, *temnein* to cut.]

Flechsig, Paul Emil (b. 1847). Leipzig neurologist.

Flechsig's areas. Three areas on each side of the medulla oblongata demarcated by the fibres passing from the hypoglossal and vagal nuclei.

Flechsig's association centres. Areas of the surface of the cerebral cortex which are the last to obtain myelin sheaths. They are extensive in man, small in lower vertebrates, and are described as the anatomical areas of higher intelligence.

Flechsig's column, fasciculus or tract. The dorsal spinocerebellar tract. *See* TRACT.

Flechsig's field. Myelinogenetic field. *See* FIELD.

Flechsig's myelinogenetic law. Functionally-related tracts in the central nervous system become myelinated at about the same time.

Flechsig's treatment. The use of opium and bromides in the treatment of epilepsy.

flection (flek·shun). Flexion.

fleece (flees). *See* STILLING. [AS *fleos.*]

Fleischer, Bruno (b. 1874). Erlangen ophthalmologist.

Fleischer's ring. In keratoconus, a line running round the base of the cone of the cornea, involving the epithelium and Bowman's membrane, and often coloured yellow or green due to haemosiderin.

Fleischer-Kayser ring, Kayser-Fleischer ring. A brown ring at the outer edge of the cornea, seen in Wilson's disease (hepatolenticular degeneration) and due to copper deposition. It may only be visible on slit-lamp examination but is a diagnostic sign of the disease.

Fleischer-Struempell ring. Kayser-Fleischer ring (see above).

Fleischmann, Friedrich Ludwig (fl. 1841). German anatomist.

Fleischmann's bursa. An occasional space between the lingual septum and the origin of the genioglossus muscle.

Fleischmann's follicle. An occasional mucous follicle in the oral mucosa covering the genioglossus muscle.

Fleischmann's hygroma. A hygroma of the bursa in the sublingual space beneath the lingual frenum.

Fleming, Sir Alexander (b. 1881). Scottish bacteriologist and immunologist in London (discoverer of penicillin and lysozyme).

Fleming's nigrosin method. A method of negative staining of bacteria to show shape, size, spores, etc.

Flemming, Walther (b. 1843). Kiel anatomist.

intermediate body of Flemming. A small acidophilic body which forms the last connection between the two cells produced by mitotic division before they separate.

Flemming's fluids, or solutions. Histological fixatives containing chromic acid, osmic acid and acetic acid. They are used for the demonstration of chromosomes, fat, mitochondria and cytoplasmic structures generally.

Flemming's triple stain. Safranine, gentian violet and orange G, used successively in the staining of chromosomes.

interfibrillar substance of Flemming. A hypothetical part of the cytoplasm lying between equally hypothetical fibres, now known to be artefacts caused by the action of fixatives.

flesh (flesh). The soft muscular tissues of the body. **Goose flesh.** Skin-coloured papules caused by the contraction of the arrectores pilorum muscles. **Proud flesh.** The granulations of new vessels and young fibrous tissue which develop in the course of the healing of a surgical incision, wound or other lesion, [AS *flaesc.*]

Fletcher, Sir William (b. 1872). London and Malaya physician.

Fletcher's culture medium. A medium prepared from sterile rabbit serum 10 to 20 ml, peptone 0.2 g, sodium chloride 0.1 g, and water 100 ml, with or without semi-solid agar: used in the cultivation of *Leptospira.*

Fletcherism (flech·er·izm). The practice of taking food only when hungry, of thoroughly masticating solids until all taste is gone and of sipping fluids. [Horace *Fletcher* (b. 1849), American writer and lecturer on nutrition.]

flex (flex). To bend a limb, such as the arm, by moving the connecting joint so as to bring the two parts into approximation; to put in a state of flexion, as with a muscle. [L *flectere* to bend.]

flexibilitas cerea (flex·ib·il·it·as **seer**·e·ah). A state seen in encephalitis lethargica or schizophrenia; it is a type of catalepsy in which the limbs are retained in any position in which they are placed or in which the patient is instructed to place them. [L waxy flexibility.]

flexibility (flex·ib·il·it·e). The quality or state of being supple or flexible; pliability. [L *flexibilitas.*]

fleximeter (flex·**im**·et·er). An instrument for measuring the degree of flexion of which a joint is capable.

flexion (**flek**·shun). 1. The act of so bending a joint that the two parts it connects approximate each other. 2. The condition of being bent at an angle. **Lateral flexion.** Flexion to one or other side, as in the spine. [L *flectere* to bend.]

Flexner, Simon (b. 1863). New York bacteriologist and pathologist.

Flexner's bacillus. *Shigella flexneri.*

Flexner's dysentery. Dysentery due to bacilli of the Flexner group; frequently the attack is a mild one.

Flexner's serum. A serum for the treatment of infections by the Flexner group of dysentery bacilli.

flexor (flex·or). A muscle which flexes a joint. [L bender.]

flexor carpi radialis muscle [musculus flexor carpi radialis (NA)] (**flex**·or **kar**·pi ra·de·a·lis). A superficially-placed flexor of the forearm, extending from the medial epicondyle to the bases of the 2nd and 3rd metacarpal bones.

flexor carpi ulnaris muscle [musculus flexor carpi ulnaris (NA)] (**flex**·or **kar**·pi ul·**na**·ris). A superficial forearm flexor muscle extending from the medial epicondyle and ulna to the pisiform bone. It has 2 heads, the humeral [caput humerale (NA)] and the ulnar [caput ulnare (NA)].

flexor digiti minimi muscle [musculus flexor digiti minimi brevis (NA)] (**flex**·or **dij**·it·i **min**·im·i). One of the muscles of the hypothenar eminence arising from the hook of the hamate and the flexor retinaculum and inserted into the base of the 1st phalanx of the 5th digit.

flexor digiti minimi brevis muscle [musculus flexor digiti minimi brevis] (**flex**·or **dij**·it·i **min**·im·i **brev**·is). A muscle arising around the base of the 5th metatarsal and inserted into the base of the 1st phalanx of the same toe.

flexor digitorum accessorius muscle [musculus quadratus plantae (musculus flexor accessorius (NA)] (**flex**·or dij·it·o·rum ak·ses·o·re·us). A muscle arising from the under-surface of the calcaneum and inserted into the main tendon of the flexor digitorum longus muscle, through which it can act as a flexor of the lateral 4 toes.

flexor digitorum brevis muscle [musculus flexor digitorum brevis (NA)] (**flex**·or dij·it·o·rum **brev**·is). A centrally-placed muscle in the sole of the foot arising at the heel and inserted by tendons into the 2nd phalanges of the lateral 4 toes. Its tendons are perforated by those of the long flexor muscles of these toes.

flexor digitorum longus muscle [musculus flexor digitorum longus (NA)] (**flex**·or dij·it·o·rum **long**·gus). The long flexor muscle of the toes. It arises deeply in the calf from the back of the shaft of the tibia, divides into 4 tendons which perforate those of the flexor digitorum brevis muscle, and is inserted into the distal phalanges of the lateral 4 toes.

flexor digitorum profundus muscle [musculus flexor digitorum profundus (NA)] (**flex**·or dij·it·o·rum pro·**fun**·dus). A deep muscle on the front of the forearm. It flexes the terminal phalanges of the lateral 4 digits, and its tendons perforate those of the flexor digitorum sublimis muscle.

flexor digitorum sublimis muscle [musculus flexor digitorum superficialis (NA)] (**flex**·or dij·it·o·rum **sub**·lim·is). The more superficial of the 2 long flexor muscles of the digits, arising from the medial epicondyle and proximal parts of the radius and ulna and inserted into the bases of the 2nd phalanges of the 2nd to the 5th fingers. Its digital tendons are perforated by the tendons of the flexor digitorum profundus muscle. It has 2 heads, the humero-ulnar [caput humero-ulnare (NA)] and the radial [caput radiale (NA)].

flexor hallucis brevis muscle [musculus flexor hallucis brevis (NA)] (**flex**·or **hal**·oo·sis **brev**·is). A deep muscle of the sole of the foot, arising from the under-side of the cuboid and lateral cuneiform bones and inserted into the base of the proximal phalanx of the big toe.

flexor hallucis longus muscle [musculus flexor hallucis longus (NA)] (**flex**·or **hal**·oo·sis **long**·gus). The flexor of the big toe, arising from the lower two-thirds of the fibula and inserted into the base of the distal phalanx of this toe.

flexor pollicis brevis muscle [musculus flexor pollicis brevis (NA)] (**flex**·or **pol**·is·is **brev**·is). One of the short muscles of the thumb arising from the flexor retinaculum and the crest on the trapezium, and inserted into the base of the proximal phalanx of the thumb.

flexor pollicis longus muscle [musculus flexor pollicis longus (NA)] (**flex**·or **pol**·is·is **long**·gus). A deep muscle on the forearm, where it lies alongside the flexor digitorum profundus muscle. Its tendon is inserted into the terminal phalanx of the thumb, which it flexes.

flexorplasty (flex·or·**plas**·te). Restoration of flexion in a joint (usually the elbow) by transplantation of tendons. [L *flexor* bender, Gk *plassein* to mould].

flexuous (**flex**·ew·us). In biology, alternately curving in opposite directions; zigzag. [L *flexus* a bending.]

flexure [flexura (NA)] (**flex**·ewr). A bend or angulation. **Basicranial flexure.** The angle made between the fore and hind parts of the base of the skull. **Cephalic flexure.** The dorsally convex bend in the embryonic brain at the level of the mid-brain. **Cervical flexure.** 1. The dorsally convex bend in the embryonic central nervous system at the junction of the brain and spinal cord. 2. The ventral convexity of the cervical part of the spine. **Flexure of the colon, left [flexura coli sinistra (NA)].** Splenic flexure; the acute bend at the junction of the transverse and descending part of the colon. **Flexure of the colon, right [flexura coli dextra (NA)].** Hepatic flexure; the bend at the junction of the ascending and transverse part of the colon. **Dorsal flexure.** The dorsal convexity of the thoracic region of the spine. **Duodenojejunal flexure [flexura duodenojejunalis (NA)].** The acute bend in the small intestine at the junction of the duodenum and jejunum. **Flexure of the duodenum, inferior [flexura duodeni inferior (NA)].** The sharp curve formed by the angulation between the second and third parts of the duodenum. **Flexure of the duodenum, superior [flexura duodeni superior (NA)].** The sharp curve formed by the angulation between the first and second parts of the duodenum. **Hepatic flexure.** Right flexure of the colon (see above). **Lumbar flexure.** The forward convexity in the spine in the lumbar region. **Mesencephalic flexure.** Cephalic flexure (see above). **Perineal flexure.** The bend in the embryo at the junction of the back and perineum. **Pontine flexure.** The ventrally convex flexure of the embryonic brain at the level of the pons. **Flexure of the rectum, perineal [flexura perinealis (NA)].** The lower smaller anteroposterior flexure with its convexity directed forwards. **Flexure of the rectum, sacral [flexura sacralis (NA)].** The larger upper antero-posterior flexure with its convexity directed backwards. **Sigmoid flexure.** The bend in the colon at the junction of its descending and pelvic portions. **Splenic flexure.** Left flexure of the colon (see above). [L *flectere* to bend.]

flicker (**flik**·er). The sensation produced by periodic light stimuli, not sufficiently rapid to create a sensation of uniform brightness. [AS *flicorian.*]

flimmerskotoma (**flim**·er·sko·**to'**·mah). Scintillating scotoma. *See* SCOTOMA. [G *Flimmer* glittering, scotoma.]

Flindt, Nicolaj (b. 1843). Danish physician.

Flindt's spots. Koplik's spots.

Flint, Austin (b. 1812). New York physician.

Flint's arcade. The arciform arteries, lying between the renal cortex and medulla, which give off the interlobular arteries of the kidney.

Austin Flint murmur, phenomenon or sign, Flint's murmur or sign. A low-pitched mid-diastolic murmur heard at the apex of the heart in patients with severe aortic-valve incompetence, but without organic stenosis of the mitral valve. It is thought to be due to relative narrowing of the mitral orifice produced by gross hypertrophy of the left ventricle; a functional mitral stenosis.

floatation (flo·**ta**·shun). 1. In colloid chemistry, the separation of mixed particles by taking advantage of differential wetting, the poorly wetted particles floating to the surface. The method has been used in the separation of valuable minerals from crushed ores, and may involve the use of a foaming agent to increase surface, collectors which are selectively adsorbed on the particles and render them less wettable, activators to induce adsorption of the collectors, and deflocculators which prevent clumping of the particles. 2. In parasitology, the method of separating for easy identification ova or cysts by raising the specific gravity of the medium in which they are lying to such a degree that they just float, e.g. by the addition of zinc sulphate solution. [Fr. *flotter to float.*]

floaters (**flo**·terz). **Vitreous floaters.** A general term used for the opacities seen floating in the vitreous. They may be degenerative, inflammatory, haemorrhagic or, rarely, neoplastic. [AS *flotian.*]

floating (**flo**·ting). 1. Unattached or detached. 2. Freely movable. 3. Unduly movable, as certain organs, e.g. spleen or kidney. [see prec.]

flocci volitantes (**flok**·si vol·it·**an**·teez). Muscae volitantes, i.e. specks floating before the eyes. [L *floccus* flock of wool, *volare* to fly.]

floccilation, floccilegium, floccitation (flok·sil·**a**·shun, flok·sil·-e·**je**·um, flok·sit·**a**·shun). The aimless plucking at the bedclothes as if picking off bits of thread or wool, which is one of the signs typical of the delirium of typhoid and other severe fevers; carphologia. [see foll.]

floccose (**flok**·oze). Woolly, loose, fluffy; applied to a deposit, precipitate or growth of organisms. [L *floccus* flock of wool.]

floccular (**flok**·ew·lar). Relating or belonging to a flocculus.

flocculation (flok·ew·**la**·shun). 1. The aggregation of the fine particles of the disperse phase in a colloidal system to form larger particles which become visible and gradually settle as a precipitate. 2. (*a*) Formation of floccules or loose masses of precipitate in a precipitation reaction; (*b*) the reaction that occurs when non-specific antibody from the serum of a syphilitic patient precipitates in a mixture with a cardiolipin antigen, as in the Kahn or VDRL tests. [L *floccus* flock of wool.]

floccule (**flok**·ewl). 1. The flocculus of the posterior lobe of the cerebellum. 2. A suspended particle aggregation. **Toxoid-antitoxin floccules, TAF.** A precipitate prepared by mixing diphtheria toxoid with diphtheria antitoxin in conditions of slight excess of the toxoid; it is used as an alternative prophylactic to alum-precipitated toxoid (APT) for immunization of older children or adults against diphtheria. [see prec.]

flocculence (**flok**·ew·lens). The condition of being flocculent.

flocculent (**flok**·ew·lent). 1. In bacteriology, containing woolly floating masses suspended in a fluid culture or deposited at the bottom. 2. Containing deposits of shreds of white material, as in urine. 3. In chemistry, applied to a liquid in which there are non-crystalline cloudy or flake-like particles. [L *floccus* flock of wool.]

flocculoreaction (**flok**·ew·lo·re·**ak'**·shun). A serum reaction marked by flocculation.

flocculus (**flok**·ew·lus). 1. [NA] The small semi-detached portion of the lateral part of the posterior lobe of the cerebellum lying immediately below the auditory nerve at the point where it enters the brain stem. 2. A small woolly tuft, like the fine curved hairs on the legs of some insects. 3. A small flake, or a shred or little tuft of something, as of wool. 4. A small mass of bacteria, variously shaped, observed floating in a culture medium. **Accessory flocculus.** Paraflocculus. [L a little tuft.]

flock (flok). Flocculus, 3rd def. [L *floccus* flock of wool.]

Flood, Valentine (b. 1800). Dublin surgeon.

Flood's ligament. The superior glenohumeral ligament of the shoulder joint.

flooding (flud·ing). Excessive menstrual discharge or copious bleeding from the uterus after childbirth. [AS *flod.*]

floor (flo·er). The lowest surface or lower boundary of any cavity or organ. [AS *flor.*]

flora (flor·ah). A collective term for the plants of any particular region, or of a geological period. It corresponds to *fauna*, the animals of the same region or period. **Intestinal flora.** The bacterial content of the lumen of the intestine. [L *flos* flower.]

Florantyrone (flor·an·ti·rone). BP Commission approved name for γ-fluoranthen-8yl-γ-oxobutyric acid; a hydrocholeretic.

Florence, Albert (b. 1851). Lyons pharmacologist.

Florence crystals. Dark-brown microcrystals formed by the addition of iodine solution (Florence's reagent) to semen. The reaction is not specific, but is nevertheless useful for the detection of seminal stains.

Florence's reagent. Dissolve 2.54 g of iodine and 1.65 g of potassium iodide in 30 ml of distilled water.

Florence test. For detection of seminal fluid; place some fluid or aqueous extract of material (if a stain) upon a glass slide, add a few drops of iodine solution and examine under the microscope. Dark-brown crystals (Florence crystals) in the form of platelets or needles will be observed if semen is present.

flores (flor·eez). 1. The flowers of a medicinal herb, e.g. flores anthemidis (chamomile flowers). 2. Crystals which occur in flower-shaped clusters, usually as the result of sublimation, e.g. camphor. **Sambuci flores.** Sambucus. **Flores sulphuris.** Flowers of sulphur; sublimed sulphur. [L flowers.]

Florey, Walter Howard, 1st Baron (b. 1895). Oxford pathologist, Nobel prizewinner for work on penicillin.

Florey unit. Oxford unit. *See* UNIT.

floribundine (flor·e·bun·deen). $C_{18}H_{19}O_2N$, a non-phenolic crystalline alkaloid extracted from the poppy, *Papaver floribundum.*

florid (flor·id). Of a lively red colour; the term is applied to the complexion and to skin lesions. [L *flos* flower.]

floripavidine (flor·e·pav·id·een). $C_{21}H_{29}O_5N$, a non-phenolic alkaloid separated from floribundine in the extraction of *Papaver floribundum.*

floripavine (flor·e·pav·een). $C_{19}H_{21}O_4N$, a crystalline phenolic alkaloid obtained from the poppy *Papaver floribundum.*

Flosdorf, Earl William (b. 1904). Philadelphia bacteriologist.

Flosdorf-Mudd apparatus. An apparatus devised for the preservation of sera, plasma, bacteria and tissues. It consists of a manifold holding ampules of the substance which is frozen by immersion in a carbon dioxide-acetone mixture and then dehydrated for some hours by a high-vacuum pump with primary and secondary condensers.

floss (flos). Untwisted silk threads. **Dental floss, Silk floss.** Untwisted fine silk used in dentistry for cleaning the surfaces of the teeth. [OFr. *flosche* down.]

flotation (flo·ta·shun). Floatation.

Flourens, Marie Jean Pierre (b. 1794). Paris physiologist and anatomist.

Flourens' law. Stimulation of a semicircular canal results in nystagmus in the plane of that canal.

flow (flo). 1. The menses. 2. Copious menstruation less profuse than flooding. 3. To menstruate freely but not so freely as to constitute flooding. 4. Any free discharge of liquid. **Aventilatory mass flow.** Term given to explain the way arterial oxygenation is maintained when apnoea takes place, in a patient whose lungs and upper airways contain pure oxygen. **Flow of ideas.** Incoherent ideation. *See* IDEATION. **Laminar flow.** The orderly, smooth flow of fluid or gas along a tube, as normally occurs in the air passages or the blood vessels. **Turbulent flow.** Disturbed, irregular or tumultuous flow of fluid or gas along a tube, as may occur in disease states in the air passages or the heart and blood vessels. [AS *flowan.*]

Flower, Sir William Henry (b. 1831). London comparative anatomist.

Flower's angle. The angle formed between the 2 lines from points where the frontonasal sutures reach the outer margins of the orbits on each side; they meet at the most depressed point of the nasal bones in the middle line. In natives of the U.K. the angle averages 135°, whereas in all persons of the Mongolian race it exceeds 140°.

Flower's bone. The pterion ossicle, a cranial sutural bone.

Flower's index. The dental index; the dental length multiplied by 100 and divided by the length of the basinasal line.

flower (flow·er). The part of a plant which consists of the essential reproductive organs, i.e. pistils and stamens, contained within a protective envelope which may be composed of 1 or more layers (petals, sepals, etc.). In materia medica, the term is often used to include part or whole of the inflorescence as well as the flowers themselves. [ME *flour.*]

flowers (flow·erz). 1. Flores. 2. Solids obtained by sublimation, i.e. the cooling of a vapour under such conditions of pressure that it passes directly into the solid state, often in flowerlike clusters of crystals, without an intermediate liquid phase. 3. The menses; a term now obsolete, but common in West Africa. **Flowers of arsenic.** Arsenic trioxide. **Flowers of benzoin.** Benzoic-acid crystals obtained by heating benzoin. **Flowers of camphor.** Sublimed camphor. **Dalmation insect flowers.** Pyrethrum Flower BPC 1954. **Elder flowers.** Sambucus BPC 1949. **Insect flowers.** Pyrethrum Flower BPC 1954. **Flowers of sulphur.** Sublimed sulphur. [see prec.]

flowmeter (flo·me·ter). A device for measuring the flow of gas, e.g. during anaesthesia. **Dry flowmeter.** An apparatus in which the rate of flow is indicated by a bobbin that is upheld by the pressure of the gas escaping through a series of holes or through the space surrounding the bobbin. **Electromagnetic flowmeter.** A flowmeter the action of which depends on the alteration of electromagnetic impedance produced by the stream. It may be used to measure the flow of blood in intact blood vessels. **Peak flowmeter.** An apparatus for measuring the peak expiratory flow rate, which is about 450-700 l/min in men and 300-500 l/min in women. **Rotameter flowmeter.** A form of dry flowmeter (see above) in which the bobbin is constantly rotating and so does not stick to the sides of the surrounding glass tube. **Sight-feed flowmeter.** A crude apparatus in which the rate of flow of the gas is roughly judged by its bubbling through a jar of water. **Water-depression flowmeter.** An apparatus in which the rate of flow of the gas through a constricted tube is indicated by the depression produced in a water manometer. [AS *flowan*, meter.]

Fluanisone (floo·an·e·sone). BP Commission approved name for 4 - fluoro - γ - [4 - (2 - methoxyphenyl)piperazin - 1 - yl]butyrophenone; a neuroleptic.

fluavil (floo·a·vil). $C_{20}H_{32}O_2$, a complex crystalline resin which occurs in gutta percha.

Fluclorolone Acetonide (floo·klor·o·lone as·e·ton·ide). BP Commission approved name for 9α, 11β - dichloro - 6α - fluoro - 21 - hydroxy - 16α, 17α - isopropylidenedioxypregna - 1,4 - diene - 3,20 - dione; a corticosteroid.

Flucloxacillin (floo·klox·ah·sil'·in). BP Commission approved name for 3 - (2 - chloro - 6 - fluorophenyl) - 5 - methylisoxazol - 4 - ylpenicillin; an antibiotic.

fluctuation (fluk·tew·a·shun). 1. A clinical physical sign consisting of an impulse transmitted to the finger or fingers of one hand by sudden pressure with the finger or fingers of the other hand. Elicited in non-tense localized fluid collections (some cysts, abscesses), soft solids (lipomata, ascites), distension of a hollow organ with fluid (the stomach), and in muscles at right angles to their long axis. 2. In biology, any non-inherited unimportant variation of structure in an organism. [L *fluctuare* to wave.]

Flucytosine (floo·si·to·seen). BP Commission approved name for 4 - amino - 5 - fluoro - 1,2 -dihydropyrimidin-2-one; an antifungal agent.

Fludrocortisone (flud·ro·kor·tis·one). BP Commission approved name for 9α-fluorohydrocortisone, the fluorosubstituted hydrocortisone. It has the actions of hydrocortisone but is much more potent, causing salt retention. **Fludrocortisone Acetate BP 1973.** 21 - Acetoxy - 9α - fluoro - 11β, 17α - dihydroxypregn - 4 - ene - 3,20 - dione; white to pale yellow, odourless, tasteless, hygroscopic crystalline powder or crystals, very slightly soluble in water, soluble in alcohol, ether and chloroform. It is used to suppress inflammation in the treatment of certain allergic dermatoses.

Flugestone (floo·**jes**·tone). BP Commission approved name for 9α - fluoro - 11β, 17 - dihydroxypregn - 4 - ene - 3,20 - dione; a progestational steroid.

Fluhrer, William Francis (b. 1870). New York physician.

Fluhrer's probe. An aluminium probe used in exploring gunshot wounds of the brain.

fluid (**floo**·id). 1. Flowing; anything that will flow. 2. A liquid. 3. A body secretion. 4. In histology, a fixative or a staining solution, **Allantoic fluid.** The contents of the allantoic sac. **Amniotic fluid.** The contents of the amniotic sac. **Ascitic fluid.** The accumulation of free fluid in the peritoneal cavity. **Cerebrospinal fluid [Liquor cerebrospinalis (NA)].** A clear fluid containing very little protein and few cells which fills the ventricles of the brain and the subarachnoid spaces of the cerebrospinal axis. **Chancre fluid.** The exudate from a chancre. The organisms *Treponema pallidum* are present in the exudate from a syphilitic chancre. **Chlorpalladium fluid.** A decalcifying agent in histology containing palladium chloride and hydrochloric acid. **Culture fluid.** Any fluid used as a medium for culturing bacteria or other micro-organisms. **Diluting fluid.** Any special mixture or solution used for diluting blood or other body fluid with the object of preventing coagulation, and of preserving certain required cellular elements, with the destruction or elimination of others, in order to facilitate enumeration or observation. Such diluting fluids are usually isotonic with blood and may incorporate particular stains. **Extracellular fluid.** The fluid bathing the outside of cells, including the blood. **Fixing fluid.** *See* FIXING FLUID. **Follicular fluid.** The contents of an ovarian graafian follicle. **Puncture fluid.** Fluid obtained from any physiological or pathological cavity by the use of a hollow needle. **Saline fluid.** Sodium chloride solution. **Seminal fluid.** Semen. **Susa fixing fluid.** A solution of mercuric and sodium chlorides, with formalin and trichloro-acetic acid, in water; it is a valuable fixative used a great deal in cytology. **Tissue fluid.** Extracellular fluid in the tissues; depleted in serious dehydration. [L *fluere* to flow.]

See also: ALTMANN, BOUIN, CALLISON, COLEY, CONDY, DISCOMBE, ERLICKI, FLEMMING, GOWERS, HAFFKINE, HAUG, HAYEM, HEIDENHAIN, HERMANN, KAISERLING, KRONECKER, MARCHI, MUELLER (H. F.), PACINI, PIAZZA, PITFIELD, RANDOLPH, REGAUD, SCARPA, THOMA, TOISON, WALDEYER-HARTZ, WEIGERT, WICKER-SHEIMER, ZENKER (K.).

fluid-level (**floo**·id **lev**·el). A radiological term indicating that fluid and air or gas are juxtaposed, classically in the maxillary antrum. [L *fluere* to flow, *levare* to lift.]

fluidism (**floo**·id·izm). Humoralism; a doctrine originally set out by Diocles (b. 350 B.C.), physician of Athens, and the interpreter of Hippocrates. He believed that the health of the individual depended upon the balance of opposites in the body, and that all diseases were attributable to disturbance of the four humours (blood, phlegm, black and yellow bile), which in their right proportions constituted health. The doctrine persisted in English mediaeval medicine and even into the 18th century. [L *fluere* to flow.]

fluke (flook). General term for all parasitic Trematoda. Those of medical importance are all internal parasites, with the asexual stage of the life cycle spent in molluscs. **Blood fluke.** *Schistosoma.* **Intestinal flukes.** Flukes of the genera *Amphistoma, Dicrocoelium, Echinostoma, Fasciolopsis, Gastrodiscoides, Haplorchis, Heterophyes, Metagonimus, Watsonius.* **Liver fluke.** A fluke of the genera *Clonorchis, Dicrocoelium, Eurytrema, Fasciola, Metorchis, Opisthorchis.* **Lung fluke.** *Paragonimus.* [AS *floc.*]

Flumedroxone (floo·med·**rox**·one). BP Commission approved name for 17α - hydroxy - 6α - trifluoromethylpregn - 4 - ene - 3,20 - dione; it is used in the treatment of migraine.

flumen (**floo**·men) (pl. *flumina*). 1. A flow. 2. Term applied to the principal cerebral commissures (*Duret*). [L stream.]

Flumethasone (floo·**meth**·az·one). BP Commission approved name for 6α,9α-difluoro-16α-methylprednisolone; a corticosteroid.

Flumethiazide (floo·meth·**i**·az·ide). BP Commission approved name for 6-trifluoromethyl-1,2,4-benzothiadiazine-7-sulphonamide 1,1-dioxide; a diuretic.

Fluocinolone (floo·o·**sin**·o·lone). BP Commission approved name for 6α,9α - difluoro - 16α - hydroxyprednisolone. **Fluocinolone Acetonide BP 1973.** 6α,9α - Difluoro-11β,21 - dihydroxy - 16α,17α - isopropylidenedioxypregna - 1,4 - diene - 3,20 - dione; an adrenocorticosteroid for topical application in skin diseases.

Fluocinonide (floo·o·**sin**·on·ide). BP Commission approved name for 21 - acetoxy - 6α,9α - difluoro - 11β - hydroxy - 16α,17α - isopropylidenedioxypregna - 1,4 - diene - 3,20 - dione; a corticosteroid.

Fluocortin Butyl (floo·o·**kor**·tin **bew**·til). BP Commission approved name for butyl 6α - fluoro - 11β - hydroxy - 16α - methyl - 3,20 - dioxopregna - 1,4 - dien - 21 - oate; an anti-inflammatory agent.

Fluocortolone (floo·o·**kor**·to·lone). BP Commission approved name for 6α-fluoro-11β,21-dihydroxy-16α-methylpregna-1,4-diene-3,20-dione. **Fluocortolone Hexanoate BP 1973.** 6α-Fluoro-21-hexanoyloxy-11β-hydroxy-16α-methylpregna-1,4-diene-3,20-dione. **Fluocortolone Pivalate BP 1973.** 6α-Fluoro-11β-hydroxy-16α-methyl-21-pivaloyloxypregna-1,4-diene-3,20-dione. Adrenocorticosteroids used topically in the treatment of skin diseases.

Fluopromazine (floo·o·**pro**·maz·een). BP Commission approved name for 10-(3 - dimethylaminopropyl) - 2 - trifluoromethylphenothiazine; it is used in the treatment of manic psychoses.

fluorane (**floo**·or·ane). A crystalline substance produced during the preparation of phenolphthalein; it is the parent of fluorescein and the fluorescein dyestuffs.

fluorcardiography (**floo**·or·kar·de·**og**'·raf·e). Electrokymography. [fluorescence, cardiography.]

fluorene (**floo**·or·een). Diphenylene methane, $(C_6H_4)_2CH_2$. A crystalline fluorescent hydrocarbon occurring in coal tar and employed in the synthesis of dyestuffs.

fluoresce (floo·or·**es**). To be or become fluorescent.

fluorescein (floo·or·**es**·e·in). Resorcinphthalein anhydride, dihydroxyfluorane. An orange-coloured dye related to eosin and prepared from phthalic anhydride and resorcinol. It dissolves in alkalis with a red colour and a green fluorescence. It is used to trace the flow of water in sewers and reservoirs, also as an absorption indicator. **Fluorescein Sodium BP 1973, Soluble fluorescein.** The disodium salt of fluorescein, used in ophthalmology to detect lesions of the cornea and foreign bodies, the damaged cornea staining and showing a strong green fluorescence.

fluoresceinuria (floo·or·**es**·e·in·**ewr**'·e·ah). The condition in which fluorescein is present in the urine.

fluorescence (floo·or·**es**·ens). The property inherent in certain substances, when illuminated, to radiate unpolarized light of a different wavelength from that of the light they absorb, e.g. transformation of ultraviolet into luminous rays. [L *fluere* to flow.]

fluorescent (floo·or·**es**·ent). 1. Displaying the phenomenon of fluorescence. 2. Exhibiting a different colour by transmitted light to that by reflected light. 3. Glowing luminously when radiated with light of a wavelength beyond the visible spectrum. **Fluorescent indicator.** *See* INDICATOR. **Fluorescent screen.** *See* SCREEN. [see prec.]

fluorescin (floo·or·**es**·in). Fluorescein.

fluoridation (**floo**·or·i·**da**'·shun). The addition of minute quantities of fluorides to water supplies to reduce dental caries in the populations served.

fluoride (**floo**·or·ide). 1. A salt of hydrofluoric acid. 2. A salt consisting of fluorine combined with another element or radical. **Hydrogen fluoride.** Hydrofluoric acid. *See* ACID.

fluorine (floo·or·een). The lightest and most active of the halogen elements. A pale-yellow gas of atomic weight 19.00, atomic number 9 and chemical symbol F. It is soluble in water to form a powerful oxidizing agent; intensely poisonous. It occurs in fluorspar, a natural calcium fluoride CaF_2, and is present in bones and teeth. [L *fluere* to flow.]

fluorite (floo·or·ite). Native calcium fluoride; also known as *fluorspar.*

fluoroacetate (floo·or·o·as′·et·ate). A derivative of acetic acid in which an atom of hydrogen has been replaced by an atom of fluorine. Its toxicity is due to its action as a precursor of fluorocitrate, a potent inhibitor of aconitate hydratase and, hence, of the citric-acid cycle. **Methyl fluoroacetate.** $CH_2FCOOCH_3$, MFA, a very poisonous substance to animals and man; it is too dangerous for use as a rodent poison. **Sodium fluoroacetate.** $CH_2FCOONa$, compound 1080, a powerful rodent poison which is also poisonous to man.

fluorocitrate (floo·or·o·sit′·rate). A potent inhibitor of aconitase hydratase. *See* FLUOROACETATE.

fluorocyte (floo·or·o·site). A reticulocyte showing a red fluorescence under certain conditions of staining. [fluorescence, Gk *kytos* cell.]

5-fluorocytosine (floo·or·o·si′·to·seen). A pyrimidine, closely related to 5-fluorouracil. It is an antimetabolite for certain pathogenic fungi but not for mammalian cells. It is effective and well tolerated when given by mouth, giving adequate antifungal concentrations in the blood, tissues, cerebrospinal fluid and aqueous of the eye. An unusual feature about the drug is that, during treatment, yeasts (e.g. *Candida albicans, Cryptococcus neoformans*) may develop resistance to it and that primary resistance in these yeasts has been reported. Thus, it is necessary that *in vitro* sensitivities should be determined on all strains isolated before and during treatment. If development of resistance during therapy is to be avoided, adequate doses of the drug must be given.

fluorodinitrobenzene (floo·or·o·di·ni·tro·ben′·zeen). FDNB; Sanger's reagent. A reagent widely used for the determination of aminoterminal residues of peptide chains.

fluorography (floo·or·og·raf·e). The photographic reproduction of a fluorescent-screen image by a camera, with a roll film of small size. Many exposures can be conveniently recorded in a short time; this technique is then called *mass miniature radiography.* The method is usually applied to chest radiography. [fluorescence, Gk *graphein* to record.]

fluorometer (floo·or·om·et·er). 1. An instrument with which the colour and intensity of fluorescence caused by radium or x-rays, can be measured. 2. A device for attachment to a fluoroscope which enables the position of the sought object to be determined with exactitude and the shadows to be correctly adjusted.

Fluorometholone (floo·or·o·meth′·o·lone). BP Commission approved name for 9α - fluoro - 11β,17α - dihydroxy - 6α - methylpregna - 1,4 - diene - 3,20 - dione; a corticosteroid. An anti-inflammatory cortisol derivative used as a suspension in ophthalmic work. Is equally potent to cortisol.

fluoroscope (floo·or·o·skope). 1. A screen coated with a substance that fluoresces in x-rays, used for direct viewing of the x-ray image. 2. An arrangement for comparing fluorescent solutions with a standard. **Biplane fluoroscope.** In x-ray work, a combination of fluorescent screens to permit examination in two planes. [fluorescence, Gk *skopein* to examine.]

fluoroscopical (floo·or·o·skop′·ik·al). Relating or belonging to fluoroscopy.

fluoroscopy (floo·or·os·ko·pe). Examination of the inner tissues of the body by means of a fluoroscope.

fluorosis (floo·or·o·sis). A chronic condition of poisoning with fluorine. **Chronic endemic fluorosis, Dental fluorosis.** A chronic fluorine poisoning that occurs naturally in certain countries and also in localities in which aluminium factories are situated; it occurs when fluorine is present in the water supply in concentrations much over one in 1 000 000. One of the signs is the mottling of the enamel of the teeth, but where it is severe there is also crippling osteosclerosis. [fluorine, Gk *-osis*, condition.]

Fluorouracil (floo·or·o·ewr′·as·il). BP Commission approved name for 5-fluorouracil; an antineoplastic agent.

fluorspar (floo·or·spar). Fluorite.

Fluoxymesterone BP 1973 (floo·ox·e·mes′·ter·one). 9α-Fluoro-11β-hydroxy-17-methyl-testosterone; an androgenic and anabolic steroid.

Flupenthixol (floo·pen·thix·ol). BP Commission approved name for 9-{3-[4-(2-hydroxyethyl)piperazin-1-yl]-propylidene}-2-trifluoromethyl-thiaxanthen; a tranquillizer.

Fluperolone (floo·per·o·lone). BP Commission approved name for 9α-fluoro-21-methylprednisolone; it is used in the treatment of skin disorders.

Fluphenazine (floo·fen·ah·zeen). BP Commission approved name for 10 - {3 - [4 - (2 - hydroxyethyl) - 1 - piperazinyl]propyl} - 2 - trifluoromethylphenothiazine. **Fluphenazine Hydrochloride BP 1973.** The dihydrochloride of fluphenazine; a tranquillizer.

Fluprednidene (floo·pred·nid·een). BP Commission approved name for 9α - fluoro - 11β,17α,21 - trihydroxy - 16 - methylene-pregna - 1,4 - diene - 3,20 - dione; a glucocorticosteroid.

Fluprednisolone (floo·pred·nis·o·lone). BP Commission approved name for 6α - fluoro - 11β,17α,21 - trihydroxypregna - 1,4 - diene - 3,20 - dione; a corticosteroid.

Fluprofen (floo·pro·fen.). BP Commission approved name for 2 - (2′ - fluoro - 4 - biphenylyl)propionic acid; an anti-inflammatory and analgesic agent.

Flurandrenolone (floo·ran·dren·o·lone). BP Commission approved name for 6α - fluoro - 16α,17α - isopropylidenedioxy - hydrocortisone; a steroid preparation similar in action to topical corticosteroids, used in the treatment of skin disorders.

Flurazepam (flewr·az·e·pam). BP Commission approved name for 7 - chloro - 1 - (2 - diethylaminoethyl) - 5 - (2 - fluorophenyl) - 1,3-dihydro - 2*H* - 1,4 - benzodiazepin - 2 - one; a hypnotic.

Flurbiprofen (fler·bi·pro·fen). BP Commission approved name for 2 - (2 - fluorobiphenyl - 4 - yl)propionic acid; an anti-inflammatory and analgesic agent.

Flurothyl (floo·ro·thile). BP Commission approved name for di-(2,2,2 - trifluoroethyl) ether; a central nervous system stimulant.

fluroxene (floo·rox·een). A volatile anaesthetic ether, trifluoroethyl vinyl ether, described by J.C. Krantz in 1953, having a boiling point of 43.2°C. Its vapour mixed with oxygen or air may be flammable and explosive.

Flury. The name of the child from whom the strain of rabies virus described below was obtained.

Flury strain. A strain of rabies virus, attenuated by passage in fertile hens' eggs and used for veterinary immunization against the disease. It has also been used, after passage through ducks' eggs and inactivation with β - propiolactone, to elicit virus antibody in man.

flush (flush). 1. Redness, usually temporary, caused by a rush of blood to the face and neck; a vasomotor disturbance for which there are many causes, physiological and pathological. It is often associated with palpitations, sweating and giddiness. 2. To exhibit such a condition. 3. To wash out a cavity or wound with a strong rapid flow of water. **Atropine flush.** Redness and dryness of the skin due to the excessive use or overdosage of atropine. **Breast flush.** Redness and tenseness of the breasts with strong marking of veins which may occur in the early puerperium. **Carcinoid flush.** The typical flushing attack associated with the carcinoid syndrome. **Hectic flush.** The bright colour of the face indicative of a rise of temperature observed in pulmonary tuberculosis, septic poisoning and similar affections. **Hot flush.** Associated with the combination of low oestrogen and high gonadotrophin levels. **Mahogany flush.** In lobar pneumonia, the brownish-red or deep-red patch occasionally seen on one cheek. **Malar flush.** The bright flush seen over the zygomatic bone in pulmonary tuberculosis. **Menopausal flush.** A condition often present during the menopausal years in which there is periodic transitory mounting of the blood to head, face and neck—in some cases a rush of blood to the whole body surface—accompanied by a sensation of heat and by sweating. [ME *fluschen.*]

Fluspirilene (floo·spi·ril·een). BP Commission approved name for 8 - [4,4 - di - (4 - fluorophenyl)butyl] - 1 - phenyl - 1,3,8 - triazaspiro[4,5]decan-4-one; a tranquillizer.

flutter (flut·er). A tremulousness. **Atrial flutter.** Rapid regular contractions of the atria of the heart independent of the activity of the sinu-atrial node due to either the circus movement round the atria of a continuously moving stimulus or the rapid regular firing of an ectopic focus. The atrial rate is usually about 300 per minute and the ventricles most commonly respond to only every other atrial beat, but other degrees of second degree heart block may occur. **Diaphragmatic flutter.** Attacks of rapid, rhythmic contractions of the diaphragm. **Flutter fibrillation.** *See* FIBRILLATION. [AS *fleotan* to move swiftly.]

flux (flux). 1. An excessive fluid discharge from the body. 2. Any substance employed in metallurgy to promote fusion. 3. The flow of any vector quantity, such as magnetic intensity, through an area. 4. The product of the number of particles or photons per unit volume and their average speed. **Alvine flux.** Diarrhoea. **Bilious flux.** Bile-stained diarrhoea. **Bloody flux.** Dysentery. **Coeliac flux.** Steatorrhoea. **Hepatic flux.** Bilious flux (see above). **Luminous flux.** The amount of light measured in lumens which passes through a given area in 1 sec. **Menstrual flux.** The discharge of blood at the menses. **Neutral flux.** Any flux which promotes fusion without exercising an oxidizing or reducing action, e.g. barium chloride. **Neutron flux.** The product of the neutron density and the average speed. The number of neutrons entering an imaginary sphere having a total area of 4π cm^2 in 1 sec. **Oxidizing flux.** Any flux which forms oxides with the metals present; it is usually a mixture of borax, sodium perborate and potassium chlorate. **Reducing flux.** Any flux which reduces metallic oxides; it usually consists of borax, argol and animal charcoal. **White flux.** Sprue. [L *fluere* to flow.]

fluxion (fluk·shun). 1. A flux. 2. A state of congestion due to unnatural flow of blood or other fluid to any particular part or area of the body.

fly (fli). 1. Insects of the order Diptera, having anterior wings only developed for flight. 2. In combinations, a general term for insects, usually flying, of many orders. **Bar fly.** *Drosophila.* **Black fly.** *Simulium.* **Blow fly.** *Calliphora, Lucilla, Wohlfahrtia.* **Bluebottle fly.** *Calliphora.* **Columbacz fly.** *Simulium.* **Deer fly.** *Chrysops.* **Eye fly.** *Hippelates, Siphunculina.* **Flesh fly.** *Sarcophaga, Wohlfahrtia.* **Fruit fly.** *Drosophila.* **Gad fly.** *Tabanus.* **Greenbottle fly.** *Lucilia.* **Horn fly.** *Haematobia irritans.* **Horse fly.** *Chrysops, Pangonia, Tabanus.* **House fly.** *Musca, Fannia.* **Latrine fly.** *Fannia.* **Lesser house fly.** *Fannia.* **Louse fly.** *Hippoboscidae.* **Mangrove fly.** *Chrysops.* **Moth fly.** *Psychodidae.* **Pipsa fly.** *Simulium indicum.* **Potu fly.** *Simulium indicum.* **Sand fly.** *Culicoides, Pericoma, Phlebotomus.* **Soldier fly.** *Hermetia.* **Spanish fly.** *Cantharis, Epicauta*; the vesicant pharmaceutical compounded from such beetles. **Stable fly.** *Stomoxys.* **Steam fly.** *Blatella germanica.* **Tsetse fly.** *Glossina.* **Tumbu fly.** *Cordylobia.* **Typhoid fly.** *Musca domestica.* **Warble fly.** *Cordylobia, Dermatobia, Hypoderma.* [AS *flyge.*]

Foa, Pio (b. 1848). Turin pathologist.

Foa-Kurlov cells. Guinea-pig mononuclear blood cells containing inclusions.

foam (fome). A mixture of fine gas bubbles in a liquid. The surface tension of the latter is lowered by the addition of substances like soap or gelatin, or even solids. **Human Fibrin Foam BP 1968.** A very porous fibrin product prepared by the interaction of human plasma thrombin and fibrinogen under controlled conditions; it is used, in conjunction with a solution of fibrinogen, as a powerful and rapid haemostatic agent that can be left in wounds from which it is gradually absorbed. [AS *fam.*]

focal (fo·kal). 1. Relating or belonging to a focus. 2. Collected at a focus.

focalization (fo·kal·i·za′·shun). Bringing together, in a single focus, or into a number of distinct foci, instead of being distributed widely.

Fochier, Alphonse (b. 1845). Lyons surgeon.

Fochier's abscess. An abscess produced artificially to attract infecting organisms to the site, and build up the defences of the patient.

focil, focile (fo·sil, fo·sil·e). Any long bone of the arm or leg. [LL from *fusillus* little spindle.]

focimeter (fo·sim·et·er). In optics: 1. An instrument with which the actinic focus of an objective lens can be found. 2. An instrument that measures the focal length of a lens or system of lenses. [focus, meter.]

focus (fo·kus) (pl. *foci*). 1. The point at which reflected rays meet. Hence, centre of activity; the point of concentration. 2. In optics, to alter the refractive power of an optical system, e.g. by manipulation of lenses, mirrors or screen relative to one another, until the image of an object produced by the system becomes clearly defined. In ophthalmology, to accommodate. **Aplanatic focus.** A focus from which the effects of spherical aberration have been eliminated. **Conjugate foci.** The points from which rays diverge and towards which, after refraction, they converge. When rays diverge from a distance greater than or equal to the focal length of the lens the conjugate focus is positive; when the distance is less than the focal length, the conjugate focus is negative. **Focus down.** To bring the object under a microscope into focus by lowering the objective; not to be recommended owing to risk of damage to the object and/or the objective lens of the microscope. **Epileptogenic focus.** The site of origin of epileptic discharges. **Focus to film distance.** The distance between the source of x-rays and the radiographic film; it is an important factor influencing definition and unsharpness. Other factors being equal, the greater the distance the sharper the radiographic image. **Focus of infection.** The point at which a pathogenic micro-organism that has gained entrance to the body settles and commences to multiply and from which it spreads. The infection may spread to other parts of the body to form other foci or become generalized as a blood infection, e.g. septicaemia. **Principal focus.** 1. The object point on the principal axis of an optical system from which parallel rays of light will be produced after passing through the system. 2. The image point of the principal axis of an optical system, produced by an object at infinity. **Protected focus.** In cardiology, a focus in the heart capable of discharging excitatory impulses whose function is not interfered with by activation of the heart from other sites because it is protected, by some form of entrance block, from being itself discharged by this activity. **Real focus.** The point at which convergent rays meet. **Focus up.** To focus a microscope by movement of the objective away from the object. **Virtual focus.** The point from which divergent rays appear to originate. [L hearth.]

See also: ASSMANN, GHON, SIMON (G.).

Fodéré, François-Emmanuel (b. 1764). French surgeon.

Fodéré's sign. Oedema of the eyelids with chloride retention.

Foeniculum (fe·nik·ew·lum). 1. A genus of plants of the family Umbelliferae. 2. Fennel, foeniculi fructus, fennel fruit; the dried ripe fruits obtained from cultivated plants of *Foeniculum vulgare* Mill. They contain a volatile oil, the main constituents of which are anethole and fenchone, and are used as a carminative. [L fennel.]

foenugreek (fe·new·greek). Foenum-Graecum BPC 1949.

Foenum-Graecum BPC 1949 (fe·num·gre′·kum). Foenugreek, the seeds of *Trigonella foenumgraecum* Linn. (family Leguminosae), used in the treatment of diabetes and as a febrifuge. [L Greek hay.]

Foerster, Otfried (b. 1873). Breslau neurosurgeon.

Foerster's operation. Intradural division of posterior nerve roots, for pain.

Foerster's cutaneous numeral test. A clinical test of topognostic sensibility: the patient closes his eyes and a number is traced out with a blunt instrument upon his skin. Repeated failure to recognize numerals so traced indicates impairment of the finer elements of sensation (tactile discrimination and topognostic sensibility) in the skin area tested and usually means a lesion in the sensory cortex or in the posterior column of the spinal cord.

Foerster–Penfield operation. Cortical scar excision for epilepsy.

Foerster, Richard (b. 1825). Breslau ophthalmologist.

Foerster's choroiditis. Areolar choroiditis.

Foerster's disease. Choroiditis.

Foerster's operation. An operation to increase the rate of ripening of a cataract; obsolete.

Foerster's photometer. Photoptometer; a device for estimating acuteness of vision by observing the least amount of light that will render objects visible.

Foerster's uveitis. Syphilitic cyclitis followed by involvement of the rest of the uveal tract.

foet-. For words beginning with **foet-**, see also FET-.

foetid (fe·tid). *See* FETID.

foetor (fe·tor). *See* FETOR.

foetus (fe·tus). *See* FETUS.

Fogarty, Thomas J. 20th century American surgeon.

Fogarty's catheter. A fine catheter with a balloon tip which is introduced into arteries to pass beyond the site of emboli. The balloon is inflated and, on withdrawal of the catheter, the embolus is removed.

fogging (fog·ing). A procedure in subjective testing for errors of refraction. In hypermetropes, fogging of the test-types is brought about by placing an excessively convex lens in front of the eye; in myopes, by placing too weak a concave lens in front of the eye, so as to prevent unconscious accommodation in either case. [etym. dub.]

foil (foil). Thin sheets of gold, platinum or tin used in dentistry. Gold foil has the power of cohesion, and is used for filling cavities in teeth. **Foil carrier.** An instrument used for conveying gold foil to a cavity in a tooth. [L *folium* leaf.]

Foix, Charles (b. 1882). Paris neurologist.

Marie–Foix sign. Forced flexion of the toes or transverse pressure on the tarsus in a severely spastic leg that is not capable of voluntary movement produces reflex withdrawal of the limb.

Fol, Hermann (b. 1845). German pathologist.

Fol's solution. A histological fixative containing picric and chromic acids, used for eggs with a large amount of yolk.

fold [plica (NA)] (fo·ld). 1. A ridge in the soft tissues, usually with reference to the external surface of the adult or fetal body, the fetal membranes, the lining of ducts and hollow viscera, or the lining of coelomic, joint and bony cavities. 2. A bend or flexure in a solid organ of the adult or embryo. 3. A sheet-like flap, reduplication or mesentery of the coelomic lining. 4. The sharp or well-defined edge of a sheet-like structure. **Alar fold [plica alaris (NA)].** A wing-like reduplication of the synovial lining of the knee joint on either side of the infrapatellar synovial fold. **Amniotic fold.** The anterior and posterior flaps of extra-embryonic ectoderm and mesoderm which grow over the dorsal aspect of the embryo of many vertebrates (not man) and coalesce to form the definitive amnion. **Aryepiglottic fold [plica aryepiglottica (NA)].** The ridge-like lateral wall of the entrance to the larynx, between the epiglottis in front and the arytenoid cartilages behind; it contains a muscle and ligament of the same name, between two layers of mucous membrane. **Axillary fold.** Either of the lower margins of the anterior [plica axillaris anterior (NA)] and posterior [plica axillaris posterior (NA)] walls of the axilla stretching between the chest wall and the arm, and containing respectively the pectoralis major and the latissimus dorsi muscles. **Body fold.** A lateral margin of the embryonic body wall (somatopleure) which is folded under to form the ventral wall. **Bulboventricular fold.** The internally-projecting ridge in the wall of the embryonic heart at the junction of the bulbus cordis and ventricle. **Fold of the buttock [sulcus gluteus (NA)].** The horizontal lower margin of the buttock at its junction with the thigh. **Caecal fold [plica cecalis (NA)].** A mesenteric sheet of peritoneum which attaches the posterolateral part of the caecum and adjoining ascending colon to the posterior abdominal wall, forming the right boundary of the caecal recess of the peritoneal cavity. **Fold of the caecum, vascular [plica cecalis vascularis (NA)].** A peritoneal fold containing the anterior caecal artery. **Caudal genital fold.** Inguinal fold; the ridge on the posterior abdominal wall running downwards from the lower pole of the embryonic testis or ovary before their descent, in which the upper part of the gubernaculum develops. **Caval fold.** A ridge in the posterior abdominal wall of the embryo through which the inferior vena cava passes to the back of the liver; it is the posterior pillar of the mesolateral fold of Brachet, and forms the posterior and superior boundaries of the epiploic foramen of Winslow. **Cholecystoduodenocolic fold.** An abnormal peritoneal fold, lying between and connecting the gall bladder, duodenum and colon. **Fold of the chorda tympani [plica chordae tympani (NA)].** The fold of mucous membrane over the chorda tympani nerve on the lateral wall of the middle ear. **Ciliary folds [plicae ciliares (NA)].** A number of ridges between the ciliary processes of the eyeball. **Circular fold [plica circularis (NA)].** A large transverse fold of mucous membrane which projects into the lumen of the small intestine. **Folds of the colon, semilunar [plicae semilunares coli (NA)].** Crescentic folds of mucous membrane which separate the sacculations. **Conjunctival fold.** 1. The plica semilunaris conjunctivae at the inner angle of the eye. 2. A ridge in the lax upper part of the conjunctiva. **Costocolic fold.** Phrenicocolic ligament, parietocolic fold; a triangular horizontal fold of peritoneum attaching the splenic flexure of the colon to the diaphragm near the 10th rib. **Cranial genital fold.** The ridge on the posterior abdominal wall of the embryo extending upwards from the upper pole of the testis or ovary; the diaphragmatic ligament. **Duodenal folds.** Folds of Jonnesco. (*a*) Inferior [plica duodenalis inferior (NA)]; a non-vascular sheet of peritoneum passing towards the left from the lower end of the fourth part of the duodenum; the inferior duodenal recess lies behind it. (*b*) Superior [plica duodenalis superior (NA)]: a sheet of peritoneum passing towards the left from the termination of the fourth part of the duodenum, usually containing part of the inferior mesenteric vein; the superior duodenal recess lies behind it. (*c*) Paraduodenal [plica paraduodenalis (NA)]: a sickle-shaped fold of peritoneum to the left of the fourth part of the duodenum, raised up by the inferior mesenteric vein and ascending branch of the left colic artery; the paraduodenal fossa lies behind it. (*d*) Duodenojejunal [plica duodenojejunalis (NA)]: a fold of peritoneum attached to the duodenojejunal flexure containing the suspensory ligament of Trietz. **Duodenojejunal fold.** *See* DUODENAL FOLDS (preceding). **Duodenomesocolic fold [plica duodenomesocolica (NA)].** A single or double peritoneal fold occasionally present between the terminal part of the duodenum and the adjacent part of the mesocolon and forming the margin of the opening into the duodenojejunal or mesocolic recess. **Fold of the duodenum, longitudinal [plica longitudinalis duodeni (NA)].** A longitudinally-placed fold of mucous membrane lying immediately distal to the duodenal papilla. **Epicanthal fold, Epicanthine fold.** Epicanthus. **Epigastric fold.** One of the ridges of the peritoneum on the lower part of the internal surface of the anterior wall caused by the underlying inferior epigastric arteries as they pass towards the rectus sheath. **Fimbriated fold [plica fimbriata (NA)].** A slightly notched laterally-placed ridge in the mucous membrane beneath the tongue, best marked in the fetus and child. **Folds of the gall bladder [plicae tunicae mucosae vesicae felleae (NA)].** The folds in the mucous membrane of the gall bladder. **Gastric folds [plicae gastricae (NA)].** The mainly longitudinal folds into which the gastric mucosa is thrown in the empty organ. **Gastropancreatic folds [plicae gastropancreaticae (NA)].** The gastropancreatic ligaments; the right and left peritoneal sheets which pass from the back of the stomach to the pancreas, bounding the isthmus of the lesser sac. The left one contains the left gastric vessels; the right may contain the hepatic artery. **Genital fold.** 1. The medial part of the urogenital ridge on the posterior abdominal wall of the embryo caused by the underlying gonad. 2. The ridge on either side of the cloacal membrane, later subdivided into inner and outer (labioscrotal and urethral) folds. **Glosso-epiglottic fold [plica glosso-epiglottica mediana (NA)].** A median fold of mucous membrane lying between the valleculae and connecting the back of the tongue to the front of the epiglottis. **Gluteal fold.** Fold of the buttock (see above). **Gonadal fold.** Genital fold (see above). **Gubernacular fold.** The ridge on the posterior abdominal wall passing from the lower pole of the testis or ovary towards the groin; it overlies the gubernaculum. Also known as *caudal genital fold, inguinal fold.* **Haversian folds.** The extrasynovial pads of fat. **Head fold.** The flexure of the anterior end of the embryonic blastoderm which appears as the brain bulges forward and ventrally, and the heart is turned through 180 degrees to reach its definitive position, **Hypogastric fold.** The lateral umbilical fold (see below). **Ileocaecal fold [plica ileocaecalis (NA)].** The bloodless or inferior ileocaecal fold of Treves; a sheet of peritoneum which passes from the antimesometrial border of the terminal ileum to the base of the appendix and neighbouring portion of the caecum. It forms the anterior wall of the inferior ileocaecal recess, and represents part of the original mesentery of the caecum. **Ileocolic fold.** The superior ileocaecal fold of Treves; a sheet of peritoneum passing from the ventral surface of the mesentery of the terminal ileum, in front of the ileocolic junction, to the anterior surface of the ascending colon near the caecum. It contains branches of the anterior caecal vessels, and forms the anterior wall of the superior ileocaecal recess. **Fold of the incus [plica incudis (NA)].** A ridge in the mucosa of the tympanic cavity descending from the roof to the upper part of the body of the incus. **Infrapatellar synovial fold [plica synovialis infrapatellaris (NA)].** A reduplication of the synovial lining of the knee joint covering the infrapatellar pad of fat and passing in the midline from the lower margin of the patella to the intercondylar notch of the femur. It is continuous on either side with the alar folds. **Inguinal fold.** Caudal genital fold (see above). **Interarytenoid fold.** A fold of mucous membrane joining the corniculate cartilages and bounding the interarytenoid notch. **Folds of the iris [plicae iridis (NA)].** Folds commencing on the posterior surface and winding round the pupillary border producing its crenated appearance. **Labioscrotal fold.** The primordia of the labia majora and scrotum of the early fetus. **Lacrimal fold [plica lacrimalis (NA)].** Hasner's fold; a valve-like fold in the lower part of the nasolacrimal duct. **Fold of the laryngeal nerve [plica nervi laryngei (NA)].** The fold of mucous membrane raised in the floor of the piriform fossa by the internal branch of the superior laryngeal nerve. **Fold of the left vena cava [plica venae cavae sinistrae (NA)].** Ligament of the left vena cava. **Malleolar folds [plicae malleares, anterior et posterior (NA)].** Ridges of the mucous membrane of the tympanic cavity passing upwards from the handle of the malleus and bordering the flaccid part of the tympanic membrane. **Mammary fold.** The inferior line of attachment of the mammary gland to the chest wall. **Medullary fold.** Neural fold (see below). **Mesolateral fold.** Brachet's mesolateral fold, the right part of the dorsal mesentery of the embryonic foregut, cut off by the development of the upper recess of the lesser sac and containing part of the inferior vena cava. **Mesonephric fold.** The ridge on the posterior abdominal wall of the embryo containing the mesonephros and the mesonephric (wolffian) and paramesonephric (muellerian) ducts. **Meso-uterine fold.** The broad ligament of the uterus. *See* LIGAMENT. **Nail fold.** The ingrowing epidermal plate overlying the distal phalanx and giving rise to the root of the nail; it is subdivided into a deep proximal nail fold, and shallow lateral nail folds. **Nasal fold, lateral.** A swelling which develops on the outer side of the nasal placode of the early embryo and forms the basis of the ala of the nostril. **Nasal fold, medial.** The globular process; the swelling which appears medial to the nasal placode of the early embryo, and which gives rise to one half of the fleshy septum of the nose. It was at one time thought to contribute to the medial portion of the upper lip. **Neural fold.** The raised edges of the neural plate of the early embryo prior to formation of the neural tube. **Opercular fold.** An adhesion between the anterior pillar of the fauces and the surface of the tonsil. **Palatine folds, transverse [plicae palatinae transversae (NA)].** The transverse corrugations in the mucoperiosteum of the hard palate. **Palmate folds.** The oblique ridges in the interior of the cervix of the uterus. **Palpebronasal fold [plica palpebronasalis (NA)].** The epicanthus. **Paraduodenal fold.** *See* DUODENAL FOLDS (above). **Parietocolic fold, Parietoperitoneal fold.** Costocolic fold (see above). **Patellar synovial fold.** Infrapatellar synovial fold (see above). **Pharyngo-epiglottic fold [plica glosso-epiglottica lateralis (NA)].** A lateral ridge of mucous membrane passing downwards from the back of the tongue on to the lateral pharyngeal wall, forming the lateral boundary of a vallecula. **Pituitary fold.** Rathke's fold; a depression in the roof of the embryonic mouth just anterior to the buccopharyngeal membrane, the walls of which give rise to the anterior lobe of the pituitary gland. **Rectal folds.** Folds of the rectum, horizontal (see below). **Recto-uterine fold [plica recto-uterinal (NA)].** Peritoneal folds containing the uterosacral ligaments which run from the cervix uteri on either side of the rectum to the posterior pelvic wall. **Rectovaginal fold.** A fold of peritoneum from the posterior fornix of the vagina to the front of the rectum. **Rectovesical fold.** Sacrogenital fold (see below). **Folds of the rectum, horizontal [plicae transversales recti (NA)].** Permanent shelf-like semilunar folds of the rectal mucosa and muscularis, usually three in number. **Sacrogenital folds.** Peritoneal folds passing from the back of the bladder to the front of the sacrum, bordering the inlet of the recto-uterine pouch of Douglas. **Salpingopalatine fold [plica salpingopalatina (NA)].** A ridge in the lateral wall of the nasopharynx passing from the eustachian orifice to the soft palate. **Salpingopharyngeal fold [plica salpingopharyngea (NA)].** A ridge in the lateral wall of the pharynx passing downwards from the inner end of the eustachian tube, caused by the salpingopharyngeus muscle. **Semilunar fold [plica semilunaris (NA)].** A curved fold connecting the palatoglossal arch with the palatopharyngeal arch; it contains lymphoid tissue and forms the upper extremity of the intratonsillar cleft. **Sexual fold.** Genital fold (see above). **Fold of the stapes [plica stapedis (NA)].** A ridge in the mucous membrane of the tympanic cavity. **Sublingual fold [plica sublingualis (NA)].** The ridge raised in the floor of the mouth by the underlying sublingual gland. **Synovial fold [plica synovialis (NA)].** A reduplication of the synovial membrane of a joint. **Tail fold.** The flexure of the posterior end of the embryonic blastoderm. **Transverse vesical fold [plica vesicalis transversa (NA)].** The fold of peritoneum which crosses the upper surface of the empty urinary bladder. **Triangular fold [plica triangularis (NA)].** In fetal life, a free fold of mucous membrane sweeping back from the anterior pillar of the fauces to cover the antero-inferior parts of the tonsil; it may persist in part into adult life. **Umbilical fold, lateral [plica umbilicalis lateralis (NA)].** A ridge on the lower part of the inner surface of the anterior abdominal wall made by the obliterated umbilical arteries. **Umbilical fold, medial [plica umbilicalis medialis (NA)].** The ridge raised by the obliterated umbilical artery. **Umbilical fold, median [plica umbilicalis mediana (NA)].** The ridge raised by the urachus, in the midline on the inner aspect of the anterior abdominal wall stretching from the apex of the bladder to the umbilicus. **Fold of the urachus.** Median umbilical fold (see above). **Ureteric fold [plica interureterica (NA)].** A prominence lateral to each internal ureteric orifice, caused by the terminal portions of the ureters lying within the bladder wall. **Urogenital fold.** The ridge raised on the posterior abdominal wall of the embryo by the underlying mesonephros and gonad. **Vascular fold.** The upper part of the fetal mesentery of the testis containing the spermatic vessels. **Ventricular fold, Vestibular fold.** The false vocal cord. *See* CORD. **Vestigial fold.** The ligament of the left superior vena cava; Marshall's fold. **Villous folds [plicae villosae (NA)].** Minute convoluted folds which subdivide the gastric areas. **Vocal folds.** The true vocal cords. *See* CORD. [AS *fealdan.*]

See also: ARNOLD (F.), BRACHET, DOUGLAS (J.), DUNCAN (J. M.), GUBARER, GUÉRIN (A. F. M.), HASNER, HEISTER, HENSING, HOUSTON, JONNESCO, KERCKRING, KOHLRAUSCH (O. L. B.), LUSCHKA, MARSHALL (J.), RATHKE, RINDFLEISCH, SCHULTZE (B. S.), TREVES, TROELTSCH, ZAUFAL.

Foley, Frederic Eugene Basil (b. 1891). St. Paul, Minnesota, urologist.

Foley catheter. A latex-rubber urethral catheter, into the wall of which is built a narrow channel that is connected to a balloon just proximal to the eye of the catheter. The balloons are of various sizes, the small size of from 5 to 30 ml capacity being distended when the catheter is used for self-retaining purposes only, Larger balloons of from 75 to 100 ml capacity may be employed when the bag is intended for haemostatic purposes to prevent postprostatectomy haemorrhage.

Foley's operation. An operation for ureteropelvic stricture in which, after division of the stricture, the ureteropelvic opening is reconstructed by a Y-plasty procedure.

folia (fo·le·ah). *See* FOLIUM.

foliaceous (fo·le·a·se·us). 1. Belonging to or having the texture of a leaf. 2. In zoology, like a leaf in form or manner of growth. [folium.]

folie (fo·le). A generic term of French psychiatry, roughly corresponding to *mental disorder.* **Folie circulaire.** Cyclothymia; a form of manic-depressive disorder in which both manic and depressive phases are shown. **Folie à deux.** The common involvement of two or more persons, usually those with a close emotional tie such as mother and daughter or husband and wife, in the same or very similar delusional beliefs. As a rule, one of the two is mentally ill, and has developed the delusional ideas spontaneously, whilst the other is fundamentally normal but has adopted the same ideas, or has become persuaded of their truth. By some authorities, the term is held to presuppose the effects of suggestion and psychological contagion, and will not be admitted if both members of the pair are genuinely psychotic. Other authorities allow its use even in the latter case, provided the nature of the delusional beliefs is the same in both members of the pair. More than two persons may be affected, hence *folie à trois, folie à quatre.* **Folie du doute.** Morbid preoccupation with doubts which are recognized to be unjustified, e.g. a persistent doubt while away from home that the bath tap has been left running. A symptom of obsessional neurosis. **Folie gémellaire.** Mental disorder involving both members of a pair of twins. **Folie musculaire.** A marked form of chorea. **Folie raisonnante.** Mental disorders with apparent sound thinking ability but lacking in self control or common sense. [Fr. insanity.]

Folin, Otto Knut Olof (b. 1867). American biochemist.

Folin's method. 1. For amino-acid nitrogen in blood: 5 ml of blood filtrate (tungstic-acid method) are neutralized to phenolphthalein with 1.25 per cent Na_2CO_3, 1 ml of freshly prepared 0.5 per cent aqueous sodium β-naphthoquinone-4-sulphonate is added; the mixture is then shaken and set aside in the dark overnight. 1 ml of 2.5 per cent crystalline sodium acetate in 25 per cent aqueous acetic acid is added, followed by 1 ml of 4 per cent aqueous sodium thiosulphate and water to 15 ml. The colour is compared with 1 ml of a standard containing 0.07 mg amino-acid nitrogen per ml treated similarly but with double the quantities of reagents and water. 2. For amino-acid nitrogen in urine: a similar procedure to that with blood (1. above), except that the urine is pretreated with "Permutit" to remove ammonia, and 5 ml of the ammonia-free urine is taken for estimation. 3. For creatine and creatinine in urine. (*a*) Free creatinine: 2 ml urine is placed in a 100 ml flask; 20 ml of saturated aqueous picric-acid solution is added, followed by 1.5 ml of 10 per cent aqueous sodium hydroxide. After 10 min the solution is diluted to 100 ml with water and the colour compared with that given by 1 ml of standard creatinine (1 mg/ml). (*b*) Total creatinine: 1 ml urine is placed with 20 ml of picric-acid solution in a 100 ml flask stoppered with tin foil and heated in an autoclave at from 115° to 120°C for 20 min. After cooling, 1.5 ml of sodium hydroxide solution are added and the colour compared with the standard, as in (*a*). The difference between the values obtained in (*b*) and (*a*) gives creatine. 4. For uric acid in blood: to 5 ml of blood filtrate are added 10 ml of urea-cyanide solution and 4 ml of uric-acid reagent (Folin). After 20 min the solution is made up to 25 ml, mixed, and the colour compared with a standard. 5. For uric acid in urine: urine is diluted 1 to 100 and 5 ml of this solution is treated as the blood filtrate in 4 (above). 6. For sulphates in urine. (*a*) Inorganic: to 25 ml urine and 100 ml water add 10 ml dilute HCl (1+4), and 10 ml of 5 per cent barium chloride. After 1 h, filter, wash, dry, ignite and weigh as $BaSO_4$. (*b*) Ethereal: to 125 ml urine add 75 ml water, 30 ml dilute HCl, and 20 ml barium-chloride solution. After 1 h, filter and boil 125 ml of filtrate for at least ½ h. Filter, wash, dry, ignite and weigh as $BaSO_4$.

Folin's reagent. For uric acid: add a solution of 30 ml of syrupy phosphoric acid in 150 ml of water gradually to 100 g of molybdate-free sodium tungstate. Boil the mixture gently under reflux for 1 h, decolorize with 0.5 ml of bromine, boil to expel the excess bromine, cool and dilute to 500 ml with water.

Folin's sugar tube. A stout glass test-tube so modified that its closed end consists of a bulb connected by a constriction to the rest of the tube. In making a sugar determination, the test solution and reagent are mixed in the bulb and during subsequent heating the mixture is protected from aerial reoxidation by the decrease in surface exposure afforded by the constriction.

Folin and Bell method. For ammonia in urine: add "Permutit" to the urine (2 ml) and shake for 5 min. Wash the "Permutit" several times with water by decantation, extract with 10 per cent sodium hydroxide and nesslerize. Compare the colour with that given by a standard ammonium sulphate solution.

Folin-Ciocalteau reagent. For phenols: dissolve 100 g of sodium tungstate and 25 g of sodium molybdate in 700 ml of water in a 1500-ml flask. Add 50 ml of phosphoric acid (S.G. 1.75) and 100 ml of concentrated hydrochloric acid. Boil under relux for 10 h. Add 150 g of lithium sulphate, 50 ml of water and a few drops of bromine and boil without reflux for 15 min. Allow to cool and dilute to 1 l with water. For use, dilute 1 volume with 2 volumes of water.

Folin and Denis method. A method for determining the total nitrogen of urine by direct nesslerization of the diluted digest obtained by the micro-Kjeldahl procedure.

Folin and Farmer method. A micro-Kjeldahl method of determining the total nitrogen in urine, the ammonia being separated by aeration and then nesslerized.

Osborne and Folin method. For total sulphur in biological material: organic matter is destroyed and sulphur converted to sulphate by fusing with sodium peroxide. The sulphate is determined by precipitation as $BaSO_4$.

Ostwald-Folin pipette. A combined bulb-capillary pipette devised for measuring blood or other viscous fluid.

Folin and Wu method. For blood sugar: a protein-free filtrate of blood is prepared with sodium tungstate sulphuric acid, and this is heated with an alkaline cupric tartrate solution, when cuprous salt is formed in proportion to the amount of glucose present. Phosphomolybdic-acid reagent (see below) is added and is reduced by the cuprous salt to give a blue compound. The intensity of the colour is compared with that given by a standard glucose solution under the same conditions. The heating procedure is carried out in a special type of tube known as *Folin's sugar tube* (see above) which is designed to minimize aerial re-oxidation of the reduced copper salt.

Folin-Wu phosphomolybdic-acid reagent. For blood sugar: dissolve 35 g of molybdic acid and 5 g of sodium tungstate in 250 ml of 8 per cent sodium hydroxide and boil for 30 min. Add water to about 350 ml, followed by 125 ml of phosphoric acid (S.G. 1.75), and dilute with water to 500 ml.

folium [NA] (fo·le um) (pl. *folia*). In biology, a leaf-like part or structure, e.g. a lobe of the cerebellum. **Folium cacuminis.** The lobulus folii of the cerebellum. **Cerebellar folium [folium cerebelli (NA)].** One of the constituent leaf-life parts of the cerebellum which are marked off one from another by fissures. **Folia linguae, Lingual folia.** Foliate papillae. *See* PAPILLA. [L leaf.]

Folius, Caecilus (b. 1615). Venice anatomist.

Folius' muscle. The anterior ligament of the malleus, originally believed to have been muscular.

Folius' process. The anterior process of the malleus.

follicle [folliculus (NA)] (fol·ikl). A small cavity or recess with an excretory or secretory function, **Atretic follicle.** The scarred remains of an ovarian follicle. **Graafian follicles.** Ovarian follicle, vesicular (see below). **Hair follicle [folliculus pili [NA].** An invaginated tube of epidermal cells lying in the corium of the skin and containing the root of a hair. **Hair follicle, fundus of a.** The base of a hair follicle. **Hair follicle, neck of a.** The narrow part of a hair follicle immediately below the surface opening. **Lingual follicles [folliculi linguales (NA)].** The individual nodules of lymphoid tissue, constituting the lingual tonsil. **Lymphatic follicle [folliculus lymphaticus (NA)].** One of the densely-packed masses of lymphocytes and lymphoblasts which compose the cortex of a lymphatic node. The follicles are more or less isolated from one another by the trabeculae of the nodes and may or may not contain a germinal centre. **Ovarian follicles, primary [folliculi ovarici primarii (NA)].** Follicles lying in the cortex under the tunica albuginea and composed of an ovum separated from the surrounding tissue by a single layer of follicular cells. Their number gradually diminishes throughout reproductive life. **Ovarian follicles, vesicular [folliculi ovarici vesiculosi (NA)].** Follicles enlarged by multiplication of follicular cells, in the midst of which a cavity, the antrum, containing liquor, appears. This liquor divides the cells into an outer stratum granulosum lining the follicle, and an inner, the cumulus ovaricus, surrounding the eccentric ovum, and by which it is attached to the outer at one point. **Palpebral follicle.** Meibomian gland. **Pilosebaceous follicle, Sebaceous follicle.** A sebaceous gland that opens into a hair follicle (see above). **Solitary follicle.** Solitary lymphatic nodule. *See* NODULE. **Thyroid follicles [folliculi glandulae thyroideae (NA)].** The secretory vesicles of the thyroid gland. [L *folliculus* a small bag.]

See also: FLEISCHMANN, FREY (H.), GRAAF, LIEBERKÜHN, MONTGOMERY, NABOTH.

folliclis (fol·ik·lis). A variety of tuberculosis papulonecrotica principally affecting the extremities. [L *folliculus* a small bag.]

follicular (fol·ik·ew·lar). 1. Relating, affecting, or belonging to a follicle or follicles. 2. Consisting of follicles.

folliculin (fol·ik·ew·lin). The hormone of the ovarian follicles, now known as *oestradiol.*

folliculinuria (fol·ik·ew·lin·ewr′·e·ah). A condition in which folliculin is present in the urine.

folliculitis (fol·ik·ew·li′·tis). Inflammation of a follicle. **Folliculitis abscedens et suffodiens.** A chronic, suppurating, burrowing perifolliculitis of the scalp, probably closely related to acne conglobata. **Agminate folliculitis.** Conglomerative pustular folliculitis (see below). **Folliculitis barbae.** Sycosis barbae. **Folliculitis cheloidalis.** Dermatitis papillaris capillitii. **Conglomerate folliculitis, Conglomerative pustular folliculitis.** Pustular ringworm caused by an ectothrix, *Trichophyton.* **Folliculitis decalvans.** 1. A chronic inflammatory infection of the hair follicles of the scalp leading to patchy cicatricial alopecia. 2. Sycosis of the scalp. **Folliculitis decalvans cryptococcica.** The name given by Castellani to a furunculous disease of the scalp, face and body, clinically indistinguishable from the common boil but caused by yeast fungi. **Folliculitis depilans.** Folliculitis with loss of hair, mostly on the legs. **Folliculitis exulcerans.** Folliclis. **Folliculitis gonorrhoeica.** Small pockets of infection on the roof of the anterior urethra, usually associated with gonococcal infection of the glands of Littré which open into the lacunae of Morgagni. **Industrial folliculitis.** Inflammation of the pilosebaceous follicles caused by substances, especially oils, encountered in industry. **Folliculitis keloidalis.** Folliculitis cheloidalis; dermatitis papillaris capillitii. **Folliculitis miliaris.** A very superficial form of follicular tuberculide. **Folliculitis narium perforans.** A chronic pustular or crusted lesion on the side of the tip of the nose due to a follicular abscess inside the nostril. **Folliculitis necrotica.** Chronic, itching, somewhat grouped folliculitis leading to scarring. **Pustular folliculitis.** Bockhart's impetigo. **Pyococcal folliculitis, Pyogenic folliculitis.** An inflammation of the skin follicles that is caused by a primary or a secondary infection by pyogenic micro-organisms, such as staphylococci. **Folliculitis rubra.** Ulerythema ophryogenes. **Seborrhoeic folliculitis.** Inflammation of the pilosebaceous follicles, attributed to a seborrhoeic process. **Superficial folliculitis.** Inflammation of the follicular orifices resulting from physical or chemical causes. It may occur beneath adhesive dressings, from occlusive treatment with topical steroids or from contact with oil or tar. The pustules are usually sterile, except in Bockhart's impetigo which is caused by *Staphylococcus aureus.* **Folliculitis ulerythematosa reticulata.** Honeycomb atrophy of the skin. **Folliculitis varioliformis.** Acne varioliformis. [follicle, Gk *-itis* inflammation.]

folliculogenesis (fol·ik·ew·lo′·gen·ee·sis.) The production of ovarian follicles, usually mature. Usually under the influence of follicle-stimulating hormone (FSH).

folliculoma (fol·ik·ew·lo′·mah). A benign (lipidique) or malignant tumour of the ovary, typically composed of granulosa and theca cells, with a cystic, tubular or adenomatous structure. [follicle, Gk *-oma* tumour.]

folliculose (fol·ik·ew·loze). 1. Containing many follicles. 2. Having resemblance to a follicle.

folliculosis (fol·ik·ew·lo′·sis). A diseased condition marked by the presence of abnormally large numbers of lymph follicles. **Conjunctival folliculosis.** A condition in which an increase in the number of lymph follicles scattered throughout the conjunctival sac gives the impression of a granular surface. There is no visual evidence of infection, and it is to be differentiated from trachoma. [follicle, Gk *-osis* condition.]

folliculus (fol·ik·ew·lus). A follicle. **Folliculus solitarius.** Solitary lymphatic nodule. *See* NODULE. [L a small bag.]

Follin, François Anthime (b. 1823). French surgeon.

Follin's grains. Remnants of mesonephric tubules within the broad ligament of the uterus.

Follman's balanitis. Inflammation of the glans penis associated with posthitis or inflammation of the prepuce. The two are usually associated in such conditions as phimosis and local uncleanliness.

Foltz, Jean Charles Eugene (b. 1822). French anatomist and physiologist.

Foltz's valve. Folds of mucous membrane at the commencement of the superior lacrimal canaliculus.

Foltz's valvules. Mucosal folds at the lower end of the nasolacrimal duct.

fomentation (fo·men·ta·shun). 1. The therapeutic application of warmth and moisture to any part of the body in order to overcome inflammation or pain. 2. Any substance or medicinal preparation applied in a warm, moist state to a part of the body in order to carry heat and moisture to it; poultice; a stupe. [L *fomentare* to apply a poultice.]

fomes (fo·meez) (pl. *fomites*). Any substance, e.g. clothing, which is able to absorb and transmit contagion. Food is not included in the term. [L tinder.]

fomite (fo·mite). Fomes.

Fomocaine (fo·mo·kane). BP Commission approved name for 4 - (3 - morpholinopropyl)benzyl phenyl ether; a local anaesthetic.

Fonio, Anton (b. 1889). Berne surgeon.

Fonio's solution. A solution containing 14 per cent of magnesium sulphate, intended to retard the agglutination and disintegration of thrombocytes during the collection of a specimen of blood for the counting of platelets. It has now been superseded by other more effective preparations.

Fonio's granulopenic thrombopathy. A disease resembling von Willebrand's constitutional thrombopathy, but showing structural abnormalities such as poorly granular cytoplasm in the platelets.

fons pulsatilis (fonz pul·sat·il·is). The anterior fontanelle. [L pulsing fountain.]

Fonsecaea (fon·se·se·ah). Generic name proposed by Negroni (1936) for fungi which cause chromoblastomycosis and are more commonly known under the generic name *Phialophora.* [O. da *Fonseca,* Brazilian physician.]

fontactoscope (fon·tak·to·skope). A form of electroscope with which the radioactivity of water can be measured. [L *fons* fountain, Gk *aktis* ray, *skopein* to watch.]

Fontana, Arturo (b. 1880). Turin dermatologist.

Fontana's method, for spirochaetes. The film is fixed in an acetic acid–formalin solution, mordanted in a solution of phenol and tannic acid, treated with hot ammoniacal silver nitrate, washed and mounted in Canada balsam. Spirochaetes stain dark brown to black against a yellow background.

Fontana, Felice (b. 1730). Italian anatomist and physiologist.

Fontana's canal, or spaces. The spaces situated in the meshwork of the fibres of the pectinate ligament situated at the angle of the anterior chamber. They are important in the drainage of the aqueous into Schlemm's canal.

fontanelle [fonticulus cranii (NA)] (fon·tan·el). An unossified space in the infant skull. **Fontanelle of the skull, anterior [fonticulus anterior (NA)].** The diamond-shaped interval, completed by membrane, at the junction of the frontal, coronal and sagittal sutures. It is normally ossified at about 18 months. **Fontanelle of the skull, anterolateral [fonticulus sphenoidalis (NA)].** An interval at the junction of the parietal and frontal bones, the squamous part of the temporal bone and the great wing of the sphenoid bone. It is normally obliterated within the first 3 months after birth, and is the site of the future pterion. **Fontanelle of the skull, posterior [fonticulus posterior (NA)].** The triangular interval at the junction of the sagittal and lambdoid sutures. It is normally ossified within 3 months after birth. **Fontanelle of the skull, posterolateral [fonticulus mastoideus (NA)].** An interval between the adjacent edges of the occipital, parietal and temporal bones. It is normally closed by 12 months. [dim. of Fr. *fontaine* fountain.]

See also: CASSERIO, GERDY.

fonticulus (fon·tik·ew·lus). 1. A fontanelle. 2. A small ulcer, artificially induced. **Fonticulus gutturis.** The slight hollowing of the skin over the suprasternal notch. **Fonticulus major.** The anterior fontanelle, *See* FONTANELLE. **Fonticulus minor.** The posterior fontanelle. *See* FONTANELLE. **Fonticulus quadrangularis.** The anterior fontanelle. *See* FONTANELLE. **Fonticulus triangularis.** The posterior fontanelle. *See* FONTANELLE. [L little fountain.]

food (food). Physiologically, that which is taken into the body to maintain its normal life and growth, i.e. to replace waste, supply energy and animal heat, and to nourish and build the tissue. **Isodynamic foods.** Those which, when expressed in joules (calories), are shown to generate or liberate the same amount of energy. **Food poisoning.** *See* POISONING. **Predigested food.** Food artificially digested through the action of different ferments. [AS *foda.*]

foot [pes (NA)] (fut). The terminal part of the leg below the ankle. Distinctive parts are the dorsum [dorsum pedis (NA)], and the sole [planta (NA)]. The borders are the medial [margo medialis (tibialis)NA], and the lateral [margo lateralis (fibularis) NA]. **Athletes' foot.** An eruption of the feet, usually consisting of maceration and fissuring of the skin of the webs and adjacent sides of the toes, particularly the outermost ones; in hot weather or after much exercise acute erythema with vesicle formation may occur. The eruption on the toes may be associated with a vesicular or hyperkeratotic rash on the soles, and may be complicated by infection of the nails. The malady is due to infection with *Epidermophyton* or *Trichophyton.* The term is often loosely applied without microscopic confirmation; it may then conceal the correct diagnosis which may be candidiasis, coccal infection, contact dermatitis, pompholyx, or pustular dermatitis, and is therefore best avoided. **Burning feet.** A well-recognized condition, especially among Indian and African women. It is now thought to be due to a dietary deficiency of pantothenic acid of the vitamin B_2 complex, since the symptoms of burning of the sole is usually accompanied by an angular cheilitis. The condition has long been regarded by the people of these countries as a specific affliction, and has been given various names. **Claw foot.** *See* CLAW-FOOT. **Cleft foot.** A deformity in which the division between the 3rd and 4th toes extends between the corresponding metatarsals. **Club foot.** *See* CLUB-FOOT. **Dancers' foot.** Painful swelling beneath the 2nd and 3rd metatarsal heads. **Dangle foot.** Drop foot due to paralysis of the peroneal nerve. **Drop foot.** A condition in which the foot is plantar-flexed, with inability to dorsiflex. **Flat foot.** *See* FLAT FOOT. **Fungus foot.** Madura foot (see below). **Hollow foot.** Pes cavus. **Hong Kong foot.** Local name for tinea pedis. **Hot foot.** A sensation of burning in the soles of the feet; one of the symptoms of beriberi. **Immersion foot.** A swollen painful condition of the feet, with redness and blistering of the skin and sometimes gangrene, caused by exposure to cold and damp, occurring, for example in shipwrecked persons who have spent long periods in waterlogged boats. **Madura foot.** Mycetoma of the foot; a fungous disease found especially in parts of India (Bengal), also in Somalia, Indonesia, Algeria, Sudan, Vietnam and South Africa. It is characterized by swelling of the affected area which is invaded by the mycelium and in which numerous sinuses form. Fungus invades skin, subcutaneous and interstitial tissue and bone, evoking a chronic granulomatous tissue response. The disease runs a protracted course and may necessitate amputation. **March foot.** Spontaneous fracture of one of the metatarsal bones, usually the 2nd. **Mossy foot.** Verrucose dermatitis of the legs and feet: lymphostatic verrucosis of South America. **Shelter foot.** Trench foot (see below). **Splay foot.** Extreme eversion of the foot. **Split foot.** Lobster-claw deformity of the feet in which the middle part is missing and the digits on either side are fused; it is autosomal dominant. **Spread foot.** Flattening of the anterior metatarsal arch. **Sucker foot.** The expanded termination of a process of an astrocyte attached to a capillary wall. **Trench foot.** Moist gangrene of the feet due to freezing of the wet skin. **Weak foot.** Flat foot. [AS *fot.*]

See also: FRIEDREICH, MORTON (T. G.).

foot, dorsal digital veins of the [venae digitales dorsales pedis (NA)]. Veins draining the sides of the toes into the dorsal metatarsal veins and thence into the dorsal venous arch.

foot, dorsal lateral cutaneous nerve of the [nervus cutaneus dorsalis lateralis (NA)]. A branch of the sural nerve supplying a narrow strip on the lateral border of the dorsum of the foot.

foot-candle (fut·kandl). A unit of intensity of illumination equal to 10.7639 lux, originally defined as the illumination produced upon a surface one foot square placed one foot from one international candle ($\frac{1}{10}$ the Harcourt pentane lamp). [AS *fot, candel.*]

foot-pound (fut·pownd). A unit of energy defined as energy required to raise a weight of one pound to a height of one foot against gravity, and equal to 4.21 mJ. **Foot-pound second.** The rate of work when a foot-pound is applied for one second equal to 1.356 W. Also applied to the system employing the units of the foot, the pound and the second (f.p.s. system). [AS *fot, pund.*]

footling (fut·ling). In obstetrics, foot presentation; feet foremost. [AS *fot.*]

forage (for·ij). 1. The operation of cutting by diathermy a V-shaped channel in a hypertrophied prostate and so enlarging the urethral channel. 2. Term used to describe an operation used in the treatment of osteoarthritis of the hip to reduce the blood supply to the head of the femur. [L *forare* to bore.]

foramen [NA] (for·a·men) (pl. *foramina*). A hole or aperture. **Apical foramen [foramen apicis dentis].** A hole in the apex of the root of a tooth transmitting the nerve and blood vessels to the pulp. **Auditory foramen, external.** The external auditory meatus. **Auditory foramen, internal.** The foramen on the cranial aspect of the petrous part of the temporal bone transmitting the 7th and 8th cranial nerves. **Caecal foramen.** A blind foramen or pit. **Foramen caecum of the frontal bone.** Foramen caecum of the skull (see below). **Foramen caecum of the medulla oblongata.** The pit at the cranial end of the anteromedian fissure, immediately caudal to the pons. **Foramen caecum of the skull**

[foramen cecum (NA)]. A depression between the crista galli of the ethmoid bone and the crest of the frontal bone. **Foramen caecum of the tongue [foramen cecum linguae (NA)].** The pit marking the point of outgrowth of the thyroid diverticulum in the embryo. **Carotid foramen.** An aperture in the petrous part of the temporal bone into which pass the internal carotid artery and sympathetic nerve fibres. **Foramen centrale.** The foramen in the modiolus transmitting the nerve fibres to the apical turn of the cochlea. **Condyloid foramen, anterior.** The foramen above the condyle of the occipital bone transmitting the 12th cranial nerve. **Condyloid foramen, posterior.** A foramen behind the occipital condyle transmitting an emissary vein. **Costotransverse foramen [foramen costotransversarium (NA)].** A foramen between the anterior and posterior transverse ligaments. **Cotyloid foramen.** The foramen formed between the notch in the acetabular rim and the transverse ligament. **Dental foramen, inferior.** Mandibular foramen (see below). **Dental foramina of the maxilla [foramina alveolaria (NA)].** The openings for the branches of the superior dental nerves on the posterior surface of the maxilla. **Foramen diaphragmatis (sellae).** The foramen in the diaphragma sellae through which passes the stalk of the pituitary. **Emissary foramina.** Foramina in the skull through which the venous sinuses communicate with diploic veins and with veins outside the skull. **Epiploic foramen.** The aditus to the lesser sac of the peritoneal cavity. **Ethmoidal foramen, anterior [foramen ethmoidale anterius (NA)].** A foramen in the medial wall of the orbit transmitting the anterior ethmoidal nerve and artery. **Ethmoidal foramen, posterior [foramen ethmoidale posterius (NA)].** A foramen in the medial wall of the orbit, transmitting the posterior ethmoidal nerve (when present) and artery. **Frontal foramen [foramen (sive incisura) frontale (NA)].** A foramen sometimes present close to the orbital margin of the frontal bone medial to the supra-orbital notch. **Fronto-ethmoidal foramina.** Ethmoidal foramina (see above). **Incisive foramina [foramina incisiva (NA)].** Foramina in the incisive fossa of the hard palate. **Incisive foramen, lateral.** Stensen's foramen; a foramen in the incisive fossa, transmitting the greater palatine artery and the long sphenopalatine nerve. **Incisive foramina, median.** Foramina sometimes present in the midline of the incisive fossa of the hard palate. **Infra-orbital foramen [foramen infraorbitale (NA)].** A foramen on the anterior aspect of the maxilla transmitting the inferior orbital nerves and vessels. **Interventricular foramen [foramen interventriculare (NA)].** The communication between the lateral and 3rd ventricles of the brain. **Intervertebral foramen of the sacrum [foramen intervertebrale (NA)].** The foramen between the pedicles of adjacent vertebrae formed by the inferior vertebral notch of the vertebra above, and the superior vertebral arch of the one below. **Ischiadic foramen.** The greater sacrosciatic foramen (see below) between the hip bone and the sacrum, completed by the sacrotuberous ligament. **Jugular foramen [foramen jugulare (NA)].** The aperture in the base of the skull transmitting the sigmoid and inferior petrosal sinus and the 9th, 10th and 11th cranial nerves. On the upper border of the foramen near its medial end is the small notch for the ganglion of the 9th (glossopharyngeal) nerve, whilst near the middle of the posterior border a small spicule of bone (the intrajugular process) projects into the foramen and may completely subdivide it. **Foramen lacerum [NA].** The irregular aperture between the petrous part of the temporal bone and the body of the sphenoid in the base of the skull; it is closed by the fibrocartilage. **Foramen lacerum anterius.** The superior orbital fissure between the wings of the sphenoid bone. **Foramen lacerum medium.** Foramen lacerum (see above). **Foramen lacerum posterius.** The jugular foramen (see above). **Foramen magnum [NA].** The aperture in the occipital bone of the skull through which the brain stem joins the spinal cord. **Mandibular foramen [foramen mandibulae (NA)].** The foramen on the medial side of the ramus of the mandible transmitting the inferior dental nerve and artery. **Mastoid foramen [foramen mastoideum (NA)].** A foramen in the mastoid part of the temporal bone which transmits an emissary vein. **Mental foramen [foramen mentale (NA)].** The foramen in the body of the mandible transmitting the mental branch of the inferior dental nerve. **Foramina for nerves [foramina nervosa (NA)].** Perforations of the spiral lamina for the cochlear nerves. **Nutrient foramen [foramen nutricium (NA)].** A foramen in a bone which transmits the nutrient artery. **Obturator foramen [foramen obturatum (NA)].** The aperture in the hip bone between the ischium and the pubic bone. **Foramen occipitale magnum.** Foramen magnum (see above). **Olfactory foramina.** Small holes in the cribriform plate of the ethmoid bone. **Optic foramen [canalis opticus (NA)].** The foramen in the root of the lesser wing of the sphenoid bone transmitting the optic nerve and the ophthalmic artery. **Foramen ovale [NA].** 1. Of the heart: an aperture in the interatrial septum of the heart which normally closes at or shortly after birth. 2. Of the greater wing of the sphenoid bone: it transmits the mandibular division of the trigeminal nerve. **Foramen ovale, patent.** Persistence of the foramen ovale after birth. Closure of the foramen normally does not occur immediately after birth so that patency is common in infants; it can be found in about 15 per cent of normal adults as a valvular-like slit of no significance. Wide patency allowing shunting of blood constitutes an ostium secundum type of atrial septal defect; valvular patency may become significant if it is complicated by a rise in right atrial pressure, when a right-to-left shunt of blood through it may occur. **Palatine foramen, greater [foramen palatinum majus (NA)].** A foramen posterolaterally situated in the hard palate transmitting the greater palatine nerve and vessels. **Palatine foramina, lesser [foramina palatina minora (NA)].** Small foramina in the posterolateral part of the hard palate transmitting the lesser palatine nerves and vessels. **Papillary foramina [foramina papillaria (NA)].** The openings of the collecting tubules on the summit of a renal papilla. **Parietal foramen [foramen parietale (NA)].** A foramen in the parietal bone near the median sagittal suture, transmitting an emissary vein. **Foramen primum.** The aperture in the septum primum of the embryonic heart. **Pterygo-alar foramen.** The vomerovaginal canal. *See* CANAL. **Pterygopalatine foramen.** The opening leading from the pterygopalatine fossa into the pterygopalatine canal. **Pterygospinous foramen.** A foramen occasionally present between the lateral pterygoid plate and the spine of the sphenoid bone, transmitting the nerve to the medial pterygoid muscle. **Foramen radicis dentis.** Apical foramen (see above). **Rivinian foramen.** A foramen sometimes present in the flaccid part of the tympanic membrane. **Foramen rotundum [NA].** The foramen in the great wing of the sphenoid transmitting the maxillary nerve. **Sacral foramina, anterior [foramina sacralia pelvina (NA)].** Holes on the anterior aspect of the sacrum transmitting the anterior primary rami of the sacral nerves. **Sacral foramina, posterior [foramina sacralia dorsalia (NA)].** Foramina on the posterior aspect of the sacrum for the posterior primary rami of the sacral nerves. **Sacrosciatic foramina.** Sciatic foramina (see following). **Sciatic foramen, greater [foramen ischiadicum majus (NA)].** The aperture between the hip bone, sacrum and sacrotuberous ligament. **Sciatic foramen, lesser [foramen ischiadicum minus (NA).** The aperture bounded by the hip bone, sacrum and sacrospinous ligament. **Foramen singulare [NA].** Morgagni's foramen; a foramen for the nerve to the ampulla of the posterior semicircular canal. **Sphenopalatine foramen [foramen sphenopalatinum (NA)].** A foramen between the palatine and sphenoid bones leading from the pterygopalatine fossa to the nasal cavity. **Foramen spinosum [NA].** A foramen in the spine of the sphenoid transmitting the middle meningeal artery. **Stylomastoid foramen [foramen stylomastoideum (NA)].** A foramen medial to the mastoid process transmitting the 7th cranial nerve. **Sub-orbital foramen.** Infra-orbital foramen (see above). **Supra-orbital foramen [foramen (sive incisura) supra-orbitalis (NA)].** A foramen sometimes present above the superior margin of the orbit transmitting the supra-orbital nerve and vessels. It occurs occasionally as a notch. **Thyroid foramen.** 1. [Foramen thyroideum (NA)]. An opening in one of the thyroid cartilages. 2. An old name for the obturator foramen. **Foramen transversarium [NA].** The foramen in the transverse process of a cervical vertebra. **Transverse accessory foramen.** A small additional foramen sometimes present in the transverse process of the cervical vertebra transmitting a vertebral vein. **Foramina venarum minimarum [NA].** The openings of the venae cordis minimae into the heart chambers. **Vertebral foramen [foramen vertebrale (NA)].** The large aperture between the neural arch and the body of a vertebra. **Vertebro-arterial foramen.** Transverse foramen (see above). **Zygomaticofacial foramen [foramen zygomaticofaciale (NA)].** A small foramen on the outer surface of the zygomatic bone transmitting a nerve of the same name. **Zygomatico-orbital foramen [foramen zygomatico-orbitale (NA)].** One or two foramina on the orbital surface of the zygomatic bone for the zygomatic nerve. **Zygomaticotemporal foramen [foramen zygomaticotemporale (NA)].** A small foramen on the temporal surface of the zygomatic bone transmitting a nerve of the same name. [L]

See also: BARTHOLIN (T.), BICHAT, BOCHDALEK, BOTALLO, BOZZI, D'AZYR, DUVERNEY, FERREIN, GALEN, HUSCHKE, KEY (E. A. H.), KNOX, LANNELONGUE, LUSCHKA, MAGENDIE, MIERZEJEWSKI, MONRO (II), MORAND, MORGAGNI, PACINI, PANIZZA, RETZIUS (M. G.), SCARPA, SCHWALBE, SOEMMERING, SPOENDLI, STENSEN, TARIN, THEBESIUS, VESALIUS, VIEUSSENS, WEITBRECHT, WINSLOW.

foraminated (for·**am**·in·a·ted). 1. Perforated. 2. Having foramina. [foramen.]

foraminiferous (**for**·am·in·**if'**·er·us). Composed of or containing foramina. [foramen, L *ferre* to bear.]

foraminulate, foraminulose, foraminulous (for·am·**in**·ew·late, for·am·**in**·ew·loze, for·am·**in**·ew·lus). Having minute perforations. [L *foraminulum* little opening.]

foraminulum (for·am·**in**·ew·lum). A minute foramen. [L]

foration (for·a·shun). The process or act of perforating, boring or trephining. [L *forare* to bore.]

Forbes' amputation. Amputation through the anterior part of the foot, disarticulating the talonavicular joint on the inner side and cutting across the cuboid on the outer side.

Forbes-Albright syndrome. *See* GALACTORRHOEA.

force (fors). 1. Strength. 2. Any external agency which produces a change in motion of a body. 3. *See* ENERGY, Kinetic. **Absolute muscular force.** The greatest power of contraction shown by a maximally stimulated muscle. **Animal force.** Muscular force. **Catabolic force.** That originating from the metabolism of ingested food. **Catalytic force.** Force initiated by a catalyzer. **Centrifugal force.** The outward force acting on a body moving with uniform velocity in a curved path. It acts in opposition, and as a reaction, to the centripetal force. **Centripetal force.** The force required to maintain a body moving in a curved path. **Chemical force.** Chemical affinity; the force which binds the atoms in the molecules of a chemical compound. **Coercive force.** The magnetic field required to reduce the intensity of magnetization of a specimen to zero. **Electromotive force.** Emf. 1. That force which tends to cause a movement of electricity along a conductor. 2. The rate at which electrical energy is drawn from the source and dissipated in the circuit when unit current is flowing. The practical unit of emf is the volt. **Field force.** In embryology, the hypothetical force at a given point in a field or territory of influence of an organizer which determines the direction of influence of an organizer. On this hypothesis each organizer is supposed to have around it a field of influence analogous to the field of magnetic force surrounding a magnetic pole, so that the degree to which cells in the neighbourhood of such an organizer are subject to its influence is determined by its distance from the organizer. **G force.** Inertial forces cause acceleration; they are measured by comparison with the inertial force of gravity at the earth's surface (*G* or *g*). A force of $+1G$ causes acceleration of 9.75 m/s^2 (32 ft/s^2). **Nerve force.** The capacity of nerve fibres to conduct impulses. **Psychic force.** Mental driving power. [L *fortis* strong.]

forceps (**for**·seps). 1. An instrument whose blades are used for holding or compressing a tissue or object, or dressing material, and which may be modified for crushing, cutting or removing tissue. 2. A structure that resembles a pair of forceps. **Adenoid forceps.** Forceps with blunt crushing blades for removing adenoids. **Advancement forceps.** Forceps for the manipulation of ocular muscle in the correction of squint. **Alligator forceps.** A strong-toothed forceps with double bite. **Alveolar forceps.** Forceps for removing portions of alveolus. **Forceps anterior.** Forceps minor. **Artery forceps.** Forceps for controlling bleeding by the compression of the divided end of a vessel. **Attic-ridge forceps.** A punch forceps for removing the attic ridge in the mastoid operation. **Aural forceps.** Forceps with short blades for manipulations and the application of dressings within the external ear. **Axis-traction forceps.** An obstetrical forceps by which traction can be exerted in the line of the pelvic axis. **Bone-cutting forceps.** A forceps with a sharp edge for cutting bone across. **Bone-holding forceps.** A strong forceps or clamp used to steady a bone during operations upon it. **Bone-nibbling forceps.** A forceps with sharp curved and often cup-shaped blades for nibbling through bone. **Broad-ligament forceps.** A clamp for controlling the broad ligament in hysterectomy. **Bronchus forceps.** A forceps for the removal of foreign bodies at bronchoscopy. **Brossage forceps.** Forceps for retracting the eyelid in removing the granulations of trachoma. **Bulldog forceps.** A cross-action clip forceps for occluding a large vessel during an operation upon it. **Bullet forceps.** Forceps for extracting bullets from wounds. **Capsule forceps.** A forceps for removing the lens capsule in membranous cataract. **Cartilage forceps.** A forceps for grasping the medial semilunar cartilage for its removal from the knee. **Chalazion forceps.** A forceps with ringed blades for removal of a meibomian cyst. **Cholecystectomy forceps.** A clamp forceps for grasping the cystic duct and cystic artery in cholecystectomy. **Cholelithotomy forceps.** A forceps for removing stones from the biliary passages. **Cilia forceps.** A forceps for grasping the eyelashes. **Clamp forceps.** Any forceps with an automatic lock. **Cleft-palate forceps.** Forceps for steadying the soft palate in repair of a cleft. **Clip-compressing forceps.** A forceps for applying silver clips to compress bleeding vessels or to oppose skin edges. **Clip-extracting forceps.** A forceps for removing clips from skin wounds. **Clot-breaking forceps.** A forceps introduced through an endoscope into the bladder to break down a blood clot for evacuation. **Craniotomy forceps.** Forceps for destruction of the fetal head. **Crocodile forceps.** A forceps with long handles and blades, only one of which is hinged for use in endoscopy. **Dental forceps.** Forceps for the extraction of teeth. **Depilatory forceps.** Forceps for the removal of hair. **Disc forceps.** A forceps for grasping the circle of sclera removed when the eyeball is trephined. **Dissection forceps.** Forceps with or without teeth and hinged terminally for grasping tissue during surgical dissection. **Double-action forceps.** A nibbling forceps with a double joint for increased force. **Dressing forceps.** A hinged forceps with a scissors action for holding surgical materials during wound dressings. **Dural forceps.** Forceps for grasping the dura mater at craniotomy. **Entropion forceps.** A forceps with one flat blade and one ringed blade, for management of the eyelid in entropion. **Failed forceps.** An unsuccessful attempt at delivery by forceps. **False-membrane forceps.** A forceps for removing the false membrane in diphtheria. **Fixation forceps.** A range of forceps for use in steadying the various parts of the eye in ophthalmic operations. **Frontal-sinus forceps.** A forceps for the removal of the bony wall from the frontal sinus. **Gall-stone forceps.** Forceps for removing stones from the gall bladder or bile ducts. **Gland forceps.** A forceps for holding diseased gland masses during their excision. **Gouge forceps.** A forceps with one or both blades curved for nibbling the surface of bone. **Haemostatic forceps.** Artery forceps (see above). **Hare-lip forceps.** A delicate flat-bladed forceps for grasping the edges of a cleft lip during its repair. **High forceps.** Forceps applied when the fetal head is at the pelvic inlet. **Inlet forceps.** High forceps (see preceding). **Intubation forceps.** Forceps used to guide a tracheal tube into the larynx under direct vision, first described by Sir Ivan Magill in 1920. **Kidney-holding forceps.** A forceps for supporting the kidney during operations upon it. **Kidney-pedicle forceps.** A forceps clamp applied to the renal vessels at nephrectomy. **Laminectomy forceps.** A forceps for dividing the laminae of the vertebral arch. **Laryngeal forceps.** A range of forceps for effecting various manoeuvres on the larynx. **Lithotomy forceps.** Forceps for removing stone from the bladder. **Low forceps.** Obstetric forceps applied when the head lies at the pelvic outlet. **Forceps major.** *See* FORCEPS MAJOR. **Median forceps, Mid forceps, Mid-plane forceps.** Forceps applied when the biparietal plane of the fetal head lies in the bispinous line. **Forceps minor.** *See* FORCEPS MINOR. **Mosquito forceps.** Light clip artery forceps with fine points. **Mouse-tooth forceps.** Light forceps with fine terminal teeth for holding delicate tissue. **Nasal forceps.** A range of forceps for intranasal manipulations, which include nasal dressing forceps, nasal-polypi forceps, nasal punch forceps, and nasal-septum forceps. **Necrosis forceps.** A forceps for removing sequestra from infected bone. **Obstetric forceps.** Forceps for applying traction to the fetal head during delivery. **Oesophageal forceps.** Forceps, usually of crocodile type, for the endoscopic removal of foreign bodies and portions of tumour tissue from the oesophagus. **Ovum forceps.** Forceps for removing uterine contents. **Pedicle forceps.** Forceps for controlling bleeding from the vascular pedicle of an organ during its removal. **Peritoneum forceps.** Forceps with delicate teeth for grasping peritoneum. **Placenta forceps.** Forceps for the removal of the placenta. **Forceps posterior.** Forceps minor. **Punch forceps.** A hinged instrument like a pincers, the blades of which when closed cut out a small disc of tissue. **Rat-tooth forceps.** Forceps with inturned pointed blades for retracting tissues. **Roller forceps.** Forceps whose blades carry a terminal roller for crushing the granulation of trachoma. **Rongeur forceps.** Bone-nibbling forceps (see above). **Sequestrum forceps.** Forceps for removing fragments of dead bone. **Sinus forceps.** Forceps with narrow tapering blades for forcing an entrance into an abscess cavity or for stretching an opening into an abscess by Hilton's operation. **Sphenoidal punch forceps.** Nibbling forceps for removing the floor of the sphenoidal sinus in operations on that sinus or on the pituitary gland. **Spring forceps.** A pincers-like instrument, the blades of which are separated by a light spring. **Strabismus forceps.** Special forceps designed for holding the muscle in squint operations, usually with a catch to keep the blades in apposition. **Tenaculum forceps.** A forceps with toothed blades, for exerting traction. **Tissue forceps.** A forceps with tiny teeth for grasping and manipulating delicate tissue. **Tongue forceps.** A forceps for drawing the tongue forward during anaesthesia. **Towl forceps.** A forceps for clipping towels to skin at the operation-wound edge. **Tracheal forceps.** Long curved forceps for the removal of foreign bodies from the trachea. **Trachoma forceps.** Roller forceps (see above). **Trephine forceps.** A forceps used for the removal of the bone disc circumscribed by the trephine. **Uterine forceps.** A long forceps devised for packing the uterus with gauze. **Volsella forceps, Vulsella forceps, Vulsellum forceps.** A forceps with hinged blades for exerting traction on structures. [L pair of tongs.]

See also: ALLIS, ASCH, CAIRNS, CHAMBERLEN, CHEATLE, CORNET, CRILE, DESJARDIN, DUNHILL, DUVAL (P.), GREEN-ARMYTAGE, HAIG FERGUSON, HALSTED, HOFFMAN (W. J.), JACKSON (C.), KJELLAND, KOCHER, LABORDE, LYON (J. A.), MURRAY (R. M.), PATERSON (D. R.), PÉAN, PRINCE, SIMPSON (J. Y.), TARNIER, TERSON, TROTTER, WALSHAM, WELLS (T. S.), WILLETT, WRIGLEY.

forceps major [NA] (for·seps ma·jor). The laterally-running fibres of the splenium of the corpus callosum which proceed posteriorly into the occipital lobe; they form a bulge in the medial wall of the posterior cornu, the *bulb.*

forceps minor [NA] (for·seps mi·nor). The laterally-running fibres of the genu of the corpus callosum which proceed forward into the frontal lobe.

Forchheimer, Frederick (b. 1853). Cincinnati physician.

Forchheimer's sign. The presence of small reddish papules on the soft palate in the early stages of rubella.

forcipal (for·sip·al). Relating to or having the character of forceps.

forcipate, forcipated (for·sip·ate, for·sip·a·ted). Shaped like forceps.

Forcipomyia (for·sip·o·mi'·e·ah). A genus of small midges of the family Ceratopogonidae. *Forcipomyia townsendi* and *F. utae* are suspected vectors of mucocutaneous leishmaniasis (uta) in Peru. [L *forceps* pair of tongs, Gk *myia* fly.]

forcipressure (fors·e·presh·er). 1. In surgery, the arrest of haemorrhage by compressing the end of a divided artery in a spring forceps for a time. 2. Compression applied with a spring forceps.

Fordyce, John Addison (b. 1858). New York dermatologist.

Fordyce's disease. Enlarged sebaceous glands in the mucosa of the lips, cheeks, gums and genitals.

Fordyce-Fox disease, Fox-Fordyce disease. An apocrine gland disorder comparable to prickly heat. Itchy follicular papules occur in the axillae, at the areolae mammae, umbilicus, pubis or labia majora.

forearm [antebrachium (NA)] (for·arm). The lower arm; the part between the elbow and the wrist. It has an anterior surface [facies anterior (NA)] and a posterior surface [facies posterior (NA)] and 2 borders, medial [margo medialis (ulnaris) NA] and lateral [margo lateralis (radialis)]. [AS.]

forearm, nerves of the. Lateral cutaneous nerve of the forearm [nervus cutaneus antebrachii lateralis (NA)]. A continuation of the musculocutaneous nerve of the upper limb to supply the skin on the lateral side of the forearm and the wrist joint. **Medial cutaneous nerve of the forearm [nervus cutaneus antebrachii medialis (NA)].** A branch of the medial cord of the brachial plexus in the axilla, carrying fibres of the 8th cervical and 1st thoracic roots to supply the skin [ramus anterior and ramus ulnaris (NA)] on the medial side of the forearm. **Posterior cutaneous nerve of the forearm [nervus cutaneus antebrachii posterior (NA)].** A branch of the radial nerve, supplying a large area of skin on the back of the arm and most of the dorsal skin of the forearm.

forearm, vein of the. Median vein of the forearm [vena mediana antebrachii (NA)]. the vein draining the plexus on the palm of the hand and passing along the front of the forearm into the basilic vein at the elbow or the median cubital vein. It may divide at the cubital fossa into a median basilic and median cephalic vein, joining the main basilic and cephalic veins respectively.

forebrain [prosencephalon (NA)] (for·brane). The part of the brain consisting of the diencephalon and the telencephalon. Cf. BRAIN. [AS *fore, bragen.*]

foreconscious (for·kon·shus). Those memories which are capable of voluntary recall. [before, conscious.]

forefinger (for·finger·ger). The index finger. [AS.]

forefoot (for·fut). The part of the foot in front of the tarsometatarsal joint. [AS *fore, fot.*]

foregilding (for·gild·ing). In histology, the treating of fresh nerve tissue with gold salts. [AS *fore, gyldan.*]

foregut (for·gut). In the early embryo, that portion of the primitive alimentary canal from which arise the pharynx, the oesophagus, the stomach and the duodenum. [AS *fore, guttas.*]

forehead [frons (NA)] (for·ed). That part of the face between the eyes and the hair-line; the brow. **Olympian forehead.** The high brow of the congenital syphilitic child. [AS *forheafod.*]

foreign (for·in). 1. Not organically connected. 2. Not naturally related. 3. Placed abnormally. 4. Irrelevant. 5. Proceeding from or originating in some other person or material. **Foreign body.** A substance present in any part of the body in which normally it is not found, and usually of external origin. [O Fr. *forain.*]

forekidney (for·kid·ne). The pronephros; in embryology, the rudimentary organ, consisting of 6 or 7 horizontal tubules, which develops earlier than the mesonephros and about the end of the fourth week disappears entirely in the mesonephric duct. [AS *fore,* ME *kydney.*]

Forel, Auguste Henri (b. 1848). Zürich psychiatrist.

bundle of Forel. Nerve fibres in the upper end of the tegmentum of the mid-brain and in the region below the thalamus; their connections are uncertain, but are probably with many neighbouring structures such as the red nucleus, thalamus, hypothalamus, subthalamic nucleus and lentiform nucleus.

Forel's decussation. The ventral tegmental decussation; the crossing of the rubrospinal tracts in the tegmentum of the mid-brain.

Forel's field. The zona incerta of the hypothalamus.

foremilk (**for**·milk). Colostrum. [AS *fore, meoluc.*]

forensic (for·**en**·sik). Referring or belonging to courts of law. [L *forum* a public place.]

forepleasure (**for**·plezh·ewr). Sexual pleasure preceding that of the orgasm. [AS *fore,* ME *plesir.*]

foreskin (**for**·skin). The prepuce. [AS *fore,* ME *skinn.*]

forewaters (**for**·waw·terz). The thin mucus discharged in hydrorrhoea gravidarum. [AS *fore, waeter.*]

Forficula (for·**fik**·ew·lah). A genus of insects of the order Dermaptera. **Forficula auricularia.** The common earwig, a species occasionally recorded from the external auditory meatus. [L *forfex* scissors.]

fork (fork). The part of the human body at which the thighs branch from the trunk and the space at the point of bifurcation. [L *furca.*]

Forlanini, Carlo (b. 1847). Pavia physician.

Forlanini's treatment. The use of artificial pneumothorax in the treatment of pulmonary tuberculosis, first used by Forlanini in 1880.

form (form). 1. The distinctive external shape or structure of the body, or of a part of the body. 2. The particular shape or appearance assumed by a tissue or organism under specified conditions. **Band form.** Term applied to a granular neutrophil polymorphonuclear leucocyte, usually a metamyelocyte, having a sausage-shaped, band-like or horseshoe-shaped nucleus; this type is usually increased in numbers with certain infections and with abnormal stimulation of blood formation in the marrow. **Involution form.** The abnormal development which a micro-organism may undergo when its cultural environment is unfavourable. **Juvenile form.** A metamyelocyte. **L forms.** Abnormal morphological forms of bacteria derived by variation, usually by laboratory procedures. They lack a rigid cell wall and consequently vary in size and shape; they are capable of growth in culture media but probably not in the host tissues; they resemble the mycoplasmata or pleuropneumonia-like organisms. **Racemic form.** Racemic compound. **Replicative form.** Following infection of bacteria by single-stranded DNA or RNA viral nucleic acid, a complementary strand is synthesized to yield double-stranded molecules capable of replication. [L *forma* form.]

form-board (**form**·bord). In testing for mental capacity, a device consisting of a wooden board in which hollows of various shapes have been cut, the corresponding blocks having to be fitted into the hollows by the person who is being tested. [L *forma* form, AS *bord.*]

formal (**for**·mal). Methylal, $CH_2(OCH_3)_2$. A compound homologous with acetal, prepared from formaldehyde and methyl alcohol. A stable liquid used as an extractive for perfumes, and in medicine as an anaesthetic and hypnotic.

formaldehyde (for·**mal**·de·hide). Formic aldehyde, methanal, HCH=O. The simplest of the aldehydes; a colourless irritating gas prepared by passing the vapour of methyl alcohol and air over a heated copper catalyst, the aqueous solution (BP 1958) thus formed (40 per cent) being known as *formalin.* It possesses the property of rendering proteins insoluble, and thus preserves them from bacterial decomposition. It is itself too toxic and corrosive for use as an antiseptic or disinfectant, and is therefore employed in the form of condensation products, mostly with carbohydrates which slowly hydrolyse in the body. It is incorporated in lozenges for throat infections, and in the polymerized solid form, metaformaldehyde, is a useful solid fuel. **Formaldehyde gelatin.** A form of enteric coating obtained by dipping gelatin capsules into formalin solution and drying, which renders the capsules impervious to the acid medium of the stomach but soluble in the alkaline medium of the small intestine. **Formaldehyde sodium bisulphite,** $HCHOSO_3Na$. A compound not used in medicine as such, but forming neutral water-soluble compounds with many otherwise insoluble drugs, e.g. with arsphenamine, to form sulpharsphenamine. **Formaldehyde sulphoxylate,** $HCHOSO_2Na$. A compound used similarly to the preceding, e.g. with arsphenamine, to form neoarsphenamine.

formalin (**for**·mal·in). A solution of formaldehyde in water (40 per cent w/v), with the addition of a little alcohol to prevent polymerization to the insoluble paraformaldehyde. It is used as a disinfectant, and also for the preservation and hardening of organic tissues. Admixture with potassium permanganate produces a rapid evolution of formaldehyde gas, a fact utilized in the fumigation of rooms. **Formalin gelatin.** Gelatin rendered insoluble by treatment with formalin and used for capsules, the contents of which are intended for liberation in the alkaline medium of the small intestine after the capsule has passed intact through the acid stomach.

formalize (**for**·mal·ize). To subject to treatment with formaldehyde.

formamide (**for**·mam·ide). 1. Methane amide, $HCONH_2$. The amide of formic acid, closely related to urea. A colourless liquid soluble in water; it decomposes on heating into ammonia and carbon monoxide. 2. General name for a compound containing the radical HCONH–.

2-formamido-5-nitrothiazole (for·**mam**·id·o·ni·tro·**thi**'·az·ole). A synthetic bacteriostatic used in pessaries for the treatment of vaginitis caused by *Trichomonas vaginalis.*

formant (**for**·mant). In phonetics, the tone of constant pitch of a vowel sound. [L *formare* to form.]

formate (**for**·mate). A salt of formic acid.

formatio (for·**ma**·she·o). Formation. **Formatio reticularis [NA].** Scattered islets of grey matter, intersected by numerous nerve fibres (white) in the ventrolateral portion of the medulla and the dorsal part of the pons. [L.]

formation [formatio (NA)] (for·**ma**·shun). An arrangement in a particular shape. **Coffin formation.** The grouping around dead nerve cells of phagocytic cells or microcytes. **Compromise formation.** A mental mechanism in which a repressed wish finds partial expression (psycho-analysis). **Hippocampal formation.** Part of the rhinencephalon, comprising the indusium griseum, longitudinal striae, dentate gyrus and hippocampus. **Palisade formation.** The arrangement of fusiform cells in a compact mass all pointing in one direction or radially. **Reaction formation.** A mental mechanism in which the ego reinforces the attitude which is the opposite of the instinctual trend that is being repressed. **Reticular formation of the pons [formatio reticularis].** Islets of cells and interspersed nerve fibres in the dorsal part of the pons. **Reticular formation of the spinal cord [formatio reticularis].** A network of cells and fibres extending laterally opposite the base of the posterior columns, especially in the cervical region. **Reticular formation of the tegmentum [formatio reticularis].** Nerve cells intermingled with bundles of nerve fibres occurring widely in the brain stem. **Rouleaux formation.** The clumping together of erythrocytes, like piles or columns of discs or coins, that may be seen in wet films of blood or in hanging-drop preparations of blood from patients in certain diseases of the blood, and particularly in myelomatosis. Such rouleaux formation may greatly increase the rate of sedimentation. **Rut formation.** The formation of a settled pattern of activity. [L *formatio.*]

See also: DEITERS.

formative (**for**·mat·iv). 1. Having relation to any developmental process. 2. Having to do with the origin of an organism or a part of an organism or with the growth and development of its structures. 3. Giving form. 4. Able to grow and develop. [L *formare* to form.]

forme fruste (form **froost**). A disease that is arrested before it has run a typical course and therefore is incomplete; an abortive or atypical type of disease. [Fr. defaced form.]

Formebolone (for·**meb**·o·lone). BP Commission approved name for 2 - formyl - 11α,17β - dihydroxy - 17α - methylandrosta - 1,4 - dien - 3 - one; an anabolic steroid.

formic (for·mik). 1. Pertaining to ants. 2. Related to formic acid. [L *formica* ant.]

formicant (for·mik·ant). Applied to a pulse that is barely perceptible, small in volume and unequal in rhythm; the thready pulse. [L *formicare* to creep like an ant.]

formication (for·mik·a·shun). A form of paraesthesia characterized by an irritating sensation as of ants or other insects creeping over the skin. [see prec.]

formiciasis (form·ik·i·as·is). The condition of swelling, inflammation and itching resulting from ant bites. The bites of the large ants of the tropics may cause fits of shivering and syncope, and even paralysis. [L *formica* ant.]

formicin (for·mis·in). Methylal acetamide, CH_3CONH_2HCHO. An additive compound formed by formaldehyde and acetamide; a syrupy liquid, miscible with water, alcohol or glycerin, and employed as a disinfectant and antiseptic.

formilase (for·mil·aze). A ferment responsible for the production of formic acid from acetic acid. [formic acid.]

Forminitrazole (for·min·i·traz·ole). BP Commission approved name for 2-formamido-5-nitrothiazole; it is used as a local application in the treatment of trichomonal vaginitis.

formocresol (for·mo·kre·sol). A mixture of equal parts of tricresol and formalin which is inserted in the root canals of teeth to eliminate the infection which occurs subsequent to necrosis of the pulp.

formolage (for·mol·**ahzh**). A method of treating hydatid cyst; it mainly comprises the flushing out of the cyst with a 2 per cent solution of formalin.

formolize (for·mol·ize). To add formalin to anything.

formonitrile (for·mo·ni·trile). Hydrocyanic acid. *See* ACID.

formose (for·moze). 1. The name given to the mixture of hexoses synthesized by the polymerization of formaldehyde with lime water. 2. α-Acrose, $C_6H_{12}O_6$, or DL-fructose, formed during the above synthesis.

formosul (for·mo·sul). Formaldehyde sulphoxylate, $OHCH_2SO_2Na$. An addition product formed by formaldehyde with sodium hyposulphite; used as a reducing agent in the dyeing industry.

formosulphabenzamide, formosulphacetamide, formosulphathiazole (for·mo·sul·fah·**ben**′·zam·ide, **for**·mo·sul·fas·**et**′·am·ide, **for**·mo·sul·fah·**thi**′·az·ole). Substances which have been used in the treatment of cholera, without, however, demonstrable benefit being conferred.

formoxyl (form·ox·il). Formyl.

formula (for·mew·lah). 1. A means of describing the composition of a substance. 2. A recipe. 3. A method. **Chemical formula.** The representation of the molecule of a chemical compound by means of chemical symbols and indices, e.g. H_2SO_4. **Constitutional formula.** Structural formula (see below). **Dental formula.** A formula indicating the number of teeth of each type in the jaws. In the human it is:

```
 2 1 2
I-C-M-
 2 1 2
```

in the deciduous dentition, and

```
 2 1  2 3
I-C-PM-M-
 2 1  2 3
```

in the permanent dentition. **Electronic formula.** A formula for an element or compound in which the valency electrons of each element are represented symbolically, and the type of bond between elements is indicated. **Empirical formula.** A chemical formula which gives the numerical proportions of the different atoms in a molecule without giving necessarily the actual number, nor any indication of structural linkages, e.g. CH_2O, for acetic acid. **Extemporaneous formula.** A prescription for a medicament to be freshly prepared, and not dispensed from a stock preparation. **Graphic formula.** Structural formula (see below). **Molecular formula.** A chemical formula which gives the actual number of the different atoms in a molecule but no indication as to linkage, e.g. $C_2H_4O_2$, for acetic acid. **Official formula.** A formula appearing in the *British Pharmacopoeia.* **Psychobiological formula.** The summing-up of the mental and biological state as determined by Meyer's system. **Rational formula.** A condensed structural formula in which the linkages of radicals are depicted, e.g. CH_3COOH, for acetic acid. **Stereochemical formula.** A formula which sets out to display the spatial arrangement of atoms in the molecule of an optically-active compound. **Stopping formula.** Any experimental or theoretical relation giving the rate of loss of energy of a charged particle passing through matter. **Structural formula.** A chemical formula in which each atom is depicted linked to neighbouring atoms by valency bonds, e.g. O=C=O, for carbon dioxide. **Systematic formula.** Structural formula (see above). **Unitary formula.** Empirical formula (see above). **Vertebral formula.** The figures denoting the number of vertebrae in the respective segments of the spinal column of a vertebra. **Viscosity formula.** 1. A formula for determining η, the coefficient of viscosity of a liquid:

$$\eta = \frac{\pi p r^4 t}{8lv},$$

where p is the pressure of the liquid, r the radius of the tube through which the liquid is passing, l the length of the tube, and v the volume of liquid delivered in time, t (Poiseuille). 2. A formula for determining the coefficient of viscosity of a colloidal sol: $\eta = \eta_0\ (1 + k\phi)$, where η_0 is the viscosity of the pure liquid forming the continuous phase, ϕ the volume of colloid per unit volume, and k a constant (Einstein). [dim. of L *forma* pattern.]

See also: ARNETH, ARRHENIUS, BAZETT, BECKMANN, BERNHARDT, BETHE (H. A.), BINET, BLACK (D. A. K.), COOKE, DEMOIVRE, EINSTEIN, EINTHOVEN, HATSCHEK, KATZ, KEKWICK, KLEIN-NISHINA, MALL, MARRIOTT (H. L.), MEEH, MOOTS, PEARSON (K.), PIGNET, POISEUILLE, POISSON (S. D.), PONDER, ROLLIER, SCHILLING.

formulary (for·mew·lar·e). A published list of formulae in general medical use. **National Formulary,** N.F. 1. A book, compiled by representatives of the medical and pharmaceutical professions, of pharmaceutical preparations and formulae suggested for use in the British National Health Service; to obviate confusion this book was renamed *British National Formulary* in the 1957 edition. 2. A book of official standards compiled by a committee of the American Pharmaceutical Association. It refers to pharmaceuticals and preparations that have not been considered of sufficient importance to be included in the current edition of the *United States Pharmacopoeia.* [see prec.]

formyl (for·mil). The monovalent group, HCO–, derived from formic acid and analogous with the acetyl group of acetic acid. **Formyl iodide.** Iodoform. **Formyl trichloride.** Chloroform. **Formyl tri-iodide.** Iodoform.

fornical (for·nik·al). Relating or belonging to a fornix, e.g. the fornix of the rhinencephalon.

fornicate (for·nik·ate). 1. Overarched; shaped like the arch of a vault. 2. To practise fornication. [L *fornix* arch, and see foll.]

fornication (for·nik·a·shun). The practice of having illicit sexual intercourse. [L *fornix* brothel (in an underground vault).]

fornicolumn (for·ne·kol·um). The anterior column of the fornix of the rhinencephalon.

fornicommissure (for·ne·**kom**·is·ewr). 1. The hippocampal commissure. 2. The anterior or posterior commissure of the pudendum feminum. [L *fornix* arch, commissure.]

fornix [NA] (for·nix) (pl. *fornices*). An arch or vault; frequently used without qualification for the fornix cerebri. **Fornix cerebri [fornix (NA)].** The continuation of the fimbria which passes down to the mamillary body of the hypothalamus; it consists of efferent projection fibres from the hippocampus. **Fornix cerebri, body of the [corpus fornicis (NA)].** The part of the fornix which lies in contact with the under-surface of the corpus callosum. **Fornix commissure.** Commissural fibres of the hippocampus which pass from the fimbria into the fornix and cross beneath the corpus callosum. **Fornix of the conjunctiva.** The line of reflection of the conjunctiva from the deep surface of the eyelid on to the bulb of the eye. It occurs above [fornix conjunctivae superior (NA)] and below [fornix conjunctivae inferior (NA)]. **Fornix of the lacrimal sac [fornix sacci lacrimalis (NA)].** The part of the lacrimal sac above the entrance of the lacrimal canaliculi. **Fornix longus.** Efferent projection fibres from the hippocampus which pass through or above the corpus callosum before joining the columns of the fornix on their way to the hypothalamus; some may pass in front of the anterior commissure, where they form the precommissural fornix. **Pharyngeal fornix [fornix pharyngis (NA)]** The vault-like upper end of the nasopharynx. **Precommissural fornix.** *See* FORNIX LONGUS (above). **Fornix uteri, Fornix of the vagina [fornix vaginae (NA)].** The spaces between the cervix uteri and the anterior, posterior and lateral vaginal walls, known respectively as the *anterior, posterior* and *lateral fornices.* [L arch.]

Foroblique (for·o·bleek). A lens system used in the telescope of the cysto-urethroscope. It resembles the direct-vision telescope, but has a deviating prism in front of the objective. The deflexion of the optical axis by means of the prism enables the operator to keep instruments passed through the sheath of a cysto-urethroscope under vision during endovascular operations. The word is a registered trade-name.

Forsaria (for·sa·re·ah). A genus of freshwater snails, intermediate hosts of *Fasciola hepatica.*

Forssell, Gösta (b. 1876). Stockholm radiologist.

Forssell's sinus. A space between mucosal folds in the pyloric antrum, seen radiographically.

Forssman, John (b. 1868). Lund pathologist.

Forssman antibody. An antibody formed against the heterophil or Forssman antigen.

Forssman's antigen, or lipoid. Heterophil antigen; an antigen present in organs from the guinea-pig and certain other animals, which on injection into the rabbit lead to the production of haemolysin for sheep red corpuscles. The antigen is widely distributed among different animal species and bacteria.

Forssman's carotid syndrome. Neurological abnormalities produced when serum containing Forssman's antibody is injected into the carotid artery of the guinea-pig.

fortran. A computer language.

Fosazepam (fos·a·ze·pam). BP Commission approved name for 7 - chloro - 1 [illegible] - nethylphosphinylmethyl - 1,3 - dihydro - 5 - phenyl - $2H$ - 1,4 - benzodiazepin - 2 - one; a hypnotic.

Fosfestrol (fos·fes·trol). BP Commission approved name for *trans-αα'*-diethylstilbene-4,4'-diol bis(dihydrogen phosphate); it is used in the treatment of carcinoma of the prostate.

Foshay, Lee (b. 1896). Cincinnati bacteriologist.

Foshay serum. A serum for use in tularaemia.

Foshay's test. An allergic skin test in which a dilute suspension of *Brucella tularensis* is injected intradermally as an aid to the diagnosis of tularaemia. A positive reaction is a local erythema.

fossa [NA] (fos·ah) (pl. *fossae*). A pit or depression below the general surface level of a part; a recess. **Acetabular fossa [fossa acetabuli (NA)].** A rough non-articular depression in the floor of the acetabulum. **Amygdaloid fossa.** Tonsillar fossa (see below). **Antecubital fossa.** The cubital fossa (see below); the term is now obsolescent. **Fossa of the antihelix [fossa anthelicis (NA)].** The triangular fossa (see below). **Articular fossa [fossa mandibularis (NA)].** A transversely-disposed hollow lying between the eminentia articularis and the external auditory meatus formed anteriorly from the squamous part of the temporal bone and posteriorly from the tympanic plate. **Fossa articularis.** A cartilage-lined depression on a bone into which fits the extremity of another bone to form a joint. **Axillary fossa [fossa axillaris (NA)].** The axilla. **Caecal fossa.** A recess in the peritoneum produced by the passage of the caecal fold from the lateral aspect of the caecum to the surface of the iliacus muscle. **Canine fossa [fossa canina (NA)].** A shallow depression on the anterior surface of the body of the maxilla, lateral to the ridge formed by the root of the canine tooth. **Fossa capitelli.** The depression in the wall of the tympanic cavity which lodges the head of the malleus. **Cerebellar fossa.** The concavity in the lateral part of the posterior cranial fossa, between the foramen magnum and the groove for the transverse sinus which lodges on each side the cerebellar hemisphere. **Cerebral fossa, lateral [fossa lateralis cerebri (NA)].** The stem of the lateral sulcus; it runs from the anterior perforated substance, outwards and backwards, and separates the orbital surface of the frontal lobe from the temporal lobe. **Condylar fossa [fossa condylaris (NA)].** The depression behind the occipital condyle. **Coronoid fossa [fossa coronoidea (NA)].** A depression on the anterior aspect of the lower end of the humerus which receives the coronoid process of the ulna during full flexion of the forearm. **Cranial fossa.** Any of the depressions on the internal aspect of the base of the skull; there are 3—anterior, middle and posterior. **Cranial fossa, anterior [fossa cranii anterior (NA)].** The most anterior of the 3 subdivisions of the floor of the cranial cavity, containing the lower parts of the frontal lobes of the cerebrum. **Cranial fossa, middle [fossa cranii media (NA)].** The intermediate one of the 3 depressions on the floor of the cranial cavity, containing the hypophyseal fossa in the midline, and in each lateral part the temporal lobes of the cerebrum. **Cranial fossa, posterior [fossa cranii posterior (NA)].** The most posterior of the 3 subdivisions of the floor of the cranial cavity, which lodges the hind-brain. **Crural fossa.** A dimple in the parietal peritoneum corresponding to the position of the femoral ring; femoral fossa. **Cubital fossa [fossa cubitalis (NA)].** The depression in the front of the elbow, bounded above by a line joining the epicondyles, medially by the pronator teres muscle and laterally by the brachioradialis muscle. It contains the termination of the brachial artery, the median nerve and the tendon of insertion of the biceps brachii muscle. **Digastric fossa [fossa digastrica (NA)].** A depression behind the lower border of the mandible at the side of the symphysis menti for the attachment of the anterior belly of the digastric muscle. **Digital fossa.** 1. The pit on the medial aspect of the lateral malleolus behind the articular facet. 2. The trochanteric fossa of the femur (see below). 3. The sinus of the epididymis. **Fossa ductus venosi [NA].** A deep groove on the postero-inferior surface of the liver to the left of the caudate lobe, occupied in the fetus by the ductus venosus and in the adult by its fibrous remnant. **Duodenal fossa, inferior.** A peritoneal recess lying posterior to a fold of peritoneum which passes from the side of the ascending portion of the duodenum to the parietal peritoneum. **Duodenal fossa, superior.** The peritoneal recess lying behind the superior duodenal fold. **Duodenojejunal fossa.** A recess lying to the left of the duodenojejunal flexure between the superior and inferior duodenal folds. **Epigastric fossa [fossa epigastrica (NA)].** The surface depression known as the pit of the stomach. **Femoral fossa.** Crural fossa (see above). **Gall-bladder fossa [fossa vesicae felleae (NA)].** The depression on the under-surface of the right lobe of the liver which lodges the gall bladder. **Glenoid fossa.** The depression on the scapula which articulates with the head of the humerus. **Fossa helicis.** The depression between the helix and the antihelix. **Fossa hemielliptica.** The depression in the wall of the vestibule of the osseous labyrinth which lodges the utricle; the elliptical recess. **Fossa hemispherica.** The depression in the wall of the vestibule which lodges the saccule; spherical recess. **Hyaloid fossa [fossa hyaloidea (NA)].** The concavity on the anterior surface of the vitreous body which receives the lens; lenticular fossa. **Hypophyseal fossa [fossa hypophysialis (NA)].** A depression on the body of the sphenoid for the pituitary gland. **Ileocolic fossa.** A peritoneal recess lying behind the ileocolic fold; Luschka's fossa. **Iliac fossa [fossa iliaca (NA)].** The smoother, concave, upper and anterior part of the sacropelvic surface of the iliac bone. It forms the lateral wall of the false pelvis. **Iliacosubfascial fossa.** A recess of the peritoneum between the psoas muscle and the iliac crest; Biesiadecki's fossa. **Incisive fossa [fossa incisiva (NA)].** A depression on the anterior surface of the body of the maxilla medial to the root of the canine tooth; also a similar depression on the mandible below the incisor teeth. **Fossa for the incus [fossa incudis (NA)].** A depression in the lower part of the posterior wall of the epitympanic recess which receives the tip of the short crus of the incus. **Infraclavicular fossa.** The triangular depression below the clavicle corresponding to the interval between the clavicular fibres of the pectoralis major and deltoid muscles; Mohrenheim's fossa. **Infraduodenal fossa.** A peritoneal recess lying below the horizontal portion of the duodenum. **Infraspinous fossa [fossa infraspinata (NA)].** The area on the dorsal surface of the scapula, below the spine, for the attachment of the infraspinatus muscle. **Infratemporal fossa [fossa infratemporalis (NA)].** The depression on the side of the skull bounded anteriorly by the posterior surface of the body of the maxilla, medially by the lateral pterygoid plate, posteriorly by the articular tubercle, and roofed over by the infratemporal surface of the greater wing of the sphenoid bone. **Inguinal fossa, external.** A peritoneal recess on the back of the anterior abdominal wall lateral to the inferior epigastric artery. **Inguinal fossa, internal.** A peritoneal recess on the back of the anterior abdominal wall situated between the obliterated umbilical artery and the urachus. **Inguinal fossa, lateral [fossa inguinalis lateralis (NA)].** The shallow peritoneal depression on the anterior abdominal wall between the medial and lateral inguinal ligaments. **Inguinal fossa, middle [fossa inguinalis medialis (NA)].** A peritoneal recess on the back of the anterior abdominal wall between the inferior epigastric and obliterated umbilical arteries. **Intercondylar fossa.** Intercondylar notch. *See* NOTCH. **Interpeduncular fossa [fossa interpeduncularis (NA)].** A depression on the ventral surface of the mid-brain, between the cerebral peduncles, which is the site of emergence of the 3rd cranial nerve. **Intrabulbar fossa.** The dilatation of the spongy part of the urethra within the bulb of the penis. **Ischiorectal fossa [fossa ischiorectalis (NA)].** A space on either side of the lower end of the rectum and anal canal bounded laterally by the obturator internus muscle and the tuberosity of the ischium. **Jugular fossa [fossa jugularis (NA)].** A fossa on the temporal bone lodging the bulb of the internal jugular vein. **Fossa for the lacrimal gland [fossa glandulae lacrimalis (NA)].** A space at the lateral angle of the roof of the orbit which lodges the lacrimal gland. **Fossa of the lacrimal sac [fossa sacci lacrimalis (NA)].** A fossa on the lacrimal bone lodging the lacrimal sac. **Fossa lateralis.** The space enclosed by the lips of the lateral cerebral fissure. **Lenticular fossa.** Hyaloid fossa (see above). **Malleolar fossa [fossa malleoli lateralis (NA)].** A depression along the posterior border of the lower articular facet of the fibula, affording attachment to ligaments of the ankle joint. **Mandibular fossa.** Articular fossa (see above). **Nasal fossa.** The atrium of the middle meatus of the nose. **Navicular fossa.** 1. The fossa terminalis (see below). 2. The vestibular fossa (see below). **Navicular fossa of the ear.** Fossa helicis (see above). **Olecranon fossa [fossa olecrani (NA)].** A deep depression on the posterior surface of the lower end of the humerus which receives the olecranon process of the ulna during extension of the elbow joint. **Fossa ovalis [NA].** 1. A depression on the septal wall of the right atrium representing the position of the foramen ovale of the fetus. 2. The saphenous opening. **Ovarian fossa.** A depression in the parietal peritoneum of the pelvis, bounded in front by the obliterated umbilical artery and behind by the ureter and uterine vessels, and in which the ovary lies; Claudius' fossa. **Paraduodenal fossa.** Paraduodenal recess. *See* RECESS. **Pararectal fossa.** A peritoneal recess lying on either side of the empty rectum. **Paravesical fossa.** A peritoneal recess lying on either side of the urinary bladder; it becomes shallower as the bladder fills. **Petrosal fossa [fossula petrosa (NA)].** A triangular depression in front of the medial part of the jugular foramen which lodges the inferior ganglion of the glossopharyngeal nerve. **Pharyngeal fossa.** An occasional pit on the under-surface of the basi-occiput in front of the pharyngeal tubercle, which marks the site of the pharyngeal bursa. **Pharyngeal fossa, lateral.** A recess in the lateral wall of the nasopharynx posterior to the opening of the pharyngotympanic tube; fossa of Rosenmueller; lateral recess. **Piriform fossa [recessus piriformis (NA)].** A depression on either side of the opening into the larynx, bounded by the aryepiglottic folds and the thyrohyoid membrane and thyroid cartilage. **Pituitary fossa.** Hypophyseal fossa (see above). **Popliteal fossa [fossa poplitea (NA)].** The diamond-shaped hollow at the back of the knee joint. It is bounded on either side below by the heads of the gastrocnemius muscle and above by the biceps femoris muscle laterally and the semimembranosus muscle medially. **Postauditory fossa.** A small depression above and behind the external auditory meatus. **Pterygoid fossa [fossa pterygoideal (NA)].** The space contained by the medial and lateral pterygoid plates of the sphenoid bone. **Pterygopalatine fossa [fossa pterygopalatina (NA)].** The space, bounded in front by the posterior surface of the maxilla, behind by the root of the pterygoid process of the sphenoid bone, and medially by the perpendicular plate of the palatine bone, in which lies the sphenopalatine ganglion. **Radial fossa [fossa radialis (NA)].** A shallow depression on the front of the lower end of the humerus, which comes into relation with the head of the radius during full flexion of the forearm. **Recto-uterine fossa.** Recto-uterine pouch. *See* POUCH. **Retrocaecal fossa.** Retrocaecal recess. *See* RECESS. **Retroduodenal fossa.** Retroduodenal recess. *See* RECESS. **Retro-ureteric fossa.** A shallow depression behind the trigone of the bladder. **Rhomboid fossa.** The floor of the 4th ventricle. **Fossa sagittalis sinistra.** A continuous fissure on the under-surface of the liver made up of the fissure for the ligamentum teres anteriorly and the fossa for the ductus venosus posteriorly. **Scaphoid fossa.** 1. [Fossa scaphoidea (NA)], a shallow depression on the posterior border of the medial pterygoid plate giving origin to the tensor palati muscle. 2. [Scapha (NA)], the depression between the helix and the antihelix. **Subarcuate fossa [fossa subarcuata (NA)].** A small depression on the posteromedial surface of the petrous part of the temporal bone between the arcuate eminence and the internal auditory meatus. **Subauricular fossa.** A surface depression below the auricle. **Subinguinal fossa.** A surface depression below the inguinal ligament. **Sublingual fossa [fovea sublingualis (NA)].** A depression on the medial surface of the mandible, above the mylohyoid line, which lodges the sublingual gland. **Submandibular fossa [fovea submandibularis (NA)].** A depression on the medial surface of the mandible, below the mylohyoid line, which lodges the lateral surface of the submandibular gland. **Subnasal fossa.** A depression on the anterior surface of the maxilla beneath the nasal spine. **Subpyramidal fossa.** The sinus tympani. **Subscapular fossa [fossa subscapularis (NA)].** The concave anterior surface of the scapula which gives origin to the subscapularis muscle. **Subspinous fossa.** Infraspinous fossa (see above). **Supinator fossa.** A shallow triangular depression distal to the radial notch of the ulna. **Supraclavicular fossa, greater [fossa supraclavicularis major (trigonum ornoclaviculare) NA].** The depression above the clavicle and lateral to the sternomastoid muscle. **Supraclavicular fossa, lesser [fossa supraclavicularis minor (NA)].** The depression between the sternal and clavicular heads of the sternomastoid muscle. **Supraspinous fossa [fossa supraspinata (NA)].** The depression on the posterior surface of the scapula above the spine, which gives origin to the supraspinatus muscle. **Suprasternal fossa.** The surface depression above the upper border of the manubrium sterni. **Supratonsillar fossa.** Intratonsillar cleft. *See* CLEFT. **Supravesical fossa [fossa supravesicalis (NA)].** The shallow peritoneal fossa which is present on either side of the median umbilical ligament when the bladder is empty. **Temporal fossa [fossa temporalis (NA)].** The area on the side of the skull below the temporal lines, which is continuous deep to the zygomatic arch with the infratemporal fossa. **Fossa terminalis [fossa navicularis urethrae (NA)].** A dilatation of the terminal part of the penile urethra. **Tonsillar fossa [fossa tonsillaris (NA)].** The space in the lateral wall of the oropharynx between the 2 pillars of the fauces, which is occupied by the tonsil; amygdaloid fossa. **Fossa transversalis hepatis.** The porta hepatis. **Triangular fossa [fossa triangularis (NA)].** The depression between the two crura of the antihelix. **Trochanteric fossa [fossa trochanterica (NA)].** A pit on the medial side of the greater trochanter of the femur for the attachment of the obturator internus muscle. **Trochlear fossa [fovea trochlearis (NA)].** A small depression or process on the orbital surface of the frontal bone, just behind the medial end of the supra-orbital margin, for the attachment of the pulley of the superior oblique muscle. **Fossa umbilicalis hepatis.** The fissure on the inferior surface of the liver, occupied by the umbilical vein in the fetus and the ligamentum teres in the adult. **Vestibular fossa [fossa vestibuli vaginae (NA)].** The part of the vestibule of the vagina immediately posterior to the vaginal orifice; the navicular fossa. [L ditch.]

See also: BICHAT, BIESIADECKI, BROESIKE, CLAUDIUS, GRUBER (W. L.), HARTMANN (R.), HUGUIER, JOBERT, JONNESCO, LANDZERT, LUSCHKA, MALGAIGNE, MERKEL (K. L.), MOHRENHEIM, MORGAGNI, POISSON (F.), ROSENMUELLER, TARIN, WALDEYER-HARTZ.

Fossarulus (fos·ar·ew·lus). A genus of molluscs, intermediate hosts of *Clonorchis sinensis.*

fossette (fos·et). 1. A dimple or small depression. 2. A small deep-centred ulcer of the cornea. [Fr. dimple.]

fossula [NA] (fos·ew·lah). A small fossa. **Fossula of the fenestra cochleae [fossula fenestrae cochleae (NA)].** The small depression forming the tractus spiralis foraminosus at the outer end of the porus acusticus internus. **Fossula of the fenestra vestibuli [fossula fenestrae vestibuli (NA)].** A small depression on the inner wall of the tympanic cavity. **Tonsillar fossulae.** Tonsillar pits. *See* PIT. [L little ditch.]

fossulate (fos·ew·late). 1. Grooved or slightly hollowed. 2. Showing a small fossa. [see prec.]

Fothergill, John (b. 1712). London physician.

Fothergill's disease. Trigeminal neuralgia; tic douloureux.

Fothergill's sore throat. An ulcerative form of sore throat found in severe scarlatina.

Fothergill, William Edward (b. 1865). Manchester gynaecologist.

Fothergill operation. An improved modification of Donald's original operation for the treatment of uterovaginal prolapse by amputation of the cervix and anterior colporrhaphy. Fothergill exposed the cardinal ligaments to greater advantage and facilitated their approximation to the front of the cervix.

Fouchet, André (b. 1894). French chemist.

Fouchet's reagent, for bilirubin in urine. Trichloro-acetic acid, 25 g, dissolved in 100 ml distilled water and 10 ml of 10 per cent ferric-chloride solution added.

Fouchet's test, for bilirubin in urine. Acidify 10 ml of urine with a few drops of dilute acetic acid, add 5 ml of 10 per cent barium-chloride solution, mix and filter. To the residue on the filter paper add a drop or two of Fouchet's reagent (see above); a green to blue colour forms, depending upon the quantity of bile present in the urine.

foudroyant (foo·drwah·yahn). Fulminant. [Fr.]

foulage (foo·lahzh). A form of massage in which the muscles are kneaded and squeezed. [Fr. pressing.]

Fouli's tourniquet. A rubber tube controlled by a doubly-curved block of wood, the grooves in the wood gripping the tourniquet after it has been drawn tight.

foulis cells. Large epithelial cells found in the fluid of malignant ovarian cysts.

fourchette (foor·shet). 1. The posterior commissure of the labia majora. 2. A surgical instrument like a fork used to lift up and support the tongue while the frenulum is being divided. [Fr. fork.]

Fourier, Jean Baptiste Joseph, Baron de (b. 1768). French mathematician.

Fourier synthesis. Synthesis of a repetitive complex waveform from a series of sine or cosine terms of different wavelength and phase. It was first applied to the solution of thermodynamic problems.

Fourmentin's thoracic index. The number obtained by multiplying the transverse thoracic diameter at the level of the xiphisternal joint by 100 and dividing the product by the anteroposterior diameter at the same level.

Fourneau (foor·no). **Fourneau 190.** Acetarsol BP 1958. **Fourneau 309.** Suramin BP 1958. **Fourneau 933.** Piperoxan hydrochloride. [Ernest *Fourneau* (b. 1872), French physician.]

Fournier, Jean Alfred (b. 1832). Paris syphilologist.

Fournier's disease, or gangrene. Gangrene of the scrotum or vulva due to an anaerobic haemolytic streptococcal infection.

Fournier's smooth patches. Glistening circular or polycyclic lesions on the tongue, not associated with ulceration, indicating a depapillating glossitis, and occurring in secondary syphilis. The lesions are best seen if the tongue is dried.

Fournier's sign. 1. The abrupt limitation of a syphilitic skin lesion. 2. The sabre-shaped shin bones of congenital syphilis.

Fournier's syphiloma. Progressive infiltration of the perirectal and perianal tissues, leading to stenosis and ulceration. It is not now thought to be due to syphilis.

Fournier test. A clinical test to demonstrate ataxia: an ataxic patient, particularly one with cerebellar ataxia, is unable to rise suddenly from the sitting position, he cannot stop suddenly while walking, nor can he turn round quickly. All of these movements, if attempted rapidly, give overbalancing and perhaps falling.

fovea [NA] (fo·ve·ah) (pl. *foveae*). A shallow pit or depression; particularly applied to a depression in the retina, 1.5 mm in diameter, situated 3 mm temporal to the optic disc and responsible for accurate central vision. **Fovea cardiaca.** The depression on the mediastinal surface of the left lung where it comes into relationship with the left ventricle of the heart. **Fovea centralis [NA].** The central area of the fovea of the retina (see above), about 400 μm in diameter. **Fovea of the head of the femur.** Pit on the head of the femur. **Fovea of the head of the radius.** The shallow superior articulating surface of the head of the radius. **Fovea hemi-elliptica.** The elliptical recess of the bony vestibule of the internal ear. **Fovea hemispherica.** The spherical recess of the bony vestibule of the internal ear. **Fovea inferior [NA].** A small pit in the lower part of the floor of the 4th ventricle at the apex of the trigonum vagi. **Fovea jugularis.** The depression at the lateral end of the jugular fossa of the skull, which houses the jugular bulb. **Fovea oblonga [NA].** A depression on the anterolateral surface of the arytenoid cartilage to which the vocalis and crico-arytenoid muscles are attached. **Fovea pharyngis.** Recess of the pharynx. **Fovea pterygoidea.** Scaphoid fossa. *See* FOSSA. **Fovea superior [NA].** A small pit in the upper part of the floor of the 4th ventricle of the brain, superolateral to the facial colliculus. **Fovea supravesicalis.** The supravesical fossa of the lower part of the anterior abdominal wall. **Fovea triangularis [NA].** The depression on the anterolateral surface of the arytenoid cartilage, to which the false vocal cord (vestibular ligament) is attached. **Fovea trigemini.** Fovea superior (see above). **Fovea vagi.** Fovea inferior (see above). [L pit.]

foveate (fo·ve·ate). 1. Pitted. 2. Of a surface, bearing foveae or depressions. [see foll.]

foveation (fo·ve·a·shun). Pitting, as of the skin in chickenpox. [L *fovea* pit.]

foveola [NA] (fo·ve·o·lah). A small fovea. **Coccygeal foveola [foveola coccygea (NA)].** The dimple on the skin which is often, but not invariably, present at the tip of the coccyx. **Gastric foveolae [foveolae gastricae (NA)].** The minute furrows between the folds which characterize the gastric mucosa when examined with a hand lens. [L a small pit.]

See also: HOWSHIP.

foveolate (fo·ve·o·late). Showing small depressions or dimples. [see prec.]

Foville, Achille Louis François (b. 1799). French psychiatrist.

Foville's oblique fasciculus. The stria semicircularis in the floor of the lateral ventricle between the caudate nucleus and the thalamus.

Foville's paralysis, or syndrome. An ipsilateral paralysis of the 6th and 7th cranial nerves, with loss of conjugate deviation to the same side, associated with contralateral hemiplegia. The lesion is situated in the pons at the level of the 6th cranial-nerve nucleus, and is usually of vascular origin.

Foville's tract. The posterior spinocerebellar tract.

Millard–Gubler–Foville paralysis. 6th cranial nerve palsy, with or without ipsilateral 7th nerve palsy, and contralateral hemiplegia.

fowl-pox (fowl·pox). A disease of fowls; yellow warty nodules appear on the head. These excrescences are due to epithelial proliferation, of which the cells develop intracytoplasmic inclusions (Bollinger bodies) which are conglomerations of the virus particles. [AS *fugel, poc.*]

Fowler, Alan William. 20th century British surgeon.

Fowler's operation. A reconstructive procedure of the forefoot used in the treatment of claw toes.

Fowler, George Ryerson (b. 1848). New York surgeon.

Fowler's operation. Decortication of the lung in chronic empyema.

Fowler's position. A position in which the trunk is raised at an angle of about 45 degrees to the horizontal and the thighs are similarly raised, so that the pelvis forms the apex of a V and is the lowest part of the body.

Fowler–Murphy treatment. Treatment of a patient with peritonitis in the sitting-up (Fowler) position to encourage the collection of pus in the pelvis. Also called *Murphy treatment.*

Fowler, Sir James Kingston (b. 1852). London physician.

Fowler's law, of spread of pulmonary tuberculosis. The disease frequently spreads from the apex of the dorsal lobe along the great fissure to the periphery and elsewhere.

Fowler, Thomas (b. 1736). York physician.

Fowler's solution. A solution of potassium arsenite containing the equivalent of 1 per cent arsenic trioxide in neutral solution; it is a convenient form of arsenic used for the oral treatment of certain blood and other diseases.

Fox, George Henry (b. 1846). New York dermatologist.

Fordyce–Fox disease, Fox–Fordyce disease. An apocrine gland disorder comparable to prickly heat. Itchy follicular papules occur in the axillae, at the areolae mammae, umbilicus, pubis or labia majora.

Fox, William Tilbury (b. 1836). London physician.

Fox's impetigo. Impetigo contagiosa.

foxglove (fox·gluv). The common name for *Digitalis purpurea* Linn. (family Scrophulariaceae). **Austrian foxglove.** Woolly foxglove leaf, Digitalis Lanata Leaf BPC 1954.

fraction (frak·shun). **Blood plasma fraction.** An individual protein component of blood plasma, e.g. globulin. **Dried Human Albumin Fraction (Saline) BP 1973.** The dried preparation of human plasma protein fraction (see below), made by freeze-drying. **Dried Human Antihaemophilic Fraction BP 1973.** A dried preparation obtained from human plasma; it is rich in clotting factor VIII and used to promote haemostasis in haemophiliacs. **Ejection fraction.** In cardiology, that fraction of the volume of blood contained in the ventricle at the end of diastole which is expelled during the subsequent systole. **Human Albumin Fraction (Saline) BP 1973.** A solution of the proteins of liquid human plasma, containing albumin and certain globulins which retain their solubility on heating. **Human Coagulation Fraction (II, IX and X).** BP Commission approved name for a preparation of human blood containing coagulation factors II, IX and X; it is used in the treatment of haemophilia B deficiency. **Mol fraction.** The ratio between the weight of a substance actually present in a litre of a solution and the weight that would be present were the solution molar. **Packing fraction.** A method of expressing the mass defect of an atom: packing fraction $f=(M-A)/A$, where M is the measured mass of an isotope of mass number A. **Radiation fraction.** An aliquot of the total dose given as part of a fractionated course of radiation treatment. [L *frangere* to break.]

See also: DAKIN, WEST (R.).

fractional (frak·shun·al). 1. Divided; carried out by repeated division. 2. Accomplished in successive stages or one part at a time. [see foll.]

fractionate (frak·shun·ate). To separate into smaller component parts. [L *frangere* to break.]

fractionation (frak·shun·a·shun). 1. Division into component parts. 2. In chemistry it usually means *fractional distillation*, the process by which liquids of differing boiling points are separated during distillation of the mixture, by collecting the fractions "coming over" at various temperatures. 3. The phenomenon that repetitive stimulation applied to an afferent nerve gives rise to a reflex tetanus involving only some of the fibres of the reacting muscle. More than one afferent nerve must be stimulated to induce reflex activity involving all the fibres to the muscle. 4. In radiotherapy, a technique for dividing a course of radiation therapy into separate aliquots. [see prec.]

fractura (frak·tewr·ah). Fracture. **Fractura surcularia.** Greenstick fracture. *See* FRACTURE. [L.]

fracture (frak·tewr). 1. To break a structure, especially a bone. 2. A break or interruption in the continuity of a bone. **Abduction fracture.** A fracture produced by the movement of abduction, especially in the neck of the femur. **Adduction fracture.** A fracture produced by the movement of adduction, especially in the neck of the femur. **Apophyseal fracture.** Separation of an apophysis. **Articular fracture.** A fracture involving the articular surface of a bone, thus communicating with the adjacent joint. **Atrophic fracture.** A fracture occurring in atrophied bone. **Avulsion fracture.** The tearing of a portion of bone away from its main mass by muscle action. **Baby-car fracture.** Multiple fractures around the elbow joint resulting from a "side-swipe" injury. **Beak fracture.** Fracture of the upper portion of the tuberosity of the calcaneum. **Birth fracture.** Fracture of the bone of an infant, produced during delivery. **Blow-out fracture.** Fracture of the orbital wall resulting from a sudden increase in intra-orbital pressure secondary to a blow on the eye. **Boxers' fracture.** Fracture of one or more metacarpal bones produced by the shock of punching. **Bucket-handle fracture.** A longitudinal tear of a semilunar cartilage in the knee joint. **Bumper fracture.** A fracture of the upper third of the tibia sustained by a blow from the bumper of a motor car. **Butterfly fracture.** A fracture of a long bone in which a triangular fragment is separated from the two main fragments. **Chauffeurs' fracture.** Fracture of the lower radius and ulna with backward displacement, originally from back-firing of a motor-car engine during cranking. **Chip fracture.** The dislodgment of a small fragment of bone by a glancing force. **Clay-shovellers' fracture.** Fracture of the spinous process of the 7th cervical or 1st dorsal vertebrae in the act of shovelling. **Closed fracture.** Fracture of a bone without concomitant skin wound. **Comminuted fracture.** A fracture producing multiple fragments. **Complex simple fracture.** A fracture not involving the skin but associated with damage to other important structures such as vessels or nerves. **Complicated fracture.** A fracture associated with damage to important neighbouring structures (a vessel or a nerve, usually). **Compound fracture.** A fracture associated with a skin wound. **Compression fracture.** Fracture of a vertebral body by vertical crushing. **Condylar fracture.** Separation of the condyle of a long bone. **Congenital fracture.** A fracture present at birth, from injury at birth, or disease or maldevelopment before it. **Cough fracture.** A fracture of the rib or ribs caused by violent coughing: it occurs most frequently when the subject coughs at a time when his diaphragm is being pressed upwards by pressure in the abdomen, e.g. when he is bending forward. **Crush fracture.** Compression fracture (see above). **Dashboard fracture.** A fracture of the patella resulting from an automobile accident in which the knee strikes the dashboard of the car. The resulting fracture is complicated by the reflex bracing of the quadriceps femoris muscle which pulls the fragments apart. **Delayed-union fracture.** A fracture which is slow to heal. **Depressed fracture.** A fracture in which an area of skull is driven inwards. **Diacondylar fracture.** Fracture of the lower end of the humerus circling the olecranon fossa. **Direct fracture.** Fracture of a bone at the site of applied violence. **Double fracture.** Two fractures in the same bone. **Epiphyseal fracture.** A fracture involving the epiphysis of a bone. **Extension fracture.** Fracture produced by sudden stretching of a part, usually the spine. **Extracapsular fracture.**

Fracture of that lower part of the neck of the femur which lies partly outside the hip joint. **Fatigue fracture.** A fine, hair-line crack appearing in a bone without injury. **Fender fracture.** Fracture of the lateral condyle of a pedestrian produced by the fender or mudguard of a car. **Fissure fracture.** A narrow split in a bone, usually of the skull. **Flexion fracture.** Fracture produced by sudden bending, especially of the spine. **Furrow fracture.** A narrow fracture of the skull. **Greenstick fracture.** Incomplete fracture of a bone of a child, the unbroken edge bending. **Gunshot fracture.** Fracture due to the impact of a bullet or other missile. **Impacted fracture.** A fracture in which one fragment is driven into the other. **Indirect fracture.** Fracture produced by violence applied to a point distant to the fracture site. **Infected fracture.** A fracture, usually compound, into which micro-organisms have gained access. **Intercondylar fracture.** Fracture of the lower end of the humerus or femur, in which the condyles are separate from each other. **Intertrochanteric fracture.** Fracture through the base of the neck and the trochanters of the femur. **Intra-articular fracture.** A fracture entirely within the capsule of a joint. **Intracapsular fracture.** Fracture of that upper part of the neck of the femur which lies wholly within the hip joint. **Intraperiosteal fracture.** A fracture within the periosteum which remains intact, e.g. a greenstick fracture (see above). **Intra-uterine fracture.** A fracture occurring to the fetus *in utero*. **Joint fracture.** A fracture involving a joint. **Linear fracture.** A fracture in which the break follows a straight line. **Longitudinal fracture.** A fracture along the length of a bone. **Malunited fracture.** A fracture which has healed with deformity or shortening. **March fracture.** Fracture of the shaft of the 2nd, 3rd or 4th metatarsal bones occurring in unaccustomed walking or marching, and not at first visible in the x-ray. **Neoplastic fracture.** Fracture through a tumour in the bone. **Neurogenic fracture.** Fracture of a bone from slight violence applied to a paralysed limb. **Oblique fracture.** A fracture whose line is not directly across the axis of the affected bone. **Open fracture.** Compound fracture (see above). **Pathological fracture.** Fracture by slight violence of a bone weakened by disease. **Periarticular fracture.** A fracture in close proximity to a joint capsule. **Pertrochanteric fracture.** Intertrochanteric fracture (see above). **Pond fracture.** A depressed fracture of the skull, usually in children, in which the depressed fragments shelve inwards to a central point. **Rosette fracture.** Pond fracture (see preceding). **Secondary fracture.** A fracture secondary to bone disease of any kind, or pathological fracture. **Shearing fracture.** Fracture due to a shearing force. **Simple fracture.** Closed fracture (see above). **Spiral fracture.** An oblique fracture (see above) whose outline gives a spiral x-ray shadow. **Splintered fracture.** Comminuted fracture (see above). **Spontaneous fracture.** Fracture in the course of a normal movement, without violence, of a bone weakened by disease. **Sprinters' fracture.** Fracture by muscular violence of the anterior superior or anterior inferior spine of the ilium sustained during running. **Stellate fracture.** A star-shaped fracture of a flat bone, usually of the scapula or patella. **Stress fracture.** Fatigue fracture (see above). **Subcapital fracture.** A fracture of the femur through the neck immediately distal to the head of the bone. **Subcutaneous fracture.** Closed fracture (see above). **Subperiosteal fracture.** Fracture without displacement of the bone ends, and without interruption of the periosteum at the site of fracture. **Subtrochanteric fracture.** Fracture of the upper end of the femur immediately below the lesser trochanter. **Supracondylar fracture.** Fracture of the lower end of the humerus or femur immediately above the condyles. **Torsion fracture.** Fracture by twisting violence, especially on the fibula at the ankle. **Transcondylar fracture.** Fracture through the condyles of the humerus or femur. **Transverse fracture.** A fracture whose line is at right angles to the axis of the affected bone. **Trimalleolar fracture.** A fracture-dislocation of the ankle, where the medial and lateral malleoli are fractured, also the posterior part of the lower articular surface of the tibia. **Ununited fracture.** A fracture which remains unhealed over a prolonged period. **Wedge fracture.** Fracture involving cancellous bone, as of the body of a vertebra, which is compressed to a wedge shape. [L *fractura*.]

See also: BARTON, BENNETT (E. H.), COLLES, DUPUYTREN, GALEAZZI, GUÉRIN (A. F. M.), LOBSTEIN, MALGAIGNE, MONTEGGIA, POTT, SMITH (R. W.), VROLIK.

fracture-dislocation (frak·tewr·dis·lo·ka'·shun). Dislocation at a joint and fracture of one of the bones concerned.

Fraenkel, Albert (b. 1848). Berlin physician.

Fraenkel's pneumococcus, Fraenkel-Weichselbaum pneumococcus. *Streptococcus pneumoniae.*

Fraenkel's sign. Hypotonia of muscles about the hip joint in tabes dorsalis.

Fraenkel, Albert (b. 1864). Heidelberg physician.

Fraenkel's treatment. The use of the strophanthin group of cardiac glycosides in the treatment of cardiac failure. Like digitalis, strophanthin strengthens the contraction of the ventricular muscle, slows the heart and increases cardiac output.

Fraenkel, Bernhard (b. 1836). Berlin laryngologist.

Fraenkel's postural test. In suppuration of the anterior group of nasal sinuses: after cleansing the nasal cavity, the head is bent forward, the suspected side uppermost. On re-examination, pus is found in the middle meatus.

Fraenkel, Carl (b. 1861). German bacteriologist.

Fraenkel's nodule. A lesion characteristic of typhus; vascular endothelial proliferation associated with perivascular infiltration, eventually leading to thrombosis, necrosis and haemorrhage, in the smaller arteries and arterioles.

Fraenkel's sign. An interruption of a peristaltic wave by a lesser-curve gastric ulcer, seen in fluoroscopy. The ulcerated area blocks the wave which begins again on the distal side of the lesion.

fraenulum (fre·new·lum). Frenulum.

fraenum (fre·num). Frenum.

fragiform (fraj·e·form). Like a strawberry in shape. [L *fraga* strawberry, form.]

fragile (fraj·ile). 1. Brittle; delicate; weak. 2. Infirm. [fragilitas.]

fragilitas (fraj·il·it·as). Fragility. **Fragilitas crinium.** A condition of the hair in which it is very brittle and breaks easily into filaments. **Fragilitas ossium congenita.** Osteogenesis imperfecta. **Fragilitas sanguinis.** Fragility of the blood. [L weakness.]

fragility (fraj·il·it·e). The quality of being fragile. **Fragility of the blood.** A condition of the erythrocytes, such as occurs in acholuric jaundice, in which there is a strong tendency for them to rupture when the saline content of the blood is diminished. The same phenomenon occurs in drawn blood when the erythrocytes are placed in hypotonic solutions. **Capillary fragility.** A weakened condition of the capillaries causing them to rupture readily, as in purpura. **Hereditary fragility of bone.** Osteogenesis imperfecta. [fragilitas.]

fragilocyte (fraj·il·o·site). A red cell that is more fragile, in varying dilutions of saline, than the normal cell; it is seen in acholuric jaundice or familial haemolytic anaemia. [L *fragilis* weak, Gk *kytos* cell.]

fragilocytosis (fraj·il·o·si·to'·sis). A condition of the blood in which the erythrocytes are abnormally fragile; the condition in which the blood contains fragilocytes. [L *fragilis* weak, cytosis.]

fragment (frag·ment). 1. A part broken off. 2. In cytogenetics, denoting a centric or an acentric chromosome segment resulting from chromosome structural changes. **Fission fragments.** *See* FISSION. **Nuclear fragments.** Howell bodies. [L *frangere* to break.]

See also: SPENGLER.

fragmentation (frag·men·ta·shun). 1. The process or act of separation into fragments. 2. In bacteriology, the process by which certain micro-organisms break at a joint and thus form a new organism. 3. Amitosis. **Fragmentation of myocardium.** Rupture in a transverse plane of the muscular fibres of the heart. [see prec.]

fraise (fraze). A smooth hemispherical or conical button with cutting edges for enlarging trephine openings or cutting osteoplastic flaps. [Fr. strawberry.]

frambesin (fram·be·sin). Cultures of *Treponema pertenue* heated at 60° C and used in a skin test for framboesia (yaws).

framboesia (fram·be·ze·ah). Yaws. **Framboesia tropica.** Yaws. [Fr. *framboise* raspberry.]

framboesides (fram·be·si·dz). Manifestations of secondary yaws. [Fr. *framboise* raspberry.]

framboesioma (fram·be·ze·o′·mah). The large primary individual lesion of yaws, which takes the form of a protruding nodule. [framboesia, Gk *-oma* tumour.]

frame (frame). 1. A supporting appliance of a skeleton nature. 2. Construct, devise, adapt. **Balkan frame.** A system of overhead bars fixed to the bed, to which pulleys are attached for the purpose of suspending splints and applying extension to the leg. Also called *Balkan beam.* **Occluding frame.** A form of articulator used in dentistry. **Sampling frame.** A list of individuals in a population at a point in time, used for drawing samples. **Trial frame.** 1. A form of spectacle frame for holding trial lenses. 2. An instrument used in testing colour perception. [AS *framian* to be helpful.]

See also: BOEHLER, BRADFORD, HIBBS, JONES (R.), WHITMAN.

framework (frame·werk). **Scleral framework.** That part of the filtration angle which is next to the sclera. **Uveal framework.** The pectinate ligament of the iris. [AS *framian* to be helpful, *weorc.*]

Framycetin (fram·i·set·in). BP Commission approved name for an antibiotic derived from *Streptomyces decaris.* **Framycetin Sulphate BP 1973.** The sulphate of the basic substance; it has an antimicrobial action similar to that of neomycin sulphate.

Franceschetti, Adolphe (b. 1896). Swiss ophthalmologist.

Franceschetti-Jadassohn syndrome. A genetically determined reticulate pigmentation of the skin, with palmoplantar keratoderma and eccrine aplasia causing disturbance of temperature regulation. The teeth may be defective.

Franceschetti-Klein syndrome. Treacher-Collins syndrome. *See* COLLINS (E. T.)

Francis, Edward (b. 1872). American bacteriologist.

Francis' disease. Tularaemia.

francium (fran·se·um). A radioactive element of the alkali-metal group, atomic number 87 and chemical symbol Fr, discovered as a disintegration product of actinium in 1939 and obtained artificially by the bombardment of thorium with protons. [*France.*]

Franck's plethysmograph. A plethysmograph composed of an erect glass container in which the wrist and hand are placed.

Francke's striae. Small dilated venules or capillaries in the neighbourhood of the 7th cervical and 1st dorsal vertebrae, which were thought to be due to a viscerocutaneous reflex from tuberculosis of the apex of a lung.

Franco, Pierre (b. 1500). French surgeon.

Franco's operation. Alleged to have been the opening of the bladder suprapubically for the removal of bladder tumours.

franconium (fran·ko·ne·um). Francium.

frangible (fran·jibl). Brittle or fragile; capable of being broken. [L *frangere* to break.]

Frangula BPC 1949 (fran·gew·lah). Alder buckthorn bark, frangula bark; the bark of *Rhamnus frangula* Linn. (family Rhamnaceae), a shrub found throughout Europe. When fresh it has emetic properties and should therefore be allowed to mature for at least a year after collection before being used medicinally. It contains anthraquinone derivatives and has a purgative action similar to that of cascara. It is usually administered in the form of the liquid extract. [L *frangere* to break.]

Frank, Alfred Erich (b. 1884). German physician.

Frank's essential thrombocytopenia. Non-thrombocytopenic purpura of unknown cause; pseudohaemophilia.

Frank, Jacob (b. 1856). Chicago surgeon.

Frank's sign. Prolongation of the clotting time of the blood associated with cirrhosis of the liver in pseudohaemophilia hepatica.

Frank's syndrome. Pseudohaemophilia hepatica.

Frank, Rudolf (b. 1862). Vienna surgeon.

Frank's operation, Ssabanejew-Frank operation. Gastrotomy performed by withdrawing a cone of stomach through the chest wall and inserting a tube in it.

Franke, Elizabeth. American biochemist.

Benedict and Franke method, for uric acid in urine. The urine is diluted about 1 in 20, and to 10 ml of this solution is added 5 ml of 5 per cent sodium cyanide, followed by 1 ml of arsenophosphotungstic-acid reagent. The colour is compared with standards after 5 min.

Frankel's glands. Small glands in the mucous membrane of the lower surface of the vocal folds.

Frankenhäuser, Ferdinand (b. 1832). Zürich and Jena gynaecologist.

Frankenhäuser's ganglion. An occasional ganglion occurring in the vaginal portion of the neck of the uterus.

Frankfeldt, Frank Meyer (b. 1891). New York surgeon.

Frankfeldt's diathermy snare. A diathermy snare for the removal of rectal polypi.

frankincense (frangk·in·sens). Olibanum: an oleo-gum-resin, related to myrrh, and obtained by incision of the bark of *Boswellia carterii* and other species. It is a bitter drug with characteristic odour, occurring in the form of glassy tears, and used in fumigating powders. **Common frankincense.** The more solid form of exudate occurring in the last stages of the tapping of crude turpentine; also known as *gum thus.* [O Fr. *franc encens* free incense.]

Frankl-Hochwart, Lothar von (b. 1862). Vienna neurologist.

Frankl-Hochwart disease. Polyneuritis cerebralis menieriformis.

Franklin, Benjamin (b. 1706). American statesman and scientist.

Franklin's spectacles, Franklin's split bifocals. Spectacles in which the upper and lower segments of the lenses are separate pieces of glass, the upper for distance, the lower for reading.

Fraunhofer, Joseph von (b. 1787). German physicist.

Fraunhofer's lines. Absorption lines in the sun's spectrum caused by the passage of light from the sun through the sun's cooler atmosphere.

Fraxinus (frax·in·us). A genus of trees which includes the manna ash (*Fraxinus ornus* Linn., family Oleaceae). [L ash.]

Frazier, Charles Harrison (b. 1870). Philadelphia neurosurgeon.

Frazier's needle. A needle used for draining the lateral ventricles of the brain.

Frazier-Spiller operation. Intracranial trigeminal nerve section in the treatment of neuralgia.

freak (freek). 1. A monstrosity, or a person or thing showing any abnormal development. 2. In popular usage, an ugly, deformed or abnormally-developed person. 3. A mental caprice. [etym. dub.]

freckle (frekl). Lentigo, ephelis; any one of the small yellow-brown spots that occur on the uncovered parts of the skin, particularly in persons of sandy complexion. **Cold freckle.** Lentigo appearing on a part of the skin not exposed to the sun's rays. [ME *frecken.*]

Freda, Vincent Charles (b. 1906). Chicago gynaecologist.

Falls, Freda and Cohen test, for pregnancy. An intradermal injection of colostrum is given and no reaction occurs if the patient is pregnant.

Frédéricq, Louis Antoine (b. 1815). Belgian physician.

Frédéricq's sign. A red line on the gums in pulmonary tuberculosis.

Fredet, Pierre (b. 1870). Paris surgeon.

Fredet-Ramstedt operation. Division by a longitudinal incision of the hypertrophied pyloric muscle for the relief of congenital hypertrophic stenosis.

free (free). In chemistry, uncombined. [AS *freo.*]

Freedman, A. 20th century London physician.
Freedman inhaler. A draw-over device for adding trichloroethylene vapour to the air inspired to give obstetric anaesthesia.

freezing (fre·zing). The process of solidifying a solution or liquid by exposing it to cold or lowering its temperature. [ME *fresen* to be cold.]

Frei, Wilhelm Siegmund (b. 1885). Berlin dermatologist.
Frei antigen. An artificial antigen used in the intradermal test for lymphopathia venereum (lymphogranuloma inguinale).
Frei test. A skin test used as an indicator of delayed hypersensitivity (tuberculin-type) in patients with lymphogranuloma venereum. A suspension of lymphogranuloma venereum virus, nowadays derived from egg yolk sac culture, injected intradermally gives an indurated erythematous papule, 7 mm in diameter, 4 days later. The test may also be positive in cases of psittacosis.

Freiberg, Albert Henry (b. 1868). Cincinnati surgeon.
Freiberg's disease, or infraction. Osteochondritis of the head of the 2nd metatarsal bone.

fremitus (frem·it·us). A vibratory sensation or thrill perceived by palpation. **Bronchial fremitus.** Rhonchal fremitus (see below). **Dental fremitus.** Teeth grinding; stridor dentium. **Echinococcus fremitus.** Hydatid fremitus (see below). **Friction fremitus.** Vibrations caused by friction of inflamed serous surfaces, especially the pleura. **Hydatid fremitus.** Hydatid thrill; a peculiar vibration sometimes felt on percussion over a hydatid cyst of the lung or liver. **Pectoral fremitus.** Vocal fremitus (see below). **Pericardial fremitus.** Vibrations due to pericardial friction. **Pleural fremitus.** Friction caused by pleurisy. **Rhonchal fremitus.** Vibrations caused by air passing through partial obstructions in the bronchi. **Subjective fremitus.** Vibrations felt by a person whilst humming with the mouth closed. **Tactile fremitus.** Vibrations perceived by palpation. **Tussive fremitus.** Vibrations felt over the chest when the patient coughs. **Vocal fremitus.** Vibrations caused by the voice and conveyed to the chest wall. [L a murmuring.]

frenal (fre·nal). Relating or belonging to a frenulum.

frenator (fre·na·tor). 1. A term for any of the muscles that control the movement of the head on the atlas and axis (Dupré). 2. Anything that inhibits, restrains or holds in check. [L *fraenum* bridle.]

frenetic (fren·et·ik). 1. Phrenetic. 2. Referring to disordered mentality, or having a part in it. [Fr. *frénétique* frenzied.]

Frenkel, Heinrich S. (b. 1860). Berlin neurologist.
Frenkel's exercises, movements, or treatment. A series of muscular exercises involving precise co-ordinated movements and used for the re-education of ataxic patients.

Frenkel, Henri (b. 1864). Paris ophthalmologist.
Bordier-Frenkel sign. An outward and upward rolling movement of the eye on attempted lid closure, in facial paralysis of lower motor neurone type; also called *Bell's phenomenon, Bell's sign.*

frenosecretory (fre·no·se·kre′·tor·e). Capable of arresting or restraining the process of secretion. [L *fraenum* bridle, secretion.]

frenotomy (fre·not·o·me). The dividing of the frenulum of the tongue for tongue-tie. [frenulum, Gk *temnein* to cut.]

frenulum [NA] (fren·ew·lum). A term originally denoting the folds of mucous membrane running from the gums to the lip or tongue and limiting undue movement; now applied to many other structures similar in appearance. **Frenulum cerebelli.** Frenulum veli (see below). **Frenulum of the clitoris [frenulum clitoridis (NA)].** The junction of the labia minora below the glans of the clitoris. **Frenulum epiglottidis.** Glosso-epiglottic fold; the fold of mucous membrane extending from the front of the epiglottis to the dorsum of the tongue in the midline. **Frenulum of the ileocolic valve [frenulum valvae ileocecalis (NA)].** The prolongation of the two labia of the ileocolic valve around the inner wall of the colon. **Frenulum labiorum [frenulum labiorum pudendi (NA)].** The connecting fold between the posterior parts of the two labia minora. **Frenulum of the lower lip [frenulum labii inferioris (NA)], Frenulum of the upper lip [frenulum labii superioris (NA)].** Folds of mucous membrane situated in the midline extending from the adjacent gum to the lower or upper lip respectively. **Frenulum of the prepuce [frenulum preputii (NA)].** A fold of skin containing small blood vessels and running from the ventral surface of the glans penis to the adjacent prepuce. **Frenulum preputii clitoridis.** Frenulum of the clitoris (see above). **Frenulum pudendi.** Frenulum labiorum (see above). **Frenulum of the tongue [frenulum linguae (NA)].** The fold of mucous membrane from the floor of the mouth to the under-surface of the tongue in the midline. **Frenulum veli [frenulum veli medullaris superioris (NA)].** A median groove on the dorsum of the mid-brain, leading to the superior medullary velum. [L *fraenum* bridle.]
See also: GIACOMINI, M'DOWEL, MORGAGNI.

frenum (fre·num). Frenulum.

frenzy (fren·ze). 1. Violent temporary mental derangement or mania. 2. Delirious rage or excitement. [Fr. *frénésie* madness.]

Freon (fre·on). A proprietary brand of fluorine hydrocarbons used in refrigeration.

frequency (fre·kwen·se). 1. In a harmonic or rhythmic motion, the number of times the motion is repeated in a given period. 2. The rate of occurrence of an event. 3. In electricity, the rate at which an alternating current changes. 4. In light, or other wave motion, the number of complete waves per second; the velocity divided by wavelength. **Audio frequency.** A sound frequency within the range of normal audible human hearing, lying between 20 and 20 000 Hz (cycles/sec), or the whole of this frequency range. **Frequency of class.** *See* CLASS. **Frequency curve.** *See* CURVE. **Frequency distribution.** *See* DISTRIBUTION. **Electromagnetic frequency.** The number of complete waves of electromagnetic radiation generated per second. **Fusion frequency.** Flicker phenomenon; the rate at which objects can be merged before the eye. **Gene frequency.** The ratio in which the numbers of a given allelomorphic pair of genes are present in a population, or the ratio of the phenotypic expression of these genes. **High frequency.** Rapidly alternating electric current. **Low frequency.** Alternating current that changes more slowly per second than a certain standard. **Radio frequency.** A frequency, or the group of frequencies, related to electric currents or phenomena, covering 30 kHz to 300 MHz or more. [L *frequens* frequent.]

Frerichs, Friedrich Theodor (b. 1819). Berlin physician.
Frerichs' theory. The theory that uraemia is really a poisoning by ammonium carbonate formed by the action on urea of a ferment contained in the blood.

fret (fret). 1. Herpes. 2. An ulcer, erosion or chafing. [ME *freten* to consume.]

fretum (fre·tum). 1. A channel. 2. A constriction. **Fretum halleri.** In the early embryo, a constriction which marks off the bulbus arteriosus from the ventricle, and which later is the dividing line in the fetus between the atria and ventricles. **Fretum oris.** The pharyngeal isthmus. *See* ISTHMUS. [L strait.]

Freud, Sigmund (b. 1856). Vienna psychiatrist.
Freud's cathartic method. Psychiatric treatment by the cathartic method, following the practice of Freud.
Freud's theory, Freudian theory. A complex and highly integrated theory containing a number of tenets. Human beings are motivated by the *pleasure principle*, and all action is aimed to obtain pleasure or abolish unpleasure, the latter being caused by stimulation either from without or within. Internal stimulation is provided by the *sex instinct* and the *death instinct.* The personality has a structure, and can be divided into *ego, superego* and *id.* Below the level of the *conscious mind* there is the *preconscious*, and below that, the *unconscious.* The superego and the id are, respectively, largely and wholly in the unconscious, and in the unconscious all instinctual activity proceeds. This activity is manifested in the *libido*, equivalent to mental energy in its most general form. Libidinal urges are asocial or antisocial, and have to be restrained by the ego and superego. This is the source of

conflict. One of the modes of defence of the ego is *repression*, by which painful experiences, ideas, etc. are forced down into the unconscious, then being unknown to the conscious mind. Constellations of repressed ideas may form a *complex*, which, though in the unconscious, may yet provide powerful motivations. As the individual grows into the adult, spontaneous instinctive activity comes increasingly under the control of the ego. Development of the personality is largely determined by the development of sexuality, from the original *polymorphous perverse* phase to the adult *genital* stage. Intermediate stages are associated with certain *erogenous zones*, oral, anal, etc. This development is critically influenced by the *Oedipus situation*, i.e. the emotional relationship between the child and his mother.

freudian (froid·e·an). 1. Belonging to or related to Sigmund Freud and his doctrines. 2. A follower of Freud. **Freudian censor.** *See* CENSOR. **Freudian theory.** *See* FREUD'S THEORY.

Freund, Hermann Wolfgang (b. 1859). German gynaecologist.

Freund's anomaly. Term applied to a narrowing of the upper thoracic opening due to shortening of the first ribs, which causes deficient expansion of the apices of the lungs, and other phenomena.

Freund's operation. 1. A type of abdominal hysterectomy (now obsolete). 2. The treatment of intractable vesicovaginal fistula by transplantation of the ureters. 3. Division of cartilages for correction of congenital funnel breast.

Freund, Wilhelm Alexander (b. 1833). German gynaecologist.

Freund's law. Applied to the position of ovarian tumours, indicating that while such tumours are small and lying in the pelvis they are generally situated behind the uterus, whereas when they enlarge into the lower abdomen their position is usually above and in front of the uterus.

Frey, Heinrich (b. 1822). Zürich histologist.

Frey's gastric follicles. The ducts of the gastric glands.

Frey, Lucie. 19th–20th century Polish physician.

Frey's syndrome. The auriculotemporal syndrome. *See* SYNDROME.

Freyer, Sir Peter Johnston (b. 1851). London surgeon.

Freyer's operation. A standard method of performing transvesical suprapubic enucleation of the hypertrophied prostate. Freyer claimed priority in having originated this method in 1900.

friable (fri·abl). Easily reduced to powder; easily crumbled. In bacteriology, term applied to a culture which is dry and brittle and falls to powder when it is shaken or touched. [L *friare* to crumble.]

Fricke, Johann Karl Georg (b. 1790). Hamburg surgeon.

Fricke's operation, for cicatricial ectropion of the upper lid. A pedicle flap is cut on the medial side of the eyebrow and swung laterally on to the upper lid to fill the gap where the scar tissue has been removed.

friction (frik·shun). 1. Attrition; the act of rubbing. 2. The act of rubbing the body, e.g. with hand or brush in order to stimulate the action of the skin. 3. The rubbing of a healing or other medicinal substance into a part. 4. In massage: (*a*) firm circular rubbing and subsequent firm centripetal stroking; (*b*) shampooing. 5. The resistance present between two bodies moving against each other. **Friction fremitus.** *See* FREMITUS. **Friction sound.** *See* SOUND. [L *fricare* to rub.]

Friderichsen, Carl (b. 1886). Copenhagen physician.

Waterhouse-Friderichsen syndrome. A feature of meningococcal septicaemia in which the adrenal glands become disintegrated by haemorrhage and an acute adrenal insufficiency develops with alarming rapidity.

Fridericia's method. For estimating the alkali reserve indirectly by measuring alveolar carbon-dioxide tension. The carbon dioxide is absorbed from a known volume of alveolar air in a special apparatus by means of potassium hydroxide, and the decrease in volume is read off from a scale calibrated in terms of per cent.

Fried's rule. A rule for calculating dosage in children: adult dose multiplied by the age in months, divided by 150.

Friederichsen's test. For vitamin-A deficiency: the weakest light stimulus that will give rise to an oculomotor reflex is determined.

Friedlaender, Carl (b. 1847). Berlin pathologist.

Friedlaender's bacillus. *Bacterium friedländeri.*

Friedlaender's decidual cell. A large, clear, connective-tissue cell found in the uterine mucosa during pregnancy.

Friedlaender's disease. Arteritis obliterans.

Friedlaender's glycerin haematoxylin. A general nuclear stain made from haematoxylin, alum and glycerin.

Friedlaender's pneumonia. A form of bronchopneumonia due to infection with Friedlaender's bacillus or pneumobacillus (*Bacterium friedländeri*). The bronchopneumonic patches tend to become confluent, and, in patients who survive the acute stage, abscesses and necrosis are likely to occur. The disease is rare, and is seen most often in the elderly; the fatality rate is high.

Friedman, Maurice Harold (b. 1903). Philadelphia physiologist.

Friedman test, for pregnancy. Injection of the urine of a pregnant woman into a mature virgin female rabbit causes rupture of mature follicles of the ovary in 48 h. It is usually about 98 per cent accurate.

Friedman-Hamburger test. *See* TEST FOR CANCER.

Friedmann, Friedrich Franz (b. 1876). Berlin physician.

Friedmann treatment. Intravenous and intramuscular inoculation of tubercle bacilli isolated from turtles, and non-virulent for man.

Friedmann, Max (b. 1858). Mannheim neurologist.

Friedmann's complex, symptom complex, or vasomotor syndrome. The clinical manifestations of chronic traumatic encephalopathy, as seen in boxers. There may be headache, vertigo, defects of memory and of intellect, fatigue, insomnia and emotional instability. If parkinsonian features occur, with slurring of speech, it is then known as the *punch-drunk syndrome*, or *Homén's syndrome.*

Friedmann's disease. Relapsing spastic spinal paralysis of infancy.

Friedreich, Nikolaus (b. 1825). Heidelberg physician.

Friedreich's ataxia. A hereditary ataxia; a familial disease, usually beginning in childhood, though it may appear in early adult life, characterized by unsteadiness of gait and other movements, absent reflexes and extensor plantar response; all due to sclerosis of the posterior and lateral columns in the spinal cord.

Friedreich's change of note. A lowering of the pitch of the percussion note over a large cavity during inspiration, owing to increase in the volume of air.

Friedreich's disease, or spasm. Paramyoclonus multiplex; a form of myoclonic epilepsy.

Friedreich's foot. Pes cavus occurring in hereditary ataxia.

Friedreich's phenomenon. Skodaic resonance or high-pitched tympanitic note on percussion of the lung above the level of a pleural effusion.

Friedreich's sign. 1. Diastolic collapse of the jugular veins in adherent pericardium. 2. Friedreich's change of note (see above).

Friedrich, Paul Leopold (b. 1864). German surgeon.

Friedrich's operation. Pneumolysis; division of pleural adhesions.

Friedrich clamp. A heavy suturing clamp of modified de Petz type.

Friend, Charlotte. 20th century American virologist.

Friend disease. Swiss mouse leukaemia.

Friend virus. The organism associated with *Friend disease.* It is probably a complex of two RNA-containing viruses about 100 nm in diameter. They can be recovered from the spleens of affected mice but may not cause the disease. The virus(es) does not affect man.

fright (frite). Sudden violent fear of short duration. **Precordial fright.** The sensations of nausea and fear experienced just before the onset of an attack of manic-depressive insanity. [ME *freyt* fear.]

frigidity (frij·id·it·e). 1. Absence of bodily heat and vigour. 2. Sexual coldness. 3. Lack of animation and vivacity; coldness of manner. [L *frigidus* cold.]

frigolabile (frig·o·la·bile). Readily affected by low temperatures; able to be destroyed by cold. [L *frigus* coldness, labile.]

frigorific (frig·or·if·ik). Chilling; cooling; producing or causing a state of coldness. [L *frigus* coldness, *facere* to make.]

frigorism (frig·or·izm). A pathological condition due to the circulation being affected by exposure to extreme cold over a considerable length of time. **Local frigorism.** Trench foot. *See* FOOT. [L *frigus* coldness.]

frigostabile, frigostable (frig·o·sta·bile, frig·o·sta·bl). Resistant to low temperatures; incapable of being destroyed by exposure to cold. [L *frigus* coldness, stabile.]

frigotherapy (frig·o·ther·ap·e). Crymotherapy; the use of extreme cold as a local therapeutic measure. [L *frigus* coldness, therapy.]

frina (fre·nah). Cutaneous leishmaniasis. *See* LEISHMANIASIS.

fringe (frinj). *See* RICHARD. [see foll.]

fringing (frin·jing). A condition of the calyx of the kidney and pelvis of the ureter observable in skiagrams taken in early cases of renal tuberculosis. Bulbous deformity and tortuous lengthening of calyx and pelvis are shown. [ME *frenge* thread.]

Fritsch, Heinrich (b. 1844). Halle and Bonn gynaecologist.

Fritsch catheter, Bozeman–Fritsch catheter. A double-channel uterine catheter.

Froehde's reagent. A 1 per cent solution of ammonium molybdate in concentrated sulphuric acid. It is an alkaloidal reagent which gives different colours with various alkaloids, and is hence used to distinguish between them.

frog (frog). An amphibian of the order Anura, tailless and usually capable of leaping. They act as hosts or vectors of *Gnathostoma spinigerum* and *Trichomonas* species. **Common frog.** In Europe, *Rana temporaria*; in North America, *R. pipiens.* **Edible frog.** In Europe, *Rana esculenta.* **Rheoscopical frog.** The nerve of a muscle-nerve preparation laid across a contracting muscle; changes of potential in the latter cause a stimulus to pass along the nerve so that the muscle of the muscle-nerve preparation contracts also. **Salt frog.** Cohnheim's frog; a frog in which physiological saline solution is substituted for blood, experimentally. [AS *frogga.*]

See also: COHNHEIM.

Fröhlich, Alfred (b. 1871). Vienna physician.

Fröhlich's syndrome. Genital under-development and obesity, due to a tumour comprising the secretory cells of the anterior pituitary gland.

Frohn, Damianus (b. 1843). German physician.

Frohn's test. A test employing a solution of potassium bismuth iodide, to detect alkaloids.

Froin, Georges (b. 1874). Vienna physician.

Froin's syndrome. The cerebrospinal fluid changes in obstruction of the theca. On performing lumbar puncture below the level of the lesion, the Queckenstedt test is negative; the pressure of the fluid is low, it is xanthochromic, coagulates easily and contains a considerable excess of protein, particularly globulin. Also called the *loculation syndrome.*

frolement (frole·mahn). 1. In auscultation, e.g. in pericardial disease, the rustling type of sound that may be heard. 2. In massage, light slow friction or brushing with the palm of the hand, alternately centripetally and centrifugally. [Fr. *frôlement* brushing.]

Froment, Jules (b. 1878). French physician.

Froment's sign. In an ulnar nerve palsy, adduction of the thumb is paralysed and a sheet of paper can be gripped between index finger and thumb only by flexion of the latter at the terminal joint.

Frommann, Carl Friedrich Wilhelm (b. 1831). Heidelberg and Jena anatomist.

Frommann's line, or stria. One of the lines across the axis-cylinder of a nerve fibre near a node of Ranvier, seen after silver impregnation.

frons (fronz). The forehead. [NA]

frontal [frontalis (NA)] (frun·tal). 1. Relating or belonging to the forehead. 2. Relating to the frontal aspect or the anterior part of a body or part. **Frontal gyrus.** *See* GYRUS. **Frontal lobe.** *See* CEREBRUM. **Frontal pole.** *See* POLE. **Frontal process.** *See* PROCESS. **Frontal sinus.** *See* SINUS. **Frontal sulcus.** *See* SULCUS. **Frontal suture.** *See* SUTURE. [see prec.]

frontal bone [os frontale (NA)]. An unpaired cranial bone forming the forehead and the greater part of the orbital roof, and lying in front of the parietals.

Nasal part [pars nasalis (NA)]. A roughened area between the medial angular processes.

Cerebral surface [facies interna (NA)]. The concave surface bearing the sagittal groove, the frontal crest and the impressions for the cerebral gyri.

Frontal surface [facies external (NA)]. That part which forms the forehead.

Orbital surface [facies orbitalis (NA)]. The smooth concave surface of the orbital plate.

Temporal surface [facies temporalis (NA)]. That part which underlies the temporalis muscle.

frontal nerve [nervus frontalis (NA)]. One of the branches of the ophthalmic nerve. It supplies the forehead, conjunctiva and upper eyelid.

frontalis (fron·ta·lis). 1. Pertaining to the forehead. 2. The frontal bellies of the occipitofrontalis muscle; they are attached above and behind to the epicranial aponeurosis, and blend in front and below with the orbicularis oculi and the procerus muscles as well as gaining attachment to the skin. [L *frons* forehead.]

frontipetal (frun·tip·et·al). 1. Directed towards the front or anterior part of a body or structure. 2. Moving towards the anterior part of a body or structure. [L *frons* front, *petere* to seek.]

frontocerebellar (frun·to·ser·e·bel′·ar). Pertaining to the frontal lobe of the brain and the cerebellum.

frontomalar (frun·to·ma·lar). Relating to the frontal and the zygomatic (malar) bones.

frontomaxillary (frun·to·max·il′·ar·e). Relating or belonging to the frontal bone and the maxilla.

frontomental (frun·to·men·tal). 1. Relating to the forehead and the chin. 2. Extending from the top of the forehead to the point of the chin. [L *frons* forehead, *mentum* chin.]

frontonasal (frun·to·na·zal). Relating to the frontal sinus and the nose. **Frontonasal suture.** *See* SUTURE. [L *frons* forehead, *nasus* nose.]

frontonuchal (frun·to·new·kal). Relating to the forehead and the nape of the neck. [L *frons* forehead, *nucha* spinal cord.]

fronto-occipital (frun·to·ok·sip′·it·al). 1. Relating or belonging to the forehead and the occiput. 2. Relating to the frontal and occipital bones. **Fronto-occipital bundle.** *See* BUNDLE. [L *frons* forehead, occiput.]

frontoparietal (frun·to·par·i′·et·al). Relating or belonging to the frontal and parietal bones.

frontopontine (frun·to·pon·tine). Pertaining to the frontal lobe of the brain and the pons.

frontotemporal (frun·to·tem·por·al). Relating or belonging to the frontal and the temporal bones.

frontozygomatic (frun·to·zi·go·mat′·ik). Pertaining to the frontal and zygomatic bones.

Froriep, August von (b. 1849). Tübingen anatomist.

Froriep's ganglion. The ganglion of the 4th occipital segment, a transient feature of the developing hind-brain, occasionally persisting into adult life as a rudimentary dorsal root ganglion of the hypoglossal nerve.

Froriep's law. The skull has evolved by successive annexations of cervical vertebrae.

Froriep, Robert (b. 1804). Berlin surgeon.

Froriep's induration. Fibrosis of muscles as the result of chronic inflammation.

Frost, William Adams (b. 1853). London ophthalmologist.

Frost–Lang operation. Insertion of a glass, ivory or plastic ball into Tenon's capsule following enucleation. Its purpose is cosmetic, though the ball is often extruded later.

frostbite (**frost**·bite). A local morbid condition of varying severity, including complete gangrene, caused by freezing or partial freezing of a part due to exposure to extreme cold. [AS *frost*, *bitan*.]

froth (froth). 1. A bubbling of saliva at the lips due to nervous stimulation or disease. 2. Foam. **Bronchial froth.** The foam that rises into the mouth when there is an affection of the bronchus such as asthma. [etym. dub.]

frottage (frot·**ahzh**). 1. In massage, the rubbing movement. 2. A form of sexual perversion in the male in which an orgasm results from rubbing against or playing with women's clothing. [Fr. rubbing.]

frotteur (frot·**er**). A male sexual pervert who is addicted to frottage. [Fr. rubber.]

frozen sperm A seminal specimen submitted to deep freezing so that it can be restored to normal temperature at a later date and used for artificial insemination.

fructofuranosan (**fruk**·to·fewr·**an**'·o·san). A polymer of fructofuranose.

fructofuranose (fruk·to·**fewr**·an·oze). In sugar nomenclature, the furanose form of fructose containing the 5-membered furane ring.

fructofuranoside (fruk·to·fewr·**an**'·o·side). A fructofuranose glycoside.

fructolysis (fruk·**tol**·is·is). The breaking-down of fructose. [fructose, Gk *lysis* a loosing.]

fructopyranose (fruk·to·**pi**·ran·oze). In sugar nomenclature, the pyranose form of fructose containing the 6-membered pyran ring.

fructosamine (fruk·**to**·sam·een). Aminofructose, $CH_2OH(CHOH)_3COCH_2NH_2$. An inactive form of glucosamine prepared from the osazone of the latter. **Fructosamine 6-phosphate.** An intermediate of glycosaminoglycan synthesis.

fructosan (**fruk**·to·san). $(C_6H_{10}O_5)_n$. Term denoting a polysaccharide composed of fructose units, e.g. inulin, or dahlia starch.

fructosazone (fruk·**to**·sa·zone). An osazone formed from fructose that is identical with glucosazone.

fructose (**fruk**·toze). Laevulose, L-fructose, fruit sugar, $CH_2OH(CHOH)_3COCH_2OH$. A ketohexose, isomeric with D-glucose, and occurring with the latter in sweet fruits, flowers and honey. It is metabolized in the liver through fructokinase and in other tissues through hexokinase. Obtained also by the inversion of cane sugar or the hydrolysis of inulin; it is given in cases of diabetes. It is laevorotatory: there is also a dextrorotatory unfermentable L-fructose, and an inactive form known as *acrose* or *formose* which is synthesized from formaldehyde. Fructose is sweeter than glucose and fermentable. It is secreted by the seminal vesicles and is present in semen. **Fructose diphosphate.** Harden–Young ester. **Fructose 1,6-diphosphate.** A glycolytic intermediate. **Fructose monophosphate.** Neuberg ester. **Fructose 1-phosphate.** The immediate product of fructose phosphorylation in the liver. **Fructose 6-phosphate.** A glycolytic intermediate held in equilibrium with glucose 6-phosphate by phosphoglucose isomerase.

fructosidase (fruk·**to**·sid·aze). An enzyme which hydrolyses a fructoside.

fructoside (**fruk**·to·side). A compound analogous to a glucoside, but containing fructose units instead of glucose.

fructosuria (fruk·to·**sewr**·e·ah). A condition in which fructose is present in the urine. **Essential fructosuria.** A rare condition in which fructose is excreted in the urine without glucose. It may be accompanied by symptoms of diabetes.

fructovegetative (fruk·to·**vej**·e·ta·tiv). Comprising fruit and vegetables, e.g. a diet. [L *fructus* fruit, vegetable.]

frugivorous (froo·**jiv**·er·us). Feeding on fruit. [L *frux* fruit, *vorare* to devour.]

fruitarian (froo·**ta**·re·an). An individual whose diet consists entirely, or almost entirely, of fruit and nuts. [L *fructus* fruit.]

frumentaceous (froo·men·**ta**·shus). 1. Made of or belonging to wheat or other grain. 2. Resembling grain. [L *frumentum* corn.]

frumentum (froo·**men**·tum). Any kind of grain. [L corn.]

Frusemide BP 1973 (**froo**·sem·ide). A powerful diuretic acting by reducing the resorption of electrolytes by the renal tubule. Used, with other drugs, to abolish the oedema of cardiac failure and in the treatment of disorders caused by arterial hypertension.

frustrate (**frus**·trate). Applied to the heart beat or to an intermission of the pulse, one that because premature contraction of the ventricle is so feeble the beat fails to reach the wrist. [L *frustra* in vain.]

frustration (frus·**tra**·shun). 1. The defeating of a purpose. 2. In psychological medicine, term meaning the inability of a subject to gratify a desire or put an urge into effect. 3. The hindering of someone from acting in the way that he wishes to act. [see prec.]

Fuchs, Ernst (b. 1851). Vienna ophthalmologist.

angle of Fuchs. The angle between the superficial and deep mesodermal layers near the pupil margin.

Fuchs' coloboma. A defect of crescent shape in the choroid at the lower part of the optic disc. The affected eye is often found to have defective vision and is usually hypermetropic and astigmatic.

Fuchs' dimple. One of several transient shallow elliptical excavations on the cornea near its margin; present in the elderly.

Fuchs' corneal dystrophy. A combined endothelial and epithelial dystrophy with stromal oedema and clouding.

Fuchs' operation. 1. Permanent tarsorrhaphy at the canthal angle, best suited for the outer: both lid margins are split and the cilia removed; a triangular portion of skin is removed from the upper lid, into which a triangular flap from the lower is stitched with a mattress suture through the tarsal plate. 2. Blepharoplasty for cicatricial ectropion of both lids: a combination of Fricke's operation for upper and Dieffenbach's operation for lower lid. 3. For iris bombé with secondary glaucoma: a Graefe knife is passed across the anterior chamber from limbus to limbus so perforating the bulging iris in four places.

Fuchs' black spot. Choroidal changes in myopia.

Fuchs' stomata. The openings of small interstitial spaces in the iris on to its anterior surface near the circumference.

Fuchs' syndrome. Heterochromic cyclitis. *See* CYCLITIS.

Dalen–Fuchs nodules. Nodules formed in the pigment epithelium of the iris and choroid in sympathetic ophthalmitis. The cells of the epithelium swell up and proliferate, and are finally invaded by lymphocytes and epithelioid cells, so forming nodules.

Fuchs, Hans J. 20th century German physician.

Fuchs' test. *See* TEST FOR CANCER.

fuchsin (**fook**·sin). Fuchsine.

fuchsine (**fook**·seen). Magenta BPC 1959, aniline red, rubine. A mixture of pararosaniline and rosaniline hydrochlorides; used in the mordantless dyeing of wool and silk, and as a stain for *Mycobacterium tuberculosis.* It is also a powerful germicide used in the treatment of varicose ulcers, burns, carbuncles and impetigo. **Acid fuchsine.** Acid magenta, a mixture of the sodium and ammonium salts of the di- and trisulphonic acids of pararosaniline and rosaniline; used as a food dye and as an indicator (Andrade) in bacteriological work. **Basic fuchsine.** A mixture of parafuchsine and rosaniline. **Carbol fuchsine.** Carbolfuchsine. **Diamond fuchsine.** Basic fuchsine (see above). **English fuchsine.** Roseine, rosaniline and pararosaniline acetates. **Fuchsine N.B.** New fuchsine (see below). **New fuchsine.** Triamino-*o*-tritolylmethane, a basic dye used as a stain. **Triphenyl fuchsine.** Aniline blue, a brilliant dye prepared from rosaniline. [Leonard *Fuchs*, 16th century German botanist.]

fuchsinophil (fook·**sin**·o·fil). Having an affinity for acid or basic fuchsine dyes, as in the case of muscle fibres, red blood cells and various cytoplasmic granules. [fuchsine, Gk *philein* to love.]

fuchsinophilic, fuchsinophilous (**fook**·sin·o·**fil**'·ik, fook·sin·**of**·il·us). Applied to any tissue which takes a fuchsine stain easily. [see prec.]

fuchsonium (fook·**so**·ne·um). Applied to a series of sulphonated derivatives of fuchsine. They are used in the treatment of vaginal discharge.

fucosan (**few**·ko·san). $(C_6H_{10}O_4)_n$, a pentosan composed of fucose units which occurs in bladderwrack, *Fucus vesiculosus*, and other species of marine algae.

fucose (**few**·kose). $CH_3(CHOH)_4CHO$, a methyl pentose which occurs in seaweeds; isomeric with rhodeose.

fucosterol (few·**kos**·ter·ol). $C_{29}H_{48}O_2$, a sterol contained in bladderwrack, *Fucus vesiculosus*, and other species of *Fucus*, *Laminaria* and *Ascophyllum*.

fucoxanthin (few·ko·**zan**·thin). $C_{40}H_{56}O_6$, a carotenoid which constitutes the brown colouring matter in marine algae.

Fucus (**few**·kus). 1. A genus of seaweeds (family Fucaceae) belonging to the Phaeophyceae (Brown Algae). *Fucus serratus* Linn. and *F. vesiculosus* Linn. are used as sources of alginic acid. 2. Fucus BPC 1949 (bladderwrack, seawrack, kelpware), *Fucus vesiculosus* Linn. gathered from growing plants and dried. It has been employed as a remedy for certain types of obesity owing to the varying small amounts of iodine which it contains. [L seaweed.]

fucusaldehyde, fucusol (few·kus·**al**·de·hide, **few**·kus·ol). C_4H_3OCHO, an oily compound obtained from seaweed.

Fuerbringer, Paul (b. 1849). Berlin physician.

Fuerbringer's sign. The respiratory movements are transmitted by a needle inserted into a subphrenic abscess but not if the abscess is above the diaphragm.

Fuerstner, Carl (b. 1848). Heidelberg and Strasbourg psychiatrist.

Fuerstner's disease. A pseudospastic paralysis with tremor.

fugacious (few·**ga**·shus). 1. In biology, lasting for only a short time, fading early, or falling-off early. 2. Fleeting; volatile. [L *fugere* to flee.]

fugitive (**few**·jit·iv). 1. Transient. 2. Volatile. 3. Inconstant. 4. Wandering, as a pain. [see prec.]

fugue (fewg). A condition in which consciousness is disturbed. The sufferer acts apparently with volition and may lead an ordinary and natural life during the duration of the state; when consciousness returns to normal he cannot remember anything about his disturbed state or about himself while he was in it. **Epileptic fugue.** A fugue that may take the place of or precede an epileptic seizure. **Hysterical fugue.** A state of hysteria under the impulse of which the patient wanders away from home and may forget, or may say he forgets, everything connected with himself—name, circumstances and so on. [L *fuga* a fleeing.]

Fukala, Vincenz (b. 1847). Vienna ophthalmologist.

Fukala's operation. Lens extraction in high myopia when postoperative uncorrected visual acuity may be adequate.

fulgurant, fulgurating (**ful**·gewr·ant, **ful**·gewr·a·ting). 1. Sudden and quickly past like a flash of lightning. 2. Of pain, intense, sudden and lancinating. [see foll.]

fulguration (ful·gewr·**a**·shun). Superficial destruction of tissue by electrical sparks contracted by a movable electrode. **Direct fulguration.** Fulguration in which the electrode is connected to a uniterminal high-frequency high-voltage apparatus and the spark passes from the electrode to the patient. **Indirect fulguration.** That in which the patient is connected to a uniterminal high-frequency high-voltage apparatus and the spark is drawn by a suitable pointed earth connection. [L *fulgur* lightning.]

fulgurize (**ful**·gewr·ize). To treat morbid tissue by fulguration. [see prec.]

fuliginous (few·**lij**·in·us). Dark or dusky like smoke, or sooty. The term may be used to denote lips which are encrusted with black scabs, typical of certain diseases. [L *fuligo* soot.]

Fuller, Eugene (b. 1858). New York urologist.

Fuller's operation. Suprapubic enucleation of the enlarged prostate. One of the earliest claimants to the suprapubic operation (1895).

Fuller cell. A two-fluid modification of the bichromate cell (*see* CELL) adapted for long-continued use. One plate is of carbon, immersed in the same fluid as used in the bichromate cell, and the other plate is of zinc cast on to a copper rod. The zinc is amalgamated with mercury, and immersed in dilute sulphuric acid.

fulminant, fulminating (**ful**·min·ant, **ful**·min·a·ting). Sudden, intense and stabbing, as the pains of tabes dorsalis; foudroyant. [L *fulminare* to flash like lightning.]

Fumagillin (few·mah·**jil**·in). BP Commission approved name for an antibiotic product of some strains of *Aspergillus fumigatus*. It has been used in the treatment of amoebiasis.

fumarase (**few**·mar·aze). Fumarate hydratase.

fumarate hydratase (**few**·mar·ate **hi**·drat·aze). An enzyme of the citric acid cycle; it catalyses the reversible hydration of fumarate with production of L-malate.

fumarine (**few**·mar·een). Protopine, $C_{20}H_{19}O_5N$. An alkaloid occurring in opium, and certain plants, particularly *Dicentra spectabilis*. It is a compound of the isoquinoline group, with local anaesthetic properties and causing convulsions of an epileptiform character.

fumigacin (few·**mig**·a·sin). An antibiotic produced by *Aspergillus fumigatus* which is active mainly against staphylococci but is too toxic for parenteral administration. It appears to be the lactone of helvolic acid.

fumigant (**few**·mig·ant). A vaporizing substance used in fumigation. [L *fumigare* to expose to smoke.]

fumigatin (few·mig·**a**·tin). Hydroxymethoxy toluquinone, $CH_3C_6HO_2(OH)OCH_3$. A substance produced in cultures of *Aspergillus fumigatus*, which has bactericidal properties.

fumigation (few·mig·**a**·shun). The process of disinfecting, e.g. a room and all its contents, by setting free the fumes of a volatile substance such as sulphur. [L *fumigare* to expose to smoke.]

function (**fungk**·shun). 1. The particular office of an organ or tissue, e.g. the function of the eye is vision. 2. In chemistry, any substance with the properties characteristic of a certain radical, e.g. an alcohol. 3. In mathematics, any variable the value of which depends upon the value of another variable; it is expressed $y = f(x)$. **Allomeric function.** The function of the spinal cord and medulla taken as a whole. **Isomeric function.** The function of any particular section of the spinal cord. [L *functio* performance.]

functional (**fungk**·shun·al). 1. Relating or belonging to a function or to function. 2. Connected with or affecting the function of an organ or part but not involving the structure; it has thus come to mean psychic rather than somatic in reference to a symptom or a symptom complex. 3. In biology, regularly performing its function.

functionating (**fungk**·shun·a·ting). With reference to any organ or part, performing full and proper function.

funda (**fun**·dah) (pl. *fundae*). A four-tailed bandage. [L sling.]

fundal (**fun**·dal). Relating or belonging to a fundus.

fundament (**fun**·dah·ment). 1. The buttocks. 2. In anatomy, the anus and the anal region. 3. The base of a part or structure. [L *fundamentum* foundation.]

fundamental (fun·dah·**men**·tal). 1. Relating or belonging to the base of a structure or part. 2. Serving as a base or foundation. 3. Essential. 4. Basic. 5. Elementary. [see prec.]

fundectomy (fund·**ek**·to·me). Surgical removal of the fundus of any organ. [fundus, Gk *ektome* a cutting out.]

fundic (**fun**·dik). Having relation or belonging to a fundus.

fundiform (**fun**·de·form). Loop-shaped, like a sling. [L *funda* sling, form.]

Fundulus (**fun**·dew·lus). A genus of marine fish; killifish. *Fundulus heteroclitus* has been used as a laboratory animal.

fundus [NA] (**fun**·dus) (pl. *fundi*). The bottom or base of an organ; the part which is farthest from the aperture. **Albinotic fundus.**

The fundus of the eye in albinism, when there is absence of choroidal and retinal pigment. **Fundus albipunctatus.** The non-progressive form of albipunctate dystrophy. **Fundus of the eye.** The inner aspect of the posterior part of the eye; it comprises the retina, optic disc and those parts of the choroid and sclera visible through the pupil. **Fundus flavimaculatus.** Yellow-white irregular-shaped spots in the fundus of the eye, stationary or very slowly progressive. There may be macular degeneration. **Fundus of the gall bladder.** *See* GALL BLADDER. **Fundus of a hair follicle.** *See* FOLLICLE. **Fundus of the internal auditory meatus.** *See* MEATUS. **Pepper and salt fundus.** Term describing a fine dusting of the peripheral retina with light and dark spots, seen in congenital syphilis. **Fundus of the stomach.** *See* STOMACH. **Tessellated fundus, Fundus tigré.** The appearance of the fundus when retinal pigment is sparse or absent, but choroidal pigment is present. The choroidal vessels are then seen as red streaks against a background of pigment. The condition may be physiological or pathological. **Fundus of the uterus.** *See* UTERUS. [L bottom.]

funduscopy (fun·dus·ko·pe). Ophthalmoscopic examination of the ocular fundus. [fundus, Gk *skopein* to view.]

fundusectomy (fun·dus·**ek**·to·me). Surgical removal of the cardiac portion of the stomach. [fundus, Gk *ektome* a cutting out.]

fungaemia (fung·ge·me·ah). A condition in which fungi are present in the blood. [fungus, Gk *haima* blood.]

fungal (fung·gal). Fungous.

fungate (fung·gate). 1. Rapidly to undergo granulation, as a sore. 2. To spring up or grow exuberantly, like a fungus; term applied to certain morbid growths. [L *fungus* mushroom.]

fungating (fung·ga·ting). Denoting ulcers or sores which have a spongy fungus-like appearance.

fungi (fung·gi). Plural of fungus. **Fungi Imperfecti.** Those fungi which have no known form of sexual reproduction, and cannot be classified in the three main groups, the Phycomycetes, Ascomycetes and Basidiomycetes. Almost all the fungi pathogenic for man and animals are imperfect. **Kefir fungi.** Grains composed of symbiotic growths of yeast cells and *Lactobacillus caucasicus*, used to produce the alcoholic fermentation of milk called *kefir*.

fungicidal (funj·e·si·dal). Destructive of fungi. [see foll.]

fungicide (funj·e·side). Any agent able to destroy fungi. [fungus, L *caedere* to kill.]

fungiform (funj·e·form). Like a mushroom in shape. [fungus, form.]

fungistasis (funj·is·tas·is). The checking or arrest of a fungus growth. [fungus, Gk *stasis* a standing still.]

fungistat (funj·e·stat). Term applied to any substance which arrests or holds in check the growth of fungi. [see foll.]

fungistatic (funj·e·**stat**·ik). Holding in check or arresting the growth of fungi. [fungus, Gk *statikos* standing.]

fungisterol (funj·is·ter·ol). $C_{25}H_{40}O$, a colourless sterol occurring in ergot.

fungoid (fung·goid). 1. Characteristic of a fungus. 2. Shaped like or having resemblance to a mushroom or fungus, as certain exuberant growths on the body surface. [fungus, Gk *eidos* form.]

fungosity (fung·**gos**·it·e). 1. A spongy fungus-like growth. 2. The quality or state of being fungous.

fungous (fung·gus). Resembling, characteristic of or belonging to a fungus or fungi; term applied to growths which appear suddenly, grow rapidly and are soft in texture.

fungus (fung·gus) (pl. *fungi*). 1. One of a group of non-vascular plants which lack chlorophyll and whose reproductive and vegetative structures do not permit them to be included in the algae or the higher plants. 2. Any growth or protrusion resembling a fungus in form. **Alpha fungus, Beta fungus, Gamma fungus.** Convenient designations for three different types of a species. Among other instances, they have been applied to the varieties of *Trichophyton schoenleinii* and *T. rubrum*. **Fungus of the brain.** Protrusion of cerebral tissue through an opening, usually traumatic, in the skull, dura and scalp. **Chignon fungus.** A fungus causing chignon disease or piedra. **Cutaneous fungus.** Any fungus which lives parasitically on the skin, e.g. ringworm fungi, and several other groups. **Disease fungus.** A pathogenic fungus. **Fungus of the dura mater.** Protrusion of cerebral tissue still in the dural covering through an opening in the skull and scalp. **Fission fungus.** Schizomycetes, or bacteria. **Foot fungus.** A name applied to fungi causing mycetoma or other foot infections, e.g. athletes' foot. **Fungus haematodes.** Name formerly applied to an ulcerating proliferative tumour. **Mosaic fungus.** An artefact seen chiefly in preparations of skin scales mounted in caustic-potash solution in which the deposition of cholesterol crystals in the margins of the cells gives the impression of a highly refractile network resembling fungal mycelium. **Mould fungus.** One with a well-developed aerial mycelium. **Ray fungus.** Actinomyces, so named because of the radial or star-like structure of the parasitic colony seen in the actinomycotic lesion. **Slime fungus.** Slime mould or myxomycete. **Fungus testis.** A protrusion from a scrotal sinus of granulation tissue which may resemble the corpus testis. The condition is a result of chronic inflammation, tuberculous or non-tuberculous, and is not to be confused with the exposure of the testis which may follow gangrene of the scrotum. **Thread fungus.** A name applied to fungi having a slender thread-like thallus. In a more restricted sense it is applied to the actinomycetes or ray fungi. **Thrush fungus.** *Candida albicans*. [L.]

funic (few·nik). 1. Referring or relating to a cord-like structure or funis. 2. Referring or belonging to the umbilical cord. [L *funis* cord.]

funicle (few·nikl). 1. Funiculus. 2. Any slender cord-like structure. [L *funiculus* little cord.]

funicular (few·**nik**·ew·lar). 1. Relating or belonging to a funiculus. 2. Having relation to the umbilical cord or the spermatic cord. 3. Funic. [see prec.]

funiculate (few·**nik**·ew·late). Having a funiculus; forming a funiculus.

funiculitis (few·**nik**·ew·li′·tis). 1. An inflamed condition of any funiculus, particularly the spermatic cord. 2. Inflammation of the root of a spinal nerve within the vertebral canal. **Endemic funiculitis.** Lymphangitis of the spermatic cord occurring in Sri Lanka, Egypt and southern India, marked by acute tenderness and swelling and inflammation of the scrotum and cord; a fatal termination is to be expected unless prompt operation is undertaken. [funiculus, Gk *-itis* inflammation.]

funiculopexy (few·**nik**·ew·lo·pex·e). The operative procedure in which the spermatic cord is sutured to the surrounding tissues in radical treatment of undescended testis. [funiculus, Gk *pexis* fixation.]

funiculus [L.] (few·**nik**·ew·lus). 1. One of the bundles of fibres surrounded by perineurium, which make up a peripheral nerve trunk. 2. The term is also used as synonymous with fasciculus. [L little cord.]

See also: ROLANDO.

funiform (few·ne·form). Rope-like, cord-like, i.e. flexible and tough. [funis, form.]

funis (few·nis). 1. The umbilical cord. 2. Any rope-like or cord-like structure. **Funis argenteus.** The spinal cord. **Funis brachii.** The median cubital vein. **Funis hippocratis.** The tendo calcaneus. [L cord.]

funnel (fun·el). A glass or porcelain cone employed in chemistry for filtering and also for pouring liquids from one container into another. **Mitral funnel.** A funnel-shaped narrowing of the mitral-valve orifice due to rheumatic endocarditis; the valve is rigid and stenotic. [L *fundere* to pour.]

fur (fer). The covering of morbid matter, mainly epithelium and mucus, observed on the tongue in various diseases and disorders, particularly those involving the alimentary tract. [ME *furre* sheath.]

fural (fewr·al). 1. Furfural. 2. The radical C_4H_3OCH=derived from furfural.

furaldehyde (fer·**al**·de·hide). Furfural.

furan (fewr·an). Furane.

furane (fewr·ane). Furfurane, $\overline{OCH{-}CHCH{-}CH}$. A colourless liquid with a smell of chloroform, obtained from wood tar or by distilling sugar with lime. It is a 5-membered ring compound, and can be regarded as the parent of the furanose sugars.

furanose (fewr·an·oze). General term in sugar nomenclature, denoting a sugar that contains a 5-membered furane ring.

Furazolidone (fewr·az·o·lid·one). BP Commission approved name for 3 - (5 - nitrofurfurylideneamino)oxazolidin - 2 - one; it is used in the treatment of diarrhoea.

furca (fer·kah). 1. A fork. 2. In embryology, the first trace of the backward ossified extension of the primary membrane from which the orbit of the eye develops. [L fork.]

furcal, furcate (fer·kal, fer·kate). 1. Forked. 2. Branching like a fork into two equal parts. [see prec.]

furcocercous (fer·ko·ser·kus). Having a bifid tail or a forked tail. [L *furca* fork, *kerkos* tail.]

furcula (fer·kew·lah). In embryology, the arched ridge or inverted U-shaped structure within which a groove develops to form the lower part of the larynx and other respiratory organs. [L little fork.]

Furethidine (fewr·eth·id·een). BP Commission approved name for ethyl - 4 - phenyl - 1 - [2 - (tetrahydrofurfuryloxy)ethyl] - piperidine - 4 - carboxylate; a narcotic analgesic.

furfur (fer·fer). 1. Dandruff. 2. Any epidermal scale. 3. Porrigo; any scalp disease such as ringworm. 4. The bran of grain. [L bran.]

furfuraceous (fer·fewr·a·shus). 1. Scurfy; scaly. 2. Having resemblance to bran or dandruff; a term applied to desquamation. [see prec.]

furfural, furfuraldehyde (fer·fewr·al, fer·fewr·al·de·hide). Fural, C_4H_3OCHO. A colourless oily liquid with the character of an aromatic aldehyde, and moderately volatile. It is readily formed by the action of strong acid on carbohydrates and those proteins containing the carbohydrate group or by the distillation of bran. Its violet colour reaction with an alcoholic solution of α-naphthol forms the basis of a test for carbohydrates and certain proteins (Molisch's). It is used as an industrial solvent. Irritant to the eyes and mucous membranes, its administration by mouth to animals causes death from pulmonary oedema. [L *furfur* bran.]

furfuran, furfurane (fer·fewr·an, fer·fewr·ane). Furan.

furfurol (fer·fewr·ol). Furfural.

furfurous (fer·fewr·us). Furfuraceous.

furfuryl (fer·fewr·il). The organic radical, $C_4H_3OCH_2$, derived from furfuryl alcohol. **Furfuryl alcohol.** $C_4H_3OCH_2OH$. An alcohol which occurs in clove oil and in roasted coffee.

furibund (fewr·e·bund). 1. Applied to certain insane persons who are subject to fits of rage or frenzy. 2. Maniacal. [L *furibundus* raging.]

furor (few·ror). 1. Fury. 2. A maniacal fit of rage. 3. Insanity; madness. **Furor amatorius.** Unrestrainable sexual desire. **Furor epilepticus.** The fit of strong or furious unprovoked anger to which epileptics may be subject during an attack. **Furor femininus.** Nymphomania. **Furor genitalis.** Erotomania. **Paroxysmal furor.** Furor epilepticus (see above). **Furor tropicus.** A fit of uncontrolled anger that may occur in the white tropical sojourner. It is a behaviouristic display, probably caused by a constitutional failure of adaptation to social and environmental conditions in tropical countries, including, but not predominantly, the climatic conditions. **Furor uterinus.** Nymphomania. [L fury.]

furred (ferd). Having a coating of dust-coloured morbid matter, mainly epithelial and mucous, e.g. the tongue. [ME *furre* sheath.]

furrow (fer·o). A groove. **Genital furrow.** A longitudinal groove on the under-surface of the genital tubercle of the early fetus. **Gluteal furrow.** Fold of the buttock. **Nuchal furrow.** The median groove at the nape of the neck. **Primitive furrow.** A groove along the middle of the primitive streak. [AS *furh.*]

See also: HARRISON (E.), JADELOT, LIEBERMEISTER, SCHMORL, SIBSON.

furuncle (fewr·ungkl). A localized infection of the skin and subcutaneous tissue with *Staphylococcus aureus,* usually through a hair follicle, and characterized by the formation of a central necrotic core. It occurs particularly in dense integuments such as the back of the neck and the back. **Lochial furuncle.** A furuncle affecting midwives and obstetrical nurses and due to infection from the lochia. **Physician's furuncle.** An abscess or ulcer affecting surgeons and physicians and caused by infection from operative procedures or the handling of a cadaver. [furunculus.]

furuncular (fewr·ung·ew·lar). Belonging or relating to, or having the character of a furuncle.

furunculoid (fewr·ung·kew·loid). Resembling a furuncle; like a boil. [furunculus, Gk *eidos* form.]

furunculosis (fewr·ung·kew·lo'·sis). 1. The unhealthy condition with which the occurrence of a number of furuncles or boils is associated. 2. A condition of being affected with furuncles. **Furunculosis blastomycetica, Furunculosis cryptococcica.** A form of blastomycosis in which the superficial nodules resemble furuncles. **Furunculosis multiplex infantum.** An impetiginous condition with multiple minute abscesses, not uncommon in neglected marasmic children. **Furunculosis orientalis.** Cutaneous leishmaniasis. *See* LEISHMANIASIS. [furunculus, Gk *-osis* condition.]

furunculous (fewr·ung·kew·lus). Marked by the presence or repeated recurrence of furuncles or boils.

furunculus (fewr·ung·kew·lus). A furuncle. **Furunculus gangraenescens, Furunculus gangraenosus, Furunculus malignus.** Anthrax. **Furunculus orientalis.** Cutaneous leishmaniasis. **Furunculus vespajus.** A large painless furuncle which, instead of a central core of suppuration, has a number of small cavities through which the pus is exuded: the cavities are supposed to resemble the openings into a wasp's nest. **Furunculus vulgaris.** Carbuncle. [L a boil.]

Fusafungine (few·sah·fun·jeen). BP Commission approved name for an antibiotic produced by *Fusarium lateritium* 437.

Fusarium (few·sa·re·um). A genus of moulds. Some of the species may act as airborne allergens. **Fusarium lateritium.** The source of the antibiotic, fusafungine. *Fusarium solani* and *F. oxysporum* can cause mycotic keratitis; *F. solani* and *F. poae* have been isolated from white grain mycetomas; *F. sporotrichoides* var. *toxica* may cause alimentary toxic anaemia in animals fed contaminated foodstuffs. [L *fusus* spindle.]

fuscin (fus·in). The dark pigment of the retinal epithelium. [L *fuscus* brown.]

Fuse's nucleus. A centre for co-ordinating the movements of the external rectus muscle of one eye with the internal rectus of the other, in lateral conjugate movements. It lies between the 6th cranial-nerve nucleus and the medial vestibular nucleus, and is also called the *pontine centre for co-ordination of the movements.*

fuse (fewz). 1. To melt. 2. A wire of low melting point inserted in an electrical circuit as a precaution against overloading: its resistance is such that, beyond a certain limit, the current will melt it, thereby causing an automatic interruption. 3. A tube containing combustible material, used to ignite an explosive charge. 4. To blend. [L *fundere* to pour.]

fuseau (few·so). A spindle-shaped spore of the genus *Trichophyton.* [Fr. spindle.]

fusible (few·zibl). Of a substance, capable of being liquefied or melted. [L *fundere* to pour.]

fusicellular (few·ze·sel·ew·lar). Fusocellular.

Fusidium coccineum (few·sid·e·um·kok·sin·e·um). A micro-organism which produces fusidic acid, from which the antibiotic substances sodium fusidate and diethanolamine fusidate are synthesized.

fusiform (few·ze·form). Shaped like a spindle, i.e. tapered at the two ends. [L *fusus* spindle, form.]

Fusiformis (few·zi·for·mis). A genus of anaerobic obligatory parasites closely related to the genera *Corynebacterium* and *Pfeifferella.* **Fusiformis fragilis.** An organism that has been found infrequently in association with acute appendicitis; it is pathogenic to guinea-pigs and rabbits. **Fusiformis fusiformis.** A species found in necrotic and ulcerating lesions in association with *Borrelia vincenti,* e.g. in ulcus tropicum. **Fusiformis necrophorus.** A species found in necrotic lesions in animals and only rarely in man. [see prec.]

fusion (few·zhun). 1. Melting; the running together of several things, as in the melting of an ore with a flux. 2. In orthopaedics, ankylosis produced by operation; arthrodesis. **Binocular fusion.** The combination into a single image of the separate ones seen by each eye. **Centric fusion, Centromeric fusion.** Translocation. **Diaphyseal-epiphyseal fusion.** An operation to obliterate the epiphyseal line and thus obtain union between the epiphyseal and diaphyseal bone. **Naviculo-cuneiform fusion.** Arthrodesis at the naviculocuneiform joint, for flat foot. **Nerve fusion.** A method of anastomosis of the cut ends of injured peripheral nerves to allow regeneration; the term is rarely used now. **Spinal fusion.** An operation to obtain bony fusion between two or more vertebrae. [L *fundere* to pour.]

fusional (few·zhun·al). Characterized by fusion.

Fusobacterium (few·zo·bak·teer'·e·um). Of the 6 members of this genus in the family Bacteroidaceae only one, *Fusobacterium fusiforme,* is pathogenic for man as an associate with *Borrelia vincenti* in Vincent's angina. It is a large cigar-shaped non-motile Gram-negative bacillus, strictly anaerobic and grown with difficulty on enriched culture media. [L *fusus* spindle, bacterium.]

fusocellular (few·zo·**sel**·ew·lar). Having cells shaped like a spindle. [L *fusus* spindle, cell.]

fusospirillary (few·zo·spi·ril'·ar·e). Designating associated fusiform and spirochaetal organisms such as those present in Vincent's angina.

fusospirillosis (few·zo·spi·ril·o'·sis). Fusospirochaetosis. [fusiform, spirochaete, Gk *-osis* condition.]

fusospirochaetal (few·zo·spi·ro·ke'·tal). Relating to infection with fusiform bacilli and spirochaetes.

fusospirochaetosis (few·zo·spi·ro·ke·to'·sis). Infection with Vincent's organisms. [fusiform, spirochaete, Gk *-osis* condition.]

fusostreptococcicosis (few·zo·**strep**·to·kok·sik·**o**'·sis). The condition of being infected with fusiform bacilli and streptococci. [fusiform, streptococcus, Gk *-osis* condition.]

fustic (fus·tik). Fustic wood; the wood of *Morus tinctoria,* and a source of a yellow colouring matter. [Ar. *fustuq.*]

fustigation (fus·tig·a·shun). A form of massage which consists in beating the surface of the body or part with light rods. **Electric fustigation.** Massage by light quick tapping of the part with the electrodes of an induced current. [L *fustigare* to cudgel.]

fustin (fus·tin). 1. Fustic. 2. A yellow glucoside which occurs in the wood of Venetian sumach, *Rhus cotinus.* 3. The yellow pigment of the male fern, *Aspidium filix-mas.*

fututrix (few·**tew**·trix). The active female partner in tribadism. [L.]

G

Gabastou's hydraulic method. The umbilical cord is injected with warm saline in cases of retained placenta, and this is said to hasten separation of the placenta.

Gabriel, William Bashall (b. 1893). London surgeon.

Gabriel's operation. Perineal excision of the rectum.

Gabriel's proctoscope. A long proctoscope for the high injection of haemorrhoids.

Gabritschewsky's vaccine. A vaccine of streptococci suspended in the broth in which they were grown, and therefore likely to contain Dick toxin. It was first used for active immunization against scarlet fever in 1907, about 16 years before the discovery of Dick toxin, but is now obsolete.

Gadberry's mixture. Spleen mixture; quinine sulphate, potassium nitrate, ferrous sulphate and a trace of nitric acid, used as a tonic, and as an antiperiodic against malaria.

gadfly (**gad**·fli). Large flies of the genus *Tabanus*, of worldwide distribution. The females alone bite, many species attacking man and causing painful wounds. None act as true secondary hosts to human parasites, but they may serve mechanically in transferring infested blood. [ME *gad* spike, AS *flyge* fly.]

gadinine (**gad**·in·een). $C_7H_{16}NO_2$, a ptomaine derived from putrefying fish, especially cod. [L *gadus* cod.]

gadolinite (gad·o·lin·ite). A mineral earth consisting of the silicates of iron, beryllium, yttrium, erbium and other rare-earth metals. It is found mainly in Scandinavia and Brazil. [see foll.]

gadolinium (gad·o·**lin**·e·um). An element of the rare-earth series with atomic weight 157.25, atomic number 64, and chemical symbol Gd. It is a metal with a valency of 3. [Johan *Gadolin* (b. 1760), Finnish chemist.]

gaduin (**gad**·ew·in). $C_{35}H_{46}O_9$, a fatty substance derived from cod-liver oil. [L *gadus* cod.]

Gadus (ga·dus). A genus of salt-water fishes; many species are important as food. **Gadus morrhua.** The cod. [L cod.]

Gaenslen, Frederick Julius (b. 1877). Milwaukee surgeon.

Gaenslen's sign. Pain on hyperextension of the hip with pelvis fixed by flexion of the opposite hip.

Gaertner, August (b. 1848). Jena hygienist.

Gaertner's bacillus. *Salmonella enteritidis.*

Gaertner, Gustav (b. 1855). Vienna pathologist.

Gaertner's phenomenon. If the arm is raised with the subject lying at 45 degrees, the level above the sternal angle at which the superficial veins collapse is a rough guide to the height of the central venous pressure, in the absence of venous obstruction or gross tricuspid incompetence.

Gaertner's tonometer. A tonometer for measuring digital blood pressure.

gafeira (gaf·a·e·rah). A name for leprosy. [South American term.]

Gaffky, Georg Theodor August (b. 1850). Berlin bacteriologist.

Gaffky scale. An arbitrary scale for assessing the number of tubercle bacilli in sputum and utilizing this information for prognosis. There are 10 grades, referred to by Roman numerals, running from I, less than 5 bacilli in the whole smear, to X, more than 100 bacilli per 1/12-in (2.1mm) oil-immersion field.

Gaffkya (**gaf**·ke·ah). A genetic name for parasitic organisms (family Coccaceae) commonly found in the respiratory tract of man. They are Gram-positive cocci, occurring in tetrads, and are of doubtful, feeble pathogenicity; not widely accepted in the UK. **Gaffkya tetragena.** *Micrococcus tetragenus*, Gram-positive spheres found on the mucous membrane of the upper respiratory tract. Also called *Staphylococcus tetragenus.* [Georg Theodor August *Gaffky.*]

gag (gag). A device for separating the jaws and opening the mouth. It is usually fitted with a ratchet or similar fixing arrangement, and is used in dentistry, surgery and the administration of anaesthetics. **Incisor gag.** A gag designed to be applied to the incisor or front teeth. **Molar gag.** A gag designed to be applied to the molar or back teeth. [name imitative of choking sound.]

See also: BOYLE (H. E. G.), DOTT, DOYEN, FERGUSON, MASON, SHADWELL, SYDENHAM, WAUGH.

gage (gaje). Gauge.

gaile (gale). Scabies.

Gaillard, François Lucien (b. 1805). Poitiers surgeon.

Gaillard-Arlt sutures. For ectropion: 2 double-armed sutures passed through the conjunctiva at the edge of the tarsus nearest the eyelid margin and then brought out through the skin well below the lid, and tied over a roll of gauze.

Gaillard's syndrome. Displacement of the heart into the right hemithorax as a result of traction from adhesions, pulmonary collapse, etc.; often called pseudodextrocardia to distinguish it from true dextrocardia resulting from congenital dextroposition of the heart with rotation of the cardiac chambers, or a complete mirror image of the normal cardiac position.

Gairdner, Sir William Tennant (b. 1824). Scottish physician.

Gairdner's test. Coin test. *See* TEST.

Gaisboeck, Felix (b. 1868). Innsbruck physician.

Gaisboeck's disease or syndrome. Polycythaemia hypertonica; polycythaemia associated with increased blood pressure, without enlargement of the spleen.

gait (gate). The manner of walking. **Antalgic gait.** The limp occurring in pseudocoxalgia. **Ataxic gait.** An unsteady gait. In sensory ataxia due to disease of the posterior columns of the cord, the feet are lifted high and are brought suddenly to the ground; the patient is much more unsteady in the dark. **Cerebellar gait.** A staggering, drunken gait, in which the subject walks on a wide base and has particular difficulty in turning; due to disease of the cerebellum or cerebellar pathways. **Dromedary gait.** The gait in cases of dystonia musculorum deformans. **Duck gait.** Myopathic gait (see below). **Equine gait.** The gait associated with drop foot. **Festinating gait.** A gait of short and accelerating steps. **Gluteal gait.** Listing of the trunk when walking, associated with paralysis of the gluteus medius muscle. **Goose gait.** A waddling gait occurring in arthritis. **Helicopod gait.** The type of gait sometimes seen in hysteria, occasionally in hemiplegia, in which the feet or affected foot describe a semicircle with each step. **Hemiplegic gait.** The gait of hemiplegia, with circumduction of the affected leg; helicopod gait (see preceding). **Multiple sclerotic gait.** The spastic gait of multiple sclerosis; there is sometimes an element of sensory and/or cerebellar ataxia. **Myopathic gait.** The gait in pseudohypertrophic muscular paralysis. **Paralytic gait, Paretic gait.** The shuffling gait, with short steps and dragging of the limbs, seen in paralysis of the lower limbs. **Reeling gait.** The drunken gait of cerebellar disease; cerebellar gait (see above). **Scissor gait.** Cross-legged progression seen in cases of spastic paraplegia. **Spastic gait.** The gait seen in spasticity of the lower limbs, in which the limbs are stiff, the feet are plantar-flexed, and each step is carried out by circumduction, often with dragging of the toes. **Stamping gait.** The gait of sensory ataxia; ataxic gait, tabetic gait. **Steppage gait.** A gait in which the legs are lifted abnormally high, occurring in cases of drop foot. **Swaying gait.** Cerebellar gait (see above). **Tabetic gait.** The high steppage gait of tabes dorsalis due to sensory ataxia; ataxic gait (see above). **Waddling gait.** Myopathic gait (see above). [Old Norse *gata* a way.]

See also: CHARCOT, OPPENHEIM (H.).

galactacrasia (gal·akt·a·**kra'**·ze·ah). A condition in which human milk is of defective composition. [Gk *gala* milk, *krasis* a mingling.]

galactaemia (gal·akt·e·me·ah). A milky appearance of the blood. [Gk *gala* milk, *haima* blood.]

galactagogue (gal·**akt**·ag·og). 1. Producing milk or increasing the secretion of it. 2. Any agent or drug which increases the secretion or the flow of milk. [Gk *gala* milk, *agogos* leading.]

galactan (gal·**ak**·tan). Galactosan, gelose, $(C_6H_{10}O_5)_n$. A polysaccharide consisting of galactose units, into which it is hydrolysed. It occurs in algae and can be prepared from agar. [Gk *gala* milk.]

galactangioleucitis (gal·akt·**an**·je·o·lew·**si'**·tis). Lymphangitis arising as a result of lactation. [Gk *gala* milk, angioleucitis.]

galactapostema (gal·akt·ap·os·**te'**·mah). Milk abscess. [Gk *gala* milk, *apostema* abscess.]

galactase (gal·**ak**·taze). A proteolytic enzyme similar to erepsin which is present in milk and activates the hydrolysis of caseinogen in digestion.

galacthaemia (gal·akt·**he**·me·ah). Galactaemia.

galacthidrosis (gal·**akt**·hid·**ro'**·sis). The secretion and excretion of milk-like sweat. [Gk *gala* milk, *hidros* sweat.]

galactic (gal·**ak**·tik). 1. Referring or belonging to milk. 2. Galactagogue. [Gk *gala* milk.]

galactidrosis (gal·**ak**·tid·**ro'**·sis). Galacthidrosis.

galactin (gal·**ak**·tin). 1. The hormone of the anterior lobe of the hypophysis cerebri which promotes lactation of the developed mammary gland: also known as *prolactin*. 2. $C_{54}H_{78}O_{45}N_4$, a white substance which can be prepared from milk. [Gk *gala* milk.]

galactischia (gal·ak·**tis**·ke·ah). Galactoschesia.

galactoblast (gal·**ak**·to·blast). A colostrum corpuscle present in the alveoli of the mammary gland. [Gk *gala* milk, *blastos* germ.]

galactocele (gal·**ak**·to·seel). 1. A milk-filled cyst formed in the mammary gland because there is obstruction of a lactiferous duct. 2. A hydrocele containing milk-like fluid. [Gk *gala* milk, *kele* hernia.]

galactocrasia (gal·**ak**·to·**kra'**·se·ah). Galactacrasia.

galactoedema (gal·**ak**·te·**de'**·mah). Distension of the breast caused by accumulation of milk. [Gk *gala* milk, oedema.]

galactofuranose (gal·**ak**·to·**few'**·ran·oze). In sugar nomenclature, the furanose form of galactose which contains the 5-membered furane ring.

galactogen (gal·**ak**·to·gen). $(C_6H_{10}O_5)_n$, the polymer of galactose that is found in the eggs of snails. [see foll.]

galactogenous (gal·ak·**toj**·en·us). Suitable for or furthering the production of milk. [Gk *gala* milk, *genein* to produce.]

galactoglycosuria (gal·**ak**·to·gli·koze·**ewr'**·e·ah). Glycosuria occurring only during lactation. [Gk *gala* milk, glycosuria.]

galactogogue (gal·**ak**·to·gog). Galactagogue.

galactoid (gal·**akt**·oid). Like milk. [Gk *gala* milk, *eidos* form.]

galactokinase (gal·**ak**·to·**ki'**·naze). The liver enzyme which catalyses the phosphorylation of galactose by ATP with production of galactose 1-phosphate.

galactolipide (gal·ak·to·**lip'**·ide). Galactolipin.

galactolipin, galactolipine (gal·**ak**·to·**lip'**·in, gal·**ak**·to·**lip'**·een). Galactolipide, glycolipide, galactoside. One of the cerebrosides or esters of a fatty acid with sphingosine and galactose, which are found in brain tissue and the myelin sheaths of nerves. [Gk *gala* milk, *lipos* fat.]

galactoma (gal·ak·**to**·mah). Galactocele. [Gk *gala* milk, *-oma* tumour.]

galactometastasis (gal·**ak**·to·met·**as'**·tas·is). Galactoplania. [Gk *gala* milk, metastasis.]

galactometer (gal·ak·**tom**·et·er). 1. A glass funnel, graded, with which the fatty content of milk can be determined. 2. Lactometer. [Gk *gala* milk, meter.]

galactoncus (gal·ak·**tong**·kus). Galactocele. [Gk *gala* milk, *ogkos* a swelling.]

galactopexic (gal·**ak**·to·**pex'**·ik). Holding galactose. [see foll.]

galactopexy (gal·**ak**·to·**pex'**·e). The fixation of galactose by the liver. [galactose, Gk *pexis* fixation.]

galactophagous (gal·akt·**of**·ag·us). Feeding or keeping alive on milk. [Gk *gala* milk, *phagein* to eat.]

galactophlebitis (gal·**ak**·to·fleb·**i'**·tis). Phlegmasia alba dolens: a condition which sometimes occurs after typhoid fever or childbirth (white leg), marked by phlebitis in the femoral vein and oedematous swelling of the leg, but usually without reddish discoloration of the skin. [Gk *gala* milk, phlebitis.]

galactophlysis (gal·ak·**tof**·lis·is). 1. A vesicular eruption characterized by the presence of milky fluid in the sacs. 2. Crusta lactea. [Gk *gala* milk, *phlysis* eruption.]

galactophora (gal·ak·**tof**·or·ah). Galactagogue. [Gk *gala* milk, *pherein* to bear.]

galactophore (gal·**ak**·to·**fore'**). 1. A lactiferous duct. 2. Galactophorous. [see prec.]

galactophoritis (gal·**ak**·to·for·**i'**·tis). An inflamed condition of the lactiferous ducts. [Gk *gala* milk, *pherein* to bear, *-itis* inflammation.]

galactophorous (gal·ak·**tof**·er·us). Lactiferous. [see foll.]

galactophorus (gal·ak·**tof**·er·us). An artificial nipple worn over the breast nipple in order to protect it, particularly when there is a crack or other lesion, and to make suckling easier. [Gk *gala* milk, *pherein* to bear.]

galactophthisis (gal·**ak**·to·**thi'**·sis). Loss of flesh and strength as the result of too prolonged lactation. [Gk *gala* milk, phthisis.]

galactophyga (gal·ak·**tof**·ig·ah). Drugs or remedies administered for the purpose of preventing the secretion of milk or arresting its flow. [Gk *gala* milk, *phyge* banishment.]

galactophygous (gal·ak·**tof**·ig·us). Lactifuge: retarding or causing the cessation of secretion of milk. [see prec.]

galactoplania (gal·**ak**·to·**plane'**·e·ah). A condition in which milk is secreted in some part of the body other than the mammary gland; galactometastasis. [Gk *gala* milk, *plane* a wandering.]

galactoplerosis (gal·**ak**·to·ple·**ro'**·sis). Galactoedema. [Gk *gala* milk, *plerosis* a filling.]

galactopoiesis (gal·**ak**·to·poi·**e'**·sis). The development of milk in the mammary gland. The maintenance of established lactation. [Gk *gala* milk, *poiein* to make.]

galactopoietic (gal·**ak**·to·poi·**et'**·ik). 1. Galactagogue. 2. Having a part in the secretion or production of milk. [see prec.]

galactoposia (gal·**ak**·to·**poze'**·e·ah). Milk cure, i.e. treatment of disease by restriction to a milk diet. [Gk *gala* milk, *posis* a drinking.]

galactopyra (gal·**ak**·to·**pi'**·rah). Milk fever, 2nd def. *See* FEVER. [Gk *gala* milk, *pyr* fire.]

galactopyranose (gal·**ak**·to·**pi'**·ran·oze). In sugar nomenclature, the pyranose form of galactose that contains a 6-membered pyran ring.

galactopyretic (gal·**ak**·to·pi·**ret'**·ik). Referring to galactopyra.

galactopyretus (gal·**ak**·to·pi·**re'**·tus). Galactopyra.

galactorrhoea (gal·**ak**·to·**re'**·ah). 1. Spontaneous secretion and discharge of milk after the period of nursing is over. 2. An excessive flow of milk. [Gk *gala* milk, *rhoia* flow.]

galactosaemia (gal·**ak**·to·**se'**·me·ah). 1. The presence of galactose in the blood. 2. An inborn error of metabolism due to the absence of galactose L-phosphate uridyltransferase, probably inherited, not usually recognized at birth, but showing its presence shortly after by the infant's failure to thrive, irritability and anorexia. The infant usually goes downhill rapidly and may become jaundiced. The urine shows albuminuria, casts and a substance that reduces Benedict's solution, which is galactose. Unless treatment, which consists mainly of a lactose-free diet, is undertaken, early death is likely, or, in the event of survival, cataract and mental deficiency. [galactose, Gk *haima* blood.]

galactosamine (gal·**ak**·to·**sam**·een). 1. 6-Aminogalactose, $NH_2CH_2(CHOH)_4CHO$, a hexosamine. 2. Chondrosamine, 2-aminogalactose, $CH_2OH(CHOH)_3CHNH_2CHO$, the amino-sugar which forms a unit in chondromucoid, the glycoprotein of cartilage.

galactosan (gal·**ak**·to·san). Galactan, gelose, $(C_6H_{10}O_5)_n$. A polysaccharide consisting of galactose units, which occurs in algae and can be prepared from agar.

galactosazone (gal·ak·**to**·saz·one). $CH_2OH(CHOH)_3C{=}(NNHC_6H_5)CH{=}(NNHC_6H_5)$, a compound derived from galactose with phenylhydrazine, that forms characteristic yellow crystals which serve to distinguish galactose from the other hexoses.

galactoschesis (gal·ak·**tos**·kes·is). A condition in which the secretion or the flow of milk is suppressed. [Gk *gala* milk, *schesis* a checking.]

galactose (gal·**ak**·toze). D-Galactose, $CH_2OH(CHOH)_4CHO$. An aldohexose, isomeric with D-glucose, which forms a unit in lactose from which it can be prepared by hydrolysis. It also occurs in the trisaccharide, raffinose, in the cerebrosides of brain and nerve tissue, and, polymerized, in the galactans of seaweeds and lichens. A white dextrorotatory substance, not as sweet as glucose and somewhat less soluble in water; it is readily fermentable and forms mucic acid on oxidation. The laevo-form is obtained from flax-seed mucilage. [Gk *gala* milk.]

galactosidase (gal·**ak**·to·**si**′·daze). An enzyme that catalyses the destruction of galactosides.

galactoside (gal·**ak**·to·side). 1. A galactolipin. 2. A compound analogous to a glucoside, but containing units of galactose instead of glucose.

galactosis (gal·ak·**to**·sis). In physiology, the secretion of milk. [Gk *gala* milk, *-osis* condition.]

galactostasia (gal·ak·to·**sta**′·ze·ah). Galactostasis.

galactostasis (gal·ak·**tos**·tas·is). 1. Arrest or stagnation in the secretion of milk. 2. The collection in the mammary gland of an abnormal quantity of milk. [Gk *gala* milk, stasis.]

galactosuria (gal·**ak**·to·**sewr**′·e·ah). The condition in which galactose is present in the urine.

galactotherapy (gal·**ak**·to·**ther**′·ap·e). 1. Milk cure; treatment by means of a diet composed exclusively or almost exclusively of milk. 2. The treatment of disease in a nursing infant by administration to the mother or foster-mother of a drug or other remedy which is subsequently excreted in part by the mammary gland. 3. Protein shock therapy by the injection of sterile milk. [Gk *gala* milk, therapy.]

galactotoxicon (gal·**ak**·to·**tox**′·ik·on). The active toxin present in milk which has become poisonous. [see foll.]

galactotoxin (gal·**ak**·to·**tox**′·in). A poisonous principle generated in milk by the action of micro-organisms, but not necessarily the same as a galactotoxicon. [Gk *gala* milk, toxin.]

galactotoxism (gal·ak·to·**tox**′·izm). A condition of poisoning resulting from drinking stale or impure milk. [see prec.]

galactotrophic (gal·**ak**·to·**trof**′·ik). Stimulating the secretion of milk. [see foll.]

galactotrophy (gal·**ak**·to·**tro**′·fe). Feeding or nourishing with milk only. [Gk *gala* milk, *trophe* nutrition.]

galactozymase (gal·**ak**·to·**zi**′·maze). A ferment in milk which is able to hydrolyse starch. [Gk *gala* milk, zymase.]

galactozyme (gal·**ak**·to·zime). 1. Milk fermented by the addition of yeast. 2. Any drink prepared from fermented milk, e.g. koumiss. [Gk *gala* milk, *zyme* yeast.]

galacturia (gal·ak·**tewr**·e·ah). Chyluria; the condition in which the urine is of a milky appearance because it contains chyle or lipoid matter. [Gk *gala* milk, urine.]

galalith (**gal**·al·ith). An absorbable material formerly used to fashion a type of anastomosis button. It was prepared from the casein of milk with formaldehyde. [Gk *gala* milk, *lithos* stone.]

galanga, galangal (gal·**ang**·gah, gal·**ang**·gal). Lesser galangal, East Indian root, China root, the dried rhizome of *Alpinia officinarum* Hance (family Zingiberaceae), obtained from China. It contains a volatile oil and a pungent principle with carminative and stimulant properties. The powdered rhizome has been employed as a snuff. [Pers. *khalanjan.*]

galanthamine (gal·**an**·tham·een). An anticholinesterase and analeptic agent derived from the Caucasian snowdrop. [*Galanthus* snowdrop.]

galbanum (**gal**·ban·um). An oleo gum resin related to ammoniacum and asafoetida and found in *Ferula galbaniflua* and other species. It is used as a stimulant in bronchitis. [Gk *chalbane*, juice of all-heal.]

Gale's formula. The basal metabolic rate can be roughly calculated by adding together the pulse rate and the pulse pressure and subtracting 111.

galea (**ga**·le·ah). 1. Epicranial aponeurosis. *See* APONEUROSIS. 2. The amnion. 3. A caul. 4. Headache involving the entire head. 5. A particular type of bandage for the head. [L helmet.]

galeamaurosis (ga·le·am·aw·**ro**′·sis). Amaurotic cat's eye; the term applied to a blind eye with a white reflex in the pupil. It is usually restricted to the appearance seen in an infant suffering from glioma retinae or from pseudoglioma. [Gk *gale* cat, amaurosis.]

galeanthropy (ga·le·**an**·throp·e). A condition in which the patient is under the insane delusion that he has turned into a cat or that a cat is living inside his body. [Gk *gale* cat, *anthropos* man.]

Galeati, Domenico Maria Gusmano (Galeazzi) (b. 1686). Bologna physician.

Galeati's glands. Intestinal glands of simple tubular type.

galeatus (ga·le·a·tus). Born with a caul. [L helmeted.]

Galeazzi, Riccardo (b. 1866). Milan orthopaedic surgeon.

Galeazzi fracture. Isolated fracture of the shaft of the radius with dislocation of the lower radio-ulnar joint.

galega (gal·e·gah). Goat's rue, *Galega officinalis* Linn. (family Leguminosae); a decoction of the herb has been employed as a stimulant and diuretic. It contains an alkaloid, galegine, reported as being of value in reducing the blood sugar in diabetes. [Gk *gala* milk, *agein* to lead.]

galegine (gal·e·jeen). $(CH_3)_2C{=}CHCH_2NHC(NH)NH_2$, an alkaloid found in goat's rue (*Galega officinalis*, family Leguminosae). It reduces the blood sugar, and has been used in diabetes, especially in insulin-resistant cases.

Galen, Claudius (c. A.D. 130–200). Greek physician in Rome.

Galen's ampulla. A dilatation of the great cerebral vein.

Galen's anastomosis. The anastomosis between the internal and external laryngeal nerves.

Galen's cerate. Cold cream. *See* CREAM.

Galen's foramen. The opening of the anterior cardiac vein into the right atrium.

Galen's nerve. The communicating branch with the recurrent laryngeal nerve.

Galen's veins. The internal cerebral veins; the great vein of Galen is formed by their union. The anterior cardiac vein is also known as Galen's vein.

Galen's great vein. The great cerebral vein.

Galen's ventricle. The saccule of the larynx (appendix of the laryngeal ventricle).

galena (gal·e·nah). The principal ore of lead; a native sulphide, PbS, found mostly in Canada and the USA in the form of metallic cubic crystals. [Gk *galene* lead ore.]

galenic (gal·**en**·ik). 1. Referring to Galen and his medical principles or methods. 2. Referring to medicines prepared by infusion and decoction as distinct from chemical preparations. [Claudius *Galen.*]

galenical (gal·**en**·ik·al). A preparation, in a form suitable for therapeutic use, of a crude drug of animal or vegetable origin. Among such are confections, creams, decoctions, elixirs, extracts, infusions, liniments, liquors, ointments, poultices, spirits, syrups, tinctures, vinegars and aromatic waters. Extemporarily prepared medicaments, and pills, tablets, injections and preparations of pure chemical substances are not classed as galenicals. [Claudius *Galen.*]

galenism (ga·len·izm). A doctrine based on Galen's teachings.

galeophilia (gal·e·o·**fil**′·e·ah). Ailurophilia; excessive fondness for cats. [Gk *gale* cat, *philein* to love.]

galeophobia (gal·e·o·**fo**′·be·ah). Ailurophobia; fear of cats exaggerated to a morbid degree. [Gk *gale* cat, phobia.]

Galeotti, Gino (b. 1867). Italian bacteriologist.

Lustig and Galeotti's vaccine. A sterile preparation of *Pasteurella pestis* in 1 per cent caustic soda neutralized by acetic acid.

galeropia, galeropsia (gal·er·o·pe·ah, gal·er·**ops**·e·ah). Abnormal clearness of vision resulting from functional derangement of the mechanism of seeing; the subjective effect is one of light. [Gk *galeros* cheerful, *ops* eye.]

Galezowski, Xavier (b. 1832). Russian ophthalmologist.

Galezowski's operation, for discission in cataract. Two sickle-shaped needles are used, one to hold the capsule tissue and the other to cut it from within outwards.

Galipea (gal·ip·e·ah). Angostura. *Galipea cusparia* and *Cusparia febrifuga* have both been given as the source of angostura bark, but in modern classification *Galipea officinalis* Hancock is the accepted name for the plant.

galipot (gal·e·pot). **French galipot.** The resin from the tree *Pinus maritima.* [Fr.]

gall (gawl). 1. The bile. [ME *gal.*] 2. (BPC 1963), gallae ceruleae, gall-nut, nutgall, blue galls, galls; excrescences on the twigs of the gall-oak, *Quercus infectoria* Olivier, resulting from the stimulus given to the tissues by deposition of the eggs of the gall wasp, *Cynips gallae tinctoriae.* They contain 50–70 per cent of gallotannic acid by virtue of which they are powerfully astringent; not used internally, but in the form of an ointment. They are an important source of tannic acid for tanning, dyeing and the manufacture of ink. **Aleppo galls.** Galls of *Quercus infectoria,* collected in Asia Minor. **Chinese galls.** Galls produced by the aphis *Schlechlendaria sinensis* on the leaves of *Rhus javanica.* **Hungarian galls.** Galls produced by the wasp *Cynips lignicola* on *Quercus robur.* **Japanese galls.** Similar to Chinese galls (see above). **Smyrna galls, Syrian galls, Turkey galls.** Similar to Aleppo galls (see above). [L *galla* gall-nut.]

gall bladder [vesica fellea (NA)] (**gawl blad**·er). A pear-shaped sac on the inferior surface of the right lobe of the liver, in which bile is stored and concentrated. It is joined by the cystic duct to the bile duct. **Body of the gall bladder [corpus vesicae felleae (NA)].** The part between the fundus and the neck which lies in the fossa for the gall bladder on the under surface of the liver. **Coat of the gall bladder, mucous [tunica mucosa vesicae felleae (NA)].** Columnar epithelium raised in folds to give a honeycomb appearance. **Coat of the gall bladder, muscular [tunica muscularis vesicae felleae (NA)].** A thin layer of muscle fibres, mostly orientated longitudinally, interspersed with many collagenous fibres. **Coat of the gall bladder, serous [tunica serosa vesicae felleae (NA)].** The peritoneal layer investing the fundus and covering the under surface and sides of the remainder of the gall bladder. **Coat of the gall bladder, subserous [tela subserosa vesicae felleae (NA)].** The thin layer of areolar tissue which lies deep to the serous coat. **Fish-scale gall bladder.** An appearance of the mucous membrane of the gall bladder, resembling fish scales, and due to multiple small mucous cysts. **Folded-fundus gall bladder.** Phrygian cap; term applied to the x-ray appearance of a gall bladder the fundus of which is folded back on the body. **Fundus of the gall bladder [fundus vesicae felleae (NA)].** The expanded terminal portion of the gall bladder, projecting beyond the inferior border of the liver to make contact with the right 9th costal cartilage. **Neck of the gall bladder [collum vesicae felleae (NA)].** The narrowed end of the gall bladder leading into the cystic duct. **Phrygian-cap gall bladder.** A congenitally abnormal kink of the gall bladder, making it resemble the liberty cap of the French Revolution. **Sandpaper gall bladder.** A condition in which the mucous membrane of the gall bladder shows a deposit of fine cholesterol crystals. **Stasis gall bladder.** Enlargement of the gall bladder due to the retardation of the outflow of bile. **Strawberry gall bladder.** A condition in which there is a chronically inflamed red mucous membrane with embedded fine grains of cholesterol. **Wandering gall bladder.** An unusually mobile gall bladder displaced from the normal position. [ME *gal,* AS *blaedre.*]

See also: COURVOISIER.

gall-stone (**gawl**·stone). A concretion which may form in the gall bladder or bile duct. Its composition most commonly is of cholesterol. **Combination gall-stone.** A stone formed from a nucleus of cholesterol over which calcium bilirubin is deposited. **Silent gall-stones.** Gall-stones that give rise to no symptoms, although they can be seen radiologically or at abdominal operation. [ME *gal* bile, stone.]

gallal (gal·al). A basic aluminium gallate used in dusting powders as an astringent.

Gallamine (gal·am·een). BP Commission approved name for 1,2,3-tri-(2-diethylaminoethoxy)benzene.

Gallamine Triethiodide BP 1973 (gal·am·een tri·eth·i·o·dide). Tri-(diethylaminoethoxy)-benzene triethyliodide. A synthetic compound which acts like curare, inhibiting the transmission across the myoneural junction of voluntary muscle; its actions are reversed by neostigmine. It has less effect on ganglia than curare and liberates less histamine. It is particularly valuable for a prolonged muscular relaxation as in abdominal surgery, but it can also be used for short-term procedures such as electric-shock therapy by countering the action when desired with neostigmine. It may produce respiratory paralysis, and artificial respiration is often necessary. It is contra-indicated in myasthenia gravis, and should be used with caution in renal insufficiency and cardiac insufficiency.

Gallamini Triethiodidum (gal·**am**·in·i **tri**·eth·i·o'·did·um). *European Pharmacopoeia* name for Gallamine Triethiodide BP 1973.

gallate (gal·ate). A salt of gallic acid.

gallein (gal·e·in). $C_{20}H_{12}O_7$, a brown dye prepared from pyrogallol or gallic acid and phthalic anhydride. It is used as an indicator.

Galli Mainini, Carlos. South American physician.

Galli Mainini test, for pregnancy. 5 ml of urine from a pregnant woman is injected into the dorsal lymph sac of the South American toad *Bufo arenareum* Hensel, and 3 h later spermatozoa can be aspirated from the cloaca of the animal with a pipette. A very high degree of accuracy is claimed (99 per cent).

gallicin (gal·is·in). Methyl gallate, $C_6H_2(OH)_3COOCH_3$. An antiseptic compound, used mostly as a dusting powder.

Gallie, William Edward (b. 1882). Toronto surgeon.

Gallie's fascial graft, or transplant. The strip of fascia employed in Gallie's operation.

Gallie's needle. A fascia needle; a needle used to carry a suture of fascia lata in fascial repair of a hernia.

Gallie operation. A method of repairing a large hernia by the use of wide strips of fascia (Gallie's fascial graft, or transplant) taken from the outer aspect of the thigh as a darn to close the defect.

gallipot (gal·e·pot). A small pot or vessel of glazed earthenware, particularly for use by druggists, for holding ointments or medicines. [etym. dub.]

gallisin (gal·is·in). One of a group of polysaccharides made up of galactose units and analogous with dextrins.

gallium (gal·e·um). A rare element of atomic weight 69.72, atomic number 31, and chemical symbol Ga. It is a silver-white metal found in zinc ores and commercial aluminium, which element it resembles closely in properties. It is di- and trivalent, and forms colourless salts many of which are poisonous. [L *Gallia* Gaul.]

gallocyanin (gal·o·**si**·an·in). A basic dye used for Nissl bodies and as a nuclear stain.

gallogen (gal·o·jen). Ellagic acid, $C_{14}H_6O_8$. A yellow crystalline compound which occurs in certain tannins. It is used as an intestinal astringent in cases of diarrhoea. [L *galla* gall-nut, Gk *genein* to produce.]

gallon (gal·on). **Imperial gallon.** A liquid measure: it equals 4.546 litres. **American gallon.** A liquid measure equal to 3.785 litres. [O Fr. *galon.*]

gallop (gal·op). In cardiology, referring to the rhythm of the heart sounds when there is tachycardia with three sounds to each cycle, this being likened to the sound of a horse galloping. **Atrial gallop.** One in which the extra sound is the fourth heart sound produced by atrial systole. **Gallop rhythm.** *See* RHYTHM.

Ventricular gallop. One in which the extra sound is the third heart sound produced by rapid early ventricular filling. [Fr. *galop.*]

Galton, Sir Francis (b. 1822). English scientist.

Galton's delta. The triangular pattern of the lines on a fingerprint.

Galton's law. The parents of an individual contribute one half each to its make-up, the grandparents one quarter each, and so on.

Galton's law of regression. Parents of average characteristics tend to produce average children, and parents of extreme characteristics tend to produce extreme children, but these children will approach or diverge from the average less than the parents.

Galton system of identification. A method based upon fingerprints, the records being the imprints of the ten digits placed in a definite order upon a card.

galuteolin (gal·ew·**te**·o·lin). $C_{21}H_{20}O_{11}$, a glycoside obtained from the seeds of *Galega officinalis* (family Leguminosae).

galvanic (gal·**van**·ik). 1. Referring or belonging to galvanism. 2. Showing the phenomena of galvanism; voltaic.

galvanism (**gal**·van·izm). 1. The name applied to galvanic, direct, current produced by chemical means. 2. The application of direct current (galvanic electricity) for therapeutic purposes, e.g. iontophoresis, electrolysis. [Luigi *Galvani* (b. 1737), Italian physician.]

galvanocautery (**gal**·van·o·**kaw**'·ter·e). 1. A cautery made by applying a direct, galvanic, current to a wire. 2. Cauterization carried out by means of a wire heated by galvanic (direct) current.

galvanochemical (**gal**·van·o·**kem**'·ik·al). [Obsolete term.] Relating to the chemical changes produced by the action of a galvanic, direct, current.

galvanochemistry (**gal**·van·o·**kem**'·is·tre). [Obsolete term.] Electrochemistry. [galvanism, chemistry.]

galvanocontractility (**gal**·van·o·kon·trak·**til**'·it·e). The degree of muscular contraction resulting from stimulation by a galvanic (direct) current.

galvanofaradic (**gal**·van·o·far·**ad**'·ik). Referring to combined galvanic (direct) and faradic (induced) electric currents.

galvanofaradization (**gal**·van·o·**far**·ad·**i**·**za**'·shun). The therapeutic application to a nerve or muscle of a galvanic (direct) and a faradic (induced) current simultaneously; galvanic faradization.

galvano-ionization (**gal**·van·o·**i**·on·i·**za**'·shun). Iontophoresis; in therapeutics, the forcible introduction of ionic medication into the body through the unbroken skin by means of a direct electric current. [galvanism, ionization.]

galvanolysis (gal·van·**ol**·is·is). [Obsolete term.] Electrolysis. [galvanism, lysis.]

galvanometer (gal·van·**om**·et·er). An instrument used in electricity to indicate the strength and direction of a current. Its action depends upon the deflexion of a magnetic needle in the field produced by the current passing through a coil: if provided with a graduated scale, it can be used as an ammeter. **Mirror galvanometer.** One in which a mirror attached to the magnet reflects a beam of light on to a graduated scale. **Moving-coil galvanometer.** A galvanometer in which the current to be measured flows in a coil suspended in a strong magnetic field between the poles of a permanent magnet. Deflexion of the coil is measured by the movement on a scale of a beam of light reflected from a small mirror attached to the coil. **String galvanometer, Thread galvanometer.** A very sensitive galvanometer consisting of a fine platinum or silvered quartz thread held taut in a powerful magnetic field; minute currents in the thread cause movements which can be observed. [galvanism, meter.]

See also: D'ARSONVAL, EINTHOVEN.

galvanomuscular (**gal**·van·o·**mus**'·kew·lar). Term applied to the results of the application of a galvanic (direct) current to a muscle.

galvanonarcosis (**gal**·van·o·nar·**ko**'·sis). Electronarcosis; narcosis or unconsciousness produced by the passage of an electric current through a patient. [galvanism, narcosis.]

galvanonervous (**gal**·van·o·**ner**'·vus). Term applied to the results of the application of a galvanic (direct) current to a nerve trunk.

galvanopalpation (**gal**·van·o·pal·**pa**'·shun). A method of determining the reactions of peripheral nerves or muscles by the application of electric currents to the skin. With the addition of faradic (induced) currents the reaction of degeneration of muscles is determined. [galvanism, palpation.]

galvanoprostatectomy, galvanoprostatotomy (**gal**·van·o·pros·tat·**ek**'·to·me, **gal**·van·o·pros·tat·**ot**'·o·me). The operation for removal of portions of hypertrophied prostate gland by galvanocautery. [galvanism, prostate, Gk *ektome* excision, *temnein* to cut.]

galvanopuncture (**gal**·van·o·**pungk**'·tcher). The closing of a galvanic (direct) circuit by means of needle electrodes introduced into the body. [galvanism, puncture.]

galvanoscope (**gal**·van·o·skope). Rheoscope; an electrical apparatus which indicates the strength and direction of an electrical current passing through it. [galvanism, Gk *skopein* to look.]

galvanosurgery (**gal**·van·o·**ser**'·jer·e). The use of galvanic (direct) electricity in surgical procedures.

galvanotaxis (**gal**·van·o·**tax**'·is). The tendency of a living structure to align itself in a certain way relative to a direct electric current passing through the surrounding medium. [galvanism, Gk *taxis* arrangement.]

galvanotherapeutics (**gal**·van·o·ther·ap·**ew**'·tix). The branch of medical science concerned with the treatment by galvanic (direct) electricity. [see foll.]

galvanotherapy (**gal**·van·o·**ther**'·ap·e). The use of galvanic (direct) current for the purpose of healing. [galvanism, therapy.]

galvanothermy (**gal**·van·o·**ther**'·me). 1. The production of heat by means of a direct current. 2. The process of applying heat to, or the burning of a part, using galvanic (direct) electricity. [galvanism, Gk *therme* heat.]

galvanotonic (**gal**·van·o·**ton**'·ik). Referring to or having the character of galvanotonus.

galvanotonus (gal·van·**ot**·o·nus). An old-fashioned word suggesting that muscle responds to direct-current stimulus by sustained contraction. Actually normal muscle twitches at make and break, but not during the passage of constant current. [galvanism, Gk *tonos* tension.]

galvanotropism (gal·van·**ot**·ro·pizm). The characteristic evinced by living cells or structures to move under the stimulus of an electric current. [galvanism, Gk *trope* a turning.]

gamasoidosis (**gam**·as·oid·**o**'·sis). Dermatitis resulting from infestation by mites of the family Gamasidae, e.g. the fowl mite.

gambir (**gam**·beer). Catechu. [Malay.]

gamboge (gam·**boje**, gam·**booj**). A yellow-coloured gum resin obtained from the stem of *Garcinia hanburyi* Hook. f. (family Guttiferae). It has been employed medicinally as a hydragogue cathartic, but is now mainly used as a pigment. [*Cambodia.*]

Gambusia (gam·**bew**·ze·ah). A genus of freshwater fish.

Gambusia affinis. The top minnow or Dixie mosquito fish; it is American in origin but has been introduced into many tropical countries to control mosquitoes. [Sp. American *gambusina* nothing.]

gametangium (gam·et·**an**·je·um). In biology, the organ or cell which produces or contains the gametes. [gamete, Gk *aggeion* small vessel.]

gamete (**gam**·eet). 1. A reproductive cell, such as an ovum or a spermatozoon, which may fuse with another of opposite sex to form a zygote. 2. In the malaria parasite, the macro- (female) or micro- (male) gamete derived in a mosquito's stomach from gametocytes sucked in with the blood of a malarial subject. Following their union, an oökinete (or travelling vermicule) is formed which penetrates the mosquito's stomach wall and there, as an oöcyst, develops a new generation of malarial sporozoites. [Gk *gametes* husband; *gamete* wife.]

gametic (gam·**et**·ik). Pertaining to gametes.

gametocide (gam·e·to·side). Any agent which destroys gametes or gametocytes, particularly those of malaria. [gamete, L *caedere* to kill.]

gametocinetic (gam·e·to·sin·et′·ik). Gametokinetic.

gametocytaemia (gam·e·to·si·te′·me·ah). The presence of malarial gametocytes in the circulating blood. [gametocyte, Gk *haima* blood.]

gametocyte (gam·e·to·site). 1. The precursor of gametes. 2. The sexual phase of the malaria parasite as developed in the blood of the intermediate host. In the mosquito's stomach they give rise to male and female gametes by the extrusion of polar bodies. [gamete, Gk *kytos* cell.]

gametogenesis (gam·e·to·jen′·es·is). The formation or origination of gametes. [gamete, Gk *genein* to produce.]

gametogenic (gam·e·to·jen′·ik). 1. Favourable to or tending towards the formation or production of gametes. 2. Referring to gametogenesis. [see prec.]

gametogeny (gam·e·toj·en·e). Gametogenesis.

gametogony (gam·e·tog·on·e). The act of fertilization of the female gamete, e.g. of the malaria parasite by the male gamete. [gamete, Gk *gone* seed.]

gametoid (gam·e·toid). Having resemblance to gametes. [gamete, Gk *eidos* form.]

gametokinetic (gam·e·to·kin·et′·ik). 1. Stimulating movement or action in gametes. 2. Causing, or tending towards, true conjugation. [gamete, Gk *kinesis* movement.]

gametophagia (gam·e·to·fa′·je·ah). The disappearance of the male or female element in true conjugation or zygosis. [gamete, Gk *phagein* to eat.]

gametophyte (gam·e·to·fite). That stage in the alternation of generations of plants in which the cell nuclei are in a haploid condition. [gamete, Gk *phyton* plant.]

Gamgee, Joseph Sampson (b. 1828). Birmingham surgeon.

Gamgee tissue. A wound dressing consisting of a thickness of cotton wool between 2 thin layers of gauze.

gamic (gam·ik). Sexual; denoting eggs in which development takes place only after they have been fertilized. [Gk *gamos* marriage.]

gamma (gam·ah). 1. Γ or γ, the third letter of the Greek alphabet. 2. 10^{-6} gram. 3. A measure of magnetic flux density equal to 10^{-9} tesla (10^{-5} gauss). **Gamma angle.** *See* ANGLE. **Gamma encephalography.** *See* ENCEPHALOGRAPHY. **Gamma fibre.** *See* FIBRE. **Gamma globulin.** *See* GLOBULIN. **Gamma granule.** *See* GRANULE. **Gamma neuron.** *See* NEURON. **Gamma particle.** Gamma ray. *See* RAY. **Gamma position.** In chemistry, the position of the third atom in a chain of carbon atoms. **Gamma ray.** *See* RAY. **Gamma rhythm.** *See* RHYTHM.

gamma-aminobutyric acid (GABA). A neurotransmitter found in the diencephalon and many nerve terminals. It releases LH presumably via the hypothalamus, but not FSH apparently possibly because insufficient LH-RH is produced to affect FSH.

Gamma Benzene Hexachloride BP 1973 (gam·ah ben·zeen hex·ah·klor·ide). $C_6H_6Cl_6$, mainly the γ-isomer, but containing other stereo-isomeric forms of the same structure. An insecticide similar in properties to DDT but more potent, and more rapid in action. It is employed in the form of a dust, spray or smoke. A 1 per cent emulsion is used for scabies, and a 1 per cent solution for head lice.

gamma-emitter (gam·ah·e·mit′·er). Any gamma-ray source or radioactive isotope emitting gamma rays.

gammacism (gam·as·izm). Guttural stammering, i.e. difficulty over the pronunciation of consonants such as *g* and *k*. [Gk *gamma*.]

gammagram (gam·ah·gram). The recorded image of emitted gamma rays. (A term not in general use; *see* SCAN.)

gammopathy (gam·o·pathy). **Benign monocloral:** a condition in which the serum shows a myeloma-like increase in immunoglobulin level, but in which there is no Bence-Jones proteinuria, and in which the abnormality does not show the progressive tendency of other paraproteinaemias so that the prognosis is good.

Gamna's disease. A form of splenomegaly with nodular thickening of the capsule.

Gamna nodules. Brown or yellow tiny fibrosiderotic nodules found in the spleen in Banti's disease and other fibrotic diseases of the spleen, composed of altered blood. Also known as *Gandy-Gamna nodules.*

gamogenesis (gam·o·jen·es·is). Sexual reproduction. [Gk *gamos* marriage, *genein* to produce.]

gamogenetic (gam·o·jen·et′·ik). Pertaining to or displaying gamogenesis.

gamomania (gam·o·ma·ne·ah). Insane longing for the married state. [Gk *gamos* marriage, mania.]

gamomorphism (gam·o·mor·fizm). The state of being sexually mature; puberty. [Gk *gamos* marriage, *morphe* form.]

gamophobia (gam·o·fo·be·ah). Unbalanced instinctive fear of marriage. [Gk *gamos* marriage, phobia.]

gampsodactylia (gamp·so·dak·til′·e·ah). Claw-foot. [Gk *gampsos* bent, *daktylos* toe.]

Gandy-Gamna nodules. Gamna nodules.

Gandy-Gamna spleen. A spleen enlarged from deposits of haemosiderin.

ganglia (gang·gle·ah). *See* GANGLION.

ganglial, gangliar (gang·gle·al, gang·gle·ar). Ganglionic.

gangliate, gangliated (gang·gle·ate, gang·gle·a·ted). Ganglionate.

gangliectomy (gang·gle·ek·to·me). Ganglionectomy.

gangliform (gang·gle·form). Having the appearance or the form of a ganglion.

gangliitis (gang·gle·i·tis). Ganglionitis.

ganglioblast (gang·gle·o·blast). In embryology, one of the primitive cells from which the spinal ganglion cells develop. [ganglion, Gk *blastos* germ.]

gangliocyte (gang·gle·o·site). A ganglion cell. [ganglion, Gk *kytos* cell.]

gangliocytoma (gang·gle·o·si·to′·mah). A neoplasm in which there are ganglion cells. [gangliocyte, Gk *-oma* tumour.]

ganglioform (gang·gle·o·form). Ganglioform.

ganglioglioma (gang·gle·o·gli·o′·mah). A glioma which contains many ganglion cells.

ganglioglioneuroma (gang·gle·o·gli·o·newr·o′·mah). A glioneuroma which contains ganglion cells.

ganglioid (gang·gle·oid). Having resemblance to a ganglion. [ganglion, Gk *eidos* form.]

ganglioma (gang·gle·o·mah). 1. A tumour of a lymph gland. 2. Any tumour affecting a ganglion, either a ganglionic glioma (ganglioneuroma or neuroblastoma) or a synovioma arising from a synovial or tendon-sheath ganglion. [ganglion, Gk *-oma* tumour.]

ganglion (gang·gle·on) (pl. *ganglia*). 1. [NA] A group of nerve cells with a common function; especially applied to a collection outside the central nervous system. 2. Cystic swelling containing myxomatous material occurring in fibrous tendon sheaths, ligaments of joints and in the lateral semilunar cartilage of the knee joint. **Accessory ganglion.** 1. A nerve ganglion found along the course of a nerve bundle where one is not normally present. 2. One of the vestigial ganglia associated with the roots of origin of the vagus, accessory and hypoglossal nerves, in the early embryo. **Acousticofacial ganglion.** A sensory ganglion of the early embryo which later divides into facial and auditory ganglia. **Aorticorenal ganglion [ganglion aorticorenale (NA)].** The lower part of each coeliac ganglion which receives the lesser splanchnic nerve. **Auditory ganglion.** An aggregation of neuroblastic tissue separated early from the acousticofacial ganglion (see above) and giving rise to the cell bodies of the spiral ganglion of the cochlear (see below) and the vestibular ganglion (see below). **Basal ganglia.** The masses of grey matter within the cerebral hemispheres, including the corpus striatum, the amygdaloid nuclei and the claustrum. **Cardiac ganglion [ganglion cardiacum (NA)].** A macroscopic collection of autonomic nerve cells in the superficial cardiac plexus. **Cervical ganglion, inferior [ganglion cervicothoracicum (stellatum) (NA)].** A large, irregular ganglion on the lowest part of the cervical

ganglion

sympathetic trunk, often fused with the 1st thoracic ganglion to form the stellate ganglion. It sends grey communicating branches to the 7th and 8th cervical nerves, and through these to the upper limb. **Cervical ganglion, inferior, cardiac branch of the [nervus cardiacus cervicalis inferior (NA)].** A branch composed of postganglionic fibres from the inferior cervical ganglion to the deep part of the cardiac plexus. **Cervical ganglion, inferior, vertebral branch of the [nervus vertebralis (NA)].** A branch from the superior aspect of the inferior cervical ganglion which runs up behind the vertebral artery to form the vertebral plexus. **Cervical ganglion, middle [ganglion cervicale medium (NA)].** The smallest, and somewhat inconstant, ganglion on the cervical part of the sympathetic trunk, placed opposite the 6th cervical vertebra. It sends grey branches to the 5th and 6th cervical nerves. **Cervical ganglion, middle, cardiac branch of the [nervus cardiacus cervicalis medius (NA)].** A large twig of postganglionic fibres from the middle cervical ganglion to the deep cardiac plexus. **Cervical ganglion, middle, thyroid branches of the.** Postganglionic branches from the middle cervical ganglion to the thyroid gland. **Cervical ganglion, superior [ganglion cervicale superius (NA)].** The largest of the sympathetic ganglia, placed just below the base of the skull and behind the carotid sheath. Connected to the upper cervical nerves (by grey communicating branches), to the cranial nerves in the neighbourhood, to the cardiac plexus by long cardiac nerves, and sending a plexus of nerve fibres into the cranium along the internal carotid artery and on to the face along the external carotid artery. **Cervical ganglion, superior, cardiac branch of the [nervus cardiacus cervicalis superior (NA)].** A branch or branches from the superior cervical ganglion and composed of postganglionic fibres to the deep cardiac plexus on the right and to the superficial or deep cardiac plexus on the left. **Cervical ganglion, superior, pharyngeal branches of the [rami laryngopharyngei (NA)].** Branches from the superior cervical ganglion to the pharyngeal nerve plexus. **Ciliary ganglion [ganglion ciliare].** A small parasympathetic ganglion in the orbit, having sensory, sympathetic and parasympathetic roots. Postganglionic fibres of the latter supply the intrinsic eye muscles. **Ciliary ganglion, motor root of the [radix oculomotoria (NA)].** The parasympathetic root of the ciliary ganglion from the inferior division of the oculomotor nerve. The fibres synapse in the ganglion and postganglionic fibres innervate the sphincter of the pupil and ciliary muscles of the pupil. **Ciliary ganglion, sensory root of the [ramus communicans cum nervo nasociliari (NA)].** The sensory root to the nasociliary nerve. Its fibres pass without interruption in the ganglion from the short ciliary nerve. **Ciliary ganglion, sympathetic root of the [ramus sympathicus ad ganglion ciliare (NA)].** Filaments of the carotid plexus to the ciliary ganglion; they may travel in the 3rd cranial nerve, the nasociliary nerve or separately. They are postganglionic fibres and hence do not relay in the ganglion. They supply the dilator of the sphincter of the pupil. **Coeliac ganglion [ganglion celiacum (NA)].** A ganglion placed on each side in front of the crura of the diaphragm, intimately connected with the coeliac plexus. **Compound ganglion.** A loculated ganglion. **Compound palmar ganglion.** Chronic infection of the common synovial sheath of the flexor tendon of the hand, usually tuberculous. **Diffuse ganglion.** A cystic swelling of several adjacent tendon sheaths. **Facial ganglion, Ganglion of the facial nerve [ganglion geniculi (NA)].** A sensory ganglion in the geniculum of the facial nerve in the medial wall of the middle ear. **Gasserian ganglion.** The trigeminal ganglion (see below). **Ganglion of the glossopharyngeal nerve, inferior [ganglion inferius (NA)].** The lower of the 2 sensory ganglia situated in the lower part of the jugular foramen. **Ganglion of the glossopharyngeal nerve, superior [ganglion superius (NA)].** The upper of the 2 sensory ganglia situated in the upper part of the jugular foramen. **Habenular ganglion.** Habenular nucleus. *See* NUCLEUS. **Ganglion impar [NA].** A small ganglion in front of the coccyx at the place of union of the right and left sympathetic trunks. **Intermediate ganglia [ganglia intermedia (NA)].** Subsidiary ganglia placed outside the sympathetic trunks, usually on the segmental spinal nerves, and excluding the named ganglia such as the coeliac, phrenic or renal. **Interpeduncular ganglion.** Interpeduncular nucleus. *See* NUCLEUS. **Lumbar ganglia [ganglia lumbalia (NA)].** A series of 4 ganglia on the lumbar part of the sympathetic trunk. The upper 2 receive white communicating branches from the corresponding lumbar nerves, and each ganglion sends grey communicating branches to a lumbar spinal nerve or nerves. **Mesenteric ganglion, inferior [ganglion mesentericum inferius (NA)].** A small collection of cells just below the inferior mesenteric artery and on the inferior mesenteric plexus. **Mesenteric ganglion, superior [ganglion mesentericum superius (NA)].** A plexus of sympathetic nerve fibres, interspersed with ganglion cells, around the superior mesenteric artery. **Otic ganglion [ganglion oticum (NA)].** A ganglion associated with and lying deep to the mandibular nerve at its exit from the skull. It is the relay station for parasympathetic fibres from the glossopharyngeal nerve to the parotid gland. **Otic ganglion, communicating branch with the auriculotemporal nerve [ramus communicans cum nervo auriculotemporali (NA)].** A branch from the otic ganglion to the nerve, which probably carries postganglionic parasympathetic fibres to the parotid gland. **Otic ganglion, communicating branch with the chorda tympani [ramus communicans cum chorda tympani (NA)].** A branch of communication between the otic ganglion and the roots of the auriculotemporal nerve near their origin. **Otic ganglion, communicating branch with the nervus spinosus [ramus communicans cum ramo meningeo (nervi mandibularis) NA].** A small twig from the otic ganglion joining the nervus spinosus. **Otic ganglion, sympathetic root of the.** Postganglionic fibres from the superior cervical ganglion, reaching the otic ganglion along the middle meningeal artery and supplying the parotid gland. **Pelvic ganglia [ganglia pelvina (NA)].** Small collections of cells incorporated in the inferior hypogastric plexus, which give rise to the postganglionic fibres of the sacral autonomic components of the plexus. **Periosteal ganglion.** A cystic swelling arising from the periosteum. **Phrenic ganglia [ganglia phrenica (NA)].** Small collections of nerve cells at the junction of the cervical plexus and phrenic nerves. **Renal ganglia [ganglia renalia (NA)].** Ganglia, some microscopic in size, incorporated in the renal plexus. The most constantly occurring one is the dorsal. **Sacral ganglia of the sympathetic system [ganglia sacralia (NA)].** The ganglia on the pelvic part of the sympathetic trunk; they are usually 4 in number. *See* SYSTEM, SYMPATHETIC NERVOUS. **Semilunar ganglion.** Trigeminal ganglion (see below). **Simple ganglion.** A single swelling arising from a joint or tendon sheath. **Sphenopalatine ganglion [ganglion pterygopalatinum (NA)].** A ganglion lying in the pterygopalatine fossa and associated with the maxillary nerve. It is the probable terminal station for preganglionic parasympathetic fibres from the greater superficial petrosal nerve; the postganglionic fibres are distributed to the nose, palate, pharynx and lacrimal gland. **Sphenopalatine ganglion, orbital branches of the [rami orbitales (NA)].** Twigs from the sphenopalatine ganglion to the orbit. They are believed to carry motor fibres to the orbitalis muscle and secretomotor fibres to the lacrimal gland. **Spinal ganglion [ganglion spinale (NA)].** A cone-shaped mass of bipolar cells on the posterior root, their principal axons consisting of the posterior root of the spinal nerve. The centrally-directed axons enter the spinal cord at the posterolateral sulcus. **Spiral ganglion of the cochlea [ganglion spirale cochleae (NA)].** Bipolar nerve cells in the spiral canal of the modiolus from which the fibres of the cochlear nerve arise. **Splanchnic ganglion [ganglion splanchnicum (NA)].** A small ganglion on the greater splanchnic nerve. **Stellate ganglion.** *See* CERVICAL GANGLION, INFERIOR (above). **Sublingual ganglion.** Occasional nerve cells on the fibres from the submandibular ganglion; Blandin's ganglion. **Submandibular ganglion [ganglion submandibulare (NA)].** A ganglion associated with the lingual nerve [rami communicantes cum nervo linguali (NA)]. It is the relay station for secretomotor impulses (parasympathetic) to the submandibular and sublingual salivary glands [rami glandulares (NA)]. **Submandibular ganglion, sympathetic root of the [ramus sympathicus ad ganglion submandibulare (NA)].** Postganglionic fibres from the superior cervical ganglion, travelling to the submandibular ganglion along the facial artery. They supply the submandibular and sublingual glands. **Ganglia of sympathetic plexuses [ganglia plexuum autonomicorum (NA)].** A small collection of nerve cells frequent at the points of union of the nerves in the great plexuses of the sympathetic system. Some of these are sufficiently long and constant to be distinguished by separate names such as the ganglion of Wrisberg in the cardiac plexus, the coeliac ganglia, the aorticorenal ganglion or the superior mesenteric ganglion. **Ganglia of the sympathetic trunk [ganglia trunci sympathici (NA)].** Collections of multipolar nerve cells found in the sympathetic nervous system, more particularly, but not exclusively, in the course of the sympathetic trunk. They are generally 3 in number in the cervical, 12 in the thoracic, 4 in the lumbar and 4 in the sacral parts of the sympathetic trunk. They are cell stations on the efferent pathway of the sympathetic system. **Synovial ganglion.** Synovial cyst. *See* CYST. **Terminal ganglion [ganglion terminale (NA)].** Groups of nerve cells which occur along the terminal nerves. **Thoracic ganglia [ganglia thoracica (NA)].** A series of some 12 ganglia on the thoracic part of the sympathetic trunk. Each ganglion is connected to the corresponding thoracic spinal nerve by white and grey communicating branches. **Thoracic ganglia, cardiac branches of the [nervi cardiaci thoracici (NA)].** Twigs from the 2nd, 3rd, 4th and 5th thoracic ganglia to the deep cardiac plexus. **Thoracic ganglia, pulmonary branches of the [rami pulmonales (NA)].** Branches from the 2nd, 3rd and 4th thoracic ganglia to the posterior pulmonary plexus. **Trigeminal ganglion [ganglion trigeminale (NA)].** A sensory ganglion containing the cells of origin of the sensory fibres of the 5th cranial nerve. It lies in the posterior part of the middle cranial fossa, alongside the posterior end of the cavernous sinus; Gasser's ganglion. **Tympanic ganglion [ganglion tympanicum (NA)].** Irregular groups of nerve cells associated with the tympanic nerve during its course in the tympanum. **Ganglion of the vagus nerve, inferior [ganglion inferius (NA)].** The main sensory ganglion of the vagus nerve, about 25 mm long, lying in the carotid sheath immediately below the skull. The pharyngeal and superior laryngeal branches of the nerve arise from it. **Ganglion of the vagus nerve, superior [ganglion superius (NA)].** A small collection of ganglion cells in the jugular foramen. **Vertebral ganglion [ganglion vertebrale (NA)].** The ganglion in front of the origin of the vertebral artery. **Vestibular ganglion [ganglion vestibulare (NA)].** A collection of bipolar cells on the vestibular nerve at the outer end of the internal auditory meatus; the cells of origin of the fibres of the vestibular nerve. **Vestibulocochlear ganglion.** Auditory ganglion (see above). **Wrist ganglion.** A ganglion arising from the carpal joints or dorsal tendon sheaths at the wrist. [Gk *gagglion* knot.]

See also: ACREL, ANDERSCH, ARNOLD (F.), AUERBACH, BEZOLD (A.), BIDDER, BLANDIN, BOCHDALEK, BOCK, BOETTCHER, CLOQUET (H.), CORTI, DARKSHEVICH, EHRENRITTER, FRANKENHÄUSER, FRORIEP (A.), GANSER, GASSER, GUDDEN, HIRSCHFELD (L. M.), LANGLEY, LAUMONIER, LEE, LOBSTEIN, LUDWIG (K. F. W.), LUSCHKA, MECKEL, MEISSNER, MEYNERT, MUELLER (J.), NEUBAUER (J. E.), REMAK (R.), RIBES, SCARPA, SCHACHER, SCHMIEDEL, SOEMMERING, TROISIER, VALENTIN, WALTHER, WINTERHALTER, WRISBERG.

ganglionate, ganglionated (gang·gle·on·ate, gang·gle·on·**a'**·ted). 1. Having ganglia. 2. Twined or mixed together. [see prec.]

ganglionectomy (gang·gle·on·**ek'**·to·me). Surgical removal of a ganglion. [ganglion, Gk *ektome* a cutting out.]

See also: HENRY (A. K.), RANEY.

ganglionervous (gang·gle·o·**ner'**·vus). Belonging to the sympathetic nervous system. [ganglion, nerve.]

ganglioneure (gang·gle·o·newr). Ganglioneurone.

ganglioneuroblastoma (gang·gle·o·**newr**·o·blast·**o'**·mah). A ganglioglioneuroma composed of immature nerve cells. [ganglion, Gk *neuron* nerve, blastoma.]

ganglioneuroma (gang·gle·o·newr·**o'**·mah). A rare tumour occurring in young adults in ganglion cells of the sympathetic nervous system. [ganglion, neuroma.]

ganglioneurone (gang·gle·o·**newr'**·one). Any neurone within the spinal or cerebral ganglia.

ganglionic (gang·gle·**on**·ik). Pertaining to or of the nature of a ganglion.

ganglionitis (gang·gle·on·**i'**·tis). Inflammation of a ganglion. **Acute posterior ganglionitis.** Herpes zoster. [ganglion, Gk *-itis* inflammation.]

ganglionostomy (gang·gle·on·**os'**·to·me). Surgical incision of a ganglion associated with the synovial sheath of a tendon. [ganglion, Gk *stoma* mouth.]

gangliopathy (gang·gle·**op**·ath·e). 1. Any diseased condition of a ganglion. 2. Any affection or disorder resulting from disease of a ganglion. [ganglion, Gk *pathos* disease.]

ganglioplegia (gang·gle·o·**ple'**·je·ah). A state of depressed activity in a ganglion resulting in failure of normal transmission of impulses. [ganglion, Gk *plege* stroke.]

ganglioplexus (gang·gle·o·**plex'**·us). A nerve plexus within a ganglion.

gangliosympathectomy (gang·gle·o·sim·path·**ek'**·to·me). Surgical excision of a sympathetic ganglion. [ganglion, sympathetic, Gk *ektome* a cutting out.]

gangosa (gan·go·sah). In tertiary yaws, an ulcerative process which attacks the nasal and palatal structures and destroys them. The condition may be found in any region in which yaws is endemic, particularly in the islands of the East Indies and the Pacific. [Sp. muffled voice.]

gangrene (gang·green). Necrosis and putrefaction of tissue due to cutting off the blood supply; the term usually refers to skin necrosis, but it may also occur in the bowel. In the dry form the skin becomes shrunken and blackened and a line of demarcation from viable tissue forms; bacterial growth is minimal. In the wet form, inflammation and venous as well as arterial obstruction are usually present; the tissue becomes swollen, soggy and infected with numerous organisms which are often anaerobic. This type spreads widely. Gangrene results from complete arterial occlusion due to emboli, atherosclerosis obliterans, thrombo-angiitis obliterans or traumatic thrombosis. **Anaemic gangrene.** Gangrene due to obstruction of the blood supply to a part. **Anaphylactic gangrene.** Gangrene due to allergic reactions following repeated injections of serum. **Arteriosclerotic gangrene.** Gangrene due to arteriosclerosis. **Carbolic gangrene.** Local gangrene caused by the direct action of carbolic acid on skin or mucous membrane. **Chemical gangrene.** Gangrene following burns by corrosive chemicals. **Circumscribed gangrene.** A gangrenous area sharply demarcated from normal tissues by an inflammatory zone. **Cold gangrene.** Gangrene not preceded by inflammation. **Congenital gangrene.** Necrosis of a limb due to intra-uterine thrombosis or fracture. **Cutaneous gangrene.** Death of an area of skin. **Decubital gangrene.** A bedsore. **Diabetic gangrene.** Gangrene of a limb due to occlusive arterial changes in an elderly diabetic patient; in uncontrolled diabetes local infection is an important factor. **Disseminated cutaneous gangrene.** Widespread areas of gangrene of the skin. **Dry gangrene.** Gangrene going on to mummification of a part, due to arterial obstruction in senile patients. It is also seen in Raynaud's disease and ergotism. **Gangrene due to ergotism.** Symmetrical gangrene of the extremities due to the ingestion of ergot which produces sustained vasoconstriction. **Embolic gangrene.** Gangrene due to arterial embolism. **Emphysematous gangrene.** Gas gangrene (see below). **Epidemic gangrene.** Ergotism. **Frost gangrene.** Frostbite. **Fulminating gangrene.** Malignant oedema. *See* OEDEMA. **Fusospirochaetal gangrene.** Gangrene due to Vincent's organisms. **Gas gangrene, Gaseous gangrene.** Spreading oedema, necrosis and gas formation, due to infection of wounds with anaerobic bacilli, especially *Clostridium welchii, C. oedematiens* and *C. septicum.* **Glycaemic gangrene.** Diabetic gangrene (see above). **Hospital gangrene.** Gangrene due to the spread of anaerobic infections to operation wounds. **Hot gangrene.** That following inflammatory lesions. **Humid gangrene.** Moist gangrene (see below). **Inflammatory gangrene.** Gangrene following an acute inflammatory condition. **Mephitic**

gangrene. Gas gangrene (see above). **Mixed gangrene.** Dry gangrene with moist patches. **Moist gangrene.** Gangrene in which the part becomes soft, moist and putrefactive. **Multiple gangrene.** Gangrene occurring in more than one part of the body. **Neurotic gangrene.** Gangrene secondary to nervous disorders such as syringomyelia or Raynaud's disease. **Nosocomial gangrene.** Hospital gangrene (see above). **Oral gangrene.** Gangrenous stomatitis. **Presenile gangrene.** An obsolete term applied to gangrene due to thrombo-angiitis obliterans. **Pressure gangrene.** Gangrene due to pressure, e.g. a plaster sore, bedsore. **Primary gangrene.** Gangrene in which the necrosis and putrefaction are due to the same infective agents. **Progressive gangrene.** That in which no line of demarcation forms. **Progressive bacterial synergistic gangrene.** An uncommon variety of spreading gangrene of skin (often beginning near the site of a drainage opening) due to a symbiosis of a microaerophilic non-haemolytic streptococcus with a haemolytic staphylococcus. **Secondary gangrene.** Gangrene in which putrefactive changes follow the primary necrosis. **Senile gangrene.** That due to arterial changes in elderly patients; an obsolete term applied to gangrene due to atherosclerosis obliterans. **Spirochaetal gangrene.** That in which spirochaetes are the infective agents. **Static gangrene.** Gangrene due to circulatory stasis. **Symmetrical gangrene.** Raynaud's disease. **Tachetic gangrene.** Gangrene with ecchymotic spots. **Traumatic gangrene.** That due to severe injuries, especially with damage to blood vessels. **Trophic gangrene.** That due to neurotrophic disturbances. **Venous gangrene.** Gangrene secondary to massive venous obstruction. **Wet gangrene.** Moist gangrene (see above). **White gangrene.** Ischaemic necrosis. *See* NECROSIS. [Gk *gaggraina.*]

See also: FOURNIER, POTT.

gangrenescent (gang·gren·es·ent). Showing the first evidence of becoming gangrenous.

gangrenopsis (gang·gren·**op**·sis). Gangrenous stomatitis. [gangrene, Gk *opsis* face.]

gangrenosis (gang·gren·**o**·sis). The presence or development of gangrene. [gangrene, Gk *-osis* condition.]

gangrenous (gang·gren·us). Pertaining to, resulting from, or affected with gangrene.

ganja, ganjah (gan·jah). The name given to the forms of Indian hemp prepared for medicinal use from the short-stemmed female inflorescences. Flat, or Bombay, ganja is the compressed form used in England, round, or Bengal, ganja is the rolled form used mainly in India, and churganja is a product consisting of powder and broken pieces. It is also known as *guaza, guaja* and *gunjah,* corruptions of the original name. [Hind.]

gannister (gan·is·ter). A hard siliceous sandstone or clay rock present in some coal seams in England and used for grinding and furnace hearths. [MHG *ganster* spark.]

ganoblast (gan·o·blast). Ameloblast. [Gk *ganos* brightness, *blastos* germ.]

Ganong, William Francis (b. 1924). American physiologist.

Lown–Ganong–Levine syndrome. The combination of a short P-R interval in the electrocardiogram with a normal QRS complex in a patient subject to paroxysmal tachycardia; thought, in some cases at least, to be due to the existence of a *James bundle.*

Ganser, Sigbert Joseph Maria (b. 1853). Dresden psychiatrist.

commissure of Ganser. A component of the postoptic commissures of the hypothalamus.

Ganser's ganglion. The interpeduncular nucleus. *See* NUCLEUS.

Ganser syndrome. A hysterical twilight state in which the clinical picture is that which a lay person might imagine to be typical of madness.

Gant, Frederick James (b. 1825). London surgeon.

Gant's operation. Subtrochanteric osteotomy of the femur, for ankylosis of the hip.

Gant, Samuel Goodwin (b. 1870). New York surgeon.

Gant's clamp. An angled clamp used in the pile operation.

Gantzer, Carol Friedrich Ludovic. 18th–19th century German anatomist.

Gantzer's accessory bundle. A variant in the origin of the flexor pollicis longus muscle when it presents an extrahumeral or ulnar head.

Gantzer's muscle. An accessory muscle given off from the flexor digitorum sublimis muscle which joins the flexor digitorum profundus muscle.

gap (gap). 1. An opening; a discontinuity. 2. A space that is not occupied by an amino-acid residue (or nucleotide unit) introduced into a protein (or nucleic acid) sequence to increase the similarities of related sequences in an alignment. **Achromatic gap.** A narrow region in the chromosome which fails to stain although it does not represent a discontinuity of the chromosome. It may be in one or, more rarely, in both the chromatids of a chromosome. **Auscultatory gap.** The silent phase between the disappearance of Korotkoff's sounds and their reappearance at a higher level of pressure during the measuring of blood pressure of hypertensive individuals with the sphygmomanometer. **Cranial gap.** A congenital skull fissure. **Quenched spark gap.** A spark gap placed under conditions, such as immersion in a bath of suitable liquid, to arrest or quench the discharge. **Silent gap.** Auscultatory gap (see above). **Spark gap.** The space separating two electrodes in a high-tension circuit, across which a disruptive discharge of electricity takes place at some prescribed potential difference. [ME.]

See also: BOCHDALEK.

gape (gape). To open the mouth wide; to yawn. [ME *gapen* to open the mouth.]

gapeworm (gape·werm). A nematode worm of the genus *Syngamus.* The adults live in the mouth, nasal cavities and pharynx, and are so called because they cause *gapes* in poultry. Several species have been recorded in humans, but man is not the normal host to any. [gape, AS *wyrm.*]

garantose (gar·an·toze). Saccharin.

garbage (gar·bij). Refuse; animal or vegetable matter and other waste material from a market or kitchen which is not disposed of by the drainage system and is distinct from ashes, manure and other similar rubbish. [O Fr. *garbe* bundle.]

Garbe, William (b. 1908). Toronto dermatologist.

Sulzberger–Garbe disease. A chronic, extensive, exudative, discoid and lichenoid eruption, mostly occurring in males.

Garcinia (gar·sin·e·ah). A genus of trees, mainly tropical, belonging to the family Guttiferae and having stems which yield a yellow resinous juice. *Garcinia hanburyi* Hook. f. is the source of gamboge. The fruits of *G. mangostana* Linn. have been used as a substitute for bael fruits. [Laurent *Garcin* (b. 1683), French botanist.]

Gardiner-Brown, Alfred. British otologist.

Gardiner-Brown test, for aural disease. If the vibrations of a tuning fork placed on the mastoid process are heard for a longer or a shorter time than they are felt by the examiner, disturbance of aural function is suspected.

Gardner, Eldon John (b. 1909). American geneticist.

Gardner's syndrome. Familial multiple polyposis of the colon associated with subcutaneous lipomata, fibromata, exostoses or osteomas of facial bones. An autosomal dominant disorder, with a marked tendency to rapid malignant change.

gargalaesthesia (gar·gal·es·**the**'·ze·ah). The condition in which the tickle sensation is present and perceived. [Gk *gargalizein* to tickle, aesthesia.]

gargalanaesthesia (gar·gal·an·es·**the**'·ze·ah). A condition in which the tickle sense is absent. [Gk *gargalizein* to tickle, anaesthesia.]

gargareon (gar·**gar**·e·on). Uvula. [Gk.]

gargarism, gargarisma (gar·gar·izm, gar·gar·**iz**·mah). A gargle. [Gk *gargarisma* a gargling.]

gargle (gar·gl). 1. A liquid preparation for irrigating the throat, not usually intended to be swallowed. 2. With the head thrown back, to hold in the pharynx a medicinal fluid, to keep it agitated by gentle breathing, so that it remains in the pharynx, irrigating the mucosa, and eventually to spit it out through the mouth. [O Fr. *gargouille* throat.]

gargoylism (gar·goil·izm). Hurler's syndrome; mucopolysaccharidosis type I. [O Fr. *gargouille* throat.]

Gariel, Maurice (b. 1812). French physician.

Gariel's pessary. An inflatable rubber pessary.

Garland, George Minot (b. 1848). Boston physician.

Garland's triangle. A triangular area of skodaic resonance found on percussion of a moderate-sized pleural effusion. It is situated between the area of absolute dullness and the vertebral spine, and is due to the underlying relaxed lung.

Ellis-Garland curve, line or sign. The S-shaped line that on percussion marks the upper limit of dullness caused by a pleural effusion.

garlic (gar·lik). Allium. The fresh compound bulb of *Allium sativum* Linn. (family Liliaceae). It contains a glucoside together with some volatile oil produced by the hydrolysis of the former. The chief constituent of the oil is allyl sulphide. The bulb has a strong odour disagreeable to many people and pungent taste, and is used as a diuretic, diaphoretic and expectorant. [AS *garleac.*]

Garré, Carl (b. 1857). Swiss surgeon.

Garré's disease, osteitis or osteomyelitis. Chronic non-suppurative sclerosing osteitis or osteomyelitis; a chronic inflammatory condition of bone, associated with sclerosis and thickening, and due to infection by pyogenic cocci.

Garrod, Sir Archibald Edward (b. 1858). English physician.

Garrod's inborn errors of metabolism. The clinical states that arise from deficiency of enzymes involved in metabolism.

Garrod, Lawrence Paul (b. 1895). London bacteriologist.

Garrod's gentian-violet agar. Blood agar containing (1:1 000 000) gentian violet, used for the isolation of streptococci, which are resistant to the dye, in the presence of staphylococci, the latter being sensitive to it in very lcw concentrations.

garrot, garotte, garrotte (gar·ot). 1. A tourniquet consisting of a band which can be fastened around a part and tightened so that the artery is compressed and the circulation arrested. 2. In forensic medicine, (*a*) to strangle manually from behind; (*b*) to strangle by means of a noose thrown over the head from behind and twisted tight with a stick. [Sp. *garrote* stick used in twisting cord tight.]

Gartner, Hermann Treschow (b. 1785). Copenhagen anatomist.

Gartner's canal or duct. The vestige of the mesonephric duct found in the broad ligament of the uterus, and sometimes extending in the wall of the vagina to the vulva. It forms the vas deferens in the male.

Gartnerian cyst. A cystic dilatation of Gartner's duct.

gartnerian (gart·ne·re·an). Pertaining to Hermann Treschow *Gartner.*

gas (gas). 1. A state of matter in which the molecules are free to move rapidly and chaotically in all directions, the distance between each being much greater than its diameter; such a fluid expands to fill completely any vessel into which it is admitted. 2. Coal or Natural gas. 3. Nitrogen monoxide. 4. To expose to noxious fumes, as, for example, in chemical warfare. **Asphyxiating gas.** Any gas, such as carbon monoxide, used to asphyxiate in chemical warfare. **Blau gas.** A fuel gas produced by cracking hydrocarbons. **Blister gas.** A vesicant such as mustard gas or Lewisite, used in chemical warfare. **Blood gases.** The partial pressure of gases dissolved in blood, e.g. oxygen and carbon dioxide. **Choking gas.** Any gas used in chemical warfare which affects the lungs, as do chlorine, or phosgene and its derivatives. **Coal gas.** A gas consisting mainly of methane, carbon monoxide and hydrogen, produced by the dry-distillation of coal, and used for heating and lighting purposes. **Ethyl gas.** Tetra-ethyl lead, $Pb(C_2H_5)_4$, a liquid mixed with petrol to reduce "knocking". **Haemolytic gas.** Arsine, arseniuretted hydrogen, AsH_3, a poisonous gas which causes haemolysis. **Inert gas.** Any of the gases, helium, neon, argon, krypton and xenon, which are present in the atmosphere and display no chemical affinity; radon is also included in this group. **Lacrimatory gas.** Tear gas (see below). **Laughing gas.** Nitrous oxide, N_2O, a gas used for short anaesthesia, so called because of the hilarity it may produce. **Lethal gas.** In chemical warfare, a gas such as phosgene used for the purpose of causing death rather than for nuisance value. **Gas liquid chromatography,** *see* CHROMATOGRAPHY. **Marsh gas.** Methane, CH_4, so called because it is formed during the decomposition of vegetation in marshes. **Mustard gas.** Dichlorodiethyl sulphide, $S(CH_2CH_2Cl)_2$, a stable blister gas used in chemical warfare. **Natural gas.** A gas found in the Earth's crust, not manufactured, usually with petroleum, and consists mostly of methane; used as a fuel. **Noble gas.** Inert gas (see above). **Nose gas.** Any gas such as adamsite or dick, irritant to the mucous membrane of the nose and used in chemical warfare. **Olefiant gas.** Ethylene, $CH_2{=}CH_2$, so called from its formation of an oil with chlorine. **Phlogisticated gas.** Name for oxygen [obsolete term]. **Poison gases.** Substances used in chemical warfare for their nuisance value or to cause casualties: they consist of tear gases, nose gases, choking gases, asphyxiating gases and blister gases. **Producer gas.** A mixture of carbon monoxide and nitrogen formed by blowing air through red-hot coke; used for industrial heating. **Sewer gas.** The effluvium of sewers, consisting of gases formed by organic decomposition. **Sneezing gas, Sternutatory gas.** A nose gas, such as diphenylchlorarsine, which causes sneezing. **Suffocating gas.** A choking gas (see above). **Sweet gas.** The poisonous white damp, or carbon monoxide, which has no smell. **Tear gas.** Any gas such as chloro-acetophenone (CAP), which affects the eyes, producing lacrimation, and used for this purpose in chemical warfare. **Vesicant gas.** Blister gas (see above). **Vomiting gas.** A choking gas, chloropicrin, which also causes vomiting. **War gas.** Any poisonous substance (gas, vapour or smoke) used in chemical warfare to harass troops or cause casualties. **Water gas.** An industrial fuel gas produced by blowing steam through white-hot coal or coke. [invented word suggested by Gk *chaos.*]

See also: CLAYTON, MOND.

gaseous, gasiform (ga·se·us, ga·se·form). Pertaining to or having the character of a gas; in chemistry, the third state of matter.

Gaskell, Walter Holbrook (b. 1847). Cambridge physiologist.

Gaskell's bridge. The atrioventricular bundle. *See* BUNDLE.

Gaskell's nerves. The accelerator nerves of the heart.

gasogenic (gas·o·**jen**·ik). Giving rise to gas. [gas, Gk *genein* to produce.]

gasometer (gas·**om**·et·er). 1. An instrument which measures the quantity of gas passing through it, or the quantity of gas present. 2. A calibrated container with which the volume of respiratory gases can be measured.

gasometric (gas·o·**met**·rik). Relating or belonging to gasometry.

gasometry (gas·**om**·et·re). 1. The determination of the relative amounts of gases present in a mixture. 2. The science of measuring gas. 3. Gasometric analysis. *See* ANALYSIS. [gas, meter.]

gasp (gahsp). 1. A convulsive catching of the breath with wide open mouth. 2. To labour for breath. [ME *gaspen* to yawn.]

Gasperini's culture medium. A suspension in water of wheat flour, salts and glucose, formerly used as a culture medium for moulds.

Gasser, Johann Laurenz (b. 1723). Vienna anatomist.

Gasser's ganglion, gasserian ganglion. The trigeminal ganglion. *See* GANGLION.

gasserectomy (gas·er·**ek**·to·me). 1. Surgical excision of the trigeminal (gasserian) ganglion. 2. Total or subtotal division of the trigeminal nerve above the trigeminal (gasserian) ganglion, for relief of trigeminal neuralgia. [Johann Laurenz *Gasser*, Gk *ektome* a cutting out.]

gasserian (gas·e·re·an). Pertaining to Johann Laurenz *Gasser.*

gasteralgia (gas·ter·**al**·je·ah). Gastralgia.

gasterangiemphraxis (gas·ter·an·je·em·**frax**'·is). 1. An obstructed and congested condition of the blood vessels of the stomach. 2. Pyloric obstruction. [Gk *gaster* stomach, *aggeion* small vessel, emphraxis.]

gasterasthenia (gas·ter·as·**the**'·ne·ah). Gastrasthenia.

gasteremphraxis (gas·ter·em·**frax**'·is). 1. A distended condition of the stomach. 2. Gasterangiemphraxis. [Gk *gaster* stomach, emphraxis.]

gasterhysterotomy (gas·ter·his·ter·**ot'**·o·me). Caesarean section. *See* SECTION. [Gk *gaster* stomach, hysterotomy.]

gasteric (gas·**ter**·rik). Gastric.

gastradenitis (gas·trad·en·**i'**·tis). Gastro-adenitis.

gastraemia (gas·**tre**·me·ah). A congested state of the coats of the stomach. [Gk *gaster* stomach, *haima* blood.]

gastral (gas·tral). Gastric.

gastralgia (gas·**tral**·je·ah). 1. Any pain in the stomach. 2. Pain of a paroxysmal nature affecting the stomach or epigastrium. **Appendicular gastralgia.** Pain referred to the stomach and caused by disease of the vermiform appendix. [Gk *gaster* stomach, *algos* pain.]

gastralgokenosis (gas·**tral**·go·ken·**o'**·sis). Paroxysmal pain in the stomach occurring when the stomach is empty and relieved by the taking of food. [Gk *gaster* stomach, *algos* pain, *kenos* empty.]

gastraneuria (gas·tran·**ewr**·e·ah). Lack of normal tone and activity of the stomach. [Gk *gaster* stomach, *a*, *neuron* nerve.]

gastraneurysma (gas·tran·ewr·**iz'**·mah). Gastrectasia. [Gk *gaster* stomach, aneurysm.]

gastrasthenia (gas·tras·**the**·ne·ah). 1. Weakness of the digestive function of the stomach. 2. Lack of tone and weakness of the muscle coats of the stomach. [Gk *gaster* stomach, asthenia.]

gastratrophia (gas·trah·**tro**·fe·ah). Atrophy of the stomach. [Gk *gaster* stomach, atrophy.]

gastrectasia, gastrectasis (gas·trek·**ta**·ze·ah, gas·**trek**·tas·is). Dilatation of the stomach. [Gk *gaster* stomach, *ektasis* a stretching.]

gastrectomy (gas·**trek**·to·me). The surgical removal of the stomach in whole or in part. **Antecolic gastrectomy.** Excision of the stomach with reconstitution by anastomosis in front of the transverse colon. **Partial gastrectomy.** Removal of a portion, usually the distal portion, of the stomach. **Physiological gastrectomy.** Ligation of all the gastric vessels without actual surgical removal of the stomach. **Subtotal gastrectomy.** Removal of all of the stomach except a small cardiac portion. **Total gastrectomy.** Removal of the whole stomach. **Transthoracic gastrectomy.** Removal of the stomach by a surgical approach through the chest and diaphragm. [Gk *gaster* stomach, *ektome* excision.]

See also: BILLROTH, FINSTERER, HOFMEISTER, PÓLYA, SCHOEMAKER.

gastric (gas·trik). Relating or belonging to the stomach. [Gk *gaster* stomach.]

gastric arteries. Left gastric artery [arteria gastrica sinistra (NA)]. A division of the coeliac artery which runs upwards and to the left behind the lesser sac to reach the cardiac end of the stomach, where it gives off branches along the lesser curvature, and oesophageal branches [rami esophagei (NA)] that anastomose with aortic oesophageal vessels. **Right gastric artery [arteria gastrica dextra].** *See* HEPATIC ARTERY, COMMON. **Short gastric arteries [arteriae gastricae breves (NA)].** *See* SPLENIC ARTERY.

gastric veins. Left gastric vein [vena gastrica sinistra (NA)]. A vein from the lesser curvature of the stomach following the artery of the same name. It communicates with the oesophageal veins (systemic system) and drains into the portal vein (hepatic portal system). **Right gastric vein [vena gastrica dextra (NA)].** A tributary of the portal vein, draining parts adjacent to the lesser curvature of the stomach in the pyloric region. **Short gastric veins [venae gastricae breves (NA)].** Tributaries of the splenic vein, about 4 in number, from the fundus and left part of the body of the stomach.

gastricism (gas·tris·izm). 1. Any disorder of the stomach. 2. A belief held by some that the majority of diseases have origin in a digestive disorder. [Gk *gaster* stomach.]

gastrin (gas·trin). A gastric hormone containing 17 amino acids, and sometimes known as G-17-I (non-sulphated) or G-17-II (sulphated). In the plasma only a small fraction is in the G-17 form ("little" gastrin). Most of the immunoreactive gastrin has a molecular weight of approximately 7000 and consists of 34 amino acids G-34 ("big" gastrin) and is either non-sulphated (I) or sulphated (II). Another form contains a very large molecule ("big, big" gastrin) and yet another is "mini gastrin" (G-13-I and G-13-II).

gastrinoma (gas·trin·**oma**). (Zollinger–Ellison syndrome). The predominant gastrin is G-34 ("big" gastrin).

gastritic (gas·**trit**·ik). 1. Referring or belonging to gastritis. 2. Suffering from gastritis.

gastritis (gas·**tri**·tis). Inflammation of the gastric mucous membrane. **Acute gastritis.** Catarrhal inflammation caused by the ingestion of irritating matter such as excess of alcohol, decomposed food or by the excessive use of condiments. It may occur with acute infectious diseases such as influenza and scarlet fever, and also in uraemia. It may be caused by drugs when it may be erosive (haemorrhagic), especially after aspirin ingestion. **Acute phlegmonous gastritis.** A widespread inflammation of the submucous coat, and the mucous coat may be completely destroyed. It can be caused by irritant poisons such as concentrated acids and alkalis, by a virulent streptococcal infection, rarely staphylococcal, and may be part of a general pyaemic infection or arise through an ulcer or wound. **Alcoholic gastritis.** Gastritis caused by the direct action of strong or relatively strong alcoholic solutions on the gastric mucosa. **Atrophic gastritis.** Chronic mucosal atrophy with failure of acid secretion, always found in cases of pernicious anaemia. **Catarrhal gastritis.** An inflammatory condition of the gastric mucosa associated with excessive secretion of mucus; clinically, there are tympanites, abdominal pain or discomfort, often with vomiting, loss of appetite and possibly low fever, especially in children. **Chronic gastritis.** A chronic inflammation of the mucous membrane due to the continual ingestion of irritating matter, defective mastication or the swallowing of septic material from the mouth, tonsils or nasopharynx. Hyperchlorhydria and achlorhydria are predisposing factors. **Corrosive gastritis.** Gastritis resulting from a corrosive substance. **Fibrinous gastritis.** Gastritis in which there is much fibrin in the exudate. **Giant hypertrophic gastritis.** Gastritis with hypertrophy of the gastric mucosal folds. **Granulomatous gastritis.** A rare form of Crohn's disease causing gastric changes like those of regional ileitis. **Haematogenous gastritis.** Gastritis caused by the action of blood-borne toxins, either bacterial or metabolic, on the gastric mucosa, possibly in the process of excretion of these toxins which would then continue their action directly until removed either by the act of vomiting or via the pylorus. [Gk *gaster* stomach, *-itis* inflammation.]

gastro-acephalus (gas·tro·a·**kef'**·al·us). A monster with an acephalic abdominal parasite. [Gk *gaster* stomach, acephalic.]

gastro-adenitis (gas·tro·ad·en·**i'**·tis). Inflammation of the gastric glands. [Gk *gaster* stomach, adenitis.]

gastro-adynamia (gas·tro·a·di·**nam'**·e·ah). A condition of loss of power in the gastric musculature, resulting in local asthenia and general prostration. [Gk *gaster* stomach, adynamia.]

gastro-albumorrhoea (gas·tro·al·bew·mo·**re'**·ah). A condition in which excessive amounts of mucin are secreted by the stomach. [Gk *gaster* stomach, albumin, Gk *rhoia* flow.]

gastro-anastomosis (gas·tro·an·as·to·**mo'**·sis). Gastrogastrostomy. [Gk *gaster* stomach, *anastomoein* to provide with a mouth.]

gastro-atonia (gas·tro·at·**o'**·ne·ah). Absence of normal tone in the stomach; atonic dyspepsia. [Gk *gaster* stomach, atony.]

gastroblennorrhoea (gas·tro·blen·o·**re'**·ah). The condition in which an abnormally large quantity of mucus is secreted by the stomach. [Gk *gaster* stomach, blennorrhoea.]

gastrobrosis (gas·tro·**bro**·sis). Corrosive and perforating gastric ulcer. [Gk *gaster* stomach, *brosis* an eating.]

gastrocamera (gas·tro·**kam**·er·ah). A very small camera which is capable of being swallowed and which takes photographs of the interior of the stomach. [Gk *gaster* stomach, camera.]

gastrocardiac (gas·tro·**kar**·de·ak). Relating or belonging to, or involving both the stomach and the heart. [Gk *gaster* stomach, *kardia* heart.]

gastrocele (gas·tro·seel). Hernia of the stomach or of a portion which has become pouched. [Gk *gaster* stomach, *kele* hernia.]

gastrochronorrhoea (gas·tro·kron·o·re′·ah). Gastrosuccorrhoea. [Gk *gaster* stomach, *chronos* time, *rhoia* flow.]

gastrocnemius muscle [musculus gastrocnemius (NA)] (gas·tro·ne·me·us). The most superficial of the calf muscles, arising by a medial [caput mediale (NA)] and a lateral [caput laterale (NA)] head from the upper parts of the corresponding condyles of the femur and inserted into a broad aponeurosis to form the tendo calcaneus with the tendon of the soleus. It is a flexor of both knee and ankle. [Gk *gastroknemia* calf of the leg.]

gastrocoele (gas·tro·se′·le). In embryology, the cavity (archenteron) within the gastrula which acts as the digestive cavity in the development of the early embryo. [Gk *gaster* stomach, coelom.]

gastrocolic (gas·tro·kol·ik). Having relation or belonging to the stomach and the colon. [Gk *gaster* stomach, colon.]

gastrocolitis (gas·tro·kol·i′·tis). An inflamed condition of the stomach and the colon. [Gk *gaster* stomach, colitis.]

gastrocoloptosis (gas·tro·kol·op·to′·sis). Downward displacement or prolapse of the stomach and colon. [Gk *gaster* stomach, colon, Gk *ptosis* fall.]

gastrocolostomy (gas·tro·kol·os′·to·me). The surgical formation of an anastomosis between the stomach and the colon. [Gk *gaster* stomach, colon, Gk *stoma* mouth.]

gastrocolotomy (gas·tro·kol·ot′·o·me). A surgical incision into the stomach and colon. [Gk *gaster* stomach, colon, Gk *temnein* to cut.]

gastrodialysis (gas·tro·di·al′·is·is). Sloughing of the mucous coat of the stomach so that there is patchy erosion and loss of continuity in the walls. [Gk *gaster* stomach, dialysis.]

gastrodiaphane (gas·tro·di·af·ane). An instrument consisting of an oesophageal tube bearing a tiny electric-light bulb for illuminating the cavity of the stomach so that its outlines are visible through the wall of the abdomen. [Gk *gaster* stomach, *dia*, *phainein* to show.]

gastrodiaphanoscopy, gastrodiaphany (gas·tro·di·af·an·os′·ko·pe, gas·tro·di·af′·an·e). Examination of the cavity of the stomach by means of a gastrodiaphane. [gastrodiaphane, Gk *skopein* to view.]

gastrodidymus (gas·tro·did·im·us). A twin monster united by a common abdominal cavity. [Gk *gaster* stomach, *didymos* twin.]

Gastrodiscidae (gas·tro·dis·id·e). A family of the trematode sub-order Amphistomata or Paramphistomoidea. The genus *Gastrodiscoides* is of medical interest. [Gk *gaster* stomach, *diskos* disc, *eidos* form.]

Gastrodiscoides (gas·tro·dis·koid′·eez). A genus of small intestinal flukes. **Gastrodiscoides hominis.** A true parasite of the pig, but common in man in the tropical Far East and occasionally the cause of diarrhoea; the molluscan secondary hosts are unknown. [see prec.]

Gastrodiscus (gas·tro·dis·kus). *Gastrodiscoides.*

gastrodisk (gas·tro·disk). In the fertilized human ovum, the germ disc, i.e. the clump of large irregularly-shaped cells which makes up the bulk of the formative mass. [Gk *gaster* stomach, disc.]

gastroduodenal (gas·tro·dew·o·de′·nal). Relating or belonging to the stomach and the duodenum. [Gk *gaster* stomach, duodenum.]

gastroduodenal artery [arteria gastroduodenalis]. *See* HEPATIC ARTERY, COMMON.

gastroduodenitis (gas·tro·dew·o·de·ni′·tis). Inflammation of the stomach and the duodenum. [Gk *gaster* stomach, duodenum, Gk *-itis* inflammation.]

gastroduodeno-enterostomy (gas·tro·dew·o·de·no·en·ter·os′·to·me). Gastroduodenostomy. [Gk *gaster* stomach, duodenum, enterostomy.]

gastroduodenoscopy (gas·tro·dew·o·de·nos′·ko·pe). Inspection of the stomach and duodenum by means of a gastroscope passed through an incision in the wall of the stomach. [Gk *gaster* stomach, duodenum, Gk *skopein* to watch.]

gastroduodenostomy (gas·tro·dew·o·de·nos′·to·me). Surgical establishment of an anastomosis between the stomach and the duodenum. [Gk *gaster* stomach, duodenum, Gk *stoma* mouth.]

gastrodynia (gas·tro·din·e·ah). Gastralgia. [Gk *gaster* stomach, *odyne* pain.]

gastro-ectasis (gas·tro·ek·tas·is). Gastrectasia.

gastro-enteralgia (gas·tro·en·ter·al′·je·ah). Pain in the stomach and intestines. [Gk *gaster* stomach, *enteron* bowel, *algos* pain.]

gastro-enteric (gas·tro·en·ter′·rik). Gastro-intestinal. [Gk *gaster* stomach, *enteron* bowel.]

gastro-enteritis (gas·tro·en·ter·i′·tis). Inflammation of the mucous coat of the stomach and intestines as a result of infection with a bacterium of the *Salmonella* genus, e.g. *S. typhimurium* and *S. enteritidis* or other allied genera. There is also a rare eosinophilic gastro-enteritis with eosinophilic infiltration of the wall of the intestine which may follow eating raw herrings infected with the parasitic worm *Eustoma rotundatum.* Viral forms of gastro-enteritis due to infection with enteroviruses are common. [Gk *gaster* stomach, *enteron* bowel, *-itis* inflammation.]

gastro-entero-anastomosis (gas·tro·en·ter·o·an·as·to·mo′·sis). The artificial passage created in gastro-enterostomy. [Gk *gaster* stomach, *enteron* bowel, anastomosis.]

gastro-enterocolitis (gas·tro·en·ter·o·kol·i′·tis). Inflammation of the stomach, the small intestine and the colon. [Gk *gaster* stomach, enterocolitis.]

gastro-enterocolostomy (gas·tro·en·ter·o·kol·os′·to·me). The surgical establishment of an anastomosis between the stomach, the small intestine and the colon. [Gk *gaster* stomach, enterocolostomy.]

gastro-enterology (gas·tro·en·ter·ol′·o·je). That branch of medical science which is concerned with the stomach and intestines, and the diseases especially affecting them. [Gk *gaster* stomach, *enteron* bowel, *logos* science.]

gastro-entero-pancreatic system. G.E.P. The system of cells found in the intestinal tract which releases the hormones characteristic of this tract.

gastro-enteropathy (gas·tro·en·ter·op′·ath·e). Any gastric or intestinal disease. [Gk *gaster* stomach, *enteron* bowel, *pathos* disease.]

gastro-enteroplasty (gas·tro·en′·ter·o·plas·te). Plastic surgery of both stomach and intestines. [Gk *gaster* stomach, *enteron* bowel, *plassein* to mould.]

gastro-enteroptosis (gas·tro·en·ter·op·to′·sis). Prolapse or downward displacement of the stomach and the intestines. [Gk *gaster* stomach, *enteron* bowel, *ptosis* fall.]

gastro-enterostomy (gas·tro·en·ter·os′·to·me). The surgical establishment of a communication between the stomach and the small intestine. [Gk *gaster* stomach, *enteron* bowel, *stoma* mouth.]

gastro-enterotomy (gas·tro·en·ter·ot′·o·me). Incision into both the stomach and the intestine through the abdominal wall. [Gk *gaster* stomach, *enteron* bowel, *temnein* to cut.]

gastro-epiploic (gas·tro·ep·e·plo′·ik). Referring or belonging to the stomach and the greater omentum. [Gk *gaster* stomach, *epiploon* caul.]

gastro-epiploic arteries. Left gastro-epiploic artery [arteria gastro-epiploica sinister]. *See* SPLENIC ARTERY. **Right gastro-epiploic artery [arteria gastro-epiploica dextra].** *See* HEPATIC ARTERY, COMMON.

gastro-epiploic veins. Left gastro-epiploic vein [vena gastro-epiploica sinistra]. A tributary of the splenic vein, from the region of the greater curvature of the stomach. **Right gastro-epiploic vein [vena gastro-epiploica dextra].** The main venous drainage of the pyloric end of the stomach, adjacent to the greater curvature, and of the greater omentum. It is a tributary of the superior mesenteric vein.

gastrofaradization (gas·tro·far·ad·i·za′·shun). The application of a faradic current to the stomach or abdomen as a therapeutic measure. [Gk *gaster* stomach, faradization.]

gastrogalvanization (gas·tro·gal·van·i·za′·shun). The use of galvanism in the treatment of disorders of the stomach or abdomen. [Gk *gaster* stomach, galvanization.]

gastrogastrostomy (gas·tro·gas·**tros**′·to·me). In treatment of hour-glass stomach, the surgical establishment of a communication between the cardiac and the pyloric portions of the stomach. [Gk *gaster* stomach, *stoma* mouth.]

gastrogavage (gas·tro·**gav**·ahzh). Artificial feeding carried out by means of a tube inserted into the stomach through an incision in the wall of the abdomen [Gk *gaster* stomach, gavage.]

gastrogenic, gastrogenous (gas·tro·**jen**·ik, gas·**troj**·en·us). 1. Formed in or produced by the stomach. 2. Originating in or arising from the stomach. [Gk *gaster* stomach, *genein* to produce.]

gastrograph (**gas**·tro·graf). An instrument which, when it is applied to the surface of the body over the stomach, records the peristaltic movements. [Gk *gaster* stomach, *graphein* to record.]

gastrohelcoma (gas·tro·hel·**ko**′·mah). Gastric ulcer. [Gk *gaster* stomach, *helkos* ulcer, *-oma* tumour.]

gastrohelcosis (gas·tro·hel·**ko**′·sis). Ulceration of the stomach. [Gk *gaster* stomach, *helkosis* ulceration.]

gastrohepatic (gas·tro·hep·**at**′·ik). Having relation or belonging to the stomach and the liver. [Gk *gaster* stomach, *hepar* liver.]

gastrohepatitis (gas·tro·hep·at·**i**′·tis). Inflammation of both the stomach and the liver. [Gk *gaster* stomach, *hepar* liver, *-itis* inflammation.]

gastrohydrorrhoea (gas·tro·hi·dro·**re**′·ah). The excretion from the stomach wall of a large quantity of watery fluid in which there is neither hydrochloric acid, rennet nor pepsin. [Gk *gaster* stomach, hydrorrhoea.]

gastrohyperneuria (gas·tro·hi·per·**newr**′·e·ah). A condition in which the nerves of the stomach are morbidly overactive. [Gk *gaster* stomach, *hyper, neuron* nerve.]

gastrohypertonic (gas·tro·hi·per·**ton**′·ik). Referring to a condition, or characterized by a condition, of over-tension or over-irritability of the stomach. [Gk *gaster* stomach, hypertonia.]

gastrohyponeuria (gas·tro·hi·po·**newr**′·e·ah). A condition in which the nerves of the stomach are defective in action. [Gk *gaster* stomach, *hypo, neuron* nerve.]

gastrohysterectomy (gas·tro·his·ter·**ek**′·to·me). Caesarean section. *See* SECTION. [Gk *gaster* stomach, hysterectomy.]

gastrohysteropexy (gas·tro·**his**′·ter·o·pex·e). Ventrofixation of the uterus. [Gk *gaster* stomach, hysteropexy.]

gastrohysterorrhaphy (gas·tro·his·ter·**or**′·af·e). Ventrofixation of the uterus. [Gk *gaster* stomach, hysterorrhaphy.]

gastrohysterotomy (gas·tro·his·ter·**ot**′·o·me). Caesarean section. *See* SECTION. [Gk *gaster* stomach, *hystera* womb, *temnein* to cut.]

gastroid (**gas**·troid). Resembling a stomach; stomach-like, either in shape or function. [Gk *gaster* stomach, *eidos* form.]

gastro-ileitis (gas·tro·i·le·**i**′·tis). Inflammation of the stomach and the ileum. [Gk *gaster* stomach, ileum, Gk *-itis* inflammation.]

gastro-ileostomy (gas·tro·i·le·**os**′·to·me). An anastomosis, made usually in error between stomach and ileum instead of stomach and jejunum. [Gk *gaster* stomach, ileum, Gk *stoma* mouth.]

gastro-intestinal (gas·tro·in·**tes**′·tin·al). Relating or belonging to the stomach and the intestine. [Gk *gaster* stomach, intestine.]

gastrojejunal (gas·tro·je·**joo**′·nal). Pertaining to the stomach and jejunum. [Gk *gaster* stomach, jejunum.]

gastrojejunitis (gas·tro·je·joo·**ni**′·tis). Inflammation of both the stomach and the jejunum. [Gk *gaster* stomach, jejunum, Gk *-itis* inflammation.]

gastrojejunocolic (gas·tro·je·joo·no·**kol**′·ik). Referring or belonging to the stomach, the jejunum and the colon. [Gk *gaster* stomach, jejunum, colon.]

gastrojejuno-oesophagostomy (gas·tro·je·**joo**·no·e·sof·ag·**os**′·to·me). The implantation of an isolated jejunal loop into the oesophagus on the one hand and the stomach on the other, to short-circuit oesophageal disease. [Gk *gaster* stomach, jejunum, oesophagus, Gk *stoma* mouth.]

gastrojejunostomy (gas·tro·je·joo·**nos**′·to·me). The surgical establishment of an anastomosis between the stomach and the jejunum. [Gk *gaster* stomach, jejunum, Gk *stoma* mouth.]

gastrokateixia (gas·tro·kat·**ix**′·e·ah). Gastroptosis. [Gk *gaster* stomach, *kata, eikein* to move.]

gastrokinesograph (gas·tro·kin·**e**′·so·graf). Gastrograph. [Gk *gaster* stomach, *kinesis* movement, *graphein* to record.]

gastrolavage (gas·tro·**lav**·ahzh). The act or process of washing out the stomach. [Gk *gaster* stomach, lavage.]

gastrolienal (gas·tro·li·**e**′·nal). Gastrosplenic. [Gk *gaster* stomach, L *lien* spleen.]

gastrolith (**gas**·tro·lith). A gastric calculus. [Gk *gaster* stomach, *lithos* stone.]

gastrolithiasis (gas·tro·lith·**i**′·as·is). The formation and presence of calculi in the stomach. [Gk *gaster* stomach, lithiasis.]

gastrology (gas·**trol**·o·je). That branch of medical science which is concerned with the structure and diseases of the stomach. [Gk *gaster* stomach, *logos* science.]

gastrolysis (gas·**trol**·is·is). The surgical separation of abnormal adhesions between the stomach and neighbouring organs. [Gk *gaster* stomach, *lysis* a loosing.]

gastromalacia (gas·tro·mal·**a**′·se·ah). A condition of morbid softness of the walls of the stomach. [Gk *gaster* stomach, malacia.]

gastromegaly (gas·tro·**meg**·al·e). Morbid enlargement of the stomach, or in some cases of the abdomen. [Gk *gaster* stomach, *megas* large.]

gastromelus (gas·**trom**·el·us). A monster having a supernumerary leg or legs attached to its abdomen. [Gk *gaster* stomach, *melos* limb.]

gastromenia (gas·tro·**men**·e·ah). Haematemesis occurring cyclically with menstrual periods and regarded as a type of vicarious menstruation. [Gk *gaster* stomach, menstruation.]

gastrometritis (gas·tro·met·**ri**′·tis). Gastritis with concomitant metritis.

gastromucous (gas·tro·**mew**·kus). Marked by gastric disorder and the secretion of an abnormally large quantity of mucus. [Gk *gaster* stomach, mucus.]

gastromycosis (gas·tro·mi·**ko**′·sis). Gastric disease induced by the presence of fungi in the stomach. [Gk *gaster* stomach, mycosis.]

gastromyeloma (gas·tro·mi·el·**o**′·mah). Giant-cell sarcoma of the stomach. [Gk *gaster* stomach, myeloma.]

gastromyotomy (gas·tro·mi·**ot**′·o·me). 1. Division of the circular layer of muscle fibres of the stomach, a procedure undertaken in some cases of gastric ulcer when complicated by pylorospasm. 2. Pylorotomy. [Gk *gaster* stomach, myotomy.]

gastromyxorrhoea (gas·tro·mix·o·**re**′·ah). Gastroblennorrhoea. [Gk *gaster* stomach, myxorrhoea.]

gastronephritis (gas·tro·nef·**ri**′·tis). Gastritis and nephritis occurring simultaneously.

gastro-oesophageal (gas·tro·e·sof·ah·**je**′·al). Relating or belonging to the stomach and the oesophagus. [Gk *gaster* stomach, oesophagus.]

gastro-oesophagitis (gas·tro·e·sof·ah·**ji**′·tis). Inflammation involving both the stomach and the oesophagus. [Gk *gaster* stomach, oesophagus, Gk *-itis* inflammation.]

gastro-oesophagostomy (gas·tro·e·sof·ag·**os**′·to·me). The surgical establishment of a communication between the stomach and oesophagus. [Gk *gaster* stomach, oesophagus, Gk *stoma* mouth.]

gastro-omental (gas·tro·o·**men**′·tal). Gastro-epiploic; referring or belonging to the stomach and the greater omentum. [Gk *gaster* stomach, omentum.]

gastropancreatic (gas·tro·pan·kre·**at**′·ik). Referring or belonging to the stomach and the pancreas. [Gk *gaster* stomach, pancreas.]

gastropancreatitis (gas·tro·**pan**·kre·at·**i**′·tis). Inflammation of the stomach and the pancreas. [Gk *gaster* stomach, pancreatitis.]

gastroparalysis (gas·tro·par·**al**′·is·is). Paralysis affecting the musculature of the stomach. [Gk *gaster* stomach, paralysis.]

gastroparesis (gas·tro·par·**e**′·sis). Paralysis of the muscles of the stomach. [Gk *gaster* stomach, *paresis* relaxation.]

gastroparietal (gas·tro·par·**i**′·et·al). 1. Relating to or connecting the stomach and the walls of the abdomen. 2. Relating to the walls of the stomach. [Gk *gaster* stomach, L *paries* wall.]

gastropathic (gas·tro·**path**·ik). Relating or belonging to any disease of the stomach; referring to gastropathy.

gastropathy (gas·**trop**·ath·e). Any disease of the stomach. [Gk *gaster* stomach, *pathos* disease.]

gastroperiodynia (gas·tro·per·e·o·**din'**·e·ah). Periodic gastralgia. [Gk *gaster* stomach, period, Gk *odyne* pain.]

gastroperitonitis (gas·tro·per·it·on·**i'**·tis). Gastritis and peritonitis occurring at the same time.

gastropexis, gastropexy (gas·tro·**pex**·is, gas·tro·pex·e). In displacement or prolapse of the stomach, the operation of raising it to the correct position and fixing it there by suturing it to the abdominal wall. [Gk *gaster* stomach, *pexis* fixation.]

Gastrophilidae (gas·tro·**fil**·i·de). A family of the Diptera. [Gk *gaster* stomach, *philein* to love, *eidos* form.]

Gastrophilus (gas·**trof**·il·us). A genus of stomach oestrid (bot) flies, of which several species cause myiasis in man. **Gastrophilus equi.** *Gastrophilus intestinalis.* **Gastrophilus haemorrhoidalis.** A species that has been recorded. **Gastrophilus intestinalis.** A horse bot which normally develops in the stomach of horses. It has been recorded subcutaneously in man in Europe and North America, causing a creeping eruption. The larvae do not mature in man. [Gk *gaster* stomach, *philein* to love.]

gastrophore (**gas**·tro·for). An appliance which holds the stomach in place and shape during operation. [Gk *gaster* stomach, *pherein* to bear.]

gastrophotography (gas·tro·fo·**tog'**·raf·e). Photography of the interior of the stomach by means of a gastrocamera. [Gk *gaster* stomach, photography.]

gastrophotor (gas·tro·**fo**·tor). A camera for photographing the gastric mucosa.

gastrophrenic (gas·tro·**fren**·ik). Pertaining to or connecting the stomach and the diaphragm. [Gk *gaster* stomach, *phren* diaphragm.]

gastrophthisis (gas·tro·**thi**·sis). 1. A condition of bodily weakness and emaciation resulting from gastric disease. 2. Reduction in size of the cavity of the stomach caused by hyperplasia and consequent thickening of the mucous and submucous coats. [Gk *gaster* stomach, phthisis.]

gastroplasty (**gas**·tro·plas·te). Plastic operation for any defect or deformity of the stomach. [Gk *gaster* stomach, *plassein* to mould.]

gastroplegia (gas·tro·**ple**·je·ah). Gastroparalysis, sometimes leading to acute dilatation of the stomach. [Gk *gaster* stomach, *plege* stroke.]

gastropleuritis (gas·tro·ploor·**i'**·tis). Concomitant gastritis and pleurisy.

gastroplication (gas·tro·plik·**a'**·shun). Operative treatment of dilatation of the stomach by stitching a longitudinal tuck in it or by suturing, so as to obliterate, an existing fold in the walls. [Gk *gaster* stomach, plication.]

gastropneumonic (**gas**·tro·new·**mon'**·ik). Having reference to the stomach and the lungs. [Gk *gaster* stomach, *pneumon* lung.]

Gastropoda (gas·tro·**po**·dah). A class of the phylum Mollusca; snails, slugs, etc. All Gastropoda of medical interest are included in the sub-class Pulmonata. [Gk *gaster* stomach, *pous* foot.]

gastroptosis (gas·trop·**to**·sis). Downward displacement of the stomach. [Gk *gaster* stomach, *ptosis* fall.]

gastropulmonary (gas·tro·**pul**·mon·ar·e). Gastropneumonic. [Gk *gaster* stomach, L *pulmo* lung.]

gastropylorectomy (gas·tro·pi·lor·**ek'**·to·me). Surgical removal of the pyloric portion of the stomach. [Gk *gaster* stomach, pylorus, Gk *ektome* a cutting out.]

gastropyloric (gas·tro·pi·**lor'**·ik). Having relation or belonging to the body of the stomach and the pylorus. [Gk *gaster* stomach, pylorus.]

gastroradiculitis (gas·tro·rad·ik·ewl·**i'**·tis). Inflammation of the posterior spinal nerve roots with resultant irritation of those of their sensory fibres which supply the stomach. [Gk *gaster* stomach, L *radicula* rootlet, Gk *-itis* inflammation.]

gastrorrhagia (gas·tro·**ra**·je·ah). Haemorrhage into or from the stomach. [Gk *gaster* stomach, *rhegnynai* to burst forth.]

gastrorrhaphy (gas·**tror**·af·e). 1. The stitching up of a perforation of the stomach. 2. Gastroplication. 3. The suturing of a wound in the abdominal wall. [Gk *gaster* stomach, *rhaphe* seam.]

gastrorrhexis (gas·tro·**rex**·is). Rupture of the stomach. [Gk *gaster* stomach, *rhexis* rupture.]

gastrorrhoea (gas·tro·**re**·ah). The secretion by the stomach of an abnormally large quantity of gastric juice or of mucus. **Gastrorrhoea continua chronica.** Continuous excessive secretion of gastric juice. [Gk *gaster* stomach, *rhoia* flow.]

gastrosalpingotomy (gas·tro·sal·ping·**got'**·o·me). Incision into the uterine tube after abdominal section. [Gk *gaster* stomach, *salpigx* tube, *temnein* to cut.]

gastroschisis (gas·**tros**·kis·is). Coelioschisis; congenital fissure of the abdominal wall, the cavity being open. [Gk *gaster* stomach, *schisis* division.]

gastroscope (gas·tro·skope). An endoscope by means of which the interior of the stomach can be examined. [Gk *gaster* stomach, *skopein* to watch.]

See also: SCHINDLER, TAYLOR (H.), WOLF.

gastroscopic (gas·tro·**skop**·ik). Having reference or belonging to a gastroscope or to gastroscopy.

gastroscopy (gas·**tros**·ko·pe). The visualization of the interior of the stomach by a flexible telescopic instrument passed through the mouth and oesophagus. **Lower gastroscopy.** Laparogastroscopy. [Gk *gaster* stomach, *skopein* to watch.]

gastrosis (gas·**tro**·sis). Any disease or disorder of the stomach alone or of the abdomen. [Gk *gaster* stomach, *-osis* condition.]

gastrospasm (gas·tro·spazm). An involuntary contraction of the stomach muscles. [Gk *gaster* stomach, spasm.]

gastrospiry (gas·tro·**spi**·re). Aerophagy: a hysterical affection which consists in the spasmodic gulping and subsequent eructation of air. [Gk *gaster* stomach, L *spirare* to breathe.]

gastrosplenic (gas·tro·**splen**·ik). Relating or belonging to the stomach and the spleen. [Gk *gaster* stomach, spleen.]

gastrostaxis (gas·tro·**stax**·is). The oozing of blood from the mucous coat of the stomach. [Gk *gaster* stomach, *staxis* a dropping.]

gastrostenosis (gas·tro·sten·**o'**·sis). Contraction or shrinking of the stomach with diminution in the size of the lumen. [Gk *gaster* stomach, stenosis.]

gastrostogavage (gas·**tros**·to·**gav'**·ahzh). Gastrogavage.

gastrostolavage (gas·**tros**·to·**lav'**·ahzh). Gastrolavage.

gastrostoma (gas·tros·**to**·mah). Gastric fistula, natural or artificial. [Gk *gaster* stomach, *stoma* mouth.]

gastrostomosis (gas·**tros**·to·**mo'**·sis). The condition in which a gastrostomy opening has been established. [gastrostomy, Gk *-osis* condition.]

gastrostomy (gas·**tros**·to·me). The establishment by abdominal operation of a communication between the interior of the stomach and the skin surface for tube feeding in patients with complete inability to swallow. [Gk *gaster* stomach, *stoma* mouth.]

See also: BECK (E. G.), JANEWAY (H. H.), STAMM, WITZEL.

gastrosuccorrhoea (**gas**·tro·sewk·o·**re'**·ah). The constant secretion of gastric juice in abnormally large quantity; Reichmann's disease. **Digestive gastrosuccorrhoea.** Secretion of an abnormally large quantity of gastric juice occurring only during digestion. [Gk *gaster* stomach, L *succus* juice, Gk *rhoia* flow.]

gastrotherapy (gas·tro·**ther**·ap·e). 1. Treatment of pernicious anaemia by administration of an extract of the mucous coat of hog stomach. 2. Any treatment of disease of the stomach. [Gk *gaster* stomach, therapy.]

gastrothoracic (**gas**·tro·thor·**as'**·ik). Relating or belonging to the abdomen and the thorax. [Gk *gaster* stomach, thorax.]

gastrothoracopagus (gas·tro·thor·ak·**op'**·ag·us). A twin monster in which there is fusion of thorax and abdomen. **Gastrothoracopagus dipygus.** An unequal twin monster; the parasite is attached to the autosite at the thorax and abdomen, and usually consists of pelvis and lower limbs (although sometimes arms are present as well) partially attached to the upper part of the thorax or the abdomen of the autosite. [Gk *gaster* stomach, thorax, Gk *pagos* fixture.]

gastrotome (gas·tro·tome). A knife used in gastrotomy.

gastrotomy (gas·**trot**·o·me). Surgical incision or opening up of stomach or abdomen. [Gk *gaster* stomach, *temnein* to cut.]

gastrotonometer (gas·tro·to·**nom**′·et·er). An instrument with which the degree of intragastric pressure can be measured. [Gk *gaster* stomach, tonus, meter.]

gastrotonometry (gas·tro·to·**nom**′·et·re). The measurement of intragastric pressure. [see prec.]

gastrotoxin (gas·tro·**tox**·in). A cytotoxin acting specifically on the cells of the mucous coat of the stomach. [Gk *gaster* stomach, toxin.]

gastrotrachelotomy (gas·tro·trak·el·**ot**′·o·me). A method of caesarean section in which the uterus is opened by a transverse incision across the cervix. [Gk *gaster* stomach, *trachelos* neck, *temnein* to cut.]

gastrotropic (gas·tro·**trop**·ik). 1. Affecting or attacking the stomach. 2. Having an affinity for the stomach. [Gk *gaster* stomach, *trope* a turning.]

gastrotubotomy (gas·tro·tewb·**ot**′·o·me). Gastrosalpingotomy. [Gk *gaster* stomach, tube, Gk *temnein* to cut.]

gastrotympanites (gas·tro·tim·pan·**i**′·teez). Distension of the stomach due to the presence of gas or air. [Gk *gaster* stomach, tympanites.]

gastroxynsis (gas·trox·**in**·sis). Hyperchlorhydria. **Gastroxynsis fungosa.** Hyperchlorhydria caused by the presence of fungi in the stomach. [Gk *gaster* stomach, *oxynein* to sharpen.]

gastrula (gas·troo·lah). A hollow vesicular stage in the development of many vertebrate and invertebrate embryos, comprising an outer layer of ectodermal cells and an inner layer of entodermal cells, with, in later stages, a layer of mesodermal cells between. The gastrula cavity, or archenteron, communicates with the outside at the posterior end through the blastopore. [Gk *gaster* stomach.]

gastrulation (gas·troo·**la**·shun). In embryology, the process undergone by a cell in developing from the stage of a blastula to that of a gastrula.

gatophilia (gat·o·**fil**·e·ah). Ailurophilia; excessive love of cats. [Gk *gatos* cat, *philein* to love.]

gatophobia (gat·o·**fo**·be·ah). Ailurophobia; morbid fear of cats. [Gk *gatos* cat, phobia.]

Gaucher, Phillipe Charles Ernest (b. 1854). Paris physician.

Gaucher's cells. Large reticulo-endothelial cells with small nuclei containing the lipid, kerasin.

Gaucher's disease or splenomegaly. A rare, chronic familial disorder of lipoid metabolism, associated with splenomegaly, some pigmentation of the skin, pingueculae of the sclera and often bone changes. The spleen, bone marrow and other organs show the characteristic large Gaucher cells which contain relatively large amounts (up to 10 per cent or more of the weight of the dried spleen) of a lipid, kerasin. The disease usually commences early in life, and was said to occur most commonly in Jews, but this is not supported by modern experience.

gauge (gaje). An instrument with which to measure the flow or the pressure of a fluid, or the dimension or calibre of an object. **Bite gauge.** *See* BITE-GAUGE. **Bourdon gauge.** A gauge used to measure the degree of compression of a gas. **Catheter gauge.** A metal plate with graduated perforations with which the outside diameter of a catheter may be measured. [O Fr.]

See also: LIVINGSTON.

Gaule's spots. Sharply defined punctate erosions of the corneal epithelium, found in neuroparalytic keratitis.

Gault's cochleopalpebral reflex. For deafness: a sudden, loud, unexpected noise is applied close to the ear under test. In the presence of any hearing, there is an involuntary wink or lid contraction in the corresponding eye. Useful in cases of suspected malingering and in cases of congenital deafness in which it is important to establish the presence of any possible sound perception.

gaultherase (**gawl**·ther·aze). An enzyme acting on the glucosides of *Gaultheria* and *Betula*; betulase.

Gaultheria (gawl·**the**·re·ah). A genus of shrubs (family Ericaceae). The leaves of *Gaultheria procumbens* Linn. were formerly used as the source of oil of wintergreen, but the oil is now obtained from the bark of *Betula lenta* Linn. (family Betulaceae). [Jean François *Gaultier* (b. 1708), Quebec botanist and physician.]

gaultherin (**gawl**·ther·in). A natural glucoside of black birch, *Betula lenta* Linn. (family Betulaceae) which undergoes enzymatic decomposition when the bark is distilled, yielding oil of wintergreen (methyl salicylate). It was originally extracted from the leaves of *Gaultheria procumbens* (family Ericaceae). [see prec.]

gauntlet (**gawnt**·let). A gauntlet bandage; a bandage round fingers and palm covering them like a glove. [Fr. *gantelet* small glove.]

Gauss, Carl Joseph (b. 1875). Würzburg gynaecologist.

Gauss' sign. Unusual mobility of the uterus in early pregnancy.

gauss (gows). A unit of magnetic induction equal to 10^{-4} tesla. [Johann Karl Friedrich *Gauss* (b. 1777), German physicist.]

Gaussel, A. French physician.

Grasset-Gaussel phenomenon. A patient with a hemiparesis, may in the supine position be unable to raise both legs together by flexion at the hip joint, though he can raise either separately.

Grasset, Gaussel and Hoover sign. If a patient with hemiplegia, lying in the supine position, attempts to raise the paralysed leg, while an observer's hand is resting beneath the sound leg, the pressure of the sound limb on the observer's hand is much greater than it would be were a normal person to raise his other leg.

gauze (gawz). A loose-meshed muslin used for surgical operations and dressings. **Antiseptic gauze.** Gauze saturated with some antiseptic fluid and subsequently dried. **Aseptic gauze.** Gauze which has been subjected to sterilization. **Medicated gauze.** Gauze which has been rendered antiseptic by impregnation with antiseptics such as thymol or iodoform; now used infrequently. **Ribbon gauze.** Narrow-woven gauze, suitable for packing orifices, small cavities and fissures. [*Gaza*, Syria, whence the muslin came originally.]

gavage (gav·ahzh). 1. The giving of food or nourishment in liquid form by means of a stomach tube. 2. Superalimentation. [Fr. *gaver* to fatten.]

Gavard, Hyacinthe (b. 1753). Paris anatomist and surgeon.

Gavard's muscle. The oblique layer of the gastric musculature.

Gay, Alexander Heinrich (b.1842). Kasan anatomist.

glands of Gay. The circumanal glands. *See* GLAND.

Gay, Frederick Parker (b. 1874). New York bacteriologist.

Gay and Claypole vaccine. A typhoid prophylactic prepared by sensitizing a typhoid vaccine with antityphoid serum, and then precipitating with alcohol and extracting with saline; it is now obsolete.

Gayer test. A method of evaluating Indian hemp, depending upon the production of anaesthesia of the rabbit cornea.

Gay-Lussac, Joseph Louis (b. 1778). Paris chemist and physicist.

Gay-Lussac's law. Gases combine in simple ratios by volume, and the products, if gaseous, have also a simple relation by volume to the original gases.

Gaza, Wilhelm von (b.1883). Gottingen surgeon.

Gaza's operation. Ramisection.

gcushuwa (**goosh**·oo·wah). A venereal disease allied to yaws and occurring among the Bantu. [Bantu name.]

Gee, Samuel Jones (b. 1839). London physician.

Gee's disease, Gee-Herter disease, Gee-Herter-Heubner disease, Gee-Thaysen disease. Coeliac disease, or the infantile form of idiopathic steatorrhoea.

Gefarnate (**jef**·ar·nate). BP Commission approved name for a mixture of stereoisomers of 3,7-dimethylocta-2,6-dienyl-5,9,13-trimethyltetradeca-4,8,12-trienoate; it is used in the treatment of peptic ulcer.

Gegenbaur, Carl (b. 1826). Heidelberg anatomist.

Gegenbaur cell. An osteoblast.

Gehuchten, Arthur van (b. 1861) Louvain anatomist.

cell of van Gehuchten. A neurone from the cerebral cortex, with short branching processes; also known as *Golgi* (Type II) *cell.*

van Gehuchten's method. A method for histological fixation in a mixture of alcohol, chloroform and acetic acid.

Geigel, Richard (b. 1859). Würzburg physician.

Geigel's reflex. In the female, stimulation of the skin over the upper and inner aspect of the thigh may cause contraction of muscular fibres in the upper part of the inguinal ligament; this reflex is analogous to the cremasteric reflex in the male.

Geiger, Hans (b. 1882). German physicist in England.

Geiger counter, Geiger-Mueller counter or tube. An instrument used for the detection of ionizing radiations. It consists of a tube filled with a gas at reduced pressure, and contains a cylindrical conducting cathode and an axial tungsten wire anode. The passage of an ionizing particle through the gas gives rise to further ionization by collision, a charge being collected on the electrodes, giving an electrical pulse of potential on the anode. The amplitude of the pulse is independent of the number of ions initially formed by the ionizing particle, so that discrimination between different types of particles is not possible.

Geiger-Mueller counting circuit. The electrical circuit which amplifies the electrical impulses from a Geiger-Mueller tube exposed to radiation, so that they may be registered by a mechanical counter or other device.

Geiger-Mueller plateau. In a curve made by plotting the count rate of a Geiger counter against the potential applied between the electrodes, the part of the curve where the slope is minimal.

Geiger-Mueller region. The range of potential applied to an ionization chamber or Geiger counter in which the amplitude of the output pulse is independent of the number of ions formed initially by the passage of the ionizing particle through the counter.

Geiger-Nuttall relation. A relation between the half-life of natural alpha-particle emitters and the disintegrating energy.

geisoma, geison (gi·so·mah, gi·son). The superciliary arch of the frontal bone. [Gk *geison* a projecting.]

Geissler, Heinrich (b. 1815). German physicist.

Geissler's tubes. Glass discharge tubes of complicated shape, often spiral, made of fluorescing glass, which are decorative in appearance when energized.

gel (jel). A liquid/solid colloidal system which occurs as a more or less elastic solid enclosing part or all of the dispersed liquid phase. Examples are colloidal ferric hydroxide, aluminium hydroxide gel, agar and starch paste. They are used for suspending insoluble drugs, for facilitating their disposal, and for their adsorbent and protective properties. **Aluminium Hydroxide Gel BP 1973.** A very effective antacid which acts by chemical neutralization, and by physical adsorption of the hydrochloric acid, gas and toxins, as well as protecting the mucous membrane of the stomach. It may also be used as an adjuvant in the preparation of vaccines. **Dried Aluminium Hydroxide Gel BP 1973.** An antacid having the same uses as the mother preparation. **Aluminium Phosphate Gel BP 1973.** A white suspension containing about 4.5 per cent of $AlPO_4$; a gastric antacid used to give relief of discomfort in hyperchlorhydria and gastric and duodenal ulceration. **Dried Aluminium Phosphate Gel BP 1973.** A dried preparation of aluminium phosphate gel with the same antacid action but used in the form of tablets. [L *gelare* to congeal.]

gelante, gelanth, gelanthum (jel·an·te, jel·anth, jel·an·thum). An ointment base prepared from tragacanth, acacia and gelatin, with glycerin and thymol as preservatives. **Cuticolous gelante.** Armenian bole, a preparation of gelante, eosin and zinc oxide.

gelase (jel·aze). An enzyme capable of hydrolysing agar.

gelasma, gelasmus (jel·az·mah, jel·az·mus). 1. The spasmodic laughter of insanity. 2. Uncontrollable or hysterical laughter. [Gk *gelasma* laughter.]

gelate (jel·ate). To cause a gel to form, or to form a gel. [L *gelare* to congeal.]

gelatification (jel·at·if·ik·a′·shun). 1. The process of conversion into gelatin. 2. Gelatination. [gelatin, L *facere* to make.]

gelatigenous (jel·at·ij·en·us). 1. In physiology, producing or forming gelatin. 2. Yielding gelatin. [gelatin, Gk *genein* to produce.]

gelatin (jel·at·in). A protein obtained from the collagens of bones, cartilage and connective tissue, by hydrolysis with acid, alkali or superheated steam. Gelatin dissolves in hot water to give a viscous solution which sets to a jelly on cooling; in cold water it swells but does not form a solution. Purified gelatin for edible purposes (BP 1973) is a colourless transparent solid, but the crude product which is used in glue-making is yellow to brown, and may be contaminated with poisonous metals. **Gelatin compound, phenolized.** Unna's paste containing phenol. **Glycerinated gelatin.** A solution of equal parts of gelatin and glycerin. **Silk gelatin.** A polypeptide obtained from silk. [L *gelare* to congeal.]

See also: BAILEY (S. F.), WHARTON.

gelatinase (jel·at·in·aze). An enzyme produced by moulds and bacteria, which will liquefy gelatin.

gelatination (jel·at·in·a′·shun). Conversion of a substance into a viscous or jelly-like mass. [gelatin.]

gelatine (jel·at·een). Gelatin.

gelatiniferous (jel·at·in·if′·er·us). Yielding or producing gelatin. [gelatin, L *ferre* to carry.]

gelatiniform (jel·at·in·e·form). Having resemblance to gelatin. [gelatin, form.]

gelatinize (jelat·in·ize). 1. To form a gel. 2. To convert into gelatin or into a substance of jelly-like consistency.

gelatinoid (jel·at·in·oid). 1. Gelatiniform. 2. Gelatinous. 3. Any nitrogenous substance such as collagen or gelatin. [gelatin, Gk *eidos* form.]

gelatinolytic (jel·at·in·o·lit′·ik). Serving to split up or dissolve gelatin. [gelatin, lysis.]

gelatinothorax (jel·at·in·o·thor′·ax). A method of producing collapse of the lung by the injection of a sterile solution of gelatin into the pleural cavity. [gelatin, thorax.]

gelatinous (jel·at·in·us). Viscous; jelly-like; of the consistency of gelatin.

gelatio (jel·a·she·o). Frostbite. [L a freezing.]

gelation (jel·a·shun). 1. The conversion of a sol into a gel. 2. Chilblain. 3. A state of freezing or of frostbite. 4. A process of cooling or solidifying. 5. Catalepsy. [see prec.]

Gelb-Goldstein test. A colour-sorting test, designed to elicit a concrete or abstract mental attitude.

gelid (jel·id). 1. Frozen. 2. Indicating the coldness of ice. [L *gelidus* frozen.]

Gelidium (jel·id·e·um). The generic name of a seaweed from which agar is obtained. [see prec.]

gelification (jel·if·ik·a′·shun). Gelatination. [gelatin, L *facere* to make.]

Gélineau, Jean Baptiste Edouard (b. 1859). French physician.

Gélineau's syndrome. Narcolepsy.

Gellé, Marie Ernest (b. 1834). Paris otologist.

Gellé's test. To determine stapes-fixation in cases of conductive deafness: a vibrating tuning-fork is placed over the mastoid process. A Siegle's speculum is inserted in the meatus. In a normal ear, compression diminishes the sound of the tuning-fork. When the stapes is fixed, as in otosclerosis, the vibrations are heard unchanged.

gelodiagnosis (jel·o·di·ag·no′·sis). A routine test for distinguishing pathogenic enteric bacteria from the non-pathogenic coliform group. When plated out on a gel containing lactose and phenol red the coliform bacteria ferment the lactose, producing acid which turns the indicator red; typhoid and other enteric bacteria grow, but remain their normal colour. [gel, diagnosis.]

gelose (jel·oze). Galactosan, galactan, $(C_6H_{10}O_5)_n$. A polysaccharide consisting of galactose units, which occurs in algae and can be prepared from agar.
gelosis (jel·**o**·sis). Any mass or lump, as hard as if it were frozen, that is present in a tissue, particularly muscular tissue. [L *gelare* to congeal.]
gelotherapy (jel·o·**ther**·ap·e). Treatment of disease by inducing hilarity or provoking laughter. [Gk *gelos* laughter, therapy.]
gelotolepsy (jel·ot·o·**lep**'·se). Loss of muscle tone during laughter, with momentary loss of consciousness. [Gk *gelos* laughter, *lepsis* a seizing.]
gelototherapy (jel·ot·o·**ther**'·ap·e). Gelotherapy.
gelotripsy (jel·o·**trip**·se). In massage, the rubbing away of an indurated swelling or a hard area in a muscle. [gelosis, Gk *tripsis* a rubbing.]
gelsemicine (jel·**sem**·is·een). $C_{20}H_{24}O_4N_2$, an alkaloid obtained from the root of yellow jasmine, *Gelsemium sempervirens* Ait (family Loganiaceae). It is extremely toxic and has a depressant effect upon the central nervous system, causing paralysis of the respiratory centre. It also lowers the arterial blood pressure, but its effect is less marked than that of gelsemine. It is present in tincture of gelsemium, which is used in the treatment of trigeminal neuralgia and migraine.
gelsemine (jel·sem·een). $C_{20}H_{22}O_2N_2$, a crystalline alkaloid obtained from the root of yellow jasmine, *Gelsemium sempervirens* Ait (family Loganiaceae). It is less toxic than gelsemicine and has a depressant effect upon the central nervous system and also upon the heart, causing a very marked fall in blood pressure. It is present in tincture of gelsemium used in the treatment of trigeminal neuralgia and migraine.
gelseminine (jel·**sem**·in·een). An amorphous mixture of alkaloids obtained from *Gelsemium sempervirens* Ait (family Loganiaceae). It contains the alkaloid, sempervirine.
gelsemism (jel·sem·izm). The condition of being poisoned with gelsemium.
Gelsemium (jel·**sem**·e·um). 1. A genus of climbing plants of the family Loganiaceae. 2. (BPC 1968), gelsemii radix, gelsemium root, yellow jasmine root; the dried rhizomes and roots of *Gelsemium nitidum*. It contains the crystalline alkaloids gelsemine, sempervirine and gelsemicine. [It. *gelsomino* jasmine.]
gelsemiumism (jel·**sem**·e·um·izm). Chronic poisoning with gelsemium; a state of habitual intoxication induced by taking preparations of gelsemium.
Gély, Jules Artistide (b. 1806). French surgeon.
Gély's suture. An intestinal suture.
gemellary (jem·el·ar·e). 1. Like twins. 2. Relating or belonging to twins. [L *gemellus* twin.]
gemellipara (jem·el·**ip**·ar·ah). A woman who has borne twins. [L *gemellus* twin, *parere* to give birth.]
gemelliparous (jem·el·**ip**·ar·us). Bearing or producing twins. [see prec.]
gemellus (jem·**el**·us) (pl. *gemelli*). A twin or double. [L.]
gemellus inferior muscle [musculus gemellus inferior (NA)] (jem·**el**·us in·**feer**·e·or). A small muscle that arises from the ischial tuberosity and lies below the obturator internus tendon.
gemellus superior muscle [musculus gemellus superior (NA)] (jem·**el**·us sew·**peer**·e·or). A small muscle arising from the spine of the ischium and inserted into the upper part of the tendon of the obturator internus muscle, through which it is attached to the medial surface of the great trochanter of the femur. [L twin.]
gemina (jem·in·ah). The quadrigeminal bodies of the midbrain. [L *geminus* twin.]
geminate (jem·in·ate). 1. Coupled. 2. Paired or occurring in pairs. 3. Of teeth, applied to 2 teeth which are joined together. [L *geminare* to double.]
gemination (jem·in·a·shun). 1. A doubling or arrangement in pairs. 2. The act of producing twins. 3. The joining together of 2 teeth. **Diphyodontic gemination.** The fusion of a deciduous tooth and its corresponding permanent tooth. **False gemination, Pathological gemination.** The fusion together of 2 completely formed teeth by the continued deposition of cementum on the roots. **True gemination.** The joining together of 2 teeth due to the fusion of the tooth germs of the teeth prior to the onset of calcification. [see prec.]
geminous (jem·in·us). Geminate.
geminus (jem·in·us) (pl. *gemini*). Twin. **Gemini aequales.** Enzygotic (identical) twins. [L.]
gemistocyte (jem·**is**·to·site). An astrocyte with swollen cytoplasm and eccentric nucleus, often seen in relationship to infarcts or areas of oedema. [G *gemätete* plump.]
gemma (jem·ah). 1. Any bud-like or bulb-like structure, e.g. a taste bud. 2. Micelle. 3. In zoology, an outgrowth which becomes a new organism. [L bud.]
gemmangioma (jem·an·je·**o**'·mah). An angioma made up of angioblasts or embryonal cells. [L *gemma* bud, angioma.]
gemmation (jem·**a**·shun). In biology, asexual reproduction in which a bud-like process is put out from or forms on the parent organism and either remains attached or breaks off; in both cases a new organism is formed. [L *gemmare* to put forth buds.]
gemmule (jem·ewl). 1. A small bud. 2. The bud first produced by the process of gemmation. 3. Any one of the number of minute round excrescences which sometimes occur on the dendrites of a nerve cell. 4. Micelle. [L *gemmula* small bud.]
gena (je·nah) (pl. *genae*). The cheek. [L.]
genal (je·nal). Relating or belonging to the cheek. [see prec.]
gene (jeen). One of a series of units arranged in linear order on a chromosome, not as a rule observable, but recognizable in position. Genes are self-reproducible at cell division, and according to gene theory are the ultimate controlling factors of the characteristics of organisms. They are presumed to be composed of nucleoproteins, are highly stable, and are seldom influenced by their neighbours or their general cellular environment. They mutate on rare occasions and then remain stable in their new form. The position of a given gene can be discovered by a genetical study of linkage, inversion and chiasma formation. **Allelomorphic gene.** One of a pair or series of gene mutants situated at the same locus on homologous chromosomes. **Gene clustering.** In bacteria, the contiguous arrangement of genes mediating different steps of the same biochemical pathway, usually forming an operon or genetic unit of transcription. **Lethal gene.** A gene whose effects kill individuals bearing it in a homozygous condition. **Mimic genes.** Different genes producing the same effect. **Recessive gene.** A gene controlling a recessive character. **Regulatory gene.** A unit of genetic material responsible for regulating some specific genetic activity, often by specifying a protein repressor. **Structural gene.** A gene which specifies the structure of polypeptide chains directly concerned with function (e.g. enzymes, haemoglobin) or cellular structure (e.g. bacterial flagella). [Gk *genein* to produce.]
geneogenous (je·ne·**oj**·en·us). Congenital, in the sense of being transmitted by the mother, e.g. an infection. [Gk *genea* birth, *genein* to produce.]
general (jen·er·al). 1. Relating or belonging to the whole of a body or structure. 2. Not localized; affecting the whole organism or many parts of it; diffuse. 3. Relating or belonging to a miscellaneous group. 4. Relating to a genus; common to a large class. 5. Belonging to the generic or the typical. [L *genus* race or class.]
generalize (jen·er·al·ize). 1. To spread throughout the body, as a disease. 2. To be converted from a primarily local affection into a general disease. [see prec.]
generate (jen·er·ate). 1. To procreate. 2. To propagate or produce a being of the same species. 3. In chemistry, to make or produce an electric current or a gas. [L *generare* to beget.]
generation (jen·er·a·shun). 1. Procreation. 2. The process of producing offspring. 3. The average period of time at which children are ready to take the place of parents, usually computed as from 30 to 33 years. **Alternate generation.** In botany and zoology, reproduction of species by alternate sexual and asexual reproduction. **Asexual generation.** Reproduction by any process not involving the union of male and female cells. **Direct generation, Non-sexual generation.** Asexual generation (see

above). **Sexual generation.** Reproduction of species by the union of male and female cells. **Spontaneous generation.** The theory that living matter originates either *de novo* or from the sudden appearance of vitality in hitherto non-living matter. **Generation time.** *See* TIME. **Virgin generation.** Parthenogenesis. [see prec.]

generative (jen·er·a·tiv). 1. Possessing the power or having the function of generating or reproducing species. 2. Relating or belonging to generation.

generator (jen·er·a·tor). An apparatus with which gases are manufactured. Also applied to a device for producing electricity, static or current. **Cascade generator.** An electrical apparatus producing high voltages by charging capacitors in parallel from a relatively low voltage supply and discharging them in series into the load. **Electrostatic generator.** A high-potential generator in which electrical charge is conveyed by movement of the element on which it is situated, not by current flow, e.g. van de Graaff and Wimshurst machines. Developments of these are used to accelerate electrons and atomic particles. **Flow generator.** An artificial ventilating machine providing a constant gas flow which is not altered by changes in the compliance of the chest and lungs. **Supervoltage generator.** An electrical apparatus producing voltages above a certain arbitrary limit, which for radiotherapy is usually taken as 1 000 000 V. [L *generare* to beget.]

generic (jen·er·ik). 1. Characteristic of a natural group as distinct from individuals. 2. Referring or belonging to a particular genus. 3. General, not specific. [genus.]

generotype (jen·er·o·tipe). The type species of a genus; genotype.

genesial, genesic (jen·e·ze·al, jen·e·zik). 1. Relating to origin. 2. Relating or belonging to generation. [Gk *genesis* origin.]

genesiology (jen·e·ze·ol′·o·je). That branch of medical science which is concerned with generation, reproduction and heredity. [Gk *genesis* origin, *logos* science.]

genesis (jen·es·is). Origin; mode of formation. [Gk.]

genetic (jen·et·ik). 1. Referring to or concerned with genesis, origin or generation. 2. Relating or belonging to birth or reproduction. 3. Inherited. 4. Congenital. 5. Any disease involving the generative organs. 6. A drug or agent which affects the generative organs. **Genetic code.** *See* CODE. **Genetic counselling.** Advice based on genetic or partly genetic information. Obviously related to many other aspects of medicine and surgery. **Genetic drift.** Changes in gene frequency from generation to generation. [Gk *genesis* origin.]

geneticist (jen·et·is·ist). One who makes a special study of natural development or genetics.

genetics (jen·et·ix). 1. That branch of biology which is concerned with heredity and individual variation and characteristics. 2. The branch of science concerned with natural development and the laws of generation and origin. [Gk *genesis* origin.]

genetopathy (jen·et·op·ath·e). Any disease that affects the normal function of reproduction. [Gk *genesis* origin, *pathos* disease.]

genetotrophic (jen·et·o·trof′·ik). Pertaining to genetics and nutrition. [genetics, Gk *trophe* nutrition.]

genetous (jen·et·us). Congenital. [Gk *genesis* origin.]

Geneva Convention (jen·e·vah kon·ven·shun). An arrangement arrived at in 1864 by representatives of the great European powers met in Geneva, establishing regulations that in war on land the wounded and those attending them (physicians, nurses, ambulance corps and chaplains), as well as ambulances and hospitals, are to be regarded as neutral. In 1868 a further convention interpreted the agreement of 1864 and applied its principles to war at sea.

Génévrier, J. (fl. 1921). French army surgeon.

Génévrier's solution. An injection of quinine and urethane used as a sclerosing agent for varicose veins.

Gengou, Octave (b. 1875). Belgian bacteriologist.

Bordet-Gengou agar or culture medium. A potato, glycerin and plain agar medium with an equal quantity of defibrinated human or rabbit blood added at 55°C. It is used for the growth of *Haemophilus pertussis*.

Bordet-Gengou bacillus. *Haemophilus pertussis*.

Bordet-Gengou phenomenon. Complement-fixation test. *See* TEST.

genial, genian (jen·i·al, jen·i·an). Relating or belonging to the chin. [Gk *geneion* chin.]

genic (jen·ik). 1. Having relation or belonging to genes. 2. Caused by genes.

genicular (jen·ik·ew·lar). Pertaining to the knee joint. [L *geniculum* little knee.]

genicular arteries. **Descending genicular artery [arteria genu descendens (NA)].** A branch of the femoral artery to the knee, via articular branches [rami articulares], the muscles on the medial side of this joint and the structures on the medial side of the upper part of the leg. **Descending genicular artery, saphenous branch of the [ramus saphenus (NA)].** A branch which accompanies the saphenous vein to the upper part of the leg. **Lateral inferior genicular artery, Lateral superior genicular artery, Medial inferior genicular artery, Medial superior genicular artery, Middle genicular artery.** *See* POPLITEAL ARTERY.

genicular veins [venae genus (NA)]. Tributaries of the popliteal vein, 5 in number, which accompany the arteries of the same name. They drain the structure of the knee joint.

geniculate, geniculated (jen·ik·ew·late, jen·ik·ew·la·ted). Abruptly angled, like a bent knee. [L *geniculum* little knee.]

geniculum [NA] (jen·ik·ew·lum). 1. An abrupt bend like a knee or a knot in any small organ or structure. 2. A small angular structure like a knee or a knot. 3. Either one of the geniculate bodies on the diencephalon, medial or lateral. **Geniculum of the facial nerve [geniculum nervi facialis (NA)].** A right-angled bend on the facial nerve in the medial wall of the middle ear, marked also by a swelling of the ganglion of the facial nerve. [L little knee.]

genin (jen·in). The aglycone or non-sugar portion of a natural glycoside.

genioglossal (je·ne·o·glos′·al). Pertaining to both the chin and the tongue. [Gk *geneion* chin, *glossa* tongue.]

genioglossus muscle [musculus genioglossus (NA)] (je·ne·o·glos′·us). A muscle of the tongue, taking origin close to the midline of the mandible from the genial tubercle. It is the main protruder of the tongue.

geniohyoglossus (je·ne·o·hi·o·glos′·us). Genioglossus muscle. [genioglossus, geniohyoid.]

geniohyoid muscle [musculus geniohyoideus (NA)] (je·ne·o·hi′·oid). A muscle arising from the inferior genial tubercle of the mandible and inserted into the body of the hyoid bone. [Gk *geneion* chin, hyoid.]

genion (jen·i·on). 1. The chin. 2. In craniometry, the apex of the lower genial tubercle. [Gk *geneion* chin.]

genioplasty (jen·i·o·plas·te). Any plastic operation undertaken to restore the structures of chin or cheek. [Gk *geneion* chin, *plassein* to mould.]

genital (jen·it·al). Relating or belonging to the generative organs, or to reproduction. **Genital organ.** *See* ORGAN. **Genital ridge.** *See* RIDGE. [L *genitalis*.]

genitalia (jen·it·a·le·ah). The organs of generation in male or female, particularly the external organs. **Indifferent genitalia.** Embryonic genitalia before sex differentiation. [L.]

genitality (jen·it·al·it·e). The ability to take part in the act of generation. [see prec.]

genitals (jen·it·alz). Genitalia.

genitocrural (jen·it·o·kroo′·ral). Genitofemoral. [genitalia, L *crus* leg.]

genitofemoral (jen·it·o·fem′·or·al). Having relation to the genitalia and the thigh. [genitalia, femur.]

genitofemoral nerve [nervus genitofemoralis (NA)]. A branch of the lumbar plexus (root value 1, 2) supplying the cremaster muscle and skin of the scrotum or labium majus through its genital branch [ramus genitalis (NA)] and the skin of the upper part of the thigh through its femoral branch [ramus femoralis (NA)].

genito-infectious (jen·it·o·in·**fek**′·shus). Venereal. [genital, infection.]

genitoplasty (jen·it·o·plas·te). Plastic surgery of the genitalia. [genitalia, Gk *plassein* to mould.]

genito-urinary (jen·it·o·**ewr**′·in·ar·e). Relating or belonging to the genitalia and the urinary organs.

genius (je·ne·us). Of disease, the distinctive or inherent character. **Genius epidemicus.** (*a*) The theory that the prevalence, virulence and characters of an endemic or epidemic disease (epidemic constitution) vary according to the telluric or atmospheric conditions prevailing throughout the world at the time (Sydenham). (*b*) The dominant characteristic of any endemic or epidemic disease in any particular outbreak. **Genius morbi.** The particular or dominant characteristic of any disease. [L tutelary deity.]

Gennari, Francesco (fl. 1782). Parma anatomist.

Gennari's band, layer, line, stria or stripe. A white stripe, line or band which is seen in the visual cortex when it is cut vertically. It is produced by a layer of nerve fibres that corresponds to the outer layer of Baillarger in other cortical regions.

Gennerich, Wilhelm (b. 1877). German naval surgeon and dermatologist.

Gennerich's treatment. The intrathecal injection of neoarsphenamine solution diluted with cerebrospinal fluid; used in cases of neurosyphilis.

genoblast (jen·o·blast). 1. A mature ovum or spermatozoon. 2. The segmentation nucleus of the fertilized ovum, in its bisexual character. [Gk *genos* birth, *blastos* germ.]

genocatachresia (jen·o·kat·ah·**kre**′·ze·ah). A state in which the sexual instincts are perverted. [Gk *genos* birth, *katachresis* a misapplying.]

genodermatosis (jen·o·der·mat·**o**′·sis). A general term for any inheritable skin disease. [Gk *genos* birth, dermatosis.]

genom, genome (je·nom, je·nome). The complex set of self-reproducing particles upon which cell inheritance depends; the gene complex. [Gk *genein* to produce.]

genometabole (jen·o·met·**ab**′·o·le). Alteration in, and in some cases disappearance of, sexual characteristics as a result of menopausal changes. [gene, Gk *metabole* change.]

genoneme (jen·o·neem). Axoneme. [gene, Gk *neme* thread.]

genophobia (jen·o·**fo**·be·ah). Pathological fear of sex and sexual activity. [Gk *genos* birth, phobia.]

genophore (jen·o·for). Connoting the genetic material or chromosome of prokaryotic cells, e.g. bacteria, which, unlike eukaryotic chromosomes, comprises naked nucleic acid, is not contained by a nuclear membrane and does not undergo mitosis or meiosis. [gene, Gk *phoros* bearer.]

genotype (jen·o·tipe). 1. The genetic constitution of an organism, as opposed to the phenotype or external appearance of the organism itself. 2. The type species of a genus; generotype. [Gk *genos* birth, *typos* mark.]

genotypical (jen·o·**tip**·ik·al). 1. Referring or belonging to heredity or to the genotype. 2. Familial. [see prec.]

Gensoul, Joseph (b. 1797). Lyons surgeon.

Gensoul's disease. Ludwig's angina.

Gensoul's operation, for stricture of the lacrimal duct (obsolete).

Gentamicin (jen·tah·**mi**·sin). BP Commission approved name for an antibiotic produced by *Micromonospora purpurea.* **Gentamicin Sulphate BP 1973.** A mixture of the sulphate of the antimicrobial substances produced by *Micromonospora purpurea.*

Gentian BP 1973 (jen·shan). Gentian root, gentianae radix; the dried fermented rhizome and root of *Gentiana lutea* (family Gentianaceae), containing bitter glycosides, sugars, enzymes and a yellow colouring matter, gentisic acid. It is used as a bitter tonic to stimulate gastric secretion and improve appetite. [*Gentius,* King of Illyria.]

Gentianae Radix. *European Pharmacopoeia* name for Gentian BP 1973.

gentianophil, gentianophile, gentianophilous (jen·shan·o·fil, jen·shan·o·file, jen·shan·**of**·il·us). Having affinity for gentian-violet dyes. [gentian, Gk *philein* to love.]

gentianophobic, gentianophobous (jen·shan·o·**fo**′·bik, jen·shan·o·**fo**′·bus). Taking the stain of gentian violet very poorly or not at all; without any affinity for gentian-violet dye. [gentian, Gk *phobos* fear.]

gentiopicrin (jen·she·o·**pik**′·rin). $C_{16}H_{20}O_9$, a bitter glucoside found in gentian root. [gentian, Gk *pikros* bitter.]

gentisin (jen·tis·in). Methoxy-dihydroxyxanthone, $(CH_3O)(OH)C_6H_2{=}COO{=}C_6H_3OH$. A yellow substance found in gentian root.

genu [NA] (jen·ew) (pl. *genua*). The knee; any bent structure resembling the knee. **Genu of the corpus callosum [genu corporis callosi (NA)].** The anterior end of the corpus callosum; it is continuous below with the rostrum, and posteriorly with the trunk. **Genu of the facial nerve [genu nervi facialis (NA)].** The loop of the facial nerve around the nucleus of the abducent nerve in the substance of the pons. **Genu of the internal capsule [genu capsulae internae (NA)].** The junction of the anterior and posterior limbs of the internal capsule. **Genu recurvatum.** Back knee; abnormal posterior angulation of the knee. **Genu valgum.** Knock knee; a deformity where the knees come together and the ankles are apart. **Genu varum.** Bow leg; outward curving of the legs. [L knee.]

genual (jen·ew·al). Relating to the knee. [see prec.]

genuclast (jen·ew·klast). An instrument with which ankylotic adhesions in the knee joint can be broken. [L *genu* knee, *klasis* a breaking.]

genucubital (jen·ew·**kew**·bit·al). 1. Relating to the knees and the elbows. 2. Designating the genucubital position. *See* POSITION. [L *genu* knee, *cubitus* elbow.]

genufacial (jen·ew·**fa**·shal). 1. Relating to the knees and the face. 2. Supported by or resting on the knees and the face. [L *genu* knee, face.]

genuflex (jen·ew·flex). 1. To bend, like a knee. 2. To bend at the knee or at any joint. [L *genu* knee, *flectere* to bend.]

genupectoral (jen·ew·**pek**·tor·al). Relating to the knees and the chest, e.g. the knee–chest position. [L *genu* knee, *pectus* breast.]

genus (je·nus) (pl. *genera*). A classificatory grouping of organisms containing 1 or more species. Generic names are substantives, printed in italic with upper case initial. [L *genus* race.]

genyantralgia (jen·e·an·**tral**′·je·ah). Pain in the maxillary sinus. [genyantrum, Gk *algos* pain.]

genyantritis (jen·e·an·**tri**′·tis). Inflammation of the maxillary sinus. [genyantrum, Gk *-itis* inflammation.]

genyantrum (jen·e·**an**·trum). The maxillary sinus. [Gk *genys* jaw, *antron* cave.]

genycheiloplasty (jen·e·**ki**·lo·plas·te). Plastic surgery undertaken for repair of the cheek and lip. [Gk *genys* jaw, *cheilos* lip, *plassein* to mould.]

genyplasty (jen·e·plas·te). 1. Reparative surgery of the cheek. 2. Plastic surgery of the lower jaw. [Gk *genys* jaw, *plassein* to mould.]

geobiology (je·o·bi·**ol**′·o·je). The science and study of terrestrial life. [Gk *ge* earth, biology.]

geochemistry (je·o·**kem**·is·tre). The chemistry of the earth; that branch of geology which is concerned with modifications of the composition of the earth's crust caused by chemical changes occurring in it. [Gk *ge* earth, chemistry.]

geode (je·ode). Any one of the minute tissue spaces which contain lymph, or any cavity related to the lymphatic system in general. [Gk *ge* earth, *eidos* form (i.e. spherical).]

geoffroyine (jef·roi·een). Surinamine; *N*-methyltyrosine: an organic base occurring naturally in plants.

geomedicine (je·o·**med**·is·in). The branch of medical science which is concerned with the distribution of health and disease according to the geographical features of the earth. [Gk *ge* earth, medicine.]

Geomys (je·o·mis). A genus of rodents, pocket gophers. **Geomys breviceps.** A species which acts as a reservoir for the rickettsia of tick-borne typhus in southern USA [Gk *ge* earth, *mys* mouse.]

geopathology (je·o·path·ol′·o·je). The study of the effect of topography, climate and other environmental conditions, on disease. [Gk *ge* earth, pathology.]

geophagia, geophagism (je·o·fa·je·ah, je·of·aj·izm). The morbid practice of eating clay and other earthy substances. [Gk *ge* earth, *phagein* to eat.]

geophagist (je·of·aj·ist). One who practises geophagia.

geophagous (je·of·ag·us). Indicating addiction to the practice of geophagia.

geophagy (je·of·aj·e). Geophagia.

Georgi, Walter (b. 1889). Frankfurt serologist.

Sachs-Georgi test. A flocculation test for the serodiagnosis of syphilis.

geotaxis (je·o·tax·is). Geotropism. [Gk *ge* earth, *taxis* arrangement.]

geotragia (je·o·tra·je·ah). Geophagia. [Gk *ge* earth, *trogein* to chew.]

geotrichosis (je·o·trik·o′·sis). A rare oral, intestinal, bronchial or pulmonary infection usually due to *Geotrichum candidum.* The mycosis is usually secondary to some abnormal condition or infection. [Gk *ge* earth, *thrix* hair, *-osis* condition.]

Geotrichum (je·ot·rik·um). A genus of yeast-like fungi. They possess septate mycelia disintegrating into arthrospores which become rounded. **Geotrichum candidum.** A species commonly isolated from man's environment but only rarely causing disease in man. [Gk *ge* earth, *thrix* hair.]

geotropic (je·o·trop·ik). Having relation to geotropism.

geotropism (je·ot·rop·izm). 1. In biology, the influence of gravity on the movement of an organism or the growth of a part. 2. In plant physiology, the influence exerted on a growing plant by gravity. **Negative geotropism.** In plant physiology, the tendency of an organ to grow upwards or away from the earth, as a shoot. **Positive geotropism.** In plant physiology, the tendency of an organ to grow towards or downwards into the earth, as a root. [Gk *ge* earth, *trope* a turning.]

gephyrophobia (jef·i·ro·fo′·be·ah). Pathological fear of crossing a bridge. [Gk *gephyra* bridge, phobia.]

geraeology (jer·e·ol·o·je). Geriatrics. [Gk *geras* old age, *logos* science.]

Geraghty, John Timothy (b. 1876). Baltimore urologist.

Geraghty's test, Rowntree and Geraghty test. Phenolsulphonephthalein test. *See* TEST.

geramorphism (jer·ah·mor·fizm). The state in which a young person has the appearance of an old person; looking prematurely aged. [Gk *geras* old age, *morphe* form.]

geranial (jer·a·ne·al). α-Citral, $CH_3C(CH_3)=CH(CH_2)_2C(CH_3)=CHCHO$; the aldehyde corresponding to geraniol, which occurs in lemon grass oil and the oils of lemon and orange; a yellow oil used in perfumery and to flavour food.

geraniol (jer·a·ne·ol). $CH_3C(CH_3)=CH(CH_2)_2C(CH_3)=CHCH_2OH$; a terpene alcohol found in Indian geranium oil, citronella, rose oils, lemon grass oils, oils of eucalyptus, lavender and other essential oils; used in perfumery and as an insect bait.

geranyl (jer·a·nil). The organic radical, $C_{10}O_{17}$, derived from geraniol. **Geranyl acetate,** $C_{10}H_{17}OOCCH_3$. An ester of geraniol which occurs in oil of lemon.

geratic (jer·at·ik). Relating or belonging to old age. [Gk *geras* old age.]

geratology (jer·at·ol·o·je). Gerontology. [Gk *geras* old age, *logos* science.]

gerbil, gerbille (jer·bil). A small burrowing rodent of open grounds of the Old World. The important genera are *Desmodillus, Gerbillus, Meriones, Rhombomys* and *Tatera.* Species of *Gerbillus* and *Tatera,* and probably others, act as reservoirs of sylvatic plague in Africa and Asia. **Great gerbil.** *Rhombomys opimus* of Central Asia which acts as a reservoir of infection for *Leishmania tropica.* [Ar. *yarbu.*]

Gerbillus (jer·bil·us). A genus of gerbils. *Gerbillus paeba* is a reservoir of sylvatic plague in South Africa. [see prec.]

Gerbode, Frank Leven Albert (b. 1907). American thoracic surgeon.

Gerbode defect. A developmental abnormality of the heart involving that part of the ventricular septum, adjacent to the tricuspid valve ring, which separates the left ventricle from the right atrium. The defect allows a shunt of blood from the left ventricle into the right atrium.

Gerdy, Pierre Nicolas (b. 1797). Paris anatomist and surgeon.

Gerdy's fibres. The superficial transverse ligament of the palm.

Gerdy's fontanelle. A supernumerary fontanelle between the two parietal bones.

Gerdy's ligament. The suspensory ligament of the axilla.

Gerdy's operation. 1. For entropion: removal of the margin of the lid (obsolete). 2. For stricture of the lacrimal duct: by incisions into the duct, and excision of a piece of bone from the inner wall of the orbit (obsolete).

Gerdy's tubercle. A tubercle on the antero-external aspect of the upper end of the tibia.

Gerhardt, Carl Christian Adolph Jacob (b. 1833). Berlin physician.

Gerhardt's change of note, phenomenon or sign. The percussion note over a hydropneumothorax becomes lower in pitch when the patient lies down.

Gerhardt's disease. Erythromelalgia.

Gerhardt law, Gerhardt-Semon law. In a progressive destructive lesion of the motor nerve supplying the intrinsic laryngeal muscles, the abductor mechanism is affected before that of adduction.

Gerhardt's triangle. A triangular area of dullness to percussion over the 3rd rib, just to the left of the sternum, described in cases of patent ductus arteriosus, and other conditions in which the main pulmonary artery is enlarged.

Gerhardt, Charles Frédéric (b. 1816). French chemist.

Gerhardt's test. For aceto-acetic acid in urine: to about 5 ml urine add 5 per cent ferric chloride solution drop by drop until no further precipitation occurs. Filter, if necessary. A port-wine colour indicates aceto-acetic acid. Aceto-acetic acid in urine indicates a rather severe degree of ketosis.

geriatric (jer·e·at·rik). Pertaining to geriatrics.

geriatrics (jer·e·at·rix). The branch of medicine that is concerned with the clinical study and treatment of old age and its manifestations, e.g. senility. [Gk *geras* old age, *iatreia* treatment.]

geriopsychosis (jer·e·o·si·ko′·sis). Any group of mental diseases due to senility or presenility. [Gk *geras* old age, psychosis.]

Gerlach, Joseph von (b. 1820). Erlangen anatomist.

Gerlach's method. The demonstration of nerve fibres with dilute gold chloride after prolonged bichromate fixation.

Gerlach's annular tendon. The fibrocartilaginous ring which occupies the tympanic groove: the thickened margin of the tympanic membrane.

Gerlach's tubal tonsil. Lymphatic tissue in the mucous membrane of the pharyngotympanic (eustachian) tube close to its pharyngeal opening.

Gerlach's valve. A mucoid fold which sometimes guards the orifice of the vermiform appendix.

Gerlier, Felix (b. 1840). Swiss physician.

Gerlier's disease or syndrome. Endemic paralytic vertigo; a disease of farmworkers and stablemen, endemic in Switzerland, and characterized by episodes of vertigo, ptosis and flaccid paralysis of neck muscles, with occasional spread to muscles of the throat and extremities. A similar condition is called *kubisagari* in Japan.

germ (jerm). 1. A microbe; a bacterium. 2. The embryonic rudiment of an organ. 3. That which is capable of developing into a new individual, e.g. the embryo of a cereal grain germ, which contains a high proportion of the vitamins in the grain. **Dental germ.** The rudiment of a tooth, consisting of dental sac, dental papilla and enamel organ. **Hair germ.** Hair follicle. **Tumour germ.** Embryonal rest. *See* REST. [L *germen* sprout.]

See also: COHNHEIM.

germanium (jer·ma·ne·um). A rare element of atomic weight 72.59, atomic number 32, and chemical symbol Ge. It is a greyish metalloid resembling tin in chemical properties, being di- and tetravalent; it occurs in silver and zinc ores, and is used to harden magnesium and aluminium. [L *Germania* Germany.]

germicidal (jer·me·si·dal). Destructive of micro-organisms. [see foll.]

germicide (jer·me·side). Any agent or substance that destroys micro-organisms. [germ, L *caedere* to kill.]

germifuge (jer·me·fewj). 1. Able to drive out micro-organisms. 2. Any agent which expels micro-organisms from the body. [germ, L *fugare* to drive away.]

germinal (jer·min·al). 1. Relating or belonging to a germ. 2. Having the characters of a germ. 3. Relating or belonging to germination. 4. Embryological. 5. Incipient. **Germinal cell.** A cell, from spermatogonium to spermatozoon, derived from the germinal epithelium lining the seminiferous tubules and taking part in spermatogenesis. **Germinal epithelium.** The epithelium lining the seminiferous tubules.

germination (jer·min·a·shun). 1. The process of formation taking place within the impregnated ovum. 2. The beginning of growth or development of a spore or seed. [L *germinare* to germinate.]

germinative (jer·min·a·tiv). 1. Belonging to a germ. 2. Belonging to germination. 3. Capable of growing or developing. [see prec.]

germogen (jer·mo·jen). A mass of protoplasm which gives rise to germ cells. [germ, Gk *genein* to produce.]

geroderma, gerodermia (jer·o·der·mah, jer·o·der·me·ah). 1. The dry wrinkled skin of old age. 2. A defective state of nutrition of the skin, particularly of the genitalia, in which it becomes thin and wrinkled as in old age. **Geroderma osteodysplastica.** A rare syndrome of stunted growth, premature ageing of the skin, osteoporosis, multiple fractures and skeletal malformations. [Gk *geron* old man, *derma* skin.]

gerodontia (jer·o·don·she·ah). The branch of dental science concerned with the teeth in old age. [Gk *geron* old man, *odous* tooth.]

geromarasmus (jer·o·mar·az′·mus). The wasting, atrophy and weakness which marks extreme old age. [Gk *geron* old man, marasmus.]

geromorphism (jer·o·mor·fizm). Weakness, decrepitude and senility occurring in young persons. **Cutaneous geromorphism.** A condition of the skin of very young people in which it has the characteristics of the skin of old age. [Gk *geron* old man, *morphe* form.]

gerontal, gerontic (jer·on·tal, jer·on·tik). 1. Senile. 2. Relating or belonging to old age or the aged. 3. Relating to an old man. [Gk *geron* old man.]

gerontology (jer·on·tol·o·je). The branch of medical science which is concerned with the physiological and pathological phenomena of senescence. [Gk *geron* old man, *logos* science.]

gerontophilia (jer·on·to·fil′·e·ah). Unusually great affection for and understanding of old people. [Gk *geron* old man, *philein* to love.]

gerontopia (jer·on·to·pe·ah). Presbyopia. [Gk *geron* old man, *ops* eye.]

gerontotherapy (jer·on·to·ther′·ap·e). Treatment in old age in accordance with the view that it is a distinct stage of life and requires specialized care. [Gk *geron* old man, therapy.]

gerontoxon (jer·on·tox·on). The arcus senilis; an opaque ring round the cornea in old people. **Gerontoxon lentis.** A clouding of the equator of the lens in old people. [Gk *geron* old man, *toxon* bow.]

Gerota, Dumitru (b. 1867). Budapest anatomist.

Gerota's capsule or fascia. The renal fascia.

Gerota's method. The injection of vessels, especially lymphatics, for anatomical demonstration, with Prussian blue dissolved in alcohol.

Gersh, Isidore (b. 1907). Chicago scientist.

Altmann-Gersh method. The preparation of tissues for sectioning by freezing followed by dehydration *in vacuo.*

Gerstmann, Josef (b. 1887). Vienna neurologist.

Gerstmann's syndrome. A syndrome due to a lesion of the dominant parietal lobe of the cerebrum. There is finger agnosia, right-left disorientation and acalculia, and often constructional apraxia, alexia and homonymous hemianopia.

Gersuny, Robert (b. 1844). Vienna surgeon.

Gersuny's phenomenon. When a faecal mass is contained in the rectum, if the finger is pressed firmly into the mass so that it sticks to the mucous membrane and the finger is then slowly removed, the separation of the mass from the mucous membrane can be detected.

Gersuny's paraffin prosthesis. A means of restoring or modifying the outline of any part of the body by a subcutaneous injection of paraffin.

Gesell, Arnold (b. 1880). Connecticut psychologist.

Gesell's developmental schedule test. An inventory of norms of development and behaviour observed in 4 categories—motor, adaptive, language and personal-social—for use with children from the age of 4 weeks upward.

gestaltism (ges·tawlt·izm). In psychology, the theory that mental objects are presented to direct experience as whole formations and cannot be analysed or broken up into component parts. [G *Gestalt* form.]

gestation (jes·ta·shun). Pregnancy. [L *gestare* to bear.]

gestogen (jes·to·jen). A compound that produces characteristics similar to those of progesterone.

gestosis (jes·to·sis). 1. Any toxaemia of pregnancy. 2. Any disorder occurring during pregnancy and due to it. [gestation, Gk *-osis* condition.]

Gestronol (jes·tro·nol). BP Commission approved name for 17-hydroxy-19-norpregn-4-ene-3,20-dione; a progestational steroid.

gesture (jes·tewr). A communicatory movement, usually of head or hands, intended to convey meaning. It is sometimes evoked without this communicatory purpose by a train of private thought. **Gesture language.** The conveyance of ideas to, or by, deaf mutes, by gestures. [L *gerere* to act.]

Getsowa's adenoma. Adenoma or adenocarcinoma of the thyroid gland in which the lining cells are large and eosinophile.

geumaphobia (gew·mah·fo·be·ah). Morbid dislike or fear of tastes. [Gk *geume* taste, phobia.]

Ghilarducci, Francesco (b. 1857). Rome physician and radiologist.

Ghilarducci's reaction. Muscles in a limb can be caused to contract when an electrical stimulus is applied at a given point not immediately over the muscles.

Ghon, Anton (b. 1866). Prague pathologist.

Ghon's focus, primary lesion or tubercle. The primary lesion in tuberculosis of the lungs in children. Situated usually well out in the periphery of the lung, it appears first on a radiograph as a small homogeneous soft shadow. Later, it shows partial or complete calcification, often with areas of calcification in the associated hilar glands.

ghost (go·st). An apparition, but commonly used to imply a manifestation which occurs repeatedly. [AS *gast.*]

Giacomini, Carlo (b. 1841). Turin anatomist.

band, bandelette, banderella, frenulum or stria of Giacomini. The anterior extremity of the dentate gyrus, running on the under surface of the uncus.

Giannuzzi, Giuseppe (b. 1839). Siena physiologist.

Giannuzzi's body, cell, crescent or demilune. Crescent cell; a parietal serous cell of a mucous gland, lying between the principal mucous cells and the basement membrane, where it is flattened in the form of a crescent.

giant (ji·ant). Any organism or structure of much greater size than normal. **Eunuchoid giant.** One whose abnormal stature is due to deficiency of gonadal secretion and consequent failure of epiphyseal union. [Gk *gigas.*]

giantism (ji·ant·izm). 1. Gigantism. 2. The state of being abnormally large in size, e.g. certain cells and nuclei. [see prec.]

Giardia (je·ar·de·ah). A genus of flagellate Protozoa. **Giardia intestinalis, Giardia lamblia.** A very common parasite of the human small intestine. It is pear-shaped with 8 flagella and 2 nuclei. Individuals normally attach themselves to the intestinal epithelium and, in heavy infections, may interfere with absorption, particularly of fat. Also called *Lamblia intestinalis.* [Alfred *Giard* (b. 1846), Paris biologist.]

giardiasis (je·ar·di·as·is). Infection with a parasite of the genus *Giardia.*

Giardinus (je·ar·di·nus). A genus of freshwater fish. **Giardinus poeciloides.** Barbados millions, an important larviphage in antimosquito campaigns.

gibber (gib·er). A hump-like or sac-like swelling or enlargement. **Gibber inferior thalami.** The pulvinar of the thalamus. Gibber ulnae. The olecranon. [L *gibbus* hump.]

gibberish (gib·er·ish, jib·er·ish). Unintelligible nonsensical speech. [onomat.]

Gibbon, John Heysham (b. 1903). Philadelphia thoracic surgeon.

Gibbon and Landis test. Reflex vasodilatation test: when the peripheral circulation is normal, heat applied to an extremity is followed by vasodilatation and increase in skin temperature in the unheated extremities. If the feet are to be tested, they are exposed to the air in a warm room and heating applied to the trunk or arms for from 60 to 90 min. The skin temperature is measured at frequent intervals. Organic vascular disease is indicated by a failure of the skin temperature to reach 30–32°C. A normal response is usually obtained in subjects with vasospastic disorders as opposed to organic vascular disease.

Gibbon oxygenator. A method of oxygenating blood during cardiopulmonary by-pass in which blood flows over a number of stainless steel screens and is exposed to oxygen. Developed at the Mayo Clinic.

Gibbon, Norman Otway Knight. 20th century Liverpool surgeon.

Gibbon's catheter. A urinary catheter made of 'Portex' tubing, 1.5 mm in diameter, with flanges on either side to enable it to be held in place. It is suitable for either male or female.

Gibbon, Quinton V. (b. 1813). American surgeon.

Gibbon's hernia or hydrocele. A large inguinal hernia associated with hydrocele.

gibbosity (gib·os·it·e). A hump. [L *gibbus* hump.]

gibbous (gib·us). 1. Protuberant; swollen, particularly on one side. 2. Humpbacked. 3. Resembling a hump. [see prec.]

Gibbs, Josiah Willard (b. 1839). Yale mathematician and physicist.

Gibbs' equation. For the concentration of any component of a system at the interface:

$$U = \frac{C}{RT}\,\frac{d\sigma}{dC},$$

where U is the surface excess of solute, C its solution concentration, R the gas constant, T the absolute temperature, and σ the surface tension.

Gibbs' phase rule. In the case of several phases in equilibrium, the degrees of freedom plus the number of phases equals the number of components increased by 2.

Gibbs' theorem. Any component of a system which tends to lower surface tension will be in greatest concentration at the interface, whilst a component which tends to raise surface tension will be less concentrated at the interface. The relationship is given by Gibbs' equation (above).

gibbus (gib·us). 1. A hump. 2. The protuberance in angular deformity of the spine; applied to the deformity present in Pott's disease. [L hump.]

Gibert, Camille Melchior (b. 1797). Paris dermatologist.

Gibert's disease or pityriasis. Pityriasis rosea; an eruption of unknown cause, often preceded by the appearance of a herald patch, usually but not invariably affecting only those parts of the trunk and limbs covered by a high-necked short-sleeved vest, and characterized by the appearance of oval or round, rosy or fawn-coloured, superficial medallions covered with furfuraceous scales.

Gibert's syrup. A syrup containing potassium mercuric iodide and used for those diseases in which mercury is indicated.

Gibney, Virgil Pendleton (b. 1847). New York surgeon.

Gibney's perispondylitis. A painful fibrositic condition of the spinalis muscles.

Gibson, George Alexander (b. 1854). Edinburgh physician.

Gibson murmur. A continuous murmur throughout the cardiac cycle, waxing at the end of systole and waning in late diastole. It is heard in the 1st and 2nd intercostal spaces to the left of the sternum in patients with a patent ductus arteriosus, often accompanied by a thrill.

Gibson's rule. In adults (not in children or the elderly) suffering from pneumonia, the blood pressure expressed in millimetres of mercury should not fall below the pulse rate expressed in beats per minute; otherwise the prognosis is bad.

Gibson's vestibule. The aortic vestibule.

Gibson's chart. A chart for use in determining a patient's resistance to infection by recording the increase in neutrophil percentage as compared with the total increase in leucocytes.

Gibson's splint. A modified Thomas splint.

giddiness (gid·e·nes). A term used loosely to imply a subjective feeling of loss of balance or disorientation in space which may arise in cases of a widely-differing character. It is non-scientific and less accurate than dizziness. [AS *gydig* mad.]

Giemsa, Gustav (b. 1867). Hamburg chemist and bacteriologist.

Giemsa stain. A differential stain for blood smears and tissues. It is a Romanovsky stain containing Azure II and eosin dissolved in glycerin and methyl alcohol. Preliminary fixing of blood smears is essential.

Gierke, Edgar von (b. 1877). Karlsruhe pathologist.

von Gierke's disease. Glycogen storage disease *Type I. See* DISEASE.

Gierke, Hans Paul (b. 1847). German anatomist.

Gierke's respiratory bundle. The tractus solitarius.

Gierke's cell. A small nerve cell from the gelatinous matter of the spinal cord, representing the cell body of a secondary sensory neurone.

Gierke's corpuscles. Nests of concentrically-arranged cells of an epithelial nature found in the thymus; more commonly known as *Hassall's corpuscles.*

Gies, William John (b. 1872). New York biochemist.

Gies' biuret reagent. For proteins: 10 per cent potassium hydroxide solution, 1 litre; 3 per cent copper sulphate solution, 25 ml.

Gifford, Harold (b. 1858). Omaha ophthalmologist.

Gifford's operation. For corneal ulcer: delimiting keratotomy. A small section is made with a small Graefe knife through the ulcer, coming out on the pupil side of the ulcer. This acts as a paracentesis and stops the ulcer advancing towards the centre.

Gifford's reflex, Gifford-Galassi reflex. When the eyelids are being held apart and an effort is made to close them, the pupil constricts. Also called *von Graefe's lid reaction* and *Westphal-Pilcz phenomenon.*

Gifford's sign. Difficulty in everting the upper lid, in thyrotoxic exophthalmos.

biological theory of Gifford. To explain the spread of sympathetic ophthalmia from one to the other eye: Gifford suggests that the causative organism acquires a greater ability to live in the uveal tissues during the affection of the first eye; this gives the organism an elective affinity for the uveal tissue of the second eye.

gigantism (ji·gant·izm). A condition of excessive tallness. Individuals whose height exceeds 1.98 m (6 ft 6 in) are usually considered to be giants. Cases of 2.59 m (8 ft 6 in) have been recorded. Gigantism is classified as simple (primary), endocrine, fetal and local. **Endocrine gigantism.** This may be either hyperpituitary or hypogonadal. **Fetal gigantism.** The infant may weigh more than 6.8 kg (15 lb) at birth. The causes are primary (see above), endocrine disorders of the mother or fetus, such as maternal diabetes or pre-diabetes and post maturity. Hyperpituitary gigantism may, but does not always, date from fetal life. Post-maturity may also result in a high birth weight. **Hyperpituitary gigantism.** This is due to excessive secretion of growth hormone before the epiphyses of the long bones have united. This may be due to an eosinophil adenoma of the pituitary. Continued over-production of growth hormone after epiphyseal closure will give rise to acromegalic gigantism. **Hypogonadal gigantism.** This is due to lack of sex hormone which activates the closure of the epiphyses of the long bones, and they consequently continue to grow in contrast to the bones of the vertebral column. The span may be as much as 15 cm (6 in) greater than the height. **Local gigantism.** This may be due to acromegaly affecting one or other of the structures usually enlarged in the classical condition, or to arachnodactyly, a congenital condition characterized by extremely long and slender fingers and toes, and other congenital manifestations. Local gigantism of individual limbs or digits may also occur. **Simple (primary) gigantism.** This may be racial or hereditary but no other specific cause can be deduced. [Gk *gigas* giant.]

Gigantobilharzia monocotylea (ji·gant·o·bil·**harts**′·e·ah mon·o·**kot**·il·e·ah). A sea-bird schistosome that has been reported as causing dermatitis in man. [Gk *gigas* giant, bilharzia, Gk *monos* single, *kotyle* hollow.]

gigantoblast, gigantochromoblast (ji·**gant**·o·blast, ji·**gant**·o·**kro**′·mo·blast). A very large erythroblast. [Gk *gigas* giant, *blastos* germ, *chroma* colour.]

gigantocyte (ji·**gant**·o·site). Megalocyte. [Gk *gigas* giant, *kytos* cell.]

gigantosoma (ji·gant·o·**so**′·mah). Normal gigantism. [Gk *gigas* giant, *soma* body.]

Gigli, Leonardo (b. 1863). Florence gynaecologist.

Gigli's operation. Section of the pubis in difficult labour, by a flexible saw.

Gigli's saw. A wire saw devised for pubiotomy but now mainly used in craniotomy for cutting between two burr-holes to allow removal of the bone flap.

Gilbert, Nicolas Augustin (b. 1858). Paris physician.

Gilbert's cholaemia. Congenital haemolytic jaundice.

Gilbert's sign. In hepatic cirrhosis, more urine is secreted during fasting than during digestion.

Gilbert's syndrome. Chronic non-haemolytic unconjugated hyperbilirubinaemia of various types.

gilbert (gil·bert). A unit of magnetism [obsolete term]. [William *Gilbert* (b. 1540), English physician and physicist.]

Gilchrist, Thomas Casper (b. 1862). Baltimore dermatologist.

Gilchrist's disease or mycosis. North American blastomycosis.

Gilchristia dermatitidis (gil·**kris**·te·ah der·mah·**tit**·id·is). A synonym (Redaelli and Ciferri 1934) for *Blastomyces dermatitidis* Gilchrist and Stokes 1898. [Thomas Casper *Gilchrist*, dermatitis.]

Gilford, Hastings (b. 1861). Reading surgeon.

Gilford-Hutchinson disease, Hutchinson-Gilford disease. Progeria.

Gill, Arthur Bruce (b. 1876). Philadelphia surgeon.

Gill's operation. 1. An operation for drop foot by the insertion of a wedge of bone to block plantar flexion. 2. Shelf operation of the hip. 3. Fusion of the shoulder.

gill (jil). A unit of liquid measure equal to 0.142 litre, equivalent to a quarter of a pint; 5 fluid ounces. [L *gilla* small flask.]

Gilles de la Tourette, Georges (b. 1857). Paris neurologist.

Gilles de la Tourette's disease. Motor inco-ordination and tics, with echolalia and coprolalia.

Gillespie, James Donaldson (b. 1823). Edinburgh surgeon.

Gillespie's operation. Excision of the wrist.

Gillette, Eugene Paulin (b. 1836). Paris surgeon.

Gillette's suspensory ligament. Longitudinal muscle fibres of the oesophagus which are attached to the back of the larynx.

Gilliam, David Tod (b. 1844). Columbus, Ohio, gynaecologist.

Gilliam's operation. Correction of retrodisplacement of the uterus by drawing a loop of each round ligament through the abdominal wall and fixing them to the sheath of the rectus abdominis muscle.

Gillies, Sir Harold Delf (b. 1882). London plastic surgeon.

Gillies needle-holder. A combined scissors and needle-holder without a ratchet lock. Used principally in plastic surgery, it allows fine and rapid control of small needles.

Gillies' operation. 1. For cicatricial ectropion: excision of all scar tissue and the lid margins returned to their normal position. A "Stent's composition" mould cover with a split-skin or Thiersch graft is sutured into the bare area. 2. For cleft palate: described in 1921 as a method of improving function in unsuccessfully-repaired cleft palate—all available palatal tissue is freed and retroposed to form the velum, thus leaving a large fistula in the hard palate. The fistula is covered by an obturator or a special denture.

Gilmer, Thomas Lewis (b. 1849). Chicago dentist.

Gilmer's splint. A wire splint used for fractures of the mandible: the teeth are fixed together by silver wire.

Gimbernat, Antonio de (b. 1734). Spanish surgeon.

Gimbernat's hernia. Hernia through Gimbernat's ligament.

Gimbernat's ligament. The pectineal part of the inguinal ligament; a triangular bundle of fibres passing horizontally backward to the pectineal line from the medial end of the inguinal ligament. Its lateral free edge forms the medial boundary of the femoral ring.

Gin's test. A test for the potency of smallpox vaccine lymph. A positive result is the development of opacity in the guinea-pig's corneal 72 h after scarification with a 1:1000 dilution of lymph.

ginger (**jin**·jer). The rhizome of *Zingiber officinale* Roscoe (family Zingiberaceae), a reed-like plant cultivated in many tropical countries. The form of the drug varies with the country of origin and the method of preparation. **Ginger BP 1973.** This is the variety known as unbleached Jamaican ginger in which the rhizome is scraped to remove the outer corky surface and dried in the sun. It contains about 3 per cent of an aromatic volatile oil and a pungent principle, gingerol, and is employed medicinally as a carminative and stimulant. Other varieties, used as a condiment, include Cochin ginger, Nigerian ginger, and African ginger. These are generally darker in colour than the BP rhizome, and less aromatic. [Gk *ziggiberis.*]

gingerin (**jin**·jer·in). An oleoresin obtained by extracting powdered ginger root with acetone.

gingerol (**jin**·jer·ol). An oily liquid consisting of homologous phenols of the type $(CH_3O)C_6H_3(OH)CH_2CH_2COCH(OH)$-$(CH_2)_3CH_3$, to which ginger owes its pungency.

gingiva [NA] (**jin**·jiv·ah) (pl. *gingivae).* The gum; the tissue covering the alveolar processes of the mandible and maxillae and surrounding the necks of the teeth. It consists of a mucous membrane, a dense connective tissue and periosteal layers, i.e. a mucoperiosteum. **Attached gingiva.** The gum covering the alveolar process and continuous with the free gingiva. **Buccal gingiva.** The gum covering the outer aspect of the dental alveolar process and teeth in the molar and premolar areas. **Free gingiva.** The free collar of gum overlapping the neck and base of the crown of a tooth. **Labial gingiva.** The gum covering the outer aspect of the dental alveolar process and teeth in the incisor and canine regions. **Lingual gingiva.** The gum covering the lingual surfaces of the teeth. **Septal gingiva.** That part of the gum which occupies the space between adjacent teeth. [L gum.]

gingival (**jin**·jiv·al). Relating or belonging to the gingiva or the gum.

gingivally (**jin**·jiv·al·e). In a direction towards the gums. [gingiva.]

gingivectomy (jin·jiv·**ek**·to·me). The surgical removal of the gum margin to eliminate pockets and improve gingival contour. [gingiva, Gk *ektome* a cutting out.]

gingivitis (jin·jiv·i·tis). Inflammation of the gingival margins around the teeth, manifested by swelling and bleeding. **Catarrhal gingivitis.** Term formerly attributed to an acute bright-red gingivitis; usually part of a herpetic stomatitis. **Haemorrhagic gingivitis.** Bleeding gums in excess of a non-specific gingivitis, e.g. blood dyscrasias and scurvy. **Herpetic gingivitis.** Part of acute gingivostomatitis due to a primary herpes simplex infection. **Hypertrophic gingivitis.** Hyperplasia of the gingival tissue of non-specific origin and also seen in cases of prolonged treatment with phenytoin sodium. **Ulceromembranous gingivitis.**

An acute ulceration of the gingival tissues leading to loss of the gingival papillae. Fusiform bacilli and *Borrelia vincenti* may be isolated from the lesions. Also known as *trench mouth* or *ulcerative gingivitis.* [gingiva, Gk *-itis* inflammation.]

gingivo-ectomy (jin·jiv·o·**ek'**·to·me). Gingivectomy.

gingivoglossitis (jin·jiv·o·glos·**i'**·tis). Inflammation of the gums and tongue. [gingiva, Gk *glossa* tongue, *-itis* inflammation.]

gingivolabial (jin·jiv·o·**la'**·be·al). Relating or belonging to the gums and the lips. [gingiva, L *labia* lip.]

gingivopericementitis (jin·jiv·o·per·e·se·ment·**i'**·tis). Pyorrhoea alveolaris. [gingiva, pericementum, Gk *-itis* inflammation.]

gingivoplasty (jin·jiv·o·**plas'**·te). The surgical correction of gingival contour. [gingiva, Gk *plassein* to mould.]

gingivostomatitis (jin·jiv·o·sto·mat·**i'**·tis). An inflammatory condition involving the gingival margins and the cheeks and palate. **Herpetic gingivostomatitis.** An acute vesicular and ulcerative inflammation of the mouth due to the herpes simplex virus. Usually the primary attack is in childhood. [gingiva, stomatitis.]

ginglyform (jing·gle·form). Ginglymoid. [Gk *gigglymos* hinge, form.]

ginglymo-arthrodial (jing·gle·mo·ar·**thro'**·de·al). Denoting a joint which has the characteristics of both hinge and plane joints. [Gk *gigglymos* hinge, *arthron* joint.]

ginglymoid (jing·gle·moid). Having resemblance to a plane joint. [Gk *gigglymos* hinge, *eidos* form.]

ginglymus (jing·gle·mus). A joint that allows movement in one plane only; a simple hinged joint. [Gk *gigglymos* hinge.]

Giordano, Davide (b. 1864). Venice surgeon.

Giordano's sphincter. A sphincter at the opening of the common bile duct in the duodenum.

Giovannini, Sabastiano (b. 1851). Turin dermatologist.

Giovannini's disease. A nodular disease of the hair, said to be caused by a fungus.

Giraldès, Joachim Albin Cardazo Cazado (b. 1808). Paris surgeon and anatomist.

Giraldès' bonnet à poil. The enlarged and frontally-broadened head of the hydrocephalic.

organ of Giraldès. The paradidymis.

Girard, Alfred Conrad (b. 1841). American army surgeon.

Girard's treatment. The administration of atrophic sulphate with strychnine sulphate for seasickness.

girdle (ger·dl). 1. A belt or binder which girds or encircles the body. 2. A roughly circular, structural arrangement of bone or other tissue, e.g. the pelvic girdle, the shoulder girdle. **Emphysematous girdle.** In emphysema there is often a girdle of dilated venules at the level of the attachment of the diaphragm: the sign is not pathognomonic. **Limbus girdle.** A ring of degenerative corneal opacity concentric with the limbus. **Pelvic girdle [cingulum membri inferioris (NA)].** The bony ring composed of the two hip bones laterally and in front, and the sacrum and coccyx behind. **Shoulder girdle [cingulum membri superioris (NA)], Thoracic girdle.** The arch formed by the scapula and clavicle. [AS *gyrdel.*]

See also: HITZIG.

Girdlestone, Gathorne Robert (b. 1881). Oxford orthopaedic surgeon.

Girdlestone's excision arthroplasty of the hip. Excision of head and neck of femur; used in the treatment of arthritis.

Girdlestone's operation. 1. For claw toes: tendon transference of the flexor to extensor tendons of the toes. 2. For hallux valgus: resection of part of the proximal phalanx of the great toe with preservation of its base and the attachment of the adductor hallucis muscle.

Girdner, John Harvey (b. 1856). New York physician.

Girdner's probe. Telephonic probe. *See* PROBE.

gitalin (jit·a·lin). 1. A mixture of digitalis glucosides used in congestive heart failure, in auricular flutter and in rapid auricular fibrillation. 2. The glucoside, $C_{35}H_{56}O_{12}$, occurring in the leaves and seeds of *Digitalis purpurea,* the purple foxglove.

githagism (gith·aj·izm). Chronic poisoning, similar to lathyrism, attributed to the eating of seeds of the corn cockle (*Lychnis githago*).

gitonin (jit·o·nin). $C_{50}H_{82}O_{23}$, a physiologically-inactive saponin occurring in the purple foxglove, *Digitalis purpurea.*

gitoxigenin (jit·ox·ij·en·in). $C_{23}H_{34}O_5$, the aglycone formed on complete acid hydrolysis of the physiologically-active cardiac glycoside, gitoxin, in which it occurs combined with digitoxose.

gitoxin (jit·ox·in). $C_{41}H_{64}O_{14}$, a glycoside composed of gitoxigenin and digitoxose, formed by the hydrolysis of the natural glycosides of *Digitalis purpurea,* the purple foxglove, and *Digitalis lanata.* It is physiologically active, increasing the cardiac output and improving the peripheral circulation by stimulation of the vagus.

gitterzellen (git·er·zel·en). Compound granular corpuscles. *See* CORPUSCLE. [G.]

Givens, Maurice Hope (b. 1888). American biochemist.

Hunter and Givens method, for purine bases in urine. The Krueger-Schmidt method is modified to permit colorimetric determination of uric acid.

gizzard (giz·ard). The thick muscular second (posterior) stomach of cereal-eating birds in which the food is broken down. [Fr. *gésier.*]

glabella [NA] (glab·el·ah). The median elevation which connects the 2 superciliary arches on the frontal bone. [L *glabellus* hairless.]

glabellar (glab·el·ar). Relating or belonging to the glabella.

glabrate (gla·brate). 1. Becoming smooth and glistening from age or from loss of hair. 2. Glabrous. [L *glaber* smooth.]

glabrous (gla·brus). Bald, smooth and glistening; hairless. [see prec.]

glacial (gla·se·al). 1. Frozen or icy. 2. Having the appearance of ice. 3. Vitreous. 4. In chemistry, having an ice-like crystalline appearance, as the solid form of a liquid compound. [L *glacies* ice.]

gladiate (glad·e·ate). Sword-shaped; ensiform. [L *gladius* sword.]

gladiolus (glad·e·o·lus). The body of the sternum. [L small sword.]

gladiomanubrial (glad·e·o·man·**ew'**·bre·al). Relating or belonging to the body of the sternum (gladiolus) and the manubrium sterni.

glair (glare). 1. White of egg. 2. Any clear, thin viscous substance like white of egg. [see foll.]

glairin (gla·er·in). A mucoid substance of supposed bacterial origin found on the waters of certain sulphur springs. [ME *glayre* white of egg.]

glairy (gla·er·e). 1. Thin and clear, like white of egg. 2. Viscous or mucoid. 3. Slimy. [see prec.]

gland [glandula (NA)] (gland). Cells or accumulation of cells which elaborate secretions or excretions. **Adrenal glands.** A pair of flattened triangular glands, one at the upper pole of each kidney, composed of a cortex and medulla differing in embryonic origin and function. The cortex is the source of a hormone or hormones with actions on electrolyte and water balance, on the metabolism of protein, fat and carbohydrate, on mesodermal tissue (including fibrous and lymphoid tissue) and its responses to a variety of stimuli, and on immunological mechanisms; also with oestrogenic and androgenic properties. The activity of the cortex is controlled by the adrenocorticotrophic hormone of the anterior lobe of the pituitary gland. The medulla is composed of tissue which stains brownish yellow with certain chromium salts, and hence is designated *chromaffin* tissue. It is the source of the sympathomimetic amines, adrenaline and noradrenaline. The medulla is controlled by preganglionic fibres of the sympathetic nervous system, with which it is richly supplied. **Alveolar gland.** A gland composed of epithelial cells arranged in groups separated by connective tissue and blood vessels, e.g. the pituitary; in the case of a gland with external secretion, e.g. the salivary gland, the cells are related to a minute duct. **Apocrine gland.** *See* APOCRINE. **Areolar glands [glandulae areolares (NA)].** Sebaceous glands on the areola of the breast. **Bronchial glands [glandulae bronchiales (NA)].** Mucous glands of the submucous tissue of the trachea and bronchi. **Buccal glands [glandulae buccales (NA)].** Small salivary glands situated between the buccinator muscle and the mucous membrane of the vestibule of the mouth. **Bulbo-urethral gland [glandula bulbo-urethralis (NA)].** Either of 2 pea-sized glands embedded in the sphincter urethrae muscle posterolateral to the membranous urethra. Their ducts [ductus glandulae bulbo-urethralis (NA)], about 3 cm long, pass obliquely downward and forward through the perineal membrane to open on to the floor of the spongy urethra. **Ceruminous glands [glandulae ceruminosae (NA)].** Glands, believed to be modified sweat glands, in the cartilaginous part of the external auditory meatus; they secrete ear wax. **Cervical glands [glandulae cervicales (uteri) NA].** *See* UTERUS, MUCOUS COAT OF THE. **Ciliary glands [glandulae ciliares (NA)].** Glands, believed to be modified sweat glands, lying close to and opening on the free margins of the eyelids close to the eyelashes. **Circumanal glands [glandulae circumanales (NA)].** Large sebaceous glands around the anus; many open in the skin independently of the hair follicles. **Coil gland.** An eccrine sweat gland. **Conjunctival glands [glandulae conjunctivales (NA)].** Follicles similar to lymph follicles at the medial angle of the eye. Also known as *trachoma glands.* **Ductless glands [glandulae sine ductibus (NA)].** A group of glands, or portions of a gland, whose secretions, having an important influence on general metabolic processes, are carried from the gland by its veins and possibly by lymphatics. **Duodenal glands [glandulae duodenales (NA)].** Small compound acinar glands, more numerous in the first and second parts of the duodenum, lying in the sub-mucous coat and opening by short ducts on the surface of the mucous membrane; Brunner's glands. **Eccrine gland.** A gland that delivers its secretion to the surface, directly or via a duct or ducts. **Endocrine glands.** Ductless glands (see above). **Exocrine gland.** A gland which secrets externally, such as the pancreas that secrets enzymes into the stomach as well as insulin, a hormone that is secreted internally into the blood stream. **Gastric glands, proper [glandulae gastricae (propriae) NA].** The glands in the mucous membrane of the stomach, comprising three structurally-different types, cardiac, fundic or oxyntic, and pyloric. **Glomiform glands [glandulae glomiformes (NA)].** Glands which are coiled like a glomus, e.g. the sweat glands. **Harderian gland.** An accessory gland in the orbit which secretes an oily fluid; rarely present in the Primates. **Haversian glands.** The extrasynovial pads of fat. **Hilar gland.** A gland in the area of the hilum of the lung. **Holocrine gland.** *See* HOLOCRINE. **Interscapular gland.** A mass of brown fat situated between the scapulae of many animals and in the human fetus; Bonnot's gland. **Intestinal glands [glandulae intestinales (NA)].** Tubular glands, rich in goblet cells, found in the mucous membrane throughout the small and large intestine; glands of Lieberkühn. **Labial glands [glandulae labiales (NA)].** Small salivary glands embedded in the lips. **Lacrimal gland [glandula lacrimalis (NA)].** A tear-secreting gland, the size and shape of an almond, in the upper lateral corner of each orbit. The main orbital part [pars orbitalis (NA)] lies in the lacrimal fossa of the frontal bone; the palpebral process [pars palpebralis (NA)] extends into the upper eyelid below the tendon of the levator palpebrae superioris muscle. Its 6–10 ducts [ductuli excretorii (glandulae lacrimalis)] open into the superior fornix of the conjunctiva. **Lacrimal glands, accessory [glandulae lacrimales accessoriae (NA)].** Small tear-secreting glands near the conjunctival fornices, especially the upper. **Laryngeal glands [glandulae laryngeae (NA)].** Mucous glands found especially upon the epiglottis, in the aryepiglottic folds, and within the sinus and saccule of the larynx. **Lingual glands [glandulae linguales (NA)].** Small salivary glands in the tongue. **Lingual gland, anterior [glandula lingualis anterior (NA)].** A small group of salivary glands under the tip of the tongue, on either side of the frenulum. **Lymph glands [nodi lymphatici (lymphonodi) NA].** Encapsulated collections of lymphoid tissue, usually arranged in groups and interposed in the course of lymphatic channels. **Lymph glands, aortic [nodi lymphatici lumbales (NA)].** An intercommunicating chain of glands surrounding the abdominal aorta. Below they are continuous with the common iliac lymph gland and their efferents form the right and left lymph trunk. Sometimes they are artificially divided into pre-, para- and retro-aortic glands. **Lymph glands, apical [nodi lymphatici apicales (NA)].** The lymph nodes in the apex of the axilla, above the pectoralis minor muscle and deep to the costocoracoid membrane. They receive lymphatics directly from the mammary gland, upper limb, and from the other axillary lymph nodes. **Lymph glands, axillary [nodi lymphatici axillares (NA)].** Numerous deep glands subdivided into 5 groups: (*a*) lateral, along the axillary vein; (*b*) anterior (pectoral) along the junction of the anterior and medial wall; (*c*) posterior (subscapular) on the posterior wall; (*d*) central, on the axillary floor; all these drain into (*e*) the apical, a continuation of (*a*). They receive lymph from the whole upper limb and superficial tissues of the upper quadrant of the trunk including the breast. Their efferents form the subclavian trunk, but some apical glands may drain into the lower lateral group of the deep cervical glands. **Lymph glands, bronchopulmonary [nodi lymphatici bronchopulmonales (NA)].** Glands around and between the vessels in the hilum of the lung, which they drain, including its pleura. **Lymph glands, buccal [nodi lymphatici buccales (NA)].** Small lymph nodes on the outer surface of the buccinator muscle close to the anterior facial vein and draining the adjacent part of the face. Their efferents pass to the submandibular lymph nodes. **Lymph glands, central [nodi lymphatici centrales (NA)].** One or two inconstant glands placed in the fat in the central parts of the axilla and close to the intercostobrachial nerve. **Lymph glands, cervical. anterior.** Glands associated with the anterior jugular vein; the lowest member often occupies the suprasternal space. Their afferents drain the superficial tissue of the anterior part of the neck below the hyoid bone.Ultimately their efferents pass to the lower deep cervical glands. **Lymph glands, cervical, deep [nodi lymphatici cervicales profundi (NA)].** A chain extending from the base of the skull to the root of the neck along the great vessels, lying mainly deep to the sternomastoid muscle; the upper medial ones spread into the anterior triangle, and the lower lateral into the posterior triangle. The omohyoid divides them into an upper and lower group, and they drain directly or indirectly the whole head and neck; their efferents form the jugular lymph trunk. **Lymph glands, cervical, superficial [nodi lymphatici cervicales superficiales (NA)].** A group of glands along the upper part of the external jugular vein, continuous with the superficial parotid glands and draining into the deep cervical group. **Lymph glands, coeliac [nodi lymphatici celiaci (NA)].** A group of glands around the origin of the coeliac artery. They receive afferents from various groups of glands along the branches of the artery, by which they drain the foregut and its derivatives. Their efferents help to form the intestinal lymph trunk. **Lymph glands, colic, left [nodi lymphatici colici sinistri (NA)].** Those members of the inferior mesenteric group which lie along the colic branches of the inferior mesenteric artery. **Lymph glands, colic, middle [nodi lymphatici colici medii (NA)].** Glands draining the large intestine supplied by the middle colic artery. They are arranged along the branches of the artery, and send efferents to the superior mesenteric group. **Lymph glands, colic, right [nodi lymphatici colici dextri (NA)].** The lymph nodes along the ascending colon and the branches of the superior mesenteric artery which supply this part. **Lymph glands, delphic.** Lymph glands in close anatomical relation with the pyramidal lobe of the thyroid gland. **Lymph glands, diaphragmatic [nodi lymphatici phrenici (NA)].** Glands on the superior surface of the diaphragm, divisible into an anterior group continuous with the retrosternal glands, a posterior continuous with the posterior mediastinal glands, and a middle around each phrenic nerve. On the right the last-named drains the adjacent posterosuperior area of the liver. **Lymph glands, epigastric [nodi lymphatici epigastrici (NA)].** A group of lymph glands along the inferior epigastric artery and draining the territory supplied by this artery. **Lymph glands, gastric, left [nodi lymphatici gastrici sinistri (NA)].** A chain of glands along the left gastric artery whose proximal members are continuous with the coeliac glands. They drain the cardia and the lesser curvature and adjacent half of the stomach. **Lymph glands, gastro-epiploic, right [nodi lymphatici gastro-epiploici dextri (NA)].** A chain of glands along the right gastro-epiploic artery, draining the right half of the greater curvature and the adjacent pyloric portion of the stomach. **Lymph glands, hepatic [nodi lymphatici hepatici (NA)].** A chain of glands along the hepatic artery in the edge of the gastrohepatic omentum, including the cystic glands. They drain the inferior part of the liver and gall bladder. The efferents join the coeliac group. **Lymph gland, hilum of a [hilus (NA)].** A depressed area on the surface of a lymph gland where the medulla comes to the surface; blood vessels enter and efferent vessels leave at this area. **Lymph glands, ileocolic [nodi lymphatici ileocolici (NA)].** A double group about the proximal and distal parts of the ileocolic artery. They drain the terminal ileum, appendix, caecum and ascending colon indirectly via glands close to these structures. Their efferents go to the superior glands of the mesentery. **Lymph glands, iliac [nodi lymphatici iliaci (NA)].** The lymph node along the common and external iliac blood vessels. They receive the lymph from the lower limbs and much of the pelvis and send their efferents to the lumbar lymph glands. **Lymph glands, iliac, common [nodi lymphatici iliaci communes (NA)].** A chain of glands surrounding the common iliac artery, continuous below with those around the external iliac artery, whose lymph they receive as well as that from the internal iliac group. **Lymph glands, iliac, external [nodi lymphatici iliaci externi (NA)].** A chain of glands grouped around the external iliac artery and receiving lymph from the inguinal glands and from the deep tissues of the lower abdominal wall. They send efferents to the common iliac lymph gland. **Lymph glands, iliac, internal [nodi lymphatici iliaci interni (NA)].** Glands on the lateral pelvic wall surrounding the internal iliac vessels. They drain the pelvic organs, the deeper parts of the perineum, and the muscles of the buttock and back of the thigh. Their efferents go to the common iliac lymph glands. **Lymph glands, inguinal, deep [nodi lymphatici inguinales profundi (NA)].** A few glands along the medial side of the femoral vein; a proximal one is found in the femoral canal. They drain the deep tissues of the leg and receive lymph from the superficial inguinal glands. Their efferents run to the external iliac group. **Lymph glands, inguinal, superficial [nodi lymphatici inguinales superficiales (NA)].** Subcutaneous glands forming a T-shaped group, consisting of a proximal set below and parallel to the inguinal ligament, and a distal set around the proximal portion of the long saphenous vein. They drain the skin below the umbilicus, the lining of the lower anal canal, the penile urethra, the vulva and lower vagina and part of the uterus via the round ligament. Efferents pass to the deep inguinal glands. **Lymph glands, innominate [nodi lymphatici mediastinales anteriores (NA)].** A few scattered glands around the innominate veins and aortic arch. They drain the thymus, upper pericardium and right side of the heart. **Lymph glands, intercostal [nodi lymphatici intercostales (NA)].** One or two glands in the posterior end of each intercostal space. They drain the posterior part of the space and parietal pleura. The upper ones drain into the thoracic duct and the lower via the descending intercostal trunk into the cisterna chyli. **Lymph gland, jugulodigastric [nodus lymphaticus jugulodigastricus (NA)].** One of the group of glands found just below the point of crossing of the internal jugular vein by the digastric muscle. It drains the posterior part of the tongue. **Lymph gland, jugulo-omohyoid [nodus lymphaticus jugulo-omohyoideus (NA)].** One of the deep cervical lymph nodes lying on or above the omohyoid muscle. It receives lymph from the tongue either directly or through the submental or submandibular lymph node. **Lymph glands, lateral [nodi lymphatici laterales (NA)].** The axillary lymph glands which lie along the second and third parts of the axillary vessels. They drain most of the upper limb and send their efferents to the apical nodes. **Lymph glands, lingual [nodi lymphatici linguales (NA)].** The lymphatic nodules in the posterior third of the tongue. They are arranged around epithelial crypts and are similar to the faucial tonsils in structure. **Lymph glands, mammary, internal [nodi lymphatici parasternales (NA)].** One or two glands in the anterior end of the upper 4 intercostal spaces. They drain the anterior parts of these as well as the medial part of the mammary gland and overlying skin via perforating afferents. They empty into the bronchomediastinal lymph trunks. **Lymph glands, mandibular [nodi lymphatici mandibulares (NA)].** Small lymph nodes on the course of the facial vein, over the body of the mandible. They drain the face and lips and send their efferents to the submandibular lymph glands. **Lymph glands, mastoid [nodi lymphatici retroauriculares (NA)].** One or two glands on the mastoid process. Afferent vessels drain the posterior surface of the auricle and the scalp behind it; efferents proceed to the upper deep cervical glands. **Lymph glands, mediastinal, posterior [nodi lymphatici mediastinales posteriores (NA)].** A few variable glands around the lower oesophagus, which they drain, as well as the back of the pericardium and adjacent diaphragm. They continue into the paratracheal lymph glands. **Lymph glands, mesenteric, inferior [nodi lymphatici mesenterici inferiores (NA)].** Glands associated with the distribution of the inferior mesenteric artery. They are arranged in groups: those along the gut; those along the left colic and superior rectal branches; and those around the origin of the artery. They drain the left part of the transverse colon, the descending and pelvic colon and the rectum, the lymph passing to the adjacent pre-aortic glands. **Lymph glands of the mesentery, superior [nodi lymphatici mesenterici superiores (NA)].** Numerous glands between the layers of the mesentery of the small intestine, arranged in 3 groups; one along the attachment of the intestine; a second about the loops of the superior mesenteric artery; and a third around the proximal part of the arterial trunk. They drain the jejunum and all but the terminal 25 cm of the ileum, and send efferents to the adjacent aortic glands. **Lymph glands, occipital [nodi lymphatici occipitales (NA)].** 1 or 2 superficial glands around the occipital vessels and on the trapezius. Afferent vessels drain from the posterior part of the scalp and efferents proceed to the upper deep cervical glands. **Lymph glands, pancreaticosplenic [nodi lymphatici pancreaticolienales (NA)].** A group of glands accompanying the splenic artery along the upper border of the pancreas. They drain the left half of the greater curvature and fundus of the stomach, also the spleen and pancreas, and send efferents to the coeliac glands. **Lymph glands, paratracheal.** Small glands along the course of the trachea, which they drain as well as the corresponding part of the oesophagus. Their efferents go to the mediastinal lymph trunk. **Lymph glands, parotid [nodi lymphatici parotidei, superficiales et profundi (NA)].** 3 or 4 deep glands embedded in the surface and substance of the parotid gland. The surface ones drain the front of the auricle, scalp and forehead, and part of the cheek. The deep ones drain the meatus, tympanum and pharyngotympanic tube, and part of the nasopharynx and soft palate. Both efferents run to the deep cervical group. **Lymph glands, pectoral [nodi lymphatici pectorales (NA)].** The anterior group of axillary lymph nodes. They lie along the lower border of the pectoralis minor muscle and drain the mammary gland, chest wall and the anterior abdominal wall. **Lymph glands, popliteal [nodi lymphatici poplitei (NA)].** Small glands in the popliteal fat around the great vessels. They drain the deep tissues of the knee, leg and foot, and the heel. Their efferents run to the inguinal glands. **Lymph glands, pulmonary [nodi lymphatici pulmonales (NA)].** Small lymph nodules in the lung substance on the larger branches of the bronchi. **Lymph glands, pyloric [nodi lymphatici pylorici (NA)].** A small group of glands around the gastroduodenal artery below the angle of the pylorus and duodenum. They receive efferents from the pyloric end of the stomach and first part of the duodenum, and the right gastro-epiploic glands. They drain into the coeliac glands. **Lymph glands, retropharyngeal [nodi lymphatici retropharyngei (NA)].** Lymphatic nodes placed behind the nasopharynx and in front of the prevertebral fascia. They drain the nasopharynx and pharyngotympanic tube and send their efferents to the deep cervical lymph glands. **Lymph glands, sacral [nodi lymphatici sacrales (NA)].** Lymph nodes behind the rectum and in front of the sacrum. They receive afferents from the rectum. **Lymph glands, submandibular [nodi lymphatici submandibulares (NA)].** 4–6 glands on and in the submandibular salivary glands around the facial artery. Afferents drain the face except the middle of the lower lip and the lateral part of the tongue; efferents run to the deep cervical glands. **Lymph glands, submental [nodi lymphatici submentales (NA)].** 1-4 superficial glands on the mylohyoid below the chin, draining the medial part of the lower lip and tip of the tongue. Efferents run to the deep cervical glands. **Lymph glands, subscapular [nodi lymphatici subscapulares (NA)].** The posterior group of axillary lymph nodes. They lie along the subscapular vessel and drain the superficial tissues of the back as low as the iliac crests. **Lymph glands, supratrochlear [nodi lymphatici cubitales (NA)].** A few superficial glands above the medial epicondyle, draining the superficial tissues on the ulnar side of the hand and forearm; efferents enter the lateral axillary group of glands. **Lymph gland, tibial, anterior [nodus lymphaticus tibialis anterior (NA)].** An occasional deep lymph node on the upper part of the crural interosseous membrane close to the anterior tibial vessels. **Lymph glands, tracheobronchial [nodi lymphatici tracheales (NA)].** A group around the tracheal bifurcation, comprising the inferior [nodi lymphatici tracheobronchiales inferiores (NA)], a single group below the bifurcation connecting the lower bronchopulmonary group of either side, and the superior [nodi lymphatici tracheobronchiales superiores (NA)], in the angle between trachea and bronchi of either side. These are continuous with the upper bronchopulmonary glands; all drain ultimately into the bronchomediastinal lymph trunk. **Mammary gland [glandula mammaria (NA)].** The milk-secreting gland of the female and the corresponding vestigial gland of the male [mamma masculina (NA)]. It is believed to be composed of much modified sebaceous glands, made up of from 15 to 20 lobes [lobi glandulae mammariae (NA)], each subdivided into lobules [lobuli glandulae mammariae (NA)]. **Mammary glands, accessory [mammae accessoriae (femininae et masculinae) NA].** Accessory mammary tissue occurring usually but not invariably along the line of the milk ridge of the embryo. **Meibomian glands.** Tarsal glands of the eyelid. **Merocrine gland.** *See* MEROCRINE. **Mesenteric glands.** Lymph glands of the mesentery (see above). **Molar glands [glandulae molares (NA)].** Small salivary glands around the termination of the parotid duct and external to the buccinator muscle. **Mucous gland [glandula mucosa (NA)].** A gland which secretes fluid rich in mucin. **Mucous bile glands [glandulae mucosae biliosae (NA)].** Mucous-secreting cells or pits in the mucous membrane of the bile duct. **Nasal glands [glandulae nasales (NA)].** Branched tubular glands secreting a serous fluid, scattered through the nasal mucous membrane. **Oesophageal glands [glandulae oesophageae (NA)].** Mucous glands in the submucous area of the oesophagus. **Olfactory glands [glandulae olfactoriae (NA)].** The mucous and serous glands in the olfactory and respiratory part of the nasal mucosa. **Palatine glands [glandulae palatinae (NA)].** Small salivary glands situated in the mucous membrane of the palate. **Parathyroid glands.** Small flattened reddish discs of glandular tissue about 5 mm in diameter, situated between the posterior surface of the lobes of the thyroid and its capsule; usually 4 in number, one superior [glandula parathyroidea superior (NA)] and one inferior [glandula parathyroidea inferior (NA)] on either side. The latter may be outside the capsule and associated with either the inferior thyroid artery or vein. **Parotid gland [glandula parotis (NA)].** The largest of the salivary glands, placed behind and partly around the ascending ramus of the mandible and close to the external auditory meatus. It is a serous gland. Differentiated parts are the deep [pars profunda (NA)] and superficial [pars superficialis]. **Parotid gland, accessory [glandula parotis accessoria (NA)].** A part of the parotid gland, which may be wholly or partly detached from the remainder, lying in front of the main gland on the masseter muscle. Its duct opens into the main parotid duct. **Glands of the pelvis of the ureter.** Some evagination of the mucous membrane, not now thought to be glands. **Pharyngeal glands [glandulae pharyngeae (NA)].** Mucous glands in the wall of the pharynx. **Pineal gland.** Pineal body. *See* BODY. **Pituitary gland.** *See* PITUITARY. **Preputial glands [glandulae preputiales (NA)].** Sebaceous glands on the corona of the glans and on the neck of the penis, secreting smegma. **Prostate gland.** *See* PROSTATE. **Pyloric glands [glandulae pyloricae (NA)].** The gastric glands found in the pyloric part of the stomach, characterized by their long ducts, short gland tubes and only occasional parietal or oxyntic cells. **Rectal glands [glandulae intestinales (NA)].** Simple tubular glands opening on the epithelial surface lined with columnar epithelium containing numerous goblet cells. **Salivary glands [glandulae oris (NA)].** Glands which secrete a liquid, saliva, into the mouth. There are three large paired glands, the parotid, submaxillary and sublingual, and numerous small glands opening on the mucous membranes of the lips, cheeks, tongue and floor of the mouth and palate. **Sebaceous glands [glandulae sebaceae (NA)].** Small alveolar glands, usually associated and connected with hair follicles. They secrete a fatty substance, sebum. **Secretory gland.** Alveolar gland (see above). **Sentinel gland.** 1. An enlarged gland in the omentum which indicates a gastric ulcer opposite to it. 2. An enlarged firm gland above the left clavicle occurring with abdominal cancer. **Seromucous gland [glandula seromucosa (NA)].** A mixed mucous and serous gland, e.g. the submandibular gland. **Serous gland [glandula serosa (NA)].** A gland which secretes a thin watery, as opposed to a sticky or mucous, fluid. **Sublingual gland [glandula sublingualis (NA)].** A small, paired, salivary gland situated in the floor of the mouth, close to the symphysis menti. **Submandibular gland [glandula submandibularis (NA)].** A mixed salivary gland lying under cover of the ramus of the mandible, partly in the floor of the mouth and partly in the neck. **Sweat glands [glandulae sudoriferae (NA)].** Tubular glands derived from the epidermis of the skin and extending into the corium and even into the subcutaneous tissue. Their distal extremities are much coiled. **Sweat gland, body of a [corpus glandulae sudoriferae (NA)].** The distal coiled portion of the gland. **Tarsal glands [glandulae tarsales (NA)].** From 20 to 30 modified sebaceous glands lying in vertical grooves on the deep surface of each tarsus. **Thymus gland.** *See* THYMUS. **Thyroid gland.** 1. Thyroid BP 1958. 2. [Glandula thyroidea (NA).] A highly vascular ductless or endocrine gland situated in the front of the neck and composed of 2 conical lobes lying on either side of, and moulded to, the larynx and lower pharynx above and the upper 4 or 5 rings of trachea and oesophagus below. They are connected near their bases by a narrow isthmus which lies across the upper trachea. A pyramidal lobe [lobus pyramidalis (NA)] connecting the isthmus to the hyoid frequently exists. The gland is composed of vesicles of various sizes lined with cubical epithelium and containing colloid. They are partially divided into lobules [lobuli glandulae thyroideae (NA)] by incomplete septa derived from a thin capsule [capsula fibrosa (NA)]. Supporting the vesicles is a reticular connective tissue, or stroma, containing the blood vessels, lymphatics and nerves. They secrete the thyroid hormones q.v. **Thyroid glands, accessory [glandulae thyroideae accessoriae (NA)].** Small detached masses of thyroid tissue which may be found in the tissue planes surrounding the main gland. **Tracheal glands [glandulae tracheales (NA)].** Mucous and serous secreting glands that lie in the submucous layer. **Trachoma glands.** Conjunctival glands (see above). **Urethral glands [glandulae urethrales (NA)].** Small mucous glands in the submucous tissue. **Uterine glands [glandulae uterinae (NA)].** *See* UTERUS, MUCOUS COAT OF THE. **Varicose groin glands.** A term used by Manson to describe enlarged filarial glands associated with lymphatic varices diagnostic of bancroftian filariasis. **Vestibular gland, greater [glandula vestibularis major (NA)].** One of a pair of small round glands situated on either side of the vaginal orifice, with their ducts opening between the hymen and the labia minora. **Vestibular glands, lesser [glandulae vestibulares minores (NA)].** Numerous small mucous glands opening into the vestibule. [L *glans* acorn.]

See also: ALBARRAN, ASELLI, BARTHOLIN (C.), BAUHIN, BAUMGARTEN (P. C.), BLANDIN, BOCHDALEK, BOERHAAVE, BONNOT, BOWMAN, BRUCH, BRUNNER, CIACCIO (G. V.), CLOQUET (J. G.), COWPER, DUVERNEY, EBNER, EGLIS, FRANKEL, GALEATI, GAY (A. H.), GLEY, GUÉRIN (A. F. M.), HARDER, HAVERS, HENLE, HOCEVAR, HUGUIER, KLEINSCHMIDT, KNOLL, KRAUSE (K. F. T.), KRAUSE (W. J.

F.), LIEBERKÜHN, LITTRÉ, LUSCHKA, MANZ, MEIBOM, MÉRY, MOLL, MONTGOMERY, MORGAGNI, NABOTH, NUHN, PACCHIONI, PECHLIN, PEYER, PHILIP, POIRIER, RIVINUS, ROSENMUELLER, SANDSTRÖM, SATTLER, SCHUELLER (K. H. A. L. M.), SERRES, SIGMUND, SKENE, SORGIUS, STAHR, SUZANNE, SWAMMERDAM, TERSON, THEILE, TIEDEMANN, TYSON, VESALIUS, VIRCHOW, WALDEYER-HARTZ, WEBER (E. H.), WEPFER, WILLIS, WOELFLER, WOLFRING, ZEIS, ZUCKERKANDL.

glandebala (glan·**deb**·al·ah) (pl. *glandebalae*). Any one of the hairs of the axilla; hircus. [L.]

glanderous (**glan**·der·us). Of the nature of, relating to, or affected with glanders.

glanders (**glan**·derz). An acute or chronic highly infectious disease due to a specific bacillus (*Pfeifferella mallei*), and probably spread to man by direct contagion from a diseased horse, mule or ass, or from a patient. The mortality in man is extremely high. The disease is characterized by inflammatory or suppurative lesions arising in the nasal mucous membrane and the subcutaneous tissues. In animals especially, lymphatic involvement may cause nodules which form abscesses (farcy buds). Arthralgia sometimes occurs. The diagnosis may be difficult: the injection of mallein is of value as a sensitivity test in animals. In prophylaxis, infected animals must be slaughtered. Treatment is symptomatic. [L *glandula* small gland.]

glandilemma (glan·dil·**em**·ah). The outer covering or capsule of a gland. [gland, Gk *lemma* sheath.]

glandula (**glan**·dew·lah) (pl. *glandulae*). A small gland. [L.]

glandular (**glan**·dew·lar). 1. Belonging or relating to, or having the characteristics of a gland. 2. Containing glands or gland cells. [L *glandula* small gland.]

glandule (**glan**·dewl). A small gland. [L *glandula*.]

glandulous (**glan**·dew·lus). Consisting of or containing many small glands or kernels. [see prec.]

glans (glanz) (pl. *glandes*). 1. Any body of the shape of an acorn. 2. A suppository. **Glans of the clitoris [glans clitoridis (NA)].** The small rounded tubercle of erectile tissue which constitutes the free end of the clitoris. **Glans penis [NA].** The terminal end of the penis covering the ends of the corpora cavernosa penis. [L gland.]

Glanzmann's disease. Hereditary haemorrhagic diathesis.

glare (glare). A strong dazzling light occasioning physical discomfort when it strikes the eye. That occurring under ordinary conditions of artificial illumination when the intensity never approaches that of daylight is best described as "light in the wrong place" and becomes evident when the ratio of the intrinsic brilliancy of the source of light to that of the surrounding field exceeds 100. In daylight and intense artificial illumination, glare may be said to occur when the light is so bright that the eye can no longer adapt itself to it and light is diffused over the retina instead of being sharply focused on it. Those with defective retinal pigment, e.g. albinos, are naturally more sensitive. [ME *glaren*.]

Glaser, Johann Heinrich (b. 1629). Basle anatomist and physiologist.

Glaser's fissure. The squamotympanic fissure.

Glasgow, William Carr (b. 1845). St. Louis physician.

Glasgow's sign. A systolic murmur over the brachial artery in aneurysm of the aorta.

glass (glahs). A hard amorphous material, brittle and splinterable, normally colourless, and invariably transparent, or at least translucent. It is manufactured by melting together sand, limestone and soda at a temperature around 1300°C, though other materials such as lead, barium, zinc and potash may be added for various special reasons. It may be coloured by the addition of metallic oxides, e.g. manganese or chromium, and in constitution is a mixture of the silicates of the alkaline earths and alkali metals. **Crown glass.** A hard glass principally composed of sodium silicate, lime and alumina. This type of glass is usually used for optical purposes, having a refractive index of 1.523. **Cupping glass.** A glass from which, when applied to the skin, the air can be exhausted so as to produce a partial vacuum. It is used to draw blood to the surface. **Flint glass.** A soft glass manufactured from potassium and lead silicates. It is occasionally used for optical purposes, as in bifocals, owing to its high refractive index, 1.62. **Lead glass.** Protective glass; glass containing a high proportion of lead compounds, which absorbs radiation passing through it. It is used as a transparent protective material. **Lithium glass.** Glass with a high lithium content, at one time used for x-ray tubes producing soft x-rays (obsolete). **Magnifying glass.** In ophthalmology, a large convex spherical lens of about 13-15 dioptres, suitably mounted, to magnify the print for patients with much reduced visual acuity. **Object glass.** That lens of a compound system of lenses (e.g. microscope) which is nearest to the object under examination. **Optical glass.** Glass used for making spectacles lenses and other specialized optical instruments. Various types of glass are used, but crown most commonly for spectacles. **Protective glass.** Lead glass (see above). **Quartz glass.** Pure fused silicon dioxide used in the manufacture of prisms and lenses. **Safety glass.** A non-splinterable glass made by cementing 2 thin layers of glass together with a non-splinterable substance. **Soluble glass.** Water-glass. **Test glass.** A conical glass used in the ward or laboratory for containing biological fluids for examination. **Water glass.** *See* WATER-GLASS. [AS *glaes*.]

See also: CROOKES, PFUND, WOOD (R. W.).

glasses (**glahs**·ez). A generic term loosely applied to optical aid for defective vision. **Bifocal glasses.** Glasses in which each lens has 2 foci; usually arranged to meet the requirements of presbyopes who do not wish to change their glasses when reading. Numerous types are described, many bearing trade names. **Bloomed glasses.** Glasses in which the front surface of the lenses is covered with a fine film of magnesium fluoride that has the effect of diminishing surface reflections and so allowing more light to pass through. **Contact glasses.** Shells made of glass or plastic material which are worn inside the lids and in contact with the eyeballs. **Crutch glasses.** Glasses used for the correction of ptosis: fairly rigid curved wires are attached to the upper margin of a spectacle frame so that when the latter is worn, the loops elevate the upper lids. If the ptosis is uni-ocular only 1 wire is needed. **Franklinic glasses.** Split bifocals; the earliest type of bifocals, consisting of two lenses, the upper being for distant vision, the lower for reading, the line of separation being usually horizontal. **Multifocal glasses.** A generic term to include glasses having lenses of more than 1 focus; it is uncommon to employ more than 3 (trifocal), namely distance, intermediate and reading. **Pantoscopic glasses.** Usually applied to reading glasses in which the top half has been cut away. **Periscopic glasses.** An ideal to which most modern spectacles approximate, in that they allow of clear vision when the patient moves his eyes rather than his head. **Photochromic glasses.** Spectacles fitted with lenses the glass of which changes colour and hence the amount of light transmitted when the light falling on it increases or decreases. **Prismatic glasses.** Glasses the lenses of which incorporate prisms to prevent diplopia from malalignment of the visual axes of the eyes. **Snow glasses.** Glasses in which the lenses are tinted and rendered opaque to ultraviolet light to prevent snow blindness. **Stenopaeic glasses.** An opaque disc in front of each eye containing a slit or minute hole; lenses may or may not be incorporated. They may be of service in special cases, e.g. high degrees of irregular astigmatism, but the visual field is markedly limited. **Sun glasses.** Glasses with coloured lenses to cut out certain of the sun's rays. **Telescopic glasses.** Glasses used in cases of defective vision to enlarge the image of objects; a galilean combination of lenses is employed. **Tinted glasses.** Glasses the lenses of which are tinted. Many varieties of tint are employed; for tropical climates a thin layer of metal, e.g. gold or platinum, is useful since this reflects the light back, instead of absorbing it and turning it into heat. Another variety is polaroid which has the effect of polarizing the light before it reaches the eyes and under certain conditions eliminates reflections. **Toric glasses.** Glasses incorporating toric lenses. A torus is the solid developed by the revolution of a circle about any axis other than its diameter, and a toric lens is one which is cut from a toric surface by a plane parallel to its axis of development. The majority of modern spectacle lenses are toric, the front surface being convex and the back concave. **Trifocal glasses.** Glasses with foci usually for distant, intermediate and reading distances. There are various designs for different purposes. [AS *glaes.*]

See also: HALLAUER.

glassy (glahs·e). 1. Vitreous. 2. Hyaline. 3. Resembling glass in appearance. 4. Without expression, as of an eye. [see prec.]

Glatzel mirror. Nasographic mirror. *See* MIRROR.

Glauber, Johann Rudolf (b. 1604). German physician and chemist.

Glauber salt. Sodium sulphate.

exsiccated Glauber salt. Exsiccated Sodium Sulphate BPC 1954.

glaucedo (glaw·se·do). Glaucoma. [Gk *glaukos* greenish-grey.]

glaucine (glaw·seen). $C_{21}H_{25}O_4N$, an optically-active alkaloid of the isoquinoline group, obtained from the yellow horned poppy, *Glaucinum flavum* (family Papaveraceae) and species of *Corydalis.* It exerts a feebly narcotic action, has a depressant effect on the heart and causes stiffening of striated muscle.

glaucoma (glaw·ko·mah). A term signifying increased intra-ocular pressure and its consequences. **Absolute glaucoma.** The end-result of untreated glaucoma, the eye being completely blind. **Acute glaucoma.** A phase in the development of closed angle glaucoma (see below). **Capsular glaucoma.** Glaucoma associated with pseudo-exfoliation of the lens capsule, and possibly due to blocking of the filtration angle with exfoliative material. **Chronic closed-angle glaucoma.** A chronic phase of closed-angle glaucoma. **Chronic simple glaucoma.** Chronic open-angle glaucoma wherein the angle is open when the tension is raised, and characterized by a lowered outflow field loss and optic atrophy. **Closed-angle glaucoma.** May be primary or secondary. The primary form affects adults and is due to natural growth of the lens, in a small hypermetropic eye, producing an undue narrowing of the angle which may then close. Attacks of raised tension may be acute or subacute initially, they are always associated with a closed angle and, if unresolved, lead to a chronic state of raised intra-ocular pressure. **Compensated glaucoma.** Glaucoma in which the circulation of the eye adapts itself to the condition of raised tension. **Congenital glaucoma.** Glaucoma due to congenital defects usually in the drainage system of the eye, and associated with stretching of the coats and enlargement of the eyeball, hence the synonyms buphthalmos (ox eye) and hydrophthalmos. **Congestive glaucoma.** Glaucoma associated with congestion of the eye and, usually, with pain. It may start *de novo,* develop on top of compensated glaucoma, or follow prodromal attacks. **Haemorrhagic glaucoma.** Glaucoma associated with intra-ocular haemorrhage. **Incompensated glaucoma.** Congestive glaucoma (see above). **Infantile glaucoma.** Glaucoma, usually the result of congenital defects, but which may arise from some of the causes of adult secondary glaucoma. **Inflammatory glaucoma.** Glaucoma complicating intra-ocular inflammation. **Inverse glaucoma.** Glaucoma due to dislocation of the lens into the anterior chamber; in such a case miotics frequently raise the tension while mydriatics reduce it. **Low tension glaucoma.** A condition with the characteristics of simple glaucoma except that the tension is not raised. **Malignant glaucoma.** Glaucoma associated with a flat anterior chamber following glaucoma surgery. **Open-angle glaucoma.** Any form of glaucoma where the angle of the anterior chamber is seen to be open on gonioscopy. **Phacolytic glaucoma.** Glaucoma associated with a hypermature cataract and caused by blockage of the trabecular meshwork by phagocytes containing lens matter. **Pigmentary glaucoma.** A form of open-angle glaucoma characterized by the deposition of uveal pigment on the corneal endothelium (Krukenberg spindle), on the surface of the lens and on the trabecular meshwork. **Postinflammatory glaucoma.** Glaucoma occurring as a sequel to changes of a lasting character produced by inflammation. **Primary glaucoma.** Glaucoma, the cause of which is unknown. **Prodromal glaucoma.** Minor attacks of closed-angle glaucoma of varying severity, duration and frequency, occurring for months or years before the final crisis. **Secondary glaucoma.** A term which comprises an unrelated group of cases in which some recognized pathological lesion is complicated by a rise of ocular tension. **Simple glaucoma.** Chronic simple glaucoma (see above). **Thrombotic glaucoma.** Glaucoma secondary to thrombosis of the central retinal vein. [Gk cataract.]

glaucomatous (glaw·ko·mat·us). 1. Relating or belonging to, or having the character of, glaucoma. 2. Affected with glaucoma.

glaucosis (glaw·ko·sis). Blindness resulting from glaucoma. [Gk.]

glaucosuria (glaw·ko·sewr·e·ah). Indicanuria. [Gk *glaukos* greenish-grey, urine.]

glaze (glaze). In prosthetic dentistry, the fused surface of an artificial porcelain tooth made to resemble the surface of a natural tooth. [ME *glasen.*]

gleet (gleet). A chronic form of urethritis after acute gonorrhoea in which a small quantity of a thin, transparent mucus is continuously discharged. [ME *glet* mucus.]

Glegg, Wilfred. 19th–20th century British physician.

Glegg's mixture. A mixture of liquid paraffin and yellow soft paraffin perfumed with rose, applied to the nasal mucosa in the treatment of colds.

Glénard, Frantz (b. 1848). French physician.

Glénard's disease. Enteroptosis.

Glénard's test, for enteroptosis. The observer stands behind the patient and with both hands placed on the lower abdomen lifts the abdomen upwards. If enteroptosis is present the patient has a sensation of relief.

Glenn, William Wallace Lumpkin (b. 1914). American cardiovascular surgeon.

Glenn's operation. The creation of an anastomosis between the superior vena cava and the right pulmonary artery to conduct venous blood to the lungs, used for the palliation of tricuspid atresia and some other forms of severe cyanotic heart disease.

glenohumeral (gle·no·hew·mer·al). Relating or belonging to the glenoid cavity and the humerus; connecting the glenoid cavity with the humerus. [Gk *glene* socket of a joint, humerus.]

glenoid (gle·noid). 1. Resembling a socket or a smooth hollow depression, e.g. the glenoid cavity. 2. Belonging to the glenoid cavity or fossa. [Gk *glene* socket of a joint, *eidos* form.]

Glenosporella (gle·no·spor·el'·ah). A genus of parasitic fungi. **Glenosporella albiciscans.** A species which causes tinea albigena, a skin disease in Indonesia. **Glenosporella loboi.** *Loboaloboi,* an agent of lobomycosis. [Gk *glene* socket, *sporos* seed.]

Gley, Marcel Eugène Emile (b. 1857). Paris physiologist.

Gley's cell. One of the interstitial cells of the testis.

Gley's glands. The parathyroid glands. *See* GLAND.

glia (gli·ah). Neuroglia; the specialized supporting tissue of the central nervous system which surrounds the cell bodies, dendrites and axons of the neurones. It is composed of several types of cell, most of which have long branching processes, including fibrous and protoplasmic astrocytes, oligodendroglia and microglia. The microglia are mesodermal in origin and are phagocytic; the others named are ectodermal. **Amoeboid glia.** Altered glial cells showing an increase in cytoplasm with few processes. **Fibrillary glia.** A type of astrocyte found mainly in the white matter of the brain; its cytoplasmic processes are fibrillary. It plays an important part in repair of cerebral lesions. [Gk glue.]

gliacyte (gli·as·ite). Any neuroglia cell. *See* CELL. [glia, Gk *kytos* cell.]

gliadin (gli·ad·in). One of the main proteins present in wheat, belonging to the class of compounds known as prolamins because of their high content of proline. It is distinguished from glutenin, another wheat protein with which it is associated in the mixture, gluten, by its solubility in 70 per cent alcohol. Both glutenin and gliadin are insoluble in water and absolute alcohol, but soluble in dilute acids and alkalis. Gliadin is also distinguished from glutenin by being deficient in the essential amino acid, lysine. It is responsible for the sticky mass with water that binds flour into dough in breadmaking. [Gk *glia* glue.]

glial (gli·al). Relating or belonging to neuroglia. [glia.]

Glibenclamide (gli·**ben**·klam·ide). BP Commission approved name for *N*-{4-[β-(5-chloro-2-methoxybenzamido)-ethyl] benzenesulphonyl}-*N′*-cyclohexylurea; an oral hypoglycaemic agent.

Glibornuride (gli·**born**·ewr·ide). BP Commission approved name for 1-[(1*R*) - 2 - *endo*-hydroxy-3-*endo*-bornyl]-3-(toluene-*p*-sulphonyl)urea; an oral hypoglycaemic agent.

glioblast (gli·o·blast). Spongioblast. [glia, Gk *blastos* germ.]

glioblastoma (gli·o·blas·**to′**·mah). A tumour or neoplasm containing neuroglia cells; spongioblastoma. **Glioblastoma multiforme.** An actively growing glioma, composed of several types of cells, which expands and destroys as it grows. [glia, blastoma.]

gliococcus (gli·o·**kok**·us). 1. A micrococcus forming jelly-like matter. 2. A micrococcus enclosed in a jelly-like mass. [Gk *glia* glue, coccus.]

gliocyte (gli·o·site). Gliacyte.

gliocytoma (gli·o·si·**to′**·mah). A neurogliocytoma. [glia, cytoma.]

gliogenous (gli·**oj**·en·us). Produced by neuroglia cells. [glia, Gk *genein* to produce.]

glioma (gli·**o**·mah). A tumour composed of neuroglia cells and fibres, most commonly found in the brain, but also in the spinal cord, and occasionally in the roots of the cranial nerves. **Glioma endophytum.** Retinoblastoma arising from the inner retinal layers and growing towards the centre of the globe. **Ependymal glioma.** Ependymoma, a glioma arising from the ependyma of the floor of the 4th ventricle of the brain, most commonly in children. **Glioma exophytum.** Retinoblastoma arising from the outer retinal layers and growing away from the centre of the globe. **Ganglionic glioma.** Neuroblastoma, ganglioneuroma; a benign tumour composed of imperfectly-formed ganglion cells and adult ganglion cells, found in the sympathetic and central nervous systems and in the suprarenal gland. **Nasal glioma.** A glioma of the olfactory bulb in children, which produces a swelling at the root or side of the nose and grows into the upper nares. **Glioma of the optic chiasma.** Causing visual disturbances and hypopituitarism. **Peripheral glioma.** Neurinoma. **Glioma retinae.** A destructive glioma of the retina which occurs almost exclusively in infants, and arising chiefly from ciliary portion or posterior segment of the retina. **Glioma sarcomatosum.** Glioblastoma multiforme, spongioblastoma; a rapidly-growing glioma of the cerebral hemispheres which behaves like a local sarcoma. **Telangiectatic glioma.** Angioma of the cerebellum or of the retina. [glia, Gk *-oma* tumour.]

gliomatosis (gli·o·mat·**o′**·sis). The overdevelopment of neuroglia, especially of the spinal neuroglia, which may occur in syringomyelia. [glia, Gk *-oma* tumour, *-osis* condition.]

gliomatous (gli·o·mat·us). Affected with, having the character of, or relating to, a glioma.

gliomyoma (gli·o·mi·**o′**·mah). A combined glioma and myoma.

gliomyxoma (gli·o·mix·**o′**·mah). A combined glioma and myxoma.

glioneuroma (gli·o·newr·**o′**·mah). A combined glioma and neuroma.

gliophagia (gli·o·**fa**·je·ah). A condition in which neuroglia cells are engulfed by phagocytes. [glia, Gk *phagein* to eat.]

gliosa (gli·**o**·sah). Substantia gliosa. [Gk *glia* glue.]

gliosarcoma (gli·o·sar·**ko′**·mah). A neoplasm containing the neuroglia cells found in glioma and the fusiform cells found in sarcoma. **Gliosarcoma retinae.** Glioma retinae.

gliosis (gli·**o**·sis). A proliferation of astrocytes which may be diffuse or focal, often seen as a reparative process following cerebral injury. **Isomorphic gliosis.** In degeneration of spinal cord tracts, the proliferating glia organize their fibrillary processes in parallel with the degenerating nerve fibres. [glioma, Gk *-osis* condition.]

gliosome (gli·o·some). A granular cytoplasmic inclusion within a neuroglial cell. [glia, Gk *soma* body.]

glischrogenous (glis·**kroj**·en·us). Causing viscidity. [Gk *glischros* viscid, *genein* to produce.]

Glisoxepide (gli·**sox**·e·pide). BP Commission approved name for 3-[4-(hexahydroazepin-1-ylureiodosulphonyl)-phenethylcarbamoyl]-5-methyl-isoxazole; an oral hypoglycaemic agent.

Glisson, Francis (b. 1597). Cambridge and London physician.

Glisson's capsule. The fibrous tissue around the lobules of the liver in which run branches of the hepatic artery, portal vein and bile duct; the hepatobiliary capsule.

Glisson's cirrhosis. Capsular cirrhosis. *See* CIRRHOSIS.

Glisson's sling. A leather halter used for extension of the cervical spine.

Glisson's sphincter. The sphincter of Oddi.

glissonitis (glis·on·**i**·tis). Inflammation of the hepatobiliary (Glisson's) capsule. [Glisson's capsule, Gk *-itis* inflammation.]

globate (glo·bate). Like a globe or sphere. [L *globus* ball.]

globin (glo·bin). 1. The protein moiety of haemoglobin. 2. One of a particular group of proteins. [see prec.]

globinometer (glo·bin·**om**·et·er). An instrument with which the percentage of oxyhaemoglobin in the blood can be determined. [globin, meter.]

globomyeloma (glo·bo·mi·el·**o′**·mah). Round-cell sarcoma. [L *globus* ball, myeloma.]

globose (glo·boze). Spherical or almost spherical. [L *globus* ball.]

globular (glob·ew·lar). 1. Erythrocytic. 2. Globe-shaped. 3. Relating to a globule.

globule (glob·ewl). A small spherical particle of a liquid or solid. **Dentine globule.** A rounded mass of calcified dentine surrounded by uncalcified dentine, present as a normal stage in development but as a permanent feature only in the peripheral dentine. **Directing globule, Directive globule.** A spherule of extruded yolk from a maturing, unfertilized egg. **Extrusion globule.** Directing globule (see above). **Milk globule.** A particle of emulsified fat in milk. **Myelin globules.** Colourless, round or oval globules of varying size, resembling fat droplets, sometimes found in mucoid sputum. **Polar globule.** Directing globule (see above). [L *globulus.*]

See also: DOBIE, MARCHI, MORGAGNI.

globulicidal (glob·ewl·is·**i′**·dal). 1. Relating to a globulicide. 2. Destructive to erythrocytes or to any blood corpuscle; haemolytic. [see foll.]

globulicide (glob·ewl·is·ide). 1. Any agent which is destructive to blood corpuscles, particularly erythrocytes. 2. Globulicidal. [globule, L *caedere* to kill.]

globuliferous (glob·ewl·**if**·er·us). 1. Taking up, bearing, or containing globules. 2. Containing any kind of corpuscle. 3. Containing erythrocytes. [globule, L *ferre* to bear.]

globulimeter (glob·ewl·**im**·et·er). 1. An instrument with which the number of blood corpuscles in a measured quantity of blood can be determined. 2. A cytometer. [globule, meter.]

globulin (**glob**·ewl·in). A class of proteins occurring widely in nature, which are generally insoluble in water, soluble in dilute salt solutions, coagulated by heat, and precipitated from solution by half-saturation with ammonium sulphate. A few examples are known of water-soluble globulins, notably in blood and milk, and these have been termed *pseudoglobulins.* **Ac globulin.** Labile factor, factor V, thrombogen; a constituent of normal blood plasma that is essential for the formation of thrombin from prothrombin. It is unstable, being oxidized during storage, but is not affected by vitamin-K deficiency or anticoagulant therapy with dicoumarol and similar substances. It is regarded as a plasma-conversion factor in the formation of thrombin. **Alpha-, Beta-, Gamma-globulins,** α-, β-, γ-globulins. Three globulin fractions separable by electrophoresis. The separation is not into truly homogenous components but into groups of protein ions of the same net charge and weight, the molecular size increasing from α to γ, so that further separation is a possibility, e.g. α_1 and α_2. **Antidiphtheritic globulin.** The globulin fractions that occur in antidiphtheritic serum. **Antihaemophilic globulin.** A globulin, associated with the fibrinogen fraction, present in small quantity in normal human blood; a hereditary deficiency of this globulin occurs in and causes haemophilia, but it is apparently present in normal amounts in the blood in Christmas disease. **Antitoxic globulin.** The globulin fractions that occur in antitoxic serum. **Beta globulin.** *See* ALPHA-, BETA-, GAMMA-GLOBULINS (above). **Cell globulin.** Globulin present in, or isolated from, blood and tissue cells. **Fibrin globulin.** Fibrinoglobulin; a globulin related to fibrinogen. **Gamma globulin, γ-globulin.** Globulin with the slowest electrophoretic mobility and those that include the majority of the antibodies present in serum. *See* ALPHA-, BETA-, GAMMA-GLOBULINS (above), IMMUNOGLOBULINS and the following. **Human Gamma Globulin BP 1963, Immune globulin.** A protein constituent of human serum first separated by electrophoresis, and later prepared on a large scale by Cohn by fractionation with ethanol, freeze-dried and reconstituted in sterile distilled water before injection. It contains many of the antibodies which may have been present in the original serum, and is used for the passive immunization of susceptible contacts of measles, infective hepatitis, acute poliomyelitis and other diseases. **Alpha$_2$-macroglobulin.** Probably acts as a carrier protein transporting hormones such as growth hormone [alpha] in the blood. **Placental globulin.** A globulin obtained from human placenta; this has a high natural antibody content and was at one time used in the prophylaxis of measles. **Rabbit anti-human globulin** (Coombs' reagent). Used in blood group serology for detecting incomplete antibodies. **Rabbit globulin.** The globulin from rabbit's blood; it has been used as a local coagulant in view of its strong thrombotic qualities. **Serum globulin.** A protein fraction of blood serum, precipitated by half-saturation with ammonium sulphate which leaves the albumin in solution. There are several fractions (α, β, γ) of this globulin, each with specific properties (see above). **Thyroid-binding globulin.** The globulin in the serum which binds the hormone until it reaches its site of action. **Globulin X.** One of the proteins of muscle plasma. [L *globulus*, small globe.]

globulinaemia (glob·ewl·in·**e'**·me·ah). The presence of free globulin in the blood. [globulin, Gk *haima* blood.]

globulinuria (glob·ewl·in·**ewr'**·e·ah). The presence of globulin or of any protein of the globulin class in the urine.

globulism (**glob**·ewl·izm). 1. Polycythaemia vera. 2. The homoeopathic administration of medicines in the form of globules.

globulolysis (glob·ewl·**ol**·is·is). 1. The dissolution or destruction of erythrocytes (haemocytolysis), or of other blood corpuscles. 2. Cytolysis. [globule, lysis.]

globulolytic (**glob**·ewl·o·**lit'**·ik). 1. Haemocytolytic. 2. Cytolytic. [see prec.]

globulus (**glob**·ewl·us). 1. A globule. 2. The nucleus globosus. 3. A globe-shaped suppository. 4. In pharmacy, a bolus or pill. [L small globe.]

globus (glo·bus). A sphere. **Globus abdominalis.** The subjective sensation of a lump in the abdomen. **Globus hystericus.** "A lump in the throat"; a sensation of suffocation as though caused by a ball in the throat. **Globus pallidus [NA].** The medial pale portion of the lentiform nucleus. [L.]

glomangioma (glo·man·je·**o'**·mah). A glomus tumour. [L *glomus* ball of thread, angioma.]

glomer (glo·mer). A conglomerate gland. [L *glomus* ball of thread.]

glomerate (**glom**·er·ate). 1. Compactly gathered into a cluster. 2. Wound up together like a ball of thread. 3. Conglomerate, a term descriptive of ordinary gland structure. [L *glomerare* to wind into a ball.]

glomerular (glom·**er**·ew·lar). Relating or belonging to, or having the character of, a glomerulus of the kidney.

glomerule (**glom**·er·ewl). Glomerulus.

glomerulitis (glom·er·ew·**li'**·tis). An inflamed condition of the glomeruli of the kidney. [glomerulus, Gk *-itis* inflammation.]

glomerulonephritis (glom·**er**·ew·lo·nef·**ri'**·tis). Nephritis which is characterized primarily by inflammation of the glomeruli of the kidney and which may appear in acute, subacute or chronic forms. **Acute glomerulonephritis.** The acute stage of nephritis, usually of acute onset. It is most frequent in children, adolescents and young adults, and follows after a latent interval on some infection, of which streptococcal infection of the tonsils or upper respiratory tract is most common; but many other infections may be the cause. **Embolic glomerulonephritis.** A form of nephritis produced by multiple minute emboli in the course of subacute bacterial endocarditis.

glomerulosclerosis (glom·**er**·ew·lo·skler·**o'**·sis). Nephrosclerosis, chronic Bright's disease; a fatal condition in which many of the glomeruli of both kidneys are replaced by old fibrous scars, whereby the glomerular function of filtration of the blood is impaired or lost. It arises as the result of past infection or arterial disease (arteriosclerosis). [glomerulus, sclerosis.]

glomerulose (glom·**er**·ew·loze). Glomerular; arranged in small clusters or glomeruli.

glomerulotrophin (glom·**er**·ew·lo·**tro**·fin). A humeral agent extracted from the region of the pineal gland that is said to stimulate aldosterone production.

glomerulus [NA] (glom·**er**·ew·lus). A compact tuft or tangled mass of branching processes. **Arterial glomeruli of the cochlea [glomeruli arteriosi cochleae (NA)].** A spirally-arranged arterial plexus between the turns of the cochlear tube, accompanied by the spiral vein of the modiolus. **Juxtamedullary glomerulus.** A glomerulus situated in the deepest part of the cortex near the corticomedullary junction, the afferent arterioles of which give rise to descending vasa recta. **Malpighian glomerulus.** The tuft of capillaries lying within a renal corpuscle which filters urine from the blood stream. **Malpighian glomerulus, capsule of the [capsula glomeruli (NA)].** The expanded end of a uriniferous tubule of the kidney that surrounds the glomerular tuft of blood vessels; Bowman's capsule. **Non-encapsulated nerve glomerulus.** A type of nerve-ending in the skin and elsewhere, composed of a tuft of axonal filaments without a special connective-tissue sheath. **Olfactory glomerulus.** The tuft of axonal and dendritic processes in the olfactory bulb where synaptic contacts are made between the first and second neurones of the olfactory pathway. [L *glomerulus* small ball.]

glomus [NA] (glo·mus) (pl. *glomera*). 1. A cluster of blood vessels. 2. A complex form of arteriovenous anastomosis, found particularly in the nail bed and consisting of a cluster of anastomotic vessels surrounded by epithelioid cells and having a rich nerve supply. *See also* SUCQUET-HOYER ANASTOMOSES. **Glomus choroideum [NA].** The enlargement of the choroid plexus at the point where the interior horn joins the body of the ventricle. **Glomus coccygeum.** The coccygeal body; a small nodule in front of the tip of the coccyx, containing sinusoidal vessels and masses of polyhedral cells. Its function is unknown. [L ball of thread.]
See also: LUSCHKA.

glonoin (glo·**no**·in). A 1 per cent solution of glyceryl trinitrate in alcohol (90 per cent), used in angina pectoris because of its dilatation of the coronary arteries. Tablets usually containing 0.5 mg (1/130 grain) of glyceryl trinitrate are also supplied for this purpose.

Gloriosa superba (glo·re·o·sah sew·**per**·bah). A plant of the family Liliaceae, the fruit of which is sometimes used as a poison in Southern India, Burma and Sri Lanka: the active principle causes gastro-intestinal irritation and cardiac failure. [L glorious, proud.]

glossa (glos·ah). The tongue. [Gk.]

glossagra (glos·**ag**·rah). Glossalgia of gouty origin. [Gk *glossa* tongue, *agra* a catching.]

glossal (glos·al). Relating or belonging to the tongue. [Gk *glossa* tongue.]

glossalgia (glos·**al**·je·ah). Pain in the tongue. [Gk *glossa* tongue, *algos* pain.]

glossanthrax (glos·**an**·thrax). Carbuncle of the tongue. [Gk *glossa* tongue, anthrax.]

glossauxesis (glos·awx·e·sis). An enlargement or swollen state of the tongue. [Gk *glossa* tongue, *auxe* increase.]

glossectomy (glos·**ek**·to·me). Amputation of the tongue. **Partial glossectomy.** Surgical removal of a portion of the tongue. **Total**

glossectomy. Excision of the whole of the tongue. [Gk *glossa* tongue, *ektome* a cutting out.]

Glossina (glos·i·nah). A genus of flies of the family Muscidae; the tsetse flies. They are confined to Africa south of the Sahara, and Arabia. Both sexes suck blood, are diurnal in habit and can be recognized by the fact that the wings at rest are folded flat and straight back. The females produce a single mature larva at a time, which immediately pupates in the ground. **Glossina brevipalpis.** A species of the Zaire and an experimental vector of *Trypanosoma gambiense.* **Glossina morsitans.** Found in dry places from the Sudan to the Transvaal, and is the main vector of *Trypanosoma rhodesiense.* **Glossina pallidipes.** Of East Africa; an experimental vector of *Trypanosoma gambiense.* **Glossina palpalis.** Found in wet places in the whole western half of tropical Africa, and is the main vector of *Trypanosoma gambiense.* **Glossina swynnertoni.** Of Tanzania; a locally important vector of *Trypanosoma rhodesiense.* **Glossina tachinoides.** Of West Africa, Southern Sahara and South-west Arabia; a vector of *Trypanosoma gambiense.* Other species which bite man, but which are not known to be vectors of pathogens are: *Glossina caliginea,* West Africa; *G. fusca,* Zaire; *G. longipalpis,* Zaire; *G. newsteadi,* Zaire; *G. nigrofusca,* Zaire and West Africa; *G. submorsitans* and *G. tabaniformis,* West Africa. [Gk *glossa* tongue.]

Glossinidae (glos·i·nid·e). A family of the dipteran suborder Cyclorrhapha, sometimes included in Muscidae. The genus *Glossina* (tsetse flies) is of medical interest. [Gk *glossa* tongue, *eidos* form.]

glossitic (glos·it·ik). 1. Referring or belonging to glossitis. 2. Suffering from glossitis.

glossitis (glos·i·tis). Inflammation of the tongue. This may be superficial and affecting the mucous membrane, or deep in the parenchyma. **Acute aphthous glossitis.** Glossitis characterized by crops of small erosions. **Glossitis areata exfoliativa.** Geographical tongue: an affection in which desquamation of the superficial epithelium occurs in circinate patches; these spread marginally whilst the centre heals. The patches may fuse and their sinuous outlines resemble a geographical map. **Chronic glossitis with anaemia.** Glossitis in which in the early stage the tongue is reddened, with vesicles breaking down to superficial ulcers; later the tongue becomes smooth and shiny with destruction of the filiform papillae. It is due to iron deficiency and may be part of the Plummer-Vinson syndrome. It occurs with hypochromic and pernicious anaemias. **Benign migratory glossitis.** Geographical tongue. *See* TONGUE. **Chronic interstitial glossitis.** Irregular lobulations of the tongue with deep fissures and leucoplakia, as seen in late syphilis. **Chronic iron deficiency glossitis.** Glossitis in which the tongue becomes smooth, red and shiny due to atrophy of the filiform papillae. It may be part of the Plummer-Vinson syndrome and is seen also in pernicious anaemias. **Chronic parenchymatous glossitis.** The bald, scarred atrophic tongue of tertiary syphilis. **Chronic superficial glossitis.** Moeller's glossitis; irregularly scattered red patches and striae on the dorsum of the tongue with severe burning pain. It occurs in attacks with alternating quiescent periods lasting for weeks or months, mainly in women. **Median rhomboid glossitis.** An area in the mid-line of the base of the tongue which is devoid of papillae, flat or elevated and irregularly nodular. It is usually discovered accidentally by the patient; it is benign, and is probably a developmental defect, a persistent tuberculum impar. **Monilial glossitis.** A fungal infection of the tongue due to *Candida albicans*; usually due to dehydration or dry mouth from any cause, long-term antibiotics, cytotoxic drugs and corticosteroids. [Gk *glossa* tongue, *-itis* inflammation.]

See also: HUNTER (W.), MOELLER (J. O. L.).

glossocele (glos·o·seel). Excessive size or oedema of the tongue so that it protrudes from the mouth. [Gk *glossa* tongue, *kele* hernia.]

glossocinaesthetic (glos·o·sin·es·thet'·ik). Having reference to the subjective sensations of motion produced in the individual by the various movements of the tongue involved in speech. [Gk *glossa* tongue, *kinein* to move, aesthesia.]

glossocoma (glos·o·ko·mah). A retracted position of the tongue. [Gk *glossa* tongue, *koma* lethargy.]

glossodesmus (glos·o·dez·mus). The frenulum of the tongue. [Gk *glossa* tongue, *desmos* band.]

glossodynamometer (glos·o·di·nam·om'·et·er). An apparatus with which the contractile power of the tongue and its capacity to resist pressure can be measured. [Gk *glossa* tongue, dynamometer.]

glossodynia (glos·o·din·e·ah). A painful burning sensation in the tongue. Usually a manifestation of neurosis or depression, occasionally due to iron or vitamin B_{12} deficiency. **Glossodynia exfoliativa.** Moeller's glossitis. [Gk *glossa* tongue, *odyne* pain.]

glosso-epiglottic, glosso-epiglottidean (glos·o·ep·e·glot'·ik, glos·o·ep·e·glot·id'·e·an). Referring or belonging to the tongue and the epiglottis. [Gk *glossa* tongue, epiglottis.]

glossograph (glos·o·graf). An instrument which records the movements of the tongue in speaking. [Gk *glossa* tongue, *graphein* to record.]

glossohyal, glossohyoid (glos·o·hi·al, glos·o·hi·oid). Relating to the tongue and the hyoid bone; hyoglossal. [Gk *glossa* tongue, hyoid bone.]

glossoid (glos·oid). Having resemblance to a tongue. [Gk *glossa* tongue, *eidos* form.]

glossokinaesthetic (glos·o·kin·es·thet'·ik). Glossocinaesthetic.

glossolabial (glos·o·la·be·al). Relating or belonging to the tongue and the lip or lips. [Gk *glossa* tongue, L *labium* lip.]

glossolalia (glos·o·la·le·ah). 1. Ecstatic utterance unintelligible to the hearers. 2. The act of speaking in jargon or in an imaginary language. 3. In somnambulism or hypnosis, talking by the patient in a foreign or unknown tongue. [Gk *glossa* tongue, *lalein* to babble like a child.]

glossolysis (glos·ol·is·is). Paralysis of the tongue. [Gk *glossa* tongue, *lysis* a loosing.]

glossomantia (glos·o·man·te·ah). In any disease, the prognostic significance of the state of the tongue. [Gk *glossa* tongue, *manteia* divination.]

glossoncus (glos·ong·kus). Any swelling of the tongue, local or general. [Gk *glossa* tongue, *ogkos* swelling.]

glossopalatine (glos·o·pal·at·ine). Relating or belonging to the tongue and the palate. [Gk *glossa* tongue, L *palatum* palate.]

glossopalatinus (glos·o·pal·at·i'·nus). The palatoglossus muscle.

glossopathy (glos·op·ath·e). Any disease or diseased condition of the tongue. [Gk *glossa* tongue, *pathos* disease.]

glossopharyngeal (glos·o·far·in'·je·al). Relating or belonging to the tongue and the pharynx, or to the glossopharyngeal nerve. [Gk *glossa* tongue, pharynx.]

glossopharyngeal nerve [nervus glossopharyngeus (NA)]. The 9th cranial nerve. A mixed nerve, having its motor nucleus in the medulla oblongata and the cells of origin of its sensory fibres in the superior and inferior petrous ganglia, and supplies motor fibres to the stylopharyngeus muscle, sensory fibres to the pharynx, including taste fibres to the posterior third of the tongue, and secretomotor fibres to the parotid gland. **Branch to the carotid sinus [ramus sinus carotici (NA)].** A branch that follows the internal carotid artery and supplies the carotid sinus and carotid body; it is often double. **Communicating branch with the auricular branch of the vagus nerve [ramus communicans cum ramo auriculari nervi vagi (NA)].** A small twig from the inferior ganglion of the glossopharyngeal nerve joining with the auricular branch of the vagus nerve near its origin. **Lingual branches [rami linguales (NA)].** Branches, usually 2 in number, to the posterior third of the tongue and the vallate papillae. **Pharyngeal branches [rami pharyngei (NA)].** Twigs to the pharyngeal plexus, entering the pharynx between the superior and middle constrictor muscles. **Branch to the pharyngotympanic tube [ramus tubalis (NA)].** A sensory branch to the pharyngotympanic tube. **Branch to the stylopharyngeus [ramus musculi stylopharyngei (NA)].** A motor branch from the glossopharyngeal nerve to the stylopharyngeus muscle. **Tonsillar**

branches [rami tonsillares (NA)]. Branches which form a plexus around the tonsil with twigs from the lesser palatine nerves. **Tympanic branch.** The tympanic nerve. **Nuclei [nuclei nervi glossopharyngei (NA)].** These include the superior salivary nucleus, the nucleus ambiguus, the nucleus of the tractus solitarius and the dorsal nucleus [nucleus dorsalis (NA)], the upper part of the vagus nerve.

glossopharyngeum (glos·o·far·in′·je·um). The tongue and the pharynx considered as one structure. [Gk *glossa* tongue, pharynx.]

glossopharyngeus (glos·o·far·in′·je·us). The glossopharyngeus muscle; the glossopharyngeal part of the superior constrictor muscle of the pharynx. [see prec.]

glossophobia (glos·o·fo·be·ah). A morbid dread of speaking or of trying to speak; the condition is often present in stutterers. [Gk *glossa* tongue, phobia.]

glossoplasty (glos·o·plas·te). Any surgical repair of or plastic operation on the tongue. [Gk *glossa* tongue, *plassein* to mould.]

glossoplegia (glos·o·ple·je·ah). Paralysis of the tongue. [Gk *glossa* tongue, *plege* stroke.]

glossoptosis (glos·op·to·sis). 1. Glossocoma. 2. Downward displacement of the tongue. 3. Macroglossia. [Gk *glossa* tongue, *ptosis* fall.]

glossopyrosis (glos·o·pi·ro′·sis). A sensation of burning in the tongue. *See* GLOSSODYNIA. [Gk *glossa* tongue, *pyr* fire, *-osis* condition.]

glossorrhaphy (glos·or·af·e). Surgical suture of a wound of the tongue. [Gk *glossa* tongue, *rhaphe* seam.]

glossoscopy (glos·os·ko·pe). Examination of the tongue, generally for diagnostic purposes. [Gk *glossa* tongue, *skopein* to watch.]

glossospasm (glos·o·spazm). Spasm of the musculature of the tongue. [Gk *glossa* tongue, spasm.]

glossosteresis (glos·o·ster·e′·sis). 1. Glossectomy. 2. Lack of the tongue. [Gk *glossa* tongue, *steresis* being in want of.]

glossotomy (glos·ot·o·me). 1. Excision of the tongue. 2. Incision of or any cutting operation on the tongue. 3. Dissection of the tongue. [Gk *glossa* tongue, *temnein* to cut.]

glossotrichia (glos·o·trik·e·ah). Hairy tongue. *See* TONGUE. [Gk *glossa* tongue, *thrix* hair.]

glottic (glot·ik). 1. Referring to the glottis. 2. Glossal.

glottidean (glot·id·e·an). Glottic.

glottis [NA] (glot·is). The gap between the vocal folds; the term is often applied to the folds themselves. [Gk.]

glottitis (glot·i·tis). Glossitis.

glow (glo). 1. A burning sensation of the skin, as after exercise or friction. 2. Brightness of colour, as of face. 3. Incandescence. **Cathode glow.** The glow in a discharge tube nearest the cathode and covering its surface with a velvety light. **Negative glow.** The glow extending at low pressures some considerable distance into the discharge tube. **Salt glow.** The slight stimulus and the bright colour of the skin of the body after it has been rubbed with moist salt. [AS *glowan.*]

glucaemia (gloo·se·me·ah). Glycaemia.

glucagon (gloo·kah·gon). A peptide hormone secreted by the α-cells of the endocrine pancreas. Administration results in hyperglycaemia due to stimulation of glycogenolysis and gluconeogenesis in the liver. *See also:* ENTEROGLUCAGON. [Gk *glykys* sweet, *agein* to lead.]

glucagonoma (gloo·kah·gon·oma). A tumour of the pancreas producing excess of glucagon associated with diabetes mellitus.

glucal (gloo·kal). $CH_2OH(CHOH)_2CH{=}CHCHO$, a syrupy unsaturated monosaccharide formed by the acetylation of glucose.

glucase (gloo·kaze). Maltase; a ferment in malt and intestinal juice which converts maltose into glucose as the end-product of starch digestion.

glucatonia (gloo·kah·to·ne·ah). Insulin shock. *See* SHOCK. [Gk *glykys* sweet, atony.]

glucide (gloo·side). A general term applied to carbohydrates, including both the sugars and those compounds (glycosides) which yield sugars on hydrolysis. [Gk *glykys* sweet.]

glucinum (gloo·sin·um). An alternative name for the element *beryllium*, the latter being the more usual.

gluciphore (gloo·si·for). Glucophore.

glucochloral (gloo·ko·klor·al). Chloralose.

glucocorticoid (gloo·ko·kor·tik·oid). An adrenal hormone which affects carbohydrate metabolism. The steroids having an oxygen atom at the C11 and C17 positions, particularly corticosterone, cortisone and cortisol (hydrocortisone), are active in this respect. [Gk *glykys* sweet, cortex, *eidos* form.]

glucofuranose (gloo·ko·few·ran·oze). In sugar nomenclature, the furanose form of glucose containing the 5-membered furane ring.

glucogen (gloo·ko·jen). Glycogen.

glucogenic (gloo·ko·jen·ik). 1. Giving rise to or producing glucose. 2. Glycogenic. [Gk *glykys* sweet, *genein* to produce.]

glucohaemia (gloo·ko·he·me·ah). Glycaemia.

glucokinase (gloo·ko·ki·naze). An enzyme occurring in liver and pancreatic islets which catalyses the phosphorylation of glucose by ATP with production of glucose 6-phosphate. It differs from hexokinase in its distribution, its low affinity for glucose, its lack of inhibition by glucose 6-phosphate and its sensitivity to induction by insulin.

glucokinetic (gloo·ko·kin·et′·ik). Maintaining the sugar level in the blood. [Gk *glykys* sweet, kinetic.]

glucolysis (gloo·kol·is·is). Glycolysis.

glucolytic (gloo·ko·lit·ik). Glycolytic.

gluconeogenesis (gloo·ko·ne·o·jen′·es·is). The synthesis of glucose in biological systems. In mammals restricted to liver and kidney. [Gk *glykys* sweet, *neos* new, *genein* to produce.]

gluconic (gloo·kon·ik). Relating to glucose.

glucopenia (gloo·ko·pe·ne·ah). Glycopenia.

glucophenetidin (gloo·ko·fen·et′·id·in). A compound of glucose and phenetidin which occurs in the form of white silky crystals.

glucophore (gloo·ko·for). An organic group which exhibits sweetness when combined with certain atoms or radicals known as *auxoglucs.* [Gk *glykys* sweet, *pherein* to bear.]

glucoprotein (gloo·ko·pro·te·in). Glycoprotein.

glucoproteinase (gloo·ko·pro·te·in·aze). An enzyme in the hydrolysis of glycoprotein.

glucopyranose (gloo·ko·pi·ran·oze). In sugar nomenclature, the pyranose form of glucose containing the 6-membered pyran ring.

glucosamine (gloo·ko·sam·een). D-glucosamine, glycosamine, aminoglucose, chitosamine, $CH_2OH(CHOH)_3CH(NH_2)CHO$. An aminosaccharide obtained by the hydrolysis of chitin and occurring widely in nature combined with proteins as glycoproteins.

glucosan (gloo·ko·san). $(C_6H_{10}O_5)_n$, a general term for the polysaccharides built of glucose units, which include cellulose, starch and glycogen.

glucosazone (gloo·ko·saz·one). $CH_2OH(CHOH)_3C{=}(NNHC_6H_5)CH{=}(NNHC_6H_5)$, a compound of glucose with phenylhydrazine which forms characteristic yellow crystals. It is identical with the osazones formed by fructose and mannose, but clearly distinguishable from galactosazone.

glucose (gloo·kose). Dextrose, grape sugar, $CH_2OH(CHOH)_4CHO$. A white crystalline solid soluble in water, the solution being dextrorotatory. It is the most widely-occurring natural sugar, being present in the blood and tissue fluids of animals and in plant and fruit juices, as well as in combined form in polysaccharides such as glycogen, starch and cellulose, and in glucosides. It appears in the urine in comparatively large quantities in diabetes mellitus, and is detected by enzymic assay and identified by its reducing action upon alkaline copper-tartrate solution, the formation of a characteristic osazone and its ready fermentation by yeast. **2-Deoxyglucose.** When administered to normal people or patients with adrenocortical deficiency there is a rise of urinary adrenaline, but if the medulla is also involved there is a poor or absent catecholamine response. **Liquid Glucose BPC 1963.** A viscous mass obtained by the incomplete acid hydrolysis of starch, and containing dextrose, maltose, dextrins and water. **Medicinal glucose.** Dextrose Monohydrate BP 1958. **Glucose 1-phosphate.** $CH_2OH(CHOH)_4COOP(OH)_2$, Cori ester; an ester of glucose and phosphoric acid which plays an important rôle in fermentation and in the breakdown of glycogen. **Glucose 6-phosphatase.** The gluconeogenic enzyme which catalyses the hydrolysis of glucose 6-phosphate with production of glucose and phosphate. **Glucose 6-phosphate.** $(OH)_2POOCH_2(CHOH)_4CHO$, Embden ester; a constituent of Robison ester that takes part in fermentation and in the breakdown of glycogen. **Purified glucose.** Dextrose monohydrate. **Glucose tolerance test.** *See* TEST. [Gk *glykys* sweet.]

See also: BRUN.

glucosene (gloo·ko·seen). Glycosene, $CH_2\overline{C(CHOH)_4O}$. An unsaturated anhydride of glucose.

glucosidase (gloo·ko·sid·aze). Any enzyme which activates the hydrolysis of glucosides. In some cases the reaction may be reversible, the same enzyme operating in the synthesis of glucosides, e.g. prunase and the glucoside of the cherry laurel.

glucoside (gloo·ko·side). A particular type of glycoside in which the carbohydrate molecule or molecules linked with one or more other chemical substances is glucose (dextrose). There is a great variety of glucosides, the most important being those derived from digitalis, strophanthus and other related plants. The carbohydrate part of the molecule can be removed by hydrolysis leaving the aglucone or genin: this is generally the most important part pharmacologically, its action being merely enhanced or facilitated by the carbohydrate portion.

glucosidolytic (gloo·ko·si·do·lit′·ik). Having the power to split up glucosides. [glucoside, Gk *lysis* a loosing.]

glucosum (gloo·ko·sum). Liquid Glucose BPC 1959.

glucosuria (gloo·ko·sewr·e·ah). Glycosuria.

glucotropic (gloo·ko·trop·ik). A term applied to any substance having an effect antagonistic to that of insulin. [Gk *glykys* sweet, *trepein* to turn.]

glucuronate (gloo·kewr·on·ate). A salt of glucuronic acid.

glue (gloo). A hard, brittle solid obtained from the hooves and hides of animals by boiling with water and evaporating the extract. On warming with water it readily forms an unpleasant-smelling gelatinous fluid that is used as an adhesive. [Gk *gloios*.]

See also: SINCLAIR.

Glueck, Themistocles (b. 1853). Berlin surgeon.

Glueck's operation, Glueck-Soerensen method or operation. Removal of the larynx performed from above downwards. The hypopharynx is entered and inspected during the early stages of the operation.

Gluge, Gottlieb (b. 1812). German histologist.

Gluge's corpuscles. Compound granular corpuscles in the nervous system.

gluside, glusidum (gloo·side, gloo·sid·um). Saccharin, *o*-benzoylsulphone-imide. A white crystalline powder having a faintly aromatic odour and an intensely sweet taste. It is about 500 times as sweet as sugar and is extensively employed as a sweetening agent, being harmless in small amounts even with repeated use. It has no food value.

glutaeus (gloo·te·us). Gluteus.

glutamate (gloo·tam·ate). Any salt of glutamic acid. **Monosodium glutamate, Sodium glutamate,** $HOOCCH(NH_2)CH_2CH_2CO$ ONa. The sodium salt of glutamic acid, used as a food flavouring.

glutaminase (gloo·tam·in·aze). An enzyme catalysing the hydrolysis of glutamine to glutamic acid and ammonia. It occurs in the brain cortex and retina of vertebrates, and in the kidney of the rabbit and guinea-pig.

glutamine (gloo·tam·een). α-Aminoglutaric acid mono-amide, $COOHCH(NH_2)CH_2CH_2CONH_2$. A compound which occurs together with asparagine in beetroot and other plants; also present in plasma and cardiac muscle. It is formed from glutaric acid by *Staphylococcus aureus* and would appear to be an accessory growth factor for certain species of *Streptococcus*. In the human body it plays an important part in detoxication.

glutaraldehyde (gloo·tar·al·de·hide). An aldehyde widely used as a 1-5 per cent buffered solution for the fixation of tissues for electron microscopy. It is usually followed by post-fixation with osmium tetroxide.

glutathionaemia (gloo·tah·thi·on·e′·me·ah). The condition in which glutathione is present in the blood. [glutathione, Gk *haima* blood.]

glutathione (gloo·tah·thi·one). α-Glutamylcysteinylglycine, $COOH$ $CH(NH_2)CH_2CH_2CONHCH(CH_2SH)CONHCH_2COOH$. A naturally-occurring tripeptide which is widely distributed in living tissues. Its importance physiologically appears to be dependent upon the very reactive sulphydryl group, -SH, which is present in the molecule, the easy oxidation of which to the corresponding disulphide, -S-S-, allows of participation in oxidation-reduction systems. It antagonizes the action of organic arsenicals against protozoal and spirochaetal infections, thereby indicating that their effect is one concerned with sulphydryl-containing proteins.

gluteal (gloo·te·al). Relating or belonging to the buttocks or a gluteus muscle. [Gk *gloutos* buttock.]

gluteal arteries. Arteries supplying the buttocks. **Inferior gluteal artery [arteria glutea inferior (NA)].** One of the terminal branches of the anterior division of the internal iliac artery; it leaves the pelvis through the greater sacrosciatic foramen to supply the muscles of the buttock and back of the thigh. **Superior gluteal artery [arteria glutea superior (NA)].** A branch of the posterior division of the internal iliac artery; it leaves the pelvis through the greater sacrosciatic foramen to supply the muscles and skin of the buttock. Its superficial branch [ramus superficialis (NA)] enters the gluteus maximus muscle; its deep branch [ramus profundus (NA)] lies under the gluteus medius muscle and has an upper and lower branch [ramus superior et inferior (NA)] which pass towards the anterior superior iliac spine and the region of the hip joint, respectively.

gluteal nerves. Branches of the sacral plexus that supply the muscles of the buttocks. **Inferior gluteal nerve [nervus gluteus inferior].** A branch of the sacral plexus (root value L5, S1, 2) to supply the gluteus maximus muscle. **Superior gluteal nerve [nervus gluteus superior].** The nerve of supply of the gluteus medius, gluteus minimus and of the tensor fasciae latae muscles. It is a branch of the sacral plexus (root value L4, 5, S1).

gluteal veins. Veins draining the buttocks. **Inferior gluteal veins [venae gluteae inferiores].** Tributaries of the internal iliac vein. **Superior gluteal veins [venae gluteae superiores].** Tributaries of the internal iliac vein from the buttock.

glutelin (gloo·tel·in). One of a group of vegetable simple proteins obtained from the seeds of cereals. They are insoluble in water but soluble in dilute acids and alkalis, and are not coagulated by heat. Mixed with gliadins, they form gluten.

gluten (gloo·ten). 1. A sticky nitrogenous substance present to the extent of about 10 per cent in wheat flour, from which it may be obtained by kneading under water in a calico bag when the starch passes through the bag leaving the gluten behind as a tenacious mass. It is a mixture of glutenin and gliadin and imparts the consistency to dough in breadmaking. 2. A nitrogen-rich extract of gluten for providing a high-protein intake in small bulk. **Gluten bread and biscuits.** Starchless edible products prepared principally from gluten and bran for diabetics. [L glue.]

gluten-casein (gloo·ten·ka·se·in). A protein preparation from wheat flour; also known as *vegetable casein*. [gluten, casein.]

glutenin (gloo·ten·in). The particular glutelin occurring in wheat flour.

gluteofascial (gloo·te·o·fash′·e·al). Relating or belonging to the fascia of the buttocks and gluteal region.

gluteofemoral (gloo·te·o·fem′·or·al). Relating or belonging to the buttocks and the thigh or femoral region. [Gk *gloutos* buttock, femur.]

gluteo-inguinal (gloo·te·o·ing′·gwin·al). Pertaining to the gluteal and inguinal regions.

gluteotrochanteric (gloo·te·o·tro·kan·ter′·ik). Referring to the gluteus muscles or region and the trochanter.

Glutethimide BP 1973 (gloo·teth·im·ide). α-Ethyl-α-phenylglutarimide. It is a rapidly-acting hypnotic of medium duration. It does not depress respiration or lower blood pressure and produces no depressing after-effects. It is indicated in insomnia.

gluteus (gloo·te·us). The buttock. [Gk *gloutos* buttock.]

gluteus maximus muscle [musculus gluteus maximus (NA)] (gloo·te·us **max**·im·us). A large muscle arising from the iliac bone, the sacrum and the sacrotuberous ligament; it is inserted into the gluteal tuberosity of the femur and into the fascia lata.

gluteus medius muscle [musculus gluteus medius (NA)] (gloo·te·us **me**·de·us). A muscle arising between the middle and posterior gluteal lines on the ilium and inserted into the greater trochanter of the femur.

gluteus minimus muscle [musculus gluteus minimus (NA)] (gloo·te·us **min**·im·us). A muscle arising between the middle and anterior gluteal lines of the ilium and inserted into the greater trochanter of the femur.

glutin (**gloo**·tin). 1. Gluten-casein. 2. A complex protein substance occurring in gelatin.

glutinous (**gloo**·tin·us). 1. Having the character of glue; viscous; adhesive; sticky. 2. In botany, indicating that a surface is moist or adhesive. [L *gluten* glue.]

glutitis (gloo·**ti**·tis). Inflammation of the gluteus muscles. [Gk *gloutos* buttock, *-itis* inflammation.]

glutoid (**gloo**·toid). The name applied to gelatin-coated capsules and pills which have been specially treated with formaldehyde (15 min in a 2 per cent solution) in order to ensure that they pass through the stomach unchanged, and undergo subsequent disintegration in the intestines in those cases where the medicament is sensitive to gastric secretions.

gluton (**gloo**·ton). A nutrient substance formed from gelatin by hydrolysis with hot acid.

glycaemia (gli·se·me·ah). A condition in which the circulating blood contains a quantity of sugar (glucose) above normal amounts. [Gk *glykys* sweet, *haima* blood.]

glycal (**gli**·kal). A general name for the unsaturated monosaccharides containing the group -CH=CH-; glucal from glucose is an example.

Glycalox (**gli**·kal·ox). BP Commission approved name for a polymerized complex of glycerol and aluminium hydroxide.

glycase (**gli**·kaze). A generic term for enzymes which split polysaccharides into simpler sugars.

glyceraldehyde (glis·er·**al**·de·hide). The simplest aldose CH_2OH $CHOHCH_2OH$. It occurs physiologically during fructose metabolism in the liver. **Glyceraldehyde 3-phosphate.** A glycolytic intermediate.

glycerate (**glis**·er·ate). A salt of glyceric acid.

glyceric (**glis**·er·ik). Pertaining to glycerin.

glyceridase (**glis**·er·id·aze). Lipase.

glyceride (**glis**·er·ide). Any ester formed by glycerol with an acid, usually a fatty acid. Most animal and vegetable fats consist of glycerides, principally tripalmitin, tristearin and triolein, or mixed glycerides (see below). **Medullary glyceride.** A bone-marrow preparation used in the treatment of anaemia. **Mixed glyceride.** An ester of the trihydric glycerol with two or three different acid radicals, e.g. oleodistearin. **Simple glyceride.** An ester of glycerol in which all the acid radicals are the same, e.g. tristearin.

glycerin (**glis**·er·in). Glycerol, 1,2,3-trihydroxypropane, CH_2OH $CHOHCH_2OH$. A clear, colourless, syrupy liquid obtained from fixed oils and fats by hydrolysis, and produced as a by-product in the manufacture of soap, and in sugar fermentation. It is tasteless, odourless and neutral, hygroscopic and a good solvent; it is itself miscible with water or alcohol, but insoluble in ether, chloroform and fixed oils. Administered orally it is a mild laxative; in pharmacy it is used as a sweetening agent in dispensing and as an ingredient of linctus on account of its syrupy nature. Applied externally as a constituent of skin preparations, it acts as an emollient by reason of its hygroscopic property. This capacity to absorb water is utilized in such preparations as Paste of Magnesium Sulphate BPC 1959 which is used in the treatment of septic wounds and staphylococcal infections. It is effective by rectal injection either as an enema or in the form of suppositories for the relief of constipation (BP 1973). **Glycerin of alum.** Glycerinum Aluminis BPC 1949. **Glycerin of Belladonna BPC 1959.** A solution of green extract of belladonna in water and glycerin which is used for local application in the relief of pain. **Glycerin of Borax BPC 1959.** A 12 per cent by weight solution of borax in glycerin used as a paint for the throat and tongue, especially in mouth infections of children. **Glycerin of boric acid.** Glycerinum Acidi Borici BP 1948. **Compound Glycerin of Thymol BPC 1959.** A solution containing principally thymol, menthol, eucalyptol, volatile oils, salts and glycerin, used as a mouth wash and gargle in the treatment of infections of the mouth and throat. **Glycerin of Ichthammol BPC 1959.** A preparation of ichthammol (10 per cent) in glycerin, used as an antiseptic in certain skin infections. **Glycerin of Lead Subacetate BPC 1954.** A solution of lead subacetate in glycerin and water, used in dilution either with glycerin or (1 to 7) in the treatment of chronic eczema. **Glycerin of pepsin.** A solution of pepsin in water and glycerin, containing hydrochloric acid, syrup and flavouring agents; used in medicine to augment digestion in the stomach due to lack of pepsin. **Phenol Glycerin BP 1958.** A 16 per cent by weight solution of phenol in glycerin, used as such or diluted with glycerin as an antiseptic in ulcerative stomatitis and tonsillitis. **Starch Glycerin BP 1958.** A mucilage prepared from wheat starch, water and glycerin, used as a protective ointment in skin infections. **Tannic Acid Glycerin BP 1958.** A 15 per cent by weight solution of tannic acid in glycerin, used as an astringent paint for infections of the mouth and throat. **Glycerin of tragacanth.** A mucilage prepared from tragacanth, glycerin and water; used mainly as a pill excipient. [Gk *glykeros* sweet.]

glycerinated (**glis**·er·in·a·ted). Mixed or treated with, or preserved in, glycerin.

glycerine (**glis**·er·een). Glycerin.

glycerinum (glis·er·i·num). Glycerin. **Glycerinum Acidi Borici BP 1948.** A 3 per cent by weight of boric-acid solution in glycerin, used as a throat paint. **Glycerinum Aluminis BPC 1949.** A solution of potassium alum in water and glycerin, used as a paint or diluted with water as a gargle in the treatment of ulcerations of the mouth and throat. [Gk *glykeros* sweet.]

glyceroborate (glis·er·o·**bor**′·ate). A substance prepared from glycerol and borax.

glycerokinase (glis·er·o·**ki**′·naze). The enzyme catalysing the phosphorylation of glycerol by ATP with production of L-glycerol 3-phosphate. Mostly in liver; small activity in kidney.

Glycerol BP 1973 (**glis**·er·ol). Glycerin. Glycerol is the more usual chemical name. **Iodinated Glycerol.** BP Commission approved name for a mixture of iodinated dimers of glycerol; an expectorant.

glycerophosphatase (glis·er·o·**fos**′·fat·aze). Lecithinase; an enzyme capable of splitting egg-yolk lecithin to liberate phosphoric acid and glycerol.

glycerophosphate (glis·er·o·**fos**′·fate). An intermediate in triglyceride synthesis, formed by reduction of dihydroxyacetone phosphate. **Calcium Glycerophosphate BPC 1959,** $CaC_3H_5(OH)_2$ $PO_4{\cdot}2H_2O$. Perhaps the most popular single glycerophosphate, but tonics usually contain mixtures of several salts. **Glycerophosphate dehydrogenase.** An enzyme occurring in yeast and, with adenosine triphosphate as co-enzyme, concerned in glycolysis in the body. **Potassium glycerophosphate,** $K_2C_3H_5(OH)_2PO_4$. A salt occurring only in solution as it is too soluble to be crystallized in the pure state; the most common strength is 50 per cent w/w (BPC 1959). **Sodium glycerophosphate,** $Na_2C_3H_5(OH)_2PO_4{\cdot}5\frac{1}{2}H_2O$. Probably a mixture of sodium α-glycerophosphate pentahydrate and sodium β-glycerophosphate hexahydrate.

glycerophosphorylcholine (glis·er·o·fos·for·il·co·line). A secretion by the epididymis into the semen.

glyceryl (**glis**·er·il). The radical, C_3H_5, derived from glycerin (glycerol); it is trivalent. **Glyceryl monostearate, self-emulsifying.** Self-emulsifying Monostearin BPC 1959, a whitish waxy substance, composed chiefly of glyceryl esters of palmitic and stearic acids together with some free fatty acids, glycerin and small amounts of other substances. It is used as an emulsifying agent for oils, fats and waxes in the preparation of creams and ointments. **Glyceryl trinitrate,** nitroglycerin, $C_3H_5(NO_3)_3$. An odourless, colourless liquid prepared by the nitration of glycerin. A solution in 95 per cent alcohol is added to granules of chocolate bars to make the tablets (Glyceryl Trinitrate Tablets BP 1968) in which form the drug is prescribed. Pharmacologically it resembles some of the nitrites in causing relaxation of smooth muscle. Its chief clinical use is in the treatment of angina pectoris. **Glyceryl triolein.** Olein.

glycide (gli·side). Glycide alcohol, a colourless liquid isomeric with propionic acid, formed by the elimination of water from glycerol.

glycinaemia (gli·sin·e·me·ah). Excess glycine in blood; types include ketosis, oxaluria and acidaemia. [glycine, Gk *haima* blood.]

glycinate (gli·sin·ate). A salt of glycine.

glycine (gli·seen). α-Amino-acetic acid, NH_2CH_2COOH. The simplest of the amino acids and a common constituent of protein. It is synthesized in the body and is a precursor of porphyrins, nucleotides, phospholipids and bile salts.

glycinin (gli·sin·in). A protein of the globulin type which is present in soya.

glycinuria (gli·sin·ewr·e·ah). Excretion of glycine in urine due to glycinaemia or to renal tubular defect.

Glyciphagus (gli·sif·ag·us). A genus of mites. **Glyciphagus buski, Glyciphagus domesticus.** A species which normally inhabits dried foods and detritus. It causes grocers' itch and has occasionally been found as a true ectoparasite in superficial ulcers and in faeces. **Glyciphagus prunorum.** A species with similar habits. [Gk *glykys* sweet, *phagein* to eat.]

glycocalyx (gli·ko·ka·lix). A very thin layer of material which covers the surface (particularly the free surface) of many, or possibly all, cells. It contains acid mucopolysaccharides and may be concerned with the selective permeability of the cell membrane. [Gk *glykys* sweet, *kalyx* shell.]

glycocholate (gli·ko·ko·late). A salt of glycocholic acid.

glycocine, glycocoll (gli·ko·seen, gli·ko·kol). Glycine. [Gk *glykys* sweet, *kolla* glue.]

glycocyamine (gli·ko·si·am·een). Guanidine acetic acid, $NH{=}C(NH_2)NHCH_2COOH$. A substance formed from cyanamide and glycine, and the parent of creatine.

glycogelatin (gli·ko·jel·at·in). A flavoured pastille base prepared from gelatin, glycerin and water.

glycogen (gli·ko·jen). Animal starch, $(C_6H_{10}O_5)_x$. A polysaccharide synthesized in the body cells from hexoses and stored as reserve carbohydrate. Its distribution in the human body is divided almost equally between the liver and muscles. It is a white compound which gives a red coloration with iodine. **Hepatic glycogen.** Glycogen synthesized and stored by the liver of which it comprises about 3 per cent of the fresh tissue in the human adult. It forms the storage carbohydrate of the body and is broken down into glucose as required by the tissues. **Muscle glycogen.** Glycogen stored in the skeletal muscles, of which it comprises about 1 per cent, and utilized as a source of energy in the contraction process, the glycogen being transformed into lactate. **Glycogen storage disease.** In which glycogen cannot be converted to glucose or in galactosaemia or hereditary fructose intolerance, neither of these sugars being able to stimulate hepatic glycogen to be converted into glucose. [Gk *glykys* sweet, *genein* to produce.]

glycogenase (gli·ko·jen·aze). 1. An enzyme which splits glycogen, e.g. that produced by *Corynebacterium diphtheriae gravis.* 2. An enzyme in muscle which takes part in the conversion of glycogen into lactic acid.

glycogenesis (gli·ko·jen·es·is). Gluconeogenesis. [Gk *glykys* sweet, *genein* to produce.]

glycogenetic (gli·ko·jen·et′·ik). Referring to glycogenesis; referring or belonging to the production of sugar.

glycogenic (gli·ko·jen·ik). 1. Referring or belonging to glycogen. 2. Glycogenetic.

glycogenolysis (gli·ko·jen·ol′·is·is). The breaking down of glycogen in animal tissue, including its final conversion into glucose. [glycogen, lysis.]

glycogenolytic (gli·ko·jen·o·lit′·ik). Referring to glycogenolysis; having the power to break down glycogen.

glycogenosis (gli·ko·jen·o′·sis). Glycogen storage disease. *See* DISEASE. Several forms have been described, including Pompe's and McArdle's. Generally due to an inborn deficiency of one of the enzymes of glycogen metabolism. [glycogen, Gk *-osis* condition.]

glycogenous (gli·koj·en·us). Of the nature of glycogen.

glycogeny (gli·koj·en·e). Glycogenesis.

glycogeusia (gli·ko·jews·e·ah). A sweet taste in the mouth. [Gk *glykys* sweet, *geusis* taste.]

glycohaemia (gli·ko·he·me·ah). Glycaemia.

glycohistechia (gli·ko·his·tek′·e·ah). Increased sugar in the tissues. **Independent cutaneous glycohistechia.** An abnormal sugar content of the skin without hyperglycaemia. [Gk *glykys* sweet, *histos* tissue, *echein* to hold.]

glycol (gli·kol). 1. Ethylene glycol, CH_2OHCH_2OH, a syrupy hygroscopic liquid manufactured from ethylene and used in anti-freeze mixtures and in the cellulose industry. 2. Name given to any member of a family of dihydric alcohols derived from the aliphatic hydrocarbons. They are chiefly used as solvents, particularly for drugs which are insoluble in water or unstable in aqueous solution. They are also used in flavouring essences and fruit juices because of the high duty on ethyl alcohol which is not recoverable in such preparations. They must all be regarded as toxic potentially, since they can cause kidney and liver damage in excessive amounts, though the amounts normally ingested are small, and the lower glycols are the least toxic, the toxicity increasing with the length of the carbon chain. **Polyethylene glycol.** Macrogol. **Propylene Glycol BP 1958.** Occurring in two isomeric forms, it is a useful medicinal solvent; the β-isomer (trimethylene glycol, $OHCH_2CH_2{=}CH_2OH$) is formed during the Schizomycetes fermentation of glycerol. [Gk *glykys* sweet.]

glycolaldehyde (gli·kol·al·de·hide). Glycollic aldehyde. *See* ALDEHYDE.

glycolic (gli·kol·ik). Derived from glycol, or belonging to glycol.

glycolipide (gli·ko·lip·ide). Galactolipide, galactolipin, galactoside. One of the cerebrosides or esters of a fatty acid with sphingosine and galactose which are found in brain tissue and the myelin sheaths of nerves: phrenosin, kerasin and nervone.

glycolipin (gli·ko·lip·in). Glycolipide.

glycollate (gli·kol·ate). A salt of glycollic acid.

glycollic (gli·kol·ik). Derived from glycol.

glycollyl (gli·kol·il). The monovalent group, CH_2OHCO-, derived from glycollic acid.

glycolysis (gli·kol·is·is). The sequence of reactions whereby the natural hexoses and their phosphate esters are converted into pyruvate and lactate or ethyl alcohol. [Gk *glykys* sweet, *lysis* a loosing.]

glycolytic (gli·ko·lit·ik). Referring to glycolysis; having the power to break up or decompose sugars such as glucose.

glycometabolic (gli·ko·met·ab·ol′·ik). Referring to glycometabolism.

glycometabolism (gli·ko·met·ab′·ol·izm). The metabolism of sugar in the animal body. [Gk *glykys* sweet, metabolism.]

glycone (gli·kone). The sugar moiety of a glycoside. [Gk *glykys* sweet.]

glyconeogenesis (gli·ko·ne·o·jen′·es·is). The formation of carbohydrates, such as grape sugar, from proteins or other substances which are not carbohydrates. [Gk *glykys* sweet, *neos* new, *genein* to produce.]

glyconucleoprotein (gli·ko·new·kle·o·pro′·te·in). A name descriptive of a nucleoprotein to emphasize the presence of sugar units in the molecule. [Gk *glykys* sweet, nucleoprotein.]

glycopectic (gli·ko·pek·tik). Glycopexic.

glycopenia (gli·ko·pe·ne·ah). Hypoglycaemia; a condition in which the sugar level in the blood is too low. [Gk *glykys* sweet, *penes* poor.]

glycopexic (gli·ko·**pex**·ik). Relating to glycopexis; storing or fixing sugar or glucose.

glycopexis (gli·ko·**pex**·is). The storage of glucose or glycogen, or the fixing of it. [Gk *glykys* sweet, *pexis* fixation.]

glycophenol (gli·ko·**fe**·nol). Saccharin, gluside, *o*-sulphobenzoic acid imide. A white crystalline compound, 500 times as sweet as sugar, and used as a sweetening agent, especially in the diet of diabetics.

glycophilia (gli·ko·**fil**·e·ah). A condition in which a very small intake of glucose produces a tendency to hyperglycaemia. [Gk *glykys* sweet, *philein* to love.]

glycopolyuria (gli·ko·pol·e·**ewr'**·e·ah). A type of diabetes mellitus in which the amount of sugar in the urine is moderate but the amount of uric acid much increased (Bouchardat). [Gk *glykys* sweet, polyuria.]

glycoprotein (gli·ko·**pro**·te·in). Glucoprotein, mucoprotein. A conjugated protein formed by a protein and a carbohydrate prosthetic group, the latter a sulphuric ester of a polysaccharide such as mucoitin or chondroitin, They include the mucins of saliva, mucous membrane and vitreous humour, and the mucoids of cartilage, bone, tendons and serum. [Gk *glykys* sweet, protein.]

glycoptyalism (gli·ko·ti·al·izm). Excretion of glucose by the salivary glands and consequent presence of this substance in the saliva. [Gk *glykys* sweet, *ptyalon* saliva.]

Glycopyrronium Bromide (gli·ko·pi·**ro'**·ne·um **bro**·mide). BP Commission approved name for 3-α-cyclopentylmandeloyloxy-1, 1-dimethylpyrrolidinium bromide; an anticholinergic.

glycorrhachia (gli·ko·**rak**·e·ah). A condition in which there is sugar in the cerebrospinal fluid. [Gk *glykys* sweet, *rhachis* spine.]

glycorrhoea (gli·ko·re·ah). The excretion of any sugary fluid from the body, as in the condition of glycosuria. [Gk *glykys* sweet, *rhoia* flow.]

glycosaemia (gli·ko·se·me·ah). Glycaemia.

glycosamine (gli·**ko**·sam·een). Glucosamine, aminoglucose, chitosamine, $CH_2OH(CHOH)_3CH(NH_2)CHO$. An aminosaccharide obtained by the hydrolysis of chitin and occurring widely in nature combined with glucuronic acid in the prosthetic group of glycoproteins.

glycosaminoglycans (**gli**·ko·sam·in·o·**gli'**·kanz). Mucopolysaccharides.

glycosecretory (**gli**·ko·se·**kre'**·tor·e). Belonging to or influencing the formation and secretion of glycogen.

glycosene (**gli**·ko·seen). Glucosene, $CH_2\overline{C(CHOH)_4O}$. An unsaturated anhydride of glucose.

glycosialia (**gli**·ko·si·**a'**·le·ah). A condition in which sugar is present in the saliva. [Gk *glykys* sweet, *sialon* saliva.]

glycosialorrhoea (**gli**·ko·si·al·o·**re'**·ah). Excessive secretion of saliva containing sugar. [Gk *glykys* sweet, *sialon* saliva, *rhoia* flow.]

glycoside (**gli**·ko·side). General term embracing the naturally-occurring substances which consist of sugars combined with non-sugar units (aglycones). They include the vegetable pigments, tannins, drugs such as digitalis and also the cerebrosides and nucleosides of animal tissue. They hydrolyse into the corresponding monosaccharides, and in plants are usually associated with a specific enzyme capable of accomplishing this. Cf. GLUCOSIDE. **Cardiac glycoside.** A glycoside that has a stimulating effect on the heart; the principal ones are obtained from species of *Digitalis, Scilla, Strophanthus* and *Thevetia*. **Cyanogenetic glycoside, Cyanophoric glycoside.** Any glycoside that yields hydrocyanic acid on hydrolysis, e.g. amygdalin, from bitter almonds. **Sterol glycoside.** One which, on hydrolysis, yields a genin containing the sterol nucleus, e.g. strophanthin. [Gk *glykys* sweet.]

glycosometer (**gli**·ko·**som**·e·ter). An instrument with which the proportion of sugar in the urine can be determined. [Gk *glykys* sweet, meter.]

glycostatic (gli·ko·**stat**·ik). Maintaining a constant level of sugar. [Gk *glykys* sweet, *stasis* a standing.]

glycosuria (gli·ko·**sewr**·e·ah). The excretion of sugar in the urine. **Alimentary glycosuria.** Glycosuria due to excessive absorption of sugar from the alimentary tract. **Anxiety glycosuria.** Temporary glycosuria caused by anxiety. **Artificial glycosuria.** The glycosuria that results from injury to the floor of the 4th ventricle in the medulla oblongata. It was first demonstrated by Claude Bernard. **Benign glycosuria.** Renal glycosuria (see below). **Diabetic glycosuria.** Excessive secretion of sugar due to diabetes mellitus. **Digestive glycosuria.** Alimentary glycosuria (see above). **Emotional glycosuria.** Glycosuria occurring temporarily from emotional disturbance. **Epinephrine glycosuria.** Glycosuria occurring after an injection of adrenaline (epinephrine). **Hyperglycaemic glycosuria.** Glycosuria due to a raised blood sugar. **Lipogenic glycosuria.** Glycosuria associated with obesity. **Magnesium glycosuria.** Glycosuria associated with increased magnesium concentration in the blood. **Nervous glycosuria.** Glycosuria experimentally produced by puncture of the floor of the 4th ventricle. **Non-diabetic glycosuria, Non-hyperglycaemic glycosuria.** Glycosuria occurring with a normal blood sugar. **Normoglycaemic glycosuria, Orthoglycaemic glycosuria.** Renal glycosuria (see below). **Pathological glycosuria.** Glycosuria due to disease of the pancreas. **Persistent glycosuria.** Diabetes mellitus. **Phloridzin glycosuria.** Glycosuria due to the administration of phloridzin. **Pituitary glycosuria.** Glycosuria due to excessive secretion of the pituitary diabetogenic hormone. **Renal glycosuria.** A familial condition in which sugar is excreted in the urine, although the blood sugar is within normal limits. It is associated with a lowering of the renal threshold to sugar. **Toxic glycosuria.** Glycosuria due to lowering of sugar tolerance by toxins. **Traumatic glycosuria.** Glycosuria occurring after cerebral injuries or haemorrhage. [Gk *glykys* sweet, urine.]

glycotaxis (gli·ko·**tax**·is). The apportioning of glucose to all the tissues of the body, carried out in the process of metabolism. [Gk *glykys* sweet, *taxis* arrangement.]

glycotropic (gli·ko·**trop**·ik). Glucotropic.

glycuresis (gli·kewr·e·sis). The passing of urine containing an abnormally large quantity of sugar. [Gk *glykys* sweet, uresis.]

glycuronate (gli·**kewr**·on·ate). A salt or ester of glycuronic acid; in the process of detoxication, any ester of glycuronic acid formed by the conjugation of the latter acid with such substances as chloral, phenols, morphine, turpentine, aspirin, etc. They are excreted in the urine and their estimation may be used as a test of liver function.

glycuronide (gli·**kewr**·on·ide). Glycuronate.

glycuronuria (gli·kewr·on·**ewr'**·e·ah). The excretion of glycuronates in the urine. Increased excretion always occurs after ingestion of antipyrin, arsenic, camphor, chloral hydrate, chloroform, morphine, phenol, salicylic acid and sulphonal, and also as a result of intestinal stasis. Glycuronates give positive reactions in the copper-reduction tests for sugar.

glycyl (**gli**·sil). An important radical, NH_2CH_2COO- derived from glycine and present in many peptide units. Also applied to the divalent radical, $-NHCH_2COO$-.

glycylglycine (gli·sil·**gli**·seen). $NH_2CH_2CONHCH_2COOH$, the simplest of the peptides.

glycyltryptophan (gli·sil·**trip**·to·fan). A dipeptide consisting of glycine and tryptophan. It is used as a reagent for the estimation of dipeptidase activity in intestinal juice.

Glycyrrhiza (glis·e·**ri**·zah). 1. A genus of perennial herbs (family Leguminosae), widely distributed over Europe and North America. 2. Liquorice BP 1958, glycyrrhizae radix, a drug having a taste, sweet and almost free from bitterness, obtained from *Glycyrrhiza glabra* Linn. and other species of *Glycyrrhiza*, and consisting of stolon and root in the peeled or unpeeled condition. The taste is due to the presence of a sweet principle, glycyrrhizin. Both in powder form and as the liquid extract it is widely used in medicine as a flavouring agent and as a mild expectorant. [Gk *glykys* sweet, *rhiza* root.]

glycyrrhizin (glis·er·**ize**·in). The principal constituent of liquorice root; a very sweet, white crystalline substance consisting of the potassium and calcium salts of glycyrrhizinic acid. **Ammoniated glycyrrhizin.** A preparation of ammonium glycyrrhizinate derived from liquorice root. [see prec.]

Glymidine (gli·mid·een). BP Commission approved name for the sodium salt of 2-benzenesulphonamido-5-(2-methoxyethoxy)pyrimidine; an oral hypoglycaemic agent.

glyoxal (gli·ox·al). Glyoxylic aldehyde, CHOCHO. A dialdehyde prepared by the oxidation of ethyl alcohol or acetaldehyde and itself oxidized to glyoxylic acid.

glyoxalase (gli·ox·al·aze) An enzyme of the oxidoreductase class which activates the conversion of ketonic aldehydes into hydroxy acids. It occurs in the liver where, in the presence of its co-enzyme, glutathione, it converts methyl glyoxal, CH_3COCHO, to lactic acid, $CH_3CHOHCOOH$.

glyoxalin, glyoxaline (gli·ox·al·in, gli·ox·al·een). Iminazole, $CH(NH)=N(CH)_2$. A cyclic compound from which is derived histidine and the pilocarpine alkaloids.

Glyptocranium gasteracanthoides (glip·to·kra·ne·um gas·ter·ak·an·thoid′·eez). A Peruvian spider whose venom causes haemorrhagic and neurotoxic symptoms and local gangrene. [Gk *glyptos* carved, *kranion* skull, *gaster* belly, *akantha* thorn, *eidos* form.]

Gmelin, Leopold (b. 1788). Heidelberg physiologist.

Gmelin's reaction. When a fluid containing bile is layered on to concentrated nitric acid in a test tube, various coloured rings are formed at the junction of the 2 liquids. The colours vary from green, blue, violet, to red.

Gmelin's test, for bile pigments. To a few ml of nitric acid in a test tube add the fluid or aqueous extract carefully to avoid mixing. Various coloured rings, green, blue, violet and red, are formed at the junction of the liquids.

Rosenbach-Gmelin test, for bile pigments. Filter from 10 to 20 ml of urine acidified with a few drops of dilute hydrochloric acid through a small heavy filter paper. Add a drop of nitric acid to the filter and note the colour changes, as in Gmelin's test.

gnat (nat). 1. Any fly of the family Culicidae; mosquito (English usage). 2. Any small biting or irritating fly (American usage). **Buffalo gnat.** *Simulium.* **Eye gnat.** *Hippelates.* **Turkey gnat.** *Simulium.* [AS *gnaet.*]

gnathalgia (nath·al·je·ah). Pain in one or both jaws. [Gk *gnathos* jaw, *algos* pain.]

gnathic (nath·ik). Relating or belonging to jaw or cheek, or to the alveolar process. [Gk *gnathos* jaw.]

gnathion (nath·e·on). In craniometry, the lowest point of the median line of junction of the lower jaw. [Gk *gnathos* jaw.]

gnathitis (nath·i·tis). An inflamed condition of the maxilla or mandible, or of both bones, or of the cheek. [Gk *gnathos* jaw, *-itis* inflammation.]

gnathocephalus (nath·o·kef·al·us). A monster lacking most of the head except a greatly enlarged lower jaw. [Gk *gnathos* jaw, *kephale* head.]

gnathodynamics (nath·o·di·nam′·ix). The science of the physical forces in mastication. [Gk *gnathos* jaw, dynamics.]

gnathodynamometer (nath·o·di·nam·om′·et·er). An instrument with which the force of the bite can be measured. It consists of 2 rubber pads upon which the teeth bite, the pressure exerted being shown by the movement of a pointer along a graduated scale. [Gk *gnathos* jaw, dynamometer.]

gnathodynia (nath·o·din·e·ah). Gnathalgia. [Gk *gnathos* jaw, *odyne* pain.]

gnathography (nath·og·raf·e). A recording of the strength of a subject's bite. [Gk *gnathos* jaw, *graphein* to record.]

gnathoneuralgia (nath·o·newr·al′·je·ah). Gnathalgia. [Gk *gnathos* jaw, neuralgia.]

gnathopagus parasiticus (nath·op·ag·us par·ah·sit·ik·us). Epignathus. [Gk *gnathos* jaw, *pagos* that which is fixed, *parasitos* parasite.]

gnathoplasty (nath·o·plas·te). Any plastic operation on the jaw or cheek. [Gk *gnathos* jaw, *plassein* to mould.]

gnathoplegia (nath·o·ple·je·ah). Paralysis of the cheek muscles. [Gk *gnathos* jaw, *plege* stroke.]

gnathorrhagia (nath·o·ra·je·ah). Haemorrhage from the mucosa of the cheeks or from the jaws. [Gk *gnathos* jaw, *rhegnynai* to burst forth.]

gnathoschisis (nath·os·kis·is). A congenital fissure in the maxilla, such as is present in cleft palate. [Gk *gnathos* jaw, *schisis* division.]

gnathostatics (nath·o·stat·ix). Measurements involving the teeth and the bones of the skull. [Gk *gnathos* jaw, *statike* weighing.]

Gnathostoma (nath·os·to·mah). A genus of nematode worms. Larval infection in human skin and subcutaneous tissues is common, giving rise to transient granulomatous, eosinophilic swelling; adult intestinal infections occasionally occur. **Gnathostoma hispidum.** A species found in pigs; it has been recorded in the human skin once. **Gnathostoma spinigerum.** A large roundworm of South-east Asia whose normal hosts are cats, and secondary hosts fish and frogs. Larval infections in human skin are common, and adult intestinal infections occasional. [Gk *gnathos* jaw, *stoma* mouth.]

gnathostomatics (nath·o·sto·mat′·ix). Physiology in its application to the jaws and mouth. [see prec.]

gnathostomiasis (nath·o·sto·mi′·as·is). Infection with the parasite *Gnathostoma.*

gnoscopine (nos·ko·peen). DL-Narcotine, $C_{22}H_{23}O_7N$. An alkaloid derived structurally from benzyl isoquinoline, and obtained during the preparation of narceine from opium.

gnosia (no·se·ah). The perceptive faculty of recognizing the nature and form of living beings and inanimate things. [Gk *gnosis* knowing.]

gnosis (no·sis). The faculty of knowing. Of the cerebral cortex, the arousing of associative memories by means of sensory impulses (Edinger). [Gk knowing.]

gnostic (nos·tik). 1. Relating to the finer and discriminative aspects of sensibility (e.g. the recognition of objects, tactile discrimination, etc.) as distinct from the cruder forms of sensory perception (crude touch, pain, temperature). 2. Relating to knowledge; occult, mystic. 3. Early Christian heretic claiming esoteric spiritual knowledge. [Gk *gnosis* knowing.]

gnotobiotics (no·to·bi·ot′·ix). The study of germ-free animals reared under sterile conditions. [Gk *gnotos* known, *bios* life.]

Godélier, Charles Pierre (b. 1813). French physician.

Godélier's law. Tuberculosis of the peritoneum is always associated with disease of the pleural membranes.

godet (god·et). 1. A drinking cup [obsolete term]. 2. Scutulum. [Fr.]

Godfrey's cordiale. A sweetened and flavoured tincture of opium, a preparation rarely prescribed in modern medicine.

Godman, John Davidson (b. 1794). Maryland and Philadelphia anatomist.

Godman's fascia. The continuation of the pretracheal fascia into the thorax.

Goethe, Johann Wolfgang von (b. 1749). German poet, philosopher and scientist.

Goethe's bone. 1. A large wormian bone at the junction of the occipital and parietal bones. 2. The premaxilla.

goitre (goi·ter). An enlargement of the thyroid gland; it is usually taken to mean a visible enlargement, but see, for example, intrathoracic goitre (below). **Aberrant goitre, Accessory goitre.** Enlargement of an accessory mass of thyroid tissue. **Acute goitre.** A goitre of sudden onset. **Adenomatous goitre.** A goitre containing adenomata. **Amyloid goitre.** Enlargement of the thyroid due to amyloid disease. **Cabbage goitre.** A goitre which develops from a diet of cabbage or other similar vegetables. **Cancerous goitre, Carcinomatous goitre.** Carcinoma of the thyroid gland. **Colloid goitre.** Enlargement of the thyroid gland due to the accumulation of large quantities of colloid substance in the acini. **Congenital goitre.** Goitre present from birth. **Cyanide goitre.** Experimental tumour of the thyroid gland produced by cyanide. **Cystic goitre.** Goitre containing cysts. **Diffuse goitre.** General enlargement of the thyroid without palpable nodules. **Endemic goitre.** Goitre occurring commonly in a particular geographical area. **Exophthalmic goitre.** Goitre associated with protrusion of the eyeballs. **Fibrous goitre.** A goitre containing a high proportion of fibrous tissue. **Follicular goitre.** Goitre in which the follicles of the gland are distended with colloid; colloid goitre. **Hyperplastic goitre.** An enlarged thyroid gland characterized by abnormal multiplication of the epithelial cells lining the acini. **Intrathoracic goitre.** A goitre wholly or partially within the thorax. **Iodine deficiency goitre.** Occurring sometimes during adolescence in girls or during pregnancy, or when the soil, water and food are low in iodine. **Goitre due to iodine excess.** Some cough mixtures contain iodine and may produce enlargement of the gland. **Lingual goitre.** A swelling on the back of the tongue due to enlargement of a thyroid gland which has failed to descend into the normal position in the neck. **Lymphadenoid goitre.** A condition in which the normal thyroid tissue has been replaced by tissue resembling lymph glands. When the whole of the normal thyroid tissue has been thus replaced, the condition is known as *Hashimoto's disease.* **Malignant goitre.** A goitre which is the seat of malignant new growth. **Nodular goitre.** A goitre containing nodules. **Non-toxic goitre.** Goitre that is not producing excess of hormone. **Parenchymatous goitre.** Enlargement of the thyroid due to increase in the epithelium without colloid accumulation. **Plunging goitre.** A substernal goitre that becomes visible on coughing or swallowing. **Retrosternal goitre.** A goitrous enlargement of a part or whole of the thyroid gland that is lying behind the sternum. **Retrovascular goitre.** An intrathoracic goitre situated behind the great vessels. **Sarcomatous goitre.** Sarcoma of the thyroid gland. **Simple goitre.** A goitre which is not producing the signs and symptoms of hyperthyroidism. **Sporadic goitre.** Non-toxic non-endemic goitre. **Substernal goitre.** A goitre which lies behind the sternum. **Thiouracil goitre.** Goitre due to administration of drugs of the thiouracil group. **Toxic goitre.** A goitre which is producing the signs and symptoms of hyperthyroidism. [L *guttur* throat.]

See also: HASHIMOTO.

goitrogen (goi·tro·jen). A substance that causes goitre. [goitre, Gk *genein* to produce.]

gold (go·ld). An element of atomic weight 196.97, atomic number 79 and chemical symbol Au (*aurum*). It is a yellow metal, highly ductile and malleable, with a melting point 1063°C and volatilizing 100°C above that. It is a good conductor of heat and electricity, resists corrosion and is unattacked by most aids and reagents. It occurs in the free state in quartz veins mainly in South Africa, North America (California, Klondike), and in Russia. It is sometimes found alloyed with silver and is a micro-constituent of sea water. Alloyed with silver and copper it is used in coinage, jewellery and dentistry; also alloyed with platinum. Its compounds are employed in medicine, mainly in rheumatoid arthritis, and in photography. **Adhesive gold.** Cohesive gold (see below). **Annealed gold.** Gold which has been heated to make it more pliable. **Gold bromide.** Auric bromide, $AuBr_3$, formerly used combined with potassium bromide as potassium bromaurate, $KAuBr_4$, in the treatment of epilepsy, hysteria, neurasthenia and whooping-cough. **Cohesive gold.** Pure gold which forms a solid mass when packed piece by piece in a cavity prepared in a tooth. **Colloidal gold.** Formed by striking an arc between gold electrodes under water, or by the reduction of gold solutions with formaldehyde; formerly used intramuscularly or intravenously. **Crystal gold.** Cohesive gold (see above) composed of a mass of crystals. **Gold cyanide.** Fused potassium cyanide for the extraction of gold. **Non-cohesive gold.** Gold which is forced piece by piece into a cavity prepared in a tooth without uniting to form a solid mass. **Platinized gold.** Gold used in dental restorations to which platinum has been added to make it harder. **Gold sodium thiomalate.** Sodium aurothiomalate. **Gold sodium thiosulphate.** Sodium aurothiosulphate. [AS.]

Goldblatt, Harry (b. 1891). Cleveland physiologist.

Goldblatt's clamp. A short clamp inserted partially to occlude the renal artery and produce experimental hypertension.

Goldblatt's hypertension. Hypertension experimentally produced by constricton of renal arteries and consequent ischaemia of the kidneys; attributed to the liberation of a pressor substance, renin.

golden rod (go·ldn rod). The herb *Solidago virgaurea* Linn. (family Compositae), an infusion of which is used as a carminative and diaphoretic. [AS *gold, rodd.*]

golden seal (go·ldn seel). The common name for *Hydrastis canadensis* Linn. (family Ranunculaceae). [AS *gold,* O Fr. *seel.*]

Goldflam, Samuel Vulfovich (b. 1852). Warsaw neurologist.

Goldflam's disease, Erb-Goldflam disease or syndrome, Goldflam-Erb disease, Hoppe-Goldflam syndrome. Myasthenia gravis.

Goldman, Victor Abraham. 20th century London anaesthetist.

Goldman's halothane vaporizer. An apparatus for vaporizing halothane in an anaesthetic machine; commonly used in dental anaesthesia.

Goldman's inhaler. An apparatus from which the vapour of vinyl ether is delivered to the patient for anaesthesia.

Goldmann, Hans (b. 1899). Swiss ophthalmologist.

Goldmann's applanation tonometer. An instrument used for measuring intra-ocular pressure; it is especially valuable in cases of suspected glaucoma. Its use eliminates the effect of scleral rigidity, which is a source of error in estimating intra-ocular pressure with the conventional form of tonometer.

Goldmann's contact lens. One containing a small mirror which also allows examination of the angle of the anterior chamber with the slit lamp and Goldmann's prism.

Goldmann's prism. A special prism that fits on to the arm of the slit lamp and, combined with Goldmann's contact lens, enables the angle of the anterior chamber to be examined, i.e. gonioscopy.

Goldscheider, Alfred (b. 1858). Berlin Physician.

Goldscheider's disease. Epidermolysis bullosa.

Goldscheider's percussion. Threshold percussion; percussion performed by tapping lightly upon a glass-rod pleximeter, one end of which is covered with a rubber cap and rests upon an intercostal space. The method confines the vibrations to a very small area, and has been used to delimit the boundaries of organs such as the heart.

Goldscheider's test. The slightly pointed end of a heated metal cylinder is applied to the skin to determine the hot spots.

Goldstein, Eugen (b. 1850). Berlin physicist.

Goldstein's rays. Positive rays; a radiation observed by Goldstein in 1886 to pass through the cathode of a discharge tube when it took the form of a metal netting. It is now known to be a stream of positive ions.

Goldstein, Hyman Isaac (b. 1887). Camden, New Jersey, physician.

Goldstein's haematemesis. Haematemesis due to bleeding from multiple telangiectases of the gastric mucous membrane.

Goldstein's sign. Wideness of the space between the 1st and 2nd toes, seen in mongolism and occasionally in cretinism.

Goldstein's operation. For lagophthalmos or exophthalmos; a recession of the levator palpebrae superioris muscle which is sutured to the skin just below the eyebrow.

Goldstein-Gelb-Weigl-Scheerer test. A test in which objects must be sorted in various categories, revealing a concrete or abstract mental aptitude.

Goldstein-Scheerer test. A performance test used for studying brain function: a test involving the arrangement of wooden blocks, used to assess the function of conceptual thought. Impairment of performance in this test is particularly common after diffuse brain injury.

Goldthwait, Joel Ernest (b. 1866). Boston surgeon.

Goldthwait brace. A device used for spinal support in ambulant patients.

Goldthwait operation. Transplantation of the patella tendon for recurrent dislocation of the patella.

Goldthwait's sign. Flexion of the straight leg at the hip elicits pain in the sacro-iliac region in sprain of the sacro-iliac ligaments.

Golgi, Camillo (b. 1844). Italian anatomist and histologist.

Golgi's apparatus or body. A specialized region of the cytoplasm, often close to the nucleus, which is composed of stacks of flattened cisternae, numerous vesicles and some larger vacuoles. In secretory cells it is concerned with packaging the secretory product. It is also probably concerned in some cells with the secretion of polysaccharides but its full range of functions has not yet been elucidated.

Golgi's cell. 1. An astrocyte. 2. Name given to 2 types of nerve cell within the grey matter of the central nervous system, one with long processes (type I), the other with short (type II).

Golgi corpuscle. A tendon spindle; a fusiform tension receptor found at the musculotendinous junction.

side fibril of Golgi. A collateral given off from an axon near the cell body.

Golgi's law. The number of parasites in the red blood cells determines the severity of an attack of malaria.

Golgi's method. For the demonstration of nerve cells and their processes; there are three variations: 1. The *quick method* in which an osmic-bichromate mixture is used on fresh tissues. 2. The *slow method* in which after prolonged bichromate fixation the tissues are treated with silver nitrate or mercuric chloride. 3. The *mixed method* in which the tissues are first fixed in bichromate mixture and then treated first by an osmic-bichromate solution and then by silver nitrate.

Golgi's organ. The nerve-ending of a muscle spindle.

rosette of Golgi. A cyst containing spores arranged in the form of a rosette.

Golgi's solution. A mixture of chromic acid and potassium dichromate used as a histological fixative.

Golgi stain. *See* GOLGI'S METHOD (above).

Golgi's theory. The theory that in the central nervous system each neurone and its processes is an anatomically-independent structure, i.e. nerve fibres from different nerve cells do not form a continuous network.

Holmgren-Golgi canal. Intracytoplasmic canal; one of a system of fine canals in the cytoplasm of many cells.

Golgi-Mazzoni bodies or corpuscles. Encapsulated sensory nerve-endings found in the superficial and deep connective tissues of the body; they resemble lamellated corpuscles but are much smaller. They are also known as *Krause's terminal bulbs.*

Golgi-Rezzonico spirals or threads. The fibrils supporting the myelin globules of the myelin sheath of a nerve fibre which appear to be arranged in spiral fashion around the axon.

golgiosome (gol·je·o·some). A cytoplasmic body, having similar staining reactions to the Golgi apparatus, and thought to represent a dispersed element of the latter. The Golgi apparatus of vertebrates may disperse in various physiological and pathological conditions; in invertebrates the dispersed condition is apparently normal. [Golgi apparatus, Gk *soma* body.]

Goll, Friedrich (b. 1829). Zürich anatomist.

column or fasciculus of Goll, Goll's tract. Fasciculus gracilis; fibres which ascend in the medial part of the posterior columns of the spinal cord; they arise from cells in the spinal ganglia from the level of the 7th thoracic segment downwards, and end in the gracile nucleus.

Goll's nucleus. A nucleus in the medulla oblongata in which the fibres of the fasciculus gracilis terminate; the gracile nucleus.

Golonbov's sign. Tenderness over the tibiae on percussion in certain blood conditions such as chlorosis.

Goltz, Friedrich Leopold (b. 1834). Königsberg and Strasbourg physiologist.

Goltz experiment. The demonstration in the frog of the reflex inhibition of the heart beat when the abdomen is tapped.

Goltz theory. The theory that the function of the semicircular canals is to be excited by changes in the position of the head, and so to aid in maintaining equilibrium.

Goltz, Robert William (b. 1923). American dermatologist.

Goltz syndrome. Dental anomalies, syndactyly and focal dermal hypoplasia; autosomal dominant.

Gombault, François Alexis Albert (b. 1844). Paris neurologist.

Gombault's degeneration or neuritis. Periaxial segmental degeneration of nerves.

Gombault's triangle, Gombault-Philippe triangular bundle, triangular tract of Gombault-Philippe. The septomarginal tract of the spinal cord in the sacral region.

Gompertz's law. A relation which can be expressed statistically exists between the probability of death from a given disease and the age of the person affected.

gomphiasis (gom·fi·as·is). A pathological condition in which the teeth become loose in their sockets, particularly the molar teeth. [Gk *gomphios* grinder tooth.]

gomphosis (gom·fo·sis). One of the suture forms of fibrous joint in which an immovable hard conical process lies within a socket. That type of attachment in which a tooth lies in a bony socket to which it is attached by the periodontal membrane, allowing limited physiological movement to occur. [Gk *gomphos* bolt.]

gonad (gon·ad) (pl. *gonads* or *gonades*). 1. A reproductive gland or group of glands. 2. An ovary. 3. A testis. **Female gonad.** Ovary. **Indifferent gonad.** In embryology, the early stage of the basic germinal epithelium before the derivation of the definitive sex cells. **Male gonad.** Testis. [Gk *gone* seed.]

gonadal (gon·ad·al). Relating or belonging to a gonad.

gonadectomy (gon·ad·ek·to·me). Surgical removal of the ovary or the testis. [gonad, Gk *ektome* a cutting out.]

gonadoblastoma (gon·ad·o·blast·oma). An ovarian tumour of ill-defined cellular origin and doubtful malignancy that secretes androgens and may therefore give rise to female pseudohermaphroditism of gonadal rather than adrenal origin.

gonadocentric (gon·ad·o·sen'·trik). Concerned with the phase of development when the libido is centred on the gonads.

gonadokinetic (gon·ad·o·kin·et'·ik). Having the power to stimulate gonadal activity. [gonad, Gk *kinesis* movement.]

gonadotherapy (gon·ad·o·ther'·ap·e). Treatment by injection of an extract (hormone) prepared from the testis or ovary. [gonad, therapy.]

gonadotrope (gon·ad·o·trope). 1. An individual whose endocrine constitution is of the gonadal type. 2. A gonadotropic substance. [gonad, Gk *tropos* a turning.]

gonadotrophic (gon·ad·o·trof'·ik). 1. Relating or belonging to gonadotrophism. 2. Pertaining to the genitalia.

gonadotrophin (gon·ad·o·trof'·in). Any substance which regulates the activity of the gonads. Such substances are present in extracts of the pituitary glands (*pituitary gonadotrophin*), in the blood (*serum gonadotrophin*), and in the urine (*chorionic gonadotrophin*) of pregnant animals or women. The known pituitary gonadotrophins are: 1. Follicle-stimulating hormone (FSH), a peptide hormone secreted by the anterior pituitary. It regulates the development of the Graafian follicle in the female and of spermatogenesis in the male. Its secretion is controlled by the activity of FSH-releasing factor, an oligopeptide hormone from the hypothalamus. 2. Luteinizing hormone (LH), a peptide hormone secreted by the anterior pituitary. It controls luteinization in the female and testosterone production in the male; with FSH it regulates oestrogen production by the ovary. Its secretion is controlled by the activity of LH-releasing factor, an oligopeptide hormone from the hypothalamus. [gonad, Gk *trophe* nutrition.]

gonadotrophism (gon·ad·o·trof'·izm). That state in which the gonads and their secretions exert a predominant influence on the bodily constitution. [gonad, Gk *trophe* nutrition.]

gonadotropic (gon·ad·o·trop'·ik). Having special affinity for the gonads; relating or belonging to gonadotropism. [gonad, Gk *tropos* a turning.]

gonadotropin (gon·ad·o·**trop**′·in). Gonadotrophin.

gonadotropism (gon·ad·**ot**·rop·izm). The type of endocrine constitution in which the secretion of the gonads exerts a predominant influence. [gonad, Gk *tropos* a turning.]

gonaduct (**gon**·ah·dukt). 1. The vas deferens. 2. The uterine tube. [gonad, duct.]

gonae (**gon**·e). The genitalia. [L fr. Gk *gone* seed.]

gonagra (gon·**ag**·rah). Gout in the knee joint. [Gk *gony* knee, *agra* a catching.]

gonalgia (gon·**al**·je·ah). Pain in the knee or knee joint. [Gk *gony* knee, *algos* pain.]

gonangiectomy (**gon**·an·je·**ek**′·to·me). Surgical excision of the vas deferens, or of a portion of it. [Gk *gone* seed, angiectomy.]

gonarthritis (gon·ar·**thri**·tis). Inflammation of the knee joint or of the knee. [Gk *gony* knee, arthritis.]

gonarthrotomy (gon·ar·**throt**·o·me). Surgical incision into the knee joint. [Gk *gony* knee, *arthron* joint, *temnein* to cut.]

gonatocele (**gon**·at·o·seel). 1. A swelling in the knee. 2. A tumour of the knee. [Gk *gony* knee, *kele* hernia.]

gonda reflex. Dorsiflexion of the big toe upon plantar flexion and sudden release of the 4th or 5th toes, analogous to the Babinski sign.

gondi (**gon**·di). A North African rodent *Ctenodactylus gundi* in which *Toxoplasma gondi* was first discovered.

gonecyst, gonecystis (**gon**·e·sist, gon·e·**sis**·tis). A seminal vesicle. [Gk *gone* seed, *kystis* bag.]

gonecystitis (**gon**·e·sis·**ti**′·tis). An inflamed condition of the seminal vesicles. [gonecyst, Gk *-itis* inflammation.]

gonecystolith (gon·e·**sis**·to·lith). A calculus present in a seminal vesicle. [gonecyst, Gk *lithos* stone.]

gonecystoncus (**gon**·e·sis·**tong**′·kus). Any tumour of a seminal vesicle. [gonecyst, Gk *ogkos* a swelling.]

gonecystopyosis (**gon**·e·sis·to·pi·**o**′·sis). A condition in which pus forms in and is discharged from a seminal vesicle. [gonecyst, pyosis.]

goneitis (gon·e·i·tis). Inflammation of the knee. [Gk *gony* knee, *-itis* inflammation.]

gonepoiesis (**gon**·e·poi·**e**′·sis). The formation of semen. [Gk *gone* seed, *poiein* to make.]

gonepoietic (**gon**·e·poi·**et**′·ik). Relating or belonging to gonepoiesis.

gongrona (gon·**gro**·nah). Goitre. [Gk *goggrone* ganglion.]

Gongylonema (**gon**·jil·o·**ne**′·mah). A genus of nematode worms. **Gongylonema hominis, Gongylonema pulchrum.** A common parasite of domestic ruminants, occurring in the oesophageal epithelium, and occasionally found in man in Southern USA and Italy. It burrows rapidly about the mouth and lips. [Gk *goggylos* round, *nema* thread.]

gongylonemiasis (**gon**·jil·o·ne·**mi**′·as·is). Infection with the nematode parasite Gongylonema.

gonic (**gon**·ik). 1. Having relation or belonging to generation. 2. Relating or belonging to the semen. [Gk *gone* seed.]

gonid, gonidium (**gon**·id, gon·**id**·e·um). 1. The algal part of a lichen. Early observers considered the algal hosts as possibly reproductive in nature and applied to them the term gonidia. The algae concerned are usually the blue-green (Myxophyceae) or the green algae (Chlorophyceae). 2. The name has also been applied to endospores of fungi, particularly the sporangiospore of *Mucor*. [Gk *gone* seed.]

Gonin, Jules (b. 1870). Lausanne ophthalmologist.

Gonin's operation, for retinal detachment. The original thermocautery operation for retinal detachment, also called *ignipuncture*. The beginning of successful surgical treatment of retinal detachment; of historical interest.

goniocheiloschisis (go·ne·o·ki·**los**′·kis·is). A congenital defect in which the mouth is abnormally wide, due to a failure of fusion between maxillary and mandibular processes. [Gk *gonia* angle, *cheilos* lip, *schisis* cleavage.]

goniocraniometry (go·ne·o·kra·ne·**om**′·et·re). Measurement of the angles of the skull. [Gk *gonia* angle, craniometry.]

gonioma (gon·e·**o**·mah). A tumour originating in the sex cells. [Gk *gone* seed, *-oma* tumour.]

goniometer (go·ne·**om**·et·er). 1. An instrument with which angles can be measured, e.g. the angle between two articulating bones. 2. In craniometry, an instrument with which the angles of the skull can be measured. 3. An appliance used in static testing of disease of the labyrinth. The patient stands on a plank one end of which is gradually raised and the degree of angulation of plank and floor at which he can no longer maintain balance is noted. 4. A device for measuring optical angles, particularly of crystals. **Vesical goniometer.** An instrument with which the angle between the long axis of the urethra and a line extending from the internal orifice to the orifice of the ureter can be measured. [Gk *gonia* angle, meter.]

gonion (**go**·ne·on). In craniometry, the outer point of the angle of the mandible. [Gk *gonia* angle.]

goniophotography (**go**·ne·o·fo·**tog**′·raf·e). Photography of the angle of the anterior chamber of the eye, with a gonioscopic contact lens. [Gk *gonia* angle, photography.]

goniopuncture (**go**·ne·o·**pungk**′·tcher). Goniotomy procedure wherein the gonio-knife incises the trabecular wall so that the point appears subconjunctivally, producing an exit for aqueous humour from the anterior chamber to the subconjunctival space. [Gk *gonia* angle, L *punctura* puncture.]

gonioscope (**go**·ne·o·skope). An instrument for rendering visible the angle of the anterior chamber. It consists of a special type of contact lens, and in one model (Goldmann's) a small mirror is incorporated. [Gk *gonia* angle, *skopein* to view.]

gonioscopy (go·ne·**os**·ko·pe). The examination of the angle of the anterior chamber of the eye with a gonioscope. **Slit-lamp gonioscopy.** Gonioscopy performed using the slit lamp for illumination and magnification. [Gk *gonia* angle, *skopein* to view.]

goniotomy (go·ne·**ot**·o·me). An operation devised by Otto Barkan for removing obstructions to the entry of aqueous into the canal of Schlemm. It is usually performed with his gonioscopic contact lens and is of especial service in hydrophthalmos (infantile glaucoma or buphthalmia). [Gk *gonia* angle, *temnein* to cut.]

gonitis (gon·i·tis). Inflammation of the knee or knee joint. [Gk *gony* knee, *-itis* inflammation.]

gonoblast (**gon**·o·blast). In biology, any reproductive cell or bud. [Gk *gonos* generation, *blastos* germ.]

gonoblennorrhoea (**gon**·o·blen·o·**re**′·ah). 1. Gonorrhoea. 2. Gonorrhoeal conjunctivitis. [Gk *gone* seed, blennorrhoea.]

gonocampsis (gon·o·**kamp**·sis). Gonycampsis.

gonocele (**gon**·o·seel). Spermatocele; a testicular tumour or a swelling of the spermatic cord resulting from retention of seminal fluid. [Gk *gone* seed, *kele* hernia.]

gonochorism (gon·**ok**·or·izm). 1. In embryology, sex differentiation. 2. In biology, separation of sex. 3. The separation of the sexes or the development of sexual distinction in racial evolution. [Gk *gone* seed, *chorisis* separation.]

gonocide (**gon**·o·side). Gonococcide.

gonococcaemia (**gon**·o·kok·**se**′·me·ah). The condition in which gonococci are present in the circulating blood. [gonococcus, Gk *haima* blood.]

gonococcal, gonococcic (gon·o·**kok**·al, gon·o·**kok**·sik). Relating or belonging to the gonoccus.

gonococcide, gonococcocide (gon·o·**kok**·side, gon·o·**kok**·o·side). Any agent which has the power to destroy the gonococcus. [gonococcus, L *caedere* to kill.]

gonococcus (gon·o·**kok**·us). *Neisseria gonorrhoeae*. [Gk *gone* seed, *kokkos* berry.]

gonocyte (**gon**·o·site). 1. A primary sex cell before sex differentiation takes place. 2. A cell from which gametes are derived. 3. Applied to a maturing ovum when it is at the stage at which the polar bodies are separated off so that it contains only the female pronucleus (Van Beneden). 4. Myeloblast. **Primary gonocyte.** A primordial germ cell arising in the wall of the yolk sac and migrating into the genital ridge. **Secondary gonocyte.** The primitive germ cell arising in the germinal epithelium covering the genital ridge. [Gk *gone* seed, *kytos* cell.]

gonocytoma (gon·o·si·to'·mah). A tumour originating from a gonocyte. [gonocyte, Gk *-oma* tumour.]

gonohaemia (gon·o·he·me·ah). Gonococcal septicaemia. [gonococcus, Gk *haima* blood.]

gonoid (gon·oid). Having resemblance to semen. [Gk *gone* seed, *eidos* form.]

gonomery (gon·om·er·e). In cytology, the condition in which the maternal and paternal chromosomes remain discrete at fertilization, instead of forming one body. [Gk *gone* seed, *meros* part.]

gonone (go·no·ne). Local name in Celebes for *Microtrombidium wichmanni*, a mite which attacks man.

gononephrotome (gon·o·nef·ro·tome). In the embryo, that differentiated part of the secondary mesoderm from which the organs of reproduction and excretion develop. [Gk *gone* seed, *nephros* kidney, *tome* section.]

gonophage (gon·o·faje). The bacteriophage which uses the gonococcus as its host. [gonococcus, Gk *phagein* to eat.]

gonophore, gonophorus (gon·o·for, gon·of·or·us). Any accessory structure of the generative organs which stores or conducts the sexual cells, e.g. uterine tube, seminal vesicle. [Gk *gone* seed, *pherein* to bear.]

gonopoiesis (gon·o·poi·e'·sis). Gonepoiesis.

gonopoietic (gon·o·poi·et'·ik). Gonepoietic.

gonoreaction (gon·o·re·ak'·shun). An old name for the gonococcal complement-fixation test. [gonococcus, reaction.]

gonorrhoea (gon·o·re·ah). An inflammatory disease of the genito-urinary passages characterized by pain on micturition and a purulent discharge and, later, by long continued chronicity with few or no symptoms. It is usually acquired during coitus, and less commonly by homosexual practice among men. The causative micro-organism is the *Neisseria gonorrhoeae* which is readily found in stained films and cultures of the discharge. Gonorrhoea is the oldest known venereal disease and is prevalent over the whole world. In males the disease may spread to involve the epididymis, prostate gland and seminal vesicles. Persistent chronic urethritis may produce a stricture. In females the urethra and cervical canal are first affected, from which the infection may spread to the uterus, uterine tubes and ovaries; the rectum may also be involved. In both sexes iritis, polyarthritis and, rarely, endocarditis, may ensue. Vulvovaginitis and proctitis occur in little girls from contaminated bedding or toilet articles or, more rarely, from sexual assault. Ophthalmia neonatorum may be of gonococcal origin and is due to contamination of the baby's eye during birth from the infected mother. Gonococcal ophthalmia from direct transference of infective discharge to the eye of the adult sufferer, or physician or nurse, is rare. **Black gonorrhoea.** Gonorrhoea with black or bloody discharge. [Gk *gone* seed, *rhoia* flow.]

gonorrhoeal (gon·o·re·al). Relating or belonging to gonorrhoea.

gonoscheocele (gon·os·ke·o·seel). Swelling of the testis due to the accumulation of seminal fluid. [Gk *gone* seed, *oscheon* scrotum, *kele* hernia.]

gonosome (gon·o·some). Sex chromosome. *See* CHROMOSOME.

gonotome (gon·o·tome). That portion of the early embryonic mesoderm lying between the somite and the lateral plate, which gives rise to the gonad and neighbouring urinary organs. [gonad, Gk *tome* section.]

gonotoxaemia (gon·o·tox·e'·me·ah). Toxaemia resulting from infection by the gonococcus.

gonotoxic (gon·o·tox·ik). Caused by gonococcus infection, or by the toxin of gonorrhoea.

Gonyaulax (gon·e·aw·lax). A genus of planktonic Protozoa. *Gonyaulax catenella* and probably other species have been shown to be the main cause of shellfish poisoning on the North American Pacific seaboard. The molluscs feed on the *Gonyaulax* which contain a toxin. The 'Red Tide' is the phenomenon seen when a massive generation of the Protozoa colour the sea, and is a warning that shellfish in the affected area will be toxic if eaten. [Gk *gony* knee, *aulax* furrow.]

gonycampsis (gon·e·kamp·sis). Ankylosis of the knee joint or any deformity of the knee caused by abnormal curvature. [Gk *gony* knee, *kampe* a bending.]

gonycrotesis (gon·e·kro·te'·sis). Genu valgum (knock knee). [Gk *gony* knee, *krotesis* a striking.]

gonyectyposis (gon·e·ek·ti·po'·sis). Genu varum (bow leg). [Gk *gony* knee, *ektyposis* displacement.]

gonyoncus (gon·e·ong·kus). A tumour swelling of the knee. [Gk *gony* knee, *ogkos* a swelling.]

Gooch, Benjamin (c. 1700–1776). Norwich surgeon.

Gooch splint. A flexible splint made of strips of wood glued to cloth or leather.

Gooch, Frank Austin (b. 1852). American chemist.

Gooch crucible. A porcelain vessel with a hole in the bottom, used for the evaporation of liquids or solutions in conjunction with the Gooch filter.

Gooch filter. A layer of asbestos upon the perforated bottom of a Gooch crucible.

good faith (gud·fathe). The term used in statutory English law on abortion to describe the attitude of mind in those properly undertaking the termination of a pregnancy: an indication of honesty of purpose, of abiding by the proper concept of the law. [AS *got* root, ME *feit* trust.]

Goodall, Edward Wilberforce (b. 1861). London physician.

Goodall's illness or infection. A mild febrile attack with malaise and a fleeting rash that may occur within a few hours of infection in certain specific fevers, notably measles.

Goodell, William (b. 1829). Philadelphia gynaecologist.

Goodell's law or sign. The softening of the cervix in pregnancy.

Goodpasture, Ernest William (b. 1886). Nashville, Tennessee, pathologist.

Goodpasture's stain. A peroxidase stain containing sodium nitroprusside, benzidine and basic fuchsine.

Goodpasture's syndrome. A rare condition which combines haemoptysis, anaemia and glomerulonephritis, leading to renal failure.

Goodsall's stitches. Interlocking mattress stitches inserted in prolapsed rectal mucosa before its excision.

Goormaghtigh, Norbert (b. 1890). Ghent pathologist.

Goormaghtigh cells. The juxtaglomerular apparatus in the wall of the afferent arteriole of the glomerulus.

Gordh, Torsten. 20th century Stockholm anaesthetist.

Gordh needle. An intravenous needle with an expanded butt bearing a small rubber diaphragm. This is left in place in a vein so that repeated intravenous injections may be given during the course of an operation.

Gordiacea (gor·de·a·se·ah). Horse-hair worms; a phylum or class of worms. Their larvae are parasitic in insects, but the adults are free living. Genera of medical interest are *Gordius*, *Parachordodes* and *Paragordius*. [see foll.]

Gordius (gor·de·us). A genus of Gordiacea, horse-hair worms. **Gordius aquaticus.** A species which resembles an animated horse-hair; it is occasionally swallowed in drinking water and later vomited. [after the Gordian knot.]

Gordon, Alfred (b. 1874). Philadelphia neurologist.

Gordon's reflex. An extensor-plantar response produced by squeezing of the calf muscles; an elaboration of the Babinski reflex, it is also called the *paradoxical flexor reflex*, and is seen in pyramidal-tract disease.

Gordon, Mervyn Henry (b. 1872). London bacteriologist.

Gordon's test. A flocculation or precipitation test for differentiating smallpox from chickenpox. Saline extracts of dried crusts are added to dilutions of serum obtained from a rabbit immunized against vaccinia. The occurrence of flocculation after a period of incubation indicates the presence of smallpox or vaccinia virus, but not of chickenpox virus.

Gordon, Walter. 20th century British surgeon.

Green-Gordon tube. An endobrachial tube designed for insertion into the right main-stem bronchus, used in anaesthesia for operations on the left lung.

gorget (gor·jet). A guiding instrument with a wide groove used in lithotomy. **Probe gorget.** A gorget with a pointed tip. [Fr. *gorge* throat.]

gorgoya (gor·goi·ah). A name used in Somalia for the tick-conveyed relapsing fever of Central Africa.

Gorham, L. Whittingham. 20th century American physician.
Gorham's disease. Massive osteolysis or vanishing-bone disease.

Gorlin, Robert J. (b. 1923). American professor of oral pathology.
Gorlin's syndrome. Disorders of the skin such as milia, basal cell naevi or carcinomata, and palmar-plantar dyskeratosis; multiple cysts of the jaws and abnormalities of the central nervous system such as calcification of the falx cerebri, absent corpus callosum and medulloblastoma; disorders of the skeletal system including bifid ribs, fused vertebrae and ocular hypertelorism.

gorondou (go·ron·doo). Goundou.

Gosselin, Léon Athanese (b. 1815). French surgeon.
Gosselin's fracture. V-shaped fracture of the distal end of the tibia.

Gossypium (gos·ip·e·um). A genus of perennial shrubs (family Malvaceae) widely cultivated for the production of cotton. A number of species are grown including *Gossypium barbadense* Linn. (West Indies). *G. herbaceum* Linn. (India, Egypt and North America), *G. hirsutum* (North America), and *G. peruvianum* (South America). Cotton is prepared from the long epidermal hairs on the seeds. **Gossypium Acidi Borici BPC 1949.** Absorbent cotton impregnated with boric acid. **Gossypium capsicum.** Absorbent cotton impregnated with capsicum and methyl salicylate. **Gossypii cortex.** Cotton root bark, the dried bark obtained from the root. It has been used as an emmenagogue. **Gossypium purificatum.** Absorbent cotton. *See* COTTON. [Gk *gossypion* cotton-tree.]

gossypol (gos·e·pol). $C_{30}H_{30}O_8$, a poisonous tannin-like substance obtained from cotton seed.

Gottinger's line. A line which lies parallel to the zygomatic arch along its superior margin.

Gottlieb, Bernhard (b. 1885). Vienna dentist.
epithelial attachment of Gottlieb. The attachment of the gingiva to a tooth, formed during eruption of the tooth by the fusion of the remains of cells of the enamel organ lying on the surface of the enamel with the deep layers of cells of the oral epithelium; initially attached to the crown, it later moves down to become attached to the root during the process of continuous eruption of the tooth.

Gottstein, Jacob (b. 1832). Breslau otolaryngologist.
Gottstein's fibres or process. An outward prolongation in the organ of Corti of any outer hair cell that connects this cell to the basilar membrane.

gouge (gowj). A surgical chisel with a strong convex blade used in operations on hard structures such as bone. [Fr. scoop.]

Gougerot, Henri (b. 1881). Paris dermatologist.
Gougerot's disease or syndrome. A syndrome consisting of nodules, erythematous macules, purpura and urticaria; blisters may also occur. The eruption is chiefly on the limb, and is thought to be an allergic phenomenon.
de Beurmann-Gougerot disease. Sporotrichosis.
Gougerot-Hailey-Hailey disease. Chronic benign familial pemphigus.

Goulard, Thomas (b. 1697). Montpellier surgeon.
Goulard's cerate. Ointment of lead subacetate.
Goulard's extract. Strong lead subacetate solution.
Goulard's powder. Lead acetate.
Goulard's water. Dilute lead subacetate solution.

goundou (goon·doo). A bilateral hyperostosis of the nasal bones which occurs in indigenous natives who have been infected with yaws, especially in West Africa. Originally sufferers were termed "the horned men of Africa". A similar disease occurs in the larger apes, chimpanzees and baboons, and has been demonstrated in ancient Inca skulls. As the tumour grows, it encroaches on the orbits and may interfere with vision. [West African name.]

Gouraud, Vincent Ollivier (b. 1772). Tours surgeon.
Gouraud's disease. Inguinal hernia. *See* HERNIA.

gout (gowt). A disease of the purine metabolism, characterized by attacks of arthritis with an associated raised serum uric acid. The big toe is the joint most commonly affected. There is often a familial history. In chronic cases renal failure may ensue and there may be deposits of uric acid in the subcutaneous tissues, forming *tophi.* These are often found in the pinna of the ear. It occurs more commonly in men than in women. **Abarticular gout.** Gout involving structures other than joints. **Calcium gout.** Acute episodes of joint pain and swelling in association with deposition of calcium salts. **Chalk gout.** The usual term for tophaceous gout (see below). **Irregular gout.** Abarticular gout (see above). **Latent gout.** Hyperuricaemia without the clinical features of gout; the gouty diathesis often found in the relatives of sufferers from gout. **Lead gout.** Gout ascribed to chronic lead poisoning. **Oxalic gout.** A perversion of the oxalate metabolism, associated with painful symptoms. **Polyarticular gout.** An unusual form of gout in which many joints are affected; it is sometimes mistaken for rheumatic fever, and attacks may last for a considerable time, passing from joint to joint. **Poor-man's gout.** Gout ascribed to hard work, exposure, wrong diet and an excess of malt liquors. **Retrocedent gout.** Term used for the type of gout in which articular symptoms alternate with the abarticular syndrome. **Rheumatic gout.** An archaic term for rheumatoid arthritis, formerly believed to be due to a gouty diathesis. **Saturnine gout.** Lead gout (see above). **Tophaceous gout.** Gout in which chalky deposits of sodium biurate occur (tophi). These are most usually situated under the skin in the cartilage of the ear, or of any of the joints, especially those of the fingers, and may ulcerate, discharging periodically their chalky content; more deeply situated tophi may be detected by x-rays. In time these tophi may almost destroy any joint with which they are associated. **Visceral gout.** 1. An 18th-century concept accounting for visceral pain of unknown origin. 2. A disease of hens and turkeys. [L *gutta* drop, from the ancient belief that the noxa was distilled drop by drop into the affected joints.]

goutte militaire (goot mil·e·tare). Gleet. [Fr. military drop.]

gouty (gow·te). Pertaining to, suffering from, or having the character of gout.

Gowers, Sir William Richard (b. 1845). London neurologist.
Gowers' tonic atrophy. A muscular wasting that occurs in progressive muscular atrophy, especially that associated with amyotrophic lateral sclerosis.
column, fasciculus or tract of Gowers. The superficial fibres in the lateral columns of the spinal cord which form the anterior spinocerebellar and the lateral spinothalamic tracts.
Gowers' contraction. Front tap contraction; contraction of the gastrocnemius muscle when the muscles of the front of the leg are tapped.
Gowers' disease. Saltatory spasm; also called *Bamberger's disease.*
Gowers' muscular dystrophy. Distal myopathy.
Gowers' diluting fluid or solution. A diluting solution containing sodium sulphate 12.5 g, acetic acid 33.3 g, distilled water 200 ml, used for the enumeration of red blood corpuscles.
Gowers' haemoglobinometer. A graduated tube with a standard colour tube for determining, as oxyhaemoglobin, the haemoglobin in the blood.
Gowers' panatrophy. Sharply-defined atrophy of the skin and subcutaneous tissue occurring without preceding inflammation and without scleroderma.
Gowers' paraplegia. Paraplegia secondary to vertebral osteitis.
Gowers' phenomenon. Pain along the course of the sciatic nerve on dorsiflexion of the foot in sciatica.
Gowers' intermediate process. The lateral grey horns of the spinal cord.
Gowers' reflex. Achilles-tendon reflex. *See* REFLEX.
Gowers' sign. 1. Early in the course of tabes dorsalis, light thrown upon the retina may cause intermittent oscillations of

the iris. 2. In weakness of proximal leg muscles, especially in muscular dystrophy, the method of rising from the ground by placing the hands on the knees.

Gowers' symptom. Gowers' sign, 1st def. (see above).

Gowers' syndrome. Vasovagal attacks. *See* ATTACK.

Goyrand, Jean Gaspard Blaise (b. 1803). Paris surgeon.

Goyrand's hernia. Funicular hernia; inguinal hernia into a partial sac.

Graaf, Reijnier (Regnier) de (b. 1641). Dutch physician and anatomist.

Graafian follicle. A follicle which matures in each ovarian cycle. It may be the follicle which in that particular cycle ruptures and discharges an ovum. It is lined with epithelial cells and surrounded by a stromal capsule; a vesicular ovarian follicle.

Graber–Duverney operation. Drilling the neck of the femur with the object of increasing the blood supply of the femoral head in osteoarthritis.

gracile (gras·ile). Slight or slender; delicate; thin. [L *gracilis* slender.]

gracilis muscle [musculus gracilis (NA)] (gras·il·is). A muscle arising from the body of the pubis and the ischiopubic ramus, and inserted on the medial side of the upper end of the tibia. [L slender.]

Gradenigo, Giuseppe (b. 1859). Naples otologist.

Gradenigo's syndrome. 6th cranial-nerve paralysis and pain in the area supplied by the 5th cranial nerve, due to infection of the apex of the petrous part of the temporal bone from otitis media on the same side.

Gradenigo's test. A test for auditory fatigue in cases of nerve deafness: a tuning-fork vibrating at about 4000 Hz is held close to the meatus. Once it ceases to be audible, it is withdrawn, and then, still vibrating, applied again to the ear. This procedure can be repeated several times in cases of auditory-nerve deafness.

gradient (gra·de·ent). 1. Inclination to the horizontal. 2. The rate at which a quantity increases or decreases with distance or time. **Axial gradient.** Any regular variation of a biological property along the axis of an organism, whether it be morphological or biochemical. **Physiological gradient.** A line of progressive increase or decrease in the intensity of any function of a part. **Pressure gradient.** The difference between the pressures of the blood on the two sides of a cardiac valve during the period when the valve is open. Normally the gradient is negligible but when valve stenosis is present it may be large and its magnitude can be used to assess the severity of the stenosis. **Ventricular gradient.** In cardiology, the axis of the mean vector of ventricular polarization and repolarization in the frontal plane. [L *gradus* step.]

grading (gra·ding). *See* BRODERS. [see prec.]

graduated (grad·ew·a·ted). 1. Progressive. 2. Divided into or marked by degrees, as a flask. 3. Arranged in steps, layers or lines. [L *gradus* step.]

Graefe, Friedrich Wilhelm Ernst Albrecht von (b. 1828). Berlin ophthalmologist.

Graefe's disease. Progressive paralysis of the extra-ocular muscles.

Graefe's knife. A narrow knife used in cataract operations.

von Graefe's operation. 1. For squint: tenotomy of the muscle through a preliminary conjunctival incision. 2. For glaucoma: broad iridectomy, originally described by von Graefe, 1857. 3. For cataract: a linear section made with a Graefe knife combined with an iridectomy, the capsule being opened with a cystotome. 4. For conical cornea: cauterizing the apex of the cone; obsolescent.

von Graefe's phenomenon. An absolute and reflex paralysis of the pupil to light on very marked abduction of the eye. There is a latent period before contraction takes place.

von Graefe's lid reaction. Westphal–Pilcz reaction.

Graefe section. Cataract section: the incision made into the eye through which the cataractous lens is extracted. Classically this is through the upper half of the limbus, and is made with a Graefe knife.

von Graefe's sign. Lagging of the upper lid behind the globe when the eye looks downwards, occurring in thyrotoxic exophthalmos.

pseudo-Graefe phenomenon or sign. Retraction of the upper lid on looking down in cases of recovering 3rd cranial-nerve paralysis.

Graefe–Saemisch operation. Saemisch operation.

Graefenberg, Ernst (b. 1881). German gynaecologist.

Graefenberg ring. A ring of coiled silver wire inserted into the uterine cavity to prevent implantation of the fertilized ovum.

Graeupner, Salo (b. 1861). German physician.

Graeupner's method. A method of measuring the work performed by a patient in turning a wheel provided with a brake and at the same time measuring the blood pressure, on the assumption that the blood pressure of a strong heart rises during exercise but that of a weak heart fails.

Graffi, Arnold. 20th century American virologist.

Graffi virus. An RNA-containing virus associated with a transmissible leukaemia in mice.

graft (grahft). 1. A portion of tissue removed from one site and placed at another, either in the same or in another individual, in order to repair a defect caused by operation, accident or disease. 2. To remove such a piece of tissue and place it in a new site. **Accordion graft.** A full-thickness graft (see below) with multiple slits cut in it so that it will stretch. **Activated graft.** Hyperplastic graft (see below). **Allograft, Allogeneic graft.** Graft from a donor who belongs to the same species as the recipient but is genetically dissimilar. **Arterial graft.** A portion of artery transplanted to replace an arterial defect. **Autodermic graft, Auto-epidermic graft.** A skin graft transferred from one site to another in the same individual. **Autogenous graft, Autoplastic graft.** A graft transplanted from one site to another in the same individual; autograft. **Blanket graft.** A thick graft. **Bone graft.** A portion of bone removed from its site and inserted to repair a defect in another bone. **Bridging graft.** A graft left attached at both ends during the first stage of its transplantation. **Bucket-handle graft.** *See* TUBE GRAFT (below). **By-pass graft.** In cardiovascular surgery, a tubular graft inserted to by-pass an obstruction in the arterial system. **Cable graft.** A graft formed by a bundle of segments from a small unimportant nerve, inserted to repair a defect in a larger important nerve. **Cadaver graft.** A graft, of cornea or artery, removed from an individual after death to repair a defect in the living body. **Calibrated graft.** Thick split-skin graft (see below). **Cancellous graft.** A bone-grafting technique using fragments of cancellous bone. **Cartilage graft.** A portion of cartilage removed from one site to repair a cartilage defect in another. **Chondrocutaneous graft.** A graft composed of cartilage and skin, e.g. from the pinna. **Chorio-allantoic graft.** A graft of fetal membrane used to repair a surface defect. **Composite graft.** A graft composed of more than one type of tissue. **Corneal graft.** A portion of cornea, usually from fresh cadaver or from enucleated eye, employed to replace a cornea rendered opaque by disease. **Coronary arterial venous by-pass graft.** The use of a length of vein (usually saphenous) taken from the patient to by-pass an obstruction in a coronary artery; one end is inserted into the aortic wall and the other end into the coronary artery distal to the obstruction. **Delayed graft.** A skin graft partially elevated and replaced again for later transfer. **Derma-fat-fascia graft.** A graft of skin together with its underlying fat and fascia. **Dermal graft, Dermic graft.** Any skin graft which contains dermis, and is therefore capable of sweating, sebum secretion, hair growth and of withstanding trauma. **Double-end graft.** Tube graft (see below). **Epidermic graft.** Split-skin graft (see below). **Fascia graft, Fascial graft.** A graft of fascia, usually of fascia lata, used for the repair of a membrane such as the abdominal wall at a hernia, or the dura mater at the site of a defect. **Fat graft.** A portion of fat removed from its site to fill a cavity, or to return movement between two abnormally-adherent surfaces. **Free graft.** A graft completely detached from its original site and replaced at a new site by a one-stage operation. **Full-thickness graft.** A skin graft which includes the whole thickness of the skin without any attached fat, first described by Lawson. **Heterodermic graft.** A heterogenous graft (see following) of skin. **Heterogenous graft.** A portion of tissue removed from a donor of one species to apply to a recipient of another species; such a graft does not "take". **Heterologous graft, Heteroplastic graft.** Heterodermic graft (see above). **Heterotopic graft.** Tissue for a graft taken from some other part of the body. **Homogenous graft, Homologous graft.** A portion of tissue removed from a donor to be applied to a recipient of the same species; such grafts survive for a very short period except in the case of cornea, artery, bone, cartilage and perhaps endocrine tissue; homograft. **Homoplastic graft.** A homogenous graft (see preceding) of skin. **Hyperplastic graft.** A graft which is in an active state of repair. **Implantation graft.** Thick split-skin graft (see below). **Inlay graft.** A bone graft inserted into a suitably-shaped excavation in the surface of the recipient bone. **Intermediate graft.** Thick split-skin graft (see below). **Intramedullary graft.** A bone graft whose ends are inserted in the narrow cavities of the recipient fragments, the defect between which it serves to repair. **Island graft.** A graft left attached only by feeding vessels passing to its deep surface. **Isogeneic graft, Isograft.** Graft of tissue from donor to genetically identical recipient, e.g. identical twin. **Isoplastic graft.** Autoplastic graft (see above). **Jump graft.** A tube graft (see below) temporarily attached to an intermediate site for carriage to a distant recipient area; for example, a tube graft from abdomen to wrist and, later, wrist to face. **Lamellar graft.** Inset corneal graft applicable to superficial corneal scars. **Mucosal graft.** A graft of mucous membrane. **Muscle graft.** A graft of muscle, usually to occlude a cavity. **Nerve graft.** The transplantation of a portion of nerve to replace a defect in a second and more important nerve. **Omental graft.** A portion of omentum transplanted to repair a defect, e.g. a perforation in a hollow viscus. **Onlay graft.** A bone graft applied directly to the unbroken surface of the recipient bone. **Organ graft.** The transplantation of a whole organ from one site to another. **Osseous graft.** Bone graft (see above). **Osteoperiosteal graft.** A portion of bone which is transplanted together with its periosteum to another site. **Ovarian graft.** The transplantation of slices of ovary from one site to another. **Parathyroid graft.** The burial of parathyroid glands, removed accidentally at thyroidectomy, in the muscles of the neck. **Pedicle graft.** A skin graft which is left attached at one end, until its free end has "taken" at the recipient site or at a desired intermediate site. **Periosteal graft.** Osteoperiosteal graft (see above). **Pinch grafts.** Small, circular, deep grafts a few millimetres in diameter, sliced off so that the centre is of whole skin, the periphery of epidermis only. **Postage-stamp grafts.** Split-skin grafts cut up into small segments. **Razor graft.** Thick split-skin graft (see below). **Rope graft.** Cable graft (see above). **Seed graft.** Implantation graft (see above). **Sieve graft.** The converse of pinch graft (see above); a sheet of thick skin raised to contain multiple perforations so that tiny islands like pinch grafts are left at the donor site for regenerative purposes. **Skin graft.** A portion of skin removed, in one or more stages, from one site, the "donor" area, to repair a defect at another site, the "recipient" area. **Sleeve graft.** An operation, now obsolete, in which a tube-like structure such as a vein is inserted into the gap between widely separated cut nerve endings, in the hope that it would serve as a guide for the regenerating nerve fibrils. **Split-skin grafts.** Grafts of part of the thickness of the skin; thick split-skin grafts are perhaps the only variety now employed. **Stent graft.** A skin graft adapted to the recipient area by the pressure upon it of a suitably-shaped mould of the malleable plastic material "Stent's composition". **Syngeneic graft.** Isogeneic graft (see above). **Tendon graft.** Transplantation of a portion of one tendon to replace a defect in another, or the transplantation of the insertion of a tendon to alter the line of pull of the muscle to which it is attached. **Testis graft.** The transplantation of a portion of testis. **Thick split-skin grafts.** Free grafts of large sheets of skin, usually by one-half to almost full thickness; the graft commonly employed to replace skin defects after burns. **Thyroid graft.** Transplantation of portions of thyroid gland for the treatment of myxoedema. **Tube graft.** A pedicle graft of skin left initially attached at both ends (bucket-handle graft), with its cutting edges sutured to each other so that the epithelial surface faces outward; at successive stages first one end and then the other are transplanted to a new site, with or without temporary attachment (jump graft) to an intermediate site. **Tunnel graft.** A skin graft used to form the lining of a cavity. **Vascular graft.** A portion of a blood vessel (artery or vein) taken from the patient (autograft) or from a donor (homograft) and used, often after preservation chemically or by freezing, to bridge a gap in a damaged blood vessel, usually an artery. **Vein graft.** A vein, usually the long saphenous vein of the patient (autograft), used to replace or by-pass an obstructed artery. **Xenogeneic graft.** Graft from a donor of a species different from the recipient. **Zooplastic graft.** Tissue removed from a donor animal to recipient man, especially kangaroo tendon, beef-bone chips and ivory inlay. [Gk *graphion* stylus, from resemblance of a plant graft.]

See also: BLAIR, BRITTAIN, BROWN (J. B.), DAVIS, DOUGLAS (B.), ESSER, GALLIE, KRAUSE (F. V.), OLLIER, REVERDIN (J. L.), THIERSCH, WOLFE.

grafting (**grahf**·ting). The preparation and application of a graft or grafts.

graft-rejection (**grahft**·re·**jek**'·shun). Cellular response by the host evoked by transplantation of genetically dissimilar tissue, leading to the destruction of the transplanted tissue. [Gk *graphion* stylus, from resemblance to a plant graft, L *rejicere* to throw back.]

Graham, Evarts Ambrose (b. 1883). St. Louis surgeon.

Graham's operation. Total removal of the lung for carcinoma. Total pneumonectomy.

Graham test. The original method of visualizing the gall bladder radiologically by oral or intravenous administration of sodium tetraiodophenolphthalein. It has been superseded by oral administration of iopanoic acid which is a contrast medium containing approximately 66 per cent iodine. It is absorbed in the small intestines, excreted by the liver in the bile, and shows maximum concentration in the gall bladder within 10-12 h. When the gall bladder contracts in response to a fatty meal, the contrast medium is expelled through the bile ducts which can then be demonstrated radiographically. It is of great value in determining the size of the gall bladder, its power of concentration and contraction, and in demonstrating the presence of filling defects due to stones or new growths within its lumen.

Graham-Cole test. Cholecystography.

Graham, George Sellers (b. 1879). Albany, New York, pathologist.

Graham's benzidine stain. A peroxidase stain with benzidine as the main constituent.

Kay-Graham pasteurization test. Phosphatase test. *See* TEST.

Graham, Sylvester. 19th century American physician.

Graham bread. Bread made from entire wheat flour.

Graham, Thomas (b. 1805). Glasgow and London chemist.

Graham's law. The velocity with which a gas diffuses is inversely proportional to the square root of its density.

Graham swab. A modified NIH swab. *See* SWAB.

grain (grane). 1. A seed of a cereal. 2. A unit of weight equal to 64.798 mg: one seven-thousandth part of a pound, the twentieth part of a scruple, symbolized gr. 437.5 grains equal 1 oz. [L *granum.*]

grains (gra·nz). 1. Any small particles or bodies, usually hard, e.g. of sand; granules. 2. Small parakeratotic cells in the vesicles, and superficial to the stratum granulosum, in ichthyosis hystrix. 3. In radiotherapy, small pieces of fine radioactive wire (usually gold, Au^{198}) encased in a β-ray screen (usually platinum) for implantation into tissues to be irradiated by γ-rays. **Cayenne-pepper grains.** Term applied to the brick-red urinary deposit of uric-acid crystals coloured by absorbed urinary pigments. **Grains of**

paradise. The seeds of *Aframomum melegueta* (Rosc.) K. Schum. (family Zingiberaceae); they contain a volatile oil and a pungent substance, and are used in veterinary medicine as a carminative. [see prec.]

See also: FOLLIN.

Gram, Hans Christian Joachim (b. 1853). Copenhagen physician.

Gram's method, for bacteria in paraffin sections. Sections are stained successively in haematoxylin, eosin and aniline methyl violet. Nuclei are stained blue, cytoplasm red and bacteria violet.

Gram's method or stain (Jensen's modification). A differential stain for bacteria. Heat-fixed films are stained with 0.5 per cent aqueous methyl violet for 1 min, treated with 1 per cent iodine in 2 per cent potassium iodide for 30 sec, decolorized with alcohol and counterstained for from 1 to 2 min with 1 per cent neutral red in 2 per cent acetic acid. Gram-positive organisms stain violet, and Gram-negative organisms stain pink.

Gram's solution. 1 g iodine and 2 g potassium iodide dissolved in 300 ml water.

Gram's stain. A staining method for differentiating and classifying micro-organisms. There are several variations of procedure, but see Gram's method (above).

Gram-Weigert method, for bacteria in celloidin sections. Sections are first stained with lithium carmine to demonstrate cell nuclei, then with aniline gentian violet, and differentiated with iodine to show bacteria. For *Trichophyton* in hair: the technique is as outlined, but the differentiation is effected very slowly by iodized aniline oil. The fungus is stained dark blue.

gram (gram). A unit of mass now defined as a thousandth part of a kilogram. [Fr.]

gram-calorie (gram·**kal**·or·e). A unit of heat; the small calorie: equal to 4.1855 J. Abbreviated, gcal.

gram-equivalent (gram·ek·**wiv**·al·ent). The chemical equivalent or combining weight of any substance in grams.

gram-ion (gram·**i**·on). The sum of the atomic weights of the atoms in an ion expressed in grams.

gram-metre (gram·**me**·ter). A unit of work defined as the work necessary to raise 1 g of weight 1 m against gravity.

gram-mole (gram·**mole**). Gram-molecule.

gram-molecular (gram·mol·**ek**·ew·lar). Pertaining to the gram-molecule.

gram-molecule (gram·**mol**·e·kewl). The molecular weight of a substance in grams.

Gram-negative, Gram-positive (gram·**neg**·at·iv, gram·**poz**·it·iv). Classificatory terms providing a most important division of the bacteria: according to the ability of the bacteria to retain the violet of Gram's stains, those that do so are designed Gram-positive, those that do not, Gram-negative.

gram-rad (gram·**rad**). In radiology, a unit of absorbed dose. 1 gram-rad equals 10 μJ (100 ergs). [gram, radiation.]

gram-roentgen (gram·**runt**·yen). In radiology, a unit of total energy absorption for ionizing radiation. 1 gram-roentgen equals 8.38 μJ (83.8 ergs). [gram, roentgen.]

gramicidin (gram·**is**·id·in). One of the antibiotics produced by *Bacillus brevis* which is specifically effective against Gram-positive bacteria. It is a polypeptide of particular interest since half of the amino-acid residues are in the D-form, a configuration rarely found naturally. [Hans Christian Joachim *Gram,* L *caedere* to kill.]

Gramineae (gram·**in**·e·e). The grass family; a large family of plants which includes the important cereals, barley, maize, oats, rice, rye, sugar cane and wheat. The plants are characterized by their long hollow stems, with simple sessile leaves, and flowers which are hermaphrodite, much reduced and arranged in spikes. The fruit is a caryopsis or grain. [L *gramen* grass.]

gramme (gram). Gram.

granatum (gran·a·tum). Pomegranate. [L.]

Grancher, Jacques Joseph (b. 1843). French physician.

Grancher's granular breathing. The irregular coarse sounds suggestive of, but not actually identifiable as, distant or fine râles, as heard over the early lesions in pulmonary tuberculosis.

Grancher's sign. Equality of pitch of the inspiratory and expiratory breath sounds when there is obstruction to breathing.

Grancher system. A system devised under the title of "Oeuvre Grancher" for protecting the young children of tuberculous parents against infection. The children are removed from infected homes and boarded out with healthy country families.

Grancher's triad. Decreased air entry, skodaic resonance and increased vocal fremitus; thought at one time to indicate early pulmonary tuberculosis.

Granger, Amedée (b. 1879). New Orleans radiologist.

Granger's line. A curved line seen in radiographs of the skull taken in Granger's position. It represents the superior surface of the sphenoid bone whereon lies the optic groove.

Granger's position. A position for obtaining an occipitofrontal view of the nasal sinuses in radiography. The patient lies prone with forehead and superior maxilla in contact with the cassette supported on a reverse 23 degree angle block. The tube is centred so that the central ray is projected through the head from above straight downward so that it will emerge at the glabella.

Granger's sign. If, in a lateral oblique radiograph of the mastoid region, the anterior wall of the lateral sinus is viewed as a hard distinct line, there is extensive acute infection of the mastoid cells. The sign occurs in infants and adults.

granoplasm (**gran**·o·plazm). Granuloplasm.

granula (**gran**·ew·lah). Any granule or other minute constituent of protoplasm. [L *granulum* little grain.]

granular (**gran**·ew·lar). 1. Having or composed of grains or granules. 2. Having the character of granules.

granulase (**gran**·ew·laze). A ferment in grain which hydrolyses starch into maltose.

granulation (gran·ew·**la**·shun). 1. The subdivision of a solid into small free-flowing particles, or the coalescence of the particles of a powder to form the same. 2. The formation of small rounded masses in tissues. 3. The development of young connective tissue and blood vessels on the surface of an ulcer or open wound. **Arachnoid granulations [granulationes arachnoideales (NA)].** Large clusters of arachnoid villi found in relation to the dural venous sinuses, especially the superior sagittal sinus. They increase in number and size with age, and may show calcification. **Cell granulation.** The appearance of numerous minute bodies in the cytoplasm of a cell. **Exuberant granulation.** Overgrowth of granulation preventing ingrowth of surrounding epithelium. **Pharmaceutical granulation.** The conversion of a powder into free-flowing granules. These granules may be used as such or they may be converted to tablets in a machine. Substances must be either crystalline or granular before they can be compressed, as fine powders, not being free-flowing, would block the machine. **Pyroninophilic granulations.** Small granules within cells, especially liver and plasma cells, that stain red with the methyl-green-pyronine stain of Pappenheim. [L *granulum* little grain.]

See also: BRIGHT, LANGLEY, PACCHIONI.

granule (**gran**·ewl). A small particle or grain; a small dry mass capable of free movement without adhering to its fellows. Granules, unlike particles of fine powders, are free-flowing because of the small surface forces involved. **Acidophil granule.** A cytoplasmic granule having an affinity for acid dyes such as eosin or acid fuchsine. **Agminated granule.** A fragment of a red blood cell present in the plasma. **Albuminous granule.** A small mass of albuminous protein in the cytoplasm of a cell. **Alpha granule.** Acidophil granule (see above) seen in leucocytes. **Amphophil granule.** A granule stainable with either acid or basic dyes. **Argentaffine granule.** A granule having an affinity for silver. **Azure granule, Azurophil granule.** A granule having a special affinity for azure dyes. **Basal granule.** The centriole at the base of a cilium or flagellum. **Basophil granule.** A granule having an affinity for basic dyes such as methylene blue. **Beta granule.** Basophil granule (see prec.) seen in leucocytes and rarely in the marrow. **Chromatic granule, Chromophilic granule.** A Nissl granule of a nerve cell. **Chromosome granule.** A gene locus on a chromosome. **Cone granule.** The nucleus of a cone retinal cell. **Cytoplasmic granule.** A granule in the cytoplasm of a cell, especially one having an affinity for acid or basic dyes. **Delta granule.** 1. A granule of a delta (δ) cell of the pancreatic islets of Langerhans. 2. A basophil granule (see above) seen in lymphocytes. **Eosinophil granule.** A cytoplasmic granule (see above) having an affinity for eosin. **Epsilon granule.** A neutrophil granule (see below) that occurs in polymorphonuclear leucocytes. **Fuchsinophil granule.** A cytoplasmic granule (see above) having an affinity for acid or basic fuchsine. **Gamma granule.** A basophil granule (see above) seen in the marrow and other tissues. **Interstitial granule.** A granule from the sarcoplasm of a striated muscle fibre. **Iodophil granule.** Bodies staining brown with iodine, seen in the polymorphonuclear cells during some acute infections. **Leucocyte granule.** One of the granules in the cytoplasm of a white blood corpuscle. **Mast-cell granule.** One of the large metachromatic granules (see below) in the cytoplasm of mast cells, believed to contain heparin. **Meningeal granules.** Pacchionian bodies. **Metachromatic granules.** Deeply-staining bodies seen in the cytoplasm of some bacteria, e.g. *Corynebacterium diphtheriae*; Babes-Ernst granules. **Neutrophil granule.** One of the granules of neutrophil polymorphonuclear leucocytes which has a slight affinity for both acid and basic dyes. **Oxyphil granule.** Acidophil granule (see above). **Pigment granule.** One of the coloured granules of a pigmented cell. **Polar granule.** Metachromatic granule (see above). **Protein granules.** Tiny masses of protein within cells. **Rod granule.** The nucleus of a retinal rod cell. **Secretory granule.** One of the zymogen granules of exocrine secretory cells. **Seminal granule.** One of the granules found in seminal fluid. **Sulphur granules.** Peculiar yellow granules found in the pus from actinomycosis lesions. **Tannophil granules.** Granules that stain specifically after treatment by a tannin mordant. **Thread granule.** A filamentous mitochrondrion. **Toxic granules.** Basophil-staining granules seen in the cytoplasm of leucocytes under the influence of toxic substances or infections. **Vitelline granule.** Yolk granule (see foll.). **Yolk granule.** One of the granular bodies found in the developing egg, from which the yolk is formed. **Zymogen granule.** One of the secretory granules (see above) found in the cytoplasm of salivary and pancreatic cells. [L *granulum* little grain.]

See also: ALTMANN, BABÈS, BENSLEY, BOLLINGER, ERNST, FAUVEL, GRAWITZ, KOELLIKER, LANGLEY, MUCH, NISSL, PANETH, PASCHEN, PLEHN, SCHRIDDE, SCHUEFFNER, ZIMMERMANN (G. H. E.).

granuliform (gran·ew·le·form). 1. Granular in structure. 2. In the form of granules or small grains. 3. Resembling granules or grains.

granulitis (gran·ew·**li**·tis). Acute miliary tuberculosis. [granule, Gk *-itis* inflammation.]

granulo-adipose (gran·ew·lo·**ad'**·e·poze). Characterized by a type of fatty degeneration in which granules of fat are present. [granule, L *adeps* fat.]

granuloblast (gran·ew·lo·blast). A stem of haemopoietic organs which gives rise to granular leucocytes (neutrophils, eosinophils and basophils). [granule, Gk *blastos* germ.]

granulocorpuscle (gran·ew·lo·**kor'**·pusl). A small corpuscle found in infected tissue in lymphopathia venereum. [granule, corpuscle.]

granulocytaemia (gran·ew·lo·si·**te'**·me·ah). An uncommon condition in which the numbers of platelets, or thrombocytes, in the blood are considerably increased, sometimes to as much as 2 000 000 per ml^3. [granulocyte, Gk *haima* blood.]

granulocyte (gran·ew·lo·site). Any cell the cytoplasm of which contains granules, particularly a leucocyte in which are basophil, eosinophil or neutrophil granules. [granule, Gk *kytos* cell.]

granulocytopenia (gran·ew·lo·si·to·**pe'**·ne·ah). A deficiency of granulocytes in the blood. [granulocyte, Gk *penia* poverty.]

granulocytopoiesis (gran·ew·lo·si·to·poi·**e'**·sis). The formation of granulocytes; in the adult this takes place in the red marrow of flat bones. [granulocyte, Gk *poiein* to make.]

granulocytopoietic (gran·ew·lo·si·to·poi·**et'**·ik). 1. Having relation to granulocytopoiesis. 2. Able to produce or excite more vigorous formation of granulocytes.

granulocytosis (gran·ew·lo·si·**to'**·sis). The presence of an unusually large number of granulocytes in the circulating blood. [granulocyte, Gk *-osis* condition.]

granulofilocyte (gran·ew·lo·**fil'**·o·site). A reticulocyte, i.e. a recently-formed circulating blood cell reticular in structure. [granule, L *filum* thread, Gk *kytos* cell.]

granuloma (gran·ew·**lo**·mah). A tumour composed of granulation tissue. **Amoebic granuloma.** A granuloma, usually in the large intestine, caused by *Entamoeba histolytica* infection and often simulating a neoplasm; an amoeboma. **Granuloma annulare.** Chronic eruption of papules which grow to form nodules and then coalesce to produce circinate or annular lesions, finally to disappear spontaneously. **Apical granuloma.** A mass of granulation tissue attached to the apex of a tooth formed as a result of infection in the root canal; a dental granuloma. **Asbestos granuloma.** A granulomatous nodule caused by implantation of asbestos in the skin. **Benign granuloma of the thyroid.** Lymphadenoma of the thyroid gland. **Beryllium granuloma.** A sarcoid-like granuloma in the skin, or in the lungs, due to occupational exposure to beryllium dust. **Coccidioidal granuloma.** The name applied to the relatively-rare progressive granulomatous stage of coccidioidomycosis. Before the commoner primary or benign stage of the disease was recognized the term was applied to all infections by *Coccidioides immitis.* **Granuloma contagiosum.** Granuloma inguinale (see below). **Dental granuloma.** Apical granuloma (see above). **Eosinophilic granuloma.** 1. A granuloma composed of eosinophilic cells, found as a localized tumour in the long bones of children. 2. Facial granuloma with eosinophilia. 3. Eosinophilic granuloma of the skin (Letterer-Christian disease, Letterer-Siwe and Jaffe-Lichtenstein's disorders). **Eosinophilic granuloma of the stomach.** A rare lesion usually in the pyloric area of the stomach, possibly of allergic origin. **Granuloma faciale.** Facial granuloma with eosinophilia; a benign, localized, red, infiltrated patch, of unknown cause, possibly an allergic vasculitis, but resistant to treatment. **Granuloma fissuratum.** A granuloma in the gingival sulcus caused by ill-fitting dentures, or in the postauricular fold from the pressure of the earpiece of spectacle frames. **Foreign-body granuloma.** The chronic inflammatory mass that collects around foreign bodies such as suture material, gravel or splinters, and contains at least one foreign-body giant cell. **Granuloma fungoides.** Mycosis fungoides. **Granuloma gangraenescens.** Progressive granuloma of the pharynx. **Histiocytic granuloma.** Histiocytosis X (Letterer-Christian disease). **Infectious granuloma.** A lumpy lesion of tuberculosis, syphilis, actinomycosis, etc. **Granuloma inguinale.** A chronic granulomatous ulceration of the skin of the genitalia and inguinal and anoperineal regions. The causal agent, *Donovania granulomatis* (Donovan body), is present in the mononuclear cells of the granulation tissue. The painless velvety ulcer spreads slowly and develops exuberant, friable, beefy-red granulations. Secondary infection leads to widespread ulceration and necrosis of the soft tissues. The disease is transmitted venereally but may be implanted on to regions distal from the primary site by the fingers. **Iodide granuloma.** A granulomatous eruption that occurs in persons on large doses of iodides: sensitivity sometimes develops, so that subsequent administration even in moderate doses will cause a recurrence. **Granuloma iridis.** Granulomatous tissue forming in the iris. It characterizes some forms of iritis, e.g. tuberculous and syphilitic. **Lipoid granuloma, Lipoid-cell granuloma.** Cholesteatoma; a granuloma that has formed around masses of lipoid material or cholesterol, e.g. a polypoid swelling in the rectum due to injection of oily preparations for the treatment of haemorrhoids. **Lipophagic granuloma.** A granuloma in which the cells have phagocytosed fat granules. **Lycopodium granuloma.** A granuloma in an operation wound caused by the spores of species of *Lycopodium*, club mosses. **Malarial granuloma.** An agglomeration of glia cells around a necrotic focus in the brain caused by a small haemorrhage in the brain; such haemorrhages are secondary to the blocking of arterioles by an aggregation of infected red blood cells that causes a localized anoxia. **Malignant granuloma, Granuloma malignum.** A malignant lymphoma, such as Hodgkin's sarcoma; a lymphosarcoma. **Midline granuloma.** A rare disease with granulomatosis of the respiratory tract, especially the nose and lungs, together with widespread vasculitis; Wegener's granuloma. **Granuloma multiforme.** A common skin condition occurring in northern Nigera, consisting of papules, nodules or plaques resembling, and possibly identical with, granuloma annulare. **Paracoccidioidal granuloma.** The South American type of blastomycosis which is caused by *Paracoccidioides* (*Blastomyces*) *brasiliensis.* **Granuloma pudendi.** Granuloma telangiectaticum (see below). **Granuloma pyogenicum.** Septic granuloma (see below). **Reticulo-endothelial systemic granuloma.** Histiocytosis X (Letterer-Christian disease). **Reticulohistiocytic granuloma.** Histiocytosis X (Letterer-Christian disease). **Sarcoid granuloma.** An epithelioid cell granuloma resembling sarcoidosis but without clinical or immunological evidence of sarcoidosis. Causes include foreign bodies, necrobiosis and granuloma annulare. **Granuloma sarcomatodes.** Mycosis fungoides. **Septic granuloma.** A fungating granuloma mass which is heavily infected. **Septic progressive granuloma.** Chronic and recurrent bacterial infections, only recorded in males, of undetermined cause, possibly genetically determined. Skin, respiratory and other infections occur repeatedly. **Swimming-pool granuloma.** Chronic infection of the skin by *Mycobacterium balnei* acquired in non-chlorinated swimming pools. **Talc granuloma.** A granuloma that may develop in the peritoneal cavity or surgical wounds as a result of the introduction of silicate of magnesium in the form of talc that has been used for treating surgical gloves. **Granuloma telangiectaticum.** 1. A highly vascular granuloma found in the nasal cavities and pharynx. 2. A bright red or bluish-black soft nodule in the skin, developing rapidly, bleeding easily and caused by proliferation of capillaries. It is benign but tends to regrow rapidly if it is incompletely removed. **Granuloma trichophyticum.** Granulomatous folliculitis and perifolliculitis on the legs from fungal infections, usually *Trychophyton rubrum.* **Granuloma tropicum.** Yaws [obsolete term]. **Ulcerating granuloma of the pudenda.** Granuloma inguinale (see above). **Umbilical granuloma.** Granulation tissue at the umbilicus persisting for 3 or 4 weeks. **Venereal granuloma, Granuloma venereum.** Granuloma inguinale (see above). **Zirconium granuloma.** A granuloma caused by a zirconium salt entering the skin, for example in the axillae from an antiperspirant. [granule, Gk *-oma* tumour.]

See also: HODGKIN, MAJOCCHI.

granulomatosis (gran·ew·lo·mat·**o**'·sis). A chronic inflammatory process leading to the formation of nodules or tumour-like masses. **Granulomatosis infantiseptica.** A generalized, highly fatal infection in babies following a symptomless intra-uterine infection by *Erysipelothrix monocytogenes* in the mother. **Lipoid granulomatosis.** Hand-Schueller-Christian syndrome. **Malignant granulomatosis.** Hodgkin's disease; lymphadenoma. **Granulomatosis siderotica.** A nodular fibrosis of the lungs due to iron-containing dusts. [granuloma, Gk *-osis* condition.]

granulopectic (gran·ew·lo·**pek**'·tik). 1. Relating or belonging to granulopexy. 2. Having the power to fix granules or granulocytes.

granulopenia (gran·ew·lo·**pe**'·ne·ah). Granulocytopenia. **Essential granulopenia.** Agranulocytosis.

granulopexy (gran·ew·lo·**pex**'·e). The process of fixation of granules. [granule, Gk *pexis* fixation.]

granulophthisis (gran·ew·lo·**thi**'·sis). A condition in which the material from which granulocytes are formed becomes degenerated or is destroyed; agranulocytosis. [granulocyte, phthisis.]

granuloplasm (gran·ew·lo·plazm). 1. That part of the protoplasm of a cell body which contains the paraplasm (granules). 2. The inner substance or cytoplasm of any unicellular organism such as an amoeba.

granuloplastic (gran·ew·lo·**plas**'·tik). Forming or producing granules. [granule, Gk *plassein* to mould.]

granulopoiesis (gran·ew·lo·poi·**e**'·sis). Granulocytopoiesis. [granulocyte, Gk *poieien* to make.]

granulopoietic (gran·ew·lo·poi·**et**'·ik). Granulocytopoietic.

granulopotent (gran·ew·lo·**po**'·tent). Possessing the power to form granules. [granule, L *potentia* power.]

granulosa (gran·ew·**lo**·sah). Membrana granulosa. [L *granulum* little grain.]

granulosarcoid, granulosarcoma (gran·ew·lo·**sar**'·koid, gran·ew·lo·sar·**ko**'·mah). Mycosis fungoides: a severe disease of the skin, particularly on the face, chest and scalp, characterized by dermatitis, infiltration and the formation of painful red tumours which later may ulcerate. The cause may be a bacterial infection and the outcome usually is fatal after an illness lasting for several years. [granule, sarcoid, sarcoma.]

granulose (gran·ew·loze). Obsolete name for the soluble starch within the starch granule; now known as *amylose.*

granulosis (gran·ew·**lo**·sis). Any morbid condition characterized by the accumulation of granules, or having the appearance of being covered with granules. **Granulosis rubra nasi.** A chronic sharply-defined erythema, with minute papules and beads of sweat, on the distal part of a child's nose. [granule, Gk *-osis* condition.]

granulosity (gran·ew·**los**·it·e). 1. A mass of any kind of minute granules. 2. A cluster of granulations. [see prec.]

granulotuberculoma (gran·ew·lo·tew·ber·kew·**lo**'mah). Any localized masses of tuberculous tissue which appear to the naked eye as minute granules. **Laryngeal granulotuberculoma.** Granules of tuberculous tissue protruding from the mucous membrane of the larynx. [granule, tuberculoma.]

granum (gra·num). Grain. [L.]

Granville, Joseph Mortimer (b. 1833). London physician.

Granville's hammer. An instrument used at one time in vibratory massage.

Graomys (gra·o·mis). A genus of South American rodents. **Graomys griseoflavus.** An Argentine species living wild and in house roofs; it is a suspected reservoir of plague. [Gk *graein* to gnaw, *mys* mouse.]

grape bark (**grape** bark). Cocillana BPC 1959. [O Fr. *grape*, Scandinavian *bark.*]

grapes (gra·ps). *See* CARSWELL. [O Fr. *grape.*]

graph (graf). 1. A continuous record upon a strip of paper or film of the variation in value of an attribute, usually obtained by a recording contrivance. 2. A diagrammatic representation upon squared paper of the relationship between two variables. [Gk *graphein* to record.]

graphaesthesia (graf·es·**the**·ze·ah). The ability to recognize letters or figures traced on the skin by blunt pressure, as in Foerster's cutaneous numeral test. [Gk *graphein* to record, *aisthesis* feeling.]

graphic (**graf**·ik). Relating or belonging to or represented by a diagram, curve or graph.

graphite (**graf**·ite). Black lead, plumbago. An allotropic form of carbon found naturally in Siberia, Sri Lanka and the USA, or made from amorphous carbon in an electric furnace. A soft dark-grey chemically-inert crystalline substance, used for lead pencils, electrodes, crucibles and as a lubricant. [Gk *graphein* to record.]

grapho-analysis (**graf**·o·an·**al**'·is·is). A form of psycho-analytic therapy in which patients write down their thoughts. [Gk *graphein* to record, analysis.]

graphocatharsis (graf·o·kath·**ar**'·sis). Grapho-analysis. [Gk *graphein* to record, catharsis.]

graphology (graf·ol·o·je). 1. The science and study of handwriting. 2. Graphopathology. [Gk *graphein* to record, *logos* science.]

graphomania (graf·o·ma·ne·ah). A morbid desire or irresistible urge to be always writing. [Gk *graphein* to record, mania.]

graphomotor (graf·o·mo·tor). 1. Affecting the movements concerned in the process of writing. 2. Relating or belonging to the movements used in writing. [Gk *graphein* to record, motor.]

graphopathology (graf·o·path·ol'·o·je). The study of handwriting for indications of disorder or disease, mental or physical. [Gk *graphein* to record, pathology.]

graphophobia (graf·o·fo·be·ah). Morbid fear of writing. [Gk *graphein* to record, phobia.]

graphorrhoea (graf·o·re·ah). In psychiatric medicine, a condition characterized by the occasional writing down of long lists of unassociated and meaningless words. [Gk *graphein* to record, *rhoia* flow.]

graphospasm (graf·o·spazm). Writers' cramp. *See* CRAMP. [Gk *graphein* to record, spasm.]

Grashey, Hubert von (b. 1839). Munich psychiatrist.

Grashey's aphasia. A form of aphasia encountered in concussion and in some acute diseases; sensory impressions last only a short time, so that association and perception cannot function properly.

grass (grahs). A general term applied to members of the family Gramineae; it also occurs in the common names of a number of plants. **Couch grass.** *Agropyron repens* Beauvois, the dried rhizome of which contains triticin. **Lemon grass.** Name given to two tropical species of *Cymbopogon*, *C. citratus* Stapf. and *C. flexuosus* Stapf. (family Gramineae) that yield an oil with a characteristic lemon-like odour, used mainly in perfumery. **Scurvy grass.** *Cochlearia officinalis* Linn., an extract of which has been used in the treatment of scurvy and other skin affections. **Timothy grass.** A common pasture grass that matures in early summer; a common cause of hay fever. [AS *graes.*]

Grasset, Joseph (b. 1849). Montpellier physician.

Grasset's law, Landouzy-Grasset law. In a unilateral cerebral lesion producing hemiplegia, the head is turned to the side of the cerebral lesion if paralysis is flaccid, and to the side of the affected limbs if spastic.

Grasset's phenomenon or sign, Grasset-Bychowski sign, Grasset-Gaussel phenomenon. A patient with a hemiparesis, in the supine position, may be unable to raise both legs together by flexion at the hip joint, though he can raise either separately.

Grasset, Gaussel and Hoover sign. If a patient with hemiplegia, lying in the supine position, attempts to raise the paralysed leg, while an observer's hand is resting beneath the sound leg, the pressure of the sound limb on the observer's hand is much greater than would be observed during the same action in a normal person.

gratification (grat·if·ik·a'·shun). The release of emotional tension which occurs when an instinctive desire or aim has been fulfilled. [L *gratificari* to cause to please.]

grating (gra·ting). A perforated frame having a geometrical pattern of holes, sometimes parallel slots. **Diffraction grating.** A glass plate, closely ruled with a series of parallel equidistant lines, which produces dispersion of white light passing through it. The lines may also be ruled on metals to produce spectra by reflection. [L *cratis* hurdle.]

Gratiola officinalis (grat·i·o·lah of·is·in·a'·lis). A perennial herb (family Scrophulariaceae) commonly known as *hedge hyssop.* The dried herb and an infusion of the root are used for their strong emetic and purgative properties. [L *gratia* grace, *officina* workshop.]

Gratiolet, Louis Pierre (b. 1815). Paris anatomist and physiologist.

ansa or ansa peduncularis of Gratiolet. The combined fibres of the ansa peduncularis and ansa lenticularis.

Gratiolet's bundle. Fibres which appear to come from the ventral surface of the thalamus and pass laterally to the cortex of the temporal lobe and insula.

Gratiolet's radiating fibres. The fibres contained in Gratiolet's radiation.

Gratiolet's radiation. The optic radiation. *See* RADIATION.

grattage (grat·ahzh). The scraping away of granulations with a stiff brush or rough sponge to stimulate the process of healing. [Fr. scratching.]

gravedo (grav·e·do). Coryza; catarrh of the nasal passages. [L.]

gravel (gravl). Very small or sand-like concretions of uric acid and other substances which constitute the basic material of calculus in the kidney. They may be voided in the urine. [Fr. *grave* sandy beach.]

graveolent (grav·e·o·lent). Fetid; having a rank odour. [L *gravis* heavy, *olere* to smell.]

Graves, Robert James (b. 1796). Dublin physician.

Graves' disease. Exophthalmic goitre. *See* GOITRE.

Graves' scapula. Scaphoid scapula. *See* SCAPULA.

gravid (grav·id). 1. Pregnant. 2. Containing a fetus. [see foll.]

gravida (grav·id·ah). A woman who is pregnant. **Gravida I.** A woman pregnant for the first time (primigravida). **Gravida II.** A woman pregnant for the second time (secundigravida). [L pregnant.]

gravidic (grav·id·ik). 1. Having relation to or occurring during pregnancy. 2. Referring to a pregnant woman. [see prec.]

gravidism (grav·id·izm). The physical and mental changes, taken as a whole, which are induced and produced by the state of pregnancy. [L *gravidus*, pregnant.]

graviditas (grav·id·it·as). Pregnancy. **Graviditas examnialis.** A condition in which the amnion has ruptured and has shrunk around the fetus. **Graviditas exochorialis.** Pregnancy in which the fetus forms outside the chorion but within the uterus. [L.]

gravidity (grav·id·it·e). The state of being pregnant. [see prec.]

gravidocardiac (grav·id·o·kar'·de·ak). Relating or referring to disorders of the heart induced by the state of pregnancy. [gravid, Gk *kardia* heart.]

gravimeter (grav·im·et·er). Gravitometer.

gravimetric (grav·e·met·rik). 1. Pertaining to measurement by weight. 2. Performed or determined by using the measurement of weight, not of capacity or size. [L *gravis* heavy, meter.]

gravistatic (grav·e·stat·ik). Relating to or caused by the force of gravitation; hypostatic. [L *gravis* heavy, Gk *statikos* standing.]

gravitation (grav·it·a·shun). 1. The force of attraction between bodies by reason of their mass. 2. The force exerted by the earth upon objects situated at a distance from its centre. [L *gravis* heavy.]

gravitol (grav·it·ol). $N(C_2H_5)_2(CH_2)_2OC_6H_3(OCH_3)C_3H_5$, the diethylamino-ethyl ether of 2-methoxy-6-allylphenol, a complex synthetic compound which on injection into animals has ergot-like action, causing weak contraction of the uterus but also marked slowing of the heart. Also known as *clavitol.*

gravitometer (grav·it·om·et·er). A special form of balance for comparing the weights of an object in air and in water, used in the determination of specific gravities. [L *gravis* heavy, meter.]

gravity (grav·it·e). 1. Weight; the forces of the earth's gravitational attraction. 2. Specific gravity; the weight of a substance compared with the weight of an equal volume of water at 4°C. [L *gravis* heavy.]

Grawitz, Paul Albert (b. 1850). Greifswald pathologist.

Grawitz's cachexia. Cachexia occurring in old people with severe anaemia.

Grawitz cell. A hypothetical undifferentiated connective-tissue cell.

Grawitz's degeneration. Basophilic degeneration. *See* DEGENERATION.

Grawitz's granules. Small granules seen in erythrocytes that show punctate basophilia following lead intoxication.

Grawitz's tumour of the kidney. A hypernephroma; the most common tumour of the renal parenchyma, now regarded as a renal carcinoma. The tumour cells have small nuclei and the protoplasm may be clear or granular, usually the former. The tumour structure is papillary or tubular, and metastases occur by the blood stream, chiefly to the bones and the lungs.

Gray, Thomas Cecil. 20th century Liverpool anaesthetist.

Gray's triad of anaesthesia. Narcosis, suppression of reflex activity and relaxation.

Greeff, Carl Richard (b. 1862). Berlin ophthalmologist.

Prowazek-Greeff bodies. Intracellular bodies found in trachomatous secretions and believed to represent a stage in the life history of the causal virus. Also called *Prowazek-Halberstaedter bodies.*

Green, John (b. 1835). St. Louis ophthalmologist.

Green's operation, for entropion. Incision through conjunctiva and tarsal plate 2 mm behind the meibomian openings; a 2-mm strip of skin is excised 1.5 mm above the lashes. Sutures are then passed from the conjunctival side of the lashes out through the skin wound and then deep and out 10 mm higher in the skin of the lid; they are tied loosely. Modified by Ewing.

Green, Ronald Alan. 20th century British anaesthetist.

Green-Gordon tube. An endobrachial tube designed for insertion into the right main-stem bronchus, used in anaesthesia for operations on the left lung.

green (green). 1. A colour of the visible spectrum, of wavelength between 492 and 575 nm; the pigment obtained by mixing yellow and blue pigments. 2. Raw; untreated. **Acid green.** The sulphonate of diethylbenzyl diaminotriphenyl carbinol used for staining plasma. **Benzaldehyde green.** Malachite green (see below). **Brilliant Green BP 1973.** A tetra-ethyl derivative of malachite green; it is a basic stain with bacteriostatic properties for Gram-positive bacteria used in differential culture media for salmonellae. **Bromcresol green.** Sodium tetrabromo-*m*-cresol sulphonephthalein, $(CH_3C_6HBr_2OH)_2CHC_6H_4SO_2ONa$, a dye used as an indicator (pH 4.5-5.5). **Brunswick green.** Copper oxychloride, $CuCl_2{\cdot}3Cu(OH)_2$, a pigment prepared from copper sulphate and bleaching powder. **Chrome green.** Chromic oxide, Cr_2O_3, used as a pigment in paint manufacture. **Diamond green.** Malachite green (see below). **Diazin green.** Janus green B (see below). **Ethyl green.** A synonym for brilliant green (see above) and for malachite green G (see below). **Imperial green.** Paris green (see below). **Iodine green.** A basic dye used as a nuclear stain; it is a phenolphthalein derivative, also used as an indicator (pH 1.0). **Janus green B.** An azo dye chiefly employed in the supravital staining of mitochondria. **Malachite green.** The oxalate of tetramethyl diaminotriphenyl carbinol $C_6H_5C(OH)[C_6H_4N(CH_3)_2]_2$, used as an antiseptic, especially against Gram-positive organisms. **Malachite green G.** A stain used as a counterstain in a modification of the Ziehl-Neelsen method for staining tubercle bacilli and in Albert's stain for *Corynebacterium diphtheriae.* Also as an inhibitory agent in the Loewenstein-Jensen medium. **Methyl green.** Chloromethyl hexamethyl-*p*-rosaniline hydrochloride, a dye used in tissue staining. **Methylene green.** A mononitromethylene blue formed by the action of nitrous acid on methylene blue; it is a green cotton dye. **Paris green.** Schweinfurt green (see below); the name is also applied sometimes to methyl green (see above). **Schweinfurt green.** Copper aceto-arsenite, $Cu(CH_3COO)_2{\cdot}3Cu(AsO_2)_2$, a poisonous arsenical used chiefly as an insecticide. **Swedish green.** Scheele's green, cupric arsenite, $Cu_3(AsO_3)_2{\cdot}2H_2O$; a green pigment, also employed as an insecticide. **Victoria green.** Malachite green (see above). [AS *grene.*]

See also: HOFMANN (A. W.), SCHEELE.

green t stoff (green te **shtoff**). A mixture of xylyl bromide and bromacetone which is powerfully lacrimatory; used in chemical warfare as a tear gas. [green, G *Stoff* substance.]

Green-Armytage, Vivian Bartley (b. 1882). Indian Medical Service and London gynaecologist.

Green-Armytage forceps. A specially designed pressure forceps for controlling haemorrhage from the uterus during caesarean section.

Green-Armytage operation. A method of transplanting the outer portions of the fallopian tubes into the uterus as a treatment for sterility due to localized tubal occlusion.

Greenberg's method. A method for estimating serum protein by the use of sodium sulphate.

Greene, Charles Lyman (b. 1863). St. Paul, Minnesota, physician.

Greene's sign. Displacement of the cardiac borders with respiration in pleural effusion.

Greenfield, Joseph Godwin (b. 1884). London neuropathologist.

Greenfield's disease. Demyelinating encephalopathy; also known as *Balo's disease.*

Greenfield manometer. A length of graduated glass tubing for the measurement of cerebrospinal-fluid pressure.

Greenfield lumbar-puncture needle. A lumbar-puncture needle with a three-way tap, designed for ease of manometry.

Greenhow, Edward Headlam (b. 1814). London physician.

Greenhow's disease. Vagabonds' disease; chronic pediculosis vestimentorum, with harsh, dry, scratched, crusted, pigmented skin.

Greenough binocular microscope. A microscope suitable only for lower powers, and giving a marked stereoscopic effect.

Greeves, Reginald Affleck (b. 1878). London ophthalmologist.

Greeves' operation. 1. For deepening the lower fornix of a deformed socket: the conjunctiva in the socket is incised, and is then stitched to the periosteum of the floor of the orbit with three mattress sutures brought out and tied on the skin of the cheek. 2. For ptosis: a modification of Motais' operation. Thin medial and lateral horizontal strips are cut from the upper border of the tarsal plate; these are left attached in the centre and sutured to the medial and lateral border of the tendon of the levator palpebrae superioris muscle.

greffotome (gref·o·tome). A surgical knife with which portions of skin or other tissue can be sliced off for use as grafts. [Fr. *greffe* graft, Gk *temnein* to cut.]

gregaloid (greg·al·oid). Applied to a colony of Protozoa which forms as the result of chance union of independent cells, or belonging to such a colony. [L *grex* herd, Gk *eidos* form.]

Gregg, Sir Norman McAlister (b. 1892). Australian ophthalmologist.

Gregg's maternal rubella syndrome. Congenital defects due to maternal infection with rubella during early pregnancy—cataract, congenital heart disease, deafness, microcephaly and mental retardation.

Gregory, James (b. 1753). Edinburgh physician.

Gregory's mixture or powder. Rhubarb, with heavy and light magnesium carbonates and ginger, used as an antacid and laxative.

Gregory's dinner pill. A pill consisting of 1 grain (65 mg) each of extract of aloes, ipecacuanha root, rhubarb and hard soap.

Gregory's sign. Rovsing's sign.

gregre (gre·gre). The tree *Erythrophloeum guineense* G. Don. (family Leguminosae), from which erythrophloeum is obtained. [African name.]

Greig, David Middleton (b. 1864). Scottish physician.

Greig's hypertelorism. Ocular hypertelorism. *See* HYPERTELORISM.

Greinacher circuit. A full-wave rectifier circuit used for x-ray machines, in which a constant potential is developed across the x-ray tube.

Grenacher, Hermann (b. 1843). German zoologist.

Grenacher's alcoholic borax carmine, for bulk staining of tissues. A concentrated solution of carmine in 4 per cent borax, diluted with 70 per cent alcohol. Nuclei are brilliantly stained.

Grenet cell. A form of bichromate cell. *See* CELL.

Greppi, Enrico (b. 1896). Italian physician.

Rietti-Greppi-Micheli disease. Thalassaemia.

Greville bath. A form of electric hot-air bath.

grey (gra). Ash colour; a mixture of black and white pigments. **Silver grey, Steel grey.** Water-soluble nigrosin; a mixture of induline (violet) with a yellow dye, used alone or in combination with other stains, e.g. haematoxylin, for algae and fungi. [AS *graeg.*]

grey-out (gra·owt). Greying of the visual field due to lack of blood supply to the retina. In aviation, a common cause is increased weight of blood due to excess *G* force during acceleration. [AS *graeg, ut.*]

Grey Turner. *See* TURNER, GEORGE GREY.

grid (grid). 1. A grating; a frame of parallel bars. 2. The ridged plate carrying the active substance in an accumulator. 3. The wire network between filament and anode of a thermionic valve, or other perforated electrode, which controls the flow of electrons. [etym. dub.]

Griesinger, Wilhelm (b. 1817). German physician.

Griesinger's disease. Ankylostomiasis.

Griesinger's sign. An oedematous swelling behind the mastoid bone over the mastoid emissary vein, which is seen in thrombosis in the transverse sinus.

Duchenne-Griesinger disease. Pseudohypertrophic muscular dystrophy.

Griesinger-Kussmaul sign. Pulsus paradoxus; paradoxical pulse: the force of the pulse wave diminishes on inspiration and increases on expiration. This phenomenon occurs occasionally in large pericardial effusions or constrictive pericarditis (i.e. any condition which hampers cardiac pulsation, particularly diastolic filling). It may also occur in cases of large pleural effusion and mediastinal disease. A recent explanation of this phenomenon is as follows: the right ventricular filling pressure increases on inspiration, but this is without effect on the left ventricle, since the fall in intrathoracic pressure on inspiration is equally applied to the pulmonary veins and the left ventricle. When the heart is compressed, however, increases in filling of the right ventricle will increase the intrapericardial pressure, and hence hinder filling of the left ventricle. This results in a fall of left ventricular output, and waning of the pulse.

griffado (grif·ah·do). An octoroon, i.e. an individual who has one-eighth part Negro blood, one of the parents being a quadroon and the other white. [Fr. *griffe* half-breed of Negro and mulatto.]

griffe des orteils (greef daze or·ta). Claw-foot. [Fr. talon toes.]

griffin-claw (grif·in·klaw). Claw-hand; *main en griffe.* [Fr. *griffe* hand, claw.]

Griffith, Frederick (d. 1941). London bacteriologist.

Griffith types. Antigenic types of haemolytic streptococci recognized by agglutinoid reactions. The method of typing was first developed by Griffith.

Griffith, Robert Eglesfeld (b. 1798). Philadelphia physician.

Griffith's mixture. Ferrous sulphate, potassium carbonate, myrrh, liquid glucose, spirit of nutmeg and rosewater. It may be used for the administration of iron in deficiency anaemia.

Griffith's method. For hippuric acid in urine: the hippuric acid is extracted with ether in a continuous-extraction apparatus, the ether is distilled off and the urea in the residue is destroyed with sodium hypobromite solution. The nitrogen is then determined by Kjeldahl's method and calculated to hippuric acid.

Grignard, Victor (b. 1871). French chemist.

Grignard compound. A compound of magnesium with an alkyl radical and a halogen, e.g. MgC_2H_5I, used in organic synthesis for the introduction of the particular alkyl radical into another organic compound.

Grignard reaction. The synthesis of hydrocarbons, acids, ketones and alcohols (particularly secondary and tertiary alcohols), by means of a Grignard reagent.

Grignard reagent. A mixture of magnesium powder and an alkyl halide in dry ether, used instead of a Grignard compound in organic synthesis.

Grimson, Keith Sanford (b. 1910). Durham, North Carolina, surgeon.

Grimson's operation. Total sympathectomy for hypertension.

Grindelia (grin·de·le·ah). A genus of flowering plants of the family Compositae. **Grindelia BPC 1949, Grindelia robusta.** Gum plant; the dried leaves and flowering tops were at one time used in hay fever, whooping-cough, bronchitis and spasmodic asthma. They contain an amorphous resin, tannin and a trace of volatile oil. [David Hieronymus *Grindel* (b. 1776), German botanist.]

grip (grip). 1. Old name for influenza. 2. A seizing. **Devil's grip.** Epidemic pleurodynia. **Grip strength.** A semi-objective means of measuring strength in the hands, using a modified sphygmomanometer cuff. [Fr. *grippe.*]

See also: PAWLIK.

gripe (gripe). To cause a severe clutching spasmodic pain in the intestine. [AS *gripan* to grasp.]

gripe-stock (gripe·stok). A tourniquet. [AS *gripan* to grasp, *stacc.*]

grippe (grip). Old name for influenza. **Grippe aurique.** The occurrence of polyneuritis as the result of therapeutic administration of gold salts. **Balkan grippe.** Q fever. **Winter grippe.** *See* INFLUENZA, ENDEMIC. [Fr.]

grisein (gri·se·in). An antibiotic obtained from a strain of *Streptomyces griseus.* It is active against certain Gram-positive and Gram-negative bacteria, and also certain fungi. Its therapeutic potentialities are under investigation.

Griseofulvin BP 1973 (gri·se·o·ful′·vin). 7-Chloro-4,6-dimethyloxycoumaran-3-one-2-spiro-1′-(2′-methoxy-6′-methylcyclohex-2′-en-4′-one), an antibiotic isolated from *Penicillium griseofulvum.* It is active against dermatophytes but inactive against bacteria, *Candida albicans, Actinomyces, Malassezia furfur* and *Corynebacterium minutissimum.*

Griseofulvinum (gri·se·o·ful′·vin·um). *European Pharmacopoeia* name for Griseofulvin BP 1973.

Grisolle, Augustin (b. 1811). Paris physician.

Grisolle's sign. The early papule of smallpox can still be felt when the affected skin is stretched, whereas the papule of measles becomes impalpable.

Grisonella ratellina (gri·son·el·ah rat·el·i·nah). A mammal of the family Mustelidae that acts as a reservoir of *Trypanosoma cruzi.*

Gritti, Rocco (b. 1828). Milan surgeon.

Gritti's amputation or operation, Gritti-Stokes amputation. Supracondylar amputation of the femur, the patella being retained, denuded of its articular cartilage and applied to the end of the stump.

Grocco, Pietro (b. 1856). Florence physician.

Grocco's sign, triangle or triangular dullness, Koranyi-Grocco triangle. A paravertebral triangular area of dullness found posteriorly on the side opposite to a pleural effusion. The apex of the triangle is at the level where the dullness due to the effusion reaches the vertebral spine, and the base is at the level of the 10th thoracic vertebra, extending outward for 25 or 50 mm.

Grocco's test. In slight cases of purpura rheumatica: the application of a ligature round the forearm below the elbow produces petechial haemorrhages in slight Henoch-Schoenlein purpura.

Orsi-Grocco method. A method of palpatory percussion of the heart.

Groenblad, Ester Elizabeth (b. 1898). Stockholm ophthalmologist.

Groenblad-Strandberg syndrome. The association of angioid streaks with pseudoxanthoma elasticum (yellow patches seen on the skin of the neck and flexures).

Groff knife. Endotherm knife; a steel needle carrying high-frequency current which seals vessels as it divides them.

groin [inguen (NA)] (groin). The external groove or depression that marks the junction of the lower part of the anterior abdominal wall and the thigh. [ME *grynde.*]

groove (groov). A long, shallow depression; a furrow; a sulcus. **Atrioventricular groove [sulcus coronarius (NA)].** A groove, separating the atria and ventricles of the heart, divided into an upper part on the sternocostal surface and a lower part which separates the base from the diaphragmatic surface. **Auricular groove.** Pre-auricular sulcus. *See* SULCUS. **Bicipital groove**

groove

[sulcus intertubercularis (NA)]. A groove between the lesser and greater tuberosities of the humerus, for the tendon on the long head of the biceps muscle. Below the tuberosities the groove is limited by well-marked lateral [crista tuberculi majoris (NA)] and medial [crista tuberculi minoris (NA)] lips which are roughened for muscular attachments, and are continuous below with the anterior and medial borders of the shaft of the humerus. **Branchial groove.** One of the grooves leading to a branchial pouch in the lateral wall of the embryonic pharynx. **Groove of the calcaneum [sulcus calcanei (NA)].** A groove on the upper surface, in front of the posterior facet. It forms with a corresponding groove on the under surface of the talus, the sinus tarsi. **Costal groove [sulcus costae (NA)].** The groove on the lower part of the inner surface of the shaft of a rib, lodging the intercostal vessels and nerve. **Deltopectoral groove.** The interval between the deltoid and pectoralis major muscles in which lies the cephalic vein. **Dental groove.** A groove along the surface of the embryonic jaw marking the site of invagination of the dental lamina. **Developmental groove.** A groove in the enamel between embryonic tooth lobes. **Ethmoidal groove [sulcus ethmoidalis (NA)].** A groove on the nasal bone lodging the anterior ethmoidal nerve. **Groove for the flexor hallucis longus tendon [sulcus tendinis musculi flexoris hallucis longi (NA)].** An oblique groove on the posterior surface of the talus between the medial and posterior tubercles. It is continued on to the sustenaculum tali of the calcaneum. **Genital groove.** A groove on the under-surface of the genital tubercle of the embryo which closes over in the male to form part of the urethra. **Groove for the greater superficial petrosal nerve [sulcus nervi petrosi majoris (NA)].** *See* PETROSAL NERVE, GREATER SUPERFICIAL. **Groove for the inferior petrosal sinus [sulcus sinus petrosi inferioris (NA)].** A groove along the petro-occipital suture. **Infra-orbital groove [sulcus infra-orbitalis (NA)].** The groove on the orbital surface of the maxilla, lodging vessels and nerves of the same name. **Interventricular groove, anterior [sulcus interventricularis cordis anterior (NA)].** The groove separating the right from the left ventricle of the heart on the sternocostal surface. **Interventricular groove, inferior [sulcus interventricularis cordis posterior (NA)].** The groove separating the right from the left ventricle of the heart on the diaphragmatic surface. **Lacrimal groove [sulcus lacrimalis (NA)].** A groove in the medial wall of the orbit composed of the lacrimal bone and the frontal process of the maxilla and lodging the lacrimal sac and the upper end of the nasolacrimal duct. **Laryngotracheal groove.** A sagittal gutter in the floor of the primitive pharynx, later closed in to form the laryngeal and tracheal cavities. **Groove for the lesser superficial petrosal nerve [sulcus nervi petrosi minoris (NA)].** *See* PETROSAL NERVE, LESSER SUPERFICIAL. **Medullary groove.** Neural groove (see below). **Meningeal grooves.** Grooves on the inner surfaces of the skull bones, occupied by the meningeal vessels. **Mentolabial groove [sulcus mentolabialis (NA)].** The skin furrow between the chin and lower lip. **Groove for the middle temporal artery [sulcus arteriae temporalis mediae (NA)].** The groove on the external surface of the squamous part of the temporal bone produced by the middle temporal artery. **Mylohyoid groove [sulcus mylohyoideus (NA)].** A groove on the inner surface of the mandible, beginning behind the lingula and passing obliquely downwards and forwards, lodging the mylohyoid nerve and vessels. **Groove of the nail bed [sulcus matricis unguis (NA)].** The groove between the nail bed and the nail wall. **Nasolabial groove [sulcus nasolabialis (NA)].** The groove between the upper lip and cheek. **Nasolacrimal groove [sulcus lacrimalis (NA)].** The groove on the nasal surface of the maxilla, converted into a canal by the lacrimal bone and inferior concha, and lodging the nasolacrimal duct. **Neural groove.** The furrow on the dorsal surface of the embryo produced by the neural plate as it begins to close over to form the neural tube. **Nuchal groove.** Nuchal furrow. *See* FURROW. **Obturator groove [sulcus obturatorius (NA)].** A groove for the obturator vessels and nerves on the under-surface of the superior pubic ramus. **Occipital groove [sulcus arteriae occipitalis (NA)].** The medial of 2 grooves on the under-surface of the mastoid portion of the temporal bone. It lodges the occipital artery. **Palatine groove, greater [sulcus palatinus major (NA)].** A groove on the perpendicular plate of the palatine bone which is completed by the maxilla in the articulated skull and lodges the greater palatine nerve. **Palatine groove of the maxilla [sulcus palatinus (NA)].** The sulcus between the nasal crests which receives the vomer. **Paracolic grooves [sulci paracolici (NA)].** Peritoneal gutters lying between the ascending and descending colons and the lateral abdominal walls. **Groove for the peroneus longus tendon [sulcus tendinis musculi peronei longi (NA)].** A diagonally-placed groove on the inferior surface of the cuboid bone. **Pharyngeal ectodermal groove.** Branchial cleft. *See* CLEFT. **Groove for the pharyngotympanic tube [sulcus tubae auditivae (NA)].** A groove on the inferior surface of the skull, between the posterior border of the greater wing of the sphenoid bone and the petrous part of the temporal bone. **Popliteal groove.** A depression on the lateral aspect of the lateral femoral condyle, lodging the tendon of the popliteus muscle when the knee is flexed. **Pre-auricular groove.** A shallow gutter forming the inferior boundary of the auricular surface of the sacro-iliac joint in female skeletons. **Primitive groove.** A sagittal furrow along the midline of the embryonic primitive streak. **Grooves of the promontory [sulci promontorii (NA)].** Grooves on the surface of the promontory which lodge the nerves of the tympanic plexus. **Sagittal groove of the frontal bone [sulcus sinus sagittalis superioris (NA)].** A groove on the cerebral surface of the frontal bone lodging the anterior portion of the superior sagittal sinus. **Sagittal groove of the occipital bone [sulcus sinus sagittalis superioris (NA)].** The groove on the internal surface of the squamous part of the occipital bone for the superior sagittal sinus. **Sagittal groove of the parietal bone [sulcus sagittalis (NA)].** A groove on the upper border of the parietal bone for the superior sagittal sinus. **Sigmoid groove [sulcus sinus sigmoidei (NA)].** A groove on the cerebral surface of the mastoid part of the temporal bone, lodging part of the sigmoid venous sinus. It is continued on to the parietal bone. **Grooves of the skin [sulci cutis (NA)].** The fine furrows on the surface of the skin. **Groove of the sphenoid bone, carotid [sulcus caroticus (NA)].** A winding groove on the lateral surface of the body, lodging the internal carotid artery. **Groove of the sphenoid bone, optic [sulcus chiasmatis].** A transverse groove lying between the tuberculum sellae and the limbus sphenoidalis. **Groove for a spinal nerve [sulcus nervi spinalis (NA)].** A groove on the lateral surface of the articular process of a cervical vertebra made by the posterior primary ramus of a spinal nerve. **Spiral groove [sulcus nervi radialis (NA)].** A shallow groove which passes obliquely downward and laterally from the posterior to the anterolateral surface of the shaft of the humerus in its middle third; it lodges the radial nerve and the profunda brachii vessels. **Groove for the subclavian artery [sulcus arteriae subclaviae (NA)].** The groove accommodating the subclavian artery on the upper surface of the 1st rib and behind the scalene tubercle. **Groove for the subclavian vein [sulcus venae subclaviae (NA)].** The groove on the first rib, in front of the scalene tubercle, which is occupied by the subclavian vein. **Groove for the superior petrosal sinus [sulcus sinus petrosi superioris (NA)].** A groove on the superior border of the petrous part of the temporal bone. **Supplemental groove.** A groove in the enamel which does not mark the junction between embryonic tooth lobes. **Groove of the talus [sulcus tali (NA)].** A roughened groove on the inferior surface of the neck which, with a similar groove on the calcaneum, forms the sinus tarsi. **Groove for the tendons of the peroneus muscles [sulcus tendinis musculori peronei (fibularis longi (NA)].** A groove on the calcaneum for the tendons of the muscles. **Groove for the tibialis posterior muscle [sulcus malleolaris (NA)].** A hollow furrow on the posterior surface of the medial malleolus of the tibia for the tendon of the tibialis posterior muscle. **Tracheobronchial groove.** The lower part of the laryngotracheal groove (see above). **Groove for the transverse sinus [sulcus sinus transversi (NA)].** The horizontal groove on either side of the squamous part of the occipital bone for the transverse sinus. **Tympanic groove [sulcus tympanicus (NA)].** The groove on the tympanic part of the temporal bone for the attachment of the tympanic membrane. **Groove for the ulnar nerve [sulcus nervi ulnaris (NA)].** A vertical groove behind the medial epicondyle of the humerus. **Groove for the umbilical vein [sulcus venae umbilicalis (NA)].** The groove on the visceral surface of the fetal liver in which lies the proximal end of the left umbilical vein. **Grooves of the upper limb, lateral bicipital, medial bicipital [sulcus bicipitalis lateralis, sulcus bicipitalis medialis (NA)].** The grooves on either side of the biceps muscle. **Groove for the vena cava [sulcus venae cavae (NA)].** A deep groove on the posterior surface of the liver; it is sometimes a tunnel enclosing the inferior vena cava completely. **Vertebral groove.** The furrow on either side of the spinous processes of the vertebral column occupied by the deep back muscles. **Groove for the vertebral artery [sulcus arteriae vertebralis (NA)].** A shallow channel on the upper surface of the posterior arch of the atlas, lodging the vertebral artery. **Visceral groove.** Branchial groove (see above). [D *groeve.*]

See also: BLESSIG, HARRISON (E.), LIEBERMEISTER, LUCAS, MADDOX, SCHMORL, SIBSON, VERGA.

Gross, Ludwik (b. 1904). New York tumour virologist.

Gross virus. An RNA-containing virus associated with a transmissible leukaemia in AK mice. Serologically distinct from other mouse leukaemia viruses.

Gross, Robert Edward (b. 1905). Boston surgeon.

Gross' operation. Ligation or division of a patent ductus arteriosus.

Gross, Samuel David (b. 1805). Philadelphia surgeon.

Gross' disease. Encysted rectum.

Gross, Samuel Weissel (b. 1837). American surgeon.

Gross' operation. A procedure in which a urethrotome, the stilette of which contains caustic potash mixed with lard, is used. This was used to cauterize a stricture after incision.

gross (grose). 1. Having large components or particles. 2. Coarse or macroscopical. 3. Burly, fat or bulky. 4. Insensitive or dull of feeling. 5. Dealing with broader aspects or distinctions, as in anatomy. [Fr. *gros* big.]

Grossman's sign. Dilatation of the heart in early pulmonary tuberculosis.

Groth's test. A test for the potency of smallpox vaccine lymph: an area of infiltration and congestion should appear 72 h after an intradermal injection of 0.1 ml of 1:1000 dilution of lymph into the depilated skin of the back of a rabbit.

Grotthus' law, Grotthus-Draper law. Absorbed radiation alone is biologically active.

group (groop). 1. A number of objects taken together, having similar characteristics. 2. In chemistry, a radical or a number of linked atoms which behave like an element, entering into combination as a unity. It is also applied to the elements with similar properties appearing in each of the vertical columns of the Periodic Table, and to elements behaving similarly towards certain reagents in systematic qualitative analysis. 3. To ascertain, by agglutination techniques or other means, to which group a biological substance, e.g. a blood sample or a micro-organism, belongs. 4. To arrange in groups. **Acid group.** The carboxyl radical, COOH, which is characteristic of all organic acids. **Alcohol group.** The group containing the hydroxyl OH which confers alcoholic properties upon a compound; it may be primary, $-CH_2OH$, secondary, =CHOH, or tertiary, ≡COH. **Azo group.** The group -N:N-; it is chromophoric and confers colour upon compounds in which it occurs. **Blood groups.** Individuals can be classified according to the following red-cell blood group systems: ABO, MNSs, P, Rhesus, Lutheran, Kell, Lewis, Duffy, Kidd, Diego, Yt, I and Xg. The ABO system (Landsteiner 1900) is of vital importance in blood transfusion practice. According to the presence or absence of the A and B antigens from the cells, α and β agglutinins from the serum, individuals are classified into the following groups: AB (agglutinogen A and B, no agglutinins), A (agglutinogen A, agglutinin β), B (agglutinogen B, agglutinin α), and O (no A or B agglutinogens, α and β agglutinins). The confusing numerical descriptions of the ABO group of Moss and Jansky are now obsolete. Groups O and A are the commonest in white persons, the former being known as the universal donor group. Subsidiary groups also exist based on the presence of agglutinogens such as A_1, A_2, A_3, M, N and P, and also upon the many Rh factors. **Characterizing group.** The group which is responsible for the characteristic properties of any class of compound, e.g. the carboxyl group, COOH, of acids, or the hydroxyl OH of alcohols. **Control group.** One kind of standard against which the truth of a conclusion may be measured. **Functional group, Functioning group.** An organic radical which confers characteristic properties on the compound into which it is introduced, e.g. the alcoholic or phenolic group, OH, the carboxyl radical, COOH, or the amino-group, NH_2. **Glucophore group.** That part of the molecule that is responsible for the sweet taste of a substance. **Haemorrhagic-septicaemia group.** A group of species of bacteria, typified by *Pasteurella pestis*, often causing septicaemia and haemorrhagic lesions. **Labile methyl group.** Name given to the CH_3 group of methionine which is transferred in biological transmethylation. **Methyl group.** The monovalent group, CH_3, derived from methane. **Osmophore group.** That part of the molecule that is responsible for the odour of a substance. **Prosthetic group.** 1. In a conjugated protein, the non-protein part which is combined with the protein, e.g. the carbohydrate in a glycoprotein. 2. The term is sometimes applied to a co-enzyme in an enzyme system, but the combination between protein enzyme and non-protein co-enzyme is looser than that existing in a conjugated protein. **QRS group.** QRS complex of the electrocardiogram. **Saccharide group.** The monosaccharide unit, $C_6H_{11}O_5$, which enters into the composition of the higher saccharides. **Sapophore group.** That part of the molecule that is responsible for the taste of a substance. **Serological groups.** Groups of specific organisms closely associated antigenically, the individuals of which are agglutinated by a common group-specific antiserum. **Sulphonic group.** The group SO_2OH; it is an auxochrome of importance in acidic dyestuffs. [Fr. *groupe.*]

See also: LANCEFIELD.

group-specific (groop·spes·if'·ik). Describing anything that is specific to a particular blood group. [Fr. *groupe*, specific.]

Grove, Sir William Robert (b. 1811). London judge and physicist.

Grove cell. A two-fluid voltaic cell in which the outer cell consists of an amalgamated zinc plate immersed in dilute sulphuric acid, and the inner cell is a porous pot containing strong nitric acid in which is a piece of platinum foil serving as a negative pole. It affords an emf of 1.9 V.

growth (gro·th). 1. The progressive development of a living being or part of an organism from its earliest stage to maturity, including the attendant increase of size. 2. A tumour or other morbid formation. **Accretionary growth.** Growth by accretion of non-living substances. **Histiotypic growth.** Profuse cell growth. **Intussusceptive growth.** Growth due to increase in the size of cells. **Meristic growth, Multiplicative growth.** Growth due to increase in the number of cells. **New growth.** Neoplasm. **Organotypic growth.** Growth that reproduces the pattern of the organ concerned. [AS *growan.*]

Gruber, Josef (b. 1827). Austrian otolaryngologist.

Gruber's test, for the sensitivity of the ear to sounds. A tuning fork is held close to the meatus until its vibrations are no longer heard. A finger is then inserted into the meatus, and if the tuning fork is now applied to the finger, in a normal hearing ear the sound is heard again.

Gruber, Max von (b. 1853). Munich bacteriologist.

Gruber reaction, Gruber-Widal reaction. Widal's reaction.

Gruber, Wenceslaus Leopold (b. 1814). Prague and St Petersburg anatomist.

Gruber's hernia. Hernia through the omentum.

Gruber-Landzert fossa. The paraduodenal fossa. *See* FOSSA.

Gruby, David (b. 1810). Austrian physician working in Paris.

Gruby's disease. Tinea capitis.

Grubyella (groo·be·el·ah). Synonym for *Trichophyton* [obsolete term]. [David *Gruby.*]

gruel (groo·el). An easily digested liquid food made of oat flour or corn flour mixed thinly with hot water and cooked. [L *grutellum* fine meal.]

Gruenfelder's reflex. A reflex which is excited by the pressure at the corner of the posterolateral fontanelle of infants and resulting in dorsiflexion of the great toe with spreading out of the other toes like a fan.

Gruening's magnet. A laminated magnet used to draw fragments of steel from the eye.

Gruenwald, Ludwig (b. 1863). Munich otorhinolaryngologist.

May-Gruenwald stain. A type of Romanovsky stain.

grume (groom). 1. Any thick glutinous fluid. 2. A clot, as of blood. [L *grumus* little heap.]

grumose, grumous (**groom**·oze, **groom**·us). 1. Lumpy, like the surface of a bacterial culture. 2. Clotted, as blood. 3. Containing or resembling grume. 4. In botany, composed of clusters of granules or grains. [see prec.]

Grünbaum (afterwards Leyton), Albert Sidney Frankau (b. 1869). British pathologist.

Grünbaum-Widal reaction or test. Widal's reaction.

Gruskin's test. A digested solution of fibrin from the blood of tuberculous guinea-pigs is injected intracutaneously. A positive reaction is indicated by weals that extend from the site of injection within 6 min.

grutum (groot·um). Any small lump present in the skin as the result of defective secretion by a sebaceous gland. [L meal.]

Grynfeltt, Joseph Casimir (b. 1840). Montpellier gynaecologist.

Grynfeltt's triangle, triangle of Grynfeltt and Lesshaft. The superior lumbar triangle through which lumbar hernia may occur. It is formed by the serratus posterior inferior muscle above and medially, the internal oblique muscle laterally, and the quadratus lumborum muscle medially. It was described by Luschka, then by Grynfeltt (1866) and 4 years later by Lesshaft.

gryochrome (gri·o·krome). Any nerve cell showing in its body stainable granules, either arranged in a definite pattern or diffused generally. An example of the former is the anterior horn cell in spinal cord, stained by Nissl's method. [Gk *gry* morsel, *chroma* colour.]

gryposis (gri·**po**·sis). 1. Abnormal curvature of any structure, particularly of the nails. 2. Arthrogryposis. **Gryposis penis.** Chordee. **Gryposis unguium.** Onychogryposis. [Gk a curving.]

guaiacene (gwi·as·een). Tiglic aldehyde, $CH_3CH{=}C(CH_3)CHO$. A colourless liquid with an almond odour, obtained from guaiacum by distillation.

guaiacin (gwi·as·in). $C_{14}H_{24}O$, a resinous alcohol extracted from guaiacum and used in perfumery.

guaiacol (gwi·ak·ol). Catechol-monomethyl ether, $C_6H_4(OH)(OCH_3)$. A colourless or yellowish oily liquid, or a crystalline substance, with a strong odour and a burning taste, obtained either from fractional distillation of creosote (from wood tar), when it is usually liquid, or prepared synthetically from catechol, when it is generally crystalline. It is the chief constituent of creosote, and is related to phenol chemically; it has antiseptic and deodorant properties, and is for this reason sometimes prescribed in cases of infected bronchiectasis. Oxidation products in the urine may reduce Fehling's solution. **Guaiacol carbonate.** $CO(OC_6H_4OCH_3)_2$, a white crystalline powder, almost without odour or taste, and prepared synthetically from guaiacol. It is much less irritant than guaiacol, and has been used in its place, but is of little clinical value. **Guaiacol glycuronate.** The oxidation product of guaiacol formed in the body and excreted in the urine. It reduces Fehling's solution. **Guaiacol oleate.** Oleoguaiacol, $CH_3OC_6H_4OCOC_{17}H_{33}$, ester of guaiacol and oleic acid, used as an internal antiseptic.

guaiacolate (gwi·ak·ol·ate). 1. A compound of a metal and guaiacol, analogous to a phenate. 2. A compound of guaiacol with an organic base.

guaiacolize (gwi·ak·ol·ize). To administer guaiacol in treatment.

guaiacum (gwi·ak·um). The resin obtained from guaiacum wood, consisting of a mixture of resin acids, saponins, vanillin and yellow colouring matter. It acts as a mild laxative and is used in chronic rheumatism and gout. **Compound confection of guaiacum.** Confectio Guaiaci Composita BPC 1949, a remedy for gout containing guaiacum together with rhubarb, sulphur and flavouring agents; also known as *Chelsea pensioner.* **Guaiaci Lignum BPC 1949.** Guaiacum wood (lignum vitae), obtained from *Guaiacum officinale* Linn., and *G. sanctum* Linn. (family Zygophyllaceae), evergreen trees indigenous to South America and the West Indies. The heart wood only is used: it yields about 25 per cent of the resin, guaiacum. **Guaiacum officinale.** An evergreen tree (family Zygophyllaceae) indigenous to the West Indian islands and the north coast of South America. From it is obtained guaiacum wood and guaiacum resin. **Guaiaci Resina BPC 1949, Guaiacum resin.** Guaiacum (see above). **Tincture of guaiacum.** A tincture used for the detection of oxidizing enzymes and in a test for the presence of blood in urine. **Guaiacum wood.** Guaiaci lignum (see above). [Sp. *guayaco.*]

Guaiphenesin (gwi·**fen**·es·in). BP Commission approved name for guaiacol glycerol ether; a cough suppressant.

guaja (goo·**ah**·jah). Ganja.

Guanacline (**gwan**·ah·kleen). BP Commission approved name for 1-(2-guanidinoethyl)-1,2,3,6-tetrahydro-4-picoline; a hypotensive agent.

guanase (**gwan**·aze). An enzyme in the liver and spleen which converts guanine into xanthine in the metabolism of the purines.

Guanecycline (gwan·e·**si**·kleen). BP Commission approved name for *N*-4-(guanidoformimidoylpiperazin-1-ylmethyl)tetracycline; an antibiotic.

Guanethidine (gwan·**eth**·id·een). BP Commission approved name for 1-(2-guanidino-ethyl)azacyclo-octane; it is used in the treatment of hypertension. **Guanethidine Sulphate BP 1973.** A colourless, almost odourless crystalline powder, soluble in water, slightly soluble in alcohol, insoluble in chloroform and in solvent ether; it is used to control hypertension.

guanidinaemia (gwan·id·in·e′·me·ah). A condition in which guanidine is present in the circulating blood. [guanidine, Gk *haima* blood.]

guanidine (**gwan**·id·een). 1. Imino-urea, $NH_2C({=}NH)NH_2$; a strongly basic crystalline compound present in sugar beet and the seeds of vetch after germination, but not occurring free in the animal body. When injected into the blood stream it causes a rise in blood pressure of about 1 h duration, and produces a lowering of blood sugar by stimulation of the pancreas to increased insulin output; it is not to be recommended in the treatment of diabetes owing to its toxicity. 2. Any member of a group of derivatives of imino-urea (above), many of which are normal constituents of muscle. **Guanidine hydrochloride.** $NH_2C({=}NH)NH_2HCl$, a compound sometimes used in the treatment of myasthenia gravis. **Monomethyl guanidine.** $CH_3NHC({=}NH)NH_2$, a substance occurring in muscle and excreted in the urine largely after parathyroidectomy.

guanine (**gwan**·een). 2-Amino-6-oxypurine. A purine base which is a constituent of all nucleic acids. **Guanine deaminase.** Guanase. **Guanine mononucleotide.** Guanylic acid. *See* ACID.

Guanoclor (**gwan**·o·klor). BP Commission approved name for 2-(2,6-dichlorophenoxy)ethyl aminoguanidine; a hypotensive agent.

guanosine (**gwan**·o·seen). The nucleoside formed from guanine and ribose. **Guanosine deaminase.** An enzyme in the purine metabolism which deaminates guanosine into xanthosine. **Guanosine hydrolase.** An enzyme in the purine metabolism which activates the hydrolysis of guanosine into guanine and ribofuranose. **Guanosine phosphates.** Precursors of nucleic acids and important metabolic intermediates.

Guanoxan (gwan·**ox**·an). BP Commission approved name for 2-guanidinomethyl-1,4-benzodioxan; a hypotensive agent.

guapi bark (gwi·ap·e bark). Cocillana BPC 1959.

Guarnieri, Giuseppi (b. 1856). Pisa pathologist.

Guarnieri's body or corpuscle. The inclusion body in the cells of the skin lesions of smallpox and vaccinia.

guavacoline (gwav·ak·o·leen). Methyl guvacine, $C_7H_{11}O_2N$. An alkaloid obtained from areca nut.

guaza (goo·az·ah). The name given to the type of Indian hemp (cannabis) met in European commerce. [A corruption of the Hindustani *ganja*.]

Gubarer (Gubarew, gubaroff), Alexander Petrovitch (b. 1855). Moscow gynaecologist.

Gubaroff's fold or valve. A valvular fold at the cardiac orifice produced by the oblique entry of the oesophagus into the stomach.

gubernacular (gew·ber·nak·ew·lar). Relating or belonging to a gubernaculum.

gubernaculum (gew·ber·nak·ew·lum). A guide. **Gubernaculum testis.** A thick cord of loose tissue rich in mucopolysaccharides, at the upper end of which lies the testis and epididymis. Its lower end lies in the region of the future scrotum. Its function is to dilate the inguinal canal, thus assisting the descent of the testis and the outgrowth of the processus vaginalis. A similar structure is present in the female but it becomes converted into the round ligament of the uterus and the ovarian ligament.

See also: HUNTER (J.).

Gubler, Adolphe Marie (b. 1821). Paris physician.

Gubler's hemiplegia or paralysis, Gubler-Millard paralysis, Millard-Gubler paralysis or syndrome, syndrome temporanea di Gubler. Paralysis of the 6th and perhaps the 7th cranial nerve on one side, with a contralateral hemiplegia; one form of crossed hemiplegia due to a pontine lesion.

Gubler's line. A line connecting the superficial origins of the roots of the trigeminal nerve.

Gubler's sign. Swelling of the wrist in lead poisoning.

Millard-Gubler-Foville paralysis. 6th cranial nerve palsy, with or without ipsilateral 7th nerve palsy, and contralateral hemiplegia.

Gubler-Robin typhus. Typhus fever with renal complications.

Weber-Gubler syndrome. Weber's syndrome.

Gudden, Bernhard Aloys von (b. 1824). Zürich and Munich psychiatrist.

commissure of Gudden. The inferior commissure of the hypothalamus.

Gudden's ganglion. A ganglion in the mamillary body.

Gudden's law. In a divided nerve, the part attached to the neuron undergoes degeneration in a cellulipetal direction.

Guedel, Arthur Ernest (b. 1883). Los Angeles anaesthetist.

Guedel's classification, of stages of anaesthesia. The various stages of surgical anaesthesia as reclassified by Guedel.

Guelpa, Guglielmo (b. 1850). Paris physician.

Guelpa therapy or treatment. An old method of treating rheumatism and gout by fasting and free purging.

Guéneau de Mussy, Nöel François Odon (b. 1813). Paris physician.

de Mussy's point. A point in the epigastrium where a horizontal line drawn along the left border of the sternum and extended downward meets a transverse line at the level of the tip of the 10th rib.

de Mussy's sign or symptom. Severe pain or pressure over de Mussy's point in diaphragmatic pleurisy.

Guenz, Justus Gottfried (b. 1714). Leipzig anatomist.

Guenz's ligament. Fibres of the superficial part of the obturator membrane.

Guenzberg, Alfred (b. 1861). Frankfurt physician.

Guenzberg's reagent, for free hydrochloric acid in gastric juice. (*a*) 10 per cent phloroglucinol in absolute alcohol; (*b*) 10 per cent vanillin in absolute alcohol. For use, mix 2 parts of (*a*) with 1 part of (*b*).

Guenzberg sign. Resonance with localized borborygmi, in the area between the gall bladder and pylorus in cases of duodenal ulcer.

Guenzberg test, for free hydrochloric acid in gastric contents. Mix a small quantity of gastric fluid with 1 or 2 drops of Guenzberg's reagent (see above) in an evaporating dish and evaporate to dryness. A red colour indicates the presence of free mineral acid.

Guérin, Alphonse François Marie (b. 1816). Paris surgeon.

Guérin's fold, sinus, valve or valvule. A reduplication of mucous membrane in the posterior part of the fossa terminalis of the male urethra.

Guérin's fracture. Horizontal separation by fracture of the palate from the upper jaw.

Guérin's glands. The para-urethral glands of the female; also called *Skene's glands.*

Guérin's operation. 1. Iridotomy; a crucial incision. 2. Subconjunctival strabotomy (obsolete).

Guérin and Desmarres operation, for correctopia (obsolete).

Guérin, Camille (b. 1872). Paris bacteriologist.

bacillus of Calmette-Guérin. The bacillus from which the antituberculosis (BCG) vaccine is made.

Calmette-Guérin test. A test for the potency of smallpox vaccine lymph. An eruption of isolated vesicles numbering from 3 to 4 per cm^2 should appear after distributing 1 ml of 1:1000 dilution of lymph over a prepared area of the skin of a rabbit.

Percutaneous Bacillus Calmette-Guérin Vaccine BP 1968. A suspension of living cells of an authentic strain of the bacillus of Calmette-Guérin with a higher viable bacterial count than the latter. A prophylactic against tuberculosis, administered by percutaneous inoculation.

Guglielmo. *See* DI GUGLIELMO.

guha (goo·hah). Guja.

guide (gide). 1. A grooved sound. 2. A grooved director for a knife or probe. 3. The tunnelled sound within which is a very slender bougie used in dilatation of urethral stricture. [ME *guiden* to guard.]

Guidi, Guido (Vidius) (b. 1500). Paris and Pisa physician.

Guidi's artery, vidian artery. The artery of the pterygoid canal.

canal of Guidi, vidian canal. The pterygoid canal. *See* CANAL.

Guidi's nerve, vidian nerve. The nerve of the pterygoid canal.

Guillain, Georges (b. 1876). Paris neurologist.

Guillain-Barré syndrome, Barré-Guillain syndrome, Guillain-Barré-Strohe syndrome. Acute infective polyneuritis. After non-specific infection, demyelination in spinal roots and peripheral nerves leads to the rapid onset of generalized weakness or paralysis, often ascending to the facial muscles and sometimes causing respiratory paralysis. Tendon reflexes are absent but sensory changes are slight. The cerebrospinal fluid protein is increased, with no increase in cells. The prognosis is generally good. Also called *acute polyradiculoneuropathy.*

Landry-Guillain-Barré syndrome. A name adopted for the conditions previously known as Landry's ascending paralysis and the Guillain-Barré syndrome, which are now recognized as clinically and pathologically identical.

Guillain-Thaon syndrome. Cerebrospinal involvement in the secondary stage of syphilis; meningovascular syphilis.

Guilland's sign. In a patient with irritation of the spinal meninges (e.g. in meningitis), pinching one quadriceps muscle produces abrupt flexion of hip- and knee-joints on the opposite side.

guillotine (gil·o·teen). A surgical instrument used in tonsillectomy and the removal of pharyngeal growths. It consists of a metal ring on a long handle through which a sliding blade runs; uvulotome. [Fr. *Guillotin,* name of doctor who invented the instrument of capital punishment adopted in France in 1789.]

See also: SLUDER.

Guinard, Aimé (b. 1856). Paris surgeon.

Guinard's treatment. The application of carbide of calcium to ulcerating tumours.

guinea-pig (gin·e·pig). 1. A small rodent, *Cavia porcellus,* South American in origin, but unknown in the wild state; extensively used as a laboratory animal. 2. The term is sometimes used semi-facetiously to indicate a willing or unwilling subject for experimentation. [*Guiana*, ME *pigge.*]

guinea-worm (gin·e·werm). The nematode worm *Dracunculus medinensis.* [*Guiana*, AS *wyrm.*]

Guinon, George (b. 1859). Paris physician.

Guinon's disease or tic. Gilles de la Tourette's disease.

Charcot-Guinon disease. Dementia complicating muscular dystrophy.

guja (goo·hah). Epidemic spasmodic bronchial asthma occurring in the Mariana, Carolina and Bonin Islands of the Pacific, particularly Guam, and apparently peculiar to these islands. Two types are known: *pneumonic*, in which there is spasmodic dyspnoea; and *enteric*, in which there is severe diarrhoea with greenish stools. Both types may occur simultaneously. [Sp.]

gula (gew·lah). Gullet; oesophagus. [L.]

gular (gew·lar). Relating or belonging to the oesophagus, throat or pharynx. [see prec.]

Guldberg, Cato (b. 1862). Norwegian chemist.

Guldberg and Waage law. Law of mass action.

gulf (gulf). *See* LECAT. [Fr. *golfe.*]

Gull, Sir William Withey (b. 1816). London physician.

Gull's disease. Myxoedema.

Gull's renal epistaxis. An unexplained renal haematuria occurring in adults, without any identifiable pathological lesion.

Gull and Sutton's disease, Sutton and Gull's disease. Arteriosclerosis.

gullet (gul·et). 1. The oesophagus. 2. The pharynx. [ME *golet.*]

Gullstrand, Allvar (b. 1862). Swedish ophthalmologist.

Gullstrand's schematic eye. A simplified and diagrammatic representation of the optical properties of the human eye.

Gullstrand's slit lamp. A lamp which projects a slit of intense illumination on to the eye and facilitates the examination of its anterior parts with a binocular corneal microscope.

gulose (gew·loze). $CH_2OH(CHOH)_4CHO$, a synthetic hexose prepared from xylose; it is an isomer of glucose, but does not ferment.

gum (gum). 1. The gingiva; the dense fibrous tissue of the alveolar processes of the upper and lower jaws with its smooth vascular mucous membrane. [AS *goma.*] 2. Any of the complex heterosaccharides constituted of pentose and hexose units with a uronic acid, usually glucuronic. They are amorphous substances formed, normally or as the result of injury, by plants. [L *gummi.*] 3. A colloidal solution of a gum or dextrin used as an adhesive. **Acacia gum.** Acacia BP 1958, the dried gummy exudate of the stem and branches of *Acacia senegal,* consisting chiefly of the calcium, potassium and magnesium salts of arabic acid. It is used in combination with sodium chloride in the preparation of intravenous injections to raise the blood volume and pressure in cases of haemorrhage; also employed as a suspending agent and emulgent in dispensing. **Gum animi.** Copal. **Gum arabic.** Acacia gum (see above). **Gum benjamin, Gum benzoin.** Benzoin BP 1958, a balsamic resin obtained by incision of the stems of species of *Styrax.* It contains free cinnamic and benzoic acids, together with their esters, and is used in the form of a compound tincture as an astringent and mild antiseptic. It is also of value as an expectorant. **British gum.** Dextrin, a yellowish powder obtained from starch by partial hydrolysis, and used as an emulsifying and binding agent. **Carob gum.** Ceratonia. **Gum dragon.** Tragacanth BP 1958. **Eucalyptus gum.** Kino eucalypti, eucalyptus kino, red gum, the dried juice obtained by incision of the stems of *Eucalyptus rostrata* and other species, containing tannin-like substances and used as an astringent in the form of lozenges, pastilles and gargles; it is sometimes administered to arrest diarrhoea. **Fermentation gum.** Dextrin. **Ghatti gum.** Indian gum (see below). **Gum guaiacum.** Guaiaci Resina BPC 1949, guaiacum resin, a resin obtained from the wood of *Guaiacum officinale* and *G. sanctum* either by extraction with alcohol or by heating until the gum runs out. It contains guaiaconic and resin acids and has laxative and diuretic properties. **Hog gum.** False tragacanth, a gum obtained from a species of *Prunus* and used as a substitute for tragacanth. **Indian gum.** Ghatti gum, a gum derived from *Anogeissus latifolia* (family Combretaceae), and forming a thick mucilage with water. It is used as an acacia substitute as a suspending and emulsifying agent. **Gum juniper.** Sandarac. **Karaya gum.** Indian tragacanth, a gum obtained from the incised stems of *Sterculia urens* and used in the treatment of constipation on account of its ability to stimulate peristalsis; also used as an adhesive in denture fixatives. **Gum opium.** An unofficial name for opium. **Gum plant.** Grindelia. **Receding gum.** A condition denoting recession of the gingival margin and the exposure of part of the root of a tooth. **Red gum.** Eucalyptus gum (see above). **Gum resin.** *See* RESIN. **Spongy gum.** A condition denoting swelling and flabbiness of the gingival margin due to oedema of the tissues. **Starch gum.** Dextrin. **Sterculia gum.** Karaya gum (see above). **Gum thus.** The end portion of the exudate in the collection of crude turpentine. **Gum tragacanth.** Tragacanth BP 1958, gum dragon, a dried gummy exudate obtained from the incised stems of *Astragalus gummifer* (family Leguminosae) and other species, known in commerce as *Persian tragacanth.* It is partly soluble in water, swelling to a gelatinous mass, which is used pharmaceutically as a suspending agent and emulgent, in the latter case with acacia. It is employed as a basis of toilet preparations in conjunction with glycerin; and in skin preparations containing medicaments such as salicylic acid, resorcinol, sulphur or ichthammol, which are required to dry out on the skin. In combination with gelatin and glycerin it is used in the preparation of Unna's paste. It is also an effective denture fixative.

gumbo (gum·bo). Okra.

gumboil (gum·boil). An abscess arising from a tooth, which is pointing on the overlying gum. [gum, AS *byl.*]

gumma (gum·ah) (pl. *gummata*). The soft degenerating tumour of gummy material (infectious granuloma) which is the characteristic lesion of tertiary syphilis. **Tuberculous gumma.** A firm, subcutaneous nodule which slowly softens, due to haematogenous dissemination of *Mycobacterium tuberculosis* from a deep focus of tuberculosis in a debilitated individual. [L *gummi* gum.]

gummate (gum·ate). Arabate. [L *gummi* gum.]

gummatous (gum·at·us). 1. Having the character of or relating to gumma. 2. Affected with gummata.

gummide (gum·ide). Name given to any substance which is hydrolysed by acids or alkalis into glucose.

gummose (gum·oze). The sweet monosaccharide solution obtained by the hydrolysis of animal gum.

gummy (gum·e). 1. Gummatous. 2. Viscous. 3. Covered with a gum-like substance. [L *gummi* gum.]

Gumprecht, Ferdinand (b. 1864). Weimar physician.

Gumprecht's shadows. Deformed cell masses sometimes seen in lymphadenosis.

gun (gun). **Electron gun.** An assembly of components producing an electron stream of defined cross-section from a thermionic source. [etym. dub.]

See also: HEAF.

gun-cotton (gun·kotn). A mixture of nitric esters of cellulose obtained by treating cotton wool with nitric and sulphuric acids in the cold. The degree of nitration depends on the concentration of the acids and the time they are allowed to act: the product, containing roughly 13 per cent nitrogen, is a powerful explosive; that prepared under milder conditions and with from 10 to 12 per cent nitrogen is known as *pyroxylin,* a solution of which in alcohol-ether mixture (collodion) is used as a plastic skin, as a basis for corn paints and in nail varnishes. [gun, Ar. *qutun.*]

gundo (goon·do). Goundou.

gunja (gun·jah). Ganja.

Gunn, Robert Marcus (b. 1850). London ophthalmologist.

Gunn's dots. White dots seen in the fundus of the eye in the region of the macula.

Gunn's crossing sign. Compression of a retinal vein by the crossing of an artery in benign hypertension.

Gunn's pupillary sign. A diminished direct-light reaction in one eye with preservation of the consensual reaction. It denotes retinal or optic nerve disease and is best demonstrated with the swinging flashlight test wherein the affected pupil dilates when the light is transferred from the sound eye. Also called *afferent pupil defect.*

Gunn's syndrome, Marcus Gunn phenomenon or syndrome. Jaw-winking syndrome. *See* SYNDROME.

inverse Marcus Gunn syndrome. Jaw-winking syndrome. *See* SYNDROME.

Gunning, Jan Willem (b. 1827). Dutch chemist.

Gunning's mixture. Concentrated sulphuric acid, potassium sulphate and copper sulphate, used for the estimation of nitrogen in urine by the Kjeldahl method.

Gunning, Thomas Brian (b. 1813). American dentist.

Gunning's splint. An interdental splint used for fractures of the mandible.

Gurvich, Alexander Gavilovich (b. 1874). Moscow pathologist.

Gurvich rays. Mitogenetic rays; rays said to be produced by dividing cells and having an effect on photographic plates. They are probably not rays but emanations of volatile chemical substances.

Gussenbauer, Carl (b. 1842). Liège and Prague surgeon.

Gussenbauer's clamp. A metal internal splint for approximating bone fragments in ununited fracture.

gustation (gus·ta·shun). The faculty, sense or act of tasting. **Coloured gustation.** The associating of a particular colour with a particular taste. [L *gustare* to taste.]

gustatism (gus·tat·izm). A condition in which a sensation of taste is produced indirectly by stimuli unrelated to the sense of taste. [see prec.]

gustatory (gus·tat·or·e). Relating or belonging to the sense and the organs of taste. [L *gustare* to taste.]

gustometry (gus·tom·et·re). The determination, by measurement, of the acuteness of the sense of taste. [L *gustare* to taste, meter.]

gut (gut). 1. The intestine. 2. Catgut. **Primitive gut.** The archenteron; that part of the gut of lower vertebrates which is formed by invagination at the blastopore. **Ribbon gut.** Catgut prepared in a flat ribbon. **Silkworm gut.** A non-absorbable suture material prepared by drawing out the silkworm cocoon to a fine strand. [AS *guttas.*]

Guterman, Henry Samuel. American physician.

Guterman's test, for measuring the urinary pregnanediol. Urine is extracted with butyl alcohol and precipitated by acetone. The pregnanediol sodium glucuronate is then weighed.

Guthrie, George James (b. 1785). London surgeon.

Guthrie's muscle. The deep transversus perinei muscle.

Guthrie-Smith, Mrs. 20th century British physiotherapist.

Guthrie-Smith apparatus. An apparatus designed to support the weight of the patient's body and limbs by means of slings running over pulleys fixed on a beam above the bed. It is used to encourage patients in rehabilitation to carry out active movement.

Gutièrrez, A. (b. 1932). Buenos Aires surgeon.

Gutièrrez sign. A method of identifying the extradural space involving the aspiration of a drop of fluid placed on the hub of a lumbar puncture needle as its point enters the extradural space, due to negative pressure therein.

Gutman and Gutman method. For serum acid phosphatase: this follows the same procedure as the King and Armstrong method for serum alkaline phosphatase, except that an acid buffer (citric-acid sodium citrate, pH 4.9) is used and the incubation is for 1 h at 37°C. Normal range, from ½ to 5 units.

Gutmann, Carl (b. 1872). Berlin physician.

Michaelis-Gutmann bodies. Pinhead, raised, brownish areas of the mucous membrane of the bladder in malacoplakia; they may be found also in the kidney, pelvis and ureter. The lesions are of unknown aetiology and may be of long duration, but do not appear to be precancerous.

Gutstein's method. A method for making permanent preparations of spirochaetes, and also of elementary bodies from smallpox vesicles; the medium consists of methyl violet and $NaCHO_3$.

gutta (gut·ah) (pl. *guttae*). A drop; usually about a minim. Drops are intended for application to the external auditory meatus or to the conjunctiva for anaesthetic, antiseptic or, in the case of the eye, mydriatic purposes. **Guttae pro auribus.** Ear-drops. **Gutta cadens.** The falling-drop sound; a sound sometimes heard on auscultation over a hydropneumothorax and due to a drop of liquid falling into the accumulated liquid at the base of the pleural cavity. **Guttae ophthalmicae.** Eye-drops. **Gutta Percha BPC 1949.** The dried, purified latex of *Palaquium oblongifolium* and other species (family Sapotaceae). It is a rubber-like substance, solutions of which in chloroform are used as substitutes for collodion in preparing plastic skins; also used as a temporary tooth-filling. **Gutta rosacea.** Rosacea. **Gutta serena.** An obsolete term applied to unexplained forms of blindness, especially glaucoma. [L.]

guttate (gut·ate). In biology, marked by or covered with drop-like spots. [L *gutta* drop.]

gutter (gut·er). **Paracolic gutter.** The vertical peritoneal trough which lies lateral to the ascending or the descending colon. [O Fr. *gutiere.*]

guttering (gut·er·ing). The surgical procedure of cutting a groove in a bone. [O Fr. *gutiere* gutter.]

guttiform (gut·e·form). Shaped like a drop. [gutta, form.]

Guttmann, Paul (b. 1834). Berlin physician.

Guttmann's sign. The humming sound heard over the thyroid in thyrotoxicosis [obsolete term].

guttural (gut·er·al). 1. Relating or belonging to the throat. 2. Of voice sounds, throaty. [L *guttur* throat.]

gutturophony (gut·er·of·on·e). A throaty quality of voice sounds. [L *guttur* throat, Gk *phone* voice.]

gutturotetany (gut·er·o·tet'·an·e). A type of laryngeal spasm which causes a stuttering difficulty in the pronouncing of gutturals, e.g. *g, k.* [L *guttur* throat, tetanus.]

Gutzeit, Max Adolf (b. 1847). Leipzig chemist.

Gutzeit test, for arsenic. Organic matter is destroyed by wet oxidation with sulphuric and nitric acids, residual nitric acid being removed by boiling with ammonium-oxalate solution. The solution is neutralized, acidified with hydrochloric acid and placed in a special wide-mouthed bottle. The bottle is fitted with a rubber bung carrying a glass tube, at the top of which are fixed 2 rubber bungs clamped together by a suitable clip. A strip of lead-acetate paper is rolled up and inserted in the tube, and a piece of mercuric-chloride paper is placed at the top of the tube clamped between the rubber bungs. To the solution in the bottle is added 10 g of arsenic-free zinc, the bung is immediately inserted and the reaction allowed to proceed for 40 min. The lead-acetate paper removes any hydrogen sulphide in the gas produced, whilst the arsine produced from any arsenic present in the material reacts with the mercuric-chloride paper to give a yellow stain. For quantitative purposes the colour of the stain is compared with that produced by known amounts of arsenic (up to 0.01 mg arsenic trioxide). All the reagents used must be arsenic-free.

guvacine (guv·as·een). Δ^3-Tetrahydropyridine-3-carboxylic acid, 1,2,5,6-tetrahydronicotinic acid, $C_6H_9O_2N$. An alkaloid occurring in areca nut; its methyl derivative is the toxic alkaloid, arecoline.

guvacoline (guv·ak·o·leen). Guavacoline.

Guye's sign. Aprosexia resulting from adenoid hypertrophy in children.

Guyon, Jean Casimir Félix (b. 1831). Paris surgeon.

Guyon's amputation or operation. Amputation of the foot, the incision used being elliptical and the bones divided just above the malleoli.

Guyon's isthmus. The isthmus of the uterus.

Guyon's sign. The fixation of a mobile kidney between the fingers on bimanual examination of the abdomen of the patient in the recumbent posture. The kidney may be allowed to slip upwards on release of the pressure of the fingers during expiration.

Gwathmey, James Taylor (b. 1865). New York anaesthetist. **Gwathmey's oil-ether anaesthesia.** General anaesthesia produced by running a mixture of olive oil and ether through the rectum into the colon; the ether is absorbed into the blood stream.

gymnasium (jim·na·ze·um). A building or place where physical exercise is performed with or without mechanical apparatus. [Gk *gymnazein* to exercise (naked).]

gymnastic (jim·nas·tik). Relating or belonging to exercise in a gymnasium.

gymnastics (jim·nas·tix). The science of the systematic exercise of the muscles with or without mechanical apparatus. **Antagonistic gymnastics.** Systematic exercises, e.g. in the Schott treatment of heart affections, in which two persons resist each other's movements. **Medical gymnastics.** Systematic exercises designed to improve the tone of muscles and to correct deformities. **Ocular gymnastics.** Systematic exercise of the muscles of the eye in order to strengthen them and ensure proper function and movement. **Resistance-antagonistic gymnastics.** Antagonistic gymnastics (see above). **Swedish gymnastics.** A form of remedial exercise in which the instructor resists the patient's movements. **Vocal gymnastics.** The expanding of the lungs and the broadening of the chest by means of systematic exercise of the voice. [Gk *gymnazein* to exercise (naked).]

Gymnema (jim·ne·mah). *Gymnema sylvestre* R. Br. (family Asclepiadaceae), an Indian plant the root of which is used in the treatment of snake bite. The fresh leaves, when chewed, have the property of temporarily destroying the sense of taste. [Gk *gymnos* naked, *nema* thread.]

Gymnoascaceae (jim·no·as·ka'·se·e). A family of fungi either saprophytic (especially on keratinized substrates) or parasitic (ringworm infections), commonly found in soil. [Gk *gymnos* naked, *askos* bag.]

Gymnoascus (jim·no·as·kus). A genus of the Gymnoascaceae, of which 1 species, *Gymnoascus setosus* Eidam (syn. *Eidamella spinosa* Matruchot and Dassonville), was isolated from ringworm-like lesions on a dog. Its relationship to the lesion is uncertain. [Gk *gymnos* naked, *askos* bag.]

gymnobacteria (jim·no·bak·teer'·e·ah). A general term for all non-motile (non-flagellate) bacteria. [Gk *gymnos* naked, bacteria.]

gymnocyte (jim·no·site). A cell without a limiting membrane or distinct cell wall. [Gk *gymnos* naked, *kytos* cell.]

gymnophobia (jim·no·fo·be·ah). Morbid aversion to the sight of a naked human body or any naked part of the body. [Gk *gymnos* naked, phobia.]

gymnoplast (jim·no·plast). 1. Gymnocyte. 2. A mass of protoplasm without a limiting membrane or distinct cell wall. [Gk *gymnos* naked, *plastos* formed.]

gymnosophy (jim·nos·o·fe). The cult of nudism. [Gk *gymnos* naked, *sophia* wisdom.]

gymnosperm (jim·no·sperm). A plant belonging to the classes in which the seeds are not contained in an ovary or are naked, e.g. the coniferous trees. [Gk *gymnos* naked, sperm.]

gymnospore (jim·no·spor). A naked spore;. one which is not provided with a protective envelope. [Gk *gymnos* naked, *sporos* seed.]

gynaecatoptron (gi·ne·kat·op'·tron). A vaginal speculum. [Gk *gynaikos* of a woman, *katoptron* mirror.]

gynaecic (gi·ne·sik). Relating or belonging to diseases of the female sex. [Gk *gynaikos* of a woman.]

gynaecium (gi·ne·se·um). The female organs of a flower. [Gk *gyne* woman, *oikos* house.]

gynaecogen (gi·ne·ko·jen). Any substance which is productive of or stimulates female characteristics, e.g. the female sex hormones. [Gk *gynaikos* of a woman, *genein* to produce.]

gynaecogenic (gi·ne·ko·jen'·ik). Productive of female characteristics. [see prec.]

gynaecography (gi·ne·kog·raf·e). The use of x-rays in the diagnosis of women's diseases, e.g. pneumoradiography of the pelvis. [Gk *gynaikos* of a woman, *graphein* to record.]

gynaecoiatry (gi·ne·ko·i'·at·re). Gyniatrics. [Gk *gynaikos* of a woman, *iatreia* treatment.]

gynaecoid (gi·ne·koid). Woman-like in form and structure. [Gk *gyanaikos* of a woman, *eidos* form.]

gynaecological (gi·ne·ko·loj'·ik·al). Relating or belonging to gynaecology.

gynaecologist (gi·ne·kol·o·jist). A physician who specializes in the diagnosis and treatment of diseases peculiar to women. [see foll.]

gynaecology (gi·ne·kol·o·je). Broadly speaking, the study of disease in the female. Generally used to indicate a disease of the pelvic organs in particular, and occasionally diseases involving adjacent organs such as the urinary tract and rectum. [Gk *gynaikos* of a woman, *logos* science.]

gynaecomania (gi·ne·ko·ma'·ne·ah). Oversexuality in the male; satyriasis. [Gk *gynaikos* of a woman, mania.]

gynaecomastia, gynaecomastism, gynaecomasty, gynaecomazia (gi·ne·ko·mas'·te·ah, gi·ne·ko·mas'·tizm, gi·ne·ko·mas'·te, gi·ne·ko·ma'·ze·ah). A condition in the male in which the mammary glands are excessively developed. The secretion of milk may be an attendant phenomenon. **Refeeding gynaecomastia.** Noticed in prisoners of war when released or having received food parcels. [Gk *gynaikos* of a woman, *mastos* breast.]

gynaecopathy (gi·ne·kop·ath·e). 1. Any disease peculiar to women. 2. Gynaecology. [Gk *gynaikos* of a woman, *pathos* disease.]

gynaecophonous (gi·ne·kof·on·us). Applied to a voice in a man that lacks maleness and sounds like a woman's voice. [Gk *gynaikos* of a woman, *phone* voice.]

gynaecophonus (gi·ne·kof·on·us). A man whose voice is like that of a woman. [Gk *gynaikos* of a woman, *phone* voice.]

gynaecophorus (gi·ne·kof·or·us). A rare synonym of *Schistosoma.* [Gk *gynaikos* of a woman, *pherein* to bear.]

gynaephobia (gi·ne·fo·be·ah). Morbid dread of women or strong aversion to their society. [Gk *gyne* woman, phobia.]

gynaeplasty (gi·ne·plas·te). Gynoplastics.

gynanatomy (gi·nan·at·o·me). Female anatomy. [Gk *gyne* woman, anatomy.]

gynander, gynandra (gi·nan·der, gi·nan·drah). 1. A female whose secondary genital organs are like those of a male; a female pseudohermaphrodite. 2. An individual who is genetically female, but in whom influences, believed to be hormonal, have produced a partial inversion towards the male sex. [Gk *gyne* woman, *aner* man.]

gynandria (gi·nan·dre·ah). Male hermaphroditism. [see prec.]

gynandrism (gi·nan·drizm). 1. Male hermaphroditism. 2. Partial female pseudohermaphroditism, the general appearance of the genital organs being that of a penis and scrotum. **Adipose gynandrism.** A familial syndrome occurring in boys, in which there is precocious development of the genitalia and obesity with a female configuration of the body. [Gk *gyne* woman, *aner* man.]

gynandroblastoma (gi·nan·dro·blas·to'·mah). A rare ovarian tumour which contains arrhenoblastomatous and granulosa-cell elements, and which is associated with masculinization of the subject. [Gk *gyne* woman, *aner* man, *blastos* germ, *-oma* tumour.]

gynandroid (gi·nan·droid). A female hermaphrodite who can pass for a man. [gynander, Gk *eidos* form.]

gynandromorph (gi·nan·dro·morf). An individual in which both male and female structural characters are present. It is a condition often met in insects, less commonly in birds and mammals, and may be the result of a deficiency of an X chromosome in one of the blastomeres. [see foll.]

gynandromorphism (gi·nan·dro·mor'·fizm). The abnormal state of having the external characteristics of both the male and the female. [Gk *gyne* woman, *aner* man, *morphe* shape.]

gynandromorphous (gi·nan·dro·mor'·fus). Having both male and female characteristics. [see prec.]

gynandry (gi·nan·dre). Gynandrism.

gynanthropia, gynanthropism (gi·nan·thro·pe·ah, gi·nan·thro·pizm). Gynandrism. [see foll.]

gynanthropus (gi·nan·thro·pus). A hermaphrodite in whom the male characteristics predominate. [Gk *gyne* woman, *anthropos* man.]

gynatresia (gi·nat·re·ze·ah). Imperforation of the vagina or occlusion of the hymen. [Gk *gyne* woman, atresia.]

gyniatrics, gyniatry (gi·ne·**at**·rix, gi·ne·**at**·re). The treatment of diseases peculiar to women. [Gk *gyne* woman, *iatreia* treatment.]

gynocardate (jin·o·**kar**·date). A salt or ester of gynocardic acid.

Gynocardia odorata (gi·no·**kar**·de·ah o·dor·a·tah). An evergreen glabrous tree with hard round fruits, found from Sikkim and the Khasia mountains eastward to Chittagong, Rangoon and Tenasserim (family Bixineae). The seeds are said to yield chaulmoogra oil, used in India for cutaneous diseases, especially leprosy, but this is not the official source of the oil. [Gk *gyne* woman, *kardia* heart, L *odoratus* fragrant.]

gynoecium (gi·**ne**·se·um). Gynaecium; the female organs of a flower. [Gk *gyne* woman, *oikos* house.]

gynogenesis (gi·no·**jen**·es·is). The development of an ovum which contains only maternal chromosomes and nuclei. [Gk *gyne* woman, *genein* to produce.]

Gynograph (gi·no·graf). A proprietary name given to an apparatus for injecting radio-opaque substances into the uterus, etc. for radiography. [Gk *gyne* woman, *graphein* to record.]

gynopathic (gi·no·**path**·ik). Relating or belonging to diseases peculiar to women. [see foll.]

gynopathy (gi·**nop**·ath·e). Any disease peculiar to women. [Gk *gyne* woman, *pathos* disease.]

gynophobia (gi·no·**fo**·be·ah). Gynaephobia.

gynoplastic (gi·no·**plas**·tik). Having relation or belonging to gynoplastics.

gynoplastics, gynoplasty (gi·no·**plas**·tix, gi·no·plas·te). Reparative or plastic surgery of the female genitalia. [Gk *gyne* woman, *plassein* to mould.]

gypsum (**jip**·sum). A natural form of hydrated calcium sulphate, $CaSO_4{\cdot}2H_2O$, which on heating to 130°C loses its water and becomes plaster of Paris, $2CaSO_4H_2O$. Mixed with water, the latter slowly hardens, forming gypsum again; the slight expansion accompanying this "setting" renders the substance ideal for the preparation of plaster casts. [Gk *gypsos*.]

gyral (**ji**·ral). Relating or belonging to a cerebral gyrus or gyri.

gyrate (**ji**·rate). 1. Convoluted or ring-shaped. 2. Circular in course. 3. Twisted in a spiral or coil. 4. To revolve round an axis. [L *gyrare* to turn round.]

gyration (ji·**ra**·shun). 1. Spiral or circular movement. 2. Rotation. 3. Arrangement in convolutions or twists, as the cerebral gyri. 4. A term for giddiness. [see prec.]

Gyraulus (ji·**raw**·lus). A genus of freshwater pulmonate snails resembling *Planorbis*. **Gyraulus prashadi.** A species which is intermediate host to the worm *Echinostoma ilocanum* in the tropical Far East. [Gk *gyros* turn, *aulos* tube.]

gyre (jire). Gyrus.

gyrectomy (ji·**rek**·to·me). Resection of a cerebral gyrus. **Frontal gyrectomy.** Topectomy. [gyrus, Gk *ektome* excision.]

gyrencephalic, gyrencephalous (ji·ren·kef·**al**'·ik, ji·ren·**kef**·al·us). Referring to a brain the surface of which has many convolutions. [Gk *gyros* turn, *egkephalos* brain.]

gyri (**ji**·ri). *See* GYRUS.

gyrochrome (**ji**·ro·krome). A nerve cell in which the tigroid (Nissl's) bodies are arranged in a ring within the cytoplasm. [Gk *gyros* turn, *chroma* colour.]

gyroma (ji·**ro**·mah). A form of ovarian tumour containing a mass of convoluted fibres. [Gk *gyros* turn, *-oma* tumour.]

gyromele (**ji**·ro·meel). 1. A catheter of flexible material to the tip of which a small piece of sponge is fixed. 2. A type of stomach tube through which can be passed a flexible rotating rod bearing attachments for the purpose of cleansing or treating the stomach, taking specimens for culture, massage and so on (Turck). [Gk *gyros* turn, *mele* a sort of cup.]

gyrometer (ji·**rom**·et·er). An instrument with which the cerebral gyri can be indirectly measured. [Gk *gyros* turn, meter.]

gyrosa (ji·**ro**·sah). Vertigo due to disease of the stomach. The patient's sensation when he is standing is that his environment is revolving and that unless he closes his eyes he will fall. [Gk *gyros* turn.]

gyrose (**ji**·roze). Bearing irregular wavy lines, undulations or circles, similar to the surface of the cerebral hemisphere. Applied to colonies of bacteria, which show such marking. [Gk *gyros* turn.]

gyrospasm (**ji**·ro·spazm). 1. Spasmodic rotary movement of the head; eclampsia rotans. 2. Nodding spasm of the head. [Gk *gyros* turn, spasm.]

gyrous (**ji**·rus). Gyrose.

gyrus[NA] (**ji**·rus) (pl. *gyri*). Convolution; an elevation of the surface of the cerebral hemisphere, usually elongated in form and bounded by irregular grooves or sulci. The formation of gyri greatly increases the extent of the area of cerebral cortex contained in the cranial cavity. **Angular gyrus.** The middle part of the inferior parietal lobule. **Annectant gyri.** Small gyri joining two larger gyri. **Cerebral gyri [gyri cerebri (NA)].** *See* MAIN DEF. (above). **Gyrus cinguli [NA].** A gyrus on the medial surface of the cerebral hemisphere surrounding the corpus callosum and bounded peripherally by the sulcus cinguli. **Gyrus cunei.** A small gyrus buried in the depth of the calcarine sulcus. **Deep gyri.** Gyri not appearing on the surface of the cerebral hemisphere but found in the walls of the deeper fissures. **Dentate gyrus [gyrus dentatus (NA)].** A small gyrus the surface of which is irregular or denticulate, running along the border of the cornu ammonis; a part of the hippocampal formation. **Gyrus descendens.** Posterior occipital gyrus. **Gyrus fornicatus.** A general term including the gyri surrounding the corpus callosum, the paraterminal, cingulate and splenial gyri and extending into the temporal lobe where it includes the hippocampal formation and uncus. Non-cortical structures, such as the olfactory peduncle and tracts, may also be included in this term. **Frontal gyrus, inferior [gyrus frontalis inferior (NA)].** The part of the frontal lobe lying below the inferior sulcus of the frontal lobe. It is divided into 3 parts, a posterior [pars opercularis (NA)], a triangular [pars triangularis (NA)] and an orbital [pars orbitalis (NA)], by the horizontal ascending ramus of the lateral sulcus of the cerebrum. **Frontal gyrus, medial.** A gyrus on the medial surface of the frontal lobe between the supermedial border and the sulcus cinguli. **Frontal gyrus, middle [gyrus frontalis medius (NA)].** The middle of 3 frontal gyri lying between the superior and inferior sulci, and divided into a superior and inferior part by an incomplete middle frontal sulcus. **Frontal gyrus, superior [gyrus frontalis superior (NA)].** The superior of the 3 horizontal gyri lying between the superomedial border of the hemisphere and the superior frontal sulcus. **Hippocampal gyrus [gyrus parahippocampalis (NA)].** A gyrus on the medial side of the temporal lobe, extending from the uncus anteriorly to the isthmus posteriorly. **Gyri of the insula, long and short [gyrus longus insulae et gyri breves insulae (NA)].** Gyri on the surface of the insula. **Intralimbic gyrus.** A part of the uncus related to the tail of the dentate gyrus. **Lingual gyrus [gyrus lingualis (NA)].** The gyrus between the collateral and calcarine sulci. **Occipital gyri, lateral.** Superior and inferior gyri formed by the lateral occipital sulcus. **Occipitotemporal gyrus, lateral [gyrus occipitotemporalis lateralis (NA)].** A gyrus on the tentorial surface, lateral to the occipitotemporal sulcus. **Occipitotemporal gyrus, medial [gyrus occipitotemporalis medialis (NA)].** A gyrus on the tentorial surface, medial to the occipitotemporal sulcus. **Orbital gyri of the orbital surface of the cerebral hemisphere [gyri orbitales (NA)].** The gyri lateral to the gyrus rectus. **Paraterminal gyrus [gyrus paraterminalis (NA)].** A small area of cortex anterior to the lamina terminalis and below the rostrum of the corpus callosum. **Postcentral gyrus [gyrus postcentralis (NA)].** The gyrus immediately posterior to the central sulcus of the cerebrum and containing the greater part of the general sensory area. **Precentral gyrus [gyrus precentralis (NA)].** The gyrus immediately anterior to the central sulcus of the cerebrum and containing the pyramidal area. **Gyrus rectus [NA].** A gyrus on the medial border of the orbital surface of the frontal lobe. **Splenial gyrus [gyrus fasciolaris (NA)].** A band of grey matter which passes round the splenium of the corpus callosum and joins the indusium griseum to the hippocampal formation; the fasciola cinerea. **Supramarginal gyrus.** The anterior part of the inferior parietal lobule. **Temporal gyrus, inferior [gyrus temporalis inferior (NA)].** The lowest of the 3 temporal gyri below the inferior temporal sulcus of the temporal lobe. **Temporal gyrus, middle [gyrus temporalis medius (NA)].** The intermediate of the 3 temporal gyri horizontal in direction and lying between the superior and inferior temporal sulci of the temporal lobe. **Temporal gyrus, superior [gyrus temporalis superior (NA)].** The gyrus lying between the lateral sulcus of the cerebrum and the superior temporal sulcus of the temporal lobe. **Temporal gyri, transverse [gyri temporales transversi (NA)].** The 3 or 4 gyri into which the floor of the posterior ramus of the lateral sulcus of the cerebrum is divided by the transverse temporal sulci of the temporal lobe. **Transitional gyri.** Transversely-running gyri in the floors of the deeper sulci. **Transverse gyrus.** A gyrus connecting pre- and post-central gyri in the depth of the central sulcus. **Uncinate gyrus.** The uncus on the medial side of the temporal pole. [Gk *gyros* turn.]

See also: BROCA, ECKER, HESCHL, RETZIUS (A. A.), RETZIUS (M. G.), ZUCKERKANDL.

H

Haab, Otto (b. 1850). Zürich ophthalmologist.

Haab's degeneration, Biber-Haab-Dimmer degeneration. A familial type of dystrophy or degeneration of the corneal epithelium, beginning about puberty and characterized by the junction of fine lines which may or may not intersect.

Haab's magnet. A heavily mounted magnet employed in eye injuries to remove embedded steel particles from the eye.

Haab's band opacity. The tears in Descemet's membrane found in cases of buphthalmia which form a band-shaped corneal opacity.

habena (hab·e·nah). Habenula. [L rein.]

habenal, habenar (hab·e·nal, hab·e·nar). Habenular.

habenula [NA] (hab·en·ew·lah). Any rein-, thong- or whip-like structure. The term is particularly applied to the fibres which appear to run posteriorly along the dorsomedial border of the thalamus to the habenular ganglia or epithalamus; the fibres on the 2 sides, taken together, have a superficial resemblance to reins. [L little rein.]

See also: HALLER.

habenular (hab·en·ew·lar). Relating to a habenula.

Habermann, Rudolf (b. 1884). Hamburg dermatologist.

Habermann's disease. Pityriasis lichenoides et varioliformis acuta.

habit (hab·it). 1. A frequent or constant practice or acquired tendency which has been fixed by frequent repetition. 2. A bodily or mental constitution or temperament; the usual behaviour or mode of life. 3. An automatic response, usually motor, produced by learning. **Apoplectic habit.** A body-build comprising a short neck, tendency to stoutness and a plethoric flushed face. **Asthenic habit.** A slender type of body-build with a long flat chest, winged scapulae and poor muscular development. **Drug habit.** Addiction to a drug. **Endothelioid habit.** The state of a cell having a small nuclear-cytoplasmic ratio. **Full habit.** Apoplectic habit (see above). **Glaucomatous habit.** The appearance of an eye predisposed to glaucoma, i.e. with a shallow anterior chamber. **Hierarchy of habits.** The elevation of simpler habits into the complex ones needed in, say, learning to play the piano. **Leucocytoid habit.** Endothelioid habit (see above). **Opium habit.** Addiction to opium. **Physiological habit.** An acquired regular response to stimulation brought about by constant repetition. **Pyknic habit.** A short stocky build. [L *habitus* state.]

habitat (hab·it·at). The natural abode of an animal or plant, as distinct from range (geographical distribution), locality (circumscribed area) and station (exact spot). [L *habitare* to dwell.]

habituation (hab·it·ew·a'·shun). 1. The process of gradually becoming accustomed to environment. 2. The process of gradually becoming adapted to a particular stimulus. 3. In drug addiction, the psychical parallel to acquired physical tolerance. [L *habituare* to make a habit of.]

habitus (hab·it·us). The general physical appearance characteristic of those with a constitutional tendency to some particular disease or disorder of metabolism; habit. **Habitus apoplecticus.** The supposed appearance of anyone with a tendency to apoplexy, i.e. square and corpulent build, short neck, prominent twisted temporal arteries and dark red complexion; apoplectic habit. **Habitus enteroptoticus.** The bodily shape significant of enteroptosis, i.e. a long and narrow abdomen and a costal angle of less than 90°. **Eurymorph habitus.** Pyknic habit. *See* HABIT. **Habitus hyposthenicus.** A physique with a long, narrow chest and an acute costal angle, usually associated with visceroptosis. **Habitus phthisicus.** The bodily characteristics of predisposition to tuberculosis, e.g. lank, dull hair, thin, shiny, white and dry skin; alar chest. **Ptotic habitus.** A general tendency to ptosis. [L state.]

habromania (hab·ro·ma·ne·ah). 1. Amoenomania. 2. A form of delusional insanity in which the delusions are pronouncedly cheerful and gay in type. [Gk *habros* graceful, mania.]

habu (hab·oo). The local name for *Trimeresurus flavoviridis*, a pit viper of the family Crotalidae. [Jap.]

hachement (ahsh·mahn). In massage, the hacking or chopping stroke carried out with the edge of the hand or of the extended fingers. [Fr. *hacher* to hack.]

Hachimycin (ha·che·mi·sin). BP Commission approved name for an antibiotic produced by *Streptomyces hachijoensis*; it is used in the treatment of trichomoniasis.

Hackenbruch, Peter Theodor (b. 1865). German surgeon.

Hackenbruch's experience. The area affected by the subcutaneous injection of a local anaesthetic solution is the shape of a rhombus.

Hacker, Viktor von (b. 1852). Vienna surgeon.

von Hacker's operation. An operation for hypospadias.

hacking (hak·ing). Hachement. [AS *haeccan.*]

Haden, Russell Landram (b. 1888). Kansas City physician.

Haden-Hausser method. An acid haematin method of estimating haemoglobin, with a special instrument in which a coloured wedge is used.

Hadfield, Geoffrey (b. 1889). London pathologist.

Clark-Hadfield syndrome, Hadfield-Clark syndrome. Infantilism due to congenital insufficiency of the pancreas, probably identical with cystic fibrosis of the pancreas (Dorothy Anderson) or fibrocystic disease of the pancreas.

Haeckel, Ernst Heinrich (b. 1834). Jena zoologist.

Haeckel's law. Embryos, during development, recapitulate the characters of the phylogenetic series to which they belong.

haem (heem). Reduced haematin; a ferroprotoporphyrin, $C_{34}H_{33}N_4O_4FeOH$, which forms the non-protein part of the molecules of haemoglobin, myoglobin and cytochrome C. **Haem "A".** The prosthetic group of cytochromes of the "a" class (cytochromes a and a_3). It differs from haem in having an aldehyde group and a 15-carbon isoprenoid side-chain in place of a methyl and a vinyl group respectively which are present in haem. *Haem-haem interaction* is the effect of binding of a molecule of oxygen to 1 haem group in a haemoglobin molecule on the rate of binding of oxygen to the remaining haem groups. [Gk *haima* blood.]

Haemachatus (he·mah·ka·tus). A genus of elapid snakes. **Haemachatus haemachatus.** The ringhals, a dangerously poisonous cobra of South Africa. The poison may be sprayed as well as injected and may cause blindness.

haemachromatosis (he·mah·kro·mat·o'·sis). Haemochromatosis.

haemachrome (he·mah·krome). Haemochrome.

haemachrosis (he·mah·kro·sis). 1. The redness of the blood. 2. Any disease in which the blood is of intensified or other abnormal redness. [Gk *haima* blood, *chrosis* colouring.]

haemacyte (he·mah·site). Haemocyte.

haemacytometer (he·mah·si·tom'·et·er). Haemocytometer.

haemacytozoon (he·mah·si·to·zo'·on). Haemocytozoon.

haemaden (he·mad·en). A ductless gland. [Gk *haima* blood, *aden* gland.]

haemadenology (he·mad·en·ol'·o·je). Endocrinology. [Gk *haima* blood, *aden* gland, *logos* science.]

Haemadipsa (he·mah·**dip**·sah). A genus of terrestrial leeches. *Haemadipsa zeylandica* is a serious blood sucker in parts of Sri Lanka; the bites are painful and may cause bacterial infection. Similar leeches occur in other parts of the tropical Far East. [Gk *haima* blood, *dipsa* thirst.]

haemadostenosis (**he**·mad·o·sten·**o**′·sis). 1. Contraction of the arteries. 2. Narrowing or obliteration of an artery or vein. [Gk *haimas* blood stream, stenosis.]

haemadosteosis (**he**·mad·os·te·**o**′·sis). Calcification or ossification of the blood vessels. [Gk *haimas* blood stream, *osteon* bone.]

haemadromograph (he·mad·**ro**·mo·graf). Haemodromograph.

haemadromometer (**he**·mad·ro·**mom**′·et·er). Haemodromometer.

haemadsorption (he·mad·**sorp**·shun). Adsorption of red blood cells. The surface of some strains of cells in culture after infection with some viruses is altered to include viral haemagglutinin. Red cells added to the culture will then adsorb to the infected cells. [Gk *haima* blood, L *ad, sorbere* to suck in.]

haemadynamic (**he**·mah·di·**nam**′·ik). Haemodynamic.

haemadynamics (**he**·mah·di·**nam**′·ix). Haemodynamics.

haemadynamometer (**he**·mah·di·nam·**om**′·et·er). Haemodynamometer.

haemafacient (he·mah·**fa**·shent). 1. Haematopoietic. 2. Any agent which improves the quality of the blood and increases the quantity of it. [Gk *haima* blood, L *facere* to make.]

haemafaecia (he·mah·**fe**·se·ah). The condition in which the stools contain blood. [Gk *haima* blood, faeces.]

haemagglutination (**he**·mag·loo·tin·**a**′·shun). The aggregation of erythrocytes by specific antibody (through antigens on the erythrocyte surface) or by viruses or bacteria or plant proteins (through receptors on the erythrocyte surface). This aggregation may be prevented (*haemagglutination inhibition*) by free antigen or by antiviral antibody, respectively. In *direct haemagglutination*, antigens naturally present on the erythrocyte are involved; in *indirect, conditioned or passive haemagglutination*, soluble antigens are attached to the erythrocyte artificially. [Gk *haima* blood, L *agglutinare* to glue.]

haemagglutinative (he·mag·**loo**·tin·at·iv). Causing the clumping together of erythrocytes. [see prec.]

haemagglutinin (he·mag·**loo**·tin·in). 1. An antibody in serum which agglutinates red blood corpuscles. It may occur naturally or be induced by the injection of red blood corpuscles from one species into a member of a different species, when the cells act as an antigen stimulating the production of the antibody. Haemagglutinins may be divided into: *autohaemagglutinins* which are contained in the serum or plasma of an individual and may under certain conditions agglutinate his own red blood cells, e.g. cold agglutinins; *iso-agglutinins* or *homologous haemagglutinins* which agglutinate the red blood cells of members of the same species and form the basis of the system of blood groups described by Landsteiner (1901); *hetero-agglutinins* which agglutinate the cells of other species of animals and which may be natural or induced. 2. A virus-specific antigen, which may be part of the virus surface or an entity separate from the virion, and which has an affinity for the surface receptors on red blood cells. Mixing of red cells and virus causes a haemagglutination which is independent of antibody but the process can be inhibited by antibody directed against the haemagglutinin. [Gk *haima* blood, agglutinin.]

haemagglutinogen (he·mag·**loo**·tin·o·jen). A substance present in erythrocytes that gives rise specifically to the haemagglutinins in the blood serum. [haemagglutinin, Gk *genein* to produce.]

haemagogue (he·mag·og). 1. An agent which causes or promotes the discharge of blood, e.g. from haemorrhoids or during the menstrual periods; an emmenagogue. 2. Promoting the discharge of blood. [Gk *haima* blood, *agogos* leading.]

Haemagogus (he·mag·**og**·us). A genus of the treetop-inhabiting mosquitoes, a species of which, *Haemagogus capricorni*, transmits yellow fever. **Haemagogus equini.** A potential mosquito vector of yellow fever. [see prec.]

haemagonium (he·mag·**o**·ne·um). An erythroblast. [Gk *haima* blood, *gone* seed.]

haemal (**he**·mal). 1. Relating or belonging to the blood or the vascular system. 2. On the same side of the body as are the heart and great blood vessels [obsolete term]. [Gk *haima* blood.]

haemalexin (he·mal·**ex**·in). An alexin of the blood. [see foll.]

haemalexis (he·mal·**ex**·is). The process by which the protective elements of the blood are formed. [Gk *haima* blood, *alexein* to ward off.]

haemalopia (he·mal·**o**·pe·ah). An effusion of blood into the eye. [Gk *haima* blood, *alaos* blind, L *ops* eye.]

haemalum (he·**mal**·um) A histological stain for cell nuclei prepared from haematoxylin and alum. It is most often used for staining in bulk.

See also: MAYER (P.).

Haemamoeba (he·mam·e·bah). Haemosporidia: an order of Protozoa belonging to the class Sporozoa. It includes the genera *Babesia, Haemogregarina, Haemoproteus, Leucocytozoon, Plasmodium* and *Theileria.* The malarial parasites are the only Haemamoeba known to cause disease in man, but many species in the genera cause disease in animals and birds. [Gk *haima* blood, amoeba.]

haemamoebiasis (**he**·mam·e·**bi**′·as·is). Infection with a blood parasite of the order Haemamoeba. [see prec.]

haemanalysis (he·man·**al**·is·is). The process of analysing the blood. [Gk *haima* blood, analysis.]

haemangiectasia, haemangiectasis (**he**·man·je·ek·**ta**′·ze·ah, **he**·man·je·**ek**′·tas·is). A state of dilatation of the blood vessels. [Gk *haima* blood, angiectasia.]

haemangioblastoma (**he**·man·je·o·blas·**to**′·mah). An angioma of the capillary vessels of the brain, consisting of angioblasts or proliferated blood-vessel cells. **Haemangioblastoma retinae.** The correct name for a form of angiomatosis retinae, or von Hippel's disease, in which there is a localized tumour made up of glial tissue situated at the retinal periphery, and large cystic blood spaces. It is also called *angiogliosis retinae* or *haemangiogliomatosis retinae.* [haemangioma, blastoma.]

haemangio-endothelioblastoma (he·**man**·je·o·en·do·**the**·le·o·blas·**to**′·mah). A neoplasm composed of proliferated endothelial cells derived from a lining of the blood vessels. [haemangioma, endothelium, blastoma]

haemangio-endothelioma (he·**man**·je·o·**en**·do·the·le·**o**′·mah). An overgrowth of the endothelial cells of the capillary vessels, variable in size and commonly found in the circulatory net of the cerebral meninges. **Haemangio-endothelioma tuberosum multiplex.** An eruption of papules and nodules due to proliferation of the endothelium of the blood vessels of the skin. [haemangioma, endothelioma.]

haemangiofibroma (he·**man**·je·o·fi·**bro**′·mah). A combined haemangioma and fibroma.

haemangiogliomatosis retinae (he·**man**·je·o·gli·o·mat·**o**′·sis **ret**·in·e). Haemangioblastoma retinae. [haemangioma, glioma, Gk *-osis* condition, retina.]

haemangiolymphangioma (he·**man**·je·o·lim·fan·je·**o**′·mah). A congenital skin growth in which both blood vessels and lymphatics are involved. [haemangioma, Gk *lympha* lymph, *-oma* tumour.]

haemangioma (**he**·man·je·**o**′·mah) (pl. *haemangiomata*). An innocent tumour composed of dilated blood vessels. **Capillary haemangioma.** Naevus. **Cavernous haemangioma.** A tumour composed of wide vascular spaces, with a close resemblance to erectile tissue. **Haemangioma congenitale.** Naevus sanguineus, strawberry mark, raspberry mark: a congenital tumour of blood vessels situated in the skin or at the surface of organs. **Haemangioma hypertrophicum cutis.** A prominent fleshy cellular angioma of the skin. **Sclerosing haemangioma.** Nodular subepidermal fibrosis. *See* FIBROSIS. **Haemangioma simplex.** A tumour composed of simple capillary-like blood vessels. [Gk *haima* blood, *aggeion* small vessel, *-oma* tumour.]

haemangiomatosis (he·man·je·o·mat·**o**′·sis). A condition characterized by the formation of multiple haemangiomata. [haemangioma, Gk *-osis* condition.]

haemangiopericytoma (he·man·je·o·per·e·si·to'·mah). A capillary tumour composed of pericytes (Rouget cells). [haemangioma, pericyte, Gk *-oma* tumour.]

haemangiosarcoma (he·man·je·o·sar·ko'·mah) A combined haemangioma and sarcoma.

Haemanthus (he·man·thus). A genus of South African plants (family Amaryllidaceae), several species of which are reported as being used medicinally both as antiseptic and soothing applications, and for their diuretic properties. The bulbs of certain members contain poisonous principles. **Haemanthus toxicarius.** A species containing an alkaloid that is employed as an arrow poison. [Gk *haima* blood, *anthos* flower.]

haemaphaein (he·mah·fe·in). Haemaphein.

haemapheic (he·mah·fe·ik). Containing haemaphein.

haemaphein (he·mah·fe·in). A brown colouring substance of the blood and urine. [Gk *haima* blood, *phaios* dusky.]

haemaphobia (he·mah·fo·be·ah). Haemophobia.

haemaphotograph (he·mah·fo·to·graf). Haemophotograph.

Haemaphysalis (he·mah·fi·sa·lis). A genus of ticks. *Haemaphysalis leachi* and the rabbit tick, *H. leporispalustris*, are important vectors of tick-borne typhus. Other species in America and Australia are reservoirs of rickettsias, though they do not bite man, e.g. *H. bispinosa* and *H. humerosa*. Females of *H. cinnabarina* in Canada and *H. punctata* in Crete are suspected causes of tick paralysis. *H. concinna* is a vector of Russian encephalitis and several species are potential vectors of tularaemia. *H. spinigua* and other species are the vectors of Kyasanur Forest disease in southern India. [Gk *haima* blood, *physalis* bubble.]

haemapoiesis (heem·ah·poi·e'·sis). Haemopoiesis.

haemarthrosis (he·mar·thro·sis). Extravasation of blood into a joint. [Gk *haima* blood, *arthron* joint.]

haemartoma (he·mar·to·mah). A tumour composed of newly-formed blood vessels. [Gk *haima* blood, artery, Gk *-oma* tumour]

haematachometer (he·mah·tak·om'·et·er). Haemotachometer.

haematal (he·mat·al). Haemal.

haematein (he·mat·e·in). $C_{16}H_{12}O_6$, a deep-violet crystalline compound resulting from the exposure to air of haematoxylin; present to a slight extent in medicinal logwood.

haematemesis (he·mat·em·es·is). Vomiting of blood. [Gk *haima* blood, emesis.]

See also: GOLDSTEIN.

haematencephalon (he·mat·en·kef'·al·on). Haemorrhage in some part of the brain; bleeding from cerebral arteries or veins. [Gk *haima* blood, *egkephalos* brain.]

haematherapy (he·mah·ther·ap·e). Haemotherapy.

haemathermal, haemathermous (he·mah·ther·mal, heem·ah·therm·us). Haematothermal.

haemathidrosis (he·mat·hid·ro'·sis). The excretion of sweat containing blood or blood pigment; sudor sanguineus. [Gk *haima* blood, *hidros* sweat.]

haemathorax (he·mah·thor·ax). Haemothorax.

haematic (he·mat·ik). 1. Haemal. 2. Contained in the blood. 3. Acting on the blood. 4. Containing or full of blood. 5. Blood-red. 6. A tonic for improving the condition or quantity of the blood. [Gk *haima* blood.]

haematicum (he·mat·ik·um). Name applied to a solution of iron salts in a mixture of alcohol and water.

haematid (he·mat·id). 1. An erythrocyte. 2. A cutaneous eruption due to some disorder of the blood. [Gk *haima* blood.]

haematidrosis (he·mat·id·ro'·sis). Haemathidrosis.

haematimeter (he·mat·im·et·er). A square-ruled microscope slide with which the number of blood corpuscles in a given volume of blood can be counted. [Gk *haima* blood, meter.]

haematimetry (he·mat·im·et·re). The process of counting the number of blood corpuscles in a given volume of blood. [see prec.]

haematin (he·mat·in). Methaem: a blue-black amorphous substance, $C_{34}H_{32}N_4O_4FeOH$, formed by the oxidation of haem, the essential feature being the conversion of iron from the ferrous to the ferric state. It is insoluble in water and most organic solvents, but in alkalis and glacial acetic acid it dissolves to form *alkaline* and *acid haematin* respectively, each with a characteristic absorption spectrum. Treated with concentrated sulphuric acid, it gives up its iron and becomes haematoporphyrin. [Gk *haima* blood.]

haematinaemia (he·mat·in·e'·me·ah). The presence of haematin in the blood. It has been reported in acute chromium poisoning. [haematin, Gk *haima* blood.]

haematinic (he·mat·in·ik). 1. Referring to or belonging to haematin. 2. Any therapeutic agent which gives rise to an increase of the haemoglobin content of the blood, but more broadly may refer to any substance having anti-anaemic properties.

haematinogen (he·mat·in·o·jen). A blood-forming or blood-producing substance. [Gk *haima* blood, *genein* to produce.]

haematinometer (he·mat·in·om'·et·er). An instrument with which the amount of haemoglobin in the blood can be measured by colorimetry. It indicates percentages of the normal quantity.

haematinuria (he·mat·in·ewr'·e·ah). Urine which is dark in colour as the result of the presence of haematin; it may also indicate haemoglobinuria.

haematite (he·mat·ite). Natural ferric oxide, Fe_2O_3; it occurs in blood-red or black crystalline or granular forms in Canada, England and Sweden principally and is one of the most important ores of iron. [Gk *haima* blood.]

haemato-aerometer (he·mat·o·a·er·om'·et·er). An instrument with which the pressure of gases in the blood can be recorded and determined. [Gk *haima* blood, *aer* air, meter.]

Haematobia (he·mat·o·be·ah). A genus of flies of the family Muscidae. **Haematobia irritans.** The horn fly; a source of great irritation to cattle but seldom biting man. **Haematobia stimulans.** Of Britain and Europe, bites man freely. It is related to the stable fly, but does not come indoors. [Gk *haima* blood, *bios* life.]

haematobium (he·mat·o·be·um). 1. A blood parasite or any other organism living in the blood. 2. The species name of a fluke, *Schistosoma haematobium.* [see prec.]

haematoblast (he·mat·o·blast). Haemocytoblast.

haematocatharsis (he·mat·o·kath·ar'·sis). 1. The process of purifying the blood by expelling harmful substances from it. 2. Blood lavage. *See* LAVAGE. [Gk *haima* blood, catharsis.]

haematocele (he·mat·o·seel). 1 A cyst or tumour filled with blood. 2. Effusion and collection of blood in a canal, cavity or part. **Parametric haematocele.** Recto-uterine haematocele (see below). **Pelvic haematocele.** An effusion of blood into the cavity of the peritoneum. **Pudendal haematocele.** A blood-filled cyst or tumour in a labium of the pudendum muliebre. **Recto-uterine haematocele.** A blood-filled tumour in the recto-uterine pouch. **Scrotal haematocele.** A blood-filled cyst or tumour in (*a*) the tunica vaginalis testis or (b) the subcutaneous tissue of the scrotum. **Vaginal haematocele.** Pachyvaginalitis. [Gk *haima* blood, *kele* hernia.]

haematocephalus (he·mat·o·kef'·al·us). 1. A fetus with a head containing a large quantity of blood which has been effused into the cerebral hemispheres. 2. Effusion of blood into the brain; haemato-encephalon. [Gk *haima* blood, *kephale* head.]

haematochromatosis (he·mat·o·kro·mat·o'·sis). Haemochromatosis.

haematochylocele (he·mat·o·ki'·lo·seel). A tumour consisting of an encysted mixture of blood and chyle, e.g. of the tunica vaginalis testis. [Gk *halima* blood, chyle, Gk *kele* tumour.]

haematochyluria (he·mat·o·ki·lewr'·e·ah). In filariasis (*Wuchereria bancrofti*), the passing of urine containing blood and chyle in varying proportions. [Gk *haima* blood, chyluria.]

haematocolpometra (he·mat·o·kol·po·met'·rah). The condition in which menstrual blood has collected in the uterus and vagina because of an obstruction such as an imperforate hymen. [Gk *haima* blood, *kolpos* vagina, *metra* womb.]

haematocolpos (he·mat·o·kol'·pos). A collection of blood or menstrual fluid in the vagina owing to an obstruction, e.g. imperforate hymen. [Gk *haima* blood, *kolpos* vagina.]

haematocrit (he·mat·o·krit). A small centrifuge used in blood analysis to separate the blood corpuscles from the plasma so that the quantity of corpuscles present may be estimated. **Haematocrit reading.** *See* VOLUME, PACKED-CELL. [Gk *haima* blood, *krinein* to separate.]

See also: WINTROBE.

haematocrystallin (he·mat·o·kris′·tal·in). Haemoglobin. [Gk *haima* blood, crystallin.]

haematocyst (he·mat·o·sist). An effusion of blood within a sac; a blood cyst. [Gk *haima* blood, *kystis* bag.]

haematocystis (he·mat·o·sis′·tis). Effusion of blood into the urinary bladder. [see prec.]

haematocyte (he·mat·o·site). Haemocyte.

haematocytoblast (he·mat·o·si′·to·blast). Haemocytoblast.

haematocytolysis (he·mat·o·si·tol′·is·is). Haemocytolysis.

haematocytometer (he·mat·o·si·tom′·et·er). Haemocytometer.

haematocytopenia (he·mat·o·si·to·pe′·ne·ah). A condition in which the number of cellular elements in the blood is decreased. [Gk *haima* blood, cytopenia.]

haematocytosis (he·mat·o·si·to′·sis). A condition of the blood in which there is a number of cellular elements. [Gk *haima* blood, *kytos* cell.]

haematocytozoon (he·mat·o·si·to·zo′·on). A protozoon parasite. *Haematocytozoon brasiliense* is a little-known blood parasite. [Gk *haima* blood, *kytos* cell, *zoon* animal.]

haematocyturia (he·mat·o·si·tewr′·e·ah). The presence of erythrocytes in the urine. [haemocyte, urine.]

haematodynamics (he·mat·o·di·nam′·ix). Haemodynamics.

haematodynamometer (he·mat·o·di·nam·om′·et·er). Haemodynamometer.

haematodyscrasia (he·mat·o·dis·kra′·ze·ah). Disease of the blood, and the state of ill health which may be associated with it. [Gk *haima* blood, dyscrasia.]

haematoedema (he·mat·e·de′·mah). Swelling of a part caused by effusion of blood into it. [Gk *haima* blood, oedema.]

haemato-encephalon (he·mat·o·en·kef′·al·on). Haemorrhage in some part of the brain; bleeding from cerebral arteries or veins. [Gk *haima* blood, *egkephalos* brain.]

haematogen (he·mat·o·jen). A substance which causes increase in the production of blood. [see foll.]

haematogenesis (he·mat·o·jen′·es·is). The development or production of the formed elements of the blood. [Gk *haima* blood, *genein* to produce.]

haematogenic, haematogenous (he·mat·o·jen′·ik, he·mat·oj·en·us). 1. Derived from or originating in blood. 2. Produced in or producing blood. 3. Transported by the blood, e.g. an infection. [see prec.]

haematoglobin (he·mat·o·glo′·bin). Haemoglobin.

haematoglobinuria (he·mat·o·glo·bn·ewr′·e·ah). Haemoglobinuria.

haematoglobulin (he·mat·o·glob′·ew·lin). Haemoglobin.

haematogone (he·mat·o·gone). Haemocytoblast. [Gk *haima* blood, *gone* seed.]

haematohidrosis (he·mat·o·hid·ro′·sis). Haemathidrosis.

haematoid (he·mat·oid). Having the characters of blood; sanguineous. [Gk *haima* blood, *eidos* form.]

haematoidin (he·mat·oid·in). A term formerly applied to the crystals of bilirubin or biliverdin which sometimes occur in blood clots, mostly of traumatic origin, or in faeces after intestinal haemorrhage. [see prec.]

haematokolpos (he·mat·o·kol′·pos). Haematocolpos.

haematokrit (he·mat·o·krit). Haematocrit.

haematolin (he·mat·o·lin). $C_{68}H_{78}O_7N_8$, an additive compound of haematin which does not contain any iron.

haematolith (he·mat·o·lith). Haemolith.

haematologist (he·mat·ol·o·jist). One who makes a special study of haematology and has the technical skill requisite for carrying out examination of the blood.

haematology (he·mat·ol·o·je). That branch of medical science which is concerned with the blood and blood-forming tissues. [Gk *haima* blood, *logos* science.]

haematolymphangioma (he·mat·o·limf·an·je·o′·mah). A tumour consisting mainly of, or involving, dilated blood vessels and lymph vessels. [Gk *haima* blood, lymph, angioma.]

haematolymphuria (he·mat·o·limf·ewr·e·ah). The passage of blood and lymph in the urine. [Gk *haima* blood, lymph, urine.]

haematolysis (he·mat·ol·is·is). Haemolysis.

haematoma (he·mat·o·mah). A tumour or swelling composed of blood, and the result of injury or of some blood disease such as leukaemia or purpura. **Aneurysmal haematoma.** The mass of blood clot which forms over a site of rupture of an aneurysm. **Haematoma auris.** An effusion of blood into the external ear as the result of rough handling or trauma, especially in various forms of insanity. **Chronic subdural haematoma.** An accumulation of blood plasma or clot beneath the dura mater, displacing the brain. Often rapidly enveloped by a thin, cellular membrane forming a cyst causing pressure symptoms. It usually results from injury, which, in the case of the elderly, can be relatively trivial. Detectable by x-ray when, as in later stages, it becomes calcified, and can readily be demonstrated by arteriography. **Dural haematoma.** A localized effusion of blood into the dura mater as the result of trauma. **Extradural haematoma.** A haematoma between the dura mater and the skull. **Intracerebral haematoma.** A haematoma within the cerebrum. **Pelvic haematoma.** An effusion of blood into the soft tissues of the pelvis during childbirth. **Peri-anal haematoma.** A haematoma in the anal region. **Pulsatile haematoma.** A blood clot through which the pulse is easily transmitted. **Retroperitoneal haematoma.** A collection of blood deep to the posterior peritoneum. **Retro-uterine haematoma.** An effusion of blood into the soft tissues adjacent to and between the rectum and the uterus. **Subumbilical haematoma.** A haematoma in the abdominal wall under the umbilicus. **Subungual haematoma.** A haematoma in the loose tissues in the floor of the mouth. [Gk *haima* blood, *-oma* tumour.]

haematomanometer (he·mat·o·man·om′·et·er). Sphygmomanometer. [Gk *haima* blood, manometer.]

haematomatous (he·mat·o·mat·us). Pertaining to or having the character of a haematoma.

haematomediastinum (he·mat·o·me·de·as·ti′·num). An effusion of blood in the mediastinum and its associated spaces. [Gk *haima* blood, mediastinum.]

haematometakinesis (he·mat·o·met·ah·kin·e′·sis). The phenomenon exhibited by the body of being able to divert (shunt) large amounts of blood from one organ or area to another in an emergency. [Gk *haima* blood, *meta*, *kinetin* to move.]

haematometer (he·mat·om·et·er). 1. Haemodynamometer. 2. Haemoglobinometer.

haematometra (he·mat·o·met′·rah). Accumulation of blood or menstrual fluid in the cavity of the uterus. [Gk *haima* blood, *metra* womb.]

haematometry (he·mat·om·et·re). Haemometry.

haematomphalocele (he·mat·om·fal·o·seel). An umbilical hernia into which an effusion of blood has occurred. [Gk *haima* blood, omphalocele.]

haematomphalos (he·mat·om·fal·os). 1. Haematomphalocele. 2. Cullen's sign: bluish discoloration around the umbilicus, considered as diagnostic of ruptured extra-uterine pregnancy; blue navel. [Gk *haima* blood, *omphalos* navel.]

haematomycosis (he·mat·o·mi·ko′·sis). A condition in which fungi are present in the blood. [Gk *haima* blood, mycosis].

haematomyelia (he·mat·o·mi·e′·le·ah). Bleeding within the substance of the spinal cord, apparently as the result of indirect trauma, usually in the cervical region. [Gk *haima* blood, *myelos* marrow.]

haematomyelitis (he·mat·o·mi·el·i′·tis). Acute haemorrhagic inflammation of the spinal cord. [Gk *haima* blood, myelitis.]

haematomyelopore (he·mat·o·mi′·el·o·por). A disease in which cavities or channels form in the substance of the spinal cord as the result of haemorrhages. [Gk *haima* blood, *myelos* marrow, *poros* passage.]

haematonephrosis (he·mat·o·nef·ro′·sis). Accumulation of blood in the pelvis of the ureter. [Gk *haima* blood, nephrosis.]

haematonic (he·mah·ton·ik). A blood tonic; a remedy which improves the condition of the blood by raising the percentage of haemoglobin. [Gk *haima* blood, tonic.]

haematonosis (he·mat·on·os·is). Any disease of the blood. [Gk *haima* blood, *nosos* disease.]

haematopathology (he·mat·o·path·ol′·o·je). That branch of medical science which is concerned with diseases of the blood. [Gk *haima* blood, pathology.]

haematopedesis (he·mat·o·ped·e′·sis). 1. Haemathidrosis. 2. Haemorrhage through the skin. [Gk *haima* blood, *pedesis* an oozing.]

haematopericardium (he·mat·o·per·e·kar′·de·um). An effusion of blood in the pericardium, unconnected with pericarditis. [Gk *haima* blood, pericardium.]

haematoperitoneum (he·mat·o·per·e·ton·e′·um). Haemoperitoneum.

haematopexin (he·mat·o·pex′·in). Haemopexin.

haematopexis (he·mat·o·pex′·is). Haemopexis.

haematophagia (he·mat·o·fa′·jeah). 1. Drinking of blood. 2. Feeding on the blood of another animal, as in the case of blood-sucking insects. 3. The destruction of erythrocytes by phagocytes. [Gk *haima* blood, *phagein* to eat.]

haematophagocyte (he·mat·o·fag′·o·site). Haemophagocyte.

haematophagous (he·mat·of·ag·us). 1. Blood-sucking. 2. Subsisting on blood. [Gk *haima* blood, *phagein* to eat.]

haematophagus (he·mat·of·ag·us). Blood-sucking insects in general; a blood eater. [see prec.]

haematophagy (he·mat·of·ah·je). Haematophagia.

haematophilia (he·mat·o·fil′·e·ah). Haemophilia.

haematophobia (he·mat·o·fo′·be·ah). Haemophobia.

haematophyte (he·mat·o·fite). Any vegetable micro-organism living in the blood. [Gk *haima* blood, *phyton* plant.]

haematopiesis (he·mat·o·pi·e′·sis). Blood pressure. [Gk *haima* blood, *piesis* pressure.]

Haematopinus (he·mat·o·pi′·nus). A genus of rat lice. [Gk *haima* blood, *pinein* to drink.]

haematoplasmopathy (he·mat·o·plaz·mop′·ath·e). Any disease in which there is any excess, deficiency or disproportion of the normal plasma proteins. [Gk *haima* blood, plasma, Gk *pathos* disease.]

haematoplast (he·mat·o·plast). Haemocytoblast. [see foll.]

haematoplastic (he·mat·o·plas′·tik). 1. Referring or belonging to the formation of blood. 2. Blood-forming. [Gk *haima* blood, *plassein* to form.]

haematopneic (he·mat·o·ne′·ik). Relating or belonging to the oxygenation of the blood. [Gk *haima* blood, *pnein* to breathe.]

haematopoiesis (he·mat·o·poi·e′·sis). Haemopoiesis.

haematopoietin (he·mat·o·poi·et·in). Haemopoietin.

haematoporphyria (he·mat·o·por·fir′·e·ah). Porphyria; disordered porphyrin metabolism, giving rise to reactions such as dermal sensitivity to light, haematoporphyrinuria and gastro-intestinal disturbance. [see foll.]

haematoporphyrin (he·mat·o·por·fir·in). A compound which is free of iron, $C_{34}H_{38}O_6N_4$, obtained by treating haemoglobin or haematin with strong acids. It is a dark-red to violet powder, insoluble in water, but dissolving readily in alkalis, alcohol and concentrated sulphuric acid. A derivative of protoporphyrin, it forms with soda lime an aetioporphyrin resembling that produced by chlorophyll. [Gk *haima* blood, *porphyra* purple.]

haematoporphyrinaemia (he·mat·o·por·fir·in·e′·me·ah). The presence of haematoporphyrin in the blood. [haematoporphyrin, Gk *haima* blood.]

haematoporphyrinism (he·mat·o·por′·fir·in·izm). Haematoporphyrinaemia and abnormal sensitivity of the skin to the rays of the sun.

haematoporphyrinuria (he·mat·o·por·fir·in·ewr′·e·ah). A condition in which haematoporphyrin is present in the urine. It may be due to the use of the sulphonamides or of sulphonal.

haematoporphyroidin (he·mat·o·por·fir·oid′·in). A substance similar in origin and character to haematoporphyrin but relatively insoluble; it may be found in the urine. [haematoporphyrin, Gk *eidos* form.]

Haematopota (he·mat·op·o·tah). An Old World genus of horse flies (family Tabanidae) many species of which bite man painfully. *Haematopota pluvialis* is the most important in Europe. [Gk *haima* blood, L *potare* to drink.]

haematoprecipitin (he·mat·o·pre·sip′·it·in). A precipitin that is specific for blood serum. [Gk *haima* blood, precipitin.]

haematorrhachis (he·mat·o·rak′·is). Haemorrhage within the dura mater or between the dura mater and the central canal of the spinal cord. [Gk *haima* blood, *rhachis* spine.]

haematorrhoea (he·mat·o·re′·ah). A profuse haemorrhage; a free and copious flow of blood. [Gk *haima* blood, *rhoia* flow.]

haematosalpinx (he·mat·o·sal′·pingx). Collection and retention of blood in a uterine tube. [Gk *haima* blood, *salpigx* trumpet.]

haematoscheocele (he·mat·os·ke·o·seel). Distension of the scrotum due to effusion of blood. [Gk *haima* blood, oscheocele.]

haematoscope (he·mat·o·skope). An instrument with which blood can be examined spectroscopically or optically. [Gk *haima* blood, *skopein* to watch.]

haematoscopy (he·mat·os·ko·pe). Examination of the blood by means of the haematoscope.

haematose (he·mat·oze). 1. Bloody. 2. Full of blood. [Gk *haima* blood.]

haematosepsis (he·mat·o·sep′·sis). Septicaemia. [Gk *haima* blood, sepsis.]

Haematosiphon (he·mat·o·si′·fon). A genus of bugs. **Haematosiphon inodora.** A chicken bug of Mexico and Central America which bites man freely and painfully; it is a potential vector of American trypanosomiasis. [Gk *haima* blood, *siphon* tube.]

haematosis (he·mat·o·sis). 1. The formation of blood; haemopoiesis. 2. Aeration of the blood in the lungs, as in respiration. [Gk *haima* blood, *-osis* condition.]

haematospectrophotometer (he·mat·o·spek·tro·fo·tom′·et·er). An apparatus with which the amount of haemoglobin in blood can be determined; the quantity of light absorbed when it is passed through the blood is measured spectroscopically. [Gk *haima* blood, spectrophotometer.]

haematospectroscope (he·mat·o·spek′·tro·skope). A specially modified spectroscope used in examination of layers of blood. [Gk *haima* blood, spectroscope.]

haematospectroscopy (he·mat·o·spek·tros′·ko·pe). Examination of the blood by means of a haematospectroscope.

haematospermatocele (he·mat·o·sper′·mat·o·seel). A spermatocele containing blood. [Gk *haima* blood, spermatocele.]

haematospermia (he·mat·o·sper′·me·ah). Haemospermia.

haematospherinaemia (he·mat·o·sfer·in·e′·me·ah). Spherocytosis. [Gk *haima* blood, *sphaira* ball, *haima* blood.]

haematostatic (he·mat·o·stat′·ik). Haemostatic.

haematosteon (he·mat·os·te·on). Haemorrhage into the medullary cavity of a bone. [Gk *haima* blood, *osteon* bone.]

haematotherapy (he·mat·o·ther′·ap·e). Haemotherapy.

haematotherma (he·mat·o·ther′·mah). The warm-blooded animals. [see foll.]

haematothermal, haematothermous (he·mat·o·ther′·mal, he·mat·o·ther′·mus). Relating or belonging to warm-blooded animals, whose temperature remains constant whatever the heat or cold of the surrounding medium. [Gk *haima* blood, *therme* heat.]

haematothorax (he·mat·o·thor′·ax). Haemothorax.

haematotoxic (he·ma·o·tox′·ik). Haemotoxic.

haematotoxicosis (he·mat·o·tox·ik·o′·sis). A toxic state of the haemopoietic system. [Gk *haima* blood, toxicosis.]

haematotoxin (he·mat·o·tox′·in). Haemotoxin.

haematotrachelos (he·mat·o·trak·e′·los). A distended condition of the neck of the uterus due to imperforation or closure of the vagina. [Gk *haima* blood, *trachelos* neck.]

haematotropic (he·mat·o·trop′·ik). Having special affinity for erythrocytes. [Gk *haima* blood, *trope* a turning.]

haematotympanum (he·mat·o·tim′·pan·um). Haemorrhage into the tympanic cavity of the ear. [Gk *haima* blood, tympanum.]

haematoxylin (he·mah·tox·il·in). $C_{16}H_{14}O_6$, a valuable histological stain prepared from logwood (*Haematoxylon campechianum* Linn.). It is a constituent of a large number of staining solutions and can be adapted to stain almost any tissue or cellular component by suitable mordanting, although it is most often employed as a nuclear stain, The best known solutions are those of Delafield, Ehrlich, Harris, Heidenhain, Mallory and Weigert. It is also used as an indicator, changing from yellow (pH 5.0) to brown (pH 6.0). **Iron haematoxylin.** A nuclear stain used in histology; it consists of haematoxylin with ferric chloride, the iron acting as a mordant.

See also: BOEHMER, DELAFIELD, EHRLICH, FRIEDLAENDER, HARRIS (H. F.), MALLORY, WEIGERT.

Haematoxylon (he·mah·tox·il·on). A genus of tropical and subtropical trees (family Leguminosae). *Haematoxylon campechianum* Linn. is the tree from which haematoxylum (logwood) is obtained. [Gk *haima* blood, *xylon* wood.]

Haematoxylum BPC 1949 (he·mah·tox·il·um). Logwood; the heartwood of *Haematoxylon campechianum* Linn.; it yields about 10 per cent of haematoxylin and is used as an astringent. [see prec.]

haematozymosis (he·mat·o·zi·mo′·sis). Fermentation of the blood, i.e. a reaction caused by an enzyme. [Gk *haima* blood, zymosis.]

haematuresis (he·mat·ewr·e′·sis). Haematuria.

haematuria (he·mat·ewr·e·ah). The presence of blood in the urine. **Haematuria aegyptica.** Endemic haematuria (see below). **Angioneurotic haematuria.** Haematuria caused by angioneurotic oedema of the urinary tract. **Endemic haematuria.** Bloody urine caused by an infection with the blood fluke *Schistosoma haematobium.* **Essential haematuria.** Haematuria occurring without a discoverable lesion. **False haematuria.** A red coloration of the urine due to the excretion of substances other than blood, such as an aniline dye. **Microscopic haematuria.** Blood in the urine, not visible to the naked eye but discovered by microscopic examination. **Renal haematuria.** Blood in the urine, derived from the kidneys. **Urethral haematuria.** Blood in the urine, due to haemorrhage from the urethra. **Vesical haematuria.** Blood in the urine, due to haemorrhage from the bladder. [Gk *haima* blood, urine.]

haemelytrometra (he·mel·it·ro·me′·trah). Haematocolpometra. [Gk *haima* blood, *elytron* sheath, *metra* womb.]

haemendothelioma (he·men·do·the·le·o′·mah). Endothelioma caused by proliferation of endothelial cells in the blood vessels. [Gk *haima* blood, endothelioma.]

Haementaria (he·men·ta·re·ah). A genus of Hirudinea. **Haementaria officinalis.** A leech used medicinally in Central and South America.

haemetaboly (he·met·ab·o·le). Metabolism of the blood. [Gk *haima* blood, metabolism.]

haemhidrosis (heem·hid·ro·sis). Haemathidrosis.

haemic (he·mik). Belonging to the blood or relating to it. [Gk *haima* blood.]

haemin (he·min). Haematin chloride, $C_{34}H_{32}O_4N_4FeCl$. A dark-brown crystalline porphyrin derivative which forms in old blood clots. It is insoluble in water but soluble in acids or alkalis, and can be prepared by the action of glacial acetic acid and sodium chloride on oxyhaemoglobin. The crystals are characteristic and serve to identify blood. [Gk *haima* blood.]

haemisotonic (he·mi·so·ton′·ik). Having the same osmotic pressure as the blood serum. [Gk *haima* blood, isotonic.]

haemo-agglutination (he·mo·ag·loo·tin·a′·shun). Haemagglutination.

haemo-agglutinin (he·mo·ag·loo′·tin·in). Haemagglutinin.

haemo-alkalimeter (he·mo·al·kal·im′·et·er). An apparatus with which the degree of alkalinity in the blood may be determined. [Gk *haima* blood, alkalimeter.]

Haemobartonella (he·mo·bar·ton·el′·ah). A sub-genus of *Bartonella.* [Gk *haima* blood, *Bartonella.*]

haemobilia (he·mo·bil·e·ah). Massive haemorrhage from the biliary tract. [Gk *haima* blood, bile.]

haemobilirubin (he·mo·bil·e·roo′·bin). The bilirubin that is normally present in blood, but which may be increased in amount in haemolytic states or as a result of liver dysfunction. [Gk *haima* blood, bilirubin.]

haemoblast (he·mo·blast). Haemocytoblast.

haemoblastosis (he·mo·blas·to′·sis). Proliferation of the haematopoietic (blood-forming) tissues and the blood cells, such as occurs in the leukaemias. [Gk *haima* blood, *blastos* germ.]

haemocatharsis (he·mo·kath·ar′·sis). 1. The process of purifying the blood by expelling harmful substances from it. 2. Blood lavage. [Gk *haima* blood, catharsis.]

haemocatheresis (he·mo·kath·er′·es·is). Haemolysis. [Gk *haima* blood, *kathairein* to bring down.]

haemocatheretic (he·mo·kath·er·et′·ik). Pertaining to or characterized by haemocatheresis.

haemocholecyst (he·mo·kol·e·sist). Haemorrhage into the gall bladder. [Gk *haima* blood, cholecyst.]

haemocholecystitis (he·mo·kol·e·sist·i′·tis). Haemorrhage and inflammation within the gall bladder. [Gk *haima* blood, cholecystitis.]

haemochorial (he·mo·kor·e·al). Concerning the maternal blood stream and the chorionic villi. [Gk *haima* blood, chorion.]

haemochromatosis (he·mo·kro·mat·o′·sis). A chronic disease in which large quantities of an iron-containing pigment, haemosiderin, form deposits in the liver and cause extensive bronze pigmentation of skin in association with cirrhosis of both liver and pancreas; also known as *bronzed diabetes.* [Gk *haima* blood, chromatosis.]

haemochrome (he·mo·krome). The oxygen-carrying colouring matter of the blood, e.g. haemoglobin. [Gk *haima* blood, *chroma* colour.]

haemochromogen (he·mo·kro·mo·jen). Any of the chromoproteins formed by haem with various nitrogenous bases: those occurring in plant and animal tissues are known as *cytochromes.* **Pyridine haemochromogen.** Formed from blood with pyridine, glucose and sodium hydroxide: small pink needles of value in the identification of blood. [Gk *haima* blood, *chroma* colour, *genein* to produce.]

haemochromometer (he·mo·kro·mom′·et·er). An instrument with which the amount of haemoglobin in the blood may be measured by colorimetry. It indicates percentages of the normal quantity. [Gk *haima* blood, *chroma* colour, meter.]

haemochromometry (he·mo·kro·mom′·et·re). The process of measuring by the colorimetric method the amount of haemoglobin in blood. [see prec.]

haemochromoprotein (he·mo·kro·mo·pro′·te·in). Any compound protein in which the prosthetic group is a haemochrome (blood pigment). [Gk *haima* blood, chromoprotein.]

haemocidal (he·mo·si·dal). Destructive of blood cells. [Gk *haima* blood, L *caedere* to kill.]

haemoclasia (he·mo·kla·ze·ah). Haemolytic crisis. [see foll.]

haemoclasis (he·mok·la·is). Haemolysis. [Gk *haima* blood, *klasis* a breaking.]

haemoclastic (he·mo·klas·tik). Haemolytic. [see prec.]

haemocoelom, haemocoeloma (he·mo·se·lom, he·mo·se·lo′·mah). 1. A blood cyst. 2. In embryology, that portion of the coelom in which the heart has its origin. [Gk *haima* blood, *koilia* cavity.]

haemoconcentration (he·mo·kon·sen·tra′·shun). Concentration of the blood by loss of water and electrolytes. This leads not only to a relative increase in the cellular elements but to an increase in the concentration of the plasma proteins; there is an increase in the viscosity of the blood with a resultant slowing of the circulation. [Gk *haima* blood, concentration.]

haemoconia (he·mo·ko·ne·ah). Minute particles present in blood, especially those from broken-down red blood cells. [Gk *haima* blood, *konis* dust.]

haemoconiosis (he·mo·ko·ne·o′·sis). A condition in which there is an unusually large number of haemoconiae in the blood. [Gk *haima* blood, *konis* dust, *-osis* condition.]

haemocryoscopy (he·mo·kri·os′·ko·pe). The process of determination of the freezing point of blood. [Gk *haima* blood, cryoscopy.]

haemocrystallin (he·mo·kris·tal·in). Haemoglobin. [Gk *haima* blood, crystallin.]

haemoculture (he·mo·kul·tcher). Bacteriological culture of the blood. [Gk *haima* blood, culture.]

haemocuprein (he·mo·kew·pre·in). A blue copper-protein compound occurring in mammalian red blood cells and serum. [Gk *haima* blood, L *cuprum* copper.]

haemocuprin (he·mo·kew·prin). A derivative of haemocyanin, the copper-containing respiratory pigment of certain cephalopods and crustacea. [see prec.]

haemocyanin (he·mo·si·an·in). A blue respiratory pigment occurring in the plasma of arthropods and molluscs. It contains copper, and its prosthetic group is probably a polypeptide. Like haemoglobin, it acts as an oxygen carrier, the oxyhaemocyanin being blue whilst the reduced form is colourless. [Gk *haima* blood, *kyanos* blue.]

haemocyte (he·mo·site). 1. A red blood corpuscle. 2. Any blood cell. [Gk *haima* blood, *kytos* cell.]

haemocytoblast (he·mo·si·to·blast). A large, non-differentiated, nucleated, reticulo-endothelial cell, having nucleoli, and from 18 to 23 μm in diameter. It is present in the bone marrow and is considered to be the common precursor of all the cellular elements of the blood (red cells, white cells and platelets). It is formed in the embryo from the blood islands of the yolk sac, and is called variously by different investigators, *lymphoidocyte, haemohistioblast* and *haematogone.* [Gk *haima* blood, *kytos* cell, *blastos* germ.]

haemocytoblastoma (he·mo·si·to·blas·to′·mah). A neoplasm containing all the cells of which typical bone marrow is composed. [Gk *haima* blood, *kytos* cell, *blastos* germ, *-oma* tumour.]

haemocytocatheresis (he·mo·si·to·kath·er′·es·is). Haemolysis. [Gk *haima* blood, *kytos* cell, catheresis.]

haemocytogenesis (he·mo·si·to·jen·es·is). The process of formation or production of blood corpuscles. [Gk *haima* blood, cytogenesis.]

haemocytology (he·mo·si·tol′·o·je). That branch of medical science which is concerned with the blood and its components. [Gk *haima* blood, cytology.]

haemocytolysis (he·mo·si·tol′·is·is). Destruction of blood corpuscles by disruption of the cell membrane. [Gk *haima* blood, cytolysis.]

haemocytolytic (he·mo·si·to·lit′·ik). Referring or belonging to, or caused by haemocytolysis.

haemocytometer (he·mo·si·tom′·et·er). An apparatus for counting the number of cells in a given volume of blood or other fluid. It consists of a diluting pipette and a slide with a counting chamber. The counting chamber is of known volume (generally 0.1 or 0.2×10^{-9}m^3) and has a ruled area in which the cells can be enumerated under a microscope. Various types are in use, differing in the pattern of the ruling, and recently electronic counters have been employed for the purpose. [Gk *haima* blood, *kytos* cell, meter.]

haemocytopoiesis (he·mo·si·to·poi·e′·sis). Haemopoiesis. [Gk *haima* blood, *kytos* cell, *poiein* to make.]

haemocytotripsis (he·mo·si·to·trip′·sis). The breaking up of blood corpuscles by subjecting them to heavy pressure. [Gk *haima* blood, *kytos* cell, *tripsis* a rubbing.]

haemocytozoon (he·mo·si·to·zo′·on). A blood parasite; any protozoal organism living in the blood cells. [Gk *haima* blood, *kytos* cell, *zoon* animal.]

haemodiagnosis (he·mo·di·ag·no′·sis). The diagnosis of disease by examination of the blood. [Gk *haima* blood, diagnosis.]

haemodialyser (he·mo·di·al·i·zer). An artificial kidney; a mechanical apparatus used in certain types of uraemia to attempt to restore to normal the chemical composition of the blood and body fluids. [Gk *haima* blood, *dia, lysis* a loosing.]

haemodialysis (he·mo·di·al′·is·is). The process of separating the crystalloids from the colloids in the blood by means of a dialyser such as an artificial kidney. [Gk *haima* blood, *dia, lysis* a loosing.]

haemodiapedesis (he·mo·di·ah·ped·e′·sis). 1. Haemathidrosis. 2. Haemorrhage through the skin. [Gk *haima* blood, *dia, pedesis* an oozing.]

haemodilution (he·mo·di·lew′·shun). A state in which the concentration of the various blood elements, especially the erythrocytes, is lowered; the reverse of haemoconcentration. [Gk *haima* blood, dilution.]

haemodromograph (he·mo·dro·mo·graf). An instrument with which changes in the velocity of the blood flow can be recorded. [Gk *haima* blood, *dromos* course, *graphein* to record.]

haemodromometer (he·mo·dro·mom′·et·er). An instrument with which the speed of the blood flow can be measured. [Gk *haima* blood, *dromos* course, meter.]

haemodromometry (he·mo·dro·mom′·et·re). The process of measuring the speed of flow of the blood by means of a haemodromometer.

haemodynamic (he·mo·di·nam′·ik). Having relation or belonging to the movements attendant upon the circulation of the blood. [Gk *haima* blood, *dynamis* force.]

haemodynamics (he·mo·di·nam′·ix). The science which is concerned with the motion of the blood and the forces involved in its circulation. [see prec.]

haemodynamometer (he·mo·di·nam·om′·et·er). An instrument with which the degree of pressure (tension) of blood in an artery or vein can be measured. [Gk *haima* blood, *dynamis* force, meter.]

haemodynamometry (he·mo·di·nam·om′·et·re). The measurement of the pressure in the blood vessels. [see prec.]

haemodystrophy (he·mo·dis·tro·fe). A poor condition of the blood due to faulty nutrition. [Gk *haima* blood, dystrophy.]

haemo-endothelioma (he·mo·en·do·the·le·o′·mah). An endothelioma caused by proliferation of endothelial cells in the blood vessels. [Gk *haima* blood, endothelioma.]

haemo-erythrin (he·mo·er·ith′·rin). A blood pigment occurring in marine worms. [Gk *haima* blood, *erythros* red.]

haemo-erythrogen (he·mo·er·ith′·ro·jen). The chromogen corresponding to haemo-erythrin.

haemofibrothorax (he·mo·fi·bro·thor′·ax). A fibrous residue following the clotting of an effusion of blood in the pleural space which may need surgical decortication to allow full re-expansion of the lung. [Gk *haima* blood, fibrothorax.]

haemoflagellate (he·mo·flaj·el·ate). Protozoa of the class Mastigophora that pass part of their life cycle in the blood, of vertebrates: the important genera are the *Leishmania* and *Trypanosoma.* [Gk *haima* blood. flagellate.]

haemoflavoprotein (he·mo·fla·vo·pro′·te·in). A class of protein which contains, as prosthetic groups, a molecule of flavin adenine dinucleotide (FAD) or flavin mononucleotide (FMN) and of haem. They are enzymes usually found bound within the lipid structure of mitochondria of eukaryotes of the respiratory particles of prokaryotes. [Gk *haima* blood, L *flavus* yellow, Gk *proteios* of first rank.]

haemofuscin (he·mo·fus·in). An iron-free yellowish-brown pigment which is found associated with haemosiderin in the tissues in haemochromatosis. [Gk *haima* blood, L *fuscus* brown.]

haemogenesis (he·mo·jen·es·is). The process of development of blood corpuscles or of blood. [Gk *haima* blood, *genesis* origin.]

haemogenia (he·mo·je·ne·ah). Pseudohaemophilia. [Gk *haima* blood, *genein* to produce.]

haemogenic (he·mo·jen·ik). Referring to haemogenesis; able to form blood.

haemoglobic (he·mo·glo·bik). Descriptive of cells which produce or contain haemoglobin.

haemoglobin (he·mo·glo·bin). The respiratory pigment of vertebrates which occurs in the red blood cells. A dark-red compound which can be obtained in crystalline form, soluble in water, insoluble in alcohol and ether, denatured by heat and has a molecular weight of 64 450. It is a tetramer of 4 polypeptide subunits with a total of 574 amino-acid residues (collectively called *globin*) and 4 haem molecules, 1 being attached to each subunit. Haemoglobindiffers in different species of animals, the variation being in the amino-acid composition of the globin and in the amino-acid sequence of the polypeptide subunits. In man and in many other animals, several haemoglobins occur, depending on the stage of development of the organism. *Embryonal haemoglobin* normally disappears before the twelfth week of gestation and occurs in 2 forms called *Gower-1* (which contains 4 subunits of the ϵ-type) and *Gower-2* (which contains a pair of α-type and a pair of ϵ-type subunits). *Fetal haemoglobin* (*haemoglobin F*) replaces the embryonal forms, is present in highest concentration at birth and disappears in most subjects before their first birthday. It contains 2 α-type and 2 γ-type subunits. Persistence of haemoglobin F may occur as a result of severe anaemia beginning early in life, of failure to switch-off production of γ-type subunits and in a variety of pathological conditions, notably sickle-cell anaemia and the thalassaemias. Haemoglobin F is more resistant to denaturation by alkali than haemoglobin A; this forms the basis for a simple procedure for its estimation. *Adult haemoglobin* is composed of a major (*haemoglobin A*, containing 2 α- and 2 β-type subunits) and a minor fraction (*haemoglobin A_2*, containing 2 α- and 2 γ-type subunits). In α-thalassaemia, tetramers containing only δ-type subunits (*haemoglobin Bart's*) or only β-type subunits (*haemoglobin H*) occur at birth and subsequently. Haemoglobin combines loosely with oxygen in the lungs, 1 molecule to the ferrous iron of each haem, to form *oxy-* (or *oxygenated*) *haemoglobin*, in which form it is carried in the arteries to the tissues where oxygen tension is low and where its oxygen is given up to form *deoxygenated* (*deoxy-* or *reduced*) *haemoglobin*. *Deoxyhaemoglobin* plays some part in the transport of carbon dioxide released from the tissues to the lungs, a portion of which penetrates the red cells and combines with the haemoglobin to form *carbaminohaemoglobin*, which reaction is reversed in the lungs as the haemoglobin becomes oxygenated, thus forming a complete cycle. The return of haemoglobin from the tissues to the lungs takes place by way of the veins. *Oxyhaemoglobin* present mainly in arterial blood is scarlet in colour. *Deoxyhaemoglobin* present mainly in venous blood has a purple hue. The absorption spectra of oxy- and deoxy- forms differ from each other as well as from those of *methaemoglobin* (which has a chocolate-brown colour and contains oxidized or ferric iron), *carbonmonoxyhaemoglobin* (in which carbon monoxide is tightly bound to the iron atoms and has a cherry-red colour characteristic of carbon-monoxide poisoning) and *sulfhaemoglobin* (poorly defined derivatives of haemoglobin containing excess sulphur). An *abnormal haemoglobin* (*S*) occurs in sickle-cell anaemia and is responsible for the characteristic abnormality of this and other disorders associated with sickling. In S, the amino acid in the sixth position of the β-polypeptide chains is valine in place of glutamic acid which occurs in normal β-chains. This change gives molecules of deoxyhaemoglobin S a strong tendency to aggregate and form intracellular filaments which are responsible for the distortion of the red cells which become sickled. Many other abnormal haemoglobins (variants) are known which arise from genetically determined structural variation in some of the polypeptide chains (α, β, γ, δ, ϵ or ζ) that occur in the physiological haemoglobins. **Anti-Lepore-type haemoglobin.** One of a class of abnormal haemoglobins which contain a type of polypeptide chain in which the H-terminal part is identical to that of the β-polypeptide chain and the C-terminal part is identical to that of the δ-polypeptide chain. **Deletion haemoglobin.** One of a class of abnormal haemoglobins which result from the loss of 1 or more nucleotide triplets in a gene for 1 of the polypeptide chains; such a variant will contain an abnormal type of polypeptide chain which lacks 1 or more amino-acid residues. **Electrophoretically-silent haemoglobin.** Silent haemoglobin variant (see below). **Fetal haemoglobin.** *See* MAIN DEF. (above). **Haemoglobin co-operativity.** The property of haemoglobin by which the binding of an oxygen molecule to 1 haem influences the affinity for the binding of additional molecules to the other haem groups. **High-affinity haemoglobin.** One of a class of abnormal haemoglobins which bind oxygen more strongly than haemoglobin A and, thus, become deoxygenated much more slowly. **Hybrid haemoglobin, Haemoglobin hybrid.** 1. One of a class of abnormal haemoglobins which contain partial sequences identical with those of 2 different polypeptide chains (Lepore-type and anti-Lepore-type haemoglobins). 2. One of a class of abnormal haemoglobins which contain 2 different types of abnormal polypeptide chains; it may arise as a result of simultaneous double heterozygosity for genes α- and β- or γ-type variants or be produced experimentally by mixing together abnormal α- and abnormal β- or γ-type chains. 3. A haemoglobin produced experimentally which contains 2 types of polypeptide chains obtained from different animal species. **Low-affinity haemoglobin.** One of a class of abnormal haemoglobins which bind oxygen more weakly than haemoglobin A and, thus, become oxygenated much more slowly. **Mean corpuscular haemoglobin.** MCH, the mean or average haemoglobin content of a single red corpuscle (erythrocyte) measured in picograms (pg); it is given by the quotient:

$$\frac{\text{Haemoglobin (grams per litre blood)}}{\text{Red blood corpuscles (millions per }\mu\text{.litre).}}$$

The normal range is from 27 to 32 pg (mean 29.5 pg). **Monomeric haemoglobin.** A type of haemoglobin composed of polypeptide chains which do not aggregate. **Multiple abnormal haemoglobin.** One of a class of haemoglobin variants which contain 2 abnormalities at different positions of the same type of polypeptide chain, or in which 2 kinds of polypeptide chain contain a structural abnormality. The latter is also called *hybrid haemoglobin*. **Muscle haemoglobin.** Myohaemoglobin. **Oxidized haemoglobin, Oxygenated haemoglobin.** Oxyhaemoglobin. **Reduced haemoglobin.** *See* MAIN DEF. (above). **Silent haemoglobin variant.** One of a class of abnormal haemoglobins which contain a structural abnormality which does not change the overall net charge of the molecule and is not detectably abnormal on electrophoresis. **Stripped haemoglobin.** Haemoglobin freed of adhering organic phosphate compounds, especially 2,3-diphosphoglycerate and ATP. **Tetrameric haemoglobin.** One of the class of haemoglobins which contain an aggregate of 4 polypeptide chains per molecule; the chains are usually of 2 different types, but under certain conditions may be of 1 type only. **Unstable haemoglobin.** One of a class of abnormal haemoglobins which may precipitate spontaneously in erythrocytes and produce Heinz bodies and which, in solution, precipitate more easily than haemoglobin A on warming to a temperature of 50°C or higher, or in the presence of isopropanol at 37°C. They are the cause of *unstable haemoglobin haemolytic anaemia* (UHHA). [Gk *haima* blood, L *globus* ball.]

haemoglobinaemia (he·mo·glo·bin·e'·me·ah). A condition in which free haemoglobin is present in the blood plasma, as in laked blood. [haemoglobin, Gk *haima* blood.]

haemoglobiniferous (he·mo·glo·bin·**if**'·er·us). Containing, transporting or yielding haemoglobin. [haemoglobin, L *ferre* to carry.]

haemoglobinocholia (he·mo·glo·bin·o·**ko**'·le·ah). A condition in which haemoglobin is present in the bile. [haemoglobin, Gk *chole* bile.]

haemoglobinogenous (he·mo·glo·bin·**oj**'·en·us). Producing haemoglobin. [haemoglobin, Gk *genein* to produce.]

haemoglobinolysis (he·mo·glo·bin·**ol**'·is·is). The destruction of haemoglobin by dissolution or digestion. [haemoglobin, lysis.]

haemoglobinometer (he·mo·glo·bin·**om**'·et·er). Any instrument used for the determination of haemoglobin in blood. Various types have been designed depending upon colorimetric procedures in which the colour of the blood itself, diluted or undiluted, or the colour produced by treating blood with various reagents is compared with a standard colour. The original forms of instrument depended upon visual comparison, but the modern trend is to employ photometers in which absorption of light is measured by means of photo-electric cells. [haemoglobin, meter.]

See also: DARE, GOWERS, HALDANE, SAHLI.

haemoglobinometry (he·mo·glo·bin·**om'**·et·re). The measuring by colorimetry of the amount of haemoglobin in blood. **Photo-electric haemoglobinometry.** The measurement of the haemoglobin concentration in the blood by a photo-electric method; the personal factor of ordinary haemoglobinometry is excluded. [see prec.]

haemoglobinopathic (he·mo·**glo**·bin·o·**path'**·ik). Relating to defects in the synthesis of haemoglobin. [haemoglobin, Gk *pathos* disease.]

haemoglobinopathy (he·mo·glo·bin·**op'**·ath·e). A disease of the blood associated with the presence of an abnormal haemoglobin in the red blood cells. [haemoglobin, Gk *pathos* disease.]

haemoglobinopepsia (he·mo·**glo**·bin·o·**pep'**·se·ah). Haemoglobinolysis. [haemoglobin, Gk *pepsis* digestion.]

haemoglobinophilia (he·mo·**glo**·bin·o·**fil'**·e·ah). 1. Of bacteria, showing preference for culture media which contain haemoglobin. 2. The state of being attracted by haemoglobin. [haemoglobin, Gk *philein* to love.]

haemoglobinorrhoea (he·mo·**glo**·bin·o·**re'**·ah). Extravasation of haemoglobin from the blood vessels. **Haemoglobinorrhoea cutis.** Effusion of haemoglobin into the skin as the result of engorgement of the veins. [haemoglobin, Gk *rhoia* flow.]

haemoglobinous (he·mo·**glo**·bin·us). Containing haemoglobin.

haemoglobinuria (he·mo·glo·bin·**ewr'**·e·ah). The presence of free haemoglobin in the urine without accompanying red corpuscles. It is always associated with free haemoglobin in the blood plasma due to disintegration of red corpuscles. **Cold haemoglobinuria.** Paroxysmal haemoglobinuria (see below). **Epidemic haemoglobinuria.** Winckel's disease; haemoglobinuria associated with anaemia and jaundice, formerly occurring in epidemics among newborn infants in institutions and probably due to a streptococcal infection. Sporadic cases are occasionally seen as a result of umbilical sepsis. **Intermittent haemoglobinuria.** Paroxysmal haemoglobinuria (see below). **Malarial haemoglobinuria.** Blackwater fever, a complication of malignant tertian malaria in hyperendemic areas; it follows heavy and repeated attacks insufficiently treated. **March haemoglobinuria.** A condition, really of myoglobinuria, in which reddish-brown pigment (myohaemoglobin) is passed in the urine following severe muscular exertion. This pigment, whose molecule is one-quarter the size of that of haemoglobin, passes much more easily through the glomerular membrane. It is recognized by spectroscopy. **Nocturnal haemoglobinuria.** Marchiafava-Micheli syndrome; paroxysms of haemoglobinuria occurring at night and associated with persistent chronic haemolytic anaemia, probably due to autohaemolysins acting when slight lowering of the hydrogen-ion concentration of the blood takes place as a result of reduced pulmonary ventilation during sleep. **Paroxysmal haemoglobinuria.** Attacks of haemoglobinuria due to intravascular haemolysis precipitated by exposure to cold. The red blood corpuscles are broken down by a haemolysin which is present in from 5 to 10 per cent of cases of tertiary syphilis and unites with the red cells at a low temperature, as when the hands are immersed in cold water; with rise of temperature the sensitized cells are lysed by the normal complement of the blood. **Toxic haemoglobinuria.** That occurring secondary to haemolysis caused by toxic agents such as arseniuretted hydrogen, potassium chlorate, ricin, saponins and certain snake venoms. It also occurs with severe burns. **Transfusion haemoglobinuria.** Haemoglobinuria due to transfusion with incompatible blood and the consequent haemolysis of the donor's cells.

See also: SCHILLING.

haemoglobinuric (he·mo·glo·bin·**ewr'**·ik). Pertaining to, suffering from, or characterized by the presence of haemoglobinuria.

haemogram (he·mo·gram). A diagrammatic or tabular correlation of data pertaining to red and white blood cells. [Gk *haima* blood, *gramma* record.]

Haemogregarina (he·mo·greg·ar·**i'**·nah). A sub-order in the Sporozoa containing a genus of the same name, several species of which have been described from human blood. Each species has been seen only once, and they are generally considered accidental or artificial. [Gk *haima* blood, L *grex* flock.]

haemohistioblast (he·mo·**his**·te·o·blast). The name given by Ferata to the primitive blood cell formed in the embryo from the blood islands of the yolk sac. *See* HAEMOCYTOBLAST. [Gk *haima* blood, *histos* tissue, *blastos* cell.]

haemohydraulics (he·mo·hi·**draw'**·lix). That branch of science which is concerned with the blood as a fluid in its passage through the blood vessels. [Gk *haima* blood, hydraulics.]

haemoid (he·moid). Haematoid; having the characters of blood. [Gk *haima* blood, *eidos* form.]

haemokonia (he·mo·**ko**·ne·ah). Haemoconia.

haemokoniosis (he·mo·kon·e·**o'**·sis). Haemoconiosis.

haemoleucocyte (he·mo·**lew**·ko·site). A leucocyte. [Gk *haima* blood, leucocyte.]

haemolith (he·mo·lith). Any hard mass or calculus present in the wall of a blood vessel. [Gk *haima* blood, *lithos* stone.]

haemology (he·**mol**·o·je). Haematology.

haemolymph (he·mo·limf). 1. The blood and lymph. 2. The blood or the nutritive fluid present in some invertebrate animals. [Gk *haima* blood, lymph.]

haemolymphadenosis (he·mo·limf·ad·en·**o'**·sis). Haemoblastosis. [Gk *haima* blood, lymphadenosis.]

haemolymphangioma (he·mo·limf·an·je·**o'**·mah). Haematolymphangioma.

haemolysin (he·**mol**·is·in, he·mo·**li**·sin). A substance which may be a chemical, an antibody (usually in conjunction with complement) or a component of a virus which is capable of damaging the wall of red blood cells, allowing leakage of the contained haemoglobin. **Bacterial haemolysin.** One produced by bacterial action. **Immune haemolysin.** One formed in the body of an animal as the result of injection of red blood cells of a different species. **Natural haemolysin.** One occurring in the serum of an animal, which haemolyses the blood of a different species. **Specific haemolysin.** Immune haemolysin (see above). [Gk *haima* blood, *lysein* to loosen.]

haemolysinogen (he·**mol**·is·**in'**·o·jen). An antigen in red blood cells which, when injected into an animal of a different species, stimulates the production of antibody-haemolysin. The haemolysin causes laking of the red blood cells. [Gk *haima* blood, *lysein* to loosen, *genein* to produce.]

haemolysis (he·**mol**·is·is). The release of haemoglobin from the red cells as a result either of osmotic effects or of the breaking-up or laking of the red blood cells. *In vivo* haemolysis occurs normally in the reticulo-endothelial system as part of haematopoiesis, but abnormal haemolysis may be brought about by various factors giving rise to the haemolytic anaemias which are classified according to the causal agent. The latter may be poisonous, such as lead, phenyl hydrazine, saponins or snake venom; infective, such as bacterial haemolysins activated by incompatible transfusion; or congenital. *In vitro* haemolysis may be induced by placing blood in a solution of lower osmotic pressure, by repeated freezing and thawing of blood, or by heating to 60°C. In bacteriology classification of streptococci is based upon the type of haemolysis produced when cultured on blood agar plates, 3 types being recognized: *α-haemolysis*, a greenish discoloration and partial haemolysis of the blood corpuscles immediately surrounding the colony; *β-haemolysis*, where the colonies are surrounded by clear colourless zones of haemolysis of sharp definition; and *γ-haemolysis*, where there is no apparent change in the medium. [Gk *haima* blood, *lysein* to loosen.]

haemolysoid (he·**mol**·is·oid). Altered haemolysin in which the toxophore group has been destroyed. It is able to unite and become fixed to the red blood cells for which it is specific, but is not capable of laking them. [haemolysin, Gk *eidos* form.]

haemolytic (he·mol·it·ik). 1. Pertaining to or causing haemolysis. 2. Any agent that has power to destroy erythrocytes.

haemolytopoietic (he·**mol**·it·o·poi·**et**′·ik). Belonging to or controlling the formation and destruction of blood corpuscles so that normal balance of blood components is maintained. [haemolysis, Gk *poien* to make.]

haemolyzation (he·mol·i·**za**′·shun). The process of producing haemolysis.

haemolyze (**he**·mol·ize). To cause or to produce haemolysis.

haemomanometer (he·mo·man·**om**′·et·er). Sphygmomanometer. [Gk *haima* blood, manometer.]

haemomediastinum (he·mo·me·de·as·**ti**′·num). Haematomediastinum.

haemometer (he·**mom**·et·er). Haemoglobinometer.

haemometra (he·mo·**met**·rah). Haematometra.

haemometry (he·**mom**·et·re). Haemoglobinometry.

haemomyelogram (he·mo·**mi**·el·o·gram). A differential analysis of the cellular contents of the bone marrow. [Gk *haima* blood, *myelos* marrow, *gramma* record.]

haemomyelosis (he·mo·mi·el·**o**′·sis). Haemoblastosis. [Gk *haima* blood, myelosis.]

Haemonchus (he·**mong**·kus). A genus of nematode worms. **Haemonchus contortus.** A stomach worm of sheep which has occasionally been recorded from man in Brazil and perhaps Australia. [Gk *haima* blood, *ogkos* hook.]

haemonephrosis (he·mo·nef·**ro**′·sis). Haematonephrosis.

haemonormoblast (he·mo·**nor**·mo·blast). Normoblast; a faintly haemoglobinized cell with a compact nucleus from which the erythrocytes develop. [Gk *haima* blood, normoblast.]

haemo-opthalmia (he·mo·of·**thal**′·me·ah). Haemophthalmia.

haemo-opsonin (he·mo·**op**·son·in). Haemopsonin.

haemopathic (he·mo·**path**·ik). 1. Relating or belonging to haemopathy. 2. Caused by disease or any disordered condition of the blood. [Gk *haima* blood, *pathos* disease.]

haemopathology (he·mo·path·**ol**′·o·je). Haematopathology; that branch of medical science which is concerned with diseases of the blood. [Gk *haima* blood, pathology.]

haemopathy (he·**mop**·ăth·e). Any diseased condition of the blood. [Gk *haima* blood, *pathos* disease.]

haemopericardium (he·mo·per·e·**kar**′·de·um). Accumulation of blood in the pericardial sac, usually from rupture of a diseased heart muscle or from rupture of the ascending aorta. Occasionally traumatic, from penetrating (e.g. stab) wounds. [Gk *haima* blood, pericardium.]

haemoperitoneum (he·mo·per·e·ton·**e**′·um). Effusion of blood into the peritoneal cavity. [Gk *haima* blood, peritoneum.]

haemopexin (he·mo·**pex**·in). 1. Any agent which can cause the blood to coagulate, e.g. a ferment. 2. A plasma protein of the β-globulin type that combines with free haemin but not with haemoglobin. [Gk *haima* blood, *pexis* fixation.]

haemopexis (he·mo·**pex**·is). 1. The process of coagulation of blood. 2. The coagulation time of blood. [see prec.]

haemophagocyte (he·mo·**fag**·o·site). A leucocyte or wandering cell which is capable of ingesting and destroying red blood cells. [Gk *haima* blood, phagocyte.]

haemophagocytosis (he·mo·fag·o·si·**to**′·sis). The ingestion of erythrocytes by phagocytes. [haemophagocyte, Gk *-osis* condition.]

haemophil, haemophile (**he**·mo·fil, **he**·mo·file). Applied to bacteria which flourish in culture media containing blood. [see foll.]

haemophilia (he·mo·**fil**·e·ah). A severe hereditary bleeding disease affecting males and transmitted by females. This recessive, sex-linked diathesis is due to a deficiency or absence of a specific antihaemophilic globulin in the blood, so that there is a failure or delay in blood thromboplastin formation with prolonged clotting time. It does occur, extremely rarely, in females who are daughters of a haemophilic father and a haemophilia-transmitting mother. **Haemophilia calcipriva.** A haemorrhagic condition resembling haemophilia, due to a gross calcium deficiency in the patient. **Hereditary haemophilia.** *See* MAIN DEF. (above). **Haemophilia neonatorum.** A haemorrhagic condition in a newborn child, resembling haemophilia clinically, but not actually a true haemophilia. **Renal haemophilia.** Gull's renal epistaxis. **Sporadic haemophilia.** A sudden haemorrhagic condition resembling haemophilia, appearing in a non-haemophilic person; not a well-recognized term. [Gk *haima* blood, *philein* to love.]

haemophiliac (he·mo·**fil**·e·ak). An individual who suffers from haemophilia.

haemophilic (he·mo·**fil**·ik). 1. Referring or belonging to haemophilia or a haemophiliac, 2. Haemophil.

haemophiliometer (**he**·mo·fil·e·**om**′·et·er). An appliance for measuring the degree of haemophilia at any one time.

Haemophilus (he·**mof**·il·us). A genus of bacteria belonging to the tribe Haemophileae (family Bacteriaceae). They are minute non-motile, non-sporing, Gram-negative rods, sometimes almost coccal, sometimes threadlike, and may be pleomorphic. They depend for growth on the presence of some factor (X factor) in blood pigment and in certain plant tissues: certain species require for growth a second factor (V factor) present in blood, yeast and in most plant tissues or in other bacterial cells. All known species appear to be obligatory parasites, inhabiting particularly the upper respiratory tract, and most of them are pathogenic or potentially pathogenic. **Haemophilus aegyptius.** A cause of acute conjunctivitis (pink eye). **Haemophilus bronchisepticus.** A minute Gram-negative bacillus which causes respiratory infections in animals, and which has been isolated from the nasopharynx of man. **Haemophilus canis.** A species in the preputial secretion of dogs, and non-pathogenic. **Haemophilus ducreyi.** A species causing soft chancre in man. **Haemophilus influenzae.** First described by Pfeiffer as the cause of influenza because of its constant presence in the purulent sputum of cases in the 1889–92 influenza pandemic, it has since become accepted as a secondary bacterial pathogen in cases of influenza (primarily caused by a group of viruses) and in other viral respiratory infections and chronic bronchitis. There are capsulate and non-capsulate strains: the former, divisible into 6 serological types, may be primary pathogens and are causally associated with (*a*) a purulent meningitis in very young children (3 months to 3 years) and (*b*) laryngo-epiglottitis (a form of croup) in slightly older children. **Haemophilus influenzae suis.** A species isolated from cases of swine influenza in which it associated with a virus. **Haemophilus para-influenzae.** A species usually non-pathogenic, but isolated from cases of ulcerative endocarditis in man. **Haemophilus parapertussis.** A species distinct from but related to *Haemophilus pertussis*, and causing whooping-cough in man. **Haemophilus pertussis.** Bordet-Gengou bacillus, the cause of whooping-cough in man. [Gk *haima* blood, *philein* to love.]

haemophobia (he·mo·**fo**·be·ah). 1. Excessive dread of the sight of blood. 2. Morbid fear of losing blood or of bleeding. [Gk *haima* blood, phobia.]

haemophoric (he·mo·**for**·ik). Conveying or carrying blood. [Gk *haima* blood, *pherein* to carry.]

haemophotograph (he·mo·**fo**·to·graf). A photograph of the corpuscles of the blood. It is used in estimating the amount of haemoglobin in blood. [Gk *haima* blood, photograph.]

haemophthalmia, haemophthalmos, haemophthalmus (he·mof·**thal**·me·ah, he·mof·**thal**·mos, he·mof·**thal**·mus). An extravasation of blood into the eye. [Gk *haima* blood, ophthalmia.]

Haemopis (he·**mo**·pis). A genus of leeches. *Haemopis sanguisuga*, the harmless false horse leech of Europe, has been confused with *Limnatis nilotica*. [Gk *haima* blood, *ops* face.]

haemoplastic (he·mo·**plas**·tik). 1. Referring or belonging to the formation of blood. 2. Blood forming. [Gk *haima* blood, *plassein* to form.]

haemopleura (he·mo·**ploor**·ah). Effusion of blood into the pleural cavity. [Gk *haima* blood, pleura.]

haemopneumopericardium (he·mo·**new**·mo·per·e·**kar**′·de·um). Pneumohaemopericardium; an accumulation of blood and air in the pericardium. [Gk *haima* blood, pneumopericardium.]

haemopneumothorax (he·mo·new·mo·**thor**′·ax). An accumulation of blood and gas in the pleural cavity. [Gk *haima* blood, pneumothorax.]

haemopoiesic (he·mo·poi·e′·sik). Haemopoietic.

haemopoiesis (he·mo·poi·e′·sis). The formation of blood cells. **Extramedullary haemopoiesis.** The formation of blood cells at centres other than the bone marrow. **Heteroplastic haemopoiesis.** The direct formation of erythrocytes from their early precursors; such formation is hypothetical. **Homoplastic haemopoiesis.** The process by which immature blood cells produce new mature blood cells of the same type. [Gk *haima* blood, *poiein* to make.]

haemopoietic (he·mo·poi·**et**′·ik). 1. Referring to haemopoiesis. 2. Taking part in, relating, or belonging to the formation of blood. [see prec.]

haemopoietin (he·mo·**poi**·et·in). Intrinsic factor; the name given by Wilkinson to the anti-pernicious-anaemia factor present in normal gastric juice. [Gk *haima* blood, *poiein* to make.]

See also: WILKINSON.

haemoprecipitin (he·mo·pre·**sip**′·it·in). Precipitin. [Gk *haima* blood, precipitin.]

haemoprotein (he·mo·**pro**·te·in) A class of conjugated protein which contain haem as a prosthetic group; examples are haemoglobin, myoglobin, cytochromes and catalase. [Gk *haima* blood, *proteios* of first rank.]

Haemoproteus (he·mo·**pro**·te·us). A genus of sporozoa that inhabit the blood of certain birds; amoeboid forms live within the erythrocytes. Species of importance are *Haemoproteus columbae* of the pigeon and *H. passeris* of the sparrow. Comparative studies with these species were carried out in the early experiments on malaria transmission. [Gk *haima* blood, *Proteus* sea-god who could change his shape.]

haemopsonin (he·**mop**·son·in). An antibody in serum which renders red blood cells more liable to phagocytosis. [Gk *haima* blood, opsonin.]

haemoptysic (he·mop·**tiz**·ik). 1. Characterized by the presence of haemoptysis. 2. Relating or belonging to haemoptysis.

haemoptysis (he·**mop**·tis·is). The expectoration of bright red blood from the lungs or bronchi and trachea. It is usually of tuberulous origin, but may occur in acute lobar pneumonia, in chronic pneumonia due to inhalation of industrial irritants such as beryllium, vanadium, etc. and in the pneumoconiosis group of lung diseases, bronchiectasis, carcinoma, rupture of an aortic aneurysm, lung abscess, parasitic disease, cardiac disease and various fungous infections of the lung. It may be seen as a rare condition in children under 16 years of age, with sudden onset of cyanosis and dyspnoea, cough and vomiting, as a result of severe disturbance of the pulmonary circulation of unknown aetiology. **Cardiac haemoptysis.** Haemoptysis occurring in mitral stenosis and pulmonary stenosis from engorgement and rupture of pulmonary or systemic capillaries, usually when cardiac failure and back pressure arises. **Endemic haemoptysis.** Manson's haemoptysis; haemoptysis due to infection with *Paragonimus westermani.* **Essential haemoptysis.** Haemoptysis occurring in a patient in whom full investigation and subsequent observation fails to reveal any serious underlying disease. **Parasitic haemoptysis.** Haemoptysis due to any parasitic infection, especially by *Paragonimus westermani* and *Echinococcus.* **Vicarious haemoptysis.** A rare form of blood spitting which occurs at or just before the onset of menstruation in some women, without any apparent cause. [Gk *haima* blood, *ptyein* to spit.]

See also: MANSON.

haemopyelectasis (he·mo·pi·el·**ek**′·tas·is). A condition in which the pelvis of the ureter is distended with accumulated blood and fluid. [Gk *haima* blood, pyelectasis.]

haemopyrrole (he·mo·**pir**·ole). Dimethylethylpyrrole, $C_8H_{13}N$. A heterocyclic compound formed by the reduction of the haematoporphyrin derived from haemoglobin, It is identical with that formed by the reduction of the phylloporphyrin from chlorophyll.

haemorrhage (**hem**·or·ij). Bleeding; the escape of blood from any part of the vascular system. **Accidental haemorrhage.** Bleeding from the placental site before the birth of the child when the placenta is situated in the upper uterine segment. **Accidental ante-partum haemorrhage.** Bleeding from the generative tract in pregnancy in the presence of a normally situated placenta. By custom the term is usually used for bleeding occurring after the 28th week of gestation. **Ante-partum haemorrhage.** Bleeding from the vagina after the 28th week of pregnancy. **Arterial haemorrhage.** Escape of blood from an artery. **Bladder haemorrhage.** Haemorrhage into the bladder. **Bronchial haemorrhage.** Bleeding into a bronchus. **Capillary haemorrhage.** Oozing of blood from capillaries. **Capsuloganglionic haemorrhage.** Bleeding into the internal and/or external capsule and the basal ganglia. **Cerebral haemorrhage.** Haemorrhage arising within the cerebral parenchyma usually the result of arterial hypertension. **Concealed haemorrhage.** Internal haemorrhage (see below) for which there is no visible evidence. **Concealed ante-partum haemorrhage.** Accidental ante-partum haemorrhage where the bleeding is entirely internal. **Consecutive haemorrhage.** A haemorrhage which does not immediately follow an injury but occurs after an interval. **Critical haemorrhage.** A haemorrhage occurring at the crisis of a disease. **Delayed haemorrhage.** A sudden, often severe, internal haemorrhage about 3–10 days after an accident; not truly a reactionary haemorrhage, but due to similar causes. **Essential haemorrhage.** Bleeding without a discoverable cause. **Essential uterine haemorrhage.** Uterine bleeding for which there is no gross pathological cause; functional uterine bleeding. **External haemorrhage.** Haemorrhage that appears externally. **Extradural haemorrhage.** Haemorrhage into the extradural space, usually due to traumatic rupture of the middle meningeal artery. **Extraperitoneal haemorrhage.** Haemorrhage from an abdominal organ or tissue but into the tissues that lie outside the peritoneal cavity. **Gastric haemorrhage.** Bleeding into the cavity of the stomach. **Gravitating haemorrhage.** Haemorrhage into the spinal canal in which the blood settles in the lowest part. **Intermediary haemorrhage, Intermediate haemorrhage.** The intermediate haemorrhages in a series of recurrent haemorrhages. **Internal haemorrhage.** A haemorrhage into a serous cavity, into a hollow viscus or into the tissues. **Intestinal haemorrhage.** Bleeding into the bowel. **Intracranial haemorrhage.** Haemorrhage within the cranium. **Intradural haemorrhage.** Subdural haemorrhage (see below). **Intrapartum haemorrhage.** Haemorrhage occurring during labour. **Intraperitoneal haemorrhage.** Haemorrhage into the peritoneal cavity. **Intrapulmonary haemorrhage.** Haemorrhage into the lung tissues. **Macular haemorrhage.** A retinal haemorrhage involving the macula. **Meningeal haemorrhage.** Haemorrhage from a meningeal artery. **Nasal haemorrhage.** Epistaxis; bleeding from the nose. **Parenchymatous haemorrhage.** Bleeding into the substance of an organ. **Petechial haemorrhage.** Small discrete haemorrhages into the skin. **Plasma haemorrhage.** Escape of the fluid portion of the blood only. **Postextraction haemorrhage.** Haemorrhage occurring from the region from which a tooth has been extracted. **Postoperative haemorrhage.** Haemorrhage after a surgical operation. **Post-partum haemorrhage.** Excessive bleeding occurring after the delivery of the child. In the UK the bleeding must be 560 g (20 oz) or more to qualify as a haemorrhage. **Post-traumatic haemorrhage.** Haemorrhage after injury. **Preretinal haemorrhage.** A haemorrhage from the inner surface of the retina and lying between it and the vitreous. It is large and roughly circular in shape and after partial absorption shows the characteristic fluid level above. **Primary haemorrhage.** That occurring immediately after injury. **Pulmonary haemorrhage.** Haemorrhage occurring into the lungs. **Punctate haemorrhage.** Petechial haemorrhage (see above). **Reactionary haemorrhage.** Haemorrhage a few hours after the primary bleeding has ceased and due mainly to the patient's improved general condition with increased blood pressure. **Reactive haemorrhage.** Haemorrhage occurring 24–48 h after initial recovery from the effects of injury or operation. **Recurring**

haemorrhage. Haemorrhage which occurs again after being stopped by clotting. **Renal haemorrhage.** Haemorrhage occurring from the kidney. **Retinal haemorrhage.** Haemorrhage in the retina. **Retro-ocular haemorrhage.** Haemorrhage into the orbit behind the eye. **Revealed ante-partum haemorrhage.** Accidental ante-partum haemorrhage where the bleeding is entirely external. **Haemorrhage per rhexin.** The flow of blood from a ruptured vessel. **Secondary haemorrhage.** Haemorrhage occurring 7-10 days after injury or operation and usually attributed to infection. **Splinter haemorrhage.** Linear haemorrhages under the nails, seen in malignant endocarditis. **Spontaneous haemorrhage.** Haemorrhage occurring without obvious exciting cause. **Subarachnoid haemorrhage.** Haemorrhage into the subarachnoid space. It may be traumatic, but if spontaneous usually results from rupture of an aneurysm of an artery of the circle of Willis. **Subdural haemorrhage.** Bleeding into the subdural space, usually due to traumatic rupture of veins crossing the space, but can be spontaneous. **Subhyaloid haemorrhage.** Preretinal haemorrhage (see above). **Subperiosteal haemorrhage.** Haemorrhage under the periosteum. **Toxaemic ante-partum haemorrhage.** Accidental ante-partum haemorrhage occurring in the presence of pre-eclampsia. **Traumatic haemorrhage.** Haemorrhage resulting from an injury. **Unavoidable haemorrhage.** The bleeding that occurs from placenta praevia. **Uterine haemorrhage.** Haemorrhage from within the uterus. **Venous haemorrhage.** Bleeding from a vein. **Vicarious haemorrhage.** Haemorrhage from some organ which is supposed to take the place of a naturally-occurring haemorrhage that is suppressed, e.g. epistaxis at the time of a supressed menstruation. [Gk *haima* blood, *rhegnynei* to gush.]

haemorrhagenic (**hem**·or·ah·**jen'**·ik). Causing haemorrhage. [haemorrhage, Gk *genein* to produce.]

haemorrhagic (hem·or·**ah**·jik). 1. Relating or belonging to haemorrhage. 2. Marked by the presence of, or accompanied by, a haemorrhage.

haemorrhagica histrionica (hem·or·**rah**·jik·ah his·tre·**on**·ik·ah). *See* MUNCHAUSEN'S SYNDROME.

haemorrhaphilia (**hem**·or·ah·**fil'**·e·ah). Haemophilia. [haemorrhage, Gk *philein* to love.]

haemorrhoea (hem·or·e·ah). Copious haemorrhage. [Gk *haima* blood, *rhoia* flow.]

haemorrhoid (**hem**·or·oid). A swelling at the anal margin; a pile. **Acute haemorrhoid.** An anal swelling from inflammation or thrombosis in the inferior rectal veins or from rupture of 1 of these veins. **External haemorrhoids.** Haemorrhoids situated outside or protruding beyond the sphincter ani externus muscle; exaggerated folds of peri-anal skin. **Internal haemorrhoid.** A redundant fold of mucous membrane of the lower rectum at the anorectal junction corresponding to the terminal branches of the inferior rectal artery and vein, caused by oedema or by dilatation of radicles of the inferior rectal vein. **Interno-external haemorrhoids.** Internal haemorrhoids which have grown downwards under the skin of the anus to protrude partly. **Prolapsed haemorrhoids.** Internal haemorrhoids that have protruded through the anal orifice. **Strangulated haemorrhoids.** Prolapsed haemorrhoids that have been gripped by the sphincter ani muscles so that they cannot be returned by pressure. [Gk *haimorrhois* vein liable to discharge blood.]

haemorrhoidal (hem·or·**oid**·al). 1. Relating or belonging to, or having the character of a haemorrhoid or haemorrhoids. 2. Suffering from haemorrhoids. 3. Term denoting structures in the anal canal such as nerves and blood vessels.

haemorrhoidal nerves, inferior [nervi rectales inferiores]. Branches of the pudendal nerve to the sphincter ani externus muscle and the skin around the anus.

haemorrhoidectomy (**hem**·or·oid·**ek'**·to·me). Surgical excision of a haemorrhoid or haemorrhoids. [haemorrhoid, Gk *ektome* a cutting out.]

haemorrhoidolysis (**hem**·or·oid·**ol'**·is·is). The dispersal and destruction of a haemorrhoid by surgical diathermy or injection of chemical solutions. [haemorrhoid, lysis.]

haemosalpinx (he·mo·**sal**·pingx). Haematosalpinx.

haemoscope (**he**·mo·skope). Haematoscope.

haemosialemesis (**he**·mo·si·al·**em'**·es·is). The discharge of bloodstained saliva. [Gk *haima* blood, *sialon* saliva, *emesis* vomiting.]

haemosiderin (he·mo·**sid**·er·in). An iron-protein compound, formed by the polymerization of ferritin, and occurring in the tissues. Large deposits are present in the liver and spleen in haemochromatosis, and it appears to be a form in which iron is stored until required for fresh haemoglobin. [Gk *haima* blood, *sideros* iron.]

haemosiderinuria (**he**·mo·sid·er·in·**ewr'**·e·ah). The presence of haemosiderin in the urine.

haemosiderosis (**he**·mo·sid·er·**o'**·sis). A condition in which a deposit of haemosiderin is present in the liver, spleen and other organs and in the tissues as the result of destruction of erythrocytes in diseases such as aplastic anaemia. **Pulmonary haemosiderosis.** Haemosiderosis caused by extravascular destruction of blood in the lung; chronic, may be fatal. [haemosiderin, Gk *-osis* condition.]

haemosozic (hem·o·**so**·zik). Antihaemolytic. [Gk *haima* blood, *sozein* to save.]

haemospasia (he·mo·**spa**·ze·ah). The drawing of blood to any particular part of the body, as by dry cupping. [Gk *haima* blood, *spasis* a drawing.]

haemospast (**he**·mo·spast). Any agent or device for effecting haemospasia; any appliance used in cupping.

haemospastic (he·mo·**spas**·tik). 1. Relating or belonging to haemospasia, or to the extraction of blood. 2. Applied to any measure that is effective in drawing blood to a part.

haemospermia (he·mo·**sper**·me·ah). A condition in which the discharged semen contains blood. [Gk *haima* blood, sperm.]

Haemosporidia (**he**·mo·spo·**rid'**·e·ah). An order of Sporozoa which includes *Plasmodium.* [Gk *haima* blood, *sporos* seed.]

haemostasia, haemostasis (he·mo·**sta**·se·ah, he·mo·**sta**·sis). 1. A slowing of the movement of the blood. 2. The arrest of haemorrhage, e.g. by ligation of an artery. 3. The stopping of circulation through the vessels of any particular part of the body. [see foll.]

haemostat (**he**·mo·stat). An agent or instrument used in the arrest of haemorrhage. [Gk *haima* blood, *stasis* a halting.]

haemostatic (he·mo·**stat**·ik). 1. Arresting haemorrhage. 2. Any drug or agent which arrests haemorrhage. These include coagulants which shorten clotting time, as in the local application of iron salts (ferric), alum, calcium salts, tannin and other astringents. When the blood-clotting mechanism is faulty, preparations containing thromboplastin and cephalin (brain extracts), or fibrin are employed externally; internally, calcium salts, vitamin K or an infusion of whole blood are effective. Adrenaline acts locally as a haemostatic by constricting the blood vessels, whilst cold itself increases the blood viscosity. Ergot and pituitary extracts are especially valuable for controlling uterine haemorrhage after labour, and the oestrogens for functional uterine bleeding. [Gk *haima* blood, *stasis* a halting.]

haemostatics (he·mo·**stat**·ix). That branch of medical science which is concerned with the equilibrium of the blood in the blood vessels. [see prec.]

haemostix (**he**·mo·stix). A sharp puncturing instrument used to withdraw a drop of blood for diagnostic purposes. [Gk *haima* blood, *stixis* puncture.]

haemostyptic (he·mo·**stip**·tik). Arresting haemorrhage. [Gk *haima* blood, *styphein* to contract.]

haemotachometer (**he**·mo·tak·**om'**·et·er). An instrument for measuring the speed of the blood flowing through the arteries; a tacheometer. [Gk *haima* blood, *tachos* speed, meter.]

See also: VIERORDT.

haemotelangiosis (**he**·mo·tel·an·je·**o'**·sis). 1. Telangiectasis. 2. A diseased condition of the smallest capillaries. [Gk *haima* blood, *telos* end, *aggeion* small vessel.]

haemotherapeutics (**he**·mo·ther·ap·**ew'**·tix). The science of haemotherapy.

haemotherapy (he·mo·**ther**·ap·e). 1. A form of treatment in which fresh blood, or blood plasma or serum, or a preparation of blood, is administered. 2. Treatment to improve the general state of the blood. [Gk *haima* blood, therapy.]

haemothorax (he·mo·**thor**·ax). Effusion of blood into the pleural cavity. **Spontaneous haemothorax.** Haemothorax without apparent cause, usually due to neoplasm. **Traumatic haemothorax.** Haemothorax due to injury. [Gk *haima* blood, thorax.]

haemothymia (he·mo·**thi**·me·ah). A state of insanity marked by homicidal impulse or irresistible desire to kill any living thing. [Gk *haima* blood, *thymos* rage.]

haemotoxic (he·mo·**tox**·ik). 1. Relating to blood poisoning. 2. Causing the destruction of erythrocytes. [see foll.]

haemotoxin (he·mo·**tox**·in). A substance which causes destruction of erythrocytes. [Gk *haima* blood, *toxikon* poison.]

haemotrophe (**he**·mo·trofe). A nutritive fluid provided by the uterus for the benefit of the early embryo. It consists chiefly of extravasated blood which is absorbed by the trophoblast. [Gk *haima* blood, *trophe* nutrition.]

haemotropic (he·mo·**trop**·ik). 1. Having a special affinity for erythrocytes. 2. In Ehrlich's side-chain theory, a term used to describe a haptophoric group. [Gk *haima* blood, *trope* a turning.]

haemotropin (he·mo·**tro**·pin). An antibody in serum which renders red blood cells more liable to phagocytosis. [see prec.]

haemotympanum (he·mo·**tim**·pan·um). The presence of blood in the tympanic cavity. [Gk *haima* blood, tympanum.]

haemovolumetry (**he**·mo·vol·**ew**'·met·re). The process of measuring the volume of the blood. [Gk *haima* blood, volume, meter.]

haemozoin (he·mo·**zo**·in). The iron-containing pigment observed in the intracorpuscular malarial parasites (trophozoites), in macrophages and in the reticulo-endothelial cells. [Gk *haima* blood, *zoon* animal.]

Haenel, Hans (b. 1874). German neurologist.

Haenel sign. Loss of pain sensation on digital compression of the eyeballs in tabes dorsalis.

Haffkine, Waldemar Mordecai Wolff (b. 1860). Bacteriologist of Russian origin and birth working in India.

Haffkine's prophylactic fluid or prophylactic. Haffkine's vaccine (see below).

Haffkine's serum or prophylactic serum. 1. An antiserum that was prepared against plague, but was of no value. 2. Haffkine's vaccine; a misnomer that has survived to the present.

Haffkine's vaccine. 1. One of the earliest vaccines used for plague prophylaxis; prepared from a 4-week broth culture of *Pasteurella pestis* and killed by heat. 2. An anticholera vaccine.

Hafnia (**haf**·ne·ah). A genus of Gram-negative bacilli belonging to the family Enterobacteriaceae and probably pathogenic for men; because of their frequent presence in the environment they need to be differentiated from other non-lactose fermenting and, possibly, pathogenic genera. [L *Hafniae* Copenhagen.]

hafnium (**haf**·ne·um). An element of atomic weight 178.50, atomic number 72 and chemical symbol Hf, discovered in the ores of zirconium, which metal it resembles closely in properties. At first it was thought to be identical with the supposed rare-earth element *celtium*, but the existence of the latter has been disproved. [L *Hafniae* Copenhagen.]

Hagedorn, Hans Christian (b. 1888). Copenhagen physician.

Hagedorn and Jensen method, for blood sugar. Precipitate the proteins from 0.1 ml blood with zinc hydroxide. Heat the filtrate with 2 ml alkaline ferricyanide reagent in boiling water for 15 min. Cool and add 3 ml of iodide reagent and 2 ml of 3 per cent acetic acid. Titrate the liberated iodine with N/200 thiosulphate.

Hagedorn, Werner (b.1831). Magdeburg surgeon.

Hagedorn's needle. A surgical needle flattened from side to side and curved on the flat.

Hageman. The name of the patient whose case was the first recorded example of the condition described below.

Hageman factor deficiency. Profound deficiency of blood coagulation factor XII without clinical abnormality.

Hagenia (ha·**je**·ne·ah). A synonym for the genus *Brayera*. *Hagenia abyssinica* Willdenow is identical with *Brayera anthelmintica* Kunth, the source of cusso.

hagiotherapy (ha·je·o·**ther**'·ap·e). 1. Treatment of disease by causing patients to take part in religious observances or visit shrines, or by placing them in contact with relics of saints. 2. Treatment carried out by a holy man and of the nature of a miracle. [Gk *hagios* holy, therapy.]

Hagner, Francis Randall (b. 1873). Washington urologist.

Hagner's bag. An inflatable rubber bag, which can be drawn through the urethra to inhibit bleeding after prostatectomy.

Hagner's operation. Aspiration by multiple punctures of pockets of pus in the epididymis following incision of the tunica vaginalis testis.

Hahn, Eugene (b. 1841). Berlin surgeon.

Hahn's cannula. A cannula with a sponge attachment used for blocking the trachea, and modified for use in endotracheal anaesthesia.

Hahnemann, Christian Friedrich Samuel (b. 1755). German physician. The founder of homoeopathy.

Hahnemann's theory, Hahnemannian theory. Like cures like, *similia similibus curantur.*

hahnemannism (**hah**·ne·man·izm). A name for homoeopathy. [C. F. S. *Hahnemann.*]

Haidinger, Wilhelm Karl von (b. 1795). Austrian mineralogist.

Haidinger's brush. A phenomenon seen when blue polarized light is thrown on the eye, which itself looks at a sheet of white paper. It appears as a series of dark-yellow double cones joined at their apices on a blue ground; these are due to the double refracting effect of the radiating nerve fibres at the macula.

Haig Ferguson, James (b. 1862). Edinburgh obstetrician.

Haig Ferguson forceps. Obstetric forceps with a pelvic and cephalic curve and an axis-traction handle fitting on to the handles of the blades.

Hailey, W. H. (b. 1898) and **Hailey, H. E.** (b. 1909). Atlanta, Georgia, dermatologists.

Hailey's disease, Hailey-Hailey disease, Gougerot-Hailey-Hailey disease. Familial benign chronic pemphigus. *See* PEMPHIGUS.

hair [pilus (NA)] (**ha**·er). An appendage of the skin, peculiar to mammals, and consisting of a root implanted in the skin and a projecting filamentous portion, the shaft. **Axillary hairs [hirci (NA)].** The hair of the armpit. **Bamboo hair.** Sparse, brittle hairs with bamboo-like nodes which telescope prior to fracture. **Bayonet hair.** Hair with spindle-shaped expansions near the pointed tip, due to thickening of the cortex. **Beaded hair.** Monilethrix. **Hairs of the ear [tragi (NA)].** The hair growing in the external auditory meatus. **Exclamation-point hair.** Short hair stump in which the distal part is more pigmented than the proximal part; found in alopecia areata. **Hairs of the eyebrows [supercilia (NA)].** The hair composing the eyebrows. **Hairs of the head [capilli (NA)].** The hair growing on the scalp. **Ingrowing hair.** Closely-shaved hair which grows into and along the skin, causing inflammation. **Kinky hair.** A genetically-determined condition of short, sparse, poorly pigmented hair, due to twists and fractures of the shafts. There is also retardation of mental and physical development. **Knotted hair.** Trichorrhexis nodosa. **Lupus hair.** Coarse, dry, fragile hair, broken off short, occurring in lupus erythematosus. **Moniliform hair.** Monilethrix. **Hairs of the nose [vibrissae (NA)].** The hairs growing in the nostrils. **Pubic hairs [pubes (NA)].** The hair of the pubic region. **Ringed hair.** Leucotrichia annularis. **Rolled hair.** Tightly coiled hairs beneath horny plugs which obstruct the ostia of follicles in ichthyosis and in keratosis pilaris. **Root of a hair [radix pili (NA)].** The part of a hair embedded in the skin. **Shaft of a hair [scapus pili (NA)].** The portion of an individual hair which projects from the surface of the skin. **Stellate hair.** Hair split at the distal end. **Terminal hair.** Postnatal, long, coarse, medullated, pigmented hair. **Twisted hair.** A congenital malformation of the hair characterized by hairs that are short, brittle and twisted. **Vellus hair.** Postnatal, soft, unmedullated hair up to 2 cm long, usually unpigmented. **Woolly hair.** Hair of negroid character. [AS *haer.*]

See also: SCHRIDDE.

haja (haj·ah). Keratoderma plantare sulcatum. [Indian name.]

hakuri (hak·oo·re). An epidemic diarrhoea of children occurring in Japan.

halation (hal·a·shun). The halo of light around the image focused on a screen when the light source is too large or too strong. [Gk *halos* the sun's disc.]

Halazone BPC 1954 (hal·az·one). $C_6H_4(COOH)SO_2NCl_2$, a chlorine antiseptic similar to chloramine and containing about 25 per cent of available chlorine. It is used for the sterilization of drinking water.

Halberstaedter, Ludwig (b. 1876). Breslau physician.

Prowazek-Halberstaedter bodies or corpuscles. Intracellular bodies found in trachomatous secretions and believed to present a stage in the life history of the causal virus.

Halcinonide (hal·sin·o·nide). BP Commission approved name for 21-chloro-9α-fluoro-11β-hydroxy-16α,17α-isopropylidenedioxy-pregn-4-ene-3,20-dione; a corticosteroid.

Haldane, John Scott (b. 1860). Oxford physiologist.

Haldane apparatus. An apparatus for the analysis of air in mines, based on the observation that a candle flame is extinguished with a certain dilution of oxygen.

Haldane chamber. A specially designed chamber in which the general metabolism of animals may be measured.

Haldane haemoglobinometer. An instrument in which blood is saturated with coal gas, and the carboxyhaemoglobin colour matched against a standard by progressive dilution, as a means of estimating the haemoglobin content.

Haldane scale. A graduated scale adapted by Haldane for use with the Gowers' haemoglobinometer with a standard colour tube, for estimating by the carbon monoxide method the amount of haemoglobin in a sample of blood; the scale is arranged so that 100 per cent is equivalent to 14.8 g of haemoglobin.

Hales, Rev. Stephen (b. 1677). English inventor and physiologist.

Hales' piesimeter. A manometer connected with an artery to measure blood pressure by the height to which the blood rises in a tube.

Halethazole (hal·eth·az·ole). BP Commission approved name for 5-chloro-2-(*p*-2-diethylamino-ethoxyphenyl)-benzothiazole; a fungicide.

Hale-White, Sir William (b. 1857). London physician.

Hale-White syndrome. Knuckle pad syndrome; fibrous pads on the dorsum of the proximal interphalangeal joints of the fingers. It may sometimes be associated with Dupuytren's contraction.

half-cycle (hahf·si·kl). In the sine-wave of an alternating current, the half of a full cycle, i.e. when the current is either fully positive or fully negative. [AS *healf*, cycle.]

half-life (hahf·life). The time in which the amount of a radioactive nuclide decays to half its initial value. The term may also be used to characterize any exponential function of the form $X = X_0e^{-at}$, whence half-life $= 0.69/a$, where a is the decay constant and t the time taken for the quantity X_0 to decay to a value X. **Antibody half-life.** The average survival time of an antibody molecule after its synthesis; it usually refers to the time in which 50 per cent of a measured dose of antibody is eliminated from the body of an inoculated animal. The half-life varies according to the type of immunoglobulin. **Biological half-life.** The time taken for the content in a biological system of a marked substance to fall to half its original value. (It is assumed that the rate of removal is exponential, which is not always true.) **Effective half-life.** When a radioactive material with a physical half-life of its radioactivity is introduced into a biological system, its stay in that system is determined not only by its biological half-life but also by its physical decay. The combination of processes gives an effective half-life. [AS *healf*, *lif.*]

half-retinal (hahf·ret·in·al). Relating to or affecting one half of the retina. [AS *healf*, retina.]

halide (hal·ide). 1. Haloid. 2. A compound of a halogen with a metal or radical. **Acid halide, Acyl halide.** An organic acid derivative in which the OH of the carboxyl group has been replaced by a halogen. **Alkyl halide.** A compound of a halogen with an alkyl radical. [Gk *hals* salt.]

halimetry (hal·im·et·re). The process of estimating the quantity of salts in a mixture or solution. [Gk *hals* salt, meter.]

halisteresis (hal·is·ter·e′·sis). Osteomalacia due to loss or lack of lime salts in bones. **Halisteresis cerea.** Waxy softening of the bones. [Gk *hals* salt, *steresis* being in want of.]

halisteretic (hal·is·ter·et′·ik). Suffering from, marked by, or having the character of halisteresis.

halite (hal·ite). Rock salt. *See* SALT. [Gk *hals* salt.]

halitosis (hal·it·o·sis). Fetid or offensive breath. [L *halitus* exhalation, Gk *-osis* condition.]

halituous (hal·it·ew·us). Having a surface coat of moisture or vapour; applied to the skin when moist. [see foll.]

halitus (hal·it·us). 1. An expiration as from the lung. 2. A warm vapour. **Halitus saturninus.** Lead breath. *See* BREATH. [L exhalation.]

Hall, Josiah Newhall (b. 1859). Colorado physician.

Hall's sign. Diastolic shock transmitted to the trachea from an aneurysm of the aorta.

Hall, Marshall (b. 1790). London physiologist.

Marshall Hall's disease. A condition of cerebral anaemia occurring in infants suffering from spurious hydrocephalus.

Marshall Hall's facies. The tall domed forehead and elongated features of infantile hydrocephalus.

Hallauer, Otto (b. 1866). Basle ophthalmologist.

Hallauer's glasses. Glasses in which the lenses are tinted a light olive green.

Hallé, Adrien Joseph Marie Noël (b. 1859). French physician.

Hallé's point. The point of intersection on the abdominal wall between a horizontal line connecting the anterior superior iliac spines and a vertical line drawn upward from the pubic tubercle, marking the point where the ureter of that side crosses the pelvic brim.

Haller, Albrecht von (b. 1708). Swiss physician and scientist.

Haller's annulus or insula. A common anomaly in which the thoracic duct is bifurcate for a variable part of its intrathoracic course.

Haller's ansa. An occasional communication lying in front of the internal jugular vein between the facial and glossopharyngeal nerves.

Haller's arches. Medial and lateral arcuate ligaments of the diaphragm.

circle of Haller. The circulus vasculosus of the optic nerve.

Haller's cone. One of the conical masses composing the head of the epididymis.

Haller's ducts. The inferior aberrant ducts of the epididymis.

Haller's fretum. In the early embryo, a constriction which marks off the bulbus arteriosus from the ventricle, and which later is the dividing line in the fetus between the atria and ventricles.

Haller's habenula. The fibrous cord representing the obliterated upper portion of the processus vaginalis of the peritoneum.

Haller's layer. Part of the vascular lamina of the choroid of the eye, made up of large blood vessels.

Haller's line. The linea splendens.

Haller's membrane. A band of peritoneum from the gall bladder and liver to the duodenum, being an extension to the right of the lesser omentum. A congenital abnormality, not often present.

Haller's network. The vascular network of the testis.

Haller's plexus. The laryngeal plexus.

Haller's tripod. The coeliac artery.

Haller's tunica vasculosa or vascular tissue. The vascular lamina of the choroid.

Haller's vas aberrans. A convoluted duct connected with the beginning of the vas deferens.

Hallervorden, Julius (b. 1882). Giessen neurologist.

Hallervorden–Spatz disease or syndrome. A progressive disease of childhood, characterized clinically by progressive rigidity, athetotic movements and mental and emotional dulling, and pathologically by degeneration of the globus pallidus and reticular part of the substantia nigra.

hallex (**hal**·ex). Hallux.

Hallion, Louis (b. 1862). Paris physiologist and pathologist.

Hallion's test. Tuffier's test.

Hallopeau, François Henri (b. 1842). Paris dermatologist.

Hallopeau's disease. 1. Lichen sclerosus et atrophicus. 2. Pyodermatitis vegetans.

hallucal (**hal**·ew·kal). Relating or belonging to the hallux.

hallucination (hal·ew·sin·a·shun). The subjective experience of a perception in the absence of the corresponding stimulus in the external real world. The experience may occur in the normal, e.g. the hallucination of hearing one's name called, especially if fatigued. Hallucinations may be in any of the senses, and be termed accordingly visual, olfactory, auditory, gustatory, tactile or kinaesthetic. **Auditory hallucination.** The commonest of all forms of hallucination, observed in a great variety of clinical syndromes, but especially in acute organic states and in schizophrenia, rather less commonly in chronic organic states and the affective psychoses and least commonly in hysterical neurotic states. **Colour hallucination.** A hallucination of colour. **Depressive hallucination.** A hallucination occurring in a state of mental depression. **Gustatory hallucination.** A false taste sensation. **Haptic hallucination.** A false tactile sensation. **Hypnagogic hallucination.** A hallucination experienced in the drowsy state preceding or succeeding sleep; many normal people have such hallucinations regularly, and they are of no known clinical significance. **Kinaesthetic hallucination.** Hallucination of the sense of movement. **Light hallucination.** A hallucination of light. **Lilliputian hallucination.** A visual hallucination of objects, persons and animals abnormally small in size. **Olfactory hallucination.** The false sensation of smell. **Reflex hallucination.** A secondary sensation aroused by a sensation of a different kind, e.g. the sensation of colour on hearing music. **Stump hallucination.** Phantom limb; the sensation of the presence of a limb which had been amputated. **Tactile hallucination.** Hallucination of touch. **Vesperal hallucinations.** Hallucinations occurring after dark. **Visual hallucination.** Hallucination in the sense of sight; less common than auditory hallucination and particularly associated with acute organic states such as toxic confusional psychoses and deliria, or the aura of epilepsy. They also occur with localizing value in focal organic disease of the brain, and are not infrequent in schizophrenic psychoses, especially early stages of acute schizophrenia. [L *alucinari* to wander in the mind.]

hallucinogen (hal·ew·**sin**·o·jen). A substance, such as a drug or a toxin, that produces hallucinosis. [L *alucinari* to wander in the mind, Gk *genein* to produce.]

hallucinosis (hal·ew·sin·**o**·sis). A state in which hallucinations are occurring constantly or at frequent intervals, as may, for instance, be the case in toxic confusional states, delirium tremens or acute schizophrenic excitements. It is usually accompanied by grave emotional upset and abnormalities of behaviour. **Paranoid hallucinosis.** Hallucinosis with a predominantly paranoid character. [L *alucinari* to wander in the mind, Gk *-osis* condition.]

hallux (**hal**·ux) (pl. *halluces*). The big toe. **Hallux flexus malleus.** A deformity of the big toe in which the interphalangeal joint is acutely flexed and the metatarsophalangeal joint extended. **Hallux rigidus.** Loss of movement at the metatarsophalangeal joint of the big toe causing pain on walking. **Hallux valgus.** Fixed displacement of the big toe towards the other toes. **Hallux varus.** Fixed displacement of the big toe away from the other toes. [L *hallex* big toe.]

Hallwachs, Franz (b. 1859). Dresden physiologist.

Hallwachs' effect. A photo-electric effect discovered by Hallwachs in 1888.

halmatogenesis (**hal**·mat·o·**jen**′·es·is). An abrupt change of type as between one generation and the next; saltatory variation. [Gk *halma* leap, genesis.]

halo (**ha**·lo). 1. The ring or rings of spectral colours seen round lights typically in glaucoma, due to oedema of the corneal epithelium, but also in cases of punctate lens opacities and sometimes in conjunctivitis. 2. The light yellow ring seen round the optic disc in cases of high myopia. 3. An areola. **Circumpapillary glaucomatous halo.** A ring of choroidoretinal atrophy seen around the optic disc in glaucoma. **Peripapillary senile halo.** A ring of choroidoretinal atrophy seen around the optic disc in old age. Also called *senile circumpapillary choroidal atrophy.* [Gk *halos* circular floor.]

haloderma (hal·o·**der**·mah). A skin eruption caused by a halogen. [Gk *hals* salt, *derma* skin.]

haloduric (hal·o·**dewr**·ik). Term applied to those bacteria which grow vigorously in salt solutions. [Gk *hals* salt, L *durare* to last.]

Halofenate (hal·o·**fe**·nate). BP Commission approved name for 2-acetamidoethyl (4-chlorophenyl)(3-trifluoromethylphenoxy)-acetate; a hypolipaemic agent.

halogen (**hal**·o·jen). Name applied to the elements fluorine, chlorine, bromine and iodine, owing to the presence of the latter 3 in sea water and their ability to form salt-like compounds with metals. [Gk *hals* salt, *genein* to produce.]

halogenic, halogenous (hal·o·**jen**·ik, hal·**oj**·en·us). 1. Producing haloid substances. 2. Producing salt. [Gk *hals* salt, *genein* to produce.]

haloid (**hal**·oid). 1. Having the character of a halide. 2. Derived from or having resemblance to halogens. 3. Having resemblance to sodium chloride (common salt). 4. Having resemblance to sea salt. [Gk *hals* salt, *eidos* form.]

halometer (ha·**lom**·et·er). 1. An instrument with which the halo surrounding the optic disc may be measured. 2. An instrument with which the size of erythrocytes can be estimated by measuring the diffraction areas, or haloes, produced by them.

halometry (ha·**lom**·et·re). 1. The process of measuring ocular haloes. 2. The measuring of the size of an erythrocyte by using a blood smear as a diffraction grating.

Halopenium Chloride (hal·o·**pe**·ne·um **klor**·ide). BP Commission approved name for 4-bromobenzyl-3-(4-chloro-2-isopropyl-5-methyl-phenoxy)propyl-dimethylammonium chloride; an antiseptic agent used in the treatment of mouth and throat infections.

Haloperidol BP 1973 (hal·o·per·id·ol). γ-[4-(4-Chlorophenyl)-4-hydroxypiperidino]-4-fluorobutyrophenone; a sedative psychotropic agent and tranquillizer. A compound which causes mammary development in rats and ewes by depression of prolactin-inhibiting factors.

halophile (**hal**·o·file). 1. A bacterium which can grow in salt culture media. 2. In botany, a salt-loving plant. 3. Being attracted by halogenic or haloid salts. [Gk *hals* salt, *philein* to love.]

Halopyramine (hal·o·**pi**·ram·een). BP Commission approved name for *N-p*-chlorobenzyl-*N′N′*-dimethyl-*N*-2-pyridylethyl-enediamine, an antihistaminic drug.

haloscope (**hal**·o·skope). An apparatus with which the quantity of salt present in a solution may be ascertained. [Gk *hals* salt, *skopein* to view.]

halosteresis (**hal**·os·ter·e′·sis). Halisteresis.

Halothane BP 1973 (**hal**·o·thane). 2-Bromo-2-chloro-1,1,1-trifluoro-ethane, the most commonly used volatile anaesthetic agent. It may cause liver damage, especially after multiple exposure, which may be fatal.

Halquinol (**hal**·kwin·ol). BP Commission approved name for a mixture of the chlorinated products of 8-hydroxyquinoline containing about 65 per cent of 5,7-dichloro-8-hydroxyquinoline; it is used in the treatment of bacillary dysentery.

Halsted, William Stewart (b. 1852). Baltimore surgeon.

Halsted's band. A metal band used for the gradual occlusion of an artery, used in the treatment of aneurysms.

Halsted forceps. A form of mosquito forceps, or small artery forceps with fine-pointed blades.

Halsted's operation. 1. Radical amputation of the breast. 2. Repair of inguinal hernia by suture of the external oblique aponeurosis behind the spermatic cord which then lies in the subcutaneous tissues.

Halsted's sign. Cyanosis around the umbilicus or over the whole abdomen, sometimes reaching the limbs, occurring in acute haemorrhagic pancreatitis.

Halsted's suture. Horizontal mattress suture. *See* SUTURE.

halzoun (hal·zun). A disease caused by the eating of the raw liver of goats infected with the common live fluke, *Fasciola hepatica.* Symptoms are due to the adherence of the flukes to the pharynx by their nucleus. It is common in Syria. [Syrian word.]

ham (ham). 1. The buttock and thigh. 2. The region at the back of the knee joint; the popliteal fossa. [AS.]

hamadryad (ham·ah·**dri**·ad). *Naia hannah. [Gk hamadryas* wood nymph.]

hamamelidin, hamamelin (ham·ah·**mel**·id·in, ham·ah·**mel**·in). The evaporated alcoholic extract of hamamelis, witch-hazel, the leaves of *Hamamelis virginiana.* It occurs as a fine brown powder containing tannins, and is used as a haemostatic and astringent, usually in suppositories.

Hamamelis (ham·ah·**me**·lis). A genus of shrubs (family Hamamelidaceae). Hamamelis BP 1958 (hamamelidis folia, witch-hazel leaves) consists of the leaves of a North American species, *Hamamelis virginiana* Linn., and hamamelis bark (hamamelidis cortex, witch-hazel bark) is the bark from the same shrub. Both the leaves and the bark contain tannins and are used as astringents and haemostatics by local application, usually in the form of extracts. [Gk *hama* together, *melon* apple tree.]

hamamelose (ham·ah·**me**·loze). $CH_2OH(CHOH)_2COH(CH_2OH)CHO$, a sugar occurring in hamamelidin and related to the hexoses.

hamartia (ham·ar·she·ah). Faulty physical development caused by failure of or defects in tissue combinations. [Gk *hamartion* bodily defect.]

hamartoblastoma (ham·ar·to·blas·**to**'·mah). An autonomous new growth originating from a hamartoma. [hamartoma, blastoma.]

hamartoma (ham·ar·**to**·mah). 1. A malformation resembling a tumour, caused by defective tissue combination. 2. A tumour composed of a new growth of blood vessels as distinct from a tumour formed by the dilatation of vessels already present (haemangioma). 3. A term for a nodule composed of redundant tissue (Albrecht). **Hypothalamic hamartoma.** A collection of nerve cells in the posterior hypothalamus which may cause precocious puberty. **Hamartoma of the lung.** Cartilaginous tumours with epithelial elements, fat and muscle fibres of bronchial origin, that occur in the lung. [Gk *hamartion* bodily defect, *-oma* tumour.]

hamartomatosis (**ham**·ar·to·mat·**o**'·sis). Multiple hamartomata. [hamartoma, Gk *-osis* condition.]

hamartoplasia (**ham**·ar·to·**pla**'·ze·ah). A condition in which a tissue, stimulated by the need to repair a defect or lesion, becomes overactive and produces an excess of tissue. [Gk *hamartion* bodily defect, *plassein* to form.]

hamate bone [os hamatum (NA)] (**ham**·ate·bone). The most medial bone in the distal row of carpal bones. [L *hamatus* hooked.]

hamatum (ham·a·tum). The hamate bone. [L hooked.]

Hamburger, Franz (b. 1874). German physician.

Hamburger's test. 0.1 ml of 1 in 10 000 dilution of old tuberculin injected subcutaneously results in a localized infiltration at the site of injection within 24 h in tuberculous subjects. Undesirable reactions may occur.

Hamburger, Hartog Jacob (b. 1859). Groningen physiologist.

Hamburger interchange. The ionic mutual reaction between the blood plasma and the blood corpuscles, as when carbon dioxide entering the red blood cells effects an increase of plasma bicarbonate and a decrease in plasma chloride.

Hamdi's solution. A preserving fluid employed in the mounting of museum specimens and the preservation of the natural colour of tissues.

Hamilton, Frank Hastings (b. 1813). Buffalo and New York surgeon.

Hamilton's pseudophlegmon. An affection of the subcutaneous tissue, characterized by a localized enlargement which in some cases becomes red and hardened but does not form or discharge pus.

Hamilton's test. In dislocation of the shoulder a ruler placed on the outer side of the arm will touch both the lateral epicondyle and the acromion process.

Hamilton Irving apparatus, or belt and box. An overflow apparatus, consisting of a belt and box, which is secured on the anterior abdominal wall over a suprapubic urinary fistula. The box is made of plastic and has a perforated lid which can be removed; this is secured over the fistula by a rubber belt which is fastened to hooks on the box. Two lateral openings in the walls of the box are provided with rubber tubes which conduct the overflow urine to a receptacle.

Hamman, Louis Virgil (b. 1877). Baltimore physician.

Hamman's disease. Spontaneous interstitial emphysema.

Hamman–Rich syndrome. Idiopathic diffuse interstitial fibrosis of the lungs, usually fatal.

Hamman's sign. Loud clicking or crunching sounds synchronous with cardiac systoles, heard along the left border of the heart in cases of mediastinal emphysema.

Hammarsten, Olof (b. 1841). Upsala physiologist.

Hammarsten's test, for bile pigments in urine. A stock reagent is prepared by mixing 1 part of dilute nitric acid (1 in 4) with 19 parts of dilute hydrochloric acid (1 in 4). The test reagent consists of 1 part stock reagent + 4 parts absolute ethyl alcohol. A few drops of urine are added to 2 ml of test reagent in a test tube. A green colour is produced if bilirubin is present.

Hammarsten's theory. The theory that blood coagulates following fibrinogen dissolution and the formation of fibrin.

hammer (**ham**·er). 1. The malleus. 2. An instrument the head of which is usually at right angles to the handle and used for beating. **Percussion hammer.** A hammer with a rubber head and flexible stem, used in percussion. **Thermal hammer.** A heated hammer used for counter-irritation. [AS *hamer.*]

See also: GRANVILLE, MAYOR, WAGNER (J. P.).

Hammerschlag, Albert (b. 1863). Vienna physician.

Hammerschlag's method. A method for the determination of the specific gravity of blood on the falling-drop principle; a mixture of benzene and chloroform of known specific gravity is used.

Hammerschlag's phenomenon. Undue fatigue in auditory appreciation induced by persistent stimulating tones of progressively less intensity.

hammock (**ham**·ok). A term occasionally applied to a sling for a fractured leg or to certain head bandages. [Sp. *hamaca.*]

Hammond, William Alexander (b. 1828). Surgeon-General, United States Army.

Hammond's disease. Congenital athetosis.

Hammond's mixture. Pepsin, wood charcoal, potassium bromide and water, used as a digestant and adsorbent.

hamose (**ham**·oze). Bent at the apex like a hook. [L *hamus* hook.]

Hampson, William (fl. 1920). London radiologist.

Hampson unit. A unit of dose of ionizing radiation formerly used.

hamster (**ham**·ster). A small burrowing rodent of the genera *Cricetus* and *Cricetulus.* They may act as reservoirs of field plague. **Chinese sand hamster.** *Cricetulus griseus*; a species readily infected with *Leishmania* and therefore used in experimental work with this organism. **Golden hamster.** *Cricetus auratus,* native to Aleppo, used as a laboratory animal. [G.]

hamstring (**ham**·string). Any one of the great tendons which bound the popliteal fossa and have their origin in the gluteal region. **Lateral hamstring.** The tendon of insertion of the biceps femoris muscle. **Medial hamstring.** The tendon of insertion of either the semitendinosus or the semimembranosus muscles. **Hamstring muscles.** The group of muscles of the lower limb comprising the biceps femoris, the semitendinosus and the semimembranosus muscles. [AS *ham, streng.*]

hamular (**ham**·ew·lar). 1. Hooked; unciform; hamate. 2. Hook-like. [L *hamus* hook.]

hamulate, hamulose (**ham**·ew·late, **ham**·ew·loze). 1. Hook-shaped. 2. Having a small hook. [L *hamus* hook.]

hamulus (**ham**·ew·lus). A little hook. **Hamulus cochleae.** Hamulus of the spiral lamina (see below). **Lacrimal hamulus [hamulus lacrimalis (NA)].** A process on the lacrimal bone. **Pterygoid hamulus [hamulus pterygoideus (NA)].** The hook-like process at the lower end of the medial pterygoid plate of the sphenoid bone. **Hamulus of the spiral lamina [hamulus laminae spiralis (NA)].** The small hooked process at the upper end of the spiral lamina. [dim. of L *hamus* hook.]

Hancock, Henry (b. 1809). London surgeon.

Hancock's amputation. A modification of Pirogoff's operation, part of the talus being retained in an anterior flap and the sawn surface of the calcaneum brought in contact with it and the tibia.

Hancock's operation. 1. Hancock's amputation. 2. For glaucoma: an obsolete method.

Hand, Alfred (b. 1868). Philadelphia paediatrician.

Hand's disease or syndrome, Hand-Schueller-Christian disease or syndrome. Schueller's disease, xanthomatosis: a non-familial disturbance of lipoid (cholesterol) metabolism seen in young children, characterized by slight anaemia, defects in membranous bone, mainly skull, exophthalmos, diabetes insipidus, often with dwarfism, and a yellowish-brown colour (xanthomatosis) of the skin. Sometimes the liver, spleen and glands are enlarged to a moderate degree.

hand [manus] (hand). The terminal part of the upper limb below the wrist. Distinctive parts are the dorsum and the palm. **Ape hand.** Describing the superficial resemblance observed between the human hand with a median and ulnar palsy and that of a brachiating ape, particularly with reference to the flattening of the thenar eminence and "rolled out" attitude of the thumb. **Apostolic hand.** A hand in which the ring and little fingers are held in flexion, the result of Dupuytren's contracture. **Battledore hand.** The large hand of acromegaly, with a wide palm and broad stubby fingers. **Beat hand.** Cellulitis of the hand caused by severe or prolonged friction or pressure. **Benediction hand.** Flexion of the ring and little fingers, as seen in ulnar paralysis or other diseases giving severe wasting of small hand muscles; also called *preachers' hand.* **Claw hand.** *See* CLAW-HAND. **Cleft hand.** 1. A congenital deformity in which there is a deep cleft in the palm extending from the space between the 3rd and 4th fingers. 2. A congenital deformity in which the middle fingers are absent. **Crab hand.** A swollen hand caused by a scratch with the shell of a crab. **Dead hand.** A condition occasionally seen in operatives using power hammers, and ascribed to repeated concussion. The hand becomes at first dark blue in colour, afterwards dead white and is painful. **Drop hand.** Wrist drop. **Flipper hand.** The deformity of ulnar deviation of the fingers which occurs as the result of chronic rheumatoid arthritis in certain individuals; seal-fin deformity. **Forceps hand.** A hand with only the thumb and little finger. **Immersion hand.** The painful, swollen condition of the hands due to long exposure to cold and damp. **Lobster-claw hand.** Cleft hand (see above). **Obstetricians' hand.** The hand in tetany, in which there are extensions at the metacarpophalangeal joints and at the interphalangeal joints, and adduction of the thumb. **Opera-glass hand.** The gross deformity of the fingers which results from absorption of the ends of the metacarpal bones in severe cases of rheumatoid arthritis. **Phantom hand.** A feeling as though the hand were still present after amputation. **Preachers' hand.** Benediction hand (see above). **Skeleton hand.** Gross atrophy of all hand muscles, as in progressive muscular atrophy; also called *main en squelette.* **Spade hand.** The hand in acromegaly. **Split hand.** Lobster-claw deformity of the hands in which the middle part is missing and the digits on either side are fused; it is autosomal dominant. **Trailing hand.** When both hands are acting synchronously, say writing together, that upon which attention is not concentrated may lag behind. **Trench hand.** Immersion hand (see above). **Trident hand.** The hand in achondroplasia. The fingers are short and thick, and nearly equal in length. The index and middle fingers are deflected to the radial side, the ring and little fingers to the ulnar side, and so with the thumb form the 3 elements of a trident. **Washerwoman's hand.** The white, sodden-looking, corrugated hand of a washerwoman or of a drowned person. **Writing hand.** The approximation of the tips of the thumb and first finger with flexion of the remaining fingers, as seen in paralysis agitans. [AS.]

See also: MARINESCO.

Handley, Richard Sampson. London surgeon.

Handley's operation. Biopsy of the internal mammary lymph nodes in cancer of the breast.

Handley, William Sampson (b. 1872). London surgeon.

Handley's method. The introduction subcutaneously of strands of silk thread in an attempt to relieve lymphoedema.

Handley's theory. Lymphatic permeation theory. *See* THEORY.

handpiece (**hand**·pees). A hand instrument provided with a chuck for holding tools used for removing tooth structure, polishing, condensing, etc. Usually has rotary, may have vibratory motion. [AS *hand,* ME *pece.*]

Hanfmann-Kasanin test. A test of conceptual or abstract thinking, modified from the Vigotsky test. The subject is presented with 22 blocks of 5 colours, 6 shapes, 2 heights and 2 widths, and is required to sort the blocks into 4 categories, namely short and narrow, tall and narrow, short and wide, tall and wide. The test is performed relatively poorly by subjects with low intelligence, with organic brain disease or with schizophrenia.

Hanger, Franklin McCue (b. 1894). New York physician.

Hanger's test, for liver function. Cephalin-cholesterol flocculation test; a colloidal suspension of a cephalin-cholesterol mixture is added to a dilution of serum in normal saline. The degree of flocculation is noted after 24 and 48 h, and affords a measure of the extent of liver impairment.

hangnail (**hang**·nale). A torn strip of skin at the side or the root of a nail, often the cause of an inflammation at the site. [AS *angnaegl* painful nail.]

Hanlon, C. Rollins (b. 1915). Chicago surgeon.

Blalock-Hanlon operation. Atrial septectomy; the surgical creation of an atrial septal defect for the palliation of transposition of the great vessels.

Hannover, Adolph (b. 1814). Copenhagen anatomist.

Hannover's canal. The space between the anterior and posterior suspensory fibres of the lens.

Hannover's intermediate membrane. Enamel membrane. *See* MEMBRANE.

Hanot, Victor Charles (b. 1844). Paris physician.

Hanot's cirrhosis or disease. Biliary cirrhosis characterized by enlargement of the liver and spleen, chronic jaundice and febrile attacks.

Hansen, Gerhard Henrik Armauer (b. 1841). Bergen physician.

Hansen's bacillus. *Mycobacterium leprae.*

Hansen's disease. Leprosy.

Hanson, Adolph Melanchton (b. 1888). American surgeon.

Hanson's extract. Thymus extract; an aqueous acid extract of the thymus glands of 2- to 6-week-old calves, said to increase the growth, development and fertility of rats.

Hanson unit. A unit of activity of an extract of parathyroid gland. It is one-hundredth of the amount required to raise the blood serum calcium by 1 mg per cent in a parathyroidectomized dog weighing 20 kg.

haouwa (hah·**oo**·wah). Cholera. [East Indian name.]

hapalonychia (hap·al·on·**ik**'·e·ah). A condition of the nails in which they have not been converted into horny tissue and therefore are soft; onychomalacia. [Gk *hapalos* soft, *onyx* nail.]

hapantismus (hap·an·**tiz**·mus). Complete adhesion of 1 surface to another or others. [Gk *hapas* entire.]

haphalgesia (haf·al·**je**·ze·ah). A condition of morbid sensitiveness of the skin when the merest touch on it occasions pain. [Gk *haphe* touch, *algesis* sense of pain.]

haphephobia (haf·e·**fo**·be·ah). The morbid fear or excessive dislike of being touched or of having to touch objects. [Gk *haphe* touch, phobia.]

haplobacteria (hap·lo·bak·**teer**'·e·ah). Bacteria which do not produce filaments during growth. [Gk *haploos* single, bacteria.]

haplodermatitis, haplodermitis (**hap**·lo·der·mat·**i**'·tis, **hap**·lo·der·**mi**'·tis). Simple inflammation of the skin. [Gk *haploos* single, dermatitis.]

haplodont (**hap**·lo·dont). Having teeth without ridges or tubercles on the crowns, i.e. simple conical crowns. [Gk *haploos* single, *odous* tooth.]

haploid (**hap**·loid). Of chromosome complements, cells or individuals with only 1 set of chromosomes. In diploid species such as man, this condition is normally found in gametes and gametocytes after the first meiotic division. Fertilization restores diploidy. [Gk *haploos* single, *eidos* form.]

haploidization (**hap**·loid·i·**za**'·shun). The reduction of the chromosome complement from the diploid to the haploid number. [Gk *haploos* single, *eidos* form.]

haploidy (**hap**·loid·e). The state characteristic of haploids. [Gk *haploos* single, *eidos* form.]

haplomycosis (**hap**·lo·mi·**ko**'·sis). Adiaspiromycosis. [Gk *haploos* single, *mykes* fungus, *-osis* condition.]

haplont (**hap**·lont). A haploid organism with a brief diploid phase represented by a zygote which undergoes meiosis and thus returns to the haploid condition. [Gk *haploos* single, *eidos* form, *on* being.]

haplopathy (hap·**lop**·ath·e). A disease without complications. [Gk *haploos* single, *pathos* disease.]

haplophase (**hap**·lo·faze). That phase in the life cycle of an organism in which nuclei are haploid. [Gk *haploos* single, *phasis* appearance.]

haplopia (hap·**lo**·pe·ah). Normal, i.e. single, vision; the opposite of diplopia. [Gk *haploos* single, *ops* eye.]

haploscope (**hap**·lo·skope). Applied to any instrument by means of which pictures shown to each eye separately are united into one. **Mirror haploscope.** An instrument in which each picture is reflected by a mirror placed at the angle of a bent tube; there is one such tube for each eye, and the angle between the tubes can be varied to suit the angle of the squint in the observer. A simple example is the amblyoscope invented by Worth, while more complex forms of this instrument are used in the training of patients with squint. [Gk *haploos* single, *skopein* to view.]

haploscopic (hap·lo·**skop**·ik). 1. Referring or belonging to a haploscope. 2. Stereoscopic.

haplosomy (hap·lo·**so**·me). Monosomy. [Gk *haploos* single, *soma* body.]

hapten (**hap**·ten). A substance which can combine specifically with antibody, but which cannot elicit a specific immune response when introduced into the body. Haptens can often be rendered immunogenic, i.e. can be made to elicit a specific immune response, if they are combined with a carrier, e.g. a protein or other large molecule. Many haptens are small molecules, e.g. dinitrophenol, but some large molecules such as pneumococcus polysaccharide are also haptenic. [Gk *haptein* to grasp.]

haptenic (hap·**ten**·ik). 1. Relating or belonging to haptens. 2. Caused by haptens.

haptic (**hap**·tik). Belonging to the sense of touch; tactile. [Gk *haptos* subject to the sense of touch.]

haptics (**hap**·tix). The science of the sense of touch. [see prec.]

haptodysphoria (**hap**·to·dis·**for**'·e·ah). The state of being unpleasantly affected by the touch of certain substances, e.g. emery paper, silk. [Gk *haptein* to grasp, dysphoria.]

haptoglobins (hap·to·**glo**·binz). Plasma proteins mainly of the α_2 globulin type that have the capacity of combining with haemoglobin liberated in the plasma, and also with isolated globin, as described first by Smythies (1955). Haemoglobin bound to haptoglobin is not excreted in the glomerular filtrate and this appears to explain the renal threshold for plasma haemoglobin, for only the surplus haemoglobin is excreted after all the combining capacity of the haptoglobin has been satisfied. The haptoglobin–haemoglobin complex is removed rapidly by the liver. The plasma haptoglobin may be very low in amount in haemolytic anaemias as it combines with the haemoglobin that is continuously released. Three main types of sera have been identified in relation to the haptoglobins and may be inherited according to a pair of genes Hp^1 and Hp^2; other phenotypes have been described. According to their genetic make-up the haptoglobins may be capable of polymerization or not, thus enabling the structure and properties of the proteins to be changed by such gene mutation. Plasma haptoglobins are increased considerably in amount following trauma or inflammation but the explanation for this is not clear. Detectable by starch gel electrophoresis haptoglobins are used in blood identification and in cases of disputed paternity, and are present in 97 per cent of infants at the age of 6 months. [Gk *haptein* to grasp, L *globus* ball.]

haptometer (hap·**tom**·et·er). An instrument with which acuteness of the sense of touch can be measured. [Gk *haptein* to grasp, meter.]

haptophil, haptophile (**hap**·to·fil, **hap**·to·file). Applied to the atom group of a receptor that tends to unite with the haptophore group of a toxin. [Gk *haptein* to grasp, *philein* to love.]

haptophore (**hap**·to·for). One of the attached groupings or side-chains of a living cell in the side-chain theory of immunity propounded by Ehrlich (1898, 1900). Theory now obsolete. [Gk *haptein* to grasp, *pherein* to bear.]

haptophoric, haptophorous (hap·to·**for**·ik, hap·**tof**·or·us). 1. Relating or belonging to a haptophore. 2. Indicating the action of a haptophore. 3. Combining.

haptotaxis (hap·to·**tax**·is). A state obtaining in particular cells and organisms so that mechanical stimuli either attract or repel them. [Gk *haptein* to grasp, *taxis* arrangement.]

haramaitism (hah·rah·**ma**·it·izm). 1. The Hindu practice of child marriage. 2. The harmful results, particularly the physical, resulting from child marriage. [Anglo-Indian term from *Haram maiti*, name of a particular Hindu exponent of the practice.]

harara (hah·**rah**·rah). A local name for an affection of the skin on the back of the hands and wrists caused by bites of sandflies of the genus *Phlebotomus*, and occurring in Israel among visitors to the country.

Harden-Young ester. Fructofuranose 1,6-diphosphate, $C_6H_{10}O_6(H_2PO_3)_2$, formed by the yeast fermentation of glucose, mannose or fructose.

hardening (**hard**·ning). The process by which tissue is made firm and compact so that it can readily be cut in thin sections for microscopical examination. [AS *heard*.]

Harder, Johann Jacob (b. 1656). Basle anatomist.

Harder's gland, Harderian gland. An accessory gland in the orbit which secretes an oily fluid, rarely present in the Primates.

hardness (**hard**·nes). 1. A term applied to water in which soap does not lather readily. It is due to dissolved calcium, magnesium and iron compounds forming insoluble salts with the fatty acids of the soap and producing a scum. Hardness varies in degree and may be reduced, i.e. the water softened, by the removing of the ions of these metals. 2. A term used in radiology to indicate the quality of radiations. The more penetrating radiations (those of short wavelengths) are called *hard*, and the less penetrating radiations (those of long wavelength) are called *soft*. **Permanent hardness.** Hardness which is not removed by boiling; it is due to the metals being present in the form of sulphates, and may be removed by precipitating the metals in question as insoluble carbonates by the addition of washing soda. **Temporary hardness.** Hardness which is removed by boiling; it is due to the metals being present as bicarbonates, the water having passed through chalk or limestone on its way, and boiling precipitates these as insoluble carbonates, e.g. fur in kettles. [AS *heard.*]

Hardy, Louis Phillipe Alfred (b. 1811). Paris physician.

Béhier–Hardy sign or symptom. Aphonia in early gangrene of the lung.

Hardy–Schultze rule. In the coagulation of a lyophobic sol, instability is increased by the addition of electrolyte, the effect being proportionately greater with doubly- and trebly-charged ions than with those bearing a single charge. The rule does not hold with lyophilic sols.

Hare, Edward Selleck (b. 1812). Stafford surgeon.

Hare's syndrome. Pancoast's syndrome.

Hare, Robert (b. 1871). American chemist.

Hare's apparatus. A specially constructed inverted glass U-tube for measuring the specific gravities of liquids.

hare-lip (ha·er·lip). A congenital malformation of the upper lip due to failure of fusion of the maxillary processes with the frontonasal process, frequently associated with cleft palate. **Acquired hare-lip.** A split upper lip acquired as the result of an accident. **Bilateral hare-lip.** Fissures present on either side of the median line. **Double hare-lip.** Two congenital fissures of the lip, one on each side of the median line, or one in each lip. **Lateral hare-lip.** Fissure on one or other side of the median line. **Median hare-lip.** Facial cleft. *See* CLEFT. **True hare-lip.** Fissure on the median line of the lip. [AS *hara, lippa.*]

harlequin (har·le·kwin). 1. Parti-coloured or variegated in colour; term applied to a fetus. 2. A scarlet and black poisonous snake of the genus *Elaps.* [It. *arlecchino* goblin.]

Harley, George (b. 1829). London physician.

Harley's disease. Recurrent haemoglobinuria.

harmaline (har·mal·een). $C_{13}H_{14}ON_2$, a crystalline alkaloid derived from the seeds and root of *Peganum harmala* (family Rutaceae) and which is oxidizable into harmine. It has anthelmintic properties and has also been proposed in malaria, nervous diseases and as a coronary dilator.

Harman, Nathaniel Bishop (b. 1869). London ophthalmologist.

Bishop Harman loupe. Prismatic operating spectacles giving a moderate magnification of the field. The lenses are sphero-prisms and the spectacles are worn at the end of the nose in ophthalmic surgery.

Bishop Harman diaphragm test. A test used in ophthalmology, indicating the capacity for fusing the visual images: a card with a row of letters or numbers is viewed through a diaphragm. When the diaphragm is wide open all the figures can be read with each eye; the diaphragm is slowly closed, until at first only the central figures are seen with both eyes, and finally none binocularly. If figures at one or other end disappear, then this eye is suppressing. If the central figures crowd, then the patient is esophoric, if the figures separate or become double, he is exophoric.

Harmer, William Douglas (b. 1873). London otolaryngologist.

Finzi–Harmer operation. Treatment of vocal-cord cancer by means of radium needles. The needles are placed in a window in the thyroid ala formed by a partial removal of a quadrilateral area of cartilage.

harmine (har·meen). An alkaloid obtained from *Peganum harmala* (family Rutaceae), and probably identical with banisterine; it has been used in the treatment of paralysis agitans.

harness (har·nes). A device for holding in position the facepiece of an anaesthetic apparatus. [O Fr. *harneis.*]

See also: CLAUSEN, CONNELL (K.).

harpoon (har·poon). An instrument with a sharply-pointed barbed head with which small portions of living muscular or other tissue can be extracted for examination. [Fr. *harpon* grappling-iron.]

Harrington, Francis Bishop (b. 1854). Boston surgeon.

Harrington's solution. An acid-alcoholic solution of mercuric chloride, $HgCl_2$, used for pre-operative treatment of the skin.

Harris, Henry Albert (b. 1886). Cambridge anatomist.

Harris' lines. Transverse lines at the growing ends of bones due to illness.

Harris, Henry Fauntleroy (b. 1867). American physician.

Harris' haematoxylin. *See* HAEMATOXYLIN.

Harris, Malcolm la Salle (b. 1862). Chicago surgeon.

Harris' band. Hepatoduodenal band. *See* BAND.

Harris' separator. An instrument used prior to ureteric catheterization in an attempt to collect from the bladder separated samples of the urine from the two kidneys.

Harris, Samuel Henry (b. 1880). Australian surgeon.

Harris' operation. Transvesical prostatectomy by the suprapubic route: adequate haemostasis and plastic reconstruction of the posterior urethra by special sutures, closure of the bladder and drainage *per urethram* by an indwelling whistle-tipped catheter.

Harrison, Edwin (b. 1789). London physician.

Harrison's curve, furrow, groove or sulcus. A transverse groove on the anterior chest wall, beginning at the xiphisternum and passing outwards towards the mid-axilla. It occurs in rickety children with some obstruction of inspiration, the chest being pressed in by external pressure at its most yielding place.

Harrison, Lawrence Whitaker (b. 1876). London venereologist.

Harrison's method. A method of manual dilatation of the cervix.

Harrison's scarifier. A surgical scarifier designed especially for scraping primary syphilitic sores.

Harrison's anterior urethroscope. A simple urethroscope for inspection of the anterior urethra by direct vision.

Harrison's whip. A long flexible bougie that tapers to a very fine calibre at one end; it is used for dilating severe urethral strictures.

Harrison–Wassermann test. A modification of the Wassermann test.

Harrower–Erickson test. A modification of the Rorschach test in which the blots are projected on a screen, and the subject writes down his responses, marks the blot reproductions on his blank and answers a series of questions on the responses.

harrowing (har·o·ing). Hersage. [ME *harwe.*]

Hart, Theodore Stuart (b. 1869). New York physician.

Hart's method, for casein in milk. The casein in 10.5 ml milk is coagulated by acidifying with acetic acid, filtered, washed thoroughly, dissolved in 10 ml 0.1M KOH solution and back titrated with 0.1M HCl to phenolphthalein. A blank is run concurrently, and the value added to volume of 0.1M HCl used in the test. The difference 10-total volume of 0.1M HCl gives the percentage of casein.

Hartel, F. German surgeon.

Hartel method or technique. The injection of the gasserian ganglion for tic douloureux, approaching the foramen ovale via the mouth.

Harting's bodies. Deposits of calcium (calcospherites) in the cerebral capillaries.

Hartley, Frank (b. 1856). New York surgeon.

Hartley–Krause operation, for trigeminal neuralgia. Excision of the gasserian ganglion and sensory 5th cranial nerve roots.

Hartley's broth. A digest nutrient broth, prepared by using a pancreatic extract as hydrolysing agent.

Hartmann, Alexis Frank (b. 1898). St. Louis paediatrician.

Hartmann's solution. Compound sodium lactate solution, an isotonic solution of salts used by injection for infantile gastro-enteritis.

Hartmann, Arthur (b. 1849). Berlin laryngologist.

Hartmann's curette. An instrument for the removal of adenoids.

Hartmann, Henri (b. 1860). Paris surgeon.

Hartmann's operation. Removal of the sigmoid or upper rectum for cancer, with closure of the rectal stump and colostomy.

Hartmann's critical point. Sudeck's point.

Hartmann's pouch. A shallow dilatation found at the junction of the neck of the gall bladder and the cystic duct.

Hartmann, Robert (b. 1831). Berlin anatomist.

Hartmann's fossa. The inferior ileocaecal recess. *See* RECESS.

Hartnup. The name of the family from which the first recorded example of the disease described below was obtained.

Hartnup disease. An inborn error of amino-acid metabolism transmitted by autosomal recessive inheritance and characterized clinically by episodic cerebellar ataxia, mental defect and a photosensitive rash.

Hartridge, Hamilton (b. 1886). London physiologist.

Hartridge reversion spectroscope. A spectroscope that gives 2 spectra of the same solution arranged so as just to make contact with 1 spectrum in the reverse direction to the other. One spectrum can be moved by turning a micrometer screw and in measuring the wavelength of an absorption band this is done so that the band in this spectrum becomes collinear with the corresponding band in the other. The wavelength can then be read from the scale of the micrometer screw.

Hartridge's cluster theory. A theory of colour vision, suggesting that as a modification to Young's theory of 3 different cones reacting to red, green and violet, these cones are arranged in clusters of similar type. This allows the visual acuity for coloured objects to equal that of white, as it in fact does.

Harveian (har·ve·an). An honorific epithet, as Harveian Oration, Harveian Society, relating to William Harvey, English physician and physiologist (b. 1578), MD Cantab. and Padua, FRCP. Discoverer of the circulation of the blood, "Father of English scientific midwifery" and pioneer in embryology. Wrote *Exercitatio de Motu Cordis et Sanguinis in Animalibus* (Movements of the Heart and Blood in Animals), 1628, *De Circulatione Sanguinis* (The Circulation of the Blood), 1649 (English translations by K. J. Franklin) and *De Generatione Animalium* (Of the Generation of Animals), 1651 (English translation by K. J. Franklin in preparation).

Harvey, Samuel Clark (b. 1886). American surgeon.

Volhard and Harvey method, for chlorides in urine. The same as the Volhard and Arnold method, except that filtration of the precipitated chloride is omitted.

haschisch, hasheesh (hash·eesh). Hashish.

Hashimoto, Hakaru (b. 1881). Japanese surgeon.

Hashimoto's disease, goitre, struma or thyroiditis. Struma lymphomatosa, a chronic thyroiditis associated with autoimmune antibodies to thyroxin in the blood serum.

hashish (hash·eesh). An Arabian name for *Cannabis sativa* Linn., applied to the plant itself and to certain of its preparations. [Ar. hay.]

Haskins, Howard Davis (b. 1871). Portland, Oregon, physician.

Osgood-Haskins test, for urinary proteins. Mix 5 ml of urine with 1 ml of 50 per cent acetic acid and 3 ml of saturated sodium-chloride solution. Proteins are precipitated immediately in the cold. If the precipitate dissolves upon boiling and reappears on cooling it is Bence-Jones protein. This test is particularly useful for the detection of Bence-Jones proteinuria, especially where the results of other tests are inconclusive.

Haslinger, F. (fl. 1931).

Haslinger bronchoscope. A form of bronchoscope in which the lighting is at the proximal end. It is self-retaining, but has no tracheal tube and is used more as a laryngoscope.

Hasner, Joseph Ritter von (b. 1819). Prague ophthalmologist.

Hasner's fold or valve. The lacrimal fold: also called the *valve of Bianchi* and the *valve of Cruveilhier.*

Hasner's operation. Canthoplasty; a modification of Blaskovics' operation. A small pedicle flap is swung medially from the temporal region, the end being shaped like a jackboot so that both lids can be repaired.

Hass, Julius (b. 1884). Vienna orthopaedic surgeon.

Hass disease. Osteochondrosis of the capital epiphysis of the humerus.

Hassall, Arthur Hill (b. 1817). London physician.

Hassall's body or corpuscle. Concentric corpuscle, thymus corpuscle; one of the small bodies found in the medulla of the thymus, formed of concentric layers of epithelial cells.

Hassall-Henle wart. Nodular thickenings of Descemet's membrane occurring after the age of from 20 to 30 years at the corneal periphery.

Hasselbalch, Karl A. (b. 1874). Copenhagen biochemist.

Henderson-Hasselbalch equation, for the determination of the pH of buffer systems. $pH = pK + \log_{10}[A]/[HA]$, where pK is the negative logarithm of the dissociation constant and [A] and [HA] the concentrations of acid ions and undissociated weak acid, respectively.

Hassin, George Boris (b. 1873). Chicago neurologist.

Hassin's sign or syndrome. In a lesion of the cervical sympathetic nerves, in addition to Horner's syndrome, there is often protrusion of the ear on the side of the lesion.

Hassin's treatment. The epidural injection of neoarsphenamine; used in cases of tabes dorsalis.

Hata, Sahachiro (b. 1873). Japanese bacteriologist and physician.

Hata phenomenon. The increase in the severity of an infection which may follow treatment with an ineffective dose of a chemotherapeutic drug.

Ehrlich-Hata treatment. Arsphenamine therapy for syphilis.

Hatchcock's sign. Tenderness on pressing upwards beneath the angle of the lower jaw in mumps.

Hatschek, Emil (b. 1868). London chemist.

Hatschek's viscosity formula.

$$\eta = \sqrt[3]{\frac{A}{A-1}}$$

a formula for η, the viscosity of a colloidal solution, in terms of A, the ratio of the volumes of the disperse and continuous phases.

Hauch (howk). In bacteriology, the name applied to the flagellated strains of certain bacteria on account of the thin spreading growth that they formed on an agar plate, in contrast to the discrete colonies of the non-flagellated variant to which the term *Ohne Hauch* was applied. The terms have been transferred to the antigens to which these strains respectively give rise, the thermolabile flagellar and the thermostable somatic antigens. [G, breath or exhalation, presumably because the appearance on the agar plate was that of exhaled breath on cold glass; *Ohne Hauch* without breath.]

Haudek, Martin (b. 1880). Vienna radiologist.

Haudek's diverticulum. The pouch-like concavity of a peptic ulcer crater.

Haudek's niche or sign. The direct radiological sign of gastric ulcer; it consists of protrusion of contrast medium into the ulcer crater. The niche may be seen in profile or *en face*; this depends on the incidence of the rays in relation to the organ examined. (In the UK this is always referred to as Haudek's niche and not as Haudek's sign.)

Haug's phloroglucin fluid. A decalcifying agent containing phloroglucinol.

haunch (hawnsh). The hips and the buttocks regarded as one structure. **Haunch bone.** The ilium. [O Fr. *hanche.*]

haustral (haws·tral). Relating to a haustrum of the colon.

haustration (haws·tra·shun). 1. The process of formation of a haustrum; sacculation. 2. A haustrum.

haustrum (haws·trum). Any one of the pouches formed by the sacculations of the colon. [L well bucket.]

haustus (haws·tus). A draught. **Haustus imperialis.** Potus Imperialis BPC 1949. **Haustus niger.** Black draught, compound senna mixture containing 25 per cent magnesium sulphate, with liquorice, cardamom, sal volatile and infusion of senna. [L.]

Haverhillia multiformis (ha·ver·hil·e·ah mul·te·for·mis). *Actinomyces muris,* a Gram-negative pleomorphic bacterium, found in association with Haverhill fever in man. It is present as a harmless commensal in the nasopharynx of rats. Also called *Streptobacillus moniliformis.* [Haverhill, Mass., where the first epidemic was recognized, L multiform.]

Havers, Clopton (c. 1650-1702). London anatomist and physician.

Havers' canals, haversian canals. The fine canals in bone which transmit blood vessels and are surrounded by concentric lamellae of bone.

Havers' glands, haversian glands. The extrasynovial pads of fat.

Havers' lamella. Concentric lamella; one of the series of lamellae arranged around the central haversian canal of the haversian system.

haversian space. A widened haversian canal resulting from bone absorption.

haversian system. An osteon; a cylindrical unit of compact bone structure built around a central, vascular canal and composed of concentric bony lamellae.

hawk (hawk). To clear the throat explosively by forcing out a current of air in order to remove phlegm or other foreign matter. [prob. onomat.]

Hay, Matthew (b. 1855). Aberdeen physician.

Hay's method. The sulphur test for bile in the urine: a little powdered sulphur is sprinkled on the surface of the urine; if bile salts are present the sulphur will sink, but with normal urine it floats. It depends upon the fact that bile salts lower the surface tension.

Hay, William Howard (b. 1866). American physician.

Hay diet. A diet in which proteins and carbohydrates are not eaten in the same meal, under the mistaken idea that to do so is unphysiological and the cause of many ailments.

Hayem, Georges (b. 1841). Paris physician.

Hayem's elementary corpuscle. A blood platelet.

Hayem's disease. Myelitis of sudden onset; apoplectiform myelitis.

Hayem's diluting fluid or solution. A diluting solution containing sodium sulphate 5 g, sodium chloride 1 g, mercuric chloride 0.5 g, distilled water 200 ml, used as a diluent in the counting of red blood corpuscles.

Hayem-Widal anaemia or syndrome. A haemolytic anaemia.

Haygarth, John (b. 1740). Chester and Bath physician.

Haygarth's nodes or nodosities. Subcutaneous nodules of the joints in rheumatoid arthritis.

Haynes, Irving Samuel (b. 1861). New York surgeon.

Haynes' operation. Drainage of the cerebellomedullary cisterna in suppurative meningo-encephalitis.

hazard (haz·ard). A risk, usually to a person, arising out of employment. **Radiation hazard.** The danger to health arising from exposure to ionizing radiation. It may be due to external radiation or to radiation from radioactive materials within the body. [O Fr. *hasard.*]

Head, Sir Henry (b. 1861). London neurologist.

Head's areas or zones. 1. Areas of reflex cutaneous hyperaesthesia and hyperalgesia due to visceral disease. 2. The segmental distribution of the sensory nerve roots, involved in the above.

head (hed). 1. [Caput (NA)] That part of the body containing the brain, special sense organs and mouth. 2. By analogy, the topmost or foremost part of anything. **After-coming head.** The head as delivered in a breech presentation. **Box head.** A term applied to the flattened head that occurs in rickets. **Floating head.** A fetal head when freely movable above the pelvic brim. **Hot-cross-bun head.** The broad cruciform depression on the infant's skull resulting from rachitic or syphilitic osteitis of the eminences of the frontal and parietal bones. **Hour-glass head.** A head with a transverse depression on the vertex corresponding to the coronal suture. **Loaf head.** Oxycephaly. **Head lock.** The locking of the fetal heads which may be seen in twin delivery. **Head nod.** A functional disorder of infancy in which rapid nodding or rotatory movements of the head occur, usually associated with nystagmus. It begins between the third and sixth months of life, and lasts a few weeks. **Powder head.** Headache occurring in persons handling explosives containing nitroglycerin. **Saddle head.** A head with a saddle-shaped depression across the vertex. **Scald head.** Old name for various scaly disorders of the scalp. **Steeple head, Tower head.** Oxycephaly. **White head.** Witkop. [AS *heafod.*]

head-cap (hed·cap). Plaster head-cap. A cap made of plaster of Paris and used in association with certain metal jaw splints. [AS *heafod, caeppe.*]

head-piece (hed·pees). *See* CRILE. [AS *heafod,* ME *pece.*]

headache (hed·ake). Pain occurring in or referred to the head. **Anoxic headache.** Headache caused by anoxaemia, as in mountain or altitude sickness. **Bilious headache, Blind headache, Cyclic headache.** Migrainous headache (see below). **Cluster headache.** Severe paroxysmal unilateral headache occurring frequently for several weeks and then remitting; migrainous neuralgia. **Cough headache.** Headache induced by coughing. **Distension headache.** Headache due to inflammation within an air sinus when the opening is obstructed. **Dynamite headache.** Severe headache occurring in persons handling high explosives. **Fibrositic headache.** Indurative headache (see below). **Helmet headache.** Headache limited to the upper half of the head. **Histamine headache.** Headache due to the vascular relaxation and lowered blood pressure following injections of histamine. **Hypertensive headache.** Sensations of throbbing or bursting in the head, associated with high blood pressure. **Indurative headache.** Headache associated with fibrositic nodular thickenings in the fasciae of the scalp. **Meningeal headache.** Severe continuous headache occurring with inflammation of the meninges. **Migrainous headache.** Severe headache, commonly unilateral, occurring in paroxysms at varying intervals. Although in mild cases headache may be the only symptom, it is usually accompanied by others, such as nausea, vomiting, visual disturbances and vertigo. **Miners' headache.** Headache caused by the explosive gases of nitroglycerin used in blasting charges. **Neuralgic headache.** Headache due to an affection of the sensory nerves of the scalp, usually paroxysmal and radiating along the course of a nerve which is tender to pressure. **Nodular headache.** Indurative headache (see above). **Organic headache.** Headache associated with gross lesions within the skull such as neoplasms, intracranial aneurysms, acute vascular lesions, and with haemorrhage, thrombosis or embolism. **Pituitary headache.** Headache caused by disorder of the pituitary gland, especially an eosinophil adenoma causing acromegaly or a chromophobe adenoma. **Psychogenic headache.** Abnormal sensations in the head occurring in neurotic or psychiatric persons and without organic basis. **Puncture headache.** That which occurs a few hours after lumbar puncture and which may be associated with nausea and vomiting. **Reflex headache.** Pain referred from distant organs such as intrathoracic or intra-abdominal viscera. **Sick headache.** Migrainous headache (see above). **Tension headache.** Headache attributed to chronic contraction of the muscles of the neck and scalp. **Toxaemic headache.** Headache which is a common symptom at the onset of many acute infectious diseases, e.g. typhoid fever, smallpox, influenza and cerebrospinal meningitis. **Uraemic headache.** Headache occurring at the onset of the cerebral type of acute uraemia. **Vacuum headache.** Headache due to absorption of air in a nasal sinus when inflammatory swelling obstructs its outlet. [AS *heafod, acan.*]

See also: HORTON.

Heaf, Frederick Rowland George (b. 1894). British physician.

Heaf's gun. An apparatus for giving multiple (6) intradermal injections of tuberculin in Heaf's test (see below); also used for giving BCG vaccine.

Heaf's intradermal multiple-puncture test. From 5 to 10 international tuberculin units of PPD are injected intradermally by means of Heaf's gun (see above). The result is read in 3 days but can be read up to 7 days: +reaction=4 or more palpable indurated papules; + +reaction=a ring of induration; + + +reaction=an indurated plateau; + + + +reaction=a plateau of induration of over 10 mm in diameter. If this is negative, 100 units are then used.

heal (heel). 1. To effect a cure or to restore to health. 2. To return to a state of soundness, said of a wound or other lesion. **Heal by**

first intention. Said of a wound when the edges adhere immediately to each other without any intervening space. **Heal by granulation.** Said of a wound which is left open, or of an ulcer the raw surface of which becomes covered first by young vascular connective tissue and later is covered from its periphery by overgrowing epithelium from the healthy edges of the defect. **Mental heal.** To heal by psychological treatment, in a broad sense. **Primary heal.** To heal by first intention (see above). **Heal by second intention.** To heal by granulation (see above). **Heal by third intention.** Said of an open wound after suppuration has occurred in it and has resolved. [AS *haelan.*]

heal-all (heel·awl). 1. A panacea or universal remedy. 2. The popular name of various plants, including *Collinsonia canadensis* and *Prunella vulgaris.* [AS *haelan, all.*]

healing (heel·ing). **Faith healing.** The regression of disease correlated with the faith of the diseased person in the power of a deity, or in some other transcendent power, to heal. To be distinguished from spiritual healing (see below). **Spiritual healing.** The regression of disease correlated with the invocation of allegedly spiritual aid to that purpose. An element of faith on the part of the sufferer is claimed not to be required. [AS *haelan.*]

health (helth). The normal physical state, i.e. the state of being whole and free from physical and mental disease or pain, so that all parts of the body carry on their proper function. [AS *haelth.*]

healthy (hel·the). 1. Sound and whole in mind and body; being without physical pain or disease. 2. Applied to a wound in which healing is proceeding satisfactorily. [see prec.]

heaped-up (heept·up). A term applied to the naked-eye, surface appearances of a growth of bacteria on solid media in stroke culture, characterized by a raised growth usually with irregular margins. [AS *heap.*]

hearing (heer·ing). The function carried out by the ear conveying sound waves to the brain. **Colour hearing.** A phenomenon whereby various different pitches of sound are associated with colours in the mind of the hearer. It is an example of synaesthesia. **Double hearing.** A double auditory impression from a single stimulus., **Double disharmonic hearing.** A double auditory impression from a single stimulus, the impressions being of a different pitch and character. **Monaural hearing.** Hearing with one ear only. **Residual hearing.** The amount of valuable hearing in a partially deaf individual. [AS *hieran.*]

hearing aid (heer·ing ade). Any appliance designed to amplify sound so that it can be heard by persons of defective hearing. **Air-conduction hearing aid.** A hearing aid utilizing the normal air-conduction pathway. **Bone-conduction hearing aid.** An aid which utilizes the normal bone-conduction mechanism. The modified or amplified sound waves picked up by the receiver are carried to the bone of the mastoid process by a special fitting. [AS *hieran,* O Fr. *aide.*]

Hearing Aid Council Act 1968. This Act provides for the establishment of a Hearing Aid Council; to register persons engaged in the supply of hearing aids; to advise on the training of persons engaged in such business and to regulate trade practices.

heart [cor (NA)] (hart). The muscular organ which maintains the circulation of the blood by its pumping action. It consists of 4 chambers (right and left atria, right and left ventricles) and 4 valves (tricuspid, mitral, pulmonary and aortic). Venous (unoxygenated) blood enters the right atrium from the superior and inferior venae cavae and passes through the tricuspid valve into the right ventricle which pumps it through the pulmonary valve into the pulmonary artery and thence into the lungs. Oxygenated blood from the lungs passes from the pulmonary veins into the left atrium and thence through the mitral valve into the left ventricle from whence it is pumped through the aortic valve into the aorta and distributed through the systemic circulation, finally returning to the right atrium after having supplied the tissues with oxygen. **Abdominal heart.** Ectopic heart within the abdominal cavity. **Apex of the heart [apex cordis (NA)].** The rounded extremity of the left ventricle at which the lower and left borders of the heart meet. It lies behind the 5th left intercostal space, 7-9 cm from the anterior midline. **Armour heart, Armoured heart.** Calcification in the pericardium as a result of pericarditis. **Athletic heart.** Hypertrophy of the heart in the absence of disease or functional disorder, said to occur in athletes; it is doubtful if the normal heart ever undergoes hypertrophy out of proportion to the body size. **Atrophic heart.** Small heart due to hypoplasia of the muscle fibres, either as a result of brown atrophy in elderly or debilitated persons, impairment of adrenal cortical function (Addison's disease) or hyperpituitarism (Simmonds' disease). **Base of the heart [basis cordis (NA)].** The flattened quadrilateral-shaped surface of the heart, directed backwards, and composed of the atria, mainly the left. **Beriberi heart.** Cardiac insufficiency due to lack of vitamin B_1; there is dilatation of the right side of the heart and the pulmonary artery, together with a hyperkinetic circulation and right-sided congestive heart failure. **Boot-shaped heart.** Cor bovinum. **Border of the heart, right [margo dexter (NA)].** The curved and somewhat indefinite right margin. It expands between the openings of the superior and inferior venae cavae and is formed by the right atrium. **Boxing-glove heart.** Term applied to the shape of the heart on radiography in mitral stenosis, in which the right ventricle, left atrium and pulmonary artery are enlarged. **Cervical heart.** Ectopic heart in the neck. **Chaotic heart.** Irregular rapid heart action due to either uncontrolled atrial fibrillation or other abnormal rhythm, or to regular rapid beating associated with hyperdynamic circulation such as occurs in severe anaemia, thyrotoxicosis, beriberi, cor pulmonale, etc. **Cottage-loaf heart.** Snowman heart (see below). **Disease of the heart.** Disease affecting the heart and involving the pericardium, myocardium or endocardium. It may result from infection, inflammation, ischaemia, hypertension, metabolic disorders, endocrine disease, infiltration, neoplasia, degeneration, deficiency states and congenital developmental defects. **Disordered action of the heart.** *See* ACTION. **Drop heart.** An extremely vertical position of the heart in tall, thin, asthenic individuals, and in asthmatic emphysematous subjects in whom the diaphragm is low and the rib spaces horizontal. **Ectopic heart.** Congenital displacement of the heart outside the thorax; it may lie in the neck (cervical heart) or within the abdominal cavity (abdominal heart). **Encased heart.** Constrictive pericarditis. *See* PERICARDITIS. **Fat heart, Fatty heart.** Tiger heart (see below). **Fibroid heart.** Myocardial fibrosis. *See* FIBROSIS. **Flask-shaped heart.** Term applied to the shape of the heart on radiography of a large pericardial effusion. **Frosted heart.** Thickening of the pericardium, giving rise to a frosted appearance, resulting from pericarditis. It occurs in constrictive mediastinopericarditis (Pick's disease) and in polyserositis (Concato's disease). **Glycogenic heart.** The heart in glycogen storage disease (von Gierke's disease); it is infiltrated with glycogen and enlarged, and sudden death is common. **Goitre heart.** The heart in thyrotoxicosis; it is characterized by tachycardia, hyperkinetic circulation, extrasystole and frequently atrial fibrillation. In young persons the heart is not usually enlarged, but in older persons cardiomegaly and congestive heart failure are frequent. **Hairy heart.** Villous heart (see below). **Ham-shaped heart.** Term applied to the radiographic appearance of the heart in thyrotoxicosis. **Hanging heart.** Drop heart (see above). **Hypertensive heart.** Hypertensive heart disease; left ventricular hypertrophy followed by dilatation and failure, in persons with systemic hypertension. **Icing heart.** Frosted heart (see above). **Irritable heart.** Disorderly action of the heart. **Kyphoscoliotic heart, Kyphotic heart.** Kyphoscoliotic cor pulmonale; in cases of severe kyphoscoliosis, inadequate ventilation, collapse of parts of the lung and compensatory emphysema may result in strain upon the right side of the heart, leading to cardiac failure, principally as a result of anoxia. The heart is usually greatly displaced and rotated within the thorax, but it is uncertain whether mechanical compression of the right side of the heart plays a part in the production of failure. **Left heart.** A term denoting the left side of the heart which supplies the tissues with oxygenated blood; it consists of the left atrium, mitral valve, left ventricle and aortic valve. **Luxus heart.** Dilatation and hypertrophy of the left ventricle, such as occurs in aortic-valve incompetence or hypertensive heart disease. **Military heart.** Disordered action of the heart. **Mobile heart.** A heart that moves freely in the chest with respiration and changes in posture. **Myxoedema heart.** Heart disease due to myxoedema; the heart is slow and enlarged. **Ox heart.** Cor bovinum. **Pear-shaped heart.** Term applied to the radiographic appearance in severe combined disease of the aortic and mitral valves; all chambers and the pulmonary artery are enlarged, with the occasional exception of the right atrium. **Pendulous heart.** Drop heart (see above). **Porpoise heart.** A heart showing right-ventricular preponderance. **Pulmonary heart.** 1. Cor pulmonale. 2. Right heart (see following). **Right heart.** Term denoting the right side of the heart which supplies the lungs with unoxygenated blood; it consists of the right atrium, right ventricle, and tricuspid and pulmonary valves. **Sabot heart.** Term applied to the radiographic appearance of the heart in the tetralogy of Fallot; the hypertrophy of the right ventricle causes upward tilting of the apex, resembling the toe of a wooden clog. Total heart size is not usually increased. **Scarlet-fever heart.** The heart in acute myocarditis due to scarlet fever. **Snowman heart.** Term applied to the radiographic appearance of the heart in totally anomalous pulmonary venous drainage through a channel running up to join the left innominate vein; the body of the snowman is represented by the main cardiac shadow, and the head by the dilated venous channel carrying the pulmonary veins to the right atrium. **Soldier's heart.** Disordered action of the heart; neurocirculatory asthenia; effort syndrome. **Stony heart.** Heart contracted in ventricular systole. **Surface of the heart, diaphragmatic [facies diaphragmatica (NA)].** The surface, composed of ventricles, which rests mainly on the central tendon of the diaphragm. **Surface of the heart, left (pulmonary) [facies pulmonalis (NA)].** The convex surface composed of the left ventricle, atrium and auricle. It is separated from the left lung by pericardium and pleura, with the phrenic nerve between. **Surface of the heart, sternocostal [facies sternocostalis (NA)].** The surface behind the body of the sternum and the medial ends of the 3rd to 6th costal cartilages on both sides. It is formed below the atrioventricular groove mainly by the right ventricle, and above the groove by the atria, which are separated from the sternum by the roots of the great vessels. **Systemic heart.** Left heart (see above). **Tabby-cat heart, Thrush-breast heart.** Tiger heart (see below). **Thyroid heart.** Involvement of the heart in disorder of the thyroid gland, e.g. thyrotoxicosis (goitre heart, see above) or myxoedema (myxoedema heart, see above). **Tiger heart, Tiger-lily heart.** The appearance of heart muscle in irregular streaks of pale friable areas of fatty degeneration resembling the stripes of a tiger; it occurs particularly in severe and prolonged anaemia, but may result from any condition which causes anoxaemia. **Tobacco heart.** The occurrence of numerous ectopic beats, produced by smoking in susceptible individuals. **Triangular heart.** Flask-shaped heart (see above). **Typhoid heart.** The heart in acute myocarditis due to typhoid fever. **Villous heart.** A heart covered with a shaggy mass of pericardial exudate. **Water-bottle heart.** Flask-shaped heart (see above). **Wooden-shoe heart.** Sabot heart (see above). [AS *heorte.*]

heart block (hart blok). A condition in which the transmission of impulses from the sinu-atrial node through the atria, atrioventricular node and bundle of His to the ventricles is delayed or interrupted in some part of its course. **Arborization heart block.** A term used to denote slight or moderate degrees of conduction defect in the finer ramifications of the bundle branches, shown cardiographically by slight increase in the QRS-complex duration without definite evidence of bundle-branch block. Since it is impossible to distinguish between block in the main bundle branch and in its ramifications, the term *intraventricular block* is to be preferred. **Atrioventricular heart block, Auriculoventricular heart block.** Heart block between the atria and the ventricles due to block at the entry to the atrioventricular node, within it, in the main bundle of His or all the branches of the bundle. It may be complete or incomplete and, although sometimes congenital, is usually due to acquired disease. Three degrees are commonly recognized: in the first, there is regular conduction between the atria and ventricles but conduction is slowed leading to prolongation of the P-R interval in the electrocardiogram; in the second, impulses from the atria are not all conducted to the ventricles and this may occur in a number of ways such that occasional beats are not conducted, only 1 of 2 or 3 are conducted, or conduction fails in a cyclical fashion (the Wenckebach phenomena); in the third degree or complete heart block, no impulses are conducted. **Bundle-branch heart block.** Failure of conduction in one of the 2 branches of the main bundle of His which may be persistent or intermittent. **Complete heart block.** Complete failure of conduction of all impulses from the atria to the ventricles so that they beat independently unless the condition results in ventricular asystole or unless accrochage occurs. **Congenital heart block.** Heart block due to imperfect development in the fetus of the conducting system of the heart. **Entrance (entry) heart block.** The phenomenon whereby a depolarization front spreading through the myocardium is prevented from entering and activating the part of the myocardium affected by the block, with the consequence that the activity of this part is uninfluenced by that of the rest of the heart. **Exit heart block.** The converse phenomenon to entrance heart block (see above) whereby a depolarization front originating from a focus of activity in the myocardium is prevented from spreading to the rest of the myocardium. It is one mechanism postulated to account for sino-atrial heart block (see below). **First degree heart block.** *See* Atrioventricular heart block (above). **Incomplete heart block.** Any form of defect of conduction of the impulses from the atria to the ventricles short of complete failure of such conduction; either first or second degree heart block (*see* Atrioventricular heart block (above)). **Intraventricular heart block.** A failure of conduction of the excitatory impulse somewhere in that part of the conducting system which lies within the ventricles; there are several varieties depending upon the exact site or sites of block. **Left bundle-branch heart block.** Failure of conduction of the exaltatory impulse in all the branches of the His bundle distributed within the left ventricle. **Monofascicular heart block.** Failure of conduction in one of the 3 or more fascicles postulated as being the final main divisions of the His bundle system. **Partial heart block.** Incomplete heart block (see above). **Peri-infarction heart block.** Impairment of conduction of the stimulating impulse in the region of a developing infarct; this is an ill-defined entity and the criteria for its electrocardiographic recognition are not generally agreed. **Retrograde heart block.** Failure of conduction of an impulse retrogradely in the conduction system from an origin in, or below, the atrioventricular node back to the atria. **Right bundle-branch heart block.** Failure of conduction of the excitatory impulse in the branch of the His bundle distributed within the right ventricle. *Incomplete right bundle-branch heart block* is a misnomer often applied to the electrocardiographic pattern with an RSR pattern in lead V_1 but with the QRS duration within normal limits, most commonly found in patients with atrial septal defect. **Second degree heart block.** *See* Atrioventricular heart block (above). **Sino-atrial (sino-auricular) heart block.** The condition in which the atria fail to be excited at the appropriate time for the current heart rhythm; this may result from delay or failure of the generation of the sinu-atrial node impulse or from failure of a generated impulse to be conducted to the atrial tissue. **Third degree heart block.** *See* Atrioventricular heart block (above). **Trifascicular heart block.** Complete heart block (see above) due to separate lesions affecting all 3 main fasciculi of the conducting system. **Unidirectional heart block.** A failure of conduction of an impulse along a pathway in one direction whilst conduction along the same pathway in the opposite direction is preserved. [AS *heorte,* Fr. *bloc.*]

heart failure (hart fa·lewr). The clinical condition caused by the failure of the heart to maintain an output of blood appropriate to the demands of the body and to the prevailing conditions affecting the cardiac performance. **Acute heart failure.** Sudden failure of heart action, commonly caused by coronary thrombosis and often fatal. **Backward heart failure.** One of the mechanisms postulated in congestive heart failure: the piling-up of blood in the venous system resulting from insufficient emptying of the right heart, producing an elevation of central and peripheral venous pressure, and the transudation of fluid from the capillaries into the tissue spaces, causing oedema, ascites, etc.; essentially a passive concept. **Chronic heart failure.** Persisting insufficiency of the circulation usually applied to congestive heart failure but also to left heart failure. **Congestive heart failure.** That form of heart failure which is characterized by venous congestion, visible in the neck veins and leading to hepatic enlargement, and fluid retention leading to oedema and ascites. **Forward heart failure.** One of the mechanisms postulated in congestive heart failure: a fall in cardiac output resulting from inefficient cardiac function, reduced renal blood flow, retention of sodium chloride and water, increase in extracellular fluid volume, increased venous pressure and the transudation of fluid from the capillaries into the tissue spaces (oedema). It is probable that both this and backward heart failure (see above) are concerned in the production of congestive failure, the forward concept being the more important, but both are over-simplifications, and many other factors also play a part. **Left heart failure.** That form of heart failure which is characterized by pulmonary venous congestion leading to exertional dyspnoea, orthopnoea and paroxysmal nocturnal dyspnoea. It may be the result of conditions interfering with left ventricular filling, such as mitral valve disease or to left ventricular failure. **Left ventricular heart failure.** Left heart failure due to impaired left ventricular function from conditions such as hypertension, aortic valve disease, coronary artery disease or cardiomyopathy. **Right heart failure.** Congestive heart failure due to conditions interfering with right ventricular filling, such as tricuspid valve disease, constrictive pericarditis and tamponade, or right ventricular failure. **Right ventricular heart failure.** Right heart failure due to impaired right ventricular function from conditions such as pulmonary stenosis or pulmonary hypertension. [AS *heorte*, O Fr. *faillir*.]

heart-lung (hart·lung). **Mechanical heart-lung.** An apparatus for carrying on the functions of the heart and lungs when the functions of either of these organs are temporarily put out of action. [AS *heorte, lungen.*]

heartburn (hart·burn). 1. A popular term for any form of indigestion in which pain, of a burning nature, occurs behind the sternum. 2. More scientifically, the burning sensation caused by regurgitation of material from the stomach, not necessarily acid, acting upon the sensitive mucous membrane of the stomach and producing an oesophagitis; pyrosis. [AS *heorte, brinnan.*]

heartworm (hart·werm). *Dirofilaria immitis*, a parasitic nematode worm belonging to the super-family Filarioidea. It is found in the right heart and veins of the dog, wolf and fox in eastern Asia and is transmitted by the bite of anopheline mosquitoes. [AS *heorte, wyrm.*]

heat (heet). 1. A form of energy due to the motion of the molecules of a body; it is transmitted to other bodies of lower temperature by conduction, convection or radiation, the latter in the form of electromagnetic waves, and may cause rise in temperature, expansion or change of state. 2. A sensation derived from hot objects and perceived by special sensory nerve-endings. 3. The period of maximum sexual desire in the oestrus cycle of animals. **Animal heat.** That heat which arises from chemical processes occurring in the living organism. **Atomic heat.** The product of the atomic weight of an element and its specific heat: approximately constant for most elements. *See* DULONG AND PETIT'S LAW. **Conductive heat.** Heat derived by contact with a hot body. **Convective heat.** Heat received on the surface of the body by convection from a heated object. **Conversive heat.** In diathermy, the heat produced in body tissues by their resistance to high-frequency electric discharges. **Delayed heat.** Recovery heat (see below). **Dry heat.** Thermal effect produced by heated dry air, especially the removal of perspiration in hyperaemization. **Initial heat.** The heat generated in muscle at the commencement of the contraction cycle. **Latent heat.** The heat absorbed by a body changing state from solid to liquid or liquid to vapour without any accompanying rise in temperature. **Molecular heat.** The product of the molecular weight of a substance and its specific heat. **Prickly heat.** Miliaria. **Radiant heat.** Electromagnetic radiation of the infrared region with wavelengths greater than those of visible red light, but less than those of radio waves; objects absorbing it exhibit a rise in temperature. **Recovery heat.** The heat generated in the second stage of muscle contraction. **Sensible heat.** Heat which produces a measurable rise in temperature of the body absorbing it. **Specific heat.** The quantity of heat necessary to raise the temperature of 1 g of a substance 1°C. [AS *haetu.*]

heater (he·ter). *See* MADDOX.

Heath, Christopher (b. 1835). London surgeon.

Heath's operation. Division of the ramus of the mandible through the mouth, for relief of ankylosis of the jaw.

Heatley, N. G. Oxford biochemist.

Heatley cups. Small glass or porcelain cylinders which, when placed on the surface of inoculated culture plates, are filled with solutions of antibacterial drugs. The drugs diffuse out into the medium producing circular zones of inhibition of growth. The diameter of these zones can be used either as a measure of the concentration of drug in a given solution or, using standard drug solutions, as a measure of the drug sensitivity of a given organism.

hebeosteotomy (he·be·os·te·ot'·o·me). Pubiotomy. [Gk *hebe* pubes, osteotomy.]

hebephrenia (he·be·fre·ne·ah). One of the 3 main forms of Kraepelin's classical description of the syndrome of dementia praecox, the other 2 being paranoid and catatonic schizophrenia, schizophrenia simplex being sometimes added as a fourth type. The main features of hebephrenia are: early onset, a florid symptomatology in which hallucinations, bizarre and unorganized delusions, and thought disorder are prominent, and a rapid deterioration of personality. [Gk *hebe* puberty, *phren* mind.]

hebephreniac (he·be·fre·ne·ak). An individual suffering from hebephrenia.

hebephrenic (he·be·fren·ik). 1. Relating or belonging to hebephrenia. 2. Suffering from hebephrenia. 3. A hebephreniac.

Heberden, William (b. 1710). London physician.

Heberden's arthritis or rheumatism. Degenerative joint disease of the terminal joints of the fingers, producing bony nodular enlargements (Heberden's nodes) and often pain. It is most common in women and in the elderly, and heredity is an important factor in its aetiology.

Heberden's disease. 1. Angina pectoris. 2. Heberden's arthritis.

Heberden's nodes, Heberden-Rosenbach nodes. Swellings of the terminal interphalangeal joints of the hands due to osteoarthrosis. These are tender in the acute stage.

hebetic (he·bet·ik). Referring or belonging to puberty or the period of adolescence; happening at the onset of or during puberty or adolescence. [Gk *hebe* puberty.]

hebetude (heb·e·tewd). 1. Stupidity or dullness. 2. The condition of lethargy and impairment of the special senses which accompanies acute fever. [L *hebeo* to be dull.]

hebetudinous (heb·e·tewd·in·us). Affected with dullness or hebetude.

heboid (he·boid). Term applied to those forms of insanity, generally schizophrenia, which appear at adolescence. [Gk *hebe* puberty, *eidos* form.]

heboid-paranoid (he·boid·par·an·oid). General term applied to such mental disorders as adolescent insanity, schizophrenia and paranoia. [heboid paranoia, Gk *eidos* form.]

hebosteotomy, hebotomy (he·bos·te·ot'·o·me, he·bot·o·me). Pubiotomy. [Gk *hebe* pubes, osteotomy, Gk *temnein* to cut.]

Hebra, Ferdinand von (b. 1816). Vienna dermatologist.

Hebra's disease or erythema. Erythema multiforme.

Hebra's eczema marginatum. Hebra gave this name (not recognizing the cause of malady) to "a peculiar form of eczema, distinguished from all others by its constant localization on the inner surface of the thighs, the pubes and the buttocks; by its centrifugal progress and simultaneous involution at the centre; by its well-defined raised border, and by its exclusive occurrence in the male sex, especially in shoemakers". It is usually due to *Epidermophyton cruris*, but can occasionally be caused by species of *Trichophyton*, and rarely by *Microsporium canis*.

Hebra nose. The nose in the nodular stage of rhinoscleroma. It has been likened to that of a rhinoceros, hippopotamus or tapir.

Hebra's ointment. Unguentum plumbi oleatis.

Hebra's pityriasis, Hebra-Jadassohn disease. Pityriasis rubra.

Hebra's prurigo. A generalized prurigo, commencing in infancy and often persisting throughout adult life. During the first year of life the malady commences as an urticarial rash, but soon the typical papules appear. Itching is severe, and secondary lesions such as excoriations, pustules, boils and abscesses may be noted. The skin becomes pigmented and thickened. In some cases the symptoms are severe (prurigo ferox), in others they are less troublesome (prurigo mitis).

hecateromeral, hecateromeric (**hek**·at·er·**om**'·er·al, **hek**·at·er·o·**mer**'·rik). Term applied to neurones of the spinal cord which send a process down each side of the cord. [Gk *hekateros* each of two, *meros* part.]

Hecht, Adolf Franz (b. 1876). Vienna paediatrician.

Hecht phenomenon. Rumpel-Leede phenomenon.

hectic (**hek**·tik). In active tuberculosis, term applied to the daily or afternoon rise of temperature, with flushing of the cheeks; also applied to pyrexia accompanying septicaemia. [Gk *hexis* habit of body.]

hectogram (**hek**·to·gram). A weight equalling 100 g. [Gk *hekaton* hundred, gram.]

hectolitre (**hek**·to·le·ter). A measure of capacity equalling 100 litres. [Gk *hekaton* hundred, litre.]

hectometre (**hek**·to·me·ter). A linear measure equalling 0.1 km or 100 m. [Gk *hekaton* hundred, metre.]

Hectopsyllidae (hek·to·**sil**·id·e). A family of the insectan order Siphonaptera. The genus *Tunga* is of medical interest. [Gk *hekaton* hundred, *psylla* flea, *eidos* form.]

Hedaquinium Chloride (hed·ah·**kwin**·e·um **klor**·ide). BP Commission approved name for hexadecamethylenebis-(2-isoquinolinium chloride), an antibacterial substance with a wide range of activity effective in local applications on the skin.

Hedeoma (hed·e·o·mah). A genus of American herbs (family Labiatae). *Hedeoma pulegioides* Pers. (American pennyroyal) yields an oil similar in composition and properties to oil of pennyroyal. [Gk *hedys* sweet, *aroma* odour.]

hederagenin (hed·er·**aj**·en·in). $C_{31}H_{50}O_4$, a non-sterol saponin derived from the common ivy, *Hedera helix*. It is related to sapotalene and is haemolytic. [L *hedera* ivy, Gk *genein* to produce.]

hederiform (**hed**·er·e·form). Resembling ivy in shape. [L *hedera* ivy, form.]

hederin (**hed**·er·in). $C_{41}H_{64}O_{11}$, a glycoside derived from species of ivy, *Hedera*.

hedonal (**hed**·on·al). Methylpropylcarbinol urethane, $C_3H_7CH(CH_3)OCONH_2$. A simple ureide used as a hypnotic in insomnia. [Gk *hedone* pleasure.]

hedonia (he·**do**·ne·ah). A state of abnormal good spirits and pleasantness. [Gk *hedone* pleasure.]

hedonic (he·**don**·ik). 1. Referring to hedonics. 2. Belonging to hedonism or the states of consciousness implicit in it. 3. Relating to adherents of hedonism.

hedonics (he·**don**·ix). In psychological medicine, the science which is concerned with painful and pleasurable states of consciousness and feeling, and their relation to the physical life of an organism. [Gk *hedone* pleasure.]

hedonism (**he**·don·izm). 1. In psychological medicine, the pursuit of a whim or a hobby to the exclusion of all else, irrespective of moral or ethical considerations. 2. Any doctrine that regards the greatest happiness of an individual or a community as the chief good in life. [see prec.]

hedratresia (hed·rah·**tre**·ze·ah). Imperforate anus. [Gk *hedra* anus, atresia.]

hedrocele (**hed**·ro·seel). 1. Prolapse of the anus or of a part of the intestine through the anus. 2. Hernia through the greater or lesser sciatic notches. [Gk *hedra* anus, *kele* hernia.]

hedrosyrinx (hed·ro·**sir**·ingx). Anal fistula. *See* FISTULA. [Gk *hedra* anus, *syrigx* pipe.]

heel [calx (NA)] (heel). The protuberance at the back of the foot. **Big heel.** Hypertrophy of the heel bone (calcaneum), probably due to yaws. **Black heel.** Dark-blue specks in the horny layer of the skin of the heels due to extravasated blood in the papillary layer of the dermis as a result of shearing stress from footwear. **Cracked heel.** Keratoderma plantare sulcata. **Gonorrhoeal heel.** Inflammation of the plantar fascia due to gonorrhoea. **Prominent heel.** Enlarged heel due to periostitis of the tuberosity of the calcaneum. **Soldier's heel.** Achilles bursitis. [AS *hela*.]

Heerfordt, Christian Frederick (b. 1871). Copenhagen ophthalmologist.

Heerfordt's disease. Uveoparotid fever. *See* FEVER.

Hefke, Hans W. (b. 1897). Milwaukee radiologist.

Hefke-Turner sign. Shenton's line.

Hegar, Alfred (b. 1830). Freiburg gynaecologist.

Hegar's dilators. A graduated series of metal sounds used to dilate the cervix.

Hegar's sign. A sign elicited on vaginal examination in the early weeks of pregnancy when the lower segment of the uterus is empty and soft thus making the fundus of the uterus seem isolated from the cervix.

Heidbrink, J. A. American anaesthetist.

Heidbrink apparatus. An American machine which gives accurate mixtures of anaesthetic gases.

Heidenhain, Rudolph Peter Heinrich (b. 1834). Breslau physiologist.

Heidenhain's cell. One of the pepsin- or acid-secreting cells of the gastric mucosa.

Heidenhain's crescent or demilune. A serous cell or collection of serous cells, at the periphery of an alveolus of mucous cells from a salivary gland.

Heidenhain's fluid. An important general histological fixative containing mercuric chloride, sodium chloride, trichloroacetic acid, acetic acid and formaldehyde.

Heidenhain's law. The process of secretion involves changes in the structures of the secreting cells.

Heidenhain's rods or striae. Columnar cells of the renal tubules.

Heidenhain's stain. An iron haematoxylin stain used for protozoa.

Ehrlich-Biondi-Heidenhain triple stain. A mixture of acid fuchsine, orange G and methyl green, used as a general connective-tissue stain.

Vulpian-Heidenhain-Sherrington phenomenon. Sherrington phenomenon; following motor denervation by section of the ventral roots of the sciatic nerve, and after allowing time for degeneration, stimulation of the sciatic nerve causes a slow contraction of the muscles. This is thought to be due to diffusion of acetylcholine from the endings of undegenerated vasodilator nerve fibres running in the sciatic-nerve trunk.

height (hite). A measurement, from the top of the head to the floor, of a person or structure. **Alveolonasal height.** The craniometric height from the nasion (the midpoint of the depression where the nasal bones join the frontal) above to the prosthion (the lowest point on the alveolus between the upper central incisors). **Auriculobregmatic height.** The craniometric height from the bregma (the junction of the coronal and sagittal sutures) above to the midpoint of an imaginary line joining the upper borders of the external auditory meatus below. **Basibregmatic height.** The craniometric height from the bregma (the junction of the coronal and sagittal sutures) above to the basion (the midpoint on the anterior border of the foramen magnum). **Gnathion-nasion height.** The craniometric height from the nasion (the midpoint of the depression where the nasal bones join the frontal) above to the gnathion (the lowest point in the midline on the lower margin of the mandible). **Orbital height.** In craniometry, the maximum measurement in a vertical direction of the external orbital opening. **Sitting suprasternal height.** An anthropometric measurement, from the surface on which the subject is sitting to the top of the manubrium sterni. **Sitting vertex height.** An anthropometric measurement, from the surface on which the subject is sitting to the top of the head. [AS *hiehtho.*]

Heim, Ernst Ludwig (b. 1747). Berlin physician.

Heim-Kreysig sign. Recession of intercostal space during ventricular systole in adherent pericarditis.

Heiman, Henry (b. 1865). New York physician.

Heiman's agar. *See* AGAR, SERUM.

Heine, Jacob von (b. 1800). Stuttgart orthopaedic surgeon.

von Heine's infantile paralysis, Heine-Medin disease. Acute anterior poliomyelitis. *See* POLIOMYELITIS.

Heine, Leopold (b. 1870). Kiel ophthalmologist.

Heine's operation, for glaucoma. Cyclodialysis; separation of the ciliary body from the sclera with a spatula. Heine was the first to describe the operation, in 1906.

Heineke, Walther Hermann (b. 1834). Erlangen surgeon.

Heineke-Mikulicz operation. Pyloroplasty; a longitudinal incision is made at the pylorus and sewn transversely.

Heinz, Robert (b. 1865). Erlangen pharmacologist.

Heinz bodies or inclusion bodies, Heinz-Ehrlich bodies. Round refractile eosinophilic particles seen in mature red blood corpuscles usually in haemolytic anaemia, but not in reticulocytes; these are produced both *in vivo* and *in vitro* by the action of substances, like phenylhydrazine, that are able to transform haemoglobin into verdoglobin. They are said to be denatured globin united with a green haem (verdoglobin) and fixed to the stroma or surface membrane by a layer of altered lipoid and stromal protein.

Heiser, Victor George (b. 1873). New York physician.

Heiser treatment. A routine for the treatment of leprosy with chaulmoogra oil; now obsolete.

Heister, Lorenz (b. 1683). Helmstadt anatomist and surgeon.

Heister's diverticulum. The sinus of the external jugular vein.

Heister's fold or valve. The spiral valve of the cystic (gall bladder) duct. *See* VALVE.

helcodermatosis (**hel**·ko·der·mat·**o**′·sis). Ulceration associated with a dermatosis. [Gk *helkos* ulcer, dermatosis.]

helcoid (**hel**·koid). Ulcerous; like an ulcer in appearance. [Gk *helkos* ulcer, *eidos* form.]

helcology (hel·**kol**·o·je). That branch of medical science which is concerned with ulcers, their cause, prevention and treatment. [Gk *helkos* ulcer, *logos* science.]

helcoma (hel·**ko**·mah). A corneal ulcer. [Gk *helkos* ulcer, *-oma* tumour.]

helcoplasty (**hel**·ko·plas·te). Plastic repair of lesions formed by ulcers. The grafting of skin on an ulcer for the purpose of aiding healing. [Gk *helkos* ulcer, *plassein* to mould.]

helcosis (hel·**ko**·sis). Ulceration. [Gk *helkos* ulcer.]

helcotic (hel·**kot**·ik). 1. Having the character of ulceration. 2. Ulcerative. [see prec.]

Held, Hans (b. 1866). Leipzig anatomist and neurologist.

Held's bundle. The tectospinal tract. *See* TRACT.

Held's decussation. Decussation of fibres arising in the cochlear nuclei and passing to the lateral lemniscus in the trapezoid body.

Held's method. For so-called neurosomes in nerve cells; sections are fixed, stained in warm erythrosin, and then in Nissl's methylene blue containing acetone, and finally differentiated in a very dilute solution of alum.

Held's ground net. A theoretical terminal reticulum of the nervous system.

vis a tergo of Held. The force proposed by Held to account for the peripheral growth of the nerve axoplasm.

helenin (**hel**·en·in). Alant camphor; a terpene derivative obtained from the oil of elecampane, used as an antiseptic and expectorant in whooping-cough and bronchitis. [Gk *helenion* elecampane.]

helianthine (he·le·**an**·theen). Dimethylamino-azobenzene-*p*-sulphonic acid, $(CH_3)_2NC_6H_4N{=}NC_6H_4SO_2OH$. An orange dye, the sodium salt of which is known as *methyl orange* and is used in volumetric analysis as an indicator (pH 3.0 to 4.4). [Gk *helios* sun, *anthos* flower.]

heliation (he·le·**a**·shun). Heliotherapy.

heliciform (hel·**is**·e·form). Spiral, like the shell of a snail. [helix, form.]

helicin (**hel**·is·in). Salicylaldehyde glucoside, $C_{13}H_{16}O_7$. A compound prepared by the oxidation of salicin.

helicine (**hel**·is·een). 1. Heliciform. 2. Belonging to the helix of the ear.

helicine arteries [arteriae helicinae (NA)]. Arterial branches which enter the corpora cavernosa of the penis and which, in the flaccid condition of the organ, have a coiled or convoluted course.

helicis major muscle [musculus helicis major (NA)] (**hel**·is·is **ma**·jor). An intrinsic muscle of the auricle on the lateral surface, running up the ascending part of the helix from the spine.

helicis minor muscle [musculus helicis minor (NA)] (**hel**·is·is **mi**·nor). An intrinsic muscle of the auricle on the lateral surface, covering the crus of the helix.

helicoid (**hel**·ik·oid). 1. Resembling a helix. 2. Like a coil or spiral in appearance. [Gk *helix* coil, *eidos* form.]

helicopod (**hel**·ik·o·pod). Term for a peculiar gait in individuals with certain forms of hysteria or paralysis in which one or both feet are swung in a half-circle. [Gk *helix* coil, *pous* foot.]

helicopodia (**hel**·ik·o·**po**′·de·ah). The condition in which the feet are dragged and swung in a half-circle during walking. [see prec.]

helicotrema [NA] (**hel**·ik·o·**tre**′·mah). A cavity in the upper turn of the cochlea, where the scala tympani and the scala vestibuli meet. [Gk *helix* coil, *trema* hole.]

See also: BRESCHET.

helide (**he**·lide). A compound of helium with a metal, the existence of which has been reported but not confirmed.

Helie, Louis Theodore (b. 1804). Paris gynaecologist and anatomist.

Helie's bundle of fibres. A bundle of longitudinally running, median placed, muscle fibres found in the uterus.

helio-aerotherapy (**he**·le·o·a·er·o·**ther**′·ap·e). Heliotherapy combined with fresh-air treatment. [Gk *helios* sun, *aer* air, therapy.]

heliomyelitis (**he**·le·o·mi·el·**i**′·tis). Myelitis resulting from exposure to the hot rays of the sun. A very doubtful entity. [Gk *helios* sun, myelitis.]

helion (**he**·le·on). A name proposed for helium to emphasize its relationship with the other inert gases. [Gk *helios* sun.]

helionosus (**he**·le·o·**no**′·sus). Heat stroke; so-called sunstroke. [Gk *helios* sun, *nosos* disease.]

heliopathia (**he**·le·o·**path**′·e·ah). Any physical disorder or disturbance caused by exposure to the hot rays of the sun. [Gk *helios* sun, *pathos* disease.]

heliophobe (**he**·le·o·fobe). One morbidly sensitive to sunlight or one who takes excessive care to avoid it. [see foll.]

heliophobia (**he**·le·o·**fo**′·be·ah). Morbid fear and avoidance of the rays of the sun. [Gk *helios* sun, phobia.]

heliosensitivity (**he**·le·o·sen·sit·**iv**′·it·e). Sensitivity to the sun's rays. [Gk *helios* sun, sensitivity.]

heliosis (he·le·**o**·sis). 1. Heat stroke; so-called sunstroke. 2. Heliotherapy. [Gk *helios* sun.]

heliostat (**he**·le·o·stat). An instrument consisting of a mirror mounted on an axis rotated by clockwork so that a ray of the sun is continuously reflected to one spot throughout the day. [Gk *helios* sun, *stasis* a standing still.]

heliotaxis (he·le·o·**tax'**·is). 1. A form of reaction on the part of living organisms, e.g. cells or micro-organisms, which causes them either to seek sunlight (positive heliotaxis) or to shun it (negative heliotaxis). 2. Heliotropism. [Gk *helios* sun, *taxis* arrangement.]

heliotherapy (he·le·o·**ther'**·ap·e). Sunbathing as a therapeutic measure. [Gk *helios* sun, therapy.]

heliotrope B (**he**·le·o·trope be). Amethyst violet, 3,7-diethyldiamino-5-phenylphenazonium chloride, $(C_2H_5)_2NC_6H_3{=}N_2(C_6H_5)Cl{=}C_6H_3N(C_2H_5)_2$. A basic safranine dye occasionally used in histology. [see foll.]

heliotropic (he·le·o·**trop'**·ik). 1. Referring to heliotropism. 2. Relating or belonging to the effect which sunlight has on protoplasm in regard to movement of the latter. [Gk *helios* sun, *trope* a turning.]

heliotropin (he·le·o·**tro'**·pin). Piperonal, methylene-protocatechuic aldehyde, $CH_2O_2{=}C_6H_3CHO$. A white crystalline solid prepared by the oxidation of safrol, the chief constituent of oil of sassafras, and used in perfumery. [see prec.]

heliotropism, heliotropy (he·le·**ot**·ro·pizm, he·le·**ot**·ro·pe). 1. The tendency of living organisms to turn towards or seek the sunlight. 2. In plant physiology, the effect exerted by sunlight on the movements of growth, as exemplified by curves in the stem of a plant. [Gk *helios* sun, *trope* a turning.]

helium (**he**·le·um). An element of the inert gas series, with atomic weight 4.003, atomic number 2 and chemical symbol He. It occurs in the natural gases of mineral springs in Canada and the USA, in occluded form in certain minerals (e.g. cleveite) and as a constituent of the atmosphere (1 part in 200 000); it is also the product of radioactive changes, being emitted in the nature of alpha particles. It is an extremely light colourless gas, inert in the body, less soluble in the blood than nitrogen and more diffusible. A mixture of 80 per cent helium and 20 per cent oxygen is more easily breathed than air or oxygen alone, and is used in obstructional types of dyspnoea such as status asthmaticus and bronchiectasis, when it is administered through a tight-fitting mask (BP 1973). The gas is also valuable for decompressing divers, reducing the incidence of bends. [Gk *helios* sun.]

helix [NA] (**he**·lix). 1. The prominent incurved rim of the auricle of the ear. 2. The coil of wire in an electromagnet. 3. The nucleocapsid of viruses with helical symmetry as seen in the electron microscope. **Alpha helix.** The coiled conformation of a polypeptide which is maintained by hydrogen bonding between the CO and NH groups of the peptide bonds of adjacent coils; in natural polypeptides the helix is right-handed. [Gk *helix* coil.]

Helkesimastix (hel·kes·e·**mas'**·tix). A genus of Mastigophora; *Helkesimastix faecicola* has been recorded from stale faeces. [Gk *helkein* to drag, *mastix* whip.]

hellebore (**hel**·e·bor). White hellebore, which consists of the rhizome and roots of a European herb *Veratrum album* Linn. (family Liliaceae). It contains jervine, veratrine and other alkaloids having a powerful depressant action on the heart and nervous system. **American hellebore.** Green hellebore (see below). **Black hellebore.** The rhizome and root of the Christmas rose, *Helleborus niger* Linn. (family Ranunculaceae). It has strong sternutatory properties and has been employed as a cathartic and emmenagogue. **False hellebore.** The name given to *Adonis vernalis* Linn. (family Ranunculaceae), a herb containing cardiac glycosides, which has been used as an alternative to digitalis. **Green Hellebore BPC 1954.** Green hellebore rhizome; the rhizome and roots of a plant similar to white hellebore, *Veratrum viride* Ait., indigenous to North America, and having constituents and properties similar to those of white hellebore. [Gk *helleboros.*]

helleborein (hel·e·**bor**·e·in). $C_{37}H_{56}O_{18}$, a saponin obtained from the black hellebore, *Helleborus niger* Linn.

helleborin (hel·e·**bor**·in). $C_{36}H_{42}O_6$, a glucoside found in the rhizome of black hellebore, *Helleborus niger* Linn. It is toxic with violent purgative action.

helleborism (**hel**·e·bor·izm). 1. Poisoning due to hellebore. 2. The therapeutic use of hellebore.

Hellenopolypus (hel·en·o·**pol'**·e·pus). A genus of contact-poisonous sea anemones.

Heller, Arnold Ludwig Gotthelf (b. 1840). Kiel pathologist.

Heller's method, for myelin sheaths. Fix in Mueller's fluid, embed in celloidin, place in 1 per cent osmic acid and reduce with alkaline pyrogallic acid. Differentiation is in potassium permanganate followed by oxalic acid.

Heller–Doehle aortitis or disease. Syphilitic aortitis. *See* AORTITIS.

Heller, Ernst (b. 1877). Leipzig surgeon.

Heller's operation. Longitudinal division of the muscle of the lower oesophagus for cardiospasm.

Heller, Johann Florenz (b. 1813). Vienna physician.

Heller bath. A form of hydro-electric bath.

Heller's plexus. A network of arteries found in the submucosa of the intestine.

Heller's test, for protein in urine. Urine is layered upon concentrated nitric acid in a test-tube. A white ring of precipitated protein forms at the junction of the liquids. Some care in interpretation of this test is required, as uric acid and urates may give a similar ring if the urine is concentrated, as also do some excretory products following administration of certain drugs.

Hellicella (hel·e·**sel**·ah). A genus of land snails, some of which are intermediate hosts of certain trematode worms that rarely infect man.

Hellin, Dyonizy (b. 1867). Warsaw pathologist.

Hellin's law. Twins occur in 1 in 80 pregnancies, triplets in 80^2 and quadruplets in 80^3 pregnancies.

Helly, Konrad (b. 1875). Swiss pathologist.

Helly's fixing fluid. A solution of potassium bichromate, mercuric chloride and formalin; used for preserving bone marrow.

Helmholtz, Hermann Ludwig Ferdinand von (b. 1821). Berlin physicist and physiologist.

Helmholtz' law. When the fixation lines of the eyes are parallel, the torsion of each eye is a function only of the angle of elevation and the angle of azimuth.

Helmholtz' ligaments. 1. *Anterior:* a band of fibres which forms part of the anterior ligament of the malleus, and which extends from the anterior aspect of the malleus to the greater tympanic spine. 2. *Posterior:* the posterior part of the lateral ligament of the malleus.

wheel rotation of Helmholtz. The rotation of the eyeball around the fixation axis; rolling; torsion.

eye speculum of Helmholtz. The instrument consisting of a number of glass slides held in a simple tube, with which Helmholtz first saw the fundus of the eye. It was therefore the first ophthalmoscope.

Helmholtz' theory. 1. As originally put forward, this suggested that the suspensory ligament of the lens was normally in a state of tension; on accommodation the ciliary muscle contracted, which relaxed the suspensory ligament and allowed the lens to become more globular by its own inherent elasticity. This has recently been modified by Fincham, in that the lens substance is mouldable, and that the capsule is elastic and differs in thickness, the thinnest parts being at the 2 poles and at the equator. On relaxation of the suspensory ligament the central part of the lens becomes more globular than the rest owing to the uneven pressure exerted by the elastic capsule on the mouldable lens. 2. Of peripheral analysis: it is implied that the cochlea acts like a resonator, the individual fibres of the basilar membrane reacting to fixed pitches, the long fibres of the basilar membrane responding to low-pitched vibration, whilst the shorter fibres react to high tones; sometimes called the *resonance theory.*

Young–Helmholtz theory. A trichromatic theory of colour vision: all colours can be reduced to the 3 primary colours, red, green and violet. Young originally suggested that there were 3 different types of cone in the retina, each reacting only to 1 of these 3 colours. Helmholtz thought the unit should be smaller and suggested that each cone would react differently to each of the 3 primary colours. Other colours would be perceived by the mixture of these 3 basic reactions, e.g. white.

helminth (hel·minth). The general term for worms of the phyla Platyhelminthes, Nematoda and Acanthocephala, especially parasites. [Gk *helmins* worm.]

helminthemesis (hel·min·them·es·is). The vomiting of intestinal worms. [helminth, emesis.]

helminthiasis (hel·min·thi·as·is). The presence of parasitic worms in some parts of the body. **Cutaneous helminthiasis.** A worm infection of the skin, e.g. larva migrans. **Helminthiasis elastica.** The condition in which the presence of parasitic worms causes elastic tumours to form in the axillae and groin. **Helminthiasis wuchereri.** A name proposed for all forms of filariasis; not generally accepted. [helminth.]

helminthic (hel·min·thik). 1. Pertaining to worms. 2. Anthelminthic. [helminth.]

helminthicide (hel·min·this·ide). Vermicide. [helminth, L *caedere* to kill.]

helminthism (hel·min·thizm). The presence of parasitic worms in the intestines. [helminth.]

helminthoid (hel·min·thoid). 1. Wormlike. 2. Like an intestinal worm. [helminth, Gk *eidos* form.]

helminthology (hel·min·thol·o·je). That branch of medical science which is concerned with parasitic worms. [helminth, Gk *logos* science.]

helminthoma (hel·min·tho·mah). A tumour due to the presence of a parasitic worm. [helminth, Gk *-oma* tumour.]

helminthophobia (hel·min·tho·fo'·be·ah). An obsession in which the patient believes that he is infested with intestinal parasitic worms; unreasoning dread of being so infested. [helminth, phobia.]

helminthous (hel·min·thus). 1. Indicating infestation with intestinal worms; wormy. 2. Belonging to worms. [helminth.]

Helmont, Jean Baptiste van (b. 1577). Brussels chemist and physician.

Helmont's mirror or speculum. The central tendon of the diaphragm.

Heloderma (he·lo·der·mah). A genus of lizards of western USA and Mexico. The 2 species *Heloderma horridum*, the Gila monster, and *H. suspectum*, are the only lizards in the world with a poisonous bite. [Gk *helos* nail, *derma* skin.]

helodermatous (he·lo·der·mat·us). In biology, a term indicating that the skin shows numerous warts, nodules or tubercles. [see prec.]

helodes (he·lo·deez). 1. Malaria. 2. Indicating a fever in which there is profuse sweating. 3. Boggy or swampy. [Gk *helos* swamp.]

heloma (he·lo·mah). A circumscribed thickening and hardening of the skin of the hand or foot; a corn or callosity. [Gk *helos* nail, *-oma* tumour.]

helonias (he·lo·ne·as). Blazing star, false unicorn, starwort, devil's bit, fairy wand; the dried rhizome and roots of *Chamaelirium luteum* (family Liliaceae). Its main constituent is a saponin; it was supposed to have a tonic action on the uterus and was used in amenorrhoea and dysmenorrhoea. It has also been employed as an anthelmintic, though its medicinal value is doubtful. [Gk *helos* swamp.]

helophilous (he·lof·il·us). Living in marshes or bogs, as do some malaria mosquitoes. [Gk *helos* swamp, *philein* to love.]

Helophilus (he·lof·il·us). A genus of hover flies. The larvae of some species, normally aquatic, have been recorded in accidental intestinal and cutaneous myiasis. [Gk *helos* swamp, *philein* to love.]

helopyra (he·lo·pi·rah). Malaria. [Gk *helos* swamp, *pyr* fire.]

helosis (he·lo·sis). The condition of having callosities or corns. [Gk *helos* nail, *-osis* condition.]

helotic (he·lot·ik). 1. Having relation to or belonging to corns. 2. Any agent that produces a blister; a vesicant. [see prec.]

helotomeia (he·lo·to·mi'·ah). The surgical treatment of corns; helotomy. [see foll.]

helotomon (he·lot·om·on). A name for a surgical knife used in the cutting or other treatment of corns. [Gk *helos* nail, *temnein* to cut.]

helotomy (he·lot·o·me). The surgical treatment of corns or callosities. [see prec.]

Helvetius, Johannis Claudius Adrian (b. 1685). Paris philosopher and anatomist.

Helvetius' ligaments. Anterior and posterior thickenings of longitudinal muscle wall of the pyloric antrum.

Helweg, Hans Kristian Saxtorph (b. 1847). Vedingborg, Denmark, psychiatrist.

bundle of Helweg, Helweg's triangular tract. The olivospinal tract. *See* TRACT.

hemanthine (he·man·theen). An alkaloid, or perhaps mixture of alkaloids, derived from the bulb of *Haemanthus toxicarius* (*Buphane disticha*), resembling hyoscine in mydriatic and hypnotic properties.

hembra (hem·brah). An ulcerative form of dermal leishmaniasis.

hemeralope (hem·er·al·ope). An individual who suffers from hemeralopia.

hemeralopia (hem·er·al·o'·pe·ah). Day blindness; in practice applied to cases when vision is better in reduced light. The term is sometimes incorrectly used for night blindness. [Gk *hemera* day, *alaos* blind, *ops* eye.]

hemeraphonia (hem·er·ah·fo'·ne·ah). Loss of voice during the hours of daylight only. [Gk *hemera* day, *a*, *phone* voice.]

hemeropathia (hem·er·o·path'·e·ah). 1. Any disease which shows an increase in severity during the day. 2. Any disease lasting only 1 day. [Gk *hemera* day, *pathos* disease.]

hemiablepsia (hem·e·a·blep'·se·ah). Hemianopia. [Gk *hemi* half, ablepsia.]

hemiacardiacus (hem·e·a·kar·di'·ak·us). One fetus of a twin monster in which the circulation is derived partly from its own heart and partly from the heart of its twin. [Gk *hemi* half, acardius.]

hemiacephalus (hem·e·a·kef'·al·us). A monster with a rudimentary head. [Gk *hemi* half, *a*, *kephale* head.]

hemiachromatopsia (hem·e·a·kro·mat·op'·se·ah). 1. Loss or absence of colour perception in one half of the field of vision. 2. Loss or absence of colour perception in corresponding halves of the field of both eyes. [Gk *hemi* half, achromatopsia.]

hemiageusia, hemiageustia (hem·e·a·gew'·se·ah, hem·e·a·gew'·ste·ah). Loss, absence or diminution of the sense of taste in one lateral half of the tongue. [Gk *hemi* half, ageusia.]

hemialbumose (hem·e·al·bew'·moze). An intermediate in protein digestion. It is found in bone marrow and occurs in the urine of patients with osteomalacia. [Gk *hemi* half, albumose.]

hemialbumosuria (hem·e·al·bew·mo·sewr'·e·ah). A condition in which hemialbumose is present in the urine.

hemialgia (hem·e·al·je·ah). Neuralgic pain affecting the right or the left side of the body or the right or left side of any part of the body, particularly the head. [Gk *hemi* half, *algos* pain.]

hemiamaurosis (hem·e·am·aw·ro'·sis). Hemianopia with associated amblyopia in the other half of the visual field. [Gk *hemi* half, amaurosis.]

hemiamblyopia (hem·e·am·ble·o'·pe·ah). Hemianopia. [Gk *hemi* half, amblyopia.]

hemiamyasthenia (hem·e·a·mi·as·the'·ne·ah). Absence or loss of power in the muscles of one side of the body. [Gk *hemi* half, amyasthenia.]

hemianacousia, hemianacusia, hemianacusis (hem·e·an·ak·oos'·e·ah, hem·e·an·ak·ews'·e·ah, hem·e·an·ak·ew'·sis). Deafness affecting only one ear. [Gk *hemi* half, anacousia.]

hemianaesthesia (hem·e·an·es·the'·ze·ah). Loss of sensation of either lateral half of the body. **Alternate hemianaesthesia.** Loss of sensation of one side of the head and of the opposite side of the body. **Cerebral hemianaesthesia.** That due to a lesion of the internal capsule. **Crossed hemianaesthesia.** Alternate hemianaesthesia (see above). **Hysterical hemianaesthesia.** Loss of sensation without organic basis, of one lateral half of the body. **Mesencephalic hemianaesthesia, Pontine hemianaesthesia.** That associated with lesions of the brain stem and which may show crossed hemiplegia also. **Spinal hemianaesthesia.** Loss of sensation due to a local lesion in the spinal cord. [Gk *hemi* half, anaesthesia.]

hemianalgesia (hem·e·an·al·je′·ze·ah). Lack of feeling, or insensibility to pain, affecting the whole of one lateral half of the body. [Gk *hemi* half, analgesia.]

hemianasarca (hem·e·an·ah·sar′·kah). A condition of oedema affecting one lateral half of the body. [Gk *hemi* half, anasarca.]

hemianopia (hem·e·an·o′·pe·ah). Loss of half the vision in each eye; hemianopsia; hemiopia [obsolete term]. The word is also applied loosely to loss of vision in a half field in one eye only, and scotomata which occupy only a part of the half fields. **Absolute hemianopia.** Hemianopia with complete visual loss, i.e. no perception of light, in the affected area. **Altitudinal hemianopia.** That in which the upper or lower half of the field is lost in each eye. **Bilateral hemianopia.** Hemianopia affecting both eyes. **Binasal hemianopia.** That in which the nasal halves are lost. **Bitemporal hemianopia.** That in which the temporal halves are lost. **Complete hemianopia.** Hemianopia of the complete half of a visual field. **Congruous hemianopia.** In homonymous hemianopia (see below), when the areas of field loss are identical in size and shape on each side, and are superimposable. **Crossed hemianopia.** In bilateral quadrantic hemianopia when one quadrant is in the upper half and the other in the lower half of the visual field. **Heteronymous hemianopia.** A bilateral hemianopia affecting either the two nasal halves of the visual field or the two temporal halves. **Homonymous hemianopia.** That in which the loss is on the same side in each eye. **Horizontal hemianopia.** Altitudinal hemianopia (see above). **Incomplete hemianopia.** Hemianopia of only a part of the half of the visual field. **Incongruous hemianopia.** In homonymous hemianopia (see above), when the areas of field loss on each side are not identical in size and shape, and are not superimposable. **Lateral hemianopia.** Homonymous hemianopia (see above). **Nasal hemianopia.** Hemianopia affecting the nasal half of the visual field. **Partial hemianopia.** Incomplete hemianopia (see above). **Quadrantic hemianopia.** That in which the field loss occurs in a quadrant bounded by a vertical and horizontal radius. It can be either upper or lower, nasal or temporal. **Relative hemianopia.** 1. Hemianopia in which objects are sometimes perceived and sometimes not in the affected field, depending on the counter stimulus in the normal field. 2. Hemianopia in which there is only partial, not absolute, visual loss in the affected area. **Temporal hemianopia.** That affecting the temporal half of the visual field. **Unilateral hemianopia.** Hemianopia affecting only one eye. [Gk *hemi* half, *a*, *opsis* vision.]

hemianopic (hem·e·an·o·pik). 1. Relating or belonging to hemianopia. 2. Suffering from or affected with hemianopia.

hemianopsia (hem·e·an·op′·se·ah). Hemianopia.

hemianoptic (hem·e·an·op′·tik). Hemianopic.

hemianosmia (hem·e·an·oz′·me·ah). Absence or loss of the sense of smell in one nostril. [Gk *hemi* half, anosmia.]

hemiapraxia (hem·e·ap·rax′·e·ah). Apraxia, i.e. loss of muscular co-ordination affecting one side of the body. [Gk *hemi* half, apraxia.]

hemiarthrosis (hem·e·ar·thro′·sis). A false synchondrosis. [Gk *hemi* half, arthrosis.]

hemiasynergia (hem·e·a·sin·er′·je·ah). Hemiasynergy.

hemiasynergy (hem·e·a·sin·er′·je). Asynergy affecting one lateral half of the body. [Gk *hemi* half, asynergy.]

hemiataxia, hemiataxy (hem·e·at·ax′·e·ah, hem·e·at·ax′·e). Ataxia affecting one lateral half of the body. [Gk *hemi* half, ataxia.]

hemiathetosis (hem·e·ath·e·to′·sis). Athetosis affecting one hand, or a foot and a hand of the same side. [Gk *hemi* half, athetosis.]

hemiatonia, hemiatony (hem·e·a·to′·ne·ah, hem·e·at·on·e). Partial or complete muscular atony of one lateral half of the body. **Hemiatonia apoplectica.** Hemihypertonia postapoplectica. [Gk *hemi* half, atony.]

hemiatrophy (hem·e·at·ro·fe). Atrophy affecting one side only of the body, or one half of an organ or part, as the tongue or face. **Cranial hemiatrophy.** Abnormal smallness of one lateral cranial cavity, due to incomplete development of the contained cerebral hemisphere as a result of damage *in utero* or in early childhood. **Facial hemiatrophy.** Atrophy of nervous origin affecting one lateral half of the face; it may be progressive. **Progressive lingual hemiatrophy.** Atrophic paralysis affecting one lateral half of the tongue. [Gk *hemi* half, atrophy.]

hemiazygous (hem·e·az·ig·us, hem·e·az·i·gus). Partially paired. [Gk *hemi* half, azygous.]

hemiballism, hemiballismus (hem·e·bal·izm, hem·e·bal·iz′·mus). Violent flinging movements of the limbs on one side, usually due to infarct involving the subthalamic nucleus. [Gk *hemi* half, *ballismos* jumping.]

Hemibia (hem·e·bi·ah). A genus of snails; 2 species, *Hemibia hupensis* and *H. quadrasi,* act as intermediate hosts for *Schistosoma japonicum.* [Gk *hemi* half, *bios* life.]

hemibilirubin (hem·e·bil·e·roo′·bin). The former name for mesobilinogen, $C_{33}H_{44}N_4O_6$, a compound formed by the reduction of bilirubin.

hemiblock (hem·e·blok). In heart block, failure of conduction in one of the two main divisions of the left branches of the conducting bundle. **Left anterior hemiblock.** Failure of conduction in the anterior division of the left branch of the conducting bundle. **Left posterior hemiblock.** Failure of conduction in the posterior division of the left branch of the conducting bundle. [Gk *hemi* half, Fr. *bloc.*]

hemicanities (hem·e·kan·ish′·e·eez). Greying or whitening of the hair on one side of the head only. [Gk *hemi* half, canities.]

hemicardia (hem·e·kar·de·ah). Either lateral half of a 4-chambered heart. **Hemicardia dextra.** The right lateral half, i.e. the right atrium and right ventricle of the heart. **Hemicardia sinistra.** The left lateral half, i.e. the left atrium and left ventricle of the heart. [Gk *hemi* half, *kardia* heart.]

hemicellulose (hem·e·sel·ew·lose). A polysaccharide, e.g. galactan, composed of monosaccharide anhydride units. With pectin substances they are present in the primary cell walls of plants, within the cellulose framework, where they form a cellulose reserve; they also occur in seeds. They hydrolyse with dilute mineral acids into monosaccharides, thus differing from cellulose. [Gk *hemi* half, cellulose.]

hemicentrum (hem·e·sen·trum). Either lateral half of the body of a vertebra. [Gk *hemi* half, *kentron* spur.]

hemicephalia (hem·e·kef·a′·le·ah). 1. Congenital absence of one lateral half of the skull and head. 2. Migraine. [Gk *hemi* half, *kephale* head.]

hemicephalus (hem·e·kef·al·us). 1. A monster with only one cerebral hemisphere. 2. Hemiacephalus. [see prec.]

hemicephaly (hem·e·kef·al·e). Hemicephalia.

hemicerebrum (hem·e·ser·e·brum). Either one of the cerebral hemispheres. [Gk *hemi* half, cerebrum.]

hemichorea (hem·e·ko·re′·ah). Chorea with unilateral movements. [Gk *hemi* half, chorea.]

hemichromatopsia (hem·e·kro·mat·ops′·e·ah). Hemiachromatopsia.

hemichromosome (hem·e·kro·mo·some). Either one of the bodies formed by the longitudinal splitting of a chromosome. [Gk *hemi* half, chromosome.]

hemicolectomy (hem·e·ko·lek′·to·me). Surgical excision of a portion of the colon. [Gk *hemi* half, colon, *ektome* a cutting out.]

hemicrania (hem·e·kra·ne·ah). Hemicephalia. [Gk *hemi* half, *kranion* skull.]

hemicraniectomy (hem·e·kra·ne·ek′·to·me). Hemicraniotomy. [Gk *hemi* half, craniectomy.]

hemicraniosis (hem·e·kra·ne·o′·sis). An enlarged condition of one half of the head or face, due to hyperostosis of the bones on that side of the skull, and involving the cerebrum. [hemicrania, Gk *-osis* condition.]

hemicraniotomy (hem·e·kra·ne·ot′·o·me). Longitudinal section of the skull near the median line and reflection of part or all of the one half so that there is exposure of half of the brain. The procedure is a preliminary to operation on the brain. [Gk *hemi* half, craniotomy.]

hemidecortication (hem·e·de·kor·te·ka′·shun). Surgical removal of one half of the cerebral cortex. [Gk *hemi* half, decortication.]

Hemidesmus (hem·e·dez·mus). A genus of climbing shrubs (family Asclepiadaceae) indigenous to India and Sri Lanka; the root obtained from *Hemidesmus indicus* R. Br. is widely used in India as a substitute for sarsaparilla. [Gk *hemi* half, *desmos* bond.]

hemidiaphoresis (hem·e·di·ah·for·e′·sis). Sweating occurring on one lateral half of the body. [Gk *hemi* half, diaphoresis.]

hemidiaphragm (hem·e·di·ah·fram). Either half of the diaphragm. [Gk *hemi* half, diaphragm.]

hemidysaesthesia (hem·e·dis·es·the′·ze·ah). Unilateral dysaesthesia. [Gk *hemi* half, dysaesthesia.]

hemidysergia (hem·e·dis·er′·je·ah). The condition in which there is motor inco-ordination of nervous origin of one lateral half of the body. [Gk *hemi* half, dysergia.]

hemidystrophia, hemidystrophy (hem·e·dis·tro′·fe·ah, hem·e·dis′·tro·fe). 1. A condition in which the two sides of the body are not equal in development. 2. A state of imperfect nourishment or semi-starvation. [Gk *hemi* half, *dys, trophe* nutrition.]

hemiectromelia (hem·e·ek·tro·me′·le·ah). The condition of having defective or imperfect limbs on one side of the body. [Gk *hemi* half, ectromelia.]

hemiencephalon (hem·e·en·kef′·al·on). Either of the lateral halves of the brain. [Gk *hemi* half, *egkephalos* brain.]

hemiencephalus (hem·e·en·kef′·al·us). 1. A monster with one cerebral hemisphere. 2. A fetus the brain of which is nearly normal but lacks the organs of sense. [see prec.]

hemiepilepsy (hem·e·ep·il·ep′·se). Epilepsy in which the convulsions involve only one side of the body. [Gk *hemi* half, epilepsy.]

hemifacial (hem·e·fa·she·al, hem·e·fa·shal). Relating to or affecting one lateral half of the face. [Gk *hemi* half, face.]

hemifornix (hem·e·for·nix). Inclusive term for that portion of the floor of either of the lateral ventricles of the brain which is composed of the hippocampus, the anterior column of the fornix and the fimbria. [Gk *hemi* half, fornix.]

hemigastrectomy (hem·e·gas·trek′·to·me). 1. Surgical excision of half of the stomach. 2. Resection of the pyloric end of an hour-glass stomach. [Gk *hemi* half, gastrectomy.]

hemigeusia (hem·e·gew·se·ah). Hemiageusia.

hemiglossal (hem·e·glos·al). Hemilingual. [Gk *hemi* half, *glossa* tongue.]

hemiglossectomy (hem·e·glos·ek′·to·me). Resection of one lateral half of the tongue. [Gk *hemi* half, glossectomy.]

hemiglossitis (hem·e·glos·i′·tis). Unilateral inflammation of the tongue. [Gk *hemi* half, glossitis.]

hemignathia (hem·e·nath·e·ah). The state of having only one jaw. [Gk *hemi* half, *gnathos* jaw.]

hemihepatectomy (hem·e·hep·at·ek′·to·me). Formal operation for removal of half of the liver after preliminary control of the corresponding branches of the hepatic artery, hepatic vein and portal vein. [Gk *hemi* half, *hepar* liver, *ektome* a cutting out.]

hemihidrosis (hem·e·hid·ro′·sis). Sweating occurring on one lateral half of the body; hemidiaphoresis. [Gk *hemi* half, hidrosis.]

hemihypaesthesia (hem·e·hi·pes·the′·ze·ah). Hemihypo-aesthesia.

hemihypalgesia (hem·e·hi·pal·je′·ze·ah). Hemihypo-algesia.

hemihyperaesthesia (hem·e·hi·per·es·the′·ze·ah). The state of having acute cutaneous sensation or excessively developed sensitiveness to pain and touch in one lateral half of the body. [Gk *hemi* half, hyperaesthesia.]

hemihyperhidrosis, hemihyperidrosis (hem·e·hi·per·hid·ro′·sis, hem·e·hi·per·id·ro′·sis). Excessive secretion and excretion of sweat on one lateral half of the body. [Gk *hemi* half, hyperidrosis.]

hemihypermetria (hem·e·hi·per·met′·re·ah). Hypermetria affecting one half only of a part, such as the tongue. [Gk *hemi* half, hypermetria.]

hemihypertonia (hem·e·hi·per·to′·ne·ah). A state of exaggerated tension in the muscles of one lateral half of the body, causing tonic contraction. **Hemihypertonia postapoplectica.** Tonic spasm occurring from time to time in different groups of muscles of one lateral half of the body and without affecting their power. [Gk *hemi* half, hypertonia.]

hemihypertrophy (hem·e·hi·per·tro′·fe). Morbid enlargement or overgrowth of one half or one side of the body or of one half of a part. **Facial hemihypertrophy.** Hypertrophy of one lateral half of the face. [Gk *hemi* half, hypertrophy.]

hemihypo-aesthesia (hem·e·hi·po·es·the′·ze·ah). Blunting of sensation down one lateral half of the body. [Gk *hemi* half, hypo-aesthesia.]

hemihypo-algesia (hem·e·hi·po·al·je′·ze·ah). Diminished sensitiveness to pain in one lateral half of the body. [Gk *hemi* half, hypo-algesia.]

hemihypogeusia (hem·e·hi·po·gew′·se·ah). Hemiageusia. [Gk *hemi* half, hypogeusia.]

hemihypothermia (hem·e·hi·po·ther′·me·ah). Unilateral hypothermia, i.e. a state in which the temperature of one side of the body is lower than that of the other. [Gk *hemi* half, hypothermia.]

hemihypotonia (hem·e·hi·po·to′·ne·ah). Unilateral hypotonia. [Gk *hemi* half, hypotonia.]

hemikaryon (hem·e·kar·e·on). A cell nucleus with the haploid number of chromosomes (half the diploid number). [Gk *hemi* half, *karyon* nucleus.]

hemilabyrinthectomy (hem·e·lab·ir·in·thek′·to·me). A partial removal of the labyrinth. [Gk *hemi* half, labyrinthectomy.]

hemilaminectomy (hem·e·lam·in·ek′·to·me). Surgical removal of the lamina of the vertebral arch on one side. [Gk *hemi* half, laminectomy.]

hemilaryngectomy (hem·e·lar·in·jek′·to·me). Resection of one lateral half of the larynx. [Gk *hemi* half, laryngectomy.]

hemilateral (hem·e·lat·er·al). Relating or belonging to or affecting one lateral half. [Gk *hemi* half, lateral.]

hemilesion (hem·e·le·zhun). A lesion on one side of the body, e.g. a unilateral lesion of the spinal cord. [Gk *hemi* half, lesion.]

hemilingual (hem·e·ling·gwal). Relating or belonging to or affecting one lateral half of the tongue; hemiglossal. [Gk *hemi* half, L *lingua* tongue.]

hemimacroglossia (hem·e·mak·ro·glos′·e·ah). An enlarged condition of one lateral half of the tongue. [Gk *hemi* half, macroglossia.]

hemimandibulectomy (hem·e·man·dib·ewl·ek′·to·me). Surgical excision of half of the mandible. [Gk *hemi* half, mandible, Gk *ektome* a cutting out.]

hemimelia (hem·e·me·le·ah). 1. The condition of having defective limbs. 2. Hemimelus. [see foll.]

hemimelus (hem·e·me·lus). 1. A fetus with imperfect, defective or stunted limbs. 2. Any individual with incomplete or defective extremities. [Gk *hemi* half, *melos* limb.]

hemimetabolic (hem·e·met·ab·ol′·ik). Of insects, describing those forms in which the immature individuals are like the adults except for the full development of genitalia and, usually, wings, as in the Exopterygota which develop by moults, e.g. the cockroach. [Gk *hemi* half, *metabole* change.]

hemimetamorphosis (hem·e·met·ah·mor′·fo·sis). In biology, imperfect or incomplete transition from one stage to the next. [Gk *hemi* half, *metamorphosis* transformation.]

hemimyasthenia (hem·e·mi·as·the′·ne·ah). Muscular debility affecting one lateral half of the body. [Gk *hemi* half, myasthenia.]

hemimyoclonus (hem·e·mi·o·klo′·nus). Clonic muscular spasm affecting one lateral half of the body. [Gk *hemi* half, myoclonus.]

heminephrectomy (hem·e·nef·rek′·to·me). Surgical removal of a portion of a kidney. [Gk *hemi* half, nephrectomy.]

hemiobesity (hem·e·o·be′·sit·e). Excessive accumulation of fat on one side of the body. [Gk *hemi* half, obesity.]

hemiopalgia (hem·e·op·al′·je·ah). Pain in one side of the head and in the eye of that side. [Gk *hemi* half, *ops* eye, *algos* pain.]

hemiopia (hem·e·o·pe·ah). Hemianopia. [see foll.]

hemiopic (hem·e·o·pik). 1. Hemianoptic; relating or belonging to hemianopia. 2. Affecting one eye only. [Gk *hemi* half, *ops* eye.]

hemipagus (hem·**ip**·ag·us). A twin monster with fused navel and thorax. [Gk *hemi* half, *pagos* fixture.]

hemipara-anaesthesia (hem·e·**par**·ah·an·es·**the**'·ze·ah). 1. Anaesthesia of one foot. 2. Anaesthesia limited to the lower half of one side of the body. [Gk *hemi* half, para-anaesthesia.]

hemiparaesthesia (**hem**·e·par·es·**the**'·ze·ah). Unilateral paraesthesia, i.e. any abnormal or perverted sensation, such as numbness, experienced on one side of the body. [Gk *hemi* half, paraesthesia.]

hemiparalysis (**hem**·e·par·**al**'·is·is). Hemiplegia. [Gk *hemi* half, paralysis.]

hemiparaplegia (**hem**·e·par·ah·**ple**'·je·ah). Paraplegia affecting only one side of the body. [Gk *hemi* half, paraplegia.]

hemiparesis (**hem**·e·par·e'·sis, hem·e·**par**·es·is). Unilateral muscular paralysis. [Gk *hemi* half, paresis.]

hemiparkinsonism (hem·e·**par**·kin·son·izm). Paralysis agitans affecting one side of the body. [Gk *hemi* half, parkinsonism.]

hemipelvectomy (**hem**·e·pel·**vek**'·to·me). Removal of one half of the pelvis together with the leg; hindquarter amputation. [Gk *hemi* half, pelvis, Gk *ektome* a cutting out.]

hemipeptone (hem·e·**pep**·tone). One of the peptone intermediates formed in proteolytic digestion [obsolete term]. [Gk *hemi* half, peptone.]

hemiphalangectomy (**hem**·e·fal·an·**jek**'·to·me). In treatment of hallux valgus, surgical excision of a portion of a phalanx. [Gk *hemi* half, phalangectomy.]

hemiphonia (hem·e·**fo**·ne·ah). The uneven voice sounds produced by exhaustion and weakness, the sounds sometimes being those of the ordinary voice and sometimes of whispering. [Gk *hemi* half, *phone* voice.]

hemiplegia (hem·e·**ple**·je·ah). Paralysis of one side of the body due to disease of or damage to the upper motor neurones at various levels in the central nervous system (cerebral cortex, internal capsule, brain stem). Lesions in the brain stem may show crossed hemiplegia (see below). **Hemiplegia alternans hypoglossica.** That due to a lesion in the medulla oblongata with paralysis of the tongue on one side of the body and limb paralysis on the other side; an example of crossed hemiplegia (see below). **Alternate hemiplegia.** Crossed hemiplegia (see below). **Ascending hemiplegia.** Hemiplegia presenting peripherally and extending upwards. **Congenital hemiplegia.** That due to cerebral damage at birth or to developmental causes during fetal life. **Crossed hemiplegia, hemiplegia cruciata.** Cranial-nerve paralysis on one side with limb paralysis on the opposite side of the body. **Flaccid hemiplegia.** Hemiplegia with lack of muscle tone instead of the usual spasticity. **Hysterical hemiplegia.** Hemiplegia without organic basis. **Infantile hemiplegia.** Hemiplegia occurring in infancy, often during a febrile illness. **Spastic hemiplegia.** Hemiplegia with increased muscle tone. **Stuttering hemiplegia.** Hemiplegia progressing in sudden episodes. **Superior alternating hemiplegia.** Weber's syndrome. [Gk *hemi* half, *plege* stroke.]

See also: GUBLER.

hemiplegic (hem·e·**ple**·jik). 1. Relating or belonging to or having the characteristics of hemiplegia. 2. Suffering from hemiplegia.

hemiprosoplegia (**hem**·e·pro·so·**ple**'·je·ah). Paralysis affecting one lateral half of the face. [Gk *hemi* half, *prosopon* face, *plege* stroke.]

hemiprostatectomy (**hem**·e·pros·tat·**ek**'·to·me). Resection of one lateral half of the prostate gland. [Gk *hemi* half, prostatectomy.]

Hemiptera (hem·**ip**·ter·ah). An order of insects, the bugs, characterized by their sucking mouth parts and, in all those of medical importance, the proximal areas of the fore wings, when present, are more highly sclerosed than the distal. Genera of medical importance are *Cimex, Reduvius, Rhodnius* and *Triatoma.* [Gk *hemi* half, *pteron* wing.]

hemipylorectomy (**hem**·e·pi·lor·**ek**'·to·me). Resection of a part of the pylorus. [Gk *hemi* half, pylorectomy.]

hemipyocyanin (**hem**·e·pi·o·**si**'·an·in). $C_6H_4N_2C_6H_3(OH)$, an antibacterial pigment produced by *Pseudomonas pyocyanea;* it is yellow in colour, but alkaline solutions are violet-red. It is also antifungal, but its therapeutic importance is still under investigation.

hemipyonephrosis (**hem**·e·pi·o·nef·**ro**'·sis). 1. A hydronephrotic tumour or sac present in a part of the kidney. 2. Pyonephrosis affecting one half of a double kidney. [Gk *hemi* half, pyonephrosis.]

hemirachischisis (**hem**·e·rak·**is**'·kis·is). Rachischisis without associated prolapse of the spinal cord. [Gk *hemi* half, *rhachis* spine, *schisis* division.]

hemisacralization (**hem**·e·sa·kral·i·**za**'·shun). Abnormal development of the transverse process on one half of the 5th lumbar vertebra, so that it appears to be a part of the sacrum. [Gk *hemi* half, sacralization.]

hemiscotosis (**hem**·e·sko·**to**'·sis). A condition of the eyes in which there is a dark blind spot or disc in the visual field of one eye. [Gk *hemi* half, *skotos* darkness, *-osis* condition.]

hemisection (hem·e·**sek**·shun). In anatomy, division along the median plane; particularly, bisection into two lateral halves. [Gk *hemi* half, section.]

hemisomus (hem·e·**so**·mus). A monster with one lateral half of the body absent or imperfectly developed. [Gk *hemi* half, *soma* body.]

hemispasm (**hem**·e·spazm). Spasm in which only one side of the body is involved. **Facial hemispasm.** *See* SPASM, FACIAL. [Gk *hemi* half, spasm.]

hemisphere (**hem**·e·sfeer). A half-sphere. **Cerebellar hemisphere [hemispherium cerebelli (NA)].** Either one of the lateral halves of the cerebellum. **Cerebral hemisphere [hemispherium (NA)].** Either one of the lateral halves of the cerebrum. **Cerebral hemisphere, inferior surface of the [facies inferior hemispherii (NA)].** A surface composed of two parts, an anterior formed of the under-surface of the frontal lobes, the orbital part, and a posterior or tentorial part formed by the under-surface of the temporal and occipital lobes. The two parts are separated by the stem of the lateral sulcus. **Cerebral hemisphere, medial surface of the.** The surface between the two cerebral hemispheres. **Cerebral hemisphere, orbital surface of the.** A surface formed by the inferior surface of the frontal lobe. **Cerebral hemisphere, tentorial surface of the.** That part of the inferior surface lying behind the stem of the lateral sulcus; it is formed of temporal and occipital lobes and lies on the floor of the middle cranial fossa and the tentorium cerebelli. **Dominant hemisphere.** In a left-handed person, the right cerebral hemisphere; in a right-handed person, the left. [Gk *hemi* half, *sphaira* sphere.]

hemispherectomy (**hem**·e·sfeer·**ek**'·to·me). Resection of one of the cerebral hemispheres. [hemisphere, Gk *ektome* a cutting out.]

hemisphygmia (hem·e·**sfig**·me·ah). A condition in which the beat of the pulse is twice as fast as that of the heart. [Gk *hemi* half, *sphygmos* pulse.]

Hemispora (hem·e·**spo**·rah). Hyphomycetes. [Gk *hemi* half, *spora* seed.]

hemisporosis (**hem**·e·spo·**ro**'·sis). A fungus infection due to *Hemispora (Hyphomycetes)* reported from cases of osteoperiostitis, cold abscesses and sporotrichoid lesions. [Gk *hemi* half, *spora* seed, *-osis* condition.]

hemistrumectomy (**hem**·e·stroo·**mek**'·to·me). 1. Resection of one half of a goitre. 2. Resection of one half of a scrofulous gland or goitrous tumour. [Gk *hemi* half, strumectomy.]

hemisynergia (**hem**·e·sin·**er**'·je·ah). Synergy of only one half of the body with inco-ordination of the other. [Gk *hemi* half, *syn, ergein* to work.]

hemisystole (hem·e·**sis**·to·le). A condition in which there is irregular contraction of the heart muscle so that there is systole of only one ventricle, the left, resulting in one beat of the pulse for every two beats of the heart. [Gk *hemi* half, systole.]

hemiterata (hem·e·**ter**·at·ah). A term for those persons who are congenitally malformed but not sufficiently so to be disabled or notably defective in physical structure, and who cannot be classed as monsters. [Gk *hemi* half, *teras* monster.]

hemiteratic, hemiteric (hem·e·ter·at′·ik, hem·e·ter·ik). Referring or belonging to hemiterata.

hemiterpene (hem·e·ter·peen). Any hydrocarbon of formula C_5H_8. Isoprene, obtained during the distillation of rubber, is the most important. [Gk *hemi* half, terpene.]

hemitetany (hem·e·tet·an·e). Tetany affecting one side of the body only. [Gk *hemi* half, tetany.]

hemithermo-anaesthesia (hem·e·ther·mo·an·es·the′·ze·ah). Unilateral loss or absence of sensitivity to heat and cold. [Gk *hemi* half, thermo-anaesthesia.]

hemithorax (hem·e·thor·ax). One half of the chest. [Gk *hemi* half, *thorax* chest.]

hemithyroidectomy (hem·e·thi·roid·ek′·to·me). Surgical removal of one lobe of the thyroid gland. [Gk *hemi* half, thyroidectomy.]

hemitomias (hem·e·to·me·as). A male with only one testis or from whom one testis has been removed. [Gk *hemi* half, *tomias* eunuch.]

hemitonia (hem·e·to·ne·ah). Hemihypertonia.

hemitremor (hem·e·trem·or). Tremor or involuntary quivering affecting the muscles of one lateral half of the body. [Gk *hemi* half, tremor.]

hemivagotonia (hem·e·va·go·to′·ne·ah). Hyperexcitability of the vagus nerve on one side of the body. [Gk *hemi* half, vagotonia.]

hemivertebra (hem·e·ver·te·brah). Defective development of a vertebra in which one of the growth centres fails to develop. [Gk *hemi* half, vertebra.]

hemizygote (hem·e·zi·gote). Describing an individual which carries only one of a pair of chromosomes, or one of an allelomorphic pair of genes, as in individuals of heterogametic sex. [Gk *hemi* half, *zygos* yoke.]

hemlock (hem·lok). The common name for *Conium maculatum* Linn. (family Umbelliferae), a plant indigenous to the UK and central Europe and containing the alkaloid coniine. Hemlock leaf consists of the leaves and flowering tops in a fresh condition. The extract has been employed as a respiratory sedative. **Hemlock spruce.** Hemlock bark, pinus canadensis, a bark obtained from a North American tree, *Tsuga canadensis* (Linn.) Carr (family Pinaceae). It is used as an astringent. **Hemlock water dropwort.** *Oenanthe crocata* Linn. (family Umbelliferae), a British plant containing in all parts a poisonous oil which acts on the spinal cord and produces convulsions. [AS *hymlic.*]

hemp (hemp). A fibrous material prepared from the stems of *Cannabis sativa* and other plants and used in the manufacture of rope, etc. **Canadian hemp.** The root and rhizome of North American species of *Apocynum* (family Apocynaceae). It contains cymarin which, in addition to its stimulant action on the heart, acts as a diaphoretic, diuretic and emetic. In the form of the tincture it is used in the treatment of cardiac dropsy. **Common hemp, Indian hemp.** *Cannabis sativa.* [AS *henep.*]

Hempel, Walther (b. 1851). German chemist.

Hempel apparatus. An apparatus with which different constituents of a gaseous mixture can be absorbed and estimated.

henbane (hen·bane). **Egyptian henbane.** *Hyoscyamus muticus.* **Henbane leaves.** Hyoscyamus BP 1958; the dried flowering tops and leaves of *Hyoscyamus niger*, a wild plant of Europe, and also cultivated. It contains the alkaloids, hyoscyamine, hyoscine and atropine. So called because of its poisonous effect upon domestic fowls. [AS *henn, bana* death.]

Hench, Philip Showalter (b. 1896). Rochester, Minnesota, physician and Nobel prizewinner.

Hench-Aldrich salivary urea index or test. A measure of the salivary urea obtained by titrating saliva with 5 per cent mercuric-chloride solution. The index is the number of millilitres of the latter solution required by 100 ml saliva, and normally lies between 30 and 50.

Hench-Rosenberg syndrome. Palindromic rheumatism. *See* RHEUMATISM.

Henderson, Lawrence Joseph (b. 1878). Boston, Mass., biochemist.

Henderson-Hasselbalch equation, for the determination of the pH of buffer systems. $pH = pK + \log_{10}[A]/[HA]$, where p*K* is the negative logarithm of the dissociation constant and [A] and [HA] the concentrations of acid ions and undissociated weak acid, respectively.

Henderson, Melvin Starkey (b. 1883). Rochester, Minnesota, orthopaedic surgeon.

Henderson-Jones disease. Synovial chondromatosis.

Henderson, William (b. 1810). Scottish pathologist.

Henderson-Paterson body. The inclusion body of molluscum contagiosum.

Henderson, Yandell (b. 1873). New Haven physiologist.

Henderson's test, for anaesthetic risk. The patient takes a deep breath and holds it as long as possible. 30 s is normal, but, in the absence of cardiac or pulmonary insufficiency, less than 20 s is said to indicate the presence of acidosis and to contra-indicate administration. This test is not commonly used in the UK.

Henke, Philipp Jakob Wilhelm (b. 1834). Tübingen anatomist.

Henke's space. The retropharyngeal space. *See* SPACE.

Henke's triangle or trigone. Inguinal triangle. *See* TRIANGLE.

Henle, Friedrich Gustav Jakob (b. 1809). Gottingen anatomist.

Henle's ampulla. The ampulla of the uterine tube.

Henle's ansa, loop, looped tube or tubule. The portion of the nephron which follows the proximal tubule. It consists of a thin descending limb which passes for a varying distance into the inner medulla, a thin ascending limb which also lies in the inner medulla and a thick ascending limb which lies in the outer medulla. The loop plays an important part in the counter-current multiplier mechanism of the medulla.

Henle's canals. Renal tubules constituting the ansa or loop of Henle.

Henle's cell. One of the supporting cells of the seminiferous tubules, lying between clumps of germinal cells and having a number of spermatids partially buried in its cytoplasm. Also known as *Sertoli's cell.*

Henle's fibres. Fibres constituting the internal elastic (fenestrated) membrane of an artery of large or medium calibre.

Henle's fissures. Spaces containing connective tissue between the fibres of cardiac muscle.

Henle's glands. Tubular glands in the palpebral part of the conjunctiva.

Henle's layer. The outer layer of cells of the inner root sheath of a hair follicle.

fibre layer of Henle. The horizontal striated appearance of the layer of cones at the fovea.

Henle's ligament. The conjoint tendon of the transversus abdominis muscle. *See* TENDON.

Henle's membrane. Bruch's membrane.

Henle's elastic membrane. The outer elastic limiting membrane between the adventitia and media of the arterial wall.

Henle's fenestrated membrane. The deepest elastic layer of the intima of the arterial wall.

Henle's reaction. The production of a brown colour with salts of chromium given by adrenaline-producing cells.

sheath of Henle. Endoneurial sheath; the delicate connective-tissue covering of individual nerve fibres, outside the sheath of Schwann.

Henle's sphincter. Annular muscle fibres surrounding the prostatic part of the male urethra.

Henle's spine. The suprameatal spine. *See* SPINE.

Henle's wart, Hassall-Henle wart. Nodular thickenings of Descemet's membrane occurring after the age of from 20 to 30 years at the corneal periphery.

henna (hen·ah). The dried leaves of *Lawsonia alba* (family Lythraceae). An aqueous extract imparts a Titian-red colour to wool, hair and other natural protein fibres; it is commonly used as a hair dye. [Ar. *hinna.*]

Henneberg, Richard (b. 1868). Berlin neurologist.

Laehr-Henneberg hard-palate reflex. When the hard palate of a patient with pseudobulbar palsy is scratched there is contraction of the orbicularis oris muscle, giving a downward movement of the lower lip.

Hennebert, Camille (b. 1867). Belgian otologist.

Hennebert's sign. Nystagmus resulting from rarefaction and compression of the air in the external auditory meatus when a fistula into one of the semicircular canals is present.

Henoch, Eduard Heinrich (b. 1820). Berlin paediatrician.

Henoch's disease or purpura. Allergic purpura; it is usually characterized by purpura with abdominal colic, and melaena due to urticarial, serous or haemorrhagic effusions into the intestinal mucosa.

Henoch-Bergeron disease. Bergeron's disease; electrical chorea.

Henoch-Schoenlein disease, purpura or syndrome, Schoenlein-Henoch disease, purpura or syndrome. Allergic purpura. The term is used to include all the features of Schoenlein's and Henoch's pupura.

henogenesis (hen·o·jen·es·is). In biology, the origin and the development of the individual organism as distinct from the development of the species. [Gk *hen* one, genesis.]

henosis (hen·o·sis). 1. The process of healing. 2. The act of uniting, a term applied particularly to union of parts that normally are separate, as the upper and lower eyelids or the eyelids to the eyeball. [Gk *hen* one, *-osis* condition.]

henotic (hen·ot·ik). 1. Relating or belonging to henosis. 2. Aiding or promoting healing.

henpue, henpuye (hen·poo·ye). Goundou. [West African, dog-nose.]

Henriques, Valdemar (b. 1864). Copenhagen biochemist.

Henriques and Sørensen method, for amino-acid nitrogen in urine. The urine is treated with barium chloride and barium hydroxide to remove carbonates and phosphates, and any large amount of ammonia distilled off *in vacuo.* The filtrate is neutralized to phenolphthalein, neutral formaldehyde solution is added and the acidity produced is titrated with standard alkali.

Henry, Adolf Felix Gerhard (b. 1894). Istanbul pathologist.

Henry's melanin reaction or melanoflocculation test. A suggested serum test for malaria that depends on the changes in the protein constituents of the serum; now discredited as a test for malaria.

Henry, Arnold Kirkpatrick (b. 1886). London and Dublin surgeon.

Henry's ganglionectomy. The posterior approach for excision of thoracic sympathetic ganglia and sympathetic trunk.

Henry, William (b. 1774). Manchester chemist.

Henry's law. The weight of a gas dissolved by a given volume of a liquid at a constant temperature is directly proportional to the pressure.

Dalton-Henry law. In the case of a mixture of gases in equilibrium with a liquid, the amount of any one particular gas dissolved is directly proportional to its partial pressure.

Henry's shoulder-strap incision. An incision in the line of the deltopectoral groove for approach to Codman's bursa.

henry (hen·re). The unit of electric inductance (self- or mutual). A circuit has a self-inductance of 1 henry when a rate of change of current of 1 ampere per second through it produces an induced electromotive force of 1 volt in the circuit. The mutual inductance of 2 circuits is 1 henry when a rate of change of current of 1 ampere per second in 1 circuit produces an electromotive force of 1 volt in the other circuit. [Joseph *Henry,* 1797–1878, American physicist.]

Hensen, Viktor (b. 1835). Kiel pathologist.

Hensen's body. The modified Golgi apparatus in the outer hair cells of the cochlea.

Hensen's canal or duct. The ductus reuniens.

Hensen's cells. Tall columnar cells forming the outer border cells of the organ of Corti.

Hensen's disc, line or plane. A light band seen in the dark segment (A disc of a striated muscle fibre. It is further subdivided by a thin dark M disc.

Hensen's knot or node. Protochordal knot; a rounded swelling at the anterior end of the primitive streak on the surface of the blastoderm from which the head process (future notochord) is derived. It is homologous with the dorsal lip of the blastopore of lower vertebrates.

Hensen's stripes. A band on the under-surface of the tectorial membrane of the internal ear; it is opposite the interval between the inner and outer rows of hair cells.

Hensing, Friedrich Wilhelm (b. 1719). Giessen anatomist.

Hensing's fold or ligament. The phrenicocolic ligament. *See* LIGAMENT.

hepar (he·par). 1. The Greek and Latin for *liver.* 2. The term was applied at one time to any substance resembling liver in colour or texture. **Hepar adiposum.** Adipohepatic liver. *See* LIVER. **Hepar induratum.** Cirrhosis of the liver. **Hepar lobatum.** The contracted and distorted nodular liver which eventually results from chronic syphilitic hepatitis. **Hepar Proteolysatum BPC 1949.** Proteolysed liver. *See* LIVER. **Hepar sulphuris.** Liver of sulphur; a deliquescent yellowish-brown mass made by melting sulphur with potassium carbonate. It is water-soluble, and contains potassium sulphide and the potassium salts of various oxy-acids of sulphur. It was formerly used in sulphur baths for scabies.

heparin (hep·ar·in). A substance allied to mucoitinsulphuric acid and a physiological anticoagulant found in most tissues of a body, especially the liver and lung. It inhibits the clotting of blood *in vivo* and *in vitro* by preventing the conversion of prothrombin to thrombin and by antagonizing the action of thrombokinase. It requires to be injected, being inactive by mouth, and is used to prevent or limit thrombosis and to stop the clotting of shed blood (BP 1973). Overdosage may be antagonized by protamine sulphate. **Heparin sodium.** The sodium salt of heparin, prepared from mammalian lung or liver tissue, and used as an anticoagulant by injection or intravenous drip. [Gk *hepar* liver.]

heparinaemia (hep·ar·in·e′·me·ah). Heparin in the circulating blood. [heparin, Gk *haima* blood.]

heparinate (hep·ar·in·ate). 1. Any heparin salt. 2. A sterile preparation of mammalian lung or liver tissue containing the sodium salt of heparin, and possessing the property of delaying the clotting of blood. Unlike dicoumarol it is useless when administered orally, but it is far swifter in its action. It is given by injection or intravenous drip.

heparinize (hep·ar·in·ize). To increase the clotting time of the blood by giving injections of heparin.

hepatalgia (hep·at·al·je·ah). Pain in the liver. [Gk *hepar* liver, *algos* pain.]

hepatalgic (hep·at·al·jik). Relating or belonging to hepatalgia.

hepatargia, hepatargy (hep·at·ar·je·ah, hep·at·ar·je). Auto-intoxication caused by hepatic insufficiency. [Gk *hepar* liver, *argia* idleness.]

hepatatrophia, hepatatrophy (hep·at·at·ro′·fe·ah, hep·at·at·ro·fe). An atrophied or wasted condition of the liver. [Gk *hepar* liver, atrophy.]

hepatauxe (hep·at·awx·e). A state of enlargement or hypertrophy of the liver. [Gk *hepar* liver, *auxe* increase.]

hepatectomize (hep·at·ek·tom·ize). Total (in experimental animals) or partial resection of the liver. [Gk *hepar* liver, *ektome* a cutting out.]

hepatectomy (hep·at·ek·to·me). The operation of resection of the liver. [see prec.]

hepatic (hep·at·ik). Relating or belonging to the liver. [Gk *hepar* liver.]

hepatic arteries. Common hepatic artery [arteria hepatica communis (NA)]. A division of the coeliac artery which runs to the right behind the lesser sac of the peritoneum, enters the lesser omentum [rami epiploici (NA)] and runs upward to the liver in its free margin, terminating by dividing into left and right branches [ramus sinister, ramus dexter (NA)], the former usually supplying a cystic branch [arteria cystica (NA)] to the gall bladder. Both right and left branches then supply segmental arteries to the hepatic segments, including branches to the caudate lobe [arteriae lobi caudati (NA)]. In addition it gives off the right gastric artery [arteria gastrica dextra (NA)] to the lesser curvature of the stomach, and the gastroduodenal artery [arteria gastroduodenalis (NA)] which itself divides into the right gastro-epiploic artery [arteria gastro-epiploica dextra (NA)] to the right half of the greater curvature and the greater omentum, and the superior pancreaticoduodenal arteries [arteriae supraduodenales superiores (NA)] to the head of the pancreas [rami pancreatici (NA)] and the duodenum [rami duodenales et arteriae retroduodenales (NA)]. **Proper hepatic artery [arteria hepatica propria (NA)].** The branch of the common hepatic artery which supplies the liver and gall bladder.

hepatic veins. Right, middle and left hepatic veins [venae hepaticae dextra, mediae et sinistrae]. The main veins draining the liver into the inferior vena cava, just below the diaphragm.

hepatica (hep·at·ik·ah). *Anemone hepatica* Linn., American liverwort (family Ranunculaceae). An infusion of the herb is reported as having tonic and astringent properties. [Gk *hepar* liver.]

hepaticocholangiojejunostomy (hep·**at**·ik·o·ko·**lan**·je·o·jej·oon·**os'**·to·me). Surgical establishment of an anastomosis between the gall bladder, the hepatic duct and the jejunum. [Gk *hepar* liver, *chole* bile, *aggeion* small vessel, jejunum, Gk *stoma* mouth.]

hepaticocolic (hep·**at**·ik·o·**kol'**·ik). Hepatocolic. [Gk *hepar* liver, colon.]

hepaticodochotomy (hep·**at**·ik·o·do·**kot'**·o·me). Hepaticotomy. [Gk *hepar* liver, choledochotomy.]

hepaticoduodenostomy (hep·**at**·ik·o·**dew**·o·de·**nos**·to·me). The establishment of an anastomosis between the hepatic duct and the duodenum. [Gk *hepar* liver, duodenum, Gk *stoma* mouth.]

hepatico-enterostomy (hep·**at**·ik·o·en·ter·**os'**·to·me). The establishment of an anastomosis between the hepatic duct and the intestine. [Gk *hepar* liver, enterostomy.]

hepaticogastric (hep·**at**·ik·o·**gas'**·trik). Relating or belonging to the liver and the stomach. [Gk *hepar* liver, *gaster* stomach.]

hepaticogastrostomy (hep·**at**·ik·o·gas·**tros'**·to·me). The establishment of an anastomosis between the hepatic duct and the stomach. [Gk *hepar* liver, gastrostomy.]

hepaticojejunostomy (hep·**at**·ik·o·jej·oon·**os'**·to·me). The establishment of an anastomosis between the hepatic duct and the jejunum. [Gk *hepar* liver, jejunostomy.]

hepaticola (hep·at·**ik**·o·lah). *Capillaria.* [Gk *hepar* liver, L *colere* to inhabit.]

hepaticoliasis (hep·**at**·ik·o·**li'**·as·is). Infestation with worms of the genus *Capillaria* (*Hepaticola*).

hepaticolithotomy (hep·**at**·ik·o·lith·**ot'**·o·me). The operation of opening the bile ducts for the purpose of removing gall-stones. [Gk *hepar* liver, lithotomy.]

hepaticolithotripsy (hep·**at**·ik·o·**lith'**·o·trip·se). The operation of crushing a stone in the hepatic duct. [Gk *hepar* liver, *lithos* stone, *tribein* to crush.]

hepaticopancreatic (hep·**at**·ik·o·pan·kre·**at'**·ik). Relating or belonging to the liver and the pancreas. [Gk *hepar* liver, pancreas.]

hepaticopulmonary (hep·**at**·ik·o·**pul'**·mon·ar·e). Hepatopulmonary. [Gk *hepar* liver, L *pulmo* lung.]

hepaticorenal (hep·**at**·ik·o·**re'**·nal). Hepatorenal. [Gk *hepar* liver, L *ren* kidney.]

hepaticostomy (hep·**at**·ik·**os'**·to·me). The surgical establishment of a permanent artificial opening into the hepatic duct. [Gk *hepar* liver, *stoma* mouth.]

hepaticotomy (hep·**at**·ik·**ot'**·o·me). Surgical incision into the hepatic duct. [Gk *hepar* liver, *temnein* to cut.]

hepatism (**hep**·at·izm). Disease or disordered function of the liver. [Gk *hepar* liver.]

hepatitic (hep·at·it·ik). Relating or belonging to hepatitis.

hepatitis (hep·at·i·tis) (pl. *hepatitides*). Inflammation of the liver. **Acute infective hepatitis.** Catarrhal jaundice; hepatitis due to infection with hepatitis A virus. The disease is generally benign with pyrexia, abnormal liver function tests, jaundice and tender enlargement of the liver. The virus is generally spread by the faecal–oral route. **Acute parenchymatous hepatitis.** Acute yellow atrophy, icterus gravis; a rare and fatal disease with acute necrosis of the liver, causing jaundice, severe gastro-intestinal and nervous symptoms, with diminution of the size of the liver. It may be due to an unknown intrinsic toxin developing during pregnancy, or to extrinsic poisons such as trinitrotoluene, chloroform, arsenic, phosphorus, carbon tetrachloride and acetanilide. **Amoebic hepatitis.** Inflammation occurring in the course of amoebic dysentery, which may go on to suppuration and the formation of an abscess. **Cytomegalic hepatitis.** Hepatitis due to a cytomegalic inclusion virus transmitted transplacentally. **Enzootic hepatitis.** Rift Valley fever; a virus disease of newborn lambs in East Africa. It is transmissible to man. **Epidemic hepatitis.** Acute infective hepatitis (see above). **Familial hepatitis.** Hepatolenticular degeneration, progressive lenticular degeneration; a progressive familial disease in which cirrhosis of the liver following attacks of acute hepatitis is associated with degeneration of parts of the brain, especially the corpus striatum. **Homologous serum hepatitis.** Homologous serum jaundice, serum hepatitis, hippy hepatitis; hepatitis due to infection with hepatitis B virus. Both virus and disease are slightly different from those of acute infective hepatitis (see above). The virus is generally spread by transfusion or injection of blood, or blood products, or by the use of contaminated instruments, particularly syringes. It may also be transmitted via faeces and urine. Development of the disease is associated with the appearance of hepatitis B antigen and, later, its antibody. The course of the disease is generally benign but a small proportion of cases are fatal in the acute stage, or else the patients become chronic carriers of the antigen. **Infective hepatitis.** Hepatitis due to a specific virus or occurring in a variety of infective diseases such as yellow fever, spirochaetosis icterohaemorrhagica, malaria, typhoid fever, influenza and streptococcal infections. **Infective necrotic hepatitis.** A fatal disease of sheep in Australasia, marked by necrotic areas in the liver. **Interstitial hepatitis.** Cirrhosis of the liver. **Serum hepatitis.** Homologous serum hepatitis (see above). **Suppurative hepatitis.** Abscess of the liver occurring in amoebic dysentery, or secondary to suppurative pylephlebitis. **Toxic hepatitis.** Hepatitis due to a toxin of chemical, parasitic or metabolic origin. **Transfusion hepatitis.** Homologous serum hepatitis (see above). **Trophopathic hepatitis.** Hepatitis due to dietary deficiency. **Virus hepatitis.** Acute infective hepatitis (see above). [Gk *hepar* liver, *-itis* inflammation.]

hepatitis-associated antigen (hep·at·i·tis as·**sosh**·i·at·ed **an**·te·gen). *See* HEPATITIS B ANTIGEN.

hepatitis b antigen (hep·at·i·tis·be·**an**·te·gen). Also known as Australia antigen, Australia/Serum Hepatitis (Au/SH) antigen and Hepatitis-associated antigen (H.A.A.) but these terms are now obsolete. It is found in association with hepatitis type B only, and consists of 20 nm spherical or bacillary bodies found in the serum of those who have, or have had, type B hepatitis. Larger 42 nm forms (Dane particles) are also found and these may be complete virus particles. All 3 forms have similar surface antigens (HBsAg). In addition to a common antigen, a, there are subtypes of surface antigens, of which there are two major alternates, d or y and w or r, and several minor ones. A distinct core antigen (HBcAg) is found on the 28 nm inner core of the Dane particle. The presence of the antigen in a patient's serum is diagnostic of present or past hepatitis B infection. It appears at or shortly before the onset of symptoms and persists for a variable period after they regress. In the majority of cases the antigen becomes undetectable rapidly but a proportion show prolonged carriage and a small number become lifelong carriers. Of these the majority show no evidence of disordered liver function but some do have evidence of chronic hepatitis. Carriage rates vary between 1:500 to 1:100 in most temperate zones to between 1:8 and 1:5 in some tropical areas. Rates also vary according to the method used to detect the antigen. Radioimmunoassay and passive haemagglutination (PHA) are the most sensitive and reliable methods currently used. The exact relationship of the antigen to the virus has yet to be established (it is thought to be self-assembled viral coat protein). It was originally discovered in the serum of an Australian aborigine as part of a search for minor serum proteins but is distributed world-wide.

Antibody to the antigen (anti-HBs) develops slowly in convalescence and probably correlates with the immunity to reinfection.

hepatitis virus (hep·at·i·tis vi·rus). Viral hepatitis is predominantly due to 2 viruses, type A and type B. Clinically the disease caused by each is very similar, but the viruses are probably entirely unrelated and neither virus is known to be related to other viruses. *Type A*, causes infections or catarrhal jaundice (hepatitis A). An RNA virus, the virions may be 27 nm particles found in the faeces during the acute stages of the disease. There is no routine diagnostic test at present. It is not known if there is more than one serotype. *Type B*, causes serum hepatitis (hepatitis B). The virion is probably the 42 nm Dane particle seen in the serum by electron microscopy. It is probably a DNA virus and the presence of the hepatitis B antigen (HBsAg) in the serum is a reliable indicator of present or past infection. Examination of HBsAg suggests that there are several subtypes of the virus. Chimpanzees and some monkeys can be infected but the virus cannot be grown in routine cell cultures. Hepatitis may be associated with infection due to cytomegalovirus and some other viruses but hepatitis is not a major or common feature of infection with them. *See also* HEPATITIS B ANTIGEN.

hepatization (hep·at·i·za'·shun). A stage in the course of lobar pneumonia in which the lung, when cut into, shows a resemblance to liver. **Grey hepatization.** A stage of lobar pneumonia when the air passages are stuffed with leucocytes and fibrin so that the lung appears solid and grey in colour. **Red hepatization.** An early stage of lobar pneumonia when the air passages are filled with red blood corpuscles and fibrin. **Yellow hepatization.** A later stage of grey hepatization (see above), when the leucocytes in the air passages contain much fat [see foll.]

hepatized (hep·at·i·zd). Converted into the consistency of liver, applied particularly to the consolidation of lung tissue in lobar pneumonia. [Gk *hepatizein* to be like the liver.]

hepatizon (hep·at·i·zon). Chloasma: a general term for pigmentary discoloration of the skin occurring in spots or patches of yellow, brown or black. [see prec.]

hepatobiliary (hep·at·o·bil'·e·ar·e). Belonging to the liver and the bile duct or bile ductules. [Gk *hepar* liver, biliary.]

hepatoblastoma (hep·at·o·blas·to'·mah). A malignant teratoma of the liver made up of cells of epithelial type, often with areas of immature cartilage and bone of mixed embryonal nature. [Gk *hepar* liver, *blastos* germ, *-oma* tumour.]

hepatocarcinogenic (hep·at·o·kar·sin·o·jen'·ik). Causing carcinoma of the liver. [Gk *hepar* liver, carcinogenic.]

hepatocele (hep·at·o·seel). Hernia of part of the liver through the diaphragm or the abdominal wall. [Gk *hepar* liver, *kele* hernia.]

hepatocellular (hep·at·o·sel'·ew·lar). Relating to or having an effect on liver cells. [Gk *hepar* liver, cell.]

hepatocholangeitis (hep·at·o·ko·lan·je·i'·tis). An inflamed condition of the liver and the bile ductules. [Gk *hepar* liver, cholangitis.]

hepatocholangiocystoduodenostomy (hep·at·o·ko·lan·je·o·sist·o·dew·o·de·nos'·to·me). The surgical establisment of drainage of the bile duct and biliary ductules through the gall bladder into the duodenum. [Gk *hepar* liver, *chole* bile, *aggeion* small vessel, *kystis* bag, duodenostomy.]

hepatocholangioduodenostomy (hep·at·o·ko·lan·je·o·dew·o·de·nos'·to·me). The surgical establishment of drainage from the bile duct and biliary ductules into the duodenum. [Gk *hepar* liver, *chole* bile, *aggeion* small vessel, duodenostomy.]

hepatocholangio-enterostomy (hep·at·o·ko·lan·je·o·en·ter·os'·to·me). The surgical establishment of drainage from the bile duct and biliary ductules into the intestine. [Gk *hepar* liver, *chole* bile, *aggeion* small vessel, enterostomy.]

hepatocholangiogastrostomy (hep·at·o·ko·lan·je·o·gas·tros'·to·me). An operation by means of which the bile duct and biliary ductules are enabled to drain into the stomach. [Gk *hepar* liver, *chole* bile, *aggeion* small vessel, gastrostomy.]

hepatocholangiostomy (hep·at·o·ko·lan·je·os'·to·me). The drainage of a hepatic duct either to the exterior (external hepatocholangiostomy) or to the intestine (internal hepatocholangiostomy). [Gk *hepar* liver, *chole* bile, *aggeion* small vessel, *stoma* mouth.]

hepatocholangitis (hep·at·o·ko·lan·ji'·tis). Hepatocholangeitis.

hepatocholecystopathy (hep·at·o·ko·le·sist·op'·ath·e). Dysfunction of the liver in which there is both parenchymal and biliary dysfunction. [Gk *hepar* liver, *chole* bile, *kystis* bladder, *pathos* disease.]

hepatocirrhosis (hep·at·o·sir·o'·sis). Cirrhosis of the liver. [Gk *hepar* liver, cirrhosis.]

hepatocolic (hep·at·o·kol'·ik). Relating or belonging to the liver and the colon. [Gk *hepar* liver, colon.]

hepatocuprein (hep·at·o·kew'·pre·in). A copper-containing protein from the liver. [Gk *hepar* liver, L *cuprum* copper.]

Hepatocystes (hep·at·o·sist'·eez). A genus of haemosporidial parasites of the monkey that were at one time classified as *Plasmodium. H. kochi* and *H. murinum* are recognized species. [see foll.]

hepatocystic (hep·at·o·sist'·ik). Having relation to or belonging to the liver, or to the liver and the gall bladder together. [Gk *hepar* liver, *kystis* bag.]

hepatocyte (hep·at·o·site). Liver cell. More specifically, parenchymal cell. [Gk *hepar* liver, *kytos* cell.]

hepatodidymus (hep·at·o·did'·im·us). A monster in which all the organs of the upper part of the body, including the liver, are duplicated. [Gk *hepar* liver, *didymos* twin.]

hepatoduodenal (hep·at·o·dew·o·de'·nal). Relating or belonging to the liver and the duodenum. [Gk *hepar* liver, duodenum.]

hepatoduodenostomy (hep·at·o·dew·o·de·nos'·to·me). The surgical establishment of an anastomosis between the liver and the duodenum. [Gk *hepar* liver, duodenostomy.]

hepatodynia (hep·at·o·din'·e·ah). Pain in the liver. [Gk *hepar* liver, *odyne* pain.]

hepatodystrophy (hep·at·o·dis'·tro·fe). Acute hepatic necrosis. [Gk *hepar* liver, dystrophy.]

hepato-enteric (hep·at·o·en·ter'·ik). Relating or belonging to the liver and the intestine. [Gk *hepar* liver, *enteron* bowel.]

hepatoflavin (hep·at·o·fla'·vin, hep·at·o·flav'·in). A lyochrome obtained from liver. [Gk *hepar* liver, flavin.]

hepatogastric (hep·at·o·gas'·trik). Relating or belonging to the liver and the stomach. [Gk *hepar* liver, *gaster* stomach.]

hepatogastritis (hep·at·o·gas·tri'·tis). An inflamed condition of both the liver and the stomach. [Gk *hepar* liver, gastritis.]

hepatogenic, hepatogenous (hep·at·o·jen'·ik, hep·at·oj·en·us). 1. Arising from or produced in the liver. 2. Caused by a condition of the liver. [Gk *hepar* liver, *genein* to produce.]

hepatoglycaemia glycogenetica (hep·at·o·gli·se'·me·ah gli·ko·jen·et'·ik·ah). Glycogen disease. *See* DISEASE. [Gk *hepar* liver, glycaemia, glycogen.]

hepatogram (hep·at·o·gram). 1. A sphygmographic tracing of the pulsations of the liver. 2. The radiograph or record made during hepatography. [Gk *hepar* liver, *gramma* record.]

hepatography (hep·at·og·raf·e). 1. A recording of the liver pulse, as in a hepatogram. 2. Radiographic or radio-isotopic visualization of the liver, covering arteriography and scintigraphy. [Gk *hepar* liver, *graphein* to record.]

hepatohaemia (hep·at·o·he'·me·ah). A condition in which the liver is congested with blood. [Gk *hepar* liver, *haima* blood.]

hepatoid (hep·at·oid). Resembling the liver in structure or in character of tissue. [Gk *hepar* liver, *eidos* form.]

hepatolenticular (hep·at·o·len·**tik**'·ew·lar). Belonging or relating to the liver and to the lentiform nucleus of the cerebrum. [Gk *hepar* liver, L *lens* lentil.]

hepatolienal (hep·at·o·**li**'·en·al). Relating or belonging to the liver and the spleen, [Gk *hepar* liver, L *lien* spleen.]

hepatolienography (hep·at·o·li·en·**og**'·raf·e). Hepatosplenography. [Gk *hepar* liver, L *lien* spleen, Gk *graphein* to record.]

hepatolienomegaly (hep·at·o·li·en·o·**meg**'·al·e). Hepatosplenomegaly. [Gk *hepar* liver, spleen, Gk *megas* large.]

hepatolith (hep·at·o·lith). A gall-stone; term applied mainly to a concretion in the liver itself. [Gk *hepar* liver, *lithos* stone.]

hepatolithectomy (hep·at·o·lith·**ek**'·to·me). Surgical removal of a gall-stone or concretion from the liver or the hepatic duct. [Gk *hepar* liver, lithectomy.]

hepatolithiasis (hep·at·o·lith·**i**'·as·is). The pathological condition in which concretions form in the liver or gall bladder. [Gk *hepar* liver, *lithos* stone.]

hepatologist (hep·at·**ol**·o·jist). One who specializes in diseases of the liver. [see foll.]

hepatology (hep·at·**ol**·o·je). That branch of medical science which is concerned particularly with the liver and its diseases. [Gk *hepar* liver, *logos* science.]

hepatolysin (hep·at·**ol**·is·in). A cytolysin which is specific for the destruction of liver cells. [Gk *hepar* liver, lysin.]

hepatolysis (hep·at·**ol**·is·is). The process of destruction by lysis of liver cells. [Gk *hepar* liver, lysis.]

hepatolytic (hep·at·o·**lit**'·ik). 1. Referring to hepatolysis. 2. Term applied to anything that is able to destroy the liver cells or substance.

hepatoma (hep·at·**o**·mah). A combined adenomatous and carcinomatous neoplasm originating in the hepatic parenchyma. [Gk *hepar* liver, *-oma* tumour.]

hepatomalacia (hep·at·o·mal·**a**'·she·ah). A condition of morbid softening or softness of the liver. [Gk *hepar* liver, malacia.]

hepatomegalia, hepatomegaly (hep·at·o·meg·**a**'·le·e·ah, hep·at·o·**meg**'·al·e). A condition of enlargement of the liver. **Hepatomegalia glycogenica.** Glycogen disease. *See* DISEASE. [Gk *hepar* liver, *megas* large.]

hepatomelanosis (hep·at·o·mel·an·**o**'·sis). A condition in which the liver is very darkly pigmented owing to abnormally large deposits of melanin. [Gk *hepar* liver, melanosis.]

hepatomphalocele (hep·at·**om**·fal·o·seel). Umbilical hernia in which a portion of the liver is extruded within the sac. [Gk *hepar* liver, omphalocele.]

hepatomphalos (hep·at·**om**·fal·os). A condition in which the liver protrudes through the abdominal wall in the region of the navel. [Gk *hepar* liver, *omphalos* navel.]

hepatomyeloma (hep·at·o·mi·el·**o**'·mah). Medullary carcinoma of the liver, the substance of the tumour being composed mostly of soft cellular material like marrow. [Gk *hepar* liver, myeloma.]

hepatoncus (hep·at·**ong**·kus). Any tumour of, or swelling in the liver. [Gk *hepar* liver, *ogkos* a swelling.]

hepatonecrosis (hep·at·o·nek·**ro**'·sis). Gangrene of the liver [Gk *hepar* liver, necrosis.]

hepatonephric (hep·at·o·**nef**'·rik). Having relation to the liver and the kidney. [Gk *hepar* liver, *nephros* kidney.]

hepatonephritic (hep·at·o·nef·**rit**'·ik). Referring or belonging to hepatonephritis.

hepatonephromegaly (hep·at·o·nef·ro·**meg**'·al·e). Enlargement of both the liver and the kidney or kidneys. **Glycogenic hepatonephromegaly.** Glycogen disease. *See* DISEASE. [Gk *hepar* liver, *nephros* kidney, *megas* large.]

hepatopathy (hep·at·**op**·ath·e). An inclusive term for diseases of the liver. [Gk *hepar* liver, *pathos* disease.]

hepatoperitonitis (hep·at·o·per·e·ton·**i**'·tis). An inflamed condition of the visceral peritoneum over the liver. [Gk *hepar* liver, peritonitis.]

hepatopexy (hep·at·o·pex·e). The surgical fixation in its proper position of a displaced, prolapsed or floating liver by anchoring it to the wall of the abdomen. [Gk *hepar liver, pexis* fixation.]

hepatophlebitis (hep·at·o·fleb·**i**'·tis). An inflamed condition of the veins of the liver. [Gk *hepar* liver, phlebitis.]

hepatophlebotomy (hep·at·o·fleb·**ot**'·o·me). The act or process of withdrawing blood from the liver by aspiration. [Gk *hepar* liver, phlebotomy.]

hepatophyma (hep·at·o·**fi**'·mah). An inclusive term for abscesses or tumours of the liver. [Gk *hepar* liver, *phyma* a growth.]

hepatopleural (hep·at·o·**ploor**'·al). Relating or belonging to or affecting the liver and the pleura, as a fistula. [Gk *hepar* liver, pleura.]

hepatopneumonic (hep·at·o·new·**mon**'·ik). Hepatopulmonary. [Gk *hepar* liver, *pneuma* breath.]

hepatoportal (hep·at·o·**port**'·al). Relating or belonging to the portal vein and its ramifications. [Gk *hepar* liver, L *porta* gate.]

hepatopostema (hep·at·o·pos·**te**'·mah). Abscess of the liver. [Gk *hepar* liver, *apostema* abscess.]

hepatoptosia, hepatoptosis (hep·at·o·**to**'·se·ah, hep·at·o·**to**'·sis). Downward displacement of the liver. [Gk *hepar* liver, ptosis.]

hepatopulmonary (hep·at·o·**pul**'·mon·ar·e). Affecting or having relation to the liver and the lungs. [Gk *hepar* liver, L *pulmo* lung.]

hepatorenal (hep·at·o·**re**'·nal). Relating or belonging to the liver and the kidneys. [Gk *hepar* liver, L *ren* kidney.]

hepatorrhagia (hep·at·o·**ra**'·je·ah). Haemorrhage from the liver. [Gk *hepar* liver, *rhegnynai* to gush.]

hepatorrhaphy (hep·at·**or**·af·e). Surgical suture of a wound of the liver. [Gk *hepar* liver, *rhaphe* seam.]

hepatorrhexis (hep·at·o·**rex**'·is). Rupture of the liver. [Gk *hepar* liver, *rhexis* rupture.]

hepatoscirrhus (hep·at·o·**skir**'·rus). Scirrhous carcinoma of the liver. [Gk *hepar* liver, *skirrhos* hard.]

hepatoscopy (hep·at·**os**·ko·pe). Diagnostic examination of the liver by laparotomy or peritoneoscopy. [Gk *hepar* liver, *skopein* to watch.]

hepatosis (hep·at·**o**·sis). Inclusive term for any non-inflammatory disorder of the liver leading to dysfunction. **Serous hepatosis.** A name suggested for a disease of young children in certain tropical countries, in which histologically there is occlusion of the blood vessels which contain a gelatinous substance, oedema, eosinophilic infiltration and finally fibrosis of the liver; clinically there is hepatomegaly, ascites and finally the classical picture of cirrhosis of the liver. The cause is probably dietary. [Gk *hepar* liver, *-osis* condition.]

hepatosplenic (hep·at·o·**splen**'·ik). Hepatolienal. [Gk *hepar* liver, spleen.]

hepatosplenitis (hep·at·o·splen·**i**'·tis). Inflammation of the liver and of the spleen occurring simultaneously. [Gk *hepar* liver, spleen, Gk *-itis* inflammation.]

hepatosplenography (hep·at·o·splen·**og**'·raf·e). Intravenous injection of an opaque substance and subsequent radiographical examination of the liver and spleen. [Gk *hepar* liver, spleen, Gk *graphein* to record.]

hepatosplenomegaly (hep·at·o·splen·o·**meg**'·al·e). An enlarged condition of the liver and the spleen. [Gk *hepar* liver, spleen, Gk *megas* large.]

hepatosplenopathy (hep·at·o·splen·**op**'·ath·e). A disease involving both the liver and the spleen. [Gk *hepar* liver, spleen, Gk *pathos* disease.]

hepatostomy (hep·at·**os**·to·me). Incision of the liver. [Gk *hepar* liver, *stoma* mouth.]

hepatotherapy (hep·at·o·**ther**'·ap·e). 1. The therapeutic use of raw liver or liver extract, as in pernicious anaemia. 2. Treatment of any disease of the liver. [Gk *hepar* liver, therapy.]

hepatothrombin (hep·at·o·**throm**'·bin). The fibrin factor, supposedly formed by the liver, which combines with leucothrombin to form thrombin. [Gk *hepar* liver, thrombin.]

hepatotomy (hep·at·**ot**·o·me). Surgical incision into the substance of the liver. **Transthoracic hepatotomy.** Radical treatment of liver abscess by resection of a rib and reaching the liver by way of the cavity of the pleura and the diaphragm. [Gk *hepar* liver, *temnein* to cut.]

hepatotoxic (**hep**·at·o·**tox**'·ik). Destructive to liver cells. [Gk *hepar* liver, toxin.]

hepatotoxin (**hep**·at·o·**tox**'·in). 1. A cytotoxin which may be present in the liver and which, if released, is able to destroy its cells. 2. An antibody derived from an experimental animal into which liver cells have been injected. [Gk *hepar* liver, toxin.]

hepatotropic (**hep**·at·o·**trop**'·ik). Term applied to a substance the action of which is specific for the liver. [Gk *hepar* liver, *trope* a turning.]

hephephilia (hef·e·**fil**·e·ah). A form of sexual perversion in which gratification is obtained by contact with soft smooth fabrics such as silk and velvet; frottage. [Gk *hephaptein* to grasp, *philein* to love.]

Heptabarbitone (hep·tah·**bar**·bit·one). BP Commission approved name for 5-ethyl-5-cyclohept-1'-enylbarbituric acid; it is used in the treatment of insomnia.

heptachromic (hep·tah·**kro**·mik). Applied to persons who possess full colour vision for all the colours of the spectrum. [Gk *hepta* seven, *chroma* colour.]

heptad (**hep**·tad). General term denoting an element or radical with a valency of 7. [Gk *hepta* seven.]

heptadactylism (hep·tah·**dak**·til·izm). The possession of 7 digits at an extremity, hand or foot. [Gk *hepta* seven, *daktylos* finger.]

heptaldehyde (hep·**tal**·de·hide). Heptyl aldehyde, oenanthal, $CH_3(CH_2)_5CHO$. A colourless liquid obtained by the distillation of castor oil under reduced pressure. [Gk *hepta* seven, aldehyde.]

Heptaminol (hep·**tam**·in·ol). BP Commission approved name for 6-amino-2-methylheptan-2-ol; a coronary vasodilator.

heptane (**hep**·tane). C_7H_{16}, a saturated hydrocarbon, seventh in the methane series, which occurs in the resin of Californian pine and in petroleum. A colourless liquid employed as a solvent and anaesthetic. [Gk *hepta* seven.]

heptaploid (**hep**·tah·ploid). Having 7 times the haploid number of chromosomes in the somatic cell nuclei. [Gk *heptaploos* sevenfold, *eidos* form.]

heptatomic (hept·at·**om**·ik). 1. Heptavalent. 2. Describing a molecule composed of 7 atoms. [Gk *hepta* seven, atom.]

heptavalent (hep·tah·**va**·lent). Having a valency of 7. [Gk *hepta* seven, valency.]

heptose (**hep**·tose). A monosaccharide of the general formula $C_7H_{14}O_7$. [Gk *hepta* seven.]

heptosuria (hep·to·**sewr**·e·ah). The condition in which a heptose is present in the urine.

heptyl (**hep**·til). The organic radical C_7H_{15} present in heptyl alcohol. [Gk *hepta* seven.]

Heracleum (her·ah·**kle**·um). A genus of plants, related to the hogweeds, some of which have the property of causing urticaria where the latex comes in contact with the skin. [Gk *Heracles* god of physical strength.]

herapathite (her·**ap**·ath·ite). $4C_{20}H_{24}O_2N_2{\cdot}3H_2SO_4{\cdot}2HI{\cdot}2I_2{\cdot}6H_2O$, a crystalline compound prepared from quinine sulphate and iodine, and used as a polarizer in polarimeters. **Cinchonine herapathite.** The analogous compound of cinchonine, used as an antiseptic.

herb (herb). 1. Botanically, a plant in which the aerial parts do not persist from year to year. 2. In materia medica, any plant which is used for culinary or medicinal purposes. 3. In drug commerce, a drug which consists of the whole plant or of all or the greater part of the aerial portions. [L *herba* grass.]

herbaceous (her·**ba**·shus). Of the nature of a herb.

herbal remedy (**her**·bal **rem**·ed·e). This is a medicinal product consisting of a substance produced by subjecting a plant or plants to drying, crushing or any other process, or of a mixture whose sole ingredients are one or more substances so produced, water or some other inert substance.

herbalist (**her**·bal·ist). 1. A dealer in medicinal herbs. 2. One who believes in the efficacy of herbs and prescribes them or preparations made from them.

herbarium (her·**ba**·re·um). A collection of dried, preserved and pressed plants arranged in order so that they may be studied. [L *herba* grass.]

Herbert, Herbert (b. 1865). Bombay and Nottingham ophthalmic surgeon.

Herbert's operation, for chronic glaucoma. A wedge-shaped trap-door area of sclera is cut, hinged at the limbus. With massage this gives a filtering cicatrix.

herbicarnivorous (her·be·kar·**niv**'·or·us). Applied to an organism that lives on both vegetable and animal food. [herb, L *caro* flesh, *vorare* to devour.]

herbivora (her·**biv**·or·ah). In zoology, name given to a group of mammals that lives mainly if not entirely on herbage. [herb, L *vorare* to devour.]

herbivorous (her·**biv**·er·us). In zoology, feeding on plants. [see prec.]

Herbst, Ernst Friedrich Gustav (b. 1803). Gottingen anatomist.

Herbst's corpuscles. Large sensory end-organs found in the beaks of ducks.

herd (herd). In bacteriology, a large colony of bacteria. [ME host.]

hereditable (her·**ed**·it·abl). Inheritable, as disease that can be transmitted from parent to child. [see foll.]

hereditary (her·**ed**·it·ar·e). Inheritable; transmitted from ancestors or parents to child, as a quality or condition of constitution. [L *hereditas* inheritance.]

hereditation (her·**ed**·it·**a**'·shun). 1. The effects on an individual of the operation of the laws of heredity. 2. The process of heredity.

hereditosyphilitic (her·**ed**·it·o·sif·il·**it**'·ik). Relating or belonging to hereditary syphilis.

heredity (her·**ed**·it·e). The total of the factors, physical and mental, present in the organism at the outset of its individual life and derived from its parents; the handing-on of such factors by parents to offspring. [L *hereditas* inheritance.]

heredo-akinesia (**her**·ed·o·a·kin·**e**'·se·ah). A familial nervous disease of unknown aetiology. It is characterized by sudden temporary attacks of paralysis, severe pain in the extremities and a feeling of general exhaustion. [L *heres* heir, Gk *a*, *kinesis* motion.]

heredo-ataxia (**her**·ed·o·at·**ax**'·e·ah). Friedreich's ataxia. [heredity, ataxia.]

heredobiological (**her**·ed·o·bi·o·**loj**'·ik·al). Relating or belonging to hereditary endogenous factors. [heredity, biological.]

heredodegeneration (**her**·ed·o·de·jen·er·**a**'·shun). Inherited degeneration caused by defective or diseased hyaloplasm of the cell body, as in Marie's ataxia. [heredity, degeneration.]

heredodiathesis (**her**·ed·o·di·**ath**'·es·is). Hereditary predisposition or constitution. [heredity, diathesis.]

heredofamilial (**her**·ed·o·fam·**il**'·e·al). Applied to diseases that are hereditary in certain families. [heredity, familial.]

heredo-immunity (**her**·ed·o·im·**ewn**'·it·e). The state of having inherited immunity from certain diseases or affections. [heredity, immunity.]

heredo-infection (**her**·ed·o·in·**fek**'·shun). Germinal infection, i.e. infection transmitted to the offspring from either the ovum or the spermatozoon of one or other parent. [heredity, infection.]

heredolues (**her**·ed·o·**lew**'·eez). Congenital syphilis. [heredity, L *lues* plague (syphilis).]

heredoluetic (**her**·ed·o·lew·**et**'·ik). Relating or belonging to congenital syphilis. [see prec.]

heredopathia (**her**·ed·o·**path**'·e·ah). Any pathological condition that has been inherited. **Heredopathia atactica polyneuritiformis.** An inborn error of metabolism transmitted by autosomal recessive inheritance and leading to storage of phytanic acid in certain tissues. Clinically there is episodic ataxia, polyneuritis, retinitis pigmentosa and other less constant features. *Refsum's disease.* [heredity, Gk *pathos* disease.]

heredosyphilis (**her**·ed·o·**sif**'·il·is). Congenital syphilis. [see foll.]

heredosyphilitic (**her**·ed·o·sif·il·**it**'·ik). 1. Pertaining to or suffering from congenital syphilis. 2. An individual who is suffering from congenital syphilis. [heredity, syphilis.]

heredosyphilology (**her**·ed·o·sif·il·**ol**'·o·je). That branch of medical science which is concerned with congenital syphilis. [heredity, syphilis, Gk *logos* science.]

heredotrophoedema (her·ed·o·trof·e·**de**'·mah). Hereditary oedema. [heredity, Gk *trophe* nutrition, oedema.]

Hering, Heinrich Ewald (b. 1866). Vienna and Cologne physiologist.

Hering's nerve. A branch of the glossopharyngeal nerve to the carotid sinus and body.

Hering's phenomenon. If the stethoscope is placed over the lower end of the sternum, a faint murmur can be heard for a short time after death.

Hering, Karl Ewald Konstantin (b. 1834). Vienna and Leipzig physiologist.

Hering's canal. The connections between the cell cords of the liver lobules and the bile duct.

Hering's law. 1. The distinctness of a sensation depends on the relation between its intensity and the total intensity of all simultaneous sensation, 2. Any central stimulation. whether excitatory or inhibitory, reaches both eyes equally, so that movement of the two eyes is never independent but takes place in the same direction to the same extent.

Hering's drop test, for stereoscopic vision. The patient looks horizontally through a tube at a thread, and states whether small balls are dropped in front of or behind the thread. Of historical interest only.

Hering's theory. A theory of colour vision, suggesting that there are 3 photochemical substances in the retina, each constantly building up or breaking down; also that there are 6 primary colours in 3 antagonistic pairs, green and red, blue and yellow, and black and white. Green, blue and black build up the photochemical substance; red, yellow and white break it down. Also called *opponent-colours theory.*

Hering-Breuer reflex. A reflex regulating respiration, the act of inspiration reflexly exciting expiration, and vice versa.

Hering-Hillebrand deviation. A physiological deviation whereby intervals on the temporal side of the field of vision seem less than on the nasal side. If an attempt is made to bisect a horizontal line uni-ocularly, the outer half tends to be too large.

Hering-Semon hypothesis, Semon-Hering theory. The mnemic theory. *See* THEORY.

Traube-Hering curve or waves. Slow rhythmical waves on the blood-pressure record of curarized or otherwise immobilized animals and corresponding in frequency with the respiratory rhythm before curarization. They are due to irradiation from the respiratory to the vasomotor centre.

heritable (**her**·it·abl). Capable of being inherited or transmitted from one generation to another, as a disease. [Fr. *héritable.*]

heritage (**her**·it·aje). All those characteristics, physical and psychical, which are transmitted from one generation to the next. [Fr. *héritage.*]

Hermann, Friedrich (b. 1859). Erlangen anatomist.

Hermann's fluid. A fixative containing platinum chloride, glacial acetic acid and osmic acid. It is a good general cytoplasmic fixative, similar in action to Flemming's fluid.

Hermann's mixture. Chloroform, eucalyptus oil and castor oil used for intestinal parasites.

hermaphrodism (her·**maf**·ro·dizm). Hermaphroditism.

hermaphrodite (her·**maf**·ro·dite). 1. A person affected with hermaphroditism. 2. In chemistry, amphoteric, i.e. having basic as well as acid properties.

hermaphroditic (her·**maf**·ro·**dit**'·ik). Referring or belonging to hermaphroditism.

hermaphroditism (her·**maf**·ro·di·tizm). A condition in which the physical characteristics of both sexes are combined in one individual. **Bilateral hermaphroditism.** The condition in which an ovary and a testicle are present on each side. **False hermaphroditism.** Pseudohermaphroditism. **Lateral hermaphroditism.** The condition in which an individual has an ovary on one side and a testicle on the other. **True hermaphroditism.** The condition in which a single individual possesses both the male and the female gonad. **Unilateral hermaphroditism.** The condition in which an individual has an ovary and a testicle on one side and either an ovary or a testicle on the other. [Gk *Hermaphroditos,* son of Hermes and Aphrodite.]

Hermetia (her·**me**·she·ah). A genus of flies of the family Stratiomyidae. The larvae of *Hermetia illucens* have occasionally been recorded in intestinal myiasis.

hermetic, hermetical (her·**met**·ik, her·**met**·ik·al). 1. Made perfectly airtight; guarded from exposure to air as the sealing of a wound. 2. Relating to occult science, especially alchemy. [*Hermes Trismegistus* (*Thoth*), reputed author of alchemical doctrines.]

hermodactyl (her·mo·**dak**·til). The name given to a colchicine-containing drug collected in Asia Minor and used there and in India instead of colchicum. The botanical source has been given as *Colchicum variegatum* Linn. (family Liliaceae). [Gk *hermodaktylos, Colchicum autumnale.*]

hernia (**her**·ne·ah). The protrusion of an internal organ through a defect in the wall of the anatomical cavity in which it lies, or into a subsidiary compartment of that cavity. **Abdominal hernia.** Protrusion of abdominal content through the abdominal wall. **Acquired hernia.** Hernia due to a defect, for example in the abdominal wall, which develops at some time after birth. **Hernia adiposa.** A protrusion of extraperitoneal fat through the abdominal wall. **Amniotic hernia.** Hernia at the umbilicus of a newborn child. **Hernia of the bladder.** Protrusion of the bladder through a defect in the abdominal wall. **Hernia of the brain.** Protrusion of the brain through a defect in the skull. **Broad-ligament hernia.** Hernia through a defect in the broad ligament of the uterus, usually the result of the Baldy-Webster operation for uterine retroversion. **Cerebellar hernia.** Displacement downwards of the cerebellum into the foramen magnum by an increase of pressure within the skull due to head injury, brain tumour or hydrocephalus. **Hernia cerebri.** Hernia of the brain through a defect in the cranium. **Complete hernia.** Protrusion of the hernial sac and abdominal contents through the abdominal wall. **Concealed hernia.** Hernia covered by an outer layer of abdominal wall so that the protrusion cannot be felt. **Congenital hernia.** A hernia due to a defect already present at birth. **Crural hernia.** Cloquet's hernia; a hernia which protrudes behind the posterior layer of the femoral sheath. **Cystic hernia.** Herniation of the bladder. **Diaphragmatic hernia.** Hernia of abdominal content upwards through the diaphragm. **Direct hernia.** Hernia through the posterior wall of the inguinal canal, medial to the deep epigastric vessels. **Dry hernia.** Hernia in which adhesions between protruding organs and sac have obliterated the cavity of the sac. **Duodenojejunal hernia.** Internal hernia (see below) at the site of the duodenojejunal junction. **Encysted hernia.** Hernia surrounded by cystic loculation of its sac. **Epigastric hernia.** Hernia through the linea alba. **External hernia.** Protrusion of an organ externally through the wall of the cavity in which it lies. **Extrasaccular hernia.** Sliding hernia (see below). **Fascial hernia.** Muscle herniation through a hiatus in the deep fascia where it is perforated by a communicating vein. A soft, compressible nodule results on the medial aspect of the leg. **Fat hernia.** Hernia adiposa (see above). **Femoral hernia.** Hernia through the femoral canal. **Foraminal hernia.** Internal hernia (see below) through the foramen of Winslow into the lesser sac of the peritoneum. **Funicular hernia.** Inguinal hernia (see below) into a partial sac. **Gastro-oesophageal hernia.** A hiatus hernia in which the lower end of the oesophagus is involved. **Hernia par glissement.** Sliding hernia (see below). **Gluteal hernia.** Hernia through the greater or lesser sciatic notch into the buttock. **Hiatus hernia.** Diaphragmatic hernia (see above) through the oesophageal hiatus. **Ileo-appendicular hernia.** An internal hernia (see below) in a fossa between the ileum and appendix. **Incarcerated hernia.** Irreducible hernia (see below) of a loop of bowel whose ends are so occluded that its solid content cannot escape. **Incisional hernia.** Hernia through an operation scar. **Indirect hernia.** Hernia through the abdominal inguinal ring. **Infantile hernia.** An inguinal hernia (see following) with the upper part of a hydrocele sac in front of it. **Inguinal hernia.** Hernia at the inguinal canal. **Inguinocrural hernia.** Holthouse's hernia; an inguinal hernia (see preceding) which has turned laterally over the groin. **Inguinofemoral hernia.** Combined femoral and inguinal hernia (see above). **Inguinolabial hernia.** An inguinal hernia (see above) which reaches the subcutaneous tissue of the labium majus. **Intermuscular hernia.** A hernia between 2 muscular layers of the abdominal wall. **Internal hernia.** Hernia into a recess, loculus or fossa of the peritoneal cavity. **Interparietal hernia.** Interstitial hernia (see below). **Intersigmoid hernia.** An internal hernia (see above) in a fossa formed at the root of the sigmoid part of the mesocolon. **Interstitial hernia.** Hernia enlarging behind, between or in front of the layers of the abdominal wall. **Intraperitoneal hernia.** Internal hernia (see above). **Hernia of the iris.** Protrusion of part of the iris. **Irreducible hernia.** Hernia which will not return to its normal situation with suitable manipulation. **Ischiatic hernia.** Gluteal hernia (see above). **Ischiorectal hernia.** Hernia downwards through the levator ani muscle into the perineum. **Labial hernia.** Inguinolabial hernia (see above). **Left duodenal hernia.** Internal hernia (see above) behind the inferior mesenteric vein in Landzert's fossa. **Hernia of the linea alba.** A small protrusion of extraperitoneal fat through a slit in the linea alba. **Lumbar hernia.** Hernia through the lumbar triangle of Petit in the loin. **Hernia of the lung.** Protrusion of lung through a defect in the chest wall. **Hernia magna.** A large congenital hernia with numerous loculi. **Mesenteric hernia.** Internal hernia (see above) through a defect in the mesentery. **Mesenterico-parietal hernia.** Hernia through an opening behind the superior mesenteric artery just below the third part of the duodenum. **Mesocolic hernia.** Hernia through a defect in the mesocolon. **Mucosal hernia.** Protrusion of the gastro-intestinal mucosa through a wound in the seromuscular coat. **Hernia of muscle.** Protrusion of muscle through a defect in its overlying fascia; usually protrusion of the vastus lateralis muscle through a defect in the fascia lata of the thigh. **Hernia of the nucleus pulposus.** Protrusion backwards of a portion of the intervertebral disc into the vertebral canal or intervertebral foramen of the sacrum. **Oblique hernia.** Inguinal hernia (see above) through the abdominal inguinal ring into the inguinal canal. **Obturator hernia.** Hernia through the upper part of the obturator foramen. **Omental hernia.** Protrusion of omentum in a hernial sac. **Hernia of an ovary.** Protrusion of an ovary in an inguinal-hernia sac. **Paracaecal hernia.** Internal hernia (see above) at the site of one of the fossae in relation to the caecum. **Paraduodenal hernia.** Left duodenal hernia (see above). **Para-oesophageal hernia.** Diaphragmatic hernia (see above) through the oesophageal hiatus. **Parasternal hernia.** Diaphragmatic hernia (see above) through a defect between the slip from the sternum and the costal portion of the diaphragm. **Para-umbilical hernia.** Hernia through the linea alba just above the umbilical orifice. **Pectineal hernia.** Femoral hernia (see above) entering the thigh behind the posterior layer of the femoral sheath. **Pelvic hernia.** Any hernia through the pelvic floor. **Perineal hernia.** Hernia through the central point of the perineum. **Pleuroperitoneal hiatus hernia.** A congenital diaphragmatic hernia (see above) through the persistent fetal communication between the peritoneal and pleural cavities. **Posterior vaginal hernia.** Hernia of the pouch of Douglas into the perineum or through the posterior vaginal wall. **Postoperative hernia.** Hernia through a defect produced in the abdominal wall by a previous operation. **Hernia of the pouch of Douglas.** A variety of pelvic hernia (see above) protruding downwards between the vagina and rectum into the perineum, or through the posterior vaginal wall, or backwards into the rectum. **Prevascular hernia.** Femoral hernia (see above) entering the thigh in front of the femoral sheath. **Prevesical hernia.** Hernia downwards between the bladder and pubis in the midline into the space of Retzius. **Properitoneal hernia.** An interstitial hernia (see above) which enlarges between the peritoneum and abdominal muscles. **Pudendal hernia.** Posterior vaginal hernia (see above). **Hernia of pulp.** Protrusion of the dental pulp through the dentine wall of the pulp cavity. **Pulsion hernia.** A hernia caused by sudden increase in pressure in the abdominal cavity, e.g. from a cough. **Rectal hernia.** Hernia of the pouch of Douglas (see above) into the rectum. **Rectovaginal hernia.** Perineal hernia (see above). **Reducible hernia.** A hernia whose contents can be returned into the abdomen by manipulation. **Retrocaecal hernia.** Internal hernia (see above) at the site of the retrocaecal fossa. **Retroduodenal hernia.** Internal hernia (see above) in the fossa behind the third part of the duodenum. **Retrograde hernia.** Return of an intermediate portion of the intestinal content of a hernial sac back into the abdomen. **Retrosternal hernia.** A variety of diaphragmatic hernia (see above) extending from abdomen to chest between the portion of diaphragm arising the xiphoid process and the portion arising from the 7th costal cartilage. **Sciatic hernia.** Hernia through the greater sciatic notch. **Scrotal hernia.** Oblique inguinal hernia which has descended into the scrotum. **Short oesophagus hernia.** Hernia of the stomach upwards through the oesophageal opening in the diaphragm in association with an abnormally short oesophagus. **Sliding hernia, Slip hernia, Slipped hernia.** 1. Hernia during the enlargement of which a partly extraperitoneal organ, usually colon or caecum, descends with the sac so that the hernia contains a sac and its contents and, outside the sac proper, the sliding viscus. 2. The displacement of the gastro-oesophageal junction together with the adjacent part of the stomach through the oesophageal hiatus into the thorax. **Spigelian hernia.** Hernia through the linea semilunaris at the lateral border of the sheath of the rectus abdominis muscle. **Strangulated hernia.** Hernia, the contents of which have their vessels of supply constricted by the neck of the hernial sac or by the edges of the defect in the abdominal wall. **Subfalcial hernia.** Herniation of part of the medial surface of the cerebral hemisphere beneath the falx cerebri, due to a space-occupying lesion. **Subpubic hernia.** Obturator hernia (see above). **Synovial hernia.** Protrusion of the synovial membrane of a joint through the joint capsule. **Tentorial hernia.** Herniation of part of the temporal lobe through the tentorial opening of the dura mater, due to raised intracranial pressure. **Tonsillar hernia.** Herniation of the tonsils of the cerebellum through the foramen magnum of the skull as a result of increase in intracranial pressure from tumour or injury. **Tunicary hernia.** Mucosal hernia (see above). **Umbilical hernia.** Hernia through the umbilical orifice. **Vaginal hernia.** Posterior vaginal hernia (see above). **Vaginolabial hernia.** Inguinolabial hernia (see above). **Ventral hernia.** Any hernia through the anterior abdominal wall. **W hernia.** Maydl's hernia; strangulation by the neck of a hernia of a loop of bowel which has re-entered the abdomen from the hernia and strangulated within the peritoneal cavity. [L rupture.]

See also: BARTH, BÉCLARD, BERGMANN (E.), BIRKETT, BRUGGISSER, CLOQUET (J. G.), COOPER (A. P.), GIBBON (Q. V.), GIMBERNAT, GOYRAND, GRUBER (W. L.), HESSELBACH, HEY (W.), HOLTHOUSE, KROENLEIN, KUESTER, LAUGIER, LITTRÉ, MAYDL, NARATH, PETIT (J. L.), RICHTER (A. G.), RIEUX, ROKITANSKY, SPIEGHEL, TEALE, TREITZ, TREVES, VELPEAU.

hernial (**her**·ne·al). Relating or belonging to hernia.

herniary (**her**·ne·ar·e). 1. Indicating any condition found in association with hernia. 2. Hernial.

herniate (**her**·ne·ate). To burst through a retaining tissue, as in a hernia.

herniation (her·ne·a·shun). The process of formation of a hernia or a protrusion. **Herniation of the nucleus pulposus.** Prolapse of the nucleus pulposus into the spinal canal.

Hernig-Lommel sign. Respiratory arrhythmia, sinus arrhythmia; increase of heart rate on inspiration and decrease on expiration. It is due to variation in the influence of vagal tone on the sinu-atrial node and occurs frequently in normal children, less often in adults.

hernio-appendicectomy (**her**·ne·o·ap·**en**·dis·**ek**′·to·me). The combined operation of herniotomy and appendicectomy.

herniocoeliotomy (**her**·ne·o·se·le·**ot**′·o·me). Incision through the abdomen for the reduction of hernia. [hernia, coeliotomy.]

hernio-enterotomy (**her**·ne·o·en·ter·**ot**′·o·me). Combined herniotomy and enterotomy.

hernioid (**her**·ne·oid). Having resemblance to hernia. [hernia, Gk *eidos* form.]

herniolaparotomy (**her**·ne·o·**lap**·ar·**ot**′·o·me). Herniocoeliotomy. [hernia, laparotomy.]

herniology (her·ne·**ol**·o·je). That branch of medical science which is concerned with hernia, its cause, diagnosis and radical treatment. [hernia, Gk *logos* science.]

hernioplasty (**her**·ne·o·plas·te). Operative reduction of hernia. [hernia, Gk *plassein* to mould.]

herniopuncture (**her**·ne·o·**pungk**′·tcher). Reduction of a hernia by the insertion of a hollow needle through which liquid or gas can be withdrawn. [hernia, puncture.]

herniorrhaphy (her·ne·**or**·af·e). The radical cure of hernia by replacement of the protruded tissue and strengthening the weakened wall by suturing it. [hernia, Gk *rhaphe* seam.]

herniotome (**her**·ne·o·tome). A surgical knife used in herniotomy.

herniotomy (her·ne·**ot**·o·me). The operation for the relief of hernia and the resultant reduction of the latter. [hernia, Gk *temnein* to cut.]

heroic (he·**ro**·ik). Term applied to the treatment of desperate illness by bold or normally unorthodox measures, either surgical or medical. [Gk *heroikos* relating to a hero.]

heroin (**her**·o·in). Diacetylmorphine, $C_{21}H_{23}O_5N$. A synthetic derivative of morphine produced by acetylation of both OH groups. It resembles morphine in its general effects but has stronger excitatory actions, and is a more powerful and quicker-acting analgesic; at the same time it is more toxic especially on the respiratory centre. Though it depresses the cough centre, the drug offers no real advantage over morphine in this respect, apart from a reduced incidence of nausea and vomiting. In view of its severe addictive properties the use of this drug has been prohibited in some countries but, since the drug is easily made, it is claimed that this measure only makes its legitimate use difficult and encourages its illegal manufacture. It causes intense euphoria together with excitation, and addiction once produced is most difficult to treat successfully. It is usually administered in the form of the hydrochloride. [etym. dub.]

heroinism (**her**·o·in·izm). 1. The habitual use of heroin. 2. The condition that is the result of addiction to heroin.

heroinomania (**her**·o·in·o·**ma**′·ne·ah). Excessive or insane addiction to heroin. [heroin, mania.]

herpangina (her·pan·**ji**·nah). A specific, mild, febrile throat infection (angina) of children. It is caused by Coxsackie group A viruses, which are enteroviruses and not members of the herpes group. Vesicles and small ulcers develop in the tonsillar region and disappear in a few days. Epidemics have occurred in summer and autumn. The mode of spread is from cases, convalescent carriers and contacts. [herpes, angina.]

herpes (**her**·peez). Inflammation of the skin or mucous membrane, with clusters of deep-seated vesicles. **Herpes B.** A natural herpes-like infection of Asiatic monkeys, including Rhesus and Cynomolgus species, which can be transmitted to those handling monkeys or monkey tissues. It causes local inflammation at the site of a bite followed by an ascending myelitis, or an encephalomyelitis. Almost all cases have been fatal; recovery is associated with residual disability. **Herpes circinatus bullosus** (Wilson, 1867). Herpes gestationis (see below). **Herpes cornealis.** A variety of herpes simplex affecting the cornea and leading to dendritic ulceration. **Herpes desquamans** (Turner). Tinea imbricata. **Herpes digitalis.** A variety of herpes simplex affecting the fingers or toes and the nails. **Herpes disseminatus.** A disseminated form of herpes simplex occurring in children with atopic dermatitis. **Herpes encephalitis.** Herpes simplex complicated by encephalitis (rare). **Herpes facialis, Herpes febrilis.** Herpes simplex (see below). **Herpes generalisatus.** 1. Herpes zoster associated with lesions identical with those of chickenpox elsewhere in the body. 2. A generalized herpetiform eruption occurring as a sequel to an acute infectious fever. **Herpes of the geniculate ganglion.** Herpes zoster oticus (see below). **Herpes genitalis.** Herpes progenitalis (see below). **Herpes gestationis.** A bulbous eruption occurring as a complication of pregnancy. Often the malady appears before the seventh month of gestation, but it may develop later in pregnancy. Retrogression may occur after delivery, but there may be recurrences in succeeding pregnancies. **Herpes iris.** A special variety of erythema multiforme in which the lesions are concentric rings of vesicles. **Herpes keratoconjunctivitis.** Herpes simplex associated with keratitis and conjunctivitis. **Herpes labialis.** Herpes simplex (see below) affecting the lip or lips. **Herpes menstrualis.** Recurrent herpes simplex, the lesions appearing at the time of menstruation. **Herpes mentalis.** Herpes of the chin. **Herpes ophthalmicus.** Herpes zoster ophthalmicus (see below). **Herpes phlyctaenodes.** Dermatitis herpetiformis. **Herpes praeputialis.** Herpes simplex (see below) involving the prepuce. **Herpes progenitalis.** Herpes simplex (see below) involving the penis or the vulva. **Herpes pyaemicus.** Impetigo herpetiformis. **Herpes recurrens, Recurrent herpes.** The recurrence of herpes simplex. **Herpes simplex.** An acute vesicular eruption which most commonly appears at mucocutaneous junctions, especially on the face, but lesions may be found anywhere on the body. Once established, usually in childhood, the disease recurs at intervals with complete healing between episodes. Recurrence is precipitated by disturbed metabolism which can be provided by febrile illnesses, ultraviolet light, menstruation or emotional stress. Strains of the causative virus, herpes simplex virus, that are isolated from the genital area are slightly different (antigenically, biochemically and in growth patterns) from those isolated from elsewhere on the body. Such strains are referred to as type II and an association has been found between the possession of antibody to the type II virus and the development of cervical cancer in women. However, a direct cause-and-effect relationship has not been established. Herpes simplex is generally a benign, if uncomfortable, infection but rare complications include encephalitis and a generalized infection in neonates, both of which carry a high mortality. Idoxuridine has been used in the treatment of *herpes keratoconjunctivitis, herpes encephalitis* and generalized herpes, and some success has been reported. Synonyms for the disease include: *cold sores, herpes febrilis, herpes genitalis, herpes labialis, herpes recurrens.* **Herpes simplex cornealis.** Dendritic ulcer. *See* ULCER. **Herpes tonsurans.** Tinea capitis. **Herpes tonsurans barbae.** Tinea barbae. **Herpes tonsurans capillitii.** Tinea capitis. **Herpes tonsurans maculosus.** Stelwagon supported Jarisch's contention that there are 2 maladies, clinically indistinguishable: the first, pityriasis rosea; the second, a type of extensively distributed ringworm. The name was therefore applicable to each disease, but connoted the second. **Herpes vacciniforme.** A vacciniform eruption occurring on the napkin area of neglected infants. **Herpes vegetans.** Pemphigus vegetans. **Herpes zoster.** Shingles, zona. An acute vesicular inflammation due to the recrudescence of chickenpox virus which has remained latent, probably in the posterior root ganglia of the spinal cord, since the initial infection. The eruption is usually unilateral, following accurately the distribution of a cutaneous sensory nerve. It may be preceded, accompanied or followed by neuralgia which may be very severe and which is more common in older people. Healing occurs without scarring even after extensive areas of involvement. Chickenpox may be caught from zoster, but not vice versa. The mechanism by which the latent virus is activated is not known; there is no specific therapy. **Herpes zoster ophthalmicus.** Herpes zoster affecting the first division of the 5th cranial nerve. The frontal, nasal and palpebral regions are involved and ocular complications are frequent, especially when the nasociliary branch is implicated, as shown by the appearance of vesicles on the ala of the nose. **Herpes zoster oticus.** A painful form of herpes said to result from a virus infection of the ganglion of the facial nerve; sometimes referred to as a herpes of the ganglion of the facial nerve or as Hunt's syndrome. The mild forms are associated with a vesicular deposit on the ear-drum, which is easily missed; in the more severe form there is widespread vesicle formation of the ear-drum, external auditory meatus and the pinna, and sometimes of the pharynx. The facial nerve may be paralysed; there may also be pronounced deafness and severe dizziness. [Gk *herpein* to creep.]

herpesvirus (her·peez·vi'·rus). The generic name for a group of DNA-containing viruses which have a very similar structure but few other properties in common, and which are dissimilar antigenically. They have a symmetrical core or capsid, 100 nm in diameter, surrounded by an outer envelope. The members of the group include herpes simplex, varicella/zoster, cytomegalovirus, Epstein-Barr virus and herpes B, all of which infect man, and numerous animal viruses which are found in a wide variety of species. [herpes, virus.]

herpetic (her·**pet**·ik). Relating, belonging to, or having the characteristics of herpes.

herpetiform (her·**pet**·e·form). Having resemblance to herpes. [herpes, form.]

herpetology (her·pet·**ol**·o·je). That branch of medical science which is concerned with diseases of the skin, particularly herpetic diseases. [herpes, Gk *logos* science.]

herpetomonad (her·pet·**om**·on·ad). A protozoon of the genus *Herpetomonas.*

Herpetomonas (her·pet·**om**·on·as). A genus of the family Trypanosomidae; species of this genus are confined to invertebrate hosts, especially arthropods. From time to time these parasites have been noted in blood-sucking arthropods and mistaken for species of other genera of this family, e.g. *Leishmania* and *Trypanosoma.* [Gk *herpeton* reptile, *monas* unit.]

herpetomoniasis (her·**pet**·o·mon·i'·as·is). Infection with any species of *Herpetomonas.*

Herrick, James Bryan (b. 1861). Chicago physician.

Herrick's anaemia. Sickle-cell anaemia. *See* ANAEMIA.

Herring, Percy Theodore (b. 1872). St. Andrews physiologist.

Herring's bodies. Masses of deeply staining material found throughout the posterior lobe of the hypophysis cerebri. They consist of accumulations of neurosecretion which have passed down the hypothalamo-hypophyseal tract.

Herring test, Herring-Binet test. A revision (1922) of the Binet test, including a grouping of tests enabling a short form to be used when required.

hersage (her·sage). In disease of any area served by a peripheral nerve, the operation of splitting the nerve sheath and so releasing the fibres, which are then teased out and left free. [Fr. harrowing.]

Herter, Christian Archibald (b. 1865). New York pathologist.

Herter's disease, Gee-Herter disease, Gee-Herter-Heubner disease, Herter-Heubner disease. Coeliac disease (*see* DISEASE) or the infantile form of idiopathic steatorrhoea (*see* STEATORRHOEA).

Herter's β-naphthoquinone test, for indole. To 10 ml of test solution add 2 drops of 2 per cent β-naphthoquinone sodium monosulphonate and 2 ml of 10 per cent sodium hydroxide. Allow to stand for 15 min, add 2 ml of chloroform and mix gently. The chloroform is coloured reddish-pink if indole is present in the test solution.

Hertig, Arthur Tremain (b. 1904). Boston pathologist and embryologist.

Hertig-Rock embryo. One of a number of beautifully-preserved and accurately-dated early human embryos, acquired and described by Hertig and Rock in 1952.

Hertig-Rock ovum. A fertilized human ovum, 7–7½ days old, described in 1945.

Hertwig, Karl Wilhelm Theodor Richard (b. 1850). Jena embryologist.

Hertwig-Magendie sign or syndrome. Skew deviation of the eyes occurring in acute cerebellar lesions; the eye on the same side looks down and in, on the opposite side it looks up and out.

Hertwig, Wilhelm August Oscar (b. 1849). Jena and Berlin anatomist.

Hertwig's sheath. Epithelial sheath; a downgrowth from the enamel organ around the root of a developing tooth which determines the form of the root.

hertz (hertz). A unit of frequency indicating number of cycles per second. Symbol Hz.

Hertz, Heinrich Rudolf (b. 1857). Bonn physicist.

hertzian wave. An electromagnetic wave of the type used in radio.

Herxheimer, Karl (b. 1861). Frankfurt dermatologist.

Herxheimer fever. Pyrexia associated with the Herxheimer reaction (see below).

Herxheimer fibres. Spirally-arranged fibres found in the stratum germinativum of the epidermis.

Herxheimer's method, for elastic fibres. After fixation with Mueller's fluid, stain in an alcoholic solution of haematoxylin containing lithium carbonate; differentiate with ferric chloride. Elastic fibres are stained black against a bluish background.

Herxheimer reaction, Jarisch-Herxheimer reaction. Intensification of a syphilitic lesion, associated with pyrexia and malaise, occurring within a few hours of an injection of a potent antisyphilitic remedy.

Pick-Herxheimer disease. Acrodermatitis chronica atrophicans.

Heryng, Théodor (b. 1847). Polish laryngologist.

Heryng's sign, Voltolini-Heryng sign. Absence of a crescentic area of light in the infra-orbital region in cases of disease of the maxillary antrum, when this sinus is illuminated from the mouth.

Herz, Max (b. 1865). German physician.

triad of Herz. Phrenocardia; a psychogenic condition characterized by palpitation, pain under the left breast and sighing.

Heschl, Richard Ladislaus (b. 1824). Graz and Vienna pathologist.

Heschl's convolutions, Transverse gyri of Heschl. Small gyri on the upper surface of the temporal operculum of the insula where the auditory radiations end.

hesperanopia (hes·per·an·o'·pe·ah). Night blindness. *See* BLINDNESS. [Gk *hespera* evening, *a*, *ops* eye.]

hesperetin (hes·**per**·et·in). $C_{16}H_{14}O_6$, the flavone which occurs as a glucoside in hesperidin.

hesperidene (hes·**per**·id·een). D-Limonene.

hesperidin (hes·**per**·id·in). $C_{22}H_{26}O_{12}$, a flavone glucoside found in lemon and orange peel, and known commercially as *citrin.* Its effect is to strengthen the capillary walls to pressure, and it is a factor against capillary haemorrhage (vitamin P).

Hess, Alfred Fabian (b. 1875). American physician.

Hess' test. Capillary resistance test; a test to measure the resistance of the capillaries to increased venous pressure. A sphygmomanometer cuff is placed on the forearm and inflated to a pressure midway between the systolic and diastolic arterial pressures for a period of 5 min. The test is positive when large numbers of petechiae appear over the forearm, indicating an abnormality of the vascular endothelium, with or without thrombocytopenia. A positive result is obtained in diseases associated with purpura.

Hess, Carl von (b. 1863). Würzburg ophthalmologist.

Hess operation, for ptosis. The upper lid is slung to the occipitofrontalis muscle above the eyebrow with silk sutures.

Hess, Germain Henri (b. 1802). German chemist.

Hess' law. In a chemical reaction the total heat evolved or absorbed is the same whether the action proceeds in stages or directly, provided that the end-products are the same.

Hess, Walter Rudolf (b. 1881). Swiss physiologist and ophthalmologist.

Hess chart. The chart on which the results of the Hess screen test (see below) for diplopia are recorded.

Hess screen and screen test. A form of tangent screen made of black cloth and marked with thin red horizontal and vertical lines forming squares subtending an angle of 5 degrees; every 15 degrees there is a red spot at the intersection. The patient, wearing red and green goggles, sits at half a metre, and places a green circle on the end of a pointer on each red dot in turn. Any error of the green pointer shows the amount of weakness or overaction of any of the ocular muscles, which is recorded on a Hess chart.

Hesselbach, Franz kaspar (b. 1759). Würzburg anatomist and surgeon.

Hesselbach's fascia. The cribriform fascia. *See* FASCIA.

Hesselbach's hernia. Hernia through the lateral part of the femoral sheath and the femoral artery, usually associated with oblique inguinal hernia.

Hesselbach's ligament. Interfoveolar ligament; the lateral portion of the conjoint tendon of the transversus abdominis muscle.

Hesselbach's triangle. Inguinal triangle; the triangle bounded by the lateral margin of the rectus abdominis muscle, the inferior epigastric vessels and the inguinal (Poupart's) ligament. It marks the site of development of a direct inguinal hernia.

Hetacillin (het·ah·sil·in). BP Commission approved name for 6-(2,2-dimethyl-5-oxo-4-phenylimidazolidin-1-yl)penicillanic acid; an antibiotic.

heteracephalus (het·er·a·kef'·al·us). Heterocephalus.

heteradelphia (het·er·ad·el'·fe·ah). Of a twin monster, the condition in which the parasite is joined to the abdomen of the autosite and is very incompletely developed. A heteradelphous teratism. [Gk *heteros* different, *adelphos* brother.]

heteradelphous (het·er·ad·el'·fus). Relating to a heteradelphus or to any monster consisting of an autosite and a parasite.

heteradelphus (het·er·ad·el'·fus). A twin monster of which the parasite is very incomplete and may lack a head; it is joined to the abdomen of the autosite. [Gk *heteros* different, *adelphos* brother.]

heteradenia (het·er·ad·e'·ne·ah). 1. Any abnormal condition or structure of a gland or of gland tissue. 2. The condition in which glandular tissue is present in parts which normally do not contain glands. [Gk *heteros* different, *aden* gland.]

heteradenic (het·er·ad·e'·nik). Referring or belonging to, or affected with heteradenia.

heteradenoma (het·er·ad·en·o'·mah). An adenoma arising in tissue normally not provided with glands. [Gk *heteros* different, adenoma.]

heteraesthesia (het·er·es·the'·ze·ah). Hetero-aesthesia. [Gk *heteros* different, aesthesia.]

heteralicus, heteralius (het·er·a·lik·us, het·er·a·le·us). A twin monster of which the parasite is so incompletely developed as to be little more than a projection on the abdomen of the autosite and without apparent connection with the umbilical cord of the autosite. [Gk *heteros* different, *alos* disc.]

heterauxesis (het·er·awx·e'·sis). In plant physiology, any unsymmetrical or irregular growth of organs or tissues. [Gk *heteros* different, *auxe* increase.]

heteraxial (het·er·ax·e·al). In zoology, having 3 axes perpendicular to each other but unequal in length, as in animals with bilateral symmetry. [Gk *heteros* different, axis.]

hetero-aesthesia (het·er·o·es·the'·ze·ah). A condition in which the sensitivity of the skin varies as between 2 adjoining areas of the body surface. [Gk *heteros* different, aesthesia.]

hetero-agglutinin (het·er·o·ag·loo'·tin·in). An agglutinin in the serum of an animal which is able to agglutinate the red blood cells of an animal of a different species. [Gk *heteros* different, agglutinin.]

hetero-albumose (het·er·o·al·bew'·moze). A hemialbumose that is insoluble in water but soluble in hydrochloric acid and solutions of sodium chloride. [Gk *heteros* different, albumose.]

hetero-albumosuria (het·er·o·al·bew·mo·sewr'·e·ah). The presence of hetero-albumose in the urine.

heteroalleles (het·er·o·al·eelz'). A pair of homologous genes having mutations at different sites (DNA base pairs). [Gk *heteros* different, *allelon* of one another.]

hetero-antibody (het·er·o·an·te·bod·e). An antibody which corresponds to an antigen from another species of animal. [Gk *heteros* different, antibody.]

hetero-atom (het·er·o·at'·om). In a heterocyclic compound, that atom of the ring structure which is not carbon. [Gk *heteros* different, atom.]

hetero-autoplasty (het·er·o·awt'·o·plas·te). In plastic surgery, the transference of a portion of skin or tissue from one part of the body to another. [Gk *heteros* different, autoplasty.]

hetero-auxin (het·er·o·awx'·in). Indole-acetic acid, indolyl β-acetic acid, $C_6H_4C(NHCH)(CH_2)_2COOH$. A product of the bacterial decomposition of tryptophan which appears in the urine. It is a hormone-like substance which promotes root growth in plants.

heteroblastic (het·er·o·blas·tik). Originating in tissue of another kind. [Gk *heteros* different, *blastos* germ.]

heterocele (het·er·o·seel). Hernia present in a prolapsed organ, as in proctocele. [Gk *heteros* different, *kele* hernia.]

heterocellular (het·er·o·sel'·ew·lar). In biology, formed of more than one kind of cell. [Gk *heteros* different, cell.]

heterocentric (het·er·o·sen'·trik). 1. Of an individual, having the focus of interest in other people, not in self. 2. Of rays of light, not meeting at a common focus. [Gk *heteros* different, centre.]

heterocephalus (het·er·o·kef'·al·us). A monster with 2 heads of which one is smaller than the other. [Gk *heteros* different, *kephale* head.]

heterocheiral (het·er·o·ki'·ral). 1. Relating to the opposite hand. 2. In physics, describing a mirror image which is identical in shape and size with the original object, but reversed. [Gk *heteros* different, *cheir* hand.]

heterochromatic (het·er·o·kro·mat'·ik). Of chromosomes or chromosome regions, showing the behaviour characteristic of heterochromatin. [Gk *heteros* different, chromatin.]

heterochromatin (het·er·o·kro'·mat·in). Chromosomes or chromosome regions which are densely packed in interphase, prophase and, possibly, telophase and stain differently from the rest of the chromatin (euchromatin) with conventional stains. The term is now often used to denote any chromosome region showing a staining and/or coiling behaviour different from the rest of the chromatin, thus embracing positive and negative heteropyknosis. Heterochromatin has important functional characteristics usually associated with the described morphological behaviour, namely: late DNA replication, reduced RNA priming activity, relative genic inertness. Although euchromatin and heterochromatin are often considered different states of the same substance, there is some evidence indicating that they may differ in the nature and association of their proteins to the DNA and that constitutive heterochromatin may be particularly rich in repetitive DNA sequences. **Constitutive heterochromatin.** Chromatin which is heterochromatic in both members of a homologous pair and which, presumably, does not revert to a euchromatic state during the life history of the organism. **Facultative heterochromatin.** Chromatin which is heterochromatic in only one member of a homologous pair and which assumes the euchromatic behaviour during some stage of the life history of the organism. [Gk *heteros* different, chromatin.]

heterochromatinization (het·er·o·kro·mat·in·i·za'·shun). The process resulting in the acquisition by chromosomes or chromosome regions of the heterochromatic properties. [Gk *heteros* different, chromatin.]

heterochromatization (het·er·o·kro·mat·i·za·shun). Heterochromatinization.

heterochromatosis (het·er·o·kro·mat·o'·sis). 1. Heterochromia. 2. Discoloration of the skin caused by foreign substances. [Gk *heteros* different, chromatosis.]

heterochromia (het·er·o·kro'·me·ah). A difference of colour in 2 structures or in 2 parts of the same structure which normally are of the same colour, as of the irides of the eye. [Gk *heteros* different, *chroma* colour.]

heterochromosome (het·er·o·kro'·mo·some). A chromosome which occurs as a homologous pair in one sex, and as an unlike pair or as a single chromosome in the other; a sex chromosome. **X heterochromosome.** A chromosome with peculiar and distinctive form of behaviour. Often used to denote the sex chromosomes.

heterochromous (het·er·o·kro'·mus). In biology, showing abnormal difference in coloration; showing heterochromia. [Gk *heteros* different, *chroma* colour.]

heterochron (**het**·er·o·kron). Relating to the development of parts or tissues at an abnormal time. [Gk *heteros* different, *chronos* time.]

heterochronia (**het**·er·o·**kro′**·ne·ah). 1. Occurring irregularly in time. 2. Differences in chronaxia amongst grouped and similar neurones. [Gk *heteros* different, *chronos* time.]

heterochronic, heterochronous (**het**·er·o·**kron′**·ik, het·er·**ok**·ron·us). 1. Referring or belonging to heterochronia. 2. Occurring at irregular times or not at the proper times. 3. Specifically, term applied to a teratoma occurring in an unusual situation.

heterochthonous (het·er·**ok**·thon·us). Arising or having its origin in some region other than that in which the particular structure is found. Applied to tumours arising in the body from cells of another individual, e.g. choriocarcinoma. [Gk *heteros* different, *chthon* ground.]

heterocinesia (het·er·o·sin·**e′**·ze·ah). A condition in which the patient makes movements the reverse of or other than those which he has been requested to make. [Gk *heteros* different, *kinesis* movement.]

heterocladic (**het**·er·o·**klad′**·ik). Term applied to anastomoses between terminal branches of different arterial trunks. [Gk *heteros* different, *klados* twig.]

heterocomplement (**het**·er·o·**kom′**·ple·ment). A complement from a different species of animal from that providing the amboceptor. [Gk *heteros* different, complement.]

heterocrania (**het**·er·o·**kra′**·ne·ah). 1. A condition in which the skull is asymmetrical. 2. Unilateral headache. [Gk *heteros* different, *kranion* skull.]

heterocrine (**het**·er·o·krine). Secreting more than one specific juice. [Gk *heteros* different, *krinein* to secrete.]

heterocrisis (**het**·er·o·**kri′**·sis). In disease, a crisis which is either irregular in time of occurrence or unusual in symptoms shown. [Gk *heteros* different, crisis.]

heterocyclic (**het**·er·o·**si′**·klik). Denoting a cyclic compound which contains in its ring structure one or more atoms of elements other than carbon. [Gk *heteros* different, cycle.]

heterocytolysin (**het**·er·o·si·**tol′**·is·in). Heterolysin. [Gk *heteros* different, *kytos* cell, lysin.]

heterocytotoxin (**het**·er·o·si·to·**tox′**·in). A toxin which has a destructive action on the cells of another species of animal. [Gk *heteros* different, cytotoxin.]

Heterodera radicicola (het·er·**od**·er·ah **rad**·is·ik·**o′**·lah). A nematode worm of edible vegetables which may survive intestinal passage and appear in human faeces. Its presence may lead to mistakes in diagnosis; a pseudoparasite. [Gk *heteros* different, *dere* neck, L *radix* root, *colere* to cultivate.]

heterodermic (**het**·er·o·**der′**·mik). Applied to the method of skin grafting (dermatoheteroplasty) in which the skin of another person is used. [Gk *heteros* different, *derma* skin.]

heterodesmotic (**het**·er·o·dez·**mot′**·ik). Applied to nerve fibres which connect nerve centres with other parts or one centre with a dissimilar centre. [Gk *heteros* different, *desmos* band.]

heterodidymus (**het**·er·o·**did′**·im·us). A double monster of which the parasite consists only of an imperfect head, neck and thorax, the last 2 parts growing out of the anterior abdominal wall of the autosite. [Gk *heteros* different, *didymos* twin.]

heterodikaryon (**het**·er·o·di·**kar′**·e·on). A cell, spore or mycelium containing 2 genetically different nuclei. [Gk *heteros* different, di-, *karyon* nut.]

heterodont (**het**·er·o·dont). In biology, having teeth of different sorts (e.g. canine, incisor), as man. [Gk *heteros* different, *odous* tooth.]

heterodrome (**het**·er·o·drome). In electricity, a current induced in the opposite direction. [see foll.]

heterodromia (**het**·er·o·**dro′**·me·ah). The condition in which conduction is better in one direction than the other, especially in nerve or muscle. [Gk *heteros* different, *dromos* course.]

heterodymus (het·er·**od**·im·us). Heterodidymus.

heteroecious (het·er·e·she·us). Applied to parasites which have different hosts at different stages of their life cycle. [see foll.]

heteroecism (het·er·**e**·sizm). In the life cycle of a parasite, the occurrence of more than one stage, each of which is passed in a different host. [Gk *heteros* different, *oikos* house.]

hetero-eroticism (**het**·er·o·er·**ot′**·is·izm, **het**·er·o·**er′**·ot·izm). Sexual desire fixed on another individual of the opposite sex. [Gk *heteros* different, eroticism.]

heterogametic (**het**·er·o·gam·**et′**·ik). Of the sex which produces male or female determining gametes. [Gk *heteros* different, gamete.]

heterogamy (het·er·**og**·am·e). Conjugation between gametes of unequal size, as in all higher animals and plants. [see prec.]

heteroganglionic (**het**·er·o·gang·gle·**on′**·ik). 1. Connecting or associated with ganglia in widely-separated position. 2. Referring to various or different ganglia. In both cases, the term is applied to the autonomic nervous system. [Gk *heteros* different, ganglion.]

heterogeneity (**het**·er·o·jen·**e′**·it·e). The state or quality of being heterogeneous.

heterogeneous (**het**·er·o·**je′**·ne·us). 1. Dissimilar in kind; having different or dissimilar characteristics and qualities. 2. Composed of different ingredients. [Gk *heteros* different, *genos* kind.]

heterogenesis (**het**·er·o·**jen′**·es·is). 1. The production of offspring having different characteristics in successive generations. 2. Asexual generation. *See* GENERATION. 3. Abiogenesis. [Gk *heteros* different, genesis.]

heterogenetic (**het**·er·o·jen·**et′**·ik). 1. Relating or belonging to, or characterized by heterogenesis. 2. Originating outside the organism. 3. Heterophil.

heterogenic, heterogenous (**het**·er·o·**jen′**·ik, het·er·**oj**·en·us). 1. Originating in a different species. 2. Derived from a different source. 3. Occurring abnormally in one of the sexes; masculine or feminine characters showing themselves in opposite sexes. [Gk *heteros* different, *genos* kind.]

heterogenote (**het**·er·o·**je′**·note). In bacterial genetics, connoting a bacterium heterozygous for a region of chromosome by carrying an F-prime factor or localized transducing phage. [Gk *heteros* different, *genein* to produce.]

heterogony (het·er·**og**·on·e). Heterogenesis. [Gk *heteros* different, *gone* seed.]

heterograft (**het**·er·o·grahft). In skin or tissue grafting, a portion of skin taken from an animal of a different species, not from the patient himself (autograft) or from another individual. [Gk *heteros* different, graft.]

heterohaemagglutinin (**het**·er·o·he·mag·**loo′**·tin·in). A blood agglutinin that causes agglutination of the red cells of other species. [Gk *heteros* different, *haima* blood, agglutinin.]

heterohaemolysin (**het**·er·o·he·**mol′**·is·in). A haemolysin which occurs naturally in the blood of an animal and can cause haemolysis in an animal of a different species. [Gk *heteros* different, haemolysin.]

heterohexosan (**het**·er·o·**hex′**·o·san). General term for the complex polysaccharides which contain non-carbohydrate units combined with hexose residues. [Gk *heteros* different, hexose.]

heterohypnosis (**het**·er·o·hip·**no′**·sis). Hypnosis induced by another individual. [Gk *heteros* different, hypnosis.]

heteroid, heteroideus (**het**·er·oid, het·er·**oid**·e·us). Indicating that 2 parts of a structure are formed of different substances, such as a sheath and the structure it encloses. [Gk *heteros* different, *eidos* form.]

hetero-immune (**het**·er·o·im·**ewn′**). Possessing immunity to an antigen from another species of animal. [Gk *heteros* different, immunity.]

hetero-infection (**het**·er·o·in·**fek′**·shun). Infection acquired from a micro-organism originating outside the body; the opposite of auto-infection. [Gk *heteros* different, infection.]

hetero-inoculation (**het**·er·o·in·ok·ew·**la′**·shun). Inoculation with a virus derived from another person or another organism. [Gk *heteros* different, inoculation.]

hetero-intoxication (**het**·er·o·in·tox·ik·**a′**·shun). A state of poisoning caused by substances introduced from outside the body; the opposite of auto-intoxication. [Gk *heteros* different, intoxication.]

heterokaryon (het·er·o·**kar**'·e·on). A multinucleated cell or organism containing genetically different nuclei. Hetero*di*karyon, hetero*tri*karyon and hetero*poly*karyon are heterokaryons with 2, 3 and more than 2 nuclei, respectively. [Gk *heteros* different, *karyon* nut.]

heterokaryotic (het·er·o·kar·e·**ot**'·ik). Referring to heterokaryons.

heterokaryotype (het·er·o·**kar**'·e·o·tipe). A karyotype showing heterozygosity for a chromosomal structural change. [Gk *heteros* different, *karyon* nut, *typos* mark.]

heterokeratoplasty (het·er·o·**ker**'·at·o·plas·te). Plastic surgery of the cornea in which a corneal graft from an animal is used. [Gk *heteros* different, keratoplasty.]

heterolalia (het·er·o·**la**'·le·ah). A variety of aphasia in which terms and words are habitually or often incorrectly used; saying one thing and meaning another. [Gk *heteros* different, *lalein* to babble like a child.]

heterolateral (het·er·o·**lat**'·er·al). Relating to or occurring on the opposite side. [Gk *heteros* different, L *latus* side.]

heteroliteral (het·er·o·**lit**'·er·al). 1. Characterized by or relating to the substitution of one letter for another in the utterance of words, as a *w* for an *r* before vowels. 2. Relating to or characterized by stammering over the pronunciation of any particular letter or word. [Gk *heteros* different, L *littera* letter.]

heterolith (het·er·o·lith). An intestinal concretion that is composed of substances other than mineral. [Gk *heteros* different, *lithos* stone.]

heterologous (het·er·**ol**·og·us). 1. In general, differing from the normal or from some other specified substance; not homologous or autologous, as serum. 2. Composed of divers proportions of like elements or of different elements. 3. Of a different species. **Heterologous transplantation.** *See* TRANSPLANTATION. [Gk *heteros* different, *logos* relation.]

heterology (het·er·**ol**·o·je). 1. An abnormality in form or derivation. 2. The development of cells in such a way that they differ from the parent cells. 3. Chemically, the relationship of substances which resemble one another in structure, but display completely different properties. [see prec.]

heterolysin (het·er·**ol**·is·in). A lysin which forms as the result of introduction into the blood of an antigen derived from an animal belonging to a different species; distinct from homolysin and autolysin. [Gk *heteros* different, lysin.]

heterolysis (het·er·**ol**·is·is). 1. The dissolution of the blood corpuscles of an animal of one species by blood serum of an animal of another species. 2. The destruction or digestion of a cell by an external agent; the opposite of autolysis. [Gk *heteros* different, lysis.]

heterolysosome (het·er·o·**li**'·so·some). A membrane-bound body within a cell resulting from the fusion of a lysosome and a heterophagosome so that the contents of the latter are exposed to the enzymes of the former. [Gk *heteros* different, *lysis* a loosing, *soma* body.]

heterolytic (het·er·o·**lit**'·ik). Having relation to or caused by heterolysis or by a heterolysin.

heteromastigote (het·er·o·**mas**'·tig·ote). A mastigote which has an anterior and a posterior flagellum. [Gk *heteros* different, mastigote.]

heteromeral, heteromeric (het·er·**om**·er·al, **het**·er·o·**mer**'·ik). Term applied to spinal neurones some processes of which pass over to the opposite side of the spinal cord. [see foll.]

heteromerous (het·er·**om**·er·us). 1. Having homologous parts differing in composition. 2. Heteromeral. 3. Unrelated or not alike in chemical composition; term applied to homoeomorphous substances. [Gk *heteros* different, *meros* part.]

heterometaplasia (het·er·o·met·ah·**pla**'·ze·ah). The development of tissue of a kind that is not natural to the part in which it is produced. [Gk *heteros* different, metaplasia.]

heterometropia (het·er·o·met·**ro**'·pe·ah). The condition in which there is a dissimilar degree of refraction as between the two eyes. [Gk *heteros* different, *metron* measure, *ops* eye.]

heterometry (het·er·**om**·et·re). Variation of a part or organ with regard to the amount of its contents. [Gk *heteros* different, *metron* measure.]

heteromorphic (het·er·o·**mor**'·fik). 1. Having different forms at different stages in the life history, as in many parasites. 2. Having, in somatic cells, an unequal pair of chromosomes, i.e. sex chromosomes, X and Y. [see foll.]

heteromorphism (het·er·o·**mor**'·fizm). 1. Variation from the normal in form. 2. In biology, (*a*) deviation from the type or standard; (*b*) the taking on of a different form at different stages of the life history. 3. In chemistry the property shown by compounds of similar composition of crystallizing in different forms. [Gk *heteros* different, *morphe* shape.]

heteromorphosis (het·er·o·mor·**fo**'·sis). 1. Any disease in which malformation or deformity is a characteristic. 2. Malformation, deformity or abnormal position of a tissue, an organ or a part. 3. The development of tissue of one type or kind from tissue of another. [Gk *heteros* different, *morphosis* a shaping.]

heteromorphous (het·er·o·**mor**'·fus). Heteromorphic.

heteronephrolysin (het·er·o·nef·**rol**'·is·in). A nephrotoxin derived from an animal and affecting the cells of animals of another species. [Gk *heteros* different, nephrolysin.]

Heteronium Bromide (het·er·o·ne·um **bro**·mide). BP Commission approved name for 1,1-dimethyl-3-(α-2-thienylmandeloyl-oxy)pyrrolidinium bromide; an anticholinergic.

heteronomous (het·er·**on**·o·mus). 1. General term indicating abnormality or deviation from type. 2. Term descriptive of the images of crossed double vision, e.g. in relative divergence of the eyes; not homonomous. 3. In biology, abnormality or diversity in a series of related structures because of specialization along different lines. 4. In psychology, under the influence of the will of another, as in the case of suggestion or hypnotism. [Gk *heteros* different, *nomos* place.]

heteronomy (het·er·**on**·o·me). 1. The condition of being subject to a law of adaptive modification. 2. The condition of being segmental in structure. [see prec.]

heteronymous (het·er·**on**·im·us). 1. Having different names; the opposite of synonymous. 2. Expressed in unlike terms. 3. In optics, referring to the 2 images of 1 object. [Gk *heteros* different, *onyma* name.]

hetero-osteoplasty (het·er·o·**os**'·te·o·plas·te). The operation of bone grafting in which a piece of bone taken from an animal is used. [Gk *heteros* different, osteoplasty.]

heteropagus (het·er·**op**·ag·us). A double monster of which the rudimentary parasite, consisting of head, hands and feet, grows out from the abdomen of the autosite. [Gk *heteros* different, *pagos* fixture.]

heteropancreatism (het·er·o·pan'·kre·at·izm). A condition in which the pancreas functions irregularly. [Gk *heteros* different, pancreatism.]

heteropathic (het·er·o·**path**'·ik). Relating or belonging to heteropathy.

heteropathy (het·er·**op**·ath·e). 1. Allopathy. 2. The condition of being abnormally or morbidly sensitive to a stimulus or irritant. [Gk *heteros* different, *pathos* suffering.]

heteropentosan (het·er·o·**pen**'·to·san). General term for the complex polysaccharides which contain non-carbohydrate units combined with pentose residues: they include the gums, mucilages, pectic substances and hemicelluloses. [Gk *heteros* different, pentose.]

heterophagosome (het·er·o·**fag**'·o·some). A membrane-bound body within a cell, containing ingested material. [Gk *heteros* different, *phagein* to eat, *soma* cell.]

heterophany (het·er·**of**·an·e). Variation in the signs and symptoms of the same disease or condition. [Gk *heteros* different, *phainein* to display.]

heterophasia (het·er·o·**fa**'·ze·ah). Heterolalia. [Gk *heteros* different, *phasis* a speaking.]

heterophemia, heterophemy (het·er·o·**fe**'·me·ah, het·er·**of**·em·e). Heterolalia. [Gk *heteros* different, *pheme* speech.]

heterophil, heterophile, heterophilic (**het**·er·o·fil, **het**·er·o·file, **het**·er·o·**fil'**·ik). Having affinity for something which is not the normal, e.g. a tissue or micro-organism which takes a stain other than the usual, or an antibody which reacts to an antigen other than the specific one. [Gk *heteros* different, philein to love.]

heterophonia, heterophony (**het**·er·o·**fo'**·ne·ah, het·er·**of**·o·ne). 1. Abnormal change in the voice or the quality of the sounds produced. 2. The change of voice that occurs at puberty. [Gk *heteros* different, *phone* voice.]

heterophoralgia (**het**·er·o·for·**al'**·je·ah). Sensation of pain or strain in the eyes in association with heterophoria. [heterophoria, Gk *algos* pain.]

heterophoria (**het**·er·o·**for'**·e·ah). A deviation of the eyes from the ortho-position that is present only when fusion is interrupted. Cf. ESOPHORIA, EXOPHORIA, HYPERESOPHORIA, HYPEREXOPHORIA, HYPERPHORIA, PHORIA [Gk *heteros* different, *phora* orbit.]

heterophoric (**het**·er·o·**for'**·ik). 1. Relating or belonging to heterophoria. 2. One suffering from heterophoria.

heterophthalmia, heterophthalmos, heterophthalmus (**het**·er·of·**thalm'**·e·ah, **het**·er·of·**thal'**·mos, **het**·er·of·**thal'**·mus). 1. A condition in which there is difference between one eye and the other, e.g. in size, in aperture between the lids, in direction of the axes; allophthalmia. 2. Heterochromia. [Gk *heteros* different, *ophthalmos* eye.]

heterophthongia (**het**·er·of·**thon'**·je·ah). 1. Heterophonia. 2. Ventriloquism. [Gk *heteros* different, *phthoggos* voice.]

heterophydiasis (**het**·er·o·fi·**di'**·as·is). Heterophyiasis.

Heterophyes (het·er·**of**·i·eez). A genus of very small intestinal flukes. *Heterophyes heterophyes* is an abundant fluke of cats, dogs and man in the Near and Far East, but it may cause diarrhoea. Intermediate hosts are brackish water snails (*Pirenella conica* in Egypt) and the cercariae encyst in marine fish (*Mugil* and *Acanthogobius* species). *H. katsuradai* is a little-known human species from Japan which also encysts in mullets. [Gk *heteros* different, *phye* form.]

heterophyiasis (**het**·er·o·fi·**i'**·as·is). Intestinal infection resulting from infestation with flukes of the family Heterophyidae, e.g. *Heterophyes* and *Metagonimus*.

Heterophyidae (**het**·er·o·**fi'**·id·e). A family of the trematode sub-order Distomata or Fascioloidea. The genera *Heterophyes* and *Metagonimus* are of medical importance.

heteroplasia (**het**·er·o·**pla'**·ze·ah). 1. Heterometaplasia. 2. The development of abnormal tissue; a condition in which normal cells are in the wrong place or position. [Gk *heteros* different, *plassein* to form.]

heteroplasm (**het**·er·o·plazm). Any tissue which is abnormal in the place in which it is found. [Gk *heteros* different, *plasma* something formed.]

heteroplastic (**het**·er·o·**plas'**·tik). 1. Abnormal or different in structure. 2. Referring to heteroplasty or to tissue used in heteroplasty. 3. Referring to heteroplasia. [Gk *heteros* different, *plassein* to form.]

heteroplastid (**het**·er·o·**plas'**·tid). The graft used in heteroplasty.

heteroplasty (**het**·er·o·plas·te). 1. Plastic surgery employing tissue removed from an individual other than the patient. 2. A reparative procedure in which the graft is taken from another species of animal. [Gk *heteros* different, *plassein* to form.]

heteroploid (**het**·er·o·ploid). Of a chromosome number which is not typical of the species in question. Also applied to cells or organisms having such a chromosome number. Heteroploid chromosome complements may be euploid or aneuploid. [Gk *heteros* different, *ploos* times, *eidos* form.]

heteroploidy (**het**·er·o·**ploid**·e). The state characteristic of heteroploids.

heteropolykaryon (**het**·er·o·pol·e·**kar'**·e·on). *See* HETEROKARYON.

heteropolyribonucleotide (**het**·er·o·**pol**·e·ri·bo·**new'**·kle·o·tide). A polynucleotide made up of more than one class of ribonucleotide units. [Gk *heteros* different, *polys* many, ribose, nucleotides.]

heteroprosopus (**het**·er·o·pro·**so'**·pus). 1. A monster having 1 head and 2 faces. 2. Janiceps. [Gk *heteros* different, *prosopon* face.]

heteropsia (het·er·**op**·se·ah). A state in which the two eyes have inequality of vision. [Gk *heteros* different, *ops* eye.]

heteropsychology (**het**·er·o·si·**kol'**·o·je). That part of psychology which is based on fact and objective experience. [Gk *heteros* different, psychology.]

Heteroptera (het·er·**op**·ter·ah). A sub-order of the Hemiptera which contains all the bugs of medical importance. [Gk *heteros* different, *pteron* wing.]

heteroptics (het·er·**op**·tix). Perversion or falsity of vision, so that things are seen which are not there or things that are seen are wrongly interpreted. [Gk *heteros* different, *optikos* belonging to the eye.]

heteropyknosis (**het**·er·o·pik·**no'**·sis). Different stainability of some chromosome or chromosome region in relation to the majority of chromatin. This is one of the properties of heterochromatin. **Positive heteropyknosis.** Higher stainability. **Negative heteropyknosis.** Lower stainability. [Gk *heteros* different, *pyknosis* thickening.]

heteropyknotic (**het**·er·o·pik·**not'**·ik). Showing heteropyknosis; heterochromatic.

heterosaccharide (**het**·er·o·**sak'**·ar·ide). General term for the complex polysaccharides which are composed of non-sugar units with saccharide residues: they include the heteropentosans, heterohexosans and mucopolysaccharides. [Gk *heteros* different, saccharide.]

heteroscope (**het**·er·o·skope). An apparatus consisting of a pair of specially-mounted fusion tubes so that deviations in strabismus can be accurately measured and the range of vision progressively determined. [Gk *heteros* different, *skopein* to view.]

heteroscopy (het·er·**os**·ko·pe). 1. A condition of unequal vision in the two eyes. 2. The use of a heteroscope in determining the range of vision in strabismus, and its progress. [see prec.]

heteroserotherapy (**het**·er·o·seer·o·**ther'**·ap·e). The therapeutic use of serum derived from an individual other than the patient or of non-specific antiserum. [Gk *heteros* different, serotherapy.]

heterosexual (**het**·er·o·**sex'**·ew·al). Relating or belonging to the opposite sex. [Gk *heteros* different, sex.]

heterosexuality (**het**·er·o·sex·ew·**al'**·it·e). Sexual attraction towards an individual of the opposite sex. [see prec.]

heteroside (**het**·er·o·side). Name applied sometimes to glycosides in view of the fact that they are constituted of saccharide and non-saccharide units. [see foll.]

heterosis (het·er·**o**·sis). Increase in size, rate of growth, fertility or viability, appearing in the offspring of a cross between 2 species or stocks of the same species; hybrid vigour. [Gk *heteros* different.]

heterosmia (het·er·**oz**·me·ah). A condition in which the sense of smell is perverted so that odours are wrongly interpreted. [Gk *heteros* different, *osme* odour.]

heterosome (**het**·er·o·some). A synonym of *allosome* and *heterochromosome*. In contraposition to *autosome* to indicate sex chromosomes. [Gk *heteros* other, *soma* body.]

heterosporous (**het**·er·o·**spo'**·rus). Having asexual spores of more than one kind; producing microspores and macrospores. [Gk *heteros* different, spore.]

heterostomy (het·er·**os**·to·me). An asymmetrical state of the mouth. [Gk *heteros* different, *stoma* mouth.]

heterosuggestion (**het**·er·o·suj·**es'**·chun). Suggestion exercised by someone else on an individual, particularly with regard to matters affecting the latter. Opposite of autosuggestion. [Gk *heteros* different, suggestion.]

heterosynkaryon (**het**·er·o·sin·**kar'**·e·on). A cell with a nucleus formed by fusion of 2 or more genetically different nuclei. [Gk *heteros* different, *syn* together, *karyon* nut.]

heterotaxia, heterotaxis, heterotaxy (**het**·er·o·**tax'**·e·ah, **het**·er·o·**tax'**·is, **het**·er·o·**tax'**·e). Displacement, abnormal arrangement or transposition of parts or organs of the body in relation one with another. [Gk *heteros* different, *taxis* arrangement.]

heterothallic (**het**·er·o·**thal'**·ik). In microbial genetics, indicating that mating is possible only between different strains or mating types. [Gk *heteros* different, *thallos* young green shoot.]

heterotherapy (het·er·o·ther'·ap·e). Treatment aimed at combating the main symptom of a disease rather than the disease itself; non-specific therapy. [Gk *heteros* different, therapy.]

heterotonia (het·er·o·to'·ne·ah). A condition of variable or abnormal tension or tonus. [Gk *heteros* different, tone.]

heterotopia (het·er·o·tope'·e·ah). 1. The development of tissue of a kind that is not natural to the part in which it is produced. 2. Malformation, deformity or abnormal position of a tissue, an organ or a part. 3. Confusion of utterance so that the various sounds in words are jumbled. [Gk *heteros* different, *topos* place.]

heterotopic (het·er·o·top'·ik). 1. Relating to heterotopia. 2. Occurring in the wrong part of the body. 3. Referring to the placing of a graft in relation to a different type of tissue, e.g. a dermal graft deep to the skin.

heterotoxic (het·er·o·tox'·ik). Relating or belonging to a heterotoxin or to heterotoxis.

heterotoxin (het·er·o·tox'·in). Any toxin introduced into the body from outside. [Gk *heteros* different, toxin.]

heterotoxis (het·er·o·tox'·is). Poisoning resulting from the introduction of external poisons into the body. [see prec.]

heterotransplant (het·er·o·trans'·plahnt). Heterograft; in skin or tissue grafting, a graft taken from another animal. [Gk *heteros* different, transplant.]

heterotransplantation (het·er·o·trans·plahnt·a'·shun). The grafting of tissue from one animal to another of different species. [see prec.]

heterotrichosis (het·er·o·trik·o'·sis). The occurrence of hair of different colours on the head and other parts of the body. **Heterotrichosis superciliorum.** Having eyebrows of different colour. [Gk *heteros* different, *thrix* hair, *-osis* condition.]

heterotrikaryon (het·er·o·tri·kar'·e·on). *See* HETEROKARYON.

heterotrophe (het·er·o·trofe). Any organism for which organic food is a necessity, as man. [Gk *heteros* different, *trophe* nutrition.]

heterotrophia (het·er·o·tro'·fe·ah). 1. Perverted nutrition; malnutrition. 2. Any abnormal means of obtaining nutrition. [see foll.]

heterotrophic (het·er·o·trof'·ik). Pertaining to heterotrophia; of micro-organisms, indicating those which require complex substances for their nutrition, as they possess limited powers of synthesizing essential proteins and carbohydrates for themselves from simpler materials. [Gk *heteros* different, *trophe* nutrition.]

heterotrophy (het·er·ot·ro·fe). Heterotrophia.

heterotropia, heterotropy (het·er·o·tro'·pe·ah, het·er·ot·ro·pe). Strabismus. [Gk *heteron* different, *trope* a turning.]

heterotypical (het·er·o·tip'·ik·al). Pertaining to a process which takes an unusual course. [Gk *heteros* different, *typos* pattern.]

heterotypus (het·er·o·ti'·pus). A double monster of which the immature parasite grows and depends from the abdominal wall of the autosite. [see prec.]

heteroxanthine (het·er·o·zan'·theen). Methylxanthine, 7-methyl-2,6-dioxypurine, $C_6H_6O_2N_4$. An exogenic base found in human urine and attributed to the caffeine and theobromine in the diet. [Gk *heteros* different, xanthine.]

heteroxenous (het·er·ox·en·us). Applied to parasites which have different hosts at different stages of their life cycle. [Gk *heteros* different, *xenos* host.]

heteroxeny (het·er·ox·en·e). In the life cycle of a parasite, the occurrence of more than one stage, each of which is passed in a different host. [see prec.]

heterozoic (het·er·o·zo'·ik). Having relation or belonging to a different animal or a different animal species. [Gk *heteros* different, *zoon* animal.]

heterozygosis (het·er·o·zi·go'·sis). The development of hybrids from the union of 2 different kinds of gamete; cross-breeding. [Gk *heteros* different, *zygosis* a joining.]

heterozygote (het·er·o·zi'·gote). An organism whose somatic cells have 2 different allelomorphic genes in the same locus on each of a pair of chromosomes. The organism may be morphologically identical with one of the homozygous forms or may show intermediate characters; it will produce 2 different types of gametes. **Structural heterozygote.** Individual heterozygous for chromosomal structural changes (interchange, translocation, heterozygote, etc.). [Gk *heteros* different, *zygotos* yoked.]

heterozygotic advantage (het·er·o·zi·go·tic ad·vant·age). When the heterozygous state produces more favourable results that the homozygous state.

heterozygous (het·er·o·zi'·gus). 1. Produced from unlike gametes, one allelomorph being dominant and the other recessive. 2. Having the characteristics of a heterozygote. [see prec.]

hettocyrtosis (het·o·ser·to'·sis). A slight degree of curvature. [Gk *hetton* less, *kyrtos* curved.]

Heublein, Arthur Carl (b. 1879). Hartford, Connecticut, radiologist.

Heublein method. Total body irradiation at low voltage and low dosage rate for cancer treatment.

Heubner, Johann Otto Leonhard (b. 1843). Leipzig and Berlin paediatrician.

Heubner's disease or specific endarteritis. Syphilitic endarteritis of the cerebral vessels.

Gee-Herter-Heubner disease, Herter-Heubner disease. Coeliac disease or the infantile form of idiopathic steatorrhoea.

Heurnius. *See* HORNE, JAN van.

Heurteloup, Charles Louis Stanislas (b. 1793). French surgeon.

Heurteloup's leech. An artificial leech.

Hevea (he·ve·ah). A genus of trees of the family Euphorbiaceae from which Para rubber is obtained. Important species yielding the latex in South America are *Hevea siberi* and *H. braziliensis.* [*heve* (South American name).]

Hewer, Christopher Langton. London anaesthetist.

Hewer's pilot balloon. An inflatable balloon communicating with the cuff of an endotracheal tube to ensure maintenance of distension.

Hewer's non-slip mattress. A corrugated mattress placed on top of an operating table to prevent a patient slipping when the table is tilted. Described in 1953.

hexabasic (hex·ah·ba·sik). 1. Denoting an acid that has 6 atoms of hydrogen replaceable by a metal or radical. 2. Of an alcohol, one containing 6 hydroxyl groups. [Gk *hex* six, base.]

hexabiose (hex·ah·bi·oze). The term for a disaccharide such as sucrose, because it is constituted of 2 hexose units.

hexacanth (hex·ak·anth). Having 6 spines. The hexacanth embryo is the oncosphere of tapeworms, which develops within the egg; it emerges from the egg and undergoes further development only in the secondary host. [Gk *hex* six, *akantha* spine.]

hexachlorocyclohexane (hex·ah·klor·o·si·klo·hex'·ane). The generic name for a group of 9 isomeric compounds all possessing the formula $C_6H_6Cl_6$. The most important is the gamma isomer, Gamma Benzene Hexachloride BP 1958, which is a potent insecticide stronger and more rapid in action than DDT. It is employed as a spray, a 1 per cent alcoholic solution being effective against head lice, and a 1 per cent emulsion for scabies. It is also used as a dust.

Hexachlorophane BP 1973 (hex·ah·klor·o·fane). Di-(3,5,6-trichloro-2-hydroxyphenyl)methane, an antiseptic employed with soap for the cleansing of surgeons' hands. Its bactericidal properties are of a very high order and the antiseptic effect is remarkably persistent.

hexachromic (hex·ah·kro·mik). Designating a person who has normal colour vision and can perceive the 6 colours of the spectrum, namely, red, orange, yellow, green, blue and violet, according to the classification of colour blindness adopted by Edridge-Green. [Gk *hex* six, *chroma* colour.]

hexacontane (hex·ah·kon·tane). $C_{60}H_{122}$, a solid saturated hydrocarbon of the methane series, found in ozocerite. [Gk *hexekonta* sixty.]

hexacosane (hex·ah·ko·sane). $C_{26}H_{54}$, a crystalline saturated hydrocarbon of the methane series, obtained from arachis oil and vegetable waxes. [Gk *hex* six, *eikosi* twenty.]

hexad (hex·ad). 1. General term denoting an element or radical with a valency of 6. 2. A crystal of the hexagonal system. [Gk *hex* six.]

hexadactylism (hex·ah·**dak**·til·izm). Having 6 fingers on a hand or 6 toes on a foot, or on both hands or feet. [Gk *hex* six, *daktylos* finger, toe.]

hexadienol (hex·ah·**di**·e·nol). 2,4-Hexadienol hexanol, sorbic alcohol, $CH_3CH=CHCH=CH_2OH$. An amber-coloured semisolid substance, insoluble in water, but which can be mixed with oils or organic solvents; it is unstable in the air or in oil. It was once used as a treatment for burns, but is now used to isolate anhidrotic areas of skin and to assess intensity of sweating after administration of drugs, etc. When it is applied to the skin, areas that sweat turn pink.

Hexadimethrine Bromide (hex·ah·di·**meth'**·reen **bro**·mide). BP Commission approved name for poly-*N,N',N',n'*-tetramethyl-*N*-trimethylenehexamethylenediammonium dibromide); a heparin antagonist.

hexa-ethyltetraphosphate (hex·ah·**eth**·il·tet·rah·**fos'**·fate). HETP, $(C_2H_5O)_2P_2O_3P_2O_4(OC_2H_5)_4$. One of a series of agricultural and horticultural insecticides containing organic phosphorus; it owes its action to its anticholinesterase effect. It is used against red spider and aphis, but like all insecticides of this class needs care in handling by humans.

hexafluorenium (hex·ah·floo·or·**en'**·e·um). A bis-quaternary ammonium compound used to potentiate the effects of suxamethonium on motor end-plates. **Hexafluorenium bromide.** Hexamethylene-bis-fluoren-9-yldimethylammonium bromide, a serum cholinesterase inhibitor used to potentiate and prolong the neuromuscular blocking action of suxamethonium.

hexahydric (hex·ah·**hi**·drik). 1. Denoting a hydrate that contains 6 molecules of water of crystallization. 2. Applied to an alcohol that has 6 hydroxyl OH groups, each attached to a different carbon atom. **Hexahydric alcohol.** A naturally-occurring alcohol such as mannitol, sorbitol or dulcitol, which gives rise to the corresponding hexose on oxidation. [Gk *hex* six, *hydor* water.]

hexahydrohaematoporphyrin (hex·ah·**hi**·dro·he·mat·o·**por'**·fir·in). $C_{34}H_{44}O_6N_4$, an iron-free derivative of haem obtained by reduction.

hexahydroxybenzene (hex·ah·hi·drox·e·**ben'**·zeen). $C_6(OH)_6$, a white substance that reduces readily to benzene and which is oxidized by nitric acid to a quinone. It forms an explosive potassium salt, $C_6(OK)_6$, potassium carboxide.

hexamethonium (hex·ah·meth·**o'**·ne·um). An organic radical derived by substitution from ammonium. It is the hexamethylene member of a series of polymethylene bis [trimethylammonium] radicals of general formula $(CH_3)_3N^+(CH_2)_nN^+(CH_3)_3$ known as methonium bases, *n* in this case being 6. The simple salts (e.g. the bromide) paralyse transmission across the ganglionic synapse; they reduce the sympathetic tone, causing vasodilatation and a fall in blood pressure, for which reason they are used therapeutically in hypertension and also during surgical operations, to reduce bleeding. They are of value in the reduction of gastric acidity and gastric mobility in peptic ulcer, and in causalgia and the relief of hiccup. Hexamethonium Bromide BPC 1959 and Hexamethonium Iodide BPC 1954 are BP Commission approved names. The tartrate is BP 1958.

hexamethylated (hex·ah·**meth**·il·a·ted). Denoting an organic compound which has 6 methyl groups in its structure. [Gk *hex* six, methyl.]

hexamethylene-amine (hex·ah·**meth**·il·een·**am'**·een). Hexamine.

hexamethylenediamine (hex·ah·**meth**·il·een·**di'**·am·een). $NH_2(CH_2)_6NH_2$, a toxic amine formed during the putrefaction of muscle and pancreas.

hexamethylenetetramine (hex·ah·**meth**·il·een·**tet'**·ram·een). Hexamine. **Hexamethylenetetramine tetra-iodide.** $(CH_2)_6N_4I_4$, an insoluble red compound administered for the same purposes as are inorganic iodides.

Hexamine BPC 1959 (**hex**·am·een). Hexamethylenetetramine, methenamine, $(CH_2)_6N_4$. A heterocyclic substance obtained by the reaction between ammonia and formaldehyde. It is a colourless crystalline solid which is readily soluble in water to give an alkaline solution. It is used in conjunction with sodium acid phosphate in the treatment of urinary infections on account of the fact that formaldehyde is liberated under such acid conditions. **Hexamine Hippurate.** BP Commission approved name for a 1,1 complex of hexamine and hippuric acid.

hexamylose (hex·**am**·il·oze). $(C_6H_{10}O_5)_6$, a polysaccharide derived from starch and believed to consist of bis- and triamyloses.

hexane (**hex**·ane). Normal hexane, C_6H_{14}. A saturated liquid hydrocarbon, sixth of the methane series, occurring in petroleum. It appears as the product of the continued reduction of glucose. [Gk *hex* six.]

hexanitrin (hex·ah·**ni**·trin). Mannitol hexanitrate, $CH_2ONO_2(CHONO_2)_4CH_2ONO_2$. A compound similar in vasodilator effect to glyceryl trinitrate but the action is milder and more prolonged; it is administered diluted with carbohydrate. By itself it is an explosive and is used in detonators.

hexanitro-inositol (hex·ah·**ni**·tro·in·**os'**·it·ol). $[CHO(NO_2)]_6$, a compound used for its hypotensive effect, as are other nitrites.

hexaploid (**hex**·ah·ploid). Polyploid with 6 chromosome sets. [Gk *hexaploos* sixfold, *eidos* form.]

Hexapoda (hex·ah·**po**·dah). A now rare synonym for Insecta by reason of their possessing 6 legs. [Gk *hex* six, *pous* foot.]

Hexaprofen (hex·ah·**pro**·fen). BP Commission approved name for 2-(4-cyclohexylphenyl)propionic acid; an anti-inflammatory, antipyretic and analgesic agent.

Hexapropymate (hex·ah·**pro**·pim·ate). BP Commission approved name for 1-prop-2'-ynylcyclohexyl carbamate; a sedative.

hexasomic (hex·ah·**so**·mik). A cell or individual having a chromosome represented 6 times, but otherwise diploid. [Gk *hex* six, *soma* body.]

hexatomic (hex·at·**om**·ik). 1. Hexavalent. 2. Describing a molecule composed of 6 atoms. 3. In the theory of immunity, capable of uniting with 6 different complements. [Gk *hex* six, atom.]

hexavalent (hex·ah·**va**·lent). *See* MULTIVALENT. [Gk *hex* six, L *valere* to be worth.]

Hexazole (**hex**·az·ole). BP Commission approved name for 3-ethyl-4-cyclohexyl-1,2,4-triazole, a compound used in the convulsion treatment of schizophrenia, usually by the intramuscular or intravenous injection of aqueous solutions.

hexenmilch (**hex**·en·milsh). The secretion of a milky fluid from the breasts of a newborn child. [G witch's milk.]

Hexetidine (hex·**et**·id·een). BP Commission approved name for 5-amino-1,3-di-(2-ethylhexyl)hexahydro-5-methylpyrimidine, an antiseptic and trichomonicidal compound used in the treatment of infections of the vagina and cervix.

hexhydric (hex·**hi**·drik). Hexahydric.

hexiology (hex·e·**ol**·o·je). The science of the relation of an organism to its environment; bionomics. [Gk *hexis* permanent condition, *logos* science.]

hexobarbital (hex·o·**bar**·bit·al). Hexobarbitone.

hexobarbitone (hex·o·**bar**·bit·one). 5-Δ'-Cyclohexenyl-5-methyl-*N*-methyl barbituric acid, $(CH_3)(C_6H_9)C(CONH)(CONCH_3)CO$. A rapidly acting intravenous anaesthetic, first used in 1932, and one of the first drugs to be used for the rapid induction of a patient into anaesthesia. **Hexobarbitone Sodium BPC 1959.** The sodium derivative of hexobarbitone, even more rapid in action than the latter.

Hexobendine (hex·o·**ben**·deen). BP Commission approved name for 1,2-di[*N*-methyl-3-(3,4,5-trimethoxybenzoyloxy)-propylamino]ethane; a coronary vasodilator.

hexobiose (hex·o·**bi**·oze). Hexabiose.

Hexocyclium methylsulphate (hex·o·**si**·kle·um meth·il·**sul**·fate). BP Commission approved name for 1-(2-cyclohexyl-2-hydroxyphenethyl)-4,4-dimethyl-piperazinium methylsulphate, a cholinergic blocking agent used in the treatment of peptic and duodenal ulcers.

hexodiose (hex·o·**di**·oze). Hexabiose.

Hexoestrol BPC 1968 (**hex**·ees·trol). Dihydrodiethylstilboestrol, 4,4'-dihydroxy-γ,δ-diphenyl-*n*-hexane, $OHC_6H_4CH(C_2H_5)CH(C_2H_5)C_6H_4OH$. A synthetic oestrogen, similar to silboestrol but better tolerated, less potent and probably seldom now used clinically. (BPC 1959). **Hexoestrol dipropionate.** The ester of hexoestrol and propionic acid; being water-soluble its use is indicated when it is desired to administer hexoestrol by intramuscular injection.

hexokinase (hex·o·**kin**·aze). An enzyme catalysing the formation of glucose 6-phosphate from glucose and ATP. Widespread in all tissues and eukaryote organisms. [hexose, Gk *kinein* to move.]

hexonic (hex·**on**·ik). Relating to the hexone bases.

Hexoprenaline (hex·o·**pren**·al·een). BP Commission approved name for *N,N′*-di-[2-(3,4-dihydroxyphenyl)-2-hydroxyethyl]hexamethylenediamine; a bronchodilator.

hexosamine (hex·o·**sam**·een). General term for the amino sugars derived from the hexoses by the substitution of an amino NH_2 group for a hydroxyl OH group. They have the formula $CH_2OH(CHOH)_3CHNH_2CHO$: glucosamine is the chief example.

hexosan (**hex**·o·san). Any of the polysaccharides formed from hexose units. They have the general formula $(C_6H_{10}O_5)_m$, and are represented principally by starch, cellulose and glycogen.

hexosazone (hex·o·**saz**·one). General term for the osazones formed by phenylhydrazine with the hexoses.

hexose (**hex**·oze). The simple sugars or monosaccharides, consisting of 6 carbon atoms in a chain, which occur widely in nature. They have the formula $C_6H_{12}O_6$, and may be divided into aldo- and keto- hexoses, glucose and fructose being respectively the principal members of the 2 groups. **Hexose diphosphate.** Fructose 1,6-diphosphate. **Hexose monophosphate.** Fructose 6-phosphate, glucose 1- and 6-phosphates.

hexose-phosphate (hex·oze·**fos**·fate). General name for the phosphoric esters of hexose sugars which are important intermediates in the metabolism of carbohydrates during sugar fermentation processes and the cycle of muscle contraction.

hexoside (**hex**·o·side). A compound saccharide composed of hexose units.

hexoxidase (hex·**ox**·id·aze). Ascorbic acid oxidase; the enzyme factor which is responsible for the oxidation of ascorbic (hexuronic) acid.

hexyl (**hex**·il). The monovalent radical C_6H_{13}-, derived from normal hexyl alcohol. [Gk *hex* six.]

Hexylresorcinol BP 1973 (**hex**·il·rez·**or**′·sin·ol). $CH_3(CH_2)_5C_6H_3(OH)_2$, an antiseptic and anthelminthic. Used as a general antiseptic in a 1 in 1000 solution in glycerin and water, it may be applied to wounds and mucous membranes, and is also employed as a gargle. Internally it may be used as a urinary antiseptic, but it is most frequently employed as an anthelminthic which is effective against roundworms and hookworms and is less toxic than male fern and carbon tetrachloride. It should be given on an empty stomach in the form of enteric-coated pills. Food is withheld for 5 h and the following morning a saline purge is given. It may also be employed as an enema. The powder itself is irritating to the skin and respiratory tract.

Hey, William (b. 1736). Leeds surgeon.

Hey's amputation or operation. Disarticulation through the tarsometatarsal joints; part of the medial cuneiform bone is removed.

Hey's internal derangement. Dislocation of the semilunar cartilages of the knee joint causing muscular spasm and intense pain.

Hey's hernia. Encysted hernia; hernia surrounded by cystic loculation of its sac.

Hey's ligament. The ligament protecting the saphenous opening in the inguinal triangle.

Hey's saw. A narrow-bladed saw for enlarging small holes in bones.

Hey, Wilson Harold. Manchester urologist.

Wilson Hey suprapubic prostatectomy operation. Transverse suprapubic prostatectomy with trigonectomy and diathermic control of bleeding. The bladder is closed and drainage provided through an indwelling urethral catheter.

Hey Groves, Ernest William (b. 1872). Bristol surgeon.

Hey Groves' director. A metal director used to guide the introduction of a Smith-Petersen nail along the neck of the femur.

Heyd, Charles Gordon (b. 1884). New York surgeon.

Heyd's syndrome. Symptoms of combined hepatolienal and renal failure.

Heyman, James (b. 1882). Swedish gynaecologist.

Heyman's technique. 1. For cancer of the neck of the uterus: the treatment of carcinoma of the neck of the uterus by means of uterine radium tubes and vaginal boxes using relatively large quantities of radium and 3 irradiations, with 1 week between the first and second and 3 weeks between the second and third. Also known as the *Stockholm technique.* 2. For cancer of the body of the uterus: the treatment of carcinoma of the body of the uterus by packing the uterine cavity with cylindrical radium applicators approximately 1.0×1.5 cm in size.

Heyman's law. The threshold value of a visual stimulus is increased in proportion to the intensity of a simultaneously existing or applied stimulus.

hiant (**hi**·ant). Gaping wide, as of a fissure; yawning. [L *hiare* to yawn.]

hiatal (hi·**a**·tal). Relating or belonging to, or affecting a hiatus.

hiation (hi·**a**·shun). 1. Yawning. 2. The state of being wide open. [L *hiare* to yawn.]

hiatopexia, hiatopexy (hi·a·to·**pex**′·e·ah, hi·a·to·**pex**′·e). Surgical repair of a hiatus. [hiatus, Gk *pexis* fixation.]

hiatus (hi·**a**·tus). An opening. **Adductor hiatus.** The opening in the adductor magnus muscle. **Aortic hiatus.** Aortic opening in the diaphragm. *See* DIAPHRAGM. **Ethmoidal hiatus [hiatus ethmoidalis (NA)].** The gap between the ethmoidal bulla and the uncinate process of the ethmoid bone. **Hiatus of the facial canal, Fallopian hiatus, Hiatus fallopii.** Hiatus for the greater superficial petrosal nerve (see below). **Hiatus femoralis.** The femoral ring lying deep to the inguinal ligament. **Hiatus for the greater superficial petrosal nerve [hiatus canalis nervi petrosi majoris (NA)].** The opening of the canal in the petrous part of the temporal bone for the greater superficial petrosal nerve. **Hiatus for the lesser superficial petrosal nerve [hiatus canalis nervi petrosi minoris (NA)].** The opening of the canal in the petrous part of the temporal bone which lies lateral to the hiatus for the greater superficial petrosal nerve and which transmits the lesser superficial petrosal nerve. **Interosseus hiatus.** The space between the radius and ulna, proximal to the interosseous membrane, through which pass the posterior interosseus vessels. **Maxillary hiatus [hiatus maxillaris (NA)].** The opening in the maxilla through which the antrum communicates with the middle meatus of the nose. **Neural hiatus.** The longitudinal opening between the neural folds, present in the early stages of development of the brain and spinal cord. This opening persists longest at the cranial and caudal ends of the body as the anterior and posterior neuropores, respectively. **Oesophageal hiatus.** Oesophageal opening in the diaphragm. *See* DIAPHRAGM. **Pleuroperitoneal hiatus.** A deficiency in the diaphragm, normally present only in the fetus, through which the pleural and peritoneal cavities communicate. **Sacral hiatus [hiatus sacralis (NA)].** The opening on the posterior aspect of the 5th segment of the sacrum, leading into the neural canal, and through which the filum terminale passes out to become attached to the coccyx. **Hiatus semilunaris [NA].** The maxillary hiatus (see above) when partially covered over by the bulla of the ethmoid bone, remaining only as a narrow semicircular opening into the middle meatus of the nose. **Vena-caval hiatus.** Vena-caval opening in the diaphragm. *See* DIAPHRAGM. [L gap.]

See also: BRESCHET, LOCKWOOD, SCARPA.

Hibbs, Russell Aubra (b. 1869). New York orthopaedic surgeon.

Hibbs' arthrodesis of the hip. An extra-articular arthrodesis using an iliofemoral graft fashioned from a large fragment of the greater trochanter. Previously used in the management of tuberculosis of the hip.

Hibbs' frame. A frame used in the application of plaster in the treatment of scoliosis.

Hibbs' operation. Arthrodesis of a tuberculous spine by division of the spinous processes and downward fracture of one half of each process to lie in contact with the process below; the intervertebral joints are also scraped out and the laminae are roughened.

hibernation (hi·ber·na·shun). Passing the winter months in a torpid or comatose state. [L *hibernare* to winter.]

hibernoma (hi·ber·no·mah). A rare, multilobular, encapsulated, benign tumour of primitive fetal fat, comparable with what is seen in the dorsal foot-pads of hibernating animals. [L *hibernus* winter, Gk *-oma* tumour.]

hiccup, hiccough (hik·up). Clonic spasm of the diaphragm causing a sudden inhalation which is interrupted by spasmodic closure of the glottis; also referred to as *singultus.* **Epidemic hiccup.** Persistent hiccup lasting without intermission for several days. It may occur in encephalitis lethargica, or may be a variant of that disease, or may occur in influenza, etc. [onomat.]

hidradenitis (hid·rad·en·i'·tis). Inflammation of the sweat glands. **Hidradenitis suppurativa.** An infection, usually staphylococcal, of the apocrine sweat glands, characterized by 1 or several subcutaneous nodules which gradually enlarge until they are about ½ cm in diameter and then soften; the overlying skin becomes red and necrotic, a small amount of purulent fluid is discharged and healing occurs by cicatrization. The malady is often chronic and deep sinus tracts may form. The usual site is the axillae but the lesions may occur in the regions of the anus, nipples, scrotum and labia majora. [Gk *hidros* sweat, *aden* gland, *-itis* inflammation.]

hidradenocarcinoma (hid·rad·en·o·kar·sin·o'·mah). A malignant tumour derived from sweat glands. [Gk *hidros* sweat, *aden* gland, carcinoma.]

hidradenoma (hid·rad·en·o'·mah). 1. Syringocystadenoma. 2. An exacerbation of inflammation occurring in an already inflamed tumour of a sweat gland. **Hidradenoma papilliferum.** A benign, rounded or warty, apocrine, glandular tumour occurring on the vulva or on the perianal skin. [Gk *hidros* sweat, adenoma.]

hidroa (hid·ro·ah). Any skin affection such as sudamina, with associated sweating. This affection is not to be confused with *hydroa.* [Gk *hidros* sweat.]

hidrocystoma (hid·ro·sis·o'·mah). Hydrocystoma.

hidromancy (hid·ro·man·se). Prognosis based on the character of the sweat and the amount secreted. [Gk *hidros* sweat, *manteia* mode of divination.]

hidropedesis (hid·ro·ped·e'·sis). Excessive secretion of sweat. [Gk *hidros* sweat, *pedesis* a leaping.]

hidropoiesis (hid·ro·poi·e'·sis). The process of formation and secretion of sweat. [Gk *hidros* sweat, *poiesis* formation.]

hidropoietic (hid·ro·poi·et'·ik). Relating or belonging to hydropoiesis.

hidrorrhoea (hid·ro·re·ah). Profuse sweating. [Gk *hidros* sweat, *rhoia* flow.]

hidrosadenitis (hid·ros·ad·en·i'·tis). Hidradenitis. **Hidrosadenitis destruens suppurativa.** Folliclis. [Gk *hidros* sweat, *aden* gland, *-itis* inflammation.]

hidroschesis (hid·ros·kes·is). 1. Retention of the sweat. 2. Suppression of the excretion of sweat. [Gk *hibros* sweat, *schesis* a checking.]

hidrosis (hid·ro·sis). 1. The process of secreting sweat. 2. Abnormally profuse sweating. 3. Primary adenitis of the sweat glands. 4. Any disease of the skin with which abnormal or disordered sweating is associated. [Gk *hidros* sweat.]

hidrotic (hid·rot·ik). 1. Relating to or causing hidrosis; sudorific; diaphoretic. 2. Any remedy or agent that causes sweating.

hidrotopathic (hid·rot·o·path'·ik). Relating or belonging to any disorder of sweating. [Gk *hidros* sweat, *pathos* disease.]

hiera picra (hi·e·rah pik·rah). Pulvis aloes et canellae, an old-fashioned emmenagogue. [Gk *hieros* sacred, *pikros* bitter.]

hieralgia (hi·er·al·je·ah). A painful condition of the sacrum. [Gk *hieron* sacrum, *algos* pain.]

hierolisthesis (hi·er·o·lis·the'·sis). Displacement of the sacrum. [Gk *hieron* sacrum, *olisthanein* to slip.]

hieromania (hi·er·o·ma'·ne·ah). Religious mania. *See* MANIA. [Gk *hieros* sacred, mania.]

hieronosus (hi·er·on·o·sus). Epilepsy. [Gk *hieros* sacred, *nosos* disease.]

hierophobia (hi·er·o·fo'·be·ah). 1. Morbid dread or awe of church ritual or of any form of religious ritual, or of sacred things. 2. A state of morbid anxiety affecting clergymen when they are conducting church or other public services. [Gk *hieros* sacred, phobia.]

hierotherapy (hi·er·o·ther'·ap·e). The therapeutic use of prayer and religious exercises and practices. [Gk *hieros* sacred, therapy.]

Higginson, Alfred (b. 1808). Liverpool surgeon.

Higginson's syringe. A firm, compressible, rubber bag with a ball-valve fitting to ensure flow in one direction only, used mainly in giving enemata.

Highmore, Nathaniel (b. 1613). Sherborne physician.

antrum of Highmore. The maxillary sinus. *See* SINUS.

Highmore's body. Mediastinum testis.

highmoritis (hi·mor·i·tis). Inflammation of the maxillary sinus (antrum of Highmore). [Nathaniel *Highmore,* Gk *-itis* inflammation.]

hilar (hi·lar). Relating or belonging to a hilum.

Hildenbrand, Johann Valentin (b. 1763). Vienna physician.

Hildenbrand's disease. Typhus fever. *See* FEVER.

Hilgenreiner, Heinrich. Czech orthopaedic surgeon.

Hilgenreiner's angle. Used in the measurement of acetabular dysplasia. This is the angle subtended between a transverse line drawn through the upper edges of the triradiate cartilages and a line from the triradiate cartilage to the outer and upper margin of the acetabulum.

hilitis (hi·li·tis). 1. Inflammation of any hilum. 2. Inflammation of the hilum of the lung. [hilum, Gk *-itis* inflammation.]

Hillebrand, Franz (b. 1863). Vienna psychiatrist.

Hering-Hillebrand deviation. A physiological deviation whereby intervals on the temporal side of the field of vision seem less than on the nasal side. If an attempt is made to bisect a horizontal line uni-ocularly, the outer half tends to be too large.

Hilliard's lupus. Lupus marginatus, a superficially scarring disease of unknown nature. [Named by Jonathan *Hutchinson* in 1890 after the patient whose case he reported.]

hillock (hil·ok). Anatomically, any small mound or raised prominence. **Anal hillock.** Anal tubercle; one of a pair of swellings flanking the embryonic proctodaeal membrane, which fuse to form the wall of the lower part of the anal canal. **Auricular hillock.** Auricular tubercle; one of a number of small elevations around the first ectodermal gill cleft, which fuse to form the external ear. **Axon hillock.** That part of the body of a nerve cell from which the axon arises. **Cloacal hillock.** Genital tubercle; a protuberance at the anterior end of the embryonic cloacal membrane, which later forms the body of the penis or clitoris. **Seminal hillock.** Seminal colliculus; an elongated swelling of the posterior wall of the prostatic urethra, on which the ejaculatory ducts open. [dim. of AS *hyll.*]

See also DOYÈRE, MUELLER (J.).

Hilton, John (b. 1804). London surgeon.

Hilton's law. The skin over, and the muscles to, a joint are innervated from the same nerve trunk.

Hilton's line or white line. Mucocutaneous junction of the anal canal.

Hilton's muscle. The aryepiglottic muscle.

Hilton's operation. The drainage of an abscess by the insertion of forceps into it.

Hilton's sac. The saccule of the larynx which lies between the vestibular fold and the thyroid cartilage.

hilum [hilus (NA)] (hi·lum) (pl. *hila*). A depression in an organ where vessels, nerves and ducts enter or emerge. **Hilum of the dentate nucleus.** *See* NUCLEUS. **Hilum of the kidney.** *See* KIDNEY. **Hilum of the lung.** *See* LUNG. **Hilum of a lymph gland.** *See*

GLAND. **Hilum of the olivary nucleus.** *See* NUCLEUS. **Hilus of the ovary.** *See* OVARY. **Hilum of the spleen.** *See* SPLEEN. **Hilum of a suprarenal gland.** *See* GLAND. [L a little thing.]

himantosis (hi·man·**to**·sis). Elongation of the uvula. [Gk *himas* thong, *-osis* condition.]

Himly, Carl (b. 1772). Gottingen ophthalmologist.

Himly's operation. 1. For corectopia. 2. For iridodialysis. 3. For symblepharon. Obsolete.

hinchazon (hinsh·az·**on**). Beriberi. [Cuban.]

hind (hi·nd). 1. In the rear. 2. Belonging to a posterior part. [ME.]

hind-brain [rhombencephalon (NA)] (hi·nd·brane). In the development of the brain of an embryo, the division which eventually becomes the medulla oblongata, the pons and the cerebellum. [ME *hind*, AS *bragen*.]

hind-gut (hi·nd·gut). In embryology, that portion of the yolk sac which is included within the tail fold and later develops into the colon and rectum. [ME *hind*, AS *guttas*.]

hind-kidney (hi·nd·kid·ne). The metanephros; the permanent kidney. It succeeds the mesonephros and develops from the mesonephric duct and the nephrogenic cord. [ME *hind*, *kydney*.]

Hines, Edgar Alphonso (b. 1906). Rochester, Minnesota, physician.

Hines-Bannick syndrome. Intermittent attacks of intense sweating, combined with low temperature.

Hines and Brown test. Cold pressor test; a test to detect subjects who may be likely to develop persistent hypertension in the future. The basal blood pressure is recorded at rest, and then the other hand of the subject is plunged into water at from 3 to 5°C for 1 min, the blood pressure being recorded at half-minute intervals. A rise of more than 2.7/2.0 kPa (20/15 mmHg) constitutes a hyper-reaction, and is shown by persons with essential hypertension or by those individuals who are likely to develop it ultimately. The test has also been suggested as a method of differentiating essential hypertension from renal and other forms of hypertension, but some doubt has been cast upon its validity.

Hinshelwood, James (b. 1859). Glasgow ophthalmologist.

Hinshelwood's theory. Congenital word blindness is due to a localized defect of development in the dominant temporal lobe of the cerebrum.

hip [coxa (NA)] (hip). The hip joint. *See* JOINT. **Observation hip.** Suspected tuberculosis of the hip. **Snapping hip.** A condition in which there is a loud snap on movement of the hip, due to a tendon slipping over the greater trochanter. [AS *hype*.]

hip bone [os coxae (NA)]. A composite bone formed by the fusion of ilium, ischium and pubis. It forms the pelvis with its fellow of the opposite side and the sacrum.

articular surface [facies lunata (NA)]. The horseshoe-shaped articular surface of the acetabulum.

hippanthropy (hip·**an**·thro·pe). A maniacal delusion (type of zoanthropy) in which the subject thinks he is a horse and imitates the movements of a horse. [Gk *hippos* horse, *anthropos* man.]

Hippel, Eugen von (b. 1867). Gottingen ophthalmologist.

von Hippel's disease, von Hippel-Lindau disease. A disease considered by von Hippel and numerous other observers to be a form of angiomatosis limited to the retina. Lindau in 1926, however, pointed out its association with cysts and angiomata elsewhere, especially in the cerebellum, medulla, cord, pancreas, liver, kidney, suprarenals and reproductive glands.

von Hippel's operation. For corneal transplantation with a rabbit's cornea; obsolete.

von Hippel trephine. One designed for keratoplasty.

Hippelates (hip·el·a·teez). A genus of small eye flies of the family Chloropidae. *Hippelates flavipes* and *H. pallipes* are suspected vectors of yaws in the West Indies and, with several other species in Central America, are a serious pest. Other species, *H. pusio*, have a high nuisance value and are suspected transmitters of conjunctivitis (California). [Gk driver of horses.]

Hippeutes cantori (hip·ew·teez kan·**tor**·i). A species of water snails that are intermediate hosts of *Fasciolopsis buski.* [Gk *hippeutes* horsemen.]

hippo (**hip**·o). An arrow poison used by certain tribes in Africa, and obtained from species of *Strychnos.* It produces vomiting, followed by tetanic convulsions with arrest of respiration.

Hippoboscidae (hip·o·**bos**·id·e). A family of the dipteran sub-order Cyclorrhapha, series Pupipara. The genus *Melophagus* is of medical interest. [Gk *hippos* horse, *boskein* to feed.]

hippocamp (**hip**·o·kamp). The hippocampus.

hippocampal (hip·o·**kam**·pal). Relating or belonging to the hippocampus.

hippocampus [NA] (hip·o·**kam**·pus). An elongated rounded elevation projecting into the temporal horn of the lateral ventricle of the brain; the cornu ammonis. It consists essentially of an atypical area of cerebral cortex (archipallium; allocortex) older in an evolutionary sense than most other areas, and covered by a layer of myelinated fibres [alveus hippocampi (NA)] on its ventricular surface. It has been thought to be concerned functionally with the sense of smell, but this is doubtful. The dentate gyrus and fimbria are sometimes included under this term as part of a general hippocampal formation. The hippocampal gyrus on the medial side of the temporal lobe of the cerebrum is not part of the hippocampus or hippocampal formation, from which it is separated by a transitional zone of cortex, the subiculum. [Gk *hippokampos* sea-horse.]

Hippocrates (c. 460–375 B.C.), of the island of Cos, in the Aegean. Called the "Father of Medicine" because he, with his followers, laid the foundation of scientific medicine in the group of writings known as the *Hippocratic corpus.* Observant, cautious and humane, basing his practice on experience, he was the ideal physician of the Greeks. He introduced the concept of the "four humours"—blood, black bile, yellow bile and phlegm. The *Hippocratic oath* has been the basis of medical ethics throughout the ages.

cord of Hippocrates. The tendo calcaneus.

Hippocrates reduction. Reduction of a dislocated shoulder by pulling on the extended arm against the counter-thrust of the operator's foot on the axilla.

hippocratic (hip·o·**krat**·ik). Pertaining to Hippocrates. **Hippocratic corpus.** An incomplete collection of writings written in Ionic dialect embodying the learning, based on exact observation, of the Greek school of medicine founded in the island of Cos by Hippocrates. **Hippocratic oath.** I swear by Apollo Physician, by Asclepius, by Health, by Heal-all, and by all the gods and goddesses, making them witnesses, that I will carry out, according to my ability and judgment, this oath and this indenture: To regard my teacher in this art as equal to my parents; to make him partner in my livelihood, and when he is in need of money to share mine with him; to consider his offspring equal to my brothers; to teach them this art, if they require to learn it, without fee or indenture; and to impart precept, oral instruction, and all the other learning, to my sons, to the sons of my teacher, and to pupils who have signed the indenture and sworn obedience to the physicians' Law, but to none other. I will use treatment to help the sick according to my ability and judgment, but I will never use it to injure or wrong them. I will not give poison to anyone though asked to do so, nor will I suggest such a plan. Similarly I will not give a pessary to a woman to cause abortion. But in purity and in holiness I will guard my life and my art. I will not use the knife either on sufferers from stone, but I will give place to such as are craftsmen therein. Into whatsoever houses I enter, I will do so to help the sick, keeping myself free from all intentional wrong-doing and harm, especially from fornication with woman or man, bond or free. Whatsoever in the course of practice I see or hear (or even outside my practice in social intercourse) that ought never to be published abroad, I will not divulge, but consider such things to be holy secrets. Now if I keep this oath and break it not, may I enjoy honour, in my life and art, among all men for all time; but if I transgress and forswear myself, may the opposite befall me. [*The Doctor's Oath* by W. H. S. Jones, M.A., Cambridge University Press.]

hippocratism (hip·ok·rat·izm). The system of treatment of the hippocratic school, in which diet, fresh air, gymnastics and the taking of medicinal waters were the chief therapeutic agents.

hippomyxoma (hip·o·mix·o′·mah). The local inflammatory lesion of glanders and farcy. [Gk *hippos* horse, myxoma.]

hippophagy (hip·of·aj·e). The practice of eating horse-flesh. [Gk *hippos* horse, *phagein* to eat.]

hippurase (hip·ewr·aze). Hippuricase.

hippurate (hip·ewr·ate). Any salt of hippuric acid.

hippuria (hip·ewr·e·ah). An excess of hippuric acid in the urine.

hippuric (hip·ewr·ik). Pertaining to horses' urine. [Gk *hippos* horse, urine.]

hippuricase (hip·ewr·ik·aze). An enzyme which acts upon hippuric acid yielding benzoic acid and glycine. It occurs in the body in the liver and kidneys, but its probable action there is to synthesize hippuric acid reversibly.

hippus (hip·us). Spasmodic alternate dilatation and contraction of the pupil. **Respiratory hippus.** A condition in which the pupils of the iris dilate during inspiration and contract during expiration; it is sometimes associated with paradoxical pulse. [Gk *hippos* horse.]

hips (hips). Rose fruit. [AS *heope.*]

hircine (her·seen). A compound which occurs in goats' fat. [L *hircus* goat.]

hircismus (her·siz·mus). An offensive strong odour like the odour of a he-goat, sometimes given off from the axillae of human beings. [see prec.]

hircus (her·kus). 1. One of the axillary hairs. 2. The tragus of the ear. 3. Hircismus. [L goat.]

Hirschberg, Julius (1843). Berlin ophthalmologist.

Hirschberg's magnet. A strong electromagnet used for the removal of particles of steel from the eye.

Hirschberg's operation. For detachment of the retina, by paracentesis of the sclera; obsolete.

Hirschberg's test. A rough test for measuring the angle of squint: the patient looks at a candle 1 ft away; the examiner looks from behind the candle at the corneal images of the flame. If that of the squinting eye is situated at the margin of the pupil, the angle =15 degrees; if at the margin of the cornea, the angle =45 degrees approximately. Nowadays a torch or mirror is used.

Hirschberg, Leonard Keene (b. 1877). Baltimore physician.

Hirschberg's reflex or sign. Inversion of the foot when its medial margin is stroked; a sign of disease of the pyramidal tract.

Hirschfeld, Felix (b. 1863). German physician.

Hirschfeld's disease. A rapidly progressive form of diabetes mellitus.

Hirschfeld, Isador (b. 1881). American dentist.

Hirschfeld's canals. Interdental vascular canals in the alveolar process of the mandible between the lateral and central incisors.

Hirschfeld, Ludwig Moritz (b. 1816). Warsaw anatomist.

Hirschfeld's ganglion. A sympathetic ganglion of the renal plexus, lying in front of the renal artery.

Hirschfeld's nerve. The communicating branch of the facial nerve with the glossopharyngeal nerve.

Hirschsprung, Harald (b. 1831). Danish physician.

Hirschsprung's disease. A form of megacolon.

Hirst, George Keble (b. 1909). New York physician.

Hirst test, Hirst and Hare test, Hirst–McLelland–Hare phenomenon. A laboratory test for detecting the presence of either influenza viruses or the corresponding antibodies. The viruses agglutinate the red blood corpuscles of fowls and certain mammals. Immune serum inhibits this agglutination specifically.

hirsute (her·sewt). 1. Bearing coarse, long, shaggy hairs. 2. Hairy. [see foll.]

hirsuties (her·sew·she·eez). 1. Excessive growth of hair. 2. A growth of hair in an unusual place. **Hirsuties papillaris penis.** Pearly penile papules. *See* PAPULE. [L *hirsutus* shaggy.]

hirsutism, hirsutismus (her·sewt·izm, her·sewt·iz·mus). Excessive hairiness, especially the condition in the female in which hair grows in places from which normally it is absent in the female but present in the male. [see prec.]

hirudicide (hir·ew·dis·ide). Any substance which kills leeches, e.g. cocaine. [L *hirudo* leech, *caedere* to kill.]

hirudin (hir·ew·din). A glycoprotein of the buccal-gland secretion of leeches. It is a strong anticoagulant, and prevents the blood from clotting whilst they are feeding. [L *hirudo* leech.]

Hirudinea (hir·ew·din·e·ah). A class of the Annelida including the genus *Hirudo,* to which belong the medicinal leeches, e.g. *Hirudo medicinalis* and *H. troctina.* [L *hirudo* leech.]

hirudiniasis (hir·ew·din·i′·as·is). Infestation by leeches. **External hirudiniasis.** Hirudiniasis from the attachment to the skin of land or water leeches. **Internal hirudiniasis.** Hirudiniasis due to the swallowing of aquatic leeches which attach themselves to the mucosa of the upper respiratory tract and sometimes of the abdominal organs. [see prec.]

hirudiniculture (hir·ew·din·e·kul′·tcher). The propagation of leeches by artificial means. [L *hirudo* leech, culture.]

hirudinization (hir·ew·din·i·za′·shun). The therapeutic application of leeches. [L *hirudo* leech.]

hirudinize (hir·ew·din·ize). To inject hirudin for the purpose of producing non-coagulability of the blood.

Hirudo (hir·ew·do). A genus of Hirudinea; leeches. **Hirudo medicinalis.** Leech BPC 1954, the European medical leech, about 12 cm long when expanded. The adults feed on blood of vertebrates, including man, injecting a powerful anticoagulant, hirudin. The species has been experimentally infected with many human pathogens. **Hirudo officinalis.** *Hirudo medicinalis* (see preceding). **Hirudo troctina.** A Mediterranean species which will bite man. [L.]

His, Wilhelm, Jnr. (b. 1863). Gottingen and Berlin physician.

bundle of His, Kent–His bundle. Atrioventricular bundle. *See* BUNDLE.

His' bundle electrogram. The graphical record of the electrical activity of the His bundle (the conducting bundle) in the heart obtained by approximating an intracardiac electrode, introduced pervenously, to the region of the bundle in the interatrial septum near the tricuspid valve.

His' disease, His–Werner disease, Werner–His disease. Trench fever. *See* FEVER.

His' spindle. A dilatation of the aorta immediately below the point of entry of the ductus arteriosus, large in fetal life, less marked in the adult.

His' bundle tachycardia. Paroxysmal tachycardia arising from a focus in the bundle of His; a form of nodal tachycardia.

His–Tawara node. Atrioventricular node. *See* NODE.

His, Wilhelm, Snr. (b. 1831). Basle and Leipzig anatomist and embryologist.

His' canal. Thyroglossal duct. *See* DUCT.

cells of His. Angioblast cells.

septum inferius of His. The embryonic ventricular septum.

septum intermedium of His. The septum formed in the embryonic heart by the fusion of the endocardial cushions in the atrioventricular orifice.

His' perivascular space. Continuations of the subarachnoid space around the vessels of the central nervous system.

His' stroma. The connective tissue of the mammary gland.

His' tubercle. Tubercle of the auricle.

zone of His. One of the 4 longitudinal thickenings of the wall of the neural tube of the embryo, comprising a dorsal (alar) and a ventral (basal) lamina (zone) on either side.

Hiss, Philip Hanson (b. 1868). New York bacteriologist.

Hiss' method, for capsules. Heat-fixed smears are stained with gentian violet and heated until steam rises. The stain is then washed off with 20 per cent copper sulphate. The capsules are stained pale violet and the bacteria deep violet.

Hiss' serum sugars. Liquid media containing serum water and sugars, for the investigation of the fermentative powers of the *Neisseria, Corynebacterium,* etc.

Hiss' serum-dextrose water. Serum-dextrose culture medium. *See* CULTURE MEDIUM.

Hiss and Russell bacillus. *Shigella flexneri.*

histaminaemia (**his**·tam·in·**e'**·me·ah). A condition in which histamine is present in the blood. [histamine, Gk *haima* blood.]

histaminase (**his**·tam·in·aze). An enzyme occurring in various body tissues, which catalyses the deamination of histamine. High serum levels are consistently present in medullary carcinoma of the thyroid.

histamine (**his**·tam·een). β-Iminazolylethylamine, $C_3H_3N_2CH_2C$-H_2NH_2. An amine related to histidine and widely distributed in plant and animal tissues. It was first isolated from ergot. The physiological significance of its presence in animal tissue is not clearly established, but it can be released in a free form by a variety of substances, e.g. morphine and curare. It produces capillary dilatation and, with larger doses, haemoconcentration. In higher animals it causes dilatation of the arterioles; the vessels of the meninges and brain are dilated and the pressure of the cerebrospinal fluid rises, both of which may account for the headache which follows its injection. The heart rate and cardiac output are increased as a result of the fall in blood pressure occasioned by these circulatory changes. It stimulates smooth muscle, producing contraction in that of the intestine, uterus and bronchi. If injected subcutaneously it evokes a copious secretion of saliva and gastric juice, the latter of high acidity, an effect which is not antagonized by antihistamine drugs. It has been injected in gastric-function tests to distinguish between true and pseudo- gastric achylia. Histamine has also been administered by iontophoresis to treat peripheral vascular disease. **Histamine Acid Phosphate BP 1973.** A white crystalline compound, soluble in water and the one most commonly used. **Histamine dihydrochloride.** A soluble white compound used for injection. **Histamine phosphate.** Histamine acid phosphate (see above). **Histamine test for phaeochromocytoma.** *See* TEST. [Gk *histos* tissue, amine.]

histaminia (his·tam·**in**·e·ah). Shock due to an excess of free histamine in the body. It may be the result of over-zealous use of histamine therapeutically.

histanoxia (his·tan·**ox**·e·ah). A condition in which there is lack of oxygen in the tissues because the supply of blood to them is diminished. [Gk *histos* tissue, anoxia.]

histic (**his**·tik). 1. Relating or belonging to tissue. 2. Having the characteristics of tissue. [Gk *histos* tissue.]

histidinaemia (**his**·tid·in·**e'**·me·ah). Lack of histidase causing histidine and iminazole-pyruvic acid to appear in urine where the latter may be detected by the ferric-chloride reaction (blue colour). There is a variable clinical picture. [histidine, Gk *haima* blood.]

histidine (**his**·tid·een). α-Amino-β-iminazole propionic acid, $C_3H_3N_2CH_2CH(NH_2)COOH$. An indispensable amino acid found in most proteins but not regarded as being essential in the human diet. It is observed in the urine during pregnancy. Chemically it is closely related to histamine and may be a precursor of this substance. It has been used in peptic ulcer, but there is no evidence of its having any significant value. **Histidine hydrochloride.** The soluble hydrochloride of histidine, formerly injected for peptic ulcer but discontinued as of doubtful efficacy. [see prec.]

histidinuria (**his**·tid·in·**ewr'**·e·ah). A condition in which histidine is present in the urine.

histin (**his**·tin). Fibrin. [Gk *histion* web.]

histioblast (**his**·te·o·blast). A tissue histiocyte. [Gk *histion* web, *blastos* germ.]

histioblastoma (**his**·te·o·blas·**to'**·mah). A reticulo-endothelioma. [histioblast, Gk *-oma* tumour.]

histiocyte (**his**·te·o·site). The macrophage of connective tissues. It is an important member of the reticulo-endothelial system of cells and plays a vital rôle in the tissue defences as a scavenger. [Gk *histion* web, *kytos* cell.]

histiocytoma (**his**·te·o·si·**to'**·mah). A neoplasm in which there are histiocytes. **Lipoid histiocytoma.** Fibroxanthoma. [histiocyte, Gk *-oma* tumour.]

histiocytomatosis (**his**·te·o·si·to·mat·**o'**·sis). A condition in which the reticulo-endothelial system is abnormal, giving rise to diseases such as lymphogranulomatosis or Niemann-Pick disease. The more modern terms are reticulo-endotheliosis and reticulosis. [histiocytoma, Gk *-osis* condition.]

histiocytosarcoma (**his**·te·o·si·to·sar·**ko'**·mah). A malignant reticulo-endothelial tumour composed of histiocytes. [Gk *histion* web, *kytos* cell, sarcoma.]

histiocytosis (**his**·te·o·si·**to'**·sis). A condition in which histiocytes are present in the blood. **Lipoid histiocytosis, Lipoidal histiocytosis.** Niemann-Pick disease. **Histiocytosis X.** Letterer-Christian disease. [histiocyte, Gk *-osis* condition.]

Histiogaster (**his**·te·o·**gas'**·ter). A genus of mites of which *Histiogaster entomophagus* causes vanillism. There is 1 record of infestation of a testicular cyst by this species. [Gk *histion* web, *gaster* stomach.]

histiogenic (**his**·te·o·**jen'**·ik). Any structure that is formed by the tissues. [Gk *histion* web, *genein* to produce.]

histioid (**his**·te·oid). Histoid.

histio-irritative (**his**·te·o·**ir'**·it·a·tiv). Histo-irritative.

histioma (his·te·**o**·mah). Any tissue tumour, such as a fibroma, myoma or osteoma. [Gk *histos* tissue, *-oma* tumour.]

histionic (his·te·**on**·ik). Belonging to or arising in a tissue. [Gk *histion* web.]

Histiotis loephotis (his·te·**o**·tis lo·**fo**·tis). A bat which is a potential host of *Trypanosoma cruzi.*

histiotrophic (**his**·te·o·**trof'**·ik). Histotrophic.

histoblast (**his**·to·blast). Histioblast.

histoblastoma (**his**·to·blas·**to'**·mah). Histioblastoma.

histochemistry (his·to·**kem**·is·tre). That branch of medical science which is concerned with applying chemical techniques to histological sections so that the reaction products can be recognized with the light or electron microscope. [Gk *histos* tissue, chemistry.]

histochemotherapy (**his**·to·kem·o·**ther'**·ap·e). Chemotherapy. [Gk *histos* tissue, chemotherapy.]

histochromatosis (**his**·to·kro·mat·**o'**·sis). Reticulo-endotheliosis. [Gk *histos* tissue, chromatosis.]

histoclasis (his·to·**kla**·sis). Tissue disintegration. [Gk *histos* tissue, *klasis* a breaking.]

histoclastic (his·to·**klas**·tik). Of cells, capable of breaking-down tissue. [see prec.]

histocompatibility (his·to·kom·pati·bility). The compatibility of the antigens of donors and recipients of transplanted tissue. **Histocompatibility antigen.** Antigen which determines compatibility of grafts; genetically determined cell-membrane iso-antigen. In man the HL-A system is the strongest of the histocompatibility antigen systems. **Histocompatibility gene.** Gene which determines formation of histocompatibility antigens.

histocyte (**his**·to·site). Histiocyte.

histocytoma (**his**·to·si·**to'**·mah). Histiocytoma.

histocytomatosis (**his**·to·si·to·mat·**o'**·sis). Histiocytomatosis.

histocytosis (**his**·to·si·**to'**·sis). Histiocytosis.

histodiagnosis (**his**·to·di·ag·**no'**·sis). Diagnosis by means of microscopical examination of pieces of tissue. [Gk *histos* tissue, diagnosis.]

histodialysis (**his**·to·di·**al'**·is·is). The dissolving or breaking-down of tissue by means of external agents. [Gk *histos* tissue, *dia*, lysis.]

histodifferentiation (**his**·to·dif·er·en·she·**a'**·shun). Development of undifferentiated stem cells into characteristic cells of special tissue. [Gk *histos* tissue, differentiation.]

histofluorescence (**his**·to·floo·or·**es'**·ens). Fluorescence of the tissues as the result of administration of a drug before x-ray treatment of any particular part of the body. [Gk *histos* tissue, fluorescence.]

histogenesis (his·to·**jen**·es·is). The origin, formation and development of body tissues from the embryological germ layer. [Gk *histos* tissue, genesis.]

histogenetic (his·to·jen·et'·ik). Relating or belonging to histogenesis.
histogenous (his·toj·en·us). Histiogenic.
histogeny (his·toj·en·e). Histogenesis.
histography (his·tog·raf·e). A description of organic tissues. [Gk *histos* tissue, *graphein* to record.]
histohaematin (his·to·he·mat·in). A former name for cytochrome. [Gk *histos* tissue, haematin.]
histohaematogenous (his·to·he·mat·oj'·en·us). Arising from both the tissues and the blood; applied to certain cells in an inflammatory exudate which partly may form from multiplication of fixed tissue cells and partly may migrate from blood vessels. [Gk *histos* tissue, *haima* blood, *genein* to produce.]
histohydria (his·to·hi·dre·ah). Waterlogging. [Gk *histos* tissue, *hydor* water.]
histoid (his·toid). 1. Having structural resemblance to normal organic tissue, e.g. in a tumour. 2. Made up of or developed from a single tissue. 3. Web-like. 4. Resembling the tissues of immediately surrounding parts. [Gk *histos* tissue, *eidos* form.]
histo-irritative (his·to·ir·it·a·tiv). Having a stimulating or irritating effect on connective tissue. [Gk *histos* tissue, irritative.]
histokinesis (his·to·kin·e'·sis). The movement which occurs in the fundamental elements of the tissue structure of the body. [Gk *histos* tissue, *kinesis* movement.]
histological (his·to·loj·ik·al). Relating or belonging to histology.
histologist (his·tol·o·jist). An expert in the science of histology.
histology (his·tol·o·je). That branch of biological science which is concerned with the anatomy of tissues and their minute cellular structure; microscopic anatomy. **Normal histology.** Histology of healthy tissue. **Pathological histology.** Histology of diseased tissue. **Topographical histology.** Histology of the formation of organs from tissue. [Gk *histos* tissue, *logos* science.]
histolysate (his·tol·is·ate). A substance formed by the process of histolysis.
histolysis (his·tol·is·is). Spontaneous breaking-down or dissolution of living organic tissue. [Gk *histos* tissue, lysis.]
histolytic (his·to·lit·ik). Pertaining to or causing histolysis.
histoma (his·to·mah). Histioma.
histometaplastic (his·to·met·ah·plas'·tik). Causing the transformation of one kind of tissue into another kind. [Gk *histos* tissue, metaplasia.]
histomorphology (his·to·morf·ol'·o·je). Histology. [Gk *histos* tissue, morphology.]
histonectomy (his·to·nek·to·me). Periarterial sympathectomy; an operation designed to produce peripheral vasodilatation in vasospastic conditions of a limb. A segment of the main artery of the limb is denervated by stripping the adventitious coat, which contains the sympathetic nerve fibres. On theoretical grounds this operation is incomplete owing to segmental innervation of arteries at different levels throughout their length, and the operation has been largely superseded by that of lumbar sympathectomy. [Gk *histos* tissue, *ektome* excision.]
histones (his·to·nz). A group of simple proteins occurring in the thymus gland, blood corpuscles and sperm cells. They are soluble in water, not coagulable by heat, strongly basic and insoluble in ammonia. They usually occur in combination with nucleic acid. [Gk *histos* tissue.]
histoneurology (his·to·newr·ol'·o·je). Histology in its application to the nervous system. [Gk *histos* tissue, neurology.]
histonomy (his·ton·o·me). The laws of tissue development. [Gk *histos* tissue, *nomos* law.]
histonuria (his·ton·ewr'·e·ah). The presence of histones in the urine.
histopathology (his·to·path·ol'·o·je). Histological description or investigation of diseased tissues. [Gk *histos* tissue, pathology.]
histophysiology (his·to·fiz·e·ol'·o·je). The physiology of healthy cells and tissues. [Gk *histos* tissue, physiology.]
Histoplasma (his·to·plaz·mah). A dimorphic fungus parasitic for man and animals. Common in soil. **Histoplasma capsulatum.** The cause of histoplasmosis in man. In its parasitic form the fungus grows as a budding, oval yeast in cells of the reticulo-endothelial system. In culture, at room temperature, it grows as a whitish, filamentous mould which reproduces by spherical, tuberculate macroconidia and smooth, round microconidia. At elevated temperatures on enriched media, the yeast form can be cultured. (Perfect state is reported to be *Emmonsiella capsulata.*) **Histoplasma duboisii.** The aetiological agent of African histoplasmosis in man. In tissue form the fungus grows as a large, budding, thick-walled yeast (approximately 4 times the size of *H. capsulatum*); in culture the form is indistinguishable from *H. capsulatum* but, like the latter species, *H. duboisii* is unable to split urea. **Histoplasma farciminosum.** The cause of epizootic lymphangitis or African farcy. [Gk *histos* tissue, *plasma* anything formed.]
histoplasmin (his·to·plaz·min). An intradermal skin testing antigen prepared from *Histoplasma capsulatum,* used in the diagnosis of histoplasmosis. [Gk *histos* tissue, *plasma* anything formed.]
histoplasmosis (his·to·plaz·mo'·sis). A highly infectious disease of the reticulo-endothelial system due to *Histoplasma capsulatum* which usually results in a primary, acute, benign pulmonary disease and, rarely, in a progressive, chronic, malignant disease. If dissemination occurs, lymphatic tissues, spleen, liver, kidneys, skin and central nervous system may be affected. **African histoplasmosis.** An infection due to *Histoplasma duboisii.* The disease may occur in any part of the body but primary lesions are usually in the skin, lymph nodes and bones. The large yeast cells are found in giant cells and must be distinguished from those of blastomycosis. The disease is at present only known from the region of Africa between latitudes 15°N and 10°S; cases have been reported in man and in monkeys. **Histoplasmosis farciminosum.** The aetiological agent of epizootic lymphangitis (African farcy) in horses and mules. The disease is characterized by the presence of subcutaneous, ulcerated lesions of the skin, especially in areas subject to trauma, e.g. neck, legs. [Gk *histos* tissue, *plasma* anything formed, *-osis* condition.]
histopsyche (his·to·si·ke). The mental factor inherent in protoplasm; the directive force which governs protoplasmic activities as such. [Gk *histos* tissue, *psyche* mind.]
histopsychology (his·to·si·kol'·o·je). Anatomy of the tissues combined with psychological investigation. [Gk *histos* tissue, psychology.]
historadiography (his·to·ra·de·og'·raf·e). X-ray photography of tissue, particularly of microscopical sections. [Gk *histos* tissue, radiography.]
historrhexis (his·to·rex·is). Destruction of circumscribed areas of nerve or other tissue by an agency other than that of infection (Southard). [Gk *histos* tissue, *rhexis* rupture.]
histotherapy (his·to·ther·ap·e). The therapeutic use of animal tissue, e.g. hog's stomach. [Gk *histos* tissue, therapy.]
histothrombin (his·to·throm·bin). Thrombin which has been derived from connective tissue. [Gk *histos* tissue, thrombin.]
histotome (his·to·tome). A microtome. [Gk *histos* tissue, *temnein* to cut.]
histotomy (his·tot·o·me). Microtomy; the process of slicing thin sections of fixed tissue for microscopical study. [see prec.]
histotoxic (his·to·tox·ik). Possessing the special characteristics of a histotoxin.
histotoxin (his·to·tox·in). A substance that is poisonous to the tissues. [Gk *histos* tissue, *toxikon* poison.]
histotribe (his·to·tribe). A strong forceps in which a mass of tissue containing blood vessels can be held in order to ensure haemostasia. [Gk *histos* tissue, *tribein* to crush.]
histotripsy (his·to·trip·se). The crushing of tissue by the use of a histotribe or an écraseur.
histotroph (his·to·trof). A nutritive fluid for the early embryo, derived from the disintegration of the uterine endometrium around the trophoblast. [Gk *histos* tissue, *trophe* nutrition.]
histotrophic (his·to·trof·ik). 1. Relating or belonging to the formation or nutrition of tissue. 2. Aiding or favouring the formation or nutrition of tissue. [Gk *histos* tissue, *trophe* nutrition.]

histotropic (his·to·**trop**·ik). Having a special affinity for tissue cells; applied to parasites, chemical compounds and stains. [Gk *histos* tissue, *trope* a turning.]

histozoic (his·to·**zo**·ik). Applied to parasites which live on or in the tissues but not within the cell body. [Gk *histos* tissue, *zoon* animal.]

histozyme (**his**·to·zime). Hippuricase. [Gk *histos* tissue, enzyme.]

histrionic, histrionical (his·tre·**on**·ik, his·tre·**on**·ik·al). 1. Affecting those muscles of the face which produce expression. 2. Marked by exaggerated gestures, speech and facial expression such as are used by actors. [L *histrio* actor.]

histrionism (**his**·tre·on·izm). Dramatic gesturing and general behaviour observed in cases of hysteria or insanity. [see prec.]

histuria (his·**tewr**·e·ah). An increased output of macromolecules in the urine after renal transplantation. [Gk *histos* tissue, *ouron* urine.]

Hitchens, Arthur Parker (b. 1877). Washington physician.

Hitchens' agar. A nutrient broth with 0.1 per cent agar.

Hittorf, Johann Wilhelm (b. 1824). German physicist.

Hittorf number. Transport number; the ratio of the migration velocity of an ion to the combined velocities of anion and cation.

Hitzig, Julius Eduard (b. 1838). Zürich and Halle psychiatrist.

Hitzig's centre. A motor area in the frontal lobe of the cerebrum, accurately defined by Hitzig in dogs and monkeys.

Hitzig's girdle. A girdle of anaesthesia, usually in the distribution of the 3rd and 6th thoracic nerves, in tabes dorsalis.

Hitzig's galvanic test, for diseases of the labyrinth and vestibular nerve. The patient standing with his eyes closed and feet together holds the cathode in his hand. The anode rests in front of his ear, and a 5 mA current is applied. In the absence of disease, the normal reaction is for the patient to lean towards the stimulated side. In diseases of the labyrinth, a stronger and possibly painful current may have to be applied to elicit the reaction. In diseases of the vestibular neural pathways, no reaction at all may be produced.

hives (**hi**·vz). Urticaria. [etym. dub.]

hoarhound (**ho**·er·hownd). Horehound.

hoarse (**ho**·ers). Of the voice, rough, grating or discordant. [ME *hors.*]

hoarseness (**ho**·ers·nes). The harsh, rough, grating quality of voice distinctive of affections or diseases of throat and larynx. [see prec.]

Hoboken, Nicolaas (b. 1632). Harderwijk and Utrecht anatomist.

Hoboken's nodules. Projections on the umbilical arteries caused by underlying dilatations of the vessels.

Hocevar's sterile glands. Mucous glands of the conjunctiva that have no secretory duct.

Hoche, Alfred Erich (b. 1865). Strasbourg and Freiburg psychiatrist.

Hoche's bandelette. A small bundle of nerve fibres in the white matter of the spinal cord, adjacent to the posterior horns.

Hoche's tract. The septomarginal tract. *See* TRACT.

Hochenegg, Julius von (b. 1859). Vienna surgeon.

Hochenegg's operation. An operation for removal of a malignant rectum by a sacral route.

Hochsinger, Karl (b. 1860). Vienna paediatrician.

Hochsinger's phenomenon or sign. Contraction of the hand when the inner side of the biceps is pressed. It is seen in tetany due to hypoparathyroidism.

Hodara, Menahem (d. 1926). Turkish physician.

Hodara's disease. Trichorrhexis nodosa.

hodegetics (hod·e·**jet**·ix). Medical ethics or etiquette. [Gk *hodegetikos* suitable for guiding.]

Hodge, Hugh Lennox (b. 1796). Philadelphia gynaecologist.

Hodge's pessary. A bakelite pessary used to hold the uterus in an anteverted position following manual correction.

Hodge's plane. A plane passing through the upper border of the symphysis pubis and the second piece of the sacrum, parallel to the plane of the pelvic inlet.

Hodgen, John Thompson (b. 1826). St. Louis, Missouri, surgeon.

Hodgen's splint. A metal splint used in the treatment of fractures of the femoral shaft.

Hodgkin, Thomas (b. 1798). London physician.

Hodgkin's cell. A giant cell of Hodgkin's disease.

Hodgkin's disease or granuloma. A disease of unknown aetiology, characterized by enlargement of the lymph glands, hyperplasia of the lymphoid tissue in the spleen, liver and other organs, and anaemia.

Hodgkin's paragranuloma. A variant of Hodgkin's disease with mature lymphocytic hyperplasia and Sternberg–Reed cells, but running a more benign course for some years at least.

Hodgkin's prurigo. Excoriated, scabbed papules resulting from pruritus in Hodgkin's disease.

Hodgkin's sarcoma. A highly malignant variety of Hodgkin's disease.

Reed–Hodgkin disease (a term confined to the USA). Lymphadenoma.

Hodgson, Joseph (b. 1788). Birmingham and London surgeon.

Hodgson's disease, maladie de Hodgson. Aneurysmal dilatation of the aorta.

hodi-potsy (ho·de·**pot**·se). Pityriasis versicolor.

Hodogenes (hod·**oj**·en·eez). A genus of South African scorpions.

hodograph (**hod**·o·graf). 1. An instrument with which the movements of locomotion can be recorded. 2. A curve showing the velocity of a moving particle. [Gk *hodos* path, *graphein* to record.]

hodology (hod·**ol**·o·je). The branch of neurology which is concerned with the pathways of the nervous system. [Gk *hodos* path, *logos* science.]

hodoneuromere (hod·o·**newr**·o·meer). In embryology, a segment of the trunk together with its 2 neurones and their branches. [Gk *hodos* path, *neuron* nerve, *meros* part.]

hody-potsy (ho·de·**pot**·se). Pityriasis versicolor.

hoe (ho). 1. An instrument for scraping, used in operative repair of cleft palate. 2. A type of chisel used in conservative dentistry for cutting or cleaving enamel and for cutting dentine walls to proper form. [O Fr. *hone.*]

Hoeve's bundle. Inferior longitudinal fasciculus consisting chiefly of itinerant fibres.

Hofbauer, Isfred Isidore (b. 1878). Austrian gynaecologist in Cincinnati.

Hofbauer cell. A histiocyte from the connective tissue of a chorionic villus.

Hofbauer's method. A method of staining iodophil granules within the leucocytes.

Hofer, Gustav (b. 1887). Austrian otorhinolaryngologist.

Hofer's nerve. A branch of the superior laryngeal nerve to the deep cardiac plexus; Cyon's nerve.

Hoff, Jacobus Henricus van't (b. 1852). Dutch chemist.

van't Hoff's law. The osmotic pressure of a solution is the same as the gas pressure which the molecules of the solution would exert if they occupied the same volume as the solution, but in gaseous form instead of in solution.

van't Hoff's rule. The velocity of a chemical reaction is roughly doubled for every 10 degrees rise in temperature.

Hoffa, Albert (b. 1859). Berlin orthopaedic surgeon.

Hoffa–Lorenz operation. Manipulative reduction of a congenital dislocation of the hip.

Hoffman, Frederick Ludwig 8b. 1865). American physician.

Hoffman bronchitis. Membranous bronchitis.

Hoffman, William Joseph (b. 1894). New York surgeon.

Hoffman laminectomy forceps. A punch-type bone forceps, one blade being fenestrated.

Hoffmann, Johann (b. 1857). Heidelberg neurologist.

Hoffmann's phenomenon or sign. Increased mechanical irritability of the peripheral nerves, as in tetany.

Hoffmann's reflex. Digital reflex, 2nd def. *See* REFLEX.

Hoffmann's syndrome. Muscular hypertrophy with weakness and delayed relaxation in hypothyroidism in adults.

Werdnig-Hoffmann disease. Familial progressive spinal atrophy of infancy.

Hoffmann, Moritz (b. 1622). Altdorf anatomist.

Hoffmann's duct. The pancreatic duct. *See* DUCT.

Hoffmann, Raoul. Swiss orthopaedic surgeon.

Hoffmann's method of osteosynthesis. A method of fracture fixation using skeletal pins inserted into the bony fragments and joined together by external metal rods.

Hofmann, August Wilhelm von (b. 1812). German chemist.

Hofmann's green. Iodine green. *See* GREEN.

Hofmann, Heinrich (b. 1909). Jena biochemist.

Hofmann's reaction or test, for tyrosine. Millon's reaction applied to the detection of tyrosine.

Hofmann Wellenhof, Georg von (d. 1890). Vienna bacteriologist.

Hofmann's bacillus. *Corynebacterium hofmannii.*

Hofmeister, Franz von (b. 1867). Stuttgart surgeon.

Hofmeister gastrectomy. Removal of the stomach with end-to-side union of the gastric remnant and jejunum, the remnant being partly closed as a valve.

Hogben test. Toad test, xenopus test: 5 ml of urine from a pregnant woman is injected into the dorsal lymph sac of the South African clawed toad, *Xenopus laevis.* Eggs are produced in large numbers in from 8 to 24 h. Seldom if ever now used.

Högyes, Endre (b. 1847). Budapest physician.

Högyes' treatment. Prophylactic treatment of rabies by the subcutaneous injection of a suspension of fixed virus, diluted from 1:100 to 1:10 000. The treatment is begun with inactive dilutions and continued with dilutions increasing in virulence.

hoist (hoist). An apparatus for lifting. **Nursing hoist.** An apparatus, fixed or mobile, which reduces the amount of energy output required to move a patient, e.g. from a lying to an upright position, into a chair, etc.

holagogue (hol·ag·og). 1. A radical remedy; a medicine that completely removes any morbid substance. 2. A panacea. [Gk *holos* whole, *agogos* leading.]

holandric (hol·an·drik). Describing genes which are carried by the Y chromosome in the heterogametic sex. [Gk *holos* whole, *aner* man.]

holarctic (hol·ark·tik). Of the geographical region north of the tropic of Cancer, but including the Cape Verde Islands and excluding the oriental region south of the Himalayas, and sometimes excluding the Sonoran region of North America. [Gk *holos* whole, *arktikos* northern.]

Holarrhena (hol·ar·e·nah). 1. A genus of trees of the family Apocynaceae. 2. The dried bark from the stem and root of a small Indian tree, *Holarrhena antidysenterica* Wall., which contain the alkaloid conessine amongst many other subsidiary alkaloids. It is used widely in India in the treatment of amoebic dysentery. Also known as *kurchi* or *conessi bark.*

holarthritic (hol·ar·thrit·ik). Relating or belonging to holarthritis.

holarthritis (hol·ar·thri·tis). Gout or arthritis affecting all the joints at the same time. [Gk *holos* whole, *arthron* joint.]

Holden, Luther (b. 1815). London surgeon.

Holden's line. A flexure line at the junction of the thigh and the abdomen. It is not always apparent in thin muscular subjects.

holder (ho·lder). Any device for securing an object in a desired position, e.g. crucibles, culture dishes, watch-glasses. **Needle holder.** A forceps for holding a needle; used in the insertion of sutures, particularly in suturing in the depths of a wound or at the bottom of a deep cavity. [AS *haldan.*]

See also: GILLIES.

holergasia (hol·er·ga·ze·ah). A term introduced by Adolf Meyer to cover the major psychoses and to distinguish them from neurotic reactions. The name signifies a *total* reaction, and was introduced in accordance with the belief that illnesses such as schizophrenia and the affective psychoses involved the whole of the personality, whereas conditions such as anxiety states are to be regarded as partial reactions (merergasias). In the meyerian system, all forms of mental illness are reactions (ergasias) between the psychobiologically unified personality and the environment. [Gk *holos* whole, *ergein* to work.]

holergastic (hol·er·gas·tik). In the system of Adolf Meyer, describing a major psychosis involving the whole personality. [Gk *holos* whole, *ergein* to work.]

Holfelder, Hans (b. 1891). Frankfurt radiologist.

Holfelder's method. Multiple-field treatment giving daily irradiation of the tumour but spaced irradiation of each skin area.

holism (ho·lizm). A philosophy in which man, his body and his mind, are considered as an indivisible unity. [Gk *holos* whole.]

holistic (ho·lis·tik). Relating to holism.

Holl, Moritz (b. 1852). Austrian anatomist.

Holl's ligament. A small ligament frequently found uniting the 2 ischiocavernosus muscles in front of the urethral opening in the female.

hollow (hol·o). In anatomy, a depression. [ME *holg.*]

See also: SEBILEAU.

hollyhock (hol·e·hok). *Althaea rosea* Linn. (family Malvaceae), common or garden hollyhock. The flowers yield a purple dye, and are stated to have properties similar to those of the marshmallow. [AS *halig* holy, *hoc* mallow.]

Holmes, Sir Gordon Morgan (b. 1876). London neurologist.

Holmes' degeneration. Primary progressive cerebellar degeneration. *See* DEGENERATION.

Holmes' phenomenon or sign. Rebound phenomenon; this is seen when a patient with a cerebellar lesion is asked to attempt movement against resistance. On withdrawing the resistance the ipsilateral limb moves forcibly in the direction in which the effort was made.

Holmes-Adie syndrome. Adie's syndrome.

Stewart-Holmes sign. Holmes' phenomenon (see above).

Holmes, Timothy (b. 1825). London surgeon.

Holmes' operation. Excision of the calcaneum.

Holmgren, Alarik Frithiof (b. 1831). Upsala physiologist.

yarns of Holmgren. Commonly called *Holmgren's wools* and employed in a matching test for colour blindness; now largely replaced by other methods, e.g. Ishihara's and lantern tests.

Holmgren, Emilie Algot (b. 1866). Stockholm histologist.

Holmgren-Golgi canal. Intracytoplasmic canal; one of a system of fine canals in the cytoplasm of many cells.

holmium (hol·me·um). A rare-earth element of atomic weight 164.93, atomic number 67 and chemical symbol Ho, found in the mineral gadolinite. It is a trivalent metal which forms rose-coloured salts. [L *Holmia* Stockholm.]

holo-acardius (hol·o·a·kar′·de·us). 1. A monster with a body that has no openings and lacks a heart. 2. A twin monster in which there are 2 hearts but the circulation is carried on by only one of them. **Holo-acardius acephalus.** A holo-acardius lacking a head. **Holo-acardius acormus.** One consisting only of a much deformed head, without trunk or limbs. **Holo-acardius amorphus.** A holo-acardius which consists only of a mass of tissue without form or shape. [Gk *holos* whole, *a, kardia* heart.]

holoblast (hol·o·blast). A pre-blastula embryo in which cleavage is total. [Gk *holos* whole, *blastos* germ.]

holoblastic (hol·o·blas·tik). Describing eggs which undergo total cleavage; it occurs in those containing relatively small amounts of yolk, e.g. man, frog. [see prec.]

holocephalic (hol·o·kef·al′·ik). Term applied to a monster of which the head is complete although other parts are not. [Gk *holos* whole, *kephale* head.]

holocrine (hol·o·krine). Applied to a gland the function of which is secretory only, or the secretion of which (as in the sebaceous glands) consists of disintegrated cells of the gland itself. [Gk *holos* whole, *krinein* to secrete.]

holodiastolic (hol·o·di·as·tol′·ik). Relating or belonging to the whole phase of diastole. [Gk *holos* whole, diastole.]

holo-endemic (hol·o·en·dem′·ik). A term used by malariologists to indicate intensely endemic areas with spleen rate of 75 per cent or over in children under 10 years of age. [Gk *holos* whole, endemic.]

holoenzyme (hol·o·en·zime). A complete enzyme composed of the protein component, or apoenzyme, together with its non-protein coenzyme. [Gk *holos* whole, enzyme.]

hologamy (hol·og·am·e). The condition in which the gametes are the same as the undifferentiated body cells in size and type of structure. [Gk *holos* whole, *gamos* marriage.]

hologastroschisis (hol·o·gas·tros′·kis·is). A congenital fissure running the whole length of the abdomen, exposing the viscera. [Gk *holos* whole, *gaster* belly, *schisis* a cleavage.]

hologenesis (hol·o·jen·es·is). The theory that the human species did not originate in any special region or regions of the earth but in all parts of the earth at the same time. [Gk *holos* whole, genesis.]

hologram (hol·o·gram). A three-dimensional image. [Gk *holos* whole, *gramma* record.]

holography (hol·og·raf·e). A type of three-dimensional photography with medical applications. Invented by Professor D. Gabor of Imperial College, London, who received the Nobel Prize in 1971 for his discovery. [Gk *holos* whole, *graphein* to record.]

hologynic (hol·o·ji·nik). Inheritance by the female line only. [Gk *holos* whole, *gyne* woman.]

Holokenius' valves. Crescentic folds of the internal lining of the umbilical vessels.

holomastigote (hol·o·mas·tig·ote). Having a scattering of flagellae over the whole surface of the body. [Gk *holos* whole, *mastigx* lash.]

holometabolic, holometabolous (hol·o·met·ab·ol′·ik, hol·o·met·ab′·ol·us). Of insects, those in which a pupal stage is intercalated between the larva and adult; they are thus said to undergo complete metamorphosis. Characteristic of the Endopterygota. [Gk *holos* whole, *metabole* change.]

holomorphosis (hol·o·mor·fo·sis). The complete renewal or regrowth of a part that has been lost. [Gk *holos* whole, *morphosis* a forming.]

holonarcosis (hol·o·nar·ko′·sis). Complete narcosis. [Gk *holos* whole, narcosis.]

holopathy (hol·op·ath·e). 1. A constitutional or generalized disease manifesting itself as a local disease or disorder. 2. The theory that any local disorder or disease is the sign of constitutional or generalized disease. [Gk *holos* whole, *pathos* disease.]

holophytic (hol·o·fi·tik). Having plant-like characteristics; applied to those protozoa which have metabolic processes similar to those of plants. [Gk *holos* whole, *phytikos* like a plant.]

holoplexia (hol·o·plex·e·ah). A term for generalized paralysis. [Gk *holos* whole, *plexis* stroke.]

holoprosencephaly (hol·o·pros·en·kef·al·e). Deficiency of the forebrain. [Gk *holos* whole, *pro, egkephalos* brain.]

holorepressor (hol·o·re·pres·or). The combination of corepressor and aporepressor to give a functional repressor. [Gk *holos* whole, L *reprimere* to press back.]

holorrachischisis (hol·o·rak·is′·kis·is). Complete spina bifida, in which the spinal column is cleft along its entire length with the vertebral canal non-existent. [Gk *holos* whole, *rhachis* spine, *schisis* division.]

holosaccharide (hol·o·sak·ar·ide). General term for polysaccharides composed of sugar units only: they consist of the pentosans and hexosans. [Gk *holos* whole, saccharide.]

holoschisis (hol·os·kis·is). Simple or direct division of a cell by cleavage of the nucleus only. [Gk *holos* whole, *schisis* division.]

holoside (hol·o·side). Name applied to the true carbohydrates which are constituted of sugar units only. [Gk *holos* whole.]

holosteosclerosis (hol·os·te·o·skler·o′·sis). Generalized osteosclerosis. [Gk *holos* whole, osteosclerosis.]

holosteous (hol·os·te·us). In biology, having a well-developed or completely bony skeleton. [Gk *holos* whole, *osteon* bone.]

holosteric (hol·o·ster·ik). Wholly solid, as an aneroid barometer, in which liquids are not used. [Gk *holos* whole, *steros* solid.]

holostomatous (hol·o·sto·mat·us). In biology and zoology, having the margin of the mouth or aperture entire; notches are absent and all parts are present. [Gk *holos* whole, *stoma* mouth.]

holosymphysis (hol·o·sim·fis·is). Complete union, e.g. between bones. [Gk *holos* whole, symphysis.]

holosystolic (hol·o·sis·tol′·ik). Relating or belonging to the whole phase of systole. [Gk *holos* whole, systole.]

holotetanus (hol·o·tet·an·us). Generalized muscular tetanus or tonic spasm. [Gk *holos* whole, tetanus.]

Holothyrus (hol·o·thi·rus). A genus of ticks, of which *Holothyrus coccinella* from Mauritius and normal to ducks and geese, bites man, giving rise to serious poisoning. [Gk *holos* whole, *thyreos* shield.]

holotomy (hol·ot·o·me). Surgical removal of an organ or part in its entirety. [Gk *holos* whole, *temnein* to cut.]

holotonia (hol·o·to·ne·ah). Holotetanus. [Gk *holos* whole, *tonos* tone.]

holotonic (hol·o·ton·ik). Having relation or belonging to holotetanus. [see prec.]

holotopic (hol·o·top·ik). Pertaining to the relationship in which any particular part of an organ stands to the organ as a whole. [Gk *holos* whole, *topos* place.]

holotopy (hol·ot·o·pe). The position of a part or organ in relation to the whole organism or body (Waldeyer). [see prec.]

holotrichous (hol·ot·rik·us). Having the body or surface more or less completely and uniformly covered with cilia, as in some infusoria. [Gk *holos* whole, *thrix* hair.]

ho-louan (ho·loo·an). Cholera. [Chinese name.]

holozoic (hol·o·zo·ik). In biology, applied to those protozoa which have metabolism like that of animals or obtain their food as animals do. [Gk *holos* whole, *zoon* animal.]

Holst, Johan Martin (b. 1892). Oslo surgeon.

Holst thoracoplasty. A one-stage thoracoplasty in which the upper ribs, except the first, and the apex of the lung are mobilized downwards and fixed, to produce relaxation and healing in pulmonary tuberculosis.

Holt, Mary. London cardiologist.

Holt-Oram syndrome. The association of skeletal deformities of the forearm with atrial septal defect.

Holt-Harris, John Evan (b. 1876). Albany, New York, physician.

Holt-Harris and Teague agar. Eosin methylene blue agar. *See* AGAR.

Holter, John W. American engineer.

Holter ventriculocaval-shunt valve. A surgical device for the control of intracranial pressure.

Holth, Sören (b. 1863). Norwegian ophthalmic surgeon.

Holth's operation, for glaucoma. 1. Iridencleisis; a radial incision of the iris including the sphincter, leaving one or two pillars included in the wound. 2. Punch sclerectomy; a modification of Lagrange's operation in which a piece of the scleral lip of the wound is removed with a punch.

Holthouse, Carsten (b. 1810). English surgeon.

Holthouse's hernia. An inguinal hernia which has turned laterally over the groin.

Holtz, Wilhelm (b. 1836). German physicist.

Holtz machine. An apparatus designed to produce high-voltage static electricity by multiplication of an induced charge.

Holzknecht, Guido (b. 1872). Vienna radiologist.

Holzknecht's space. A radiographically translucent area, 25–50 mm wide, between the posterior border of the heart shadow and the spine, in the right anterior oblique position.

Holzknecht stomach. The extreme form of hypertonic or steerhorn stomach in which, seen radiographically, the pylorus forms the lowest point of the diagonal.

Holzknecht unit. A unit of dose of ionizing radiation formerly used; one-fifth of an erythema dose.

Holzmann, Willy (b. 1878). Munich physician.

Much-Holzmann reaction. Psychoreaction; the inhibition of the haemolytic action of cobra venom on the red blood corpuscles in schizophrenia and affective psychosis. It is now discredited.

homalocephalus (hom·al·o·kef′·al·us). An individual with a flat skull (Lissauer). [Gk *homalos* flat, *kephale* head.]

homalocoryphus (hom·al·o·kor′·e·fus). In craniometry, a skull in which the angle formed by the meeting of 2 lines drawn from the occipital point and the bregma to the highest point of the skull, is between 132 and 142 degrees (Lissauer). [Gk *homalos* flat, *koryphe* crown of head.]

homalographic (hom·al·o·graf′·ik). Relating or belonging to homalography.

homalography (hom·al·og·raf·e). Anatomy studied by means of plane sections of the various parts, or by means of sectional drawings. [Gk *homalos* flat, *graphein* to record.]

homalometopus (hom·al·o·met·o′·pus). In craniometry, a skull in which the frontal angle is between 130.5 and 141 degrees (Lissauer). [Gk *homalos* flat, *metopon* forehead.]

homalopisthocranius (hom·al·o·pis·tho·kra′·ne·us). In craniometry, a skull in which the angle formed by the meeting of 2 lines drawn from the inion and the occipital point to the highest point of the skull, is between 140 and 154 degrees (Lissauer). [Gk *homalos* flat, *opisthe* behind, *kranion* skull.]

homalosternal (hom·al·o·ster′·nal). In biology, having a level or keelless sternum, as some birds. [Gk *homalos* flat, sternum.]

homaluranus (hom·al·ewr·a′·nus). In craniometry, a skull in which the angle formed by the meeting of 2 lines drawn from the occipital point and the bregma to the highest point of the skull is between 147.5 and 163.5 degrees (Lissauer). [Gk *homalos* flat, *ouranos* palate.]

Homans, John (b. 1877). Boston surgeon.

Homans' sign. Pain in the calf and popliteal region on passive dorsiflexion of the foot with the knee flexed. It occurs in venous thrombosis of the deep calf veins, and is a valuable sign since it may be present before there is any complaint of pain, swelling or tenderness in the leg.

homarecoline (hom·ar·ek·o·leen). Homo-arecoline.

homatropine (hom·at·ro·peen). $C_6H_5CH(OH)COOC_8H_{14}N$, the tropine ester of mandelic acid (BPC 1954). **Homatropine Hydrobromide BP 1973.** A soluble salt of homatropine with actions similar to those of atropine but less powerful and of shorter duration. It is seldom used internally, but is employed chiefly as a mydriatic and cycloplegic especially valuable for ophthalmoscopic examination and in refraction, where it shows less tendency to increase the intra-ocular pressure and to have a less prolonged action than atropine. It is used in solution or in the form of lamellae, and may be potentiated by cocaine. **Homatropine methylbromide.** A compound used internally as an inhibitor of secretions and as an antispasmodic. It acts like atropine but is less toxic, and is administered chiefly for disorders of the gastro-intestinal tract. [Gk *homos* same, atropine.]

homaxial, homaxonal, homaxonic (hom·ax·e·al, hom·ax·on·al, hom·ax·on·ik). 1. In morphology, having all the axes equal. 2. In bacteriology. cocci which grow equally in all directions. [Gk *homos* same, *axon* axle.]

Home, Sir Everard (b. 1756). London surgeon.

Home's lobe. The third or middle lobe of the prostate gland, which lies between the neck of the bladder and the verumontanum.

homedric (hom·ed·rik). Term applied to a structure, all the facets of which are equal. [Gk *homos* same, *hedra* base.]

Homén, Ernst Alexander (b. 1851). Finnish physician.

Homén's syndrome. A syndrome due to a lesion of the lentiform nucleus, often due to chronic trauma. There is slurring of speech, unsteadiness of gait and rigidity of limbs, impairment of memory and intellect, and progressive dementia. The traumatic form often occurs in boxers; the punchdrunk syndrome.

homeo-. For words beginning **homeo-**, *see also* HOMOEO-.

homeochrome (ho·me·o·krome). Term applied to certain apparently serous cells of the salivary glands which give staining reactions for mucus after bichromate fixation. [Gk *homoios* similar, *chroma* colour.]

homeokinesis (ho·me·o·kin·e′·sis). Normal mitotic division in which the daughter cells have similar numbers of chromosomes. [Gk *homoios* similar, *kinesis* motion.]

homergy (hom·er·je). The process of normal metabolism with its results. [Gk *homos* same, *ergon* work.]

homicidal (hom·e·si·dal). Relating or belonging to homicide.

homicide (hom·e·side). 1. In general, the killing of one human being by another. 2. In forensic medicine, colloquially murder; but homicide may be *justifiable* (approved by law), *excusable* including accidental (excused by law) or *criminal* which would include murder, manslaughter or infanticide (punishable by law). [L *homo* man, *caedere* to kill.]

Hominoidea (hom·in·oid·e·ah). A super-family of the primate sub-order Anthropoidea. It includes gibbons, apes and man. [L *homo* man, Gk *eidos* form.]

homme rouge (om·roozh). The second stage in mycosis fungoides in which the red and scaly lesions become infiltrated, raised above the surface of the skin and coalescent. [Fr. red man.]

Homo (ho·mo). 1. A genus of catarrhine apes of Old World origin; *Homo sapiens* is man. Various races or structural groups have from time to time been described under different names, but it is in general customary to treat all mankind under the one name without further specific or sub-specific distinction. Several fossil hominids are also placed in *Homo.* 2. A slang term to denote a male homosexual.

homoalleles (hom·o·al·eelz). A pair of homologous genes having independent mutations at the same site. [Gk *homos* same, *allelon* of one another.]

homo-arecoline (hom·o·ar·ek′·o·leen). $CH_3NC_5H_7COOC_2H_5$, an arecoline alkaloid synthesized by the esterification of arecaidine with ethyl alcohol. The hydrobromide is employed as a taenicide and miotic.

homoblastic (hom·o·blas·tik). 1. Having direct embryonic development. 2. Arising from like cells or germs. [Gk *homos* same, *blastos* germ.]

homocentric (hom·o·sen·trik). Having the same focus or centre. [Gk *homos* same, centre.]

homochelidonine (hom·o·kel·id·on′·een). $C_{21}H_{23}NO_5$, an alkaloid obtainable from *Chelidonium majus* and from bloodroot (*Sanguinaria canadensis*). [Gk *homos* same, *Chelidonium.*]

Homochlorcyclizine (ho·mo·klor·si′·kliz·een). BP Commission approved name for 1-(4-chlorobenzhydryl)-4-methyl-1,4-diazacycloheptane; an antihistaminic drug.

homochrome (hom·o·krome). Applied to a type of serous cell of a salivary gland which stains a similar colour to that of the dye employed. [Gk *homos* same, *chroma* colour.]

homochronous (hom·ok·ron·us). 1. Occurring at the same time. 2. Occurring in successive generations at the same period or age. [Gk *homos* same, *chronos* time.]

homocinchonicine (hom·o·sin·kon′·is·een). An impure form of cinchonine.

homocinchonidine (hom·o·sin·kon′·id·een). $C_{19}H_{22}ON_2$, one of the less important cinchona alkaloids, and thought by some to be identical with cinchonine.

homocinchonine (hom·o·sin·kon·een). An impure form of cinchonine.

homocladic (hom·o·klad·ik). Anastomosis occurring between twigs of the same artery. [Gk *homos* same, *klados* twig.]

homococaine (hom·o·ko·kane′). Cocaethyline.

homocyclic (hom·o·si·klik). Denoting an organic cyclic compound the ring of which consists of similar atoms, usually carbon. [Gk *homos* same, cycle.]

homocysteine (hom·o·sis·te·een). $HSCH_2CH_2CH(NH_2)COOH$, the next higher homologue of cysteine which occurs in the catabolism of methionine as the result of the demethylation of the latter. **Adenosyl homocysteine.** A compound in which the adenosyl group is attached to homocysteine through the terminal thiol group; its function is as an acceptor of methyl groups with formation of adenosyl methionine (*see* METHIONINE).

homocystine (hom·o·sis·teen). $(SCH_2CH_2CHNH_2COOH)_2$, the homologue of cystine formed by the condensation of homocysteine during the catabolism of methionine.

homocystinuria (hom·o·sist·in·ewr·e·ah). A rare inborn error of amino-acid metabolism presenting with mental deficiency, epilepsy, dislocation of the lens, growth-disturbance, thromboses and defective hair growth. [Gk *homos* same, cystinuria.]

homodesmotic (hom·o·dez·mot′·ik). Applied to certain fibres which join similar structures of the central nervous system. [Gk *homos* same, *desmos* band.]

homodikaryon (ho·mo·di·kar·e·on). A cell, spore or mycelium containing 2 genetically identical nuclei. [Gk *homos* same, *di-*, *karyon* nut.]

homodont (hom·o·dont). In biology, having all the teeth similar in form. [Gk *homos* same, *odous* tooth.]

homodromous (hom·od·ro·mus). Moving in the same direction or having action directed towards the same end. [Gk *homos* same, *dromos* course.]

homoeograft (hom·e·o·grahft). Homograft.

homoeologous (hom·e·ol·o·gus). In genetics, of chromosomes which are only partially homologous. [Gk *homoios* similar, *logos* relation.]

homoeology (hom·e·ol·o·je). Imperfect, incomplete homology. [Gk *homoios* similar, *logos* relation.]

homoeomorphous (hom·e·o·mor′·fus). Nearly similar in form and structure. [Gk *homoios* similar, *morphe* shape.]

homoeopath (hom·e·o·path, ho·me·o·path). 1. Anyone who believes in homoeopathy. 2. A physician who practises homoeopathy. [Gk *homoios* similar, *pathos* disease.]

homoeopathic (hom·e·o·path′·ik, ho·me·o·path′·ik). Referring or belonging to homoeopathy.

homoeopathist (hom·e·op·ath·ist, ho·me·op·ath·ist). Homoeopath.

homoeopathy (hom·e·op·ath·e, ho·me·op·ath·e). A system of therapeutics based on the law, *similia similibus curentur.* Partly anticipated by Hippocrates and Paracelsus (1658), but introduced by Samuel Hahnemann (1755–1843) in 1796. Its essential principle is that the cure of disease is effected by drugs "proved" to be capable of producing in a healthy subject symptoms similar to those of the disease to be treated. The dosage is usually minute. [Gk *homoios* similar, *pathos* disease.]

homoeoplasia (hom·e·o·pla′·ze·ah). The formation of new tissue similar to the normal tissue of the part. [Gk *homoios* similar, *plassein* to form.]

homoeoplastic (hom·e·o·plas′·tik). Relating to homoeoplasia.

homoeoplasty (hom·e·o·plas′·te). Homoeoplasia.

homoeosis (hom·e·o·sis). 1. The assimilation of nourishing substances. 2. In biology, the taking on of the characters proper to one of a series of parts by another of the series to which these characters are not proper. [Gk *homoios* similar.]

homoeostasis (hom·e·os·tas·is). 1. The dynamic processes by which an organism maintains a state of equilibrium of its various functions and tissue chemistry. 2. The state of equilibrium so maintained. [Gk *homoios* similar, *stasis* a standing still.]

homoeostatic (hom·e·o·stat′·ik). Referring or belonging to homoeostasis.

homoeothermal (hom·e·o·ther′·mal). Homothermal.

homoeotoxin (hom·e·o·tox′·in). A toxin derived from one individual and toxic for others of the same species. [Gk *homoios* similar, toxin.]

homoeotransplant (hom·e·o·trans′·plahnt). Homograft. [Gk *homoios* similar, transplant.]

homoeotransplantation (hom·e·o·trans·plan·ta′·shun). Homotransplantation.

homoeotypical (hom·e·o·tip′·ik·al). Resembling the normal type, or of the usual type, e.g. the second meiotic division of germ cells. [Gk *homoios* similar, type.]

homo-erotic (hom·o·er·ot′·ik). Homosexual. [Gk *homos* same, *eros* love.]

homo-eroticism (hom·o·er·ot′·is·izm). Homosexuality. [see prec.]

homogametic (hom·o·gam·et′·ik). Producing only one kind of gamete with respect to sex determination. [Gk *homos* same, gamete.]

homogenate (hom·oj·en·ate). A homogenous tissue suspension.

homogeneity (hom·o·jen·e′·it·e). The state of being homogeneous.

homogeneization (hom·o·je·ne·i·za′·shun). Homogenization.

homogeneous (hom·o·je·ne·us). 1. Having the same nature or being of the same kind. 2. In chemistry, of uniform or similar quality and nature in all parts. [Gk *homos* same, *genos* kind.]

homogenesis (hom·o·jen·es·is). In biology, the production of the same characteristics in successive generations. [see prec.]

homogenitality (hom·o·jen·it·al′·it·e). The state in which interest is directed to the genitals of the same sex as the subject. [Gk *homos* same, genitals.]

homogenization (hom·oj′·en·i·za′·shun). 1. The process or act of making homogeneous. 2. The process or act of reducing to a common standard. 3. In microscopy, the process of making objects for examination fixed and clear.

homogenize (hom·oj·en·ize). To make homogeneous.

homogenizer (hom·oj·en·i·zer). An apparatus for breaking up fat particles so that they make a homogeneous mixture in the fluid and do not tend to separate out, or for making a homogeneous mixture of a fluid containing other solid matter. Also called *viscolizer.*

homogenote (hom·o·je·note). In bacterial genetics, connoting a partially diploid bacterium, carrying an F-prime factor or localized transducing phage, in which the diploid chromosomal regions are identical. [Gk *homos* same, *genein* to produce.]

homogenous (hom·oj·en·us). Relating or belonging to homogeny.

homogentisuria (hom·o·jen·tiz·ewr′·e·ah). Alkaptonuria. [homogentisic acid, urine.]

homogeny (hom·oj·en·e). 1. In biology, correspondence between organs or parts due to common ancestry or the inheritance of a common part. 2. Homogenesis. [Gk *homos* same, *genos* race.]

homoglandular (hom·o·glan·dew·lar). Relating or belonging to the same gland. [Gk *homos* same, gland.]

homograft (hom·o·grahft). A portion of tissue removed from a donor to be applied to a recipient of the same species; such grafts survive for a very short period except in the case of cornea, artery, bone, cartilage and perhaps endocrine tissue; homotransplant. [Gk *homos* same, graft.]

homografting (hom·o·grahft·ing). Homotransplantation. [see prec.]

homohaemotherapy (hom·o·he·mo·ther′·ap·e). The therapeutic measure of injecting blood withdrawn from one human being into another. [Gk *homos* same, *haima* blood, therapy.]

homoioplasia (hom·oi·o·plaze′·e·ah). Homoeoplasia.

homoiosis (hom·oi·o·sis). Homoeosis.

homoiostasis (hom·oi·os·tas·is). Homoeostasis.

homoiothermal (hom·oi·o·ther′·mal). Homothermal.

homoiotoxin (hom·oi·o·tox′·in). Homoeotoxin.

homokaryon (ho·mo·kar·e·on). A multinucleated cell or organism containing nuclei of the same genetic constitution, Homo*di*karyon, homo*tri*karyon and homo*poly*karyon are homokaryon with 2, 3 or more than 2 nuclei, respectively. [Gk *homo* same, *karyon* nut.]

homokaryotype (hom·o·kar·e·o·tipe). In contraposition to heterokaryotype; a karyotype not showing structural heterozygosity. [Gk *homos* same, *karyon* nut, *typos* mark.]

homokeratoplasty (hom·o·ker·at·o·plas·te). Reparative surgery of the cornea in which corneal tissue from another individual is used. [Gk *homos* same, keratoplasty.]

homolateral (hom·o·lat·er·al). Relating to, or on, the same side. [Gk *homos* same, L *latus* side.]

Homolle, Augustin Eugène (b. 1808). Paris physician.

Homolle's digitalin. A mixture of digitalis glycosides, mainly digitalin; it is almost insoluble in water.

homologous (hom·ol·og·us). 1. Having a similar embryological origin, even if serving a different function and being different in structure in the adult, e.g. the wing of a bird and the forelimb of a mammal, since both are derived from the anterior limb bud which is common to all vertebrates. 2. In chemistry, similar in structure. 3. In bacteriology, related, e.g. a species of bacterium and the immune serum prepared from it. 4. In cytogenetics, of chromosome or chromosome regions carrying the same gene loci. *See* TRANSPLANTATION. [see foll.]

homologue (**hom**·o·log). 1. Any organ which is homologous to another in a different organism. 2. In chemistry, any member of a series possessing the general properties and structure of the other members, but differing from its neighbours by some regular and constant uniformity such as the CH_2 group. 3. In cytogenetics, a chromosome which carries the same gene loci of another. [Gk *homos* same, *logos* relation.]

homology (hom·**ol**·o·je). 1. In biology: (*a*) correspondence in structural type between different parts of the same individual or between corresponding parts in 2 individuals of different species; (*b*) structural correspondence between organs or parts of different organisms due to descent from a common ancestor. 2. In molecular biology, the correspondence of amino-acid residues in different polypeptides, or of nucleotide sequences in nucleic acids. 3. In chemistry, the relationship between organic compounds which are members of a series that progresses structurally by the regular addition of a constant group such as CH_2. 4. In cytogenetics, the condition of chromosomes or chromosome regions carrying the same gene loci. [Gk *homos* same, *logos* science.]

homolysin (hom·**ol**·is·in). A lysin formed by injection into the body of an antigen obtained from an animal belonging to the same species. [Gk *homos* same, lysin.]

homolysis (hom·**ol**·is·is). Isohaemolysis. [Gk *homos* same, lysis.]

homomorphic (hom·o·**mor**·fik). Having in somatic cells equal pairs of chromosomes. [see foll.]

homomorphism (hom·o·**mor**·fizm). 1. In biology, superficial resemblance (e.g. in external characters) between organisms of one group and those of another. 2. Adaptive mimicry. [Gk *homos* same, *morphe* form.]

homomorphosis (**hom**·o·mor·**fo**'·sis). Replacement of a lost part by the formation and growth of a similar part. [Gk *homos* same, morphosis.]

homomorphous (hom·o·**mor**·fus). Belonging to or manifesting homomorphism.

homonomous (hom·**on**·o·mus). 1. Applied to a series of parts of similar structure or form, such as toes. 2. Under the influence of the same law. 3. On the same side or in the same place. [Gk *homos* same, *nomos* law, place.]

homonymous (hom·**on**·im·us). 1. Having the same sound, designation or name, or expressed in the same terms. 2. In the same relationship, such as uncrossed images in diplopia. [Gk *homos* same, *onyma* name.]

homo-organic (**hom**·o·or·**gan**'·ik). Homorganic.

homophil (**hom**·o·fil). An antibody that reacts with or has affinity for a specific antigen only. [Gk *homos* same, *philein* to love.]

homophleine (hom·o·**fle**·een). $C_{56}H_{90}O_9N_2$, an amorphous alkaloid with anaesthetic properties similar to erythrophloeine and found with the latter in sassy bark.

homoplasmy (hom·o·**plaz**·me). Analogy or mimetic resemblance of organs or parts. [Gk *homos* same, *plasma* something formed.]

homoplast (**hom**·o·plast). 1. One of two or more plastids. 2. A homologous or homomorphous organ or part. [Gk *homos* same, *plassein* to form.]

homoplastic (hom·o·**plas**·tik). 1. Referring or belonging to homoplasty. 2. Referring to a tissue graft taken from another individual belonging to the same species. 3. Applied to neoplasms such as glioma, the cells of which resemble those of the surrounding tissue.

homoplastid (hom·o·**plas**·tid). An organism consisting of cells, each of which is capable of reproducing the species. [Gk *homos* same, plastid.]

homoplasty (**hom**·o·plas·te). Surgical replacement of lost tissues by the grafting on of similar tissues from another of the same species. [Gk *homos* same, *plassein* to mould.]

homopolykaryon (**ho**·mo·pol·e·**kar**'·e·on). *See* HOMOKARYON.

homopolyribonucleotide (**hom**·o·pol·e·ri·bo·**new**'·kle·o·tide). A polynucleotide which is made up of only one class of ribonucleotide units (e.g. polyadenylic acid). [Gk *homos* same, *polys* many, ribose, nucleotide.]

homoquinine (hom·o·**kwin**·een). $C_{20}H_{24}O_2N_2C_{19}H_{22}O_2N_2 \cdot 4H_2O$, a molecular compound of quinine and cupreine which separates out from the alkaloids of cuprea bark. [Gk *homos* same, quinine.]

homorganic (hom·or·**gan**·ik). Produced by or derived from the same or homologous organs. [Gk *homos* same, organ.]

homosaligenin (**hom**·o·sal·**ij**'·en·in). Methyl saligenin, $CH_3C_6H_3(OH)CH_2OH$. The methyl derivative of salicyl alcohol.

homoserine (hom·o·**ser**·een). α-Amino-γ-hydroxybutyric acid, $CH_2OHCH_2CH(NH_2)COOH$. An amino acid which occurs as its derivatives, canaline and canavanine, in the proteins of soy bean and jack bean, although it has not itself been isolated. It is belived to occur as an intermediate in the biosynthesis of threonine and methionine.

homosexual (hom·o·**sex**·ew·al). 1. Relating or belonging to or directed towards the same sex. 2. An individual whose sexual feelings are aroused only by others of the same sex. [Gk *homos* same, sex.]

homosexuality (**hom**·o·sex·ew·**al**'·it·e). The form of sexual perversion in which there is attraction only to others of the same sex. **Female homosexuality.** Lesbiansm; sapphism. [see prec.]

homosporous (hom·o·**spo**·rus). Having asexual spores of only one kind. [Gk *homos* same, spore.]

homostimulant (hom·o·**stim**·ew·lant). An organic extract which, when injected into the body, stimulates the gland or organ of the same kind as that from which the extract was prepared. [Gk *homos* same, stimulant.]

homostimulation (**hom**·o·stim·ew·**la**'·shun). 1. The use of a homostimulant in treatment of disease. 2. The intensifying of the action of a gland by administering an extract of the same gland taken from an animal.

homosulphanilamide (**hom**·o·sul·fan·**il**'·am·ide). 4-Amino-2-methylbenzenesulphonamide, $NH_2CH_2C_6H_4SO_2NH_2$. An antibacterial drug closely related to sulphanilamide: its mode of action is, however, different as it is not competitively antagonized by *para*-aminobenzoic acid.

homosynkaryon (**hom**·o·sin·**kar**'·e·on). In contradistinction with heterosynkaryon; a cell with the nucleus formed by fusion of genetically identical nuclei. [Gk *homos* same, *syn* together, *karyon* nut.]

homothallic (hom·o·**thal**·ik). In microbial genetics, indicating that mating is possible between cells of the same strain. [Gk *homos* same, *thallos* young green shoot.]

homothermal, homothermic (hom·o·**ther**·mal, hom·o·**ther**·mik). Applied to warm-blooded animals whose temperature normally is always the same and is unaffected by environmental conditions. [Gk *homos* same, *therme* heat.]

homotonic (hom·o·**ton**·ik). 1. Uniform in course. 2. Unvarying in tone or tension. [Gk *homos* same, tonus.]

homotransplant (hom·o·**trans**·plant). Homograft; a portion of tissue taken from an individual for grafting on to another individual of the same species. [Gk *homos* same, transplant.]

homotransplantation (**hom**·o·trans·plan·**ta**'·shun). The grafting on to an individual of one species, tissue taken from another individual of the same species. [see prec.]

homotrikaryon (**ho**·mo·tri·**kar**·e·on). *See* HOMOKARYON.

homotropism (hom·**ot**·rop·izm). The property inherent in a cell of a certain order by which it attracts like cells. [Gk *homos* same, *trope* a turning.]

homotype (**hom**·o·tipe). Any part or structure which is in reversed symmetry with its fellow, such as the hand. [Gk *homos* same, type.]

homozoic (hom·o·**zo**·ik). Pertaining to the same species or to an animal of the same kind. [Gk *homos* same, *zoon* animal.]

homozygosis (**hom**·o·zi·**go**'·sis). The production of a zygote by the union of gametes which have identical genes at any given locus. [see foll.]

homozygote (hom·o·**zi**·gote). An organism whose somatic cells have identical genes in the same locus on one of the chromosome pairs. The organism will always show the characters produced by this gene. [Gk *homos* same, *zygon* yoke.]

homozygous (hom·o·zi·gus). Having identical genes in the same locus on one of the chromosme pairs. [see prec.]

Homprenorphine (hom·pren·or·feen). BP Commission approved name for *N*-cyclopropylmethyl-7-α-[1(R)-hydroxy-1-methylpropyl]-6, 14-*endo*ethenotetrahydronorthebaine; an analgesic.

homunculus (ho·mun·kew·lus). 1. An individual who is a dwarf but is perfectly proportioned. 2. A fetus. [L little man.]

honey (hun·e). A mixture of invert sugars and compound saccharides produced from the nectar of flowers by enzyme action in the honey sac of the bee *Apis mellifica.* It is esteemed as a food and sweetening agent. **Purified Honey BPC 1968.** Honey which has been purified by melting, straining and then adjusting to a definite specific gravity with distilled water. Its quality is further controlled by tests for optical rotation and for the absence of added invert sugar. [AS *hunig.*]

honeydew (hun·e·dew). A sweet exudate from plants produced by the punctures of aphides, leaf-hoppers and other insects. [AS *hunig, deaw.*]

honk (hongk). **Precordial honk.** A systolic murmur of unusual quality, as indicated by the name, usually found in children and probably arising from the mitral valve apparatus.

hood (hud). A covering or protection of a part or structure. **Tooth hood.** The soft tissue of the gingiva which covers the occlusal surface of a partially erupted tooth such as a lower third molar tooth. [AS *hod.*]

hook (huk). A metal surgical instrument with a hook at one end used to pull aside structures and to improve access. The hook may be single or double, it may have a sharp or blunt end or it may have other special characteristics (see below). **Blunt hook.** A metal hook used to facilitate delivery by groin traction in an impacted breech presentation. It is only used when the child is dead. **Dural hook.** A handled hook with a delicate sharp point used for fixing and retracting the margins of an incision in the dura mater. **Fixation hook.** A very slender instrument with a hook only a few millimetres long, used specially in ophthalmic surgery and in handling split-skin grafts. **Hook of the hamate bone [hamulus ossis hamati (NA)].** A process projecting from the anterior surface of the hamate bone. It gives attachment to the flexor retinaculum. **Nerve hook.** A delicate blunt hook used to pull nerves to one side. **Palate hook.** A form of retractor used to draw the soft palate forward to facilitate posterior rhinoscopy. **Retraction hook.** A sharp or blunt, single or double hook for retraction of tissues. **Squint hook.** A blunt-ended hook used for slipping under an extra-ocular muscle in squint surgery. **Surgical hook.** Ancistrum. **Tracheotomy hook.** A stout hook designed for fixation of the margins of the incision in the trachea made at tracheotomy. [AS *hok.*]

See also: BRAUN (G. A.), CHAVASSE, JARDINE, KILNER, MALGAIGNE, PAJOT, RAMSBOTHAM, TYRRELL.

Hooker-Forbes' test. A sensitive test for progesterone, dependent upon its capacity to restore to normal the shrunken endometrial stromal nuclei of oöphorectomized mice. Seldom if ever now used because progesterone can be identified and synthesized chemically.

hookworm (huk·werm). A roundworm with conspicuous buccal teeth. Two species are serious intestinal parasites of man, *Ancylostoma duodenale,* mainly northern and Old-World in distribution, and *Necator americanus,* common throughout the tropics. *A. brasiliense,* the dog hookworm, occasionally infests man in tropical countries. [AS *hok, wyrm.*]

hoolamite (hoo·lam·ite). An absorbent used in the detection and estimation of carbon monoxide. It is a mixture of fuming sulphuric acid and iodine pentoxide in a base of pumice; the carbon monoxide reduces the iodine pentoxide to free iodine.

Hoorweg, Jan Leendert (b. 1841). Utrecht biophysicist.

Hoorweg's law. In order to cause a neuromuscular response, an electrical stimulus of given voltage must endure for a minimal time. If it endures indefinitely, there is no relationship between its intensity and duration.

Hoover, Charles Franklin (b. 1865). Cleveland physician.

Hoover's sign. 1. In organic paralysis of the lower limbs, firm voluntary pressure of one leg upon the bed results in a slight lifting movement of the other leg; this is not seen in hysterical paralysis. *See* GRASSET, GAUSSEL AND HOOVER SIGN (below). 2. The lower ribs are drawn inwards during inspiration on the side of the lesion owing to rigidity and flattening of the diaphragm resulting from empyema, pleural thickening after pleurisy or any organized effusion of long standing. In emphysema it may occur bilaterally, e.g. in children after whooping-cough.

Grasset, Gaussel and Hoover sign. If a patient with hemiplegia, lying in the supine position, attempts to raise the paralysed leg while an observer's hand is resting beneath the sound leg, the pressure of the sound limb on the observer's hand is much greater than would be observed during the same action in a normal person.

Hopf, Gustav (fl. 1931). Hamburg dermatologist.

Hopf's disease. Acrokeratosis verruciformis.

Hopkins, Sir Frederick Gowland (b. 1861). Cambridge biochemist.

Hopkins-Cole test, for tryptophan or proteins containing tryptophan. A glyoxylic-acid reagent is prepared by adding 4 g of magnesium powder slowly to 100 ml of saturated oxalic-acid solution. When the reaction is complete the solution is filtered and diluted to 400 ml with water. To 3 ml of test solution add 2 ml of reagent and layer with 3 ml of concentrated sulphuric acid. If tryptophan is present, a deep purple ring forms at the junction of the liquids.

Hoplopsyllus (hop·lop·sil·us). A genus of fleas; *Hoplopsyllus anomalus* is a vector of plague. [Gk *hoplon* weapon, *psylla* flea.]

Hoppe, Hermann Henry (b. 1867). Cincinnati neurologist.

Hoppe-Goldflam syndrome. Myasthenia gravis.

Hoppe-Seyler, Ernst Felix Immanuel (b. 1825). German biochemist.

Hoppe-Seyler's test, for carbon monoxide. Add sodium hydroxide (sp. gr. 1.34) to blood. In the presence of carbon monoxide a bright-red colour develops; if the blood is normal, a dirty-green colour.

hops (hops). The fruits of *Humulus lupulus* Linn. (family Cannabinaceae). *See* LUPULUS. **Hop tree.** The wafer ash or shrubby trefoil, *Ptelea trifoliata* Linn. (family Rutaceae). The fruits have been used as a substitute for hops and the root bark is employed as a tonic and stomachic. [ME *hoppe.*]

hordein (hor·de·in). One of the simple proteins of the gliadin or prolamin class found in barley. It is insoluble in water or alcohol but will dissolve in from 70 to 80 per cent aqueous alcohol. It has a large proportion of proline. [L *hordeum* barley.]

hordenine (hor·den·een).Parahydroxyphenylethyldimethylamine, $OHC_6H_4CH_2CH_2N(CH_3)_2$. An alkaloid found in malted barley. Chemically it is related to adrenaline and has the same sympatheticomimetic properties. It stimulates the heart, constricts the blood vessels and relaxes the bronchioles and intestine. [L *hordeum* barley.]

hordeolum (hor·de·o·lum). Sty. **External hordeolum.** An acute localized infection occurring at the eyelid margin, in a lash follicle and the associated gland of Zeis. It is usually staphylococcal. **Internal hordeolum.** An acute infection, usually staphylococcal, of the meibomian gland, going on to suppuration. [dim. of L *hordeum* barley.]

hordeum (hor·de·um). Barley, the seeds of *Hordeum distichon.* **Hordeum decorticatum.** Pearl barley; dehusked barley such as is used in the preparation of barley water. [L.]

horehound (ho·er·hownd). Marrubium; white horehound; a herb, *Marrubium vulgare* Linn. (family Labiatae), indigenous to Britain and central Europe. It is used in the form of the infusion or syrup as an expectorant, laxative and bitter tonic. **Black horehound, Spanish horehound.** *Ballota hirsuta* Benth. (family Labiatae), which is stated to have stimulant and antispasmodic properties. [AS *har* hoar, *hune* a plant.]

horismascope (hor·iz·mah·skope). An instrument designed to facilitate ring tests by showing clearly against a background the junction between the liquid under examination and the reagent. [Gk *horisma* boundary, *skopein* to view.]

horizocardia (hor·i·zo·kar'·de·ah). The state in which the heart is in a horizontal position on the diaphragm. It may be due to dilatation of both ventricles or to their considerable eccentric hypertrophy. [horizon, Gk *kardia* heart.]

horizon (hor·i·zon). **Retinal horizon.** The horizontal plane which passes through the transverse axis of the eyeball (Helmholtz). [Gk *horizein* to encircle.]

horizontal [horizontalis (NA)] (hor·iz·on·tal). Flat, or on a level, as of a surface; at a right angle to a vertical plane; parallel to a horizon. [see prec.]

horme (hor·me). The nerve centre in which instincts originate (Monakow). [Gk the point of starting.]

hormesis (hor·me·sis). The stimulating effect of small doses of substances which in larger doses are inhibitory. [Gk *hormaein* to set in motion.]

hormic (hor·mik). Referring to the theory that phenomena of organic type have origin in stimuli springing from urges and various congenital tendencies peculiar to each individual. [see prec.]

hormion (hor·me·on). In craniology, the median point of the line of union of the posterior border of the vomer with the sphenoid bone. [Gk *hormos* chain.]

hormodendrum (hor·mo·den·drum). A fungus which occurs frequently in soil and as a spoiling agent in dairy products, raw cotton, wood, etc. Some species are pathogenic for man. **Hormodendrum algeriense.** A species reported from lesions resembling sporotrichosis. **Hormodendrum compactum.** A species isolated from cases of chromoblastomycosis. **Hormodendrum fontoynonti.** The causative agent of hodi-potsy in Madagascar. **Hormodendrum langeroni.** A species isolated from ulceronodular lesions of the leg. **Hormodendrum pedrosoi,** Brumpt 1921. A species isolated from cases of chromoblastomycosis; also known as *Phialophora pedrosoi.* [Gk *hormos* chain, *dendron* tree.]

hormonagogue (hor·mon·ag·og). 1. Stimulating the production of hormones. 2. Any agent which increases the production of hormones. [hormone, Gk *agogos* leading.]

hormonal (hor·mo·nal). Pertaining to or having the character of a hormone.

hormone (hor·mone). A chemical substance formed in one part of the body and transmitted by the blood stream to another part of the body where it has an effect on function. Most hormones are formed by the endocrine glands but some, such as secretin, are not. In character it may be steroid (e.g. the adrenal cortical hormones or the sex hormones), phenolic (e.g. adrenaline) or protein (e.g. the pituitary hormones), and as a rule is thermostabile, highly potent, with temporary and local specific effect, and not evoking immunity or anaphylactic phenomena in animals of the species from which it has been derived. **Adrenal cortical hormone.** Any hormone secreted by the adrenal cortex. All are steroids; some are glucocorticoid, others mineralocorticoid. **Adrenal medullary hormone.** Adrenaline and noradrenaline. **Adrenocorticotropic hormone.** Adrenocorticotrophin (ACTH), a polypeptide hormone secreted by the anterior pituitary and regulating the steroid output of the adrenal cortex. **Adrenotrophic hormone, Adrenotropic hormone.** A hormone secreted by the anterior part of the pituitary gland which stimulates the secretion of adrenal cortical hormones by the adrenal cortex. The only such hormone positively identified is corticotrophin. **Allosteric hormone.** A class of hormones which function as allosteric effectors for enzymes. **Anabolic hormones.** Derivates of testosterone, in the form of 19-nortestosterone, which retain the anabolic effects of testosterone without its androgenic effects. **Androgenic hormone.** Testosterone and related male sex hormones. **Anterior pituitary hormone.** Any hormone secreted by the anterior part of the pituitary gland; 4 such hormones have been isolated in pure form (prolactin, somatotrophin, corticotrophin and interstitial-cell-stimulating hormone), whilst there is adequate evidence of the existence of 2 others (thyrotrophin and follicle-stimulating hormone). **Anterior pituitary-like hormone.** A description used of hormones isolated from body fluids or tissues other than the anterior pituitary, the actions of which are similar to those of hormones isolated from the anterior pituitary gland itself, e.g. chorionic gonadotrophin, serum gonadotrophin. **Antidiuretic hormone.** Vasopressin. **Cardiac hormone.** A substance which, it has been suggested, occurs in heart muscle; *in vitro* it is said to stimulate the amplitude of cardiac contractions. **Circulatory hormone.** A term used to describe any of the tissue extracts which possess vasodilating properties; their hormonal nature has not been established. **Corpus luteum hormone.** Progesterone, $C_{21}H_{30}O_2$, a steroid hormone which regulates the endometrium prior to menstruation, inhibits ovulation during pregnancy and controls the embedding of the fertilized ovum. **Diabetogenic hormone.** A hormone formerly believed present in extracts of the anterior pituitary gland or which rendered experimental animals diabetic; this action is now considered to be due to the presence in the extracts of somatotrophin. **Follicle-stimulating hormone** (FSH). A gonadotrophin produced by the pituitary which maintains the spermatogenic epithelium in the male and is responsible for the early growth of the ovarian follicles in the female. **Galactopoietic hormone.** Prolactin, a hormone secreted by the anterior pituitary which stimulates the production of milk; also called *mammotrophin.* **Gastric hormone.** Gastrin. **Glucocorticoid hormones.** Steroid hormones from the adrenal cortex whose primary action is upon carbohydrate metabolism. **Gonadotrophic hormones.** Gonadotrophin. **Growth hormone.** A polypeptide hormone secreted by the anterior pituitary. Its functions are ill-defined but it appears to act on bone growth, carbohydrate and nitrogen metabolism. An excess of the hormone during development is associated with acromegaly. **Interstitial-cell-stimulating hormone** (ICSH). Luteinizing hormone (see below). **Luteinizing hormone** (LH). A gonadotrophin produced by the pituitary gland which is trophic to Leydig cells and causes release of testosterone in the male. In the female it causes final maturation of the ovarian follicles and stimulates oestrogen secretion. It is also responsible for ovulation and the initial formation of the corpus luteum and the secretion of progesterone. **Mammotrophic hormone.** Mammotrophin, prolactin, a hormone secreted by the anterior pituitary which stimulates the production of milk. **Melanocyte-stimulating hormone.** Intermedin. **Melanophoric hormone.** Intermedin. **Mineral corticoid hormones.** Hormones produced by the adrenal cortex under the stimulation of adrenocorticotrophic hormones (ACTH) of the anterior pituitary. They control electrolytes and fluid balance, produce retention of sodium and water and lead to the elimination of potassium. Their excessive production may cause severe renal damage, progressing to nephrosclerosis and arteriosclerosis. **N. hormone.** A fraction of the secretion of the cortex of the suprarenal gland which has androgenic and nitrogen-retaining properties. **Neurohypophyseal hormone.** Posterior pituitary hormone (see below). **Oestrogenic hormones.** One of the oestrogens, or female sex hormones. **Ovarian hormone.** Any hormone secreted by the ovaries. Such hormones have either folliculoid (oestrogenic) activity or luteoid (progestogenic); actual ovarian secretion is probably confined to oestradiol in the former class and progesterone in the latter. **Pancreatic hormone.** A term incorrectly applied to a number of substances other than insulin derived from the pancreas, e.g. vagotonin, lipocaic. **Parathyroid hormone.** Parathormone, the polypeptide hormone produced by the parathyroid gland. It controls the overall balance of calcium and phosphate in the body. **Pregnant-mare's serum hormone.** The hormone present in the serum of a pregnant mare which is identical in action with follicle-stimulating hormone. **S. hormone.** A fraction of the secretion of the suprarenal gland which increases glyconeogenesis. **Sebotrophic hormone.** A postulated pituitary hormone which stimulates the sebaceous glands. **Sex hormones.** The androgens and oestrogens. **Steroid hormones.** Secretions of ductless glands whose chemical formulae contain the steroid nucleus. **Testis hormone.** Any hormone secreted by the testis; normally applied only to testosterone, but strictly should also include an oestrogenic hormone derived from the testis. **Thyroid hormone.** Thyroxine. **Thyroid-stimulating hormone** (TSH). Thyrotropic hormone (see below). **Thyrotrophic hormone, Thyrotropic hormone.** A polypeptide hormone secreted by the anterior pituitary and regulating the secretion of thyroxine by the thyroid gland. [Gk *hormaein* to set in motion.]

hormonic (hor·**mon**·ik). Pertaining to, acting as, or having the stimulative effect of a hormone.

hormonogenesis (**hor**·mon·o·**jen**′·es·is). Hormonopoiesis. [hormone, Gk *genein* to produce.]

hormonogenic (**hor**·mon·o·**jen**′·ik). Hormonopoietic [see prec.]

hormonology (hor·mon·**ol**·o·je). The science of hormones. [hormone, *logos* science]

hormonopexic (**hor**·mon·o·**pex**′·ik). An agent which is able to fix hormones chemically. [hormone, Gk *pexis* fixation.]

hormonopoiesis (**hor**·mon·o·**poi**·e′·sis). The producing of a hormone or an internal secretion. [hormone, Gk *poiein* to make.]

hormonopoietic (**hor**·mon·o·poi·**et**′·ik). Referring or belonging to hormonopoiesis, applied to glands which produce hormones or internal secretions.

hormonotherapy (**hor**·mon·o·**ther**′·ap·e). The therapeutic use of hormones.

hormopoiesis (**hor**·mo·poi·**e**′·sis). Hormonopoiesis.

hormopoietic (**hor**·mo·poi·**et**′·ik). Hormonopoietic.

horn (horn). 1. A protuberance on the head, noted in many mammals, principally used for offence or defence. 2. [Cornu (NA).] In anatomy, the name includes several types of structures, sometimes median in position but often lateral and paired. 3. An angular extension of the pulp chamber of a tooth towards a cusp. **Cicatricial horn.** A cutaneous horn arising from scar tissue. **Cutaneous horn.** Cornu cutaneum; a horny cutaneous outgrowth occasionally seen in human beings which usually grows slowly and is formed by localized hyperkeratosis. Cutaneous horns vary in diameter from one-eighth of an inch to 4 or 5 inches and are wider at their bases than at their extremities; in shape they may be conical, cylindrical, straight or twisted. Epitheliomatous degeneration may occur at the base. D. W. Montgomery classified the tumours as *filiform horns*, horns arising from an open atheroma (i.e. the *sebaceous horn* of earlier writers), horn formed by the cornification of a papilloma or wart (*warty horn*), horn arising from a naevus and horn arising from mucous membrane. **Grey horns of the spinal cord [columnae griseae (NA)].** The crescentic projections of grey matter within the spinal cord, seen as horns [cornu anterius, cornu laterale and cornu posterius (NA)] in transverse sections but actually consisting of solid columns, projecting backwards, posterior columns, laterally, lateral columns, or anteriorly, anterior columns. The posterior column is differentiated into an apex [apex cornus posterioris (NA)] capped by the gelatinous matter, and a neck. **Horn of the hyoid bone, greater [cornu majus (NA)].** Either of the slender processes extending backward from each end of the body of the hyoid bone. **Horn of the hyoid bone, lesser [cornu minus (NA)].** Either of 2 small conical eminences attached at their bases to the angles of junction of the body and the greater cornua. **Iliac horn.** Conical bony projections arising from the posterolateral aspects of the blades of the ilium, occurring in hereditary onycho-osteodysplasia (nail-patella syndrome). **Nail horn.** Onychogryphosis. **Horn of pulp.** That part of the tooth pulp which occupies a horn of the pulp chamber; a pulp cornu. **Horns of the thyroid cartilage.** *See* CARTILAGE. [AS.]

See also: AMMON.

Horne (Heurnius), Jan van (b. 1621). Amsterdam surgeon and anatomist.

saccus of van Horne. The cisterna chyli.

Horner, Johann Friedrich (b. 1831). Zürich ophthalmologist.

Horner's law. Colour blindness is transmitted from the male through an unaffected female to the male, i.e. a sex-linked recessive transmission.

Horner's ptosis. The slight degree of ptosis seen in Horner's syndrome due to weakness of the palpebral muscle of Mueller.

Horner's syndrome, Claude Bernard–Horner syndrome, Horner–Bernard syndrome. Slight enophthalmos, miosis, and slight ptosis, with narrowing of the palpebral fissure, with sometimes decrease of sweating, vasodilatation of the conjunctival, retinal and facial vessels, and rise in the skin temperature. It is due to interference with the cervical sympathetic fibres on the affected side.

Horner, William Edmonds (b. 1793). Philadelphia anatomist.

Horner's muscle. The lacrimal part of the orbicularis oculi muscle.

hornification (**horn**·if·ik·**a**′·shun). The process of degeneration of stratified squamous epithelial cells, whereby they become horny and cast off from the surface, as in the mouth. [horn, L *facere* to make.]

horny (**horn**·e). 1. Hard and callous like horn, or having the character and appearance of horn; corneous. 2. Composed of horn.

horopter (hor·**op**·ter). The locus of those points in space which form images upon corresponding points of the two retinae. [Gk *horos* limit, *opter* observer.]

See also: MUELLER (J.).

horopteric (hor·op·ter·ik). Referring or belonging to a horopter.

horrida cutis (**hor**·id·ah **kew**·tis). Cutis anserina; goose flesh. [L *horridus* rough, *cutis* skin.]

horripilation (hor·ip·il·a′·shun). Erection of the hairs of the skin caused by cutis anserina. [L *horridus* rough, *pilus* hair.]

Horrocks, Peter (b. 1852). British obstetrician.

Horrocks' maieutic. A rubber bag tied over the end of a catheter used in dilatation of the neck of the uterus.

horror fusionis (**hor**·or **few**·shun·is). Incapacitating diplopia following operation for squint. [L a trembling in fusion.]

horse-chestnut (hors·**ches**·nut). *Aesculus hippocastanum* Linn. (family Sapindaceae), a tree widely distributed. An infusion of the bark is used as a febrifuge, and an extract made from the fruits is stated to be of value in rheumatic and neuralgic conditions. A tincture prepared from the seeds alone has been used in the treatment of haemorrhoids. [AS *hors*, Gk *kastanon* chestnut, AS *hnutu*.]

horse-foot (**hors**·fut). Talipes equinus. [AS *hors, fot.*]

horse-hair (**hors**·ha·er). The hair of the horse used for surgical ligature, e.g. of the skin, from whence it can be subsequently removed since it is not absorbed. [AS *hors, haer.*]

horse-mint (**hors**·mint). An American herb, *Monarda punctata* Linn. (family Labiatae). A hot infusion is stated to have diuretic properties and is also used as an emmenagogue. [AS *hors, minte.*]

horse-nettle (**hors**·netl). *Solanum carolinense* Linn. (family Solanaceae). The fruits have been used as an antispasmodic. [AS *hors, netele.*]

horsepower (**hors**·pow·er). A unit of power or rate of work; it is defined as a rate of 33 000 foot-pounds per minute and is equivalent to 746 watts. [AS *hors*, ME *poer.]*

horseradish (**hors**·rad·ish). Armoracia, consisting of the fresh root of *Cochlearia armoracia* Linn. (family Cruciferae), collected from plants cultivated in Great Britain. It is used externally as a vesicant and counter-irritant, and internally as a digestive stimulant. [AS *hors*, L *radix* root.]

horsetail (**hors**·tale). The common name for *Equisetum*, a genus of cryptogamic plants belonging to the family Equisetaceae. *Equisetum arvense* Linn. has been used as a diuretic and astringent and in the treatment of dyspepsia. All plants of the genus contain large amounts of silica. [AS *hors, taegl.*]

Horsley, Sir Victor Alexander Haden (b. 1857). London neurosurgeon.

Horsley's operation, for trigeminal neuralgia. Preganglionic trigeminal root section for neuralgia.

Horsley's putty or wax. A plastic preparation of yellow beeswax, phenol and olive oil. At about 40°C it can be manipulated easily and is used in surgery.

Horsley's sign. In a case of middle meningeal haemorrhage the temperature in the axilla on the paralysed side may be higher than that on the normal side.

Horsley's trephine. A trephine which takes to pieces for cleaning.

Hortega, Pio del Rio (b. 1882). Spanish histologist in Buenos Aires.

Hortega cell. A microglial cell. *See* CELL.

Hortega method, for microglia. A complicated silver carbonate method for the impregnation of microglia.

Horton, Bayard Taylor (b.1895). Rochester, Minnesota, physician.

Horton's headache or syndrome. Histamine headache; histamine cephalalgia. *See* CEPHALALGIA.

hospital (hos·pit·al). An institution which is equipped and organized for the care of the sick, usually possessing facilities for the diagnosis, treatment and cure of disease. Formerly, a place which provided hospitality for the sick and aged poor. **General hospital.** 1. A hospital that provides for all the medical and surgical treatment that the population of a town or area may require. Such hospitals usually have a large range of specialist departments but they seldom accommodate patients suffering from infectious diseases or mental patients, though they may have a psychiatric outpatient department. 2. An army hospital in the field; its staff and equipment can be adjusted to the number of beds required. Common requirements are for hospitals of 600 or 1200 beds. [L *hospes* guest.]

hospitalism (hos·pit·al·izm). 1. An aura of morbidity—the effect of concentrating many diseased or sick persons in a hospital. 2. A psychoneurosis which impels the subject to go on attending the outpatient department of a hospital and, usually, to seek admission.

hospitalization (hos·pit·al·i·za'·shun). The act or process of being or becoming hospitalized.

hospitalize (hos·pit·al·ize). 1. To refer a patient to a hospital; to send him into hospital or cause him to be received in hospital. 2. In the past tense, for a patient to become hospitalized means that he has been in hospital for so long that he has no desire to go out and that for this reason, and others, hospital treatment is having little or no beneficial effect on him. This second meaning was the only one current in the UK before World War II; the first is an importation from the USA and is now well established in this country.

host (ho·st). 1. Any organism upon which another organism can live parasitically; e.g. in typhoid fever, the host is the patient and the parasite is the typhoid bacillus. The host harbouring the adult stage of a parasite is known as the *definitive* or *final host*; the host harbouring larval forms of the parasite is known as the *intermediate host*, and these may be primary or secondary when there is more than one larval stage. A *reservoir* host is the source from which new hosts are infected. 2. Any animal that receives a transplanted graft. [L *hospes.*]

hot-box (hot·box). **Japanese hot-box.** An appliance used in the application of dry heat to the eyes or other parts of the body. [AS *hat*, L *buxum* boxwood.]

hottentotism (hot·en·tot·izm). A variety of stammering. [D *hottentot* a stammerer.]

Hotz, Ferdinand Carl (b. 1843). German ophthalmologist in Chicago.

Hotz-Anagnostakis operation, for entropion, usually upper lid. Excision of orbicularis fibres along the length of the lid, followed by suture of the skin margins to the tarsal plate high up, so everting the lid margin and straightening out the deformed tarsus.

Houghton's law. When a muscle or group of muscles does work to the point of fatigue, then the total work done multiplied by the rate of work is constant.

Houssay, Bernardo Alberto (b. 1887). Buenos Aires physiologist.

Houssay animal. An experimental animal from which both the pancreas and the whole pituitary gland have been removed.

Houssay phenomenon. The apparent disappearance of diabetes mellitus in a depancreatized animal on removal of the hypophysis cerebri.

Houssay's syndrome. A natural syndrome resulting from lesions comparable to those produced experimentally in the Houssay animal (see above); a number of instances of the syndrome have been recorded since Houssay originally reported his experiments. The development of a destructive anterior-pituitary lesion in a subject with diabetes mellitus produces a varied clinical picture in which the signs due to hypoglycaemia predominate. The condition is usually rapidly fatal.

Houston, John (b. 1802). Dublin surgeon.

Houston's folds or valves. Horizontally-placed crescentic folds in the wall of the rectum.

Houston's muscle. An inconstant portion of the ischiocavernosus muscle passing to the dorsum of the penis.

Hovius, Jacobus (b. c. 1675). Utrecht ophthalmologist.

canals of Hovius. Anastomoses between the venae vorticosae of the eye, present in some mammals but not in man.

circle of Hovius. An intrascleral anastomosis of the ciliary veins at the sclerocorneal junction.

Hovius' membrane. The internal layer of the choroid coat of the eye.

Hovius' plexus. An intrascleral circular anastomosis, formed by the ciliary veins close to the corneoscleral margin, which is found only in mammals.

Howard, Benjamin Douglas (b. 1840). New York physician.

Howard's method. *See* RESPIRATION, ARTIFICIAL.

Howard-Jones, W. 20th century London anaesthetist.

Howard-Jones technique of spinal analgesia. Injection of a volume of hypobaric local analgesic solution, turning the patient into the prone, then the supine position. Described in 1930.

Howard-Jones spinal needle. A fine flexible needle with stilette, used for lumbar puncture.

Howarth, Walter Goldie (b. 1879). London otolaryngologist.

Howarth's operation. An external and radical operation for frontal sinus suppuration; the anterior wall of the sinus is left undisturbed. It is claimed that the cosmetic result after this method of treatment is better than after other radical procedures.

Howell, William Henry (b. 1860). Baltimore physiologist.

Howell's bodies, Howell-Jolly bodies. Spherical, eccentrically-placed granules or nuclear remnants about 1 μm in diameter, occasionally seen in red blood corpuscles, usually very numerous in haemolytic or toxic anaemias and after splenectomy.

Howells, Thomas Hilary. London anaesthetist.

Howells' ventilator. A gas-operated volume-cycled artificial ventilator used either in the ward or operating theatre. Described in 1960.

Howship, John (b. 1781). London surgeon.

Howship's foveolae, lacunae or pits. Absorption lacunae; any small spaces in a bone where resorption is taking place.

Howship's sign, Howship-Romberg sign, Romberg-Howship sign. Pain due to an obturator hernia may be referred along the obturator nerve into the medial part of the thigh; often accompanied by tenderness in the adductor region.

Hoyer, Heinrich Friedrich (b. 1834). Warsaw surgeon.

Hoyer's canals, Sucquet-Hoyer anastomoses or canals. Communications between preterminal branches (glomic branches) of cutaneous arterioles and venules found in the digits.

Hoyer's method, for Nissl substance. The staining of nerve cells with thionin,with mercuric chloride as a mordant.

Hoyle's (tellurite) culture medium A medium prepared from "Lab.-Lemco" 10 g, proteose peptone 10 g, sodium chloride 5 g, potassium tellurite 0.35 g, sterile laked horse blood 50 ml, agar 20 g and water 1000 ml.

Hruby lens. A −54 dioptre preset lens with an anterior surface of

+5.0 dioptres, through which the posterior segment of the eye can be examined with a slit lamp.

Hubbard, Leroy Watkins (b. 1857). Warm Springs, Georgia, orthopaedic surgeon.

Hubbard tank. A tank containing water in which patients perform exercises, the buoyancy of the water assisting weakened muscles.

Hubl's iodine solution. A solution of iodine monochloride in glacial acetic acid, used for determining the iodine value of fixed oils.

Hubrecht, Ambrosius Arnold Willon (b. 1853). Leyden and Utrecht anatomist, embryologist and zoologist.

Hubrecht's protochordal knot. A rounded swelling at the anterior end of the primitive streak on the surface of the blastoderm from which the head process is derived. It is homologous with the dorsal lip of the blastopore of lower vertebrates.

Huchard, Henri (b. 1844). Paris physician.

Huchard's disease. Arterial hypertension.

Huchard's sign. When a patient with hypertension changes from standing to lying down, the usual slowing of the pulse does not occur.

Huchard's treatment. A dietetic treatment for dilatation of the stomach that includes strict limitation of liquids.

hucklebone (**hukl·bone**). The talus. [ME *huccle-bone* the astragalus.]

Huddleson, I. Forest (b. 1893). American bacteriologist.

Huddleson's test. Opsonocytophagic test. *See* TEST.

Hudson, Claude Silbert (b. 1881). American chemist.

Hudson's lactone rule, as applied to the crystalline lactones obtained from monosaccharides. When the lactone ring is formed on the right side of the carbon chain the optical rotation of the compound is towards the right; when formed on the left side the compound rotates to the left.

Hudson, William H. (b. 1862). Alabama surgeon.

Hudson brace. A brace and drill for use in trephination, with an automatic stop to prevent dural injury.

Hudson's line. A pigmented brown line sometimes found in the superficial layers of the cornea of the eyes of old people.

Hueck, Alexander Friedrich (b. 1802). Dorpat anatomist.

Hueck's ligament. The pectinate ligament of the iris.

Huenefeld, Friedrich Ludwig (b. 1799). Greifswald chemist.

Huenefeld's mixture. Acetic acid, water, turpentine, alcohol and chloroform, used as a liniment.

Huerthle, Karl Wilhelm (b. 1860). Breslau histologist.

Huerthle's adenoma. Huerthle-cell tumour (see below).

Huerthle cell. A large eosinophilic cell within the thyroid gland, possibly of parathyroid origin.

Huerthle-cell tumour. A tumour arising from eosinophilic Huerthle cells of the thyroid gland.

Hüet, G. J. Dutch physician.

Pelger–Hüet anomaly, of the granulocytes. An anomaly inherited as a mendelian dominant in otherwise apparently well persons. It is characterized by an increase in the numbers of juvenile or band forms of granulocytes or polymorphonuclear leucocytes which have dumb-bell, kidney-shaped or bilobed nuclei. These cells may sometimes exceed the numbers of ordinary segmented granulocytes, and may be associated with certain infections or with very active cell-formation in the marrow.

Hueter, Karl (b. 1838). Greifswald surgeon.

Hueter's manoeuvre. While inserting the stomach tube the patient's tongue is pulled downwards and forwards by the left forefinger.

Vogt–Hueter point. Vogt's point.

Hufeland, Christoph Wilhelm (b. 1762). Berlin physician.

Hufeland's powder. A mixture of rhubarb, magnesium carbonate and oil of fennel, used as a laxative and carminative.

Hughes, Charles Hamilton (b. 1839). American neurologist.

Hughes' reflex. Virile reflex: contraction of the bulbospongiosus muscle in response to stimulation of the glans penis.

Hughes, Wendell Lochead (b. 1900). New York ophthalmologist.

Hughes' operation. Used in the reconstruction of a full-thickness loss of an eyelid: the normal lid is divided in 2 layers between the tarsus and the skin; the deep layer containing conjunctiva and tarsus is advanced and sewn to the conjunctival edge of the lid defect and the skin cover is obtained by advancing the adjacent cheek after it has been undermined. The new palpebral fissure is made by dividing the lids 2 months later.

Huguenin, Gustav (b. 1841). Zürich physician.

Huguenin's projection systems. Systems of motor and sensory activities.

Huguier, Pierre Charles (b. 1804). Paris surgeon.

Huguier's canal. The canal from which the chorda tympani emerges in the petrotympanic fissure.

Huguier's circle. An arterial anastomosis in the region of the neck of the uterus that is only occasionally present; although it has been attributed to Huguier, it was not described by him.

Huguier's fossa or sinus. A fossa on the medial wall of the middle-ear cavity.

Huguier's gland. The greater vestibular gland. *see* GLAND.

Huguier's operation, for iridodialysis; obsolete.

Huhner, Max (b. 1873). New York surgeon.

Huhner test. Postcoital test for motility of spermatozoa: the patient is advised to have intercourse at or about the time of ovulation, and within a few hours a specimen of cervical mucus is taken and the number and motility of spermatozoa present is noted.

Huldschinsky, Kurt (b. 1883). German physician.

Huldschinsky's radiation. A course of 3 months' ultraviolet light therapy, the radiation being produced from a quartz mercury-vapour lamp.

hum (hum). A continuous murmuring sound or note. **Venous hum.** A continuous high-pitched murmur throughout systole and also to be heard to the right of the sternum and in the neck, usually in children. It is probably due to the swirling of blood in large veins, and can be abolished by compressing the jugular vein or by rotating the neck. [onomat.]

Human, John Urban. London physician.

Human's sign. Tracheal tug. *See* TUG.

human placental lactogen (H.P.L.). An estimation of this in maternal serum indicates whether the patient is likely to abort, in which case she has a low level; or not, in which case she has a normal level. It is a polypeptide which appears in maternal serum from about the 8th week of gestation onwards.

Human Tissue Act 1961. This Act makes provision for the use of parts of bodies of deceased persons for therapeutic purposes and purposes of medical education and research.

humanized (**hew·man·i·zd**). 1. Applied to viruses from an animal source that have passed through a human being. 2. Applied to milk which has been treated so that it has the properties of human milk. [L *humanus* human.]

humanol (**hew·man·ol**). Liquid human fat placed in surgery around nerves or tendons to prevent adhesion formation. [see prec.]

Humber, John Davis (b. 1895). San Francisco physician.

Coffey–Humber treatment. The treatment of cancer by injections of an extract of the suprarenal cortex of sheep.

Humby, Thomas. British surgeon.

Humby's knife. A skin-grafting knife with a 23 cm (9 in) blade which has a metal roller parallel to the cutting edge. This roller determines the thickness of the graft that the instrument will cut.

Humby's procedure, for reconstruction of the urethra. An operation for hypospadias, in which the buried skin graft is introduced on a bougie.

humectant (**hew·mek·tant**). 1. Moistening; supplying moisture to a part as by a poultice applied to it. 2. A diluent. [L *humectare* to moisten.]

humectation (hew·mek·**ta**·shun). 1. The act of wetting or moistening, or the condition of being wetted or moistened. 2. Infiltration of the tissues by serous fluid. [see prec.]

humeral (**hew**·mer·al). Relating or belonging to the humerus.

humeroradial (**hew**·mer·o·**ra**′·de·al). Relating or belonging to the humerus and the radius.

humeroscapular (**hew**·mer·o·**skap**′·ew·lar). Relating or belonging to the humerus and the scapula.

humero-ulnar (**hew**·mer·o·**ul**′·nar). Relating or belonging to the humerus and the ulna.

humerus [NA] (**hew**·mer·us). The longest and largest bone of the arm; it articulates above with the glenoid cavity of the scapula; below, in conjunction with the radius and the ulna, it forms the elbow joint. **Head of the humerus [caput humeri (NA)].** The rounded surface at the upper end of the humerus, articulating with the glenoid cavity of the scapula. **Neck of the humerus, anatomical [collum anatomicum (NA)].** The slight constriction immediately adjoining the head. **Neck of the humerus, surgical [collum chirurgicum (NA)].** The portion of the shaft of the humerus immediately distal to the tuberosities. **Shaft of the humerus [corpus humeri (NA)].** The main, almost straight, part of the bone carrying the upper and lower ends and supporting the arm. It is somewhat triangular in cross-section and presents anterior, medial [margo medialis (NA)] and lateral [margo lateralis] borders separating anteromedial [facies anterior medialis (NA)], anterolateral [facies anterior lateralis (NA)] and posterior [facies posterior (NA)] surfaces, the last-named giving attachment to the triceps brachii muscle. The brachialis and deltoid muscles attach to the remaining surfaces. The borders and surfaces are easily identified only in the lower half of the shaft. **Humerus varus.** A condition in which the humerus is bent. [L shoulder.]

humidifier (hew·**mid**·if·i·er). An apparatus with which the moisture in the air of a room or breathing circuit can be maintained at any desired level. [L *humidus* moist, *facere* to make.]

humidity (hew·**mid**·it·e). Moisture, dampness; the state of the air in respect of moisture content, the saturation point depending on the temperature of the air. **Absolute humidity.** The actual weight of moisture present in a unit volume of air. **Relative humidity.** The percentage amount of moisture in the air, regarding saturation as 100. [L *humidus* moist.]

Hummelsheim, Eduard Karl Marie Joseph (b. 1868). German ophthalmologist.

Hummelsheim's operation, for 6th cranial nerve paralysis. A strip of tendon from the superior and inferior rectus muscles of the orbit is dissected free from the temporal side and sutured to the upper and lower border of the external rectus muscle of the orbit.

humoral (**hew**·mor·al). Relating or belonging to the bodily humours. **Humoral immunity.** Antibody-mediated immunity, cf. cell-mediated immunity.

humoralism, humorism (**hew**·mor·al·izm, **hew**·mor·izm). The humoral theory. *See* HUMOURS.

humour (**hew**·mor). 1. Any fluid of the body, e.g. lymph, blood. 2. Any chronic cutaneous disease. 3. Any morbid animal fluid. 4. (Humor (NA).] Any fluid or semifluid hyaline substance. 5. The disposition or state of mind. 6. A state of mind; uncertainty or vagary. **Aqueous humour [humor aquosus].** The clear fluid which fills the anterior chamber of the eye. **Crystalline humour.** The lens of the eye. **Ocular humour.** The aqueous or vitreous humour or the lens of the eye. **Thunder humour.** A chronic skin disease popularly supposed to be due to lightning stroke. **Vitreous humour [humor vitreus (NA)].** The thin, transparent, jelly-like substance which fills the concavity of the retina and is enclosed in the hyaloid membrane. [L *humor* moisture.]

See also: MORGAGNI.

humours (**hew**·morz). The theory of humours was the mainstay of all pathology and physiology from the time of Hippocrates for more than 2000 years up to the 17th century. According to the ideas of Empedocles and Pythagoras in ancient Greece, it was thought that all nature was compounded of 4 elements: earth, air, fire and water. Similarly it was taught that the body has 4 corresponding humours: black bile (earth), blood (air), yellow bile (fire) and phlegm (water). When these were in perfect balance the body was healthy; an imbalance produced ill-health. Linked with the humours were the corresponding temperaments: melancholic, plethoric, choleric and phlegmatic. There are many traces of the theory of humours in modern medical terminology and even in popular speech, in the phrases "good humour" and "bad humour". [see prec.]

humpback (**hump**·bak). Popular name for kyphosis. [D *homp* thick slice, AS *baec.*]

Humphry, Sir George Murray (b. 1820). Cambridge anatomist and surgeon.

Humphry's ligament. A variable ligament attached to the anterior surface of the posterior cruciate ligament of the knee.

humulene (**hew**·mew·leen). The chief constituent of the volatile oil of lupulin, derived from hops (*Humulus lupulus*).

humulon (**hew**·mew·lon). An antibacterial substance extracted from hops (*Humulus lupulus*).

humulus (**hew**·mew·lus). A synonym for the hop, *Humulus lupulus* Linn. [LL.]

humus (**hew**·mus). Partially decomposed vegetable matter. It is used in remedial baths. [L earth.]

hunchback (**hunsh**·bak). One who suffers from kyphosis; popular name for kyphosis. [hunch, etym. dub., AS *baec.*]

hundfieber (**hoont**·fe·ber). Sandfly fever. *See* FEVER. [G dog fever.]

hunger (**hung**·ger). A physical sensation associated with rhythmical contractions of an empty stomach. The term is also used for the craving for any physical or mental satisfaction. **Air hunger.** The hyperpnoea of diabetic coma. [AS *hungor.*]

Hunner, Guy Leroy (b. 1868). Baltimore urologist.

Hunner's stricture. A localized ureteric spasm, ureteritis or constriction of the ureter, described by Hunner in 1911. The histological changes associated with the condition are minimal, but may lead to alterations in the sensitivity of the ureter which may give rise to pain.

Hunner's ulcer. An intractable and extremely painful form of ulcer in the bladder, associated usually with inflammation in its wall.

Hunt, Howard Francis (b. 1918). Chicago psychologist.

Hunt-Minnesota test. A test of intellectual impairment, based on the comparison of scores on a vocabulary sub-test with those on a variety of other sub-tests. [*Minnesota University.*]

Hunt, H. Lyons. American surgeon.

Hunt-Tansley operation, for ptosis. A horizontal band of skin brought to a point at each end is removed from the upper lid but leaving the centre part intact as a vertical strip attached below. This is passed subcutaneously up to the eyebrow and stitched to the occipitofrontalis muscle.

Hunt, James Ramsay (b. 1874). New York neurologist.

Hunt's atrophy. Atrophy of the small muscles of the hand; it is nervous in origin and is unassociated with any impairment of sensation.

Hunt's disease. 1. Juvenile paralysis agitans resulting from progressive degeneration of the globus pallidus. 2. Herpes zoster of the ganglion of the facial nerve; usually called the *Ramsey Hunt syndrome. See* HUNT'S NEURALGIA OR SYNDROME (following).

Hunt's neuralgia or syndrome. Herpes zoster of the ganglion of the facial nerve; there may be pain in the ear, followed by a serosanguineous discharge, due to vesicles on the tympanic membrane. This is followed by homolateral facial paralysis of lower motor neurone type, with loss of taste sensibility on the anterior two-thirds of the affected side of the tongue. Occasionally other cranial nerves may be involved, particularly the 8th, giving nerve deafness; usually called the *Ramsay Hunt syndrome* and sometimes *Hunt's disease.*

Hunt's paradoxical phenomenon. In torsion spasm, attempted passive plantar flexion of the foot results in accentuation of dorsiflexion spasm, whereas attempted voluntary dorsiflexion may result in plantar flexion.

Hunt's palaeostriatal syndrome. Hunt's striatal syndrome, 1st def. (see following).

Hunt's striatal syndrome. 1. Juvenile paralysis agitans, due to degeneration of the globus pallidus (palaeostriatum). 2. Chorea syndrome, due to degeneration of the neostriatum. 3. Mixed striatal syndromes due to degeneration of both the neostriatum and palaeostriatum; characterized by evidence of muscular rigidity and involuntary movements of many types in a variety of combinations. Clinical syndromes that may fall into the group include athetosis, torsion spasm and Wilson's disease.

Hunt's tremor. The intention tremor of cerebellar disease.

Hunt, Reid (b. 1870). Baltimore and New York pharmacologist.

Hunt's method. A method of assaying thyroid preparations based on the reduction of toxicity to acetonitrile of mice treated with a thyroid preparation for a week previously.

Hunter, George (b. 1894). Canadian biochemist.

Hunter and Givens method, for purine bases in urine. The Krueger and Schmidt method is modified to permit colorimetric determination of uric acid.

Hunter, John (b. 1728). Scottish surgeon and anatomist in London.

Hunter's canal. The subsartorial canal. *See* CANAL.

hunterian chancre. The characteristic hard chancre of syphilis.

Hunter's gubernaculum. Gubernaculum testis.

hunterian ligation. *See* HUNTER'S METHOD (following).

Hunter's method. Treatment of peripheral aneurysm by high proximal ligation: it applies especially to ligation of the femoral artery in the subsartorial (Hunter's) canal in the treatment of popliteal aneurysm.

Hunter's operation, for trichiasis; obsolete.

Hunter, William (b. 1718). Scottish anatomist and obstetrician in London; brother of John Hunter.

Hunter's ligament. The round ligament of the uterus; a fibromuscular band attached to the lateral margin of the uterus below and in front of the uterine tube. It passes laterally in the broad ligament and traverses the inguinal canal to become attached to the skin of the labium majus.

Hunter's line. The linea alba.

Hunter's membrane. The decidua.

Hunter, William (b. 1861). London physician.

Hunter's glossitis. The smooth glazed, atrophic condition of the tongue seen characteristically in pernicious anaemia and described by Hunter; it also occurs in patients with achlorhydric, microcytic, hypochromic anaemia, and is essentially associated with the achlorhydria or achylia gastrica rather than with the anaemia.

hunterian (hun·te·re·an). Associated with John Hunter.

Huntington, George Sumner (b. 1851). New York physician.

Huntington's chorea or disease. A degenerative disease of the brain, transmitted by dominant inheritance and characterized by progressive chorea and dementia.

Hunyadi János (**hoon**·yah·dee **yah**·nosh). A mineral water, imported from Hungary. It contains principally the sulphates of sodium and magnesium and is a mild aperient. [Hunyadi *János*, Hungarian war-captain, d. 1456.]

Huppert, Karl Hugo (b. 1832). Prague physician.

Huppert's disease. Multiple myelomatosis.

Huppert's test, for bile pigments in urine. To 10 ml of urine add 5 ml of a 1.5 per cent suspension of calcium hydroxide in water, mix and filter, and wash the filter with water. Moisten the residue on the filter with about 10 drops of concentrated hydrochloric acid, pour 10 ml of alcohol on to the filter. Collect and warm the filtrate. A green colour indicates bile pigment.

Hurler, Gertrud (fl. 1920). Munich paediatrician.

Hurler's disease or syndrome. Mucopolysaccharidosis type I; gargoylism or lipochondrodystrophy. Bones, liver, spleen, cornea and brain are especially involved by infiltration with mucopolysaccharide. An autosomal recessive, inborn disorder of carbohydrate metabolism.

pseudo-Hurler's disease. Neurovisceral lipidosis. *See* LIPIDOSIS.

Huschke, Emil (b. 1797). Jena anatomist.

Huschke's canal or foramen. A canal present in the floor of the bony part of the external auditory meatus during early childhood.

Huschke's cartilage. The subvomerine cartilage. *See* CARTILAGE.

auditory tooth of Huschke. A thickened, periosteal swelling resembling a cock's comb, found on the inner portion of the osseous spiral lamina of the cochlea. It roofs over the internal spiral sulcus, and has a ridge from which some 7000 prominences, shaped like incisor teeth, project, in the direction of the inner hair cells of the organ of Corti.

Huschke's valve. The valve guarding the lower lip of the opening of the lacrimal ducts into the lacrimal sac.

Hutchinson, Sir Jonathan (b. 1828). London surgeon.

Hutchinson's changes. Degeneration of the macula which is surrounded by a ring of bright white spots. It tends to occur in the aged, and is probably caused by small haemorrhages in the outer retinal layers; this condition is also called *circinate retinopathy*.

Hutchinson's choroiditis. Tay's central guttate choroiditis. Although this choroiditis was originally described by Hutchinson, in his description he took in several other conditions, so that Tay's choroiditis is a more specific description.

Hutchinson's disease. 1. Prurigo aestivalis. 2. Cheiropompholyx. 3. Infective or serpiginous angioma (*see* ANGIOMA). Other conditions that he also first described include: 4. Arsenical keratosis (*see* KERATOSIS); 5. Erythema elevatum diutinum; 6. Recurrent lymphangitis (*see* LYMPHANGITIS) leading to chronic lymphoedema and elephantiasis; and 7. Degeneration of the macula. *See* HUTCHINSON'S CHANGES (above).

Hutchinson's mask. A feeling as if a mask were constricting the skin of the face; it occurs in tabes dorsalis.

Hutchinson's patch. Salmon patch; a pinkish area seen in the cornea during the course of specific interstitial keratitis. It is one of the diagnostic features of this disease.

Hutchinson's pill. A pill composed of mercury with chalk and opium, used formerly in the treatment of syphilis.

Hutchinson's prurigo. An erythematous and papular eruption commencing at or about puberty and becoming worse during the summer months; it occurs mainly on the face and limbs. It usually persists throughout adolescence, but during adult life it tends to decrease in intensity. It is less itchy than Hebra's prurigo.

Hutchinson's pupil. A pupil which is widely dilated and completely inactive to all stimuli, associated with lesions of the central nervous system.

Hutchinson's tooth. One of the permanent teeth, especially one of the upper incisors, which has a narrowed and notched cutting edge. It is recognized as a stigma of congenital syphilis, but does occur otherwise.

Hutchinson's triad. Found in congenital syphilis and comprises interstitial keratitis, deafness from labyrinthine disease and Hutchinson's teeth.

Hutchinson–Boeck disease. Cutaneous sarcoidosis.

Gilford–Hutchinson disease, Hutchinson–Gilford disease. Progeria.

Hutchison, Sir Robert (b. 1871). London physician.

Hutchison's syndrome. Sarcoma of the adrenals in infants, with secondary growths in the orbits causing marked exophthalmos.

Hutinel, Victor Henri (b. 1849). Paris physician.

Hutinel's disease. 1. Fibrosis of the liver and pericardium frequently due to tuberculosis. The symptoms follow an unresolved pneumonia, with residual bronchitis, and the signs are gradual enlargement of the liver, with ascites and oedema.

2. Erythema accompanying infectious fevers such as typhoid, pneumonia, etc.

Huxley, Thomas Henry (b. 1825). English biologist.

Huxley's layer or membrane. The inner layer of the inner root sheath of a hair follicle.

Huyghens, Christiaan (b. 1629). Dutch physicist.

Huyghens' ocular, huyghenian ocular. An eyepiece composed of 2 planoconvex lenses mounted with their convex surfaces towards the objective.

hyaenanchin (hi·e·**nan**·kin). A substance obtained from the fruits and seeds of a South African plant, *Toxicodendron capense* Thunb. (family Euphorbiaceae). It resembles strychnine in action, and has been used medicinally and as an arrow poison.

hyal (**hi**·al). Hyoid: 1. Shaped like a Y or a U. 2. The hyoid bone, or belonging to it. [Greek letter Υ (upsilon.]

hyalin (**hi**·al·in). 1. A glassy, homogeneous material derived from collagen and deposited around blood vessels and scars. 2. The chitinous material in the wall of a hydatid cyst. **Haematogenous hyalin.** Hyalin found in the walls of arteries and capillaries with advancing age, or as a sequel to fibrosis. [Gk *hyalos* glass.]

hyaline (**hi**·al·een). 1. Nearly or entirely transparent like glass. 2. Crystalline. [see foll.]

hyalinization (**hi**·al·in·i·**za**′·shun). The development into an albuminoid mass, or the development of such masses, e.g. within a cell. [Gk *hyalos* glass.]

hyalinogen (hi·al·**in**·o·jen). 1. The precursor of hyalin. 2. A mucoid substance occurring in cartilage. 3. A substance found in the walls of hydatid cysts. [hyalin, Gk *genein* to produce.]

hyalinosis (**hi**·al·in·**o**′·sis). Hyaline or amyloid degeneration. *See* DEGENERATION, AMYLOID. **Hyalinosis cutis et mucosae.** Lipoid proteinosis. *See* PROTEINOSIS. [hyaline, Gk *-osis* condition.]

hyalinuria (**hi**·al·in·**ewr**′·e·ah). The presence of hyaline casts in the urine.

hyalitis (hi·al·**i**·tis). Inflammation of the vitreous body or of the hyaloid membrane of the eye. **Asteroid hyalitis.** Inflammation of the vitreous body in which globular or stellate masses form; Benson's disease. **Hyalitis punctata.** Inflammation of the vitreous body accompanied by the formation of minute opacities. **Hyalitis suppurativa.** Inflammation of the vitreous body accompanied by the formation of pus. [Gk *hyalos* glass, *-itis* inflammation.]

hyalo-enchondroma (**hi**·al·o·en·kon·**dro**′·mah). A cartilaginous (chondromatous) neoplasm, consisting of hyaline cartilage. [hyaline, enchondroma.]

hyaloid (**hi**·al·oid). 1. Hyaline. 2. Having a glassy appearance. [Gk *hyalos* glass, *eidos* form.]

hyaloid artery [arteria hyaloidea (NA)]. A vessel present in the vitreous of the embryonic eye. It is a branch of the central artery of the retina which atrophies before birth, its position being marked in the adult by the hyaloid canal.

hyaloidin (hi·al·**oid**·in). The name given to a complex carbohydrate, $C_{26}H_{46}N_2O_{20}$, related to chondroitic acid and isolated from the wall of a hydatid cyst.

hyaloiditis (**hi**·al·oid·**i**′·tis). 1. Hyalitis. 2. Inflammation of the hyaloid membrane. [hyaloid, Gk *-itis* inflammation.]

hyaloma (hi·al·**o**·mah). 1. Colloid milium; degeneration of the skin resulting in the formation of yellow gelatinous papules. 2. The mass of hyalin into which the eye can be converted by degeneration. [Gk *hyalos* glass, *-oma* tumour.]

hyalomere (**hi**·al·o·meer). The colourless homogeneous cytoplasm of a blood platelet as distinct from the stainable granules. [Gk *hyalos* glass, *meros* part.]

hyalomitome (**hi**·al·o·**mi**′·tome). Hyaloplasm. [Gk *hyalos* glass, *mitos* thread.]

Hyalomma (hi·al·**om**·ah). A genus of ticks. **Hyalomma aegyptium impressum.** A vector of tick-borne typhus. [Gk *hyalos* glass, *omma* eye.]

hyalomucoid (**hi**·al·o·**mew**′·koid). A glycoprotein (mucoid) which may be present in the vitreous body of the eye. [Gk *hyalos* glass, mucoid.]

hyalonyxis (**hi**·al·o·**nix**′·is). The surgical procedure of puncturing the vitreous body of the eye. [Gk *hyalos* glass, *nyxis* a pricking.]

hyalophagia, hyalophagy (**hi**·al·o·**fa**′·je·ah, hi·al·**of**·ah·je). The practice of eating glass, a characteristic of certain types of insanity. [Gk *hyalos* glass, *phagein* to eat.]

hyalophobia (**hi**·al·o·**fo**′·be·ah). A morbid fear of coming in contact with glass. [Gk *hyalos* glass, phobia.]

hyaloplasm (**hi**·al·o·plazm). 1. The fluid-like constituent of the cytoreticulum of the cell body. 2. The portion of the axon which is concerned with the actual passage of impulses. **Nuclear hyaloplasm.** Karyolymph. [Gk *hyalos* glass, *plasma* something formed.]

hyaloserositis (**hi**·al·o·seer·o·**si**′·tis). Inflammation of a serous membrane, marked by the formation of a fibrinous exudate which undergoes hyaline transformation and takes on the appearance of porcelain, as in perihepatitis chronica hyperplastica. **Progressive multiple hyaloserositis.** Progressive malignant inflammation of the serous membranes; polyorrhomenitis. [Gk *hyalos* glass, serositis.]

hyalosis (hi·al·o·sis). **Asteroid hyalosis.** The presence of multiple, spherical, white bodies suspended in the vitreous. They consist of calcium salts. [Gk *hyalos* glass, *-osis* condition.]

hyalosome (**hi**·al·o·some). A body resembling the nucleolus of a cell and taking only a slight stain. [Gk *hyalos* glass, *soma* body.]

hyalotome (**hi**·al·o·tome). Hyaloplasm. [Gk *hyalos* glass, *mitos* thread.]

Hyaluronidase BP 1973 (**hi**·al·ewr·**on**′·id·aze). An enzyme which destroys hyaluronic acid. It is present in the filtrates of several bacterial species, and is associated with their invasion and spread through the tissues by decomposing the hyaluronic acid in intercellular spaces. It is used to add to solutions of local analgesics to increase their spread in the tissues.

hybrid (**hi**·brid). The product of a cross between genetically unlike individuals. **DNA hybrid.** One of a class of DNA molecules produced by the joining (end-to-end) of 2 strands of DNA obtained from different sources (e.g. from different animal species or from a eukaryote and a virus). **DNA–RNA hybrid.** One of a class of double-helical nucleic acids in which a strand of DNA and one of RNA, having complementary base sequences, are held together by hydrogen bonding between the base-pairs. **Interspecific hybrid.** The product of a cross between individuals of different species. **Intraspecific hybrid.** The product of a cross between individuals of the same species. **Hybrid molecule.** *See* MOLECULE. **Numerical hybrid.** A hybrid formed by a cross between gametes differing in the number of chromosomes. **Somatic hybrid.** A cell produced by fusion of somatic cells with different genotypes from individuals of either the same or different species. **Structural hybrid.** A hybrid formed by a cross between gametes differing in the chromosomal arrangement of their loci (structural heterozygote). [L *hybrida* offspring of tame sow and wild boar.]

hybridism (**hi**·brid·izm). 1. A disease which is a composite of various diseases. 2. The state of being crossbred. [see prec.]

hybridization (**hi**·brid·i·**za**′·shun). 1. The process or act of hybridizing or crossbreeding. 2. The state of being hybridized. 3. The production of hybrid offspring. **Cell hybridization.** The process leading to the formation of viable products from the fusion of cells with different genotypes.

hydaleous (hi·**da**·le·us). Dropsical. [Gk *hydaleos* watery.]

hydantoin (hi·**dan**·to·in). $CH_2(NHCO)_2$, the inner anhydride of hydantoic acid, related to allantoin, and also derived from creatinine. **Diphenyl hydantoin,** $(C_6H_5)_2C(NHCO)_2$. A hydantoin derivative, the sodium salt of which is used as an anticonvulsant in the treatment of epilepsy. **Phenylethyl hydantoin,** $(C_6H_5)(C_2H_5)C(NHCO)_2$. A compound also used in epilepsy.

hydantoinate (hi·**dan**·to·in·ate). Any salt derived from hydantoin, e.g. diphenylhydantoin sodium.

hydatenterocele (hi·dat·**en**·ter·o·seel). Hydrocele and intestinal hernia combined. [Gk *hydor* water, *enteron* bowel, *kele* hernia.]

hydatic (hi·**dat**·ik). Containing hydatids.

hydatid (hi·**dat**·id). 1. A vesicle; a cystic stage in the life history of *Echinococcus granulosus.* 2. A tiny congenital vesicle attached to the uterine tube or to the epididymis in the male. **Alveolar**

hydatid. One that has many loculi resulting from the development of daughter hydatids. **Secondary hydatid.** A daughter hydatid cyst. **Sessile hydatid, Stalked hydatid.** A pedunculated hydatid cyst of Morgagni. **Sterile hydatid.** A hydatid cyst containing no daughter or granddaughter cysts. [Gk *hydatis* drop of water.]

See also: MORGAGNI.

hydatidiform (hi·dat·**id**·e·form). Having the appearance or form of a hydatid.

hydatidocele (hi·dat·**id**·o·sel). A tumour of the scrotum or testis containing hydatid cysts. [hydatid, Gk *kele* hernia.]

hydatidoma (**hi**·dat·id·**o**′·mah). 1. A tumour composed of or containing hydatid cysts. 2. A tumour caused by the presence of hydatids. [hydatid, Gk *-oma* tumour.]

hydatidosis (**hi**·dat·id·**o**′·sis). The morbid condition resulting from the presence of hydatid cysts. [hydatid, Gk *-osis* condition.]

hydatidostomy (**hi**·dat·id·**os**′·to·me). The surgical evacuation and drainage of a hydatid cyst. [hydatid, Gk *stoma* mouth.]

hydatiform (hi·**dat**·e·form). Hydatidiform.

hydatism (**hi**·dat·izm). The sound caused by the movement of pathological fluid in any body cavity. [Gk *hydor* water.]

hydatogenesis (**hi**·dat·o·**jen**′·es·is). The formation of water or fluid within the body cavities or tissues. [Gk *hydor* water, genesis.]

hydatoid (**hi**·dat·oid). 1. The hyaloid membrane of the eye. 2. The aqueous humour of the eye. 3. Relating or belonging to the aqueous humour. 4. Resembling water, or watery. 5. Hydatidiform. [Gk *hydor* water, *eidos* form.]

hydatoncus (hi·dat·**ong**·kus). Any tumour or cyst the contents of which are watery. [Gk *hydor* water, *ogkos* a swelling.]

hydatorrhoea (**hi**·dat·o·**re**′·ah). A strong flow or copious discharge of water or fluid. [Gk *hydor* water, *rhoia* flow.]

Hyde, James Nevin (b. 1840). Chicago dermatologist.

Hyde's disease. Prurigo nodularis.

hydnocarpate (hid·no·**kar**·pate). A salt of hydnocarpic acid.

Hydnocarpus (hid·no·**kar**·pus). A genus of Indian trees (family Flacourtiaceae). The seeds of *Hydnocarpus wightiana* Blume are the official source of hydnocarpus oil. Several other species, including *H. anthelmintica* Pierre and *H. kurzii* Warb. (*Taraktogenos kurzii* King), yield a similar oil. [Gk *hydnein* to nourish, *karpos* fruit.]

hydracetin (hi·**dras**·et·in). Acetylphenylhydrazine, C_6H_5NHNH $COCH_3$, a powerful antipyretic. Its use is, however, dangerous, since it destroys the red blood cells. Also known as *pyrodine.*

hydracid (hi·**dras**·id). Term denoting a binary acid which does not contain any oxygen; it usually consists of 2 elements only, of which hydrogen is one: hydrochloric acid is an example.

hydradenitis (**hi**·drad·en·**i**′·tis). 1. Hidradenitis. 2. Lymphadenitis. [Gk *hydor* water, *aden* gland, *-itis* inflammation.]

hydradenoma (**hi**·drad·en·**o**′·mah). Syringocystadenoma; a disease of the skin characterized by the appearance of multiple nodular papular lesions, caused by hypertrophy and dilatation of the sweat glands. [Gk *hydor* water, adenoma.]

hydraemia (hi·**dre**·me·ah). A condition in which the blood is abnormally watery. [Gk *hydor* water, *haima* blood.]

hydraeroperitoneum (hi·**dra**·er·o·per·e·ton·**e**′·um). The presence of water and air or gas in the peritoneal cavity; hydropneumoperitoneum. [Gk *hydor* water, *aer* air, peritoneum.]

hydragogue (**hi**·drag·og). 1. A cathartic which produces profuse watery stools. 2. Any agent which produces a watery discharge or expels water. 3. Producing water or a watery discharge. [Gk *hydor* water, *agogos* leading.]

Hydrallazine (hi·**dral**·az·een). BP Commission approved name for 1-hydrazinophthalazine, an antihypertensive drug, the exact pharmacological action of which is not known. It antagonizes the hypertensive actions of serotonin and noradrenaline, and it also has antihistamine actions. There is evidence of a central action on the hypothalamus and on the peripheral arterioles. It increases the renal blood flow without increasing the glomerular filtration rate. **Hydrallazine Hydrochloride BP 1963.** 1-Hydrazinophthalazine hydrochloride; an antipressor drug which reduces both systolic and diastolic blood pressure and improves the renal blood flow. Its action is similar to that of the base (see above).

hydramine (**hi**·dram·een). Name applied to the amines derived from glycols in which one of the hydroxyl OH groups present in the latter is replaced by an amino NH_2 group: hydroxyethylamine, $OHC_2H_4NH_2$, is an example.

hydramnion, hydramnios (hi·**dram**·ne·on, hi·**dram**·ne·os). Excessive accumulation of amniotic fluid; a dropsical condition of the amnion. [Gk *hydor* water, amnion.]

hydranencephaly (**hi**·dran·en·**kef**′·al·e). Internal hydrocephalus. *See* HYDROCEPHALUS. [Gk *hydor* water, *egkephalos* brain.]

Hydrangea (hi·**dran**·je·ah). A genus of shrubs (family Saxifragaceae). An infusion of the root of *Hydrangea arborescens* Linn. has been used as a cathartic and diuretic. [Gk *hydor* water, *aggeion* small vessel.]

hydrangeion (hi·**dran**·je·on) (pl. *hydrangeia*). A lymph vessel. [Gk *hydor* water, *aggeion* small vessel.]

Hydrargaphen (hi·**drar**·gah·fen). BP Commission approved name for phenylmercury 2,2′-dinaphthylmethane-3,3′-disulphonate; a fungicide.

hydrargyrate (hi·**drar**·ji·rate). Containing or pertaining to mercury. [see foll.]

hydrargyria, hydrargyriasis (hi·drar·**ji**·re·ah, **hi**·drar·ji·**ri**′·as·is). Chronic mercurial poisoning. [L *hydrargyrum* mercury.]

hydrargyric (hi·drar·**ji**·rik). Mercuric. [see prec.]

hydrargyrism (hi·**drar**·ji·rizm). Chronic mercurial poisoning. [L *hydrargyrum* mercury.]

hydrargyromania (hi·**drar**·ji·ro·**ma**′·ne·ah). Insanity resulting from mercurialism (hydrargyria). [hydrargyrum, mania.]

hydrargyrophobia (hi·**drar**·ji·ro·**fo**′·be·ah). Unreasoning or morbid dread of using any preparation of mercury. [hydrargyrum, phobia.]

hydrargyrophthalmia (hi·**drar**·ji·rof·**thal**′·me·ah). Ophthalmia resulting from mercurial poisoning (hydrargyria).

hydrargyrosis (**hi**·drar·ji·**ro**′·sis). Chronic mercurial poisoning. [hydrargyrum, Gk *-osis* condition.]

hydrargyrum (hi·**drar**·ji·rum) (gen. *hydrargyri*). **Hydrargyrum ammoniatum.** Ammoniated Mercury BP 1958. *See* MERCURY. **Hydrargyri Cyanidum BPC 1949.** Mercuric cyanide, a colourless or white crystalline substance, soluble in water, with potent antiseptic properties. **Hydrargyrum oleatum.** Oleated Mercury BP 1958. *See* MERCURY. **Hydrargyri oxidum flavum.** Yellow Mercuric Oxide BP 1958. *See* MERCURIC. **Hydrargyri Oxidum Rubrum BPC 1949.** Red mercuric oxide, an orange-red powder, insoluble in water and used in ointment form for certain skin diseases. **Hydrargyri oxycyanidum.** Mercuric Oxycyanide BP 1953. **Hydrargyri perchloridum.** Mercuric Chloride BP 1953. **Hydrargyri Salicylas BPC 1949.** Mercuric salicylate, a compound employed in the form of a dusting powder and ointment as an antiseptic and antisyphilitic. **Hydrargyri subchloridum.** Mercurous Chloride BP 1953. [L mercury.]

hydrarthrodial (hi·drar·**thro**·de·al). Relating or belonging to hydrarthrosis.

hydrarthrosis (hi·drar·**thro**·sis). A watery effusion into the cavity of a joint. **Intermittent hydrarthrosis.** Periodical accumulation of water or other fluid within the cavity of a joint. [Gk *hydor* water, *arthron* joint.]

hydrastidis rhizome (hi·**dras**·tid·is **ri**·zome). Hydrastis.

hydrastine (hi·**dras**·teen). $C_{21}H_{21}O_6N$, an alkaloid, closely related to narcotine, and obtained from the golden seal (*Hydrastis canadensis*). It depresses the heart rate and raises the blood pressure; solutions of the hydrochloride are injected hypodermically for this purpose (BPC 1949).

hydrastinine (hi·**dras**·tin·een). $C_{11}H_{13}O_3N$, an alkaloid produced by the oxidation of hydrastine. It is little used in medicine. **Hydrastinine hydrochloride.** $C_{11}H_{11}O_2NHCl$, a salt, solutions of which are injected hypodermically to contract the uterus, and also applied to the eye to dilate the pupil.

Hydrastis BPC 1949 (hi·**dras**·tis). Hydrastis rhizome, golden seal, yellow root; the rhizome and roots of *Hydrastis canadensis*

Linn. (family Ranunculaceae), a plant indigenous to North America. Two alkaloids, hydrastine and berberine, form the main active constituents; these and the drug itself cause uterine contraction and have been employed in menorrhagia. In the form of the tincture or extract it is also widely used as a bitter tonic and, by local application, to allay inflammation of mucous membranes. [Gk *hydor* water, *dran* to do.]

hydrate (**hi**·drate). 1. A hydroxide. 2. A chemical compound formed by a substance with 1 or more molecules of water. 3. A crystalline compound in molecular proportions of a salt with water, the latter being known as *water of crystallization.* 4. In aqueous solutions, the complex formed by molecules or ions of the solute with water molecules. [Gk *hydor* water.]

hydrated (hi·**dra**·ted). Transformed into a hydrate by combination with water.

hydration (hi·**dra**·shun). The process of chemical combination with water in which the latter is taken up without disruption of the molecule. [Gk *hydor* water.]

hydraulics (hi·**draw**·lix). The practical science of hydrodynamics. [Gk *hydor* water, *aulos* pipe.]

hydrazine (**hi**·draz·een). 1. Diamine, NH_2NH_2, a colourless liquid used in organic synthesis, and the parent of important derivatives. 2. General name for bases derived from hydrazine; they may be primary, secondary, tertiary or quaternary, according to the number of hydrogen atoms of hydrazine replaced by alkyl radicals.

hydrazone (**hi**·draz·one). General term for compounds formed by hydrazines with aldehydes or ketones; they contain the group =C=NNH-. Of particular importance are those formed by aldoses and ketoses with phenylhydrazine, which in turn give rise to osazones.

hydrectasis (hi·**drek**·tas·is). The state of being distended with any thin fluid such as water. [Gk *hydor* water, *ektasis* a stretching.]

hydrelatic (hi·dre·**lat**·ik). Relating to the action of nerves on glands, causing a watery secretion. [Gk *hydor* water, *elaunein* to drive.]

hydremesis (hi·**drem**·es·is). Vomiting of thin or watery material, in single or multiple occurrence. [Gk *hydor* water, emesis.]

hydrencephalitis (**hi**·dren·kef·al·**i**'·tis). Hydrocephalus with inflammation of the meninges. [Gk *hydor* water, encephalitis.]

hydrencephalocele (hi·dren·**kef**·al·o·seel). Hernia, through a fissure in the skull, of brain substance distended in the form of a sac containing watery or cerebrospinal fluid. [Gk *hydor* water, encephalocele.]

hydrencephalomeningocele (hi·dren·**kef**·al·o·men·**ing**'·go·seel). Hydrencephalocele in which the sac contains brain tissue as well as watery fluid. [Gk *hydor* water, encephalomeningocele.]

hydrencephalus (hi·dren·**kef**·al·us). Hydrocephalus. [Gk *hydor* water, *egkephalos* brain.]

hydrenterocele (hi·**dren**·ter·o·seel). Hernia of the intestine with escaped fluid in the sac. [Gk *hydor* water, enterocele.]

hydrenterorrhoea (hi·**dren**·ter·o·**re**'·ah). Diarrhoea of very watery type. [Gk hydor water, enterorrhoea.]

hydrepigastrium (**hi**·drep·e·**gas**'·tre·um). An accumulation of fluid between the muscular wall of the abdomen and the peritoneal lining. [Gk *hydor* water, epigastrium.]

hydriatic, hydriatric (hi·dre·**at**·ik, hi·dre·**at**·rik). Referring or belonging to hydrotherapy. [Gk *hydor* water, *iatreia* treatment.]

hydriatrics (hi·dre·**at**·rix). Hydrotherapeutics. [see prec.]

hydriatrist (hi·**dri**·at·rist). A practitioner who specializes in hydrotherapy. [Gk *hydor* water, *iatreia* treatment.]

hydriatry (hi·**dri**·at·re). Hydrotherapeutics. [see prec.]

hydric (**hi**·drik). 1. Hydro-; related to water; containing water. 2. Combined with, or related to hydrogen. 3. Possessing hydrogen which is available for replacement. [Gk *hydor* water.]

hydride (**hi**·dride). Name for any binary compound of hydrogen with an element or radical, such as calcium hydride, CaH_2.

hydriodate (hi·**dri**·o·date). Hydriodide.

hydriodide (hi·**dri**·o·dide). A compound formed by an organic base, usually an alkaloid, with hydriodic acid.

hydrion (hi·**dri**·on). The hydrogen ion, H^+.

hydroa (hi·**dro**·ah). Any eruption characterized by small blisters. **Hydroa aestivale.** Recurrent summer eruption; a recurring, usually vesicular eruption, beginning in early life and often disappearing when the patient becomes adult. Generally the lesions are found only on the parts exposed to sunlight, and these are eventually replaced by scars. In some cases there is an abnormal porphyrin metabolism. **Hydroa gestationis, Hydroa gravidarum.** Herpes gestationis; an eruption during pregnancy or the puerperium. **Hydroa herpetiforme.** Dermatitis herpetiformis. **Hydroa puerorum.** Hydroa aestivale (see above); originally the malady was thought to occur only in males, and as it was noted in early life the name seemed appropriate. **Hydroa vacciniforme.** Hydroa aestivale (see above). **Hydroa vesiculosum.** Herpes iris. [Gk *hydor* water, *oon* egg.]

hydro-adipsia (**hi**·dro·a·**dip**'·se·ah). Absence of thirst. [Gk *hydor* water, adipsia.]

hydro-aeric (hi·dro·a·er·ik). Applied to the sound heard when body cavities containing water or air are being examined by auscultation. [Gk *hydor* water, *aer* air.]

hydro-aeroperitoneum (**hi**·dro·a·er·o·per·e·ton·e'·um). Hydraeroperitoneum.

hydro-aestivale (**hi**·dro·es·tiv·a'·le). Hydroa aestivale. [Gk *hydor* water, L *aestivus* relating to summer.]

hydro-anencephaly (**hi**·dro·an·en·**kef**'·al·e). Internal hydrocephalus. *See* HYDROCEPHALUS. [Gk *hydor* water, *a*, *egkephalos* brain.]

hydro-angiography (**hi**·dro·an·je·**og**'·raf·e). A description of the anatomy and physiology of the lymphatic system. [Gk *hydor* water, *aggeion* small vessel, *graphein* to write.]

hydro-angiology (**hi**·dro·an·je·**ol**'·o·je). Dissection of the lymph vessels and glands. [Gk *hydor* water, *aggeion* small vessel, *logos* science.]

hydro-appendix (**hi**·dro·ap·**en**'·dix). A vermiform appendix that is distended by serous fluid. [Gk *hydros* water, appendix.]

hydro-arthrodial (hi·dro·ar·**thro**'·de·al). Hydrarthrodial.

hydro-arthrosis (**hi**·dro·ar·**thro**'·sis). Hydrarthrosis.

hydrobilirubin (**hi**·dro·bil·e·**roo**'·bin). A substance obtained by the reduction of bilirubin with sodium amalgam. It has been stated to consist of a mixture of mesobilinogen, mesobilirubin and a non-crystalline substance.

Hydrobiodes (hi·dro·**bi**·o·deez). A genus of molluscan hosts of *Clonorchis sinensis.* [Gk *hydor* water, *bios* life, *eidos* form.]

hydrobiosis (**hi**·dro·bi·o'·sis). In biology, the origin of life in fluid media and its maintenance therein. [Gk *hydor* water, *bios* life.]

hydroblepharon (hi·dro·**blef**·ar·on). Oedema of the eyelids. [Gk *hydor* water, *blepharon* eyelid.]

hydrobromate (hi·dro·**bro**·mate). Hydrobromide.

hydrobromic (hi·dro·**bro**·mik). Pertaining to hydrogen bromide.

hydrobromide (hi·dro·**bro**·mide). A compound formed by an alkaloid or other organic base with hydrobromic acid.

hydrocalycosis (**hi**·dro·ka·lik·**o**'·sis). A later stage in calycectasis, when there is actual expansion and dilatation of the calyx, or group of calyces, as a result of obstruction. [Gk *hydor* water, *kalyx* cup, *-osis* condition.]

hydrocarbon (hi·dro·**kar**·bon). Any organic compound of carbon and hydrogen only. They are classified in homologous series according to structure and the proportions of carbon and hydrogen of which they are composed. **Aliphatic hydrocarbon.** One in which the carbon atoms are in open chains. **Aromatic hydrocarbon.** One in which the carbon atoms are in a ring or rings. **Bivalent hydrocarbon.** An unsaturated hydrocarbon such as an olefine, which can act as a bivalent radical by rupture of the double bond. **Carcinogenic hydrocarbon.** One of a series of hydrocarbons, mostly derivatives of benzanthracene, which are liable to produce cancer. **Cyclic hydrocarbon.** One containing a ring or rings of carbon atoms; usually an aromatic hydrocarbon. **Fatty hydrocarbon.** A hydrocarbon derived from fats; a paraffin. **Saturated hydrocarbon.** One that has the valency bonds of all carbon atoms combined with hydrogen. **Univalent hydrocarbon.** Term applied loosely to the monovalent alphyl radicals.

Unsaturated hydrocarbon. One in which carbon atoms are linked by double or triple bonds.

See also: DIELS.

hydrocarbonism (hi·dro·**kar**·bon·izm). A state of poisoning induced by the use of or exposure to hydrocarbons, e.g. in those who take preparations of kerosene internally, those who work in kerosene refineries or who are exposed to petroleum fumes in any way.

hydrocardia (hi·dro·**kar**·de·ah). An excessive accumulation of fluid in the pericardium. [Gk *hydor* water, pericardium.]

hydrocele (**hi**·dro·seel). A circumscribed collection of fluid, particularly a collection of fluid in the tunica vaginalis testis. **Cervical hydrocele.** The name formerly applied to lymphangioma of the neck. **Chylous hydrocele.** A hydrocele with milky content. **Hydrocele colli.** Cervical hydrocele (see above). **Congenital hydrocele.** Hydrocele already present at birth. **Diffuse hydrocele.** A collection of fluid interspersed in the tissue spaces of the spermatic cord. **Encysted hydrocele.** Hydrocele in the unobstructed remnant of the processus vaginalis of the peritoneum in the spermatic cord, between the abdominal inguinal ring and the upper pole of the testis. **Hydrocele of the epididymis.** Spermatocele; a cyst, or usually multiple cysts, of the epididymis. **Funicular hydrocele.** An incompletely encysted hydrocele which retains a narrow connection with the cavity of the peritoneum. **Hernial hydrocele.** A collection of fluid in a hernial sac. **Intermittent hydrocele.** Funicular hydrocele (see above). **Interstitial hydrocele.** Diffuse hydrocele (see above). **Hydrocele muliebris.** Hydrocele of the canal of Nuck. **Hydrocele of the neck.** Cervical hydrocele (see above). **Scrotal hydrocele.** Hydrocele of the tunica vaginalis testis. **Spermatic hydrocele.** Spermatocele. **Hydrocele spinalis.** Meningocele; myelomeningocele or syringomyelocele. [Gk *hydor* water, *kele* hernia.]

See also: DUPUYTREN, GIBBON (Q. V.), MAUNOIR, NUCK.

hydrocelectomy (**hi**·dro·se·**lek'**·to·me). The surgical removal of any kind of hydrocele, particularly of the tunica vaginalis testis, the round ligament of the uterus or the canal of Nuck. [Gk *hydor* water, *kele* hernia, *ektome* a cutting out.]

hydrocelodes (**hi**·dro·se·**lo'**·deez). A tumour containing extravasated urine and resembling a hydrocele. [Gk *hydor* water, *kele* hernia, *eidos* form.]

hydrocenosis (**hi**·dro·sen·**o'**·sis). The removal or withdrawal of water or dropsical fluid by surgical puncture or by the administration of hydragogues or other medicinal means. [Gk *hydor* water, *kenosis* an emptying.]

hydrocephalic (hi·dro·kef·**al'**·ik). 1. Pertaining to or causing hydrocephalus. 2. Suffering from hydrocephalus.

hydrocephalocele (hi·dro·**kef**·al·o·seel). Hernia, through a fissure in the skull, of brain substance distended in the form of a sac containing watery or cerebrospinal fluid. [Gk *hydor* water, encephalocele.]

hydrocephaloid (hi·dro·**kef**·al·oid). 1. Having resemblance to or belonging to hydrocephalus. 2. A condition resembling hydrocephalus but attended with depression of the fontanelles; it is often associated with marasmus and premature weaning and there may be diarrhoea with resultant anaemia and debility (Marshall Hall's disease). There is no excessive accumulation of cerebrospinal fluid. [Gk *hydor* water, *kephale* head, *eidos* form.]

hydrocephalus, hydrocephaly (hi·dro·**kef**·al·us, hi·dro·**kef**·al·e). An abnormal increase of cerebrospinal fluid within the skull. **Acquired hydrocephalus.** That secondary to obstruction in the cerebrospinal-fluid circulation, most commonly by adhesions due to posterior basic meningitis, thrombosis of intracranial venous sinuses or intracranial neoplasms. It may also follow head injuries and infection of the bones of the skull. **Acute acquired hydrocephalus.** A rapid and severe obstruction to the flow of cerebrospinal fluid in patients whose skulls cannot expand, so that there is increased intracranial pressure without enlargement of the skull. **Communicating hydrocephalus.** Hydrocephalus in which the increase involves the ventricles and the general subarachnoid space. **Compensating hydrocephalus.** Increased volume of cerebrospinal fluid without increased pressure; the excess of fluid is compensatory to atrophy of the brain. **Congenital hydrocephalus.** That due to congenital malformations causing obstruction at some point in the circulatory channels. It is often associated with other congenital malformations such as spina bifida, hare-lip, club-foot, or imperforate anus. **Hypertonic hydrocephalus.** An increased volume of cerebrospinal fluid with increased pressure. **Internal hydrocephalus.** Hydrocephalus in which the increased fluid is confined within the ventricles which become greatly distended. **Low pressure hydrocephalus, Normal-pressure hydrocephalus.** Dilatation of the cerebral ventricles due to obstruction of absorption of cerebrospinal fluid, without apparent rise in pressure. **Otitic hydrocephalus.** Raised intracranial pressure occurring in cases of otitis media, probably due to thrombosis of cortical veins or venous sinuses. [Gk *hydor* water, *kephale* head.]

hydrochinone (hi·dro·**kin**·one). Hydroquinone.

hydrochinonuria (**hi**·dro·kin·o·**newr'**·e·ah). The presence of hydroquinone in the urine as the result of administration of any derivative or preparation of the drug.

hydrochloric (hi·dro·**klor**·ik). Pertaining to hydrogen chloride.

hydrochloride (hi·dro·**klor**·ide). A compound of an alkaloid or other organic base with hydrochloric acid. It is an additive combination, and in the case of alkaloids is achieved by the nitrogen atom becoming pentavalent as in ammonium compounds.

Hydrochlorothiazide BP 1973 (**hi**·dro·klor·o·**thi'**·az·ide). 6-Chloro-3,4-dihydro-7-sulphamoylbenzo-1,2,4-thiadiazine 1,1-dioxide; a diuretic.

hydrocholecystis (**hi**·dro·ko·le·**sist'**·is). Distension of the gall bladder by an inflammatory exudate, fluid or water. [Gk *hydor* water, cholecystis.]

hydrocholeresis (**hi**·dro·ko·ler·**e'**·sis). An increased flow of water bile of low specific gravity and viscosity. [Gk *hydor* water, choleresis.]

hydrocholeretic (**hi**·dro·ko·ler·**et'**·ik). Applied to any substance or influence that increases the volume of the bile without stimulating secretion of its solid constituents. [see prec.]

hydrocinchonidine (**hi**·dro·sin·**kon'**·id·een). Dihydrocinchonidine, cinchamidine, $C_{19}H_{24}ON_2$. An alkaloid isomeric with cinchotine, which occurs in certain cinchona barks.

hydrocirsocele (hi·dro·**ser**·so·seel). Combined hydrocele and varicocele. [Gk *hydor* water, cirsocele.]

Hydrocodone (hi·dro·**ko**·done). BP Commission approved name for 7,8-dihydro-O^3-methylmorphinone.

hydrocollidine (hi·dro·**kol**·id·een). $C_8H_{13}N$, a ptomaine resulting from the putrefaction of the albumin in decayed fish and flesh. [Gk *hydor* water, *kolla* glue.]

hydrocolpos (hi·dro·**kol**·pos). A retention cyst of the vagina filled with a clear fluid. [Gk *hydor* water, *kolpos* vagina.].

hydrocoridine (hi·dro·**kor**·id·een). $C_{10}H_{17}N$, a ptomaine produced from decaying onions.

Hydrocortisone BP 1968 (**hi**·dro·**kor'**·tiz·one). 11β-17α,21-Trihydroxypregn-4-ene-3,20-dione, a compound secreted by, and isolated from, the cortex of the suprarenal gland. It has also been synthesized and has been tried in the treatment of rheumatic diseases and in inflammatory and allergic conditions, as has Cortisone (BP 1968). **Hydrocortisone Acetate BP 1973.** 21-Acetoxy-11β,17α-dihydroxypregn-4-ene-3,20-dione, the acetate ester of Hydrocortisone, used in the form of intra-articular injection or ointment. **Hydrocortisone Hydrogen Succinate BP 1973.** 21-(3-Carboxypropionyloxy)-11β,17α-dihydroxypregn-4-ene-3,20-dione. This compound is used in the form of intravenous injection. **Hydrocortisone Sodium Succinate BP 1973.** Chemically akin to Hydrocortisone Hydrogen Succinate (see above) but, as it is soluble in water, it can be given intravenously to obtain the therapeutic effects of steroid immediately in patients in Addisonian crisis or in status asthmaticus. [Gk *hydor* water, cortisone.]

hydrocortisonum (**hi**·dro·kor·tiz·**o'**·num). *European Pharmacopoeia* name for Hydrocortisone BP 1973. **Hydrocortisoni acetas.**

European Pharmacopoeia name for Hydrocortisone Acetate BP 1973.

hydrocotarnine (hi·dro·ko·**tar**′·neen). $C_{12}H_{15}O_3N$, an alkaloid obtained by the acid hydrolysis of narcotine, and also found in opium.

Hydrocotyle (hi·dro·**kot**·il·e). A genus of herbs (family Umbelliferae). *Hydrocotyle asiatica* Linn. is widely used in India in the treatment of leprosy and other skin affections. *Hydrocotyle vulgaris* Linn., a European species, has been employed as a purgative and diuretic. [Gk *hydor* water, *kotyle* cup.]

hydrocrania (hi·dro·**kra**·ne·ah). Hydrocephalus. [Gk *hydor* water, *kranion* skull.]

hydrocupreidine (hi·dro·kew·**pre**′·id·een). Dihydrocupreidine, a synthetic alkaloid isomeric with hydrocupreine and prepared from quinidine.

hydrocupreine (hi·dro·**kew**·pre·een). Dihydrocupreine, $C_{19}H_{24}O_2N_2$. An alkaloid not found in nature, but prepared by the demethylation of dihydroquinine, or by the reduction of cupreine.

hydrocyanism (hi·dro·**si**·an·izm). A condition of poisoning with hydrocyanic acid.

hydrocyst (**hi**·dro·sist). 1. A cyst filled with water or a watery fluid. 2. Hydatid. [Gk *hydor* water, cyst.]

hydrocystadenoma (hi·dro·**sist**·ad·en·**o**′·mah). Syringocystadenoma. [Gk *hydor* water, cystadenoma.]

hydrocystoma (hi·dro·sist·**o**′·mah). 1. A cystic tumour originating in a sweat gland. 2. A syringoma with dilatation of the ducts, usually occurring on the eyelids and cheeks. The lesions feel cystic and enlarge on exposure to heat. [Gk *hydor* water, cystoma.]

hydrodictyotomy (hi·dro·dik·te·**ot**′·o·me). Incision of the retina to allow escape of fluid. [Gk *hydor* water, *diktyon* retina, *temnein* to cut.]

hydrodiffusion (hi·dro·dif·**ew**′·zhun). 1. Diffusion in which the solvent is water. 2. Term applied to the diffusion of one liquid through another. [Gk *hydor* water, diffusion.]

hydrodipsomania (hi·dro·dip·so·**ma**′·ne·ah). An abnormal desire to be continually drinking water. [Gk *hydor* water, *dipsa* thirst, *mania* madness.]

hydrodiuresis (hi·dro·di·ewr·**e**′·sis). The passing of an abnormal amount of watery urine. [Gk *hydor* water, diuresis.]

hydrodynamics (hi·dro·di·**nam**′·ix). The theoretical and mathematical study of the energy and pressure of liquids in motion. [Gk *hydor* water, dynamics.]

hydro-electric (hi·dro·el·**ek**′·trik). 1. Relating to the generation of electricity by water power. 2. Connected with the use of water and electricity in medical treatment. [Gk *hydor* water, electricity.]

hydro-electrization (hi·dro·el·ek·tri·**za**′·shun). The application of the galvanic or faradic current to 1 or more limbs, or occasionally to the entire body, whilst immersed in suitable metal-lined baths. [see prec.]

hydro-encephalitis (hi·dro·en·kef·al·**i**′·tis). Hydrencephalitis.

hydro-encephalomeningocele (hi·dro·en·kef·al·o·men·**ing**′·go·seel). Hydrencephalomeningocele.

hydro-enterocele (hi·dro·**en**·ter·o·seel). Hydrenterocele.

hydro-enterorrhoea (hi·dro·**en**·ter·o·**re**′·ah). Hydrenterorrhoea.

hydro-epigastrium (hi·dro·ep·e·**gas**′·tre·um). Hydrepigastrium.

hydro-epiplocele (hi·dro·ep·**ip**′·lo·seel). An epiplocele the sac of which contains water. [Gk *hydor* water, epiplocele.]

hydro-ergotinine (hi·dro·er·**got**′·in·een). Ergotoxine.

hydroferrocyanate, hydroferrocyanide (hi·dro·fer·o·**si**′·an·ate, hi·dro·fer·o·**si**′·an·ide). Names given indiscriminately to compounds of hydroferrocyanic acid.

Hydroflumethiazide BP 1973 (hi·dro·floo·meth·**i**′·az·ide). 3,4-Dihydro-6-trifluoromethyl-1,2,4-benzo-thiadiazine-7-sulphonamide 1,1-dioxide; a diuretic.

hydrofluosilicate (hi·dro·floo·o·**sil**′·ik·ate). A salt of hydrofluosilicic acid.

hydrogalvanic (hi·dro·gal·**van**′·ik). Hydro-electric. [Gk *hydor* water, galvanism.]

hydrogel (**hi**·dro·jel). Denoting a gel in which water is the disperse phase. [Gk *hydor* water, gel.]

hydrogen (**hi**·dro·gen). The lightest of the chemical elements, with atomic weight 1.0079, atomic number 1 and chemical symbol H. It is a colourless inflammable gas without taste or smell, present in volcanic gases, to a small extent in the earth's atmosphere and to a large extent in that of the sun. It occurs combined in water and in all animal and vegetable matter. It has three isotopes: protium, deuterium and tritium; molecular hydrogen exists in *ortho-* and *para-* forms. **Activated hydrogen.** Atomic hydrogen (see below). **Arseniuretted hydrogen.** Arsine. **Atomic hydrogen.** H, produced by the disruption of the hydrogen molecule in an intense electromagnetic field. **Hydrogen chloride.** HCl, a colourless gas forming a concentrated solution in water. **Hydrogen dioxide.** Hydrogen peroxide (see below). **Hydrogen disulphide.** Hydrogen persulphide (see below). **Hydrogen fluoride.** Hydrofluoric acid. *See* ACID. **Heavy hydrogen.** Deuterium, ^2H, the isotope of hydrogen with mass 2; it forms *heavy water.* **Hydrogen monoxide.** Water, H_2O. **Nascent hydrogen.** Highly reactive hydrogen at the moment of formation of the gas. **Hydrogen peroxide.** H_2O_2, a strongly oxidizing liquid used as a bleach and disinfectant. **Hydrogen persulphide.** H_2S_2, a yellow liquid with a disagreeable odour, used as a bleach and antiseptic. **Radioactive hydrogen.** Tritium. **Hydrogen selenide.** H_2Se, a poisonous gas which affects the mucous membrane causing coryza and destroying the sense of smell. **Hydrogen sulphide, Sulphuretted hydrogen.** H_2S, a colourless gas with the odour of bad eggs, used to precipitate metallic sulphides. [Gk *hydor* water, *genein* to produce.]

hydrogenase (**hi**·dro·gen·aze). A bacterial enzyme catalysing reduction by molecular hydrogen.

hydrogenate (**hi**·dro·jen·ate). To introduce hydrogen into a compound.

hydrogenation (hi·dro·jen·**a**′·shun). The process of chemically saturating or reducing a compound with hydrogen. It is achieved by means of heat or pressure in the presence of suitable catalysts: it is used industrially to harden animal and vegetable oils, crack hydrocarbons, produce oil from coal and to convert fatty acids and glycerides into alcohols.

hydrogenide (**hi**·dro·jen·ide). Hydride. A binary compound of hydrogen with an element or radical.

Hydrogenii Peroxidum. *European Pharmacopoeia* name for Strong Hydrogen Peroxide Solution BP 1973.

hydrogenize (**hi**·dro·jen·ize). Hydrogenate.

hydrogenoid (**hi**·dro·jen·oid). In homoeopathy, a bodily constitution in which there is excess of water in the blood; one which will not tolerate much moisture. [Gk *hydor* water, *genein* to produce, *eidos* form.]

Hydrogenomonas (hi·dro·jen·**om**′·on·as). A genus of soil microorganisms capable of deriving energy from the oxidation of hydrogen to water. [hydrogen, Gk *monas* unit.]

hydrogenous (hi·**droj**·en·us). 1. Relating or belonging to hydrogen. 2. Of the nature of hydrogen. 3. Containing hydrogen.

hydrogerous (hi·**droj**·er·us). Containing water or conveying water. [Gk *hydor* water, L *gerere* to bear.]

hydroglossa (hi·dro·**glos**·ah). Ranula. [Gk *hydor* water, *glossa* tongue.]

hydrogymnasium (hi·dro·jim·**na**′·ze·um). A pool in which remedial exercises under water can be carried out. [Gk *hydor* water, gymnasium.]

hydrogymnastic (hi·dro·jim·**nas**′·tik). Referring or belonging to exercises in a hydrogymnasium.

hydrogymnastics (hi·dro·jim·**nas**′·tix). Physical exercises carried out in water. [Gk *hydor* water, gymnastics.]

hydrohaematocele (hi·dro·**he**·mat·o·seel). Combined haematocele and hydrocele. [Gk *hydor* water, *haima* blood, *kele* hernia.]

hydrohaematonephrosis (hi·dro·**he**·mat·o·nef·**ro**′·sis). Dilatation of the pelvis and calyces of the ureter due to a collection of blood and urine. [Gk *hydor* water, *haima* blood, *nephros* kidney.]

hydrohaemia (hi·dro·**he**·me·ah). A condition in which the blood is abnormally watery. [Gk *hydor* water, *haima* blood.]

hydrohaemostat (hi·dro·**he**·mo·stat). An apparatus for arresting haemorrhage by means of hydrostatic pressure. [Gk *hydor* water, *haima* blood, *stasis* a standing still.]

hydrohaemothorax (**hi**·dro·he·mo·**thor**'·ax). The extravasation of haemorrhagic fluid into the cavity of the pleura. [Gk *hydor* water, *haima* blood, thorax.]

hydrohymenitis (**hi**·dro·hi·men·**i**'·tis). Any inflammatory condition of a serous surface or membrane. [Gk *hydor* water, *hymen* membrane, *-itis* inflammation.]

hydrohystera (hi·dro·**his**·ter·ah). Hydrometra. [Gk *hydor* water, *hystera* womb.]

hydroid (**hi**·droid). 1. Like water. 2. In zoology, living in water. [Gk *hydor* water, *eidos* form.]

hydrokinetics (**hi**·dro·kin·**et**'·ix). The science of the movement of fluids under force, as in hydraulics and hydrodynamics. [Gk *hydor* water, kinetics.]

hydrol (**hi**·drol). 1. Hydrone; the unassociated molecule of water, H_2O, as in steam. 2. The mother liquor in the manufacture of corn syrup.

hydrolabile (hi·dro·**la**·bile). Having a tendency to lose weight because of loss of body fluids as the result of gastro-intestinal disorder or febrile disease or because of smaller intake of salt or carbohydrate. [Gk *hydor* water, L *labilitas* changefulness.]

hydrolability (**hi**·dro·la·**bil**'·it·e). Any state or condition in which the quantity of fluids in the tissues varies, as in febrile disease. [see prec.]

hydrolabyrinth (hi·dro·**lab**·ir·inth). Hydrops of the labyrinth; increase in the amount of endolymph in the labyrinth, believed to be the underlying pathology in aural vertigo.

hydrolactometer (**hi**·dro·lak·**tom**'·et·er). An apparatus for determining the water content of milk. [Gk *hydor* water, L *lac* milk, meter.]

hydrolase (**hi**·dro·laze). General term for enzymes which activate specific linkages in a substrate and bring about hydrolysis.

hydrolith (**hi**·dro·lith). Calcium hydride, CaH_2. So called because it evolves hydrogen with water, and is used for this purpose to generate hydrogen for small balloons. [hydrogen, Gk *lithos* stone.]

hydrology (hi·**drol**·o·je). The science which is concerned with the properties, phenomena, solutions and uses of water and its geological distribution. [Gk *hydor* water, *logos* science.]

hydrolysate (hi·**drol**·is·ate). The product of hydrolysis. **Protein hydrolysate.** The amino-acid product of a protein that has been split up by hydrolysis. Such a product is sometimes more suitable as a food than the original protein.

hydrolyse (**hi**·dro·lize). To produce hydrolysis; to subject to the process of hydrolysis.

hydrolysis (hi·**drol**·is·is). The splitting of a substance by molecules of water which themselves split, contributing hydrogen atoms and hydroxyl groups to the respective products. **Reversible hydrolysis.** The process whereby substances combine with the formation of a new product and accompanying molecules of water. [Gk *hydor* water, *lysis* a loosing.]

hydrolyst (**hi**·dro·list). Any substance, such as a hydrolase, which catalyses hydrolysis.

hydrolyte (**hi**·dro·lite). Term applied to the substance or substrate which is being hydrolysed.

hydrolytic (hi·dro·**lit**·ik). Relating to, or capable of producing hydrolysis.

hydroma (hi·**dro**·mah). 1. Hygroma. 2. A cyst-like distension of a lymph vessel of the neck. 3. A tumour which contains water or any swelling in which there is a large quantity of water. [Gk *hydor* water, *-oma* tumour.]

hydromania (hi·dro·**ma**·ne·ah). 1. An intense morbid craving for liquids, particularly water. 2. Insanity in which there is a tendency to commit suicide by drowning. [Gk *hydor* water, mania.]

hydromassage (**hi**·dro·mas·**ahzh**'). Massage by the use of water. [Gk *hydor* water, massage.]

hydromeningitis (**hi**·dro·men·in·**ji**'·tis). 1. Internal hydrocephalus. *See* HYDROCEPHALUS. 2. Inflammation of the meninges of the brain accompanied by profuse serous exudation. [Gk *hydor* water, meningitis.]

hydromeningocele (**hi**·dro·men·**ing**'·go·seel). 1. Spina bifida in which the meningeal sac contains cerebrospinal fluid. 2. A meningocele filled with watery fluid. 3. Encephalocele. [Gk *hydor* water, *menigx* membrane, *kele* hernia.]

hydrometer (hi·**drom**·et·er). An instrument consisting of a suitable weighted float with a graduated stem, used for the direct reading of the specific gravities of liquids. [Gk *hydor* water, meter.]
See also: BEAUMÉ.

hydrometra (hi·dro·**me**·trah). An accumulation of watery fluid or thin mucus in the cavity of the uterus. [Gk *hydor* water, *metra* womb.]

hydrometrectasia (**hi**·dro·me·trek·**ta**'·ze·ah). Distension of the uterus by a large accumulation of watery fluid. [Gk *hydor* water, *metra* womb, *ektasis* a stretching.]

hydrometric (hi·dro·**met**·rik). Relating or belonging to a hydrometer or to hydrometry.

hydrometrocolpos (hi·dro·me·tro·**kol**'·pos). Distension of the uterus and vagina by a collection of fluid. [Gk *hydor* water, *metra* womb, *kolpos* vagina.]

hydrometry (hi·**drom**·et·re). The act of measuring the specific gravity of a fluid by means of a hydrometer.

hydromicrencephalia, hydromicrencephaly, hydromicrocephaly (**hi**·dro·mi·kren·kef·**a**'·le·ah, **hi**·dro·mi·kren·**kef**'·al·e, **hi**·dro·mi·kro·**kef**'·al·e). Micrencephalia complicated by the collection of serum-like fluid in the cerebral cavity. [Gk *hydor* water, micrencephalia.]

Hydromorphinol (hi·dro·**mor**·fin·ol). BP Commission approved name for 14-hydroxydihydromorphine; an analgesic.

hydromorphone (hi·dro·**mor**·fone). BP Commission approved name for dihydromorphinone, a narcotic and analgesic with morphine-like actions.

hydromphalocele (hi·drom·**fal**·o·seel). An umbilical hernia the sac of which contains a cystic tumour. [Gk *hydor* water, omphalus, Gk *kele* hernia.]

hydromphalus (hi·**drom**·fal·us). An umbilical cyst or tumour containing watery fluid. [Gk *hydor* water, omphalus.]

hydromyelia (**hi**·dro·mi·e'·le·ah). 1. Distension of the central canal of the spinal cord with fluid, due to inflammation of the cord with an increased accumulation of fluid, or (as demonstrated experimentally) through blocking of the upper, medullary end of the canal. 2. Congenital cavities, filled with fluid, distending the cord substance. [Gk *hydor* water, *myelos* marrow.]

hydromyelocele (**hi**·dro·mi·**el**'·o·seel). A type of spina bifida in which the protrusion is caused by a spinal cord that has been widened by a hydromyelia, and has penetrated through the meninges (myelocystocele) or caused the meninges also to protrude (myelocystomeningocele). Such malformation may be combined with a defect of the spinal cord itself, e.g. persistence of an embryonic fissure, resulting from excessive proliferation of connective tissue or dermoid cysts that prevented a closing of the open tube. [Gk *hydor* water, *myelos* marrow, *kele* hernia.]

hydromyelus (hi·dro·mi·**el**'·us). The condition of hydromyelia.

hydromyoma (**hi**·dro·mi·**o**'·mah). A myoma containing fluid-filled cysts and found usually in the uterus. [Gk *hydor* water, myoma.]

hydromyringa, hydromyrinx (**hi**·dro·mir·**ing**'·gah, hi·dro·**mir**'·ingx). 1. Distension of the tympanic membrane with watery fluid. 2. Term sometimes used for hydrotympanum. [Gk *hydor* water, myrinx.]

hydroncus (hi·**drong**·kus). Any swelling or dilatation caused by a collection of water. [Gk *hydor* water, *ogkos* a swelling.]

hydrone (**hi**·drone). 1. Hydrol; the single reactive molecule of water, H_2O, which occurs unassociated in steam. 2. An alloy of sodium (35 per cent) and lead (65 per cent) used to generate hydrogen from water.

hydronephrectasia, hydronephros (**hi**·dro·nef·rek·**ta**'·ze·ah, hi·dro·**nef**·ros). An enlargement of the kidney due to abnormal accumulation of fluid in its substance and cavities. [Gk *hydor* water, nephrectasia.]

hydronephrosis (hi·dro·nef·**ro**'·sis). A cyst-like distension of the calyces and pelvis of the ureter with non-infected urine. Ureteral or urethral obstruction is the cause and the pressure of the fluid produces atrophy of the structure of the kidney. **Intermittent hydronephrosis.** Hydronephrosis in which occasional escape of urine through the ureter causes temporary reduction in the size of the cyst. [Gk *hydor* water, nephrosis.]

hydronephrotic (hi·dro·nef·**rot**'·ik). Pertaining to or affected with hydronephrosis.

hydro-oligocythaemia (hi·dro·ol·ig·o·si·**the**'·me·ah). A secondary anaemia in which the ratio of plasma to blood corpuscles is increased and the erythrocytes are few. [Gk *hydor* water, oligocythaemia.]

hydropancreatosis (hi·dro·**pan**·kre·at·**o**'·sis). A condition in which an abnormally large quantity of fluid is present in the pancreas. [Gk *hydor* water, pancreas, Gk *-osis* condition.]

hydroparasalpinx (hi·dro·par·ah·**sal**'·pingx). The name given to small cysts which have a solid pedicle uniting them to the uterine tube. They are muellerian in origin. [Gk *hydor* water, *para, salpigx* tube.]

hydroparesis (hi·dro·par·**e**'·sis). A type of paresis, such as occurs in beriberi, in which there is oedema of the subcutaneous tissues as well as effusion into the serous cavities. [Gk *hydor* water, paresis.]

hydroparotitis (hi·dro·par·o·**ti**'·tis). Distension of the parotid gland with fluid. [Gk *hydor* water, parotid gland, Gk *-itis* inflammation.]

hydropathic (hi·dro·**path**·ik). Relating or belonging to hydropathy or hydrotherapeutics. [Gk *hydor* water, *pathos* disease.]

hydropathy (hi·**drop**·ath·e). 1. Hydrotherapy. 2. A non-scientific system of treatment based on the copious use of water internally and externally; the water cure. [see prec.]

hydropedesis (hi·dro·ped·**e**'·sis). Excessive secretion of sweat. [Gk *hydor* water, *pedesis* an oozing.]

hydropenia (hi·dro·**pe**·ne·ah). A state of water deficiency. [Gk *hydor* water, *penia* poverty.]

hydropericarditis (hi·dro·per·e·kar·**di**'·tis). Pericarditis with copious serous effusion into the pericardium. [Gk *hydor* water, pericarditis.]

hydropericardium (hi·dro·per·e·**kar**'·de·um). Excessive accumulation of serous fluid in the pericardium. [Gk *hydor* water, pericardium.]

hydroperinephrosis (hi·dro·per·e·nef·**ro**'·sis). An accumulation of serous fluid in the connective tissues surrounding the kidney, often accompanied by effusion into the calyces and pelvis of the ureter. [Gk *hydor* water, *peri, nephros* kidney.]

hydroperion (hi·dro·**per**·e·on). In the early stages of gestation, the nourishing fluid held to be present between the decidua basalis and the decidua parietalis. [Gk *hydor* water, *peri, oon* egg.]

hydroperitoneum, hydroperitonia (hi·dro·per·e·ton·**e**'·um, hi·dro·per·e·**to**'·ne·ah). Ascites. [Gk *hydor* water, peritoneum.]

hydroperitonitis (hi·dro·per·e·ton·**i**'·tis). Peritonitis with associated serous effusion. [Gk *hydor* water, peritonitis.]

hydropexia, hydropexis (hi·dro·**pex**·e·ah, hi·dro·**pex**·is). The property of fixing water or of retaining it. [Gk *hydor* water, *pexis* fixation.]

hydrophagocytosis (hi·dro·fag·o·si·**to**'·sis). The engulfing by phagocytes of droplets of plasma. [Gk *hydor* water, phagocytosis.]

hydrophallus (hi·**drof**·al·us). Distension of the penis due to accumulation of water in the tissues. [Gk *hydor* water, *phallos* penis.]

Hydrophidae (hi·**drof**·id·e). A family of sea snakes, mostly poisonous. [Gk *hydor* water, *ophis* serpent.]

hydrophil, hydrophile (hi·dro·fil, hi·dro·file). A substance that has a strong attraction for water; one easily wetted by water. Applied particularly to emulsoids. [Gk *hydor* water, *philein* to love.]

hydrophilia (hi·dro·**fil**·e·ah). Hydrophilism.

hydrophilic (hi·dro·**fil**·ik). Having the properties of a hydrophil.

hydrophilism (hi·**drof**·il·izm). The ability of colloids and tissues to absorb and retain water. [see foll.]

hydrophilous (hi·**drof**·il·us). 1. Hygroscopic; able to absorb moisture. 2. Denoting organisms which are fertilized through the medium of water. [Gk *hydor* water, *philein* to love.]

Hydrophinae (hi·**drof**·in·e). A sub-family of sea snakes. [Gk *hydor* water, *ophis* serpent.]

hydrophlegmasia (hi·dro·fleg·**ma**'·ze·ah). An inflammatory condition associated with a serous exudate. [Gk *hydor* water, phlegmasia.]

hydrophlogosis (hi·dro·flo·**go**'·sis). Any inflammatory condition associated with serous effusion. [Gk *hydor* water, *phlogosis* inflammation.]

hydrophobe (hi·dro·fobe). An individual suffering from rabies. [see foll.]

hydrophobia (hi·dro·**fo**·be·ah). 1. Rabies. 2. Exaggerated fear of water, as in rabies. [Gk *hydor* water, phobia.]

hydrophobic (hi·dro·**fo**·bik). 1. Rabid; relating or belonging to or having the character of rabies. 2. Adversely affected by water or tending not to absorb water, as a colloid. 3. Molecules, and the side chains of amino acids, which are poorly soluble in water because of their hydrocarbon structure, being composed of carbon and hydrogen and having no charged or polar groups. [Gk *hydor* water, *phobein* to fear.]

hydrophobin (hi·dro·**fo**·bin). Lyssin. [see prec.]

hydrophobophobia (hi·dro·fo·bo·**fo**'·be·ah). Morbid dread of rabies in which symptoms of the true disease may be simulated. [hydrophobia, Gk *phobein* to fear.]

hydrophone (hi·dro·fone). An instrument used in auscultation, the percussion note being conveyed through a column of water. [Gk *hydor* water, *phone* sound.]

hydrophore (hi·dro·for). A short, grooved catheter for use in simultaneous dilation and irrigation of the urethra. [Gk *hydor* water, *phoros* bearer.]

hydrophorograph (hi·dro·**for**·o·graf). An instrument by means of which the flow of urine through the ureter or the pressure of spinal fluid in lumbar puncture is recorded on a graph. [Gk *hydor* water, *phora* range, *graphein* to record.]

hydrophthalmia, hydrophthalmos (hi·drof·**thal**·me·ah, hi·drof·**thal**·mos). Congenital glaucoma. *See* GLAUCOMA. **Anterior hydrophthalmia.** A condition in which the dilatation of the eyeball may be limited to the anterior portion of the eye containing aqueous. **Posterior hydrophthalmia.** One in which the dilatation is limited to the vitreous cavity. **Total hydrophthalmia.** Hydrophthalmia in which the dilatation affects the whole eyeball. [Gk *hydor* water, *ophthalmos* eye.]

hydrophthalmoscope (hi·drof·**thal**·mo·skope). A small watchmaker's glass filled with saline and worn by the patient. Corneal refraction is thus eliminated and the fundus rendered more easily visible. Its principal use nowadays is for keeping fluids in contact with the cornea and it is seldom employed in ophthalmoscopy. In a sense it was a forerunner of the contact lens; originally introduced by Czermak and modified by Batten. [Gk *hydor* water, ophthalmoscope.]

See also: BATTEN.

hydrophthalmus (hi·drof·**thal**·mus). Hydrophthalmia.

hydrophysocele (hi·dro·**fiz**·o·seel). A sac which contains both gas and liquid. [Gk *hydor* water, *physa* breath, *kele* hernia.]

hydrophysometra (hi·dro·fiz·o·**me**'·trah). The presence of liquid and gas in the cavity of the uterus. [Gk *hydor* water, *physa* breath, *metra* womb.]

hydropic (hi·**drop**·ik). Relating or belonging to dropsy; dropsical; suffering from dropsy. [Gk *hydrops* dropsy.]

hydropigenous (hi·dro·**pij**·en·us). Applied to diseases which cause dropsy, e.g. renal and cardiac diseases. [Gk *hydrops* dropsy, *genein* to produce.]

hydroplasm (hi·dro·plasm). The fluid part of protoplasm or of any other plasma. [see foll.]

hydroplasma (hi·dro·**plaz**·mah). 1. Oedema; a dropsical or waterlogged condition of the tissues. 2. A watery or diluted condition of the blood plasma. [Gk *hydor* water, plasma.]

hydroplasmia (hi·dro·plaz·me·ah). The process by which the blood plasma becomes diluted because of increase in the water content. [see prec.]

hydropleuritis (hi·dro·ploor·i′·tis). Pleurisy with effusion. [Gk *hydor* water, *pleura* lung, *-itis* inflammation.]

hydropneumatic (hi·dro·new·mat′·ik). Relating or belonging to a combination of water and air or gas. [Gk *hydor* water, *pneuma* air.]

hydropneumatosis (hi·dro·new·mat·o′·sis). The accumulation of fluid and gas in the tissues; combined oedema and emphysema. [Gk *hydor* water, pneumatosis.]

hydropneumogony (hi·dro·new·mog′·on·e). The procedure of injecting air into a joint in order to determine whether or not water or other extravasated fluid is present. [Gk *hydor* water, *pneuma* air, *genein* to produce.]

hydropneumonia (hi·dro·new·mo′·ne·ah). 1. Pneumonia with pleural effusion. 2. Pulmonary oedema due to serous extravasation into the lung. [Gk *hydor* water, pneumonia.]

hydropneumopericardium (hi·dro·new·mo·per·e·kar′·de·um). The presence of gas or air and fluid in the pericardial cavity. [Gk *hydor* water, *pneuma* air, pericardium.]

hydropneumoperitoneum (hi·dro·new·mo·per·e·ton·e′·um). The accumulation of water or other fluid and air or gas in the cavity of the peritoneum. [Gk *hydor* water, *pneuma* air, peritoneum.]

hydropneumothorax (hi·dro·new·mo·thor′·ax). The accumulation of serous fluid and air or gas in the cavity of the pleura. [Gk *hydor* water, *pneuma* air, thorax.]

hydroposia (hi·dro·po·ze·ah). The drinking of only water as a beverage. [Gk *hydor* water, *posis* a drinking.]

hydropotherapy (hi·dro·po·ther′·ap·e). The therapeutic injection of ascitic fluid. [Gk *hydrops* dropsy, therapy.]

hydrops (hi·drops). Dropsy. **Hydrops of the abdomen, Hydrops abdominis.** Ascites. **Hydrops antri.** An effusion of fluid in the antrum of Highmore. **Hydrops articuli.** Serous effusion in a joint. **Hydrops capitis.** Hydrocephalus. **Hydrops cellularis.** Fluid secretion in the nasal air sinuses. **Hydrops cystidis felleae.** Dropsy of the gall bladder. **Endolymphatic hydrops.** An excess of fluid in the labyrinthine canals as occurs in Ménière's disease. **Hydrops foetalis.** The excessive oedema of the fetus which sometimes occurs in cases of Rhesus incompatibility. It may occur in other conditions also. **Hydrops folliculi.** An excessive collection of fluid in a graafian follicle. **Hydrops gravidarum.** Oedema due to pregnancy. **Hydrops hypostrophos.** Angioneurotic oedema. *See* OEDEMA. **Labyrinthine hydrops.** Ménière's disease. **Hydrops ad matulam.** Polyuria. **Hydrops peritonaei.** Ascites. **Hydrops spurius.** Fluid in the cavity of the peritoneum, from a ruptured cyst or other source, that simulates ascites. **Hydrops tubae.** A collection of fluid in the uterine tube. **Hydrops tubae profluens.** A collection of fluid in one or both uterine tubes, which discharges intermittently through the uterine cavity. **Hydrops vesicae felleae.** Fluid swelling of the gall bladder. [Gk.]

hydropyonephrosis (hi·dro·pi·o·nef·ro′·sis). A condition in which the pelvis of the ureter is distended by accumulation of purulent urine or of other fluid and pus, as a result of obstruction of the ureter. [Gk *hydor* water, pyonephrosis.]

hydropyopneumothorax (hi·dro·pi·o·new·mo·thor′·ax). The accumulation of pus in association with hydropneumothorax. [Gk *hydor* water, *pyon* pus, pneumothorax.]

hydropyosalpinx (hi·dro·pi·o·sal′·pingx). The distension of a uterine tube by serous fluid and pus. [Gk *hydor* water, *pyon* pus, *salpigx* tube.]

hydropyretic (hi·dro·pi·ret′·ik). Relating or belonging to miliaria (hydropyretos). [Gk *hydor* water, *pyretos* burning heat.]

hydropyretos (hi·dro·pi·re′·tos). Miliaria. [see prec.]

hydroquinine (hi·dro·kwin·een). $C_{20}H_{26}O_2N_2$, an alkaloid base which occurs in *Cinchona ledgeriana* and is also obtained by the catalytic hydrogenation of quinine.

hydroquinone (hi·dro·kwin·one). $C_6H_4(OH)_2$, a dihydric phenol prepared by reducing quinone with sulphur dioxide; it occurs naturally as the glucoside, arbutin, in bearberry leaves. Used mainly as a photographic developer, but it has also certain antiseptic properties.

hydrorenal (hi·dro·re·nal). Relating or belonging to a dropsical condition of the kidney. [Gk *hydor* water, L *ren* kidney.]

hydrorrhachiocentesis (hi·dro·rak·e·o·sen·te′·sis). The treatment of hydrorrhachitis by puncture of the spinal meninges. [Gk *hydor* water, *rhachis* spine, *kentesis* a pricking.]

hydrorrhachitis (hi·dro·rak·i′·tis). Inflammation of the spinal cord or membranes, with marked exudation. [Gk *hydor* water, *rhachis* spine.]

hydrorrheostat (hi·dro·re·o·stat). In electricity, an instrument used to control current by means of water resistance. [Gk *hydor* water, *rheos* anything flowing, *statos* standing.]

hydrorrhoea (hi·dro·re·ah). A copious discharge of thin watery fluid from any part. **Hydrorrhoea gravidarum.** During pregnancy, the discharge from the vagina of watery fluid or thin mucus due to excessive secretion by the uterine glands. **Nasal hydrorrhoea.** Rhinorrhoea. [Gk *hydor* water, *rhoia* flow.]

hydrosalpinx (hi·dro·sal·pingx). A uterine tube distended with fluid. This is now held to be the end result of previous inflammation. **Intermittent hydrosalpinx.** Hydrops tubae profluens. [Gk *hydor* water, *salpigx* tube.]

hydrosarca (hi·dro·sar·kah). Anasarca. [Gk *hydor* water, *sarx* flesh.]

hydrosarcocele (hi·dro·sar·ko·seel). Combined hydrocele and sarcocele.

hydrosaturnism (hi·dro·sat·ern·izm). Lead poisoning from water containing lead. [Gk *hydor* water, *Saturn*, identified by alchemists with lead.]

hydroscheocele (hi·dros·ke·o·seel). Scrotal hernia complicated by the presence of serous fluid in the sac. [Gk *hydor* water, *oscheon* scrotum, *kele* hernia.]

hydroscope (hi·dro·skope). 1. Any device which demonstrates the presence of water in the atmosphere; a hygroscope. 2. A water clock. [Gk *hydor* water, *skopein* to watch.]

hydroscopic (hi·dro·skop·ik). Able to absorb moisture from the air. [see prec.]

hydroscopy (hi·dros·ko·pe). Examination of water or watery fluids. [Gk *hydor* water, *skopein* to watch.]

hydrosol (hi·dro·sol). A colloidal suspension of a solid in water. **Gold hydrosol.** Colloidal gold in water, once used by alchemists as a cure-all, is now employed in the examination of cerebrospinal fluid. [Gk *hydor* water, sol.]

hydrosoluble (hi·dro·sol·ew·bl). Water-soluble. [Gk *hydor* water, soluble.]

hydrospermatocyst (hi·dro·sper·mat·o·sist). A hydrocele containing spermatozoa. [Gk *hydor* water, spermatocyst.]

hydrosphygmograph (hi·dro·sfig·mo·graf). A sphygmograph in which the pulse beat is transmitted through a column of water to the recorder. [Gk *hydor* water, sphygmograph.]

hydrospirometer (hi·dro·spi·rom′·et·er). A spirometer in which the force of the air is indicated by the rise and fall of a column of water. [Gk *hydor* water, L *spirare* to breathe, meter.]

hydrostabile (hi·dro·sta·bile). Applied to a patient who has a tendency to preserve an even weight in spite of suffering from gastro-intestinal disease or of being on a restricted diet. [Gk *hydor* water, L *stabilis* steadfast.]

hydrostat (hi·dro·stat). A device which maintains the level of water at a predetermined height. [see foll.]

hydrostatic (hi·dro·stat·ik). Describing a liquid at rest or in equilibrium. [Gk *hydor* water, *statos* standing.]

hydrostatics (hi·dro·stat·ix). The theoretical and mathematical study of the pressures in liquids at rest or in equilibrium. [see prec.]

hydrostomia (hi·dro·sto·me·ah). A condition in which water is constantly dribbling out of the mouth. [Gk *hydor* water, *stoma* mouth.]

hydrosulphite (hi·dro·**sul**·fite). A salt of hydrosulphuric acid $H_2S_2O_4$, e.g. $Na_2S_2O_4$, sodium hydrosulphite. Sometimes called *hyposulphite*, but the latter has also been applied to sodium thiosulphate $Na_2S_2O_3$ (hypo), and hence causes confusion.

hydrosynthesis (hi·dro·**sin**·thes·is). Any reaction between chemical compounds in the course of which molecules of water are produced. [Gk *hydor* water, synthesis.]

hydrosyringomyelia (**hi**·dro·sir·**ing**·go·mi·e'·le·ah). Degeneration of and cavity formation in the spinal cord with distension of the central canal owing to effusion of fluid. [Gk *hydor* water, syringomyelia.]

Hydrotaea (hi·dro·**te**·ah). A genus of small flies of the family Muscidae. The larvae of *Hydrotaea meteorica*, and perhaps of other species, have occurred in intestinal myiasis.

Hydrotalcite (hi·dro·**tal**·site). BP Commission approved name for aluminium magnesium hydroxide carbonate hydrate; an antacid.

hydrotaxis (hi·dro·**tax**·is). The influence exerted by moisture on the direction of movement of small organisms or cells. [Gk *hydor* water, *taxis* arrangement.]

hydrotherapeutics (**hi**·dro·ther·ap·**ew**'·tix). The science and practice of the treatment of disease by means of water. [Gk *hydor* water, therapeutics.]

hydrotherapy (hi·dro·**ther**·ap·e). The treatment of disease by means of water. [Gk *hydor* water, therapy.]

hydrothermostat (hi·dro·**ther**·mo·stat). A device for keeping water at an even temperature. [Gk *hydor* water, thermostat.]

hydrothion (hi·dro·**thi**·on). Name applied to sulphuretted hydrogen, H_2S. [hydrogen, Gk *theion* sulphur.]

hydrothionaemia (**hi**·dro·thi·on·**e**'·me·ah). The presence of hydrogen sulphide in the blood. [Gk *hydor* water, *theion* sulphur, *haima* blood.]

hydrothionammonaemia (**hi**·dro·**thi**·on·am·on·**e**'·me·ah). The presence of ammonium sulphate in the blood. [Gk *hydor* water, *theion* sulphur, ammonium, Gk *haima* blood.]

hydrothionuria (**hi**·dro·thi·on·**ewr**'·e·ah). The presence of hydrogen sulphide in the urine. [hydrothion, urine.]

hydrothoracic (**hi**·dro·thor·**as**'·ik). Relating or belonging to hydrothorax.

hydrothorax (hi·dro·**thor**·ax). A non-inflammatory transudation of fluid in the pleural cavity as contrasted with an inflammatory exudate: the transudate has a lower specific gravity and less protein, whilst the cells present are few and of endothelial origin. It occurs with the oedema of congestive heart failure and renal disease, and may also be caused by obstruction of the thoracic veins and lymphatics from the pressure of enlarged glands at the root of the lung. **Chylous hydrothorax.** Chylothorax; a condition in which the fluid is opalescent from fat globules. It follows rupture of the thoracic duct from trauma or increased pressure due to obstruction usually by a malignant growth. **Pseudochylous hydrothorax.** Hydrothorax in which the opalescent appearance of the fluid is not due to chyle but to a lecithin-globulin compound or to cholesterol from the breakdown of cells shed into the pleural cavity. [Gk *hydor* water, thorax.]

hydrotimeter (hi·dro·**tim**·et·er). A device for estimating the hardness of water, using a soap solution. [Gk *hydor* water, meter.]

hydrotis (hi·**dro**·tis). An effusion of serous fluid into the ear. [Gk *hydor* water, *ous* ear.]

hydrotomy (hi·**drot**·o·me). In dissection, the act of separating tissues by forcibly injecting water. [Gk *hydor* water, *temnein* to sever.]

hydrotoxicity (**hi**·dro·tox·**is**'·it·e). A pathological condition resulting from the drinking of excessive quantities of water. [Gk *hydor* water, toxicity.]

hydrotropic (hi·dro·**trop**·ik). Pertaining to hydrotropy.

hydrotropism (hi·dro·**trop**·izm). In biology, the tendency of growing plants or organs to turn either towards moisture (positive hydrotropism) or away from moisture (negative hydrotropism). [Gk *hydor* water, *trope* a turning.]

hydrotropy (hi·**drot**·ro·pe). The phenomenon whereby substances insoluble in water under ordinary conditions are brought into solution by means of hydrotropic substances. Thus fats, normally insoluble in water, are rendered so by the action of bile salts. The action is specific, and would appear to be due to the formation of complexes, with reduction of surface tension. [see prec.]

hydrotympanum (hi·dro·**tim**·pan·um). An effusion of serous fluid into the middle ear. [Gk *hydor* water, tympanum.]

hydro-ureter, hydro-ureterosis (**hi**·dro·ewr·e'·ter, **hi**·dro·ewr·e·ter·**o**'·sis). Distension of the ureter with watery fluid or urine owing to an obstruction or stricture. [Gk *hydor* water, ureter.]

hydro-uria (hi·dro·**ewr**·e·ah). The secretion of an abnormally large quantity of urine the solid constituents of which may be either normal in amount or reduced. [Gk *hydor* water, urine.]

hydrous (**hi**·drus). Containing water, or of a watery consistency. [Gk *hydor* water.]

hydrovarium (hi·dro·**va**·re·um). 1. Dropsy affecting the ovary. 2. Cystoma of the ovary. [Gk *hydor* water, ovary.]

Hydroxamethocaine (hi·**drox**·am·**eth**'·o·kane). BP Commission approved name for 2-dimethylaminoethyl 4-*n*-butylaminosalicylate, a local anaesthetic, less toxic than amethocaine. It has been used clinically in Germany for tracheobronchial anaesthesia.

hydroxide (hi·**drox**·ide). General term denoting a compound which contains the hydroxyl, OH, group. Metallic hydroxides are usually basic, non-metallic hydroxides acidic.

hydroxidion (hi·**drox**·id·**i**'·on). The hydroxyl ion.

Hydroxocobalamin BP 1973 (hi·drox·o·ko·bal·am·in). Vitamin B_{12a},α-(5,6-dimethylbenzimidazol-2-yl)hydroxocobamide. It is "an important member of a group of similar compounds which influence erythropoiesis and represent the anti-pernicious anaemia principle of purified liver extracts" (BPC 1968). The standard preparation is used in the treatment of subacute combined degeneration of the spinal cord. It is administered intramuscularly, maintenance doses being required every 3 or 4 weeks.

hydroxyacetone (hi·**drox**·e·**as**'·et·one). Acetyl carbinol, CH_2OH $COCH_3$. A ketol obtained by fusing cane sugar; also known as *acetol*.

11-hydroxyaetiocholanolone. A 17-ketosteroid which is an excretion product of cortisol and is therefore absent in cases of congenital adrenal hyperplasia.

Hydroxyamphetamine (hi·**drox**·e·am·**fet**'·am·een). BP Commission approved name for 2-amino-1-*p*-hydroxyphenylpropane, a sympatheticomimetic used in the treatment of acute and chronic rhinitis.

hydroxyanisole (hi·**drox**·e·**an**'·e·sole). **Butylated Hydroxyanisole BP 1973.** 2-*tert*-Butyl-4-methoxyphenol, an anti-oxidant for preserving oils and fats.

hydroxyanthraquinone (hi·**drox**·e·an·thrah·**kwin**'·one). A general class of hydroxy derivatives of anthraquinone. They occur in rhubarb and buckthorn, and when prepared synthetically are used in the manufacture of dyestuffs.

hydroxyapatite (hi·**drox**·e·**ap**'·at·ite). $3Ca_3(PO_4)_2Ca(OH)_2$, the form of calcium phosphate from which bone salts are derived.

hydroxybenzene (hi·**drox**·e·**ben**'·zeen). Phenol, C_6H_5OH. A colourless crystalline compound, slightly soluble in water; used as an antiseptic and disinfectant.

hydroxycaffeine (hi·**drox**·e·**kaf**'·e·een). Caffuric acid, $C_8H_{10}O_3N_4$. A white crystalline substance employed as a diuretic.

hydroxycarotene (hi·**drox**·e·**kar**'·o·teen). A general class of hydroxy derivatives of the carotenes. They include the xanthophylls or phytoxanthins.

Hydroxychloroquine (hi·**drox**·e·**klor**'·o·kwin). BP Commission approved name for 7-chloro-4-[4-(*N*-ethyl-*N*-2-hydroxyethyl-amino)-1-methylbutylamino]-quinoline. **Hydroxychloroquine Sulphate BP 1973.** The sulphate of hydroxychloroquine, an antimalarial with actions similar to those of chloroquine phosphate but erythematosus, both the discoid and systemic forms. to those of chloroquine phosphate but used principally in the treatment of rheumatoid arthritis and lupus erythematosus, both the discoid and systemic forms.

1α-hydroxychorecalciferol. 1α-OHCC is a synthetic Vitamin D analogue which may be given by mouth to increase calcium absorption from the intestinal tract and the calcium content of bone. It is effective in cases of metabolic bone disease associated with chronic renal failure.

17-hydroxycorticosterone (hi·**drox**·e·kor·tik·o·**steer**'·one). Hydrocortisone.

hydroxycyclohexane (hi·**drox**·e·si·klo·**hex**'·ane). Cyclohexanol.

Hydroxydione Sodium Succinate (hi·drox·e·**di**·one **so**·de·um **sux**·in·ate). BP Commission approved name for sodium 21-hydroxypregnane-3,20-dione succinate, a steroid, injected intravenously, used as a general anaesthetic. It has no hormone-like actions.

hydroxyethylamine (hi·**drox**·e·eth·il·**am**'·een). Ethanolamine, $CH_2OHCH_2NH_2$. A base which occurs in cephalin, and which can be regarded as the parent of choline. It is employed as a sclerotizing agent for varicose veins, being injected with oleic acid.

hydroxyethylapocupreine (hi·**drox**·e·eth·il·ap·o·**kew**'·pre·een). A derivative of quinine obtained from the latter by altering 2 of the groupings; it has been used in pneumonia.

hydroxyethylapoquinine (hi·**drox**·e·eth·il·ap·o·**kwin**'·een). A synthetic alkaloid obtained from quinine, and used in pneumococcal infections.

hydroxyethylhydrocupreine (hi·**drox**·e·eth·il·hi·dro·**kew**'·pre·een). A derivative of hydrocupreine, which has been employed in pneumonia and empyema.

hydroxykynureninuria (hi·**drox**·e·ki·**newr**·en·in·**ewr**'·e·ah). A defect of kynureninase in the tryptophan pathway of catabolism to nicotinic acid, with deficiency causing pellagra.

hydroxyl (hi·**drox**·il). The monovalent radical, OH, which forms hydroxides with elements or radicals.

hydroxylamine (hi·drox·il·**am**'·een). 1. NH_2OH, a compound used as a reducing agent. 2. Any of a series of organic compounds of general formula NH_2OR, where R is an alkyl radical.

hydroxylysine (hi·**drox**·e·**li**'·seen). An amino acid, β-ϵ-di-amino-β-hydroxy-*n*-caproic acid, $CH_2(NH_2)CH_2CH_2CH(OH)CH(NH_2)COOH$. It is found in collagen.

hydroxymalonate (hi·**drox**·e·**mal**'·on·ate). An inhibition of mitochondrial malate transport.

Hydroxypethidine (hi·**drox**·e·**peth**'·id·een). BP Commission approved name for ethyl 4-*m*-hydroxyphenyl-1-methylpiperidine-4-carboxylate, a derivative of pethidine, which has about the same analgesic activity as the latter, and has been reported to have given promising clinical results when used as a general anaesthetic by intravenous injection.

hydroxyphenol (hi·drox·e·**fe**'·nol). Resorcinol.

hydroxyphenylethylamine (hi·**drox**·e·fe·nil·eth·il·**am**'·een). Tyramine, $OHC_6H_4CH_2CH_2NH_2$. A toxic amine formed from tyrosine during putrefaction, and found in ergot and mouldy cheese. It is a pressor base and ecbolic.

Hydroxyprocaine (hi·**drox**·e·**pro**'·kane). BP Commission approved name for the hydrochloride of diethylamino-ethanol 4-aminosalicylate; a local anaesthetic rather similar to procaine, but said to be quicker acting and of slightly longer duration. It has been used clinically in Germany.

Hydroxyprogesterone (hi·**drox**·e·pro·**jes**'·ter·one). BP Commission approved name for 17α-hydroxypregn-4-ene-3,20-dione. **Hydroxyprogesterone Hexanoate BP 1973.** 17α-hexanoyloxy-pregn-4-ene-3,20-dione; a progestational steroid.

hydroxyproline (hi·**drox**·e·**pro**'·leen). Hydroxy pyrrolidine carboxylic acid, an amino acid which is glucogenic. It is found in collagen.

hydroxyquinoline (hi·**drox**·e·**kwin**'·o·leen). A derivative of quinoline produced by the hydroxylation of the pyridine nucleus. **α-Hydroxyquinoline, 2-Hydroxyquinoline.** Carbostyril.

hydroxysteroids (hi·**drox**·e·**steer**'·oidz). **3α-,3β-Hydroxysteroids.** More correctly named 3(α)-*hydroxy*-17-*ketosteroids* and 3(β)-*hydroxy*-17-*ketosteroids.* The 2 main fractions of neutral 17-ketosteroids excreted in urine. (α) and (β) denote the spatial position of the hydroxyl group attached to the C_3 carbon in the sterol configuration: in the latter the OH group projects frontally in beta compounds and towards the rear in alpha compounds. Normally urinary excretion consists mainly of alpha compounds, the beta fraction amounting to up to 15 per cent of the total 17-ketosteroids. In certain pathological conditions, notably adrenal tumour, the beta fraction is greatly increased. The beta fraction is separated from the alpha fraction by precipitation with digitonin. Characteristic steroids are androsterone (alpha) and dehydro-androsterone (beta).

Hydroxystilbamidine (hi·**drox**·e·stil·**bam**'·id·een). BP Commission approved name for 4,4'-diamidino-2-hydroxystilbene, a drug very similar to stilbamidine; it has been used in the treatment of kala-azar in India and good results have been claimed. It is less toxic than stilbamidine.

hydroxytetracaine (hi·**drox**·e·**tet**'·rah·kane). Hydroxamethocaine.

hydroxytoluene (hi·**drox**·e·**tol**'·ew·ene). **Butylated Hydroxytoluene BP 1973.** 2,6-Di-*tert*-butyl-*p*-cresol, an anti-oxidant for preserving oils and fats.

hydroxytryptamine (hi·**drox**·e·**trip**'·tam·een). Serotonin; a substance released from blood platelets by an antigen–antibody reaction. It can be isolated from the blood, and is capable of producing adrenaline-like effects when administered to a patient.

Hydroxyurea (hi·**drox**·e·ewr·e·ah). An antineoplastic agent. BP Commission approved name.

hydroxyvaline (hi·**drox**·e·**va**'·leen). Dimethylserine, $(CH_3)_2C(OH)CHNH_2COOH$. An amino acid which occurs in protein.

Hydroxyzine (hi·**drox**·iz·een). BP Commission approved name for a substituted piperazine having central sedative action in anxiety states.

hydruria (hi·**droor**·e·ah). 1. Polyuria. 2. Diabetes insipidus. [Gk *hydor* water, urine.]

hydruric (hi·**droor**·ik). Pertaining to or marked by hydruria.

hyetometry (hi·et·**om**·et·re). The measurement of rain. [Gk *hyetos* rain, meter.]

hygeiolatry, hygieiolatry (hi·je·**ol**·at·re, **hi**·je·e·**ol**'·at·re). 1. Obsession with the state of one's own health. 2. Strict and excessive observance of the laws of health. [Gk *hygieia* health, *latreia* worship.]

hygieist (hi·**je**·e·ist). Hygienist.

hygiene (**hi**·je·een). 1. The science of health. 2. The principles and laws of the preservation of health. **Industrial hygiene.** The branch of preventive medicine which is concerned with the preservation and protection of the health of workers in industry. **Mental hygiene.** That branch of psychological medicine which is concerned with the development and preservation of health of mind. **Oral hygiene.** The care of the teeth and mouth. **Sex hygiene.** Hygiene associated with sex organs and sex behaviour. **Social hygiene.** A term popularly used to denote the prevention of venereal disease and the care of those suffering from it. [Gk *hygieia* health.]

hygienic (hi·je·**en**·ik). Referring or belonging to hygiene or to health.

hygienics (hi·je·**en**·ix). The science of health or hygiene.

hygienist (**hi**·je·en·ist). One who specializes in hygiene and the application of its laws.

hygienization (**hi**·je·en·i·**za**'·shun). The application of the rules of hygiene to environment or conditions of living.

hygraemometry (hi·gre·**mom**·et·re). The estimation of the proportion of haemoglobin in the blood by measuring the amount of the dried substance. [Gk *hygros* moist, *haima* blood, meter.]

hygrechema (hi·grek·e·mah) (pl. *hygrechemata*). The characteristic sound heard on auscultation when liquid is present in a cavity or tissue. [Gk *hygros* moist, *echema* sound.]

hygric (**hi**·grik). Moist, or connected with moisture. [Gk *hygros* moist.]

hygroblepharic (hi·gro·**blef**·ar·ik). Applied to any structure which serves to bring moisture to the eyelids, as the lacrimal canaliculi. [Gk *hygros* moist, *blepharon* eyelid.]

hygrodermia (hi·gro·**der**·me·ah). An affection of the skin in which there is oedema but no inflammation. [Gk *hygros* moist, *derma* skin.]

hygrol (**hi**·grol). A colloidal form of mercury.

hygrology (hi·**grol**·o·je). That branch of medical science which is concerned with the fluids of the body. [Gk *hygros* moist, *logos* science.]

hygroma (hi·**gro**·mah) (pl. *hygromas, hygromata*). A cystic lymphangioma; a swelling with serous fluid. **Hygroma colli, Cystic hygroma, Hygroma cysticum colli congenitum.** A congenital cystic lymphangioma of the neck. **Hygroma praepatellare.** A cystic lymphangioma arising within the prepatellar bursa. **Subdural hygroma.** A collection of cerebrospinal fluid in the subdural space. [Gk *hygros* moist, *-oma* tumour.]

See also: FLEISCHMANN.

hygromatous (hi·gro·**mat**·us). Relating or belonging to, or having the character of a hygroma.

hygromedry (hi·**grom**·ed·re). Estimation of the quantity of vapour given off from any particular superficial area of the body. [Gk *hygros* moist.]

hygrometer (hi·**grom**·et·er). 1. An apparatus for the estimation of the amount of water vapour in the air. 2. An instrument to determine the dew point and thence the relative humidity of the air. **Chemical hygrometer.** An indicator which changes colour or becomes cloudy in damp air. **Hair hygrometer.** One which depends upon the lengthening of a hair in a humid atmosphere. **Physical hygrometer.** Wet-and-dry-bulb hygrometer (see following). **Wet-and-dry-bulb hygrometer.** A pair of thermometers mounted side by side; one is cooled by evaporation, and the difference in readings gives relative humidity from appropriate tables. [Gk *hygros* moist, meter.]

See also: DANIELL, SAUSSURE.

hygrometric (hi·gro·**met**·rik). 1. Hygroscopic. 2. Referring or belonging to the hygrometer or to hygrometry.

hygrometry (hi·**grom**·et·re). The estimation of the amount of moisture in the air by determination of relative humidity or dew point. [Gk *hygros* moist, meter.]

hygrophobia (hi·gro·**fo**·be·ah). A morbid or obsessional dread of liquids in any form, particularly wine and water. [Gk *hygros* moist, phobia.]

hygroscope (**hi**·gro·skope). A device which estimates the amount of moisture in the air. [Gk *hygros* moist, *skopein* to watch.]

hygroscopic (hi·gro·**skop**·ik). 1. Absorbing moisture from the atmosphere. 2. Relating to hygroscopy.

hygroscopy (hi·**gros**·ko·pe). The estimation of the quantity of moisture in the atmosphere by means of a hygroscope.

hygrostomia (hi·gro·**sto**·me·ah). Ptyalism; a condition in which there is increased secretion or flow of saliva. [Gk *hygros* moist, *stoma* mouth.]

hyle (**hi**·le). The raw material or primitive undifferentiated substance of all matter. [Gk *hyle* stuff.]

hylephobia (hi·le·**fo**·be·ah). A morbid dread of materialism and its mechanical doctrines. [Gk *hyle* matter, phobia.]

hylergography (hi·ler·**gog**·raf·e). With regard to cells, the process of recording the effects of environmental influences. [Gk *hyle* matter, *ergon* work, *graphein* to record.]

hylic (**hi**·lik). 1. Corporeal. 2. Descriptive of the primal animal tissues of the embryo (Adami). 3. Having relation to pulp tissues or primitive matter. [Gk *hyle* matter.]

hylogenesis, hylogeny (hi·lo·**jen**·es·is, hi·**loj**·en·e). The origination and formation of matter. [Gk *hyle* matter, genesis.]

hylology (hi·**lol**·o·je). The science of the primitive substance or raw material of matter, or of elementary matter. [Gk *hyle* matter, *logos* science.]

hyloma (hi·**lo**·mah). A tumour arising in the primal tissues of the embryo (Adami). **Mesenchymal hyloma.** A tumour derived from mesenchymal tissue. **Mesothelial hyloma.** A tumour derived from mesothelial tissue. [Gk *hyle* matter, *-oma* tumour.]

hylopathism (hi·**lop**·ath·izm). 1. The theory that the cause of disease lies in disordered arrangement of or changes in animal matter. 2. Any disease which stems from disorder of or defect in the tissue substance. 3. The theory that matter is sentient. [Gk *hyle* matter, *pathos* disease.]

hylopathist (hi·**lop**·ath·ist). A believer in the theory of hylopathism.

hylotropic (hi·lo·**trop**·ik). Denoting a substance the composition of which remains the same although its form can change, e.g. a solid which can be melted or distilled. [Gk *hyle* matter, *trope* a turning.]

hylozoism (hi·lo·**zo**·izm). The theory that all matter in the universe possesses, in one form or another, life or sensation. [Gk *hyle* matter, *zoon* animal.]

hymen [NA] (**hi**·men). The fold of mucous membrane which during virginity partially or entirely closes the external orifice of the vagina. **Annular hymen.** Circular hymen (see below). **Bifenestrate hymen, Hymen bifenestratus, Hymen biforis.** A hymen with 2 parallel openings separated by a broad dividing wall. **Bilobate hymen.** One with 2 lobes. **Circular hymen.** One with a small round foramen. **Crescentic hymen.** One in the form of a crescent moon. **Cribriform hymen.** One in which there are a number of small perforations. **Denticular hymen.** A hymen in which the edges of the foramen are serrated. **Falciform hymen.** One crescentic in shape. **Fenestrated hymen.** Cribriform hymen (see above). **Fimbriate hymen.** One in which the edges of the foramen are fringed. **Horseshoe hymen.** Crescentic hymen (see above). **Imperforate hymen.** One which entirely closes the external orifice of the vagina. **Infundibuliform hymen.** A hymen the opening of which is central, with sloping sides. **Lunar hymen.** Crescentic hymen (see above). **Ruptured hymen.** A hymen which has been torn as the result of injury or coitus. **Sculptured hymen.** One in which the edge of the opening is irregularly curved as if it had been carved out. **Septate hymen, Hymen septus.** One in which the opening is divided into 2 not necessarily equal parts by a narrow separating wall. **Subseptate hymen, Hymen subseptus.** A partial hymen covering the anterior and posterior portions of the vaginal orifice but not extending across from one side to the other. [Gk membrane.]

hymenal (**hi**·men·al). Relating or belonging to the hymen.

hymenectomy (hi·men·**ek**·to·me). 1. Surgical excision of the hymen. 2. Surgical excision of any membrane. [hymen, Gk *ektome* a cutting out.]

hymenitis (hi·men·**i**·tis). 1. Inflammation of the hymen. 2. Inflammation of any membrane or membranous structure. [hymen, Gk *-itis* inflammation.]

hymenography (hi·men·**og**·raf·e). Hymenology. [Gk *hymen* membrane, *graphein* to record.]

hymenolepiasis (**hi**·men·ol·ep·**i**′·as·is). Infestation with *Hymenolepis.*

hymenolepididae (**hi**·men·ol·ep·**id**′·id·e). A family of the cestode order Cyclophyllidea. The genera *Drepanidotaenia* and *Hymenolepis* are of medical interest. [Gk *hymen* membrane, *lepis* rind, *eidos* form.]

Hymenolepis (hi·men·**ol**·ep·is). A genus of tapeworms. **Hymenolepis diminuta.** Normally a parasite of the rat, rarely infests man. **Hymenolepis nana.** A small form, of world-wide distribution, and often the commonest human tapeworm; it is unique in normally having no intermediate host. The eggs must be ingested, but develop to cysticercoids in the intestinal villi; when fully developed they move into the lumen and mature. Development may also occur in secondary hosts such as meal worms (*Tenebrio*) or fleas. A morphologically indistinguishable form (var. *fraterna*), of rats and mice, has been considered specifically identical. [Gk *hymen* membrane, *lepis* rind.]

hymenology (hi·men·**ol**·**o**·je). That branch of anatomy and physiology which is concerned with the membranous structures of the body. [Gk *hymen* membrane, *logos* science.]

Hymenoptera (hi·men·**op**·ter·ah). An order of insects which includes ants, bees and wasps and characterized by 2 pairs of membranous wings which hook together in flight. Some members are social, forming a highly organized community with sterile female workers. Many have the ovipositor modified as a sting. Life histories are very various but many are phytophagous, including gall makers; in others the larvae are parasitoids, mostly on other insects. [Gk *hymen* membrane, *pteron* wing.]

hymenopterism (hi·men·**op**·ter·izm). Poisoning resulting from the stings or bites of insects of the order Hymenoptera, e.g. wasp or bee.

hymenorrhaphy (hi·men·**or**·af·e). 1. The surgical suturing of the hymen to procure partial or entire closure of the vagina. 2. The surgical suturing of any membranous structure. [Gk *hymen* membrane, *rhaphe* seam.]

hymenotome (hi·**men**·o·tome). A knife used to divide any membrane. [Gk *hymen* membrane, *temnein* to sever.]

hymenotomy (hi·men·**ot**·o·me). 1. In surgery, incision of the hymen. 2. In anatomy, dissection of membranes. [see prec.]

Hynes' desoxycholate citrate agar. A medium prepared from agar 22.5 g, "Lab.-Lemco" 5 g, proteose peptone 5 g, lactose 10 g, sodium citrate 8.5 g, sodium thiosulphate 8.5 g, ferric citrate 1 g, sodium desoxycholate 5 g, neutral red as an indicator, and water to 1 litre.

hyobasioglossus (hi·o·ba·se·o·**glos**'·us). The lower posterior part of the hyoglossus muscle of the tongue. [hyoid, basioglossus.]

hyocholalic (hi·o·kol·**al**'·ik). Relating to hog bile. [Gk *hys* swine, *chole* bile.]

hyo-epiglottic, hyo-epiglottidean (hi·o·ep·e·**glot**'·ik, hi·o·ep·glot·**id**'·e·an). Relating to the hyoid bone and the epiglottis, e.g. the ligament connecting them.

hyoglossal (hi·o·**glos**·al). 1. Relating or belonging to the hyoid bone and the tongue, e.g. the aponeurosis connecting them. 2. Relating to the hyoglossus. [hyoid, Gk *glossa* tongue.]

hyoglossus (hi·o·**glos**·us). The hyoglossus muscle. [see prec.]

hyoglossus muscle [musculus hyoglossus (NA)]. A muscle of the tongue arising from the hyoid bone and passing vertically to the organ. It is a depressor of the organ.

hyoid (**hi**·oid). 1. Shaped like a Y or a U. 2. The hyoid bone, or belonging to it. [Gk *hyoeides* like the letter Υ (upsilon).]

hyoid bone [os hyoideum (NA)]. A U-shaped bone situated at the base of the tongue, consisting of a body with 2 greater and 2 lesser cornua.

body [corpus (NA)]. The middle part of the hyoid bone, giving attachment posteriorly to the cornua.

hyolaryngeal (hi·o·lar·**in**'·je·al). Relating or belonging to or connected with the hyoid bone and the larynx.

hyomandibular (hi·o·man·**dib**'·ew·lar). Relating or belonging to the hyoid bone and the mandible.

hyomental (hi·o·**men**·tal). Relating or belonging to the hyoid bone and the chin. [hyoid, L *mentum* chin.]

hyopharyngeus (hi·o·far·**in**'·je·us). The middle constrictor muscle of the pharynx. [hyoid, pharynx.]

hyoscine (**hi**·o·seen). Scopolamine, $C_{17}H_{21}NO_4$. An alkaloid obtained from several solanaceous plants, particularly henbane (*Hyoscyamus niger*) and species of *Datura* and *Scopolia.* It is an oily liquid, but the hydrobromide (BP 1973), in which form it is normally used, is a colourless crystalline substance, soluble in water and alcohol. Pharmacologically it resembles atropine, apart from its action on the central nervous system. It often causes amnesia. It relaxes smooth muscle generally, particularly that of the respiratory and gastro-intestinal tracts, and of the urinary tract and bladder. It diminishes the secretory activity of the respiratory mucous glands, of the salivary glands and of the sweat glands. It dilates the pupil and paralyses accommodation. In contrast to atropine it has a depressant action on the central nervous system as a rule, though occasionally it causes excitement, probably a form of idiosyncrasy. It is used as a central depressant in some manic and hypomanic states, such as delirium tremens; together with morphine as pre-anaesthetic medication; in the treatment of extrapyramidal rigidity in man; occasionally to relieve smooth-muscle spasm of the alimentary and urinary tracts; and sometimes as a mydriatic. **Hyoscine *N*-butylbromide.** The *N*-butylbromide (quaternary ammonium) derivative of hyoscine. It has the mild anticholinergic and spasmolytic actions of atropine and stronger ganglionic blocking and curariform actions than atropine. It does not cause central stimulation like atropine, and is at present under clinical trials. **Hyoscine Hydrobromide BP 1973.** $C_{17}H_{21}NO_4HBr·3H_2O$, the form in which hyoscine is dispensed. **Hyoscine Methobromide.** A substance having the actions and uses of hyoscine; it lacks the central actions of atropine and is used in the control of gastric ulcers. BP Commission approved name.

Hyoscyami Folium. *European Pharmacopoeia* name for Hyoscyamus BP 1973.

hyoscyamine (hi·o·si·am·een). $C_{17}H_{23}NO_3$, an alkaloid obtained mainly from Egyptian henbane, but present also in other solanaceous plants. It occurs in D- and L- forms, atropine being the racemic form. **Hyoscyamine hydrobromide, Hyoscyamine sulphate.** Water-soluble salts of hyoscyamine given in neuralgia, mental excitement and mania. Their mydriatic action is greater than atropine, though of equal duration. [see foll.]

Hyoscyamus (hi·o·si·am·us). 1. A genus of herbs (family Solanacea). 2. Hyoscyamus BP 1973. Hyoscyami folia, hyoscyamus leaves, consists of the leaves and flowering tops of *Hyoscyamus niger* Linn., a biennial species distributed throughout Europe and widely cultivated. It contains the alkaloids hyoscyamine, atropine and hyoscine, and in the form of the extract or tincture is used as a sedative in nervous conditions, also in the relief of griping caused by drastic purgatives. *Hyoscyamus muticus* Linn., a perennial species of Egypt and India, yields a drug (Egyptian henbane) the constituents, action and uses of which are similar. [Gk *hys* swine, *kyamos* bean.]

hyosternal (hi·o·**ster**·nal). Relating or belonging to the hyoid bone and the sternum.

hyothyroid (hi·o·**thi**·roid). Belonging to the hyoid bone and the thyroid cartilage.

hypacidaemia (hi·pas·id·e'·me·ah). Subacidity of the blood. [Gk *hypo,* acid, *haima* blood.]

hypacidity (hi·pas·**id**·it·e). Hypo-acidity.

hypaemia (hi·**pe**·me·ah). Hyphaemia.

hypaesthesia (hi·pes·**the**·ze·ah). Lessened or impaired sensibility to touch; hypo-aesthesia. [Gk *hypo,* aesthesia.]

hypaesthetic (hi·pes·**thet**·ik). Relating or belonging to hypaesthesia.

hypalbuminosis (hi·pal·bew·min·**o**'·sis). Deficiency of albumin in the blood. [Gk *hypo,* albumin, Gk *-osis* condition.]

hypalgesia (hi·pal·**je**·ze·ah). Diminished sensibility to pain. [Gk *hypo,* algesia.]

hypalgesic (hi·pal·**je**·zik). Referring or belonging to hypalgesia; showing diminished sensibility to pain.

hypamnion (hi·**pam**·ne·on). The presence of an abnormally small quantity of amniotic fluid. [Gk *hypo,* amnion.]

hypaphorine (hi·**paf**·or·een). $C_{14}H_{18}O_2N_2$, a base isolated from *Erythrina hypaphorus* and other species. It increases reflex irritability and tetanic convulsions in frogs. Chemically it is a derivative of tryptophan.

hypaphrodisia (hi·paf·ro·**diz**'·e·ah). Diminution or deficiency of sexual desire. [Gk *hypo,* aphrodisia.]

hyparterial (hi·par·**teer**·e·al). Hypo-arterial.

hypasthenia (hi·pas·**the**·ne·ah). Slight loss of strength. [Gk *hypo,* asthenia.]

hypatonia (hi·pat·o·ne·ah). Slight loss of tone or tension. [Gk *hypo,* atony.]

hypaxial (hi·**pax**·e·al). Lying beneath or towards the ventral aspect of the body axis. [Gk *hypo,* axis.]

hypazoturia (hi·paz·o·**tewr**'·e·ah). An unusually small amount of nitrogenous material in the urine. [Gk *hypo,* azoturia.]

hypencephalon (hi·pen·**kef**·al·on). 1. The embryonic cerebellum. 2. The quadrigeminal bodies, the pons and the medulla oblongata regarded as one structure. [Gk *hypo,* encephalon.]

hypenchyme (hi·**pen**·kime). In embryology, the primitive tissues which form in the archenteron. [Gk *hypo,* enchyma.]

hypeosinophil (hi·pe·o·**sin**'·o·fil). 1. Those leucocyte granules from which eosin stain can be removed by the action of acid or alkali. 2. Any primitive or other structure or cell which does not readily take eosin dye. [Gk *hypo,* eosin, Gk *philein* to love.]

hyper-. Prefix, from the Greek preposition *hyper,* meaning *above, excessive.*

hyperabduction (hi·per·ab·**duk'**·shun). Superabduction; abnormal abduction of a limb. [Gk *hyper*, abduction.]

hyperacanthosis (hi·per·ak·an·**tho'**·sis). Hypertrophy of the prickle-cell layer of the epidermis, e.g. in condylomata and warts. [Gk *hyper, akantha* prickle, *-osis* condition.]

hyperacid (hi·per·**as**·id). More than normally acid. [Gk *hyper*, acid.]

hyperacidaminuria (hi·per·**as**·id·am·in·**ewr'**·e·ah). An excess of amino acids in the urine. [Gk *hyper*, acidaminuria.]

hyperacidity (hi·per·as·**id'**·it·e). Abnormally acid. **Gastric hyperacidity.** Hyperchlorhydria. **Larval hyperacidity.** Larval hyperchlorhydria. *See* HYPERCHLORHYDRIA. [Gk *hyper*, acidity.]

hyperacousia (hi·per·ak·**oo'**·se·ah). Excessive acuteness of hearing; auditory hyperaesthesia. [Gk *hyper, akouein* to hear.]

hyperaction (hi·per·**ak**·shun). Increase of activity beyond normal. [Gk *hyper*, action.]

hyperactivity (hi·per·ak·**tiv'**·it·e). 1. Hyperaction. 2. The mental state in which there is aggressiveness, talkativeness, optimism and a leaning towards exaltation.

hyperacuity (hi·per·ak·**ew'**·it·e). Abnormal sharpness of sight or other special sense. [Gk *hyper*, acuity.]

hyperacusia, hyperacusis (hi·per·ak·**ew'**·ze·ah, **hi**·per·ak·**ew'**·sis). Hyperacousia.

hyperacute (hi·per·ak·**ewt'**). Applied to any of the senses indicating that they are very acute or excessively so. [Gk *hyper*, acute.]

hyperadenoma (hi·per·ad·en·**o'**·mah). An enlarged gland, particularly a lymph gland. [Gk *hyper, aden* gland, *-oma* tumour.]

hyperadenosis (hi·per·ad·en·**o'**·sis). A condition in which the glands are enlarged. [Gk *hyper, aden* gland, *-osis* condition.]

hyperadiposis, hyperadiposity (hi·per·ad·ip·**o'**·sis, **hi**·per·ad·ip·**os'**·it·e). A state of excessive fatness or obesity. [Gk *hyper*, adiposis.]

hyperadrenalism (hi·per·ad·**re'**·nal·izm). Abnormal increase in the secretory activity of the suprarenal glands either before or after birth. [Gk *hyper*, adrenalism.]

hyperadrenocorticism (hi·per·ad·re·no·**kor'**·tis·izm). Hypersecretion of the cortex of the suprarenal gland. [Gk *hyper*, adrenal cortex.]

hyperaemia (hi·per·e·me·ah). An excess of blood in any part of the body. **Active hyperaemia.** That due to an increased flow of blood into a part. **Collateral hyperaemia.** Increased flow of blood through the collateral circulation. **Inflammatory hyperaemia.** Hyperaemia due to dilatation of arterioles and capillaries, occurring as part of the tissue response to noxious agents. **Reactive hyperaemia.** Increased flow of blood after temporary ischaemia. **Stauungs hyperaemia.** Bier's hyperaemia; a method of producing passive hyperaemia of a limb by constriction with a rubber band. [Gk *hyper, haima* blood.]

See also: BIER.

hyperaemization (hi·per·e·mi·**za'**·shun). The artificial production of hyperaemia, as in Bier's method.

hyperaeration (hi·per·a·er·**a'**·shun). Hyperventilation. [Gk *hyper, aer* air.]

hyperaesthesia (hi·per·es·**the'**·ze·ah). Excessive sensitiveness of the skin, due to local causes or to peripheral nerve trouble. **Acoustic hyperaesthesia, Auditory hyperaesthesia.** Abnormally acute sense of hearing. **Cerebral hyperaesthesia.** A condition due to a cerebral lesion. **Gustatory hyperaesthesia.** Abnormally acute sense of taste. **Muscular hyperaesthesia.** Undue sensitiveness of muscles, due to local disease or to peripheral neuritis. **Olfactory hyperaesthesia.** Excessive sensitiveness to odours. **Optic hyperaesthesia.** Over-sensitiveness to light. **Sexual hyperaesthesia.** Abnormal increase of sexual impulse. **Tactile hyperaesthesia.** Increased tactile sensibility. [Gk *hyper, aesthesis* sensitivity.]

hyperaesthetic (hi·per·es·**thet'**·ik). Relating or belonging to or affected with hyperaesthesia.

hyperaffectivity (hi·per·af·ek·**tiv'**·it·e). Acute sensibility to mild stimuli. [Gk *hyper*, affectivity.]

hyperalbuminaemia (hi·per·al·bew·min·**e'**·me·ah). The presence of an excessive amount of albumin, or an abnormally high albumin/globulin ratio in the blood. [Gk *hyper*, albuminaemia.]

hyperalbuminosis (hi·per·al·bew·min·**o'**·sis). The occurrence in increased amount in the blood and other body fluids of albumin. [Gk *hyper*, albuminosis.]

hyperaldosteronism (hi·per·al·do·**steer'**·on·izm). The excessive production of aldosterone in the body. **Primary hyperaldosteronism.** Conn's syndrome, hyperaldosteronism resulting from adenomatous growth in the adrenal cortex, usually associated clinically with hypertension, polyuria that is not affected by vasopressin, and episodes of muscular weakness, but no oedema. **Secondary hyperaldosteronism.** Hyperaldosteronism occurring in nephrosis and certain other conditions. [Gk *hyper*, aldosterone.]

hyperalgesia (hi·per·al·**je'**·ze·ah). Exaggerated pain sensitivity. **Acoustic hyperalgesia, Auditory hyperalgesia.** A condition in which noise causes acute pain; an extreme form of hyperacousia. **Muscular hyperalgesia.** A condition of muscle fatigue, when slight movement produces pain. **Olfactory hyperalgesia.** A painful sensation in the nose, produced by certain odours. [Gk *hyper, algos* pain.]

hyperalgesic, hyperalgetic (hi·per·al·**je'**·zik, **hi**·per·al·**jet'**·ik). Relating or belonging to or marked by hyperalgesia.

hyperalgia (hi·per·**al**·je·ah). Hyperalgesia.

hyperalimentation (hi·per·al·im·en·**ta'**·shun). Superalimentation; treatment of an individual with neurasthenia, tuberculosis or other wasting disease by enforced feeding in excess of the demands of the appetite. [Gk *hyper*, alimentation.]

hyperalimentosis (hi·per·al·im·en·**to'**·sis). The pathological condition induced by either over-eating or superalimentation. [Gk *hyper*, aliment, Gk *-osis* condition.]

hyperalkalinity (hi·per·al·kal·**in'**·it·e). Superalkalinity; a state of excessive alkalinity. [Gk *hyper*, alkalinity.]

hyperallantoinuria (hi·per·**al**·an·to·in·**ewr'**·e·ah). The presence in the urine of an excessive amount of allantoin. [Gk *hyper*, allantoin, urine.]

hyperalonaemia (hi·per·al·on·**e'**·me·ah). Excess of salts in the blood. [Gk *hyper, als* salt, *haima* blood.]

hyperamino-acidaemia (hi·per·**am**·in·o·as·id·**e'**·me·ah). The presence of an excessive amount of amino acids in the blood. [Gk *hyper*, amino acid, Gk *haima* blood.]

hyperamylasaemia (hi·per·am·il·a·**ze'**·me·ah). Increased blood amylase. [Gk *hyper*, amylase, Gk *haima* blood.]

hyperanabolism (hi·per·an·**ab'**·ol·izm). Excess of growth, producing hypertrophy of a part or a tissue. [Gk *hyper, anaballein* to throw up.]

hyperanacinesia (hi·per·an·ah·sin·**e'**·ze·ah). Excessive functional activity of a part or organ, as of the stomach or intestine. **Hyperanacinesia ventriculi.** Excessive activity of the stomach. [Gk *hyper, anakinesis* a swinging to and fro.]

hyperaphia (hi·per·**af**·e·ah). Marked acuteness of the sense of touch. [Gk *hyper, haphe* touch.]

hyperaphic (hi·per·**af**·ik). Pertaining to or characterized by hyperaphia.

hyperaphrodisia (hi·per·af·ro·**diz'**·e·ah). Excessive sexual appetite. [Gk *hyper*, aphrodisia.]

hyperarithmous (hi·per·ar·**ith'**·mus). In excess of the normal number; supernumerary. [Gk *hyper, arithmos* number.]

hyperauxesis (hi·per·awx·**e'**·sis). Abnormal increase in size of any part, as by haemorrhage or effusion of fluid into it. [Gk *hyper, auxe* increase.]

hyperazotaemia (hi·per·az·o·**te'**·me·ah). The presence in the blood of an abnormally large amount of nitrogenous matter, e.g. urea. [Gk *hyper*, azotaemia.]

hyperazoturia (hi·per·az·o·**tewr'**·e·ah). The presence in the urine of an abnormally large amount of nitrogenous matter. [Gk *hyper*, azoturia.]

hyperbaric (hi·per·**bar**·ik). Heavier than its environment; describing an anaesthetic solution for intrathecal injection which has a specific gravity greater than that of normal cerebrospinal fluid. **Hyperbaric oxygen.** *See* OXYGEN. [Gk *hyper, baros* weight.]

hyperbarism (hi·per·bar·izm). *See* DYSBARISM. [Gk *hyper, baros* weight.]

hyperbilirubinaemia (hi·per·bil·e·roo·bin·e′·me·ah). The presence in the blood of an abnormally large quantity of bilirubin. [Gk *hyper*, bilirubin, Gk *haima* blood.]

hyperblastosis (hi·per·blas·to′·sis). Hypertrophy of any particular kind of tissue. [Gk *hyper, blastos* germ.]

hyperbrachycephalic (hi·per·brak·e·kef·al′·ik). 1. Relating or belonging to hyperbrachycephaly. 2. Markedly brachycephalic. [Gk *hyper, brachys* short, *kephale* head.]

hyperbrachycephaly (hi·per·brak·e·kef′·al·e) An extreme degree of brachycephaly, i.e. with a cephalic index of over 85. [see prec.]

hyperbulia (hi·per·bew·le·ah). 1. Abnormal display of will power. 2. Wilfulness almost to the point of psychiatric illness. [Gk *hyper, boule* will.]

hypercalcaemia (hi·per·kal·se′·me·ah). Excess of calcium in the blood. **Infantile hypercalcaemia.** Hypercalcaemia occurring in the early months of life, with osteosis at growing points, unusual facies (epicanthus, large nasolabial folds, pug nose, longer upper lip without philtrum), hypertension and mental defect. [Gk *hyper*, calcium, Gk *haima* blood.]

hypercalcipexy (hi·per·kal·se·pex·e). Calcium fixation in excess. [Gk *hyper*, calcium, Gk *pexis* fixation.]

hypercalciuria (hi·per·kal·se·ewr′·e·ah). Excess of calcium in the urine.

hypercapnia, hypercarbia (hi·per·kap·ne·ah, hi·per·kar·be·ah). The presence of a raised carbon dioxide content or tension in the blood. [Gk *hyper, kapnos* vapour.]

hypercarbia (hi·per·kar·be·ah). A high concentration of carbon dioxide in the blood. [Gk *hyper*, L *carbo* coal.]

hypercardia, hypercardiotrophy (hi·per·kar·de·ah, hi·per·kar·de·ot′·ro·fe). Morbid enlargement of the heart. [Gk *hyper, kardia* heart, *trophe* nourishment.]

hypercarotenaemia (hi·per·kar·ot·en·e′·me·ah). The presence in the blood of an excessive amount of carotene. [Gk *hyper*, carotene, Gk *haima* blood.]

hypercatabolism (hi·per·kat·ab′·ol·izm). Excessive wasting or destruction of a part or tissue. [Gk *hyper*, catabolism.]

hypercatharsis (hi·per·kath·ar′·sis). Excessive purging; excessive movements of the bowels. [Gk *hyper*, catharsis.]

hypercathartic (hi·per·kath·ar′·tik). 1. Relating or belonging to hypercatharsis. 2. Applied to any agent that effects excessive purging.

hypercathexis (hi·per·kath·ex′·is). An excessive concentration of psychic energy directed towards an object. [Gk *hyper, kathexis* retention.]

hypercementosis (hi·per·se·ment·o′·sis). Overgrowth of the cementum of the teeth. [Gk *hyper*, cementosis.]

hyperchloraemia (hi·per·klor·e′·me·ah). An excessive amount of chloride in the blood. [Gk *hyper*, chloride, Gk *haima* blood.]

hyperchlorhydria (hi·per·klor·hi′·dre·ah). The presence in the stomach of an excessive amount of hydrochloric acid as a result of overactivity of the secreting cells. **Larval hyperchlorhydria.** A masked state of hyperchlorhydria, the symptoms not being apparent. [hyperchloride, Gk *hydor* water.]

hyperchloridation (hi·per·klor·id·a′·shun). The giving of excessive amounts of sodium chloride and thereby producing an excess in the blood. [Gk *hyper*, chloridation.]

hyperchloride (hi·per·klor·ide). A perchloride; one which contains more chlorine atoms than does the normal chloride. [Gk *hyper*, chloride.]

hyperchloruria (hi·per·klor·ewr′·e·ah). The presence of an excessive amount of chlorides in the urine. [Gk *hyper*, chloride, urine.]

hypercholesterolaemia (hi·per·ko·les·ter·ol·e′·me·ah). Excess of cholesterol in the blood. [Gk *hyper*, cholesterol, Gk *haima* blood.]

hypercholesterolia (hi·per·ko·les·ter·o′·le·ah). Excess of cholesterol in the bile. [Gk *hyper*, cholesterol.]

hypercholia (hi·per·ko·le·ah). Excessive secretion of bile. [Gk *hyper, chole* bile.]

hyperchondroma (hi·per·kon·dro′·mah). Chondroma; a neoplasm composed of cartilaginous tissue. [Gk *hyper, chondros* cartilage, *-oma* tumour.]

hyperchondroplasia (hi·per·kon·dro·pla′·ze·ah). The formation of cartilage in abnormal amount. [Gk *hyper, chondros* cartilage, *plassein* to form.]

hyperchroma (hi·per·kro·mah). Excessive formation of pigment in the skin, as in syphilitic lesions. [Gk *hyper, chroma* colour.]

hyperchromaemia (hi·per·kro·me′·me·ah). A condition of the blood in which the colour index is high because of increased average amount of haemoglobin per corpuscle. [Gk *hyper, chroma* colour, *haima* blood.]

hyperchromaffinism (hi·per·kro·maf′·in·izm). Over-secretion from the chromaffin cells of the medulla of the suprarenal glands with resultant paroxysmal arterial hypertension. [Gk *hyper*, chromaffin.]

hyperchromasia (hi·per·kro·ma′·ze·ah). Hyperchromatism.

hyperchromatic (hi·per·kro·mat′·ik). 1. Highly coloured or over-pigmented. 2. Showing hyperchroma. 3. Containing a greater number of chromosomes than is normally the case. [Gk *hyper, chroma* colour.]

hyperchromatin (hi·per·kro·mat·in). That part of the chromatin which takes a blue aniline dye. [Gk *hyper*, chromatin.]

hyperchromatism (hi·per·kro·mat·izm). A degenerated state of the nucleus of the cell body in which it is filled with chromatin-like particles of pigment. **Macrocytic hyperchromatism.** Hyperchromatic macrocythaemia. *See* MACROCYTHAEMIA. [Gk *hyper, chroma* colour.]

hyperchromatopsia (hi·per·kro·mat·op′·se·ah). Abnormality of vision in which every object seen appears to be coloured. [Gk *hyper*, chromatopsia.]

hyperchromatosis (hi·per·kro·mat·o′·sis). Hyperchromatism.

hyperchromia (hi·per·kro·me·ah). 1. Hyperchromatism. 2. A condition of the blood in which the amount of haemoglobin in the erythrocytes is greatly increased. [Gk *hyper, chroma* colour.]

hyperchromic (hi·per·kro·mik). 1. Showing hyperchroma. 2. Intensely coloured.

hyperchylia (hi·per·ki·le·ah). Superabundance of chyle. [Gk *hyper, chylos* juice.]

hypercoenaesthesia (hi·per·se·nes·the′·ze·ah). Unfounded and over-emphasized feeling of well-being, typical of maniacal states and of general paralysis of the insane. [Gk *hyper, koinos* affable, aesthesia.]

hypercompensation (hi·per·kom·pen·sa′·shun). Excess of compensatory activity, e.g. in healing processes, the formation of more tissue than is required. [Gk *hyper*, compensation.]

hypercorticalism (hi·per·kor·tik·al·izm). Excessive functioning of the cortex of the suprarenal gland. [Gk *hyper*, cortex.]

hypercritical (hi·per·krit·ik·al). Applied to a crisis of extreme or unusual severity. [Gk *hyper*, crisis.]

hypercryaesthesia (hi·per·kri·es·the′·ze·ah). Acute or excessive sensitivity to cold. [Gk *hyper, kryos* cold, aesthesia.]

hypercryalgesia (hi·per·kri·al·je′·ze·ah). Hypercryaesthesia. [Gk *hyper, kryos* cold, *algos* pain.]

hypercupraemia (hi·per·kew·pre′·me·ah). An excess of copper present in the blood, e.g. in pregnancy. [Gk *hyper*, L *cuprum* copper, Gk *haima* blood.]

hypercusis (hi·per·kew·sis). Increased sensitivity to sound. [Gk *hyper, akouein* to hear.]

hypercyanotic (hi·per·si·an·ot′·ik). Marked by an extreme degree of cyanosis. [Gk *hyper*, cyanosis.]

hypercyesis (hi·per·si·e′·sis). Superfetation. [Gk *hyper, kyesis* pregnancy.]

hypercythaemia (hi·per·si·the′·me·ah). A condition of the blood in which there is formation of an excessive number of erythrocytes; an increase in the ratio of blood corpuscles to plasma. [Gk *hyper, kytos* cell, *haima* blood.]

hypercytochromia (hi·per·si·to·kro′·me·ah). The condition of a blood cell in which its capacity to take stain is increased. [Gk *hyper, kytos* cell, *chroma* colour.]

hypercytosis (hi·per·si·**to**′·sis). An excessive number of cells in any body fluid. [Gk *hyper, kytos* cell.]

hyperdacryosis (hi·per·dak·re·**o**′·sis). Excessive secretion of tears with continual lacrimation. [Gk *hyper, dakryon* tear.]

hyperdactylia, hyperdactylism (hi·per·dak·**til**′e·ah, hi·per·**dak**′·til·izm). The abnormal condition in which a hand or a foot has more than 5 fingers or toes. [Gk *hyper, daktylos* finger or toe.]

hyperdermatosis (hi·per·der·mat·**o**′·sis). A condition in which there is overgrowth of the skin. [Gk *hyper,* dermatosis.]

hyperdesmosis (hi·per·dez·**mo**′·sis). A condition in which there is overgrowth of the connective tissue. [Gk *hyper, desmos* band.]

hyperdiaemorrhysis (hi·per·di·em·**or**′·is·is). 1. Hyperaemia affecting the capillaries. 2. Increase in the flow of blood through the veins. [Gk *hyper, dia, haima* blood, *rhysis* a flowing.]

hyperdiastole (hi·per·di·**as**′·to·le). Extreme dilatation during the diastolic stage of the cardiac cycle. [Gk *hyper,* diastole.]

hyperdicrotic (hi·per·di·**krot**′·ik). Pronouncedly dicrotic. [Gk *hyper, dikrotos* double beat.]

hyperdicrotism (hi·per·**di**·krot·izm). 1. A state of pronounced or extreme dicrotism. 2. The quality of being pronouncedly dicrotic. [see prec.]

hyperdiploid (hi·per·**dip**·loid). *See* HYPERPLOID. [Gk *hyper, diploos* double, *eidos* form.]

hyperdistension (hi·per·dis·**ten**′·shun). Extreme degree of distension. [Gk *hyper,* distension.]

hyperdiuresis (hi·per·di·ewr·**e**′·sis). Abnormal increase in the quantity of urine excreted. [Gk *hyper,* diuresis.]

hyperdontogeny (hi·per·don·**toj**′·en·e). A shedding of teeth of the permanent dentition and their replacement by a third series of teeth. [Gk *hyper, odous* tooth, *genein* to produce.]

hyperdynamia (hi·per·di·**nam**′·e·ah). Abnormally great muscular or nervous activity; extreme functional energy. **Hyperdynamia uteri.** Excessively strong uterine contractions in labour. [Gk *hyper, dynamis* power.]

hyperdynamic (hi·per·di·**nam**′·ik). Referring or belonging to or marked by hyperdynamia.

hypereccrisis (hi·per·**ek**·ris·is). Excessive excretion of faeces. [Gk *hyper, ekkrisis* excrement.]

hypereccritic (hi·per·ek·**rit**′·ik). Referring or belonging to excessive excretion of faeces. [see prec.]

hyperechema (hi·per·ek·**e**′·mah). Exaggeration of a normal sound. [Gk *hyper, echema* sound.]

hyperekplexia (hi·per·ek·**plex**′·e·ah). Myoclonic jerking in response to startle. [Gk *hyper, ek, plessein* to strike.]

hyperemesis (hi·per·**em**·es·is). Excessive vomiting. **Hyperemesis gravidarum.** The uncontrollable vomiting of pregnancy. **Hyperemesis lactentium.** The vomiting to which infants are subject. [Gk *hyper,* emesis.]

hyperemetic (hi·per·em·**et**′·ik). Referring to or marked by excessive vomiting. [see prec.]

hyperemotivity (hi·per·e·mo·**tiv**′·it·e). 1. The capacity for more than normal response to mild stimuli. 2. Excessive capacity for emotion. [Gk *hyper,* emotivity.]

hyperencephalus (hi·per·en·**kef**′·al·us). A monster of which the sinciput is lacking so that the brain substance is exposed. [Gk *hyper, egkephalos* brain.]

hyperendemic (hi·per·en·**dem**′·ik). A term applied to a highly endemic area; in malariology it indicates a spleen rate of 50 per cent or over in children under 10 years of age. [Gk *hyper,* endemic.]

hyperenergia, hyperenergy (hi·per·en·**er**′·je·ah, hi·per·**en**·er·je). 1. Excessive energy. 2. Excessive activity or action. [Gk *hyper,* energy.]

hypereosinophilia (hi·per·e·o·sin·o·**fil**′·e·ah). A marked degree of eosinophilia. [Gk *hyper,* eosinophilia.]

hyperephidrosis (hi·per·ef·id·**ro**′·sis). Long-continued perspiration or the secretion of an excessive quantity of sweat. [Gk *hyper, epi, hidros* sweat.]

hyperepinephria (hi·per·ep·e·**nef**′·re·ah). Hyperadrenalism. [Gk *hyper, epi, nephros* kidney.]

hyperepinephrinaemia (hi·per·ep·e·nef·rin·**e**′·me·ah). The presence of an abnormally large amount of suprarenal secretion in the blood. [Gk *hyper,* epinephrinaemia.]

hyperepithymia (hi·per·ep·e·**thi**′·me·ah). Excessive desire. [Gk *hyper, epithymia* desire.]

hyperequilibrium (hi·per·e·kwil·**ib**′·re·um). A tendency to vertigo when the subject makes even slight revolving movements. [Gk *hyper,* equilibrium.]

hypererethism (hi·per·**er**·e·thizm). 1. A condition of excessive irritability of the nerves. 2. A state of extreme mental irritation. [Gk *hyper, erethisma* excitation.]

hyperergasia (hi·per·er·**ga**′·ze·ah). Increased or excessive functional activity. [Gk *hyper, ergon* work.]

hyperergia (hi·per·**er**·je·ah). 1. The condition of being extremely allergic. 2. Hyperergasia. [Gk *hyper, ergon* work.]

hyperergic (hi·per·**er**·jik). 1. Relating or belonging to hyperergia. 2. More than normally active.

hypererythrocythaemia (hi·per·er·**ith**·ro·si·**the**′·me·ah). An excess of erythrocytes in the blood, as in polycythaemia vera. [Gk *hyper,* erythrocythaemia.]

hyperesophoria (hi·per·e·so·**for**′·e·ah). The tendency on the part of an eye to deviate upward and inward because of muscular insufficiency; a type of heterophoria. [Gk *hyper, eso* inward, *pherein* to bear.]

hypereuryopia (hi·per·ewr·e·**o**′·pe·ah). Having abnormally widely-opened eyes. [Gk *hyper, eurys* wide, *ops* eye.]

hyperexcretory (hi·per·ex·**kre**′·tor·e). Characterized by excessive excretion. [Gk *hyper,* excretion.]

hyperexophoria (hi·per·ex·o·**for**′·e·ah). The tendency on the part of an eye to deviate upward and outward because of muscular insufficiency; a type of heterophoria. [Gk *hyper, exo* outward, *pherein* to bear.]

hyperextend (hi·per·ex·**tend**′). To extend forcibly beyond the normal limits, e.g. a limb in orthopaedic treatment. [see foll.]

hyperextension (hi·per·ex·**ten**′·shun). In orthopaedics, the forcible over-extending of a limb for the purpose of correcting deformity. [Gk *hyper,* extension.]

hyperfecundation (hi·per·fek·un·**da**′·shun). The successive fertilization by separate acts of coitus of 2 or more ova produced during the same ovulation. [Gk *hyper,* L *fecundare* to fertilize.]

hyperflexion (hi·per·**flek**·shun). The forcible bending of a limb to a degree greater than normal. [Gk *hyper,* flexion.]

hyperfunction (hi·per·**fungk**·shun). 1. Excessive functional activity on the part of any organ. 2. To manifest excessive function. [Gk *hyper,* function.]

hypergammaglobulinaemia (hi·per·gam·ah·glob·ew·lin·**e**′·me·ah). An increase above normal of the blood γ-globulins. [Gk *hyper,* γ-globulin, Gk *haima* blood.]

hypergasia (hi·per·**ga**·ze·ah). Lessened functional activity. [Gk *hypo, ergon* work.]

hypergenesis (hi·per·**jen**·es·is). 1. Hyperplasia. 2. Superfluity or excess of parts or organs of the body. 3. Over-production or over-development. [Gk *hyper, genesis* origin.]

hypergenetic (hi·per·jen·**et**′·ik). 1. Describing the condition in which there is congenital enlargement of 1 or more organs or parts. 2. Relating or belonging to hypergenesis. [see prec.]

hypergenitalism (hi·per·**jen**·it·al·izm). The condition resulting from over-activity of the internal secretions of the genital glands, e.g. precocious puberty and over-development of the genitalia. [Gk *hyper,* L *genitalis* productive.]

hypergeusia (hi·per·**gew**·se·ah). More than normal acuteness or too great acuteness of the sense of taste. [Gk *hyper, geusis* taste.]

hypergigantosoma (hi·per·ji·**gant**·o·**so**′·mah). A marked degree of gigantism. [Gk *hyper, gigas* huge, *soma* body.]

hyperglandular (hi·per·**glan**·dew·lar). Characterized by excessive activity of the endocrine glands. [Gk *hyper,* gland.]

hyperglobulinaemia (hi·per·**glob**·ewl·in·**e**′·me·ah). An excess of globulin in the blood. [Gk *hyper,* globulin, Gk *haima* blood.] *See also:* WALDENSTRÖM (J. G.).

hyperglobulism (hi·per·**glob**·ewl·izm). A condition in which the production of erythrocytes is abnormally great; erythrocytosis; polycythaemia. [Gk *hyper*, globule.]

hypergluconeogenesis (hi·per·**gloo**·ko·ne·o·**jen**′·es·is). Excessive conversion of protein into carbohydrate, a characteristic of suprarenal cortical over-activity. [Gk *hyper*, *glykys* sweet, *neos* new, *genein* to produce.]

hyperglycaemia (hi·per·gli·**se**′·me·ah). An excessive amount of sugar in the blood. [Gk *hyper*, glycaemia.]

hyperglycodermia (hi·per·gli·ko·**der**′·me·ah). An excess of sugar in the skin; a condition that is reputed to be associated with certain chronic skin diseases which respond to therapy directed to adjust this condition. [Gk *hyper*, *glykys* sweet, *derma* skin.]

hyperglycogenolysis (hi·per·gli·ko·jen·**ol**′·is·is). Excessive glycogenolysis. [Gk *hyper*, glycogenolysis.]

hyperglyconeogenesis (hi·per·**gli**·ko·ne·o·**jen**′·es·is). Hypergluconeogenesis.

hyperglycoplasmia (hi·per·gli·ko·**plaz**′·me·ah). The condition in which the blood plasma contains an excessive amount of sugar. [Gk *hyper*, *glykys* sweet, plasma.]

hyperglycorrhachia (hi·per·gli·ko·**rak**′·e·ah). A condition in which the cerebrospinal fluid contains an excessive amount of sugar. [Gk *hyper*, glycorrhachia.]

hyperglycosaemia (hi·per·gli·ko·**se**′·me·ah). Hyperglycaemia. [Gk *hyper*, glycosaemia.]

hyperglycosuria (hi·per·gli·ko·**sewr**′·e·ah). High excess of sugar in the urine. [Gk *hyper*, glycosuria.]

hyperglycystia (hi·per·gli·**sist**′·e·ah). The presence in the tissues of an abnormally large amount of sugar. [Gk *hyper*, *glykys* sweet, *histos* web.]

hypergnosia, hypergnosis (hi·per·**no**·se·ah, hi·per·**no**·sis). Exaggerated or distorted perception influenced by the unconscious projection of subjective emotional experience. [Gk *hyper*, *gnosis* knowing.]

hypergonadism (hi·per·**gon**·ad·izm). Excessive secretory activity by the ovary or testis. [Gk *hyper*, *gone* seed.]

hyperguanidinaemia (hi·per·**gwan**·id·in·**e**′·me·ah). An excessive amount of guanidine in the circulating blood. [Gk *hyper*, guanidine, Gk *haima* blood.]

hyperhaemoglobinaemia (hi·per·**he**·mo·glo·bin·**e**′·me·ah). A condition in which the quantity of haemoglobin in the blood is in excess of the normal. [Gk *hyper*, haemoglobin, Gk *haima* blood.]

hyperhaploid (hi·per·**hap**·loid). *See* HYPERPLOID. [Gk *hyper*, *haploos* single, *eidos* form.]

hyperhedonia (hi·per·he·**do**′·ne·ah). A morbid condition in which there is a feeling of great pleasure attached to any sense perception, or in which any act, in itself an agreeable one, induces a feeling of intense gratification. [Gk *hyper*, *hedone* pleasure.]

hyperhedonism (hi·per·**he**·don·izm). 1. Sexual erethism. 2. Hyperhedonia. [see prec.]

hyperheparinaemia (hi·per·hep·ar·in·**e**′·me·ah). Excess of heparin in the blood. [Gk *hyper*, heparin, Gk *haima* blood.]

hyperhepatia (hi·per·hep·**at**′·e·ah). Excessive liver function. [Gk *hyper*, *hepar* liver.]

hyperhidrosis (hi·per·hid·**ro**′·sis). The secretion of an abnormally large quantity of sweat. **Gustatory hyperhidrosis.** Sweating on the forehead, nose and lips, usually after eating hot, spicy food. **Hyperhidrosis lateralis.** Excessive sweating on one lateral half of the body. **Hyperhidrosis nudorum.** An exacerbation of sweating caused by the sudden effect of cold air causing contraction of the muscles associated with the sweat glands, especially in the axilla. [Gk *hyper*, *hidros* sweat.]

hyperhistaminaemia (hi·per·his·tam·in·**e**′·me·ah). Excess of histamine in the blood. [Gk *hyper*, histamine, Gk *haima* blood.]

hyperhormonal (hi·per·**hor**·mon·al). 1. Relating or belonging to excess of hormone. 2. Having excess of hormone. 3. Caused by excess of hormone. [Gk *hyper*, hormone.]

hyperhydraemia (hi·per·hi·**dre**′·me·ah). An abnormally large water content in the blood. [Gk *hyper*, *hydor* water, *haima* blood.]

hyperhydration (hi·per·hi·**dra**′·shun). The condition of containing too much fluid. **Cellular hyperhydration.** A syndrome in which there is an increase of intracellular fluid without necessarily an increase of extracellular fluid. It is characterized clinically by nausea and anorexia, weakness, headache, cramps and convulsions, and in the absence of associated extracellular hyperhydration it responds to hypertonic saline transfusions. **Extracellular hyperhydration.** Hyperhydration in which the excess fluid is confined to the extracellular tissues. [Gk *hyper*, *hydor* water.]

hyperhydrochloria, hyperhydrochloridia (hi·per·hi·dro·**klor**′·e·ah, hi·per·hi·dro·klor·**id**′·e·ah). Hyperchlorhydria. [Gk *hyper*, hydrochloride.]

hyperhydropexia, hyperhydropexis (hi·per·hi·dro·**pex**′·e·ah, hi·per·hi·dro·**pex**′·is). The fixation or the holding of an abnormally large amount of water. [Gk *hyper*, hydropexia.]

hyperhypnosis (hi·per·hip·**no**′·sis). A constantly recurring state of sleepiness; excessive sleepiness. [Gk *hyper*, *hypnos* sleep.]

hyperhypocytosis (hi·per·hi·po·si·**to**′·sis). Leucopenia in which there is an abnormally large proportion of neutrophil cells. [Gk *hyper*, hypocytosis.]

hypericin (hi·**per**·is·in). A complex polyhydroxy-polycyclic compound occurring in many species of St. John's wort which causes photosensitization; this has been mainly observed in cattle. [see foll.]

Hypericum (hi·**per**·ik·um). A genus of plants of the family Hypericaceae. **Hypericum perforatum Linn.** St. John's wort, a species from which an infusion has been employed as a remedy for coughs and as a healing application to wounds. [Gk *hypo*, *erike* heather.]

hyperidrosis (hi·per·id·**ro**′·sis). Hyperhidrosis.

hyperimmunity (hi·per·im·**ewn**′·it·e). Immunity greater than that usually present in the particular circumstances under consideration. [Gk *hyper*, immunity.]

hyperimmunization (hi·per·**im**·ewn·i·**za**′·shun). 1. Immunization to a very high degree. 2. The immunizing of a convalescent patient by inoculation with active virus of the disease. [Gk *hyper*, immunization.]

hyperingestion (hi·per·in·**jes**′·chun). Over-eating or over-drinking, either as a single incident or, more commonly, as a habit. [Gk *hyper*, ingestion.]

hyperinosaemia (hi·per·in·o·**se**′·me·ah). 1. An excess of fibrinogen or a strong tendency to form fibrin in the blood. 2. Extreme coagulability of the blood. [Gk *hyper*, *is* fibre, *haima* blood.]

hyperinosis (hi·per·in·**o**′·sis). 1. Hyperinosaemia. 2. Increase in the fibrin-forming elements in the blood. [Gk *hyper*, *is* fibre, *-osis* condition.]

hyperinotic (hi·per·in·**ot**′·ik). Pertaining to or marked by hyperinosis.

hyperinsulinaemia (hi·per·in·sew·lin·**e**′·me·ah). Hypoglycaemia resulting from excess of insulin secretion. [Gk *hyper*, insulin, Gk *haima* blood.]

hyperinsulinism (hi·per·**in**′·sew·lin·izm). 1. Hypoglycaemia resulting from excess of insulin secretion. 2. A state of shock induced by overdosage of insulin (insulin shock). [Gk *hyper*, insulin.]

hyperinter-renal (hi·per·in·ter·**re**′·nal). Relating or belonging to or caused by hyperfunction of the cortex of the suprarenal gland. [Gk *hyper*, inter-renal.]

hyperinter-renalopathy (hi·per·in·ter·re·nal·**op**′·ath·e). Any disease resulting from too great activity of the cortex of the suprarenal gland. [Gk *hyper*, inter-renalopathy.]

hyperinvolution (hi·per·in·vol·**ew**′·shun). Too great involution of any organ after it has undergone enlargement; e.g. the uterus after childbirth may become smaller than it was before the occurrence of pregnancy. [Gk *hyper*, involution.]

hyperiodaemia (hi·per·i·od·**e**′·me·ah). The existence of too much iodine in the blood. [Gk *hyper*, iodine, Gk *haima* blood.]

hyperisotonic (hi·per·i·so·**ton**′·ik). 1. Term applied to a solution of more than 0.45 per cent sodium chloride in which erythrocytes become crenated owing to exosmosis. 2. Denoting a solution which has an osmotic pressure greater than an isotonic solution; one more concentrated than an isotonic solution. [Gk *hyper*, isotonicity.]

hyperisotonicity (hi·per·i·so·ton·is′·it·e). The state of being hyperisotonic.

hyperkalaemia, hyperkaliaemia (hi·per·kal·e′·me·ah, hi·per·kal·e·e′·me·ah). Excess of potassium in the blood. [Gk *hyper*, L *kalium* potassium, Gk *haima* blood.]

hyperkeratinization (hi·per·ker·at·in·i·za′·shun). The horny thickening of the epithelium, e.g. of palms and soles, which is characteristic of chronic arsenical poisoning or due to vitamin-A deficiency. [Gk *hyper*, keratinization.]

hyperkeratomycosis (hi·per·ker·at·o·mi·ko′·sis). Thickening of the horny layer of the skin caused by the presence of a fungus. [Gk *hyper*, *keras* horn, mycosis.]

hyperkeratosis (hi·per·ker·at·o′·sis). Hypertrophy of the stratum corneum of the skin without parakeratosis and usually associated with thickening of the underlying transitional layers. It may be congenital or acquired, diffuse or limited in extent; and follicular in character. Harlequin fetus is an example of diffuse congenital hyperkeratosis. The malady can affect mucosae as in leucoplakia. **Hyperkeratosis eccentrica** (Respighi). Porokeratosis of Mibelli. **Hyperkeratosis follicularis et parafollicularis in cutem penetrans** (Kyrle). A rare malady resembling Darier's disease in which horny plugs form in the follicles on limited areas and penetrate the corium leading to the development of small foreign-body granulomata. **Hyperkeratosis lenticularis perstans** (Flegel). A condition of warty keratoses on the trunk and limbs with pin-point keratotic depressions on the palms and soles, with no history of ingestion of inorganic arsenic. **Hyperkeratosis linguae.** Lingua nigra; black hairy tongue (*see* TONGUE). **Perifollicular hyperkeratosis.** Localized accumulations of horny cells around the pilosebaceous follicles of the skin. **Precancerous hyperkeratosis.** Any persistent, localized hyperkeratosis affecting the skin or mucous membrane, which may be a precursor of cancer. **Hyperkeratosis subungualis.** Hyperkeratosis affecting the nail beds. [Gk *hyper*, keratosis.]

hyperketonuria (hi·per·ke·ton·ewr′·e·ah). The presence in the urine of an excess of ketone. [Gk *hyper*, ketone, urine.]

hyperketosis (hi·per·ke·to′·sis). The forming of ketone in excessive quantity. [Gk *hyper*, ketone, Gk *-osis* condition.]

hyperkinaemia (hi·per·kin·e′·me·ah). The condition in which an abnormally large quantity of blood is pumped through the heart while the subject is at rest. [Gk *hyper*, *kinein* to move, *haima* blood.]

hyperkinesia, hyperkinesis (hi·per·kin·e′·se·ah, hi·per·kin·e′·sis). A condition in which there is abnormally great strength of movement, as in muscular spasm. **Essential hyperkinesia.** Hyperkinesia in children in which movements are excessive and repeated, but are not dissociated as in chorea. **Professional hyperkinesia.** Occupational neurosis. *See* NEUROSIS. [Gk *hyper*, *kinesis* movement.]

hyperkinetic (hi·per·kin·et′·ik). Relating or belonging to hyperkinesia.

hyperlactacidaemia (hi·per·lak·tas·id·e′·me·ah). Excess of lactic acid in the blood. [Gk *hyper*, lactacidaemia.]

hyperlecithinaemia (hi·per·les·ith·in·e′·me·ah). The presence in the blood of an excessive quantity of lecithin. [Gk *hyper*, lecithinaemia.]

hyperlethal (hi·per·le·thal). A term applied to a dose of a drug which is more than strong enough to cause death. [Gk *hyper*, lethal.]

hyperleucocytosis (hi·per·lew·ko·si·to′·sis). Great increase in the number of leucocytes in the blood. [Gk *hyper*, leucocytosis.]

hyperleydigism (hi·per·li′·dig·izm). Excessive activity of the interstitial (Leydig) cells of the testicles. [Gk *hyper*, Leydig cells.]

hyperlipaemia (hi·per·lip·e′·me·ah). An excessive amount of neutral fat or of lipoids in the blood. **Carbohydrate-induced hyperlipaemia.** Hyperlipaemic and hypercholesterolaemic xanthomatosis induced by excessive consumption of carbohydrates. **Essential hyperlipaemia, Familial idiopathic hyperlipaemia.** A familial condition in which there is an increase in the neutral fat in the plasma sufficient to cause turbidity associated usually with an increase in blood cholesterol. [see foll.]

hyperlipidaemia (hi·per·lip·id·e′·me·ah). The condition in which lipids are present in excess in the blood. [Gk *hyper*, *lipos* fat, *haima* blood.]

hyperlipoidaemia (hi·per·lip·oid·e′·me·ah). Hyperlipidaemia. [Gk *hyper*, lipoid, Gk *haima* blood.]

hyperlipoproteinaemia (hi·per·lip·o·pro·te·in·e′·me·ah). The condition in which protein-bound lipids are present in excess in the blood. [Gk *hyper*, *lipos* fat, *proteios* of first rank, *haemia* blood.]

hyperliposis (hi·per·lip·o′·sis). The condition in which the blood contains an excess of lipase (lipolytic enzyme). [Gk *hyper*, lipase.]

hyperlithic (hi·per·lith·ik). Relating to or containing excess of uric (lithic) acid. [Gk *hyper*, lithic acid.]

hyperlithuria (hi·per·lith·ewr′·e·ah). Excess of uric (lithic) acid in the urine. [Gk *hyper*, lithic acid, urine.]

hyperlogia (hi·per·lo·je·ah). 1. Excessive loquacity. 2. Maniacal babbling. [Gk *hyper*, *logos* discourse.]

hyperlordosis (hi·per·lor·do′·sis). Excessive lordosis. [Gk *hyper*, lordosis.]

hyperluteinization (hi·per·lew·te·in·i·za′·shun). A condition occurring in the ovaries in hydatidiform mole and chorionepithelioma in which there is excessive luteinization of the follicular cysts. [Gk *hyper*, luteinization.]

hyperlymphia (hi·per·limf·e·ah). Increase in the quantity of lymph in the bodily tissues. [Gk *hyper*, L *lympha* water.]

hyperlysinaemia (hi·per·li·sin·e′·me·ah). A metabolic disorder with increased diaminocaproic acid in the blood, in which the hair is fine and sparse. [Gk *hyper*, lysine, Gk *haima* blood.]

hypermagnesaemia (hi·per·mag·neez·e′·me·ah). An abnormally large amount of magnesium in the plasma. [Gk *hyper*, magnesium, Gk *haima* blood.]

hypermastia (hi·per·mas·te·ah). 1. Excessive development of the breasts. 2. The formation and development of one or more supernumerary breasts. [Gk *hyper*, *mastos* breast.]

hypermature (hi·per·mat·ewr′). 1. Applied to anything which has progressed beyond the state of maturity. 2. Over-ripe, as a cataract. [Gk *hyper*, mature.]

hypermedication (hi·per·med·ik·a′·shun). Excess therapeutic administration or use of drugs. [Gk *hyper*, medication.]

hypermegalia, hypermegaly (hi·per·meg·a′·le·ah, hi·per·meg·al·e). The state or condition of being excessively enlarged. [Gk *hyper*, *megas* large.]

hypermegasoma (hi·per·meg·ah·so′·mah). A stage of general overgrowth affecting height, breadth and bulk of the body. [Gk *hyper*, megasoma.]

hypermegasthenic (hi·per·meg·as·then′·ik). 1. Having abnormal or excessive strength. 2. Relating or belonging to abnormal or excessive strength. [Gk *hyper*, megasthenic.]

hypermelanosis (hi·per·mel·an·o′·sis). Excessive brown pigmentation of the skin due to increased melanin production. [Gk *hyper*, *melas* black, *-osis* condition.]

hypermenorrhoea (hi·per·men·o·re′·ah). Menstruation in which the flow is excessive. [Gk *hyper*, menorrhoea.]

hypermesosoma (hi·per·mes·o·so′·mah). Stature exceeding the normal. [Gk *hyper*, mesosoma.]

hypermetabolism (hi·per·met·ab′·ol·izm). Increased metabolism. [Gk *hyper*, metabolism.]

hypermetamorphosis (hi·per·met·ah·mor′·of·sis). 1. The distraction and confusion of mind characteristic of maniacal states and resulting from constant change and drift of ideas. 2. In biology, the mode of development of some insects in which they pass through more marked, rapid or frequent changes than is normally the case. [Gk *hyper*, metamorphosis.]

hypermetaplasia (hi·per·met·ah·pla′·ze·ah). Excessive metaplasia or abnormal increase in metaplasia. [Gk *hyper*, metaplasia.]

hypermetria (hi·per·me·tre·ah). 1. Abnormally wide range of movement. 2. The abnormal extension of a part in any particular direction. [Gk *hyper*, *metron* measure.]

hypermetrope (hi·per·**met**·rope). An individual who has a long range of sight. [Gk *hyper*, *metron* measure, *ops* eye.]

hypermetropia (hi·per·met·**ro**′·pe·ah). A condition in which the image of an object viewed by the eye is formed behind the retina. **Absolute hypermetropia.** The amount of hypermetropia that cannot be overcome by accommodation. If this is present, clear vision will not be obtained without glasses. **Acquired hypermetropia.** That occurring with age, due to the lens becoming more homogeneous and slightly flatter in curvature as the new lens fibres keep on being formed. **Axial hypermetropia.** That due to the anteroposterior length of the eye being shorter than normal. **Curvature hypermetropia.** Hypermetropia in which the curvature of 1 or more of the refracting surfaces of the eye is insufficient. **Facultative hypermetropia.** That amount of the manifest hypermetropia that can be overcome by accommodation. **Index hypermetropia.** Hypermetropia in which the refractive index of the lens is too low. **Latent hypermetropia.** That amount of the total hypermetropia which is constantly corrected by the tone of the ciliary muscle. It can only be estimated by refraction under a mydriatic. **Manifest hypermetropia.** That amount of the total hypermetropia that is not overcome by the tone of the ciliary muscle, i.e. the total minus the latent. It is estimated by the strongest convex lens that gives normal vision when no mydriatic has been used. **Refractive hypermetropia.** That due to the curvature of the cornea or lens, or that due to the refractive indices of the media, i.e. curvature or index hypermetropia (see above). **Senile hypermetropia.** Acquired hypermetropia (see above). **Total hypermetropia.** The whole amount of hypermetropia present. It can only be estimated under a mydriatic, and is the latent plus the manifest. [Gk *hyper*, *metron* measure, *ops* eye.]

hypermetropic (hi·per·met·**ro**′·pik). Affected with, characterized by, belonging or having relation to hypermetropia.

hypermicrosoma (hi·per·mi·kro·**so**′·mah). Extreme dwarfism; extreme smallness of stature. [Gk *hyper*, *mikros* small, *soma* body.]

hypermimia (hi·per·**mim**·e·ah). The use of exaggerated gestures or of an excessive amount of gesticulation when speaking. [Gk *hyper*, *mimeomai* to mimic.]

hypermineralization (hi·per·min·er·al·i·**za**′·shun). An excess of mineral elements in the body. [Gk *hyper*, mineralization.]

hypermnesia (hi·per·**mne**·ze·ah). 1. An abnormally acute state of the memory. 2. The extraordinary power of memory that may be present in states of exaltation. [Gk *hyper*, *mnesis* memory.]

hypermnesic (hi·per·**mne**·zik). 1. Relating or belonging to hypermnesia. 2. A term for disorders of the psyche accompanied by over-activity of the mind, e.g. obsession (Meyer).

hypermnesis (hi·per·**mne**·sis). Hypermnesia.

hypermorph (hi·per·morf). A person with arms and legs disproportionately long in relation to the slender narrow trunk, and whose head, face and features are narrow. [Gk *hyper*, *morphe* form.]

hypermotility (hi·per·mo·**til**′·it·e). Excessive motility or motility of an abnormal kind. [Gk *hyper*, motility.]

hypermyelohaemia (hi·per·mi·el·o·**he**′·me·ah). Hyperaemia affecting the spinal marrow. [Gk *hyper*, *myelos* marrow, *haima* blood.]

hypermyotonia (hi·per·mi·o·**to**′·ne·ah). A state of excessive muscular tension. [Gk *hyper*, *mys* muscle, *tonos* tone.]

hypermyotrophia, hypermyotrophy (hi·per·mi·o·**tro**′·fe·ah, hi·per·mi·**ot**′·ro·fe). Overgrowth of muscular tissue. [Gk *hyper*, *mys* muscle, *trophe* nourishment.]

hypernatraemia (hi·per·nat·**re**′·me·ah). Excess of sodium in the blood. [Gk *hyper*, natron, Gk *haima* blood.]

hyperneocytosis (hi·per·ne·o·si·**to**′·sis). Hyperleucocytosis characterized by the presence of many immature forms of leucocytes. [Gk *hyper*, *neos* new, *kytos* cell.]

hypernephritis (hi·per·nef·**ri**′·tis). Inflammation of the suprarenal gland. [Gk *hyper*, *nephros* kidney, *-itis* inflammation.]

hypernephroid (hi·per·**nef**·roid). Having resemblance to the suprarenal gland. [Gk *hyper*, *nephros* kidney, *eidos* form.]

hypernephroma (hi·per·nef·**ro**′·mah). A renal carcinoma which arises from the tubules at the upper pole of the kidney, and resembles adrenal tissue in its naked-eye appearance; Grawitz's tumour. [Gk *hyper*, *nephros* kidney, *-oma* tumour.]

hypernephrotrophy (hi·per·nef·**rot**′·rof·e). Morbid enlargement or overgrowth of the kidney. [Gk *hyper*, *nephros* kidney, *trophe* nourishment.]

hyperneuroma (hi·per·newr·**o**′·mah). A nerve tumour in which neural elements predominate to an unusual degree and in which growth of such elements is abnormally rapid and widespread. [Gk *hyper*, *neuron* nerve, *-oma* tumour.]

hyperneurotization (hi·per·newr·ot·i·**za**′·shun). The procedure of increasing the working force of a muscle, which already has the normal supply of nerves, by implanting in it an exogenous motor nerve. [Gk *hyper*, neurotization.]

hypernidation (hi·per·nid·**a**′·shun). Abnormal proliferation of the cells of the endometrium during menstruation, which sometimes causes membranous dysmenorrhoea. [Gk *hyper*, L *nidus* nest.]

hypernitraemia (hi·per·ni·**tre**′·me·ah). Excess of nitrogen in the circulating blood. [Gk *hyper*, nitrogen, Gk *haima* blood.]

hypernoea, hypernoia (hi·per·**ne**·ah, hi·per·**noi**·ah). 1. Excessive imagination or activity of mind. 2. Extreme rapidity of thought. [Gk *hyper*, *nous* mind.]

hypernomic (hi·per·**no**·mik). Above the law; exaggerated. [Gk *hyper*, *nomos* law.]

hypernormal (hi·per·**nor**·mal). 1. Above the normal or more than the normal. 2. Relating to a state that is beyond normal. [Gk *hyper*, normal.]

hypernormocytosis (hi·per·nor·mo·si·**to**′·sis). A more than normal proportion of neutrophil cells in the blood. [Gk *hyper*, normocytosis.]

hypernutrition (hi·per·new·**trish**′·un). Over-feeding, with its resultant effect on the body generally. [Gk *hyper*, nutrition.]

hyperodontogeny (hi·per·o·don·**toj**′·en·e). A shedding of teeth of the permanent dentition and their replacement by a third series of teeth. [Gk *hyper*, *odous* tooth, *genein* to produce.]

hyperoestrogenaemia (hi·per·e·sto·jen·**e**′·me·ah). The presence of an excessive amount of oestrogen in the blood. [Gk *hyper*, oestrogen, Gk *haima* blood.]

hyperoestrogenism (hi·per·e·stro·jen·izm). The bodily condition resulting from an excess of oestrogen in the circulating blood. [Gk *hyper*, oestrogen.]

hyperoestrogenuria (hi·per·e·stro·jen·**ewr**′·e·ah). The presence in the urine of an excessive quantity of oestrogen. [Gk *hyper*, oestrogen, urine.]

hyperoic (hi·per·o·ik). Relating or belonging to the palate. [Gk *hyperoa* palate.]

hyperoitis (hi·per·o·**i**′·tis). Inflammation of the palate. [Gk *hyperoa* palate, *-itis* inflammation.]

hyperol (hi·per·ol). $CO(NH_2)_2H_2O_2$, an addition compound of urea and hydrogen peroxide which yields H_2O_2 with water.

hyperoncosis (hi·per·ong·**ko**′·sis). The state of being excessively swollen, as that of a tumour. [Gk *hyper*, *ogkos* a swelling.]

hyperonychia, hyperonychosis (hi·per·on·**ik**′·e·ah, hi·per·on·ik·**o**′·sis). Hypertrophy of the nails. [Gk *hyper*, *onyx* nail, *-osis* condition.]

hyperope (hi·per·ope). Hypermetrope.

hyperopia (hi·per·o·pe·ah). Hypermetropia.

hyperopic (hi·per·o·pik). Hypermetropic.

hyperorchidism (hi·per·**or**·kid·izm). Excessive activity of the endocrine function of the testes. [Gk *hyper*, *orchis* testis.]

hyperorexia (hi·per·o·**rex**′·e·ah). Bulimia. [Gk *hyper*, *orexis* appetite.]

hyperorthocytosis (hi·per·**or**·tho·si·**to**′·sis). A general hyperleucocytosis affecting all types of leucocytes and without disturbance of the normal ratio among the various categories of leucocyte; the differential count is normal. [Gk *hyper*, *orthos* exact, *kytos* cell.]

hyperosmia (hi·per·**oz**·me·ah). Abnormal acuteness of the sense of smell; sensitiveness to odour of such degree that it amounts to morbidity. [Gk *hyper*, *osme* odour.]

hyperosmotic (hi·per·oz·**mot**·ik). 1. Relating to increased osmosis. 2. Caused by or producing extremely rapid osmosis. [Gk *hyper*, osmosis.]

hyperosphresia, hyperosphresis (hi·per·os·**fre**′·ze·ah, hi·per·os·**fre**′·sis). Hyperosmia. [Gk *hyper*, *osphresis* sense of smell.]

hyperosteogeny (hi·per·os·te·**oj**′·en·e). Overgrowth of bone. [Gk *hyper*, *osteon* bone, *genein* to produce.]

hyperosteopathy (hi·per·os·te·**op**′·ath·e). Widespread and advanced disease of a bone or bones. [Gk *hyper*, *osteon* bone, *pathos* disease.]

hyperostosis (hi·per·os·**to**′·sis). Exostosis; an overgrowth of bone. **Hyperostosis frontalis interna.** A common variety of osteoma, often multiple, arising from the inner surface of the frontal bone. **Infantile cortical hyperostosis.** A benign syndrome in infants consisting in bony swellings, especially of the mandible, which radiographically appear to be subperiosteal new bone. The involved parts are tender and the child is irritable and pyrexial. The condition is familial and possibly an autosomal dominant. Syn. Caffey's disease. [Gk *hyper*, *osteon* bone, *-osis* condition.]

See also: MORGAGNI.

hyperostotic (hi·per·os·**tot**′·ik). Having relation or belonging to hyperostosis.

hyperovaria, hyperovarianism (hi·per·o·**va**′·re·ah, hi·per·o·**va**′·re·an·izm). A condition affecting young girls, in which overdevelopment of the ovaries leads to excessive secretion and therefore to sexual precocity. [Gk *hyper*, ovary.]

hyperoxaemia (hi·per·ox·**e**′·me·ah). Extreme acidity of the blood. [Gk *hyper*, *oxys* sour, *haima* blood.]

hyperoxia (hi·per·**ox**·e·ah). The condition in which there is too much oxygen in the body.[Gk *hyper*, oxygen.]

hyperoxidation (hi·per·ox·id·**a**′·shun). Over-oxidation; the presence of more than the normal amount of oxygen. [Gk *hyper*, oxidation.]

hyperoxygenation (hi·per·ox·e·jen·**a**′·shun). Excess of dissolved or combined oxygen, e.g. in blood, as a result of hyperventilation. [Gk *hyper*, oxygenation.]

hyperpallaesthesia (hi·per·pal·es·**the**′·ze·ah). Increased perception of vibration. [Gk *hyper*, pallaesthesia.]

hyperparasite (hi·per·**par**·ah·site). A parasite parasitic in or on another parasite. **Second-degree hyperparasite.** A parasite living on or in a hyperparasite. [Gk *hyper*, parasite.]

hyperparasitism (hi·per·**par**·ah·sit·izm). Infestation of a parasite by another parasite. [see prec.]

hyperparathyroidism (hi·per·par·ah·**thi**′·roid·izm). Abnormally increased activity of the parathyroid glands due to a neoplasm or to hyperplasia. The main signs are raised calcium secretion, bending of long bones and deformity of the jaw; there are also gastro-intestinal symptoms and polyuria. [Gk *hyper*, parathyroid.]

hyperparotidism (hi·per·par·**ot**′·id·izm). The condition resulting from extreme activity of the parotid gland. [Gk *hyper*, parotid gland.]

hyperpathia (hi·per·**path**·e·ah). 1. Excessive sensory sensibility. 2. A condition of extreme illness. [Gk *hyper*, *pathos* suffering.]

hyperpepsia (hi·per·**pep**·se·ah). 1. Dyspepsia marked by the presence of an excessive amount of chlorides in the gastric juice although the amount of free hydrochloric acid is normal. 2. Term applied to abnormally rapid digestion. [Gk *hyper*, *pepsis* digestion.]

hyperpepsinia (hi·per·pep·**sin**′·e·ah). Secretion in the stomach of an abnormally large amount of pepsin. [Gk *hyper*, pepsin.]

hyperperistalsis (hi·per·per·is·**tal**′·sis). Exaggerated muscular spasm of the stomach causing discomfort on account of the persistent rapid contractions after food has been ingested. [Gk *hyper*, peristalsis.]

hyperpermeability (hi·per·per·me·ab·**il**′·it·e). Abnormal permeability. [Gk *hyper*, permeability.]

hyperpexia, hyperpexis, hyperpexy (hi·per·**pex**·e·ah, hi·per·**pex**·is, hi·per·**pex**·e). The fixation on the part of a tissue of an excessively large amount of any particular substance. [Gk *hyper*, *pexis* fixation.]

hyperphagia (hi·per·**fa**·je·ah). Overeating, gluttony. [Gk *hyper*, *phagein* to eat.]

hyperphalangia (hi·per·fal·**an**′·je·ah). The condition in which one or more phalanges on a finger or toe are of more than usual length. [Gk *hyper*, phalanges.]

hyperphalangism (hi·per·fal·**an**′·jizm). The condition of having more than the usual number of phalanges on a finger or toe. [see prec.]

hyperphasia (hi·per·**fa**·ze·ah). Hyperlogia. [Gk *hyper*, *phasis* speech.]

hyperphlebosis (hi·per·fleb·**o**′·sis). Hypervenosity. [Gk *hyper*, *phlebe* vein.]

hyperphlogosis (hi·per·flo·**go**′·sis). A condition of acute or violent inflammation. [Gk *hyper*, phlogosis.]

hyperphonesis (hi·per·fo·**ne**′·sis). Increased percussion sound, or increased intensity of the voice sound in auscultation. [Gk *hyper*, *phone* voice.]

hyperphonia (hi·per·**fo**·ne·ah). 1. Explosive energy in utterance, such as that which characterizes stuttering. 2. The stuttering or stammering which is the result of extreme irritability of the vocal muscles. [Gk *hyper*, *phone* voice.]

hyperphoria (hi·per·**for**·e·ah). A type of heterophoria in which the visual axis of one eye tends to deviate above that of the other eye. [Gk *hyper*, *pherein* to bear.]

hyperphoric (hi·per·**for**·ik). Relating or belonging to hyperphoria.

hyperphosphataemia (hi·per·fos·fat·**e**′·me·ah). Hyperphosphoraemia.

hyperphosphaturia (hi·per·fos·fat·**ewr**′·e·ah). A condition in which the urine shows an extremely high percentage of phosphates. [Gk *hyper*, phosphaturia.]

hyperphrasia (hi·per·**fra**·ze·ah). The incoherent and over-stressed vocal sounds produced in certain forms of insanity. [Gk *hyper*, *phrasein* to utter.]

hyperphrenia (hi·per·**fre**·ne·ah). 1. Hypernoea. 2. A state of extreme mental excitement or exaltation, such as occurs in insanity. [Gk *hyper*, *phren* mind.]

hyperpiesia (hi·per·pi·**e**′·ze·ah). Essential arterial hypertension. [Gk *hyper*, *piesis* pressure.]

hyperpiesis (hi·per·pi·**e**′·sis). A condition of abnormally high pressure, especially of the blood. [see prec.]

hyperpietic (hi·per·pi·**et**′·ik). Relating or belonging to hyperpiesia.

hyperpigmentation (hi·per·pig·men·**ta**′·shun). Superpigmentation; excess of pigment in tissue. [Gk *hyper*, pigmentation.]

hyperpinealism (hi·per·**pin**·e·al·izm). Excessive activity of the pineal body. [Gk *hyper*, pineal body.]

hyperpituitarism (hi·per·pit·**ew**′·it·ar·izm). Over-activity of the pituitary gland. The term is invariably used to imply over-activity of the anterior part of the gland. **Basophilic hyperpituitarism.** Over-activity of the basophilic cells of the anterior pituitary gland, such as occurs in Cushing's syndrome; pituitary basophilism. **Eosinophilic hyperpituitarism.** Over-activity of the eosinophil cells of the anterior pituitary gland, such as occurs in gigantism and acromegaly. [Gk *hyper*, pituitary.]

hyperplasia (hi·per·**pla**·ze·ah). Any condition in which there is an increase in the number of cells in a part. **Cementum hyperplasia.** An over-development of the bone which forms in the dental follicle over the root of the tooth. **Dysgenetic epithelial hyperplasia.** A term used by Cheatle for the precancerous condition of epitheliosis of the breast. **Fibromuscular hyperplasia.** Hyperplasia of fibrous and muscular tissue; one of the causes of narrowing of the renal artery. **Focal epithelial hyperplasia.** A familial condition characterized by nodular areas of epithelial hyperplasia of the oral mucosa. **Inflammatory hyperplasia.** The cell infiltration typical of inflammation. **Irritation hyperplasia.** Chronic inflammation of the gums with excessive collagen formation, caused by ill-fitting dentures. **Lipoid-cell hyperplasia.** An increase in lipoid-containing cells. **Neoplastic hyperplasia.** Neoplasia; abnormal increase in cells of a tissue, typical of a tumour. **Pseudo-epitheliomatous hyperplasia.** Benign, persistent hyperplasia of the epidermis, clinically and histologically resembling squamous epithelioma, and caused by chronic inflammation in the underlying dermis. **Swiss-cheese hyperplasia.** Adenomyosis of the uterus. [Gk *hyper, plassein* to form.]

hyperplastic (hi·per·**plas**·tik). Relating or belonging to or marked by hyperplasia.

hyperplerosis (hi·per·pler·**o**′·sis). Excessive fullness. [Gk *hyper, plerosis* filling.]

hyperploid (hi·per·ploid). A chromosome complement cell or organism with 1 or more extra chromosomes or chromosome centric fragments. According to the ploidy one can distinguish beween hyperhaploid, hyperdiploid, hypertriploid, hypertetraploid and so on. [Gk *hyper, eidos* form.]

hyperploidy (hi·per·**ploid**·e). The state of hyperploids.

hyperpnoea (hi·per·**pne**·ah). Overbreathing, hyperventilation. [Gk *hyper, pnoe* a blowing.]

hyperpolarization (hi·per·po·lar·i·**za**′·shun). The development of a transmembrane potential greater than the normal resting potential; it can be induced in cardiac muscle by the effects of catecholamines. [Gk *hyper*, L *polus* pole.]

hyperpolypeptidaemia (hi·per·pol·e·pep·tid·**e**′·me·ah). Excess of polypeptides in the blood. [Gk *hyper*, polypeptide, Gk *haima* blood.]

hyperporosis (hi·per·pr·**o**′·sis). The formation of bone callus in excess. [Gk *hyper, poros* callus.]

hyperpotassaemia (hi·per·pot·as·**e**′·me·ah). Excess of potassium in the blood. [Gk *hyper*, potassium, Gk *haima* blood.]

hyperpragia (hi·per·**pra**·je·ah). Hyperpraxia.

hyperpragic (hi·per·**pra**·jik). Referring or belonging to, or characterized by hyperpraxia.

hyperpraxia (hi·per·**prax**·e·ah). In psychiatry, a condition of extreme mental activity characterized by great restlessness, as in the manic phase of manic-depressive insanity. [Gk *hyper, praxis* action.]

hyperpresbyopia (hi·per·prez·be·**o**′·e·ah). Hypermetropia as associated with the presbyopic state. [Gk *hyper*, presbyopia.]

hyperprochoresis (hi·per·pro·kor·**e**′·sis). Any abnormal increase in motor propulsive function, but generally of the gastrointestinal tract. [Gk *hyper, pro, choreia* a dancing.]

hyperprosexia (hi·per·pro·**sex**′·e·ah). Mental disorder in which the whole attention is occupied by and the entire mind concentrated on one idea or mental process. [Gk *hyper, prosexein* to heed.]

hyperproteinaemia (hi·pe·pro·te·in·**e**′·me·ah). Excess of protein in the blood plasma. [Gk *hyper*, protein, Gk *haima* blood.]

hyperproteosis (hi·per·pro·te·**o**′·sis). The bodily condition resulting from a diet in which there is an excessive amount of protein. [Gk *hyper*, protein, Gk *-osis* condition.]

hyperpselaphesia (hi·per·sel·af·**e**′·ze·ah). Excessive development of the sense of touch; abnormal sensitivity to touch. [Gk *hyper, pselaphema* touch.]

hyperpsychosis (hi·per·si·**ko**′·sis). Abnormal mental activity resulting in a rapid flow of ideas. [Gk *hyper, psyche* mind, *-osis* condition.]

hyperpyretic (hi·per·pi·**ret**′·ik). Relating to or affected with hyperpyrexia.

hyperpyrexia (hi·per·pi·**rex**′·e·ah). 1. Body temperature of extremely high degree, generally 41°C (106°F) or over. 2. A degree of body temperature abnormally high for any given disease. **Heat hyperpyrexia.** Hyperpyrexia leading to convulsions and coma, due to exposure to great heat especially in a humid atmosphere. **Malignant hyperpyrexia.** A serious condition associated with general anaesthesia in which there is greatly increased formation of heat from abnormal muscle metabolism. [Gk *hyper*, pyrexia.]

hyperpyrexial (hi·per·pi·**rex**′·e·al). Relating to hyperpyrexia.

hyper-reflexia (hi·per·re·**flex**′·e·ah). A condition in which reflexes are unduly exaggerated. [Gk *hyper*, reflex.]

hyper-resonance (hi·per·**rez**·on·ans). Increase of resonance elicited by percussion. [Gk *hyper*, resonance.]

hyper-rhinencephalia (hi·per·ri·nen·kef·**a**′·le·ah). Congenital deformity consisting in marked prominence of the frontal lobes of the cerebrum and excessive development of the olfactory bulbs. [Gk *hyper, rhis* nose, *egkephalos* brain.]

hyper-rhinolalia (hi·per·ri·no·**la**′·le·ah). *See* VOICE, NASAL. [Gk *hyper, rhis* nose, *lalein* to speak.]

hyper-rhinoplaty (hi·per·**ri**·no·plat·e). Deformity consisting in marked breadth of the nose. There may be, in association, hypertrophy of the nasal bone. **Interocular hyper-rhinoplaty.** Ocular hypertelorism. *See* HYPERTELORISM. [Gk *hyper, rhis* nose, *platys* broad.]

hypersalaemia (hi·per·sal·**e**′·me·ah). A condition in which the salt content of the blood is increased. [Gk *hyper*, L *sal* salt, Gk *haima* blood.]

hypersaline (hi·per·**sa**·line). Applied to treatment, term indicating the use of large quantities of sodium chloride. [Gk *hyper*, saline.]

hypersalivation (hi·per·sal·iv·**a**′·shun). Excessive secretion of saliva. [Gk *hyper*, salivation.]

hypersarcosis (hi·per·sar·**ko**′·sis). 1. Hypertrophy. 2. The formation of excess of granulation tissue. 3. Obesity. [Gk *hyper*, sarcosis.]

hypersecretion (hi·per·se·**kre**′·shun). Secretion greatly in excess of the normal. **Gastric hypersecretion.** Hyperchlorhydria. [Gk *hyper*, secretion.]

hypersensibility (hi·per·sen·sib·**il**′·it·e). 1. Anaphylaxis. 2. Hyperaesthesia. [Gk *hyper*, sensibility.]

hypersensitive (hi·per·**sen**·sit·iv). Abnormally sensitive; term applied to subjects who when exposed, superficially or otherwise, to particular allergens, react to an amount too small to evoke any response in persons of normal sensitivity. [Gk *hyper*, sensitivity.]

hypersensitivity (hi·per·sen·sit·**iv**′·it·e). 1. A state of abnormally strong responsiveness to the action of any external agent. 2. An immunological term used to describe excessive host reaction resulting from a dose of an antigen, e.g. foreign protein (horse-serum, etc.), or pathogenic bacteria, or their products, when the host's tissues have already been sensitized from previous injection or infection by these antigens. The reaction may be *immediate* (*see* ANAPHYLAXIS (Syn. Arthus' reaction)) or *delayed* when it represents a cell-mediated response as in the tuberculin test. Hypersensitivity reactions are characterized by tissue damage. They have been divided into 4 types by Gell and Coombs as follows: Type I reactions—anaphylaxis, immediate hypersensitivity mediated by IgE antibody; Type II reactions—allergic cytotoxicity mediated by cytotoxic or cytolytic antibody; Type III reactions—mediated by immune complexes; Type IV or delayed reactions—mediated by primed lymphocytes. [Gk *hyper*, L *sentire* to feel.]

hypersensitization (hi·per·**sen**·sit·i·**za**′·shun). 1. The condition of reacting in an abnormally sensitive degree. 2. The process of producing a state of abnormal sensitivity as in a laboratory animal. [Gk *hyper*, sensitivity.]

hypersialosis (hi·per·si·al·**o**′·sis). Hypersalivation. [Gk *hyper, sialon* saliva.]

hyperskeocytosis (hi·per·**ske**·o·si·**to**′·sis). Hyperneocytosis. [Gk *hyper, skaios* left, *kytos* cell.]

hypersomia (hi·per·**so**·me·ah). Gigantism. [Gk *hyper, soma* body.]

hypersomnia (hi·per·**som**·ne·ah). A pathological condition in which periods of excessively long-lasting sleep occur, with normal hours of sleep in the intervening periods. [Gk *hyper*, L *somnus* sleep.]

hypersomy (hi·per·**so**·me). The state of a cell or organism having an excessive number of either 1 or a few chromosomes. [Gk *hyper, soma* body.]

hypersphyxia (hi·per·**sfix**·e·ah). A condition in which there is increased blood pressure and circulatory activity greater than normal. [Gk *hyper, sphyxis* pulse.]

hypersplenia, hypersplenism (hi·per·**sple**·ne·ah, hi·per·**sple**·nizm). A condition in which there is greatly increased haemolytic action of the spleen: more especially a blood condition characterized by splenomegaly. a refractory anaemia, leucopenia and thrombocytopenia, in spite of an active, often hyperplastic, bone marrow; there is usually poor response to treatment. [Gk *hyper*, spleen.]

hypersplenotrophy (**hi**·per·splen·**ot**'·ro·fe). Splenomeagaly. [Gk *hyper*, spleen, Gk *trophe* nourishment.]

hypersteatosis (**hi**·per·ste·at·**o**'·sis). A condition in which there is marked increase in the secretion of the sebaceous glands. [Gk *hyper*, *stear* fat, *-osis* condition.]

hyperstereoroentgenography (hi·per·**steer**·e·o·runt·yen·**og**'·raf·e). Hyperstereoskiagraphy. [Gk *hyper*, stereoroentgenography.]

hyperstereoskiagraphy (hi·per·**steer**·e·o·ski·**ag**'·raf·e). Stereoskiagraphy with wider than normal separation between the 2 points from which the rays are projected, so that a better perspective is obtained in the stereogram. [Gk *hyper*, stereoskiagraphy.]

hypersthenia (hi·per·**sthe**·ne·ah). A condition of excessive or unusual tone or strength of the body or of any part of it. [Gk *hyper*, *sthenos* strength.]

hypersthenic (hi·per·**sthen**·ik). Relating or belonging to or characterized by hypersthenia.

hypersthenuria (**hi**·per·sthen·**ewr**'·e·ah). The passing of a highly concentrated urine with a raised specific gravity as a result of restriction of fluid intake, or fluid loss from perspiration, etc. [Gk *hyper*, *sthenos* strength, urine.]

hypersusceptibility (**hi**·per·sus·sep·tib·**il**'·it·e). 1. A condition in which the subject falls a ready prey to infection or poisons. 2. The state of allergy. 3. Anaphylaxis. [Gk *hyper*, susceptibility.]

hypersympathicotonus (**hi**·per·sim·**path**·ik·o·**to**'·nus). A condition marked by increased tone of the sympathetic nervous system. [Gk *hyper*, sympathetic, Gk *tonos* tone.]

hypersynchrony (hi·per·**sin**·kron·e). In electro-encephalography, a discharge, usually paroxysmal, of high-amplitude waves of any frequency. [Gk *hyper*, *synchronein* to be in time with.]

hypersystole (hi·per·**sis**·to·le). A state of extreme contraction during the systolic phase of the cardiac cycle. [Gk *hyper*, systole.]

hypersystolic (**hi**·per·sis·**tol**'·ik). 1. Relating or belonging to hypersystole. 2. An individual who has excessivly strong contractions of the heart.

hypertarachia (hi·per·tar·**ak**'·e·ah). A condition marked by exaggerated irritability of the nervous system. [Gk *hyper*, *tarache* tumult.]

hypertelorism (hi·per·**tel**·or·izm). A condition marked by abnormal width between the 2 members of a pair of organs or parts. **Ocular hypertelorism.** A developmental congenital deformity in which the lesser wings of the sphenoid bone are greatly enlarged so that there is excessive breadth of the bridge of the nose and immoderate width between the orbits of the eyes. There may be associated mental deficiency and optic atrophy, divergent squint and exophthalmos. [Gk *hyper*, *tele* far, *horizo* to separate.]

See also: GREIG.

hypertensin (hi·per·**ten**·sin). Angiotensin. [Gk *hyper*, tension.]

hypertensinogen (hi·per·ten·**sin**'·o·jen). Angiotensinogen. [Gk *hyper*, tension, Gk *genein* to produce.]

hypertension (hi·per·**ten**·shun). High arterial blood pressure. **Adrenal hypertension.** Hypertension of adrenal origin. **Benign hypertension.** High blood pressure of whatever cause, with a relatively benign prognosis; the term is used to distinguish other degrees of hypertension from *malignant hypertension* (see below). **Climacteric hypertension.** Hypertension developing during the climacteric, which may disappear spontaneously after a variable period or become permanent. **Episodic hypertension.** Paroxysmal hypertension (see below). **Essential hypertension.** Hypertension which cannot be shown to be secondary to other pathological conditions, such as renal disease; this is the commonest type of hypertension. **Idiopathic arterial hypertension.** Essential hypertension (see above). **Labile hypertension.** Hypertension, usually of relatively mild degree, which shows great variation in the level of pressure measured at different times. **Malignant hypertension.** Severe hypertension of whatever cause, with a very bad prognosis, characterized by optic papilloedema with retinal haemorrhages and exudates, and progressive impairment of renal function. **Neuromuscular hypertension.** Excessive reflex response. **Paroxysmal hypertension.** Paroxysmal attacks of hypertension associated with pallor, palpitation, nausea, vomiting, headache and other symptoms; during an attack the systolic blood pressure may rise to as much as 30 mmHg. They are caused by the excessive secretion of adrenaline by a phaeochromocytoma of the medulla of the suprarenal gland. **Pituitary hypertension.** High blood pressure associated with basophil adenomata of the pituitary (Cushing's syndrome). **Pregnancy hypertension.** High blood pressure occurring in the toxaemia of pregnancy (eclampsia). **Pulmonary hypertension.** Increased blood pressure in the pulmonary arteries, usually secondary to diseases of the lungs such as emphysema or fibrosis, or to mitral stenosis. **Renal hypertension.** Hypertension accompanied by renal artery abnormality. Ischaemia and hypertension may follow when there is greater diminution of blood supply than there is of functioning renal parenchyma. **Saturnine hypertension.** Hypertension due to lead poisoning especially in children and young persons, associated with lead encephalopathy. **Suprarenal hypertension.** Paroxysms of hypertension occurring with tumours of the chromaffin cells of the medulla of the suprarenal gland (phaeochromocytomata) due to the release of large quantities of adrenaline. [Gk *hyper*, L *tendere* to stretch.]

See also: GOLDBLATT.

hypertensive (hi·per·**ten**·siv). Marked by increase in blood pressure or causing such an increase. [see prec.]

hypertensor (hi·per·**ten**·sor). Anything which produces a rise of blood pressure. [Gk *hyper*, L *tendere* to stretch.]

hypertetraploid (hi·per·**tet**·rah·ploid). *See* HYPERPLOID. [Gk *hyper*, *tetraploos* fourfold, *eidos* form.]

hyperthelia (hi·per·**the**·le·ah). The state of having supernumerary nipples, generally bilaterally. [Gk *hyper*, *thele* nipple.]

hyperthermal (hi·per·**ther**·mal). Relating or belonging to or characterized by hyperthermia.

hyperthermia (hi·per·**ther**·me·ah). Very high body temperature. **Malignant hyperthermia.** A serious and apparently increasing complication of modern anaesthesia, in which there is greatly increased heat formation from abnormal muscle metabolism, usually associated with the use of either halothane or suxamethonium, in patients with a hereditary abnormality. [Gk *hyper*, *therme* heat.]

hyperthermo-aesthesia (hi·per·**ther**·mo·es·**the**'·ze·ah). Increased sensitivity to heat. [Gk *hyper*, *therme* heat, *aisthesis* sensation.]

hyperthermo-algesia (**hi**·per·ther·mo·al·**je**'·ze·ah). A condition in which sensitiveness to heat is so extreme that even slight heat causes pain. [Gk *hyper*, *therme* heat, algesia.]

hyperthermy (hi·per·**ther**·me). Hyperthermia. [Gk *hyper*, *therme* heat.]

hyperthrombinaemia (**hi**·per·throm·bin·**e**'·me·ah). An abnormal increase of thrombin in the blood, with resultant tendency to intravascular clotting. [Gk *hyper*, thrombin. Gk *haima* blood.]

hyperthrombocythaemia (hi·per·**throm**·bo·si·**the**'·me·ah). A condition of the blood marked by the presence of an excessively large number of blood platelets. [Gk *hyper*, *thrombos* clot, *kytos* cell, *haima* blood.]

hyperthymergasia (hi·per·thi·mer·**ga**'·ze·ah). In psychiatry, a term for an overactive state of mind the characteristic signs of which are agitation, elation, excitement and ergasiomania. [Gk *hyper*, *thymos* spirit, *ergasia* work.]

hyperthymia (hi·per·**thi**·me·ah). 1. Excessive emotionalism or mental excitability. 2. A state of morbid over-sensitivity. 3. Foolish venturesomeness or impetuous cruelty regarded as symptom of disease of the mind. [Gk *hyper*, *thymos* spirit, passion.]

hyperthymic (hi·per·**thi**·mik). Relating or belonging to hyperthymia.

hyperthymism, hyperthymization (hi·per·**thi**·mizm, **hi**·per·thi·mi·**za**'·shun). A toxaemic condition produced by excessive activity of the thymus gland. [Gk *hyper*, thymus gland.]

hyperthyroid (hi·per·**thi**·roid). Caused or characterized by hyperthyroidism.

hyperthyroidism, hyperthyroidosis (hi·per·**thi**·roi·dizm, **hi**·per·thi·roi·**do**′·sis). A condition caused by over-activity of the thyroid gland, e.g. exophthalmic goitre or toxic adenoma. **Masked hyperthyroidism.** Hyperthyroidism the presenting feature of which appears to indicate a different disease, e.g. heart disease. [Gk *hyper*, thyroid gland.]

hyperthyroxinaemia (**hi**·per·thi·rox·in·**e**′·me·ah). The condition resulting from an excess of thyroxine in the blood. [Gk *hyper*, thyroxine, Gk *haima* blood.]

hypertonia (hi·per·**to**·ne·ah). 1. Excessive tension, as of arteries or muscles. 2. Excessive activity, as of muscles. 3. A state of increased intra-ocular tension. **Hypertonia polycythaemica.** Polycythaemia with increase of blood pressure. [Gk *hyper*, *tonos* tone.]

hypertonic (hi·per·**ton**·ik). 1. Showing excessive tension; relating or belonging to hypertonia. 2. A saline solution of strength above normal; describing a solution with an osmotic pressure greater than that of an isotonic solution. 3. One affected with hypertonia. [see prec.]

hypertonicity, hypertonus (**hi**·per·ton·**is**′·it·e, hi·per·**to**·nus). Hypertonia.

hypertoxic (hi·per·**tox**·ik). Extremely poisonous. [Gk *hyper*, toxic.]

hypertoxicity (**hi**·per·tox·**is**′·it·e). The condition or quality of being extremely poisonous. [Gk *hyper*, toxicity.]

hypertrichiasis (**hi**·per·trik·**i**′·as·is). Hypertrichosis.

hypertrichophobia (hi·per·trik·o·**fo**′·be·ah). The morbidly worried state which affects those suffering from hypertrichosis. [Gk *hyper*, trichophobia.]

hypertrichophrydia (**hi**·per·trik·o·**frid**′·e·ah). Growth of the eyebrows to excessive length. [Gk *hyper*, *thrix* hair, *ophrys* eyebrow.]

hypertrichosis (**hi**·per·trik·**o**′·sis). An excessive growth of hair on the body or on a part of the body, particularly that occurring on surfaces covered usually with lanugo hairs, e.g. the face in women. **Circumscribed acquired hypertrichosis.** Localized overgrowth of the hair secondary to chronic or repeated trauma, or due to persistent hyperaemia. **Idiopathic hypertrichosis.** Hypertrichosis of unknown origin. **Hypertrichosis lanuginosa.** Excessive growth of lanugo. **Naevoid hypertrichosis.** Excessive growth of hair in a naevus, e.g. pigmented fleshy mole. **Hypertrichosis partialis.** Patchy growth of hair on a normally hairless part, as the back. **Hypertrichosis universalis.** Hairiness affecting the whole of the body and all limbs. [Gk *hyper*, trichosis.]

hypertriploid (hi·per·**tri**·ploid). *See* HYPERPLOID. [Gk *hyper*, *triploos* triple, *eidos* form.]

hypertrophia (hi·per·**tro**·fe·ah). Hypertrophy. **Hypertrophia musculorum vera.** A condition of generalized muscular hypertrophy with normal or increased strength.

hypertrophic (hi·per·**trof**·ik). Relating or belonging to or marked by hypertrophy.

hypertrophy (hi·**per**·tro·fe). An increase in the number or size of the cells of which a tissue is composed as the result of increase in function of that tissue. **Adaptive hypertrophy.** An increase in the amount of tissue consequent upon loss of a similar or allied tissue, the idea being that this process is a compensation for an impairment of function. **Cardiac hypertrophy.** Enlargement of the heart muscle as the result of more work being thrown upon it. **Cicatricial hypertrophy.** Enlargement of a tissue or organ because of increase of its fibrous tissue support. **Compensatory hypertrophy.** Adaptive hypertrophy (see above). **False hypertrophy.** Hyperplasia. **Functional hypertrophy.** Adaptive hypertrophy (see above). **Haemangiectatic hypertrophy.** Haemangiomatous and, often, lymphangiomatous hyperplasia of a limb, with varicosities and diffuse hypertrophy of the affected limb. **Numerical hypertrophy.** Hyperplasia. **Physiological hypertrophy.** Adaptive hypertrophy (see above). **Pseudomuscular hypertrophy.** Fatty infiltration of a muscle, with atrophy of the fibres but gross enlargement of the muscle as a whole. **Simple hypertrophy, True hypertrophy.** Adaptive hypertrophy (see above). **Ventricular hypertrophy.** Enlargement of the heart muscle of the ventricles as the result of valvular disease or hypertension. [Gk *hyper*, *trophe* nourishment.]

See also: MARIE.

hypertropia (hi·per·**tro**·pe·ah. Hypermetropia; a term used in the USA.

hyperuresis (**hi**·per·ewr·**e**′·sis). 1. Polyuria. 2. Enuresis. [Gk *hyper*, uresis.]

hyperuricacidaemia (**hi**·per·**ewr**·ik·as·id·**e**′·me·ah). Hyperuricaemia.

hyperuricaciduria (**hi**·per·**ewr**·ik·as·id·**ewr**′·e·ah). Hyperuricuria.

hyperuricaemia (**hi**·per·ewr·ik·**e**′·me·ah). The presence in the blood of an excessive amount of uric acid. [Gk *hyper*, uric acid, Gk *haima* blood.]

hyperuricuria (**hi**·per·ewr·ik·**ewr**′·e·ah). The presence in urine of an excessively large amount of uric acid. [Gk *hyper*, uric acid, urine.]

hypervaccination (**hi**·per·vak·sin·**a**′·shun). 1. A subsequent inoculation or inoculations of a person already immunized. 2. Repeated inoculations of an immunized animal for the purpose of obtaining a potent antitoxin. [Gk *hyper*, vaccination.]

hypervascular (hi·per·**vas**·kew·lar). Applied to any part that contains an abnormally large number of blood vessels. [Gk *hyper*, vascular.]

hypervenosity (**hi**·per·ven·**os**′·it·e). 1. The condition in which the venous system is excessively developed. 2. A state of the blood in which it has become abnormally venous in character. [Gk *hyper*, venosity.]

hyperventilation (**hi**·per·ven·til·**a**′·shun). Increased pulmonary ventilation which usually leads to hypocapnia. It may be associated with dizziness and tetany if severe. [Gk *hyper*, L *ventilare* to wave.]

hyperviscosity (hi·per·vis·**kos**′it·e). An exaggeratedly viscous condition, e.g. of the blood. [Gk *hyper*, viscosity.]

hypervitaminosis (**hi**·per·vi·tam·in·**o**′·sis). The bodily condition resulting from an excess of synthetic vitamins in the diet or when these are administered as therapeutic agents. The symptoms vary according to the particular vitamin in question; excess of vitamin D, for instance, causes hypercalcaemia. **Hypervitaminosis A.** Lethargy, dry rough skin, patchy pigmentation, follicular keratoses, diffuse alopecia, purpura, bone and joint pains, hepatomegaly; in extreme cases, headache, vomiting and papilloedema. [Gk *hyper*, vitaminosis.]

hypervitaminotic (**hi**·per·vi·tam·in·**ot**′·ik). 1. Relating to or arising from too free ingestion of a vitamin or vitamins. 2. Characterized by hypervitaminosis. [see prec.]

hypervolaemia (**hi**·per·vol·**e**′·me·ah). Plethora. [Gk *hyper*, volume, Gk *haima* blood.]

hypha (**hi**·fah) (pl. *hyphae*). One of the thread-like elements of the mycelium of a fungus. **Aerial hyphae.** Those hyphae which occur above the mycelial mat on the surface of the substratum on which the fungus is growing. The organs of vegetative reproduction are usually produced on aerial hyphae. **Non-septate hypha.** A filamentous, vegetative element of certain fungi, which is not divided by transverse septa or cross walls, so that the protoplasmatic contents of the whole hypha are continuous and multinuclear. It is found in the vegetative mycelium of the class of Phycomycetes among the fungi, and in the Algae. **Septate hypha.** A filamentous fungal element (thallus) which is divided by transverse septa or cross walls into a series of separate cells which may be uninuclear or multinuclear. [Gk *hyphe* web.]

hyphaemia (hi·**fe**·me·ah). 1. Oligohaemia. 2. Anaemia. 3. Effusion of blood into the anterior chamber of the eye. **Intertropical hyphaemia, Tropical hyphaemia.** Ancylostomiasis. [Gk *hypo*, *haima* blood.]

hyphal (**hi**·fal). Pertaining to a hypha, the filamentous thallus of a fungus.

hyphedonia (hipe·he·**do**·ne·ah). A morbid mental condition in which pleasure in performing certain acts is very much modified. [Gk *hypo*, *hedone* pleasure.]

hyphidrosis (hipe·hid·**ro**·sis). Hypohidrosis.

hyphology (hi·**fol**·o·je). An alternative name for histology. [Gk *hyphe* web, *logos* science.]

Hyphomyces (hi·fo·**mi**·seez). A genus of fungi of which 1 species, *Hyphomyces destruens*, is known to cause subcutaneous infections in horses and mules. [Gk *hyphe* web, *mykes* fungus.]

Hyphomycetes (hi·fo·mi·**se**′·teez). One of the 3 main groups of Fungi Imperfecti, and the only one of the 3 involved in human pathology. The complete life cycle is not yet known and classification is confused. The ringworm (tinea) and favus fungi, and *Aspergillus*, *Madurella* and *Sporotrichum* genera among others, belong to this group. [Gk *hyphe* web, *mykes* fungus.]

hyphomycetic (hi·fo·mi·**se**′·tik). 1. Relating or belonging to hyphomycetes. 2. Resulting from the presence of mould fungi.

hyphomycetoma (hi·fo·mi·se·**to**′·mah). A subcutaneous tumour caused by infection with *Hyphomyces destruens*. [Gk *hyphe* web, *mykes* fungus, *-oma* tumour.]

hyphomycosis (hi·fo·mi·**ko**′·sis). The disease in horses and mules caused by *Hyphomyces destruens*. [Gk *hyphe* web, *mykes* fungus, *-osis* condition.]

hyphostroma (hi·fo·**stro**·mah). Mycelium. [Gk *hyphe* web, *stroma* mattress.]

hypinosis (hi·pi·**o**·sis). 1. A decrease in the amount of fibrin normally present in blood. 2. Lessened power of coagulability of blood. [Gk *hypo*, *is* fibre, *-osis* condition.]

hypinotic (hi·pin·**ot**·ik). Relating or belonging to, or marked by hypinosis.

hypisotonic (hipe·i·so·**ton**′·ik). A term applied to a solution which is more dilute than an isotonic solution; one with lower osmotic pressure, e.g. a solution of much less than 0.85 per cent sodium chloride (isotonic) in which haemolysis of erythrocytes takes place. Haemolysis usually occurs below 0.4 per cent. [Gk *hypo*, isotonicity.]

hypisotonicity (hipe·i·so·ton·**is**′·it·e). The state of being hypisotonic.

hypnaesthesia (hip·nes·**the**·ze·ah). Drowsiness. [Gk *hypnos* sleep, aesthesia.]

hypnagogic (hip·nag·**oj**·ik). 1. Inducing or producing sleep; hypnotic. 2. Term applied to the visual images or delusions which present themselves during transition from the waking to the sleeping state. [Gk *hypnos* sleep, *agogos* leading.]

hypnagogue (**hip**·nag·og). 1. Hypnotic. 2. Belonging to sleepiness or drowsiness. [see prec.]

hypnal (**hip**·nal). A mixture of chloral and phenazone used as an antipyretic and hypnotic. [Gk *hypnos* sleep.]

hypnalgia (hip·**nal**·je·ah). Pain occurring and recurring during sleep. [Gk *hypnos* sleep, *algos* pain.]

hypnapagogic (**hip**·nap·ag·**oj**′·ik). Causing wakefulness. [Gk *hypnos* sleep, *apo*, *agogos* leading.]

hypnic (**hip**·nik). 1. Hypnotic. 2. Belonging to sleep. [Gk *hypnos* sleep.]

hypno-analysis (**hip**·no·an·**al**′·is·is). A psychotherapeutic technique by which the patient is first put into a hypnotic trance, induced to relate events and describe feelings which might be too painful for discussion in a fully conscious state and is finally provided with therapeutic suggestions. [hypnosis, analysis.]

hypnobat, hypnobate (**hip**·no·bat, **hip**·no·bate). One who walks in his sleep. [Gk *hypnos* sleep, *bainein* to walk.]

hypnobatia (hip·no·**ba**·she·ah). Somnambulism; sleep walking. [see prec.]

hypnocinematograph (**hip**·no·sin·e·**mat**′·o·graf). An apparatus for recording the movements of a sleeper. [Gk *hypnos* sleep, *kinema* movement, *graphein* to record.]

hypnocyst (**hip**·no·sist). 1. A cyst in the non-active phase. 2. In zoology, an encysted resting stage undergone by protozoa, e.g. during times of drought or hibernation. [Gk *hypnos* sleep, cyst.]

hypnogenesis (hip·no·**jen**·es·is). The process of inducing sleep or hypnosis. [Gk *hypnos* sleep, *genein* to produce.]

hypnoid, hypnoidal (**hip**·noid, hip·**noi**·dal). 1. Pertaining to or resembling hypnosis. 2. Having the form or character of the hypnotic state; like sleep. [Gk *hypnos* sleep, *eidos* form.]

hypnoidization (**hip**·noi·di·**za**′·shun). The production of a hypnoidal state.

hypnolepsy (**hip**·no·lep·se). A state of abnormal sleepiness which may amount to morbidity. [Gk *hypnos* sleep, *lepsis* seizure.]

hypnology (hip·**nol**·o·je). That branch of medical science which is concerned with sleep, particularly hypnotic sleep, or with hypnotism. [Gk *hypnos* sleep, *logos* science.]

hypnonarco-analysis (**hip**·no·nar·ko·an·**al**′·is·is). The method of conducting a psychiatric interview when the patient is in a form of hypnotic state following the intravenous injection of a narcotic. [Gk *hypnos* sleep, narcotic, psycho-analysis.]

hypnonarcosis (**hip**·no·nar·**ko**′·sis). Combined light hypnosis and narcosis.

hypnophobia (hip·no·**fo**·be·ah). Morbid fear of sleep. [Gk *hypnos* sleep, phobia.]

hypnophrenosis (**hip**·no·fren·**o**′·sis). Sleep disturbance. [Gk *hypnos* sleep, *phren* mind, *-osis* condition.]

hypnopompic (hip·no·**pom**·pik). Of dreams, visual images that persist into the half-waking state before full awakening occurs, or that are present at the moment of full awakening. [Gk *hypnos* sleep, *pompe* procession.]

hypnosia (hip·**no**·ze·ah). Morbid drowsiness that defies efforts to overcome it. [see foll.]

hypnosis (hip·**no**·sis). 1. The state of being hypnotized and in a condition of suggestibility. 2. The process of inducing sleep. 3. The gradual change over from wakefulness to sleep. [Gk *hypnos* sleep.]

hypnosophy (hip·**nos**·o·fe). The sum of knowledge regarding the phenomena of sleep. [Gk *hypnos* sleep, *sophia* wisdom.]

hypnotherapy (hip·no·**ther**·ap·e). 1. Hypnotism used as a method of treatment. 2. The induction of prolonged sleep as a therapeutic measure. [Gk *hypnos* sleep, therapy.]

hypnotic (hip·**not**·ik). 1. Relating or belonging to hypnotism. 2. Having the character of hypnotism. 3. Any drug or other remedy which has the property of inducing nomal sleep or has an anodyne effect. **Indirect hypnotic.** A remedy which indirectly induces sleep by curing the condition causing the wakefulness.

hypnotism (**hip**·no·tizm). 1. Hypnosis. 2. A technique designed to bring about in the subject an altered state of consciousness and greatly increased suggestibility, most usually for a psychotherapeutic purpose. In a fully-developed hypnotic trance, the subject is aware only of the hypnotist and of his commands, to which he is almost completely responsive, so that he may be imperceptive of other stimuli, even painful ones. Apart from analgesia, other physiological changes, such as alterations of muscular tone, may be produced or abolished at will by the hypnotist. Posthypnotic suggestions may also be given in the trance state, to take effect at a later time. [Gk *hypnos* sleep]

hypnotist (**hip**·no·tist). One who practises hypnotism or makes use of it in treatment.

hypnotization (**hip**·no·ti·**za**′·shun). The process of placing a person in a state of hypnotism.

hypnotize (**hip**·no·tize) To place a person in the state of hypnotism, or to bring him under the influence of hypnotism.

hypnotoid (**hip**·no·toid). 1. Having resemblance to hypnotism. 2. Resulting from hypnotism, e.g. vasomotor changes. [hypnotism, Gk *eidos* form.]

hypnotoxin (hip·no·**tox**·in). A hypothetical soporific substance claimed to be produced by the brain; it is advanced in a chemical theory of sleep. [Gk *hypnos* sleep, toxin.]

hypo-. Prefix from the Greek preposition *hypo*, meaning *under*, *deficient*.

hypo-acidity (hi·po·as·**id**′·it·e). A condition in which acid constituents are deficient. [Gk *hypo*, acidity.]

hypo-activity (hi·po·ak·**tiv**′·it·e). A state of lessened activity. [Gk *hypo*, activity.]

hypo-adenia (hi·po·ad·**e**′·ne·ah). A condition in which there is defective or diminished activity on the part of the glands. [Gk *hypo*, *aden* gland.]

hypo-adrenalaemia (hi·po·ad·re·nal·**e**′·me·ah). The presence in the blood of an abnormally small amount of suprarenal secretion. [Gk *hypo*, adrenal, Gk *haima* blood.]

hypo-adrenalism (**hi**·po·ad·**re'**·nal·izm). Suprarenal deficiency such as occurs in certain infections. [Gk *hypo*, adrenal.]

hypo-adrenocorticism (**hi**·po·ad·re·no·**kor'**·tis·izm). Insufficency of the secretion of the cortex of the suprarenal gland, e.g. Addison's disease. [Gk *hypo*, adrenal cortex.]

hypo-aesthesia (**hi**·po·es·**the'**·ze·ah. Diminished sensibility to touch. [Gk *hypo*, aesthesia.]

hypo-aesthetic (hi·po·es·**thet'**·ik). Relating or belonging to hypo-aesthesia; showing diminished sensibility to touch.

hypo-affective (hi·po·af·**ek'**·tiv). Deficient in emotional reaction. Describing anyone whose power to react to emotional stimulus is abnormally slight. [Gk *hypo*, affect.]

hypo-albuminaemia (hi·po·al·bew·min·**e'**·me·ah). The presence in the blood of an abnormally small quantity of albumin. [Gk *hypo*, albuminaemia.]

hypo-aldosteronism. A clinical condition due to deficiency of aldosterone.

hypo-algesia (hi·po·al·**je'**·ze·ah). Diminished sensibility to pain. [Gk *hypo*, algesia.]

hypo-alimentation (hi·po·al·im·en·**ta'**·shun). The condition resulting from insufficient food or a diet that is inadequate in nourishment. [Gk *hypo*, alimentation.]

hypo-alkaline (hi·po·**al**·kal·ine). Denoting a condition of less alkalinity than is normal. [Gk *hypo*, alkaline.]

hypo-alkalinity (hi·po·al·kal·**in'**·it·e). The state or property of being less alkaline than is normal. [see prec.]

hypo-alonaemia (**hi**·po·al·on·**e'**·me·ah). A deficiency of salts in the blood. [Gk *hypo*, *als* salt, *haima* blood.]

hypo-androgenism (hi·po·**an**·dro·jen·izm). Insufficiency in the secretion of androgen hormone. [Gk *hypo*, androgen.]

hypo-arterial (**hi**·po·ar·**teer'**·e·al). Indicating structures lying beneath an artery, e.g. the branches of the bronchi. [Gk *hypo*, artery.]

hypo-azoturia (**hi**·po·az·o·**tewr'**·e·ah). A condition in which there is less than the normal amount of nitrogenous material in the urine. [Gk *hypo*, azoturia.]

hypobaric (hi·po·**bar**·ik). Describing substances (fluids and gases) which have less density than a standard substance of the same kind. In anaesthetic practice, a hypobaric solution (injected intrathecally) has a specific gravity less than that of cerebrospinal fluid. A hypobaric gas has a density less than that of the atmosphere. [Gk *hypo*, *baros* weight.]

hypobarism (hi·po·**bar**·izm). *See* DYSBARISM. [Gk *hypo*, *baros* weight.]

hypobaropathy (**hi**·po·bar·**op'**·ath·e). Anoxaemia resulting from the low atmospheric pressure prevalent at high altitudes in mountainous areas or in aviation. There are distressing mental, muscular and respiratory effects. [Gk *hypo*, *baros* weight, *pathos* disease.]

hypobilirubinaemia (hi·po·bil·e·roo·bin·**e'**·me·ah). Decrease in the normal blood bilirubin. [Gk *hypo*, bilirubinaemia.]

hypoblast (hi·po·blast). Entoderm. [Gk *hypo*, *blastos* germ.]

hypoblastic (hi·po·**blas**·tik). Entodermal. [see prec.]

hypobromite (hi·po·**bro**·mite). Any salt of hypobromous acid; sodium hypobromite is used in the estimation of urea in urine.

hypobulia (hi·po·**bew**·le·ah). 1. A markedly indecisive mental state. 2. Defective power of will. 3. Lack of power of motor innervation. [Gk *hypo*, *boule* determination.]

hypocalcaemia (hi·po·kal·**se'**·me·ah. Abnormally low calcium content of the blood. [Gk *hypo*, calcium, Gk *haima* blood.]

hypocalcia (hi·po·**kal**·se·ah). A deficiency of calcium in the body. [Gk *hypo*, calcium.]

hypocalcification (hi·po·kal·sif·ik·**a'**·shun). Deficient calcification. [see prec.]

hypocalcipexic (hi·op·kal·se·**pex'**·ik). Pertaining to or characterized by hypocalcipexis.

hypocalcipexis (hi·po·kal·se·**pex'**·is). Deficient fixation of calcium in organic tissue. [Gk *hypo*, calcipexis.]

hypocalciuria (hi·po·kal·se·**u**·**ria**). Diminished quantities of calcium in the urine.

hypocapnia (hi·po·**kap**·ne·ah). A diminished amount of carbon dioxide in the blood. [Gk *hypo*, *kapnos* vapour.]

hypocatharsis (hi·po·kath·**ar'**·sis). Mild purgation. [Gk *hypo*, catharsis.]

hypocathexis (hi·po·kath·**ex'**·is). A diminished concentration of psychic energy directed towards an object. [Gk *hypo*, *kathexis* retention.]

hypochloraemia (hi·po·klor·**e'**·me·ah). The condition in which the chloride content of the blood is lowered. [Gk *hyo*, chloride, Gk *haima* blood.]

hypochloraemic (hi·po·klor·e'·mik). Relating or belonging to, or marked by hypochloraemia.

hypochlorhydria (hi·po·klor·**hi'**·dre·ah). A condition in which there is abnormal decrease in the secretion of hydrochloric acid by the stomach. [Gk *hypo*, hydrochloric acid.]

hypochloridaemia (hi·po·klor·id·**e'**·me·ah). Hypochloraemia.

hypochloridation (hi·po·klor·id·**a'**·shun). Systemic deficiency of chloride. [Gk *hypo*, chloride.]

hypochlorite (hi·po·**klor**·ite). Any salt of hypochlorous acid. Many hypochlorites are used as disinfectants and antiseptics.

hypochlorization (hi·po·klor·i·**za'**·shun). The giving of half the normal quantity of sodium chloride in the diet as a therapeutic measure, e.g. in Bright's disease. [Gk *hypo*, chloride.]

hypochloruria (hi·po·klor·**ewr'**·e·ah). The presence of an abnormally small amount of chlorides in the urine. [Gk *hypo*, chloride, urine.]

hypocholesterolaemia (hi·po·ko·**les**·ter·ol·**e'**·me·ah). Lowering of the cholesterol content of the blood. [Gk *hypo*, cholesterol, Gk *haima* blood.]

hypocholia (hi·po·**ko**·le·ah). Deficiency or lack in the secretion of bile. [Gk *hypo*, *chole* bile.]

hypochondria (hi·po·**kon**·dre·ah). A state of mind in which the sufferer is so preoccupied with his health or with symptoms of ill-health that this preoccupation is itself a disability. The term is most commonly employed when no physical cause for the symptoms can be discovered. [Hypochondrium, the region to which such anxiety is commonly referred.]

hypochondriac (hi·po·**kon**·dre·ak). 1. Anyone suffering from hypochondria. 2. Relating or belonging to the hypochondrium.

hypochondriacal (hi·po·kon·**dri'**·ak·al). 1. Affected with or relating or belonging to hypochondria. 2. Relating or belonging to the hypochondrium.

hypochondriasis (hi·po·kon·**dri'**·as·is). Hypochondria.

hypochondrium (hi·po·**kon**·dre·um). Either of the lateral regions in the upper zone of the abdomen, below the level of the floating ribs. [Gk *hypo*, *chondros* cartilage.]

hypochordal (hi·po·**kor**·dal). On the ventral side of the spinal cord. [Gk *hypo*, cord.]

hypochromaemia (hi·po·kro·**me'**·me·ah). A condition of the blood in which the colour index is abnormally low. **Idiopathic hypochromaemia.** Idiopathic hypochromic anaemia. *See* ANAEMIA. [Gk *hypo*, *chroma* colour, *haima* blood.]

hypochromasia (hi·po·kro·**ma'**·ze·ah). 1. Hypochromatism. 2. Taking stain less readily and intensely than is normally the case.

hypochromatic (hi·po·kro·**mat'**·ik). 1. Deficient in pigment, so that in any individual tissue there is less than the normal amount. 2. Of a cell nucleus, containing too little chromatin. [Gk *hypo*, *chroma* colour.]

hypochromatism (hi·po·**kro**·mat·izm). A state of the nucleus of the cell body in which it contains too little chromatin. [see prec.]

hypochromatosis (hi·po·kro·mat·**o'**·sis). A pathological condition in which the chromatin of a cell nucleus gradually diminishes and disappears. [Gk *hypo*, *chroma* colour, *-osis* condition.]

hypochromia (hi·po·**kro**·me·ah). 1. A condition of the blood in which the amount of haemoglobin is abnormally decreased. 2. The more than normal transparency and paleness of the skin which is present in some diseases. 3. Hypochromatism. [Gk *hypo*, *chroma* colour.]

hypochromic (hi·po·**kro**·mik). 1. Pertaining to hypochromia. 2. Lightly stained or coloured.

hypochromotrichia (**hi**·po·kro·mo·**trik**′·e·ah). A decrease in the colour of the scalp hair. [Gk *hypo, chroma* colour, *thrix* hair.]

hypochylia (hi·po·**ki**·le·ah). A condition in which the secretion of chyle is deficient or in which the amount of gastric juice is lessened. [Gk *hypo,* chyle.]

hypocoelom (hi·po·**se**·lom). The ventral part of the body cavity of the embryo. [Gk *hypo,* coelom.]

hypocoenaesthesia (**hi**·po·se·nes·**the**′·ze·ah). Lessening or loss of the sense of well-being normal to human beings, such as is present in hypochondria. [Gk *hypo,* coenaesthesia.]

hypocolasia (**hi**·po·kol·**a**′·ze·ah). Hypokolasia.

hypocomplementaemia (hi·po·com·pli·ment·e·me·ah). Low level of serum complement. Seen either in conditions where complement is used rapidly *in vivo* by antigen–antibody reactions, e.g. in acute glomerulonephritis, or in various inherited complement deficiency states, e.g. C3 deficiency.

hypocondylar (**hi**·po·kon·**di**′·lar). Situated below a condyle. [Gk *hypo,* condyle.]

hypocone (**hi**·po·kone). In the tritubercular theory of evolution, the name given to the postero-internal cusp of an upper molar tooth. [see foll.]

hypoconid (hi·po·**ko**·nid). In the tritubercular theory of evolution, the name given to the postero-external cusp of a lower molar tooth. [Gk *hypo, konos* cone.]

hypoconule (hi·po·**kon**·ewl). The distal (fifth) cusp of an upper molar tooth. [Gk *hypo, konos* cone.]

hypoconulid (hi·po·**kon**·ew·lid). In the tritubercular theory of evolution, the name given to the distobuccal cusp of a lower molar tooth. [see prec.]

hypocorticalism (hi·po·**kor**·tik·al·izm). The condition resulting from abnormally deficient functioning of the cortex of the suprarenal gland. [Gk *hypo,* cortex.]

hypocuprinaemia (**hi**·po·kew·prin·**e**′·me·ah). Deficiency in the copper content of the blood. [Gk *hypo,* L *cuprum* copper, Gk *haima* blood.]

hypocyclosis (**hi**·po·si·**klo**′·sis). In optics, deficiency of accommodation. **Ciliary hypocyclosis.** That caused by weakness of the ciliary muscle. **Lenticular hypocyclosis.** Hypocyclosis caused by lack of elasticity of the lens. [Gk *hypo, kyklos* circle.]

hypocystotomy (**hi**·po·sist·**ot**′·o·me). In surgery, incision of the perineal region in order to reach the bladder. [Gk *hypo, kystis* bag, *temnein* to cut.]

hypocythaemia, hypocytosis (**hi**·po·si·**the**′·me·ah, **hi**·po·si·**to**′·sis). A deficiency of blood cells in the blood. [Gk *hypo, kytos* cell, *haima* blood.]

hypodactylia (**hi**·po·dak·**til**′·e·ah). A condition in which there is a lack of 1 or more fingers or toes. [Gk *hypo, daktylos* finger.]

hypoderm (**hi**·po·derm). The subcutaneous connective tissue. [Gk *hypo, derma* skin.]

Hypoderma (hi·po·**der**·mah). A genus of warble flies of the family Oestridae. The larvae of *Hypoderma bovis* and *H. lineatum* normal to cattle, and very rarely *H. diana* normal to deer, have been recorded from human skin, causing cutaneous myiasi known as larva migrans since they move about. [Gk *hypo, derma* skin.]

hypodermatic (**hi**·po·der·**mat**′·ik). Hypodermic.

hypodermatoclysis (**hi**·po·der·mat·**ok**′·lis·is). The injection beneath the skin of large quantities of physiological saline and other fluids for the purpose of replacing sudden loss such as occurs in haemorrhage. [Gk *hypo, derma* skin, *klysis* a washing out.]

hypodermatomy (**hi**·po·der·**mat**′·o·me). Subcutaneous incision or section of parts. [Gk *hypo, derma* skin, *temnein* to cut.]

hypodermiasis (**hi**·po·der·**mi**′·as·is). Infestation with worms of the genus *Hypoderma*; larva migrans.

hypodermic (hi·po·**der**·mik). Introduced beneath the skin, as an injection. [Gk *hypo, derma* skin.]

hypodermis (hi·po·**der**·mis). 1. The subcutaneous connective tissue. 2. The entoderm. [see prec.]

hypodermoclysis (**hi**·po·der·**mok**′·lis·is). Hypodermatoclysis.

hypodermolithiasis (hi·po·**der**·mo·lith·**i**′·as·is). The condition in which calcareous nodules form or are present beneath the skin. [Gk *hypo, derma* skin, *lithos* stone.]

hypodiaphragmatic (**hi**·po·di·ah·frag·**mat**′·ik). Subdiaphragmatic. [Gk *hypo,* diaphragm.]

hypodiploid (hi·po·**dip**·loid). *See* HYPOPLOID. [Gk *hypo, diploos* double, *eidos* form.]

hypodipsia (hi·po·**dip**·se·ah). The taking of such a small amount of fluid or water that the health becomes impaired. [Gk *hypo, dipsios* dry.]

hypodontia (hi·po·**don**·she·ah). Diminished development or even absence of teeth, which are often also imperfectly formed. [Gk *hypo, odous* tooth.]

hypodynamia (**hi**·po·di·**nam**′·e·ah). 1. Diminished muscular or nervous energy. 2. Reduced functional energy. **Hypodynamia cordis.** Heart failure. [Gk *hypo, dynamis* force.]

hypodynamic (hi·po·di·**nam**′·ik). 1. Relating or belonging to hypodynamia. 2. Diminished in power.

hypodynia (hi·po·**din**·e·ah). A slight degree of pain. [Gk *hypo, odyne* pain.]

hypo-eccrisis (hi·po·**ek**·ris·is). Deficient excretion of waste material. [Gk *hypo,* eccrisis.]

hypo-eccritic (**hi**·po·ek·**rit**′·ik). Relating or belonging to hypo-eccrisis or defiency of excretion.

hypo-endemic (**hi**·po·en·**dem**′·ik). A term applied to areas with a low degree of endemicity; in malariology it indicates spleen rates in children of under 10 per cent. [Gk *hypo,* endemic.]

hypo-eosinophilia (**hi**·po·e·o·sin·o·**fil**′·e·ah). The presence of an abnormally small number of eosinophil leucocytes in the blood. [Gk *hypo,* eosin, Gk *philein* to love.]

hypo-epinephria, hypo-epinephry (**hi**·po·ep·e·**nef**′·re·ah, **hi**·po·ep·e·**nef**′·re). A condition in which the suprarenal glands do not secrete a sufficient quantity of hormone. [Gk *hypo, epi, nephros* kidney.]

hypo-equilibrium (hi·po·e·kwil·**ib**·re·um). A state of decreased sensitivity of the labyrinth; in this condition, movements which would produce vertigo in a normal individual are without effect. [Gk *hypo,* L *aequus* equal, *libra* balance.]

hypo-ergasia (**hi**·po·er·**ga**′·ze·ah). A condition in which functional activity is diminished. [Gk *hypo, ergon* work.]

hypo-ergia (hi·po·**er**·je·ah). 1. A condition in which response to a stimulus is unusually weak. 2. A condition of weak allergy because of less active reaction. [Gk *hypo, ergon* work.]

hypo-ergic (hi·po·**er**·jik). Relating or belonging to hypoergia. [see prec.]

hypo-erythrocythaemia (**hi**·po·er·**ith**·ro·si·**the**′·me·ah). The presence of less than the normal number of erythrocytes. [Gk *hypo,* erythrocyte, Gk *haima* blood.]

hypo-esophoria (**hi**·po·es·o·**for**′·e·ah). A condition in which when one eye is covered it deviates downwards and inwards, but when both eyes are open they can be directed to the same point. [hypophoria, esophoria.]

hypo-evolutism (**hi**·po·e·**vol**′·ewt·izm). The condition in which there is less than normal development and growth of the body. [Gk *hypo,* L *e, volvere* to roll.]

hypo-exophoria (**hi**·po·ex·o·**for**′·e·ah). A condition similar to hypo-esophoria except that the eye when covered turns downwards and outwards. [hypophoria, exophoria.]

hypoferraemia (**hi**·po·fer·**e**′·me·ah). Deficiency of blood iron. [Gk *hypo,* L *ferrum* iron, Gk *haima* blood.]

hypoferrism (hi·po·**fer**·izm). Deficiency of iron in the body. [Gk *hypo,* L *ferrum* iron.]

hypofibrinogenaemia (**hi**·po·fi·brin·o·jen·**e**′·me·ah). Deficiency in blood fibrogen. **Congenital hypofibrinogenaemia.** A congenital reduction in blood fibrinogen resembling congenital afibrinogenaemia. [Gk *hypo,* fibrinogen, Gk *haima* blood.]

hypofunction (hi·po·**fungk**·shun). Too little or diminished functional activity on the part of an organ. [Gk *hypo,* function.]

hypogalactia (**hi**·po·gal·**ak**′·she·ah). The secretion of too small a quantity of milk. [Gk *hypo, gala* milk.]

hypogammaglobulinaemia (**hi**·po·gam·ah·**glob**·ewl·in·é·me·ah). Low level of gamma globulin, and usually also of antibody, in serum. Maybe inherited as in Bruton type hypogammaglobulinaemia in which there is a failure of development of the B-lymphocyte system and therefore a diminished capacity to mount humoral immune responses. [Gk *hypo, gamma*, L *globulus* small globe, Gk *haima* blood.]

hypogastralgia (**hi**·po·gas·**tral**'·je·ah). Sensation of pain in the hypochondriac region. [Gk *hypo, gaster* stomach, *algos* pain.]

hypogastric (hi·po·**gas**·trik). Having relation or belonging to the hypogastrium.

hypogastric nerve, right and left [nervus hypogastricus (dexter et sinister)NA]. A branch of the hypogastric plexus to the pelvic viscera on each side.

hypogastrium (hi·po·**gas**·tre·um). The median region of the lower zone of the abdomen. [Gk *hypo, gaster* stomach.]

hypogastrodidymus, hypogastropagus (**hi**·po·gas·tro·**did**'·im·us, **hi**·po·gas·**trop**'·ag·us). A twin monster in which fusion has taken place at the hypogastrium. [hypogastrium, Gk *didymos* twin, *pagos* fixture.]

hypogastrorrhexis (**hi**·po·gas·tro·**rex**'·is). Protrusion of the intestines through the abdominal walls. [Gk *hypo, gaster* stomach, *rhexis* rupture.]

hypogenesis (hi·po·**jen**·es·is). 1. Hypoplasia. 2. The non-development of parts or organs of the body. 3. In biology, the normal process of development in which there is no alteration of generation. **Polar hypogenesis.** In embryology, incomplete development at one or other extremity of the body resulting in a form of monstrosity, either with incomplete head development or lack of legs. [Gk *hypo*, genesis.]

hypogenetic (**hi**·po·jen·**et**'·ik). 1. Marked by congenital defective development. 2. Relating or belonging to hypogenesis.

hypogenitalism (hi·po·**jen**·it·al·izm). Lack of development of the sexual organs. [Gk *hypo*, L *genitalis* producing.]

hypogenous (hi·**poj**·en·us). In biology, growing on the under-surface of another structure, like a fungus on the under-surface of a leaf. [Gk *hypo, genein* to produce.]

hypogeusia (hi·po·**gew**·se·ah). Under-development or weakening of the sense of taste. [Gk *hypo, geusis* taste.]

hypoglandular (hi·po·**glan**·dew·lar). Characterized by subnormal activity of the glands, particularly the endocrine glands. [Gk *hypo*, glandular.]

hypoglobulia (**hi**·po·glob·**ew**'·le·ah). A condition in which there is a decrease in the number of blood corpuscles produced. [Gk *hypo*, globule.]

hypoglossal (hi·po·**glos**·al). Lying beneath the tongue, e.g. the hypoglossal nerve. [Gk *hypo, glossa* tongue.]

hypoglossal artery. An embryonic artery, accompanying the hypoglossal nerve, which may persist into adult life to form an anastomosis between the internal carotid and basilar arteries.

hypoglossal nerve [nervus hypoglossus (NA)]. The 12th and last cranial nerve. It is probably purely motor, arising from the medulla oblongata and distributed solely to the muscles of the tongue (terminal branches [rami linguales (NA)]). It has complicated connections in the neck with the upper cervical nerves.

descending branch. A branch which leaves the nerve in the neck and courses along the carotid sheath to join the descendens cervicalis nerve from the 2nd and 3rd cervical nerve trunks to form the ansa hypoglossi. It supplies the omohyoid muscle.

branch to the thyrohyoid. A branch from the hypoglossal nerve in the neck, deriving its fibres from the 1st cervical nerve through a connection at the base of the skull.

nucleus [nucleus nervi hypoglossi (NA)]. A long nucleus situated in the dorsal part of the medulla on either side of the midline, extending from the level of the lower third of the 4th ventricle to below the level of the olive.

hypoglossitis (**hi**·po·glos·**i**'·tis). Inflammation of the tissues underlying the tongue. [Gk *hypo, glossa* tongue, *-itis* inflammation.]

hypoglossus (hi·po·**glos**·us). The hypoglossal nerve.

hypoglottis (hi·po·**glot**·is). The inferior surface of the tongue. [Gk *hypo, glotta* tongue.]

hypoglycaemia (**hi**·po·gli·**se**'·me·ah). A low blood sugar concentration. **Spontaneous hypoglycaemia.** Hypoglycaemia due to an internal cause, i.e. not due to the injection of insulin. [Gk *hypo, glykys* sweet, *haima* blood.]

hypoglycaemic (**hi**·po·gli·**se**'·mik). Relating or belonging to, or bringing about hypoglycaemia.

hypoglycaemosis (**hi**·po·gli·se·**mo**'·sis). The sum of the effects of hypoglycaemia on the body. [hypoglycaemia, Gk *-osis* condition.]

hypoglycogenolysis (**hi**·po·gli·ko·jen·**ol**'·is·is). The deficient or defective splitting up of glycogen in the body resulting in decreased formation of dextrose. [Gk *hypo*, glycogenolysis.]

hypoglycorrhachia (**hi**·po·gli·ko·**rak**'·e·ah). The presence in the cerebrospinal fluid of an abnormally small quantity of sugar. [Gk *hypo*, glycorrhachia.]

hypognathous (hi·po·**nath**·us). 1. Having a lower jaw that is longer than the upper and protrudes. 2. Having the characteristics of a hypognathus. [Gk *hypo, gnathos* jaw.]

hypognathus (hi·po·**nath**·us). A twin monster the incomplete parasite of which is attached to the mandible of the autosite. [see prec.]

hypogonadism (hi·po·**go**·nad·izm). 1. Eunuchoidism. 2. Diminished secretory activity by the glands of the ovary or testis. **Hypergonadotrophic hypogonadism.** Hypogonadism due to deficient function of the gonads, and therefore with an increased production of gonadotrophin by the anterior pituitary gland. **Hypogonadotrophic hypogonadism, Secondary hypogonadism.** Hypogonadism due to anterior-pituitary deficiency, and therefore with a deficient production of anterior-pituitary gonadotrophin and consequent gonadal activity. [Gk *hypo*, gonad.]

hypogranulocytosis (**hi**·po·gran·ew·lo·si·**to**'·sis). A lowering in the granulocytes in the blood. [Gk *hypo*, granulocyte, Gk *-osis* condition.]

hypohaemia (hi·po·**he**·me·ah). Anaemia. [Gk *hypo, haima* blood.]

hypohaemoglobinaemia (**hi**·po·**he**·mo·glo·bin·**e**'·me·ah). A condition in which there is an inadequate amount of haemoglobin in the blood. [Gk *hypo*, haemoglobinaemia.]

hypohaploid (hi·po·**hap**·loid). *See* HYPOPLOID. [Gk *hypo, haploos* single, *eidos* form.]

hypohepatia (**hi**·po·hep·**at**'·e·ah). Under-function or deficient function of the liver. [Gk *hypo, hepar* liver.]

hypohepatic (**hi**·po·hep·**at**'·ik). Relating or belonging to hypohepatia.

hypohidrosis (**hi**·po·hid·**ro**'·sis). The state in which there is too scanty secretion and excretion of sweat. [Gk *hypo, hidros* sweat.]

hypohidrotic (**hi**·po·hid·**rot**'·ik). Relating to hypohidrosis.

hypohormonal, hypohormonic (hi·po·**hor**·mon·al, **hi**·po·hor·**mon**'·ik). 1. Caused by deficiency of hormone. 2. Having decreased quantity of hormone. [Gk *hypo*, hormone.]

hypohormonism (hi·po·**hor**·mon·izm). Hypofunction of the hormonal or endocrine glands. [see prec.]

hypohydraemia (**hi**·po·hi·**dre**'·me·ah). A condition in which the watery elements of the blood are abnormally decreased. [Gk *hypo, hydor* water, *haima* blood.]

hypohydration (**hi**·po·hi·**dra**'·shun). A state in which the amount of water in the body is abnormally decreased. [Gk *hypo, hydor* water.]

hypohydrochloria (**hi**·po·hi·dro·**klor**'·e·ah). Hypochlorhydria.

hypohypnosis (**hi**·po·hip·**no**'·sis). 1. Imperfect or light sleep. 2. A state of partial hypnosis. [Gk *hypo, hypnos* sleep.]

hypohypnotic (**hi**·po·hip·**not**'·ik). 1. Characterized by light sleep or partial hypnosis. 2. Relating or belonging to hypohypnosis. [see prec.]

hypo-idrosis (**hi**·po·id·**ro**'·sis). Hypohidrosis.

hypo-immunity (**hi**·po·im·**ewn**'·it·e). A low state of immunity. [Gk *hypo*, immunity.]

hypo-inosaemia (**hi**·po·in·o·**se**'·me·ah). 1. Decrease in the quantity of fibrinogen in the blood. 2. Lessened coagulability of the blood. [Gk *hypo, is* fibre, *haima* blood.]

hypo-insulinism (hi·po·in·sew·lin·izm). Deficient secretion of insulin by the pancreas and associated diabetic symptoms and signs. [Gk *hypo*, insulin.]

hypo-isotonic (hi·po·i·so·ton'·ik). Hypisotonic.

hypo-isotonicity (hi·po·i·so·ton·is'·it·e). Hypisotonicity.

hypokalaemia, hypokaliaemia (hi·po·kal·e'·me·ah, hi·po·kal·e·e'·me·ah). Low blood potassium. [Gk *hypo*, L *kalium* potassium, Gk *haima* blood.]

hypokinaemia (hi·po·kin·e'·me·ah). A condition in which the output of the heart is less than normal. [Gk *hypo*, *kinein* to move, *haima* blood.]

hypokinesia, hypokinesis (hi·po·kin·e'·se·ah, hi·po·kin·e'·sis). Diminished power of movement or motor function; slight paralysis. [Gk *hypo*, *kinesis* movement.]

hypokinetic (hi·po·kin·et'·ik). 1. Marked by diminished power of movement or function. 2. Relating to hypokinesia. [see prec.]

hypokolasia (hi·po·kol·a'·ze·ah). Abnormal weakness of the inhibitory powers of the body. It is a nervous affection marked by the early appearance of fatigue. [Gk *hypo*, *kolasis* hindering.]

hypolarynx (hi·po·lar·inx). That part of the larynx extending from the vocal folds to the first tracheal cartilage. [Gk *hypo*, larynx.]

hypolemma (hi·po·lem·ah). In biology, a state of deficiency or defect of a sheath. [Gk *hypo*, *lemma* sheath.]

hypolepidoma (hi·po·lep·id·o'·mah). A tumour derived from hypoblast (entoderm). [Gk *hypo*, *lepis* scale, *-oma* tumour.]

hypolethal (hi·po·le·thal). Term applied to a dose of a drug that is not quite enough to cause death. [Gk *hypo*, lethal.]

hypoleucocytosis, hypoleukaemia (hi·po·lew·ko·si·to'·sis, hi·po·lew·ke'·me·ah). Leucopenia. [Gk *hypo*, leucocyte, Gk *haima* blood.]

hypoleydigism (hi·po·li·dig·izm). Diminution in the amount of androgen secreted by the interstitial (Leydig) cells of the testicles. [Gk *hypo*, Leydig cells.]

hypolipaemia (hi·po·lip·e'·me·ah). Deficiency of fat in the blood. [Gk *hypo*, *lipos* fat, *haima* blood.]

hypoliposis (hi·po·lip·o'·sis). A condition which results from the lack of the normal amount of fat in the blood or tissues. [Gk *hypo*, *lipos* fat.]

hypologia (hi·po·lo·je·ah). Defective speech or the lack of the normal powers of speech. [Gk *hypo*, *logos* discourse.]

hypolymphaemia (hi·po·limf·e'·me·ah). A blood condition in which the lymphocytes are considerably diminished in numbers. [Gk *hypo*, lymphocyte, Gk *haima* blood.]

hypomagnesaemia (hi·po·mag·ne·se'·me·ah). A condition in which there is too little magnesium in the blood plasma. [Gk *hypo*, magnesium, Gk *haima* blood.]

hypomania (hi·po·ma·ne·ah). An affective disorder consisting of maniacal excitement to a minor degree. [Gk *hypo*, mania.]

hypomaniac (hi·po·ma·ne·ak). Anyone suffering from hypomania.

hypomanic (hi·po·man·ik). Relating or belonging to hypomania.

hypomastia, hypomazia (hi·po·mas·te·ah, hi·po·ma·ze·ah). Deficient development of the breasts. [Gk *hypo*, *mastos*, *mazos* breast.]

hypomegasoma (hi·po·meg·ah·so'·mah). Very tall stature although considerably less than that of gigantism. [Gk *hypo*, *megas* large, *soma* body.]

hypomelancholia (hi·po·mel·an·ko'·le·ah). A moderate degree of melancholia, i.e. without much disorder of mind. [Gk *hypo*, melancholia.]

hypomelanosis (hi·po·mel·an·o'·sis). Reduced pigmentation of the skin due to diminished formation of melanin. [Gk *hypo*, *melas* black, *-osis* condition.]

hypomenorrhoea (hi·po·men·o·re'·ah). Menstruation characterized by unusually small flow. [Gk *hypos*, menorrhoea.]

hypomere (hi·po·meer). The ventral muscle-forming mass of tissue derived from the myotome of a mesodermal somite. It forms the musculature of the body wall. [Gk *hypo*, *meros* part.]

hypomesosoma (hi·po·me·zo·so'·mah). A stature that is rather below that of middle height. [Gk *hypo*, *mesos* middle, *soma* body.]

hypometabolism (hi·po·met·ab'·ol·izm). Low metabolic rate. [Gk *hypo*, metabolism.]

hypometria (hi·po·met·re·ah). 1. An abnormally narrow range of movement, as of the tongue. 2. Abnormally diminished extension of a part so that it does not reach as far as it was intended to reach. [Gk *hypo*, *metron* measure.]

hypometropia (hi·po·met·ro'·pe·ah). Myopia. [Gk *hypo*, *metron* measure, *ops* eye.]

hypomicron, hypomicrone (hi·po·mi·kron, hi·po·mi·krone). A submicron; an ultramicroscopic particle ranging from 5 to 200 nm in size, occurring in colloidal solutions and as a molecular aggregate when crystals dissolve. [Gk *hypo*, micron.]

hypomicrosoma (hi·po·mi·kro·so'·mah). The smallest stature that is included in the category of the normal. [Gk *hypo*, *mikros* small, *soma* body.]

hypomineralization (hi·po·min·er·al·i·za'·shun). A state of deficiency of mineral elements in the body. [Gk *hypo*, mineral.]

hypomnesia, hypomnesis (hi·po·mne·ze·ah, hi·po·mne·sis). A weak or defective state of the memory. [Gk *hypo*, *mnesis* memory.]

hypomorph (hi·po·morf). An individual whose legs are disproportionately short so that the sitting height is tall in relation to the standing height. [Gk *hypo*, *morphe* form.]

hypomotility (hi·po·mo·til'·it·e). Lack of the power of movement, or a state in which motility is reduced. [Gk *hypo*, motility.]

hypomyosthenia (hi·po·mi·os·the'·ne·ah). A state in which the muscles lack power or are deficient in power. [Gk *hypo*, *mys* muscle, *sthenos* strength.]

hypomyotonia (hi·po·mi·o·to'·ne·ah). A state of deficient or diminished muscular tone. [Gk *hypo*, *mys* muscle, *tonos* tension.]

hypomyxia (hi·po·mix·e·ah). A condition in which there is decrease in the secretion of mucus. [Gk *hypo*, *myxa* mucus.]

hyponanosoma (hi·po·nan·o·so'·mah). A state of marked dwarfishness. [Gk *hypo*, nanosoma.]

hyponatraemia (hi·po·nat·re'·me·ah). Deficiency of the sodium content of the blood. [Gk *hypo*, L *natron* sodium, Gk *haima* blood.]

hyponeocytosis (hi·po·ne·o·si·to'·sis). Leucopenia in which the blood contains many undeveloped types of leucocyte. [Gk *hypo*, *neos* new, *kytos* cell.)

hyponeuria (hi·po·newr·e·ah). A state of diminished nervous energy. [Gk *hypo*, *neuron* nerve.]

hyponitraemia (hi·po·ni·tre'·me·ah). A condition in which the nitrogen content of the blood is less than normal. [Gk *hypo*, nitrogen, Gk *haima* blood.]

hyponoderma, hyponodermia (hi·po·no·der'·mah, hi·po·no·der'·me·ah). Creeping eruption; larva migrans. [Gk *hyponomos* underground, *derma* skin.]

hyponoetic (hi·po·no·et'·ik). Relating or belonging to or under intellectual or voluntary control. [Gk *hypo*, *noein* to think.]

hyponoia (hi·po·noi·ah). Mental slowness or sluggishness; dullness of imagination. [Gk *hypo*, *nous* intellect.]

hyponomoderma (hi·po·no·mo·der'·mah). Hyponoderma.

hyponychial (hi·po·nik·e·al). Relating or belonging to the hyponychium.

hyponychium [NA] (hi·po·nik·e·um). The narrow fold of the horny zone of a nail which overlaps the lunula. [Gk *hypo*, *onyx* nail.]

hyponychon (hi·pon·ik·on). Subungual ecchymosis. [see prec.]

hypo-orthocytosis (hi·po·or·tho·si·to'·sis). Leucopenia in which the differential count is normal. [Gk *hypo*, *orthos* right, *kytos* cell.]

hypo-osmia (hi·po·oz·me·ah). An abnormally dull sense of smell; abnormal insensitivity to odours. [Gk *hypo*, *osme* odour.]

hypo-osmosis (hi·po·oz·mo'·sis). Osmosis proceeding at a slower rate than is normally the case. [Gk *hypo*, osmosis.]

hypo-oxaemia (hi·po·ox·e'·me·ah). A condition in which the blood contains too little oxygen. [Gk *hypo* oxygen, *haima* blood.]

hypopallaesthesia (hi·po·pal·es·the'·ze·ah). A condition in which the perception of vibration is diminished. [Gk *hypo*, pallaesthesia.]

hypopancreatism (hi·po·**pan**·kre·at·izm). A state of decreased activity of the pancreas. [Gk *hypo*, pancreatism.]

hypoparathyroidism, hypoparathyrosis (**hi**·po·par·ah·**thi**'·roid·izm, **hi**·po·par·ah·thi·**ro**'·sis). A form of tetany set up either as a result of parathyroid hypofunction leading to a subnormal concentration of serum calcium, or of the removal of the parathyroid glands. [Gk *hypo*, parathyroid gland.]

hypopepsia (hi·po·**pep**·se·ah). 1. Dyspepsia caused by deficiency of the gastric juice, particularly of pepsin. 2. Abnormal slowness and weakness of the process of digestion. [Gk *hypo*, *pepsis* digestion.]

hypopepsinia (hi·po·pep·**sin**'·e·ah). The secretion of an abnormally small amount of pepsin in the stomach. [Gk *hypo*, pepsin.]

hypoperistalsis (**hi**·po·per·is·**tal**'·sis). Abnormally slow peristaltic action of the alimentary canal. [Gk *hypo*, peristalsis.]

hypopermeability (**hi**·po·per·me·ab·**il**'·it·e). Diminished permeability. [Gk *hypo*, permeability.]

hypophalangism (hi·po·fal·**an**'·jizm). The congenital state of having less than the normal number of phalanges in a finger or toe. [Gk *hypo*, phalanx.]

hypophamine (hi·**pof**·am·een). Oxytocin.

hypopharyngoscope (**hi**·po·far·**ing**'·go·skope). A form of pharyngoscope used in examination of the laryngeal part of the pharynx. [Gk *hypo*, pharynx, Gk *skopein* to watch.]

hypopharyngoscopy (**hi**·po·far·ing·**gos**'·ko·pe). Examination of the laryngeal part of the pharynx by means of a hypopharyngoscope.

hypopharynx (hi·po·**far**·ingx). The laryngeal part of the pharynx. [Gk *hypo*, pharynx.]

hypophobia (hi·po·**fo**·be·ah). Absence of fear in circumstances that ordinarily would induce fear in a normal person. [Gk *hypo*, *phobos* fear.]

hypophonesis (**hi**·po·fo·**ne**'·sis). In auscultation or percussion, abnormal faintness of the sounds elicited. [Gk *hypo*, *phonema* sound.]

hypophonia (hi·po·**fo**·ne·ah). A condition in which the voice is weak or whispering as the result of inco-ordination of the muscles concerned in the production of vocal sounds. [Gk *hypo*, *phone* voice.]

hypophoria (hi·po·**for**·e·ah). A condition in which an affected eye turns downwards on covering. [Gk *hypo*, *pherein* to bear.]

hypophosphataemia (**hi**·po·fos·fat·**e**'·me·ah). A condition in which the blood serum contains less than the normal amount of phosphates. [Gk *hypo*, phosphate, Gk *haima* blood.]

hypophosphatasia (**hi**·po·fos·fat·**a**'·ze·ah). A deficiency of alkaline phosphatase; it occurs in a form of rickets. [Gk *hypo*, phosphatase.]

hypophosphate (hi·po·**fos**·fate). Any salt of hypophosphoric acid.

hypophosphaturia (**hi**·po·fos·fat·**ewr**'·e·ah). Deficiency in the amount of phosphates excreted in the urine. [Gk *hypo*, phosphate, urine.]

hypophosphite (hi·po·**fos**·fite). Any salt of hypophosphorous acid. They are prescribed as nerve tonics in neurasthenia and anaemia.

hypophrenia (hi·po·**fre**·ne·ah). Feebleness of mind. [Gk *hypo*, *phren* understanding.]

hypophrenic (hi·po·**fren**·ik). 1. Mentally subnormal; feebleminded. 2. A feebleminded person. 3. Subphrenic; lying below the diaphragm. [Gk *hypo*, *phren* understanding, diaphragm.]

hypophrenium (hi·po·**fre**·ne·um). A space in the peritoneum between the pelvic diaphragm and the transverse colon. [Gk *hypo*, *phren* diaphragm.]

hypophrenosis (**hi**·po·fren·**o**'·sis). Any mental state included in the group of hypophrenia, e.g. subnormality, imbecility. [Gk *hypo*, *phren* understanding, *-osis* condition.]

hypophyseal (hi·**pof**·iz·**e**'·al). Relating or belonging to the hypophysis cerebri.

hypophysectomize (hi·**pof**·iz·**ek**'·to·mize). To excise the hypophysis cerebri. [hypophysis, Gk *ektome* a cutting out.]

hypophysectomy (hi·**pof**·iz·**ek**'·to·me). The surgical excision of the hypophysis cerebri. [see prec.]

hypophyseotrophic (hi·**pof**·iz·e·o·**tro**·fik). Concerning that area of the hypothalamus that produces the hypophyseal-releasing hormones.

hypophysial (hi·**pof**·iz·e·al). Hypophyseal.

hypophysiectomy (hi·po·fiz·e·**ek**'·to·me). Hypophysectomy.

hypophysin (hi·**pof**·is·in). A now little-used term for the posterior pituitary hormone. [hypophysis.]

hypophysis (hi·**pof**·is·is). 1. An outgrowth. 2. Hypophysis cerebri; the pituitary body. **Hypophysis cerebri [hypophysis (glandula pituitaria) (NA)].** The most important endocrine gland, situated in the hypophyseal fossa of the sphenoid bone and attached to the floor of the 3rd ventricle by the infundibulum. About 8 by 12 mm, it consists of 2 lobes. The anterior lobe [lobus anterior (adenohypophysis) (NA)] comprises a large anterior part [pars distalis (NA)], a small middle part [pars intermedia (NA)] and an upward prolongation [pars infundibularis (NA)] which surrounds the infundibulum. The anterior lobe is sometimes known as the adenohypophysis and it contains chromophil cells which may be either eosinophil (α-cells) or basophil (β-cells) and chromophobe cells which only stain lightly. The posterior (neural) lobe [lobus posterior (neurohypophysis) (NA)] is derived from the floor of the forebrain and consists of neuroglial cells and fine nerve fibres. The infundibulum is covered by the tuberal part [pars infundibularis (NA)]. **Pharyngeal hypophysis [pars pharyngea (NA)].** A remnant of the entodermal pouch of Rathke beneath the mucous membrane of the pharynx, which shows pituitary tissue. [Gk *hypo*, *phyein* to grow.]

hypophysitis (hi·**pof**·iz·**i**'·tis). Inflammation of the hypophysis cerebri. [hypophysis, Gk *-itis* inflammation.]

hypopiesia, hypopiesis (**hi**·po·pi·**e**'·ze·ah, **hi**·po·pi·**e**'·sis). A condition of abnormally diminished blood pressure not due to any basic organic disease. [Gk *hypo*, *piesis* pressure.]

hypopigmentation (**hi**·po·pig·men·**ta**'·shun). Abnormally light pigmentation. [Gk *hypo*, pigmentation.]

hypopinealism (hi·po·**pin**·e·al·izm). Diminished activity of the pineal body with resultant deficiency of its secretion, or the condition caused by such defective activity. [Gk *hypo*, pineal body.]

hypopituitarism (**hi**·po·pit·**ew**'·it·ar·izm). A clinical condition due to a deficiency in secretion of the anterior pituitary gland. It may refer to deficiency of one particular secretion, e.g. of thyrotrophin, leading to thyroid deficiency, or of gonadotrophin, producing sexual deficiency, but more usually it is applied to the condition of panhypopituitarism (Simmonds' disease) in which all anterior pituitary functions are depressed. [Gk *hypo*, pituitary.] *See also:* BERGMANN (G.).

hypoplasia (hi·po·**pla**·ze·ah). Defective formation or underdevelopment of a tissue or part. **Cartilage-hair hypoplasia.** An autosomal recessive syndrome with dwarfism, skeletal abnormalities and sparse, brittle, fine, light hair, bow legs and short stature. [Gk *hypo*, *plasis* a forming.]

hypoplastic (hi·po·**plas**·tik). Pertaining to or characterized by hypoplasia.

hypoplasty (**hi**·po·plas·te). 1. Hypoplasia. 2. A condition in which the power to form or to cause development is deficient.

hypoploid (**hi**·po·ploid). A chromosome complement cell or organism missing 1 or more chromosome centric fragments. According to the ploidy one can distinguish between *hypohaploids, hypodiploids, hypotriploids, hypotetraploids* and so on. [Gk *hypo*, *eidos* form.]

hypoploidy (hi·po·**ploid**·e). The state of hypoploids.

hypopnoea (hi·po·**ne**·ah). Shallow and rapid breathing. [Gk *hypo*, *pnoia* breath.]

hypoporosis (**hi**·po·por·**o**'·sis). A condition in which there is insufficient formation of callus, e.g. after fracture of a bone. [Gk *hypo*, *poros* callus.]

hypopotassaemia (**hi**·po·pot·as·**e**'·me·ah). Diminution in the amount of potassium in the blood. [Gk *hypo*, potassium, Gk *haima* blood.]

hypopraxia (hi·po·**prax**·e·ah). 1. A condition in which activity is diminished and ineffective. 2. In psychiatry, listlessness and disinclination for exertion. [Gk *hypo, praxis* action.]

hypoproteinaemia (hi·po·pro·te·in·e'·me·ah). A condition in which there is an abnormally diminished quantity of protein in the blood plasma, such as occurs in nephrosis, hepatic dysfunction or as the result of too little protein in the diet. **Prehepatic hypoproteinaemia.** Hypoproteinaemia due to the prolonged intake of a diet low in protein. [Gk *hypo,* protein, Gk *haima* blood.]

hypoproteinosis (hi·po·pro·te·in·o'·sis). A condition in which there is deficiency in dietary protein. [Gk *hypo,* protein, Gk *-osis* condition.]

hypoprothrombinaemia (hi·po·pro·throm·bin·e'·me·ah). Prothrombinopenia; a congenital or acquired condition in which there is a deficiency of prothrombin in the blood, causing haemorrhagic manifestations. It may follow excessive treatment with dicoumarol or similar anticoagulants, or a deficient intake or absorption of vitamin K, while disease of the liver and bile ducts may be causal factors. It is relieved by treatment with vitamin K or its analogues. [Gk *hypo,* prothrombin, Gk *haima* blood.]

hypopselaphesia (hi·po·sel·af·e'·ze·ah). Partial loss or diminution of the sense of touch. Insensitiveness to touch. [Gk *hypo, pselaphema* touch.]

hypopsychosis (hi·po·si·**ko**'·sis). Mental slowness or sluggishness; dullness of imagination. [Gk *hypo, psyche* mind, *-osis* condition.]

hypoptyalism (hi·po·ti·al·izm). A condition in which the secretion of saliva is diminished. [Gk *hypo, ptyalon* spittle.]

hypopus (hi·**po**·pus). A nymphal stage of certain mites, e.g. species of *Tyroglyphus,* in which the mouth parts are absent and the legs reduced. Hypopi attach themselves to insects, etc. and are thus passively distributed. [Gk *hypo, pous* foot.]

hypopyon, hypopyum (hi·**po**·pe·on, hi·**po**·pe·um). Accumulation of pus or a pus-like fluid in the anterior chamber of the eye. [Gk *hypo, pyon* pus.]

hypoquebrachine (hi·po·ke·**brah**'·keen). $C_{21}H_{26}N_2O_2$, one of the less important of the yohimbé alkaloids, derived from quebracho bark. [Gk *hypo,* quebrachine.]

hyporeflexia (hi·po·re·**flex**'·e·ah). A condition in which there is only weak reflex action. [Gk *hypo,* reflex.]

hyporhinolalia (hi·po·ri·no·**la**'·le·ah). *See* VOICE, NASAL. [Gk *hypo, rhis* nose, *lalein* to speak.]

hyposalaemia (hi·po·sal·e'·me·ah). A condition in which the quantity of blood salts is abnormally small. [Gk *hypo,* L *sal* salt, Gk *haima* blood.]

hyposalivation (hi·po·sal·iv·a'·shun). A condition in which the secretion of saliva is so diminished that the mouth is dry. [Gk *hypo,* salivation.]

hyposarca (hi·po·**sar**·kah). Anasarca; oedema of the cellular tissues of the body, characterized by soft and pallid but inelastic swelling. [Gk *hypo, sarx* flesh.]

hyposcheotomy (hi·po·ske·**ot**'·o·me). Surgical incision or puncture into a hydrocele at the lower dependent part of the tunica vaginalis testis. [Gk *hypo, oscheon* scrotum, *temnein* to cut.]

hyposcleral (hi·po·**skleer**·al). Beneath the sclera of the eyeball. [Gk *hypo,* sclera.]

hyposecretion (hi·po·se·**kre**'·shun). Secretion in quantity below the normal. [Gk *hypo,* secretion.]

hyposensitive (hi·po·**sen**·sit·iv). Applied to the patient in a case of allergy when he shows great power of resistance to the allergen because repeated increasing doses of it have been administered or when his response is delayed or diminished. [Gk *hypo,* sensitive.]

hyposensitivity (hi·po·sen·sit·**iv**'·it·e). Diminished sensitivity. [see prec.]

hyposensitization (hi·po·sen·sit·i·**za**'·shun). Loss or reduction of susceptibility to infection. For immunological meaning *see* DESENSITIZATION. [Gk *hypo,* sensitization.]

hyposexuality (hi·po·sex·ew·**al**'·it·e). Deficient or lessened sexuality. [Gk *hypo,* sexuality.]

hyposialadenitis (hi·po·si·al·ad·en·i'·tis). Inflammation of the submandibular salivary gland. [Gk *hypo, sialon* saliva, adenitis.]

hyposkeocytosis (hi·po·ske·o·si·**to**'·sis). Hyponeocytosis. [Gk *hypo, skaios* left, *kytos* cell.]

hyposmia (hi·**poz**·me·ah). Hypo-osmia.

hyposmosis (hi·poz·**mo**·sis). Hypo-osmosis.

hyposomatotrophic (hi·po·**so**·ma·to·**tro**·fik). Deficient in somatotrophin (growth hormone).

hyposomia (hi·po·**so**·me·ah). Under-development of the body. [Gk *hypo, soma* body.]

hyposomnia (hi·po·**som**·ne·ah). Insomnia. [Gk *hypo,* L *somnus* sleep.]

hyposomy (hi·po·**so**·me). The state of a cell or organism with 1 or few chromosomes present in numbers lower than normal. [Gk *hypo, soma* body.]

hypospadia (hi·po·**spa**·de·ah). Hypospadias.

hypospadiac (hi·po·**spa**·de·ak). Relating or belonging to, or affected with hypospadias.

hypospadias (hi·po·**spa**·de·as). A congenital defect of the wall of the male urethra or of the vagina so that instead of the normal external orifice there is an opening for a greater or lesser distance on the under-side of the penis or in the vagina. [Gk *hypo, spadon* a rent.]

hyposphresia (hi·pos·**fre**·ze·ah). Hypo-osmia. [Gk *hypo, osphresis* sense of smell.]

hyposphyxia (hi·po·**sfix**·e·ah). Diminished circulatory activity and lowered pressure of the blood combined with extreme viscosity. [Gk *hypo, sphyxis* pulse.]

hypostasis (hi·**pos**·tas·is). 1. A condition due to feebleness of circulation, in which the blood gravitates to and remains in a dependent part of an organ of the body. 2. The forming of a deposit, e.g. of the solid elements of the blood due to stagnation of blood. 3. A sediment or deposit. [Gk *hypo, stasis* a standing still.]

hypostatic (hi·po·**stat**·ik). 1. Relating or belonging to, or caused by hypostasis. 2. In mendelian laws, a term applied to those characters hidden by others superimposed and determined by genes at other loci.

hyposteatolysis (hi·po·ste·at·**ol**'·is·is). Defective splitting of fats during the process of digestion. [Gk *hypo, stear* fat, lysis.]

hyposteatosis (hi·po·ste·at·o'·sis). Diminished formation of skin fats due to developmental abnormality, ageing, xeroderma or the use of powerful skin cleansers. [Gk *hypo, stear* fat, *-osis* condition.]

hyposthenia (hi·po·**sthe**·ne·ah). Subnormal strength of body; an enfeebled or weak condition. [Gk *hypo, sthenos* strength.]

hyposthenia nt, hyposthenic (hi·po·**sthe**·ne·ant, hi·po·**sthen**·ik). 1. Having power to depress the vital forces; debilitating. 2. Any medicine or other agent that tends to weaken. 3. Any remedy or drug that depresses the action of the heart but leaves the rhythm unimpaired. 4. Referring or belonging to, or marked by hyposthenia. [see prec.]

hyposthenuria (hi·po·sthen·**ewr**'·e·ah). The passing of urine of low specific gravity as a result of defective concentrating power of the kidneys. [Gk *hypo, sthenos* strength, urine.]

hypostosis (hi·**pos**·to·sis). A deficiency in bony development. [Gk *hypo, osteon* bone, *-osis* condition.]

hypostypsis (hi·po·**stip**·sis). A mild degree of astringency. [Gk *hypo, styptikos* astringent.]

hypostyptic (hi·po·**stip**·tik). Moderately styptic or mildly astringent. [see prec.]

hyposulphite (hi·po·**sul**·fite). Any salt of hyposulphurous acid. Also applied to photographers' "hypo", sodium thiosulphate, $Na_2S_2O_3$.

hyposympathicotonus (hi·po·sim·**path**·ik·o·to'·nus). Hypotonia of the sympathetic nervous system. [Gk *hypo,* sympathetic system, tone.]

hyposynergia (hi·po·sin·**er**'·je·ah). A state of defective or impaired co-ordination. [Gk *hypo,* synergy.]

hyposystole (hi·po·**sis**·to·le). Abnormally weak contraction in the systolic phase of the cardiac cycle. [Gk *hypo,* systole.]

hypotaxia, hypotaxis (hi·po·tax·e·ah, hi·po·tax·is). A condition of weak co-ordination of will and action such as that which marks the early stage of hypnotism. [Gk *hypo, taxis* arrangement.]

hypotension (hi·po·ten·shun). A fall in blood pressure below the normal range. **Controlled hypotension.** A reduction of blood pressure produced by drugs during an operation, to diminish bleeding. **Induced hypotension.** Deliberate lowering of the blood pressure to reduce bleeding during surgery. **Intracranial hypotension.** A lower than normal pressure of the cerebrospinal fluid. **Orthostatic hypotension, Postural hypotension.** A condition in which the blood pressure falls, often to the extent of producing syncope, when the subject assumes the erect posture. It is due to failure of the normal autonomic responses to the change of posture and may result from the effect of drugs or from disease of the autonomic nervous system. [Gk *hypo,* tension.]

hypotensive (hi·po·ten·siv). 1. Term applied to those diseases in which the blood pressure falls, e.g. infective diseases. 2. A subject with a low blood pressure. [Gk *hypo,* tension.]

hypotensor (hi·po·ten·sor). Any substance the administration of which causes a fall of blood pressure. [see prec.]

hypotetraploid (hi·po·tet·rah·ploid). *See* HYPOPLOID. [Gk *hypo, tetraploos* fourfold, *eidos* form.]

hypothalamotomy (hi·po·thal·am·ot′·o·me). The surgical production of lesions in the hypothalamus. [hypothalamus, Gk *temnein* to cut.]

hypothalamus [L.] (hi·po·thal·am·us). The part of the diencephalon which lies below the thalamus and forms the floor and the side walls of the 3rd ventricle below the hypothalamic sulcus. Macroscopically it contains the tuber cinereum and mamillary bodies, and nuclei containing "releasing factors" or hormones that cause the pituitary to release its specific hormones. [Gk *hypo,* thalamus.]

Hypothalmichthys nobilis (hi·po·thal·mik′·this no·bil·is). A fish host of *Clonorchis sinensis.* [Gk *hypo, thalamos* chamber, *ichthys* fish, L noble.]

hypothenar (hi·po·the·nar). 1. Referring to the hypothenar eminence. 2. Describing any structure in relation with the hypothenar eminence. [Gk *hypo, thenar* palm.]

hypothermal (hi·po·ther·mal). 1. Relating or belonging to, or characterized by hypothermia. 2. Tepid or slightly warm. [Gk *hypo, therme* heat.]

hypothermia, hypothermy (hi·po·ther·me·ah, hi·po·ther·me). 1. A condition in which the temperature of the body is markedly subnormal; deficiency of bodily heat. 2. The technique of artificially reducing body temperature in order to reduce oxygen requirements of tissues and thus allow more time for operations involving the heart or brain. **Deep hypothermia, Profound hypothermia.** Lowering of the body temperature to less than 28°C. Because of the risk of producing ventricular fibrillation, this usually requires extracorporeal circulation. **Renal hypothermia.** Reduction of the temperature of a kidney at operation so that the blood supply may be safely occluded for a longer period of time than at normal temperature. [Gk *hypo, therme* heat.]

hypothesis (hi·poth·es·is). A conclusion as to the underlying process, drawn from observed facts. It lacks the breadth of a theory, but like the latter should be able to stand the test of experiment and should predict the outcome of other experiments. **Adaptor hypothesis.** The hypothesis that amino acids recognize the sequence of nucleic acid bases coding for them (codons) through the intermediary of oligonucleotide "adaptors" (F.H.C. Crick). **Cardionecteurs hypothesis.** A cardiological term referring to the 2 specialized nodes of conducting tissue in the heart, the sinu-auricular node (atrionecteur) and the atrioventricular node (ventriculonecteur) [obsolete term]. **Inactive X-chromosome hypothesis.** Lyon hypothesis. **One gene-one enzyme hypothesis,** states that the function of genes is to determine the synthesis of specific enzymes; now confirmed in the more general sense that genes determine the structure of polypeptide chains. **Sequence hypothesis,** now confirmed, states that the sequence of amino acids in polypeptide chains is determined by the sequence of nucleotide bases in nucleic acids (the genetic material); *see* COLINEARITY. **Unitarian hypothesis.** A hypothesis advanced by some immunologists that after an injection of, say, a bacterial antigen or infection by a pathogenic micro-organism, a single antibody with multiple functions (agglutination, precipitation, complement fixation, etc.) was produced rather than that each manifestation was due to separate antibodies. This hypothesis is now rendered obsolete by recent studies on immunoglobulins. [Gk foundation.]

See also: ARRHENIUS, AVOGADRO, EINTHOVEN, HERING (K. E. K.), MAKEHAM, PLANCK, SELYE, SEMON (R. W.).

hypothrepsia (hi·po·threp·se·ah). 1. A state of malnutrition. 2. Deficiency in nutrition. [Gk *hypo, threpsis* nutrition.]

hypothrombinaemia (hi·po·throm·bin·e′·me·ah). An abnormal decrease of thrombin in the blood with resultant tendency to bleed easily. [Gk *hypo,* thrombin, Gk *haima* blood.]

hypothymergasia (hi·po·thi·mer·ga′·ze·ah). In psychiatry, a term for an under-active state of mood, the characteristic signs of which are anxiety, sadness, depression and stupor (Meyer). [Gk *hypo,* thymergasia.]

hypothymia (hi·po·thi·me·ah). 1. A state of marked despondency or depression of spirits. 2. A low state of emotional tone. 3. A diminished state of feeling tone. [Gk *hypo, thymos* spirit.]

hypothymic (hi·po·thi·mik). Referring or belonging to, or characterized by hypothymia.

hypothymism (hi·po·thi·mizm). Great impairment of the activity of the thymus gland. [Gk *hypo,* thymus gland.]

hypothyroid (hi·po·thi·roid). Caused by or characterized by hypothyroidism.

hypothyroidism (hi·po·thi·roi·dizm). A condition caused by under-activity of the thyroid gland; thyroid deficiency. **Primary hypothyroidism.** Hypothyroidism due directly to loss of thyroid substance through removal or atrophy. **Secondary hypothyroidism.** Hypothyroidism due to defects of stimulation of the thyroid. [Gk *hypo,* thyroid gland.]

hypotonia (hi·po·to·ne·ah). 1. Lessened tone or tension, generally, or applied to any body structure. 2. Arterial hypotension. 3. Deficient intra-ocular tension. **Affective hypotonia.** A form of temporary paralysis provoked by startle. [Gk *hypo,* tone.]

hypotonic (hi·po·ton·ik). 1. Relating or belonging to hypotonia. 2. Of a solution, less than isotonic strength. 3. Anyone affected with hypotonia.

hypotonus, hypotony (hi·po·to·nus, hi·pot·on·e). Hypotonia.

hypotoxicity (hi·po·tox·is′·it·e). 1. The condition or quality of being mildly poisonous. 2. Of a toxic agent, decrease of the poisonous properties. [Gk *hypo,* toxicity.]

hypotrichosis (hi·po·trik·o′·sis). Deficiency of hair on the head or body. [Gk *hypo, thrix* hair, *-osis* condition.]

hypotrichous (hi·po·trik·us). Having cilia almost entirely confined to the under-side of the body. [Gk *hypo, thrix* hair.]

hypotriploid (hi·po·tri·ploid). *See* HYPOPLOID. [Gk *hypo, triploos* triple, *eidos* form.]

hypotrophy (hi·pot·rof·e). 1. Abiotrophia. 2. Defective assimilation of nourishment. [Gk *hypo, trope* nutrition.]

hypotropia (hi·po·tro·pe·ah). A condition in which an affected eye turns downwards, even when both eyes are open. [Gk *hypo, trepein* to turn.]

hypotryptophanic (hi·po·trip·to·fan′·ik). Relating to or resulting from the presence of too little of the amino acid, tryptophan, in the diet. [Gk *hypo,* tryptophan.]

hypotympanic (hi·po·tim·pan′·ik). In a position below the tympanum. [Gk *hypo,* tympanum.]

hypo-uraemia (hi·po·ewr·e′·me·ah). The condition in which there is a subnormal quantity of urea in the blood. [Gk *hypo,* urea, Gk *haima* blood.]

hypo-uresis (hi·po·ewr·e′·sis). Daily output of urine below normal levels. [Gk *hypo,* uresis.]

hypo-uricuria (hi·po·ewr·ik·ewr′·re·ah). Diminished uric acid in the urine. [Gk *hypo,* uric acid, urine.]

hypo-urocrinia (hi·po·ewr·o·krin′·e·ah). Diminished amount of total secretion of urine as compared with the normal output for a similar period. [Gk *hypo,* urine, Gk *krinein* to secrete.]

hypovarianism (hi·po·va·re·an·izm). Deficiency of ovarian secretion.

hypovenosity (hi·po·ven·os′·it·e). A condition in which there is, in any particular area, under-development of the venous system with resultant muscular atrophy and degeneration. [Gk *hypo,* venous system.]

hypoventilation (hi·po·ven·til·a′·shun). A lower pulmonary ventilation than normal; it usually results in a raised blood CO_2 content. [Gk *hypo,* L *ventilare* to wave.]

hypovitaminosis (hi·po·vi·tam·in·o′·sis). Insufficiency of an essential vitamin or vitamins in the diet. [Gk *hypo,* vitaminosis.]

hypovolaemia (hi·po·vol·e′·me·ah). A condition in which the volume of the blood in the body is diminished. [Gk *hypo,* volume, Gk *haima* blood.]

hypoxaemia (hi·pox·e·me·ah). Hypo-oxaemia; a condition in which the blood contains too little oxygen. [Gk *hypo* oxygen, *haima* blood.]

hypoxanthine (hi·po·zan·theen). 6-Oxypurine, $C_5H_4ON_4$. A purine derivative related to uric acid and occurring in various human organs, such as the liver and spleen; it also occurs in tea, with caffeine. It is oxidized to uric acid in the liver, but appears in the urine in leukaemia.

hypoxanthine-guanine phosphoribosyl-transferase (hi·po·zan·theen·gwan·een fos·fo·ri·bo·sil·trans′·fer·aze). Hg-PRTase; the enzyme catalysing the breakdown of hypoxanthine and guanine to their nucleotides. Absent in the Lesch–Nyhan syndrome.

hypoxia (hi·pox·e·ah). A supply of O_2 to the tissues which is inadequate to maintain normal tissue respiration. This is reflected by an alteration in the redox state of the respiratory enzymes systems to a more reduced state and a reduction in the concentration of high energy phosphates in the tissue. **Diffusion hypoxia.** Reduction of the partial pressure of oxygen in the alveoli of the lung due to outward diffusion from the plasma of nitrous oxide, following a prolonged period of nitrous oxide anaesthesia. **Histotoxic hypoxia.** A condition occurring when the tissue cells are unable to utilize the normal supply of oxygen brought to them, e.g. in cyanide poisoning. First described by Peters and Van Slyke in 1932. **Stagnant hypoxia.** Reduction of the oxygen tension of the blood due to a retarded rate of circulation. [Gk *hypo,* oxygen.]

Hypromellose (hi·pro·mell·ose). BP Commission approved name for a partial mixed methyl and hydroxypropyl ether of cellulose; a surface acting agent.

hypsarrhythmia (hips·a·rith·me·ah). A severe generalized disorganization of the electroencephalogram in children, usually accompanying infantile convulsions of the Salaam type. (Syn. West syndrome.) [Gk *hypsi* high, *a, rhythmos* rhythm.]

hypsibrachycephalic (hip·se·brak·e·kef·al′·ik). Applied to a broad and high skull, as that of the Malays. [Gk *hypsi* high, *brachys* short, *kephale* head.]

hypsicephalic (hip·se·kef·al′·ik). Applied to a skull the cranial index of which is above 75.1 degrees. [Gk *hypsi* high, *kephale* head.]

hypsicephaly (hip·se·kef·al·e). A craniometrical term for a head that is high. [Gk *hypsi* high, *kephale* head.]

hypsiconchous (hip·se·kong·kus). In craniometry, a skull that shows an orbital index above 85. [Gk *hypsi* high, *kogche* shell.]

hypsiloid (hip·sil·oid). In the shape of the Greek letter *upsilon;* U- or V-shaped. [Gk letter φ, *eidos* shape.]

hypsiphobia (hip·se·fo·be·ah). Hypsophobia.

hypsistaphylia (hip·se·staf·il′·e·ah). A palate that is narrow and high. [Gk *hypsi* high, *staphyle* palate.]

hypsistenocephalic (hip·se·sten·o·kef·al′·ik). Applied to a skull which is extremely high and narrow, as in the Abyssinian. The jaws are prognathous and the zygomatic bones prominent. [Gk *hypsi* high, *stenos* narrow, *kephale* head.]

hypsocephalic, hypsocephalous (hip·so·kef·al′·ik, hip·so·kef·al·us). Hypsicephalic.

hypsocephaly (hip·so·kef·al·e). Hypsicephaly.

hypsokinesis (hip·so·kin·e′·sis). A disorder of the gait due to the displacement of the centre of gravity in diseases such as paralysis agitans; any interference with the forward movement causes the patient to sway forwards, backwards or sideways, or to fall according to the force and direction of the counter-stroke. [Gk *hypsos* height, *kinesis* movement.]

hypsonosus (hip·so·no·sus). Aviators' disease. *See* DISEASE. [Gk *hypsos* height, *nosos* disease.]

hypsophobia (hip·so·fo·be·ah). Morbid fear of being at a great height or of high places. [Gk *hypsos* height, phobia.]

hypsotherapy (hip·so·ther·ap·e). Treatment of disease by sending the patient to live, temporarily or permanently, at a high altitude. [Gk *hypsos* height, therapy.]

hypurgia (hi·poor·je·ah). The aggregate of certain minor or subordinate factors which favour recovery in a patient's illness. [Gk *hypourgia* service.]

Hyrtl, Joseph (b. 1811). Vienna anatomist.

Hyrtl's anastomosis or loop. An anastomosis between the hypoglossal nerves across the midline in the submental region.

Hyrtl's recess. The epitympanic recess. *See* RECESS.

Hyrtl's sphincter. A localized thickening of circular muscle fibres in the upper part of the ampulla of the rectum.

hyssop (his·op). The common name for *Hyssopus officinalis* Linn. (family Labiatae). An infusion or extract prepared from the herb is employed as a carminative and in the treatment of coughs. **Hedge hyssop.** *Gratiola officinalis.* [Gk *hyssopos* an aromatic plant.]

hystera (his·ter·ah). The uterus. [Gk womb.]

hysteralgia (his·ter·al·je·ah). Pain affecting the uterus. [hysteria, Gk *algos* pain.]

hysteranesis (his·ter·an·es·is). Lessened or entire lack of tension of the uterus. [hystera, Gk *anesis* a relaxing.]

hysteratresia (his·ter·at·re′·ze·ah). A completely closed and imperforate state of the os uteri. [hystera, atresia.]

hysterauxesis (his·ter·awx·e′·sis). An enlarged condition of the uterus which may be either pathological or normal (due to pregnancy). [hystera, Gk *auxesis* increase.]

hysterectomy (his·ter·ek·to·me). Removal of the whole, or the body, of the uterus. **Abdominal hysterectomy.** Removal of the uterus via the abdomen. **Caesarean hysterectomy.** Total or subtotal hysterectomy following caesarean section. **Radical abdominal hysterectomy.** Wertheim's hysterectomy; removal of the uterus and its appendages, with as much cellular tissue of the pelvis and as many regional glands as possible, together with an ample vaginal cuff. **Subtotal hysterectomy, Supracervical hysterectomy, Supravaginal hysterectomy.** Removal of the body of the uterus, leaving the cervix. **Total hysterectomy.** The removal of the whole uterus (usually by the abdominal route); sometimes referred to as *panhysterectomy.* **Vaginal hysterectomy.** Removal of the whole uterus by the vaginal route. [hystera, Gk *ektome* excision.]

See also: PORRO, WERTHEIM.

hysterelcosis (his·ter·el·ko′·sis). An ulcerated condition of the uterus. [hystera, Gk *helkosis* ulceration.]

hysteremphysema (his·ter·em·fi·se′·mah). A condition in which the uterus is distended with air or gas. [hystera, emphysema.]

hysteresis (his·ter·e·sis). 1. The phenomenon of an effect failing to keep up with its cause. 2. A tendency for magnetism to lag behind in an iron core after the magnetic field has been reversed: this causes serious energy loss in alternating electromotors. [Gk *hysterein* to come too late.]

hystereurynter (his·ter·ewr·in′·ter). Any instrument used to dilate the os uteri. [hystera, Gk *eurynein* to dilate.]

hystereurysis (his·ter·ewr·is·is). Dilatation of the cervix uteri. [hystera, Gk *eurynein* to dilate.]

hysteria (his·teer·e·ah). A neurotic disorder the symptoms of which may take almost any imaginable form, but have arisen most usually by a process of suggestion or autosuggestion and involve some degree of dissociation of consciousness. The symptom may take the form of a loss of function, paresis of a limb, mutism or loss of memory, the patient being so convinced that he cannot carry out these functions that in fact he cannot, although no physical or physiological bar to his capacity can be found. Alternatively, the symptom may take the form of an uncontrolled or excessive activity, a tremor, hyperkinesia, paraesthesia or feeling of pain, again with no known physiological cause. The actual form of the symptom frequently corresponds to an idea in the patient's mind, an analgesic area for instance having limits which do not correspond to the distribution of neuronic pathways. A hysterical symptom may also be shown in a wholly mental field, as a trance or ecstatic state, an apparent dementia, a fit of wandering or other disorder of behaviour, and then commonly has a theatrical, dramatized quality. Other common, but not invariable, features of hysterical symptoms are their psychogenic origin, and their purposeful meaning when related to the patient's emotional life. A frequent but incorrect lay usage of the term is to signify a state of heightened emotional response, or an emotional display, excitement, laughter or tears, especially when dramatic or likely to attract attention. **Anxiety hysteria.** A neurotic illness in which symptoms both of anxiety and of hysteria are shown. The term was also used by Freud with a very special and precise meaning, as a hysterical illness traceable to the anxiety derived from sexual frustration or deprivation. **Conversion hysteria.** A hysterical state in which a functional maladjustment has been translated from one field into another, especially from a mental form into a physical one, e.g. the home-sickness of an adolescent girl placed among strangers, expressed as mutism in their presence. **Convulsive hysteria.** A variety of hysteria characterized by the occurrence of convulsions. **Traumatic hysteria.** A hysterical disorder that may appear after an injury, in which the patient is convinced that he is still disabled and suffering although in fact he is again in normal health. [Gk *hystera* womb, which was once considered to be the seat of all such disorders.]

hysteriac (his·**teer**·e·ak). Anyone suffering from hysteria.

hysteric (his·**ter**·ik). 1. Hysterical. 2. A hysteriac.

hysterical (his·**ter**·ik·al). 1. Relating or belonging to hysteria. 2. Showing hysteria or characterized by its presence.

hystericism (his·**ter**·is·izm). A condition tending towards hysteria and the manifestation of hysterical symptoms; a predisposition to hysteria; the hysterical diathesis.

hystericoneuralgia (his·**ter**·ik·o·newr·**al**'·je·ah). Neuralgic pain of hysterical origin.

hysterics (his·**ter**·ix). Popular term for an emotional display.

hysteriform (his·**ter**·e·form). Like hysteria; having the characteristics of hysteria. [hysteria, form.]

hysterism (**his**·ter·izm). The state of being hysterical.

hysteritis (his·ter·**i**·tis). A condition of inflammation of the uterus. [hystera, Gk *-itis* inflammation.]

hysterobubonocele (**his**·ter·o·bew·**bon**'·o·seel). An incomplete inguinal hernia the sac of which contains the uterus. [hystera, bubonocele.]

hysterocarcinoma (**his**·ter·o·kar·sin·**o**'·mah). Carcinoma of the uterus. [hystera, carcinoma.]

hysterocatalepsy (**his**·ter·o·**kat**'·al·ep·se). A state of hysteria with cataleptic symptoms in association.

hysterocele (**his**·ter·o·seel). Hernia of a part or the whole of the uterus. [hystera, Gk *kele* hernia.]

hysterocervicotomy (**his**·ter·o·ser·vik·**ot**'·o·me). The procedure, carried out in difficult labour, of incising the lower segment and the neck of the uterus. [hystera, cervix, Gk *temnein* to cut.]

hysterocleisis (**his**·ter·o·**kli**'·sis). The sealing up of the uterus by suturing the edges of the os uteri. [hystera, Gk *kleisis* closure.]

hysterocolpectomy (**his**·ter·o·kol·**pek**'·to·me). Surgical removal of the uterus and vagina. [hystera, Gk *kolpos* vagina, *ektome* a cutting out.]

hysterocolposcope (**his**·ter·o·**kol**'·po·skope). An instrument with a small electric bulb attached used in examination of the cavity of the uterus. [hystera, Gk *kolpos* vagina, *skopein* to watch.]

hysterocyesis (**his**·ter·o·si·**e**'·sis). Uterine pregnancy. [hystera, cyesis.]

hysterocystic (**his**·ter·o·**sist**'·ik). Relating or belonging to the uterus and the urinary bladder. [hystera, Gk *kystis* bag.]

hysterocystocele (**his**·ter·o·**sist**'·o·seel). Combined hysterocele and cystocele, complete or partial.

hysterocystocleisis (**his**·ter·o·sist·o·**kli**'·sis). The operation carried out for relief of ureterovaginal or vesicovaginal fistula. The neck of the uterus is turned into the bladder and fastened into its wall. [hystera, Gk *kystis* bag, *kleisis* closure.]

hysterocystopexia, hysterocystopexy (**his**·ter·o·sist·o·**pex**'·e·ah, **his**·ter·o·**sist**'·o·pex·e). An operation carried out for the relief of prolapse, by means of which the uterus and bladder are fastened to the abdominal wall. [hystera, Gk *kystis* bag, *pexis* fixation.]

hysterodemonopathy (**his**·ter·o·de·mon·**op**'·ath·e). Demonomania occurring in a hysterical person.

hysterodynamometer (**his**·ter·o·di·nam·**om**'·et·er). An apparatus for measuring the frequency and intensity of uterine contractions. [hystera, Gk *dynamis* force, meter.]

hysterodynia (**his**·ter·o·**din**'·e·ah). Sensation of pain in the uterus. [hystera, Gk *odyne* pain.]

hysteroedema (**his**·ter·e·**de**'·mah). Oedema of the uterus. [hystera, oedema.]

hystero-epilepsy (**his**·ter·o·ep·il·**ep**'·se). Convulsive hysteria. *See* HYSTERIA. [hysteria, epilepsy.]

hystero-epileptogenic, hystero-epileptogenous (**his**·ter·o·ep·il·ep·to·**jen**'·ik, **his**·ter·o·ep·il·ep·**toj**'·en·us). Giving rise to convulsive hysteria. [hystero-epilepsy, Gk *genein* to produce.]

hystero-erotic (**his**·ter·o·er·**ot**'·ik). 1. Marked by hysterical eroticism. 2. Relating to a state that is both hysterical and erotic.

hysterofrenatory, hysterofrenic (**his**·ter·o·fre·**na**'·tor·e, **his**·ter·o·**fre**'·nik). 1. Applied to certain areas or points on the surface of the body, pressure on which arrests an attack of hysteria. 2. Preventing, arresting or delaying hysteria. [hystera, L *fraenum* bridle.]

hysterogastrorrhaphy (**his**·ter·o·gas·**tror**'·af·e). The operation of fastening the uterus to the wall of the stomach. [hystera, Gk *gaster* stomach, *rhaphe* suture.]

hysterogenic, hysterogenous (**his**·ter·o·**jen**'·ik, his·ter·**oj**·en·us). 1. Applied to certain areas or points on the surface of the body, pressure on which induces an attack of major hysteria. 2. Causing hysteria or the appearance of hysterical symptoms. [hysteria, Gk *genein* to produce.]

hysterogeny (his·ter·**oj**·en·e). The setting up of a paroxysm of hysteria or of the hysterical state. [see prec.]

hysterogram (**his**·ter·o·gram). An x-ray photograph of the uterus. [hystera, Gk *gramma* a record.]

hysterograph (**his**·ter·o·graf). An instrument by which the power of uterine contractions can be assessed. [hystera, Gk *graphein* to record.]

hysterography (his·ter·**og**·raf·e). The use of x-rays in examination of the uterus. [see prec.]

hysteroid (**his**·ter·oid). Having resemblance to hysteria or a hysterical attack. [hysteria, Gk eidos form.]

hysterokataphraxis (**his**·ter·o·kat·ah·**frax**'·is). An operation for replacement of the uterus in which the latter is supported in a framework composed of metal ligatures passed through the walls of the abdomen and around the organ. [hystera, Gk *kataphrasein* to fence in.]

hysterolaparotomy (**his**·ter·o·lap·ar·**ot**'·o·me). Abdominal hysterectomy. *See* HYSTERECTOMY. [hystera, Gk *lapara* flank, *temnein* to cut.]

hysterolith (**his**·ter·o·lith). A calculus or stone formed within the uterus. [hystera, Gk *lithos* stone.]

hysterolithiasis (**his**·ter·o·lith·**i**'·as·is). A condition in which there is formation of calculi or stones (hysteroliths) within the uterus.

hysterology (his·ter·**ol**·o·je). That branch of medical science which is concerned with the uterus and all associated structures. [hystera, Gk *logos* science.]

hysteroloxia (**his**·ter·o·**lox**'·e·ah). Flexion or version of the uterus in an oblique direction. [hystera, Gk *loxos* crosswise.]

hysteromalacia (**his**·ter·o·mal·**a**'·she·ah). A condition of morbid softening of the uterus. [hystera, malacia.]

hysteromania (**his**·ter·o·**ma'**·ne·ah). 1. Nymphomania. 2. Insanity of hysterical origin; anxiety hysteria. [hystera, hysteria, mania.]

hysterometer (his·ter·**om**·et·er). Any instrument with which the cavity of the uterus can be measured; e.g. a graduated uterine sound with which the depth of the cavity of the organ can be determined. [hystera, meter.]

hysterometry (his·ter·**om**·et·er. The taking of measurements of the uterus with regard to length and dimensions. [hystera, meter.]

hysteromucography (**his**·ter·o·mew·**kog'**·raf·e). The injection of a radio-opaque substance into the cavity of the uterus for the purpose of coating the mucosa, and the examination of the cavity thereafter by means of x-rays. [hystera, mucus, Gk *graphein* to record.]

hysteromyoma (**his**·ter·o·mi·**o'**·mah). A fibromyoma or a myoma formed within the uterus. [hystera, myoma.]

hysteromyomectomy (**his**·ter·o·mi·o·**mek'**·to·me). Surgical removal of that part of the uterus containing a leiomyofibroma together with the tumour itself. [hystera, myomectomy.]

hysteromyotomy (**his**·ter·o·mi·**ot'**·o·me). Incision of the uterus with a view to removal of a solid tumour. [hystera, Gk *mys* muscle, *temnein* to cut.]

hysteronarcolepsy (**his**·ter·o·**nar'**·ko·lep·se). Narcolepsy originating in hysteria.

hysteroncus (his·ter·**ong**·kus). Any swelling or tumour of the uterus. [hystera, Gk *ogkos* a swelling.]

hysteroneurasthenia (**his**·ter·o·newr·as·**the'**·ne·ah). The presence of neurasthenia in association with a hysterical condition, or in a hysterical subject.

hysteroneurosis (**his**·ter·o·newr·**o'**·sis). Any neurosis caused by disorder or disease of the uterus. [hystera, neurosis.]

hystero-oöphorectomy (**his**·ter·o·o·of·or·**ek'**·to·me). Surgical excision of the uterus as well as the ovaries. [hysterectomy, oöphorectomy.]

hystero-ovariotomy (**his**·ter·o·o·va·re·**ot'**·o·me). Hystero-oöphorectomy. [hystera, ovariotomy.]

hysteropathy (his·ter·**op**·ath·e). Any disordered condition or disease of the uterus. [hystera, Gk *pathos* disease.]

hysterope (**his**·ter·ope). Applied to anyone suffering from hysteropia.

hysteropexia (**his**·ter·o·**pex'**·e·ah). Histeropexy.

hysteropexy (**his**·ter·o·pex·e). Surgical fixation of a displaced, or too freely movable, uterus. **Abdominal hysteropexy.** Fixation of the uterus to the wall of the abdomen. **Vaginal hysteropexy.** Fixation of the uterus to the wall of the vagina. [hystera, Gk *pexis* fixation.]

hysterophilia (**his**·ter·o·**fil'**·e·ah). A group of disorders including asthma, epilepsy and migraine, considered by Lewandowsky to resemble hysteria. [hysteria, Gk *philein* to love.]

hysterophore (**his**·ter·o·fore). A support, such as a pessary, for a uterus that is prolapsed or displaced. [hystera, Gk *pherein* to carry.]

hysteropia (his·ter·o·pe·ah). Disorder or defect of vision of hysterical origin. [hysteria, Gk *ops* eye.]

hysteropnix (his·ter·**op**·nix). Globus hystericus. [hysteria, Gk *pnixai* to stifle.]

hysteropsychopathy (**his**·ter·o·si·**kop'**·ath·e). Any disease of the mind secondary to uterine disease. [hystera, psychopathy.]

hysteropsychosis (**his**·ter·o·si·**ko'**·sis). A hysterical form of psychosis.

hysteroptosia, hysteroptosis (**his**·ter·op·**to'**·ze·ah, **his**·ter·op·**to'**·sis). Prolapse of the uterus; displacement downwards or inversion of the uterus. [hystera, Gk *ptosis* a falling.]

hysterorrhaphy (his·ter·**or**·af·e). 1. Hysteropexy. 2. The suturing together of the cut or torn edges of a wound of the uterus or neck of the uterus. [hystera, Gk *rhaphe* suture.]

hysterorrhexis (**his**·ter·o·**rex'**·is). Rupture of the uterus, in the non-gravid or gravid state. [hystera, Gk *rhexis* rupture.]

hysterorrhoea (**his**·ter·o·**re'**·ah). A discharge of any kind from the uterus. [hystera, Gk *rhoia* flow.]

hysterosalpingectomy (**his**·ter·o·sal·pin·**jek'**·to·me). Surgical removal of the body of the uterus and the uterine tubes. [hystera, salpinx, Gk *ektome* a cutting out.]

hysterosalpingography (**his**·ter·o·sal·ping·**gog'**·raf·e). Injection of radio-opaque material into the uterus and uterine tubes and subsequent x-ray examination of the organs. [hystera, salpinx, Gk *graphein* to record.]

hysterosalpingo-oöphorectomy, hysterosalpingo-oöthecectomy (**his**·ter·o·**sal**·ping·go·o·of·or·**ek'**·to·me, **his**·ter·o·**sal**·ping·go·o·o·the·**sek'**·to·me). Excision of the uterus, uterine tubes and ovaries. [hystera, salpinx, oöphoron, Gk *ektome* a cutting out.]

hysterosalpingostomy (**his**·ter·o·sal·ping·**gos'**·to·me). The establishment by surgical means, when there is occlusion of a part of a uterine tube, of communication between the uterus and that portion of the tube beyond the excised occluded part. [hystera, salpinx, Gk *stoma* mouth.]

hysterosalpinx (**his**·ter·o·**sal'**·pingx). The uterine tube. *See* TUBE.

hysteroscope (**his**·ter·o·skope). A form of speculum fitted with an electric bulb and reflector, used for examining the cavity of the uterus. [hystera, Gk *skopein* to watch.]

hysteroscopy (his·ter·**os**·ko·pe). Examination of the cavity of the uterus by means of a hysteroscope.

hysterospasm (**his**·ter·o·spazm). Spasmodic contraction of the uterus. [hystera, spasm.]

hysterostat (**his**·ter·o·stat). A device in which tubes of radium are so held that they can be distributed in any given direction. It is used in treatment of carcinoma of the uterus. [hystera, Gk *statikos* standing still.]

hysterostomatocleisis (**his**·ter·o·**sto**·mat·o·**kli'**·sis). The operation of closing the canal of the cervix and establishing a communication between the urinary bladder and the uterus so that together they form one cavity. It is performed for vesicovaginal fistula. [hystera, Gk *stoma* mouth, *kleisis* closure.]

hysterostomatome (**his**·ter·o·**sto'**·mat·ome). A type of surgical knife used in hysterostomatotomy.

hysterostomatotomy (**his**·ter·o·**sto**·mat·**ot'**·o·me). Opening up the os uteri by incision of the cervix uteri. [hystera, Gk *stoma* mouth, *temnein* to cut.]

hysterosyphilis (**his**·ter·o·**sif'**·il·is). Hysteroneurosis resulting from syphilis.

hysterosystole (**his**·ter·o·**sis'**·to·le). In the cardiac cycle, a heart beat delayed beyond the time of its normal occurrence. [Gk *hysteros* too late, systole.]

hysterotabetism (**his**·ter·o·**ta'**·bet·izm). Hysteria and tabes occurring simultaneously.

hysterotome (**his**·ter·o·tome). A type of surgical knife used for incision of the uterus. [hystera, Gk *temnein* to cut.]

hysterotomotocia (**his**·ter·o·to·mo·**to'**·se·ah). Caesarean section. [hystera, Gk *temnein* to cut, *tokos* birth.]

hysterotomy (his·ter·**ot**·o·me). 1. Surgical incision of the uterus. 2. Caesarean section. 3. Hysterostomatotomy undertaken for the purpose of removing a fibroid growth of the uterus and leaving the uterus intact. **Vaginal hysterotomy.** Hysterotomy through the vagina. [hystera, Gk *temnein* to cut.]

hysterotrachelectasia (**his**·ter·o·trak·el·ek·**ta'**·ze·ah). Dilatation of the cervical canal and the cavity of the uterus. [hystera, Gk *trachelos* neck, *ektasis* a stretching.]

hysterotrachelectomy (**his**·ter·o·trak·el·**ek'**·to·me). Amputation of the neck of the uterus. [hystera, Gk *trachelos* neck, *temnein* to cut.]

hysterotracheloplasty (**his**·ter·o·**trak'**·el·o·plas·te). Reparative surgery of the neck of the uterus. [hystera, Gk *trachelos* neck, *plassein* to mould.]

hysterotrachelorrhaphy (**his**·ter·o·trak·el·**or'**·af·e). Repair of a laceration of the neck of the uterus by means of sutures. [hystera, Gk *trachelos* neck, *rhaphe* suture.]

hysterotrachelotomy (**his**·ter·o·trak·el·**ot'**·o·me). Incision of the neck of the uterus. [hystera, Gk *trachelos* neck, *temnein* to cut.]

hysterotraumatic (**his**·ter·o·traw·**mat'**·ik). Relating or belonging to, or found in association with hysterotraumatism.

hysterotraumatism (his·ter·o·traw′·mat·izm). Symptoms of hysteria initiated by a condition of severe shock after injury. [hysteria, trauma.]

hysterotrismus (his·ter·o·triz′·mus). 1. Hysterospasm. 2. Lockjaw of hysterical origin. [hystera, hysteria, Gk *trimos* a creaking.]

hysterotubography (his·ter·o·tew·bog′·raf·e). Hysterosalpingography. [hystera, tube, Gk *graphein* to record.]

hysterovagino-enterocele (his·ter·o·vaj·i·no·en′·ter·o·seel). Hernia in which portions of the uterus, vagina and intestine are contained in the sac. [hystera, vagina, Gk *enteron* bowel, *kele* hernia.]

hystrichiasis (his·trik·i·as·is). 1. A diseased condition of the hair in which it stands out erect and stiffly from the head like spines. 2. Ichthyosis hystrix. [Gk hedgehog.]

hystrix (his·trix). Ichthyosis hystrix. [Gk hedgehog.]

hyther (hi·ther). A term denoting the influence exerted on human beings by atmospheric temperature and humidity. [Gk *hydor* water, *therme* heat.]

hyzone (hi·zone). Name given to a triatomic hydrogen molecule.

iamatology (i·am·at·**ol**′·o·je). That branch of medicine concerned with remedies; therapeutics. [Gk *iama* remedy, *logos* science.]

ianthinopsia (i·**an**·thin·**op**′·se·ah). A condition in which all objects appear to be coloured or tinged with violet. [Gk *ianthinos* violet, *opsis* sight.]

iasis (i·a·sis). Treatment, either medical or surgical. [Gk, cure.]

iateria (i·at·**eer**·e·ah). Therapeutics. [Gk, modes of cure.]

iatraliptic (i·at·rah·**lip**′·tik). Referring or belonging to treatment by inunction and friction. [Gk *iatrikos* the art of healing, *aleiphein* to anoint.]

iatraliptics (i·at·rah·**lip**′·tix). The method of treatment by inunction and friction. [see prec.]

iatrarchy (i·at·rar·ke). The system of government by physicians. [Gk *iatros* physician, *arche* rule.]

iatreusiology (i·at·roo·se·**ol**′·o·je). Therapeutics. [Gk *iatreusis* healing, *logos* science.]

iatreusis (i·at·**roo**·sis). Treatment, either medical or surgical. [Gk, healing.]

iatric (i·**at**·rik). Referring or belonging to the science of medicine or to physicians. [Gk *iatros* physician.]

iatrochemical (i·at·ro·**kem**′·ik·al). Relating or belonging to iatrochemistry.

iatrochemist (i·at·ro·**kem**′·ist). Anyone who subscribes to the doctrines or follows the practice of alchemistic medicine (iatrochemistry). [Gk *iatros* physician, chemist.]

iatrochemistry (i·at·ro·**kem**′·is·tre). The system of treatment of which Paracelsus was the chief exponent, that life and health are founded on the proper chemical balance in and action of the organs and fluids of the body, and that disease should be treated chemically. [see prec.]

iatrogenic (i·at·ro·**jen**′·ik). 1. Term commonly applied to disorders directly attributable to medical or surgical procedures. 2. Term applied to disorders which can be traced to fears implanted in the patient's mind by the examining physician's manner or injudicious remarks (Hurst). [Gk *iatros* physician, *genein* to produce.]

iatrology (i·at·**rol**·o·je). The science of medicine and healing. [Gk *iatros* physician, *logos* science.]

iatromathematical, iatromechanical (i·at·ro·math·em·**at**′·ik·al, i·at·ro·mek·**an**′·ik·al). Iatrophysical. [Gk *iatros* physician, mathematics, mechanics.]

iatrophysical (i·at·ro·**fiz**′·ik·al). Relating or belonging to iatrophysics.

iatrophysicist (i·at·ro·**fiz**′·is·ist). Anyone who subscribes to the doctrines or follows the practice of iatrophysics.

iatrophysics (i·at·ro·**fiz**′·ix). 1. Physical medicine or physiotherapy. 2. An Italian school of medicine of the 17th century which applied the laws of mechanics and physics in the treatment of disease and interpreted physiological and pathological phenomena according to physical laws. [Gk *iatros* physician, physics.]

iatrosophist (i·at·ro·**so**′·fist). A physician having profound knowledge of the principles of medicine and medical treatment. [Gk *iatros* physician, *sophia* skill.]

iatrotechnics, iatrotechnique (i·at·ro·**tek**′·nix, i·at·ro·tek·**neek**′). The practical application of the arts of medicine and surgery. [Gk *iatros* physician, surgeon, *techne* craft.]

Ibufenac (i·**bew**·fen·ak). BP Commission approved name for 4-isobutylphenylacetic acid; an anti-inflammatory agent.

Ibuprofen (i·bew·**pro**·fen). BP Commission approved name for 2-(4-isobutylphenyl)propionic acid; an anti-inflammatory agent.

ice (ise). The solid state of water produced by a reduction of temperature to 0°C (32°F). The freezing is accompanied by expansion, and hence ice is less dense than water. It is used to reduce body temperature, to soothe bruised inflamed tissues, and to arrest haemorrhage. **Camphor ice.** Unguentum Camphorae Durum BPC 1949. **Dry ice.** 1. Solid carbon dioxide. 2. Ice washed with strong alcohol. [ME *is.*]

Iceland spar (**ise**·land **spar**). Crystalline calcite showing optical double refraction; used in the manufacture of Nicol prisms. [*Iceland,* LG *spar.*]

ichnogram (**ik**·no·gram). In forensic medicine, an imprint of the sole of the foot made by the subject when he is standing. [Gk *ichnos* footprint, gramma a writing.]

ichor (i·kor). The thin, acrid, watery fluid discharged from a sore or ulcer. [Gk, ethereal fluid (class. mythol.).]

ichoraemia (i·kor·e·me·ah). Septicaemia. [ichor, Gk *haima* blood.]

ichoroid (i·kor·oid). Like pus or ichor; descriptive of a thin discharge containing pus. [ichor, Gk *eidos* form.]

ichorous (i·kor·us). Serous; thin and watery; like or relating to ichor.

ichorrhaemia (i·kor·e·me·ah). Septicaemia. [ichor, Gk *haima* blood.]

ichorrhoea (i·kor·e·ah). A profuse discharge of ichorous fluid. [ichor, Gk *rhoia* flow.]

Ichthammol BP 1958 (**ik**·tham·ol). The mixture of ammonium salts of the sulphonic acids prepared from the oily substance obtained by destructively distilling the fossilized remains of fish and marine animals. It forms a black viscous liquid with a characteristic odour, soluble in water, glycerin, and fixed oils; it is used in the treatment of skin affections, either in ointments or in aqueous applications such as calamine lotion. Its efficacy is supposed to be due to organic sulphur compounds. [Gk *ichthys* fish, ammonia, L *oleum* oil.]

ichtholsulphonate (ik·thol·**sul**·fon·ate). Ichthyolsulphonate.

ichthyiasis (ik·the·i·as·is). Ichthyosis. [Gk *ichthys* fish.]

ichthyism (**ik**·the·izm). Ichthyismus.

ichthyismus (ik·the·**iz**·mus). 1. Poisoning due to eating stale fish. 2. Ichthyotoxism. **Ichthyismus exanthematicus.** Scarlatiniform rash appearing in association with ichthyismus. [Gk *ichthys* fish.]

Ichthyocolla BPC 1949 (**ik**·the·o·**kol**′·ah). Isinglass; the dried and prepared swimming bladder of the sturgeon, *Acipenser huso* Linn. and other species of *Acipenser* (family Acipenseridae). It consists mainly of collagen material and is readily soluble in boiling water, in which form it is used as an adhesive for the preparation of court plaster and other similar types of plaster. Also employed to clarify liquids, e.g. wines. [Gk *ichthys* fish, *kolla* glue.]

ichthyoid (**ik**·the·oid). Having resemblance to or shaped like a fish. [Gk *ichthys* fish, *eidos* form.]

ichthyolsulphonate (**ik**·the·ol·**sul**′·fon·ate). 1. A salt of ichthyolsulphonic acid. 2. A loose term for the constituents of ichthammol.

ichthyophagous (ik·the·**of**·ag·us). Subsisting on a fish diet. [Gk *ichthys* fish, *phagein* to eat.]

ichthyophagy (ik·the·**of**·aj·e). The habit of living on fish or of including fish in the diet. [see prec.]

ichthyophobia (**ik**·the·o·**fo**′·be·ah). Intense dislike of or morbid aversion to the taste of fish or to eating fish. [Gk *ichthys* fish, phobia.]

ichthyosis (ik·the·**o**·sis). Fish-skin disease (mild forms receive the name xeroderma): an incurable, congenital, cutaneous abnormality, characterized by generalized dryness, harshness, and scaling of the skin; often the flexor surfaces of the large joints are not affected. The malady is commonly noted during the first or second year of life, and occurs in varying degrees of severity in different persons. In many cases a family history of ichthyosis can be obtained. **Acquired ichthyosis.** Ichthyosis developing in Hodgkin's disease, reticulosis, carcinomatosis, gross nutritional deficiency, or leprosy. **Ichthyosis congenita.** Harlequin fetus; keratosis universalis congenita: a very rare condition in which, *in utero,* there is great universal thickening of the horny zone of the epidermis, and the child when born is covered with a carapace of horny plates separated by furrows into variously-shaped plaques, rendering existence impossible. A milder variety is recognized in which the infant lives and the skin may become normal. **Ichthyosis congenitalis palmare et plantare (Thost).** Keratosis palmaris et plantaris. **Ichthyosis fetalis.** Ichthyosis congenita (see above). **Ichthyosis follicularis (Macleod).** Generalized ichthyosis associated with follicular keratosis and absence of hair on some parts. Trachoma and conjunctivitis may co-exist. **Ichthyosis hystrix.** Linear naevus; naevus unius lateris: a cutaneous abnormality in which bands or lines of thick, rough, warty, hypertrophic papillary excrescences are noted. Commonly the lesions are unilateral. **Ichthyosis hystrix gravior.** Gross lesions similar to those of ichthyosis hystrix (see prec.) occurring on large areas of the skin. The "porcupine man" of the freak show is an example of this malady. **Intra-uterine ichthyosis.** Ichthyosis congenita (see above). **Lamellar ichthyosis.** A rare, inherited form of ichthyosis resembling ichthyosiform erythroderma but with recurrent lamellar desquamation. **Ichthyosis linearis circumflexa.** A form of ichthyosiform erythroderma with serpiginous and polycyclic lesions slowly changing in pattern. **Ichthyosis linearis neuropathica.** Ichthyosis hystrix (see above). **Ichthyosis linguae.** Leucoplakia of the tongue. **Ichthyosis nacrée.** Ichthyosis nitida (see below). **Ichthyosis nigricans.** Ichthyosis with brown-grey, green, or black scales. **Ichthyosis nitida.** Ichthyosis characterized by shiny, translucent scales. **Ichthyosis palmaris et plantaris.** Keratosis palmaris et plantaris. **Ichthyosis serpentina.** Ichthyosis in which the scales are thick plates resembling crocodile skin. **Ichthyosis simplex.** Xeroderma. **Ichthyosis thysanotrichica.** Trichostasis spinosa. **Ichthyosis vulgaris.** Xeroderma. [Gk *ichthys* fish, *-osis* condition.]

ichthyotic (ik·the·ot·ik). Relating or belonging to, suffering from, or having the characteristics of ichthyosis.

ichthyotoxic (ik·the·o·tox'·ik). Relating or belonging to or caused by the toxic principle present in certain kinds of fish. [Gk *ichthys* fish, toxic.]

ichthyotoxism, ichthyotoxismus (ik·the·o·tox'·izm, ik·the·o·tox·iz'·mus). 1. Poisoning caused by eating fish infected with certain forms of bacteria, e.g. the proteus group. 2. Ichthyismus. [see prec.]

iconolagny (i·kon·o·lag'·ne). Sexual stimulation through looking at suggestive pictures and statuary. [Gk *eikon* likeness, *lagneia* lust.]

iconomania (i·kon·o·ma'·ne·ah). Abnormal interest in images and symbolism. [Gk *eikon* likeness, mania.]

icteric (ik·ter·ik). Relating or belonging to, suffering from, or characterized by jaundice. [icterus.]

ictero-anaemia (ik·ter·o·an·e'·me·ah). The combination of jaundice and anaemia which occurs in the group of haemolytic anaemias. The most important examples are congenital and due to abnormalities of the red blood cells, as in achloluric jaundice, Cooley's anaemia, and sickle-cell anaemia. The group, however, includes chronic acquired haemolytic jaundice or Hayem–Widal anaemia, and the acute haemolytic anaemia of Lederer. [icterus, anaemia.]

icterode (ik·ter·ode). Icteroid.

icterogenic (ik·ter·o·jen'·ik). Causing jaundice. [icterus, Gk *genein* to produce.]

icterogenicity (ik·ter·o·jen·is'·it·e). The quality of being able to cause jaundice. [icterus, Gk *genein* to produce.]

icterogenous (ik·ter·oj·en·us). Icterogenic.

icterohaematuria (ik·ter·o·he·mat·ewr'·e·ah). Jaundice associated with the passing of blood in the urine. [icterus, Gk *haima* blood, urine.]

icterohaematuric (ik·ter·o·he·mat·ewr'·ik). Relating or belonging to, or indicating icterohaematuria.

icterohaemoglobinuria (ik·ter·o·he·mo·glo·bin·ewr'·e·ah). A condition in which jaundice and haemoglobinuria are present at the same time. [icterus, haemoglobin, urine.]

icterohepatitis (ik·ter·o·hep·at·i'·tis). Inflammation of the liver with jaundice as an outstanding symptom. [icterus, hepatitis.]

icteroid (ik·ter·oid). Having resemblance to jaundice. [icterus, Gk *eidos* form.]

icterus (ik·ter·us). Jaundice. **Icterus castrensis.** Spirochaetosis icterohaemorrhagica. **Icterus catarrhalis.** Catarrhal jaundice. *See* JAUNDICE. **Congenital familial icterus.** Acholuric familial jaundice. *See* JAUNDICE. **Epidemic catarrhal icterus.** Infective hepatitis. *See* HEPATITIS. **Familial haemolytic icterus.** Acholuric familial jaundice. *See* JAUNDICE. **Icterus gravis.** Acute yellow atrophy. *See* ATROPHY. **Icterus gravis neonatorum.** Haemolytic jaundice of the newborn. *See* JAUNDICE. **Icterus infectiosus.** Spirochaetosis icterohaemorrhagica. **Icterus neonatorum.** Simple physiological jaundice of infants. **Spirochaetal icterus.** Spirochaetosis icterohaemorrhagica. **Icterus viridans.** Green jaundice. *See* JAUNDICE. [Gk *ikteros.*]

ictometer (ik·tom·et·er). An instrument with which the force of the apex beat of the heart can be determined. [L *ictus* stroke, meter.]

ictus (ik·tus). A sudden attack or stroke. **Ictus cordis.** 1. A sudden heart attack. 2. A powerful widespread cardiac impulse without a definite point of maximum intensity. **Ictus epilepticus.** An epileptic fit. **Ictus laryngeus.** An attack of unconsciousness during a severe paroxysm of coughing; so-called *laryngeal epilepsy.* **Ictus paralyticus.** A paralytic stoke. **Ictus sanguinis.** Cerebral haemorrhage; apoplexy. **Ictus solis.** Sunstroke. [L, stroke.]

id (id). 1. Any one of the structural units of a chromosome, each one of which contains a gene. 2. An allergic skin lesion, e.g. tuberculid. 3. The Freudian term for the totality of instincts which compose the unconscious. [L, it.]

idea (i·de·ah). A concept; a mental image formed independently of any actual sensory perception. **Autochthonous idea.** A notion, e.g. a belief, fear, or desire, entering the mind without ideational antecedent, and appearing to arise *de novo,* and therefore due to introspection. Autochthonous delusions are a common and highly pathognomonic symptom of schizophrenia. **Compulsive idea.** A notion which, at the time of its appearance in the mind, seems absurd or unpleasant, calls forth resistance and an ineffectual attempt at suppression, and so, with recurrence, seems to be experienced under compulsion. **Dominant idea.** An idea which predominantly influences all other thoughts and actions; an obsession. **Fixed idea.** Largely the same as dominant idea (see prec.); an idea, belief, wish, fear, valuation, etc., out of harmony with reality, but maintained contrary to reason and uninfluenced by argument. **Hyperquantivalent idea.** Dominant idea (see above). **Imperative idea.** Largely the same as compulsive idea (see above); an idea (often morbid) which seems to call insistently for corresponding action. **Idea of reference.** A symptom, common in paranoid schizophrenia and other paranoid states, but also occurring in neurotic syndromes: the patient feels that the actions of others have some reference to him although this objectively is highly improbable, e.g. that strangers in the street are talking about him, that others smile, sneer, or sniff at his approach, that he is being referred to over the radio or in newspapers. **Ruminative idea.** An idea which is persistently and unprofitably ruminated upon. [Gk, form.]

ideal (i·de·al). Relating to an idea or a fantasy; not real. **Ego ideal.** That standard of perfection which each individual sets unconsciously for himself and towards the attainment of which he strives. [see prec.]

ideation (i·de·a·shun). 1. The function of the cerebrum which is concerned in the forming of ideas. 2. The capacity of the mind to harbour ideas and form mental concepts. **Incoherent ideation.** A condition of mental disorder in which there is a continual uprush of ideas into consciousness so that before any particular idea can be expressed in words it is thrust aside by another. [Gk *idea* form.]

ideational (i·de·a·shun·al). Relating or belonging to ideation.

identical (i·**den**·tik·al). Exactly alike, equal or corresponding in kind, characteristic, or quality. [L *idem* the same.]

identification (i·**den**·tif·ik·**a**′·shun). 1. The recognition and proof of a person as a definite individual, or the recognition of a thing as belonging to a certain class, species, or variety. 2. In psychiatry, the mechanism by which an emotional tie with a person leads to the unconscious moulding of the personality after the model. **Anthropometric identification.** The method of identifying a person by means of certain measured and recorded physical items peculiar to himself. **Cosmic identification.** A delusion in which the subject identifies himself with the universe. [L *idem* the same, *facere* to make.]

ideodynamism (i·**de**·o·di·**nam**′·izm). The action motivated by an idea or by a suggestion made under hypnosis. [idea, Gk *dynamis* force.]

ideogenetic, ideogenous (i·de·o·jen·**et**′·ik, i·de·**oj**·en·us). 1. Referring to a condition the origin of which is in the mind and without reference to the body. 2. Produced by a mental concept or image. [idea, Gk *genein* to produce.]

ideology (i·de·**ol**·o·je). 1. The science of ideas or thought. 2. A scheme of ideas, a philosophy. [idea, Gk *logos* science.]

ideometabolic (i·de·o·met·ab·**ol**′·ik). Relating or belonging to ideometabolism.

ideometabolism (i·de·o·met·**ab**′·ol·izm). Metabolism induced by a mental activity or process. [idea, metabolism.]

ideomotion (i·de·o·**mo**′·shun). Muscular movement induced or produced by the influence of or in connection with thought, and neither reflex nor voluntary. [idea, motion.]

ideomotor, ideomuscular (i·de·o·**mo**′·tor, i·de·o·**mus**′·kew·lar). 1. Indicating involuntary muscular movement produced by or carried out in connection with thought. 2. Belonging to both ideation and motor activity. [idea, motor, muscle.]

ideophrenia (i·de·o·**fre**′·ne·ah). Insanity characterized by disordered or perverted ideation. [idea, Gk *phrenetikos* frantic.]

ideophrenic (i·de·o·**fren**′·ik). Relating or belonging to ideophrenia, marked by disorder or perversion of ideas.

ideoplastia (i·de·o·**plas**′·te·ah). That stage in hypnosis in which the subject is entirely receptive to suggestions made to him by the hypnotist and is ready to carry out any action required of him. [idea, Gk *plassein* to mould.]

ideoplasty (i·de·o·**plas**′·te). The process of influencing the subject's mind by suggestion from the hypnotist. [see prec.]

ideosynchysia, ideosynchysis (i·de·o·sin·**ki**′·ze·ah, i·de·o·**sin**′·kis·is). 1. A state in which the ideas are in confusion. 2. Delirium. [idea, Gk *sygchysis* a confounding.]

ideovascular (i·de·o·**vas**′·kew·lar). Relating or belonging to change in circulation brought about by the influence of any particular mental activity such as a recollection or a ruling idea. [idea, vascular.]

idioblast (id·e·o·blast). 1. One of the sub-microscopic aggregates of parallel long fibrous-protein molecules found in colloidal sols and gels. 2. In biology, a tissue cell which is different in kind or composition from the surrounding parenchyma. [Gk *idios* own, *blastos* germ.]

idiochromosome (id·e·o·**kro**′·mo·some). Sex chromosome. [Gk *idios* own, *soma* body.]

idiocrasia, idiocrasis, idiocrasy (id·e·o·**kra**′·ze·ah, id·e·**ok**·ras·is, id·e·**ok**·ras·e). Idiosyncrasy. [Gk *idios* own, *krasis* mixture.]

idiocratic (id·e·o·**krat**′·ik). Relating to or characterized by temperamental or constitutional idiosyncrasy. [see prec.]

idioctonia (id·e·ok·**to**′·ne·ah). Suicide. [Gk *idios* own, *ktonos* murder.]

idiocy (id·e·o·se). Grossly abnormal and incomplete development of intellectual functions; legally defined as the state of a "person so deeply defective in mind from birth or from an early age as to be unable to guard himself against common physical dangers" (Henderson and Gillespie). As idiocy implies arrest of development, rather than regression from a higher level (dementia), it must be due to causes genetical, traumatic, infective, etc., arising either before or within two or three years after birth. A physical basis is practically invariably found in gross disease, agenesis, or abnormal development of the brain or damage to it. *See* IDIOT. **Amaurotic family idiocy.** Cerebromacular degeneration. *See* DEGENERATION. Two distinct forms are known, both incorrectly termed idiocy, as the condition in each case is a dementia rather than an arrest of development. In the infantile form the condition begins within the first few months of life, and the blindness is accompanied by a cherry-red spot at the site of the macula in the retina. The juvenile form begins much later, but still in childhood, and no cherry-red spot is seen. They are quite distinct, and both due to distinct sex-linked recessive genes. **Athetotic idiocy.** Idiocy accompanied by disease of the basal ganglia causing athetosis. **Aztec idiocy.** Microcephalic idiocy (see below) with receding forehead and chin. **Cretinoid idiocy.** Idiocy accompanying cretinism: the condition is directly attributable to the basic disease of the thyroid gland, and, unlike most forms of idiocy, may be cured, held in check, or alleviated, by the administration of thyroid extract in sufficient dosage from an early age. **Developmental idiocy.** Idiocy due to failure of brain development. **Diplegic idiocy.** Idiocy accompanying cerebral diplegia (Little's disease). **Eclamptic idiocy.** Idiocy which has supervened in the infant after eclampsia in the mother. **Epileptic idiocy.** Idiocy complicated by the occurrence of epileptic fits, and due to a lesion of the brain that causes both conditions. **Genetous idiocy.** Idiocy due to causes arising before birth. **Hemiplegic idiocy.** Idiocy produced by an early (mostly vascular) lesion, which has also produced hemiplegia. **Hydrocephalic idiocy.** Idiocy accompanying hydrocephalus. **Intrasocial idiocy.** Idiocy which nevertheless permits the following of an occupation. **Kalmuk idiocy.** *See* DOWN'S SYNDROME. **Microcephalic idiocy.** Idiocy accompanying such a deficient degree of cerebral development that the brain, cerebral cavity, and skull itself are abnormally small. **Mongolian idiocy.** *See* DOWN'S SYNDROME. **Moral idiocy.** Inadequate or perverse development of the moral and ethical aspects of the personality, and liable to lead to habitual criminality, recidivism, or crimes of exceptional cruelty or callousness. **Paralytic idiocy.** Idiocy accompanied by paralysis. **Paraplegic idiocy.** Idiocy accompanying a lesion which has also caused paraplegia. **Plagiocephalic idiocy.** Idiocy associated with distortion of the skull. **Porencephalic idiocy.** Idiocy due to porencephalia. **Scaphocephalic idiocy.** Idiocy associated with scaphocephaly. **Sensorial idiocy.** Mental deficiency attributable to lack of one or more of the senses. [Gk *idiotes* ignoramus.]

idiogamist (id·e·o·**gam**′·ist). One who is sexually impotent with all but one or a few partners. [Gk *idios* own, gamete.]

idiogenesis (id·e·o·**jen**′·es·is). Term applied to the origin of any apparently spontaneous (idiopathic) disease. [Gk *idios* own, genesis.]

idiogenic (id·e·o·**jen**′·ik). Pertaining to idiogenesis.

idioglossia (id·e·o·**glos**′·e·ah). 1. Defective or imperfect articulation in which sounds not belonging to any language are produced, the same sound being always used to express the same idea. 2. The use by a child, from the first beginnings of speech, of three or four consonants for the whole series, so that he may come to speak a language peculiarly his own. [Gk *idios* own, *glossa* tongue.]

idioglottic (id·e·o·**glot**′·ik). Relating or belonging to idioglossia.

idiogram (id·e·o·gram). Graphic, diagrammatic representation of the karyotype of a species, variety, individual, or cell. [Gk *idios* own, *gramma* record.]

idiohypnotism (id·e·o·**hip**′·not·izm). Self-hypnotism. *See* SELF-HYPNOSIS. [Gk *idios* own, hypnotism.]

idio-iso-agglutinin (id·e·o·i·so·ag·**loo**′·tin·in). 1. An iso-agglutinin present in normal blood which agglutinates the red blood cells of other animals of the same species. 2. An iso-agglutinin present in fetal blood through immunization communicated from the mother to the child and vice versa. [Gk *idios* own, iso-agglutinin.]

idio-isolysin (id·e·o·i·**sol**′·is·in). A haemolysin present in normal blood which lyses the cells of other animals of the same species. [Gk *idios* own, isolysin.]

idiokinetic (id·e·o·kin·**et**′·ik). Ideomotor. [Gk *idios* own, *kinesis* movement.]

idiolalia (id·e·o·**lal**′·e·ah). A condition in which the subject speaks a language invented by himself. [Gk *idios* own, *lalein* to babble like a child.]

idiologism (id·e·**ol**·o·jizm). A form of utterance or an expression peculiar to and habitually used by a particular person in certain types of insanity. [Gk *idios* own, *logos* discourse.]

idiolysin (id·e·**ol**·is·in). A lysin which is not produced by external stimulus and is present in normal blood. [Gk *idios* own, lysin.]

idiomere (id·e·o·meer). Any one of the structural units of a chromosome, each one of which contains a gene. [Gk *idios* own, *meros* part.]

idiometritis (id·e·o·met·**ri**′·tis). Inflammation of the muscular coat of the uterus. [Gk *idios* own, *metra* womb.]

idiomiasma (id·e·o·mi·**az**′·mah). Any offensive odour exhaled from the body. [Gk *idios* own, *miasma* pollution.]

idiomuscular (id·e·o·**mus**′·kew·lar). Pertaining to the function of muscle only, without any reference to nerve stimulus. [Gk *idios* own, muscle.]

idioneural (id·e·o·**newr**′·al). Relating or belonging exclusively to the nervous system or to one nerve only. [Gk *idios* own, *neuron* nerve.]

idioneurosis (id·e·o·newr·**o**′·sis). Any neurosis of unknown causation originating in the nerves themselves; idiopathic or simple neurosis. [Gk *idios* own, neurosis.]

idioparasite (id·e·o·**par**′·ah·site). A parasitic growth originating within the body of its host. [Gk *idios* own, parasite.]

idiopathetic (id·e·o·path·**et**′·ik). Idiopathic.

idiopathic (id·e·o·**path**′·ik). 1. Relating or belonging to an idiopathy. 2. Describing any pathological condition of unknown aetiology or which is not secondary to any other disease.

idiopathy (id·e·**op**·ath·e). 1. Any morbid condition occurring without apparent external cause. 2. A primary disease. **Toxic idiopathy.** Any disease of the group due to hypersensitivity to various proteins, e.g. urticaria, certain eczemas and asthmas, and disorders of the stomach and intestine. [Gk *idios* own, *pathos* disease.]

idiophonia (id·e·o·**fo**′·ne·ah). A distinctive character or timbre of voice which has an unpleasant effect on the listener. [Gk *idios* own, *phone* voice.]

idiophrenic (id·e·o·**fren**′·ik). 1. Referring or belonging to the brain or mind exclusively. 2. Neither reflex nor secondary but caused by or originating in the brain or mind exclusively, as some forms of insanity. [Gk *idios* own, *phren* mind.]

idioplasm (id·e·o·plazm). The substance which represents the physical basis of heredity. [Gk *idios* own, *plasma* something formed.]

idiopsychological (id·e·o·si·ko·**loj**′·ik·al). Relating or belonging to a person's own mind and the ideas developed within it independently of any outside influence. [see foll.]

idiopsychology (id·e·o·si·**kol**′·o·je). The psychological study by a person of his own mind and mental operations. [Gk *idios* own, psychology.]

idioreflex (id·e·o·re′·flex). Reflex action occurring in an organ as the result of a stimulus originating in the same organ. [Gk *idios* own, reflex.]

idioretinal (id·e·o·**ret**′·in·al). Peculiar to or characteristic of the retina, or coming from the retina itself. [Gk *idios* own, retina.]

idiospasm (id·e·o·spazm). Spasm limited to one part or area. [Gk *idios* own, spasm.]

idiospastic (id·e·o·**spas**′·tik). Relating or belonging to idiospasm.

idiosthenia (id·e·o·**sthe**′·ne·ah). The possession of inherent force or strength. [Gk *idios* own, *sthenos* strength.]

idiosyncrasy (id·e·o·**sin**′·kras·e). 1. A susceptibility to an article of diet, a drug or any other agent, and peculiar to any particular individual. 2. An individual characteristic; a particular quality or habit of mind or bodily constitution or temperament peculiar to a certain individual. [Gk *idios* own, *sygkrasis* a mixing together.]

idiosyncratic (id·e·o·sin·**krat**′·ik). 1. Marked by an idiosyncrasy. 2. Relating or belonging to idiosyncrasy.

idiot (id·e·ot). Obsolete term, now a person suffering from a mental disorder involving a state of arrested or incomplete development of the mind, which includes subnormality of intelligence and is such that the patient is, and will continue to be, incapable of living an independent life or of guarding himself against serious exploitation. *See* MENTAL HEALTH ACT 1959. **Erethistic idiot.** An idiot exhibiting restlessness. **Mongolian idiot.** A person in a state of mongolian idiocy. *See* IDIOCY. **Pithecoid idiot.** An idiot with apelike features. **Profound idiot.** An idiot of very low mentality and usually of small physique. **Idiot savant.** A mental defective, never of such low degree as an idiot, who maintains some faculties preserved to a normal or even superior degree. The abilities which may be shown in this enhanced form by persons otherwise of feeble-minded intelligence have included a phenomenal memory for dates, calculations based on the calendar, other arithmetical abilities, music, mechanical ingenuity, etc. **Superficial idiot.** An idiot of a degree higher than a profound idiot (see above). **Torpid idiot.** An idiot characterized by inactivity. [Gk *idiotes* ignoramus.]

idiotism (id·e·ot·izm). 1. The condition of being an idiot. 2. The state of idiocy.

idiotopie, idiotopy (id·e·**ot**·op·e). The mapping-out of an organ of the body to show the inter-relation of its parts. [Gk *idios* own, *topos* place.]

idiotoxin (id·e·o·**tox**′·in). An antigen which induces allergic reaction; an allergen. [Gk *idios* own, toxin.]

idiotrophic (id·e·o·**trof**′·ik). Applied to an organism which selects its own nourishment. [Gk *idios* own, *trophe* nutrition.]

idiotropic (id·e·o·**trop**′·ik). Of personality, that type which does not seek external emotional or intellectual experiences but is content with those originating within itself. [Gk *idios* own, *trope* a turning.]

idiotype (id·e·o·tipe). 1. The complex of the hereditary factors: chromosomal (genotype) and extrachromosomal (plasmatype). 2. An obsolete term in chemistry for any one of several substances referred to a common type. [Gk *idios* own, type.]

idioventricular (id·e·o·ven·**trik**′·ew·lar). 1. Belonging to or affecting only the ventricle of the heart. 2. Having reference to the ventricle of the heart when it is dissociated from the atrium. [Gk *idios* own, ventricle.]

idiozome (id·e·o·zome). In spermatogenesis, the modified protoplasmic substance from which the head cap of a spermatozoon develops. [Gk *idios* own, *soma* body.]

iditol (i·dit·ol). $CH_2OH(CHOH)_4CH_2OH$; the hexahydric alcohol corresponding to the hexose, idose. It occurs in the berry of the mountain-ash.

idolum (i·**do**·lum). 1. A phantasm. 2. A mental image or illusion. [Gk *eidolon* image in the mind.]

idorgan (id·or·gan). In biology, a structural unit composed of two or more cells but without the positive character of an individual or colony (Haeckel). [id, organ.]

idose (i·doze). $CH_2OH(CHOH)_4CHO$; an aldohexose isomeric with glucose and occurring in two optically-active forms.

Idoxuridine BP 1973 (i·dox·**ewr**·id·een). 5-Iodo-2′-deoxyuridine, $C_9H_{11}IN_2O_5$; an iodine-containing nucleoside which is an analogue of thymidine. It is incorporated in cells into new DNA to produce malfunctioning molecules. It has been used in the treatment of severe infections due to herpes simplex, e.g. keratoconjunctivitis, encephalitis.

idromania (id·ro·**ma**·ne·ah). Hydromania.

Idus melanotus (i·dus mel·an·o·tus). The chub, a fish host of *Opisthorchis felineus.* [Gk *eidos* form, *melas* black, *notos* back.]

ignatia (ig·**na**·she·ah). Ignatia amara, St. Ignatius bean; the seeds of a climbing plant indigenous to the Philippine Islands, *Strychnos ignatii* Berg. (family Loganiaceae). They contain about 3 per cent of strychnine and brucine and are similar in action to nux vomica.

igni-extirpation (ig·ne·ex·ter·**pa'**·shun). The removal of an organ by cauterization. [L *ignis* fire, extirpation.]

igni-operation (ig·ne·op·er·**a'**·shun). The use of a cautery knife in any operation. [L *ignis* fire, operation.]

ignipedites (ig·ne·ped·**i'**·teez). A sensation of burning pain in the soles of the feet, caused by peripheral neuritis; burning feet, one of the symptoms of vitamin-B_2-complex deficiency. [L *ignis* fire, *pes* foot.]

ignipuncture (ig·ne·**pungk**·tcher). The cauterizing of tissues by the insertion of needles at red heat. [L *ignis* fire, puncture.]

ignis (ig·nis). Cautery; moxa. **Ignis sacer.** Erysipelas, or herpes zoster. **Ignis Sancti Antonii.** Erysipelas, or anthrax. **Ignis Sancti Ignatii.** Erysipelas. [L, fire.]

ignisation (ig·niz·a·shun). The state of having an abnormally high body temperature resulting from exposure to artificial heat. [L *ignis* fire.]

ignition (ig·**nish**·un). 1. Setting on fire; the application of a flame to a combustible substance. 2. Strong heating, as when substances are burnt to ash in a muffle furnace. 3. In chemical analysis, the burning-off of organic compounds in an atmosphere of oxygen. 4. A system, usually electrical, for firing combustible gases in an enclosed space, as in the internal combustion engine. [L *ignis* fire.]

Ihle's paste. Resorcinol, zinc oxide, and starch, in soft paraffin.

ikota (i·**ko**·tah). A form of palmus or lata prevalent as a type of religious exercise among the women of the Samoyeds, a race of Siberian Mongols.

ileac (i·le·ak). 1. Belonging to the ileum. 2. Having the character of ileus.

ileal (i·le·al). Pertaining to the ileum.

ileal arteries [arteriae ilei]. *See* MESENTERIC ARTERY, SUPERIOR.

ileectomy (i·le·**ek**·to·me). Surgical excision of the ileum. [ileum, Gk *ektome* a cutting out.]

ileitis (i·le·i·tis). Inflammation of the ileum or of a part of it. **Regional ileitis, terminal ileitis.** A disease in which the ileum is attacked by chronic inflammation, ulceration, and eventual obstruction. The condition may be of infective origin, but the nature of the infection is not known. [ileum, Gk *-itis* inflammation.]

ileocaecal (i·le·o·**se'**·kal). Relating or belonging to both the ileum and the caecum.

ileocaecostomy (i·le·o·se·**kos'**·to·me). The surgical establishment of an anastomosis between the ileum and the caecum. [ileum, caecum, Gk *stoma* mouth.]

ileocaecum, ileocaecus (i·le·o·**se'**·kum, i·le·o·**se'**·kus). The ileum and the caecum taken as one organ.

ileocolectomy (i·le·o·kol·**ek'**·to·me). Excision of the terminal ileum and whole colon in ulcerative colitis. [ileum, colon, Gk *ektome* excision.]

ileocolic (i·le·o·**kol'**·ik). Referring or belonging to the ileum and the colon together.

ileocolic artery [arteria ileocolica]. *See* MESENTERIC ARTERY, SUPERIOR.

ileocolic vein [vena ileocolica (NA)]. A tributary of the superior mesenteric vein draining the terminal ileum, the caecum, and the adjacent part of the ascending colon and the veins from the appendix.

ileocolitis (i·le·o·ko·**li'**·tis). Inflammation of the ileum and the colon. **Acute ileocolitis.** Epidemic diarrhoea in children. **Ileocolitis ulcerosa chronica.** Chronic ileitis in which there is intermittent mild pyrexia and slight diarrhoea, with anorexia and anaemia and dull pain in the right iliac or inguinal region. [ileum, colon, Gk *-itis* inflammation.]

ileocolonic (i·le·o·ko·**lon'**·ik). Ileocolic.

ileocolostomy (i·le·o·ko·**los'**·to·me). The surgical establishment of a communication between the ileum and the colon. [ileum, colon, Gk *stoma* mouth.]

ileocolotomy (i·le·o·ko·**lot'**·o·me). Any operation which involves incision of the ileum and colon. [ileum, colon, Gk *temnein* to cut.]

ileocystoplasty (il·e·o·**sist'**·o·plas·te). The use of a segment of ileum to form a urinary bladder. [ileum, Gk *kystis* bag, *plassein* to mould.]

ileo-ileostomy (i·le·o·i·le·**os'**·to·me). The surgical establishment of communication between two non-continuous parts of the ileum. [ileum, Gk *stoma* mouth.]

ileoparietal (i·le·o·par·**i'**·et·al). Relating or belonging to the wall of the ileum. [ileum, L *paries* wall.]

ileoproctostomy (i·le·o·prok·**tos'**·to·me). Surgical anastomosis between the ileum and the rectum. [ileum, Gk *proktos* rectum, *stoma* mouth.]

ileorectostomy (i·le·o·rek·**tos'**·to·me). Ileoproctostomy. [ileum, rectum, Gk *stoma* mouth.]

ileorrhaphy (i·le·**or**·af·e). Surgical suture of the ileum. [ileum, Gk *rhape* seam.]

ileosigmoid (i·le·o·**sig'**·moid). Belonging to the ileum and the pelvic colon (sigmoid flexure).

ileosigmoidostomy (i·le·o·sig·moid·**os'**·to·me). Surgical anastomosis between the ileum and the pelvic colon (sigmoid flexure). [ileum, sigmoid, Gk *stoma* mouth.]

ileostomy (i·le·**os**·to·me). The establishment of an artificial opening of the ileum onto the abdominal wall. **Permanent ileostomy.** The bringing out of the cut end of the distal ileum onto the abdominal wall; performed in the treatment of ulcerative colitis, usually accompanied by coloproctectomy. **Temporary ileostomy.** An operation rarely performed in small bowel obstruction. **Terminal ileostomy.** Permanent ileostomy (see above). [ileum, Gk *stoma* mouth.]

ileotomy (i·le·**ot**·o·me). Surgical incision of the ileum through the wall of the abdomen. [ileum, Gk *temnein* to cut.]

ileotransversostomy (i·le·o·trans·vers·**os'**·to·me). Surgical anastomosis between the ileum and the transverse colon. [ileum, transverse colon, Gk *stoma* mouth.]

ileum [NA] (i·le·um). The lower three-fifths of that part of the small intestine which extends between the duodenojejunal flexure and the ileocolic valve. **Angulation of the ileum.** Lane's kink. **Duplex ileum.** Doubling of the ileum present from birth. [L *ilia* intestines.]

ileus (i·le·us). Originally any form of intestinal obstruction, but now restricted usually to intestinal distension from loss of the muscular action of the bowel, in the absence of any direct mechanical occlusion. **Adynamic ileus.** Ileus from paralysis of intestinal muscle. It may follow shock, trauma, or surgical operation, or be associated with peritonitis. **Angiomesenteric ileus, arteriomesenteric ileus, duodenal ileus.** Distension of that part of the duodenum proximal to the root of the mesentery and the superior mesenteric artery. **Ileus duplex.** Adynamic ileus (see above) affecting the small intestine and the large intestine at two separate levels, in peritonitis. **Dynamic ileus.** Spastic ileus (see below). **Gall-stone ileus.** Obstruction of the intestinal lumen by a gall-stone. **Gastromesenteric ileus.** Angiomesenteric ileus (see above). **Hyperdynamic ileus.** Spastic ileus (see below). **Mechanical ileus.** Mechanical intestinal obstruction. **Meconium ileus.** Inspissation and impaction of meconium causing intestinal obstruction in the newborn suffering from cystic fibrosis. **Occlusive ileus.** Mechanical intestinal obstruction. **Paralytic ileus.** Adynamic ileus (see above). **Postoperative ileus.** Adynamic ileus occurring after operation. **Spastic ileus.** Ileus due to spasm in a segment of intestine. **Ileus subparta.** Ileus due to pressure of the pregnant uterus on the pelvic colon. **Verminous ileus.** Ileus due to obstruction by masses of parasites. [Gk *eilein* to twist.]

Ilex (i·lex). A genus of shrubs (family Aquifoliaceae) distributed over Europe, Asia, and America. The leaves and berries of *Ilex* *acquifolium* Linn., the common holly, are a domestic remedy for rheumatism and fevers. *I. paraguayensis* St. Hilaire is the source of Paraguay tea, or maté. [L, holm-oak.]

iliac (il·e·ak). Relating or belonging to the ilium. **Iliac bone.** Ilium.

iliac arteries. Common iliac artery [arteria iliaca communis (NA)]. A terminal branch of the abdominal aorta carrying most of the blood to the lower limbs and the pelvic walls and viscera. **External iliac artery [arteria iliaca externa (NA)].** The larger of the two branches of the common iliac artery. It leaves the abdomen and becomes the femoral artery under the inguinal ligament, and supplies the muscles in the false pelvis and of the lower abdominal wall. **Internal iliac artery [arteria iliaca interna (NA)].** One of the two terminal branches of the common iliac artery which descends into the true pelvis where it divides into anterior and posterior divisions. It constitutes the main blood supply to the pelvic organs, gluteal region, perineum, and medial side of the thigh.

iliac veins. Common iliac vein [vena iliaca communis (NA)]. A main vein, formed by the union of the external and internal iliac veins, draining the lower limb and pelvis and uniting in front of the 5th lumbar vertebra to form the inferior vena cava. **External iliac vein [vena iliaca externa (NA)].** An upward continuation of the femoral vein, draining also part of the lower abdominal wall and iliac fossa. It joins the internal iliac vein to form the common iliac vein. **Internal iliac vein [vena iliaca interna (NA)].** A tributary of the common iliac vein, draining the pelvic walls and organs and the gluteal and perineal regions.

iliacus muscle [musculus iliacus (NA)] (il·i·ak·us musl). The muscle arising from the inner surface of the iliac bone of the pelvis, and which, becoming closely associated with the psoas major muscle, runs under the inguinal ligament to be inserted just below the lesser trochanter of the femur.

iliadelphus (il·e·ad·**el**′·fus). A monster which has a single head and body and two arms but which has two pairs of legs. [ilium, Gk *adelphos* brother.]

ilial (il·e·al). Iliac.

iliococcygeal (il·e·o·kok·**sij**′·e·al). Relating or belonging to the ilium and the coccyx.

iliococcygeus muscle [musculus iliococcygeus (NA)] (il·e·o·kok·**sij**′·e·us musl). Those fibres of the levator ani muscle which arise from the fascia over the obturator internus muscle and the ischial spine and insert into the median raphe and coccyx.

iliocolotomy (il·e·o·kol·**ot**′·o·me). The surgical procedure of incising the colon in the iliac (inguinal) region. [ilium, colon, Gk *temnein* to cut.]

iliocostal (il·e·o·**kos**′·tal). 1. Relating or belonging to the ilium and the ribs. 2. Connecting the ilium with the ribs. [ilium, L *costa* rib.]

iliocostalis (il·e·o·kos·**ta**′·lis). The iliocostalis muscle.

iliocostalis muscle [musculus iliocostalis lumborum (NA)]. A part of the iliocostocervicalis muscle.

iliocostocervicalis muscle [musculus iliocostalis (NA)] (il·e·o·**kos**·to·ser·vik·**a**′·lis musl). A muscle which forms the lateral column of the sacrospinalis muscle and is composed of three muscles, iliocostalis, costalis, and costocervicalis.

iliodorsal (il·e·o·**dor**′·sal). Relating or belonging to the surface of the ilium. [ilium, L *dorsum* back.]

iliofemoral (il·e·o·**fem**′·or·al). Relating or belonging to the ilium and the femur.

iliofemoroplasty (il·e·o·**fem**′·or·o·plas·te). Extra-articular fixation of the hip by a bone graft running from the ilium to the greater trochanter. [ileum, femur, Gk *plassein* to mould.]

iliohypogastric (il·e·o·hi·po·**gas**′·trik). Relating or belonging to the ilium and the hypogastrium.

iliohypogastric nerve [nervus iliohypogastricus (NA)]. A sensory branch of the 1st lumbar nerve to the skin of the side of the buttock (lateral cutaneous branch [ramus cutaneus lateralis] NA) and lower abdomen (anterior cutaneous branch [ramus cutaneus anterior] NA).

ilio-inguinal (il·e·o·**ing**′·gwin·al). 1. Relating or belonging to the ilium and the inguinal region. 2. Situated in part within the inguinal region and in part within the region round the ilium.

ilio-inguinal nerve [nervus ilio-inguinalis (NA)]. A mixed motor and sensory branch of the 1st lumbar nerve, supplying part of the internal oblique muscle and the skin on the upper and medial side of the thigh and the adjacent parts of the external genital organs [nervi scrotales anteriores, nervi labiales anteriores (NA)].

iliolumbar (il·e·o·**lum**′·bar). 1. Belonging to the iliac and lumbar regions. 2. Belonging to the flank and the loin.

iliolumbar artery [arteria iliolumbalis (NA)]. A branch of the internal iliac artery which ascends in front of the sacro-iliac joint and supplies the iliacus [ramus iliacus (NA)], psoas, and the quadratus lumborum [ramus lumbalis (NA)] muscles, and also the cauda equina [ramus spinalis (NA)].

iliolumbar vein [vena iliolumbalis (NA)]. A tributary of the common iliac vein. It accompanies the artery of the same nerve, and drains the muscles on the posterior abdominal wall and in the iliac fossa.

iliolumbocosto-abdominal (il·e·o·lum·bo·**kos**·to·ab·**dom**′·in·al). Relating or belonging to the iliac, lumbar, costal, and abdominal regions.

iliometer (il·e·**om**·et·er). An instrument for determining the relative height of the iliac spines and their relative distance from the centre of the vertebral column. [ilium, meter.]

ileopectineal (il·e·o·pek·**tin**′·e·al). Iliopubic. [ilium, L *pecten* comb.]

iliopelvic (il·e·o·**pel**′·vik). 1. Relating or belonging to the iliacus muscle and the pelvis. 2. Referring or belonging to the iliac region and the pelvic cavity.

ilioperoneal (il·e·o·per·o·**ne**′·al). Relating or belonging to the ilium and the fibula or the peroneal region.

iliopsoas (il·e·o·**so**′·as). The iliopsoas muscle.

iliopsoas muscle [musculus iliopsoas (NA)]. The combined muscle formed by the iliacus and psoas muscles. These insert by a common tendon, but are separable above this.

iliopubic (il·e·o·**pew**′·bik). Relating or belonging to the ilium and the pubis.

iliosacral (il·e·o·**sa**′·kral). Relating or belonging to the ilium and the sacrum.

iliosciatic (il·e·o·si·**at**′·ik). Referring or belonging to the ilium and the ischium. [ilium, sciatic.]

ilioscrotal (il·e·o·**skro**′·tal). Relating or belonging to the ilium and the scrotum.

iliospinal (il·e·o·**spi**′·nal). Relating or belonging to the ilium and the vertebral column. [ilium, spine.]

iliothoracopagus (il·e·o·thor·ak·**op**′·ag·us). A twin monster of which the ilium of one fetus is fused with the sternum of the other. [ilium, thorax, Gk *pagos* hardened.]

iliotibial (il·e·o·**tib**′·e·al). 1. Relating or belonging to the ilium and the tibia. 2. Connecting the ilium to the tibia or extending from the one to the other.

iliotrochanteric (il·e·o·tro·kan·**ter**′·ik). Relating or belonging to the ilium and a trochanter, particularly the greater trochanter of the femur.

ilioxiphopagus (il·e·o·zif·**op**′·ag·us). Xiphopagus. [ilium, xiphopagus.]

ilium [os ilium (NA)] (il·e·um). 1. That part of the hip bone which supports the flank and includes the upper part of the acetabulum and wide flattened area of bone above it. 2. The flank. [L *ilia* flank.]

Body [corpus ossis ilii (NA)]. The lower end which enters into the formation of the acetabulum.

Inner lip [labium internum (NA)]. The inner edge of the iliac crest. It gives attachment in its ventral two-thirds to the transversus abdominis muscle.

Outer lip [labium externum (NA)]. The outer edge of the iliac crest. It gives attachment in its ventral half to the external oblique muscle of the abdomen. Between this and the inner lip lies the intermediate area.

Auricular surface [facies auricularis (NA)]. A part of the sacropelvic surface of the ilium; the area shaped like an auricle on the ilium which articulates with the lateral mass of the sacrum.

Gluteal surface [facies glutea (NA)]. The surface of the ilium directed backward and laterally and giving attachment to the gluteal muscles.

Sacropelvic surface [facies sacropelvina (NA)]. The posterior and lower part of the inner surface of the ilium.

ill (il). 1. Not healthy; diseased. 2. Indisposed. 3. An illness or disease. **Foehn ill.** The condition of depression with headache and lassitude which attacks people exposed to the hot dry wind that often blows up the valleys of the northern Alps and other parts of the world. Relief is experienced when washed air is breathed. **Navel ill.** Omphalophlebitis. [ME.]

illacrimation (il·ak·rim·a′·shun). Continuous accumulation and overflow of tears, the result of excessive secretion, or obstruction of the lacrimal passages. [L *in*, lacrimation.]

illaqueation (il·ak·we·a·shun). An ancient operation for correcting the position and direction of an ingrowing eyelash by drawing it, with a loop of thread, through a tract made by a needle. [L *in*, aqueous.]

illegitimacy (il·e·jit·im·as·e). The state of being illegitimate.

illegitimate (il·e·jit·im·ate). 1. Abnormal. 2. Not born in lawful wedlock. 3. Not authorized by statutory law. [L *in*, legitimate.]

Illicium (il·is·e·um). A genus of evergreen shrubs or small trees (family Magnoliaceae). *Illicium verum* Hook, f., the star anise, is the main commercial source of anise oil. [L *illicire* to allure.]

illinition (il·in·ish·un). Inunction. [L *illinere* to smear.]

illness (il·nes). The condition of being ill. **Compressed-air illness.** Caisson disease. *See* DISEASE. **Illness of infection.** A mild febrile attack with malaise and a fleeting rash that may occur within a few hours of infection in certain specific fevers, notably measles. [ME.]

See also: GOODALL.

illumination (il·ew·min·a′·shun). 1. The lighting of a surface or an object. 2. The quantity of light falling on unit area of surface in unit time. 3. In microscopy, the light thrown upon an object, which varies in quality, quantity, and direction. **Axial illumination.** In microscopy, illumination such that the axis of the illuminating cone is coincident with the optical axis of the objective and eyepiece. **Central illumination.** In microscopy, illumination of the object by rays of light passing perpendicularly through it. **Contact illumination.** Illumination obtained when the source of light is placed in contact with the eyeball. **Critical illumination.** In microscopy, illumination such that the image of the source of light is formed by the condenser coincident with the object. **Dark-field illumination, dark-ground illumination.** In microscopy, illumination of the object by a hollow cone of light from the condenser such that light passing rectilinearly through the object plane cannot enter the objective. Thus the object may only be seen by light which is scattered, reflected, or refracted by it, and appears bright on a dark background. Such illumination is obtained by using a central stop beneath the condenser, or by the use of a special condenser. **Direct illumination.** In microscopy, illumination by a beam of light falling upon an object from above the microscope stage; also called *vertical illumination* or *surface illumination.* **Focal illumination.** Illumination of an object by light focused upon it by the lens of a concave mirror. **Lateral illumination.** Illumination of an object or surface by rays that are not coincident with the line of sight; in microscopy, illumination of an object by a cone of rays the axis of which is not coincident with the optic axis of the microscope. **Oblique illumination.** Lateral illumination (see prec.). **Orthogonal illumination.** Illumination of an object by light which is at right angles to the direction of vision. **Stroboscopic illumination.** Intermittent illumination of a moving part such as a rotating wheel which, when of the correct frequency, produces an apparent stillness of the part. **Surface illumination.** Direct illumination (see above). **Through illumination.** Transillumination. **Vertical illumination.** Direct illumination (see above). [L *illuminare* to make light.]

illuminism (il·ew·min·izm). A hallucinatory state in which hallucinations take the form of messages from supernatural beings. [L *illuminare* to make light.]

illusion (il·ew·zhun). A false interpretation of a genuine percept, e.g. seeing an overcoat hanging on a hook and thinking it to be a man. Illusions are most likely to be experienced when the sensory stimulus is itself vague or ambiguous, e.g. when lights are dim, or when the mind of the subject is fatigued, or confused, or is being affected by suggestion. They may occur in any of the five senses. **Optical illusions.** 1. Erroneous visual perceptions usually of movement which may occur in flight. 2. Any disorder of visual perception, e.g. metamorphopsia. 3. *Oculogravic* (*optogravic*)—during linear acceleration, objects with fixed relation to the observer appear to change position. During acceleration, objects appear to move upwards; during deceleration they appear to move downwards. 4. *Oculogyral* (*optogyral*)—during angular acceleration, objects fixed in relation to the observer appear to move in the same direction as the angular movements of the observer. 5. *Autokinetic*—if a small source of light is viewed against a featureless background, it appears to move slowly in an irregular path. 6. *Agravic* (*oculoagravic* or *octoagravic*)—the apparent movement of an object in the visual field when the gravitational force changes from 1 G to zero G. It is thought to be due to the effect of zero G on the otolith. [L *illudere* to mock.]

See also: KUNDT.

illusional (il·ew·zhun·al). 1. Marked by illusions. 2. Relating or belonging to an illusion, or having the character of one.

illutation (il·ew·ta·shun). 1. The therapeutic use of mud baths. 2. A mud bath. [L *in*, *lutum* mud.]

Ilosvay, Lajos de (b. 1851). Budapest chemist and Cabinet Minister.

Ilosvay's reagent, for nitrites; (*a*) Dissolve 0.5 g of sulphanilic acid in 30 ml of glacial acetic acid, add 100 ml water, and filter. (*b*) Dissolve 0.1 g of α-naphthylamine in 100 ml boiling water, cool, add 30 ml glacial acetic acid, and filter. For testing, add 2 ml of each reagent to 50 ml of the approximately neutral test solution and match any red colour against a standard (0.001 mg nitrite N per ml) after 15 min.

image (im·ij). 1. The portrayal of an object. 2. The picture of an object formed by a lens or mirror. 3. The appearance in the mind of a picture representing an object, in the absence of that object. **Accidental image.** After-image. **Acoustic image.** An image or concept excited by sound. **Aerial image.** A real image (see below) formed in the air by a lens system, as in indirect ophthalmoscopy. **After image.** *See* AFTER-IMAGE. **Auditory image.** Acoustic image (see above). **Body image.** The elements of the body schema accessible to consciousness. **Direct image.** An image whose orientation is the same as that of the object. **Double image.** 1. The two images as seen in physiological diplopia, e.g. when a near object is fixed a distant object will fall on non-corresponding retinal points in each eye, and so give a double image. 2. The two images seen in a deviation of the visual axes, as in squint. In the undeviated eye the image will fall on the macula (true image), while in the squinting eye the image will fall away from the macula and so stimulate a non-corresponding retinal point (false image). 3. The two images seen in uni-ocular diplopia, due usually to early cataract or dislocated lens. **Erect image.** Direct image (see above). **False image.** In deviation of the visual axes, the image which comes from the deviated, or squinting, eye, and therefore falls off the macula and on to a non-corresponding retinal point. It is less well defined than the true image (see below). **Heteronymous image.** Diplopia in which the image on the right side is seen by the left eye, and that on the left by the right. It occurs when the eyes are divergent or not sufficiently convergent. **Homonymous image.** Diplopia in which the right image is seen with the right eye, and the left with the left. It occurs in cases of convergence excess. **Incidental image.** After-image. **Inverted image.** An image which is reversed, e.g. that seen on the ground-glass screen of a camera. **Memory image.** The recollection of an object by picturing it in the mind. **Mental image.** The mental picture of an absent object. **Mirror image.** Usually applied to the image of the source of light obtained with the slit lamp from the reflecting surfaces of the cornea or lens; it may also be applied to the image formed by a plane mirror. **Negative image.** Negative after-image. *See* AFTER-IMAGE. **Ocular image.** The mental appreciation of the image formed by one eye. **Optical image.** An image formed by optical means, e.g. by lenses and mirrors. **Positive image.** Positive after-image. *See* AFTER-IMAGE. **Real image.** An image formed by the meeting of convergent rays of light. **Retinal image.** The impression formed on the retina. **Sensory image.** A conception of the outer world due to the functioning of one or more sense organs. **Specular image.** Mirror image (see above). **Tactile image.** The conception of an object formed by the sense of touch. **True image.** In deviation of the visual axes the image which comes from the undeviated eye and therefore falls on the macula. It is sharper and more defined than the false image, which comes from the deviated eye. **Virtual image.** An image having no real existence in space, e.g. that seen in a plane mirror. **Visual image.** The mental interpretation of something seen. **Window image.** The reflection of a window by the anterior surface of the cornea. [L *imago.*]

See also: PURKINJE, SANSON, STIERLIN.

image-intensifier (**im**·ij·in·**ten'**·se·fi·er). An instrument used in diagnostic radiology to intensify many times the fluorimetric image which would otherwise be obtained by a given exposure to x-rays. [L *imago, intensus* stretched tight.]

imagination (im·**aj**·in·**a'**·shun). 1. The mental power of being able to picture material objects not present to the senses. 2. The faculty of being able to create in the mind ideal constructions based on recombined past experiences, or of seeing the future as in the mirror of an idealized past. 3. In zoology, changing into an imago. [L *imaginari* to picture to oneself.]

imago (im·**a**·go). 1. In analytical psychology, a picture or fanciful image of someone loved which persists in adult life. 2. In zoology, the final adult stage of an insect. [L, likeness.]

imagocide (im·**a**·go·side). A substance that kills insects in the imago (adult) stage. [imago, L *caedere* to kill.]

imbalance (**im**·bal·ans). 1. Lack of equality of power as between two sets of opposing muscles. 2. The state of being powerless to stand upright. **Autonomic imbalance.** Any disturbed condition of the autonomic nervous system, e.g. autonomic ataxia. **Chromosome imbalance.** *See* CHROMOSOME. **Gene imbalance.** A condition of abnormal development due to lack of proportion between the genes transmitted. **Sympathetic imbalance.** Vagotony. **Vasomotor imbalance.** Autonomic imbalance (see above). [L *in,* balance.]

imbecile (**im**·bes·eel). 1. Defective or deficient in mental power. 2. Feebleminded from birth and of mental age between 2 and 7 years. **Moral imbecile.** An individual of almost negligible moral as well as mental development. (Obsolete term.) [L *imbecillus* feeble.]

imbecility (im·**bes**·il·it·e). 1. The condition or state of being an imbecile. 2. Congenital mental deficiency less in degree than idiocy. 3. Feeblemindedness. **Acquired imbecility.** Dementia praecox. **Phenylpyruvic imbecility.** Phenylpyruvic oligophrenia. *See* OLIGOPHRENIA.

imbed (im·**bed**). Embed.

imbibe (im·**bibe**). To absorb; to suck in; to inhale or to assimilate. [L *imbibere* to drink in.]

imbibition (im·bib·**ish**·un). 1. The process of assimilation; sucking up of moisture. 2. The absorption of liquid by a gel or solid body. **Haemoglobin imbibition.** The absorbing of free haemoglobin by tissue. [see prec.]

imbricated (**im**·brik·a·ted). Overlapping alternately, like tiles or shingles on a roof. [L *imbrex* hollow roofing tile.]

imbrication (im·brik·**a**·shun). 1. In surgery, the closing of a wound or repair of a defect by the fixing of layers of tissue so that one overlaps the other. 2. In dentistry, the overlapping of one tooth on another in the same arch. [L *imbrex* hollow roofing tile.]

Imhoff, Karl (b. 1876). German hygienist.

Imhoff tank. A form of digestion tank for the treatment of sewage.

imidazole (im·id·**a**·zole). Glyoxalin, $CH(NH){=}N(CH)_2$. A cyclic compound derived from glyoxal, and the parent of histidine and histamine.

imide (**im**·ide). Name applied to any compound containing the imino group, =NH.

iminazole (im·in·a·zole). Imidazole.

β-iminazolylethylamine (be·tah·**im**·in·a·zol·il·eth·il·**am'**·een). The systematic chemical name for histamine.

imino-urea (**im**·in·o·ewr·**e'**·ah). Guanidine.

Imipramine (i·**mip**·ram·een). BP Commission approved name for 1 - (3 - dimethylaminopropyl) - 4,5 - dihydro - 2,3 - 6,7 - di-benzazepine. **Imipramine Hydrochloride BP 1973.** The hydrochloride of the base; a white, odourless crystalline powder with a burning taste followed by a sensation of numbness, soluble in water, alcohol and chloroform, and almost insoluble in ether. It is an antidepressant used in psychiatric therapy, its effects developing in 2 to 3 weeks.

imipramini (i·mip·**ram'**·in·i). Imipramine. **Imipramini Hydrochloridum.** *European Pharmacopoeia* name for Imipramine Hydrochloride BP 1973.

imitation (im·it·a·shun). A copy of any particular process or object. **Morbid imitation.** The reproduction by one person of a spasmodic or mental affection seen in another. [L *imitari* to copy.]

Imlach, Francis (b. 1819). Scottish surgeon in Liverpool.

Imlach's fat plug. A mass of fat sometimes seen at the mesial side of the superficial inguinal ring.

immaculate (im·**ak**·ew·late). 1. Without blemish or flaw; spotless. 2. In zoology and botany, without coloured spots or other marks. [L *in, macula* spot.]

immature (im·at·**ewr**). Not fully developed; unripe; not fully grown; not yet adult. [L *in,* mature.]

immediate (im·e·de·ate). 1. Direct and without reference to or intervention of anything else. 2. Direct or close connection in time or space. 3. Urgent. [L *in,* mediate.]

immedicable (im·**ed**·ik·abl). Incurable, or cannot be remedied. Applied to wounds that cannot heal or be healed. [L *immedicabilis* that cannot be healed.]

immersion (im·**er**·shun). The submerging of a solid in a liquid. **Homogeneous immersion.** In microscopy, the use of a liquid with a refractive index the same as that of glass. **Oil immersion.** The use of oil to cover the objective and the object in microscopy. **Water immersion.** The use of water to connect the objective and the object in microscopy. [L *in, mergere* to dip.]

See also: ABBÉ.

imminence (**im**·in·ens). The condition or state of constituting a threat or of being about to happen. **Morbid imminence.** The interval of time immediately before the stage of incubation of an infection sets in. [L *imminere* to overhang.]

immiscible (im·**is**·ibl). Of liquids, incapable of mixing or of being caused to mix with one another, e.g. oil and water. [L *in, miscere* to mix.]

immobilization (im·o·bil·i·za'·shun). The act of rendering incapable of movement. In surgery, the fixation of a joint, limb, or fracture so that it cannot move or be moved. [L *in,* mobilize.].

immobilize (im·**o**·bil·ize). To render immobile; in surgery, the use of splints to hold immovable a normally mobile part, or the fragments of a fracture. [see prec.]

immune (im·**ewn**). 1. Protected against an attack of any particular infective or allergic disease. 2. Incapable of being harmed by a pathogenic agent. 3. In a state in which lymphocytes show a specific alteration in reactivity to an antigen such that they are capable of mounting a humoral or cell-mediated immune response to it. **Immune adherence.** Adherence of immune complexes or antibody-coated bacteria to red cells in the presence of bound complement component C3. **Immune**

complex. Complex of antigen and antibody molecules bound together by reactions between determinants and combining sites. May form a precipitate if the number of molecules involved is large, or, especially in antigen excess, may form a soluble complex. Circulating soluble complexes are important in hypersensitivity states (type III) such as glomerulonephritis. **Immune elimination.** Elimination of antigen as a result of a specific immune response against it. **Immune response.** A specific adaptive response to the introduction of antigen into the body, by which antibody, or antigen-reactive lymphocytes, which can react specifically with the antigen are formed. In tolerance, the response takes the form of specific failure to mount such a response to a given antigen. [L *immunis* free from.]

immune-electro-osmophoresis (im·**ewn**′·el·ec·tro·**oz**·mo·for·e·sis). IEOP, counter-current electrophoresis. A method of detecting antigens by causing them to migrate in an agar or agarose gel towards the anode by electrophoresis while antibody moves in the reverse direction towards the antigen by endosmosis. The effect is to cause precipitation where the antigen meets antibody with a considerable increase in sensitivity over the otherwise very similar immuno-diffusion. The technique has been widely used in the detection of hepatitis B antigen.

immunifacient (im·**ewn**·e·**fa**′·shent). A prophylactic serum or vaccine, or an attack of a particular disease, which renders an individual immune, at least for a time, from a further attack of the disease in question. [immune, L *facere* to make.]

immunifaction (im·**ewn**·e·**fak**′·shun). Immunization. [see prec.]

immunisin (im·ewn·is·in). Amboceptor.

immunity (im·**ewn**·it·e). The state of resistance of the animal body to disease, especially to a particular disease. It includes resistance to infection, to progress of the disease after infection, and the influence of all those factors that may raise or lower the resistance of the body. These factors may be classified into general or local. General factors may be natural, dependent on the species, the race, or the individual; in the latter case they may be inherent or genetic (e.g. resistant or susceptible strains of animals), active acquired (e.g. subclinical infection), or passive acquired (e.g. maternal antibodies in the blood). Artificial general immunity may be attributed to non-specific factors (e.g. nutrition, shock), or acquired actively, passively, or chemotherapeutically. Tissue defences constitute natural factors of local immunity, while artificial local factors include tissue injury. **Acquired immunity.** Immunity acquired during life, not inherited; it may be active or passive. **Active immunity.** Protection acquired by contact with antigen. *See also:* PREMUNITION. **Adoptive immunity.** Transfer of passive cell-mediated immunity to unimmunized host by immunologically active lymphocytes from an immunized donor. **Antibacterial immunity.** The ability to resist infection by bacteria or microbes. **Antitoxic immunity.** Immunity to the action of a toxin. **Antiviral immunity.** Immunity to infection by a virus. **Artificial immunity.** Immunity produced artificially, in contrast to natural immunity; it may be active or passive. **Athreptic immunity.** An obsolete theory that immunity might be caused by exhaustion of bacterial food-stuffs. **Cell-mediated immunity.** Graft-rejection. Specific immunity mediated by the action of products of thymus-derived lymphocytes. **Cellular immunity.** Immunity due to increased capacity of macrophages, activated during an immune response, to destroy pathogenic or antigenic agents. Often also used as a synonym for all-mediated immunity. **Chemoprophylactic immunity.** Immunity due to a chemotherapeutic agent in the blood stream (e.g. sulphonamide prophylaxis). **Community immunity.** Herd immunity (see below). **Congenital immunity.** Immunity possessed at birth. **Cross immunity.** Immunity produced by one agent (usually bacterium or virus) to another closely related but not identical infection. **Familial immunity, genetic immunity.** Inherited immunity (see below). **Herd immunity.** The level of resistance of a community or group of people to a particular disease. **Humoral immunity.** Immunity in which the reacting substance is present in the plasma, in contrast to cellular immunity (see above). **Inborn immunity.** Racial immunity (see below). **Individual immunity.** Immunity due to factors in the life or circumstances of the individual. **Infection immunity.** Resistance against infection which is only maintained during active infection (e.g. syphilis). **Inherent immunity.** Immunity due to genetic constitution, or natural immunity (see below). **Inherited immunity.** Immunity due to the genetic constitution of the individual. **Innate immunity.** Racial immunity (see below). **Intra-uterine immunity.** Congenital immunity (see above). **Local immunity.** Immunity of a particular organ or tissue. **Maturation immunity.** Immunity that develops with advancing age. **Natural immunity.** Immunity inherited or passively acquired *in utero* or via the maternal milk, or obtained actively by clinical or subclinical infection. **Non-specific immunity.** Immunity or protection other than that conferred by the specific reaction of lymphocytes with antigen. This includes general genetic and constitutional effects, non-specific agents such as interferon or lysozyme and the protective action of phagocytic cells, neutrophils, mononuclear phagocytes and eosinoplints. **Opsonic immunity.** Immunity assisted by the presence of opsonins. **Passive immunity.** That obtained as a result of the transfer of some immune mechanism (e.g. serum-containing antibodies) from another animal. **Phagocytic immunity.** Immunity due to the activity of phagocytes in engulfing and destroying the disease-producing agent. **Placental immunity.** Congenital immunity (see above). **Postoncolytic immunity.** Immunity that develops as a result of lysis of a tumour and protects against a subsequent development of a similar tumour. **Pre-emptive immunity.** Immunity to infection with a virus, dependent not upon the formation of antibodies but upon the interference phenomenon. (The term was proposed by C. H. Andrewes.) **Racial immunity.** Immunity peculiar to a particular race. **Species immunity.** Resistance of a particular species, e.g. rabbits to human tuberculosis. **Specific immunity.** Immunity resulting from the specific recognition of antigen by lymphocytes. Includes humoral and cell-mediated immunity. **Superinfection immunity.** Of bacteria, immunity conferred by carriage of plasmid or prophage, against reinfection by the same or closely-related agent. **Theories of immunity** (instructive, and template). *See* THEORY. **Tissue immunity.** Local immunity (see above). **Toxoid-antitoxin immunity.** Immunity produced by injection of a mixture of toxin and its specific antitoxin (first used by Behring for the prevention of diphtheria). [L *immunis* free from.]

See also: BEHRING, COLLES, PROFETA.

immunization (im·ewn·i·**za**·shun). The production of immunity by specific means: this may be the production of active immunity by the injection (or other modes of administration) of antigenic materials, or passive immunity by the injection of antibodies, in serum or serum fractions, preformed in another animal or human.

immunizator (im·ewn·i·**za**′·tor). Anything which sets up immunity in an organism against disease or infection.

immunize (im·ewn·ize). To make immune; to produce immunity.

immunoassay (im·ewn·o·**as**′·a). The technique by which proteins or protein-bound molecules may be measured, using the high affinity between antigens and their specific antibodies. The antigen-antibody complexes are isolated by filtration, centrifugation, specific adsorption or electrophoresis. The radioactivity associated with each such complex is dependent on (1) the amount of radioactive protein added, and (2) the ratio of the concentrations of the known radioactive protein and the same protein in the "unknown" sample. *See also:* RADIO-IMMUNOASSAY. [immunity, assay.]

immunochemistry (im·ewn·o·**kem**′·is·tre). The study of biochemical and molecular aspects of immunology, especially the nature of antibody, antigen and their interactions. [immunity, chemistry.]

immunoconglutinin (im·ewn·o·kon·**gloo**′·tin·in). Auto-antibody against fixed complement components, especially C3 and C4; not to be confused with *conglutinin.* [L *immunis* free from, *conglutinare* to glue together.]

immunocyte (im·ewn·o·site). A cell concerned in immunity, especially antibody formation (reticulo-endothelial cells, lymphocytes, plasma cells, and their precursors). [L *immunis* free from, Gk *kytos* cell.]

immunodeficiency (im·**ewn**·o·de·**fish**·en·se). Clinical condition in which there is a deficiency of humoral immunity (such as the antibody deficiency syndromes), cell-mediated immunity (such as thymic hypoplasia) or phagocytic function (as in chronic granulomatous disease). May result from genetic abnormalities, often manifest in childhood, or from acquired disease, especially of lymphoid tissue (e.g. Hodgkin's disease).

immunodiagnosis (im·ewn·o·di·ag·**no**′·sis). In diagnosis, the use of immune reactions exhibited by blood serum; serum diagnosis.

immunodiffusion (im·ewn·o·dif·**ew**·zhun). Gel diffusion; a precipitation test in which antigen and antibody are placed in a gel of agar, or similiar substance, and allowed to diffuse towards each other to form a precipitate as shown by a white line. Single or double diffusions in one or two dimensions are obtained by different techniques. [L *immunis* free from, *diffundere* to pour out.]

immunofluorescence (im·ewn·o·floo·or·**es**′·ens). A technique of labelling specially prepared antibodies with fluorescent dyes and applying them to a histological preparation in order to view and localize specific proteins. [immunity, fluorescence.]

immunogen (im·**ewn**·o·**jen**). A substance which, when introduced into the body, stimulates a specific immune response.

immunogenic (im·ewn·o·**jen**′·ik). Giving rise to or capable of stimulating a specific immune response. [immunity, Gk *genein* to produce.]

immunoglobulins (im·ewn·o·**glob**′·ew·linz). Proteins endowed with known antibody activity and certain other proteins, mostly gamma globulins, related to them by chemical structure and, hence, antigenic specificity. Six distinct classes of immunoglobulins (Ig) are known to occur in man and analogous proteins occur in animals. They are found in the blood plasma (and in serum) and other fluids and tissues of normal and immunologically stimulated individuals, and as paraproteins in various diseases. The basic pattern of the Ig molecule contains four polypeptide chains: two heavy (H or A chains) and two light (L or B chains). IgA and IgM molecules are multiples of the four-chain unit as found in IgG; in addition, all Ig classes contain carbohydrate in different amounts and secretory IgA has an additional T chain. H chains are distinctive for each Ig: L chains are the same in all Ig classes but can exist in the same individual in two forms, α and β, giving Ig types K and L. Immunoglobulins are heterogeneous also in their allotypes, their ability to cross membranes such as the placenta, their affinity for cells, their stability to reducing agents (mercaptoethanol) and to heat (56–65°C for 30 min), and especially in their serological activities including antibody valence. Sub-classes can exist in some Ig classes, differing in H chain structure, electrophoretic mobility and serological properties. Papain and pepsin split the Ig molecule into fragments with recognizable Ig features. [L *immunis* free from, *globulus* small globe.]

immunological (im·ewn·**ol**·o·je·cal). **Immunological enhancement.** Enhancement of growth of tumours due to antibody which reacts with antigen on the surface of the tumour cells, thus blocking T-lymphocytes from exerting a cytotoxic effect on the tumour cells. **Immunological paralysis.** Synonym for acquired immunological tolerance. **Immunological rejection.** Rejection of grafted tissue due to an immune reaction against it. **Immunological surveillance.** Hypothesis suggested by Sir MacFarlane Burnet that lymphocytes monitor the cells of the body and destroy any cells which have undergone antigenic change due to somatic mutation. The early development of neoplasms may be arrested by this mechanism. **Immunological unresponsiveness.** Failure to respond to challenge with antigen due either to immunological tolerance or to a general unresponsiveness, such as may occur in immunodeficiency.

immunologist (im·ewn·**ol**·o·jist). One who has special knowledge of immunology and the application of its principles.

immunology (im·ewn·**ol**·o·je). That branch of science which is concerned with immunity and its phenomena. [immunity, Gk *logos* science.]

immunopolysaccharide (im·**ewn**·o·pol·e·**sak**′·ar·ide). Any polysaccharide of bacterial origin, which has specific immunological properties.

immunoprotein (im·**ewn**·o·**pro**′·te·in). Immune protein. *See* PROTEIN.

immunoradiometric (im·ewn·o·**ra**·de·o·**met**′·rik). A form of saturation analysis where the radioactive label is attached to the binding agent rather than to a preparation of the substance to be assayed, as is the case with radio-immunoassay. [immunity, radiation, Gk *metron* measure.]

immunoreaction (im·ewn·o·re·**ak**′·shun). The mutual reaction of antigen and antibody. [immunity, reaction.]

immunoserum (im·**ewn**·o·**seer**′·um). Antitoxin. **Immunoserum Antibotulinum.** *European Pharmacopoeia* name for Botulinum Antitoxin BP 1973. **Immunoserum Anticlostridium Mixtum.** *EP* name for Mixed Gas-gangrene Antitoxin BP 1973. **Immunoserum Anticlostridium Oedematiens.** *EP* name for Gas-gangrene Antitoxin (Oedematiens) BP 1973. **Immunoserum Anticlostridium Perfringens.** *EP* name for Gas-gangrene Antitoxin (Perfringens) BP 1973. **Immunoserum Anticlostridium Septicum.** *EP* name for Gas-gangrene Antitoxin (Septicum) BP 1973. **Immunoserum Antidiphthericum.** *EP* name for Diphtheria Antitoxin BP 1973. **Immunoserum Antirabicum.** *EP* name for Rabies Antiserum BP 1973. **Immunoserum Antitetanicum.** *EP* name for Tetanus Antitoxin BP 1973.

immunosuppression (im·ewn·o·sup·**resh**′·un). The suppressing, wholly or in part, of the formation of protective substances generated by a living organism as a sequel to the incorporation into the organism's tissues of a foreign protein—such as the proteins of an organ transplant. A drug that acts as an immunosuppressant may therefore be administered to reduce the tendency of the living organism to reject tissues or an organ (e.g. kidney or heart) from a donor. [immunity, L *supprimere* to press down.]

immunosurgery (im·**ewn**·o·**ser**′·jer·e). The use of specific antigenic substances in surgical treatment. [immunity, surgery.]

immunotherapy (im·**ewn**·o·**ther**′·ap·e). The production of immunity as a therapeutic measure; immunization therapy.

immunotoxin (im·**ewn**·o·**tox**′·in). An antitoxin of any kind. [immunity, toxin.]

immunotransfusion (im·**ewn**·o·trans·**few**′·shun). Transfusion with blood, plasma, or serum containing immune bodies.

Imolamine (i·**mol**·am·een). BP Commission approved name for 4-(2-diethylaminoethyl)-5-imino-3-phenyl-1,2,4-oxadiazoline; it is used in the treatment of angina pectoris.

impact (**im**·pakt). 1. Sudden and forcible contact of one body against another. 2. To drive one particle, e.g. of bone into another so that the two are firmly locked together. 3. To wedge together. [L *impactus* struck together.]

impacted (im·**pak**·ted). 1. Driven strongly against and held, as one fragment of bone on another. 2. Firmly lodged, as faeces in the bowel. 3. Wedged closely together, as calculi or unerupted teeth. [see prec.]

impaction (im·**pak**·shun). The state or condition of being impacted. **Ceruminal impaction.** An impacted aggregation of cerumen in the external auditory meatus. **Dental impaction.** So close retention of a tooth in its socket that eruption is not possible. **Faecal impaction.** A condition in which a mass of hardened faeces is retained in some part of the bowel.

impalpable (im·**pal**·pabl). A state or condition that cannot be appreciated by the sense of touch, e.g. a very faint pulse, or a powder so finely ground that there is no perception of grit. [L *in*, *palpare* to touch.]

impaludation (im·**pal**·ew·**da**′·shun). Malarial therapy. *See* THERAPY. [L *in*, *palus* marsh.]

impaludism (im·**pal**·ew·dizm). Chronic malaria. *See* MALARIA. [see prec.]

impar (**im**·par). Unpaired; odd. [L, unequal.]

impardigitate (im·par·**dij**·it·ate). Having an odd number of digits. [impar, digit.]

impatency (im·pa·ten·se). The state of being impatent, i.e. closed.

impatent (im·pa·tent). Closed; not patent. [L *in, patere* to be open.]

impedance (im·pe·dans). 1. The total resistance of an electrical circuit to the passage of an alternating current. This may be due to the electrical resistance, capacitance, or inductance of the circuit, and is obtained by vector addition of the total resistance and the total reactance of the circuit. 2. It may be used when referring to the flow of blood through the cardiovascular system. This recognizes the fact that flow in the major arteries is pulsatile and the vessels offer reactive, as well as purely resistive, obstruction to flow. **Vascular impedance.** By analogy with an electrical circuit the total resistance offered by a vascular system to the flow of blood through it. The concept of impedance in a vascular system takes into account the pulsatile nature of blood flow in arteries. [L *impedire* to entangle the feet.]

imperative (im·per·at·iv). 1. Not under the control of the will. 2. Dominant, as a concept. [L *imperare* to command.]

imperception (im·per·sep·shun). 1. Lack or imperfect powers of perception. 2. Inability to form a mental picture of an object from the sensations to which it gives rise or the stimulus it effects. [L *in,* perception.]

imperforate (im·per·for·ate). 1. Without an opening or aperture. 2. Abnormally occluded, as the anus. [L *in,* perforated.]

imperforation (im·per·for·a′·shun). The condition of being closed or occluded; the term is used particularly in relation to structures which normally are open, as the vagina. **Otic imperforation.** Complete stenosis of the external ear passage. [see prec.]

Imperial Drink (im·peer·e·al dringk). Potus Imperialis BPC 1949. [L *imperium* dominion.]

impermeable (im·per·me·abl). Not allowing passage of fluid or air. [L *in, per, meare* to pass.]

impervious (im·per·ve·us). 1. Not permitting passage through; impenetrable. 2. Impermeable. [L *impervius.*]

impetigination, impetiginization (im·pet·ij·in·a′·shun, im·pet·ij·in·i·za′·shun). The occurrence of impetigo on a part of the skin on which previously there had been a different skin lesion.

impetiginoid, impetiginous (im·pet·ij·in·oid, im·pet·ij·in·us). 1. Having the character of impetigo or resembling impetigo. 2. Relating or belonging to impetigo. [impetigo, Gk *eidos* form.]

impetigo (im·pet·i·go). An inflammation of the skin associated with discrete vesicles or bullae, generally attributed to streptococcal infection. **Chronic symmetrical impetigo.** Pityriasis alba. **Impetigo circinata.** A form of impetigo, usually bullous, in which the lesions heal in the centre, so that the patient presents several annular lesions. **Impetigo contagiosa.** An acute, contagious, inflammatory skin disease, characterized by the formation of discrete lesions covered with vesicles; the latter burst and their serous contents coagulate to form typical thin, honey-coloured crusts. **Impetigo contagiosa bullosa.** A less acute variety of impetigo in which the primary lesions are bullae and not vesicles. The crusts seen in this malady are thin and of a greenish-yellow hue. **Impetigo contagiosa gyrata.** A less acute variety of impetigo in which the lesions heal in the centre, spread at the periphery, and by fusion with adjacent lesions form gyrate patterns. **Impetigo follicularis.** Bockhart's impetigo. **Furfuraceous impetigo.** Pityriasis alba. **Impetigo herpetiformis.** An acute, often fatal, febrile malady, usually seen in pregnant women, commencing with the eruption of irregularly-shaped or circinate groups of small pustules which tend to coalesce; it originates on the genitofemoral area and then spreads widely. **Impetigo neonatorum.** Pemphigus neonatorum; an acute widespread bullous eruption of growing infants, usually developing before the umbilical stump has healed, attributed to staphylococci or streptococci. In the pre-antibiotic era the disease was often fatal. **Impetigo parasitica.** Impetigo contagiosa (see above). **Impetigo pityroides.** Pityriasis alba. **Impetigo rodens.** Acne varioliformis. **Sigilliform impetigo.** Yellowish-brown "stuck-on" crusts as seen in the form of impetigo contagiosa. **Impetigo simplex.** Impetigo staphylogenes (see below). **Impetigo sparia.** Impetigo contagiosa (see above). **Impetigo staphylogenes.** Impetigo in which primary lesions are vesicles or bullae; as the acute stage passes, folliculitis or boils may develop on the affected zones. **Impetigo streptogenes.** Impetigo contagiosa (see above). **Impetigo syphilitica.** A former name for impetiginous syphilid. *See* SYPHILID. **Impetigo varicellosa.** A variety of varicella in which large, flat bullae or pustules form. **Impetigo vulgaris.** Impetigo contagiosa (see above). [L *impetus* attack.]

See also: BOCKHART, FOX (W. T.).

impetus (im·pet·us). 1. The onset of paroxysm of an illness or disease. 2. In psychological medicine, the amount of individual energetic force expended by instinctive impulses. [L, attack.]

impilation (im·pil·a·shun). Rouleaux formation. *See* FORMATION. [L *in,* pile.]

impinger (im·pin·jer). A device for estimating the number of particles of dust in a measured sample of air. The sample is sent through an underwater jet and impinges on an upright plate. The water containing the dust is then placed in a shallow receptacle and its particles counted microscopically. Cf. JET DUST COUNTER, KONIMETER. [L *impingere* to strike against.]

Implacentalia (im·plas·en·ta′·le·ah). A sub-division of the class Mammalia which includes those in which there is no placenta. [L *in,* placenta.]

implant (im·plant, im·plant). 1. To insert or graft in securely. 2. Any piece of tissue for use as a graft. 3. A small cylindrical container in which a radioactive isotope, to be imbedded in the tissues, is placed for interstitial radiotherapy. **Basket implant.** In ophthalmology, a cup-shaped implant, made of a plastic or inert material, for inserting into Tenon's capsule following enucleation of the eyeball. The cup has a number of holes to which are sutured the four recti muscles; this gives a moving stump to which can be fitted the prosthesis. **Carcinomatous implant.** Formation of a secondary carcinomatous nodule as a result of direct implantation of free cells from the primary tumour. It occurs in surgical wounds and the body cavities. **Endometrial implant.** Implants of endometrial tissue on intrapelvic structures or in the lower genital tract after it has been spilled spontaneously through the fallopian tubes or the cervix uteri, or after it has been spilled during operations on the uterus and tubes. **Hormone implant.** A tablet or cylinder of fused or compressed hormone, intended for subcutaneous or intramuscular implantation. The BP 1973 lists Deoxycortone Acetate Implant and Testosterone Implant. **Permanent implant.** An implant of radioactive material, usually of short half-life (radon seeds, gold grains), which is left permanently in the tissues. **Planar implant.** A radioactive implant in which the sources are arranged in planes (single-plane implant, two-plane implant, multiple-plane implant). **Volume implant.** A radioactive implant in which the sources are arranged throughout a specified volume of tissue the whole of which can be implanted. [see foll.]

See also: SAMPSON.

implantation (im·plan·ta·shun). 1. In therapeutics, the introduction of a drug in solid form, usually in the subcutaneous tissues of the abdominal wall to ensure local action and or sustained action. 2. In surgery, the introduction of one tissue or structure into another, e.g. divided ureter into bladder, or one nerve into another. 3. In radiotherapy, the insertion of solid radioactive sources directly into the tissues of the body. 4. In bacteriology, the introduction of bacteria into blood, blood serum, or blood plasma *in vitro,* in order to test the bactericidal power or growth inhibition. 5. The embedding of the fertilized ovum in the uterine mucous membrane. **Arterial implantation.** The operation of implanting the bleeding, cut end of an internal mammary artery into an ischaemic area of ventricular myocardium with the object of achieving anastomotic communication with the coronary blood vessels. **Filigree implantation.** Filigree repair; a method of hernial repair, involving the insertion of a mesh of (silver) wire in the parietes at the point of weakness. **Hypodermic implantation.** The introduction of a solid medicine under the skin, usually in the form of a small tablet, so as to permit of the slow absorption of a drug. **Parenchymatous**

implantation. The introduction of a solid medicine into the substance of a tumour so as to produce a local and sustained action, e.g. of testosterone in treating widespread mammary cancer. **Teratic implantation, teratological implantation.** Union of a fetal monster with a normal fetus. [L *implantare* to set into.]

imponderable (im·**pon**·der·abl). Without appreciable weight; so light as to be incapable of being weighed. [L *in, pondus* weight.]

importation (im·por·**ta**·shun). The transference, as of a contagious disease, from one country or region into another. [L *importare* to bring in.]

impotence, impotency (**im**·po·tens, im·**po**·ten·se). Inability to perform the sexual act (in contradistinction to sterility—inability to reproduce), owing to failure of the reflex mechanism. As the female can perform the sexual act even without activation of the normal reflexes, impotence is correctly used, in a strict sense, only of the male. **Functional impotence.** Impotence in the healthy and fully matured male, invariably due to psychological causes. **Organic impotence.** Impotence due to disease or abnormality of development, e.g. extreme hypospadias, infantilism, tabes, etc. **Primary impotence.** Impotence due to psychogenic causes; also used to denote relative or total failure of the primary sexual urge with resulting incapacity, e.g. the impotence which comes on with advancing age. **Psychic impotence, psychogenic impotence.** Functional impotence (see above). **Relative impotence.** Inability to perform the sexual act with one or more particular women, though not generally. **Secondary impotence.** Impotence due to organic causes; organic impotence (see above). [L *in, potentia* power.]

impotentia (im·po·**ten**·she·ah). Impotence. **Impotentia coeundi.** Sexual impotence in the male. **Impotentia erigendi.** Sexual impotence due to lack of the power of erection of the penis. **Impotentia generandi.** Inability to reproduce. [L, impotence.]

impregnate (im·**preg**·nate). 1. To make pregnant. 2. In biology, to fertilize. 3. In chemistry, to charge or saturate with a gas or liquid. [L *impregnare* to render pregnant.]

impregnation (im·preg·**na**·shun). 1. Insemination. 2. The act of fertilization. 3. The act or process of saturating with a protective material, as in waterproofing. **Artificial impregnation.** Impregnation effected by instrumental injection of seminal fluid in the uterus. [see prec.]

impression (im·**presh**·un). 1. The mental effect of afferent sensory stimulation. 2. In dentistry, a mould taken of the mouth, into which is poured a substance which sets, giving a model upon which a crown, bridge, or artificial denture is constructed. 3. [Impressio.] A mark of depression on an organ or structure to accommodate another organ or structure. **Basilar impression.** 1. *Primary*—congenital upward displacement of basilar and condylar portions of the occipital bone causing deformity of the foramen magnum and posterior fossa, often with neurological disability. 2. *Secondary*—similar deformity resulting from softening of bone by disease. **Cardiac impression [impressio cardiaca].** 1. A shallow concavity near the centre of the upper surface of the liver, underlying the heart. 2. An impression on the mediastinal part of the lung in contact with the pericardium. **Centrifugal impression.** A nerve impulse travelling from the central nervous system to the periphery of an organism. **Centripetal impression.** A nerve impulse travelling from the periphery of an organism to the central nervous system. **Impressions for the cerebral gyri [impressiones digitatae].** *See* CALVARIA. **Impression for the costoclavicular ligament [impressio ligamenti costoclavicularis].** A roughened triangular impression on the inferior surface of the sternal end of the clavicle. **Impressions on the liver.** *See* LIVER, LOWER (OR VISCERAL) SURFACE. **Mental impression.** The mental picture that remains as the result of an incident. **Oesophageal impression [impressio esophagea (NA)].** A groove on the posterior surface of the left lobe of the liver, lodging the oesophagus. **Petrous impression.** The area in contact with the anterior surface of the petrous part of the temporal bone. **Sensory impression.** The effect produced on an organ of sense, or on a single sensory ending, by an external stimulus. **Impressions on the spleen.** *See* SPLEEN, VISCERAL SURFACE. **Trigeminal impression [impressio trigemini (NA)].** A shallow depression on the anterior surface of the petrous part of the temporal bone near its apex, lodging the trigeminal ganglion. [L *imprimere* to press into.]

impressorium (im·pres·**or**·e·um). Sensorium, i.e. the seat of sensation. [see prec.]

imprinting (**im**·print·ing). A species-specific type of irreversible learning occurring during a *critical period* early in life. [OFr. *empreinter* impress.]

impulse (**im**·puls). 1. A sudden force; a thrust. 2. An urge to act in a specified way. **Cardiac impulse.** The thrust which the contracting heart makes against the chest wall. The site of the maximal impulse of the apex of the heart constitutes the apex beat, formed normally by the left ventricle and lying in the 5th intercostal space in, or just to the right of, the midclavicular line. The position and character of the apex impulse may be altered by dilatation or displacement of the heart, hypertrophy of either or both ventricles, by pericardial effusion or constriction, and by disease of the lungs. **Enteroceptive impulses.** Afferent nerve impulses arising from stimulation of internal organs. **Episternal impulses.** Pulsation in the suprasternal notch due to the impulse of the aorta and the innominate or right common carotid arteries. Increase in the normal pulsation occurs in aortic aneurysm, coarctation of the aorta, innominate aneurysm, and in kinking of an atherosclerotic carotid artery in elderly persons. Rarely, pulsations may be due to a tumour in the mediastinum. **Morbid impulse.** An impulse which has a cause in some disordered mental mechanism, or which has a morbid end in view. **Nerve impulse, nervous impulse, neural impulse.** That activity in a nerve fibre that causes a stimulus applied at one end to be propagated to the other end and induce activity there. The stimulus necessary for this propagation may originate in the nerve cell from which the fibre arises, or at that end of the fibre distant from the nerve cell, according to the function of the nerve. **Voluntary impulse.** An impulse determined by the will. [L *impellere* to drive before.]

impulsion (im·**pul**·shun). 1. The act of impelling or driving forward mentally or physically. 2. Sudden abnormal passion to perform certain (usually unlawful or unpleasant) acts. **Wandering impulsion.** A fugue. [see prec.]

impunctate (im·**pungk**·tate). 1. Unmarked with dots or points. 2. Unpunctured. [L *in, punctum* point, puncture.]

impurity (im·**pewr**·it·e). 1. The quality or condition of being unclean or impure. 2. Lack of clarity in heart sounds but not enough to constitute a murmur. 3. In chemistry, a condition of adulteration of a substance. 4. The object or substance the presence of which causes adulteration or uncleanness. **Respiratory impurity.** The quantity of carbon dioxide present in a room that is proportionately in excess of the quantity present in the open air. [L *impurus* filthy.]

imputability (im·**pewt**·ab·**il**'·it·e). 1. In forensic medicine, the condition of being sound enough mentally to be responsible for actions. 2. The quality of being completely responsible and sound in mind. [L *imputare* to give credit or blame.]

im-pyeng (**im**·pi·eng). Collapsing typhus. *See* TYPHUS. [Korean word.]

Imre, Josef (b. 1884). Budapest ophthalmologist.

Imre's operation. The use of curved sliding skin flaps, with a Burow's triangle at the end, to close lid defects, especially of the lower.

imu (e·moo). A disease endemic among the Ainu race of Japan. The precipitating factor is emotional shock, which causes mental disorder and liability to attacks of psychomotor disturbance.

imvic (**im**·vik). A mnemonic for the five tests used to distinguish coliform organisms: indole production, methyl-red test, Voges-Proskauer test, and the ability to utilize citrate as a sole source of carbon. Typical faecal *Bacterium coli* are indole positive, methyl-red positive, and negative for the other two characters; the inability to ferment citrate is true only for the true faecal strains.

in-. Prefix, from the Latin preposition *in,* meaning *in, intensive action, not.*

in articulo mortis (in ar·**tik**·ew·lo **mor**·tis). At the instant of death. [L.]

in extremis (in ex·**tre**·mis). At the point of death. [L.]

in-knee (**in**·nee). Genu valgum; knock knee. [L *in,* AS *cneow.*]

in situ (in **si**·tew). 1. In the normal, natural or original position. 2. In a given place. [L, in place.]

in-toe (**in**·to). Hallux valgus. [L *in,* AS *ta.*]

in-toeing (**in**·to·ing). A manner of walking, particularly observed in very young children, in which the feet are so far turned inwards that when running is attempted the subject is apt to fall because the toes of the one foot strike against the toes of the other. [see prec.]

in utero (in **ew**·ter·o). Within the uterus. [L.]

in vacuo (in **vak**·ew·o). In a vacuum. [L.]

in vitro (in **vi**·tro). Within a glass vessel, e.g. a test-tube; applied to changes taking place in the test-tube method of investigation; extended to include any changes occurring under experimental conditions outside the body of a living organism. Cf. IN VIVO [L, in glass.]

in vivo (in **vi**·vo). Within the living organism; applied to chemical processes and changes taking place in the body. Cf. IN VITRO. [L, in the living being.]

inacidity (in·as·**id**·it·e). Lack or absence of acidity, i.e. the absence of a sufficient quantity of hydrochloric acid in the gastric juice. [L *in,* acidity.]

inaction (in·**ak**·shun). 1. A condition in which there is very little response (or none at all) to normal stimuli. 2. Inertness; want of energy. 3. Rest; inactivity. [L *in,* action.]

inactivate (in·**ak**·tiv·ate). To render physically inactive; to destroy the active principle. [see foll.]

inactivation (in·**ak**·tiv·**a**'·shun). The act or process of destroying the activity of any of the body fluids, e.g. serum or other substance, by exposing it to heat or some other physical or chemical force. **Inactivation of the complement.** Destruction of the complement of serum by heating it to about 56°C, and keeping it at that temperature for 30 min. **X chromosome inactivation.** Lyon hypothesis. [L *in,* activation.]

inadequacy (in·**ad**·e·kwas·e). Insufficiency or incompetence; the inability to carry out an allotted function. [L *in,* adequate.]

inaemia (in·e·me·ah). The presence of formed fibrin in the blood plasma. [Gk *is* fibre, *haima* blood.]

inagglutinable (in·ag·**loo**·tin·abl). Not agglutinable. [L *in,* agglutinate.]

inanagenesis, inanaphysis (**in**·an·ah·**jen**'·es·is, in·an·**af**·is·is). Repair or renewal of muscular fibre. [Gk *is* fibre, *ana, genein* to produce, *physis* natural origin.]

inangulate (in·**ang**·gew·late). Without angles. [L *in,* angle.]

inanimate (in·**an**·im·ate). Not alive; dead. [L *in,* animate.]

inanition (in·an·**ish**·un). The physical condition of exhaustion and wasting that is the result of complete lack of or non-assimilation of food; a state of starvation. [L *inanis* empty.]

inankyloglossia (in·**ang**·kil·o·**glos**'·e·ah). A congenital or acquired condition of the tongue in which it cannot be moved. [L *in,* Gk *agkyle* a bending, *glossa* tongue.]

inappetence (in·**ap**·et·ens). 1. Want or loss of appetite. 2. Lack of desire. [L *in, appetere* to seek.]

inarticulate (in·ar·**tik**·ew·late). 1. Without joints or articulations or distinct body segments. 2. Incapable of intelligible speech. 3. Without the power of clear or distinct expression in speech. [L *in,* articulate.]

inassimilable (in·as·**im**·il·abl). Not able to be assimilated and therefore incapable of being used for nourishment. [L *in,* assimilable.]

inborn (**in**·born). Acquired by or engrafted in mind or body during the process of development *in utero,* e.g. any constitutional peculiarity or mental trait; innate or inherent; natural. [L *in,* AS *beran* to bear.]

inbreeding (**in**·breed·ing). The act of breeding from a male and female very closely related the one to the other, having the same parents or grandparents. [L *in,* AS *breden.*]

inca bone (**inc**·kah bone). Incarial bone.

incallosal (in·kal·o·sal). Lacking the corpus callosum. [L *in,* corpus callosum.]

incanate (in·**ka**·nate). Hoary white. [L *incanus* quite grey.]

incandescent (in·kan·**des**·ent). The condition of a substance glowing white-hot; emitting intense light rays at high temperatures. [L *incandescere* to begin to glow.]

incanous (in·**ka**·nus). Incanate.

incarcerated (in·kar·ser·a·ted). 1. Constricted. 2. Held abnormally fast, as an irreducible hernia. 3. Confined within something. [L *in, carcerare* to imprison.]

incarceration (**in**·kar·ser·**a**'·shun). The imprisonment or unnatural confinement of a part, as the placenta or a hernia. [see prec.]

incarial bone (ing·**ka**·re·al bone). A small bone lying in the suture between the two parietal bones of the skull. It is so called from its occurrence as a separate bone in the skulls of ancient Incas.

incarnant (in·**kar**·nant). 1. Producing flesh; flesh-forming. 2. Promoting or hastening the granulation of a wound. 3. Any agent which hastens or aids the process of granulation, or which is flesh-forming. [see foll.]

incarnatio (in·kar·**na**·she·o). The process of being converted into flesh. **Incarnatio unguis.** The ingrowing of a nail; onychogryphosis. [L *incarnare* to make flesh.]

incarnation (in·kar·**na**·shun). 1. The process of forming granulations. 2. Conversion into flesh. [see prec.]

incarnative (in·**kar**·nah·tiv). 1. Taking part in the forming of granulations. 2. Incarnant, 3rd def. [L *incarnare* to make flesh.]

inceal (in·se·al). Incudal.

incest (**in**·sest). Cohabitation or sexual intercourse between persons so closely related by blood that their marriage is prohibited by law. [L *incestum* unchastity.]

incidence (**in**·sid·ens). 1. The act of affecting or falling on. 2. The rate of occurrence of new cases (or manifestations) in a defined population in a period of time. *See also:* PREVALENCE. **Angle of incidence.** *See* ANGLE. **Point of incidence.** *See* POINT. [L *incidere* to fall on, to happen.]

incident (**in**·sid·ent). 1. Afferent, or going towards. 2. Happening with, or falling or impinging upon. 3. A happening or occurrence. [see prec.]

incineration (in·**sin**·er·**a**'·shun). Cremation; the process of burning organic substance to ashes. [L *incinerare* to burn to ashes.]

incipient (in·**sip**·e·ent). 1. Beginning to show itself. 2. Beginning to exist. 3. Initial, as a stage of a disease. [L *incipire* to begin.]

incisal (in·**si**·zal). Relating or belonging to a cutting edge, e.g. of a tooth. [see foll.]

incise (in·**size**). To cut into, e.g. with a knife. [L *incidere.*]

incised (in·**si**·zd). 1. Having undergone incision. 2. Made by the process of cutting, as a wound; notched, as a leaf. [L *incidere* to cut into.]

incision (in·**sizh**·un). 1. A linear cut or wound made by a sharp cutting edge or instrument. 2. The act of cutting. **Buttonhole incision.** A small drainage incision made by the removal of an ellipse of skin. **Coeliotomy incision.** An incision through the abdominal wall to open the peritoneal cavity. **Gridiron incision.** For appendicectomy: an abdominal incision in the line of the fibres of the external oblique muscle with its centre at the junction of the middle and outer third of a line joining the umbilicus to the anterior superior iliac spine; the external oblique, internal oblique, and transversus abdominis muscles are split successively in the line of their fibres. **Median incision.** An incision in the midline of the anterior abdominal wall. **Paramedian incision.** An incision about one inch from the midline of the anterior abdominal wall with displacement of the rectus abdominis muscle laterally. **Rectus incision.** Transrectus incision (see below). **Relief incision.** An incision made at a distance from a wound to relax the tension on the skin which is used to close it. **Stab incision.** A puncture incision made for drainage. **Suprapubic incision.** A transverse or vertical incision between umbilicus and pubis. **Transrectus incision.** A paramedian incision with splitting of the rectus abdominis muscle in the line of incision. **Transverse incision.** A horizontal incision through the abdominal wall with transverse division of one or both rectus abdominis muscles, and, if necessary, splitting of the lateral muscles of the outer border of the rectus sheath. [L *incidere* to cut into.]

See also: ALEXANDER, AUVRAY, BAR, BATTLE, BERGMANN (E.), BEVAN, CHIENE, CODMAN, COURVOISIER, EDEBOHLS, HENRY, JALAGUIER, KAMMERER, KEHR, KOCHER, KUESTNER (O. E.), LILIENTHAL, MCBURNEY, MCLAUGHLIN, MORISON, PERTHES, PFANNENSTIEL, ROLLET (E.), WHIPPLE (A. O.).

incisive (in·si·siv). 1. Having the power to cut or penetrate. 2. Having the quality of cutting. 3. Belonging to or situated near the incisor teeth. [see prec.]

incisive bone of the maxilla [os incisivum (NA)]. A bone incorporated in the anterior part of the maxilla, and often distinct on the palate. It is a separate bone in many lower vertebrates, and also during development in man; the premaxilla; intermaxillary bone.

incisor (in·si·zor). 1. Anything adapted for cutting. 2. Any one of the four front teeth in each jaw. **Incisor tooth.** *See* TOOTH. [L *incidere* to cut into.]

incisura (in·si·**sewr**·ah). 1. A notch or indrawing, causing an angular outline of an organ. It may be organic or spastic in origin. 2. [NA] In anatomy, a notch. **Incisura apicis cordis [NA].** A small notch on the anterior border of the heart where the anterior interventricular groove turns around the border to become continuous with the inferior interventricular groove. **Incisura of the cartilage of the auditory meatus [incisura cartilaginis meatus acustici (NA)].** The deficiency in the upper and posterior part of the cartilaginous external auditory meatus. It is filled by fibrous tissue. **Incisura intertragica [NA].** The notch, open superiorly, between the tragus and antitragus. **Posterior incisura.** An inconstant infolding of the gastric wall caused by the pancreatic ridge when a patient is in the supine position, shown radiologically in a lateral view of the stomach. **Incisura rivini.** The notch of Rivinus, or Rivinus' incisura; tympanic notch (*see* NOTCH). **Incisura terminalis of the auricle [incisura terminalis auris (NA)].** A deep fissure between the commencement of the helix and the cartilage of the external auditory meatus. [L *incidere* to cut into.]

See also: DUVERNEY, RIVINUS.

incisure (in·si·zhewr). A notch. **Radiological incisure.** Any notch or indentation that is seen in an x-ray film of a hollow organ containing an opaque meal. [see prec.]

See also: LANTERMANN, RIVINUS, SANTORINI, SCHMIDT (H. D.).

incitogram (in·si·to·gram). The group of conditions or impelling urges in the central nervous system which originates and sets in motion efferent impulses. [L *incitare* to rouse up, Gk *gramma* a writing.]

inclination (in·klin·a·shun). 1. A deviation or propensity; a leaning. 2. In dentistry the deviation of a tooth from its normal vertical position. **Inclination of the pelvis [inclinatio pelvis (NA)].** The angle of the plane of the pelvic inlet to the horizontal in the erect posture, normally about 55°. [L *inclinare* to incline.]

inclinometer (in·klin·**om**·et·er). An instrument with which the direction of the visual axes can be determined. [inclination, meter.]

inclusion (in·**klew**·zhun). Anything enclosed within another thing; the act of enclosing such. **Cell inclusion.** Any foreign substance contained within a cell. **Fetal inclusion.** A monster in which one fetus is enclosed within another. **Intranuclear inclusion.** Any foreign substance contained within the nucleus of a cell. **Owl's-eye inclusion.** The inclusion body, or bodies, found in giant cells formed in cytomegalovirus infection. **Viral inclusion.** Aggregates of virus material which may contain virus particles, found in the nucleus and/or cytoplasm of virus-infected cells. [L *in*, *claudere* to shut.]

See also: WALTHARD.

incoagulable (in·ko·ag·ew·labl). Applied to a substance that is incapable of clotting and will not curdle. [L *in*, *coagulare* to curdle.]

incoercible (in·ko·**ers**·ibl). 1. That cannot be restrained, overcome or stopped, such as hiccup. 2. In physics, incapable of being reduced to a liquid state by pressure. [L *in*, coercible.]

incoherence (in·ko·**he**·rens). 1. The lack of coherence or adherence. 2. Incongruity or inconsistency. 3. A mental condition in which ideas are unconnected. 4. Lack of relevance and connection in phrasing and wording, or the utterance of disjointed words and phrases. [see foll.]

incoherent (in·ko·**he**·rent). 1. Without consistency or connection. 2. Lacking in sequence; disconnected; incongruous. [L *in*, *cohaerere* to hold together.]

incombustibility (in·kom·bust·ib·il'·it·e). The state or quality of being incapable of burning, or of being uninflammable, as is asbestos. [L *in*, combustible.]

incompatibility (in·kom·pat·ib·il'·it·e). The quality or state of being incompatible. **Chemical incompatibility.** A state in which substances have mutual reaction, with the production of new substances when they are mixed. **Physiological incompatibility.** Applied to substances, such as drugs, which have the property of being mutually antagonistic in their effects on the body. **Therapeutic incompatibility.** Descriptive of drugs which, when given, say in a mixture, to the patient, lose their intrinsic effect because they neutralize each other. [L *in*, compatible.]

incompatible (in·kom·**pat**·ibl). 1. Applied to substances which cannot be put together in a mixture because they undergo chemical change and consequently the therapeutic effect of one or both is lost. 2. Of two or more drugs, unsuitable for administration to the same patient at the same time because of mutual antagonism. 3. Of a blood transfusion, whereby the donor blood produces harmful effects when transfused into the recipient because the two bloods are of incompatible groups. [see prec.]

incompetence, incompetency (in·**kom**·pet·ens, in·**kom**·pet·en·se). Applied to a valve or sphincter, failure to close. **Aortic incompetence.** Aortic insufficiency, aortic regurgitation; failure of the aortic valves to close completely during ventricular diastole, with the result that blood leaks back into the left ventricle. It is often combined with some degree of stenosis, and is usually due to rheumatic infection or to syphilis. A congenital bicuspid and incompetent aortic valve may be associated with coarctation of the aorta, or become the seat of bacterial endocarditis. Rarely, trauma may cause rupture of one of the aortic-valve cusps causing acute and gross incompetence, while slight aortic incompetence may occur in severe systemic hypertension or in old age, due to dilatation of the aorta. **Free incompetence.** Incompetence of a considerable degree without stenosis. **Ileocaecal incompetence, ileocolic incompetence.** Failure of the ileocolic valve to prevent the flow of faeces from the colon backward into the ileum. **Mitral incompetence.** Mitral insufficiency, mitral regurgitation; incompetence of the mitral valve, most commonly the result of rheumatic carditis, when it is usually associated with some stenosis; it also occurs as the result of a variety of congenital abnormalities, from ischaemic disease of the papillary muscles, rupture of the chordae, cardiomyopathy, bacterial endocarditis, and other non-infective inflammatory diseases. **Organic incompetence of the cardiac valves.** A failure of a valve to close completely so that blood leaks back into the proximal chambers during contraction of the distal chamber. It may affect any or all of the four cardiac valves and is the result of acquired disease (rheumatic fever, syphilis, or bacterial endocarditis), or congenital maldevelopment; very rarely, trauma is responsible. **Paravalvar incompetence, paravalvular incompetence.** Paravalvular regurgitation; regurgitation of blood between a cardiac valve prosthesis and the natural valve ring due to partial detachment of the valve. **Pulmonary incompetence.** Pulmonary valvular insufficiency, pulmonary regurgitation; incompetence of the pulmonary valve. It is nearly always functional or relative, due to dilatation of the main pulmonary artery and stretching of the valve ring as a result of pulmonary hypertension. It can occur in extreme hypertension in mitral stenosis (Graham Steell murmur), and is also seen in association with atrioseptal defects; occasionally it may be due to abnormality of the valve itself. Acquired organic pulmonary-valve lesions are exceptional. **Pyloric incompetence.** The failure of the pyloric sphincter to hold back undigested food from entering the duodenum. **Relative incompetence of the cardiac valves.** Incompetence (functional) of a valve due to stretching of the valve ring as a result of enlargement of the chamber proximal or distal to the valve. It is usually reversible. **Tricuspid incompetence.** Tricuspid insufficiency, tricuspid regurgitation; incompetence of the tricuspid valve. It may be functional (relative) due to stretching of the valve ring as a result of enlargement and failure of the right ventricle (e.g. in severe pulmonary stenosis, pulmonary hypertension, rheumatic heart disease), and disappears with resolution of the failure. It may become permanent (organic) after repeated episodes of functional incompetence; organic incompetence may also be due to rheumatic infection, and is then combined with some degree of stenosis. [L *incompetens* insufficient.]

inconsistency (in·kon·**sis**·ten·se). *See* ZINSSER. [L *in, consistere* to exist.]

incontinence (in·**kon**·tin·ens). 1. The lack of voluntary control over the discharge of faeces or urine. 2. The absence of self-restraint in sexual relations. **Active incontinence.** The involuntary evacuation of faeces or urine at regular intervals. **False incontinence.** The leakage of urine which occurs when the bladder is over-distended. **Intermittent incontinence.** Incontinence of urine on muscular effort or pressure on the bladder. **Incontinence of milk.** The uncontrollable leakage of milk from the breast which may occur post partum. **Overflow incontinence.** The overflow of urine from a greatly distended paralysed bladder. **Paradoxical incontinence, paralytic incontinence, passive incontinence.** Overflow incontinence (see preceding). **Stress incontinence.** Incontinence of urine in women when the intra-abdominal pressure is raised by such efforts as coughing, sneezing, or lifting weights. [L *incontinentia* inability to retain anything.]

incontinentia pigmenti (in·**kon**·tin·**en**'·she·ah **pig**·men·ti). A syndrome consisting of vesicular, verrucose and pigmented lesions of the skin, and varied anomalies of the eye, central nervous system, bones, and teeth. The condition is inherited as a dominant, sex-linked trait which is lethal in the male.

inco-ordination (in·ko·or·din·**a**'·shun). 1. A condition in which the muscles involved in the carrying out of movements do not work together harmoniously. 2. The failure of any group of organs to work well together. **Jerky inco-ordination.** Muscular inco-ordination causing markedly sudden and irregular movement. [L *in*, co-ordinate.]

incorporation (in·**kor**·por·**a**'·shun). 1. The union of two or more ingredients in a single mass. 2. The act of combining or the condition of being combined into a homogeneous mass. [L *in, corpus* body.]

incostapedial (in·ko·stap·**e**'·de·al). Incudostapedial.

incrassate (in·**kras**·ate). Thickened or swollen. [L *incrassare* to become thick.]

incrassation (in·kras·**a**·shun). 1. The enlargement of an organ or part due to fatty deposit. 2. The act of becoming or making thick or thicker. [see prec.]

increment (**in**·kre·ment). 1. The act or process of enlarging or increasing. 2. Augmentation, e.g. of a disease. 3. An addition; that which is added. 4. The state of augmentation of an electrical discharge. [L *increscere* to grow.]

incremental (in·kre·**men**·tal). 1. Relating or belonging to increment or growth. 2. Resulting from the process of growth.

incretin (in·**kre**·tin). Secretin. [see foll.]

incretion (in·**kre**·shun). 1. An internal secretion. 2. That which is produced by activity of an endocrine gland. 3. The functional activity of endocrine glands. **Negative incretion.** Any internal secretion which has no endocrine activity but appears to neutralize toxins present in the blood. [L *in*, secretion.]

incretodiagnosis (in·**kre**·to·di·ag·**no**'·sis). Diagnosis in its relation to disorders or diseases of the internal secretions. [incretion, diagnosis.]

incretogenous (in·kre·**toj**·en·us). Originating in or due to a hormone or other internal secretion. [incretion, Gk *genein* to produce.]

incretology (in·kre·**tol**·o·je). Endocrinology. [incretion, Gk *logos* science.]

incretopathy (in·kre·**top**·ath·e). Any disease which affects the internal secretions. [incretion, Gk *pathos* disease.]

incretory (in·**kre**·tor·e). 1. Endocrine. 2. Belonging to the process or the products of the functional activity of the endocrine glands. [incretion.]

incretotherapy (in·**kre**·to·**ther**'·ap·e). Endocrinotherapy. [incretion, therapy.]

incrustation (in·krus·**ta**·shun). 1. The forming of a hard crust or scab or scale, e.g. on a lesion. 2. The formation of a coating of exudate or some other accidental material, e.g. a mineral salt. 3. A crust, scab, or scale. [L *incrustare* to cover with a crust.]

incubate (**in**·kew·bate). To maintain animal embryos or bacteria in any kind of apparatus in which there is a steady warm temperature most favourable to their development and growth. [L *incubare* to lie on.]

incubation (in·kew·**ba**·shun). 1. The act or process of incubating. 2. The process of development and growth that takes place in a fertilized ovum. **Incubation period.** The period of time elapsing between the moment when the organisms of an infective disease are implanted in the host and the appearance of the first clinical symptoms of the disease. [see prec.]

incubator (**in**·kew·ba·tor). 1. A box-like, specially ventilated apparatus in which a prematurely born infant is placed in an even, warm temperature and in conditions favourable to its further development until it is strong enough to bear ordinary room temperatures and less specialized feeding and care. 2. An apparatus in which bacterial cultures are kept at a constant temperature favourable to growth, usually 37 °C. **Cool incubator.** An incubator in which certain protozoal cultures are incubated at 22 °C. [L *incubare* to lie on.]

incubus (**in**·kew·bus). 1. Anything that is a heavy burden on the mind. 2. Nightmare. [see prec.]

incudal (**in**·kew·dal). Relating or belonging to the incus.

incudectomy (in·kew·**dek**·to·me). Operative removal of the incus. [incus, Gk *ektome* a cutting out.]

incudiform (in·**kew**·de·form). Like an anvil in shape. [incus, form.]

incudius (in·**kew**·de·us). The anterior ligament of the malleus, running between the neck of the malleus and the anterior wall of the tympanic cavity. [incus.]

incudomalleal, incudomalleolar (in·**kew**·do·**mal**'·e·al, in·**kew**·do·mal·e·**o**'·lar). Relating or belonging to the incus and the malleus. **Incudomalleal joint.** *See* JOINTS OF THE AUDITORY OSSICLES.

incudostapedial (in·**kew**·do·stap·**e**'·de·al). Relating or belonging to the incus and the stapes.

inculturing (in·**kul**·tcher·ing). In bacteriology, the introduction of bacteria into the blood, blood serum, or blood plasma *in vitro*, in order to test the bactericidal power or growth inhibition. [L *in*, culture.]

incuneation (in·**kew**·ne·**a**'·shun). 1. Gomphosis. 2. Impaction of the head of the fetus. 3. Impaction of a fractured portion of bone. [L *in, cuneus* wedge.]

incurable (in·**kewr**·abl). 1. Not admitting of cure. 2. A person suffering from an incurable disease. [L *in*, cure.]

incurvate (in·**ker**·vate). Curved inwards. [see foll.]

incurvation (in·ker·**va**·shun). 1. The state of being curved or bent inwards. 2. An inward curvature. [L *incurvare* to bend.]

incurvorecurved (in·**ker**·vo·re·**kervd**'). Curved backwards after being curved inwards. [L *incurvare* to bend, *recurvare* to bend backwards.]

incus [NA] (**in**·kus). The bone situated in the middle ear between and articulating with the malleus and stapes, i.e. the central one of the three auditory ossicles. The body [corpus incudis (NA)] bears the facet for the malleus. [L, anvil.]

incustapedic (in·kew·stap·e′·dik). Incudostapedial.

incwadi (ink·wad·e). An African name for *Burphane disticha* Herb. (family Amaryllidaceae), a South African plant allied to the genus *Haemanthus.* The bulb is reported to contain toxic alkaloids which resemble colchicine in action. It is used medicinally as a soothing application.

incyclophoria (in·si·klo·fo′·re·ah). A condition in which an affected eye on covering rotates inwards on its anteroposterior axis (i.e. the 12 o'clock position on the corneal margin turns inwards towards the nose). [L *in*, cyclophoria.]

incyclotropia (in·si·klo·tro′·pe·ah). A condition in which an affected eye is rotated inwards on its anteroposterior axis, even when both eyes are open. [L *in*, cyclotropia.]

incyclovergence (in·si·klo·ver′·jens). Disjunctive reciprocal motion of the eyes in which the upper poles of the cornea are rotated inwards; adtorsion. [L in, Gk *kyklos* circle, L *vergere* to bend.]

indagation (in·dag·a·shun). 1. Searching investigation with the finger. 2. Close examination. 3. Careful examination of the external sexual organs at the end of the puerperium. [L *indagare* to investigate.]

indamine (in·dam·een). 1. A class of synthetic organic dyestuffs. 2. Phenylene blue, $NH_2C_6H_4N{=}C_6H_4NH_2Cl$, a synthetic dye prepared from aniline and paraphenylenediamine.

indecent (in·de·sent). In forensic medicine, descriptive of sexual behaviour lewd or libidinous in character which constitutes an offence at law. [L *indecens* unseemly.]

indecision (in·des·izh·un). A state of vacillation or hesitation of mind; morbid weakness of will; hypobulia. [L *in, decisio* decision.]

indehiscent (in·de·his·ent). In botany, descriptive of a fruit or seed-pod which remains closed at maturity, such as a berry. [L *in, dehiscere* to gape.]

indenization (in·den·i·za′·shun). The process of cell proliferation that occurs in different parts of the body after metastasis has occurred. [L *in*, OFr *denzein* one living within (a city or country).]

indentation (in·den·ta·shun). 1. The condition of being dented or notched or of bearing a depression. 2. A recess or depression in a surface. 3. The act of pitting, as when the finger is pressed down on a yielding surface. [L *in, dens* tooth.]

independent assortment (in·de·pen·dent as·ort·ment). In genetics, the distribution in the gametes of the members of allelomorphic pairs such that the distribution of one pair will not affect or be affected by the distribution of other pairs. It is an observed fact that the combinations of two or more pairs of contrasted characters in the individuals will follow the laws of chance. This is a necessary concomitant of Mendel's second law, and will only hold good if the pairs of allelomorphic genes controlling the characters are not on the same chromosome pairs, i.e. linked. [L *in*, dependent.]

inderal (in·der·al). *See* PROPANOLOL.

index (in·dex). 1. A formula expressing the ratio of one measurement to another, e.g. an anthropometric index. 2. Forefinger or second digit. **ACH index.** An index of the state of nutrition of a child based on Arm girth, Chest depth, and Hip width. **Acidosis index.** An index based upon the estimation of the alkali reserve in cases of acidaemia. **Alpha index.** In electroencephalography, a measure of the proportion of time during which the record shows alpha rhythm as compared with other rhythms. **Alveolar index.** Gnathic index (see below). **Anaesthetic index.** An abstract factor said to evaluate the safety of an anaesthetic. It is defined as the units of an agent required to produce anaesthesia, divided by the number of units needed to cause respiratory cessation, but as anaesthesia is a progressive state the first number can hardly be calculated with accuracy. **Anthropometric index.** An index used in anthropometry. **Anthropophilic index.** The ratio of *Anopheles* mosquitoes, or other blood-sucking insects, containing human blood as against animal blood, sometimes expressed as a percentage. **Antibacterial index.** Of antimetabolites: the minimal ratio of analogue to metabolite which will prevent multiplication of a test organism dependent upon the metabolite for growth. **Antitryptic index.** Used as a serum test for cancer in a patient: it is determined by incubating a casein solution with trypsin and the patient's serum, and comparing the viscosity of this reaction mixture with a similar one obtained simultaneously using normal blood serum. **Articular index.** A semiquantitative method of measuring joint tenderness in rheumatic diseases. **Auricular index.** A hundred times the breadth of the ear, the distance between two lines parallel to the long axis of the ear (one of these lines being tangential to the anterior, the other to the posterior, border of the helix) divided by the maximum length of the ear, the distance from the highest point on the border of the helix to the lowest point on the lobule. **Auricular-height index (of the skull).** A hundred times the auricular-bregmatic height, from the bregma above to the midpoint of an imaginary line joining the upper borders of the external auditory meati below, divided by the maximum length of the skull, the distance from the most prominent point of the glabella to the opisthocranion (see CEPHALIC INDEX below). **Bacterial index.** In leprology, a method of assessing the degree of bacterial skin infection. Smears are assessed as 6+ when many clumps of *Mycobacterium leprae* are seen in each oil-immersion field, 5+ when one or two only are seen, 4+ when one or more isolated *M. leprae* are seen in every field, 3+ when at least one bacterium is seen in 10 fields, 2+ in 20 fields, and 1+ in 50 fields. The interpretation is subject to slight variation by individual leprologists, but it makes findings of different individuals roughly comparable. **Baric index.** A hundred times the body weight divided by the cube of the height. **Basilar index.** The ratio between the basiprosthionic length and the total length of the cranium, expressed as a percentage. **Biochemical racial index.** The ratio of the number of people in any population belonging to Blood Group A (II), compared to the number of people whose red blood cells are Group B (III). **Body-build index.** The body weight divided by the square of the stature. **Brachial index.** A hundred times the length of the forearm, the distance from the radiale (the upper border of the head of the radius) to the stylion (the tip of the styloid process), divided by the length of the arm, the distance from the acromion (acromial angle) to the radiale. **Buffer index.** A measure of the buffer capacity of a solution, given by the expression dB/dpH, where dB represents a small addition of acid or alkali in gram-equivalents added per litre, and dpH the corresponding change in pH produced. **Calcium index.** The relative amount of calcium in the blood when compared with a standard solution (1/6 000 CaO). **Cardiac index.** The minute volume of blood passing round the circulatory system in each minute per square meter of the body surface; there is a wide normal range varying with age and sex around a value of 3.6 litres per minute. **Cardiothoracic index.** The ratio between the greatest transverse diameter of the heart shadow on an x-ray screen and the greatest diameter of the chest. **Centromeric index.** The ratio of the short arm to the total chromosome length, usually expressed as a percentage. **Cephalic index.** A hundred times the maximum breadth of the head, the greatest horizontal transverse diameter of the vault of the head above the supramastoid crest, divided by the maximum length of the head, the distance from the most prominent point of the glabella (the midpoint between the two supra-orbital ridges on the frontal bone) to the opisthocranion (that point on the back of the head in the midline which is the most distant from the glabella). **Cephalic-height index.** A hundred times the height of the head, the distance from the vertex above to the upper border of the auditory opening below, divided by the maximum length of the head, the distance from the glabella to the opisthocranion (see CEPHALIC INDEX prec.). **Cephalorrhachidian index, cerebrospinal index.** The amount of cerebrospinal fluid removed by lumbar puncture multiplied by the final pressure and divided by the initial pressure. **Chemotherapeutic index.** Originally defined as the ratio of the minimal curative dose of a drug to the maximum tolerated dose per kg of body weight, now more often assessed in terms of a ratio of a percentage lethal dose to a percentage curative dose in the experimental animal. **Colour index.** The ratio of the percentage of haemoglobin compared with a normal of 100 per cent to the percentage of the number of red blood corpuscles also compared with a normal 100 per cent; thus, if 5 000 000 is arbitrarily fixed as the normal 100 per cent for red blood corpuscles, and 14.8 g of haemoglobin per cent is the normal 100 per cent hb, then the colour index is given by:

$$\frac{\text{per cent haemoglobin (calculated as 14.8 g per cent} = \text{100 per cent)}}{\text{per cent red blood corpuscles (calculated as } 5\times10^{6} = \text{100 per cent)}}$$

$$= \frac{\text{haemoglobin coefficient}}{\text{red-blood-corpuscular coefficient}}$$

$$= \frac{\text{per cent haemoglobin}}{20\times\text{red-blood-corpuscle count in millions per mm}^3}.$$

This colour index also expresses the mean corpuscular haemoglobin content as compared with the normal red-blood corpuscular content of haemoglobin. (*See* HAEMOGLOBIN COEFFICIENT, RED-BLOOD-CORPUSCULAR COEFFICIENT, MEAN CORPUSCULAR HAEMOGLOBIN.) The colour index is also given by dividing the mean corpuscular haemoglobin by the average normal mean corpuscular haemoglobin, which latter is 29.5×10^{-12} g, i.e.

$$\frac{\text{MCH}}{29.5\times10^{-12}\,\text{g}}$$

The normal range is 0.85–1.15. **Cornification index.** The percentage of cornified cells (flat cells with no nuclei or pyknotic nuclei) found in 200 cells counted in a vaginal smear to determine the extent of oestrogenic stimulation. **Corpuscular thickness index.** Obtained by dividing the mean corpuscular average thickness by the normal mean corpuscular average thickness (2.1 μm). **Cranial index.** This and the cephalic index (see above) relate similar measurements on the skull and head, respectively. **Cranial-height index (of the skull).** A hundred times the basibregmatic height, from the bregma above to the midpoint on the anterior border of the foramen magnum below (the basion), divided by the maximum length of the skull, the distance from the most prominent point of the glabella to the opisthocranion (see CEPHALIC INDEX above). **Craniometric index.** An index used in craniometry which expresses one linear cranial measurement as a percentage of another, e.g. cranial-height index (see above). **Cytophagic index.** The phagocytic power of particular white blood corpuscles as compared with normal or standard white blood corpuscles. **Dental index.** A hundred times the length of the premolar and molar teeth divided by the length from the basion to the prosthion (see GNATHIC INDEX below). **Effective temperature index.** An index of temperature derived from estimation of the temperature, movement, and humidity of the air. **Empathic index.** An estimate of the degree of empathy. **Endemic index.** In an outbreak of disease in a country, area, or locality, the percentage of persons suffering from the disease. **Index of excursion of uterus.** The distance, expressed in centimetres, that the uterus can be displaced upwards and downwards by pressure and traction. **Facial index, total.** A hundred times the total height of the face, from the trichion (the midpoint of the hair line at the upper limit of the forehead) to the gnathion (the lowest point in the midline on the lower margin of the mandible), divided by the bimalar diameter, the maximum distance between the two most lateral points on the malar bones. **Facial index, total (of the skull).** A hundred times the gnathion-nasion height, from the nasion (the midpoint of the depression where the nasal bones join the frontal) above to the gnathion (the lowest point in the midline on the lower margin of the mandible), divided by the maximum bizygomatic breadth, the most widely separated points on the external surfaces of the zygomatic arches. **Facial index, upper.** A hundred times the nasio-alveolar height, from the nasion (the midpoint of the depression where the nasal bones join the frontal) to the prosthion or alveolar point (the lowest point on the gum line between the upper central incisors) divided by the bimalar diameter (see TOTAL FACIAL INDEX preceding). **Facial index, upper (of the skull).** A hundred times the alveolonasal height, from the nasion (the midpoint of the depression where the nasal bones join the frontal) above to the prosthion or alveolar point (the lowest point on the gum line between the upper central incisors), divided by the maximum bizygomatic breadth, the most widely separated points on the external surfaces of the zygomatic arches. **Femorohumeral index.** A hundred times the arm length, the distance from the acromion (acromial angle) above to the radiale (the upper border of the head of the radius) below, divided by the thigh length, the distance from the trochanterion (the upper border of the greater trochanter) above to the tibiale (the upper border of the medial condyle of the tibia) below. **Flea index.** A term used in plague surveying; the number of fleas per rat. **Forearm-hand index.** A hundred times the length of the hand, the distance from the stylion (the tip of the styloid process) above to the most distal point of the middle finger, divided by the length of the forearm, from the radiale (the upper border of the head of the radius) above to the stylion below. **Frontal index.** A hundred times the minimum frontal breadth of the head, the distance between the most medial points on the curvature of the two temporal ridges, divided by the maximum breadth, the greatest horizontal transverse diameter of the head above the supramastoid crest. **Generation index.** The logarithm to the base of which multiplication is taking place in a culture. **Gnathic index.** A hundred times the length from the basion (the midpoint on the anterior margin of the foramen magnum) to the prosthion (the lowest point on the gum line between the upper central incisors), divided by the length from the basion to the nasion (the midpoint of the depression where the nasal bones join the frontal). **Gono-opsonic index.** The opsonic index (see below) estimated by using *Neisseria gonorrhoeae* as the test organism. **Habitus index.** A hundred times the sum of the chest girth and abdominal girth divided by the stature. **Haematopnoeic index.** A measure of the degree of oxygenation of the whole blood. **Haemophagocytic index.** Opsonocytophagic index (see below). **Hand index.** A hundred times the breadth of the hand, from the metacarpale radiale (the most prominent point upon the radial margin of the head of the metacarpale bone of the index finger) to a corresponding point on the head of the metacarpal bone of the little finger (the metacarpaleulnare) measured across the palm of the hand with the fingers extended, divided by the length of the hand, from the stylion (the tip of the styloid process) above to the tip of the middle finger below. **Icteric index, icterus index.** A measure of the degree of yellow colour in the blood plasma or blood serum when compared with the colour of standard yellow solution, potassium dichromate being usually used for this purpose; while this test is non-specific and only measures the yellow colour that may be due to any yellow colouring matter (e.g. carotene, bilirubin) in the blood, it is usually used to detect increased amounts of bilirubin. The normal value is 4–7 units. **Iron index.** A relatively inaccurate ratio or index of the blood iron, obtained by dividing the total whole blood iron value (mg) by the red-blood-corpuscular count (in millions per mm³). Obsolete. **Leucopenic index** (Vaughan). A test of sensitivity to certain foods in allergic individuals; the fasting and resting patient is given the test food and total leucocyte counts are made before, at 15-min intervals in the first hour, and at 30-min intervals in the second hour. A decrease in the leucocyte count by 1 000 cells per mm³ indicates a positive incompatibility. **Limb index.** A hundred times the arm and forearm length, from the acromion (acromial angle) above to the stylion (the tip of the styloid process) below, divided by the thigh and leg length, from the trochanterion (the upper border of the greater trochanter) above to the sphyrion (the lowest point on the medial malleolus). **Lymphocyte-monocyte index.** Lymphocyte-monocyte ratio; the proportion of lymphocytes to monocytes in the blood. **Maxillo-alveolar index.** A hundred times the maximum breadth of the alveolar border, i.e. the maximum width of the palate measured to the external surface of the alveolar border on each side, divided by the length of the alveolar arch, from the prosthion (the lowest point on the gum line between the upper central incisors) anteriorly to the midpoint of a line joining the posterior extremities of the alveolar border. **Mitotic index.** The fraction of a cell population which is found in mitosis. This is a measure of the proliferative activity of the cell population in question. **Monocyte-leucocyte index.** Monocyte-leucocyte ratio; the number obtained by dividing the number of monocytes by the total number of white blood corpuscles (leucocytes). **Nasal index.** A hundred times the breadth of the nose, the maximum breadth between the alaria (the external surfaces of the alae of the nose) divided by the height of the nose, from the nasion (the midpoint of the depression where the nasal bones join the frontal) to the subnasale (the apex of the angle formed by the lower border of the nasal septum and the philtrum). **Nasal index (of the skull).** A hundred times the nasal breadth, the widest separation of the nasal borders in the horizontal plane, divided by the nasal height, from the nasion (the midpoint of the depression where the nasal bones join the frontal) superiorly to the midpoint of a line connecting the lowest limits of each nasal fossa. **Obesity index.** The body weight divided by the body volume. **Index of operability.** *See* MOOTS-MCKESSON RATIO (under MOOTS). **Opsonic index.** The ratio of organisms phagocytosed by normal leucocytes in the presence of serum from a subject infected with the homologous organism, to the number phagocytosed in serum from a normal individual. **Opsonocytophagic index.** The ratio of organisms ingested by normal leucocytes in the presence of their own serum, to the number phagocytosed by leucocytes from the blood of a patient infected by the organisms under test in the presence of normal serum. **Optical index.** A constant applied to microscope objectives for purposes of comparison. The magnification of the lens and also the numerical aperture is taken into account. **Orbital index.** A hundred times the mean height of the orbits (the measurement of the maximum separation of the upper and lower borders of the orbit in any sagittal plane) divided by the mean breadth of the orbits, from the dacryon (the point on the medial wall of the orbit where the frontal, maxillary, and lacrimal bones meet) to the lateral border of the orbit in the horizontal plane. **Oscillometric index.** The number of divisions on the scale of an oscillometer over which the needle moves when recording the arterial pulsations in a limb. **Palatal index.** A hundred times the breadth of the palate, the distance between the inner margins of the alveolar borders between the second molar teeth, divided by the length of the palate (measured from, anteriorly, the median point of a line tangential to the posterior alveolar border of the central incisors, to, posteriorly, the median point of a transverse line connecting the most anterior points of the notches in the posterior margin of the palate). **Parasite index.** The percentage of individuals who show (malarial) parasites in the blood. **Pelvic index.** The ratio of the pelvic conjugate and transverse diameters. **Phagocytic index.** Measure of mononuclear phagocyte function by determining the ability of the body to clear particles from the circulation. Term also used to indicate the ratio of average number of bacteria ingested by test leucocytes *in vitro* to the average number ingested by control leucocytes. **Polymorphonuclear lymphocyte index.** Polymorphonuclear lymphocyte ratio; the ratio of the number of polymorphonuclear leucocytes to the lymphocytes in the differential white-cell count. It is of importance in detecting overexposure to radioactive agents, especially if the relative numbers are reversed. **Ponderal index.** A hundred times the cube root of the body weight divided by stature. **Prothrombin index.** A somewhat misleading measure of the plasma prothrombin concentration calculated from the determined prothrombin time according to the formula,

$$\frac{\text{normal prothrombin time} \times 100}{\text{patient's prothrombin time}}$$

Radiographic splenic index. A radiological measurement of the spleen. **Refractive index.** The ratio of the velocity of light *in vacuo* to the velocity of light in the medium. **Sacral index.** A hundred times the breadth of the sacrum divided by its length. **Salivary urea index.** *See* HENCH-ALDRICH SALIVARY UREA INDEX. **Saturation index.** An index obtained by dividing the colour index (see above) by the volume index (see below), or dividing the mean corpuscular haemoglobin concentration, MCHC, by the normal average MCHC (34 per cent), and is a measure of the haemoglobin content of red blood corpuscles compared with the normal value. **Sedimentin index.** The measurement of certain products of tissue destruction which when present in blood plasma cause an increase in the rate of red-cell sedimentation. This index is obtained from the logarithm of the maximal velocity of sedimentation expressed in mm per 100 min during 2 hours; the normal sedimentin index is 0.5 or less. **Spleen index.** The percentage of children, between the ages of 2 and 10 years, who show enlargement of the spleen on palpation. **Splenometric index.** A method of indicating the endemicity of malaria by which both the spleen index (see prec.) and the average size of the spleens measured are employed in combination. **Sporozoite index.** The percentage of female mosquitoes showing sporozoites in their salivary glands. **Stroke index.** In cardiology, the stroke volume of the heart divided by the surface area of the body expressed in square metres. **Tension-time index.** The mean pressure in the ventricle during ejection multiplied by the ejection time, used to provide a measure of the ventricular work and oxygen demand. **Thickness index.** The ratio of the mean corpuscular average thickness to the normal mean corpuscular average thickness (2.1 μm). **Thoracic index.** A hundred times the transverse diameter of the thorax, measured in the horizontal plane at the mesosternale (the midpoint of the sternum), divided by the sagittal diameter of the thorax, measured at the junction of the horizontal plane at the level of the mesosternale and the median plane. **Tibiofemoral index.** A hundred times the length of the leg, from the tibiale (the upper border of the medial condyle of the tibia) above to the sphyrion (the lowest point on the medial malleolus) below, divided by the length of the thigh, from the trochanterion (the upper border of the greater trochanter) above to the tibiale below. **Tibioradial index.** A hundred times the forearm length, the distance from the radiale (the upper border of the radius) to the stylion (the tip of the styloid process), divided by the length of the leg (see TIBIOFEMORAL INDEX prec.). **Trunk index.** A hundred times the biacromial breadth, the maximum diameter between the two acromial points (the acromial angles) divided by the sitting suprasternal height, from the suprasternale (the middle of the suprasternal notch) above to the flat surface on which the subject is seated. **Tuberculo-opsonic index.** The opsonic index (see above), estimated by using *Mycobacterium tuberculosis* as the test organism. **Uricolytic index.** The ratio, expressed as a percentage, of allantoin nitrogen to (allantoin + uric acid) nitrogen excreted in urine. The index represents the power of the animal to destroy uric acid, and is thus a measure of uricase activity. It varies with species, from almost nil in man to 96-98 in dogs, cats, and pigs. An exception in dogs is the Dalmatian which excretes almost as high a proportion of uric acid as man. **Ventilation index.** An index found by dividing the pulmonary ventilation per minute by the vital capacity. **Vertical index.** Cranial-height index (see above). **Vital index.** Birth-death ratio: the proportion of the number of births to the number of deaths in a population estimated over a period of time, e.g. one year. **Volume index.** The ratio of mean corpuscular volume divided by the normal average mean corpuscular volume, i.e. MCV/86; the normal value is 1.0. **Xanthoproteic index.** Mulder's test. **Zoophilic index.** The percentage of mammalian-blood-containing mosquitoes in which the blood-meal is from an animal, as shown by negative precipitin reaction for human blood. **Zygomatico-auricular index.** The ratio between the zygomatic and auricular diameters of the skull. [L, pointer.]

See also: ALDRICH (M.), ARNETH, AYALA, BARACH, BAZETT, BECKER, BODECKER, BOUCHARD, BRODERS, BROWN (G. E.), COOKE,

FLOWER, FOURMENTIN, HENCH, KREBS (M.), LENNHOFF, MACDONALD, MUELENGRACHT, SCHILLING.

indexometer (in·dex·**om**·et·er). An instrument with which the refractive index of a liquid can be determined. [index, meter.]

indian hemp (**in**·de·an hemp). Cannabis indica, Cannabis BPC 1949, consisting of the dried flowering and fruiting tops of the female plants of *Cannabis sativa* Linn. (family Cannabinaceae). The plant is indigenous to central and western Asia and is cultivated in tropical India, Africa, and North America. In temperate countries it does not produce the narcotic resin, but is cultivated for hemp fibre and hemp seed. Guaza and ganja are names given to forms of the drug as produced in India. Bhang, churrus, and hashish are products of *Cannabis sativa* used by orientals for smoking and the preparation of electuaries; dagga is the material used by addicts in South Africa. Marihuana is the Mexican name for the drug. Cannabis contains a soft resin from which cannabinol has been isolated. The drug acts on the central nervous system, often producing pleasurable excitement, hallucinations, distortion of the sense of time and space, followed by lethargy and sleep. Addicts to the drug may become psychotic. It has been used as a sedative in nervous disorders and spasmodic coughs, but is unreliable in use. [*India*, AS *henep*.]

indiarubber (**in**·de·ah·**rub**'·er). Caoutchouc: the coagulated juice, or latex, of species of Euphorbiaceae grown in South America, India, Malaya, and elsewhere, and consisting of a polymerized hydrocarbon, polyisoprene, $(C_5H_8)_n$, related to the terpenes, in a colloidal solution of protein, resins, and mineral salts; it is soluble in chloroform and carbon disulphide, and combines with sulphur to form vulcanized rubber. [*India*, ME *rubben* to rub.]

indican (**in**·dik·an). 1. Indoxyl-β-glucoside, a naturally-occurring glucoside present in indigo, which is hydrolysed by acids or enzymes producing the colouring matter, indigotin. 2. The potassium salt of indoxylsulphuric acid, the conjugated form in which indoxyl, from the decomposition of tryptophan, is excreted in the urine (*urinary indican*). [Gk *indikon* indigo.]

indicanaemia (**in**·dik·an·e'·me·ah). The presence of indican in the blood. [indican, Gk *haima* blood.]

indicanhidrosis, indicanidrosis (**in**·dik·an·hid·**ro**'·sis, **in**·dik·an·id·**ro**'·sis). The excretion of blue-coloured sweat due to the presence of indican. [indican, Gk *hidros* sweat.]

indicant (**in**·dik·ant). That which draws attention to or points out anything; a symptom pointing to a particular disease; any fact or symptom that indicates the proper treatment for any particular disease. [L *indicare* to draw.]

indicanuria (**in**·dik·an·**ewr**'·e·ah). The presence of an abnormally large quantity of indican in the urine.

indicarminum (in·de·kar·**mi**'·num). Indigo Carmine BP 1958.

indicatio, indication (in·dik·a·she·o, in·dik·**a**·shun). Any symptom, sign, circumstance, or occurrence that indicates the presence (*indicatio morbi*), the aetiology and pathology (*indicatio causalis*), the diagnosis (*indicatio symptomatica*), and the treatment and prognosis (*indicatio curativa*) of a disease. [see foll.]

indicator (**in**·dik·a·tor). Any substance employed in a chemical operation to indicate by a colour change the completion of a reaction or the attainment of a desired state, e.g. neutralization. **Anaerobic indicator.** A chemical solution used to indicate the presence or absence of oxygen in an anaerobic culture of micro-organisms, e.g. a solution of equal parts of 6 per cent M/10 sodium hydroxide in water, 0.015 per cent methylene blue in water, and 6 per cent dextrose in water. **Complex indicator.** In psycho-analysis, any observation from which the influence of a *complex* may be inferred. Main usage in relation to word-association tests (Jung). **Indicator dilution.** *See* DILUTION. **Fluorescent indicator.** An indicator used for the titration by ultraviolet light of highly-coloured or turbid liquids which would mask the use of an ordinary indicator. **Oxidation-reduction indicator.** Any compound which, by a change in colour and intensity of the latter, serves as an indication of potential in an oxidation-reduction system; thus, methylene blue, which is reduced to a colourless compound, or ferrous salts, which change from green to yellow (ferric) on oxidation. **pH indicator.** An indicator employed either in the titration of acids and alkalis to denote end-point, or, by a change in coloured ions, in estimating the pH value of a solution. **Radioactive indicator.** A radioactive isotope of an element used to trace the course of that element in the metabolism. **Redox indicator.** Oxidation-reduction indicator (see above). **Universal indicator.** A mixture of indicators chosen for the easily recognized colour each displays for a certain value of pH; such an indicator affords a rapid means of colorimetric estimation of hydrogen-ion concentration. **Vegetable indicator.** Any colouring matter, such as litmus, extracted from plants and used for its different colour in acid and alkaline media. [L *indicare* to indicate.]

See also: ANDRADE, SCHNEIDER (E. C.).

indictment (in·**dite**·ment). The written or printed counts (each one set out separately) of accusations against the accused person or persons read out by the Clerk at the beginning of a trial. [OFr. *enditer* to make known.]

Indiella (in·de·**el**·ah). Madurella. *Indiella brumpti* (*I. mansoni*) causes white mycetoma of the foot. [*India*.]

indifference (in·**dif**·er·ens). Absence of interest or concern. **Belle indifference.** A manifestation of hysteria in which there is a lack of concern shown by the patient for his illness. [L *indifferens* neither good nor bad.]

indifferent (in·**dif**·er·ent). 1. Neutral, e.g. in intensity or size. 2. Without any particular affinity. 3. Without preponderating weight or influence. 4. Not tending in any particular direction. 5. Of tissues or cells, undifferentiated. 6. Not responding easily or reacting readily to stimulus. 7. Mentally uninterested. [L *indifferens* neither good nor bad.]

indifferentism (in·**dif**·er·ent·izm). 1. Without any particular differentiation. 2. A mental state of systematic lack of interest. [see prec.]

indigenous (in·**dij**·en·us). Arising, living, or growing naturally in a particular country or locality; autochthonous. [L *indigena* belonging to one's own country.]

indigestible (in·dij·**est**·ibl). Not easily convertible into a form suitable to be absorbed as nourishment; not capable of being easily acted on by the gastric juice; not digestible. [see foll.]

indigestion (in·dij·**est**·chun). Any disturbance of the normal process of digestion. **Acid indigestion.** Hyperchlorhydria. **Fat indigestion.** Imperfect digestion of fat. **Gastric indigestion.** Indigestion due to failure of the gastric functions. **Intestinal indigestion.** Imperfect digestion in the intestines. **Nervous indigestion.** Indigestion due to functional nervous causes. **Psychic indigestion.** Indigestion of psychic origin. **Sugar indigestion.** Discomfort produced by an excess of sugar in the diet. [L *in*, *digerere* to separate.]

indigitation (**in**·dij·it·a'·shun). Intussusception; the invagination of one part of the intestine into another part immediately below. [L *in*, *digitus* finger.]

indiglucin (in·dig·**loo**·sin). The sweet substance obtained in the hydrolysis of indican, the glucoside of the indigo plant. It owes its sweetness to the glucose so produced. [indigo, Gk *glykys* sweet.]

indigo (**in**·dig·o). A vat dye, used for dyeing woollens, formerly obtained from the indigo plant, *Indigofera tinctoria*, and woad, *Isatis tinctoria*, but now synthesized, e.g. from naphthalene. The commercial natural product contains indican, a glucoside of indoxyl from which the colouring matter is developed by oxidation. **Indigo blue.** Indigotin $C_6H_4(CONH)C{=}C(CONH)C_6H_4$, an insoluble blue colouring matter obtained by air oxidation of the indican of commercial indigo. It is not itself used in medicine. **Indigo Carmine BP 1973.** The sodium salt of the disulphonic acid of indigotin, a water-soluble blue dye used for testing the efficiency of the kidneys. **Indigo red.** Indoxyl red indirubin; a synthetic compound closely related to indigotin. **Red indigo.** Cudbear; Persio BPC 1949. **Indigo white.** The compound obtained from indigo blue by reduction; it is the form in which indigo is introduced into fabrics which are subsequently oxidized to develop the colour. **Wild indigo.** *Baptisia tinctoria.* [Gk *indikon.*]

indigotin (in·dig·o·tin). Indigo blue, $C_6H_4(CONH)C{=}C(CONH)C_6H_4$. The essential dye of indigo, produced by the hydrolysis of indican and subsequent oxidation of the freed indoxyl. It is a dark-blue insoluble substance which can be reduced to the compound, indigo white.

indigo-uria, indiguria (in·dig·o·ewr'·e·ah, in·dig·ewr·e·ah). The presence of indigo in the urine due to the decomposition of indican.

indirect (in·di·rekt). 1. Not immediate, as results. 2. Not leading obviously in a certain direction or towards a particular aim. 3. Acting in a roundabout way, i.e. through an intervening medium. 4. Not in a direct line, as heredity. [L *in, directus* straight.]

indirubin (in·de·roo·bin). $C_6H_4(CONH)C{=}C(CONH)C_6H_4$, a red pigment, a minor constituent of natural indigo, and sometimes occurring in the urine in association with indican as a result of oxidation of some of the indoxyl to isatin which thereupon combines with unaltered indoxyl. It is isomeric with indigotin.

indirubinuria (in·de·roo·bin·ewr'·re·ah). The presence of indirubin in the urine so that it is of a red colour.

indiscriminate (in·dis·krim·in·ate). 1. Belonging to or affecting a number of unrelated parts, as lesions. 2. Promiscuous; confused. [L *in, discrimen* difference.]

indisposition (in·dis·po·zish'·un). A slightly disordered state of health; malaise. [L *in, dispositus* in proper order.]

indium (in·de·um). A rarer element of atomic weight 114.82, atomic number 49, and chemical symbol In. It is a metal closely related to aluminium, with some application in low-melting alloys. [indigo.]

individuation (in·div·id·ew·a'·shun). The emergence during development, of individual and specific structures and functions. [L *individuus* indivisible.]

indococcus (in·do·kok·us). A micrococcus found in the mouth, detected by means of iodine which tinges the organism blue. [indigo, Gk *kokkos* berry.]

indolaceturia (in·dole·as·et·ewr'·e·ah). The presence of a considerable amount of indole-acetic acid in the urine as a consequence of some disorder of the intestinal tract.

indole (in·dole). A crystalline substance with a characteristic faecal odour, soluble in hot water, alcohol, and ether. It is formed in the intestine by the action of certain bacteria upon tryptophan and is excreted in faeces. A small amount is absorbed daily and excreted in the urine as the potassium sulphate compound of its oxidation product, indoxyl (indican). Conjugation is thought to occur mainly in the liver, but attempts to use this reaction as a test of liver function have not been successful. It has also been found in jasmine oil and can be regarded as the parent of indigo. [indigo.]

indolent (in·do·lent). 1. Sluggish; inactive. 2. Painless, or almost so, as an ulcer or tumour. [L *in, dolere* to suffer pain.]

indoloemia (in·dol·e·me·ah). Cholera. [Gk *Indos* an Indian, *loimos* pestilence.]

indologenous (in·do·loj·en·us). 1. Leading to the production of indole. 2. Producing indole. [indole, Gk *genein* to produce.]

indoluria (in·dole·ewr·e·ah). The presence of indole in the urine.

Indomethacin BP 1973 (in·do·meth·as·in). 1-(4-Chlorobenzoyl)-5-methoxy-2-methylindol-3-ylacetic acid; an analgesic and anti-inflammatory agent.

indophenolase (in·do·fe·nol·aze). Indophenoloxidase.

indophenoloxidase (in·do·fe·nol·ox'·id·aze). Cytochrome oxidase; an enzyme distributed widely in animal and plant tissues, which re-oxidizes reduced cytochrome in the processes of tissue respiration.

indophenols (in·do·fe·nolz). General name for dyestuffs which are amino derivatives of phenylquinone mono-imine, $C_6H_5N{=}C_6H_4{=}O$.

Indoramin (in·dor·am·in). BP Commission approved name for 3 - [2 - (4 - benzamidopiperidino)ethyl]indole; an antihypertensive agent.

indoxyl (in·dox·il). β-Hydroxy-indole, $C_6H_4NHCH{=}COH$. A toxic phenolic derivative of indole formed by the breakdown of tryptophan, and excreted in the urine as potassium indoxyl sulphate (indican). It is easily transformed into indigo blue on exposure to air, or oxidation with acid hydrogen peroxide. **Indoxyl sulphate.** Any salt of indoxylsulphuric acid, particularly the potassium salt which appears in urine as urinary indican.

indoxylaemia (in·dox·il·e'·me·ah). The presence of indoxyl in the blood. [indoxyl, Gk *haima* blood.]

indoxyluria (in·dox·il·ewr'·e·ah). 1. The presence of an excessive quantity of indoxyl in the urine. 2. Indicanuria.

induced (in·dewst). 1. Brought on by indirect methods. 2. Artificially produced, as labour. 3. Caused or produced by induction, as electricity. [L *inducere* to lead in.]

inducer (in·dew·ser). A compound the effect of which is to increase either the concentration of another molecule, frequently a protein, or the rate of a metabolic process. In micro-organisms, the inducer is that molecule which combines directly with the corresponding repressor protein and thereby prevents binding to the operator gene. In higher animals, inducers are frequently hormones. [L *inducere* to lead in.]

inducibility (in·dews·ib·il'·it·e). The property by which a living cell produces larger amounts of an enzyme when a particular compound (called an *inducer*) is present within it in appropriate amounts. [L *inducere* to lead in.]

inductance (in·duk·tans). The property of an electric circuit by virtue of which an increase or decrease of current through the circuit exercises an inductive effect upon itself (*self-inductance*) or upon a neighbouring circuit (*mutual inductance*), this effect being due to the change in the magnetic field surrounding the varying current. The unit of inductance is the henry. [L *inducere* to lead in.]

induction (in·duk·shun). 1. The act of initiating a phenomenon. 2. The process of inferring general laws from particular instances. 3. The process whereby a changing electromagnetic field produces an electric current in a conductor within that field. 4. In biology, the process whereby tissue and cellular differentiation is initiated as a result of influences emanating from neighbouring cells of a different type, or as the result of artificial stimuli. Also, the initiation of any cellular process, such as enzyme synthesis or latent virus reproduction, as a result of either a specific or non-specific stimulus. 5. The production of an effect at a distance. 6. In genetics, the process by which there is an increase in concentration of an enzyme in a living cell as the result of the presence, in suitable amounts, of a compound of low molecular weight called an *inducer*. 7. The process whereby an inducer exerts its metabolic effect. **Induction of abortion.** Abortion induced intentionally. **Induction of anaesthesia.** The method of administering a general anaesthetic agent so that the patient passes from consciousness to unconsciousness. **Electromagnetic induction.** *See* MAIN DEF. 3 (above). **Induction of enzyme synthesis.** A rise in the rate of specific enzyme synthesis from basal to maximal level, invoked by the presence of substrate or substrate analogues (inducer); usually due to allosteric inactivation of a protein repressor which prevents transcription of the gene specifying the enzyme. **Induction of labour.** Labour brought on by artificial means. **Magnetic induction.** The production of an electromotive force in a conductor by change of intensity or direction of the magnetic field in which it is placed. **Medical induction.** The production of labour by medicinal means. **Induction of mutations.** By chemical or physical agents (mutagens), as opposed to their spontaneous generation. **Induction of prophage.** Release of prophage from its chromosomal, or other, location in lysogenic bacteria followed by vegetative reproduction, either spontaneously or as a result of treatment with agents such as ultraviolet light. **Somatic induction.** The hypothetical effects of the general body cells on the germ cells, whereby the genes of the latter are changed so that acquired somatic characteristics can be inherited. **Spinal induction.** Term introduced by Sherrington to describe that process in the spinal cord whereby activity in one nerve cell, or a group or nerve cells, lowers the threshold to activity in other functionally-related nerve cells. **Surgical induction.** The production of labour by surgical interference such as rupture of the membranes or the insertion of a foreign body into the lower uterine segment. **Zygotic induction.** Induction of a prophage following transfer to the cytoplasm of a non-lysogenic (non-immune) bacterium by conjugation or transduction. [L *inducere* to lead in.]

See also: SPEMANN.

inductometer (in·duk·**tom**·et·er). A device used to measure the electricity induced in a conductor. [induction, meter.]

inductopyrexia (in·**duk**·to·pi·**rex**′·e·ah). Electropyrexia; the artificial raising of the body temperature to fever height by passing electric currents through the tissues (pyrexial or fever therapy). [induction, pyrexia.]

inductor (in·**duk**·tor). Any substance which will induce cells exposed to its action to differentiate into an organized tissue. The term is most often applied to substances which will induce the formation of a neural tube from indifferent ectoderm in amphibian embryos. [L *inducere* to lead in.]

inductorium (in·duk·**tor**·e·um). An apparatus for the production of high-voltage electrical discharges by induction; an induction coil. [L *inducere* to lead in.]

See also: DUBOIS-REYMOND.

inductothermy (in·**duk**·to·**ther**′·me). A method of producing deep heating in the tissues by the high-frequency (short-wave diathermy) current, the inductothermy cable being used in place of the normal electrodes. [induction, Gk *therme* heat.]

induline (**in**·dew·leen). Any one of a group of complex dyestuffs related to the safranines; they are occasionally used in histology as counterstains, and in bacteriology for the negative staining of micro-organisms.

indulinophil, indulinophile, indulinophilic (in·dew·**lin**·o·fil, in·dew·**lin**·o·file, **in**·dew·lin·o·**fil**′·ik). Applied to substances that stain readily with induline. [induline, Gk *philein* to love.]

indurated (**in**·dewr·a·ted). Having become hardened or having been made hard. [see foll.]

induration (in·dewr·**a**·shun). The hardening of a tissue or organ because of pathological change within its texture. **Black induration.** Anthracosis of the lungs. **Brown induration.** Fibrosis and pigmentation of the lungs, resulting from chronic venous congestion of the organs. **Cyanotic induration.** Chronic passive venous congestion of organs, especially the spleen and kidneys, in which cyanosis of the tissues develops because of pronounced slowing of the blood flow. **Fibroid induration.** Fibrosis. **Granular induration.** Fibrosis of an organ, such as the liver or kidney, whereby the normal smooth architectural pattern is broken up into a series of minute localized areas or granules. **Grey induration.** Chronic pneumonia with fibrosis of the air spaces. **Penile induration.** Fibrosis and distortion of the penis as the result of a chronic inflammation or neoplasm. **Plastic induration.** Fibrosis. **Red induration.** Chronic interstitial pneumonia with severe congestion of the lung vessels. [L *indurare* to make hard.]

See also: FRORIEP (R.).

indurative (**in**·dewr·a·tiv). Pertaining to, characterized, or caused by induration.

indurescent (in·dewr·**es**·ent). Going through a process of gradual hardening. [L *indurescere* to become hard.]

indusium (in·**dew**·se·um) (pl. *indusia*). 1. In botany, a membranous covering or investment. 2. The amnion. **Indusium griseum** [NA]. The thin sheet of grey matter covering the upper surface of the corpus callosum and continuous with the cortex of the gyrus cinguli. [L *induere* to clothe.]

inebriant (in·e·bre·ant). 1. An intoxicant. 2. Causing intoxication or drunkenness. [L *inebriare* to make drunk.]

inebriation (in·e·bre·a′·shun). 1. A condition of habitual intoxication or drunkenness. 2. The condition of being so exhilarated that the sense of proportion and judgment is absent. [see prec.]

inebriety (in·e·**bri**·et·e). The habit or state of being drunk frequently. [L *inebriare* to make drunk.]

Inermicapsifer (in·er·me·**kap**′·sif·er). A genus of tapeworms. **Inermicapsifer cubensis.** A species which has been recorded in children in the West Indies. Rodents are the usual primary hosts, but the secondary hosts are not known. [L *inermis* defenceless, *capsifer* carrying a box.]

inert (in·**ert**). 1. Without active properties. 2. Sluggish or indolent in body or mind. 3. Without the power to move itself; without active resistance to motion applied. 4. In chemistry, unreactive, or resisting chemical action. [L *iners* idle.]

inertia (in·**er**·she·ah). 1. A state of complete inactivity. 2. A condition of indolence or sluggishness of body or mind. 3. In physics: (*a*) the tendency of matter to remain at rest unless external force is applied; (*b*) a negative property of force, e.g. electrical force, by which it tends to keep on acting in the same direction. **Psychic inertia.** The tendency to resist change in ideas, attitudes, or neurotic symptoms involving resistance to progress and reconstruction, and to fixation of ideas. **Inertia uteri, uterine inertia.** In labour, lack of activity of the uterus, i.e. when the contractions have ceased or nearly ceased. [L, idleness.]

infancy (**in**·fan·se). 1. Early childhood: the period of complete dependency prior to the acquisition of competence in walking, talking and self-feeding; generally accepted as the first two years of life. 2. In law, the period of minority; under the age of 18. **Natural infancy.** In law, the first 7 years of life during which the child is not legally responsible. [L *infans* unable to speak.]

infant (**in**·fant). 1. A child under the age of two years. 2. In law, one who has not reached the age of 18 years. [see prec.]

infanticide (in·**fan**·te·side). In law, it is infanticide when a woman, by a wilful act or omission, causes the death of her child, it being under the age of one year at the time, having the balance of her mind disturbed (*a*) by reason of not having recovered from the effect of giving birth to such a child, or (*b*) as the effect of lactation. In such circumstances she is charged with the offence of infanticide, which is the same as manslaughter, and not with murder. [infant, L *caedere* to kill.]

infanticulture (in·**fan**·te·**kul**′·tcher). The science and art of rearing and training children. [infant, culture.]

infantile (**in**·fan·tile). 1. Relating to an infant or to the state or period of infancy. 2. Childish; characteristic of an infant.

infantilism (in·**fan**·til·izm). A condition in which infantile characteristics persist into adult life; the retardation of bodily growth and retention of infantile proportions and contour is associated with delayed or absent development of the secondary sexual characters. **Cardiac infantilism.** Infantilism secondary to severe congenital or acquired cardiac disease. **Coeliac infantilism.** Retarded development due to coeliac disease. Some patients may eventually reach a normal standard after arrest of the disease, though some permanent stunting is usual. **Hepatic infantilism.** Rare cases of infantilism associated with cirrhosis of the liver. **Hypothyroid infantilism.** Sometimes referred to as the Brissaud type of infantilism, occurring mostly in cretins and in cases of juvenile myxoedema. **Ovarian infantilism.** The condition of short stature and absence of secondary female characteristics, due to ovarian deficiency or Turner's syndrome. **Pancreatic infantilism.** Infantilism associated with pancreatic disease and steatorrhoea acquired in early life. Many cases described under this heading are probably instances of coeliac disease. **Pituitary infantilism.** Owing to the lack of growth hormone the child does not grow but is perfectly formed although all the proportions are symmetrically diminished. The adult at first sight resembles a child, but the shape is that of an adult in miniature. Sexual organs are immature but intelligence is not impaired. Another type of pituitary infantilism is associated with obesity (Froehlich's syndrome or dystrophia adiposogenitalis. This is a rare condition too often diagnosed. A lesion of the hypothalamus or the pituitary is essential for diagnosis.). Infantilism of pituitary origin may also occur with diabetes insipidus. **Primary infantilism.** Ateleiosis, infantilism in which the lack of growth is the most apparent defect and the cause often obscure. **Pulmonary infantilism.** Infantilism secondary to severe disease of the lungs occurring in early life. **Renal infantilism.** Infantilism associated with excessive secretion of urine and excessive thirst, due to chronic interstitial nephritis which may be congenital. **Secondary infantilism.** Retarded growth secondary to severe organic disease of important organs, occurring at an early age. **Sexual infantilism.** Infantile state of the sexual organs beyond the normal age of puberty. **Syphilitic infantilism.** Infantilism secondary to congenital syphilis. **Thyroid infantilism.** Infantilism due to hypothyroidism, occurring in cretinism or juvenile myxoedema. [L *infans* unable to speak.]

See also: BRISSAUD, LÉVI, LORAIN.

infarct (in·farkt). A wedge-shaped area of dead tissue, with or without haemorrhage, produced by the obstruction of an end artery. **Anaemic infarct.** An infarct which is white in colour because of the absence of haemorrhage. **Aseptic infarct.** An infarct free from infection and showing no suppuration. **Bilirubin infarct.** A renal infarct containing bilirubin crystals. **Bland infarct.** Aseptic infarct (see above). **Bone infarct.** An area of sclerosis sometimes found in the medulla of long bones. **Calcareous infarct.** An old infarct which has become fibrosed and calcified. **Cardiac infarct.** An infarct of the heart muscle due to inadequacy of blood supply which most commonly results from atheromatous disease of the coronary arteries, often with superimposed thrombotic occlusion of a vessel. Small patchy infarcts, leading to scattered fibrosis, may occur in conditions in which the coronary perfusion is inadequate even though the coronary arteries are patent, as for example in aortic stenosis. **Cerebral infarct.** An infarct of cerebral tissue due to failure of blood supply resulting from vascular thrombosis, embolism, or spasm. **Cicatrized infarct.** An infarct in which the dead tissue has been completely replaced by scar tissue. **Cystic infarct.** An infarct from which most of the dead tissue has been absorbed, leaving a cavity. **Embolic infarct.** An infarct produced by the impaction of an embolus in an end artery. **Haemorrhagic infarct.** An infract which is red in colour because of much effusion of blood into its substance. **Healed infarct.** Cicatrized infarct (see above). **Infected infarct.** An infarct which is in process of conversion into an abscess. **Marginal infarct.** An infarct situated at the edge of an organ such as the lung or the spleen. **Myocardial infarct.** Cardiac infarct (see above.). **Pale infarct.** Anaemic infarct (see above). **Recent infarct.** One which has just been produced. **Red infarct.** Haemorrhagic infarct (see above). **Remote infarct.** One which was produced at some distant time. **Septic infarct.** Infected infarct (see above). **Sterile infarct.** Aseptic infarct (see above). **Thrombotic infarct.** An infarct produced by thrombosis of an end artery. **Uric-acid infarct.** The deposition of uric acid and urate crystals in a wedge-shaped area of renal tubules in the newborn child. **White infarct.** Anaemic infarct (see above). [L *infarcire* to stuff.]

infarction (in·fark·shun). 1. The process of formation of an infarct. 2. An infarct. **Cardiac infarction.** The process of the formation of a cardiac infarct. **Infarction of the lung.** The condition resulting from occlusion of a branch of the pulmonary artery by embolism or thrombosis. **Myocardial infarction.** The process of the formation of a myocardial infarct. **Uterine infarction.** 1. Haemorrhagic necrosis of the uterine wall as the result of arteriosclerosis of its vessels. 2. Red degeneration in a fibroid. [see prec.]

infect (in·fekt). 1. To contaminate with disease-producing micro-organisms or toxic factors. 2. To transmit infection, e.g. the specific virus of any particular disease. [L *inficere* to stain.]

infectible (in·fekt·ibl). In a state in which infection can be communicated and harboured.

infection (in·fek·shun). The invasion of the body by pathogenic or potentially pathogenic organisms, and their subsequent multiplication in the body. **Aerial infection.** Air-borne infection (see below). **Agonal infection.** Terminal infection (see below). **Air-borne infection.** Infection by micro-organisms suspended in the air. They may reach the body directly by inspiration of the infected air, or indirectly on food; the former route is usually implied. **Apical infection.** 1. An infection of the apex of the root of a tooth. 2. An infection of the apex of a lung. **Autochthonous infection.** An infection indigenous or native to a locality. **Consecutive infection.** A secondary infection superimposed on a primary one. **Contact infection.** An infection transmitted by direct contact with an infected person. **Cross infection.** The infection of a patient in hospital from a case of infectious disease in the same ward. **Cryptogenic infection.** An infection of which the site of entrance is unknown. **Diaplacental infection.** Infection via the placenta. **Direct infection.** Contact infection (see above). **Droplet infection.** An infection by air-borne droplets of saliva or sputum. **Dust infection.** Infection by inhaled infected dust particles. **Endogenous infection.** Infection arising from some focus within the body. **Exogenous infection.** An infection of which the source lies outside the body. **Focal infection.** An active infection which exists in a small circumscribed focus in some part of the body, such as the tonsils, dental roots, nasal sinuses, prostate, etc., and which spreads periodically or continuously therefrom. **Germinal infection.** Infection transmitted to the fetus through the agency of a germ cell. **Hand-borne infection.** Infection conveyed by contaminated hands. **Inapparent infection.** An infection which does not show itself by signs or symptoms. **Indirect infection.** An infection transmitted from one person to another by an intermediate agent such as food or water. **Latent infection.** An infection that usually, but not necessarily, after a period of activity becomes quiescent, the micro-organisms persisting but ceasing to multiply. **Mass infection.** An infection by a large number of organisms at the same time extensively distributed throughout the body. **Mixed infection.** One in which more than one species of organism is present. **Phytogenic infection.** Infection derived from plants. **Pyogenic infection.** Infection by organisms that cause suppuration. **Secondary infection.** An infection added to a pre-existing infection. **Septic infection.** Pyogenic infection (see above). **Silent infection.** Either a latent or a subclinical infection. **Simple infection.** A pure infection by one kind of micro-organism. **Subclinical infection.** An infection which does not cause clinically-recognizable symptoms. **Terminal infection.** An infection occurring shortly before death. **Water-borne infection.** Infection caused by the agency of water containing pathogenic organisms. **Zoogenetic infection.** An infection derived from lower animals. [L *inficere* to stain.]

See also: GOODALL.

infectiosity (in·fek·she·os′·it·e). The degree of infectiousness of a bacterium or other toxic agent. [see foll.]

infectious (in·fek·shus). 1. As applied to a parasitic micro-organism, having the property of invading and multiplying in the tissues of a host thereby causing harm. 2. Of a disease, one caused by pathogenic parasitic micro-organisms and transmissible to other persons by direct means. 3. Of a person, one who is suffering from an infectious disease which can be transmitted to another person. [L *inficere* to stain.]

infective (in·fek·tiv). Of a disease, one that is caused by parasitic micro-organisms but not necessarily directly transmissible to other persons. [see prec.]

infectivity (in·fek·tiv·it·e). The quality of being infective.

infecundity (in·fek·un·dit·e). 1. Barrenness in woman. 2. The state of being sterile or infertile. [L *infecunditas* barrenness.]

inferent (in·fer·ent). Afferent. [L *in, ferre* to bear.]

inferior (in·feer·e·or). 1. [NA] Situated lower down in relation to another structure when the body is in the anatomical position; directed downward. 2. Poorer in quality or value; less useful. [L, lower.]

inferocostal (in·fer·o·kos′·tal). Relating or belonging to the region beneath the lower border of a rib or to the lower border itself. [inferior, L *costa* rib.]

inferofrontal (in·fer·o·frun′·tal). Relating or belonging to the inferior part of the frontal lobe of the cerebrum.

inferolateral (in·fer·o·lat′·er·al). In a position below and to one side of another structure. [inferior, L *latus* side.]

inferomedian (in·fer·o·me′·de·an). Below and closer to the midline than another structure. [inferior, L *medius* middle.]

inferoposterior (in·fer·o·pos·teer′·e·or). In relation to another structure, in a position below and at the back of or behind. [inferior, posterior.]

infertile (in·fer·tile). Not fertile; barren; sterile. [L *in*, fertile.]

infertility (in·fer·til·it·e). The state or quality of being infertile.

infestation (in·fes·ta·shun). 1. The state of harbouring animal parasites on the surface of or within the body. 2. Invasion of the body by animal parasites. [L *infestare* to attack.]

infested (in·**fes**·ted). Harbouring parasites: the term should be confined to ectoparasites and to arthropod endoparasites, but it is sometimes used with reference to the harbouring of helminths, and even of protozoa. [see prec.]

infestment (in·**fest**·ment). Infestation.

infibulation (in·**fib**·ew·**la'**·shun). The stitching together of or the attaching of a ring or clasp to the male prepuce or the labia majora in the female in order to prevent coitus from taking place. [L *in, fibula* buckle.]

infiltrate (in·**fil**·trate). 1. To enter by penetrating the pores of or by filtering through a substance. 2. Any substance which seeps into the tissues and accumulates there. **Corneal infiltrate.** A corneal opacity caused by infiltration, or scarring after infiltration, of the cornea, resulting from damage or disease. [see foll.]

See also: ASSMANN.

infiltration (in·fil·tra·shun). A condition of the tissue cells in which various waste or other materials are brought to and deposited in the cells or in the space around them. **Adipose infiltration.** Either the accumulation of large amounts of fat within the cells of a tissue or organ, without appreciable change in the function of the latter, or the ingrowth of fatty tissue at the expense of the cells. **Calcareous infiltration, calcium infiltration.** The deposition of calcium and other mineral salts in the tissues. **Circumferential infiltration.** The surgical process of segregating an operation area from its nerve supply by a ring of anaesthetizing tissue infiltration. **Epituberculous infiltration.** Assmann's focus; a transient allergic tuberculous lesion in the upper portion of the lung. **Fatty infiltration.** Adipose infiltration (see above). **Gelatinous infiltration.** Mucoid degeneration. *See* DEGENERATION. **Glycogenic infiltration.** Abnormal accumulation of glycogen within tissue cells. **Inflammatory infiltration.** The appearance within a tissue or organ of the products and cells of inflammation. **Mineral infiltration.** Calcareous infiltration (see above). **Myocardial infiltration.** A general term embracing infiltrative conditions such as leukaemia, sarcoidosis, etc. **Paraneural infiltration.** Analgesia produced by injection of an analgesic into the immediate neighbourhood of a nerve. **Peripheral annular infiltration.** Circumferential infiltration (see above). **Pigmentary infiltration.** Pigmentation of a tissue from deposition of a pigment in its cells or intercellular spaces. **Purulent infiltration.** Pus formation. **Saline infiltration.** The introduction of a physiological salt solution into the tissues by some sort of device. **Sanguineous infiltration.** Diffuse haemorrhage within a tissue. **Serous infiltration.** Oedema. **Tuberculous infiltration.** Tuberculous tissue. **Urinous infiltration.** Extravasation of urine. **Waxy infiltration.** Zenker's degeneration of muscle. [L *in, filtrare* to strain through.]

infiltrator (in·fil·**tra**·tor). *See* JAMES (N. R.). [see prec.]

infirm (in·**ferm**). 1. Physically unsound or frail, or of low vitality, particularly on account of old age; feeble. 2. Irresolute or weak of will or character. Both conditions may be the result of disease. [L *infirmus* weak.]

infirmary (in·**fer**·mar·e). 1. Originally that part of a monastery used for the care of the sick or infirm. 2. A hospital or institution where sick or infirm persons are maintained or treated. 3. Under the obsolete Poor Law system, the institution or place in a workhouse reserved for the care and treatment of necessitous sick persons. [see prec.]

infirmity (in·**fer**·mit·e). 1. Weakness or feebleness of the body or mind as the result of old age or disease. 2. A malady of body or mind, resulting in weakness. 3. A defect or failing peculiar to a particular individual. [L *infirmitas* weakness.]

inflame (in·**flame**). To produce inflammation. [L *inflammare* to set on fire.]

inflammation (in·flam·a·shun). The reactive state of hyperaemia and exudation from its blood vessels, with consequent redness, heat, swelling, and pain, which a tissue enters in response to physical or chemical injury or bacterial invasion. **Acute inflammation.** Inflammation of rapid development. **Adhesive inflammation.** Inflammation of serous cavities, characterized by the fusion of apposed serous surfaces within them. **Allergic inflammation.** The inflammatory response to a protein towards which the affected tissues are sensitive. **Bacterial inflammation.** Inflammation in response to bacterial invasion. **Catarrhal inflammation.** Inflammation of a mucous surface with the formation of a surface discharge of mucus, pus, and desquamated epithelial cells. **Chemical inflammation.** Inflammation in response to chemical injury. **Chronic inflammation.** Inflammation of slow development and course, with overgrowth usually of fibrous tissue. **Croupous inflammation.** Diphtheritic inflammation (see below). **Diffuse inflammation.** Inflammation spreading over a wide area and with no tendency to localization. **Diphtheritic inflammation.** Inflammation of a mucous or raw surface with the formation of a fibrinous pseudomembrane over it. **Disseminated inflammation.** Inflammation spreading from its primary site to distant organs or tissues. **Exudative inflammation.** Inflammation of a serous or raw cavity, characterized by the outpouring of fluid from the inflamed surface. **Fibrinous inflammation.** Inflammation characterized by the aggregation of deposits of fibrin. **Fibroid inflammation.** Inflammation characterized by extensive deposits of fibrous tissue. **Focal inflammation.** Inflammation developing from one or more small areas initially infected. **Follicular inflammation.** Inflammation, characterized by local overgrowth within the inflamed area, of lymphatic follicles. **Granulomatous inflammation.** Chronic inflammation in which there is a deposit of abundant granulation tissue, especially in such diseases as tuberculosis, syphilis, yaws, and in actinomycosis and other mycelial infections. **Hyperplastic inflammation.** Inflammation productive of a gross overgrowth of young fibrous tissue. **Hypertrophic inflammation.** Inflammation affecting primarily the stroma of an organ. **Metastatic inflammation.** Inflammation occurring as a result of spread of the causative agent from its primary focus to a distant part by way of the blood stream or lymph stream. **Necrotic inflammation.** Inflammation associated with the death of part of the tissue affected. **Obliterative inflammation.** Inflammation of a hollow organ or cavity wherein anatomical spaces are obliterated by adhesions. **Parenchymatous inflammation.** Inflammation wherein the epithelial or glandular elements of an organ or tissue are primarily affected. **Plastic inflammation.** Adhesive inflammation (see above). **Productive inflammation, proliferous inflammation.** Hyperplastic inflammation (see above). **Purulent inflammation.** Inflammation attended by the formation of pus. **Reactive inflammation.** Inflammation in response to a foreign body or portion of dead tissue. **Sclerosing inflammation.** Inflammation associated with the production of fibrous tissue throughout the affected part. **Seroplastic inflammation.** Inflammation of a serous cavity, attended both by the outpouring of serous fluid and by adhesion formation. **Serous inflammation.** Inflammation of a serous cavity such as pleura, pericardium, peritoneum, or of synovial membrane. **Specific inflammation.** Inflammation due to a particular variety of micro-organism, particularly the spirochaete of syphilis. **Subacute inflammation.** Inflammation of gradual onset, proceeding to a severe or chronic form. **Toxic inflammation.** Inflammation produced by chemical poisons, or by the toxic products of bacterial action rather than by the bacteria themselves. **Traumatic inflammation.** Inflammation consequent upon injury. [L *inflammare* to set on fire.]

inflammatory (in·**flam**·at·or·e). Belonging to, having the characteristics of, or marked by inflammation.

inflation (in·fla·shun). 1. Distension of an organ or part with fluid, air, or a gas. 2. The process of filling with air or a gas in order to produce distension. [L *in, flare* to blow.]

See also: VALSALVA.

inflator (in·**fla**·tor). An apparatus with which a part or organ can be filled with air for the purpose of diagnosis or treatment. [see prec.]

inflected (in·**flek**·ted). 1. Curved or bent downwards or inward. 2.

Diffracted. 3. Colourful, of the voice; not monotonous. [L *in, flectere* to bend.]

inflection (in·**flek**·shun). Inflexion.

inflexed (in·**flexd**). Inflected.

inflexion (in·**flek**·shun). 1. The state of being inflected or diffracted. 2. The act of bending inward or downward. 3. Change in pitch or tone of the speaking voice so that there is not monotony of sound. [L *in, flectere* to bend.]

inflorescence (in·flor·**es**·ens). In botany, the disposition and arrangement of flowers on an axis and their manner of development. [L *in, florescere* to come into flower.]

influenza (in·floo·**en**·zah). An acute infectious disease due to influenza virus (*see* VIRUS). Infection is of the upper respiratory tract with general constitutional symptoms of fever, malaise, and muscular aches. In otherwise healthy children and adults the disease, though uncomfortable, is not serious and resolves in two or three days. Physical weakness and depression may persist longer. In the elderly and those with chronic respiratory impairment, the disease can precipitate severe and sometimes fatal complications. Influenza is endemic in most parts of the world, with highest incidence in the winter months. The virus undergoes antigenic variation, with new strains replacing the old. When there is a major alteration in antigenic structure, the virus becomes effectively a new virus to which there is no pre-existing immunity; consequently an epidemic and, periodically, a pandemic occurs. There is no specific treatment, though amantadine has been used prophylactically and reductions in the incidence and severity of the disease have been reported. Antibiotics are used in those with chronic respiratory diseases to prevent secondary bacterial infection, but they do not affect the virus. Vaccines, using virus inactivated by formalin, have been used and confer limited protection. Live attenuated vaccines have also shown promise but require more evaluation. The symptoms and signs of influenza may be mimicked by several other virus diseases in the early stages, as well as by some bacterial ones. **Abdominal influenza.** Gastric influenza; influenza with gastro-intestinal symptoms, which is readily confused with *Salmonella* infections (food poisoning, typhoid fever), and with other causes of abdominal pain, and diarrhoea. Laboratory aids are necessary for differentiation. **Asian influenza.** Influenza due to a strain of virus having no apparent antigenic relationship to older strains. It first appeared in Hong Kong and Singapore in April 1957 and spread through India into several western countries. **Clinical influenza.** An infection resembling influenza clinically, from which the specific virus has not been isolated. **Endemic influenza.** An obsolete description for the catarrhal fevers (influenza nostras or winter grippe), that occur during the winter months, and are relatively milder than true epidemic influenza. **Spanish influenza.** A name given to the great pandemic of 1918–19; this did not originate in Spain (a popular misconception at that time). [It., influence.]

influenza virus (in·floo·**en**·zah **vi**·rus). The causative viruses of influenza. They are RNA-containing viruses of the family orthomyxoviridae, pleomorphic in appearance, about 90 nm in size. There are 3 influenza viruses, each entirely separate antigenically, called A, B and C. *Influenza A:* The virus of epidemic influenza, due to its ability to undergo periodic antigenic alteration. The virus has two surface antigens, a haemagglutinin and a neuraminidase both of which undergo independent variation. This variation shows two forms. A gradual and progressive alteration of antigenic identity is called *drift.* Periodically there is a major alteration, probably by genetic reassortment with animal or bird strains, resulting in the acquisition of entirely new antigens and this phenomenon is called *shift.* Influenza virus is unique among viruses in that new antigenic variants replace the old completely, making existing vaccines and immunity obsolete. All influenza A types possess a similar internal nucleoprotein antigen, which does not elicit any protective antibody in the host, and they have been isolated from numerous species of birds, horses and swine as well as man. Generally there is a barrier to spread from one species to another but haemagglutinin and neuraminidase antigens indistinguishable from some human strains have been found in animal strains. Influenza A types sufficiently different from previous strains to cause pandemics may acquire names of their own, e.g. Spanish influenza in 1918 and Asian influenza in 1957. *Influenza B:* Morphologically identical with influenza A but antigenically distinct. It has haemagglutinin and neuraminidase surface antigens which show a gradual alteration (drift), but major changes (shift) are not seen, probably because there are no animal strains. Influenza B has therefore not been the cause of pandemics. *Influenza C:* Differs slightly but significantly in morphology from influenzas A and B, and is quite different antigenically. It has been associated with influenza-like illnesses but may not readily cause clinical influenza. Consequently its designation as a true influenza virus still has to be established. Its surface haemagglutinin and neuraminidase antigens show some drift but no shift.

influenzal (in·floo·**en**·zal). Pertaining to, characterized, or caused by influenza.

informational (in·form·**a**·shun·al). Information-bearing. Used of some nucleic acids (DNA, mRNA and tRNA) and of most proteins. [L *informationem* information.]

informosome (in·**form**·o·some). A class of particles which contain ribonucleic acid and protein; they are thought to be the form in which mRNA is transported between the genetic material and the protein-synthesizing apparatus in living cells. [inform, Gk *soma* body.]

infra-. Prefix, from the Latin preposition *infra,* meaning *below, under.*

infra-axillary (in·frah·ax·**il**′·ar·e). In a position below the axilla. [L *infra,* axilla.]

infrabranchial (in·frah·**brang**·ke·al). In zoology, below the gills. [L *infra,* branchial.]

infraclavicular (in·frah·klav·**ik**′·ew·lar). Below the clavicle or the level of the clavicle. [L *infra,* clavicle.]

infraclusion (in·frah·**kloo**·zhun). In dentistry, the position of a tooth when its occluding surface is below the normal place of occlusion. [L *infra,* occlusion.]

infracommissure (in·frah·**kom**·is·ewr). The inferior commissure of the hypothalamus. [L *infra,* commissure.]

infraconscious (in·frah·**kon**·shus). Subconscious. [L *infra,* conscious.]

infraconstrictor (in·frah·kon·**strik**′·tor). The inferior constrictor muscle of the pharynx. *See* PHARYNX, CONSTRICTOR MUSCLES OF THE. [L *infra,* constrictor.]

infracortical (in·frah·**kor**·tik·al). Situated beneath the cortex of the brain or kidney. [L *infra,* cortex.]

infracostal (in·frah·**kos**·tal). In a position under the ribs or a rib. [L *infra, costa* rib.]

infracostales (in·frah·kos·**ta**′·leez). The subcostal muscles. [see prec.]

infracotyloid (in·frah·**kot**·il·oid). Beneath the acetabulum (cotyloid cavity). [L *infra,* cotyloid.]

infracristal (in·frah·**kris**·tal). Below the crista of the right heart. [L *infra, crista* ridge.]

infraction, infracture (in·**frak**·shun, in·**frak**·tewr). 1. A fracture of a bone without displacement. 2. An incomplete fracture. [L *infractio* a breaking.]

See also: FREIBERG.

infradentale (in·frah·den·**ta**′·le). The point of transition from the crown of the most prominent mandibular central incisor to the alveolar projection. [L *infra, dens* tooth.]

infradiaphragmatic (in·frah·di·ah·frag·**mat**′·ik). Situated below the diaphragm. [L *infra,* diaphragm.]

infraduction (in·frah·**duk**·shun). The turning downwards or underneath of any part of the eye; rotation of the eyeball downwards on its transverse axis. [L *infra, ducere* to lead.]

infragenual (in·frah·**jen**·ew·al). Pertaining to a part beneath the patella; lying beneath the patella. [L *infra, genu* knee.]

infraglenoid (in·frah·**gle**·noid). Placed below the glenoid cavity. [L *infra,* glenoid.]

infraglottic (in·frah·**glot**·ik). In a position below the glottis. [L *infra*, glottis.]

infrahyoid (in·frah·**hi**·oid). In place below the hyoid bone. [L *infra*, hyoid.]

infrahyoid muscles [musculi infrahyoidei (NA)]. A group of muscles lying below the hyoid bone and attaching to it. They include the sternohyoid, omohyoid, thyrohyoid, and levator glandulae thyreoideae muscles.

infra-inguinal (in·frah·**ing**·gwin·al). Situated below the inguinal region. [L *infra*, inguinal.]

inframamillary (in·frah·**mam**·il·ar·e). Situated below the nipple of the breast. [L *infra*, mamilla.]

inframammary (in·frah·**mam**·ar·e). Situated below the breast. [L *infra*, *mamma* breast.]

inframandibular (in·frah·man·**dib**'·ew·lar). Below the mandible. [L *infra*, mandible.]

inframarginal (in·frah·**mar**·jin·al). Placed beneath any edge or margin. [L *infra*, margin.]

inframaxillary (in·frah·max·**il**'·ar·e). Situated under the maxilla. [L *infra*, maxilla.]

inframicrobe (in·frah·**mi**·krobe). A filtrable virus. [L *infra*, microbe.]

infranuclear (in·frah·**new**·kle·ar). Situated under a nucleus. [L *infra*, nucleus.]

infra-occipital (in·frah·ok·**sip**'·it·al). Below the occipital bone or below the occiput. [L *infra*, occiput.]

infra-occlusion (in·frah·ok·**loo**'·zhun). That form of occlusion where one or more teeth fail to rise to the normal occlusal level. [L *infra*, occlusion.]

infra-orbital (in·frah·**or**·bit·al). Situated below the level of the floor of the orbit. **Infra-orbital canal.** *See* CANAL. **Infra-orbital groove.** *See* GROOVE. **Infra-orbital margin.** *See* MARGIN. [L *infra*, orbit.]

infra-orbital artery [arteria infra-orbitalis (NA)]. *See* MAXILLARY ARTERY.

infra-orbital nerve [nervus infra-orbitalis (NA)]. The continuation of the maxillary nerve in the infra-orbital groove and canal, and on to the face.

infra-orbital vein. A vessel draining from the face through the infra-orbital canal to the pterygoid plexus.

infrapatellar (in·frah·pat·**el**'·ar). Situated below the level of the patella. **Infrapatellar bursa.** *See* BURSA. [L *infra*, patella.]

infraplacement (in·frah·**plase**·ment). In dentistry, the downward displacement of a tooth. [L *infra*, displacement.]

infrapsychic (in·frah·**si**·kik). Below the level of consciousness, i.e. automatic. [L *infra*, Gk *psyche* mind.]

infrapubic (in·frah·**pew**·bik). Relating or belonging to parts below the pubis. [L *infra*, pubis.]

infrarectus (in·frah·**rek**·tus). The inferior rectus muscle of the orbit. *See* RECTUS MUSCLES OF THE ORBIT. [L *infra*, rectus.]

infrared (in·frah·**red**). That part of the electromagnetic spectrum beyond the red end of the visible spectrum; within it lie the heat-producing rays with wavelengths from 7 500 Å (750 nm) to a few mm. Helpful as an adjunct in the treatment of acute and chronic traumatic and inflammatory conditions. [L *infra*, red.

infrascapular (in·frah·**skap**·ew·lar). In a position below the scapula. [L *infra*, scapula.]

infrasonic (in·frah·**son**·ik). Sounds of a frequency below those audible to the human ear. [L *infra*, *sonus* sound.]

infraspinatus (in·frah·spi·**na**'·tus). The infraspinatus muscle of the upper limb. [L *infra*, spine.]

infraspinatus muscle [musculus infraspinatus (NA)]. A muscle which extends from the infraspinous fossa on the scapula to the greater tuberosity of the humerus.

infraspinous (in·frah·**spi**·nus). 1. Situated below the scapular spine. 2. Below the spine of a vertebra. [L *infra*, spine.]

infrastapedial (in·frah·stap·e'·de·al). Situated below the stapes. [L *infra*, stapes.]

infrasternal (in·frah·**ster**·nal). Below the sternum. [L *infra*, sternum.]

infratemporal (in·frah·**tem**·por·al). Situated below the temporal fossa of the skull. [L *infra*, temporal.]

infrathoracic (in·frah·thor·**as**'·ik). Situated below the thorax. [L *infra*, thorax.]

infratonsillar (in·frah·**ton**·sil·ar). Situated in the pharynx below the tonsil. [L *infra*, tonsil.]

infratracheal (in·frah·trak·e'·al). In a position beneath the trachea. [L *infra*, trachea.]

infratrochlear (in·frah·**trok**·le·ar). Below the trochlea. [L *infra*, trochlea.]

infratrochlear nerve [nervus infratrochlearis (NA)]. A branch from the nasociliary nerve in the orbit to the skin of the medial side of the eyelids and the adjacent part of the side of the nose. **Palpebral branches [rami palpebrales (NA)].** The branches to the skin of the eyelids from the infratrochlear nerve.

infratubal (in·frah·**tew**·bal). Situated beneath a tube. [L *infra*, tube.]

infraturbinal (in·frah·**ter**·bin·al). The inferior nasal concha. [L *infra*, turbinate bone.]

infra-umbilical (in·frah·um·**bil**'·ik·al). Below the umbilicus. [L *infra*, umbilicus.]

infravaginal (in·frah·vaj·**i**'·nal). 1. Below the fornix of the vagina. 2. Below any sheath. [L *infra*, vagina.]

infravergence (in·frah·**ver**·jens). Disjunctive reciprocal motion of the eyes in which one eye is turned downward. [L *infra*, *vergere* to bend.]

infraversion (in·frah·**ver**·shun). A downward deviation of the eye. [L *infra*, *vertere* to turn.]

infriction (in·**frik**·shun). Medication by rubbing ointments, liniments, and other preparations into the skin. [L *in*, *fricare* to rub.]

infundibular (in·fun·**dib**·ew·lar). 1. Relating to the infundibulum of the hypothalamus. 2. Having the character of or resembling an infundibulum or funnel.

infundibuliform (in·fun·**dib**·ew·le·form). Funnel-shaped; having the form of a cone. [L *infundibulum* funnel, form.]

infundibuloma (in·fun·dib·ew·**lo**'·mah). A neoplasm of the infundibulum of the hypothalamus. [infundibulum, Gk *-oma* tumour.]

infundibulo-ovarian (in·fun·**dib**·ew·lo·o·**va**'·re·an). Relating or belonging to the infundibulum of the uterine tube and the ovary.

infundibulopelvic (in·fun·**dib**·ew·lo·**pel**'·vik). Referring or belonging to any two structures named infundibulum and pelvis, e.g. the expanded calyx and pelvis of the ureter.

infundibulum [NA] (in·fun·**dib**·ew·lum). Any funnel-shaped structure or passage, particularly the funnel-shaped depression in the floor of the 3rd ventricle of the brain immediately above the attachment of the stalk of the hypophysis cerebri (pituitary gland). **Infundibulum of the ethmoid [infundibulum ethmoidale (NA)].** A depression in the lateral wall of the middle meatus of the nose, into which the anterior ethmoidal air cells and, usually, the frontonasal duct from the frontal air sinus open. **Infundibulum of the frontal air sinus.** Infundibulum of the ethmoid (see prec.). **Infundibulum of the heart [conus arteriosus (infundibulum) (NA)].** The part of the right ventricle from which the trunk of the pulmonary artery arises. **Infundibulum of the lung.** The expanded termination of bronchioles into which the pulmonary alveoli open. **Infundibulum of the uterine tube [infundibulum tubae uterinae (NA)].** The funnel-shaped opening at the lateral end of a uterine tube. [L, funnel.]

infused (in·**fewzd**). Of substances, steeped in water or other fluid so that the soluble properties are extracted. [L *in*, *fundere* to pour.]

infusible (in·**fewz**·ibl). 1. Incapable of being fused or melted. 2. Able to undergo infusion. [L *in*, *fundere* to pour.]

infusion (in·**few**·zhun). 1. A saline or other solution given intravenously for therapeutic purposes. 2. A dilute solution containing the water-soluble extract of a vegetable drug; it is obtained by macerating the drug with water, usually boiling, and straining the liquid without pressing the residue. Cold water is employed for drugs containing readily soluble active principles, e.g. quassia, and for those containing much starch, e.g. calumba. As infusions are aqueous extracts, they are readily fermented;

they have therefore always to be freshly prepared, and for that reason are being replaced by *concentrated infusions* which are extracts containing alcohol (usually 25 per cent) as a preservative, and which are anything up to eight times the strength of fresh infusions, requiring to be diluted with water before use. **Infusion of calumba.** A simple bitter. **Cold infusion.** An infusion made with cold water (*see* MAIN DEF. 2 above). **Compound Gentian Infusion BP 1958.** The commonest bitter containing the water-soluble parts of gentian, orange, and lemon. **Drop infusion.** A drip. **Dural infusion.** An obsolete term for intrathecal medication. **Meat infusion.** A watery extract of raw beef, veal, etc., used as the base for bacteriological media, e.g. 500 g lean, fat-free meat, minced and added to 1 litre of water, gradually heated to boiling point, filtered, and allowed to cool. **Infusion of Quassia, Concentrated BPC 1959.** A simple bitter. **Saline infusion.** An infusion made with saline solution (*see* MAIN DEF. 1 above). [L *in, fundere* to pour.]

infusor (in·**few**·sor). An apparatus through which any medicinal liquid can be run slowly into a vein or into the parenchyma. [see prec.]

infusoria (in·few·**sor**·e·ah). 1. Microscopic organisms which develop in infusions of hay and other organic materials; mostly Protozoa, but also Rotifera, unicellular algae, etc. 2. Protozoa of the class Ciliata. [L *in, fundere* to pour.]

infusoriotoxin (in·few·**sor**·e·o·**tox**′·in). Any poisonous substance that has the power to destroy infusoria. [infusoria, toxin.]

infusum (in·**few**·sum). Infusion. Before 1953 all BP infusions were classified as Infusa. [L.]

ingesta (in·**jes**·tah). Any nourishment that reaches the body tissues by way of the alimentary canal. [L *in, gerere* to carry.]

ingestant (in·**jes**·tant). Food or other substance taken in by the mouth. **Sensitizing ingestant.** One which conditions a person for allergic reactions. [L *in, gerere* to carry.]

ingestion (in·**jes**·chun). 1. The taking of substances, either nourishing or medicinal, into the body. 2. The phagocytic process by which a foreign body such as a bacillus is surrounded and assimilated by a cell. [L *in, gerere* to carry.]

ingestive (in·**jes**·tiv). 1. Having the function of ingestion. 2. Relating or belonging to the function of ingestion.

ingluvin (in·**glew**·vin). An enzyme found in the gizzard of the hen. It is a pepsin-like ferment which has been used for the vomiting of pregnancy. [L *ingluvies* gizzard.]

Ingrassia, Giovanni Filippo (b. 1510). Naples and Padua anatomist.

Apophysis of Ingrassia, Ingrassia's process. The lesser wing of the sphenoid bone.

Wings of Ingrassia. Wings of the sphenoid bone.

ingravescent (in·grav·**es**·ent). Increasing gradually in severity, as a pathological condition. [L *ingravescere* to grow worse.]

ingravidation (in·**grav**·id·**a**′·shun). Impregnation. [L *ingravidare* to impregnate.]

ingredient (in·**gre**·de·ent). Any substance that is one of the components of a mixture. [L *ingredi* to enter in.]

inguen (ing·gwen). The groin. [L.]

inguinal (ing·gwin·al). Relating or belonging to the groin, or in the region of the groin. [L *inguen* groin.]

inguino-abdominal (ing·gwin·o·ab·**dom**′·in·al). Relating or belonging to both the groin and the abdomen. [L *inguen* groin, abdomen.]

inguinocrural (ing·gwin·o·**kroo**′·ral). Relating or belonging to both the groin and the thigh. [L *inguen* groin, *crus* leg.]

inguinodynia (ing·gwin·o·**din**′·e·ah). Pain felt in the groin, often hysterical in origin. [L *inguen* groin, Gk *odyne* pain.]

inguino-interstitial (ing·gwin·o·in·ter·**stish**′·al). Occurring or situated within the tissues of the inguinal region. [L *inguen* groin, interstice.]

inguinolabial (ing·gwin·o·**la**′·be·al). Relating or belonging to the groin and a labium majus, e.g. a hernia which passes down into the labium from the canal. [L *inguen* groin, *labium* lip.]

inguinoscrotal (ing·gwin·o·**skro**′·tal). Relating or belonging to the groin and the scrotum, or to the inguinal canal and the scrotum, e.g. a hernia that descends into the scrotum from the canal. [L *inguen* groin, scrotum.]

ingulation (in·gew·**la**·shun). The act or process of introducing something into the throat. [L *in, gula* gullet.]

ingurgitation (in·**ger**·jit·**a**′·shun). 1. The act of swallowing or gulping greedily. 2. Any material so swallowed. 3. Over-eating and over-drinking. [L *ingurgitare* to gormandize.]

inhalant (in·**ha**·lant). A liquid preparation of one or more volatile medicaments intended to be inhaled. Dry inhalants are inhaled as such from a handkerchief or a sponge, and are usually alcoholic solutions; wet inhalants are normally added to hot water and the steam inhaled. Among the former are the volatile oils of eucalyptus, pine, and solutions of menthol and thymol: the chief wet inhalants are friars' balsam and menthol. The seats of action are the nasal passages, throat, and lungs where large and rapid absorption occurs. [L *in, halare* to breathe.]

inhalation (in·hal·**a**·shun). 1. Inhalant. 2. The inspiration of air or vapour.

inhale (in·**hale**). 1. To breathe in, to draw air into the lungs by breathing. 2. To draw in air impregnated by some medicinal substance in the form of steam, vapour, or powder. [L *in, halare* to breathe.]

inhaler (in·**ha**·ler). 1. A device for administering vapour, volatile substances, or fine powder, by inhalation. 2. An apparatus for cleansing inhaled air of dust, etc., or for warming inhaled air. **Cardiff inhaler.** An apparatus introduced in 1969 for self-administration of methoxyflurane in obstetrics. **Ether inhaler.** An apparatus in which anaesthetic ether is vaporized before its inhalation. **HH inhaler.** An apparatus for inhaling oxygen, used for gassed patients. It is named after Henderson and Haggard. **Oxford inhaler.** Oxford vaporizer. *See* VAPORIZER. [see prec.]

See also: FREEDMAN, GOLDMAN, MARRETT.

inherent (in·**heer**·ent). Existing as a permanent attribute or settled function of an organism; part of the essential character of a person. Innate; intrinsic to the organism. [L *inhaerere* to be always connected with.]

inheritance (in·**her**·it·ans). The derivation of characters from parents and ancestors; the total of such characters derived. **Alternative inheritance.** That in which all the characters are derived from one parent only. **Amphigonous inheritance.** That in which some of the characters are derived from each parent. **Blending inheritance.** That in which opposing characters of the parents appear as a blend in the offspring. **Chromosome inheritance.** The inheritance of genetic information contained in the chromosomes or the mode of inheritance characteristics of the genetic factors carried by the chromosomes (mendelian inheritance). **Criss-cross inheritance.** That in which maternal characters are shown by male offspring and paternal by female. **Dominant inheritance.** Inheritance in which the distribution of a characteristic to the offspring will follow mendelian principles for a dominant. **Holandric inheritance.** Inheritance in which the distribution of a characteristic to the offspring will follow mendelian principles for a gene on a Y chromosome. **Hologynic inheritance.** That in which a character appears in all the female offspring but in none of the males. **Maternal inheritance.** That in which the characters are derived from the female parent, either genetically or by the uterine environment. **Mendelian inheritance.** That in which the appearance of the characters in the offspring follows Mendel's laws or other laws based on mendelian principles. **Particulate inheritance.** That in which a character is inherited in a particulate (presence or absence) manner: mendelian inheritance. **Paternal inheritance.** That in which characters are derived from the male parent. **Recessive inheritance.** Inheritance in which the distribution of a characteristic to the offspring will follow mendelian principles for a recessive. **Sex-limited inheritance.** Inheritance in which the distribution of a characteristic to the offspring will be such that it will appear in one or other sex only. **Sex-linked inheritance.** Inheritance in which the distribution of a characteristic to the offspring will follow mendelian principles for a gene on an X chromosome. **Unilinear inheritance.** The inheritance of a character along only one line of descent, i.e. at each cellular division only one of the two daughter cells inherits the character. Characterized by abortive transduction of bacteria. [L *in, hereditare* to inherit.]

inherited (in·**her**·it·ed). Applied to a quality or trait that is present as a natural inheritance, derived from ancestors, e.g. constitution. [see prec.]

inhibin (in·**hib**·in). A hypothetical substance said to be secreted by the testis, having the power to suppress the production of the luteinizing hormone of the anterior pituitary gland. It is improbable that it exists as a separate hormone. [see foll.]

inhibit (in·**hib**·it). 1. To hinder the appearance of or to check or arrest a functional process; to restrain or stop a chemical action. 2. In psychological medicine, to suppress any thought or idea to which a sense of guilt is attached. [L *inhibere* to restrain.]

inhibition (in·hib·**ish**·un). 1. The prevention or attenuation of a reaction, activity or function. 2. The prevention of the emergence from the unconscious mind into the conscious mind of an instinctive impulse. **Autogenous inhibition.** A reflex inhibition occurring at the site of stimulation. **Competitive inhibition.** Inhibition of acetylcholine at the myoneural junction; the action of non-depolarizing or anti-depolarising muscular relaxants, e.g. tubocurarine. **End-product inhibition.** The inhibition of activity of the first enzyme of a biochemical pathway by the end-product of the pathway; a widespread cellular mechanism for regulating biochemical activity. **Feed-back inhibition.** End-product inhibition (see prec.). **Haemadsorption inhibition.** The inhibition of virus-specific haemadsorption by antiserum to the virus. **Haemagglutination inhibition.** *See* HAEMAGGLUTINATION. **Reflex inhibition.** A reflex which prevents activity from occurring in a related nerve centre, so that an appropriate stimulus apparently evokes no response. On the other hand, the reflex prevention of nervous activity may induce a visible response, as when removal of constrictor tone results in vasodilatation. **Selective inhibition.** The displacement of an active substance by a similar but inactive one, so that a given physiological function is abolished or reduced. **Specific inhibition.** Excessive saturation of an antibody by its specific antigen. **Vagal inhibition.** Vagal reflex. *See* REFLEX. [L *inhibere* to restrain.]

See also: WEDENSKY.

inhibitive (in·**hib**·it·iv). Inhibitory.

inhibitor (in·**hib**·it·or). 1. A nerve which decreases or stops the activity of the part supplied by it. 2. A mechanical device which prevents breathing through the mouth. 3. In embryology, any chemical substance which restrains or stops altogether the activity of a tissue organizer in determining the line of development of the fetus. 4. In chemistry, any substance which stops or arrests action or reaction. **Allosteric inhibitor.** A compound which, when bound to an allosteric site of an allosteric enzyme, produces a decrease in catalytic activity; negative allosteric effector. **Carbonic anhydrase inhibitor.** A substance assumed to inhibit renal tubular anhydrase, causing increased excretion of water and alkali. **Competitive inhibitor.** An inactive or blocking substance which can occupy the receptor site in a cell or at its surface by virtue of the fact that part of its molecular configuration is similar to that of an active substance. **Mitotic inhibitor.** A substance that inhibits karyokinesis or mitosis. **Mono-amine oxidase inhibitors.** Substances which diminish the action of the enzyme and thus lead to a higher concentration of mono-amines in the tissues; many drugs used as antidepressants are mono-amine oxidase inhibitors, for example iproniazid. **Specific inhibitor.** A substance which combines with, and so inactivates, an active substance. **Viral inhibitor.** Any substance which inhibits replication of a virus within the host cell, without inactivating the virus directly. [L *inhibere* to restrain.]

inhibitory (in·**hib**·it·or·e). Putting a restraint on function or hindering the carrying out of a process. [see prec.]

inhibitrope (in·**hib**·e·trope). Any individual in whom function is arrested by the application of certain kinds of stimuli. [inhibit, Gk *trope* a turning.]

inhomogeneity (in·**ho**·mo·jen·**e**′·it·e). Absence of uniformity of quality, so that samples taken in different places may show wide variations, e.g. of blood taken simultaneously from different parts of the circulation. [L *in*, homogeneity.]

iniac, inial (**in**·e·ak, **in**·e·al). In craniology, belonging to the inion.

iniencephalus (**in**·e·en·**kef**′·al·us). A monster in which the substance of the brain protrudes through a fissure in the occiput, generally associated with fissure of the vertebral column. [inion, Gk *egkephalos* brain.]

iniencephaly (**in**·e·en·**kef**′·al·e). The condition found in an iniencephalus. [see prec.]

iniodymus (in·e·**od**·im·us). A twin monster in which the backs of the heads of the two fetuses are fused but there are two separate bodies. [inion, Gk *didymos* twin.]

iniofacial (**in**·e·o·**fa**′·shal). Relating or belonging to the inion and the face.

inioglabellar (**in**·e·o·**glab**·**el**′·ar). 1. Relating or belonging to the inion and the glabella. 2. Uniting the inion and the glabella.

iniomesial (**in**·e·o·**me**′·ze·al). Relating or belonging to the inion and the median line of the body. [inion, Gk *mesos* middle.]

inion [NA] (**in**·e·on). In craniology, the most prominent point in the median plane of the external occipital protuberance. [Gk, the back of the head.]

iniopagus (in·e·**op**·ag·us). A twin monster in which the backs of the two heads are united. [inion, Gk *pagos* fixed.]

iniops (**in**·e·ops). A double monster joined from the thorax upwards, with a single head having anteriorly one complete face and posteriorly only a suggestion of a face or one feature of a face, e.g. an eye. [inion, Gk *ops* eye.]

inirritative (in·**ir**·it·a·tiv). Not capable of being irritant; soothing. [L *in*, irritative.]

initial (in·**ish**·al). Relating or belonging to the beginning or the first stage of any process, e.g. the primary stage of a disease. [L *initium* a beginning.]

initiation (in·**ish**·e·a·shon). **Chain initiation.** *See* CHAIN.

initiator (in·**ish**·e·a·tor). In molecular biology, a protein postulated to initiate DNA synthesis by acting on a site termed the *replicator*. [L *initium* a beginning.]

initis (in·**i**·tis). 1. Fibrositis. 2. Myositis. 3. Tendinitis. [Gk *is* fibre, *-itis* inflammation.]

inject (in·**jekt**). 1. To pass fluid into a blood vessel, a hollow viscus, a body cavity, or any body tissue. 2. In anatomy, to force a fluid into a blood vessel, a cavity or tissue of the body, usually for the purpose of colouring, preserving, or hardening. 3. In pathology, to distend the capillaries with blood. Hence, *injected.* [L *in, jacere* to throw.]

injectio (in·**jek**·she·o). Injection. Before 1953 all the BP Injections were classed as Injectio. [L.]

injection (in·**jek**·shun). 1. The act of propelling a fluid into the body, especially by the use of a hollow needle. 2. A sterile fluid preparation of a medicament intended to be used parenterally, i.e. by injection subcutaneously, intramuscularly, intravenously, or intrathecally. 3. A state of visible hyperaemia (e.g. of the conjunctiva). **Booster injection.** Booster dose. *See* DOSE. **Capillary injection.** Undue visibility of the small blood vessels of the skin, especially of the face, due to capillary dilatation. **Endermic injection.** Intradermal injection (see below). **Epidural injection.** Injection of local anaesthetics or other substances into the extradural (epidural) space. **Epifascial injection.** Injection of a substance on the surface of a fascia, used, especially formerly, for irritant substances. **Exciting injection.** Sensitizing injection (see below). **Gaseous injection.** Injection of air or other gas for diagnostic (e.g. ventriculography) or therapeutic (e.g. pneumothorax) purposes. **Gelatin injection.** A preservative injection containing gelatin. **Hypodermatic injection, hypodermic injection.** Subcutaneous injection (see below). **Intra-articular injection.** Injection into a joint. **Intracardiac injection.** An injection directly into the heart (e.g. adrenaline in cardiac arrest). **Intradermal injection, intradermic injection.** Injection into the substance of the skin (e.g. in the Mantoux test). **Intramuscular injection.** Injection into the substance of a muscle. **Intravascular**

injection. Injection into a bloodvessel lumen. **Intravenous injection.** Injection into a vein. **Macrisalb (^{131}I) Injection.** BP 1973 macro-aggregated iodinated (^{131}I) human albumin injection; it is used in the examination of pulmonary perfusion. **Opacifying injection, opaque injection.** Injection of a radio-opaque substance for diagnostic purposes. **Parenchymatous injection.** Injection into the substance of an organ. **Plaster injection.** Injection of a gypsum and water paste into vessels, in making anatomical preparations. **Preparatory injection.** Sensitizing injection (see below). **Reacting injection.** Reacting dose. *See* DOSE. **Sclerosant injection.** Injection of an irritant fluid to induce fibrous reaction and sclerosis. **Sclerosing injection.** Injection of a substance into a blood vessel to obliterate it (e.g. ethanolamine into varicose veins). **Sensitizing injection.** The first, or sensitizing, dose of an antigen. **Subcutaneous injection.** An injection into the loose fascia immediately under the skin. [L *in, jacere* to throw.]

See also: BROWN-SÉQUARD, SCHLOESSER.

injector (in·**jek**·tor). An instrument or apparatus with which injections are made into the body.

See also: DUSSEAU.

injury (in·jur·e). 1. Hurt done to or damage suffered by the body. 2. A wound of any kind. **Birth injury.** Injury caused at birth. **Blast injury.** Lung blast. *See* BLAST. **Charley-horse injury.** Rupture of some fibres of hamstrings; common in footballers, cricket bowlers, and sprinters. **Cold injury.** 1. Injury to tissues caused by exposure to reduced temperatures, not necessarily very low. Hypothermia in the elderly, when sustained for hours, causing stasis, skin blebbing, cyanosis and oedema, sometimes ulceration patches or gangrene, also internal ulceration of the oesophagus and stomach, and pancreatic necroses with fat necrosis. 2. Frank freezing and tissue death; frostbite and gangrene of ears, fingers and toes. **Compression injury.** Any injury resulting from prolonged compression that produces ischaemic necrosis and may, if extensive, lead to the compression syndrome. **Crush injury.** 1. Any injury that results from a crushing of the body tissues, e.g. of a finger. 2. An injury that results in the crushing of any considerable mass of the body tissues, and gives rise to the compression syndrome. **Decompression injury.** The damage sustained in caisson disease. **Egg-white injury.** The toxic effect of a diet rich in egg-white due to the presence of avidin which combines with biotin and thus deprives the body of the benefit of the latter. **Internal injury.** Injury to internal organs or viscera. **Occupational injury.** An injury occurring solely as the result of a person's occupation, which may or may not be an industrial one. **Whiplash injury.** An injury to the cervical spine (and sometimes to the spinal cord) produced by a sudden acceleration or deceleration of the head, usually resulting from a road traffic accident. **Wringer injury.** A severe injury to the hand and arm due to their being drawn between the rollers of an automatic wringer. [L *injuria.*]

inlay (in·la). 1. Anything which is cut to shape and embedded to fit a space. 2. A restoration which is made and cemented to a tooth to replace tissue which has been lost owing to caries or injury. **Bone inlay.** A method of bone grafting whereby the graft is sunk into a gutter cut in the host bone. **Cast inlay.** An inlay, cast in molten metal which solidifies on cooling, made to the required size and shape. **Epithelial inlay.** A method of grafting using a split-skin graft usually wrapped round a mould of "Stent's composition", and buried in the tissues in order to fashion a skin-lined cavity, e.g. in recreating the gingivolabial sulcus, to allow of the wearing of a denture. **Gold inlay.** A cast inlay made of gold. **Gold-shell inlay.** A cast-gold inlay in the form of a hollow shell. **Porcelain inlay.** An inlay made of fused porcelain. [L *in,* MA *leien.*]

inlet (in·let). 1. [Aditus (NA).] A passage or opening by which a cavity can be entered, e.g. larynx. 2. In ventilation of a room, the space through which the air enters. **Pelvic inlet, inlet of the pelvis.** *See* PELVIS. **Thoracic inlet.** The upper bony margin of the thoracic cage. [L *in,* ME *leten.*]

Inman, Thomas (b. 1820). Bristol physician.

Inman's disease. Myalgia.

innate (in·**ate**). 1. Inborn; existing in an individual from birth; congenital. 2. Natural, like any particular quality. [L, *innatus.*]

innervation (in·er·**va**·shun). 1. Of a part or organ, the nerves supplying that part or organ. 2. The nervous stimulus or energy in any part the supply of which is necessary for the life and function of the part. 3. Discharge of nervous force. **Double innervation.** Having a double nerve supply, the nerve fibres supplying the part coming from two different nerves or nerve systems. **Reciprocal innervation.** The state of innervation of muscles attached to a joint by which the contraction of one muscle causes relaxation or loss of tension in its antagonist. [L *in,* nerve.]

innidation, innidiation (in·id·a·shun, in·id·e·**a**′·shun). Cell proliferation at any part of the body to which the cells concerned have been transported in a metastatic process. [L *in, nidus* nest.]

innocent (in·o·sent). Free from harmful effect; benign. Of a tumour, one which is not of a nature to threaten life and is not liable to recur. [L *innocens* harmless.]

innocuous (in·**ok**·ew·us). Causing neither injury nor ill effect; innocent. [L *innocuus* harmless.]

innominata (in·**om**·in·**a**′·tah). 1. The innominate artery. 2. The innominate bones. [L *innominatum* nameless.]

innominatal (in·**om**·in·**a**′·tal). Relating or belonging to the innominate artery or the innominate bone.

innominate (in·**om**·in·ate). Nameless or unnamed. **Innominate bone.** Hip bone. [L *innominatum* nameless.]

innominate artery [truncus brachiocephalicus (NA)]. The largest branch of the arch of the aorta, passing upward and to the right for 5 cm before dividing into its terminal branches (the right common carotid and right subclavian arteries).

innominate veins, right and left [venae brachiocephalicae (dextra et sinistra) NA]. Venous trunks formed by the union of the internal jugular and subclavian veins on each side.

innominatum (in·**om**·in·**a**′·tum). The hip bone; innominate bone. [L, nameless.]

innoxious (in·ox·e·us). Innocuous. [L *innoxius* harmless.]

innutrition (in·ew·**trish**·un). 1. A state in which there is absence or lack of nourishment. 2. Failure in the process of nourishment. [L *in,* nutrition.]

inoblast (**in**·o·blast). Any one of the mesenchymal cells from which connective tissue develops. [Gk *is* fibre, *blastos* germ.]

inoccipitia (**in**·ok·sip·**it**′·e·ah). Lack or defect of the occipital lobe of the cerebrum. [L *in,* occiput.]

inochondritis (in·o·kon·**dri**′·tis). 1. Inflammation of a fibrocartilage. 2. An inflamed condition of both tendons and cartilages. [Gk *is* fibre, *chondros* cartilage, *-itis* inflammation.]

inochondroma (**in**·o·kon·**dro**′·mah). A tumour of which the elements are fibrous and cartilaginous. [Gk *is* fibre, *chondros* cartilage, *-oma* tumour.]

inoculability (in·**ok**·ew·lab·**il**′·it·e). 1. Susceptibility to disease communicated by inoculation. 2. The quality of being inoculable.

inoculable (in·**ok**·ew·labl). 1. That can be passed on by inoculation. 2. Susceptible to inoculation. 3. Sensitive to any disease that can be transmitted by inoculation.

inoculate (in·**ok**·ew·late). To transfer or implant material containing micro-organisms or their products. In preventive medicine such material is introduced in order to stimulate the production of immunity, as in the prevention of smallpox or typhoid fever; with different materials different methods may be used, e.g. scarification of the skin, instillation into the nose, or injection by subcutaneous, intradermal, intravenous, intramuscular, intraperitoneal or other routes. In bacteriology, to transfer from one nutrient medium to another for the purposes of subculture. [L *inoculare* to graft.]

inoculation (in·ok·ew·**la**·shun). The act or process of inoculating. The introduction of micro-organisms or infective or toxic material into the tissues for the purpose of studying the specific reactions to a particular micro-organism, investigating the toxicity of bacterial products in the living animal, identifying an unknown infection, or for the production of antisera. It is also used as a method of producing active immunization by the introduction of attenuated living organisms or toxins. Inoculation may be performed by scarification of the skin, by subcutaneous injection, by intraperitoneal injection, by intravenous injection, or by injection into special regions. [L *inoculare* to graft.]

inoculator (in·**ok**·ew·la·tor). 1. A syringe or other instrument used in inoculation. 2. An individual who carries out inoculation.

inoculum (in·**ok**·ew·lum). The material introduced into the body by inoculation.

inocyst (in·o·sist). A capsule of fibrous material. [Gk *is* fibre, cyst.]

inocystoma (in·o·sis·**to**′·mah). A fibrous neoplasm in which cystic degeneration is present. [Gk *is* fibre, cystoma.]

inocyte (in·o·site). Fibroblast. [Gk *is* fibre, *kytos* cell.]

inogen (in·o·jen). A hypothetical substance in muscle tissue the decomposition of which causes muscular contraction. [see foll.]

inogenesis (in·o·**jen**·es·is). The process of formation of muscular or fibrous tissue. [Gk *is* fibre, *genein* to produce.]

inogenous (in·**oj**·en·us). 1. Forming or producing tissue. 2. Derived or produced from tissue. [see prec.]

inoglia (in·**o**·gli·ah). The supporting tissue of fibroblasts corresponding to the neuroglia of neuroblasts. [Gk *is* fibre, *glia* glue.]

inoglioma (in·o·gli·**o**′·mah). Fibroglioma. [Gk *is* fibre, *glia* glue, *-oma* tumour.]

inohymenitis (in·o·hi·men·**i**′·tis). Inflammation of any kind of fibrous membrane or tissue. [Gk *is* fibre, *hymen* membrane, *-itis* inflammation.]

inoleiomyoma (in·o·li·o·mi·**o**′·mah). A myoma which is composed of, or in which there are, fibres of unstriped muscular tissue. [Gk *is* fibre, *leios* smooth, *mys* muscle, *-oma* tumour.]

inolith (in·o·lith). A concretion of fibrous material or one formed in fibrous tissue. [Gk *is* fibre, *lithos* stone.]

inoma (in·o·mah). Fibroma. [Gk *is* fibre, *-oma* tumour.]

inomyoma (in·o·mi·**o**′·mah). Fibromyoma. [Gk *is* fibre, myoma.]

inomyositis (in·o·mi·o·**si**′·tis). Fibromyositis. [Gk *is* fibre, myositis.]

inomyxoma (in·o·mix·**o**′·mah). Fibromyxoma. [Gk *is* fibre, myxoma.]

inoneuroma (in·o·newr·**o**′·mah). Fibroneuroma. [Gk *is* fibre, neuroma.]

inopectic (in·o·**pek**·tik). Relating or belonging to inopexia.

inoperable (in·**op**·er·abl). 1. Applied to a tumour, one that is not suitable for radical treatment or on which operation is precluded by the risk involved. 2. Referring to a condition or state in which operative measures would not bring relief. [L *in*, operable.]

inopexia (in·o·**pex**·e·ah). A condition of the blood in which spontaneous coagulation may occur. [Gk *is* fibre, *pexis* a fixation.]

inophragma (in·o·**frag**·mah). The Z line in striated muscle. [Gk *is* fibre, *phragmos* enclosure.]

inorganic (in·or·**gan**·ik). 1. That branch of chemistry concerned with all substances other than organic ones. 2. Not natural or appropriate to the structure or normal development of an organism. 3. Referring to or composed of matter which is neither animal nor vegetable. 4. Without bodily organs. [L *in*, organic.]

inosaemia (in·o·se·me·ah). 1. An excess of fibrin in the blood. [Gk *is* fibre, *haima* blood.] 2. A condition in which inositol (muscle sugar) is present in the blood. [inositol, Gk *haima* blood.]

inosclerosis (in·o·skler·**o**′·sis). 1. A condition in which there is increase in density of fibrous tissue. 2. Sclerosis due to indurated fibrous tissue. [Gk *is* fibre, sclerosis.]

inoscopy (in·**os**·ko·pe). The peptic digestion of a fluid, e.g. blood, with the object of removing cells and fibrin preliminary to centrifuging-out suspended bacteria. [Gk *is* fibre, *skopein* to view.]

inosculate (in·**os**·kew·late). 1. To unite two tubular vessels by placing their cut ends in apposition. 2. To make an anastomosis between, for example, two organs. [L *in*, *osculum* little mouth.]

inosculation (in·**os**·kew·**la**′·shun). In reference to arteries and veins, a condition in which there is anastomosis or direct union. [see prec.]

inose (**in**·oze). Inositol.

inosinate (in·**o**·sin·ate). Any salt or ester of inosinic acid.

inosine (**in**·o·seen). The nucleoside, 7-hypoxanthine-D-riboside, produced by the elimination of phosphoric acid from inosinic acid.

inosite (in·o·site). Inositol.

inositis (in·o·**si**·tis). An inflamed condition of fibrous tissue. [Gk *is* fibre, *-itis* inflammation.]

inositol (in·o·sit·ol). Muscle sugar, $(CHOH)_6$. A compound with a slight sweetness, found in many body tissues particularly muscle, and, in the form of a phytate, in the phytin of certain cereal grains. It is a member of the bios complex, deficiency of it in rats leading to retarded growth and dermatitis. It has also been shown to prevent fatty livers in rats fed experimental diets. It appears to have a rôle in nutrition associated with the vitamins. Therapeutically, it is being used in the treatment of cirrhosis of the liver, toxic hepatitis, and functional liver impairment; it is generally given in conjunction with choline and methionine, and in various skin diseases; also, in conjunction with tocopherol, in the treatment of progressive muscular dystrophy. **Inositol hexaphosphate.** Phytic acid. *See* ACID. **Inositol Nicotinate.** BP Commission approved name for *meso*-inositol hexanicotinate; a peripheral vasodilator. [Gk *is* fibre.]

inositoluria, inosituria (in·o·sit·ol·**ewr**′·e·ah, in·o·sit·**ewr**′·e·ah). The presence of inositol in the urine; it occurs occasionally in albuminuria, diabetes mellitus and insipidus, and has been stated to be caused by copious water drinking.

inosteatoma (in·o·ste·at·**o**′·mah). A steatoma which contains fibres or fibrous elements. [Gk *is* fibre, *stear* fat, *-oma* tumour.]

inostosis (in·os·**to**·sis). After bony tissue has been destroyed, the production of similar tissue in the affected area. [L *in*, Gk *osteon* bone.]

inotropic (in·o·**trop**·ik). Of nerve fibres, influencing the contractility of muscles and muscular tissue, particularly of the heart. **Negatively inotropic.** Weakening muscular action and contraction. **Positively inotropic.** Strengthening muscular action and contraction. [Gk *is* fibre, *trope* a turning.]

inotropism (in·**ot**·rop·izm). Modification of or interference with muscular action and contraction. [see prec.]

inplantation (in·plan·**ta**′·shun). The process of insertion of a natural tooth into the socket from which another tooth has been removed. [L *in*, *plantare* to set.]

Inproquone (**in**·pro·kwone). BP Commission approved name for 2,5-di-(aziridin-1-yl)-3,6-dipropoxy-1,4-benzoquinone; an antineoplastic agent.

inquest (**in**·kwest). In forensic medicine, an inquiry held by a coroner or other official with or without a jury into the cause, manner, and circumstances of an unexpected, sudden, or violent death. [L *in*, *quaerere* to seek.]

inquiline (**in**·kwil·ine). A parasite which lives in the nest of some other animal, and feeds on the latter's food; e.g. a cuckoo. [L *inquilinus* inhabitant.]

inructation (in·ruk·**ta**·shun). The unnatural swallowing of air in a noisy and gulping manner. [L *in*, *ructare* to belch.]

insaccation (in·sak·a·shun). 1. The state of being enclosed in a sac. 2. Encystment. [L *in*, *saccus* bag.]

insalivation (in·sal·iv·**a**′·shun). The process by which food becomes well mixed with saliva in mastication. [L *in*, saliva.]

insalubrious (in·sal·ew·bre·us). 1. Unhealthy, as a climate. 2. Unwholesome or insanitary, as air or environment. [L *in*, salubrious.]

insalubrity (in·sal·**ew**·brit·e). 1. Of climate, unhealthiness. 2. Of environment, an insanitary state. [see prec.]

insane (in·**sane**). 1. Unsound, diseased or deranged of mind. 2. Legally, not only mentally disordered but also in need of care and control to protect either the patient himself or the public. [L *in*, *sanus* sound.]

insanitary (in·**san**·it·ar·e). Not conducive to the preservation of, or injurious to, health. [L *in*, sanitary.]

insanitation (in·san·it·a′·shun). A condition in which sanitation is deficient or defective. [see prec.]

insanity (in·san·it·e). 1. Mental disease of a grave kind; one of the psychoses, as distinct from a neurotic state. Now termed psychotic disorder, a persistent disorder or disability of mind, whether or not including subnormality of intelligence, which results in abnormally aggressive or seriously irresponsible conduct on the part of the patient, and requires medical treatment. 2. The state of being legally certifiable as insane. **Adolescent insanity.** An obsolescent term signifying any grave mental disorder affecting the adolescent; in its old use as a clinical category it corresponded, as a rule, to the schizophrenic psychoses of the young, but was very loosely applied. **Affective insanity.** One of the affective psychoses, such as manic-depressive insanity, or involutional depression. **Alternating insanity.** Circular insanity (see following). **Circular insanity.** A form of mental disorder in which attacks of manic excitement and depression follow one another; one of the clinical forms of manic-depressive insanity. **Climacteric insanity.** An obsolescent term, signifying mental disorder occurring at the time of the climacteric without other known cause. **Communicated insanity.** Folie à deux. **Confusional insanity.** A mental disorder accompanied by clouding of consciousness, disorientation and affections of memory and intellectual processes, and nearly always traceable to an identifying organic cause, such as infection, poisoning, cardiac decompensation, or epilepsy. **Cyclic insanity.** Circular insanity (see above). **Delusional insanity.** An obsolescent term, used as a clinical category to comprehend all forms of mental disorder, however caused, in which delusions are prominent. **Depressive insanity.** A mental disorder in which depression of the spirits, or melancholy, is the most prominent symptom; melancholia. **Hereditary insanity.** An obsolete term for a mental disorder, of whatever type, which is known to have been shared by another member of the same family. **Homicidal insanity.** A non-medical term for a mental disorder with marked and dangerous aggressive tendencies. **Hysterical insanity.** A self-contradictory term for states of excitement or confusion of a psychogenic, reactive, and recoverable kind. **Intermittent insanity.** Periodic insanity (see below). **Manic-depressive insanity.** A syndrome described by Kraepelin, characterized by recurrent attacks of illness of a manic or depressive kind, with a very strong tendency towards spontaneous recovery; individual patients may be liable to only one form of the illness, manic or depressive, or at different times to both. **Melancholic insanity.** Melancholia. **Moral insanity.** A term first used by Pritchard to describe the condition of an individual, usually of dull or defective intelligence, who appears to have no appreciation of right and wrong and so may be guilty of crimes, even of an inhuman kind, and be recalcitrant to punishment or reform. **Periodic insanity.** A form of mental disorder, not otherwise characterized, in which there are recurrent remissions and relapses; as a rule a disorder falling within the manic-depressive syndrome. **Polyneuritic insanity.** Mental disorder accompanying polyneuritis, i.e., as a rule, Korsakoff's syndrome. **Primary insanity.** Primary dementia. *See* DEMENTIA. **Puerperal insanity.** A term, obsolescent if used as a clinical category, which includes all forms of mental disorder occurring in about the first 3 months after the birth of a child. **Recurrent insanity.** Periodic insanity (see above). **Senile insanity.** One of the mental disorders, aetiologically many and various, which may affect the aged, inclusive of senile dementia and recoverable senile depressive states. **Stuporous insanity.** Insanity accompanied by stupor, i.e., as a rule, a catatonic form of schizophrenia. **Toxic insanity.** A mental disorder attributable to some form of poisoning, as a rule taking the form of a confusional state. The poisons most commonly involved are the exotoxins of micro-organisms, the products of disordered metabolism, drugs such as alkaloids and barbiturates, alcohol, carbon monoxide, lead, and mercury. **Volitional insanity.** The impairment of will-power observed in certain psychoses. [L *in, sanus* sound.]

inscription (in·skrip·shun). The main part of a prescription, giving the names of the drugs and other ingredients and the quantities of each to use. [L *inscribere* to write on.]

insect (in·sekt). Any member of the arthropodan class Insecta.

Insecta (in·sek·tah). A class of the Arthropoda characterized by the division of the adult body into a head, a thorax which bears six legs and, usually, two pairs of wings, and an abdomen. Members of the following orders contain species of medical interest: Anoplura (lice), Coleoptera (beetles), Diptera (flies), Hemiptera (bugs), Hymenoptera (ants, bees, and wasps), Orthoptera (locusts, cockroaches), Siphonaptera (fleas), and Thysanura (silver fish). [L *in, secare* to cut.]

insectary (in·sek·tar·e). A place where mosquitoes and other insects are kept in captivity.

insecticide (in·sek·tis·ide). Any agent which kills or destroys insects. [insect, L *caedere* to kill.]

insectiform (in·sek·te·form). In zoology, having resemblance to an insect. [insect, form.]

insectifuge (in·sek·te·fewj). Insect repellent. [insect, L *fugare* to put to flight.]

insectivore (in·sek·tiv·or). A feeder on insects. [insect, L *vorare* to swallow.]

insemination (in·sem·in·a′·shun). 1. Fertilization of an ovum by the penetration of a spermatozoon. 2. The deposition of semen in the vagina during coitus or by artificial means. 3. Impregnation. **Artificial insemination.** The introduction of viable spermatozoa into the canal of the cervix other than through the act of coitus with the object of producing pregnancy. **Donor insemination, heterologous insemination.** Insemination of semen from a person other than the subject's husband. **Homologous insemination.** Insemination of semen from the subject's husband. [L *in, seminare* to impregnate.]

insenescence (in·sen·es·ens). 1. The process of becoming old; the drawing near of old age. 2. A state in which the approach of old age is not accompanied by the usual signs of infirmity but on the contrary normal vigour still persists. [L *in, senescere* to become old, to lose strength.]

insensibility (in·sen·sib·il′·it·e). 1. Loss of consciousness from whatever cause; a state of anaesthesia. 2. The condition of being without or being temporarily deprived of normal sense perceptions, or in which the senses are blunted. 3. Stupidity or apathy. [L *in, sentire* to feel.]

insensible (in·sen·sibl). 1. Deprived of consciousness. 2. Unendowed with or deprived of sense perception, or with this blunted. 3. Lacking in sense or intelligence. 4. Apathetic. [see prec.]

insertion (in·ser·shun). 1. The process or act of setting or thrusting in. 2. Something thrust or placed within. 3. The point on a bone at which the distal end of a muscle is attached. 4. The point at or the manner in which an organ is attached to its support. 5. In cytogenetics, a chromosomal structural change resulting in the intercalation of a segment of a chromosome into another member of the complement. **Parasol insertion.** A type of attachment of the umbilical cord in the placenta, in which there is separation of the cord vessels, resembling the ribs of a parasol, before they pass to different places of insertion in the placenta. **Velamentous insertion.** The attachment of the umbilical cord to the placenta by insertion into the membranes. [L *inserere* to connect in.]

insidious (in·sid·e·us). Applied to a disease with few signs or symptoms of its presence, and which furtively increases in severity. [L *insidiosus* cunning.]

insight (in·site). Discernment; mental vision. In psychiatry, the patient's appreciation of the extent and nature of his mental illness. [L *in*, AS *gesihth.*]

insipid (in·sip·id). 1. Without taste; stale. 2. Lacking animation and spirits. [L *insipidus* tasteless.]

insolation (in·sol·a·shun). 1. Sunbathing regarded as a therapeutic measure. 2. Sunstroke or heat stroke. **Asphyxial insolation.** Heat stroke with associated fall of temperature, weak pulse, and chilly skin. **Hyperpyrexial insolation.** Heat stroke with associated hyperpyrexia, capillary congestion, and coma. [L *insolare* to expose to the sun.]

insolubility (in·sol·ew·bil′·it·e). 1. The state of being unable to be dissolved in a liquid. 2. The quality of being insoluble. [see foll.]

insoluble (in·sol·ewbl). Applied to any substance that cannot be dissolved in a liquid. [L *in*, soluble.]

insomnia (in·som·ne·ah). The condition of being unable to sleep. [L *in, somnus* sleep.]

insomniac (in·som·ne·ak). An individual who suffers from insomnia.

inspection (in·spek·shun). Close and careful scrutiny or examination by looking. [L *inspectare* to look at.]

inspectionism (in·spek·shun·izm). A form of sexual behaviour in which pleasure is experienced by looking at the sexual organs or at any object connected with sex. [see prec.]

inspergation, inspersion (in·sper·ga·shun, in·sper·shun). The process or act of dusting over a surface with fine powder. [L *inspergere* to besprinkle.]

inspiration (in·spir·a·shun). The act of breathing air into the lungs; inhalation. [L *inspirare* to breathe in.]

inspirator (in·spir·a·tor). 1. A type of respirator. 2. An inhaler. [see prec.]

inspiratory (in·spi·rah·tor·e). 1. Relating or belonging to or aiding the act of inspiration. 2. Characterized by inspiration. 3. Used for inspiration.

inspirometer (in·spi·rom·et·er). An instrument with which the volume, force, and frequency of inspirations can be measured. [inspiration, meter.]

inspissant (in·spis·ant). 1. Having the effect of thickening or diminishing the fluidity of any of the body fluids. 2. Any agent that causes the blood or any other body fluid to become thicker. [L *inspissare* to thicken.]

inspissate (in·spis·ate). To cause to condense or to increase in consistence by means of absorption or evaporation of fluid; hence inspissated. [see prec.]

inspissation (in·spis·a·shun). 1. The process or act of causing a liquid to become thick by subjecting it to a process of evaporation. 2. The condition of being condensed by evaporation. **Uratic inspissation.** A uric-acid infarct. [L *inspissare* to thicken.]

inspissator (in·spis·a·tor). An apparatus by means of which the thickness of the blood or other body fluids can be increased by evaporation. [see prec.]

instar (in·star). Of arthropods, a larval stage of which there may be several. [L, image.]

instauration (in·staw·ra·shun). 1. The institution or first beginnings of a physiological condition or of a new function. 2. The process of becoming restored after decay. 3. Repair. [L *instauratio* renewal.]

instep (in·step). The highest part of the foot (the dorsum) which corresponds to the medial longitudinal arch. [L *in*, AS *staepe*.]

instillation (in·stil·a·shun). The act of introducing a liquid into a cavity, or on to a surface, drop by drop. [L *instillare* to pour in by drops.]

instillator (in·stil·a·tor). A dropper or other apparatus for pouring a liquid in by drops. [see prec.]

instinct (in·stingkt). An inherent tendency of the organism to react in a precise though complex way to a particular constellation of environmental circumstances, this mode of reaction serving the adaptation of the organism to the circumstances and having a purpose when seen against the background of the individual or of the race. Instinctive behaviour in animals, notably birds, may be defined down to the last detail and be subject to very little variation; in man, though instincts may be the mainspring of behaviour, the behaviour itself is much more plastic and variable. Most psychologists accept instincts of self-preservation and of racial perpetuation, the former being the source of such reactions as flight from danger, the latter the source of sexual and parental instincts. McDougall built a system of psychology on the basis of the instincts, defining fourteen different ones. The freudian theory is based on two, the sex instinct and the death instinct. **Ego instinct.** Any instinct unconnected with sex. **Herd instinct.** The tendency to gregariousness; the need experienced by man and other social animals for the companionship of his fellows, and (secondary) the tendency to conform to the standards, behaviour, or attitude of mind of one's fellows. [L *instinctus* impulse.]

instinctive (in·stingk·tiv). 1. Belonging or relating to or of the character of an instinct. 2. Determined by natural impulsion or propensity. 3. Prompted by or derived from instinct.

instrument (in·stroo·ment). 1. Any mechanical device, appliance, or apparatus for performing work or achieving an effect; a tool. 2. An agent or means. [L *instrumentum* tool.]

See also: FELEKI.

instrumental (in·stroo·men·tal). 1. Relating to an instrument. 2. Performed by means of any mechanical appliance, as certain types of work. 3. Conducive to a result or serviceable for a purpose.

instrumentation (in·stroo·men·ta′·shun). 1. The use of instruments in any operative or other procedure. 2. A task carried out by means of instruments. 3. Agency or means.

insuccation (in·suk·a·shun). The soaking of a crude drug. The expressed juice may then be used in making standardized pharmaceutical preparations. [L *succus* juice.]

insufficiency (in·suf·ish·en·se). The state of being inadequate to perform normal functions. *See also* INCOMPETENCE. **Adrenal insufficiency.** Addison's disease. **Aortic insufficiency.** Aortic incompetence. *See* INCOMPETENCE. **Basilar insufficiency.** Temporary failure of midbrain functioning from temporary vascular depletion. **Capsular insufficiency.** Failure of function of the cortex of the suprarenal gland. **Cardiac insufficiency.** Failure of the heart to meet the physiological demands made upon it. This may be due to disturbed function or disease of the myocardium, endocardium, pericardium, or the conducting tissue. **Insufficiency of the cardiac valves.** Incompetence of the cardiac valves. **Coronary insufficiency.** An insufficient blood supply through the coronary arteries, such as occurs in angina pectoris. **Insufficiency of the externi.** Weakness of the external rectus muscles of the orbit, causing esophoria or esotropia particularly in distant vision. **Insufficiency of the eyelids.** A condition in which the eyes remain open, except when closed by a conscious effort. **Gastric insufficiency, gastromotor insufficiency.** Atony of the gastric musculature. **Hepatic insufficiency.** Failure or partial failure of liver function. **Insufficiency of the interni.** Weakness of the internal rectus muscles of the orbit, causing exophoria or exotropia, particularly in near vision. **Insufficiency of mesenteric arteries.** Atheromatous changes of mesenteric arteries leading to ischaemia with enteritis or colitis, or sudden occlusion with symptoms of acute intestinal obstruction. **Mitral insufficiency.** Mitral incompetence. *See* INCOMPETENCE. **Muscular insufficiency.** Muscular weakness. **Myocardial insufficiency.** Failure of the myocardium to meet the physiological demands made upon it. It may be secondary to the effects of valvular lesion, or to systemic or pulmonary hypertension; it may also result directly from disease of the muscle' (ischaemia, myocarditis, or cardiomyopathy). **Ocular insufficiency.** A generic term describing weakness of any or all of the extra-ocular muscles. **Ovarian insufficiency.** A condition which may be primary, with failure of the normal development at puberty, or secondary, with absence or scantiness of menstruation. **Parathyroid insufficiency.** Failure of parathyroid secretion. **Pituitary insufficiency.** Total or partial absence of one or all of the pituitary hormones. **Proteopexic insufficiency.** A severe neutrophilic leucopenia (neutropenia) that may be temporary in duration, produced as a result of protein shock following the introduction of toxic or sensitizing protein substances into the blood stream. It may occur after transfusion of blood, plasma, serum, protein solutions, and preparations of many types which produce anaphylactic shock, or sometimes after high-protein meals in patients suffering from severe liver disease. **Pseudo-aortic insufficiency.** An obsolete term used to describe aortic insufficiency due to supposedly arteriosclerotic changes in the valve. **Pulmonary valvular insufficiency.**

Pulmonary incompetence. *See* INCOMPETENCE. **Pyloric insufficiency.** Dysfunction of the pylorus, allowing too rapid escape of gastric contents. **Renal insufficiency.** Failure of kidney function; the term usually implies partial failure of excretion. **Thyroid insufficiency.** Hypothyroidism. **Tricuspid insufficiency.** Tricuspid incompetence. *See* INCOMPETENCE. **Uterine insufficiency.** Ineffectual or weak contractions of the uterine muscle during labour. **Valvular insufficiency.** Incompetence of the cardiac valves. **Vertebrobasilar insufficiency.** Relative failure of blood flow through the vertebral and basilar arteries causing symptoms of brain-stem and occipital-lobe dysfunction. [L *in, sufficere* to suffice.]

insufficientia vertebrae (in·suf·ish·e·en′·she·ah ver·te·bre). Pain in the back as the result of trauma insufficient to damage the spine. [L, insufficiency of the spine.]

insufflation (in·suf·la·shun). The act of blowing air, gas, or powder into a body cavity. **Cranial insufflation.** The forcing of air into the ventricles or the subdural space. **Intratracheal insufflation.** The procedure of forcing air into the lungs by way of a tracheotomy or intratracheal tube. **Insufflation of the lungs.** Artificial respiration carried out by actively forcing air into the lungs. **Mouth-to-mouth insufflation.** Artificial respiration carried out by blowing directly into the mouth of the subject. **Perirenal insufflation.** The injection of air around the kidneys; used in investigation of suspected adrenal tumours. **Tubal insufflation, uterotubal insufflation.** The passage of a gas, usually carbon dioxide, through a cervical cannula, to determine the patency of the uterine tubes. [L *insufflare* to blow into.]

insufflator (in·suf·la·tor). An apparatus used for insufflation.

insula [NA] (in·sew·lah). An island: applied to an area of cortex surrounded by the circular sulcus and lying in the depth of the lateral sulcus. [L.]

See also: HALLER'S ANNULUS (under HALLER).

insular (in·sew·lar). 1. Relating or belonging to the insula. 2. Relating or belonging to the islands of Langerhans. 3. Characterized by the presence of isolated spots or patches. 4. Applied to any eruption that is arranged in isolated groups of spots or in patches. [see foll.]

insulate (in·sew·late). 1. To separate anything from contact with its neighbours by completely enclosing it. 2. To protect a conductor of heat or electricity with a suitable non-conducting material, thereby preventing loss of energy. [L *insula* island.]

insulation (in·sew·la·shun). 1. The state of being insulated. 2. The act or process of insulating. 3. Any non-conducting material or substance which prevents the escape or transference of heat or electricity. [see prec.]

insulin (in·sew·lin). A pancreatic hormone which controls glucose, fat, and amino-acid metabolism. Injection of the hormone leads to hypoglycaemia, and increases the amounts of stored carbohydrate, fat and protein. It is secreted by the β-cells of the islets of Langerhans; this secretion is controlled by a number of factors including the blood glucose concentration. It is a protein of molecular weight 5 700; the two polypeptide chains, A and B, are linked by disulphide bridges. It is synthesized primarily as a precursor, *proinsulin*, which consists of a single polypeptide chain. Proteolytic removal of the "C" chain fragment releases insulin. The sequence of insulin has been determined and the hormone has been synthesized. Absence of insulin leads to diabetes. It is frequently administered to diabetics, but does not cure the disease. **Amorphous insulin.** Uncrystallized pure insulin. **Crystalline insulin.** The crystalline product formed when insulin is precipitated in the presence of zinc. **Depot insulin.** A loose term for any form of insulin which is slowly absorbed from the site of injection. **Globin zinc insulin.** Insulin modified by the addition of globin (from the haemoglobin of beef blood) and zinc chloride. **Hexamine insulin.** A combination of hexamethylenetetramine and insulin; no longer in use. **Histone insulin.** A combination of histone from the thymus with insulin; no longer in use. **Histone zinc insulin.** Histone insulin (see preceding) with zinc added. **Isophane Insulin.** BP Commission approved name for NPH insulin. **NPH insulin.** A crystalline insulin used in buffered aqueous suspension and containing 0.03 mg zinc and 0.4 mg protamine per 100 units. **Pectin insulin.** A preparation of insulin with pectin; no longer in use. **Protamine insulin.** A preparation of insulin with protamine, but without zinc; no longer in use. **Insulin tolerance test.** *See* TEST. **Vegetable insulin.** Any substance prepared from plant sources, especially yeast, which lowers the blood sugar of experimental animals. **Zinc protamine insulin.** A combination of insulin with protamine and zinc; one of the most valuable preparations of insulin, with prolonged action of gradual onset. **Insulin Zinc Suspension BP 1973.** *See* SUSPENSION. [L *insula* island; island of Langerhans.]

insulinaemia (in·sew·lin·e′·me ah). Excess of insulin in the blood. [insulin, Gk *haima* blood.]

insulinase (in·sew·lin·aze). An enzyme that inactivates insulin.

insulinization (in·sew·lin·i·za′·shun). The therapeutic use of insulin; insulin therapy.

insulinlipodystrophy (in·sew·lin·lip·o·dis′·tro·fe). The loss of fat occurring in certain regions in patients with diabetes mellitus, resulting from treatment with insulin. [insulin, Gk *lipos* fat, dystrophy.]

insulinogenesis (in·sew·lin·o·jen′·es·is). The formation of insulin. [see foll.]

insulinogenic (in·sew·lin·o·jen′·ik). Resulting from therapeutic administration of insulin. [insulin, Gk *genein* to produce.]

insulinoid (in·sew·lin·oid). Of a substance, having properties resembling those of insulin; like insulin. [insulin, Gk *eidos* form.]

insulinoma (in·sew·lin·o′·mah). A neoplasm composed of tissue from the islands of Langerhans. [insulin, Gk *-oma* tumour.]

insulitis (in·sew·li·tis). A rare condition involving an inflammation of the islands of Langerhans. [L *insula* island, Gk *-itis* inflammation.]

insulogenic (in·sew·lo·jen′·ik). Originating in disorder of the endocrine function of the pancreas. [insulin, Gk *genein* to produce.]

insulopathic (in·sew·lo·path′·ik). Pertaining to or caused by any abnormality of insulin secretion. [insulin, Gk *pathos* disease.]

insusceptibility (in·sus·sep·tib·il′·it·e). Immunity; lack of susceptibility to infection or disease. [L *in*, susceptible.]

integration (in·teg·ra·shun). 1. The unification of a whole by the functional amalgamation of its parts. There are two fundamentally distinct modes of integration; nervous, through the agency of the central and autonomic nervous systems, and humoral, by the agency of hormones released into the blood stream and exerting effects on distant organs. 2. In psychiatry, the organization of components into a complex whole. 3. In mathematics, a process (calculus) for the summation of a series of infinitesimal parts; it is of value in calculating the area beneath a curve, and is denoted by the symbol $\int$. **Primary integration.** The process by which a person recognizes himself as a unit distinct from the environment. **Secondary integration.** The organization of pregenital components into a psychosexual unit. [L *integrare* to make whole.]

integrity (in·teg·rit·e). 1. The quality or state of being complete, sound, or entire. 2. Wholeness. 3. Virginity. [L *integritas* unimpaired condition.]

integument (in·teg·ew·ment). A covering, coating, or capsule of a part. **Common integument [integumentum commune (NA)].** The skin, regarded as the entire covering of the body. **Fetal integument.** The fetal membranes. [L *integumentum* a covering.]

integumentary (in·teg·ew·men′·tar·e). 1. Belonging to or composed of skin. 2. Relating to or used as a covering, e.g. the skin. [see prec.]

intellect (in·tel·ekt). 1. The cognitive faculty of the mind as it operates at higher abstract and conceptual levels. 2. The faculty of the mind by which one knows and reasons. [L *intellectus* discernment.]

intellection (in·tel·ek·shun). 1. Cognition; exercise of the intellect. 2. A specified intellectual act. 3. The intellect.

intelligence (in·tel·ij·ens). 1. The faculty of understanding and comprehension; the capacity of comprehending. 2. The quality originating in the ability to perceive objectively, and sagaciously to work towards an envisaged end. 3. Sagacity; mental acuteness. **Intelligence quotient.** *See* QUOTIENT. **Intelligence test.** *See* TEST. [L *intelligentia* perception.]

intemperance (in·**tem**·per·ans). Lack of moderation in or excessive indulgence of any appetite: immoderation in eating and drinking, especially over-indulgence in the taking of alcohol in any form. [L *in, temperare* to moderate.]

intensification (in·**ten**·sif·ik·**a**'·shun). 1. An increase in intensity of any kind. 2. The process of becoming increased in strength. 3. The act or process of concentration of force. **Image intensification.** The process of increasing the intensity or brightness of a visual image, often a fluoroscopic x-ray picture, by electronic means. [L *intensus* stretched tight, *facere* to make.]

intensifier (in·**ten**·se·fi·er). An instrument used to bring about intensification. **Image intensifier.** An instrument used to achieve image intensification. [L *intensus* stretched tight, *facere* to make.]

intensimeter (in·ten·**sim**·et·er). An electrical apparatus incorporating a selenium cell, used for the comparison and measurement of x-ray intensities. [intensity, meter.]

intensity (in·**ten**·sit·e). 1. The quality or state of being intense, i.e. in an extreme state of activity, tension, or energy. 2. Magnitude of a phenomenon such as light. 3. In electricity, the density or strength of an electric field. 4. In psychology, the degree of effectiveness of a sensation. **Electric intensity.** The force in magnitude and direction exerted upon a unit positive charge placed at a point in an electric field. **Intensity of illumination.** The amount of light falling on unit area of a surface in one second. **Magnetic intensity.** The force in magnitude and direction exerted on a unit magnetic pole placed at a point in a magnetic field. **Intensity of radiation.** The total amount of radiation passing in one second through a unit area placed at right angles to the central axis of the beam. **X-ray intensity.** The amount of energy passing in one second through a unit area placed at right angles to the direction of the rays. [L *intensus* stretched tight.]

See also: UNITS.

intensive (in·**ten**·siv). 1. Characterized by gradually increased strength, as of a substance introduced into the system in successive inoculations. 2. Marked by increase of force or strength. **Intensive care.** Term used to describe the treatment of severe medical and surgical disorders. [see prec.]

intention (in·**ten**·shun). 1. A manner or process of healing of wounds and other injuries. *See* HEAL. 2. A process or operation, natural or otherwise. 3. The aim or purpose in view. [L *intendere* to direct towards.]

inter-. Prefix, from the Latin preposition *inter*, meaning *between, among, mutual.*

interaccessory (in·ter·ak·**ses**'·or·e). Denoting certain muscles which connect the accessory processes of the vertebrae. [L *inter, accedere* to go to.]

interacinar, interacinous (in·ter·as·in·ar, in·ter·**as**·in·us). In a position between acini. [L *inter*, acinus.]

interagglutination (in·ter·ag·**loo**·tin·**a**'·shun). The process by which one kind of cell is agglutinated by the agglutinins of another closely-related kind of cell. [L *inter*, agglutination.]

interalveolar (in·ter·al·**ve**'·o·lar). Situated between alveoli. [L *inter*, alveolus.]

interangular (in·ter·**ang**·gew·lar). 1. Occurring between angles. 2. Lying in a position between angles. [L *inter*, angle.]

interannular (in·ter·**an**·ew·lar). Placed between two ring-like structures, e.g. the tracheal rings. [L *inter, annulus* ring.]

interarticular (in·ter·ar·**tik**'·ew·lar). Situated between the articular surfaces of a joint or between two joints. [L *inter, articulus* joint.]

interarytenoid (in·ter·ar·**it**'·en·oid). Situated between the arytenoid cartilages of the larynx. [L *inter*, arytenoid.]

interarytenoideus muscle (in·ter·ar·it·en·**oid**'·e·us musl). A conjoint name for the arytenoid muscles. [see prec.]

interatrial (in·ter·**at**·re·al). In a position between the atria of the heart. [L *inter*, atrium.]

interauricular (in·ter·aw·**rik**'·ew·lar). Interatrial. [L *inter*, auricle.]

interbrain (**in**·ter·brane). The thalamencephalon. [L *inter*, brain.]

intercadence (in·ter·**ka**·dens). 1. The occurrence of a supernumerary beat between the normal beats of the heart; extreme dicrotism. 2. A supernumerary beat of the heart. [L *inter, cadere* to fall.]

intercadent (in·ter·**ka**·dent). Marked by an irregular rhythm; having a supernumerary beat. [see prec.]

intercalary, intercalated (in·ter·**kal**·ar·e, **in**·ter·kal·**a**'·ted). Interposed; inserted among others at regular intervals, as an upstroke occurring between two normal heart beats in a cardiogram. [L *intercalare* to insert.]

intercalation (in·ter·kal·**a**'·shun). A type of neurosis in which some sound or word is uttered between any two other words and phrases. [see prec.]

intercalatum (in·ter·kal·**a**'·tum). The substantia nigra of the brain. [L, inserted.]

intercanalicular (in·ter·kan·al·**ik**'·ew·lar). Situated between canaliculi, or occurring between canaliculi. [L *inter*, caniliculus.]

intercapillary (in·ter·kap·**il**'·ar·e). Situated between capillaries or among them. [L *inter*, capillary.]

intercapitular veins [venae intercapitales (NA)] (in·ter·**kap**'·it·ew·lar va·nz). The connections between the palmar digital veins and the dorsal venous arch. They pass dorsally between the heads of the metacarpal bones. [L *inter, caput* head, vein.]

intercarotid (in·ter·kar·**ot**'·id). In a position between the external and internal carotid arteries, like the carotid body. [L *inter*, carotid.]

intercarpal (in·ter·**kar**·pal). Situated between the carpal bones. [L *inter*, carpal.]

intercartilaginous (in·ter·kar·til·**aj**'·in·us). Connecting cartilages or lying between them. [L *inter*, cartilage.]

intercavernous (in·ter·kav·**ern**'·us). 1. Denoting either one of the two sinuses through which the cavernous sinuses of the dura mater communicate with each other. 2. Situated between two antra or cavities. [L *inter, caverna* cave.]

intercellular (in·ter·**sel**·ew·lar). Placed between the cells of a structure, or among them. [L *inter*, cell.]

intercentral (in·ter·**sen**·tral). Connecting nerve centres or placed between them. [L *inter*, centre.]

intercerebral (in·ter·**ser**·e·bral). Situated between the right and left cerebral hemispheres of the brain. [L *inter*, cerebrum.]

interchange (**in**·ter·cha·nj). 1. Mutual exchange. 2. Chromosomal structural change resulting in the exchange of a segment between two chromosomes and, therefore, also called *reciprocal translocation.* **Chromatid interchange.** Interchange where the translocation involves chromatids rather than chromosomes. **Interchange trisomic.** *See* TRISOMIC. [L *inter, cambire* to change.]

See also: HAMBURGER (H. J.).

interchondral (in·ter·**kon**·dral). 1. Intercartilaginous. 2. Of ligaments, those that connect the costal cartilages of the lower ribs. [L *inter, chondros* cartilage.]

interchromomere (in·ter·**kro**·mo·meer). The regions intercalated between adjacent chromomeres. [L *inter*, Gk *chroma* colour, *meros* part.]

intercidence (in·ter·sid·ens). Intercadence.

intercident (in·**ter**·sid·ent). 1. Intercadent. 2. Intercalary.

intercilium (in·ter·**sil**·e·um). 1. The glabella. 2. That part of the forehead lying over the glabella between the eyebrows. [L *inter, cilium* eyelid.]

interclavicular (in·ter·klav·**ik**'·ew·lar). Between the clavicles. [L *inter*, clavicle.]

interclinoid (in·ter·**kli**·noid). Between the posterior and the anterior clinoid processes of the sphenoid bone. [L *inter*, clinoid.]

intercoccygeal, intercoccygean (in·ter·kok·**sij**'·e·al, in·ter·kok·**sij**'·e·an). Between segments of the coccyx. [L *inter*, coccyx.]

intercolumnar (in·ter·kol·**um**'·nar). Between any two pillars or columns. [L *inter*, column.]

intercondylar, intercondyloid (in·ter·kon·**di**'·lar, in·ter·kon·**di**'·loid). Situated between two condyles. **Intercondylar area.** *See*

TIBIA. **Intercondylar line.** *See* LINE. **Intercondylar notch.** *See* NOTCH. **Intercondylar tubercle.** *See* TUBERCLE. [L *inter*, condyle.]

intercornual (in·ter·**kor**·new·al). Between cornua. **Intercornual ligament.** *See* LIGAMENT. [L *inter*, cornu.]

intercoronoideal (in·ter·kor·on·**oid**'·e·al). Referring to the space between the two coronoid processes of the mandible. [L *inter*, coronoid.]

intercostal (in·ter·**kos**·tal). Between the ribs. **Intercostal lymph gland.** *See* GLAND. **Intercostal membrane.** *See* MEMBRANE. **Intercostal space.** *See* SPACE. [L *inter*, *costa* rib.]

intercostal arteries. Anterior intercostal arteries [rami intercostales anteriores (NA)]. Two small arteries running laterally in each of the upper nine intercostal spaces. Six spaces are supplied from the internal mammary artery; the other three from the musculophrenic artery. **Posterior intercostal arteries (I and II) [arteriae intercostales posteriores (I et II) NA].** *See* SUPERIOR INTERCOSTAL ARTERY (below). **Posterior intercostal arteries (III–XI) [arteriae intercostales posteriores (III–XI) NA].** Nine pairs of arteries supplying the lower nine intercostal spaces. Their branches correspond to those of the intercostal nerves, namely, posterior branch [ramus dorsalis (NA)] to the back muscles [rami musculares] and, usually, the skin [rami cutanei, medialis et lateralis (NA)]; a spinal branch [ramus spinalis (NA)]; a collateral branch [ramus collateralis (NA)] running in the lower part of the intercostal space; the lateral cutaneous branch [ramus lateralis cutaneus (NA)], and, in the female, a mammary branch [ramus mammarius (NA)]. **Superior intercostal artery [arteria intercostalis suprema (NA)].** A division of the costocervical trunk which descends to supply the back of the first two intercostal spaces [arteriae intercostales posteriores I et II (NA)].

intercostal muscles. External intercostal muscles [musculi intercostales externi (NA)]. Thin sheets of muscle extending from the tubercle to the anterior end of a rib, the fibres of which run downward and forward, continuous with the anterior intercostal membranes which lie between adjacent costal cartilages. **Internal intercostal muscles [musculi intercostales interni (NA)].** Thin sheets of muscle attached to the adjacent ribs and costal cartilages and extending from the angle of the rib to the sternum, the fibres of which run downward and backward. They are continuous posteriorly with the posterior intercostal membranes.

intercostal nerves [nervi intercostales (NA)]. The anterior primary rami of the upper 11 thoracic nerves; they run between the ribs and supply the intercostal muscles, the underlying pleura, and the skin. The lower 5 run on to the abdominal wall and supply the muscles and skin here while the lower 6 or 7 supply the diaphragm also.

intercostal veins. Anterior intercostal veins [venae intercostales anteriores (NA)]. Veins in the anterior parts of the intercostal spaces; they are tributaries of the internal mammary and musculophrenic veins. **First (posterior) intercostal vein [vena intercostalis suprema].** The vein draining the 1st intercostal space into the innominate or the vertebral vein. **Posterior intercostal veins [venae intercostales posteriores (IV–XI) NA].** Veins draining the posterior and lateral parts of the intercostal spaces and muscle of the back into the vena azygos, vena hemiazygos, except the 1st, 2nd, and 3rd intercostal spaces on both sides, the 4th on the right, and occasionally the 4th on the left. **Posterior intercostal vein, posterior tributary of the [ramus dorsalis (NA)].** A tributary from the muscles and skin of the back and the vertebral (venous) plexus. It accompanies a similarly named artery. **Posterior intercostal vein, spinal tributary of the [ramus spinalis (NA)].** A tributary draining the spinal medulla and its membranes. **Superior intercostal vein, left [vena intercostalis superior sinistra (NA)].** The venous drainage of the 2nd, 3rd, and often the 4th intercostal spaces on the left. It is a tributary of the left innominate vein. **Superior intercostal vein, right [vena intercostalis superior dextra].** A tributary of the vena azygos, draining the 2nd, 3rd, and 4th intercostal spaces.

intercostales intimi muscles [musculi intercostales intimi (NA)] (in·ter·kos·**ta**'·leez **in**·tim·i muslz). Part of the transversus thoracis muscle and similarly arranged to the internal intercostal muscles, but separated from them by the intercostal nerves and vessels. Some fibres may pass over a rib.

intercostobrachial nerve [nervus intercostobrachialis (NA)] (in·ter·kos·to·**bra**'·ke·al nerv). The lateral cutaneous branch of the 2nd intercostal nerve. It communicates with the medial cutaneous nerve of the arm, and supplies the skin on the medial side of the upper part of the arm.

intercostohumeral (in·ter·kos·to·**hew**'·mer·al). Relating or belonging to the arm and an intercostal space, as the nerve which supplies the skin of the arm. [intercostal, L *humerus* shoulder.]

intercoupler (in·ter·**kup**·ler). A system of conductors arranged to prevent differences of electric potential between anaesthetist, patient, anaesthetic apparatus, and operating table. This device lessens the risk of inflammable anaesthetics being ignited or exploding by the accidental discharge of static electricity. [L *inter*, *copula* bond.]

intercourse (**in**·ter·kors). Coitus. **Carnal intercourse, sexual intercourse.** Coitus. [L *intercursus* interposition.]

intercoxal (in·ter·**cox**·al). Between the hips. [L *inter*, *coxa* hip.]

intercranial (in·ter·**kra**·ne·al). Endocranial. [L *inter*, cranium.]

intercricothyrotomy (in·ter·**kri**·ko·thi·**rot**'·o·me). Incision of the larynx made through the cricovocal membrane. [L *inter*, cricothyroid, Gk *temnein* to cut.]

intercristal (in·ter·**kris**·tal). Situated between two crests, e.g. of a bone or process. [L *inter*, *crista* ridge.]

intercrural (in·ter·**kroo**·ral). 1. Situated between any two crura. 2. Between the legs. [L *inter*, *crus* leg.]

intercuneate, intercuneiform (in·ter·**kew**·ne·ate, in·ter·kew·**ne**'·e·form). Between or among the cuneiform bones. [L *inter*, *cuneus* wedge, form.]

intercurrent (in·ter·**kur**·ent). 1. Intervening between or among. 2. Applied to a disease which intervenes in and alters the course of a disease already existing in any individual. 3. Applied to diseases the occurrence of which is not limited to any particular season of the year. [L *intercurrere* to run between.]

intercuspal (in·ter·**kus**·pal). As between the cusps of the teeth of one jaw and those of the teeth of the opposing jaw. [L *inter*, cusp.]

intercusping (in·ter·**kus**·ping). The relationship between the cusps of the teeth of one jaw and the depressions between the cusps of the teeth of the opposing jaw. [see prec.]

intercutaneomucous (in·ter·kew·**ta**·ne·o·**mew**'·kus). Occurring between the skin and a mucous membrane, or situated between them, e.g. between the cheek and lip. [L *inter*, *cutis* skin, mucous membrane.]

intercutaneous (in·ter·kew·**ta**'·ne·us). Within the skin; situated at one or other of the strata. [L *inter*, *cutis* skin.]

interdeferential (in·ter·def·er·**en**'·shal). Lying between the vasa deferentia. [L *inter*, vas deferens.]

interdental (in·ter·**den**·tal). Between teeth. [L *inter*, *dens* tooth.]

interdentium (in·ter·**den**·she·um). The space between adjacent teeth; interdental space. [see prec.]

interdigit (in·ter·**dij**·it). The part of the hand or foot situated between any two adjacent fingers or toes. [see foll.]

interdigital (in·ter·**dij**·it·al). Situated or occurring between two adjacent fingers or toes. [L *inter*, *digitus* finger, toe.]

interdigitation (**in**·ter·dij·it·**a**'·shun). 1. The interlocking of finger-like processes, e.g. of muscle. 2. In dentistry, the closure of the cusps of the teeth into the depressions in the teeth of the opposite jaw. [see prec.]

intereruptive (**in**·ter·e·**rup**'·tiv). Separating or occurring between two eruptive attacks. [L *inter*, eruption.]

interface (**in**·ter·fase). Interspace, interphase; the junction of two phases. Many important biological processes depend upon the phenomena associated with an interface, e.g. concentration of dissolved substances, orientation of molecules, adsorption, etc. **Dineric interface.** The interface between two liquids in contact, so-called because of the forces set up at such a junction. [L *inter*, face.]

interfacial (in·ter·**fa**·she·al). Relating or belonging to an interface.

interfascicular (**in**·ter·fas·**ik**'·ew·lar). Lying between fasciculi or tracts. [L *inter*, fasciculus.]

interfeminium (**in**·ter·fem·**in**'·e·um). 1. The inside of the thighs. 2. The space between the thighs. [L *inter*, femur.]

interfemoral (in·ter·**fem**·or·al). Situated between the thighs. [see prec.]

interfemus (in·ter·**fe**·mus). Interfeminium.

interference (in·ter·**feer**·ens). 1. In physics, a phenomenon peculiar to wave motion (light, sound) whereby the waves of one beam interfere with and extinguish the waves of another in certain positions of coincidence. 2. In the heart, the extinction of a wave of excitation by another. 3. Electrical signals obscuring the desired signal, e.g. atmospherics in radio. 4. Combination of wave trains leading to a wave pattern of regularly varying amplitude. 5. In pathology, the action of a pathogen in establishing itself at the expense of another invading pathogen. 6. In genetics, *chromosome interference.* The influence that a crossing-over event has on the incidence of another in its vicinity (*positive interference* is lower incidence of second crossing-over; *negative interference* is higher incidence of second crossing-over). **Dissociation by interference.** When a nodal rhythm occurs at a fast rate, the sinu-auricular node may activate the auricles at a slower rate; this produces auriculoventricular dissociation. Although retrograde conduction is thus blocked, anterograde conduction can occur, and, if an auricular impulse reaches the ventricle when the latter is not refractory, a premature ventricular beat may result. **Negative interference.** Indicating an excess in the number of double cross-overs over that expected, frequently observed in micro-organisms when the distance between loci is very small. **Virus interference.** The phenomenon whereby infection of a cell with one virus will generally prevent superinfection with another. [L *inter, ferire* to strike.]

interferometer (**in**·ter·feer·**om**'·et·er). An optical instrument depending for its action on the interference of two beams of light, by means of which the superfine structure of spectral lines can be examined, standard lengths determined in terms of wavelengths of light, and prisms or lenses tested for faults; it has also been used for many other purposes, such as the investigation of the speed of the earth through the ether, and the measurement of star diameters. [interference, meter.]

interferometry (**in**·ter·feer·**om**'·et·re). The measuring of small movements, displacements, or distances with an interferometer.

interferon (in·ter·**feer**·on). A small basic protein produced in cells as a response to a variety of agents. Viruses are the most potent inducers but some bacteria, their by-products (endotoxins, statolon), nucleic acids (naturally occurring and synthetic polynucleotides), phytohaemagglutinin and some co-polymers can also induce its formation. Interferon inhibits viral replication and is active against a wide range of viruses. It acts only in cells from the same species as those in which it was produced. It has not yet proved to be useful therapeutically. [L *inter, ferire* to strike.]

interfibrillar, interfibrillary (in·ter·**fi**·bril·ar, in·ter·**fi**·bril·ar·e). Situated between or among fibrils. [L *inter*, fibril.]

interfibrous (in·ter·**fi**·brus). Between fibres. [L *inter*, fibre.]

interfilamentous (**in**·ter·fil·am·**en**'·tus). Situated between filaments. [L *inter*, filament.]

interfilar (in·ter·**fi**·lar). Occurring between the filaments of a reticulum, as the substance of protoplasm. [see prec.]

interfollicular (**in**·ter·fol·**ik**'·ew·lar). Situated between two follicles. [L *inter*, follicle.]

interfrontal (in·ter·**frun**·tal). Situated between the two halves of the frontal bone before they have fused. [L *inter*, frontal.]

interganglionic (**in**·ter·gang·gle·**on**'·ik). 1. In a position between two ganglia or among ganglia. 2. Extending as a connection from one ganglion to another. [L *inter*, ganglion.]

intergemmal (in·ter·**jem**·al). 1. Between two or more bulb-like bodies. 2. Situated between the taste buds, as a nerve-ending. [L *inter, gemma* bud.]

interglandular (in·ter·**glan**·dew·lar). In a position between glands. [L *inter*, gland.]

interglobular (in·ter·**glob**·ew·lar). Found among or between globules. The term is applied to the minute irregular cavities (Czermak's spaces) in dentine due to imperfection in the process of calcification; such cavities are surrounded by dentine globules. **Interglobular spaces.** *See* SPACE. [L *inter*, globule.]

intergluteal (in·ter·**gloo**·te·al). Between the buttocks. [L *inter*, Gk *gloutos* buttock.]

intergonial (in·ter·**go**·ne·al). Between the gonion on one side of the jaw and the gonion on the other side. [L *inter*, gonion.]

intergrade (**in**·ter·grade). A transitional stage merging with the stage before and the stage after. [L *inter, gradus* a step.]

intergranular (in·ter·**gran**·ew·lar). Between granules; between the granule cells of the cerebellum and the cerebrum. [L *inter*, granule.]

intergyral (in·ter·**ji**·ral). Placed or occurring between the cerebri gyri. [L *inter*, gyrus.]

interhaemal (in·ter·**he**·mal). Between the haemal arches. [L *inter, haima* blood.]

interhemicerebral (**in**·ter·hem·e·**ser**'·e·bral). Intercerebral. [L *inter*, hemicerebrum.]

interhemispheric (**in**·ter·hem·e·**sfer**'·ik). Situated between any two hemispheres. [L *inter*, hemisphere.]

interictal (in·ter·**ik**·tal). Occurring in the interval between convulsions or seizures. [L *inter, ictus* stroke.]

interinhibitive (**in**·ter·in·**hib**'·it·iv). Having an inhibitive effect on one another. [L *inter*, inhibitive.]

interior (in·**teer**·e·or). 1. Situated on the inner side. 2. Remote from the surface. [L, inner.]

interischiadic (**in**·ter·is·ke·**ad**'·ik). Situated between the two ischia, more particularly between the two ischial tuberosities. [L *inter*, ischium.]

interjugal (in·ter·**joo**·gal). Between the zygomatic processes. [L *inter, jugum* yoke.]

interkinesis (**in**·ter·kin·**e**'·sis). The interval between the first and second meiotic division. Sometimes (less appropriately) used to indicate the interval between two mitoses. [L *inter*, Gk *kinein* to move.]

interlabial (in·ter·**la**·be·al). 1. Between the labia. 2. Between the lips. [L *inter, labium* lip.]

interlamellar (**in**·ter·lam·**el**'·ar). Between lamellae. [L *inter*, lamella.]

interlaminar (in·ter·**lam**·in·ar). Between laminae. [L *inter*, lamina.]

interligamentary, interligamentous (**in**·ter·lig·am·**en**'·tar·e, **in**·ter·lig·am·**en**'·tus). Situated between ligaments or among them. [L *inter*, ligament.]

interlobar (in·ter·**lo**·bar). Situated between the lobes of any organ or structure, or occurring between them. [L *inter*, lobe.]

interlobar arteries [arteriae interlobares renis (NA)]. Paired branches of the lobar arteries running towards the cortex on each side of a renal pyramid, accompanied by a corresponding vein.

interlobar veins [venae interlobares (NA)]. The veins accompanying the interlobar arteries.

interlobitis (**in**·ter·lo·**bi**'·tis). Interlobular pleurisy. [L *inter*, lobe, Gk *-itis* inflammation.]

interlobular (in·ter·**lob**·ew·lar). Between lobules. [L *inter*, lobule.]

interlobular arteries [arteriae interlobulares (NA)]. 1. Straight branches of the arcuate arteries, running in a radial direction and supplying afferent capillaries to the glomeruli of the kidney; the vasa afferentia. 2. The smallest branches of the hepatic artery, running between the liver lobules in a fibrous capsule, the hepatobiliary capsule (of Glisson).

interlobular veins [venae interlobulares (NA)]. 1. Veins of the kidney running with the interlobular arteries and receiving the stellate veins. 2. Branches of the portal vein accompanying the interlobular arteries and sending sinusoids between the liver columns to reach the central veins.

intermalar (in·ter·**ma**·lar). Situated between the zygomatic (malar) bones. [L *inter, mala* jawbone.]

intermalleolar (in·ter·**mal**·e·o·lar). Between the malleoli. [L *inter*, malleolus.]

intermamillary (in·ter·mam·**il**'·ar·e). 1. Intermammary. 2. Between the nipples, as an imaginary line drawn between the two. [L *inter, mamilla* nipple.]

intermammary (in·ter·**mam**·ar·e). Between the breasts. [L *inter, mamma* breast.]

intermarginal (in·ter·**mar**·jin·al). Occurring or situated between two margins or edges. [L *inter*, margin.]

intermarriage (in·ter·**mar**·ij). 1. Inbreeding; marriage of individuals having the same parents or grandparents. 2. Marriage between individuals of whom one is of a different race from the other. [L *inter*, Fr. *mariage*.]

intermastoid (in·ter·**mas**·toid). Between the mastoid processes of the temporal bone, or connecting the one process with the other. [L *inter*, mastoid.]

intermaxilla (in·ter·max·**il**'·ah). In embryology, the premaxilla. [L *inter*, maxilla.]

intermaxillary (in·ter·max·**il**'·ar·e). Between the maxilla and the mandible. [see prec.]

intermaxillary bone. The premaxilla or incisive bone of the maxilla.

intermediary (in·ter·**me**·de·ar·e). 1. Coming, occurring or performed neither early nor late but at or in a median stage. 2. Intermediate in time or place. [L *inter, mediare* to divide.]

intermediate [intermedius (NA)] (in·ter·**me**·de·ate). Between two limits or extremes; in the middle; interposed or intervening. [see prec.]

intermedin (in·ter·**me**·din). Chromatophorotropic hormone, melanophoric hormone; a substance secreted by the intermediate part of the pituitary which expands the pigment cells of the skin of certain reptiles, amphibians, and fish. A term now seldom used. Thought to be produced by the pars intermedia of the pituitary. Is probably identical with MSH (melanocyte stimulating hormone).

intermediolateral (in·ter·**me**·de·o·**lat**'·er·al). Intermediate and lying to one side. [intermediate, L *latus* side.]

intermembral (in·ter·**mem**·bral). Existing or occurring between the limbs or members of any particular organism. [L *inter*, member.]

intermembranous (in·ter·**mem**·bran·us). Between membranes. [L *inter*, membrane.]

intermeningeal (in·ter·men·**in**'·je·al). Between any two of the three meninges of the brain, or occurring among or between the three. [L *inter*, meninx.]

intermenstrual (in·ter·**men**·stroo·al). Occurring between the periods of menstruation, or between any two menstrual periods. [L *inter*, menstruum.]

intermenstruum (in·ter·**men**·stroo·um). The length of time between the end of one menstrual period and the beginning of the next. [see prec.]

intermesenteric (in·ter·mes·en·**ter**'·ik). Between or among any of the mesenteries. [L *inter*, mesentery.]

intermesoblastic (in·ter·mez·o·**blas**'·tik). In embryology, between the layers of mesoblast or mesoderm. [L *inter*, mesoblast.]

intermetacarpal (in·ter·met·ah·**kar**'·pal). In a position between or among the metacarpal bones. **Intermetacarpal joint.** *See* JOINT. [L *inter*, metacarpal.]

intermetameric (in·ter·met·am·**er**'·ik). Pertaining to the region between adjacent segments (metameres) of the animal body, particularly in its embryonic stages. [L *inter*, metamere.]

intermetatarsal (in·ter·met·ah·**tar**'·sal). In a position between or among the metatarsal bones. **Intermetatarsal joint.** *See* JOINT. [L *inter*, metatarsal.]

intermission (in·ter·**mish**·un). 1. Temporary interruption or cessation, e.g. of paroxysms of pain, or of the heart beat. 2. Temporary subsidence of a feverish condition. 3. Interval. [L *inter, mittere* to send.]

intermittent (in·ter·**mit**·ent). 1. Recurrent; coming and going at intervals, as an interval of complete inactivity occurring between two periods of activity. 2. Missing occasionally, as a heart beat. **Intermittent flow machines.** *See* MACHINE. **Intermittent positive pressure ventilation.** *See* VENTILATION. **Postponing intermittent.** A form of intermittent fever in which the onset of the attack occurs at a later hour every day. [see prec.]

intermolecular (in·ter·mol·**ek**'·ew·lar). Occurring between the molecules of a substance. [L *inter*, molecule.]

intermural (in·ter·**mewr**·al). Between the walls of an organ of the body. [L *inter, murus* wall.]

intermuscular (in·ter·**mus**·kew·lar). Between muscles or among the muscles. **Intermuscular septum.** *See* SEPTUM. [L *inter*, muscle.]

intern (in·tern). A USA term: a medical graduate who prior to registration as a qualified practitioner resides and serves in a hospital. There is no exact equivalent in the UK. [see foll.]

internal [internus (NA)] (in·ter·nal). 1. Occurring on the inside. 2. In a position within, e.g. a part or organ. 3. Interior, away from the surface. 4. Towards the median axis. [L *internus* inward.]

internarial (in·ter·**na**·re·al). In a position between the nostrils. [L *inter, naris* nostril.]

internasal (in·ter·**na**·zal). 1. Between the nasal bones, cartilages or passages. 2. Internarial. [L *inter, nasus* nose.]

internatal (in·ter·**na**·tal). Between the buttocks. [L *inter*, nates.]

interneural (in·ter·**newr**·al). Between the vertebral (neural) arches. [L *inter*, Gk *neuron* nerve.]

interneuronal (in·ter·**newr**·on·al). Occurring between neurons. [see foll.]

interneuron (in·ter·**newr**·one). A neuron with short processes, acting as an intermediate link in a nervous pathway between two neurons with longer processes. The term is applied especially to any neuron in the grey matter of the spinal cord between the afferent and efferent neurons subserving a simple reflex arc. [L *inter*, neuron.]

internist (in·ter·nist). A USA term: a physician who specializes in internal medicine; a medical specialist.

internodal (in·ter·**no**·dal). 1. Between two nodes. 2. Belonging or relating to an internode. [see foll.]

internode (in·ter·node). An internodal segment of a nerve fibre. [L *inter, nodus* knot.]

internodular (in·ter·**nod**·ew·lar). Occurring between two nodes; internodal. [see prec.]

internuclear (in·ter·**new**·kle·ar). 1. Between nuclei, or situated among nuclei. 2. Between the outer and inner nuclear layers of the retina. [L *inter*, nucleus.]

internuncial (in·ter·**nun**·she·al). Serving as a messenger between two parties, e.g. internuncial neurone, or a nerve cell and its processes which serve as a link between other nerve cells. [L *internuntius* messenger between.]

internus (in·ter·nus). The medial rectus muscle of the orbit. [L, inward.]

interoceptive (in·ter·o·**sep**'·tiv). The term applied by Sherrington to the internal surfaces of an organism (e.g. the alimentary canal) and its receptor organs. As used by Cannon the term includes the nerves of the autonomic nervous system as a whole. [L *internus* inward, *capere* to take.]

interoceptor (in·ter·o·**sep**'·tor). Any nerve-ending concerned with the reception of stimuli from the internal organs, as distinguished from an exteroceptor, which is concerned with stimuli from outside the body, e.g. in vision, or a proprioceptor, which is concerned with stimuli from muscles and joints. [see prec.]

interofective (in·ter·o·**fek**'·tiv). Descriptive of the autonomic nervous system, i.e. affecting the inside of an organism. [L *internus* inward, *facere* to make.]

interolivary (in·ter·**ol**·iv·ar·e). Between the olives of the medulla oblongata. [L *inter*, olive.]

interoptic (in·ter·**op**·tik). Between the quadrigeminal bodies or the optic tracts or nerves of the brain. [L *inter*, optic.]

interorbital (in·ter·**or**·bit·al). Situated or occurring between the orbits. [L *inter*, orbit.]

interosculate (in·ter·**os**·kew·late). To form an anastomosis between two structures. [L *inter*, *osculum* little mouth.]

interosseal (in·ter·**os**·e·al). Interosseous.

interossei muscles of the foot, dorsal [musculi interossei dorsales (NA)], and plantar [musculi interossei plantares (NA)] (in·ter·**os**·e·i muslz). A group of small muscles, four placed dorsally and three towards the plantar side of the intervals between the metacarpal bones, and inserted into the base of the phalanges and into the dorsal extensor expansion. They act as abductors and adductors of the toes, respectively. By means of their insertions into the extensor expansions they cause flexion of the metacarpophalangeal joints and extensors of the interphalangeal joints, thus preventing the toes buckling under the action of the long flexors and keeping the toes in contact with the ground.

interossei muscles of the hand, dorsal [musculi interossei dorsales (NA)], and palmar [musculi interossei palmares (NA)]. A series of deep muscles of the palm of the hand. They arise from one of the adjacent metacarpals and insert into the bases of the phalanges and into the dorsal extensor expansion. They produce abduction and adduction of the fingers, respectively, and, via their insertion into the extensor expansion, they produce flexion at the metacarpophalangeal joint and extension at the interphalangeal joints.

interosseous (in·ter·**os**·eus). 1. Placed between bones or occurring between bones. 2. Connecting bones, as ligaments. [L *inter*, *os* bone.]

interosseous arteries. *See* ULNAR ARTERY.

interosseous nerves. Anterior interosseous nerve [nervus interosseus (antebrachii) anterior (NA)]. A branch of the median nerve which runs along the anterior aspect of the interosseous membrane and supplies the flexor digitorum profundus, the flexor pollicis longus, and the pronator quadratus muscles and the wrist-joint. **Posterior interosseous nerve [nervus interosseus (antebrachii) posterior (NA)].** A branch of the radial nerve given off at the level of the elbow and winding to the back of the forearm through the supinator muscle; it supplies this muscle and the deep extensor muscles in the forearm.

interosseus (in·ter·**os**·e·us). Any one of the interosseous muscles. [L *inter*, *os* bone.]

interpalpebral (in·ter·**pal**·pe·bral). Between the eyelids. [L *inter*, *palpebra* eyelid.]

interpapillary (in·ter·pap·**il**'·ar·e). Occurring between papillae. [L *inter*, papilla.]

interparietal (in·ter·par·**i**'·et·al). 1. Placed between the parietal bones. 2. Situated between the walls of a part. 3. Between any two parts of the parietal lobe of the cerebrum. [L *inter*, *paries* wall.]

interparietal bone [os interparietale (NA)]. The portion of the squamous part of the occipital bone above the highest nuchal line, which ossifies separately and may remain separate throughout life.

interparoxysmal (in·ter·par·ox·**iz**'·mal). Occurring between any two paroxysms. [L *inter*, paroxysm.]

interpediculate (in·ter·ped·**ik**'·ew·late). From one pedicle of the vertebral arch to another. [L *inter*, pedicle.]

interpeduncular (in·ter·ped·**ung**'·kew·lar). Between the peduncles of cerebellum or cerebrum. **Interpeduncular nucleus.** *See* NUCLEUS. [L *inter*, peduncle.]

interphalangeal (in·ter·fal·**an**'·je·al). Between two phalanges. **Interphalangeal joints.** *See* JOINTS OF THE HAND, JOINTS OF THE TOES. [L *inter*, phalanx.]

interphase (**in**·ter·faze). 1. Interface; interspace; the zone where two phases contact, e.g. liquid/liquid or liquid/gas, in which the phenomena of molecular concentration and orientation take place. 2. The stage of a cell between divisions; the resting stage. [L *inter*, phase.]

interphyletic (in·ter·fi·**let**'·ik). Of cells, transitional types that occur during the process of metaplasia. [L *inter*, *phyle* class.]

interpial (in·ter·**pi**·al). Between the layers of the pia mater. [L *inter*, pia mater.]

interplacental (in·ter·plas·**en**'·tal). Between the placental lacunae. [L *inter*, placenta.]

interpleural (in·ter·**ploor**·al). Between the two pleurae. [L *inter*, pleura.]

interpleuricostal (in·ter·ploor·e·**kos**'·tal). Situated between the pleura and the ribs. [L *inter*, pleura, L *costa* rib.]

interpolated (in·ter·**pol**·a·ted). Intercalary; inserted in or introduced among. [see foll.]

interpolation (in·ter·pol·**a**'·shun). 1. The transfer of tissue such as occurs in plastic operations. 2. In statistics, the introduction of intermediate, estimated values of a variable between known values of the variable. [L *interpolare* to form anew.]

interpositum (in·ter·**poz**·it·um). The velum interpositum (the tela choroidea of the 3rd ventricle). [L, insertion.]

interpretation (in·ter·pret·**a**'·shun). The description or formulation of the deeper meaning of a patient's productions during psychotherapy. **Direct interpretation.** The giving of interpretations of the patient's thinking and actions by the therapist in an authoritative, challenging manner in positive terms. **Dream interpretation.** The meaning given to a dream. The kind used in psychiatric practice is that originated by Freud. The manifest content is made up of hidden disguised material based on wishes, conflicts, emotions, etc. The method used in free association of the manifest content to reveal the underlying processes in the deeper meaning of the latent content. **Premature interpretation.** The giving of a description or formulation of a patient's symptoms or behaviour before he is emotionally ready. **Transference interpretation.** In psychotherapy, the process whereby the patient projects his wishes, emotions, thoughts and attitudes to the therapist who has come during treatment to represent someone from the patient's past. An important part of treatment is the interpretation and resolution of transference. [Fr. to spread abroad.]

interproximal, interproximate (in·ter·**prox**·im·al, in·ter·**prox**·im·ate). Lying between adjacent surfaces; in dentistry referring to the spaces between adjacent teeth. [L *inter*, *proximus* nearest.]

interpterion (in·ter·**teer**·e·on). In craniology, situated between the two pteria. [L *inter*, pterion.]

interpterygoid (in·ter·**ter**·ig·oid). Between the two pterygoid processes of the sphenoid bone. [L *inter*, pterygoid.]

interpubic (in·ter·**pew**·bik). Between the two pubic bones. [L *inter*, pubis.]

interpupillary (in·ter·**pew**·pil·ar·e). Between the pupils of the eyes. [L *inter*, pupil.]

interpyramidal (in·ter·pir·**am**'·id·al). 1. Between the pyramids of the medulla oblongata. 2. Situated between any two pyramid-like structures or processes. [L *inter*, pyramid.]

inter-renal (in·ter·**re**·nal). In a position between the kidneys. [L *inter*, *ren* kidney.]

inter-renalin (in·ter·re·nal·in). A word originally coined for the principle of the cortex of the suprarenal gland, so essential to life, and now proved to be a group of glucocorticoid hormones. [see prec.]

inter-renalism (in·ter·**re**·nal·izm). The condition of hyperplasia of the cortex of the suprarenal gland. [Obsolete term.] [L *inter*, *ren* kidney.]

inter-renalopathy (in·ter·re·nal·**op**'·ath·e). Any functional disorder of the cortex of the suprarenal gland. [inter-renal, Gk *pathos* disease.]

inter-renalotropic, inter-renotropic (in·ter·re·nal·o·**trop**'·ik, in·ter·re·no·**trop**'·ik). 1. Showing affinity for the cortex of the suprarenal gland. 2. Having a stimulating effect on the cortex of the suprarenal gland. [inter-renal, Gk *trope* a turning.]

interrupted (in·ter·**up**·ted). Discontinuous; characterized by intermissions; not regular; broken. [L *interrumpere* to sever.]

interrupter (in·ter·**up**·ter). Any appliance which automatically at regular intervals breaks a direct current. [see prec.]

See also: WEHNELT.

interscapilium (in·ter·skap·**il**′·e·um). Interscapulum.

interscapular (in·ter·**skap**·ew·lar). Between the scapulae. [see foll.]

interscapulum (in·ter·**skap**·ew·lum). The region between the shoulder blades. [L *inter*, scapula.]

intersciatic (in·ter·si·**at**′·ik). Interischiadic; situated between the two ischia, more particularly, between the two ischial tuberosities. [L *inter*, sciatic.]

intersection (in·ter·**sek**·shun). A division. **Tendinous intersection [intersectio tendinea (NA)].** A fibrous band which passes transversely or obliquely across the belly of a muscle, as in the rectus abdominis muscle. [L *inter, secare* to cut.]

intersegment (in·ter·**seg**·ment). A metamere. [L *inter*, segment.]

intersegmental (in·ter·seg·**men**′·tal). 1. Relating to an intersegment (metamere). 2. Lying between two segments. **Intersegmental tract.** *See* TRACT. [see prec.]

intersegmental arteries (in·ter·seg·**men**′·tal **ar**·ter·es). In the embryo, the dorsal branches of the aorta which pass between the somites and originally supply the neural tube. [L *inter*, segment.]

intersegmental veins [venae intersegmentales]. *See* PULMONARY VEINS, RIGHT AND LEFT.

interseptal (in·ter·**sep**·tal). Situated between two septa. [L *inter*, septum.]

interseptum (in·ter·**sep**·tum). The diaphragm. [L, division.]

intersex (**in**·ter·sex). A condition in which anatomical features of both sexes are evident. [L *inter*, sex.]

intersexual (in·ter·**sex**·ew·al). Relating to sex intergrade. [see prec.]

intersexuality (in·ter·sex·ew·**al**′·it·e). The condition of being intermediate between the typical male and the typical female, i.e. having both the male and the female characters of intersex. [L *inter*, sexuality.]

interspace (**in**·ter·spase). 1. A space or interval between two similar objects or structures, as costal interspace. 2. Interface, interphase; the region between two phases. **Dineric interspace.** The surface existing between two liquids in contact. [L *inter*, space.]

interspinal (in·ter·**spi**·nal). Placed between the processes of the spine of a vertebra, or between any two spines of any kind. [L *inter*, spine.]

interspinales muscles [musculi interspinales (NA)] (in·ter·spi·**na**′·leez muslz). Muscles situated between the contiguous borders of adjacent vertebral spines mainly in the cervical and lumbar regions, and consisting of a slip on either side of the interspinous ligament. They are cervical [musculi interspinales cervicis (NA)], thoracic [musculi interspinales thoracis (NA)], and lumbar [musculi interspinales lumborum (NA)].

interspinalis (in·ter·spi·**na**′·lis). One of the interspinales muscles of the back. [L *inter*, spine.]

interspinous (in·ter·**spi**·nus). Interspinal.

intersternal (in·ter·**ster**·nal). Occurring between the sternal segments. [L *inter*, sternum.]

interstice (in·**ter**·stis). 1. Any small space or crevice present between parts of the body. 2. One of the small chinks in the structure of areolar tissue. 3. A pore. [L *interstitium* a space between.]

interstitial (in·ter·**stish**·al). 1. Relating or belonging to an interstice or interstices. 2. Situated or occurring within the tissues or the tissue spaces. **Interstitial-cell stimulating hormone, ICHS.** *See* HORMONE.

interstitialoma (in·ter·stish·al·**o**′·mah). Any mass or neoplasm composed of connective tissue. [interstitial, Gk *-oma* tumour.]

intersuperciliary (in·ter·sew·per·**sil**′·e·ar·e). Between the superciliary arches of the frontal bone. [L *inter*, superciliary.]

intersystole (in·ter·**sis**·to·le). The slight pause which occurs between the atrial and the ventricular systoles of the cardiac cycle. [L *inter*, systole.]

intertarsal (in·ter·**tar**·sal). In a position between adjacent tarsal bones. **Intertarsal joint.** *See* JOINT. [L *inter*, tarsus.]

intertendinous (in·ter·**ten**·din·us). Situated between tendons. [L *inter*, tendon.]

intertinctus (in·ter·**tingk**·tus). Indicating that there is differential coloration, especially in skin lesions. [L *inter, tingere* to dye.]

intertragicus (in·ter·**traj**·ik·us). An intrinsic muscle of the pinna of the external ear. [L *inter*, tragicus.]

intertransversalis (in·ter·trans·ver·**sa**′·lis). Any one of the intertransverse muscles of the back.

intertransverse (in·ter·**trans**·vers). Between the transverse processes of the vertebrae. [L *inter*, transverse.]

intertransverse muscles [musculi intertransversarii (NA)]. Muscles lying between adjacent transverse processes in the cervical, lower thoracic [musculi intertransversarii thoracis (NA)], and lumbar regions, and usually consisting of an anterior and posterior slip. **Anterior intertransverse muscles [musculi intertransversarii anteriores cervicis (NA)].** Anterior slips of intertransverse muscles. **Lateral intertransverse muscles [musculi intertransversarii laterales lumborum (NA)].** Muscular slips in the lumbar region connecting the transverse process and accessory processes. **Medial intertransverse muscles [musculi intertransversarii mediales lumborum (NA)].** Muscular slips in the lumbar region connnecting the accessory process of one vertebra to the mamillary process of the next. **Posterior intertransverse muscles [musculi intertransversarii posteriores cervicis (NA)].** Posterior slips [pars lateralis, pars medialis (NA)] of intertransverse muscles.

intertriginous (in·ter·**tri**·jin·us). 1. Suffering from intertrigo. 2. Having the character of intertrigo.

intertrigo (in·ter·**tri**·go). Erythema or dermatitis of contiguous cutaneous or mucocutaneous surfaces. **Intertrigo podicis.** Intertrigo of the natal cleft. **Retro-auricular intertrigo.** An inflammatory skin condition that develops in the fold where the pinna joins the scalp: a crack appears and is very persistent. **Seborrhoeic intertrigo.** A condition similar to retro-auricular intertrigo (see above), which may appear under the breasts or in the folds of the buttocks. [L *inter, terere* to rub.]

intertrochanteric (in·ter·tro·kan·**ter**′·ik). In a position between the greater and the lesser trochanter of the femur, or drawn between the trochanters, as an intertrochanteric line. [L *inter*, trochanter.]

intertubercular (in·ter·tew·**ber**′·kew·lar). Situated between tubercles, or drawn between tubercles. [L *inter*, tubercle.]

intertubular (in·ter·**tew**·bew·lar). Between tubules or tubes, or among them. [L *inter*, tubule.]

interureteral, interureteric (in·ter·ewr·e′·ter·al, in·ter·ewr·e′·ter·ik). Between the ureters. **Interureteric ridge.** *See* RIDGE. [L *inter*, ureter.]

interuteroplacental (in·ter·ew·ter·o·plas·**en**′·tal). Referring to structures or occurrences between the uterus and the placenta. [L *inter*, uterus, placenta.]

intervaginal (in·ter·vaj·**i**′·nal). Occurring between sheaths. [L *inter, vagina* sheath.]

interval (**in**·ter·val). 1. The space between two things, or the lapse of time between two events. 2. Any break in a continuous flow. 3. In physics, the difference in the frequencies of two sounded notes. **A-C interval.** Intersystolic period; the interval between the "a" wave and the "c" wave of the atrial pressure curve, approximately representing the period between atrial and ventricular systole. The "a" wave is due to atrial contraction and the "c" wave is said to be due to the increase in pressure in the atrium caused by contraction of the ventricle against closed atrioventricular valves. **Atriocarotid interval.** The interval between the contraction of the atrium, as noted by the atrial systolic wave of the jugular venous pulse, and the carotid arterial pulse. It approximately measures the interval between atrial and ventricular systole. *See* A-C INTERVAL (prec.). **Atrioventricular interval.** The interval between the contractions of the atrium and the ventricle. **Auriculocarotid interval.** Atriocarotid interval (see above). **Auriculoventricular interval, A-V interval.** Atrioventricular interval (see above). **C-A interval, cardio-arterial interval.** The interval between the ejection period of ventricular contraction (apex beat) and the arterial pulse. It measures the rate of propagation of the arterial pulse wave. **Coupling interval.**

The time between the onset of the QRS complex of a normally conducted beat and the onset of the QRS complex of a coupled ectopic beat succeeding it. **Focal interval.** The interval between two foci of the eye; this is sometimes used as a synonym for Sturm's interval. **Induction-delivery interval.** The time between the induction of labour and the delivery of the child. **Isometric interval.** Presphygmic period, period of isometric contraction; the first period of ventricular systole in which the muscle fibres are contracting against closed semilunar valves; the fibres are not shortening since they are contracting upon an incompressible mass of blood. The isometric interval ends with the opening of the aortic and pulmonary valves which heralds the onset of the ejection or sphygmic period of systole. **Lucid interval.** A period of mental clarity between two periods of mental abnormality: applied, for example, to the period of mental clarity between concussion and the impairment of consciousness resulting from a haemorrhage from the middle meningeal artery. **Passive interval.** The period of the heart cycle when no contraction is occurring (atrial and ventricular diastole). **Postsphygmic interval.** Postsphygmic period. *See* PERIOD. **P–R interval.** The period of the electrocardiogram between the P wave and the R wave, representing the atrioventricular conduction time. **Presphygmic interval.** Presphygmic period; isometric interval (see above). **Protodiastolic interval.** Protodiastole. **QRST interval.** The electrocardiographic period covering ventricular systole (see Q–T interval, foll.). **Q–T interval.** The period of the electrocardiogram between the onset of the Q wave (commencement of ventricular depolarization) and the end of the T wave (termination of ventricular repolarization). It measures the duration of electrical ventricular systole, and varies inversely with the heart rate. **S–T interval.** S–T segment; the period of the electrocardiogram between the S wave and the T wave, representing the interval between ventricular depolarization and repolarization. [L *intervallum* space between ramparts.]

See also: STURM.

intervallary (in·ter·**val**·ar·e). Occurring or appearing between one paroxysm of a disease and another. [interval.]

intervalvular (in·ter·**val**·vew·lar). In a position between valves. [L *inter*, valve.]

intervascular (in·ter·**vas**·kew·lar). Situated between vessels, e.g. blood vessels. [L *inter*, *vasculum* little vessel.]

interventricular (in·ter·ven·**trik**′·ew·lar). Between ventricles, as a septum. [L *inter*, ventricle.]

intervertebral (in·ter·**ver**·te·bral). Between two adjacent vertebrae, e.g. intervertebral disc. [L *inter*, vertebra.]

intervertebral vein [vena intervertebralis (NA)]. A vein issuing through the intervertebral foramen, draining the vertebral plexuses. It terminates in the vertebral, intercostal, lumbar, or lateral sacral veins.

intervillous (in·ter·**vil**·us). Placed between villi or among them. [L *inter*, villus.]

intestinal (in·**tes**·**tin**·al). Relating or belonging to the intestine.

intestine (in·**tes**·tin). The part of the digestive tract that extends from the stomach (pylorus) to the anus. **Large intestine [intestinum crassum (NA)].** That part of the intestine which includes the caecum, the colon, and the rectum. **Small intestine [intestinum tenue (NA)].** That part of the intestine which includes the duodenum, the jejunum, and the ileum. **Small intestine, mucous coat of the [tunica mucosa (NA)].** The inner coat of the small intestine, characterized by the presence of villi on its fine surface. **Small intestine, muscular coat of the [tunica muscularis (NA)].** A coat consisting of inner circular [stratum circulare (NA)] and outer longitudinal layers [stratum longitudinale (NA)] of smooth muscle. **Small intestine, serous coat of the [tunica serosa (NA)].** The peritoneal investment of the small intestine. **Small intestine, submucous coat of the [tela submucosa (NA)].** The layer of areolar tissue between the muscular and mucous coats. [L, *intestinum.*]

intestinotoxin (in·**tes**·tin·o·**tox**′·in). 1. A toxin originating in the intestine. 2. A cytotoxin specific for the cells of the mucous coat of the intestine. [intestine, Gk *toxikon* poison.]

intestinulum (in·tes·**tin**·ew·lum) (pl. *intestinula*). 1. The small intestine. 2. The umbilical cord. 3. A cerebral gyrus. [L, little bowel.]

intestinum (in·tes·**ti**·num) (pl. *intestina*). Intestine. [L.]

intima (**in**·tim·ah). The tunica intima of a blood vessel, i.e. the innermost coat. [L *intimus* inmost.]

intima-pia (**in**·tim·ah·**pi**′·ah). The structure formed by the tunica intima of the blood vessels of the brain combined with the cerebral pia mater.

intimal (**in**·tim·al). Relating or belonging to the tunica intima of a blood vessel.

intimectomy (in·tim·**ek**·to·me). Removal of the diseased intima of an artery. [intima, Gk *ektome* a cutting out.]

intimitis (in·tim·**i**·tis). Inflammation of the tunica intima of a blood vessel. **Proliferative intimitis.** A condition of the skin resulting from intimitis of the small cutaneous arteries and veins and characterized by discoloured patches and ulcers. [intima, Gk *-itis* inflammation.]

intine (**in**·tine). The transparent inner sheath (endosporium) of a pollen grain. [L *intus* within.]

intolerance (in·**tol**·er·ans). 1. Inability to endure, e.g. light or pain. 2. Responding with an unfavourable reaction to a drug. 3. Impatience. **Fructose intolerance.** An inherited disorder of autosomal dominant type due to absence of enzymes, causing digestive symptoms with vomiting and failure to grow in infants. [L *in*, *tolerare* to bear.]

intonation (in·to·**na**·shun). 1. The pitch and tone of the voice in pronouncing words. 2. The sound produced by the movement of flatus in the bowels. [L *in*, *tonus* tone.]

intorsion (in·**tor**·shun). Rotation of the eye inwards round its anteroposterior axis, so that 12 o'clock on the corneal margin approaches the nose. [see foll.]

intort (in·**tort**). To deviate or turn inwards. [L *in*, *torquere* to twist.]

intorter (in·**tor**·ter). An internal rotatores muscle. [see prec.]

intoxation (in·tox·**a**·shun). A state of poisoning by any toxic product of bacteria or insects. [L *in*, toxin.]

intoxicant (in·**tox**·ik·ant). 1. Intoxicating or poisoning. 2. Any agent which produces a state of intoxication or poisoning.

intoxication (in·tox·ik·a′·shun). The general condition resulting from the absorption and diffusion in the body of a soluble poison. **Acid intoxication.** Acidosis. **Alkaline intoxication.** Alkalosis. **Anaphylactic intoxication.** The reaction of an allergic subject to a substance to which he is sensitized. **Bongkrek intoxication.** Poisoning from bongkrek, a Javanese dish that is normally non-poisonous but which exceptionally through a fault in preparation becomes very poisonous and leads to vomiting, sweating, muscular cramps, and coma. **Bromide intoxication.** Brominism. **Citrate intoxication.** Deleterious effect on the heart from an excess of citrate in the plasma, e.g. following massive blood transfusions. Due to reduction of ionized calcium concentration of the plasma. **Intestinal intoxication.** Poisoning by toxins absorbed from the intestines. **Menstrual intoxication.** General symptoms associated with menstruation, at one time attributed to toxic absorption. **Roentgen intoxication.** A general toxic reaction to the application of roentgen rays (x-rays), leading to lassitude, nausea, and vomiting; usually known as *x-ray sickness.* **Septic intoxication.** The absorption of septic products. **Water intoxication.** Symptoms caused by excessive water retention in the body; they comprise headache, nausea, asthenia, and muscular inco-ordination. [L *in*, Gk *toxikon* poison.]

intoxications (in·**tox**·ik·a′·shunz). Diseases which result from administration of exogenous poisons. [see prec.]

intra-. Prefix, from the Latin preposition *intra*, meaning *within.*

intra vitam (**in**·trah **vi**·tam). During life. [L.]

intra-abdominal (**in**·trah·ab·**dom**′·in·al). Situated or occurring within the cavity of the abdomen. [L *intra*, abdomen.]

intra-acinar, intra-acinous (in·trah·**as**·in·ar, in·trah·**as**·in·us). Occurring, or in a position, within an acinus. [L *intra*, acinus.]

intra-appendicular (in·trah·ap·en·**dik**'·ew·lar). Situated within the vermiform appendix. [L *intra*, appendix.]
intra-arachnoid (in·trah·ar·**ak**'·noid). Beneath or within the arachnoid mater of the brain or the spine. [L *intra*, arachnoid.]
intra-arterial (in·trah·ar·**teer**'·e·al). Within an artery. [L *intra*, artery.]
intra-articular (in·trah·ar·**tik**'·ew·lar). Within a joint or inside the cavity of a joint. **Intra-articular ligament.** *See* LIGAMENT. [L *intra, articulatio* joint.]
intra-atomic (in·trah·at·**om**'·ik). 1. Within the atom. 2. Relating or belonging to atomic structure. [L *intra*, atom.]
intra-atrial (in·trah·**at**·re·al). Inside an atrium of the heart. [L *intra*, atrium.]
intra-aural (in·trah·**aw**·ral). Within the ear. [L *intra, auris* ear.]
intra-auricular (in·trah·aw·**rik**'·ew·lar). 1. On the inside of or within an auricle of the ear. 2. Within an auricle or an atrium of the heart. [L *intra*, auricle.]
intrabronchial (in·trah·**brong**·ke·al). Within a bronchus. [L *intra*, bronchus.]
intrabuccal (in·trah·**buk**·al). 1. Within the substance of the cheek. 2. Within the mouth. [L *intra, bucca* cheek.]
intracanalicular (in·trah·kan·al·**ik**'·ew·lar). Situated or occurring within a canaliculus or canaliculi. [L *intra*, canaliculus.]
intracapsular (in·trah·**kap**·sew·lar). Within a capsule. Of fractures (e.g. of the head of the humerus), occurring within the confines of the capsular ligament of a joint. [L *intra*, capsule.]
intracardiac (in·trah·**kar**·de·ak). Within the cavity of the heart. [L *intra*, Gk *kardia* heart.]
intracarpal (in·trah·**kar**·pal). Situated or occurring within the wrist or among the carpal bones. [L *intra*, carpus.]
intracartilaginous (in·trah·kar·til·**aj**'·in·us). Formed or situated within cartilaginous tissue or cartilage, as ossification; endochondral. [L *intra*, cartilage.]
intracavitary (in·trah·**kav**·it·ar·e). Within the cavity of a hollow organ. [L *intra*, cavity.]
intracellular (in·trah·**sel**·ew·lar). Relating to the contents of a cell. [L *intra*, cell.]
intracephalic (in·trah·kef·**al**'·ik). Within the head or brain. [L *intra*, Gk *kephale* head.]
intracerebellar (in·trah·ser·e·**bel**'·ar). Within the cerebellum. [L *intra*, cerebellum.]
intracerebral (in·trah·**ser**·e·bral). Within the cerebrum. [L *intra*, cerebrum.]
intracervical (in·trah·**ser**'·vik·al). Situated within any cervical canal. [L *intra*, cervix.]
intrachange (in·trah·cha·nj). Chromosome mutation resulting from the exchange of segments within the same chromosome. [L *intra, cambire* to change.]
intrachondral (in·trah·**kon**·dral). Intracartilaginous; endochondral. [L *intra*, chondrus.]
intrachordal (in·trah·**kord**·al). Occurring or situated within the notochord. [L *intra*, chord.]
intracistern, intracisternal (in·trah·**sis**·tern, in·trah·sis·**ter**'·nal). 1. Within any cistern or open space. 2. Within the cerebellomedullary cisterna of the arachnoid mater of the brain. [L *intra*, cistern.]
intracoelial (in·trah·**se**·le·al). Within a cavity of the body. [L *intra, koilia* cavity.]
intracolic (in·trah·**kol**·ik). Inside the colon. [L *intra*, colon.]
intracordal (in·trah·**kord**·al). 1. Within the heart; endocardiac. 2. Originating within the cavity of the heart. [L *intra, cor* heart.]
intracorpuscular (in·trah·kor·**pus**'·kew·lar). Situated within or occurring within a corpuscle, particularly an erythrocyte. [L *intra*, corpuscle.]
intracostal (in·trah·**kos**·tal). On the inner surface of a rib or ribs. [L *intra, costa* rib.]
intracranial (in·trah·**kra**·ne·al). Within the skull. [L *intra*, cranium.]
intracutaneous (in·trah·kew·**ta**'·ne·us). Within the structure of the skin. [L *intra, cutis* skin.]
intracystic (in·trah·**sist**·ik). Lying within a bladder or cyst or occurring within it. [L *intra*, cyst.]
intracytoplasmic (in·trah·si·to·**plaz**'·mik). Within the cell cytoplasm. [L *intra*, cytoplasm.]
intradermal, intradermic (in·trah·**der**·mal, in·trah·**der**·mik). Intracutaneous. [L *intra*, Gk *derma* skin.]
intraduct (in·trah·dukt). Within a duct or the ducts of a secreting gland. [L *intra*, duct.]
intraduodenal (in·trah·dew·o·**de**'·nal). On the inner surface of the duodenum or within the duodenum. [L *intra*, duodenum.]
intradural (in·trah·**dewr**·al). Within the dura mater. [L *intra*, dura mater.]
intra-epidermal, intra-epidermic (in·trah·ep·e·**der**'·mal, in·trah·ep·e·**der**'·mik). Within the substance of the epidermis. [L *intra*, epidermis.]
intra-epiphyseal, intra-epiphysial (in·trah·ep·e·**fiz**'·e·al). Within an epiphysis. [L *intra*, epiphysis.]
intra-epithelial (in·trah·ep·e·**the**'·le·al). Within the epithelium or situated among its cells. [L *intra*, epithelium.]
intrafaradization (in·trah·**far**·ad·i·**za**'·shun). The use of the surged induced (faradic) current on the inner surface of any viscus (e.g. the vagina), for the purpose of stimulating muscle; endofaradism. [L *intra*, faradic current.]
intrafascicular (in·trah·fas·**ik**'·ew·lar). Occurring or situated within the fasciculi of a structure or tissue. [L *intra*, fasciculus.]
intrafebrile (in·trah·**fe**·brile). Occurring during the course of the febrile stage of a disease. [L *intra*, febrile.]
intrafetation (in·trah·fe·**ta**'·shun). The development of a parasitic fetus within the body of the autosite. [L *intra*, fetus.]
intrafilar (in·trah·**fi**·lar). 1. Within a network. 2. Lying within reticular tissue. [L *intra, filum* thread.]
intrafissural (in·tra·**fish**·ewr·al). Lying within a fissure of the brain. [L *intra*, fissure.]
intrafistular (in·trah·**fis**·tew·lar). Within a fistula. [L *intra*, fistula.]
intrafollicular (in·trah·fol·**ik**'·ew·lar). Within a follicle. [L *intra*, follicle.]
intrafusal (in·trah·**few**·zal). Relating or belonging to the striated fibres of a muscle spindle. [L *intra, fusus* spindle.]
intragalvanization (in·trah·**gal**·van·i·**za**'·shun). The application of a direct galvanic current to the inner surface of any organ or body cavity for therapeutic purposes. [L *intra*, galvanic current.]
intragastric (in·trah·**gas**·trik). Situated within the stomach or occurring within it. [L *intra*, Gk *gaster* stomach.]
intragemmal (in·trah·**jem**·al). 1. Within any bulb-like or bud-like body, e.g. a taste bud. 2. Relating or belonging to the nerve terminal fibrils within an end-organ. [L *intra, gemma* bud.]
intraglandular (in·trah·**glan**·dew·lar). Within glandular tissue or inside a gland. [L *intra*, gland.]
intraglobular (in·trah·**glob**·ew·lar). Intracorpuscular. [L *intra*, globule.]
intragyral (in·trah·**ji**·ral). Within a cerebral gyrus. [L *intra*, gyrus.]
intrahepatic (in·trah·hep·**at**'·ik). Inside the liver or within the substance of the liver. [L *intra*, Gk *hepar* liver.]
intrahyoid (in·trah·**hi**·oid). Lying within the hyoid bone, e.g. referring to accessory thyroid glandular tissue which may be within the substance of the bone or in one of its hollows. [L *intra*, hyoid.]
intra-intestinal (in·trah·in·**tes**'·tin·al). Within the intestine or any part of it. [L *intra*, intestine.]
intrajugular (in·trah·**jug**·ew·lar). Inside or internal to the jugular notch or process, or to the jugular vein. [L *intra*, jugular.]
intralamellar (in·trah·lam·**el**'·ar). Within lamellae. [L *intra, lamella* small leaf.]
intralaryngeal (in·trah·lar·**in**'·je·al). Situated or occurring within the larynx. [L *intra*, larynx.]
intraleucocytic (in·trah·lew·ko·**sit**'·ik). Within a leucocyte. [L *intra*, leucocyte.]
intraligamentous (in·trah·lig·am·**en**'·tus). Situated or occurring within any ligament. [L *intra*, ligament.]

intralingual (in·trah·**ling**·gwal). 1. Within the tongue. 2. Referring to the substance of the tongue. [L *intra, lingua* tongue.]

intralobar (in·trah·**lo**·bar). Situated or occurring within a lobe of any structure. [L *intra*, lobe.]

intralobular (in·trah·**lob**·ew·lar). Situated or occurring within a lobule. [see prec.]

intralocular (in·trah·**lok**·ew·lar). Within the small spaces or cavities (loculi) of any tissue. [L *intra*, loculus.]

intralumbar (in·trah·**lum**·bar). Within the lumbar enlargement of the spinal cord. [L *intra*, lumbar.]

intraluminal (in·trah·**lew**·min·al). Within the lumen of any tubular structure or organ. [L *intra*, lumen.]

intralymphatic (in·trah·limf·**at**·ik). Inside a lymph vessel. [L *intra, lympha* water.]

intramammary (in·trah·**mam**·ar·e). Within the mammary gland. [L *intra, mamma* breast.]

intramarginal (in·trah·**mar**·jin·al). Situated or occurring within the margin of any organ or structure. [L *intra*, margin.]

intramastoiditis (in·trah·mas·toid·i′·tis). Inflammation of the tympanic antrum and the mastoid air cells. [L *intra*, mastoiditis.]

intramatrical (in·trah·**ma**·trik·al). Within a matrix. [L *intra*, matrix.]

intramedullary (in·trah·med·**ul**′·ar·e). 1. Occurring or situated within the medulla oblongata. 2. Within the bone marrow. 3. Within the spinal cord. [L *intra*, medulla.]

intramembranous (in·trah·**mem**·bran·us). Formed, occurring, or situated between the layers of a membrane. [L *intra*, membrane.]

intrameningeal (in·trah·men·**in**′·je·al). Situated or occurring within the cerebral meninges or within those of the spinal cord. [L *intra*, meninx.]

intramolecular (in·trah·mol·**ek**′·ew·lar). 1. Occurring within the molecules of a substance. 2. Belonging to molecular structure. [L *intra*, molecule.]

intramural (in·trah·**mewr**·al). 1. Situated or occurring within the substance of the wall of any hollow organ or cavity of the body, as a fibroid. 2. Within the boundaries of an organ or structure. [L *intra, murus* wall.]

intramuscular (in·trah·**mus**·kew·lar). Occurring within the substance of a muscle. [L *intra*, muscle.]

intramyocardial (in·trah·mi·o·**kar**′·de·al). Within the myocardium. [L *intra*, myocardium.]

intranarial (in·trah·**na**·re·al). Inside the nostrils. [L *intra, naris* nostril.]

intranasal (in·trah·**na**·zal). Occurring or situated within the nose or the cavity of the nose. [L *intra, nasus* nose.]

intranatal (in·trah·**na**·tal). 1. At the time of birth. 2. Occurring during the process of birth. [L *intra, natalis* of birth.]

intraneural (in·trah·**newr**·al). Within a nerve. [L *intra*, Gk *neuron* nerve.]

intranidal (in·trah·**ni**·dal). Occurring before birth, i.e. during growth within the nidus of the uterus. [L *intra*, nidus.]

intranuclear (in·trah·**new**·kle·ar). Inside a nucleus. [L *intra*, nucleus.]

intra-ocular (in·trah·**ok**·ew·lar). Occurring or situated within the eyeball. [L *intra, oculus* eye.]

intra-oral (in·trah·**or**·al). Inside the mouth. [L *intra, os* mouth.]

intra-orbital (in·trah·**or**·bit·al). Occurring or situated within the orbit. [L *intra*, orbit.]

intra-ossal, intra-osseous, intra-osteal (in·trah·**os**·al, in·trah·**os**·e·us, in·trah·**os**·te·al). In bony substance; within a bone. [L *intra, os* bone.]

intra-ovarian (in·trah·o·**va**′·re·an). Within an ovary or within its stroma. [L *intra*, ovary.]

intraparenchymatous (in·trah·par·en·**ki**′·mat·us). Within the parenchymal elements of a tissue or organ. [L *intra*, parenchyma.]

intraparietal (in·trah·par·**i**′·et·al). 1. Within the parietal region or lobe of the cerebrum. 2. Intramural. **Intraparietal sulcus.** *See* SULCUS OF PARIETAL LOBE, INTRAPARIETAL. [L *intra, paries* wall.]

intrapartum (in·trah·**par**·tum). During the process of delivery. [L *intra, partus* a bringing forth.]

intrapelvic (in·trah·**pel**·vik). 1. Situated in the pelvic girdle. 2. Occurring within the pelvic cavity. [L *intra*, pelvis.]

intrapericardiac, intrapericardial (in·trah·per·e·**kar**′·de·ak, in·trah·per·e·**kar**′·de·al). Within the pericardium. [L *intra*, pericardium.]

intraperineal (in·trah·per·in·**e**′·al). Within the tissues of the perineum. [L *intra*, perineum.]

intraperitoneal (in·trah·**per**·e·ton·**e**′·al). Occurring within the cavity of the peritoneum. [L *intra*, peritoneum.]

intrapial (in·trah·**pi**·al). Within the pia mater. [L *intra*, pia mater.]

intraplacental (in·trah·plas·**en**′·tal). Within the substance of the placenta. [L *intra*, placenta.]

intrapleural (in·trah·**ploor**·al). Within the pleura or the cavity of the pleura. [L *intra*, pleura.]

intrapontine (in·trah·**pon**·tine). Situated or occurring within the substance of the pons. [L *intra*, pons.]

intraprostatic (in·trah·pros·**tat**′·ik). Situated or occurring within the prostate gland. [L *intra*, prostate.]

intraprotoplasmic (in·trah·pro·to·**plaz**′·mik). Within the protoplasm. [L *intra*, protoplasm.]

intrapsychic, intrapsychical (in·trah·**si**·kik, in·trah·**si**·kik·al). 1. Arising or taking place within the mind. 2. Having to do with both unconscious and conscious processes. [L *intra*, Gk *psyche* mind.]

intrapulmonary (in·trah·**pul**·mon·ar·e). Within the tissue of the lung. [L *intra, pulmo* lung.]

intrapyretic (in·trah·pi·**ret**′·ik). Occurring during the course of the febrile stage of a disease. [L *intra*, Gk *pyr* fire.]

intrarachidian (in·trah·rak·**id**′·e·an). Intraspinal. [L *intra, rhachis* spine.]

intrarectal (in·trah·**rek**·tal). Within the rectum. [L *intra*, rectum.]

intrarenal (in·trah·**re**·nal). Within the kidney. [L *intra, ren* kidney.]

intraretinal (in·trah·**ret**·in·al). Within the tissues of the retina. [L *intra*, retina.]

intrarhachidian (in·trah·rak·**id**′·e·an). Intraspinal. [L *intra, rhachis* spine.]

intrascleral (in·trah·**skleer**·al). 1. Situated or occurring within the sclera. 2. Carried out within the sclera, as an operation. [L *intra*, sclerum.]

intrascrotal (in·trah·**skro**·tal). Within the scrotum. [L *intra*, scrotum.]

intrasellar (in·trah·**sel**·ar). In the interior of the sella turcica. [L *intra*, sella turcica.]

intraserous (in·trah·**seer**·us). Contained or occurring within the blood serum. [L *intra*, serum.]

intraspinal (in·trah·**spi**·nal). 1. Within the substance of the vertebral column. 2. Within the vertebral canal. [L *intra*, spine.]

intrasplenic (in·trah·**splen**·ik). Within the spleen. [L *intra*, spleen.]

intrasternal (in·trah·**ster**·nal). Within the sternum or into the myeloid cavity of the sternum. [L *intra*, sternum.]

intrastitial (in·trah·**stish**·al). Situated or occurring within the fibres or cells of a tissue. [L *intra, sistere* to sit.].

intrastromal (in·trah·**stro**·mal). Situated within the framework of an organ. [L *intra, stroma* mattress.]

intrasynovial (in·trah·si·**no**′·ve·al). Within the cavity of a synovial joint. [L *intra*, synovial.]

intratesticular (in·trah·tes·**tik**′·ew·lar). Within a testis. [L *intra*, testis.]

intrathecal (in·trah·**the**·kal). 1. Within a sheath or coat. 2. Within the intradural or subarachnoid space. [L *intra, theke* sheath.]

intrathenar (in·trah·**the**·nar). Applied to the slight depression present between the thenar and hypothenar eminences of the palm of the hand. [L *intra*, thenar.]

intrathoracic (in·trah·thor·**as**′·ik). In a position or occurring inside the cavity of the thorax. [L *intra*, thorax.]

intratonsillar (in·trah·**ton**·sil·ar). Situated or occurring within the tonsil. **Intratonsillar cleft.** *See* CLEFT. [L *intra*, tonsil.]
intratrabecular (in·trah·trab·**ek**′·ew·lar). Within trabeculae. [L *intra*, trabecula.]
intratracheal (in·trah·**trak**·e·al). In the inside of or inserted into the trachea. [L *intra*, trachea.]
intratubal (in·trah·**tew**·bal). 1. Occurring within or situated within the uterine (fallopian) tube. 2. In the interior of any tube-like organ. [L *intra*, tube.]
intratubular (in·trah·**tew**·bew·lar). Situated or occurring within or among the tubes or tubules of any organ. [L *intra*, tubule.]
intratympanic (in·trah·tim·**pan**′·ik). Situated or occurring within the tympanic cavity. [L *intra*, tympanic cavity.]
intra-ureteral (in·trah·ewr·**e**′·ter·al). Inside the ureter. [L *intra*, ureter.]
intra-urethral (in·trah·ewr·**e**′·thral). Inside the urethra. [L *intra*, urethra.]
intra-uterine (in·trah·**ew**·ter·ine). Within the uterus. [L *intra*, uterus.]
intravaginal (in·trah·vaj·**i**′·nal). Within the vagina. [L *intra*, vagina.]
intravasation (in·trah·vas·**a**′·shun). The introduction or the entrance of exogenous material (e.g. pus) into a vein, artery, or other vessel. [L *intra*, *vas* vessel.]
intravascular (in·trah·**vas**·kew·lar). Situated in or occurring within a vessel or vessels of the body, particularly the blood vessels. [L *intra*, *vasculum* little vessel.]
intravenous (in·trah·**ve**·nus). Within or introduced into a vein. [L *intra*, vein.]
intraventricular (in·trah·ven·**trik**′·ew·lar). Situated in or occurring within a ventricle, e.g. of the heart or brain. [L *intra*, ventricle.]
intravertebral (in·trah·**ver**·te·bral). Within the substance of the vertebral column; intraspinal. [L *intra*, vertebra.]
intravesical (in·trah·**ves**·ik·al). Within the urinary bladder, or within any other bladder. [L *intra*, vesicle.]
intravillous (in·trah·**vil**·us). Within a villus. [L *intra*, villus.]
intravital (in·trah·**vi**·tal). Occurring during life. [L *intra*, *vita* life.]
intravitelline (in·trah·vi·**tel**′·een). In embryology, within the yolk of an egg. [L *intra*, *vitellus* yolk.]
intravitreous (in·trah·**vit**·re·us). Within the vitreous body or humour. [L *intra*, vitreous.]
intrinsic (in·**trin**·sik). 1. Relating or belonging to the essential nature of an organism. 2. Peculiar to any particular organic structure. 3. Included entirely within an organ or part. 4. Inherent; essential. [L *intrinsecus* inside.]
introcession (in·tro·**sesh**·un). An inward sinking of a part or parts so that there is superficial depression. [L *introcedere* to move into.]
introcision (in·tro·**sizh**·un). The tribal practice among aborigines of intentional rupture of the hymen of every female when puberty is reached. [L *intro* inside, *caedere to cut.]*
introducer (in·tro·**dew**·ser). 1. Intubator. 2. Any instrument used for inserting therapeutic appliances and other agents in places within the body. [L *intro* inside, *ducere* to lead.]
See also: BAILEY (H.), RICHES.
introflexion (in·tro·**flek**·shun). 1. The state of being flexed or bent inwards. 2. The act of bending in or flexing inwards. [L *intro* inside, *flectere* to bend.]
introgastric (in·tro·**gas**·trik). 1. Leading into the stomach. 2. Passed or conveyed into the stomach. [L *intro* inside, Gk *gaster* stomach.]
introitus (in·**tro**·it·us). The entrance into any hollow organ or canal; an aperture. **Introitus oesophagi.** The inlet into the stomach from the oesophagus. **Introitus pelvis.** The pelvic inlet, i.e. the communication between the false pelvis and the true pelvis. **Introitus vaginae.** The vulva; the entrance into the vagina. [L *intro* inside, *ire* to go.]
introjection (in·tro·**jek**·shun). A term peculiar to freudian theory and not otherwise employed, meaning a mental process by which the individual identifies himself with another person or object, feeling the latter to be part of himself. [L *intro* inside, *jacere* to throw.]
intromission (in·tro·**mish**·un). The insertion or the admission of one body into another body, as the penis into the vagina. [L *intro* inside, *mittere* to send.]
introspection (in·tro·**spek**·shun). Examination by a person of his own feelings, thoughts, and mental state. **Morbid introspection.** Morbid preoccupation with one's own thoughts and feelings. [L *introspicere* to look inside.]
introsusception (in·tro·sus·**ep**′·shun). Intussusception. [L *intro* inside, *suscipere* to receive.]
introversion (int·tro·**ver**·zhun). 1. A turning of anything within itself. 2. One of the two forms of general psychological orientation and attitude of an individual; that determined by subjective factors, and characterized by a negative attitude to the object. [L *intro* inside, *vertere* to turn.]
introvert (**in**·tro·vert). 1. To bend or turn inwards, as toes. 2. To investigate. 3. An intussusception. 4. In psychology, an individual who is given to introversion. [see prec.]
introvision (in·tro·**vizh**·un). Preoccupation on the part of any person with his own feelings, their meaning and their analysis. [L *intro* inside, vision.]
intrude (in·**trood**). To project in upon or to thrust between. [L *intrudere* to thrust in.]
intrusion (in·**troo**·zhun). Inward projection or penetration. [L *intrudere* to thrust in.]
intubate (**in**·tew·bate). To insert a tube into any organ or part of the body; to catheterize. [see foll.]
intubation (in·tew·**ba**·shun). 1. The therapeutic use of a tube. 2. The introduction of a tube into the larynx through the glottis in order to permit air to pass in and out, as in anaesthesia, diphtheria or in oedema of the glottis. 3. Catheterization. **Blind intubation.** A technique of inserting a tracheal tube from the nose into the larynx without the use of a laryngoscope. First described by Ivan Magill and Stanley Rowbotham in 1920. **Nasotracheal intubation.** A technique of introducing a tube from the naris into the trachea, either under direct vision via a laryngoscope, or "blind". First described in 1920 by Magill and Rowbotham. **Tracheal intubation.** The passage of a breathing tube from either the mouth or the nose into the trachea. Also known as *endotracheal intubation*, and *intratracheal intubation.* [L *in*, tube.]
intubator (**in**·tew·ba·tor). An instrument for passing a tube in the process of intubation.
intumesce (in·tewm·**es**). 1. To enlarge by swelling out. 2. In chemistry, an obsolete term, to expand with heat. [L *intumescere* to swell.]
intumescence (in·tewm·**es**·ens). 1. A swelling of an organ or part of the body. 2. The process of becoming swollen. [see prec.]
intumescent (in·tewm·**es**·ent). Becoming swollen or expanded; enlarging; inflating. [L *intumescere* to swell.]
intussusception (in·tus·sus·**ep**′·shun). The invagination or telescoping of one segment of the gastro-intestinal tract into an adjacent and usually lower segment, commonly with the production of obstruction and strangulation of the invaginated portion. **Agonal intussusception.** Intussusception occurring at death in the course of the exaggerated intestinal movement which may occur terminally. **Appendicular intussusception.** The invagination or inversion of the appendix into the caecum. **Chronic intussusception.** Long-standing or repeated intussusception, usually without sufficient constriction of the telescoped part to produce the effects of strangulation. **Colon intussusception, colonic intussusception.** Invagination of one segment of colon into an adjacent segment. **Compound intussusception.** Invagination into an adjacent loop of bowel of a fully formed intussusception, to give a swelling which includes five layers of bowel wall. **Double intussusception.** Compound intussusception (see prec.). **Enteric intussusception.** Invagination of a loop of small intestine into an adjacent loop of small intestine. **Gastroduodenal intussusception.** Telescoping of the pyloric antrum of the stomach into the first part of the duodenum. **Ileocaecal**

intussusception. Invagination of the ileum into the caecum and ascending colon, the ileocolic valve forming the apex of the telescoping loop. **Ileocolic intussusception.** Intussusception of a loop of ileum through the ileocolic valve into the caecum and ascending colon. **Jejunogastric intussusception.** Invagination distoproximally of a jejunal loop through a gastrojejunostomy stoma into the stomach. **Multiple intussusception.** Simultaneous occurrence of telescoping at several levels in the intestinal canal, usually either a sequel of gastro-enteritis, or agonal (see above). **Postmortem intussusception.** Invagination of a loop of small intestine into an adjacent loop after the moment of death, death of the intestine being delayed for a little after death of the individual. **Retrograde intussusception.** Invagination of a segment of the gastro-intestinal tract into an adjacent and proximal segment. **Secondary intussusception.** Intussusception secondary to a tumour of the bowel, which is passed onwards as if it were a foreign body, drawing after it the loop of intestine to which it is attached. [L *intus* within, *suscipere* to receive.]

See also: WOODHALL.

intussusceptum (in·tus·sus·**ep**'·tum). In intussusception, the segment of bowel that is invaginated into the other part. [L *intus* within, *susceptus* received.]

intussuscipiens (in·tus·sus·**ip**'·e·enz). In intussusception, the segment of bowel into which the other part is invaginated. [L *intus* within, *suscipiens* receiving.]

Inula (in·ew·lah). A genus of herbs (family Compositae). The rhizome and roots of *Inula helenium* Linn. (elecampane) have antiseptic properties, and are used in the form of the extract as a remedy for coughs and bronchitis. [L, elecampane.]

Inulin BP 1973 (in·ew·lin). A polysaccharide; a white, amorphous, granular powder obtained from the tubers of *Dahlia variabilis, Helianthus tuberosus* and other genera of the family Compositae. It is a dignostic agent used as Inulin Injection (BP) for the measurement of glomerular filtration rate. [*Inula*.]

inunction (in·**ungk**·shun). 1. The process or act of rubbing an ointment or oily substance into the skin. 2. Any ointment or oily substance so employed. [L *in, unguere* to smear.]

inunctum (in·**ungk**·tum). Any ointment or oily substance used for rubbing into the skin. [see prec.]

inustion (in·**us**·chun). 1. The act of applying actual cautery. 2. Deep cauterization. [L *in, urere* to burn.]

invaccination (in·**vak**·sin·**a**'·shun). The accidental inoculation with the virus of some other disease while vaccination against smallpox is being carried out. [L *in,* vaccination.]

invaginate (in·**vaj**·in·ate). To push back one portion of a tube or fold into another portion, so that the former is ensheathed by the latter. [L *in, vagina* sheath.]

invaginated (in·**vaj**·in·a·ted). Inserted or folded in as into a sheath. [see prec.]

invagination (in·vaj·in·**a**'·shun). 1. Intussusception. 2. Operative treatment of a hernia by reducing it and preventing its recurrence by forming a sheath of tissue which obliterates the opening. [L *in, vagina* sheath.]

invaginator (in·**vaj**·in·a·tor). In the surgical treatment of hernia, an instrument used to turn in the tissues. [see prec.]

invalid (**in**·val·id). 1. Feeble. 2. Suffering from ill health, particularly chronic ill health. 3. An infirm and weak person. 4. Denoting anything designed or arranged for the needs of a person suffering from ill health, as diet, chair, etc. [L *in, validus* strong, healthy.]

invalidism (**in**·val·id·izm). 1. The condition of being a chronic invalid; infirmity. 2. A state of permanent ill health.

invasion (in·**va**·zhun). The first attack or onset of a disease or the entrance and establishment of parasites into the body of a host, whether producing ill-effects or not. [L *in, vadere* to go.]

invasiveness (in·**va**·siv·nes). The ability of a micro-organism to gain a footing and spread within the tissues of the host. [see prec.]

inversion (in·**ver**·shun). 1. A reversal of the normal relations of an organ, such as turning inside out or upside down; transposition of the viscera. 2. The reversal of the sexual instincts; homosexuality. 3. The turning round of a part of a chromosome so that the genes on it are in reverse linear order. 4. A temperature record in which the highest temperatures are in the morning. 5. In chemistry, the changing of an optically-active compound into its opposite isomer, or the changing of a compound into its geometrical isomer, e.g. *cis-* to *trans-*, or *anti-* to *syn-*. 6. In cytogenetics, an intrachromosomal structural change leading to an inverted arrangement of the loci belonging to a segment of the chromosome in relation to all the others. **Inversion of the bladder.** A rare condition which occurs only in females, when the whole bladder may be inverted into the urethra. The part projecting beyond the orifice of the ureter appears pedunculated and is covered by mucous membrane which bleeds easily. Occasionally the ureteric orifice may be seen. The protrusion is increased on coughing and straining and there is incontinence. **Carbohydrate inversion.** The hydrolysis of a compound saccharide into monosaccharides with accompanying reversal of optical activity; thus cane sugar (dextrorotatory) is hydrolysed into a mixture of glucose and fructose which is laevorotatory. **Lateral inversion.** The inversion observed when an object is viewed in a plane mirror. **Paracentric inversion.** Inversion involving a chromosome region which does not contain the centromere. **Pericentric inversion.** Inversion involving a region containing the centromere; this may produce a change in the chromosome arm ratio. **Sexual inversion.** Homosexuality. **Inversion of the uterus.** The turning out of the uterus. [L *invertere* to turn upside down.]

See also: WALDEN.

inversive (in·**ver**·siv). Describing the enzyme which brings about the hydrolysis of sucrose into the mixture of glucose and fructose known as *invert sugar.* [see foll.]

invert (**in**·vert). 1. An individual who is a homosexual or tends towards homosexuality. 2. In organic chemistry, to subject to inversion. [L *invertere* to turn upside down.]

invertase (in·**ver**·taze). Sucrase, saccharase; an enzyme occurring widely in plants, fungi, bacteria, yeasts, and the intestinal secretions of animals, which hydrolyses cane sugar (sucrose) producing fructose and glucose in equimolecular proportions. The hydrolysis is commonly known as *inversion* and the product as *invert sugar,* the terms arising from the change in optical rotation from positive to negative which occurs as the reaction proceeds. The enzyme has an optimum pH value of 4.5. [invert.]

invertebral (in·**ver**·te·bral). Without a vertebral column. [L *in, vertebra* joint.]

invertebrata (in·ver·te·**bra**'·tah). In zoology, a collective designation for animals without a vertebral column. [see foll.]

invertebrate (in·**ver**·te·brate). 1. Without a vertebral column. 2. Relating to the invertebrata. [L *in, vertebra* joint.]

invertin (in·**ver**·tin). Invertase.

invertor (in·**ver**·tor). A muscle which is responsible for inward rotation of a part. [L *in, vertere* to turn.]

invertose (**in**·ver·toze). Invert sugar.

investing (in·**ves**·ting). The process of embedding crowns, bridges, and dentures in a plaster-like substance during their fabrication. [L *investire* to clothe.]

investiture (in·**vest**·it·ewr). Investment.

investment (in·**vest**·ment). An external covering or sheath, e.g. of a cell or part. **Fibrous investment.** A fibrous sheath formed from connective tissue around an anatomical structure, but distinct from its capsule. **Myelin investment.** Medullary sheath. *See* SHEATH. [L *investire* to clothe.]

inveterate (in·**vet**·er·ate). Deep-rooted; of long standing; chronic; confirmed; habitual; difficult to cure. [L *in, vetus* old.]

invious (**in**·ve·us). Not allowing passage; that cannot be penetrated. [L *in, via* way.]

inviscation (in·vis·**ka**·shun). The mixing of saliva with food during mastication; insalivation. [L *in, viscum* bird-lime.]

involucre, involucrum (in·vol·ew·ker, in·vol·ew·krum). 1. In necrosis, the sheath of new bone which forms about a sequestrum. 2. In botany and zoology, a sheath or enveloping membrane. [L *involvere* to roll up.]

involuntary (in·**vol**·un·tar·e). Independently of the will, e.g. a movement so performed; in psychology, any action performed in opposition to or independently of the will or choice. [L *in, voluntas* will.]

involute (**in**·vol·ewt). Having the edges turned in. [L *involvere* to roll up.]

involuted (**in**·vol·ew·ted). Reduced to normal size after distension or enlargement. [See foll.]

involution (in·vol·**ew**·shun). 1. A turning inward. 2. The reduction of an organ in size; the shrinking of an organ to its original size. 3. The physiological degeneration of organs or tissues. 4. The appearance of abnormal forms of micro-organisms in old cultures or in unfavourable conditions. **Buccal involution.** The infolding of ectoderm to form the embryonic mouth cavity. **Pituitary involution.** The formation of a recess in the roof of the embryonic buccal cavity whose walls will give rise to the anterior lobe of the pituitary gland. **Senile involution.** The slow degenerate changes in senility, causing the shrinking of organs. **Sexual involution.** Cessation of the menstrual flow. **Involution of the uterus.** The process by which the uterus returns to its normal state following pregnancy. [L *involvere* to roll up.]

involutional (in·vol·**ew**·shun·al). 1. Relating or belonging to involution. 2. Occurring during involution. 3. Caused by the process of involution.

iodaemia (i·od·e·me·ah). The presence of iodides in the blood. [iodide, Gk *haima* blood.]

iodalbumin (i·od·**al**·bew·min). Albumin in which iodine has been chemically incorporated. It has properties similar to, but far weaker than, thyroglobulin.

Iodamide (i·o·dam·id). BP Commission approved name for α,5-di(acetamido)-2,4,6-tri-iodo-*m*-toluic-acid; a contrast medium.

Iodamoeba (i·od·am·**e**′·bah). A genus of Amoebae (synonym *Pseudolimax*) of which *Iodamoeba bütschlii* is a not uncommon parasite of the large intestine. The adults reach about 20 μm and resemble *Entamoeba coli*, except in the nuclei. The cysts are known as iodine cysts; they contain volutin and also glycogen which can be demonstrated with iodine solution. This species is widely distributed and is probably non-pathogenic. [iodine, amoeba.]

iodate (i·o·date). Applied to any salt of iodic acid.

iodated, iodatum (i·o·da·ted, i·o·**da**·tum). Iodized.

iodeosin (i·o·**de**·o·sin). Erythrosin, tetraiodofluorescein, $C_{20}H_8O_5I_4$. A yellowish-red fluorescent dyestuff, the iodine analogue of eosin. It is used as a pH indicator (1.5–2.5).

iodide (i·o·dide). Any salt of hydriodic acid; those usually employed in medicine are of sodium or potassium. Iodides are readily absorbed from the intestine and rapidly excreted, partly by the kidneys and partly through the salivary and mucous glands, the secretions of which are thereby increased. They are administered as expectorants and in the treatment of some forms of asthma on account of their action on the mucous glands of the bronchi. Similar action on the mucous glands of the nose and throat leads to their employment in catarrh. They are also used as a source of iodine in the treatment of endemic goitre.

iodimetric (i·o·de·**met**′·rik). Relating to iodimetry.

iodimetry (i·o·**dim**·et·re). 1. The volumetric determination of free iodine in a mixture by titration with standard solutions of sodium thiosulphate, with starch as an indicator. 2. The indirect estimation of other substances which displace iodine, the latter being determined in turn by the above method. [iodine, meter.]

iodination (i·o·din·a′·shun). 1. The treatment of a substance with iodine. 2. The addition of iodine to a mixture, or its compounding.

iodine (i·o·deen). A halogen non-metallic element, of atomic weight 126.90, atomic number 53, and chemical symbol I. It is a black substance occurring in scales that are readily volatile, forming a violet vapour with a pungent odour. It is obtained commercially from seaweed, and from the heavy deposits of sodium iodate found with the nitrate in Chile. The element occurs in plants and animals to a minute extent, in man principally in the thyroid gland as thyroxine. It is soluble in alcohol and in solutions of iodides, such solutions being applied externally to the skin as an antiseptic and sterilizer; as it is an irritant it is of value as a counter-irritant. It is essential in the diet; deficiency produces colloid goitre, often endemic in localities, and indirectly cretinism. Iodine (BP 1973) is used in the prophylaxis of goitre, in the pre-operative treatment of thyrotoxicosis, and in expectorants. **Butanol-extractable iodine (BEI).** *See* DYSHORMOGENESIS. **Iodine bromides.** Iodine tribromide, IBr_3, and iodine pentabromide, IBr_5; fluids which have been used as throat sprays. **Iodine chloride.** Iodine trichloride (see following). **Iodine trichloride.** ICl_3, a yellowish-brown crystalline substance with a pungent odour, soluble in water and organic solvents; it has been used in a 1 per cent solution as an antiseptic. [Gk *ioeides* violet-like.]

iodine-basedow (i·o·deen·**bas**′·e·dow, **bas**·e·dove). A name given by Continental writers to hyperthyroidism that has been caused by the administration of iodine in excess to persons with endemic goitre. [K. A. von *Basedow*.]

iodinophil, iodinophile (i·o·**din**·o·fil, i·o·**din**·o·file). Iodophil.

iodinophilous (i·o·din·**of**′·il·us). Iodophil.

Iodipamide (i·o·**dip**·am·ide). BP Commission approved name for *NN′* - di - (3 - carboxy - 2,4,6 - tri - iodophenyl)adipdiamide; a contrast medium.

iodism (i·o·dizm). A morbid condition caused by the continuous use of iodine or iodine compounds, characterized *inter alia* by frontal headache, excessive salivation, sensation of cold in the head, skin eruptions and glandular disorders.

iodize (i·o·dize). 1. To treat with iodine. 2. To charge with iodine.

iodoacetate (i·o·do·**as**′·et·ate). ICH_2COOH, an inhibitor of thiol-containing enzymes and carrier proteins. Classically associated with the elucidation of the glycolytic sequence through its inhibition of glyceraldehyde 3-phosphate dehydrogenase.

iodochlorhydroxyquin (i·o·do·klor·hi·**drox**′·e·kwin). Clioquinol.

iodochlorhydroxyquinoline (i·o·do·klor·hi·drox·e·**kwin**′·o·leen). C_9H_5NOClI. An amoebacide; also used as an antiseptic dusting powder.

iododerma (i·o·do·**der**′·mah). Any eruption of the skin which is caused by the internal administration of iodine. [iodine, Gk *derma* skin.]

Iodoform BPC 1954 (i·o·do·form). Tri-iodomethane, CHI_3. A yellow crystalline substance, with a pungent odour and unpleasant taste. It is only very slightly soluble in water, but soluble in fixed and volatile oils, and has been used as an antiseptic, particularly as a wound dressing, in the form of a paste. It has very weak germicidal powers, and has been largely superseded nowadays in view of its toxicity on absorption. [iodine, chloroform.]

iodoformism (i·o·do·**form**′·izm). Poisoning caused by the absorption of excessive amounts of iodoform.

iodoformize (i·o·do·**form**′·ize). 1. To treat with iodoform. 2. To charge or combine with iodoform.

iodohydrargyrate (i·o·do·hi·**drar**′·ji·rate). Name applied to a compound of mercuric iodide with the iodide of another metal, e.g. $HgI_2{\cdot}2KI$.

iodolography (i·o·do·**log**′·raf·e). Radiographic examination of an organ or part of the body by injection into it of iodized oil. [iodized oil, Gk *graphein* to write.]

iodometry (i·o·**dom**·et·re). Iodimetry.

iodophil, iodophile (i·o·do·fil, i·o·do·file). 1. Readily taking an iodine stain. 2. Combining easily with iodine. 3. Any tissue that takes an iodine stain. [iodine, Gk *philein* to love.]

Iodophthalein BP 1953 (i·o·do·**thal**·e·in). Tetraiodophenolphthalein, $COONaC_6H_4C(C_6H_2I_2O)(C_6H_2I_2ONa)$. A yellow disodium salt formed by the iodination of phenolphthalein in a solution of sodium hydroxide, and used as a contrast medium for radiography of the gall bladder and bile duct, since it is excreted in the bile and is opaque to x-rays. There is a certain danger of necrosis in its use, necessitating caution.

iodopsin (i·o·**dop**·sin). Visual violet, a visual pigment found in the cones of the retina. [Gk *ioeides* violet-like, *optikos* sight.]

iodopyracet (i·o·do·pi'·ras·et). The non-proprietary title for a solu- of the British product diodone, used as a contrast medium, chiefly for intravenous pyelography.

iodopyrin (i·o·do·pi·rin). Antipyrin iodide, $C_{11}H_{11}N_2OI$. A colourless crystalline substance containing about 40 per cent of iodine, and administered as a source of iodide ions.

iodostick (i·o·do·stik). An applicator tipped with a mixture of iodine and potassium iodide. [iodine, AS *sticca*.]

iodoterpene (i·o·do·ter'·peen). Terpene hydriodide, $C_{10}H_{16}{\cdot}HI$. A compound employed as an antiseptic.

iodotherapy (i·o·do·ther'·ap·e). The treatment of a disease by the administration of iodine or of an iodide. [iodine, therapy.]

Iodothiouracil (i·o·do·thi·o·ewr'·as·il). BP Commission approved name for 5-iodo-2-thiouracil, the iodine derivative of the antithyroid drug thiouracil with the advantage over the latter than no pre-operative iodine administration is necessary. It is administered orally as the sodium salt.

iodothyroglobulin (i·o·do·thi·ro·glob'·ew·lin). Thyroglobulin; an iodine-containing protein present in the colloid matter of the thyroid gland; it may be isolated by saline extraction of thyroid tissue and precipitation of the extract with saturated ammonium sulphate solution. Hydrolysis yields thyroxine and di-iodotyrosine. Thyroglobulin is regarded as the natural thyroid hormone, which plays an important rôle in determining the level of tissue metabolism.

iodotyrosine (i·o·do·tir·o·sen). The tyrosine molecule with one iodine substituent (monoiodotyrosine) or two substituents (diiodotyrosine). Condensation of one molecule of monoiodotyrosine and one molecule of diiodotyrosine produces triiodothyronine (T_3) and of two molecules of diiodotyrosine produces tetraiodothyronine (14, thyroxine).

iodoventriculography (i·o·do·ven·trik·ew·log'·raf·e). Contrast visualization by x-rays of the ventricles of the brain after injection into them of iodized oil. [iodized oil, ventricle, Gk *graphein* to write.]

Iodoxyl BP 1958 (i·o·dox·il). $C_3H_3O_5NI_2Na_2$, the disodium salt of *N*-methyl-3,5-di-iodo-4-pyridone-2,6-dicarboxylic acid, used mainly in intravenous pyelography for examination of the kidneys and urinary tract.

Iodum. *European Pharmacopoeia* name for Iodine BP 1973.

ioduria (i·o·dewr·e·ah). The presence of iodides in the urine.

ion (i·on). An atom or group of atoms bearing an electrical charge, a positive ion (cation) having shed one or more electrons, a negative ion (anion) having gained them. Ions may be created by dissociation in solution, or in gases by the passage of an electrical discharge, ionizing rays (e.g. x-rays, γ-rays), or ultraviolet light. **Acid ion.** An electronegative atom or radical produced by the dissociation of an acid in solution. **Amphoteric ion, dipolar ion.** Zwitterion. **Ion exchange.** *See* ION-EXCHANGE. **Gram-ion.** *See* GRAM-ION. **Hydrogen ion.** H^+, the proton; the hydrogen atom deprived of an electron and therefore positively charged. Its presence confers acid properties on a solution. **Hydronium ion, hydroxonium ion.** The hydrogen ion associated with a molecule of water, H_3O^+. It occurs in acid solutions. **Hydroxyl ion.** OH^-. **Sulphide ion.** The negative ion, S^{2-}, of divalent sulphur. **Sulphite ion.** The negative divalent ion, SO_3^{2-}. [Gk *ion* going.]

ion-exchange (i·on·ex·cha'·nj). A phenomenon in which labile ions, positive or negative, in solution, may replace ions of similar charge in material with which the solution comes in contact. The process has been used widely in water softening, the "hardness" (calcium and magnesium ions) being replaced by sodium ions. Many synthetic resins have been prepared which exhibit the property, and these have been used in medicine to reduce the sodium ions in the body in cases of oedema, or to replace potassium ions by sodium ions in anuria. They have also been found of value in removing the calcium ion from blood to prevent coagulation during storage in blood banks. Excess acid in the stomach can be reduced by ion-exchange without the production of excess alkalinity, as would be the case in the use of sodium bicarbonate for the purpose. *See* RESINS, ION-EXCHANGE. [ion, OFr. *eschangier.*]

ion-protein (i·on·pro·te·in). The zwitterion of a protein united to an inorganic ion when above or below the iso-electric point.

ionic (i·on·ik). Relating to or having the properties of ions.

ionium (i·o·ne·um). A natural radioactive isotope of thorium having a mass number of 230. [Gk *ion* going.]

ionization (i·on·i·za'·shun). 1. Ionic dissociation; the splitting of molecules of electrolytes in aqueous solutions into atoms or groups of atoms bearing electrical charges of opposite sign. 2. The production of charged atoms or molecules in a gas by x-rays, nuclear radiation or electric discharge. **Medical ionization.** Iontophoresis. **Specific ionization of an ionizing particle.** The linear density of the ions along the path of an ionizing particle. Specific ionization varies as the square of the charge of the particle, and is a complicated function of its speed. In general, large differences in specific ionization occur between x-rays and β-rays on the one hand, and heavy particle radiation (α-rays, protons, neutrons, etc.) on the other.

ionize (i·on·ize). 1. To split into ions. 2. To gain or lose electrons, thereby becoming charged electrically.

ionocolorimeter (i·on·o·kol·or·im'·et·er). A colorimetric range of standard tubes containing solutions with appropriate indicators, used for the rapid determination of pH value by comparison. [ion, colorimeter.]

ionogen (i·on·o·jen). Formerly applied to any substance that produces ions in solution; an electrolyte. [ion, Gk *genein* to produce.]

ionogenic (i·on·o·jen'·ik). Capable of producing ions; dissociating in solution. [see prec.]

ionometer (i·on·om·et·er). Iontoquantimeter.

ionone (i·o·none). A terpene with an odour of violets, occurring in two isomeric forms, α- and β-, and both isomeric with irone. It is used as an artificial perfume. [Gk *ion* violet.]

ionophoresis (i·o·no·for·e'·sis). Iontophoresis.

ionophose (i·on·o·foze). A phose with which the colour violet is associated. [Gk *ion* violet, phose.]

ionotherapy (i·on·o·ther'·ap·e). 1. Treatment of disease by the application of ultraviolet rays. 2. Iontophoresis. [ion, therapy.]

iontherapy (i·on·ther·ap·e). Iontophoresis. [ion, therapy.]

iontophoresis (i·on·to·for·e'·sis). The introduction of therapeutic ions into the tissues by direct current, the selection of the active electrode depending on the charge carried by the ion to be introduced, e.g. histamine is driven in from the positive pole, and the iodine ion from the negative pole. Also known as *galvano-* or *medical ionization.* [ion, Gk *pherein* to carry.]

iontoquantimeter (i·on·to·kwon·tim'·et·er). Ionometer; an instrument for measuring the quantity or intensity of an x-ray beam. The beam ionizes air in a closed chamber and the current so produced is proportional to the intensity of the x-rays. [ion, L *quantus* how much, meter.]

iontoradiometer (i·on·to·ra·de·om'·et·er). Iontoquantimeter. [ion, radiation, meter.]

iontotherapy (i·on·to·ther'·ap·e). The treatment of certain bodily conditions by the introduction of therapeutic ions into the tissues by a constant current (iontophoresis). [ion, therapy.]

Iophendylate (i·o·fen·di·late). BP Commission approved name for ethyl-10-*p*-iodophenylundecanoate; a contrast medium.

iophobia (i·o·fo·be·ah). Morbid fear of poisons; toxicophobia. [Gk *ios* poison (particularly of snakes), phobia.]

iopropane (i·o·pro·pane). Di-iodohydroxypropane, $C_3H_5(OH)I_2$. An oily substance with a high iodine content, used for inunction.

Iopydol (i·o·pi·dol). BP Commission approved name for *N*-(2,3-dihydroxypropyl)-3,5-di-iodo-4-pyridone; a radio-opaque substance.

Iopydone (i·o·pi·done). BP Commission approved name for 3,5-di-iodo-4-pyridone; a radio-opaque substance.

iotacism (i·o·tas·izm). 1. Defective speech characterized by the repeated and incorrect use of the *ee* sound. 2. Speech defect consisting of lack of ability to produce the sound of *ee.* [Gk letter *iota.*]

ipecacuanha (ip·e·kak·ew·**an'**·ah). Ipecacuanhae radix, ipecacuanha root, the dried root, or rhizome and root, of the shrubs *Cephaëlis ipecacuanha* (Brot.) A. Rich, or *C. acuminata* Karsten, which are found in South America, and in Malaya and Burma. Many different varieties are described, commonly by names indicating their country of origin. The chief constituents are the two alkaloids, emetine and cephaeline, of which emetine is the more important. Ipecacuanha irritates the alimentary canal, causing nausea, vomiting and diarrhoea, and reflexly increasing the sweat- and bronchial-gland secretions. It was considered formerly that doses less than that required for emesis would still increase bronchial secretion, but there is no sure evidence for this theory. In spite of this, the drug is still widely used in expectorant cough medicines (BP 1973), but is rarely used now as an emetic. **Ipecacuanha Liquid Extract BP 1973.** An extract containing 2 per cent of total ipecacuanha alkaloids, calculated as emetine. **Ipecacuanha and Opium Powder BP 1963.** Dover's powder, a powder containing 10 per cent each of prepared ipecacuanha and powdered opium. It has mild sedative, analgesic, and diaphoretic properties, and is widely used in coryza and other mild febrile states. **Prepared Ipecacuanha BP 1973, Ipecacuanha pulverata.** Light-grey or yellowish-brown powder, with a bitter taste, containing 2 per cent of ipecacuanha alkaloids, calculated as emetine. **Ipecacuanha Tincture BP 1973.** A tincture containing 0.1 per cent of total ipecacuanha alkaloids, calculated as emetine. **Ipecacuanhae Pulvis Normatus.** *European Pharmacopoeia* name for Prepared Ipecacuanha BP 1973. **Ipecacuanhae Radix.** *European Pharmacopoeia* name for Ipecacuanha BP 1973. [Port. from local Brazilian name.]

ipecacuanhin (ip·e·kak·ew·**an'**·in). A glycoside in ipecacuanha root. It has little pharmacological action.

ipecine (**ip**·e·seen). Emetine.

ipoh (**ee**·po). An arrow poison used in Malaya, derived from *Antiaris toxicaria* Lesch and causing vomiting, prostration and convulsions. Another poison from *Derris elliptica* Benth. is also used under this name for tipping arrows and killing fish under water; it acts by paralysis of respiration. **Ipoh aker.** An arrow poison from *Strychnos wallichiana* Benth. causing paralysis of peripheral nerves. [Malay.]

Ipomoea (i·po·**me**·ah). 1. A genus of tropical and subtropical climbing herbs and shrubs (family Convolvulaceae) in which the roots or tubers contain a resin having purgative properties. Several species are used medicinally, the most important being *Ipomoea orizabensis* (Pellet.) Ledanois (Ipomoea BPC 1963), and *I. purga* Hayne (Jalap BPC 1963). Others include *I. simulans* Hanbury (Tampico jalap) and *I. tuberosa* Linn. (Brazilian jalap). 2. Ipomoea (BPC 1963), ipomoeae radix, Orizaba jalap root, Mexican scammony root, the dried root of *I. orizabensis* (Pellet.) obtained from Mexico. It is usually administered as ipomoea resin, of which it yields about 12 to 18 per cent. **Ipomoea Resin BPC 1963.** Scammony resin, the crude resin obtained from Ipomoea by extraction with alcohol. It is a complex mixture consisting chiefly of glycosides of jalapinolic acid and its derivatives. It is a rapidly-acting drastic purgative. [Gk *ips* woodworm, *homoios* like.]

Ipratropium Bromide (ip·rah·**tro**·pe·um **bro**·mide). BP Commission approved name for 8-isopropyl-3-(±)-tropoyloxy-1αH,5αH-tropanium bromide; a bronchodilator.

Iprindole (i·**prin**·dole). BP Commission approved name for 5-(3-dimethylaminopropyl)-6,7,8,9,10,11-hexahydrocyclo-oct[*b*]-indole; an antidepressant.

Iproclozide (i·**pro**·klo·zide). BP Commission approved name for *N*-4-chlorophenoxyacetyl -*N'*-isopropylhydrazine; a monoamine oxidase inhibitor.

Iproniazid (i·pron·i·az·id). BP Commission approved name for *N*-isonicotinoyl-*N*-isopropylhydrazine; the isopropyl derivative of isoniazid. A monoamine oxidase inhibitor.

ipsation (ip·**sa**·shun). Sexual pleasure from stimulation of various parts of the body, e.g. breasts, external genitalia, anus. [Gk *ipse* same.]

ipselateral, ipsilateral, ipsolateral (ip·se·**lat**·er·al, ip·so·**lat**·er·al). Occurring or located on the same side; denoting symptoms of paralysis or other disorder which are present on the same side as the cerebral lesion which has caused them. [L *ipse* same, *latus* side.]

iralgia (ir·**al**·je·ah). Iridalgia.

irascibility (ir·**as**·ib·**il'**·it·e). Morbid irritability, particularly the irritability or choleric temper that is often present in neurasthenia and in certain types of insanity. [L *irasci* to be wrathful.]

iridadenosis (ir·id·ad·en·**o'**·sis). The production of adenomatous growths by an iris. [iris, adenosis.]

iridaemia (ir·id·e·me·ah). Haemorrhage from the iris. [iris, Gk *haima* blood.]

iridal (**ir**·id·al). Iridic.

iridalgia (ir·id·**al**·je·ah). Pain in the iris, or pain referred to the iris. [iris, Gk *algos* pain.]

iridauxesis (**ir**·id·awx·**e'**·sis). Thickened or swollen iris. [iris, Gk *auxe* increase.]

iridavulsion (ir·id·av·**ul'**·shun). Irido-avulsion.

iridectome (ir·id·**ek**·tome). An instrument with a cutting edge used in excision of a portion of the iris. [iris, Gk *ektome* a cutting out.]

iridectomesodialysis (ir·id·**ek**·to·**mez**·o·di·**al'**·is·is). The making of an artificial pupil by removal of the iris from the ciliary ligament. [iris, Gk *ektome* a cutting out, *mesos* middle, *dialysis* a loosing.]

iridectomize (ir·id·**ek**·tom·ize). To perform the operation of iridectomy; to remove a portion of the iris.

iridectomy (ir·id·**ek**·to·me). Removal of a portion of the iris. There are several types of iridectomy, e.g. *basal* or *peripheral*, when a small portion is removed from the base of the iris; *buttonhole*, when only a small piece of the iris is removed; *complete*, when the portion removed includes the whole width of the iris; *glaucoma iridectomy*, when a wide iridectomy is performed for relief of congestive glaucoma; *optical*, to provide a new pupil, when the cornea overlying the original pupil is deformed or opaque; *preliminary*, usually to be followed in 4–6 weeks by cataract extraction; and *therapeutic*, to prevent recurrences of iritis. **Basal iridectomy.** Peripheral iridectomy (see below). **Broad iridectomy.** Excision of a large area of the iris, including the pupillary margin, leaving a key-hole type deficit. **Buttonhole iridectomy.** Peripheral iridectomy (see below). **Complete iridectomy.** Broad iridectomy (see above). **Glaucoma iridectomy.** *See* MAIN DEF. (above). **Optical iridectomy.** One performed to make a new pupil and improve vision when there are central opacities of the cornea or lens present preventing light beams reaching the retina through the normal pupil. **Peripheral iridectomy.** Excision of a small area of the iris at its periphery and not including the pupillary border. **Preliminary iridectomy.** One proposed as a preliminary operation before extraction of a cataract; the object is to see how the eye reacts to the more minor procedure before embarking on the major. It was used in cases of secondary or complicated cataracts, but is rarely used nowadays. **Therapeutic iridectomy.** Iridectomy performed to prevent recurrences of iritis. **Wide iridectomy.** Peripheral iridectomy (see above). [iris, Gk *ektome* excision.]

iridectropium (ir·id·ek·**tro'**·pe·um). Eversion of the iris. [iris, ectropion.]

iridencleisis (ir·id·en·**kli'**·sis). A filtering operation first described by Holth. A scleral incision is made at the angle of the anterior chamber, and a meridianal cut is made in the iris through the sphincter and either one or both pillars are left in the wound to help form a filtering cicatrix. Also called *iris inclusion operation.* [iris, Gk *egklein* to shut in.]

iridentropium (ir·id·en·**tro'**·pe·um). Inversion of the iris or of a portion of it. [iris, entropion.]

irideremia (ir·id·e·**re'**·me·ah). Congenital absence of a part or of the whole of the iris. [iris, Gk *eremia* want of.]

iridescence (ir·id·**es**·ens). 1. The play of rainbow-like interference colours on the surface of a substance. 2. The property of being able to break light up into the colours of the spectrum. [L *iridescere* to gleam like a rainbow.]

iridescent (ir·id·es·ent). Displaying a combination of rainbow colours; gleaming like mother of pearl. [see prec.]

iridesis (ir·id·e·sis). A method of making an artificial pupil by fixing a small strip of iris tissue to the site of incision in the cornea. Obsolete. [iris, Gk *desis* a binding together.]

iridiagnosis (ir·e·di·ag·**no**′·sis). Iridodiagnosis.

iridial, iridian (ir·**id**·e·al, ir·**id**·e·an). Iridic.

iridic (ir·**id**·ik). Relating or belonging to the iris.

iridicolour (ir·**id**·e·kul·or). Iridescent. [iris, colour.]

Iridis Rhizoma BPC 1949 (ir·**id**·is ri·**zo**·mah). Orris.

iridium (ir·**id**·e·um). An element of atomic weight 192.2, atomic number 77, and chemical symbol Ir, found with platinum in alluvial sands. It is a hard silvery metal, unattacked by aqua regia; used in platinum alloys for tipping gold pen-nibs, and for the manufacture of incorrodible chemical ware, also for thermocouples. It forms salts of many colours. The radioactive isotope is used for curietherapy. [Gk *iris* rainbow.]

iridization (ir·id·i·**za**′·shun). The visualization of an iridescent halo round objects by anyone suffering from glaucoma. [see prec.]

irido-avulsion (ir·id·o·av·**ul**′·shun). Surgical avulsion of the iris.

iridocapsulitis (ir·id·o·kap·sew·**li**′·tis). A condition of inflammation in which the iris and the capsule of the lens are involved. [iris, capsule, Gk *-itis* inflammation.]

iridocele (ir·**id**·o·seel). Herniation of a portion of the iris through a defect in the cornea. [iris, Gk *kele* hernia.]

iridochoroiditis (ir·id·o·kor·oid·**i**′·tis). Iritis and choroiditis occurring in combination.

iridocinesia, iridocinesis (ir·id·o·sin·e′·ze·ah, ir·id·o·sin·**e**′·sis). Iridokinesia.

iridocoloboma (ir·id·o·kol·o·**bo**′·mah). 1. A coloboma of the iris. 2. That part of the iris which is excised in iridectomy.

iridoconstrictor (ir·id·o·kon·**strik**′·tor). An agent, usually a drug, producing contraction of the sphincter of the iris. [iris, constriction.]

iridocorneosclerectomy (ir·id·o·**kor**·ne·o·skleer·**ek**′·to·me). In the treatment of glaucoma, the excision of a part of the iris, cornea, and sclera. [iris, cornea, sclera, Gk *ektome* a cutting out.]

iridocyclectomy (ir·id·o·si·**klek**′·to·me). The operation of removing the iris and the ciliary body. [iris, Gk *kyklos* circle, *ektome* a cutting out.]

iridocyclitis (ir·id·o·si·**kli**′·tis). Inflammation involving the iris and the ciliary body. [iris, Gk *kyklos* circle, *-itis* inflammation.]

iridocyclochoroiditis (ir·id·o·si·klo·kor·oid·**i**′·tis). Inflammation in which the iris, the ciliary body, and the choroid are involved. [iris, Gk *kyklos* circle, choroid, Gk *-itis* inflammation.]

iridocystectomy (ir·id·o·sist·**ek**′·to·me). An operation devised by Knapp for removal of a cyst of the iris. [iris, cyst, Gk *ektome* a cutting out.]

iridodesis (ir·id·o·**de**′·sis). Iridesis. [iris, Gk *desis* a binding together.]

iridodiagnosis (ir·id·o·di·ag·**no**′·sis). Determination of the nature or existence of disease by examination of the iris. [iris, diagnosis.]

iridodialysis (ir·id·o·di·**al**′·is·is). Detachment of the iris from its insertion; usually traumatic in origin. [iris, Gk *dialysis* a loosing.]

iridodiastasis (ir·id·o·di·**as**′·tas·is). A colobomatous defect of the peripheral part of the iris, leaving the pupillary border intact, rarely multiple; iris diastasis. [iris, Gk *diastasis* a separating.]

iridodilator (ir·id·o·di·**la**′·tor). Effecting dilatation of the pupil, as the radiating muscular fibres of the iris.

iridodonesis (ir·id·o·do·**ne**′·sis). Tremulousness of the iris, due to lack of support by the lens in high myopia, or to its absence or dislocation. [iris, Gk *donesis* tremor.]

iridokeratitis (ir·id·o·ker·at·**i**′·tis). Iritis in association with keratitis.

iridokinesis (ir·id·o·kin·**e**′·sis). Any movement of expansion and contraction of the iris. [iris, Gk *kinesis* movement.]

iridokinetic (ir·id·o·kin·**et**′·ik). Relating or belonging to iridokinesis.

iridoleptynsis (ir·id·o·lep·**tin**′·sis). Wasting or atrophic thinning of the iris. [iris, Gk *leptynein* to thin.]

iridology (ir·id·**ol**·o·je). The special branch of ophthalmology which concerns the iris, normal and abnormal, but especially with regard to changes in colour, shape, and other physical characteristics in disease. [iris, Gk *logos* science.]

iridomalacia (ir·id·o·mal·**a**′·she·ah). Pathological softening of the iris. [iris, Gk *malakia* softness.]

iridomedialysis, iridomesodialysis (ir·id·o·me·di·**al**′·is·is, ir·id·o·mes·o·di·**al**′·is·is). Division of adhesions around the pupillary border of the iris. [iris, L *medius* middle, Gk *mesos* middle, *dialysis*.]

iridomotor (ir·id·o·**mo**′·tor). Relating to or concerned with movement occurring in the iris, e.g. contraction; iridokinetic. [iris, L *movere* to move.]

iridoncosis (ir·id·ong·**ko**′·sis). Iridauxesis. [iris, Gk *ogkos* a swelling.]

iridoncus (ir·id·**ong**·kus). A tumour or oedematous swelling of the iris, causing general thickening. [iris, Gk *ogkos* a swelling.]

iridoparalysis (ir·id·o·par·**al**′·is·is). Iridoplegia. [iris, paralysis.]

iridoparelkysis (ir·id·o·par·**el**′·kis·is). Prolapse of the iris brought about by surgical means, in order to effect displacement of the pupil. [iris, Gk *parelkein* to draw aside.]

iridoparesis (ir·id·o·par·**e**′·sis). A state of incomplete paralysis of the iris. [iris, paresis.]

iridopathy (ir·id·**op**·ath·e). Disease of the iris. [iris, Gk *pathos* disease.]

iridoperiphacitis, iridoperiphakitis (ir·id·o·per·e·fas·**i**′·tis, ir·id·o·per·e·fak·**i**′·tis). Iritis associated with inflammation of the anterior portion of the lens capsule. [iris, Gk *peri, phakos* lens, *-itis* inflammation.]

iridoplania (ir·id·o·**pla**′·ne·ah). Hippus. [iris, Gk *plane* a wandering.]

iridoplegia (ir·id·o·**ple**′·je·ah). A generic term applied to paralysis of the sphincter of the iris, the dilator muscle, or both. It may or may not be accompanied by paralysis of the ciliary muscle. **Complete iridoplegia.** A state in which the pupil does not react to light or accommodation (convergence). **Reflex iridoplegia.** Iridoplegia where the pupil does not react directly or consensually to light, but contracts on convergence of the visual axes. A common example is the Argyll Robertson pupil in tabes. **Sympathetic iridoplegia.** A condition in which the dilator muscle of the iris supplied by sympathetic fibres is paralysed, resulting in defective dilatation of the pupil in reduced illumination, or after instillation of cocaine. [iris, Gk *plege* stroke.]

iridoptosis (ir·id·op·**to**′·sis). Prolapse of the iris. [iris, Gk *ptosis* a falling.]

iridopupillary (ir·id·o·**pew**′·pil·ar·e). Relating or belonging to the iris and the pupil.

iridorrhexis (ir·id·o·**rex**′·is). Tearing of the iris. [iris, Gk *rhexis* rupture.]

iridoschisis, iridoschisma (ir·id·**os**·kis·is, ir·id·o·**skiz**′·mah). Separation of the iris stroma into two layers with disintegration of the anterior layer. [Gk *iris* rainbow, *schisis* a cleft.]

iridosclerotomy (ir·id·o·skler·**ot**′·o·me). Operative treatment of glaucoma by puncturing the sclera and dividing the border of the iris. [iris, sclera, Gk *temnein* to cut.]

iridoscope (ir·**id**·o·skope). A particular type of ophthalmoscope used in examination of the interior of the eye. [iris, Gk *skopein* to watch.]

iridoscopy (ir·id·**os**·ko·pe). Eye examination by means of an iridoscope.

iridosis (ir·id·**o**·sis). Iridesis.

iridosteresis (ir·id·o·ster·**e**′·sis). Removal of a portion of or the whole of the iris. [iris, Gk *steresis* being in want of.]

iridotasis (ir·id·**ot**·as·is). In glaucoma, operative dilatation or stretching of the iris as an alternative treatment to iridotomy. Borthen's operation. [iris, Gk *tasis* a stretching.]

iridotome (ir·id·o·tome). An instrument for cutting the iris. [iris, Gk *temnein* to cut.]

iridotomy (ir·id·ot·o·me). Incision of the iris, with or without the formation of an artificial pupil. [see prec.]

iridotromos (ir·id·ot·rom·os). Hippus. [iris, Gk *tromos* a quivering.]

irinic (ir·in·ik). Iridic.

iris (i·ris) (pl. *irises* or *irides*). 1. [NA] A thin circular disc, perforated, usually a little to its nasal side, by the pupil. It contains a sphincter muscle near its margin for contraction of the pupil and radiating muscle fibres for its dilatation, and is backed by densely pigmented cells derived from the most anterior part of the fetal optic cup. 2. A genus of plants of the family Iridaceae. *See* ORRIS. **Iris bombé.** A bulging forward of the iris by aqueous which cannot escape into the anterior chamber because the pupillary border is adherent all the way round to the anterior surface of the lens capsule. **Border of the iris, ciliary [margo ciliaris (NA)].** The attached border, continuous with the ciliary body and choroid. **Border of the iris, pupillary [margo pupillaris (NA)].** The free border, encircling the pupil. **Iris collarette.** Iris frill (see following). **Iris frill.** An irregular line on the surface of the iris, representing the attachment of the fetal pupillary membrane. Outside this line is the ciliary zone, and inside it the pupillary zone, which often differ in colour. **Surface of the iris, anterior [facies anterior (NA)].** The surface towards the cornea. **Surface of the iris, posterior [facies posterior (NA)].** The surface towards the ciliary processes and the lens. **Tremulous iris.** 1. A condition in which, when the support of the lens is absent, the iris is free to make tremulous movements as the eye moves. Otherwise the iris is normal. 2. Hippus; pathological exaggeration of the normal pupillary excursions, often associated with epilepsy. **Umbrella iris.** Iris bombé (see above). [Gk, rainbow.]

Irish moss (i·rish mos). Carrageen, Chondrus BPC 1959; the dried seaweed, *Chondrus crispus* Stackh. (family Gigartinaceae), mainly collected from the northern shores of Brittany, from Northern Ireland, and the eastern seaboard of the United States of America. The fresh seaweed is washed, bleached in the sun, and finally dried. The chief constituents are mucilaginous polysaccharides in combination with metallic salts of sulphuric acid. It has slight nutritive value, and, being easily digested and readily administered in the form of a decoction, occasionally forms a useful article of diet. The decoction is also used as a demulcent in the treatment of coughs, and as a soothing application to the skin. It is employed commercially as an emulsifying agent, especially for cod-liver oil. [AS *Iras, mos.*]

irisopsia (i·ris·op·se·ah). A defect in vision in which the patient sees circles of coloured light around objects. [iris, Gk *opsis* vision.]

iritic (i·rit·ik). Relating or belonging to, or having the characteristics of iritis.

iritis (i·ri·tis). Inflammation of the iris. It is rare for this structure to be involved alone, hence the terms *iridocyclitis*, when the ciliary body is also affected, or *uveitis* when the uveal tract, comprising iris, ciliary body, and choroid, are implicated. **Endogenous iritis.** Iritis coming from some source within the body; it may be classified into *granulomatous* and *non-granulomatous*. Granulomatous iritis is usually chronic and characterized pathologically by the presence of macrophages, epithelioid cells and giant cells; important causes are tuberculosis, syphilis, sarcoidosis, toxoplasmosis, fungi, sympathetic iritis, and lens-induced iritis. Non-granulomatous iritis is usually acute and recurrent, and is characterized pathologically by the presence of plasma cells and lymphocytes and the absence of a granulomatous reaction; important causes are ankylosing spondylitis, virus infections, genital infections, Reiter's syndrome, and heterochromia. However, many cases are idiopathic. **Exogenous iritis.** Iritis following introduction of microbes or of toxic substances from without as the result of trauma or operation. **Granulomatous iritis.** *See* ENDOGENOUS IRITIS (above). **Metabolic iritis.** Iritis occurring in the course of general metabolic disorders, but it is probable that these act by lowering general resistance to infective processes. Such diseases are diabetes, gout, renal disease, and rheumatism. **Non-granulomatous iritis.** *See* ENDOGENOUS IRITIS (above). **Serous iritis.** 1. Chronic cyclitis. [Obsolete term.] *See* CYCLITIS. 2. The acute type of iritis caused by an allergic reaction with few keratic precipitates or permanent posterior synechia. Also called *non-granulomatous iritis* in contradistinction to the plastic or granulomatous type. **Sympathetic iritis.** Nearly always a uveitis affecting both eyes, and almost invariably following a perforating wound or ulcer involving uveal tissue. The injured eye is called the *exciting eye*, the uninjured, which may develop a more severe inflammation, the *sympathetic* or *sympathizing eye*. It may result in the loss of both eyes. [iris, Gk *-itis* inflammation.]

irito-ectomy (i·rit·o·ek'·to·me). In treatment of cataract, the operation of excising a part of the iris when the pupil has been occluded by the products of inflammation. [iris, Gk *ektome* a cutting out.]

iritomy (i·rit·o·me). Iridotomy.

irkintja (er·kint·jah). Australian boomerang leg. *See* LEG.

iron (i·ern). 1. An element of atomic weight 55.85, atomic number 26, and chemical symbol Fe (*ferrum*). It is a hard grey metal, the colour, ductility, and malleability of which can be varied by alloying with other metals and the admixture of carbon. It occurs widely in nature, principally as the minerals magnetite and haematite, and in all animal tissue and in that of certain plants. As a constituent of the respiratory pigments (haemoglobin in the higher animals) it is concerned with oxygen transference in the tissues; in plants it is found in the chlorophyll-bearing organelle. It has two valencies, Fe^{2+} forming ferrous salts, and Fe^{3+} forming ferric compounds. Its main use (Iron BPC 1968) in medicine is in the treatment of anaemia; also as an astringent and styptic. 2. A semi-popular name applied to a variety of iron surgical appliances which correct anatomical defects or allow or aid walking. **Iron acetate.** $Fe(O_2CCH_3)_3$, an astringent salt. **Iron adenylate.** An iron preparation used for intramuscular injection. **Iron albuminate.** Includes a number of preparations made from egg albumin and ferric chloride which have been used in the treatment of anaemias. **Alcoholized iron.** Pulverized iron (see below). ("Alcoholized" iron is a survival of the original Arabic, meaning "very finely divided".) **Iron alginate, alginoid iron.** The compound $C_{76}H_{77}Fe_3N_2O_{22}$, containing 10.12 per cent iron. **Iron and aluminium sulphate.** An astringent salt little used now. **Iron and ammonium acetate.** A preparation used in solution in anaemia. **Iron and ammonium citrate.** Ferric Ammonium Citrate BP 1958, a preparation in scale form, used widely in the treatment of anaemia. **Iron and ammonium citrate, green.** A scale preparation now being replaced by simpler iron salts. **Iron and ammonium citro-arsenite.** A scale preparation now being replaced by simpler iron salts. **Iron and ammonium sulphate.** Ammonio-ferric alum, $FeNH_4(SO_4)_2{\cdot}12H_2O$, an astringent and styptic salt. **Iron and ammonium tartrate.** A scale preparation which can be used in anaemia. **Iron arsenate.** $Fe_3(AsO_4)_2{\cdot}6H_2O$, a preparation used in the treatment of skin diseases. It is insoluble in water. **Iron arsenite.** A basic iron salt of variable composition. **Iron arsenotartrate.** A preparation formerly used in the treatment of anaemia. **Iron ascorbate.** A soluble salt formed by reduced iron and ascorbic acid. It can be given parenterally in the treatment of anaemia. **Available iron.** The proportion of iron in food which is absorbed, and therefore available for haemoglobin formation, after digestion. **Iron benzoate.** $Fe(O_2CC_6H_5)_3$, a salt in powder form used in iron preparations. **Iron bromide.** Ferrous bromide, $FeBr_2$, a soluble salt, very styptic, formerly used in chorea. **Iron cacodylate.** $Fe[(CH_3)_2AsO_2]_3$, an arsenic-containing compound formerly used in various blood diseases and reticuloses. It can be given orally or parenterally. **Iron carbonate.** Ferrous carbonate, $FeCO_3$, a salt used in the treatment of anaemia, e.g. in Blaud's pill or as saccharated ferrous carbonate. **Iron caseinate, caseinated iron.** A preparation of casein and iron; also known as *iron nucleo-albuminate*. **Iron cevitaminate.** Iron ascorbate (see above). **Iron**

chloride. Ferric chloride, $FeCl_3$; iron perchloride. A very astringent salt, too irritant for effective internal use. It may be used externally for its styptic and astringent properties, in the form of the tincture. **Iron citrate.** A compound similar to iron and ammonium citrate (see above), but not now in general use. **Iron citrate, green.** A compound similar to citrate which used to be given subcutaneously or intramuscularly. **Iron citro-pyrophosphate.** A scale preparation which is soluble, and has been used in the treatment of anaemia. **Dialysed iron.** A solution of ferric oxychloride prepared by dialysis; a dark-red liquid miscible with water. **Iron gallotannate.** Iron tannate (see below). **Iron gluconate.** An iron preparation used in the treatment of anaemia. **Iron glycerophosphate.** Ferric Glycerophosphate BPC 1959, a preparation made from ferric hydroxide and glycerophosphoric acid, used for its reputed tonic properties. **Iron haematoxylin.** *See* HAEMATOXYLIN. **Iron hydroxide.** $Fe(OH)_3$, a compound used, freshly prepared, as an antidote for arsenic poisoning. Its value is disputed and it is now obsolete. **Iron hypophosphite.** Ferric Hypophosphite BPC 1959, a compound reputed to have tonic properties. **Iron iodate.** $Fe(IO_3)_3$, a compound of variable composition. **Iron iodide.** FeI_2, an unstable compound sometimes used in tonic medicines, especially formerly in tuberculosis. **Iron iodobehenate.** An amorphous powder preparation, formerly much used in a number of diseases (e.g. anaemias and rickets). **Iron lactate.** Ferrous lactate, $Fe(C_3H_5O_3)_2{\cdot}3H_2O$, a mild sweetish-tasting salt, sometimes used in anaemia. **Iron magnesium sulphate.** $FeSO_4$ $MgSO_4{\cdot}H_2O$, a salt used in anaemia. **Iron malate.** A preparation made from iron and apple juice and containing a varying amount of iron. **Iron and manganese citrate.** A scale preparation now being replaced by simpler iron salts. **Masked iron.** Organic compounds of iron, formerly preferred to organic iron in anaemia but of no therapeutic advantage. **Iron nucleo-albuminate.** Iron caseinate (see above). **Iron oleate.** A waxy solid preparation, used as an astringent. **Iron oxalate.** $FeC_2O_4{\cdot}H_2O$, an ineffective salt formerly used in anaemias. **Iron oxide.** A term including various oxides, e.g. native ferric oxide (Fe_2O_3), magnetic iron oxide (Fe_3O_4), iron subcarbonate, etc. **Iron oxide, saccharated.** Soluble ferric oxide; a mixture of ferric saccharate and some sodium saccharate with sugar. It is soluble in water and is now in common use in intravenous iron therapy. **Iron perchloride.** Iron chloride (see above). **Iron pheophytin.** A chlorophyll derivative of iron. **Iron Phosphate BPC 1968.** Ferric and ferrous phosphates which have been used in anaemia. **Iron phosphate, saccharated.** A scale preparation now being replaced by simpler iron salts. **Iron phosphate, soluble.** $FePO_4$, rendered soluble by sodium citrate. It can be used in solution in anaemia. **Iron and potassium tartrate.** A scale preparation only slightly astringent. **Pulverized iron.** Metallic iron mechanically powdered. **Iron pyrophosphate.** $Fe_4(P_2O_7)_3{\cdot}9H_2O$, a salt insoluble in water, soluble in mineral acids, available commercially as a good additive affording an alternative to iron phosphate. **Iron and quinine citrate.** A scale preparation, considered to be a tonic on account of its bitter properties. **Iron quinine and strychnine citrate.** A scale preparation that has been replaced by simpler iron salts. **Reduced iron.** A greyish-black powder, consisting mainly of metallic iron with some ferric oxide, formerly used in anaemia. **Iron and strychnine citrate.** A scale preparation now being replaced by simpler iron salts. **Iron subcarbonate.** Precipitated iron oxide, a brown powder made by precipitating ferrous sulphate with sodium carbonate, and drying. It consists mainly of ferric hydroxide and some ferric and ferrous carbonates. **Iron subsulphate.** Ferric subsulphate, $Fe_4O(SO_4)_5$, used in the textile industry, and in medicine as a styptic. **Iron succinate.** Ferric or ferrous succinate, a salt of variable composition with no special therapeutic uses. **Iron sulphate.** Ferrous Sulphate BP 1958, $FeSO_4{\cdot}7H_2O$, green crystals (hence green vitriol), soluble in water, and highly effective in iron-deficiency anaemias (probably the compound in widest use today). It is astringent, and large doses may cause gastro-intestinal irritation. **Iron tannate.** Iron gallotannate, a compound of variable composition; a blue-black powder, insoluble in water. **Iron valerianate.** Ferric valerate, $FeC_5H_9O_2(OH)_2$; a salt insoluble in water, which has been used in anaemia. **Iron vitellinate.** A preparation of egg yolk and iron. **Walking iron.** An iron (see MAIN DEF. 2 above) which aids or allows walking. [AS *iren.*]

See also: QUEVENNE.

irone (i·rone). $(CH_3)_2C_6H_6(CH_3)CH{=}CHCOCH_3$, a naturally-occurring alicyclic ketone having an intense odour of violets, especially in high dilution. It is obtained from the essential oil of orris root, *Iris germanica* Linn., *I. pallida* Lam., and *I. florentina* Linn. (family Iridaceae), also from other plant products, and is used as a perfume base.

irotomy (i·rot·o·me). Iridotomy.

irradiate (ir·a·de·ate). 1. To subject to the action of x-rays or rays from a radioactive substance for diagnostic or therapeutic purposes. 2. To radiate; to spread out from a central point. [L *irradiare* to emit rays in all directions.]

irradiating (ir·a·de·a·ting). Spreading out like rays from a central point; applied especially to pain. [see prec.]

irradiation (ir·a·de·a′·shun). 1. A spread from a common centre, as of nerve impulses in both normal and abnormal conditions. 2. Treatment of disease by the various forms of radiant energy. 3. A condition in which an object appears larger than it really is owing to the difference in illumination between it and its background, the effect being increased when accommodation is relaxed. It is caused by diffraction of light and irregular astigmatism in the eye. 4. The application of rays to an object, e.g. the ultraviolet irradiation of ergosterol. **Heterogeneous irradiation.** Uneven dose distribution in the tissues in radiotherapy. **Homogeneous irradiation.** Even dose distribution in the tissues in radiotherapy. **Interstitial irradiation.** Treatment by the insertion into the tissues of naturally-radioactive materials in the form of radium needles, or radon seeds, or of artificially-radioactive materials such as cobalt-60, tantalum or gold, usually in the form of needles or wire. **Intracavitary irradiation.** Treatment by the insertion into body cavities of radium, radon, or other radioactive isotopes in solid or fluid form. **Sieve irradiation.** Treatment of cancer through a sieve grid, which allows for the use of larger dosage. **Surface irradiation.** The application of radioactive sources to the surface of the body. [L *irradiare* to emit rays in all directions.]

See also: ROENTGEN.

irreducible (ir·e·dew·sibl). Not permitting of reduction, e.g. fracture or hernia. [L *in, reducere* to bring back.]

irregular (ir·eg·ew·lar). 1. Asymmetrical; not straight. 2. Abnormal; not conforming to natural law or rule. 3. Not recurring at regular intervals, as beats of the pulse. [see foll.]

irregularity (ir·eg·ew·lar·it·e). Any variation from a normal rhythm. **Phasic irregularity.** Irregularity of the rhythm of the heart, occurring at regular intervals, usually due to phasic alteration in vagal tone (sinus arrhythmia) related to respiration. Such an irregularity may also be produced by premature contractions occurring at regular intervals, or by atrioventricular dissociation which varies in degree at regular intervals. **Irregularity of pulse.** Arrhythmia. [L *in, regula* rule.]

irrespirable (ir·es·pir·abl). Unsuitable for respiration because of danger to life; applied to air or gases. [L *in,* respiration.]

irresuscitable (ir·e·sus·it·abl). Incapable of being resuscitated. [L *in, resuscitare* to rouse again.]

irrhythmia (ir·ith·me·ah). Arrhythmia. [L *in,* rhythm.]

irrigant (ir·ig·ant). The fluid used in irrigation.

irrigate (ir·ig·ate). To wash out with water or other liquid. [L *irrigare* to conduct water to any place.]

irrigation (ir·ig·a·shun). The act of washing out a cavity such as the vagina, bladder, etc., or of cleansing the surface of a wound, by a constant or intermittent stream of lotion or water. [see prec.]

irrigator (ir·ig·a·tor). An apparatus used in irrigation. [L *irrigare* to conduct water to any place.]

See also: WELLS (C. A.).

irrigoradioscopy, irrigoscopy (ir·ig·o·ra·de·**os**′·ko·pe, ir·ig·**os**·ko·pe). Radiographic examination of the intestines by means of an enema containing an opaque medium, usually barium sulphate. [irrigation, radioscopy.]

irritability (ir·it·ab·**il**′·it·e). 1. The quality of being excitable and responding to stimuli. 2. A condition of abnormal excitability or sensitivity of an organ. **Irritability of the bladder.** Abnormal sensitiveness of the mucous membrane of the bladder, causing frequent micturition. **Chemical irritability.** Responsiveness of a tissue to a chemical stimulus. **Contact irritability.** The condition of being excitable in response to mechanical stimulation such as touch. **Electric irritability.** The response of nerve or muscle to stimulation by an electric current. **Faradic irritability.** The response of nerve or muscle to the faradic (induced) current. **Galvanic irritability.** The condition in which muscle may respond to the galvanic (continuous) current. **Mechanical irritability.** Irritability resulting from a mechanical stimulus. **Muscular irritability.** An abnormal responsiveness of a muscle to a slight stimulus. **Myotatic irritability.** The contraction of a muscle as a response to stretching. **Nervous irritability.** 1. Hypernormal excitability of the nervous system. 2. The property of a nerve to respond to stimulation. **Specific irritability.** The power of responding to only one type of stimulation and of being inert towards all other types. **Irritability of the stomach.** Vomiting produced by small amounts of food. **Tactile irritability.** Hyperaesthesia. [L *irritare* to tease.]

irritable (ir·it·abl). 1. Responding readily or able to respond to stimulus. 2. Reacting unduly to stimulation. [see prec.]

irritant (ir·it·ant). 1. Causing or producing irritation. 2. An agent which causes irritation. **Primary irritant.** A chemical substance that will cause dermatitis in all who come into contact with it, provided the exposure is long enough and strong enough. Examples include acids, alkalis, fat solvents, detergents, skin cleansers, oxidizing and reducing agents, animal and vegetable products, and many other chemicals including some used topically in treatment. Even water can have an irritant effect. Physical and mechanical damage can also cause primary irritant effects.

irritation (ir·it·a·shun). 1. The act of exciting or stimulating. 2. A condition of hypersensitivity of an organ, especially of the central nervous system. **Cerebral irritation.** The symptoms produced by over-activity of a part of the brain, due to a local lesion or a general abnormal state. **Direct irritation.** That irritation caused by direct excitation of an organ. **Functional irritation.** Over-activity of the functions of an organ. **Meningeal irritation.** The symptoms of inflammation of the meninges due to infection or haemorrhage. **Spinal irritation.** Over-activity of the spinal cord, due to an irritative lesion. **Sympathetic irritation.** Over-activity of the sympathetic nervous system. [L *irritare* to tease.]

irritative (ir·it·at·iv). 1. Arousing irritation or excitement. 2. Caused by irritation; contingent on a state of irritation. 3. Produced or accompanied by increased action.

irrumation (ir·ew·**ma**·shun). Fellatio. [L *irrumare* to give suck.]

Isaacs, Charles Edward (b. 1811). New York physiologist.

Isaacs–Ludwig arteriole. A branching of the afferent glomerular arteriole which appears to communicate directly with the capillary plexus.

isaconitine (i·sak·**on**·it·een). Benzoyl aconine, benzaconine, picraconitine, $C_{32}H_{45}O_{10}N$. A constituent alkaloid of aconite, formed from aconitine by loss of an acetyl group. It is less toxic than aconitine.

isafgul (is·af·gul). Ispaghula.

Isambert, Emile (b. 1827). Paris physician.

Isambert's disease. Tsutsugamushi disease: Japanese river fever; mite-borne typhus.

isamine blue (i·sam·een **bloo**). Naphthylpararosaniline; a dye which has been used experimentally in treatment of various types of neoplasm in man and animals, administered intravenously or by direct injection into the tumour. The results have, however, been unsatisfactory. It is also used as a stain in histology.

isatin (i·sat·in). $C_8H_5NO_2$, the lactam of *o*-aminobenzoylformic acid, obtained by the oxidation of indigo. It is a reddish crystalline solid employed in the synthesis of dyestuffs.

ischaemia (is·**ke**·me·ah). Insufficient blood supply to a part of the body relative to the local needs, usually the result of disease of the blood vessels supplying the part affected. **Ischaemia cordis intermittens.** Angina pectoris. **Coronary ischaemia.** Ischaemia resulting from disease of the coronary arteries. **Myocardial ischaemia.** Insufficiency of the blood supply to the myocardium, usually the result of coronary artery disease but also occurring with syphilitic aortitis, aortic stenosis and congenital arterial abnormalities. Clinically the condition is principally manifested by original pain but there is associated impairment of myocardial function. **Ischaemia retinae.** A temporary deficiency of blood in the retina (von Graefe). [Gk *ischein* to hold back, *haima* blood.]

ischaemic (is·**ke**·mik). Relating or belonging to, affected with, or characterized by ischaemia.

ischeocele (is·ke·o·seel). Ischiocele.

ischesis (is·**ke**·sis). 1. The arrest or the retention of a discharge. 2. A condition in which any normal secretion is stopped. [Gk *ischein* to hold back.]

ischiac, ischiadic (is·ke·ak, is·ke·**ad**·ik). Ischiatic.

ischiadelphus (is·ke·ad·**el**′·fus). Ischiodidymus. [Gk *ischion* hip joint, *adelphos* brother.]

ischiagra (is·ke·**ag**·rah). Gout of the hip joint. [Gk *ischion* hip joint, *agra* a catching.]

ischial (is·ke·al). Ischiatic: pertaining to the hip joint. **Ischial bursa.** *See* BURSA. **Ischial spine.** *See* SPINE.

ischialgia (is·ke·**al**·je·ah). Sciatica. [Gk *ischion* hip joint, *algos* pain.]

ischialgic (is·ke·**al**·jik). Relating or belonging to, affected with, or characterized by ischialgia.

ischias, ischiasis (is·**ke**·as, is·**ki**·as·is). Ischialgia. **Ischias scoliotica.** A temporary scoliosis which is caused by neuralgic or muscular pain in the back. [Gk *ischion* hip joint.]

ischiatic (is·ke·**at**·ik). Belonging to the ischium; sciatic.

ischiatitis (is·ke·at·**i**′·tis). Inflammation of the sciatic nerve. [Gk *ischion* hip joint, *-itis* inflammation.]

ischiatocele (is·ke·**at**·o·seel). Ischiocele.

ischidrosis (is·kid·**ro**·sis). Arrest of secretion of sweat. [Gk *ischein* to hold back, *hidros* sweat.]

ischidrotic (is·kid·**rot**·ik). Checking the secretion of sweat. [see prec.]

ischigalactic (is·ke·gal·**ak**′·tik). 1. Retarding or causing the cessation of secretion of milk. 2. An agent that arrests lactation. [Gk *ischein* to hold back, *gala* milk.]

ischiitis (is·ke·**i**·tis). Inflammation around the ischium, often due to a bursa induced by pressure. [ischium, Gk *-itis* inflammation.]

ischio-anal (is·ke·o·**a**′·nal). Relating or belonging to the ischium and the anus.

ischiobulbar (is·ke·o·**bul**′·bar). Relating to the ischium and the bulb of the penis.

ischiocapsular (is·ke·o·**kap**′·sew·lar). Belonging to the ischium and the capsular ligament of the hip joint.

ischiocavernosus (is·ke·o·kav·ern·**o**′·sus). The ischiocavernosus muscle. [Gk *ischion* hip joint, corpus cavernosum.]

ischiocavernosus muscle [musculus ischiocavernosus (NA)]. The muscle which covers the crus of the penis.

ischiocavernous (is·ke·o·**kav**′·ern·us). Belonging to the ischium and the corpora cavernosa penis or the clitoris.

ischiocele (is·ke·o·seel). Hernia through either the greater or the lesser sciatic foramen. [Gk *ischion* hip joint, *kele* hernia.]

ischiococcygeal (is·ke·o·kok·**sij**′·e·al). Relating or belonging to the ischium and the coccyx.

ischiococcygeus (is·ke·o·kok·**sij**′·e·us). 1. The coccygeus muscle. 2. The posterior portion of the levator ani muscle. [Gk *ischion* hip joint, coccyx.]

ischiodidymus (is·ke·o·**did**′·im·us). A twin monster joined at the hips. [Gk *ischion* hip joint, *didymos* twin.]

ischiodymia (is·ke·o·**dim**'·e·ah). A twin monster in which union occurs at the ischia. [see prec.]

ischiodynia (is·ke·o·**din**'·e·ah). Ischialgia. [Gk *ischion* hip joint, *odyne* pain.]

ischiofemoral (is·ke·o·**fem**'·or·al). 1. Belonging to the ischium and the femur. 2. The adductor magnus muscle. **Ischiofemoral ligament.** *See* LIGAMENT.

ischiofibular (is·ke·o·**fib**'·ew·lar). Relating or belonging to the ischium and the fibula.

ischiohebotomy (is·ke·o·he·**bot**'·o·me). The operation of dividing the ischium and pubis. [Gk *ischion* hip joint, *hebe* pubes, *ektome* a cutting out.]

ischiomenia (is·ke·o·**me**'·ne·ah). Arrest of the menstrual discharge. [Gk *ischein* to hold back, *menes* menses.]

ischiomyelitis (is·ke·o·mi·el·**i**'·tis). Lumbar myelitis. [Gk *ischion* hip joint, myelitis.]

ischioneuralgia (is·ke·o·newr·**al**'·je·ah). Sciatica; ischialgia. [Gk *ischion* hip joint, neuralgia.]

ischionitis (is·ke·on·**i**'·tis). Inflammation of the ischial tuberosity. [Gk *ischion* hip joint, *-itis* inflammation.]

ischiopagia (is·ke·o·**pa**'·je·ah). Of twin monsters, fusion by the hips. [see foll.]

ischiopagus (is·ke·**op**·ag·us). A twin monster fused end-to-end at the hips and having a head on each pair of shoulders, four arms and usually four legs. **Ischiopagus tetrapus.** An ischiopagus with four legs. **Ischiopagus tripus.** An ischiopagus which has only three legs. [Gk *ischion* hip joint, *pagos* fixed.]

ischioperineal (is·ke·o·per·in·**e**'·al). 1. Relating or belonging to the ischium and the perineum. 2. The urogenital region in the male. 3. The superficial transversus perinei muscle.

ischioprostatic (is·ke·o·pros·**tat**'·ik). 1. Relating or belonging to the ischium and the prostate. 2. The superficial transversus perinei muscle.

ischiopubic (is·ke·o·**pew**'·bik). Relating to the ischium and the pubic bone.

ischiopubiotomy (is·ke·o·pew·be·**ot**'·o·me). Incision of the pubic bone with a saw, in order to enlarge the pelvic cavity in cases such as outlet contraction. It is a little-used manoeuvre, symphyseotomy being usually employed in suitable cases. [ischium, pubis, Gk *temnein* to cut.]

ischiorectal (is·ke·o·**rek**'·tal). Relating to the ischium and rectum.

ischiosacral (is·ke·o·**sa**'·kral). Relating or belonging to the ischium and the sacrum.

ischiovaginal (is·ke·o·**vaj**'·in·al). Relating or belonging to the ischium and the vagina.

ischiovertebral (is·ke·o·**ver**'·te·bral). Relating to the ischium and the vertebral column.

ischium [os ischii (NA)] (is·ke·um). Of the three fetal pelvic bones, the one that after fusion forms the inferior and posterior portion of the hip bone. [Gk *ischion* hip joint.]

Body [corpus ossis ischii (NA)]. That part of the bone which enters into the formation of the acetabulum and bears the tuberosity.

Dorsal surface. The surface of the ischium directed posteriorly and continuous above with the gluteal surface of the ilium. It is raised and rough in its lower part to form the ischial tuberosity which gives attachment to the hamstring or flexor muscles of the thigh.

Femoral surface. The surface of the ischium directed towards the thigh.

Pelvic surface. The surface of the ischium directed towards the pelvic cavity; part of the side wall of the true pelvis.

ischocenosis (is·ko·sen·**o**'·sis). Ischesis. [Gk *ischein* to hold back, *kenosis* an emptying.]

ischocholia (is·ko·**ko**·le·ah). Arrest of the secretion of bile. [Gk *ischein* to hold back, *chole* bile.]

ischochymia (is·ko·**ki**·me·ah). Arrest of the process of digestion of the gastric contents, causing characteristic dilatation of the stomach because of the accumulation and retention of food in it (Einhorn). [Gk *ischein* to hold back, chyme.]

ischogalactia (is·ko·gal·**ak**'·te·ah). Arrest of normal lactation. [Gk *ischein* to hold back, *gala* milk.]

ischogalactic (is·ko·gal·**ak**'·tik). 1. Retarding or causing the cessation of secretion of milk. 2. Any agent that arrests lactation. [see prec.]

ischogyria (is·ko·**ji**·re·ah). 1. A condition characterized by a jagged appearance of the cerebral gyri and found in some cases of sclerosis. 2. A condition, resulting from senile atrophy, in which the cerebral gyri are abnormally small. [Gk *ischein* to hold back, *gyros* ring.]

ischolochia (is·ko·**lo**·ke·ah). Arrest of the lochial discharge. [Gk *ischein* to hold back, lochia.]

ischomenia (is·ko·**me**·ne·ah). Ischiomenia; arrest of the menstrual discharge. [Gk *ischein* to hold back, *menes* menses.]

ischopyosis (is·ko·pi·**o**'·sis). Arrest in the discharge of purulent material. [Gk *ischein* to hold back, *pyon* pus.]

ischospermia (is·ko·**sper**·me·ah). Arrest of the secretion of semen. [Gk *ischein* to hold back, *sperma* seed.]

ischuretic (isk·ewr·**et**·ik). Relating to ischuria. [Gk *ischein* to hold back, urine.]

ischuria (isk·**ewr**·e·ah). Suppression or retention of the urine. **Ischuria paradoxa.** Abnormal distention of the urinary bladder, although micturition does not cease. **Ischuria spastica.** Suppression or retention of the urine due to spasmodic contraction of the sphincter of the bladder. [Gk *ischein* to hold back, urine.]

iseiconia (i·si·**ko**·ne·ah). Iso-iconia.

iseiconic (i·si·**kon**·ik). Iso-iconic.

isethionate (i·seth·**i**·on·ate). Any salt or ester of isethionic acid.

Ishihara, Shinobu (b. 1879). Tokio ophthalmologist.

Ishihara's colour-vision test. The patient is shown a number of plates made up of coloured circular dots. In each plate a number is picked out in dots of one colour with a background of a confusion colour. The patient with normal colour vision reads the number correctly, while the colour-blind patient sees another number.

Isidora (i·**sid**·or·ah). A genus of snails which are potential intermediate hosts of *Schistosoma.*

isinglass (i·sing·glas). Ichthyocolla. **Japanese isinglass.** Agar. [Old Dutch, *huysenblas* sturgeon-bladder.]

island (i·land). In anatomy, a relatively small area or mass of tissue clearly separated from surrounding structures or tissues. **Blood island.** A small localized area of blood formation found on the wall of the yolk sac in the early embryo. **Bone island.** A term sometimes used to describe a small area of sclerosis within the medullary cavity of bone. **Tonal islands.** A condition which occurs in cases of congenital and acquired deafness in which the hearing loss is patchy and incomplete. Some hearing may still be present at isolated frequencies at intensities above threshold. [AS *igland.*]

See also: CALLEJA, LANGERHANS, PANDER, REIL.

islet (i·let). A small island. **Blood islet.** Blood island. *See* ISLAND. **Islet of the pancreas.** Any of the small clumps of cells in the pancreas having no functional connection with the duct system of that organ; they form an internal secretion, insulin, which is passed directly to the blood stream. Also known as *intra-alveolar cell-islets* or *islets of Langerhans.* [OFr. *islette.*]

See also: CALLEJA, LANGERHANS, WALTHARD.

iso-agglutination (i·so·ag·loo·tin·**a**'·shun). Agglutination brought about by the activities of iso-agglutinins.

iso-agglutinative (i·so·ag·**loo**'·tin·at·iv). Relating or belonging to, or effecting iso-agglutination.

iso-agglutinin (i·so·ag·**loo**'·tin·in). An agglutinin in the blood of an individual which will agglutinate the red blood cells of another member of the same species. Such agglutinins are of value in blood grouping and tests for differentiating species. [Gk *isos* equal, agglutinin.]

iso-agglutinogen (i·so·ag·**loo**'·tin·o·jen). An agglutinogen (either A or B) present in red blood corpuscles and causing agglutination of those corpuscles when brought into contact with a plasma containing the corresponding α- or β-agglutinin. [Gk *isos* equal, agglutinogen.]

iso-alcohol (i·so·**al**·ko·hol). *See* ALCOHOL. [Gk *isos* equal, alcohol.]

iso-alloxazine (i·so·al·**ox'**·az·een). The isomer of alloxazine which is the parent of riboflavine. **Iso-alloxazine adenine dinucleotide.** An ester of riboflavine phosphate (cytoflavin) and adenylic acid. **Iso-alloxazine mononucleotide.** Cytoflavin, riboflavine phosphate; the prosthetic group of Warburg's ferment (yellow enzyme).

Isoaminile (i·so·**am**·in·ile). BP Commission approved name for 4-dimethylamino-2-isopropyl-2-phenylvaleronitrile; a cough suppressant.

iso-amylamine (i·so·am·**il'**·am·een). $(CH_3)_2CHCH_2CH_2NH_2$, an alkaloid base occurring naturally in the leaf of the tobacco plant, and also formed by the decomposition of protein. It is derived from the amino acid, leucine.

iso-amylene (i·so·**am**·il·een). Trimethylethylene, pental, β-isoamylene, $(CH_3)_2C{=}CHCH_3$. A compound formerly used as a general anaesthetic but found to be too toxic.

iso-androsterone (i·so·an·dro·**steer'**·one). $C_{19}H_{30}O_2$, an androgenic substance occurring in the urine of women with adrenal hyperplasia or certain ovarian neoplasms, and that of men in some cases of carcinoma. The systematic chemical name is androstane-3(β)-ol-17-one.

iso-antibody (i·so·**an**·te·bod·e). An antibody produced in the body against one of the animal's own cells or cell constituents which, serving as a stimulus to the production of an iso-antibody, are termed iso-antigens. Thus, in acquired haemolytic anaemia, the haemolysis may be due to the appearance in the patient's serum of an iso-antibody active against the patient's own red blood cells (the iso-antigen). [Gk *isos* equal, antibody.]

iso-antigen (i·so·**an**·te·jen). The cell or cell constituent serving as a stimulus to the production of an iso-antibody. [Gk *isos* equal, antigen.]

iso-apiole (i·so·a·pe·ole). 1-Propenyl-2,5-dimethoxy-3,4-methylenedioxybenzene, $C_{12}H_{14}O_4$. A compound obtained by molecular rearrangement of apiole (parsley camphor). It is similar to apiole which is employed in dysmenorrhoea and other uterine disorders.

isobar (i·so·bar). A line drawn on a meteorological map connecting places with equal barometric pressure at any given moment. [Gk *isos* equal, *baros* weight.]

isobare (i·so·ba·er). An element which has the same atomic weight as another element but different chemical properties, and almost invariably a different atomic number. Cf. ISOTOPE. [see foll.]

isobaric (i·so·**bar**·ik). Of the same specific gravity as the solution with which it is to come in contact, e.g. an analgesic solution for intrathecal injection of specific gravity equal to that of normal cerebrospinal fluid. [Gk *isos* equal, *baros* weight.]

isobolism (i·so·bo·lizm). The tendency of a motor nerve fibre to respond maximally to excitation. [Gk *isos* equal, *ballein* to throw.]

isoborneol (i·so·**bor**·ne·ol). $C_{10}H_{17}OH$, a stereoisomer of borneol. A secondary alcohol obtained by the catalytic reduction of camphor, not occurring naturally, and existing in two optically-active forms.

Isobuzole (i·so·bew·zole). BP Commission approved name for 5 - isobutyl - 2 - *p* - methoxybenzenesulphonamido - 1,3,4 - thiadiazole; it is used in sulphonamide therapy.

Isocarboxazid BP 1973 (i·so·kar·**box'**·az·id). 3 - *N* - Benzylhydrazinocarbonyl - 5 - methyliso - oxazole; an antidepressant drug which acts by inhibiting monoamine oxidase. Its uses are similar to those of Phenelzine sulphate.

isocellular (i·so·**sel**·ew·lar). Composed of cells which are similar in character and equal in size. [Gk *isos* equal, L *cellula* cell.]

isochromatic (i·so·kro·**mat'**·ik). Uniform in colour throughout, or of the same colour. [Gk *isos* equal, *chroma* colour.]

isochromatophil, isochromatophile (i·so·kro·**mat'**·o·fil, i·so·kro·**mat'**·o·file). Describing tissues which absorb an equal amount of the same stain or have equal affinity for the same dye. [Gk *isos* equal, *chroma* colour, *philein* to love.]

isochromosome (i·so·**kro**·mo·some). A chromosome with arms that are morphologically identical and contain the same loci (isogenic). Isochromosomes are the product of structural changes involving the centromere region and resulting in deficiency of the loci of one chromosome arm and duplication of those of the other. Chromosomes with unequal arms may give rise to isochromosomes for the long or the short arms; these are formed by two long or two short arms, respectively. [Gk *isos* equal, *chroma* colour, *soma* body.]

isochronal (i·so·**kro**·nal). Performed in equal times; said of the oscillations of a pendulum when the time of oscillation is the same for all amplitudes of vibration. Also applied to muscles or nerves which have the same chronaxie. [Gk *isos* equal, *chronos* time.]

isochronia (i·so·**kro**·ne·ah). The condition where a muscle and its nerve have identical chronaxies (Lapicque). Lapicque believed that unless this condition exists within a near approximation, excitation will not be transmitted (the law of isochronism): thus curare, which increases muscle chronaxie without a corresponding increase of that of nerve, upsets the isochronism and blocks neuromuscular transmission. The theory is not now accepted. [Gk *isos* equal, chronaxie.]

isochronic (i·so·**kron**·ik). Isochronal.

isochronism (i·so·**kro**·nizm). Isochronia.

isochronous (i·so·**kro**·nus). Isochronal.

isochroous (i·so·**kro**·us). Isochromatic.

isocitrate (i·so·**sit**·rate). An intermediate of the citric-acid cycle; formed from citrate through the action of aconitate hydratase. [Gk *isos* equal, citrate.]

isocoria (i·so·**ko**·re·ah). Uniformity in size of the pupils of the eyes. [Gk *isos* equal, *kore* pupil.]

isocortex (i·so·**kor**·tex). Neopallium; that part of the cerebral cortex in which the outermost stratum is grey. It forms the bulk of the cortex in man. [Gk *isos* equal, cortex.]

isocyanide (i·so·**si**·an·ide). Isonitrile; carbylamine: a compound of the general formula RNC, where R is a monovalent radical. Isocyanides are poisonous, colourless liquids with an offensive smell.

isocyclic (i·so·**si**·klik). Describing a cyclic compound, the ring of which is composed entirely of atoms of the same element, usually carbon (carbocyclic). Cf. HETEROCYCLIC. [Gk *isos* equal, *kyklos* circle.]

isocytolysin, isocytolysine (i·so·si·**tol'**·is·in, i·so·si·**tol'**·is·een). A cytolysin which produces its effect on the cells of animals belonging to the same species as that from which it has originated. [Gk *isos* equal, cytolysin.]

isocytosis (i·so·si·**to'**·sis). Equality in size of cells, particularly erythrocytes. [Gk *isos* equal, *kytos* cell.]

isocytotoxin (i·so·si·to·**tox'**·in). A cytotoxin which has a toxic effect on similar cells of animals of the same species as that from which it is derived. [Gk *isos* equal, cytotoxin.]

isodactylism (i·so·**dak**·til·izm). A condition of the hand or foot in which the fingers or toes are of about equal length. [Gk *isos* equal, *daktylos* finger, toe.]

isodactylous (i·so·**dak**·til·us). Applied to a hand or foot the fingers or toes of which are about equal in length. [see prec.]

isodiagnosis (i·so·di·ag·**no'**·sis). A diagnostic measure which consists in inoculating a susceptible animal with blood from a patient who is thought to be suffering from a particular infection. [Gk *isos* equal, diagnosis.]

isodiametric (i·so·di·am·**et'**·rik). 1. Of equal dimensions, as cells of parenchymatous tissue. 2. Of structures, having all diameters of equal length. [Gk *isos* equal, diameter.]

isodicentric (i·so·di·**sen'**·trik). A dicentric chromosome or chromatid whose free arms are identical morphologically and contain the same loci (isogenic). [Gk *isos* equal, *di-*, *kentron* centre.]

isodihydro-androsterone (i·so·di·**hi**·dro·an·dro·**steer'**·one). $C_{19}H_{32}O_2$, a synthetic androgen which is isomeric with androstanediol.

isodisperse (i·so·**dis**·pers). A colloidal sol in which the colloid is dispersed in particles of the same size. An example of such is a solution of haemoglobin in which all particles are of molecular weight 68 000. [Gk *isos* equal, disperse.]

isodont, isodontic (i·so·dont, i·so·**don**·tik). Having all teeth alike in shape and size. [Gk *isos* equal, *odous* tooth.]

isodoses (i·so·do·sez). Isodose curves; lines joining points receiving equal doses. [Gk *isos* equal, dose.]

isodulcite (i·so·**dul**·site). Rhamnose.

isodulcitol (i·so·**dul**·sit·ol). Rhamnose.

isodynamia (i·so·di·**nam**'·e·ah). The state of having equal power or strength, e.g. food materials. [Gk *isos* equal, *dynamis* force.]

isodynamic (i·so·di·**nam**'·ik). 1. Being of equal force. 2. Of food materials, liberating or generating equal amounts of energy or force in heat units or calories during the process of digestion. [see prec.]

isodynamogenic (i·so·di·nam·o·**jen**'·ik). Iso-energetic. [Gk *isos* equal, *dynamis* force, *genein* to produce.]

iso-electric, iso-electrical (i·so·el·**ek**'·trik, i·so·el·**ek**'·trik·al). 1. Being at the same electric potential. 2. Ionically in a state of electrical balance, determined by the pH of the solution in which the substance is present. **Iso-electric point.** *See* POINT. [Gk *isos* equal, electricity.]

iso-energetic (i·so·en·er·**jet**'·ik). 1. Isodynamic. 2. Equally active. [Gk *isos* equal, energy.]

isoenzyme (i·so·**en**·zime). A term applied to protein enzymes of different chemical constitution which are separable by electrophoresis and which catalyse the same reaction. [Gk *isos* equal, enzyme.]

isoephedrine (i·so·ef·ed·reen). The stereoisomer of ephedrine.

iso-erythro-agglutinin (i·so·er·**ith**·ro·ag·**loo**'·tin·in). Iso-agglutinin. [Gk *isos* equal, erythrocyte, agglutinin.]

Isoetharine (i·so·**eth**·ar·een). BP Commission approved name for 1 - (3,4 - dihydroxyphenyl) - 2 - isopropylaminobutan - 1 - ol; a bronchodilator.

isoeugenol (i·so·ew·jen·ol). $OHC_6H_3(OCH_3)CH{=}CHCH_3$, a compound obtained from eugenol by heating with alcoholic potassium hydroxide, and an intermediary in the synthesis of vanillin. It is used in perfumery, on account of its penetrating carnation-like odour.

isogame (i·sog·am·e). Isogamy.

isogamete (i·so·**gam**·eet). 1. One of the two uniting cells in reproduction by isogamy. 2. A type of gamete in which there is no differentiation. [Gk *isos* equal, gamete.]

isogamous (i·**sog**·am·us). 1. Reproducing by conjugation of gametes similar in all respects. 2. Indicating male and female gametes which in organic form and structure are identical. [see foll.]

isogamy (i·**sog**·am·e). In protozoology and botany, reproduction in which the two uniting cells are similar in all respects, including size; conjunction between two gametes equal in size. [Gk *isos* equal, gamete.]

isogeneic (i·so·jen·**e**'·ik). Of the same genetic constitution, e.g. identical twins, pure-bred animal strains. **Isogeneic graft.** Graft of tissue between isogeneic individuals. [Gk *isos* equal, *genein* to produce.]

isogenesis (i·so·**jen**·es·is). In morphology, identity of developmental processes. [Gk *isos* equal, genesis.]

isogenous (i·**soj**·en·us). Having the same origin or developing from the same cell. [see prec.]

isograft (i·so·grahft). A graft of tissue from one animal to another genetically identical animal. In man, limited to identical twins. In animals grafts between members of pure-bred strains. [Gk *isos* equal, graft.]

isohaemagglutination (i·so·he·mag·loo·tin·**a**'·shun). Iso-agglutination. [Gk *isos* equal, *haima* blood, agglutination.]

isohaemagglutinin (i·so·he·mag·**loo**'·tin·in). Iso-agglutinin. [see prec.]

isohaemolysin (i·so·he·**mol**'·is·in). A haemolysin derived from the blood of one animal which affects the erythrocytes of another animal of the same species. [Gk *isos* equal, haemolysin.]

isohaemolysis (i·so·he·**mol**'·is·is). Haemolysis of the erythrocytes in the blood of an animal when serum taken from the blood of another animal of the same species is used. [see prec.]

isohydria (i·so·**hi**·dre·ah). A condition of fluid balance in the body. [Gk *isos* equal, *hydor* water.]

isohypercytosis (i·so·hi·per·si·**to**'·sis). A condition of the blood in which the percentage of polymorphonuclear leucocytes remains stable although the total number of leucocytes is increased. [Gk *isos* equal, hyperleucocytosis.]

isohypocytosis (i·so·hi·po·si·**to**'·sis). A state of the blood in which the percentage of polymorphonuclear leucocytes remains stable although there is a decrease in the total number of leucocytes. [Gk *isos* equal, hypoleucocytosis.]

iso-iconia (i·so·i·**ko**'·ne·ah). A state in which the ocular images in the two eyes are equal in size and shape. [Gk *isos* equal, *eikon* image.]

iso-iconic (i·so·i·**kon**'·ik). Relating to or characterized by iso-iconia.

iso-idiolysin (i·so·id·e·**ol**'·is·in). Idio-isolysin; a haemolysin which may be present normally in blood but which acts harmfully on the cells of other animals of the same species. [Gk *isos* equal, *idios* own, lysin.]

iso-ikonia (i·so·i·**ko**'·ne·ah). Iso-iconia.

iso-ikonic (i·so·i·**kon**'·ik). Iso-iconic.

iso-immunization (i·so·im·ewn·i·**za**'·shun). Immunization of an animal or person with antigens derived from the same species; the development of iso-antibodies. [Gk *isos* equal, immunization.]

iso-ionia (i·so·i·**o**'·ne·ah). A condition in which the concentration of ions in a solution remains constant. [Gk *isos* equal, ion.]

isolate (i·so·late). 1. Of individuals, to keep from contact with the rest of the community. 2. In chemistry, to separate from any foreign substance or prepare in a pure condition. 3. In bacteriology, to derive from any source a pure culture of an organism. [It. *isolare* to detach.]

isolation (i·so·**la**·shun). 1. The process of isolating. 2. In psychoanalysis, either the loss of the emotional aspects of memories or the blocking of a wish or memory as in *repression* but without the lack of awareness characteristic of the latter process. [see prec.]

isoleucine (i·so·**lew**·seen). γ-Methylvaline, 2-amino-3-methylpentanoic acid, $CH_3CH_2CH(CH_3)CH(NH_2)COOH$. An amino acid essential in diet for the maintenance of health and occurring in protein hydrolysates.

isoleucocytosis, isoleukocytosis (i·so·**lew**·ko·si·**to**'·sis). Leucocytosis, the blood film of which shows normal distribution of leucocytes. [Gk *isos* equal, leucocytosis.]

isologous (i·**sol**·og·us). Term applied to animals which are genetically identical. In man, limited to identical twins. In animals, pure-bred strains. [Gk *isos* equal, *logos* relation.]

isologue (i·so·log). Any compound which resembles another in structure and general chemical properties, the only difference being that a particular element in the one is replaced by an element of the same group in the Periodic Table. Thus, hydrochloric acid, HCl, is an isologue of hydrobromic acid, HBr. [Gk *isos* equal, *logos* relation.]

isolophobia (i·so·lo·**fo**'·be·ah). Morbid fear of being alone. [isolation, phobia.]

isolysin (i·**sol**·is·in). Isohaemolysin.

isolysis (i·**sol**·is·is). Isohaemolysis.

isolytic (i·so·**lit**·ik). Relating or belonging to or caused by an isohaemolysin (isolysin) or isohaemolysis (isolysis).

isomaltose (i·o·**mawlt**·oze). Dextrinose, $C_{12}H_{22}O_{11}$. An isomer of maltose, glucose β-glucoside, which occurs naturally in beer and honey, and is synthesized by the action of enzymes or hydrochloric acid on glucose. It is dextrorotatory and non-fermentable.

isomastigote (i·so·**mas**·tig·ote). A protozoal organism which has two or four equal flagella at the anterior end. [Gk *isos* equal, *mastigx* lash.]

isomer (i·so·mer). 1. In chemistry, any compound which is isomeric with another. 2. In zoology, any organ or function that is homologous. [Gk *isos* equal, *meros* part.]

isomerase (i·so·mer·aze). An enzyme catalysing the isomerization of its substrates. *Phosphoglucose isomerase* interconverts glucose and fructose 6-phosphates; *phosphomannose isomerase* interconverts glucose and mannose 6-phosphates; *triosephosphate isomerase* catalyses the interconversion of glyceraldehyde 3-phosphate and dihydroxyacetone phosphate. [Gk *isos* equal, *-ase* enzyme.]

isomeric (i·so·**mer**·ik). Displaying isomerism.

isomeride (i·**so**·mer·ide). An isomer. [Obsolete term.]

isomerism (i·**so**·mer·izm). A phenomenon in chemistry, whereby two or more compounds having the same percentage composition and molecular weight differ widely in chemical and physical properties owing to differences in the arrangement of the atoms within their respective molecules. **Chain isomerism.** Isomerism arising in the higher paraffins owing to differences in the linkage of the carbon atoms in chains, e.g. straight, or branched. **Dynamic isomerism.** Tautomerism. **Geometrical isomerism.** A form of stereoisomerism in which compounds have identical structure but differ in the orientation of groups about an axis or plane (*cis-* and *trans-* forms). **Labile-stable isomerism.** Geometrical isomerism (see prec.). **Nuclear isomerism.** A form of structural isomerism (see below) due to differences in the arrangement of carbon nuclei. **Optical isomerism.** Stereoisomerism due to one or more asymmetric carbon atoms, and characterized by optical activity. **Place isomerism, position isomerism.** Isomerism due to a difference in position of a substituting element or radical in the same chain or ring of carbon atoms. **Space isomerism.** *See* STEREOISOMERISM. **Structural isomerism.** Isomerism of the chain or position type (see above). [Gk *isos* equal, *meros* part.]

isomerous (i·**so**·mer·us). Isomeric.

Isomethadone (i·so·**meth**·ad·one). BP Commission approved name for 6-dimethylamino-5-methyl-4,4-diphenylhexan-3-one. A compound chemically related to methadone, and obtained in the L-, D-, and DL- forms. The L- form is a potent analgesic and is about as active as morphine. The DL- form is only about one-third as active as morphine, while the D- form is practically inactive. The pharmacological properties of Isomethadone are very similar to those of methadone, but with fewer side-effects, although this does not appear to be true with equally active analgesic doses in man. It has addictive properties, like methadone.

isomethheptene (i·so·meth·**hep**'·teen). A sedative and antispasmodic in smooth muscle spasm complicated by nervous tension and pain. It is used in vesical, ureteral, and biliary colic, spasmodic dysmenorrhoea, and migraine headaches.

isometric (i·so·**met**·rik). Having equal dimensions; isodiametric. [Gk *isos* equal, *metron* measure.]

isometropia (i·so·met·**ro**'·pe·ah). Equality in the refractive condition of the two eyes. [Gk *isos* equal, *metron* measure, *ops* eye.]

isomicrogamete (i·so·mi·kro·**gam**'·eet). In protozoa, a small sexual cell of equal size with the cell with which it conjugates. [Gk *isos* equal, *mikros* small, gamete.]

isomolar (i·so·**mo**·lar). Equimolar; having the same number of moles in solution. [Gk *isos* equal, L *moles* mass.]

isomorphic (i·so·**mor**·fik). Displaying isomorphism; isomorphous.

isomorphism (i·so·**mor**·fizm). 1. In morphology, equality or similarity in form or shape. 2. The ability of certain compounds of different but chemically related elements to crystallize in the same form. [Gk *isos* equal, *morphe* form.]

isomorphous (i·so·**mor**·fus). Isomorphic.

isonaphthol (i·so·**naf**·thol). β-Naphthol, $C_{10}H_7OH$. White crystals or powder with faint phenolic odour. It has been used as an intestinal antiseptic and anthelminthic; externally in skin diseases as 5 to 15 per cent ointment. Its toxic effects resemble phenol poisoning and limit its internal use. Also employed in the manufacture of dyestuffs.

isonephrotoxin (i·so·nef·ro·**tox**'·in). A nephrotoxin which, derived from one animal of a particular species, affects the cells of other animals of the same species. [Gk *isos* same, nephrotoxin.]

Isoniazid BP 1973 (i·so·**ni**'·az·id). Isonicotinic acid hydrazide, $C_5H_4NCONHNH_2$. A compound with a high activity against *Mycobacterium tuberculosis, in vitro. In vivo* it is undergoing extensive clinical trials which at present indicate that the drug is as active as streptomycin, but there is evidence that resistance to it may develop. It can be readily administered orally and is rapidly absorbed, and there are few toxic effects: its use should be avoided in epileptic cases. Treatment with isoniazid is frequently combined with streptomycin therapy.

Isoniazidum. *European Pharmacopoeia* name for Isoniazid BP 1973.

isonicotinyl hydrazine (i·so·nik·o·**tin**'·il **hi**·draz·een). Isoniazid.

isonitrile (i·so·**ni**·trile). Isocyanide.

isonomic (i·so·**nom**·ik). Relating to substances that crystallize in the same form and are very similar in chemical composition. [Gk *isos* equal, *nomos* law.]

isonormocytosis (i·so·**nor**·mo·si·**to**'·sis). Normal condition of the leucocytes in the blood; dinormocytosis. [Gk *isos* equal, normocytosis.]

Iso-odon torosus (i·so·o·don tor·**o**·sus). The Australian bandicoot; a marsupial that is the natural host of the rickettsiae of Q fever. [Gk *isos* equal, *odous* tooth, L *torosus* fleshy.]

iso-osmotic (i·so·oz·**mot**'·ik). With equal osmotic pressures. [Gk *isos* equal, osmosis.]

Isoparorchidae (i·so·par·**or**'·kid·e). A family of the trematode sub-order Distomata or Fascioloidea. The genus *Isoparorchis* is of medical interest. [Gk *isos* equal, *para, orchis* testicle, *eidos* form.]

Isoparorchis (i·so·par·**or**'·kis). A genus of liver flukes whose normal hosts are freshwater fish. *Isoparorchis hypselobagri* and *I. trisimilitubis* have been recorded in temporary infestations in man in India and the tropical Far East. [Gk *isos* equal, *para, orchis* testicle.]

isopathotherapy, isopathy (i·so·path·o·**ther**'·ap·e, i·**sop**·ath·e). Isotherapy. [Gk *isos* equal, *pathos* disease, therapy.]

isopentaquine (i·so·**pen**·tah·kween). 8-[4-Isopropylamino-amyl-amino]-6-methoxyquinoline. An antimalarial drug which acts on gametocytes and, in combination with quinine, on the exo-erythrocytic stage of the malaria parasite. It is slightly less toxic than pentaquine.

isophagy (i·**sof**·aj·e). 1. The self-digestion or self-destruction of the cells of an organism by its own serum. 2. The self-disintegration of tissue cells, a condition encountered in certain pathological conditions and occurring after death. [Gk *isos* equal, *phagein* to eat.]

isophan (i·so·fan). A hybrid, the germinal constitution of which is different from that of other hybrids, although its appearance is similar to theirs. [Gk *isos* equal, *phanein* to show.]

isophoria (i·so·**for**·e·ah). The condition in which the visual axes of the two eyes are on the same horizontal plane, so that there is neither hyperphoria nor hypophoria. [Gk *isos* equal, *pherein* to bear.]

isopia (i·**so**·pe·ah). A term implying identical vision in the two eyes; not commonly used in the UK. [Gk *isos* equal, *ops* eye.]

isopilocarpine (i·so·pi·lo·**kar**'·peen). The stereoisomer of pilocarpine. It is formed from the latter by heating, and occurs naturally in *Pilocarpus microphyllus.*

isoplastic (i·so·**plas**·tik). In reconstructive surgery, descriptive of tissue and other transplants taken from an individual of the same species as the one under treatment. [Gk *isos* equal, *plassein* to form.]

isopleural (i·so·**ploor**·al). Symmetrical on both sides, especially with regard to the thorax. [Gk *isos* equal, *pleura* rib.]

Isoprednidene (i·so·**pred**·nid·een). BP Commission approved name for 11β, 17α,21 - trihydroxy - 16 - methylenepregna - 4,6 - diene - 3,20 - dione; an ACTH inhibitor.

Isoprenaline (i·so·**pren**·al·een). $C_6H_3(OH)_2CHOHCH_2NH(C_3H_7)$. The BP Commission approved name for isopropyl noradrenaline, a homologue of adrenaline having a similar action. It is usually employed as the sulphate. **Isoprenaline Sulphate BP 1973.** $C_6H_3(OH)_2CHOHCH_2NH(C_3H_7)\cdot\frac{1}{2}H_2SO_4\cdot H_2O$; a stable synthetic analogue of adrenaline, used mainly for the relief of bronchitic asthma. Unlike adrenaline, it is active when administered sublingually.

isoprene (i·so·preen). $CH_2=C(CH_3)CH=CH_2$, a compound formed during the distillation of rubber. Rubber itself is a polymer of isoprene.

Isopropamide Iodide (i·so·**pro**·pam·ide i·o·dide). BP Commission approved name for (3-carbamoyl-3,3-diphenylpropyl) methyldi-isopropyl-ammonium iodide; it is used in the treatment of peptic ulcer.

isopropanol (i·so·**pro**·pan·ol). Isopropyl alcohol. *See* ALCOHOL.

isopropyl (i·so·**pro**·pil). The monovalent radical, $(CH_3)_2CH-$.

Isopropyl Myristate BPC 1968 (i·so·**pro**·pil·**mi**·ris·tate). A synthetic, prepared by the esterification of myristic acid with isopropyl alcohol; it is used in external applications in place of vegetable oils.

isopropylarterenol (i·so·**pro**·pil·ar·ter·**e'**·nol. Isoprenaline sulphate.

isopropylbenzanthracene (i·so·**pro**·pil·benz·**an'**·thrah·seen). $(CH_3)_2CHC_{18}H_{11}$, a derivative of 1,2-benzanthracene, and known to possess carcinogenic activity.

isopropylepinephrine (i·so·**pro**·pil·ep·e·**nef'**·reen). Isopropyl-adrenaline, isoprenaline, $C_6H_3(OH)_2CHOHCH_2NH(C_3H_7)$. A synthetic analogue of adrenaline; the sulphate is isoprenaline sulphate.

isoproterenol (i·so·pro·**ter'**·en·ol). Isoprenaline BPC.

isopters (i·**sop**·terz). Lines drawn on a chart of the field of vision which pass through points of equal visual acuity. [Gk *isos* equal, *opter* observer.]

isoquinoline (i·so·**kwin**·o·leen). $\overline{CH=CHN=CHC}_6H_4$, a basic substance from which many alkaloids are derived. It is an isomer of quinoline, and occurs in coal tar.

isoriboflavine (i·so·ri·bo·**fla'**·veen). An isomer of the vitamin riboflavine, claimed to be more efficient at reducing cytochrome C.

isorrhopic (i·so·**rop**·ik). Equal in value. [Gk *isorrhopos* in equipoise.]

isoserotherapy (i·so·seer·o·**ther'**·ap·e). The therapeutic use of an isoserum.

isoserum (i·so·seer·um). Serum taken from a person suffering from or who has suffered from the disease which is affecting the patient under treatment. [Gk *isos* equal, serum.]

isosmotic (i·soz·**mot**·ik). With similar osmotic pressure. [Gk *isos* equal, osmotic.]

Isospora (i·**sos**·po·rah). A genus of Sporozoa. *Isospora belli* is a well-known parasite of the intestinal epithelium in warm countries. It is relatively non-pathogenic, but heavy infections may cause dysentery. *I. bigemina*, common in cats, has been recorded from man. *I. hominis*, very similar to *I. belli*, is the more common intestinal parasite in temperate countries. *I. natalensis* is a species that is a relatively common infection among the African peoples of Durban and probably elsewhere. The differentiation of these species is not very clear and some parasitologists recognize only one species, *I. belli* or *hominis*. [Gk *isos* equal, spore.]

isospore (i·so·spore). A non-sexual spore that is produced from plants possessing only one kind of spore and that grows to maturity without conjugation. [see prec.]

isostere (i·so·steer). 1. A competitive inhibitor. 2. In chemistry, any atom, radical, or compound which possesses the same number and arrangement of electrons as another atom, radical, or compound, and hence displays similar physical properties. [Obsolete term.] [Gk *isos* equal, *stereos* solid.]

isosthenuria (i·so·sthen·**ewr'**·e·ah). A condition occurring in chronic renal disease with renal insufficiency in which there is regular secretion of urine of the same specific gravity as protein-free plasma. The specific gravity remains stable (about 1.010) irrespective of the fluid intake. [Gk *isos* equal, *sthenos* strength, urine.]

isostimulation (i·so·stim·ew·**la'**·shun). A method of stimulating functional activity by injecting into the body cells of the same kind as those of the organ under treatment, e.g. injection of liver cells in order to increase liver function. [Gk *isos* equal, stimulation.]

isotel (i·so·tel). A food factor that replaces another otherwise essential. [Gk *isoteles* bearing the same burden.]

isotherapeutics (i·so·ther·ap·**ew'**·tix). The science of isotherapy.

isotherapy (i·so·**ther**·ap·e). A method of treatment in which the active causal agent or the products of the disease are administered. [Gk *isos* equal, therapy.]

isotherm (i·so·therm). A line drawn on a map connecting places that have the same mean temperature. [see foll.]

isothermal (i·so·**ther**·mal). Having the same temperature. [Gk *isos* equal, *therme* heat.]

isothermognosis (i·so·ther·mog·**no'**·sis). A state of disordered sense perception in which cold, heat, and pain are all felt as heat. [Gk *isos* equal, *therme* heat, *gnosis* a recognizing.]

isothiocyanate (i·so·thi·o·**si'**·an·ate). Any salt or ester of isothiocyanic acid. **Acrinyl isothiocyanate.** $OHC_6H_4CH_2NCS$, a product of the hydrolysis of sinalbin, the glucoside contained in white mustard seeds. **Allyl isothiocyanate.** $CH_2=CHCH_2NCS$, a compound produced by the hydrolysis of sinigrin, the glucoside of black mustard, and a constituent of mustard oil. It is a strong rubefacient and vesicant when applied to the skin, and is employed, diluted with alcohol and oil, as a counter-irritant for sprains, rheumatism, and the relief of deep-seated pain. **Butyl isothiocyanate, isobutyl isothiocyanate.** $(CH_3)_2CHCH_2NCS$, an oily compound occurring in horse-radish and other species of *Cochlearia*. **Phenyl isothiocyanate.** A reagent used in the determination of terminal amino residues in peptides. **Phenylethyl isothiocyanate.** $C_6H_5(C_2H_5)NCS$, a compound derived from oil of mignonette.

Isothipendyl (i·so·thi·**pen'**·dil). BP Commission approved name for 9 - (2 - dimethylaminopropyl) - 10 - thia - 1,9 - diaza - anthracene; an antihistamine. **Isothipendyl Hydrochloride BPC 1968.** The hydrochloride of isothipendyl; it is potent but its action is of short duration and it is less liable than many other antihistamines to cause drowsiness.

isothymol (i·so·**thi**·mol). Carvacrol, methylisopropylphenol, $CH_3C_6H_3(OH)CH(CH_3)_2$. A colourless liquid present in the oils of thyme and caraway and isomeric with thymol. It has been used as a deodorant in chronic lung infections, but is not now of therapeutic importance.

isotonia (i·so·to·ne·ah). 1. The resistance normally shown to any outside pressure, influence, or stimulation. 2. A condition in which the osmotic pressure in two solutions or constituents of a solution is the same. [Gk *isos* equal, tone.]

isotonic (i·so·**ton**·ik). 1. Of uniform or equal tension or tonicity. 2. Of equal tonus; in solutions applied to those exerting equal osmotic pressures whatever their composition. 3. In muscle physiology, referring to a contraction in which the muscle length alters, but not the tension exerted. [see prec.]

isotonicity (i·so·ton·**is'**·it·e). 1. The state or quality of having and maintaining normal and uniform resistance or tension. 2. Of fluids, having the same osmotic pressure. [Gk *isos* equal, tone.]

isotope (i·so·tope). A nuclide of a particular chemical element which has the same atomic number as but a different mass number from other nuclides of the same element. **Carbon-labelled isotope.** A compound labelled with a radioactive isotope of carbon. **Carrier-free isotope.** An element or compound containing an isotope in which all the atoms of the radioactive component are active, and no inactive atoms isotopic with the active component are present. **Double isotope derivative dilution.** A method of estimating very small quantities of hormones, such as testosterone in blood or urine. **Hydrogen isotopes.** The two isotopes, deuterium and tritium. **Radio-isotope, radioactive isotope.** An isotope with a nuclear composition that is unstable; nuclei undergoing spontaneous disintegration with the emission of α, β, or γ radiation. They are widely used as tracers. **Stable isotope.** An isotope which is not radioactive. **Tritiated isotope.** Isotope labelled with tritium. [Gk *isos* equal, *topos* place.]

isotoxic (i·so·tox·ik). Relating or belonging to an isotoxin.

isotoxin (i·so·tox·in). A toxin in the blood which has a harmful effect on other individuals or animals of the same species. [Gk *isos* equal, toxin.]

isotransplant (i·so·trans·plahnt). In plastic surgery, tissue or other structures taken from one individual for repair of lesions in another individual of the same species. Isogeneic graft. [Gk *isos* equal, transplant.]

isotransplantation (i·so·trans·plan·ta′·shun). The process of taking an isotransplant from one individual and applying it to another.

isotrimorphism (i·so·tri·mor′·fizm). The phenomenon in which the three forms of crystals of a trimorphous substance are similar to those of another trimorphous substance. [Gk *isos* equal, trimorphism.]

isotrimorphous (i·so·tri·mor′·fus). Belonging to or having the quality of isotrimorphism.

isotron (i·so·tron). A device in which ions are accelerated in pulses which are synchronous with a deflecting field. Since the acceleration of an isotope is dependent on its mass, a mixture of isotopes can be separated into its constituents by the use of such a device. [Obsolete term.] See MASS SPECTROMETER. [Gk *isos* equal.]

isotropic (i·so·trop·ik). 1. Possessing the same properties uniformly throughout. 2. Having the same appearance and shape from all viewpoints. 3. In physics, having the same refractive index along any axis. 4. In biology, not having any predetermined axes. [Gk *isos* equal, *trope* a turning.]

isotypical (i·so·tip·ik·al). Relating to or being of the same type. [Gk *isos* equal, type.]

isouretin (i·so·ewr·e′·tin). $NH_2CH{=}NOH$, a compound formed by hydrocyanic acid and ammonia: it is an isomer of urea.

isovolumic (i·so·vol·ew′·mik). The state of having equal or unchanging volume. In cardiology, applied to those phases of ventricular systole during which both the atrioventricular and semilunar valves are closed. [Gk *isos* equal, volume.]

Isoxsuprine (i·sox·sew·preen). BP Commission approved name for 1 - *p* - hydroxyphenyl - 2 - (1 - methyl - 2 - phenoxyethylamino) - 1 - propanol; a vasodilator.

ispaghula (is·pag·ew·lah). Spogel seeds, the ripe seeds obtained from *Plantago ovata* Forsk. (family Plantaginaceae), a herb indigenous to India and Iran. They contain mucilage, and swell on contact with water to form a gelatinous mass; used in diarrhoea as a demulcent, and in the treatment of intestinal atony (BPC 1968). **Ispaghula husk.** The separated mucilage-containing outer layer of the seed only, and therefore more powerful in action than the whole seeds. [Indonesian name.]

Israel, James Adolf (b. 1848). Berlin surgeon.

Israel's actinomycosis. Actinomycosis due to *Actinomyces bovis* (*israeli*).

issue (is·ew). 1. Offspring. 2. A discharge. 3. An exit or vent. 4. An artificial sore or fistula kept open for the purpose of counter-irritation or for the discharge of pus in order to relieve congestion in or pressure on a part. **Paternity issues.** Cases of disputed paternity requiring investigation of the blood system, including the blood groups, haptoglobins, and latterly the enzyme systems, inheritable on a Mendelian basis. Exclusion, rather than proof, of paternity is the object of such tests, now acceptable in most courts of law. **Issue pea.** A pellet of some irritating material such as orris root placed in an artificial sore for the purpose of maintaining the flow of pus. (Obsolete.) [OFr. *issir* to go out.]

isthmectomy (is·mek·to·me). 1. Median strumectomy; in goitre, excision of the thyroid isthmus. 2. Surgical excision of any isthmus. [isthmus, Gk *ektome* a cutting out.]

isthmian, isthmic (is·me·an, is·mik). Relating or belonging to any isthmus.

isthmitis (is·mi·tis). Inflammation of the oropharyngeal isthmus. [isthmus, Gk *-itis* inflammation.]

isthmocholosis (is·mo·ko·lo′·sis). Catarrh of the fauces with synchronous disorganization of biliary flow. [isthmus, Gk *chole* bile, *-osis* condition.]

isthmoid (is·moid). Having resemblance to an isthmus. [isthmus, Gk *eidos* form.]

isthmoparalysis (is·mo·par·al′·is·is). Isthmoplegia. [isthmus, paralysis.]

isthmoplegia (is·mo·ple·je·ah). A paralysed condition of the oropharyngeal isthmus. [isthmus, Gk *plege* stroke.]

isthmopolypus (is·mo·pol·e·pus). A polypus growing in the oropharyngeal isthmus.

isthmospasm (is·mo·spazm). Spasm of any isthmus, as of the uterine tube.

isthmus [NA] (is·mus, isth·mus). In anatomy, a short narrow part or constriction in an elongated cavity or canal; a narrow band of tissue joining two larger masses of similar tissue. **Aortic isthmus [isthmus aortae (NA)].** A slight constriction of the aorta between the site of the left common carotid artery and the ductus arteriosus. **Isthmus of the auricular cartilage [isthmus cartilaginis auris (NA)].** The strip of cartilage linking the cartilage of the auricle to that of the external auditory meatus. **Isthmus of the external auditory meatus.** A constriction in the bony part of the meatus, about 2 cm from the bottom of the concha. **Isthmus of the gyrus cinguli [isthmus gyri cinguli (NA)].** A narrow connection between the gyrus cinguli and hippocampal gyrus. **Oropharyngeal isthmus [isthmus faucium (NA)].** A slight constriction between the mouth and pharynx, bounded by the palate, tongue, and the palatoglossal arches. **Pharyngeal isthmus.** A slight constriction between the nasal and oral parts of the pharynx. **Isthmus of the pharyngotympanic tube [isthmus tubae auditivae (NA)].** The narrowest part of the tube, which occurs at the junction of the bony and cartilaginous parts. **Isthmus of the prostate [isthmus prostatae (NA)].** A connection between the right and left lobes of the prostate in front of the urethra. **Isthmus rhombencephali [NA].** A constriction in the neural tube of the embryo, situated at the anterior end of the hind-brain (rhombencephalon) where it joins the mid-brain. **Isthmus of the thyroid gland [isthmus glandulae thyroideae (NA)].** The part of the thyroid anterior to the trachea, which joins the two lateral lobes. **Isthmus of the uterine tube [isthmus tubae uterinae (NA)].** The narrow medial third of the uterine tube. **Isthmus of the uterus [isthmus uteri (NA)].** The narrow region at the junction of the body and neck of the uterus; the term is also used to denote the upper third of the cervix which is taken up into the body during pregnancy. [Gk *isthmos.*]

See also: GUYON, KROENIG.

isuria (i·sewr·e·ah). A condition in which the rate of excretion of urine does not vary. [Gk *isos* equal, urine.]

Itard, Jean Marie Gaspard (b. 1775). Paris otologist.

Itard's catheter. A type of eustachian catheter.

Itard-Cholewa sign. Anaesthesia of the tympanic membrane and external auditory meatus in otosclerosis.

itch (itsh). 1. Any sensation of irritation in the skin or mucous membranes that gives rise to a desire to scratch or rub. 2. Scabies. **Alkali itch.** A dermatitis from alkalis, occurring in those handling chemicals. **Bakers' itch.** A rash usually occurring on the hands and anterior aspect of the forearms of bakers; it may be mechanical in origin, or due to sensitivity to flour improvers or to sugar. It is sometimes caused by the mite *Tyroglyphus* or by *Pediculoides ventricosus.* **Barbers' itch.** Tinea barbae. **Barley itch.** 1. Grain itch (see below). 2. A sensitivity to the plant *Mucuna pruriens,* which grows among the barley, and sheds irritant hairs. **Bath itch.** The sensation of itching or burning immediately after taking a bath. **Bedouin itch.** Miliaria rubra or prickly heat. **Bricklayers' itch.** A dermatitis occurring among bricklayers, due to lime. **Cavalryman's itch.** An atypical form of scabies caused by *Sarcoptes scabiei* var. *equi.* **Cheese itch.** Grocers' itch (see below). **Coolie itch.** 1. An irritating rash in coolies in low-lying tropical regions, caused by nematode worms. 2. Infestation of workers in Indian tea plantations with *Rhizoglyphus parasiticus.* **Copra itch.** An itching papular or papulovesicular eruption, chiefly affecting the limbs but sometimes found on the trunk of those handling copra; it is caused by the mite, *Tyroglyphus longior.* **Cotton-seed itch.**

An eruption in those handling in bulk, cotton seed infested with *Pediculoides ventricosus.* **Cuban itch.** 1. An eruption reported from Cuba during the Spanish-American war; probably alastrim. 2. Scabies. **Dew itch.** Ground itch (see below). **Dhobie itch.** Tinea cruris; in India it was thought to be due to the spread of tinea by washermen (dhobies) wearing their customers' clothes and infecting them. **Dogger Bank itch.** Seaweed dermatitis. *See* DERMATITIS. **Dry-salters' itch.** A dermatitis from sugar. **Farmers' itch.** Scabies. **Filarial itch.** An eruption due to the filarial parasite *Onchocerca.* **Foot itch.** Cutaneous ancylostomiasis. **Frost itch.** Pruritus hiemalis. **Grain itch.** Dermatitis caused by *Pediculoides ventricosus,* a parasite on the wheat-straw worm, the joint worm, and the grain moth; the lesions are weals, papules, minute vesicles, and sometimes pustules. Also known as *acarodermatitis urticaroides* (*Schamberg*). **Grocers' itch.** 1. Parasitic dermatitis due to mites in grain, *Pediculoides ventricosus,* cheese mites, *Carpoglyphus passularum,* or *Glyciphagus domesticus* which infests dried foods. 2. Dermatitis from sugar. **Ground itch.** Ancylostomiasis cutis, a cutaneous eruption caused at the point of entry of ancylostoma larvae: irritating blisters form: when they are ruptured the lesion may become secondarily infected and an eczematous condition may follow. In the case of *Ancylostoma braziliense* infections, not normally a parasite of man, the larvae are unable to reach the deeper tissues and migrate laterally causing a migrating lesion, one form of larva migrans. **Haberswein itch.** An eruption resembling dermatitis herpetiformis, occurring in the Haberswein area of northern Kenya; it is caused by the shed hairs of certain Lepidoptera. **Harvest itch.** Scrub itch (see below). **Jock itch.** Tinea cruris. **Lumbermen's itch.** Scabies. **Mad itch.** Pseudorabies. **Malabar itch.** Tinea imbricata. **Mattress itch.** Grain itch (see above). **Millers' itch.** Grain itch (see above). **Miners' itch.** Cutaneous ancylostomiasis. **Mite itch.** Scrub itch (see below). **Norway itch.** Norwegian scabies. *See* SCABIES. **Philippine itch.** 1. Alastrim. 2. Scabies. **Poultrymen's itch.** A rash on the hand and forearms caused by *Dermanyssus gallinae,* the poultry mite. **Prairie itch.** 1. Grain itch (see above). 2. Irritation of the skin caused by the fine dust of the prairies. 3. Scabies. **Scrub itch.** An eruption on the lower limbs occurring in the Far East, especially during and just after the monsoon; caused by *Trombicula* (harvest mites) which sometimes carry *Rickettsia orientalis,* causing scrub typhus. **Straw itch, straw-bed itch.** Grain itch (see above). **Sugar itch.** Contact dermatitis from sugar. **Swamp itch.** 1. Grain itch (see above). 2. Scabies. **Swimmers' itch.** Cercarial dermatitis produced in man by blood flukes, especially of aquatic birds. **Tar itch.** Diffuse dermatitis from contact with tar. **Warehousemen's itch.** Irritation of the skin of warehousemen, caused by the goods they carry. **Washerwomen's itch.** An eruption of the hands due to constant use of detergents and soda. **Water itch.** 1. Cutaneous ancylostomiasis. 2. An eruption of the feet of coolies in Indian tea gardens; due to *Rhizoglyphus.* **Wet-weather itch.** Cutaneous ancylostomiasis. **Winter itch.** Pruritus hiemalis. [AS *giccan.*]

See also: BOECK (C. W.).

itching (it·ching). Any irritation or tickling sensation of the skin; pruritus. [see prec.]

iter (i·ter). A passage or tunnel. **Iter a tertio ad quartum ventriculum.** Aqueduct of the mid-brain. **Iter chordae anterius.** Anterior canaliculus of the chorda tympani. **Iter chordae posterius.** Posterior canaliculus of the chorda tympani. **Inter dentis.** The route by which a tooth erupts. [L, a way.]

See also: SYLVIUS.

iteral (i·ter·al). Relating or belonging to an iter.

ithykyphosis (ith·e·ki·fo'·sis). Backward angular projection of the vertebral column without any lateral displacement. [Gk *ithys* straight, *kyphosis* hump-back.]

ithylordosis (ith·e·lor·do'·sis). Forward angular projection of the vertebral column without any lateral displacement. [Gk *ithys* straight, lordosis.]

itinerarium (i·tin·er·a'·re·um). A lithotomy staff. *See* STAFF. [L *iter* a way.]

Ito, Hayazo (fl. 1913). Japanese physician.

Ito's naevus. A dermal melanocytic naevus in the acromioclavicular region and upper chest, occurring mostly in the Japanese.

Ito-Reenstierna test. A test for chancroid infection by intradermal injection of a suspension of killed *Haemophilus ducreyi.* An inflammatory papule developing within 48 hours indicates present or past infection. The skin does not react until about 14 days after infection, and the test is believed to remain positive for the remainder of the patient's life.

Itramin Tosylate (i·tram·in tos·il·ate). BP Commission approved name for 2-nitrato-ethylamine toluene-*p*-sulphonate; a vasodilator.

ivory (i·vor·e). 1. Dentine. 2. The fine-grained bony substance of which the teeth and tusks of elephants and other large mammals are composed. **Black ivory.** Animal charcoal. *See* CHARCOAL. [L *ebur.*]

Iwanoff (Iwanow), Wladimir P. (b. 1861). Russian ophthalmologist.

Iwanoff's retinal oedema. The appearance of cystic spaces at the extreme periphery of the retina in early adult life; these increase in number with age.

Ixodes (ix·o·deez). A genus of ticks of world-wide distribution, many species of which bite man and cause various diseases. *Ixodes ricinus,* the dog or sheep tick of Europe, a vector of Russian encephalitis; *Ixodes holocyclus* of Australia and *Ixodes pilosus* of South Africa may cause tick paralysis. *Ixodes persulcatus* is a reservoir for the virus of spring-summer encephalitis in the temperate Far East, and also of Q fever. *Ixodes rubicundus* causes tick paralysis. Several species are potential vectors of tularaemia. [Gk, sticky.]

ixodiasis (ix·o·di·as·is). 1. Infestation with ticks. 2. Any of the tick-borne fevers or any wound or other lesion caused by tick bites. [*Ixodes.*]

ixodic (ix·od·ik). Due to, relating to, or derived from ticks. [see prec.]

ixodism (ix·o·dizm). Ixodiasis.

Ixodoidea (ix·o·doid·e·ah). A superfamily of Acarina, the ticks, characterized by the large size and thick cuticle of the adults. All are parasitic at some stage. [*Ixodes,* Gk *eidos* form.]

ixomyelitis (ix·o·mi·el·i'·tis). Inflammation of the lumbar segment of the spinal cord. [Gk *ixys* waist, myelitis.]

ixovotoxin (ix·o·vo·tox'·in). Name for a theoretical substance which causes tick paralysis, produced by gravid female ticks of several species. [*Ixodes,* L *ovum* egg, Gk *toxikon* poison.]

J

jaba (jah·bah). Joba.

jaborandi (jab·o·ran·de). 1. A name given to several plants belonging to the families Rutaceae and Piperaceae, which have diaphoretic and salivant properties. 2. Jaborandi leaves, the leaflets from a Brazilian shrub, *Pilocarpus microphyllus* (family Rutaceae). It contains about 0.5 per cent of the alkaloid, pilocarpine, upon which the main therapeutic action of preparations of the drug depends. It is also reputed to stimulate the growth of hair, and in the form of the extract or tincture it is added to hair tonics for this purpose. Its main use is as the source of pilocarpine. [Brazilian.]

Jaboulay, Mathieu (b. 1860). Lyons surgeon.

Jaboulay's amputation. Interpelvi-abdominal amputation; amputation of the thigh and removal of the hip bone.

Jaboulay's operation. 1. For hydrocele: eversion of the sac of a hydrocele so that it lies inside out within the scrotum. 2. Jaboulay's amputation (see above).

Jacaranda (jak·ah·ran·dah). A genus of South American trees (family Bignoniaceae). The leaves of *Jacaranda procera* Spreng (caroba) have been used in syphilitic conditions and in the treatment of epilepsy. [Brazilian.]

Jaccoud, Sigismond (b. 1830). Paris physician.

Jaccoud's dissociated fever. The paradoxically slow pulse rate in febrile patients with meningitis; it was first applied to adult cases of tuberculous meningitis.

Jaccoud's sign. A suprasternal prominence of the aorta, said to indicate the presence of a leukaemic condition.

jacket (jak·et). A piece of apparatus or clothing, usually designed to be worn or applied to the upper part of the trunk. **Cotton jacket.** A jacket made from cotton wool or gamgee tissue, worn as extra protection against operative shock, or by patients with chest diseases. **Leather jacket.** An orthopaedic appliance for the correction of deformities. **Localizer jacket.** A corrective plaster jacket used in the treatment of scoliosis. **Minerva jacket.** A plaster-of-Paris spinal support which also incorporates a plaster helmet, thus supporting the chin and immobilizing the cervical spine. **Plaster-of-Paris jacket.** An encasement made of plaster of Paris, moulded to fit the trunk. It is used to immobilize the spine and sometimes the hip joints, thus promoting healing by rest, to prevent deformity in active disease of the spine or to correct established deformity. **Pneumonia jacket.** A gamgee or cotton-wool jacket. **Polyethylene jacket.** A stiff moulded surgical jacket made of the plastic substance, polyethylene. **Poroplastic-felt jacket.** A jacket which is manufactured from porous and plastic felt, and used in orthopaedic conditions. **Strait jacket.** An appliance made from strong material and having long sleeves which extend beyond the hands, by which control may be exerted, when necessary, to restrain violently insane persons from acts of violence to themselves or to others. [Fr. *jaquette.*]

See also: RISSER, SAYRE.

jackscrew (jak·skroo). A device used for expanding the dental arch. [O Fr. *Jacques, escroue.*]

Jackson, Chevalier (b. 1865). Philadelphia laryngologist.

Chevalier Jackson forceps. A bronchoscopic forceps having a distally controlled, hinged, basket-shaped cutting beak for the removal of portions of tissue from the trachea or bronchi for biopsy.

Chevalier Jackson oesophagoscope. An instrument with distal lighting and circular in cross-section, used for examining the oesophagus.

Jackson's sign. A wheezing expiratory sound over a tuberculous area of the lung.

Chevalier Jackson safety triangle. The triangle formed by the medial borders of the sternocleidomastoid muscles, which meet below to form the apex; the base is formed by a horizontal line at the level of the lower border of the thyroid cartilage.

Jackson, Ian. 20th century London anaesthetist.

Bowen-Jackson laryngoscope blade. A long, curved blade occupying little room in the mouth.

Jackson, Jabez North (b. 1868). Kansas City surgeon.

Jackson's membrane or veil. Bands of peritoneum, probably congenital in origin, passing across the front of the caecum to the parietes; they may be of some aetiological significance in appendicitis.

Jackson, James, Jnr. (b. 1810). Boston physician.

Jackson's sign. Pulse deficit; in rapid auricular fibrillation, the pulse at the wrist is slower than the apex beat. This is due to failure of many of the weaker beats to reach the radial pulse.

Jackson, John Hughlings (b. 1835). London neurologist.

Jacksonian convulsion. A unilateral focal convulsion, beginning at the angle of the mouth, the thumb or great toe, and spreading in a motor march (*Jacksonian motor march*) corresponding to the order of representation of movement in the cortex, the march being centripetal in the limb first involved, centrifugal in the other. Consciousness is lost only if the opposite limbs are involved. *See* JACKSONIAN EPILEPSY (below).

Jacksonian epilepsy. Epileptic phenomena of motor or sensory nature due to epileptic discharge of focal onset and spreading to the contralateral prerolandic or postrolandic cortex. The attack starts in one bodily segment and spreads. It may then become generalized and it may be attended by loss of consciousness. syn. *Bravais-Jacksonian epilepsy.*

Jackson's law or rule. In disease of the brain, complex highly-developed, that is the most recently developed, processes are the first to be lost and the last to recover.

Jackson's paralysis or syndrome, Hughlings Jackson syndrome. Syndrome of vago-accessory hypoglossal paralysis: unilateral paralysis of palatal, pharyngeal and intrinsic laryngeal muscles, of the sternocleidomastoid and trapezius muscles, and of one half of the tongue. It is usually due to a medullary lesion, but can result from infranuclear damage.

Bravais-Jackson epilepsy. Jacksonian epilepsy (see above).

Jacob, Arthur (b. 1790). Dublin ophthalmic surgeon.

Jacob's membrane. A layer of rods and cones in the retina.

Jacob's triad. Amaurosis, ophthalmoplegia and trigeminal neuralgia.

Jacob's ulcer. Rodent ulcer. *See* ULCER.

Jacobaeus, Hans Christian (b. 1879). Stockholm surgeon.

Jacobaeus operation. Pneumolysis; the cautery division of pleural adhesions by way of a thoracoscope.

jacobine (jak·o·been). $C_{18}H_{25}O_6N$, an alkaloid obtained from *Senecio jacoboea* and other species. It is highly toxic to the liver.

Jacobsohn's reflex. The patient's forearm rests on its ulnar side with the fingers semi-extended; the extensor aspect of the lower end of the radius is then tapped sharply and finger flexion results. This reflex is an elaboration of the finger jerk and of Hoffman's sign, and occurs in pyramidal-tract disease. Its specific nature has been questioned as it occurs in normal individuals, but it is at least a sign of hyper-irritability.

Jacobson, Julius (b. 1828). Königsberg ophthalmologist.

Jacobson's operation, for cataract. A scleral flap incision below the lower corneal limbus was used with iridectomy; of historical interest.

Jacobson's retinopathy. Syphilitic retinopathy; the affection of the retina and optic nerve in different ways, most commonly the infection of the underlying choroid.

Jacobson, Ludwig Levin (b. 1783). Copenhagen anatomist and physician.

Jacobson's canal. The canaliculus for the tympanic nerve.

Jacobson's cartilage. The subvomerine cartilage. *See* CARTILAGE.

Jacobson's nerve. The tympanic nerve.

Jacobson's organ. The vomeronasal organ. *See* ORGAN.

Jacobson's plexus. The tympanic plexus. Sometimes incorrectly called *Jacobson's anastomosis.*

Jacobson's sulcus. A groove on the promontory of the tympanic cavity which contains the tympanic nerve.

Jacquart, Henri. 19th century French physician and anthropologist.

Jacquart's angle. The ophryospinal angle. *See* ANGLE.

Jacquemet, Marcel (b. 1872). French physician.

Jacquemet's recess. A peritoneal recess between the liver and gall bladder formed as a result of the complete investment of the organ with peritoneum.

Jacquemier, Jean Marie (b. 1806). French obstetrician.

Jacquemier's sign. Violet coloration of the vaginal skin (due to increased vascularity) as a sign of early pregnancy.

Jacques' plexus. A plexus of nerves in the muscular wall of the uterine tube.

Jacquet, Leonard Marie Lucien (b. 1860). Paris dermatologist.

Jacquet's dermatitis or erythema. A form of napkin (or diaper) rash attributed to irritation from ammonia formed in urine by bacteria.

Jacquet's disease. 1. Alopecia caused reflexively by dental disease. 2. Jacquet's dermatitis (see above).

Jacquet's syndrome. Alopecia attributed to dental abnormalities.

jactation (jak·ta·shun). Jactitation. [L *jactare* to toss.]

jactitation (jak·tit·a·shun). 1. Restlessness and tossing of the body occurring in acute illness. 2. Twitching of muscles or sets of muscles, such as occurs in epilepsy. 3. Anoxic spasms of muscles, formerly sometimes seen during dental anaesthesia. **Periodic jactitation.** Chorea. [L *jactitare* to toss about.]

jaculiferous (jak·ew·lif·er·us). In zoology, covered with sharp spines or prickles. [L *jaculum* dart, *ferre* to bear.]

Jaculus gordoni (jak·ew·lus gor·don·i). The white-rumped gerbil which can be infected with *Leishmania.* [L *jaculari* to throw.]

Jadassohn, Josef (b. 1863). Breslau dermatologist.

Jadassohn's disease. 1. Anetoderma. 2. Granulosis rubra nasi. 3. Cutis rhomboidalis nuchae.

Jadassohn's test. Irrigation test. *See* TEST.

Jadassohn-Bloch test. Patch test. *See* TEST.

Hebra-Jadassohn disease. Pityriasis rubra.

Jadassohn-Lewandowsky syndrome. Pachyonychia congenita.

Jadelot, Jean François Nicolas (b. 1766). Paris physician.

Jadelot's furrows, lines or traits. Characteristic lines of the facies associated with problematical but not necessarily proven disease, e.g. the labial line, extending from the corner of the mouth downwards in chronic respiratory disease, the nasal line extending from the ala of the nose to the corner of the mouth in inflammation of the paranasal sinuses or chronic alimentary disease, and the ocular line extending from the inner canthus downwards.

Jaeger, Eduard Ritter von Jastthal (b. 1818). Vienna ophthalmologist.

Jaeger's operation. Five operations are described, all of which are now obsolete. 1. For cataract extraction. 2. and 3. For ectropion. 4. For entropion. 5. For trichiasis.

Jaeger's test-type. A test for near vision, consisting of paragraphs in ordinary printer's type of varying sizes, the smallest labelled "Brilliant" = J_1, the next "Pearl" = J_2, and so on, increasing in size. The smallest type read at the closest distance is then recorded.

Jaeger, Heinrich (b. 1856). German bacteriologist.

Jaeger's meningococcus. *Diplococcus crassus.*

Jaesche, George Emanuel (b. 1815). German surgeon.

Jaesche-Arlt operation, for trichiasis. The lid margin is split just behind the lash margin; a crescentic area of skin is excised from the lid about 3-4 mm from the margin. This is sutured, so pulling the lash margin up, and the excised skin is trimmed and inserted into the gaping raw area below the lash margin where the lid was originally split. Of historical interest.

Jaffe, Henry L. 20th century New York physician.

Jaffe-Lichtenstein disease. Eosinophilic granuloma of bone; a solitary slow-growing lesion in older children. It is considered to be, with Letterer-Siwe and Hand-Schueller-Christian diseases, part of a group of diseases to which the name *Letterer-Christian disease* has been given. The term has also been applied to cystic osteofibromatosis, a fibrous dysplasia involving the medullary cavities of many bones.

Jaffé, Karl (b. 1854). German surgeon.

Jaffé's sign. From a sinus connected with a subphrenic abscess, pus tends to be expressed during inspiration, whereas if it is connected with an empyema, pus will tend to be expressed during expiration.

Jaffé, Max (b. 1841). Königsberg biochemist.

Jaffé reaction. The production of a red colour by creatinine with picric acid in alkaline solution.

Jaffé's test, for indican. To 5 parts of urine add 6 parts of concentrated hydrochloric acid and mix. Add 3 ml of chloroform and mix by repeated inversion. A blue colour in the chloroform indicates indican. Add 1 drop of 1 per cent potassium chlorate and mix again. If the chloroform becomes colourless, only a minute amount of indican is present. If the chloroform is coloured a deeper blue, add further drops with mixing as before until it finally becomes colourless. The greater the number of drops required the greater is the amount of indican in the urine.

Jakob, Alfons Maria (b. 1884). Hamburg neurologist.

Jakob's disease, Jakob-Creutzfeldt disease. Pseudosclerosis spastica; a progressive disease of middle life, with dementia, peripheral muscular wasting and degeneration of the pyramidal and extrapyramidal systems, giving spasticity and tremor or other involuntary movements. Transmission experiments in chimpanzees suggest that the disease may be due to a slow virus of, as yet, unknown characteristics.

Jaksch, Rudolf von (b. 1855). Prague physician.

von Jaksch anaemia, disease or syndrome. Originally described as a specific disease, "anaemia pseudoleukaemica infantum", seen in children under the age of 3 years; it is now considered to be a symptom complex and not a disease entity, associated with many factors such as malnutrition, tuberculosis, gastrointestinal disorders and many infections leading to severe anaemia, leucocytosis, relative lymphocytosis, splenomegaly, hepatomegaly and lymphadenopathy, among others. Gaucher's and Niemann-Pick diseases were originally included in this group.

Jalaguier, Adolphe (b. 1853). French surgeon.

Battle-Jalaguier-Kammerer incision, for appendicectomy. A vertical incision medial to the outer border of the right rectus abdominis muscle, with divisions of the rectus sheath and retraction of the muscle inwards.

Jalap (jal·ap). (BPC 1963.) The dried tubers obtained from a Mexican climbing plant, *Ipomoea purga* Hayne (family Convolvulaceae). It contains about 8-12 per cent of a resin similar in action to that obtained from ipomoea but differing from it in chemical constitution. The powdered drug, and the tincture prepared from it, are used as purgatives. **Brazilian jalap.** Obtained from the root of *Ipomoea tuberosa* Linn.; it yields a purgative resin allied to that obtained from ipomoea. **Orizaba jalap.** Ipomoea. **Jalap Resin BPC 1963.** The crude resin obtained from jalap by extraction with alcohol. The action and uses are the same as those of jalap. **Tampico jalap.** The root of *Ipomoea simulans* Hanbury. It contains a purgative resin similar to, but not identical with, that obtained from jalap. [*Jalapa*, town in Mexico.]

jalapa (jal·ap·ah). Jalap.

Jalapin BPC 1954 (jal·ap·in). That portion of jalap resin precipitated from an alcoholic solution by the addition of ether. It is usually administered in pill form as a purgative.

jamais vu (zham·a vew). The sensation that familiar objects have never been seen before. [Fr. never seen.]

James, Norman Reynolds 20th century Dallas anaesthetist.

James' pressure infiltrator. An apparatus by which supplies of a solution of local anaesthetic are fed by pressure through the infiltrating needle.

James, Robert (b. 1705). London physician.

James' powder. Antimonial powder. *See* POWDER.

James, Sidney Price. 20th century India and London malariologist.

James' classification. A classification of attacks of malaria into primary attack, recrudescence, relapse and recurrence.

James, William (b. 1842). American psychologist.

James-Lange theory. The theory of the emotions which postulates that the conscious emotional experience is a consequence of the visceral changes. According to the famous argument advanced by James, we do not run because we are afraid but are afraid because we run. (*See also* CANNON THEORY.)

Jamin, Jules Celèstin (b. 1818). French physicist.

Jamin's refractometer. An instrument for measuring the refractive index of a gas by the interference of 2 light beams produced by reflection and refraction in a rectangular block of glass.

Janet, Pierre Marie Fèlix (b. 1859). Paris psychiatrist.

Janet's disease. Psychasthenia.

Janet's test. A clinical test for differentiating between functional and organic superficial anaesthesia: the patient's skin is touched lightly and the patient, whose eyes are closed, is asked to say "yes" or "no". The answer "no" is taken to indicate functional anaesthesia, since the patient with organic loss of sensation will make no response when an anaesthetic area is touched.

Janeway, Edward Gamaliel (b. 1841). New York physician.

Janeway's spots. Small, raised, nodular, purple lesions on the palms of the hands and the soles of the feet in subacute bacterial endocarditis. They are due to infected emboli, and are similar to Osler's nodes which occur on the tips of the fingers from the same cause.

Janeway, Henry Harrington (b. 1873). New York surgeon.

Janeway's operation, Lepage-Janeway gastrostomy. The establishment of a communication from skin to stomach by a tube formed from the anterior stomach wall.

janiceps (jan·e·seps). A twin monster, the backs of the heads of which are fused together, the 2 faces looking in opposite directions. **Janiceps asymmetrus.** A janiceps one face of which is more incompletely developed than the other. [L *Janus* a two-faced Roman deity, *caput* head.]

Janin, Jospeph (b. 1864). Paris physician.

Janin's tetanus. Head tetanus; tetanus following a wound of the head, especially of the eyebrow region. It is characterized by trismus, facial paralysis on one side and marked dysphagia. The symptoms superficially resemble those of rabies.

Janker, Robert (b. 1894). Bonn radiologist.

Janker's apparatus. An apparatus for cineradiography of the heart with a 32 mm film in which 18–24 frames are taken per second with a skin exposure of 50 roentgens in a period of about 8 s.

Jansen, Albert (b. 1859). Berlin otologist.

Jansen's operation. A method of draining the internal ear in suppurative labyrinthitis.

Jansen, W. Muerk (b. 1867). Leyden orthopaedic surgeon.

Jansen's test. A patient who is unable to cross his legs with a point just above the ankle resting upon the opposite knee is likely to be suffering from osteo-arthritis of the hip joint on the affected side.

Janský, Jan (b. 1873). Prague physician.

Janský's classification. A classification of blood groups suggested by Janský, similar to the Moss classification but numbered from I to IV, corresponding to Moss groups IV, II, III and I, and to Landsteiner's groups O, A, B and AB respectively [obsolete].

Bielschowsky-Janský disease, Janský-Bielschowsky disease. The late infantile form of cerebromacular degeneration.

Janthinosoma (jan·thin·o·so″·mah). A genus (or sub-genus of *Psorophora*) of mosquitoes. The adults of several species act as passive carriers of the eggs of *Dermatobia hominis.* [Gk *ianthinos* violet-coloured, *soma* body.]

janus (ja·nus). Janiceps. [L a two-faced Roman deity.]

Jaques, James Archibald (b. 1815). British india-rubber manufacturer.

Jaques' catheter. A catheter originally made of soft red india rubber. Modern catheters are made of plastic.

jar (jar). A vessel, usually made of glass and cylindrical in form. **Leyden jar.** An electrical condenser composed of a glass vessel which is coated inside and outside with tinfoil. (Described in 1746 in Leyden, Holland.) [Ar. *jarrah.*]

jararaca (jar·ah·rak·ah). A very poisonous crotaline snake of tropical South America (*Bothrops atrox*). [Brazilian name.]

Jardine's hook. A combined hook and knife used for decapitation of the fetus.

jargon (jar·gon). 1. The babbling talk and incomprehensible words uttered by certain idiots and by insane persons; gibberish. 2. The terminology used by scientists, artists and others, not generally comprehended. [Fr. *jargonner* to utter indistinctly.]

Jarisch, Adolf (b. 1850). Vienna and Innsbruck dermatologist.

Jarisch-Herxheimer reaction. Intensification of a syphilitic lesion, associated with pyrexia and malaise, occurring within a few hours of an injection of a potent antisyphilitic remedy.

Jarjavay, Jean François (b. 1815). Paris anatomist and surgeon.

Jarjavay's ligaments. The rectovaginal and recto-uterine folds.

Jarjavay's muscle. A slender muscle which is a common abnormality found associated with the bulbospongiosus muscle.

Jarotzky, Alexander (b. 1866). Moscow physician.

Jarotsky's treatment. The treatment of a gastric ulcer with white of egg, bread and milk, and fresh butter.

Jarvis, William Chapman (b. 1855). New York laryngologist.

Jarvis' operation. A turbinectomy carried out by means of a specially-designed snare.

Jarvis' snare. A wire snare which is tightened by means of a screw in the handle and is used to remove polypi in the nose and throat.

jasmine (jaz·min). *Gelsemium.* **Yellow jasmine.** A plant of South America, *Gelsemium nitidum.* The dried roots and rhizomes constitute the gelsemium of pharmacy. [Pers. *yasmin.*]

Jateorhiza (ja·te·o·ri″·zah). A genus of tropical plants (family Menispermaceae). *Jateorhiza palmata* Lamarck is the source of calumba root. [Gk *iatros* physician, *rhiza* root.]

Jatropha (jat·ro·fah). A genus of tropical plants (family Euphorbiaceae), several species of which are employed in native medicine. The leaves of *Jatropha curcas* Linn. are used as a rubefacient, and the juice from the stem has haemostatic properties. The seeds of the same plant yield a strongly purgative oil reported as intermediate in action between castor oil and croton oil. *Jatropha glandulifera* Roxb. has similar properties. *Jatropha manihot* Willd. (=*Manihot utilissima* Pohl) is the source of tapioca. [Gk *iatros* physician, *trophe* nutrition.]

jaundice (jawn·dis). Icterus; a syndrome characterized by an excess of bile pigment in the blood (hyperbilirubinaemia) and consequent deposition of bile pigment in the skin, conjunctivae, mucous membranes, and generally in the urine. **Acholuric**

jaundice. The presence of jaundice without the appearance of bile pigment in the urine. Normally bilirubin appears in the urine when the concentration in the blood has risen to 1 in 50 000, but in haemolytic jaundice the concentration may reach 1 in 12 000 without escape of pigment into the urine. **Acholuric familial jaundice.** Familial haemolytic icterus, congenital haemolytic anaemia, spherocytosis: a hereditary disease characterized by jaundice, anaemia and splenomegaly; the red blood cells are more spherical than normal and less resistant to haemolysis. The jaundice is variable and of the acholuric type. **Acquired acholuric jaundice.** Acholuric jaundice beginning in adult life and running a more severe course than the congenital form. **Black jaundice.** Epidemic haemoglobinuria; jaundice associated with haemoglobinuria and anaemia which formerly occurred in epidemics among newborn infants in institutions, and was due to infection of the umbilical cord. The colour of the skin was dark slaty with underlying jaundice. **Catarrhal jaundice.** Synonymous with acute infective hepatitis; in rare cases it may be due to obstruction of the common bile duct following gastroduodenal catarrh. **Congenital obliterative jaundice.** That due to congenital obliteration of the bile ducts. **Dissociated jaundice.** The independent retention or excretion of bile pigments and bile salts: in haemolytic jaundice bilirubin accumulates in the blood, but the bile salts are excreted normally into the intestine and their blood concentration does not increase. **Green jaundice.** The greenish colour of the skin occurring in cases of long-standing obstructive jaundice. **Haemolytic jaundice.** Jaundice caused by excessive destruction of red blood corpuscles in the circulation, and the consequent formation of bilirubin in larger amounts than the hepatic cells can excrete. **Haemolytic jaundice of the newborn.** Icterus gravis neonatorum, erythroblastosis fetalis; jaundice occurring in the fetus or newborn infant in connection with the haemolytic anaemia due to incompatibility between the mother's serum and the red blood corpuscles of the child. It most often occurs when the child has inherited the Rh factor from the father while the mother is Rh-negative. **Homologous serum jaundice.** Jaundice due to hepatitis B virus following parenteral transmission of human blood products contaminated with the virus. The virus may also be spread by the faecal-oral route and by the communal use of any instrument penetrating the skin. The virus is distinct from that of infectious hepatitis. **Idiopathic dyserythropoietic jaundice.** A very rare hyperbilirubinaemia due to faulty red-cell synthesis in the bone marrow or liver. **Infective jaundice.** The jaundice due to an infective agent, commonly the viruses of hepatitis (types A or B) or the spirochaetes of leptospirosis. **Intrahepatic cholestatic jaundice.** Cholestasis due to drugs, chemicals or toxins without bile duct obstruction; it may occur in late pregnancy. **Latent jaundice.** A condition in which hyperbilirubinaemia occurs without visible jaundice. This may be present in pernicious anaemia and with slight degrees of biliary obstruction. A positive van den Bergh reaction is given, but the bilirubin is below a concentration of 1 in 50 000. **Leptospiral jaundice.** Leptospirosis associated with jaundice. Besides Weil's disease, several other types of leptospirosis occur. **Nuclear jaundice.** Kernicterus. **Obstructive jaundice.** Jaundice in which excreted bile is reabsorbed into the blood through hepatic blood capillaries or lymphatics owing to obstruction in the bile ducts. The obstruction may occur within the ducts, through changes in their walls or as the result of pressure from without. **Physiological jaundice.** Simple jaundice of infants (see following). **Simple jaundice of infants.** Icterus neonatorum, physiological jaundice, which occurs in about 50 per cent of newborn infants. It is haemolytic in type and due to the breaking down of the excessive number of red blood corpuscles present at birth. **Spirochaetal jaundice.** Spirochaetosis icterohaemorrhagica, Weil's disease; an acute febrile disease with jaundice due to infection with the *Leptospira icterohaemorrhagiae* which is excreted in the urine of rats. In man it generally occurs in persons working in rat-infested places. **Syphilitic jaundice.** Jaundice which very occasionally results from diffuse changes in the liver in congenital syphilis, the hepatitis of secondary syphilis or the gummata of tertiary syphilis. **Syringe-transmitted jaundice.** An infection due to the transmission of the virus of infective hepatitis by the employment of an insufficiently sterilized hypodermic or serum syringe. **Toxic jaundice.** Infective jaundice (see above). **Xanthochromic jaundice.** Yellow patches in the skin due to deposits of cholesterol, occasionally associated with chronic jaundice. [Fr. *jaune* yellow.]

jaw (jaw). A bone of the face supporting the teeth and concerned with mastication. The upper jaw comprises the two superior maxillae and the lower jaw the mandible. **Hapsburg jaw.** The prognathous jaw of members of the Hapsburg family. **Locked jaw.** Trismus; tonic spasm of the masseter muscles so that the jaw is clenched and cannot be opened. **Lumpy jaw.** Cervicofacial actinomycosis. **Parrot jaw.** A marked protrusion of the upper jaw beyond the lower. **Phossy jaw.** Phosphonecrosis. **Wolf jaw.** Cleft palate. *See* PALATE. [etym. dub.]

jaw chattering (**jaw chat**·er·ing). Clonic spasms of the jaw which may occur with a rigor or as a habit spasm. [etym. dub.]

jaw winking (**jaw wing**·king). A congenital abnormality in which partial ptosis at rest is associated with exaggerated elevation of the lid on movement of the jaw; *Marcus Gunn phenomenon. Hemifacial spasm. See* SPASM. [etym. dub.]

Jaworski, Valery (b. 1849). Cracow physician.

Jaworski's bodies. Spiral masses of mucus described in cases of hyperchlorhydria.

Jeanselme, Antoine Edouard (b. 1858). French dermatologist.

parasitic achromia of Jeanselme. Pityriasis versicolor.

jecoral, jecorary (**jek**·or·al, **jek**·or·ar·e). Hepatic. [see foll.]

jecorin (**jek**·or·in). A sugar-containing phospholipide isolated from the liver. It is of doubtful constitution, the sugar possibly being present merely as contaminant. [L *jecur* liver.]

jecorize (**jek**·or·ize). To impart to a food or preparation the therapeutic virtues of fish-liver oil. It is applied particularly to the treatment of milk by ultraviolet irradiation in order to confer vitamin-D activity upon it. [L *jecur* liver.]

jecorose (**jek**·or·oze). Hepatic. [see prec.]

jecur (**jek**·er). The liver. [L.]

Jeghers, Harold Joseph (b. 1904). Jersey City, New Jersey, physician.

Peutz-Jeghers syndrome. A rare condition in childhood, although more frequent in later life, said to be inherited through a Mendelian dominant gene of high penetration. A child with brown pigmented spots on the circumoral skin and on the intra-oral mucous membrane presents with abdominal pain associated with marked borborygmi. The pigmented spots show melanin deposits in the basal-cell layer. Intestinal intussusception caused by polyposis is found at operation, sometimes in multiple areas; polypi are not found in other areas common to their development.

jejunal (jej·**oon**·al). Belonging to the jejunum.

jejunal and ileal arteries [arteriae jejunales et ilei (NA)]. Jejunal and ileal branches of the superior mesenteric artery. *See* MESENTERIC ARTERIES.

jejunal and ileal veins [venae jejunales et ilei (NA)]. Veins accompanying the corresponding arteries to the jejunum and ileum; tributaries of the superior mesenteric vein.

jejunectomy (jej·oon·**ek**·to·me). The operation of excising the whole or a portion of the jejunum. [jejunum, Gk *ektome* a cutting out.]

jejunitis (jej·oon·**i**·tis). Inflammation affecting the jejunum. [jejunum, Gk *-itis* inflammation.]

jejunocaecostomy (jej·**oon**·o·se·**kos**'·to·me). Anastomosis between the jejunum and caecum. [jejunum, caecum, Gk *stoma* mouth.]

jejunocolostomy (jej·**oon**·o·kol·**os**'·to·me). Anastomosis between the jejunum and the colon. [jejunum, colon, Gk *stoma* mouth.]

jejuno-ileitis (jej·**oon**·o·i·le·**i**'·tis). Inflammation affecting the jejunum and ileum simultaneously. [jejunum, ileum, Gk *-itis* inflammation.]

jejuno-ileostomy (jej·**oon**·o·i·le·**os**'·to·me). Anastomosis between the jejunum and the ileum. [jejunum, ileum, Gk *stoma* mouth.]

jejuno-ileum (jej·oon·o·i′·le·um). The portion of the small intestine which extends from the end of the duodenum to the caecum. [jejunum, ileum.]

jejunojejunostomy (jej·**oon**·o·jej·oon·**os**′·to·me). Anastomosis between 2 segments of the jejunum. [jejunum, Gk *stoma* mouth.]

jejunorrhaphy (jej·oon·**or**·af·e). Suture of the jejunum. [jejunum, Gk *rhaphe* seam.]

jejunostomy (jej·oon·**os**·to·me). The establishment of an opening into the jejunum through the wall of the abdomen. [jejunum, Gk *stoma* mouth.]

jejunotomy (jej·oon·**ot**·o·me). The operation of incising the jejunum. [jejunum, Gk *temnein* to cut.]

jejunum [NA] (jej·**oon**·um). The proximal two-fifths of the small intestine extending from the end of the duodenum to the ileum, situated for the most part in the umbilical region but on occasion reaching into any of the neighbouring areas. [L *jejunus* empty.]

Jelks, John Lemuel (b. 1870). American surgeon.

Jelks' operation. An operation for perirectal abscess.

Jellinek, Stefan (b. 1871). Vienna physician.

Jellinek's sign. Abnormal pigmentation of the upper lid in thyrotoxic exophthalmos.

jelly (**jel**·e). 1. A non-liquid colloidal solution or gel. 2. A mixture of solids and liquids to form a semi-solid mass, e.g. petroleum jelly. **Contraceptive jelly.** A jelly for introduction into the vagina as a contraceptive. **Enamel jelly.** In the enamel organ of a forming tooth, that part of the stellate reticulum which lies between the cells. **Glycerin jelly.** A colloidal solution of gelatin, glycerin and water, which melts at body temperature and is used as a basis for pastilles or suppositories. By varying the gelatin content the melting point may be altered. **Mineral jelly, Petroleum jelly.** Soft paraffin. **Tuberculin jelly.** A tuberculin preparation used for a percutaneous tuberculin test. **Vaginal jelly.** Any jelly for introduction into the vagina for contraceptive or other purposes. [L *gelare* to congeal.]

See also: WHARTON.

jelly-leaf (**jel**·e·leef). The leaf of *Sida rhombifolia* (family Malvaceae). It contains a quantity of mucilage and is used in Australia as a demulcent, also in the preparation of poultices. A fluid extract is said to have expectorant properties. [jelly, AS *leaf.*]

Jena Nomenclature (ya·nah no·**men**·klah·tcher). The anatomical terminology agreed upon and incorporated in the *Jena Nomina Anatomica.* [see foll.]

Jena Nomina Anatomica (ya·nah **nom**·in·ah an·at·**om**·ik·ah). JNA. The anatomical terminology adopted at Jena, by a committee of German anatomists in 1933. [L *nomen* name, Gk *anatome* dissection.]

Jendrassik, Ernst (b. 1858). Budapest physician.

Jendrassik's manoeuvre. The patient hooks the fingers of the two hands together and pulls them one against the other forcibly; a method of reinforcing the knee and ankle jerks.

Jendrässik, Eugen (b. 1824). Budapest physician.

Jendrässik's sign. Thyrotropic exophthalmos [obsolete].

Jenkin's filter. A bacterial filter prepared from porcelain; now obsolete.

jenkol (**jen**·kol). Djenkol.

Jenner, Edward (b. 1749). Gloucestershire physician.

Jenner's vaccination, jennerian vaccination. Arm-to-arm vaccination with cowpox, the forerunner of modern vaccination for the prevention of smallpox.

Jenner's vaccine, jennerian vaccine. Cowpox vaccine. *See* VACCINE.

Jenner, Louis Leopold (b. 1866). London physician.

Jenner's stain. A type of Romanovsky stain.

Jensen, B. N. 20th century Danish biochemist.

Hagedorn and Jensen method, for blood sugar. Precipitate the proteins from 0.1 ml blood with zinc hydroxide. Heat the filtrate with 2 ml alkaline ferricyanide reagent in boiling water for 15 min. Cool and add 3 ml of iodide reagent and 2 ml of 3 per cent acetic acid. Titrate the liberated iodine with M/200 thiosulphate.

Jensen, Carl Oluf (b. 1864). Copenhagen veterinary pathologist.

Jensen's sarcoma. A transplantable sarcoma of rats.

Jensen, Edmund Zensten (b. 1861). Copenhagen ophthalmologist.

Jensen's choroidoretinitis juxtapapillaris, disease or retinopathy. Choroidoretinitis near the disc margin. It is associated with the production of vitreous opacities and of a scotoma, often radiating from the blind spot to the periphery owing to the involvement of the retinal nerve fibres. The cause is unknown, and the age onset is from 20 to 34.

Jensen, Orla. 20th century Danish bacteriologist.

Jensen's classification. A classification of all bacteria, based on their nutrititive requirements and biochemical characteristics.

Jensen's modification of Gram's method or stain. A differential stain for bacteria. Heat-fixed films are stained with 0.5 per cent aqueous methyl violet for 1 min, treated with 1 per cent iodine in 2 per cent potassium iodide for 30 s, decolorized with alcohol and counterstained for from 1 to 2 min with 1 per cent neutral red in 2 per cent acetic acid. Gram-positive organisms stain violet and Gram-negative organisms stain pink.

Jephson, Henry (b. 1798). Leamington physician.

Jephson's powder. A mixture of powdered guaiacum and precipitated sulphur, used as a mild laxative and diuretic, especially in rheumatism.

jequiritin (jek·**kwir**·it·in). A mixture of poisonous proteins obtained from the seeds of jequirity; also known as *abrin.*

jequirity (je·**kwir**·it·e). *Abrus precatorius.* [Port. *jequiriti.*]

jerboa (jer·**bo**·ah). A desert rodent that is a potential carrier of plague infection. [Ar. *yarbu.*]

jerk (jerk). The muscular contraction evoked when a tendon overlying a bone is tapped, e.g. knee jerk; the production of the jerk indicates that the local reflex nervous arc, afferent sensory and descending motor, is intact. **Ankle jerk.** Contraction of the calf muscles produced by the tapping of the stretched tendo calcaneus. **Biceps jerk.** A contraction produced by the tapping over the lower end of the radius when the elbow will flex owing to the contraction of the biceps and supinator muscles. **Crossed jerk.** Movement produced in the opposite leg when an infrapatellar tendon is tapped. **Finger jerk.** Digital reflex. *See* REFLEX. **Jaw jerk.** That produced by the tapping of the lower jaw with the mouth open. **Knee jerk.** Contraction of the quadriceps femoris muscle on the tapping of an infrapatellar tendon; usually present in health. Absence of the reflex is seen in any affection where the local reflex arc is not intact, e.g. tabes dorsalis, peripheral neuritis, poliomyelitis. Increase of the reflex is seen in spastic conditions. **Triceps jerk.** Contraction of the triceps brachii muscle produced by the tapping of the triceps tendon just above the olecranon. [onomat.]

jerks (jerx). A type of choromania sometimes associated with religious emotion. [see prec.]

jervine (**jer**·veen). $C_{26}H_{37}O_3N$, an alkaloid occurring in white and green hellebore.

jessur (**jes**·er). The Bengali name for *Vipera russelli* (Russell's viper).

Jesuit bark (**jez**·ew·it bark). Cinchona bark. [Society of *Jesus,* bark.]

Jianu, Amza. Bucharest surgeon.

Jianu's operation. Use of a loop of small intestine in gastrostomy as a canal from the surface to the stomach.

jigger (**jig**·er). *Tunga penetrans,* the sand flea.

jinja-fly (**jin**·jah·fli). *Simulium damnosum.*

joba (**jo**·bah). The local name for the shoe flower, *Hibiscus rosasinensis* Linn. (family Malvaceae). It is used in India as a demulcent and in the treatment of menorrhagia.

Jobert de Lamballe, Antoine Joseph (b. 1799). Paris surgeon.

Jobert's fossa. The groove in the intact limb, seen just above the knee joint, bounded by the adductor magnus muscle anteriorly, and the gracilis and sartorius muscles posteriorly.

Jobert's operation. Plastic closure of a vesicovaginal fistula.

Jochmann, Georg (b. 1874). Berlin physician.

Jochmann's serum. Antimeningococcus serum. *See* SERUM.

Joffroy, Alexis (b. 1844). Paris neurologist and psychiatrist.

Joffroy's reflex. When the lower limbs are the seat of spastic paralysis, pressure against the buttocks produces reflex contraction of the gluteus muscles.

Joffroy's sign. Lack of the usual creasing of the skin of the forehead on looking up, as seen in thyrotoxic exophthalmos.

Johne, Heinrich Albert (b. 1839). Dresden bacteriologist.

bacillus of Johne. *Mycobacterium johnei.*

Johne's disease. A chronic pseudotuberculous enteritis due to an acid-fast bacillus, probably avian in origin, affecting bovines in which the tuberculin reaction is negative; it is not known to affect human beings. Also called *paratuberculosis.*

johnin (yo·nin). An extract prepared from cultures of Johne's bacillus and used in the diagnosis, and sometimes for the prevention, of Johne's disease in cattle.

Johnson, Frank Bacchus (b. 1919). American pathologist.

Dubin–Johnson syndrome. Chronic jaundice due to difficulty in getting conjugated bilirubin out of the hepatic cell, which contains dark pigment granules.

Johnson, F. C. (b. 1894). American physician.

Stevens–Johnson disease or syndrome. Erythema multiforme with a purulent conjunctivitis, complicated often by corneal ulceration and perforation, associated with fever and vesicles in the mouth (stomatitis), nose, genito-urinary orifices and anal canal.

Johnson, Sir George (b. 1818). British physician.

Johnson's test, for glucose in urine. A test based on the reduction of yellow picric acid to red picramic acid when the urine is boiled with picric acid and potassium hydroxide. It is also known as *Braun's test.*

joint [articulatio (junctura ossium) NA] (joint). A junction of 2 or more bones, especially one that allows relative movement to occur between them [articulatio (NA)]. **Acromioclavicular joint [articulatio acromioclavicularis (NA)].** The plane joint between the acromial end of the clavicle and the medial margin of the acromion. **Ankle joint [articulatio talocruralis (NA)].** A synovial hinge joint; the lower end of the tibia, its malleolus, and the lateral malleolus of the fibula form a mortise which receives the upper surface of the talus and its medial and lateral surfaces. **Atlanto-axial joints [articulationes atlanto-axiales, mediana et lateralis (NA)].** The articulation between each lateral mass of the atlas and the corresponding facet of the axis and between the odontoid process and the anterior arch of the atlas. **Atlanto-occipital joint [articulatio atlanto-occipitalis (NA)].** The joint between the superior articular facet of the lateral mass of the atlas and the condyle of the occipital bone; nodding of the head mainly occurs here. **Joints of the auditory ossicles [articulationes ossiculorum auditus (NA)].** Two joints, one a saddle-shaped synovial joint [articulatio incudomallearis (NA)] between the head of the malleus and the body of the incus; it is surrounded by a capsule from the inner surface of which a wedge-shaped disc projects, partially dividing the joint. The second joint is between the lentiform nodule of the incus and the head of the stapes [articulatio incudostapedia (NA)] and is probably a ball-and-socket joint. **Ball-and-socket joint [articulatio cotylica (NA)].** A synovial joint in which a globular surface is received into a cup-like cavity. **Bleeders' joint.** Haemorrhage into a joint in haemophilia. **Calcaneocuboid joint [articulatio calcaneocuboidea (NA)].** A saddle-shaped joint, usually continuous with the talonavicular joint, together forming the transverse tarsal joint. **Carpometacarpal joints [articulationes carpometacarpeae (NA)].** The joints between the distal row of carpal bones and the bases of the metacarpals; the first joint is saddle-shaped and mobile, the remainder plane and relatively immobile. **Cartilaginous joint [junctura cartilaginea (NA)].** A joint where the bony surfaces are connected by intervening cartilage. **Cartilaginous joint, primary [synchondrosis (NA)].** A temporary joint where there is an intervening plate of hyaline cartilage which is converted in the adult into bone. **Cartilaginous joint, secondary [symphysis (NA)].** A joint where the opposed bones are permanently connected by a flattened disc of fibrocartilage. **Compound joint [articulatio composita (NA)].** A joint involving more than 2 bones. **Condyloid joint [articulatio condylaris (NA)].** Ellipsoid joint (see below). **Costochondral joint [articulationes costochondrales (NA)].** The junction between a rib and its costal cartilage. **Costotransverse joint [articulatio costotransversaria (NA)].** The joint between the tubercle of a rib and the transverse process of the corresponding vertebra. **Costovertebral joints [articulationes costovertebrales (NA)].** Joints of the ribs with the vertebral column, comprising joints of the heads of the ribs (see below) and costotransverse joints (see prec.). **Crico-arytenoid joint [articulatio crico-arytenoidea (NA)].** A synovial joint allowing rotation of the arytenoid cartilage about a vertical axis as well as to-and-fro sliding. **Cricothyroid joint [articulatio cricothyreoidea (NA)].** A synovial joint between each inferior horn of the thyroid cartilage and the corresponding facet on the cricoid cartilage. **Cuneonavicular joint [articulatio cuneonavicularis (NA)].** The joint between the navicular bone and the 3 cuneiform bones. **Elbow joint [articulatio cubiti (NA)].** The hinge joint between the trochlea of the humerus and the trochlear notch of the ulna, and between the capitulum of the humerus and the head of the radius. **Ellipsoid joint [articulatio ellipsoidea (NA)].** A modified ball-and-socket joint in which the articular surfaces are ellipsoid, a shape which prevents axial rotation while permitting all other movements of a ball-and-socket joint. **False joint.** A joint which arises at the site of an old fracture; pseudarthrosis. **Fibrous joint [junctura fibrosa (NA)].** A joint in which the bony surfaces are united by intervening fibrous tissue, allowing only slight movements if any. **Flail joint.** A joint in which the controlling muscles are paralysed. **Fringe joint.** A joint affected with menopausal arthritis; an archaic term. **Haemophilic joint.** Bleeders' joint (see above). **Joints of the hand, interphalangeal [articulationes interphalangeae manus (NA)].** Hinge joints between the proximal and middle, and middle and distal, phalanges. **Joint of the head of a rib [articulatio capitis costae (NA)].** The joint between the head of a rib and, typically, the bodies of 2 adjacent vertebrae and the intervening intervertebral disc. **Hinge joint [ginglymus (NA)].** A synovial joint in which the articular surfaces allow movement in 1 plane only. **Hip joint [articulatio coxae (NA)].** A very stable joint of the ball-and-socket type, formed by the acetabulum of the hip bone and the head of the femur. **Humeroradial joint [articulatio humeroradialis (NA)].** The part of the elbow joint formed by the articulation between the capitulum of the humerus and the head of the radius. **Humero-ulnar joint [articulatio humero-ulnaris (NA)].** The part of the elbow joint formed by the articulation between the trochlea of the humerus and the trochlear notch of the ulna. **Intercarpal joints [articulationes intercarpeae (NA)].** The joints between the small bones of the carpus; they communicate freely with each other except for the joint between the pisiform and triquetral bones. **Interchondral joints [articulationes interchondrales (NA)].** The joints between the contiguous borders of the 6th and 7th, 7th and 8th, and 8th and 9th costal cartilages. **Intermetacarpal joints [articulationes intermetacarpeae (NA)].** The plane joints between the bases of the 2nd, 3rd, 4th and 5th metacarpal bones. **Intermetatarsal joints [articulationes intermetatarseae (NA)].** Synovial joints between the lateral 4 metatarsal bases and continuous with the tarsometatarsal joints. **Interphalangeal joint.** *See* JOINTS OF THE HAND, INTERPHALANGEAL (above) and JOINTS OF THE TOES, INTERPHALANGEAL (below). **Intertarsal joints [articulationes intertarseae (NA)].** Four joints consisting of: the talocalcanean; the talocalcaneonavicular; the joint between the talus and calcaneum posteriorly and the cuboid and navicular anteriorly; and the joint between the navicular, cuboid and 3 cuneiform bones. **Irritable joint.** An inflamed joint in which all movements are limited by the associated muscle spasm. **Knee joint [articulatio genu (NA)].** A modified hinge joint composed of 3 articulations, 2 between the femoral condyles, menisci and tibia, and 1 between the femur and patella. **Lax joints.** Abnormal joint mobility found either in congenital connective-tissue disorders such as Ehlers-Danlos syndrome and Marfan's syndrome or in otherwise normal people, sometimes with a familial tendency. The condition may lead to premature osteoarthritis. **Lumbosacral joint [junctura lumbosacralis (NA)].** The joint between the fifth lumbar vertebra and the first piece of the sacrum, lying immediately above the promontory of the sacrum. **Mandibular joint [articulatio temporomandibularis (NA)].** The joint between the head of the mandible and the articular fossa of the temporal bone. The synovial cavity is divided into 2 compartments by a complete disc of fibrocartilage (the articular disc). **Manubriosternal joint [synchondrosis manubriosternalis (NA)].** The joint between the manubrium and the body of the sternum; it is usually cartilaginous but sometimes contains a synovial cavity. **Metacarpophalangeal joints [articulationes metacarpophalangeae (NA)].** The condyloid joints between the metacarpal heads and the proximal phalanges. **Metatarsophalangeal joints [articulationes metatarsophalangeae (NA)].** Condyloid joints between the convex heads of the metatarsals and the shallow cavities on the proximal ends of the phalanges. That of the great toe has 2 sesamoid bones in the plantar metatarsal ligament. **Midcarpal joint [articulatio mediocarpea (NA)].** The joint between the proximal and distal rows of carpal bones. **Midtarsal joint.** *See* TARSAL JOINT, TRANSVERSE (below). **Neurocentral joint.** The primary cartilaginous joint between the centrum of the vertebra and vertebral arch. **Petro-occipital joint [synchondrosis petro-occipitalis (NA)].** The cartilaginous joint between the lateral part of the petrous temporal bone and the jugular process of the occipital bone. **Pisiform joint [articulatio ossis pisiformis (NA)].** The plane joint between the pisiform and triquetral bones. **Pivot joint [articulatio trochoidea (NA)].** A synovial joint in which a pivot of bone rotates within a ring formed partly of bone and partly of ligament. **Plane joint [articulatio plana (NA)].** A synovial joint between plane surfaces, allowing gliding movement only. **Prosthetic joint.** An artificial joint used either as an internal replacement or in combination with an external prosthesis used to replace a limb. **Radiocarpal joint [articulatio radiocarpea (NA)].** The wrist joint; a condyloid joint, between the lower end of the radius and the articular disc above, and the scaphoid, lunate and triquetral bones below. **Radio-ulnar joint, inferior [articulatio radio-ulnaris distalis (NA)].** The pivot joint between the head of the ulna and the ulnar notch of the radius. **Radio-ulnar joint, superior [articulatio radio-ulnaris proximalis (NA)].** The pivot joint between the head of the radius and the osseofibrous ring formed by the annular ligament and the radial notch of the ulna. **Sacrococcygeal joint [junctura sacrococcygea (NA)].** A secondary cartilaginous joint between the lower end of the sacrum and the base of the coccyx, becoming ossified in the aged. **Sacro-iliac joint [articulatio sacro-iliaca (NA)].** A synovial joint between the auricular surfaces of the ilium and sacrum; it is very irregular, to ensure stability. **Saddle joint [articulatio sellaris (NA)].** A synovial joint the opposing surfaces of which are reciprocally concavo-convex. **Shoulder joint [articulatio humeri (NA)].** The ball-and-socket joint between the rounded head of the humerus and the shallow glenoid cavity of the scapula. **Simple joint [articulatio simplex (NA)].** A joint formed by 2 bones only. **Joints of the skull.** Primary cartilaginous joints between certain skull bones, of importance in aiding moulding of the fetal head during parturition. **Joints of the skull, cartilaginous [synchondroses cranii (NA)].** Temporary cartilage unions in the base of the skull persisting until the completion of growth. **Spheno-occipital joint [synchondrosis spheno-occipitalis (NA)].** The cartilaginous joints between the bodies of the sphenoid and occipital bones. **Sphenopetrous joint [synchons drosis sphenopetrosa (NA)].** The cartilage filling in the lower lateral part of the foramen lacerum, between the greater wing of the sphenoid bone and the petrous part of the temporal bone. **Spheroid joint [articulatio spheroidea (cotylica) NA].** A joint such as a ball-and-socket joint (see above) where the surfaces are somewhat spherical. **Sternoclavicular joint [articulatio sternoclavicularis (NA)].** The joint between the rounded sternal end of the clavicle and the concavity formed by the clavicular notch of the manubrium and 1st costal cartilage. **Sternocostal joints [articulationes sternocostales (NA)].** The joints between the costal cartilages of true ribs and the sternum; they are all synovial except the first. **Subastragaloid joint, Subtalar joint.** Talocalcanean joint (see below). **Synovial joint [junctura synovialis (articulatio) NA].** A joint where the opposed bones are separated by a space containing a fluid, synovial fluid, to nourish and lubricate the surfaces. It is usually freely mobile. **Talocalcanean joint [articulatio subtalaris (NA)].** The joint between the inferior surface of the body and the talus and the large posterior facet on tne upper surface of the calcaneum. **Talocalcaneonavicular joint [articulatio talocalcaneonavicularis (NA)].** A modified ball-and-socket joint between the head and under-surface of the neck of the talus and the sustentaculum tali, plantar calcaneonavicular ligament, and the navicular bone. **Talonavicular joint.** A part of the transverse tarsal joint, common to it and the talocalcaneonavicular joint. **Tarsal joint, transverse [articulatio tarsi transversa (NA)].** The midtarsal joint between the talus and calcaneum posteriorly and the navicular and cuboid bones anteriorly; Chopart's joint. **Tarsometatarsal joints [articulationes tarsometatarseae (NA)].** Three joint cavities between the 3 cuneiform bones and cuboid bone posteriorly and the metatarsal bases anteriorly. The oblique joint line runs laterally and posteriorly. The 2nd metatarsal base is mortised between the 3 cuneiform bones. **Temporomandibular joint.** Mandibular joint (see above). **Joint of the thumb, carpometacarpal [articulatio carpometacarpea pollicis (NA)].** The saddle joint between the 1st metacarpal bone and the trapezium. **Tibiofibular joint, inferior [syndesmosis (articulatio) tibiofibularis (NA)].** A syndesmosis between the rough opposed surfaces of the lower ends of the tibia and fibula. **Tibiofibular joint, superior [articulatio tibiofibularis (NA)].** A plane synovial joint between the lateral tuberosity of the tibia and the head of the fibula. **Joints of the toes, interphalangeal [articulationes interphalangeae pedis (NA)].** Hinge joints in which the proximal articular surface is rounded and the distal one a shallow depression. **Trochoid joint.** A pivot joint (see above). **Wrist joint.** Radiocarpal joint (see above). **Xiphisternal joint [synchondrosis xiphosternalis (NA)].** The secondary cartilaginous joint between the xiphoid process and the body of the sternum; it usually fuses soon after puberty. **Zygapophyseal joints [juncturae zygapophyseales (NA)].** Joints between the articular processes of vertebrae (zygapophysis). [L *jungere* to join.]

See also: BUDIN, CHARCOT, CHOPART, CLUTTON, CRUVEILHIER, LISFRANC, VON GIES.

Jolles, Adolf (b. 1863). Vienna biochemist.

Jolles' test, for indican in urine. A few thymol crystals are added to the urine and Jaffé's test or Obermayer's test is then carried out as described under these headings. The addition of thymol increases the sensitivity of these tests.

Jolly, Friedrich (b. 1844). Würzburg and Berlin neurologist.

Jolly's reaction. A reaction said to occur in certain amyotrophies, in which a voluntarily exhausted muscle can be made to contract in response to faradic stimulation, and a faradically exhausted muscle can contract under the influence of the will.

Jolly, Justin Marie Jules (b. 1870). Paris histologist.

Jolly bodies, Howell-Jolly bodies. Spherical, eccentrically-placed granules or nuclear remnants about 1 μm in diameter, occasionally seen in red blood corpuscles, usually very numerous in haemolytic or toxic anaemias and after splenectomy.

Joly, John Swift (b. 1876). London urologist.

Swift Joly urethroscope. An irrigating urethroscope with an indirect lens system for combining cystoscopy with urethroscopy.

Jonas, August Frederick (b. 1858). Omaha surgeon.

Jonas' operation. Excision of the transverse tarsal joint for the treatment of deformities of the feet.

Jonas, Siegfried (b. 1874). Vienna physician.

Jonas' symptom. Pyloric spasm in rabies.

Jones, Ernest (b. 1879). Toronto and London psychiatrist.
Ross-Jones test. A test similar to the Nonne-Apelt reaction.

Jones, Hugh Toland (b. 1892). Los Angeles orthopaedic surgeon.
Henderson-Jones disease. Synovial chondromatosis.

Jones, Sir Robert (b. 1858). British orthopaedic surgeon.
Jones' frame, for immobilization of fractures. A metal frame for immobilization of the hip.
Jones' pseudarthrosis. An operation designed to restore movement to a fixed hip by producing a pseudarthrosis at the subtrochanteric level [obsolete].
Jones' cock-up splint. A metal splint used to hold the wrist in dorsiflexion.
Jones' spinal support. A metal and leather spinal brace.

Jones, Thomas Wharton (b. 1808). British ophthalmologist.
Jones' operation, for ectropion. Also called the V-Y *operation*: a V-shaped area of skin is excised below the lower lid with apex downwards. The edges are undermined and sutured in the form of a Y.

Jongck test. The squatting test for vitamin B_1 deficiency.

Jonnesco, Thoma (b. 1860). Bucharest surgeon.
Jonnesco's anaesthesia. A method of spinal analgesia by which the whole body may be rendered insensitive.
Jonnesco's folds. Duodenal folds. *See* FOLD.
Jonnesco's fossa. Duodenojejunal fossa; a recess lying to the left of the duodenojejunal flexure between the superior and inferior duodenal folds.
Jonnesco operation. Removal of cervical ganglia of the sympathetic trunk.

Jonston, John (b. 1603). Scottish surgeon in Poland.
Jonston's alopecia. Alopecia areata.

Jordan, Edwin Oakes (b. 1866). Boston bacteriologist.
Jordan's tartrate agar. A medium containing sodium potassium tartrate 10 g, sodium chloride 5 g, peptone 10 g, agar 20 g, phenol red (0.4 per cent aqueous solution) 6 ml, and water to 1 litre.

Jorgensen, N. B. 20th century American dentist.
Jorgensen's technique. The intravenous injection of such sedatives as pentobarbitone, hyoscine and pethidine together with local analgesia, for dental treatment.

Jorissen's test. For formaldehyde in milk: to 10 ml of milk in a test-tube add several drops of 10 per cent aqueous phloroglucin. Shake, and then add a few drops of sodium hydroxide solution. A flesh-pink coloration indicates formaldehyde.

Jorissenne, Gustav (b. 1846). Belgian physician.
Jorissenne's sign. A sign of pregnancy characterized by a failure of the woman's pulse rate to increase on standing after previously lying down.

Joule, James Prescott (b. 1818). British physicist.
Joule effect. The heating of a conductor by the passage through it of an electric current, due to the resistance of the conductor.
Joule's equivalent. The mechanical equivalent of heat, i.e. the amount of work that will produce unit quantity of heat. In the SI system of units all energy or work is measured in the same units, joules, and therefore there is direct equivalence. In c.g.s. units, 4.185×10^7 ergs produce 1 calorie.
Joule's law. 1. At constant temperature the internal energy of a gas does not vary with its volume. 2. The molecular heat of a solid compound is the sum of the atomic heats of its constituents. 3. The heat produced by a current is proportional to the square of the latter multiplied by the time the current passes.
Joule-Thomson effect. The change in temperature which occurs when a gas passes through a porous plug which separates 2 regions at different pressures.

Joule (jowl, jool). The unit of work, defined as the work done when the point of application of one newton (unit of force) moves a distance of 1 metre in the direction of the force. [James Prescott *Joule.*]

Jourdain's disease. *See* BERCHILLET-JOURDAIN.

juccuya (yoo·koo·yah). Cutaneous leishmaniasis due to infection with *Leishmania tropica,* a zoonotic infection of gerbils and marmots transmitted to man by *Phlebotomus japatasi.* The lesions tend to be ulcerative or "wet".

judam (joo·dam). Arabic name for leprosy.

Judet, Robert Louis (b. 1909). French orthopaedic surgeon.
Judet's prosthesis. A prosthesis made of acrylic resin and used to replace the head of the femur in the operation of arthroplasty.

Juengling, Otto Adolf (b. 1884). Tübingen and Flensburg surgeon.
Juengling's disease. Multiple tuberculous infection of bones, characterized by cysts.

juga (joo·gah). *See* JUGUM.

jugal (joo·gal). 1. Attaching; yoked together. 2. Pertaining to the zygomatic bone. **Jugal bone.** Zygomatic bone. [L *jugum* yoke.]

jugale (joo·ga·le). The jugal point. *See* POINT.

jugate (joo·gate). 1. Joined together. 2. Ridged. 3. In biology, paired. [L *jugum* yoke.]

Juglans (jug·lans). A genus of trees (family Juglandaceae). The bark of *Juglans cinerea* Linn. (butternut, white walnut), an American species, acts as a cathartic and hepatic stimulant. *Juglans regia* Linn. is the common European walnut. Preparations of the bark and the leaves have been used as an antispasmodic and as an external application to wounds and ulcers. [L walnut.]

juglone (jug·lone). 5-Hydroxy-1,4-naphthaquinone, $C_{10}H_6O_3$. A derivative of α-naphthaquinone, occurring in the leaves of various species of walnut (*Juglans*).

jugomaxillary (joo·go·max·il'·ar·e). 1. Belonging to the zygomatic (jugal) bone and the maxilla. 2. Pertaining to the jugular vein and the maxilla.

jugular (jug·ew·lar). Relating or belonging to the throat or neck. **Jugular arch.** *See* ARCH. **Jugular foramen.** *See* FORAMEN. **Jugular notch.** *See* NOTCH. **Jugular venous pressure.** *See* PRESSURE. **Jugular trunk.** *See* TRUNK. [L *jugulum* neck.]

jugular nerve [nervus jugularis (NA)]. A branch from the superior cervical ganglion to the inferior ganglion of the glossopharyngeal nerve and to the superior ganglion of the vagus nerve.

jugular veins. Anterior jugular vein [vena jugularis anterior (NA)]. A superficial vein of the front of the neck, commencing in the submental region and draining at the lower end of the neck into the external jugular or subclavian veins. **External jugular vein [vena jugularis externa (NA)].** The main superficial vein in the neck, formed behind the angle of the mandible, and draining the tissues of the face and scalp. It ends just above the clavicle by piercing the deep fascia and joining the subclavian vein. **Internal jugular vein [vena jugularis interna (NA)].** The chief vein of the head and neck, commencing at the base of the skull as the continuation of the sigmoid sinus, and joining the subclavian vein at the root of the neck to form the innominate veins. **Posterior external jugular vein.** A tributary of the external jugular vein, draining the occipital region.

jugulocephalic (jug·ew·lo·kef·al'·ik). Belonging or relating to the throat and the head. [L *jugulum* neck, Gk *kephale* head.]

jugulum (jug·ew·lum). 1. The clavicle. 2. The throat or neck. [L neck, collarbone.]

jugum [NA] (joo·gum) (pl. *juga*). A ridge or furrow connecting 2 points or 2 structures. **Alveolar juga [juga alveolaria (NA)].** Depressions on the anterior part of the alveolar process of the maxilla between the ridges of the roots of the incisor teeth. Similar juga occur in the body of the mandible. **Jugum petrosum.** The arcuate eminence. *See* EMINENCE. **Jugum sphenoidale (NA).** The anterior part of the cerebral surface of the body of the sphenoid bone which separates the anterior cranial fossa from the sphenoidal sinus. [L yoke.]

juice [succus] (joos). Any fluid secretion of animal or plant tissues. **Appetite juice.** Gastric secretion stimulated by appetite and the sight, taste or smell of food. **Apple juice.** The juice obtained from apples by expression contains sugars, malic acid and tannins; certain varieties are used in the making of cider. The active constituent is pectin, and it is used in the treatment of infantile diarrhoea and enteritis. **Cancer juice.** The milky fluid obtained by scraping the surface of a cancer. **Gastric juice.** A clear, colourless, acid fluid secreted by the stomach under the stimulus of food. **Intestinal juice.** A colourless, alkaline fluid secreted by the small intestine during digestion of food. It contains various enzymes which assist in completing the digestion of food. **Pancreatic juice.** A clear, colourless, alkaline fluid secreted by the pancreas into the duodenum during digestion of food. The chief constituents are proteins and the enzymes, trypsin, amylase and lipase. **Press juice.** Any fluid obtained from animal or plant tissues by submitting them to mechanical pressure. **Testicular juice.** Sperm. [L *jus* broth.]

jujube (**joo**·joob). The berries of *Zizyphus vulgaris* Lamk. (family Rhamnaceae). They are mucilaginous and sweet tasting, and the genuine *jujube paste* was originally prepared from them and used in the manufacture of lozenges. [Gk *zizyphon*.]

Julliard, Gustave (b. 1836). Geneva surgeon.

Julliard's mask. A mask formerly used in anaesthetics.

jumentous (joo·**men**·tus). Having a strong odour like that of the urine of a horse; applied to human urine in certain abnormal states. [L *jumentum* beast of burden.]

jumper (**jum**·per). Applied to persons in certain neurotic and weak-willed states who carry out any movement they are ordered to do and leap and jump suddenly. A sufferer from jumping disease or latah. [onomat.]

jumps (jumps). 1. Chorea. 2. Term for delirium tremens. [onomat.]

junction (**jungk**·shun). A joining; a meeting place; an interface. **Amelodentinal junction.** The junction between the enamel and dentine in the crown of a tooth. **Cemento-enamel junction.** The junction between the cementum and enamel of a tooth. **Corticomedullary junction.** The junctional region between the deeper part of the cortex and the outer medulla. The arcuate vessels lie in this region. **Dentino-enamel junction.** Amelodentinal junction (see above). **Dentocemental junction.** The junction of dentine and cementum in the root of a tooth. **Junction of the lips.** The junction of the upper and lower lip at their lateral margin; the angles of the mouth. **Mucocutaneous junction.** The junction between mucous membrane and skin, e.g. lip margin. **Myoneural junction.** The microscopic area of contact between a nerve-end and the muscle fibre it innervates. **Neuromuscular junction.** Motor end-plate. **R(S)-T junction.** *See* SEGMENT R(S)-T. **Sclerocorneal junction.** The junction of the cornea and sclera, sometimes called the limbus. It is not an exact line, since the cornea is let into the sclera like a watch-glass. **Synaptic junction.** The microscopic area of proximity between 2 neurones, i.e. between axon and dendrite or axon and cell body. **Tight junction.** Zonula occludens. [L *jungere* to join.]

junctional (**jungk**·shun·al). At, or associated with, a junction, e.g. of different anatomical structures or types of tissue (mucocutaneous).

junctura (jungk·**tewr**·ah). A joining or union; a joint. Any qualified use of this term is obsolete in British anatomy. [L.]

Jung, Carl Gustav (b. 1875). Zürich psychiatrist.

Jung's method. Psychiatric treatment according to the doctrines of Jung.

Jung, Karl Gustav (b. 1793). German anatomist in Basle.

Jung's muscle. An occasional slip from the tragicus muscle which has attachment to the helix of the auricle.

Jungbluth, Hermann. 20th century German physician.

Jungbluth's vasa propria. Vessels associated with the early amnion.

Juniper, Juniperus (**joo**·nip·er, **joo**·nip·er·us). A genus of evergreen shrubs or trees (family Pinaceae), widely distributed. *Juniperus sabina* Linn. is the source of sabina. The fruits obtained from *J. communis* Linn. are used in veterinary practice and yield about 1 per cent of juniper oil. **Gum juniper.** Sandarac. **Oil of juniper.** An oil distilled from the fruits of *Juniperus communis* Linn. It is used as a carminative, stimulant and antiseptic. **Juniper tar oil.** Cade oil. [L *juniperus*.]

junk (jungk). 1. Oakum, sometimes used in surgical dressings. 2. Slang for narcotic drug especially heroin. [L *juncus* bulrush.]

Junker, Ferninand Ethelbert (b. 1828). Austrian surgeon in London and Kyoto.

Junker's apparatus or bottle. A simple anaesthetic apparatus; air is pumped by hand through a quantity of chloroform in the bottom of a bottle and the resulting mixture of air and vapour is led to the patient's air-passages.

junket (**jung**·ket). Curds and whey produced by the coagulation of milk with rennet. [L *juncus* bulrush.]

jurisprudence (joor·is·**proo**·dens). **Medical jurisprudence.** 1. The science which deals with the application of medicine to various branches of criminal and civil law. 2. The legal inter-relation between medical and dental practitioners on the one hand, and patients and the community as a whole on the other. [L *juris* of law, *prudentia* knowledge of any subject.]

jury-mast (**joor**·e·mahst). A support for the head and trunk used in cases of tuberculous disease of the spine. It consists of an upright steel bar to which are attached curved iron rods to go round the body and an open-hook-shaped rod curving over the head from which a sling passes under the chin. [etym. dub.]

Juster, Emile. 20th century Paris neurologist.

Juster reflex. Extension rather than flexion of the fingers when the palm is stimulated.

justo major (**jus**·to **ma**·jor). Descriptive of a pelvis of which the diameters and all dimensions are greater than normal. [L *justus* sufficient, *major* greater than.]

justo minor (**jus**·to **mi**·nor). Descriptive of a pelvis of which the diameters and all dimensions are less than normal. [L *justus* sufficient, *minor* less than.]

jute (joot). The strands of lignified phloem fibres obtained from the stem of various species of *Corchorus* (family Tiliaceae). It is used in the manufacture of tow. [Bengali, matted hair.]

Jutte, Max Ernest (b. 1875). New York physician.

Jutte tube. A form of duodenal tube.

juvantia (joo·**van**·she·ah). Medicines or appliances which are palliative or adjuvant. [L *juvare* to assist.]

juvenile (**joo**·ven·ile). Relating or belonging to childhood or youth; characteristic of a child; youthful. [L *juvenis* youth.]

juxta-articular (**jux**·tah·ar·**tik'**·ew·lar). In close proximity to a joint; in the neighbourhood of a joint. [L *juxta* near, *articulus* joint.]

juxtacortical (jux·tah·**kor**·tik·al). Near the cortex of an organ or tissue, e.g. bone. [L *juxta* near, *cortex* bark.]

juxta-epiphyseal (**jux**·tah·ep·e·**fiz'**·e·al). Situated close to or contiguous with an epiphysis. [L *juxta* near, epiphysis.]

juxtaglomerular (**jux**·tah·glom·**er'**·ew·lar). The area in the renal cortex between afferent and efferent arterioles of a glomerulus. Cells in this area are responsible for the secretion of renin. [L *juxta* near, *glomerulus* small ball.]

juxtangina (juxt·an·**ji**·nah). Inflammation of the muscles of the pharynx. [L *juxta* near, *angina* quinsy.]

juxtapapillary (**jux**·tah·pap·**il'**·ar·e). Situated close, or adjacent, to the optic disc. [L *juxta* near, *papilla* nipple.]

juxtaposition (**jux**·tah·po·**zish'**·un). Apposition; a side-by-side position. [L *juxta* near, position.]

juxtapyloric (**jux**·tah·pi·**lor'**·ik). Close to the pylorus or the prepyloric vein. [L *juxta* near, pylorus.]

juxtaspinal (jux·tah·**spi**·nal). Situated near to the vertebral column. [L *juxta* near, spine.]

K

kaalkop (kahl·kop). An African name for a condition of atrophic scarring that results from witkop, a syphilitic lesion of the scalp occurring in Africans.

Kabatschnik's hearing test. A vibrating tuning fork is applied to the external auditory meatus until no longer heard. Still vibrating, it is then placed on the nail of the examiner's forefinger which is inserted so as to occlude the meatus. A normal hearing ear again perceives the sound of the fork.

kadamba (kad·am·bah). *Anthocephalus cadamba* Miq. (family Rubiaceae), the bark of which is used in India as a febrifuge and tonic.

Kader, Bronislaw (b. 1863). Breslau surgeon.

Kader's operation, Kader–Senn operation. Gastrostomy by the inversion of the stomach wall around the gastrostomy tube in the form of an invertible ink-well.

Kaes, Theodor (b. 1852). German neurologist.

Kaes' layer, Kaes–Bechterew layer. A horizontal layer of fibres in the cerebral cortex just deep to the outer granular layer.

kafindo (kaf·in·do). Onyalai.

Kahlbaum, Karl Ludwig (b. 1828). Gorlitz psychiatrist.

Kahlbaum's disease. Catatonia.

Kahler, Otto (b. 1849). Prague and Vienna physician.

Kahler's disease. Lymphomatosis of the bones or multiple myeloma.

Kahler's law. After entering the spinal cord the ascending branches of the posterior roots of the spinal nerves pass successively from the root zone towards the mesial plane.

Kahn, Herbert 20th century Karlsruhe physician.

Kahn's test. *See* TEST FOR CANCER.

Kahn, Reuben Leon (b. 1887). Lansing, Michigan, serologist.

Kahn test. A serological precipitation test for syphilis: the serum is first inactivated by heating as in the Wassermann test; to 0.3 ml of serum 0.05 ml of the antigen dilution is added, the tube is shaken and incubated at 37° overnight. A positive reaction is one in which clumps of precipitate appear. It is an important and widely used test.

kaif (kife). The drowsy, sensuous, languorous condition that is produced by absorption of drugs such as hashish.

kainite (ka·in·ite). $K_2SO_4MgSO_4MgCl_2 \cdot 6H_2O$, a natural mineral obtained principally from deposits in Stassfurt (Saxony) and Poland. It is a valuable source of potassium and magnesium. [Gk *kainos* new.]

kainophobe (ki·no·fobe). One who dreads anything new and is morbidly averse to its introduction. [Gk *kainos* new, phobia.]

kainophobia (ki·no·fo·be·ah). Dread of or morbid aversion to anything new. [see prec.]

Kaiser, Eduard. German biologist.

Kaiser's nucleus. One of the cell columns of the anterior horn of the spinal grey matter.

Kaiserling, Karl (b. 1869). Königsberg pathologist.

Kaiserling's fluids or solutions. There are 3: (*a*) a tissue fixative consisting of 15 g potassium nitrate, 30 g potassium acetate, 200 ml formalin, and water to 1000 ml; (*b*) a colour restorative consisting of 80 per cent alcohol; (*c*) a preservative consisting of 100 g potassium acetate, 50 g sodium arsenate, 200 ml glycerin, and water to 1000 ml.

Kaiserling's method. For preserving natural colours in museum specimens. Specimens are fixed in a mixture of formaldehyde, potassium acetate and potassium nitrate (Kaiserling solution *a*), then partially dehydrated in alcohol (solution *b*), and finally preserved in 20 per cent glycerin containing potassium acetate and sodium arsenate (solution *c*).

kakaesthesia (kak·es·the·ze·ah). Cacaesthesia.

kakergasia (kak·er·ga·ze·ah). Cacergasia.

kakidrosis (kak·id·ro·sis). Cacidrosis.

kakosmia (kak·oz·me·ah). Cacosmia.

kala-azar (kah·lah·ah·zar'). Visceral leishmaniasis; a febrile infective disease due to a parasitic protozoon, *Leishmania donovani*, which is found in the reticulo-endothelial cells. The parasite can be cultured from the blood, bone marrow, or spleen pulp on a special (NNN) culture medium in which it develops into a flagellate form. The name, *black fever*, is derived from a darkening of the skin which often occurs in the course of the disease. It is most prevalent in India, Pakistan, China, East Africa, the Sudan, southern USSR, South America and on the Mediterranean littoral. It is transmitted by sandflies of various species in various countries, e.g. by *Phlebotomus argentipes* in India, and is amenable to treatment by compounds of antimony and by aromatic amidines. The disease, which in the absence of chemotherapy is generally fatal, is usually ushered in by a typhoid-like fever without marked toxaemia, followed by characteristically irregular fever with a double rise in 24 h; the spleen and liver are enlarged, the patient is anaemic and there is great diminution in the white blood cell count with a relative increase in large mononuclear cells. An alteration occurs in the albumin–globulin ratio in the serum: this can be detected by the aldehyde and antimony tests. An allied, if not identical, disease occurs in dogs in the Mediterranean littoral (canine kala-azar); its relation to the human disease (infantile or Mediterranean kala-azar) prevalent amongst infants in Greece and Portugal has not yet been determined, but the protozoa are morphologically and serologically identical. [Hind. *kala* black; *azar* Assamese dialect word for fever.]

kaladana (kal·ah·da·nah). The seeds of *Ipomoea hederacea* Jacq. (family Convolvulaceae), a climbing plant indigenous to India. It contains about 2 per cent of a resin similar to, but not identical with, jalap resin, and has been used in India as a purgative instead of jalap.

kaliaemia (kal·e·e·me·ah). The presence of potassium in the blood. [G *Kali* potash, Gk *haima* blood.]

kaligenous (kal·ij·en·us). Yielding potash. [G *Kali* potash, Gk *genein* to produce.]

kalimeter (kal·im·e·ter). Alkalimeter. [G *Kali* potash, meter.]

Kalischer, Otto (b. 1842). German physician.

Sturge–Kalischer disease, Sturge–Kalischer–Weber disease. Naevoid amentia; the combination of meningeal and facial angioma.

kalium (ka·le·um). Potassium. **Kalii Bromidum.** *European Pharmacopoeia* name for Potassium Bromide BP 1973. **Kalii Chloridum.** *European Pharmacopoeia* name for Potassium Chloride BP 1973. **Kalii Iodidum.** *European Pharmacopoeia* name for Potassium Iodide BP 1973. **Kalii Permanganas.** *European Pharmacopoeia* name for Potassium Permanganate BP 1973. [G *Kali* potash.]

kaliuresis (kal·e·ewr·e'·sis). Excretion of potassium in the urine in excess. [G *Kali* potash, Gk *ouresis* uresis.]

kallak (kal·ak). An inflammatory condition of the skin characterized by the presence of pustules, affecting Eskimos living on the coast of Labrador. [Eskimo disease of the skin.]

kallidin (kal·id·in). A mixture of 2 polypeptides, the nonapeptide bradykinin and the lysyl-bradykinin, but now synonymous with the latter compound. The kinins act mainly as local hormones.

kallikrein (kal·ik·re·in). An enzyme secreted by the salivary gland which, when injected intravenously, causes a fall in blood pressure. It facilitates the formation of bradykinin (kallidin) from a plasma protein.

Kallius' method. The preservation of Golgi stains by reduction with a photographic type of developer.

Kallmann, Franz Josef (b. 1897). New York psychiatrist.

Kallman's syndrome. A familial disorder of hypogonadism with loss of the sense of smell, thought to be due to hormonal dysfunction of the hypothalamus, often with testicular degeneration.

kalmegh (kal·meg). A drug on the *Indian Pharmacopoeial List.* It contains not less than 1 per cent andrographolide and is used in Indian medicine as a bitter: it is reputed to have antimalarial properties.

kalopsia (kal·op·se·ah). A state in which things seen appear to be more elegant or lovely than in fact they are. [Gk *kalos* beautiful, *opsis* appearance.]

Kalt, Eugene S. (b. 1861). French ophthalmologist.

Kalt's corneoscleral suture. A corneoscleral suture inserted, after the section has been completed, with a very fine needle.

kaluresis (kal·ewr·e·sis). Kaliuresis.

kamala (kam·a·lah). The hairs and glands of the fruits of *Mallotus philippinensis* (family Euphorbiaceae), a tree indigenous to India, Australia and the Malay Archipelago. It is an effective taenicide and purgative. [Sanskrit.]

kamalin (kam·al·in). Rottlerin. [see prec.]

kamela (kam·e·lah). Kamala.

Kammerer, Frederic (b. 1856). New York surgeon.

Battle-Jalaguier-Kammerer incision, for appendicectomy. A vertical incision medial to the outer border of the right rectus abdominis muscle, with division of the rectus sheath and retraction of the muscle inwards.

Kanamycin (kan·am·i·sin). BP Commission approved name for an antibiotic produced by *Streptomyces kanamyceticus.* **Kanamycin Sulphate BP 1973.** The sulphate salt of Kanamycin, a water-soluble, thermostabile, polybasic antibiotic, active against many aerobic Gram-positive bacteria including strains of *Staphylococcus* and *Mycobacterium tuberculosis,* and Gram-negative bacteria such as strains of *Aerobacter, Bacterium coli, Klebsiella pneumoniae, Neisseria, Proteus vulgaris, Salmonella* and *Shigella,* and various acid-fast organisms. It is used only in serious systemic infections and when the infecting organism is resistant to other antibiotics.

Kanavel, Allen Buckner (b. 1874). Chicago surgeon.

Kanavel's sign. In infections of the ulnar bursa in the hand there is a point of maximum tenderness (*Kanavel's point*) in the line of the 4th interdigital cleft and between the 2 transverse palmar creases.

Kanavel's spaces. The mid-palmar and thenar fascial spaces.

Kanavel's splint. A splint to correct finger deformities.

Kanavel's triangle. The surface marking on the palm of the hand of the fibrous flexor sheath.

Kandinsky, Viktor Chrisanfovich (b. 1825). Russian psychiatrist.

Clérambault-Kandinsky complex or syndrome. In a psychotic state the occurrence of paranoid ideas of reference or control.

kaninloma (ka·nin·lo·mah). Gangosa; in tertiary yaws, an ulcerative process which attacks the nasal and palatal structures and destroys them. The condition may be found in any region in which yaws is endemic, particularly in the islands of the East Indies and the Pacific. [Javanese name.]

Kanter, Aaron Elias (b. 1893). Chicago gynaecologist.

Kanter's sign. An unreliable method of testing for viability of the fetus in a cephalic presentation by examining the patient rectally or vaginally and exerting pressure on the fetus: if the child is alive it should move.

Kanthack, Alfredo Antunes (b. 1863). Brazilian pathologist in London.

Kanthack and Stephens serum agar. *See* AGAR, SERUM.

Kantor, John Leonard (b. 1890). New York physician.

Kantor's sign. In radiography, also known as the *string sign*; the shadow of a narrow streak of barium seen in regional ileitis or Crohn's disease. A similar shadow is also seen in colitis; in neither instance is it specific.

kanyemba (kan·yem·bah). Chiufa.

kaodzera (ka·od·ze·rah). The form of trypanosomiasis found in Rhodesia.

kaolin (ka·o·lin). China clay, potters' clay, argilla, $Al_2O_3{\cdot}2SiO_2{\cdot}2H_2O$. A hydrated aluminium silicate found naturally as a fine deposit, and used as a filler for paper and in the manufacture of porcelains and earthenwares. Purified, it is employed medically, Heavy Kaolin (BP 1968) and Light Kaolin (BP 1973), as an absorbent, a protective, a dusting powder and as a constituent of poultices; also for filtering and clarifying liquids. **Light Kaolin (Natural) BP 1973.** A purified native hydrated aluminium silicate containing a suitable dispersing agent. An adsorbent, given by mouth for its action in infections of the alimentary tract and in food poisoning. It is also applied externally as a poultice and in compound dusting powders. **Kaolin Poultice BP 1968.** A poultice of light kaolin mixed with glycerin, and containing boric acid and small amounts of oils of wintergreen, peppermint and thymol. It is applied hot for the relief of inflammation. [Chinese *Kao-ling* High Ridge, where it was found.]

kaolinosis (ka·o·lin·o'·sis). A type of pneumoconiosis which results from the inhalation of kaolin dust. [kaolin, Gk *-osis* condition.]

Kaposi, Moritz Kohn (b. 1837). Vienna dermatologist.

Kaposi's dermatosis, disease or xeroderma. Xeroderma pigmentosum; a rare infection of the skin which commences in infancy or very early childhood. It involves chiefly the exposed parts, and is characterized at first by erythema and vesiculation after exposure to sunlight, followed by freckle-like pigmentation and telangiectasia, later by superficial ulcerations, warty growths and the formation of small areas of atrophy, and finally by malignant epitheliomata and death.

Kaposi's varicelliform eruption. A severe generalized pock-like disease of eczematous infants caused by the virus of herpes simplex, or following intentional or accidental vaccination against smallpox by vaccinia virus.

Kaposi's compound ointment. Compound betanaphthol ointment; a mixture of betanaphthol, chalk, soft soap and lard.

Kaposi's sarcoma. Multiple haemorrhagic sarcomata, especially affecting the skin of the extremities.

kappa (kap·ah). K or κ, the tenth letter of the Greek alphabet, used in chemistry as a prefix to denote the tenth carbon atom in a chain. **Kappa chain.** One of the 2 classes of immunoglobulin light chains.

Kappis, Max 20th century German surgeon.

Kappis' method of splanchnic block. The approach to the coeliac plexus from the back. Described in 1914.

Karell, Philip Jakob (b. 1806). St. Petersburg physician.

Karell's diet. A diet recommended for congestive heart failure; it consists solely of 800 ml of milk given in 4 meals of 200 ml each.

Karell's treatment. A treatment for heart and kidney disease by rest in bed, and Karell's diet (see above) for 12 days.

karezza (kah·rez·ah). Coitus reservatus.

Karplus, Johann Paul (b. 1866). Vienna physician.

Karplus' sign. Aegophony heard over a pleural effusion.

Karr, Walter Gerald (b. 1892). Philadelphia biochemist.

Karr's method, for urea in blood. Incubate blood filtrate with a urease solution at 50°C for 15 min. Add some ghatti-gum solution followed by Nessler reagent, and compare the colour with that given by a standard urea solution similarly treated.

Karr's salt mixture. Sodium chloride, calcium lactate, magnesium citrate, ferric nitrate and a few drops of Lugol solution, used as an aperient and tonic saline solution.

Kartagener, Manes (b. 1897). Zürich physician.

Kartagener's syndrome or triad. A hereditary syndrome in which there is bronchiectasis, maldevelopment of the sinuses and transposition of the viscera.

karyapsis (kar·e·**ap**·sis). In karyogamy, nuclear union after cell conjugation. [Gk *karyon* nut, *apsis* juncture.]

karyenchyma (**kar**·e·en·**ki**′·mah). Karyolymph. [Gk *karyon* nut, *en, chymos* juice.]

karyoblast (**kar**·e·o·blast). A developing erythrocyte having a circular nucleus with nucleoli and a cloudy cytoplasm which may not contain haemoglobin. [Gk *karyon* nut, *blastos* germ.]

karyochromatophil, karyochromatophile (**kar**·e·o·**kro**′·mat·o·fil, **kar**·e·o·**kro**′·mat·o·file). Referring to a cell which has a nucleus that is readily stainable. [Gk *karyon* nut, chromatophil.]

karyoclasis (kar·e·**ok**·las·is). Karyorrhexis. [Gk *karyon* nut, *klasis* a breaking.]

karyocyte (**kar**·e·o·site). Normoblast. [Gk *karyon* nut, *kytos* cell.]

karyogamy (kar·e·**og**·am·e). The fusion (conjugation) of cell nuclei. [Gk *karyon* nut, *gamos* marriage.]

karyogenesis (**kar**·e·o·**jen**′·es·is). The formation of the cell nucleus. [Gk *karyon* nut, *genein* to produce.]

karyogenic (**kar**·e·o·**jen**′·ik). Relating or belonging to karyogenesis; producing the cell nucleus.

karyogonad (**kar**·e·o·**gon**′·ad). Gonad nucleus. *See* NUCLEUS. [Gk *karyon* nut, gonad.]

karyokinesis (**kar**·e·o·kin·**e**′·sis). The division of a somatic cell nucleus into two, without a reduction in chromosome number. In contradistinction to division of the cytoplasm or cytokinesis. *See* MITOSIS. [Gk *karyon* nut, *kinesis* motion.]

karyokinetic (**kar**·e·o·kin·**et**′·ik). Pertaining to, or having the characteristics of karyokinesis.

karyolobic (**kar**·e·o·**lo**′·bik). Having a lobe-shaped nucleus. [see foll.]

karyolobism (**kar**·e·o·**lo**′·bizm). A condition of the cell nucleus, especially that of the leucocyte, in which it takes on a lobe-shaped form. [Gk *karyon* nut, lobe.]

karyolymph (**kar**·e·o·limf). The fluid substance in the nucleus of a cell. [Gk *karyon* nut, lymph.]

karyolysis (kar·e·**ol**·is·is). The apparent destruction by lysis of the cell nucleus so that the chromatin no longer takes basic dyes. [Gk *karyon* nut, lysis.]

karyolytic (**kar**·e·o·**lit**′·ik). Relating or belonging to karyolysis.

karyomere (**kar**·e·o·meer). 1. Chromomere. 2. Chromosomal vesicles seen at telophase of certain mitoses. 3. The head of a spermatozoon. [Gk *karyon* nut, *meros* part.]

karyometry (kar·e·**om**·et·re). Measurement of the nucleus of a cell. [Gk *karyon* nut, *metron* measure.]

karyomicrosome (**kar**·e·o·**mi**′·kro·some). 1. Any one of the small particles of the karyoplasm. 2. Any one of the small segments or tangible bodies of which a chromatin fibre is composed. [Gk *karyon* nut, microsome.]

karyomit (**kar**·e·o·mit). A chromosome. [Gk *karyon* nut, *mitos* thread.]

karyomitome (**kar**·e·o·**mi**′·tome). The nuclear network. [see prec.]

karyomitosis (**kar**·e·o·mi·**to**′·sis). Karyokinesis. [Gk *karyon* nut, mitosis.]

karyomitotic (**kar**·e·o·mi·**tot**′·ik). Relating or belonging to karyomitosis (karyokinesis).

karyomorphism (**kar**·e·o·**mor**′·fizm). The form assumed by the nucleus of a cell, in particular, a leucocyte. [Gk *karyon* nut, *morphe* form.]

karyon (**kar**·e·on). 1. The cell nucleus. [obsolete term.] 2. An extract of the leaves of the walnut tree, *Juglans regia* (family Juglandaceae), which was introduced as a remedy for tuberculosis, but proved clinically ineffective. [Gk nut.]

karyophage, karyophagus (**kar**·e·o·faje, kar·e·**of**·ag·us). A cytozoon which causes phagocytosis of the nucleus. [Gk *karyon* nut, *phagein* to eat.]

karyoplasm (**kar**·e·o·plazm). The semifluid substance (protoplasm) which fills the meshes of the chromatin network of the cell nucleus. [Gk *karyon* nut, *plasma* something formed.]

karyoplasmic (**kar**·e·o·**plaz**′·mik). Relating or belonging to karyoplasm.

karyoplast (**kar**·e·o·plast). The cell nucleus. [Gk *karyon* nut, *plassein* to form.]

karyoplastin (**kar**·e·o·**plas**′·tin). The chromatin substance which forms the chromatic fibrils during indirect division of cells. [see prec.]

karyoreticulum (**kar**·e·o·ret·**ik**′·ew·lum). The part of the nucleus which consists of fibrils arranged in a network. [Gk *karyon* nut, reticulum.]

karyorrhexis (**kar**·e·o·**rex**′·is). Disintegration of the nucleus of a cell; the chromatin is distributed in the cytoplasm in shapeless granules which are finally thrust out from the cell. [Gk *karyon* nut, *rhexis* rupture.]

karyosoma (**kar**·e·o·**so**′·mah). Karyosome.

karyosome (**kar**·e·o·some). 1. Minute spheres to be found in the nucleus and said to consist of fragments of chromatin; often confused with a nucleolus. 2. Chromosome. 3. The cell nucleus. [Gk *karyon* nut, *soma* body.]

karyospherical (**kar**·e·o·**sfer**′·ik·al). Having a globular nucleus. [Gk *karyon* nut, spherical.]

karyostasis (kar·e·**os**·tas·is). The resting condition of a cell nucleus, as apposed to karyokinesis. [Gk *karyon* nut, *stasis* a standing still.]

karyostatic (**kar**·e·o·**stat**′·ik). Relating or belonging to karyostasis.

karyostenosis (**kar**·e·o·sten·**o**′·sis). Simple or direct division of a cell by simple cleavage of the nucleus. [Gk *karyon* nut, *stenos* a strait.]

karyota (**kar**·e·o·tah). Nucleated cells. [Gk *karyon* nut.]

karyotheca (**kar**·e·o·**the**′·kah). The nuclear-investing membrane. [Gk *karyon* nut, *theke* sheath.]

karyotin (**kar**·e·o·tin). The basophilic or acidophilic substance of the nuclear framework. [Gk *karyon* nut.]

karyotype (**kar**·e·o·tipe). The chromosome complement of a cell, an individual or a group of related individuals. Each karyotype is characterized by the number and morphology of its chromosomes. The diagrammatic representation of a karyotype is called an *idiogram.* [Gk *karyon* nut, *typos* mark.]

karyozoic (**kar**·e·o·**zo**′·ik). Living in or present in the cell nucleus of its host; applied to a protozoal parasite. [Gk *karyon* nut, *zoon* animal.]

Kashida's sign. Hyperaesthesia to heat and cold, sometimes seen in tetany.

kassa (**kas**·ah). Leprosy. [Jap.]

Kassowitz, Max (b. 1842). Vienna physician.

Kassowitz's law. Diday's law.

Kastle, Joseph Hoeing (b. 1864). American chemist.

Kastle–Meyer reagent. Dissolve 2 g of phenolphthalein and 20 g of potassium hydroxide in 100 ml of water. Add about 100 g of zinc dust and boil until the pink colour has completely disappeared. Decant from the zinc and make up to 100 ml. This reagent does not keep well.

Kastle–Meyer test, for blood in urine, faeces, etc. To 3 ml of Kastle–Meyer reagent, add 10 drops of 10 volume hydrogen peroxide. Add 3 ml of urine or aqueous extract of material. If blood is present, a pink colour develops.

kata-. 1. Prefix from the Greek preposition *kata,* meaning *down, entirely, wrongly, according to, alongside, thoroughly, back, against.* 2. For words beginning **kata-** *see also* CATA-.

katabolic (kat·ab·**ol**·ik). Catabolic.

katabolism (kat·**ab**·ol·izm). Catabolism.

katachromasis (kat·ah·**kro**·mas·is). The process by which there is reconstruction of the daughter nuclei by the daughter chromosomes. [Gk *kata,* chromosome.]

katadyn (**kat**·ah·din). An activated form of silver used to coat the quartz sand grains of a filter, having bactericidal value for the sterilization of water. The method was devised by Krause of Munich in 1929. [Gk *kata, dynamis* power.]

kataphoria (kat·ah·**for**·e·ah). Cataphoria.

kataphraxis (kat·ah·**frax**·is). The surgical procedure of investing an organ with metallic supports in order to maintain it in position. [Gk *kataphrassein* to fence in.]

kataphrenia (kat·ah·**fre**·ne·ah). Cataphrenia.

kataphylaxis (**kat**·ah·fil·**ax**'·is). Cataphylaxis.

katathermometer (**kat**·ah·ther·**mom**'·et·er). An instrument to measure the cooling power of air on the human body. It consists of 2 alcohol thermometers, one with a dry bulb, the other with a wet bulb; both, after being heated to a temperature of 110°F (43°C), are exposed to the air, and the time taken by each to fall from 100° to 90°F (38° to 32°C) is noted. [Gk *kata, therme* heat, meter.]

Katayama, Kuniyoshi (b. 1855). Tokyo physician.

Katayama's test, for carbon monoxide. To dilute blood add a few drops of ammonium-sulphide solution and acidify with acetic acid. If carbon monoxide is present, a rose-red colour appears; with normal blood, a dirty greenish-grey.

Katayama (kat·ah·**yah**·mah). A genus of snails. **Katayama nosophora.** *Oncomelania nosophora*; a molluscan intermediate host of the oriental schistosome, *Schistosoma japonicum*. [*Katayama*, a district in Japan.]

katharometer (kath·ar·**om**·et·er). A device by which the basal metabolic rate is estimated electrometrically. [Gk *katharos* clean, *metron* measure.]

katharophore (kath·**ar**·o·for). An instrument used for washing out the urethra. [Gk *katharos* clean, *pherein* to carry.]

kathode (**kath**·ode). Cathode.

katine (**kat**·een). $C_{10}H_{18}ON_2$, an alkaloid from *Catha edulis* which acts as a stimulant to the central nervous system.

kation (**kat**·i·on). Cation.

katipo (**kat**·e·po). A poisonous spider of New Zealand, *Latrodectus hasselti*.

katolysis (kat·**ol**·is·is). Intermediate or partial breaking-down of complex chemical bodies into more simple ones; applied particularly to processes of digestion. [Gk *kato* down, lysis.]

Katz, Johann Rudolf (b. 1880). German chemist.

Katz formula. A formula for obtaining the average erythrocyte sedimentation rate:

$$\frac{S_1 + \frac{S_2}{2}}{2}$$

where S_1 and S_2 are the heights of the column of clear fluid plasma in mm at the end of 1 and 2 h, respectively.

Kaufmann, Fritz (b. 1875). Mannheim neurologist.

Kaufmann's method or treatment. Psychiatric treatment according to the doctrines of Kaufmann, using vigorous suggestion, persuasion and encouragement.

kava, kava-kava (**kah**·vah, kah·vah·**kah**·vah). 1. The rhizome of a tropical shrub, *Piper methysticum* Forst. (family Piperaceae). It has a local action similar to pepper and has been administered in the form of the liquid extract as a diuretic and antiseptic in genito-urinary infections. 2. A Polynesian beverage made from the rhizome of *Piper methysticum*; it is drunk on festive occasions, and produces a condition of excitement and eventually loss of use of the legs. Habitual use causes debility and a roughening of the skin. [Hawaiian name.]

kavaism (**kah**·vah·izm). A morbid condition resembling absinthism; it is caused by addiction to kava.

Kay, Herbert Davenport (b. 1893). Canadian biochemist.

Kay-Graham pasteurization test. Phosphatase test. *See* TEST.

Kayser, Bernhard (b. 1869). Stuttgart ophthalmologist.

Kayser's disease. A form of hepatolenticular degeneration.

Fleischer-Kayser ring, Kayser-Fleischer ring. A brown ring at the outer edge of the cornea, seen in Wilson's disease (hepatolenticular degeneration) and due to the deposition of copper-containing pigment of unknown constitution. It may only be visible on slit-lamp examination, but is a diagnostic sign of the disease.

Kayser, Heinrich (b. 1876). Weimar physician.

Brion-Kayser disease. Paratyphoid fever. *See* FEVER.

Keegan, Denis Francis (b. 1840). British surgeon.

Keegan's operation. Rhinoplasty.

Keen, William Williams (b. 1837). Philadelphia surgeon.

Keen's point. A point 3 cm above and 3 cm behind the external auditory meatus for needling the lateral ventricle.

Keetley, Charles Robert Bell (b. 1848). London surgeon.

Keetley-Torek operation. Correction of undescended testis by implanting it temporarily in the subcutaneous tissue of the thigh.

kefir, kefyr (**kef**·eer). A preparation of curdled fermented milk originating from the Caucasus and formed by the addition of kefir grains. **Kefir grain.** A small granule of dried ferment consisting of a yeast (*Torula kefir*) and bacteria of the *Lactobacillus* genus, added to goats' milk in the preparation of the food. [Caucasian name.]

Kehr, Hans (b. 1862). Gotha and Halberstadt surgeon.

Kehr's incision. An extensive incision for opening the abdomen widely; it is carried from the xiphoid cartilage to the umbilicus, then obliquely downwards to the right or left of the umbilicus, and then vertically downwards again.

Kehr's sign. The presence of pain over the tip of the left shoulder in rupture of the spleen.

O'Connell's modification of Kehr's shoulder sign, of rupture of the spleen. Pain in the tip of the left shoulder when the foot of the bed is raised.

Kehrer, Ferdinand Adalbert (b. 1883). Münster neurologist.

Kehrer's reflex. Kisch's reflex; closure of the eye as a result of stimulation of the top part of the auditory meatus.

Kehrer's sign. In a tumour of the posterior cranial fossa, pressure over the lower occiput where the greater occipital nerve emerges gives severe pain and involuntary backward jerking of the head.

Kehrer, Ferdinand Adolph (b. 1837). Heidelberg gynaecologist.

Kehrer's operation. An operation to correct a depressed nipple, the skin around the nipple being excised.

keiro-. For words beginning with **keiro-**, *see* CHEIRO-.

Keith, Sir Arthur (b. 1866). London anatomist and anthropologist.

Keith's node, node of Keith and Flack. Sinu-atrial node. *See* NODE.

Keith, Thomas (b. 1827). Edinburgh surgeon.

Keith's drain. A glass tube with perforations at one extremity and a narrow collar at the other.

Kekwick, Alan (b. 1909). London physician.

Marriott-Kekwick apparatus. An apparatus for giving drip transfusions, in which the blood is kept stirred by oxygen bubbling through it.

Marriott and Kekwick formula, in blood transfusion. A formula for calculating the volume of blood in millilitres required to produce the desired rise in haemoglobin in adults or infants; it assumes that the normal blood volume is 40 ml per lb (88 ml per kg) body weight:

$$\frac{\text{Percentage rise haemoglobin required} \times \text{patient's normal blood volume}}{100}$$

Marriott and Kekwick U-tube regulator. A regulator for use in blood transfusions, designed to avoid the constriction, and therefore easy blocking, that results from lateral compression of a rubber tube. It consists of 4 lengths of glass tubing each bent in a U and their ends connected by a short-circuiting tube. Blood can be caused to flow along the short circuit or along one or more of the U tubes; in passing through the tubes the blood is slowed by frictional resistance. The rate of flow can be further regulated by raising or lowering the reservoir in relation to the U tubes.

kelectome (**ke**·lek·tome). Celectome.

kelis (**ke**·lis). 1. Keloid. 2. Localized scleroderma. [Gk spot.]

kell *See* Blood GROUP.

Keller, Philipp (b. 1891). Freiburg dermatologist.

Keller's ultraviolet test, for determining the presence of erythema-producing waves in compound radiations. A test whereby the proportion of ultraviolet radiation in combined radiations is determined by the use of photographic paper.

Keller, William Lordan (b. 1874). American surgeon.

Keller's arthroplasty or operation. Excision arthroplasty of the 1st metatarsophalangeal joint in which the base of the phalanx is removed.

Kellgren, Henry (b. 1827). Swedish physician.

Kellgren treatment. A system of active and passive movements combined wtih massage.

Kelling, Georg (b. 1866). Dresden surgeon.

Kelling's test, for lactic acid in gastric contents. A very dilute ferric-chloride solution is prepared by adding 2 drops of 10 per cent solution to about 10 ml of water. Divide this into equal parts; to one add a little strained gastric juice and to the other an equal amount of water. If lactic acid is present a distinct yellow colour is produced immediately in the tube containing the gastric juice.

Kelly, Adam Brown (b. 1865). Scottish laryngologist.

Kelly–Paterson syndrome, Paterson–Kelly syndrome. Plummer–Vinson syndrome.

Kelly, Howard Atwood (b. 1858). Baltimore gynaecologist.

Kelly's operation. A method of treating stress incontinence by repairing and supporting the bladder neck; probably the first satisfactory operation devised for this condition.

Kelly's sign. The muscular contractions induced by pinching the ureter with forceps when exposed on the operating table.

Kelly's speculum. A cylindrical handled speculum with an obturator, used in examining the rectum.

Kelly's urethral speculum. A narrow hollow cylinder with an obturator, used in the examination of the female urethra.

Kelly's test, to differentiate between saphenous varix and femoral hernia. The veins below the knee are compressed by the left hand whilst the right hand squeezes sharply the inner side of the thigh above the knee. Blood will be forced through the great saphenous vein and cause the swelling to quiver if it is due to a varix.

Kelly, Joseph Dominic (b. 1888). New York otolaryngologist.

Kelly's operation. A cordopexy operation for the displacement and fixing of a paralysed vocal cord in the position of abduction; a method of restoring the airway in bilateral paralysis of the vocal cords.

keloid (ke·loid). The cellular overgrowth of fibrous tissue in a scar at the site of a skin injury, frequent in negroes and in pregnant women of all races. **Acne keloid.** Keloid formation in the scars of acne pustules. [Gk *kelis* spot, *eidos* form.]

See also: ADDISON (T.).

keloidosis (ke·loid·o·sis). A condition characterized by the presence of a crop of keloids. [keloid, Gk *-osis* condition.]

keloma (ke·**lo**·mah). Keloid. [Gk *kelis* spot, *-oma* tumour.]

keloplasty (ke·lo·plas·te). Plastic surgery performed on scars and scar tissue. [Gk *kelis* spot, *plassein* to mould]

kelos (ke·los). Keloid.

kelotome (ke·lo·tome). A particular type of surgical knife used in herniotomy. [Gk *kele* hernia, *temnein* to cut.]

kelotomy (ke·**lot**·o·me). Section of the constriction causing strangulated hernia and the resultant reduction of the latter. [see prec.]

kelp (kelp). The ashes of seaweeds, the red wracks, species of *Laminaria* which are cast up on the coasts of Scotland, Normandy and Spain, and burnt in a process for the extraction of their iodine content. In Normandy the ashes are known as *varec.* [ME *culp.*]

kelpware (kelp·wa·er). Fucus.

Kelser, Raymond Alexander (b. 1892). American pathologist.

Kelser vaccine. An antirabic vaccine prepared from inoculated rabbit brain.

Kelvin, Lord. *See* THOMSON, WILLIAM.

kelvin (kel·vin). An electrical unit; a kilowatt-hour. [Lord *Kelvin* (b. 1824), Glasgow physicist.]

Kendall, Edward Calvin (b. 1886). Connecticut biochemist at the Mayo Clinic.

Kendall's compound A. 11-Deoxycorticosterone.

Kendall's compound E. Cortisone.

Kendall's compound F. 17-Hydroxycorticosterone.

Kendrick, Pearl. 20th century Michigan bacteriologist.

Kendrick mouse intracerebral test. A laboratory method of comparative testing of the potency of whooping-cough vaccines. Mice are immunized with pertussis vaccine and the level of immunity is determined by the intracerebral challenge injection of virulent *Haemophilus pertussis.*

Kennedy, Foster (b. 1884). British and New York neurologist.

Foster Kennedy syndrome, Kennedy's syndrome. Ipsilateral optic atrophy, often with central scotoma, and contralateral papilloedema, due to a tumour compressing the ipsilateral optic nerve; it usually occurs in meningiomata of the sphenoid ridge.

Kenny, Elizabeth (b. 1886). Brisbane nurse.

Kenny method or treatment. A method used in the treatment of cases of infantile paralysis. During the acute stage, the affected muscles are wrapped with hot moist packs; when pain and muscular spasm have eased, passive movements and muscular re-education are introduced.

kenophobia (ken·o·**fo**·be·ah). Morbid dread of large open spaces. [Gk *kenos* empty, phobia.]

kenotoxin (ken·o·**tox**·in). Fatigue toxin. *See* TOXIN. [Gk *kenos* empty, toxin.]

Kent, Albert Frank Stanley (b. 1863). Bristol and London physiologist.

Kent's bundle, Kent–His bundle, Stanley Kent bundle. The atrioventricular bundle; also known as the *bundle of His.* The term *Kent bundle* is also used by electrophysiologists in the sense of a bundle of conducting tissue in the heart which totally bypasses the normal atrioventricular node and bundle of His, producing in the electrocardiogram a short P-R interval with widening of the QRS complex without a delta wave (the Wolff–Parkinson–White syndrome).

Kent syndrome. A condition in which the duration of the QRS complex of the electrocardiogram is greater than 0.1/s (bundle-branch block), in association with a short P-R interval. It is thought to be due to early excitation of one or other ventricle, the impulse from the sinu-atrial node being short circuited through anomalous conducting tissue in the bundle of Kent (see above). The condition is congenital and is associated with a liability to paroxysmal tachycardia. The heart is generally normal but cases may occur in association with congenital heart disease. The syndrome may also complicate acquired heart disease. An alternative explanation is that a nodal rhythm is the cause of the syndrome. More usually known as the *Wolff–Parkinson–White syndrome* or *pre-excitation syndrome.*

Kent, Grace Helen (b. 1875). American psychologist.

Kent tests. A series of brief oral tests designed to provide a preliminary measure of intelligence.

kephalepsalis (kef·al·**ep**·sal·is). Shears designed for use in embryotomy operations. [Gk *kephale* head, *psalis* pair of shears.]

kephir, kephyr (**kef**·eer). Kefir.

Kepler, Johannes (b. 1571). German natural philosopher.

Kepler's theory of accommodation. That accommodation was brought about by movement of the lens forward. This was disproved, as in order to attain the amount of accommodation necessary the lens would have to be in front of the cornea.

Kérandel, Jean François (b. 1873). French physician in Indo-China and Africa.

Kérandel's sign. In sleeping sickness (trypanosomiasis), a delayed but severe deep pain after a moderate or slight blow on the skin or other bony prominence.

kerasin (ker·as·een). A cerebroside in brain tissue; it is a galactolipide composed of galactose, sphingosine and lignoceric acid.

keratalgia (ker·at·al·je·ah). Pain in the cornea. [Gk *keras* horn, *algos* pain.]

keratectasia (ker·at·ek·ta′·ze·ah). A protrusion of the cornea. [Gk *keras* horn, *ektasis* a stretching.]

keratectomy (ker·at·ek·to·me). Operative removal of a part or the whole of the cornea. [Gk *keras* horn, *ektome* a cutting out.]

keratiasis (ker·at·i·as·is). A skin condition marked by the development of horny wart-like excrescences. [see foll.]

keratic (ker·at·ik). 1. Horny. 2. Belonging to the cornea. [Gk *keras* horn.]

keratin (ker·at·in). A class of scleroprotein derived from the surface ectoderm that forms the horny layer of the skin, and the major component of hair, nails, feathers and superficial scales. Keratins are insoluble in water, dilute acids or alkalis, and are unaffected by proteolytic enzymes, e.g. pepsin, trypsin. They are rich in the amino acid, cystine. A solution of keratins in ammoniated alcohol is used in pharmacy for preparing enteric-coated pills, capsules, etc., intended to pass through the stomach unchanged, though their value in this respect is erratic. [see prec.]

keratinization (ker·at·in·i·za′·shun). 1. The appearance of horny characteristics in a tissue. 2. The process of covering pills with a coating of keratin. [see foll.]

keratinize (ker·at·in·ize). Of tissue, to make or become horny. [Gk *keras* horn.]

keratinoid (ker·at·in·oid). 1. Having keratin-like properties. 2. Keratin-coated, so as to pass through the stomach unchanged and dissolve in the intestine. [Keratin, Gk *eidos* form.]

Keratinomyces (ker·at·in·o·mi′·seez). A fourth genus of the dermatophyte fungi. Now considered synonymous with *Trichophyton.* [Gk *keras* horn, *mykes* fungus.]

keratinous (ker·at·in·us). 1. Horny. 2. Relating or belonging to keratin.

keratitic (ker·at·it·ik). Pertaining to keratitis.

keratitis (ker·at·i·tis). Inflammation of the cornea. **Acne-rosacea keratitis.** Keratitis associated with acne rosacea of the skin and conjunctiva. It produces vascularized scars and an uneven surface, tends to relapse and to interfere seriously with vision, and is frequently bilateral. **Actinic keratitis.** That due to exposure to ultraviolet rays and characterized by numerous punctate erosions of the epithelium. **Alphabet keratitis.** The appearance of double contoured lines raised above the surface of the cornea and due to folds in Bowman's membrane, associated with lowering of intra-ocular pressure. It may occur spontaneously or follow trauma. **Anaphylactic keratitis.** If one cornea is sensitized by intracorneal injection of protein, subsequent injection of the other cornea causes violent parenchymatous (interstitial) keratitis, identical with that due to congenital syphilis. **Annular keratitis.** A form of congenital syphilitic keratitis (see below) in which a plastic exudate forms a hazy ring on the back of the cornea. **Artificial-silk keratitis.** Probably due to hypersensitivity to chemical fumes formed during manufacture of artificial silk; it is characterized by oedema and desquamation of corneal epithelium, redness of the eye and photophobia. **Band keratitis, Band-shaped keratitis, Keratitis bandalette.** Occurring in 2 forms: (*a*) usually in elderly people, a subepithelial encrustation of lime salts in the exposed part of the cornea, tending to involve both eyes; (*b*) a horizontal, greyish-brown band of opacity developing in an old blind eye, in the lower third of the cornea. **Keratitis bullosa.** Formation of epithelial bullae upon the cornea of an eye, the subject of old iridocyclitis, glaucoma or interstitial keratitis. **Deep keratitis.** A greyish opacity in the deep layers of the cornea, associated with an anterior uveitis; of varied and doubtful aetiology. **Dendriform keratitis, Dendritic keratitis.** A branching form of ulcer affecting the corneal epithelium, due to infection with the virus of herpes simplex. **Keratitis disciformis.** A delicate grey disc occupying nearly the middle of the cornea, non-suppurative and chronic; due to infection from without by a virus or by mildly virulent bacteria. **Epithelial diffuse keratitis.** Keratitis which may be due to deficiency of vitamin B_2: both corneae are covered by minute grey epithelial opacities. **Epithelial punctate keratitis.** Superficial punctate keratitis (see below). **Exfoliative keratitis.** Keratitis in which large areas of cornea are denuded of epithelium. It occurs in association with exfoliative dermatitis in arsenical hypersensitiveness. **Exposure keratitis.** That which occurs when the cornea cannot be covered by the lids, e.g. in proptosis or in facial palsy. The epithelium desiccates, exfoliates and the way is open for microbic invasion. **Fascicular keratitis.** A form of phlyctenular keratitis (see below) in which the ulcer progresses across the cornea in linear fashion, followed by a small leash of vessels. **Filamentary keratitis, Keratitis filamentosa.** That associated with the formation of fine epithelial filaments. It occurs in keratitis sicca (see below), and after abrasions or herpetic lesions. (Cf. KERATOCONJUNCTIVITIS SICCA.) **Furrow keratitis.** A degenerative process in which the area of the arcus senilis becomes thin, and a groove or gutter is formed which eventually bulges to form a marginal ectasia. **Herpetic keratitis.** 1. Keratitis due to herpes febrilis, usually causing dendritic keratitis (see above). 2. That due to herpes zoster, beginning as widespread epithelial oedema and going on to severe, deep infiltration with keratitic precipitates. If the cornea becomes anaesthetic, neuroparalytic keratitis (see below) may develop. **Hypopyon keratitis.** Serpiginous ulcer; keratitis associated with an exudate of pus, usually sterile, into the bottom of the anterior chamber. The ulcer is frequently pneumococcal. **Interstitial keratitis.** A diffuse chronic keratitis involving the whole thickness of the cornea, associated with superficial and deep vascularization, but almost always without ulceration. Eighty to 90 per cent of cases are due to congenital syphilis, the remainder to tuberculosis and, more rarely, to other infections. **Lagophthalmic keratitis.** Exposure keratitis (see above). **Lattice keratitis.** A folding of Bowman's membrane, associated with inflammation and occurring after trauma. **Leprotic keratitis.** Various forms of keratitis associated with leprosy, of which the commonest are nodules on the limbus and a milky appearance in the substantia propria with minute white spots. **Marginal keratitis.** Furrow keratitis (see above). **Mustard-gas keratitis.** Keratitis due to mustard gas; the immediate reaction may be slight or severe, leaving corneal opacities. It is associated with the development of ampullary dilatations of vessels on the bulbar conjunctiva which grow into the cornea. Years later the opacities break down into ulcers causing more disability. **Mycotic keratitis.** Ulceration and inflammation of the cornea due to injury and subsequent invasion by fungi, e.g. *Aspergillus fumigatus, Fusarium* species, *Candida albicans.* **Neuroparalytic keratitis.** That which occurs when the cornea is anaesthetic. It begins with fine stippling of the epithelium, going on to vesiculation, exfoliation and secondary infection. **Neuropathic keratitis.** A term applied to any lesion associated with the nerves supplying the cornea, including the gasserian ganglion, e.g. herpes zoster ophthalmicus, neurotrophic keratitis. **Neurotrophic keratitis.** A condition thought at one time to be due to disturbance of trophic nerves of the cornea. It occurs when there is disturbance of the corneal nerve supply, probably caused by unregulated accumulation of metabolites. **Nodular keratitis.** Reticular keratitis (see below). **Nummular keratitis.** Dimmer's keratitis, a characteristic finding in ocular onchocerciasis. **Oyster-shuckers' keratitis.** Keratitis caused by small particles of oyster shell striking the cornea. **Parenchymatous keratitis.** Interstitial keratitis (see above). **Keratitis petrificans.** Band keratitis (see above). **Phlyctenular keratitis.** Keratitis associated with conjunctival involvement and known as *phlyctenular keratoconjunctivitis.* It starts usually at the limbus as 1 or more small nodules, and is essentially an allergic phenomenon, in which the allergen is most commonly tuberculous protein. Associated with photophobia, blepharospasm and epiphora, it may affect vision seriously owing to formation of corneal opacities and vascularization. **Keratitis profunda.** The formation of a greyish opacity in the deeper layers of the cornea, unassociated with ulceration. Irritative symptoms may or may not occur, but there is usually some iridocyclitis. It probably has an allergic bacterial basis. **Keratitis punctata.**

Formerly applied to the punctate deposit on the back of the cornea occurring in anterior uveitis. Since there is no associated keratitis, the condition is now termed *keratitic precipitates*, or more shortly, K.P. **Keratitis punctata leprosa.** The commonest form of keratitis occurring in leprosy, and consisting of minute white spots. **Keratitis punctata profunda.** A rare manifestation of late syphilis, appearing as circumscribed, pinhead-sized, greyish spots in the the substantia propria. **Keratitis punctata subepithelialis.** Superficial or epithelial punctate keratitis, which has been ascribed to various causes, e.g. virus, nutritional, bacterial, neuropathic. Onset is acute, usually with catarrhal conjunctivitis, and manifests itself by the development of numerous small infiltrates on both sides of Bowman's membrane. It is commonly binocular. **Punctate keratitis.** Keratitis punctata (see above). **Purulent keratitis.** Severe keratitis, usually starting from a trifling injury, in elderly patients or those with depressed nutrition. Secondary infection occurs most commonly with pneumococci from an infected lacrimal sac. It causes a large spreading ulcer, with pus in the anterior chamber, and purulent disintegration of the cornea. **Keratitis pustuliformis profunda.** An uncommon condition in which yellowish deposits surrounded by greyish opacity form in the deep layers of the cornea. Some cases are syphilitic; in others the cause is unknown. It usually occurs in elderly men. **Reticular keratitis.** A familial disease consisting of multiple opacities in, or deep to, Bowman's membrane, and affecting both corneae, especially the axial region; the onset is usually in adolescence. Also known as *nodular, superficial linear* or *alphabet keratitis.* **Ribbon-like keratitis.** Band keratitis (see above). **Rosacea keratitis.** Keratitis occurring in association with facial rosacea, blepharitis and conjunctivitis. It begins as vascular infiltrates at the limbus, which advance into the superficial layers of the cornea; ulceration occurs over them with resultant scarring. It usually involves both eyes. **Sclerosing keratitis.** Includes 2 types of disease: (*a*) in which nodular infiltrates appear near the margin of the cornea in association with a ring of anterior scleritis and anterior uveitis. Relapses tend to occur and sight is frequently lost. Most cases are probably tuberculous in origin; (*b*) *Sclerosing keratitis proper*; a triangular opacity in the deeper layers of the cornea with its base towards the patch of scleritis which has caused it. It is frequently of tuberculous aetiology. **Scrofulous keratitis.** Phlyctenular keratitis (see above). **Secondary keratitis.** Keratitis which is dependent on disease in some other part of the eye, e.g. the conjunctiva. **Serpiginous keratitis.** *Acute*; a purulent ulcerative keratitis which spreads over the surface and into the depths of the cornea. it is usually pneumococcal, may cause hypopyon and in one-third of the cases is associated with an infected lacrimal sac. *Chronic*; rodent or Mooren's ulcer of the cornea. **Keratitis sicca.** A chronic condition of the cornea associated with absence of lacrimal and mucous secretions. There are photophobia, numerous small opacities in the exposed part of the cornea and usually filaments. It may be due to trauma, but is more commonly spontaneous, occurring in women at the menopause and associated with a dry mouth and arthritis (Sjögren's syndrome). **Striate keratitis.** A term erroneously applied to the folds in Descemet's membrane, sometimes seen after trauma or operation, especially cataract extraction, and as a result of excessively tight and prolonged bandaging. **Superficial linear keratitis.** Alphabet keratitis (see above). **Superficial punctate keratitis.** One in which the cornea shows many small circular erosions of the epithelium. It is often associated with acute conjunctivitis and is then known as epidemic keratoconjunctivitis, caused by a virus. **Suppurative keratitis.** A term applied to ulceration as opposed to non-ulcerative keratitis or to the formation of pustules in the cornea as in smallpox, other exanthemata or pyaemia. **Syphilitic keratitis.** Syphilis may effect the cornea: (*a*) very rarely as a primary infection; (*b*) by direct spread from gummatous scleritis or cyclitis; (*c*) as interstitial keratitis (see above). **Trachomatous keratitis.** Corneal ulcers occurring during the course of trachoma and associated with pannus. **Traumatic keratitis.** Reaction of the cornea to injury, which includes among other possibilities, foreign bodies, concussion, wounds, burns, noxious fumes, chemicals and radiations. The reaction varies according to the type of injury and to the presence or absence of micro-organisms, and of hypersensitivity. **Trophic keratitis.** A term applied to keratitis following lesions of the trigeminal nerve. The presence of trophic fibres has never been established, however, so it is doubtful if such a condition exists. **Keratitis urica.** A rare condition, the substantia propria becoming infiltrated with crystalline urea and sodium urate in non-gouty patients: probably a form of dystrophy. Deposition of crystals occasionally occurs in gouty patients, associated with widespread intra-ocular inflammation. **Vascular keratitis.** A term which can be applied to any form of keratitis in which new vessels are formed, e.g. trachomatous pannus or phlyctenular disease. It was originally used to describe a form of vascularization thought to be a clinical entity but subsequently found to be a variety of interstitial keratitis (see above). **Vasculonebulous keratitis.** Keratitis associated with opacities and new vessel formation; pannus. **Vernal keratitis.** A complication of spring catarrh which occurs as a direct spread of the jelly-like elevations at the limbus or as a dystrophy due to interference with nutrition. **Vesicular keratitis.** Keratitis which may be an early stage of keratitis bullosa, and associated with oedema of the epithelium, or occur as a neurotropic manifestation, e.g. in herpes febrilis, recurrent erosions, etc. **Xerotic keratitis.** That due to dryness of the conjunctiva causing ulceration of the cornea. It is due to malnutrition and especially to deficiency of vitamin A; it is commonest in infants. [Gk *keras* horn, *-itis* inflammation.]

See also: DIMMER.

kerato-acanthoma (ker·at·o·ak·an·**tho'**·mah). Molluscum pseudocarcinomatosum, molluscum sebaceum; a small innocent tumour of the skin, usually on the face, which heals spontaneously. Histologically it resembles a squamous-celled epithelioma in certain respects and has been confused with this in the past. [Gk *keras* horn, acanthoma.]

kerato-angioma (ker·at·o·an·je·**o'**·mah). An angiomatous patch on the skin, usually of the legs and feet of children, with characteristic warty outgrowths. [Gk *keras* horn, angioma.]

keratocele (ker·at·o·seel). Descemetocele; hernia of Descemet's membrane through the floor of an ulcer which has destroyed the layers of the cornea anterior to the posterior elastic lamina. [Gk *keras* horn, *kele* hernia.]

keratocentesis (ker·at·o·sen·**te'**·sis). Puncture of the cornea. [Gk *keras* horn, *kentesis* a pricking.]

keratochromatosis (ker·at·o·kro·mat·**o'**·sis). A condition in which the cornea becomes pigmented. [Gk *keras* horn, *chroma* colour, *-osis* condition.]

keratoconjunctivitis (ker·at·o·kon·jungk·tiv·**i'**·tis). The syndrome of keratitis associated with conjunctivitis. **Artificial-silk keratoconjunctivitis.** An acute irritant inflammation of the conjunctiva and cornea found in workers in artificial-silk factories. It is characterized by corneal oedema. The cause is unknown. **Epidemic keratoconjunctivitis.** An acute epidemic conjunctivitis due to an adenovirus, almost invariably type 8. Spread mainly by contaminated materials or instruments in eye clinics, particularly where minor eye injuries are common, e.g. among shipyard workers—hence the alternative name *shipyard eye.* **Flash keratoconjunctivitis.** An acute inflammation of the conjunctiva with watering, photophobia and pain, associated with small punctate corneal ulceration; it is caused by the ultraviolet rays in the flash of arc welding or from sunlight in snow blindness. **Mustard-gas keratoconjunctivitis.** An acute inflammation of the cornea and conjunctiva following the use of mustard gas in wartime. In severe cases the corneal lesions reappear often 20 years later and cause an intractable vascularizing keratitis which shows small lakes of blood or dilated vessels, diagnostic of the disease. **Phlyctenular keratoconjunctivitis.** An acute inflammation of the conjunctiva associated with the formation of raised nodules astride the limbus (phlyctens) which often ulcerate. These may spread towards the centre and become vascularized. It is allergic in nature, most commonly to tuberculous protein.

Keratoconjunctivitis sicca. Sjögren's syndrome; a condition associated with diminution of lacrimal and salivary secretion. It occurs principally in women at the menopause and is usually accompanied by formation of the fine filaments adhering to the cornea and composed of desquamated cells of the corneal epithelium, hence sometimes called *filamentary keratitis.* The syndrome is often associated with rheumatoid arthritis and other collagen disorders.

keratoconometer (ker·at·o·kon·**om'**·et·er). An instrument for estimating the degree of conicity of the cornea; usually a camera which photographs the corneal image of a Placido's disc or a keratoscope. [Gk *keras* horn, *konos* cone, meter.]

keratoconus (ker·at·o·**ko'**·nus). A conical protrusion of the cornea with central thinning; conical cornea. [Gk *keras* horn, *konos* cone.]

keratocyst (ker·at·o·sist). A thin-walled dental cyst lined by keratinizing epithelium, characterized by its tendency to recur after enucleation. It probably arises from undifferentiated cell rests of the dental lamina. [Gk *keras* horn, cyst.]

keratoderma (ker·at·o·**der'**·mah). A local or generalized hardening of the skin due to changes in the horny layer of the epidermis. **Arsenical keratoderma.** Keratoderma due to chronic arsenical poisoning. **Keratoderma blennorrhagica.** Keratotic, scaly rash occurring on the soles of the feet in about 10 per cent of patients with Reiter's syndrome, especially in the venereal form of the disease. **Climacteric keratoderma, Keratoderma climactericum.** A disease marked by localized hyperkeratosis of the skin of the palms and soles of women during the menopause. **Keratoderma disseminatum.** Keratoderma punctata (see below). **Keratoderma eccentrica.** Porokeratosis. **Gonorrhoeal keratoderma.** The occurrence in gonorrhoea of horny nodules in the skin of the palms and soles. **Lymphoedematous keratoderma.** A velvety papillomatous thickening of the skin over the lymphoedematous area. **Mutilating keratoderma.** A genetically-determined condition of palmoplantar keratoderma with irregular keratoses elsewhere and ainhum-like constricting bands on the fingers or toes. **Keratoderma palmaris et plantaris.** Symmetrical keratoderma of the palms and soles. **Keratoderma palmoplantaris transgrediens.** Mal de Meleda. **Keratoderma plantare sulcata.** A disease of the tropics, seen in adults who go barefooted. At one time it was considered to be due to tertiary yaws, but often the cause is obscure. The soles of the feet become thickened and pitted. Cf. KERATOMA PLANTARE SULCATUM; pitted KERATOLYSIS. **Keratoderma punctata.** Diffuse circumscribed hyperkeratoses, somewhat resembling the keratoses of chronic arsenical poisoning; probably a naevoid condition. **Symmetrical keratoderma.** Keratoderma of the palms and soles. **Syphilitic keratoderma.** A rare manifestation of tertiary syphilis in which, quite often, only one sole is affected. [Gk *keras* horn, *derma* skin.]

keratodermatitis (ker·at·o·der·mat·**i'**·tis). An inflamed condition of the horny layer of the skin. [Gk *keras* horn, *derma* skin, *-itis* inflammation.]

keratodermatocele (ker·at·o·**der'**·mat·o·seel). Keratocele. [Gk *keras* horn, *derma* skin, *kele* hernia.]

keratodermatosis (ker·at·o·der·mat·**o'**·sis). A morbid condition of the skin in which there is some change in the tissue of the horny layer. [Gk *keras* horn, *derma* skin, *-osis* condition.]

keratodermia (ker·at·o·**der'**·me·ah). Keratoderma. While originally the word *keratodermia* was reserved for deep-seated conditions, both names are now used indiscriminately. Cf. KERATODERMA. [Gk *keras* horn, *derma* skin.]

kerato-ectasia (ker·at·o·ek·**ta'**·ze·ah). Corneal protrusion. [Gk *keras* horn, *ektasis* a stretching out.]

keratogenesis (ker·at·o·**jen'**·es·is). The development or origination of horn-like tissue. [Gk *keras* horn, *genein* to produce.]

keratogenetic (ker·at·o·jen·**et'**·ik). Relating or belonging to keratogenesis.

keratogenous (ker·at·**oj**·en·us). Developing horny tissue or causing a growth of it. [Gk *keras* horn, *genein* to produce.]

keratoglobus (ker·at·o·**glo'**·bus). Distension of the eyeball or of the anterior segment of the eye. [Gk *keras* horn, globe.]

keratoglossus (ker·at·o·**glos'**·us). That part of the hyoglossus muscle which arises from the greater cornua of the hyoid bone. [Gk *keras* horn, *glossa* tongue.]

keratohaemia (ker·at·o·**he'**·me·ah). An accumulation of blood in the cornea. [Gk *keras* horn, *haima* blood.]

keratohelcosis (ker·at·o·hel·**ko'**·sis). Ulceration of the cornea. [Gk *keras* horn, *helkosis* ulceration.]

keratohyalin (ker·at·o·**hi'**·al·in). Eleidin; the substance composing the granules of the granular layer of the epidermis. It stains with eosin and haematoxylin. [Gk *keras* horn, hyalin.]

keratohyaline (ker·at·o·**hi'**·al·een). Descriptive of tissue which is both horny and hyaline. [Gk *keras* horn, *hyalos* transparent.]

keratoid (ker·at·oid). 1. Horny. 2. Having resemblance to corneal tissue. [Gk *keras* horn, *eidos* form.]

keratoiditis (ker·at·oid·**i'**·tis). Keratitis. [Gk *keras* horn, *eidos* form, *-itis* inflammation.]

kerato-iridocyclitis (ker·at·o·ir·id·o·si·**kli'**·tis). Inflammation affecting the cornea, ciliary body and iris simultaneously. [Gk *keras* horn, iridocyclitis.]

kerato-iritis (ker·at·o·i·**ri'**·tis). Keratitis present in association with iritis. **Hypopyon kerato-iritis, Suppurative kerato-iritis.** Suppuration involving the cornea and iris.

keratoleptynsis (ker·at·o·lep·**tin'**·sis). The operation performed for cosmetic purposes on an eye that has lost its function; it consists in removing the anterior surface of the cornea so that adhesion to the bulbar conjunctiva takes place. [Gk *keras* horn, *leptynein* to make thin.]

keratoleucoma (ker·at·o·lew·**ko'**·mah). Leucoma; a dense, white opacity of the cornea. [Gk *keras* horn, *leukos* white, *-oma* tumour.]

keratolysis (ker·at·**ol**·is·is). A morbid condition characterized by the periodical shedding of the epidermis, which peels off whole like a glove or stocking; it affects in particular the soles and the palms; deciduous skin. **Keratolysis exfoliativa.** Small areas of superficial desquamation on the sides of the fingers, a mild form of pompholyx. **Keratolysis neonatorum.** Dermatitis exfoliativa infantum. **Pitted keratolysis.** A condition of the hyperkeratotic regions of the palms and soles in which areas of erosion occur, often with characteristic pitting. Gram-positive, filamentous organisms are associated with the base of the pits. Aetiology is unproven, but may be due to species of *Streptomyces* or *Corynebacterium.* Cf. KERATODERMA PLANTARE SULCATA, KERATOMA PLANTARE SULCATUM. **Keratolysis plantare sulcatum.** A superficial infection of the plantar skin with erosion and bromhidrosis. [Gk *keras* horn, *lysis* a loosing.]

keratolytic (ker·at·o·**lit'**·ik). 1. Relating or belonging to, or causing keratolysis. 2. A substance having the capacity to dissolve epidermis.

keratoma (ker·at·**o**·mah). A hard, thickened, epidermal patch due to hypertrophy of the horny zone of the skin. The word has been used as a synonym for a callosity, and also to denote an epithelial cyst. **Keratoma auriculare.** Chondrodermatitis nodularis chronica helicis. **Keratoma diffusum, Keratoma hereditarium mutilans** (Vohwinkel). A term applied to spontaneous amputation due to encircling bands in association with palmar hyperkeratosis. **Keratoma malignum.** A variant of erythroderma ichthyosiform congenitum. **Keratoma palmare et plantare** (Hebra; Thost). Diffuse, congenital hyperkeratosis of the palms and soles. **Keratoma plantare sulcatum.** Plantar keratosis with fissuring, seen in those Asiatics who seldom wear shoes. Some of the horny keratoses become detached, causing characteristic punched-out cavities. Cf. KERATODERMA PLANTARE SULCATUM; pitted KERATOLYSIS. **Keratoma senile.** A slightly-raised, flat-topped, discrete, brown or black lesion, usually occurring on exposed skin, particularly on the face or on the backs of the hands of elderly persons; frequently the lesions are multiple. Ormsby and Montgomery suggested the name *pre-epitheliomatous keratosis,* as true epithelioma often commences in such a lesion. [Gk *keras* horn, *-oma* tumour.]

keratomalacia (ker·at·o·mal·a'·she·ah). 1. Softening of the horny layer of the skin. 2. A soft condition of the cornea. [Gk *keras* horn, *malakia* softness.]

keratome (ker·at·ome). An instrument with a sharp edge for making an incision into the cornea. [Gk *keras* horn, *temnein* to cut.]

keratometer (ker·at·om·et·er). An instrument with which the degrees of curvature of the corneal surface may be measured. [Gk *keras* horn, meter.]

keratometry (ker·at·om·et·re). The process or act of measuring the curvature of the corneal surface. [see prec.]

keratomileusis (ker·at·o·mil·ew'·sis). A form of refractive keratoplasty; a deep lamella disc is removed, then frozen and ground to a new curvature before being replaced. [Gk *keras* horn, *smileusis* carving.]

keratomycosis (ker·at·o·mi·ko'·sis). Disease of the cornea caused by a fungus. **Keratomycosis linguae.** Black tongue. *See* TONGUE. **Keratomycosis nigricans palmaris.** Tinea nigra. [Gk *keras* horn, *mykes* fungus, *-osis* condition.]

keratoncus (ker·at·ong·kus). Keratoma. [Gk *keras* horn, *ogkos* a swelling.]

keratonosis (ker·at·o·no'·sis). Any abnormal condition of the horny layer of the skin. [Gk *keras* horn, *-osis* condition.]

keratonosus (ker·at·o·no'·sus). Any diseased condition of the cornea. [Gk *keras* horn, *nosos* disease.]

keratonyxis (ker·at·o·nix'·is). The operation of puncturing the cornea; puncture of the cornea for the purpose of needling the lens in cases of soft cataract. [Gk *keras* horn, *nyssein* to pierce.]

keratophagia (ker·at·o·fa'·je·ah). Disease of the nails characterized by thickness, softness, brittleness and opacity, caused by the presence of parasitic fungi such as trichophyton. [Gk *keras* horn, *phagein* to eat.]

keratoplasia (ker·at·o·pla'·ze·ah). The formation of a new horny layer of the skin. [Gk *keras* horn, *plassein* to form.]

keratoplastic (ker·at·o·plas'·tik). Relating or belonging to keratoplasty.

keratoplasty (ker·at·o·plas·te). Plastic surgery of the cornea; corneal grafting. **Optic keratoplasty.** Removal of a scar which obstructs vision and the grafting on of a portion of corneal tissue. **Tectonic keratoplasty.** Transference of a portion of corneal tissue to a part from which it has been lost. [Gk *keras* horn, *plassein* to form.]

keratorrhexis (ker·at·o·rex'·is). Rupture of the cornea caused by the formation of an ulcer or by injury. [Gk *keras* horn, *rhexis* rupture.]

keratoscleritis (ker·at·o·skler·i'·tis). Keratitis present in association with scleritis.

keratoscope (ker·at·o·skope). Placido's disc; a disc upon which are drawn concentric black circles on a white background with a slight hole in the centre. It is used in the diagnosis of deformities of the anterior surface of the cornea, e.g. conical cornea in which there is a distortion of the corneal reflection of the circles. [Gk *keras* horn, *skopein* to view.]

keratoscopy (ker·at·os·ko·pe). 1. Inspection of the cornea by means of a keratoscope. 2. Retinoscopy (Cuignet).

keratose (ker·at·oze). Horny. [Gk *keras* horn.]

keratosic (ker·at·o·sik). Relating to or marked by keratosis.

keratosis (ker·at·o·sis). A lesion of the skin or of a mucocutaneous junction caused by many different aetiological factors and essentially degenerative in type. The epidermis is usually atrophic and shows hyperkeratosis and parakeratosis. Vascular dilatation and degenerative changes are often to be seen in the corium and the condition must often be regarded as premalignant. In industry, keratoses may be noted after long-continued exposure to substances such as coal tar, pitch, asphalt, soot and lampblack. **Actinic keratosis.** A premalignant lesion caused by much exposure to sunlight or actinic rays. Keratoma senile is more frequently a form of actinic keratosis than due merely to old age. **Arsenical keratosis.** Keratosis due to chronic arsenical poisoning. **Keratosis blennorrhagica.** Keratoderma blennorrhagica. **Keratosis circumscripta.** Circumscribed keratoses of the elbows, knees, hips, dorsa of the hands, palms and soles occurring in Nigerian children. **Keratosis diffusa fetalis.** Ichthyosis congenita. **Keratosis extremitatum hereditaria progrediens** (Kogoj). Mal de Meleda. **Inverted follicular keratosis.** A benign tumour of the face, apparently a seborrhoeic wart of the hair follicle. **Follicular keratosis, Keratosis follicularis.** A name applied to several conditions, the most important being Darier's disease which in the UK has been named *dyskeratosis.* Phrynoderma is characterized by follicular keratosis and by certain pathological conditions of the eyes. Also applied to more severe types of keratosis pilaris (Unna). **Keratosis follicularis contagiosa** (Brooke). A follicular keratosis occurring chiefly in children, affecting the extensor aspects of the limbs and sometimes the neck and face. The condition is not contagious. **Keratosis follicularis serpiginosa.** Perforating elastoma. **Keratosis labialis, Keratosis linguae.** Archaic terms, probably denoting leucoplakia of the lips and of the tongue. **Keratosis nigricans.** Acanthosis nigricans. **Keratosis palmaris et plantaris, Keratosis palmoplantaris.** Tylosis palmarum et plantarum, ichthyosis palmaris et plantaris, keratoma palmare et plantare; a congenital abnormality characterized by dense thickening of the horny layer of the palms and soles. Very occasionally the malady is complicated by keratoma hereditarium mutilans. **Keratosis pharyngis.** Stalactite-like excrescences of horny deposits found anywhere in the lymphoid tissue of the pharynx or in the tonsillar ring of Waldeyer. **Keratosis pilaris** (Brocq). Lichen spinulosus (Devergie), lichen pilaris (Bazin), pityriasis pilaris; an abnormality of the skin characterized by the presence of small horny plugs in the pilosebaceous follicles, associated with perifollicular hyperkeratosis. MacLeod and Muende state that Unna named the mild variety of this malady *keratosis suprafollicularis* and the more severe types *keratosis follicularis.* **Keratosis pilaris rubra atrophicans faciei.** Ulerythema ophryogenes. **Pre-epitheliomatous keratosis.** *See* KERATOMA SENILE. **Keratosis punctata.** Keratoderma punctata; a malady of the palms and soles characterized by circumscribed hyperkeratosis at the orifices of the sweat pores. The condition may be idiopathic or may follow the administration of arsenic. **Keratosis rubra figurata.** Erythrokeratoderma variabilis. **Keratosis seborrhoeica.** Seborrhoeic wart; a lesion sometimes confused with keratoma senile which usually develops on the trunk in middle-aged or elderly persons; *acanthotic naevus* is probably the most suitable name. Seborrhoeic warts are usually multiple, superficial, sharply circumscribed, sessile, round or oval, yellowish or brown thickenings of the epidermis, and seldom undergo malignant change. **Keratosis senilis.** Keratoma senile. **Solar keratosis.** Keratoma senile associated with long-continued exposure to the sun. **Keratosis spinulosa.** Lichen spinulosus. **Keratosis suprafollicularis.** A mild variety of keratosis pilaris (Unna). **Keratosis universalis congenita.** Ichthyosis congenita or harlequin fetus. **Keratosis vegetans.** Dyskeratosis (Darier's disease). **X-ray keratosis.** A keratosis that develops from chronic x-ray dermatitis, frequently affecting the hands and finger nails; the condition predisposes to malignant changes. [Gk *keras* horn, *-osis* condition.]

keratotic (ker·at·ot·ik). Keratosic.

keratotome (ker·at·o·tome). An instrument with a sharp edge for making an incision into the cornea. [Gk *keras* horn, *temnein* to cut.]

keratotomy (ker·at·ot·o·me). Division of the cornea. This is the first step in many intra-ocular operations; it is also used occasionally in the treatment of ulcers, e.g. Saemisch's section and Gifford's operation. [see prec.]

keraunographic (ker·awn·o·graf'·ik). In cases of lightning stroke, applied to the impressions sometimes found on the body of the victim or elsewhere, of external objects in the vicinity, e.g. arborization, in which a tree-like or branch-like pattern is impressed. [Gk *keraunos* thunder and lightning, *graphein* to record.]

keraunoneurosis (ker·awn·o·newr·o'·sis). Neurosis due to the effects of lightning stroke, or terror induced by a thunderstorm. [Gk *keraunos* thunder and lightning, neurosis.]

keraunoparalysis (ker·awn·o·par·al'·is·is). Lightning stroke. *See* STROKE. [Gk *keraunos* thunder and lightning, paralysis.]

keraunophobia (ker·awn·o·fo'·be·ah). Abnormal fear of lightning or thunderstorms. [Gk *keraunos* thunder and lightning, phobia.]

Kerckring, Theodor (b. 1640). German anatomist in Amsterdam.

Kerckring's folds, valves or valvules. Circular mucosal folds of the small intestine.

Kerckring's ossicle. A small ossification sometimes present at the posterior margin of the foramen magnum.

kerectasis (ker·ek·tas·is). Protrusion of the cornea. [Gk *keras* horn, *ektasis* a stretching.]

kerectomy (ker·ek·to·me). Keratectomy.

kerion (ke·re·on). A painful, elevated, boggy, erythematous and localized tumefaction caused by ringworm infection generally of the scalp, but occasionally elsewhere (e.g. beard); deep-seated pustules are usually seen on its surface. [Gk honeycomb.]

keritherapy (ker·e·ther·ap·e). Treatment by wax baths. [Gk *keros* wax, *therapeia* treatment.]

Kerley, Peter James. 20th century British radiologist.

Kerley's lines. Linear shadows in the lung fields on the chest x-ray which are found in pulmonary venous congestion. There are 2 types: the *A lines* are fairly thick linear shadows radiating from the hila, and are less common than the *B lines* which are well-defined slender lines arranged parallel to each other and perpendicular to the pleural surface, occurring at the bases of the lungs especially in costodaphragmatic angles.

kerma (ker·mah). The energy transfer from photons to secondary electrons within the same mass. [*k*inetic *e*nergy *r*eleased in *ma*terial.]

kermes (ker·meez). An insect, *Coccus ilicis,* of the family Coccidae, found on the leaves of the kermes-oak, *Quercus coccifera*; the dried bodies furnish a red dye of great antiquity.

Kermes mineral. A natural sulphide of antimony used formerly in medicine and as a red pigment. Cf. COCHINEAL. [Ar. *qirmiz.*]

kernel (ker·nel). In atomic theory, the atom considered with its outer valency electrons removed. [obsolete term.] [AS *cyrnel.*]

kernicterus (kern·ik·ter·us). Degenerated yellow pigmentation of basal ganglia and other nerve cells in the spinal cord and brain, found in association with extrapyramidal motor disorders and in children with icterus gravis. Kernicterus shows itself about the second or third day of life by convulsions or neuromuscular irritability, drowsiness and anorexia. Death usually occurs at the end of the first week, but in non-fatal and less severe cases, athetosis, spasticity and mental defects may appear at a later date. [G *Kern* kernel, icterus.]

Kernig, Vladimir Mikhailovich (b. 1840). St. Petersburg physician.

Kernig's sign. In irritation of the spinal meninges, if the patient lies supine with the hip flexed, passive extension of the knee joint gives pain behind the knee and spasm of the hamstring muscles.

kernschwund (karn·shwoond). Congenital maldevelopment or lack of nuclei in the cells of the brain and spinal cord, such as is found in congenital ophthalmoplegia (Moebius). [G atrophy of the kernel.]

Kerodon rupestris (ker·o·don roo·pest·ris). The wild cavy, a reservoir of *Trypanosoma cruzi.* [Gk *keras* horn, *odous* tooth, *rupes* rock.]

keroid (ker·oid). Keratoid.

kérose (ka·roze). Darier's name for Barber's seborrhoeic state. [Gk *keros* wax.]

kerosene (ker·o·seen). A liquid distilled from petroleum; the domestic paraffin used in oil lamps. It is used for destroying mosquito larvae by floating it on the surface of water. It is also used as a solvent for oily medicinal substances intended for external application, e.g. for insect repellants. [Gk *keros* wax.]

kerotherapy (ker·o·ther·ap·e). Keritherapy.

kesso (kes·o). Japanese valerian. *See* VALERIAN.

Ketamine (ket·am·een). BP Commission approved name for 2-(2-chlorophenyl)-2-methylaminocyclohexanone, an intravenous agent for the production of dissociative anaesthesia. Its use may lead to postoperative psychic disturbances, especially in adults.

keten, ketene (ke·ten, ke·teen). 1. Carbomethane, $CH_2{=}CO$, a colourless gas obtained from acetic anhydride. It is the simplest of the ketones and is used as an acetylating agent, especially in the industrial production of cellulose acetate. 2. Name applied to a group of derivatives of the above, of value in organic synthesis.

keto- (ke·to). In chemistry, denoting the presence of the carbonyl group.

Ketobemidone (ke·to·bem·id·one). BP Commission approved name for 4-*m*-hydroxyphenyl -1-methyl-4-propionyl-piperidine, a derivative of pethidine which has about 20 times its activity. Clinical trials have shown it to have excellent analgesic properties, but it has proved to be a powerful drug of addiction, comparable with heroin in this respect, and its clinical use has been abandoned.

ketogenesis (ke·to·jen·es·is). The formation or production of ketone bodies. [ketone, Gk *genein* to produce.]

ketogenetic, ketogenic (ke·to·jen·et'·ik, keto·jen·ik). Now more often referred to as oxogenic. 1. Producing or forming ketone. 2. Having the quality of being convertible into ketone. [see prec.]

ketoheptose (ke·to·hep·toze). General term for the isomeric heptoses which contain a keto group, =CO. They have the formula $CH_2OH(CHOH)_4COCH_2OH$.

ketohexose (ke·to·hex·oze). General term for the isomeric hexoses which contain a keto group, =CO. They have formula $CH_2OH(CHOH)_3COCH_2OH$; fructose is an example.

ketohydroxyoestratriene (ke·to·hi·drox·e·e·strah·tri'·een). Oestrone.

ketohydroxyoestrin (ke·to·hi·drox·e·e'·strin). Oestrone.

ketol (ke·tol). Ketone alcohol; the name given to any alcohol which contains, in addition to its hydroxyl group, the keto group, =CO.

ketole (ke·tole). Indole.

ketolysis (ke·tol·is·is). The dissolution of acetone bodies. [ketone, Gk *lysis* a loosing.]

ketolytic (ke·to·lit·ik). Pertaining to ketolysis.

ketonaemia (ke·ton·e·me·ah). A morbid condition marked by the existence of ketone (acetone) bodies in the blood. [ketone, Gk *haima* blood.]

ketone (ke·tone). General term for an organic compound which has in its structure the carbonyl (keto) group, =CO, attached to 2 alkyl groups. They are produced by the oxidation of secondary alcohols and are themselves oxidized to simpler acids due to the rupture of the carbon chain. **Dimethyl ketone.** Acetone. **Methyl phenyl ketone.** Acetophenone. **Mixed ketone.** A ketone in which the alkyl groups attached to the carbonyl radical are different, e.g. methyl ethyl ketone, $CH_3COC_2H_5$. **Naphthyl methyl ketone.** Acetonaphthone. **Phenyl methyl ketone.** Acetophenone.

ketonic (ke·ton·ik). Relating or belonging to, or produced from a ketone.

ketonization (ke·ton·i·za'·shun). The process of being converted into a ketone.

ketonuria (ke·ton·ewr·e·ah). The excretion of ketone (acetone) substances in the urine.

ketoplasia (ke·to·pla·ze·ah). The production of ketone bodies. [ketone, Gk *plassein* to form.]

ketoplastic (ke·to·plas·tik). Causing the production or formation of ketones. [see prec.]

Ketoprofen (ke·to·pro·fen). BP Commission approved name for 2-(3-benzoylphenyl)propionic acid; an anti-inflammatory agent.

ketose (ke·toze). General name for monosaccharides which contain in their structure the keto group, =CO.

ketoside (ke·to·side). Applied to a glycoside, the carbohydrate portion of which is a ketose.

ketosis (ke·to·sis). The presence of excessive quantities of ketone bodies in the tissues. [ketone, Gk *-osis* condition.]

ketosteroid (ke·to·**steer**·oid). Now more often referred to as oxosteroid; e.g. 17-oxosteroid instead of 17-ketosteroid. A steroid in which 1 of the carbon atoms of the basic cyclopentenophenanthrene structure has attached to it a ketonic oxygen. This type of compound is particularly associated with sex hormones or their catabolites, the keto group occurring at the carbon in either the 3-position, as in testosterone and progesterone, or the 17-position, as in androsterone and oestrone. The urinary excretion of neutral 17-ketosteroids has considerable significance in the diagnosis of hyperplasia or tumour of the adrenal cortex, being above normal in both conditions and very high in the latter; a low excretion of these compounds has been observed in Addison's disease, whilst in Simmonds' disease excretion drops almost to zero.

ketosuria (ke·toze·**ewr**·e·ah). The excretion of ketose in the urine.

ketotetrahydrophenanthrene (ke·to·**tet**·rah·hi·dro·fen·**an**'·threen). $C_{14}H_{13}CO$, a phenanthrene derivative with carcinogenic properties.

ketotetrose (ke·to·**tet**·roze). A tetrose which contains a keto group, =CO. Only one exists, erythrulose, with the formula $CH_2OH(CHOH)COCH_2OH$.

kettle (ketl). A metal container for boiling liquids. **Bronchitis kettle.** A kettle with a very long spout, designed to humidify the atmosphere in an enclosed space for the treatment of acute pulmonary conditions; called also *croup kettle.* **Copper kettle.** An apparatus used to vaporize a volatile anaesthetic liquid in which microbubbles of oxygen take up the vapour. Made of copper because of its high specific heat and thermal conductivity. Described by Lucien Morris, an American anaesthetist, in 1952. [AS *cetel.*]

Key, Charles Aston (b. 1793). British surgeon.

Key's operation. A lateral operation for lithotomy done with a straight staff.

Key, Ernst Axel Henrik (b. 1832). Stockholm anatomist and physician.

Key and Retzius corpuscles. Sensory nerve-endings in the skin.

Key-Retzius foramen. The lateral aperture of the 4th ventricle: also called *Luschka's foramen.*

Key and Retzius sheath. A single layer of cuboidal cells in the inner layer of the hair follicle; Henle's sheath.

Key, John Albert (b. 1890). American orthopaedic surgeon.

Key's arthrodesis. Arthrodesis of the knee using a large, central autogenous bone peg.

key (ke). 1. An appliance for opening a lock. 2. Any metaphorical application of the above. **Dental key.** An instrument formerly used for removing teeth. **Tetanizing key.** An electrical appliance consisting of a reed made up of electrically-conducting material which can be adjusted to vibrate over a certain range of frequency, and one end of which has a terminal for the attachment of a wire and source of current. The other end has a copper tip which dips in and out of a pool of mercury as the reed vibrates, and so intermittently and regularly completes and breaks the circuit. **Tooth key.** Dental key (see above). [AS *caeg.*] *See also:* DUBOIS-REYMOND.

khellin (kel·in). Visammin, $C_{14}H_{12}O_5$. A smooth-muscle relaxant and coronary dilator extracted from the powdered fruits of *Ammi visnaga* or prepared synthetically. It is administered for angina pectoris and bronchial asthma. [Ar. *khella.*]

kibe (kibe). A cracked or ulcerated chilblain, or any crack in the flesh caused by cold. [Welsh *cibwst* chilblain.]

kibisitome (ki·**bis**·e·tome). A cystitome. [Gk *kibisis* pouch, *temnein* to cut.]

kick sorter (kik sor·ter). Pulse Height analyser. *See* ANALYSER.

Kidd, Francis (Frank) Seymour (b. 1878). London urological surgeon.

Kidd's cystoscope. An operating cystoscope with an insulated sheath, the point of which forms the electrode. The instrument may be used in the endoscopic diathermy treatment of bladder tumours.

Kidd's suprapubic trocar and cannula. One in which the trocar may be introduced and withdrawn from the main cannula by a side channel. The catheter is inserted to the bladder through the central channel.

Kidd's U-tube. A simple apparatus incorporating the U-shaped tube for gradual decompression of the bladder after catheterization.

Kidd. *See* Blood GROUP.

kidney [ren (NA)] (**kid**·ne). One of the paired organs, right and left, in the lumbar region below the diaphragm lateral to the spine in the retroperitoneal tissue plane. Each is bean-shaped with the convexity to the lateral side and measures in the adult 12 × 6 × 3 cm, and weighs about 150 g. Each lies obliquely so that the *upper end* [extremitas superior (NA)] is nearer the midline than the *lower* [extremitas inferior (NA)] and one surface is antero-external, the other postero-internal. The outer lateral margin [margo lateralis (NA)] is convex and the inner medial margin [margo medialis (NA)] concave. Posteriorly [facies posterior (NA)] each kidney rests from above downwards on the diaphragm, the psoas major, quadratus lumborum and the transversus abdominis muscles. Anteriorly [facies anterior (NA)] on the right side, the kidney lies in relation to the liver, the second part of the duodenum and the right flexure of the colon; on the left side the anterior relations are the stomach, pancreas, spleen and left flexure of the colon. The right and left suprarenal glands are immediate superior relations to the kidneys. The *hilum* [hilus renalis (NA)] at the inner border of the kidney is a notch which receives the upper expanded portion of the ureter where it forms the renal pelvis; the renal arteries and veins enter and leave at the hilum. Each kidney is enclosed in a fibrous and a fatty capsule. The delicate *fibrous capsule* is intimately attached to the kidney, but strips easily unless the kidney is diseased. The *fatty capsule* surrounds the kidney, so that the kidney lies comparatively loosely within the fatty capsule, which is enclosed in the renal fascia. The parenchyma of the kidney is divided into the medulla and cortex. The *cortex* lies immediately beneath the capsule, the *medulla* lies adjacent to the expanded renal pelvis which breaks up into 12 or more divisions to form the *calyces.* The terminations of the minor calyces are cup-shaped and receive the apices of the cone-shaped segments of the medulla which are termed the *pyramids.* The cortex dips down between the segments of medulla. The function of the kidney is to regulate normal concentrations of the constituents of the blood by the excretion of water, the soluble end-products of nitrogen metabolism and the electrolytes necessary to maintain the electrolyte balance of the blood. This is brought about by a combination of filtration, excretion and reabsorption. The functioning unit in the kidney is termed the *nephron,* which is made up of a *renal corpuscle* and a series of joined tubules, the contents of which drain into the calyces at the apex of the medullary pyramid. There are about 1 million nephrons in each human kidney. The renal corpuscle is formed by the *glomerulus* [NA], which is a tuft of minute capillary channels supplied individually by the terminal branches of the renal artery, and an enclosing capsule, the *capsule of the malpighian glomerulus.* The inner layer of this capsule is intimately associated with the loops of the vessels of the glomerulus, and its outer layer forms a collecting funnel which is continuous with the renal tubule. The glomerulus functions as an ultra-filter. The renal tubules are divided into the *proximal convoluted tubule, Henle's loop, the distal convoluted tubule* and a system of *collecting tubules* which open into the renal pelvis at the apex of the renal papilla where it enters the calyx. The glomerular filtrate as it passes through the tubular system of the nephron is subject to an active reabsorption of high-threshold substances, e.g. glucose, whereas the low-threshold substances are highly concentrated in the urine, e.g. urea. **Amyloid kidney.** A pathological condition in which the blood vessels of the kidney, the tunica of the tubules and the interstitial tissue have undergone amyloid degeneration. **Arteriosclerotic kidney.** The granular contracted kidney caused by renal ischaemia and consequent fibrosis of the renal parenchyma, due to hyaline and fatty degeneration of the smaller arteries and arterioles. **Artificial kidney.** An apparatus in which the patient's circulating blood is subjected to dialysis extracorporeally by means of which some of the non-protein nitrogen and other toxic substances are removed; it is resorted to where there is suppression of kidney function. **Atrophic kidney.** Atrophy of the renal parenchyma due to congenital hypoplasia, or acquired when there is shrinkage of the renal tissues as a result of backpressure, as in hydronephrosis, or to sclerosis associated with chronic nephritis. **Branny kidney.** Opaque projecting granules on the kidney surface when there is fatty degeneration. **Cadaver kidney.** The name applied to a kidney which has been removed immediately after death with a view to transplanting it into a renoprival man. **Cake kidney.** Fusion of the two kidneys. **Cicatricial kidney.** The shrunken, scarred kidney subsequent to chronic infection, frequently associated with stone. **Cirrhotic kidney, Contracted kidney.** Arteriosclerotic kidney (see above). **Cyanotic kidney.** Renal anoxia from passive congestion. **Cystic kidney.** Renal cysts occurring as solitary cysts, congenital polycystic disease of the kidney, and as cortical cysts usually associated with nephrosclerosis. **Definitive kidney.** The metanephros or permanent adult kidney of amniota. **Disc kidney.** Congenital anomaly in which the two kidneys are fused, one lying posterior to the other. **Embryonic kidney.** One of the 3 renal organs which appear in succession in development, viz. pronephros, mesonephros and metanephros. **Fatty kidney.** 1. Kidney in which the deposition of peripelvic and intrahilar fat is excessive, as in the chronic irritation of stone. 2. Fatty degeneration of the epithelial cells in chronic inflammatory or arterial disease of the kidney. **Flea-bitten kidney.** Arteriosclerotic kidney (see above). **Floating kidney.** Mobile kidney (see below). **Fused kidney.** A condition in which the two kidneys are fused, the lower pole of one to the upper pole of the other, the ureter crossing the midline from a normal ureterovesical orifice. **Gouty kidney.** Red granular kidney (see below). **Head kidney.** The pronephros or primitive kidney, or early embryonic kidney. **Hind kidney.** The metanephros or definitive kidney which develops caudal to the pronephros. **Horseshoe kidney.** A congenital anomaly produced by fusion of the upper or lower poles of the two kidneys, usually the latter, across the midline, so that the kidney assumes the general shape of a horseshoe. **Lardaceous kidney.** Amyloid kidney (see above). **Large red kidney.** The condition when the kidney is the site of acute nephritis, whether from bacterial inflammation, chemical irritation or from some toxin. **Large white kidney.** An enlarged kidney which is pale in colour from nephrosis. **Leaky kidney.** A term which has been employed when abnormal constituents appear intermittently in the urine without evidence of renal or systemic disease, e.g. albuminuria after exercise or sugar following a large carbohydrate meal; renal glycosuria when the blood sugar concentration is normal. **Lobe of the kidney.** *See* LOBE, RENAL. **Medullary sponge kidney.** Dilatation of the distal tubules of the kidney, probably congenital and often accompanied by stone formation. **Middle kidney.** The mesonephros or wolffian body of embryonic life, which develops caudal to the pronephros. The wolffian body is destined to form the sex organ, but the cephalic mesonephric tubules persist to form the efferent ducts of the epididymis. **Mobile kidney, Movable kidney.** A kidney that is mobile owing to inadequate support from the fatty capsule and the perinephric fascia. In normal healthy people who are thin, the lower pole of the right kidney may be palpated through the abdominal wall on inspiration; in a mobile kidney the normal ascent of the kidney during expiration may be retarded by bimanual palpation. The mobility should be such as to produce symptoms. *See* NEPHROPTOSIS. **Myelin kidney.** Abnormal fatty substances lodged in the cells of the kidney as a result of degenerative changes. They may be chemical combinations of lipoids. **Palpable kidney.** In normal individuals who are thin, the lower poles of both kidneys may be palpable through the abdominal wall: when the greater part of any kidney may be palpated through the abdominal wall, either the kidney is enlarged or there is an abnormal mobility. **Pelvic kidney.** A congenital anomaly in which the metanephros, or permanent kidney, has failed to ascend to its normal lumbar position during embryonic life. The kidney is situated in the pelvis, the ureter is short and the renal blood vessels spring from the aorta or the iliac vessels. Not to be confused with nephroptosis. **Polycystic kidney.** A congenital anomaly in which, owing to a failure of the fusion of the secreting with the collecting tubules, multiple cysts occur throughout the substance of both kidneys. Clinical evidence of the condition may not appear until adult life, when both kidneys are enlarged. **Pregnancy kidney.** A loose term covering any type of renal disease associated with pregnancy, varying in severity from true nephritis or pyelonephritis to the transient hydronephrosis and hydro-ureter of pregnancy. **Primitive kidney, Primordial kidney.** The pronephros of early embryonic life, which is transitory in appearance and consists of a series of pronephric tubules which have a segmental distribution. The tubules unite to form the primary excretory duct. **Red contracted kidney.** Arteriosclerotic kidney (see above). **Red granular kidney.** The chronic stage of arteriosclerotic kidney; gouty kidney. **Sacculated kidney.** An advanced hydronephrotic dilatation of the kidney. **Sclerotic kidney.** Arteriosclerotic kidney (see above). **Sigmoid kidney.** Fused kidney (see above). **Small red kidney.** Arteriosclerotic kidney (see above). **Small white kidney.** Secondary contracted kidney (*see* ARTERIOSCLEROTIC KIDNEY above) of chronic glomerulonephritis. **Soapy kidney.** A swollen pale kidney, with depositions of amyloid in the pyramids, and fatty degeneration of the epithelial cells of the tubules. **Solitary kidney.** A single kidney which may be present on one or other side, either due to congenital absence of the contralateral kidney or to its surgical removal. **Sponge kidney.** The condition (bilateral, unilateral or localized to a part of one kidney) in which multiple small cysts arise in the renal parenchyma adjacent to the termination of the calyces. **Succenturiate kidney.** The suprarenal or adrenal gland, so termed from the likeness in shape of the adrenal gland to a Roman helmet. **Sulpha kidney.** A term of modern usage applied to the pathological state of the kidney when, following the administration of sulpha drugs, there is distal tubular obstruction in the kidney from a crystalline deposit of the sulpha preparation within the tubules, which may have led to oliguria or anuria. **Supernumerary kidney.** A rare congenital anomaly in which two kidneys of equal size may occur on one side, each complete with separate blood supply and ureter. The poles of the two kidneys may be fused. **Surgical kidney.** Unilateral suppurative pyelonephritis with abscess formation in the renal parenchyma, so-called because the only practicable treatment is nephrectomy. **Tandem kidney.** A congenital anomaly in which the two kidneys are present on the same side, the lower pole of the one fused to the upper pole of the other; fused kidney (see above). **Wandering kidney.** Mobile kidney (see above). **Waxy kidney.** Amyloid kidney (see above). [etym. dub.]

See also: ROKITANSKY.

kidney, arteries of the [arteriae renis (NA)]. Branches of the abdominal aorta to the kidneys, suprarenal glands, ureter and surrounding tissue. They enter the sinus of the kidney, mainly anterior to the pelvis of the ureter, and divide into lobar arteries. Accessory renal arteries to the upper or lower poles of the kidney are common.

kidney, veins of the [venae renis (NA)]. Main renal veins formed by the union of the lobar veins within the renal sinus, lying in front of the renal arteries and joining the inferior vena cava. The left receives the left suprarenal and left testicular (ovarian) veins.

Kielland, Christian (b. 1871). Oslo obstetrician.

Kielland's forceps. Obstetrical forceps with a short handle and a joint which allows a gliding movement between the blades.

Kienboeck, Robert (b. 1871). Vienna radiologist.

Kienboeck's atrophy. An osteochondrosis affecting the lunate bone, which undergoes extensive aseptic necrosis as a result of inflammation or ischaemia.

Kienboeck's disease. 1. Traumatic myelomalacia; owing to the central situation of the cavities that form, a clinical picture resembling syringomyelia develops. 2. Kienboeck's atrophy (see above).

Kienboeck's phenomenon. Paradoxical movement of the diaphragm observed in pyopneumothorax. The affected side rises with inspiration and falls with expiration.

Kienboeck-Adamson method or technique and points. In epilation of the scalp, the hair is cut very short all over the scalp, and 5 points are then marked as follows: Point A, 1½-2 in (35-50 mm) behind the frontal margin of the hair; Point B, 1-1½ in (25-35 mm) above the centre of the flat area which forms the upper part of the occiput; Point C, 1 in (25 mm) above the lower border of the scalp at the lower part of the occiput; Point D, on the right side just above and in front of the ear; Point E, on the left side just above and in front of the ear. Points A, B and C are in the mid-sagittal plane of the scalp: the distance between any 2 of the points is 5 in (125 mm). An x-ray beam is focused on each of the points in turn and a sufficient exposure is given (about 400 R) to cause epilation. During the exposures, the glabrous skin is protected by lead.

Kiernan, Francis (b. 1800). Irish surgeon in London.

Kiernan's spaces. The intervals between the lobules of the liver which are occupied by prolongations of Glisson's capsule containing interlobular lymphatics.

kieselguhr (**ke**·zel·goor). Diatomite. [G gravel sediment.]

Kiesselbach, Wilhelm (b. 1839). Erlangen laryngologist.

Kiesselbach's area. The anterior part of the nasal septum; it is often covered with a small vascular varicosity and is sometimes called the *bleeding area of the nasal septum, Little's area.*

Kilian, Hermann Friedrich (b. 1800). Bonn gynaecologist.

Kilian's line. The transverse line formed by the promontory of the sacrum.

Kiliani, Heinrich (b. 1855). Freiburg chemist.

Kiliani's digitalin. The original "true digitalin"; an amorphous mixture of digitalis glycosides that are soluble in alcohol.

Killian, Gustav (b. 1860). Berlin otolaryngologist.

Killian's bundle. The lowest fibres of the inferior constrictor muscle of the pharynx.

Killian's dehiscence. The midline triangular area between the lower horizontal fibres and the oblique fibres of the inferior constrictor muscle of the pharynx. It may be the site of a pharyngeal diverticulum.

Killian's operation. A radical operation on a frontal air sinus carried out through an incision in the eyebrow. The anterior wall and the floor of the sinus are removed, but the bony orbital ridge is left *in situ.*

Kilner, Thomas Pomfret (b. 1890). London plastic surgeon.

Kilner hook. A fine sharp hook for atraumatic handling of skin edges. The hook is made detachable from the handle for ease of replacement.

kilo- (**kil**·o). A prefix used to signify one thousand (10^3). [Gk *chilioi* a thousand.]

kilocalorie (kil·o·**kal**·or·e). Large calorie equal to 4186 joules. *See* CALORIE. [Gk *chilioi* a thousand, calorie.]

kilocycle (**kil**·o·si·kl). A measure of the frequency of electromagnetic waves: 1000 Hertz. [Gk *chilioi* a thousand, cycle.]

kilogram (**kil**·o·gram). The unit of mass, equal to the mass of the international prototype of the kilogram. This international prototype is made of platinum-iridium and kept at the International Bureau of Weights and Measures. The *weight* of a body is the product of its mass and the acceleration due to gravity. [Gk *chilioi* a thousand, gram.]

kilometre (**kil**·o·me·ter). A unit of length equivalent to 1000 m (3280.89 ft.) [Gk *chilioi* a thousand, metre.]

kilonem (**kil**·o·nem). A unit of nutrition, equivalent to 667 calories, provided by 1 litre of milk. [obsolete term.] [Gk *chilioi* a thousand, *nemein* to feed.]

kilostere (**kil**·o·steer). A unit of volume; equivalent to 1000 cubic metres. [obsolete term.] [Gk *chilioi* a thousand, *stereos* solid.]

kilovolt (**kil**·o·**volt**′). A unit of electrical potential equal to 1000 volts. [Gk *chilioi* a thousand, volt.]

kilovoltmeter (kil·o·**volt**·me·ter). A voltmeter which is graduated in kilovolts.

kilowatt (**kil**·o·wat). A unit of electrical power equivalent to 1000 watts. **Kilowatt hour.** The unit of work done in 1 hour by 1 kilowatt. [Gk *chilioi* a thousand, watt.]

Kimmelstiel, Paul (b. 1900). Boston pathologist.

Kimmelstiel's disease, Kimmelstiel-Wilson disease or syndrome. Nephrotic symptoms, gross oedema and albuminuria combined with glycosuria, caused by intercapillary nephrosclerosis.

kinaemia (kin·e·me·ah). The amount of blood circulated by the heart; cardiac output. [Gk *kinein* to move, *haima* blood.]

kinaemic (kin·e·mik). Relating or belonging to kinaemia.

kinaesthesia, kinaesthesis (kin·es·**the**·ze·ah, kin·es·**the**·sis). 1. The sum of sensations by which weight, position and muscular motion are perceived. 2. The force which compels an individual to throw himself to the ground when looking down from a great height. [Gk *kinein* to move, aesthesia.]

kinanaesthesia (**kin**·an·es·**the**′·ze·ah). Derangement of deep sensibility causing inability to perceive the sensation of movement. [Gk *kinein* to move, anaesthesia.]

kinase (**ki**·naze). A group of enzymes which catalyse reactions involving the transfer of phosphate moieties from ATP to sugars and other substrates. **Protein kinase.** An enzyme, or enzymes, which catalyses the phosphorylation of proteins by ATP. In animal tissues a protein kinase, or kinases, is activated by cyclic 3′5′ AMP and phosphorylate; it activates glycogen phosphorylase and hormone-sensitive lipase and phosphorylate, and inactivates glycogen synthetase. It thus forms an essential link in the chain of events by which the metabolic actions of adrenaline and some other hormones are brought about. **Pyruvate kinase.** An enzyme which catalyses the phosphorylation of ADP by phosphoenolpyruvate to give ATP and pyruvate in glycolysis. This reaction is virtually irreversible and, in gluconeogenesis, phosphoenolpyruvate is synthesized by other reactions involving pyruvate carboxylase and phosphoenolpyruvate carboxykinase. [Gk *kinesis* motion.]

kinematics (kin·e·**mat**·ix). Cinematics.

kineplastics, kineplasty (kin·e·**plas**·tix, kin·e·**plas**·te). Cineplastics.

kinepock (**kine**·pok). Vaccinia. [cowpox.]

kineradiotherapy (**kin**·e·ra·de·o·**ther**′·ap·e). Otherwise known as moving-beam therapy; radiotherapy with either the tube or the patient in motion, in order to reduce the skin dose while allowing a full depth dose. [kinesis, radiotherapy.]

kinesalgia (kin·es·**al**·je·ah). Cinesalgia.

kinesia (kin·e·ze·ah). Cinesia. **Kinesia paradoxa.** The ability of some patients with Parkinson's disease to run quickly while only able to walk with difficulty.

kinesi-aesthesiometer (kin·e·ze·es·the·ze·**om**′·et·er). An instrument for determining or measuring the extent of muscle sense. [kinesis, aesthesia, meter.]

kinesiatrics (kin·e·ze·**at**′·rix). Cinesitherapy.

kinesic (kin·e·zik). Kinetic.

kinesimeter (kin·e·**sim**·et·er). 1. A device used to determine quantitatively the degree of movement in a part. 2. A device for examination of the body surface in order to measure the degree of sensibility of the skin. [kinesis, meter.]

kinesiodic (kin·e·se·**od**′·ik). Referring to the pathways of the motor nerves. [kinesis, Gk *odos* way.]

kinesiology (kin·e·ze·**ol**′·o·je). Cinesiology.

kinesiometer (kin·e·ze·**om**′·et·er). Kinesimeter.

kinesioneurosis (kin·e·ze·o·newr·**o**′·sis). A neurosis or disorder of nervous function which is allied with some motor disorder, e.g. spasm, tic. **External kinesioneurosis.** Kinesioneurosis in which the external muscles are affected. **Internal kinesioneurosis.** Kinesioneurosis in which the muscles of the viscera are affected. **Vascular kinesioneurosis.** Vasomotor neurosis; angioneurosis. **Visceral kinesioneurosis.** Internal kinesioneurosis (see above). [kinesis, neurosis.]

kinesiotherapy (kin·e·ze·o·**ther**′·ap·e). Cinesitherapy.

kinesis (kin·e·sis). General term for physical movement or force; with regard to the human being, the sum of bodily potential. **Kinesis paradoxa.** The type of walking and running observed in patients with paralysis agitans; owing to the festinating gait, in which the patient appears to be chasing his own centre of gravity, he may walk very quickly with marked over-exertion, in striking contrast to his immobility and poverty of muscular movement when at rest. [Gk movement.]

kinesitherapy (kin·e·ze·**ther**′·ap·e). Cinesitherapy.

kinesodic (kin·e·**sod**·ik). Relating or belonging to the transmission of impulses along the motor pathways. [kinesis, Gk *odos* way.]

kinesophobia (kin·e·so·**fo**′·be·ah). Fear of movement. [Gk *kinesis* motion, *phobus* fear.]

kinesotherapy (kin·e·so·**ther**′·ap·e). Cinesitherapy.

kinesthesiometer (kin·es·the·ze·**om**′·et·er). Kinesi-aesthesiometer.

kinetia (kin·e·she·ah). Cinesia.

kinetic (kin·et·ik). Belonging or relating to motion, or producing it. [see foll.]

kinetics (kin·et·ix). That branch of science which deals with the motion produced in bodies by the forces acting upon them. [Gk *kinesis* motion.]

kinetism (kin·e·tizm). The capacity to arouse activity in muscles or to perform muscular movements. [see prec.]

kinetocardiogram (kin·e·to·**kar**·de·o·gram). A record of the lower frequency precordial vibrations. [Gk *kinesis* motion, *kardia* heart, *gramma* record.]

kinetocardiograph (kin·e·to·**kar**·de·o·graph). The instrument used to record the kinetocardiogram. [Gk *kinesis* motion, *kardia* heart, *graphein* to record.]

kinetocardiography (kin·e·to·kar·de·**og**′·raf·e). The graphic registration of the lower frequency precordial vibrations. The technique is related to phonocardiography but the major vibrations recorded are below the audible range. [Gk *kinesis* motion, *kardia* heart, *graphein* to record.]

kinetochore (kin·e·to·kore). Centromere. [Gk *kinesis* motion, core.]

kinetogenic (kin·e·to·**jen**′·ik). Inducing or producing motion. [Gk *kinesis* motion, *genein* to produce.]

kinetographic (kin·e·to·**graf**′·ik). Cinetographic.

kinetonucleus (kin·e·to·**new**′·kle·us). Kinetoplast. [Gk *kinesis* motion, nucleus.]

kinetoplasm (kin·e·to·plazm). That part of a cell which is the most highly contractile. [Gk *kinesis* motion, *plasma* anything formed.]

kinetoplast (kin·e·to·plast). The organelle in flagellate Protozoa consisting of the blepharoplast and parabasal body, believed to co-ordinate movement. [Gk *kinesis* motion, *plassein* to mould.]

kinetoscope (kin·e·to·skope). An optical device which produces the illusion of objects in motion by the presentation of a succession of photographs, sometimes stereoscopically. [Gk *kinesis* motion, *skopein* to watch.]

kinetoscopy (kin·e·**tos**·ko·pe). The use of the kinetoscope, particularly for purposes of diagnosis and in physiology.

kinetosis (kin·e·**to**·sis). Cinesia. [Gk *kinesis* motion, *-osis* condition.]

kinetotherapeutic (kin·e·to·ther·ap·**ew**′·tik). Relating or belonging to kinetotherapy.

kinetotherapy (kin·e·to·**ther**′·ap·e). A type of therapeutics in which systematic movements, either active or passive, are employed. [kinesis, therapy.]

King, Brien Thaxton (b. 1886). Seattle, Washington, surgeon. **King's operation.** A form of chordopexy operation.

King, Earl (b. 1901). Toronto biochemist. **King and Armstrong method,** for serum alkaline phosphatase. Equal volumes of a barbitone sodium buffer (pH 9.0) and disodium phenylphosphate substrate solution are mixed and incubated at 37°C, 0.5 ml of serum is added and, after exactly 30 min, diluted Folin-Ciocalteau's reagent and the mixture filtered. Sodium carbonate solution is added to the filtrate and the blue colour developed by incubating at 37°C for 15 min. A control is prepared by omitting incubation to determine preformed phenol. The reading of the control is subtracted from that of the test and the result is compared with the reading of a standard phenol and reagent mixture. 1 unit of phosphatase activity is defined by King and Armstrong as 1 mg of phenol liberated by 100 ml of serum. Normal range from 3 to 13 units.

King–Armstrong unit. A phosphatase (alkaline) activity of 1 unit per 100 ml of serum or plasma liberates 1 mg of phenol at 37°C in 30 min from a substrate of disodium phenylphosphate at pH 9.

King, Joseph Eggleston Johnson (b. 1886). New York surgeon. **King's operation.** Direct opening of a brain abscess by removal of the overlying cerebral tissue followed by controlled herniation of the abscess wall.

king's evil (kingz e·vil). Scrofula; the royal touch was held to have healing powers. [AS *cynig, yfel.*]

Kingsley, Norman William (b. 1829). American dentist. **Kingsley's extra-oral bars.** Metal bars, usually of German silver, attached to a Kingsley splint (see below) or modified upper denture. They protrude from each side of the mouth and curve back along the cheek where they are fastened to a head halter or plaster head-cap, and thus support a fractured upper jaw.

Kingsley's splint. An appliance that fits over the upper teeth; it has 2 arms (Kingsley's extra-oral bars, above) which protrude from the mouth and are fixed to a cap to immobilize a fractured maxilla.

kinin (ki·nin). Peptide with activity in increasing vascular permeability, vasodilatation and contraction of smooth muscle, formed as an end product of the kinin enzyme cascade which is activated in various types of tissue injury including anaphylaxis. A major factor in producing the carcinoid flushes. *See also* BRADYKININ, CASCADE, KALLIKREIN.

kininogen (ki·**nin**·o·jen). A substance which, when exposed to appropriate enzyme action, yields a kinin. The kinin-releasing enzymes are kallikreins and they occur widely in the body fluids—plasma, lymph, cerebrospinal fluid, saliva, tears, urine and sweat. [Gk *kinesis* motion, *genein* to produce.]

kink (kingk). Angulation; an unnatural angle in a tubular organ such as the intestine or ureter. An intestinal kink may follow a surgical operation for resection. **Ileal kink.** A bend or twist in the last part of the ileum, with external adhesions of the folded gut, causing obstruction. [Dutch.]

See also: LANE (W. A.).

Kinmonth, John Bernard. 20th century London surgeon. **Kinmonth's technique.** Of lymphography, direct injection of a trunk lymphatic vessel with a radio-opaque medium after preliminary identification of the vessel by interstitial injection of trypan blue.

Kinney's law. In persons previously possessing normal speech who become totally deaf, the length of time before speech changes develop is in direct relation to the length of time speech was previously present.

Kinnier Wilson. *See* WILSON, S. A. KINNIER.

kino (ki·no). East Indian, Malabar, Madras or Cochin kino; the dried juice obtained by incision of the trunk of *Pterocarpus marsupium* Roxb. (family Leguminosae). It consists principally of kinotannic acid and related substances. It is a powerful astringent and is used in the treatment of diarrhoea and dysentery (BPC 1949); in this respect it is more efficient than tannic acid internally, since it liberates the latter only on reaching the intestine and hence does not upset the stomach. **Kino Eucalypti BPC 1949, Eucalyptus kino.** Eucalyptus gum. *See* GUM. [West African name.]

kinocentrum (kin·o·**sen**·trum). Centrosome (Zimmerman). [Gk *kinein* to move, *kentron* centre.]

kinohapt (**kin**·o·hapt). An aesthesiometer for initiating a number of tactile stimulations at predetermined intervals of space or time. [Gk *kinein* to move, *haptein* to touch.]

kinoin (ki·**no**·in). $C_{14}H_{12}O_6$, a colourless crystalline non-astringent resin present in kino.

kinology (kin·**ol**·o·je). Cinesiology.

kinometer (kin·**om**·et·er). An instrument used to determine the extent of uterine displacement when a tumour is present or in a case of pelvic cellulitis. [Gk *kinein* to move, meter.]

kinomometer (kin·o·**mom**·et·er). An instrument with which the range of movement in a joint may be measured. [Gk *kinein* to move, meter.]

kinoplasm (**kin**·o·plazm). The specific kinetic or functional substance of the cell. [Gk *kinein* to move, *plassein* to mould.]

kinosphere (**kin**·o·sfeer). Aster. [Gk *kinein* to move, sphere.]

kinotoxin (kin·o·**tox**·in). Fatigue toxin. *See* TOXIN. [Gk *kinein* to move, toxin.]

kionorrhaphy (ki·on·**or**·af·e). Staphylorrhaphy; reparative surgery of the uvula. [Gk *kion* pillar, *rhaphe* suture.]

kiotome (**ki**·o·tome). A uvulotome. [Gk *kion* pillar, *temnein* to cut.]

kiotomy (ki·**ot**·o·me). Uvulotomy. [see prec.]

Kirchner, Wilhelm (b. 1849). Würzburg otologist.

Kirchner's diverticulum. A small pouch in the lower portion of the pharyngotympanic tube.

Kirk, Norman Thomas Kirk (b. 1888). American surgeon.

Kirk's amputation. A supracondylar tenoplastic amputation.

Kirklin, Byrl Raymond (b. 1888). Minnesota radiologist.

Kirklin's sign. Meniscus sign. *See* SIGN. In the USA the sign is attributed to *Carman* and not to *Kirklin.*

Kirmisson, Edouard (b. 1848). Paris surgeon.

Kirmisson's operation. Transplantation of the tendo calcaneus to the peroneus longus muscle.

kirrhonosis (kir·on·**o**·sis). Cirrhonosus.

Kirschmann's law. The greatest contrast in colour is seen when the difference in luminosities is small.

Kirschner, Martin (b. 1879). Tübingen and Heidelberg surgeon.

Kirschner's apparatus. A series of instruments employed to pass and tighten a piece of piano wire through a bone end for the application of traction to a fracture; these include a special caliper and a weight suspended from it.

Kirschner wire. Wire used in skeletal traction (see above).

Kirschner's culture medium. A medium for the culture of *Mycobacterium tuberculosis.*

Kirstein, Alfred (b. 1863). Berlin physician.

Kirstein's method. A means of examining the larynx by extending the head and depressing the tongue with a specially designed spatula.

Kisch, Bruno (b. 1890). German physiologist.

Kisch's reflex. Kehrer's reflex; closure of the eye as a result of stimulation of the top part of the auditory meatus.

Kitasato, Shibasaburo, Baron (b. 1852). Tokyo bacteriologist.

Kitasato's glucose formate agar. A nutrient agar containing 2 per cent glucose and 0.4 per cent sodium formate.

Kitasato's bacillus. The plague bacillus, first observed by Kitasato and accurately described by Yersin.

Kitasato's glucose formate bouillon. A nutrient broth containing glucose 2 per cent and sodium formate 0.4 per cent [obsolete].

Kitasato's filter. A cylindrical porcelain bacterial filter through which the filtrate is drawn by suction.

Kitasato's serum. Anti-cholera serum: of very doubtful value.

kitol (**kit**·ol). A substance from whale-liver oil, a source of vitamin A.

Kittel, M. J. (fl. 1900). German physician.

Kittel's treatment. Treatment of gouty joints by manipulation and massage, with the object of resolving deposits of uric acid.

Kjeldahl, Johan Gustav Christoffer (b. 1849). Copenhagen chemist.

Kjeldahl apparatus. A distillation apparatus designed for the determination of small quantities of nitrogen derived from organic nitrogen compounds in the form of ammonia.

Kjeldahl's method, for nitrogen in organic material. The sample is boiled with sulphuric acid, potassium sulphate and a catalyst such as copper sulphate, mercury or selenium, until a colourless digest is obtained. This is diluted, made alkaline, and the liberated ammonia distilled into standard acid. Many modifications of this procedure are in use.

Klapp, Rudolf (b. 1873). Marburg surgeon.

Klapp's creeping treatment. A method of exercising the spine in scoliosis.

Klebs, Theodor Albrecht Edwin (b. 1834). Zürich and Chicago bacteriologist.

Klebs' disease. Glomerulonephritis.

Klebs–Loeffler bacillus. *Corynebacterium diphtheriae.*

Klebsiella (kleb·se·**el**·ah). A bacterial genus belonging to the family Enterobacteriaceae. They are short, plump, Gram-negative, non-motile and encapsulated rods, give profuse mucoid growth on solid media, are aerobic and actively fermentative with the production of acid and gas. They are found in the respiratory tract of man and animals and in the environment, associated with respiratory, urinary and other infections in man, particularly in warm-climate countries. **Klebsiella aerogenes.** Found in the environment, in water supplies and in the intestine of man and certain animals, associated with urinary-tract infections. **Klebsiella ozaenae.** Found in cases of ozaena but not necessarily causally related. **Klebsiella pneumoniae.** *Bacterium friedlanderi*; associated with respiratory infections and, rarely, a cause of pneumonia. **Klebsiella rhinoscleromatis.** Situated in the nose or oropharynx and associated with chronic granuloma, particularly in South East Europe. [Theodor Albrecht Edwin *Klebs.*]

Klein, Edward Emanuel (b. 1844). Hungarian histologist in London.

Klein's muscle. The marginal muscle bundle of the orbicularis oris muscle which lies next to the mucous membrane of the lips.

Kleine–Levin syndrome. A syndrome comprising periodic attacks of somnolence, compulsive eating, motor unrest and confused behaviour.

Kleinschmidt's glands. Accessory lacrimal glands of the upper eyelid.

Kleist, Karl (b. 1879). Frankfurt neurologist.

Kleist's sign. Exaggerated finger flexion elicited by slight extension of the fingers with the hand in the position of rest; seen especially in frontal lesions.

Klemm, Paul (b. 1861). Riga surgeon.

Klemm's tetanus. Head tetanus; tetanus following a wound of the head, especially of the eyebrow region. It is characterized by trismus, facial paralysis on one side and marked dysphagia. The symptoms superficially resemble those of rabies. Also called *Janin's tetanus.*

Klemperer, Georg (b. 1865). German physician.

Klemperer's disease. Banti's syndrome.

kleptolagnia (klep·to·**lag**·ne·ah). Thieving as a perverted means of sexual satisfaction. [Gk *kleptein* to steal, *lagneia* lust.]

kleptomania (klep·to·**ma**·ne·ah). An uncontrollable impulse to steal, without the existence of any need or desire for the object stolen. [Gk *kleptein* to steal, mania.]

kleptomaniac (klep·to·**ma**·ne·ak). A sufferer from kleptomania.

kleptophobia (klep·to·**fo**·be·ah). A morbid fear of thieves or of suffering loss by theft. [Gk *kleptein* to steal, phobia.]

Klimmer, Martin (b. 1873). Dresden and Leipzig veterinary pathologist.

Klimmer's vaccine. A vaccine prepared from killed tubercle bacilli [obsolete].

Klinefelter, Harry Fitch (b. 1912). Baltimore physician.

Klinefelter's syndrome. Testicular dysgenesis with aspermatogenesis associated with a high output of gonadotrophins and sometimes gynaecomastia. An X chromatin negative and positive variety can be distinguished, the former having usually a normal male karyotype and the latter showing an excess of X chromosomes. The most common karyotype of the X chromatin positive variety is 47,XXY. Other possible chromosome complements are: 46,XY/47,XXY; 46,XX/47,

XXY; 46,XX; 48,XXXY; 46,XY/47,XXY/48,XXXY; 47,XXY/48,XXXY; 48,XXYY; 47,XXY/48,XXYY. Cases with more than two X chromosomes are generally mentally defective, and subjects with two Y chromosomes have characteristics of the double Y syndrome.

Klippel, Maurice (b. 1858). Paris neurologist.

Feil-Klippel syndrome, Klippel-Feil disease or syndrome. Shortness of the neck and limitation of neck movements due to congenital fusion of the cervical vertebrae; the growth of hair on the back of the neck reaches an abnormally low level.

Klippel-Trenauney-Weber syndrome. Haemangiectatic hypertrophy.

Klippel-Weil sign. In disease of the pyramidal tract with flexion contracture of the fingers, passive extension of the fingers produces flexion and adduction of the thumb.

klopemania (klop·e·ma·ne·ah). Kleptomania. [Gk *klope* theft, mania.]

Klotz, Oskar (b. 1878). Pittsburgh physician.

Klotz's stain. A complex method for demonstrating fatty-acid crystals in sections.

Klumpke. *See* DÉJÉRINE-KLUMPKE.

Knapp, Hermann Jakob (b. 1831). Berlin and New York ophthalmologist.

Knapp's operation. 1. For squint: a method of combined advancement and tucking of the muscle concerned. 2. For symblepharon: 2 quadrangular flaps are cut vertically from the conjunctiva and sutured horizontally to meet in the centre and cover the bare excised area. 3. For pterygium: the pterygium is dissected off the cornea and the sclera, split horizontally, each half being buried under the mobilized conjunctiva above and below, and the conjunctiva sutured. 4. For cataract: a method of extraction of the lens within its capsule by dislocation of the lower pole with traction by capsule forceps and then removing the forceps and tumbling the lens out by pressure from below with a hook.

Celsus-Knapp blepharoplasty. A sliding skin flap is pulled horizontally from the temporal area to fill lid defects, upper or lower. It is associated with two Burow's triangles at its base.

kneading (ne·ding). Pétrissage, one of the movements carried out in massage, in which the muscles are grasped in the masseur's hand and rolled and pressed. [AS *cnedan.*]

knee (nee). That part of the lower limb between the thigh and the leg. **Back knee.** Genu recurvatum; hyperextension of the knee, often following paralysis of the thigh. **Beat knee.** Bursitis or cellulitis at the knee caused by severe or prolonged friction or pressure. **Football knee.** A chronic synovitis often seen in football players and sometimes due to tears of the semilunar cartilage. **Housemaids' knee.** Prepatellar bursitis. *See* BURSITIS. **Knee joint.** *See* JOINT. **Knock knee.** Genu valgum; a deformity where the knees come together and the ankles are apart. **Lock knee.** A condition in which the knee cannot be fully extended, usually due to a tear of the semilunar cartilage. **Out knee.** Bow leg; genu varum. **Rugby knee.** Chronic traumatic synovitis seen in rugby players. **Septic knee.** Infection of the knee joint due to pyogenic organisms. [AS *cneow.*]

kneippism (ni·pizm). Hydrotherapy in the form of cold baths of various kinds, vapour baths, wet packs, compresses, douches and walking barefoot in the early morning dew. [Sebastian *Kneipp* (b. 1821), German priest.]

Knemidokoptes (ne·mid·o·kop′·teez). Fowl mites which may infest man. *Knemidokoptes mutans* causes scaly leg in poultry while *K. laevis* is the depluming mite.

knife (nife). A cutting instrument with a sharp blade used in surgical operations and other procedures. **Amputating knife.** A knife for dividing the soft tissues in amputations. **Cataract knife.** A knife for cutting the cornea in operations for cataract. **Cautery knife.** A knife whose blade is connected to the electric battery of a cautery machine, so that blood vessels are closed by heat and bleeding is prevented during its use. **Electric knife, Electro-surgical knife, Endotherm knife.** A steel needle carrying high-frequency current which seals vessels as it divides them. **Hernia knife.** A knife formerly used for the release of the constriction of a strangulated hernia. **Meniscectomy knife.** A knife used in the removal of the cartilages of the knee. [AS *cnif.*]

See also: BARD, BEER, BLAIR, GRAEFE, GROFF, HUMBY, LANG, PARKER (W.), TAYLOR (C. B.), WHEELER.

knismogenic (nis·mo·jen·ik). Causing a sensation of tickling. [Gk *knismos* tickling of the skin, *genein* to produce.]

knitting (nit·ing). A popular term applied to a fractured bone, indicating the process of repair. [AS *cnyttan.*]

knob (nob). A small rounded swelling or protuberance. **Basal knob.** One of several small node-like swellings at the point of attachment of the cilia to the free margin of the cell. [ME.]

knock (nok). A hard beat or stroke. **Pericardial knock.** A distinct metallic click that may be heard on auscultation over the precordium when there is a penetrating wound in the area of the pericardium. It has been assumed to be due to the presence of free air in the interstitial connective tissue of the lung or to emphysema of the mediastinal connective tissue. [AS *cnocian.*]

Knoepfelmacher, Wilhelm (b. 1866). Vienna paediatrician.

Knoepfelmacher's meal. Butter meal. *See* MEAL.

Knoll, Philipp (b. 1841). Prague and Vienna physiologist.

Knoll's glands. Glands in the false vocal cords.

Knoop, Franz (b. 1875). Freiburg physiologist.

Knoop's theory. The formation of aceto-acetic acid and β-hydroxybutyric acid in the liver occurs by oxidation of fatty acids at the carbon atom in the beta position with respect to the terminal carboxyl group.

Knopf, Sigard Adolphus (b. 1857). New York physician.

Knopf's method or treatment. The encouragement, by practice, of diaphragmatic respiration and limitation of intercostal muscular movement in order to limit the expansion of the apices in upper-lobe tuberculosis.

knot (not). 1. In surgery, a methodical intertwining of flexible material by which advantage is taken of its frictional resistance to provide a secure grip. 2. A disorderly entanglement of flexible material. 3. A cluster of vessels or fibres. **Clove-hitch knot.** A knot consisting of 2 loops which are placed one behind the other, thereby providing a sling which may be used for purposes of traction in the reduction of fractures and dislocations. **Double knot.** Surgeons' knot (see below). **False knot.** Granny knot (see below). **Friction knot.** Surgeons' knot (see below). **Granny knot.** A knot which is similar to a reef knot (see below), except that the second tie is in the opposite line to the first and is thus liable to slip. **Protochordal knot.** Hensen's knot; a rounded swelling at the anterior end of the primitive streak on the surface of the blastoderm from which the head process (future notochord) is derived. It is homologous with the dorsal lip of the blastopore of lower vertebrates. **Reef knot.** A knot consisting of a double tie, the second tie being in the same line as the first. **Sailor's knot.** Reef knot (see prec.). **Square knot.** Reef knot (see above). **Staffordshire knot.** A method of securing a pedicle: a double-threaded needle is passed through the stump, leaving a loop of thread which is passed round the stump. One end of the thread is passed through the loop and the other round the pedicle, and they are tied in a reef knot (see above). **Stay knot.** A knot used for ligating large blood vessels. It is made by tying 2 or more separate ligatures one above the other, and then tying all the ends of one side to all the ends of the other as a reef knot (see above). **Surgeons' knot.** A surgical knot which is a modification of the reef knot (see above), the ends of the thread being passed 2 or more times through the same loop. **Syncytial knot.** One of the multinucleated swellings of the chorion epithelium covering the villi of the mature human placenta. [AS *cnotta.*]

See also: HENSEN, HUBRECHT, TAIT.

Knox, Robert (b. 1791). Edinburgh anatomist.

Knox's foramen. Supracondylar foramen of the humerus: normally present in the carnivora and some other animals. The supracondylar process which is occasionally found in human anatomy is looked on as representing the front wall of the bony foramen.

knuckle (nukl). 1. A prominence produced by the head of any of the metacarpal bones. 2. Term used to describe any part of the viscera which has been forced out of the abdominal cavity, e.g. a loop of intestine or part of omentum in a hernia. [ME *knokel.*]

Kobelt, Georg Ludwig (b. 1804). Freiburg anatomist.

Kobelt's cyst. A distension of Kobelt's tubules (see below).

Kobelt's muscle. Part of the ischiocavernosus muscle passing to the dorsum of the penis: also called *Houston's muscle.*

Kobelt's network. A venous network formed by the veins of the bulbs of the vestibule inferior to the clitoris.

Kobelt's tube or tubule. One of the vestigial tubes of the broad ligament, near the ovary, derived from the mesonephros.

Kober, Philip Adolph (b. 1884). American biochemist.

Kober test, for oestrogens in urine extracts. The test is applied to purified urinary phenolic fractions. To the dry residue add 2 ml of phenolsulphonic-acid reagent and heat for 10 min at 100°C. Cool, dilute to 4 ml with 5 per cent sulphuric acid. A pink colour is given by oestrogens. The phenolsulphonic-acid reagent is prepared by mixing 36 parts of redistilled phenol with 56 parts of concentrated sulphuric acid and warming to 60°C.

Kobus (ko·bus). The generic name of the water buck, a reservoir host of *Trypanosoma rhodesiense.*

Koch, Frederick Conrad (b. 1876). American biochemist.

Koch and McMeekin method. A micro-Kjeldahl method for nitrogen determination, employing direct nesslerization of the diluted digest.

Koch, Lewis Alfred (b. 1900). Brooklyn, New York, paediatrician.

Koch's test, for haemorrhagic diathesis. Bleeding and ecchymoses may occur in the subcutaneous tissues around a number of needle points made into those tissues.

Koch, Robert (b. 1843). Berlin bacteriologist.

Koch's bacillus. *Mycobacterium tuberculosis.*

Koch's circuit, law or postulates. To incriminate any organism as the causal agent of a particular disease the following conditions should be met: (*a*) the organism must be demonstrable in all cases of the disease; (*b*) it must be cultivated in pure culture; (*c*) re-inoculation of such a culture into a susceptible animal must reproduce the disease; and (*d*) the organism must be re-isolated from the infected animal and cultivated in pure culture.

Koch's lymph. Old Tuberculin BP 1958; a crude product obtained by concentrating a 6-8 weeks' culture of tubercle bacilli in glycerin-veal broth to 1/10 volume at 100°C and filtering to free it from bacilli. Formerly recommended for the treatment of tuberculosis, it is now used in modified forms for the diagnosis of tuberculosis in the nature of a skin test.

Koch phenomenon, *See* KOCH'S REACTION (following).

Koch's reaction. A tuberculin reaction which follows the injection of a culture of tubercle bacilli into animals already infected with tuberculosis (Koch phenomenon). In man a positive tuberculin reaction indicates sensitization as a result of tuberculous infection.

Koch's coagulated blood serum. Serum coagulated at 75°C and intermittently sterilized.

Koch's postulates. *See* KOCH'S CIRCUIT, LAW OR POSTULATES (above).

Koch's vibrio. *Vibrio cholerae.*

Koch–Weeks bacillus. *Haemophilus aegyptius.*

Koch–Weeks conjunctivitis. An acute epidemic mucopurulent bilateral form of conjunctivitis caused by Koch–Weeks bacillus, very contagious and commonly seen in schools and institutions: also known as *acute epidemic mucopurulent conjunctivitis,* or *pink eye.*

Koch, Walter (b. 1880). Berlin and Freiburg pathologist and cardiologist.

Koch's node. Atrioventricular node. *See* NODE.

Koch's triangle. The part of the wall of the right atrium which overlies the atrioventricular node.

Kocher, Emil Theodor (b. 1841). Berne surgeon.

Kocher's forceps. A forceps with serrated blades bearing interlocking terminal teeth, for controlling bleeding during operation.

Kocher's incision. For exposure of the gall bladder; an incision from the tip of the xiphoid process to the tip of the 9th costal cartilage parallel to the rib margin and 25 mm (1 in) below it. Also called *Courvoisier's incision.*

Kocher's method or shoulder dislocation. A method of reducing dislocation of the shoulder by adduction of the arm followed by internal rotation.

Kocher's operation. 1. A type of excision applicable to several joints and performed through an anterolateral incision. 2. Excision of the tongue through an incision from the symphysis of the jaw to the hyoid bone and backwards to the mastoid process. 3. Excision of the ankle joint.

Kocher's point. A point 35 mm in front of the bregma and 25 mm from the midline. It is the point for trephining for ventricular puncture.

Kocher's reflex. Contraction of the muscles of the abdominal wall when a testis is squeezed; also called *testicular-compression reflex.*

Kocher's sign. 1. The increase of upper lid retraction on fixing an object with attention, occurring in thyrotoxic exophthalmos. 2. The upper lid moving faster and ahead of the globe, when the eye looks up, as seen in thyrotoxic exophthalmos.

Koebner, Heinrich (b. 1838). Breslau dermatologist.

Koebner's disease. Epidermolysis bullosa.

Koebner's phenomenon. The development of lesions of psoriasis on areas of skin which have been irritated by mechanical, physical or chemical agents, provided the trauma has involved the papillary layer. The phenomenon is noted during the efflorescence of an attack of psoriasis, but cannot be produced in the cleared centre of a psoriasis plaque.

Koehler, Alban (b. 1874). German physician.

Koehler's disease, bone disease or scaphoiditis. 1. An obscure degenerative condition of the tarsal scaphoid in children. 2. Osteochondritis of the head of the 2nd metatarsal occurring in adolescents.

Koelliker, Rudolf Albert von (b. 1817). Zürich and Würzburg anatomist and histologist.

Koelliker's dental crest. The incisive portion of the developing maxilla; the part on which the incisor teeth develop.

Koelliker's granule. Interstitial granule. *See* GRANULE.

Koelliker's membrane. The reticular lamina of the cochlea.

Koelliker's nucleus. The medial nucleus of the thalamus.

Koenig, Charles Joseph (b. 1868). California otologist.

Koenig's rods. Steel bars which, when struck, produce a note of a given pitch.

Koenig, Franz (b. 1832). Gottingen and Berlin surgeon.

Koenig's operation. The shelf operation in congenital dislocation of the hip, an osteoperiosteal flap being turned downwards from the dorsum of the ilium.

Koenig, Fritz (b. 1866). Würzburg surgeon.

Koenig's syndrome. Alternating diarrhoea and constipation, with abdominal pain, distension and gurgling in the right iliac fossa, occurring in tuberculosis of the caecum.

Koenig's manometer. A gas flame controlled by a diaphragm which is sensitive to the pressure variations set up by musical notes of a certain pitch.

Koenig–Rutzen bag. A removable rubber bag which is attached by adhesive to the skin; it is used in the control of a permanent ileostomy. [*Koenig,* the name of a patient who devised this bag.]

Koeppe, Leonhard (b. 1884). Saxony ophthalmologist.

Koeppe lens. A contact lens for examining the angle of the anterior chamber.

Koeppe's nodule. Deposit seen on the pupillary border of the iris in cases of low-grade uveitis, somewhat similar to keratitic precipitates and composed of epithelioid cells and lymphocytes.

Koerte, Emil Werner (b. 1853). Berlin surgeon.

Koerte-Ballance operation. Hypoglossal-facial-nerve anastomosis.

Koga, Kensai. 20th century Kioto physician.

Koga treatment. Treatment of peripheral vascular disease (including thrombo-angiitis obliterans) by the intravenous infusion of hypertonic saline solution which increases blood volume and produces vasodilatation.

Kohlrausch, Friedrich (b. 1840). German physicist.

Kohlrausch's law. A law relating to the migration of ions: the conductivity of a salt at infinite dilution depends upon 2 parts, one relating specifically to the cation, the other to the anion.

Kohlrausch, Otto Ludwig Bernhard (b. 1811). Hanover physician.

Kohlrausch's folds. Horizontal folds of the rectum.

Kohlrausch's muscle. The longitudinal muscular tissue of the rectum.

Kohlrausch's valves. Rectal valves; more properly named *Houston's valves.*

Kohlrausch's veins. The superficial veins of the penis, passing round the sides of the organ from its under surface to reach the superficial dorsal vein.

Kohn, Alfred (b. 1867). Prague histologist.

Kohn's bodies. Bodies of the chromaffin system.

Kohn, Hans (b. 1866). Erlangen and Berlin pathologist.

pores of Kohn. Openings in the interalveolar septa of the lungs connecting adjacent alveoli. There is much evidence that they are present only in pathological material.

Kohnstamm, Oskar (b. 1871). German physician.

Kohnstamm's phenomenon. Following release of pressure exerted by the extended arm against a rigid object, the arm muscles contract in such a way that the arm is involuntarily raised away from the body.

Kohs, Samuel Calmin (b. 1890). American psychologist.

Kohs' blocks. *See* KOHS' TEST (below).

Kohs' test. A test which requires the subject to reproduce a pattern made of coloured cubes (Kohs' blocks). The score is a measure of intelligence, and impairment on the test is found particularly in persons with lesions of the parietal lobes of the cerebrum.

koilonychia (koi·lon·**ik**·e·ah). A condition in which the sides of the nail are raised and there is a concavity in the centre of the nail; spoon nail. [Gk *koilos* hollow, *onyx* nail.]

koilorrhachic (koi·lo·**rak**·ik). A reversed curvature of the lumbar part of the vertebral column, the concavity being anterior. [Gk *koilos* hollow, *rhachis* spine.]

koilosternia (koi·lo·**ster**·ne·ah). Cobblers' chest. [Gk *koilos* hollow, sternum.]

koinotropic (koi·no·**trop**·ik). Denoting a personality that is normal, well balanced and shows natural social proclivities (Meyer). [Gk *koinos* kindred, *trope* a turning.]

Kola BPC 1949 (**ko**·lah). Kola nuts, cola seeds, bissy nuts, gooroo nuts; the kernels separated from the seeds of *Cola nitida* A. Chev. and *C. acuminata* Schott and Endl. (family Sterculiaceae), trees indigenous to tropical Africa. They contain about 2 per cent of caffeine and traces of theobromine and tannin. They are used as a nerve stimulant and general tonic. [dialect word from Temne, West Africa.]

Koller, F. 20th century Swiss haematologist.

factor VII of Koller. A prothrombin conversion factor present in a pro-form in the plasma and found in the active form in the serum following the clotting of blood. Its concentration is decreased by the addition of the dicoumarol group of drugs.

kollonema (kol·on·e·mah). Myxoma. [Gk *kolla* glue, *nema* tissue.]

kolyone (**ko**·le·one). Colyone.

kolypeptic (ko·le·**pep**·tik). Hindering digestion. [Gk *kolyein* to hinder, *peptein* to digest.]

kolyphrenia (ko·le·**fre**·ne·ah). Colyphrenia.

kolyseptic (ko·le·**sep**·tik). Colyseptic; antiseptic. [Gk *kolyein* to hinder, *sepsis* decay.]

kolytic (ko·**lit**·ik). Colytic.

kombé (**kom**·ba). An arrow poison derived from *Strophanthus kombé* and containing the glycosides, kombé strophanthin and cymarin. **Kombé strophanthin.** A glucoside of strophanthidin occurring in kombé. [African.]

Kondoleon, Emmanuel (b. 1879). Athens surgeon.

Kondoleon operation. The removal of strips of deep fascia to permit subcutaneous lymph to drain into muscle in the treatment of elephantiasis of a limb.

koniantron (ko·ne·**an**·tron). An instrument with which medicaments may be sprayed into the tympanic cavity. [Gk *konis* dust, *antron* cave.]

konimeter (ko·**nim**·et·er). Coniometer.

koniocortex (**ko**·ne·o·**kor**′·tex). Coniocortex.

koniology (ko·ne·**ol**·o·je). Coniology.

koniosis (ko·ne·**o**·sis). Coniosis.

konometer (ko·**nom**·et·er). Konimeter.

Konstantinowich, Vikentiz Bonifatiyevich (b. 1845). Russian surgeon.

Konstantinowich's artery. A branch of the superior rectal artery to the rectum.

Konstantinowich's vein. The marginal vein of the anus.

kophemia (ko·**fe**·me·ah). Auditory aphasia; word deafness. [Gk *kophos* dull of hearing, *pheme* speech.]

kopiopia (ko·pe·**o**·pe·ah). Copiopia.

Koplik, Henry (b. 1858). New York paediatrician.

Koplik's sign or spots. Filatov's spots, Flindt's spots; bluish-white specks, usually surrounded by a red areola, seen on the mucous membrane of the mouth in the period of invasion of measles. They are of value in early diagnosis.

kopophobia (ko·po·**fo**·be·ah). Pathological fear of fatigue. [Gk *kopos* fatigue, *phobein* to fear.]

koprosterin (kop·ro·**steer**·in). Coprosterol, normal dehydrocholesterol, $C_{27}H_{47}OH$. A fully saturated sterol formed in the intestine by the bacterial reduction of cholesterol and excreted in the faeces. [Gk *kopros* dung, sterol.]

Korányi, Alexander von (b. 1866). Hungarian physician.

Korányi's treatment. The treatment of chronic leukaemias with benzene.

Korányi, Baron Friedrich von (Sandor) (b. 1829). Budapest physician.

Korányi-Grocco triangle. Grocco's triangle.

Korff's fibres. Irregularly spiralling fibres in the dental pulp of a developing tooth. Either they are continuous with pulpal fibres or they fuse with the membrana preformativa. They are concerned in the formation of dentine.

koro (**ko**·ro). A hysterical manifestation that occurs among the Macassars and the Buginese in the Celebes, and in China; the patient has a morbid fear that his penis is retracting into his abdomen.

koronion (ko·**ro**·ne·on). Coronion.

koroscopy (kor·**os**·ko·pe). Coroscopy.

Korotkoff, Nikolai Sergeyevich (b. 1874). Moscow physician.

Korotkoff's method. The auscultatory method of estimating blood pressure.

Korotkoff's sounds. The sounds heard with the stethoscope in the auscultatory method of estimating blood pressure.

Korotkoff's test. If pulsation remains in vessels distal to an aneurysm when the main proximal artery is compressed, the collateral circulation is adequate.

Korsakoff, Sergei Sergeyevich (b. 1854). Moscow psychiatrist.

Korsakoff's disease, psychosis or syndrome. A disorder identified by confusion, disorientation with regard to time and place, retro-active amnesia, confabulation and polyneuritis. It is seen most commonly in alcoholism and in other disorders in which deficiency of the B vitamins occurs; it may also develop as a manifestation of many intracranial pathological changes.

Korthof's culture medium. A medium prepared from peptone-salt solution (peptone 0.8 g, sodium chloride 0.4 g, sodium bicarbonate 0.02 g, potassium chloride 0.04 g, calcium chloride 0.04 g, monopotassium phosphate 0.24 g, disodium phosphate

0.88 g, and redistilled water to 1 litre), sterile inactivated rabbit serum and haemoglobin solution (equal parts of haemolysed rabbit red cells and distilled water sterilized by filtration), in the proportions of 100 ml peptone-salt solution, 8 ml serum and 0.8 ml haemoglobin solution.

Kortzeborn's operation. An operation for median-nerve paralysis in the hand: the thumb is fixed by tenodesis.

Koser, Stewart Arment (b. 1894). Chicago bacteriologist.

Koser's citrate culture medium. A synthetic medium which contains citrate as the sole source of carbon. It is used in the examination of water to differentiate soil coliforms, which can grow in it, from faecal coliforms which cannot.

kosin (ko·sin). A mixture of 2 inactive crystalline substances, α-kosin and β-kosin, obtained from kousso, and thought to be artefacts.

kosotoxin (ko·so·tox·in). $C_{26}H_{34}O_{10}$, a yellow amorphous substance isolated from kousso and thought to be the active principle responsible for its anthelminthic action. It is a butyrate of phloroglucinol.

Kossa's stain. *See* MAGYARY-KOSSA.

koumiss (koo·mis). A substance used for the fermentation of milk and probably containing a number of micro-organisms including yeast, *Saccharomyces cerevisiae, Lactobacillus caucasicus* and *Bacterium acidi lactici.* Kefir, obtained by the action of koumiss on cow's milk, is sometimes used in specialized dietetic treatments. [Tartar *kumiz.*]

koussin (koo·sin). Kosotoxin.

kousso (koo·so). Cusso BPC 1949. [Abyssinian.]

koussotoxin (koo·so·tox·in). Kosotoxin.

Kovalevski, Nikolaus Osipovich (b. 1840). Kasan physiologist.

canal of Kovalevski. The archenteric canal. *See* CANAL.

Kozhevnikoff, Alexei Yakovlevich (b. 1836). Moscow neurologist.

Kozhevnikoff's disease or epilepsy. Continuous partial epilepsy. *See* EPILEPSY.

Krabbe, Knud H. (b. 1885). Copenhagen neurologist.

Krabbe's disease. Familial diffuse infantile cerebral sclerosis; galactocerebroside β-galactosidase deficiency.

Kraepelin, Emil (b. 1856). Heidelberg and Munich psychiatrist.

Kraepelin's classification. A classification of mental disorders introduced by Kraepelin.

Kraepelin–Morel disease, Morel-Kraepelin disease. Dementia praecox.

krait (krate). A small venomous Indian snake of the genus *Bungarus.* [Hind. *karait.*]

Kramer, Benjamin (b. 1888). Baltimore physician.

Kramer and Tisdall method, for calcium in serum. Calcium is precipitated directly from diluted serum by the addition of ammonium-oxalate solution. After standing for half an hour, the precipitate is separated and washed with dilute ammonia by centrifugation, dissolved in hot dilute sulphuric acid and titrated with N/100 potassium permanganate.

Krameria (kram·eer·e·ah). 1. A genus of South American shrubs (family Krameriaceae). 2. Krameria BPC 1954 (krameria root, rhatany root), the root of *Krameria triandra* Ruiz. and Pav. It is strongly astringent due to the presence of about 10 per cent of tannin, and is used in lozenges and mouth washes, as a haemostatic, and in the treatment of diarrhoea. [Johann Georg Heinrich *Kramer* (d. 1742), Austrian military surgeon and botanist.]

Kraske, Paul (b. 1851). Freiburg surgeon.

Kraske's operation. Removal of a malignant rectum to which access is gained by excision of part of the sacrum and coccyx.

Kraske's position. A prone position with the head and legs inclined downwards, for sacral excision of the rectum.

krauomania (kraw·o·ma·ne·ah). A tic the characteristic of which is a rhythmical movement.

kraurosis (kraw·ro·sis). Dryness and shrivelling of a part. **Kraurosis penis.** Balanitis xerotica obliterans. **Kraurosis vulvae.** That which affects the vulva. [Gk *krauros* dry.]

Krause, Fedor Victor (b. 1857). Berlin surgeon.

Krause's operation, for trigeminal neuralgia. Excision of the gasserian ganglion extradurally.

Hartley-Krause operation, for trigeminal neuralgia. Excision of the trigeminal ganglion and sensory 5th cranial-nerve roots.

Wolfe-Krause graft. A free graft of skin completely removed from one part of the body surface and sutured to repair a defect.

Krause, Karl Friedrich Theodor (b. 1797). Hanover anatomist.

Krause's glands. Accessory lacrimal glands of the upper eyelid.

Krause's muscle. The marginal muscle bundle of the lips.

Krause, Wilhelm Johann Friedrich (b. 1833). Gottingen and Berlin anatomist.

Krause's bone. The os acetabuli.

Krause's bulbs, end-bulbs, terminal bulbs or corpuscles. Encapsulated nerve-endings widely distributed in superficial, e.g. skin and cornea, and deep, e.g. genital organs, tissues.

Krause's bundle. The tractus solitarius.

Krause's glands. Glands in the mucous membrane of the tympanic cavity.

Krause's line or membrane. Z line.

Krause's nerve. The ulnar collateral branch of the radial nerve.

Krause's valve. A valve at the junction of the lacrimal sac and duct: also called *Béraud's valve.*

Krause's ventricle. An extension of the central canal of the spinal cord at its lower end.

Krauss' precipitin reaction. The precipitation of a suitable extract of typhoid bacilli by an antibody called precipitin present in typhoid serum.

kreat (kre·at). Creat.

kreatine (kre·at·een). Creatine.

kreatinine (kre·at·in·een). Creatinine.

Krebs, Hans Adolf (b. 1900). British biochemist.

Krebs' cycle. Citric-acid cycle. *See* CYCLE.

Krebs' urea cycle. Ureagenesis.

Krebs, Martin (b. 1895). Leipzig physician.

Krebs' leucocyte index. An index obtained by dividing the percentage of neutrophils by the percentage of lymphocytes.

kreotoxicon (kre·o·tox·ik·on). A ptomaine formed by the infection of meat by bacteria. [Gk *kreas* flesh, *toxikon* poison.]

kreotoxin (kre·o·tox·in). Any poisonous substance formed in meat by bacterial action. [Gk *kreas* flesh, toxin.]

kreotoxism (kre·o·tox·izm). Creatotoxism; poisoning caused by the eating of tainted or rotten meat. [see prec.]

Kretschmann, Friedrich (b. 1858). Halle and Magdeburg otologist.

Kretschmann's space. A space lined with mucous membrane which lies in the epitympanic recess of the middle ear.

Kretschmer, Ernst (b. 1888). German physician.

Kretschmer type. The type of physique according to Kretschmer, i.e. pyknic, asthenic, athletic or dysplastic.

Kreysig, Friedrich Ludwig (b. 1770). Dresden pathologist, physician and surgeon.

Kreysig's sign, Heim-Kreysig sign. Recession of intercostal spaces during ventricular systole in adherent pericarditis.

krinosin (kri·no·sin). An aminolipide isolated from alcoholic extracts of brain. It contains an amino group and no phosphorus, otherwise its composition is unknown.

Krishaber, Maurice (b. 1836). Hungarian physician in Paris.

Krishaber's disease. A neuropathic disorder of sensory and autonomic nerves, giving tachycardia, hyperaesthesia and vertigo, and sometimes illusions of abnormal sensation.

Kristeller, Samuel (b. 1820). Berlin gynaecologist.

Kristeller expression, manoeuvre, method or technique. Expression of the fetus by applying the hands to the sides of the uterus during a contraction, and pushing.

Kroenig, Georg (b. 1856). Berlin physician.

Kroenig's area, field or isthmus. A narrow band of resonance uniting the anterior and posterior areas of resonance found on percussion over the apices of the lungs above the clavicles. This normally is 40–60 mm in width, but in apical tuberculosis the isthmus is reduced in width or may disappear owing to the contraction of the underlying lung.

Kroenig's percussion. Percussion over the upper border of the trapezius muscle to determine the band of resonance (see preceding) which overlies the apex of the lung.

Kroenlein, Rudolf Ulrich (b. 1847). Zürich surgeon.

Kroenlein's hernia. An inguinal hernia which enlarges between the transversalis fascia and the abdominal wall.

Kroenlein's operation. Exploration of the orbit through the lateral wall by turning back a bone flap.

Krogh, August (b. 1874). Danish physiologist.

Krogh apparatus. A closed-circuit apparatus for measuring the basal metabolism by oxygen consumption, similar in principle to the Benedict–Roth method but with a wedge-shaped instead of a cylindrical spirometer.

Kromayer, Ernst Ludwig Franz (b. 1862). Berlin dermatologist.

Kromayer's lamp. A mercury-vapour lamp employed for local ultraviolet irradiation. It is water-cooled and is used in contact with the skin.

Kromayer treatment. Treatment of localized areas of skin (usually for lupus vulgaris) by ultraviolet light emanating from a water-cooled mercury-vapour lamp (see prec.).

Krompecher, Edmund (b. 1870). Budapest pathologist.

Krompecher's tumour. Basal-cell carcinoma; rodent ulcer. *See* ULCER.

Kronecker, Karl Hugo (b. 1839). Swiss physiologist.

Kronecker's centre. That part of the cardiac centre concerned with slowing of the heart; its activity is mediated via the vagus nerve.

Kronecker's mounting fluid. A simple suspending fluid for cells, containing sodium chloride and sodium carbonate.

Krueger, Martin. Berlin biochemist.

Krueger and Schmidt method. Uric acid and purine bases are determined in urine by precipitation with copper, and the copper precipitate decomposed with sodium sulphide. Uric acid is then precipitated by adding hydrochloric acid and concentrating; the purine bases in the filtrate are precipitated as copper or silver compounds. The nitrogen in both the uric-acid and purine-base precipitates is determined by Kjeldahl's method.

Krukenberg, Adolf (b. 1816). Brunswick and Halle anatomist.

Krukenberg's vein. The central vein of a lobule of the liver.

Krukenberg, Friedrich Ernst (b. 1870). Halle ophthalmologist.

Krukenberg spindle, Axenfeld–Krukenberg spindle. A vertical narrow fusiform deposition of pigment on the corneal endothelium which may be associated with pigmentary glaucoma.

Krukenberg, Georg Peter Heinrich (b. 1856). Bonn gynaecologist.

Krukenberg tumour of the ovary. Mucinous carcinoma; a tumour of the ovary almost invariably bilateral and commonly secondary to carcinoma in the gastro-intestinal tract.

Krukenberg, Hermann (b. 1863). Elberfeld surgeon.

Krukenberg's amputation. Cineplastic amputation; an amputation so fashioned that the stump can be used to make movements, e.g. a gripping action between a mobilized radius and ulna.

Krukenberg's arm. A claw appendage produced by a special cineplastic amputation.

Krumweide, Charles (b. 1879). New York physician.

Krumweide agar. Brilliant-green agar. *See* AGAR.

Kruse, Walther (b. 1864). Bonn and Leipzig bacteriologist.

Shiga–Kruse bacillus. *Shigella shigae.*

krymotherapy (kri·mo·**ther**·ap·e). Crymotherapy. [Gk *krymos* frost, therapy.]

kryoscopy (kri·**os**·ko·pe). Cryoscopy. [Gk *kryos* cold, *skopein* to watch.]

krypton (**krip**·ton). An element of atomic weight 83.80, atomic number 36 and chemical symbol Kr. It is a colourless gas of the inert series, occurring in the atmosphere to the extent of 1 part in 670 000 by volume, and is used in fluorescent lighting tubes. [Gk *kryptos* hidden.]

kryptopyrrole (krip·to·**pir**·ole). *See* DIMETHYLETHYLPYRROLE.

kryptoxanthin (krip·to·**zan**·thin). Cryptoxanthin, 3-hydroxy-β,β'-carotene, $C_{40}H_{55}OH$. A provitamin which is converted in the body into vitamin A. It is a yellow pigment, occurring in yellow corn, paprika and in various red blossoms and fruits.

KSK (**ka**·es·**ka'**). The common name for the war gas, ethyliodoacetate.

K-stoff (**ka**·shtof). Chloromethylchloroformate, $CH_2ClCOOCl$. A lacrimatory liquid used in chemical warfare. Also known as *palite*.

kubisagari (**koo**·bi·sag·**ah'**·re). A form of paralytic vertigo that is endemic in Japan: it is very similar to the Swiss disease, Gerlier's disease or syndrome. [Jap. hang-head.]

Kuder preference record test. A test of the subject's interests based on selections.

Kuechler, Heinrich (b. 1811). German physician.

Kuechler's operation, for cataract extraction. The incision passes through the centre of the cornea [obsolete].

Kuehne, Heinrich. 20th century German histologist.

Kuehne's methylene blue. A preparation of methylene blue 1.5 parts, absolute alcohol 10 parts and 5 per cent phenol solution 100 parts; it is used as a microscopic stain for *Pfeifferella mallei.*

Kuehne, Willy (b. 1837). Amsterdam and Heidelberg physiologist.

Kuehne's phenomenon. Porret's phenomenon; on passing a continuous current through a muscle fibre, a wave of contraction arises at the positive pole and passes towards the negative pole.

Kuehne's terminal plate. The motor end-plate of a striated muscle fibre, formed about the terminal ramifications of a motor nerve fibre.

Kuehne's spindle. Muscle spindle. *See* SPINDLE.

Kuelz, Rudolph Eduard (b. 1845). Marburg physiologist.

Kuelz's cast or cylinder. A hyaline or granular cast thought to be diagnostic of impending diabetic coma; coma cast.

Kuemmell, Hermann (b. 1852). Hamburg surgeon.

Kuemmell's disease or spondylitis. A compression fracture, a wedge-shaped deformity of the body of a vertebra, generally considered to be the late result of fracture of that vertebra.

Kuemmell's point. A point 1 or 2 cm below and to the right of the umbilicus which is tender in chronic appendicitis.

Kuess, Emil (b. 1815). Strasbourg physiologist.

Kuess' experiment. The demonstration that substances are not absorbed through the epithelium of the urinary bladder by the lack of symptoms produced when drugs are injected into that organ.

Kuester, Ernst Georg Ferdinand von (b. 1839). Berlin surgeon.

Kuester's hernia. Inguinal hernia which enlarges upwards between the abdominal muscles and subcutaneous fascia.

Kuester's operation. 1. Resection and re-implantation of the ureter to the renal pelvis in hydronephrosis. 2. Osteoplastic opening of the mastoid process of the temporal bone. It consists of forming a tongue-shaped postauricular flap containing skin, periosteum and a large bony plate of mastoid cortex. The base of the flap is level with the superior bony meatal wall, the apex with the mastoid tip. The flap is replaced after surgical clearance of the mastoid process. 3. The Kuester–Bergmann radical mastoid operation or Schwartze's operation for chronic mastoiditis: the mastoid process, tympanic antrum and middle-ear cavity are cleaned of diseased tissue and converted into a single cavity draining into the external auditory meatus. 4. Kuester's operation on the maxillary antrum: removal of the anterior osseous wall of the sinus through a gingivolabial incision. Diseased mucosa and bony sequestra are removed. The incision is kept open until the cavity ceases to suppurate.

Kuester–Bergmann radical mastoid operation. Kuester's operation 3 (above).

Kuestner, Heinz (b. 1897). Breslau gynaecologist.

Prausnitz-Kuestner reaction or test. Production of local passive sensitization by an intradermal injection of serum from a hypersensitive subject. Kuestner himself was hypersensitive to certain fish, and the reaction was first demonstrated with his serum.

reversed Prausnitz-Kuestner reaction or test. The reaction, a weal, that appears when the antibody is given after the administration of the antigen, instead of before, as in the Prausnitz-Kuestner reaction.

Kuestner, Otto Ernst (b. 1849). Breslau gynaecologist.

Kuestner's incision. A curved incision convex downwards in the suprapubic region and in the line of the vertical abdominal skin folds.

Kufs' disease. The late juvenile variety of cerebromacular degeneration.

Kuhlmann, Frederick (b. 1876). American psychologist.

Kuhlmann test. A modification of the Binet-Simon test.

Kuhlmann-Anderson test. A series of intelligence tests for children.

Kuhn, Ernst (b. 1873). Berlin physician.

Kuhn's mask. A mask used over the nose and mouth with the object of impeding expiration and inducing an artificial hyperaemia of the lung in cases of tuberculosis, on the same principle as Bier's passive hyperaemia.

Kuhnt, Hermann (b. 1850). Bonn ophthalmologist.

Kuhnt's operation. 1. For ectropion: a triangle of conjunctiva and tarsal plate is excised from the lower lid with its base at the lid margin. The edges are then securely sutured through the skin. It was modified later by Dimmer and Szymanowski. 2. Canthoplasty: the filling of a conjunctival defect following canthoplasty, with a flap of skin from the lower lid. 3. For lower lid defects: a bridge skin flap from outside the outer canthus to inside the inner canthus is fashioned and lined with cartilage from the ear to form a new tarsal plate. 4. For symblepharon: defects of conjunctiva are made good by skin pedicles or flaps taken from nearby skin. 5. An operation for the complete obliteration of the frontal sinus.

Kuhnt's recesses. Pouches between the ciliary zonule and the ciliary body which open into the posterior chamber of the eye.

Antyllus-Kuhnt operation. Kuhnt's operation 1 (above).

Kuhnt-Szymanowski operation. An operation for transverse shortening of the eyelid in cases of ectropion: the lateral half of the lid is split between the tarsal and cutaneous layers, a triangle of tarsus from the medial part and a similar triangle of skin from the lateral part are removed and the wounds are sutured. The lid is shortened by an amount equal to the base of these triangles.

Kulchitsky, Nikolai (b. 1856). Russian anatomist.

cell of Kulchitsky. One of the argentaffin connective-tissue cells in the depths of the intestinal mucosa, between the crypts of Lieberkühn.

kumiss (**koo**·mis). Koumiss.

Kundrat, Hans (b. 1845). Vienna pathologist.

Kundrat's disease or lymphosarcoma. A variety of lymphosarcoma which arises from groups of lymph nodes, not from single nodes, and from the lymphoid tissue of mucous membranes. Leukaemic features are absent, and the spleen, marrow and liver are rarely involved.

Kundt, August Adolph Eduard Aberhardt (b. 1838). Berlin physicist.

Kundt's illusion. When a horizontal line is bisected by a person with one eye closed, the half on the side of the open eye is always the longer.

Kunkel's test. For carbon monoxide: dilute blood with 9 parts of water and add a few drops of a 3 per cent aqueous solution of tannin. In the presence of carbon monoxide, a pinkish-white precipitate forms; in normal blood, a brownish-white.

Kuntscher, Gerhard (b. 1902). Kiel surgeon.

Kuntscher nail. A long steel nail used for the intramedullary fixation of fractures.

Kupffer, Karl Wilhelm von (b. 1829). Munich anatomist.

Kupffer's canals. The ureteric buds from the mesonephric ducts.

Kupffer's cell. One of the phagocytic endothelial cells lining the venous sinusoids of the liver.

Kupressoff, J. (fl. 1870). St. Petersburg physician.

Kupressoff's centre. The spinal centre concerned with the control of micturition and of bladder activity.

kurchi (**koor**·che). Holarrhena. [Sanskrit *kurca* bundle of grass.]

kurchine (**koor**·cheen). $C_{23}H_{38}N_2$, an alkaloid isolated from kurchi bark, *Holarrhena antidysenterica.* It is of limited value in the treatment of amoebic dysentery.

Kurie plot. A graphical method of exhibiting the spectral distribution of a continuous beta-ray spectrum, which in most cases leads to an approximately straight line.

Kurlov, Mikhail Georgievich (b. 1859). Russian physician.

Kurlov's body. A granule of unknown origin, sometimes seen in the mononuclear leucocytes of some animals and variously thought to be the early stage of formation of an amoeboid body or an eosinophil leucocyte.

Foa-Kurlov cells. Guinea-pig mononuclear blood cells containing inclusions.

Kurthia (**koor**·te·ah). A genus of micro-organisms, occurring as Gram-positive rods in chains. They are non-sporing aerobic and non-pathogenic, and are found in decomposing material. The earlier generic name, *Zopfius,* is preferred by most British bacteriologists. *Kurthia zenkeri* and *K. zopfi,* differentiated by their growth in gelatin media, are considered to be identical by some workers. [Heinrich *Kurth* (b. 1860), Bremen bacteriologist.

kuru (**koo**·roo). A form of progressive brain damage confined to the Fore tribe of New Guinea. It involves the cerebellum and the higher intellectual symptoms leading to ataxia and dementia. It is believed to be due to a slow virus allied to that of scrapie in sheep, and has been transmitted experimentally to chimpanzees. Cannibalism of the brain of a victim is the probable mode of transmission.

Kussmaul, Adolf (b. 1822). Strasbourg physician.

Kussmaul's aphasia. The non-use of speech as typical in some forms of insanity.

Kussmaul's breathing or respiration, sign or symptom. Extreme hyperpnoea; seen in diabetic coma.

Kussmaul's disease, Kussmaul-Maier disease. Polyarteritis nodosa.

Kussmaul's paralysis, Kussmaul-Landry paralysis. Acute ascending paralysis; usually called *Landry's paralysis.*

Kussmaul's pulse, Griesinger-Kussmaul sign. Paradoxical pulse; the force of the pulse wave diminishes on inspiration and increases on expiration. This phenomenon occurs occasionally in large pericardial effusions or constrictive pericarditis (i.e. any condition which hampers cardiac pulsation, particularly diastolic filling). It may also occur in cases of large pleural effusion and mediastinal disease. A recent explanation of this phenomenon is as follows: the right ventricular filling pressure increases on inspiration, but this is without effect on the left ventricle, since the fall in intrathoracic pressure on inspiration is equally applied to the pulmonary veins and the left ventricle. When the heart is compressed, however, increases in filling of the right ventricle will increase the intrapericardial pressure and hence hinder filling of the left ventricle. This results in a fall of left ventricular output and waning of the pulse.

kutch (kuch). Black catechu.

Kutscher, Karl. German bacteriologist.

Kutscher's modification of Gram's method. Sections are floated on the surface of a dilute solution of gentian violet before being treated with Lugol's solution. It is used to demonstrate the staining characteristics of bacteria in the tissues.

Kveim, Morten Ansgar (b. 1892). Oslo physician.

Kveim test. A test for sarcoidosis, by the intradermal injection of material from a gland of a person known to have Boeck's sarcoid.

kwashiorkor (kwosh·e·**or**·kor). Chronic malignant malnutrition in children observed mostly in tropical Africans, but occurring also in the East and West Indies. The characteristic signs are stunting of growth, reddening of the hair, crazy-pavement appearance of the skin with oedema of the face, feet and hands. There is a pancreatic defect and extensive fatty degeneration of the liver. [An African word that indicates "the disease the child gets when the next baby is born".]

kymatism (**ki**·mat·izm). Myokymia. [Gk *kyma* wave.]

kymocyclograph (ki·mo·**si**·klo·graf). An apparatus for the graphic recording of movement. [Gk *kyma* wave, *kyklos* circle, *graphein* to record.]

kymogram (**ki**·mo·gram). The graphic tracing made by a kymograph.

kymograph (**ki**·mo·graf). An apparatus on which can be recorded arterial or other waves and, in particular, variations in blood pressure. **X-ray kymograph.** A metal grid in which are transverse slits of equal width, equidistant from each other. The grid is placed between the patient and the film cassette. Two types are in use: in one the grid moves at right angles to the slits during the exposure; in the other the grid is stationary and the cassette moves. [Gk *kyma* wave, *graphein* to record.]

kymography (ki·**mog**·raf·e). The process of recording arterial and other pressure variations by means of the kymograph. **X-ray kymography.** Radiokymography; the recording on one x-ray film of the several movements of a structure or organ. [see prec.]

kymoscope (**ki**·mo·skope). An apparatus used to study the blood current, e.g. variations in blood pressure; it may be employed also in the measurement of pulse waves. [Gk *kyma* wave, *skopein* to watch.]

kymotrichous (ki·**mot**·rik·us). With wavy hair. [Gk *kyma* wave, *thrix* hair.]

kynocephalous (ki·no·**kef**·al·us). Cynocephalous.

kynocephalus (ki·no·**kef**·al·us). Cynocephalus.

kynophobia (ki·no·**fo**·be·ah). Cynophobia.

kynurin (ki·**newr**·in). γ-Hydroxyquinoline, C_9H_7NO. A compound derived from kynurenic acid, and isomeric with carbostyril.

kynurinuria (ki·newr·in·**ewr**'·e·ah). Sclerodermia with products of tryptophane in urine, probably due to partial block of kynurenine hydroxylase. [kynurin, Gk *ouron* urine.]

kyogenic (ki·o·**jen**·ik). Serving to produce pregnancy. The term is usually used to indicate something which will produce changes similar to those occurring during pregnancy. Thus, if a frog's egg is pricked with a needle it will segment; this is said to be a kyogenic effect, although fertilization has not taken place. [Gk *kyesis* pregnancy, *genein* to produce.]

kyphorrachitis (ki·fo·rak·**i**'·tis). A rachitic hunch-back deformity. [Gk *kyphos* hunch-backed, *rhachis* spine.]

kyphos (**ki**·fos). The hump of the vertebral column which is present in kyphosis. [Gk *kyphos* hunch-backed.]

kyphoscoliorrachitic (ki·fo·sko·le·o·rak·**it**'·ik). Kyphoscoliotic. [see foll.]

kyphoscoliorrachitis (ki·fo·sko·le·o·rak·**i**'·tis). An angular kyphotic deformity with scoliosis, due to rickets. [Gk *kyphos* hunch-backed, *skolios* curved, *rhachis* spine.]

kyphoscoliosis (ki·fo·sko·le·**o**'·sis). Forward and lateral curvature of the spine. Some rotational deformity is also present. [Gk *kyphos* hunch-backed, *skolios* curved.]

kyphoscoliotic (ki·fo·sko·le·**ot**'·ik). Relating or belonging to or affected with kyphoscoliosis.

kyphosis (ki·**fo**·sis). The excessive forward curvature of the spine. **Adolescent kyphosis, Kyphosis dorsalis juvenilis, Juvenile kyphosis.** Scheuermann's disease. **Senile kyphosis.** A common tendency in old age. [Gk *kyphos* hunch-backed.]

See also: SCHEUERMANN.

kyphotic (ki·**fot**·ik). Pertaining to, marked by, or affected with kyphosis.

kyphotone (**ki**·fo·tone). An apparatus for reducing deformity in Pott's disease. [Gk *kyphos* hunch-backed, *tonos* stretching.]

kyrin (**ki**·rin). The term applied by Siegfried to any of the tripeptides isolated during slow hydrolysis of proteins, in which 2 molecules of a basic amino acid are linked with 1 molecule of a mono-amino acid.

kyrtorrhachic (ker·to·**rak**·ik). Relating or belonging to kyphosis of the lumbar portion of the vertebral column. [Gk *kyrtos* curved, *rhachis* spine.]

kysthitis (kis·**thi**·tis). Vaginitis. [Gk *kysthos* vagina, *-itis* inflammation.]

kysthoproptosis, kysthoptosis (kis·tho·prop·**to**'·sis, kis·thop·**to**'·sis). Vaginal prolapse. [Gk *kysthos* vagina, *proptosis* a falling forward.]

L

lab (lab). The German designation for the enzyme rennin, occurring in the secretion of the stomach and causing the coagulation of milk. [G, rennet.]

Labat, Louis Gaston (b. 1877). French surgeon.

Labat-type syringe. A glass and metal syringe with a device for locking the needle on to its mount, and with a convenient finger hold.

Labbé, Charles (b. 1852). Paris anatomist.

Labbé's vein. The inferior anastomotic vein; it connects the superficial middle cerebral vein with the transverse sinus of the dura mater.

Labbé, Leon (b. 1832). Paris surgeon.

Labbé's triangle. A triangular area between the line of the false ribs on the left side, the inferior border of the liver, and a horizontal line drawn through the lower border of the 9th costal cartilage.

labdacism (lab·dah·sizm). Lambdacism.

labia (la·be·ah). *See* LABIUM.

labial (la·be·al). Relating or belonging to the lips or a labium, as the labial glands. [L *labium* lip.]

labial arteries. Inferior labial artery [arteria labialis inferior (NA)]. *See* FACIAL ARTERY. **Superior labial artery [arteria labialis superior (NA)].** *See* FACIAL ARTERY.

labial veins. Inferior labial veins [venae labiales inferiores (NA)]. Tributaries of the anterior facial vein. **Superior labial vein [vena labialis superior (NA)].** A tributary of the anterior facial vein.

labialism (la·be·al·izm). A speech defect in which the labial consonants are used too frequently; tendency to labialize sounds, and in which any one labial consonant may be confused with any other.

labially (la·be·al·e). Towards the lips. [L *labium* lip.]

Labiatae (la·be·a·te·e). The mint family, a large family of plants, mostly herbs, few shrubs, and rarely trees. Most are aromatic, and include a great variety of garden herbs. [L *labiatus* lipped.]

labichorea (la·be·ko·re′·ah). Labiochorea.

labidometer (lab·id·**om**·et·er). Forceps used for measuring the diameter of the fetal head; an American term. [Gk *labis* pincers, meter.]

labile (la·bile). 1. Unstable; easily destroyed or altered, e.g. by heat or oxidation; applied to chemical substances, vitamins, and antibodies. 2. Of electrodes, moving over the surface of the skin during the passage of an electric current. 3. In psychology, unstable, fluctuating, and uncontrolled expression of the emotions. **Heat labile.** Thermolabile. [L *labilis* liable to slip.]

lability (la·**bil**·it·e). The quality of being labile.

labimeter (lab·**im**·et·er). Labidometer.

labio-alveolar (la·be·o·al·ve′·o·lar). 1. Relating or belonging to the lip and the dental alveoli. 2. Belonging to the labial surface of a dental alveolus. [L *labium* lip, alveolus.]

labiocervical (la·be·o·ser′·vik·al). Referring to the labial surface of the neck of a tooth. [L *labium* lip, *cervix* neck.]

labiochorea (la·be·o·ko·re′·ah). Choreal spasm of the lips leading to stammering. [L *labium* lip, chorea.]

labioclination (la·be·o·klin·a′·shun). In dentistry, the deviation of a tooth from its normal vertical position towards the labial side. [L *labium* lip, inclination.]

labiodental (la·be·o·den′·tal). 1. Relating or belonging to the labial surface of a tooth. 2. Applied to certain letters the pronunciation of which involves co-operation of lips and teeth, for example *f*, *v*. [L *labium* lip, *dens* tooth.]

labiogingival (la·be·o·jin′·jiv·al). Pertaining to the lips and gums. [L *labium* lip, *gingiva* gum.]

labioglossolaryngeal (la·be·o·glos·o·lar·in′·je·al). Relating to the lips, the tongue, and the larynx, e.g. bulbar paralysis involving these structures. [L *labium* lip, Gk *glossa* tongue, larynx.]

labioglossopharyngeal (la·be·o·glos·o·far·in′·je·al). Belonging to the lips, the tongue, and the pharynx, e.g. bulbar paralysis involving these structures. [L *labium* lip, Gk *glossa* tongue, pharynx.]

labiograph (la·be·o·graf). An instrument with which the movement of the lips during speech may be recorded. [L *labium* lip, Gk *graphein* to record.]

labiolingual (la·be·o·ling′·gwal). Relating or belonging to the lips and the tongue. [L *labium* lip, *lingua* tongue.]

labiology (la·be·**ol**·o·je). The science which is concerned with the lips and their movements in singing and speaking. [L *labium* lip, Gk *logos* science.]

labiomancy (la·be·o·man·se). Lip reading. [L *labium* lip, Gk *manteia* divination.]

labiomandibular (la·be·o·man·**dib**′·ew·lar). Relating to the lip and the mandible. [L *labium* lip, *mandere* to chew.]

labiomental (la·be·o·men′·tal). Relating or belonging to the lips and the chin. [L *labium* lip, *mentum* chin.]

labiomycosis (la·be·o·mi·ko′·sis). Any morbid condition of the lips which is caused by infection with a fungus, e.g. thrush. [L *labium* lip, Gk *mykes* fungus, *-osis* condition.]

labionasal (la·be·o·na′·zal). Relating or belonging to the upper lip or to both lips and the nose; applied to a letter, such as *m*, the pronunciation of which requires co-operation of lips and nose. [L *labium* lip, *nasum* nose.]

labiopalatine (la·be·o·pal′·at·ine). Relating or belonging to the lip and the palate, considered as one structure. [L *labium* lip, palate.]

labioplacement (la·be·o·plase′·ment). Displacement towards the cheeks or lips, e.g. a tooth lying outside the normal arch. [L *labium* lip, displacement.]

labioplasty (la·be·o·plas′·te). Cheiloplasty; plastic surgery for repair of defect or injury of the lip. [L *labium* lip, Gk *plassein* to mould.]

labiotenaculum (la·be·o·ten·ak′·ew·lum). An instrument for seizing and holding any lip or labium in a given position during an operation. [L *labium* lip, tenaculum.]

labioversion (la·be·o·ver′·shun). The condition of being twisted or rotated in a labial direction, e.g. a tooth. [L *labium* lip, *vertere* to turn.]

labitome (lab·e·tome). A forceps the blades of which are sharp enough to cut. [Gk *labis* pincers, *temnein* to cut.]

labium [NA] (la·be·um) (pl. *labia*). Literally, a lip. Applied to various structures shaped like a lip. **Labium majus [labium majus pudendi (NA)].** One of a pair of prominent cutaneous folds bounding the pudendal cleft in a woman. **Labium minus [labium minus pudendi (NA)].** One of a pair of small cutaneous folds within the labium majus bounding the vestibule of the vagina. **Labium urethrae.** The modified skin around the external urethral orifice. **Labium uteri.** The opening of the external os uteri. The anterior lip is separated from the posterior lip only in those who have borne children. [L.]

Lab-Lemco (lab·**lem**·ko). A proprietary meat extract used as a substitute for the extract of fresh meat in the preparation of bacterial culture media.

laboratory (lab·or·at·or·e, **lab**·or·at·or·e). A room or building given over to experimental study of the sciences. [L *laborare* to work.]

Laborde, Jean Baptiste Vincent (b. 1830). Paris physiologist.

Laborde's forceps. A forceps for effecting artificial respiration by intermittent traction on the tongue.

Laborde's method. Rhythmical traction on the tongue to stimulate breathing.

Laborde's sign. Cloquet's sign.

labour (la·bor). The process by which the fetus and placenta are expelled from the uterus. It is usually divided into four stages. *First stage*: from the commencement of painful regular contractions of the uterus to full dilatation of the cervix. *Second stage*: from full dilatation of the cervix to delivery of the fetus. *Third stage*: from delivery of the child to delivery of the placenta. *Fourth stage*: following delivery of the placenta, when post-partum haemorrhage may occur. **Artificial labour.** Induced labour (see below). **Atonic labour.** Inert labour (see below). **Complicated labour.** A labour in which there has been some deviation from the normal. **Dry labour.** A labour in which there has been premature rupture of the membranes, and most of the liquor has drained away. **False labour.** Labour in which the patient has contractions of the uterus not unlike those of true labour, but there are no other signs that the patient is actually in labour, and the contractions eventually pass off. Also known as *missed labour* or *spurious labour.* **Induced labour.** Labour which has been started by drugs or mechanical means. Also known as *artificial labour.* **Inert labour.** Labour in which the uterus never contracts efficiently. Also known as *atonic labour.* **Instrumental labour.** Labour in which the use of instruments, such as forceps or perforators, is necessary for its completion. **Missed labour.** False labour (see above). **Obstructed labour.** Labour in which there is some mechanical obstruction which makes delivery of the child impossible. **Precipitate labour.** A very rapid labour; usually referring to those cases in which it is complete within an hour. **Premature labour.** Labour coming on before the expected date of delivery. **Prolonged labour, protracted labour.** Generally used to describe labour lasting 48 hours or longer. **Spontaneous labour.** Labour which comes on and is completed without any operative interference. **Spurious labour.** False labour (see above). **Test of labour.** A labour which is allowed to continue after the cervix has been fully dilated for a period of 2 hours. At the end of this time a final assessment is made as to the probability of vaginal delivery. **Trial labour.** Labour in which there is some doubt as to whether the head will pass through the brim of the pelvis. Therefore the patient is observed carefully during labour to see if the head descends progressively into the pelvic cavity, persistent non-engagement of the head, or fetal or maternal distress, being an indication for immediate delivery. [L *labor* work.]

labrocyte (lab·ro·site). A mast cell. [Gk *labros* gluttonous, *kytos* cell.]

labrum (la·brum). Literally a brim or lip. The term is applied to two structures only, the acetabular labrum and the glenoidal labrum. **Labrum acetabulare [NA].** The fibrocartilaginous rim attached to the margin of the acetabulum, deepening its concavity. **Labrum glenoidale [NA].** The fibrocartilaginous rim attached to the margin of the glenoid cavity, deepening its concavity. [L.]

labyrinth (lab·ir·inth). An interconnecting system of cavities, applied especially to the internal ear. **Acoustic labyrinth, aural labyrinth.** The cochlea of the inner ear, the vestibule, and the semicircular canals. **Bony labyrinth [labyrinthus osseus (NA)].** The bony framework of the internal ear. **Cortical labyrinth (NA).** The system of blood vessels and tubules of the cortex of the kidney. **Ethmoidal labyrinth [labyrinthus ethmoidalis (NA)].** The ethmoidal sinuses, made up of many air cells. **Membranous labyrinth [labyrinthus membranaceus (NA)].** The structures contained within the bony labyrinth. **Osseous labyrinth.** Bony labyrinth (see above). [Gk *labyrinthos* maze.]

labyrinthectomy (lab·ir·in·**thek'**·to·me). The operation of excising the aural labyrinth. [labyrinth, Gk *ektome* a cutting out.]

labyrinthine (lab·ir·in·thine). Relating or belonging to a labyrinth.

labyrinthitis (lab·ir·in·**thi'**·tis). Otitis interna; a condition of inflammation of the labyrinth. **Primary labyrinthitis.** Voltolini's disease. **Traumatic labyrinthitis.** Labyrinthitis due to accidental trauma, e.g. fracture of the skull, or to trauma during operation, e.g. fenestration. [labyrinth, Gk *-itis* inflammation.]

labyrinthotomy (lab·ir·in·**thot'**·o·me). The operation of incising the aural labyrinth. [labyrinth, Gk *temnein* to cut.]

labyrinthus (lab·ir·in·thus). Labyrinth.

lac (lak). 1. The Latin for *milk* (gen. *lactis*). 2. Name given to any milk-like preparation. **Lac caninum.** Dog's milk. **Lac coactum.** Curdled milk. **Lac defloratum.** Skimmed milk. **Lac sulphuris.** Precipitated sulphur. **Lac vaccinum.** Cow's milk.

Lacassagne, Antoine Marcelin (b. 1884). French physician.

Regaud and Lacassagne technique for cancer of the cervix uteri. The treatment of carcinoma of the neck of the uterus by means of uterine radium tubes and vaginal cork containers retained by a colpostat, using relatively small quantities of radium and continuous irradiation for 5 days. Also known as *Paris technique.*

lacca (lak·ah). Shellac; a resinous material prepared from a secretion that encrusts the bodies of *Tachardia lacca* Kerr, a scale insect that lives on the stems of various plants, some of which are cultivated especially for the purpose. It contains 70–80 per cent of resin, and a red colouring matter, laccaic acid; it is used in the manufacture of varnishes, polishes, and sealing wax, and for the enteric coating of pills and tablets. [It., varnish.]

lacerated (las·er·a·ted). Torn. [see foll.]

laceration (las·er·a·shun). 1. A rent or tear. 2. The act of tearing the tissues. **Laceration of the perineum.** Laceration, which may occur during labour, of the wall which separates the lower extremity of the vagina and the rectum. **Stellate laceration.** A star-shaped laceration, as of the neck of the uterus. [L *lacerare* to tear.]

lacertus (las·er·tus). In its original sense, the arm from shoulder to elbow; in the anatomical sense, a fibrous arm or band. **Lacertus of the lateral rectus muscle of the orbit [lacertus musculi recti lateralis (NA)].** A tendon forming part of the origin of the lateral rectus muscle of the orbit, attached to the orbital surface of the great wing of the sphenoid bone lateral to the common tendinous ring. [L.]

Lachesine Chloride BPC 1968 (lak·es·een klor·ide). E3; β-benziloyloxyethyldimethylethylammonium chloride. A mydriatic that is sometimes used instead of atropine.

Lachesis (lak·e·sis). A genus of Crotaline snakes of America: *Lachesis mutus*, the bushmaster, and *L. lanceolatus*, the fer-de-lance, are both very poisonous. [Gk, fate.]

lachrymal (lak·rim·al). Lacrimal.

lacinia (las·in·e·ah). Fimbria. **Laciniae tubae.** The fimbriae of the uterine tubes. [L, fringe.]

laciniate (las·in·e·ate). In zoology and botany, term descriptive of division into flaps, deep irregular parts, or segments coarser than fimbriae; fringed, jagged. [see prec.]

lacmoid (lak·moid). $C_{12}H_9O_4N$, a blue dye derived from resorcinol, soluble in alcohol and used as a pH indicator (4.4–6.4), being red in acid and blue in alkaline solution. **Lacmoid tincture.** A solution of lacmoid in a mixture of water and alcohol, employed as an indicator.

lacmus (lak·mus). Litmus. [G *Lackmus.*]

lacrima (lak·rim·ah). Tear. [L.]

lacrimal (lak·rim·al). Relating or belonging to or having the characteristics of tears. **Lacrimal apparatus.** *See* APPARATUS. **Lacrimal crest.** *See* CREST. **Lacrimal fascia.** *See* FASCIA. **Lacrimal groove.** *See* GROOVE. **Lacrimal papilla.** *See* PAPILLA. **Lacrimal process.** *See* PROCESS. **Lacrimal puncta.** Puncta lacrimalia. **Lacrimal sac.** *See* SAC. [L *lacrima* tear.]

lacrimal artery [arteria lacrimalis (NA)]. *See* OPHTHALMIC ARTERY.

lacrimal bone [os lacrimale (NA)]. A small delicate bone forming the anterior part of the medial wall of the orbit and part of the side wall of the nose. It articulates with the frontal bone, the maxilla, the inferior concha, and the orbital plate of the ethmoid bone.

lacrimal nerve [nervus lacrimalis (NA)]. A branch of the ophthalmic nerve, supplying sensory fibres to the lacrimal gland and conjunctiva and to the lateral part of the upper eyelid. **Communicating branch of the lacrimal nerve with the zygomatic nerve [ramus communicans cum nervo zygomatico (NA)].** A small nerve which runs from the zygomatic branch of the maxillary nerve to the lacrimal nerve, and thence to the lacrimal gland which it supplies with secretomotor fibres.

lacrimal vein [vena lacrimalis (NA)]. A tributary of the superior ophthalmic vein.

lacrimale (lak·rim·a·le). The point where the frontolacrimal suture and posterior lacrimal crest coincide.

lacrimation (lak·rim·a·shun). The secretion and flow of tears. [see foll.]

lacrimator (lak·rim·a·tor). A substance that causes the excessive secretion of tears. [L *lacrima* tear.]

lacrimatory (lak·rim·a·tor·e). Causing the secretion of tears. [see prec.]

lacrimonasal (lak·rim·o·na′·zal). Relating or belonging to the nose and the lacrimal apparatus; nasolacrimal. [L *lacrima* tear, *nasum* nose.]

lacrimotome (lak·rim·o·tome). A cutting instrument used in incisions of the lacrimal canaliculi or lacrimal sac. [lacrimal, Gk *temnein* to cut.]

lacrimotomy (lak·rim·ot·o·me). The operation of incising the lacrimal gland, canaliculus, or sac. [see prec.]

lactacidaemia (lakt·as·id·e′·me·ah). The presence of lactic acid in the blood. [lactic acid, Gk *haima* blood.]

lactaciduria (lakt·as·id·ewr′·e·ah). The presence of lactic acid in the urine.

lactagogue (lakt·ag·og). Galactagogue. [L *lac* milk, Gk *agogos* leading.]

lactalbumin (lakt·al·bew·min). A soluble heat-coagulable protein of the albumin class occurring in milk. In human milk it normally constitutes a much higher proportion of the total protein than in cows' milk. [L *lac* milk, albumin.]

lactam (lak·tam). The keto form of ring compound created by the elimination of a molecule of water from an aminocarboxylic acid. It contains the grouping NHCO. Cf. LACTIM.

lactamide (lak·tam·ide). Lactic acid amide, $CH_3CH(OH)CONH_2$. A colourless compound with alcoholic properties: an isomer of lactamine.

lactase (lak·taze). An enzyme occurring in the small intestine of mammals, in emulsin (from almonds), and in certain yeasts, which hydrolyses lactose yielding a mixture of glucose and galactose.

lactate (lak·tate). A salt of lactic acid.

lactation (lak·ta·shun). 1. The secretion of milk. 2. The period succeeding childbirth during which milk is secreted. [L *lac* milk.]

lactational (lak·ta·shun·al). Relating or belonging to lactation.

lacteal (lak·te·al). 1. Consisting of milk, or resembling milk; milky. 2. The lymph vessels of the small intestine which convey chyle. [L *lac* milk.]

lactescence (lak·tes·ens). 1. Milky appearance or quality. 2. The state of resembling milk; the quality of becoming milky. [L *lactescere* to become milky.]

lactic (lak·tik). 1. Relating or belonging to milk. 2. Derived from sour milk or whey, as lactic fermentation. [L *lac* milk.]

lacticaemia (lak·tis·e·me·ah). Lactacidaemia.

lactiferous (lak·tif·er·us). Secreting, yielding or conveying milk. **Lactiferous sinus.** *See* SINUS. [L *lac* milk, *ferre* to bear.]

lactific (lak·tif·ik). Milk-producing. [L *lac* milk, *facere* to make.]

lactiform (lak·te·form). Milk-like; having resemblance to milk. [L *lac* milk, form.]

lactifuge (lak·te·fewj). 1. Retarding or causing cessation of the secretion of milk. 2. An agent which lessens or causes cessation of the secretion of milk. [L *lac* milk, *fugare* to drive away.]

lactigenous (lak·tij·en·us). Producing milk; secreting milk. [L *lac* milk, Gk *genein* to produce.]

lactigerous (lak·tij·er·us). Lactiferous. [L *lac* milk, *gerere* to carry.]

lactim (lak·tim). The enol form of ring compound created by the elimination of a molecule of water from an aminocarboxylic acid. It contains the grouping N=C(OH). Cf. LACTAM.

lactimorbus (lak·te·mor·bus). Milk sickness. *See* SICKNESS. [L *lac* milk, *morbus* disease.]

lactinated (lak·tin·a·ted). Prepared with, or containing lactose (milk sugar).

lactiphagous (lak·tif·ag·us). Consuming milk. [L *lac* milk, Gk *phagein* to consume.]

lactipotous (lak·tip·o·tus). Milk-drinking. [L *lac* milk, *potare* to drink.]

lactisugium (lak·te·sew·je·um). A breast pump. [L *lac* milk, *sugere* to suck.]

lactivorous (lak·tiv·or·us). Subsisting or living on a diet of milk. [L *lac* milk, *vorare* to devour.]

Lactobacillus (lak·to·bas·il′·us). A bacterial genus belonging to the family Lactobacillaceae; they are Gram-positive, non-sporing rods, highly resistant to acid and are present in the intestine of man and other mammals, particularly during the suckling period. **Lactobacillus acidophil-aerogenes.** Micro-aerophilic organisms widely distributed in nature in soil, faeces, and fermenting plant material; a large group characterized by a vigorous fermentation of pentoses, especially arabinose. **Lactobacillus acidophilus.** A micro-aerophilic organism found in milk, faeces of bottle-fed infants and adults, and in saliva and carious teeth. **Lactobacillus arabinosus.** A species used in the microbiological assay of niacin (nicotinic acid). **Lactobacillus bifidus.** Anaerobic or micro-aerophilic, constitutes the predominant bacterial flora in the intestine. **Lactobacillus brevis.** *L. acidophil-aerogenes* (see above). **Lactobacillus bulgaricus.** Massol's bacillus; used for the production of yoghurt (a fermented milk). **Lactobacillus casei.** A species found in cheese. It is of medical importance since it can be used for the identification of a growth factor, the *L. casei* factor, a liver fraction which is apparently identical with folic acid. **Lactobacillus caucasicus.** A micro-aerophilic organism found in cheese and fermenting milk products. **Lactobacillus exilis.** A species similar to *L. acidophilus*, but more slender and constant in morphology. **Lactobacillus helveticus.** An organism originally found in Swiss cheese. **Lactobacillus odontolyticus.** An aerobic organism which may be causally associated with dental caries. **Lactobacillus panis, Lactobacillus pastorianus.** Poorly defined species found in fermenting animal and plant material. **Lactobacillus thermophilus.** An aerobic organism from pasteurized milk; it grows best at from 55° to 62°C. [L *lac* milk, bacillus.]

See also: BOAS, OPPLER.

lactobiose (lak·to·bi·oze). Lactose, milk sugar, $C_{12}H_{22}O_{11}$. A crystalline soluble disaccharide which occurs in the milk of all animals.

lactobutyrometer (lak·to·bew·tir·om′·et·er). An apparatus for estimating the proportion of cream in a sample of milk. [L *lac* milk, butyrometer.]

lactocele (lak·to·seel). Galactocele. [L *lac* milk, Gk *kele* hernia.]

lactocholin (lak·to·ko·lin). A derivative of bile prepared by heating an aqueous solution of it. [L *lac* milk, Gk *chole* bile.]

lactochrome (lak·to·krome). The yellow-coloured, water-soluble, naturally-occurring pigment found in the whey of milk, and belonging to the class of nitrogenous water-soluble pigments known as *lyochromes*. Lactochrome, so defined, had been identified chemically as riboflavine, a substance formerly called lactoflavine, and observed to possess vitamin-B_2 activity. The term *lactochrome* is, in consequence, now little used. [L *lac* milk, Gk *chroma* colour.]

lactoconium (lak·to·ko·ne·um). A term applied to the minute particles in milk, seen under the ultramicroscope. [Obsolete term.] [L *lac* milk, Gk *konis* dust.]

lactocrit (**lak**·to·krit). An instrument with which the fat content of milk may be determined. [L *lac* milk, *krites* judge.]

lactodensimeter (**lak**·to·den·**sim**'·et·er). Lactometer. [L *lac* milk, *densus* thick, meter.]

lactofarinaceous (**lak**·to·far·in·a'·shus). Consisting of milk and starch. [L *lac* milk, *farina* flour.]

lactoflavine (lac·to·**fla**·veen). Riboflavine, the name applied to a particular flavin, or water-soluble yellow pigment, belonging to the lyochrome class, which was first found to occur in milk, and then in various other foods and animal tissues, and was subsequently observed to possess vitamin-B_2 activity. The term *lactoflavine* is consequently now obsolete, and has been replaced by riboflavine. [L *lac* milk, *flavus* yellow.]

lactogen (**lak**·to·jen). Any agent that stimulates the secretion of milk. *See* PLACENTA. [L *lac* milk, Gk *genein* to produce.]

lactogenic (lak·to·**jen**·ik). Suitable for, or furthering, the production of milk. [see prec.]

lactoglobulin (lak·to·**glob**·ew·lin). A heat-coagulable protein which is insoluble in water and occurs with lactalbumin in milk. [L *lac* milk, globulin.]

lactometer (lak·**tom**·et·er). An instrument used in the estimation of the specific gravity of milk. [L *lac* milk, meter.]

lactone (**lak**·tone). A ring compound formed by the elimination of water from an organic hydroxyacid. [L *lac* milk.]

lactophosphate (lak·to·**fos**·fate). Any salt of lactic and phosphoric acids combined with the same base.

lactoprecipitin (**lak**·to·pre·**sip**'·it·in). A substance produced in the serum of an animal by injection of milk from a different species; it precipitates the milk casein. [L *lac* milk, precipitin.]

lactorrhoea (lak·to·**re**·ah). Galactorrhoea. [L *lac* milk, *rhoia* flow.]

lactosazone (lak·**to**·sa·zone). The osazone derived from lactose with phenylhydrazine: yellow crystals of very characteristic appearance which serve to identify lactose.

lactose (**lak**·toze). Lactobiose, milk sugar, $C_{12}H_{22}O_{11}$. A crystalline soluble disaccharide (α-glucose-β-galactoside) which occurs in the milk of all animals, and is manufactured from whey in cheese-making. It is less soluble and less sweet than sucrose, and is non-fermentable by ordinary yeasts, but in the lactic fermentation of milk is converted into lactic acid. It is hydrolysed by lactase into glucose and galactose, and is used as a base in tablet making (BP 1973). **Beta lactose.** A more soluble form of lactose obtained by crystallizing from a hot solution of ordinary milk sugar. [L *lac* milk.]

lactoserum (lak·to·**se**·rum). The serum of an animal which has received injections of milk from a different species. The serum contains lactoprecipitin which precipitates the milk casein. [L *lac* milk, serum.]

lactosin (**lak**·to·sin). $C_{36}H_{62}O_{31}$, a complex polysaccharide built of lactose units.

Lactosum (lak·**to**·sum). *European Pharmacopoeia* name for Lactose BP 1973.

lactosuria (lak·to·**sewr**·e·ah). Excretion of lactose in the urine.

lactotherapy (lak·to·**ther**·ap·e). 1. Treatment by the administration of a diet consisting exclusively or almost exclusively of milk; milk cure. 2. Protein shock by injection of milk. [L *lac* milk, therapy.]

lactotoxin (lak·to·**tox**·in). A name applied to any of the toxic bases occurring in milk as the result of the decomposition of protein. [L *lac* milk, Gk *toxikon* poison.]

lactovegetarian (**lak**·to·vej·e·**ta**'·re·an). 1. An individual whose diet consists of eggs, milk, and vegetables. 2. Composed of milk and vegetables. [L *lac* milk, vegetarian.]

Lactuca (lak·**tew**·kah). A genus of plants of the family Compositae. **Lactuca sativa.** The common garden lettuce. **Lactuca scariola.** Prickly lettuce; a species used in medicine like wild lettuce (see following). **Lactuca virosa.** Wild lettuce, strong-scented lettuce; the dried latex was known as *lactucarium* or *lettuce opium*, the reddish or greyish-brown irregular pieces having a bitter taste and odour similar to opium. It contains the crystalline substance, lactucerin, and various bitter principles, and has from earliest times been credited with soporific properties. It has been used to allay cough and quiet nervous irritation, but its value is purely psychological. There is also doubt about its mydriatic properties. [L, lettuce.]

lactucarium (lak·tew·**ka**·re·um). The dried latex obtained from *Lactuca virosa* Linn., also known as *lettuce opium*. It is used as an anodyne and hypnotic, and as a sedative for coughs.

lactucerin (lak·**tew**·ser·in). A crystalline compound occurring in wild lettuce, *Lactuca virosa*.

lactucerol (lak·**tew**·ser·ol). $C_{18}H_{30}O$, a monohydroxy alcohol obtained from lactucarium.

lactucism (**lak**·tew·sizm). Poisoning caused by excessive dosage of preparations of various species of *Lactuca*. Headache, dyspnoea, giddiness, dilatation of the pupils and ataxic gait are the characteristic symptoms of the condition.

lactucol (**lak**·tew·kol). $C_{13}H_{20}O$, a crystalline compound prepared from lactucerin.

Lactulose (**lak**·tew·loze). BP Commission approved name for 4-*O*-β-D-galactopyranosyl-D-fructose; it is used in the treatment of hepatic coma and chronic constipation.

lactulum unguis (**lak**·tew·lum **ung**·gwis). The nail bed. [L, nourishing bed of the nail.]

lactyl (**lak**·til). The organic grouping, $CH_3CHOHCO$, corresponding to lactic acid.

lacuna [NA] (lak·**ew**·nah). Literally, a small pit or depression; it is also applied to any small space, actual or potential, or small defect. **Absorption lacuna.** Howship's lacuna; any small space in a bone where resorption is taking place. **Air lacuna.** Any small space filled with air. **Blood lacuna.** Any small space lined with epithelium and filled with blood; it is usually reserved for use in connection with an embryo. **Intervillous lacunae.** The blood spaces within which the villi of the placenta lie. **Lacuna lateralis [NA].** One of the small sinuses in the dura mater that communicate with the superior sagittal sinus. **Lacuna magna.** A small recess in the terminal part of the penile part of the male urethra. **Lacuna musculorum [NA].** The lateral part of the space between the inguinal ligament and the hip bone. It is occupied by the iliacus and pectineus muscles. **Parasinoidal lacuna.** Lacuna lateralis (see above). **Lacunae urethrales [NA].** Morgagni's lacunae; the numerous small depressions in the urethral mucous membrane into each of which a urethral gland opens; they are most common in the bulbous urethra. **Lacuna vasorum [NA].** The medial part of the space between the inguinal ligament and the hip bone. It is occupied by the femoral vessels and nerve and the femoral canal. **Venous lacuna.** Lacuna lateralis (see above). [L.]

See also: HOWSHIP, MORGAGNI.

lacunar (lak·**ew**·nar). Relating or belonging to, or characterized by the presence of lacunae.

lacunose (lak·**ew**·noze). Having depressions, pits, recesses, or spaces; full of hollows. [L *lacuna* pit.]

lacunula, lacunule (lak·**ew**·new·lah, lak·**ew**·newl). A very small lacuna; one of the air spaces to be observed microscopically in a grey hair. [dim. of lacuna.]

lacus lacrimalis [NA] (**lak**·us lak·rim·**a**·lis). A triangular area at the medial angle of the eye, bounded above and below by the hairless portion of the margin of the eyelid, and containing the lacrimal caruncle. [L, lake of tears.]

Ladd-Franklin, Christine (b. 1847). Baltimore psychologist.

Ladd-Franklin's theory. An evolutionary theory of colour vision: in the first stage of development it is suggested that there is a light-sensitive substance in the rods which is stimulated by light to liberate a reactive product which causes the sensation of white light. In the next stage this substance becomes more specific and liberates two reactive products, one for each end of the spectrum, and causing the sensation of yellow and blue, e.g. peripheral cones in man. In the final stage, the reactive product giving the sensation of yellow becomes two products giving the sensation of red and green, e.g. the central cones in man.

Laelaps (le·laps). A genus of mites. **Laelaps jettmari.** A mite of the common house mouse suspected as a vector of epidemic haemorrhagic disease. **Laelaps stabularis.** A species of nymphs which have been recorded as human parasites in Europe, causing pruritus. They are found in farm buildings. [Gk *lailaps* hurricane.]

laemoparalysis (le·mo·par·al′·is·is). Paralysis of the oesophagus. [Gk *laimos* gullet, paralysis.]

laemostenosis (le·mo·sten·o′·sis). Stricture of the oesophagus or pharynx. [Gk *laimos* gullet, stenosis.]

Laënnec, René Théophile Hyacinthe (b. 1781). Paris physician.

Laënnec's catarrh. Asthmatic bronchitis with a viscous sputum.

Laënnec's cirrhosis. Cirrhosis of the liver.

Laënnec's disease. 1. Dissecting aneurysm. *See* ANEURYSM. 2. Laënnec's cirrhosis: cirrhosis of the liver.

Laënnec's pearls. Small pellets, resembling boiled sago grains, expectorated during a paroxysm of asthma. They consist of a central refractive nucleus of mucinoid material with threads of mucus coiled spirally around it.

Laënnec's sign. The presence of Laënnec's pearls in the sputum in asthma.

laevo- (le·vo). A prefix indicating *left* in contradistinction to *right* (dextra); used in the nomenclature of organic chemistry it indicates a compound which, in solution, rotates to the left the plane of a beam of polarized light passed through it. In modern nomenclature L is not an abbreviation for 'laevo' and therefore does not necessarily mean that a substance is laevorotatory: it is purely a configurational symbol. Optical activity is indicated by a plus or minus sign following the prefix, e.g. L(−)-glyceraldehyde. [L *laevus* left.]

laevoangiocardiogram (le·vo·an·je·o·kar′·de·o·gram). The radiographs made during laevoangiocardiography. [L *laevus* left, angiocardiogram.]

laevoangiocardiography (le·vo·an·je·o·kar·de·og′·raf·e). The study of the left chambers of the heart by x-ray means after injection of radio-opaque contrast medium into the left ventricle. [L *laevus* left, angiocardiography.]

laevocardia (le·vo·kar·de·ah). The situation in which the apex of the heart is directed towards the left; with normal visceral situs this is the normal state of affairs. **Isolated laevocardia.** Laevocardia occurring with situs inversus; the heart is always grossly abnormal. [L *laevus* left, Gk *kardia* heart.]

laevocardiogram (le·vo·kar·de·o·gram). 1. The complex derived from a unipolar electrode facing the left ventricle, consisting of a small Q wave and a large R wave. Cf. DEXTROCARDIOGRAM. 2. The terms laevocardiogram and dextrocardiogram have been used to describe the appearances in the three standard leads in horizontal hearts with left axis deviation, and in vertical hearts with right axis deviation, respectively. The laevocardiogram would thus consist of a tracing showing a predominant R wave in lead I, and a predominant S wave in lead III, while the dextrocardiogram would show a large S in lead I, and a large R in lead III. 3. *See* LAEVOANGIOCARDIOGRAM. [L *laevus* left, electrocardiogram.]

laevoclination (le·vo·klin·a′·shun). A turning or twisting to the left; in particular, involuntary intorsion of the right eye and extorsion of the left eye. [L *laevus* left, *clinatus* bent.]

laevocycloduction (le·vo·si·klo·duk′·shun). In ophthalmology, the amount by which the eyes can be rotated to the left on their anteroposterior axes. [L *laevus* left, Gk *kyklos* circle, L *ducere* to lead.]

laevoduction (le·vo·duk·shun). In ophthalmology, the amount in degrees by which the eye or eyes can be moved to the left from the primary position. [L *laevus* left, *ducere* to lead.]

laevoglucose (le·vo·gloo·kose). Laevulose, fruit sugar, fructose, $C_6H_{12}O_6$. A monosaccharide which occurs with D-glucose in fruit and honey. It is laevorotatory, sweeter than glucose and fermentable.

laevogram (le·vo·gram). Laevocardiogram.

laevogyrate, laevogyric, laevogyrous (le·vo·ji·rate, le·vo·ji·rik, le·vo·ji·rus). Laevorotatory. [L *laevus* left, *gyrare* to turn.]

Laevolosum (le·vew·lo·sum). *European Pharmacopoeia* name for Laevulose BP 1973.

laevophobia (le·vo·fo·be·ah). Abnormal fear of objects situated at the left side of the body. [L *laevus* left, phobia.]

laevophoria (le·vo·for·e·ah). Tendency of the visual lines to turn to the left. [L *laevus* left, *pherein* to bear.]

laevorotation (le·vo·ro·ta′·shun). 1. The rotation of the plane of polarized light to the left in a counter-clockwise direction. 2. In cardiology, isolated laevocardia supposedly due to rotation to the left about the long axis of the body of a heart, of which the development had commenced normally for situs inversus. [L *laevus* left, *rotare* to turn.]

laevorotatory (le·vo·ro·tat·or·e). Having the power, when in solution, of rotating to the left in a counter-clockwise direction the plane of a beam of polarized light passed through it. [see prec.]

laevothyroxine (le·vo·thi·rox′·een). Synthetic laevorotatory thyroxine. [L *laevus* left, thyroxine.]

laevotorsion (le·vo·tor·shun). Laevoclination. [L *laevus* left, torsion.]

laevoversion (le·vo·ver·shun). 1. Turning to the left, e.g. of the eyes. 2. In cardiology, laevorotation. [L *laevus* left, *vertere* to turn.]

laevulin (le·vew·lin). Synanthrose, $(C_6H_{10}O_5)_n$. A carbohydrate isomeric with inulin, which occurs in the rhizomes of *Helianthus tuberosus.*

laevulosaemia (le·vew·lo·se′·me·ah). The presence of laevulose in the blood. [laevulose, Gk *haima* blood.]

laevulosan (le·vew·lo·san). Fructosan, $(C_6H_{10}O_5)_n$. Term denoting a polysaccharide such as inulin, composed of laevulose units.

laevulosazone (le·vew·lo·sa·zone). An osazone formed from laevulose with phenylhydrazine; it is identical with glucosazone.

Laevulose BP 1973 (le·vew·loze). D-Fructose, $C_6H_{12}O_6$, a diagnostic agent in assessing hepatic insufficiency. Injected intravenously in preference to dextrose as a source of carbohydrate in the treatment of renal failure. It is also used in the management of neonatal hypoglycaemia of newborn infants of diabetic mothers who have received a large dose of insulin.

laevulosuria (le·vew·lo·sewr′·e·ah). The presence of laevulose in the urine.

Laewen, Georg Arthur (b. 1876). Königsberg surgeon.

Buedinger-Ludloff-Laewen disease. Osteomalacia of the patella.

lag (lag). 1. The time elapsing between the application of a stimulus and the appearance of the resulting reaction. 2. Lag period. *See* PERIOD. **Genotypic lag.** In bacteria which contain more than one chromosome copy, the time elapsing between the occurrence of a mutation in one chromosome, or the formation of a recombinant chromosome, and the segregation of a bacterium carrying only altered chromosomes. **Phenotypic lag.** The time required for the expression of an allelic gene, arising in a haploid cell by mutation or introduced by sexual transfer; usually occurring only with recessive alleles and depending on segregation of a cell devoid of wild-type chromosomes. **Quadriceps lag.** Inability of the quadriceps femoris muscle to produce the final stage of extension at the knee joint in which lateral rotation of the tibia occurs. [etym. dub.]

lagaena (laj·e·nah). The termination of the duct of the cochlea. It is more commonly used in comparative anatomy for the representative of the whole cochlea in primitive vertebrates. [L, flask.]

lageniform (laj·en·e·form). Shaped like a flask, i.e. increasing from a slender neck to a dilatation below. [L *lagaena* flask, form.]

lagging (lag·ging). The loss of a chromosome, usually a sex-chromosome because it lags behind the other chromosome in meiotic division and therefore fails to appear in the resulting sex-chromosome pattern.

lagnesis, lagnosis (lag·**ne**·sis, lag·**no**·sis). Pathological increased heterosexual desire in the male. **Lagnesis furor.** Uncontrollable sexual desire. [Gk *lagneia* lust.]

Lagochilascaris (la·go·kil·**as**′·kar·is). A genus of round worms of which *Lagochilascaris minor,* found normally in wild cats, has been recorded rarely in abscesses in man in central America. [Gk *lagos* hare, *cheilos* lip, *askaris* pinworm.]

lagophthalmia, lagophthalmos, lagophthalmus (lag·of·**thal**·-me·ah, lag·of·**thal**·mos, lag·of·**thal**·mus). An abnormal condition in which the eyes cannot be entirely closed because, owing to involvement of the facial nerve, the upper eyelid cannot descend; hare eye. [Gk *lagos* hare, *ophthalmos* eye.]

Lagrange, Pierre Felix (b. 1857). Bordeaux ophthalmologist.

Lagrange's operation, or sclerectomy. A drainage procedure for chronic glaucoma: a sclerecto-iridectomy is performed by making a small scleral section between 10 o'clock and 2 o'clock with a conjunctival flap. A cigar-shaped piece of sclera is excised from the scleral flap and a complete iridectomy performed. It has many modifications. *See* BERENS' OPERATION, HOLTH'S OPERATION.

Lahey, Frank Howard (b. 1880). Boston surgeon.

Lahey's operation. Two-stage excision of pharyngeal diverticulum.

Laigret, J. 19th century French Colonial physician.

Laigret-Durand vaccine. A living vaccine, dried, suspended in egg yolk and in olive oil.

Laimer-Haeckermann area. A small, roughly triangular area on the posterior pharyngeal wall, through which the lining of the pharynx may herniate and produce a branchial pouch. It is a weak spot, since it lacks the support of fibres of the constrictor muscle, being in fact an interval between the oblique and the horizontal fibres of the inferior constrictor muscle of the pharynx.

Lain, Everett Samuel (b. 1876). Oklahoma dermatologist.

Lain's disease. Burning of the soft tissues of the mouth produced by galvanic action due to the use of dissimilar metals in dentistry.

laiose (la·e·oze). The name given by Hans Leo to a sugar which he discovered in a specimen of urine of a diabetic. It is believed to be a heptose, the occurrence of which in urine is extremely rare.

laira (la·rah). An epidemic hysteria, characterized by the utterance of barking sounds, which affected a large number of women at Arnon, France, in 1613 and at Blackthorn, Oxfordshire, in 1700.

lake (lake). A small cavity or depression containing fluid. **Lacrimal lake.** Lacus lacrimalis, the prolongation inward of the palpebral fissure of the eyelids. [L *lacus* lake.]

Lake, Norman Claudius (b. 1888). London surgeon.

Lake's technique. A technique of spinal analgesia using light cinchocaine solution. Described in 1938.

laked (la·kt). Describing blood which has become transparent and dark red in colour as the result of the release of the haemoglobin from the erythrocytes, effected by various chemical and physical agencies. [Fr. *laque* deep red colouring matter.]

lakmoid (lak·moid). Lacmoid.

lalia (lal·e·ah). Speech. [Gk.]

laliatry (lal·i·at·re). The science which is concerned with speech disorders and their treatment. [Gk *lalia* speech, *iatreia* treatment.]

lallation (lal·a·shun). A speech defect in which the subject avoids the use of all difficult consonants and speaks like a baby. [L *lallare* to babble like a child.]

Lallemand, Claude François (b. 1790). Montpellier surgeon.

Lallemand's body, Lallemand-Trousseau body. A cylindrical body in coagulated seminal-vesicle secretion.

lalling (lal·ing). Lallation.

lalognosis (lal·og·no·sis). The science of understanding speech, particularly lallation. [Gk *lalia* speech, *gnosis* a knowing.]

laloneurosis (lal·o·newr·o′·sis). Any nervous disorder which is characterized by incoherence or other defect of speech. [Gk *lalia* speech, neurosis.]

lalopathology (lal·o·path·**ol**′·o·je). That banch of medicine concerned with speech disorders. [Gk *lalia* speech, pathology.]

lalopathy (lal·**op**·ath·e). Any disorder which gives rise to speech defect. [Gk *lalia* speech, *pathos* disease.]

lalophobia (lal·o·**fo**·be·ah). A morbid dread of speaking or of even trying to speak, leading to muscular spasm; the condition is often present in stutterers. [Gk *lalia* speech, phobia.]

laloplegia (lal·o·**ple**·je·ah). A condition of paralysis, not of the tongue but of the muscles concerned in speaking. [Gk *lalia* speech, *plege* stroke.]

lalorrhoea (lal·o·**re**·ah). A condition characterized by an excessive or abnormal flow of words; abnormal talkativeness. [Gk *lalia* speech, *rhoia* flow.]

Lalouette, Pierre (b. 1711). Paris physician.

Pyramid of Lalouette. The pyramidal or median lobe of the thyroid gland.

Lamarck, Jean Baptiste Pierre Antoine de Monet, Chevalier de (b. 1744). French naturalist.

Lamarck's theory. Characters acquired by parents during their life can be inherited by the offspring and later generations.

lamarckism (lah·**mark**·izm). The advocacy of Lamarck's theory.

lambda (**lam**·dah). 1. The eleventh letter of the Greek alphabet. 2. The point of junction of the sagittal and lambdoid sutures, and the site of the posterior fontanelle of the skull. **Lambda chain.** One of the two classes of immunoglobulin light chains. **Lambda wave.** *See* ELECTRO-ENCEPHALOGRAPH. [Gk, letter l.]

lambdacism, lambdacismus (**lam**·dah·sizm, lam·dah·**siz**·mus). 1. A type of stammering in which the letter *r* is pronounced as *l*; too frequent use of the letter *l* in speaking. 2. Inability to produce the sound of the letter *l*, or difficulty in producing it. [Gk *lambda*, letter *l*.]

lambdoid, lambdoidal (**lam**·doid, lam·**doid**·al). In shape like the Greek letter *lambda* (Λ, λ). [Gk *lambda* letter *l*, *eidos* form.]

Lambert, Alexander (b. 1861). New York physician.

Lambert's treatment. For opium addicts: the amount of opium is reduced daily by one-tenth of the amount the patient had been taking and replaced by gradually increasing amounts of codeine from 0.03 g every 4 hours to 0.3 g every 4 hours. The administration of codeine is continued for 4 days after the opium has been discontinued, and is then tapered off.

Towns-Lambert treatment. For drug addiction: systematic purging, gradual withdrawal of the drug, and the prescribing of belladonna, hyoscyamus, and xanthoxylum.

Lambert, E. H. (b. 1915). American neurologist.

Eaton-Lambert syndrome. Myasthenia occasionally accompanying bronchial carcinoma.

Lambert, Johann Heinrich (b. 1728). German physicist and mathematician.

Lambert's cosine law. The intensity of radiation falling on a surface is directly proportional to the cosine of the angle of incidence of the ray.

Lambert's law of light absorption. The percentage of light transmitted by a homogeneous medium decreases in geometrical progression as the thickness of the medium increases in arithmetical progression. The relationship is given by the formula $I = I_0 \exp(-ax)$, where I and I_0 are the respective intensities of the light entering and leaving the medium, x the thickness of the medium, and a the absorption coefficient of the medium for the particular wavelength. *See also:* BEER'S LAW.

Lambert, Victor Francis. British otolaryngologist.

Lambert-Watson operation. A method of treating malignant disease of the larynx by the application of x-rays direct to the growth, after the removal of the thyroid ala on the affected side.

lambert (**lam**·bert). In physics, a unit of luminance (or intensity per unit area), being the brightness of a perfectly diffusing surface, whether self-luminous or lighted by an outside source, emitting or reflecting one lumen per square centimetre. [Johann Heinrich *Lambert*.]

Lambl's excrescences. Tiny delicate warty polyps attached to the left atrioventricular or aortic valves of the heart; most likely the result of organization of thrombi, but sometimes due to mucoid degeneration of part of a valve.

lamblia intestinalis (**lam**·ble·ah in·**tes**·tin·**a'**·lis). *Giardia intestinalis.* [Wilhelm Dusan *Lambl*, b. 1824, Czechoslovakian physician.]

lambliasis (lam·**bli**·as·is). A condition in which there is infestation with the intestinal flagellate *Giardia intestinalis* (*Lamblia intestinalis*); giardiasis.

lambliogenic (**lam**·ble·o·**jen'**·ik). Produced by *Giardia intestinalis* (*Lamblia intestinalis*). [*Lamblia*, Gk *genein* to produce.]

Lambrinudi, Constantine (b. 1890). London surgeon.

Lambrinudi's disease. Metatarsus primus elevatus.

Lambrinudi's drop-foot operation. Midtarsal and subastragalar arthrodesis: the astragalus is placed in the full equinus position; the head is shaped to a sharp edge which is placed in a deep groove cut in the inferior half of the tarsal navicular bone.

lamella (lam·**el**·ah). 1. A thin plate or layer. 2. A thin disc of glycogelatin, 3 mm in diameter, containing medicament and intended to be applied to the eyeball; the glycogelatin dissolves and the medicament is absorbed. **Lamella of bone.** The structural unit of mature bone in the form of a thin shell-like plate of bone matrix. **Concentric lamella.** One of a series of lamellae arranged around the central haversian canal of cortical bone. **Enamel lamella.** A band of organic matter running from the enamel surface towards the dentine of a tooth. **Intermediate lamella.** A bony lamella lying between haversian systems of concentric lamellae. **Interstitial lamellae.** Curved plates of bone lying between the definitive haversian systems of cortical bone. They represent persisting fragments of older haversian systems which have been partly resorbed to make way for new. **Osseous lamella.** Lamella of bone (see above). **Periosteal lamella, peripheral lamella.** A bony lamella lying near the surface of a bone, adjacent to the periosteum. **Triangular lamella.** The pial covering of the roof of the 3rd ventricle of the brain between the choroid plexuses. **Vascular lamella.** A thin sheet of well vascularized tissue. **Vitreous lamella.** The innermost layer of the choroid adjoining the retina. [L, a small plate.]

See also: HAVERS.

lamellar (lam·**el**·ar). Arranged in, composed of, or characterized by lamellae.

lamina [NA] (**lam**·in·ah). A thin plate. **Lamina affixa [NA].** That part of the medial wall of the telencephalic vesicle which has been invaginated by the dorsal surface of the thalamus and in the adult lies in the floor of the lateral ventricle and overlies the thalamus. **Alar lamina [lamina alaris].** The posterolateral part of the embryonic neural tube into which the sensory nerves enter. **Basal lamina [lamina basalis (NA)].** 1. The anterolateral part of the embryonic neural tube from which motor nerve roots emerge. 2. Basal (basement) lamina, the layer of material, 50–80 nm thick, which lies adjacent to the plasma membrane of the basal surfaces of epithelial cells. It contains collagen and certain carbohydrates. It is often called "basement membrane" but this term is best reserved for the apparent membrane which is seen with the light microscope. **Basal lamina of the choroid [lamina basalis (NA)].** A thin, structureless membrane covering the inner surface of the choroid. **Basal lamina of the ciliary body [lamina basalis (NA)].** A thin, apparently structureless lamina between the stroma of the ciliary body and the pigment layer on its deep surface. It is continuous behind with the basal lamina of the choroid. **Basement lamina.** Basal lamina (see above). **Basilar lamina [lamina basilaris (NA)].** The basilar membrane. **Choriocapillary lamina [lamina choroidocapillaris (NA)].** The middle layer of the choroid, in which lie many capillary blood vessels. **Choroid lamina.** Any part of the epithelial lining of the ventricles of the brain from which a choroid plexus is formed. **Lamina cribrosa sclerae [lamina episcleralis (NA)].** That part of the sclera pierced by the optic nerve. **Lamina of the cricoid cartilage.** *See* CARTILAGE. **Dental lamina.** An invagination of the ectoderm in the embryonic mouth, from which the enamel organs of the teeth are formed. **Elastic lamina, anterior [lamina limitans anterior (NA)].** Bowman's lamina; a thin tough membrane immediately beneath the corneal epithelium. **Elastic lamina, external.** The outer of two compact layers of elastic fibres found in the walls of arteries. **Elastic lamina, internal.** The inner of the two layers of elastic fibres found in the walls of arteries. **Elastic lamina, posterior [lamina limitans posterior (NA)].** A membrane lining the inner aspect of the substantia propria of the cornea. **Lamina elastica.** A layer of elastic tissue found in the walls of the trachea and bronchi. **Lamina epithelialis [NA].** The layer of modified epithelial cells which cover the choroid plexuses. **Lamina fusca sclerae [NA].** A thin loose areolar tissue, brown in colour on the inner surface of the sclera, connecting it to the choroid. **Labiogingival lamina.** An ectodermal invagination which in the embryo separates the lips from the gums. **Medullary laminae of the thalamus [laminae medullares thalami (NA)].** A layer of collagenous fibres separating some of the thalamic nuclei. **Medullary lamina of the thalamus, external [lamina medullaris lateralis (NA)].** A layer of white matter on the lateral surface of the thalamus. **Medullary lamina of the thalamus, internal [lamina medullaris medialis (NA)].** A vertical Y-shaped layer of white matter which subdivides the thalamus into the medial, anterior, and lateral nuclei. **Lamina of the modiolus [lamina modioli (NA)].** Osseous spiral lamina (see below). **Lamina muscularis mucosae [NA].** A smooth muscle layer responsible for movements of the mucous membrane on the oesophagus, stomach, small intestine, colon, and rectum. It lies in the deepest part of the mucous membrane. **Neural lamina.** Lamina of the vertebral arch (see below). **Osseous spiral lamina [lamina spiralis ossea (NA)].** A spiral flange of bone projecting from the modiolus of the cochlea, to which the basilar membrane is attached. **Lamina of the pharyngotympanic tube, lateral [lamina (cartilaginis) lateralis (NA)].** The lateral slope of the cartilaginous part of the pharyngotympanic tube. It is united above to the medial lamina. **Lamina of the pharyngotympanic tube, medial [lamina (cartilaginis) medialis (NA)].** The medial slope of the cartilaginous part of the pharyngotympanic tube. It is wider than the lateral lamina, to which it is united above. **Lamina of the pharyngotympanic tube, membranous [lamina membranacea (NA)].** The fibrous membrane which joins the lower margin of the medial and lateral laminae of the pharyngotympanic tube and completes the tube below. **Lamina propria, Lamina propria mucosae [NA].** The connective tissue of a mucous membrane, containing blood vessels, lymphatics, etc. **Pterygoid lamina, lateral.** The lateral pterygoid plate of the sphenoid bone. **Pterygoid lamina, medial.** The medial pterygoid plate of the sphenoid bone. **Quadrigeminal lamina.** Tectal lamina (see below). **Reticular lamina of the cochlea, reticular lamina of the spiral organ.** A net-like membrane in the spiral organ having holes in it for the outer hair cells. **Secondary spiral lamina [lamina spiralis secundaria (NA)].** A ridge projecting from the outer wall of the bony spiral canal of the cochlea towards the osseous spiral lamina. It is present only in the first half-turn of the cochlea. **Laminae of the septum lucidum [laminae septi pellucidi (NA)].** Two thin sheets making up the septum lucidum which separates the cavities of the lateral ventricles anteriorly. **Spiral lamina.** Osseous spiral lamina (see above). **Suprachoroid lamina [lamina suprachoroidea (NA)].** The outer pigmented layer of the choroid. **Tectal lamina [lamina tecti (NA)].** The thin plate of grey and white matter, forming the roof of the mid-brain, from which project the quadrigeminal bodies. **Lamina terminalis [NA].** The anterior wall of the 3rd ventricle of the brain. **Lamina of the thyroid cartilage.** *See* CARTILAGE. **Lamina of the tragus [lamina tragi (NA)].** A cartilaginous lamina forming the commencement of the cartilage of the external auditory meatus. **Vascular lamina of the choroid [lamina vasculosa (NA)].** The outer vascular layer of the choroid. **Lamina of the vertebral arch [lamina arcus vertebrae (NA)].** The posterolateral part on each side of the vertebral arch between the roots of the spine and transverse process. **Vestibular lamina.** Labiogingival lamina (see above). **Lamina vitrea.** Basal lamina of the choroid (see above). **White laminae [laminae albae (NA)].** White matter forming the cores of the folia of the cerebellum. [L, thin plate.]

See also: BOWMAN.

laminagram (**lam**·in·ah·gram). A radiograph of a selected layer of the body taken by means of laminagraphy (or tomography).

laminagraph (**lam**·in·ah·graf). An x-ray apparatus which will reproduce a selected layer of the body sharply on a radiograph. [L *lamina* thin plate, Gk *graphein* to record.]

laminagraphy (lam·in·**ag**·raf·e). Radiography of selected layers of the body by means of a laminagraph (or tomograph).

laminar (**lam**·in·ar). Arranged in laminae, or composed of them.

Laminaria (lam·in·a·re·ah). A genus of seaweeds (family Laminariaceae), belonging to the Brown Algae. Several species, particularly *Laminaria cloustoni* Edm., are used as a source of alginic acid and alginates. The dried stalks of *L. digitata* Lam. have been employed surgically to dilate cavities. [L *lamina* thin plate.]

laminated (**lam**·in·a·ted). Laminar.

lamination (lam·in·a·shun). 1. Arrangement in the form of laminae or thin flat plates. 2. In embryotomy, the cutting of the fetal head in slices. 3. The action of laminating.

laminectomy (lam·in·**ek**·to·me). The operation of removing the laminae of a vertebral arch. [lamina, Gk *ektome* a cutting out.]

laminitis (lam·in·i·tis). Inflammation affecting any lamina. A term more frequently used in veterinary science. [lamina, Gk *-itis* inflammation.]

laminogram (**lam**·in·o·gram). Laminagram.

laminograph (**lam**·in·o·graf). Laminagraph.

laminography (lam·in·**og**·raf·e). Laminagraphy.

laminotomy (lam·in·**ot**·o·me). Division of the laminae of a vertebral arch. [lamina, Gk *temnein* to cut.]

lamp (lamp). A device for provision of artificial illumination. **Annealing lamp.** A spirit lamp used to anneal the gold foil intended as a filling for a cavity prepared in a tooth. **Arc lamp.** A low-voltage, high-current, electrical discharge between electrodes, the incandescent ends of the electrodes and the gas between them giving an intense source of light rich in ultraviolet light. **Carbon arc lamp.** An open-flame arc lamp (see prec.) employing carbon electrodes. It is used as a source of ultraviolet light. **Cold quartz mercury-vapour lamp.** A source of ultraviolet rays of low pressure and requiring a low amperage. **Halide lamp.** An alcohol burner with a copper filament, used in the detection of organic halides in the presence of which the flame becomes green. **Mercury-vapour lamp.** An evacuated quartz lamp containing a trace of mercury which is vaporized when an arc is struck; it is a powerful source of ultraviolet radiations. There are many types, air- and water-cooled. **Mignon lamp.** A tiny electric lamp used in cystoscopy. **Pentane lamp.** A lamp burning pentane, once used as a standard of illumination. **Pointolite lamp.** A small homogeneous source of light produced by a glowing tungsten ball. It is used for the examination of the eye in ophthalmoscopy. **Quartz lamp.** A mercury-vapour lamp constructed of quartz which transmits ultraviolet light. **Slit lamp.** Any of the many modifications of Gullstrand's original model. In the latest types, the beam can be made to coincide with the axis of a microscope, thus allowing the examination of the fundus of the eye in addition to the cornea, lens, and vitreous. **Sun lamp.** A source of light with a spectrum similar to the sun; the carbon-arc lamp (see above) possesses these characteristics. **Ultraviolet lamp.** 1. A source of ultraviolet radiation such as a carbon arc or mercury-vapour lamp (see above). 2. An electric-light bulb made of a glass that transmits ultraviolet light. **Uviol lamp.** A trade name for a lamp producing a light of high ultraviolet content. [Gk *lampas* torch.]

See also: BIRCH-HIRSCHFELD (A.), BURDICK, DUKE-ELDER, EDRIDGE-GREEN, FINSEN (N. R.), GULLSTRAND, KROMAYER, LISTER (W.), LOMHOLT, NERNST, REYN.

lampblack (**lamp**·blak). Carbon black. A form of fine carbon prepared by burning oil, tar, resin, or other substances rich in carbon, in a deficiency of air. Used as a filler in rubber manufacture, and as a pigment in inks and paint. [lamp, AS *blac.*]

Lampropedia (lam·pro·**pe**·de·ah). A genus of bacteria with cells united in tetrads, forming flat tubular masses containing sulphur globules and yellow and red carotenoids. Species occur in stagnant water and decomposing effluent from sugar refineries. They are non-pathogenic. [Gk *lampros* clear, *paidia* children.]

lamprophonia (lam·pro·**fo**·ne·ah). Unusual distinctness and clarity of tonal sound; a sonorous quality of voice. [Gk *lampros* clear, *phone* sound.]

lamprophonic (lam·pro·**fon**·ik). Applied to a clear sonorous voice. [see prec.]

lampsis (**lamp**·sis). Brilliance. [Gk *lampein* to shine brilliantly.]

lana (**la**·nah). Animal wool: wool prepared from the fleece of the sheep *Ovis artis* Linn. (family Bovidae) by a process of cleaning and degreasing. It is used in the manufacture of flannel and flannel bandages, and in chiropody to protect inflamed parts from pressure. [L.]

lanatoside (la·**na**·to·side). A glycoside obtained from *Digitalis lanata* Ehrh. **Lanatoside C BP 1973.** A glycoside used for the same purpose as digitalis and said to be less cumulative than digitoxin. It has a bigger therapeutic index than most other digitalis glycosides.

Lancaster, Walter Brackett (b. 1863). American ophthalmologist.

Lancaster projection test. For investigating diplopia and oculomotor paralysis: the patient wearing red and green glasses looks at a linear red light on a screen and himself holds a torch with which he projects a similar green light on to the screen and attempts to superimpose his green light on the red. The lights are moved to different positions on the screen and the separation of the lights is marked on a chart.

lance (lahns). 1. A small surgical knife, usually pointed and having a double cutting edge, commonly used in the days before anaesthesia for the rapid incision of abscesses; a lancet. 2. To cut with a lancet. [L *lancea* spear.]

Lancefield, Rebecca Craighill (b. 1895). New York bacteriologist.

Lancefield's classification. An orderly serological arrangement of the Streptococceae.

Lancefield groups. Labelled A–R, they represent a serological classification of β-haemolytic streptococci based on the carbohydrate somatic antigen. Group A streptococci (*Streptococcus pyogenes*) constitute most of the β-haemolytic streptococci causing infection in man; other groups occasionally pathogenic to man are B, C, D and G (*see* STREPTOCOCCUS).

lanceolate (**laņ**·se·o·late). Resembling a lance in shape.

Lancereaux, Étienne (b. 1829). Paris physician.

Lancereaux's law. Thrombosis associated with marasmus is most likely to occur at sites where the blood flow is most sluggish, especially outside the thorax.

Lancereaux-Mathieu disease. Leptospiral jaundice. *See* JAUNDICE.

lancet (**lahn**·set). A small, pointed, double-edged surgical knife. This was formerly used specifically for the opening of abscesses but is seldom required in present-day surgery. [Fr. *lancette.*]

lancinate (**lan**·sin·ate). To cut or tear; to lacerate; to pierce. [L *lancinare* to tear to pieces.]

Lancisi, Giovanni Maria (b. 1654). Italian physician.

Lancisi's nerves, or striae. The longitudinal striae on the upper surface of the corpus callosum.

Landeker, Alfons (b. 1886). German physicist.

Landeker-Steinberg light. Light similar to that emitted from the sun, with the exception of the ultraviolet rays which have been absorbed.

Landerer, Albert Sigmund (b. 1854). Leipzig surgeon.

Landerer treatment. The treatment of tuberculosis with injections of cinnamic acid.

Landis, Eugene Markley (b. 1901). Boston physiologist.

Gibbon and Landis test. Reflex vasodilatation test; when the peripheral circulation is normal, heat applied to an extremity is followed by vasodilatation and increase in skin temperature in the unheated extremities. If the feet are to be tested, they are exposed to the air in a warm room and heating applied to the trunk or arms for 60-90 min. The skin temperature is measured at frequent intervals. Organic vascular disease is indicated by a failure of the skin temperature to reach 30-32°C. A normal response is usually obtained in subjects with vasospastic disorders as opposed to organic vascular disease.

landmarks (land·marx). Noticeable markings in the form of grooves or prominences on the surface of the body which act as guides to the position of underlying structures or organs. [AS *land, meark.*]

Landolfi, Niccolo (fl. 1845). Naples physician.

Landolfi's caustic, or paste. A mixture of the chlorides of antimony, gold, and zinc, with bromine; used as a caustic application.

Landolt, Edmund (b. 1846). Zürich and Paris ophthalmologist.

Landolt's bodies, or clubs. Branches of some of the bipolar nerve cells in the retinae of birds, amphibia, and reptiles; they are given off in the outer plexiform layer and extend as far as the membrana limitans externa where they end in club-shaped enlargements.

Landolt's operation. A blepharoplasty for eyelid defects, by sliding a flap from the lateral side and filling the raw defect with a small temporal flap.

Landolt's rings. Broken black rings on a white background as a test for visual acuity. *See* LANDOLT'S RING TEST (following).

Landolt's ring test. A test for visual acuity, useful in illiterates and young children: similar to Snellen's test type, but the letters are replaced by black circles on a white background, each circle having a gap similar to the letter "C", the gap measuring one-fifth the diameter of the circle. The circles are of diminishing size with different positions of the gap. This position has to be accurately indicated by the patient.

Landouzy, Louis Théophile Joseph (b. 1845). Paris physician.

Landouzy's disease. Leptospiral jaundice. *See* JAUNDICE.

Landouzy type, Déjérine-Landouzy atrophy, myopathy, or type, Landouzy-Déjérine atrophy, dystrophy, myopathy, or type. Facioscapulohumeral muscular dystrophy; a heredofamilial form, probably an incomplete mendelian dominant. It is a slowly progressive disease, producing weakness and wasting of the facial and shoulder-girdle muscles and later affecting the pelvic girdle. A characteristic smooth facies with pouting lips develops, lumbar lordosis is accentuated, and there is a waddling gait.

Erb-Landouzy disease. Progressive muscular dystrophy.

Landouzy-Grasset law. In a unilateral cerebral lesion producing hemiplegia, the head is turned to the side of the cerebral lesion if paralysis is flaccid, and to the side of the affected limbs if spastic.

Landry, Jean Baptiste Octave (b. 1826). Paris physician.

Landry's disease, palsy, paralysis, or syndrome, Kussmaul-Landry paralysis. Acute ascending paralysis; a syndrome of flaccid paralysis beginning in the lower limbs and ascending to involve the upper limbs, and bulbar and respiratory muscles.

Landry-Guillain-Barré syndrome. A name adopted for the conditions previously known as Landry's ascending paralysis and the Guillain-Barré syndrome, which are now recognized as clinically and pathologically identical.

Landsberg, J. W. (b. 1907). Baltimore haematologist.

Wintrobe and Landsberg method. A method for the determination of packed-cell volume and sedimentation rate of blood, with a small graduated haematocrit tube (*Wintrobe's tube.*)

Landsteiner, Karl (b. 1868). Vienna and New York pathologist.

Landsteiner classification. A system of blood groups, the so-called ABO system, the four groups being A, B, AB, and O, according to the different combinations of the agglutinogens A and B in the cells, and the agglutinins α (anti-A) and β (anti-B) in the sera.

Landsteiner's method. A method for establishing non-paternity by means of inherited blood-group factors. The preliminary observations on which this test was made were based on the work of von Dungern, of Hirszfeld, and of Bernstein.

Donath-Landsteiner phenomenon. When blood taken from a patient with paroxysmal haemoglobinuria is cooled to 5°C, a cold haemolysin in the plasma combines with the red blood cells; when the temperature is allowed to rise the sensitized red cells are then haemolysed by the complement normally present in the blood.

Landström, John (b. 1869). Stockholm surgeon.

Landström's muscle. The peribulbar musculature; an ill-defined mass of smooth muscle fibres stretching round the anterior part of the eyeball and fused with the palpebral muscles. It was said by Landström to be one of the factors entering into the causation of exophthalmos.

Landzert, Theodor (d. 1889). St. Petersburg anatomist.

Landzert's canal. The craniopharyngeal canal. *See* CANAL.

Landzert's fossa, Gruber-Landzert fossa. The paraduodenal recess. *See* RECESS.

Lane, Clayton Arbuthnot (b. 1868). British helminthologist in India.

Lane's direct centrifugal flotation technique. A procedure for examination of the faeces for helminthic ova. A tap-water emulsion of faeces is subjected to preliminary removal of debris and concentration by centrifugalization. A 33 per cent solution of zinc sulphate is added, and by further centrifugalization the ova are floated to the top of the tube; after the surface of the fluid has been raised to form a meniscus, by the pipetting of further zinc-sulphate solution into the tube, a coverglass is placed over the tube. The ova (of most helminths) adhere to this; it is examined after being placed face downward on a microscope slide.

Lane, Sir William Arbuthnot (b. 1856). London surgeon.

Lane's band. Genitomesenteric band. *See* BAND.

Lane's clamp. A double (twin) clamp for lateral anastomosis.

Lane's kink. A bend or twist in the last few centimetres of the ileum, with external adhesions of the folded gut, causing obstruction; ileal kink.

Lane needle. A half-curved needle, half of its shaft being straight and half curved.

Lane's plate. A metal plate used for the internal fixation of fractures.

Lane-Lannelongue operation. Removal of a portion of the skull to allow cerebral decompression.

Lang, W. 19th century British ophthalmologist.

Lang's dissector and scoop. An instrument used in excision of the lacrimal sac; a blunt dissector at one end and a sharp spoon at the other. The latter is used for scraping the nasolacrimal duct.

Lang's knives. Blunt or sharp-ended knives used for cutting synechiae in the eye.

Lang's operation. For anterior synechiae: twin Lang's knives are used, one sharp-pointed and the other blunt. The sharp twin is used to make the entry into the anterior chamber at the limbus and this is then withdrawn and the synechia divided.

Lang's eye speculum. One in which the retracting portion is solid and not fenestrated, and so keeps the lashes out of the field of operation.

Frost-Lang operation. Insertion of a glass, ivory, or plastic ball into Tenon's capsule following enucleation. It gives good cosmetic result, though the ball is often extruded later.

Langdon-Down, John Langdon Haydon (b. 1828). British physician.

Down's disease or syndrome. Mongolism.

Lange, Carl Friedrich August (b. 1883). Berlin physician.

Lange's colloidal gold test. Into the first of 10 small clean test-tubes place 0.9 ml of 0.4 per cent saline (prepared with redistilled water) and in each of the other 9 tubes place 0.5 ml. To the first tube add 0.1 ml serum, mix, and transfer 0.5 ml to the second tube. Continue the serial dilution, discarding 0.5 ml from the tenth tube. To each tube add 2.5 ml of colloidal-gold solution, stopper and leave for 16-24 h. The reaction is read as follows: 5, complete precipitation, colourless supernatant; 4, partial precipitation, light blue supernatant; 3, deep blue; 2, lilac to purple; 1, reddish blue; 0, no change from original red. Normal spinal fluids cause no change in any of the tubes. When maximum reaction occurs in the first tubes it is termed a *paretic curve*, in tubes 3 to 5 a *luetic curve*, and in tubes 5 to 8 a *meningitic curve*. A paretic curve is given in general paralysis of the insane and in disseminated sclerosis; a luetic curve in tabes; and a meningitic curve in coccal and tuberculous meningitis.

Lange, Carl G. (b. 1834). Danish psychologist.

James-Lange theory. The theory of the emotions which postulates that the conscious emotional experience is a consequence of the visceral changes. According to the famous argument advanced by James, we do not run because we are afraid but are afraid because we run. (*See also* CANNON'S THEORY.)

Lange, Fritz (b. 1864). Munich orthopaedic surgeon.

Lange's operation. Tendon transplantation: the tendon is replaced by strands of silk (obsolete).

Langenbeck, Bernhard Rudolf Konrad von (b. 1810). Berlin surgeon.

Langenbeck's amputation. Amputation with anterior and posterior flaps.

Langenbeck's operation. Closure of a cleft palate with the use of lateral incisions.

Langenbeck's triangle. The area which overlies the head of the femur between the piriformis and gluteus medius muscles.

Langenbeck, Konrad Johann Martin (b. 1776). Würzberg and Gottingen anatomist and surgeon.

Langenbeck's nerve. 1. The lateral supraclavicular nerve. 2. An offset from the nasociliary nerve to the frontal sinus and ethmoid cells.

Langendorff, Oskar (b. 1853). Rostock physiologist.

Langendorff's cells. Epithelial cells forming the walls of the vesicles of the thyroid gland.

Langer, Carl Ritter von Edenburg (b. 1819). Vienna anatomist.

Langer's axillary arch, or muscle. An inconstant slip from the latissimus dorsi muscle which crosses the axillary vessels and is inserted into the pectoralis major muscle.

Langer's line. The underlying orientation of the dermal fibrous tissue which gives rise to visible tension or cleavage lines on the surface of the skin. *See also:* SIMON'S LINES.

Langerhans, Paul (b. 1847). Freiburg pathologist.

Langerhans' body, island of Langerhans. Islets of Langerhans (see below).

Langerhans' cell. 1. Langerhans' stellate corpuscle (see below). 2. A corneal histiocyte. 3. Cell of the island of Langerhans.

islets of Langerhans. Islets of the pancreas: small clumps of cells in the pancreas having no functional connection with the duct system of that organ; they synthesize, store and release the hormones insulin (β-cells), glucagon (A_2 cells) and gastrin (A_1 or D cells).

Langerhans' stellate corpuscles. Stellate cells in the interstitial spaces of the epidermis. Langerhans thought that nerve fibres could be traced to these; improved methods of staining have not brought confirmation of his findings.

Langerhans' layer. The granular layer of the skin.

Langhans, Theodor (b. 1839). Berne pathologist.

Langhans' cell. A cytotrophoblastic cell of a chorionic villus, lying deep to the syncytiotrophoblast.

Langhans' giant cell. An inflammatory giant cell found in chronic lesions such as those of tuberculosis.

Langhans' layer. The cytotrophoblast of a chorionic villus.

Langhans' method. The use of origanum oil as a mountant in order to preserve iodine-stained tissue components such as glycogen.

Langhans' stria. A band of fibrinoid in the chorionic plate of the human placenta.

Langley, John Newport (b. 1852). Cambridge physiologist.

Langley's ganglion. A ganglion in the hilum of the submandibular gland in some animals; not usually present in man.

Langley's granulations. Intracellular granules apparent in serous glands during secretion.

Langley's granules. The granules within salivary glands.

Langley's nerves. The nerves to the arrectores pilorum muscles.

Langmuir, Irving (b. 1881). American physical chemist.

Langmuir atom. The atom imagined as shells of electrons grouped concentrically about the nucleus.

lanigallol (lan·e·gal·ol). Pyrogallol triacetate. $(CH_3COO)_3C_6H_3$. A thick, dark, viscid liquid used in the treatment of skin diseases.

Lannelongue, Odilon Marc (b. 1840). Paris pathologist.

Lannelongue's foramina. The largest of the foramina venarum minimarum of the right atrium.

Lannelongue's ligament. An extension of the anterior attachment of the superior sternopericardial ligament to the 1st costal cartilage, sometimes described as a separate ligament, the costopericardiac ligament.

Lannelongue's tibia. A syphilitic tibia.

Lane-Lannelongue operation. Removal of a portion of the skull to allow cerebral decompression.

lanolin (lan·o·lin). Hydrous Wool Fat BP 1958: wool fat containing 25-30 per cent of purified water; a yellowish white greasy mass used as an emollient ointment and as a basis for other ointments, being readily absorbed by the skin. **Poloxyl Lanolin.** BP Commission approved name for a polyoxyethylene condensation product of anhydrous lanolin; an emollient. [L *lana* wool, *oleum* oil.]

Lanosterol (lan·o·steer·ol). $C_{30}H_{50}O$, a tetracyclic terpene alcohol, derived from picene and present in the form of its esters as a constituent of wool fat.

Lantana (lan·ta·nah). A genus of tropical and sub-tropical shrubs (family Verbenaceae). A lotion prepared from *Lantana salvifolia* Jacq. is used in South Africa for wounds and sores. [It., viburnum.]

Lantermann, A. J. (fl. 1877). Strasbourg anatomist.

incisures of Lantermann, Schmidt-Lantermann clefts or incisures. Numerous irregular oblique notches or interruptions in the myelin sheath of a nerve fibre between the nodes of Ranvier.

Lantermann's segment, Schmidt-Lantermann segment. That portion of the myelin sheath of a nerve fibre that lies between successive incisures of Lantermann.

lantern (lan·tern). *See* EDRIDGE-GREEN, THOMSON (W.), WILLIAMS (H. W.). [L *lanterna*.]

lanthanide (lan·than·ide). Any member of the first rare-earth series of chemical elements in the Periodic Table which begins with lanthanum.

lanthanum (lan·than·um). A rare-earth element of atomic weight 138.91, atomic number 57, and chemical symbol La. It is a grey trivalent metal, occurring in the rare-earth minerals lanthanite and cerite, and closely resembling cerium. [Gk *lanthanein* to elude notice.]

lanthionine (lan·thi·o·neen). Betacarboxyaminoethyl sulphide, a diamino acid containing sulphur.

lanuginose, lanuginous (lan·ew·jin·oze, lan·ew·jin·us). In biology, covered with lanugo; downy; woolly.

lanugo (lan·ew·go). 1. The downy hair which appears on the body of the fetus during the fourth month of pregnancy and is later shed. 2. The fine downy growth of hair present on most parts of the body with the exception of the palms and soles and those parts, e.g. the head, on which long hair grows. It may be prominent on the faces of girls and women. [L, down.]

lanulous (lan·ew·lus). Having a covering of short hair. [L *lana* wool.]

lanum (la·num). Lanolin.

Lanz, Otto (b. 1865). Berne and Amsterdam surgeon.

Lanz's line. The line between the anterior superior iliac spines.

Lanz's operation. 1. The insertion of strips of fascia lata into the femur for the relief of elephantiasis. 2. Appendicectomy through a transverse incision.

Lanz's point. A point on the line drawn between the superior iliac spines and one-third of the distance from the right spine; it indicates the position of the appendix.

lapara (**lap**·ar·ah). The loins or flank; less properly, the abdomen in general. [Gk, loin.]

laparacolpotomy (**lap**·ar·ah·kol·**pot'**·o·me). Laparo-elytrotomy. [Gk *lapara* loin, colpotomy.]

laparectomy (lap·ar·**ek**·to·me). Removal of strips of tissue from the wall of the abdomen in order to correct laxity of the abdominal muscles and to provide support. [Gk *lapara* loin, *ektome* a cutting out.]

laparelytrotomy (**lap**·ar·el·e·**trot'**·o·me). Laparo-elytrotomy.

laparocele (**lap**·ar·o·seel). Hernia in the lumbar or the abdominal region. [Gk *lapara* loin, *kele* hernia.]

laparocholecystotomy (**lap**·ar·o·ko·le·sist·**ot'**·o·me). Laparotomy combined with cholecystotomy.

laparoclysis (**lap**·ar·o·**kli'**·sis). Peritoneal irrigation; peritoneoclysis. [Gk *lapara* loin, *klysis* a washing out.]

laparocolectomy (**lap**·ar·o·ko·**lek'**·to·me). Colectomy; resection of the colon. [Gk *lapara* loin, colectomy.]

laparocolostomy (**lap**·ar·o·ko·**los'**·to·me). Colostomy by means of an incision in the anterolateral wall of the abdomen; abdominal colostomy. [Gk *lapara* loin, colostomy.]

laparocolotomy (**lap**·ar·o·ko·**lot'**·o·me). Abdominal colotomy. [Gk *lapara* loin, colotomy.]

laparocolpohysterotomy (**lap**·ar·o·**kol**·po·his·ter·**ot'**·o·me). Caesarean section by means of a laparotomy and an incision into the vagina. [Gk *lapara* loin, colpohysterotomy.]

laparocolpotomy (**lap**·ar·o·kol·**pot'**·o·me). Laparo-elytrotomy. [Gk *lapara* loin, *kolpos* vagina, *temnein* to cut.]

laparocystectomy (**lap**·ar·o·sist·**ek'**·to·me). 1. The operation of removing a cyst through an incision made in the wall of the abdomen. 2. In advanced ectopic pregnancy, surgical removal of the fetus and the complete sac. [Gk *lapara* loin, cystectomy.]

laparocystidotomy (**lap**·ar·o·sist·id·**ot'**·o·me). Suprapubic cystotomy. [Gk *lapara* loin, *kystis* bag, *temnein* to cut.]

laparocystotomy (**lap**·ar·o·sist·**ot'**·o·me). 1. Evacuation of an ectopic fetus without removal of the enveloping sac. 2. Suprapubic cystotomy. *See* CYSTOTOMY. [Gk *lapara* loin, cystotomy.]

laparocystovariohysterotomy (**lap**·ar·o·**sist**·o·va·re·o·his·ter·**ot'**·o·me). The combined operation of hysterotomy and ovariotomy performed through an incision in the abdominal wall. [Gk *lapara* loin, *kystis* bag, ovary, Gk *hystera* womb, *temnein* to cut.]

laparo-elytrotomy (**lap**·ar·o·el·it·**rot'**·o·me). A type of caesarean section in which an incision is made above the inguinal ligament; the peritoneum is divided as far as the vagina, in which a transverse incision is made, with subsequent delivery of the child through the enlarged os uteri. [Gk *lapara* loin, elytrotomy.]

laparo-enterostomy (**lap**·ar·o·en·ter·**os'**·to·me). Incision into the intestine through the wall of the abdomen in order to make an artificial opening. [Gk *lapara* loin, enterostomy.]

laparo-enterotomy (**lap**·ar·o·en·ter·**ot'**·o·me). Incision of the intestine by means of an incision in the lumbar region or abdominal wall. [Gk *lapara* loin, enterotomy.]

laparogastroscopy (**lap**·ar·o·gas·**tros'**·ko·pe). Exploratory incision of the stomach. [Gk *lapara* loin, gastroscopy.]

laparogastrostomy (**lap**·ar·o·gas·**tros'**·to·me). The operation to create an artificial opening in the stomach. [Gk *lapara* loin, gastrostomy.]

laparogastrotomy (**lap**·ar·o·gas·**trot'**·o·me). The operation of opening the stomach through an abdominal incision. [Gk *lapara* loin, gastrotomy.]

laparohepatotomy (**lap**·ar·o·hep·at·**ot'**·o·me). The operation of incising the liver through an abdominal incision. [Gk *lapara* loin, *hepar* liver, *temnein* to cut.]

laparohysterectomy (**lap**·ar·o·his·ter·**ek'**·to·me). Incision of the abdominal wall and excision of the uterus. [Gk *lapara* loin, hysterectomy.]

laparohystero-oöphorectomy (**lap**·ar·o·**his**·ter·o·o·of·or·**ek'**·to·me). Combined hysterectomy and oöphorectomy performed through an incision in the abdominal wall. [Gk *lapara* loin, *hystera* womb, oöphorectomy.]

laparohysteropexy (**lap**·ar·o·**his'**·ter·o·pex·e). Ventrofixation of the uterus. [Gk *lapara* loin, hysteropexy.]

laparohysterosalpingo-oöphorectomy (**lap**·ar·o·**his**·ter·o·**sal**·ping·go·o·of·or·**ek'**·to·me). Combined hysterectomy, salpingectomy and oöphorectomy through an abdominal incision. [Gk *lapara* loin, hysterosalpingo-oöphorectomy.]

laparohysterotomy (**lap**·ar·o·his·ter·**ot'**·o·me). The operation of incision of the uterus through an abdominal opening. [Gk *lapara* loin, hysterotomy.]

laparo-ileotomy (**lap**·ar·o·i·le·**ot'**·o·me). Ileotomy performed through an abdominal incision. [Gk *lapara* loin, ileotomy.]

laparomonodidymus (**lap**·ar·o·mon·o·**did'**·im·us). A twin monster the bodies of which are fused below the pelvis and separate above it. [Gk *lapara* loin, *monos* standing alone, *didymos* twin.]

laparomyomectomy, laparomyomotomy (**lap**·ar·o·mi·o·**mek'**·to·me, **lap**·ar·o·mi·o·**mot'**·o·me). Myomectomy performed through an incision in the abdominal wall. [Gk *lapara* loin, myomectomy.]

laparomyositis (**lap**·ar·o·mi·os·**i'**·tis). Inflammation of the abdominal muscles. [Gk *lapara* loin, myositis.]

laparonephrectomy (**lap**·ar·o·nef·**rek'**·to·me). Removal of a kidney through a lumbar incision. [Gk *lapara* loin, nephrectomy.]

laparorrhaphy (lap·ar·**or**·af·e). The suturing of a wound in the wall of the abdomen. [Gk *lapara* loin, *rhaphe* suture.]

laparosalpingectomy (**lap**·ar·o·sal·pin·**jek'**·to·me). Removal of a uterine tube through an abdominal incision. [Gk *lapara* loin, salpingectomy.]

laparosalpingo-oöphorectomy (**lap**·ar·o·**sal**·ping·go·o·of·or·**ek'**·to·me). Removal of the uterine tube and the ovary through an abdominal incision. [Gk *lapara* loin, salpingo-oöphorectomy.]

laparosalpingotomy (**lap**·ar·o·sal·ping·**got'**·o·me). Incision of a uterine tube through an abdominal opening. [Gk *lapara* loin, salpingotomy.]

laparoscope (**lap**·ar·o·skope). A type of trocar provided with an illuminating mechanism with which the cavity of the peritoneum, the abdominal viscera, and in particular the surface of the peritoneum and the liver, can be examined. [Gk *lapara* loin, *skopein* to watch.]

laparoscopy (lap·ar·**os**·ko·pe). The act or process of examining the peritoneal cavity and its contents by means of a laparoscope.

laparosplenectomy (**lap**·ar·o·splen·**ek'**·to·me). The operation of removing the spleen through an abdominal incision. [Gk *lapara* loin, splenectomy.]

laparosplenotomy (**lap**·ar·o·splen·**ot'**·o·me). Incision of the spleen through an abdominal opening, e.g. in order to drain a splenic abscess or cyst. [Gk *lapara* loin, splenotomy.]

laparotome (**lap**·ar·o·tome). A type of knife used in laparotomy.

laparotomophilia migrans (**lap**·ar·o·to·mo·**fil'**·e·ah **mi**·granz). *See* MUNCHAUSEN'S SYNDROME. [laparotomy, Gk *philein* to love, L *migrans* wandering.]

laparotomy (lap·ar·**ot**·o·me). 1. Properly, the operation of incising the flank or loin. 2. By common usage the term has come to mean an incision into any part of the abdominal wall. [Gk *lapara* loin, *temnein* to cut.]

laparotrachelotomy (**lap**·ar·o·trak·el·**ot'**·o·me). A type of caesarean section in which the neck of the uterus and the lower uterine segment are incised with as little involvement as possible of the peritoneum; cervical caesarean section. [Gk *lapara* loin, *trachelos* neck, *temnein* to cut.]

laparotyphlotomy (**lap**·ar·o·tif·**lot'**·o·me). The surgical procedure of making a lateral abdominal opening in order to expose the caecum and incise it. [Gk *lapara* loin, typhlotomy.]

laparovaginal (**lap**·ar·o·vaj·**i'**·nal). Abdominovaginal. [Gk *lapara* loin, vagina.]

lapathin (lap·ath·in). Chrysophanic acid. *See* ACID.

Lapicque, Louis (b. 1866). Paris physiologist.

Lapicque's constant. The factor 0.37 for converting non-inductive resistance into the equivalent direct current.

Lapicque's law. In a nerve fibre, chronaxia is inversely related to the diameter.

lapilliform (lap·il·e·form). Resembling small stones in form. [L *lapillus* little stone, form.]

lapinization (lap·in·i·za·shun). The cutaneous passage of smallpox virus through rabbits to maintain the quality of the seed lymph for vaccination of calves or sheep in preparation of vaccine lymph. [Fr. *lapin* rabbit.]

lapis (lap·is). The Latin for *stone*, and therefore applied by alchemists to all substances which did not volatilize. **Lapis albus.** Native calcium silicofluoride, and also the precipitated compound. **Lapis calaminaris.** Calamine. **Lapis causticus.** Caustic potash. **Lapis dentalis.** Tartar of the teeth. **Lapis divinus.** Cuprammonium sulphate. **Lapis imperialis, lapis infernalis.** Silver nitrate. **Lapis lazuli.** A rare mineral, sodium aluminium silicate, of a beautiful blue colour, used in ancient times as an amulet, and internally as an emetic and purgative. **Lapis lunaris.** Silver nitrate. **Lapis mitigatus.** Dilute silver nitrate solution. **Lapis ophthalmicus.** Cuprammonium sulphate.

Laplace, Pierre Simon, Marquis de (b. 1749). French mathematician, astronomer and physicist.

Laplace's law. The relationship between the pressure within a sphere and the tension in its wall, defined as $T = P \times R$, where T = wall tension, P = cavity pressure, and R = radius of the sphere. This relation has many applications in biological systems.

Laportea (lap·or·te·ah). A genus of tropical herbs or woody plants (family Urticaceae). *Laportea stimulans* Miq. is used in Malaya for poultices. *L. crenulata* Gand., the fever or devil nettle, yields seeds which are used in India as a carminative.

lappa (lap·ah). The burdock, *Arctium lappa* Linn. (family Compositae). A decoction prepared from the whole plant, or the root alone, has been used as a diuretic and diaphoretic. [L, burr.]

lapsus (lap·sus). Ptosis; a falling of a part. **Lapsus palpebrae superioris.** Ptosis of the upper eyelid. **Lapsus pilorum.** Alopecia. **Lapsus unguium.** Shedding of the nails. [L, fall.]

Larat, Jules Louis François Adrien (b. 1857). Paris physician.

Larat's treatment. Treatment of palatal paralysis in diphtheria, by faradism.

larch (larch). *See* LARIX. [L *larix*.]

lard (lard). Adeps, prepared lard; the purified internal fat of the hog, *Sus scrofa* Linn. It is a white unctuous mass, melting between 34 and 41°C, and consisting of glycerides, mainly of oleic acid. It is used in ointment bases (BPC 1963), but is being replaced by more stable vehicles. **Benzoinated lard.** Lard which has been heated to 60°C for one hour with 3 per cent its weight of benzoin, and then strained. The aromatic acids and esters thus extracted from the benzoin act as preservatives. It is used as an ointment base. [L *laridum*.]

lardacein (lar·da·se·in). Amyloid; a chemical substance of protein origin which is deposited on the surface of fibres and cells of tissues when there is prolonged and profuse suppuration, or the secondary infection of tuberculous or syphilitic lesions. It is recognized in the kidneys, liver, spleen, and intestines through its reaction with iodine and the dye, methyl violet. [see prec.]

lardaceous (lar·da·shus). 1. Having resemblance to lard. 2. Consisting of or containing lardacein.

Lardennois, Henri (b. 1872). Paris surgeon.

Lardennois' manoeuvre, or method, Lardennois-Pauchet method. The avascular separation of the greater omentum by its division close to its attachment to the transverse colon.

Larix (la·rix). 1. A genus of deciduous trees, the larches (family Pinaceae). 2. The bark of *Larix decidua* Mill., the European larch. It contains tannin and a bitter principle, and is used as an expectorant. It yields an oleoresin known as *Venice turpentine.* [L, larch.]

larixin (lar·ix·in). Laricic acid. *See* ACID.

larkspur (lark·sper). 1. The common name for the genus *Delphinium* (family Ranunculaceae). 2. The seeds of *D. consolida* Linn., used in the form of the tincture as a parasiticide and insecticide. [AS *lawerce, spura.*]

Larrey, Dominique Jean, Baron (b. 1766). Paris surgeon.

Larrey's amputation, or operation. Disarticulation of the humerus at the shoulder by a lateral racket amputation.

Larrey's cleft, or space. The interval between the sternal and costal origins of the diaphragm. Also called Morgagni's *foramen.*

Larroussius (lar·oos·e·us). A sub-genus of *Phlebotomus.*

Larsen, Loren Joseph (b. 1914). American orthopaedic surgeon.

Larsen's syndrome. Flat facies, multiple dislocation of joints, and short metacarpals.

larva (lar·vah). 1. General term for a pre-adult form of an animal where that form differs more or less markedly from the adult; metamorphosis to the adult is usually rapid. Larvae are important as distributional forms; further they use a part of the general environment that is not available to the adult, so that the two are not in competition. 2. In insects specifically, the young stages of the Holometabola, in which a pupal stage occurs. Cf. NYMPH. **Larva currens.** A linear urticarial rash on the perianal skin caused by rhabditiform larvae of *Strongyloides stercoralis* which moult to become invasive filariform larvae, penetrating the skin and wandering through it. **Larva migrans.** Creeping eruption due to a larval nematode (e.g. *Ancylostoma braziliensis, Strongyloides stercoralis*) burrowing under the skin; the term has also been applied to a somewhat similar migrating lesion caused by the larvae of species of *Hypoderma, Gastrophilus,* and *Gnathostoma.* **Larva migrans, visceral.** Visceral enlargement with eosinophilia of blood, usually assumed to be due to infection with *Toxocara.* [L, mask.]

larvaceous (lar·va·shus). Larvate.

larval (lar·val). 1. Relating or belonging to the stage of a larva; in the stage of being a larva. 2. Larvate.

larvate (lar·vate). Masked; term applied to a disease or to symptoms which are hidden or atypical. [L *larva* mask.]

larvicide (lar·ve·side). An agent which destroys larvae. [larva, L *caedere* to kill.]

larviparous (lar·vip·ar·us). Of certain insects, depositing larvae instead of laying eggs. [larva, L *parere* to give birth.]

larviphage (lar·ve·faje). Fish or insects that feed on larva. [larva, Gk *phagein* to eat.]

larviposition (lar·ve·po·zish'·un). The depositing of larvae by a larviparous insect. [larva, L *ponere* to place.]

larvivorous (lar·viv·or·us). Feeding on larvae, i.e. applied to certain fish. [larva, L *vorare* to swallow.]

laryngalgia (lar·in·gal·je·ah). A condition in which there is sensation of pain in the larynx. [larynx, Gk *algos* pain.]

laryngeal (lar·in·je·al). Pertaining to the larynx.

laryngeal arteries. Inferior laryngeal artery [arteria laryngea inferior]. *See* THYROID ARTERY, INFERIOR. **Superior laryngeal artery [arteria laryngea superior].** *See* THYROID ARTERY, SUPERIOR.

laryngeal nerves. External laryngeal nerve [ramus externus (NA)]. The motor branch of the superior laryngeal nerve to the cricothyroid muscle. **Internal laryngeal nerve [ramus internus (NA)].** The sensory branch of the superior laryngeal nerve to the larynx and the mucous membrane in and around the piriform fossa of the pharynx. The communicating branch with the recurrent laryngeal nerve [ramus communicans cum nervo laryngeo inferiore (NA)] is known as *the nerve of Galen.* **Recurrent laryngeal nerve [nervus laryngeus recurrens (NA)].** A branch of the vagus nerve carrying motor fibres to the intrinsic muscles of the larynx, to the inferior constrictor muscle of the pharynx and the trachea, bronchi, and oesophagus, with sensory fibres to the mucous membrane of the larynx below the vocal folds, the trachea, bronchi, and oesophagus. The right nerve hooks around the subclavian artery, and the left around the arch of the aorta and the ligamentum arteriosum. It has a communicating branch with the internal laryngeal nerve [ramus communicans cum ramo laryngeo interno (NA)]. **Superior laryngeal nerve [nervus laryngeus superior (NA)].** A branch from the inferior ganglion of the vagus nerve which supplies sensory fibres to the mucous membrane of the larynx above the vocal folds, and of the pharynx in and around the piriform fossa (internal laryngeal nerve). It also supplies a motor branch to the cricothyroid muscle (external laryngeal nerve).

laryngeal veins. Inferior laryngeal veins [venae laryngeae inferiores (NA)]. Veins accompanying the arteries of the same name; they are tributaries of the inferior thyroid vein. **Superior laryngeal vein [vena laryngea superior (NA)].** A tributary of the superior thyroid vein; it emerges from the larynx through the thyrohyoid membrane.

laryngectomy (lar·in·**jek**·to·me). Complete excision of the larynx, usually carried out for malignant disease. **Partial laryngectomy.** Removal of only a portion of the larynx. [larynx, Gk *ektome* excision.]

laryngemphraxis (lar·inj·em·**frax**′·is). A condition in which the larynx has become blocked or closed. [larynx, emphraxis.]

laryngendoscope (lar·in·**jen**·do·skope). An endoscope for examining the larynx. It is sometimes used to describe an optical instrument resembling a cystoscope, and is used for examining the less accessible parts of the larynx such as the subglottic region.

laryngismal (lar·in·**jiz**·mal). Relating or belonging to laryngismus.

laryngismus (lar·in·**jiz**·mus). Spasmodic contraction of the larynx. **Laryngismus stridulus.** A condition occurring in children, particularly rachitic children, and similar to glottic spasm. It is characterized by short, noisy inspirations, a cessation of breathing, and finally long crowing inspirations. [Gk *laryggismos* a whooping.]

laryngitic (lar·in·**jit**·ik). Relating or belonging to laryngitis.

laryngitis (lar·in·**ji**·tis). Inflammation of the larynx. **Acute catarrhal laryngitis.** Catarrhal inflammation of the larynx, as encountered in the common cold and the like. **Atrophic laryngitis.** Laryngitis resulting from atrophy of the mucous membrane, similar to laryngitis sicca (see below). **Chronic catarrhal laryngitis.** A chronic form of inflammation of the larynx. **Croupous laryngitis.** An acute laryngitis of childhood. Symptomatically it may resemble diphtheritic laryngitis (see following). **Diphtheritic laryngitis.** Inflammation of the larynx caused by infection of the larynx with the Klebs–Loeffler bacillus. Formation of a false membrane may produce a fatal laryngeal obstruction. **Dry laryngitis.** Laryngitis sicca (see below). **Membranous laryngitis.** Diphtheritic laryngitis (see above). **Oedematous laryngitis.** A localized oedema of the larynx most commonly caused by trauma from corrosive fluids or gases, but also associated with diseases such as typhoid, pneumonia, and syphilis. **Phlegmonous laryngitis.** Acute inflammation of the larynx found in debilitated people, or resulting from an infection from a virulent streptococcus; it is often associated with great oedema. **Laryngitis sicca.** Chronic inflammation of the larynx causing atrophy of the mucous membrane, and resulting in the formation of crusts. **Spasmodic laryngitis.** Acute laryngitis of the same type as the croupous laryngitis (see above). **Laryngitis stridulosa.** Laryngeal stridor most commonly encountered in children, with sudden onset and without signs of infection. **Subglottic laryngitis.** Inflammation of the subglottic region of the larynx, associated with oedema of a varying degree. **Syphilitic laryngitis.** Laryngitis resulting from invasion of *Treponema pallidum.* **Tuberculous laryngitis.** That due to inflammation of the larynx resulting from infection by *Mycobacterium tuberculosis.* [larynx, Gk *-itis* inflammation.]

laryngocatarrh (lar·**ing**·go·kat·**ar**′). Mucous congestion and catarrh of the larynx.

laryngocele (lar·**ing**·go·seel). An air-containing cavity connected to the laryngeal ventricle. It is a normal structure in certain animals, including the higher apes, but regarded as pathological in man. [larynx, Gk *kele* hernia.]

laryngocentesis (lar·**ing**·go·sen·**te**′·sis). Puncture of, or the making of a short incision into the larynx. [larynx, centesis.]

laryngo-epiglottitis (lar·**ing**·go·ep·e·glot·**i**′·tis). A form of croup in children caused by *Haemophilus influenzae.* [larynx, epiglottis, Gk *-itis* inflammation.]

laryngofissure (lar·**ing**·go·**fish**′·ewr). The splitting of the larynx in the middle line surgically, usually through the thyroid cartilage, to expose the contents of the larynx. [larynx, fissure.]

laryngogram (lar·**ing**·go·gram). X-ray picture of the larynx, the internal surface of which has been made visible by the application of a contrast medium. [larynx, Gk *graphein* to record.]

laryngograph (lar·**ing**·go·graf). An instrument with which a tracing of movements of the larynx in speech can be made. [larynx, Gk *graphein* to record.]

laryngography (lar·in·**gog**·raf·e). X-ray examination of the larynx after application of a contrast medium. [see prec.]

laryngologic, laryngological (lar·**ing**·go·**loj**′·ik, lar·**ing**·go·**loj**′·ik·al). Relating or belonging to laryngology.

laryngologist (lar·in·**gol**·o·jist). One who specializes in the science of laryngology.

laryngology (lar·in·**gol**·o·je). That branch of medical science which is concerned with the larynx, its anatomy, and its diseases and their treatment. [larynx, Gk *logos* science.]

laryngometry (lar·in·**gom**·et·re). Measurement of the larynx.

laryngoparalysis (lar·**ing**·go·par·**al**′·is·is). Laryngeal paralysis. *See* PARALYSIS.

laryngopathy (lar·in·**gop**·ath·e). Any disease or disordered condition of the larynx. [larynx, Gk *pathos* suffering.]

laryngophantom (lar·**ing**·go·**fan**′·tom). A model of the larynx for use in anatomical study of its structures; it may also be used for practice in laryngoscopy. [larynx, Gk *phantasma* image.]

laryngopharyngeal (lar·**ing**·go·far·**in**′·je·al). Belonging or relating to both the larynx and the pharynx or to the laryngopharynx.

laryngopharyngectomy (lar·**ing**·go·far·in·**jek**′·to·me). Surgical removal of both the larynx and the pharynx. [larynx, pharynx, Gk *ektome* a cutting out.]

laryngopharyngeus (lar·**ing**·go·far·**in**′·je·us). The inferior constrictor muscle of the pharynx. *See* PHARYNX, CONSTRICTOR MUSCLES OF THE. [larynx, pharynx.]

laryngopharyngitis (lar·**ing**·go·far·in·**ji**′·tis). An inflammatory condition of both the larynx and the pharynx; inflammation of the laryngopharynx. [larynx, pharynx, Gk *-itis* inflammation.]

laryngopharynx (lar·**ing**·go·**far**′·ingx). The inferior or laryngeal part of the pharynx.

laryngophony (lar·in·**gof**·on·e). The voice sounds heard through a stethoscope applied to the larynx. [larynx, Gk *phone* voice.]

laringophthisis (lar·**ing**·go·**thi**′·sis). Tuberculosis of the larynx. [larynx, Gk *phthisis* a wasting.]

laryngoplasty (lar·**ing**·go·plas·te). Plastic surgery or repair of the larynx. [larynx, Gk *plassein* to mould.]

laryngoplegia (lar·**ing**·go·**ple**′·je·ah). Laryngeal paralysis. *See* PARALYSIS. [larynx, Gk *plege* stroke.]

laryngoptosis (lar·**ing**·go·**to**′·sis). Downward displacement of the larynx with exceptional mobility, as may be noted in elderly persons. [larynx, ptosis.]

laryngopyocele (lar·**ing**·go·**pi**′·o·seel). A laryngocele containing pus. [laryngocele, Gk *pyon* pus.]

laryngorhinology (lar·**ing**·go·ri·**nol**′·o·je). That branch of medical science which is concerned with the larynx and the nose, and their anatomy, diseases, and treatment. [larynx, Gk *rhis* nose, *logos* science.]

laryngorrhagia (lar·**ing**·go·**ra**′·je·ah). Haemorrhage from the larynx. [larynx, Gk *rhegnynein* to gush forth.]

laryngorrhaphy (lar·in·**gor**·af·e). The surgical procedure of suturing the larynx. [larynx, Gk *rhaphe* suture.]

laryngorrhoea (lar·**ing**·go·**re**′·ah). A condition in which there is excessive secretion from the mucous membrane of the larynx, particularly while the person affected is speaking. [larynx, Gk *rhoia* flow.]

laryngoscleroma (lar·**ing**·go·skler·**o**′·mah). Scleroma of the larynx.

laryngoscope (lar·ing·go·skope). An apparatus for viewing the larynx. [larynx, Gk *skopein* to view.]

laryngoscopic (lar·ing·go·**skop'**·ik). Relating or belonging to laryngoscopy.

laryngoscopy (lar·in·**gos**·ko·pe). The use of the laryngoscope. **Direct laryngoscopy.** A subdivision of peroral endoscopy; examination of a larynx by means of a suitably illuminated tube introduced through the mouth. **Suspension laryngoscopy.** A method of exposing the larynx for examination and operation; a long spatula attached to a suspension mechanism displaces the tongue and holds up the epiglottis, thus exposing the larynx.

laryngospasm (lar·ing·go·spazm). Muscular spasm of the larynx, with associated closure.

laryngostasis (lar·in·**gos**·tas·is). Croup. [larynx, Gk *stasis* a standing still.]

laryngostat (lar·**ing**·go·stat). An apparatus with which a capsule of radium can be held in position inside the larynx. [larynx, Gk *stasis* a standing still.]

laryngostenosis (lar·ing·go·sten·**o'**·sis). Stricture or other narrowing of the lumen of the larynx. [larynx, stenosis.]

laryngostomy (lar·in·**gos**·to·me). The creation of a permanent opening into the larynx through an incision of the neck and trachea. [larynx, Gk *stoma* mouth.]

laryngostroboscope (lar·ing·go·**stro'**·bo·skope). A stroboscope specially adapted for use in the larynx to enable accurate observations to be made on cord movement and vibration.

laryngostroboscopy (lar·**ing**·go·stro·**bos'**·ko·pe). The use of the laryngostroboscope.

laryngosyrinx (lar·**ing**·go·**sir'**·ingx). A tube used for maintenance of the laryngeal airway. [larynx, Gk *syrygx* pipe.]

laryngotomy (lar·in·**got**·o·me). An opening into the larynx through the cricovocal membrane; it is of a temporary nature, and is usually carried out in an emergency where a tracheotomy cannot be performed. [larynx, Gk *temnein* to cut.]

laryngotracheal (lar·**ing**·go·trak·**e'**·al). Relating or belonging to both larynx and trachea.

laryngotracheitis (lar·ing·go·trak·e·**i'**·tis). An inflammatory condition of both the larynx and trachea. [larynx, trachea, Gk *-itis* inflammation.]

laryngotracheobronchitis (lar·**ing**·go·**trak**·e·o·brong·**ki'**·tis). Inflammation of the larynx, trachea, and bronchi. [larynx, trachea, bronchitis.]

laryngotracheobronchoscopy (lar·**ing**·go·**trak**·e·o·brong·**kos'**·ko·pe). Inspection of the interior of the trachea and bronchi through a bronchoscope. [larynx, trachea, bronchus, Gk *skopein* to watch.]

laryngotracheoscopy (lar·ing·go·trak·e·**os'**·ko·pe). Tracheoscopy by way of the mouth and larynx. [larynx, trachea, Gk *skopein* to watch.]

laryngotracheotomy (lar·**ing**·go·trak·e·**ot'**·o·me). 1. The operation of incising the larynx and trachea. 2. Tracheotomy in which one or several of the cartilaginous rings of the trachea are incised as well as the cricoid cartilage. [larynx, trachea, Gk *temnein* to cut.]

laryngovestibulitis (lar·**ing**·go·ves·tib·ew·**li'**·tis). An inflammatory state of the vestibule of the larynx. [larynx, vestibule, Gk *-itis* inflammation.]

laryngoxerosis (lar·**ing**·go·zer·**o'**·sis). A dry state of the laryngeal mucosa. [larynx, Gk *xerosis* dryness.]

larynx [NA] (**lar**·ingx). The organ situated at the upper end of the trachea and concerned with the production of the voice. It is composed of a cartilaginous outer structure, made up of the following cartilages, held together by ligaments: single thyroid and cricoid, paired arytenoid, corniculate and cuneiform, and a single epiglottis. The whole structure is lined on its inner side by mucous membrane, which also covers over two pairs of elastic ligaments stretching from the arytenoid cartilages behind to the thyroid cartilages in front, the upper (false) and the lower (true) vocal cords. Sounds are produced by air passing through the true vocal cords. Variation in the sound is produced by tensing the vocal cords, and by separating or bringing them together (abduction and adduction respectively). This effect on the vocal cords is achieved by movement of the cartilages on one another, which is itself the result of the action of the muscles on the cartilages. The epiglottis acts during swallowing to prevent foodstuff finding its way into the trachea. **Inlet of the larynx [aditus laryngis (NA)].** The aperture bounded by the epiglottis anteriorly, the aryepiglottic folds laterally, and the mucous membrane stretching between the arytenoids posteriorly. [Gk.]

lascivia (las·iv·e·ah). Satyriasis or nymphomania. [L, wantonness.]

Lasègue, Ernest Charles (b. 1816). Paris physician.

Lasègue's disease. Anorexia nervosa.

Lasègue's law. Reflexes are enhanced in the presence of functional disorders but diminished in the presence of organic lesions.

Lasègue's sign, or test. 1. Painful straight leg raising in sciatica; it is usual to record the result of the test as the angle to which the leg can be raised without giving pain. 2. A patient with loss of postural sensibility in a limb may be able to move and use it when the eyes are open, but when the eyes are closed it becomes useless, since the patient does not know where it is.

laser (**la**·ser). A device containing certain substances, which, when stimulated with light energy of sufficient intensity, emit a beam of light which has the following properties: it is coherent, monochromatic, highly directional, and of great intensity. Lasers are used in ophthalmology to treat retinal and choroidal disease, and also in dentistry, skin surgery and cancer therapy. [*L*ight *A*mplification by the *S*timulated *E*mission of *R*adiation.]

Lassaigne's test. For organic nitrogen: a small bright piece of sodium is placed in a long narrow hard-glass test-tube with a little of the substance to be tested. The tube is heated gently until charring commences, and then to dull red heat for 30 s. The tube is then plunged whilst still hot into about 10 ml of water, when the tube shatters and the residual sodium reacts with the water. The solution is boiled and filtered. To 5 ml of filtrate is added 0.5 ml of a saturated ferrous sulphate solution, which has been boiled and cooled to form some ferric salt, and the solution is boiled for 30 s, cooled rapidly and concentrated hydrochloric acid added drop by drop until the precipitate dissolves. If the substance tested contains nitrogen, the solution will be bluish-green and a precipitate of Prussian blue will gradually form; if nitrogen is absent the solution remains yellow.

Lassar, Oskar (b. 1849). Berlin dermatologist.

Lassar's paste. Salicylic acid 2 per cent, zinc oxide 24 per cent, starch 24 per cent, soft paraffin 50 per cent; one of the best known of all medicinal pastes.

lata, lâtah (**lah**·tah). A psychoneurotic condition peculiar to members of the Malay race and characterized by clouding of the consciousness with impulsive, mimetic and repetitive tendencies, i.e. echolalia and echopraxia. [Malay, ticklish.]

Latarget, André (b. 1877). Lyons anatomist.

Latarget's nerve. The hypogastric plexus. *See* PLEXUS.

Latarget's vein. The prepyloric vein, or vein of Mayo; it serves to demarcate the pylorus.

latency (**la**·ten·se). The quality or the state of appearing to be inactive; the latent period intervening between the moment of application of a stimulus and the moment at which the response begins. It is also applied to a bacterial or other parasitic infection: in this case reactivation may occur after a long period of latency. **Latency period.** *See* PERIOD. [L *latere* to keep out of sight.]

latent (**la**·tent). 1. Dormant; existing but not manifest. 2. Potential. [L *latere* to keep out of sight.]

lateral (**lat**·er·al). 1. Towards, at, or belonging to, the side. 2. [LATERALIS (NA)] Relating or belonging to structures which are on the outer side of the median plane. 3. Radiographic projection in which the x-ray beam is directed from one side of the body, e.g. left lateral decubitus (*cross-table lateral*) when the x-rays enter the side of the recumbent patient and penetrate the body in a horizontal direction. [L *latus* side.]

latericeous (lat·er·**ish**·us). Having the appearance and quality of brick dust. [L *later* brick.]

latericumbent (lat·er·e·**kum'**·bent). Descriptive of a person lying on his side. [L *latus* side, *cumbere* to lie.]

laterigrade (lat·er·e·grade). Laterograde.

lateritious (lat·er·**ish**·us). Latericeous.

lateriversion (lat·er·e·**ver'**·shun). Lateroversion.

latero-abdominal (lat·er·o·ab·**dom'**·in·al). Relating or belonging to the abdomen and the sides, flanks, or loins, or to the sides of the abdomen. [L *latus* side, abdomen.]

lateroduction (lat·er·o·**duk'**·shun). Muscular action or movement to one or the other side, with special reference to the eye. [L *latus* side, *ducere* to draw.]

lateroflexion (lat·er·o·**flek'**·shun). Lateral flexion; the condition of being bent or curved to one or other side. [L *latus* side, flexion.]

laterograde (lat·er·o·grade). Moving or advancing towards the side. [L *latus* side, *gradi* to step.]

lateromarginal (lat·er·o·**mar'**·jin·al). Situated on the lateral margin or border. [L *latus* side, margin.]

lateroposition (lat·er·o·po·**zish'**·un). The state of being displaced to one side. [L *latus* side, position.]

lateropulsion (lat·er·o·**pul'**·shun). Lateral pulsion; movement of involuntary kind to one side, e.g. in walking. [L *latus* side, *pellere* to drive.]

laterotorsion (lat·er·o·**tor'**·shun). Lateral torsion; twisting to one side, especially with reference to the eye in which the vertical meridian is diverted to one or the other side. [L *latus* side, torsion.]

lateroversion (lat·er·o·**ver'**·shun). Lateral version; turning or being deflected to one or other side. [L *latus* side, version.]

latex (la·tex). An emulsion or suspension produced in special cells or vessels contained in the tissues of certain plants. The latex exudes from the plant when the tissue is cut. [L, liquid.]

lathyrism (lath·ir·izm). A disease that occurs, particularly in times of famine, among peoples that have vetches of the genus *Lathyrus* as their staple diet, e.g. India and Spain. There are several theories as to its cause: that certain conditions favour poisonous changes in the vetch; that a poisonous contaminating weed, *Vicia sativa*, which is very like *Lathyrus* in appearance, is responsible; and that the disease is due to a conditioned vitamin deficiency. The main symptoms are muscular weakness and a spastic paraplegia that is irreversible. [Gk *lathyros* a pulse.]

Lathyrus (lath·i·rus). A genus of vetches, the consumption of which has been associated with lathyrism. The species involved include *Lathyrus cicera*, *L. odoratus* and *L. sativus*. [see prec.]

latissimus colli muscle (lat·is·im·us **kol**·i musl). The platysma muscle. [L, widest of the neck.]

latissimus dorsi muscle [musculus latissimus dorsi (NA)] (lat·is·im·us **dor**·si musl). A large, flat, triangular muscle covering the lumbar region and lower part of the chest, arising from the lumbar fascia and iliac crest, and inserted on the upper third of the humerus. [L, widest of the back.]

latissimus dorsi muscle, nerve to the [nervus thoracodorsalis (NA)]. A branch of the posterior cord of the brachial plexus to this muscle. [see prec.]

latitude (lat·it·ewd). A term used in radiology to describe the range of exposure of an x-ray film that is compatible with an adequate diagnostic result. [L *latitudinis* broad.]

latrine (lat·**reen**). A privy, or place used for urination or defaecation; applied especially to military sanitary offices, permanent and temporary, in barracks and camps. [L *latrina*.]

Latrodectus (lat·ro·**dek**·tus). A genus of spiders. The numerous species are black with white or red markings, and the bite of several is dangerous and occasionally fatal. *Latrodectus tredecimguttatus*, from Southern Europe and Asia Minor, *L. hasselti*, from Australia, and *L. mactans*, the black widow, from the Americas, are the best known. [L *latro* robber, Gk *dekein* to bite.]

lattice (lat·is). A regular geometrical arrangement of units over an area or in space; the atom arrangement in a crystal is an example of a lattice. [OFr. *lattis*.]

Latzko, Wilhelm (b. 1863). Viennese obstetrician.

Latzko's operation. 1. A type of extra-peritoneal caesarean section where the bladder is retracted laterally. 2. A method of treating a small vesicovaginal fistula by local excision and suturing in two layers. 3. An extended abdominal hysterectomy for the treatment of carcinoma of the cervix (obsolete).

Laubry, Charles (b. 1872). French physician.

Laubry, Routier, and van Bogaert sign. Presystolic gallop rhythm (atrial gallop). *See* RHYTHM, GALLOP.

laudable (lawd·abl). Healthy; at one time used to describe thick, creamy, inoffensive pus, which was regarded as an indication of the healthy state of a wound. [L *laudare* to praise.]

laudanum (law·dan·um). Tincture of opium; a tincture prepared from raw opium by maceration, first with water and subsequently with alcohol (50 per cent). It contains one per cent of anhydrous morphine, and was used as a narcotic. [etym. dub.]

Laudet's tinnitus. A ticking sound resulting from spasm of the tensor palati muscle.

Laudexium Methylsulphate (law·**dex**·e·um meth·il·**sul**·fate). BP Commission approved name for a complex synthetic muscle relaxant closely resembling D-tubocurarine, but producing a relaxation lasting about 30 per cent longer for an equipotent dose.

Laue, Max von (b. 1879). German physicist.

Laue method. A method of obtaining an x-ray diffraction pattern from a crystal, using a heterogeneous x-ray beam and a stationary crystal.

laugh (lahf). 1. To make the sounds and facial movements which are expressive of amusement, scorn, or exultation and associated with laughter; hence *laughing*. 2. The sound of laughing. **Canine laugh, sardonic laugh.** Risus caninus, risus sardonicus. [AS *hlehhan*.]

laughter (lahf·ter). A series of irregular and often involuntary expirations associated with vibratory movements of the vocal cords which are usually expressive of amusement; laughter may also be a sign of hysteria or a reflex action set up by tickling. **Compulsive laughter, obsessive laughter.** The loud laughter for which there is no cause, which is sometimes a symptom of schizophrenia. [AS *hleahtor*.]

Laugier, Stanislas (b. 1799). Paris surgeon.

Laugier's hernia. Hernia through the lacunar ligament.

Laumonier, Jean Baptiste (b. 1749). Rouen surgeon.

Laumonier's ganglion. A collection of ganglion cells in the carotid nerve.

Launois, Pierre-Emile (b. 1856). Paris physician.

Launois' syndrome, Launois-Clérat syndrome. Acromegalic gigantism. Obsolete.

Laura, Giovanni Battista (fl. 1882). Turin anatomist.

Laura's nucleus. The lateral vestibular nucleus, or Deiters' nucleus.

Laurence, John Zachariah (b. 1830). London ophthalmologist.

Laurence-Biedl syndrome. More generally known as the Laurence-Moon-Biedl dystrophy, or syndrome (see foll.).

Laurence-Moon-Biedl syndrome. (Sometimes also known as the Laurence-Moon-Bardet-Biedl syndrome.) The combination of obesity, sexual under-development, retinitis pigmentosa, mental deficiency, and polydactylism or syndactylism.

Laurens, Georges. 20th century French surgeon.

Laurens' operation. A plastic operation for the closure of a fistula in the region of the mastoid.

Laurocerasus BPC 1949 (law·ro·**ser**·as·us). Cherry laurel, laurocerasi folia; the leaves of the cherry laurel, *Prunus laurocerasus* Linn. (family Rosaceae). When fresh they yield hydrocyanic acid on hydrolysis, and a solution prepared from them, known as cherry-laurel water, is used as a mild sedative and carminative. [L *laurus* laurel, *cerasus* cherry.]

Laurolinium Acetate (law·ro·**lin**·e·um **as**·et·ate). BP Commission approved name for 4-amino-1-dodecylquinaldinium acetate; an antiseptic.

Laurus (law·rus). A genus of shrubs (family Lauraceae). The leaves and fruits of the bay laurel, *Laurus nobilis* Linn., yield a volatile oil used as a stimulating application in rheumatism. [L, laurel.]

lauryl (law·ril). 1. The group $C_{12}H_{25}$, derived from lauryl alcohol. 2. The acyl group $CH_3(CH_2)_{10}CO$, derived from lauric acid. **Lauryl alcohol.** *See* ALCOHOL. **Lauryl thiocyanate.** $C_{12}H_{25}CNS$, a compound used in a 10 per cent emulsion in pediculosis pubis.

Lauth, Ernest Alexandre (b. 1803). Strasbourg physiologist.

Lauth's canal, or sinus. The sinus venosus sclerae.

Lauth, Thomas (b. 1758). Strasbourg anatomist and surgeon.

Lauth's ligament. A fibrous slip derived from the alar ligaments of the occipito-axoid articulation which passes from one side of the foramen magnum to the other behind the odontoid process of the axis. It is superior to the transverse ligament.

Lautier J. T. 20th century French physician.

Lautier's test. Two to three drops of 1 per cent dilution of Old Tuberculin BP 1958 are dried on the skin of the forearm and covered for 48 hours with adhesive plaster. A red papular reaction is produced in tuberculous subjects; only a negative reaction is of any clinical value.

lavage (lav·**ahzh**, **lav**·ahzh, **lav**·ij). The act of washing-out or irrigating an organ (e.g. the stomach). **Lavage of the blood, blood lavage.** A process in use at one time of adding serum to the circulating blood to dilute circulating toxic substances. **Colonic lavage.** Lavage of the colon. **Ether lavage.** An obsolete process of washing out the cavity of the peritoneum with ether in cases of peritonitis or pelvic infection. **Gastric lavage.** Lavage of the stomach, e.g. to remove poisons. **Peritoneal lavage.** A continuous infusion of saline into the cavity of the peritoneum combined with an outflow, for removal of metabolites, e.g. in uraemia. **Pleural lavage.** Lavage of the pleural cavity following paracentesis. **Systemic lavage.** Lavage of the blood (see above). [Fr.]

lavation (lav·a·shun). Lavage; irrigation or washing out.

lavender (lav·en·der). A widely cultivated shrub, *Lavandula officinalis* Chaix (family Labiatae). [LL *lavendula.*]

Laveran, Charles Louis Alphonse (b. 1845). French pathologist and parasitologist in Algeria.

Laveran's corpuscle. A term at one time used to describe the malaria parasite which Laveran discovered.

Laverania (lav·er·a·ne·ah). A generic name given to the parasites of malaria and still employed by some French writers, but the name *Plasmodium* is now generally used. [C. L. A. *Laveran.*]

laveur (lah·**ver**). An appliance used in irrigation of an organ. [Fr., one that washes.]

lavipedium (lav·e·**pe**·de·um). A foot bath. [L *lavare* to wash, *pes* foot.]

law (law). 1. Any rule laid down by a recognized authority and enforced by prescribed sanctions. 2. In science, a concise general statement of facts or principles, as applied to natural phenomena, which has been tested and tried so as to render it practically beyond doubt. **All-or-none law.** In cardiac and skeletal muscle the weakest stimulus capable of producing a contraction will produce the maximal one possible in the circumstances. **Law of anticipation.** Mott's law of anticipation. **Law of avalanche.** The hypothesis that a single peripheral stimulus might give rise to multiple sensory responses centrally (Ramón y Cajal). **Law of average localization.** Visceral pain is best localized in the least mobile viscera. **Biogenetic law.** Haeckel's law. **Law of combining weights.** Law of reciprocal proportions (see below). **Law of constant composition.** Any specific chemical compound always contains the same elements combined in the same proportions by weight. **Law of constant energy consumption.** Rubner's law. 1. **Law of constant growth quotient.** Rubner's law 2. **Law of constant proportions.** Law of constant composition (see above). **Law of contrary innervation.** A nerve the stimulation of which causes flexion also contains inhibitory fibres for the extensors. **Law of definite proportions.** Law of constant composition (see above). **Law of denervation.** Denervation of an organ sometimes increases its sensitivity to certain chemical stimulants. **Law of diffusion.** Any process set up in the nerve centres affects the organism as a whole. **Law of equivalents.** Law of reciprocal proportions (see below). **Law of excitation.** Dubois-Reymond law. **Law of facilitation.** A series of neurones through which an impulse has once passed are altered in some way so that there is less resistance to the next impulse. Consequently a given impulse will always tend to take the same path. **Law of fatigue.** Houghton's law. **Law of frequency of error.** *See* VARIANCE. **Gas laws.** Laws relating the volume of a gas to its temperature and pressure; examples are Boyle's law and Charles' law. **Gaussian distribution law.** In statistics, the normal frequency distribution curve that is bell-shaped. **Law of gravitation.** Newton's law. **Law of the heart.** Starling's law. **Law of independent assortment.** The genetic expression of Mendel's second law: the distribution of one pair of allelomorphic genes is independent of the distribution of any other pair, provided that the two pairs do not lie on the same pair of chromosomes. **Law of initial value.** The more nearly an organ is working at maximal capacity the less easily can it be stimulated to do further work, though it may be depressed or inhibited without difficulty. **Law of inverse squares.** The intensity of any effect (e.g. radiation, gravitation, etc.) at a point varies inversely as the square of the distance of the point from the source of the effect. **Law of isochronism.** Normally the chronaxia of a muscle and that of its nerve are of the same order. **Law of isolated conduction.** A nerve impulse in one neurone passes to other neurones only through the terminal synaptic connections. **Linkage law.** Genes situated on the same chromosome tend to segregate together, in contradiction of the law of independent assortment (see above). The strength of this tendency is, in general, inversely proportional to the linear distance between the gene loci. **Law of mass action.** In a chemical reaction, the rate of chemical change is proportional to the molecular concentrations of the interacting substances. **Law of multiple proportions.** When two elements combine to form more than one compound, the different weights of one element which combine with a given weight of the other bear a simple whole-number relationship to one another. **Myelinogenetic law.** Flechsig's myelinogenetic law. **Law of ocular movements.** The movements of the two eyes are equal and symmetrical. This law is correct except for extreme lateral movements, when the fixation line of one eye is interfered with by the nose. Also called *Hering's law.* **Periodic law.** The principle enunciated by Mendeléeff in 1869 that if the elements are arranged in order of their atomic weights their properties, being functions of the latter, show a regular periodicity and the elements themselves fall into related groups. The modern Periodic Table is based on order of atomic number. **Psychophysical law.** In order that a sensation may increase in intensity by arithmetical progression, the stimulus must increase by geometrical progression. **Law of reciprocal proportions.** The weights of elements which individually combine with a given weight of a particular element are also the weights with which they combine with one another, or a simple whole-number multiple of them. **Law of referred pain.** Morley's law. **Laws of reflection.** 1. The incident ray, the normal to the surface at the point of incidence, and the reflected ray lie in the same plane. 2. The incident and reflected rays are equally inclined to the normal and lie on opposite sides of it, i.e. the angle of incidence is equal to the angle of reflection. **Laws of refraction.** 1. The incident ray, the normal to the surface at the point of incidence, and the refracted ray lie in the same plane. 2. The sine of the angle of refraction bears a constant relation to the sine of the angle of incidence, this ratio depending on the nature of the two media and the incident light. Also called *Snell's law.* **Law of refreshment.** A fatigued muscle recovers at a rate depending on its blood supply. **Law of regression.** Galton's law of regression. **Law of relativity.** Simultaneous and successive sensations modify each other. **Law of segregation.** The genetic expression of Mendel's first law: the two members of an allelomorphic pair of genes segregate during meiotic cell division. **Law of specific irritability.** Mueller's law: normally each type of sensory nerve responds to its specific stimulus only, and gives rise to a specific sensation. Abnormally, it may respond to an unusual stimulus, but the induced sensation is of the same type as before. [AS *lagu.*]

See also: ABNEY, ALLEN (F. M.), AMPÈRE, ÅNGSTRÖM, ARAN,

ARNDT, ARRHENIUS, AVOGADRO, BABINSKI, BAER (K. E.), BASTIAN, BAUMÉS (P. P. F.), BEER, BEHRING, BELL (C.), BERGONIÉ, BERTHOLLET, BLAGDEN, BORDET, BOUDIN, BOWDITCH, BOYLE (R.), BRETON, BREWSTER, BRUNS, BUHL, BUNSEN, CAMERER, CHARLES, CLAPEYRON, COLLES, COPE (E. D.), COULOMB, COURVOISIER, CURIE (P.), CUSHING (HARVEY W.), DALTON, DASTRE, DESCARTES, DIDAY, DITTRICH, DOLLO, DONDERS, DRAPER, DUBOIS-REYMOND, DULONG, EDINGER, ELLIOTT (T. R.), FAGET, FAJANS, FARADAY, FARR, FECHNER, FICK, FITZ (R. H.), FLATAU, FLECHSIG, FLOURENS, FOWLER (J. K.), FRORIEP (A.), GALTON, GAY-LUSSAC, GERHARDT (C. C. A. J.), GODÉLIER, GOLGI, GOMPERTZ, GOODELL, GRAHAM (T.), GRASSET, GROTTHUS, GUDDEN, GULDBERG, HAECKEL, HEIDENHAIN, HELLIN, HELMHOLTZ, HENRY (W.), HERING (K. E. K.), HESS (G. H.), HEYMAN, HILTON, HOFF, HOORWEG, HORNER (J. F.), HOUGHTON, JACKSON (J. H.), JOULE, KAHLER, KASSOWITZ, KINNEY, KIRSCHMANN, KOCH (R.), KOHLRAUSCH (F.), LAMBERT (J. H.), LANCEREAUX, LANDOUZY, LAPICQUE, LASÈGUE, LE CHATELIER, LENZ, LISTING, LOSSEN, LOUIS, MACH, MAGENDIE, MAREY, MARIOTTE, MAXWELL (J. C.), MELTZER, MENDEL (G. J.), MENDELÉEFF, METCHNIKOFF, MORAT, MORLEY, MOTT, MUELLER (J.), MURPHY (J. B.), NAEGELI, NASSE, NERNST, NEUMANN (F. E.), NEWLANDS, NEWTON (I.), NYSTEN, OHM, PASCAL, PETER (C. F. M.), PETIT (A. T.), PFLUEGER, PLATEAU, POISEUILLE, POISSON (S. D.), PRENTICE, PREVOST, PROFETA, PROUST (L. J.), RAOULT, RITTER (J. W.), ROSCOE, ROSENBACH (O.), RUBNER, SCHROEDER VAN DER KOLK, SCHULZ, SEMON (F.), SHERRINGTON, SNELL (S.), SPALLANZANI, STARLING, STOKES (G. G.), STOKES (WILLIAM), TAIT, TALBOT (W. H. F.), TOYNBEE, TRIBONDEAU, VALLI, VIRCHOW, VULPIAN, WAAGE, WALLER, WALTON, WEBER (E. H.), WEIGERT, WIEN, WILDER, WOLFF (J.), WUNDERLICH.

Lawford, John Bowring (b. 1858). London ophthalmologist.

Lawford's corneal splitter. An instrument designed for a similar purpose to Tooke's corneal splitter, but shaped like a narrow-bladed knife with a slight convex curve to the cutting edge and a rounded tip.

Lawford's eye speculum. One in which the upper retracting part is solid and the lower fenestrated.

lawrencium (law·ren·se·um). The transuranic element of atomic number 103, and chemical symbol Lr. [named after Ernest Orlando *Lawrence* inventor of the cyclotron and 1939 Nobel Prize winner for Physics.]

lax (lax). Relaxed; loose. **Cardia lax.** Cardio-oesophageal relaxation. *See* RELAXATION. [L *laxus* loose.]

laxarthrus (lax·ar·thrus). Dislocation of a joint. [L *laxus* loose, Gk *arthron* joint.]

laxation (lax·a·shun). An evacuation of the bowels, natural or induced by various agents. [see foll.]

laxative (lax·at·iv). 1. Aperient. 2. An aperient remedy. [L *laxare* to loosen.]

laxator (lax·a·tor). Anything that has a relaxing effect. [see prec.]

laxitas (lax·it·as). Looseness or lack of compactness or tone. **Laxitas alvi.** Diarrhoea. **Laxitas gingivarum.** Spongy gums. **Laxitas ventriculi.** Atony of the stomach. [L, looseness.]

laxity (lax·it·e). Atony; looseness. [see prec.]

layer [stratum (NA)] (la·er). A covering of even thickness spread over an area. **Adamantine layer.** The layer of enamel on a tooth. **Anterior limiting layer of the iris.** A modified stroma consisting mostly of chromatophores, and the most anterior layer except for endothelium. **Bacillary layer of the retina.** The layer of rods and cones, and the outermost layer. **Basal layer.** Stratum basale; the deepest layer of the uterine mucosa which is not involved in menstruation or parturition. **Basal-cell layer of the epidermis [stratum basale (cylindricum) (NA)].** The basal layer of the epidermis, abutting on the basement membrane, from which all other cells of the epidermis are derived by mitotic division of its cells. **Basement layer.** Basement membrane; a fibrous or hyaline membrane connecting an epithelium to the underlying connective tissue. **Blastodermic layer.** Germ layer (see below). **Buffy layer.** Buffy coat. *See* COAT. **Layers of the cerebellar cortex.** *See* CORTEX. **Cerebral layer of the retina [stratum cerebrale (NA)].** The inner five layers. **Circular layer of the colon [stratum circulare (NA)].** The circular muscle coat of the colon. **Circular layer of the eardrum.** The circular elastic fibres of the middle layer of the tympanic membrane. **Clear layer of the epidermis [stratum lucidum (NA)].** The layer of clear cells beneath the horny layer. **Columnar layer.** The rod-and-cone layer of the retina. **Compact layer.** The most superficial layer of the uterine mucosa containing the narrow necks of the uterine glands. It is most prominent in the luteal phase of the menstrual cycle and in early pregnancy. **Cuticular layer.** A cuticle; a horny layer at the free end of a cell. **Cuticular layer of the tympanic membrane.** The outer or skin layer of the tympanic membrane. **Dermic layer.** Cuticular layer of the tympanic membrane (see prec.). **Ependymal layer.** The inner of the three zones in the wall of the neural tube of the embryo. Now known as the matrix layer. **Epitrichial layer.** The outermost cellular layer of the embryonic epidermis. **Fatty layer of the perineum.** The loose fatty layer of the superficial fascia of the perineum. **Ganglionic layer of the retina [stratum ganglionare nervi optici (NA)].** The layer of ganglion cells; the innermost layer of retina except for nerve fibres. **Germ layer.** One of the three layers of cells comprising the early embryo, viz. ectoderm, mesoderm, and entoderm. **Germinative layer.** The deeper layers of the stratified epithelium of the epidermis which show cell division and are responsible for the renewal of the epithelium as it is denuded from the surface. **Granular layer.** The middle zone of the cerebellar cortex, containing many small nerve cells. **Granular layer of the epidermis [stratum granulosum (NA)].** The layer of flattened cells containing granules which stain with carmine. **Half-value layer.** The thickness of a material required to reduce the intensity of an x-ray beam to half its original value. **Horny layer of the epidermis [stratum corneum (NA)].** The superficial layer of the epidermis containing keratinized cells. **Inner molecular layer of the retina.** Inner plexiform layer of the retina (see below). **Inner neuroblastic layer.** An embryonic retinal layer which gives rise to ganglion cells, amacrine cells, and nuclei of Mueller's fibres. **Inner nuclear layer of the retina [stratum ganglionare retinae (NA)].** A layer of nerve nuclei consisting of bipolar cells, amacrine and horizontal cells, and nuclei of Mueller's fibres. **Inner plexiform layer of the retina.** Synapses of the nerve fibres of the bipolar and amacrine cells with those of the ganglion cells. **Mantle layer.** The middle zone of the wall of the neural tube of the embryo. **Marginal layer.** A superficial embryonic layer of cells of the optic cup forming later the nerve-fibre layer and layer of Chievitz; the outer zone of the wall of the neural tube. **Matrix layer.** The innermost layer of the embryonic neural tube, the cells of which give rise to the ependyma and to the cells of the mantle and marginal layers. **Membranous layer of the perineum.** The thin aponeurotic layer of the superficial fascia of the perineum, lying deep to the fatty layer and attached to the rami of the pubis and ischium laterally, the posterior border of the perineal membrane behind, and continuous in front through the dartos muscle with a similar layer over the lower abdomen. **Nerve-fibre layer of the retina.** The innermost layer of the retina, consisting of nerve fibres running to the disc to form the optic nerve. **Neurodermal layer.** The ectoderm. **Neuro-epithelial layer of the retina [stratum neuro-epitheliale (NA)].** The outermost layer of the retina. **Osteoblastic layer, osteogenetic layer.** The deepest layer of the periosteum, lying adjacent to the bone, and containing osteoblasts or potential osteoblasts. **Outer molecular layer.** Outer plexiform layer of the retina (see below). **Outer neuroblastic layer.** An embryonic retinal layer giving rise to nuclei of rods and cones, bipolar cells, and horizontal cells. **Outer nuclear layer of the retina.** A layer of nerve nuclei deep to rods and cones. **Outer plexiform layer of the retina.** Synapses of the nerve fibres of the inner nuclear layer with those of the outer nuclear layer of the retina. **Pigmented layer [stratum pigmenti (NA)].** The internal layer of the eye comprising the pigmented layers of the ciliary body, iris, and retina. **Pigmented layer of the ciliary body [stratum pigmenti corporis ciliaris (NA)].** A double layer of cuboidal pigmented cells on the posterior surface of the ciliary body; it is the forward continuation of the retina. **Pigmented**

layer of the iris [stratum pigmenti iridis (NA)]. The forward continuation of the retina on to the iris, consisting of a double layer of pigmented cells. **Pigmented layer of the retina [stratum pigmenti retinae (NA)].** The outer layer of the retina, composed of pigmented cuboidal cells extending as a double layer on to the surface of the ciliary body and iris. **Prickle-cell layer of the epidermis [stratum spinosum (NA)].** Several layers of the epidermis immediately superficial to the basal-cell layer of the epidermis, where the individual cells are connected by cell bridges. When a single cell is examined, the incomplete bridges on its borders appear as prickles. **Primary blastodermic layer.** The single-layered embryo before the appearance of the definitive germ layers. **Primitive layer.** A deep embryonic layer of neuro-epithelium of the optic cup forming later the inner and outer neuroblastic layer. **Layer of rods and cones.** The outermost layer of the retina. **Skeletogenous layer.** That portion of the mesoderm from which bone and cartilage will arise. **Sluggish layer, still layer.** The blood nearest the vessel wall where white cells tend to accumulate. **Submantle layer.** The layer of orthodentine around the tooth pulp; circumpulpar dentine. **Transient fibre layer.** *See* CHIEVITZ LAYER. **Trophic layer.** Old term for the entoderm. **Vegetative layer.** Entoderm. **Vessel layer of the iris.** A layer almost entirely made up of blood vessels running in a meridional direction. **Yellow layer.** Buffy coat. *See* COAT. [AS *lecgan.*]

See also: BAILLARGER, BECHTEREW, BERNARD (C.), BOWMAN, CHIEVITZ, DÉBOVE, DOBIE, GENNARI, HALLER, HENLE, HUXLEY, KAES, LANGERHANS, LANGHANS, MALPIGHI, MAUTHNER, MEYNERT, NITABUCH, OEHL, OLLIER, PANDER, PURKINJE, RAUBER, RENAUT, ROHR, SATTLER, TOMES (J.), UNNA, WALDEYER-HARTZ, WEIL (L. A.), ZEISSL.

layette (la·et). Inclusive term for the set of clothes, bed, furniture, toilet, and other articles required for the newborn child. [Fr., baby-linen.]

Leach's test. For formaldehyde in milk: 10 ml of milk are mixed in a porcelain dish with 10 ml of concentrated hydrochloric acid containing 0.2 ml of 10 per cent ferric chloride solution per 100 ml. On warming the mixture nearly to boiling point with constant agitation to break up the curd, a violet colour appears if formaldehyde is present, and a brown colour if absent.

leaching (le·ching). Lixiviation; the process of washing out the soluble contents of a mixture, leaving the insoluble portion behind. [AS *leccan.*]

lead (led). An element of atomic weight 207.2, atomic number 82, and chemical symbol Pb (*plumbum*). It is a relatively soft and malleable metal, found naturally in the form of ores, principally galena, PbS, and is used in low-melting alloys, plumbing, chemical plant, and, in its compounds, in the manufacture of paint. It is di- and trivalent, forming respectively *plumbous* and *plumbic* salts. Minute traces are found in grasses, crustacea, and molluscs. Therapeutically its compounds are employed mainly as astringent lotions, but its importance medically lies in its toxic effects, lead poisoning being a serious risk in industrial processes. The risk has, however, been much reduced by the adoption of various protective measures. The chief features of lead poisoning are abdominal colic with constipation, anaemia with punctate basophilia, and wrist drop; a bluish punctate line near the gum margins occurs when lead is absorbed in sufficient quantity. Individual susceptibility shows considerable variation. Lead compounds have been used to procure abortion, and several deaths have been caused in this way. **Lead Acetate BP 1963.** Sugar of lead, $(CH_3COO)_2Pb{\cdot}3H_2O$, a white, crystalline, soluble substance which has astringent properties when employed in dilute solution. **Lead azide.** PbN_3, an unstable compound used in detonators. **Black lead.** Graphite. **Lead carbonate.** Plumbi Carbonas BPC 1949. **Lead chloride.** $PbCl_2$, an insoluble white compound, important as a pigment and reagent. **Lead Chromate.** Chrome yellow, $PbCrO_4$, a yellow pigment. **Lead Monoxide BP 1963.** Litharge, massicot, PbO, a reddish-brown powdery substance, used to prepare Solutions of Lead Subacetate BP 1958, and emplastrum plumbi. **Lead oleate.** $(C_{17}H_{33}COO)_2Pb$, the chief component of lead plaster, which is used for its astringent properties, particularly in the treatment of corns and bunions. **Lead oxide.** Lead monoxide (see above). **Plastermass of Lead BPC 1954.** Diachylon, a preparation made from lead monoxide, arachis oil, and water; it is used for its mildly astringent properties. **Red lead.** Minium, Pb_3O_4, a compound used in the manufacture of glass. **Stable lead.** Radium G. **Lead subacetate.** $Pb_2O(OOCCH_3)_2$, a compound employed as a lotion. **Tetraethyl lead.** $Pb(C_2H_5)_4$, a clear, oily liquid added to petrol to prevent premature ignition. It may be absorbed through the skin as well as by the lungs and alimentary canal, causing lead poisoning with predominance of nervous symptoms and signs. **Lead tetroxide.** Red lead (see above). **White lead.** Lead carbonate (see above). [AS.]

lead (leed). An electrocardiographic record which varies in accordance with the placing of the two electrodes on the body: *Lead I,* right arm and left arm; *Lead II,* right arm and left leg; *Lead III,* left arm and left leg. **Chest lead.** The electrocardiographic lead from the chest wall overlying the heart. Such a lead is formed either by coupling the precordial electrode with a remote electrode on a limb (*bipolar precordial lead*), or with a central terminal to which electrodes on the left arm, right arm, and left leg are connected (*unipolar precordial lead*). Single precordial leads have now been abandoned in favour of multiple leads, each of which has an exact position on the chest wall (1 to 7). The number of the lead is prefixed by the letter V in the case of unipolar lead, and CF, CR, or CL, according to whether the remote electrode is on the left leg, right arm, or left arm, respectively, in the case of bipolar leads. Positions 1 and 2 are on the 4th intercostal space at the right and left sternal borders respectively; position 4 is at the intersection of the midclavicular line with the 5th intercostal space, and position 3 is at the midpoint of a straight line drawn between positions 2 and 4. Position 5 lies at the intersection of a horizontal line drawn laterally from position 4 with the anterior axillary line. Position 6 lies at the intersection of a horizontal line drawn laterally from position 5 with the midaxillary line, whilst position 7 lies at the same level in the posterior axillary line. Additional leads in analogous positions to the right of the sternum are often used (V_3R, V_4R, V_6R). **Direct lead.** The electric potentials recorded from an electrode placed directly on the source of electrical activity (heart, brain, etc.), and paired with another electrode at the periphery. In experimental electrocardiography, a direct lead is obtained when an electrode is placed directly upon the surface of the heart muscle and paired with a remote electrode placed at a sufficient distance from the exploring electrode to render negligible the influence of the remote upon the central electrode. When this exploring electrode is connected to a central terminal to which have been connected the right arm, left arm, and left leg electrodes, the influence of the remote electrode is neutralized, the central terminal being at zero, and the exploring electrode records faithfully the potentials beneath it. **Indirect lead.** That obtained when the exploring electrode cannot be placed directly on the source of electrical activity, but at a distance. The surrounding tissues form an electrolyte solution which allows spread of the current from the source in three directions, thus acting as a volume conductor. The exploring electrode is placed as close to the source as possible and paired with a central terminal or with a direct lead. That placed upon the precordium and connected to the central terminal records an almost true picture of the changes in electric potential beneath it, distortion due to the volume conductor being minimal. This is an indirect or semidirect unipolar precordial lead. **Oesophageal lead.** The record obtained with one electrode on the oesophagus. **Precordial lead.** *See* CHEST LEAD (above). **V lead, voltage lead.** A record using an indifferent electrode of minimal potential charge, obtained by connecting the right arm, left arm, and left leg in a central terminal; the second, or exploring, electrode may be placed on the precordium or other part of the body. [AS *laedan.*]

Leadbetter, Guy Whitman (b. 1893). Washington orthopaedic surgeon.

Leadbetter manoeuvre. Reduction of the deformity from fracture of the neck of the femur by traction inflexion, internal rotation and abduction of the hip.

leader (le·der). A tendon; the term is obsolescent, but is used by the layman. [AS *laedan.*]

leading (led·ing). Chronic lead poisoning. *See* POISONING. [AS *lead.*]

leaflet (leef·let). In cardiology, a valve cusp, especially of the mitral or tricuspid valves. [AS *léaf* leaf.]

leak (leek). **Natural leak.** The rate of loss of charge of a capacitor due to cosmic rays, or possibly radioactive contamination or faulty insulators. In measuring instruments such as electrometers the natural leak must be subtracted from the observed leak to obtain the true rate of discharge. [Old Norse *leka* drip.]

leakage (le·kij). A term used in psycho-analysis; it describes any discussion the patient may have in regard to his analysis, with an individual other than the psycho-analyst in charge of the case. [see prec.]

Leake and Guy method. A method for counting blood platelets by suspending them in a diluting fluid containing formalin (6 ml), sodium oxalate (1.6 g), and crystal violet (0.01 g) in water (94 ml).

lean body mass. Cell solids, extracellular and intracellular water and mineral mass.

leans (leenz). An illusion of leaning to one side sometimes experienced by aviators; a form of disorientation. [ME *lenen* to lean.]

leash (leesh). A term which refers to bands or bundles of nerves, fibres, veins, arteries, or other cordlike structures. [OFr. *lesse.*]

leben (leb·en). A fermented sour milk preparation made by Arabs. [Ar.]

Leber, Theodor von (b. 1840). Gottingen and Heidelberg ophthalmologist.

Circle of Leber, or Leber's venous plexus. An intrascleral anastomosis of the ciliary veins at the sclerocorneal junction.

Leber's congenital amaurosis. A recessive disorder characterized by blindness, or near blindness, in infants with normal fundi. Later, the appearance of pigmentary retinal degeneration develops.

Leber's congenital retinal miliary aneurysms. Congenital vascular malformations which may be stationary, cause vitreous haemorrhages, or progress into classical Coats' disease.

Leber's corpuscle. Hassall's corpuscle.

Leber's disease, von Leber's optic atrophy. A hereditary form of optic atrophy, usually affecting young males, and preceded by transient signs of optic neuritis.

Leber's optic atrophy. A disease with a unique form of hereditary transmission, usually affecting males but not transmitted through the male line. The onset is often subacute and vision is impaired by bilateral central scotomata, but visual loss is not usually progressive.

Lebistes (leb·is·teez). A genus of freshwater fish. **Lebistes reticulatus.** The millions fish, or guppy, native to the West Indies. It has been used extensively in the control of mosquitoes and as a laboratory animal. [Gk.]

Lecat, Claude Nicolas (b. 1700). Rouen surgeon and anatomist.

Lecat's gulf. The dilated bulb of the anterior urethra which lies immediately in front of its membranous portion.

Le Chatelier, Henri Louis (b. 1850). French physical chemist.

Le Chatelier's law, or principle. Any stress applied to a system in equilibrium produces a reaction that tends to annul the stress.

leche de higueron (la·cha da e·ga·rone). The latex of a wild fig tree, *Ficus glabrata* or *F. dolaria,* which grows in Central and South America; it has a great local reputation as a vermifuge. It has to be used fresh, so that it is only exceptionally available for use in countries other than its source of origin. [Sp., fig-milk.]

lecithal (les·ith·al). With a yolk. [Gk *lekithos* yolk.]

lecithalbumin (les·ith·al·bew′·min). A protein composed of albumin and lecithin found in the stomach, liver and kidneys. [Gk *lekithos* yolk, L *albus* white.]

lecithigenous (les·ith·ij·en·us). Yielding lecithin. [lecithin, Gk *genein* to produce.]

lecithin (les·ith·in). A member of a class of phospholipides formed by combination of glycerol with two fatty acids, one of which is saturated and the other unsaturated, and with choline phosphate. The difference between individual lecithins is due to the difference in the particular fatty acids contained in the molecule. Two series of lecithins exist which are termed alpha- (α-) and beta- (β-) lecithins according to whether the phosphoric-acid group is attached to the α-carbon or to the β-carbon of the glycerol. The general formula of the α-lecithins may be written, $RCOOCH_2CHOCOR^1CH_2OPO(OH)OCH_2CH_2N(CH_3)_3OH$ where R and R^1 are fatty-acid chains. The general formula for the β-lecithins is similar except that the choline phosphate is attached to the middle carbon atom of the glycerol molecule. Lecithins are essential constituents of all living cells, animal and vegetable, and appear to be intimately concerned with the absorption and transport of fats. [Gk *lekithos* yolk.]

lecithinaemia (les·ith·in·e′·me·ah). The presence of lecithin in the blood. [lecithin, Gk *haima* blood.]

lecithinase (les·ith·in·aze). 1. An enzyme in kidney and other tissue which catalyses the hydrolysis of lecithin. 2. A toxic enzyme produced by *Clostridium welchii.* It hydrolyses lecithin, is haemolytic, dermonecrotic, and lethal for laboratory animals. 3. An active constituent of certain snake venoms. Its activity is neutralized by specific antitoxin. **Lecithinase A.** A lecithinase which liberates only one fatty-acid molecule, forming lysolecithins and cephalins which are powerful haemolysins. **Lecithinase B.** A lecithinase which liberates both fatty-acid molecules.

lecithoblast (les·ith·o·blast). Obsolete term for the early embryonic entoderm. [Gk *lekithos* yolk, *blastos* germ.]

lecithoid (les·ith·oid). Like lecithin. [lecithin, Gk *eidos* form.]

lecithoprotein (les·ith·o·pro′·te·in). Any one of a number of compounds formed by combination of lecithins with proteins and occurring in cytoplasm.

lecithovitellin (les·ith·o·vi·tel′·in). A suspension of egg yolk in normal saline. It is used to test strains of *Clostridium welchii* for the production of the toxin, lecithinase. [Gk *lekithos* yolk, vitellin.]

Leclainche, Emmanuel (b. 1861). Paris veterinarian.

Leclainche–Vallée serum. A serum used for anthrax.

Leclanché, Georges (b. 1839). Paris chemist.

Leclanché cell. A two-fluid voltaic cell in which the outer cell consists of a zinc rod immersed in a solution of ammonium chloride and the inner cell is a porous pot containing carbon surrounded by broken carbon and black oxide of manganese which serves as a depolarizer. It furnishes an electromotive force of 1.4 V.

lectual (lek·tew·al). Referring to a bed or a couch; applied to certain states of health which make it necessary for the patient to stay in bed, e.g. lectual diseases. [L *lectus* bed.]

lectulum (lek·tew·lum). The nail bed. [L, little bed.]

Lederer, Max (b. 1885). Brooklyn, New York, pathologist.

Lederer's anaemia, or disease. An acute haemolytic anaemia.

Leduc, Stéphane Armand Nicolas (b. 1853). Paris physicist.

Leduc current. An interrupted direct current whose pulses are of constant strength and duration. It produces unconsciousness lasting for just so long as the current is applied.

Lee, John Alfred. 20th century British anaesthetist.

Lee's needle. A spinal needle onto which have been engraved marks 4, 5 and 6 cm from the point to enable an anaesthetist to estimate the distance of the tip from the skin. Used in extradural analgesia.

Lee, Robert (b. 1793). London gynaecologist.

Lee's ganglion. A sympathetic ganglion which lies in relation to the neck of the uterus.

leech (leech). 1. Any member of the class Hirudinea. Many leeches feed on body fluids of vertebrates; most are freshwater, a few land or marine animals. 2. By extension, a physician: now obsolete except jocular. 3. To apply leeches. Several species, chiefly *Hirudo medicinalis,* were used formerly to remove small quantities of blood by local application; they are now only applied occasionally (BPC 1954). **Artificial leech.** An old device for removal of blood by suction. **Horse leech.** Any large leech, particularly *Haemopis sanguisuga* in Europe, which does not feed on man or horses, and *Limnatis nilotica.* **Land leech.** Any terrestrial leech, particularly *Haemadipsa zeylanica.* **Medicinal leech.** In Europe *Hirudo medicinalis,* in North America *Macrobdella decora,* and other suitable species throughout the world. [AS *laece.*]

See also: HEURTELOUP.

Leede, Carl Stockbridge (b. 1882). Seattle, Washington, physician.

Leede-Rumpel phenomenon, Rumpel-Leede phenomenon, or sign. The production of minute subcutaneous haemorrhages or petechiae by applying a tourniquet for 10–15 min to the upper arm of a patient with a scarlatinal rash on the forearm. The test is positive in scarlet fever, purpura, and certain other blood diseases.

Lees' inhalation treatment. An inhalation for tuberculosis consisting of a mixture of creosote, phenol, weak iodine solution, spirit of ether, and chloroform spirit, dropped on to a mask, 6 drops an hour, continuously.

lees (leez). Term for sediment or any more solid substance that sinks to the bottom, e.g. the lees of wine. [see foll.]

leet (leet). Of an eczematous lesion, to ooze. [Fr. *lie* dregs.]

leeting (leet·ing). The exudate found on the skin surface in cases of eczema. [see prec.]

Leeuwenhoekia australiensis (ler·wen·**ho**·ke·ah **aw**·stra·le·**en**′-sis). A parasite which causes mite dermatitis (scrub itch). [A. *van Leeuwenhoek,* 1632–1723, Dutch microscopist.]

Le Fort, Léon Clément (b. 1829). Paris surgeon.

Le Fort's amputation. A modification of Pirogoff's amputation in which the calcaneum is divided horizontally to leave a large lower part in the flap.

Le Fort's fractures. Fractures of the facial bones, classified into three types according to the bony parts involved.

Le Fort's operation. Strips of epithelium are removed from the anterior and posterior vaginal walls and the raw areas united; occasionally used in uterovaginal prolapse in elderly women.

Le Fort, René (b. 1869). French surgeon.

Le Fort's classification of facial fractures. Simplified—Type 1 involves the maxilla only, Type 2 involves the anterior orbit, and Type 3 involves the posterior orbit—there being complete craniofacial disjunction.

left [sinister (NA)] (left). Relating or belonging to the left, as opposed to the right. [ME.]

left-footed (left·**fut**·ed). Applied to persons who use the left foot in preference to the right, in carrying out certain movements or actions. [ME *left,* AS *fot.*]

left-handed (left·**han**·ded). Referring to a person who gives priority to the left hand rather than the right in carrying out certain movements. [ME *left,* AS *hand.*]

leg [crus (NA)] (leg). The lower extremity. Named surfaces are the anterior [facies anterior (NA)], posterior [facies posterior (NA)], medial [facies medialis (tibialis) (NA)], and lateral [facies lateralis (fibularis) (NA)]. **Bakers' leg.** Genu valgum. **Bandy leg.** Genu varum. **Barbados leg.** Elephantiasis of the leg. **Black leg.** Symptomatic anthrax; a fatal disease of cattle and sheep characterized by a crepitant fluctuating swelling on one of the quarters. In cattle it is usually caused by *Clostridium chauvoei* and in sheep more usually by *Clostridium septicum.* The latter is one of the causes of gas gangrene in man. **Boomerang leg.** Australian boomerang leg; a leg with a forward bulge between knee and ankle, observed in Australia. **Bow leg.** Genu varum. **Deck legs.** A somewhat ill-defined condition observed among passengers, especially women, during a voyage in tropical waters. The aetiological factors are probably sunburn, decreased activity under hot conditions, posture, endocrine imbalance, and sweating with loss of electrolytes. It should not be confused with *deck ankle* but the conditions may be coincident to some extent. **Elephant leg.** Elephantiasis. **Fidgety legs.** Restless legs (see below). **Milk leg.** Phlegmasia alba dolens. **Phantom leg.** Persistent sensation of the presence of the leg after amputation. **Restless legs.** A condition in which there is intolerable discomfort in the legs at rest, relieved by movement; *Ekbom's syndrome.* **Scissor leg.** Crossed legs due to adduction deformity of the hip or spasm of the adductor muscles. **White leg.** Phlegmasia alba dolens. [Old Norse *leggr.*]

leg, lateral cutaneous nerve of the calf of the [nervus cutaneus surae lateralis (NA)]. A sensory branch of the lateral popliteal nerve to the skin of the lateral side of the leg.

Legal, Emmo (b. 1859). Breslau physician.

Legal's test. For acetone bodies in urine: a nitroprusside test similar to that of Rothera.

Le Gendre, François Laurent (b. 1812). Paris physician.

Le Gendre's node, or nodosity. A nodular enlargement of the midphalangeal joint described in patients with gastric dilatation, but also found in other conditions.

Le Gendre's sign. In facial paralysis of upper motor neurone type, although weakness is apparently limited to the lower half of the face there is greater resistance to passive raising of the upper eyelid on the normal side.

Legg, Arthur Thornton (b. 1874). Boston surgeon.

Legg's disease, Legg-Calvé disease, Legg-Calvé-Perthes disease, Legg-Calvé-Waldenström disease. Coxa plana; osteochondritis of the upper femoral epiphysis.

leghaemoglobin (leg·he·mo·**glo**′·bin). A type of monomeric haemoglobin formed in the root nodules of leguminous plants; it is the product of two symbiotic organisms, the host plant supplying the globin polypeptide chain of 140 amino-acid residues, the bacteroid synthesizing the haem moiety. [L *legumen* pulse, Gk *haima* blood, L *globus* ball.]

legitimacy (le·**jit**·im·as·e). The condition of being born in lawful wedlock. [L *legitimus* lawful.]

Legueu, Felix (b. 1863). Paris surgeon.

Signe de Legueu. In bilateral upper urinary tract obstruction, renal tenderness and muscular resistance are most marked on the more recently obstructed side.

legumelin (leg·**ew**·mel·in). A water-soluble, heat-coagulable protein of the albumin class found in the seeds of leguminous plants such as the pea, bean, and lentil.

legumin (leg·**ew**·min). A heat-coagulable protein of the globulin class, insoluble in water, and found in the seeds of leguminous plants such as the pea, bean, lentil, and vetch.

leguminivorous (leg·**ew**·min·**iv**′·or·us). Subsisting on a diet of peas, beans, and other leguminous vegetables. [L *legumen* pulse, *vorare* to eat.]

Leguminosae (leg·**ew**·min·**o**′·se). A large family of plants characterized by usually having fruit in a pod (legume). The family contains the bean and the pea, and many medicinal plants. [see foll.]

leguminous (leg·**ew**·min·us). Of the nature of pulses: of the nature of *Leguminosae.* [L *legumen* pulse.]

leiasthenia (li·as·**the**·ne·ah). Asthenia or undue fatigue of unstriped muscle. [Gk *leios* smooth, asthenia.]

Leichtenstern, Otto Michael (b. 1845). Cologne physician.

Leichtenstern's phenomenon, or sign. Wincing produced by tapping a bone of the arm or leg in a patient with meningitis.

Struempell-Leichtenstern disease. Struempell's disease.

Leifson, Einar (b. 1902). Scandinavian bacteriologist.

Leifson desoxycholate citrate agar. An inhibitory selective medium used to isolate *Salmonellae* and *Shigellae* from faeces.

Leifson's selenite culture medium. Sodium selenite and peptone in a phosphate buffer. It is an enrichment selective medium used for the isolation of *Salmonellae.* There are three formulae: F. for faeces, M. for milk, and S. for sewage.

Leigh, A. Denis (b. 1915). London psychiatrist.

Leigh's disease. Subacute necrotizing encephalopathy;

inherited by autosomal recessive transmission, it affects infants and causes increasing dementia, spasticity and optic atrophy leading to death within a year. Possibly due to an enzyme defect.

Leiner, Karl (b. 1871). Vienna paediatrician.

Leiner's disease. Erythrodermia desquamativa.

leiodermatous (li·o·**der**·mat·us). Marked by an abnormally glossy, smooth skin. [Gk *leios* smooth, *derma* skin.]

leiodermia (li·o·**der**·me·ah). A skin affection characterized by abnormal smoothness and glossiness, and by atrophy. [see prec.]

leiodystonia (li·o·dis·**to'**·ne·ah). Dystonia of unstriped muscle. [Gk *leios* smooth, dystonia.]

leiomyoblastoma (li·o·mi·o·blas·**to'**·mah). Leiomyoma. [Gk *leios* smooth, *mys* muscle, blastoma.]

leiomyofibroma (li·o·mi·o·fi·**bro'**·mah). A mixed leiomyoma and fibroma. [Gk *leios* smooth, *mys* muscle, fibroma.]

leiomyoma (li·o·mi·**o'**·mah). A tumour composed of unstriped muscular elements. **Leiomyoma cutis.** A disease of the skin characterized by the presence of many small translucent nodules on the extensor surfaces of the limbs; these nodules contain bundles of unstriped muscular elements. **Leiomyoma of the stomach.** A benign tumour of the muscular coat of the stomach, often causing bleeding. [Gk *leios* smooth, *mys* muscle, *-oma* tumour.]

leiomyosarcoma (li·o·mi·o·sar·**ko'**·mah). A sarcoma in which large spindle cells of unstriped muscle are to be found. [Gk *leios* smooth, *mys* muscle, sarcoma.]

leiotriches (li·**o**·trik·eez). One of Haeckel's two main types of mankind, indicating races with straight hair. Cf. ULOTRICHES. [see foll.]

leiotrichous (li·o·trik·us). Having smooth or straight hair. Cf. ULOTRICHOUS. [Gk *leios* smooth, *thrix* hair.]

leiotrichy (li·o·trik·e). Having straight hair. [see prec.]

leipomeria (li·po·**meer**·e·ah). A monster fetus in which one or more extremities are absent. [Gk *leipein* to fail, *meros* part.]

leipostomatous (li·po·**sto**·mat·us). Not having a mouth. [see foll.]

leipostomosis (li·po·sto·**mo'**·sis). Absence of the mouth. [Gk *leipein* to fail, *stoma* mouth.]

leipostomy (li·**pos**·to·me). Atrophy of the mouth. [see prec.]

leipothymia (li·po·**thi**·me·ah). Syncope. [Gk *leipein* to fail, *thymos* mind.]

leipothymic (li·po·**thi**·mik). Syncopal. [see prec.]

leipotrichia (li·po·**trik**·e·ah). Gradual loss of the hair. [Gk *leipein* to fail, *thrix* hair.]

leipyria (li·**pi**·re·ah). The coldness of the limbs which is experienced during a febrile attack. [Gk *leipein* to fail, *pyr* fire.]

Leishman, Sir William Boog (b. 1865). British Army pathologist.

Leishman's anaemia. Kala-azar.

Leishman's stain. An alcoholic differential stain for blood smears, useful for identifying malarial parasites in which it stains the chromatin a dark red and the cytoplasm a light blue. It is a Romanovsky stain containing 1 per cent methylene blue, and 0.1 per cent eosin, in methyl alcohol. Preliminary fixing is unnecessary.

Leishman-Donovan body. The round or resting stage of the protozoon *Leishmania donovani*, the causal organism of kala-azar; this is the stage in which the parasites occur in the tissues of the vertebrate host. The term is also, not inappropriately, applied to the similar stage of other species of *Leishmania* which is morphologically identical, e.g. that of *L. tropica*.

Leishmania (leesh·**ma**·ne·ah). The generic name of protozoa which, though morphologically similar, cause three clinically differing diseases in humans and also infect animals. Their distribution is both tropical and subtropical. **Leishmania americana, Leishmania braziliensis.** An organism which causes the severe illness known as *espundia*, with an initial cutaneous sore followed after a relatively long interval by ulceration of mouth and palate, extending through to the nose. **Leishmania donovani.** The type species which causes a febrile illness known as *kala-azar* with, as a possible sequel, dermal leishmaniasis. **Leishmania furunculosa.** *Leishmania tropica* (see below). **Leishmania infantum, Leishmania mediterranea.** A variety or subspecies of *Leishmania donovani* (see above), which is found around the Mediterranean and appears especially to infect children. **Leishmania nilotica.** *Leishmania tropica* (see foll.). **Leishmania tropica.** A species that causes cutaneous leishmaniasis. The parasites are present in the base of the ulcers. [Sir W. B. *Leishman*.]

leishmaniacides (leesh·man·i·as·i·dz). Chemical substances used in the treatment of leishmaniasis.

leishmaniasis (leesh·man·**i'**·as·is). The general name given to a group of diseases caused by infection with protozoal parasites of the genus *Leishmania*, which are transmitted to man by sand flies (*Phlebotomus*) of several species, from human or animal reservoirs of infection. Three disease entities occur, visceral leishmaniasis or kala-azar, mucocutaneous leishmaniasis, and cutaneous leishmaniasis or oriental sore. **American leishmaniasis, Brazilian leishmaniasis.** Mucocutaneous leishmaniasis (see below). **Cutaneous leishmaniasis, dermal leishmaniasis.** A specific granulomatous lesion that usually ulcerates; it occurs on the face or other parts of the body exposed to the bites of sand flies. It is encountered in many tropical and subtropical countries mostly in the Near and Middle East; it is also known as *oriental sore, Baghdad boil, Aleppo boil, Sart sore, Delhi boil, Bouton de Biskra,* and by many other qualifying place-names. **Leishmaniasis diffusa.** A rare form of chronic dermal leishmaniasis simulating lepromatous leprosy, in which a dense aggregation of histiocytes containing innumerable *Leishmania* distend the dermis. It is associated with impaired cellular immunity. **Framboesoid leishmaniasis.** Leishmaniasis resembling late (tertiary) yaws. **Lupoid leishmaniasis.** Cutaneous leishmaniasis with nodules and scarring clinically resembling lupus vulgaris. **Mucocutaneous leishmaniasis.** A form found in South and Central America; the initial lesions are like oriental sores, and these skin ulcers may or may not be followed by severe ulceration of the mouth and nose; the disease is also known as *espundia* or *uta*. **Naso-oral leishmaniasis, nasopharyngeal leishmaniasis.** Mucocutaneous leishmaniasis (see prec.). **Leishmaniasis nodosus.** The nodular, early-ulcerating or moist type of cutaneous leishmaniasis. Russian writers recognize this as a distinctive form of cutaneous leishmaniasis and believe that it is caused by a different strain of *Leishmania tropica* from that which causes the more chronic, late-ulcerating or dry form, which they call leishmaniasis recidivus. **Post-kala-azar dermal leishmaniasis.** A sequel to visceral leishmaniasis or kala-azar developing usually from one to two years after cure or spontaneous remission of the latter disease. Nodular and other non-ulcerating eruptions occur on many parts of the body, especially on the face; these are relatively resistant to treatment, but do eventually respond to the antimony compounds that are used in the treatment of kala-azar. It is sometimes called *leishmanoid*. **Leishmaniasis recidivus.** *See* LEISHMANIASIS NODOSUS (above). **Leishmaniasis tropica.** Cutaneous leishmaniasis (see above). **Visceral leishmaniasis.** More commonly known as *kala-azar*, a disease occurring in many hot countries, notably India and China, with a subtropical, infantile, or Mediterranean variety attacking children. The illness is in the nature of a prolonged fever with enlargement of the spleen and liver, and it usually ends fatally unless treated.

leishmanioma (leesh·man·e·**o'**·mah). Primary chancre of kala-azar seen in Kenya and caused by bites of infected sand flies. [leishmaniasis, Gk *-oma* tumour.]

leishmaniosis (leesh·man·e·**o'**·sis). Leishmaniasis.

leishmanoid (leesh·man·oid). Post-kala-azar dermal leishmaniasis. *See* LEISHMANIASIS. [leishmaniasis, Gk *eidos* form.]

Leiter, Joseph (d. 1892). Austrian instrument maker.

Leiter's coil, or tube. A coiled flexible lead tube through which iced water can be passed.

Leloir, Henri Camille Chrysostome (b. 1855). Lille dermatologist.

Leloir's disease. Lupus vulgaris erythematodes.

lema (le·mah). The secretion of the tarsal glands. [Gk *leme* rheum.]

Lembert, Antoine (b. 1802). Paris surgeon.

Lembert's suture. A suture used in intestinal anastomosis which includes all layers from the serous down to and including the submucous coat. It may be continuous or interrupted.

Czerny–Lembert suture. A haemostatic two-layer intestinal suture consisting of a mucosal in addition to a Lembert (seromuscular) suture (see prec.).

lemma (lem·ah). 1. General term for any membrane that encloses or defines a bodily structure. 2. In embryology, the membranous envelope of the nucleus (germinal vesicle) of the ovum. [Gk, sheath.]

lemmoblast (lem·o·blast). A primitive neurilemmal or Schwann cell. [Gk *lemma* sheath, *blastos* germ.]

lemmoblastic (lem·o·blas·tik). Producing neurilemmal tissue. [see prec.]

lemmoblastoma (lem·o·blast·o'·mah). Spongioblastoma. [Gk *lemma* sheath, blastoma.]

lemniscus [NA] (lem·nis·kus). A band or strip: the term is commonly applied to crossed ascending fibres which are the axons of secondary sensory neurones and which end in the thalamus. **Lateral lemniscus [lemniscus lateralis (NA)].** Fibres ascending after decussation from the cochlear nuclei to the inferior quadrigeminal body and the medial geniculate body. Some fibres are relayed by the nucleus of the lateral lemniscus [nucleus lemnisci lateralis]. **Medial lemniscus [lemniscus medialis (NA)].** Fibres ascending after decussation from the cuneate and gracile nuclei of the medulla to the thalamus. **Spinal lemniscus [lemniscus spinalis (NA)].** The upward continuation of the lateral spinothalamic tract into the brain stem. The term is sometimes used to denote the combined upward continuation of both lateral and anterior spinothalamic tracts in the brain stem. **Trigeminal lemniscus [lemniscus trigeminalis (NA)].** The tract formed by the axons of secondary neurones which arise in the sensory nuclei of the trigeminal nerve and terminate in the ventral nucleus of the thalamus. [Gk *lemniskos* fillet.]

See also: BECHTEREW.

lemnoblast (lem·no·blast). Lemmoblast.

lemon (lem·on). The fruit of *Citrus limonia* Osbeck. (family Rutaceae), a tree widely cultivated in the Mediterranean countries. **Lemon juice.** The expressed juice of the ripe fruit of the lemon. It may be preserved with sulphur dioxide, and contains citric acid, a small quantity of sugar, and ascorbic acid (25-95 mg per 100 ml). Since the introduction of synthetic vitamin C, lemon juice is used mainly as a flavouring agent. **Lemon Oil BP 1953.** Oleum limonis, a volatile oil expressed from the fresh peel; the oil itself, and the fresh (Fresh Lemon Peel BP 1958), or dried peel (Dried Lemon Peel BP 1968), are used as flavouring agents in certain official preparations. [Ar. *laymun.*]

Lempert, Hyme (b. 1906). Manchester clinical pathologist.

Lempert's solution. A diluting fluid used in the direct method for enumerating blood platelets, and containing sodium citrate 1.0 g, mercuric chloride 0.002 g, brilliant cresyl blue 0.2 g, distilled water 100 ml, added at a temperature of 45°C; it is kept in the dark until required, and then before use is mixed with an equal quantity of a 20 per cent solution of urea (A.R.) in distilled water, buffered to pH 7.2.

Lempert, Julius (b. 1890). New York otologist.

Lempert's operation. A form of fenestration operation for the treatment of chronic deafness resulting from otosclerosis.

Lenard, Philipp Eduard Anton (b. 1862). German physicist.

Lenard rays. Cathode rays emitted from a vacuum tube furnished with a window of aluminium.

Lenard tube. An evacuated discharge tube with a thin window to permit the passage of the electrons (cathode rays) into the air.

length (length). A measurement of extension, or of the distance between two points. **Basinasal length.** The craniometric length from the basion (the midpoint of the anterior margin of the foramen magnum) to the nasion (the midpoint of the depression where the nasal bones join the frontal). **Basiprosthionic length.** The craniometric length from the basion (the midpoint of the anterior margin of the foramen magnum) to the prosthion (the lowest point on the alveolus between the upper central incisors). **Crown-rump length.** The greatest overall length of a fetus measured in its natural flexed position from the top of the head to the prominence of the buttocks. **Dental length.** The distance between the anterior border of the upper first premolar tooth and the posterior border of the last molar tooth. **Focal length.** *Of a spherical mirror,* the distance along the principal axis from the principal focus to the pole or vertex of the mirror. *Of a lens,* the distance along the principal axis from the principal focus to the optical centre of the lens, or, in a system of lenses, to the principal point of the system. **Sitting length.** The length measured from the vertex to the tip of the coccyx. **Stem length.** The length from the vertex to a a line joining the ischial tuberosities. **Tube length.** In a microscope, the distance between adjacent focal planes of the objective and eyepiece. [AS *lengthu.*]

Lenhartz, Hermann Albert Dietrich (b. 1854). Hamburg physician.

Lenhartz diet, or treatment. For peptic ulcer: from the first the patient has an abundant diet of high-protein value, mainly of eggs and milk, to which later chopped meat is added. The patient is kept in bed for 4 weeks.

Lenhossék, Mihály (Michael) (b. 1863). Budapest anatomist.

Lenhossék's processes. The central processes of the gustatory cells of the tongue.

Lennander, Karl Gustave (b. 1857). Upsala surgeon.

Lennander's operation. Excision of the inguinal and iliac lymph glands.

Lennhoff, Rudolf (b. 1866). Berlin physician.

Lennhoff's index, Becker-Lennhoff index. The distance between the top of the sternum and the pubic symphysis in centimetres is multiplied by 100 and divided by the greatest circumference of the abdomen. An index above 75 indicates an atonic habitus.

Lennhoff's sign. A transverse furrow on inspiration, seen below the last rib and above a hydatid of the liver.

Lennox's syndrome. An epileptic encephalopathy with diffused slow spike-and-wave electro-encephalographic discharges.

Lenoir, Camille Alexandre Henri (b. 1867). French surgeon.

Lenoir's facet. The facet on the most medial part of the articular surface of the patella.

lens (lenz). 1. A portion of a refracting medium bounded by two curved surfaces. 2. [NA] The crystalline lens of the eye. **Achromatic lens.** A lens having the same focal length for red and blue light. **Acrylic lens.** An artificial plastic lens sometimes inserted into the eye to replace the extracted cataractous lens. **Anamorphote lens.** A lens with a cylindrical element incorporated, used to produce or correct a distorted image. **Aniseikonic lens.** One which has no refractive power and yet can cause magnification; used in aniseikonia to correct the difference in size of the retinal images; also called *size lens.* **Aplanatic lens.** A lens corrected for errors due to spherical aberration. **Apochromatic lens.** A lens having the same focal length for red, green, and blue light. **Biconcave lens.** A lens bounded by two concave surfaces. **Biconvex lens.** A lens bounded by two convex surfaces; it is used to correct hypermetropia and presbyopia. **Bicylindrical lens.** A lens bounded by two cylindrical surfaces. **Bifocal lens.** A spectacle lens designed for presbyopes in which a lens of greater converging power for near vision is incorporated in the lower part of the lens for distance vision. **Bispherical lens.** A lens bounded by two spherical surfaces. **Cataract lens.** A convex spectacle lens used after cataract operation to replace the refractive power of the crystalline lens. **Cataractous lens.** The crystalline lens of the eye when it becomes opaque. **Compound lens.** A combination of more than one lens which is used as a single optical unit, e.g. microscope objective. **Concave lens.** A lens of which the surfaces have a concave curve which diverges rays of light; used to correct myopia. **Concave dispersing lens.** A lens which produces divergence of light. **Concavoconcave lens.** Biconcave lens (see above). **Condensing lens.** A strong convex spherical lens of large size used to focus available light on to the eye for examination purposes. **Contact lens.** A lens fitted in contact with the front of the eye. Used for refractive errors, protection, cosmetic purposes, examination, diagnosis, and treatment. Types include: *Corneal contact lens* designed to be worn in front of the cornea only; *Hard contact lens* which, under normal conditions, substantially retains its form without support; *Hydrophilic contact lens* made from a material which can absorb water; *Scleral contact lens* consisting of an optic portion in front of the cornea and a haptic surround lying in front of the sclera; *Soft contact lens* made of a material which, in its final form, readily yields to pressure. Most are hydrophilic. Advantages are comfort and long wearing time, since oxygen can diffuse through the lens to the corneal epithelium. **Converging lens.** A lens producing convergence of light. **Convex lens.** Biconvex lens (see above). **Convexoconcave lens.** A lens bounded by one convex and one concave surface. **Crossed lens.** A simple convergent lens designed to have minimal spherical aberration. **Crystalline lens of the eye.** That made up of transparent fibres enclosed in a capsule and focusing the image seen on the retina. The anterior surface [facies anterior lentis (NA)] is related to the aqueous chamber, and the posterior surface [facies posterior lentis (NA)] faces the vitreous chamber. **Cylindrical lens.** A lens in the form of a segment of a cylinder. It has no refractive power in one meridian, its axis, and its greatest refractive power is in the meridian at right angles. Its principal focus is a line, not a point, and it is used to correct astigmatism. **Decentred lens.** A spectacle lens in which the optical centre is not in line with the centre of the pupil of the eye. This causes a prismatic effect which can be used to overcome a small degree of muscle imbalance. **Dislocated lens.** A gross displacement of the crystalline lens of the eye from its normal position. **Diverging lens.** Concave lens (see above). **Fenestrated lens.** A contact lens in which a small hole has been cut at a point where it does not interfere with vision; this hole allows the escape of carbon dioxide and the entry of air, and thereby prevents the haziness of the cornea known as *Sattler's veil.* **Flat lens.** A spectacle lens in which the curve is equal on both sides. **Fluorite lens.** A microscope objective lens containing a certain amount of fluorite to improve the optical performance towards that of the apochromatic lens. **Immersion lens.** A lens system in which the space between the lens and object is liquid, filled usually with oil of the same refractive index as the lens. **Lenticular lens.** A spectacle lens which is ground only in the central portion, the periphery being flat; used in lenses of high power in order to reduce weight. **Magnifying lens.** A powerful convex spherical lens which enlarges objects; used as an assistance to reading in low visual acuity. **Meniscus lens.** A spherical spectacle lens which has a concave curve towards the eye, the outer curve of which is increased or decreased to compensate for this; this causes less distortion when the wearer looks obliquely. **Minus lens.** Concave lens (see above). **Nucleus of the lens [nucleus lentis (NA)].** The firm central portion of the lens, surrounded by the softer cortex. **Orthoscopic lens.** A spectacle lens which is a combination of spherical lens to relieve accommodation and prism to relieve an equal amount of convergence. **Periscopic lens.** A form of meniscus lens (see above) with a base of 1.25 D. **Plane lens.** A spectacle lens with no curve and no refractive power. **Planoconcave lens.** A lens bounded by one plane and one concave surface. **Planoconvex lens.** A lens bounded by one plane and one convex surface. **Plus lens.** Converging lens (see above). **Size lens.** Aniseikonic lens (see above). **Spherical lens.** A refracting medium, one or both surfaces being curved like a sphere the principal focus of which is a point. **Spherical afocal lenses.** Those with spherical surfaces which have no focal power. The term usually refers to a type of contact lens that has no focal power in air. **Subluxated lens.** Minor displacement of the crystalline lens of the eye from its normal position. **Telescopic lens.** A system of lenses made up in the form of spectacles which magnifies the object on the principle of the galilean telescope. **Toric lens.** A spectacle lens similar to a meniscus, with the addition of a cylinder ground on to the outer surface. **Trial lens.** One of a set of lenses of varying strengths and types used in testing for spectacles. **Trifocal lens.** Similar to a bifocal lens (see above), three different lens powers are incorporated, for distance, intermediate, and near. **Wandering lens.** Dislocation of the crystalline lens. [L, a lentil.]

See also: ABBÉ, CROOKES, GOLDMANN, HRUBY.

lenticel (**len**·te·sel). A lentiform gland; in particular one found at the root of the tongue. [L *lenticella* small lentil.]

lenticonus (len·te·**ko**·nus). Abnormal curvature of the lens or its nucleus, usually affecting the posterior surface. Anterior lenticonus is rare, except in so far as it occurs, normally, in accommodation. [lens, Gk *konos* cone.]

lenticula (len·**tik**·ew·lah). 1. The lentiform nucleus. 2. A freckle. [dim. of L *lens* lentil.]

lenticular (len·**tik**·ew·lar). 1. Referring to, or shaped like a lentil. 2. Referring to the lens of the eye. 3. Relating to the lentiform nucleus. [see prec.]

lenticulate (len·**tik**·ew·late). Lenticular.

lenticulo-optic (len·**tik**·ew·lo·**op**'·tik). Referring to the lentiform nucleus and the optic tract or optic radiation. [lenticula, optic.]

lenticulostriate (len·**tik**·ew·lo·**stri**'·ate). Belonging to the lentiform nucleus and the corpus striatum. [lenticula, corpus striatum.]

lenticulothalamic (len·**tik**·ew·lo·thal·**am**'·ik). Pertaining to the lentiform nucleus and the thalamus. [lenticula, thalamus.]

lentiform (**len**·te·form). Lenticular. **Lentiform nodule.** *See* NODULE. **Lentiform nucleus.** *See* NUCLEUS. [lens, form.]

lentigines (len·**tij**·in·eez). *See* LENTIGO.

lentiginose, lentiginous (len·**tij**·in·oze, len·**tij**·in·us). Marked with lentigines.

lentiginosis (len·**tij**·in·**o**'·sis). A condition characterized by the presence of numerous lentigines. [lentigo, Gk *-osis* condition.]

lentiglobus (len·te·**glo**·bus). An extremely rare condition, in which there is an anterior spherical protrusion of the lens substance. [lens, L *globus* sphere.]

lentigo (len·**ti**·go) (pl. *lentigines*). 1. A brownish or yellowish spot found on the skin, most often on the hands, arms, or face, often caused by exposure to sunlight; a freckle. Fair-complexioned persons are most susceptible. 2. A small avascular naevus. **Lentigo aestiva.** The freckle associated with summer and which may soon fade. **Lentigines leprosae.** The macular eruption which may be present in leprosy. **Lentigo maligna.** A superficial malignant melanoma presenting as a dark, shiny plaque which spreads laterally and ultimately invades in depth. [L, freckle.]

lentigomelanosis (len·**ti**·go·mel·an·**o**'·sis). A malignant condition of the skin arising from lentigines. [lentigo, melanosis.]

lentitis (len·**ti**·tis). Inflammation of the crystalline lens; phacitis. [lens, Gk *-itis* inflammation.]

Lentocebus chrysomelas (len·to·**se**·bus kris·**om**·el·as). A marmoset, a reservoir of yellow-fever virus.

lentoptosis (len·top·**to**·sis). Dislocation of the crystalline lens; phacocele. [lens, Gk *ptosis* fall.]

lentor (**len**·tor). The sluggishness of any function or reaction. [L *lentus* slow.]

Lenz, Heinrich Friedrich Emil (b. 1804). German physicist.

Lenz's law. If an electric current moves in a magnetic field the current induced will itself produce a magnetic field that tends to halt the motion.

Lenzmann, Richard (b. 1856). Duisburg physician.

Lenzmann's point. A point similar to Lanz's point.

Leo, Hans (b. 1854). Bonn physician.

Leo's sugar. A sugar identified in a specimen of urine. It is believed to be a heptose, and its occurrence in urine is extremely rare.

Leonardo da Vinci (b. 1452). Italian artist.

Leonardo's moderator band. The moderator band of the right ventricle of the heart; it was first figured by Leonardo da Vinci.

Leonotis (le·o·**no**·tis). A genus of tropical plants (family Labiatae), several species of which are reputed to have narcotic properties. Various parts of the plants are widely used in South Africa, both internally and in the form of external applications for the relief of pain.

leontiasis (le·on·**ti**·as·is). Nodulation and thickening of the skin of the face that occurs in leprosy; leonine facies. **Leontiasis ossea.** Overgrowth of the bones of the face and sometimes of the cranial bones as well, resulting in a generalized hypertrophy of the parts and the assumption of a lion-like expression. [Gk *leon* lion.]

leotropic (le·o·**trop**·ik). Wound in a spiral from right to left. [Gk *laios* left, *tropos* a turning.]

Leotta, Nicolo (b. 1878). Italian surgeon.

Leotta's sign. Pain produced by downward pressure in the right upper quadrant of the abdomen, due to the traction on a colon adherent to the liver or gall bladder.

leper (**lep**·er). Any person suffering from leprosy. The word is usually avoided in medical connections, because of the stigma attached. [Gk *lepis* scale.]

lepidic (lep·**id**·ik). Scaly; an obsolete adjective, applied particularly to describe the embryonic lining membranes. [Gk *lepis* scale.]

lepidoid (lep·id·oid). Squamous. [Gk *lepis* scale, *eidos* form.]

lepidoma (lep·id·**o**·mah). A tumour derived from lepidic (scaly) tissue.

lepidoplastic (lep·id·o·**plas**'·tik). Referring to any condition in which scales are developed. [Gk *lepis* scale, *plassein* to form.]

Lepidoptera (lep·id·**op**·ter·ah). An order of insects which includes the moths and butterflies. [Gk *lepis* scale, *pteron* wing.]

lepidosarcoma (lep·id·o·sar·**ko**'·mah). A sarcoma coated with scales and occurring inside the mouth. [Gk *lepis* scale, sarcoma.]

lepidosis (lep·id·**o**·sis). Any eruption which consists of scales; leprosy; pityriasis. [Gk *lepis* scale, *-osis* condition.]

lepocyte (**lep**·o·site). Any nucleated cell with a distinct cell wall. [Gk *lepos* husk, *kytos* cell.]

lepothrix (**lep**·o·thrix). Trichomycosis. [Gk *lepos* husk, *thrix* hair.]

lepra (**lep**·rah). An obsolete term for leprosy, now used only in connection with the defensive mechanism. **Lepra alphos.** Psoriasis. **Lepra arabum.** Tuberculoid leprosy. *See* LEPROSY. **Lepra graecorum.** Psoriasis. **Lepra tuberosa.** Nodular leprosy. *See* LEPROSY. [Gk, leprosy.]

lepraphobia (lep·rah·**fo**·be·ah). Morbid fear of leprosy. [Gk *lepra* leprosy, phobia.]

leprechaunism (**lep**·re·kawn·izm). A genetically determined condition of broad nose and widely spaced eyes, low-set large ears, facial hypertrichosis, excessive folded skin, bone dystrophy, large phallus or ovarian cysts, retarded growth and susceptibility to infections. [Old Irish *lu* small, *corp* body.]

leprelcosis (lep·rel·**ko**·sis). Ulceration which occurs in leprosy. [Gk *lepra* leprosy, *helkosis* ulceration.]

lepriasis (lep·**ri**·as·is). Leprosy; psoriasis; a term, now obsolete, employed to indicate certain affections of the skin characterized by the presence of a scaly eruption. [Gk *lepra* leprosy.]

lepric (**lep**·rik). Referring to lepra.

leprid, lepride (**lep**·rid, **lep**·ride). Any skin lesion of leprosy. Usually termed the *indeterminate macule*, the patch is pink or hypopigmented and is hypo-aesthetic. *Mycobacterium leprae* can be demonstrated within terminal nerve fibrils. **Maculo-anaesthetic lepride.** An anaesthetic macular lesion occurring in tuberculoid leprosy. **Major lepride.** A raised and infiltrated lesion of tuberculoid leprosy. **Minor lepride.** A hypopigmented irregularly infiltrated lesion of tuberculoid leprosy. **Polyneuritic lepride.** A leprotic lesion involving nerves, a very mutilating form of tuberculoid leprosy, with paralysis and contractions. [Gk *lepros* scaly.]

leprology (lep·**rol**·o·je). The study of leprosy. [leprosy, Gk *logos* science.]

leproma (lep·**ro**·mah). The characteristic granulomatous lesion of lepromatous leprosy, usually nodular but it may be macular; histologically it shows foamy cells and lepra bacilli, *Mycobacterium leprae*. [leprosy, Gk *-oma* tumour.]

lepromatous (lep·**ro**·mat·us). Of or referring to a leproma. The word is used to qualify that form of leprosy in which host resistance is low and the lesion shows abundant lepra bacilli, *Mycobacterium leprae*.

lepromin (**lep**·ro·min). A sterile antigen prepared from lepromatous tissue rich in *Mycobacterium leprae*.

leprophobia (lep·ro·**fo**·be·ah). Lepraphobia.

leprophthalmia (lep·rof·**thal**·me·ah). Ophthalmia which is due to leprosy.

leprosarium, leprosary (lep·ro·**sa**·re·um, **lep**·ro·sar·e). A leper colony or hospital.

leprosy (**lep**·ro·se). A chronic infective disease of man due to invasion of the body by the leprosy bacillus, *Mycobacterium leprae*, which is active mainly in the skin and peripheral nerve trunks. The disease is characterized clinically by a wide range of lesions in the skin and nerves. Owing to the varying degree of resistance offered to the invading bacillus by different races and individuals, the main presenting feature in any particular case may be due to (*a*) the formation of sharply demarcated anaesthetic skin tumours (*tuberculoid leprosy*); (*b*) damage to sensory, motor, and trophic nerves on account of a strangulating defensive fibrosis, resulting in thickening of the nerves (*nerve leprosy*), anaesthetic patches (*anaesthetic leprosy*), or perforating ulcers (*trophoneurotic leprosy*); or (*c*) ill-defined blemishes or macules in the skin (*macular leprosy*), or soft multiple nodules (*nodular leprosy*), both macules and nodules teeming with bacilli and being examples of low resistance or *lepromatous leprosy*. Before recognition of *Mycobacterium leprae* as the specific factor in the causation of leprosy, numerous other skin lesions were confused with the disease, e.g. leucoderma or vitiligo (*white leprosy*) and pellagra (*Asturian leprosy*). **Borderline leprosy.** Leprosy which is intermediate between the nodular and tuberculoid forms. The immunological status is unstable and the condition tends to swing either to the lepromatous or to the tuberculoid form. Subgroups are borderline-lepromatous and borderline-tuberculoid. **Closed leprosy.** Leprosy in which there are no skin or mucosal lesions in which *Mycobacterium leprae* can be demonstrated. **Intermediate leprosy.** Borderline leprosy (see above). **Lazarine leprosy.** Mutilating, scarred and ulcerated leprosy. **Murine leprosy.** Rat leprosy (see following). **Rat leprosy.** A disease in rats caused by a *Mycobacterium* very similar to that of human leprosy; this organism has been used extensively in experimental work. [Gk *lepra*.]

leprotic (lep·**rot**·ik). Leprous.

leprous (**lep**·rus). Relating to, caused by, or infected with leprosy.

leptandra (lep·**tan**·drah). The root of a North American plant, *Veronica virginica* Linn. (family Scrophulariaceae), used as a cathartic. [Gk *leptos* thin, *aner* man, stamen.]

Leptazol BP 1958 (**lep**·taz·ol). Pentamethylenetetrazole, $C_6H_{10}N_4$. A respiratory and medullary stimulant formerly used in cases of narcotic poisoning (especially by barbiturates), collapse during anaesthesia, and to restore the apparently drowned. With ephedrine, it is used for bronchitic asthma.

lepthymenia (lep·thi·**me**·ne·ah). Thinness of a membrane. [Gk *leptos* thin, *hymen* membrane.]

leptocephalia (lep·to·kef·**a**'·le·ah). The condition of being leptocephalic.

leptocephalic, leptocephalous (lep·to·kef·**al**'·ik, lep·to·**kef**·al·us). Having a small, narrow head. [Gk *leptos* thin, *kephale* head.]

leptocephalus (lep·to·**kef**·al·us). A monster in which premature union of the frontal and sphenoid bones produces an abnormally small and narrow head. [see prec.]

leptocephaly (lep·to·**kef**·al·e). Leptocephalia.

leptochroa (lep·to·**kro**·ah). Unusual thinness of the skin. [Gk *leptos* thin, *chroa* skin.]

leptochromatic (**lep**·to·kro·**mat**'·ik). Having a chromatin network of unusually delicate texture. [Gk *leptos* thin, chromatin.]

Leptoconops (lep·to·**ko**·nops). A genus of biting midges. [Gk *leptos* thin, *konops* gnat.]

leptocyte (**lep**·to·site). An erythrocyte that is unusually thin. [Gk *leptos* thin, *kytos* cell.]

leptocytosis (**lep**·to·si·**to**′·sis). The presence of leptocytes in the blood. [leptocyte, Gk *-osis* condition.]

leptodactylous (lep·to·**dak**·til·us). Having long and slender toes or fingers; both conditions may be found in one person. [Gk *leptos* thin, *daktylos* finger or toe.]

leptodermic, leptodermous (lep·to·**der**·mik, lep·to·**der**·mus). Having a thin, easily injured skin. [Gk *leptos* thin, *derma* skin.]

leptodontous (lep·to·**don**·tus). Having narrow teeth. [Gk *leptos* thin, *odous* tooth.]

leptomeningioma (**lep**·to·men·in·je·**o**′·mah). A tumour of the leptomeninges. [leptomeninx, Gk *-oma* tumour.]

leptomeningitis (**lep**·to·men·in·**ji**′·tis). Inflammation of the finer membranes, pia and arachnoid, of the brain and spinal cord. [leptomeninx, Gk *-itis* inflammation.]

leptomeningopathy (**lep**·to·men·in·**gop**′·ath·e). A diseased condition of the leptomeninges. [leptomeninx, Gk *pathos* disease.]

leptomeninx (lep·to·**men**·ingx) (pl. *leptomeninges*). 1. The pia mater of the brain. 2. The arachnoid mater of the brain. 3. In the plural, pia mater and arachnoid mater regarded as one membrane. [Gk *leptos* thin, *menigx* membrane.]

Leptomicrurus (**lep**·to·mi·**kroo**′·rus). A genus of poisonous coral snakes found in America. [Gk *leptos* thin, *mikros* small, *oura* tail.]

Leptomitus (lep·**tom**·it·us). A class of sheath-producing bacteria, causing pollution of the effluents from sugar factories, and associated with the presence of sucrose. They are non-pathogenic. [Gk *leptos* thin, *mitos* thread.]

Leptomonas (lep·to·**mo**·nas). A genus of the class Mastigophora, the members of which are haemoflagellates. [Gk *leptos* thin, *monas* unit.]

leptonema (lep·to·**ne**·mah). A fine elongated spireme thread; the form taken by the chromosomes in the presynaptic stage of meiosis. [Gk *leptos* thin, *nema* thread.]

leptonomorphology (**lep**·to·no·mor·**fol**′·o·je). The science of the constitution and morphology of membranes. [Gk *leptos* thin, morphology.]

leptopellic (lep·to·**pel**·ik). Applied to the condition in which there is an unusually narrow pelvis. [Gk *leptos* thin, *pella* bowl.]

leptophonia (lep·to·**fo**·ne·ah). A condition in which the vocal power is weak, with the result that the voice is small and feeble. [Gk *leptos* thin, *phone* sound.]

leptophonic (lep·to·**fon**·ik). Marked by a weak voice. [see prec.]

leptoprosope (lep·to·**pro**·sope). An individual with a narrow face and elongated cranium; the nose is long in proportion and the orbital spaces are unduly large. [Gk *leptos* thin, *prosopon* face.]

leptoprosopia (**lep**·to·pro·**so**′·pe·ah). Abnormal narrowness and length of the face; the condition typical of the leptoprosope.

leptoprosopic (**lep**·to·pro·**so**′·pik). Having a long narrow face; showing the characteristics of leptoprosopia. [Gk *leptos* thin, *prosopon* face.]

Leptopsylla (lep·to·**sil**·ah). A genus of fleas which are arthropod hosts of the small tapeworm, *Hymenolepis diminuta*. **Leptopsylla segnis.** A vector of plague and of flea-borne (murine) typhus. [Gk *leptos* thin, *psylla* flea.]

leptorrhinia (lep·to·**rin**·e·ah). Narrowness of the nasal bones; with a nasal index below 48. [Gk *leptos* thin, *rhis* nose.]

leptosomatic (**lep**·to·so·**mat**′·ik). Term indicative of slight physique; smallness and slenderness of bodily framework. [Gk *leptos* thin, *soma* body.]

leptosome (**lep**·to·some). An individual of slight physique. [see prec.]

Leptosphaeria (lep·to·**sfer**·e·ah). A fungus caused by black-grain mycetoma in man, e.g. *Leptosphaeria senegalensis*. [Gk *leptos* thin, *sphaira* sphere.]

Leptospira (lep·to·**spi**·rah). A genus of small spirochaetes of the family Treponemataceae. Although there are differences between the parasitic and saprophytic strains, the genus is presently considered to have only one species composed of two broadly based complexes, one containing the saprophytic strains *biflexa* and the other containing the parasitic strains *interrogans*. Within the *interrogans* complex there are 16 serological groups comprising over 100 different serological types isolated from animals and man. Leptospires have numerous closely-set spirals and hooked ends, and are 7–14 μm long and 0.1 μm broad; they are actively motile. A wide variety of wild and domestic mammals and some other species (e.g. toads, hedgehogs, waders and snakes) are natural hosts, but the most important of these are rodents and other small mammals; of domestic animals, dogs, pigs, goats and cattle may also be important sources of infection for man, who usually becomes infected through the skin from water, sludge, etc., contaminated by animal carriers of the leptospires (zoonosis). Some of the more common pathogenic types for man are *Leptospira icterohaemorrhagicae*, present most commonly in rodents and causing a febrile illness which, in its most severe form, is associated with a haemorrhagic jaundice (Weil's disease); *Leptospira pomona*, found in cattle and pigs; *Leptospira canicola*, found mostly in dogs and associated with a form of meningitis in man. The natural infection in animals is globally distributed and, in man, is often an occupational disease, e.g. among rice-field, cane-field, and other agricultural workers, miners, sewer workers, fish handlers, etc., where there is high risk from rat or other animal carriers. **Leptospira autumnalis.** A species that produces a relatively mild non-icteric leptospirosis in man, e.g. Fort Bragg fever. **Leptospira biflexa.** A non-pathogenic member of the group, often found in water. **Leptospira canicola.** A species which causes Stuttgart disease of dogs and canicola fever in man. **Leptospira celledoni.** A strain that appears to be antigenetically distinct from the other recognized strains. It has been found in Queensland and Malaya, but the infections reported in man have not been of the severe type. **Leptospira grippotyphosa.** A species causing swamp fever. **Leptospira hebdomadis.** The cause of the 7-day fever of Japan. **Leptospira icterohaemorrhagiae.** The type species that is the cause of Weil's disease. **Leptospira icteroides.** The name given to a leptospira isolated from a supposed case of yellow fever: it is possible that the case was one of leptospirosis, and that the organism was in fact *Leptospira icterohaemorrhagiae* (see preceding). **Leptospira pomona.** A species responsible for swineherds' disease in which signs of meningeal irritation may be severe; it also causes a serious disease in cattle. **Leptospira pyrogenes.** A species frequently isolated in leptospirosis in Malaya. **Leptospira sejroe.** A species related to *Leptospira hebdomadis* (see above), isolated from patients in Denmark. [Gk *leptos* thin, *speira* coil.]

leptospirosis (**lep**·to·spi·**ro**′·sis). A group of diseases caused by spirochaetal micro-organisms of the genus *Leptospira*. **Leptospirosis canicola.** A disease similar to, but usually milder than Weil's disease. The infection is transmitted from dogs which suffer a more severe, frequently fatal illness (Stuttgart disease). **Leptospirosis hebdomadis.** Seven-day fever of Japan caused by *Leptospira hebdomadis*; a similar disease has been reported in other countries. **Leptospirosis icterohaemorrhagica.** Weil's disease; an acute, potentially fatal, febrile infection caused by *Leptospira icterohaemorrhagiae*, transmitted from rats in their urine, often via food or water, and in its severer forms associated with jaundice. [*Leptospira*, Gk *-osis* condition.]

leptostaphyline (lep·to·**staf**·il·ine). Referring to a type of palate in which the arch is higher and narrower than normal. [Gk *leptos* thin, *staphyle* palate.]

leptotene (**lep**·to·teen). The first stage of the prophase of meiosis; during this stage chromosomes become visible and are not yet paired. [Gk *leptos* thin, *tainia* ribbon.]

leptothricosis (**lep**·to·thrik·**o**′·sis). Any diseased condition due to infection with a species of *Leptothrix*. **Leptothricosis conjunctivae.** Parinaud's conjunctivitis. [*Leptothrix*, Gk *-osis* condition.]

Leptothrix (**lep**·to·thrix). A genus of the family Chlamydobacteriaceae (order Chlamydobacteriales) consisting of filamentous, non-branching, colourless, algae-like bacteria with a ferric-hydroxide sheath; false branching may occur. They are usually found in water, and are non-pathogenic for man. The name was proposed by Kuetzing (1843). **Leptothrix buccalis.** The name applied to a filamentous unbranched organism found in the mouth, by Robin (1847); it was transferred by Trevisan (1874) to a new genus *Leptotrichia*, the validity of which is now questioned. [Gk *leptos* thin, *thrix* hair.]

Leptotrichia buccalis (lep·to·trik·e·ah buk·a·lis). A species of filamentous Gram-positive organisms found in the mouth and believed to be associated with dental caries. Also called *Leptothrix buccalis*. Their taxonomic position is uncertain. [Gk *leptos* thin, *thrix* hair, L *bucca* cheek.]

leptotrombicula (lep·to·trom·bik'·ew·lah). The larva of a *Trombicula* mite. [Gk *leptos* thin, *Trombicula*.]

Leptus (lep·tus). 1. A pseudogenus of trombidiiform mites which are known only as larvae. Several species in the tropical New World cause intense pruritus. 2. A genus of trombidiiform mites of no medical interest. 3. A name misapplied as a generic name to certain mites of medical interest. **Leptus akamushi.** *Trombicula akamushi.* **Leptus autumnalis.** *Trombicula autumnalis.* [Gk *leptos* thin.]

Lepus brachyurus (lep·us brak·e·ewr·us). A Japanese rabbit; a supposed reservoir of tularaemia. [L *lepus* hare, Gk *brachys* short, *oura* tail.]

leresis (ler·e·sis). The talkativeness which is characteristic of senility or insanity. [Gk, silly talk.]

Leri, André (b. 1875). Paris physician.

Leri's melorheostosis. A rare bone disease of unknown origin presenting as a hyperostosis of a long bone and usually affecting only one limb. The dense and irregular cortical overgrowth has been likened to the flow of candle grease down the limb.

Leri's pleonosteosis. An uncommon hereditary condition characterized by broadening and deformity of the thumbs, flexion contracture of the fingers, deformity of the toes, short stature, and Mongoloid features.

Leri's sign. In a normal subject passive flexion of hand and wrist causes some flexion of the elbow; in a hemiplegic subject this does not occur on the affected side.

Leriche, René (b. 1879). Strasbourg surgeon.

Leriche's compression. Scalenus anticus syndrome. *See* SYNDROME.

Leriche's operation. Partial sympathectomy.

Leriche's syndrome. Occlusion of the abdominal aorta by saddle embolus or thrombus.

Leriche's treatment. Injection of a local anaesthetic solution into the periarticular structures in the treatment of joint sprains.

Sudeck-Leriche syndrome. Acute atrophy of bone at the site of an injury showing radiographically as an area of osteoporosis and probably caused by reflex local vasospasm. It occurs most commonly in the small bones of the hand or foot.

Lermoyez, Marcel (b. 1858). Paris otolaryngologist.

Lermoyez's syndrome. Sudden attacks of dizziness and tinnitus, associated with hyperacousia and not with deafness as in the case of Ménière's disease.

lesbian (lez·be·an). A female homosexual; one who practises sapphism. [see foll.]

lesbianism (lez·be·an·izm). Sapphism. [Gk island of *Lesbos* on which Sappho lived.]

Leschke, Erich Friedrich Wilhelm (b. 1887). Berlin physician.

Leschke syndrome. Hyperglycaemia with asthenia and brown pigmented spots on the skin.

Leser, Edmund (b. 1853). German surgeon.

Leser-Trélat sign. A sign dependent on the (quite incorrect) belief that senile angiomata, seborrhoeic warts, and pigmented areas are evidence of carcinoma.

Lesieur, Charles (b. 1876). Lyons physician.

Lesieur-Privey sign. The presence of albumin in the sputum. It is positive in tuberculosis and in acute or subacute congestive conditions of the lungs, such as pneumonia, but it is not specific.

Lesieur-Privey test. For albumin in sputum in cases of suspected tuberculosis, emphysema with cardiac dilatation, and pneumonia. An equal quantity of 3 per cent acetic acid is well shaken up with the sputum and allowed to stand for some time, then filtered. If albumin is present, this clear filtrate becomes cloudy on boiling.

lesion (le·zhun). A pathological disturbance, such as an injury, an infection, or a tumour. **Degenerative lesion.** A disturbance which results in loss of function; degeneration. **Depressive lesion.** A lesion that reduces functional activity. **Destructive lesion.** A disturbance which leads to the death of a tissue or organ. **Diffuse lesion.** One that involves all portions of an extensive area of tissue. **Discharging lesion.** One in the central nervous system which causes sudden abnormal episodic discharge of nerve impulses; used especially by Hughlings Jackson in contrast to destructive lesion (see above) in which all function is absent. **Disseminated lesion.** A scattered lesion involving several sites. **Focal lesion.** One that picks out circumscribed or restricted areas of a tissue. **Functional lesion.** Disturbance of the function of cells or organs without obvious structural changes. **Gross lesion.** Damage of tissue that can be seen with the naked eye. **Histological lesion.** Damage of tissue that can be detected only by means of the microscope. **Indiscriminate lesion.** A lesion which attacks different tissues or organs instead of selecting a particular one. **Initial syphilitic lesion.** The chancre which develops at the site of inoculation of the disease. **Irritative lesion.** One that stimulates the functions of the part affected. **Macroscopical lesion.** Gross lesion (see above). **Microscopical lesion.** Histological lesion (see above). **Mixed lesion.** Indiscriminate lesion (see above). **Molar lesion.** Macroscopical lesion (see above). **Molecular lesion.** Functional lesion (see above). **Naked-eye lesion.** Gross lesion (see above). **Organic lesion.** A disturbance of the structure of a tissue or organ. **Partial lesion.** One that does not affect the whole of an organ. **Peripheral (nerve) lesion.** Interruption (usually traumatic) of normal nerve conduction at a point distal to nerve roots and/or plexuses. **Precancerous lesion.** A lesion predisposing to malignant changes. **Primary lesion.** In dermatology, the initial lesion of a skin eruption; Besnier termed such lesions the essential primary eruptive elements. Maculae, papules, nodules, vesicles, pustules, and weals are included in this group. **Primary syphilitic lesion.** Initial syphilitic lesion (see above). **Ring-wall lesion.** The slight purpuric lesions sometimes seen in thrombocytopenia. **Secondary lesion.** A late or retrogressive stage of a primary lesion (see above), or the result of adventitious influences acting upon it or in the course of its evolution (MacLeod). Occasionally, a lesion may be primary in one skin affection and secondary in another. Crusts, excoriations, fissures, scars, scales, and ulcers are examples in this group. **Secondary syphilitic lesion.** The manifestations of syphilis which appear within the first 2 years in areas separate from that of the primary lesion. **Structural lesion.** Organic lesion (see above). **Systemic lesion.** One that involves a system of tissues with a common function. **Total lesion.** One which affects the whole of an organ or tract. **Toxic lesion.** A disturbance in the tissues produced by bacterial toxins as the result of infection. **Traumatic lesion.** Disturbance in tissues or organs produced by mechanical injury such as crushing. **Trophic lesion.** One caused by interference with the nutrition of a part. **Vascular lesion.** A lesion of a blood vessel. **Wire-loop lesion.** The appearance of the smaller blood vessels in the glomeruli of the kidney of a patient who has died from lupus erythematodes. [L *laesio* a hurting.]

See also: COUNCILMAN, DURET, GHON, MELENEY.

Lespinasse, Victor Darwin (b. 1878). Chicago urologist.

Lespinasse suture. Suture of the vas deferens to the epididymis in vaso-epididymostomy for sterility.

Lesser's triangle. A triangle subtended by the hypoglossal nerve and the anterior and posterior bellies of the digastric muscle.

Lesshaft, Pyotr Frantsovich (b. 1836). Kasan and St. Petersburg anatomist.

Lesshaft's muscles. The deep transversus perinei muscles.

Lesshaft's triangle, triangle of Grynfelt and Lesshaft. The superior lumbar triangle through which lumbar hernia may occur. It is formed by the serratus posterior inferior muscle above and medially, the internal oblique muscle laterally, and the quadratus lumborum muscle medially. It was described by Luschka, then Grynfelt (1866), and 4 years later by Lesshaft.

lethal (le·thal). 1. Fatal; causing death. 2. Genetic. A genotype which is fatal to its possessor. [L *lethum* death.]

lethargic (leth·ar·jik). Pertaining to, or characterized by lethargy.

lethargogenic (leth·ar·go·**jen**′·ik). Causing lethargy. [lethargy, Gk *genein* to produce.]

lethargy (**leth**·ar·je). 1. Morbid drowsiness. 2. Mental torpor. **Hysterical lethargy.** Lethargy in hysteria. **Induced lethargy.** Lethargy caused by suggestion. **Lucid lethargy.** Lethargy in a setting of clear consciousness. **Negro lethargy.** African trypanosomiasis. [Gk *lethargia* drowsiness.]

lethe (**le**·the). Amnesia. [Gk, forgetfulness.]

letheomania (le·the·o·**ma**′·ne·ah). Morbid craving for narcotics. [Gk *lethe* forgetfulness, mania.]

letheral (le·ther·al). Of or referring to lethe.

lethiferous (le·**thif**·er·us). 1. Causing death. 2. Inducing sleep. [L *lethum* death, *ferre* to bear.]

lethologica (le·tho·**loj**·ik·ah). Inability to remember the appropriate word. [Gk *lethe* forgetfulness, *logos* discourse.]

Letterer, Erich (b. 1895). Tübingen pathologist.

Letterer-Christian disease. A name given to a group of diseases that includes Hand-Schueller-Christian, Letterer-Siwe, and Jaffe-Lichtenstein diseases. *Histiocytosis X* has also been suggested as a name.

Letterer-Siwe disease. Systemic aleukaemic reticulo-endotheliosis or non-lipoid reticulo-endotheliosis in young children; it is characterized by a fatal progressive anaemia with haemorrhagic manifestations, splenomegaly, hepatomegalia, lymphadenopathy, and a generalized hyperplasia of the reticulo-endothelial cells, resembling leukaemia clinically, but it is related in many ways to Hand-Schueller-Christian disease and to eosinophilic granuloma.

lettuce (**let**·is). Lactuca; the herb *Lactuca virosa* (family Compositae). **Lettuce opium.** Lactucarium. **Wild lettuce.** *Lactuca virosa.* [L *lactuca.*]

Leube, Wilhelm Olivier von (b. 1842). Würzburg physician.

Leube treatment. For gastric ulcer: rest in bed, daily saline laxatives, compresses to the abdomen, and a diet principally of increasing amounts of milk to which later cereals and minced meat are added.

Leube-Riegel test-dinner. A test-meal used occasionally to study gastric function. It consists of beef soup, beef steak, white bread, and water.

leuc-. For words beginning with *leuc-, see also* LEUK-.

leucaemia (lew·se·me·ah). Leukaemia. [Gk *leukos* white, *haima* blood.]

leucaethiops (lew·**ke**·the·ops). An albino of the Negro race. [Gk *leukos* white, *Aithiops* Ethiopian.]

leuceine (lew·**se**·een). A dehydro- compound formed by the reduction of leucine.

leucine (lew·seen). 2-Amino-4-methylpentanoic acid, $(CH_3)_2CH$ $CH_2CH(NH_2)COOH$. An amino acid essential in diet for the maintenance of health and occurring in most protein hydrolysates. It may occur, with tyrosine, in urinary deposits, but is normally broken down into aceto-acetic acid in the metabolism. [Gk *leukos* white.]

leucinethylester (**lew**·sin·eth·il·**es**′·ter). Ethyl ester of 2-amino-4-methylpentanoic acid, $(CH_3)_2CHCH_2CH(NH_2)COOC_2H_5$. An oily liquid derived from leucine.

leucinimide (lew·**sin**·im·ide). Di-isobutyldiketopiperazine, C_4H_9 $CH(CONH)_2CHC_4H_9$. The anhydride of leucine formed by condensation of two molecules of the amino acid with elimination of water. The reaction occurs readily and some leucinimide is formed when a solution of leucine is evaporated to dryness.

leucinosis (lew·sin·**o**·sis). A morbid condition in which there is an excessive quantity of leucine in the liver or other part of the body, leucine appearing in the urine. [leucine, Gk *-osis* condition.]

leucinuria (lew·sin·**ewr**·e·ah). The excretion of leucine in the urine.

leucitis (lew·**si**·tis). Scleritis. [Gk *leukos* white, *-itis* inflammation.]

Leuckart, Karl Georg Friedrich Rudolf (b. 1823). Leipzig anatomist.

Leuckart's canal. An unpaired canal formed by fusion of the paramesonephric ducts; the uterovaginal canal from which the uterus and the upper part of the vagina are developed.

leucoblast (**lew**·ko·blast). A leucocyte not fully developed. **Granular leucoblast.** A promyelocyte. [Gk *leukos* white, *blastos* germ.]

leucoblastosis (**lew**·ko·blas·**to**′·sis). A general term for a dyscrasia of the white-cell elements of the blood-forming tissues, e.g. myelosis, lymphadenosis. [Gk *leukos* white, *blastos* germ, *-osis* condition.]

leucocidin (lew·ko·**si**·din). Any toxin which causes destruction (cytolysis) of leucocytes. [Gk *leukos* white, L *caedere* to kill.]

leucocyte (**lew**·ko·site). White blood corpuscle; any of the various colourless amoeboid cells found in normal blood to the number of approximately 8000 per mm^3. They are classified as *granular leucocytes* (*neutrophils, eosinophils,* and *basophils*), small and large *lymphocytes,* and *monocytes.* Of these, the neutrophils possess numerous fine granules which are neither distinctly eosinophilic nor basophilic; they typically contain lobed or segmented nuclei and are sometimes called *polymorphonuclear leucocytes* or *polymorphs.* Eosinophils possess large conspicuous granules in their cytoplasm, and a bilobed nucleus; the granules are basophilic and the nucleus is non-lobed in the basophils. Lymphocytes are small round cells with a large spherical nucleus and little cytoplasm, whilst the large lymphocyte possesses more cytoplasm, has a reniform nucleus, and is not readily distinguished from a monocyte, which is also a large cell with a clear cytoplasm and has a large reniform nucleus. **Acidophil leucocyte.** Eosinophil leucocyte (see above). **Lazy leucocyte syndrome.** Clinical defect of leucocyte chemotaxis associated with an increased tendency to infection. [Gk *leukos* white, *kytos* cell.]

leucocytic (lew·ko·**sit**·ik). Of or relating to leucocytes.

leucocytoblast (lew·ko·**si**·to·blast). A cell from which a leucocyte is formed. [leucocyte, Gk *blastos* germ.]

leucocytoclasis (**lew**·ko·si·to·**kla**′·sis). Disintegration of leucocytes. [leucocyte, Gk *klassein* to break.]

leucocytoclastic (**lew**·ko·si·to·**klas**′·tik). Pertaining to leucocytoclasis.

leucocytogenesis (**lew**·ko·si·to·**jen**′·es·is). The production of leucocytes. [leucocyte, Gk *genein* to produce.]

leucocytoid (**lew**·ko·si·toid). Like a leucocyte. [leucocyte, Gk *eidos* form.]

leucocytology (**lew**·ko·si·**tol**′·o·je). The science dealing with leucocytes. [leucocyte, Gk *logos* science.]

leucocytolysin (**lew**·ko·si·**tol**′·is·in). A lysin which causes the disintegration of leucocytes.

leucocytolysis (**lew**·ko·si·**tol**′·is·is). The dissolution of leucocytes. **Venom leucocytolysis.** The breaking down of leucocytes with snake venom. [leucocyte, Gk *lysis* a loosing.]

leucocytolytic (**lew**·ko·si·to·**lit**′·ik). 1. Pertaining to leucocytolysis. 2. Causing dissolution of leucocytes.

leucocytoma (**lew**·ko·si·**to**′·mah). A mass having the general appearance of a tumour and composed of numbers of leucocytes. [leucocyte, Gk *-oma* tumour.]

leucocytopenia (**lew**·ko·si·to·**pe**·ne·ah). Leucopenia. [leucocyte, Gk *penes* poor.]

leucocytoplania (**lew**·ko·si·to·**pla**′·ne·ah). The migration of leucocytes from the blood vessels or their transition through a membrane. [leucocyte, Gk *plane* a wandering.]

leucocytopoiesis (lew·ko·si·to·poi·e′·sis). Formation of leucocytes in the body. [leucocyte, Gk *poiein* to make.]

leucocytosis (lew·ko·si·to′·sis). An increase in the total number of leucocytes in the blood above the normal upper limit of 11 000 per mm^3, irrespective of the type or types of leucocytes involved. The increase may be *generalized* and affect all types of cells equally, or be confined to one or more types of cells only. Thus, *neutrophilic leucocytosis* (neutrophilia) is an increase in neutrophils above the normal adult upper limit of 7 500 per mm^3 and similarly *eosinophilic leucocytosis* (eosinophilia) exists when eosinophils rise above 400 per mm^3; *basophilic leucocytosis* (basophilia) is when basophils rise above 200 per mm^3, *lymphocytic leucocytosis* (lymphocytosis) when lymphocytes rise above 4 500 per mm^3, and *mononuclear leucocytosis* (monocytosis) when monocytes rise above 800 per mm^3. A leucocytosis is *absolute* when the maximum total figure for a specific type of cell is exceeded, or *relative* when the proportion of a type of cell is increased, more particularly when there is no associated increase in the total numbers of all circulating leucocytes. A leucocytosis is *physiological* when associated with natural functions, thus: *digestion leucocytosis* occurring normally after taking food; *pregnancy leucocytosis*; *emotional leucocytosis*. A *terminal* (*agonal*) *leucocytosis* occurs in moribund states. Numerous pathological conditions cause leucocytosis, notably inflammation, infection, trauma, haemorrhage, certain intoxications and drugs, and leukaemia. [leucocyte, Gk *-osis* condition.]

leucocytotactic (lew·ko·si·to·tak′·tik). Referring to or characterized by leucocytotaxia.

leucocytotaxia, leucocytotaxis (lew·ko·si·to·tax′·e·ah, lew·ko·si·to·tax′·is). The movement of leucocytes, either away from or towards a focus, e.g. damaged and/or inflamed tissue. **Negative leucocytotaxia.** The movement of leucocytes away from a focus. **Positive leucocytotaxia.** The movement of leucocytes towards a focus. [leucocyte, Gk *taxis* arrangement.]

leucocytotherapy (lew·ko·si·to·ther′·ap·e). Treatment of a disease by administration of leucocytes. **Preventive leucocytotherapy.** Leucoprophylaxis. [leucocyte, therapy.]

leucocytotic (lew·ko·si·tot′·ik). Relating to or characterized by leucocytosis.

leucocytotoxic (lew·ko·si·to·tox′·ik). Pertaining to leucocytotoxin.

leucocytotoxin (lew·ko·si·to·tox′·in). A toxin which causes disintegration of leucocytes.

leucocytotropic (lew·ko·si·to·trop′·ik). Having a specific attraction for leucocytes. [leucocytes, Gk *trope* a turning.]

leucocytozoon (lew·ko·si·to·zo′·on). The generic name of certain blood parasites of birds. [leucocyte, Gk *zoon* living thing.]

leucocyturia (lew·ko·si·tewr′·e·ah). The presence of leucocytes in the urine.

leucoderma (lew·ko·der·mah). 1. Any white area of skin. 2. Vitiligo. **Acquired leucoderma.** Vitiligo. **Leucoderma acquisitum centrifugum.** Rounded areas of leucoderma with a pigmented naevus in the centre of each; also known as *Sutton's disease, perinaevic vitiligo,* or *halo naevus.* **Leucoderma colli.** Syphilitic leucoderma (see below). **Congenital leucoderma.** Albinism. **Halo leucoderma.** Leucoderma acquisitum centrifugum (see above). **Occupational leucoderma.** Areas of depigmentation of skin due to contact with rubber; caused by an anti-oxidant, the monobenzyl ether of hydroquinone. **Leucoderma psoriaticum.** Depigmented areas of skin, occurring on the sites of healed lesions of psoriasis. **Leucoderma solare.** White areas of skin caused by the sun's rays. **Syphilitic leucoderma.** Macular depigmentation of the skin of the neck and shoulder occurring in late syphilis. [Gk *leukos* white, *derma* skin.]

leucodermia (lew·ko·der·me·ah). Whiteness in the skin, as distinguished from leucoderma, which means white skin. Nevertheless, often used as a synonym of leucoderma. [see prec.]

leucodermic, leucodermatous (lew·ko·der·mik, lew·ko·der·mat·us). Pertaining to, characterized by, or resembling leucoderma.

leucodiagnosis (lew·ko·di·ag·no′·sis). Determination of the nature of a disease (e.g. leukaemia) by examination, enumeration, and typing of the leucocytes. [leucocyte, diagnosis.]

leucodystrophy (lew·ko·dis·tro·fe). Disturbance of cerebral white matter with demyelination. **Metachromatic leucodystrophy.** A fatal demyelinating disease of infancy with metachromatic material in the brain, peripheral nerves and viscera, also often in urine. Deficient aryl sulphatase A causes disturbance of sulphatide metabolism. It is autosomal recessive. [Gk *leukos* white, *dys-*, *trophe* nourishment.]

leucoencephalitis (lew·ko·en·kef·al·i′·tis). Inflammation of the cerebral white matter. **Acute haemorrhagic leucoencephalitis.** An acute fatal form of encephalitis of unknown cause characterized pathologically by cerebral patechial haemorrhages with demyelination and intense inflammation. **Subacute sclerosing leucoencephalitis.** An inflammatory disease of the brain affecting children and adolescents characterized by increasing mental deterioration, myoclonus, rigidity and sometimes blindness, with a fatal outcome after several months. Probably a chronic form of measles encephalitis. [Gk *leukos* white, *egkephalos* brain, *-itis* inflammation.]

leucoencephalopathy (lew·ko·en·kef·al·op′·ath·e). Disease of the cerebral white matter. **Acute necrotizing haemorrhagic leucoencephalopathy.** Acute haemorrhagic leucoencephalitis. *See* LEUCOENCEPHALITIS. **Metachromatic leucoencephalopathy.** An inborn deficiency of aryl sulphatase A, transmitted by autosomal recessive inheritance and characterized pathologically by accumulation of metachromatic material throughout the brain and peripheral nervous system, and in the kidneys and gut. From about the age of 3, there is a progressive weakness and mental deterioration leading to death in a year or two. **Progressive multifocal leucoencephalopathy.** A rare demyelinating disorder occurring as a terminal event in patients with reticuloses. Severe progressive paralysis, ataxia and blindness cause death in a few months. [Gk *leukos* white, encephalon, Gk *pathos* disease.]

leuco-erythroblastosis (lew·ko·er·ith·ro·blas·to′·sis). The occurrence in the circulating blood of a large number of erythrocytes and leucocytes. [leucocyte, erythrocyte, Gk *blastos* germ.]

leucogenic (lew·ko·jen·ik). Forming leucocytes. [leucocyte, Gk *genein* to produce.]

leucokeratosis (lew·ko·ker·at·o′·sis). Leucoplakia: white thickening of patches of mucosa, especially in the mouth (leucokeratosis buccalis, leukokeratosis oris); it is autosomal dominant. [Gk *leukos* white, keratosis.]

leucolysin (lew·kol·is·in). Leucocytolysin.

leucolysis (lew·kol·is·is). Leucocytolysis.

leucolytic (lew·ko·lit·ik). Leucocytolytic.

leucoma (lew·ko·mah). A white scar of the cornea. **Leucoma adherens.** A dense white corneal scar following a perforation, in which the iris is incarcerated. [Gk *leukos* white, *-oma* tumour.]

leucomainaemia (lew·ko·ma·in·e′·me·ah). A morbid condition characterized by the presence or retention of excessive quantities of leucomaines in the blood. [leucomaine, Gk *haima* blood.]

leucomaine (lew·ko·ma·een). A toxic amine or other nitrogenous base produced in the body in the course of the metabolism. [Gk *leukoma* whiteness.]

leucomainic (lew·ko·ma·in′·ik). Referring to or due to the presence of leucomaines.

leucomyelitis (lew·ko·mi·el·i′·tis). Inflammation in the white matter of the spinal cord. [Gk *leukos* white, myelitis.]

leucomyelopathy (lew·ko·mi·el·op′·ath·e). Any morbid condition of the white matter of the spinal cord. [Gk *leukos* white, myelopathy.]

leucomyoma (lew·ko·mi·o′·mah). Lipomyoma. [Gk *leukos* white, myoma.]

Leuconostoc (lew·ko·nos·tok). A genus of saprophytic bacteria belonging to the tribe Streptococceae (family Coccaceae) and consisting of spherical or ovoid cells, arranged in pairs and chains surrounded by a gelatinous envelope which unites them into zoogloeal masses. They are usually Gram-positive, but decolorize easily. **Leuconostoc citrovorum, leuconostoc dextranicum.** Species which are found in milk and dairy products. **Leuconostoc mesenteroides.** A species found in fermenting vegetable and other plant materials, and in sugar-cane solutions. [Gk *leukos* white, *Nostoc* a genus of algae.]

leuconychia (lew·ko·**nik**·e·ah). Patchy white discoloration of the nails caused by air which is present between the nail and the nail bed; leucopathia unguium. **Leuconychia punctata.** Leuconychia with small white dots. **Leuconychia striata.** Leuconychia with small white striae. **Leuconychia totalis.** Leuconychia involving the whole nail. **Leuconychia trichophytica.** Whitening of a nail plate from *Trichophyton* infection. [Gk *leukos* white, *onyx* nail.]

leucopathia, leucopathy (lew·ko·**path**·e·ah, lew·**kop**·ath·e). 1. Leucoderma. 2. A morbid state of the leucocytes or one caused by an accumulation of dead leucocytes. **Symmetrical progressive leucopathy.** A punctate leucoderma of the trunk and limbs reported from Japan and Brazil. **Leucopathia unguium.** Leuconychia. [Gk *leukos* white, *pathos* disease.]

leucopedesis (**lew**·ko·ped·**e**′·sis). The passage of leucocytes through the walls of blood vessels. [leucocyte, Gk *pedesis* an oozing.]

leucopenia (lew·ko·**pe**·ne·ah). A diminution in the number of leucocytes normally present in the blood; a count of less than 5 000 per mm^3. **Basophil leucopenia, basophilic leucopenia.** A diminution in the number of basophil leucocytes in the blood. **Malignant leucopenia, pernicious leucopenia.** Agranulocytosis. [leucocyte, Gk *penes* poor.]

leucopenic (lew·ko·**pe**·nik). Relating to or affected with leucopenia.

leucophlegmasia (**lew**·ko·fleg·**ma**′·ze·ah). A type of white oedema without any generalized dropsy, e.g. phlegmasia alba dolens (white leg). **Leucophlegmasia dolens puerperarum.** Phlegmasia alba dolens. [Gk *leukos* white, phlegmasia.]

leucophthalmous (lewk·of·**thal**·mus). Applied to a condition in which the sclera of the eye is abnormally white. [Gk *leukos* white, *ophthalmos* eye.]

leucoplakia (lew·ko·**pla**·ke·ah). A chronic inflammatory lesion resulting in the formation of smooth, dry, white, thickened patches in the mucous membrane, especially of the mouth, where it may occur on the tongue, inside of the cheeks, or gums. It is apparently due to chronic irritation such as from heavy smoking, excessive alcohol, highly spiced foods, or tertiary syphilis, not infrequently a precursor of epithelioma. **Leucoplakia penis.** An induration of the mucous membrane of the prepuce, glans, or urethral meatus, in which there is oedema of the superficial portion of the dermis and hypertrophy of the prickle-cell layer of the epithelium. **Leucoplakia vesicae.** A rare condition in which white plaques appear in the mucous membrane at the base of the bladder and sometimes become malignant. **Leucoplakia vulvae.** A chronic inflammation of the vulva, in which there occur patches of white, sodden or dry, and often fissured epithelium. It appears to follow chronic irritation such as scratching due to pruritus, and may be a precursor of epithelioma. [Gk *leukos* white, *plax* plate.]

leucoplania (lew·ko·**pla**·ne·ah). Leucocytoplania.

leucoplasia (lew·ko·**pla**·ze·ah). Leucoplakia. [Gk *leukos* white, *plasis* a moulding.]

leucopoiesis (**lew**·ko·poi·**e**′·sis). Leucocytopoiesis.

leucoprophylaxis (**lew**·ko·pro·fil·**ax**′·is). The attempt to procure immunity to surgical infection by increasing artificially the number of polymorphonuclear leucocytes circulating in the blood, e.g. by the injection of sodium pentanucleotide. [leucocyte, prophylaxis.]

leucopsin (lew·**kop**·sin). Visual yellow. [Gk *leukos* white, *opsis* sight.]

leucoria (lew·**kor**·e·ah). A white pupil due to retinoblastoma, cataract, retrolental fibroplasia, developmental abnormalities, or inflammatory masses. [Gk *leukos* white, *kore* pupil.]

leucoriboflavine (**lew**·ko·ri·bo·**fla**′·veen). A colourless dihydro-compound of riboflavine, produced by reduction. [Gk *leukos* white, riboflavine.]

leucorrhagia (lew·ko·**ra**·je·ah). Profuse leucorrhoea. [Gk *leukos* white, *rhegnynein* to gush forth.]

leucorrhoea (lew·ko·**re**·ah). A discharge of whitish, viscid fluid from the cavity of the uterus and the vagina, commonly known as the *whites.* **Menstrual leucorrhoea, periodic leucorrhoea.** Leucorrhoea which occurs at the menstrual period or just before the onset of menstruation. [Gk *leukos* white, *rhoia* flow.]

leucosarcoma (**lew**·ko·sar·**ko**′·mah). Lymphosarcoma-cell leukaemia; a form of lymphosarcoma having a leukaemoid type of blood picture. [Gk *leukos* white, sarcoma.]

leucosarcomatosis (**lew**·ko·sar·ko·mat·**o**′·sis). A condition in which there are present multiple leucocytic sarcomata, probably intermediate between myelomatosis and myeloid leukaemia. [leucocyte, sarcoma, Gk *-osis* condition.]

leucoscope (**lew**·ko·skope). An instrument devised by Helmholtz (modified by A. Koenig) used in the investigation of colour vision. [Gk *leukos* white, *skopein* to view.]

leucosin (**lew**·ko·sin). A water-soluble, heat-coagulable protein of the albumin class found in wheat, rye, barley, and other cereals. [Gk *leukos* white.]

leucosis (lew·**ko**·sis). A condition of overgrowth of the tissue from which leucocytes form, such as is seen in myelosis and lymphadenosis. **Lymphoid leucosis.** Leucosis chiefly involving lymphocytes. **Myeloblastic leucosis.** Leucosis involving mainly myeloblasts. **Myelocytic leucosis.** Leucosis chiefly involving the myelocytes. [Gk *leukos* white.]

leucotactic (lew·ko·**tak**·tik). Chemotactic for leucocytes.

leucotaxine (lew·ko·**tax**·een). A nitrogenous, crystalline principle, probably a polypeptide, found in inflammatory exudates, which increases capillary permeability allowing the free escape of plasma proteins, and which induces migration of leucocytes through the capillary wall. [leucocyte, Gk *taxis* arrangement.]

leucotherapy (lew·ko·**ther**·ap·e). Leucocytotherapy.

leucothrombin (lew·ko·**throm**·bin). A coagulation factor in the blood, said to originate from leucocytes and associated with prothrombin in the formation of thrombin.

leucothrombopenia (**lew**·ko·thromb·bo·**pe**′·ne·ah). A condition in which the leucocyte and the thrombocyte counts of the blood are lower than is normally the case. [leucocyte, thrombocyte, Gk *penes* poor.]

leucotome (**lew**·ko·tome). An instrument used in leucotomy, consisting of a loop of wire that can be passed through a cannula.

leucotomy (lew·**kot**·o·me). An operation for cutting pathways in the anterior parts of the frontal lobes of the cerebrum which lie in the subcortical and central white matter (originated by Moniz of Portugal). It is resorted to in the treatment of severe mental disease and, more recently, in unendurable states of chronic pain. The term is commonly qualified by the adjective *frontal* or *prefrontal.* Derived operations used for the same purpose are: *lobotomy,* a USA variant for a similar operation; *topectomy,* the excision of limited areas of the frontal cortex; *cortical undercutting,* the severing of downward connections of limited areas of the frontal cortex; and *thalamotomy,* the electrocoagulation of parts of thalamic nuclei assumed to be end-stations of fronto-thalamic pathways. [Gk *leukos* white, *temnein* to cut.]

leucotoxic (lew·ko·**tox**·ik). Leucocytotoxic.

leucotoxin (lew·ko·**tox**·in). Leucocytotoxin.

leucotrichia (lew·ko·**trik**·e·ah). Whiteness of the hair. **Leucotrichia annularis.** A condition in which the hairs show alternate white and pigmented patches. [Gk *leukos* white, *thrix* hair.]

leucotrichous (lew·ko·**trik**·us). Characterized by, or having white hair. [see prec.]

Leudet, Théodore Emile (b. 1825). Rouen physician.

Leudet's sign. Tinnitus auscultated through a stethoscope placed in the neighbourhood of the ear.

leuk-. For words beginning with *leuk-* see *also* LEUC-.

leukaemia (lew·**ke**·me·ah). A fatal disease of unknown aetiology, showing gross disturbances of the leucocytopoietic tissues, first in the bone marrow and then affecting the blood and other organs. Any or several of the types of white blood cells may be involved, thus characterizing the particular leukaemia. Usually in the chronic leukaemias there may be a marked increase in the number of leucocytes, involving the granular, lymphocytic, or monocytic series, and later showing an increasing number of immature white-cell precursors in the marrow and blood; in the acute leukaemias, which are rapidly fatal, there may be a diminished number (leucopenia), or only a slight increase, while later the primitive cells become very prominent in number and immaturity. The chronic sufferers have an expectation of life of from one to sixteen years, but the acute cases, which have entirely different aetiologies, show a very bad prognosis, rarely living longer than a few weeks or months irrespective of treatment. Leukaemias show a variety of non-specific chromosome abnormalities, with the exception of chronic myeloid leukaemia, which is nearly always associated with the presence in the bone-marrow cells of a deletion of the long arm of a G group chromosome, presumably No. 22 (*see* Philadelphia CHROMOSOME). Also known as *leucaemia,* or *leucosis.* **Acute leukaemia.** A very progressive fatal form of unknown aetiology, commencing acutely with severe anaemia, usually a leucopenia, and increasing numbers of immature, often undifferentiated cells of the myeloid, lymphatic, and monocytic series. Sometimes one type of cell predominates and a special form of leukaemia is recognizable, though without any improvement in prognosis. There is no satisfactory treatment. **Acute lymphatic leukaemia, acute lymphoblastic leukaemia.** An acute leukaemia with lymphoblasts or lymphocytes as the main cells concerned. **Acute monocytic leukaemia.** A rare acute leukaemia involving the monoblasts and monocytes, with a very characteristic hyperplasia of the gums, often associated with bleeding from them. **Acute myeloblastic leukaemia, acute myelocytic leukaemia, acute myeloid leukaemia.** Acute myelosis, an acute leukaemia in which the main cellular disturbance concerns the myeloblasts and myelocytes. **Acute primitive (haemocytoblastic, stem-cell, or undifferentiated) leukaemia.** An acute leukaemia characterized by the presence of very primitive undifferentiated cells. **Aleukaemic leukaemia, aleukocythaemic leukaemia.** Aleukaemic lymphadenosis, a leukaemia with typical changes in marrow and other organs, usually in its early stages showing a low or normal leucocyte count, often with few abnormal white cells present; later the chronic forms develop marked leucocytosis which the acute forms do not. **Basophilic leukaemia, basophilocytic leukaemia.** A form of leukaemia said to occur with a greatly increased number of basophilic leucocytes in the bone marrow and blood; it is not generally accepted as a definite entity, and is probably a chronic myeloid leukaemia with an increase in the number of basophilic leucocytes. **Leukaemia cutis.** Cutaneous lesions occurring in acute, chronic, and aleukaemic phases of any of the leukaemias. Nodules in the skin and subcutaneous tissues which develop during chronic lymphatic leukaemia are the most common. In myeloid leukaemia, maculae, slightly elevated patches, and nodules occasionally develop. In acute lymphatic leukaemia, petechial and diffuse haemorrhages into the skin and mucosae may be seen, also ulcers and necrotic lesions including noma. Terminal toxic manifestations include urticaria and intracutaneous haemorrhages. Erythroderma and exfoliative dermatitis occasionally occur, more usually in lymphatic than in myeloid leukaemia. In acute myeloid leukaemia, and rarely in acute lymphatic leukaemia, chloroma may develop in children. In monocytic leukaemia, maculae and papules imitating the lesions of secondary syphilis may develop, but after a while the lesions become slate-blue in colour; deeply-seated, pale, shot-like papules have been noted. Purpuric and bullous lesions are not uncommon. **Embryonal leukaemia.** Acute primitive leukaemia (see above). **Eosinophilic leukaemia, eosinophilocytic leukaemia.** A chronic myeloid leukaemia in which the predominating cell may be the mature eosinophilic polymorphonuclear leucocyte, or an eosinophilic myelocyte. **Fowl leukaemia.** A leukaemic condition occurring in fowls and transmissible by a filtrable virus. **Histiocytic leukaemia.** Acute primitive leukaemia (see above). **Intestinal leukaemia.** A leukaemia in which the main features are due to leukaemic deposits in the mucous membranes of the intestines. **Leukopenic leukaemia.** Aleukaemic leukaemia (see above). **Lienomyelogenous leukaemia.** Myeloid leukaemia (see below). **Lymphatic leukaemia, lymphocytic leukaemia, lymphogenous leukaemia, lymphoid leukaemia.** A chronic (3–15 years) fatal disease with a variable degree of enlargement of the spleen and lymph glands, occasionally skin lesions, and a great increase in lymphocytes in the blood and bone marrow. It may follow exposure to toxic and radioactive agents, but is usually of unknown aetiology. **Lymphosarcoma-cell leukaemia.** Leucosarcoma, a form of lymphosarcoma having a leukaemoid type of blood picture. **Mast-cell leukaemia.** Basophilic leukaemia (see above). **Medullary leukaemia.** Myeloid leukaemia (see below). **Megakaryocytic leukaemia.** A leukaemic condition associated with a megakaryocytic hyperplasia of bone marrow, and sometimes with an increase of megakaryocytes in the blood. It is usually seen in chronic myeloid leukaemia or myelophthisic anaemias. **Micromyeloblastic leukaemia.** An acute leukaemia with increase in the number of micromyeloblasts, which is often confused with, or thought identical with, acute lymphoblastic leukaemia (see above). **Mixed leukaemia.** A so-called mixed leukaemia, with myeloid and lymphatic changes in the blood and marrow, but not now generally accepted, as it is thought that the cells have been incorrectly identified. **Monocytic leukaemia.** A severe leukaemic condition characterized by a disturbance of the monocytic series of white cells, usually causing a rapidly fatal acute monocytic leukaemia; very rarely a more chronic monocytic leukaemia may be observed in older people, usually females, with a prognosis of 1–3 years. **Myeloblastic leukaemia, myelogenic leukaemia, myelogenous leukaemia, myeloid leukaemia.** Chronic myelosis, a chronic form of leukaemia with mild to very great splenomegaly and hepatomegalia, and usually of relatively slow progress (3–16 years); it usually shows a very high myeloid leucocytosis in blood and bone marrow when first diagnosed. It may follow exposure to toxic and radioactive agents, and certain other diseases of the blood, but is usually of unknown aetiology. **Neutrophilic leukaemia.** A form of leukaemia associated with a great increase in the neutrophil myelocytes or leucocytes. **Paramyeloblastic leukaemia.** Rieder-cell leukaemia. **Plasma-cell leukaemia.** A rapidly fatal condition in which plasma cells are present in large numbers in the marrow, blood, and other organs; the condition may be associated with myelomatosis and plasmacytoma. **Pseudosplenic leukaemia.** A term used to describe a variety of conditions with glandular enlargement, but without leukaemic changes in the blood. **Leukaemia of the skin.** Leukaemia cutis (see above). **Splenic leukaemia, splenomedullary leukaemia, splenomyelogenous leukaemia.** Myeloid leukaemia (see above). **Subleukaemic leukaemia.** Aleukaemic leukaemia (see above). [Gk *leukos* white, *haima* blood.]

See also: NÄGELI (O.), RIEDER, SCHILLING.

leukaemic (lew·ke·mik). Referring to or suffering from leukaemia.

leukaemid (lew·ke·mid). A lesion of the skin which is sometimes present in cases of leukaemia. The term has been used to describe both non-specific and specific leukaemic lesions, especially necrotic and purpuric lesions, prurigo-like papules, and erythrodermias.

leukaemogen (lew·ke·mo·jen). A substance which induces or causes leukaemia. [see foll.]

leukaemogenesis (lew·ke·mo·jen′·es·is). The origin and development of leukaemia. [leukaemia, Gk *genein* to produce.]

leukaemogenic (lew·ke·mo·jen′·ik). Inducing or causing leukaemia. [see prec.]

leukaemoid (lew·ke·moid). Resembling leukaemia. [leukaemia, Gk *eidos* form.]

leukanaemia (lew·kan·e·me·ah). A condition in which the blood picture resembles leukaemia and pernicious anaemia; it may be due to leukaemoid changes in the marrow and blood in pernicious anaemia, or, in chronic myeloid leukaemia, to disturbances of the bone marrow by a proliferating myeloid tissue interfering with red-cell erythropoiesis, leading to anaemia often macrocytic in type. [Gk *leukos* white, anaemia.]

leukin (lew·kin). A name given to bactericidal substances extracted from polymorphonuclear leucocytes (Schneider). They are thermostabile, withstanding a temperature of 56°C but destroyed in 30 min at 75°C, thus differing from complement. Those derived from the leucocytes of rabbits, dogs, and guinea-pigs are active against *Bacillus anthracis* and species of *Proteus,* but not against *Salmonella typhi* or *Vibrio cholerae.* [Gk *leukos* white.]

leukocorea (lew·ko·**re**·ah). White pupil secondary to, e.g. cataract, retrolental fibroplasia, retinoblastoma. [Gk *leukos* white, *kore* pupil.]

leukodystrophy (lew·ko·**dis**·tro·fe). A condition in which there is faulty myelination with secondary gliosis. [Gk *leukos* white, *dys-, trophe* nourishment.]

Levaditi, Constantin (b. 1874). Rumanian bacteriologist in Paris.

Levaditi's method. For *Spirochaeta pallida* (*Treponema pallidum*) in tissue sections. After fixation in 10 per cent formalin, and dehydration in 98 per cent alcohol, the tissue is placed in 1.5 per cent silver nitrate solution and kept at 37°C in the dark for 3 days. It is then washed in water and reduced with a pyrogallic-acid-formalin mixture for 48 h in the dark. The mixture is then dehydrated, embedded in paraffin and sections are cut. The spirochaetes appear dark brown or black and the tissue cells a yellowish brown.

Levallorphan (le·val·**or**·fan). BP Commission approved name for (−)-*N*-allyl-3-hydroxymorphinan. **Levallorphan Tartrate BP 1973.** The hydrogen tartrate dihydrate of levallorphan, an antagonist of morphine and similar drugs. Its action resembles that of nalorphine but it is more potent.

Levamisole (le·**vam**·is·ole). BP Commission approved name for (−) - 2,3,5,6 - tetrahydro - 6 - phenylimidazo[2,1 - *b*]thiazole; an anthelmintic.

Levamphetamine (le·vam·**fet**·am·een). BP Commission approved name for (−)-2-aminopropylbenzene; a sympathomimetic drug.

levan (**le**·van). A polymer of fructose produced by the action of *Bacillus mesentericus* or *Bacillus subtilis* on cane sugar (sucrose). It is similar to inulin, but differs in the linkage of the fructose units.

levansucrase (le·van·**sew**·kraze). An enzyme secreted by certain bacteria which catalyses the synthesis of levan from sucrose.

Levant berries (lev·**ant ber**·iz). *Cocculus indicus,* the fruits of *Anamirta paniculata* (family Menispermaceae). [*Levant,* an area of the Mediterranean, berry.]

Levant wormseed (lev·**ant werm**·seed). Santonica, the dried flower heads of *Artemesia cina* Berg. (family Compositae). [*Levant,* an area of the Mediterranean, wormseed.]

levarterenol (lev·ar·**ter**·en·ol). Noradrenaline.

levator (lev·**a**·tor). Any muscle which has a raising or lifting action. [L, lifter.]

levator anguli oris muscle [musculus levator anguli oris] (lev·**a**·tor **ang**·gew·li **or**·is musl). A muscle attached above to the canine fossa of the maxilla and below to the angle of the mouth, decussating with the depressor anguli oris and orbicularis oris muscles.

levator ani muscle [musculus levator ani] (lev·**a**·tor **a**·ni musl). The chief muscle of the pelvic floor, attached above within the lesser pelvis and below to the perineal body, the wall of the anal canal, the anococcygeal raphe, and the coccyx.

levator glandulae thyroideae muscle [musculus levator glandulae thyroideae (NA)] (lev·**a**·tor **glan**·dew·le thi·**roid**·e·e musl). An occasional unpaired slip running from the hyoid bone to the isthmus or pyramidal lobe of the thyroid gland.

levator labii superioris muscle [musculus levator labii superioris (NA)] (lev·**a**·tor **la**·be·i sew·peer·e·**or**·is musl). A muscle attached to the maxilla above the infra-orbital foramen and to the skin of the upper lip.

levator labii superioris alaeque nasi muscle [musculus levator labii superioris alaeque nasi (NA)] (lev·**a**·tor **la**·be·i sew·peer·e·**or**·is a·**le**·kwe **na**·zi musl). A muscle attached above to the frontal process of the maxilla, and below by two slips to the skin of the ala of the nose and upper lip.

levator palati muscle [musculus levator veli palatini (NA)] (lev·**a**·tor **pal**·at·i musl). The elevator of the soft palate, arising from the under-surface of the petrous part of the temporal bone and the pharyngotympanic tube.

levator palpebrae superioris muscle of the orbit [musculus levator palpebrae superioris (NA)] (lev·**a**·tor **pal**·pe·bre sew·peer·e·**or**·is musl). A thin triangular muscle arising from the lesser wing of the sphenoid bone above the origin of the superior rectus muscle and fanning out anteriorly into the superior tarsus, the skin of the eyelid, and the superior conjunctival fornix. The upper of the two lamellae [lamina superficialis (NA)] is attached to the upper edge of the upper tarsal plate and to the skin of the upper eyelid; the lower [lamina profunda (NA)] is attached to the margin of the upper tarsal plate and to the fornix of the conjunctiva and consists of unstriped muscle fibres.

levator prostatae muscle [musculus levator prostatae (musculus pubovaginalis) NA] (lev·**a**·tor **pros**·ta·te musl). The fibres of the levator ani muscle which pass back around the prostate gland to be inserted into the perineal body.

levator scapulae muscle [musculus levator scapulae (NA)] (lev·**a**·tor **skap**·ew·le musl). A muscle which arises from the upper four cervical transverse processes, and is inserted into the superior angle of the scapula.

levatores costarum muscles [musculi levatores costarum (NA)] (lev·a·**tor**·eez kos·**ta**·rum muslz). Small fan-shaped muscles arising from the transverse processes of the 7th cervical to the 11th thoracic vertebrae inclusive, and inserting into the external surface of the ribs medial to their angles [musculi levatores costarum breves (NA)]. The four lower muscles each give rise to additional muscles [musculi levatores costarum longi (NA)], which run from one rib to the second one below.

level (**lev**·el). 1. Standard, e.g. of conscious behaviour in the infant or adult. 2. A stage in a series of heights, distances, processes, etc. 3. The position or plane in an organ at which a given physiological or pathological activity or function is localized. 4. In psychiatry, one of a series of planes of increasing complexity and organization. **Levels of anaesthesia.** The stages and planes of anaesthesia from full consciousness to death. Systematized by A. E. Guedel in the years following 1920. **Iso-electric level.** Iso-electric line; the zero baseline of the galvanometer string of the electrocardiogram from which all deflexions are referred. **Metastable levels.** States of a system, e.g. a nucleus or molecule, with energy higher than that of the ground state, but for which the probability of transition to a state of lower energy is unusually small. **Neurological level.** A term used with reference to the part of the nervous system engaged in the integration of the nervous impulses involved in a particular physiological activity. **Psychological level.** A term used with reference to the conscious, preconscious, and unconscious aspects of mental activity. **Sensation level.** A scale of subjective auditory threshold stimuli; usually applied to the appreciation of sound, and recorded in decibels. **Tolerance level.** The daily or weekly dose of ionizing radiation, or the concentration of a radioactive or toxic substance in air or water, exposure to which is considered not likely to lead to significant impairment of health. [OFr. *livel.*]

Leventhal, Michael Leo (b. 1901). American obstetrician and gynaecologist.

Stein-Leventhal syndrome. Bilateral enlargement of the ovaries associated with menstrual abnormalities, sterility, hirsutism and obesity. The enlargement is due to the excessive number of ripening follicles and overgrowth of the stroma.

lever (**le**·ver). A mechanical appliance operating upon a fulcrum, designed to gain mechanical advantage in direct proportion to the perpendicular distance of the applied force from the fulcrum. [L *levare* to lift.]

See also: DAVY (R.).

Lévi, Leopold (b. 1868). Paris endocrinologist.

Lévi's syndrome, Lévi-Lorain disease, dwarfism, infantilism, or type, Lorain-Lévi syndrome. Pituitary infantilism, a condition in which a child does not grow, but is perfectly formed with all the proportions symmetrically diminished. The adult at first sight resembles a child, but the shape is that of an adult in miniature. Sexual organs are immature, but intelligence is not impaired.

levicellular (lev·e·**sel**·ew·lar). Smooth-celled; as applied to a muscle fibre, indicating absence of striation. [L *levis* smooth, *cellula* little cell.]

levidulinose (lev·**id**·ew·lin·oze). $C_{18}H_{32}O_{16}$, a trihexoside formed of glucose and mannose units, which occurs naturally in manna.

levigate (**lev**·ig·ate). To subdivide finely, usually with a mortar and pestle; to reduce to a firm, smooth powder; occasionally, to make into a paste with water or oil by triturating in a mortar or with a knife on a slab. [L *levigare* to make smooth.]

levigation (lev·ig·**a**·shun). The process of levigating.

Levin, Abraham Louis (b. 1880). New Orleans physician.

Levin tube. A stomach tube for passing through the nose.

Levinthal-Coles-Lillie body. A minute body in infected tissues in psittacosis; it resembles the Paschen granule.

Levisticum (lev·**is**·tik·um). A genus of European herbs of the family Umbelliferae. **Levisticum officinale.** Lovage, a Mediterranean herb the root and leaves of which have been used as a diuretic, carminative, and febrifuge. [Gk *ligystikon.*]

levitation (lev·it·**a**·shun). 1. A subjective sensation of rising and floating in the air, as experienced in dreams. 2. In psychical research, the term used for the particular case of telekinesis where the paranormal movement of an object is in such a direction as would imply that the gravitational force acting on the object has been temporarily overcome. [L *levitas* lightness.]

Levodopa BP 1973 (le·vo·**do**·pah). (−)-3-(3,4-Dihydroxyphenyl)-L-alanine; it is used in the treatment of Parkinson's syndrome.

Levomethorphan (le·vo·meth·**or**′·fan). BP Commission approved name for L-3-methoxy-*N*-methylmorphinan, a powerful synthetic analgesic based on the morphine skeleton.

Levomoramide (le·vo·**mor**·am·ide). BP Commission approved name for (−)-1-(3-methyl-4-morpholino-2,2-diphenylbutyryl)-pyrrolidine; a narcotic analgesic.

Levophenacylmorphan (le·vo·fen·as·il·**mor**′·fan). BP Commission approved name for (−)-3-hydroxy-*N*-phenacylmorphinan; a narcotic analgesic.

Levopropoxyphene (le·vo·pro·**pox**′·e·feen). BP Commission approved name for α - (−) - 4 - dimethylamino - 3 - methyl - 1,2 - diphenyl - 2 - propionyloxybutane; it is used in the treatment of cough.

Levorphanol (lev·**or**·fan·ol). BP Commission approved name for (−)-3-hydroxy-*N*-methylmorphinan. **Levorphanol Tartrate BP 1973.** The hydrogen tartrate dihydrate of levorphanol, a powerful analgesic comparable with morphine in its actions, uses and side-effects. By contrast with morphine, it is almost as effective by mouth as by injection.

levosin (**le**·vo·sin). $(C_6H_{10}O_5)_n$, a holosaccharide found in wheat flour, bran, and rye. When hydrolysed it splits into glucose and fructose. [L *laevus* left.]

levulan (**le**·vew·lan). Fructosan. [L *laevus* left.]

levurid, levuride (**lev**·ew·rid, **lev**·ew·ride). Moniliid; any sterile lesion, usually vesicular, localized or wide-spread, due to dissemination through the blood of the products of *Candida albicans.* So called because of the yeast-like nature of the organism. [Fr. *levure* yeast.]

Lévy, Fernand (b. 1881). Paris neurologist.

Roussy-Lévy disease, or syndrome. Peroneal muscular atrophy associated with cerebellar ataxia and scoliosis; it is familial.

Lewandowsky, Felix (b. 1879). Bern and Hamburg dermatologist.

Lewandowsky's disease. Rosaceous tuberculid. *See* TUBERCULID.

Lewandowsky's naevus. Pseudoxanthoma elasticum.

Jadassohn-Lewandowsky syndrome. Pachyonychia congenita.

Lewandowsky-Lutz disease. Epidermodysplasia verruciformis.

Lewis. *See* Blood GROUP.

Lewis, Gilbert Newton (b. 1875). American physical chemist.

Lewis atom. The static atom in which the electrons are believed to oscillate about centres situated at the corners of cubes or tetrahedra. [Obsolete term].

Lewis, Sir Thomas (b. 1881). British physician.

Lewis' reaction. The triple response: name given to the vasomotor reaction occurring in skin when a pointed, but not sharp, instrument is drawn heavily across it. First stage, local reddening; second stage, more widespread flush or flare; third stage, development of a weal. The response is probably due to the liberation of a histamine-like (H) substance from the tissues as a result of the noxious stimuli. The H substance is released both directly and as the result of an axon reflex.

Lewis and Pickering test. Reactive hyperaemia test: a test to detect organic arterial occlusion in a limb. Full vasodilatation in the limb is obtained by immersion in hot water, the limb is elevated to drain venous blood, and a sphygmomanometer cuff is then applied and inflated to above the systolic blood pressure. After 5 min the cuff is removed. In a normal limb a flush spreads down to the toes in 2-5 s, but when organic vascular disease is present, the flush spreads slowly, and is patchy in distribution.

lewisite (**loo**·is·ite). A mixture of the vesicants, dichlorodivinylchloroarsine and chlorovinyldichloroarsine, used as a blister gas in chemical warfare. [Winford Lee *Lewis,* 1878-1943, American chemist.]

Lewisohn, Richard (b. 1875). New York surgeon.

Lewisohn's method. A technique of indirect blood transfusion by the prior administration of sodium citrate.

Lexer, Erich (b. 1867). Munich surgeon.

Lexer's vessels. Small juxta-epiphyseal vessels derived from the anastomosis round a joint which pierce the metaphysis at the line of attachment of the joint capsule.

Leyden, Ernst Victor von (b. 1832). Berlin physician.

Leyden's cells. Leydenia gemmipara; the large mononuclear phagocytic cells discovered by Leyden in the ascitic fluid associated with peritoneal carcinomatosis.

Leyden's disease. A form of periodic vomiting.

Leyden's duct. The wolffian or mesonephric duct.

Leyden's neuritis. Lipomatous neuritis, a form of neuritis in which nerve fibres are destroyed and replaced by fibrous tissue with an added deposition of fat.

Leyden's serum. The blood serum of scarlet-fever convalescents used in treatment by Leyden.

Charcot-Leyden crystals. Diamond-shaped crystals occurring in the sputum in asthma. Similar crystals have been observed in the faeces in various pathological states, and in leukaemic spleens.

Leyden-Moebius dystrophy, or type, Moebius-Leyden dystrophy, or type. The atrophic type of progressive childhood muscular dystrophy, first affecting muscles of the pelvic girdle.

leydenia gemmipara (li·**de**·ne·ah jem·**ip**·ar·ah). Leyden's cells. [E. V. von *Leyden,* L *gemma* bud, *parere* to give birth.]

Leydig, Franz von (b. 1821). Bonn anatomist and zoologist.

Interstitial cell of Leydig. One of the epithelial cells lying between the seminiferous tubules of the testis, and held responsible for the production of testosterone.

Leydig cell tumour of the ovary. Hilus cell tumour.

Sertoli-Leydig tumour. An ovarian tumour which usually causes masculinization and has varied histological structure.

Lhermitte, Jacques Jean (b. 1877). Paris neurologist.

Lhermitte's sign. Sudden shooting paraesthesiae, like electric shocks running down the trunk and limbs, on sudden flexion of the neck. It is seen in disease of the cervical part of the spinal cord, disseminated sclerosis, and other demyelinating conditions.

Lhermitte and McAlpine syndrome. A syndrome in which there are signs due to a combination of lesions affecting the pyramidal and extrapyramidal motor systems.

Lian, Camille (b. 1882). Paris physician.

Lian's point. A point of election for paracentesis situated on a line joining the umbilicus and the left anterior superior iliac spine at the junction of the outer and middle one-thirds.

Lian's sign. Echo sign; echolalia.

libidinal (lib·id·in·al). Erotic; belonging to the libido.

libidinous (lib·id·in·us). Lustful. [L *libidinosus.*]

libido (lib·i·do), (pl. *libidines*). 1. Sexual desire. 2. Peculiar to psycho-analysis: the energy derived from the sexual instinct; by inhibition or displacement from its immediate object, it may be diverted into other channels and provide the driving power of aims and tendencies of an infinitely varied kind. **Ego libido.** Narcissism. [L, lust.]

Libman, Emanuel (b. 1872). New York physician.

Libman-Sacks disease, or syndrome. Progressive anaemia in young people, with slight persistent fever and purpuric and erythematous rash.

Libman-Sacks endocarditis. Non-bacterial verrucose endocarditis associated with systemic lupus erythematosus.

Osler-Libman-Sacks syndrome. Libman-Sacks endocarditis (see above).

libra (li·brah). 1. Pound (lb). 2. Balance. [L.]

lice (lise). *See* LOUSE.

lichen (li·ken). 1. Botanically, a cryptogram which forms a thallus that is either shrubby, leafy, crustaceous, or powdery. A symbiosis of hyphal filaments with algal gonidia, i.e. a symbiotic association of alga and fungus. It is often found attached to medicinal barks such as cinchona. 2. A papular cutaneous eruption; an old term originally applied to skin affections which seemed to spread on the skin like the lichen on trees, used to designate a group of maladies in which the elements are papules and remain as such throughout the whole course of the malady. This convention was long retained, but the term came to be used by various writers for eruptions in which the papules developed into vesicles or pustules. Consequently *lichen* qualified by an adjective has been used to denote a number of affections which differ in nature and aetiology. **Lichen acuminatus.** Lichen ruber acuminatus (see below). **Lichen agrius.** Obsolete term; probably either papular eczema or Hebra's prurigo. **Lichen albus** (von Zumbusch). Lichen sclerosus et atrophicus (see below). **Lichen amyloidosus** (Freudenthal). Localized widespread eruption of itching papules, nodules, or plaques, due to deposits of amyloid in the skin, but not associated with generalized amyloidosis. **Lichen annularis.** 1. Granuloma annulare (Galloway). 2. Lichen planus annularis (see below). **Lichen annularis et serpiginosus.** Obsolete term used by Wilson for a variety of seborrhoeic dermatitis. **Lichen atrophicus.** Lichen planus atrophicus (see below). **Lichen aureus.** A bruise-like collection of lichenoid papules of a rusty colour, of unknown cause. **Lichen axillaris.** Fordyce-Fox disease; an eruption of discrete, itching, dome-shaped papules in the axillae. The papules are associated with the aprocrine glands, and may develop also in the pubic area, areolae of the nipples, and near the navel. Almost invariably, the patients are females between the ages of 15 and 48. **Lichen circinatus.** Obsolete term for seborrhoeic dermatitis. **Lichen circumscriptus.** Lichen simplex chronicus (Vidal) (see below). **Lichen corneus hypertrophicus** (Darier). 1. Lichen planus verrucosus (see below). 2. An unusual complication of eczema crustosum. **Lichen diabeticorum.** Obsolete term for a form of xanthoma, associated with diabetes, in which the lesions are small and papular. **Lichen eczematodes.** Obsolete term for eczema papulosum. **Lichen fibromucinodosis.** Lichen myxoedematosus (see below). **Lichen framboesianus.** Pian datre; a secondary manifestation of yaws. **Lichen haemorrhagicus.** Various forms of papules, in which small haemorrhages have occurred, or small purpuric lesions at the orifices of hair follicles. **Lichen hypertrophicus.** Lichen planus hypertrophicus; lichen planus verrucosus (see below). **Lichen infantum.** Lichen urticatus (see below). **Lichen islandicus.** Iceland moss. *See* MOSS. **Lichen lividus.** Obsolete term for a form of lichen scrofulosus (see below) in which there is slight haemorrhage into the lesions. **Lichen myxoedematosus.** A lichenoid eruption with excessive deposition of acid mucopolysaccharide in the skin lesions. **Lichen nitidus.** A rare cutaneous malady of unknown aetiology, usually occurring in males, the lesions being small, discrete papules, flesh-coloured or pinkish in hue. The distribution is limited in the majority of cases; the genitalia, abdomen, breast, flexors of the elbows and palms are the sites of election. **Lichen nuchae.** Lichen simplex of the nape of the neck. **Lichen obtusus.** Lichen planus obtusus (see below). **Lichen obtusus corneus.** Prurigo nodularis. **Lichen pilaris.** Lichen spinulosus (see below). **Lichen planopilaris.** A form of lichen planus in which shiny follicular papules are noted, as well as the typical plane papules of the disease. **Lichen planus.** A cutaneous disease of unknown aetiology, characterized by an eruption of multiple flat-topped papules, with an angular contour, and a characteristic waxy appearance when observed obliquely. The malady is usually associated with severe itching, and the eruption may be widespread. **Lichen planus actinicus.** Lichen planus induced by exposure to sunlight. **Lichen planus et acuminatus atrophicans.** A follicular type of lichen planus affecting the scalp and leading to cicatricial alopecia. **Lichen planus annularis.** A type of lichen planus in which annular lesions are noted. These are formed either from the peripheral spread of a large papule or from an aggregation of close-set papules. **Lichen planus atrophicus.** A rare form of lichen planus in which the papules in the centre of a plaque of lichen become atrophic; fresh papules form at the periphery. Many cases so diagnosed are probably examples of lichen sclerosus et atrophicus (see below). **Lichen planus bullosus.** A rare form of lichen planus in which large vesicles or bullae form on the top of some of the rapidly evolving papules. **Lichen planus erythematosus.** A rare condition of uncertain nature indeterminate between lichen planus and poikiloderma vascularis atrophicans of Jacobi. **Lichen planus erythrodermia.** A lichenoid eruption resulting from mepacrine, gold, or amiphenazole, and appearing when the initial erythroderma subsides. **Lichen planus hypertrophicus.** Lichen planus verrucosus (see below). **Lichen planus linearis.** A rare form of lichen planus, usually seen in children, in which the eruption occurs as a long line of papules, usually on a limb. **Lichen planus moniliformis.** Large, somewhat verrucose lesions of lichen planus, arranged like the beads of a necklace. **Lichen planus morphoeicus.** Lichen sclerosus et atrophicus (see below). **Lichen planus obtusus.** A form of lichen planus in which round or oval, flat or convex, large papules develop. **Lichen planus pemphigoides.** Lichen planus bullosus (see above). **Lichen planus pilarus** (Pringle). A form of lichen planus (see above) in which shiny follicular papules are noted, as well as the typical plane papules of the disease. **Lichen planus verrucosus.** A variety of lichen planus in which the predominant lesions, specially about or near the ankle, are confluent plaques, thickened, sometimes quite dark in colour, hard, rough, and wart-like. **Lichen purpuricus.** Lichen aureus (see above). **Lichen ruber** (Hebra). 1. Pityriasis rubra pilaris. 2. Lichen planus (see above). **Lichen ruber acuminatus** (Kaposi). Pityriasis rubra pilaris. **Lichen ruber moniliformis.** 1. Lichen planus moniliformis (see above). 2. Morbus moniliformis lichenoides. **Lichen ruber pemphigoides.** Lichen planus bullosus (see above). **Lichen ruber planus.** Lichen planus (see above). **Lichen sclerosus et atrophicus.** An eruption of irregular, often polygonal, flat-topped, ivory-white papules, which may be discrete or grouped. On the surface of each papule are either comedo-like plugs, or follicular puncta where these plugs have been present. The malady is chronic. It may cause intractable pruritus if the lesions develop on the anal area or vulva, and may be associated with balanitis xerotica obliterans. **Lichen scorbuticus.** A papulo-follicular rash, sometimes seen in scurvy. There is usually slight haemorrhage into the lesions. **Lichen scrofulosorum, lichen scrofulosus.** Tuberculosis lichenoides; an eruption of tiny, punctiform, reddish-brown papules, grouped in patches or circles, seen usually in children suffering from some form of surgical tuberculosis. The trunk is the site of election, and the malady is a tuberculid. **Lichen simplex.** Eczema papulosum. **Lichen simplex aigu** (Vidal). Lichen urticatus (see below). **Lichen simplex chronicus.** Lichenification, lichen vidal, neurodermatitis, névrodermite: a circumscribed prurigo in which, as a result of rubbing, the skin becomes thickened and pigmented. Often three distinct zones may be noted: the outermost shows some pigmentation and a few papules; the middle, lozenge-shaped papules, exaggeration of the natural lines of the skin, and pigmentation; the centre, more thickening and pigmentation, with gross exaggeration of the natural lines which enclose the lozenge-shaped papules. **Lichen simplex circumscriptus.** Lichen simplex chronicus (see prec.). **Lichen spinulosus** (Devergie). Keratosis follicularis spinulosa (Unna), lichen pilaris seu spinulosus (Crocker), acné cornée (Hardy, Leloir), kératose pilaire engainante (Audry); a skin affection characterized by groups or patches of follicular, acuminate, pinkish papules, each surmounted by a filiform spine. **Lichen striatus.** A linear dermatosis with pink lichenoid papules but with an eczematoid histology, lasting for 3 to 12 months or more. **Lichen strophulosus.** Archaic term, probably referring to papular urticaria, or to the papular stage of miliaria rubra. **Lichen syphiliticus.** A lichenoid eruption of the skin occurring in the secondary stage of syphilis. **Lichen trichophyticus.** A dermatophytid consisting of small red papules on the back and shoulders, occasionally associated with tinea capitis. **Lichen tropicus.** Miliaria rubra; prickly heat. **Lichen urticatus.** Lichen simplex aigu (Vidal), prurigo simplex (Brocq); papular urticaria of infants and children. **Lichen variegatus** (Crocker). Parakeratosis variegata. **Lichen verrucosus.** Lichen planus verrucosus (see above). **Lichen vidal.** Lichen simplex chronicus (see above). [Gk *leichen.*]

See also: WILSON (W. J. E.).

licheniasis (li·ken·i·as·is). 1. The growth and development of lichen. 2. The state of a person affected by lichen. **Licheniasis strophulus.** Strophulus.

lichenification (li·ken·if·ik·a′·shun). A thickening and hardening of the skin which is the site of an eczematous or other eruption, so that there is set up a lesion very much akin to that of lichen. **Pebbly lichenification.** Lichenification with discrete or confluent, smooth, pebbly nodules. **Secondary lichenification.** Lichenification secondary to hypostatic eczema, discoid eczema, atopic dermatitis, contact dermatitis, psoriasis, lichen planus, or fungal infection. [lichen, L *facere* to make.]

lichenin (li·ken·in). $(C_6H_{10}O_5)_n$, a complex carbohydrate (polysaccharide) contained in Iceland moss, *Cetraria islandica.* It yields glucose on hydrolysis. Isolichenin, found associated with lichenin, hydrolyses to produce mannose, galactose, and glucose. [lichen.]

lichenization (li·ken·i·za′·shun). The process of development of lesions of lichen on the skin.

lichenoid (li·ken·oid). 1. Resembling lichen. 2. A condition of the tongue which affects young children, and is characterized by the presence of whitish spots circumscribed by yellow rings. [lichen, Gk *eidos* form.]

Lichtenstein, Louis. 20th century Los Angeles physician.

Jaffe-Lichtenstein disease. Eosinophilic granuloma of bone; a solitary slow-growing lesion in older children. It is now considered to be, with Letterer-Siwe and Hand-Schueller-Christian diseases, part of a group of diseases to which the name of *Letterer-Christian disease* has been given. The term has also been applied to cystic osteofibromatosis, a fibrous dysplasia involving the medullary cavities of many bones.

Lichtheim, Ludwig (b. 1845). Königsberg and Bonn physician.

Lichtheim's aphasia, phenomenon, or sign, Dejerine-Lichtheim phenomenon. Expressive dysphasia in which the patient, though speechless, may be able to indicate with his fingers the number of syllables in a word.

Lichtheim's disease, or syndrome. Any disease in which there is combined degeneration of the posterior and lateral columns of the spinal cord; applied particularly to subacute combined degeneration as a manifestation of pernicious anaemia. As first described, the syndromes included splenomegaly (due to the pernicious anaemia).

Lichtheim's plaques. Areas of demyelination found in the cerebral white substance in pernicious anaemia.

lichtheimia (likt·hi·me·ah). Absidia. [Ludwig *Lichtheim.*]

licorice (lik·or·is). Liquorice.

lid (lid). Eyelid. **Granular lid.** Trachoma. **Lid lag.** The upper eyelid comes down in jerks instead of smoothly when the patient is asked to follow the examiner's down-moving finger, a characteristic of Graves' disease. **Lid retraction.** Indicated by the presence of sclera between the retracted upper eyelid and the cornea, a characteristic of Graves' disease. [AS *hlid.*]

See also: COLLIER.

Liddell, Edward George Tandy (b. 1895). British physiologist.

Liddell and Sherrington reflex. Stretch reflex. *See* REFLEX.

lidocaini (lid·o·ka·ni). Lignocaine. **Lidocaini Hydrochloridum.** *European Pharmacopoeia* name for Lignocaine Hydrochloride BP 1973.

Lidoflazine (lid·o·fla·zeen). BP Commission approved name for *N* - {4 - [4,4 - di - (4 - fluorophenyl)butyl]piperazin - 1 - ylacetyl}-2,6 - xylidine; a cardiac stimulant.

lie (li). The direction or position. **Longitudinal lie.** The normal position of the fetus in the uterus, in which the fetus lies in the axis of the birth canal. The breech or the head may present. [AS *licgan.*]

Lieben, Adolf (b. 1836). Vienna chemist.

Lieben's test. For acetone bodies in urine: the iodoform test (*see* TEST) carried out on the distillate from the urine.

Lieberkühn, Johann Nathanael (b. 1711). Berlin anatomist.

Crypts, follicles, or glands of Lieberkühn. Simple tubular glands opening between the bases of the villi of the small intestine, and also on the surface of the epithelium of the large intestine; the intestinal glands.

Liebermann, L. von Szentlorincz (b. 1852). Hungarian physician and biochemist.

Liebermann-Burchard reaction, or test. For cholesterol: to 5 ml of a chloroform solution of cholesterol are added 2 ml of acetic anhydride and 0.1 ml of concentrated sulphuric acid. A violet colour changing to green upon standing is produced.

Liebermeister, Carl von (b. 1833). Tübingen physician.

Liebermeister's furrows. Transverse grooves on the upper surface of the liver corresponding to the ribs, and caused by external pressure such as tight lacing.

Liebermeister's grooves. Developmental grooves on the surface of the liver running anteroposteriorly.

Liebermeister's rule. In febrile conditions the pulse rate increases approximately 8 beats for every 1°C rise in temperature.

Liebermeister's sign. A pale area of the tongue as an early sign of air embolism.

Liebig, Justus von (b. 1803). Giessen and Munich chemist.

Liebig's extract. An extract of meat; the first one of its kind to be prepared.

Liebreich, Richard (b. 1830). Königsberg ophthalmologist.

Liebreich's lacrimal probe. A straight, double-ended, fine metal probe, with flattened grip in the centre, designed for passing down the lacrimal passages.

lien (li·en). The spleen. [L.]

lienal (li·en·al). Splenic. [L *lien* spleen.]

lienculus (li·en·kew·lus). An accessory spleen. [L, little spleen.]

lienectomy (li·en·ek·to·me). Splenectomy. [L *lien* spleen, Gk *ektome* a cutting out.]

lienitis (li·en·i·tis). Splenitis. [L *lien* spleen, Gk *-itis* inflammation.]

lienocele (li·en·o·seel). Hernial protrusion of the spleen. [L *lien* spleen, Gk *kele* hernia.]

lienogram (li·en·o·gram). The radiograph made during lienography. [L *lien* spleen, Gk *gramma* record.]

lienography (li·en·og·raf·e). Radiographic or radio-isotopic visualization of the spleen. [L *lien* spleen, radiography.]

lieno-intestinal (li·en·o·in·tes′·tin·al). Pertaining to the spleen and intestine. [L *lien* spleen, intestine.]

lienomalacia (li·en·o·mal·a′·she·ah). Splenomalacia. [L *lien* spleen, Gk *malakia* softness.]

lienomedullary (li·en·o·med·ul′·ar·e). Splenomedullary. [L *lien* spleen, medulla.]

lienomyelogenous (li·en·o·mi·el·oj′·en·us). Splenomedullary. [L *lien* spleen, Gk *myelos* marrow, *genein* to produce.]

lienomyelomalacia (li·en·o·mi·el·o·mal·a′·she·ah). Splenomyelomalacia. [L *lien* spleen, Gk *myelos* marrow, *malakia* softness.]

lienopancreatic (li·en·o·pan·kre·at′·ik). Splenopancreatic. [L *lien* spleen, pancreas.]

lienopathy (li·en·op·ath·e). Splenopathy. [L *lien* spleen, Gk *pathos* disease.]

lienorenal (li·en·o·re′·nal). Splenonephric. [L *lien* spleen, *ren* kidney.]

lienotoxin (li·en·o·tox′·in). Splenotoxin. [L *lien* spleen, toxin.]

lienteric (li·en·ter·ik). Referring to, or characterized by a type of diarrhoea in which the faeces consist mainly of undigested food (lientery).

lientery (li·en·ter·e). A form of diarrhoea characterized by the passage of undigested food in the stools. [Gk *leios* smooth, *enteron* bowel.]

lienunculus (li·en·ung·kew·lus). A portion of the spleen which has become detached and which is functioning independently. [L, little spleen.]

Liepmann, Hugo Carl (b. 1863). Breslau and Berlin psychiatrist.

Liepmann's apraxia. Apraxia.

Liesegang, Raphael Eduard (b. 1860). Frankfurt colloid chemist.

Liesegang's phenomenon. If a reagent in solution is allowed to diffuse into a gel and react with another reagent contained in the gel, any insoluble product is deposited in the form of rings (*Liesegang's rings*) or bands (*Liesegang's bands, or striae*) interspaced by clear gel.

Lieutaud, Joseph (b. 1703). Aix and Paris physician.

Lieutaud's triangle, or trigone. The trigone of the bladder.

life (life). The energy which is essential to existence, or the force which endows organized beings with power to exercise such functions as growth, metabolism, reproduction, evolution, and so on. **Animal life.** In contradistinction from vegetative life, that in which there are spontaneous acts of conscious exercise of will-power and the voluntary use of the senses. **Antenatal life.** Life before birth; that is, within the uterus. **Average life.** A term applied to a thing or substance decaying or being eliminated, and equal to the average value of the intervals elapsing between a given instant and the decay or elimination of the individual constituents initially present at that instant. **Catheter life.** A life which relies for its continued existence on the discharge of urine through a catheter. **Change of life.** The menopause. **Embryonic life.** The earlier stages in the life history of an organism, when it is contained within an egg or uterus and before it is capable of independent existence. In man, embryonic life is arbitrarily succeeded by fetal life at the end of the 8th week of gestation. **Intellectual life.** That which is manifested by exercise of the will, impulses, and reason. **Intra-uterine life.** Life within the uterus. **Mean life.** Average life (see above). **Mental life, psychical life.** Intellectual life (see above). **Uterine life.** Intra-uterine life (see above). **Vegetative life.** That which is represented by metabolic, reproductive, and other automatic activities which are essential for continued existence. [AS *lif.*]

ligament [ligamentum (NA)] (lig·am·ent). 1. A thickened band of white fibrous tissue which connects bones and forms the capsule of joints. 2. A single or double layer of peritoneum connecting one abdominal viscus to another, or to the abdominal wall. 3. A localized condensation of subperitoneal fibrous and smooth-muscle tissue which serves to support a viscus. 4. The fibrous remnant of a disused fetal structure. 5. Any condensation of fascia subserving a supporting function. **Accessory ligament.** A ligament, usually distinct from the joint capsule, which serves to strengthen the union between two bones. **Accessory atlanto-axial ligament.** A narrow band which extends obliquely upwards and laterally from the back of the body of the axis to the back of the lateral mass of the atlas. **Accessory plantar ligament.** Ligament of the metatarsophalangeal joint, plantar (see below). **Accessory volar ligament.** Ligament of the metacarpophalangeal joint, palmar (see below). **Acromioclavicular ligament [ligamentum acromioclaviculare (NA)].** The thickened superior portion of the capsule of the acromioclavicular joint. **Adipose ligament.** A fat-containing fold of the synovial membrane of the knee joint. **Alar ligament of the odontoid process [ligamentum alare (NA)].** One of two strong bands which extend upwards and laterally from the sides of the apex of the odontoid process of the axis to be attached to the inner aspect of each occipital condyle; odontoid ligament. **Alveodental ligament.** The fibrous tissue which connects the cementum of a tooth with the bone of the alveolar wall; periodontal membrane. **Ligament of the ankle joint, anterior.** The thin and lax anterior portion of the capsular ligament. **Ligament of the ankle joint, lateral.** A capsular thickening composed of three separate bands radiating from the lateral malleolus: the anterior and posterior talofibular ligaments with a calcaneofibular ligament between them. **Ligament of the ankle joint, medial.** Deltoid ligament (see below). **Ligament of the ankle joint, posterior.** The thin and lax posterior portion of the capsular ligament. **Annular ligament of the base of the stapes [ligamentum anulare stapedis (NA)].** A fibro-elastic ring attaching the base of the stapes to the circumference of the fenestra vestibuli. **Annular ligament of the radius [ligamentum anulare radii (NA)].** A circumferential band forming four-fifths of a circle which surrounds the head of the radius, and is attached to the ends of the radial notch of the ulna. **Annular ligaments of the trachea [ligamenta anularia (trachealia) NA].** The fibro-elastic membranes which enclose and connect the individual rings of the trachea and complete the tube posteriorly. **Anococcygeal ligament.** Anococcygeal body. *See* BODY. **Apical ligament of the odontoid process [ligamentum apicis dentis (NA)].** A thin band which may contain notochordal remnants connecting the apex of the odontoid process of the axis with the anterior edge of the foramen magnum. **Appendiculo-ovarian ligament.** A fold of peritoneum connecting the appendix with the broad ligament of the uterus. **Arcuate ligament [ligamentum arcuatum (NA)].** Any ligament having an arched form. **Arcuate ligament, lateral [ligamentum arcuatum lateralis (NA)].** A fibrous arch which spans the quadratus lumborum muscle and provides the origin for the diaphragm; the lateral lumbocostal arch. **Arcuate ligament, medial [ligamentum arcuatum medialis (NA)].** A fibrous arch which spans the psoas muscle and provides an origin for the diaphragm; the medial lumbocostal arch. **Arcuate ligament, median [ligamentum arcuatum medianum (NA)].** A tendinous band which spans the aortic opening of the diaphragm and joins with the crura on either side. **Arcuate ligament of the knee [ligamentum popliteum arcuatum (NA)].** A bundle of fibres from the lateral condyle of the femur arching over the tendon of the popliteus muscle to blend with the capsule posteriorly. **Arcuate popliteal ligament.** Arcuate ligament of the knee (see preceding). **Arcuate pubic ligament.** *See* PUBIC LIGAMENTS (below). **Auricular ligaments [ligamenta auricularia (NA)].** 1. Extrinsic: the ligaments connecting the auricular cartilage to the temporal bone [ligamenta auricularia, anterius, posterius et superius (NA)]. 2. Intrinsic: those connecting the various parts of the cartilage. **Bifurcated ligament [ligamentum bifurcatum (NA)].** A band attached posteriorly to the front of the dorsum of the calcaneum, which divides anteriorly into the calcaneonavicular and calcaneocuboid ligaments, attached respectively to the navicular and cuboid bones. **Broad ligament of the eye.** The orbital septum. **Broad ligament of the uterus [ligamentum latum uteri (NA)].** A double fold of peritoneum extending on either side from the lateral border of the uterus to the side wall of the pelvis, and containing the ovary, uterine tube, ligaments, and vessels. **Calcaneocuboid ligaments.** 1. Calcaneocuboid medial part of the bifurcated ligament [ligamentum calcaneocuboideum (NA)]: that extending between the anterior part of the dorsum of the calcaneum and the dorsomedial aspect of the cuboid bone. 2. Dorsal: a weak band connecting the dorsal aspects of the two bones. 3. Plantar [ligamentum calcaneocuboideum plantare (NA)]: the short plantar ligament of the tarsus. **Calcaneofibular ligament**

ligament

[ligamentum calcaneofibulare (NA)]. A strong narrow bundle which connects the tip of the lateral malleolus with the lateral surface of the calcaneum. **Calcaneonavicular ligaments.** 1. Calcaneonavicular lateral part of the bifurcated ligament [ligamentum calcaneonaviculare (NA)]: that extending between the anterior part of the dorsum of the calcaneum and the lateral angle of the navicular. 2. Dorsal: a weak band connecting the dorsal aspects of the two bones. 3. Plantar [ligamentum calcaneonaviculare plantare (NA)]: a strong fibrocartilaginous band extending between the sustentaculum tali and the plantar and medial surfaces of the navicular bone; spring ligament. **Calcaneotibial ligament.** That portion of the deltoid ligament of the ankle which is attached below to the sustentaculum tali and the spring ligament. **Capitular ligament of the head of a rib.** A short bundle extending between the crest of the head of a rib and the adjacent intervertebral disc. **Capsular ligament [membrana fibrosa (NA)].** An investing sleeve for synovial joints composed of white fibrous tissue. It usually has a linear attachment to the component bones at or near the borders of their articular cartilage. It commonly has two or more localized thickenings which form the ligaments [ligamenta extracapsularia et intracapsularia (NA)] of the joints. **Cardinal ligament.** A condensation of the parametrial tissue extending on each side from the side wall of the pelvis to the cervix uteri. An important support of the uterus; Mackenrodt's ligament. **Carpal ligaments.** 1. Dorsal: the extensor retinaculum, an oblique fascial band on the dorsum of the wrist attached laterally to the lower end of the radius and medially to the styloid process of the ulna, the pisiform bone, and the triquetral bone. The extensor tendons pass beneath it. 2. Radiate [ligamentum carpi radiatum (NA)]: a group of fibres radiating from the head of the capitate bone to the volar aspects of the other bones of the carpus. 3. Transverse: the flexor retinaculum, a broad flat band attached laterally to the tubercle of the scaphoid and the crest of the trapezium, and medially to the pisiform and the hamate bones, beneath which the flexor tendons enter the palm. 4. Volar: the superficial part of the flexor retinaculum. **Carpometacarpal ligaments.** A series of ligaments, palmar [ligamenta carpometacarpea palmaria (NA)] and dorsal [ligamenta carpometacarpea dorsalia (NA)], connecting the distal row of carpal bones with the metacarpal bones from the 2nd to the 5th. **Central ligament.** The filum terminale. **Ceratocricoid ligaments.** Three bands, anterior, posterior, and lateral, which extend from the inferior horns of the thyroid cartilage to the lamina of the cricoid cartilage. **Check ligament.** 1. Of the atlas: the alar ligament of the odontoid process (see above). 2. Of the extra-ocular muscles: fibrous expansions from the sheaths of the extra-ocular muscles which extend to the walls of the orbit and allegedly check their actions. **Collateral ligaments [ligamenta collateralia (NA)].** 1. Fibular: ligament of the knee, lateral (see below). 2. Interphalangeal: ligaments of the interphalangeal joints, collateral (see below). 3. Metacarpophalangeal: ligaments of the metacarpophalangeal joints, collateral (see below). 4. Metatarsophalangeal: ligaments of the metatarsophalangeal joints, collateral (see below). 5. Radial of the elbow: ligament of the elbow, radial collateral (see below). 6. Radial of the wrist: ligament of the wrist, lateral (see below). 7. Tibial: ligament of the knee, medial (see below). 8. Ulnar, of the elbow: ligament of the elbow, ulnar collateral (see below). 9. Ulnar, of the wrist: ligament of the wrist, medial (see below). **Conoid ligament [ligamentum conoideum (NA)].** The conoid part of the coracoclavicular ligament; a strong band extending between the upper surface of the coracoid process of the scapula and the conoid tubercle on the under surface of the clavicle. **Coraco-acromial ligament of the shoulder girdle [ligamentum coraco-acromiale (NA)].** A triangular horizontally placed band attached by its apex to the acromial tip and by its base to the lateral border of the coracoid process. **Coracoclavicular ligament [ligamentum coracoclaviculare (NA)].** A strong ligament connecting the coracoid process of the scapula with the under surface of the clavicle, and divided into conoid and trapezoid parts. **Coracohumeral ligament [ligamentum coracohumerale (NA)].** A bundle of fibres arising from the root of the coracoid process, more or less blending with the capsule of the shoulder joint before becoming attached to the neck and greater tuberosity of the humerus. **Corniculopharyngeal ligament.** The cricopharyngeal ligament (see below). **Coronary ligament of the liver [ligamentum coronarium hepatis (NA)].** The folds of peritoneum connecting the posterior surface of the liver to the inferior surface of the diaphragm, and consisting of an upper and a lower layer enclosing the bare area of the liver. **Costoclavicular ligament [ligamentum costoclaviculare (NA)].** A strong band connecting the superior surface of the 1st costal cartilage with the costal tubercle of the clavicle. **Costocoracoid ligament.** A thickening of the clavipectoral fascia, extending between the 1st costal cartilage and the coracoid process. **Costopericardiac ligament.** A band which connects the 1st costal cartilage to the pericardium. **Costosternal ligaments.** Sternocostal ligaments (see below). **Costotransverse ligament, inferior [ligamentum costotransversarium (NA)].** A strong ligament connecting adjacent surfaces of a transverse process and the neck of the corresponding rib. **Costotransverse ligament, lateral [ligamentum costotransversarium laterale (NA)].** The ligament from the apex of a thoracic transverse process to the non-articular portion of the tubercle of the corresponding rib. **Costotransverse ligament, superior [ligamentum costotransversarium superius (NA)].** The ligament connecting the neck of a rib with the transverse process of the preceding vertebra. It is composed of two layers, anterior and posterior. **Costoxiphoid ligaments [ligamenta costoxiphoidea (NA)].** Fibres binding the 6th and 7th costal cartilages to the xiphoid process. **Cotyloid ligament.** The labrum glenoidale of the shoulder joint. **Crico-arytenoid ligament, posterior [ligamentum crico-arytenoideum posterius (NA)].** An elastic band attached above the medial part of the base of the arytenoid cartilage and below to the upper margin of the lamina of the cricoid cartilage. **Cricopharyngeal ligament [ligamentum cricopharyngeum (NA)].** A Y-shaped ligament connecting the corniculate and cricoid cartilages. **Cricosantorinian ligament.** The cricopharyngeal ligament (see above). **Cricothyroid ligament [ligamentum cricothyroideum (NA)].** The median part of the cricothyroid membrane which extends between the lower border of the thyroid and the upper border of the cricoid cartilage. **Cricotracheal ligament [ligamentum cricotracheale (NA)].** The fibrous ring connecting the cricoid cartilage with the 1st tracheal cartilage. **Cruciate ligament of the atlas [ligamentum cruciforme atlantis (NA)].** A cruciform structure, the horizontal part of which is formed by the transverse ligament of the atlas (see below), the vertical limb being formed by two bands, the superior and inferior crura, which pass respectively from the transverse ligament to the anterior margin of the foramen magnum and the back of the body of the axis. **Cruciate ligaments of the knee [ligamenta cruciata genus (NA)].** The anterior and posterior cruciate ligaments of the knee. **Cruciate ligament of the knee, anterior [ligamentum cruciatum anterius (NA)].** A strong band within the capsule of the knee joint, attached below to the area in front of the intercondyloid eminence of the tibia and above to the posterior part of the medial aspect of the lateral condyle of the femur. **Cruciate ligament of the knee, posterior [ligamentum cruciatum posterius (NA)].** A strong band within the capsule of the knee joint, attached below to the area behind the intercondylar eminence of the tibia and above to the anterior part of the lateral aspect of the medial condyle of the femur. **Cruciate ligament of the leg.** The inferior extensor retinaculum. **Cubonavicular ligaments.** Bands, dorsal [ligamentum cuboideonaviculare dorsale (NA)], interosseous, and plantar [ligamentum cuboideonaviculare plantare (NA)], uniting the cuboid and navicular bones. **Cuneocuboid ligaments.** Bands, dorsal [ligamentum cuneocuboideum dorsale (NA)], interosseous [ligamentum cuneocuboideum interosseum (NA)], and plantar [ligamentum cuneocuboideum plantare (NA)], uniting the cuboid and 3rd cuneiform bones. **Cuneonavicular ligaments.** Bands, dorsal [ligamenta cuneonavicularia dorsalia (NA)] and plantar [ligamenta cuneonavicularia plantaria], uniting the navicular with the cuneiform bones. **Cutaneophalangeal ligaments.** A series of fascial slips connecting the skin of a finger to the underlying phalanges. **Cysticoduodenal ligament.** A fold of peritoneum connecting the gall bladder with the duodenum. **Deltoid ligament [ligamentum mediale (deltoideum) deltoideum (NA)].** The medial ligament of the ankle joint. The apex of the delta attaches to a pit on the tip of the medial malleolus. The base is attached continuously from before backwards; to the tuberosity of the navicular bone medially [pars tibionavicularis (NA)]; to the medial borders of the calcaneonavicular ligament and the sustentaculum tali [pars tibiocalcanea (NA)]; to the lateral surface of the body of the talus behind the articular facet [pars tibiotalaris posterior (NA)]. Deep to the anterior fibres of the above is a band attached to the neck of the talus [pars tibiotalaris anterior (NA)]. **Dentate ligament.** Ligamentum denticulatum. **Ligament of the elbow, anterior.** The slight thickening of the anterior part of the capsule of the elbow joint. **Ligament of the elbow, lateral.** Ligament of the elbow, radial collateral (see below). **Ligament of the elbow, medial.** Ligament of the elbow, ulnar collateral (see below). **Ligament of the elbow, posterior.** The slight thickening of the posterior part of the capsule of the elbow joint. **Ligament of the elbow, radial collateral [ligamentum collaterale radiale (NA)].** A triangular band attached proximally to the lateral epicondyle of the humerus, and distally to the margins of the radial notch of the ulna and the annular ligament. **Ligament of the elbow, transverse.** A portion of the ulnar collateral ligament of the elbow joint (see following) which connects the medial sides of the coronoid and olecranon processes. **Ligament of the elbow, ulnar collateral [ligamentum collaterale ulnare (NA)].** That extending between the medial epicondyle of the humerus and the coronoid and olecranon processes of the ulna. It is divisible into anterior, posterior, and transverse bands. **Epididymal ligaments.** Two folds of the tunica vaginalis testis which pass from the sides of the testis to the head [ligamentum epididymidis superius (NA)] and tail [ligamentum epididymidis inferius] of the epididymis. They form the upper and lower boundaries of the entrance to the sinus of the epididymis. **Falciform ligament of the liver [ligamentum falciforme hepatis (NA)].** A median crescentic fold of peritoneum connecting the liver with the diaphragm and anterior abdominal wall as far as the umbilicus, and containing between its layers the round ligament of the liver. **False ligaments.** A term applied to the peritoneum reflected from the vertex and lateral borders of the bladder to the walls of the pelvis. Each consists of a single layer, and their value as support is practically nil. **Fundiform ligament of the penis [ligamentum fundiforme penis (NA)].** The extension in the midline of the deep layer of superficial fascia of the lower abdomen from the lower end of the linea alba to the dorsum of the penis. **Gastrocolic ligament [ligamentum gastrocolicum (NA)].** A part of the greater omentum. **Gastropancreatic ligaments.** Gastropancreatic folds. *See* FOLD. **Gastrophrenic ligament [ligamentum gastrophrenicum (NA)].** A fold of peritoneum extending between the cardiac end of the stomach and the under surface of the right side of the diaphragm. **Gastrosplenic ligament [ligamentum gastrolienale (NA)].** A fold of peritoneum connecting the upper part of the greater curvature of the stomach with the hilum of the spleen. **Genito-inguinal ligament [ligamentum genito-inguinale (NA)].** The precursor of the gubernaculum testis. **Glenohumeral ligaments [ligamenta glenohumeralia (NA)].** Thickened bands, superior, middle, and inferior, on the inner aspect of the anterior portion of the capsule of the shoulder joint attached proximally to the anterior margin of the glenoid cavity and labrum, and distally to the lesser tuberosity and neck of the humerus. **Glenoid ligament.** The labrum glenoidale of the shoulder joint. **Ligament of the head of the femur [ligamentum capitis femoris (NA)].** An intra-articular ligament of the hip joint, attached proximally to the transverse ligaments of the acetabulum and the margins of the acetabular notch, and distally to the pit on the head of the femur. **Ligaments of the head of the fibula.** 1. Anterior [ligamentum capitis fibulae anterius (NA)]: a thickening of the anterior aspect of the capsule of the tibiofibular joint. 2. Posterior [ligamentum capitis fibulae posterius (NA)]: a thickening of the posterior aspect of the capsule of the tibiofibular joint. **Hepatocolic ligament [ligamentum hepatocolicum (NA)].** An occasional extension to the right of the lesser omentum, extending from the gall bladder to the right flexure of the colon. **Hepatoduodenal ligament [ligamentum hepatoduodenale (NA)].** The right portion of the lesser omentum extending between the duodenum and the liver. **Hepatogastric ligament [ligamentum hepatogastricum (NA)].** A part of the lesser omentum stretching between the liver and the stomach. **Hepatorenal ligament [ligamentum hepatorenale (NA)].** The peritoneal fold connecting the inferior surface of the liver to the front of the right kidney; the lower layer of the coronary ligament of the liver, if it happens to be reflected on to the upper pole of the right kidney instead of on to the diaphragm. **Hyaloideocapsular ligament.** Fibres passing between the vitreous body and the capsule of the crystalline lens. **Hyo-epiglottic ligament [ligamentum hyo-epiglotticum (NA)].** An elastic band which connects the upper border of the hyoid bone with the anterior aspect of the cartilage of the epiglottis. **Hyothyroid ligaments.** Thyrohyoid ligaments (see below). **Iliofemoral ligament [ligamentum iliofemorale (NA)].** A triangular band, the central part of which is thin, giving the appearance of an inverted Y, attached by its apex to the anterior inferior iliac spine and acetabular margin, and by its base to the intertrochanteric line of the femur. **Iliolumbar ligament [ligamentum iliolumbale (NA)].** The thickened, lower border of the anterior lamella of the lumbar fascia, which extends between the 5th lumbar transverse process and the inner lip of the iliac crest. **Iliotrochanteric ligament.** 1. A fascial band associated with the anterior fibres of the gluteus minimus muscle, which passes from the dorsum ilii to the greater trochanter of the femur. 2. The lateral part of the iliofemoral ligament (see above). **Ligaments of the incus.** 1. Posterior [ligamentum incudis posterius (NA)]: that which connects the tip of the short process of the incus to the fossa for the incus. 2. Superior [ligamentum incudis superius (NA)]: a fold of mucous membrane which passes from the incus to the roof of the tympanic cavity. **Infundibulopelvic ligament [ligamentum suspensorium ovarii (NA)].** The superolateral portion of the broad ligament of the uterus, which passes from the tubal end of the ovary to the peritoneum over the external iliac vessels. It contains the ovarian vessels and nerves. **Inguinal ligament [ligamentum inguinale (NA)].** The thickened lower edge of the aponeurosis of the external oblique muscle, which spans the gap between the anterior superior iliac spine and the pubic tubercle. **Inguinal ligament, pectineal part of the [ligamentum lacunare (NA)].** A triangular bundle of fibres passing horizontally backwards to the pectineal line from the medial end of the inguinal ligament. Its lateral free edge forms the medial boundary of the femoral ring. **Inguinal ligament, reflected part of the [ligamentum reflexum (NA)].** A triangular band derived from the aponeurosis of the external oblique muscle, which crosses the midline to be attached to the pectineal line of the opposite side. **Intercarpal ligaments.** A series of ligaments, palmar [ligamenta intercarpea palmaria (NA)], dorsal [ligamenta intercarpea dorsalia (NA)], and interosseous [ligamenta intercarpea interossea (NA)], binding the carpal bones together. **Interclavicular ligament [ligamentum interclaviculare (NA)].** A band of fibres connecting the sternal ends of the clavicles across the clavicular notch. **Interclinoid ligaments.** Bands connecting the clinoid processes of the sphenoid bone, to which the diaphragma sellae is attached. **Intercornual ligaments.** Ligaments connecting the sacral cornu to the coccyx. **Intercostal ligaments.** The anterior and posterior intercostal membranes. **Intercuneiform ligaments.** Bands, dorsal [ligamenta intercuneiformia dorsalia (NA)], interosseous [ligamenta intercuneiformia interossea (NA)], and plantar [ligamenta intercuneiformia plantaria (NA)], binding the cuneiform bones together. **Interfoveolar ligament [ligamentum interfoveolare (NA)].** The lateral portion of the conjoint tendon of the transversus abdominis muscle. **Interlaminar ligaments.** Ligamenta flava. **Intermetacarpal ligaments.** Bands, palmar, dorsal, and interosseous, connecting together the bases of the medial four metacarpal bones. **Intermetatarsal ligaments.** Bands, dorsal, plantar, and interosseous, connecting the bases of the lateral four metatarsal bones. **Ligaments of the interphalangeal joints, collateral.** Strong obliquely running bands at the sides of the joints; they extend between the dorsal aspect of the lateral surface of the distal end of the proximal bone and the anterolateral aspect of the base of the distal bone. **Ligament of the interphalangeal joint, palmar.** A stout ligament resembling that of the metacarpophalangeal joint. **Ligament of the interphalangeal joint, plantar.** A disc of fibrocartilaginous consistency developed in the plantar surface of the articular capsule. **Interspinous ligaments [ligamenta interspinalia (NA)].** A series of ligaments connecting together the vertebral spinous processes. **Intertransverse ligaments [ligamenta intertransversaria (NA)].** A series of weak bands, mainly in the lumbar region, connecting together the vertebral transverse processes. **Intra-articular ligament.** Any ligament lying within the articular capsule of a joint. **Intra-articular ligament of the joint of the head of a rib [ligamentum capitis costae intra-articulare (NA)].** The ligament joining the head of a rib to the corresponding intervertebral disc. **Intra-articular ligament of a sternocostal joint [ligamentum sternocostale intra-articulare (NA)].** A ligament from the cartilage of the second rib to the sternum. **Ischiofemoral ligament [ligamentum ischiofemorale (NA)].** A triangular band blending with the articular capsule of the hip joint. Its base is attached to the ischium close to the acetabulum, and its apex to the medial surface of the greater trochanter. **Ligament of the knee, lateral [ligamentum collaterale fibulare (NA)].** The fibular collateral ligament; a cord-like band on the lateral aspect of the knee joint, attached above to the lateral condyle of the femur, and below to the head of the fibula anterior to the styloid process. **Ligament of the knee, medial [ligamentum collaterale tibiale (NA)].** A flat band from the medial epicondyle of the femur to the tibia. **Laciniate ligament.** The flexor retinaculum of the ankle; a strong wide band of the deep fascia which stretches between the medial malleolus and the medial tubercle of the calcaneum. The long flexor tendons pass beneath it on their way to the sole of the foot. **Lacunar ligament.** The pectineal part of the inguinal ligament (see above). **Ligament of the left vena cava [plica venae cavae sinistrae (NA)].** A fold of pericardium containing a fibrous cord, running from the oblique vein of the left atrium to the superior intercostal vein; it is a remnant of the left duct of Cuvier. **Lienophrenic ligament.** Phrenicolienal ligament (see below). **Lienorenal ligament [ligamentum phrenicolienale (ligamentum lienorenale) NA].** A double fold of peritoneum which passes from the anterior surface of the right kidney to the hilum of the spleen. It contains the splenic vessels. **Longitudinal ligaments.** 1. Anterior [ligamentum longitudinale anterius (NA)]: a strong broad band which extends along the anterior aspects of the vertebral bodies and intervertebral discs, from the anterior tubercle of the atlas to the front of the sacrum. 2. Posterior [ligamentum longitudinale posterius (NA)]: a similar though narrower band on the posterior aspect, within the vertebral canal, and continuous above with the membrana tectoria. **Lumbocostal ligament [ligamentum lumbocostale (NA)].** The ligament joining the neck of the 12th rib to the base of the transverse process of the 1st lumbar vertebra. **Lumbosacral ligament.** A ligament which connects the 5th lumbar transverse process with the ala of the sacrum. **Ligaments of the malleus.** 1. Anterior [ligamentum mallei anterius (NA)]: consists of two portions, Meckel's ligament, which passes from the anterior process through the petrotympanic fissure to the spine of the sphenoid bone, and the anterior ligament of Helmholtz, which passes from the anterior aspect of the malleus above the anterior process, to the greater tympanic spine. 2. Lateral [ligamentum mallei laterale (NA)]: a fan-shaped band extending between the posterior margin of the tympanic notch and the head of the malleus. 3. Superior [ligamentum mallei superius (NA)]: a band connecting the head of the malleus to the roof of the epitympanic recess. **Medial ligament.** Deltoid ligament (see above). **Meniscofemoral ligament, anterior [ligamentum meniscofemorale anterius (NA)].** An occasional tendinous slip running from the posterior end of the lateral meniscus (lateral semilunar cartilage) in the knee in front of the posterior cruciate ligament to end in the anterior cruciate ligament. **Meniscofemoral ligament, posterior [ligamentum meniscofemorale posterius (NA)].** A tendinous slip arising from the posterior end of the lateral meniscus (lateral semilunar cartilage) in the knee and passing up behind the posterior cruciate ligament to attach to the medial condyle of the femur just posterior to it. **Mesentericomesocolic ligament.** A fold of peritoneum which forms the inferior boundary of the paraduodenal recess. **Metacarpal ligaments, deep transverse.** Ligaments of the palm, deep transverse (see below). **Metacarpal ligaments, dorsal [ligamenta metacarpea dorsalia (NA)].** Thickenings of the dorsal aspect of the carpometacarpal joint capsules. **Metacarpal ligaments, interosseous [ligamenta metacarpea interossea (NA)].** Ligaments connecting the adjacent margins of the capitate and hamate bones to the corresponding parts of the bases of the 3rd and 4th metacarpal bones. **Metacarpal ligaments, palmar [ligamenta metacarpea palmaria (NA)].** Thickenings of the palmar aspect of the carpometacarpal joint capsules. **Metacarpal ligament, superficial transverse [ligamentum metacarpeum transversum superficiale (NA)].** A band of fascia in the palm running transversely across the superficial aspects of the fibrous flexor sheaths. **Ligaments of the metacarpophalangeal joints, collateral.** Strong obliquely running bands at the sides of the joints; they extend between the dorsal aspect of the lateral surface of the distal end of the proximal bone and the anterolateral aspect of the base of the distal bone. **Ligaments of the metacarpophalangeal joint, palmar [ligamenta palmaria (NA)].** Thick fibrocartilaginous structures attached firmly to the base of each proximal phalanx, deepening the socket for the head of the corresponding metacarpal. They blend with the collateral ligaments, deep transverse ligaments of the palm, and the fibrous flexor sheaths. **Metatarsal ligaments, dorsal [ligamenta metatarsea dorsalia (NA)].** Thin transverse bands uniting the bases of the four lateral metatarsals in their dorsal surfaces. **Metatarsal ligaments, interosseous [ligamenta metatarsea interossea (NA)].** Dense bands uniting the contiguous surfaces of the four lateral metatarsal bases distal to the joints. **Metatarsal ligaments, plantar [ligamenta metatarsea plantaria (NA)].** Dense transverse bands uniting the bases of the four lateral metatarsals on their plantar surfaces. **Metatarsal ligaments, superficial transverse [ligamenta metatarsea transversa superficialia (NA)].** Transverse fibres in the superficial fascia of the sole of the foot which connect the webs of the toes. **Ligaments of the metatarsophalangeal joints, collateral.** Strong obliquely running bands at the sides of the joints; they extend between the dorsal aspect of the lateral surface of the distal end of the proximal bone and the anterolateral aspect of the base of the distal bone. **Ligament of the metatarsophalangeal joints, plantar [ligamentum plantare (NA)].** A plate of fibrocartilaginous consistency, strengthening the plantar aspect of the capsule. It is firmly attached to the phalanx, but lightly to the metatarsal. That for the great toe has two sesamoid bones developed in it. **Mucosal ligament.** The infrapatellar synovial fold. **Nephrocolic ligaments.** Fibrous strands connecting the kidneys with the ascending and descending colons. **Nuchal ligament.** Ligamentum nuchae. **Oblique ligament.** The oblique cord. *See* CORD. **Oblique posterior ligament of the knee [ligamentum popliteum obliquum (NA)].** A contribution from the tendon of insertion of the semimembranosus muscle to the posterior portion of the capsule of the knee joint. **Odontoid ligament.** Alar ligament of the odontoid process (see above). **Orbicular ligament.** The annular ligament of the radius (see above). **Ligament of the ovary [ligamentum ovarii proprium (NA)].** A cord-like band which connects the uterine end of the ovary with the side of the uterus behind and below the point of attachment of the uterine tube. **Ligaments of the palm, deep transverse [ligamenta metacarpea transversa profunda (NA)].** A composite ligament made up of the three bands which connect the accessory volar ligaments of the medial four metacarpophalangeal joints. **Ligament of the palm, superficial transverse [fasciculus transversus (NA)].** A band of fibrous tissue stretching across the bases of the lateral four digits, superficial to the digital vessels and nerves. **Palpebral ligaments.** 1. Lateral [ligamentum palpebrale laterale (NA)]: a thin band which connects the lateral ends of the tarsal plates of the eyelids to the zygomatic bones. 2. Medial [ligamentum palpebrale mediale (NA)]: a strong band passing between the medial ends of the tarsal plates and the anterior and posterior lacrimal crests. **Patellar ligament.** Ligamentum patellae. **Pectinate ligament of the iris [ligamentum pectinatum anguli iridocornealis (NA)].** A triangular (on section) open meshwork of fibres situated at the angle of the iris, and continuous with the posterior elastic lamina of the cornea. **Pectineal ligament [ligamentum pectineale (NA)].** A triangularly-shaped ligament stretching between the medial end of the inguinal ligament and the pectineal line of the pubis. **Petroclinoid ligament, petrosphenoid ligament.** A dural band connecting the apex of the petrous part of the temporal bone with the posterior clinoid process, and beneath which the 6th cranial nerve passes. **Phrenicocolic ligament [ligamentum phrenicocolicum (NA)].** A triangular fold of peritoneum which extends between the diaphragm and the left flexure of the colon. It supports the spleen. **Phrenicolienal ligament, phrenicosplenic ligament.** Lienorenal ligament (see above). **Pisohamate ligament [ligamentum pisohamatum (NA)].** A ligamentous extension from the tendon of insertion of the flexor carpi ulnaris muscle, which passes from the pisiform bone to the hook of the hamate bone. **Pisometacarpal ligament [ligamentum pisometacarpeum (NA)].** A band similar to the pisohamate ligament, which passes from the pisiform bone to the base of the 5th metacarpal bone. **Pterygomandibular ligament [raphe pterygomandibularis (NA)].** A fibrous band attached superiorly to the medial pterygoid plate of the sphenoid bone, and inferiorly to the mandible just behind the last molar tooth. The buccinator and superior constrictor muscles derive part of their origins from it. **Pterygospinous ligament [ligamentum pterygospinale (NA)].** A weak band connecting the spine of the sphenoid bone with the posterior border of the lateral pterygoid plate. **Pubic ligaments.** Bands, anterior, posterior, superior [ligamentum pubicum superius (NA)], and inferior or arcuate [ligamentum arcuatum pubis (NA)], binding the two pubic bones together at the symphysis. **Pubofemoral ligament [ligamentum pubofemorale (NA)].** A triangular thickening in the capsule of the hip joint on its inferior aspect. The base is attached to the iliopubic eminence and adjacent pubic ramus, and its apex to the inferior aspect of the femoral neck. **Puboprostatic (pubovesical) ligaments [ligamenta puboprostatica (pubovesicalia) NA].** 1. Lateral: an expansion of the pelvic fascia which extends from the lateral aspect of the sheath of the prostate to the side wall of the pelvis. 2. Medial: a similar expansion connecting the anterior aspect of the sheath with the back of the pubic bone close to the symphysis. **Pulmonary ligament [ligamentum pulmonale (NA)].** A double fold of pleura, below the root of the lung, which connects the medial surface of the lung to the pericardium. **Quadrate ligament of the superior radio-ulnar joint [ligamentum quadratum (NA)].** The thin band of fibres of annular ligament from the radial notch of the ulna to the neck of the radius. **Radiate ligaments.** 1. Of the carpus: radiate carpal ligament (*see* CARPAL LIGAMENTS, above). 2. Of the head of a rib [ligamentum capitis costae radiatum (NA)]: a fan-shaped band which connects the head of a rib to the vertebrae and disc with which it articulates. **Radiocarpal ligaments.** 1. Anterior [ligamentum radiocarpeum palmare (NA)]: the anterior ligament of the radiocarpal joint, which extends from the anterior aspects of the lower ends of the radius and ulna to the proximal row of carpal bones. 2. Posterior [ligamentum radiocarpeum dorsale (NA)]: the posterior ligament of the radiocarpal joint, which extends from the posterior edge of the lower end of the radius to the proximal row of carpal bones. **Radio-ulnar ligaments.** Bands, anterior and posterior, which form the capsule of the inferior radio-ulnar joint. **Rhomboid ligament.** The costoclavicular ligament (see above). **Round ligament of the femur.** Ligament of the head of the femur (see above). **Round ligament of the liver [ligamentum teres hepatis (NA)].** A fibrous band, the remains of the left umbilical vein of the fetus, which passes from the umbilicus in the free edge of the falciform ligament to the left branch of the portal vein. **Round ligament of the uterus [ligamentum teres uteri (NA)].** A fibromuscular band attached to the lateral margin of the uterus below and in front of the uterine tube. It passes laterally in the broad ligament and traverses the inguinal canal to become attached to the skin of the labium majus. It is a remnant of the gubernaculum testis. **Sacrococcygeal ligaments.** 1. Anterior [ligamentum sacrococcygeum ventrale (NA)]: a band which passes from the anterior aspect of the last piece of the sacrum to the front of the coccyx. 2. Lateral [ligamentum sacrococcygeum laterale (NA)]: a band which passes from the lateral aspect of the lower end of the sacrum to the first segment of the coccyx. 3. Posterior: a composite band, consisting of superficial [ligamentum sacrococcygeum dorsale superficiale (NA)] and deep [ligamentum sacrococcygeum dorsale profundum (NA)] fibres, which passes from the back of the lower edge of the sacrum to the back of the coccyx. **Sacro-iliac ligaments.** 1. Anterior [ligamentum sacro-iliacum ventralium (NA)]: a band which connects the anterior aspect of the ala of the sacrum with the adjacent portion of the ilium. 2. Interosseous [ligamenta sacro-iliaca interossea (NA)]: a group of strong fibres which connects the adjacent surfaces of the sacrum and ilium posterior to their articular surfaces. 3. Posterior [ligamenta sacro-iliaca dorsalia (NA)]: a set of fibres situated posterior to the previous ligament. One group (long posterior sacro-iliac ligament) passes from the posterior superior iliac spine to the transverse tubercles of the 3rd and 4th sacral segments; another group (short posterior sacro-iliac ligament) passes from the posterior inferior iliac spine and adjacent portion of the ilium to the back of the sacrum. **Sacrosciatic ligament, lesser.** Sacrospinous ligament (see foll.). **Sacrospinous ligament [ligamentum sacrospinale (NA)].** A triangular band attached by its apex to the ischial spine and by its base to the lateral margins of the lower sacral and upper coccygeal segments. **Sacrotuberous ligament [ligamentum sacrotuberale (NA)].** A considerable band attached proximally to the posterior inferior iliac spine, the posterior and lateral aspects of the lower part of the sacrum, and the side of the coccyx. Distally it is attached to the medial edge of the ischial tuberosity; a prolongation anteriorly of this attachment is the falciform process. **Sheath ligament.** A sheath enclosing the flexor tendon of a finger or toe. **Ligaments of the skull.** A group of ligaments including the pterygospinous, stylohyoid, stylomandibular, and sphenomandibular ligaments. **Ligaments of the sole, deep transverse [ligamenta metatarsea transversa profunda (NA)].** Strong fibrous bands connecting the contiguous borders of the plantar ligaments of all the metatarsophalangeal joints. **Ligaments of the sole, superficial transverse [fasciculi transversi (NA)].** Transverse bands linking the five main subdivisions of the plantar aponeuroses, at the base of the toes. **Sphenomandibular ligament [ligamentum sphenomandibulare (NA)].** A fibrous band which extends between the spine of the sphenoid bone and the lingula of the mandible. It is a remnant of Meckel's cartilage. **Spinoglenoid ligament [ligamentum transversum scapulae inferius].** A weak bundle of fibres which bridges the suprascapular notch. **Spiral ligament of the cochlea [ligamentum spirale cochleae (NA)].** A thickening of the periosteum of the outer wall of the duct of the cochlea to which the basilar membrane is attached. **Spring ligament.** Calcaneonavicular ligament, plantar (see above). **Stapedial ligament.** The annular ligament of the base of the stapes (see above). **Sternoclavicular ligaments.** Bands, anterior [ligamentum sternoclaviculare anterius (NA)], and posterior [ligamentum sternoclaviculare posterius (NA)], which connect the medial end of the clavicle to the sternum. **Sternocostal ligaments [ligamenta sternocostalia radiata (NA)].** Broad bands radiating from the sternal ends of the cartilages of the true ribs to the sternum. **Sternopericardial ligaments [ligamenta sternopericardiaca (NA)].** Two fibrous bands, superior and inferior, which connect the pericardium to the back of the sternum. **Stylohyoid ligament [ligamentum stylohyoideum (NA)].** A fibrous band which passes from the tip of the styloid process of the temporal bone to the lesser horn of the hyoid bone. It is a remnant of the cartilage of the hyoid arch. **Stylomandibular ligament [ligamentum stylomandibulare (NA)].** A condensation of the deep cervical fascia attached above to the styloid process and below to the lower part of the posterior border of the ramus of the mandible. **Subpubic ligament.** The inferior, or arcuate, pubic ligament (*see* PUBIC LIGAMENTS above). **Suprascapular ligament of the shoulder girdle [ligamentum transversum scapulae superius (NA)].** The ligament from the base of the coracoid process to the medial end of the suprascapular notch, which it converts into a foramen. **Supraspinous ligaments [ligamenta supraspinalia (NA)].** A series of fibrous bands connecting the tips of the spinous processes of the vertebrae. In the cervical region they help to form the ligamentum nuchae. **Suspensory ligament of the axilla.** An extension of the clavipectoral fascia below the lower border of the pectoralis minor muscle to join the fascial floor of the axilla. **Suspensory ligaments of the breast [ligamenta suspensoria mammae (NA)].** Bands of fibrous tissue that anchor the breast to the overlying skin and to the underlying fascia on the pectoralis major muscle; Cooper's suspensory ligaments. **Suspensory ligament of the clitoris [ligamentum suspensorium clitoridis (NA)].** A fibrous band which passes from the pubic symphysis to the body of the clitoris. **Suspensory ligament of the dens.** The apical ligament of the odontoid process (see above). **Suspensory ligament of the duodenum.** A fibromuscular band which passes from the right crus of the diaphragm to the duodenojejunal flexure. **Suspensory ligament of the eyeball.** A portion of the fascial sheath of the eyeball derived from the sheaths of the lateral, medial, and inferior rectus muscles, which is slung like a hammock beneath the eyeball. **Suspensory ligament of the lens.** The anterior portion of the ciliary zonule of the vitreous body, which blends with the capsule of the crystalline lens of the eye. **Suspensory ligament of the ovary.** Infundibulopelvic ligament (see above). **Suspensory ligament of the penis [ligamentum suspensorium penis (NA)].** A band of fibrous tissue which extends from the front of the pubic symphysis to the fibrous capsule of the penis. **Sutural ligament.** The fibrous tissue joining two bones at a suture. **Talocalcanean ligaments.** Bands, anterior, interosseous [ligamentum talocalcaneum interosseum], lateral [ligamentum talocalcaneum laterale (NA)], medial [ligamentum talocalcaneum mediale (NA)], and posterior, which connect the adjacent surfaces of the talus and the calcaneum. The interosseous ligament is the strongest of them all, and occupies the sinus tarsi between the two bones. **Talofibular ligaments.** 1. Anterior [ligamentum talofibulare anterius (NA)]: a band which passes from the anterior border of the lateral malleolus to the lateral aspect of the neck of the talus. 2. Posterior [ligamentum talofibulare posterius (NA)]: a strong band which passes from the pit on the posteromedial aspect of the lateral malleolus to the posterior process of the talus. **Talonavicular ligament [ligamentum talonaviculare (NA)].** A band which passes from the dorsal aspect of the neck of the talus to the corresponding aspect of the navicular bone. **Talotibial ligaments.** Two subdivisions of the deltoid ligament of the ankle joint, the anterior of which passes to the medial side of the neck of the talus, and the posterior to the medial side of the body of the talus below the posterior part of the medial articular area. **Tarsometatarsal ligaments.** 1. Dorsal and plantar [ligamenta tarsometatarsea dorsalia et plantaria (NA)]: bands connecting the dorsal and plantar aspects respectively of the distal tarsal and metatarsal bones. 2. Interosseous [ligamenta cuneometatarsea interossea (NA)]: two bands, one of which passes from the 1st cuneiform bone to the base of the 2nd metatarsal, and the other from the 3rd cuneiform bone to the base of the 4th metatarsal. **Ligaments of the tarsus, dorsal [ligamenta tarsi dorsalia (NA)].** An inclusive name for the following ligaments on the dorsal aspect of the intertarsal joints: talonavicular, intercuneiform, cuneocuboid, cuboideonavicular, bifurcated, and cuneonavicular. **Ligaments of the tarsus, interosseous [ligamenta tarsi interossea (NA)].** An inclusive term for the interosseous ligaments between contiguous surfaces of the tarsal bones comprising the cuneocuboid, intercuneiform, and talocalcaneal interosseous ligaments. **Ligaments of the tarsus, plantar [ligamenta tarsi plantaria (NA)].** 1. Long [ligamentum plantare longum (NA)]: a strong bundle of fibres attached posteriorly to the plantar surface of the calcaneum, and anteriorly to the cuboid and the bases of the lateral four metatarsal bones. 2. Short [ligamentum calcaneocuboideum plantare (NA)]: a stout bundle extending between the anterior end of the plantar surface of the calcaneum and the plantar surface of the cuboid bone. It lies deep to the long plantar ligament. **Temporomandibular ligament [ligamentum laterale (NA)].** An oblique band which passes downward and backward from the tubercle and inferior border of the zygomatic process, to be attached to the posterior and lateral aspects of the neck of the mandible. **Thyro-epiglottic ligament [ligamentum thyro-epiglotticum (NA)].** A strong band attached proximally to the lower end of the epiglottic cartilage, and distally to the back of the thyroid cartilage below the notch. **Thyrohyoid ligament, lateral [ligamentum thyrohyoideum (NA)].** The thickened posterior margin of the thyrohyoid membrane, connecting the tip of the superior horns of the thyroid cartilage to the posterior ends of the hyoid bone. **Thyrohyoid ligament, median [ligamentum thyreohyoideum medianum (NA)].** The midline thickening of the thyrohyoid membrane, extending between the notch of the thyroid cartilage and the posterior aspect of the upper border of the body of the hyoid bone. **Tibiofibular ligaments.** 1. Interosseous: a strong band which unites the opposed surfaces of the lower ends of the tibia and the fibula. 2. Proximal weak bands, anterior and posterior, uniting the corresponding surfaces of the head of the fibula with the adjoining parts of the tibia. 3. Anterior inferior [ligamentum tibiofibulare anterius (NA)]: an oblique band connecting adjacent margins of the tibia and fibula in front of the interosseous ligaments. 4. Posterior inferior [ligamentum tibiofibulare posterius (NA)]: a similar band to the anterior inferior, situated posteriorly. Its lower and deeper part, the transverse ligament, articulates with the talus. **Tibionavicular ligament.** That portion of the deltoid ligament of the ankle joint which is attached to the dorsal and medial aspects of the navicular bone. **Transverse ligament of the acetabulum [ligamentum transversum acetabuli (NA)].** A fibrous band which spans the acetabular notch. **Transverse ligament of the atlas [ligamentum transversum atlantis (NA)].** A strong transverse band which passes behind the odontoid process of the axis, and is attached on each side to the lateral mass of the atlas. **Transverse humeral ligament.** That portion of the capsule of the shoulder joint, beneath which the long tendon of the biceps brachii muscle emerges to enter the bicipital groove. **Transverse ligament of the knee [ligamentum transversum genus (NA)].** A bundle of fibres which passes between the anterior extremities of the menisci of the knee joint. **Transverse ligament of the pelvis [ligamentum transversum perinei (NA)].** The thickened anterior portion of the perineal membrane. **Transverse scapular ligament.** Suprascapular ligament (see above). **Transverse tibiofibular ligament.** A stout band, articular on its anterior face, which passes between the posteromedial aspect of the lateral malleolus and the inferior border of the posterior surface of the tibia. **Trapezoid ligament [ligamentum trapezoideum (NA)].** The trapezoid part of the coracoclavicular ligament (see above); a flat band attached below to a ridge on the upper surface of the coracoid process of the scapula and above to the trapezoid line of the clavicle. **Triangular ligament.** The fasciae, superior and inferior, of the urogenital diaphragm. **Triangular ligaments of the liver.** 1. Left [ligamentum triangulare sinistrum (NA)]: a triangular fold forming the left extremity of the coronary ligament of the liver. It extends from the upper surface of the left lobe to the diaphragm. 2. Right [ligamentum triangulare dextrum (NA)]: the double fold of peritoneum which forms the right free border of the coronary ligament of the liver. **Ligament of the tubercle of a rib.** Costotransverse ligament, lateral (see above). **Ulnocarpal ligament [ligamentum ulnocarpeum palmare (NA)].** A fibrous band passing downwards and laterally from the styloid process of the ulna and the articular disc to the proximal row of carpal bones. **Umbilical ligaments.** 1. Medial [ligamentum umbilicale mediale (NA)]: the obliterated umbilical artery. 2.

Median [ligamentum umbilicale medianum (NA)]: a fibrous band which extends upwards from the apex of the bladder to the umbilicus; the urachus. **Uterosacral ligaments.** Fibromuscular bands which extend backwards on either side from the uterus to the front of the sacrum. They lie beneath the recto-uterine folds. **Uterovesical ligament.** The fold of peritoneum which is reflected from the anterior surface of the uterus to the upper surface of the bladder. **Vaginal ligament.** The fibrous remnant of the obliterated processus vaginalis: it is found in the inguinal canal. **Vaginal ligaments of the fingers and toes.** Fibrous sheaths which keep the flexor tendons of the fingers and toes closely applied to the volar aspects of the phalanges. They are weakest opposite the interphalangeal joints. **Vertebropelvic ligaments.** An inclusive term for the iliolumbar, sacrotuberous and sacrospinous ligaments (see above). **Vertebropericardial ligament.** A band of fibrous tissue which connects the upper part of the pericardium with the 3rd thoracic vertebra and the disc below it. **Vestibular ligament [ligamentum vestibulare (NA)].** A fibrous band which underlies the ventricular fold of the larynx. It is attached anteriorly to the lamina of the thyroid cartilage, and posteriorly to the anterolateral aspect of the arytenoid cartilage. **Vocal ligament [ligamentum vocale (NA)].** The superior border of the cricovocal membrane which underlies the vocal cord. It is attached anteriorly to the back of the lamina of the thyroid cartilage close to the midline, and posteriorly to the vocal process of the arytenoid cartilage. **Ligament of the wrist, lateral [ligamentum collaterale carpi radiale (NA)].** The ligament running from the tip of the styloid process of the radius to the scaphoid bone, a few fibres being prolonged to the trapezium. **Ligament of the wrist, medial [ligamentum collaterale carpi ulnare (NA)].** A bundle extending between the styloid process of the ulna and the pisiform and triquetral bones. **Y ligament.** The iliofemoral ligament (see above). **Zonular ligament.** The common tendinous ring; a fibrotendinous ring surrounding the optic foramen which gives origin to the rectus muscles of the orbit. [L *ligare* to bind.]

See also: ARANZIO (ARANTIUS), BARDINET, BARKOW, BELLINI, BÉRAUD, BERRY (J.), BERTIN, BICHAT, BIGELOW, BOTALLO, BOURGERY, BRODIE (C. G.), BURNS (A.), CALDANI, CAMPBELL (W. F.), CARCASSONE, CASSERIO, CIVININI, CLADO, CLELAND, CLOQUET (J. G.), COLLES, COOPER (A. P.), DENUCÉ, DICKEY (J. S.), DOUGLAS (J.), FLOOD, GERDY, GILLETTE, GIMBERNAT, GUENZ, HELMHOLTZ, HELVETIUS, HENLE, HENSING, HESSELBACH, HEY (W.), HOLL, HUECK, HUMPHRY, HUNTER (W.), JARJAVAY, LANNELONGUE, LAUTH (T.), LISFRANC, LOCKWOOD, LUSCHKA, MACKENRODT, MECKEL, PETIT (A.), POUPART, RETZIUS (A. A.), SEBILEAU, SOEMMERING, STANLEY, STRUTHERS, TEUTLEBEN, TOYNBEE, TREITZ, VALSALVA, WEITBRECHT, WINSLOW, WRISBERG, YOUNG (R. B.), ZAGLAS, ZINN.

ligamentary (lig·am·en·tar·e). Ligamentous.

ligamentopexis, ligamentopexy (lig·am·en·to·**pex**′·is, lig·am·en·to·**pex**′·e). Hysteropexy by fixation or shortening of the round ligament of the uterus. [ligament, Gk *pexis* a fixing.]

ligamentous (lig·am·en·tus). Referring to, or having the characteristics of a ligament.

ligamentum (lig·am·**en**·tum) (pl. *ligamenta*). Ligament. Most ligaments are now referred to by their anglicized names, but a few retain their Latin names in common usage. **Ligamentum arteriosum [NA].** The fibrous remnant of the ductus arteriosus of the fetus. It connects the left pulmonary artery to the under aspect of the arch of the aorta. **Ligamentum denticulatum [NA].** A lateral extension from the spinal pia mater, which connects with the dura mater in the intervals between the spinal nerves by means of its serrated lateral border. It extends from the foramen magnum to the 1st lumbar vertebra. **Ligamenta flava [NA].** A series of yellow elastic ligaments which bind the vertebral laminae together. **Ligamentum nuchae [NA].** A median, more or less triangular, ligamentous septum at the back of the neck. Its base is attached to the external occipital crest, its apex to the 7th cervical vertebra; its anterior margin is attached to the cervical spinous processes, while its posterior edge almost reaches the surface. **Ligamentum patellae [NA].** The strong flattened tendon of the quadriceps femoris muscle, attached above to the apex and adjacent margins of the patella and below to the lower rough area on the tubercle of the tibia. **Ligamentum teres.** Round ligament. *See* LIGAMENT. **Ligamentum transversale colli.** Cardinal ligament; Mackenrodt's ligament. **Ligamentum venosum [NA].** The fibrous remnant of the ductus venosus of the fetus. It occupies the deep fissure between the caudate and left lobes of the liver and connects the left branch of the portal vein with the inferior vena cava. [L.]

ligand (li·gand). In chemistry, a molecule which is bonded, usually to transition-metal elements, by means of electron-donor bonds. The term is applied to a molecule which is bound specifically to one site on a protein or nucleic acid. [L *ligare* to bind.]

ligase (lig·ase). **DNA ligase, polynucleotide ligase.** A class of enzymes that can join the ends of two DNA chains, or join the two ends of a single DNA chain to form a circular molecule. [L *ligare* to bind, *-ase* enzyme.]

ligate (li·gate). To tie with a ligature, e.g. a blood vessel or the pedicle of a tumour. [L *ligare* to bind.]

ligation (li·ga·shun). The tying of a knot or ligature round a blood vessel or other hollow structure or round a pedicle. **Distal ligation.** Ligation of a vessel on the distal side of a lesion, e.g. of an artery on the side of an aneurysm farther from the heart to reduce the blood-flow through the aneurysm. **Immediate ligation.** Ligation of an artery without the inclusion in the ligature of any adjacent tissue. **Mediate ligation.** Ligation of an artery together with adjacent tissue. **Pole ligation.** Ligation of the two superior thyroid arteries at the upper pole of the lateral lobe of the thyroid gland on each side, as a stage of thyroidectomy. **Proximal ligation.** Ligation of a vessel on the proximal side of a lesion, e.g. of an artery on the side of an aneurysm nearer to the heart to slow the circulation of blood in it, and induce clotting. **Saphenous ligation.** Ligation of the long saphenous vein in the treatment of varicose veins. **Terminal ligation.** The ligation of the divided end of the artery. **Triple ligation.** Ligation of the common, internal, and external carotid arteries at the carotid bifurcation. [L *ligare* to bind.]

See also: HUNTER (J.).

ligator (lig·a·tor). An instrument used for the passing of a ligature round a vessel. [L *ligare* to bind.]

ligature (lig·at·ewr). 1. Any material tied around a structure with the intention either of occluding its vessels, or of obstructing its lumen, e.g. in obliterating the neck of a hernial sac. 2. To apply such a ligature. 3. In dentistry, a piece of silk or wire used to fasten a tooth to an orthodontic appliance or to an adjacent tooth. **Absorbable ligature.** Soluble ligature (see below). **Chain ligature.** A method of tying off a pedicle by a chain of ligatures. **Ligature in continuity.** The occlusion of the lumen of a vessel completely by ligature but without its division, e.g. of the external carotid artery to diminish bleeding in mouth operations. **Distal ligature.** Treatment of peripheral aneurysm by ligation of the artery on the distal side of the sac, especially where it is inaccessible, e.g. innominate aneurysm. **Double ligature.** Two ligatures applied as a safety measure to secure the cut end of large and inaccessible vessels, e.g. left gastric and superior thyroid arteries. **Immediate ligature.** The prompt control of bleeding by the ligation forthwith of the main vessel. **Interlacing ligature, interlocking ligature.** A safe method of tying a large vessel by two interlocking ligatures. **Intermittent ligature.** Any method of occluding a vessel so that its flow can be released from time to time during the course of an operation. **Lateral ligature.** A ligature applied to the side of a vessel, commonly a large vein, to close a tear in its wall, but without occlusion of the lumen. **Non-absorbable ligature.** A ligature that is not absorbed, e.g. silk. **Occluding ligature.** A ligature which arrests completely the flow of blood along a vessel. **Provisional ligature.** A ligature applied for an initial trial period, e.g. on the common carotid artery: at any hint of hemiparesis it is removed forthwith. **Proximal ligature.** Treatment of peripheral aneurysm by ligation of the artery on the proximal side of the aneurysm, either close to the sac (Anel) or at a distance from it (Hunter). **Soluble ligature.** A ligature of absorbable material, e.g. catgut. **Suboccluding ligature.** A ligature which does not completely occlude a vessel but reduces the lumen to some degree. **Terminal ligature.** A ligature applied to the cut end of a vessel. [L *ligare* to bind.]

See also: STANNIUS.

light (lite). Electromagnetic radiation of wavelength 4 000–8 000 Å (400–800 nm), giving the sensation of vision. **Actinic light.** Light having a strong chemical and biological action, having a high ultraviolet content. **Light adaptation.** The various alterations which take place in the eye when changing from a low to a high intensity of light. **Axial light.** A beam of light converging on the axis of an optical instrument, e.g. the light from the condenser of a microscope in correct adjustment. **Light chaos.** Also called *entopic phenomena, luminous dust,* and *intrinsic light of the retina*: the sensation of light in the form of spots, lines, etc., that takes place in complete darkness when all after-images have faded. **Light coagulation.** *See* COAGULATION. **Light difference.** The smallest alteration of the intensity of light that can be appreciated by the eye. **Diffused light.** That in which the source of light cannot be seen, the apparent area of the source being increased, for example, by diffusion of light through ground glass. **Infrared light.** Infrared radiation; invisible radiation beyond the red end of the spectrum, which exhibits a heating effect. **Intrinsic light of the retina.** Light chaos (see above). **Light minimum.** The lowest intensity of light that can be appreciated by the eye. **Monochromatic light.** Light of one wavelength. **Neon light.** 1. Light having a characteristic orange-red colour, emitted from a discharge tube containing neon. 2. A small discharge tube containing neon. **Polarized light.** Plane-polarized light; light in which the vibration direction is confined to one plane. It may be produced by reflection, or by the passage of light through a sheet of polarizing material, such as "Polaroid". The eye cannot distinguish between normal and polarized light. **Light projection.** A rough test for the normality of the fundus of the eye when this is obscured, as in cataract. It consists of the correct placing of a source of light in different positions. **Reflected light.** Light which has been reflected from a surface. **Refracted light.** Light which has been refracted by passage across an interface of two media in which the velocity of light is different. **Refrigerated light.** Finsen light. **Transmitted light.** Light which has passed through a transparent medium, generally solid. **Ultraviolet light.** Invisible radiation of wavelength between approximately 2 000 and 3 200 Å (200–320 nm) which is responsible for biological reactions such as sunburn, and destruction of bacteria. [AS *leoht.*]

See also: FINSEN (N. R.), LANDEKER, MININ, SIMPSON (W. S.), TYNDALL, WOOD (R. W.).

lightening (li·ten·ing). A popular term used to describe the sensation of diminished distension of the abdomen caused by the lowering of the uterus into the pelvic cavity during the last three weeks of pregnancy. [see prec.]

Lightwood, Reginald (b. 1898). British paediatrician.

Lightwood's syndrome. Hyperchloraemic renal acidosis in the first year of life, later with nephrocalcinosis and sometimes rickets.

ligneous (lig·ne·us). Conveying the impression of a woody texture; applied to certain lesions of the body, especially those of inflammatory origin. [L *lignum* wood.]

Lignières, Joseph Léon Marcel (b. 1868). French physician in Buenos Aires.

Lignières' test. A cutaneous reaction in which the skin is shaved and a drop of raw tuberculin rubbed in. In tuberculosis cases papules arise in a few hours with pink or deep-red colouring.

lignin (lig·nin). A characteristic constituent of wood, resembling cellulose. [L *lignum* wood.]

lignite (lig·nite). A form of soft peat-like coal found in Germany and the USA [see prec.]

Lignocaine (lig·no·kane). BP Commission approved name for diethylaminoacet-2,6-xylidine. A compound which, in weak solutions (under 1 per cent), is a more powerful local anaesthetic than procaine, with the same degree of toxicity. **Lignocaine Hydrochloride BP 1973.** A compound which has an action similar to that of the base.

lignosulphite (lig·no·sul·fite). A by-product which occurs in the sulphite process of wood pulping: used in tanning, as a fumigant, and medically as an inhalant. [L *lignum* wood, sulphite.]

lignum vitae (lig·num vi·te). Guaiaci lignum. [L, tree of life.]

ligula, ligule (lig·ew·lah, lig·ewl). A thin strip of white matter at the lateral extremity of the floor of the 4th ventricle which passes upwards from the gracile tubercle to the inferior cerebellar peduncle. [L *ligula* strap.]

Ligusticum (li·gus·tik·um). A genus of herbs (family Umbelliferae), widely distributed. *Ligusticum scoticum* Linn., the Scotch lovage, is used as a pot herb, and the aromatic seeds have been employed medicinally as a carminative and stimulant. [L *Ligusticus* from Liguria.]

Lilienthal, Howard (b. 1861). New York surgeon.

Lilienthal's parotid incision. A curved incision whose upper part, convex forwards, extends downwards from the zygoma in front of the ear, and whose lower part, convex backwards, extends round the angle of the mandible.

limatura (li·mat·ewr·ah). Filings. **Limatura ferri.** Iron filings. [L.]

limb (lim). 1. [Membrum (NA)] A leg [membrum inferius (NA)] or arm [membrum superius (NA)]. 2. Any structure which has fundamental resemblance to a leg or arm. **Anacrotic limb.** The part of a sphymographic tracing representing the upstroke. **Artificial limb.** A prosthesis replacing a limb lost in war, by accident, or as a result of an operation. **Limb of the internal capsule, anterior [crus anterius capsulae internae (NA)].** The anterior part of the internal capsule, between the lentiform nucleus and the head of the caudate nucleus. **Limb of the internal capsule, posterior [crus posterius capsulae internae (NA)].** The fibres lateral to the thalamus. The anterior (lentiform) part is medial to, and the posterior part is posterior to, the lentiform nucleus. **Limb of a microscope.** The shaped metal carrying the tube in which is mounted the optical system, and supported on a swivel at the top of the pillar. It is by means of this that the instrument is usually handled. **Pectoral limb.** An arm. **Pelvic limb.** A leg. **Phantom limb.** A feeling that an amputated arm or leg is still present; painful, paraesthetic, or other sensations may be experienced in it. **Limb of the stapes, anterior [crus anterius (NA)].** The shorter and less curved of the two limbs connecting the neck to the base. **Limb of the stapes, posterior [crus posterius (NA)].** The longer and more curved of the two limbs connecting the neck to the base. **Thoracic limb.** An arm. [AS *lim.*]

Limberg operation. For cleft palate: the soft palate and mucoperiosteum of the hard palate is displaced backwards.

limbic (lim·bik). 1. Marginal. 2. Existing at the junction of the cornea and conjunctiva. **Limbic system.** *See* SYSTEM. [limbus.]

limbous (lim·bus). Overlapping. [limbus.]

limbus [NA] (lim·bus). An edge, or border. **Corneal limbus [limbus corneae (NA)].** The edge of the cornea adjoining the sclera. **Limbus laminae spiralis [limbus laminae spiralis osseae (NA)].** The thickened modified periosteum on the upper surface of the osseous spiral lamina, from the outer edge of which the vestibular and tympanic lips project. **Limbus sphenoidalis.** The anterior edge of the optic (chiasmatic) groove on the upper surface of the body of the sphenoid bone. **Limbus thorn.** A term used to describe the labrum acetabulare as it appears in an arthrogram of the hip. [L.]

lime (lime). 1. Quicklime, calcium oxide, CaO. A white powder prepared by the calcination of limestone, which readily absorbs carbon dioxide and water. It is used in the preparation of caustic pastes. 2. The fruit of *Citrus acida,* rich in vitamin C and employed as an antiscorbutic. **Chlorinated Lime BP 1968.** A product obtained by the action of chlorine on slaked lime. It is a dull white powder containing not less than 30 per cent of available chlorine, and partly soluble in water or alcohol. It is used as a deodorant and disinfectant, its action being dependent upon the liberation of chlorine in the presence of water and organic matter. Solutions obtained by shaking with water and filtering were formerly used for wound disinfection, but have now been replaced by substances which give less alkaline solutions and hence cause less irritation It is also a powerful bleaching agent. **Slaked lime.** Calcium hydroxide, a white powder obtained by the action of water on quicklime. It is slightly soluble in water (1 in 900) to give an alkaline solution which readily absorbs carbon dioxide from the atmosphere, forming a white precipitate of calcium carbonate. It is more soluble in glycerin and sugar solutions, and is used as a mild antacid in the treatment of diarrhoea and sickness in infants. It is also used as a constituent of various ointments and lotions for application externally to the skin. **Soda Lime BP 1973.** Slaked lime which has been treated with sodium or potassium hydroxide and dried; it is usually obtained in the form of hard granules and is used for the absorption of carbon dioxide, e.g. in closed-circuit anaesthetic apparatus. **Sulphurated lime.** Calx sulphurata, a mixture of calcium sulphide (CaS) and calcium sulphate ($CaSO_4$) obtained by igniting the latter with charcoal. It is administered internally, usually in the form of tablets, pills, or capsules, in the treatment of boils and carbuncles; its value is, however, doubtful. **Lime water.** Calcium hydroxide solution, a solution of slaked lime (see above) in water; used as an antacid. [AS *lim.*]

limen [NA] (li·men). A threshold. **Limen insulae [NA].** The cortex which forms a threshold to the insula and over which the middle cerebral artery passes to reach the surface of the insula. **Limen nasi [NA].** A curved ridge bounding the vestibule of the nose. The stratified squamous epithelium of the latter changes to ciliated columnar epithelium at the limen. **Limen of twoness.** The threshold distance apart at which simultaneous stimulation with two points can be discriminated at any one area of the skin. [L.]

limes (li·meez). Limit. **Limes death.** Limes tod (see below). **Limes of flocculation.** The amount of toxin (or toxoid) that, when mixed with one unit of a chosen antitoxin, flocculates more rapidly under the same conditions than all other mixtures containing other amounts of the same toxin (or toxoid) per unit of the same antitoxin. The *in vitro* equivalent of antitoxin is the equivalent of one limes of flocculation dose of toxin tested by the flocculation method. It is symbolized L_f. **Limes nul.** Ehrlich's name for the largest amount of toxin that, when mixed with one unit of antitoxin and injected subcutaneously into a 250 g guinea-pig, will give rise to no observed reaction. It is symbolized L_0. **Limes of reaction.** The least amount of toxin that, when mixed with one unit of antitoxin, forms a mixture of which 0.2 ml will cause a minimal skin reaction when injected subcutaneously into a guinea-pig. It is symbolized L_r. **Limes tod.** Ehrlich's name for the smallest amount of toxin that, when mixed with one unit of antitoxin and injected subcutaneously into a 250 g guinea-pig, will kill the animal within 96 h. It is symbolized L_+. [L, limit.]

limic (lim·ik). Relating to hunger. [Gk *limos* hunger.]

liminal (lim·in·al). A term used in physiology; it concerns the stimuli which are only just perceptible to the senses. [L *limen* threshold.]

limit (lim·it). A boundary or fixed point. **Limit of audibility.** The upper and lower limits of sound frequencies heard by the human ear, the lower being in the region of 16 Hz, and the upper in the region of 18 000 Hz. **Limit of perception.** The smallest object that can be differentiated by the eye. Normally this object must subtend a visual angle of one minute to produce a retinal image just larger than the diameter of a cone (0.004 mm) for differentiation to take place; more correctly *normal limit of visual acuity.* **Quantum limit.** The minimum wavelength existing in the continuous spectrum of an X-ray tube, which may be shown by Planck's hypothesis to be inversely proportional to the maximum potential across the tube. [L *limes* limit.]

limitans (lim·it·anz). The membrana limitans of the retina. [L, limiting.]

limitation (lim·it·a·shun). The condition of being limited or restricted. **Eccentric limitation.** Loss of the visual field varying in degree over the periphery. [see prec.]

limitrophic (lim·e·trof·ik). Concerned with the regulation of nutrition; describing the sympathetic nervous system, its nerves or its ganglia. [limit, Gk *trophe* nourishment.]

limnaemia (lim·ne·me·ah). Malarial cachexia. [Gk *limne* marsh, *haima* blood.]

limnaemic (lim·ne·mik). Pertaining to malarial cachexia. [see prec.]

Limnatis (lim·na·tis). A genus of leeches. *Limnatis nilotica* is the horse leech of the Mediterranean and Middle East. The young often enter the mouth with drinking water and attach themselves in the pharynx, where they feed. [Gk *limne* marsh.]

limoctonia (lim·ok·to·ne·ah). Death or suicide the result of starvation. [Gk *limos* hunger, *kteinein* to kill.]

limonene (lim·on·een). A naturally occurring monocyclic terpene of wide distribution. The dextrorotatory form, carvene, a colourless liquid with an odour of lemons, is the main constituent of the essential oils of orange, lemon rind, lavender, bergamot, and caraway. L-Limonene is found with L-pinene in pine needles and fir cones, and in the oils of peppermint and spearmint. There is also a racemic form known as *dipentene*, which occurs naturally in turpentine, citronella oil and oil of cubebs; it may be synthesized from isoprene. [L *limo* lemon.]

limonin (lim·on·in). A glucoside found in citrus fruits. [see prec.]

limophoitos, limophoitosis (lim·o·fo·it·os, lim·o·fo·it·o'·sis). Insanity caused by starvation. [Gk *limos* hunger, *phoitos* madness.]

limophthisis (lim·of·this·is). Emaciation caused by starvation. [Gk *limos* hunger, *phthisis* a wasting.]

limopsora (lim·op·so·rah). A type of skin irritation, resembling pruritus or scabies, with which human beings and animals are believed to be affected after long-continued starvation. [Gk *limos* hunger, *psora* a cutaneous disease.]

limosis (lim·o·sis). 1. Abnormal hunger. 2. A disease characterized by perverted or unusually great appetite. [Gk *limos* hunger.]

limosphere (li·mo·sfeer). An ovoid body adjacent to the nucleus in certain of the developing male germ cells. [L *limus* sidelong, Gk *sphaira* sphere.]

limotherapy (lim·o·ther·ap·e). The treatment of disease by absolute fasting or by limitation of the quantity of food; hunger therapy. [Gk *limos* hunger, therapy.]

limp, limping (limp, limp·ing). Claudication; walking lamely. **Antalgic limp.** A limp due to pain. **Gluteal limp.** Dipping gait due to weakness of the gluteus medius and minimus muscles. **Intermittent limping.** Intermittent claudication. *See* CLAUDICATION. [ME.]

linalool (lin·al·o·ol). Coriandrol, $(CH_3)_2C{=}CH(CH_2)_2C(CH_3)(OH)CH{=}CH_2$. An unsaturated terpene alcohol, or mixture of isomers, which is found in oil of linaloe from the wood of the Mexican tree *Ocotea caudata*, and the oils of rose, bergamot, coriander, and orange.

linalyl acetate (lin·al·il as·et·ate). Linalool acetic ester, $CH_3COC_{10}H_{17}$. A volatile oil which occurs in bergamot, and is used in perfumery.

linamarin (lin·am·ar·in). A poisonous glycoside which occurs in flax and the lima bean *Phaseolus lunatus*; it yields hydrocyanic acid, glucose, and acetone, on hydrolysis. [L *linum* flax, *amarus* bitter.]

Lincomycin (lin·ko·mi·sin). BP Commission approved name for $C_{18}H_{34}N_2O_6S$, an antibiotic produced by *Streptomyces lincolnensis* var. *lincolnensis.* **Lincomycin Hydrochloride BP 1973.** The monohydrate of the hydrochloride of methyl 6-8 - dideoxy - 6 - (1 - methyl - 4 - propyl - 2 - pyrrolidine-carboxamide) - 1 - thio - D - erythro - D - galacto-octapyranoside, an antimicrobial substance produced by *Streptomyces lincolnensis* var. *lincolnensis* or by other means.

lincture (lingk·tewr). Linctus.

linctus (lingk·tus). A syrupy liquid medicament, usually having sucrose as a basis, used in the treatment of irritating throaty coughs. It should not be diluted with water and is intended to be swallowed in sips. [L *lingere* to lick.]

Lindau, Arvid (b. 1892). Lund pathologist.

Lindau's disease, or syndrome, von Hippel-Lindau disease. A disease considered by von Hippel and numerous other observers to be a form of angiomatosis limited to the retina. Lindau in 1926, however, pointed out its association with cysts and angiomata elsewhere, especially in the cerebellum, medulla, cord, pancreas, liver, kidney, suprarenals, and reproductive glands.

Lindbergh, Charles Augustus (b. 1902). New York technician and former aviator.

Lindbergh pump, Carrel-Lindbergh perfusion apparatus. An apparatus for keeping alive intact organs, such as the thyroid gland or kidney after removal from the body.

Lindemann, Edward E. (b. 1883). New York surgeon.

Lindemann's method. A direct method of whole-blood transfusion using a two-way syringe.

Lindemann, Frederick Alexander, Lord Cherwell (b. 1886). British physicist.

Lindemann electrometer. An electrometer in which the electric potential is measured in terms of the angle of twist produced in a quartz fibre by the electrostatic forces acting between a quartz rod attached to the fibre and fixed metallic plates. The rod is in electrical communication with the unknown potential via the metallized quartz fibre, while the fixed plates are maintained at definite potentials.

Lindemann apparatus. An apparatus for the rapid determination of oxygen in the air.

Linder's sign. In sciatica, if the patient sits with outstretched legs, passive flexion of the neck may cause pain in the lumbar region or in sciatic distribution.

Lindner, Karl David (b. 1883). Vienna ophthalmologist.

Lindner's initial body. The early stage of development of a trachoma body; it resembles a coccus and is located in the periphery of the conjunctival epithelial cell.

line (line). 1. The connection between two points. 2. [Linea (NA)] A ridge or mark. **Absorption line.** A black line in the continuous spectrum of light passing through an absorbing medium, caused by the absorption of light of that particular wavelength in the medium. **Accretion line.** One of the many microscopic lines seen in a ground section of the enamel of a tooth marking the successional layers of calcification; brown stria of Retzius. **Adrenal line.** A white line which appears if the skin, e.g. of the abdomen, is lightly stroked with the finger nail. It appears after a short latent period, and after a minute or two it gradually fades. **Alveonasal line.** A line joining the prosthion and the nasion. **Anocutaneous line.** A bluish-white stripe seen in the mucosa of the anal canal, representing the boundary between the ectodermal and entodermal components of the embryonic canal. It lies a little way below the anal valves, and is an important lymphatic, blood vascular, and nervous watershed. Also known as *Hilton's white line.* **Anthropological base line.** Frankfurt horizontal line (see below). **Arcuate line (of Vogt).** A small white crescentic line seen at the posterior pole of the lens of the eye, thought to represent the reflection of Cloquet's canal. **Arcuate line of the ilium [linea arcuata (NA)].** The curved line close to the lower and posterior border of the ilium which in the complete hip bone is the backward continuation of the pubic pecten. It lies at the junction of the true and false pelves. **Arcuate line of the pelvis [linea terminalis (NA)].** A curved line passing laterally and then forward from the promontory of the sacrum to the crest of the pubis. It forms the boundary between the true and false pelves. Its pubic part is formed by the pectineal line and the pubic crest, its iliac part separates the iliac fossa from the true pelvis, and its sacral part is formed by the lower or anterior margin of the ala of the sacrum. **Arcuate line of the rectus abdominis muscle [linea arcuata (NA)].** The curved lower end of the posterior wall of the sheath of the rectus abdominis muscle, situated midway between the umbilicus and the pubic symphysis. **Axillary line [linea axillaris (NA)].** The vertical line on the body wall passing through the point midway between the anterior and posterior folds of the axilla. **B lines.** Short, transverse lines in the lungs about 1-2 cm long, touching the pleura and more prominent at the bases. They are composed of interlobular septa filled with lymphatic oedema—a form of chronic interstitial oedema. It is best seen in mitral stenosis but also in pneumoconiosis, carcinomatosis, and any form of heart failure giving rise to oedema. **Basinasal line.** The line from the basion to the nasion. **Bi-auricular line.** A line drawn across the vertex of the skull which joins the two external auditory meatuses. **Blue line.** A bluish discoloration of the gingival margin—only seen when gingivitis is present—in cases of chronic lead (and occasionally bismuth) poisoning; the pigment is the sulphide of the metal being excreted in the saliva. **Calcification line.** Accretion line (see above). **Canthomeatal line.** Orbitomeatal line (see below). Syn. Reid's base line. **Central pupillary line.** A straight line passing through the centre of the pupil and perpendicular to the cornea. **Cervical line.** The undulating line formed at the neck of a tooth by the junction of the enamel and cementum. **Cleavage lines.** The lines along which the skin will most readily split, because of the arrangement of the subcutaneous collagen fibres. **Lines of communication.** A term used in warfare for describing the means of communicating that a military headquarters maintains between the scene of active operations and the base, and by which intelligence, supplies, etc., are transmitted, and sick and wounded conveyed from the front line to the base. **Contour line.** One of the microscopic markings in dentine produced by the superimposition of interglobular spaces. **Copper line.** The green line at the base of the teeth due to copper. **Deadly mesenteric line.** The small triangular space at the mesenteric border of the intestine which is uncovered by peritoneum. **Line of demarcation.** The boundary between gangrenous and healthy tissue in gangrene of a limb, or a line indicating a change in condition of the tissues. **Ectental line.** The junction between the entoderm and the ectoderm. **Embryonic line.** The primitive streak. *See* STREAK. **Epiphyseal line [linea epiphysialis (NA)].** The cartilaginous plate between the epiphysis and the diaphysis of a long bone. **Facial line.** A line touching tangentially the glabella and passing downwards to the lower border of the face; a line that is said to indicate abdominal disease in a child. **Fixation line.** A straight line passing through the centre of rotation of the eyeball and the object of vision; also called *fixation axis.* **Focal line.** The line to which the rays of light passing through a cylindrical lens will be brought to a focus. **Frankfurt horizontal line.** A base line of the skull made by joining the infra-orbital point to the superior border of the external auditory meatus. **Genal line.** A line passing from the nasal line near the mouth towards the zygomatic bone. **Gingival line.** The line formed by the gingival margin at the neck of a tooth. **Gluteal line, inferior [linea glutea inferior (NA)].** A curved line on the gluteal surface of the iliac bone just above the acetabulum and marking the lower limit of attachment of the gluteus minimus muscle. **Gluteal line, middle [linea glutea anterior (NA)].** A curved line on the gluteal surface of the ilium running from the greater sciatic notch to a point about 5 cm along the iliac crest from the anterior superior iliac spine. It marks the lower and anterior attachment of the gluteus medius muscle. **Gluteal line, posterior [linea glutea posterior (NA)].** A short curved line on the gluteal surface of the ilium commencing at the greater sciatic notch and extending to the iliac crest about 5 cm in front of the posterior superior iliac spine. It marks the anterior limit of attachment of the gluteus maximus muscle. **Gum line.** Gingival line (see above). **Imbrication line.** One of the lines on the enamel surface of a tooth which indicates the periodicity of deposition of the tissue. **Incremental line.** One of the lines seen in a microscopic section of enamel (brown striae of Retzius) and cementum (incremental lines of Salter) indicating the periodic deposition of these tissues. **Intercondylar line [linea intercondylaris (NA)].**

The border separating the popliteal and intercondylar areas on the femur. It is the posterior limit of the intercondylar notch, and the site of attachment of the posterior part of the articular capsule of the knee joint. **Intertrochanteric line.** Trochanteric line (see below). **Iso-electric line, isopotential line.** The base line of the electrocardiogram at a period of the cardiac cycle when neither positive nor negative potentials are recorded, and the galvanometer string is still. Also known as *iso-electric level.* **Isothermal line.** Isotherm; a line placed on a meteorological map of a country, or continent, or of the earth, connecting places which have the same mean annual temperature. **K, L, M, N, O, P lines.** Spectral lines emitted in the x-ray spectra of the elements, having wavelengths characteristic of the element and not of the exciting potential. **Labial line.** A line which passes outwards from the angle of the mouth and is said to indicate disease of the lung. **Lateral sinus line.** A surface marking which outlines an approach to the lateral sinus; it is a line dividing the angle formed by the anterior border of the mastoid process and the temporal line. **Lead line.** Blue line (see above). **Lower lung line.** In radiology, a line representing the lower posterior pleural boundary; not in use in the UK. **M line.** M disc, the dark transverse line seen in stained preparations of striated muscle at the centre of the H band. It is situated at the midpoint of the myosin filaments of the sarcomere. **Magnetic line of force.** A line showing the direction of the magnetic field at a point. Its direction at a point is that of the force exerted on a north pole placed at that point. The line of force may also be used quantitatively, the number of lines of force crossing unit area at right angles to the direction of a magnetic field being numerically equal to the strength of the field at that point. **Mamillary line [linea mamillaris (linea medioclavicularis) NA].** The vertical line passing through the nipple. **Mammary line.** A horizontal line through the nipples. **Median line, anterior [linea mediana anterior (NA)].** The line along which the median plane meets the anterior surface of the body. **Median line, posterior [linea mediana posterior (NA)].** The line along which the median plane meets the posterior surface of the body. **Milk line.** One of two ridges on either side of the ventral aspect of the trunk of an embryo from which the mammary glands are developed. **Mylohyoid line [linea mylohyoidea (NA)].** An oblique ridge on the inner surface of the mandible from the region of the last molar tooth to the base of the symphysis menti. **Nasal line.** A line running from the ala of the nose in a semicircle around the mouth. **Nasobasilar line.** A line joining the basion and the nasion. **Nasosubnasal line.** A line joining the subnasal point and the nasion. **Neonatal line.** A microscopic line in enamel and dentine marking the junction between those parts of the tissues formed prenatally and postnatally. **Nuchal line, highest [linea nuchae suprema (NA)].** The higher of the two curved lines running laterally from the external occipital protuberance. **Nuchal line, inferior [linea nuchae inferior (NA)].** A line running laterally on the occipital bone midway between the external occipital protuberance and the back of the foramen magnum. **Nuchal line, superior [linea nuchae superior (NA)].** The lower of the two curved lines running laterally from the external occipital protuberance. **Oblique line of the body of the mandible.** *See* MANDIBLE. **Oblique line of the thyroid cartilage [linea obliqua (NA)].** A line running downwards and forwards on the outer surface of each thyroid lamina. It gives attachment to the sternothyroid, thyrohyoid, and inferior constrictor muscles. **Oblique orbital line.** A radiological landmark seen in the postero-anterior skull radiograph, indicating the boundary of the middle cranial fossa. **Line of occlusion.** The line formed by teeth which are in normal occlusion. **Ocular line, oculozygomatic line.** A line from the inner canthus of the eye outwards towards the zygoma and supposed to indicate nervous disease. **Omphalospinous line.** A line from the umbilicus to the anterior superior iliac spine. McBurney's point lies on this line. **Orbitomeatal line.** A radiographic base line made by joining the outer cathus of the eye to the central point of the external auditory meatus. **Pectinate line.** The line of the anal valves; it indicates the site of junction of the proctodaeum and hind-gut of the fetus. **Pectineal line [pecten ossis pubis (NA)].** A sharp ridge forming the upper and posterior border of the superior pubic ramus. It gives attachment to the conjoint tendon and part of the inguinal ligament. **Primitive line.** The primitive streak. *See* STREAK. **Pure line.** A series of generations of an organism which are theoretically homozygous for all characters. Although such a state cannot perhaps be achieved, pure-line stocks are very valuable when uniformity of response to experimental procedure is required. **Red line.** A stage of the skin reaction to irritants, described by Lewis; primary dilatation of the capillaries. **Regression line.** A term applied in forensic dentistry to the limit of extension of translucency in the root, as an indication of age. **Respiratory line.** A line uniting the bases of the upstrokes on a sphygmographic curve. **Scapular line [linea scapularis (NA)].** The vertical line passing through the inferior angle of the scapula. **Line of sight.** A straight line passing through the object of vision and the centre of the pupil. **Soleal line [linea musculi solei (NA)].** An obliquely placed rough ridge crossing the upper part of the posterior surface of the tibia and giving part origin to the soleus muscle. **Spino-umbilical line.** A line joining the anterior superior iliac spine to the umbilicus. **Spiral line [linea pectinea (NA)].** A low roughened ridge from the upper end of the linea aspera on the femur to the lower end of the anterior trochanteric line; it forms the line of insertion of the pectineus muscle. **Supracondylar lines.** Rough ridges forming the inner and outer boundaries of the popliteal surface of the femur. They are continuous above with the lips of the linea aspera. **Temporal line, inferior [linea temporalis inferior (NA)].** The lower of two curved lines on the external surface of the parietal bone at the upper limit of the temporal muscle. **Temporal line, superior [linea temporalis superior (NA)].** The upper of two curved lines on the external surface of the parietal bone which gives attachment to the temporal fascia. **Temporal lines of the frontal bone [lineae temporales (NA)].** Continuations of the temporal lines from the parietal bone. They join anteriorly to form a single line terminating at the zygomatic process. **Temporary atropic line.** A line normal to the secondary axis plane of the eye. **Trapezoid line [linea trapezoidea (NA)].** A ridge on the inferior surface of the clavicle, near its acromial end, to which is attached the trapezoid part of the coracoclavicular ligament. **Trochanteric line [linea intertrochanterica (NA)].** A rough ridge anteriorly between the neck and the shaft of the femur. It gives attachment to the capsular and iliofemoral ligaments. **Vertical line.** A vertically placed ridge on the middle part of the shaft of the tibia, giving attachment to the fascia which separates the tibialis posterior and flexor digitorum muscles in the leg. **Visual line.** A line passing through the macula and nodal point of the eye, thence to the object of vision, also called *visual axis.* **White line.** A white line on the skin due to capillary contraction and produced by light stroking; adrenal line. **Z line.** Z disc; Krause's membrane; the thin dark line which traverses the I band in stained preparations of striated muscle. It is composed of filaments of tropomyosin to which the actin filaments of the muscle are attached. [L *linea.*]

See also: AMBERG, AMICI, BAILLARGER, BEAU, BORSIERI DE KANILFELD, BRIDGETT, BRÖDEL, BRUECKE, BRYANT, BURTON, CAMPER, CHAUSSIER, CHIENE, CLAPTON, CONRADI (A. C.), CORRIGAN, CRAMPTON (P.), CZERMAK (J. N.), DAMOISEAU, DAUBENTON, DE SALLE, DOBIE, DOUGLAS (J.), DUHOT, EBERTH, ELLIS (C.), FARRE (A.), FRAUNHOFER, FROMMANN, GARLAND, GENNARI, GOTTINGER, GRANGER, GUBLER, HALLER, HARRIS (H. A.), HENSEN, HILTON, HOLDEN, HUDSON, HUNTER (W.), JADELOT, KILIAN, KRAUSE (W. J. F.), LANGER, LANZ, MCKEE, MONRO (II), NÉLATON, OWEN, PASTIA, PICKERILL, POIRIER, POUPART, REID, RETZIUS (M. G.), RICHTER (A. G.), ROLANDO, ROSER, SALTER (S. J. A.), SCHOEMAKER, SCHREGER, SERGENT, SHENTON, SIMON (O.), SKINNER, SPIEGHEL (SPIGELIUS), STAEHLI, THOMPSON (T.), TOPINARD, TRUEMMERFELD, VIRCHOW, VOGT (A.), VOIGT, WALDEYER-HARTZ, WALLACE (A. R.), WRISBERG, ZAHN, ZOELLNER.

linea (lin·e·ah) (pl. *lineae*). A line. **Linea alba [L].** A tendinous raphe formed by the interlacing of the aponeurosis of the flat abdominal muscles and stretching between the xiphoid process and the pubic symphysis. **Lineae albicantes.** White lines on the abdomen, commonly seen during and after pregnancy. They may occur in any condition giving rise to abdominal distension. **Linea aspera [NA].** A roughened ridge at the posterior border of the femur, giving attachment to the adductor muscles, the vastus lateralis and medialis muscles, the short head of the biceps femoris muscle, and the medial and lateral intermuscular septa. It is bounded laterally and medially by distinct lips, the lateral lip [labium laterale (NA)] and medial lip [labium mediale (NA)], to which the corresponding vasti muscles and intermuscular septa are attached. **Lineae atrophicae.** The cutaneous striae or lines of skin atrophy seen particularly on the abdominal wall in cases of Cushing's syndrome. **Linea corneae senilis.** A tenuous brown line running horizontally in the cornea below the midline and not extending to the limbus, found in normal corneae of old people. Also called *Hudson's line* or *Staehli's line.* **Lineae distensae.** Lines, white or red according to the acuteness of the condition, which occur on the skin as a result of stretching due to swelling from adiposity or other causes. **Linea mensalis.** Lines on the palm caused by flexion of the middle, ring, and little fingers. **Linea nigra.** A black line on the abdomen seen in the later months of pregnancy. It extends from the pubes to the region of the umbilicus. **Linea semilunaris [NA].** The curved groove on the anterior abdominal wall marking the lateral edge of the rectus abdominis muscle. **Linea splendens.** A band on the pia mater of the spinal cord. **Linea vitalis.** The line on the palm curving round the base of the thumb. [L.]

lineal (lin·e·al). Linear.

lineament (lin·e·a·ment). 1. The distinguishing characteristics or features of the face. 2. An outline of the embryo. 3. Any of the main bodily outlines or contours. [L *linea* line.]

linear (lin·e·ar). Relating to a line or lines. **Linear accelerator.** *See* ACCELERATOR.

Ling, Per Henrik (b. 1776). Swedish poet and gymnast.

Ling's system. A system of gymnastic exercises performed without employing apparatus.

lingism (ling·izm). The treatment of disease by means of callisthenics or other types of active and passive movement. [P. H. *Ling.*]

lingua (ling·gwah). Tongue. **Lingua dissecta.** Scrotal tongue. *See* TONGUE. **Lingua fraenata.** Tongue-tie. **Lingua geographica.** Geographical tongue. *See* TONGUE. **Lingua nigra.** Black tongue. *See* TONGUE. **Lingua plicata.** Scrotal tongue. *See* TONGUE. **Lingua villosa nigra.** Black tongue. *See* TONGUE. [L.]

lingual (ling·gwal). 1. Belonging to the tongue; glossal. 2. Shaped like the tongue. **Lingual follicles.** *See* FOLLICLE. **Lingual tonsil.** *See* TONSIL. [L *lingua* tongue.]

lingual artery [arteria lingualis (NA)]. A branch of the external carotid artery supplying the tongue; where it runs forward beneath the tongue it is called the profunda artery [arteria profunda linguae (NA)]. Its branches are the small suprahyoid artery [ramus suprahyoideus (NA)] along the upper border of the hyoid bone, two or three dorsales linguae branches [rami dorsales linguae (NA)] to the back of the tongue and the adjoining pharyngeal wall, and a sublingual branch [arteria sublingualis (NA)] to the sublingual gland and the floor of the mouth.

lingual nerve [nervus lingualis (NA)]. A sensory branch from the mandibular nerve to the mucous membrane of the anterior two-thirds of the tongue [rami linguales (NA)] and the floor of the mouth [nervus sublingualis (NA)]. It also carries taste fibres from the facial nerve to the same region of the tongue and mouth, and secretomotor fibres for the salivary glands related to the floor of the mouth. It communicates with the hypoglossal nerve [rami communicantes cum nervo hypoglosso (NA)]. There are also branches to the anterior pillars of the fauces [rami isthmi faucium (NA)].

lingual vein [vena lingualis (NA)]. The main venous drainage of the tongue; a tributary of the common facial vein.

linguale (ling·gwa·le). The point at the upper end of the symphysis menti on its lingual surface.

lingually (ling·gwal·e). In a direction towards the tongue. [L *lingua* tongue.]

Linguatula (ling·gwat·ew·lah). A genus of the arthropod class Pentastomida. The nose worm of the dog, *Linguatula serrata,* occurs as a larva in human mesentery not uncommonly. Human infestation with the adult is very rare. There is a resistant free-living egg. [L *linguatus* tongued.]

linguatuliasis (ling·gwat·ew·li′·as·is). Infestation with a species of the genus *Linguatula.*

Linguatulida (ling·gwat·ew′·lid·ah). A class of worm-like arthropods. *See* PENTASTOMIDA. [see foll.]

Linguatulidae (ling·gwat·ew′·lid·e). A family of the arthropod class Pentastomida. The genus *Linguatula* is of medical interest. [L *linguatus* tongued, Gk *eidos* form.]

linguatulosis (ling·gwat·ew·lo′·sis). Linguatuliasis.

linguiform (ling·gwe·form). Lingulate; shaped like a tongue. [L *lingua* tongue, form.]

linguistics (ling·gwis·tiks). The scientific enterprise of investigating the languages and dialects which are in use, or have been used, by various speech communities throughout the world. **Contrastive linguistics.** The general comparison of features of language-systems. [L *lingua* tongue.]

lingula (ling·gew·lah). Any structure or process resembling a tongue in shape. **Lingula of the cerebellum [lingula cerebelli (NA)].** The tongue-shaped portion of the vermis which overlies the superior medullary velum. **Lingula of the lung [lingula pulmonis sinistri (NA)].** A projection from the costal surface of the upper lobe of the left lung just below the cardiac notch. **Lingula of the mandible [lingula mandibulae (NA)].** A triangular spur of bone overhanging the mandibular foramen, to which the sphenomandibular ligament is attached. **Lingula of the sphenoid bone [lingula sphenoidalis (NA)].** A spur of bone which projects from the medial part of the posterior border of the greater wing of the sphenoid close to the body of the bone. [L, small tongue.]

See also: WRISBERG.

lingular (ling·gew·lar). Relating to a lingula or small tongue-shaped structure.

lingulate (ling·gew·late). Linguiform.

lingulectomy (ling·gew·lek·to·me). Surgical incision of the lingula of the lung. [lingula, Gk *ektome* excision.]

linguoclination (ling·gwo·klin·a′·shun). In dentistry, the deviation of a tooth from its normal vertical position, towards the lingual side. [L *lingua* tongue, inclination.]

linguodental (ling·gwo·den·tal). Referring to the tongue and the teeth. [L *lingua* tongue, *dens* tooth.]

linguodistal (ling·gwo·dis·tal). Appertaining to the lingual and the distal surfaces of a tooth.

linguogingival (ling·gwo·jin·jiv·al). Pertaining to the tongue and the gums. [L *lingua* tongue, *gingiva* gum.]

linguo-occlusion (ling·gwo·ok·loo′·zhun). That form of occlusion when one or more teeth are occluded lingually to their normal position in the arch.

linguopapillitis (ling·gwo·pap·il·i′·tis). A condition in which small painful ulcers form about the papillae at the edges of the tongue. [L *lingua* tongue, papillitis.]

linguoplacement (ling·gwo·plase·ment). Displacement to the lingual side, e.g. a tooth which is lying inside the normal arch. [L *lingua* tongue, displacement.]

linguotrite (ling·gwo·trite). An instrument for grasping the tongue and pulling it forward. [L *lingua* tongue, *terere* to crush.]

linguoversion (ling·gwo·ver·shun). The condition of being rotated or twisted in a lingual direction, e.g. a tooth. [L *lingua* tongue, *vertere* to turn.]

lini semina (li·ni sem·in·ah). Linseed. **Lini semina contusa.** Crushed linseed. [L, seeds of flax.]

liniment (lin·im·ent). A preparation intended for application to the skin, either by friction or upon lint or other surgical dressing. Liniments often contain alcohol, and some medicaments such as camphor to increase their rubefacient action. The inclusion of soaps and oils in such preparations is to facilitate their being rubbed into the surface. **ABC liniment.** Liniment of aconite, belladonna, and chloroform (see below). **Liniment of Aconite BPC 1959.** Aconite root percolated with 90 per cent alcohol, and camphor dissolved in the percolate. **Liniment of Aconite, Belladonna, and Chloroform BPC 1959.** A liniment prepared by mixing chloroform and liniment of belladonna. **Liniment of ammonia.** Linimentum ammoniae. **Liniment of Belladonna BPC 1959.** Belladonna root percolated with 80 per cent alcohol and camphor added. **Liniment of belladonna and chloroform.** Linimentum belladonnae cum chloroformo. **Camphor Liniment BP 1958.** A liniment made by dissolving camphor in arachis oil. **Liniment of Camphor, Ammoniated, BP 1953.** A liniment of camphor and lavender oil in alcohol with strong ammonia added. **Liniment of cantharidin.** Linimentum cantharidini. **Liniment of chloroform.** Linimentum chloroformi. **Liniment of Methyl Salicylate BPC 1959.** A liniment prepared by mixing methyl salicylate (25 per cent) with ether, arachis, cotton seed or rape oil. **Liniment of Methyl Salicylate and Eucalyptus BPC 1954.** A liniment prepared from menthol, eucalyptus oil, rectified camphor oil, and methyl salicylate. **Liniment of mustard.** Linimentum sinapis. **Liniment of opium.** Linimentum opii. **Liniment of potassium iodide with soap.** Linimentum potassii iodidi cum sapone. **Soap Liniment BP 1958.** A solution of soap, camphor, and rosemary oil in alcohol. **Turpentine Liniment BP 1973.** A liniment prepared by triturating camphor and soap with turpentine oil and adding water. **Liniment of Turpentine, Acetic BPC 1954.** A liniment prepared by mixing glacial acetic acid with liniment of camphor and turpentine oil. **White Liniment BPC 1959.** A liniment prepared from oleic acid, dilute ammonia solution, ammonium chloride, turpentine oil, and water. [L *linere* to smear.]

linimentum (lin·im·en·tum). Liniment. **Linimentum aconiti oleosum.** Liniment of aconite, belladonna, and chloroform. **Linimentum album.** White liniment. *See* LINIMENT. **Linimentum Ammoniae BPC 1949.** Liniment of ammonia, a liniment prepared from dilute solution of ammonia, oleic acid, and liquid paraffin. **Linimentum Belladonnae cum Chloroformo BPC 1949.** Liniment of belladonna and chloroform, a liniment prepared by mixing chloroform and liniment of belladonna. **Linimentum Cantharidini BPC 1949.** Liniment of cantharidin, a liniment prepared from acetone, alcohol (90 per cent), and castor oil, containing 0.23 per cent of cantharidin. **Linimentum Chloroformi BPC 1949.** Liniment of chloroform, a liniment prepared by mixing equal parts of chloroform and liniment of camphor. **Linimentum Opii BPC 1949.** Liniment of opium, a liniment prepared by mixing equal parts of tincture of opium and liniment of soap. **Linimentum Potassii Iodidi cum Sapone BPC 1949.** Liniment of potassium iodide with soap, a liniment prepared from potassium iodide (15 per cent) and curd soap, glycerin, lemon oil, and water. **Linimentum Sinapis BPC 1949.** Liniment of mustard, a liniment prepared from volatile oil of mustard (3.5 per cent), camphor, castor oil, and alcohol. [see prec.]

linin (li·nin). 1. An amaroid, $C_{23}H_{22}O_9$, believed to be the active constituent of purging flax, *Linum catharticum.* 2. The substance of the faintly stained threads seen in the nucleus of fixed cells to which the chromatin granules appear to be attached.

linitis (li·ni·tis). Inflammation of the gastric cellular tissue; used only in the term *linitis plastica,* which describes an infiltrating variety of carcinoma of the stomach. [Gk *linon* web, *-itis* inflammation.]

linkage (lingk·ij). 1. In chemistry, the lines employed in structural formulae to denote valency connections between atoms. 2. The association of gene effects such that they pass from parent to offspring without showing independent assortment: this is because their genes lie on the same chromosome. Such effects may be separated only by crossing over within chromosome pairs during meiosis. If the genes are very near to each other on the chromosomes, they are said to be closely linked, and the nearer they are the less their likelihood of being separated. 3. In psychology, the association of a stimulus with its response. **Linkage group.** All the genes present in any one chromosome, which consequently show linkage. **Linkage map.** A topographical representation of the spatial relationships between genetic loci on a linkage group, as derived by recombination analysis. **Peptide linkage.** =CHCONHCH=, the grouping which unites amino acids into peptide chains to form proteins. [ME *linke.*]

linked (lingkt). In heredity, describing characters which are associated in order to be transmitted. [see prec.]

linolein (lin·o·le·in). Linoleic glyceride; a neutral fat contained in linseed oil, which is responsible for the drying properties of the latter. [L *linum* flax, *oleum* oil.]

linoxanthine (lin·o·zan·theen). The yellow colouring matter produced by *Sarcina aurantiaca.* [L *linum* flax, Gk *xanthos* yellow.]

linseed (lin·seed). The seeds of the flax, *Linum usitatissimum* Linn. (family Linaceae), widely cultivated. It contains about 30 to 40 per cent of fixed oil together with mucilage and proteins, and the infusion is used as a demulcent drink (BPC 1954). **Crushed Linseed BPC 1954.** A form employed as a poultice to apply warmth in bronchitis and other conditions. [AS *linsaed.*]

Linser, Paul (b. 1871). Tübingen dermatologist.

Linser's method. The treatment of varicose veins by the injection of mercuric chloride.

lint (lint). Cotton lint, unmedicated lint, linteum absorbens, Absorbent Lint BPC 1959. A cotton cloth of plain weave, with the nap raised from the warp yarns on one side only. It is used for direct application to wounds or infected tissues, or to assist the application of other medicaments such as ointments, lotions, and liniments. **Boric Acid Lint BPC 1959.** Absorbent lint which has been impregnated with boric acid. It is usually tinted pink to distinguish it from absorbent lint. **Euflavine Lint BPC 1959.** Absorbent lint impregnated with euflavine. [L *linum* flax.]

linteum (lin·te·um). Lint.

lintin (lin·tin). A loose cotton fabric for wound dressing. [lint.]

lintine (lin·teen). An absorbent fat-free cotton material. [lint.]

Linton's test. A test for varicose veins: the leg is elevated to empty the superficial veins and a tourniquet is applied below the knee. If the valves of the deep veins are incompetent, the superficial veins rapidly refill when the patient stands.

Linum (li·num). 1. Flax. 2. A genus of plants (family Linaceae); the seeds of *Linum usitatissimum* Linn. are known as *linseed,* and the fibres from the stem of the same plant are manufactured into linen thread. 3. Linseed. **Linum contusum.** Crushed linseed. *See* LINSEED. [L.]

Linzenmeier, Georg (b. 1882). Karlsruhe physician.

Linzenmeier's blood sedimentation tube. A tube designed for measuring the sedimentation rate of erythrocytes in terms of the time taken for the level of erythrocytes to fall a specified distance.

lio-. For words beginning with *lio- see also* LEIO-.

Liothyronine (li·o·thi·ro·neen). BP Commission approved name for L - 2 - amino - 3 - [4 - (4 - hydroxy - 3 - iodophenoxy) - 3,5 - di - iodophenyl]propionic acid. **Liothyronine Sodium BP 1973.** The sodium derivative of liothyronine, one of the active principles of thyroid gland. Its action is that of thyroxine sodium, but it acts more rapidly and is indicated in the first phase of treatment of severe hypothyroidism.

lip [labium oris (NA)] (lip). Either of two fleshy folds, upper and lower [labium superius, labium inferius (NA)], bordering the external entrance to the cavity of the mouth. **Lips of the bicipital groove.** *See* GROOVE. **Cleft lip.** Hare-lip. **Double lip.** A redundant fold of mucous membrane within the mouth, on either side of the midline of the lip. **Hapsburg lip.** The overdeveloped thick lower lip which accompanies the Hapsburg jaw. **Lips of the iliac crest.** *See* ILIUM. **Lips of the linea aspera.** *See* LINEA ASPERA. **Lips of the neck of the uterus.** *See* UTERUS, NECK OF THE. **Rhombic lip.** The lateral edge of the embryonic hind-brain to which the roof of the 4th ventricle is attached and whose cells migrate to give rise to the vestibular and olivary nuclei and the nuclei of the cerebellum. **Tympanic lip [labium limbi tympani-**

cum (NA)]. A tapering projection from the lower part of the limbus laminae spiralis, to which the inner margin of the basilar membrane is attached. It is perforated by the foramina for nerves for the numerous branches of the cochlear nerve. **Vestibular lip [labium limbi vestibulare (NA)].** An overhanging ledge projecting from the upper part of the limbus laminae spiralis, giving attachment to the membrana tectoria. [AS *lippa.*]

lip, incisive muscles of the lower. Slips of the orbicularis oris muscle which attach to the mandible.

lip, incisive muscles of the upper. Slips of the orbicularis oris muscle which attach to the maxilla.

lip reading (lip re·ding). The appreciation by a deaf person of what is being spoken, by observing the movement of the lips and associated facial muscles. [AS *lippa, raedan.*]

lipacidaemia (lip·as·id·e'·me·ah). The presence of one or more fatty acids in the blood. [Gk *lipos* fat, acid, Gk *haima* blood.]

lipaciduria (lip·as·id·ewr'·e·ah). The presence of fatty acids in the urine. [Gk *lipos* fat, acid, urine.]

lipaemia (lip·e·me·ah). The presence of abnormal quantities of fats or lipoids in the blood, e.g. in such conditions as hypercholesterolaemia, xanthomatosis, and other types of hyperlipaemia. **Alimentary lipaemia.** Lipaemia caused by the excessive ingestion of fat. **Lipaemia retinalis.** Lipaemic infiltration of the retinae and retinal blood vessels in cases of hyperlipaemia. [Gk *lipos* fat, *haima* blood.]

liparia (lip·ar·e·ah). Excess of fat; obesity. [Gk *liparos* fatty.]

liparocele (lip·ar·o·seel). 1. A fatty tumour of the scrotum. 2. Adipocele. [Gk *liparos* fatty, *kele* hernia.]

liparodyspnoea (lip·ar·o·disp·ne'·ah). The dyspnoea experienced by excessively fat individuals. [Gk *liparos* fatty, dyspnoea.]

liparoid (lip·ar·oid). Lipoid; like fat. [Gk *liparos* fatty, *eidos* like.]

liparomphalos, liparomphalus (lip·ar·**om**·fal·os, lip·ar·**om**·fal·us). A fatty tumour of the umbilicus. [Gk *liparos* fatty, *omphalos* navel.]

liparoscirrhus (lip·ar·o·skir'·us). A fatty tumour with scirrhus invasion. [Gk *liparos* fatty, *skirros* hard.]

liparotrichia (lip·ar·o·trik'·e·ah). An excessively greasy condition of the hair. [Gk *liparos* fatty, *thrix* hair.]

liparous (lip·ar·us). Obese. [Gk *liparos* fatty.]

lipases (lip·a·zez). Enzymes of the esterase type which hydrolyse glycerides to fatty acids and glycerol or other organic esters to the alcohol and acid. Lipases occur not only in the exocrine secretion of the pancreas but are widely distributed in different animal cells, releasing fatty acids for respiration from storage glycerides. Of particular physiological significance is the hormone sensitive lipase of adipose tissue which undergoes activation by cyclic 3′,5′-adenosine monophosphate (*see also*: PROTEIN KINASE). Lipases also occur widely in plants and micro-organisms. **Lipoprotein lipase** (*clearing factor lipase*). An enzyme associated with a wide variety of animal tissues, especially muscle and adipose tissue which hydrolyses the triglycerides of chylomicrons and low density lipoproteins to glycerol and fatty acids. The enzyme is under hormonal control by insulin and can be released into blood plasma from tissues by heparin. [Gk *lipos* fat.]

lipasuria (lip·a·**zewr**·e·ah). The presence of lipase in the urine.

lipectomy (lip·**ek**·to·me). Operative removal of fatty-tissue neoplasms or of the subcutaneous fatty tissue. [Gk *lipos* fat, *ektome* a cutting out.]

lipid (lip·id). A member of the family of fats, or fat-like compounds, which occur in living tissues, either structurally as the tissue fat of cells or deposited for nutritional purposes as in adipose tissue and seeds. They are esters of fatty acids, or related to such, and are insoluble in water but soluble in fat solvents such as benzene, chloroform, or ether. They may be classified into: (*a*) *simple lipids,* which include the true fats, oils, and waxes; (*b*) *compound lipids,* which consist of phospholipids, glycolipids, aminolipids, and sulpholipids; (*c*) *derived lipids,* being the various fatty acids and sterols. [Gk *lipos* fat.]

lipidaemia (lip·id·e·me·ah). Lipaemia.

lipide (lip·ide). Lipid.

lipidic (lip·id·ik). Referring to or composed of lipids.

lipidol (lip·id·ol). Any of the lipid alcohols such as glycerol and the higher solid alcohols.

lipidosis (lip·id·o·sis). Any abnormality of the metabolism of lipids. **Neurovisceral lipidosis.** Gangliosidosis of the brain with mucopolysaccharidosis of viscera; a fatal disease starting in infancy. It may be familial. [lipid, Gk *-osis* condition.]

lipidtemns (lip·id·**temz**). A general term for the products of fat hydrolysis; glycerol and fatty acids. [Gk *lipos* fat, *temnein* to cut.]

lipin, lipine (lip·in, lip·een). Lipid.

lipo-arthritis (lip·o·ar·**thri'**·tis). A form of arthritis in which there is inflammation of the fatty tissue around a joint. [Gk *lipos* fat, arthritis.]

lipo-atrophy (lip·o·at·ro·fe). A condition in which there is failure of deposition of fat in the subcutaneous tissues; it has been described in diabetics. Cf. LIPODYSTROPHY, in which there is selective failure of fat deposition, e.g. above the level of the umbilicus. **Circumscribed lipo-atrophy.** Localized areas of subcutaneous fatty atrophy occurring in dermatolysis (cutis laxa). **Partial lipo-atrophy.** Loss of fat from the face and the upper part of the body (Weir-Mitchell type) or also with hypertrophy of the subcutaneous fat of the lower part of the body (Laignel-Lavastine-Viard type). **Total lipo-atrophy.** Generalized loss of subcutaneous and visceral fat with hepatomegaly, diabetes, hyperlipaemia and increased bone growth; lipo-atrophic diabetes. [Gk *lipos* fat, atrophy.]

lipoblast (lip·o·blast). A fat cell originating as a connective-tissue cell and becoming specialized. [Gk *lipos* fat, *blastos* germ.]

lipoblastoma (lip·o·blas·**to'**·mah). A lipomatoid tumour composed of lipoblasts. [Gk *lipos* fat, blastoma.]

lipocardiac (lip·o·**kar**·de·ak). Referring to a fatty heart, or to the person affected with the condition of fatty heart. [Gk *lipos* fat, *kardia* heart.]

lipocele (lip·o·seel). Adipocele. [Gk *lipos* fat, *kele* hernia.]

lipoceratous (lip·o·**ser**·at·us). Adipoceratous. [see foll.]

lipocere (lip·o·seer). Adipocere. [Gk *lipos* fat, L *cera* wax.]

lipochondrodystrophy (lip·o·kon·dro·**dis'**·tro·fe). A congenital syndrome in which a storage defect produces raised blood cholesterol, enlarged liver and spleen, thickened subcutaneous tissues, cloudy corneae, and deposits in the central nervous system. The abnormal substance, formerly described as a lipoid, is a carbohydrate/protein dysfunction. Skeletal changes comprise flexion deformities of the extremities producing dwarfism; deformity of the skull which is large, square, or scaphocephalic; facial abnormalities due to a varying degree of hypertelorism, guttering of the frontal bones and defects of the sphenoid bone; and deformity of one or more lumbar vertebrae due to defects of the upper and anterior parts of the bodies, producing lumbar kyphosis. Forme fruste may be occasionally seen, and there is mental defect. [Gk *lipos* fat, *chondros* cartilage, *dys* ill, *trophe* nutrition.]

lipochondroma (lip·o·kon·**dro'**·mah). A tumour consisting of cartilaginous and fatty tissue. [Gk *lipos* fat, *chondros* cartilage, *-oma* tumour.]

lipochromaemia (lip·o·kro·**me'**·me·ah). An excessive amount of lipochrome in the blood. [lipochrome, Gk *haima* blood.]

lipochrome (lip·o·krome). Any of the fat-soluble pigments which give the yellow colour to fats. They are unsaturated hydrocarbons, those in animal tissues being the carotenes and xanthophylls which in turn are derived from plant sources. [Gk *lipos* fat, *chroma* colour.]

lipochromogen (lip·o·**kro**·mo·jen). Term applied to the phytol derivatives which are the precursors of the lipochromes. [lipochrome, Gk *genein* to produce.]

lipoclasis (lip·**ok**·las·is). Lipolysis. [Gk *lipos* fat, *klasis* a breaking.]

lipoclastic (lip·o·**klas**·tik). Lipolytic. [see prec.]

lipocorticoid (lip·o·**kor**·tik·oid). The property of corticosteroids of laying down fat. [Gk *lipos* fat, cortex, Gk *eidos* form.]

lipocyanine (lip·o·si·an·een). The transient blue-violet compound formed by lipochromes with concentrated sulphuric acid, the appearance of which serves as a test for carotenoids and vitamin A. [Gk *lipos* fat, *kyanos* blue.]

lipocyte (**lip**·o·site). A fat cell. [Gk *lipos* fat, *kytos* cell.]

lipodiaeresis (**lip**·o·di·**er**'·es·is). The loss of accumulated fat from an organ, especially by splitting of fatty elements and general disintegration. [Gk *lipos* fat, *diairesis* separation.]

lipodystrophia (**lip**·o·dis·**tro**'·fe·ah). Lipodystrophy.

lipodystrophy (lip·o·**dis**·tro·fe). A disorder of fat metabolism. **Intestinal lipodystrophy.** A disease that occurs mostly in middle-aged men, characterized clinically by cough, dyspepsia, loss of weight, steatorrhoea and diarrhoea, and polyarthritis. Pathologically, there is swelling of the intestinal villi and submucosa, with deposits of fat and fatty acids in much enlarged intestinal glands. A high-protein low-fat diet with hydrocortisone by mouth often produces improvement. **Progressive lipodystrophy.** A rare disease of unknown origin in which there is a symmetrical and progressive (eventually complete) loss of fat from the subcutaneous tissues of the upper part of the body above the pelvis, whilst the subcutaneous fat of the buttocks and lower limbs is unaffected or may be increased: the general health remains unimpaired. It occurs almost exclusively in females, and usually begins between the ages of 5 and 15. [Gk *lipos* fat, dystrophy.]

lipoedema (lip·e·**de**·mah). A type of oedema which is characterized by the presence of abnormal deposits of fat beneath the skin. [Gk *lipos* fat, oedema.]

lipoferous (lip·**of**·er·us). Carrying or containing fat. [Gk *lipos* fat, *ferre* to carry.]

lipofibroma (**lip**·o·fi·**bro**'·mah). A mixed lipoma and fibroma.

lipofuscin (lip·o·**fus**·in). The colouring matter produced by the solution of a pigment in fat. [Gk *lipos* fat, fuscin.]

lipogenesis (lip·o·**jen**·es·is). Production or deposition of fat. [Gk *lipos* fat, *genein* to produce.]

lipogenetic, lipogenic, lipogenous (**lip**·o·jen·**et**'·ik, lip·o·**jen**·ik, lip·**oj**·en·us). Relating to or resulting from the formation or deposition of fats. [see prec.]

lipogranuloma (**lip**·o·gran·ew·**lo**'·mah). The low-grade inflammatory reaction to fat necrosis, sometimes multiple. **Lipogranuloma of kidney.** A rare, parenchymal tumour containing friable material like an atheromatous plaque. **Sclerosing lipogranuloma.** Fat necrosis, particularly affecting the penis and scrotum; a lipogranuloma, either infective or due to injection of oil. [Gk *lipos* fat, granuloma.]

lipogranulomatosis (**lip**·o·gran·ew·lo·mat·**o**'·sis). Defective lipoid metabolism characterized by the deposition of yellow nodules containing fatty matter in the skin, mucous membranes, or muscle perimysia, resulting in the development of numerous granulomata. **Disseminated lipogranulomatosis.** Farber's disease; originally thought to be a disorder of lipid metabolism, now known to be a disorder of mucopolysaccharides. Characterized by nodular periarticular swellings, ankylosis, joint contractures and mental retardation in infants; the voice is often hoarse and the subjects are liable to recurrent infections. [Gk *lipos* fat, granulomatosis.]

lipohaemangioma (**lip**·o·he·man·je·**o**'·mah). A haemangioma with fatty tissue incorporated in its substance. [Gk *lipos* fat, haemangioma.]

lipohaemia (lip·o·**he**·me·ah). Lipaemia.

lipohistiodiaeresis (**lip**·o·his·te·o·di·**er**'·es·is). Absence of fat in the tissues. [Gk *lipos* fat, *histos* tissue, *diairesis* separation.]

lipoid (**lip**·oid). An indefinite term which has been applied to compound lipids and also to biological substances which show some similarity in physical properties to the true lipids. **Acetone-insoluble lipoid.** The material, mainly lecithin, obtained on the addition of excess acetone to an ethereal extract of dried ox heart. It is the basis of antigens used in the Wassermann reaction. **Congenital adrenal lipoid hyperplasia.** The adrenal glands contain large amounts of cholesterol because the enzymes that convert it to the normal adrenocortical hormones are congenitally absent. [Gk *lipos* fat, *eidos* form.]

See also: FORSSMAN.

lipoidaemia (lip·oid·**e**·me·ah). The presence of lipoids in the blood. [lipoid, Gk *haima* blood.]

lipoidolytic (**lip**·oid·o·**lit**'·ik). The decomposition or splitting of lipoids. [lipoid, Gk *lysis* a loosing.]

lipoidosis (lip·oid·**o**·sis). A group of diseases in which there is reticulo-endothelial hyperplasia associated with an abnormal deposit of lipoids in the cells, e.g. in spleen, liver, and bone marrow. **Arterial lipoidosis.** Atherosclerosis. **Cerebroside lipoidosis.** Gaucher's disease; a rare familial disease beginning in early life and of great chronicity, in which the reticulo-endothelial cells are packed with the cerebroside, kerasin, with consequent great enlargement of the spleen and liver and a tendency to fragility of bone and spontaneous fractures. Haemorrhages occur from the skin and mucous membranes; the skin shows a brownish pigmentation, and the eyes show pingueculae. **Cholesterol lipoidosis.** Hand-Schueller-Christian disease; a disease of early childhood, characterized by local deposits of a cholesterol ester in the bones, especially in those of the skull. Invasion of the orbit causes exophthalmos, and involvement of the pituitary leads to diabetes insipidus; the blood cholesterol is raised. **Lipoidosis cutis et mucosae.** Xanthoma tuberosum; deposits of cholesterol causing yellow nodules in the skin: the mucous membranes, bones, tendons, and viscera may also be involved. In the skin the nodules are numerous and mainly on the extensor surfaces of the limbs; some may form tumours the size of a small orange. In xanthoma diabeticorum the nodules are the size of lentils and come out in crops; they disappear with effective treatment for the diabetes. **Kerasin lipoidosis.** Disturbance of the metabolism of lipoids with the deposition of kerasin. **Phosphatide lipoidosis.** 1. Niemann-Pick disease; a generalized familial disease of the reticulo-endothelial system, beginning in infancy and becoming fatal within 2 years. The affected cells are packed with a phosphatide lipoid; the spleen, liver, bone marrow, and lymph glands are enlarged, and the skin shows a yellow-brown pigmentation. 2. Tay-Sachs disease, amaurotic family idiocy, cerebromacular degeneration; a familial disease of infancy in which there is a progressive degeneration of nerve cells throughout the whole nervous system and retinae. The degenerating nerve cells are filled with a lipoid similar to that in Niemann-Pick disease, but there is no enlargement of the liver and spleen. **Renal lipoidosis.** Lipoid degeneration of renal cells, occurring in lipoid nephrosis. [lipoid, Gk *-osis* condition.]

lipoidproteinosis (**lip**·oid·pro·te·in·**o**'·sis). A disease the characteristic signs of which are the presence on the mucosae and skin of small yellowish nodes, horny growths on hands and feet, and defective lipoid metabolism indicated by hoarseness of voice. The condition is familial and occurs in latent diabetes mellitus. [lipoid, protein, Gk *-osis* condition.]

lipoiduria (lip·oid·**ewr**·e·ah). A condition characterized by the presence of lipoids in the urine.

lipolipoidosis (**lip**·o·lip·oid·**o**'·sis). Infiltration of lipoids and neutral fats into the cells. [Gk *lipos* fat, lipoidosis.]

lipolysis (lip·**ol**·is·is). The chemical disintegration or splitting of fat. [Gk *lipos* fat, lysis.]

lipolytic (lip·o·**lit**·ik). Pertaining to or causing lipolysis.

lipolytic hormone (lip·o·**lit**·ik **hor**·mone). (LPH lipotrophin, fat-mobilizing hormone). Found in pituitary extracts but not yet established as a pure hormone.

lipoma (lip·o·mah). An innocent tumour composed of fatty tissue. **Lipoma annulare colli.** A localized overgrowth of the fatty tissue of the neck, producing great enlargement of that structure. **Lipoma arborescens.** An extensive papillary outgrowth from the fatty tissues of the synovial membrane and articular capsule of the knee joint, which fills the joint spaces. **Lipoma capsulare.** A localized overgrowth of the fatty tissue in the capsule of organs, especially when these are atrophying. **Lipoma cavernosum.** A vascular fatty tumour. **Diffuse lipoma.** Lipomatosis. **Lipoma diffusum renis.** 1. Partial or complete replacement of the kidney by fatty tissue. 2. Liposarcoma of the kidney. **Lipoma durum, lipoma fibrosum.** A fibrolipoma. **Granular cell lipoma.** Hibernoma. **Lipoma myxomatodes.** A combination of myxoma and lipoma often resulting in a large malignant tumour, especially in the retroperitoneal region. **Naevoid lipoma.** A soft mole containing much fat. **Lipoma ossificans, lipoma petrificans, lipoma petrificum ossificans.** A lipoma showing calcification with or without ossification of its substance. **Lipoma sarcomatodes.** Liposarcoma. **Telangiectatic lipoma, lipoma telangiectodes.** Lipoma cavernosum (see above). [Gk *lipos* fat, *-oma* tumour.]

lipomatoid (lip·o·mat·oid). Lipomatous.

lipomatosis (lip·o·mat·o'·sis). The excessive deposition of fat in tissues in the form of tumour-like masses. **Lipomatosis atrophicans.** Localized masses of fat in certain parts, associated with wasting elsewhere. **Diffuse symmetrical lipomatosis of the neck.** This occurs chiefly in adult males. It is characterized by diffuse and symmetrical masses of fat around the neck and occasionally on the trunk. There may be pain, tenderness, asthenia, and mental changes, but usually the general health is not affected. **Lipomatosis dolorosa.** Adiposis dolorosa, a disease mainly occurring in middle-aged women, characterized by the formation of diffuse symmetrical masses of fat in various parts of the body, especially around the shoulder girdle, the abdomen, buttocks, and thighs; the forearms and lower legs may be affected but the hands and feet escape. The masses are painful and very tender on pressure; asthenia and psychical disturbances are usually also present. **Nodular circumscribed lipomatosis.** Multiple circumscribed nodules or tumours of varying size, few or many, in various sites scattered throughout the body. They may be painful or tender, and associated with asthenia and mental changes. **Renal lipomatosis.** A great increase of fat surrounding the kidney, in association with calculous pyelitis or other conditions causing atrophy. **Visceral lipomatosis.** Lipomata occurring within or surrounding any of the internal organs in which fat is normally present. The most important forms are those connected with the kidneys, breasts, and peritoneum. [lipoma, Gk *-osis* condition.]

lipomatous (lip·o·mat·us). Pertaining to or resembling a lipoma. [lipoma, Gk *eidos* form.]

lipometabolic (lip·o·met·ab·ol'·ik). Pertaining to lipometabolism.

lipometabolism (lip·o·met·ab'·ol·izm). Metabolism of fat. [Gk *lipos* fat, metabolism.]

lipomphalus (lip·om·fal·us). A fat hernia at the umbilicus. [Gk *lipos* fat, *omphalos* navel.]

lipomyoma (lip·o·mi·o'·mah). A mixed lipoma and myoma.

lipomyxoma (lip·o·mix·o'·mah). A mixed lipoma and myxoma.

liponephrosis (lip·o·nef·ro'·sis). Lipoid nephrosis. *See* NEPHROSIS.

liponeurocyte (lip·o·newr·o·site). A term used to describe certain cells in the pituitary of rats (Cramer). [obsolete term]. [Gk *lipos* fat, neurocyte.]

Liponyssus (lip·o·nis·us). A common synonym of *Bdellonyssus.* The tropical rat mite, *Bdellonyssus* (= *Liponyssus*) *bacoti*, is a serious nuisance in rat-infested premises in temperate as well as tropical countries. The larvae cause mite dermatitis (a vesicular and intensely irritating dermatitis) in industrial workers. *Liponyssus nagayoi, bursa,* and *silviarum* also cause mite dermatitis. [Gk *lipos* fat, *nyssein* to pierce.]

lipopectic (lip·o·pek·tik). Pertaining to or marked by lipopexia.

lipopenia (lip·o·pe·ne·ah). A reduction in the amount of lipids in the body. [Gk *lipos* fat, *penes* poor.]

lipopenic (lip·o·pe·nik). Pertaining to lipopenia.

lipopexia (lip·o·pex·e·ah). The stabilization or storage of fats in the tissues. [Gk *lipos* fat, *pexis* fixation.]

lipophage (lip·o·faje). A cell which takes up or absorbs fat. [see foll.]

lipophagia (lip·o·fa·je·ah). 1. Lipolysis. 2. Fat absorption. **Lipophagia granulomatosis.** A disease in which the enlarged intestinal and mesenteric lymph spaces are filled with fat and fatty acids. [Gk *lipos* fat, *phagein* to eat.]

lipophagic (lip·o·fa·jik). Lipolytic. [see prec.]

lipophagy (lip·of·ah·je). Lipophagia.

lipophil (lip·o·fil). Capable of absorbing fat. [see foll.]

lipophilia (lip·o·fil·e·ah). 1. A tendency to absorb fat. 2. A peculiarity of metabolism in adipose persons. [Gk *lipos* fat, *philein* to love.]

lipophrenia (li·po·fre·ne·ah). Mental failure. [Gk *leipein* to fail, *phren* mind.]

lipopolysaccharide (lip·o·pol·e·sak'·ar·ide). A term used bacteriologically to denote lipopolysaccharide as component of O antigen (endotoxin) of Gram-negative bacteria, especially enterobacteria, e.g. *Escherichia, Salmonella, Shigella* spp. and probably *Bordetella* and *Haemophilus.* When injected intravenously, bacterial lipopolysaccharides produce shock, leucopenia followed by leucocytosis and pyrexia (hence called *pyrogens*). They also act as antigen adjuvants, probably because of the lipid A fraction. [Gk *lipos* fat, *polys* many, *sakcharon* sugar.]

lipoproteins (lip·o·pro·te·inz). Complexes of lipids with protein that have the solubility characteristics of proteins. Covalent linkages are rarely involved in such complexes. In cells, lipoproteins are especially important in the structural and catalytic activities of membranes. In blood plasma, lipoproteins have been separated and classified by physical techniques employing centrifugation or electrophoresis into α (high density), β (low density) and pre-β (very low density) lipoproteins and chylomicrons.

liposarcoma (lip·o·sar·ko'·mah). A mixed lipoma and sarcoma; the cells of the latter are of primitive embryonic type.

lipose, liposin (lip·oze, lip·o·sin). A lipase that may be present in the blood. [Gk *lipos* fat.]

liposis (lip·o·sis). Lipomatosis.

liposoluble (lip·o·sol·ewbl). Fat-soluble. [Gk *lipos* fat, soluble.]

liposteatosis (lip·o·ste·at·o'·sis). Any lipoid-storage disease. The word is not favoured in the UK. [lipoid, Gk *stear* fat, *-osis* condition.]

lipotamponade (lip·o·tam·pon·ade). The use of an autogenous mass of fatty tissue inserted in the extrapleural space to immobilize a diseased area of lung. It is normally used in conjunction with a thoracoplasty in the same area to improve the immobilization of the lung, but the fat tends to be absorbed too soon to be of much value. [Gk *lipos* fat, Fr. *tampon* pack.]

lipotrophic (lip·o·trof·ik). Increasing the amount of fat present in the body tissues. [see foll.]

lipotrophin (li·po·trow·fin). (LPH). May be a larger pro-hormone of B-melanocyte-stimulating hormone both of which are found in excess in chronic renal failure and in Addison's disease and Nelson's disease.

lipotrophy (lip·ot·ro·fe). An increase in the amount of fat present in the body tissues. [Gk *lipos* fat, *trophe* nourishment.]

lipotropic (lip·o·trop·ik). Having an attraction for oils or fats and so influencing fat metabolism. [see foll.]

lipotropism, lipotropy (lip·ot·ro·pizm, lip·ot·ro·pe). Affinity (e.g. of basic dyes) for fats, oils, or fatty tissue. [Gk *lipos* fat, *trope* a turning.]

lipotuberculin (lip·o·tew·ber'·kew·lin). A tuberculin preparation which includes the fatty fraction of *Mycobacterium tuberculosis* in solution or emulsion. [Gk *lipos* fat, tuberculin.]

lipovaccine (lip·o·vak·seen). A vaccine made by suspending the organisms in vegetable oil in order to delay absorption of the antigenic material. [Gk *lipos* fat, vaccine.]

lipoxenous (li·pox·en·us). Describing a parasitic organism which deserts its host when development is complete. [see foll.]

lipoxeny (li·pox·en·e). Abandonment of the host by a parasitic organism on completion of its development. [Gk *leipein* to forsake, *xenos* host.]

lipoxidaemia (lip·ox·id·e'·me·ah). Lipacidaemia. [Gk *lipos* fat, *oxys* sour, *haima* blood.]

lipoxysm (lip·ox·izm). Oleic acid poisoning. [Gk *lipos* fat, *oxys* sour.]

lippa (lip·ah). Marginal blepharitis. *See* BLEPHARITIS. [L *lippus* blear-eyed.]

lipping (lip·ing). An overgrowth of bone which projects beyond the margin of the affected joints in osteoarthritis, and can be seen on x-ray examination. [AS *lippa.*]

lippitude (lip·it·ewd). A late stage of blepharitis in which the lid margins are rounded, swollen, everted, and deprived of lashes. [L *lippus* blear-eyed.]

Lipschuetz, Benjamin (b. 1878). Vienna dermatologist.

Lipschuetz bodies. Small or large eosinophilic bodies within the basophilic nuclei of the early forms of "balloon cells" (described by Unna in the deeper part of the rete of the epidermis in cases of zoster), and sometimes in the nuclei of swollen connective-tissue cells and of endothelial cells in the corium. These are not now considered to be degenerated nucleoli or parasitic cell inclusions.

Lipschuetz cell. A type of cell with granular cytoplasm, found in certain forms of skin lesion, such as lichen planar.

Lipschuetz's acute ulcer of the vulva. Ulcus vulvae acutum; there are several varieties, including a venereal and a non-venereal; the former is indolent, and not associated with constitutional disturbance, and the latter, which may be severe, even gangrenous, and accompanied by fever and other constitutional symptoms, is associated with a variety of micro-organisms, including *Lactobacillus acidophilus.*

lipsis (lip·sis). Cessation. **Lipsis animi.** Syncope. [Gk *leipsis* a failing.]

lipsotrichia (lip·so·**trik**·e·ah). Falling out of the hair. [Gk *leipein* to fail, *thrix* hair.]

lipuria (lip·**ewr**·e·ah). The presence or excretion of an oily emulsion or fat in the urine. [Gk *lipos* fat, urine.]

lipuric (lip·**ewr**·ik). Pertaining to or marked by the presence of an oily emulsion or fat in the urine. [see prec.]

liquamen (**lik**·wah·men). The flux which can be drained away in the melting of solids. [L *liquare* to make liquid.]

liquefacient (lik·we·**fa**·shent). 1. Having the power to cause a solid substance to become liquid. 2. An agent which has the property of liquefying a hard growth or deposit. [liquid, L *facere* to make.]

liquefaction (lik·we·**fak**·shun). Conversion of a solid substance into liquid. [see prec.]

liquefactive (lik·we·**fak**·tiv). Relating to, or causing liquefaction.

liquescent (lik·**wes**·ent). Liable to become liquid or fluid. [L *liquescere* to become liquid.]

liquid (**lik**·wid). A substance in that state of matter where it acquires the shape of the containing vessel but, unlike a gas, is bounded on its upper surface by an interphase. Certain substances attain the shape of the containing vessel only very slowly, e.g. shellac, pitch, and are therefore liquids. **Blistering liquid.** Liquor Epispasticus BPC 1949. **Dutch liquid.** Ethylene chloride. [L *liquere* to flow.]

See also: BONAIN, CADET, EBNER, PICTET.

Liquidambar (lik·wid·**am**·bar). A genus of trees (family Hamamelidaceae), which yield a fragrant balsam. **Liquidambar orientalis.** A species which is the source of storax. [L *liquidus* liquid, LL *ambar* amber.]

liquiform (**lik**·we·form). Like a liquid. [liquid, form.]

liquiritae (lik·ir·it·e). Liquorice. **Liquiritae Radix.** *European Pharmacopoeia* name for Liquorice BP 1973.

liquogel (**lik**·wo·jel). Any gel which liquefies on heating to form a sol of low viscosity.

liquor (**li**k·er, li·kwor). 1. A solution, usually aqueous but sometimes alcoholic, of pure substances. 2. [NA] A secretion. 3. A solution in a chemical manufacturing process. **Liquor amaranthi.** Solution of Amaranth BPC 1959. **Liquor ammoniae dilutus.** Dilute Ammonia Solution BP 1958. **Liquor ammoniae fortis.** Strong Ammonia Solution BP 1958. **Liquor ammonii acetatis dilutus.** Dilute Solution of Ammonium Acetate BP 1953. **Liquor ammonii anisatus.** An alcoholic solution of ammonia and anise oil. **Liquor amnii.** The amniotic fluid. **Liquor amnii spurius.** The allantoic fluid. **Liquor arseni acidus.** A dilute hydrochloric acid solution containing 1 per cent of arsenic trioxide. **Liquor arsenicalis.** Arsenical Solution BP 1953. **Liquor Arsenii et Hydrargyri Iodidi BPC 1949.** Donovan's solution; an aqueous solution of red mercuric iodide and arsenic tri-iodide. **Liquor calcii hydroxidi, liquor calcis.** Calcium Hydroxide Solution BP 1968. **Liquor carbonis detergens.** A solution of coal tar in soap solution. **Liquor chloridorum trium isotonicus.** Ringer's solution. **Liquor chorii.** The fluid contained between the amnion and chorion of the early embryo. **Liquor corneae.** The tissue fluid of the cornea. **Liquor cotunnii.** Perilymph. **Liquor cresolis saponatus.** Cresol Soap Solution BP 1968. **Liquor entericus.** The secretion of the intestinal glands. **Liquor Epispasticus BPC 1949.** Blistering liquid; a solution of cantharidin in a mixture of acetone, castor oil, and colophony. **Liquor folliculi.** The fluid contents of an ovarian follicle. **Liquor formaldehydi.** Formaldehyde Solution BP 1968. **Liquor hamamelidis.** Hamamelis water. *See* WATER. **Liquor hepatis.** A liquid preparation from fresh liver. **Liquor hydrogenii peroxidi.** Hydrogen Peroxide Solution BP 1968. **Liquor iodi fortis.** Strong Iodine Solution BP 1958. **Malt liquor.** A solution obtained by allowing barley to germinate in warm water. **Liquor morphinae acetatis.** A 1 per cent solution of morphine acetate. **Liquor morphinae hydrochloridi.** Morphine Hydrochloride Solution BP 1968. **Mother liquor.** The saturated solution from which crystallization has taken place. **Liquor pancreaticus.** The secretion of the pancreas. **Liquor pericardii.** The fluid within the pericardial cavity. **Liquor pituitarii posterii.** An aqueous extract of the posterior lobe of the pituitary body. **Liquor plumbi subacetatis dilutus.** Dilute Lead Subacetate Solution BP 1963. **Liquor plumbi subacetatis fortis.** Strong Lead Subacetate Solution BP 1963. **Liquor potassii arsenatis.** A 1 per cent solution of arsenious oxide in an aqueous solution of potassium hydroxide. **Liquor potassii hydroxidi.** Potassium Hydroxide Solution BP 1968. **Liquor sanguinis.** Blood plasma. **Liquor scarpae.** Endolymph. **Liquor seminis.** Semen. **Liquor sodii chloridi isotonicus.** A 0.9 per cent solution of sodium chloride; it is isotonic with blood serum. [L, liquid.]

See also: MORGAGNI.

Liquorice BP 1973 (**lik**·or·is). Glycyrrhiza, a drug having a taste, sweet and almost free from bitterness, obtained from *Glycyrrhiza glabra* Linn. and other species of *Glycyrrhiza* and consisting of a shoot and root in the peeled or unpeeled condition, The taste is due to the presence of a sweet principle, glycyrrhizin. Both in powder form and as the liquid extract it is widely used in medicine as a flavouring agent and a mild expectorant. [Gk *glykyrrhiza* sweet-root.]

Lisfranc, Jacques (b. 1790). Paris surgeon.

Lisfranc's amputation, or operation. 1. Removal of the foot at the tarsometatarsal joint. 2. Removal of the arm at the shoulder joint; also called *Dupuytren's operation.*

Lisfranc's joint. The tarsometatarsal joints.

Lisfranc's ligament. The interosseous ligament connecting the 1st cuneiform bone with the base of the 2nd metatarsal.

Lisfranc's tubercle. The scalene tubercle of the 1st rib. It is for the attachment of the scalenus anterior muscle.

lisp (lisp). In speaking, to substitute the *th* sounds for sibilants. Hence *lisping.* [AS *wlisp.*]

Lissauer, Heinrich (b. 1861). Breslau neurologist.

Lissauer's column, fasciculus, or tract. The posterolateral tract of the spinal cord. It lies at the apex of the posterior horn of the spinal grey matter.

Lissauer's paralysis. General paralysis of rapid onset and progression; similar to galloping paralysis.

Lissauer's zone. A bridge of white matter between the apex of the posterior horn and the periphery of the spinal cord.

Column of Spitzka–Lissauer. Lissauer's column (see above).

lissencephalia (lis·en·kef·a′·le·ah). Hypoplasia of the brain characterized by partial or total absence of the gyri. [Gk *lissos* smooth, *egkephalos* brain.]

lissencephalic, lissencephalous (lis·en·kef·**al**′·ik, lis·en·**kef**·al·-us). Having a brain in which the gyri are partially or completely absent. [see prec.]

Lister, Joseph, Baron (b. 1827). Glasgow, Edinburgh, and London surgeon.

Lister's antiseptic. A solution of mercuric and zinc cyanides.
Lister's tubercle. The dorsal tubercle of the radius. *See* TUBERCLE.

Lister, Sir William Tindall (b. 1868). London ophthalmologist.
Lister ophthalmic lamp. A specially designed electric lamp partially blacked on the outside and silvered on the inside, in common use for the examination of the eye. It provides two circular apertures, one larger than the other, either to be used as a source of light for retinoscopy or ophthalmoscopy, and one large aperture for use in direct illumination of the anterior part of the eye.
Lister perimeter. A simple self-recording perimeter in common use.

Listerella (lis·ter·el·ah). A genus of Gram-positive rod-shaped organisms, motile, aerobic or micro-aerophilic; in the *rough* form long filaments may predominate, They form no spores, and are parasitic and usually pathogenic: infections are characterized by a monocytosis. **Listerella monocytogenes.** A widespread animal parasite, occasionally causing in man a generalized infection with local lesions in the liver, myocardium, or central nervous system, and related to *Erysipelothrix.* Since the genus *Listerella* is not valid, species of this genus are placed in either the genus *Erysipelothrix* or the genus *Listeria* by different bacteriologists. [Joseph, Baron *Lister.*]

listerellosis (lis·ter·el·**o'**·sis). Infection with *Listerella.* [*Listerella,* Gk *-osis* condition.]

Listeria (lis·**teer**·e·ah). A bacterial genus in the family Corynebacteriaceae. Gram-positive, short, non-sporing motile rods, often in pairs, sometimes as elongated filaments; the rods readily become Gram-negative in older cultures. It closely resembles *Erysipelothrix.* **Listeria monocytogenes.** *Erysipelothrix monocytogenes;* in man the infection may manifest as a meningo-encephalitis in adults or as a generalized, highly fatal, infection in babies (granulomatosis infantiseptica) following a symptomless intra-uterine infection in the mother. [Joseph, Baron *Lister.*]

listerism (lis·ter·izm). The application of an antiseptic technique in surgery, so named after Joseph Lister who introduced the antiseptic method and made modern surgery possible.

Listing, Johann Benedict (b. 1808). Göttingen physicist and physiologist.
Listing's law. When the line of fixation of the eye passes from its primary position to any other position, the angle of torsion of the eye in this second position is the same as if the eye had arrived at this position by turning about a fixed axis perpendicular to the initial and final positions of the line of fixation.
Listing's plane. That which passes through the equator and centre of rotation of the eyeball when this is directed straight ahead in the primary position. The vertical and transverse axes of rotation of the eyeball run in this plane, and the anterior-posterior plane runs perpendicular to it.

Liston, Robert (b. 1794). Scottish surgeon in London.
Liston's operation. Excision of the upper jaw.
Liston's scissors. Plaster scissors; strong scissors for removing plaster casts.
Liston's splint. A long, straight, wooden splint used for fractures of the femur.

lithaemia (lith·e·me·ah). Uricacidaemia. [Gk *lithos* stone, *haima* blood.]

lithagogue (**lith**·ag·og). 1. Causing the expulsion of calculi. 2. An agent which causes the dislodgment or expulsion of calculi. [Gk *lithos* stone, *agogein* to lead forth.]

litharge (**lith**·arj). Lead monoxide, PbO. [Gk *lithos* stone, *argyros* silver.]

lithate (**lith**·ate). A urate; from *lithic acid* the old name for uric acid.

lithectasy (lith·**ek**·tas·e). Removal of calculi through the urethra after the canal has been instrumentally dilated. [Gk *lithos* stone, *ektasis* a stretching.]

lithectomy (lith·**ek**·to·me). Lithotomy. [Gk *lithos* stone, *ektome* a cutting out.]

lithia (**lith**·e·ah). Lithium oxide.

lithiasic (lith·i·as·ik). Relating to lithiasis.

lithiasis (lith·i·as·is). The tendency to form calculi or concretions; the gouty diathesis. **Appendicular lithiasis.** The formation of concretions in the lumen of the appendix, which they may obstruct. **Lithiasis conjunctivae.** Small, hard, white concretions formed in the palpebral part of the conjunctiva. **Pancreatic lithiasis.** Concretions in the pancreatic duct. **Urinary lithiasis.** A calculus occurring in the urinary tract. [Gk *lithos* stone.]

lithiatry (lith·i·at·re). The treatment of urinary calculus by medicinal, as opposed to operative, measures. [Gk *lithos* stone, *iatreia* treatment.]

lithic (**lith**·ik). 1. Relating to calculi. 2. Relating to lithium. [Gk *lithos* stone.]

lithicosis (lith·**ik**·**o**·sis). Pneumoconiosis. [Gk *lithikos* made of stone.]

lithium (**lith**·e·um). An element of the alkaline metals group, with atomic weight 6.941, atomic number 3, and chemical symbol Li. It occurs in minute quantities in bone, muscle, and lung tissue and somewhat resembles potassium in its actions, though more toxic; continued use may cause gastro-enteritis. The salts were formerly used in the treatment of gout, due to their reputation for ready combination with uric acid, but it has since been shown that under the conditions prevailing in the body lithium urate is not formed. **Lithium acetylsalicylate.** $CH_3COOC_6H_4COOLi$, a compound formerly used in rheumatism. **Lithium bromide.** LiBr, a deliquescent white crystalline powder with the general therapeutic properties of a bromide, but liable to cause alimentary upset. **Lithium Carbonate BP 1973.** Li_2CO_3, used in the prophylaxis and treatment of manic-depressive disorders. Its mode of action is obscure. Excessive doses cause serious toxic effects, including encephalopathy and renal damage. **Lithium chloride.** LiCl, a compound which has been used as a substitute for sodium chloride in salt-restricted diets; its toxic effects include drowsiness, weakness, and tremors. **Lithium citrate.** $Li_3C_6H_5O_7{\cdot}4H_2O$, a deliquescent white compound with properties similar to the carbonate. **Lithium oxide.** LiO_2, a white oxide formed by the combustion of lithium. It dissolves slowly in water to form the hydroxide. **Lithium salicylate.** $LiOOCC_6H_4OH$, a compound resembling the other salicylates in pharmacological action. It has also been used in the local sclerosing treatment of varicose veins. [Gk *lithos* stone.]

lithocenosis (**lith**·o·sen·**o'**·sis). Evacuation of the crushed fragments of a calculus or calculi from the urinary bladder. [Gk *lithos* stone, *kenosis* an emptying.]

lithoclast (**lith**·o·klast). A lithotrite. [Gk *lithos* stone, *klaein* to break in pieces.]

lithoclysma (lith·o·**kliz**·mah). The injection into the urinary bladder of a liquid which is capable of dissolving calculi. [Gk *lithos* stone, *klysma* a drenching.]

lithoconion (lith·o·**ko**·ne·on). An instrument used for the crushing of vesical calculi. [Gk *lithos* stone, *konis* dust.]

lithocystotomy (**lith**·o·sis·**tot'**·o·me). Lithotomy. [Gk *lithos* stone, cystotomy.]

lithocysturia (**lith**·o·sist·**ewr'**·e·ah). An affection of the bladder which results from the existence of lithuria. [Gk *lithos* stone, *kystis* bag, urine.]

lithodialysis (**lith**·o·di·**al'**·is·is). 1. Litholysis. 2. Lithotripsy. [Gk *lithos* stone, *dialysis* a loosing.]

lithodialytic (**lith**·o·di·al·**it'**·ik). Pertaining to lithodialysis.

lithogenesis (lith·o·**jen**·es·is). The origination and formation of calculi. [Gk *lithos* stone, *genein* to produce.]

lithogenous (lith·**oj**·en·us). Pertaining to lithogenesis.

lithogeny (lith·**oj**·en·e). Lithogenesis.

lithoid, lithoidal (**lith**·oid, lith·**oid**·al). Like a stone. [Gk *lithos* stone, *eidos* form.]

lithokelyphopaedion (**lith**·o·kel·e·fo·**pe'**·de·on). A lithopaedion in which the membranes also have become petrified. [lithopaedion, *kelyphos* shell.]

lithokelyphos (lith·o·**kel**·if·os). An embryonic mass in which only the fetal membranes are petrified, the fetus being unaffected. [Gk *lithos* stone, *kelyphos* shell.]

litholabe (**lith**·o·labe). An instrument used to grasp and hold a calculus in the urinary bladder during an operation for its extraction. [Gk *lithos* stone, *labein* to grasp.]

litholapaxy (lith·o·lap·**ax**′·e). The evacuation of the fragments of a vesical calculus after the stone has been crushed by a lithotrite. [Gk *lithos* stone, *lapaxis* evacuation.]

lithology (lith·**ol**·o·je). The science which is concerned with calculi in any of the organs of the body. [Gk *lithos* stone, *logos* science.]

litholysis (lith·**ol**·is·is). The dissolving of vesical calculi *in situ* by the use of drugs. [see foll.]

litholyte (**lith**·o·lite). An instrument of catheter pattern for the injection of calculary solvents into the urinary bladder. [Gk *lithos* stone, lysis.]

litholytic (lith·o·**lit**·ik). Relating to the solution of calculi in the bladder. [see prec.]

lithomalacia (**lith**·o·mal·**a**′·she·ah). Softening of a calculus in the urinary bladder or in any other bodily organ. [Gk *lithos* stone, *malakia* softness.]

lithometer (lith·**om**·et·er). A device for measuring the size of calculi of the bladder or of any other organ of the body. [Gk *lithos* stone, *metron* measure.]

lithometra (lith·o·**me**·trah). Conversion of the uterus in whole or in part into calcified matter, often referred to as *ossification.* [Gk *lithos* stone, *metra* womb.]

lithomyl (**lith**·o·mil). A lithotrite. [Gk *lithos* stone, *myle* mill.]

lithonephria (lith·o·**nef**·re·ah). The syndrome resulting from the existence of a calculus in the kidney. [Gk *lithos* stone, *nephros* kidney.]

lithonephritis (**lith**·o·nef·**ri**′·tis). Nephritis having origin in the irritation resulting from the presence of renal calculi. [Gk *lithos* stone, nephritis.]

lithonephrosis (**lith**·o·nef·**ro**′·sis). A condition characterized by the presence of gravel or of renal calculi. [Gk *lithos* stone, nephrosis.]

lithonephrotomy (lith·o·nef·**rot**′·o·me). Removal of a renal calculus by means of an incision into the kidney. [Gk *lithos* stone, *nephros* kidney, *temnein* to cut.]

lithopaedion (lith·o·**pe**·de·on). A dead fetus which has undergone calcification. [Gk *lithos* stone, *paidion* child.]

lithoscope (**lith**·o·skope). A device used in the inspection of vesical calculi. [Gk *lithos* stone, *skopein* to watch.]

lithosis (lith·o·sis). Grinders' rot. The type of pneumoconiosis which results from the occupation of steel-grinding and which is caused by exposure to fine particles of silica or other similar matter in the atmosphere of the workshop. [Gk *lithos* stone.]

Lithospermum ruderale (lith·o·**sper**·mum roo·der·**a**·le). A plant, the juice of which has been used by American Indians to reduce fertility. [Gk *lithos* stone, *sperma* seed, LL *ruderalis* growing in waste places.]

lithotome (**lith**·o·tome). A knife used in performing lithotomy.

lithotomist (lith·**ot**·o·mist). One expert in lithotomy.

lithotomy (lith·**ot**·o·me). Incision of the bladder for the removal of stone. **Bilateral lithotomy.** Transverse perineal incision with deep incisions through the lateral lobes of the prostate. **High lithotomy.** Suprapubic lithotomy (see below). **Lateral lithotomy.** The operation for the removal of stone from the bladder by incision of the perineum to one side of the midline. **Marian lithotomy, median lithotomy.** A perineal lithotomy practised by Mariano Santo di Barletta in the 16th century: the lithotomist employed a grooved staff, a knife with a sharp point and broad blade, and dilators which were the forerunners of the gorget. **Perineal lithotomy.** The usual approach in the operation for the cutting for stone as practised by lithotomists from the earliest times; it has been entirely replaced by suprapubic lithotomy. **Suprapubic lithotomy.** The approach normally used now for the removal of all bladder stones which are unsuitable for crushing, or which are contained in diverticula. [Gk *lithos* stone, *temnein* to cut.]

lithotony (lith·**ot**·o·ne). The establishment of an artificial fistula in the urinary bladder; this is dilated so that a calculus may be extracted. [Gk *lithos* stone, *teinein* to stretch.]

lithotresis (lith·o·**tre**·sis). The operation of drilling holes in a calculus preparatory to crushing and subsequent evacuation of the fragments. [Gk *lithos* stone, *tresis* a boring.]

lithotripsy (**lith**·o·trip·se). The operation of crushing a vesical calculus *in situ.* [Gk *lithos* stone, *tribein* to wear away.]

lithotriptic (lith·o·**trip**·tik). 1. Pertaining to lithotripsy. 2. Causing solution of calculi in the urinary bladder. 3. An agent which causes solution of calculi.

lithotriptor (lith·o·**trip**·tor). Lithotrite. [Gk *lithos* stone, *tribein* to wear away.]

lithotriptoscope (lith·o·**trip**·to·skope). A device used in lithotriptoscopy operations.

lithotriptoscopy (**lith**·o·trip·**tos**′·ko·pe). The operation of crushing, under direct visual control, a calculus in the urinary bladder, the lithotriptoscope being used. The fragments are subsequently removed. [Gk *lithos* stone, *tribein* to wear away, *skopein* to watch.]

lithotrite (**lith**·o·trite). An instrument used in performing lithotrity. **Cystoscopic lithotrite.** A lithotrite combined with a cystoscope. [Gk *lithos* stone, L *terere* to rub.]

See also: THOMPSON (G. R.).

lithotritic (lith·o·**trit**·ik). Relating to lithotrity.

lithotrity (lith·**ot**·rit·e). The operation of crushing a vesical calculus with the lithotrite. [Gk *lithos* stone, L *terere* to rub.]

lithous (**lith**·us). Stony in quality or with the constitution and features of a calculus. [Gk *lithos* stone.]

lithoxiduria, lithoxyduria (**lith**·ox·id·**ewr**′·e·ah). The presence of xanthine in the urine. [Gk *lithos* stone, oxide, urine.]

lithuresis (lith·**ewr**·e·sis). The passage of gravel during micturition. [Gk *lithos* stone, uresis.]

lithuria (lith·**ewr**·e·ah). A morbid condition marked by the presence of excessive amounts of uric acid or of urates in the urine. [lithium, urine.]

litmus (**lit**·mus). A blue colouring matter prepared from lichens, especially those of *Roccella* species, by treatment with ammonia. It contains azolitmin, erythrolitmin, and erythrolein: used as an indicator (pH 4.5–8.5), being red in acids and blue in alkalis. [corruption of G *Lakmus.*]

Litomosoides carinii (li·to·mo·**soi**′·deez kar·**in**·e·i). A filarial worm that infects the cotton rat *Sigmodon hispidus*: it has been used extensively in the experimental therapeutics of filariasis.

litrameter (le·**tram**·et·er). An instrument used to determine the specific gravity of a liquid. [Gk *litra* pound, meter.]

litre (**le**·ter). A unit of volume being 10 cubic decimetres (1.76 pints). Defined as the volume occupied by a mass of 1 kilogram of pure water, at its maximum density and at standard atmospheric pressure. [F.]

Litten, Moritz (b. 1845). Berlin physician.

Litten's diaphragm phenomenon, or sign. In a thin person lying on a bed with his feet towards a window, when he breathes slowly and deeply, a shadow can be seen passing down the lateral aspect of the chest between the lower ribs. It is produced by the diaphragmatic movement causing the intercostal spaces to fall in slightly on inspiration.

litter (**lit**·er). A couch fitted with handles which is used for carrying sick and wounded persons; a more elaborate form of stretcher. [Fr. *liter* to place in beds.]

Little, James Laurence (b. 1836). Vermont surgeon.

Little's area. The site of normal anastomosis, on the anterior part of the septum of the nose; it is the commonest site for epistaxis. The area is sometimes also called *Kiesselbach's area,* or the *tache anastomotique.*

Little, William John (b. 1810). London orthopaedic surgeon.

Little's disease. 1. A term used to cover all forms of congenital cerebral diplegia. 2. Little's paralysis (see below).

Little's paralysis. 1. Cerebral diplegia. 2. Acute anterior poliomyelitis; sometimes called *Little's disease,* more often *Heine-Medin disease.*

Stromeyer–Little operation. Evacuation of a chronic liver abscess which is located by a cannula and incised by a knife introduced along the cannula.

Littré, Alexis (b. 1658). Paris anatomist.

Littré's colotomy. Littré's operation (see below).

Littré's glands. Urethral glands. *See* GLAND.

Littré's hernia. Meckel's diverticulum in a hernia sac.

Littré's operation. Left inguinal colotomy.

Littré's sinus. The most anterior of the basilar group of venous sinuses of the cerebral cavity.

littreitis, littritis (lit·re·i·tis, lit·ri·tis). A condition of inflammation affecting the urethral (Littré's) glands. [Littré's gland, Gk *-itis* inflammation.]

Littrow spectograph. A special instrument in which, by means of mirrors, the same system of lenses serves both to collimate the light and focus the spectrum on the photographic plate.

Litzmann, Karl Conrad Theodor (b. 1815). Kiel obstetrician.

Litzmann's obliquity. Posterior parietal presentation in which the posterior parietal line of the fetal head presents over the brim of the pelvis. It is sometimes seen in patients with a flat pelvis.

livedo (liv·e·do). A livid mottling of the skin. **Livedo annularis.** Ring-shaped mottling due to cold. **Livedo calorica, livedo frigore.** Livedo due to heat or cold. **Livedo mechanica.** Livedo due to vascular stasis. **Livedo with nodulation.** Cutaneous polyarteritis nodosa. **Livedo racemosa.** Livedo reticularis (see below). **Livedo reticularis.** Reticular mottling due to cold. **Livedo reticularis annularis a frigore.** Livedo frigore (see above) with reticular and annular lesions. **Livedo reticularis idiopathica.** A reticular or annular purplish mottling of the skin, occurring in young people, chiefly on the limbs and more noticeable in the cold. **Livedo reticularis symptomatica.** A reticular or annular purplish mottling of the skin which may become persistent, seen in certain debilitating diseases, especially tuberculosis, syphilis, rheumatism, alcoholism, and hypothyroidism. **Livedo telangiectatica.** A permanent mottling of the skin due to widespread telangiectasia of the capillaries. **Livedo with ulceration.** A painful condition, usually affecting middle-aged women on the legs. There is livedo with painful purpura which ulcerates. It is disabling but not a threat to life. [L, a mottled spot.]

livedoid (liv·e·doid). Describing a type of dermatitis which resembles livedo. [livedo, Gk *eidos* form.]

liver [hepar (NA)] (liv·er). The largest gland in the body, occupying the upper part of the abdomen especially on the right side. It is reddish-brown in colour and friable in consistency, and roughly pyramidal in form. It has an investing peritoneal coat [tunica serosa (NA)] and an inner connective-tissue capsule [tunica fibrosa (NA)]. Its rounded upper surface is in contact with the diaphragm [pars superior (NA)]; its triangular anterior surface [pars anterior (NA)] with the diaphragm, lower chest wall and upper abdominal wall; its right surface [pars dextra (NA)] with the right side of the diaphragm; its posterior surface [pars posterior (NA)] is deeply concave due to the forward projection of the vertebral column, and its lower (visceral) surface faces downwards, backwards, and to the left, making contact with the upper abdominal organs and containing the porta hepatis. Its average weight in the adult is 1 800 g. It has many functions: it is the central organ of metabolism of carbohydrates, proteins, and fat; it stores glycogen and takes part in regulating blood sugar, and stores other essential substances such as vitamins and factors concerned in haemopoiesis. It synthesizes fibrinogen, prothrombin, heparin, and plasma proteins; it is a site of destruction of deteriorated red blood cells and it secretes bile. It is also the chief detoxicating organ of the body, rendering unwanted substances innocuous by conjugation with glucuronic acid or glycine, or with radicals such as acetyl or sulphate, or by oxidation or reduction. **Adipohepatic liver.** Fatty change of the liver cells. **Albuminous liver, amyloid liver.** The deposition of amyloid on the surface of, and eventually within, the liver cells, as the result of long-continued sepsis. **Beaver-tail liver.** A liver with an unusually large left lobe. **Biliary cirrhotic liver.** Biliary cirrhosis; an increase of fibrous tissue in the liver as the result of chronic infection or obstruction of the bile passages. **Border of the liver, lower [margo inferior (NA)].** The margin between the right and anterior surfaces above, and the lower surface below. **Bronze liver.** Pigmented changes in the liver, due to malaria. **Cardiac liver.** The liver of chronic venous congestion, as in cases of congestive heart failure or pressure on the upper part of the inferior vena cava. **Cirrhotic liver.** A liver showing overgrowth of the supporting connecting tissue from whatever cause. **Cod liver.** The liver of the cod, *Gadus morrhua*; it is of value for its content of fixed oil, rich in vitamin A. **Corset liver.** Tight-lace liver (see below). **Degraded liver.** A human liver that possesses an abnormal number of lobes. **Fatty liver.** Adipohepatic liver (see above). **Floating liver.** A dropped, unduly mobile liver. **Foamy liver.** An infection of the liver by anaerobes, leading to the development of a honeycomb appearance due to the formation of gas. **Frosted liver.** Chronic perihepatitis, resulting in the liver becoming covered with a shaggy fibrous layer resembling the icing on a cake; a form of polyserositis. **Gas-gangrene liver.** Foamy liver (see above). **Gin-drinkers' liver, hobnail liver.** Atrophic cirrhosis. *See* CIRRHOSIS. **Icing liver.** Frosted liver (see above). **Infantile liver.** Biliary cirrhosis of children. **Iron liver.** The liver in haemochromatosis; bronzed diabetes. **Lardaceous liver.** Amyloid liver (see above). **Lobe of the liver, caudate [lobus caudatus (NA)].** Part of the right lobe of the liver, lying between the fissure for the ligamentum venosum and the bare area of the liver. It projects into the upper recess of the lesser sac of the peritoneum. **Lobe of the liver, left [lobus hepatis sinister (NA)].** That part of the liver to the left of the falciform ligament, the fissure for the round ligament, and the fissure for the ligamentum venosum. **Lobe of the liver, quadrate [lobus quadratus (NA)].** The part of the right lobe enclosed between the gall bladder, the porta hepatis, the round ligament, and the lower border of the liver. **Lobe of the liver, right [lobus hepatis dexter (NA)].** That part of the liver to the right of the falciform ligament, the fissure for the round ligament, and the fissure for the ligamentum venosum. **Nutmeg liver.** Passive venous congestion, with fatty change, of the liver, which on section shows resemblance to a nutmeg. **Pigmented liver.** The deposition of pigment in the liver, as in haemochromatosis, malaria, or melanotic carcinoma. **Proteolysed liver.** A proteolysed liver preparation which has largely replaced ordinary liver extracts for oral administration in anaemia. **Sago liver.** A variety of amyloid liver (see above). **Scrofulous liver.** Amyloid liver (see above). **Stasis liver.** A passively congested liver from obstruction to venous outflow. **Sugar-icing liver.** Frosted liver (see above). **Surface of the liver, lower (or visceral) [facies visceralis (NA)].** The surface facing downwards and backwards. Part of the left lobe is in contact with the anterior surface of the stomach [impressio gastrica (NA)]. To the right of this is the tuber omentale which is in contact with the pancreas, lesser omentum intervening. The left lobe is separated from the right by the fissure for the round ligament in which lies the obliterated umbilical vein. Between this and the fossa for the gall bladder lies the quadrate lobe, above which is the porta hepatis. To the right of the gall bladder the ventral surfaces of the duodenum, right flexure of the colon, right suprarenal gland, and kidney make correspondingly named impressions on the inferior surface [impressiones duodenalis, colica, suprarenalis, renalis (NA)]. **Surface of the liver, upper (or diaphragmatic) [facies diaphragmatica (NA)].** The rounded upper surface of the liver in contact with the diaphragm. **Syphilitic liver.** The contracted and distorted nodular liver which eventually results from chronic syphilitic hepatitis. **Tight-lace liver.** A liver deformed by tight lacing. **Tropical liver.** A hepatotic, enlarged liver possibly induced by lack of exercise, over-eating, and alcohol, in the tropics. **Wandering liver.** Floating liver (see above). **Waxy liver.** Amyloid liver (see above). [AS *lifer.*]

liverwort (liv·er·wert). A member of a group of lower green plants, the non-vascular cryptogams, which reproduce by spores.

American liverwort. Hepatica. **English liverwort.** The lichen, *Peltigera canina* Hoffm., with demulcent properties and reputed to be of value in liver complaints. [liver, AS *wyrt* plant.]

livetin (li·vet·in). A phosphoglobulin, heat-coagulable and insoluble, which occurs in egg yolk, of which it constitutes about 25 per cent of the total protein.

livid (liv·id). Congested and discoloured as by a contusion. [L *lividus* bluish.]

lividity (liv·id·it·e). The condition of being livid; blue or red discoloration due to venous congestion in the dependent parts. **Cadaveric lividity, post-mortem lividity.** The livid staining of the skin in underlying parts owing to accumulation of fluid blood in the subcutaneous vessels.

Livingston binocular gauge. An instrument for measuring the power of convergence of the visual axis; a convergiometer.

livor (li·vor). Lividity. **Livor mortis.** A bluish-red spot or area caused by venous congestion of the dependent parts of a cadaver. [L, livid spot on the body.]

lixiviation (lix·iv·e·a'·shun). The process of washing out the soluble components of a mixture, leaving the insoluble portion behind. [L *lixivius* made of lye.]

lixivium (lix·iv·e·um). 1. Any solution obtained by lixiviation. 2. In particular, the solution of potash obtained by leaching wood ash. [see prec.]

Lizars, John (b. 1787). Edinburgh surgeon.

Lizars' operation. Excision of the upper jaw.

Lloyd-Davies, Oswald Vaughan (b. 1905). London surgeon.

Lloyd-Davies operation. Simultaneous combined removal of the pelvic colon, rectum and anus for carcinoma, one surgeon performing the abdominal part and another the perineal part.

Loa (lo·ah). A genus of filarial roundworms. **Loa inquirenda.** A species of doubtful authenticity, found in India in man. **Loa loa.** The eye worm, a common human parasite in tropical Africa. The adult female moves about in the subcutaneous tissues and intermuscular planes, sometimes round the eyes, while the embryos (microfilariae) are found in superficial blood vessels in the daytime. Intermediate hosts are flies of the genus *Chrysops*, the larvae developing in the muscles and migrating to the proboscis from which they enter the primary hosts. Calabar swellings are patches of giant urticaria which develop at sites where the adult worm has been damaged by pressure and has released allergenic body proteins. [West African name.]

loasis (lo·a·sis). Loiasis.

lobar (lo·bar). Relating to a lobe.

lobate (lo·bate). Having or arranged in lobes or rounded divisions.

lobe [lobus (NA)] (lobe). 1. A structural (morphological) division or subdivision of an organ, often demarcated by connective tissue or a fissure. 2. A projection, e.g. the appendicular lobe (see below). 3. A cusp on the crown of a tooth. **Appendicular lobe.** A tongue-shaped downward projection of the right lobe of the liver; Riedel's lobe. **Azygos lobe.** A small accessory lobe on the medial aspect of the apex of the right lung; a developmental anomaly in which the vena azygos with a fold of pleura becomes deeply embedded in the apex. Seen radiographically, the fissure forms a curved hair line, convex outwards, ending inferiorly in a pear-shaped shadow formed by the vena azygos. **Lobes of the cerebellum.** *See* CEREBELLUM. **Lobes of the cerebrum [lobi cerebri (NA)].** *See* CEREBRUM. **Flocculonodular lobe.** The posterior subdivision of the cerebellum, consisting of the nodulus centrally with a flocculus on either side. It is anatomically and functionally related to the vestibular apparatus, and is regarded as, phylogenetically, the oldest portion of the cerebellum. **Lobe of the hypophysis cerebri.** *See* HYPOPHYSIS. **Lacing lobe.** A lobe-like portion of the liver separated by a depression, caused by tight lacing, from the rest of the liver. **Linguiform lobe.** Appendicular lobe (see above). **Lobes of the liver.** *See* LIVER. **Lobes of the lung.** *See* LUNG. **Olfactory lobe.** A structure seen only in lower animals; in man its remnants are widely distributed in the cerebral hemispheres. **Optic lobes of the mid-brain.** The superior quadrigeminal bodies. *See* BODY. **Lobes of the prostate.** *See* PROSTATE. **Renal lobes [lobi renales (NA)].** A part of the kidney corresponding to a single renal pyramid, represented in the fetus and infant by a rounded elevation of the cortex, visible on the surface of the kidney. **Supplemental lobe.** An extra cusp on the crown of a tooth. **Lobe of the testis.** *See* TESTIS. **Lobes of the thymus.** *See* THYMUS. **Lobes of the thyroid gland.** *See* GLAND, THYROID. [Gk *lobos*.]

See also: HOME, RIEDEL, SPIEGHEL (SPIGELIUS).

lobectomy (lo·bek·to·me). The operation of excising one of the lobes of an organ such as the lung, brain, or thyroid gland. [lobe, Gk *ektome* a cutting out.]

lobelanidine (lo·bel·an·id·een). $C_{22}H_{29}O_2N$, a minor alkaloidal constituent of lobelia; the *nor*-alkaloid which occurs with it has the formula $C_{21}H_{27}O_2N$.

lobelanine (lo·bel·an·een). $C_{22}H_{25}O_2N$. A minor alkaloidal constituent of lobelia and next in importance to lobeline from which it may be produced by oxidation. The *nor*-alkaloid has the formula $C_{21}H_{23}O_2N$.

Lobelia (lo·be·le·ah). 1. A genus of herbs (family Campanulaceae), having an acrid milky juice. 2. (BPC 1968) Lobelia herb, Indian tobacco; the dried herb *Lobelia inflata* Linn., indigenous to North America. It contains a mixture of alkaloids of which the most important is lobeline. In small doses it is expectorant, and is used in the treatment of spasmodic asthma and bronchitis; larger doses are emetic and may cause paralysis of the medulla. [Mathias de *Lobel*, 1538–1616, Flemish botanist.]

lobeline (lo·bel·een). $C_{22}H_{27}O_2N$, the principal alkaloid of lobelia with pharmacological actions rather like nicotine, being first a stimulant and then a depressant of autonomic ganglia. It is occasionally used as an expectorant in bronchitis. **Lobeline Hydrochloride BPC 1968.** The hydrochloride of α-lobeline, used in the treatment of respiratory depression caused by poisoning. It has also been employed in the treatment of asthma. Owing to its unreliability and toxicity, its use is limited.

lobelism (lo·be·lizm). Lobelia poisoning.

lobi (lo·bi). *See* LOBUS.

lobite (lo·bite). Confined to a lobe; used in describing certain forms of pulmonary tuberculosis.

lobitis (lo·bi·tis). A condition of inflammation affecting the lobe of an organ, in particular one of the lobes of a lung. [lobe, Gk *-itis* inflammation.]

Loboa loboi (lo·bo·ah lo·bo·i). The causal organism of lobomycosis.

lobocyte (lo·bo·site). An obsolete name for a granular leucocyte. [Gk *lobos* lobe, *kytos* cell.]

lobomycosis (lo·bo·mi·ko'·sis). A chronic infection of the skin resulting in fibrous tumours or keloids. Although the keloids are filled with catenulate, round, budding, thick-walled cells, the organism has never been isolated in culture, nor has it yet been possible to infect laboratory animals with the organism using macerated, infected tissue from human cases. The organism has been tentatively named *Loboa loboi*.

lobopodium (lo·bo·po·de·um). A pseudopodium which is fluid within the confining membrane, as in the amoeba. Cf. AXOPODIUM. [Gk *lobos* lobe, *pous* foot.]

lobose (lo·boze). Lobate.

lobotomy (lo·bot·o·me). Literally, the cutting of a lobe; but referring specifically to the cutting of the connections of the anterior part of the frontal lobe of the cerebrum by the passage of a blunt instrument, such as a brain needle, spatula, or similar instrument (leucotome) specially designed for the purpose, and introduced through a burr-hole in the skull. The operation has been undertaken for certain forms of mental disease and for diseases with a hopeless prognosis accompanied by severe pain (e.g. carcinomatosis). It is a USA synonym for *leucotomy*, both words being commonly used with the prefix *prefrontal* or *frontal*. [lobe, Gk *temnein* to cut.]

lobous (lo·bus). Lobate.

Lobstein, Jean Georges Chrétien Frédéric Martin (b. 1777). Strasbourg surgeon.

Lobstein's cancer. Retroperitoneal sarcoma. *See* SARCOMA.

Lobstein's fracture. Osteogenesis imperfecta of the post-natal type.

Lobstein's ganglion. A small nerve ganglion on the greater splanchnic nerve.

Lobstein's syndrome. Osteogenesis imperfecta.

lobster-claw (lob·ster·klaw). Split hand or split foot. *See* HAND, FOOT.

lobular (lob·ew·lar). Referring to, made up of, or like lobules.

lobulated (lob·ew·la·ted). Composed of or arranged in lobules.

lobule [lobulus (NA)] (lob·ewl). A lobe, or subdivision of a part (macro- or microscopic) circumscribed by more or less obvious boundaries such as sulci or septa. **Ansiform lobule [lobulus simplex (NA)].** The lobule forming part of the cerebellum. **Ansiform lobule, inferior surface of the [lobulus semilunaris inferior (NA)].** The posterior three-quarters of the under-surface of the cerebellar hemispheres, lying behind and lateral to the tonsil. **Ansiform lobule, superior surface of the [lobulus semilunaris superior (NA)].** The posterior part of the upper surface of the cerebellar hemispheres, behind the postlunate fissure. **Lobule of the auricle [lobulus auriculae (NA)].** The fleshy portion of the ear below the antitragus. **Biventral lobule [lobulus biventer (NA)].** A lobule on the lower surface of the cerebellum. **Central lobule [lobulus centralis (NA)].** The intermediate part of the vermis portion of the anterior lobe of the cerebellum, between the postlingual and postcentral fissures. **Cerebellar lobule.** Any one of the subdivisions of the vermis and lateral hemispheres of the cerebellum. With a few exceptions, they have no functional significance. Included are, biventral lobule, central lobule, lobulus clivi, crescentic lobule, lobulus culminis, ensiform lobule, floccular lobule, lobulus folii, lunate lobules, paracentral lobule, senilunar lobule, and lobulus tuberis. **Cortical lobules of the kidney [lobuli corticales (NA)].** Polygonal areas on the surface of the renal cortex; they are the surface indication of underlying medullary rays with their attendant malpighian corpuscles and tubules. **Lobules of the epididymis [lobuli epididymidis (coni epididymidis) NA].** Tubules, continuous with the efferent ductules of the testis, which form small conical coiled masses in the head of the epididymis. **Lobule of the liver [lobulus hepatis (NA)].** A histological subdivision of the liver, consisting of columns of cells radiating from a central vein. In man, they merge with one another. **Lunate lobule, anterior [lobulus quadrangularis (NA)].** The lateral extension of the lobulus culminis on to the cerebellar hemispheres. **Lunate lobule, posterior.** The region of the superior surface of the lateral lobes of the cerebellum between the fissura prima and the post-lunate fissure. **Lobules of the lung.** Subdivisions of the lung, produced by the passage into its interior of septal processes from the surface layer of fibrous tissue. **Lobule of a mammary gland.** *See* GLAND, MAMMARY. **Paracentral lobule [lobulus paracentralis (NA)].** A subdivision of the medial surface of the cerebral hemisphere bounded below by the sulcus cinguli and above by the superomedial border. The upper end of the central sulcus may cut into it. **Parietal lobule.** Any one of two, superior [lobulus parietalis superior (NA)], and inferior [lobulus parietalis inferior (NA)], divisions of the superolateral surface of the parietal lobe of the cerebrum, lying respectively above and below the intraparietal sulcus. The inferior lobule has an anterior part [gyrus supramarginalis (NA)], middle part [gyrus angularis (NA)], and posterior part. **Quadrate lobule.** The precuneus. **Lobule of the testis.** Lobe of the testis. *See* TESTIS. **Lobule of the thymus.** *See* THYMUS. **Lobules of the thyroid gland.** *See* GLAND, THYROID. [L *lobulus* small lobe.]

See also: MALL.

lobulet, lobulette (lob·ew·let). 1. A very small lobule. 2. One of the primary divisions of a lobule. [Fr., small lobule.]

lobulose, lobulous (lob·ew·loze, lob·ew·lus). Disposed in, or provided with lobules.

lobulus (lob·ew·lus). Lobule. **Lobulus clivi [declive (NA)].** The anterior of the two parts of the middle lobe of the cerebellum that extend on to the superior vermis. **Lobulus culminis [culmen (NA)].** The region of the vermis portion of the anterior lobe that is visible on the upper surface of the cerebellum, lying between the postcentral fissure and the fissura prima. **Lobulus folii.** The posterior of the two parts of the middle lobe of the cerebellum that extend on to the superior vermis. **Lobulus tuberis [tuber vermis (NA)].** The most posterior part of the four subdivisions of the middle lobe of the cerebellum that lie in the inferior vermis. [L.]

lobus (lo·bus) (pl. *lobi*). A lobe. **Lobus placentae.** One of the polygonal areas visible on the maternal surface of the shed placenta. [Gk *lobos*.]

See also: SPIEGHEL (SPIGELIUS).

local (lo·kal). Not generally or systemically distributed; confined to one part or spot. [L *locus* place.]

localization (lo·kal·i·za'·shun). 1. The assignment of a function or lesion to a particular site in an organ, or in the body as a whole. 2. The determination of the site of a biological function. 3. The determination of the position of any x-ray-opaque object in the body by radiography. **Cerebral localization.** 1. The assignment to a defined position in the brain of a given faculty or function. 2. The determination of the site in the brain at which control is exercised over given physiological functions. **Elective localization.** Selective localization (see below). **Experimental localization.** Determination of the position of nerve centres by means of experiment. **Selective localization.** The predilection which certain micro-organisms have for certain tissues, e.g. *Shigella* for the large intestine, virus of poliomyelitis for the central nervous system. [L *locus* place.]

localize (lo·kal·ize). To restrict to one definite part or place. [see prec.]

localizer (lo·kal·i·zer). A term applied to any of the various devices for localizing the position of intra-ocular or other foreign bodies, generally from x-ray films taken in different positions. [L *locus* place.]

locative (lok·at·iv). Noting the position of any item in relation to another in a series. [L *locare* to place.]

lochia (lo·ke·ah). The normal discharge from the cavity of the uterus following either delivery or abortion. It is made up of blood, mucus, leucocytes, fibrin, and necrotic tissue. **Lochia alba.** The white discharge which occurs about a fortnight after delivery, and persists for about 3 weeks. **Lochia purulenta.** Lochia alba (see above). **Lochia rubra.** The red discharge from the uterus, which occurs for about 4 to 5 days after delivery or abortion. It may persist longer in some cases. **Lochia serosa.** Later in the puerperium, the lochia which has turned from a red to a brown colour. [Gk *lochos* childbirth.]

lochial (lo·ke·al). Referring to the lochia.

lochiocolpos (lo·ke·o·kol'·pos). A state of distension in the vagina caused by arrested discharge of the lochia. [lochia, Gk *kolpos* pocket.]

lochiometra (lo·ke·o·me'·trah). Congestion of the cavity of the uterus caused by non-evacuation or retention of the lochia. [lochia, Gk *metra* womb.]

lochiometritis (lo·ke·o·me·tri'·tis). Metritis occurring after childbirth. [lochia, metritis.]

lochioperitonitis (lo·ke·o·per·e·ton·i'·tis). Puerperal peritonitis. *See* PERITONITIS. [lochia, peritonitis.]

lochiopyra (lok·e·o·pi'·rah). Puerperal fever. *See* FEVER. [lochia, Gk *pyr* fire.]

lochiorrhagia, lochiorrhoea (lo·ke·o·ra'·je·ah, lo·ke·o·re'·ah). A copious discharge of lochia. [lochia, Gk *rhegnynein* to gush forth, *rhoia* flow.]

lochioschesis (lo·ke·os·ke·sis). Non-discharge of the lochia. [lochia, Gk *schesis* a holding fast.]

lochiostasis (lo·ke·os·tas·is). Retention of the lochia. [lochia, Gk *stasis* a standing still.]

Locke, Frank Spiller (b. 1871). London physiologist.

Locke's solution, Ringer-Locke solution. An aqueous solution of the following percentage composition: sodium chloride 0.9, potassium chloride 0.042, calcium chloride 0.024, sodium bicarbonate 0.01 to 0.03, glucose 0.1 to 0.25, water to 100. This solution is useful for experiments on the mammalian heart, and other physiological experiments.

Locke's citrated solution. A solution of the following composition: sodium chloride 9.2 g, potassium chloride 0.5 g, calcium chloride 0.1 g, sodium citrate 10 g, distilled water to 1 000 ml. It is autoclaved and adjusted to pH 7.4.

Lockhart-Mummery, John Percy (b. 1875). British surgeon.

Lockhart-Mummery perineal excision. Perineal excision of the rectum with permanent colostomy.

lockjaw (**lok**·jaw). Tetanus. [AS *loc*, jaw.]

Lockwood, Charles Barrett (b. 1856). British surgeon and anatomist.

Lockwood's hiatus muscularis. A series of deficiencies in the muscle coats of the vermiform appendix through which the lymphatics of the submucosa pass into the meso-appendix.

Lockwood's ligament. The suspensory ligament of the eyeball; a portion of the fascia of the orbit derived from the sheaths of the lateral, medial, and inferior rectus muscles which is slung like a hammock beneath the eyeball.

locoism (lo·ko·izm). Loco poisoning. *See* POISONING. [Sp. *loco* mad.]

locomotion (lo·ko·**mo**·shun). Motion or the power of motion from one place to another. **Locomotion of an artery.** The uncurving of an artery under the influence of the pulse wave. **Quadruped locomotion.** Locomotion on hands and feet, the only means of locomotion available to persons suffering from certain very severe forms of tuberculosis of the vertebral column. [L *locus* place, *motio* movement.]

locomotive (lo·ko·**mo**·tiv). Relating to locomotion.

locomotor (lo·ko·**mo**·tor). Of or relating to locomotion.

locomotorial (lo·ko·mo·**tor**'·e·al). Belonging to the locomotorium.

locomotorium (lo·ko·mo·**tor**'·e·um). The locomotor system; the mechanism in any organism concerned with movement.

locomotory (lo·ko·**mo**·tor·e). Relating to or having locomotion.

locular (**lok**·ew·lar). Relating to a loculus; possessed of cells or loculi.

loculate, loculated (**lok**·ew·late, **lok**·ew·la·ted). Having loculi or separated into a number of loculi.

loculation (lok·ew·**la**·shun). The presence of numerous loculi.

loculus (**lok**·ew·lus) (pl. *loculi*). A small cavity or space. [L, little place.]

locum tenens (**lo**·kum **te**·nens). A medical practitioner who acts as deputy for another. [L *locus* place, *tenens* holding.]

locus (**lo**·kus). 1. General term for the place at which anything is present or any action occurs. 2. In genetics, the position on a chromosome at which one of a series of allelomorphs will be present. **Locus ceruleus [locus ceruleus (NA)].** A groove along the lateral boundary of the eminentia medialis. **Locus minoris resistentiae.** The place of least resistance; an organ or tissue most likely to be attacked by a particular disease. [L, place.]

locust (**lo**·kust). A member of one of a number of large species of grasshoppers, which under certain circumstances form aggregations and migrate over long distances either as nymphs, called *hoppers*, or as winged adults. [L *locusta*.]

lodestone (**lode**·stone). *See* MAGNET. [AS *lad* journey, *stan* stone.]

Loeb, Leo (b. 1869). Washington pathologist.

Loeb's deciduoma. The production in an experimental animal of the maternal part of the placenta as the result of administration of progesterone.

Loeffler, Friedrich August Johannes (b. 1852). Berlin bacteriologist.

Loeffler's blue or methylene-blue solution. A saturated alcoholic solution of methylene blue 30 ml, 1:10 000 potassium hydroxide in water 100 ml.

Loeffler's serum medium. Three parts serum (ox, sheep or horse) to one part nutrient broth, sterilized in an inspissator or a steam sterilizer; useful for cultivation of the diphtheria bacillus which grows rapidly and shows characteristic staining by Neisser's or Albert's methods.

Klebs–Loeffler bacillus. *Corynebacterium diphtheriae.*

Schuetz–Loeffler bacillus. *Pfeifferella (Malleomyces) mallei.*

Loeffler, Wilhelm (b. 1887). Basle physician.

Loeffler's eosinophilia, pneumonia, or syndrome. A syndrome characterized clinically by cough, breathlessness, loss of appetite and loss of weight, but seldom any definite physical signs or fever; radiologically there are small soft shadows not unlike those seen in silicosis, but quite transient; and there is always a marked eosinophilia.

Loefflerella (lef·ler·**el**'·ah). A bacterial genus in the family Pseudomonadaceae; slender, pleomorphic, Gram-negative, non-motile and non-sporing rods. There are two pathogenic species: *Loefflerella mallei*, the causal organism of glanders in equines, and *L. pseudomallei*, the causal organism of a glanders-like disease in rodents, particularly in South-East Asia. Man may be infected by rat-contaminated food or possibly the rat flea, and the disease manifests as an acute lung infection followed by widespread miliary abscesses. [Friedrich A. J. *Loeffler*.]

loeffleria (lef·**leer**·e·ah). A morbid condition in which the *Corynebacterium diphtheriae* (Klebs–Loeffler bacillus) is present, although the characteristic symptoms of diphtheria are absent.

loemaemia (le·**me**·me·ah). The presence of *Pasteurella pestis* organisms in the blood, plague of septicaemic type. [Gk *loimos* plague, *haima* blood.]

loemic (**le**·mik). Pertaining to plague or any other epidemic disease. [Gk *loimos* plague.]

loemology (le·**mol**·o·je). The branch of medical science which is concerned with epidemic and contagious diseases, such as plague. [Gk *loimos* plague, *logos* science.]

loempe (**lem**·pe). Beriberi.

loeschia (**le**·she·ah). A rare synonym of *Entamoeba.*

loeschiasis (le·**shi**·as·is). Amoebiasis.

Loewe, Karl Friedrich (b. 1874). Berlin optician.

Loewe's ring. A circle of light which appears in the visual field when illumination is changed from blue to white. It surrounds the position of the macula lutea.

Loewenberg, Benjamin Benno (b. 1836). Vienna and Paris otologist.

Loewenberg's canal or scala. The duct of the cochlea.

Loewenstein, Ernst (b. 1878). Vienna pathologist.

Loewenstein's ointment. *See* LOEWENSTEIN'S VACCINATION (below).

Loewenstein's vaccination. An attempt to produce immunity against diphtheria by inunction with *Loewenstein's ointment*, a preparation of dead bacilli and toxoid.

Loewenstein–Jensen culture medium. A medium containing egg, potato, and malachite green. It is used for the culture of *Mycobacterium tuberculosis.*

Loewenthal, Nathan (fl. 1885). Lausanne histologist.

Loewenthal's marginal bundle. Part of the anterolateral white column of the spinal cord. Loewenthal considered that there is a bundle in this situation that consists of fibres running from the homolateral cerebellar cortex to the spinal cord; such a bundle is not generally considered to exist.

Loewenthal's tract. The tectospinal tract.

Loewi, Otto (b. 1873). Graz and New York pharmacologist.

Loewi reaction, or sign. Three drops of 1 in 1 000 adrenaline solution are instilled on to the conjunctiva: dilation of the pupil in from half to one hour suggests irritability of the sympathetic system, and is frequent in both pancreatic disease and hyperthyroidism.

Loewit, Moritz (b. 1851). Innsbruck pathologist.

Loewit's formic acid method. A method employing formic acid and gold chloride for the demonstration of nerve endings.

Lofepramine (lo·**fee**·pram·een). BP Commission approved name for 5 - (3[*N* - (4 - chlorophenacyl)methylamino]propyl) - 10,11 - dihydrodibenz[*b,f*]azepine; an antidepressant.

logadectomy (log·ad·**ek**·to·me). Partial excision of the conjunctiva. [Gk *logades* whites of the eyes, *ektome* a cutting out.]

logades (**log**·ad·eez). The whites of the eyes; the sclera. [Gk.]

logaditis (log·ad·**i**·tis). Scleritis. [Gk *logades* whites of the eyes, *-itis* inflammation.]

logadoblennorrhoea (log·ad·o·blen·or·e′·ah). Conjunctival blennorrhoea. [Gk *logades* whites of the eyes, blennorrhoea.]

logagnosia (log·ag·no·se·ah). Alexia. [Gk *logos* word, agnosia.]

logagraphia (log·a·graf·e·ah). Agraphia; inability to put into written words ideas present in the mind; loss of the writing power. [Gk *logos* word, agraphia.]

logamnesia (log·am·ne·ze·ah). Auditory or visual aphasia; word deafness, word blindness. [Gk *logos* word, amnesia.]

logaphasia (log·af·a·ze·ah). Motor aphasia; generally caused by a cerebral lesion. [Gk *logos* word, aphasia.]

logasthenia (log·as·the·ne·ah). Impairment of the mental faculty which is concerned with understanding of the spoken word. [Gk *logos* word, asthenia.]

logoclonia (log·o·klo·ne·ah). Irregular repetition of the last syllable of a word. [Gk *logos* word, *klonein* to agitate.]

logographic (log·o·graf·ik). Relating to written words. [Gk *logos* word, *graphein* to record.]

logokophosis (log·o·ko·fo′·sis). Auditory aphasia; loss of power of understanding what is said. [Gk *logos* word, *kophos* deaf.]

logomania (log·o·ma·ne·ah). 1. Garrulity so excessive that it constitutes a form of mania; in many cases new words are invented to keep up the flow of talk. 2. Aphasia. [Gk *logos* word, mania.]

logoneurosis (log·o·newr·o′·sis). 1. Any neurotic condition which is associated with a speech defect. 2. A neurotic condition associated with impaired mental faculties. [Gk *logos* word, neurosis.]

logopaedia, logopaedics (log·o·pe·de·ah, log·o·pe·dix). That branch of medical science which is concerned with the general physiological and pathological aspect of the speech organs and with the study and correction of defects of speech. [Gk *logos* word, *pais* child.]

logopathy (log·op·ath·e). 1. Any speech disorder which is caused by a central-nerve lesion. 2. Logoneurosis. [Gk *logos* word, *pathos* disease.]

logophasia (log·o·fa·ze·ah). Loss of ability to articulate correctly. [Gk *logos* word, *phasis* utterance.]

logoplegia (log·o·ple·je·ah). 1. Any type of paralysis which affects the organs of speech. 2. Failure to utter words although the latter are not actually forgotten; a defect of the mechanism of word production. [Gk *logos* word, *plege* stroke.]

logorrhoea (log·o·re·ah). Garrulity to an excessive degree. [Gk *logos* word, *rhoia* flow.]

logospasm (log·o·spazm). A condition in which words are produced in spasms; speech tending to be of explosive type and stuttering in character. [Gk *logos* word, spasm.]

logwood (log·wud). 1. The tree *Haematoxylon campechianum* Linn. 2. Haematoxylum. [ME *logge, wudu.*]

Lohmann, Karl (b. 1898). Berlin biochemist.

Lohmann reaction. The high-energy transfer of a phosphate radical from adenosine triphosphate to creatine, or to adenosine diphosphate from creatine phosphate.

loiasis (lo·i·as·is). The condition caused by infection with the helminth *Loa loa*, conveyed by bites of flies of the genus *Chrysops*, and found especially in the Cameroons.

loin [lumbus (NA)] (loin). That portion of the body on both sides of the spine which is between the false ribs and the upper plane of the pelvis; the flank. [OFr. *logne.*]

loliism, lolism (lo·le·izm, lo·lizm). Poisoning by the seeds of *Lolium temulentum* which is said to contain an alkaloid, although it has also been stated that the toxicity is due to a fungus. Symptoms of vertigo, dizziness, headache, and impaired vision are produced.

Lombard, Etienne (b. 1868). French physician.

Lombard's test. For simulated unilateral deafness: a Bárány noise box is applied to the allegedly good ear. The patient is asked to read aloud from a newspaper. The noise box is switched on. A patient with a severe degree of deafness in the opposite ear will immediately raise his voice and may even shout; a malingerer will continue to read in the same even tone.

Lombardi, Antonio (fl. 1910). Naples physician.

Lombardi's sign. Dilated venules over the spines of the 7th cervical and first three dorsal vertebrae in early pulmonary tuberculosis.

Lomholt, Svend (b. 1888). Copenhagen dermatologist.

Lomholt's ointment. Unguentum potassii polysulphidi.

Finsen–Lomholt lamp. A lamp that emits ultraviolet rays of wavelength mainly from 3 300 to 3 600 Å (330–360 nm); the light rays are all filtered out and the heat rays absorbed. The ultraviolet rays constitute 75 per cent of the total, and the irradiation time is only one-third of that required with the Finsen lamp.

Finsen–Lomholt treatment. Treatment of lupus vulgaris by filtered ultraviolet rays emanating from a Finsen–Lomholt lamp; obsolescent.

lonchocarpus (long·ko·kar′·pus). Cube root, barbasco, timbo; the dried root of species of *Lonchocarpus* (family Leguminosae). It contains about 3 per cent of the insecticide, rotenone, and is used for the same purposes as derris root; it is also employed in scabies. [Gk *lonche* spear, *karpos* fruit.]

long-acting thyroid stimulator (LATS). An IgG immunoglobulin which binds to thyroid membranes at a site close to or identical with the TSH receptor. It is found in the serum of patients with Graves' disease and it, rather than TSH, is probably the cause of the hyperthyroidism in this condition. **LATS absorbing activity (LAA).** A neutralizing factor which is found in thyroid microsomes and cell sap. **LATS protector** (LATS P). An immunoglobulin found in the serum of hyperthyroid patients with Graves' disease. It inhibits the absorption of LATS by LAA (LATS absorbing activities) and can pass through the placenta and induce neonatal hyperthyroidism similar to that produced by LATS in hyperthyroid mothers. This new type of neonatal hyperthyroidism is associated with absence of LATS in the maternal serum.

longevity (lon·jev·it·e). Long life. [L *longus* long, *aevum* age.]

longilineal (lon·je·lin·e·al). Referring to a slight and long type of bodily build. [L *longus* long, line.]

longimanous (lon·je·man·us). Having long, slender hands. [L *longus* long, *manus* hand.]

longing (long·ing). An eager desire or craving, very often for some unusual kind of food, or even for inedible material, as is often observed in pregnancy. Some form of abnormal longing may also be noted in persons who are neurotic or mentally unstable. [AS *langian.*]

longipedate (lon·je·ped·ate). Having long, narrow feet. [L *longus* long, *pes* foot.]

longissimus muscle [musculus longissimus (NA)] (lon·jis·im·us musl). A muscle which forms the intermediate column of the sacrospinalis muscle and is composed from below upwards of the longissimus thoracis, longissimus cervicis, and longissimus capitis muscles. [L, longest.]

longissimus capitis muscle [musculus longissimus capitis (NA)] (lon·jis·im·us kap·it·is musl). A part of the longissimus muscle attached to the skull. [L, longest of the head.]

longissimus cervicis muscle [musculus longissimus cervicis (NA)] (lon·jis·im·us ser·vis·is musl). A part of the longissimus muscle attached to the cervical vertebrae. [L, longest of the neck.]

longissimus thoracis muscle [musculus longissimus thoracis (NA)] (lon·jis·im·us thor·as·is musl). One of the elements of the longissimus muscle mass which is inserted by two series of slips; medially into the transverse processes of the thoracic vertebrae and the transverse and accessory processes of the lumbar vertebrae, and laterally into the ribs. It is supplied by posterior rami of thoracic and lumbar nerves, and is an extensor of the spine. [L, longest of the thorax.]

longitudinal [longitudinalis (NA)] (lon·je·tew·din·al). Running lengthwise; in a direction parallel to the long axis of the body. [L *longitudo* length.]

longitypical (lon·je·tip·ik·al). Longilineal. [L *longus* long, type.]

Longmire, William Polk (b. 1913). Los Angeles surgeon.

Longmire's operation. The use of the left hepatic duct, after resection of the left lobe of liver, to replace a congenitally obliterated common hepatic duct.

longus capitis muscle [musculus longus capitis (NA)] (**long**·gus **kap**·it·is musl). One of the prevertebral muscles. It arises from the anterior tubercles of the transverse processes of the 3rd, 4th, 5th, and 6th cervical vertebrae, and is inserted into the inferior surface of the basilar portion of the occipital bone, lateral to the pharyngeal tubercle. It is supplied by the 2nd, 3rd, and 4th cervical nerves. [L, long of the head.]

longus cervicis muscle [musculus longus colli] (**long**·gus **ser**·vis·is musl). One of the prevertebral muscles, divisible into three portions. The inferior oblique portion arises from the front of the bodies of the upper three thoracic vertebrae and is inserted into the anterior tubercles of the 5th and 6th cervical vertebrae. The vertical portion arises from the bodies of the upper three thoracic, and lower three cervical vertebrae, and is inserted into the 2nd, 3rd, and 4th cervical vertebrae. The superior oblique portion arises from the anterior tubercles of the 3rd, 4th, and 5th cervical vertebrae and is inserted into the anterior tubercle of the atlas. The three parts are supplied by the cervical nerves from the 2nd to the 8th inclusive. [L, long of the neck.]

Loomis, Alfred Lebbeus (b. 1831). New York pathologist.

Loomis' mixture. A diarrhoea mixture containing sassafras oil, tincture of opium, tincture of rhubarb, tincture of gambir, and lavender oil.

loop (loop). 1. A turn or bend in a thread or line; a bend in a wire. 2. One of the patterns formed by the dermal ridges on the finger tips. This is characterized by the presence of a triradius and a central core. The loop may be open laterally or medially and can therefore be called *radial* or *ulnar*. **Bulboventricular loop.** A U-shaped loop of the embryonic heart tube, comprising the bulbus cordis on the right and the primitive ventricle on the left. It lies in front of the primitive atrium and sinus venosus. **D-loop, dextro-loop.** Terms used to describe the normally developing primitive cardiac tube which loops to the right so that the morphological right ventricle forms on that side. **L-loop, laevo-loop.** Terms used to describe an abnormally developing primitive cardiac tube which loops to the left, instead of the normal right, so that the morphologically right ventricle develops on the left side of the heart, forming the apex. **Platinum loop.** A platinum wire, bent to form a loop at the end and mounted in a holder; used to transfer bacterial cultures. **X-loop.** The term applied to the developing primitive cardiac tube which has given rise to a form of ventricular and great-vessel anatomy which cannot be explained in terms of a postulated D-loop or L-loop (see above). [ME *loupe*.]

See also: HENLE, HYRTL.

loopful (**loop**·ful). The amount of liquid which can be retained within the platinum loop employed in the transference of bacterial cultures. [see prec.]

Looser, Emil (b. 1877). Zürich surgeon.

Looser's transformation zone. A transverse translucent band up to 1 cm in width, seen radiographically in bones affected with osteomalacia or certain other deficiency diseases, often symmetrical.

Loperamide (lo·**per**·am·ide). BP Commission approved name for 4 - (4 - *p* - chlorophenyl - 4 - hydroxypiperidino) - *N,N* - dimethyl - 2,2 - diphenylbutyramide; an antidiarrhoeal agent.

lophocomi (lo·**fok**·o·me). In anthropology, a subdivision of ulotriches, one of Haeckel's two main types of mankind, indicating races with tufted hair, e.g. Hottentots. [Gk *lophos* tuft, *kome* the hair of the head.]

lophodont (lo·fo·dont). A cheek tooth which has transverse ridges on its occlusal surface. [Gk *lophos* tuft, *odous* tooth.]

Lophophora (lo·**fof**·or·ah). A genus of Mexican cactus.

Lophophora williamsii. A species of cactus from which many alkaloids have been recovered, some of which have been used medicinally. [Gk *lophos* tuft, *pherein* to carry.]

lophotrichate, lophotrichous (lo·**fot**·rik·ate, lo·**fot**·rik·us). Terms used to describe a micro-organism with a tuft of flagella at one pole or at both poles. [Gk *lophos* tuft, *thrix* hair.]

loquacity (lo·**kwas**·it·e). The habit of being excessively garrulous; extreme talkativeness. The condition is often present in persons with certain types of disordered mentality. [L *loquacitas* talkativeness.]

Lorain, Paul Joseph (b. 1827). Paris physician.

Lorain disease, or syndrome, Lévi-Lorain disease, dwarfism, infantilism, type, Lorain-Lévi syndrome. Pituitary infantilism; a condition in which a child does not grow, but is perfectly formed with all the proportions symmetrically diminished. The adult at first sight resembles a child, but the shape is that of an adult in miniature. Sexual organs are immature, but intelligence is not impaired. Due to lack of growth hormone. The eponymous description is seldom now used.

Lorazepam (lor·**az**·e·pam). BP Commission approved name for 7 - chloro - 5 - (2 - chlorophenyl) - 1,3 - dihydro - 3 - hydroxy - 1,4 - benzodiazepin - 2 - one; a tranquillizer.

Lord, Jere Williams (b. 1910). New York surgeon.

Blakemore-Lord operation. Vascular anastomosis with use of a vitallium cuff, the *Blakemore-Lord tube*, the proximal vascular segment being passed through the cuff, which is then inserted in the distal segment; the method is particularly applicable to venous anastomosis, e.g. portacaval shunt.

Blakemore-Lord tube. A vitallium tube devised to facilitate vascular suture, by approximating intima to intima without any intervening foreign body in the Blakemore-Lord operation.

lordoma (lor·**do**·mah). Lordosis.

lordoscoliosis (**lor**·do·sko·le·o′·sis). Combined lordosis and scoliosis.

lordosis (lor·**do**·sis). A form of spinal curvature in which the curve is in a forward direction, generally in the lumbar region. [Gk *lordos* bent so as to be convex in front.]

lordotic (lor·**dot**·ik). Pertaining to lordosis.

Lorenz, Adolf (b. 1854). Vienna orthopaedic surgeon.

Lorenz's method, Hoffa-Lorenz operation. A manipulative procedure for the reduction of congenital dislocation of the hip.

Lorenz's operation, or osteotomy. An operation for unreduced congenital dislocation of the hip: an oblique subtrochanteric osteotomy of the femur is performed, and the lower fragment displaced into the acetabulum.

Loriga's disease. Pneumatic-hammer disease. *See* DISEASE.

Loring, Edward Greely (b. 1837). New York ophthalmologist.

Loring's ophthalmoscope. An ophthalmoscope incorporating a disc of graduated lenses together with a supplemental quadrant of lenses which can be introduced when desired.

Lorrain Smith, James (b. 1862). Edinburgh pathologist.

Lorrain Smith stain. The use of Nile-blue sulphate as a fat stain in frozen sections.

loss (los). **Dissociated sensory loss.** Loss of pain and thermal sensation with retention of touch, as in a lesion of the spinothalamic tract.

Lossen, Herman Friedrich (b. 1842). Heidelberg surgeon.

Lossen's law, or rule. Only females transmit, and only males inherit, haemophilia.

Lossen's operation. Section of the second division of the 5th cranial nerve for trigeminal neuralgia.

Lotheissen, Georg (b. 1868). Innsbruck and Vienna surgeon.

Lotheissen's operation. Repair of femoral hernia through an incision above the inguinal ligament.

Lotheissen's point. A point situated 5 cm below McBurney's point at right angles to the right spino-umbilical line. It is tender in appendicitis.

lotio (lo·she·o). Lotion. **Lotio acidi salicyli et hydrargyri perchloridi.** Lotion of Salicylic Acid and Mercuric Chloride BPC 1959. **Lotio Acidi Sulphurosi BPC 1949.** A lotion prepared by mixing equal parts of sulphurous acid, tannic acid, glycerin, and water. **Lotio Acidi Tannici BPC 1949.** A lotion prepared freshly for use, from tannic acid (4 per cent), mercuric chloride, and water; used in the treatment of burns. **Lotio alba.** Lotio Potassae Sulphuratae cum Zinco BPC 1949 (see below). **Lotio calaminae oleosa.** Lotion of Calamine, Oily, BPC 1959. **Lotio Calcii Hydroxidi Oleosa BPC 1949.** A lotion prepared by shaking together equal parts of linseed oil and lime water; used at one time in the treatment of burns. **Lotio cupri et zinci sulphati.** Lotion of Copper and Zinc Sulphates BPC 1959. **Lotio evaporans.** Evaporating Lotion BPC 1954. **Lotio phenolis.** Lotion of Phenol BPC 1954. **Lotio plumbi.** Lotion of Lead BPC 1959. **Lotio Plumbi et Glycerini BPC 1949.** A lotion which should be freshly prepared by mixing strong solution of lead subacetate, glycerin, and freshly boiled and cooled distilled water. **Lotio plumbi cum opio.** Lotion of Lead with Opium BPC 1959. **Lotio Potassae Sulphuratae cum Zinco BPC 1949.** Lotio alba, white lotion, a lotion which should be freshly prepared from zinc sulphate, sulphurated potash, and water; used in the treatment of acne vulgaris. **Lotio Sulphuris Composita BPC 1949.** A lotion prepared from precipitated sulphur, alcohol, glycerin, tincture of quillaia, and calcium hydroxide solution. **Lotio zinci sulphatis.** Lotion of Zinc Sulphate BPC 1959. [L, a washing.]

lotion (lo·shun). A wash; a liquid preparation for application to the skin without friction; usually of a cooling or antiseptic action. Certain lotions are specially prepared for irrigation of the ears, eyes, nose, and throat. **Calamine Lotion BP 1968.** A cooling lotion prepared from calamine, zinc oxide, glycerin, and rose water; used as an application for the relief of sunburn. **Lotion of Calamine, Oily, BPC 1959.** A water-in-oil emulsion containing calamine, oleic acid, wool fat, arachis oil, and calcium hydroxide solution. **Lotion of Copper and Zinc Sulphates BPC 1959.** Alibour water, a solution of copper and zinc sulphates in camphor water; diluted with water it has been used as a wet dressing in eczema. **Evaporating Lotion BPC 1954.** A lotion prepared from alcohol, ammonium chloride, and distilled water. **Lotion of Lead BPC 1959.** A lotion prepared by dilution of strong solution of lead subacetate (2.5 per cent) with freshly boiled and cooled water (to 10 parts); it is useful for application to bruises. **Lotion of Lead with Opium BPC 1959.** A lotion which should be freshly prepared from tincture of opium, strong solution of lead subacetate, and freshly boiled and cooled distilled water. **Lotion of Phenol BPC 1954.** A solution of liquefied phenol and amaranth in water. **Lotion of Salicylic Acid and Mercuric Chloride BPC 1959.** A solution of salicylic acid and mercuric chloride in alcohol added to castor oil and acetone, and made up with alcohol (95 per cent). **White lotion.** Lotio Potassae Sulphuratae cum Zinco BPC 1949. **Lotion of Zinc Sulphate BPC 1959.** A solution of zinc sulphate and amaranth in water. [L *lotio* a washing.]

See also: CASTELLANI.

lotoflavine (lo·to·fla·veen). A yellow pigment derived from species of *Lotus.* [lotus, L *flavus* yellow.]

lotus (lo·tus). Name given to the genus *Zizyphus*; jujube is the fruit of *Zizyphus vulgaris.* **Sacred lotus.** An Eastern water-lily, *Nelumbium speciosum* Willd. (family Nymphaeaceae), various parts of which are used in native medicine as astringent applications and in the treatment of dysentery and fevers. [Gk *lotos* a shrub with sweet fruit.]

Louis, Pierre Charles Alexandre (b. 1787). Paris physician.

Angle of Louis. The angle between the manubrium and the body of the sternum.

Louis' law. Tuberculosis usually begins in the left lung, and a tuberculous focus anywhere in the body is accompanied by a lesion in the lung.

loupe (loop). A magnifying lens particularly used in ophthalmology. **Binocular loupe.** A binocular instrument used for magnification, usually only up to 3 times, and giving depth perception. Prisms are incorporated to assist convergence. **Binocular telescopic loupe (of Zeiss).** Telescopic glasses used in ophthalmic surgery to magnify the field of operation. **Corneal loupe.** A magnifying lens for examination of the cornea and anterior segment of the eye giving a magnification of 8 to 10 times; usually uni-ocular but often binocular. [Fr, magnifying glass.]

See also: BEEBE, HARMAN, ZEISS.

louping-ill (low·ping·il). A virus encephalomyelitis of sheep which can be transmitted to man either as sheep-handler or laboratory worker. The virus is a group B arbovirus and is transmitted by a tick, *Ixodes ricinus.* It is the only arbovirus indigenous to the UK. [Old Norse *hloupa* to lope, ME *ill.*]

louse (lows) (pl. *lice*). A general name applied to insects of the order Anoplura, consisting of small wingless forms without metamorphosis. All are ectoparasites of birds and mammals, the whole life cycle being spent on the host, whilst eggs are attached to the hair or the feathers. Transfer from host to host is normally by direct contact. Lice of the sub-order Mallophaga have biting mouth parts and are mostly from birds; those of the sub-order Siphunculata have piercing and sucking mouth parts, and are peculiar to mammals. Three forms infect man: the head louse (*Pediculus humanus capitis*), the body or clothes louse (*Pediculus humanus corporis*), and the crab louse (*Phthirus pubis*). Typhus, trench fever, Brill's disease, relapsing fever, and perhaps other diseases, may be louse-borne. [AS *lus.*]

lousicide (lows·e·side). Any substance that will kill lice. [louse, L *caedere* to kill.]

lousiness (low·ze·nes). Pediculosis. [louse.]

lousy (low·ze). Infested with lice. [louse.]

lovage (luv·ij). A Mediterranean herb, *Levisticum officinale* Koch. (family Umbelliferae), having a characteristic aromatic odour; the root and also the leaves have been used as a diuretic, carminative, and febrifuge. **Scotch lovage.** *Ligusticum scoticum* Linn., a pot herb the aromatic seeds of which have been employed medicinally as a carminative and stimulant. [L *Ligusticus* Ligurian.]

Lovén, Otto Christian (b. 1835). Stockholm physiologist.

Lovén reflex. Local vasodilatation with generalized vasoconstriction.

Lovibond unit. An arbitrary unit of red, yellow, or blue colour contained in the standardized glass screens of an instrument used for measuring all shades of colour in terms of these primary colours. The instrument is known as the *Lovibond tintometer.*

Løvset, Jørgen. 20th century Bergen obstetrician.

Løvset manoeuvre. In a breech presentation when the fetus is born to beyond the umbilicus the body is gently rotated to bring the posterior scapula anteriorly; during this procedure the body is drawn slightly downward and away from this shoulder with the result that the arm delivers spontaneously or can be easily hooked down. The fetal trunk is now rotated in the opposite direction until the other scapula appears below the pubes and the other arm can be delivered in a similar manner.

Low, George Carmichael (b. 1872). London physician.

Castellani-Low sign. Fine tremor of the tongue in trypanosomiasis.

Lowe, Charles Upton (b. 1921). American paediatrician.

Lowe's syndrome. Oculocerebrorenal dystrophy; a disease of male children, with hypotonia, loss of reflexes, mental deterioration, glaucoma, cataracts, and excretion of organic and amino acids in urine.

Lower, Richard (b. 1631). London physician.

Lower's rings. The tendinous rings which form the fibrous rings of the heart and also those which surround the roots of the pulmonary artery and aorta.

Lower's sac. The bulb of the jugular vein.

Lower's tubercle. A small eminence said to lie between the openings of the superior and inferior venae cavae into the right atrium and behind the upper part of the fossa ovalis; its presence has been much disputed.

Lowsley, Oswald Swinney (b. 1884). New York urologist.

Lowsley's operation. An operation for impotence resulting from an insufficiently maintained erection of the penis: the bulbospongiosus muscle is plicated with ribbon gut and the ischiocavernosus muscles on each side are similarly shortened by ribbon gut. The object of the operation is to increase the resistance to the return of blood through the efferent veins of the erectile tissue.

Lowy, Otto (b. 1879). Newark, New Jersey, pathologist.

Lowy's sign. Dilatation of the pupil caused by the instillation of adrenaline solution into the conjunctival sac, seen in pancreatic insufficiency.

loxa bark (lox·ah bark). *Cinchona officinalis.*

Loxapine (lox·ah·peen). BP Commission approved name for 2 - chloro - 11 - (4 - methylpiperazin - 1 - yl)dibenz[*b,f*][1,4]-oxazepine; a tranquillizer.

loxarthrosis (lox·ar·**thro**·sis). Deformity of a joint, the result of congenital or developmental factors, and not traumatic. [Gk *loxos* oblique, *arthron* joint.]

loxia (lox·e·ah). Torticollis. [Gk *loxos* oblique.]

loxic (lox·ik). Deformed; in a state of being twisted. [see prec.]

loxocyesis (lox·o·si·e′·sis). A condition in which the pregnant uterus is displaced in an oblique direction. [Gk *loxos* oblique, *kyesis* pregnancy.]

loxophthalmos, loxophthalmus (lox·of·**thal**·mos, lox·of·**thal**·mus). Squint. [Gk *loxos* oblique, *ophthalmos* eye.]

loxotic (lox·ot·ik). Slanting at an angle.

loxotomy (lox·ot·o·me). Elliptical amputation. [Gk *loxos* oblique, *temnein* to cut.]

lozenge (loz·enj). A medicinal sweet, prepared from a flavoured and sweetened base with which the medicament is incorporated. They are intended for medication of the mouth and throat and should be allowed to dissolve slowly in the mouth, thus providing a steady release of medicament to the affected part. **Compound Lozenges of Bismuth BPC 1968.** Lozenges containing bismuth, magnesium, and calcium carbonates with oleum rosae in the usual base. **Lozenges of Penicillin BPC 1968.** Lozenges containing benzylpenicillin with sucrose or lactose and binding agents. [Fr.]

See also: TROCHISCUS.

luargol (loo·ar·gol). Diaminohydroxyarsenobenzene silver bromide antimonyl sulphate, $[C_{12}H_{12}O_2N_2As_2]_2AgBrSbO(H_2SO_4)_2$. An arsenical derivative which has been used in the treatment of syphilis and trypanosomiasis.

Lubarsch, Otto (b. 1860). German pathologist.

Lubarsch's crystals. Crystals occasionally seen in the testis and thought to be derived from seminal fluid.

lubb (lub). In auscultation, the term expressive of the first sound of the heart. It is lower in pitch and slightly longer than the second sound, dupp. [onomat.]

lubb-dupp (lub·dup). In auscultation, the two sounds which represent each cardiac cycle. [onomat.]

lubricant (lew·brik·ant). 1. Having the quality of rendering smooth or slippery. 2. An agent, such as an ointment or a fluid, which diminishes friction and renders a surface slippery or smooth. [L *lubricans* making slippery.]

lubrication (lew·brik·a·shun). Application of a lubricant in order to render a surface slippery or smooth.

Luc, Henry (b. 1855). Paris otolaryngologist.

Luc's operation. Any of several operations for the relief of diseases of the frontal and maxillary air sinuses, designed by Luc.

Caldwell-Luc operation. A radical operation on the maxillary antrum carried out through an incision in the gingivolabial fold; the antral cavity is then explored after removal of the bone in the region of the canine fossa.

Ogston-Luc operation. An external operation on the frontal sinus.

Lucae, August Johann Constanz (b. 1835). Berlin otologist.

Lucae's probe. A means of massaging the pharyngotympanic tube.

Lucae-Teuber test. For simulated unilateral deafness: a rubber tube is inserted into each auditory meatus. Each tube connects with a metal pipe leading through a wall beyond which an examiner speaks first into one tube and then the other. The patient is asked to repeat what he hears. A person with true unilateral deafness reiterates only the words heard in one ear. A malingerer becomes confused by the rapid alteration and repeats words heard in both ears.

Lucanthone (lew·**kan**·thone). BP Commission approved name for 1-2′-diethylamino - ethylamino - 4 - methylthiaxanthone. **Lucanthone Hydrochloride BP 1968.** A schistosomicidal drug more effective against *Schistosoma haematobium* than *S. mansoni* and with very little effect on *S. japonicum.* It may cause vomiting, and impaired renal function is a contra-indication.

Lucas, Richard Clement (b. 1846). London anatomist and surgeon.

Lucas' groove. A groove on the medial side of the spine of the sphenoid bone which is occasionally produced by the close proximity of the chorda tympani.

Lucas' sign. Abdominal distension in early rickets.

Lucas-Championnière, Just Marie Marcellin (b. 1843). Paris surgeon.

Lucas-Championnière's disease. Pseudomembranous bronchitis.

lucerne (lew·sern). A plant of the family Leguminosae, *Medicago sativa,* grown for fodder. It is also called *alfalfa.* [Fr. *luzerne.*]

Luciani, Luigi (b. 1840). Rome physiologist.

Triad of Luciani. The three major manifestations of cerebellar disease: asthenia, atony, and astasia.

lucid (lew·sid). Clear; intelligible; used particularly in the expression, lucid interval. *See* INTERVAL. [L *lucidus* clear.]

lucidity (lew·**sid**·it·e). Clarity of mind; intelligibility. [see prec.]

luciferase (lew·**sif**·er·aze). An enzyme present in glow-worms (*Lampyris*), fireflies (*Pyrophorus*), certain bacteria and fungi, and many marine plants and animals, all of which emit luminescence. It receives from activated oxyluciferin a quantum of energy which it subsequently releases in the form of light. [L *lux* light, *ferre* to bear.]

luciferin (lew·**sif**·er·in). A substance present in glow-worms, fireflies, in certain bacteria and fungi, and in marine plants and animals, all of which emit luminescence. Activated by the enzyme luciferase, it combines with ozygen to produce *oxyluciferin,* which, in turn, passes a quantum of energy to the enzyme itself. It is the emission of this energy as light by the enzyme that is responsible for the luminescence. [see prec.]

luciform (lew·sif·orm). Having a resemblance to, or of the nature of, light. [L *lux* light, form.]

lucifugal, lucifugous (lew·sif·ew·gal, lew·**sif**·ew·gus). Having the tendency to avoid exposure to bright light or to be repulsed by it. [L *lux* light, *fugare* to flee.]

Lucilia (lew·**sil**·e·ah). A genus of greenbottle flies of the family Calliphoridae. **Lucilia sericata.** The common greenbottle fly. Its larvae, normally carrion feeders, are a common cause of sheep strike. It may occur in neglected human sores and will attack healthy tissues, for which reason it has been widely used as a surgical maggot. Occasional cases of intestinal myiasis have occurred. Adult flies act as mechanical transmitters of infection. Other species that cause myiasis include *Lucilia caesar* and *Lucilia cuprina.* [L *lux* light.]

lucotherapy (lew·ko·**ther**·ap·e). Phototherapy; x-ray therapy. [L *lux* light, therapy.]

Ludloff, Karl (b. 1864). Breslau orthopaedic surgeon.

Ludloff's operation. Osteotomy of the 1st metatarsal to correct hallux valgus.

Buedinger-Ludloff-Laewen disease. Osteomalacia of the patella.

Ludwig, Karl Friedrich Wilhelm (b. 1816). Vienna and Leipzig anatomist and physiologist.

Ludwig's ganglion. Clumps of ganglion cells in the atrial septum of the frog are collectively known as Ludwig's ganglion.

Ludwig's theory. That the glomerulus of the kidney acted as a filter to remove water and all substances other than protein from the plasma. Concentration of the filtrate occurred by diffusion of the greater part of the water back to the blood through the tubular lumen.

Isaacs-Ludwig arteriole. A branch of the afferent glomerular arteriole of the kidney which appears to communicate directly with the capillary plexus.

Ludwig, Wilhelm Friedrich von (b. 1790). Tübingen surgeon.

Ludwig's angina. Cellulitis of the floor of the mouth and soft parts of the neck, usually streptococcal in origin, producing marked swelling and displacement of the tongue and hyoid bone downwards. It may obstruct the airway, whence the name *angina* (strangling).

Luer (d. 1883). German instrument maker in Paris.

Luer's syringe, Luer-Lok syringe. An all-glass syringe with a device which facilitates rapid and secure fixation of the needle.

lues (lew·eez). 1. Syphilis. 2. Plague. **Lues hepatis.** Syphilitic affection of the liver. **Lues nervosa.** Syphilis characterized by strongly marked lesions of the nervous system. **Lues venerea.** Syphilis. [L, plague.]

luetic (lew·et·ik). Syphilitic. [see prec.]

luetin (lew·et·in). An extract of what were claimed to be cultures of *Treponema pallidum*, employed in a skin test for syphilis. It is no longer used. [L *lues* plague.]

Luffa (luf·ah). A genus of tropical climbing plants (family Cucurbitaceae), of which two species, *Luffa acutangula* Roxb. and *Luffa cylindrica* Roem., are used medicinally. They contain in all parts, particularly in the ripe fruits, a bitter purgative juice. They also have diuretic properties. [Ar.]

Lugol, Jean Guillaume Auguste (b. 1786). Paris physician.

Lugol's caustic, or solution. A solution of 5 per cent w/v of iodine and 10 per cent of potassium iodide in water.

lumbago (lum·ba·go). A generic term for pain affecting the lumbar or lumbosacral region; it may be acute or chronic. Many cases are now recognized as being caused by a lesion of one of the intervertebral discs in this region. It may progress to sciatica. **Ischaemic lumbago.** An archaic term applied to cases in which muscular spasm is prominent, this being believed to result from vascular ischaemia. [L *lumbus* loin.]

lumbar (lum·bar). Relating to the loins. [L *lumbus* loin.]

lumbar arteries [arteriae lumbales (NA)]. Four paired arteries in series with the posterior intercostal and subcostal arteries: each gives off a posterior branch [ramus dorsalis (NA)] to the back muscles and skin, and a spinal branch [ramus spinalis (NA)]. They ramify freely with each other and with neighbouring arteries. **Fifth lumbar artery [arteria lumbalis ima (NA)].** An occasional paired branch from the median sacral artery at the level of the lumbosacral disc.

lumbar nerves [nervi lumbales (NA)]. Segmental nerves, five in number, from the lumbar portion of the spinal cord; each emerges from the vertebral canal below the corresponding vertebra. The anterior primary rami [rami ventrales (NA)] of the first three and part of the fourth form the lumbar plexus; the remainder of the fourth and the whole of the fifth form the lumbosacral trunk. The posterior primary rami [rami dorsales (NA)] divide into medial and lateral branches [rami mediales, rami laterales (NA)] which supply the muscles of the back and the skin of the buttocks [nervi clunium superiores].

lumbar veins. Veins draining the posterior abdominal wall into the inferior vena cava [venae lumbales (3 and 4) NA], or the ascending lumbar vein [venae lumbales (1 and 2) NA]. **Ascending lumbar vein [vena lumbalis ascendens (NA)].** A longitudinally running vein in the abdomen, deep to the psoas major muscle, ending with the subcostal vein in the vena azygos or inferior vena hemiazygos, and communicating with the common iliac and lumbar veins.

lumbarization (lum·bar·i·za'·shun). Fusion of the 1st sacral vertebra with the transverse processes of the 5th lumbar vertebra.

lumbo-abdominal (lum·bo·ab·dom'·in·al). Belonging to the lumbar region and the abdomen.

lumbocolostomy (lum·bo·ko·los'·to·me). Lumbar colostomy. *See* COLOSTOMY.

lumbocolotomy (lum·bo·ko·lot'·o·me). Lumbar colotomy. *See* COLOTOMY.

lumbocostal (lum·bo·kos·tal). Belonging to the lumbar region and the ribs. [L *lumbus* loin, *costa* rib.]

lumbocrural (lum·bo·kroo·ral). Relating to the lumbar and iliac (crural) regions.

lumbodorsal (lum·bo·dor·sal). Belonging to the lumbar and dorsal regions.

lumbodynia (lum·bo·din·e·ah). Lumbago; myalgia or fibrositis of the lumbar region, [L *lumbus* loin, *odyne* pain.]

lumbo-iliac (lum·bo·il·e·ak). Relating to the lumbar and iliac regions.

lumbo-inguinal (lum·bo·ing·gwin·al). Lumbo-iliac. [L *lumbus* loin, inguinal.]

lumbo-ischial (lum·bo·is·ke·al). Pertaining to the lumbar vertebrae and the ischium.

lumbo-ovarian (lum·bo·o·va'·re·an). Belonging to the lumbar region and the ovary.

lumbosacral (lum·bo·sa·kral). Relating to the lumbar vertebrae and the sacrum.

lumbrical (lum·brik·al). Lumbricoid; vermiform; like a worm. [L *lumbricus* earthworm.]

lumbrical muscles [musculi lumbricales (NA)]. 1. Of the foot: four slender muscles in the sole of the foot arising from the tendons of the flexor digitorum longus muscle and inserted into the extensor expansions on the dorsum of the corresponding toe. 2. Of the hand: a series of four tapering muscles in the palm of the hand running from the tendons of the flexor digitorum profundus muscle and winding through the clefts between the fingers to the extensor expansion on the dorsum of the first phalanx. They flex the metacarpophalangeal joints and extend the interphalangeal joints.

lumbricales (lum·brik·a·leez). The four lumbrical muscles of the hand or foot.

lumbricide (lum·bre·side). 1. Destructive to lumbricoid worms. 2. An agent which destroys lumbricoid worms. [L *lumbricus* earthworm, *caedere* to kill.]

lumbricoid (lum·brik·oid). 1. Relating or having a resemblance to a species of the genus *Lumbricus.* 2. A term sometimes used to describe the worm, *Ascaris lumbricoides.* [L *lumbricus* earthworm, *eidos* form.]

lumbricosis (lum·brik·o·sis). Infestation with round intestinal worms, especially *Ascaris lumbricoides.* [L *lumbricus* earthworm, Gk *-osis* condition.]

Lumbricus (lum·brik·us). A genus of oligochaete annelids; earthworms. *Lumbricus terrestris* and probably other species are intermediate hosts of the nematode worm *Metastrongylus elongatus.* [L, earthworm.]

lumen (lew·men) (pl. *lumina*). 1. The bore of a tube such as a duct or artery. 2. The unit of light flux: the amount of light emitted in unit solid angle (steradian) by a source of luminous intensity equal to one candela. [L, light.]

lumichrome (lew·me·krome). Dimethyl iso-alloxazine, $C_{12}H_{10}N_4O_2$. A crystalline substance obtained when riboflavine is irradiated.

lumiflavine (lew·me·fla·veen). A lyochrome obtained from Warburg's yellow enzyme by irradiation with ultraviolet light. [L *lumen* light, *flavus* yellow.]

lumina (lew·min·ah). *See* LUMEN.

luminescence (lew·min·es·ens). The phenomenon of light being produced by a body without any appreciable accompanying rise in temperature, as with electric discharges in low-pressure tubes, decaying wood, and glow-worms. [L *lumen* light.]

luminiferous (lew·min·if·er·us). Descriptive of a medium which will transmit light, e.g. luminiferous ether, the ether or medium which transmits light. [L *lumen* light, *ferre* to bear.]

luminophore (lew·min·o·for). 1. Any substance which displays luminescence. 2. Any chemical grouping in a molecule which is responsible for the luminescence of the compound. [L *lumen* light, Gk *pherein* to bear.]

luminosity (lew·min·os·it·e). The ability to give out light. [L *lumen* light.]

luminous (lew·min·us). Producing light; glowing, especially in the dark. [see prec.]

lumisterol (lew·mis·ter·ol). $C_{28}H_{44}O$, one of the isomeric steroids produced as a precursor of vitamin D_2 when ergosterol is irradiated with ultraviolet light.

lump (lump). 1. A small collection, aggregation, or mass, regarded as a whole. 2. A protuberant swelling. 3. A person who is sluggish or dull; a thickset, sturdy person. [ME.]

Lumsden, Thomas William (b. 1874). London pathologist.

Lumsden's centre. Pneumotaxic centre. *See* CENTRE.

lunacy (lew·nas·e). Insanity. The origin of this term is to be found in the old idea that mental disease may be associated with the lunar changes. [see foll.]

lunar (lew·nar). 1. Pertaining to the moon. 2. Relating to silver, owing to the association of that metal with the moon by alchemists. [L *luna* moon.]

lunare (lew·nar·e). The lunate bone.

lunate (lew·nate). Crescent-shaped. [L *luna* moon.]

lunate bone [os lunatum (NA)]. The middle bone in the proximal row of carpal bones.

lunatic (lew·nat·ik). 1. Insane. 2. Obsolete term for a person suffering from psychopathic disorder within the meaning of the Mental Health Act 1959. [L *luna* moon.]

lunatism (lew·nat·izm). 1. A disease which alters with the changes of the moon. 2. Somnambulism during moonlight. [see prec.]

lunatomalacia (lew·na·to·mal·a′·she·ah). Osteochondrosis of the lunate bone (Kienboeck). [lunate bone, Gk *malakia* softening.]

Lund, Frederic Bates (b. 1865). Boston surgeon.

Lund's operation. Talectomy.

Lundsgaard sclerotome. A special knife designed for making gutter-like incisions into the sclera for inserting sutures before cutting the section in cataract extraction.

Lundvall, Alvar. 20th century Swedish physician.

Lundvall's blood crisis. The transition from leucopenia to leucocytosis in cases of schizophrenia.

lung [pulmo (NA)] (lung). The paired organ of respiration, situated on each side of the mediastinum. It is spongy in texture due to the presence of air in its minute air sacs (the alveoli) and is covered by a smooth glistening membrane, the pleura. **Apex of the lung [apex pulmonis (NA)].** The highest point on the lung which extends into the root of the neck to the level of the neck of the 1st rib. **Arc-welders' lung.** Siderosis. **Artificial lung.** *See* DRINKER RESPIRATOR. **Base of the lung [basis pulmonis (NA)].** The concave inferior surface of the lung, resting upon the diaphragm. **Bird fancier's lung.** Hypersensitivity state of immune complex disease type seen especially in pigeon and budgerigar fanciers. Characterized by acute attacks of breathlessness shortly after exposure to avian antigens, e.g. in droppings, in confined spaces such as pigeon lofts. **Border of the lung, anterior [margo anterior (NA)].** The thin sharp anterior edge of the lung overlapping the front of the pericardium. **Border of the lung, inferior [margo inferior (NA)].** The sharp edge separating the base from the costal surface of the lung. **Border of the lung, posterior.** The indefinite line where the costal and medial surfaces of the lung meet. **Cardiac lung.** Venous engorgement of the lung secondary to heart disease. When long-standing, the lung shows brick-red rough areas of induration. **Carnified lung.** A solid, airless, flesh-like lung due to fibrous induration following acute lobar penumonia or collapse. **Coal-miners' lung.** Anthracosis, miners' lung, silicosis; a form of pneumoconiosis due to the heavy deposit of particles of coal dust in the lungs of coalminers. In all cases there is some associated fibrosis, more so in miners of hard coal or anthracite. Chronic bronchitis and emphysema may be associated with the condition, and, in hard-coal miners, respiratory tuberculosis may supervene. **Farmers' lung.** A clinicoradiological syndrome of uncertain aetiology, occurring most commonly among farmers harvesting damp hay. A hypersensitivity reaction in the bronchopulmonary tissues due to inhalation of vast numbers of spores of the thermophilic actinomycete *Micromonospora faeni.* The symptoms are distressing dyspnoea, cyanosis, and a dry cough; radiologically there are increased lung markings and superimposed soft shadows. Spontaneous recovery usually occurs in 1-2 months, and there may be some residual fibrosis. **Fibroid lung.** Fibrosis of the lung occurring as a sequel to various inflammatory or irritative processes. **Hilum of the lung [hilus pulmonis (NA)].** A triangular depression on the medial surface of each lung where the structures forming the root of the lung enter. **Honeycomb lung.** A radiological term descriptive of multiple small cysts or cavities suggestive particularly of bronchiectasis, mycotic disease or tuberculosis. **Iron lung.** A rigid chamber into which the body of an apnoeic patient can be placed so that artificial ventilation can be maintained by changes in pressure within the chamber. **Lobe of the lung, lower [lobus inferior (NA)].** The part of each lung below the oblique fissure. **Lobe of the lung, upper [lobus superior (NA)].** The part of the left lung above the oblique fissure; the part of the right lung above the oblique and horizontal fissures. **Masons' lung.** Pneumoconiosis in stone-masons, due to the absorption by their lungs of lime, gypsum, and other dusts. **Middle lobe [lobus medius (pulmonis dextri) (NA)].** The part of the right lung between the horizontal and oblique fissures. **Miners' lung.** Coal-miners' lung (see above). **Root of the lung [radix pulmonis (NA)].** Structures connecting the lung to the heart and trachea, namely the bronchi, the pulmonary and bronchial arteries and veins, the pulmonary nerve plexuses, and the lymph vessels. **Saccular lung.** Honeycomb lung (see above). **Surface of the lung, costal [facies costalis (NA)].** The surface of the lung in contact with the ribs. **Surface of the lung, diaphragmatic [facies diaphragmatica (NA)].** The base of the lung. **Surfaces of the lung, interlobar [facies interlobares (NA)].** The surfaces of the lobes in contact in the oblique and horizontal fissures. **Surface of the lung, medial [facies medialis (NA)].** This surface is divided into a posterior area [pars vertebralis (NA)] in contact with the vertebral column, and an anterior area [pars mediastinalis (NA)], in contact with the pericardium and the vessels and tubes behind and above it. **Trench lung.** Hysterical dyspnoea in soldiers. **White lung.** Diffuse syphilitic infiltration in stillborn infants. [AS *lungen.*]

Lunge, George (b. 1839). German chemist.

Lunge nitrometer. A burette containing mercury in which sulphuric acid is allowed to act on a solution of the given substance, and the nitric oxide measured.

Reich-Lunge apparatus. An absorption apparatus where the non-absorbed gaseous remainder is measured after each absorption treatment; used in gas analysis.

lungmotor (lung·mo·tor). An apparatus for pumping air, or a mixture of air and oxygen, into the lungs of an asphyxiated individual. [lung, motor.]

lungwort (lung·wert). 1. Name given to a lichen, *Stricta pulmonaria* Linn., an extract of which is reputed to be of value in the treatment of coughs and bronchial affections. 2. A common name for *Pulmonaria officinalis* Linn. (family Boraginaceae), which is stated to have similar properties, medicinally, but is now rarely used. [lung, AS *wyrt* herb.]

lunula (lew·new·lah). Lunule. **Lunula of the nail [lunula (NA)].** The whitish half-moon at the root of the nail. [L dim. of *luna* moon.]

lunule (lew·newl). A crescent moon. **Lunules of the aortic valve [lunulae valvularum semilunarium aortae (NA)].** Two narrow crescentic parts of the cusp of the aortic valve on either side of the nodule. **Lunule of the nail.** Lunula of the nail. **Lunules of the pulmonary valve [lunulae valvularum semilunarium (NA)].** Two narrow crescentic parts of the cusp of the pulmonary valve on either side of the nodule. [L *lunula* small moon.]

lupanine (lew·pan·een). $C_{15}H_{24}ON_2$, an alkaloid occurring in the seeds of *Lupinus albus* Linn. and other species of *Lupinus.*

lupiform (lew·pe·form). 1. Lupoid. 2. Like a sebaceous cyst. [lupus, form.]

lupinidine (lew·pin·id·een). An alkaloid isolated from *Lupinus* species and identical with sparteine.

lupinosis (lew·pin·o·sis). Lathyrism. [lupinus, Gk *-osis* condition.]

Lupinus (lew·pin·us). A genus of herbs, the lupins (family Leguminoseae), the seeds of several species of which, particularly *Lupinus albus* Linn. and *Lupinus perennis* Linn., are reputed to have anthelminthic and diuretic properties. They have also been used in external applications. [L.]

lupoid (lew·poid). 1. Resembling lupus. 2. Boeck's sarcoid; a granulomatous lesion of the skin which, under glass-pressure, shows grey-yellow specks similar to the "apple-jelly" nodules of lupus vulgaris. There may be only a solitary lesion, or large numbers which appear as papules, nodules, or plaques; all are sarcoid forms. **Disseminated miliary lupoid.** Multipapular sarcoidosis. **Lupoid pernio.** Lupus pernio of Besnier. [lupus, Gk *eidos* form.]

See also: BOECK (C. P. M.).

lupoma (lew·po·mah). One of the miliary tubercles which form a nodule of lupus vulgaris. [lupus, Gk *-oma* tumour.]

lupomania (lew·po·ma·ne·ah). Rabies. [L *lupus* wolf, mania.]

lupous (lew·pus). Relating to or having the characteristics of lupus.

lupulin (lew·pew·lin). A yellowish-brown powder which consists of the glandular hairs separated from the fruits of the hop, *Humulus lupulus* Linn. It is occasionally used as a tonic and mild hypnotic. [L *lupulus* hop.]

lupulus (lew·pew·lus). The fruits of the common hop, *Humulus lupulus* Linn. (family Cannabinaceae), a climbing plant widely cultivated. It contains a volatile oil with sedative properties, also a bitter principle, and an infusion is used as a tonic. [L.]

lupus (lew·pus). Originally any chronic progressive ulcerating skin disease; now, particularly, lupus vulgaris (see below). **Acne rosacea lupus.** Any rosacea-like tuberculid. **Lupus acneiformis.** Lupus erythematosus (see below). **Lupus acutus.** Rapidly spreading lupus vulgaris. **Agminate lupus.** A common type of lupus of closely aggregated lupomata with central dense scarring. **Lupus annularis.** Lupus vulgaris with central involution and peripheral spread. **Lupus atrophicus.** A special self-descriptive form of lupus vulgaris. **Bat's-wing lupus.** Lupus erythematosus (see below). **Butterfly lupus.** Lupus erythematosus affecting the nose and cheeks. **Lupus carcinoma.** Epithelioma arising in a patch of lupus vulgaris. **Chilblain lupus.** Lupus erythematosus in a patient with poor circulation, affecting nose, ears, hands, or feet (Hutchinson); the term is incorrectly used to denote lupus pernio (Besnier). **Lupus crustosus.** Lupus vulgaris with ulceration and crusting. **Lupus discretus.** Lupus disseminatus (see below). **Disseminated follicular lupus.** Lupus miliaris disseminatus faciei (see below). **Lupus disseminatus.** Lupus vulgaris with widely distributed lesions. **Lupus elephantiacus.** Lupus vulgaris of a limb, resulting in gross oedema. **Lupus elevatus.** Lupus vulgaris with raised lesions without ulceration. **Lupus endemicus.** Cutaneous leishmaniasis. *See* LEISHMANIASIS. **Lupus erythematosus.** An inflammatory condition in which a characteristic rash is associated with widespread internal pathology particularly causing fever, arthritis, vasculitis, glomerulonephritis and changes in the central nervous system. **Lupus erythematosus acutus.** An acute systemic disease characterized by changes in blood vessels and collagen; it occurs chiefly in young adult women. **Lupus erythematosus chronicus.** A skin disease characterized by sharply demarcated red lesions with follicular plugging and resulting in scarring; it occurs chiefly on the face and forehead. **Lupus erythematosus discoides.** Lupus erythematosus chronicus with coin-shaped lesions. **Lupus erythematosus disseminated.** Lupus erythematosus (see above). **Lupus erythematosus migrans.** A superficial variety of lupus erythematosus discoides. **Lupus erythematosus nodularis.** A rare variety of lupus erythematosus of the face, with nodules. **Lupus erythematosus profundus.** A variety of lupus erythematosus chronicus with deep infiltrated plaques. **Lupus erythematosus, systemic.** An immunological disorder, believed to be auto-allergic, affecting the connective tissue and vessels of the skin, nervous system, heart, lungs, kidneys, joints and other organs. **Lupus erythematosus tumidus.** A superficial type of lupus erythematosus with raised lesions. **Lupus erythematosus unguium mutilans.** Lupus erythematosus affecting the fingers, with severe changes in the nails. **Lupus exedens.** An ulcerating variety of lupus vulgaris. **Lupus exfoliativus.** Lupus vulgaris in which the nodules flatten, the centres become scarred, and scaling appears. **Lupus exuberans.** Lupus hypertrophicus (see below). **Lupus exulcerans.** Lupus exedens (see above). **Lupus fibrosus.** Lupus sclerosus (see below). **Follicular lupus.** Lupus miliaris disseminatus faciei (see below). **Lupus fungoides.** Ulcerating lupus vulgaris with great overgrowth of granulation tissue. **Lupus gangrenosus.** Ulcerating lupus vulgaris with a gangrenous base. **Lupus hypertrophicus.** Lupus vulgaris with great overgrowth of infiltrated tissue. **Lupus keloid, lupus keloides.** Lupus vulgaris with overgrowth of scar tissue. **Lupus leishmaniasis.** Cutaneous leishmaniasis. *See* LEISHMANIASIS. **Lupus lymphaticus.** Lymphangioma circumscriptum. **Lupus maculosus.** The early flat lesions of lupus vulgaris. **Lupus marginatus.** A superficially scarring disease of unknown nature described by Hutchinson, **Lupus miliaris disseminatus faciei.** Large brown or brown-violet papules occurring chiefly around the eyes and mouth; usually regarded as a tuberculid. **Lupus mutilans.** Lupus vulgaris of the extremities causing loss of fingers or toes. **Myxomatous lupus.** Soft, tumour-like masses of lupus vulgaris. **Lupus nodosus.** Lupus vulgaris with nodules. **Lupus nonexedens, lupus nonulcerosus.** Lupus vulgaris without ulceration. **Lupus oedematosus.** Lupus vulgaris with raised oedematous lesions. **Lupus papillomatosus.** 1. Warty crusted lesions of lupus vulgaris especially around the genitalia, ankles, and dorsum of the foot. 2. Pyodermatitis vegetans. **Lupus pernio.** 1. Hutchinson type: a variety of lupus erythematosus; chilblain lupus (see above). 2. Besnier type: a variety of sarcoidosis chiefly affecting the nose. **Lupus phagedaenicus.** A widespread tuberculous ulceration of the skin. **Lupus planus.** Lupus maculosus (see above). **Post-exanthematic lupus.** Lupus disseminatus following an acute specific fever: it occurs in children. **Lupus profundus.** A deep variety of ulcerating lupus vulgaris. **Lupus psoriasiformis.** Lupus exfoliativus (see above). **Lupus rodens.** A progressively ulcerating type of lupus vulgaris. **Lupus rupoides.** Lupus crustosus (see above). **Lupus sclerosus.** Lupus vulgaris in which there is much contracted fibrous tissue. **Lupus sebaceus.** Lupus erythematosus (see above). **Lupus seborrhagicus.** Lupus erythematosus (see above). **Lupus serpiginosus.** Gyrate lesions formed by the coalescence of two or more patches of lupus vulgaris. **Lupus superficialis.** Lupus erythematosus (see above). **Syphilitic lupus.** An ulcerating gumma. **Telangiectatic lupus, telangiectatic lupus erythematosus.** Lupus erythematosus with red superficial plaques containing many small dilated blood vessels. **Lupus tumidus.** Lupus vulgaris with raised lesions. **Lupus vegetans.** Lupus fungoides (see above). **Lupus verrucosus.** Warty skin lesions due to local exogenic inoculation of *Mycobacterium tuberculosis.* **Lupus vorax.** Rapidly and severely ulcerating lupus vulgaris. **Lupus vulgaris.** A granulomatous variety of tuberculosis of the skin, characterized by the presence of "apple-jelly" nodules. **Lupus vulgaris erythematosus.** Flat red patches of lupus vulgaris without nodules; it closely resembles lupus erythematosus. **Lupus vulgaris fibromatosus.** Lupus sclerosus (see above). [L, wolf.]

See also: BESNIER, HILLIARD, WILLAN.

lupuscarcinoma (lew·pus·kar·sin·o′·mah). Carcinoma developed in the scar tissue of lupus vulgaris.

Luschka, Hubert von (b. 1820). Tübingen anatomist.

Luschka's bursa. The pharyngeal bursa; a pouch that lies behind Rathke's fold and is produced by traction of the notochord on the entoderm in the roof of the developing pharynx.

Luschka's cartilage. The interarytenoid and other accessory cartilages of the larynx.

Luschka's crypts. Congenitally abnormal channels in the outer layer of the gall bladder.

Luschka's fold, or ligament. Sternopericardial ligament; any one of two fibrous bands, superior and inferior, that connect the pericardium to the back of the sternum.

Luschka's foramen. The aperture of the lateral recess of the 4th ventricle of the brain.

Luschka's fossa. Ileocolic fossa; a peritoneal recess lying behind the ileocolic fold.

Luschka's ganglion, gland, or glomus. The glomus coccygeum; a small vascular body in relation to the median sacral artery.

Luschka's muscle. Plain muscle fibres in the uterosacral ligaments.

Luschka's nerve. The posterior ethmoidal nerve, a branch of the nasociliary nerve in the orbit.

Luschka's sinus. A venous sinus lying within the petrosquamous suture in the fetus; it may persist into adult life.

Luschka's tonsil. The nasopharyngeal tonsil. *See* TONSIL.

Lusk, William Thompson (b. 1838). New York physician.

Lusk's ring. Bandl's ring.

lusoria (lew·sor·e·ah). **Arteria lusoria.** A right subclavian artery which arises as the last major branch of the arch of the aorta. It passes behind the oesophagus and may cause dysphagia. It is the result of persistence of the distal part of the embryonic right dorsal aorta which normally disappears. **Dysphagia lusoria.** Difficulty in swallowing, usually found in the newborn or infants, due to an abnormal right subclavian artery pressing on the oesophagus. [L, deceitful.]

Lust's phenomenon, reflex, or sign. A phenomenon of increased neuromuscular excitability (spasmophilia): tapping the lateral popliteal nerve produces dorsiflexion and eversion of the foot.

Lustig, Alessandro (b. 1857). Italian bacteriologist.

Lustig and Galeotti vaccine. A sterile preparation of *Pasteurella pestis* in 1 per cent caustic soda neutralized by acetic acid.

lusus naturae (lew·sus na·tewr·e). A teratism or other freak of nature. [L, sport of nature.]

luteal (lew·te·al). Pertaining to or having the characteristics of the corpus luteum or of its constituents. [L *luteus* yellow.]

lute-ectomy (lew·te·ect·omy). Surgical removal of corpora lutea.

lutein (lew·te·in). $C_{40}H_{56}O_2$, a yellow xanthophyll pigment occurring in yolk of egg, in green leaves, and in the follicle during luteinization. [L *luteus* yellow.]

luteinization (lew·te·in·i·za′·shun). The formation of the corpus luteum from the vesicular ovarian follicle after the extrusion of the ovum, by the hypertrophy of the follicular lutein cells and the ingrowth of connective tissue and blood vessels.

luteinizing hormone-releasing hormone (lew·te·in·i·zing hor·mone re·lees·ing hor·mone). LRH is a decapeptide causing rapid release of luteinizing hormone with a concomitant increase of follicle-stimulating hormone, though it is smaller and occurs later. It might therefore restore fertility and regulate menstruation in a non-ovulating female. It does not release testosterone in the male.

Lutembacher, René (b. 1884). Paris physician.

Lutembacher complex, disease, or syndrome. The combination of mitral valve disease with an ostium secundum type of atrial septal defect.

luteoid (lew·te·oid). Any substance having the physiological activity of the secretion of the corpora lutea, e.g. progesterone. [corpus luteum, Gk *eidos* form.]

luteoma (lew·te·o·mah). Represents luteinization in a granulosa or theca cell tumour; secretes oestrogen and progesterone. [corpus luteum, Gk *-oma* tumour.]

luteose (lew·te·oze). The polysaccharide from which luteic acid is derived.

lutetium (lew·te·she·um). A rare-earth element of atomic weight 174.97, atomic number 71, and chemical symbol Lu, which occurs in the gadolinite earths. It is a metal, mainly trivalent, which gives colourless salts. [L *Lutetia* Paris.]

lutheran. *See* Blood GROUP.

Lutz, Henri Charles (fl. 1860). French physician.

Lewandowsky-Lutz disease. Epidermodysplasia verruciformis.

Lutz-Splendore-Almeida disease. Paracoccidioido-mycosis (South American blastomycosis).

Lutzia (lut·ze·ah). A subgenus of *Phlebotomus.*

lux (lux). A unit of illumination defined as one lumen per square metre of surface at right angles to the direction of the light (0.0929 foot candles). [L, light.]

luxatio, luxation (lux·a·she·o, lux·a·shun). Dislocation. **Luxatio coxae congenita.** Congenital dislocation of the hip. **Luxatio erecta.** Dislocation downwards of the head of the humerus, so that the arm is fixed in full elevation. **Luxation of the globe.** Displacement of the eyeball forward so that the lids close behind it. [L *luxare* to dislocate.]

Luys, Georges (b. 1870). Paris urologist.

Luys' separator. An instrument used prior to ureteric catheterization in an attempt to collect from the bladder separated samples of the urine from the two kidneys.

Luys, Jules Bernard (b. 1828). Paris neurologist.

Luys' body, or nucleus. The subthalamic nucleus. *See* NUCLEUS.

Body of Luys syndrome. Apoplectic chorea due to a lesion of the subthalamic nucleus or body of Luys; violent hemichorea occurs on the opposite side of the body, the affected limbs are hypotonic, and there may be gross dysarthria.

Luzet, Charles (fl. 1891). French physician.

Luzet's anaemia. Anaemia pseudoleukaemia infantum.

lyase (li·aze). A class of enzyme which disrupts the linkage between carbon atoms and brings about the cleavage of organic substances in such vital processes as respiration and glycolysis. [Gk *lyein* to loosen.]

lycanthropy (li·kan·thro·pe). A type of delusion in which the individual believes that he or she is a wolf. [Gk *lykos* wolf, *anthropos* man.]

lycine (li·seen). Betaine.

lycodes (li·ko·deez). A variety of chronic tonsillitis. [Gk *lykos* wolf.]

lycoid (li·koid). Wolf-like; having resemblance to a wolf. [Gk *lykos* wolf, *eidos* form.]

lycomania (li·ko·ma·ne·ah). Lycanthropy. [Gk *lykos* wolf, mania.]

lycopene (li·ko·peen). $C_{40}H_{56}$, a carotenoid pigment which occurs in tomatoes and other plants. A red compound isomeric with the carotenes. [Gk *lykopersikon* tomato.]

Lycoperdon (li·ko·per·don). A genus of fungi, the puff balls, contained in the group Gasteromycetes. *Lycoperdon bovista* Linn. has been dried and used as a styptic. [Gk *lykos* wolf, *perdesthein* to break wind.]

lycopin (li·ko·pin). A lipochrome pigment produced by certain chromogenic bacteria. [obsolete term.] [lycopus.]

lycopodine (li·ko·po·deen). $C_{16}H_{25}ON$, an alkaloid obtained from a number of species of *Lycopodium,* which acts as a respiratory stimulant.

Lycopodium (li·ko·po·de·um). 1. A genus of the Lycopodiales, known as the club mosses. 2. A fine mobile powder which consists of the spores of a widely distributed species, *Lycopodium clavatum* Linn., and which is used as a diluent in snuffs, and as a dusting powder. In the form of a tincture it has been employed internally in the treatment of urinary disorders. *L. complanatum* Linn., the American ground pine, has similar uses. [Gk *lykos* wolf, *pous* foot.]

Lycopus (li·ko·pus). A genus of herbs (family Labiatae). *Lycopus europaeus* Linn., the gypsywort, common throughout Europe, and *L. virginicus* Linn., bugleweed, an American species, have both been used in the treatment of coughs, as astringents, and as mild sedatives. [see prec.]

lycorexia (li·ko·rex·e·ah). Bulimia; perpetual and voracious appetite for food in large quantities, as a result of increased hunger sense, to a morbid degree. [Gk *lykos* wolf, *orexis* appetite.]

Lycosa (li·ko·sah). A genus of hunting spiders. The species are often large and the bites painful. The poison of some species has a strong necrotic effect and can be fatal. **Lycosa raptoria.** A dangerous species in Brazil. **Lycosa tarantula.** A species of southern Italy which is supposed to cause high fever accompanied by delirious dancing, but it is probably fairly harmless. [Gk *lykos* a predatory spider.]

lycostoma (li·**kos**·to·mah). Cleft palate. *See* PALATE. [Gk *lykos* wolf, *stoma* mouth.]

lye (li). 1. The lixivium obtained by leaching wood ash; a solution of potash used formerly to make soap. 2. A solution of caustic soda and washing soda used for domestic cleaning. [AS *leah.*]

lyencephalous (li·en·**kef**·al·us). Denoting cerebral hemispheres that are united by thin or weak connections. [Gk *lyein* to loosen, *egkephalos* brain.]

lygophilia (li·go·**fil**·e·ah). An affection, so strong that it constitutes a form of mania, for places from which light is excluded, or generally for being in the dark. [Gk *lyge* gloom, *philein* to love.]

lying-in (**li**·ing·**in**'). 1. Parturition. 2. The puerperium. [AS *licgan.*]

Lymecycline BP 1973 (li·me·**si**·kleen). Tetracycline-L-methylenelysine, an antibiotic used for the same purposes as tetracycline hydrochloride. Readily soluble in water, it is easily absorbed from the upper alimentary tract; it can also be injected (with procaine hydrochloride) intramuscularly.

Lymnaea (lim·**ne**·ah). A genus of fresh-water, pulmonate snails. *Lymnaea truncatula* is the usual intermediate host of *Fasciola hepatica*, but several other species may serve. *Echinostoma revolutum* has been recorded from several species. [Gk *limne* marsh.]

lymph (limf). 1. [Lympha (NA)] A pale-yellow clear, or cloudy, fluid that flows in the lymphatic channels. Its composition varies according to its site, e.g. that in the liver lymphatics contains more protein than that from the limbs, and that in the thoracic duct may contain much fat when it is very milky and is known as *chyle*, but generally its composition is similar to plasma except for the lower percentage of protein. Strictly, it should be distinguished from tissue fluid, which has a very similar composition. 2. Any pale-yellow transudate. **Animal lymph.** Lymph from an animal. **Bovine lymph.** Lymph from the ox. **Calf lymph.** A preparation derived from the exudate of the skin lesions of cowpox and used to immunize human beings against smallpox. **Croupous lymph.** An inflammatory exudate tending to produce a membrane. **Euplastic lymph, fibrinous lymph.** An obsolete and inaccurate term for coagulable tissue fluid exuded from permeable capillaries during inflammation. **Lymph glands.** *See* GLAND. **Glycerinated lymph.** Calf lymph (see above) mixed with glycerin in order to destroy bacteria. **Humanized lymph.** Lymph obtained from the skin lesion of cowpox in the human subject. **Inflammatory lymph.** An old term for the inflammatory exudate from a sore, wound, or inflamed serous surface. This exudate becomes organized by the development in it of connective-tissue cells and blood vessels. **Intercellular lymph.** An inaccurate term for tissue fluid. **Intravascular lymph.** True lymph contained within lymph vessels. **Lymph node.** Lymph gland. *See* GLAND. **Plastic lymph.** Inflammatory lymph (see above). **Tissue lymph.** An inaccurate term for tissue fluid. **Vaccine lymph.** Calf lymph (see above). **Lymph vessel.** *See* VESSEL. [L *lympha* water.]

See also: KOCH (R.).

lymph vascular (limf **vas**·kew·lar). Having lymph vessels, or relating to lymph vessels. [lymph, L *vasculum* little vessel.]

lymphaden (**limf**·ad·en). A lymph gland. *See* GLAND. [lymph, Gk *aden* gland.]

lymphadenectasis (**limf**·ad·en·**ek**'·tas·is). Dilatation of a lymph gland. [lymphaden, Gk *ektasis* a stretching.]

lymphadenectomy (**limf**·ad·en·**ek**'·to·me). The operation of excising a lymph gland. [lymphaden, Gk *ektome* a cutting out.]

lymphadenhypertrophy (**limf**·ad·en·hi·**per**'·tro·fe). Morbid enlargement of the lymph glands. [lymphaden, hypertrophy.]

lymphadenia (limf·ad·e·ne·ah). Hyperplasia of the lymph tissue. **Lymphadenia ossea, lymphadenia ossium.** Multiple myeloma. *See* MYELOMA. [lymphaden.]

lymphadenism (limf·**ad**·en·izm). The symptoms which are characteristic of lymphadenoma. [lymphaden.]

lymphadenitis (**limf**·ad·en·**i**'·tis). Inflammation of lymph glands. **Lymphadenitis calculosa.** Lymphadenitis associated with calcareous degeneration. **Dermatopathic lymphadenitis.** Lipomelanic reticulosis. *See* RETICULOSIS. **Paratuberculous lymphadenitis.** Inflammation in the lymph glands associated with tuberculous reaction in another area but not showing the presence of *Mycobacterium tuberculosis* in the lymph glands. **Scrofulous lymphadenitis.** Suppurative or small-celled caseous hyperplasia of the lymph glands. **Tuberculous lymphadenitis.** Lymphadenitis characterized by the presence of *Mycobacterium tuberculosis* in the glands. [lymphaden, Gk *-itis* inflammation.]

lymphadenocyst (limf·**ad**·en·o·sist). Great dilatation of the lymph sinuses of lymph glands, especially in the mesentery, some fusing to form cysts. [lymphaden, cyst.]

lymphadenogram (limf·ad·**en**'·o·gram). The radiograph made during lymphadenography. [lymphaden, Gk *gramma* record.]

lymphadenography (**limf**·ad·en·**og**'·raf·e). Radiological visualization of a lymph gland (usually pathologically enlarged) after injection of a radio-opaque contrast medium directly into its substance. [lymphaden, Gk *graphein* to record.]

lymphadenoid (limf·**ad**·en·oid). Like lymphatic tissue or a lymph gland. [lymphaden, Gk *eidos* form.]

lymphadenoma (**limf**·ad·en·**o**'·mah). Hypertrophy of a lymph gland. **Malignant lymphadenoma.** Lymphosarcoma. **Multiple lymphadenoma.** Hodgkin's disease. [lymphaden, Gk *-oma* tumour.]

lymphadenomatosis (**limf**·ad·en·o·mat·**o**'·sis). Lymphomatosis. **Lymphadenomatosis of bones.** Multiple myeloma. *See* MYELOMA. [lymphaden, Gk *-oma* tumour, *-osis* condition.]

lymphadenopathy (**limf**·ad·en·**op**'·ath·e). Any morbid condition of the lymph glands. **Dermatopathic lymphadenopathy.** Widespread, rubbery lymphadenopathy secondary to erythroderma. **Giant follicular lymphadenopathy.** A slow-growing lymphoma of lymph glands in which the follicles enlarge enormously. [lymphaden, Gk *pathos* disease.]

lymphadenosis (**limf**·ad·en·**o**'·sis). Generalized enlargement of the lymph glands and lymphatic tissue of the organs, due to leukaemia, Hodgkin's disease, and other varieties of lymphomatosis. The term is also used for innocent enlargements or hyperplasias of lymphoid tissue. **Acute lymphadenosis.** Acute Hodgkin's disease. **Aleukaemic lymphadenosis.** A vague term which generally means a slow-growing lymphosarcoma or an atypical leukaemia. **Chronic lymphadenosis.** Chronic lymphatic leukaemia. **Leukaemic lymphadenosis.** Lymphatic leukaemia with especially prominent lymph nodes. [lymphaden, Gk *-osis* condition.]

lymphadenotomy (**limf**·ad·en·**ot**'·o·me). The operation of removal of a lymphatic gland. [lymphaden, Gk *ektome* a cutting out.]

lymphadenovarix (**limf**·ad·en·o·**va**'·rix). Hypertrophy of the lymph nodes due to the exertion of pressure by dilated lymph vessels. [lymphaden, L *varix* a varicose vein.]

lymphaemia (limf·e·me·ah). Lymphatic leukaemia.

lymphagogue (**limf**·ag·og). 1. Any substance, e.g. sugar, sodium chloride, commercial peptone, which when introduced into the circulation stimulates the secretion of lymph. 2. Promoting the secretion of lymph. [lymph, Gk *agogos* leading.]

lymphangectodes (limf·an·**jek**·to·deez). Lymphangioma circumscriptum. [lymph, Gk *aggeion* vessel, *ektasis* dilatation, *eidos* form.]

lymphangeitis (**limf**·an·je·**i**'·tis). Lymphangitis.

lymphangial (limf·**an**·je·al). Relating to a lymph vessel. [lymph, Gk *aggeion* vessel.]

lymphangiectasia (**limf**·an·je·ek·**ta**'·ze·ah). Lymphangiectasis.

lymphangiectasis (**limf**·an·je·**ek**'·tas·is) (pl. *lymphangiectases*). Dilatation of the smaller branches of lymph vessels resulting from obstruction in the larger lymph vessels when the superficial lymphatics are involved; this produces small isolated groups of vesicles, but when the deeper ones are involved, elephantiasis may result. It may also result from a congenital deficiency in the valves of the major lymph trunks. [lymph, Gk *aggeion* vessel, *ektasis* a stretching.]

lymphangiectatic (limf·an·je·ek·tat′·ik). Referring to or of the nature of lymphangiectasis.

lymphangiectodes (limf·an·je·ek′·to·deez). Lymphangioma circumscriptum. [lymph, Gk *aggeion* vessel, *ektasis* dilatation, *eidos* form.]

lymphangiectomy (limf·an·je·ek′·to·me). Excision of a lesion involving the lymph vessels. [lymph, Gk *aggeion* vessel, *ektome* a cutting out.]

lymphangiitis (limf·an·je·i′·tis). Lymphangitis.

lymphangio-endothelioblastoma (limf·an·je·o·en·do·the·le·o·b-las·to′·mah). A malignant tumour with the characteristics of a sarcoma, arising from the endothelial lining cells of lymphatics, and showing little evidence of differentiation to form lymph spaces. [lymph, Gk *aggeion* vessel, endothelioblastoma.]

lymphangio-endothelioma (limf·an·je·o·en·do·the·le·o′·mah). A malignant tumour arising from the endothelial lining cells of lymphatics, with a definite tendency to differentiate into lymph spaces. [lymph, Gk *aggeion* vessel, endothelioma.]

lymphangiofibroma (limf·an·je·o·fi·bro′·mah). An innocent tumour rich in lymphatics and fibrous tissue. [lymph, Gk *aggeion* vessel, fibroma.]

lymphangiogram (limf·an·je·o·gram). The radiograph made during lymphangiography. [lymph, Gk *aggeion* vessel, *gramma* record.]

lymphangiography (limf·an·je·og′·raf·e). Radiographic visualization of the lymphatic system, utilizing radio-opaque contrast medium introduced into the lymphatic vessels. [lymph, Gk *aggeion* vessel, *graphein* to record.]

lymphangiology (limf·an·je·ol′·o·je). The science which is concerned with the lymphatic system. [lymph, Gk *aggeion* vessel, *logos* science.]

lymphangioma (limf·an·je·o′·mah). Lymphatic naevus; a tumour analogous to haemangioma but formed of lymphatic tissue. **Lymphangioma capillare varicosum, lymphangioma cavernosum, lymphangioma circumscriptum.** A dilated and cystic condition of the lymphatic vessels, leading to the formation of deep-seated vesicles in the skin, resembling frog-spawn; sometimes the surface is verrucose. In some instances the lesions are subcutaneous, in which case, small, rounded, compressible, circumscribed tumours may be noted; the overlying skin may be normal in colour, pink, yellowish, or sometimes telangiectatic. **Congenital lymphangioma.** Lymphatic naevus. *See* NAEVUS. **Cystic lymphangioma.** Multilocular lymphatic cysts, usually congenital in origin. **Fissural lymphangioma.** Lymphangioma which forms at the site of choroid fissures. **Simple lymphangioma.** Lymphangioma formed by dilatation and hypertrophy of lymphatic vessels. Macroglossia and macrocheilia may be symptomatic of the condition. **Lymphangioma tuberosum multiplex** (Kaposi). Syringocystadenoma. **Xanthomatous polycystic lymphangioma.** A lymphangioma with cholesterol depositions causing yellow patches in the skin. [lymph, Gk *aggeion* vessel, *-oma* tumour.]

lymphangiomyoma (limf·an·je·o·mi·o′·mah). A tumour formed of unstriated muscular and lymphatic elements, forming a sessile or pedunculated growth, from 1 to 3 cm in size, or larger, usually situated on the scrotum, vulva, or nipple. Occasionally, more than one tumour develops. [lymph, Gk *aggeion* vessel, *mys* muscle, *-oma* tumour.]

lymphangiophlebitis (limf·an·je·o·fleb·i′·tis). Lymphangitis associated with phlebitis. [lymph, Gk *aggeion* vessel, phlebitis.]

lymphangioplasty (limf·an·je·o·plas′·te). The Handley method; an attempt to encourage the lymphatic drainage of a limb, the seat of chronic oedema, by the implantation of silk threads in the subcutaneous tissue of the affected limb and of the adjacent part of the trunk. [lymph, Gk *aggeion* vessel, *plassein* to mould.]

lymphangiosarcoma (limf·an·je·o·sar·ko′·mah). A malignant tumour arising from the endothelial lining cells of lymphatics and showing characteristics of sarcoma, e.g. lymphangio-endothelioblastoma, lymphangio-endothelioma. [lymph, Gk *aggeion* vessel, sarcoma.]

lymphangiotomy (limf·an·je·ot′·o·me). 1. The dissection and anatomy of the lymph vessels. 2. Any surgical operation in which lymph vessels are incised. [lymph, Gk *aggeion* vessel, *temnein* to cut.]

lymphangitis (limf·an·ji·tis). Inflammation of lymphatic vessels. **Acute lymphangitis.** Lymphangitis which is the result of the spread of infection from a septic focus, most commonly streptococcal in origin; it is a prominent lesion in many other infections with a primary site in the skin, e.g. malignant pustule, rat-bite fever, mite-borne typhus. In farcy, the lymphatic vessels are much enlarged. **Chronic lymphangitis.** That which occurs in tuberculosis and is well seen in the subperitoneal lymphatics in cases of tuberculous ulcer of the bowel. It may also be the result of syphilis or glanders. **Filarial lymphangitis.** That due to the presence of filarial parasites in the vessels, causing mechanical obstruction and inflammatory reaction with resultant varicose lymphatics and lymphatic oedema. Recurrent attacks lead to elephantiasis. **Sclerosing lymphangitis of the penis.** A cord-like thickening proximal to the corona glandis due to hypertrophy and sclerosis of the lymphatic vessels. [lymph, Gk *aggeion* vessel, *-itis* inflammation.]

lymphatic (limf·at·ik). 1. Relating to, secreting or conveying lymph. 2. A lymph vessel. 3. Describing a dull, apathetic temperament; phlegmatic. **Afferent lymphatic.** A lymph vessel leading to a lymph gland. **Efferent lymphatic.** A lymph vessel leading from a lymph gland. **Lymphatic nodules.** *See* NODULE.

lymphaticosplenic (limf·at·ik·o·splen′·ik). Pertaining to the lymph glands and the spleen.

lymphaticostomy (limf·at·ik·os′·to·me). The operative insertion of a drain in the thoracic duct. It was formerly used, but only for a short period, as a form of treatment of peritonitis. [lymphatic, Gk *stoma* mouth.]

lymphatism (limf·at·izm). 1. Status lymphaticus. 2. The lymphatic temperament. *See* TEMPERAMENT.

lymphatitis (limf·at·i·tis). Inflammation of any part of the lymphatic system, including lymphangitis. [lymphatic, Gk *-itis* inflammation.]

lymphatocele (limf·at·o·seel). A tumour composed of dilated lymph vessels. [lymph vessel, Gk *kele* hernia.]

lymphatolysin (limf·at·ol·is·in). A lysin acting on lymphatic tissue.

lymphatolysis (limf·at·ol·is·is). The dissolution of lymph tissue. [lymph tissue, Gk *lysis* a loosing.]

lymphatolytic (limf·at·o·lit′·ik). Having the power of destroying lymph tissue. [see prec.]

lymphatome (limf·at·ome). Lymphotome.

lymphectasis (limf·ek·tas·is). Lymphangiectasis.

lymphendothelioma (limf·en·do·the·le·o′·mah). Lymphangio-endothelioma.

lymphenteritis (limf·en·ter·i′·tis). 1. Enteritis associated with serous infiltration. 2. Peritonitis. [lymph, enteritis.]

lympherythrocyte (limf·er·ith·ro·site). Lympho-erythrocyte.

lymphexosmosis (limf·ex·oz·mo′·sis). Osmotic transference of lymph throughout the coats of the lymph vessels. [lymph, exosmosis.]

lymphitis (limf·i·tis). Lymphangitis.

lymphization (limf·i·za·shun). Lymphogenesis.

lympho-adenoma (limf·o·ad·en·o′·mah). Lymphadenoma.

lymphoblast (limf·o·blast). Lymphoblast-like cells are formed by lymphocyte transformation on contact with antigen or mitogens. They are found normally in the germinal centres of paracortical areas of lymphatic tissue in which an immune response is taking place. Abnormally, they occur in large numbers in the peripheral blood and lymphatic tissue in acute lymphatic leukaemia. A typical cell is 15-20 μm in size with a round or oval chromatin-deficient nucleus containing one or two nucleoli and with a distinct nuclear membrane. It is basophilic. [lymph, Gk *blastos* germ.]

lymphoblastic (limf·o·**blas**·tik). 1. Referring to lymphoblasts. 2. Forming lymphocytes.

lymphoblastoma (**limf**·o·blas·**to**′·mah). A malignant variety of lymphoma in which single or multiple tumours arise from the lymphoblasts of lymph glands, and which is sometimes associated with acute lymphatic leukaemia. **Lymphoblastoma malignum.** Hodgkin's disease.

See also: BRILL.

lymphoblastomatous (**limf**·o·blas·**to**′·mat·us). Pertaining to or having the characteristics of a lymphoblastoma.

lymphoblastomid (limf·o·**blas**·to·mid). Any skin manifestation of lymphoblastoma.

lymphoblastosis (**limf**·o·blas·**to**′·sis). A morbid condition characterized by the presence of excessive numbers of lymphoblasts in the blood. **Acute benign lymphoblastosis.** Infectious mononucleosis; glandular fever. *See* MONONUCLEOSIS. [lymphoblast, Gk *-osis* condition.]

lymphocele (**limf**·o·seel). Lymphocyst. [lymph, Gk *kele* hernia.]

lymphocerastism (**limf**·o·ser·**as**′·tizm). The production of lymphoid cells. [lymph, Gk *kerastos* mingled.]

lymphocyst (**limf**·o·sist). A cystic tumour containing lymph.

lymphocystosis (**limf**·o·sist·**o**′·sis). The development of lymphocysts. [lymphocyst, Gk *-osis* condition.]

lymphocyte (**limf**·o·site). A mature leucocyte derived through the intermediate stage of lymphoblast from the reticulo-endothelium found in lymphatic tissue in glands and in the nodes present in most organs. Normal adult blood contains 1 500–2 500 large and small lymphocytes per mm^3, or some 20–25 per cent of circulating leucocytes, but the cells, especially large cells, are far more numerous in infancy and childhood. *Large lymphocytes*, which comprise 1–5 per cent of all leucocytes in the adult, are 12–15 μm in size, with a large round nucleus sometimes containing relics of nucleoli, and a cytoplasm which is abundant and stains clear blue; they are assumed to be young mature lymphocytes that give rise to the more numerous small lymphocytes. *Small lymphocytes*, which constitute 20–25 per cent of all leucocytes in the adult, and are small round cells about the same size as red cells (6–7 μm), contain a round deeply-staining nucleus occupying nearly the whole of the cell. **Plasmacytoid lymphocyte.** Plasma cell. *See* CELL. [L *lympha* water, Gk *kytos* cell.]

lymphocythaemia (**limf**·o·si·**the**′·me·ah). Lymphocytosis. [lymphocyte, Gk *haima* blood.]

lymphocytic (limf·o·**sit**·ik). Relating to lymphocytes.

lymphocytoblast (limf·o·**si**·to·blast). Lymphoblast. [lymphocyte, Gk *blastos* germ.]

lymphocytoma (**limf**·o·si·**to**′·mah). A tumour composed chiefly of lymphocytes and occurring in the lymphatic system. **Aleukaemic nodular lymphocytoma.** Lymphocytic lymphoma. *See* LYMPHOMA. [lymphocyte, Gk *-oma* tumour.]

lymphocytomatosis (**limf**·o·si·to·mat·**o**′·sis). A generic term for any condition in which lymphocytes collect in the tissues as localized masses, as in leukaemia or the various forms of lymphoma and lymphosarcoma. [lymphocytoma, Gk *-osis* condition.]

lymphocytopenia (**limf**·o·si·to·**pe**′·ne·ah). Absolute or relative diminution in the number of lymphocytes present in the blood. [lymphocyte, Gk *penes* poor.]

lymphocytopoiesis (**limf**·o·si·to·poi·**e**′·sis). The formation of lymphocytes. [lymphocyte, Gk *poiein* to make.]

lymphocytopoietic (**limf**·o·si·to·poi·**et**′·ik). Pertaining to lymphocytopoiesis.

lymphocytosis (**limf**·o·si·**to**′·sis). An increase in the number of lymphocytes present in the blood or in any serous effusion. **Acute infectious lymphocytosis.** An acute non-fatal infection characterized by a lymphocytic leucocytosis which may reach 150 000 normal lymphocytes per mm^3, a pyrexia, malaise, and no glandular enlargement; it usually clears up spontaneously in a few weeks. [lymphocyte, Gk *-osis* condition.]

lymphocytotic (**limf**·o·si·**tot**′·ik). Relating to lymphocytosis.

lymphocytotoxin (**limf**·o·si·to·**tox**′·in). Any toxin which has the specific effect of damaging lymphocytes.

lymphodermia (limf·o·**der**·me·ah). Any morbid condition affecting the lymph glands or associated lymph vessels of the skin. **Lymphodermia perniciosa.** Leukaemia cutis. [lymph, Gk *derma* skin.]

lymphoduct (**limf**·o·dukt). A lymph vessel. [lymph, duct.]

lymphoedema (limf·e·**de**·mah). Lymphatic oedema. *See* OEDEMA. **Congenital lymphoedema.** Oedema of the lower limbs due usually to congenital deficient development (aplasia) of lymph vessels, or to congenital deficiency in the valves of the lymph trunks with resulting lymphangiectasis. Commonest in young females. Milroy's disease. **Filarial lymphoedema.** Chronic oedema due to the blocking of large lymphatics such as those of the lower extremity or scrotum by the filarial parasites, with associated lymphangitis. **Infantile lymphoedema.** An early sign of Turner's syndrome. **Primary lymphoedema.** Congenital lymphoedema (see above). **Lymphoedema tarda.** Lymphoedema developing late in life.

lympho-epithelioma (**limf**·o·ep·e·the·le·**o**′·mah). A radiosensitive mixed tumour of the tonsillar and nasopharyngeal region, partly epithelioma, partly lymphoma.

lympho-erythrocyte (**limf**·o·er·**ith**′·ro·site).A misleading synonym for an anerythrocyte, being a red blood corpuscle without haemoglobin. [lymph, erythrocyte.]

lymphogenesis (limf·o·**jen**·es·is). The formation of lymph. [lymph, Gk *genein* to produce.]

lymphogenic, lymphogenous (limf·o·**jen**·ik, limf·**oj**·en·us). 1. Derived from lymph, lymph vessels, or lymph glands. 2. Producing lymph. [see prec.]

lymphogonia (limf·o·**go**·ne·ah). Large lymphocytic cells with a large chromatin-deficient nucleus and a basophilic non-granular cytoplasm, found in lymphatic leukaemia. [lymph, Gk *gonos* seed.]

lymphogram (**limf**·o·gram). The radiograph made during lymphography. [lymph, Gk *gramma* record.]

lymphogranuloma (**limf**·o·gran·ew·**lo**′·mah). Any one of an ill-defined group of diseases which in some ways are intermediate between the inflammatory granulomata and sarcomata. They include lymphadenoma, sarcoidosis, mycosis fungoides, and reticulosis. **Lymphogranuloma benignum.** A disease of the reticulo-endothelial system in which characteristic granulomatous inflammation may occur in many organs. Various syndromes have been described under various names as separate conditions, but are now included under the term *sarcoidosis* or *Besnier-Boeck-Schaumann disease.* The lesions comprise lupus pernio and sarcoids of the skin, nodular and reticular changes with glandular enlargement in the lungs, areas of rarefaction of bones, iridocyclitis and uveoparotitis, enlarged lymph glands, and lesions in the viscera, most frequently in the spleen. Different combinations of these lesions occur, giving a very varied picture. The lesions do not necrose or caseate, but fibrous infiltration may occur. The prognosis is generally good, unless vital organs are affected. **Lymphogranuloma inguinale.** Lymphogranuloma venereum. **Malignant lymphogranuloma.** Lymphadenoma. **Venereal lymphogranuloma.** Climatic or tropical bubo, poradenitis nostras, Durand–Nicolas–Favre disease: a virus infection of the genitalia of adults in tropical areas, characterized by a transient small papule or erosion and subsequently by inguinal buboes which slowly suppurate. Sinuses may form in the groins and may persist for months or years. In women, proctitis frequently ensues and a stricture of the rectum may develop later. The intracutaneous reaction of Frei becomes positive in the third week and may persist for many years. The condition is believed to be of venereal origin and is sometimes termed *the fourth venereal disease.* [lymph, L *granulum* small grain, Gk *-oma* tumour.]

lymphogranulomatosis (**limf**·o·gran·ew·lo·mat·**o**′·sis). Lymphogranuloma. **Benign lymphogranulomatosis.** Sarcoidosis. **Lymphogranulomatosis cutis.** A group of diseases of the skin, comprising cutaneous sarcoidosis, lymphadenoma of the skin, and mycosis fungoides. **Lymphogranulomatosis inguinalis.** Venereal lymphogranuloma. **Lymphogranulomatosis maligna.**

Hodgkin's disease; lymphadenoma. [lymphogranuloma, Gk *-osis* condition.]

lymphography (limf·og·raf·e). Radiographic visualization of the regional lymphatic vessels following the injection of a radio-opaque contrast medium. [lymph, Gk *graphein* to record.]

lymphoid (limf·oid). 1. Resembling lymph. 2. Adenoid. [lymph, Gk *eidos* form.]

lymphoidectomy (limf·oid·ek·to·me). The operation of excising lymphoid tissue; tonsillectomy; adenoidectomy. [lymphoid, Gk *ektome* a cutting out.]

lymphoidocyte (limf·oid·o·site). The name given by Pappenheim to the primitive blood cell formed in the embryo from the blood islands of the yolk sac. *See* HAEMOCYTOBLAST. [lymph, Gk *eidos* form, *kytos* cell.]

lymphoidotoxaemia (limf·oid·o·tox·e′·me·ah). Status lymphaticus. [lymph, Gk *eidos* form, toxaemia.]

lymphokinesis (limf·o·kin·e′·sis). 1. The passage of lymph through the body. 2. A term used to describe the activities of the endolymph in the semicircular canals of the ear. [lymph, Gk *kinesis* movement.]

lymphology (limf·ol·o·je). Lymphangiology.

lymphoma (limf·o·mah). A general term comprising tumours, and conditions allied to tumours, arising from some or all of the cells of lymphoid tissue. Modern usage includes the lymphatic leukaemias, Hodgkin's disease, and reticuloses in this group. A convenient classification, due to the American workers Gall and Mallory, recognizes the following varieties of lymphoma: (1) *stem cell,* composed of primitive mesenchymal cells; (2) *clasmatocytic,* in which the cells of the tumour and associated monocytic leukaemia resemble large mononuclear cells or clasmatocytes; (3) *lymphoblastic,* with cells of the lymphoblastic type predominating in the tumour and overflowing into the blood as acute lymphatic leukaemia; (4) *lymphocytic,* a tumour and a leukaemia marked by mature lymphocytes; (5) *Hodgkin's lymphoma and sarcoma,* in which both monocytic and lymphocytic cells are concerned; and (6) *giant follicular lymphadenopathy,* a lymphoma which reproduces all of the features of lymphoid follicles. Generally speaking, these tumours reflect in their histology the clinical course of the disease, since those composed of immature lymphocytes or monocytes are more malignant than the ones made up of mature cells. **African lymphoma.** A rapidly fatal lymphoblastic reticulotic tumour affecting the maxillae, mandibles, spleen, liver, adrenals, kidneys, coeliac lymph nodes, gastro-intestinal tract, and testes or ovaries; Burkitt's tumour. **Giant follicular lymphoma.** Giant follicular reticulosis. *See* RETICULOSIS. [lymph, Gk *-oma* tumour.]

lymphomatoid (limf·o·mat·oid). Like a lymphoma. [lymphoma, Gk *eidos* form.]

lymphomatosis (limf·o·mat·o′·sis). A condition of multiple lymphomata, or a leucosis due to lymphocytes. **Lymphomatosis granulomatosa.** Lymphogranulomatosis; Hodgkin's disease. [lymphoma, Gk *-osis* condition.]

lymphomatous (limf·o·mat·us). Relating to or having the characteristics of a lymphoma.

lymphomyeloma (limf·o·mi·el·o′·mah). A multiple bone-marrow tumour affecting the flat bones and the vertebrae, in which many of the cells resemble lymphocytes. [lymphocyte, myeloma.]

lymphomyxoma (limf·o·mix·o′·mah). Any innocent soft tumour which consists of adenoid tissue. [lymphoid tissue, myxoma.]

lymphoncus (limf·ong·kus). A hard swelling of the lymph glands. **Lymphoncus iridis.** Iridauxesis. [lymph, Gk *ogkos* swelling.]

lymphopathia venereum (limf·o·path·e·ah ven·e·re·um). Old term for lymphogranuloma venereum. [lymphopathy, venereal.]

lymphopathy (limf·op·ath·e). Any morbid condition of the lymph vessels or glands. **Ataxic lymphopathy.** Enlargement of the lymph glands which sometimes occurs during the pain crisis associated with tabes dorsalis. [lymph, Gk *pathos* disease.]

lymphopenia (limf·o·pe·ne·ah). Lymphocytopenia.

lymphoplasm (limf·o·plazm). 1. Karyomitome; the nuclear network. 2. The granular cells of an axon. [lymph, plasma.]

lymphoplasty (limf·o·plas·te). Lymphangioplasty.

lymphopoiesis (limf·o·poi·e′·sis). The process of formation of lymphoid tissue or of lymphocytes. [lymphoid, Gk *poiein* to make.]

lymphopoietic (limf·o·poi·et′·ik). Relating to lymphopoiesis.

lymphoprotease (limf·o·pro·te·aze). A ferment present in lymphocytes with a capacity for splitting proteins. [lymphocyte, protease.]

lymphoreticulosis (limf·o·re·tik·ew·lo′·sis). **Benign lymphoreticulosis.** A subacute granulomatous lymphadenitis transmitted by cat scratches. There is an ulcerated papule about 10 days after the scratch, with fever and tender lymphadenopathy, sometimes proceeding to suppuration. The causative organism has not been identified. [lymph, reticulosis.]

lymphorrhage (limf·o·raje). A collection of lymphocytes in part of a muscle. [lymphocyte, Gk *rhegnynein* to gush forth.]

lymphorrhagia (limf·o·ra·je·ah). Lymphorrhoea. [see prec.]

lymphorrhoea (limf·o·re·ah). An escape of lymph from ruptured or severed lymph vessels. [lymph, Gk *rhoia* flow.]

lymphosarcoleukaemia (limf·o·sar·ko·lew·ke′·me·ah). A fatal leukaemoid condition having the features of a leucosarcoma (lymphosarcoma) with infiltrating glandular enlargement and a blood picture resembling lymphatic leukaemia. There are large numbers of a mononuclear type of cell, which cell is considered to be a specific lymphosarcoma cell though it has many of the characteristics of a lymphocyte.

lymphosarcoma (limf·o·sar·ko′·mah). Malignant lymphatic and lymphoblastic lymphoma; a malignant tumour with the features of sarcoma, arising from lymphocytes and their cells of origin in the lymph glands. Some varieties are associated with a lymphocytic leukaemia blood picture, and the dividing line between lymphosarcoma, Hodgkin's disease, and the leukaemias is very narrow.

See also: KUNDRAT.

lymphosarcomatosis (limf·o·sar·ko·mat·o′·sis). The disease due to and associated with the presence of multiple lymphosarcomata. [lymphosarcoma, Gk *-osis* condition.]

lymphoscrotum (limf·o·skro·tum). Lymph scrotum. *See* SCROTUM.

lymphosis (limf·o·sis). The development and production of lymph.

lymphostasis (limf·os·tas·is). Cessation of the flow of lymph. [lymph, Gk *stasis* a standing still.]

lymphotaxis (limf·o·tax·is). The power of attraction or repulsion exerted on lymphocytes. [lymphocyte, Gk *taxis* arrangement.]

lymphotism (limf·o·tizm). A morbid condition which is associated with the growth of adenoids. [lymphoid.]

lymphotome (limf·o·tome). The generic name for instruments used for excising lymphoid tissue in the throat and post-nasal space. [lymph, Gk *temnein* to cut.]

lymphotoxaemia (limf·o·tox·e′·me·ah). Status lymphaticus. [lymphoid, toxaemia.]

lymphotoxic (limf·o·tox·ik). Applied to a substance which has a toxic effect on lymphatic tissue.

lymphotoxin (limf·o·tox·in). 1. A toxin destructive to cells, particularly lymphoid cells. 2. A toxin present in lymph glands.

lymphotrophy (limf·ot·ro·fe). Nutrition of the cells by lymph in parts deficient in blood supply. [lymph, Gk *trophe* nourishment.]

lymphous (limf·us). Filled with, or pertaining to lymph.

lymphuria (limf·ewr·e·ah). The presence of lymph in the urine. **Filarial lymphuria.** A condition caused by lymphatic obstruction around the kidney by a filarial worm.

Lynn Thomas tourniquet. Forceps tourniquet; a clamp with one flat blade and one probe-pointed. The former lies externally; the latter is passed deep to the femoral artery which is controlled by closure of the two blades. It is employed in disarticulation of the hip.

Lynoestrenol BP 1973 (lin·e·stren·ol). 17α-ethynyloestr-4-en-17-β-ol; the action is that of progesterone. It is chiefly used in conjunction with an oestrogen such as mestranol to prevent ovulation, as a contraceptive procedure. It is also used in the treatment of endometriosis.

lyochrome (li·o·krome). A class of coloured, water-soluble, naturally occurring substances, related to iso-alloxazine, and distinguished by their yellow colour, insolubility in fat, fluorescence in ultraviolet light, and their reduction to colourless leuco-compounds. They are to be found in plant and animal tissues, and are designated *flavins* according to their source, e.g. lactoflavine, from milk. [Gk *lyein* to dissolve, *chroma* colour.]

lyo-enzyme (li·o·en·zime). An enzyme which is not confined to the parent cell. It is soluble and may pass out from the cell wall. [Gk *lyein* to dissolve, enzyme.]

lyogel (li·o·jel). A gel which contains a great deal of water or dilute solution in the disperse phase. [Gk *lyein* to dissolve, gel.]

Lyon, Bethuel Boyd Vincent (b. 1880). Philadelphia surgeon.

Lyon's method. Duodenal intubation with administration of 50–100 ml of 25 per cent magnesium sulphate solution which stimulates secretion of bile from the bile passages and this can be drawn off in three fractions (A from the bile ducts, B from the gall bladder, and C from the liver) which are examined microscopically, bacteriologically, and chemically. The test is designed for the diagnosis of disease of the biliary tract, particularly with regard to the site of the lesion.

Lyon, James Alexander (b. 1882). Washington physician.

Lyon forceps. A heavy-toothed forceps for grasping bone, particularly that of the upper jaw, during its excision.

Lyon, Mary (b. 1925). English (Harwell) geneticist.

Lyon hypothesis. A hypothesis formulated to explain the phenomenon of dosage compensation (Müller) and the behaviour of the X chromosome in mammals. This stipulates that in the female one of the two X chromosomes is inactivated at random during embryogenesis and becomes heterpyknotic; such inactive X chromosome is maintained in this state throughout the progeny of the cell so that in the adult individual only one X chromosome is active in each cell and, barring cell selection, half of these, on the average, have the paternal and half the maternal X in the active state.

lyophil, lyophile (li·o·fil, li·o·file). Water- or solvent-loving: applied to a colloid which forms stable colloidal solutions and is not easily precipitated, readily dissolving again to form a colloidal solution. Emulsoids are of this type. [Gk *lyein* to dissolve, *philein* to love.]

lyophilic (li·o·fil·ik). Having the properties of a lyophil.

lyophilization (li·of·il·i·za′·shun). A method used for the preservation of sera, plasma, bacteria, viruses, or tissues by drying them from the frozen state *in vacuo*. *See* FLOSDORF-MUDD. [Gk *lyein* to dissolve, *philein* to love.]

lyophobe (li·o·fobe). Water- or solvent-fearing: applied to a colloid that is easily precipitated by salts which neutralize the charges carried by the particles; such precipitate is not readily brought back into colloidal solution again. Suspensoids are of this nature. [Gk *lyein* to dissolve, *phobos* fear.]

lyophobic (li·o·fo·bik). Having the properties of a lyophobe.

lyosol (li·o·sol). A sol in which the continuous phase is liquid. [Gk *lyein* to dissolve, sol.]

lyosorption (li·o·sorp·shun). An adsorption effect in a colloidal solution whereby a layer of the solvent or continuous phase is held on the surface of the particles of the disperse phase. [Gk *lyein* to dissolve, adsorption.]

lyotrope (li·o·trope). 1. An easily soluble substance. 2. A member of a lyotropic series. [Gk *lyein* to dissolve, *trepein* to turn.]

lyotropic (li·o·trop·ik). Entering easily into solution. [Gk *lyein* to dissolve, *trope* a turning.]

lypemania (li·pe·ma·ne·ah). Melancholia. [Gk *lype* grief, mania.]

Lyponyssus (li·po·nis·us). *Bdellonyssus.* [Gk *lipos* fat, *nyssein* to prick.]

Lypressin (li·pres·in). BP Commission approved name for 8-lysinevasopressin; an antidiuretic hormone.

lyra, lyre (li·rah, lire). A structure bearing a supposed resemblance to a lyre. **Lyra davidis.** The appearance presented by the posterior columns and commissure of the fornix when viewed from above and behind. **Lyra of the uterus.** The arbor vitae of the mucous membrane of the canal of the cervix of the uterus. [Gk *lyra* lyre.]

lysate (li·sate). 1. Hydrolysate; the products of hydrolysis, usually of proteins. 2. The product of solution of tissue or microbial cells by the action of chemicals, enzymes, bacteriophage, supersonic waves, etc. [Gk *lysein* to dissolve.]

lyse (lize). To produce or cause lysis.

Lysergide (li·ser·jide). BP Commission approved name for *N,N*-diethyl-lysergamide (lysergic acid diethylamide); a psychotomimetic drug.

lysidine (lis·id·een). A condensation product of ethylene and ethylidene diamine which is supposed to have a solvent action on uric acid and is hence used in the treatment of gout. It is soluble in water or alcohol, but is incompatible with acids and alkaloids.

lysimeter (li·sim·et·er). An arrangement for estimating the solubility of a substance in a certain solvent. [Gk *lysis* a loosing, meter.]

lysin (li·sin). 1. An antibody which causes partial or complete dissolution of the cell against which it is directed; it requires the presence of a suitable fresh complement for its action. The term also includes haemolysins, bacteriolysins, cytolysins, etc. 2. A toxin that causes lysis of cells. **Beta lysin.** A relatively thermostabile naturally occurring non-specific bactericidal substance in the serum of certain animals, e.g. β-lysin of rat serum for *Bacillus anthracis*. [Gk *lysein* to loosen.]

lysinaemia (li·sin·e·me·ah). High plasma lysine level with lysine in urine, which may be associated with mental defect. [lysin, Gk *haima* blood.]

lysine (li·seen). 2,6-Diamino-hexanoic acid, $NH_2(CH_2)_4CH(NH_2)COOH$. An amino acid indispensable to animal nutrition and occurring in casein, gelatin, and certain protamines.

lysine-vasopressin (li·seen·va·zo·pres·in). A synthetic compound, sometimes referred to as syntopressin, is the form in which the posterior pituitary hormone is administered as a nasal spray for the treatment of diabetes insipidus. It stimulates pituitary ACTH output in patients with hypothalamic damage whose pituitary glands are intact. It can also stimulate the output of growth hormone from the pituitary. It is used to differentiate hypothalamic from pituitary function. *See also:* VASOPRESSIN.

lysinogen (li·sin·o·jen). An antigen that causes the production of a lytic antibody. [lysin, Gk *genein* to produce.]

lysinogenesis (li·sin·o·jen′·es·is). The production of lysins. [lysin, Gk *genein* to produce.]

lysinogenic (li·sin·o·jen′·ik). Forming lysins or effecting lysis. [see prec.]

lysis (li·sis). 1. The recovery from an infectious disease by a gradual fall in temperature and disappearance of symptoms. 2. The solution of cellular material by chemicals, physical agents, enzymes, bacteriophage, specific lytic sera, etc. **Hot-cold lysis.** Lysis of cells produced by the alternating application of heat and cold. [Gk, a loosing.]

lysocephalin (li·so·kef·al·in). Partly hydrolysed cephalin, produced by the action of the lecithinase present in the venom of certain snakes, in the course of which the unsaturated acid is removed from the cephalin molecule. [Gk *lysis* a loosing, cephalin.]

lysogen (li·so·jen). 1. Lysinogen. 2. A lysogenic bacterium which carries a prophage and, therefore, has the heritable potentiality to produce phage and to lyse.

lysogenesis (li·so·jen·es·is). Lysinogenesis.

lysogenic (li·so·jen·ik). 1. Lysinogenic. 2. Applied to a bacterium which carries a prophage.

lysogeny, lysogenicity (lie·soj·en·ie). The carriage, by a bacterium, of the genetic material of a bacteriophage, in an inactive integrated form. The integrated material, prophage, may be reactivated after certain treatments of the bacteria, e.g. ultraviolet irradiation. The presence of prophage may alter the properties of the host bacterium. Toxin production by *Corynebacterium diphtheriae*, for example, is due to a lysogenic bacteriophage.

lysolecithin (li·so·**les**·ith·in). A haemolytic substance produced by removal of the unsaturated fatty acid of lecithin when lecithinase A of cobra venom acts on the lecithin in blood. It is antagonized by cholesterol, forming a non-haemolytic compound. [Gk *lysis* a loosing, lecithin.]

lysosomes (li·so·so·mz). Intracellular particles, frequently isolated with the mitochondrial fraction, particularly abundant in the liver and kidney. They contain degradative enzymes which are ultimately responsible for cellular autolysis. [Gk *lysis* a loosing, *soma* body.]

lysozyme (il·so·zime). An enzyme present in tears, nasal secretion, the skin and other tissues, and in egg white (uncooked), which induces lysis in certain bacteria. It acts by splitting the linkage between *n*-acetylmuramic acid and *N*-acetylglucosamine whose repeated sequence constitutes muramic acid, a principal constituent of mucoprotein which gives rigidity to bacterial cell walls. Lysozyme is the first enzyme whose three-dimensional structure and molecular mode of action was elucidated by x-ray diffraction analysis. [Gk *lysis* a loosing, enzyme.]

lyssa (**lis**·ah). Rabies. [Gk, frenzy.]

lyssic (**lis**·ik). Relating to or caused by rabies (lyssa).

lyssin (**lis**·in). The infecting agent of hydrophobia. [Gk *lyssa* frenzy.]

lyssodexis (lis·o·**dex**·is). The bite of a dog infected with rabies. [lyssa, Gk *dexis* bite.]

lyssoid (**lis**·oid). Like rabies. [lyssa, Gk *eidos* form.]

lyssophobia (lis·o·**fo**·be·ah). 1. A morbid fear of being affected with rabies. 2. Imitative neurosis caused by such fear in persons who have had a dog bite. 3. Pseudorabies. [lyssa, Gk *phobein* to fear.]

Lyster, William John L. (b. 1869). American army surgeon.

Lyster's tube. A glass tube containing calcium hypochlorite, employed in the sterilization of drinking water in temporary encampments.

Lysuride (li·sewr·ide). BP Commission approved name for 9 - (3,3 - diethylureido) - 4,6,6a,7,8,9 - hexahydro - 7 - methylindolo[4,3 - *f,g*]quinoline; it is used in the prophylaxis of migraine.

lyterian (li·**teer**·e·an). Showing evidence of the abatement of disease symptoms. [lysis.]

lytic (**lit**·ik). Lysinogenic.

lytta (**lit**·ah). 1. Rabies; *lyssa* is the more usual form. 2. A genus of vesicant beetles. [Gk, frenzy.]

lyxose (**lix**·oze). $CH_2OH(CHOH)_3CHO$, an aldopentose which is a stereoisomer of arabinose.

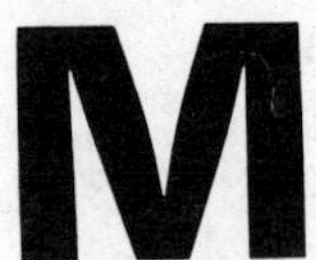

Macaca (mah·kah·kah). A genus of old-world monkeys. **Macaca mulatta, Macaca rhesus.** A species of South-east Asia that is used as a laboratory animal most frequently. [Congolese name.]

McArdle, Brian. London biochemist.
McArdle's disease. An inborn error of metabolism probably transmitted by autosomal recessive inheritance and comprising absence of phosphorylase in skeletal muscle. Cramp and weakness occur on exercise.

macaroni (mak·ar·o·ne). Wheat paste moulded into tubes or sticks, for use as a food. It is made from a special variety of wheat rich in gluten to give it sufficient viscidity for moulding, and is essentially a carbohydrate food though also a fairly good source of protein. It is, however, devoid of vitamins and low in roughage, leaving little residue in the intestines. [It.]

McArthur, Louis Linn (b. 1858). Chicago surgeon.
McArthur's method. Repair of inguinal hernia using, as a darn, a strip of fascia cut from the edge of the incision in the external oblique muscle, and left attached at one end.

McBurney, Charles (b. 1845). New York surgeon.
McBurney's incision, or operation. Gridiron incision for appendicectomy, an abdominal incision in the line of the fibres of the external oblique muscle with its centre at the junction of the middle and outer third of a line joining the umbilicus to the anterior superior iliac spine; the external oblique, internal oblique and transversus abdominis muscles are split successively in the line of their fibres.
McBurney's point. A point which indicates the normal position of the appendix. It is a point on the line between the right anterior superior iliac spine and the umbilicus, roughly two inches (or one-third of the distance) from the former point.
McBurney's sign. A valuable sign in the diagnosis of acute appendicitis; tenderness on pressure over McBurney's point (see above).

McCarthy, Daniel Joseph (b. 1874). Philadelphia neurologist.
McCarthy's reflex. Contraction of the orbicularis oculi muscle on tapping the forehead above the eyebrow.
McCarthy's sign. McCarthy's reflex is exaggerated in pyramidal-tract disease.

McCarthy, Joseph Francis (b. 1874). New York urologist.
McCarthy's cystoscope. A panendoscope.
McCarthy's prostatic electrotome. A resectoscope which incorporates the McCarthy foroblique visual system, a bakelite non-conducting sheath, and a loop electrode which cuts from within the bladder outwards. The electric current furnished by the McCarthy surgical units cuts very easily under water, owing to its undamped oscillations of high frequency.
McCarthy's foroblique visual system. One in which the telescope is similar to a direct-vision instrument. The optical system consists of eighteen lenses and one prism, and the deviating prism is placed in front of the objective, so that an erect image is obtained.
McCarthy surgical unit. The series of endoscopic instruments incorporating the panendoscope, resectoscope, and prostatic electrotome, in all of which the foroblique telescope is of the direct-vision type.

McClure, William Bradbury (b. 1884). American physician.
McClure-Aldrich test. A biological test for the rate of absorption of fluid from the skin. A 0.8 per cent solution of sodium chloride is injected into the skin. The rate of disappearance of the resulting weal is noted.

McCollum, Elmer Verner (b. 1879). American biochemist.
Prebluda and McCollum test. For vitamin B_1: diazotized *p*-aminoacetophenone is added to the test solution and the red colour produced is extracted with xylene and compared with standards obtained with pure aneurine hydrochloride treated similarly.

MacConkey, Alfred Theodore (b. 1861). London bacteriologist.
MacConkey's bile-salt agar. *See* AGAR, BILE-SALT.
MacConkey's bile-salt broth or MacConkey's bouillon. A differential medium containing bile salts, lactose, and an acid indicator in order to distinguish between intestinal lactose-fermenting organisms and the pathogenic non-lactose-fermenting *Salmonellae*, etc.

McCord, Carey Pratt (b. 1886). American physician.
McCord's stain. For basophilic stippling of red cells in lead poisoning. It contains borax and methylene blue.

MacCormac, William (b. 1836). Irish surgeon in London.
MacCormac's reflex. Adduction of the opposite leg on eliciting the patellar reflex (percussing the ligamentum patellae).

McCrudden, Francis Henry (b. 1879). Boston physician.
McCrudden's method. For calcium and magnesium in urine: calcium is precipitated as oxalate, ignited, and weighed as CaO or titrated with potassium permanganate. Nitric acid is added to the filtrate which is then evaporated and ignited. The residue is dissolved in hydrochloric acid and the magnesium precipitated as magnesium ammonium phosphate, which is washed, dried, ignited, and weighed as $Mg_2P_2O_7$.

McCune, Donovan James (b. 1902). New York paediatrician.
McCune-Albright syndrome. Polyostotic fibrous dysplasia with cutaneous melanotic patches and, in the female, precocious puberty.
Albright-McCune-Sternberg syndrome. Albright's syndrome [obsolete term].

Macdonald, George (b. 1903). London and cosmopolitan malariologist.
Macdonald index. The percentage of young children with enlarged spleens and malaria parasites in the blood.

MacDougal, Daniel Trembly (fl. 1906).
MacDougal's theory. The hypothesis that animal and plant variation is due to the direct influence of the environment on the germ cells.

McDougall, William (b. 1871). Oxford psychologist.
McDougall's theory. A theory of colour vision which suggests that, as in the Young-Helmholtz theory, there is a trichromatic mechanism in the retinal cones and also one for white in the rods. The impulses from these four retinal mechanisms are integrated and redistributed at cortical level, where there are four separate centres for each eye.

M'Dowel, Benjamin George (b. 1829). Dublin anatomist and surgeon.
Frenulum of M'Dowel. An aponeurotic sheet passing from the pectoralis major muscle insertion across the bicipital groove.

McDowell, Ephraim (b. 1771). American surgeon.
McDowell's operation. Abdominal ovariotomy [obsolete].

mace (mase). The oil-containing external covering of the seed of the nutmeg, *Myristica fragrans* Houtt. It is used as an aromatic spice and flavouring agent. [Gk *maker* spice.]

maceration (mas·er·a·shun). The act of steeping a solid substance in liquid to produce softening, and to allow soluble matter to dissolve. The process is used for the preparation of certain tinctures, e.g. tincture of orange, compound tincture of benzoin, and tincture of capsicum. **Neonatal maceration.** The softening of the fetus that ensues when, having died *in utero*, it remains immersed in the amniotic fluid; an increasing flabby limpness of the fetus, and peeling of the moist dead skin where handled, are characteristic. Neither infection nor decomposition is concerned in these changes. [L *macerare* to soften.]

macerative (**mas**·er·ate·iv). Describing the changes undergone by a solid subjected to maceration.

MacEwen, Sir William (b. 1848). Glasgow surgeon.

MacEwen's operation, or osteotomy. Subcutaneous supra condylar osteotomy of the femur for knock knee and bow leg.

MacEwen's sign. In cases of hydrocephalus or cerebral abscess, percussion of the skull gives an unusually resonant note; this may be particularly evident on simultaneous auscultation.

MacEwen's triangle. The suprameatal triangle of the temporal bone; it marks the position of the mastoid antrum.

McGill, Arthur Fergusson (b. 1846). English surgeon.

McGill's operation. Suprapubic transvesical prostatectomy. *See* PROSTATECTOMY.

Mach, Ernst (b. 1838). Prague psychologist.

Mach's law. A uniform movement has no effect on the statokinetic reflexes of the eyes. The only effective stimulus is its positive or negative variation, e.g. starting, accelerating, or slowing.

machado-guerreiro reaction. A diagnostic complement-fixation test for American trypanosomiasis; the antigen is either prepared from a culture of *Trypanosoma cruzi*, or is a glycerin extract of a heavily infected organ, e.g. the heart, of an animal infected with *Trypanosoma cruzi.*

Mache, Heinrich (b. 1876). Vienna physicist.

Mache unit. The saturation current produced in air by 1 curie of radium emanation in equilibrium with its products, measured under conditions to include total alpha-particle ionization [obsolete].

Machek (fl. 1914). Lemberg surgeon.

Machek's operation. For ptosis: a horizontal strip of skin is dissected up 4 mm wide nearly the whole length of the upper lid and 3 mm above the lid margin. This strip is divided vertically in the centre and left attached at the ends. The two strips are passed up subcutaneously on each side and then sutured to the occipitofrontalis muscle just above the eyebrow.

Machek-Blaskovics operation. For entropion of the upper lid: a 3 mm wide bridge of skin and orbicularis oculi muscle fibres, taking in the lash margin, is dissected off the tarsal plate. A second narrower bridge is dissected off above the first and passed under it, so that it heals in position between the first bridge and the eyelid margin.

machine (mash·**een**). **Continuous flow machines.** Anaesthetic machines in which the flow of gases is continuous and not dependent on the patient's respiration, which are termed *intermittent flow machines.* **Intermittent flow machines.** Anaesthetic machines which deliver gas only when the patient inspires. **Pressure generator artificial ventilating machine.** A machine which maintains a constant outlet pressure independent of flow changes. [L *machina.*]

See also: HOLTZ, VAN DE GRAAFF, WIMSHURST.

Machray, Robert (b. 1906). London anaesthetist.

Machray's endobronchial tube. A rubber-cuffed endobronchial tube to be inserted into the left main-stem bronchus for surgery on the right lung. Described in 1958.

macies (**ma**·se·eez). Leanness, thinness, meagreness; implying wasting or emaciation. [L wasting.]

McIndoe, Sir Archibald Hector (b. 1900). London plastic surgeon.

Nové-Josserand-McIndoe procedure. For reconstruction of the urethra: a dermo-epidermal urethral tube is used as a graft, the latter being wrapped round a bougie and introduced subcutaneously on a specially assembled trocar.

McIntosh, James. 20th century London pathologist and bacteriologist.

McIntosh and Fildes jar or method. A method used to obtain oxygen-free conditions for the growth of anaerobic bacteria.

McIntosh, John Forbes (b. 1897). Montreal physician.

Møller, McIntosh and Van Slyke test. Urea clearance test. *See* TEST.

McIntyre, William.

McIntyre's splint. A metal splint in the form of two inclined planes, used to support the leg and thigh.

McKee, George Kenneth. Norwich orthopaedic surgeon.

McKee pin and plate. An appliance used in the fixation of peritrochanteric fracture of neck of the femur.

McKee-Farrar arthroplasty. A prosthesis for total hip replacement, consisting of a false acetabulum and a false femoral head, both fixed in position with acrylic cement.

McKee's line. A line drawn from the tip of the 11th costal cartilage to a point one and a half inches to the inner side of the anterior superior iliac spine and then curving downwards and inwards to just above the superficial inguinal ring; it marks the iliac artery.

Mackenrodt, Alwin Karl (b. 1859). Berlin gynaecologist.

Mackenrodt's ligament. The cardinal ligament of the uterus, a condensation of the parametrial tissue extending on each side from the side wall of the pelvis to the neck of the uterus; an important support of the uterus.

Mackenrodt's operation. 1. A three-layer repair of vesico-vaginal fistula. 2. Vaginal shortening of the round ligaments for uterine retrodisplacement [obsolete].

Mackenzie, Sir James (b. 1853). Scottish cardiologist and physician in Burnley and London.

Mackenzie's disease. A state of ill health associated with various functional disturbances of digestion, respiration, and circulation, described by Mackenzie under the term *X disease.*

Mackenzie's phlebograph. Mackenzie's ink polygraph (see following) adapted to the recording of venous pulsations.

Mackenzie's ink polygraph. An improved polygraph by which tracings are recorded on a moving roll of paper. The essential components are a small shallow cup placed over the part of which the pulsations are to be recorded, tubes for transmitting the variations in air pressure to tambours, and levers with pens.

Mackenzie, Richard James (b. 1821). Edinburgh surgeon.

Mackenzie's amputation. A modification of that of Syme, the flap being made from the skin of the inner side of the ankle.

Mackenzie, Sir Stephen (b. 1844). London physician.

Mackenzie's syndrome. Unilateral paralysis of the vagus and hypoglossal nerves, giving rise to paralysis of palatal, pharyngeal, and intrinsic laryngeal muscles.

Mackenzie's point. A point of tenderness in the upper segment of the right rectus abdominis muscle present in disease of the gall bladder.

McKesson, Elmer Isaac (b. 1881). American anaesthetist.

McKesson apparatus. An American anaesthesia apparatus which gives intermittent flow of a controlled mixture of nitrous oxide and oxygen.

McKesson mouth-prop. A rubber appliance for separating the teeth during dental surgery.

Moots-McKesson ratio. *See* MOOTS' FORMULA.

McKinnon, Neil E. (b. 1894). Toronto physician.

McKinnon's test. A laboratory test for the differential diagnosis of smallpox and chickenpox. Variolous material inoculated intracutaneously into rabbits produces a characteristic lesion, whereas material from varicella, as a rule, gives rise to no reaction.

mackintosh (**mak**·in·tosh). 1. Originally macintosh, a waterproof outer garment, bearing the name of its manufacturer. 2. Waterproof sheeting, made of rubberized material or similar synthetic product, and used extensively in nursing for the protection of bedding, etc.

MacLagan, Noel Francis (b. 1904). British pathologist.

MacLagan's test. Thymol-turbidity test. *See* TEST.

McLaughlin's incision. For approach to Codman's bursa; an incision in the line of the shoulder-strap extending forward from the acromion.

Maclean, Hugh (b. 1879). London pathologist.

Maclean-De Wesselow test. Urea concentration test. *See* TEST.

McLean, John Milton (b. 1909). Baltimore ophthalmologist.

McLean's corneoscleral suture. For cataract extraction: a suture inserted, before the section is made, through the anterior and posterior lips of a small cut through only half the depth of the sclera, placed at the limbus under a conjunctival flap. The suture is pulled out of the cut and looped to the side while the section is made and the lens extracted.

McLean tonometer. A tonometer in which the scale reads directly in mm of Hg (Pa); the footplate is of smaller diameter than in the Schiøtz tonometer and there is only one fixed weight. Readings are higher than with the Schiøtz model.

McLeod, James Walter (b. 1887). Leeds bacteriologist.

McLeod's tellurite heated-blood agar. A medium composed of low-temperature meat extract, peptone, 0.04 per cent potassium tellurite, and 10 per cent rabbit blood heated ten minutes at 75°C. It is used for isolation of *Corynebacterium diphtheriae.*

McLeod's culture media. 1. Tellurite heated-blood agar (as above). 2. Low-temperature meat extract, peptone agar, and with 20 per cent rabbit blood heated ten minutes at 75°C, for growth of gonococci.

McMeekin, Thomas Leroy (b. 1900). American biochemist.

Koch and McMeekin method. A micro-Kjeldahl method for nitrogen determination, employing direct nesslerization of the diluted digest.

McMurray, Thomas Porter (b. 1887). Liverpool orthopaedic surgeon.

McMurray's operation. For osteoarthritis of the hip: subtrochanteric osteotomy with displacement of the femoral shaft directly below the head of the femur.

McMurray's sign. For tears of the semilunar cartilages: rotation of the tibia with the knee flexed produces an audible and palpable thud in the knee.

McNaghten, Daniel. The name of the person accused in 1843 of the murder of Sir Robert Peel's secretary.

McNaghten's Rules on Insanity at Law. A defence of insanity at law on a charge of murder, based on answers to questions put to Judges after the trial of McNaghten in 1843. The Jury returned a verdict of insanity. The rules are as follows: 1. Every man is presumed to be sane and to possess a sufficient degree of reason to be responsible for his crimes until the contrary is proved to the satisfaction of the Jury. 2. To establish a defence on the ground of insanity, it must be clearly shown that, at the time of committing the act, the accused was labouring under such defect of reason from disease of the mind as not to know the nature and quality of the act he was doing, or if he did know this, that he did not know that what he was doing was wrong. 3. If the accused knew the particular act he committed was one which he ought not to do, he is punishable. 4. If the accused suffers from delusions it will depend upon the nature of these in relation to his crime as to what responsibility the accused must bear; he will be under the same degree of responsibility as if the facts were actually as he imagined them to be. 5. A medical man, though not seeing the prisoner prior to trial but who was present during the whole trial and the examination of the witnesses can, where the facts of the case are not in dispute and the question of deceased's responsibility becomes one of science only, give his opinion on the state of the prisoner's mind at the time of the crime. The Homicide Act 1957 introduced an alternative "abnormality of mind as substantially impaired" the mental responsibility of an accused.

McNeal, Ward J. (b. 1881). New York pathologist.

Novy-Nicolle-McNeal culture medium. A saline rabbit's-blood agar used for growing *Leishmania donovani*; NNN medium.

MacPhail, Frank L. (b. 1899). Canadian obstetrician.

MacPhail test. A method of estimating progesterone biologically, based on the proliferating effect of progesterone on the endometrium of the immature rabbit uterus previously treated with an oestrogen.

McPheeters, Herman Oscar (b. 1891). Minneapolis surgeon.

McPheeters' treatment. The treatment of a varicose ulcer by bandaging a rubber sponge over the area and encouraging the patient to walk as much as possible.

Macracanthorhynchus (**mak**·rak·an·tho·**ring**′·kus). A genus of acanthocephalan worms. *Macracanthorhynchus hirudinaceus* is a very large species of Eastern Europe and Asia found in the intestines of pigs. It was recorded more than a hundred years ago as common in man in parts of Russia where cockchafer larvae, the secondary hosts, were eaten. [Gk *makros* large, *akantha* prickle, *rhynchos* nose.]

macrencephalia, macrencephaly (**mak**·ren·kef·**a**′·le·ah, mak·ren·-**kef**·al·e). Abnormal enlargement of the brain. [Gk *makros* large, *egkephalos* brain.]

McReynolds, John Oliver (b. 1865). American otolaryngologist.

McReynolds' operation, or transplant. An operation for pterygium; the latter, after being freed from the cornea, is tucked under the lower lip of the conjunctival wound.

macro-aesthesia (**mak**·ro·es·**the**′·ze·ah). Subjective sensation caused by abnormality of the sense of touch and of tactile perception, according to which any object fingered or handled gives the impression that it is greater in size than in fact it is. [Gk *makros* large, aesthesia.]

Macrobdella (mak·ro·**del**·ah). A genus of Hirudinea. **Macrobdella decora.** A leech used medicinally in North America. [Gk *makros* large, *bdella* leech.]

macrobiosis (**mak**·ro·bi·**o**′·sis). Longevity. [Gk *makros* long, *bios* life.]

macroblast (**mak**·ro·blast). Megaloblast. [Gk *makros* large, *blastos* germ.]

macroblepharia (**mak**·ro·blef·**ar**′·e·ah). A condition in which the eyelids are of unusually large size. [Gk *makros* large, *blepharon* eyelid.]

macrobrachia (mak·ro·**bra**·ke·ah). A condition in which the arms are of abnormal length or size. [Gk *makros* large, *brachion* arm.]

macrocardius (mak·ro·**kar**·de·us). A fetal monster having an abnormally large heart. [Gk *makros* large, *kardia* heart.]

macrocephalia (**mak**·ro·kef·**a**′·le·ah). Macrocephaly.

macrocephalic, macrocephalous (**mak**·ro·kef·**al**′·ik, mak·ro·**kef**·-al·us). Having, or pertaining to, a head which is abnormally large. [see foll.]

macrocephalus (mak·ro·**kef**·al·us). A fetus with an abnormally large head. [Gk *makros* large, *kephale* head.]

macrocephaly (mak·ro·**kef**·al·e). Excessive size of the head. The condition may be associated with idiocy. [see prec.]

macrocheilia (mak·ro·**ki**·le·ah). A condition of unusually large lips so that they are out of proportion to the rest of the face; the enlargement is normal in Negroes, but abnormal in white races and generally indicates cretinism and lymphangioma. [Gk *makros* large, *cheilos* lip.]

macrocheiria (mak·ro·**ki**·re·ah). Excessive largeness of the hands. [Gk *makros* large, *cheir* hand.]

macroclitoris (mak·ro·**klit**·or·is). Enlargement of the clitoris. [Gk *makros* large, clitoris.]

macrocnemia (mak·ro·**ne**·me·ah). A condition in which the legs from the knee downwards are of excessive size. [Gk *makros* large, *kneme* leg.]

macrococcus (mak·ro·**kok**·us). A coccus of excessive size. [Gk *makros* large, coccus.]

macrocolon (mak·ro·**ko**·lon). A condition in which the descending colon and pelvic colon are of unusually great length. [Gk *makros* long, *kolon* colon.]

macrocomous (mak·ro·**ko**·mus). Having fibres or hairs of abnormal length. [Gk *makros* long, *kome* hair of the head.]

macroconidium (**mak**·ro·ko·**nid**′·e·um). The large, generally multinucleate, asexual spore, e.g. the fuseaux of the ringworm fungi. [Gk *makros* large, *konidion* a particle of dust.]

macrocornea (mak·ro·**kor**·ne·ah). A cornea of abnormally large size; sometimes referred to as *megalocornea* or *keratoglobus.* [Gk *makros* large, cornea.]

macrocyst (**mak**·ro·sist). A cyst of large size. [Gk *makros* large, *kystis* bag.]

macrocyte (**mak**·ro·site). A red blood cell that is larger than normal (over 9 μm in diameter), seen in the peripheral blood in macrocytic anaemias such as pernicious anaemia. [Gk *makros* large, *kytos* cell.]

macrocythaemia (**mak**·ro·si·**the**′·me·ah). The presence of macrocytes in the blood. **Hyperchromatic macrocythaemia.** Macrocytic hyperchromatism; the occurrence of macrocytes which have an abnormally large amount of haemoglobin. [Gk *makros* large, *kytos* cell, *haima* blood.]

macrocytic (mak·ro·**si**·tik). Characterized by macrocytes. [Gk *makros* large, *kytos* cell.]

macrocytosis (**mak**·ro·si·**to**′·sis). Macrocythaemia. [Gk *makros* large, *kytos* cell, *-osis* condition.]

macrodactylia, macrodactylism, macrodactyly (**mak**·ro·dak·-**til**′·e·ah, mak·ro·**dak**·til·izm, mak·ro·**dak**·til·e). Hypertrophy of the fingers and toes. [Gk *makros* large, *daktylos* finger or toe.]

macrodont (**mak**·ro·dont). Having teeth which are larger than the normal size. [Gk *makros* large, *odous* tooth.]

macrodontia, macrodontism (mak·ro·**don**·she·ah, mak·ro·**don**·-tizm). A condition in which the teeth are excessively large. [see prec.]

macro-erythroblast (**mak**·ro·er·**ith**′·ro·blast). A large nucleated erythrocyte. [Gk *makros* large, erythroblast.]

macrofistula (mak·ro·**fis**·tew·lah). Fistula of macroscopic size. [Gk *makros* large, L *fistula* pipe.]

macrogamete (mak·ro·**gam**·eet). Of plasmodia, the female gamete, larger than the microgamete or male gamete, which develops into an oökinete on fertilization. [Gk *makros* large, gamete.]

macrogametocyte (**mak**·ro·gam·e′·to·site). The female sexual stage of the malaria parasite, or of any species of *Plasmodium,* which, after extrusion of polar bodies, gives rise to the macrogamete. [Gk *makros* large, gametocyte.]

macrogamy (mak·**rog**·am·e). Fusion of two mature cells of the protozoa. [Gk *makros* large, *gamein* to marry.]

macrogastria (mak·ro·**gas**·tre·ah). Enlargement of the stomach by dilatation. [Gk *makros* large, *gaster* stomach.]

macrogenesis (mak·ro·**jen**·es·is). Abnormal development in size of any organ or part of the body. [Gk *makros* large, *genein* to produce.]

macrogenesy (mak·ro·**jen**·es·e). Gigantism. [see prec.]

macrogenitosomia (**mak**·ro·jen·it·o·**so**′·me·ah). Generalized premature development of the body, the genitalia especially being of abnormal size. **Macrogenitosomia praecox.** Precocious sexual and somatic development usually due to congenital adrenal hyperplasia. [Gk *makros* large, genital, Gk *soma* body.]

macrogingivae (mak·ro·**jin**·jiv·e). Hypertrophy of the gums. [Gk *makros* large, L *gingiva* gum.]

macroglia (mak·**rog**·le·ah). The large type of neuroglial cell as opposed to the microglia. [Gk *makros* large, neuroglia.]

macroglobulin (mak·ro·**glob**·ew·lin). High-molecular weight globulin. The two most important macroglobulins in serum are α_2-macroglobulin and IgM. [Gk *makros* large, globulin.]

macroglobulinaemia (**mak**·ro·glob·ew·lin·e′·me·ah). Increase in serum level of macroglobulins, usually of IgM. The best-studied form is Waldenstrom's macroglobulinaemia which occurs usually in elderly men and is associated with paraproteinaemia of IgM type, lassitude, lymphoid tissue enlargement, splenomegaly and haemorrhagic tendency. **Primary macroglobulinaemia.** A clinically recognizable syndrome, somewhat similar to lymphosarcomatosis, that is associated with disorder of the plasma cell and lymphocyte systems. [Gk *makros* large, globulin, Gk *haima* blood.]

macroglossia (mak·ro·**glos**·e·ah). Enlargement of the tongue; hypertrophy may be (*a*) of lymphangiectatic type or (*b*) of muscular hypertrophic type (megaloglossia). [Gk *makros* large, *glossa* tongue.]

macrognathia (mak·ro·**nath**·e·ah). A condition in which the jaw is larger than normal. [Gk *makros* large, *gnathos* jaw.]

macrognathic (mak·ro·**nath**·ik). Referring to either jaw which is larger than normal. [see prec.]

macrogol (**mak**·ro·gol). Mixtures of the polycondensation products of ethylene and water obtained under controlled conditions. **Macrogol 300 BP 1973.** A surface-active agent with the formula $CH_2(OH)(CH_2OCH_2)_mCH_2OH$ where m may be 5 or 6. **Macrogol 1540 BP 1973.** A surface-active agent analogous to macrogol 300 (see above) but in the formula m may be 28 to 36. **Macrogol 4000 BP 1973.** A surface-active agent analogous to macrogol 300 (see above) but in the formula m may be 69 to 84.

macrographia, macrography (mak·ro·**graf**·e·ah, mak·**rog**·raf·e). The forming, during the process of writing, of letters larger than those usually formed by the individual. [Gk *makros* large, *graphein* to record.]

macrogyria (mak·ro·**ji**·re·ah). Excessive size of the gyri of the cerebral cortex. [Gk *makros* large, gyrus.]

macrolabia (mak·ro·**la**·be·ah). Macrocheilia. [Gk *makros* large, L *labium* lip.]

macroleucoblast (mak·ro·**lew**·ko·blast). An immature leucocyte of abnormally large size. [Gk *makros* large, leukoblast.]

macrolymphocyte (mak·ro·**lim**·fo·site). A large lymphocyte. [Gk *makros* large, lymphocyte.]

macromania (man·ro·**ma**·ne·ah). 1. A form of mania in which the subject is possessed of the grandiose belief that his body and everything about him is greater in size than in fact it is. 2. Megalomania. [Gk *makros* large, mania.]

macromastia, macromazia (mak·ro·**mas**·te·ah, mak·ro·**ma**·ze·ah). Over-development of the breasts. [Gk *makros* large, *mastos, mazos* breast.]

macromelia (mak·ro·**me**·le·ah). Abnormal largeness of one or more limbs. **Macromelia paraesthetica.** In the first stage of acromegaly and in atypical forms of hyperpituitarism, a sensation experienced by the patient that the extremities are lengthening and that the head is becoming larger. [Gk *makros* large, *melos* limb.]

macromelus (mak·**rom**·el·us). 1. A monster with limbs of unusually great size or length. 2. Macromelia. [see prec.]

macromere (**mak**·ro·mere). A blastomere of abnormally large size. [Gk *makros* large, *meros* part.]

macromerozoite (**mak**·ro·mer·o·**zo**′·ite). A merozoite of abnormal size. [Gk *makros* large, merozoite.]

macromimia (mak·ro·**mim**·e·ah). Mimicry of exaggerated pattern, generally in association with abnormal mental condition. [Gk *makros* large, *mimos* mime.]

macromolecular (**mak**·ro·mol·**ek**′·ew·lar). Having molecules of a large size. [Gk *makros* large, molecule.]

macromonocyte (mak·ro·**mon**·o·site). A monocyte of abnormally large size. [Gk *makros* large, monocyte.]

macromyeloblast (mak·ro·**mi**·el·o·blast). A myeloblast of large size. [Gk *makros* large, myeloblast.]

macronormoblast (mak·ro·**nor**·mo·blast). A large normoblast. [Gk *makros* large, normoblast.]

macronormochromoblast (**mak**·ro·nor·mo·**kro**′·mo·blast). Macro-erythroblast. [Gk *makros* large, L *norma* pattern, chromoblast.]

macronormocyte (mak·ro·**nor**·mo·site). A giant erythrocyte. [Gk *makros* large, normocyte.]

macronucleus (mak·ro·**new**·kle·us). In ciliated Protozoa, the larger of the two nuclei. Macronuclei divide amitotically during fission and disappear during conjugation, being reconstituted in the offspring from the micronucleus. [Gk *makros* large, nucleus.]

macronychia (mak·ro·**nik**·e·ah). Excessive length or size of the nails. [Gk *makros* large, *onyx* nail.]

macropathology (mak·ro·path·ol'·o·je). The section of pathology which deals with gross morbid changes in the body. [Gk *makros* large, pathology.]

macrophage (mak·ro·fage). A large phagocytic cell found in the connective tissues, especially in areas of inflammation. It is a member of the mononuclear phagocyte system. Plays an important role in clearance of inflammatory tissue and also in carrying antigen and assisting contact of antigen with lymphocytes. During specific immune responses, macrophages may become activated so that this bactericidal activity is enhanced. **Macrophage cytophilic antibody.** Antibody with affinity for a receptor on the cell-membrane of macrophages, and capable of reacting with antigen on the macrophage surface. **Fixed macrophage.** Non-motile mononuclear phagocytes in liver sinuses (Kupffer cells), spleen, lymph glands, bone marrow and other tissues. **Free macrophage.** Motile macrophage, derived from the blood monocyte, which responds to chemotactic factors and migrates out of the blood vessels into tissue spaces such as the pulmonary alveoli or the peritoneum or into inflammatory sites. **Macrophage migration inhibition factor.** A lymphokine produced by primed lymphocytes on contact with antigen which immobilizes migrating macrophages. [Gk *makros* large, *phagein* to eat.]

macrophagocyte (mak·ro·fag·o·site). Macrophage. [Gk *makros* large, phagocyte.]

macrophallus (mak·ro·fal·us). Abnormal size of the penis. [Gk *makros* large, *phallos* penis.]

macrophthalmous (mak·rof·thal·mus). Having eyes of abnormally large size. [Gk *makros* large, *ophthalmos* eye.]

macropia (mak·ro·pe·ah). Macropsia.

macroplasia, macroplastia (mak·ro·pla·ze·ah, mak·ro·plas·te·ah). Over-development of tissue or of a part. [Gk *makros* large, *plasis* a forming.]

macropodia (mak·ro·po·de·ah). Abnormally large size of the feet. [Gk *makros* large, *pous* foot.]

macropolycyte (mak·ro·pol·e·site). An abnormally large leucocyte (up to 25 μm in diameter), having numerous lobes in its nucleus and sometimes seen in pernicious anaemia. It arises from the giant metamyelocyte in the bone marrow. [Gk *makros* large, *polys* many, *kytos* cell.]

macropromyelocyte (mak·ro·pro·mi'·el·o·site). A promyelocyte of abnormally large size. [Gk *makros* large, promyelocyte.]

macroprosopia (mak·ro·pro·so'·pe·ah). Over-development of the face. [Gk *makros* large, *prosopon* face.]

macroprosopus (mak·ro·pro·so'·pus). A monster with a face of abnormally large size. [see prec.]

macropsia, macropsy (mak·rop·se·ah, mak·rop·se). An abnormal visual state in which objects appear to be larger than in fact they are. [Gk *makros* large, *opsis* vision.]

macroradiograph (mak·ro·ra·de·o·graf). The radiograph made during macroradiography.

macroradiography (mak·ro·ra·de·og'·raf·e). The technique of producing an enlarged radiographic image of an organ or region of the body. [Gk *makros* large, radiograph.]

macrorrhinia (mak·ro·ri·ne·ah). Nasal hypertrophy, congenital in origin. [Gk *makros* large, *rhis* nose.]

macroscopic, macroscopical (mak·ro·skop·ik, mak·ro·skop·ik·al). Visible without the aid of a microscope; gross. [see foll.]

macroscopy (mak·ros·ko·pe). Examination of any object with the naked eye. [Gk *makros* large, *skopein* to watch.]

macrosigma, macrosigmoid (mak·ro·sig·mah, mak·ro·sig·moid). Hypertrophy of the sigmoid colon. [Gk *makros* large, sigmoid.]

macrosis (mak·ro·sis). An increase in size or volume. [Gk *makros* large.]

macrosmatic (mak·ros·mat·ik). Possessing an abnormally acute sense of smell. [Gk *makros* large, *osmaomein* to scent.]

macrosomatia (mak·ro·so·mah'·she·ah). The condition of having a body greatly exceeding the normal size. **Macrosomatia adiposa congenita.** A form of precocious development, marked by obesity; the cause may be overactivity of the cortex of the suprarenal gland. [Gk *makros* large, *soma* body.]

macrosome (mak·ro·some). One of the larger particles observed in the nuclei of some cells. [Gk *makros* large, *soma* body.]

macrosomia (mak·ro·so·me·ah). Macrosomatia. **Macrosomia praecox.** Macrosomatia adiposa congenita.

macrosplanchnic (mak·ro·splangk·nik). Possessing viscera of large size; a term used for the type of physical frame in which the horizontal diameters are increased as compared with the vertical diameters. [Gk *makros* large, *splagchna* viscera.]

macrospore (mak·ro·spore). A spore of excessive size. [Gk *makros* large, *sporos* seed.]

macrostereognosia (mak·ro·steer·e·og·no'·se·ah). The abnormal perception of objects felt as being larger than they are. [Gk *makros* large, *stereos* solid, *gnosis* knowledge.]

macrostoma (mak·ros·to·mah). Old name for *Chilomastix.* [Gk *makros* large, *stoma* mouth.]

macrostomia (mak·ro·sto·me·ah). General increase in size of the mouth, the oral fissure being of much greater width than in the normal person. [Gk *makros* large, *stoma* mouth.]

macrotia (mak·ro·she·ah). Abnormal largeness of the ears. [Gk *makros* large, *ous* ear.]

macrotome (mak·ro·tome). A cutting apparatus used for making gross sections of organs such as the brain. [Gk *makros* large, *temnein* to cut.]

macrotomogram (mak·ro·to·mo·gram). The radiograph made during macrotomography. [macrotome, Gk *gramma* record.]

macrotomography (mak·ro·to·mog'·raf·e). The technique of producing an enlarged radiographic image of a particular level of the body. [macrotome, Gk *graphein* to record.]

macrotys (mak·ro·tis). Cimicifuga. [Gk *makros* large, *ous* ear.]

macula (mak·ew·lah) (pl. *maculae*). 1. A transient or permanent, congenital or acquired, small or large, circumscribed alteration in the colour of the skin, without any change in the consistence of the skin or disturbance of its surface. Petechiae, telangiectases, and freckles are examples of maculae. 2. [NA] In anatomy, a circumscribed spot in any tissue. **Macula adherens.** Desmosome; a component of the junctional complex between cells. It consists of a pair of localized plaques on adjacent cell membranes, with underlying cytoplasmic filaments; it is believed to help to maintain contact between adjacent cells. **Macula albida.** Milk patch; tache laiteuse; small localized white areas of adhesion in the serous membranes, especially the pericardium, or small collections of reticulo-endothelial cells in the peritoneum and pleura. **Maculae atrophicae.** Small circumscribed areas of cutaneous atrophy, symptomatic of atrophoderma maculatum. **Maculae caeruleae.** Bluish macules from 0.2 to 3.0 cm in diameter, irregular in outline, which are sometimes noted at the site where *Phthirus pubis* has bitten the skin. They have been produced experimentally by injections of the crushed reniform salivary glands of the louse. **Cerebral macula.** Taches cérébrales; flushing of the skin in response to stroking. It is seen with meningitis, but is not pathognomonic. **Macula corneae.** A dense, usually circumscribed, corneal opacity. **Maculae cribrosae [NA].** Minute holes in the wall of the vestibule of the internal ear penetrated by nerves from the membranous labyrinth. **Macula cribrosa inferior [NA].** Perforations through which pass nerves to the inferior ampulla of the posterior semicircular ducts. **Macula cribrosa media [NA].** Perforations through which pass nerves to the saccule. **Macula cribrosa superior [NA].** Perforations through which pass nerves to the utricle and the ampullae of the superior and lateral semicircular ducts. **Macula densa.** A thickening in the wall of a distal tubule of the kidney which occurs where it comes into contact with the afferent glomerular arteriole. It is a component of the juxtaglomerular apparatus and may form part of a feedback mechanism for sodium. **False macula.** Found in certain cases of squint, when the squinting eye is grossly amblyopic: the area of retina of the squinting eye on which the image of the object which is being fixed by the straight eye falls. When the straight eye is covered, the squinting eye does not move to fix on the normal macula, but remains fixing on the false. Also called *eccentric fixation.* **Macula folliculi.** The place in the wall of a vesicular ovarian follicle where rupture will eventually take place. **Macula germinativa.** The blastodisc or germinal area of large-yolked eggs. **Macula gonorrhoeica.** A red spot encircling and involving the orifice of the duct of the greater vestibular gland due to gonococcal infection of the duct. **Macula lactea.** Macula albida (see above). **Macula lutea [macula (NA)].** That area of the retina containing yellow luteal pigment. It is a horizontal oval, 2-5 mm in diameter, lying 3 mm lateral to the optic disc, and having at its centre the *fovea centralis* which is responsible for accurate central vision. **Maculae of the membranous labyrinth [maculae (NA)].** Special sensory areas within the saccule, utricle, and semicircular ducts, containing hair cells in contact with calcareous otoliths. **Mongolian macula.** Mongolian spot; bluish spots on the lower sacral area seen in mongolism and occurring in certain Mongolian races. **Macula of the saccule [macula sacculi (NA)].** The macule on the anterior wall of the saccule. **Macula solaris.** Freckle. **Macula tendinea.** Macula albida (see above). **Macula of the utricle [macula utriculi (NA)].** The macula on the inferolateral wall of the utricle. [L spot.]

See also: SAENGER (M.).

macular (mak·ew·lar). Resembling or marked by or with reference to maculae.

maculate (mak·ew·late). Stained or spotted; marked by maculae.

maculation (mak·ew·la·shun). 1. The development of spots or maculae. 2. A condition in which spots are present. **Pernicious maculation.** The formation of purpuric spots in severe types of malignant malaria.

macule (mak·ewl). Macula. **Indeterminate macule.** Leprid, any skin lesion of leprosy. The patch is pink or hypopigmented and is hypoaesthetic. *Mycobacterium leprae* can be demonstrated within terminal nerve fibrils.

maculocerebral (mak·ew·lo·ser′·e·bral). Cerebromacular.

maculopapular (mak·ew·lo·pap′·ew·lar). Characterized by maculae and papules. [see foll.]

maculopapule (mak·ew·lo·pap′·ewl). A spot which has the characteristics between those of a macula and a papule. [L *macula* spot, *papula* pimple.]

madarosis (mad·ar·o·sis). Congenital hypotrichosis. [Gk *madaros* a falling off (hair), *-osis* condition.]

madder (mad·er). The name given to two plants of the genus *Rubia* (family Rubiaceae), *Rubia tinctoria* Linn., a European species, and *Rubia cordifolia* Linn., indigenous to India, the roots of which yield a red dye known as *Turkey red.* Both plants are reputed to be medicinally active and have been employed as tonics and astringents. [AS *maedere.*]

Maddox, Ernest Edmund (b. 1860). Bournemouth ophthalmologist.

Maddox groove. A lens ground in the form of a row of parallel double prisms which produces the same optical effect as the Maddox rod (see below).

Maddox heater. A small electrically-heated pad for applying heat to the eyeball.

Maddox needle. A small cutting needle used in advancing the muscle in squint operations.

Maddox prism, Maddox double-prism test. A test for cyclophoria or rotation of the eyeball on the anteroposterior axis: a double prism base to base is placed in front of one eye and the patient looks at a horizontal line at the reading distance. If the three lines seen are parallel, then no cyclophoria exists; if the centre line is tilted, this shows cyclophoria of the eye not covered by the double prism.

Maddox rod. One, or a number of parallel red or green glass cylinders in the shape of rods and mounted in the form of a lens. This alters a spot light into a coloured line, when placed before one eye, and so breaks up binocular vision by removing the desire for fusion. Used in a test for manifest or latent squint. *See* MADDOX ROD TEST below.

Maddox hand-frame test. A method of performing the Maddox rod test (see below) with a frame which, held before the patient's eyes, places a Maddox rod, either vertical or horizontal, in front of one eye and a rotating prism in front of the other. A spot light is then fixed and the prism rotated until the line of the Maddox rod is over the spot light. The number of prism dioptres of heterophoria can then be estimated from the amount of rotation of the prism.

Maddox rod test. For testing distance muscle balance of the eyes by removing the stimulus to binocular vision: a spot light is fixed, and one eye is covered with a glass containing a row of red cylinders which turn the light into a red line, either vertical or horizontal. The distance, vertical or horizontal, between the line and the light as seen by the other eye, is measured in prism doptres or on a tangent scale and gives the amount of esophoria, exophoria, or hyperphoria.

Maddox wing test. For testing near muscle balance of the eyes by removing the stimulus to binocular vision: the left eye sees a row of numbers while the right eye sees an arrow. The figure to which the arrow points gives the measurement in prism doptres of esophoria, exophoria, or hyperphoria.

Maddox prism verger. Two rotating prisms mounted in a frame, one in front of each eye.

madefaction (mad·e·fak·shun). The process in which any substance is made wet or moist. [L *madefacere* to moisten.]

Madelung, Otto Wilhelm (b. 1846). Gottingen surgeon.

Madelung's deformity. Displacement of the hand to the radial side, the result of relative overgrowth of the ulna.

Madelung's neck. Diffuse symmetrical lipomatosis of the neck.

Madelung's sign. A greater difference than normal between the axillary and rectal temperatures as a sign of purulent peritonitis.

madescent (mad·es·ent). Becoming moist. [L *madescere* to become moist.]

madidans (mad·id·anz). Descriptive of a lesion the surface of which exudes moisture ("weeping"). [L *madidus* moist.]

madisterion, madisterium (mad·is·teer·e·on, mad·is·teer·e·um). An instrument for the extraction of hairs. [Gk *madizein* to pluck bare.]

madness (mad·nes). Insanity. [AS *gemad.*]

madra buba (mad·rah boo·bah). Mother yaw, the primary lesion of yaws. [Port. *madra* mother, Brazilian *bubas* yaws.]

madura foot (mad·ewr·ah fut). Mycetoma of the foot; a fungous disease, found especially in parts of India (Bengal), also in Algeria, Indonesia, Somalia, South Africa, South America and Vietnam. It is characterized by enlargement of the feet, more rarely of the hands, with oily degeneration and fusion of the affected tissues. The disease is chronic and neglected cases may necessitate amputation. Various species of *Nocardia, Streptomyces* and filamentous fungi (e.g. *Madurella*) are the infecting agents. [*Madura*, a district in India.]

Madurella (mad·ewr·el·ah). A genus of fungi causing mycetoma, e.g. *Madurella mycetomi* (syn. *M. americana, M. ikedae, M. lackawanna, M. tabarkae, M. tozeuri*), and *Madurella grisea.* The grains produced are of the black variety. [dim. of *Madura*, a district in India].

maduromycetoma (mad·ewr·o·mi·se·to′·mah). Mycetoma caused by filamentous fungi as opposed to actinomycetes causing actinomycotic mycetoma. Both types produce granulomas and abscesses which suppurate and drain through sinus tracts. Pus contains granules pigmented black, red or white. Granules of maduromycetoma are composed of aggregates of septate hyphae with hyphal swellings. [*Madura*, a district in India, Gk *mykes* fungus, *-oma* tumour.]

maduromycosis (mad·ewr·o·mi·ko′·sis). Maduromycetoma, especially with reference to the type in which there are grains of black or white or red, these being composed of filaments of mycelium. [*Madura*, a district in India, mycosis.]

maedi (may·di). A haemorrhagic pneumonia of sheep, originally endemic to Iceland and due to a virus. The virus is one of the *slow viruses* or *lentivirinae*, and is serologically related to that of another disease of sheep, *visna.* The disease occurred naturally only in the Karakul breed of sheep, but is no longer found in the wild. It is maintained in laboratories as a model for slow viruses.

Mafenide (maf·en·ide). BP Commission approved name for a sulphonamide used in the treatment of burns and infected wounds, but too soluble and too rapidly excreted for oral use. It is applied as a powder, solution or ointment and, unlike the usual sulpha drugs, its action is not inhibited by *p*-aminobenzoic acid.

Maffucci, Angelo (b. 1845) Italian physician.

Maffucci's syndrome. Cavernous haemangioma with enchondromas of skeleton, producing deformities.

Magendie, François (b. 1783). Paris physician and physiologist.

Magendie's foramen. The median aperture in the roof of the 4th ventricle of the brain.

Magendie law, Bell-Magendie law. In a reflex arc the impulse can be conducted in one direction only.

Magendie's spaces. The subarachnoid cisternae; they contain cerebrospinal fluid.

Hertwig-Magendie sign, or syndrome. Skew deviation of the eyes occurring in acute cerebellar lesions; the eye on the same side looks down and in, on the opposite side it looks up and out.

magenta (mah·jen·tah). A red dyestuff consisting of a mixture of pararosaniline, rosaniline, and other aniline dyes; also known as *basic fuchsine.* It is widely used in histology and bacteriology as a stain (BPC 1968). When decolorized with sulphurous acid it constitutes Schiff's reagent. **Acid magenta.** Acid fuchsine, a mixture of the sodium and ammonium salts of sulphonic acids of pararosaniline and rosaniline used as an indicator (Andrade's) in bacteriology and as a constituent of several histological stains. [discovered soon after the battle of *Magenta,* Italy (1859).]

maggot (mag·ot). The larva of any (usually cyclorrhaphous) Diptera, characterized by the absence of head and legs, and usually dirty-white in colour; particularly that of blow, flesh, and house flies. **Congo floor maggot.** The larva of *Auchmeromyia luteola.* **Rat-tailed maggot.** The larva of species of *Eristalis,* which bears an elongate anal respiratory tube. [ME *mathek.*]

Magill, Sir Ivan Whitehouse. British anaesthetist.

Magill's forceps. Intubation forceps used to guide a tracheal tube into the larynx under direct vision. Described in 1920.

magistery (maj·is·ter·e). 1. An unusual remedy specially prescribed by a physician. 2. A term used formerly to describe a chemical precipitate. **Magistery of bismuth.** Bismuth subnitrate. **Magistery of tin.** Stannous oxide. [L *magister* master.]

Magitot, Emile (b. 1833). Paris surgeon and dentist.

Magitot's disease. The resorption of the apex of a tooth and its replacement by bone.

Magnan, Valentin Jacques Joseph (b. 1835). Paris psychiatrist.

Magnan's movement. Trombone tremors of the tongue as seen in general paralysis of the insane.

Magnan's symptom. The subjective sensation of small foreign bodies under the skin. It may occur in cocainism.

magnesaemia (mag·ne·se·me·ah). The presence of magnesium in the blood. [magnesium, Gk *haima* blood.]

magnesia (mag·ne·she·ah). Strictly, magnesium oxide, MgO, but loosely applied to various preparations or compounds of magnesium. **Magnesia alba.** Magnesium carbonate (Obsolete term). **Black magnesia.** Manganese dioxide, MnO_2 (Obsolete term). **Calcined magnesia.** Magnesium oxide, MgO, so called because it is prepared by calcining magnesium carbonate. **Cream of magnesia.** Magnesium Hydroxide Mixture BP 1973. **Fluid magnesia.** Magnesium bicarbonate solution. **Heavy magnesia.** Heavy Magnesium Oxide BP 1958. **Magnesia levis, Light magnesia.** Light Magnesium Oxide BP 1973. **Milk of magnesia.** Magnesium Hydroxide Mixture BP 1973. **Magnesia ponderosa.** Heavy Magnesium Oxide BP 1958. **Magnesia usta.** Magnesium oxide (Obsolete term). **White magnesia.** An obsolete name formerly used to distinguish light or heavy magnesium oxide from manganese dioxide. [*Magnesia,* a district in ancient Greece.]

magnesic (mag·ne·sik). Containing, or relating to magnesium or a magnesium compound.

magnesii. Magnesii Oxidum Leve, *European Pharmacopoeia* name for Light Magnesium Oxide BP 1973. **Magnesii Subcarbonas Levis,** *European Pharmacopoeia* name for Light Magnesium Carbonate BP 1973. **Magnesii Subcarbonas Ponderosus,** *European Pharmacopoeia* name for Heavy Magnesium Carbonate BP 1973. **Magnesii Sulfas,** *European Pharmacopoeia* name for Magnesium Sulphate BP 1973.

magnesite (mag·ne·site). $MgCO_3$, a naturally-occurring form of magnesium carbonate, used in medicine for the same purposes as plaster of Paris.

magnesium (mag·ne·ze·um). An element of atomic weight 24.305, atomic number 12, and chemical symbol Mg. It is a silvery lustrous metal of comparatively low melting point, tarnishing easily in air and burning readily with an intense white flame. It occurs widely in mineral deposits and in sea water, and is a microconstituent of lower plants, and an essential metal in chlorophyll. It is present in many of the body tissues and in the plasma and extracellular fluid where it helps to maintain osmotic equilibrium. It has an important role in metabolism being required for many enzyme catalysed reactions, especially those in which nucleotides participate where the reactive species is the magnesium salt (e.g. $MgATP^{2-}$). Lack of magnesium is associated with abnormal irritability of muscle and convulsions, excess of it with depression of the central nervous system and of peripheral neuromuscular transmission. Various salts are used in therapeutics, principally for their local action on the alimentary canal as antacids and purgatives; the salts have also on occasion been administered intravenously to produce depression of the central nervous system, an action which is immediately abolished by calcium salts similarly given. **Magnesium bicarbonate solution.** Fluid magnesia; a clear colourless liquid which effervesces on warming. It contains not less that 2.5 per cent $Mg(HCO_3)_2$, and has antacid and mild laxative properties. **Magnesium borocitrate.** A compound used as a urinary antiseptic. **Magnesium Carbonate, Heavy, BP 1973.** $Mg(OH)_2 \cdot 3MgCO_3 \cdot 4H_2O$, a white granular powder, odourless and almost tasteless; used as an antacid, often admixed with others. **Magnesium Carbonate, Light, BP 1973.** $Mg(OH)_2 \cdot 3MgCO_3 \cdot 3H_2O$, a light white powder, odourless and almost tasteless, with antacid and laxative properties. **Magnesium Chloride BP 1973.** $MgCl_2 \cdot 6H_2O$, used in solution for peritoneal dialysis and haemodialysis. **Magnesium Glycerophosphate BPC 1963, Magnesium glycerylphosphate.** $C_3H_7O_3 \cdot MgPO_3$, a white amorphous powder with a bitter taste, sometimes incorporated in so-called "nerve tonics" but without rational basis. **Magnesium hydrate.** Magnesium Hydroxide (see foll.). **Magnesium Hydroxide BPC 1963.** $Mg(OH)_2$, a white, amorphous, odourless, tasteless powder, almost insoluble in water. It is used as an antacid in hyperchlorhydria and in the treatment of peptic ulcer; also as an antacid and mild laxative for children. Unlike the carbonates, it does not form carbon dioxide, but produces magnesium chloride which has a mild laxative effect. It may be administered in the form of tablets, alone or in conjunction with other antacids such as magnesium trisilicate, or as an aqueous suspension. **Magnesium Hydroxide Mixture BP 1973.** Cream of magnesia; a suspension in water of hydrated magnesium oxide, containing about 8.25 per cent of $Mg(OH)_2$. It is used as an antacid and mild laxative. **Magnesium Oxide, Heavy, BP 1958.** MgO, a white powder, almost insoluble in water, used as an antacid and mild laxative. **Magnesium Oxide, Light, BP 1973.** A very light white insoluble powder prepared from magnesium carbonate and used as an antacid. **Magnesium peroxide.** MgO_2, a white powder with mild antiseptic properties due to the release of nascent oxygen and used particularly in mouth-washes and tooth-pastes. **Magnesium phosphate.** $Mg_3(PO_4)_2 \cdot 4H_2O$, an insoluble white powder with antacid and mildly laxative properties. **Magnesium Stearate BP 1973.** The magnesium salt of a commercial stearic acid the main constituents of which are stearic and palmitic acids. It is useful in the treatment of certain dermatoses. **Magnesium Sulphate BP 1973.**

Epsom salts; $MgSO_4 \cdot 7H_2O$, a colourless crystalline compound with a bitter taste. It is soluble in water, especially if warm; as it is only slightly absorbed from the alimentary canal it acts as a fairly rapid and powerful purgative. **Magnesium Sulphate, Dried, BP 1973.** A white, odourless powder with a bitter taste prepared by drying magnesium sulphate at 100 °C until it has lost about 25 per cent in weight. **Magnesium Trisilicate BP 1973.** $2MgO \cdot 3SiO_2 \cdot xH_2O$, a tasteless, odourless, white powder with adsorbent and antacid properties. It does not cause alkalosis and so may be given in comparatively large amounts. [see foll.]

magnet (**mag**·net). 1. Piece of iron, steel, alloy, ore, etc., that has the power of attracting iron and which, when suspended, turns in the direction of the earth's poles. 2. Natural magnet, lodestone. 3. Electromagnet, a core of soft iron wound with insulated copper wire, which becomes magnetic when an electric current is passed through the coil. **Horseshoe magnet.** A magnet bent like a horseshoe so that the poles are brought together. **Permanent magnet.** A magnet that retains its magnetism long after the magnetizing influence has been removed. **Temporary magnet.** A piece of soft iron that is temporarily magnetized by an electric current or by induction from a nearby permanent magnet. [Gk *Magnesia*, a district in ancient Greece where lodestone was mined.]

See also: GRUENING, HAAB, HIRSCHBERG (J.), MELLINGER.

magnetic (mag·**net**·ik). 1. Relating to or derived from a magnet. 2. Having the property of magnetism. 3. Referring to any substance that can be magnetized.

magnetism (**mag**·net·ism). The property of a magnet or a magnetic field to attract or repel a magnetic pole. **Animal magnetism.** Hypnotism.

magnetization (**mag**·net·i·**za**′·shun). The process of rendering a substance magnetic.

magnetoconstriction (mag·**ne**·to·kon·**strik**′·shun). The alteration in length or breadth of a body during magnetization due to the reorientation of its molecules along the direction of the lines of force. [magnet, constriction.]

magneto-electricity (mag·**ne**·to·el·ek·**tris**′·it·e). Generation of electricity by means of a magnetic field.

magnetograph (mag·**ne**·to·graf). An instrument which is used in the determining of the strength and power of any magnetic field. [magnet, Gk *graphein* to record.]

magneto-induction (mag·**ne**·to·in·**duk**′·shun). Magnetic induction. *See* INDUCTION.

magnetology (mag·net·**ol**·o·je). The science of magnetism. [magnet, Gk *logos* science.]

magnetometer (mag·net·**om**·et·er). An apparatus for determining the intensity of magnetic forces. [magnet, Gk *metron* measure.]

magneton (**mag**·net·on). The unit of nuclear magnetic moment. **Nuclear magneton.** Magneton (see above).

See also: BOHR, WEISS (G.)

magnetotherapy (mag·**ne**·to·**ther**′·ap·e). Magnetism used therapeutically.

magnetropism (mag·ne·**tro**·pizm). In an organism, a change of direction in its development caused by magnetic influence. [magnet, Gk *trope* a turning.]

magnification (**mag**·ne·fik·**a**′·shun). The apparent enlargement or increase in the size of an object when viewed through a lens or arrangement of lenses, as in a microscope. [L *magnus* great, *facere* to make.]

magnify (**mag**·ne·fi). To amplify the size of an object by a single lens or by the microscope so that it appears to be much greater than it is. [see prec.]

Magnolia (mag·**no**·le·ah). A genus of trees (family Magnoliaceae), which are widely cultivated. Several species have been used medicinally, including *Magnolia virginiana* Linn., the bark of which forms a popular remedy for rheumatism and fevers, and *Magnolia acuminata* Linn., employed as a bitter tonic. [Pierre *Magnol*, 1635–1715, French physician and botanist.]

Magnus, Heinrich Gustav (b. 1802). German physician.

Magnus' sign. A ligature around a finger after death produces no visible alteration in the appearance of the distal part.

Magnus and de Kleijn neck reflex. A sign of decerebrate rigidity, first described in cases of tuberculous meningitis in children. Passive rotation of the head to one side causes extention of the limbs and increase of tonus on the side towards which the head is turned, and limb flexion with decrease of tonus on the opposite side.

Magyary-Kossa, Julius von. Budapest physician.

Kossa's stain. For lime salts: sections are immersed in silver nitrate solution in the presence of sunlight; lime salts reduce the silver nitrate to black metallic silver.

mahamari (mah·hah·**mah**·re). A form of plague which is found amongst the inhabitants of the southern slopes of the Himalayan mountains.

ma-huang (mah·hoo·ang). Ephedra BPC 1954; the dried stem of the Chinese herbs *Ephedra sinica* Stapf. and *Ephedra equisetina* Bunge, and also of the Indian species *Ephedra gerardiana* Wall. (family Ephedraceae). It contains the alkaloids ephedrine and pseudo-ephedrine which are responsible for its action as a vasoconstrictor and cardiac stimulant. It is administered as a liquid extract, and is used as a source of ephedrine.

maidalakri (mi·dah·**lak**·re). The local name for an Indian evergreen tree, *Litsea sebifera* Pers. (family Lauraceae), the bark of which is used as an astringent in diarrhoea and dysentery. The oil obtained from the fruit is employed as a remedy for rheumatism.

maidism, maidismus (ma·id·izm, ma·id·**iz**·mus). Pellagra. [Cuban *mahiz* maize.]

Maier, Rudolf Robert (b. 1824). Freiburg pathologist.

Maier's sinus. A depression in the wall of the lacrimal sac which is adjacent to the openings of the lacrimal canaliculi.

Kussmaul-Maier disease. Polyarteritis nodosa.

maieusiomania (mi·ew·se·o·**ma**′·ne·ah). Insanity occurring during the puerperium. [Gk *maieusis* delivery, mania.]

maieusiophobia (mi·**ew**·se·o·**fo**′·be·ah). Unnatural fear of the ordeal of bearing a child. [Gk *maieusis* delivery, phobia.]

maieutic (mi·**ew**·tik). Relating or belonging to obstetrics. [Gk *maieusis* delivery.]

See also: HORROCKS.

maieutics (mi·**ew**·tix). The science of obstetrics. [see prec.]

maim (mame). To disfigure or deform by injury. In law: to inflict disabling or deforming injury such as might prevent the victim, even after recovery, serving the Crown as a member of the armed force. [ME *maimem*.]

main (mahn). Hand. **Main d'accoucheur.** Obstetricians' hand. *See* HAND. **Main en crochet.** A hand in which the ring and little fingers are fixed in flexion. **Main en griffe.** A deformity of the hand in which the proximal phalanges of the middle, ring, and little fingers are hyperextended and the terminal phalanges flexed as a result of low ulnar paralysis. **Main en lorgnette.** The result of severe destructive arthritis of the hands, rheumatoid arthritis or psoriatic arthropathy, in which the fingers can be shortened and lengthened by the examiner like the sections of a telescope. **Main en squelette.** Skeleton hand. *See* HAND. **Main succulente.** Marinesco's succulent hand. **Main des tranchées.** Immersion hand; swollen, red, painful hands due to exposure to damp and cold. Analogous with trench foot. [Fr.]

maisin (ma·zin). A protein-like product found in maize seeds.

Maisonneuve, Jacques Gilles Thomas (b. 1809). Paris surgeon.

Maisonneuve's amputation. A method in which the bone is fractured first and the soft tissues are subsequently cut.

Maisonneuve's fracture. An external rotation fracture of the ankle with a spiral fracture of the upper shaft of the fibula and a tibiofibular diastasis.

Maisonneuve's operation. Internal urethrotomy by a guarded triangular knife blade introduced along a specially designed staff or urethrotome.

Maisonneuve's urethrotome. A urethrotome in which a concealed knife travels to the tip of the instrument; the flat apex of the blade pushes aside healthy mucous membrane and the knife-edge divides the stricture.

Walker's modification of Maisonneuve's urethrotome. An

internal urethrotome in which the triangular knife in its passage through the groove in the staff is firmly controlled within the groove, and the face of the stricture only is engaged and divided. The apex of the triangular knife is bevelled and non-cutting.

Maissiat, Jacques Henri (b. 1805). Paris anatomist.

Maissiat's band, bandelette, or tract. The iliotibial tract. *See* TRACT.

maize (maze). Indian corn; the American graminaceous plant *Zea mays*, or more particularly the grain produced by it, the eating of which as a staple food is aetiologically associated with pellagra. [Cuban *mahiz.*]

Majocchi, Domenico (b. 1849). Bologna dermatologist.

Majocchi's disease, or purpura. Purpura annularis telangiectodes.

trichophytic granuloma of Majocchi. An allergic granulomatous infiltration of the dermis provoked by infection with species of *Trichophyton.*

Makeham's hypothesis. The hypothesis that death is due to two co-existing factors: chance, which is constant, and the inability to resist destructive factors, which progresses geometrically.

Makkas, M. 19th–20th century Bonn surgeon.

Makkas' operation. An operation for ectopia of the bladder in which the caecum is utilized as a bladder and the appendix as a urethra.

mal (mal). Disease. **Mal d'aviateur.** Anoxaemia due to high altitude. **Mal de bassine.** Silk-winders' dermatitis; an eruption of the hands and forearms occurring in those who wind silk from cocoons softened in hot alkaline water. **Mal de cayenne.** Filarial elephantiasis. *See* ELEPHANTIASIS. **Mal comitial.** Epilepsy. **Grand mal, Haut mal.** Major epilepsy. *See* EPILEPSY. **Mal de Meleda.** Congenital symmetrical hyperkeratosis of palms, soles, elbows and knees, endemic on the Adriatic island of Meleda; it is autosomal recessive. **Mal de mer.** Seasickness. **Mal de misère.** Pellagra. **Mal perforans.** Neurogenic ulcer. *See* ULCER. **Mal perforant.** Perforating ulcer of the foot, due to trophic changes such as occur in tabes, diabetes, anaesthetic leprosy, etc. **Mal perforant palatin.** Perforation of the hard palate due to the breaking down of a syphilitic gumma. **Petit mal.** Minor epilepsy. *See* EPILEPSY. **Mal del pinto, Mal de los pintos.** Pinta. **Mal de quebracho.** Paaj; a contact dermatitis caused by the leaves of the red quebracho, *Schinopsis lorenzii*, of the Argentine. **Mal de la rosa, Mal rosso, Mal del sole.** Pellagra. **Mal de vers.** Silk-winders' dermatitis; mal de bassine (see above). [Fr.]

See also: BOECK (C. P. M.).

mala (ma·lah). The zygomatic bone. [L cheek bone.]

malabsorption (mal·ab·**sorp**·shun). 1. Defective absorption of fluids or of any other nutritive substances. 2. Defective anabolism. [L *malus* bad, absorption.]

Malacarne, Michele Vincenzo Giacintos (b. 1744). Italian surgeon and anatomist.

Malacarne's pyramid. The projection formed by the pyramid of the cerebellum on the inferior vermis.

Malacarne's space. The part of the interpeduncular fossa which contains the posterior perforated substance.

malacia (mal·a·she·ah). Pathological softening of an organ or tissue. **Malacia cordis.** Softening of the wall of the heart resulting from an infarct caused by coronary obstruction. **Metaplastic malacia.** Softening of bone due to secondary malignant deposits. **Myeloplastic malacia.** Softening of the bones due to multiple myelomatosis. **Porotic malacia.** Softening of a tissue accompanied by fibrous proliferation. **Malacia traumatica.** Softening of bone following injury. **Vascular malacia.** Softening of an artery due to degenerative changes in its wall. [Gk *malakia* softness.]

malacic (mal·a·sik). Pertaining to morbid softness or malacia.

malacologist (mal·ah·**kol**·o·jist). One who makes a special study of malacology.

malacology (mal·ah·**kol**·o·je). The branch of zoology that is concerned with molluscs. **Medical malacology.** The branch of malacology that is concerned with those molluscs that act as intermediate hosts of helminthic parasites of man, e.g. of the snail genera *Bulinus, Physopsis, Planorbis, Segmentina*, that are intermediate hosts of schistosomes. [Gk *malakos* soft, *logos* science.]

malacoma (mal·ah·**ko**·mah). 1. Abnormal softness of any organ or part. 2. A spot or part which has become softened by disease. [Gk *malakos* soft, *-oma* tumour.]

malacopathia (mal·ah·ko·**path**′·e·ah). Epidermolysis bullosa. [Gk *malakos* soft, *pathos* disease.]

malacophonous (mal·ah·**kof**·on·us). Possessing a soft voice. [Gk *malakos* soft, *phone* sound.]

malacoplakia (mal·ah·ko·**pla**′·ke·ah). The presence of soft patches on the mucous membrane of a hollow viscus, e.g. of the stomach. **Malacoplakia vesicae.** Soft fungus-like growth occurring on the mucous membrane of the ureters and bladder. [Gk *malakos* soft, *plax* flat place.]

malacosarcosis (mal·ah·ko·sar·**ko**′·sis). A softened condition of tissues, especially muscular tissues. [Gk *malakos* soft, *sarx* flesh, *-osis* condition.]

malacosis (mal·ah·**ko**·sis). Malacia.

malacosomous (mal·ah·ko·**so**′·mus). In biology, having a soft body. [Gk *malakos* soft, *soma* body.]

malacosteon, malacosteosis (mal·ah·**kos**·te·on, mal·ah·kos·te·**o**′·sis). Osteomalacia.

malacotic (mal·ah·**kot**·ik). 1. Relating or subject to malacia. 2. Applied to teeth which, through imperfect calcification, are abnormally prone to caries. They are often white in appearance. [Gk *malakos* soft.]

malacotomy (mal·ah·**kot**·o·me). An incision of the wall of the abdomen. [Gk *malakos* soft, *temnein* to cut.]

maladie (mal·ad·e). A disease or illness. **Maladie bleue.** Congenital heart disease. *See* HEART. **Maladie bronzée.** Addison's disease. **Maladie de Carrion.** Oroya fever. *See* FEVER. **Maladie cystique.** Cystic degeneration of the breast. **Maladie des jambes.** A disease described in rice growers in Lousiana which was probably a form of beriberi. **Maladie du sommeil.** African trypanosomiasis. *See* TRYPANOSOMIASIS. [Fr.]

See also: HODGSON, ROGER (H. L.), WOILLEZ.

maladjustment (mal·ad·**just**·ment). In psychiatry, indicating a state in which the subject cannot or will not fit into his environment, and is subject to irritability, anxiety, melancholia, and other psychopathic reactions. [L *malus* bad, adjustment.]

malady (mal·ad·e). A disease or illness.

malaise (mal·aze). An indefinite sensation of discomfort, indicative to the sufferer of disturbance of the normal bodily equilibrium. [Fr. uneasiness.]

malalignment (mal·al·**ine**·ment). The state of lying in imperfect alignment, e.g. teeth which do not conform to the normal arch. [L *malus* bad, alignment.]

malar (ma·lar). Relating to the cheek or cheek-bone (zygomatic bone). [L *mala* cheek.]

malaria (mal·a·re·ah). A disease characterized clinically by periodic paroxysms of shivering, fever, and profuse sweating, formerly attributed to "bad air" or the noxious emanations from swamps, but caused by the injection into the human body, by the bites of the females of certain species of anopheles mosquitoes, of infective forms (sporozoites) of one or more of at least four different species of *Plasmodium*. These invade the liver and subsequently the red blood cells, giving rise to periodic shivering, pyrexia, and sweating, with enlargement of the spleen, severe anaemia, and, in *malignant tertian malaria*, with local blocking of capillaries in individual organs. The species identified in man so far are *Plasmodium malariae* causing *quartan malaria*, *Plasmodium vivax* causing *benign tertian malaria*, *Plasmodium ovale* causing *ovale malaria*, and *Plasmodium falciparum* causing *malignant tertian malaria*. Closely allied, if not identical, forms of the disease occur in monkeys in tropical forests. The malaria cycle may be said to commence with the appearance in the red blood cells of special sexual forms of the parasites (gametocytes): the male or microgametocyte and the female or macrogametocyte. These heavily pigmented non-motile sexual cells circulate inertly until sucked up by a female anopheline mosquito of an appropriate species. In the stomach of the mosquito the microgametocyte throws off a number of wriggling thread-like microgametes which penetrate the female cell, now after certain changes a macrogamete. The cell resulting from the fusion is an oökinete or travelling vermicule, an actively motile cell which burrows through the stomach wall and then settles down under the lining of the abdomen to form an oöcyst within which large numbers of threadlike sporozoites develop. The oöcyst eventually ruptures into the abdominal cavity and sporozoites make their way to the salivary glands so that the mosquito becomes infective to human beings. On injection by mosquito bite, the sporozoites rapidly leave the blood stream, invade the parenchymatous cells of the liver (pre-erythrocytic stage) and after about a week rupture into the blood sinuses of the liver. Some of the young parasites are then destroyed by phagocytes, others enter red blood corpuscles to commence the asexual erythrocytic stage, whilst yet others (except in *Plasmodium falciparum*) re-enter fresh liver cells, producing the cryptic exo-erythrocytic phase. The young parasites which invade the red cells assume a ring form, but soon develop into growing feeding forms (trophozoites) with active amoeboid movement. They then commence to segment (schizonts) and eventually produce a number of individual merozoites clustered round a deposit of pigment (haemozoin). The infected corpuscles rupture and the individual merozoites invade fresh corpuscles to commence the asexual cycle anew. Untreated and undertreated cases of malaria tend to become chronic with recrudescence (recurrence of pyrexia within two months of the primary fever) and relapse (recurrence of pyrexia after an interval of some months). The blocking of brain capillaries by the schizonts of malignant tertian malaria produces *cerebral malaria*, a variety of pernicious malaria which is characteristic of *Plasmodium falciparum* infection, as only that species of parasite sporulates in the deep vital organs of the body. As a result, pernicious malaria may mimic acute disease of any organ of the body. In *algid malaria* the appearance of the patient is that of profound shock with peripheral vascular failure. Ineffectively treated malignant malaria in hyperendemic areas may produce a form of *haemolytic malaria* with resulting haemoglobinuria (blackwater fever). Dementia paralytica is often treated by pyretotherapy (fever treatment), and *induced malaria* may be used to cause the pyrexia; it may be produced by the bites of infective mosquitoes or by the injection of blood from a malaria patient. **Aestivo-autumnal malaria.** Malignant tertian malaria (see above). **Algid malaria.** *See* MAIN DEF. (above). **Avian malaria.** A plasmodial infection in birds; there are many species of avian plasmodia that are used extensively in experimental malariology and chemotherapy. **Benign tertian malaria.** Malaria caused by *Plasmodium vivax*; also called *simple tertian* or *vivax malaria.* **Bromeliad malaria.** Malaria transmitted by anopheles that breed in certain bromeliaceous plants which grow in South America and the West Indies. **Cerebral malaria.** Infection by *Plasmodium falciparum* in which there is blocking of the cerebral arterioles by parasites, with resultant cerebral symptoms. Such infections may be fatal unless specific and general treatment is given promptly. **Chronic malaria.** A vague term that is best avoided; strictly, any malarial manifestation after the primary attack, but most frequently applied to malaria occurring in a native of a malarious country who has been repeatedly infected, suffers from irregular and frequent febrile attacks, marked anaemia, and has an enlarged and fibrotic spleen (ague cake). **Cold malaria.** Algid malaria (*see* MAIN DEF. above). **Falciparum malaria.** Malignant tertian malaria (see above). **Latent malaria.** A persisting infection giving rise to no clinical symptoms, due to a biological balance developing between the parasite and the defence mechanism of the body. Small numbers of parasites survive, but are not demonstrable unless blood is inoculated into a non-immune person. Immunity due to a persisting latent infection is known as premunition. It tends to disappear if the latent infection dies out. **Malignant tertian malaria.** Malaria caused by *Plasmodium falciparum*; also called *aestivo-autumnal, subtertian*, or *falciparum malaria.* **Monkey malaria.** A plasmodial infection of monkeys; there are numerous varieties of which some are used in laboratory studies, the parasite employed being mainly *Plasmodium cynomolgi.* The possible relationship between human malaria and some kinds of African monkey malaria is still under investigation. **Ovale malaria.** A benign form of malaria caused by *Plasmodium ovale.* **Quartan malaria.** Malaria in which the paroxysms occur every fourth day, that is at 72-hourly intervals, caused by *Plasmodium malariae.* **Quotidian malaria.** Malaria in which the paroxysm occurs at 24-hourly intervals. **Simian malaria.** Monkey malaria (see above). **Simple tertian malaria.** Benign tertian malaria (see above). **Subtertian malaria.** Malaria in which the tertian periodicity may be partially obscured by some degree of pyrexia between the true paroxysms caused by *Plasmodium falciparum.* Also called *aestivo-autumnal, malignant tertian*, and *falciparum malaria.* **Tertian malaria.** Malaria in which the paroxysm recurs every third day, that is at 48-hourly intervals. It includes both *benign tertian* and *malignant tertian malaria* (see above). **Vivax malaria.** Benign tertian malaria (see above). [It. *mala aria* bad air.]

malariacidal (mal·a·re·ah·si'·dal). Having the power to destroy the malaria parasite. [malaria, L *caedere* to kill.]

malarial (mal·a·re·al). Relating to or caused by malaria.

malarialization (mal·a·re·al·i·za'·shun). Malarial therapy. *See* THERAPY.

malarialize (mal·a·re·al·ize). To induce malaria; more particularly to inject malarial plasmodia into the blood as a type of treatment in general paresis.

malariatherapy (mal·a·re·ah·ther'·ap·e). Malarial therapy. *See* THERAPY.

malariology (mal·a·re·ol'·o·je). The science of the study of malaria. [malaria, Gk *logos* science.]

malariometry (mal·a·re·om'·et·re). The application of quantitative measurements to the study of malaria.

malariosis (mal·a·re·o'·sis). A neurotic condition observed in members of the fighting forces whose health is restored after an attack of malaria but who regard themselves as permanent invalids with a right to a pension and medical care. [malaria, neurosis.]

malariotherapy (mal·a·re·o·ther'·ap·e). Malarial therapy. *See* THERAPY.

malarious (mal·a·re·us). Characterized by the presence of malaria, mainly used with reference to a geographical area.

Malassez, Louis Charles (b. 1842). Paris physiologist.

epithelial debris of Malassez, Malassez's rests. The unatrophied remains of the epithelial sheath of Hertwig found in the periodontal membrane which may contribute to the formation of cysts associated with a tooth.

Malassez's disease. Cyst of the testicle.

Malassez's method. A method for staining neuroglia with ammoniacal picrocarmine.

Malassezia (mal·as·e·ze·ah). A group of fungi imperfecti. **Malassezia furfur.** The causal agent in tinea versicolor. **Malassezia ovale.** A commensal of man, often associated with dandruff. **Malassezia tropica.** Malassezia furfur (see above). [L. C. *Malassez.*]

malassimilation (mal·as·im·il·a'·shun). Faulty assimilation. [L *malus* bad, assimilation.]

malate (mal·ate). Any salt or ester of malic acid.

malathon (mal·ah·thon). *s*-(1,2-Dicarbethoxyethyl)-1,1,1-trichloroethane. An insecticide of very low toxicity and high efficiency; it is particularly useful against DDT-resistant strains.

malaxation (mal·ax·a·shun). Pétrissage, one of the movements carried out in massage, in which the muscles are grasped in the masseur's hands and rolled and pressed; kneading. [L *malaxare* to soften.]

male (male). 1. Designating a human being or other organism of the sex that begets young or performs the act of fecundation. 2. Of the male sex, as distinct from the female sex. 3. Applied to that part of an instrument which fits into the other and hollow (or female) part. **XX male.** In man, a male with a46, XX karyotype and phenotype corresponding to Klinefelter's syndrome. **XXY male.** A male disomic for the X chromosome. In man, males with this chromosome constitution form the majority of the X-chromatin-positive cases of Klinefelter's syndrome. **XXXY male.** A male trisomic for the X chromosome. In man, males with this chromosome constitution show Klinefelter's syndrome with mental retardation. **XXXXY male.** A male tetrasomic for the X chromosome. In man, individuals with such chromosome constitution represent an extreme form of Klinefelter's syndrome. However, since they show some distinctive features such as characteristic facies, skeletal abnormalities, severe mental deficiency and extreme hypogenitalism, they are considered to be a somewhat distinct clinical group. **XXYY male.** A male disomic for the X and the Y chromosomes. In man, males with this chromosome constitution have the features of Klinefelter's syndrome (testicular dysgenesis) with stature and psychological traits similar to those of XYY males. **XYY male.** A male disomic for the Y chromosome. In man, individuals with such chromosome constitution may have a normal phenotype or one of the characteristic somatic and psychological anomalies which result in the YY or double Y syndrome [L *mas.*]

Malécot, Achille-Etienne (b. 1852). French surgeon.

Malécot's catheter. A type of self-retaining catheter.

malemission (mal·e·**mish**·un). In coitus, non-ejaculation of the semen. [L *malus* bad, *emissio* a sending out.]

maleruption (mal·e·**rup**·shun). The eruption of a tooth in an abnormal position. [L *malus* bad, eruption.]

Malethamer (mal·**eth**·am·er). BP Commission approved name for maleic anhydride-ethylene polymer; an antiperistaltic agent.

Malfatti, Hans. German biochemist.

Malfatti's method. For ammonia+amino-acid nitrogen in urine: powdered potassium oxalate is added to 2.5 ml urine and is then neutralized to phenolphthalein with 0.1 M NaOH; 10 ml neutral formaldehyde solution is added, and the solution titrated with 0.1 M NaOH.

malformation (mal·for·**ma**·shun). Faulty development of a structure; congenital deformity. [L *malus* bad, *formatio* a forming.] *See also:* ARNOLD (J.), CHIARI.

Malgaigne, Joseph François (b. 1806). Paris surgeon.

Malgaigne's amputation. Subtalar amputation. *See* AMPUTATION.

Malgaigne's fossa, or triangle. The carotid triangle of the neck.

Malgaigne's fracture. Bilateral vertebral fracture of the pelvis.

Malgaigne's hook. An apparatus for holding the fragments of a fractured patella in apposition.

Malgaigne's operation. An operation for the repair of hare-lip.

Malgaigne's pad. A fatty pad in the knee joint immediately above the articular surface of the femur and lateral to the upper end of the patella.

maliasmus (mal·e·**az**·mus). Glanders. [Gk *maliasmos* a disease of horses and asses.]

malice (**mal**·is). Harmful intention. **Malice aforethought.** In law, malicious intention which must precede the act intended; this does not necessarily mean premeditation. *Expressed malice aforethought* is that in which a person deliberately lies in wait or has uttered threats or menaces before, or who has shown a former grudge. *Implied malice aforethought* is that in which a deliberate cruel act is committed by a person against another, e.g. by poisoning. [L *malitia* badness.]

malignancy (mal·**ig**·nan·se). 1. In reference to neoplasms, indicative of danger to life, in contradistinction to the term *benign.* 2. A state in which there is malignant new growth. [L *malignus* of bad disposition.]

malignant (mal·**ig**·nant). 1. Threatening life or tending to cause death; the opposite of benign. 2. Virulent, 3. Recurrent, even after careful extirpation; this is in special reference to neoplasms. [see prec.]

malignin (mal·**ig**·nin). A hypothetical ferment which is supposed to endow cancer cells with their malignant character.

malignogram (mal·**ig**·no·gram). Graphic representation of the factors determining the malignancy of a tumour. [L *malignus* of bad disposition, Gk *gramma* record.]

malingerer (mal·**ing**·ger·er). An individual who feigns disease or illness. [Fr. *malingre* sickly.]

malingering (mal·**ing**·ger·ing). Feigning illness or disease or pretending inability to undertake work or service. [see prec.]

malinterdigitation (mal·**in**·ter·dij·it·**a**′·shun). The condition of abnormal intercuspal relationship between upper and lower teeth. [L *malus* bad, *inter, digitus* digit.]

Mall, Franklin Paine (b. 1862). Baltimore anatomist.

Mall's formula. The age of a fetus can be estimated by taking the square root of the length of the fetus from breech to vertex in millimetres and multiplying by 100. The result is expressed in days.

Mall's lobules. Small compartments bounded by branches of the splenic trabeculae. A spherule of splenic capillaries lies in the centre of each.

Mall's method. A method for the demonstration of reticulin fibres with acid fuchsine, after preliminary digestion of collagen fibres with pancreatic extract.

Mall's ridge. The pulmonary ridge; it is a ridge of mesenchyme, found in the embryo, connecting the dorsal end of the septum transversum with the wolffian body and is the anlage of both the pleuropericardial and pleuroperitoneal membranes.

malleal, mallear (**mal**·e·al, **mal**·e·ar). Belonging to the malleus.

malleation (mal·e·**a**·shun). Spasmodic tic-like twitching of the hands; the typical pattern is one of beating the thighs with the closed fists at regular intervals. [L *malleare* to hammer.]

malleiform (**mal**·e·e·form). Shaped like a hammer. [malleus, form.]

mallein (**mal**·e·in). An extract of *Pfeifferella mallei,* used in testing for glanders infection in man and animals: a febrile reaction follows injection in infected subjects. [L *malleus* glanders.]

malleo-incudal (**mal**·e·o·**in**′·kew·dal). Relating or belonging to the malleus and the incus.

malleolar (mal·e·o·lar). Relating or belonging to a malleolus.

malleolar arteries. Arteries arising from the posterior tibial, the anterior tibial [arteriae malleolares anterior lateralis et medialis (NA)] and the peroneal arteries.

malleolus (mal·e·o·lus). A rounded bony prominence on either side of the ankle joint. **External malleolus, Malleolus fibulae.** Lateral malleolus (see below). **Inner malleolus, Internal malleolus.** Medial malleolus (see below). **Lateral malleolus [malleolus lateralis (NA)].** A conspicuous prominence on the outer surface of the ankle joint; on its medial surface is a large articular facet for the lateral side of the talus. **Medial malleolus [malleolus medialis (NA)].** A rounded process on the internal surface of the ankle joint. **Outer malleolus.** Lateral malleolus (see above). **Malleolus radialis.** The styloid process of the radius. **Malleolus tibiae.** Medial malleolus (see above). **Malleolus ulnaris.** The styloid process of the ulna. [L little hammer.]

malleotomy (mal·e·**ot**·o·me). In cases of ankylosis of the ossicles of the middle ear, the division of the malleus. [malleus, Gk *temnein* to cut.]

malleus [NA] (**mal**·e·us). The largest auditory ossicle, club shaped with a rounded head [caput mallei (NA)] joined to a long handle [manubrium mallei (NA)] by a neck [collum mallei (NA)], and having an anterior [processus anterior (NA)] and a lateral [processus lateralis (NA)] process. The head articulates with the incus, the lateral process and handle are attached to the tympanic membrane, and a ligament attaches the anterior process to the squamotympanic fissure. [L hammer.]

mallochorion (mal·o·**kor**·e·on). The primitive chorion of a mammal. [Gk *mallos* wool, *chorion* skin.]

Mallory, Frank Burr (b. 1862). Boston pathologist.

Mallory body. A protozoon-like organism claimed to have been seen in the skin in scarlet fever.

Mallory's phosphomolybdic-acid haematoxylin. A method for staining the grey matter of central nervous system sections, or gross specimens, with a ripened mixture of haematoxylin, phosphomolybdic acid, and chloral hydrate.

Mallory's stain. For elastic fibres: the use of phosphotungstic-acid haematoxylin after alcohol fixation.

Mallory's differential stain. For neuroglial fibres: fibres are mordanted with trinitrophenol and then stained with phosphotungstic-acid haemotoxylin.

Mallory, G. Kenneth (b. 1926). American pathologist.

Mallory-Weiss syndrome. Massive haematemesis due to acute rupture of the mucosa at the gastro-oesophageal junction after straining and vomiting. Hiatus hernia may be associated.

mallotoxin (mal·o·**tox**·in). Rottlerin. [*Mallotus philippinensis* (Kamala tree), toxin.]

Mallotus (mal·**o**·tus). A genus of trees (family Euphorbiaceae). *Mallotus philippinensis* Muell. Arg. is the source of kamala. [Gk *mallotus* fleecy.]

mallow (**mal**·o). The name given to the genus *Malva* and certain other plants of the family Malvaceae. **Blue mallow, Common mallow.** *Malva sylvestris* Linn. **Dwarf mallow.** *Malva rotundifolia* Linn. **Marsh mallow.** Marshmallow. [L *malva.*]

malnutrition (mal·new·**trish**·un). Faulty nutrition due to imperfect or incomplete assimilation, faulty feeding or starvation, disease, or any other cause. **Malignant malnutrition.** Kwashiorkor, a state of dietetic insufficiency found in African infants and young children. It is frequently associated with malaria and other parasitic infection. The findings include pancreatic changes, adipohepatic liver, macrocytic anaemia, and hypoproteinaemia. Skin changes are a prominent clinical feature. [L *malus* bad, nutrition.]

malocclusion (mal·ok·**lew**·zhun). The lack of occlusion, or the abnormal occlusion, existing between the teeth of opposite jaws either when the jaws are at rest or during their physiological movements. **Close-bite malocclusion.** That form of malocclusion in which there is gross vertical overbite of the upper over the lower incisor teeth on closure of the mouth. **Open-bite malocclusion.** That form of malocclusion in which the cheek teeth prevent the incisor teeth from meeting one another on closure of the mouth. [L *malus* bad, occlusion.]

malomaxillary (ma·lo·max·**il**'·ar·e). Related or belonging to the malar bone and the maxilla.

malonal (**mal**·on·al). Diethylbarbituric acid. *See* ACID.

malonate (**mal**·on·ate). $CH_2(COOH)_2$, an inhibitor of succinate dehydrogenase.

malonyl (**mal**·on·il). The bivalent group or radical, $-COCH_2CO-$, the residue of malonic acid and an important feature in the structure of the barbiturates. **Malonyl coenzyme A.** An intermediate in the biosynthesis of fatty acids being formed by the incorporation of carbon dioxide into acetyl coenzyme A by acetyl CoA carboxylase. **Malonyl urea.** Barbituric acid, $CH_2(CONH)_2CO$, a compound formed by the union of malonic acid and urea with the elimination of two molecules of water. By replacement of the two hydrogen atoms of the CH_2 group with various combinations of alkyl radicals, a wide range of compounds may be produced with hypnotic properties.

maloplasty (**ma**·lo·plas·te). Plastic surgery performed on the cheek. [L *mala* cheek, Gk *plassein* to mould.]

Malpighi, Marcello (b. 1628). Rome and Bologna anatomist, physician and physiologist.

Malpighian corpuscle. 1. A lymphoid germinal centre of the spleen. 2. Renal corpuscle. *See* CORPUSCLE.

Malpighian glomerulus. The tuft of capillaries within a renal corpuscle which filters urine from the blood stream.

Malpighi's layer. The stratum germinativum of the epidermis.

pyramids of Malpighi. Renal pyramids; conical masses of tissue which form the medulla of the kidney, the apices of which project into the lesser calyces.

Malpighi's vesicles. The pulmonary alveoli.

malpighian (mal·**pig**·e·an). Associated with Malpighi.

malposition (mal·po·**zish**·un). Faulty or wrong position, a term used especially with regard to the fetus *in utero*, or to fractured bones under treatment. [L *malus* bad, position.]

malpractice, malpraxis (mal·**prak**·tis, mal·**prax**·is). The failure of employment of reasonable skill or attention on the part of a medical attendant, thereby endangering the health or even the life of a patient. A civil offence often referred to as professional negligence and liable to action for damages. A more serious criminal lack of care arising from a deliberate disregard for the care and safety of other persons constitutes *manslaughter.* [L *malus* bad, OFr. *practiser*, Gk *praxis* action.]

malpresentation (mal·pres·en·**ta**'·shun). Abnormal presentation of the fetus. [L *malus* bad, presentation.]

malrotation (mal·ro·**ta**·shun). Abnormal rotation, a term used especially of the vertebral column. [L *malus* bad, *rotare* to turn.]

malt (mawlt). Grain, usually barley, which has been softened by soaking and allowed to sprout. It has digestive and nutritive properties by virtue of the carbohydrate and enzyme it contains and has been employed in the treatment of wasting diseases such as cholera infantum and tuberculosis. [AS *mealt.*]

maltase (**mawlt**·aze). An enzyme associated with amylase in animal and plant cells, which completes the breakdown of starch and glycogen by converting each molecule of maltose, the end-product of amylase action, to two molecules of glucose. It acts upon other α-glucosides and is also referred to as *α-glucosidase.* Its optimal pH varies to some extent with its source, ranging between 4 and 7.

Malthus, Thomas Robert (b. 1766). English political economist and divine.

doctrine of Malthus. Malthusianism.

malthusianism (mal·**thew**·ze·an·izm). The belief that the population increases faster than the means of subsistence, and the increase in population should be limited by sexual continence and late marriage. [T. R. *Malthus.*]

maltobiose (mawlt·o·**bi**·oze). Maltose.

maltose (**mawlt**·oze). Malt sugar, $C_{12}H_{22}O_{11}$. A soluble disaccharide (α-glucose-α-glucoside) formed by the hydrolysis of starch or glycogen. It occurs in germinated barley (malt) and is itself split into glucose by the enzyme, maltase. It is highly soluble in water, is dextrorotatory, and gives the reactions of a reducing sugar. It is employed chiefly in bacteriological culture media, and is sometimes used, mixed with dextrins, for infant feeding.

maltosuria (mawlt·o·**zewr**·e·ah). The presence of maltose in the urine.

malturned (mal·**ternd**). In dentistry, the condition of a tooth which is rotated around its long axis in either a lingual direction, linguoversion, or in a labial direction, labioversion; a term little used in English practice. [L *malus* bad, turn.]

malum (**mal**·um). Disease. This Latin word has survived in a number of obsolescent terms, mainly but not solely those indicating osteo-arthritic changes in the hip joints of the aged. **Malum aegypticum.** Diphtheria. **Malum arteriarum senile.** Senile arteriosclerosis. **Malum caducum.** Epilepsy. **Malum cotunni.** Cotugno's disease. **Malum coxae.** Hip-joint disease; usually applied to tuberculosis of the hip. **Malum perforans pedis.** Perforating ulcer of the foot. **Malum primarium.** A primary disease. **Malum venereum.** Syphilis. [L bad.]

malunion (mal·**ew**·ne·on). Incomplete or incorrect union of the fragments or ends of a fractured bone. [L *malus* bad, union.]

Malva (**mal**·vah). A genus of herbs (family Malvaceae). The leaves and flowers of the two British species, *Malva sylvestris* Linn., the common or blue mallow, and *M. rotundifolia* Linn., the dwarf mallow, are used in cough mixtures for their demulcent properties. [L mallow.]

mamanpian (mah·mahn·pe·**ahn**). A mother yaw. *See* YAWS. [Fr. *maman* mother, *pian* yaw.]

mamba (**mam**·bah). An African snake, *Dendroaspis angusticeps.* [S. Afr. *m'namba.*]

mamelon (**mam**·el·on). One of the three cusps which are present on the incisive edges of incisor teeth when they erupt but which wear away with use. [L *mammilla* nipple.]

mamelonated (mam·el·on·a·ted). Having rounded prominences on the surface; nodulated. [mamelon.]

mamelonation (mam·el·on·a′·shun). The development of rounded teat-like prominences on bony or other structures. [mamelon.]

mamilla (mam·il·ah). The nipple; any teat-like structure. [L *mammilla* nipple.]

mamillary (mam·il·ar·e). Belonging to or resembling a nipple. [mamilla.]

mamillate, mamillated (mam·il·ate, mam·il·a·ted). Studded with nipple-like projections. [mamilla.]

mamillation (mam·il·a·shun). 1. A mamilliform prominence. 2. The state of being mamillated.

mamilliform (mam·il·e·form). Nipple-shaped. [mamilla, form.]

mamilliplasty (mam·il·e·plas·te). A plastic procedure for the correction of depressed nipple. [mamilla, Gk *plassein* to mould.]

mamillitis (mam·il·i·tis). Inflammation of the nipple. [mamilla, Gk *-itis* inflammation.]

mamilloid (mam·il·oid). Mamilliform. [mamilla, Gk *eidos* form.]

mamillopeduncular (mam·il·o·ped·ung′·kew·lar). Referring to the mamillary body and the peduncle.

mamillose (mam·il·oze). Having many teats or teat-shaped processes. [mamilla.]

mamillotegmental (mam·il·o·teg·men′·tal). Referring to the mamillary body and the tegmentum.

mamillothalamic (mam·il·o·thal·am′·ik). Referring to the mamillary body and the thalamus.

mamma (mam·ah). A mammary gland; the breast. **Mamma aberrans, Accessory mamma.** Supernumerary mamma (see below). **Mamma areolata.** Protuberance of the areola of the breast. **Mamma erratica.** Supernumerary mamma (see foll.). **Supernumerary mamma.** An abnormal number of mammary glands. [L breast.]

mammal (mam·al). Any individual or species of the Mammalia.

mammalgia (mam·al·je·ah). Mastalgia. [L *mamma* breast, Gk *algos* pain.]

Mammalia (mam·a·le·ah). A class of the phylum Chordata; mammals, characterized by the presence of mammary glands and hair, homothermal blood, and, usually, viviparous reproduction. Living Mammalia are divided into Prototheria, the monotremes, and Theria, the marsupials and placentals. [L *mamma* breast.]

mammary (mam·ar·e). Belonging or relating to the mammary gland. **Mammary gland.** *See* GLAND. [L *mamma* breast.]

mammary artery, internal [arteria thoracica interna (NA)]. A branch from the first part of the subclavian artery descending behind the upper six costal cartilages to end by dividing into the musculophrenic and superior epigastric arteries. It supplies perforating branches [rami perforantes (NA)] to the front of the chest (the 2nd, 3rd, and 4th entering the mammary gland [rami mammarii] NA) and twigs to the thymus [rami thymici (NA)], anterior mediastinum [rami mediastinales (NA)], pericardium, intercostal muscles, and diaphragm. Bronchial branches [rami bronchiales (NA)] anastomose with the bronchial arteries and usually also give branches which ramify on the sternum. Sternal branches [rami sternales (NA)] are distributed to the sternocostalis muscle and posterior surface of the sternum, and anastomose with vessels in the adjacent part of the mediastinum. There is also a lateral costal branch [ramus costalis lateralis (NA)].

mammary veins, internal [venae thoracicae internae (NA)]. Veins, usually two, accompanying the artery of the same name and draining the anterior intercostal spaces, diaphragm, abdominal wall, and pericardium. They end in the subclavian vein.

mammate (mam·ate). Having mammary glands.

mammectomy (mam·ek·to·me). Mastectomy. [L *mamma* breast, Gk *ektome* a cutting out.]

mammiform (mam·e·form). Shaped like a mammary gland. [L *mamma* breast, form.]

mammilingus (mam·e·ling·gus). The sucking or licking of the breast. [L *mamma* breast, *lingua* tongue.]

mammilla (mam·il·ah). Mamilla. [L.]

mammillary bodies. The breast-shaped structures that are situated behind the third ventricles of the brain.

mammitis (mam·i·tis). Mastitis. [L *mamma* breast, Gk *-itis* inflammation.]

mammogen (mam·o·jen). Prolactin. [L *mamma* breast, Gk *genein* to produce.]

mammogram (mam·o·gram). A radiograph of the mammary gland.

mammography (mam·og·raf·e). The study of the mammary gland by a specialized soft-tissue radiographic technique without injection of a radio-opaque contrast medium. [L *mamma* breast, Gk *graphein* to record.]

mammoplasty (mam·o·plas·te). An operation to reduce the size of the female breasts, usually employed when they are pendulous and hypertrophic. [L *mamma* breast, Gk *plassein* to mould.]

mammose (mam·oze). Having full or large mammary glands.

mammotomy (mam·ot·o·me). Mastotomy. [L *mamma* breast, Gk *temnein* to cut.]

mammotrophic (mam·o·trof·ik). Affecting the nutrition of the mammary gland, e.g. stimulating mammary development or milk production. [L *mamma* breast, Gk *trophe* nourishment.]

mammotrophin (mam·o·trof·in). Prolactin, galactin, galactopoietic hormone. A hormone isolated as a pure substance from the anterior pituitary, which stimulates milk secretion by the mammary glands previously brought to full development by the ovarian hormones. [L *mamma* breast, Gk *trophe* nourishment.]

mammotropic (mam·o·trop·ik). Having a stimulating effect on, or having affinity for, the mammary gland. [L *mamma* breast, Gk *trepein* to turn.]

mammotropin (mam·o·trop·in). Mammotrophin. [see prec.]

manchester brown (man·ches·ter brown). Triaminoazobenzene, $NH_2C_6H_4N{=}NC_6H_3(NH_2)_2$. A basic dye used for staining mucin, cartilage matrix and other basophilic substances.

manchineel (man·kin·eel). A tropical American tree, *Hippomane mancinella* Linn. (family Euphorbiaceae), which contains in all parts a poisonous and acrid juice.

mancinism (man·sin·izm). Left-handedness. [L *mancus* defective.]

mand (man·d). In spoken language a self-limiting statement concerning the needs of the speaker. Intransitive speech.

mandama (man·dam·ah). Severe hyperkeratosis of the mouths of the pilosebaceous follicles, giving a rough skin which has been likened to toad skin; it is often due to deficiency of vitamin A. [East Indian name for phrynoderma.]

mandible [mandibula (NA)] (man·dibl). The bone shaped like a horseshoe which forms the lower jaw. [L *mandere* to chew.]

angle [angulus mandibulae (NA)]. The junction of the base of the mandible with the posterior border of the ramus.

base [basis mandibulae (NA)]. The lower border of the body of the mandible.

body [corpus mandibulae (NA)]. The horizontal portion of the mandible. With its fellow of the opposite side it forms a horseshoe-shaped bone, flattened from without inwards and presenting two surfaces, the outer and the inner, and by an upper and lower margin. The inner surface is marked by a ridge, the oblique line [linea obliqua (NA)] or mylohyoid line, from behind forward and downward, giving attachment to the mylohyoid muscle which forms the floor of the mouth. The alveolar part [pars alveolaris (NA)] is the upper, tooth-bearing portion.

head [caput mandibulae (NA)]. The expanded upper part of the condyloid process of the mandible.

neck [collum mandibulae (NA)]. A constriction immediately below the head of the mandible.

mandible, articular veins of the [venae articulares temporomandibulares (NA)]. Small veins draining the temporomandibular joint which open into the pterygoid plexus.

mandibular (man·dib·ew·lar). Relating to the mandible, or resembling a mandible.

mandibular nerve [nervus mandibularis (NA)]. The third division of the trigeminal nerve. It is a mixed nerve supplying sensory fibres to the temple, auricle, skin over the lower jaw, mucous membrane of the anterior two-thirds of the tongue, floor of the mouth, lower teeth, and dura mater. Its motor root supplies nerves to the masseter [nervus massetericus (NA)], medial pterygoid [nervus pterygoideus medialis (NA)], lateral pterygoid [nervus pterygoideus lateralis (NA)], temporal, and mylohyoid muscles.

mandibulectomy (man·**dib**·ew·**lek**·to·me). Excision of the mandible. [L *mandere* to chew, Gk *ektome* excision.]

mandibulofacial (man·**dib**·ew·lo·**fa'**·shal). Relating to the mandible and to the facial bones.

mandibulopharyngeal (man·**dib**·ew·lo·far·**in'**·je·al). Relating to the mandible and to the pharynx.

Mandl, Louis (b. 1812). Hungarian physician in Paris.

Mandl's paint, or solution. A throat paint of iodine in glycerin, flavoured with peppermint oil.

mandler filter. A domestic filter constructed of earth and composed of the shells of diatoms.

Mandragora (man·**drag**·or·ah). A genus of herbs, the mandrakes (family Solanaceae), having emetic, purgative, and narcotic properties, but now rarely used. Owing to their poisonous nature many superstitions were formerly connected with them. [Gk *mandragoras*.]

mandragorine (man·**drag**·or·een). $C_{15}H_{19}O_2N$, an alkaloid found in mandrake root with properties similar to atropine.

mandrake (**man**·drake). Any herb of the genus *Mandragora*. **American mandrake.** *Podophyllum peltatum* Linn. **English mandrake.** *Bryonia alba* Linn. [Gk *mandragoras*.]

mandrel (**man**·drel). An axis with which a rotating, cutting or polishing device is attached to a dental handpiece.

mandrin (**man**·drin). A guide or stylet for a catheter, generally used in soft catheters. [Fr. a punching tool.]

manducation (man·dew·**ka**·shun). The mastication of food. [L *manducare* to chew.]

manducatory (man·dew·**ka**·tor·e). 1. Relating to manducation. 2. Masticating.

manganese (**mang**·gan·eez). An element of atomic weight 54.94, atomic number 25, and chemical symbol Mn. It is a reddish-grey hard and brittle metal, with a very high melting point, which occurs in Spain, India, and Brazil as the ore, pyrolusite, MnO_2, and is used in alloys for hard tough steel and (with copper and zinc) for resistance alloys. It is present in many foods and in the tissues of most plants and animals; traces are necessary for normal development and for the proper functioning of the body's enzyme systems. It is essential for haemoglobin formation. Poisoning has occurred among those exposed to manganese in industry, producing a syndrome somewhat resembling parkinsonism. In therapeutics it is only employed in the form of the permanganates which have germicidal properties, and traces of manganese salts are sometimes added to haematinics, without justification, as deficiency does not occur. **Manganese butyrate.** $(C_3H_7COO)_2Mn$, a compound used in the treatment of boils, carbuncles, and other staphylococcal skin infections; it is injected intramuscularly, but its value is uncertain. **Manganese chloride.** $MnCl_2 \cdot 4H_2O$, a compound used in the treatment of staphylococcal infections by hypodermic injection; small amounts may be included in iron preparations as a trace element in the treatment of microcytic anaemia. **Manganese dioxide.** MnO_2, an insoluble black compound used in the form of precipitated manganese dioxide with iron salts in the treatment of anaemia, usually as pills. **Manganese Hypophosphite BPC 1963.** $Mn(H_2PO_2)_2 \cdot H_2O$, a compound with the properties of other hypophosphites, and a constituent of compound syrup of hypophosphites used as a "nerve tonic" in debilitated conditions. It may be employed as a trace element with iron in microcytic anaemia. **Manganese peptonate.** A constituent of solution of iron peptonate with manganese, consisting of iron peptonate with manganese chloride; it is used orally in the treatment of microcytic anaemia. **Manganese saccharate.** A preparation of manganese sometimes used with iron in microcytic anaemia. **Manganese Sulphate BPC 1968.** $MnSO_4 \cdot 4H_2O$, a compound used in the treatment of microcytic anaemia. [corruption of magnesia.]

manganism (**mang**·gan·izm). A condition of poisoning affecting individuals who work with manganese.

manganous (**mang**·gan·us). 1. Characterized by or containing manganese, e.g. an ore or alloy. 2. Describing a salt of manganese in which the latter is bivalent.

mange (**ma**·nj). An infectious skin disease of domestic animals, especially dogs. **Demodectic mange.** Infestation of an animal with *Demodex*. **Sarcoptic mange.** An infection with a sarcoptic mite, common in dogs and rarely affecting man. [Fr. *manger* to eat.]

mangifera indica (mang·**gif**·er·ah **in**·dik·ah). The mango tree; an Indian tree of the family Anacardiaceae, and the source of the fruit, mango, and of mango gum. [mango, L *ferre* to bear, *Indicus* Indian.]

mango (**mang**·go). The ripe fruit of the mango tree, *Mangifera indica* (family Anacardiaceae), which is cultivated chiefly for this purpose. It is nourishing, and a valuable source of vitamin C. The powdered kernel of the seed is occasionally used as an astringent in diarrhoea; the bark of the tree contains tannic acid and from it exudes a gum (mango gum) which occurs as amber or reddish-yellow transparent lumps and is approximately 40 per cent soluble in water. [Tamil *mankay*.]

mangosteen (**man**·go·steen). The common name for *Garcinia mangostana* Linn. A tropical fruit. [Malay *mangustan*.]

mania (**ma**·ne·ah). 1. A loose term frequently applied to any form of mental disorder or even a dominant preoccupation (e.g. mania for collecting stamps), seen in derivatives such as *homicidal mania* and *religious mania*. 2. As an obsolete diagnostic term, any form of mental disorder accompanied by very florid symptoms and some degree of excitement. 3. Precisely, a manic phase of a manic-depressive psychosis, i.e. a state in which there is elevation of mood, increased output of energy, speeding up of association even to the point of flight of ideas, and an enhanced opinion of the self, e.g. delusions of grandeur. **Acute hallucinatory mania.** An obsolete diagnostic term used to describe states of excitement accompanied by florid hallucinosis, and inclusive of catatonic excitement, confusional psychoses with much excitement, and genuine manic attacks of such an extreme degree or accompanied by sufficient somatic upset for hallucinations to be seen. **Akinetic mania.** An unusual form of mania in which retardation and inhibition, rather than overactivity, accompany elevation of mood; in its extreme form it becomes manic stupor. **Dancing mania.** Term specifically applied to several epidemics of mass hysteria in the Middle Ages with powerful religious motivations, in which dancing to the point of exhaustion affected members of crowds, and spread by suggestion. **Delirious mania.** An extreme manic excitement, in which there is also confusion, incoherence, and hallucinosis; Bell's mania. **Epileptic mania.** An epileptic twilight state in which there is much excitement; obsolete as a diagnostic term. **Homicidal mania.** A state of excitement in which homicidal tendencies are present. **Hysterical mania.** Hysterical insanity. *See* INSANITY. **Mania mitis.** The obsolete equivalent of hypomania. **Periodic mania.** A manic-depressive recurrent illness, in which the phases are predominantly manic. **Mania à potu.** State of excitement, especially if accompanied by marked aggressiveness, supervening on a drinking bout; more precisely, in a now obsolescent diagnostic use, such a state supervening on the imbibing of a trifling amount of alcohol. **Puerperal mania.** Puerperal insanity; more precisely a manic episode precipitated by childbirth. *See* INSANITY. **Religious mania.** A non-medical term for any mental disorder with delusions or preoccupations of religious content. **Singing mania.** Melomania; a type of mental disease in which the patient is given to singing for long periods. **Unproductive mania.** An ambiguous term used to describe mania in which there is little elaboration of positive symptoms, or mania in which the tendency to overactivity is blocked by inhibitory processes or by excessive distractibility, so that sentences are not completed in conversation, and acts are broken off before performance. [Gk madness.]

See also: BELL (L. V.).

maniac (ma·ne·ak). One afflicted with violent insanity or mania.

maniacal (man·i·ak·al). Relating to, or affected with mania.

manic (man·ik). Pertaining to mania.

manic-depressive (man·ik·de·pres′·iv). A person suffering from a psychosis, classified as an affective disorder, in which excitement and mania alternate with periods of depression: delusions are prominent and suicide is a relatively common termination.

manikin (man·e·kin). A model of the human body with movable parts and limbs, used in the teaching of anatomy; a model used in teaching obstetrics or surgery. [D *manneken* little man.]

manioc (man·e·ok). Cassava. [Tupi (South American) name.]

maniphalanx (man·e·fa·langx). A phalanx of the hand. [L *manus* hand, Gk *phalagx* a line of soldiers.]

manipulation (man·ip·ew·la′·shun). Adroit treatment carried out with the hands, especially in obstetrics. In physiotherapy, a term used to denote the forced passive movement of a joint beyond its active extent of movement. When the use of the hands is applied as a sole therapeutic agency, the treatment should be regarded as consisting of *manipulation*; applied to the soft parts, it is customary to refer to the treatment as *massage*, whilst when applied for the purpose of restoring lost mobility of joints the term *joint manipulation* is often used, but in recent years it has been customary to abbreviate further to the single word *manipulation*. **Conjoined manipulation.** Obstetric manipulative treatment in which both hands are employed, one on the abdomen and one in the vagina. [L *manipulare* to handle.]

Manley, Roger Edward Wentworth. English physician.

Manley ventilator. An apparatus for artificial ventilation, operated by the gas flow delivered to it, the tidal volume being preset.

Mann, Frank Charles (b. 1887). Rochester, Minnesota, surgeon.

Mann–Bollman fistula. Experimental diversion of duodenal juice into the ileum for the production of peptic ulcer in animals.

Mann, Gustav (b. 1864). German physiologist at Oxford and New Orleans.

Mann's methylene-blue eosin stain. For Negri bodies and other virus inclusion bodies. The stain is made up of 35 parts of 1 per cent aqueous methylene blue, 45 parts of 1 per cent aqueous eosin, and 100 parts of distilled water. Tissue sections previously fixed in Zenker's or Bouin's fluid are stained with the solution for twelve hours at 37° C, differentiated in 70 per cent alcohol containing 1 drop of orange G solution per ml, dehydrated, and mounted in Canada balsam.

Mann, John Dixon (b. 1840). Manchester physician.

Mann's sign, Dixon Mann's sign. A change in electrical resistance of the skin, thought to be associated with certain neuroses.

Mann, Ludwig (b. 1866). German neurologist.

Wernicke–Mann type. Partial hemiplegia; hemiparesis.

manna (man·ah). 1. A term applied to the sweetish exudations obtained from a number of different plant and animal sources. 2. The sweetish juice or exudate obtained from incisions in the bark of the manna ash tree, *Fraxinus ornus* Linn. (family Oleaceae), a small tree indigenous to Southern Europe and cultivated in Sicily. It contains about 50 per cent of mannitol and has a gentle laxative action. Similar exudates from other trees are known individually as Australian, Armenian, tamarisk (etc.) mannas. [Hebrew *man*.]

mannan (man·an). A polymer of mannose.

manninositose (man·in·o′·sit·oze). A compound of mannose and inositol isolated from the phosphatide fraction of *Mycobacterium tuberculosis* by alkaline saponification.

mannite (man·ite). Mannitol.

mannitol (man·it·ol). Hexahydroxyhexane, $CH_2OH(CHOH)_4CH_2OH$. A hexahydric alcohol found in many plants, such as sugar cane, celery, and the larch, also in manna from the manna ash *Fraxinus ornus*. It has been used to produce a forced diuresis and in kidney function tests to measure glomerular filtration rate as it is not reabsorbed by the tubules (BP 1973). **Mannitol hexanitrate.** $CH_2ONO_2(CHONO_2)_4CH_2ONO_2$, a compound which in the pure state is explosive. Diluted with carbohydrate, it is used as a vasodilator because of the nitrite ion it frees.

Mannkopf, Emil Wilhelm (b. 1833). Marburg physician.

Mannkopf's sign, Mannkopf-Rumpf sign. The pulse rate increases on pressure over a painful area if the pain is genuine.

Mannomustine (man·o·mus·teen). BP Commission approved name for the mannitol complex of mustine; it is a cytotoxic agent, and is used in the treatment of leukaemias. **Mannomustine Hydrochloride BPC 1968.** 1,6-di(2-chloroethylamino)-1,6-dideoxy-D-mannitol dihydrochloride, a cytotoxic agent used in the treatment of neoplastic disease, particularly of lymphoid and haemopoietic tissues. Its action and side-effects are those of mustine hydrochloride.

mannose (man·ose). D-mannose, $CH_2OH(CHOH)_4CHO$. An aldohexose found as a glycoside in certain plants, as a unit in compound saccharides, in mucoproteins, and, polymerized, as mannan in vegetable ivory nut; it can also be synthesized. It is a stereo-isomer of glucose, but is of little significance in nutrition. [manna.]

mannosidosis (man·o·sid·o′·sis). A rare disease with absence of D-mannosidase and accumulation of mannoside in tissues. [mannoside, Gk *-osis* condition.]

mannosocellulose (man·o·so·sel′·ew·loze). A variety of cellulose differing from the usual kind in yielding on hydrolysis a mixture of both mannose and glucose instead of glucose only. It is present in coffee.

manoeuvre (man·oo·ver). A skilled method of manipulation; a procedure employed at operation. **Prague manoeuvre.** A manoeuvre to extract posterior positions of the occiput in breech presentations if there is delay with the aftercoming head. Two fingers of one hand grasp the shoulders from below and the other hand draws the feet of the fetus up over the abdomen of the mother. Thus the occiput is born first. [Fr.]

See also: ADELMANN, BURNS (J. W.), BUZZARD, CREDÉ, DE LEE, HUETER, JENDRASSIK (EUGEN), KRISTELLER, LARDENNOIS, LØVSET, MARSHALL (C. M.), MAURICEAU, MUELLER (A.), MUNRO KERR, NAEGELI, PAJOT, PAUCHET, PINARD, SANTE, SAXTORPH, SCANZONI, SCHATZ, SCHREIBER, SMELLIE, THORN (W.), VALSALVA, VEIT, WIGAND, WILKIE.

Manoiloff, E. O. 19th–20th century Russian physician.

Manoiloff's reaction. 1. A test for comparing the bloods of alleged parents and child to determine the paternity of the latter. 2. A pregnancy test involving the decolorization of 2 per cent aqueous theobromine and sodium salicylate solution and Nile blue by blood serum from a pregnant woman.

manometer (man·om·et·er). An apparatus employed to measure the pressure of gases or liquids. **Aneroid manometer.** A manometer the action of which depends on the movement of a diaphragm forming the lid of an evacuated metal box which is subjected to the pressure to be measured. The diaphragm is connected to a pointer which moves on a scale and gives a direct reading. **Capacitance manometer.** An instrument for the measurement of pressure changes in which the pressure-sensitive element alters the spacing between the plates of an electrical capacitor. In some instruments the pressure-sensitive element is itself the moving capacitor plate. The capacitance change is detected and displayed electrically. **Flame manometer.** A manometric flame used to determine variations in gas pressure. **Mercury manometer.** A U-tube containing mercury, one arm of which is connected to the gas or liquid system; the difference in the mercury levels is a measure of the pressure. **Optical manometer.** A special manometer that will record changes in pulse pressure visually and photographically. **Piezo-electric manometer.** An instrument for the measurement of pressure changes, in which the piezo-electric effect is used. The electrical charge produced on the surface of a disc of piezo-electric material such as quartz is proportional to the pressure applied to the disc: if the surfaces of the disc are conducting, a potential is developed between opposite surfaces which may be measured and is proportional to the applied pressure. **Spring manometer.** A thin coiled tube into which gas or liquid is admitted; the pressure is indicated by the uncoiling of the tube. [Gk *manos* thin, meter.]

See also: GREENFIELD, KOENIG, WARBURG (O. H.).

manometric (man·o·**met**·rik). 1. Relating to a manometer or to the measurements obtained by its use. 2. Sensitive to variations in gas or liquid pressure. **Manometric flame.** A gas flame sensitive to the variations in atmospheric pressure caused by sound waves of certain frequency.

manometry (man·**om**·et·re). The science of pressure measurement of liquids and gases. [Gk *manos* thin, *metron* measure.]

manoptoscope (man·**op**·to·skope). An instrument used to demonstrate ocular function. [L *manus* hand, Gk *optos* seen, *skopein* to watch.]

manoscope (**man**·o·skope). An apparatus for measuring the volume of gases in gas analysis and density determinations. [Gk *manos* thin, *skopein* to watch.]

manoscopy (man·**os**·ko·pe). 1. The analysis of gases by volume. 2. The determination of gas densities by use of the manoscope.

manslaughter (**man**·slaw·ter). The reduced criminal charge that may follow upon operation of the Homicide Act 1957 in connection with the crime of killing. It is the *unintended* killing of a person by some act itself unlawful, e.g. assault, killing by dangerous driving. *See also* HOMICIDE. [AS *man, slean.*]

Manson, Sir Patrick (b. 1844). Hongkong and London physician.

Manson's disease, or schistosomiasis. Intestinal schistosomiasis, caused by *Schistosoma mansoni.*

Manson's haemoptysis. Haemoptysis due to infection with *Paragonimus westermani.*

Manson's mycetoma. *See* MYCETOMA, WHITE.

Manson's pyosis. Pemphigus contagiosus; a staphylococcal infection of the skin, producing bullous lesions; this tropical form of bullous impetigo can, and often does, spread quickly, hence the Japanese name tobichi, which means "sparks flying across".

Manson's solution. Borax methylene blue; the stain used by Manson in his earlier work on malaria.

Mansonella (man·son·**el**·ah). A genus of filarial nematodes. **Mansonella ozzardi.** A common, apparently harmless, parasite of man in the West Indies, Central America, and Northern Argentine. The adults live in visceral mesenteries, the larvae in the blood; intermediate hosts are midges of the genus *Culicoides.* [Sir Patrick *Manson.*]

mansonelliasis (man·son·el·**i**′·as·is). Infection with *Mansonella ozzardi.*

mansonia (man·**so**·ne·ah). The old name for *Taeniorhynchus.* [Sir Patrick *Manson.*]

Mansonioides (man·son·e·**oid**′·eez). A subgenus of *Taeniorhynchus.* [*Mansonia*, Gk *eidos* form.]

mantissa (man·**tis**·ah). In mathematics, the decimal following the whole number (characteristic) in a logarithm. [Etruscan, makeweight.]

mantle (**man**·tl). The pallium. **Acid mantle.** The surface film of the epidermis (pH 4.2–5.6) which can neutralize small amounts of alkali or acid. **Myo-epicardial mantle.** The layer of condensed mesenchyme surrounding the endothelial heart tubes of the early embryo, from which the heart muscle and visceral pericardium are derived. [L *mantellum.*]

Mantoux, Charles (b. 1877). French physician.

Mantoux conversion. The change from a negative to a positive reaction to the Mantoux tuberculin test following tuberculous infection or artificial immunization with BCG vaccine.

Mantoux reversion. The change from Mantoux-positive to Mantoux-negative sometimes seen with the lapse of time in persons immunized with BCG vaccine; the opposite of Mantoux conversion, may be an indication for revaccination with BCG vaccine.

Mantoux test. 0.1 ml of 1 in 10 000 Old Tuberculin BP 1973 is injected intracutaneously to raise a small cuticular bleb. A positive reaction is recorded if a raised reddened swelling of more than 5 mm diameter appears in from 2 to 3 days. A modification was later used: in this 1 international tuberculin unit (or 0.00002 mg of PPD) was used for the first test, and if negative this was followed by 10 units and eventually 100 units. A variation of this test using a multiple puncture apparatus with very short fine needles may be used. *See* HEAF'S TEST.

manubrial (man·**ew**·bre·al). 1. Belonging to the manubrium sterni. 2. Shaped like a manubrium.

manubriate (man·**ew**·bre·ate). Having a handle-shaped process. [L *manubrium* handle.]

manubriosternal (man·**ew**·bre·o·**ster**′·nal). Relating to the manubrium and the sternum.

manubrium (man·**ew**·bre·um). A handle. **Manubrium sterni [NA].** The upper portion of the sternum. [L]

manuduction (man·ew·**duk**·shun). 1. In obstetrical and surgical practice, operations performed by the hands. 2. Guidance, or introduction, as by the hand. [L *mandus* hand, *ducere* to lead.]

manudynamometer (**man**·ew·di·nam·**om**′·et·er). An apparatus used for measuring the extent of thrust. [L *manus* hand, Gk *dynamis* force, meter.]

manus (**man**·us). Hand. **Manus extensa.** Fixed dorsiflexion of the hand. **Manus flexa.** Fixed palmar flexion of the hand. **Manus valga.** Club-hand where the hand is deviated to the radial side. **Manus vara.** Club-hand where the hand is deviated to the ulnar side. [L]

manustupration (**man**·ew·stew·**pra**′·shun). Masturbation. [L *manus* hand, *stuprare* to defile.]

Manz, Wilhelm (b. 1833). Freiburg ophthalmologist.

Manz utricular glands. Glandular depressions in the ocular part of conjunctiva around the limbus: it has been suggested that they are no more than artefacts.

Schmidt and Manz theory. To explain swelling of the optic disc: accumulation of fluid in the intervaginal space causes a stasis of lymph in the trunk of the optic nerve, especially in the region of the lamina cribrosa sclerae; this causes compression of the central vessels, particularly the vein. This outflow of blood being obstructed, the disc becomes increasingly swollen.

Manzullo, Alfredo. 20th century Buenos Aires physician.

Manzullo's test. Tellurite test: a clinical test used as an aid to the diagnosis of diphtheria; 2 per cent potassium tellurite applied to the diphtheritic membrane or exudate produces blackening in from 5 to 10 minutes. Obsolete.

map (map). **Genetic map.** A gene and/or chromosome map.

mapping (**map**·ing). *Genetic.* Determining the position of genes on chromosomes. [L *mappa.*]

Maprotiline (map·**ro**·ti·leen). BP Commission approved name for 3-(9,10-dihydro-9,10-ethanoanthracen-9-yl)-propylmethylamine; an antidepressant.

Maragliano, Edoardo (b. 1849). Genoa physician.

Maragliano body, endoglobular degeneration. A round or elliptical body, resembling an inclusion body or nuclear remnant, looking like a vacuole in an erythrocyte; this appearance may be due to a partial degeneration of the latter.

Maragliano's serum. An antituberculosis serum prepared in animals. [obsolete.]

Marañon, Gregorio (b. 1887). Madrid physician.

Marañon's sign. Blushing of the skin of the throat on palpation, occurring in thyrotoxicosis.

Marañon's syndrome. The association of ovarian insufficiency with scoliosis and flat foot.

maransis (mar·**an**·sis). Marasmus. [Gk *marainein* to waste away.]

Maranta (mar·**an**·tah). A group of American tropical herbs. The roots of several species yield the starchy product, arrowroot, especially the variety *Maranta arundinacea.* [Bartolomeo *Maranta*, d. 1554, Italian physician and botanist.]

marantic (mar·**an**·tik). Of the nature of, relating to, or resulting from marasmus. [Gk *marainein* to waste away.]

marasmic (mar·az·mik). 1. Of the nature of, or relating to marasmus. 2. Affected with marasmus.

marasmoid (mar·az·moid). Resembling marasmus. [marasmus, Gk *eidos* form.]

marasmus (mar·az·mus). Infantile atrophy; a condition of severe and chronic malnutrition, resulting in lack of growth and failure to gain weight. The aetiology is often obscure. Primary or congenital causes may be: prematurity; congenital defects of the gastro-intestinal tract; congenital morbus cordis; congenital abnormality of the urinary tract; mental deficiency; or congenital fibrocystic disease of the pancreas. Secondary or acquired causes may be: infection, such as congenital syphilis; infection of the urinary tract, which may also show a congenital defect; parenteral infection associated with gastro-enteritis or chronic indigestion, usually associated with abnormal protein or fat metabolism; parasitic infestation; or neoplasms in the hypothalamic region of the brain. Underfeeding, whether dietetic or consequent on one of the above disturbances, causes the physical findings, which are: gross underweight for age; retardation of skeletal growth; complete loss of subcutaneous fat; inelastic, wrinkled skin; eyes sunken owing to lack of orbital fat; anterior fontanelle (if still open) depressed; muscular and mental lethargy; acidosis and hypoproteinaemia due to excessive metabolism of fat and protein destruction. If fluids are lost to a severe degree, whether from vomiting or diarrhoea, the above signs are present, together with dehydration fever, interference with circulatory and respiratory control resulting in cold blue extremities, failure to keep warm, irregular respirations and almost inevitable respiratory infection, blood concentration, oedema of hands and feet, excessive loss of nitrogen and salt, and, later, purpuric eruptions (cachectic purpura) over the trunk. Frequently the abdomen is distended, which enhances the appearance of wasting of the rest of the body. Treatment aims at dealing with the primary cause after any superadded infection has been dealt with. If this is not possible, correction of the dietetic deficiency must be undertaken with extreme care, fluid and salt correction being made by intravenous saline mixtures, plasma, fresh blood or packed red cell transfusions; protein derivatives may be given by the intravenous or the oral route. Care must be taken that protein given by the mouth is easily digestible (acidification of milk helps this) and that fat and carbohydrate intake are well balanced. Vitamins should be added to all regimens, as growth will begin as soon as the causative factors have been corrected. Sometimes good results are achieved by the judicious use of insulin covered by an adequate carbohydrate intake, if infection and congenital abnormalities are not present. **Enzootic marasmus.** A disease affecting sheep and cattle which arises from cobalt deficiency in soil and pasture. [Gk *marasmos* a wasting.]

Marcacci, Arturo (b. 1854). Perugia, Palermo, and Pavia physiologist.

Marcacci's muscle. A sheet of muscle fibres which lies beneath the areola and nipple.

Marchand, Felix Jacob (b. 1846). Leipzig pathologist.

Marchand's cell. A phagocytic cell from the adventitia of blood vessels.

Marchant, Gerard (b. 1850). Paris surgeon.

Marchant's zone. A zone within the skull where the dura mater is easily detached by extradural haemorrhage from a torn middle meningeal artery. The zone extends from the level of the lesser wings of the sphenoid bone anteriorly to a point from 2 to 3 cm from the internal occipital protuberance posteriorly; superiorly it reaches the superior sagittal sinus of the dura mater and inferiorly it is bounded by a transverse line at the level of the lesser wing of the sphenoid bone.

Marchi, Vittoria (b. 1851). Italian physician.

Marchi's ball, or globule. A particle of degenerating myelin.

Marchi's fluid. A mixture of Mueller's fluid and osmic acid used as a fixative for the central nervous system.

Marchi's method. After prolonged fixation in Mueller's fluid the portions of the central nervous system are placed in Marchi's fluid (see above). Recently-degenerated myelin sheaths stain black.

Marchi's reaction. The staining of degenerating myelin sheaths with osmic acid after prolonged treatment with potassium dichromate.

Marchiafava, Ettore (b. 1847). Rome physician.

Marchiafava disease, or syndrome, Marchiafava–Bignami disease. Primary degeneration of the corpus callosum, giving rise to mental symptoms, convulsions, and variable motor weakness.

Marchiafava–Micheli disease, or syndrome. A rare chronic haemolytic anaemia with paroxysmal nocturnal haemoglobinuria, first described by Struebing (1882), but usually associated with the names of Marchiafava (1911) and Micheli (1931). It occurs during sleep (day or night) when the blood pH is reduced.

marcid (mar·sid). 1. Wasted. 2. Exhausted. 3. In a state of general emaciation. [L *marcidus* faded.]

Marcille, Maurice (b. 1871)

Marcille's triangle. The lumbosacral triangle; a triangular space bounded by the body of the 5th lumbar vertebra, the ala of the sacrum, and the medial border of the psoas major muscle.

marcor (mar·kor). Marasmus. [L decay.]

Marcus Gunn. *See* GUNN, ROBERT MARCUS.

marcussen's ointment. Potassium polysulphide ointment.

Marcy, Henry Orlando (b. 1837). Boston surgeon.

Marcy's cobbler stitch. Cobblers' suture. *See* SUTURE.

mareo (mah·ra·o). Seasickness. **Mareo de la cordillera.** Mountain sickness; anoxia. [Sp.]

Marey, Etienne Jules (b. 1830). Paris physiologist.

Marey's law, or reflex. The cardiac rate is inversely proportional to the blood pressure, an adjustment mediated through the reflexes in the aortic arch and the carotid sinus, or more simply, the high-tension pulse is slow.

Marfan, Bernard-Jean Antonin (b. 1858). Paris paediatrician.

Marfan's disease. Syphilitic progressive spastic paraplegia of childhood.

Marfan's method, or epigastric puncture. A method of aspirating the pericardial sac in cases of pericardial effusion. A needle or trocar is introduced through the skin, under local analgesia, immediately below and to the left of the xiphoid process and diverted obliquely upward and slightly to the left, passing beneath the posterior surface of the sternum, for a distance of from 2 to 4 cm, when it pierces the base of the pericardial sac. In this way the peritoneum and diaphragm are avoided, and the most dependent portion of the pericardial sac where small effusions tend to accumulate may be drained.

Marfan's sign. A small triangular, clean and glazed area at the point of a furred tongue in typhoid fever.

Marfan's syndrome. A congenital mesodermal disturbance of hereditary nature, probably dominant but which does also occur sporadically, with variable clinical presentation. Common features are tall stature, increased span, long thin digits (arachnodactyly), subluxation of the lens of the eyes, weakness of the arterial walls leading to dissecting aneurysms or rupture of the aorta, or globular dilatation of the aortic root with aortic regurgitation. The term has also been extended to cover abnormalities of the mitral valve in which there is prolapse of a cusp into the atrium.

margarate (mar·gar·ate). Any salt or ester of margaric acid.

margarid (mar·gar·id). Having resemblance to a pearl. [Gk *margaron* pearl.]

margarine (mar·gar·een, mar·jer·een). Oleomargarine; a substitute for butter, or an imitation of butter. It is prepared from suitable vegetable and animal fats by emulsifying them with water and adding small amounts of milk (the bacterial action of which contributes flavour), salt and colouring matter; when vitamins A and D are added, as is compulsory in the UK, the nutritive value is indistinguishable from that of butter. In composition it is essentially fat with about 15 per cent of water. [Gk *margaron* pearl.]

margaritoma (mar·gar·it·o′·mah). Cholesteatoma of the auditory canal. [Gk *margaron* pearl, *oma* tumour.]

margin [margo (NA)] (mar·jin). The edge or border of a structure. **Cervical margin.** An undulating line, being the junction of enamel and cementum at the neck of a tooth. **Ciliary margin (of the iris).** Ciliary border of the iris. *See* IRIS. **Falciform margin [margo falciformis (NA)].** The curved lateral edge of the saphenous opening in the deep fascia of the thigh. Its upward extension is the superior cornu [cornus superius (NA)], and its downward extension the inferior cornu [cornu inferius (NA)]. **Infra-orbital margin [margo infra-orbitalis (NA)].** The lower margin of the orbital opening, formed by the maxillary and zygomatic bones. **Nasal margin [margo nasalis (NA)].** The serrated mid-portion of the lower border of the nasal part of the frontal bone between the medial angular processes. **Parietal margin [margo parietalis (NA)].** The thick serrated border of the frontal bone joining the parietal bone, and articulating below with the greater wing of the sphenoid bone. **Pupillary margin (of the iris).** Pupillary border of the iris. *See* IRIS. **Supra-orbital margin [margo supra-orbitalis (NA)].** The boundary between the frontal and orbital surfaces of the frontal bone. The rounded medial third is separated from the lateral two-thirds by the supra-orbital notch. It forms the upper margin of the orbital opening. **Margin of the tongue [margo linguae (NA)].** The lateral border of the tongue. [L *margo*.]

marginal (mar·jin·al). 1. Relating or belonging to, or situated at a margin or edge. 2. In psychology, belonging to the fringe of consciousness, i.e. to those contents of consciousness that, although obscurely and faintly felt, are not present to the attention. **Marginal artery of the colon.** A composite vessel composed of the proximal and distal branches of the ileocolic, right colic, superior and inferior left colic, and branches of the superior rectal arteries. These form an anastomotic chain parallel to and near to the colon, which is important in maintaining the collateral circulation when one or more of the colic arteries is occluded.

margination (mar·jin·a·shun). A circulatory condition occurring in the preliminary stages of an inflammatory process in which there is adherence of leucocytes to the walls of the blood vessels. **Margination of the placenta.** Placenta marginata. [L *margo* margin.]

marginoplasty (mar·jin·o·plas·te). Plastic renewal of a border, such as that of the eyelid. [margin, Gk *plassein* to mould.]

margo (mar·go) (pl. *margines*). Margin. [L]

Mariano Santo di Barletta (b. 1490). Neapolitan surgeon.

Mariano's operation, Marian operation. A perineal median operation for stone in the bladder.

Marie, Pierre (b. 1853). Paris neurologist.

Marie's ataxia. A bilateral symmetrical cortical atrophy of the upper anterior parts of the cerebellum resulting in symptoms and signs similar to those of Friedreich's disease but with increased reflexes and greater tendency to optic atrophy; it is usually noted at a later age than Friedreich's disease. Cases of Friedreich's and Marie's ataxia have occurred in the same family.

Marie's disease, or syndrome. 1. Clubbing of the fingers in suppurative diseases of the lungs. 2. Acromegaly. [obsolete term.]

Marie's hypertrophy. Hypertrophic pulmonary osteopathy.

Marie's sign, Charcot–Marie symptom. Tremor of thyrotoxicosis. [obsolete term.]

Marie's test. A test in which the subject is given three pieces of paper, and is told to put one in a waste-paper basket, another on a table, and return the third to the examiner. A test of memory.

Bamberger–Marie disease. Marie's disease 1st def. (see above).

Brissaud–Marie sign, or syndrome. Unilateral spasm of lips and tongue due to hysteria.

Charcot–Marie–Tooth atrophy, disease, or type, Marie–Tooth disease. Peroneal muscular atrophy; a familial disease of the spinal cord characterized by wasting and weakness of distal muscles in the lower and upper limbs; there is usually pes cavus, and appreciation of vibration and position may be impaired in the lower limbs.

Marie–Foix sign. Forced flexion of the toes or transverse pressure on the tarsus in a severely spastic leg that is not capable of voluntary movement produces reflex withdrawal of the limb.

Marie–Robinson syndrome. Laevulosuric syndrome. *See* SYNDROME.

Marie–Strümpell arthritis, disease, or spondylitis, Strümpell–Marie's disease. Ankylosing spondylitis, spondylitis ankylopoietica; sometimes known as *rheumatoid spondylitis.*

Marié Davy cell. A two-fluid voltaic cell the two electrodes of which are zinc and carbon immersed respectively in zinc sulphate and mercuric sulphate, the latter acting as a depolarizer. It yields an emf of 1.4 volts.

marihuana (mar·e·wah·nah). The Spanish Mexican name for the drug, cannabis, usually made into cigarettes and smoked by addicts. The drug acts on the higher nerve centres producing excitement, hallucinations, and euphoria, followed by deep sleep; excessive use may lead to insanity. It has been employed in medicine as a hypnotic to relieve pain, and to induce sleep, but there is great danger of addiction. The name has been corrupted variously to *mariguana, mariahuana, mariajuana, marijuana, Mary Jane,* and *Mary Warner.* [Sp.]

Marinesco, Georges (b. 1863). Bucharest neurologist.

Marinesco's succulent hand, or sign. A hand showing oedema, cyanosis, sluggish circulation, and other trophic changes, as in syringomyelia.

marinotherapy (mar·e·no·ther′·ap·e). The treatment of convalescents and those suffering from various diseases by the stimulatory influence of the climate at the seaside. [L *mare* sea, Gk *therapeia* treatment.]

Marion, G. 20th century Paris surgeon.

Marion's sign. In prostatic disease, the appearance of the margin of the prostate together with the ureteric orifices in the same cystoscopic field in the earlier stages of simple prostatic hypertrophy.

Mariotte, Edmé (b. 1620). French physicist.

Mariotte's experiment. A method of demonstrating the blind spot: with the left eye closed a cross on a card is fixated; a black spot to the right of the cross on the card will disappear when the card is held at the correct distance, about 22 cm.

Mariotte's law. *See* BOYLE'S LAW.

Mariotte's blind spot. *See* SPOT, BLIND.

marisca (mar·is·kah) (pl. *mariscae*). A haemorrhoid: the plural is generally used in order to indicate the disease, haemorrhoids. [L pile.]

mariscal (mar·is·kal). Haemorrhoidal. [see prec.]

maritonucleus (mar·it·o·new′·kle·us). The nucleus of the ovum immediately after fusion with a spermatozoon has occurred, and therefore descriptive of the earliest embryo. [L *maritus* conjugal, nucleus.]

Marjolin, Jean Nicolas (b. 1780). Paris surgeon.

Marjolin's ulcer. A squamous carcinoma developing in a chronic benign ulcer, e.g. varicose ulcer, an old unhealed burn, or a wound scar.

mark (mark). A spot; a birthmark. **Cafe-au-lait marks.** Oval, light brown patches in the skin in neurofibromatosis. **Longing mark.** Naevus. **Mulberry mark.** Strawberry naevus. **Port-wine mark.** Naevus flammeus. **Powder marks.** The residue of a firearm discharge on the hands or the forearm and on the body or clothing of the target. (*See* Paraffin glove TEST.) **Raspberry mark, Strawberry mark.** Haemangioma simplex. **Supra-segmental mark.** Used to indicate such features of articulated utterance as stress, pitch levels and terminal contours which would otherwise remain unexpressed. [AS *mearc.*]

marker (mark·er). *See* AMSLER, MARC.

marmoration (mar·mor·a·shun). Becoming veined, like marble. [L *marmor* marble.]

marmoreal (mar·mor·e·al). Resembling marble. [see prec.]

Marmorek, Alexander (b. 1865). Austrian physician in Paris.

Marmorek's serum. A serum prepared in horses; it was used against both tuberculosis and streptococcal infections; now obsolete.

marmorekin (mar·mor·ek·in). A serum for use in streptococcal infections. [Alexander *Marmorek.*]

marmot (mar·mot). A rodent of the genus *Arctomys.* It is an important reservoir of sylvatic plague in South Africa, North America, and Asia. **Siberian marmot.** The tarabagan *Arctomys bobac.* [L *mus montis* mountain rat.]

marochetti's blisters. The small blisters which form below the tongue in hydrophobia.

Marquis' test. For opium alkaloids: add 1 ml of concentrated sulphuric acid containing 1 drop of formalin to a little of the alkaloid. A purple colour is produced.

Marrett, Henry Rex, Coventry anaesthetist.

Marrett's bottle, or inhaler. A "draw-over" type of anaesthesia apparatus in which the air inspired by a patient is impregnated with vapour trichloroethylene and/or ether.

Marriott, Hugh Leslie (b. 1900). London physician.

Marriott-Kekwick apparatus. An apparatus for giving drip transfusions, in which the blood is kept stirred by oxygen bubbling through it.

Marriott and Kekwick formula. In blood transfusions: a formula for calculating the volume of blood in millilitres required to produce the desired rise in haemoglobin in adults or infants; it assumes that the normal blood volume is 88 ml per kg (40 ml per lb) body weight:

$$\frac{\text{Percentage rise haemoglobin required} \times \text{patient's normal blood volume}}{100}$$

Marriott and Kekwick U-tube regulator. A regulator for use in blood transfusions designed to avoid the constriction, and therefore easy blocking, that results from lateral compression of a rubber tube. It consists of four lengths of glass tubing each bent in a U, and their ends connected by a short-circuiting tube. Blood can be caused to flow along the short circuit or along one or more of the U tubes; in passing through the tubes the blood is slowed by frictional resistance. The rate of flow can be further regulated by raising or lowering the reservoir in relation to the U tubes.

Marriott, Williams McKim (b. 1885). American paediatrician.

Marriott's method. For alkali reserve: air is rebreathed into a rubber bag until the CO_2 tension equals that of venous blood. The alveolar air is then bubbled through a solution of sodium bicarbonate containing indicator until colour change ceases. The colour is then matched against standard tubes.

Shaffer and Marriott method. For acetone bodies in urine: urine is treated with basic lead acetate and the filtrate distilled. Acetone is determined in the filtrate iodimetrically; β-hydroxybutyric acid in the residue from distillation is oxidized with dichromate to acetone which is distilled off and estimated as before.

marrow [medulla ossium (NA)] (mar·o). The soft material found in the hollow centre of the long bones and in the cancellous spaces of all bones. It consists of a basic mesh of reticular fibres and reticular cells supporting a rich vascular network, with variable proportions of haemopoietic and fat cells. The characteristic histological feature is the sinusoid, a modified capillary, lined with specialized endothelial cells. Red and white cells are manufactured from germinal centres in and around the walls of the sinusoids. **Gelatinous marrow.** A brownish translucent tissue which replaces the normal bone marrow in certain wasting diseases. **Red marrow [medulla ossium rubra].** The marrow in late fetal and early post-natal life, being red owing to its high content of developing red blood cells. **Yellow marrow [medulla ossium flava].** The marrow of the limb bones in adult life, which loses its haemopoietic function and then consists largely of yellowish fat. [AS *mearh.*]

marrowbrain (mar·o·brane). Myelencephalon. [AS *mearh, bragen.*]

marrubiin (mar·oo·be·in). $C_{21}H_{28}O_4$, the bitter principle found in horehound (*Marrubium vulgare*). Horehound itself has been employed as an expectorant and stomachic, but is now little used.

Marrubium (mar·oo·be·um). A genus of plants of the family Labiatae; the dried leaves and flowering tops of *Marrubium vulgare* Linn. contain a volatile oil, resin and tannin, also a bitter principle, marrubin. [L horehound.]

Marsh, James (b. 1794). English chemist.

Marsh test, Marsh-Berzelius test. For arsenic: the arsenic in the prepared solution is reduced to arsine by zinc and dilute sulphuric acid and the gas is passed through a heated tube. A mirror of metallic arsenic is deposited and may be estimated by comparison with standard deposits prepared from known amounts of arsenic. A similar stain is given by antimony, but the latter may be differentiated from arsenic by its insolubility in sodium hypochlorite solution.

Marshall, Charles McIntosh (b. 1901). Liverpool gynaecologist.

Burns-Marshall manoeuvre, or method. Delivery of the aftercoming head by allowing the child to hang from the vulva by its own weight. When the head has entered the pelvis the legs are lifted downward and then forward; thus gradually the head is delivered.

Marshall, Eli Kennerly (b. 1889). Baltimore pharmacologist.

Marshall's method. A simple method for estimating urea in urine by urease, with direct titration of the liberated ammonia with standard acid.

Bratton and Marshall method. For sulphonamides in blood and urine: blood is deproteinized with trichloroacetic acid and the filtrate treated successively with sodium nitrite, ammonium sulphamate (to destroy excess nitrite) and *N*-(l-naphthyl)-ehtylenediamine dihydrochloride. The red colour produced is compared with standards: this gives free sulphonamide. Total sulphonamide is determined similarly after hydrolysis of the blood filtrate by heating with hydrochloric acid in boiling water for one hour. Urine is diluted 1 to 25 and the dilution treated in the same way as blood.

Marshall, John (b. 1818). London surgeon and anatomist.

Marshall's fold (ligament). The fibrous remnant of the left superior vena cava connecting the oblique vein of the left atrium to the left superior intercostal vein.

Marshall's vein. The oblique vein of the left atrium.

marshmallow (marsh·mal·o). Althaea; marshmallow root, the root of *Althaea officinalis* from which a mucilaginous demulcent solution may be made; useful in the symptomatic treatment of coughs and inflammation of the membrane of the mouth and throat. It is not, however, commonly used nowadays. [AS *mersc,* mallow.]

marsupial (mar·sew·pe·al). 1. Possessing a pouch. 2. One of the primitive mammals of Australasia and South America, in most of which the young are carried in a pouch. [L *marsupium* pouch.]

marsupialization (mar·sew·pe·al·i·za′·shun). The external drainage of a cavity, usually a cyst, by opening the cavity widely and suturing its edges to the edges of the skin wound. [L *marsupium* pouch.]

marsupium (mar·sew·pe·um) (pl. *marsupia*). 1. The scrotum. 2. A pouch or sac, e.g. in marsupials. **Marsupia patellaris.** The alar folds of the knee. [L pouch.]

Martegiani, J. (fl. 1814). Italian ophthalmologist.

area of Martegiani. The funnel-shaped beginning of the hyaloid canal anterior to the optic disc.

martial (mar·shal). Ferruginous; relating to or containing iron, known to the ancients as *Mars.*

Martin, August (b. 1847). Berlin gynaecologist.

Martin's pelvimeter. A caliper with a measuring scale, for determining the external measurements of the pelvis.

Martin, Henry Austin (b. 1824). Roxbury, Massachusetts, surgeon.

Martin's operation. 1. A type of vaginal hysterectomy (now obsolete). 2. A flap-splitting method of repairing vesicovaginal fistulae (now obsolete). 3. Vaso-epididymostomy for inflammatory occlusion of the epididymis.

Martin's syringe. For aspiration in empyema: a metal and glass syringe with a three-way tap, for aspiration and lavage of a pleural exudate or intrapleural blood through the intercostal space.

Martinotti, Giovanni (b. 1857). Bologna pathologist.

Martinotti's cell. A fusiform nerve cell from the deepest layer of the cerebral cortex, whose axon ascends into the layer of pyramidal cells.

Martinotti's vaccine. A vaccine prepared from killed *Mycobacterium tuberculosis*; now obsolete.

martonite (mar·ton·ite). A mixture of bromo- and chloro-acetones, used in chemical warfare as a tear gas.

Marwedel, Georg. German surgeon.

Marwedel's operation. A type of gastrostomy similar to Witzel's.

marx stain. A mixture of eosin, quinine and potassium hydroxide used in histology.

maschaladenitis (mas·kal·ad·en·i′·tis). Inflammation of the axillary lymph glands. [Gk *maschale* armpit, adenitis.]

maschale (mas·ka·le). Axilla. [Gk armpit.]

maschalephidrosis (mas·kal·ef·e·dro′·sis). Excessive sweating in the axillae. [maschale, ephidrosis.]

maschaliatria, maschaliatry (mas·kal·i·at′·re·ah, mas·kal·i·at′·re). Treatment of general or local conditions by inunction of the axilla, from which area absorption is rapid. [maschale, Gk *iatreia* treatment.]

maschalister (mas·kal·is·ter). The axis, or 2nd cervical vertebra. [obsolete term] [Gk band.]

maschaloncus (mas·kal·ong·kus). A tumour of the axillary region. [maschale, Gk *ogkos* tumour.]

masculation (mas·kew·la·shun). Masculinization.

masculinity (mas·kew·lin·it·e). The sum of characteristics inherent in the male of a species. [see foll.]

masculinization (mas·kew·lin·i·za′·shun). The development in woman of characteristics and qualities appropriate to man. [L *masculinus* male.]

masculinize (mas·kew·lin·ize). To cause or develop masculine traits or characteristics (virilism) in the female.

masculinovoblastoma (mas·kew·lin·o·vo·blas·to′·mah). Arrhenoblastoma; a testiculo-ovarian adenoma associated with masculinization. [L *masculinus* male, ovum, blastoma.]

maser (ma·zer). A device similar to a laser but operating with electromagnetic waves in the microwave region. [*m*icrowave *a*mplification by *s*timulated *e*mission of *r*adiation.]

masesis (mas·e·sis). Mastication. [Gk *masaomein* to chew.]

Masini. 20th century Italian physician.

Masini's sign. Hypo-extension of the digits in mental defectives.

mask (mahsk). 1. An appliance, commonly made of gauze and properly incorporating some impermeable material, used to cover the mouth and nose in the prevention of droplet infection. It is used at operations, and during the dressing of wounds. 2. A metal frame covered with gauze or lint on to which volatile anaesthetic liquids are dropped so that the vapour may be inhaled. 3. The facies, in certain conditions. **BLB mask.** An apparatus for the administration of oxygen designed in 1938 by Boothby, Lovelace and Bulbulian. A small nasal mask fitted snugly to the face is connected by an aluminium tube (the connecting device) with a rubber bag of about 700 ml capacity. The connecting device has three ports at its upper end which can be opened or closed by rotation of a metal collar with corresponding holes. An oxygen inlet tube enters lower down exactly opposite an expiratory valve. A length of rubber tubing is attached to this so that the oxygen is delivered within the bag. When the three air ports are closed the patient inspires entirely from the bag into which oxygen is flowing at a rate to prevent its collapse; by opening one or more air ports, more air and less oxygen is inspired. **Death mask.** A plaster of Paris cast of the face of a recently dead person. **Ecchymotic mask.** The violet-blue discoloration of the face with petechial haemorrhages, found in traumatic asphyxia. **Edinburgh mask.** A simple, semi-rigid, oxygen mask worn by the patient in bed, designed to give an alveolar oxygen concentration of between 20 and 40 per cent. Described in 1963. **Face mask.** A malleable appliance which fits over the nose and mouth to enable the patient to inhale a gas or vapour. **Meter mask.** A mask connected with a meter which measures the flow of oxygen. **Mask of pregnancy.** The pigmentation sometimes seen in pregnancy over the forehead, nose, and cheeks. **Tabetic mask.** Hutchinson's mask. **Uterine mask.** Mask of pregnancy (see above); chloasma uterinum. [Fr. masque.]

See also: ESMARCH, HUTCHINSON, JULLIARD, KUHN, OMBRÉDANNE, PARKINSON (J.), SCHIMMELBUSCH, WANSCHER.

masked (mahskd). 1. Disguised or overshadowed, e.g. a sign or symptom by another more prominent but possibly less relevant sign or symptom, or by the action of a drug; the action of a drug by that of another drug; a heart sound by another sound of unlike frequency. 2. In chemistry, applied to an element or radical the presence of which in a compound is concealed so far as its usual reactions are concerned owing to the peculiar manner of its combination, as in the case of the iron in haemoglobin. [see prec.]

masochism (mas·o·kizm). A type of sexual perversion in which an individual experiences a heightened enjoyment when being treated cruelly and subjected to humiliation and degradation. [Leopold von Sacher-*Masoch*, 1836–1895, Austrian author who depicted this type of character.]

masochist (mas·o·kist). One who indulges in masochism.

mason gag. A type of molar gag.

mass (mas). 1. Anything made up of coherent particles. 2. A cohesive mixture for making into pills. 3. The property of matter which endows it with inertia. The acceleration produced in any body by a given force is inversely proportional to its mass; the latter is to be distinguished from weight, which depends upon the force of gravitation. Cf. WEIGHT. 4. [Massa (NA)]. A bulky portion of bone. **Achromatic mass.** The unstained protoplasm surrounding the chromosomes during cell division. **Appendix mass.** An abdominal tumour consisting mainly of omentum and intestine, bound together closely to wall off infection in the appendix. Its presence is sometimes taken as the indication for the non-operative treatment of appendicitis. **Mass of the atlas.** *See* ATLAS. **Atomic mass.** The mass of the atom of any element; the atomic weight (C = 12) multiplied by the mass of the hydrogen atom. **Blue mass.** Blue pill. *See* PILL. **Electronic mass.** The mass of the electron; 9.107×10^{-28} g, approximately 1/1840 the mass of the hydrogen atom. **Filar mass.** The hypothetical spongy or reticular material of protoplasm; spongioplasm. [obsolete term.] **Interfilar mass.** The structureless fluid component of protoplasm, supposed to be present between the meshes of the spongioplasm; hyaloplasm. [obsolete term.] **Intermediate cell mass.** That part of the mesoderm which lies between the somites and the lateral plates on either side of the early embryo, from which the greater part of the urogenital apparatus is developed. **Mulberry mass.** Morula. **Pill mass, Pilular mass.** Bulk pill; a mass ready to be rolled and cut to form pills of any required size. **Relativistic mass.** The increase of the mass of a body with increase of its velocity relative to the laboratory co-ordinates, as given by the equation $m = m_0/\sqrt{(1 - v^2/c^2)}$ where m is the mass, m_0 the rest mass, v the velocity of the body, and c the velocity of light. This effect is of importance in calculating the motion of the atomic particles, the velocity of which may approach that of light. **Rest mass.** The mass of a body that is at rest relative to the laboratory co-ordinates. **Mass of the sacrum.** *See* SACRUM. **Tigroid mass.** Nissl substance. **Ventrolateral mass.** That portion of the myotome which gives rise to the ventrolateral musculature of the neck, thorax, and abdomen. [L *massa*.]

See also: PRIESTLEY.

massa (mas·ah). Mass; applied in pharmacy to the mass for pills. **Massa ferri carbonatis.** The mass for Blaud's pill. **Massa hydrargyri.** The mass for blue pill. **Massa kaolini.** Unguentum kaolini. [L]

massage (mas·ahzh). The treatment of disease or injury by skilful manual manipulation of the bodily tissues. It is employed in the relief of pain and spasm, to produce relaxation, to promote the absorption of exudates, to stretch adhesions, and to increase metabolism. The basic manipulations include effleurage, pétrissage, frictions, tapôtement, and vibrations. **Abdominal massage.** That sometimes used in the relief of chronic constipation. **Auditory massage.** Massage to the drum of the ear. **Cardiac massage.** The technique of rhythmically compressing the heart in order to maintain the circulation when spontaneous cardiac contraction has ceased. *External cardiac massage.* Cardiac massage performed by rhythmic compression of the chest, used when circulatory arrest occurs in circumstances other than those when the chest has been opened for an operation. *Internal cardiac massage.* Cardiac massage performed by rhythmic manual squeezing of the ventricles of the heart, used when cardiac arrest occurs after the chest has been opened for an operation. **Douche massage.** Massage given in conjunction with a douche. **Electrovibratory massage.** Massage given by electrical vibrators. **Inspiratory massage.** Diaphragmatic breathing employed to massage the liver indirectly. **Spray massage.** Massage given in conjunction with the Vichy douche. *See* DOUCHE. [Fr.]

massalis (mas·a·lis). A name for mercury. [L *massa* mass.]

Masselon, Michel Julien (b. 1844). Paris ophthalmologist.

Masselon's spectacles. Crutch glasses. *See* GLASSES.

Masselon test. A test of imagination and intelligence: the patient is required to compose a sentence in which three given words are included; this is one of the many projection intelligence tests.

masseter muscle [musculus masseter (NA)] (mas·e·ter musl). One of the muscles of mastication. It consists of superficial [pars superficialis (NA)] and deep [pars profunda (NA)] fibres, which arise from the anterior two-thirds of the inferior margin and the whole of the deep surface of the zygomatic arch. It is inserted into the coronoid process, lateral surface of the ramus, and angle of the mandible, and is supplied by the mandibular division of the 5th cranial nerve. An elevator of the mandible. [Gk one who chews.]

masseter, nerve to the [nervus massetericus (NA)]. *See* MANDIBULAR NERVE.

masseteric (mas·et·er·ik). Relating to the masseter muscle.

masseteric artery [arteria masseterica]. *See* MAXILLARY ARTERY.

masseteric veins [rami parotidei (NA)]. Veins which drain into the pterygoid plexus.

masseur (mas·er). 1. A man who practises massage. 2. An instrument used for the purpose of giving mechanical massage. [Fr.]

masseuse (mas·erz). A woman who practises massage. [Fr.]

massicot (mas·e·kot). The yellow powdery form of lead monoxide, PbO, obtained by heating lead in air at medium temperature: fusing converts it into litharge. [Fr.]

massive (mas·iv). Weighty; heavy; large in volume; of solid bulky shape. [L *massa* mass.]

Massol, Léon (b. 1837). Geneva bacteriologist.

Massol's bacillus. *Lactobacillus bulgaricus.*

massolin (mas·o·lin). An application introduced into the nose, throat, and body cavities in chronic inflammation, consisting of a pure culture of *Lactobacillus bulgaricus.* The line of treatment has mostly been discredited. [Léon *Massol.*]

Masson, James Carruthers (b. 1881). Rochester, Minnesota, surgeon.

Masson's fascia stripper. An instrument for the subcutaneous removal of strips of fascia lata required for transplantation. It consists of two metal tubes, one inside the other; the inner tube is longer and has an eye at its end through which the fascia is drawn. The instrument is thrust down the line of the fascia and withdrawal of the inner tube severs the fascial strand at the required point.

mastaden (mast·ad·en). The mammary gland. [Gk *mastos* breast, *aden* gland.]

mastadenitis (mast·ad·en·i′·tis). A condition of inflammation in the mammary gland. [mastaden, Gk *-itis* inflammation.]

mastadenoma (mast·ad·en·o′·mah). A tumour of the mammary gland. [mastaden, Gk *-oma* tumour.]

mastalgia (mast·al·je·ah). Pain in the mammary gland. [Gk *mastos* breast, *algos* pain.]

mastatrophia, mastatrophy (mast·at·ro·fe·ah, mast·at·ro·fe). A condition of atrophy of the mammary gland. [Gk *mastos* breast, atrophy.]

mastauxe, mastauxy (mast·aux·e). Hypertrophy of the mammary gland. [Gk *mastos* breast, *auxe* increase.]

mastectomy (mast·ek·to·me). Amputation of the breast. **Radical mastectomy.** Surgical removal of the breast, pectoral muscles and axillary lymph nodes in continuity. **Radical mastectomy, extended.** Radical mastectomy with, in addition, removal of internal mammary lymph nodes and sometimes supraclavicular nodes. **Radical mastectomy, modified.** Surgical removal of the breast and axillary lymph nodes in continuity but without removal of the pectoralis major muscle, and sometimes also of the pectoralis minor muscle. **Simple mastectomy.** Removal of the breast without the axillary lymph nodes. [Gk *mastos* breast, *ektome* a cutting out.]

Master, Arthur Morris (b. 1895). New York physician.

Master's tolerance test, Master's two-step test. 1. Of myocardial reserve: a test which measures the response of the heart rate and blood pressure to a standardized amount of exercise. The subject performs a variable number of ascents of two steps (each 23 cm (9 in) high) for 1½ min, the number of climbs being previously calculated from tables based on age, weight, and height. In normal persons the pulse rate should not rise more than 10 beats/minute, and the blood pressure not more than 1.3 kPa (10 mm Hg), and both should return to the pre-exercise level within two minutes. An increase in pulse rate or blood pressure in excess of the normal range may indicate cardiac disease, but emotional factors, cardiac neurosis, obesity, anaemia, disease of the lungs, and poor general physical condition may all produce an increase in pulse rate irrespective of cardiac disease. Furthermore, patients with cardiac disease but without cardiac insufficiency may have a normal exercise tolerance. 2. For myocardial ischaemia: during, or as soon as possible after, the same exercise routine as in 1 (above) an electrocardiogram is recorded; the presence of ST segment depression, especially in the central anterior chest leads, may indicate the development of myocardial ischaemia or exercise and assist the recognition of anginal pain.

masthelcosis (mast·hel·ko·sis). An ulcerative condition of the mammary gland. [Gk *mastos* breast, *helkosis* ulceration.]

Mastic BPC 1968 (mas·tik). A concrete resinous exudation from the tree *Pistacia lentiscus* Linn. (family Anacardiaceae), occurring in small pear-shaped tears. It contains resenes and resin acids, and an essential oil. [Gk *mastiche.*]

masticate (mas·tik·ate). To chew food. [L *masticare* to chew.]

mastication (mas·tik·a·shun). The act of chewing food. [see prec.]

masticatory (mas·tik·a·tor·e). 1. Having an effect on the muscles of mastication. 2. A remedy to be chewed only and not swallowed.

mastich, mastiche (mas·tik, mas·tik·e). Mastic.

Mastigophora (mas·tig·of·or·ah). A class of protozoa characterized by the presence of one or more flagella, by means of which the animals move. Flagellate unicellular algae may also be included. Species of the genera *Bodo, Cercomonas, Chilomastix, Craigia, Embadomonas, Enteromonas, Giardia, Leishmania,*

Trichomonas, and *Trypanosoma* are of medical importance. Flagellata constitute a sub-class. [Gk *mastix* whip, *pherein* to bear.]

mastigophorous (mas·tig·**of**·o·rus). 1. Relating to the Mastigophora. 2. Flagellate; a term applied to micro-organisms bearing cilia. [see prec.]

mastigote (**mas**·tig·ote). A member of the protozoon class Mastigophora; a flagellate. [Gk *mastix* whip.]

mastitis (mas·**ti**·tis). Inflammation, or changes resembling inflammation, in the mammary gland. **Acute mastitis.** Infection of the mammary gland by pyogenic organisms. **Mastitis carcinosa.** Cancer of the breast so rapidly growing that it resembles inflammation. **Chronic mastitis.** Literally a chronic inflammation of the breast. An obsolete concept to explain pain in the breasts without evidence of organic disease, often psychological in origin, and vague variations in consistency of the breast, often physiological in origin. **Chronic cystic mastitis.** A term used to describe the paraphysiological condition of multiple involution cysts of the breast under the obsolete concept of chronic mastitis (see above), according to which the cysts were wrongly regarded as obstructive from fibrosis. **Glandular mastitis.** Parenchymatous mastitis (see below). **Interstitial mastitis.** Inflammation of the supporting tissue which lies between the ducts of the breast. **Mastitis neonatorum.** Inflammation of the breast in newborn babies. **Mastitis obliterans.** An abscess-like enlargement of one of the duct systems of the breast. **Parenchymatous mastitis.** Inflammation of the secreting tissue of the breast. **Phlegmonous mastitis.** Spreading pyogenic inflammation of the breast. **Plasma-cell mastitis.** A form of chronic cystic mastitis (see above). **Puerperal mastitis.** A form of acute mastitis in a nursing mother. **Retromammary mastitis.** Inflammation between the breast and chest wall. **Stagnation mastitis.** Mastitis occurring after lactation. **Submammary mastitis.** Retromammary mastitis (see above). **Suppurative mastitis.** Mastitis proceeding to abscess formation. [Gk *mastos* breast, *-itis* inflammation.]

mastocarcinoma (**mas**·to·kar·sin·o′·mah). Carcinoma of the mammary gland. [Gk *mastos* breast, carcinoma.]

mastochondroma, mastochondrosis (mas·to·kon·**dro**′·mah, **mas**·to·kon·**dro**′·sis). A cartilaginous tumour, or chondroma, of the mammary gland. [Gk *mastos* breast, chondroma.]

mastocyte (**mas**·to·site). A mast cell. *See* CELL. [G *Mast* fattening, Gk *kytos* cell.]

mastocytoma (**mas**·to·si·**to**′·mah). A neoplastic tumour containing mast cells. [mastocyte, Gk *-oma* tumour.]

mastocytosis (**mas**·to·si·**to**′·sis). Neoplastic proliferation of the mast cell components of the reticulo-endothelial system. Manifestations include urticaria pigmentosa, telangiectasia, flushing, pruritus, dermographia, with deposits in liver, spleen, bone and gastro-intestinal tract; but in the vast majority of cases urticaria pigmentosa alone occurs. [mastocyte, Gk *-osis* condition.]

mastodynia (mas·to·**din**·e·ah). Pain in the mammary gland. [Gk *mastos* breast, *odyne* pain.]

mastoid (**mas**·toid). 1. Shaped like a nipple. 2. The mastoid part of the temporal bone. 3. Belonging to the mastoid part of the temporal bone. [Gk *mastos* breast, *eidos* form.]

mastoidal (mas·**toid**·al). Belonging to the mastoid part of the temporal bone.

mastoidale (mas·toid·**a**·le). In craniometry, the tip of the mastoid process.

mastoidalgia (mas·toid·**al**·je·ah). Pain in the mastoid part of the temporal bone. [mastoid, Gk *algos* pain.]

mastoideal, mastoidean (mas·**toid**·e·al, mas·**toid**·e·an). Mastoidal.

mastoidectomy (mas·toid·**ek**·to·me). An operation for the drainage and toilet of the mastoid or tympanic antrum, and the mastoid air cells. When the operation is limited to these structures it is known as the *simple* or *cortical mastoidectomy.* Where the operation is extended to drain the tympanic cavity as well as the mastoid antrum, it is known as a *radical mastoidectomy.* There is an intermediate stage between these two operations, known as a *modified radical mastoidectomy,* or sometimes, a *conservative mastoidectomy.* [mastoid, Gk *ektome* excision.]

mastoideocentesis (mas·**toid**·e·o·sen·**te**′·sis). Surgical opening, by puncture, chiselling, or drilling, of the mastoid air cells. [mastoideum, centesis.]

mastoideum (mas·**toid**·e·um). The mastoid part of the temporal bone.

mastoiditis (mas·toid·**i**·tis). Inflammation of the mastoid antrum and air cells; it may be acute or chronic. **Sclerosing mastoiditis.** Inflammation of the mastoid bone which results in thickening of the bone and obliteration of the air cells in it. **Silent mastoiditis.** Inflammation or suppuration within the mastoid antrum and air cells or mastoid bone, of a subacute or chronic character, without obvious general or local signs or symptoms, even sometimes without discharge from the ear. [mastoid, Gk *-itis* inflammation.]

See also: BEZOLD (F.).

mastoidotomy (mas·toid·**ot**·o·me). Incision of the mastoid air cells or of the tympanic antrum. [mastoid, Gk *temnein* to cut.]

mastoidotympanectomy (mas·**toid**·o·tim·pan·**ek**′·to·me). Total excision of the tympanic antrum or of the mastoid air cells. [mastoid, tympanum, Gk *ektome* a cutting out.]

mastology (mas·**tol**·o·je). That branch of medicine which deals with the study or the science of the mammary glands. [Gk *mastos* breast, *logos* science.]

mastomenia (mas·to·**me**·ne·ah). A vicarious menstrual discharge from the mammary gland. [Gk *mastos* breast, *menes* menses.]

mastomys coucha (mas·**to**·mis **kow**·chah). The multimammate mouse; a host-reservoir of *Pasteurella pestis* infection. [Gk *mastos* breast, *mys* mouse.]

mastoncus (mast·**ong**·kus). A tumour of the mammary gland, or nipple; the term may also refer to general swelling of the breast. [Gk *mastos* breast, *ogkos* tumour.]

masto-occipital (**mas**·to·ok·**sip**′·it·al). Belonging to the mastoid part of the temporal bone and the occipital bone.

mastoparietal (**mas**·to·par·**i**′·et·al). Relating or belonging to the mastoid part of the temporal bone and the parietal bone, e.g. the parietomastoid suture.

mastopathia, mastopathy (mas·to·**path**·e·ah, mas·**top**·ath·e). Any diseased condition of the mammary gland. [Gk *mastos* breast, *pathos* disease.]

mastopexy (**mas**·to·pex·e). The surgical readjustment of a pendulous mammary gland. [Gk *mastos* breast, *pexis* fixation.]

mastoplasia (mas·to·**pla**·ze·ah). Hyperplasia of breast tissue. [see foll.]

mastoplastia (mas·to·**plas**·te·ah). Hyperplasia affecting the mammary gland. [Gk *mastos* breast, *plassein* to mould.]

mastoplasty (**mas**·to·plas·te). The use of plastic surgery in lesions or abnormalities of the mammary gland. [see prec.]

mastoptosis (mas·top·**to**·sis). A condition in which the mammary glands are abnormally pendulous. [Gk *mastos* breast, *ptosis* fall.]

mastorrhagia (mas·to·**ra**·je·ah). Haemorrhage of sudden occurrence from the mammary gland. [Gk *mastos* breast, *rhegnynein* to gush forth.]

mastoscirrhus (mas·to·**skir**·us). A scirrhous tumour of the mammary gland. [Gk *mastos* breast, *skirrhos* hard.]

mastosis (mas·**to**·sis). Enlargement of the breast. [Gk *mastos* breast, *-osis* condition.]

mastospargosis (**mas**·to·spar·**go**′·sis). A condition of enlargement of the breast, in particular that caused by an excessive secretion of milk. [Gk *mastos* breast, *spargaein* to be full to bursting.]

mastosquamous (mas·to·**skwa**·mus). Belonging to or affecting the mastoid and squamous parts of the temporal bone. [Gk *mastos* breast, L *squama* scale.]

mastostomy (mas·**tos**·to·me). Incision and drainage of the mammary gland. [Gk *mastos* breast, *stoma* mouth.]

mastosyrinx (mast·o·**sir**·ingx). A fistula in the mammary gland. [Gk *mastos* breast, *syrigx* tube.]

mastotic (mas·**tot**·ik). Referring to or marked by mastosis.

mastotomy (mas·**tot**·o·me). Incision of a mammary gland. [Gk *mastos* breast, *temnein* to cut.]

mastous (mas·tus). Having large mammary glands. [Gk *mastos* breast.]

masturbation (mas·ter·**ba**·shun). The production of an orgasm by manual or mechanical friction of the genitalia. [L *masturbatio*.]

Matas, Rudolph (b. 1860). New Orleans surgeon.

Matas' aneurysmorrhaphy. *See* ANEURYSMORRHAPHY, *also* Matas' operation (below).

Matas' band. An aluminium band used to occlude temporarily a large blood vessel in order to observe the state of the collateral circulation.

Matas' operation. Endo-aneurysmorrhaphy; repair of an aneurysm by obliteration or excision with ligation of branches arising from it and reconstruction of the artery by a plastic approximation of the walls of the sac.

Matas' test. A test similar to Moschcowitz's test, but with the addition of compression of the main artery to the limb during the test.

Matas' treatment. The treatment of neuralgia by the injection of absolute alcohol into sensory ganglia; applied particularly to injection of the trigeminal ganglion in tic douloureux.

matching (mach·ing). A comparison of two or more things which are in accord. **Matching of blood.** The comparison of the blood of an intended donor with that of the recipient patient in order to determine whether or not both samples of blood are of the same ABO group and Rh type (i.e. Rh positive or negative). *Cross matching,* the method of determining whether transfusion of the donor blood to the recipient will be safe. The recipient's serum is tested by more than one technique, for the presence of antibodies capable of reacting with the donor's red cells; if no reaction occurs, the two bloods are compatible. [AS *gemaecca*.]

maté (**mat**·a). Paraguay tea; the leaves of the shrub *Ilex paraguayensis* St. Hilaire, growing wild in Brazil and cultivated in the Argentine. It contains tannin, approximately 1 per cent of caffeine and traces of aneurine; it is used like tea in South America as a stimulant infusion. [Sp. Amer.]

materia (mat·**eer**·e·ah). Matter; substance. **Materia alba.** White matter around the root of the tooth consisting of epithelial debris, bacteria, and moulds, indicating poor oral hygiene. **Materia Medica.** Originally applied to the study of the botanical and chemical properties of drugs, together with a description of the diseases in which they had proved of value, the term now includes *pharmacognosy* (the study of the natural history, physical characters, and chemical properties of drugs; materia medica proper), *pharmacy* (the art of preparation and compounding of drugs), *pharmacology* (the study of the actions of drugs on the body both in health and disease), and *therapeutics* (the art of applying drugs in disease). **Materia peccans.** Materies morbi. [L]

material (mat·eer·e·al). The matter from which anything is made. **Air-equivalent material.** A material having the same effective atomic number as air for x-ray absorption, used as a wall material for cavity ionization chambers. **Cross-reacting material (CRM).** Two distinguishable antigens, such as wild-type protein and a non-functional mutant derivative of it, each of which interacts with an antiserum prepared against the other. **Enriched material.** Material containing an element in which the abundance of one of the isotopes has been increased above that found in the naturally-occurring material. [L *materia* stuff.]

materies (mat·eer·e·eez). Material; substance. **Materies morbi, Materies peccans.** Any substance, whether it be a chemical entity or an organism such as a virus, which directly causes disease. [L]

Mathieu, Albert (b.1855). Paris physician.

Mathieu's disease, Lancereaux-Mathieu disease. Leptospiral jaundice. *See* JAUNDICE.

Mathieu's sign. In complete intestinal obstruction, a splashing sound can be produced by rapid percussion over the umbilical area.

mating (ma·ting). The process of sexual union. **Interrupted mating.** In bacterial genetics, the separation of conjugal pairs of mating bacteria, usually by violent agitation, thus preventing further chromosome transfer; by interrupting at intervals and analysing those donor genes which appear among recombinants as a function of time, the order of transfer of genes on the donor chromosome, and their distance apart in "time units", may be ascertained. **Random mating.** When an individual has an equal chance of mating with those of other genetic constitutions. [ME]

matlazahuatl (mat·laz·ah·**watl**). The Mexican name for tabardillo, or the epidemic typhus of that country.

matrass (**mat**·ras). A long-necked glass vessel formerly used in distillation. [Fr. *matras*.]

matrical (ma·trik·al). Belonging or referring to a matrix.

Matricaria (mat·rik·a·re·ah). 1. A genus of plants of the family Compositae. 2. The dried flowering heads of *Matricaria chamomilla* Linn. contain an essential oil composed of azulene and sesquiterpenes, and also a bitter principle. [L *matrix* womb.]

matrices (**mat**·ris·eez). *See* MATRIX.

matricial (ma·**trish**·al). Matrical.

matriclinous (mat·**rik**·lin·us). Matroclinous.

matrix (**ma**·trix) (pl. *matrices*). 1. The womb. 2. Any medium in which a thing is formed; a setting, e.g. intercellular tissue. 3. A mould in which a restoration for a tooth is cast. **Amalgam matrix.** A thin strip of metal which is fitted around a tooth to support and shape an amalgam filling which is being inserted in a compound cavity. **Interterritorial matrix.** The matrix between groups of cartilage cells. **Territorial matrix.** The matrix encapsulating a small group of cartilage cells. [L womb.]

matroclinous (mat·**rok**·lin·us). Having traits which have been transmitted from the mother. [L *mater* mother, Gk *klinein* to incline.]

matt (mat). Dull; lustreless; applied to the finely granular appearance of certain bacterial colonies. The condition was first described in the streptococci and is associated there with virulence; as the strain becomes less virulent the colonies tend to acquire a glossy surface, an important example of bacterial variation. [O Fr. *mat* dull.]

matte (mat). Coarse metal, white metal; a mixture of metallic sulphides, usually of copper and iron or copper and nickel, produced in the smelting of copper ores. [see prec.]

matter (**mat**·er). 1. Any liquid, solid, or gaseous substance that occupies space; material; elements. 2. A lay term for pus. **Central grey matter of the mid-brain [substantia grisea centralis (NA)].** An area around the aqueduct containing the nuclei of the 3rd and 4th cranial nerves and the mesencephalic nucleus of the 5th, in addition to the scattered nerve cells. **Central grey matter of the spinal cord [substantia grisea (NA)].** The fluted column of grey matter, H-shaped in cross-section, running the length of the spinal cord. **Gelatinous matter [substantia gelatinosa (NA)].** A translucent, cap-like region of grey matter at the apex of the posterior horn of the grey matter of the spinal cord. **Grey matter [substantia grisea (NA)].** Grey nervous tissue consisting largely of non-medullated nerve fibres and nerve cells. **Radiant matter.** 1. Radioactive material. 2. A gas at a very low pressure the atoms of which are emitting radiant energy in an electrical discharge. **White matter [substantia alba (NA)].** White nervous tissue consisting largely of medullated nerve fibres. [L *materia*.]

mattoid (**mat**·oid). A person whose mentality fluctuates between the brilliant and the mediocre; to this category belong the cranks and eccentrics. There is general instability of the mind, and conduct is therefore unpredictable. [L *mattus* drunken, Gk *eidos* form.]

mattress (**mat**·res). **Non-slip mattress.** A corrugated rubber mattress fitted to the top of an operating table to prevent the patient from slipping when the table is tilted. (*See* PUTTI.)

maturate (**mat**·ewr·ate). 1. To suppurate. 2. To bring to maturity. [see foll.]

maturation (mat·ewr·**a**·shun). 1. Ripening: commonly applied to the final stages in the development of the ovarian follicles. 2. Used by biologists to denote the division of the germ cells which leads to halving of the number of their chromosomes. 3. The emergence of personal and behavioural characteristics through growth processes. [L *maturare* to make ripe.]

mature (mat·ewr). 1. Completely developed or grown by natural process; fully grown; ripe. 2. Grown and developed to the point of being fit for any appropriate action, function, or state. 3. Relating or belonging to the condition of full development. 4. The forensic term applied to the developing fetus in the region of full term. Sometimes used by obstetricians for fetuses of over 2.5 kg (5½ lb) weight, but not used by the law which dates viability from the seventh month.

maturity (mat·ewr·it·e). 1. Puberty. 2. Those years of life during which the organs of reproduction best fulfil their function. 3. The state of being fully developed or grown. [see prec.]

Mauclaire's disease. Osteochondrosis of the heads of the metacarpal epiphyses.

Maumené, Edmé Jules (b. 1818). French chemist.

Maumené's test. For temperature reaction of oils and fats: to 50 g of sample in a tall beaker, surrounded by cotton wool to avoid heat loss, are added 10 ml of 97 per cent sulphuric acid (standardized by titration), the addition being made with constant stirring and taking about 60 s. The difference between the initial temperature and the highest temperature noted after the addition is taken as the *temperature reaction* of the oil or fat.

Maunoir, Jean Pierre (b. 1768). Geneva surgeon.

Maunoir's hydrocele. Cervical hydrocele; lymphangioma of the neck.

Maunoir's operation. For iridotomy. [obsolete.]

Maunsell, Henry Widenham (b. 1847). New Zealand surgeon.

Maunsell's operation. Removal of the gangrenous inner part of an intussusception through an incision in its outer sheath.

Maurer, Georg. 19th-20th century German physician in Sumatra.

Maurer's clefts, dots or stippling. A coarse irregular spotting of the erythrocyte characteristic of *Plasmodium falciparum* infections.

Mauriac, Charles (b. 1832). Paris physician.

Mauriac's disease. Syphilitic erythema nodosum.

Mauriceau, François (b. 1637). Paris obstetrician.

Mauriceau-Smellie-Veit manoeuvre, Smellie-Mauriceau-Veit manoeuvre, or method. To deliver the aftercoming head: the child is placed astride one arm and the middle and forefingers are placed over the upper jaw on each side of the nose, or the forefinger is placed in the mouth. This maintains the head in an attitude of flexion. The ring and little finger of the other hand are applied over the child's right shoulder and the thumb is placed over the left shoulder. Traction is now exerted in a downward and backward direction until the head is brought into the pelvis. Gentle pressure suprapubically facilitates this manoeuvre. The child's body is now carried up towards the mother's abdomen and the head delivered slowly over the perineum.

Mauthner, Ludwig (b. 1840). Vienna ophthalmologist.

Mauthner's layer, membrane, or sheath. A thin layer inside the myelin of a nerve fibre which is said to be in immediate contact with the axon; it is probably a fixation artefact.

mauveine (mo·ve·een). Aniline purple, $C_{24}H_{19}N_4Cl$. A violet safranine dye used for mordanted cotton, and as an indicator (pH 0.1–2.9). The first organic dye to be synthesized. [Fr. *mauve* mallow.]

Maxcy, Kenneth Fuller (b. 1889). Baltimore physician and bacteriologist.

Maxcy's disease. A variety of typhus fever. [obsolete term.]

maxilla [NA] (max·il·ah). One of the bones of the face which, with its fellow of the opposite side, forms the upper jaw. It consists of a body [corpus maxillae (NA)], containing an air space (the maxillary sinus or antrum) and four processes: the alveolar process projecting downward and bearing the teeth; the frontal process extending upward to articulate with the frontal and nasal bones; the palatine process projecting medially to join with the corresponding process of the opposite side in forming the anterior two-thirds of the hard palate; and the zygomatic process extending laterally to articulate with the zygomatic bone. The maxilla also articulates with the lacrimal bone, ethmoid bone, inferior concha, sphenoid bone, and the vomer. [L jaw.]

Anterior surface [facies anterior (NA)]. The surface of the body of the maxilla facing forward and laterally. It is bounded above by the infra-orbital margin, below by the alveolar process, and laterally by the zygomatic process and a ridge which runs from this to the roots of the first molar tooth. The medial boundary is the nasal notch, the sharp curved border separating the anterior from the nasal surface. This terminates below in a spicule of bone which, with its fellow on the opposite maxilla, forms the anterior nasal spine. There are a number of elevations in the lower part of this surface which overlie the sockets of the incisor, canine, and premolar teeth. That over the root of the canine tooth (canine eminence) is especially prominent and separates two shallow depressions, the incisive fossa above the incisor roots and a larger and more marked one, the canine fossa, above the premolar roots. Between the latter and the orbital margin is the infra-orbital foramen transmitting the infra-orbital vessels and nerve. Between this and the orbital margin in the infant there is a suture, the infra-orbital suture.

Nasal surface [facies nasalis (NA)]. The medial surface separated from the anterior surface by the nasal notch and contiguous with the posterior surface. The hard palate bounds it below. There is a large deficiency, the maxillary hiatus, in the posterosuperior part of the surface where the medial wall is lacking. In front of this the surface is continuous superiorly with the nasal process [margo lacrimalis (NA)]. Between the latter and the hiatus in the upper part of the medial surface there is a short groove, the nasolacrimal groove, whose overhanging edges almost meet; this lodges the nasolacrimal duct. The lower end of the anterior edge is continued into a rough ridge running downward and forward which gives attachment to the anterior end of the inferior concha. The roughened surface behind the hiatus is traversed by a groove running downward and forward from the posterior border. This is converted into the greater palatine canal by the coaptation of a similar groove in the perpendicular plate of the palatine bone which articulates with the roughened area.

Orbital surface [facies orbitalis (NA)]. The surface of the maxilla forming the floor of the orbit and also the roof of the maxillary sinus. Medially and in front it is notched for the nasolacrimal duct (lacrimal notch); behind this it articulates with the lacrimal, ethmoid, and palatine bones. The anterior border forms the infra-orbital margin. Laterally it slopes into the lateral wall of the orbit in front and forms the margin of the infra-orbital foramen behind. Its surface is grooved for the infra-orbital vessels and nerves, which enter a canal in the bone in front (infra-orbital groove and canal).

Posterior surface [facies infratemporalis (NA)]. The surface contiguous to the anterior surface laterally and to the nasal surface medially. Superiorly it is bounded by the margin of the inferior orbital fissure which separates it from the orbital surface. At the medial end of this border there is a notch leading into the infra-orbital groove. This surface is generally convex, the upper, wider part being smooth and forming the anterior wall of the infratemporal fossa laterally and the pterygopalatine fossa medially. There are two or three foraminae (dental foraminae) near the centre of this area which transmit the posterior superior dental nerves and vessels. The lower and narrower part of this surface forms the maxillary tuberosity. It is roughened for articulation with the tubercle of the palatine bone and the lower part of the anterior border of the lateral pterygoid plate.

maxillary (max·il·ar·e). Relating to the maxilla.

maxillary artery [arteria maxillaris (NA)]. The larger terminal branch of the external carotid artery, running forward medial to the neck of the mandible to enter the pterygoid fossa, which it leaves by passing through the pterygomaxillary fissure. It supplies multiple branches to the external auditory meatus (deep auricular artery [arteria auricularis profunda (NA)]), the tympanic membrane and cavity (anterior tympanic artery [arteria tympanica anterior (NA)]), the dura mater of the middle cranial fossa [ramus meningeus accessorius (NA)], the upper and the lower teeth [arteriae alveolares superiores (anteriores et posterior) and arteria alveolaris inferior (NA)], with dental branches [rami dentales (NA)] of the inferior alveolar artery to the lower teeth and mylohyoid muscle [ramus mylohyoideus (NA)], and of the superior alveolar artery to the upper teeth, the muscles of mastication, buccal artery [arteria buccalis (NA)], the mandibular joint, the pterygoid muscles [rami pterygoidei (NA)], the nasal cavity [arteria sphenopalatine (NA)] with posterior, lateral, and septal nasal branches [arteriae nasales posteriores, laterales, et septi (NA)], the palate [arteriae palatinae (major et minores) NA], the masseter artery [arteria masseterica (NA)], the lower part of the orbit [arteria infra-orbitalis (NA)], and the front of the cheek and chin [arteria mentalis (NA)].

maxillary nerve [nervus maxillaris (NA)]. The second division of the trigeminal nerve. It is sensory to the teeth [nervi alveolares superiores (NA)] with anterior, middle, and posterior superior dental branches, the face (zygomatic, palpebral, nasal, and labial branches [nervus zygomaticus, rami palpebrales inferiores, rami nasales interni et externi, et rami labiales superiores] NA), the mucous membrane of the nose and paranasal sinuses (anterior, middle, and posterior dental and palatine nerves), and the mucous membrane of the palate and pharynx (palatine and pharyngeal branches of the sphenopalatine ganglion). It also supplies the dura mater (meningeal branch [ramus meningeus (medius) NA]).

Ganglionic branches [nervi pterygopalatini (NA)]. Branches, usually two, from the maxillary nerve to the sphenopalatine ganglion. They carry sensory fibres which are not relayed in the ganglion.

maxillary vein, or veins [vena (venae) maxillaris (NA)]. A vein (or veins) draining the pterygoid plexus, and joining the commencement of the posterior facial vein.

maxillate (max·il·ate). Having jaws. [L *maxilla* jaw.]

maxillitis (max·il·i·tis). Inflammation of the maxilla. [L *maxilla* jaw, Gk *-itis* inflammation.]

maxillodental (max·il·o·den′·tal). Relating to the jaws and the teeth. [maxilla, L *dens* tooth.]

maxillofacial (max·il·o·fa′·she·al). Relating to the jaws and the face. [maxilla, face.]

maxillojugal (max·il·o·joo′·gal). Relating to the maxilla and the zygomatic bone. [maxilla, L *jugum* yoke.]

maxillolabial (max·il·o·la′·be·al). Relating to the maxilla and the lips. [maxilla, L *labium* lip.]

maxillomandibular (max·il·o·man·dib′·ew·lar). Relating to the maxilla and the mandible.

maxillopalatine (max·il·o·pal′·at·ine). Relating to the maxilla and the palatine bone.

maxillopharyngeal (max·il·o·far·in′·je·al). Relating to the maxilla and the pharynx.

maxilloturbinal (max·il·o·ter′·bin·al). Relating to the maxilla and the inferior nasal concha. [maxilla, L *turbo* spinning top.]

maximal (max·im·al). Used in the sense of "probably in the region of the maximum" where the available data are insufficient to state the precise value of the maximum. The term is often used in reporting clinical or physiological studies where successive values of a significant parameter are recorded and the maximum value of this data is of interest but cannot precisely be determined from the recorded observations. It is not synonymous with *maximum.* [L *maximus* greatest.]

maximum (max·im·um). 1. The greatest quantity or effect or the highest attainable value. 2. The crisis of a disease or process. 3. Utmost; greatest or largest. [L *maximus* greatest.]

Maxwell, James Clerk (b. 1831). British physicist.

Maxwell's law. The square of the refractive index of a medium equals its dielectric constant (specific inductive capacity).

Maxwell, Patrick William (b. 1856). Irish ophthalmologist.

Maxwell's ring. A circle of light which may appear in the visual field around the position of the macula; it is similar to Loewe's ring.

maxwell (max·wel). The cgs unit of magnetic flux; the flux through 1 cm^2 at right angles to a magnetic field of 1 gauss intensity and equal to 10^{-8} weber. [James Clerk *Maxwell.*]

May, Charles Henry (b. 1861). New York ophthalmologist.

May's ophthalmoscope. A simple and efficient self-illuminating electric instrument; the light is reflected into the eye by means of a prism, and the lenses are mounted in a rotating disc.

May, Richard (b. 1863). Munich physician.

May-Gruenwald stain. A type of Romanovsky stain.

Maydl, Karel (b. 1853). Vienna and Prague surgeon.

Maydl's hernia. Strangulation by the neck of a hernia of a loop of bowel which has re-entered the abdomen from the hernial sac and strangulated within the peritoneal cavity.

Maydl's operation. 1. Colostomy in which the colon is exposed and drawn out of the wound, being kept in place by means of a glass rod placed beneath it, until adhesions have formed. 2. Insertion of the extroverted bladder into the rectum.

Mayer, Ferdinand F. 19th-20th century American pharmaceutical chemist.

Mayer's reagent. A solution of mercuric chloride 13.5 g, and potassium iodide 49.8 g, made up to one litre with distilled water. It is used for the detection of alkaloids.

Mayer's solution. A solution of calcium phosphate, magnesium sulphate, and potassium hydrogen phosphate, used for synthetic media.

Mayer's test. For detecting alkaloids: most alkaloids yield white or yellow precipitates with Mayer's reagent (see above).

Tanret-Mayer test. A modification of the Tanret test adapted for testing for quinine in urine in order to check whether the patient is actually taking quinine that has been prescribed: a solution of 1.45 g of mercuric chloride in 80 ml of undistilled water is added to a solution of 5 g of potassium iodide in 20 ml of distilled water, the mixture being agitated during the process. The urine is first boiled and filtered, and to 5 ml of the filtrate a few drops of reagent is added; an immediate precipitate forms if the alkaloid is present in the urine.

Mayer, Karl (b. 1862). Austrian neurologist.

Mayer's reflex. Adduction of the thumb produced on firm flexion of the second finger into the palm.

Mayer, Paul (b. 1848). German histologist.

Mayer's carmalum. *See* CARMALUM.

Mayer's carmalum and indigo carmine. A mixture of carmalum and indigo carmine, used as a general tissue stain, especially for staining in bulk. Nuclei are stained red, cytoplasm blue.

Mayer's haemalum. A stain prepared from haematoxylin, sodium iodate, and alum. It is a powerful nuclear stain, admirable for staining in bulk.

Mayer's acid haemalum. Haemalum with 2 per cent glacial acetic acid used as a nuclear stain, especially for staining in bulk.

Mayer's haemalum and indigo carmine. A mixture of haemalum and indigo carmine, used as a general tissue stain. Nuclei are stained blue-black and cytoplasm a light blue.

Mayer's glycerin-albumin mixture. A mixture of white of egg, glycerin, and sodium salicylate, used for fixing sections to glass slides.

Mayer's muchaematein. A mixture of haematein, aluminium chloride, and glycerin in water; it stains mucus blue.

Mayer's paracarmine. A mixture of carminic acid, aluminium chloride, calcium chloride, and alcohol. It is used as a nuclear stain, especially for bulk staining.

Mayer's waves. Slow waves, not related to respiratory frequency, sometimes seen on the blood-pressure record when the blood supplying the medulla is deficient in oxygen; the waves are due to periodic variations in the tone of the vasomotor centre. They are sometimes incorrectly called *Traube-Hering waves.*

Maylard-Sonnenburg method. A method of intestinal anastomosis. The introduction of a temporarily occluded bowel end through an incision in the wall of a distal loop of the bowel; the proximal end is then released and fixed in place by mattress sutures. The advantages claimed are freedom from soiling, early return of peristalsis, and simplicity.

Mayo, Charles Horace (b. 1865). Rochester, Minnesota, surgeon.

Mayo's method, or treatment. The treatment of tic douloureux by resection of the affected division, followed by occlusion of the foramen ovale with a silver screw [obsolete term.]

Mayo's operation. For varicose veins: removal by stripping around them with a ring carried on a long narrow handle.

Mayo's gall-stone probe. A flexible probe consisting of a spiral of metal with a central removable wire which makes it more rigid, for the detection of stones in the bile passages.

Mayo's scissors. A variety of scissors with specially shaped blunt points, valuable in scissor dissection.

Mayo, William James (b. 1861). Rochester, Minnesota, surgeon.

Mayo's operation. Repair of umbilical hernia by excision of the sac and overlapping of the rectus sheath transversely over the closed peritoneum.

Mayo's vein. The prepyloric vein.

Mayo-Robson, Sir Arthur William (b. 1853). Leeds surgeon.

Robson's point. A point of maximum tenderness present in cases of inflammation of the gall bladder. It is situated at the junction of the middle and lower third of a line drawn from the right nipple to the umbilicus.

Mayo-Robson's position. A position on the operating table in which access to the gall bladder and bile ducts is facilitated by arching the back over a support, the patient being supine.

Mayor, Mathias Louis (b. 1775). Lausanne surgeon.

Mayor's hammer. A metal hammer used for counter-irritation by heating in boiling water and then applying to the skin.

Mayou, Marmaduke Stephen (b. 1876). London ophthalmologist.

Batten-Mayou disease. The juvenile form of cerebromacular degeneration; usually called *Spielmeyer-Vogt disease.*

maza (ma·zah). The placenta. [Gk *maza* cake.]

mazalgia (ma·zal·je·ah). Mastalgia. [Gk *mazos* breast, *algos* pain.]

mazalysis (ma·zal·is·is). Placental retention. [Gk *maza* cake, *a*, *lysis* a loosing.]

mazamorra (maz·am·or·ah). Ground itch. [Puerto Rico name.]

maze (maze). A network or intercommunicating system of paths. **Radiation maze.** A system of protective walls giving access to rooms containing sources of radiation. [etym. dub.]

mazic (ma·zik). Placental; belonging to the placenta. [Gk *maza* cake.]

mazocacothesis (ma·zo·kak·o·the″·sis). Faulty situation of the placenta. [Gk *maza* cake, *kakos* bad, *thesis* position.]

mazodynia (ma·zo·din·e·ah). Mastodynia. [Gk *mazos* breast, *odyne* pain.]

mazoitis (ma·zo·i·tis). Mastitis. [Gk *mazos* breast, *-itis* inflammation.]

mazology (ma·zol·o·je). Mastology. [Gk *mazos* breast, *logos* science.]

mazolysis (ma·zol·is·is). Placental detachment. [Gk *maza* cake, *lysis* a loosing.]

mazolytic (ma·zo·lit·ik). Referring to mazolysis.

mazopathy (ma·zop·ath·e). Any diseased condition of the placenta. [Gk *maza* cake, *pathos* disease.]

mazopexy (ma·zo·pex·e). Mastopexy. [Gk *mazos* breast, *pexis* fixation.]

mazoplasia (ma·zo·pla·ze·ah). Hyperplasia of breast tissue; cystic hyperplasia of the breast. [Gk *mazos* breast, *plassein* to mould.]

mazun (ma·zun). An Armenian form of *Lactobacillus*-treated milk, similar to yoghurt.

Mazzoni, Vittori (b. 1823). Rome physician.

Mazzoni's corpuscles, Golgi-Mazzoni bodies, or corpuscles. Encapsulated sensory nerve-endings found in the superficial and deep connective tissues of the body; they resemble pacinian corpuscles, but are much smaller. Also known as *Krause's terminal bulbs.*

mbundu (mboon·doo). A substance used in West Africa as an "ordeal" poison and also for tipping arrows. It is prepared from the root of a species of *Strychnos,* and some authorities say that it contains both narcotic and convulsant drugs.

meal (meel). The food taken on one occasion or at a stated time. **Barium meal.** An emulsion of barium sulphate taken before x-ray examination of the stomach and intestines as a contrast medium. **Bismuth meal.** A meal, for instance bread and milk, containing an insoluble bismuth salt, which is used in the x-ray examination of the alimentary canal. **Butter meal.** A meal containing butter, milk, flour, and sugar. **Liver meal.** A meal consisting mainly of liver with flavouring ingredients, for patients on a liver diet. **Opaque meal.** A meal containing a substance opaque to x-rays. **Oslo meal.** A meal given to schoolchildren, containing unskimmed milk, wholemeal bread, margarine, cheese from goats' milk, and half an apple or orange. **Test meal.** *See* TEST-MEAL. [AS *melo.*]

See also: BOYDEN, KNOEPFELMACHER.

mean (meen). 1. Intermediate; occurring between the limits or extremes of a structure or organ. 2. Average; moderate. 3. In mathematics, a quantity having an intermediate value between several others of which it expresses the mean value. **Weighted mean.** A mean treated by a statistical method to take into account certain special outside factors. [ME *mene* in the middle.]

measles (me·zlz). Morbilli; an acute virus exanthem, predominantly of early childhood. The incubation period is 10 to 12 days followed by an initial period of fever (which may be high) with coryza, cough and conjunctivitis. Koplik's spots, small bluish-white spots with a red areola, appear on the buccal mucosa at this stage. As they fade, the main maculopapular rash appears, initially on the head and spreading downwards. With full development of the rash the fever goes and recovery follows. Complications include pneumonia, otitis media and, rarely (one case in 1000), encephalomyelitis. A very rare and late complication is subacute sclerosing panencephalitis. Treatment is symptomatic but immunoglobulin (containing measles antibody) may be used to diminish the severity of the disease, particularly in young children, if given in the incubation period. Live attenuated vaccines are available and give a high degree of protection. **Black measles.** Haemorrhagic measles (see below). **German measles.** Rubella. **Haemorrhagic measles.** A severe form with haemorrhages into the skin and mucous membranes. May be confused with haemorrhagic smallpox or meningococcal septicaemia. **Pork measles** (bladder worms). The name given to the intermediate host stage (cysticercus cellulosae) of *Taenia solium* in the muscles of the pig. The muscles so affected are 'measly pork'. [OHG *masala* blister.]

measly (me·zle). Like measles; spotted or mottled, like the rash of measles. Used to describe pork when it is infected with cysticerci, the larval stage of *Taenia solium.*

meatal (me·a·tal). Of, or relating to a meatus.

meatome (me·at·ome). Meatotome.

meatometer (me·at·om·et·er). A device employed in measuring the size of a meatus, especially the external orifice of the urethra.

meatoplasty (me·a·to·plas·te). Plastic operation on a meatus, especially the urinary meatus. [meatus, Gk *plassein* to mould.]

meatorrhaphy (me·at·or·af·e). Suture of the mucous membrane of the urethra to the epithelium of the glans penis after meatotomy, in order to prevent subsequent contracture of the enlarged meatus. [meatus, Gk *rhaphe* suture.]

meatoscope (me·at·o·skope). A urethroscope. [meatus, *skopein* to watch.]

meatoscopy (me·at·os·ko·pe). The inspection of a meatus by means of the meatoscope. **Ureteral meatoscopy.** Inspection of the orifice of a ureter by means of a cystoscope.

meatotome (me·at·o·tome). A surgical instrument with a short cutting edge employed in performing a meatotomy. [meatus, Gk *temnein* to cut.]

meatotomy (me·at·ot·o·me). Incision of the urethral meatus for the purpose of enlarging it. [see prec.]

meatus [NA] (me·a·tus). A passage; an opening. **Auditory meatus, external [meatus acusticus externus (NA)].** A sinuous channel connecting the auricle with the tympanum and closed at its inner end by the tympanic membrane, set in an oblique plane so that the anterior wall and floor are longer than the posterior wall and roof. The meatus consists of a shorter cartilaginous portion [meatus acusticus externus cartilagineus (NA)] laterally continuous with the cartilage of the auricle and fused to the circumference of the longer bony portion medially. The axis of the former is upward, backward, and medially, and the latter downward, forward, and medially. There is a constriction, the isthmus, near the inner end of the bony portion. It is lined with skin which, in the cartilaginous portion, contains ceruminous glands and hairs. The greatest diameter is nearly vertical in the cartilaginous and nearly horizontal in the bony portion. The canal is much shorter in the newborn as the bony portion has not developed from the tympanic ring and the tympanic membrane is nearly horizontal. **Auditory meatus, internal [meatus acusticus internus (NA)].** A short passage opening on the posterior surface of the petrous part of the temporal bone and closed at its lateral end, the fundus [fundus meatus acustici interni (NA)], by a vertical plate of bone (the cribriform plate). The facial nerve area [area nervi facialis (NA)] is the upper anterior part of the vertical plate closing the fundus of the internal auditory meatus, and transmits the facial nerve. The cochlear area [area cochleae (NA)] is the lower anterior part of the vertical plate closing the fundus of the internal auditory meatus, and is perforated by small spirally arranged holes that transmit the fibres of the cochlear division of the auditory nerve, constituting the tractus spiralis foraminosus. The inferior vestibular area [area vestibularis inferior (NA)] is the shallow depression posterior to the cochlear area in which are the orifices of several small canals transmitting fibres of the vestibular nerve to the saccule. The superior vestibular area [area vestibularis superior (NA)] is the shallow depression posterior to the facial canal with several small apertures transmitting fibres of the vestibular nerves to the superior and lateral semicircular canals and the utricle. **Meatus of the nose, inferior [meatus nasi inferior (NA)].** The part of the nasal cavity below and lateral to the inferior concha. **Meatus of the nose, middle [meatus nasi medius (NA)].** The part of the nasal cavity below and lateral to the middle concha. **Meatus of the nose, superior [meatus nasi superior (NA)].** The part of the nasal cavity below and lateral to the superior concha. **Urinary meatus.** The external opening of the urethra. [L passage.]

Mebanazine (meb·an·az·een). BP Commission approved name for α-methylbenzylhydrazine; a monoamine oxidase inhibitor.

Mebendazole (me·ben·daz·ole). BP Commission approved name for methyl 5-benzoylbenzimidazol-2-ylcarbamate; an anthelmintic.

Mebeverine (meb·ev·er·een). BP Commission approved name for 7-(3,4-dimethoxybenzoyloxy)-3-ethyl-1-(4-methoxyphenyl)-2-methyl-3-azaheptane; an antispasmodic.

Mebezonium Iodide (meb·ez·o·ne·um i·o·dide). BP Commission approved name for 4,4′-methylenedi(cyclohexyltrimethylammonium iodide); a neuromuscular blocking agent.

Mebhydrolin (meb·hi·dro·lin). BP Commission approved name for 5-benzyl-1,2,3,4-tetrahydro-2-methyl-γ-carboline. **Mebhydrolin Napadisylate BPC 1968.** The naphthalene-1-5-disulphonate of mebhydrolin, an antihistamine with the actions, uses and side-effects of mepyramine maleate.

Mebutamate (meb·ew·tam·ate). BP Commission approved name for 2,2-di(carbamoyloxymethyl)-3-methylpentane; it is used in the treatment of hypertension.

Mecamylamine (mek·am·il·am·een). BP Commission approved name for 3-methylaminoisocamphane, a potent ganglion-blocking drug with a hypotensive action. It is used in the treatment of hypertension, where it combines the advantages of a high activity with a good absorption by the oral route. **Mecamylamine Hydrochloride BP 1968.** The hydrochloride of the base; a white, odourless, crystalline powder, soluble in water, alcohol and glycerin. A ganglion-blocking agent with a strong inhibitory effect on the transmission of nerve impulses in autonomic ganglia, it is used in the treatment of moderate to severe hypertension.

mechanicoreceptor (mek·an·ik·o·re·sep′·tor). *See* MECHANORECEPTOR.

mechanics (mek·an·ix). The branch of physics which deals with the action of forces upon matter: it includes the sciences of dynamics and statics. **Animal mechanics.** The study of the mechanical principles involved in animal physiology, such as levers and stresses. [Gk *mechane* machine.]

mechanism (mek·an·izm). 1. The arrangement and action of the parts of a machine by which it functions. 2. In biological sciences, the fundamental physical or chemical changes by which a function is exercised. **Defence mechanism, Escape mechanism.** In psychology, mental strategies employed, often unconsciously, to avoid recognition of unacceptable aspects of the self and hence to reduce anxiety. **Mental mechanism.** The mental pathway taken by a reaction pattern. **Outgoing mechanism.** The effector apparatus externalizing thoughts, effects, and intuitions. [Gk *mechane* machine.]

mechanist (mek·an·ist). An individual who regards all biological phenomena as being founded on a purely chemical and physical basis. [see prec.]

mechanogram (mek·an·o·gram). A tracing made by an instrument which records the movements of such organs as the stomach or the heart. [Gk *mechane* machine, *gramma* record.]

mechanogymnastics (mek·an·o·jim·nas′·tix). Gymnastics performed or assisted by mechanical means, e.g. slings, pulleys, weights and springs.

mechanoreceptor, mechanicoreceptor (mek·an·o·re·sep′·tor, mek·an·ik·o·re·sep′·tor). A receptor which responds to a mechanical stimulus, e.g. carotid-sinus baroreceptors. [Gk *mechane* machine, L *recipere* to receive.]

mechanotherapy (mek·an·o·ther′·ap·e). The treatment of disease or injury by mechanical measures, e.g. massage, exercises, or by apparatus. Assisted, active and resisted movements may be carried out on the Guthrie-Smith suspension apparatus; weak or paralysed muscles may be exercised by electrical stimulation, and the use of the iron lung in paralysis of the respiratory muscles is a striking example. [Gk *mechane* machine, therapy.]

mèche (mashe). A plug of soft material such as gauze or lint, employed as a drain or surgical tent. [Fr. wick.]

mecism (me·sizm). A condition characterized by abnormal lengthening of a part or parts of the body. [Gk *mekos* length.]

Meckel, Johann Friedrich (b. 1714). Berlin anatomist.

Meckel's band, or ligament. One of the two parts of the anterior ligament of the malleus: it is a band of fibres attached to the base of the long process of the malleus and it passes through the petrotympanic fissure to reach the spine of the sphenoid bone.

Meckel's cave, or cavity. A small pocket of the dura mater above the petrous part of the temporal bone, containing the trigeminal ganglion.

Meckel, Johann Friedrich (b. 1781). Halle surgeon and anatomist.

Meckel's cartilage, or rod. The cartilage that develops in the mandibular part of the first visceral arch of the embryo. In mammals, the malleus is formed by ossification at its posterior end: its middle part persists as the sphenomandibular ligament; its anterior part disappears, or may be incorporated in the mandible.

Meckel's diverticulitis. Inflammation of a Meckel's diverticulum: a condition that may simulate appendicitis.

Meckel's diverticulum. A small pouch, comparable in size with the vermiform appendix, which projects from the ileum about 90 cm (3 ft) from the ileocolic junction in about 2 per cent of people; it is a persistent part of the embryonic connection between the gut and the yolk sac (vitello-intestinal duct).

Meckel's ganglion. The sphenopalatine ganglion. *See* GANGLION.

Meckel's plane. A plane passing through the auricular points and the prosthion.

meckelectomy (mek·el·**ek**·to·me). Surgical excision of the sphenopalatine (Meckel's) ganglion. [Meckel's ganglion, Gk *ektome* a cutting out.]

Meclofenoxate (**mek**·lo·fen·**ox**′·ate). BP Commission approved name for 2-dimethylaminoethyl 4-chlorophenoxyacetate; a cerebral stimulant.

Meclozine (**mek**·lo·zeen). BP Commission approved name for 1-*p*-chlorobenzhydryl-4-*m*-methylbenzylpiperazine, an antihistaminic used in the treatment of hay fever and other allergic conditions. **Meclozine Hydrochloride BP 1973.** The dihydrochloride of 1-(4-chloro-benzhydryl)-4-(3-methylbenzyl)piperazine, a white, almost odourless, tasteless crystalline powder, slightly soluble in water and in alcohol. An antihistaminic agent which is effective in the treatment of motion sickness, nausea, vomiting and vertigo.

Mecobalamin (me·ko·**bal**·am·in). BP Commission approved name for α-(5,6-dimethylbenzimidazol-2-yl)cobamide methyl; it is used in the treatment of vitamin B_{12} deficiency.

mecocephalic (me·ko·kef·**al**′·ik). Dolichocephalic. [Gk *mekos* length, *kephale* head.]

mecometer (me·**kom**·et·er). An instrument resembling a pair of calipers with a scale attachment, used for the determination of the length of a newborn infant or of a fetus. [Gk *mekos* length, *metron* measure.]

meconalgia (me·kon·**al**·je·ah). A neuralgic or other painful condition which ensues when the administration of opium has been discontinued. [Gk *mekon* poppy, *algos* pain.]

meconate (**me**·kon·ate). Any salt or ester of meconic acid. They are particularly important, being the form in which most of the opium alkaloids occur naturally. [Gk *mekon* poppy.]

meconeuropathia (me·ko·newr·o·**path**′·e·ah). A psychoneurotic condition brought on by the misuse of opium or of any of its derived substances. [Gk *mekon* poppy, *neuron* nerve, *pathos* disease.]

meconic (me·**kon**·ik). Referring to, containing, or composed of opium. [Gk *mekon* poppy.]

meconidine (me·**kon**·id·een). $C_{21}H_{23}O_4N$, a minor constituent alkaloid of opium, which has a weak tetanizing effect.

meconine (me·kon·een). $(CH_3O)_2C_6H_2{=}CO(CH_2){=}O$, a neutral principle found in opium, and *Hydrastis canadensis*; also synthesized. It is the lactone of 6-hydroxymethyl-2,3-dimethoxybenzoic acid.

meconiorrhoea (me·**ko**·ne·or·**e**′·ah). An abnormally profuse discharge of meconium. [meconium, Gk *rhoia* flow.]

meconism (**me**·kon·izm). 1. Opium addiction. 2. Poisoning through the use of opium. [Gk *mekon* poppy.]

meconium (me·**ko**·ne·um). 1. The first matter, dark green in colour and consisting of bile, mucoid debris, and epithelial elements, discharged from the bowels of a newborn infant. 2. Opium. [Gk *mekon* poppy.]

meconophagism (me·kon·**of**·aj·izm). The practice of taking opium. [Gk *mekon* opium, *phagein* to eat.]

mecystasis (me·**sis**·tas·is). A phenomenon in which a muscle maintains its initial tension despite an increase in length. [Gk *mekos* length, *stasis* a standing still.]

medallion (med·**al**·e·on). A raised rose-coloured patch of pityriasis rosea. [Fr. *medallion.*]

Medazepam (med·a·ze·pam). BP Commission approved name for 7-chloro-2,3-dihydro-1-methyl-5-phenyl-1*H*-1,4-benzodiazepine; a tranquillizer.

media (**me**·de·ah). 1. *See* MEDIUM. 2. The middle coat of an artery or vein; the tunica media. 3. The transparent media of the eye (see below). **Diophtric media, Refracting media.** In ophthalmological examination, the transparent optic fluids and tissues through which the rays of light pass, are refracted, and brought to a focal point. **Transparent media of the eye.** The aqueous humour, the lens, the vitreous body, and the cornea. [L *medius* middle.]

medial [medialis (NA)] (**me**·de·al). 1. Of or belonging to the middle. 2. Nearer to the median plane. [L *medius* middle.]

median (**me**·de·an). 1. [Medianus (NA)] Placed in the middle; mesial. 2. An average or centre value of a series of observations taken in order from the lowest value to the highest: if the observations constitute an even number the mean of the two central ones is taken. 3. The mid-point which separates the area of a frequency curve into two equal halves. [L *medius* middle.]

median artery [arteria mediana (NA)]. A branch of the anterior interosseous artery accompanying the median nerve. Occasionally it is of large size.

median eminence. Situated in the pituitary stalk and contains a capillary bed into which humoral agents are released into the portal veins leading to the sinusoids bathing the cells of the anterior lobe.

median nerve [nervus medianus (NA)]. One of the main nerves of the forearm and hand, formed at the lower end of the axilla by the union of medial and lateral roots and deriving fibres from all the roots of the brachial plexus. It travels down the front of the arm, forearm, and hand, and it supplies most of the anterior muscles of the forearm [rami musculares (NA)], all the thenar muscles except the adductor pollicis, the lateral two lumbrical muscles, and the skin of the anterior aspects of the lateral three and a half digits and the corresponding part of the palm of the hand. There is a communicating branch with the ulnar nerve [ramus communicans cum nervo ulnari (NA)].

Palmar cutaneous branch [ramus palmaris nervi mediani (NA)]. A branch of the median nerve arising in the lower part of the forearm and passing superficial to the flexor retinaculum to supply the skin of the palm of the hand.

Lateral root [radix lateralis (NA)]. The root of the median nerve from the lateral cord of the brachial plexus.

Medial root [radix medialis (NA)]. The root of the median nerve derived from the medial cord of the brachial plexus.

median vein. *See* FOREARM, VEIN OF THE.

mediastinal (me·de·as·**ti**′·nal). Belonging or referring to the mediastinum.

mediastinal veins [venae mediastinales (NA)]. Tributaries of the azygos vein and the internal mammary vein.

mediastinitis (me·de·as·tin·**i**′·tis). Inflammation affecting the cellular substance of the mediastinum. **Indurative mediastinitis.** A condition preceded by acute mediastinitis in which there is increased mediastinal fibrosis, often associated with adherent pericarditis. [mediastinum, Gk *-itis* inflammation.]

mediastinopericarditis (**me**·de·as·**ti**·no·per·e·kar·**di**′·tis). 1. An inflammatory condition of the mediastinum and the pericardium. 2. Indurative mediastinitis. **Callous mediastinopericarditis.** A combined inflammatory condition of the mediastinum and pericardium associated with fibrous pericardial thickening. [mediastinum, pericardium, Gk *-itis* inflammation.]

mediastinoscope (**me**·de·as·**ti**′·no·skope). A tubular instrument of the same pattern as a cystoscope, used for inspecting the mediastinum. [mediastinum, Gk *skopein* to view.]

mediastinoscopy (me·de·as·tin·**os**′·ko·pe). Examination of the mediastinum through a small suprasternal incision by means of a tubular instrument fitted with a system of lenses and a terminal electric light bulb. [mediastinum, Gk *skopein* to view.]

mediastinotomy (me·de·as·tin·**ot**′·o·me). Surgical incision into the mediastinum, from the neck or dorsal regions. [mediastinum, Gk *temnein* to cut.]

mediastinum [NA] (me·de·as·**ti**′·num). A median septum occupying the interval between two parts of an organ, or two subdivisions of a region. Specifically, the space between the two pleural sacs. This presents four subdivisions. The *superior mediastinum* [mediastinum superius (NA)] lies above the pericardium and is bounded in front by the manubrium sterni, behind by the upper four thoracic vertebrae, and laterally by the mediastinal pleura. It contains the trachea, oesophagus, thoracic duct, the aortic arch and its branches, the innominate veins and superior vena cava, phrenic nerve, left recurrent laryngeal nerve, vagus nerve and cardiac branches, lymphatic glands, and the thymus. The *anterior mediastinum* [mediastinum anterius (NA)] lies between the sternum and the pericardium, and contains areolar tissue, lymphatic glands, and small branches of the internal mammary artery. The *middle mediastinum* [mediastinum medium (NA)] contains the heart and pericardium together with the phrenic nerves and vessels. The *posterior mediastinum* [mediastinum posterius (NA)] lies behind the pericardium and in front of the lower eight thoracic vertebrae. It contains the oesophagus, thoracic duct, the descending aorta and some of its intercostal branches, the vena azygos and vena hemiazygos, the vagus and greater splanchnic nerves, and some lymphatic glands. **Mediastinum testis.** A thickening of the tunica albuginea along the posterior border of the testis, from the front and sides of which fibrous septa radiate forward into the gland to divide it into lobules. It contains the rete testis. [L *mediastinus* midway.]

mediate (**me**·de·ate). 1. Not direct; brought about by means of an intervening agent. 2. In a position between two parts; intermediate. [L *medius* middle.]

mediation (me·de·**a**·shun). 1. The action of an intermediary in bringing about some desired effect between two bodies or parts. 2. The transmission of a state of excitation, either by electrical changes (*electrical mediation*), or by the liberation of a chemical substance of high potency at the point of mediation, e.g. at a nerve-ending (*chemical mediation*). [L *mediare* to divide in the middle.]

mediator (**me**·de·a·tor). Any agent which brings about mediation. **Chemical mediator.** Any chemical substance of high biological potency released at a point where it activates physiological changes, as in the neuromuscular transmission of impulses. They may be of two types, sympathetic, in which the mediation is by adrenaline or noradrenaline, and para-sympathetic, in which the mediation is performed by acetylcholine. Having transmitted the state of excitation from nerve to effector organ, e.g. muscle, the chemical mediator is rapidly destroyed by an enzyme, in this case cholinesterase.

medical (**med**·ik·al). 1. Belonging to the science of medicine. 2. Belonging to the treatment of pathological conditions by other than surgical means. **Medical expert.** *See* EXPERT. **Medical police.** A term for public health administration, used by Andrew Duncan, W. P. Alison, and others in Scotland in the early 19th century. It is a translation of the term *Medizinische Polizei*, used by J. P. Frank (1745–1821), German physician, teacher and health administrator, in the sense of medical polity or state medicine. [L *medicare* to heal.]

medicament (med·**ik**·am·ent). Any medicinal substance or agent used in the treatment of disease or for the healing of wounds. [L *medicamentum* drug.]

medicamentosus (med·**ik**·am·ent·**o'**·sus). Relating to a drug; a term descriptive of, for instance, an eruption caused by a drug. [see prec.]

medicated (**med**·ik·a·ted). Impregnated with a drug or a medicinal substance. [see foll.]

medication (med·ik·**a**·shun). The method of treatment by the administration of drugs. **Conservative medication.** The use of medicines to conserve the vital powers of the body. **Dialytic medication.** The administration of artificial mineral waters composed of watery solutions of the required salts. **Endermic medication.** The injection of drugs into the skin. **Hypodermatic medication, Hypodermic medication.** The injection of drugs subcutaneously. **Ionic medication.** The introduction of electrolytes into the body by means of an electric current. **Sublingual medication.** The absorption of drugs by the mucous membrane beneath the tongue. **Substitutive medication.** The substitution, in cases of hormone deficiency, of a product from another animal, or of one artificially produced, e.g. thyroid extract in myxoedema, insulin in diabetes. **Transduodenal medication.** The administration of drugs through a duodenal tube. [L *medicare* to heal.]

medicator (**med**·ik·a·tor). An instrument for the therapeutic application of medicines to the cavities or deeper parts of the body. [see prec.]

medicerebellar (me·de·ser·e·**bel'**·ar). Relating to the central part of the cerebellum. [L *medius* middle, cerebellum.]

medicerebral (me·de·**ser**·e·bral). Relating to the central portion of the cerebrum. [L *medius* middle, cerebrum.]

medicinal (med·**is**·in·al). 1. Having curative or healing properties. 2. Belonging to or of the nature of a medicine. [see foll.]

medicine (**med**·is·in). 1. The science and art of the treatment of disease and maintenance of health. In particular, the branch concerned with the non-surgical aspects of treatment of disease. 2. Any drug or other substance given or taken for the above purpose. **Aerospace medicine.** Space medicine (see below). **Air medicine.** Aviation medicine (see below). **Anatomical medicine.** The post-mortem study of the changes in structure produced by disease in organs of the body, and the correlation of these changes with symptoms observed while the patient was alive. **Aviation medicine.** A specialized branch of medicine dealing with the physiological, pathological, psychological and clinical conditions, as seen in aviators and persons transported by air; applied particularly to the medical study of men engaged in aviation warfare. **Clinical medicine.** 1. The study of medicine at the bedside as opposed to special laboratory investigation. 2. Instruction given to medical students by a physician in the wards or outpatient department of a hospital by examination of patients as opposed to theoretical instruction in the absence of a patient. **Domestic medicine.** The treatment at home of maladies and injuries, usually of a minor character, without medical advice or supervision. **Dosimetric medicine.** The administration of medicine in definite and prescribed doses. **Environmental medicine.** The application of medical knowledge to improving, controlling and modifying the external surroundings and influences, in the interests of health, of the community generally, or of the individual in particular. **Experimental medicine.** A system of treatment derived from conveying a disease to animals or human beings by inoculation or otherwise, then noting the symptoms produced and the efficacy of remedial measures. **Forensic medicine.** The study of medicine as related to the needs of the law. *See also* PATHOLOGY, Forensic. **Galenic medicine.** A comprehensive compilation of the state of the science and art of medicine in the second century of the Christian era. On these writings of Galen medical education in the West was based for nearly 1700 years. **Geriatric medicine.** Geriatrics; a specialized branch of medicine concerned with the prevention, diagnosis and treatment of disease in old age. **Group medicine.** The association of a number of medical practitioners together for the purpose of bringing all forms of medical knowledge to bear upon the diagnosis and treatment of disease in their patients. **Hermetic medicine.** Spagyric medicine; a medical doctrine current in the 17th century under the name of Hermes, the Thrice Great. Its tenets included magic and alchemy, and its origin is often attributed to Paracelsus. **Holistic medicine.** The aspect of the science of medicine that considers man as an integrated functioning whole, rather than as a collection of separate systems. **Internal medicine.** A USA term for the division of medicine concerned with the non-surgical aspects of diseases. **Juridical medicine, Legal medicine.** Forensic medicine (see above). **Mental medicine.** Psychiatry; the diagnosis and treatment of mental diseases or disturbances. **Military medicine.** The branch of the science of medicine that is concerned with those conditions and diseases that are influenced or caused by military service (in peace or war). Cf. WAR MEDICINE (below). **Nuclear medicine.** The application of nuclear physics in medical diagnosis and investigation. Sometimes a wider definition is used so that unsealed-source radiotherapy is included as part of nuclear medicine. **Osteopathic medicine.** Medicine as practised by osteopaths. **Patent medicine.** A term used for a medicine usually advertised to the public. The ingredients of these remedies must, by Act of Parliament, be stated on the label or wrapper. **Physical medicine.** That branch of medicine which deals with locomotor disorders and is particularly concerned with physical methods of treatment including physiotherapy, manipulation and rehabilitation. **Preclinical medicine.** The study in the medical curriculum of the sciences of chemistry, physics, biology, anatomy, physiology, and pharmacology, preliminary to clinical studies in the wards of a teaching hospital. **Preventive medicine.** The application of human knowledge to the prevention of disease. Its objects are to develop and fortify the physique of the individual and thus increase his capacity and powers of resistance, and those of the community; to prevent or remove the causes and conditions of disease or of its propagation; to prolong the span of man's life. **Proprietary medicine.** Term including any therapeutic preparation (chemical, vegetable, drug, etc.), sold either directly to the public or solely on prescription by the medical profession. By patent, trade mark, or some other method, such preparation is protected against imitation or competition, until such protection lapses; even then, such a preparation would still be known as a proprietary medicine. **Psychological medicine.** The application of the science of psychology to the diagnosis and treatment of mental diseases or disorders, or in relation to the mental condition of patients generally. **Psychosomatic medicine.** A modern branch of medicine which evaluates both the mental and physical conditions of the patient and studies their interdependence. **Quack medicine.** A medicine of little or no therapeutic value, which is recommended or advertised to the public as a cure for all or specified diseases. **Social medicine.** A comprehensive term including (*a*) research into social conditions which favour disease or affect health; (*b*) study of the social effects of disease, especially of the family unit; (*c*) health education and advice to those responsible for housing, employment, and social policy; (*d*) provision of social services, and their co-ordination with public health and the medical treatment of disease. **Space medicine.** A special branch of aviation medicine (see above) which deals with stresses experienced outside the earth's atmosphere (agravic state, radiation, isolation, etc.) and the derangements of vital function such stresses produce. **Spagyric medicine.** Hermetic medicine (see above). **State medicine.** The conservation and care of the health of the individuals comprising the community by a government. In UK this is done through an administrative system based upon a number of Acts of Parliament and upon the machinery of the Civil Service and local government. **Suggestive medicine.** A method of treatment in which hypnotic suggestion is employed, as in cases of functional or obsessional disorder. **Tropical medicine.** The branch of medical science concerned with diseases that are more prevalent, or display special features, in hot countries. **Veterinary medicine.** The application of medicine to the diagnosis and treatment of diseases of animals, more especially those of domestic animals. **War medicine.** The branch of medical science that is concerned with those conditions and diseases (among the civil or military population) that are caused or aggravated by war. Cf. MILITARY MEDICINE (above). [L *medicina*.]

medicinerea (me·de·sin·**eer'**·e·ah). The grey matter of the lentiform nucleus and claustrum. [L *medius* middle, *cinereus* ashen.]

medicodental (med·ik·o·**den'**·tal). Pertaining to both medical and dental sciences.

medicolegal (med·ik·o·**le'**·gal). Belonging or relating to forensic medicine. **Medicolegal expert.** *See* EXPERT. [medicine, L *lex* law.]

medicomechanic, medicomechanical (med·ik·o·mek·**an'**·ik, med·ik·o·mek·**an'**·ik·al). In therapeutics, relating to medical and mechanical measures.

medicophysical (med·ik·o·**fiz'**·ik·al). Medical and physical; relating to disease and to the general bodily condition.

medicophysics (med·ik·o·**fiz'**·ix). The application of the science of physics to medicine.

medicopsychological (med·ik·o·si·ko·**loj'**·ik·al). Belonging to the realms of medicine and psychology; referring to medicopsychology or to the relation of psychology to medicine.

medicopsychology (med·ik·o·si·**kol'**·o·je). Medicine in its relation to the study of mental disorder. [medicine, psychology.]

medicostatistical (med·ik·o·stat·**is'**·tik·al). Belonging to the domains of medicine and statistics.

medicothorax (med·ik·o·**thor'**·ax). An artificial pneumothorax into which some medicated vapour has been introduced.

medicotopographical (med·ik·o·top·o·**graf'**·ik·al). Concerning the association between diseases and anatomical regions. [medical, Gk *topos* place, *graphein* to record.]

medicozoological (med·ik·o·zo·o·**loj'**·ik·al). Concerning zoology in its connection with medicine.

Medin, Karl Oskar (b. 1847). Stockholm physician.

Medin's disease, Heine-Medin disease. Acute anterior poliomyelitis. *See* POLIOMYELITIS.

mediocarpal (me·de·o·**kar'**·pal). Midcarpal.

medioccipital (me·de·ok·**sip'**·it·al). Midoccipital.

mediodorsal (me·de·o·**dor'**·sal). Median and dorsal.

mediofrontal (me·de·o·**frun'**·tal). Relating to the centre of the forehead. [L *medius* middle, *frons* forehead.]

mediolateral (me·de·o·**lat'**·er·al). Relating to the median plane and one side. [L *medius* middle, *latus* side.]

medionecrosis (me·de·o·nek·**ro'**·sis). Necrosis affecting the tunica media of the aorta, which, on occasion, is succeeded by spontaneous rupture of the aorta. [L *medius* middle, necrosis.]

mediopalatine (me·de·o·**pal'**·at·ine). Belonging to the middle portion of the palate. [L *medius* middle, palate.]

mediopeduncle (me·de·o·ped·**ungkl'**). The middle cerebellar peduncle. *See* PEDUNCLE. [L *medius* middle, peduncle.]

mediopontine (me·de·o·**pon'**·tine). Belonging to the middle portion of the pons. [L *medius* middle, *pons* bridge.]

medioscalenus (me·de·o·ska·**le'**·nus). The scalenus medius muscle.

mediosylvian (me·de·o·**sil'**·ve·an). Relating to the central part of the lateral sulcus of the cerebral hemisphere (Sylvius' fissure). [L *medius* middle, Franciscus *Sylvius*.]

mediotarsal (me·de·o·**tar'**·sal). Belonging to the central portion of the tarsus. [L *medius* middle, tarsus.]

mediotemporal (me·de·o·**tem'**·por·al). Belonging to the central part of the temporal lobe of the cerebral hemisphere. [L *medius* middle, *tempora* temples.]

medisection (me·de·sek·shun). Hemisection. [L *medius* middle, section.]

medium (me·de·um) (pl. *media*). 1. Average; midway between extremes. 2. A substance through which anything acts, or one which conveys anything. 3. In bacteriology, a *culture medium*, a substance used for the culture of organisms. *See also:* CULTURE MEDIUM. 4. In psychical research, a person claiming to have parapsychological perception. **Assay medium.** A medium usually composed of synthesized chemicals and deficient in one substance (vitamin or amino acid) essential for the growth of a particular strain of organism. The amount of growth supported by the medium after the addition of a fluid containing this substance is used for its estimation. **Clearing medium.** A medium for increasing the transparency of histological or parasitological specimens. **Contrast medium.** A substance used in radiography to visualize structures which, without its use, might not be visible. Contrast media may have a density greater (e.g. barium) or less (e.g. air) than that of body tissues. **Disperse medium, Dispersion medium.** The phase of a colloidal solution corresponding to the solvent of a true solution. The term is synonymous with *continuous phase* or *external phase*. **Passive medium.** A medium that does not change the shape or size of objects placed in it. [L *medius* middle.]

See also: BEIJERINCK, BOECK (W. C.), BREWER (J. H.), BROWNING, DIEUDONNÉ, WICKERSHEIMER, WILSON (W. J.).

medius (me·de·us). 1. The middle. 2. The third digit of the hand. 3. Lying intermediately between two other structures or parts. [L]

medoblennorrhoea (me·do·blen·o·re'·ah). 1. Gonorrhoea. 2. Gleet. [Gk *medos* penis, *blennos* mucus, *rhoia* flow.]

medorrhoea (me·do·re·ah). A discharge from the urethra. [obsolete term.] **Medorrhoea urethralis.** Gonorrhoea. **Medorrhoea virilis.** A gonorrhoeal infection of the male urethra. [Gk *medos* penis, *rhoia* flow.]

Medroxyprogesterone (med·**rox**·e·pro·**jes'**·ter·one). BP Commission approved name for 17α-hydroxy-6α-methylpregn-4-ene-3,20-dione; a progestational steroid used as a contraceptive by

3-monthly injection with oral administration of stilboestrol daily for a week every month.

medulla [NA] (med·ul·ah). 1. The marrow of bones. 2. The medulla oblongata; the posterior truncated portion of the brain stem between the spinal cord and the pons and cerebellum. 3. Any structure that has a similarity to marrow. 4. That part of an organ that lies more centrally than the cortex. **Adrenal medulla.** The medulla of a suprarenal gland (see below). **Medulla of the kidney [medulla renis (NA)].** That portion of the parenchyma of the kidney which lies deep to the cortex and contains no (or very few) glomeruli. It is subdivided into the inner medulla (which includes the papilla) and the outer medulla (which extends out as far as the arcuate vessels and contains *inter alia,* the thick ascending limbs of the loop of Henle). **Medulla of a lymph gland [medulla (NA)].** The central portion of a lymph gland, composed of branching and uniting strands of lymphoid tissue (the lymphoid cords). Between the cords are the lymph sinuses. **Medulla of a suprarenal gland [medulla (NA)].** The internal part of the gland, containing masses of granular chromaffin cells permeated by venous sinusoids. It is richly supplied with medullated preganglionic nerve fibres, and contains scattered sympathetic ganglion cells. It elaborates adrenaline. [L marrow.]

medulla oblongata [NA] (med·ul·ah ob·long·gah·tah). The tapering caudal portion of the hind-brain, extending from the posterior border of the pons to the first segment of the spinal cord. The wider rostral part underlies the caudal part of the 4th ventricle which is bounded here by the inferior cerebellar peduncles diverging from the dorsal surface, and behind these by the two eminences, the gracile nucleus medially and the cuneate nucleus laterally. Into the caudal aspect of these lead afferent tracts of similar names separated by a groove [sulcus medianus posterior (NA)]. On the lateral surface is a swelling, the olive. The ventral surface presents a median sulcus [fissura mediana anterior (NA)] on either side of which lies an elongated swelling, the pyramid, formed by the corticospinal pathway. The decussating fibres of these tracts can be seen in the ventral sulcus caudal to the pyramid. The grey matter of the medulla contains the nucleus of the 12th cranial nerve whose fibres emerge as a series of rootlets in the groove between the olive and the pyramid; the nuclei of the 10th, 12th, and cranial part of the 11th cranial nerves whose fibres emerge as a linear series of rootlets on the lateral surface dorsal to the olive; the caudal part of the vestibular complex; and the nucleus associated with the spinal tract of the 5th cranial nerve. These nuclei are arranged in the order named from medial to lateral. Within the medulla oblongata lie the involuntary centres, controlling the heart, the blood vessels and the respiratory organs. [L elongated marrow.]

medullary (med·ul·ar·e). 1. Belonging to any medulla or to the marrow. 2. Similar in substance to marrow.

medullated (med·ul·a·ted). Enclosed by medullary substance; having a medullary sheath, as a nerve.

medullation (med·ul·a·shun). The process of formation of a medulla; a term used particularly of the development of the medullary sheath of a nerve fibre.

medullectomy (med·ul·ek·to·me). Surgical removal of the medulla of an organ. [medulla, Gk *ektome* excision.]

medullispinal (med·ul·e·spi'·nal). Belonging to the spinal cord. [medulla, spine.]

medullitis (med·ul·i·tis). 1. Myelitis. 2. Osteomyelitis. [L *medulla* marrow, Gk *-itis* inflammation.]

medullization (med·ul·i·za'·shun). In rarefying osteitis, a state of hypertrophy of the Haversian canals, which later are converted into marrow channels, the bone cells being replaced by marrow cells. [L *medulla* marrow.]

medullo-adrenal (med·ul·o·ad·re'·nal). Relating to the medullary part of the suprarenal glands.

medulloblast (med·ul·o·blast). An undifferentiated type of nerve cell, found in certain malignant tumours of the central nervous system, which preserves the embryonic capacity for differentiating into either a neurone or a neuroglial cell. [L *medulla* marrow, Gk *blastos* germ.]

medulloblastoma (med·ul·o·blas·to'·mah). A fourth-ventricular neuroglial tumour of children, which arises from the medulloblasts which may stem from Obersteiner's layer in the cerebellum of infants or from the posterior medullary velum. [medulloblast, Gk *-oma* tumour.]

medullocell (med·ul·o·sel). A myelocyte. [medulla, cell.]

medulloculture (med·ul·o·kul'·tcher). A culture medium containing bone marrow. [L *medulla* marrow, culture.]

medullo-epithelioma (med·ul·o·ep·e·the·le·o'·mah). A growth which consists mainly of neuro-epithelium and of primitive retina epithelium. [medulla, epithelioma.]

medullosis (med·ul·o·sis). Myelocythaemia. [medulla, Gk *-osis* condition.]

medullosuprarenoma (med·ul·o·sew·prah·re·no'·mah). A neoplasm having its origin in the medullary portion of the suprarenal glands. [medulla, suprarenoma.]

medullotherapy (med·ul·o·ther'·ap·e). A prophylactic treatment, devised by Pasteur, of rabies in man, in which the spinal cords of animals are used. [medulla, therapy.]

Meduna, Ladislaus von. (b. 1896). Budapest psychiatrist.

Meduna's method. 1. The treatment of schizophrenia by epileptiform convulsions induced chemically by camphor intramuscularly or leptazol intravenously. 2. The treatment of patients with neurotic states by the inhalation of carbon dioxide.

medusa (me·dew·sah). The free-living generation in the life history of many Coelenterata. The larger forms are called jellyfish, and can cause painful stings with their nematocysts. [L *Medusa* the snake-haired Gorgon.]

Meeh, K. (fl. 1879). Tübingen physiologist.

Meeh's formula. The surface area of the body in square decimetres $= 12.3 \times$ (weight in kilograms$^{2/3}$).

Meek's operation. For entropion of the lower eyelid: a horizontal strip of orbicularis oculi muscle is dissected free at the ends and left attached centrally. These two strips are then sutured to the periosteum of the lower orbital margin, one down and nasally, the other down and temporally.

Mees' lines or stripes. White lines or nail plate striations seen in chronic arsenical poisoning, and sometimes in leprosy.

Mefruside (mef·roo·side). BP Commission approved name for 4-chloro-N^1-methyl-N^1 - (2 - methyltetrahydrofurfuryl) - benzene - 1,3 - disulphonamide; a diuretic.

mega- (meg·ah). A prefix indicating that the quantity which follows is to be multiplied by 10^6. Thus, a megarad $= 10^6$ rads; a megacurie $= 10^6$ curies. [Gk *megas* large.]

megabacterium (meg·ah·bak·teer'·e·um). A bacterium of unusually large size. [Gk *megas* large, bacterium.]

megacaecum (meg·ah·se·kum). A caecum of excessive size. [Gk *megas* large, caecum.]

megacardia (meg·ah·kar·de·ah). Enlargement of the heart. [Gk *megas* large, *kardia* heart.]

megacephalic, megacephalous (meg·ah·kef·al'·ik, meg·ah·kef·al·us). Large-headed; generally with a cranial capacity of more than 1450 ml. [see foll.]

megacephaly (meg·ah·kef·al·e). Unusual largeness of the head. [Gk *megas* large, *kephale* head.]

megacholedochus (meg·ah·ko·le'·do·kus). Pathological enlargement of the bile duct. [Gk *megas* large, choledochus.]

megacoccus (meg·ah·kok·us). A large-sized coccus. [Gk *megas* large, *kokkos* berry.]

megacolon (meg·ah·ko·lon). A condition, usually congenital, in which there is great dilatation and hypertrophy of part or the whole of the large intestine. Recently, a distinction has been made by radiological investigation between Hirschsprung's disease and *idiopathic megacolon.* In the former the rectum is small or normal, with narrowing of the sigmoid colon immediately above, and above this, great dilatation of the colon, wholly or limited to a part. Histological investigation shows absence of the parasympathetic ganglion cells in the plexuses of the wall of the narrowed part and in the lowest part of the dilated area, which allows uninterrupted action of the sympathetic ganglia, whereby spasticity and consequent dilatation above the affected area results. In idiopathic megacolon there is a simple gross dilatation of the lower bowel, forming a pear-shaped swelling above the anus, or a massive tubular dilatation, involving the rectum and lower colon. Symptoms are those associated with chronic constipation: the bowels may be opened only once in several weeks, or constipation with overflow and incontinence may be present. Interference with appetite, failure to grow, and psychopathic tendencies may develop. Treatment depends upon the type of disability present, but should always seek to lessen the degree of anxiety associated with the infrequent bowel action. Mild idiopathic cases do well with medical treatment and improve with increasing age. Many cases can be cured by surgical removal of the aganglionic segment of the bowel. **Secondary megacolon.** A condition resulting from narrowing of part of the intestine, either at the anus or in the colon itself. It may be congenital or acquired, following organic obstruction. Symptoms usually do not date from a very early age, except in the case of anal disability. [Gk *megas* large, colon.]

megacoly (meg·ah·**ko**·le). Megacolon.

megacycle (**meg**·ah·si·kl). A million cycles per second. Now called a megahertz. [Gk *megas* large, cycle.]

megacystis (meg·ah·**sist**·is). Non-obstructive dilatation of the bladder. [Gk *megos* large, *kystis* bag.]

megadolichocolon (**meg**·ah·dol·e·ko·**ko**′·lon). Pathological elongation and dilatation of the colon. [Gk *megas* large, *dolichos* long, colon.]

megadont, megadontic (**meg**·ah·dont, meg·ah·**dont**·ik). Having dentition in which the teeth are larger than average size. [Gk *megas* large, *odous* tooth.]

megadontism (meg·ah·**dont**·izm). Excessive size of the teeth. [see prec.]

megaduodenum (**meg**·ah·dew·o·**de**′·num). Duodenum of abnormally large size. [Gk *megas* large, duodenum.]

megadyne (**meg**·ah·dine). A unit of work: a million dynes, [Gk *megas* large, dyne.]

megafarad (meg·ah·**far**·ad). A unit of electrical capacity: a million farads. [Gk *megas* large, farad.]

megagamete (meg·ah·**gam**·eet). Macrogamete. [Gk *megas* large, gamete.]

megagnathus (meg·ah·**nath**·us). Having large jaws. [Gk *megas* large, *gnathos* jaw.]

megahertz (**meg**·ah·her·tz). A unit of frequency equal to a million hertz.

megakaryoblast (meg·ah·**kar**·e·o·blast). A primitive cell seen in the bone marrow, and having an unsegmented nucleus. It is the precursor of the megakaryocyte. [Gk *megas* large, karyoblast.]

megakaryoblastoma (**meg**·ah·**kar**·e·o·blas·**to**′·mah). Hodgkin's disease; an old term used on the basis of an unproven hypothesis. [Gk *megas* large, karyoblast, Gk *-oma* tumour.]

megakaryocyte (meg·ah·**kar**·e·o·site). The mother cell from which blood platelets are derived. There may be an immature megakaryocyte with a segmented nucleus and non-granular cytoplasm, a more mature type with granular cytoplasm, and a lymphoid type usually seen in thrombocytopenic purpura. [Gk *megas* large, karyocyte.]

megakaryocytopenia (**meg**·ah·kar·e·o·si·to·**pe**′·ne·ah). Poverty of megakaryocytes in the blood. [megakaryocyte, Gk *penes* poor.]

megakaryocytosis (meg·ah·**kar**·e·o·si·**to**′·sis). The presence of megakaryocytes in the blood. [megakaryocyte, Gk *-osis* condition.]

megakaryophthisis (meg·ah·**kar**·e·o·**thi**′·sis). A condition in which there is a deficiency of megakaryocytes in the marrow. [megakaryocyte, Gk *phthein* to consume.]

megalecithal (meg·ah·**les**·ith·al). Large-yolked. [Gk *megas* large, *lekithos* yolk.]

megalencephalia (**meg**·al·en·kef·**a**′·le·ah). Congenital parenchymatous hyperplasia of the cerebral hemispheres, characterized by mental deficiency; a very rare disorder. [Gk *megas* large, *egkephalos* brain.]

megalencephalon (meg·al·en·**kef**′·al·on). A brain of unusually large size. [see prec.]

megalerythema (**meg**·al·er·e·**the**′·mah). Erythema infectiosum; fifth disease. [Gk *megas* large, *erythainein* to redden.]

megalgia (meg·**al**·je·ah). Acute pain, particularly in cases of muscular rheumatism. [Gk *megas* large, *algos* pain.]

megaloblast (**meg**·al·o·blast). A large haemoglobinized primitive nucleated erythroblast or nucleated red cell, described by Ehrlich, and produced by the pro-erythroblast instead of early normoblast under certain pathological conditions in which anti-anaemic factors are deficient; it leads to the formation of an abnormal macrocyte or large red blood cell. It possesses a characteristic nuclear pattern which differentiates the early, intermediate, and late forms and is seen almost exclusively in pernicious anaemia or related macrocytic anaemias, but not in normal blood or bone marrow, since it plays no part in normal adult erythropoiesis. [Gk *megas* large, *blastos* germ.]

See also: EHRLICH.

megalobulbus (meg·al·o·**bul**′·bus). An enlarged duodenal cap, demonstrated radiographically with a barium meal. It may be either congenital in origin, or secondary to distal duodenal obstruction or to hypotonia of the cap. [Gk *megas* large, L *bulbus* bulb.]

megalocardia (**meg**·al·o·**kar**′·de·ah). Hypertrophy of the heart. [Gk *megas* large, *kardia* heart.]

megalocephalia, megalocephaly (**meg**·a·lo·kef·**a**′·le·ah, **meg**·a·lo·**kef**′·al·e). 1. Abnormal largeness of the head. 2. Leontiasis ossea. [Gk *megas* large, *kephale* head.]

megalocerus (**meg**·al·o·**seer**′·us). A monster having horny projections on the forehead. [Gk *megas* large, *keras* horn.]

megalocheirous (**meg**·al·o·**ki**′·rus). Having hands of abnormally large size. [Gk *megas* large, *cheir* hand.]

megaloclitoris (meg·al·o·**klit**′·or·is). Enlargement of the clitoris. [Gk *megas* large, clitoris.]

megalocornea (**meg**·al·o·**kor**′·ne·ah). A condition of distension of the eyeball or of the anterior segment of the eye. [Gk *megas* large, cornea.]

megalocystis (**meg**·al·o·**sist**′·is). Hypertrophy of the bladder, often with great increase in capacity owing to over-distension. [Gk *megas* large, *kystis* bag.]

megalocyte (**meg**·al·o·site). An erythrocyte of large size, in diameter measuring 12–16 μm. [Gk *megas* large, *kytos* cell.]

megalocytosis (meg·al·o·si·**to**′·sis). The presence of megalocytes in the blood. [megalocyte, Gk *-osis* condition.]

megalodactylia, megalodactylism (**meg**·al·o·dak·**til**′·e·ah, **meg**·al·o·**dak**′·til·izm). A condition in which the toes or fingers are of abnormally large size. [Gk *megas* large, *daktylos* finger or toe.]

megalodactylous (**meg**·al·o·**dak**′·til·us). Having toes and fingers of abnormally large size. [see prec.]

megalodactyly (**meg**·al·o·**dak**′·til·e). Megalodactylia.

megalodont (**meg**·al·o·dont). Having teeth which are larger than the normal size. [Gk *megas* large, *odous* tooth.]

megalodontia (**meg**·al·o·**don**′·she·ah). A condition in which the teeth are excessively large. [see prec.]

megalo-enteron (**meg**·al·o·**en**′·ter·on). An intestine of unusually large size. [Gk *megas* large, *enteron* bowel.]

megalo-erythema (**meg**·al·o·er·e·**the**′·mah). Megalerythema.

megalogastria (**meg**·al·o·**gas**′·tre·ah). Abnormal enlargement of the stomach, or a stomach of unusually large size. [Gk *megas* large, *gaster* stomach.]

megaloglossia (**meg**·al·o·**glos**′·e·ah). Enlargement of the tongue of muscular hypertrophic type. [Gk *megas* large, *glossa* tongue.]

megalographia (**meg**·al·o·**graf**′·e·ah). Macrographia. [Gk *megas* large, *graphein* to record.]

megalohepatia (**meg**·al·o·hep·**at**′·e·ah). Hepatic enlargement; hepatomegalia. [Gk *megas* large, *hepar* liver.]

megalokaryoblast (**meg**·al·o·**kar**′·e·o·blast). Megakaryoblast.

megalokaryoblastoma (**meg**·al·o·kar·e·o·blas·**to**′·mah). Megakaryoblastoma.

megalokaryocyte (**meg**·al·o·**kar**′·e·o·site). Megakaryocyte.

megalomania (meg·al·o·**ma**′·ne·ah). A mental condition in which the patient has grandiose delusions about himself and an unwarranted belief in his own goodness, power, greatness, intellect, or importance. [Gk *megas* large, mania.]

megalomaniac (meg·al·o·**ma**′·ne·ak). An individual afflicted with megalomania.

megalomelia (meg·al·o·**me**′·le·ah). Abnormal largeness of one or more limbs. [Gk *megas* large, *melos* limb.]

megalonychosis (meg·al·on·ik·**o**′·sis). Hypertrophy of the nails. [Gk *megas* large, *onyx* nail, *-osis* condition.]

megalo-oesophagus (meg·al·o·e·**sof**′·ag·us). Hypertrophy of the oesophagus. [Gk *megas* large, oesophagus.]

megalopenis (meg·al·o·**pe**′·nis). Abnormal size of the penis. [Gk *megas* large, penis.]

megalophthalmus (meg·al·of·**thal**′·mus). Excessive largeness of the eyes. [Gk *megas* large, *ophthalmos* eye.]

megalopia (meg·al·**o**·pe·ah). An abnormal visual state in which objects appear to be larger than in fact they are. [Gk *megas* large, *ops* eye.]

megalopodia (meg·al·o·**po**′·de·ah). Abnormally large size of the feet. [Gk *megas* large, *pous* foot.]

megalopsia (meg·al·**op**·se·ah). Megalopia.

megaloscope (meg·al·o·skope). A large endoscope fitted with a magnifying lens. [Gk *megas* large, *skopein* to watch.]

megalosplanchnic (meg·al·o·**splangk**′·nik). Descriptive of the state in which the abdominal part of the body is large in proportion to the thoracic part. [Gk *megas* large, *splagchna* viscera.]

megalosplenia (meg·al·o·**sple**′·ne·ah). Enlargement of the spleen. [Gk *megas* large, spleen.]

megalosporon, megalospore (meg·al·o·**spo**′·ron, meg·al·o·spore). Obsolete terms for *Trichophyton*. [Gk *megas* large, *sporos* seed.]

megalosyndactylia, megalosyndactyly (meg·al·o·sin·dak·**til**′·e·ah, meg·al·o·sin·**dak**′·til·e). Syndactylia associated with a condition of enlargement of the fingers or toes. [Gk *megas* large, syndactylia.]

megalothymus (meg·al·o·**thi**′·mus). Hypertrophied thymus. [Gk *megas* large, thymus.]

megalo-ureter (meg·al·o·ewr·**e**′·ter). Mega-ureter. [Gk *megas* large, ureter.]

megalo-urethra (meg·al·o·ewr·**e**′·thrah). A rare condition of grossly dilated anterior urethra usually associated with gross redundancy of the skin of the penis. [Gk *megas* large, urethra.]

megamerozoite (meg·ah·mer·o·**zo**′·ite). A large-sized merozoite. [Gk *megas* large, merozoite.]

meganucleus (meg·ah·**new**·kle·us). Macronucleus. [Gk *megas* large, nucleus.]

megaphone (meg·ah·fone). A device which magnifies and directs sounds and so enables the voice to be heard over long distances. [Gk *megas* large, *phone* sound.]

megaphonia (meg·ah·**fo**·ne·ah). Abnormal loudness of the voice. [see prec.]

megaprosopous (meg·ah·**pros**′·o·pus). Having a face of abnormally large size. [Gk *megas* large, *prosopon* face.]

megarectum (meg·ah·**rek**·tum). An extremely dilated rectum. [Gk *megas* large, rectum.]

megascope (meg·ah·skope). Megaloscope.

Megaselia (meg·ah·**se**·le·ah). A genus of flies whose larvae may cause intestinal myiasis.

megasigmoid (meg·ah·**sig**·moid). A condition in which the third part of the loop of the pelvic (sigmoid) colon is greatly dilated. [Gk *megas* large, sigmoid.]

megasoma (meg·ah·**so**·mah). A degree of stature and size which although abnormal does not reach the proportions of gigantism. [Gk *megas* large, *soma* body.]

megasome (meg·ah·some). Macrosome. [see prec.]

megaspore (meg·ah·spore). Macrospore. [Gk *megas* large, spore.]

megasthenic (meg·as·**then**·ik). Having great power. [Gk *megas* large, *sthenos* strength.]

megastria (meg·as·tre·ah). Megalogastria.

megatrichophyton (meg·ah·trik·o·**fi**′·ton). Obsolete term for *Trichophyton*. [Gk *megas* large, *thrix* hair, *phyton* plant.]

mega-ureter (meg·ah·ewr·**e**′·ter). Megalo-ureter. Non-obstructive dilatation of the ureter. [Gk *megas* large, ureter.]

megavolt (meg·ah·volt). A unit of electric potential: a million volts. [Gk *megas* large, volt.]

Megestrol (me·**jes**·trol). BP Commission approved name for 17α-hydroxy-6-methylpregna-4,6-diene-3,20-dione. **Megestrol Acetate BP 1973.** 17α-acetoxy-6-methylpregna-4,6-diene-3,20-dione, a progestational steroid.

Méglin, J. A. (b. 1756). Colmar physician.

Méglin's palatine point. The point where the greater palatine branch of the sphenopalatine ganglion leaves the greater palatine foramen.

Meglumine BP 1973 (meg·loo·meen). *N*-methylglucamine, an organic base used for the preparation of salts of iodinated organic acids required as contrast media in radiological practice.

megohm (meg·ome). A unit of electrical resistance: a million ohms. [Gk *megas* large, ohm.]

megophthalmus (meg·of·**thal**·mus). Megalophthalmus.

megoxycyte (meg·**ox**·e·site). Megoxyphil. [Gk *megas* large, *oxys* acid, *kytos* cell.]

megoxyphil, megoxyphile (meg·**ox**·e·fil, meg·**ox**·e·file). A large granular eosinophil leucocyte. [Gk *megas* large, *oxys* acid, *philein* to love.]

megrim (me·grim). Migraine. [ME *migrym*.]

Meibom, Heinrich (b. 1638). Helmstadt physician.

Meibomian cyst. A cystic distension of a meibomian gland due to obstruction of its duct.

Meibom's glands, Meibomian glands. Tarsal glands of the eyelid.

meibomian (mi·**bo**·me·an). Associated with Heinrich Meibom.

Meige, Henri (b. 1866). Paris physician.

Meige's disease, Nonne-Milroy-Meige syndrome. Milroy's disease; chronic hereditary oedema of the legs.

Meigs, Arthur Vincent (b. 1850). Philadelphia surgeon.

Meigs' capillaries. Capillaries in the myocardium.

Meigs, Joe Vincent (b. 1892). Boston gynaecologist.

Meigs' syndrome. The combination of a fibroma of the ovary with a pleural effusion.

Meinicke, Ernst (b. 1878). German immunologist.

Meinicke antigen. An artificial antigen used in the diagnosis of syphilis, composed of an alcoholic extract of horse heart with 2 per cent sodium chloride.

meiosis (mi·o·sis). 1. The process of cell division which results in the production of haploid cells from diploid parents; reduction division. In almost all animals meiosis takes place during gametogenesis. Two divisions of the mother cell are involved. The first, preceded by chromosome replication, begins with a long prophase which can be divided into a series of stages according to the characteristic appearance of the chromosomes. At first these are long single threads (*leptotene stage*) then, in diploid species, the homologues begin to pair leading to the formation of bivalents (*zygotene stage*). As the chromosomes continue to pair along their whole length, they contract and their chromatids become visible and so do the exchanges between chromatids presumably resulting from crossing-over and leading to chiasma configurations (*pachytene stage*). The chromosomes then begin to come apart from each other as they continue to contract and are held together at chiasmata (*diplotene stage*). When chromosome contraction has reached a maximum the nucleolus disappears (*diakinesis*). This marks the end of prophase. During metaphase the paired homologue co-orient on the spindle so that homologous centromeres come to lie on opposite sides of the equatorial plane. At anaphase members of homologous pairs move to opposite poles where they group together at telophase. This may or may not be followed by an interphase stage (*interkinesis*) during which chromosome replication does not occur. The second division starts and proceeds like a mitotic division where the chromatids of each chromosome migrate to opposite poles. The meiotic division of a diploid gametocyte leads to the formation of four haploid cells. In the human male all such cells may differentiate into functional gametes, while in females unequal cytoplasmic division leads to a larger and functional gamete (the egg) and to smaller non-functional gametes (the polar bodies). Meiosis secures the maintenance of the species-specific chromosome number in organisms with a sexual type of reproduction; it determines the accurate segregation of alleles, the random assortment of unlinked genes (that is chromosomes) and the non-random recombination of linked genes. **C-meiosis.** A meiosis in which the spindle has been poisoned at one or both divisions by colchicine or other poisons. 2. Contraction of the pupil. [Gk diminution.]

meiotic (mi·**ot**·ik). Pertaining to, or resulting from, meiosis. Meiotic drive. *See* DRIVE.

Meisen, Valdemar (b. 1878). Copenhagen surgeon.

Meisen mixture. A 50 per cent solution of dextrose, used for the obliteration of varicose veins.

Meissner, Georg (b. 1829). German anatomist and physiologist.

Meissner's corpuscle. An encapsulated sensory nerve-ending found in the dermal papillae of the skin of the palm, fingers, sole of the foot, and toes. It is thought to be a receptor for tactile stimuli.

Meissner's ganglia. The ganglia found in the submucous plexus.

Meissner's plexus. The submucous plexus.

mel (mel). Honey; a mixture of invert sugars and compound saccharides produced from the nectar of flowers by enzyme action in the honey sac of the bee *Apis mellifica.* It is esteemed as a food and sweetening agent. **Mel boracis.** Borax and honey, a solution of borax (10 per cent) in glycerin and purified honey. **Mel depuratum.** Purified Honey BPC 1973. [L]

Meladrazine (mel·ad·**ra**·zeen). BP Commission approved name for 2,4-di(diethylamino)-6-hydrazino-1,3,5-triazine; a polysynaptic inhibitor.

melaena (mel·**e**·nah). The passage of black tarry stools, due to altered blood pigment derived from haemorrhage into the bowel. **Melaena neonatorum.** Melaena occurring within the first few days after birth; it is generally due to hypoprothrombinaemia in the so-called *haemorrhagic disease of the newborn,* and may be associated with haemorrhage from other parts. **Melaena spuria.** Melaena in nurslings, in which the blood is derived from the fissured nipples of the nurse. [Gk *melas* black.]

melaenic (mel·**e**·nik). Belonging or referring to melaena.

melagra (mel·**ag**·rah). A condition of pain affecting the muscles of the extremities. [Gk *melos* limb, *agra* a catching.]

Melaleuca (mel·al·**ew**·kah). A genus of trees of the family Myrtaceae, one species of which (*Melaleuca leucadendron*) yields cajuput. [Gk *melas* black, *leukos* white.]

melalgia (mel·**al**·je·ah). A painful neuralgic condition of the limbs. [Gk *melos* limb, *algos* pain.]

melamphonous (mel·**am**·fon·us). Hoarse-voiced. [Gk *melas* obscure, *phone* sound.]

melanaemia (mel·an·**e**·me·ah). Haemochromatosis. [melanin, Gk *haima* blood.]

melancholia (mel·an·**ko**·le·ah). A mental illness in which the predominant symptom is melancholy, depression of spirits, unhappiness, misery; frequently accompanying symptoms are disturbance of sleep, anergia, retardation, self-reproach. More specifically, an endogenous illness of this type, without detectable physical or psychogenic cause. Two aetiologically distinct types of the endogenous psychosis are recognized: the melancholic phase of a manic-depressive psychosis, and involutional melancholia (see below). **Acute melancholia.** Melancholia with acute onset. **Melancholia agitata, Agitated melancholia.** Any melancholic illness in which agitation (i.e. fidgety, ineffective restlessness accompanied by emotions of anxiety and tension) is predominant, and the more usual retardation, though it may still be present, is apparently submerged; such states are especially frequent in involutional melancholia. **Melancholia attonita.** A mild form of melancholia. **Climacteric melancholia.** Melancholia appearing at the time of the climacterium, now commonly regarded as merely an involutional melancholia with an unusually close association with the menopause, although there is some evidence to suggest that endocrine causation is involved. **Involutional melancholia.** A term sometimes loosely applied to any severe depressive illness occurring in the involutional period of life (approximately from 45 to 65), and therefore inclusive of manic-depressive depressions occurring at this time, and depressions due to organic changes such as cerebral arteriosclerosis. More precisely, a clinical syndrome now widely recognized as distinct (though originally included by Kraepelin in the manic-depressive disorders), characterized by prepsychotic rigidity of personality, insidious onset, protracted course sometimes even to complete chronicity, tendency to delusion formation in later stages, and to tension and agitation from early on, and, as a rule, satisfactory to response to convulsive shock therapy. **Paranoid melancholia.** A melancholic illness, otherwise unspecified, in which delusions, especially persecutory delusions, are prominent. **Paretic melancholia.** Melancholia accompanying general paresis, of which it may sometimes be the first sign. **Recurrent melancholia.** A manic-depressive psychosis in which most of the phases are predominantly depressive rather than manic or hypomanic. **Simple melancholia, Melancholia simplex.** Melancholia unaccompanied by any unusual or anomalous symptom. **Stuporous melancholia.** A melancholic illness in which stupor occurs. [Gk *melas* black, *chole* bile.]

melancholiac (mel·an·**ko**·le·ak). An individual afflicted with melancholia.

melancholic (mel·an·**kol**·ik). Affected with melancholia.

melanemesis (mel·an·**em**·es·is). Black vomit. *See* VOMIT. [Gk *melas* black, *emesis* vomiting.]

melanhidrosis (mel·an·hid·**ro'**·sis). The exudation of black sweat. [Gk *melas* black, *hidrosis* sweat.]

Melania (mel·a·ne·ah). A genus of snails which includes the species *Melania libertina* and *M. ebenina,* that act as intermediate hosts for the flukes *Paragonimus westermani* and *Metagonimus yokogawai.* [Gk *melas* black.]

melaniferous (mel·an·**if**·er·us). Bearing a black pigment such as melanin or similar matter. [melanin, L *ferre* to bear.]

melanin (**mel**·an·in). The black or dark-brown shapeless pigments found in melanotic tumours, the hair, the skin, the substantia nigra of the brain, and the choroid coat of the eye. It is formed from tyrosine by oxidative metabolism and polymerization. [Gk *melas* black.]

melanism (**mel**·an·izm). Melanosis.

melanistic (mel·an·**is**·tik). Melanotic.

melanoblast (**mel**·an·o·blast). A cell of epithelial tissue containing melanin granules. [Gk *melas* black, *blastos* germ.]

melanoblastoma (**mel**·an·o·blas·**to'**·mah) A tumour composed of poorly differentiated cells that produce or store melanin. [melanoblast, Gk *-oma* tumour.]

melanoblastosis (**mel**·an·o·blas·**to'**·sis). A tumour composed of melanoblasts. [melanoblast, Gk *-osis* condition.]

melanocancroid (**mel**·an·o·**kang'**·kroid). Any epithelial sore characterized by dark pigmentation. [Gk *melas* black, cancer, Gk *eidos* form.]

melanocarcinoma (**mel**·an·o·kar·sin·**o'**·mah). A darkly pigmented carcinoma; melanoid carcinoma. [Gk *melas* black, carcinoma.]

melanochroic, melanochroid, melanochrous (**mel**·an·o·**kro'**·ik, mel·an·**ok**·roid, mel·an·**ok**·rus). Having a dark skin. [Gk *melas* black, *chroa* complexion.]

melanocyte (**mel**·an·o·site). Any pigment-bearing cell such as that found in the skin, or in the choroid coat of the eye. [Gk *melas* black, *kytos* cell.]

melanocytoma (**mel**·an·o·si·**to'**·mah). A rare, benign tumour of the optic disc. [Gk *melas* black, *kytos* cell, *-oma* tumour.]

melanocyte-stimulating hormone (**mel**·an·o·site **stim**·u·lay·ting **hor**·mone). MSH; a peptide hormone secreted by the pituitary gland that causes dispersion of melanin with melanophores, resulting in darkening of the skin.

melanoderma (**mel**·an·o·**der**′·mah). 1. A condition in which there is an unusually large accumulation of melanin in the skin. 2. A general term for pigmentary discolorations of the skin occurring in spots or patches of yellow, brown, or black. **Melanoderma cachecticorum.** Pigmentation of the skin occurring in cachectic conditions. **Parasitic melanoderma.** Pigmentation of the skin occurring in long-standing infestations with pediculi. **Senile melanoderma.** Pigmentation of the skin occurring in old age. [Gk *melas* black, *derma* skin.]

melanodermatitis toxica lichenoides (**mel**·an·o·der·mat·**i**′·tis **tox**·ik·ah li·ken·**oid**·eez). An exogenous, inflammatory, pigmentary disorder of the skin, with brown or slaty discoloration, lichenoid papules, and hyperkeratosis. It is thought by many to be a variety of Riehl's melanosis. [Gk *melas* black, *derma* skin, *-itis* inflammation, L *toxicus* poisonous, Gk *leichen* lichen, *eidos* form.]

melanodermic (**mel**·an·o·**der**′·mik). Dark-skinned. [Gk *melas* black, *derma* skin.]

melanodes (mel·an·o·deez). Melanoid.

melano-epithelioma (**mel**·an·o·ep·e·the·le·**o**′·mah). A squamous-celled carcinoma, usually of the skin or its derivatives, in which melanin is produced. [Gk *melas* black, epithelioma.]

melanoflocculation (**mel**·an·o·flok·ew·**la**′·shun). Henry's melanoflocculation test for the diagnosis of malaria, based upon the precipitation of melanin from ox eyes. The reaction is non-specific, depending upon the increase of euglobulin in the serum. [Gk *melas* black, flocculation.]

melanogen (**mel**·an·o·jen). An uncoloured chromogen found in the urine, a forerunner of melanin, into which it can be converted by appropriate treatment. [see foll.]

melanogenesis (**mel**·an·o·**jen**′·es·is). The process by which melanin is produced. [Gk *melas* black, *genein* to produce.]

melanoglossia (**mel**·an·o·**glos**′·e·ah). Black tongue. *See* TONGUE. [Gk *melas* black, *glossa* tongue.]

melanohidrosis (**mel**·an·o·hid·**ro**′·sis). Dark brown or black sweat. [Gk *melas* black, *hidros* sweat.]

melanoid (**mel**·an·oid). 1. Dark in colour. 2. Having resemblance to melanosis. 3. Artificial melanin. [Gk *melas* black, *eidos* form.]

Melanolestes (**mel**·an·o·**les**′·teez). A genus of bugs of the family Reduviidae. **Melanolestes picipes.** The black corsair or common kissing bug of the USA, sometimes very abundant and the bites of which are painful. [Gk *melas* black, *lestes* robber.]

melanoleucoderma (**mel**·an·o·lew·ko·**der**′·mah). Cutis marmorata. **Melanoleucoderma colli.** Vitiligo of the neck. A manifestation of secondary syphilis, it may be temporary or permanent, is more often seen in women than men, and appears within a year of contracting the disease; venereal collar. [Gk *melas* black, leucoderma.]

melanoma (mel·an·**o**·mah). A tumour consisting of darkly pigmented cells. **Amelanotic melanoma.** Melanoma in which pigment is poorly developed or absent. **Juvenile melanoma.** A benign, melanocytic and vascular tumour of children; it is reddish-brown, soft or firm, and sometimes warty. Its histological appearance of bizarre shaped cells with some mitoses may wrongly suggest malignancy. **Malignant melanoma.** Melanotic sarcoma or carcinoma. **Subungual melanoma.** A small painful melanoma of the nail bed. [Gk *melas* black, *-oma* tumour.]

melanomalignancy (**mel**·an·o·mal·**ig**′·nan·se). A malignant tumour consisting of melanin-pigmented cells. [Gk *melas* black, malignancy.]

melanomatosis (**mel**·an·o·mat·**o**′·sis). The development of numerous metastases of malignant melanomata throughout the body. [melanoma, Gk *-osis* condition.]

melanonychia (**mel**·an·on·**ik**′·e·ah). Dark pigmentation of the nail, most pronounced at the growing ends. [Gk *melas* black, *onyx* nail.]

melanopathia, melanopathy (**mel**·an·o·**path**′·e·ah, mel·an·**op**·ath·e). Any disorder accompanied by excessive skin or other tissue pigmentation, such as melanoderma, melasma, melanosis, melanoma. [Gk *melas* black, *pathos* disease.]

melanophage (**mel**·an·o·faje). A cell which engulfs melanin. [Gk *melas* black, *phagein* to eat.]

melanophore (**mel**·an·o·fore). A chromatophore cell whose enclosed pigment is a melanin. [melanin, Gk *pherein* to bear.]

melanoplakia (**mel**·an·o·**pla**′·ke·ah). A condition in which dark-coloured plaques are developed on the mucous membrane of the mouth, e.g. in jaundice, stomatitis. [Gk *melas* black, *plax* plate.]

melanoprecipitation (**mel**·an·o·pre·sip·it·**a**′·shun). Melanoflocculation. [Gk *melas* black, precipitation.]

melanorrhagia (**mel**·an·o·**ra**′·je·ah). Profuse melaena. [Gk *melas* black, *rhegnynein* to gush forth.]

melanorrhoea (**mel**·an·o·**re**′·ah). Melaena. [Gk *melas* black, *rhoia* flow.]

melanosarcoma (**mel**·an·o·sar·**ko**′·mah). A type of darkly pigmented sarcoma of great malignancy. [Gk *melas* black, sarcoma.]

melanosarcomatosis (**mel**·an·o·sar·ko·mat·**o**′·sis). The widespread development of melanosarcomata. [melanosarcoma, Gk *-osis* condition.]

melanoscirrhus (**mel**·an·o·**skir**′·us). A type of scirrhous cancer in which there is marked pigmentation. [Gk *melas* black, *skirrhos* hard.]

melanosis (mel·an·**o**·sis). 1. An abnormal deposition of the black pigment, melanin, in the skin or other tissues. 2. A condition of general staining of all the tissues of the body with melanin found in cases of generalized melanotic carcinoma. **Melanosis bulbi.** A congenital anomaly of the eyes in which there is great increase in the pigment of the uveal tissues, iris, ciliary body, choroid, and also in the sclera. **Melanosis coli.** Pigmentation of the mucous membrane of the colon by deposits of melanin. **Melanosis of the conjunctiva.** A congenital pigmentation of the conjunctiva either in the form of spots or, more rarely, diffuse. **Melanosis iridis.** Infiltration of the iris by melanoblasts. **Melanosis lenticularis progressiva.** Xeroderma pigmentosum. **Neurocutaneous melanosis.** Melanocytic cutaneous naevi with melanocytic infiltrations of the meninges, brain or spinal cord, and a fatal outcome. **Occupational melanosis.** Toxic melanodermatitis from exposure to coal-tar products or mineral oil. The exposed skin is pigmented, atrophic, telangiectatic, with lichenoid papules and, later, keratoses and epitheliomata. **Precancerous circumscribed melanosis.** Xeroderma pigmentosum. **Melanosis of the retina.** A congenital anomaly in which there is hyperplasia of the pigment epithelium of the retina; small dark spots often in the form of cats' paw marks are seen. **Melanosis of the sclera.** A congenital pigmentary anomaly of the sclera in which there are blue-grey spots, especially round the exit of the ciliary vessels. **Tar melanosis.** Reticular pigmentation of the exposed skin of tar workers. [Gk *melas* black, *-osis* condition.]

See also: RIEHL.

melanosity (mel·an·**os**·it·e). 1. The state of melanosis. 2. Darkness of complexion. [see prec.]

melanosome (**mel**·an·o·some). One of the intracellular bodies containing melanin near the Golgi material in melanocytes. [Gk *melas* black, *soma* body.]

melanotic (mel·an·**ot**·ik). Relating to, characterized by, or affected with melanosis. [Gk *melas* black.]

melanotrichia linguae (**mel**·an·o·**trik**′·e·ah **ling**·gwe). Black tongue. *See* TONGUE. [Gk *melas* black, *thrix* hair, L *lingua* tongue.]

melanotropic (**mel**·an·o·**trop**′·ik). 1. Having an affinity for melanin. 2. Giving rise to melanin deposits. [Gk *melas* black, *trope* a turning.]

melanous (**mel**·an·us). Dark-skinned. [Gk *melas* black.]

melanuria (mel·an·**ewr**·e·ah). 1. The excretion of urine containing dark pigment. 2. A condition in which urine becomes black after being allowed to stand for some time. It is due to the conversion of colourless melanogen to melanin and occurs in cases of generalized malignant melanoma. [Gk *melas* black, urine.]

melanuric (mel·an·**ewr**·ik). Characterized by or referring to melanuria.

melanurin (mel·an·**ewr**·in). A substance, very dark in colour, and occurring rarely in urine in certain diseased conditions. [Gk *melas* black, urine.]

melarsen (mel·ar·sen). Disodium 2,4-diamino-6-(arsenoanilino)-triazine. An arsenical preparation that has been used with limited success in trypanosomiasis; it has proved very toxic. **Melarsen oxide/BAL.** Melarsoprol.

Melarsonyl Potassium (mel·ar·son·il pot·as·e·um). BP Commission approved name for dipotassium 2 - [4 - (4,6 - diamino - 1,3,5 - triazin - 2 - ylamino)phenyl]-1,3,2-dithiarsolan-4,5-dicarboxylate; it is used in the treatment of trypanosomiasis.

Melarsoprol BP 1968 (mel·ar·so·prol). Melarsen oxide/BAL, *p* - (2,4 - diamino - 1,3,5 - triazinyl - 6) - aminophenylarseno - α β - dithiopropanol, a trivalent organic arsenical combined with BAL on the theory that the latter reduces the toxicity of the arsenic. It is used in the treatment of advanced cases of human trypanosomiasis.

melasma (mel·az·mah). A general term for pigmentary discolorations of the skin, yellow, brown, or black, and occurring in macular form. **Melasma addisonii.** Addison's disease. **Melasma gravidarum.** A dark pigment observed on the skin of pregnant women. **Melasma suprarenale.** Addison's disease. **Melasma universale.** A disease marked by dark pigmentation of almost all the body surface. [Gk black spot.]

melatonin (mel·a·tone·in). A compound synthesized by the pineal gland. It affects the activity of 4-reductase which is responsible for the conversion of testosterone to dihydrotestosterone.

melatrophy (mel·at·ro·fe). Atrophy of the limbs. [Gk *melos* limb, atrophy.]

Meleney, Frank Lamont (b. 1889). New York surgeon.

Meleney's burrowing lesion. A progressive gangrene of the skin at the site of an accidental skin abrasion, due to anaerobic streptococci.

Melengestrol (mel·en·jes·trol). BP Commission approved name for 17α-hydroxy - 6 - methyl - 16 - methylenepregna - 4,6 - diene - 3,20 - dione; a progestogen.

melezitose (mel·ez·it·oze). A trisaccharide, α-glucose-2-β-fructose-6-α-glucoside, which occurs in the manna of Douglas fir and is a constituent of honeydew; on hydrolysis it yields glucose and the disaccharide turanose. [Gk *meli* honey.]

meliatin (mel·e·at·in). A glycoside found in buckbean or marsh trefoils, *Menyanthes trifoliata.*

melibiose (mel·e·bi·oze). $C_{12}H_{22}O_{11}$, a dextrorotatory disaccharide, β-glucose-6-α-galactoside, found in Australian manna and hydrolysed into glucose and galactose. Condensed with fructose it forms the trisaccharide, raffinose, which occurs in beetroot and molasses. [Gk *meli* honey.]

melicera, meliceris (mel·e·seer·ah, mel·e·seer·is). A cyst containing a syrupy or honey-like substance. [Gk *meli* honey, *keros* wax.]

melilotin (mel·e·lo·tin). A glucoside of coumarin obtained from species of *Melilotus.*

melilotoxin (mel·e·lo·tox'·in). A name given to dicoumarin which is produced by the spoiling of sweet clover, *Melilotus officinalis,* and which has a toxic effect on cattle.

Melilotus (mel·e·lo·tus). A genus of herbs of the family Leguminosae; the clovers. The dried leaf and flowering tops of *Melilotus officinalis* contain coumarin combined with melilotic and coumaric acids. Spoiled sweet clover is poisonous to cattle owing to the formation in it of the anticoagulant, dicoumarol. [Gk *meli* honey, lotus.]

melin (mel·in). Rutin. [Gk *meli* honey.]

melioidosis (mel·e·oid·o'·sis). A rare glanders-like disease occurring in Burma, Malaysia, Sri Lanka and Guam, and recognized in 1947 in Berlin. It is due to *Pfeifferella whitmori,* and produces many and various symptoms, mainly diarrhoea, septicaemia and multiple abscesses of the liver. [Gk *melis* glanders, *eidos* form, *-osis* condition.]

melissic (mel·is·ik). Describing anything that has been derived or obtained from beeswax or honey. [Gk *melissa* bee.]

melissophobia (mel·is·o·fo'·be·ah). An unnaturally acute fear of wasps, bees and other stinging insects, and of being stung by them. [Gk *melissa* bee, phobia.]

melissotherapy (mel·is·o·ther'·ap·e). A type of treatment, e.g. for rheumatism, in which bees are used to sting a particular part or in which bee venom is injected or administered in the form of ointment. [Gk *melissa* bee, therapy.]

melitaemia (mel·it·e·me·ah). Glycaemia. [Gk *meli* honey, *haima* blood.]

melitagra (mel·it·ag·rah). Eczema or eczematous dermatitis with honeycomb crusting. [Gk *meli* honey, *agra* seizure.]

melitensis (mel·it·en·sis). Malta fever; undulant fever in which the infection is transmitted from goats in milk or milk products. [L of Malta.]

melitin, melitine (mel·it·in, mel·it·een). The filtrate of a 20-day-old broth culture of *Brucella melitensis,* which has been used in one form of the brucellin test in the diagnosis of undulant fever. Abortin is a similar filtrate from *Brucella abortus.* When either preparation is injected intradermally into the arm, an allergic skin reaction may develop, denoting that infection with *Brucella* has taken place, possibly some months or years previously. The interpretation of a positive reading may be very difficult.

melitis (mel·i·tis). An inflammatory condition of the cheek. [Gk *melon* cheek, *-itis* inflammation.]

melitococcosis (mel·it·o·kok·o'·sis). Melitensis. [melitensis, coccus, Gk *-osis* condition.]

melitococcus (mel·it·o·kok'·us). *Brucella melitensis;* the name is now obsolete. [L *Melitaeus* of Malta, coccus.]

melitoptyalism, melitoptyalismus (mel·it·o·ti'·al·izm, mel·it·o·ti·al·iz'·mus). The secretion of glucose in the saliva. [Gk *meli* honey, *ptyalon* saliva.]

melitoptyalon (mel·it·o·ti'·al·on). Salivary glucose secreted in certain conditions. [see prec.]

melitose, melitriose (mel·it·oze, mel·e·tri·oze). Raffinose, $C_{18}H_{32}O_{16}$. A dextrorotatory trisaccharide, fructose-β-glucose-6-α-galactoside, found in sugar beet, beetroot, molasses, eucalyptus manna, cotton seeds and in certain cereals and fungi. Hydrolysis yields fructose and melibiose. [Gk *meli* honey.]

Melittangium (mel·it·an·je·um). A genus of bacteria of the order Myxobacteriales. The type species, *Melittangium boletum,* is found in soil and animal faeces and is non-pathogenic. [Gk *meli* honey, *aggeion* vessel.]

melituria (mel·it·ewr·e·ah). The existence of sugar of any kind in the urine. **Melituria inosita.** Inositoluria. [Gk *meli* honey, urine.]

melituric (mel·it·ewr·ik). Affected with or relating to melituria.

Meller, Josef. Vienna ophthalmologist.

Meller's operation. Extirpation of the lacrimal sac through an incision over the lacrimal crest of the maxilla.

Mellinger magnet. A giant magnet for extracting metallic fragments from the eye.

mellitum (mel·i·tum). Oxymel BPC 1973. [L *mellitus* honeyed.]

melodidymus (mel·o·did·im·us). A monster with two sets of limbs. [Gk *melos* limb, *didymos* twin.]

melomania (mel·o·ma·ne·ah). 1. An inordinate passion for music. 2. Singing mania; a type of mental disease in which the patient is given to singing for long spells. [Gk *melos* song, mania.]

melomaniac (mel·o·ma·ne·ak). An individual affected with melomania.

melomelus (mel·om·el·us). A fetal monstrosity with normal limbs and accessory rudimentary limbs. [Gk *melos* limb.]

meloncus (mel·ong·kus). Any neoplasm affecting the cheek, more especially on the outer surface. [Gk *melon* cheek, *ogkos* tumour.]

melonoplasty (mel·on·o·plas·te). Plastic repair of the cheek. [Gk *melon* cheek, *plassein* to mould.]

Melophagus (mel·of·ag·us). A genus of pupiparous Diptera. **Melophagus ovinus.** The sheep ked, a wingless form sometimes found on man. It has no vector importance. [Gk *melon* sheep, *phagein* to eat.]

meloplastic (mel·o·plas·tik). Relating or belonging to meloplasty.

meloplasty (mel·o·plas·te). 1. Melonoplasty. 2. A plastic operation performed on the extremities. [Gk *melon* cheek, *melos* limb, *plassein* to mould.]

melorheostosis (mel·o·re·os·**to**'·sis). A rare disease of long bones which assume an appearance similar to that of a lighted candle in which the wax has flowed down the sides. [Gk *melos* limb, *rheos* current, *osteon* bone.]

melosalgia (mel·os·**al**·je·ah). A painful condition of the lower limbs. [Gk *melos* limb, *algos* pain.]

meloschisis (mel·**os**·kis·is). Macrostomia. [Gk *melon* cheek, *schisis* a cleaving.]

melotia (mel·o·she·ah). A congenital deformity in which an ear is situated on the cheek. [Gk *melon* cheek, *ous* ear.]

melotridymus (mel·o·**trid**·im·us). A fetal monster with one pair of supernumerary limbs. [Gk *melos* limb, *tridymos* triple.]

Melotte, George W. (b. 1835). American dentist.

Melotte's metal. A fusible alloy used in dentistry, containing bismuth, lead and tin.

melotus (mel·o·tus). Melotia.

Melphalan BP 1973 (**mel**·fal·an). 4-di-(2-Chloroethyl)amino-L-phenylalanine, used as a cytotoxic agent in the treatment of neoplastic disease.

Melrose, Dennis Graham (b. 1921). London physiologist and medical scientist.

Melrose pump oxygenator. An apparatus used in cardiac by-pass employing a disc oxygenator. First described in 1954.

melting (**mel**·ting). Liquefaction by heat. **DNA melting.** The disruption of the double-helical structure of DNA on heating. [AS *meltan*.]

Meltzer, Samuel James (b. 1851). New York physician.

Meltzer's law. Law of contrary innervation.

Meltzer's treatment. For tetanus, by intraspinal injections of a solution of magnesium sulphate.

melung (**me**·lung). A macular exanthem of yaws.

member [membrum (NA)] (**mem**·ber). Any organ or other part of the body, in particular an extremity or a limb. [L *membrum* a limb.]

membrana (mem·**bra**·nah). Membrana. **Membrana adamantina.** Nasmyth's membrane. **Membrana adventitia.** The outer coat of an artery or vein. **Membrana caduca.** The decidua. **Membrana decidua.** The uterine endometrium in pregnancy. **Membrana eboris.** The layer of odontoblast cells lying in the periphery of the tooth pulp. **Membrana epipapillaris.** A fibrous membrane seen sometimes on the optic disc and connected with the fibrous sheath around the vessels. **Membrana gliae superficialis.** A delicate, glial, superficial covering of the optic nerve and the rest of the central nervous system. **Membrana granulosa.** The cells lining a graafian follicle of an ovary. **Membrana limitans externa, Membrana limitans interna.** *See* RETINA. **Membrana performativa.** A line appearing in histological sections of developing teeth between the internal enamel epithelium and the dental papilla. **Membrana propria.** Basement membrane. *See* MEMBRANE. **Membrana pupillaris.** A layer of mesoderm closing the pupillary opening in the fetus. Remnants of this often remain, and are known as the *persistent pupillary membrane.* **Membrana serosa.** The lining of a serous cavity, e.g. the peritoneum and pleura. **Membrana serotina.** The decidua basalis or maternal placenta. **Membrana tectoria [NA].** A spiral membrane, fusiform in cross-section, projecting from the vestibular lip above the spiral organ of Corti. **Membrana tectoria of the atlanto-occipital joint [membrana tectoria (NA)].** A broad, strong band covering the odontoid process, running from the upper surface of the basilar part of the occipital bone to the posterior surface of the body of the axis. It is continuous inferiorly with the posterior longitudinal ligament of the vertebral column. **Membrana vitellina.** The membrane surrounding the fertilized ovum, enclosing the yolk. [L]

membranaceous (mem·bran·a·shus). Relating to, or of the nature of a membrane. [L *membranaceus.*]

membranate (**mem**·bran·ate). Of membranous type.

membrane (**mem**·brane). 1. [Membrana (NA)] A thin layer of tissue which covers a surface or divides a space or organ. 2. [Meninges (NA)] Any of the coverings of the brain and spinal cord. **Accidental membrane.** A rare synonym for false membrane (see below) or pseudomembrane. **Adventitious membrane.** A membrane arising *de novo*, as in scar tissue or inflammatory adhesions. **Adventitious hyaloid membrane.** A term used for the slight thickening of the hyaloid membrane or posterior capsular membrane following extracapsular cataract extraction. **Alveo-dental membrane.** Periodontal membrane (see below). **Anal membrane.** The posterior part of the cloacal membrane of the early embryo, separating the hind-gut from the proctodaeum. **Anhistous membrane.** The uterine decidua. **Animal membrane.** A thin membrane of animal tissue, such as bladder, used in dialysing. **Atlanto-occipital membrane, anterior, of the atlanto-occipital joint [membrana atlanto-occipitalis anterior (NA)].** A broad, strong membrane running from the anterior margin of the foramen magnum to the upper border of the anterior arch of the atlas. **Atlanto-occipital membrane, posterior, of the atlanto-occipital joint [membrana atlanto-occipitalis posterior (NA)].** A broad, thin membrane running from the posterior margin of the foramen magnum to the upper border of the posterior arch of the atlas. **Basal membrane of the semicircular duct [membrana basalis ductus semicircularis (NA)].** The outer of the three layers of the semicircular duct, consisting mainly of fibrous tissue. **Basement membrane.** The interface between epithelial cells and the underlying connective tissue which can be seen by light microscopy after suitable staining such as the periodic acid-Schiff reaction. It is a composite structure and includes the basal lamina which can be recognized by electron microscopy. **Basilar membrane [membrana spiralis].** A membrane extending from the osseous spiral lamina to the outer wall of the bony cochlea. **Birth membrane.** The fused amnion and chorion of the after-birth. **Brood membrane.** Brood capsule of *Echinococcus granulosus.* **Buccopharyngeal membrane.** The temporary membrane between the foregut and stomatodaeum of the early embryo. **Capsulopupillary membrane.** The vascular membrane ensheathing the lens of the early embryonic eye. **Cell membrane.** Plasma membrane (see below). **Chorio-allantoic membrane.** Chorio-allantois. **Cloacal membrane.** A thin membrane, composed of ectoderm and entoderm without mesoderm, separating the lumen of the hind-gut from the exterior in the early embryo. **Complex membrane.** A membrane composed of several differing layers. **Compound membrane.** A membrane composed of two or more separate layers. **Costocoracoid membrane.** Clavipectoral fascia. *See* FASCIA. **Cricovocal membrane [conus elasticus (NA)].** A fibro-elastic membrane made up of an anterior part (cricothyroid ligament) and a lateral part, attached between the thyroid angle anteriorly and the arytenoid cartilage posteriorly, with a thickened upper free margin, the vocal ligament. **Croupous membrane.** The false membrane of diphtheria. **Cyclitic membrane.** A membrane formed by inflammatory products, just behind the lens on the front of the vitreous, in some cases of cyclitis. **Decidual membrane.** Decidua capsularis. **Diphtheritic membrane.** A membrane consisting of coagulated fibrin with bacteria and leucocytes (coagulation necrosis). It is typically dead-white or greyish-yellow with well-defined margins; if forcibly removed, a little bleeding results. **Dysmenorrhoeal membrane.** The cast of the uterus sometimes shed in membranous dysmenorrhoea. **Egg membrane.** Any membrane surrounding the egg, whether or not it is derived from the ovum. **Elastic membrane.** A membrane chiefly composed of elastic fibres. **Elastic membrane of the larynx [membrana fibro-elastica laryngis (NA)].** A sheet of fibro-elastic tissue underlying the mucous membrane of the larynx, attached to the arytenoid cartilage behind, the thyroid and epiglottic cartilages in front, and the cricoid cartilage below. The part above the sinus is ill-defined. The lower part, the cricovocal membrane (see above), has a stout anterior part, the cricothyroid ligament, and a free upper border, the vocal ligament, which lies in the vocal fold. It is thickened and composed mainly of elastic fibres. **Enamel membrane.** The atrophied remains of the enamel organ attached to the surface of the enamel of a newly-formed tooth; Nasmyth's membrane.

membrane

Endoneural membrane. A delicate connective-tissue sheath around an individual nerve fibre, sometimes confused with the neurilemma. **Epicytial membrane.** The plasma membrane investing an animal cell or protozoon. **External limiting membrane.** An apparent membrane which the light microscope shows to be present between the rods and cones of the retina and the outer nuclear layer. The appearance is actually caused by a row of junctional complexes between the rods and cones and the supporting cells of Mueller. **Extra-embryonic membrane.** Any membrane surrounding the embryo at birth. **False membrane.** A pathological membrane of which diphtheritic membrane (see above) is a typical example. **Fenestrated membrane.** A membrane containing a large number of pores, such as the elastic membranes of the walls of arteries. **Fetal membrane.** One of the appendages serving for the protection, support and nourishment of the fetus. They comprise the chorion, amnion, yolk sac, allantois, placenta and umbilical cord. **Fibrous membrane.** A membrane composed of interlacing collagenous fibres. **Germinal membrane.** The blastoderm of large-yolked eggs. **Glassy membrane.** Any hyaline membrane, but especially the basement membrane of a graafian follicle, hair follicle, or the innermost layer of these choroid of the eye. **Gradocol membrane.** A thin membrane of collodion or similar substance made in graded porosities from 3 to 10 μm and used in ultrafiltration. By means of these collodion membranes it has been possible to determine the size of many of the viruses: gradocol filter. **Ground membrane.** One of the membranes placed across a striated muscle fibre between adjacent sarcomeres, e.g. Krause's membrane. **Homogeneous membrane.** The syncytiotrophoblastic covering of placental villi. **Hyaline membrane.** An acidophil fibrinous exudate found covering the epithelium of terminal broncheoles in stillborn and neonatal deaths, sometimes attributed to high oxygen tensions in the perinatal period. **Hyaloid membrane [membrana vitrea (NA)].** The surface layer of the vitreous body in the eye. It was formerly considered to be an actual membrane, but is now known to be merely a condensation on the surface of the vitreous. **Intercostal membrane, anterior [membrana intercostalis external (NA)].** Any of the thin connective-tissue sheets occupying the interchondral spaces, and continuous with the external intercostal muscles. **Intercostal membrane, posterior [membrana intercostalis interna (NA)].** Any of the thin connective-tissue sheets occupying the intercostal spaces medial to the angle of the ribs, and continuous with the internal intercostal muscles. **Internal limiting membrane.** The innermost layer of the retina of the eye separating it from the vitreous body. **Interosseous membrane of the forearm [membrana interossea antebrachii (NA)].** A thin sheet of fibres running downwards and medially from the interosseous border of the radius to that of the ulna. **Interosseous membrane of the leg [membrana interossea cruris (NA)].** A membrane whose fibres run distally and laterally, uniting the lateral border of the tibia to the anteromedial border of the fibula. **Ivory membrane.** Membrana eboris. **Meconic membrane.** A layer of mucus and desquamated epithelium enclosing the fetal meconium. **Medullary membrane.** The membrane lying between the marrow and cortex of a long bone; the endosteum. **Mucocutaneous membrane.** A compound membrane of which the inner layer is mucous and the outer skin-like, such as the tympanic membrane. **Mucous membrane.** The lining of the alimentary, respiratory and genito-urinary passages, composed of an epithelium resting upon a connective-tissue layer containing plain muscle, glands, blood vessels, nerve fibres, etc. **Mucous membrane of the larynx [tunica mucosa (NA)].** The lining of the larynx, thick, vascular, containing glands, and lined with columnar ciliated epithelium, except where it is adherent to the vocal ligaments, where it is stratified squamous in type. **Mucous membrane of the mouth [tunica mucosa oris (NA)].** The lining layer of the mouth. **Mucous membrane of the nose.** The vascular moist epithelium directly applied to the bone or cartilage forming the nose. **Mucous membrane of the tongue [tunica mucosa linguae (NA)].** The whole tongue is covered with stratified epithelium. The dorsum of the anterior two-thirds bears numerous papillae; the posterior third contains numerous lymphatic follicles and serous glands, and the orifices of mucous glands. At the borders and inferior surface of the tip the mucous membrane is thin and lacks papillae. **Mucous membrane of the tympanic cavity [tunica mucosa cavi tympani (NA)].** The lining of the tympanic cavity, continuous with that of the pharynx through the pharyngotympanic tube. It covers the ossicles and other tympanic contents, and is consequently thrown into folds forming recesses such as the anterior [recessus membranae tympani anterior (NA)] and posterior [recessus membranae tympani posterior (NA)], separated by the fold for the chorda tympani lying in front of and behind the handle of the malleus. The superior recess [recessus membranae tympani superior (NA)] lies between the neck of the malleus and the flaccid part of the tympanic membrane (see below). The lining extends into the antrum and air cells. This part is non-ciliated, but elsewhere the mucous membrane is formed of ciliated columnar epithelium, and near the opening of the pharyngotympanic tube it contains mucous glands. **Nictitating membrane.** A third eyelid found in the lower vertebrates. The plica semilunaris conjunctivae is the vestigial remains in man. **Nuclear membrane.** Nuclear envelope. **Obturator membrane [membrana obturatoria (NA)].** An interlacing sheet of white fibres attached to the margin of the obturator foramen, deficient above where it bounds the obturator canal and giving attachment to parts of the obturator muscles. **Obturator membrane of the stapes [membrana stapedis (NA)].** A membrane filling the arch between the limbs and the base of the stapes. **Oral membrane.** Buccopharyngeal membrane (see above). **Oronasal membrane.** The membrane separating the nasal and oral cavities in the early embryo. It later forms part of the palate. **Membrane of otoliths [membrana statoconiorum (NA)].** The layer of gelatinous tissue in the saccule and utricle which contains the statoconia (otoliths) and which is penetrated by the hair-like ends of the receptor cells. **Ovular membrane.** The innermost egg membrane lying immediately adjacent to the surface of the ovum. **Perineal membrane [fascia diaphragmatis urogenitalis inferior (memmbrana perinei) NA].** The more superficial of the two laminae of deep fascia in the urogenital portion of the pelvic outlet. It stretches between the two pubic rami. **Perineal membrane, pelvic layer of the [fascia diaphragmatis urogenitalis superior (NA)].** The deep layer of the membrane. **Periodontal membrane.** A thin, connective-tissue structure attaching the cementum of a tooth to the surrounding tissues. **Persistent pupillary membrane.** Embryonic remnants of the pupillary membrane often seen as thin strands stretching across the pupil. **Pharyngeal membrane.** Buccopharyngeal membrane (see above). **Placental membrane.** The layer of tissue between the maternal and fetal blood streams in the placenta, very thin in the haemochorial placentas of man, rodents, etc., thick in the epitheliochorial placentas of ungulates. The placental membrane regulates the diffusion of materials between the two circulations. **Plasma membrane.** The trilaminar membrane which encloses the cytoplasm of a cell, sometimes known as the *cell membrane.* It is composed of lipids and protein and has a carbohydrate component incorporated into its outer lamina. **Pleuropericardial membrane.** The membrane which separates the pleural and pericardial cavities of the fetus and which contains the phrenic nerve and common cardinal vein. **Proligerous membrane.** The ovarian cumulus of the graafian follicle. **Proper membrane of the semicircular duct [membrana propria ductus semicircularis (NA)].** The middle coat of the semicircular duct. It consists of fibrous tissue and has papilliform projections towards the epithelial surface of the duct. **Pseudoserous membrane.** A smooth, glistening membrane similar in appearance to the lining of a serous cavity, but differing in microscopic structure. **Pupillary membrane [membrana pupillaris (NA)].** A transient membrane closing in the pupil of the embryonic eye. **Purpurogenous membrane.** The pigmented layer of the retina. **Quadrangular membrane [membrana quadrangularis (NA)].** A sometimes poorly defined fibro-elastic membrane extending from the arytenoid cartilages to the epiglottis and lying deep to the mucous membrane of the larynx. **Reticular membrane [membrana reticularis (NA)].** The netlike membrane covering the hair cells or neuro-epithelium of the organ of Corti. The hairs of the neuro-epithelium project through it. **Ruyschian membrane.** The choriocapillary lamina. *See* LAMINA. **Schneiderian membrane.** The mucous membrane lining the nasal cavities. **Secondary membrane.** A membrane present in the pupil area of the eye following cataract extraction, usually composed of capsule or lens matter. **Semipermeable membrane.** A membrane which will allow certain substances to pass through in solution but not others; for example, electrolytes may pass but the larger molecules or colloid particles are held back. A finer membrane will allow only solvent (e.g. H_2O) molecules to pass but hold back all solutes, even simple electrolytes. **Serous membrane.** The lining membrane of the pleural, peritoneal and pericardial cavities. **Spore membrane.** The membrane surrounding a developing spore or group of spores. **Sternal membrane [membrana sterni (NA)].** The membrane on the anterior surface of the sternum formed from the interweaving of the anterior sternocostal ligaments. **Striated membrane.** The zona striata of the ovum. **Subepithelial membrane.** Basement membrane (see above). **Subzonal membrane.** The outer layer of the amnion. **Suprapleural membrane [membrana suprapleuralis (NA)].** The thickened portion of the endothoracic fascia superiorly which attaches to the medial border of the first rib. **Synaptic membrane.** The membrane between the termination of an axon and the cell body or dendrite of the neurone with which it is in synaptic relation. It controls the passage of the nerve impulse from one neurone to another. **Synovial membrane [membrana synovialis (NA)].** A membrane lining the capsular ligament of a joint and usually covering all structures within the joint. It secretes a lubricating fluid, synovia. **Tectorial membrane.** 1. The membrana tectoria. 2. The membrana tectoria of the atlanto-occipital joint. **Thyrohyoid membrane [membrana thyrohyoidea (NA)].** A broad, fibro-elastic membrane running from the upper margins of the laminae of the thyroid cartilage to the upper margin of the posterior surface of the hyoid bone. **Tympanic membrane [membrana tympani (NA)].** An almost circular sheet of tissue separating the external auditory meatus from the tympanic cavity. Obliquely placed, it is set at an angle of 55 degrees to both the anterior wall and the floor of the meatus. The handle of the malleus is attached to its depressed centre. The outer of its three layers, the cuticular [stratum cutaneum (NA)], is derived from the lining of the meatus. The middle, fibrous layer, deficient in the flaccid part, is composed of outer radial [stratum radiatum (NA)] and inner circular [stratum circulare (NA)] fibres. The inner, mucous, layer [stratum mucosum (NA)] is continuous with the lining of the tympanic cavity. The bony groove lodging the periphery, the fibrocartilaginous ring [anulus fibrocartilagineus (NA)], of the membrane is notched superiorly and from the ends of these two folds, the malleolar folds, run to the lateral process of the malleolus. The portion enclosed between them is the flaccid part of the membrane [pars flaccida (NA)]; the remainder is the tense part [pars tensa (NA)]. **Tympanic membrane, secondary [membrana tympani secundaria].** The membrane closing the fenestra cochleae. **Undulant membrane, Undulating membrane.** The wavy membrane of trypanosomes associated with motility. **Urethral membrane, Urogenital membrane.** The front part of the cloacal membrane after separation of the anal canal from the urogenital sinus. It separates the cavity of the latter from the exterior in the early embryo. **Utero-epichorial membrane.** The decidua vera or parietalis. **Vestibular membrane [paries vestibularis ductus cochlearis (membrana vestibulares) NA].** A thin membrane from the osseous spiral lamina to the wall of the cochlea. **Vitelline membrane, Yolk membrane.** The innermost of the egg membranes, lying immediately in contact with the ovum. [L *membrana*.]

See also: ASCHERSON, BAER (K. E.), BECCARI, BICHAT, BOGROS (A.), BOWMAN, BRUCH, BRUNN, CORTI, DÉBOVE, DEMOURS, DESCEMET, DUDDELL, ELFORD, FIELDING, HALLER, HANNOVER, HENLE, HOVIUS, HUNTER (W.), HUXLEY, JACKSON (J. N.), JACOB, KOELLIKER, KRAUSE (W. J. F.), MAUTHNER, NASMYTH, PAYR, PRITCHARD, RANVIER, REICHERT (K. B.), REISSNER, RIVINUS, SCARPA, SCHNEIDER (K. V.), SCHULTZE (M. J. S.), SCHWANN, SHRAPNELL, SLAVIANSKI, TENON, TOLDT, TOURTUAL, TRAUBE (L.), WACHENDORF, ZEISSL, ZINN.

membraniform (mem·**bran**·e·form). Having the appearance or showing the characteristics of a membrane. [membrane, form.]

membranocartilaginous (mem·bran·o·kar·til·**aj**'·in·us). 1. Applied generally to osseous structures and indicating that origin is partly membranous and partly cartilaginous. 2. Consisting of membrane and cartilage.

membranocranium (mem·bran·o·**kra**'·ne·um). The membranous or blastemic skull of the fetus before the appearance of bone and cartilage. [membrane, cranium.]

membranoid (mem·bran·oid). Of the nature of, or similar to a membrane. [membrane, Gk *eidos* form.]

membranous (mem·bran·us). Resembling or consisting of a membrane.

memory (mem·or·e). The recall into present consciousness of past experience, or of knowledge acquired through past experience. The memory system is considered to consist of two components, a *short-term memory* of limited capacity, and a more permanent *long-term memory* into which a selection of items from short-term memory is transferred. **Affect memory.** Recall of emotion associated with a past event. **Anterograde memory.** Memory of the senile type which is able to recall events of the distant past but not those which have happened recently. **Aural memory.** The ability to recall things heard. **Eye memory.** Visual memory (see below). **Immunological memory.** The capacity of antibody-producing cells to respond much faster and in greater degree to subsequent stimuli than they did to the primary stimulus. **Kinaesthetic memory.** Recall of a past event in terms of the muscular action or effort associated with that event. **Visual memory.** The power to recall images seen. [L *memoria*.]

menacme (men·**ak**·me). The phase of a woman's life during which she menstruates. [menses, Gk *akme* highest point.]

menadione (men·ah·**di**·one). Menaphthone.

Menadoxime (men·ah·**dox**·ime). BP Commission approved name for ammonium 2-methylnaphthaquinone-4-oxime *O*-carboxymethyl ether. A vitamin-K analogue, used in haemorrhagic conditions in which the prothrombin level is low.

menagogue (men·ag·og). Emmenagogue. [menses, Gk *agogos* leading.]

menalgia (men·**al**·je·ah). Painful menstruation. [menses, Gk *algos* pain.]

menaphthone (men·**af**·thone). 2-Methyl-1,4-naphthaquinone. A synthetic compound related chemically to natural vitamin K; it is insoluble in water but soluble in fixed oils, and is absorbed from the intestine only in the presence of bile salts. It acts like vitamin K after absorption and helps to maintain the prothrombin content of the blood. It is administered by intramuscular injection (BP 1963) in conditions where the prothrombin content is below normal, as in haemorrhagic disease of the newborn, obstructive jaundice, and in certain malabsorptive syndromes; it may also be used as prophylaxis in the last days of pregnancy, or in the newborn child, to prevent haemorrhagic disease. **Menaphthone Sodium Bisulphite BP 1963.** An addition product of menaphthone with sodium bisulphite; it is soluble in water and is absorbed from the intestine even in the absence of bile salts.

menarche (men·**ar**·ke). The establishment of the menses. The mean age in UK is 12.9 years with a normal range extending from 10 to 16½ years. *Cf.* TELARCHE. [menses, Gk *archaios* from the beginning.]

Mendel, Felix (b. 1862). Essen physician.

Mendel's test. 0.05 ml diluted Old Tuberculin BP 1973 is injected intracutaneously and produces a reddened swelling in persons already infected with tuberculosis.

Mendel, Gregor Johann (b. 1822). Abbot of Brünn.

Mendel's first law. In a cross between individuals, contrasted characters will segregate and not blend.

Mendel's second law. The distribution to the offspring of one pair of contrasting characters is independent of the distribution of any other pair.

Mendelian theory. The theory that the characters of sexually reproducing organisms are handed on to the offspring in fixed ratios and without blending.

Mendel, Kurt (b. 1874). Berlin neurologist.

Mendel's dorsal reflex of the foot, Bechterew-Mendel reflex. In normal subjects percussion of the dorsum of the foot may produce dorsiflexion of the 2nd to 5th toes; in pyramidal-tract disease plantar flexion occurs (Bechterew's reflex, 4th def.). The normal reflex has also been called the *tarsophalangeal reflex, dorsocuboidal reflex, cuboidodigital reflex.*

Mendel-Bechterew sign. 1. The paradoxical pupillary reaction; dilatation on exposure to light in early cases of tabes dorsalis. 2. Mendel's dorsal reflex (see above).

Mendel, Lafayette Benedict (b. 1872). New Haven, Connecticut, biochemist.

Osborne and Mendel salt mixture. Calcium carbonate, magnesium carbonate, sodium carbonate, potassium iodide, potassium carbonate, phosphoric acid, hydrochloric acid, manganese sulphate, citric acid and iron citrate, with sodium fluoride and aluminium potassium sulphate. It is used as a tonic salt mixture to supply mineral salts.

Mendeléeff, Dimitri Ivanovich (b. 1834). Russian chemist.

Mendeléeff's law. Periodic law. *See* LAW.

mendelevium (men·del·ev·e·um, men·del·e·ve·um). The transuranic element of atomic number 101, atomic weight 256 and chemical symbol Md. [Named in honour of the Russian chemist *Mendeléeff,* discoverer of the periodic law.]

mendelian (men·**de**·le·an). Associated with G. J. Mendel.

mendelism (**men**·del·izm). Mendel's laws.

Mendelsohn, Martin (b. 1860). Berlin physician.

Mendelsohn's test. Of cardiac reserve: after exertion the heart rate returns to the pre-exercise rate more rapidly in the normal person than in a subject with cardiac insufficiency.

Mendelson, C. L. American obstetrician.

Mendelson's syndrome. The pulmonary acid aspiration syndrome due to acid gastric contents being aspirated into the air passages, especially in obstetric patients. Described in 1954.

menelipsis (men·el·**ip**·sis). Menolipsis.

Ménétrièr, Pierre (b. 1859). French physician.

Ménétrièr's disease. Pseudohyperplasia of the gastric mucosa, with giant hypertrophy of the rugae, associated with exudative enteropathy.

menhidrosis (men·hid·**ro**·sis). Periodic haemorrhage from the skin coinciding with menstruation and sometimes regarded as vicarious menstruation. [menses, Gk *hidros* sweat.]

Menière, Prosper (b. 1799). Paris physician.

Menière's disease, or syndrome. Paroxysmal labyrinthine vertigo; a condition characterized by severe bouts of vertigo with vomiting, tinnitus and progressive deafness in the affected ear, and caused by over-distension of the membranous labyrinth, possibly through hypersecretion.

meningeal (men·**in**·je·al). Of or relating to the meninges.

meningeal arteries. Accessory meningeal artery [ramus meningeus accessorius]. *See* MAXILLARY ARTERY. **Middle meningeal artery [arteria meningea media (NA)].** The largest of the meningeal arteries, arising from the maxillary artery, and entering the skull through the foramen spinosum. The anterior of its two divisions [ramus frontalis (NA)] crosses the pterion, then runs upward and backward, overlying the precentral gyrus; the posterior division [ramus parietalis (NA)] is directed towards the vertex of the skull. It gives a branch, the superior tympanic artery [arteria tympanica superior (NA)] to the tensor tympani muscle. A superficial branch [ramus petrosus (NA)] communicates with the posterior auricular artery. The orbital branch [ramus anastomoticus cum arteria lacrimali (NA)] passes through the orbital fissure to anastomose with a recurrent meningeal branch of the lacrimal artery.

meningeal veins [venae meningeae (NA)]. Veins draining the meninges into the venous sinuses of the dura mater, the diploic veins, or the emissary veins. **Middle meningeal veins [venae meningeae mediae (NA)].** Veins accompanying the middle meningeal artery, and ending in the pterygoid plexus, sphenoparietal sinus, or cavernous sinus of the dura mater.

meningeocortical (men·**in**·je·o·**kor**'·tik·al). Of or relating to the cortex and meninges of the brain.

meningeorrhaphy (men·**in**·je·**or**'·af·e). Closure of a persisting wound or defect in the dura mater. [Gk *menigx* membrane, *rhaphe* suture.]

meninges (men·**in**·jeez). The membranes (pia mater, arachnoid mater, and dura mater) which form the coverings or sheaths of the spinal cord and brain. *See* MENINX. [Gk *menigx* membrane.]

meningina (men·in·**ji**·nah). The cerebral part of the arachnoid mater and the pia mater regarded as one membrane. [see prec.]

meninginitis (men·**in**·jin·**i**'·tis). Leptomeningitis. [meningina, Gk *-itis* inflammation.]

meningioma (men·**in**·je·**o**'·mah). A benign meningeal tumour, thought to arise from the arachnoidal villi. **Angioblastic meningioma.** A meningioma rich in blood vessels. **Cutaneous meningioma.** A tumour in the skin of cells histologically characteristic of meningioma, usually occurring on the scalp or near the spine. **Endotheliomatous meningioma.** A meningioma rich in primitve blood vessels. **Fibroplastic meningioma.** A meningioma that forms much fibrous tissue. **Myxomatous meningioma.** A meningioma undergoing mucoid degeneration. **Olfactory groove meningioma, Parasagittal meningioma, Sphenoidal wing** or **ridge meningioma.** Meningiomata arising from the dura mater in these sites. (Formerly known as *endotheliomata.* If gritty particles are included, the word *psammomata* was often used.) **Suprasellar meningioma.** A meningioma located near to or within the suprasellar space. **Xanthomatous meningioma.** A meningioma rich in cholesterol and other lipids. [Gk *menigx* membrane, *-oma* tumour.]

meningiomatosis (men·**in**·je·o·mat·o'·sis). Diffuse meningioma. [meningioma, Gk *-osis* condition.]

meningion (men·**in**·je·on). 1. The arachnoid mater or membrane, which lies under the dura mater and over the pia mater of the cerebrospinal system. 2. Referring to any membranous structure. [Gk *menigx* membrane.]

meningism, meningismus (men·in·jizm, men·in·**jiz**·mus). A condition in which there are signs of meningeal irritation suggesting the presence of meningitis, but the cerebrospinal fluid, though under increased pressure, shows no pathological change. It is found in cases of acute fever in children, especially in pneumonia. [see prec.]

meningitic (men·in·**jit**·ik). Relating to, affected with, or marked by meningitis.

meningitides (men·in·**jit**·id·eez). *See* MENINGITIS.

meningitiform (men·in·**jit**·e·form). Having resemblance to meningitis. [meningitis, form.]

meningitis (men·in·**ji**·tis) (pl. *meningitides*). Inflammation of the membranes of the brain or spinal cord, i.e. of the dura mater (pachymeningitis) or of the arachnoid and pia mater (leptomeningitis). **Acute aseptic meningitis.** Benign lymphocytic meningitis (see below). **Acute pyogenic meningitis.** That caused by numerous organisms; it is seen in septicaemia, and also occurs by direct extension from inflammatory areas (e.g. mastoid disease, sinusitis). **African meningitis.** Infection by one of the trypanosomes (trypanosomiasis). **Aseptic meningitis.** Term usually referring to meningitis due to infection with a virus, most commonly an enterovirus. **Bacteroides meningitis.** Infection by anaerobic micro-organisms of the genus *Bacteroides*; pathogenic micro-organisms of the genera are mostly placed in the genus *Fusiformis* by British bacteriologists. **Meningitis of the base, Basilar meningitis.** Meningitis affecting chiefly the base of the brain. **Benign lymphocytic meningitis.** Meningitis with a mainly lymphocytic response in the cerebrospinal fluid, usually the result of viral infection. **Carcinomatous meningitis.** Invasion of the leptomeninges by carcinoma. **Cerebral meningitis.** Inflammation of the meninges of the brain showing fever, slow pulse, headache, vomiting and also ptosis, squint, facial paralysis and optic neuritis due to implication of the cranial nerves at the base of the brain. **Cerebrospinal meningitis.** That due to infection of the membranes of the brain and spinal cord by various micro-organisms. The term is more frequently used to mean epidemic cerebrospinal meningitis (see below). **Cryptococcal meningitis.** Meningitis due to *Cryptococcus neoformans* (*Torula hystolytica*), a chronic infection usually occurring in patients with reticuloses. **Eosinophilic meningitis.** A low-grade meningitis, accompanied by high eosinophilic exudate in the cerebrospinal fluid, caused by invasion of the brain by the rat lung worm of which the garden slug is the intermediary host. Infection is acquired by eating raw lettuce which harbours these slugs in certain Pacific islands, especially Hawaii, Tahiti and New Caledonia. **Epidemic cerebrospinal meningitis.** Infection by *Neisseria meningitidis*, showing the usual symptoms of meningitis with skin rashes; spotted fever. **External meningitis.** Affection of the dura mater of the brain or cord; pachymeningitis. **Gummatous meningitis.** Affection of the meninges by *Treponema pallidum*; syphilitic meningitis. **Influenzal meningitis.** Meningitis due to *Haemophilus influenzae.* **Internal meningitis.** Internal pachymeningitis. **Leptospiral meningitis.** Meningitis due to *Leptospira icterohaemorrhagiae* or *L. canicola.* **Listerial meningitis.** Meningitis due to *Listerella monocytogenes*, occurring in infancy. **Lymphocytic meningitis.** Benign lymphocytic meningitis (see above). **Meningococcal meningitis, Meningococcic meningitis.** Infection by *Neisseria meningitidis.* **Metastatic meningitis.** Infection of the meninges secondary to a remote septic focus. **Occlusive meningitis.** Meningitis in which Magendie's foramen is sealed by serous exudate (possibly leading to hydrocephalus). **Otitic meningitis.** Meningitis secondary to otitis media. **Parameningococcus meningitis.** Infection by an organism resembling *Neisseria meningitidis* but differing from it biologically and resistant to antimeningitis serum [obsolete term]. **Plague meningitis.** Meningitis due to *Pasteurella pestis.* **Plasmodial meningitis.** Meningitis associated with a malarial infection. **Pneumococcal meningitis.** Meningitis due to the pneumococcus (*Streptococcus pneumoniae*). **Post-basic meningitis of infants.** A form of meningococcal meningitis occurring in infants. **Posterior meningitis.** Meningitis whose chief incidence is in the cerebellar region. **Post-traumatic meningitis.** Meningitis resulting from injury. **Pseudotyphoid meningitis.** Bouchet's disease. **Purulent meningitis, Pyogenic meningitis.** That due to one of the pyogenic organisms. **Rheumatic meningitis.** Meningitis due to haemolytic streptococci during an attack of acute rheumatism. **Ricksettsial meningitis.** Meningitis attributed to organisms of the genus *Rickettsia.* It is doubtful if they produce a primary meningitis: as their insect hosts are always associated with insanitary conditions, other organisms may be the cause of any associated meningitis. **Septicaemic meningitis.** Acute pyogenic meningitis (see above). **Meningitis serosa.** Meningitis with an exudate over the areas involved. **Meningitis serosa circumscripta, Meningitis serosa circumscripta cystica.** Meningitis with localized serous exudation shut off by adhesions, causing a cystic accumulation. **Serous meningitis.** Meningitis with inflammation of the cranial air sinuses, especially the mastoid; a condition with features of meningitis may develop, but with normal cerebrospinal fluid (except for increased pressure), and with a favourable prognosis. **Simple meningitis.** Benign lymphocytic meningitis (see above). **Spinal meningitis.** That in which the membranes of the cord are affected primarily. **Sterile meningitis.** Benign lymphocytic meningitis (see above). **Streptococcus meningitis.** Meningitis due to streptococci, usually secondary to bone infection. **Suppurative meningitis.** Meningitis due to a pyogenic micro-organismal infection secondary to bone disease. **Meningitis sympathica.** Meningitis with changes in the cerebrospinal fluid due to affections of neighbouring structures. **Syphilitic meningitis.** Gummatous meningitis (see above). **Traumatic meningitis.** Meningitis which is the result of trauma to the skull or spine. **Tuberculous meningitis.** Meningitis resulting from infection of the meninges by the tubercle bacillus, with a classical clinical picture, headache, vomiting, slow pulse and cranial-nerve palsies. Formerly invariably fatal, it can now often be treated successfully. **Typhoid meningitis.** Meningitis occurring as a complication of typhoid fever. **Viral meningitis.** Meningitis due to viral infection. [Gk *menigx* membrane, *-itis* inflammation.]

See also: WALLGREN.

meningitophobia (men·in·jit·o·**fo**′·be·ah). A neurotic state in which dread of being affected with meningitis causes a condition simulating meningitis to develop. [meningitis, phobia.]

meningium (men·**in**·je·um). Meningion.

meningo-arteritis (men·ing·go·ar·ter·**i**′·tis). Inflammation of the meningeal arteries. [meningeal artery, Gk *-itis* inflammation.]

meningoblastoma (men·**ing**·go·blas·**to**′·mah). A highly cellular, rather rapidly growing variety of meningioma, sometimes producing melanin. [meningioma, blastoma.]

meningocele (men·**ing**·go·seel). A hernial protrusion of the meninges of the spinal cord or brain caused by a defect in the vertebral column or skull. [Gk *menigx* membrane, *kele* hernia.]

meningocephalitis (men·**ing**·go·kef·al·**i**′·tis). Meningo-encephalitis.

meningocerebritis (men·**ing**·go·ser·e·**bri**′·tis). Meningo-encephalitis. [meningitis, cerebritis.]

meningococcaemia (men·**ing**·go·kok·**se**′·me·ah). A condition in which meningococci (*Neisseria meningitidis*) are present in the blood. **Acute fulminating meningococcaemia.** Acute adrenal failure due to severe infection, most commonly meningococcal. [meningococcus, Gk *haima* blood.]

meningococcosis (men·**ing**·go·kok·**o**′·sis). A comprehensive word for meningococcal diseases. [meningococcus, Gk *-osis* condition.]

meningococcus (men·**ing**·go·**kok**′·us). *Neisseria meningitidis.* [Gk *menigx* membrane, *kokkos* berry.]

See also: JAEGER (H.).

meningocortical (men·ing·go·**kor**′·tik·al). Pertaining to the meninges and the cerebral cortex.

meningocyte (men·**ing**·go·site). A potentially phagocytic cell found in the pia-arachnoid lining the subarachnoid spaces. [Gk *menigx* membrane, *kytos* cell.]

meningo-encephalitis (men·**ing**·go·en·kef·al·**i**′·tis). An inflammatory condition of the brain and its meninges. **Chronic meningo-encephalitis, Syphilitic meningo-encephalitis.** Dementia paralytica. [Gk *menigx* membrane, encephalitis.]

meningo-encephalocele (men·**ing**·go·en·**kef**′·al·o·seel). The condition in which part of the meninges and brain protrude as a hernia. [Gk *menigx* membrane, encephalocele.]

meningo-encephalomyelitis (men·**ing**·go·en·**kef**·al·o·mi·el·**i**′·tis). A combined inflammatory condition of the meninges, brain and spinal cord. [Gk *menigx* membrane, encephalomyelitis.]

meningo-encephalopathy (men·ing·go·en·kef·al·**op**′·ath·e). A non-inflammatory disease of the membranes and of the brain. [Gk *menigx* membrane, encephalopathy.]

meningofibroblastoma (men·**ing**·go·fi·bro·blas·**to**′·mah). Meningioma. [Gk *menigx* membrane, fibroblastoma.]

meningoma (men·in·**go**·mah). Meningioma.

meningomyelitis (men·**ing**·go·mi·el·**i**′·tis). Inflammation of the spinal cord and its surrounding membranes, the pia mater and dura mater sometimes being affected. **Actinomycotic meningomyelitis.** Meningomyelitis due to invasion by mould-like organisms belonging to the genus *Actinomyces.* **Chronic meningomyelitis.** Any chronic form of meningomyelitis; also, one of the commonest varieties of spinal syphilis. **Mycotic meningomyelitis.** Meningomyelitis caused by *Blastomyces dermatitidis, Coccidioides immitis, Cryptococcus neoformans, Histoplasma capsulatum, Paracoccidioides brasiliensis, Sporothrix schenckii.* [Gk *menigx* membrane, myelitis.]

meningomyelocele (men·**ing**·go·**mi**′·el·o·seel). A hernia of some portion of the spinal cord and its meninges caused by a defective condition in the vertebral column. [Gk *menigx* membrane, myelocele.]

meningomyeloradiculitis (men·ing·go·mi·el·o·rad·ik·ew·li′·tis). Inflammation of the membranes, spinal cord and nerve roots. [Gk *menigx* membrane, myeloradiculitis.]

meningomyelorrhaphy (men·ing·go·mi·el·or′·af·e). Surgical repair of a meningomyelocele. [Gk *menigx* membrane, myelorrhaphy.]

meningopathy (men·in·gop·ath·e). Any diseased condition of the meninges. [meninges, Gk *pathos* disease.]

meningopneumonitis (men·ing·go·new·mon·i′·tis). A disease of animals caused by a virus of the psittacosis-lymphopathia-venereum group and characterized by inflammation of the meninges and the lungs. [Gk *menigx* membrane, pneumonitis.]

meningorachidian (men·ing·go·rak·id′·e·an). Of or relating to the spinal cord and meninges. [Gk *menigx* membrane, *rhachis* spine.]

meningoradicular (men·ing·go·rad·ik′·ew·lar). Relating to the membranes and roots of the spinal and cranial nerves. [Gk *menigx* membrane, L *radix* root.]

meningoradiculitis (men·ing·go·rad·ik·ew·li′·tis). Inflammation of the membranes of the nerve roots. [Gk *menigx* membrane, L *radix* root, Gk *-itis* inflammation.]

meningorécidive aigu (men·ing·go·res′·id·iv a·gew). An acute gummatous meningitis during the secondary stage, that occurs shortly after inadequate treatment, especially with arsenicals. [Gk *menigx* membrane, L *recidivus* recurring.]

meningorrhagia (men·ing·go·ra′·je·ah). Meningeal haemorrhage. [Gk *menigx* membrane, *rhoia* flow.]

meningosis (men·in·go·sis). The joining together of bones by a membranous attachment. [Gk *menigx* membrane, *-osis* condition.]

meningotyphoid (men·ing·go·ti′·foid). Typhoid fever in which symptoms of meningeal irritation are prominent. These may be due to meningism, or, rarely, to a true meningitis with pathological changes in the cerebrospinal fluid in which the typhoid bacillus can be found.

meningovascular (men·ing·go·vas′·kew·lar). Of or relating to the meningeal blood vessels. [Gk *menigx* membrane, L *vasculum* little vessel.]

meninguria (men·in·gewr·e·ah). The presence of shreds of membrane in the urine, derived as a rule from the bladder. [Gk *menigx* membrane, urine.]

meninx (men·ingx) (pl. *meninges*). A membrane; more commonly used in the plural (meninges) for the membranes surrounding the brain and spinal cord. **Meninx fibrosa.** A fibrous membrane; the term is applied to the dura mater. **Meninx primitiva.** The connective tissue surrounding the brain in primitive vertebrates, which is not differentiated into pia mater and arachnoid membranes. **Meninx serosa.** A serous membrane. **Meninx tenuis.** A thin, delicate membrane; the arachnoid membrane. **Meninx vasculosa.** A vascular membrane; the pia mater. [Gk *menigx* membrane.]

meniscectomy (men·is·ek·to·me). Excision of the semilunar cartilages of the knee joint (menisci). [Gk *meniskos* crescent, *ektome* a cutting out.]

meniscitis (men·is·i·tis). Inflammation of the semilunar cartilage of the knee joint (menisci). [Gk *meniskos* crescent, *-itis* inflammation.]

meniscocyte (men·is·ko·site). A sickle cell or drepanocyte, being the peculiar sickle- or crescent-shaped red cell characteristic of sickle-cell (African) anaemia. [Gk *meniskos* crescent, *kytos* cell.]

meniscocytosis (men·is·ko·si·to′·sis). A haemolytic anaemia in which there are meniscocytes or sickle cells in the blood; sickle-cell anaemia. [meniscocyte, Gk *-osis* condition.]

meniscoid (men·is·koid). Shaped like a crescent; resembling a meniscus. [Gk *meniskos* crescent, *eidos* form.]

meniscus (men·is·kus). 1. The curved surface of separation between liquid and gas in a capillary tube. 2. A lens having one concave and one convex surface. 3. A semilunar cartilage of the knee. **Articular meniscus.** Interarticular fibrocartilage. *See* FIBROCARTILAGE. **Converging meniscus.** A meniscus lens producing convergence of light. **Diverging meniscus.** A meniscus lens producing divergence of light. **Negative meniscus.** Diverging meniscus (see above). **Positive meniscus.** Converging meniscus (see above). **Slipped meniscus.** Displacement of the whole or part of the medial semilunar cartilage of the knee. **Tactile meniscus [meniscus tactus (NA)].** A touch receptor of the skin in the form of a curved plate. [Gk *meniskos* crescent.]

Menkin, Valy (b. 1901). American physician.

Menkin's leucocytosis-promoting factor. A pseudoglobulin isolated from inflammatory exudates which causes a leucocytosis when injected experimentally.

Mennell, James Beaver (b. 1880). London physician.

Mennell's sign. In fibrositis, tenderness on pressure over and to the sides of the posterior superior iliac spine.

Mennell, Z. (b. 1876). London anaesthetist.

Mennell's bottle. A modification of Junker's chloroform bottle (1868) in which air can be blown through chloroform and so arranged that no liquid anaesthetic can be delivered to the patient.

menolipsis (men·o·lip·sis). Amenorrhoea, generally of temporary character. [menses, Gk *leipien* to fail.]

menopausal (men·o·pawz·al). Of or relating to the menopause.

menopause (men·o·pawz). Literally, the cessation of spontaneous menstrual periods. The period at which normal menstrual life ceases; the climacteric or change of life. **Artificial menopause.** Termination of menstruation by artificial method such as irradiation or a surgical procedure. [menses, Gk *pauein* to cease.]

menophania (men·o·fa·ne·ah). The first showing of the menses at puberty. [menses, Gk *phainein* to appear.]

menophyma (men·o·fi·mah). Hyperplasia of the connective tissue and sebaceous glands of the chin, comparable to *rhinophyma*. [L *mentum* chin, Gk *phyma* tumour.]

menoplania (men·o·pla·ne·ah). A haemorrhagic discharge at the time of menstruation but originating in some region of the body other than the uterus. [menses, Gk *plane* a wandering.]

menorrhagia (men·or·a·je·ah). Excessively profuse discharge of the menses, or their excessive prolongation. [menses, Gk *rhegynein* to burst forth.]

menorrhalgia (men·or·al·je·ah). Dysmenorrhoea. [menorrhoea, Gk *algos* pain.]

menorrhoea (men·o·re·ah). The normal flow of the menses. [menses, Gk *rhoia* flow.]

menorrhoeal (men·o·re·al). Relating to menorrhoea.

menoschesis (men·os·kis·is). Retention or suppression of the menstrual flow. [menses, Gk *schesis* a holding fast.]

menostasia, menostasis (men·o·sta·se·ah, men·os·tas·is). 1. Suppression of the menstrual discharge; amenorrhoea. 2. The termination of menstruation; the menopause. [menses, Gk *stasis* a standing still.]

menoxenia (men·o·ze·ne·ah). Any menstrual irregularity. [menses, Gk *xenos* strange.]

mens rea (menz re·ah). A guilty mind; in Law, a person cannot be committed in a criminal proceeding unless it can be shown that he had a guilty mind. [L]

menses (men·sez). The monthly discharge of blood (catamenia) from the uterus. [L *mensis* month.]

menstrual (men·stroo·al). Relating to menstruation. [L *menstrualis* monthly.]

menstruate (men·stroo·ate). To have the periodical menstrual flow or to discharge the menses. [L *menstruare.*]

menstruation (men·stroo·a·shun). The periodic discharge of blood from the uterus occurring at more or less regular monthly intervals throughout the active reproductive life of women. **Anovular menstruation.** Menstruation which has not been preceded by ovulation, the formation of a corpus luteum and a progestational or secretory endometrium. **Regurgitate menstruation.** Retrograde menstruation (see foll.). **Retrograde menstruation.** That in which blood flows along the tubes and is deposited in the peritoneal cavity. **Vicarious menstruation.** Menstruation from other sites than the uterus. [see prec.]

menstruum (men·stroo·um). A term used in connection with the preparation of official tinctures, to describe the liquid which is employed in the extraction of active principles from the crude drug; a solvent. [L menstrual fluid, at one time thought to have a solvent action.]

See also: PITKIN.

mensuration (men·sewr·a·shun). Measurement; the process or the act of measuring. [L *mensurare* to measure.]

mentagra (ment·ag·rah). Sycosis. [mentum, Gk *agra* a catching.]

mental (**men**·tal). 1. Of or relating to the mind. [L *mens* mind.] 2. Of or relating to the chin. [L *mentum* chin.]

Mental Health Act 1959. This Act makes provision with respect to the treatment and care of mentally disordered persons and with respect to their properties and affairs. The Act defines mental disorder into four specific forms: mental illness; arrested or incomplete development; psychopathic disorder; and other disorder or disability of mind. A state of arrested or incomplete development of mind which includes subnormality of intelligence and is such that the patient is, and will continue to be, incapable of living an independent life or of guarding himself against serious exploitation is classed as 'severe subnormality', while such a state which includes subnormality of intelligence and is such as to require or be susceptible to medical treatment or other special training is classed as "subnormality".

mental artery [arteria mentalis (NA)]. *See* MAXILLARY ARTERY.

mental nerve [nervus mentalis (NA)]. The terminal branch of the inferior dental nerve to the skin of the chin and lower lip.

mentalia (men·ta·le·ah). Psychalia. [L *mens* mind.]

mentalis (men·ta·lis). The mentalis muscle. [L *mentum* chin.]

mentalis muscle [musculus mentalis (NA)]. A muscle attached to the incisive fossa of the mandible and below to the skin of the chin.

mentality (men·**tal**·it·e). The nature of the activity of the mind or intellect. The term is extended to mean the disposition or character of a person, and sometimes, rather loosely, his intelligence. [L *mens* mind.]

Mentha (**men**·thah). A genus of plants of the family Labiatae; the mints. **Mentha arvensis.** Japanese peppermint, a species yielding an oil which contains up to 80 per cent of menthol but not so esteemed as the American or English oil. **Mentha piperita.** American or English peppermint; the aerial parts of the plant yield a volatile oil (Peppermint Oil BP 1973) containing menthol. There are two varieties, *vulgaris* (black mint) and *officianalis* (white mint). **Mentha pulegium.** Pennyroyal. **Mentha viridis.** Spearmint; the flowering tops yield the volatile oil (spearmint oil) containing 50 per cent of carvone. [L mint.]

menthene (**men**·theen). $C_{10}H_{18}$, an unsaturated liquid hydrocarbon with a fragrant odour, obtained by the dehydration of menthol. **Menthene carbonate.** $(C_{10}H_{18})CO_3$, a white compound used in medicine similarly to menthol.

menthenone (**men**·then·one). Any of the isomeric ketones of formula $C_{10}H_{16}O$, derived from menthene and occurring in various essential oils.

Menthol BP 1973 (**men**·thol). *p*-Menthan-3-ol, $C_{10}H_{20}O$, a colourless crystalline substance with a strong odour resembling peppermint, and an aromatic taste associated with first a warm, followed by a cold, sensation. It may be obtained from the volatile oils of various species of *Mentha*, when it is laevorotatory, or prepared synthetically from thymol, when it may be laevorotatory or racemic. It is insoluble in water, but soluble in alcohol, olive oil and volatile oils. Applied locally to the skin or mucous surfaces, menthol produces a cold sensation and a degree of analgesia, accompanied by local vasodilatation. It is employed as a topical application, in the form of a liniment or ointment, in muscular rheumatism, or as a vapour-rub to the chest in tracheobronchitis. It is used as an inhalation (in hot water), or incorporated in tablets or pastilles, in upper respiratory infections.

menthone (**men**·thone). $C_{10}H_{18}O$, the ketone corresponding to menthol from which it is obtained by oxidation; it occurs in peppermint oil.

menthyl (**men**·thil). The monovalent radical $C_{10}H_{19}$–, derived from menthol.

mento-anterior (**men**·to·an·**teer**'·e·or). Describing the anterior position of the chin in the pelvis in a face presentation. [L *mentum* chin, *anterior* before.]

mentobregmatic (**men**·to·breg·**mat**'·ik). Extending from the chin to the bregma. [mentum, bregma.]

mentohyoid (men·to·**hi**·oid). Pertaining to the chin and to the hyoid bone. [mentum, hyoid.]

mentolabial (men·to·**la**·be·al). Relating to the chin and to the lip. [mentum, L *labium* lip.]

mentolabialis (**men**·to·la·be·**a**'·lis). The mentalis muscle and the depressor labii inferioris muscle considered as one muscle. [see prec.]

menton (**men**·ton). The pogonion. [L *mentum* chin.]

mentoposterior (**men**·to·pos·**teer**'·e·or). Describing the posterior position of the chin in the pelvis in a face presentation. [L *mentum* chin, *posterior* behind.]

mentum (**men**·tum). The chin. [L]

Menyanthes (men·e·**an**·theez). 1. A genus of plants of the family Gentianaceae. 2. Buckbean, marsh trefoil; the dried leaves of *Menyanthes trifoliata*, containing the glycosides menyanthin and meliatin. [Gk *men* mouth, *anthos* flower.]

menyanthin (men·e·**an**·thin). $C_{33}H_{50}O_{14}$, a glycoside found in buckbean or marsh trefoil, *Menyanthes trifoliata*. It is cathartic.

Menzer, Arthur August Ludwig (b. 1872). German bacteriologist.

Menzer's serum. A serum used for rheumatic fever.

mepacrine (**mep**·ah·kreen). 2 - Chloro - 5 - (4 - diethylamino - 1 - methylbutylamino) - 7 - methoxyacridine, $C_{23}H_{30}ON_3Cl$, an odourless, bitter-tasting, crystalline powder of a bright yellow colour, first used in the treatment of malaria in 1931. **Mepacrine Hydrochloride BP 1973.** A compound 0.5 g of which corresponds approximately to 0.4 g of mepacrine base. Its main action is on the parasites of the asexual cycle of the erythrocytic phases in all three species of plasmodium. In *Plasmodium vivax* and *Plasmodium malariae* infection it also has some action on the gametocytes of this phase. In *Plasmodium falciparum* infection it has some action in the exo-erythrocytic stage, and will effect complete eradication of the infection. Its action is slower than that of quinine, but the difference can be overcome by an increase of the initial doses of mepacrine and thereby an effective blood level is rapidly built up. It causes a yellow pigmentation of the skin if taken regularly, and in therapeutic doses may cause gastro-intestinal disturbance, a dermatitis, and a mild psychosis in susceptible subjects. It was used extensively in World War II as a malaria suppressive and prophylactic. **Mepacrine Methanesulphonate BP 1963, Mepacrine musonate.** A compound soluble in 3 parts of water, useful for parenteral injection; 0.3 g corresponds to 0.18 g of mepacrine base.

Mepenzolate Bromide (mep·en·zo·late **bro**·mide). BP Commission approved name for 3-benziloyloxy-1,1-dimethylpiperidinium bromide; a parasympatholytic agent.

Mephenesin BPC 1973 (mef·**en**·ez·in). 3-(2-Methylphenoxy) propane-1,2-diol, $CH_3C_6H_4OCH_2CHOHCH_2OH$, a compound which causes temporary paralysis of striped muscle, superficially resembling that caused by curare but arising in a fundamentally different way. Its site of action lies in the basal ganglia, the brain stem and the thalamus; it relieves certain types of muscular tremor, especially in parkinsonism and acute alcoholism, but the relief is only temporary. Its selective action on the spinal cord antagonizes the convulsions produced by strychnine but not those of leptazol. It has been used as a muscular relaxant in surgery, but does not give as good a result as curare, and its action is variable. Therapeutically it is given by mouth for the treatment of spastic, hypertonic and hyperkinetic conditions, e.g. parkinsonism, cerebral palsy, chorea and athetosis; for surgery, intravenously by slow injection or as an intravenous drip. Overdosage is treated by artificial respiration, and the injection of methylamphetamine hydrochloride.

mephentermine (mef·**en**·ter·meen). $N\alpha\alpha$-trimethylphenethylamine. **Mephentermine Sulphate BP 1973.** The dihydrate of the sulphate of the base; a white, odourless, crystalline powder or colourless crystals, soluble in water and slightly soluble in alcohol. A sympathetic amine with predominantly beta-stimulating effects on adrenergic receptors, used in the treatment of hypertension and as a nasal decongestant.

mephitic (mef·it·ik). Exhaling an effluvium. [L *mephiticus* pestilential.]

mephitis (mef·i·tis). A foul odour. [L a foul ground emanation.]

mephobarbital (mef·o·bar·bit·al). A barbiturate drug used in conjunction with diphenyl hydantoin to control epilepsy.

Mepiprazole (mep·ip·raz·ole). BP Commission approved name for 1-(3-chlorophenyl)-4-[2-(5-methylpyrazol-3-yl)ethyl]piperazine; a psychotropic agent.

Mepivacaine (mep·iv·ak·ane). BP Commission approved name for 1-methyl-2-(2,6-xylylcarbamoyl)piperidine; a local analgesic.

Meprobamate BP 1973 (mep·ro·bam·ate). 2,2-di(Carbomoylmethyl)pentane; a tranquillizing substance used in the treatment of anxiety states.

Meprochol (mep·ro·kol). BP Commission approved name for *N*-(2-methoxyprop-2-enyl)trimethylammonium bromide; a muscarine-like cholinergic stimulant used in atony of the gut, and in cases of retention of urine.

Meprothixol (mep·ro·thix·ol). BP Commission approved name for 9 - (3 - dimethylaminopropyl) - 9 - hydroxy - 2 - methoxythiaxanthen; an analgesic and anti-inflammatory agent.

Meptazinol (mep·taz·in·ol). BP Commission approved name for 3 - ethyl - 3 - (3 - hydroxy) - 5 - (4 - chlorophenyl) - 2,5 - dihydro - 3*H* - imidazo[2,1 - a]isoindol - 5 - ol; an appetite suppressant.

Mepyramine (mep·ir·am·een). BP Commission approved name for 2-[(2-dimethylaminoethyl) (*p*-methoxybenzyl) amino] pyridine. **Mepyramine Maleate BP 1973.** $C_{17}H_{23}ON_3C_4H_4O_4$, an antihistaminic used in anaphylactic and allergic conditions, especially hay fever and urticaria.

meralgia (mer·al·je·ah). Pain in the thigh. **Meralgia paraesthetica.** Sensation of pain of a burning or tingling character in the outer surface of the thigh in the area supplied by the lateral cutaneous nerve of the thigh; *Bernhardt's syndrome.* [Gk *meros* thigh, *algos* pain.]

Meralluride (mer·al·ewr·ide). BP Commission approved name for methoxyoxymercuripropylsuccinyl urea and theophylline; a mercurial diuretic that may be given intramuscularly, intravenously, or by mouth.

meramaurosis (mer·am·aw·ro'·sis). Partial amaurosis. [Gk *meros* part, *amauros* dark.]

meranaesthesia (mer·an·es·the'·ze·ah). 1. Local anaesthesia. 2. Partial anaesthesia. [Gk *meros* part, anaesthesia.]

mercaptal (mer·kap·tal). Any of the group of compounds analogous with acetals, formed by the condensation of aldehydes and mercaptan.

mercaptan (mer·kap·tan). 1. A family of organic compounds analogous to the alcohols in which the oxygen of the OH group is replaced by sulphur. Weak acids, forming salts known as *mercaptides.* 2. Ethyl hydrosulphide, C_2H_5SH, a light liquid insoluble in water and with a smell of garlic. It forms a crystalline compound with metallic mercury. [L *mercurium captans* seizing mercury.]

mercaptide (mer·kap·tide). A thio-alcohol derivative in which the hydrogen of the -SH group has been replaced by a metal or basic group. The use of BAL in cases of arsenical poisoning is based on the formation of an arsenical mercaptide, which removes the toxic metal from the readily poisoned enzyme surfaces.

2-mercapto-imidazole (mer·kap·to·im·id·a'·zole). An antithyroid drug of the thiouracil type, regarded as about five times as potent as methylthiouracil.

mercaptol (mer·kap·tol). Any of the group of compounds formed by the condensation of ketones and mercaptans.

mercaptomerin (mer·kap·to·mer'·in). A synthetic mercurial diuretic which is virtually non-toxic and painless when given subcutaneously. **Mercaptomerin Sodium.** BP Commission approved name for the disodium salt of *N*-(3-carboxymethylthiomercuri-2-methoxypropyl)camphoramic acid; a diuretic.

Mercaptopurine BP 1973 (mer·kap·to·pewr'·een). 6-Mercaptopurine, an immunosuppressant which has also been used in the treatment of leukaemia.

Mercier, Louis Auguste (b. 1811). Paris urologist.

Mercier's bar. A ridge on the inner surface of the bladder, between the ureteral openings, forming the superior boundary of the trigone.

Mercier's operation. Endoscopic division of a fibrous median bar or hypertrophied interureteric ridge.

Mercier's valve. An occasional fold of mucous membrane partially occluding the orifice of the ureter.

Merck, L. Italian physician.

hyperkeratotic border of Merck. The sharply defined pigmented border of a typical pellagrous lesion.

mercurammonium (mer·kewr·am·o'·ne·um). Term applied to a series of salts obtained by the action of ammonia on mercuric compounds. **Mercurammonium chloride.** NH_2HgCl, a white compound precipitated from mercuric chloride solution by ammonia.

mercurgan (mer·ker·gan). Mersalyl.

mercurial (mer·kewr·e·al). 1. Relating to mercury. 2. Any drug or compound containing mercury.

mercurialism (mer·kewr·e·al·izm). Chronic poisoning caused by the excessive use of mercury, by breathing its fumes, or in mining or smelting processes.

mercurialization (mer·kewr·e·al·i·za'·shun). The state of being mercurialized or the process of subjecting a patient to the therapeutic influence of mercury.

mercurialize (mer·kewr·e·al·ize). To impregnate with mercury or to contain it.

mercuriate (mer·kewr·e·ate). A loose designation applied to compounds of mercury.

mercuric (mer·kewr·ik). The term applied to ions or salts of mercury to denote that the mercury is in the bivalent form. **Mercuric benzoate.** $(C_6H_5COO)_2Hg{\cdot}H_2O$, a white crystalline compound, sparingly soluble in water but soluble in a solution of ammonium benzoate, formerly given by mouth, intramuscularly, and by urethral injection, in the treatment of gonorrhoea and syphilis. **Mercuric Chloride BPC 1973.** Corrosive sublimate, perchloride of mercury, $HgCl_2$; a white crystalline powder, soluble in water. Strong solutions are caustic to tissues, but are used as disinfectants; weak solutions are used sometimes as antiseptic and astringent lotions. There is a danger of mercury poisoning in its employment. **Mercuric cyanide,** $Hg(CN)_2$, a colourless or white crystalline substance, soluble in water. It has potent antiseptic properties. **Mercuric Iodide, Red, BPC 1954.** Mercury biniodide, HgI_2, a scarlet, odourless, tasteless powder, insoluble in water but soluble in alcohol, solutions of iodides, a solution of mercuric chloride and in oils. It is extremely poisonous, and is used as an antiseptic in a solution of potassium iodide for application to wounds, and for the skin and hands. It is also employed as a vaginal douche, as an ointment for ringworm, lupus, and syphilitic lesions, and in germicidal soap. **Mercuric nitrate.** $Hg(NO_3)_2$, a white compound, soluble in water, used as an antiseptic. **Mercuric oxide, red.** HgO, an orange-red powder or scales, insoluble in water; used in ointment form for some skin diseases. **Mercuric Oxide, Yellow, BPC 1973.** HgO, a yellow amorphous powder, insoluble in water. It has antiseptic properties, and is used in ointment form in skin and eye infections. **Mercuric Oxycyanide BPC 1968.** $HgO{\cdot}3Hg(CN_2)$, a compound formed by the interaction of mercuric oxide and an excess of mercuric cyanide. It has strong antiseptic properties and is less irritant than mercuric chloride. It is used for irrigation of the conjunctiva in ophthalmia neonatorum, and in conjunctivitis, also for irrigation of the urinary bladder. Its solution may be employed for sterilizing surgical instruments. **Mercuric salicylate.** A compound formed by boiling a solution of salicylic acid with yellow mercuric oxide. It is employed, in the form of a dusting powder and ointment, as an antiseptic and antisyphilitic. It is also injected intramuscularly as an oily suspension in syphilis. **Mercuric succinimide.** $[C_2H_4(CO)_2N]_2Hg$, a white powder, soluble in water, injected subcutaneously in the treatment of syphilis. Its solutions are relatively non-irritant. **Mercuric sulphate, yellow.** $HgSO_4{\cdot}2HgO$, a compound formed when water is mixed with mercuric sulphate; it has been used as a rapid emetic, and in ointment form for ringworm and seborrhoea capitis. **Mercuric sulphide.** HgS, a compound occurring as a brilliant red powder. It has been used in the form of an ointment in chronic skin diseases. Also known as *Chinese red, vermilion, cinnabar.*

mercuricum (mer·**kewr**·ik·um). Bivalent mercury in its compounds. [L]

Mercurochrome BPC 1954 (mer·**kewr**·o·krome). Disodium dibromohydroxymercurifluorescein, $C_{20}H_7O_5Br_2HgOHNa_2$. A water-soluble phthalein dye used as an antiseptic. Now obsolescent.

Mercurophylline Sodium (**mer**·kewr·o·**fil**′·een **so**·de·um). BP Commission approved name for a combination of the organic mercurial β-methoxy-γ-hydroxymercuripropylamide of trimethylcyclopentane dicarboxylic acid with theophylline in approximately equimolecular amounts. It is a rapidly-acting mercurial diuretic, usually administered by intramuscular or intravenous injection. The object of the theophylline is to reduce the local irritant action.

mercurosum (mer·kewr·o·sum). Monovalent mercury in its compounds.

mercurous (**mer**·kewr·us). The term applied to ions or salts of mercury to denote that the mercury is in the monovalent form. **Mercurous acetate.** A white crystalline salt formerly used in ointments for the treatment of syphilitic sores. **Mercurous Chloride BPC 1959.** Calomel, HgCl, a tasteless white powder, insoluble in water. It is used as a purgative, prescribed as a powder, tablet, or pill. In the form of an ointment it is used in the local prophylaxis of syphilis. **Mercurous iodide, yellow.** HgI, a compound prepared by the interaction of mercurous nitrate with potassium iodide. It is a yellow heavy powder, chiefly used in the form of an ointment in chronic skin diseases and for application to enlarged glands. It has been employed orally in the treatment of the later stages of syphilis, and is non-irritant to the stomach. **Mercurous tannate.** A compound occurring as a dull brownish-green powder or scales, used at one time in the form of pills or tablets in the treatment of syphilis, producing a mild mercurial reaction without derangement of digestion.

mercury (**mer**·kewr·e). An element of atomic weight 200.59, atomic number 80, and chemical symbol Hg (*hydrargyrum*). It occurs naturally as the sulphide, HgS, in the ore cinnabar, found in Spain, Italy, California and elsewhere. At ordinary temperatures it is a heavy, silvery, mobile, liquid metal, used principally as an indicator in thermometers and manometers of various kinds. It can exist in monovalent or bivalent forms, giving rise respectively to mercurous and mercuric compounds. The mercury ion is a protoplasmic poison, and may cause death. The vapour is absorbed by the respiratory system, whilst finely dispersed mercury is absorbed through the skin and alimentary canal, as are some of its inorganic salts. The chief routes of mercury excretion are via the kidneys and the colon, and these are the organs mainly damaged in mercury poisoning; the main features of the latter are nephritis with blood and albumin in the urine, colitis, amd stomatitis. In therapeutics, mercury is used mostly in combined form, both organic and inorganic compounds being employed. It is occasionally prescribed in elemental form, in a finely dispersed state (BPC 1963). Preparations of mercury were the chief therapeutic weapons against syphilis from the end of the 15th century until the introduction of the arsphenamines: they are still used in prophylaxis. At the present day, the chief uses of mercury and its compounds are: locally, as antiseptics, parasiticides and fungicides; internally, as purgatives; and, by injection, as diuretics. **Ammoniated Mercury BP 1973.** White precipitate, a white powder, NH_2HgCl, employed in an ointment base as a mild antiseptic and fungicide in some skin diseases. **Mercury bichloride.** Mercuric Chloride BPC 1973. **Mercury biniodide.** Red Mercuric Iodide BPC 1954. **Mercury carbolate.** $(C_6H_5O)_2Hg{\cdot}H_2O$, a crystalline salt of mercury and phenol with antiseptic properties. **Colloidal mercury.** A solution of colloidal mercury sulphide stabilized with a hydrolysed protein, used as an antisyphilitic of low toxicity. **Oleated Mercury BPC 1959.** An oily mass containing 20 per cent of yellow mercuric oxide; used in ointment form in some chronic skin diseases. **Mercury peroxide.** Red mercuric oxide. **Mercury and potassium iodide.** Potassium mercuric iodide, K_2HgI_4, a complex salt formed by the combination of mercuric iodide and potassium iodide. It is a powerful germicide, and has been used for skin disinfection and the disinfection of instruments and excreta. It was also used as an irrigation solution, and is a constituent of Mayer's reagent for alkaloids, and of Nessler's reagent for ammonia. **Mercury subsulphate.** Basic mercuric sulphate, $HgSO_4{\cdot}2HgO$; a yellow powder formerly used in ointment for ringworm. [L *Mercurius*, messenger of the gods.]

merergasia (mer·er·ga·ze·ah). The term coined by Adolf Meyer, and not generally employed by others than his own students, to characterize a partial psychobiological reaction not involving the whole of the personality, and theoretically identifiable with the neuroses, psychoneuroses and psychosomatic disorders of other schools. [Gk *meros* part, *ergein* to work.]

merergastic (mer·er·**gas**·tik). Neurotic, psychoneurotic, or psychosomatic; of the nature of merergasia.

meridian (mer·**id**·e·an). 1. Any great circle of a sphere that passes through the poles. 2. Midday; or the highest point of the sun. Hence, the height of achievement. **Meridian of the cornea.** Any line drawn across the cornea passing through the anterior pole and if continued also passing through the posterior pole of the eyeball, and at right angles to its equator. **Meridian of the eye [meridianus (NA)].** A circle drawn around the eyeball, passing through the two poles and at right angles to the equator. **Magnetic meridian.** A vertical plane containing the direction in which a compass-needle points. [L *meridianus* of midday.]

meridional (mer·**id**·e·on·al). Of or relating to a meridian.

Mérieux-Baillon test. Serum from a known case of tuberculosis is injected subcutaneously into the forearm of a suspected case. A reddened swelling indicates tuberculosis. This is very unreliable.

merinthophobia (mer·in·tho·**fo**′·be·ah). A morbid fear of bonds or of being tied up. [Gk *merinthos* cord, phobia.]

Meriones (mer·e·o·neez). A genus of gerbils of which certain species act as host-reservoirs of *Leishmania tropica* and possibly the virus of Q fever. [Gk companion of Cretan chief *Idomeneus.*]

merism (**mer**·izm). The recurrence of parts of a similar structure in an organism, making a consistent and regular pattern. [Gk *meros* part.]

merispore (**mer**·e·spore). A secondary spore arising from the division of another (compound or septate) spore. [Gk *meros* part, *sporos* seed.]

meristem (**mer**·is·tem). Applied to the plant embryo, indicative of its homogeneous composition and undifferentiated structure. [Gk *merizein* to divide into parts.]

meristematic (mer·is·tem·**at**′·ik). Relating to or consisting of meristem.

meristic (mer·**is**·tik). Symmetrical; having parts that are divided evenly. [Gk *merizein* to divide into parts.]

meristoma (mer·is·**to**·mah). A tumour composed of meristematic tissue. [meristem, Gk *-oma* tumour.]

Merkel, Friedrich Siegmund (b. 1845). German anatomist.

Merkel's touch cell, corpuscle, or disc. A modified epithelial cell in the deeper layers of the epidermis, closely associated with a tactile disc formed by the terminal expansion of an axis-cylinder, the whole serving as a touch receptor.

lesser ring of Merkel. Pupillary zone. *See* ZONE.

Merkel-Ranvier cell. A melanoblast of the skin.

Merkel, Karl Ludwig (b. 1812). Leipzig anatomist and laryngologist.

Merkel's fossa. A shallow groove between the cuneiform and corniculate cartilages in the posterolateral wall of the vestibule of the larynx.

Merkel's muscle. A muscle passing from the lower border of the cricoid cartilage to the inferior horn of the thyroid cartilage.

mero-anencephalia (mer·o·an·en·kef·**a'**·le·ah). Partial anencephalia. [Gk *meros* part, *a*, *egkephalos* brain.]

meroblastic (mer·o·**blas**·tik). Referring to cleavage of those animal eggs in which, as a result of the large amount of yolk contained in them, the formation of cells is restricted to one part of their surface. Cleavage is meroblastic in birds, reptiles, and many fish. [Gk *meros* part, *blastos* germ.]

merocele (**mer**·o·seel). Femoral hernia. [Gk *meros* thigh, *kele* hernia.]

merocoxalgia (**mer**·o·kox·**al'**·je·ah). A painful condition of the thigh and hip. [Gk *meros* thigh, L *coxa* hip, Gk *algos* pain.]

merocrania (mer·o·**kra**·ne·ah). In monsters, congenital absence of a portion of the cranium. [Gk *meros* part, *kranion* skull.]

merocrine (**mer**·o·krine). Pertaining to the type of secretion in which the active cell remains intact whilst forming and discharging the secretory product. [Gk *meros* part, *krinein* to separate.]

merodiastolic (**mer**·o·di·as·**tol'**·ik). Denoting or referring to a part of the cardiac diastole. [Gk *meros* part, diastole.]

mero-ergasia (**mer**·o·er·**ga'**·ze·ah). Merergasia.

merogamete (mer·o·**gam**·eet). In protozoa, a gamete which is smaller than the organism which produces it. [Gk *meros* part, *gamos* marriage.]

merogamy (mer·**og**·am·e). In protozoa, conjugation between merogametes. [see prec.]

merogastrula (mer·o·**gas**·troo·lah). A gastrula formed from an ovum exhibiting partial cleavage owing to its high yolk content. [Gk *meros* part, gastrula.]

merogenesis (mer·o·**jen**·es·is). Segmentation of an ovum. [Gk *meros* part, *genein* to produce.]

merogenetic, merogenic (**mer**·o·jen·**et'**·ik, mer·o·**jen**·ik). 1. Segmental. 2. Relating or belonging to merogenesis.

merogony (mer·**og**·on·e). The development of fragments of ova. Such development is usually the result of experimental procedure and does not occur naturally. **Andro- merogony.** Development of egg fragments without female pronuclei after fertilization with sperm. **Diploid merogony.** Development of egg fragments with female pronuclei after fertilization with sperm. **Gyno- merogony.** Development of egg fragments with female pronuclei after fertilization with sperm and subsequent removal of male pronuclei. **Parthenogenetic merogony.** Development of egg fragments without female pronuclei after artificial activation, [Gk *meros* part, *gone* seed.]

merology (mer·**ol**·o·je). In anatomy, the science dealing with the fundamental rudimentary tissues. [Gk *meros* part, *logos* science.]

meromicrosomia (**mer**·o·mi·kro·**so'**·me·ah). A condition in which there is abnormal smallness of some portion of the body. [Gk *meros* part, *mikros* small, *soma* body.]

meromorphosis (**mer**·o·mor·**fo'**·sis). Partial regeneration of the tissues of a part lost by disease or accident. [Gk *meros* part, morphosis.]

meromyerial (**mer**·o·mi·**eer'**·e·al). In nematode worms, having very few muscle cells attached to the body wall. At one time of classificatory importance. [Gk *meros* part, *mys* muscle.]

meromyosin (mer·o·**mi**·o·sin). *Heavy* and *light*, the constituent proteins of the myosin contractile filament. [Gk *meros* part, *mys* muscle.]

meronecrobiosis, meronecrosis (**mer**·o·nek·ro·bi·**o'**·sis, **mer**·o·nek·**ro'**·sis). Cellular necrosis. [Gk *meros* part, necrobiosis, necrosis.]

meroparaesthesia (**mer**·o·par·es·**the'**·ze·ah). A condition in which changes have occurred with regard to the sense of touch in arms or legs. [Gk *meros* thigh, paraesthesia.]

meropia (mer·o·pe·ah). Partial loss of sight. [Gk *meros* part, *ops* seeing.]

merorachischisis (**mer**·o·ra·**kis'**·kis·is). Partial fissure of the spinal cord. [Gk *meros* part, *rhachis* spine, *schisis* a cleaving.]

meros (**me**·ros). 1. The femur. 2. The thigh. 3. Any part of the human body. [Gk thigh, part.]

meroscope (**mer**·o·skope). An apparatus employed in meroscopy.

meroscopy (mer·**os**·ko·pe). Dissociated auscultation of various fractions of the heart cycle. [Gk *meros* part, *skopein* to watch.]

merosmia (mer·**oz**·me·ah). A disordered sense of smell in which the patient cannot detect some odours. [Gk *meros* part, *osme* odour.]

merosystolic (**mer**·o·sis·**tol'**·ik). Relating to a part of the systole of the cardiac cycle. [Gk *meros* part, systole.]

merotomy (mer·**ot**·o·me). Division into parts; segmentation. [Gk *meros* part, *temnein* to cut.]

merozoite (mer·o·**zo**·ite). In sporozoan protozoa, a product of schizogony. The nucleus of the schizont divides many times without division of the cytoplasm; these nuclei migrate to the periphery and bud off as merozoites, leaving residual cytoplasm. [Gk *meros* part, *zoon* animal.]

merozygote (mer·o·**zi**·gote). An incomplete zygote which contains only part of the genetic material from one of the two parents; usual in bacterial genetics, where part of the donor chromosome is excluded from the zygote by the mechanism of transfer. [Gk *meros* part, *zygon* yoke.]

Merrill, Maud Amanda (b. 1888). American psychologist.

Merrill-Palmer test. A test for the estimation of intelligence of children between the ages of two and five years.

Terman-Merrill test. A later revision of the Stanford test.

Mersalyl BP 1953 (**mer**·sal·il). $HgOHCH_2CH(OCH_3)CH_2NH COC_6H_4OCH_2COONa$; one of the earliest of the mercurial diuretics, which are considered to be the most efficient type of diuretic and find favour in cases of cardiac oedema and nephrosis. They are usually administered with theophylline to reduce the local irritant action, and the diuretic effect is often enhanced by prior administration of an oral diuretic such as ammonium chloride.

Merulius lacrimans (mer·**ew**·le·us **lak**·re·manz). Obsolete synonym for *Serpulia lacrimans.* [L *merula* blackbird, *lacrimare* to weep.]

Méry, Jean (b. 1645). Paris surgeon and anatomist.

Méry's glands. The bulbo-urethral glands.

merycism (**mer**·e·sizm). Rumination. [Gk *merykismos* to chew cud.]

Merzbacher, Ludwig (b. 1875). German physician in Buenos Aires.

Merzbacher-Pelizaeus disease, Pelizaeus-Merzbacher disease. Familial centrolobar sclerosis, also called *aplasia axialis extracorticalis congenita*: a progressive disorder of infancy with dementia, spasticity, cerebellar disturbances and involuntary movements of the head and eyes; it is related to Schilder's disease, Krabbe's disease and Scholz's disease.

mesal (**me**·zal). Mesial.

mesaortitis (**mes**·a·or·**ti'**·tis). Inflammation of the muscular coat of the aorta. [Gk *mesos* middle, aortitis.]

mesaraic, mesaroeic (mes·ar·a·ik, mes·ar·e·ik). Mesenteric. [Gk *mesos* middle, *araia* belly.]

mesarteritis (**mes**·ar·ter·**i'**·tis). Inflammation of the muscular or middle coat of an artery. [Gk *mesos* middle, arteritis.]

See also: MOENCKEBERG.

mesaticephalic (mes·at·e·kef·**al'**·ik). In craniometry, having a head of medium proportions, with a cephalic index of between 75 and 80. [Gk *mesatos* middle, *kephale* head.]

mesaticephalus (mes·**at**·e·**kef'**·al·us). A skull with a cephalic index of between 75 and 80. [see prec.]

mesaxon (mes·**ax**·on). The region of apposed portions of the cell membrane of a Schwann cell produced by the enveloping of an axon by the cell. [Gk *mesos* middle, *axon* axle.]

mescal (**mes**·kal). An intoxicant spirit prepared in Mexico from pulque, the fermented juice of *Agave* species. The dried tops of *Lophophora williamsii* (family Cactaceae) are known as *mescal* *buttons*, and contain a number of narcotic alkaloids. Its remedial value is doubtful. [Mexican *mezcal.*]

mescaline (mes·kal·een). $C_{11}H_{17}O_3N$, an alkaloid occurring in mescal buttons. It is a trimethoxy compound related to adrenaline, and gives rise to heightened perception and visual hallucinations when taken. [see prec.]

mescalism (mes·kal·izm). Mescaline addiction in which colourful hallucinations of great beauty are experienced.

mesectic (mes·ek·tik). Referring to the power of cells, and tissues, to take up an average amount of oxygen. [Gk *mesos* middle, *hexis* habit.]

mesectoblast (mes·ek·to·blast). An ectodermal cell, particularly of the neural crest, which contributes to the head mesenchyme. [Gk *mesos* middle, *ektos* out, *blastos* germ.]

mesectoderm (mes·ek·to·derm). That part of the head mesenchyme which is derived from the ectoderm, particularly of the neural crest, and which is thought to give rise to the meninges, melanophores and, in part, to the branchial cartilages. [Gk *mesos* middle, ectoderm.]

mesencephalic (mes·en·kef·al′·ik). Relating to the mesencephalon.

mesencephalitis (mes·en·kef·al·i′·tis). Inflammation of the mesencephalon. [mesencephalon, Gk *-itis* inflammation.]

mesencephalohypophyseal (mes·en·kef·al·o·hi·po·fiz′·e·al). Relating to the mesencephalon and the hypophysis cerebri.

mesencephalon (mes·en·kef·al·on). The mid-brain. [Gk *mesos* middle, *egkephalos* brain.]

mesencephalotomy (mes·en·kef·al·ot′·o·me). The surgical operation of placing an incision in the midbrain, usually interrupting the spinothalamic tract, in the treatment of persistent pain. [mesencephalon, Gk *temnein* to cut.]

mesenchyma (mes·en·ki·mah). Mesenchyme.

mesenchymal (mes·en·ki·mal). Relating to the mesenchyme.

mesenchyme (mes·en·kime). The embryonal connective tissue, derived chiefly from the mesoderm, which gives rise to bone, cartilage and other connective tissues as well as to the lymphatic and blood vessels. It consists of stellate cells embedded in a gelatinous ground substance containing a network of reticular fibres. [Gk *mesos* middle, *egchyma* infusion.]

mesenchymoma (mes·en·ki·mo′·mah). A tumour consisting of mesenchymal tissue. [mesenchyme, Gk *-oma* tumour.]

mesenterectomy (mes·en·ter·ek′·to·me). Excision of the mesentery. [mesentery, Gk *ektome* a cutting out.]

mesenteric (mes·en·ter·ik). Relating to the mesentery.

mesenteric arteries. Ventral branches of the abdominal aorta that supply blood to various parts of the mesentery. **Inferior mesenteric artery [arteria mesenterica inferior (NA)].** A ventral branch of the abdominal aorta supplying the terminal part of the transverse colon, the descending colon, the pelvic colon, and most of the rectum by means of superior left colic [arteria colica sinistra (NA)], multiple inferior left colic [arteriae sigmoideae (NA)] and superior rectal [arteria rectalis superior (NA)] branches. **Superior mesenteric artery [arteria mesenterica superior (NA)].** The ventral branch of the abdominal aorta supplying the alimentary canal from the second part of the duodenum to beyond the middle of the transverse colon. Its branches are named after the parts supplied: inferior pancreaticoduodenal [arteria pancreaticoduodenalis inferior (NA)], jejunal and ileal [arteriae jejunales et ilei (NA)], ileocolic [arteria ileocolica (NA)], ascending colon [arteria ascendens (NA)], caecal [arteria cecalis anterior et posterior (NA)], appendicular [arteria appendicularis (NA)], right colic [arteria colica dextra (NA)], and middle colic [arteria colica media (NA)] arteries.

mesenteric veins. Veins that receive blood from the mesentery. **Inferior mesenteric vein [vena mesenterica inferior (NA)].** The main vein of the hind-gut in the fetus, later a tributary of the splenic vein, draining the pelvic and descending colons and most of the rectum. **Superior mesenteric vein [vena mesenterica superior (NA)].** The venous drainage from the second part of the duodenum to the distal third of the colon. It is a tributary of the portal vein.

mesentericomesocolic (mes·en·ter·ik·o·mes·o·kol′·ik). Pertaining to the mesentery and the mesocolon.

mesenteriolum (mes·en·ter·e·o·lum). A small mesentery; particularly a mesentery of the vermiform appendix or of a diverticulum of the intestine. [dim. of mesentery.]

mesenteriopexy (mes·en·ter·e·o·pex·e). The operative procedure of fixing an incised or lacerated mesentery. [mesentery, Gk *pexis* fixation.]

mesenteriorrhaphy (mes·en·ter·e·or′·af·e). The process of suturing the mesentery. [mesentery, Gk *rhaphe* suture.]

mesenteriplication (mes·en·ter·e·pli·ka′·shun). The procedure of taking up redundant length of the mesentery by making folds and suturing. [mesentery, L *plicare* to fold.]

mesenteritic (mes·en·ter·it′·ik). Affected with or relating to mesenteritis.

mesenteritis (mes·en·ter·i′·tis). Inflammation of the mesentery. [mesentery, Gk *-itis* inflammation.]

mesenteron (mes·en·ter·on). The mesentery of the embryonic hind-gut and its derivatives.

mesentery [mesenterium (NA)] (mes·en·ter·e). A double layer of peritoneum connecting the intestine to the posterior abdominal wall. Nerves, vessels, and lymphatics pass between the two layers. **Common mesentery [mesenterium dorsale commune (NA)].** The mesentery proper. **Root of the mesentery [radix mensenterii (NA)].** The attached border opposite to the visceral border. **Mesentery of the vermiform appendix [mesoappendix (NA)].** A small triangular fold, having one free border and the others attached to the length of the appendix and to the under surface of the mesentery of the small intestine at its right extremity. [Gk *mesos* middle, *enteron* intestine.]

mesentoderm (mes·en·to·derm). Mesenchyme of entodermal origin.

mesentorrhaphy (mes·en·tor·af·e). Mesenteriorrhaphy.

mesepithelium (mes·ep·e·the′·le·um). Epithelium of mesodermal origin, such as that lining the urinary and genital passages above the cloaca.

mesial (me·ze·al). 1. Towards the middle plane or line of the body or of any structure. 2. Towards the apex of the dental arch. [Gk *mesos* middle.]

mesiobuccal (me·ze·o·buk·al). Pertaining to the mesial and the buccal surfaces of a tooth.

mesiobucco-occlusal (me·ze·o·buk·o·ok·loo′·zal). Pertaining to the angle formed by the mesial, buccal, and occlusal surfaces of a tooth.

mesiobuccopulpal (me·ze·o·buk·o·pul′·pal). Relating to the mesial and buccal walls and the floor adjacent to the pulp in a cavity prepared in a tooth.

mesiocervical (me·ze·o·ser′·vik·al). Pertaining to the mesial surface and the cervical margin of a tooth.

mesiodistal (me·ze·o·dis′·tal). In dentistry, pertaining to the mesial and distal surface of a tooth.

mesio-incisal (me·ze·o·in·si′·zal). Pertaining to the mesial and incisal surfaces of a tooth.

mesiolabial (me·ze·o·la′·be·al). Pertaining to the mesial and labial surfaces of a tooth.

mesiolingual (me·ze·o·ling′·gwal). Pertaining to the mesial and lingual surfaces of a tooth.

mesiolinguo-occlusal (me·ze·o·ling·gwo·ok·loo′·zal). Pertaining to the angle formed by the junction of the mesial, lingual and occlusal surfaces of a tooth.

mesiolinguopulpal (me·ze·o·ling·gwo·pul′·pal). Relating to the mesial and lingual walls and to the floor adjacent to the pulp chamber in a cavity prepared in a tooth.

mesion (me·ze·on). The median vertical longitudinal plane dividing the body into left and right superficially symmetrical halves; meson. [Gk *mesos* middle.]

mesio-occlusal (me·ze·o·ok·loo′·zal). Pertaining to the angle formed by the mesial and occlusal surfaces of a tooth.

mesio-occlusion (me·ze·o·ok·loo′·zhun). That form of malocclusion in which the lower teeth lie in a position in front of that which they normally occupy in relation to the upper teeth; antero-occlusion. [Gk *mesos* middle, occlusion.]

mesiopulpal (me·ze·o·pul′·pal). Pertaining to the mesial wall and to the floor adjacent to the pulp chamber in a cavity prepared in a tooth.

mesitylene (mes·it·il·een). Symmetrical trimethylbenzene, $C_6H_3(CH_3)_3$. A colourless liquid with a pleasant smell, occurring in coal tar, or prepared from acetone by condensation.

mesmeric (mes·mer·ik). Induced by or relating to mesmerism.

mesmerism (mes·mer·izm). A method and practice of hypnotism in which the patient becomes subject to the will and suggestions of the operator. It was attributed by Mesmer to animal magnetism. [Franz Anton *Mesmer*, 1734–1815, Austrian physician.]

meso-. 1. A prefix meaning *middle*, used in medicine to denote anything intermediate. 2. In organic chemistry, denoting the attachment of a radical to a carbon atom in a heterocyclic ring that is situated between two atoms of elements other than carbon; such a compound is distinguished by the prefix μ-. [Gk *mesos* middle.]

meso-aortitis (mes·o·a·or·ti′·tis). Inflammation of the middle coat of the aorta. **Meso-aortitis syphilitica.** Inflammation of the middle coat of the aorta caused by a syphilitic infection. [Gk *mesos* middle, aortitis.]

meso-appendicitis (mes·o·ap·en·dis·i′·tis). Inflammation of the mesentery of the vermiform appendix. [meso-appendix, Gk *-itis* inflammation.]

meso-appendix (mes·o·ap·en′·dix). The fold of the peritoneum which joins the vermiform appendix to the ileum; the mesentery of the vermiform appendix. [Gk *mesos* middle, appendix.]

meso-arial (mes·o·a·re·al). Relating to the mesovarium.

meso-arium (mes·o·a·re·um). Mesovarium. [Gk *mesos* middle, *oarion* small egg.]

mesobilin (mes·o·bi·lin). $C_{33}H_{42}N_4O_6$, a compound formed by the reduction of bilirubin with hydriodic acid or with sodium amalgam. [Gk *mesos* middle, urobilin.]

mesobilinogen (mes·o·bi·lin′·o·jen). $C_{33}H_{44}O_6N_4$, one of the reduction products of bilirubin formed by the action of sodium amalgam. It is also formed in the intestine by bacterial reduction of bilirubin and probably occurs in the urine in liver disease. Oxidation converts it to urobilin. [mesobilin, mesobilirubin, Gk *genein* to produce.]

mesobilirubin (mes·o·bil·e·roo′·bin). $C_{33}H_{40}N_4O_6$, a compound formed by the gentle reduction of bilirubin. [Gk *mesos* middle, bilirubin.]

mesobilirubinogen (mes·o·bil·e·roo·bin′·o·jen). Mesobilinogen.

mesoblast (mes·o·blast). Mesoderm. [Gk *mesos* middle, *blastos* germ.]

mesoblastic (mes·o·blas·tik). Derived from or relating to the mesoblast.

mesobronchitis (mes·o·brong·ki′·tis). Inflammation of the middle or muscular coats of the bronchi. [Gk *mesos* middle, bronchitis.]

mesocaecal (mes·o·se·kal). Relating to the mesocaecum.

mesocaecum (mes·o·se·kum). The occasionally persisting mesentery of the caecum.

mesocardia (mes·o·kar·de·ah). A condition in which the heart is placed centrally in the thorax, as is the case in early fetal life. [see foll.]

mesocardium (mes·o·kar·de·um). The mesentery of the embryonic heart. **Arterial mesocardium.** The persisting upper end of the dorsal mesentery of the embryonic heart, which surrounds the ascending aorta and pulmonary trunk between the heart and the fibrous pericardium. **Dorsal mesocardium.** A transient dorsal mesentery of the heart in all vertebrate embryos. **Venous mesocardium.** The persisting lower part of the mesentery of the embryonic heart, which surrounds the inferior and superior venae cavae and the four pulmonary veins between the heart and the fibrous pericardium. **Ventral mesocardium.** A transient ventral mesentery of the heart, found in lower vertebrates. [Gk *mesos* middle, *kardia* heart.]

mesocarpal (mes·o·kar·pal). Midcarpal. [Gk *mesos* middle, carpus.]

mesocephalic (mes·o·kef·al′·ik). 1. Mesencephalic. 2. Mesaticephalic.

mesocephalon (mes·o·kef·al·on). Mesencephalon.

Mesocestoides (mes·o·ses·toid′·eez). A genus of Cestoda. **Mesocestoides variabilis.** A species which occurs in dogs and other mammals in North America, and has recorded once from a child. [Gk *mesos* middle, *kestos* girdle, *eidos* form.]

Mesocestoididae (mes·o·ses·toid′·id·e). A family of the cestode order Cyclophyllidea. The genus *Mesocestoides* and pseudogenus *Tetrathyridea* are of medical interest. [see prec.]

mesochondrium (mes·o·kon·dre·um). The matrix holding the cells of the hyaline cartilage. [Gk *mesos* middle, *chondros* cartilage.]

mesochord (mes·o·kord). A fold of amnion which sometimes connects the umbilical cord to the placenta. [Gk *mesos* middle, cord.]

mesochoroidea (mes·o·kor·oid′·e·ah). The choriocapillary lamina. *See* LAMINA. [Gk *mesos* middle, choroid.]

mesocoele, mesocoelia (mes·o·seel, mes·o·se·le·ah). The aqueduct of the mid-brain. [Gk *mesos* middle, *koilia* cavity.]

mesocolic (mes·o·kol·ik). Relating to the mesocolon.

mesocolon [NA] (mes·o·ko·lon). The mesentery of the colon; it is usually restricted, in the adult, to the transverse and sigmoid portions of the colon. **Ascending mesocolon [mesocolon ascendens (NA)].** A short double layer of peritoneum by which the ascending colon is occasionally attached to the posterior abdominal wall. **Descending mesocolon [mesocolon descendens (NA)].** A short double layer of peritoneum by which the descending colon is occasionally attached to the posterior abdominal wall. **Pelvic mesocolon [mesocolon sigmoideum (NA)].** The mesentery of the sigmoid colon. **Transverse mesocolon [mesocolon transversum (NA)].** The mesentery of the transverse colon. [Gk *mesos* middle, colon.]

mesocolopexy (mes·o·ko·lo·pex·e). Mesocoloplication. [mesocolon, Gk *pexis* fixation.]

mesocoloplication (mes·o·ko·lo·pli·ka′·shun). A procedure for shortening the length and correcting abnormal mobility of the bowel by making a fold in the mesocolon and suturing it. [mesocolon, plication.]

meso-compound (mes·o·kom·pound). An isomer of an optically-active compound which displays no optical rotation by reason of the internal opposition of its asymmetric carbon atoms. [Gk *mesos* middle, compound.]

mesocord (mes·o·kord). Mesochord.

mesocranium (mes·o·kra·ne·um). The vertex of the skull. [Gk *mesos* middle, cranium.]

mesocuneiform (mes·o·kew·ne′·e·form). The intermediate cuneiform bone of the tarsus. [Gk *mesos* middle, cuneiform.]

Mesocyclops (mes·o·si·klops). A genus of small crustaceans of which several species act as intermediate hosts of the guinea-worm, *Dracunculus medinensis.* [Gk *mesos* middle, cyclops.]

mesocyst (mes·o·sist). The peritoneal fold that joins the gall bladder to the liver. [Gk *mesos* middle, *kystis* bag.]

mesocyte (mes·o·site). Mesolymphocyte.

mesocytoma (mes·o·si·to′·mah). A tumour made up of connective tissue; a sarcoma. [Gk *mesos* middle, *kytos* cell, *-oma* tumour.]

mesoderm (mes·o·derm). The middle germ layer of the embryo, lying between the ectoderm and the entoderm. From it are derived the muscles, bones, cartilages, fibrous connective tissues, the dermis, gonads, kidneys, upper genital and urinary ducts, spleen, cortex of the suprarenal gland and the connective-tissue component of all organs and tissues, as well as the whole of the cardiovascular and lymphatic systems. **Somatic mesoderm.** That part of the lateral embryonic mesoderm which is applied to the ectoderm outside the coelomic cavity. **Splanchnic mesoderm.** That part of the lateral embryonic mesoderm which is applied to the entoderm on the inner side of the coelomic cavity. [Gk *mesos* middle, *derma* skin.]

mesodermal, mesodermic (mes·o·**der**·mal, mes·o·**der**·mik). Relating to or originating from the mesoderm.

mesodermopath (mes·o·**der**·mo·path). A person who is supposed to have a constitutional predisposition towards diseases of those tissues which are derived from the embryonic mesoderm. [mesoderm, Gk *pathos* disease.]

mesodiastole (mes·o·di·**as'**·to·le). In the middle of diastole. [Gk *mesos* middle, diastole.]

mesodiastolic (mes·o·di·as·**tol'**·ik). Relating to the middle of the diastolic period. [see prec.]

mesodont, mesodontic (**mes**·o·dont, mes·o·**don**·tik). Having dentition in which the teeth are of average size. [Gk *mesos* middle, *odous* tooth.]

mesoduodenal (mes·o·dew·o·**de'**·nal). Relating to the mesoduodenum.

mesoduodenum (mes·o·dew·o·**de'**·num). A fold which joins the duodenum to the abdominal wall in fetal and early life and occasionally continues to exist in later life; sometimes referred to as the *duodenal mesentery.* [Gk *mesos* middle, duodenum.]

meso-epididymis (mes·o·ep·e·**did'**·im·is). A fold of tunica vaginalis testis that joins the epididymis to the testicle in a certain percentage of individuals. [Gk *mesos* middle, epididymis.]

mesoform (**mes**·o·form). Describing an isomer of an optically-active compound, which displays no optical rotation by reason of the internal opposition of its asymmetric carbon atoms. [Gk *mesos* middle, form.]

mesogaster (mes·o·**gas**·ter). Mesogastrium.

mesogastric (mes·o·**gas**·trik). Relating to the mesogastrium.

mesogastrium [NA] (mes·o·**gas**·tre·um). A mesentery of the embryonic stomach. **Dorsal mesogastrium.** An embryonic mesentery of the stomach which is attached ventrally to the greater curvature and dorsally to the posterior abdominal wall. It gives rise to the spleen, gastrosplenic and lienorenal ligaments, and most of the greater omentum. **Ventral mesogastrium.** An embryonic mesentery of the stomach attached dorsally to the lesser curvature and ventrally to the anterior abdominal wall. Part of the liver is developed in it, whilst the lesser omentum and falciform ligament are derived from it. [Gk *mesos* middle, *gaster* belly.]

mesoglia (mes·**og**·le·ah). Phagocytic neuroglial cells of mesodermal origin. [Gk *mesos* middle, neuroglia.]

mesoglioma (mes·o·gli·**o'**·mah). A tumour of the oligodendroglia. [mesoglia, Gk *-oma* tumour.]

mesogluteal (mes·o·**gloo**·te·al). Relating to the gluteus medius muscle. [see foll.]

mesogluteus (mes·o·**gloo**·te·us). The gluteus medius muscle. [Gk *mesos* middle, gluteus.]

mesognathic (mes·og·**nath**·ik). 1. Relating to the mesognathion. 2. Having slightly projecting jaws and a gnathic or alveolar index of between 98 and 103. [Gk *mesos* middle, *gnathos* jaw.]

mesognathion (mes·og·**nath**·e·on). The premaxilla or incisive bone of the maxilla. [see prec.]

mesohyloma (mes·o·hi·**lo'**·mah). A tumour originating in and developing from the mesothelium. [Gk *mesos* middle, *hyle* substance, *-oma* tumour.]

meso-ileum (mes·o·i·le·um). The mesentery of the ileum.

mesojejunum (mes·o·jej·**oon'**·um). The mesentery of the jejunum.

mesolepidoma (mes·o·lep·id·**o'**·mah). A tumour composed of tissue derived from persistent embryonic mesothelium. [Gk *mesos* middle, *lepis* scale, *-oma* tumour.]

mesologic (mes·o·**loj**·ik). Relating or belonging to mesology.

mesology (mes·**ol**·o·je). Ecology. [Gk *mesos* middle, *logos* science.]

mesolymphocyte (mes·o·**limf**·o·site). A lymphocyte of moderate size. [Gk *mesos* middle, lymphocyte.]

mesomelic (mes·o·**mel**·ik). Relating to the middle portion of a limb. [Gk *mesos* middle, *melos* limb.]

mesomere (**mes**·o·meer). A rod of mesodermal cells, lying between the epimere and the mesothelium, from which the renal tubules are derived. [Gk *mesos* middle, *meros* part.]

mesomerism (mes·**om**·er·izm). In chemistry, a state in which a compound can exist in a form intermediate between two tautomeric forms. The state is not one of equilibrium in the ordinary sense, but one of electronic strain, and is also known as *resonance.* [see prec.]

mesometritis (mes·o·me·**tri'**·tis). An inflammatory condition of the muscular coat of the uterus. [Gk *mesos* middle, metritis.]

mesometrium [L.] (mes·o·**me**·tre·um). The muscular coat of the uterus. [Gk *mesos* middle, *metra* womb.]

mesomorph (**mes**·o·morf). An individual of average height and stocky build with broad features. [see foll.]

mesomorphic (mes·o·**mor**·fik). 1. Applied to anyone who is of medium height. 2. In chemistry, being in a state of matter intermediate between liquid and crystal and displaying anisotropic properties. [Gk *mesos* middle, *morphe* form.]

mesomorphy (**mes**·o·mor·fe). The body type of the stocky individual whose height is average but whose features are broad. [see prec.]

meson (**mes**·on). 1. Mesion. 2. A heavy sub-atomic particle. [Gk *mesos* middle.]

mesonasal (mes·o·**na**·zal). Relating to the central portion of the nose. [Gk *mesos* middle, nose.]

mesonephric (mes·o·**nef**·rik). Relating to the mesonephros.

mesonephroma (mes·o·nef·**ro'**·mah). A tumour derived from the mesonephros. **Mesonephroma ovarii.** A mixed papillary cystadenoma of the ovary, doubtfully attributed to the mesonephros. [mesonephros, Gk *-oma* tumour.]

mesonephron (mes·o·**nef**·ron). The coiled tubular secretory unit of the mesonephros. It consists of a Bowman's capsule and a convoluted tubule somewhat similar to the uriniferous tubule of the permanent mammalian kidney (the metanephros). [see foll.]

mesonephros [NA] (mes·o·**nef**·ros). The secondary kidney or wolffian body, found as a transient structure in all higher vertebrate embryos, but persisting as the permanent kidney in fish and amphibia. **Caudal mesonephros.** That part of the mesonephros below the gonad, which persists in part as the paradidymis or the paroöphoron. **Cranial mesonephros.** That part of the mesonephros above the gonad, which persists as the appendix of the epididymis in the male. **Genital mesonephros.** The middle part of the mesonephros opposite the gonad, which persists as the efferent ductules of the testis and epididymis in the male. In the female it forms the epoöphoron. [Gk *mesos* middle, *nephros* kidney.]

mesoneuritis (mes·o·newr·**i'**·tis). Inflammation of the interstitial tissue of a nerve. **Nodular mesoneuritis.** Hyperplastic inflammation of the interstitial tissue of a nerve, causing the development of node-like thickenings. [Gk *mesos* middle, neuritis.]

meso-oesophagus (mes·o·e·**sof'**·ag·us). The embryonic dorsal mesentery of the oesophagus, which lies between the developing pleural cavities. It persists as the double layer of pleura and intervening connective tissue which surrounds the structures in the posterior mediastinum. In part the crura of the diaphragm are developed in it. [Gk *mesos* middle, oesophagus.]

meso-omentum (mes·o·o·**men'**·tum). The fold of peritoneum by which the omentum is fixed to the wall of the abdomen. [Gk *mesos* middle, omentum.]

mesopexy (**mes**·o·pex·e). Mesenteriopexy. [Gk *mesos* middle *pexis* fixation.]

mesopharynx (mes·o·**far**·ingx). The oropharynx. [Gk *mesos* middle, pharynx.]

mesophilic (mes·o·**fil**·ik). Describing organisms which grow best at medium temperatures, usually about 37°C. [Gk *mesos* middle, *philein* to love.]

mesophlebitis (mes·o·fleb·**i'**·tis). Inflammation of the middle coat of a vein. [Gk *mesos* middle, phlebitis.]

mesophryon (mes·**of**·re·on). The median point of the glabella. [Gk *mesos* middle, *ophrys* eyebrow.]

mesopneumon, mesopneumonium (mes·o·**new**·mon, **mes**·o·new·**mo'**·ne·um). The junction of the pleural strata at the hilum of the lung. [Gk *mesos* middle, *pneumon* lung.]

mesoporphyrin (mes·o·**por**·fir·in). $C_{32}H_{36}N_4(COOH)_2$, one of the iron-free porphyrins obtained from haemin by a process of reduction: a large number of isomeric compounds have been synthesized.
mesoprosopic (**mes**·o·pro·**so'**·pik). Having a face of medium proportion or width. [Gk *mesos* middle, *prosopon* face.]
mesopulmonum (mes·o·**pul**·mo·num). The mesentery of the lung, which contains the structures entering at the root, and below these forms the pulmonary ligament. [Gk *mesos* middle, L *pulmo* lung.]
mesorachischisis (**mes**·o·ra·**kis'**·kis·is). Merorachischisis. [Gk *mesos* middle, rachischisis.]
mesorchial (mes·**or**·ke·al). Relating to the mesorchium.
mesorchium [NA] (mes·**or**·ke·um). The mesentery of the testis, present throughout life in those mammals which exhibit seasonal descent of the testis, but found only in fetal life in animals such as man with permanently descended testes. [Gk *mesos* middle, *orchis* testis.]
mesorhine (**mes**·o·rine). Having a nasal index of between 48 and 53. [Gk *mesos* middle, *rhis* nose.]
Mesoridazine (mez·o·**rid**·az·een). BP Commission approved name for 10 - [2 - (1 - methyl - 2 - piperidyl)ethyl] - 2 - (methylsulfinyl)phenothiazine; a tranquillizer.
mesoropter (mes·or·**op**·ter). The usual position of the eyes when the muscles are relaxed. **Muscular mesoropter.** The angle made by the visual axes of the eyes when the external ocular muscles are relaxed. [Gk *mesos* middle, *horos* boundary, *opterios* belonging to sight.]
mesorrhaphy (mes·**or**·af·e). Mesenteriorrhaphy. [Gk *mesos* middle, *rhaphe* suture.]
mesosalpinx (mes·o·**sal**·pingx). The upper portion of the broad ligament which envelops the uterine tube. [Gk *mesos* middle, *salpigx* tube.]
mesoscapula (mes·o·**skap**·ew·lah). The spine of the scapula. [Gk *mesos* middle, scapula.]
mesoseme (**mes**·o·seem). Having an orbital index of between 84 and 89. [Gk *mesos* middle, *sema* sign.]
mesosigmoid (mes·o·**sig**·moid).The pelvic mesocolon. [Gk *mesos* middle, sigmoid.]
mesosigmoiditis (**mes**·o·sig·moid·**i'**·tis). Inflammation of the pelvic mesocolon. [mesosigmoid, Gk *-itis* inflammation.]
mesosigmoidopexy (**mes**·o·sig·**moid'**·o·pex·e). Surgical fixation or shortening of the pelvic mesocolon in cases of rectal prolapse. [mesosigmoid, Gk *pexis* fixation.]
mesosoma (mes·o·**so**·mah). Medium height. [Gk *mesos* middle, *soma* body.]
mesosomatous (mes·so·**so**·mat·us). Having medium height. [see prec.]
mesosome (**mes**·o·some). Convoluted membranous bodies found in (especially Gram-positive) bacteria, formed by involutions of the cytoplasmic membrane. [Gk *mesos* middle, *soma* body.]
mesosternale (**mes**·o·ster·**na'**·le). An anthropometric point; the mid-point of the sternum. [see foll.]
mesosternum (mes·o·**ster**·num). The body of the sternum. [Gk *mesos* middle, sternum.]
mesosthenic (mes·o·**sthen**·ik). Having a moderate degree of muscular strength. [Gk *mesos* middle, *sthenos* strength.]
mesosystolic (**mes**·o·sis·**tol'**·ik). Relating to the middle of the systolic phase; occurring during the systolic phase. [Gk *mesos* middle, systole.]
mesotarsal (mes·o·**tar**·sal). Midtarsal. [Gk *mesos* middle, tarsus.]
mesotendon [mesotendineum (NA)] (mes·o·**ten**·don). The part of the synovial membrane which connects the layer lining the fibrous sheath to that investing the tendon. [Gk *mesos* middle, tendon.]
mesothelial (mes·o·**the**·le·al). Relating to the mesothelium.
mesothelioma (**mes**·o·the·le·**o'**·mah). A tumour of the mesothelium of the pleura, pericardium or peritoneum, arising as a result of the presence of asbestos bodies. A locally malignant spreading tumour diagnostic of exposure to asbestos. [mesothelium, Gk *-oma* tumour.]
mesothelium [NA] (mes·o·**the**·le·um). The layer of cells lining the coelomic cavities. **Mesothelium of the anterior chamber [endothelium camerae anterioris (NA)].** A layer of flat, endothelial-like cells covering the inner surface of the cornea and helping to line the anterior chamber of the eye. [Gk *mesos* middle, epithelium.]
mesothorium (mes·o·**thor**·e·um). The first two disintegration products of thorium. Mesothorium-I is a radioactive isotope of radium and has a half-life of 6.7 years. It decays into mesothorium-II which is an isotope of actinium with a half-life of 6.13 hours, which decays to radiothorium. Radium salts may contain mesothorium as an impurity. [Gk *mesos* middle, thorium.]
mesotron (**mes**·o·tron). Obsolete synonym for meson (def. 2). [Gk *mesos* middle, electron.]
mesotropic (mes·o·**trop**·ik). Turned towards or situated in the median plane. [Gk *mesos* middle, *tropos* a turning.]
mesoturbinal, mesoturbinate (mes·o·**ter**·bin·al, mes·o·**ter**·bin·ate). The middle nasal concha. [Gk *mesos* middle, turbinal bone.]
mesovarium [NA] (mes·o·**va**·re·um). A fold of peritoneum forming a connection between the mesovarian border and the broad ligament of the ovary. [Gk *mesos* middle, ovary.]
mesoxalyl urea (mes·**ox**·al·il ewr·**e**·ah). Alloxan, CO(NH CO)$_2$CO. A compound produced by the oxidation of uric acid. It causes diabetes when experimentally given to animals, by bringing about necrosis of the β-cells of the islands of Langerhans.
messenger (**mes**·en·jer). In molecular biology, referring to ribonucleic acid (RNA) molecules which are synthesized (transcribed) from a chromosomal DNA template and thence carry the genetic messages to the ribosomes where they are translated into specific protein structures. **Messenger "first".** A hormone of polypeptide or amine constitution which attaches itself to a specific receptor site on a cell membrane of a responsive cell and activates adenyl cyclase in the cell membrane to form cyclic AMP in the cell. AMP is often referred to as the "second" messenger. The "third" messenger may be cortisol which AMP may help to produce and which may stimulate the synthesis of protein. **Polycistronic messenger.** A molecule of messenger-RNA which carries the genetic information of a number of adjacent genes (cistrons). [ME *messager* the bearer of.]
Messinger's test. Of myocardial reserve: a test which depends upon the alteration of the normal ratio between respiratory and cardiac rates on exercise in normal persons and in patients with cardiac disease. In the former the ratio increases with exercise, while in the latter the reverse occurs.
Mestanolone (mes·**tan**·o·lone). BP Commission approved name for 17β-hydroxy-17-methyl-5α-androstan-3-one; it is used in the treatment of menstrual disorders.
Mesterolone (mes·ter·o·lone). BP Commission approved name for 17β-hydroxy-1α-methyl-5α-androstan-3-one; an androgen that does not suppress endogenous testosterone but improves the sperm count and fructose and prostaglandin content of semen of infertile men. Some pregnancies have been recorded.
Mestranol BP 1973 (**mes**·tran·ol). 17α-Ethynyl-3-methoxy-oestra-1,3,5(10)-trien-17β-ol, an oestrogen with the same actions as oestradiol; it is widely used with lynoestrenol in contraceptive tablets.
Mesulphen BPC 1968 (me·**sul**·fen). Dimethyldiphenylene disulphide, a yellow viscous oil containing about 25 per cent of sulphur in organic combinations; it is a parasiticide used in acne, scabies, impetigo, especially in the treatment of hairy regions.
meta. Greek preposition with a wide range of meaning, e.g. *among, between, besides, in addition to, after, beyond, together with.* Used as a prefix it implies a change of position, order, shape, kind, etc.
meta (**met**·ah). A proprietary solid form of metaldehyde used for heating purposes, like methylated spirits.
meta-. In chemistry, denoting the attachment of atoms or radicals to a benzene ring in positions such that one carbon atom

of the ring intervenes between them: the 1,3 position. [see under *Meta*, Gk preposition.]

metabasis (met·**ab**·as·is). 1. A change from one disease to another. 2. Metastasis, or the transference of disease from one part of the body to another. [Gk alteration.]

metabiosis (met·ah·bi·o'·sis). The relationship of one organism to another when the first depends on the second for its existence. [Gk *meta, biosis* manner of life.]

metabolic (met·ab·**ol**·ik). Pertaining or belonging to metabolism.

metabolimeter (met·ab·ol·**im'**·et·er). A calorimetric device for estimating the basal metabolic rate. [metabolism, Gk *metron* measure.]

metabolimetry (met·ab·ol·**im'**·et·re). The estimation of the basal metabolic rate. [see prec.]

metabolin (met·**ab**·ol·in). Metabolite.

metabolism (met·**ab**·ol·izm). The chemical processes participating in and essential for the phenomena of life. They may be denoted individually by the class of substance involved, e.g. *carbohydrate, protein,* or *fat metabolism,* and can be subdivided into processes building-up larger molecules from small (*anabolism*), or the breaking-down of complex molecules into the more simple (*catabolism*). **Acid-base metabolism.** The processes underlying the regulation of the [H^+] of body tissues. **Basal metabolism.** The sum total of the chemical changes concerned in keeping the body functioning and its temperature normal, at rest in the postabsorptive state. It is proportional to the area of body surface, and thus to the rate of heat loss, and may be expressed either as energy, e.g. in joules (kilocalories) per square metre per hour, or in terms of oxygen used, in litres per square metre per hour, the two being related. **Constructive metabolism.** Anabolism. **Endogenous metabolism.** The chemical changes confined to the body itself, especially those concerned with the formation of end-products from body constituents as distinct from those formed more directly from food substances, e.g. endogenous uric acid from the nucleoproteins of tissue cells. **Energy metabolism.** The chemical changes which liberate energy in a form available for work (nucleoside triphosphates, especially adenosine triphosphate) and biosyntheses (nucleoside triphosphates or reduced forms of the nicotinamide coenzymes), and also as heat. **Exogenous metabolism.** The formation of end-products directly from ingested food substances which have not been previously incorporated as tissue constituents, e.g. uric acid from ingested nucleoprotein. **Inborn error of metabolism.** A hereditary disorder in which a structural abnormality occurs in a catalytic protein so that its activity is reduced or absent. Abnormal metabolites may accumulate and produce disease. Examples are: galactosaemia, alkaptonuria, albinism, phenylketonuria and the glycogen storage disorders. [Gk *metabole* change.]

metabolite (met·**ab**·ol·ite). In physiology, any product yielded by, or taking part in, metabolic processes. **Essential metabolite.** A substance that is essential for normal metabolism, e.g. a vitamin.

metabolize (met·**ab**·ol·ize). To alter the character of any substance by means of metabolism; to subject to metabolism.

metabolon (met·**ab**·o·lon). Matter having only a transient existence and formed in the course of the disintegration of radioactive substances. [Gk *metabole* change.]

metacarpal (met·ah·**kar**·pal). 1. A metacarpal bone. 2. Relating to the metacarpus.

metacarpal arteries. Dorsal metacarpal arteries [arteriae metacarpeae dorsales (NA)]. Three branches from the posterior carpal arch together with a branch of the radial artery itself (the 1st dorsal metacarpal artery) which run longitudinally on the surface of the dorsal interosseous muscles and bifurcate at the finger webs into the dorsal digital arteries. They anastomose with the deep palmar arch by the superior perforating arteries and with the palmar digital branches of the superficial palmar arch by the inferior perforating arteries. **Palmar metacarpal arteries [arteriae metacarpeae palmares (NA)].** *See* RADIAL ARTERY.

metacarpal bones [ossa metacarpalia I-V (NA)]. Any of the bones of the palm. Each consists of an expanded proximal end, the base [basis (NA)] for articulation with the carpus, a somewhat rounded intermediate part, the shaft [corpus (NA)], giving origin to the interosseous muscles of the hand, and a rounded distal end or head [caput (NA)] for articulation with the proximal phalanx of the digit. The third metacarpal bone [os metacarpale III (NA)] bears the styloid process.

metacarpal veins. Dorsal metacarpal veins [venae metacarpeae dorsales (NA)]. A series of three veins draining the adjacent sides of the lateral four digits into the dorsal venous network of the hand. **Palmar metacarpal veins [venae metacarpeae palmares].** Veins accompanying the palmar metacarpal arteries to the deep venous arch of the palm of the hand.

metacarpale radiale (met·ah·kar·pa'·le ra·de·a·le). An anthropometric point; the most prominent point on the radial margin of the head of the metacarpal bone of the index finger.

metacarpale ulnare (met·ah·kar·pa'·le ul·nar·e). An anthropometric point; the most prominent point on the ulnar margin of the head of the metacarpal bone of the little finger.

metacarpectomy (met·ah·kar·**pek'**·to·me). Excision of a bone of the metacarpus. [metacarpus, Gk *ektome* a cutting out.]

metacarpophalangeal (met·ah·**kar**·po·fal·**an'**·je·al). Relating to the metacarpal bones and the phalanges, particularly to the joint between them.

metacarpus [NA] (met·ah·**kar**·pus). The set of five bones connecting the carpus to the digits; also the region of the hand in which the metacarpal bones are situated. [Gk *meta, karpos* wrist.]

metacele (**met**·ah·seel). The true coelom, or body cavity, which is surrounded on all sides by mesoderm. [Gk *meta, koilia* hollow.]

metacentric (met·ah·**sen**·trik). Of a chromosome or chromatid, with the centromere in a median position and therefore having arms of approximately equal length. [Gk *meta, kentron* centre.]

metacercaria (met·ah·ser·**ka'**·re·ah). A late cercaria of a trematode fluke in the encysted stage. [Gk *meta,* cercaria.]

Metacetamol (met·as·**et**·am·ol). BP Commission approved name for 3-acetamidophenol; an analgesic.

metachemical (met·ah·**kem**·ik·al). Relating to or having the properties associated with the sub-atomic, as in the case of radioactive elements. [Gk *meta,* chemistry.]

metachloral (met·ah·**klor**·al). $(CCl_3CHO)_3$, a polymer analogous with metaldehyde, obtained by treating anhydrous chloral with sulphuric acid. It is insoluble in water, and little used in medicine.

metachromasia (met·ah·kro·**ma'**·ze·ah). A staining reaction exhibited by various tissue components towards certain basic dyes, whereby they are stained a different colour from that of the dye employed. Thus, cartilage and other mucopolysaccharide-containing tissues are stained red by toluidine blue. This effect is due to polymerization of the dye by molecules of high molecular weight containing numerous acidic radicals. [Gk *meta, chroma* colour.]

metachromatic (met·ah·kro·**mat'**·ik). Displaying metachromasia.

metachromatin (met·ah·**kro**·mat·in). The basophilic element of nuclear chromatin. [Gk *meta,* chromatin.]

metachromatism (met·ah·**kro**·mat·izm). Metachromasia.

metachromatophil, metachromatophile (met·ah·**kro**·mat·o·fil, met·ah·**kro**·mat·o·file). A cell which does not stain normally when treated with a particular dye. [Gk *meta,* chromatophil.]

metachromia (met·ah·**kro**·me·ah). Metachromasia.

metachromic (met·ah·**kro**·mik). Metachromatic.

metachromophil, metachromophile (met·ah·**kro**·mo·fil, met·ah·**kro**·mo·file). Metachromatophil.

metachrosis (met·ah·**kro**·sis). An alteration in colour [Gk *meta, chrosis* colour.]

metacism (**met**·ah·sizm). A defect of utterance in which the letter *m*, or its representative sound, is used excessively or wrongly. The defect may be evident as well in writing. [corruption of Gk *mytakismos* fondness for the letter *mu*.]

metacoele (**met**·ah·seel). Metacele.

metacone (**met**·ah·kone). In the tritubercular theory of evolution, the name given to the postero-external cusp of an upper molar tooth. [Gk *meta, konos* cone.]

metaconid (met·ah·**ko**·nid). In the tritubercular theory of evolution, the name given to the antero-internal cusp of a lower molar tooth. [see prec.]

metacresalol (met·ah·**kre**·sal·ol). $OHC_6H_4COOC_6H_4CH_3$, one of the three isomeric salicylic esters of the cresols with this formula. It is a white powder with antiseptic properties.

metacresol (met·ah·**kre**·sol). $CH_3C_6H_4OH$, an isomeric cresol found in the cresol obtained from coal tar. As a disinfectant it is more effective than ortho- or paracresol, and, being only sparingly soluble in water, is usually prepared as a soapy solution or in the form of an emulsion. The halogen derivative *parachlorometacresol* has greater activity (about 10 times), and is relatively less toxic; it is a constituent of a number of proprietary disinfectant solutions. **Metacresol acetate.** $CH_3C_6H_4OCOCH_3$, an anaesthetic and analgesic used in infections of the ear, nose and throat. **Metacresol purple, Metacresol sulphonephthalein.** A compound used as a pH indicator, its range being 1.5 (red) to 2.5 (yellow).

metacryptomerozoite (met·ah·**krip**·to·mer·o·**zo'**·ite). A merozoite of the second generation of the liver phase of the malaria parasite. [Gk *meta, kryptos* hidden, merozoite.]

metacryptozoite (met·ah·**krip**·to·**zo'**·ite). In malariology, an exo-erythrocytic stage that immediately follows the cryptozoite and precedes the erythrocytic trophozoite stage. [Gk *meta,* cryptozoite.]

metacyesis (**met**·ah·si·**e'**·sis). Ectopic pregnancy. *See* PREGNANCY. [Gk *meta,* cyesis.]

metadrasis (met·ah·**dra**·sis). Over-exertion of mind or body. [Gk *meta, draein* to do.]

metadysentery (met·ah·**dis**·en·ter·e). An obsolete term for dysentery-like attacks due to the meta- or para- dysentery bacilli (organisms other than the well-defined Shiga and Flexner types). As bacteriological knowledge has increased many of these organisms have been classified as Newcastle or other types of *Salmonella,* or as Schmitz or Sonne types of dysentery bacilli. [Gk *meta,* dysentery.]

metafemale (met·ah·**fe**·male). An individual with a greater dose of female determining genes than a normal female. The term is synonymous to, but less misleading than, *superfemale.* [Gk *meta,* L *femella* little woman.]

metagglutinin (met·ag·**loo**·tin·in). Partial agglutinin; an agglutinin present in an agglutinating serum that will act in lower dilutions on organisms or antigens closely related to the original antigen. [Gk *meta,* agglutinin.]

metagonimiasis (**met**·ah·gon·im·**i'**·as·is). An invasion by the trematode of the genus *Metagonimus.*

Metagonimus (met·ah·**gon**·im·us). A genus of Trematoda. **Metagonimus ovatus, Metagonimus yokogawai.** A very small fluke occurring in the duodenum of many mammals in temperate Asia. Human infections, harmless except in large numbers, are recorded from Siberia, China and Japan. Secondary hosts are snails, particularly of the genus *Melania.* The cercariae encyst in fish. [Gk *meta, gonimos* productive.]

metagranulocyte (met·ah·**gran**·ew·lo·site). A cell, characteristic of the phase in the development of the granular leucocyte intermediate between the myelocyte and granulocyte, containing neutrophilic, eosinophilic or basophilic granules and an indented bean-shaped nucleus. Also known as *metamyelocyte, progranulocyte* or *juvenile cell.* [Gk *meta,* granulocyte.]

metagrippal (met·ah·**grip**·al). Occurring as a sequel to influenza; postinfluenzal. [Gk *meta,* grippe.]

Metahexamide (met·ah·**hex**·am·ide). BP Commission approved name for 1-(3-amino-4-methylbenzenesulphonyl)-3-cyclohexylurea; it is used in the treatment of diabetes.

meta-icteric (**met**·ah·ik·**ter'**·ik). Occurring as a result of jaundice. [Gk *meta,* icterus.]

meta-infective (**met**·ah·in·**fek'**·tiv). Superseding an infection; in particular, denoting a febrile condition that occurs during the convalescent stage of an infectious disease. [Gk *meta,* infection.]

metakentrin (met·ah·**ken**·trin). The anterior pituitary luteinizing factor. [Gk *meta, kentron* goad.]

metakinesis (**met**·ah·kin·**e'**·sis). The movements of the asters towards opposite poles of a dividing cell. [Gk *meta, kinein* to move.]

metal (**met**·al). An element that is malleable, ductile, often lustrous and a conductor of electricity and heat. **Alkali metal.** Generic name for the monovalent metals including lithium, sodium, potassium, rubidium and caesium. **Bell metal.** An alloy of tin and copper. **Cliche metal.** A fusible alloy used in dentistry containing tin, lead, antimony and bismuth. **Colloidal metal.** A solution in which finely-divided metallic electrically-charged particles are dispersed; such a colloidal solution has catalytic properties of value in medicine. **Fusible metal.** A metal which melts at a relatively low temperature, round about the temperature of boiling water. They usually consist of a mixture of bismuth, lead and tin. [Gk *metallon* a mine.]

See also: BABBITT, D'ARCET, MELOTTE, WOOD.

metalbumin (met·al·**bew**·min). The mucin found in ovarian cysts. [Gk *meta,* albumin.]

metaldehyde (met·**al**·de·hide). $(CH_3CHO)_x$, a polymer of acetic aldehyde; a very inflammable white solid and used in tablet form for heating purposes. It is poisonous when taken internally.

metalepsy (met·al·**ep**·se). Chemical substitution; the replacement in a compound of atoms or groups of atoms by other atoms or groups. [obsolete term.] [Gk *metalepsis* alteration.]

metaleptic (met·al·**ep**·tik). 1. Relating or belonging to metalepsy. 2. Of muscle movement, interaction with another or others.

metalinguistics (**met**·ah·**ling'**·gew·is·tiks). The study of the cultural systems of behaviour patterns, its special correspondences with language structure and meaning; a theory of languages about languages.

metallaxis (met·al·**ax**·is). Alteration by a morbid process. [Gk *meta, allassein* to alter.]

metallocyanide (**met**·al·o·**si'**·an·ide). General name applied to the complex cyanides formed by metallic salts with an excess of a cyanide; argentocyanides and ferrocyanides are typical examples.

metalloid (**met**·al·oid). 1. Of the nature of a metal. 2. An element such as arsenic, which can be regarded as both a metal and a non-metal in properties. 3. Sometimes applied to a purely non-metallic element. [metal, Gk *eidos* form.]

metallophobia (**met**·al·o·**fo'**·be·ah). A morbid dread of metals and metal objects. [metal, phobia.]

metalloporphyrin (**met**·al·o·**por'**·fir·in). Any compounds formed by the combination of a porphyrin with a metal such as iron, copper, or magnesium, the metallic atom being attached to the nitrogen atoms in the structure of the porphyrin. These compounds are active biologically in promoting catalysis, and are widely distributed in nature, e.g. haem (iron) and chlorophyll (magnesium).

metallotherapy (**met**·al·o·**ther'**·ap·e). The treatment of disease, particularly that of nervous origin, by the application of various metals in the form of discs to the skin. [metal, therapy.]

metallurgy (met·al·er·je). The science and practice of using metals. [metal, Gk *ergein* to work.]

metaluetic (**met**·ah·lew·**et'**·ik). Metasyphilitic. [Gk *meta,* L *lyes* syphilis.]

metamer (**met**·ah·mer). In organic chemistry, applied to any compound which is metameric with another.

metamere (**met**·ah·meer). One of the series of more or less similar segments into which the embryo may be subdivided. [Gk *meta, meros* part.]

metameric (met·ah·**mer**·ik). Of or relating to a metamere, or marked by metamerism.

metamerism (met·**am**·er·izm). 1. In organic chemistry, a particular type of isomerism in which two compounds have the same percentage composition and empirical formulae, but differ widely in properties owing to dissimilarity in the constituent radicals. 2. The different disposition of metameres. [Gk *meta, meros* part.]

metameter (**met**·ah·me·ter). A quantity derived from an observation and conveying the magnitude of the phenomenon. [Gk *meta*, *metron* measure.]

metamorphic (met·ah·**mor**·fik). Exhibited by, or relating to metamorphosis.

metamorphology (met·ah·mor·**fol**′·o·je). The branch of biology that is concerned with the formal changes undergone by an organism during the course of its life. [Gk *meta*, *morphe* form, *logos* science.]

metamorphopsia (met·ah·mor·**fop**′·se·ah). The distortion of objects due to disturbance of retinal elements, usually by inflammation of the subjacent choroid. In *macropsia*, objects appear larger than normal owing to crowding together of retinal elements; in *micropsia*, objects appear smaller than normal owing to separation of retinal elements. **Cerebral metamorphopsia.** Distortion of the visual image due to a cerebral lesion. [metamorphosis, Gk *opsis* sight.]

metamorphosis (met·ah·**mor**·fo·sis). Change of form or structure, particularly the change of larvae into adult form, as with insects. **Fatty metamorphosis.** Fatty change; adipose degeneration. **Ovulational metamorphosis.** The changes that occur during ovulation. **Regressive metamorphosis, Retrograde metamorphosis, Retrogressive metamorphosis.** A degeneration. **Reversionary metamorphosis.** Anaplasia, or reversion to an embryonic type. **Metamorphosis sexualis paranoica.** The delusion that one has changed one's sex. **Tissue metamorphosis.** A change in the form or composition or habits of a tissue. **Viscous metamorphosis.** The building-up of platelet masses on a damaged blood vessel preliminary to thrombosis. [Gk change of form.]

metamorphotic (met·ah·mor·**fot**′·ik). Marked by, or relating to metamorphosis.

metamorphous (met·ah·**mor**·fus). Being in a state between the amorphous and the crystalline. [Gk *meta*, *morphe* form.]

metamyelocyte (met·ah·**mi**·el·o·site). An immature myelocyte; a primitive white cell that is intermediate between the myelocyte and the later granular leucocyte with lobed nuclei. Its nucleus is indented but not segmented or lobulated, whilst the cytoplasm has a brownish tint. [Gk *meta*, myelocyte.]

metanephric (met·ah·**nef**·rik). Relating to the metanephros.

metanephron (met·ah·**nef**·ron). A secretory unit of the metanephros, consisting of a Bowman's capsule, convoluted tubules and loop of Henle. [Gk *meta*, *nephros* kidney.]

metanephros (met·ah·**nef**·ros). The permanent kidney of reptiles, birds and mammals. [see prec.]

metaneutrophil, metaneutrophile (met·ah·**new**·tro·fil, met·ah·**new**·tro·file). Not giving a true stain with neutral dyes. [Gk *meta*, neutrophil.]

metaphase (**met**·ah·faze). That stage in meiotic or mitotic cell division at which the chromosomes lie on the equatorial plate of the spindle. **Metaphase plate.** *See* PLATE. **Metaphase spread.** *See* SPREAD. [Gk *meta*, phase.]

metaphrenia (met·ah·**fre**·ne·ah). A condition of mind in which the patient's attention is directed away from his relatives or associates, and turned towards his personal enrichment. [Gk *meta*, *phren* mind.]

metaphrenon (met·ah·**fren**·on). The area between the shoulders. [Gk *meta*, *phren* diaphragm.]

metaphyseal, metaphysial (met·ah·**fiz**·e·al). Relating to a metaphysis.

metaphysis (met·**af**·is·is). 1. The region of a long bone corresponding to the termination of the epiphysis and the beginning of the diaphysis. 2. Metamorphosis. [Gk *meta*, *phyein* to grow.]

metaphysitis (met·ah·fiz·**i**′·tis). Inflammation of the metaphysis of a long bone. [metaphysis, Gk *-itis* inflammation.]

metaplasia (met·ah·**pla**·ze·ah). The transformation of one tissue into another during adult life, as in the case of certain tumours. **Agnogenic myeloid metaplasia.** A group of blood disorders, related to myelophthisic anaemia, having immature myeloid white blood corpuscles and nucleated erythrocytes in large numbers in the circulating blood, together with severe anaemia, usually a hypoplastic fibrotic or sclerotic bone marrow, enlarged spleen and liver showing myeloid metaplasia, and occasionally jaundice resembling haemolytic anaemia. **Myeloid metaplasia.** The development of marrow tissue in a place normally free from such tissue. **Metaplasia of the pulp.** The state of a tooth pulp when it forms osteoid tissue instead of dentine. [Gk *meta*, *plassein* to mould.]

metaplasis (met·ah·**pla**·sis). In biology, the period of completed development in an individual or in an organism. [see prec.]

metaplasm (**met**·ah·plazm). Deutoplasm. [Gk *meta*, *plasma* something formed.]

metaplastic (met·ah·**plas**·tik). Pertaining to, or produced by metaplasia.

metaplex, metaplexus (**met**·ah·plex, met·ah·**plex**·us). The choroid plexus of the 4th ventricle. [Gk *meta*, plexus.]

metapneumonic (met·ah·new·**mon**′·ik). Occurring after pneumonia. [Gk *meta*, pneumonia.]

metapodalia (met·ah·pod·**a**′·le·ah). The metacarpal and metatarsal bones considered together. [Gk *meta*, *pous* foot.]

metapophysis (met·ah·**pof**·is·is). The mamillary process found on the superior articular process in certain vertebrae. [Gk *meta*, apophysis.]

metapore (**met**·ah·pore). The median aperture of the 4th ventricle (Magendie's foramen). [Gk *meta*, pore.]

metapsyche (met·ah·**si**·ke). The metencephalon. [Gk *meta*, *psyche* mind.]

metapsychics (met·ah·**si**·kix). Psychical research; parapsychology. [see prec.]

metapsychology (**met**·ah·si·**kol**′·o·je). In Freudian psycho-analysis, the skeletal outline of a theory to classify and explain the facts discovered by analytic procedures such as free association and dream interpretation. [Gk *meta*, psychology.]

metaptosis (met·ah·**to**·sis). Metastasis. [Gk *meta*, *ptosis* fall.]

Metaraminol (me·tar·**am**·in·ol). BP Commission approved name for (−)-2-amino-1-(3-hydroxyphenyl)propan-1-ol. **Metaraminol Tartrate BP 1973.** The hydrogen tartrate of metaraminol, a vasopressor agent given parenterally to combat arterial hypotension in emergencies.

metarteriole (met·ar·**teer**·e·ole). The terminal region of an arteriole. It is surrounded by isolated smooth muscle fibres and gives rise directly to capillaries. [Gk *meta*, arteriole.]

metarubricyte (met·ah·**roo**·bre·site). A normoblast in its later stage; a name suggested by Osgood but not widely accepted. [Gk *meta*, L *ruber* red, Gk *kytos* cell.]

metasellar (met·ah·**sel**·ar). At a distance from the sella turcica; descriptive of the site of an intracranial lesion, e.g. a neoplasm. [Gk *meta*, sella turcica.]

metasomatome (met·ah·**so**·mat·ome). One of the constrictions separating protovertebrae. [Gk *meta*, *soma* body, *temnein* to cut.]

metastable (met·ah·**sta**·bl). Capable of change under special conditions. [Gk *meta*, stable.]

metastasis (met·**as**·tas·is). The transfer of disease from its primary site to distant parts of the body by way of natural passages, blood vessels, lymphatics, or direct continuity. **Biochemical metastasis.** Metastasis of an abnormal biochemical product such as a hormone or an immune body. **Calcareous metastasis.** Metastatic calcification, the deposition of lime salts in such organs as the kidneys, lungs, or stomach, as the result of hyperparathyroidism or absorptive disease of bone. **Contact metastasis.** Transfer of disease across surfaces in contact. **Crossed metastasis.** The passage of material directly from the venous to the arterial circulation through a patent foramen ovale; paradoxical metastasis or embolism. **Direct metastasis.** Blood or lymph embolism **Implantation metastasis.** Transfer of tumour and other cells, including bacteria, by fluid or through the action of gravity, and their eventual lodgement in a distal situation. **Paradoxical metastasis, Retrograde metastasis.** Metastasis in a direction opposite to that of the blood flow. **Transplantation metastasis.** Transfer of cells or bacteria from one tissue to another. [Gk *meta*, *stasis* a standing.]

metastasize (met·as·tas·ize). To disseminate; to spread to a distant part, as, for example, in the case of an infection or a malignant tumour. [see prec.]

metastatic (met·ah·**stat**·ik). Of the nature of, caused by, or relating to metastasis.

metasternum (met·ah·**ster**·num). The xiphoid process of the sternum. [Gk *meta*, sternum.]

Metastrongylidae (**met**·ah·stron·**jil**'·id·e). A family of the nematode super-family or sub-order Metastrongyloidea. The genus *Metastrongylus* is of medical interest. [Gk *meta*, *stroggylos* round, *eidos* form.]

Metastrongyloidea (**met**·ah·stron·jil·**oid**'·e·tah). A super-family or sub-order of nematodes, classified either in the sub-order Strongylata of the order Rhabditata or as a sub-order of the order Strongylata. The family Metastrongylidae is of medical interest. [see prec.]

Metastrongylus (met·ah·**stron**·jil·us). A genus of round nematode worms. **Metastrongylus elongatus.** A cosmopolitan lung parasite of pigs, occasionally found in man. Intermediate hosts are earthworms. [Gk *meta*, *stroggylos* round.]

metastructure (**met**·ah·**struk**'·tcher). The fine structure of protoplasm, beyond the resolution of the microscope, consisting of orientated aggregates of molecules. [Gk *meta*, structure.]

metasyphilitic (**met**·ah·sif·il·**it**'·ik). 1. Following or occurring as a result of syphilis. 2. Relating to congenital syphilis. [Gk *meta*, syphilis.]

metatarsal (met·ah·**tar**·sal). 1. A metatarsal bone. 2. Relating to the metatarsus or a metatarsal bone.

metatarsal arteries. Dorsal metatarsal arteries [arteriae metatarseae dorsales (NA)]. Branches of the dorsalis pedis artery and of the arcuate artery which pass to the clefts between the toes, where they divide into dorsal digital vessels to the toes. **Plantar metatarsal arteries [arteriae metatarseae plantares (NA)].** Branches of the plantar arch which run to the clefts between the toes, where they divide into plantar digital arteries. At the base of the toes they send perforating branches [rami perforantes (NA)] upward to join the corresponding dorsal metatarsal arteries.

metatarsal bones [ossa metatarsalia I–V (NA)]. Five long bones forming the skeleton of the anterior part of the foot, articulating posteriorly with the tarsus and anteriorly with the phalanges.

Base [basis (NA)]. The proximal extremity.

Head [caput (NA)]. The rounded distal end.

Shaft [corpus (NA)]. The main part of the bone supporting the head distally and the base proximally. Except for that of the 1st metatarsal which is stout, these are long, slender, and tapering. They give attachment to the interosseous muscles.

metatarsal veins. Dorsal metatarsal veins [venae metatarseae dorsales pedis (NA)]. Veins formed in the clefts between the toes by the union of adjacent dorsal digital veins. They are tributaries of the dorsal venous arch of the foot. **Plantar metatarsal veins [venae metatarseae plantares (NA)].** The veins receiving the digital veins in the sole of the foot. They unite to form a plantar venous arch which is drained by the medial and lateral plantar veins.

metatarsalgia (**met**·ah·tars·**al**'·je·ah). Pain in the region of the heads of the metatarsal bones which occurs on walking and is associated with anatomical abnormalities of the toes, such as clawed toes; it may be a symptom of rheumatoid or some other acute arthritis. [metatarsus, Gk *algos* pain.]

See also: MORTON (T. G.).

metatarsectomy (met·ah·tars·**ek**'·to·me). Resection of one or more metatarsal bones. [metatarsus, Gk *ektome* a cutting out.]

metatarsometatarsal (met·ah·**tar**·so·met·ah·**tar**'·sal). Pertaining to the bones of the metatarsus in their relationship to each other.

metatarsophalangeal (met·ah·**tar**·so·fal·**an**'·je·al). Relating to the metatarsal bones and the phalanges, particularly to the joint between them.

metatarsus [NA] (met·ah·**tar**·sus). The bones of the foot between the tarsus and the toes. They consist of the five metatarsal bones. **Metatarsus adductocavus.** Metatarsus adductus combined with pes cavus. **Metatarsus adductovarus.** Metatarsus adductus combined with metatarsus varus. **Metatarsus adductus.** Medial deviation of the anterior part of the foot. **Metatarsus atavicus.** Congenital short 1st metatarsal. **Metatarsus latus.** Prolapse of the anterior metatarsal arch, causing a broad fore-foot. **Metatarsus primus elevatus.** A congenital deformity of the metatarsal of the big toe. **Metatarsus varus.** Fixed deflexion of the metatarsals inwards; a congenital deformity. [Gk *meta*, tarsus.]

metathalamus [NA] (met·ah·**thal**·am·us). The medial and lateral geniculate bodies. [Gk *meta*, thalamus.]

metathesis (met·**ath**·es·is). 1. The artificial shifting of a pathological process to another part. 2. In chemistry, the exchange of atoms between the molecules of different compounds; double decomposition. [Gk *meta*, *thesis* a placing.]

metathrombin (met·ah·**throm**·bin). Thrombin inactivated by standing. It is postulated to be a modified form produced by reversible dissociation of the components of thrombin. [Gk *meta*, thrombin.]

metatrophia, metatrophy (met·ah·**tro**·fe·ah, met·**at**·ro·fe). Atrophy of organs from malnutrition. [Gk *meta*, atrophy.]

metatuberculosis (**met**·ah·tew·ber·kew·**lo**'·sis). Positive tuberculin reactors in which no other clinical evidence of tuberculosis has been found. [Gk *meta*, tuberculosis.]

metatypical (met·ah·**tip**·ik·al). Term used to describe tissue which is formed of elements identical to that normal for the site, but atypical in that the components are not arranged in the normal pattern. [Gk *meta*, *typos* type.]

Metaxalone (met·**ax**·al·one). BP Commission approved name for 5-(3-5-xylyloxymethyl)oxazolidin-2-one; a muscle relaxant.

metaxylem (met·ah·**zi**·lem). In the development of xylem in a plant, the elements with thickened lignified vessels. [Gk *meta*, xylem.]

Metazoa (met·ah·**zo**·ah). A sub-kingdom of the Animalia which contains all multicellular forms except the Parazoa (sponges) and the Mesozoa. [Gk *meta*, *zoon* animal.]

metazoal, metazoan (met·a·**zo**·al, met·a·**zo**·an). Pertaining to or due to the metazoa.

Metazocine (met·**az**·o·seen). BP Commission approved name for 1,2,3,4,5,6 - hexahydro - 8 - hydroxy - 3,6,11 - trimethyl - 2,6 - methano - 3 - benzazocine; a narcotic analgesic.

Metchnikoff, Elie (b. 1845). Russian biologist in Paris.

Metchnikoff's law. When the body is attacked by bacteria, the polymorphonuclear leucocytes and monocytes become phagocytic.

Metchnikoff's theory. The cellular hypothesis of immunity and inflammation. According to this the phenomena of inflammation and immunity should be attributed to the phagocytic cells of the body rather than to humoral changes.

Metchnikoff's treatment. Treatment of intestinal disorder by a dietetic regimen of sour milk.

metencephalic (**met**·en·kef·**al**'·ik). Relating to the metencephalon.

metencephalon [NA] (met·en·**kef**·al·on). The part of the hindbrain which lies between the medulla oblongata and the midbrain; it consists of the pons, tegmental region of the pons, and the cerebellum. [Gk *meta*, *egkephalos* brain.]

metencephalospinal (**met**·en·kef·al·o·**spi**'·nal). Relating to the cerebellum and the spinal cord. [metencephalon, spine.]

meteoric (me·te·**or**·ik). 1. Relating or belonging to meteorism. 2. Belonging to the atmosphere. [Gk *meteoros* high in the air.]

meteorism (**me**·te·or·izm). A condition in which gas is present in the abdomen or intestines, with resultant distension and associated symptoms and signs. [Gk *meteorizein* to buoy up.]

meteorograph (me·te·**or**·o·graf). A device which produces a record of the variations in value of meteorological phenomena. [Gk *meteoros* high in the air, *graphein* to write.]

meteoropathology (**me**·te·or·o·path·**ol**'·o·je). The study of the effect of weather conditions on disease. [Gk *meteoros* high in the air, pathology.]

meteoropathy (me·te·or·**op'**·ath·e). Disease caused by climatic conditions. [Gk *meteoros* high in the air, *pathos* suffering.]

meteorophobia (me·te·or·o·**fo'**·be·ah). A morbid dread of meteors, and of natural phenomena in general. [Gk *meteoros* high in the air, phobia.]

meteororesistant (me·te·or·o·re·**zis'**·tant). Only slightly sensitive to atmospheric conditions. [Gk *meteoros* high in the air, resistant.]

meteorosensitive (me·te·or·o·**sen'**·sit·iv). Exceptionally sensitive to change of weather and to atmospheric conditions. [Gk *meteoros* high in the air, sensitive.]

meteorotropic (me·te·or·o·**trop'**·ik). Affected by weather conditions; applied to diseases as bearing on their inception and course. [Gk *meteoros* high in the air, *trope* a turning.]

meter (me·ter). 1. Any apparatus for the measurement of a physical quantity, usually by direct reading. 2. Metre, the unit of length. **Acuity meter.** An instrument used in the determination of the degree of acuteness, as well as the accuracy, of hearing. **Constancy meter.** An instrument used to maintain a controllable quantity at a constant desired value, e.g. for monitoring the dose rate at a point in an x-ray beam. **Counting-rate meter.** An instrument in which a meter indicates the average rate of arrival of electrical pulses, usually from a Geiger counter. **Dose-rate meter.** An instrument in which a meter indicates the x-ray or γ-ray dose rate at the detecting ionization chamber in roentgen or milliroenten/hour. It is used for protection in sites where a health hazard arises. **Electronic pH meter.** An instrument for the determination of the pH of a solution by the electronic measurement of an electromotive force dependent upon the pH. **Exposure meter.** A commercial photometer using a photoelectric cell, the current meter being calibrated to indicate directly the photographic exposure required for the measured light conditions. **Hot-wire meter.** One which measures direct or alternating electric current, the current heating a fine wire which alters in length and moves a pointer. **Light meter.** An instrument for the measurement of illuminance. **Phon meter.** An instrument for measuring the volume of sounds. **Rate meter.** *See* RATEMETER. [Gk *metron* measure.]

metergasia, metergasis (met·er·ga·ze·ah, met·er·ga·sis). An alteration in function. [Gk *meta, ergon* work.]

Metformin (met·for·min). BP Commission approved name for N^1N^1-dimethylbiguanide. **Metformin Hydrochloride BP 1973.** The hydrochloride of metformin, an antidiabetic agent with actions and uses similar to those of phenformin hydrochloride.

methacholine (meth·ah·**ko**·leen). **Methacholine bromide.** A compound with similar properties to the chloride, but not so hygroscopic and therefore more useful for oral use in tablet form. **Methacholine Chloride BPC 1973.** Acetyl-β-methylcholine chloride, $(CH_3)_3NCl{=}CH_2CH(CH_3)OCOCH_3$; a compound which, by mouth or by injection, has the muscarinic effects of acetylcholine, with the advantage of greater stability. It stimulates the parasympathetic nerve receptors, reducing the heart rate, lowering blood pressure and dilating the peripheral blood vessels; also it increases intestinal tone and the activity of the salivary and sweat glands. It is injected subcutaneously in selected cases of paroxysmal auricular tachycardia not responding to the usual therapeutic measures. For the prevention of attacks it is inferior to quinidine, and is of no apparent value in other forms of tachycardia or in auricular fibrillation. It is dangerous by the intravenous route as it may cause cardiac arrest, and is contra-indicated in bronchitic asthma or coronary occlusion. It may be used subcutaneously or by iontophoresis in the treatment of rheumatoid (atrophic) arthritis, Raynaud's disease, scleroderma, and other similar conditions of the extremities. Eye drops (2.5 per cent) are used in the diagnosis of Adie's pupil. Clinically, the value of this drug in the treatment of bladder dysfunction, atonic constipation, glaucoma, and hypertension has not been striking. Overdosage is counteracted by atropine.

Methacycline (meth·ah·**si**·kleen). BP Commission approved name for 4 - dimethylamino - 1,4,4a,5,5a,6,11,12a - octahydro - 3,5,10,12,12*a* - pentahydroxy - 6 - methylene - 1,11 - dioxonaphthacene - 2 - carboxamide. An antibiotic. **Methacycline Hydrochloride BP 1973.** The hydrochloride of methacycline, an antibiotic produced by synthesis from oxytetracycline.

methadol (meth·ad·ol). Dimepheptanol.

Methadone Hydrochloride BP 1973 (meth·ad·one hi·dro·**klor'**·ide). Amidone hydrochloride, $(CH_3)_2NCH(CH_3)CH_2C(C_6H_5)_2COC_2H_5HCl$. A synthetic analgesic resembling morphine in properties, but causing less severe withdrawal symptoms. For this reason it is often used to combat the symptoms produced by the withdrawal of morphine. Another advantage is its lesser effect on the alimentary canal and consequently smaller tendency to cause constipation.

Methadyl Acetate (meth·ad·il as·et·ate). BP Commission approved name for 6-dimethylamino-4,4-diphenyl-5-heptyl acetate. An analgesic compound synthesized from methadone hydrochloride and having a delayed morphine-like action. It is not in general use.

methaem (met·heem). Haematin, oxidized haem, $C_{34}H_{32}N_4O_4FeOH$. A blue-black amorphous substance formed by the oxidation of haem, the essential feature of the oxidation being the conversion of iron from the ferrous to the ferric state. It is insoluble in water and many organic solvents, but dissolves in alkalis and glacial acetic acid to give solutions of *alkaline* and *acid haematin* respectively. [Gk *meta*, haem.]

methaemalbumin (met·he·mal·**bew'**·min). A haemoglobin derivative having a similar structure to methaemoglobin, but containing plasma-albumin in place of globulin. It is produced from extracorpuscular haemoglobin in certain haemolytic anaemias, and has no oxygen-carrying function. [Gk *meta, haima* blood, albumin.]

methaemalbuminaemia (met·he·mal·bew·min·**e'**·me·ah). The presence of methaemalbumin in the blood.

methaemoglobin (met·he·mo·**glo'**·bin). *See* HAEMOGLOBIN.

methaemoglobinaemia (met·he·mo·glo·bin·**e'**·me·ah). The presence of methaemoglobin in the blood; the clinical condition resulting from the presence of abnormal amounts of methaemoglobin in the circulation, that is, when more than 1 per cent of the total haemoglobin is present as methaemoglobin. [methaemoglobin, Gk *haima* blood.]

methaemoglobinuria (met·he·mo·glo·bin·**ewr'**·e·ah). Methaemoglobin in the urine. [methaemoglobin, urine.]

Methallibure (meth·**al**·ib·ewr). BP Commission approved name for *N*-methylthiocarbamoyl-*N* - (1 - methylallylthiocarbamoyl) hydrazine; it is used in the suppression of pituitary, ovarian and adrenal function.

Methamphazone (meth·**am**·faz·one). BP Commission approved name for 4-amino-6-methyl-2-phenyl-3-pyridazone; an analgesic and antirheumatic agent.

methamphetamine (meth·am·**fet**·am·een). Methylamphetamine.

Methandienone BP 1973 (meth·an·**di**·en·one). 17β-Hydroxy-17α-methylandrosta-1,4-dien-3-one; an anabolic agent.

methane (me·thane). CH_4, the simplest of the hydrocarbons; a colourless odourless gas burning with a clear flame. It occurs naturally in the gas from oil wells, and occluded in coal seams (firedamp); the decomposition of vegetable matter in swamps also produces the gas. It is an important constituent of wood gas and coal gas, obtained by the distillation of wood and coal respectively. **Methane series.** The paraffins, a series of saturated hydrocarbons of general formula C_nH_{2n+2}, the first member of which is methane.

methanol (meth·an·ol). Methyl alcohol.

Methanomonas (meth·an·**om**·on·as). A genus of bacteria of the family Pseudomonadaceae, consisting of monotrichous cells capable of obtaining energy from the oxidation of methane to carbon dioxide and water. The type species is *Methanomonas methanica.* [methane, Gk *monas* unit.]

methantheline (meth·**an**·thel·een). β-Diethylmethylaminoethyl-9-xanthene carboxylate, $CH_2(C_6H_4)_2CHCOOCH_2CH_2N(CH_3)(C_2H_5)_2$. A parasympathetic drug having effects on the parasympathetic nerve receptors like atropine but also combining a ganglionic blocking action like tetraethylammonium chloride; toxic doses have a curare-like action at the neuromuscular junction. The drug reduces the motility of the gastro-intestinal tract and reduces secretions of saliva, gastric and pancreatic juices, also perspiration; it also causes mydriasis and cycloplegia in the eye. It is used clinically for its anticholinergic spasmolytic action, and as a valuable adjunct in the treatment of peptic ulcer, chronic hypertrophic gastritis, pylorospasm, hyperemesis gravidarum, biliary dyskinesia, pancreatitis, hypermotility of the small intestine, spastic colon, urethral and urinary-bladder spasm, hyperhidrosis, and control of salivation. Side-effects include dryness of the mouth, and some cycloplegia. It is administered orally or parenterally by the intramuscular or intravenous route. **Methantheline bromide.** β-diethylmethylaminoethyl-9-xanthene carboxylate bromide; an anti-parasympathomimetic agent with the peripheral action of atropine and the ganglionic blocking effect of the methonium drugs. It is useful as an adjunct in peptic ulcer and gastritis, and is usually administered orally.

Methanthelinium Bromide (meth·**an**·thel·e′·ne·um **bro**·mide). BP Commission approved name for methantheline bromide.

Methaphenilene (meth·ah·**fen**·il·een). BP Commission approved name for *N,N*-dimethyl-*N′*-phenyl-*N*-(2-thienylmethyl)-ethylenediamine, $C_4H_3SCH_2N(C_6H_5)CH_2CH_2N(CH_3)_2$. An antihistamine drug which is therapeutically effective, and shows a low incidence of side-effects. It is used in the treatment of allergic conditions such as seasonal hay fever, perennial vasomotor rhinitis, urticaria, angioneurotic oedema, serum sickness, and reactions to antibiotics.

Methapyrilene (meth·ah·**pir**·il·een). BP Commission approved name for *NN′*-dimethyl-*N′* - (2 - pyridyl)-*N′* - (2 - thenyl)ethylenediamine. **Methapyrilene hydrochloride.** The hydrochloride of the base, an antihistamic drug of moderate therapeutic effect.

Methaqualone BP 1973 (meth·**ak**·wal·one). 2-Methyl-3-*o*-tolylquinazolin-4-one; a hypnotic.

Metharbitone (meth·**ar**·bit·one). BP Commission approved name for 5,5-diethyl-1-methylbarbituric acid; an anticonvulsant.

Methazolamide (meth·az·**ol**·am·ide). BP Commission approved name for 5-acetylimino-4-methyl-2-sulphamoyl-1,3,4-thiadiazoline; it is used in the treatment of glaucoma.

Methdilazine (meth·**dil**·az·een). BP Commission approved name for 10-(1-methylpyrrolidin-3-ylmethyl)phenothiazine; an antihistaminic agent.

methelepsia (meth·e·**lep**·se·ah). Irresistible urge to take alcohol. [Gk *methe* strong drink, *lambanein* to take.]

methenamine (meth·**en**·ah·**meen**′). USA synonym for Hexamine.

Methenolone (meth·**en**·o·lone). BP Commission approved name for 17β-hydroxy-1-methyl-5α-endrost-1-en-3-one; an anabolic agent.

Methetoin (meth·et·**o**·in). BP Commission approved name for 5-ethyl-1-methyl-5-phenylhydantoin; an anticonvulsant.

Methicillin (meth·e·**sil**·in). BP Commission approved name for 6-(2,6-dimethoxybenzamido)penicillanic acid; an antibiotic. **Methicillin Sodium BP 1973.** The sodium monohydrate of methicillin, a white microcrystalline powder, soluble in water and in alcohol, insoluble in fixed oils and in liquid paraffin; an antibiotic which is effective against penicillinase-producing strains of staphylococci.

Methimazole (meth·**im**·az·ole). BP Commission approved name for 1-methyl-2-mercaptoimidazole, $C_6H_6N_2S$. A powerful antithyroid drug, said to be one hundred times as active as thiouracil in its ability to block the natural conversion of iodine to thyroxine.

Methiodal Sodium (meth·**i**·o·dal **so**·de·um). BP Commission approved name for sodium iodomethanesulphonate, CH_2ISO_3Na, used as an opaque medium in the genito-urinary tract; it is given intravenously or directly into the kidney pelvis by a catheter. It has a diuretic action which reaches its peak within half an hour of injection.

methioninaemia (meth·**i**·o·nin·e·me·ah). Raised level of methionine in plasma, observed in many metabolic disorders. [methionine, Gk *haima* blood.]

methionine (meth·**i**·o·neen). α-Amino-γ-methylmercaptobutyric acid, $CH_3SCH_2CH_2CH(NH_2)COOH$. An amino acid essential in diet for the maintenance of health, and occurring in protein hydrolysates. It is especially important in nutrition as one of the chief dietary sources of methyl groups necessary for the biological methylation processes of the body, the only other sources being choline and betaine. **Adenosyl methionine.** A compound in which an adenosyl residue is attached to the sulphur atom of the amino acid, methionine; it serves as an important methyl donor, for example in the synthesis of choline phospholipids and in the synthesis of the catecholamine, noradrenaline. The removal of a methyl group leaves *adenosyl homocysteine* which may, in turn, be re-methylated. **Methionine-S^{35}.** Containing radioactive sulphur by which the presence and concentration of methionine can be detected and estimated in tissues.

Methisazone (meth·**i**·saz·one). BP Commission approved name for 1-methylindoline-2,3-dione-3-thiosemicarbazone, $C_{10}H_{10}N_4OS$; an antiviral agent used in the chemical prophylaxis of smallpox and the treatment of progressive lesions due to vaccinia virus. The mode of action is unknown but thought to occur late in the viral replication cycle.

Methixene (meth·**ix**·een). BP Commission approved name for 9-(1-methylpiperid-3-ylmethyl)thiaxanthen; it is used in the treatment of parkinsonism.

methmyoglobin (meth·mi·o·**glo**′·bin). *See* MYOGLOBIN.

Methocarbamol (meth·o·**kar**·bam·ol). BP Commission approved name for 2-hydroxy-3-*o*-methoxyphenoxypropyl carbamate; it is used for the relief of muscle spasm and pain.

method (**meth**·od). 1. A scheme of classification. 2. A systematic procedure for the achievement of any end, e.g. a treatment of disease, a surgical operation, a chemical process, or an analytical test. *See* OPERATION, STAIN, TEST, TREATMENT. **A.B.C. (alum, blood, clay) method.** A rough method of treating crude sewage by adding to it alum, blood, clay, charcoal, or other substances. These precipitate the sludge and deodorize the sewage. It has been superseded by modern methods of sewage purification. **Absorption method.** A method used in serology to obtain a single antibody by absorbing the crude antisera with various bacteria to remove all the other antibodies. **Acid-haematin method.** Any method of haemoglobin estimation in which the blood is diluted with normal hydrochloric acid in order to change the haemoglobin into acid haematin, the yellow colour of which is more easily compared with a standard. **Antiserum method.** The precipitin reaction for blood. *See* REACTION. **Brine floatation method.** A method for separating metazoal ova from faecal matter by emulsifying it in saturated sodium chloride or other salt solution so that the ova float, whereas most other matter sinks. **Cat method.** A method for the assay of digitalis. **Cathartic method.** Treatment by mental purification by the release of repressed complexes and emotions. **Copenhagen method.** Holger Nielsen method of artificial respiration. *See* RESPIRATION, ARTIFICIAL. **Copper-sulphate method.** A method for specific gravity of blood. **Cubicle method.** The treatment of patients suffering from an infectious or contagious disease, by isolation or segregation in a chamber or cell ward (sometimes called a *cubicle ward*). **Direct method.** Of ophthalmoscopy; a method of examining the fundus of the eye. A reflecting or self-illuminating ophthalmoscope is used, nowadays almost exclusively the latter. A bright concentrated beam of light is reflected through the patient's pupil by a mirror or prism and the fundal details brought into focus by a battery of lenses which can be moved in front of the examiner's eye. An erect picture is obtained with a magnification of some 14 diameters. **Erlangen method.** Single massive tumour dose irradiation treatment delivered through multiple fields. **Falling-drop method.** 1. A method of determining specific gravity, for example, of plasma, by dropping the plasma for assay into a series of liquids of known specific gravity (e.g. copper-sulphate solutions of increasing concentrations) or into a layered solution of two liquids which results in a gradient of increasing specific gravity with depth. 2. Method of determining the electronic charge by observing the rate of fall of electrically-charged minute oil drops under the combined influence of gravity and an applied electric field of known strength. **Flame-photometer method.** For sodium and potassium in blood: this method by reason of its speed and accuracy has now largely replaced chemical methods for determining sodium and potassium. In the simplest form of instrument an accurately measured dilution of serum in water is sprayed by means of an atomizer into a colourless flame, and the characteristic sodium and potassium light produced is measured by means of a photo-electric cell and galvanometer after removal of non-specific light by passage through narrow-band light filters. The instrument is calibrated by spraying standard sodium and potassium solutions. **Flash method.** A method of pasteurizing milk by raising the temperature to 81°C and then rapidly chilling. **Floatation method.** A method for examining faeces for metazoal ova and protozoal cysts, dependent upon the fact that the various ova and cysts have fairly constant specific gravities. When faecal material is added to solutions of specific gravities just above these, the ova and cysts float and can be propelled off or otherwise separated for examination, e.g. brine floatation (see above). **Fogging method.** In refraction of the eye: an attempt to relax the accommodation during subjective testing by placing a much stronger convex lens than is required in front of both eyes, and then gradually reducing the strength until the best vision is just obtained. **Hippocratic method.** A method of reducing dislocation of the shoulder by leverage over the surgeon's foot in the axilla. **Holding method.** A method of pasteurizing milk by heating to 65°C and keeping it at that temperature for from 30 to 45 minutes. **Indirect method.** Of ophthalmoscopy: a method of examining the fundus of the eye. The examiner, looking through a central hole in a concave mirror, reflects a bright light into the pupil of the patient's eye from a distance of about 50 cm. In his other hand he holds a strong convex lens about 16 dioptres in front of the patient's eye at a distance equal to its focal length. The examiner will then see an inverted aerial image of the fundus with a magnification of 4 diameters. Not used now, except for retinal-detachment work. **Japanese method.** A method for fixing paraffin sections to glass slides in which a thin layer of glycerin albumin is first applied to the slide and coagulated by heat before the sections are floated on with water. **Least-squares method.** A method for combining discrepant observations of one or more unknown constants, according to which the best estimate is that for which the sum of the squared deviations of the observations from the values expected on this estimate is least. **Light-field method.** A method of dust counting using the ordinary microscope illumination in which light is transmitted through the glass slide or cover-glass. **Metatrophic method.** A procedure that entails the modification of nutrition so as to determine or increase the action of a drug taken concomitantly. **No-touch method.** In treatment of wounds: a method of cleaning and dressing a wound without introducing the fingers into it, all manipulations being performed with sterile instruments. **Open drop method.** A method of dropping volatile anaesthetic on to gauze covering a metal frame during induction and maintenance of anaesthesia. First used by Sir James Young Simpson in 1847. **Oscillating-crystal method.** A method of x-ray spectrometry in which monochromatic x-rays are used and Bragg reflection obtained by oscillating the crystal so that it passes through the reflecting angles. **Oxford cup method.** A method of assaying penicillin developed at Oxford, based on the inhibition of bacterial growth on a solid medium. **"Permutit" method.** *See* FOLIN AND BELL METHOD. **Powder method.** A method of x-ray spectrometry in which the crystal is powdered so that the orientation of the powdered crystalline fragments is random, some being at the correct angle to produce Bragg reflection. **Prussian blue method.** A histochemical technique for the demonstration of iron deposits in tissues. **Rotating-crystal method.** A method of x-ray spectrometry similar to the oscillating-crystal method except that the crystal is rotated. **Seminal-vesicle method.** An assay method for androgenic activity, in which castrated rats are used. **Spot method.** Of localizing pulmonary abscess: 0.2 ml of Iodized Oil BP 1973 and 0.2 ml of 0.5 per cent methylene blue are injected together into an intercostal space at the site selected for drainage (from study of postero-anterior and lateral radiographs). A fresh syringe containing only methylene blue is now attached to the needle still in position and, as the needle is withdrawn, it is injected into the overlying tissues of skin to leave a guide for the operator. Further radiographs will then show the relation of the iodized oil spot to the abscess and the dye will confirm the position of the spot at the time of operation after the incision is made. Measurements taken from the radiographs can then be applied to localize accurately the abscess at operation. **Staining methods.** *See* STAINS AND STAINING METHODS. **Thick-film method.** A method of examining blood for malaria parasites, in which a drop of blood is spread thickly with a needle on a slide and dried; it is then dehaemoglobinized, fixed, and stained, usually by Giemsa's method. **Uranium-acetate method.** For total phosphates in urine: urine is titrated with standard uranium-acetate solution, using potassium-ferrocyanide solution as external indicator. The end point is shown by the appearance of a reddish colour in the indicator. **Urease method.** The determination of urea in body fluids by any procedure employing the specific enzyme urease which converts urea to ammonium carbonate. [Gk *methodos* pursuit of knowledge.]

See also: ABBE, ABBOTT (A. C.), ABBOTT (E. G.), ACHUCARRO, ADAMS, ADAMSON, ADDIS, AHLFELD, ALTMANN, ANJESKY, ANTYLLUS, ARCHER, ARMSTRONG (A. R.), ARNOLD, ASKENSTEDT, AYER (S. H.), BABCOCK (M. J.), BACELLI, BAER (W. S.), BANG (B. L. F.), BANG (I. C.), BARÉTY, BARKER (S. B.), BARRAQUER (I.), BECK (E. G.), BENARIO, BENDA (C.), BENEDICT (S. R.), BERGONIÉ, BERNHEIM, BETHE (A.), BETHEA, BIELSCHOWSKY, BIER, BIRCH-HIRSCHFELD (F. V.), BIVINE, BLACK (O. F.), BLOOR, BODANSKY, BODIAN, BONNAIRE, BOUCHUT, BRAND, BRATTON, BRAUER, BREHMER, BREISKY, BROCQ, BUELAU, BUIST (R. C.), BURNS (J. W.), BUTLER, CARREL, CHERVIN, CHITTY, CHRISTIANSEN, CIACCIO (C.), CINISELLI, CLARK (E. P.), COLLIP, COOKE, CORLEY, COUTARD, COX (W. H.), CREDÉ, CULLEN (G. E.), DAKIN, DARE, DEFER, DENIS (W. G.), DIAMOND, DORNER, DRUMMOND (J. C.), DRURY, DUBOIS (P. C.), DUKE, DUNCAN (C. H.), EGGLESTON, EHRLICH, EICKEN, EINHORN, ESBACH, EVANS, EVE, EXNER, FARMER, FARRANT, FAUST, FILDES, FISKE, FITZ (R.), FOLIN, FONTANA (A.), FRANKE, FREUD, FRIDERICIA, GABASTOU, GEHUCHTEN, GERLACH, GEROTA, GERSH, GIVENS, GLUECK, GOLGI, GRAEUPNER, GRAM, GREENBERG, GRIFFITH, GROCCO, GUTMAN, GUTSTEIN, HADEN, HAGEDORN (H. C.), HAMMERSCHLAG, HANDLEY (W. S.), HARRISON (L. W.), HART, HARTEL, HARVEY, HAY (M.), HELD, HELLER (A. L. G.), HENRIQUES, HERXHEIMER, HEUBLEIN, HISS, HOFBAUER, HOLFELDER, HORTEGA, HOWARD, HOYER, HUNT (R.), HUNTER (G.), HUNTER (J.), JENSEN (B. N.), JENSEN (O.), JUNG (C. G.), KAISERLING, KALLIUS, KARR, KAUFMANN, KENNY, KIENBOECK, KING (E. J.), KIRSTEIN, KJELDAHL, KNOPF, KOCH (F. C.), KOCHER, KOROTKOFF, KRAMER, KRISTELLER, KRUEGER, KUTSCHER, LABORDE, LANDSBERG, LANDSTEINER, LANGHANS, LARDENNOIS, LAUE, LEAKE, LEVADITI, LEWISOHN, LINDEMANN (E. E.), LINSER, LOEWIT, LORENZ, LYON (B. B. V.), MCARTHUR, MCCRUDDEN, MCINTOSH, MCMEEKIN, MALASSEZ, MALFATTI, MALL, MARCHI, MARFAN, MARRIOTT (W. M.), MARSHALL (C. M.), MARSHALL (E. K.), MAURICEAU, MAYLARD-SONNENBURG, MAYO (C. H.), MEDUNA, METT, MILNE, MOELLER (A.), MORESTIN, MORISON, MUELENGRACHT, MUELLER (A.), MUIR (R.), MURPHY (J. B.), MYERS, NAEGELI, NEELSEN, NEILL (J. M.), NEISSER (M.), NEWTON (W. H.), NICOLLE, NIKIFOROFF, NIRENSTEIN, NISSL, NOCHT, O'BRIEN, OCHSNER, OERTEL, OGATA, ORR, ORSI, OSBORNE, OSTERBERG, OTTO (F. W. R.), PACHON, PAJOT, PAL, PARKER (H. M.), PATERSON (J. R. K.), PAUCHET, PAVLOV, PEDLEY, PELKAN, PÉRIER, PERTHES, PETROFF, PFAHLER, PFIFFNER, PICKWORTH, PONDER, PRICE-JONES, RAMÓN Y CAJAL, RANVIER, RASORI, REHFUSS, REINHOLD, REVERDIN (J. L.), RIBBERT, RICHARDSON, RIDEAL ROBINOW, ROE, ROMANOVSKY, ROSENHEIM (O.), SACKETT, SAHLI, SATTERTHWAITE, SCHAFER, SCHALES, SCHIFF (A.), SCHILLING, SCHLOESSER, SCHOENHEIMER, SCHUELLER (K. H. A. L. M.), SCHWENINGER, SEMPLE, SENDROY, SHAFFER, SHERREN, SHIELS, SHOHL, SIPPY, SLUDER, SMELLIE,

SMITH (H.), SNELL (E. E.), SOERENSEN, SØRENSEN, SOULIGOUX, SPERRY, STAS, STEHLE, STEINACH, STEIDA (L.), STODDARD, STOLL, STROEBE, STRONG (F. M.), SUBBAROW, SUMMERSON, SUMNER, TELEMANN, THANE, THEIS, THIERSCH, THOMA, TISDALL, TRUETA, TUTHILL, UNNA, VAN GIESON, VAN SLYKE, VEIT, VOLHARD (F.), WALDEYER-HARTZ, WALKER, WALLACE (G. B.), WALLHAUSER, WARDELL, WARING, WATSON (B. P.), WEIGERT, WEIGL (R.), WEINBACH, WELCKER, WESTERGREN, WHEAL, WHITEHEAD (J. M.), WHITEHORN, WILLIS, WINTROBE, WOHLGEMUTH, WONG, WU, WYETH, YAMAGIWA, YOUNGBURG, ZIEHL.

methodism (meth·od·izm). The school or teaching of the Methodists.

Methodists (**meth**·od·ists). Members of a school of medicine founded by Themison, a famous physician of Laodicea, about 50 BC. He introduced exact rules and theories (methods) for the practice of medicine, in contrast to the systems of the empiricists and dogmatists.

methoestrol (meth·e·strol). *αβ*-Diethyl-4,4′-dihydroxy-3,3′-dimethylstilbene, a synthetic oestrogen.

Methohexitone (meth·o·**hex**·it·one). BP Commission approved name for *α*-(±)-5-allyl-1-methyl-5-(1-methylpent-2-ynyl)barbituric acid; a short-acting agent used for intravenous anaesthesia.

Methoin BP 1973 (meth·**o**·in). 5-Ethyl-3-methyl-5-phenyl-hydantoin, an anticonvulsant of the hydantoin group, used in epilepsy.

methol (**meth**·ol). Methyl alcohol.

methomania (meth·o·**ma**·ne·ah). Insanity due to alcoholic excess. [Gk *methe* strong drink, mania.]

methondienone. (meth·on·**di**·en·on). An anabolic steroid used to improve athletic performance and used both in men and women because it is said to have little if any androgenic effect.

methonium (meth·o·ne·um). General name for organic bases which are members of a polymethylene bis [trimethylammonium] series of formula $(CH_3)_3N^+(CH_2)_nN^+(CH_3)_3$. The important homologues are pentamethonium where $n=5$, hexamethonium where $n=6$, and decamethonium where $n=10$. Salts of the penta- and hexamethonium bases are most active in blocking autonomic ganglia, while those of the decamethonium base produce neuromuscular block and are used as muscle relaxants. [methylene, ammonium.]

methorphinan (meth·**or**·fin·an). Levorphanol.

Methoserpidine BP 1973 (meth·o·**ser**·pid·een). 10-Methoxydeserpidine, used in the treatment of mild arterial hypertension (usually in conjunction with more powerful hypotensive drugs). Its action and uses are similar to those of reserpine; excessive doses cause Parkinsonism and depression, sometimes with suicidal tendencies.

Methotrexate BP 1968 (meth·o·**trex**·ate). A mixture of 4-amino-10-methylfolic acid and related substances, a cytotoxic drug used in the treatment of neoplastic disease. It is also an immunosuppressant, and a folic acid suppressant used in the treatment of severe psoriasis.

Methotrimeprazine (**meth**·o·tri·**mep**′·raz·een). BP Commission approved name for 10-(3-dimethylamino-2-methyl-propyl)2-methoxyphenothiazine; it is used in the treatment of neuroses.

Methoxamine (meth·**ox**·am·een). BP Commission approved name for 2-amino-1-(2,5-dimethoxyphenyl)propan-1-ol. **Methoxamine Hydrochloride BPC 1973.** The hydrochloride of Methoxamine, a synthetic sympathomimetic amine which produces prolonged vasoconstriction of peripheral vessels and a rise of arterial blood pressure. It is used to raise blood pressure in surgical shock during major operations, and in hypotensive states including the excessive hypotension produced by ganglion blockade.

Methoxyflurane BP 1973 (meth·**ox**·e·**floo**′·rane). 2,2-Dichloro-1,1-difluoroethyl methyl ether, a potent non-flammable non-explosive volatile anaesthetic with a high boiling point (103.5°C); useful for the production of analgesia, but in large amounts may cause renal damage.

methoxyl (meth·**ox**·il). The organic monovalent group, CH_3O–.

Methoxyphenamine (meth·**ox**·e·**fen**′·am·een). BP Commission approved name for 1-*o*-methoxyphenyl-2-methylamino-propane, an agent used as an antispasmodic.

methscopolamine bromide (**meth**·sko·**pol**′·am·een **bro**·mide). An anti-parasympathomimetic agent used for peptic ulcer, gastric disorders, etc.

Methsuximide (meth·**sux**·im·ide). BP Commission approved name for N*α*-dimethyl-*α*-phenylsuccinimide; an anticonvulsant.

Methyclothiazide (**meth**·e·klo·**thi**′·az·ide). BP Commission approved name for 6-chloro - 3 - chloromethyl - 3,4 - dihydro - 2 - methyl - 7 - sulphamoylbenzo - 1,2,4 - thiadiazine 1,1-dioxide; it is used in the treatment of hypertension.

methyl (**meth**·il). The monovalent radical, CH_3–, derived from methyl alcohol. **Methyl acetanilide.** $CH_3C_6H_4NHCOCH_3$, a compound which has been used as an antipyretic and analgesic. **Methyl acetylsalicylate.** $CH_3COOC_6H_4COOCH_3$, the methyl ester of acetylsalicylic acid, used as a fixative in perfumes. **Methyl alcohol.** A colourless liquid of characteristic odour and burning taste, obtained by the destructive distillation of wood, or synthesized from water gas. It is more slowly oxidized in the body than ethyl alcohol, and the process is incomplete, formic acid and formaldehyde being produced. It depresses the central nervous system, and its toxic oxidation products cause optic atrophy and acidosis. It is used only as a solvent, and never administered internally. **Methyl aldehyde.** Formaldehyde. **Methyl anthranilate.** Methyl-2-amino-benzoate, $NH_2C_6H_4COOCH_3$, a constituent present in a number of essential oils, but usually prepared synthetically. It is used as a perfume. **Methyl cacodylate.** $[(CH_3)_2AsO_2]_2Hg$, a compound which was used in the treatment of syphilis, the cacodylic acid radical being said to enhance the action of the mercury. **Methyl cellulose.** Cellulose methyl ether; a compound prepared from wood pulp or cotton by methylation. It is soluble in cold water, and is used as a water-soluble gum in the preparation of adhesives, and as a thickening agent and protective colloid in emulsions. Medicinally it has value as a bulk laxative as it swells and increases the intestinal contents. *See* METHYLCELLULOSE. **Methyl chloride.** CH_3Cl, a gas prepared by distilling methyl alcohol with hydrochloric acid; it has narcotic properties and may cause hepatic damage. **Methyl cyanide.** Acetonitrile. **Methyl ether.** $(CH_3)_2O$, a colourless gas with anaesthetic properties. **Methyl eugenol.** $C_6H_3(OCH_3)_2C_3H_5$, a compound present in oleum myrciae; it has aromatic properties. **Methyl hydrate.** Methyl alcohol. **Methyl hydride.** Methane. **Methyl Hydroxybenzoate BP 1973.** $C_6H_4(OH)COOCH_3$, a white crystalline substance, lightly soluble in water, used to deter bacterial growth in solutions or emulsions of drugs. It is also employed with the propyl analogue in solution for eye drops. **Methyl iodide.** CH_3I, a colourless transparent liquid used in methylation and in microscopy. It has also been used as a vesicant. **Methyl morphine.** Codeine. **Methyl orange.** Sodium *p*-dimethylamino-azobenzenesulphonate, an indicator over the range pH 3.1 to 4.4, being yellow in alkaline solutions and red in acid. **Methyl oxide.** Methyl ether. **Methyl paraben, Methyl parahydroxybenzoate.** Methyl Hydroxybenzoate BP 1973 (see above). **Methyl Phenidate.** BP Commission approved name for *α*-phenyl-*α*-(2 piperidyl)- acetic acid methyl ester, a stimulant for the treatment of exhaustion, depression, narcolepsy and emaciation. *See* METHYLPHENIDATE. **Methyl phenol.** Cresol. **Methyl red.** *p*-Dimethylamino-azobenzene-*o*-carboxylic acid, an indicator over the range pH 4.4 to 6.2. It is red in acid solutions and yellow in alkaline. **Methyl rosaniline chloride.** Methyl, crystal, or gentian violet, being a mixture of methyl derivatives of pararosaniline hydrochloride. **Methyl Salicylate BP 1973.** $C_6H_4(OH)COOCH_3$, a colourless or pale-yellow liquid with an aromatic odour and taste. It has a local irritant and rubefacient action, and is used as a local application to inflamed joints, or as a liniment in non-articular rheumatism. **Methyl tyrosine.** An alkaloid found in cabbage plant. **Methyl violet.** One of the rosaniline dyes; it is used as a bacterial stain, and has germicidal properties towards some Gram-positive organisms. **Methyl yellow.** Dimethylamino-azobenzene; a compound used as an indicator (pH 2.9 to 4.0) in analysis of the gastric contents. [Gk *methy* wine, *hyle* matter.]

methylacetylcholine (**meth**·il·as·et·il·**ko**′·leen). Acetyl-β-methylcholine, $CH_3COOCH(CH_3)CH_2N(CH_3)_3OH$. The β-methyl derivative of acetylcholine. It has the muscarinic but not the nicotinic actions of acetylcholine, is much more stable, and can be given orally; its effects are abolished by atropine. Clinically it is used in cardiac arrhythmias, especially paroxysmal tachycardia, in various vascular diseases such as Raynaud's disease, in varicose ulcers by iontophoresis, and also, by the same method, as a palliative in chronic arthritis. While it stimulates the gastro-intestinal tract and the bladder, it is not as effective as neostigmine for postoperative ileus and urine retention.

methylal (**meth**·il·al). Formal, $CH_2(OCH_3)_2$. A compound formed by the condensation of methyl alcohol and formaldehyde; used as a soporific.

methylamine (meth·il·**am**·een). CH_3NH_2. The simplest member of the primary aliphatic amine series. It is a colourless gas with a fishy ammoniacal odour, which occurs in the distillation of bones and wood, and the decomposition of fish protein.

methyl-*p*-aminophenol sulphate (**meth**·il·par·ah·**am**·in·o·**fe**′·nol·**sul**·fate). A photographic developing substance which causes a severe haemolytic anaemia when ingested by mistake.

methylamphetamine (**meth**·il·am·**fet**′·am·een). $C_6H_5CH_2CH(CH_3)NH(CH_3)$, a sympathomimetic amine chemically related to ephedrine, but having properties very similar to amphetamine; the laevorotatory isomer is less active than the D-form. It is a powerful cerebral stimulant, causing increased wakefulness, elevation of mood, and a lessening of fatigue. It tends, however, to be habit-forming and, like amphetamine, may be subject to abuse. In common with other sympathomimetic amines it causes a rise in blood pressure, but has a long duration of action. It is a valuable pressor agent, and is used to restore blood pressure during and after operations; its central actions are used to postpone sleep and to relieve mental depression (BPC 1959). The toxic effects to which it gives rise are headaches, dizziness, and sleeplessness. It is also a volatile vasoconstrictor used in inhalers. **Methylamphetamine Hydrochloride BP 1973.** The hydrochloride of the base.

methylandrostenediol (**meth**·il·an·dro·**steen**′·di·ol). $C_{19}H_{27}(CH_3)(OH)_2$, a steroid chemically related to testosterone, and used in disorders accompanied by loss of protein, when the patient does not respond to diet and remains underweight. It has the advantage over testosterone in that the virilizing effects are slighter.

methylantipyrin (**meth**·il·an·te·**pi**′·rin). 1-Phenyl-2,3,4-trimethylpyrazolone, $(CCH_3)_2N(CH_3)(CO)NC_6H_5$. A derivative of antipyrine with analgesic properties.

methylarsinate (meth·il·**ar**·sin·ate). Any salt of methylarsinic acid.

methylate (**meth**·il·ate). 1. To introduce the methyl group, CH_3, into a compound. 2. To add crude methyl alcohol and naphtha to rectified spirit to render the latter unfit for drinking. 3. An alcoholate type of compound formed by methyl alcohol with metals and having the general formula CH_3OM.

methylation (meth·il·a·shun). 1. The introduction of a methyl CH_3 group into a compound. 2. The addition of crude methyl alcohol and naphtha to a mixture with the object of the denaturing of rectified spirit for industrial purposes.

methylatropine hydrobromide (meth·il·**at**·ro·peen hi·dro·**bro**′·mide). $C_{18}H_{25}O_3NHBr$, a compound with actions similar to those of atropine. It is used as a mydriatic and for congenital pyloric stenosis in infants.

methylbenzene, methylbenzol (meth·il·**ben**·zeen, meth·il·**ben**′·zol). $C_6H_5CH_3$, a colourless volatile liquid distilled from coal tar, and used in organic synthesis and as a solvent.

Methylbenzethonium Chloride (**meth**·il·ben·zeth·**o**′·ne·um **klor**′·ide). BP Commission approved name for benzyldimethyl-2-{2-[4-(1,1,3,3-tetramethylbutyl)-tolyloxy]ethoxy}ethylammonium chloride; an anti-infective agent.

methylbenzoylecgonine (**meth**·il·ben·zo·il·**ek**′·go·neen). Cocaine.

Methylcellulose 450 BP 1973 (meth·il·**sel**·ew·lose). A methyl ether of cellulose. The number following the name indicates the approximate viscosity of a 2.0 per cent solution.

methylcephaeline (**meth**·il·sef·**a**′·el·een). $C_{29}H_{40}O_4N_2$, a compound formed by the methylation of cephaeline, a toxic alkaloid of ipecacuanha; it is identical with emetine.

methylchloroformate (**meth**·il·klor·o·**form**′·ate). CH_3COOCl, a volatile liquid with lacrimatory properties used in chemical warfare as a tear gas; admixed with hydrocyanic acid it serves to indicate the presence of the latter in fumigation.

methylchlorosulphonate (**meth**·il·klor·o·**sul**′·fon·ate). CH_3SO_3Cl, a compound used in chemical warfare as a poison gas and also for the production of fog-screens.

Methylchromone (meth·il·**kro**·mone). BP Commission approved name for 3-methylchromone; it is used in the treatment of angina pectoris.

methylcreosol (meth·il·**kre**·o·sol). $CH_3C_6H_3(OCH_3)_2$, a phenolic compound obtained from wood tar creosote; it has strong disinfectant properties.

methylcytosine (meth·il·**si**·to·seen). 5-Methyl-6-amino-2-oxypyrimidine, an amino derivative of pyrimidine which occurs combined with a pentose in nucleoprotein.

methyldehydrotestosterone (meth·il·**de**·hi·dro·tes·**tos**′·ter·one). A powerful synthetic androgen.

Methyldesorphine (meth·il·dez·**or**′·feen). BP Commission approved name for 6-methyl-Δ^6-deoxymorphine, a breakdown product of morphine.

methyldichlorarsine (**meth**·il·di·klor·**ar**′·seen). CH_3AsCl_2, a poisonous vapour, irritant to the nasal mucous membrane, and used in chemical warfare: closely related to *Dick.*

Methyldopa BP 1973 (meth·il·**do**·pah). (−)-β-(3,4-dihydroxyphenyl)-α-methylalanine; it is used in the treatment of hypertension.

Methyldopate (meth·il·**do**·pate). BP Commission approved name for (−)-3-(3,4-dihydroxyphenyl)-2-methylalanine ethyl ester; a hypotensive agent.

methylene (**meth**·il·een). The radical CH_2; it has been demonstrated in the free state but is extremely unstable. **Methylene blue.** *See* BLUE. **Methylene chloride, Methylene dichloride.** CH_2Cl_2, a colourless volatile liquid resembling chloroform and tried at one time as an inhalation anaesthetic. [Gk *methy* wine, *hyle* matter.]

methylenophil, methylenophilous (meth·il·**een**·o·fil, **meth**·il·een·**of**′·il·us). Having an affinity for methylene blue. [methylene blue, Gk *philein* to love.]

Methylergometrine (**meth**·il·er·go·**met**′·reen). BP Commission approved name for D-1-hydroxy-2-butylamide of D-lysergic acid. It produces rhythmical contractions of the uterus, especially the puerperal uterus. Its use is confined to gynaecology and obstetrics, and it is particularly valuable in post-partum haemorrhage. The official preparation is Methylergometrine Maleate BP 1973.

ββ-methylethylglutarimide (meth·il·**eth**·il·gloo·**tar**′·im·ide). $(CH_3)(C_2H_5)C(CH_2CO)_2NH$; a barbiturate antagonist. Its molecular shape is very similar to that of the barbiturates, but the antagonism is of the competitive type.

methylguanidine (meth·il·**gwan**·id·een). $CH_3NHC(NH)=NH_2$, a ptomaine produced in decaying protein. It occurs in minute quantity in muscle, and appears in the urine, particularly after excision of a parathyroid gland.

methylimine (meth·il·**im**·een). The organic radical, $CH_3N=$, the introduction of which into the structure of a drug makes it liable to cause liver damage.

methylindole (meth·il·**in**·dole). C_9H_9N, a putrefaction product formed by the action of certain bacteria upon tryptophan in the intestines, and excreted in the faeces.

methylis (meth·**il**·is). Methyl. **Methylis Salicylas,** *European Pharmacopoeia* name for Methyl Salicylate BP 1973.

6α-methyllynoestrenol (**meth**·il·**lin**·es·tren·ole). An oral progestogenic compound said to inhibit libido in the human male.

methylmania (meth·il·**ma**·ne·ah). Methomania.

methylmercaptan (**meth**·il·mer·**kap**′·tan). CH_3SH, a foul-smelling gas arising in the intestines from the decomposition of certain amino acids, e.g. cysteine.

methylmethane (meth·il·**me**·thane). Ethane.

methyloestrenolone (**meth**·il·e·**stren**·ol·one). A derivative of the oestrogens claimed to inhibit libido in the human male.

methylparafynol (**meth**·il·par·ah·**fin**′·ol). A name in the USA for methylpentynol.

methylpentose (meth·il·**pen**·toze). A group of methylated pentoses of the general formula $C_5H_9(CH_3)O_5$, of which L-rhamnose is the principal example.

Methylpentynol (meth·il·**pen**·tin·ol). BP Commission approved name for 3-methylpent-1-yn-3-ol, a sedative and hypnotic drug which is relatively non-toxic and is broken down in the body fairly rapidly. Clinically it is effective in producing sleep, but in only a percentage of cases, and it is rather short-acting: its most valuable property is to relieve apprehension and nervous tension. It has come into prominence for its value in allaying apprehension before all kinds of medical and surgical procedures, particularly before dental operations. The drug has few side-effects, and there are no contra-indications to its use. In small doses there is no drowsiness and the patient remains co-operative. It has been safely administered for long periods of time, both in adults and children.

methylphenidate (meth·il·**fen**·id·ate). α-Phenyl-D-pyridyl-2-acetic acid methylester monohydrochloride, a psychomotor and non-specific respiratory stimulant. It has also been used to counteract postoperative shivering.

Methylphenobarbital (**meth**·il·fe·no·**bar**′·bit·al). *The International Pharmacopoeia* name for methylphenobarbitone.

Methylphenobarbitone BPC 1963 (**meth**·il·fe·no·**bar**′·bit·one). $C_{13}H_{14}O_3N_2$, a barbiturate similar to phenobarbitone in action, but a better antispasmodic and a weaker hypnotic. It is also a safer drug for continued administration.

methylphenyl laevulosazone (meth·il·**fe**·nil le·vew·**lo**·sa·zone). $CH_2OH(CHOH)_3C[=NN(CH_3)C_6H_5]CH[=NN(CH_3)C_6H_5]$, a crystalline compound formed by laevulose with methylphenylhydrazine. As the latter forms osazones only with ketoses it is useful in separating them from the aldoses.

methylphenylhydrazine (**meth**·il·fe·nil·**hi**′·draz·een). $C_6H_5(CH_3)NNH_2$, a reagent sometimes used for distinguishing between fructose and glucose: fructose forms an osazone with this reagent more rapidly than glucose.

N-methyl-α-phenylsuccinamide (meth·il·**fe**·nil·sux·**in**′·am·ide). An anticonvulsant used in epilepsy of the petit-mal type.

Methylprednisolone BP 1973 (**meth**·il·pred·**nis**′·o·lone). 6α-Methylprednisolone; it is used in corticosteroid therapy.

Methylprylone (meth·il·**pri**·lone). BP Commission approved name for 3,3-diethyl-5-methyl-2,4-dioxopiperidine, a sedative for use in the treatment of insomnia.

methylpsychotrine (meth·il·**si**·ko·treen). $C_{29}H_{38}O_4N_2$, a constituent alkaloid of ipecacuanha. It is inactive as an amoebacide.

methylpyridine (meth·il·**pir**·id·een). $C_5H_4N(CH_3)$, a basic compound occurring in coal tar and bone distillate; it is used to denature spirit for industrial purposes. **Methylpyridine thiocyanate.** $C_5H_4N(CH_3)HCNS$, a crystalline substance with mild antiseptic properties.

methylresorcinol (**meth**·il·rez·**or**′·sin·ol). $CH_3C_6H_3(OH)_2$, a compound which occurs naturally in certain lichens, and also prepared from aloes. Its chief importance is its use as Bial's reagent for the detection of pentose sugars.

methylrosaniline (**meth**·il·ro·**zan**′·il·een). A name applied to any of the mixtures of tetra-, penta-, and hexamethylpararosanilines which go under the titles, *gentian violet, methyl violet,* and *crystal violet.* **Methylrosaniline chloride.** Crystal violet, an antiseptic used on wounds and mucous membranes, and against certain staphylococcal infections.

Methyltestosterone BP 1973 (**meth**·il·tes·to·**steer**′·one). $C_{20}H_{30}O_2$, a crystalline androgen similar in properties to testosterone but having the advantage of being active when administered orally.

Methyltestosteronum (**meth**·il·tes·tos·ter·**o**′·num). *European Pharmacopoeia* name for Methyltestosterone BP 1973.

methyltheobromine (**meth**·il·the·o·**bro**′·meen). Caffeine.

Methylthionine Chloride (meth·il·**thi**·o·neen **klor**·ide). *The International Pharmacopoeia* name for methylene blue.

Methylthiouracil BP 1973 (**meth**·il·thi·o·**ewr**′·as·il). $C_5H_6ON_2S$, an antithyroid drug similar to thiouracil but more active and said to be less toxic.

methyltyrosine (meth·il·**ti**·ro·seen). $C_{10}H_{13}O_3N$, an alkaloid from surinam bark (*Andira retusa*).

methyluramine (meth·il·**ewr**·am·een). Methylguanidine.

methylxanthine (meth·il·**zan**·theen). 7-Methyl-2,6-dioxypurine, $C_6H_6O_2N_4$. An exogenous base found in the human urine and attributed to the caffeine and theobromine in the diet.

Methyprylone BP 1973 (meth·e·**pri**·lone). $C_{10}H_{17}NO_2$, 3,3-diethyl-5-methyl-2,4-dioxopiperidine; a white crystalline powder with a slight odour and a bitter taste, soluble in water, alcohol, ether and chloroform. A hypnotic useful in the treatment of insomnia.

Methysergide (meth·e·**ser**·gide). BP Commission approved name for 1-(hydroxymethyl)propylamide of 1-methyl-(+)-lysergic acid; a serotonin antagonist.

methysis (**meth**·is·is). Habitual intoxication. [Gk *methysis* drunkenness.]

Metiamide (met·i·am·ide). BP Commission approved name for 1-methyl-3-[2-(5-methylimidazol-4-ylmethylthio)ethyl]thiourea; a histamine H_2-receptor blocking agent.

Metoclopramide (met·o·**klo**·pram·ide). BP Commission approved name for 4-amino-5-chloro-*N*-(2-diethylaminoethyl)-2-methoxybenzamide; a derivative of procaine amide used as an anti-emetic and agent for speeding gastric emptying time in radiology and therapeutics. It can be administered orally or by injection.

metoecius (met·e·shus). Applied to parasites which have different hosts at different stages of their life. [Gk *meta, oikos* house.]

metoestrus (met·e·strus). The interval between ovulation periods of some animals. [Gk *meta,* oestrus.]

Metofoline (met·o·**fo**·leen). BP Commission approved name for 1-(4-chlorophenethyl)-1,2,3,4-tetrahydro-6,7-dimethoxy-2-methylisoquinoline; an analgesic.

Metolazone (met·**ol**·az·one). BP Commission approved name for 7-chloro-1,2,3,4-tetrahydro-2-methyl-4-oxo-3-*o*-tolyl-6-quinazolinesulphonamide; a diuretic.

metonymy (met·**on**·im·e). Disordered thinking in which an expression or word is used in a wrong sense. [Gk *meta, onyma* name.]

metopagus (met·**op**·ag·us). A twin monster joined at the forehead. [Gk *metopon* forehead, *pagos* joined.]

metopantralgia (**met**·o·pan·**tral**′·je·ah). A painful condition of the frontal sinuses. [metopantron, Gk *algos* pain.]

metopantritis (**met**·o·pan·**tri**′·tis). Inflammation of the frontal sinuses. [metopantron, Gk *-itis* inflammation.]

metopantron, metopantrum (met·o·**pan**·tron, met·o·**pan**·trum). The frontal sinus. [Gk *metopon* forehead, antrum.]

metopic (met·o·pik). Relating to the forehead; belonging to the frontal region. [see foll.]

Metopimazine (met·o·**pim**·az·een). BP Commission approved name for 10-[3-(4-carbamoylpiperidino)propyl]-2-methane-sulphonylphenothiazine; an anti-emetic.

metopion (met·**o**·pe·on). A point situated in the middle line between the frontal eminences of the skull. [Gk *metopon* forehead.]

metopism (**met**·o·pizm). A condition in which the frontal suture persists in adults. [see prec.]

metopium toxiferum (me·**to**·pe·um tox·**if**·er·um). A poison wood that causes a severe dermatitis on contact: it occurs in the USA.

metopodynia (**met**·o·po·**din**′·e·ah). Frontal headache. [Gk *metopon* forehead, *odyne* pain.]

Metopon (**met**·o·pon). 1. BP Commission approved name for dihydromethylmorphinone, a modified morphine compound having powerful analgesic and narcotic actions. 2. The old term for *forehead.* [Gk]

metopoplasty (met·o·po·plas·te). Plastic surgery of the forehead. [Gk *metopon* forehead, *plassein* to mould.]

metoposcopy (met·o·**pos**·ko·pe). That branch of science which deals with the study of physiognomy. [Gk *metopon* forehead, *skopein* to watch.]

Metorchis (met·**or**·kis). A genus of liver flukes. **Metorchis truncatus.** A common fluke of fish-eating mammals in Canada, which has occasionally been found in man. The primary intermediate hosts are fresh-water snails; secondary intermediate hosts are sucker fish. [Gk *meta, orchis* testicle.]

metoxenous (met·**ox**·en·us). Metoecius. [Gk *meta, xenos* stranger.]

metra (**me**·trah). The uterus. [Gk womb.]

metraemia (me·**tre**·me·ah). Uterine congestion. [Gk *metra* womb, *haima* blood.]

metralgia (me·**tral**·je·ah). Pain in the uterus. [Gk *metra* womb, *algos* pain.]

metranaemia (me·tran·**e**·me·ah). An anaemic condition of the uterus. [Gk *metra* womb, anaemia.]

metranastrophe (me·tran·**as**·tro·fe). Inversion of the uterus. [Gk *metra* womb, *anastrophe* an upsetting.]

metrapectic (me·trah·**pek**·tik). Denoting a disease, such as haemophilia, which, although transmitted by the mother, does not usually affect her. [Gk *metra* womb, *apechein* to avoid.]

metratome (**me**·trah·tome). An instrument used for making an incision into the uterus. [Gk *metra* womb, *temnein* to cut.]

metratomy (me·**trat**·o·me). Hysterotomy. [see prec.]

metratonia (me·trah·**to**·ne·ah). Atony of the uterus. [Gk *metra* womb, atony.]

metratresia (me·trah·**tre**·ze·ah). An atresic or imperforate condition of the uterus. [Gk *metra* womb, atresia.]

metratrophia (me·trah·**tro**·fe·ah). An atrophied state of the uterus. [Gk *metra* womb, atrophy.]

metrauxe (me·**trawx**·e). Uterine enlargement. [Gk *metra* womb, *auxe* increase.]

metre (**me**·ter). The unit of length defined as equal to 1 650 763.73 wavelengths in vacuum of the radiation corresponding to the transitions between the levels $2p_{10}$ and $5d_5$ of the krypton-86 atom (39.37 in). [Gk *metron* measure.]

metre-candle (**me**·ter·kan·dl). A unit of intensity of illumination being equal to that on a surface placed at right angles to the light falling on it from one international candle placed at one metre distance.

metrectasia (me·trek·**ta**·ze·ah). A dilated condition of the non-gravid uterus. [Gk *metra* womb, *ektasis* a stretching.]

metrectatic (me·trek·**tat**·ik). Relating to or affected with metrectasia.

metrectomy (me·**trek**·to·me). Hysterectomy. [Gk *metra* womb, *ektome* a cutting out.]

metrectopia, metrectopy (me·trek·**to**·pe·ah, me·**trek**·to·pe). Displacement of the uterus. [Gk *metra* womb, *ektopos* out of the way.]

metrelcosis (me·trel·**ko**·sis). A condition of ulceration of the uterus. [Gk *metra* womb, *helkosis* ulceration.]

metreurynter (me·trewr·**in**·ter). A collapsible bag capable of being dilated by water or air, employed in dilatation of the uterine cervical canal. [Gk *metra* womb, *eurynein* to dilate.]

metreurysis (me·**trewr**·is·is). The process by which the neck of the uterus is dilated with the metreurynter.

metria (**me**·tre·ah). A term used to describe comprehensively the general inflammatory diseases likely to be met with during the puerperium, e.g. pelvic cellulitis, puerperal fever. [Gk *metra* womb.]

metriocephalic (**met**·re·o·kef·**al**′·ik). Describing a skull whose vault is of moderate convexity, being neither pointed nor flat. [Gk *metrios* moderate, *kephale* skull.]

metritic (me·**trit**·ik). Affected with or relating to metritis.

metritis (me·**tri**·tis). Inflammation of the myometrium. **Acute metritis.** An acute inflammation of the myometrium, secondary to an acute endometritis. **Chronic metritis.** A vague term little used today; it describes the appearance of the myometrium in chronic pelvic inflammatory disease. **Puerperal metritis.** An inflammation of the uterine muscle, occurring in the puerperium secondary to an endometritis. [Gk *metra* womb, *-itis* inflammation.]

metrocace (me·**trok**·as·e). 1. Gangrene or ulceration of the uterus. 2. Uterine carcinoma. [Gk *metra* womb, *kakia* badness.]

metrocampsis (me·tro·**kamp**·sis). Flexion of the uterus. [Gk *metra* womb, *kampsis* a curving.]

metrocarcinoma (**me**·tro·kar·sin·**o**′·mah). Uterine carcinoma. [Gk *metra* womb, carcinoma.]

metrocele (**me**·tro·seel). Herniation of the uterus. [Gk *metra* womb, *kele* hernia.]

metrocolpocele (me·tro·**kol**·po·seel). Prolapse of the uterus, with herniation into the vagina. [Gk *metra* womb, *kolpos* pocket, *kele* hernia.]

metrocystosis (**me**·tro·sis·**to**′·sis). Cystic formation in the uterus. [Gk *metra* womb, *kystis* bag, *-osis* condition.]

metrocyte (**me**·tro·site). An obsolete term for megaloblast. [Gk *metra* womb, *kytos* cell.]

metrodynamometer (**me**·tro·di·nam·**om**′·et·er). An apparatus for measuring the strength of uterine contractions. [Gk *metra* womb, dynamometer.]

metrodynia (me·tro·**din**·e·ah). Uterine pain. [Gk *metra* womb, *odyne* pain.]

metrodystocia (**me**·tro·dis·**to**′·se·ah). Dystocia caused by some disorder of the uterus. [Gk *metra* womb, dystocia.]

metro-ectasia (**me**·tro·ek·**ta**′·ze·ah). Metrectasia.

metro-endometritis (**me**·tro·en·do·me·**tri**′·tis). Widespread inflammation of the uterine body and the lining membranes. [Gk *metra* womb, endometritis.]

metrofibroma (**me**·tro·fi·**bro**′·mah). A uterine fibroma. [Gk *metra* womb, fibroma.]

metrogenous (me·**troj**·en·us). Originating in the uterus. [Gk *metra* womb, *genein* to produce.]

metrography (me·**trog**·raf·e). Radiographic visualization of the uterus by the injection into it of contrast medium. [Gk *metra* womb, radiography.]

metroleucorrhoea (**me**·tro·lew·ko·**re**′·ah). Leucorrhoea originating in the uterus. [Gk *metra* womb, leucorrhoea.]

metroloxia (me·tro·**lox**·e·ah). Oblique displacement of the uterus. [Gk *metra* womb, *loxos* oblique.]

metrolymphangitis (**me**·tro·limf·an·**ji**′·tis). Inflammation of the uterine lymph vessels. [Gk *metra* womb, lymphangitis.]

metromalacia, metromalacoma (**me**·tro·mal·**a**′·she·ah, me·tro·mal·ah·**ko**′·mah). Pathological softening of the uterus. [Gk *metra* womb, *malakos* soft, *-oma* tumour.]

metromania (me·tro·**ma**·ne·ah). 1. Nymphomania. [Gk *metra* womb, mania.]. 2. (met·ro·**ma**·ne·ah). A state in which there is an obsessional urge to write poetry. [Gk *metron* measure, mania.]

metromenorrhagia (**me**·tro·men·or·**a**′·je·ah). Menorrhagia. [Gk *metra* womb, menorrhagia.]

metronania (me·tro·**nan**·e·ah). Unusually small size of the uterus. [Gk *metra* womb, *nanos* dwarf.]

metroncus (me·**trong**·kus). Any swelling or tumour of the uterus. [Gk *metra* womb, *ogkos* swelling.]

Metronidazole BP 1973 (met·ron·**id**·az·ole). 1-(2-Hydroxyethyl)-2-methyl-5-nitro-imidazole; it is used in the treatment of *Trichomonas vaginalis* infestation and for giardiasis (*Giardia lamblia*).

metronoscope (met·**ron**·o·skope). An apparatus which exercises the eyes rhythmically to promote co-ordinated ocular movements. [Gk *metron* measure, *skopein* to view.]

metroparalysis (**me**·tro·par·**al**′·is·is). A condition of uterine paralysis. [Gk *metra* womb, paralysis.]

metropathia, metropathy (me·tro·**path**·e·ah, me·**trop**·ath·e). Any disease or disordered condition affecting the uterus. **Metropathia haemorrhagica.** Essential uterine haemorrhage. [Gk *metra* womb, *pathos* suffering.]

metroperitonitis (**me**·tro·per·it·on·**i**′·tis). Inflammation of the uterus and associated peritoneal membranes. [metritis, peritonitis.]

metrophlebitis (**me**·tro·fleb·**i**'·tis). Inflammation of the uterine veins. [Gk *metra* womb, phlebitis.]

metrophyma (me·tro·**fi**·mah). A uterine tumour. [Gk *metra* womb, *phyma* a growth.]

metroptosia, metroptosis (me·trop·**to**·se·ah, me·trop·**to**·sis). Prolapse of the uterus. [Gk *metra* womb, *ptosis* fall.]

metrorrhagia (me·tro·**ra**·je·ah). Irregular intermenstrual bleeding superimposed on a normal menstrual cycle. [Gk *metra* womb, *rhegnynai* to burst forth.]

metrorrhexis (me·tro·**rex**·is). Rupture of the uterus. [Gk *metra* womb, *rhexis* rupture.]

metrorrhoea (met·ro·**re**·ah). A flow of fluid from the uterus. [Gk *metra* womb, *rhein* to flow.]

metrosalpingitis (**me**·tro·sal·pin·**ji**'·tis). Inflammation of the uterus and uterine tubes. [Gk *metra* womb, salpingitis.]

metrosalpingography (**me**·tro·sal·ping·**gog**'·raf·e). Radiographic visualization of the uterus and uterine tubes by the injection into them of contrast medium. [Gk *metra* womb, *salpigx* tube, radiography.]

metrosalpinx (me·tro·**sal**·pingx). A uterine tube. [Gk *metra* womb, *salpigx* tube.]

metroscirrhus (me·tro·**sir**·us). A scirrhous carcinoma of the uterus. [Gk *metra* womb, *skiros* hard tumour.]

metrostasis (met·ro·**sta**·sis). A state in which a muscle contracts and relaxes at a fixed length, that is, an isometric contraction and relaxation. [Gk *metron* measure, *stasis* a standing still.]

metrostaxis (me·tro·**stax**·is). Continuous haemorrhage from the uterus of small amount, due either to leakage from an ulcer or to oozing from a more widespread area. [Gk *metra* womb, *staxis* a trickling.]

metrostenosis (**me**·tro·sten·**o**'·sis). Narrowing or contraction of the cavity of the body of the uterus. [Gk *metra* womb, stenosis.]

metrotherapy (met·ro·**ther**·ap·e). The employment of measurement in treatment, e.g. indicating by measurement the increase in the range of joint movement. [Gk *metron* measure, therapy.]

metrotome (**me**·tro·tome). A hysterotome; an instrument used for incising the uterus, particularly the neck. [see foll.]

metrotomy (me·**trot**·o·me). Hysterotomy: surgical incision of the uterus. [Gk *metra* womb, *temnein* to cut.]

Mett, Emil Ludwig Paul. 19th century German physician.

Mett's method. For peptic activity in gastric juice: small glass tubes containing coagulated egg albumen are placed in a solution of gastric juice in 0.05M HCl and incubated for 24 hours. The decrease in the length of the albumen column is measured at both ends to give an estimation of the peptic activity of the juice.

Mett's tube. A thin-walled open-ended glass tube containing coagulated egg albumen, used in Mett's method of determining peptic activity in gastric juice.

Metyrapone BP 1973 (met·**ir**·ah·pone). 2-Methyl-1,2-di(3-pyridyl) propan-1-one. A compound that inhibits 11-β-hydroxylase and thus prevents the biosynthesis of cortisol. This releases maximal quantities of ACTH. Metyrapone is used in assessing the functional efficiency of the pituitary in stimulating the adrenal cortex.

Metyzoline (met·**i**·zo·leen). BP Commission approved name for 2-(2-methylbenzo[*b*]thien-3-yl)methyl-2-imidazoline; a vasoconstrictor.

Meulengracht, Einar (b. 1887). Copenhagen physician.

Meulengracht diet. A high-calorie diet, rich in vitamins, for bleeding peptic ulcer.

Meulengracht icteric index. *See* MEULENGRACHT'S METHOD (below).

Meulengracht's method. For the icteric index of serum: 1 ml of serum is diluted with 5 per cent sodium-citrate solution until the colour matches that of 0.01 per cent potassium-dichromate solution.

Meunier, Leon (b. 1856). Paris physician.

Meunier's sign. A progressive loss of weight in measles, observed for several days before the onset of symptoms.

Mexenone BPC 1973 (**mex**·en·one). 2-Hydroxy-4-methoxy-4'-methylbenzophenone; it is used to protect the skin from sunlight.

Mexiletine (mex·**il**·et·een). BP Commission approved name for 1-methyl-2-(2,6-xylyloxy)ethylamine; an anti-arrhythmic agent.

Meyer, Adolf (b. 1866). Baltimore psychiatrist.

Meyer's system. In psychology: the study of the individual's overt and implicit behaviour in its biological aspects.

Meyer (Mayer), Edmund Victor (b. 1864). Berlin laryngologist.

Meyer's cartilages. Minute nodules of elastic cartilage in the anterior extremities of the vocal ligaments.

Meyer, Georg Hermann (b. 1815). German anatomist.

Meyer's sinus. A fossa in the external auditory meatus.

Meyer, Hans Horst (b. 1853). German pharmacologist.

Meyer-Overton theory. A theory referring to the action of anaesthetic agents and suggesting that this depends on the different affinities between the anaesthetic and the lipoid and other constituents of the nerve cell.

Meyer, Hans Wilhelm (b. 1824). Copenhagen otologist.

Meyer's disease. Adenoid hypertrophy of the postnasal space.

Meyerholtz's muscle. Plain muscle fibres which are radially disposed in the area immediately subjacent to the areola and nipple.

Meynert, Theodor Hermann (b. 1833). Vienna neurologist and psychiatrist.

Meynert's bundle, fasciculus, or tract. The fasciculus retroflexus; fibres from the habenular nuclei which pass to the interpeduncular nucleus in the tegmentum of the mid-brain.

Meynert's cell. An isolated giant pyramidal cell of the visual cortex, which sends its axon into the pretectal region of the mid-brain.

commissure of Meynert. A component of the postoptic commissure.

Meynert's decussation. The decussation of the tectospinal fibres in the mid-brain; fountain decussation.

Meynert's fibres. A tract of fibres running from the superior quadrigeminal body to the oculomotor nuclei.

Meynert's ganglion. The optic basal ganglion of the hypothalamus.

Meynert's layer. The pyramidal cell layer of the cerebral cortex.

Meynet, Paul Claude Hyacinthe (b. 1831). Paris physician.

Meynet's nodes. Nodules which occur in the course of acute rheumatic fever in or around the capsules and tendons of the affected joints.

mezereum (me·**zeer**·e·um). The dried bark of *Daphne mezereum* Linn., *Daphne gnidium* Linn., or *Daphne laureola* Linn. (family Thymeleaceae). It contains a bitter glycosidal principle. [Ar. *mazariyun.*]

mho (mo). A unit of electrical conductivity, the reciprocal of the ohm: defined as the conductance of a cubic centimetre of substance through which a current of one ampere passes when a potential difference of one volt is applied to opposite faces. Now called a siemens, S. [*ohm* spelt backwards.]

miasm (**mi**·azm). Miasma.

miasma (mi·**az**·mah). An unwholesome effluvium. [Gk defilement.]

miasmal, miasmatic (mi·**az**·mal, mi·az·**mat**·ik). Relating or belonging to miasma.

Mibelli, Vittorio (b. 1860). Parma dermatologist.

Mibelli's disease. Porokeratosis.

angiokeratoma of Mibelli. Angiokeratoma occurring on the hands and feet, sometimes on the elbows and knees, with acrocyanosis.

mica (**mi**·kah). A mineral which occurs in thin laminated scales. It is composed of the hydrated silicate of aluminium with silicates of other metals, and is used as an insulator and lubricant. [L crumb.]

micaceous (mi·**ka**·she·us). Of the nature of mica; crumbly.
mication (mi·**ka**·shun). A rapid movement such as blinking of the eye. [L *micare* to glitter.]
micella (mi·**sel**·ah). Micelle.
micelle (mi·**sel**). 1. One of the submicroscopic aggregates of parallel long fibrous-protein molecules found in colloidal sols and gels. 2. The hypothetical submicroscopic particles, capable of growth and self-multiplication, thought to be the essential living elements of protoplasm. [dim. of L *mica* crumb.]
Michaelis, Gustav Adolf (b. 1798). Kiel gynaecologist.
Michaelis rhomboid. A diamond-shaped depression seen in well-formed women on the posterior aspect of the pelvis. It is outlined by joining the following points: the tip of the spinous process of the 5th lumbar vertebra, the dimples over the posterior superior iliac spines, and the junction of the lines formed by the medial edge of the gluteus maximus muscle.
Michaelis, Leonor (b. 1875). Berlin and New York biochemist.
Michaelis constant (K_m). The concentration of substrate which gives one-half maximum velocity in an enzyme catalysed reaction; $K_m = S[V/v - 1]$ where v is reaction velocity at substrate concentration S and V is maximum velocity.
Michaelis-Gutmann bodies. Pinhead, raised, brownish areas of the mucous membrane of the bladder in malacoplakia; they may be found also in the kidney, pelvis, and ureter. The lesions are of unknown aetiology and may be of long duration, but do not appear to be precancerous.
Michel, Gaston (b. 1875). Nancy surgeon.
Michel's clamps, or suture clips. Soft metal clips with sharp teeth, used to fix the skin edges of a wound.
Micheli, F. 19th–20th century Italian physician.
Marchiafava-Micheli disease, or syndrome. A rare chronic haemolytic anaemia with paroxysmal nocturnal haemoglobinuria, first described by Struebing (1882), but usually associated with the names of Marchiafava (1911) and Micheli (1931). It occurs during sleep (day or night) when the blood pH is reduced.
Miconazole (mi·**kon**·az·ole). BP Commission approved name for 1-[2,4-dichloro-β-(2,4-dichlorobenzyloxy)-phenethyl]imidazole; an antifungal agent.
micracoustic (mi·krak·**oos**·tik). A device which so magnifies faint sounds that they are audible. [Gk *mikros* small, *akouein* to hear.]
micranatomy (mi·kran·**at**·o·me). Micro-anatomy; histology.
micrangiopathy (**mi**·kran·je·**op**'·ath·e). Micro-angiopathy.
micrangium (mi·**kran**·je·um). A capillary. [Gk *mikros* small, *aggeion* vessel.]
micrencephalia (**mi**·kren·kef·**a**'·le·ah). Micrencephaly.
micrencephalon (mi·kren·**kef**·al·on). 1. Abnormally small size of the brain. 2. The cerebellum. [Gk *mikros* small, *egkephalos* brain.]
micrencephalous (mi·kren·**kef**·al·us). Having a small brain. [see prec.]
micrencephaly (mi·kren·**kef**·al·e). A condition in which the brain is of unusually small size. [Gk *mikros* small, *egkephalos* brain.]
micro- (**mi**·kro). A prefix indicating that the quantity which follows is to be multiplied by 10^{-6}. One millionth part. [Gk *mikros* small.]
micro-adenopathy (**mi**·kro·ad·en·**op**'·ath·e). Any diseased condition of the small lymph glands. [Gk *mikros* small, *aden* gland, *pathos* disease.]
micro-aerophile, micro-aerophilic, micro-aerophilous (**mi**·kro·a'·er·o·fil, **mi**·kro·a·er·o·**fil**'·ik, **mi**·kro·a·er·**of**'·il·us). Applied to micro-organisms which grow best at reduced oxygen tensions. [Gk *mikros* small, aerophile.]
micro-aerotonometer (**mi**·kro·a·er·o·ton·**om**'·et·er). An instrument for measuring small amounts of gases dissolved or combined in fluid, e.g. in blood. [Gk *mikros* small, *aer* air, *tonos* tension, meter.]
micro-aleuriospore (**mi**·kro·al·**ewr**·e·o·spor). Microconidium. [Gk *mikros* small, *aleuron* flour, *sporos* seed.]
micro-ampere (mi·kro·**am**·pare). A unit of electric current; one millionth of an ampere. [Gk *mikros* small, ampere.]
micro-analysis (**mi**·kro·an·al'·is·is). 1. The recognition of constituents by means of their appearance under the microscope. 2. Analysis of minute quantities of materials by a specially modified technique. [Gk *mikros* small, analysis.]
micro-anatomy (**mi**·kro·an·**at**'·o·me). Histology. [Gk *mikros* small, anatomy.]
micro-angiopathy (**mi**·kro·an·je·**op**'·ath·e). Any disease or disorder of the capillary vessels. **Thrombotic micro-angiopathy.** Thrombotic micro-angiopathic haemolytic anaemia; a rare condition of acute haemolytic anaemia with thrombocytopenic purpura, pyrexia, and varying neurological disturbances. [Gk *mikros* small, angiopathy.]
micro-angioscopy (**mi**·kro·an·je·**os**'·ko·pe). Microscopical examination of the capillary vessels of the skin. [Gk *mikros* small, *aggeion* small vessel, *skopein* to watch.]
micro-arteriography (**mi**·kro·ar·teer·e·**og**'·raf·e). Radiography of microscopic sections of animal tissue which has previously been injected with radio-opaque material to demonstrate arterioles and capillaries. [Gk *mikros* small, arteriography.]
Microbacterium (**mi**·kro·bak·**teer**'·e·um). A genus of bacteria of the family Lactobacteriaceae (Bergey). They are small, non-motile, Gram-positive rods, which produce lactic acid from carbohydrates. The type species is *Microbacterium lacticum*, found in dairy products, faecal matter, and soil. [Gk *mikros* small, bacterium.]
microbalance (mi·kro·**bal**·ans). A balance designed for use in weighing minute quantities. [Gk *mikros* small, balance.]
microbe (**mi**·krobe). A lay term for a minute organism; a micro-organism. [Gk *mikros* small, *bios* life.]
microbiaemia (**mi**·kro·bi·**e**'·me·ah). The condition in which micro-organisms are present in the circulating blood.
microbial, microbian (mi·**kro**·be·al, mi·**kro**·be·an). Having the character of a micro-organism; belonging to a micro-organism. [microbe.]
microbic (mi·**kro**·bik). Relating or due to micro-organisms. [microbe.]
microbicide (mi·**kro**·be·side). Any agent that is destructive to micro-organisms. [microbe, L *caedere* to kill.]
microbid (mi·**kro**·bid). Any allergic skin lesion of micro-organismal origin, but in which the causal micro-organism is not present in the lesion itself. [microbe.]
microbiohaemia (**mi**·kro·bi·o·**he**'·me·ah). A disease caused by bacteraemia or the presence of organisms in the blood. [microbe, Gk *haima* blood.]
microbiological (**mi**·kro·bi·o·**loj**'·ik·al). Relating to microbiology.
microbiologist (**mi**·kro·bi·**ol**'·o·jist). One who is expert in the science of microbiology. [Gk *mikros* small, *bios* life, *logos* science.]
microbiology (**mi**·kro·bi·**ol**'·o·je). The study of micro-organisms, especially bacteria, rickettsiae, viruses, protozoa, and yeasts. [Gk *mikros* small, biology.]
microbionation (mi·**kro**·be·on·a'·shun). 1. The inoculation of bacterial vaccine as a method of treatment. 2. The inoculating of an individual with bacteria. [microbe.]
microbiophobia (**mi**·kro·bi·o·**fo**'·be·ah). Morbid fear of micro-organisms. [microbe, phobia.]
microbism (**mi**·kro·bizm). Infection caused by a micro-organism. **Latent microbism.** The presence of pathogenic micro-organisms in the body which remain inert until conditions are favourable to their activity. [microbe.]
microblast (**mi**·kro·blast). A small-sized erythroblast. [Gk *mikros* small, *blastos* germ.]
microblepharia, microblepharism, microblepharon, microblephary (**mi**·kro·blef·**a**'·re·ah, mi·kro·**blef**·ar·izm, mi·kro·**blef**·ar·on, mi·kro·**blef**·ar·e). Abnormal smallness of the eyelids. [Gk *mikros* small, *blepharon* eyelid.]
microbrachia (mi·kro·**bra**·ke·ah). A congenital condition in which the arms are of abnormally small size. [Gk *mikros* small, *brachion* arm.]
microbrachius (mi·kro·**bra**·ke·us). A fetus with abnormally small

arms, more particularly a monster the arms of which are mere buds. [see prec.]

microbrachycephaly (mi·kro·brak·e·**kef**'·al·e). A combined condition of microcephaly and brachycephaly. [Gk *mikros* small, *brachys* short, *kephale* head.]

microburet (mi·kro·bew·**ret**'). A buret used for the measurement of minute amounts of fluid or gases. [Gk *mikros* small, buret.]

microcalculus (mi·kro·**kal**·kew·lus). A tiny non-palpable calculus often demonstrated by radiography or histological examination. [Gk *mikros* small, L *calculus* pebble.]

microcalorie (mi·kro·**kal**·or·e). The small calorie or gram calorie; the amount of heat required to raise the temperature of one gram of water 1°C from 14.5°C to 15.5°C. It is equal to 4.1855 joules. [Gk *mikros* small, calorie.]

microcardia (mi·kro·**kar**·de·ah). Abnormal smallness of the heart. [Gk *mikros* small, *kardia* heart.]

microcardius (mi·kro·**kar**·de·us). A monster with a heart of abnormally small size. [see prec.]

microcaulia (mi·kro·**kawl**·e·ah). Abnormally small size of the penis. [Gk *mikros* small, *kaulos* stalk.]

microcentrum (mi·kro·**sen**·trum). An obsolete term for the centrosome. [Gk *mikros* small, *kentron* centre.]

microcephalia (mi·kro·kef·**a**'·le·ah). Microcephaly.

microcephalic (mi·kro·kef·**al**'·ik). Having a small head. [Gk *mikros* small, *kephale* head.]

microcephalism (mi·kro·**kef**·al·izm). Microcephaly.

microcephalon (mi·kro·**kef**·al·on). A head which is abnormally small. [Gk *mikros* small, *kephale* head.]

microcephalous (mi·kro·**kef**·al·us). Microcephalic.

microcephalus (mi·kro·**kef**·al·us). 1. A person with an unusually small size of head; generally a microcephalic idiot. 2. A monster, the head of which is not properly developed. [see foll.]

microcephaly (mi·kro·**kef**·al·e). Unusual smallness of the head. [Gk *mikros* small, *kephale* head.]

microcheilia (mi·kro·**ki**·le·ah). A condition in which the lips are abnormally small. [Gk *mikros* small, *cheilos* lip.]

microcheiria (mi·kro·**ki**·re·ah). A condition of abnormal smallness of the hands. [Gk *mikros* small, *cheir* hand.]

microchemical (mi·kro·**kem**·ik·al). Relating to microchemistry.

microchemistry (mi·kro·**kem**·is·tre). Chemical experiments conducted with minute quantities of substances, entailing the use of special apparatus or the microscope. [Gk *mikros* small, chemistry.]

microcinematography (mi·kro·sin·e·mat·**og**'·raf·e). Cinematomicrography.

microclimate (mi·kro·**kli**·mate). A small and circumscribed environment that differs from the general environment in which it occurs: e.g. inside a warm house in a cold country. [Gk *mikros* small, climate.]

microcnemia (mi·kro·**ne**·me·ah). A condition in which the length of the leg below the knee is unusually short. [Gk *mikros* small, *kneme* leg.]

Micrococcaceae (mi·kro·kok·**a**'·se·e). A family of Gram-positive cocci which includes the pathogenic genus *Staphylococcus* and non-pathogenic genera *Gaffkya, Micrococcus* and *Sarcina.* [Gk *mikros* small, *kokkos* berry.]

micrococcin (mi·kro·**kok**·sin). A fluorescent antibiotic from a micrococcus found in sewage. It was used in the early experimental work on antibiotics.

Micrococcus (mi·kro·**kok**·us). A genus of bacteria commonly found in the air and in milk. They are characterized by spherical cells arranged in pairs, tetrads, or groups, and are usually Gram-positive. They grow steadily on ordinary media. Three members of this genus are mostly non-pathogenic to animals and man, but the name has in the past been applied to many pathogens which are now transferred to other genera (see below). **Micrococcus albus.** *Staphylococcus albus.* **Micrococcus aureus.** *Staphylococcus aureus.* **Micrococcus buccalis.** A small Gram-positive coccus isolated from the mouth; it is an obligatory anaerobe, and is non-pathogenic to animals. **Micrococcus catarrhalis.** *Neisseria catarrhalis.* **Micrococcus citreus.** *Staphylococcus citreus.* **Micrococcus gonorrhoeae.** *Neisseria gonorrhoeae.* **Micrococcus intracellularis meningitidis.** *Neisseria meningitidis.* **Micrococcus lysodeikticus.** A species described by Fleming; it is readily attacked by the enzyme lysozyme. **Micrococcus melitensis.** *Brucella melitensis.* **Micrococcus meningitidis.** *Neisseria meningitidis.* **Micrococcus tetragenus.** A species isolated by Koch from the lung cavities of patients with tuberculosis. It consists of Gram-positive cocci arranged in tetrads, is highly pathogenic to mice, and very occasionally causes septicaemia in man. Bergey classifies it as *Gaffkya tetragena.* [Gk *mikros* small, *kokkos* berry.]

microcolon (mi·kro·**ko**·lon). A colon of abnormal smallness. [Gk *mikros* small, colon.]

microcolony (mi·kro·**kol**·on·e). A microscopic colony of bacteria.

microconidium (mi·kro·kon·**id**'·e·um). Micro-aleuriospore; the smaller of two types of asexual spore produced by a fungus. [Gk *mikros* small, *konis* dust.]

microcoria (mi·kro·**ko**·re·ah). A congenital bilateral condition of the iris in which the diameter of the pupils is less than 2 mm on distant vision in daylight. It is due to an undeveloped or absent dilator muscle. [Gk *mikros* small, *kore* pupil.]

microcornea (mi·kro·**kor**·ne·ah). A condition in which the cornea is smaller, thinner and flatter than the normal. [Gk *mikros* small, cornea.]

microcoulomb (mi·kro·**koo**·lom). One millionth of a coulomb; a unit of quantity of electricity. [Gk *mikros* small, coulomb.]

microcrith (mi·kro·krith). A unit used to denote the weight of one atom of hydrogen. [obsolete term.] [Gk *mikros* small, *krithe* barleycorn.]

microcrystal (mi·kro·**kris**·tal). A crystal of minute size. [Gk *mikros* small, crystal.]

microcrystalline (mi·kro·**kris**·tal·ine). Made up of crystals of minute size. [see prec.]

microcurie (mi·kro·kewr·e). One millionth of a curie. [Gk *mikros* small, curie.]

microcystometer (mi·kro·sis·**tom**'·et·er). An instrument for measuring intravesical pressures, and small enough for general clinical use. [Gk *mikros* small, *kystis* bladder, meter.]

microcyte (mi·kro·site). 1. A red blood cell which is smaller than the normal erythrocyte (less than 6 μm diameter) and is usually seen in the blood in microcytic anaemias. 2. Occasionally applied to a small polymorphonuclear leucocyte. [Gk *mikros* small, *kytos* cell.]

microcythaemia (mi·kro·si·**the**'·me·ah). The presence of an excess of microcytes in the blood. [microcyte, Gk *haima* blood.]

microcytosis (mi·kro·si·**to**'·sis). Microcythaemia. [microcyte, Gk *-osis* condition.]

microdactylia (mi·kro·dak·**til**'·e·ah). Abnormal smallness or shortness of the fingers and toes. [Gk *mikros* small, *daktylos* finger or toe.]

microdentism (mi·kro·**den**·tizm). Microdontism. [Gk *mikros* small, L *dens* tooth.]

microdetermination (mi·kro·de·ter·min·**a**'·shun). The quantitative chemical analysis of substances of which only very small quantities are available. [Gk *mikros* small, determination.]

microdissection (mi·kro·dis·**ek**'·shun). The act of dissecting a cell or tissue with the aid of the microscope.

microdont, microdontic (mi·kro·dont, mi·kro·**don**·tik). Having dentition in which the teeth are smaller than average size. [Gk *mikros* small, *odous* tooth.]

microdontism (mi·kro·**don**·tizm). Smallness of the teeth. [see prec.]

micro-electrometer (mi·kro·el·ek·**trom**'·et·er). An extremely sensitive electrometer used to measure weak electrical charges. [Gk *mikros* small, electrometer.]

micro-electrophoresis (mi·kro·el·ek·tro·for·**e**'·sis). A method of protein electrophoresis with only a small amount of fluid; a simple clinical method is that in which as little as 0.1 ml of serum is absorbed on blotting paper. [Gk *mikros* small, electrophoresis.]

micro-encephaly (mi·kro·en·**kef'**·al·e). The possession of an unusually small brain. [Gk *mikros* small, *egkephalos* brain.]

micro-erythrocyte (mi·kro·er·**ith'**·ro·site). A microcyte, i.e. a red blood corpuscle the diameter of which is outside the normal range at the small end. [Gk *mikros* small, erythrocyte.]

micro-estimation (mi·kro·es·tim·**a'**·shun). Microdetermination, [Gk *mikros* small, estimation.]

microfarad (mi·kro·**far**·ad). The unit of electrostatic capacity most convenient for practical purposes: one millionth of a farad. [Gk *mikros* small, farad.]

microfilaraemia (mi·kro·fil·a·**re'**·me·ah). Microfilariae in the blood, as occurs in bancroftian filariasis and in several other filarial infections. [microfilariae, Gk *haima* blood.]

microfilaria (mi·kro·fil·**a'**·re·ah). A term used to designate the larval form of a filaria circulating in the blood or existing in the ocular or cutaneous tissues in man or in the body cavity or tissues of the insect vector. Certain microfilariae are contained in a structureless sheath which is longer than the embryo within. **Microfilaria bancrofti.** A sheathed microfilaria which is the embryo of *Wuchereria bancrofti.* It is found in the blood in the skin during the night, but migrates to the lung capillary vessels during the day. In certain regions of the Pacific this nocturnal periodicity is not found. Complete development can occur in a large number of the tribes of mosquitos of Anophelini and Culicini. **Microfilaria streptocerca.** A sheathless microfilaria found in the skin, but not in the blood, of natives of the Cameroons and in Ghana. The extremity of the tail has a characteristic "walking-stick handle" appearance. [Gk *mikros* small, filaria.]

microfistula (mi·kro·**fis**·tew·lah). Fistula of microscopic size. [Gk *mikros* large, L *fistula* pipe.]

microflora (mi·kro·**flor**·ah). The microscopic flora of a region.

microfracture (mi·kro·**frak**·tcher). A minute fracture. [Gk *mikros* small, fracture.]

microgamete (mi·kro·**gam**·eet). 1. In malariology the thread-like flagellate structure liberated from the microgametocyte in the stomach of the mosquito to form the male fertilizing element. 2. A gamete which is smaller than the organism producing it. [Gk *mikros* small, *gametes* husband.]

microgametocyte (mi·kro·gam·**e'**·to·site). The non-motile male sexual cell which circulates in the human blood in malaria. In malignant tropical malaria (*Plasmodium falciparum*) the gametocytes have a characteristic crescent shape, and the nucleus of the microgametocyte is large and diffuse. [Gk *mikros* small, *gametes* husband, *kytos* cell.]

microgamy (mi·**krog**·am·e). In Protozoa, conjugation between microgametes. [Gk *mikros* small, *gamos* marriage.]

microgastria (mi·kro·**gas**·tre·ah). A congenital condition in which the stomach is smaller than the average. [Gk *mikros* small, *gaster* stomach.]

microgenesis (mi·kro·**jen**·es·is). Unusually small growth of a part. [Gk *mikros* small, *genein* to produce.]

microgenia (mi·kro·**je**·ne·ah). A condition in which the chin is of unusually small size. [Gk *mikros* small, *geneion* chin.]

microgenitalism (mi·kro·**jen**·it·al·izm). Abnormal smallness of the external genitalia. [Gk *mikros* small, genitalia.]

microglia (mi·**krog**·le·ah). Potentially phagocytic neuroglial cells of mesodermal origin. [Gk *mikros* small, neuroglia.]

microgliacyte, microgliocyte (mi·kro·**gli**·as·ite, mi·kro·**gli**·o·site). A microglial cell. [Gk *mikros* small, neuroglia, *kytos* cell.]

microgliomatosis (mi·kro·gli·o·mat·**o'**·sis). A condition in which there is proliferation of the microglia or cerebral histiocytes. These are branching cells of mesoblastic origin which can become amoeboid and wandering. [microglia, Gk *-oma* tumour, *-osis* condition.]

microglossia (mi·kro·**glos**·e·ah). Smallness of the tongue. [Gk *mikros* small, *glossa* tongue.]

micrognathia (mi·kro·**nath**·e·ah). Undersize of the jaw; particularly applied to the mandible. [Gk *mikros* small, *gnathos* jaw.]

microgonioscope (mi·kro·**go**·ne·o·skope). An apparatus for observing an angle of the anterior chamber of the eye. It has a binocular microscope and source of light attached to it. [Gk *mikros* small, *gonia* angle, *skopein* to view.]

microgram (mi·kro·gram). 1. A unit of weight employed in micro-analysis; one millionth of a gram, symbolized γ or μg. 2. A photograph or tracing of an extremely small object. [Gk *mikros* small, *gramma* letter.]

micrograph (mi·kro·graf). 1. Microgram 2nd def. 2. An apparatus designed to record photographically and in magnified form, movements of an extremely small amplitude. [see foll.]

micrographia (mi·kro·**graf**·e·ah). Small handwriting; decrease in the size of written characters as compared with the writer's usual hand. [Gk *mikros* small, *graphein* to write.]

micrography (mi·**krog**·raf·e). 1. The practice of very small handwriting. 2. Microscopical examination. 3. A description of minute objects; any histological findings. [see prec.]

microgyria, microgyrus (mi·kro·**ji**·re·ah, mi·kro·**ji**·rus). An abnormally small cerebral cortical gyrus, usually a congenital anomaly. [Gk *mikros* small, *gyros* circle.]

microhepatia (mi·kro·hep·**at'**·e·ah). Abnormally small size of the liver. [Gk *mikros* small, *hepar* liver.]

microhm (mi·krome). A unit of electrical resistance; one millionth of an ohm. [Gk *mikros* small, ohm.]

micro-incineration (mi·kro·in·sin·er·**a'**·shun). The incineration of small quantities of material in order to proceed to chemical analysis of the ash so produced. Specifically, the ashing of microscopic sections. [Gk *mikros* small, incineration.]

microkinesis (mi·kro·kin·**e'**·sis). Muscular movements of involuntary type to be found especially in very young children. [Gk *mikros* small, *kinesis* movement.]

microkymatotherapy, microkymotherapy (mi·kro·ki·mat·o·**ther'**·ap·e, mi·kro·ki·mo·**ther'**·ap·e). The generation of heat in the tissues by radiations of about 10 cm wavelength, of extremely high frequency of about 3000 MHz (megacycles per second). [Gk *mikros* small, *kyma* wave, *therapeia* treatment.]

microlentia (mi·kro·**len**·she·ah). A condition of abnormal smallness of the crystalline lens. [Gk *mikros* small, lens.]

microleucoblast (mi·kro·**lew**·ko·blast). Micromyeloblast. [Gk *mikros* small, leucoblast.]

microlith (mi·kro·lith). A minute calculus; when many are present, e.g. in the kidney, the condition is referred to as gravel. [Gk *mikros* small, *lithos* stone.]

microlithiasis (mi·kro·lith·**i'**·as·is). The presence or aggregation of microscopical calculi in an organ such as the kidney. **Pulmonary alveolar microlithiasis.** A rare disease of unknown cause in which alveoli become filled with calculi. [Gk *mikros* small, lithiasis.]

microlitre (mi·kro·le·ter). A unit of volume employed in micro-analysis: one millionth of a litre, one cubic millimetre. [Gk *mikros* small, litre.]

microlymphoblast (mi·kro·**limf**·o·blast). A small lymphoblast often seen in acute leukaemias. [Gk *mikros* small, lymphoblast.]

microlymphoidocyte (mi·kro·limf·**oid'**·o·site). A lymphoidocyte which is small and undeveloped. [Gk *mikros* small, lymphoidocyte.]

micromandibulare (mi·kro·man·dib·ew·**la'**·re). Possession of a small lower jaw. [Gk *mikros* small, L *mandibula* jaw.]

micromania (mi·kro·**ma**·ne·ah). A delusion held by an individual that his body or parts of it has decreased in size or that the importance of his personality has become less; general delusional belief of self-depreciation. [Gk *mikros* small, mania.]

micromanipulation (mi·kro·man·ip·ew·**la'**·shun). The dissection of cells under the microscope in biology, or the handling of minute quantities of substances in microchemistry. [Gk *mikros* small, manipulation.]

micromastia, micromazia (mi·kro·**mas**·te·ah, mik·kro·**ma**·ze·ah). Abnormal smallness of the mammary glands, generally associated with lack of development and absence of functional activity. [Gk *mikros* small, *mastos* breast, *mazos* breast.]

micromegalopsia (mi·kro·meg·al·**op'**·se·ah). A condition in which objects are not seen to be of their actual size, but as larger or smaller or as larger and smaller by turns. [Gk *mikros* small, *megas* large, *opsis* appearance.]

micromelia (mi·kro·**me**·le·ah). A condition in which the arms and legs are abnormally small. [Gk *mikros* small, *melos* limb.]

micromelus (mi·**krom**·el·us). In teratism, a monster the limbs of which are rudimentary, imperfectly developed, or abnormally small. [see prec.]

micromere (**mi**·kro·meer). A small cell of the blastula, characteristic of the animal pole. [Gk *mikros* small, *meros* part.]

micromerozoite (**mi**·kro·mer·o·**zo'**·ite). A merozoite of small size. [Gk *mikros* small, merozoite.]

micrometer (mi·**krom**·et·er). Any instrument used to measure very small objects, or to within very fine limits. **Diffraction micrometer.** A micrometer which makes use of light interference fringes. **Eyepiece micrometer.** A micrometer scale fitted within the eyepiece of a microscope and used for comparative measurements of the image. After calibration against a stage micrometer, e.g. a haemocytometer, at a particular magnification, it can be used for the rapid direct measurement of an object. **Filar micrometer.** An eyepiece micrometer in which a cross-wire is moved over the field of vision by a graduated screw. **Micrometer screw.** A screw so graduated round the circumference of the head that fine movements of the pitch may be measured. **Stage micrometer.** A glass slide engraved with a scale and fitted to the stage of a microscope. **Vernier-scale micrometer.** A glass slide engraved with a vernier for use in microscopic measurement. [Gk *mikros* small, meter.]

micrometre (mi·kro·**me**·ter). One millionth of a metre. [Gk *mikros* small, metre.]

micrometry (mi·**krom**·et·re). The measurement of very small lengths. [Gk *mikros* small, meter.]

micromicrofarad (**mi**·kro·**mi'**·kro·far·ad). A picofarad. [Gk *mikros* small, microfarad.]

micromicrogram (**mi**·kro·**mi'**·kro·gram). Picogram. [Gk *mikros* small, microgram.]

micromicron (mi·kro·**mi**·kron). Picometre. [Gk *mikros* small, micron.]

micromil (**mi**·kro·mil). Micromillimetre.

micromilligram (mi·kro·**mil**·e·gram). Nanogram. [Gk *mikros* small, milligram.]

micromillimetre (mi·kro·**mil**·e·me·ter). Nanometre. [Gk *mikros* small, millimetre.]

Micromonospora (**mi**·kro·mon·o·**spor'**·ah). A thermophilic actinomycete found in mouldy, overheated hay. Inhalation of spores of one species, *Micromonospora faeni*, cause the condition farmer's lung in agricultural workers. [Gk *mikros* small, *monos* single, *spora* spore.]

micromonosporin (mi·kro·mon·o·**spor'**·in). An antibiotic from *Micromonospora.*

micromotoscope (mi·kro·**mo**·to·skope). A device for the photographic recording of the movements of microscopical objects. [Gk *mikros* small, motion, Gk *skopein* to view.]

micromyelia (**mi**·kro·mi·**e'**·le·ah). General reduction in size of the spinal cord. [Gk *mikros* small, *myelos* marrow.]

micromyeloblast (mi·kro·**mi**·el·o·blast). A small myeloblast. [Gk *mikros* small, myeloblast.]

micromyelocyte (mi·kro·**mi**·el·o·site). A small myelocyte seen in leukaemic conditions. [Gk *mikros* small, myelocyte.]

micromyelolymphocyte (mi·kro·**mi**·el·o·**limf'**·o·site). Myeloblast. [Gk *mikros* small, myelolymphocyte.]

micron (**mi**·kron). 1. Micrometre: one millionth of a metre. 2. Microne. [Gk *mikros* small.]

microne (**mi**·krone). A particle such as occurs in a fine suspension, which is not visible to the unaided eye but is within the range of the ordinary microscope. [Gk *mikros* small.]

microneedle (**mi**·kro·ne·dl). A very fine glass needle used in microdissection and micromanipulation; its movements are usually effected by remote mechanical control, with micrometer adjustment. [Gk *mikros* small, needle.]

micronemous (mi·**kron**·em·us). Having short threads or filaments. [Gk *mikros* small, *nema* thread.]

micronodular (mi·kro·**nod**·ew·lar). Formed of or containing small nodules. [Gk *mikros* small, node.]

micronucleus (mi·kro·**new**·kle·us). A small nucleus. [Gk *mikros* small, nucleus.]

micronychia (mi·kro·**nik**·e·ah). The possession of a small nail or nails. [Gk *mikros* small, *onyx* nail.]

micro-orchidia (**mi**·kro·or·**kid'**·e·ah). Abnormal smallness of one or both testes. [Gk *mikros* small, *orchis* testis.]

micro-organism (mi·kro·**or**·gan·izm). Any plant or animal of microscopical size; a protozoon, fungus, bacterium, or virus. [Gk *mikros* small, organism.]

micro-organismal (**mi**·kro·or·gan·**iz'**·mal). Pertaining to a micro-organism.

microparasite (mi·kro·**par**·ah·site). A micro-organism which is parasitic in action.

micropathological (**mi**·kro·path·o·**loj'**·ik·al). Relating to or belonging to micropathology.

micropathology (**mi**·kro·path·**ol'**·o·je). 1. That branch of science which deals with the study of minute pathological changes. 2. The pathology of those conditions that are due to micro-organisms. [Gk *mikros* small, pathology.]

micropenis (mi·kro·**pe**·nis). Smallness of the penis. [Gk *mikros* small, penis.]

microphage (**mi**·kro·fage). A small phagocyte; a small actively phagocytic polymorphonuclear leucocyte. [Gk *mikros* small, *phagein* to eat.]

microphagocyte (mi·kro·**fag**·o·site). A form of phagocyte that is smaller than the average. [Gk *mikros* small, phagocyte.]

microphakia (mi·kro·**fa**·ke·ah). Undue small size of the lens of the eye. [Gk *mikros* small, *phakos* lens.]

microphallus (mi·kro·**fal**·us). Smallness of the penis. [Gk *mikros* small, phallus.]

microphobia (mi·kro·**fo**·be·ah). 1. Microbiophobia. 2. An insane fear of minute objects. [Gk *mikros* small, phobia.]

microphone (**mi**·kro·fone). An instrument for the conversion of sound waves to electrical oscillations, the electrical signal from the microphone being proportional to the sound pressure reaching the microphone, and being capable of conversion back to reproduce the original sound. [Gk *mikros* small, *phone* sound.]

microphonia, microphony (mi·kro·**fo**·ne·ah, mi·**krof**·o·ne). Faintness of vocal sounds. [see prec.]

microphotograph (mi·kro·**fo**·to·graf). A photomicrograph; a photograph taken through the lens system of a microscope.

microphotometer (**mi**·kro·fo·**tom'**·et·er). An instrument for measuring small units of transmitted light, e.g. from an object under the microscope. [Gk *mikros* small, *phos* light, *metron* measure.]

microphthalmia, microphthalmos (mi·krof·**thal**·me·ah, mi·krof·**thal**·mos). A condition in which the eyes are of abnormally small size, generally because of degenerative disease or lack of proper development; the condition may be unilateral. [Gk *mikros* small, *ophthalmos* eye.]

microphthalmoscope (mi·krof·**thal**·mo·skope). An apparatus used in the performance of fundus microscopy. [Gk *mikros* small, *ophthalmos* eye, *skopein* to view.]

microphthalmus (mi·krof·**thal**·mus). 1. An individual whose eyes are of abnormally small size. 2. Microphthalmia. [Gk *mikros* small, *ophthalmos* eye.]

microphyte (**mi**·kro·fite). A minute plant or bacterium. [Gk *mikros* small, *phyton* plant.]

microphytic (mi·kro·**fit**·ik). Caused by or pertaining to microphytes.

micropia (mi·kro·**pe**·ah). Micropsia.

micropipette (**mi**·kro·pip·**et'**). A very fine pipette for transferring minute quantities of fluid. [Gk *mikros* small, pipette.]

microplasia (mi·kro·**pla**·ze·ah). Dwarfism; stunting of growth. [Gk *mikros* small, *plassein* to form.]

microplastocyte (mi·kro·**plas**·to·site). A very small blood platelet. [Gk *mikros* small, plastocyte.]

microplethysmography (mi·kro·pleth·iz·**mog'**·raf·e). The assessment of minute changes in the volume of organs. [Gk *mikros* small, *plethynein* to increase, *graphein* to record.]

micropodia, micropody (mi·kro·**po**·de·ah, mi·**krop**·o·de). A condition in which the feet are abnormally small. [Gk *mikros* small, *pous* foot.]

microprojection (mi·kro·pro·**jek'**·shun). The throwing of an image of microscopic preparations upon a screen by means of a projection microscope.

microprosopa (mi·kro·pro·**so'**·pah). Congenital smallness of the face. [Gk *mikros* small, *prosopon* face.]

microprosopus (mi·kro·pro·**so'**·pus). A monster with an imperfectly developed or abnormally small face. [see prec.]

micropsia (mi·**krop**·se·ah). A condition in which objects are seen to be smaller than in fact they are. [Gk *mikros* small, *opsis* sight.]

micropsychia (mi·kro·**si**·ke·ah). Feeblemindedness. [Gk *mikros* small, *psyche* mind.]

microptic (mi·**krop**·tik). Affected with or relating to micropsia.

micropus (**mi**·kro·pus). An individual with undersized feet. [Gk *mikros* small, *pous* foot.]

micropyle (**mi**·kro·pile). Any minute canal or pore. In flowering plants, a minute pore in the seed-coat through which water enters; in insects, a pore in the egg membrane through which sperm enters; in Sporozoa a pore in the cyst wall of the macrogamete through which the microgamete enters. [Gk *mikros* small, *pyle* gate.]

microradiograph (mi·kro·**ra**·de·o·graf). An x-ray film of microscopic structures. [Gk *mikros* small, radiograph.]

microradiography (mi·kro·ra·de·**og'**·raf·e). Radiography of microscopic structures. The basic principle is enlargement of radiographic images on very fine-grained photographic emulsion, Biological tissues may first be stained with absorbing materials of varying density, or their internal structure alone may provide the necessary differential densities.

microrefractometer (mi·kro·re·frak·**tom'**·et·er). An instrument for measuring the indices of refraction of substances in cells and tissues, with particular reference to the changes in structure of the blood cells. [Gk *mikros* small, refractometer.]

microrespirometer (mi·kro·res·pir·**om'**·et·er). An apparatus devised originally for the purpose of determining the uptake of oxygen (and the output of CO_2) by fragments or slices of living tissue, by small organs, or by small animals such as insects; the best-known forms were devised by Barcroft, Krogh, Thunberg and Warburg. In principle it consists of a small closed vessel containing the tissue, and an alkali to absorb CO_2: it is filled with oxygen and a manometer is connected to the vessel; as oxygen is absorbed the manometer shows a fall of pressure, from which the oxygen used up in a given time can be calculated. Its use can be extended to the determination of gas absorbed or evolved in many reactions. [Gk *mikros* small, respiration, meter.]

microroentgen (mi·kro·**runt**·yen). A millionth of a roentgen. [Gk *mikros* small, roentgen.]

microrrhinia (mi·kro·**ri**·ne·ah). Undersize of the nose. [Gk *mikros* small, *rhis* nose.]

microrutherford (mi·kro·**ruth**·er·ford). A unit of radioactivity: the millionth part of a rutherford. [obsolete term.] [Gk *mikros* small, rutherford.]

microscelous (mi·kro·**skel**·us). Short-legged. [Gk *mikros* small, *skelos* leg.]

microscope (**mi**·kro·skope). An instrument for magnifying the size of small objects. **Binocular microscope.** A microscope designed for the simultaneous use of both eyes; this enables objects to be seen in perspective. **Compound microscope.** A microscope consisting of two or more simple or complex systems of lenses. **Corneal microscope.** A high-power lens for examining details of the cornea and iris. **Dissecting microscope.** A well-corrected aplanatic lens mounted at the end of an adjustable arm carried on a heavy base. **Electron microscope.** A microscope in which a beam of electrons replaces the beam of light of a light microscope. Electromagnetic lenses focus the electrons on to the specimen, and further lenses form a magnified image on a phosphorescent screen or a photographic negative. The wavelength of the electron beam is very much shorter than that of visible light making resolution of 0.2 nm (2Å) possible, and instrumental magnifications of up to 500 000×. Due to the low penetrations of electrons, special preparation techniques are required and a very high vacuum has to be maintained inside the microscope column. **Fluorescence microscope.** An optical microscope with a suitable light source and filters to examine specimens which have been stained with dyes which fluoresce in ultraviolet or blue light, or which have been treated with antibody to which a fluorescent dye has been coupled. **Flying-spot microscope.** Light is passed through a microscope from the eyepiece to the objective and is focused by the objective to a small spot in the object plane. The light is produced by a moving spot on a cathode-ray tube tracing a rectangular "raster" which is reproduced diminished in size on the examined transparent object. Light passing through the specimen is converted to an electrical signal by a photo-cell and the enlarged image of the object formed on the screen of a television tube, the raster of which is synchronized with the scanning raster. **Micrometer microscope.** Vernier microscope (see below). **Phase microscope, Phase-contrast microscope, Phase-difference microscope.** A microscope in which a phase difference is arranged between the light passing through and the light passing round the object, thus enabling the object itself to be seen. *See also* MICROSCOPY. **Projection microscope.** An arrangement by which the image formed in a microscope is thrown on a screen, or upon a photographic plate, thus producing a photo-micrograph for permanent record. **Reading microscope.** A microscope provided with a micrometer eyepiece scale for the accurate measurement of the dimensions and movements of objects. **Simple microscope, Single microscope.** A magnifying glass, being a simple lens or an achromatic combination of lenses cemented together. **Slit-lamp microscope.** A binocular microscope with slit illumination for examination of the eye. **Stereoscopic microscope.** Binocular microscope (see above). **Travelling microscope.** Vernier microscope (see below). **Ultrapaque microscope.** A microscope used to examine the structure of opaque organs. **Ultraviolet microscope.** A microscope furnished with quartz lenses, for use with ultraviolet light. **Vernier microscope.** A microscope mounted on a movable slide, to measure accurately the dimensions of large objects. The movements of the slide may be in one direction or in two directions at right angles to each other. **X-ray microscope.** An apparatus in which the magnifying power of the microscope is combined with the penetrating power of x-rays for the detailed examination of non-opaque structures. [Gk *mikros* small, *skopein* to view.]

See also: GREENOUGH.

microscopic, microscopical (mi·kro·**skop**·ik, mi·kro·**skop**·ik·al). 1. Relating or belonging to a microscope. 2. Applied to objects or detail too small to be seen without the aid of a microscope.

microscopy (mi·**kros**·ko·pe). The science of the use of the microscope. **Bright-field microscopy.** Microscopy by direct transillumination. **Clinical microscopy.** The use of the microscope for the examination of clinical material, e.g. urinary deposits, sputa, etc. **Corneal microscopy.** Examination of the cornea of the eye by means of a binocular microscope with a Gullstrand type of slit-lamp illumination. **Dark-field microscopy.** Dark-ground microscopy [see foll.]. **Dark-ground microscopy.** A method of microscopical examination used for micro-organisms which are too transparent or too small to be seen by transmitted light. Illumination is only by light which enters obliquely through a special condenser. Objects are seen by rays which are reflected to the eye, and appear silvery against a black background. **Electron microscopy.** The use of the electron microscope. **Fluorescence microscopy.** A technique involving the observation of the re-emitted visible light from a specimen which has been illuminated by and has absorbed light of a different wavelength. It is widely used in the fluorescent antibody technique. **Fundus microscopy.** Examination of the fundus of the eye by means of a binocular microscope fitted with a Hruby lens (strong concave) illuminated by a slit lamp fitted with a suitable prism. **Phase microscopy, Phase-contrast microscopy, Phase-difference microscopy.** A method of microscopy by which the internal structures of unstained cells can be seen. The method involves the use of an annular diaphragm or some other device in the condenser, and a phase-retarding plate in the back focal plane of the objective; by this means phase differences are converted into differences of light intensity, and objects having a higher refractive index than the material around them appear dark against a lighter background while objects of lower refractive index than their surroundings appear light against a darker background. **Polarized light microscopy.** The use of a polarizing microscope to examine crystalline material, for example the crystals of calcium pyrophosphate dihydrate and uric acid found in pyrophosphate arthropathy and gout.

microsecond (mi·kro·**sek**·ond). One millionth part of a second. [Gk *mikros* small, second.]

microseme (**mi**·kro·seem). Having a skull with an orbital index of less than 84. [Gk *mikros* small, *sema* mound.]

microslide (**mi**·kro·slide). Histology slide; a thin glass plate on which tissue sections are mounted prior to microscopical examination. [Gk *mikros* small, slide.]

microsmatic (mi·kros·**mat**·ik). Having a poorly developed sense of smell. [Gk *mikros* small, *osmaeomein* to smell.]

microsomes (**mi**·kro·so·mz). The name given to the fragments of endoplasmic reticulum associated with ribosomes that are obtained by tissue homogenization and ultracentrifugation. The ribosomes are subsequently released by treatment with mild detergents. [Gk *mikros* small, *soma* body.]

microsomia (mi·kro·**so**·me·ah). Abnormal smallness of the body. [see prec.]

microspectroscope (mi·kro·**spek**·tro·skope). 1. A spectroscope used in conjunction with a microscope to examine the absorption spectra of tissues. 2. A microscope eyepiece fitted to a spectroscope in order to examine closely the spectral lines. [Gk *mikros* small, spectroscope.]

microsphere (**mik**·kro·sfeer). Centrosome. [Gk *mikros* small, sphere.]

microspherocyte (mi·kro·**sfeer**·o·site). A small, very fragile, more globular type of red blood cell. It is characteristically observed in the blood in certain acute and chronic haemolytic anaemias, in congenital haemolytic anaemia (acholuric jaundice), and in familial spherocytosis. [Gk *mikros* small, spherocyte.]

microspherocytosis (mi·kro·**sfeer**·o·si·**to**′·sis). A condition of the blood in which there is an excessive number of microspherocytes in circulation. Such diseases include acholuric jaundice, chronic spherocytosis and certain acute haemolytic anaemias. [Gk *mikros* small, spherocytosis.]

microsphygmia, microsphygmy, microsphyxia (mi·kro·**sfig**·me·ah, mi·kro·**sfig**·me, mi·kro·**sfix**·e·ah). Diminished strength of pulse. [Gk *mikros* small, *sphygmos* pulse.]

Microspira (mi·kro·**spi**·rah). A synonym for the genus *Vibrio* [obsolete term]. [Gk *mikros* small, *speira* coil.]

Microspironema pallidum (mi·kro·spi·ro·**ne**′·mah **pal**·id·um). A synonym for *Treponema pallidum* [obsolete term]. [Gk *mikros* small, *speira* coil, *nema* thread, L *pallidum* pale.]

microsplanchnic (mi·kro·**splangk**·nik). Having small intestines. [Gk *mikros* small, *splagchnon* viscera.]

microsplenia (mi·kro·**sple**·ne·ah). Unusual smallness of the spleen. [Gk *mikros* small, spleen.]

microspore (**mi**·kro·spore). A small spore; especially when a fungus bears spores of two distinct sizes the smaller is the microspore. [Gk *mikros* small, *sporos* seed.]

microsporid (mi·kro·**spo**·rid). A skin eruption, often vesicular, due to specific allergic hypersensitivity provoked by infection with species of *Microsporum.*

microsporidia, microsporidium (mi·kro·spo·**rid**′·e·ah, **mi**·kro·spo·**rid**′·e·um). A protozoal parasite of insects: e.g. one species of the genus *Nosema* infects bees, another silkworms. [Gk *mikros* small, *sporos* seed, *eidos* form.]

microsporin (mi·kro·**spo**·rin). An extract from the fungus *Microsporum.*

microsporosis (**mi**·kro·spo·**ro**′·sis). A disease caused by the small-spored ringworm fungi. *Microsporum audouinii* is a common cause of scalp ringworm (in UK), attacking principally children before puberty. It is an anthropophilic species. *Microsporum canis* infects cats and dogs, *Microsporum equinus* infects horses; both species can infect man. *Microsporum gypseum* occurs naturally in the soil, but infections in man and animals have occurred. [Gk *mikros* small, *sporos* seed, *-osis* condition.]

Microsporum (mi·kro·**spo**·rum). A member of the dermatophyte fungi causing ringworm of the hair, skin and, rarely, the nails. Hair invasion is characterized by the production of an external sheath of small, polyhedral-shaped spores arranged in a mosaic over the hair shaft. *Microsporum audouinii* and *M. canis* will produce hair infections that fluoresce under Wood's light. Fluorescence in other species is variable, depending on the extent of hair invasion. *M. distortum,* a pathogenic fungus reported from the USA and New Zealand. *M. equinum,* a fungus which is pathogenic to horse but rarely, if ever, to man. *M. nanum,* a fungus which causes scalp ringworm. It only occasionally fluoresces under Wood's rays. *M. praecox,* a fungus pathogenic to man. *M. purpurea,* the source of the antibiotic, gentamicin. *M. vanbreuseghemii,* a fungus pathogenic to man. Species once endemic to the Far East (*M. ferrugineum*) and Africa (*M. rivalierii, M. langeronii, M. ferrugineum*) are now being isolated in Europe and elsewhere as a result of population movements. Recently the perfect (sexual) states of some species have been discovered and classified in the genus *Nannizzia* (Ascomycetes). [Gk *mikros* small, *sporos* seed.]

microstereognosia (**mi**·kro·steer·e·og·**no**′·se·ah). The abnormal perception of objects felt as being smaller than they are. [Gk *mikros* small, *stereos* solid, *gnosis* knowledge.]

microsthenic (mi·kro·**sthen**·ik). Having weak muscular power. [Gk *mikros* small, *sthenos* strength.]

microstomia (mi·kro·**sto**·me·ah). Unusual smallness of the mouth. [Gk *mikros* small, *stoma* mouth.]

microsurgery (mi·kro·**ser**·jer·e). Microdissection; micro-manipulation. [Gk *mikros* small, surgery.]

microsyringe (**mi**·kro·sir·**inj**′). Micrometer syringe; a hypodermic syringe fitted with a micrometer screw, and utilized in the measurement and delivery of minimal quantities of fluid for injection, e.g. into a living cell in micromanipulation.

microteeth (**mi**·kro·teeth). Unusually small teeth. [Gk *mikros* small, tooth.]

microthelia (mi·kro·**the**·le·ah). Abnormal smallness of the nipples. [Gk *mikros* small, *thele* nipple.]

microtia (mi·**kro**·she·ah). Abnormal smallness of the external ear. [Gk *mikros* small, *ous* ear.]

microtome (**mi**·kro·tome). An instrument for cutting sections of tissue for examination under the microscope. **Freezing microtome.** A microtome to which is attached a device for the artificial freezing, by means of solid or liquid carbon dioxide, of the tissue to be cut. **Rocking microtome.** One used for cutting serial sections of tissue embedded in a wax cube; the latter is fixed to the end of a lever, and is moved upwards and downwards on to a stationary knife. [Gk *mikros* small, *temnein* to cut.]

microtomy (mi·**krot**·o·me). The process of cutting thin sections of tissue for microscopical examination; use of the microtome.

microtonometer (**mi**·kro·to·**nom**′·et·er). A small apparatus employed in the determination of carbon dioxide and oxygen tensions in arterial blood (Krogh). [Gk *mikros* small, *tonos* tone, meter.]

microtrauma (mi·kro·**traw**·mah). An injury or lesion that is slight or insignificant. [Gk *mikros* small, trauma.]

microtrichia (mi·kro·**trik**·e·ah). Abnormal fineness or shortness of the hair. [Gk *mikros* small, *thrix* hair.]

Microtrombidium (**mi**·kro·trom·**bid**′·e·um). A genus of mites. **Microtrombidium akamushi.** *Trombicula akamushi.* **Microtrombidium wichmanni.** A mite whose larva, the gonone, is a jigger of

Celebes transmitting a typhus-like disease. [Gk *mikros* small, *trombodes* timid.]

microtropia (mi·kro·**tro**·pe·ah). A small-angle concomitant squint of less than 5 degrees often associated with abnormal retinal correspondence and/or eccentric fixation. [Gk *mikros* small, *trepein* to turn.]

Microtus (mi·**kro**·tus). A genus of small rodents, the field voles. **Microtus agrestis.** The British species which has been used as a laboratory animal. **Microtus montebelli.** A vole which acts as a reservoir of infection for the rickettsia of tsutsugamushi disease in Japan. [Gk *mikros* small, *ous* ear.]

microvillus (mi·kro·**vil**·us). A minute finger-like process, visible with the electron microscope, which is a feature of the surface of many cells. Numerous, closely-packed microvilli form a brush border. [Gk *mikros* small, villus.]

microvivisection (mi·kro·viv·e·**sek'**·shun). Microdisection of living tissues. [Gk *mikros* small, vivisection.]

microvolt (**mi**·kro·volt). A unit of electric potential: one millionth of a volt. [Gk *mikros* small, volt.]

microvoltometer (**mi**·kro·volt·**om'**·et·er). An apparatus for detecting minute changes in electric potential. [Gk *mikros* small, volt, meter.]

microzoon (mi·kro·**zo**·on). An animal organism that can be seen only by means of a microscope; a protozoon. [Gk *mikros* small, *zoon* animal.]

microzyme (**mi**·kro·zime). Micelle. [Gk *mikros* small, *zyme* leaven.]

micrurgy (mi·**krer**·je). Micromanipulation. [Gk *mikros* small, *ergon* work.]

Micruroides (mi·kroo·**roi**·deez). A genus of poisonous coral snakes. [Gk *mikros* small, *oura* tail, *eidos* form.]

micturate (**mik**·tewr·ate). Urinate. [see foll.]

micturition (mik·tewr·**ish**·un). Urination; the act of passing urine. [L *micturire* to desire to make water.]

midaxilla (mid·ax·**il**·ah). The centre of the axilla. [AS *midd*, axilla.]

mid-brain [mesencephalon (NA)] (**mid**·brane). That part of the brain containing the tectum, the tegmentum and the cerebral peduncles. [AS *midd*, brain.]

midcarpal (mid·**kar**·pal). Between the two rows of carpal bones; generally with reference to the articulation of the midcarpal region. [AS *midd*, carpal.]

mid-cycle peak. Using radioimmunoassays it has been shown that apart from the peak in serum FSH at mid-cycle in the menstrual cycle there is an even more marked peak in serum LH just preceding it which indicates that LH (or progesterone) plays an important part in inducing ovulation.

Middeldorpf, Albrecht Theodor von. (b. 1824). Breslau surgeon.

Middeldorpf's splint, or triangle. A splint in the form of a wooden triangle, used for fractures of the humerus; now obsolete.

middle [medius (NA)] (midl). Placed intermediately. [AS *middel.*]

Middlebrook, Gardener (b. 1915). New York bacteriologist.

Middlebrook-Dubos reaction. A reaction based on a positive allergic effect that can be induced in persons either exposed to or suffering from leprosy, by injection of lepromin prepared from a heat-killed suspension of triturated leprous skin nodules. Exposure to tuberculous infection in which a positive tuberculin reaction has occurred may also render the subject lepromin-positive. Both reactions appear to indicate a degree of immunity to leprosy. BCG vaccination results in lepromin conversion, and is being considered as a prophylactic measure against leprosy in exposed subjects. There appears to be a cross-sensitivity as well as a cross-immunity which can be induced by lepromin, tuberculin, or BCG, but it is not constant and other common factors may be concerned.

midfrontal (mid·**frun**·tal). Pertaining to the centre of the frontal bone or in certain cases to the frontal lobe of the brain. [AS *midd*, frontal.]

midge (mij). General name for small flies of the families Ceratopogonidae, Chironomidae, and Psychodidae. Biting midges include the species *Culicoides, Forcipomyia, Pericoma* and *Phlebotomus.* [AS *mycge.*]

midget (**mij**·et). A properly formed individual of diminutive size. [dim. of AS *mycge.*]

midgetism (**mij**·et·izm). The state of being a midget.

mid-gut (**mid**·gut). That portion of the embryonic alimentary canal which is formed from the roof of the yolk sac after the formation of the foregut and hind-gut diverticula. In man it gives rise to the distal half of the duodenum, the jejunum, the ileum, the caecum and appendix, the ascending colon and most of the transverse colon (the territory of supply of the superior mesenteric artery). [AS *midd*, gut.]

midoccipital (mid·ok·**sip**·it·al). Relating to the central point of the occipital bone or of the occiput. [AS *midd*, occiput.]

midperiphery (mid·per·**if**·er·e). The zone of fundus halfway between the macula and the most peripheral portion visible, usually from 8 to 9 mm from the corneal margin. [AS *midd*, periphery.]

midphalangeal (mid·fal·**an**·je·al). Referring to the middle phalanx. [AS *midd*, phalanx.]

midpiece (**mid**·pees). The euglobulin fraction of complement which is precipitated by the removal of electrolytes from the serum. It unites directly with sensitized red blood cells, though it will not produce haemolysis unless another fraction of complement, so-called *end-piece*, is also present. [AS *midd*, ME *pece.*]

midriff (**mid**·rif). The diaphragm. [AS *midd*, *hrif* belly.]

midsternum (mid·**ster**·num). The body of the sternum, formerly called the *gladiolus.* [AS *midd*, sternum.]

midtarsal (mid·**tar**·sal). Situated between the two rows of tarsal bones. [AS *midd*, tarsal.]

midtegmentum (mid·teg·**men**·tum). The central portion of the tegmentum. [AS *midd*, tegmentum.]

midventricle (mid·**ven**·trikl). The cavity of the mid-brain. [AS *midd*, ventricle.]

midwife (**mid**·wife). A person who is qualified to attend women in childbirth. The title is protected by law, and may only be used by persons who have undergone a specified period of training in an approved school of midwifery, and have passed the examination entitling their names to be on the State Roll of Certified Midwives. [AS *midd*, *wif.*]

midwifery (mid·**wif**·er·e). Obstetrics; particularly the more practical aspects. [see prec.]

Mierzejewski, Johann Lucian (b. 1839). St. Petersburg neurologist and psychiatrist.

Mierzejewski's foramen. The lateral aperture of the 4th ventricle.

Miescher, Johann Friedrich (b. 1811). Basle pathologist.

Miescher's tube, or tubule. Sarcocyst; the elongated cyst-like body of *Sarcocystis lindemanni.*

migraine (me·grane, **mi**·grane). A periodic condition with localized headaches, frequently associated with vomiting and sensory disturbances, and symptoms related to vision (flashes of light, amblyopia, etc.). The cause is ascribed to vasomotor disturbance of the cerebral circulation (dilatation or spasm of cerebral arteries). **Abdominal migraine.** Periodic attacks of abdominal pain, especially in children regarded as an atypical form of migraine. **Basilar migraine.** Attacks which culminate in loss of consciousness. **Fulgurating migraine.** Violent and rapidly-developing migraine. **Hemiplegic migraine.** Migraine accompanied by recurring hemiplegia, often transmitted by dominant inheritance. **Ophthalmic migraine.** That due to errors of refraction. **Ophthalmoplegic migraine.** Migraine accompanied by transient weakness of an eye muscle. [Fr. from Gk *hemi* half, *kranion* skull.]

migrate (**mi**·grate). To wander from one place to another, often used to describe cellular movement. [L *migrare* to wander.]

migrateur (me·grat·**er**). An individual having an obsessive urge to wander. [Fr. wanderer.]

migration (mi·gra·shun). An active or passive movement leading to a change of position. **External migration.** The passage of the ovum through the peritoneal cavity from one ovary to the other uterine tube. **Internal migration.** The passage of an ovum from one uterine tube to the other via the uterine lumen. **Migration of the leucocytes.** The passage of white cells through the wall of a blood vessel, especially during inflammation. **Migration of the ovum.** The passage of the ovum from the ovary to the uterus. **Transperitoneal migration.** External migration (see above). [L *migrare* to wander.]

Mikamycin (mi·kah·mi·sin). BP Commission approved name for an antibiotic produced by *Streptomyces mitakaensis.*

Mikulicz-Radecki, Johann von. (b. 1850). Breslau surgeon.

Mikulicz's angle. The angle of femoral torsion.

Mikulicz's aphthae. Chronic intermittent recurrent aphthae; recurrent ulcers on the tongue and oral mucosa, associated with leucopenia, and which disappear with improvement in the blood picture. The granulocytes are most severely affected, and secondary infection may retard the usual return to normality. Sulphonamides should be avoided in treatment.

Mikulicz's cell. A special variety of histiocyte or allied cell found in rhinoscleroma.

Mikulicz's clamp, enterotome, or enterotribe. A two-bladed clamp used to crush the spur of a double-barrelled colostomy, as in the Paul-Mikulicz operation (see Mikulicz's operation, 2nd def. below) for colon resection.

Mikulicz's disease, or syndrome. Bilateral symmetrical enlargement of the lacrimal and salivary glands. Now regarded to be of the same nature as Sjögren's disease.

Mikulicz's drain. A means of drainage obtained by introducing a single layer of gauze as a lining to a wound cavity which is then packed with thick gauze wicks.

Mikulicz's operation. 1. Stretching of the cardiac orifice by way of an incision in the stomach to relieve cardiospasm. 2. Stage resection of colon, which is withdrawn as a loop on the surface of the abdomen and removed some days later to leave a double colostomy, the colostomy being finally closed after crushing of the spur which forms between the two ends of the extruded loop. Also called *Paul's operations.* 3. An intranasal method of draining the maxillary sinus, a modification of which is still used.

Heineke-Mikulicz operation. Pyloroplasty; a longitudinal incision is made at the pylorus and sewn transversely.

Vladimiroff-Mikulicz amputation, or operation. An osteoplastic resection of the heel; the talus and the calcaneum are removed and to the lower end of the tibia is apposed the anterior row of tarsal bones.

mildew (mil·dew). A term applied to saprophytic fungal growths on fabrics and fibres which result in discoloration and weakening of the material. There are numerous species, many brightly coloured. The powdery mildews [Erysiphaceae] are plant parasites damaging flowering plants, particularly roses, also grapes, gooseberries, and hops. [AS *meledeaw.*]

Miles, William Ernest (b. 1869). London surgeon.

Miles' clamp. An angled clamp for controlling the pelvic colon in the operation for removal of the rectum.

Miles' operation. Abdominoperineal resection of the distal colon and rectum for carcinoma.

Miles' cone test. A hollow cone used for testing ocular dominance.

Milian, Gaston (b. 1871). Paris dermatologist.

Milian's ninth-day erythema, reaction, or syndrome. A morbilliform or scarlatiniform eruption associated with fever and other constitutional symptoms, lasting only a few days, occurring about the ninth day after the administration of a drug, particularly arsphenamine. The eruption is probably a biotropic phenomenon.

Milian's citrine skin. Yellow, thickened, wrinkled skin due to prolonged exposure to the sun.

Milian's sign. If the head, face, and ears are involved by an inflammatory process, the primary malady is a skin disease; whereas if the ears escape, the primary malady is subcutaneous inflammation.

white atrophy of Milian. Progressive fibrosis with telangiectasia. White sclerotic plaques on the ankle or foot with telangiectasia nearby and hyperpigmentation; a manifestation of local vascular insufficiency, often both venular and arteriolar.

miliaria (mil·e·a·re·ah). A papular or vesicular affection of the skin which accompanies profuse sweating, and is due to blocking of the ducts of sweat glands. **Miliaria alba.** Miliaria with white papules. **Miliaria crystallina.** An eruption of small vesicles which contain sweat, due to blocking of the sweat ducts at the level of the horny layer of the epidermis. **Miliaria papulosa.** Miliaria in which papules predominate. **Miliaria profunda.** Asymptomatic sweat-containing papules, due to blocking of the sweat ducts in the corium. **Miliaria propria.** Miliaria rubra [see foll.]. **Miliaria rubra.** An inflammatory form of miliaria consisting of bright-red papules surmounted by a minute vesicle, and clear vesicles with an erythematous halo around them. **Miliaria vesiculosa.** Miliaria in which vesicles predominate. [L *milium* millet.]

miliary (mil·e·ar·e). 1. Similar to, or of the size of a millet seed, or marked by the presence of lesions of this nature. 2. In zoology, of small size and numerous, as of tubercles. [L *milium* millet.]

milium (mil·e·um). 1. Pearly white pinhead-sized tumours occurring on the upper two-thirds of the face in adults, and unconnected with the sebaceous glands. 2. Lesions of similar appearance to 1. (above) on the genitalia; retention cysts of sebaceous glands. 3. Retention cysts of sebaceous glands in infants. 4. Epidermal cysts occurring in epidermolysis bullosa and, rarely, in other dermatoses such as pemphigus. **Colloid milium.** A degeneration of the dermal connective tissue presenting as yellow translucent papules or plaques on areas of skin exposed to sunlight. **Milium congenitale.** A rare congenital disorder consisting of a pale reddish-yellow plaque with scaly surface and comedones at the edges, found on the head or face. **Milium en plaques.** Milium congenitale [see prec.]. [L millet.]

milk (milk). 1. A fluid secreted by mammals for feeding their young until such time as they can feed themselves. It is an almost perfect food, containing not only fat, protein and carbohydrate, but also the necessary inorganic salts and vitamins. 2. The name has long been applied to any fluid resembling milk, e.g. the milk of a coconut, or an insoluble white compound, such as magnesia suspended in water (milk of magnesia). **Acidophilous milk.** Milk curdled by the addition of a culture of *Lactobacillus acidophilus*; prescribed for digestive disorders. Cf. YOHOURT. **Adapted milk.** Modified milk (see below). **Albumin milk.** A specially prepared milk, rich in casein and fat. It is of value in diabetes and in high-protein diets. **Milk of asafoetida.** A liquid prepared by triturating asafoetida with water and straining. It is given as an enema for abdominal distension in pneumonia and post-operative cases. **Milk of bismuth.** Bismuth hydroxide and bismuth carbonate suspended in water. It is a form of administering bismuth hydroxide, of value in treating enteritis in children. **Butter milk.** 1. Milk left after churning and removing the butter. 2. Milk treated with certain organisms. **Cancer milk.** The milky fluid which exudes when a cancer is squeezed or scraped. **Casein milk.** A milk specially prepared to contain little salts and sugar and a large amount of fat and casein. It is used in diabetes, or when a high-protein and fat diet is required. **Centrifugalized milk.** Milk with cream removed by centrifugalization. **Certified milk.** Specially designated milk: *Pasteurized* milk the temperature of which has been raised to not less than 72°C and retained there for at least 15 seconds, and then immediately cooled to not more than 13°C; *Sterilized,* milk raised to the boiling point for 15 minutes in a steam chamber; *Tuberculin Tested,* milk from cows regularly submitted to tuberculin tests and isolated from other cattle. **Citric-acid milk.** Milk with added citric acid, the calcium salts forming non-ionized citrates and the milk thus gives finer clots in the stomach. **Condensed milk.** Milk partially evaporated in vacuum pans at temperatures not exceeding 55°C. The fat is evenly distributed by homogenizing, and it may be sweetened or unsweetened. If from skimmed milk, it must be labelled unfit for babies. Unsweetened condensed milk correctly diluted is suitable for infant feeding, but the sweetened variety has a relatively high carbohydrate with low-protein content and should only be used in emergency. **Diabetic milk.** Milk containing a small percentage of lactose, for use in diabetes. **Dialysed milk.** Milk from which the sugar has been removed by dialysis through a semipermeable membrane. **Dried milk.** Defined by the Public Health Regulations as milk, partly skimmed milk, or skimmed milk, which has been concentrated to the form of a powder or solid by removal of water. Only the powder prepared from full-cream milk is suitable for babies. The two chief methods of manufacture are: drying in a thin layer at high temperature on a revolving drum (*roller-dried milk*), and condensing and spraying in a fine stream under pressure into a hot-air chamber (*spray-dried milk*). Milk powder is used extensively in the baking, confectionery, and ice-cream industries, and also in infant feeding. **Evaporated milk.** Condensed milk (see above). **Fat milk.** A modified milk containing more fat than human milk. **Fortified milk.** Milk made extra nutritious by the addition of cream or white of egg. **Homogenized milk.** Milk in which the fat globules have been reduced to a small size by passing through a homogenizer. **Humanized milk.** Cows' milk, the composition of which has been modified to resemble human milk, the former containing more protein and less lactose than the latter. It can be prepared by the addition of an equal amount of whey to cows' milk and then by adding lactose and cream. In the preparation of baby foods, extra vitamins and mineral salts, particularly iron, may be added. The caseinogen of cows' milk forms a larger clot than human milk and is less easily digested. **Hydrochloric-acid milk.** Milk to which a little hydrochloric acid has been added; of use in hypochlorhydria. **Lactic-acid milk.** Milk to which lactic acid (40 drops to the pint) has been added: this breaks up the fat globules and makes it more digestible. **Lemon-juice milk.** Milk to which lemon juice has been added, thereby contributing vitamin C. **Litmus milk.** A nutrient, bacteriological medium prepared from milk in which litmus is used as an indicator. **Milk of magnesia.** An aqueous suspension of hydrated magnesium hydroxide; it is used as an antacid and milk laxative in hypochlorhydria and dyspepsia. **Metallized milk.** Milk with an added metallic salt such as iron, copper, or magnesium; of value in anaemia. **Modified milk.** Cows' milk in which the constituents have been modified to correspond to the amounts present in human milk. The basic constituents of cows' milk are separated and reassembled in different proportions, lactose is added, and then the mixture is dried. **Pasteurized milk.** *See* CERTIFIED MILK (above). **Peptonized milk.** Milk subjected to partial digestion by the addition of pepsin. **Perhydrase milk.** Milk to which hydrogen peroxide has been added; it is thus sterilized, and then the oxygen is driven off by heating. It has the grave disadvantage that vitamin C is destroyed and the properties of the milk are otherwise adversely affected; the procedure has been largely abandoned. **Protein milk.** A modified milk with a low fat and carbohydrate content and high-protein value; it is used in diets which demand it, e.g. in diabetes. **Red milk.** Milk which has been turned red by the presence of blood, by ingestion of madder root, or by the growth of *Chromobacterium prodigiosum*. **Roller-dried milk.** *See* DRIED MILK (above). **Separated milk.** Skimmed milk [see foll.]. **Skimmed milk.** Milk from which the cream has been removed, usually by centrifugal separators; it contains little fat, and rather more solids than ordinary milk. **Soft-curd milk.** Milk, the curd of which has been made soft by boiling or by the addition of cream and sodium citrate. **Sour milk.** Milk allowed to ferment by bacteria, such as yohourt, made from curdled cows' milk and containing *Lactobacillus bulgaricus*. **Spray-dried milk.** *See* DRIED MILK (above). **Sterilized milk.** *See* CERTIFIED MILK (above). **Tuberculin-tested milk.** *See* CERTIFIED MILK (above). **Uterine milk.** The albuminous secretion between the villi of the chorion and the crypts of the decidua. **Uviol milk.** Milk sterilized by the action of ultraviolet rays. **Vegetable milk.** A synthetic milk prepared from vegetables. **Vinegar milk.** Milk with vinegar added. **Virgin's milk.** Tincture of benzoin and rose water used for toilet purposes. **Vitamin-D milk.** Milk with added vitamin D, or milk exposed to ultraviolet light. **Witch's milk.** The secretion sometimes expressed from the breast of a newborn child. [AS *meoluc.*]

See also: BUDDE, FINKELSTEIN.

milk-crust (milk·krust). The yellow seborrhoeal adherent crusts often seen on the scalp of infants. [milk, crust.]

milking (milk·ing). The action of obtaining milk from the udder by rhythmical squeezing of the teat; hence, the withdrawal by pressing out with the finger of the contents of a compressible tube such as the urethra. [AS *meoluc.*]

Milkman, Louis Arthur (b. 1895). Scranton. Pennsylvania, radiologist.

Milkman's disease, or syndrome. Multiple spontaneous idiopathic symmetrical fractures of the Looser zone type, occurring in hypocalcified bones and seen radiographically. Long bones, pelvis and scapula may be affected.

Millar, John (b. 1733). Scottish physician in England.

Millar's disease. Laryngismus stridulus.

Millard, Auguste Louis Jules (b. 1830). Paris physician.

Millard-Gubler paralysis, or syndrome, Gubler-Millard paralysis. Paralysis of the 6th and perhaps the 7th cranial nerve on one side, with a contralateral hemiplegia; one formed of crossed hemiplegia due to a pontine lesion.

Millard-Gubler-Foville paralysis. 6th cranial nerve palsy, with or without ipsilateral 7th nerve palsy, and contralateral hemiplegia.

Miller, J. W. Berlin obstetrician.

Miller ovum. A fertilized human ovum, ten to eleven days old.

Miller, Thomas Grier (b. 1886). Philadelphia physician.

Miller-Abbott tube. A long rubber tube with a double lumen, one of which passes to an inflatable bag at the leading end of the tube, the second being used for suction. It is passed through the mouth or nose and guided into the intestine to relieve intestinal obstruction.

Milletia sericea (mil·e·she·ah ser·**is**·e·ah). A poisonous plant of Indonesia.

milli- (mil·e). A prefix indicating that the quantity which follows is to be multiplied by 10^{-3}. Thus, a milligram $= 10^{-3}$ gram. One thousandth part. [L *mille* thousand.]

milliammeter (mil·e·**am**·et·er). A sensitive ammeter which measures milliamperes. [milliampere, meter.]

milliampere (mil·e·**am**·pare). A unit of electric current: one thousandth of an ampere. **Milliampere hour.** A unit of x-ray dose in therapy, superseded by the roentgen, being the product of the tube current in milliamperes and the exposure in hours. **Milliampere minute.** A unit of electrical quantity; the amount passed by one milliampere in one minute. **Milliampere second.** A measurement of radiographic dose, being the product of the exposure in seconds and tube current in milliamperes. It is used for very short exposures where, although the exposure time may be accurately known, the tube current cannot be easily determined owing to the mechanical inertia of the meter. [L *mille* thousand, ampere.]

milliamperemeter (mil·e·**am**·pare·**me**′·ter). Milliammeter.

milliatom (mil·e·**at**·om). One thousandth part of the atomic weight of the element in grams. [Obsolete term.] [L *mille* thousand, atom.]

millibar (**mil**·e·bar). A unit used in meteorology to measure atmospheric pressure: one thousandth of a bar; 100 pascals. [L *mille* thousand, bar.]

millibarn (**mil**·e·barn). A unit of cross section $= 10^{-27}$ cm^2.

millicurie (**mil**·e·kewr·e). A unit of radioactivity, being defined as one thousandth of a curie, or the amount of radon (radium emanation) in equilibrium with one milligram of radium element. So that the definition may be applicable to any radioactive element, the millicurie is now laid down as the activity of a source that disintegrates at the rate of 3.7×10^7 disintegrations per second. **Millicurie hour.** A millicurie acting for an hour, or the amount of radon produced by one milligram of radium in one hour. **Intensity millicurie.** The intensity of γ-radiation at a distance of 1 cm from a 1 mg point source of radium filtered by 0.5 mm of platinum; it is equivalent to 8.4 r/hour. [L *mille* thousand, curie.]

millicurie-destroyed (mil·e·kewr·e·dis·**troid**'). A unit of radiological dose by γ-radiation, used in the estimation of treatment by radon, where the half-life of the isotope is short. 1 millicurie-destroyed of radon is equivalent to 130 mg hours of radium. [millicurie, L *destruere* to demolish.]

milli-equivalent (mil·e·ek·**wiv**'·al·ent). One thousandth of a gram-equivalent of a substance. [L *mille* thousand, equivalent.]

milligram (mil·e·gram). One thousandth of a gram (0.0154 grains). It is symbolized *mg.* **Milligram hour.** A measure of exposure to gamma rays expressed as the product of the number of milligrams of radium element in the source and the time of exposure in hours; it has now been largely superseded in radiotherapy by statement as to dose delivered in roentgens at different points throughout the tissue irradiated. **Milligram per cent.** Milligram per 100 ml. [L *mille* thousand, gram.]

Millikan, Robert Andrews (b. 1868). Pasadena, California, physicist.

Millikan rays. Cosmic rays; a very penetrating radiation of uncertain origin arriving from outer space and detected on earth by its ionizing effects.

millilambert (mil·e·lam·bert). A unit of illumination, one thousandth of a lambert, equal to 10 lux. [L *mille* thousand, lambert.]

millilitre (mil·e·le·ter). One thousandth of a litre, a cubic centimetre. [L *mille* thousand, litre.]

millimetre (mil·e·me·ter). A unit of length: one thousandth of a metre (0.0394 inches). [L *mille* thousand, metre.]

millimicron (mil·e·**mi**·kron). An obsolete term for *nanometre.* [L *mille* thousand, micron.]

millimol (mil·e·mol). One thousandth part of a mole. Symbol *mmol.* [L *mille* thousand, mol.]

Millin, Terence John. Irish urologist in London.

Millin's operation. Retropubic prostatectomy through a lower abdominal incision, without opening of the bladder.

milling (mil·ing). In dentistry, the obtaining of perfect occlusion of artificial dentures by placing an abrasive substance on the occlusal surfaces of the teeth and letting the patient perform normal grinding movements. [AS *mylen.*]

millinormal (mil·e·**nor**·mal). Denoting the concentration of a solution that has one thousandth of the normal solution. [L *mille* thousand, normal.]

millions (mil·e·onz). The freshwater fish, *Lebistes reticulatus,* used as a larviphage in antimosquito campaigns. The name is also applied to other small freshwater fish (*see* GIARDINUS POECILOIDES). [It. *millione.*]

milliphot (mil·e·fot). A unit of intensity of illumination: one thousandth of a phot, equal to 10 lux. [L *mille* thousand, phot.]

millirad (mil·e·rad). One thousandth of a rad. [L *mille* thousand, rad.]

millirem (mil·e·rem). One thousandth of a rem. [L *mille* thousand, rem.]

milliroentgen (mil·e·**runt**·yen). One thousandth of a roentgen. [L *mille* thousand, roentgen.]

millirutherford (mil·e·**ruth**·er·ford). A unit of radioactivity: a thousandth part of a rutherford. [obsolete term.] [L *mille* thousand, rutherford.]

millivolt (mil·e·volt). A unit of electric potential: one thousandth of a volt. [L *mille* thousand, volt.]

Millon, Auguste Nicolas Eugène (b. 1812). Paris chemist.

Millon's reaction, or test. 1. For protein: to 5 ml of solution add a few drops of Millon's reagent, and boil. A white precipitate which turns red upon boiling indicates proteins containing tyrosine. If excess of chloride is present, the test, if negative, should be repeated after addition of more reagent. 2. For phenols in urine: Millon's reagent is added to urine until no further white precipitation is obtained. The precipitate turns red on standing if phenols are present.

Millon's reagent. 10 grams of mercury are dissolved in 20 ml of nitric acid; equal parts of water are added, and after 24 hours the clear supernatant fluid is decanted.

Mills, Charles Karsner (b. 1845). Philadelphia neurologist.

Mills' disease. Progressive ascending hemiplegia.

Mills' test. For tennis elbow: with the wrist flexed and the forearm pronated, extension of the elbow produces pain over the external epicondyle of the humerus.

Milne, Robert (b. 1849). British physician.

Milne's method. An obsolete method of preventing infection by veiling the patient in gauze sprayed with antiseptic, and applying antiseptic to the throat and nose every 3 hours.

milphae, milphosis (mil·fe, mil·**fo**·sis). Loss of either or both eyebrows and eyelashes. [Gk *milphosis* baldness.]

Milroy, William Forsyth (b. 1855). Omaha physician.

Milroy's disease, or oedema, Nonne-Milroy-Meige syndrome. Chronic hereditary oedema of the legs.

Milton, John Laws (b. 1820). London dermatologist.

Milton's disease or urticaria. Giant urticaria or angioneurotic oedema.

milzbrand (milts·brahnt). Anthrax. [G *Milz* spleen, *Brand* a burning.]

mimesis (mim·e·sis). Mimicry. The imitation of one disease by another; applied also to the copying of the organic disease pattern by the hysterical subject. [Gk imitation.]

mimetic, mimic (mim·et·ik, **mim**·ik). Pertaining to mimesis; characterized by imitation of another disease. [Gk *mimetikos* imitative.]

mimicry (**mim**·i·kry). The facial phenomena sub-served by the autonomic system which are the unwilled (and largely uncontrolled) expression of feeling and ideas.

mimmation (mim·**a**·shun). The frequent but incorrect use of the *m* sound in speech. [Ar. *mim* letter M.]

mimochasmesis (mim·o·kaz·**me**'·sis). Yawning which may be a form of mimicry, but which is generally set up as a sympathetic response and beyond control. [Gk *mimos* mimic, *chasmaomein* to yawn.]

mimography (mim·**og**·raf·e). The language of signs as used by deaf-mutes. [Gk *mimos* mimic, *graphein* to write.]

mimosis (mim·**o**·sis). Mimesis.

mind (mi·nd). Consciousness; reasoning, understanding. [AS *gemynd.*]

Minderer, Raimond (b. 1570). Augsburg physician.

Minderer's spirit. An aqueous solution containing 7.2 per cent of ammonium acetate; used as a stimulant, diaphoretic and diuretic.

Minepentate (min·e·**pen**·tate). BP Commission approved name for 2-(2-dimethylaminoethoxy)ethyl 1-phenyl-cyclopentanecarboxylate; it is used in the treatment of Parkinson's disease.

mineral (min·er·al). Essentially any inorganic substance found in the earth and obtained by mining; extended to include purely organic substances like coal and petroleum. **Crystal mineral.** Fused potassium nitrate. **Mineral glycerin.** Petroleum. **Kermes mineral.** Natural sulphide of antimony. **Turpeth mineral.** Basic mercuric sulphate, $HgSO_4{\cdot}2HgO$, a heavy yellow powder. [L *minera* mine.]

mineral spring (min·er·al spring). A source of water with a high mineral content; many such are reputed to be of medicinal value. [mineral, AS *springan.*]

mineralization (min·er·al·i·**za**'·shun). The addition of any mineral substance to the body.

mineralocorticoid (min·er·al·o·**kor**'·tik·oid). A hormone such as aldosterone and deoxycorticosterone secreted by the cortex of the suprarenal gland, the main function of which is the control of electrolyte and water metabolism. [mineral, cortex.]

minim (min·im). A unit of fluid measure; one sixtieth of a fluid drachm, approximately one drop. It is the volume at 16.7°C of 0.971 grains of water, equivalent to 0.0592 ml, and is symbolized in prescriptions by ♏. [L *minimum* smallest.]

minimal (**min**·e·mal). The least or smallest; indicating the smallest amount or quantity. [see foll.]

minimum (**min**·e·mum). The lowest intensity or level; the smallest amount. **Minimum audibile.** The auditory threshold; the least sound that can be heard. **Minimum cognoscibile.** The visibility threshold for recognizing shapes. **Minimum legibile.** The visibility threshold for recognizing letters. **Light minimum.** The least possible intensity of light that can be seen in dark surroundings. **Minimum sensibile.** The threshold of consciousness. **Minimum separable.** The least distance separating two objects and yet permitting them to be still identified as two objects. **Minimum visibile.** Light minimum (see above). [L smallest.]

Minin, A. V. (fl. 1900). St. Petersburg army surgeon.

Minin light. Light which is emitted from a bulb of coloured glass giving out only violet and ultraviolet rays.

minium (**min**·e·um). Red lead, lead tetroxide, Pb_3O_4. A scarlet powder obtained by roasting lead carbonate in air; used in glass-making, in paint manufacture as a pigment and drier, and, mixed with oil, as a jointing cement. [L]

Minkowski, Oskar (b. 1858). Lithuanian pathologist and physician in Wiesbaden.

Minkowski-Chauffard syndrome, Chauffard-Minkowski syndrome. Acholuric familial jaundice. *See* JAUNDICE.

Minnitt, Robert James (b. 1892). Liverpool anaesthetist.

Minnitt's apparatus. An anaesthetic apparatus giving an intermittent supply of nitrous oxide and air in sufficient concentration to produce obstetrical analgesia.

Minocycline (min·o·**si**·kleen). BP Commission approved name for 4,7 - bis(dimethylamino) - 1,4,4a,5,5a,6,11,12a - octahydro - 3,10,12,12a - tetrahydroxy - 1,11 - dioxonaphthacene - 2 - carboxamide; an antibiotic agent.

Minor, Lazar Salomovich (b. 1855). Moscow neurologist.

Minor's disease. Central haematomyelia.

Minor's sign. A patient with sciatica rises from the sitting position with one hand on the affected side of the back; he balances on the healthy leg and supports himself with the arm on the healthy side.

Minor's tremor. Essential tremor; a familial tremor that is exaggerated by stress and tends to increase with age. It is unassociated with any other nervous symptoms.

minor (**mi**·nor). 1. Lesser or smaller; of less importance comparatively. 2. In forensic medicine, anyone who is not yet "of age" in the country of domicile (18 years in England), and is still subject to the discipline of parents or guardians. [L less.]

Minot, George Richards (b. 1885). Boston physician.

Minot's disease, or purpura haemorrhagica with lymphocytosis. A rare acute but benign thrombocytopenic purpura associated with lymphocytosis and sometimes abnormal lymphocytes in the blood, without splenomegaly, adenopathy, or abnormal agglutinin in the blood.

Minot-Murphy treatment. The first effective treatment introduced for pernicious anaemia, being the oral administration of raw or lightly-cooked liver or of crude extracts of fresh calf liver.

Minsky's circle. A chart used for recording lesions of the eye.

minuthesis (min·ew·**the**·sis). The progressive loss of sensitivity of a sensory organ produced by continued excitation; fatigue. [L *minus* less, Gk *aisthesis* feeling.]

miocardia (mi·o·**kar**·de·ah). Systole; the phase representing the lessening of the capacity of the chambers of the heart. [Gk *meion* less, *kardia* heart.]

miodidymus (mi·o·**did**·e·mus). A fetal monster with two heads fused at the occipital regions. [Gk *meion* less, *didymos* twin.]

mionectic (mi·o·**nek**·tik). Referring to the inability of tissue cells and blood cells to take up the average amount of oxygen they normally require. [Gk *meion* less, *hexis* habit.]

mioplasmia (mi·o·**plaz**·me·ah). An abnormal diminution in the quantity of blood plasma. [Gk *meion* less, plasma.]

miopragia (mi·o·**pra**·je·ah). Lessening of functional activity. [Gk *meion* less, *prassein* to act.]

miopus (**mi**·o·pus). A monster with two fused heads, one rudimentary face, and in some cases two ears and three eyes. [Gk *meion* less, *ops* eye.]

miosis (mi·**o**·sis). 1. Abnormal contraction of the pupils of the eye to less than 2 mm. 2. The USA spelling of *meiosis* (reduction division of germ cells). **Congenital miosis.** A rare condition in which the contraction of the pupil is due to congenital absence of the dilator muscle. **Hysterical miosis.** A spastic contraction of the pupil usually associated with a spasm of accommodation found in hysteria. **Paralytic miosis.** Contraction of the pupil due to a paretic lesion of the sympathetic pathways, e.g. in Horner's syndrome. **Spastic miosis.** Contraction of the pupil due to irritative lesions of parasympathetic centres or pathways, e.g. pontine haemorrhage. **Spinal miosis.** A contraction of the pupil due to a paretic lesion of the sympathetic fibres in the cervical portion of the cord, e.g. tabes. [Gk *meiosis* a lessening.]

miosphygmia (mi·o·**sfig**·me·ah). A state in which the pulse beats are less in number than the heart beats. [Gk *meion* less, *sphygmos* pulse.]

miotic (mi·**ot**·ik). 1. Any agent causing contraction of the pupil of the eye. Those in common use are pilocarpine, eserine (physostigmine), prostigmine, morphine and dyflos. 2. Causing contraction of the pupil of the eye; as applied to a pupil, one that is contracted. 3. The USA spelling of *meiotic* (pertaining to the process of reduction division of germ cells). [Gk *meion* less.]

mipafox (**mi**·pah·fox). *bis*-(Mono-isopropylamino)-fluoro-phosphine oxide. An insecticide that has produced poisoning similar to that caused by triorthocresyl phosphate (ginger paralysis).

miracidioscope (mi·ras·**id**·e·o·skope). An apparatus consisting of a specially constructed wooden rack for holding centrifuge tubes. This is painted a dull black, and is partially closed in front but open above so that the light falls obliquely on the tubes and shows up the swimming miracidia. A hand lens of 65 mm focal length is used; this may be fixed to the apparatus. The apparatus is used in the diagnosis of schistosomiasis. [miracidium, Gk *skopein* to view.]

miracidium (mi·ras·**id**·e·um). The first larva of digenean flukes, a ciliated, and active stage which, in some species, is free-living, actively seeking a snail host into which it bores. In others it hatches within the snail intestine after ingestion. [Gk *meirakidion* youth.]

miracil D (**mir**·as·il **de**). Lucanthone hydrochloride.

mirage (mir·**ahzh**). *See* ATMOSPHERIC REFRACTION (under REFRACTION).

Mirault, Germanicus (b. 1796). French surgeon.

Mirault's operation. An operation for the repair of hare-lip.

mires (meerz). The targets used in the ophthalmometer (keratometer). One is cut in steps, the other is rectangular; both are illuminated and produce reflections in the cornea which are viewed through a telescopic magnifier. In some models, one mire is green and the other red. [L *mirare* to look at.]

mirror (**mir**·or). A regular smooth surface having a high reflectivity, usually for visible light. Also describing any arrangement for the production of reflection of any type of radiation. **Concave mirror.** A curved mirror in which the polished surface faces towards the centre of curvature. **Convex mirror.** One in which the polished surface faces away from the centre of curvature. **Dental mirror.** A mirror used in the performance of dental operations. **Mirror drill.** Practice before a mirror in the endeavour to control facial tics. **Frontal mirror.** A mirror strapped to the forehead, by which light from a fixed source is reflected into the cavities of the body, particularly the upper respiratory tract. **Head mirror.** Frontal mirror (see prec.). **Laryngoscopic mirror.** A mirror used for indirect examination of the larynx; invented by Manuel Garcia. **Mouth mirror.** Dental mirror (see above). **Nasographic mirror.** A cold piece of polished metal which is held below the nose to compare the patency of the nasal airways by the pattern produced by the condensed air as it is exhaled through the nasal passages. **Ophthalmoscopic mirror.** One used in an ophthalmoscope to reflect the source of light into the pupil of the eye and so illuminate the fundus tor examination. **Plane mirror.** A mirror having a flat polished surface. **Retinoscopy mirror.** One used to reflect the source of light into the pupil of the eye and when tilted to give the shadow movements on which the test relies. It may be plane or concave. **Rhinoscopic mirror.** A reflecting mirror used for the examination of the postnasal space in posterior rhinoscopy. [L *mirare* to look at.]

See also: GLATZEL, HELMONT.

misandria, misandry (mis·**an**·dre·ah, mis·**an**·dre). An abnormal aversion to men. [Gk *misein* to hate, *aner* man.]

misanthrope (**mis**·an·thrope). Anyone who hates mankind, or who is of melancholic temperament and avoids the society of others. [Gk *misein* to hate, *anthropos* human being.]

misanthropy (mis·**an**·thro·pe). Detestation of mankind; negative outlook on human affairs. [see prec.]

miscarriage (mis·**kar**·ij). Abortion; expulsion of the fetus before it is viable. [AS *mis-*, O Fr. *carier*.]

miscarry (mis·**kar**·e). To give birth to a fetus before it is capable of maintaining an independent life outside the womb. [see prec.]

miscegenation (**mis**·e·jen·**a′**·shun). The interbreeding or intermarriage of different races, especially the black with white races. [L *miscere* to mix, *genus* race.]

miscible (**mis**·ibl). Mixable, capable of being mixed. [L *miscere* to mix.]

misocainia (mis·o·**ki**·ne·ah). Dread or hatred of innovation. [Gk *misein* to hate, *kainos* new.]

misogamy (mis·**og**·am·e). Hatred of marriage. [Gk *misein* to hate, *gamos* marriage.]

misogynist (mis·**og**·in·ist). A man who has dislike amounting to hatred for women in general and particular; a woman-hater. [see foll.]

misogyny (mis·**og**·in·e). Hatred of women. [Gk *misein* to hate, *gyne* woman.]

misologia, misology (mis·ol·**o**·je·ah, mis·**ol**·o·je). Hatred of discussion or conversation, or of intellectual activity. [Gk *misein* to hate, *logos* word.]

misoneist (mis·**on**·e·ist). Applied to anyone who is morbidly afraid of anything new or of innovation of any kind. [Gk *misein* to hate, *neos* new.]

misopaedia, misopaedy (mis·o·**pe**·de·ah, mis·**op**·e·de). Dislike of children or young people amounting to hatred. [Gk *misein* to hate, *pais* child.]

misopsychia (mis·o·**si**·ke·ah). A morbid aversion of life in all its aspects. [Gk *misein* to hate, *psyche* life.]

mistletoe (**misl**·to). A parasitic plant growing on trees, particularly the apple, plum, oak and poplar. The leaves and branches contain a glutinous substance, viscin, gum and tannin. The European species, *Viscum album* and the American, *Viscum flavescens*, possess pharmacological properties said to be antispasmodic, oxytocic and vasodilator. [AS *misteltān*.]

mistura (mis·**tewr**·ah). A liquid pharmaceutical preparation, intended for oral administration, consisting of a mixture of drugs either in solution or suspension in water, usually with the addition of a flavouring agent. [L mixture.]

Misuse of Drugs Act 1971. This Act restricts the production, supply, sale and possession of dangerous or otherwise harmful drugs and related matters. These "controlled drugs" are classified into three groups according to their relative harmfulness. Class A includes mescaline, cocaine, methadone, morphine, opium, pethidine and poppy straw; Class B includes amphetamine, cannabis and codeine; Class C includes benzphetamine, pemoline and pipradol. It is unlawful for a person to be in possession of one or any of the controlled drugs unless he has obtained it on a lawful prescription or is a doctor, dentist, veterinary practitioner or veterinary surgeon, pharmacist or person lawfully conducting a retail pharmacy business. The Act has also established an Advisory Council on the Misuse of Drugs whose function is to review the situation on drug misuse and its consequent social problem, and to advise on measures for (*a*) restricting the availability of drugs, (*b*) providing services for the treatment, rehabilitation and after-care of drug users, (*c*) educating the public in the dangers of misusing such drugs, (*d*) promoting research into drug-related matters.

Mitchell, James Vincent. Oxford anaesthetist.

Mitchell needle. A needle so designed that, when inserted into a vein, it prevents clotting of blood in the lumen.

Mitchell, Silas Weir (b. 1829). Philadelphia neurologist.

Mitchell's disease, Weir Mitchell disease. Erythromelalgia.

Weir Mitchell lipo-atrophy. Partial lipo-atrophy, with loss of facial fat and subcutaneous fat from the upper half of the body.

Weir Mitchell treatment. A treatment for neurasthenia consisting of isolation, absolute rest in bed, abundant feeding, massage and electrical treatment.

mite (mite). A general term for all small members of the Acarina. The adults have eight legs and, usually, piercing and sucking mouth parts; their life histories are complex with, usually, a six-legged larva and an eight-legged nymph. Many are parasitic and carriers of pathogens; the free-living forms may cause grocers' itch and similar complaints. **Cheese mite.** *Tyroglyphus siro.* **Chicken mite.** *Dermanyssus gallinae.* **Copra mite.** *Tyroglyphus longior.* **Face mite.** *Demodex folliculorum hominis.* **Flour mite.** *Tyroglyphus farinae.* **Follicle mite.** *Demodex folliculorum hominis.* **Grain mite.** *Tyroglyphus, Tyrophagus.* **Hair-follicle mite.** *Demodex folliculorum hominis.* **Harvest mite.** *Eutrombicula, Trombicula.* **Itch mite.** *Chorioptes, Notoëdres, Sarcoptes.* **Kedani mite.** *Trombicula akamushi.* **Louse mite.** *Pediculoides.* **Mange mite.** *Notoëdres.* **Mowers' mite.** Chigger. **Red mite.** *Eutrombicula, Trombicula.* **Scabies mite.** *Sarcoptes.* **Tropical rate mite.** *Bdellonyssus.* [AS *mite*.]

mitella (mi·**tel**·ah). An arm sling. [L]

Mithramycin (mi·thrah·**mi**·sin). BP Commission approved name for an antibiotic produced from *Streptomyces argillaceus* and *Streptomyces tanashiensis.*

mithridatism (mith·**rid**·at·izm). Immunity against poisoning by administration of doses, steadily increasing in amount, of the poisons. [*Mithridates* VI, King of Pontus, 1st century B.C., who is believed to have produced immunity in himself by this means.]

miticidal (mi·tis·i·dal). Destructive to mites. [see foll.]

miticide (**mi**·tis·ide). 1. A substance that kills mites. 2. Miticidal. [mite, L *caedere* to kill.]

mitigate (**mit**·e·gate). To make or to grow milder or mild; to alleviate, as symptoms; to moderate or lessen. [L *mitigare* to soften.]

mitis (**mi**·tis). Mild; a word used to denote the weaker preparation, where there are two of the same thing, differing only in strength. [L]

Mitobronitol (mi·to·**bron**·it·ol). BP Commission approved name for 1,6-dibromo-1,6-dideoxy-D-mannitol; an antineoplastic agent.

mitochondria (mit·to·**kon**·dre·ah). Filamentous rod-shaped organelles found in the cytoplasm of all respiring cells enclosed by an outer and an inner mitochondrial membrane which is folded into shell-like structures (cristae). They are responsible for cell respiration and respiratory chain phosphorylation and contain the enzymes of the citrate cycle, of β-oxidation of fatty acids, the respiratory chain components, and other enzymes and substrate carrier systems. They may be isolated and studied by cell fractionation. [Gk *mitos* thread, *chondros* cartilage.]

Mitoclomine (mi·**to**·klo·meen). BP Commission approved name for *NN* - di - (2 - chloroethyl) - 4 - methoxy - 3 - methyl - 1 - naphthylamine; an antineoplastic agent.

mitogen (**mi**·to·jen). A substance capable of stimulating cells to enter mitosis. [Gk *mitos* thread, *genein* to produce.]

mitogenesis (mi·to·**jen**·es·is). Origination or development during the karyokinetic process. [mitosis, genesis.]

mitogenetic (**mi**·to·jen·**et′**·ik). Mitogenic. [see foll.]

mitogenic (mi·to·**jen**·ik). Referring to the ability of inducing mitosis. [Gk *mitos* thread, *genein* to produce.]

mitoplasm (**mi**·to·plazm). The chromatic nuclear reticulum of the thread-like framework of the cell. [Gk *mitos* thread, plasm.]

Mitopodozide (mi·to·**po**·do·zide). BP Commission approved name for *N′*-ethylpodophyllohydrazide; an antineoplastic agent.

mitoschisis (mi·tos·kis·is). Karyokinesis. [Gk *mitos* thread, *schisis* a clearing.]

mitosis (mi·to·sis). The process by which a cell nucleus divides into two daughter nuclei with chromosome numbers and genetic make-up identical to that of the parent cell. At the beginning of mitotic division (*prophase*) the chromosomes, which have reduplicated during the preceding interphase, become visible as long threads consisting of two chromatids. At the end of prophase the nuclear membrane disappears and the spindle is formed. The chromosomes converge to the equatorial plane of the spindle (*metaphase*). Then the two chromatids of each chromosome (*sister chromatids*) migrate to opposite poles (*anaphase*) and a new nuclear membrane forms around each one of these two groups of daughter chromosomes which elongate and cease to be optically distinct (*telophase*). Mitosis is normally followed by cytoplasmic fission (*cytokinesis*). **C mitosis.** Abnormal mitosis resulting from the action of colchicine or other poisons on the mitotic apparatus. **Multipolar mitosis.** Mitosis with more than two spindle poles. This type of mitosis often arises in multinucleated cells and often results in aberrant chromosome distribution. **Unipolar mitosis.** Mitosis with only one spindle pole. [Gk *mitos* thread.]

Mitotenamine (mi·to·ten·am·een). BP Commission approved name for 5-bromo-3-[*N*-(2-chloroethyl)ethylaminoethyl]-benzo-[*b*]thiophen; an antineoplastic agent.

mitotic (mi·tot·ik). Relating to or characterized by mitosis. **Mitotic apparatus.** *See* APPARATUS. **Mitotic index.** *See* INDEX.

mitral (mi·tral). 1. Similar in shape to a mitre. 2. Relating to the left atrioventricular (mitral) valve. *See* VALVE. **Fishmouth mitral.** A mitral valve with an extreme degree of stenosis. [L *mitra* turban.]

mitralism (mi·tral·izm). A predisposition to lesions of the left atrioventricular (mitral) valve.

mitro-arterial (mi·tro·ar·teer'·e·al). Relating to or concerning the left atrioventricular (mitral) valve and arteries.

Mitscherlich, Eilhardt (b. 1794). German chemist.

Mitscherlich's test. For white phosphorus in gastro-intestinal contents in acute phosphorus poisoning: the material is acidified with sulphuric acid and distilled in the dark. If the vapour in the condenser is luminous, phosphorus is present. A negative result does not exclude phosphorus, as the phosphorescence is inhibited by certain substances such as turpentine, alcohol and ether.

Mitsuda, K. Japanese physician.

Mitsuda test, Mitsuda–Rost test. Lepromin test. *See* TEST.

mittelschmerz (mit·el·shmertz'). Dysmenorrhoea intermenstrualis. [G intermediate pain.]

Mittermaier, Richard. 20th century Freiburg otologist.

Mittermaier's test. For labyrinthine disease: the patient is asked to stand up marking time with his feet. In hypo-active or paretic lesions of the labyrinth, turning will be towards the diseased side.

mittor (mit·or). Neuromittor.

mixing (mix·ing). **Phenotypic mixing.** In virus genetics, an association of the phenotype of one parent with the genotype of the other among the progeny particles of a mixed infection, e.g. in mixed infection of bacteria with two related phage types, genomes of one type may become incorporated into protein coats of the other during assembly of progeny particles. [L *miscere* to mix.]

mixoploid (mix·o·ploid). An individual, or cell population, whose cells differ in their chromosome number. [L *miscere* to mix, Gk *eidos* form.]

mixoscopia, mixoscopy (mix·o·sko·pe·ah, mix·os·ko·pe). A form of perversion in which sexual satisfaction is derived from the observation of others occupied in the sexual act. [Gk *mixis* copulation, *skopein* to watch.]

mixture (mix·tewr, mix·tcher). A preparation of two or more ingredients mixed together; pharmaceutically, it is applied to liquid medicines. **A.C.E. mixture.** Alcohol 1 part, chloroform 2 parts, and ether 3 parts, once popular as an inhalation anaesthetic. Very similar to C_2E_3 mixture. *See* C-E MIXTURE (below). **Alkali blood mixture.** A mixture of defibrinated blood, 1 part, and normal potassium hydroxide, 1 part. **Antifoaming mixture.** A mixture prepared by saponifying spermaceti in an alcoholic solution of sodium hydroxide. **Azeotropic mixture.** A mixture of two or more volatile liquids in such proportions that they cannot be separated by fractional distillation; for example, a mixture of diethyl ether 32 parts with halothane 68 parts. **Baryta mixture.** A mixture of 1 volume of a saturated solution of barium nitrate and 2 volumes of a saturated solution of barium hydroxide; a chemical reagent. **Brown mixture.** Opium and liquorice mixture, a mixture consisting of liquid extract of liquorice, antimony potassium tartrate, camphorated tincture of opium, spirit of nitrous ether, glycerin, and water. It is a diaphoretic and febrifuge used in the treatment of colds, coughs, and feverish conditions. **Carminative mixture.** Any mixture that relieves local abdominal pain or discomfort, especially flatulence. It usually contains opiates. **C-E mixture.** A mixture of chloroform and ether, usually denoted C_xE_y, used at one time in anaesthesia. It was regarded as a chloroform dilution in which the ether served to maintain blood pressure and facilitate induction; the proportions varied, and sometimes alcohol was also incorporated (A.C.E.). The chloroform-ether mixture C_2E_3 had wide popularity early in the century, being given on open mask either as a sole anaesthetic agent or as a preliminary to ether. **E-C mixture.** Mitigated chloroform, a mixture of ether and chloroform used as an anaesthetic; more usually denoted *C-E mixture.* **E.C.C.O. mixture.** A mixture of hydnocarpus oil, camphor, creosote, and olive oil, at one time injected intramuscularly in the treatment of leprosy. **Expectorant mixture.** 1. Ammonium carbonate, fluid extract of senega with squill, camphorated tincture of opium, and syrup of tolu, used to loosen and increase bronchial secretion. 2. Mixture of ammonia and ipecacuanha; ammonium bicarbonate, tincture of ipecacuanha, extract of liquorice, aniseed water, and camphor water, used as an expectorant to increase bronchial secretion. **Freezing mixture.** A mixture, such as ice and salt water, used for producing cold. **Magnesium Hydroxide Mixture BP 1958.** An aqueous suspension of hydrated magnesium hydroxide which is used as an antacid and mild laxative. **Oleobalsamic mixture.** An alcoholic solution of balsam of Peru with aromatic oils, used as a local stimulant. **Pectoral mixture.** Expectorant mixture (see above). **Phosphate-carbonate-thiocyanate mixture.** Sodium acid phosphate, sodium thiocyanate, and monohydrated sodium carbonate; it has been used in the treatment for hypertension. **Phosphoric-sulphuric acid copper-sulphate mixture.** A mixture of concentrated sulphuric acid and syrupy phosphoric acid with copper sulphate, used to digest protein in the estimation of nitrogen. **Saline Mixture BPC 1959.** An effervescent solution of potassium citrate, used as a diaphoretic. **Mixture of Senna, Compound, BPC 1959.** Black draught; a liquid extract of senna, with magnesium sulphate, liquid extract of liquorice, compound tincture of cardamon and aromatic spirit of ammonia. It is used as a brisk purgative. **Spleen mixture.** Gadberry's mixture. **T.A. mixture, Toxin-antitoxin mixture, Toxoid-antitoxin mixture.** A mixture of a bacterial toxoid, or toxin, with its specific antitoxin in almost neutralizing amounts. A mixture of diphtheria toxoid and antitoxin was formerly used in active immunization of children against diphtheria in the UK, whereas a toxin-antitoxin mixture was used in the USA; both are now obsolete. **Vienna mixture.** Chloroform 1 part and ether 3 parts, formerly used as an anaesthetic. [L *miscere* to mix.]

See also: AGGAZZOTTI, ALDRICH (R. H.), ARKÖVY, BACELLI, BASHAM, BERTRAM, BESTUCHEFF, BIEDERT, BILLROTH, BONAIN, CARREL, CASTELLANI, COLEY, COWGILL, ELZHOLZ, ERLENMEYER, GADBERRY, GLEGG, GREGORY, GRIFFITH (R. E.), GUNNING (J. W.), HAMMOND, HERMANN, HUENEFELD, KARR, LOOMIS, MAYER (P.), MEISEN, MENDEL (L. B.), OSBORNE, PARRISH, RINGER, TELLYESNICZKY, THIELMANN, TOISON, TOWNSEND (J.), VELPEAU, VINCENT, WEIGERT.

mnemasthenia (ne·mas·**the**·ne·ah). Inherent weakness of the faculty of remembering. The state does not depend upon organic disease. [Gk *mneme* memory, asthenia.]

mneme (**ne**·me). Memory. [Gk.]

mnemic (**ne**·mik). 1. Relating or belonging to memory. 2. Bearing the elements of memory. **Mnemic hypothesis.** The theory that a long-lasting stimulus or irritant produces in the cells concerned a change that persists, even after removal of the stimulus or irritation, thus tending to the creation of habit. [Gk *mneme* memory.]

mnemism (**ne**·mizm). Mnemic hypothesis.

mnemonics (ne·**mon**·ix). 1. An educative system of memory training by which the faculty may be developed, assisted and improved. 2. Literal or pictorial combinations to aid remembering the facts which they represent. [Gk *mnemonikos* for remembrance.]

moan (mone). 1. A continuous low murmuring sound, which may be either articulate or inarticulate, and is significant of a state of physical or mental suffering. 2. To utter such a sound; to complain. [ME *mone.*]

mobility (mo·**bil**·it·e). Freedom of movement. **Electrophoretic mobility.** A measure of behaviour on electrophoresis; the degree and direction of movement of a particle during electrophoresis. [L *mobilis* movement.]

mobilization (**mo**·bil·i·**za**′·shun). The act or process of bringing back, e.g. an ankylosed part, into a state of mobility, or of freeing structures that are not normally mobile. [L *mobilis* movable.]

mobilometer (mo·bil·**om**·et·er). An apparatus for measuring the viscosity of oils and liquid fats by observing the time it takes for a weighted disc to sink a measured distance in the liquid. [L *mobilis* movable, meter.]

moccasin (**mok**·as·in). The water moccasin, *Agkistrodon piscivorus,* a poisonous snake of the southern parts of North America. [Amer. Ind. *mockasin.*]

mode (mode). In vital statistics the maximum point on the curve which most closely describes an observed frequency distribution, i.e. the measurement which occurs most frequently. [L *modus* measure.]

modem (**mo**·dem). A device which transforms the signals from a data terminal so that they can be transmitted over ordinary telephone lines to be handled by a computer. By its use, medical and other data logging equipment does not become uniquely dependent on any one computer. The collected data can, in principle, be handled by any computer which is connected to the telephone system.

moderator (**mod**·er·a·tor). A substance used for slowing fast neutrons by elastic collisions with its atoms, e.g. anything containing a high percentage of hydrogen. [L *moderari* to restrain.]

modification (**mod**·if·e·**ka**′·shun). **Host-induced modification, Phenotypic modification.** Host-controlled variation. *See* VARIATION. [L *modus* measure.]

modioliform (mo·de·**o**·le·form). Of a shape similar to that of the hub of a wheel. [modiolus, form.]

modiolus [NA] (mo·**de**·o·lus). The cone-shaped central axis of the cochlea. The broad base [basis modioli (NA)] is towards the internal auditory meatus. [L hub.]

modiolus, spiral vein of the [vena spiralis modioli (NA)]. The vein accompanying the arterial glomeruli of the cochlea.

Moebius, Paul Julius (b. 1853). Leipzig neurologist.

Moebius' disease. Ophthalmoplegic migraine.

Moebius' sign. Weakness of convergence in thyrotoxic exophthalmos.

Moebius' syndrome. 1. Akinesia algera, a form of hysterical paralysis. 2. Paralysis of ocular muscles and of the facial musculature, due to aplasia of cranial-nerve nuclei.

Leyden–Moebius dystrophy, or type, Moebius–Leyden dystrophy, or type. The atrophic type of progressive childhood muscular dystrophy, first affecting muscles of the pelvic girdle.

Moeller, Alfred (b. 1868). Frankfort bacteriologist.

Moeller's method. A spore stain for bacteria. The spores are stained red by carbol fuchsine, and the bacterial bodies blue, by methylene blue.

Moeller's reaction. The local reaction produced by applying tuberculin to the nasal mucous membrane of persons infected with tuberculosis. The method is obsolete.

Moeller, Julius Otto Ludwig (b. 1819). Königsberg surgeon.

Moeller's disease. Acute rickets (infantile scurvy).

Moeller's glossitis. Chronic superficial glossitis with irregularly scattered red patches and striae on the dorsum of the tongue with severe burning pain. Probably a manifestation of iron or vitamin B_{12} deficiency. It occurs in attacks with alternating quiescent periods lasting for weeks or months, mainly in women.

Moenckeberg, Johann Georg (b. 1877). Bonn pathologist.

Moenckeberg arteriosclerosis, medial calcification mesarteritis, degeneration, or sclerosis. A patchy calcification of the media of arteries, particularly those of the lower limbs. The opened artery has a trachea-like appearance.

Moerner, Karl Axel Hampus (b. 1854). Stockholm physician and chemist.

Moerner's reagent. For tyrosine: mix cautiously, with cooling, 55 volumes of concentrated sulphuric acid with 45 volumes of distilled water and 1 volume of formalin.

Moerner's test. For tyrosine: to a little of the substance add 3 ml of Moerner's reagent (see above), and heat gradually to boiling. A green colour is given by tyrosine.

Moffett, Arthur James. British anaesthetist.

Moffett's method. A technique of producing analgesia within the nasal cavities by the instillation of a solution of local analgesic drug. Described in 1947.

mogiarthria (moj·e·**ar**·thre·ah). A type of dysarthria in which the involved muscles are imperfectly co-ordinated. [Gk *mogis* with toil and trouble, *arthron* joint.]

mogigraphia (moj·e·**graf**·e·ah). Writers' cramp. [Gk *mogis* with toil and trouble, *graphein* to write.]

mogilalia (moj·e·**lal**·e·ah). Speech difficulty or defect; stuttering; stammering. [Gk *mogis* with toil and trouble, *lalein* to make an inarticulate sound.]

mogiphonia (moj·e·**fo**·ne·ah). Difficulty or pain in using the voice. [Gk *mogis* with toil and trouble, *phone* voice.]

mogitocia (moj·e·**to**·se·ah). Dystocia. [Gk *mogis* with toil and trouble, *tokos* birth.]

Mohr, Karl Friedrich (b. 1806). Coblenz and Bonn pharmaceutical chemist.

Mohr's salt. Ferrous ammonium sulphate.

Mohrenheim, Baron Joseph Jacob von. (d. 1799). Vienna and St. Petersburg gynaecologist and ophthalmologist.

Mohrenheim's fossa, or space. Infraclavicular fossa; the triangular depression below the clavicle corresponding to the interval between the clavicular fibres of the pectoralis major and the deltoid.

moiety (**moi**·et·e). 1. Either of two equal parts; a half. 2. In biochemistry, any distinct component molecule of a compound molecule. [L *medietatem* middle point.]

mol (mol). The symbol for mole, the amount of a substance.

molality (mol·**al**·it·e). The expression of the strength of a solution in terms of the number of moles of solute per kilogram of solvent. Cf. MOLARITY.

molar (**mo**·lar). 1. Molar tooth; a broad-topped tooth used for grinding; one of the two back teeth in the deciduous dentition, or one of the three back teeth in the permanent dentition, situated on each side of the jaws. 2. In chemistry, referring to moles. Of solutions containing 1 mole of solute per litre. **Bud molar.** Mulberry molar (see below). **Deciduous molar.** One of the two teeth at the back of the jaws on each side up to the age of about 6 years. Each is shed and followed by a premolar tooth. **Dome-shaped molar.** A molar tooth which is wider at the neck than at the occlusal surface. **First molar.** A first permanent molar tooth which erupts at about the age of 6 years. **Impacted molar.** A molar tooth that encounters an obstruction which prevents its eruption. **Mulberry molar.** A first permanent molar tooth whose occlusal surface is nodular and pitted due to hereditary syphilis. **Permanent molar.** One of the three most posterior teeth on each side of the jaws. **Second molar.** A second permanent molar tooth which erupts at about the age of 12 years. **Sixth-year molar.** A first permanent molar tooth. **Third molar.** A third permanent molar tooth; a wisdom tooth. **Twelfth-year molar.** A second permanent molar tooth. [L *mola* mill.]

See also: MOON (H.).

molariform (mo·lar·e·form). Like a molar tooth in shape. [molar, form.]

molarity (mol·ar·it·e). The expression of the strength of a solution in terms of the number of moles of solute per litre of solution. Cf. MOLALITY.

molasses (mol·as·ez). Treacle; the thick, dark, uncrystallizable syrup remaining after the removal of crystalline sugar in the commercial process of manufacture of the latter from sugar cane or sugar beet. It is used in making rum, also in the production of alcohol for fuel purposes. [L *mel* honey.]

mole (mole). 1. The unit of the amount of substance, and is defined as the amount of substance of a system which contains as many elementary units as there are carbon atoms in 12 grams of carbon-12. When the mole is used the elementary entities must be specified and may be atoms, molecules, ions, electrons, or other particles, or specified groups of such particles. 2. A fleshy naevus, usually pigmented, although white moles (amelanotic naevi) have been described. Flat moles (naevus spilus), hairy moles (naevus pilosus), warty moles (naevus verrucosus), and moles with a papilliferous surface and an offensive secretion (naevus papillomatosus) have been described. 3. A mass in the uterus resulting from a poorly developed or degenerating ovum. **Blood mole, Carneous mole.** An ovum which has been killed by multiple haemorrhages between the decidua and chorion in the first twelve weeks of pregnancy; variously termed a *fleshy, tuberous,* or *haemorrhagic mole.* **Cellular mole.** A soft tumour of the skin, which may or may not be pigmented, consisting of a mass of naevus cells in the dermis. **Cystic mole.** Hydatidiform mole (see below). **False mole.** A mass of blood clot in the uterus, formed from a tumour. **Fleshy mole.** Blood mole (see above). **Haemorrhagic mole.** Blood mole (see above). **Hairy mole.** Naevus pilosus. **Hydatid mole.** Hydatidiform mole (see foll.). **Hydatidiform mole.** A conceptus in which the chorionic villi have undergone cystic degeneration. It is usually non-malignant, but may be known as a *malignant hydatidiform mole* if it perforates the wall of the uterus, but this must be distinguished from the truly malignant chorionepithelioma; also referred to as a *cystic hydatid* and *vesicular mole.* **Invasive mole, Malignant mole.** A malignant melanoma, usually pigmented, but not necessarily so. **Pigmented mole.** Found almost invariably in cases of Turner's syndrome. **Soft mole.** Cellular mole (see above). **Tubal mole.** A fallopian pregnancy which has been dislodged from its attachment by haemorrhage between the tube wall and the trophoblast. **Tuberous mole.** Blood mole (see above). **Vesicular mole.** Hydatidiform mole (see above). **Warty mole.** A hard, hyperkeratotic, naevus condition of the epidermis, synonymous with *naevus verrucosus,* or *hard naevus.* **White mole.** A hypopigmented mole resembling a fibroma. [AS *mal.*]

molecular (mol·ek·ew·lar). Relating to, produced by, or consisting of molecules.

molecule (mol·e·kewl). The smallest mass of a substance that can retain its independent existence and preserve its characteristic properties. It is constituted of atoms of elements bound in chemical combination and oriented in a specific pattern, alteration of which would modify the compound or even disrupt it entirely. **Biatomic molecule, Diatomic molecule.** A molecule consisting of two atoms. **Hexatomic molecule.** One consisting of 6 atoms. **Hybrid molecule.** 1. A species of molecule which is formed by the aggregation together of sub-units obtained from different macromolecules (usually sub-units of proteins or polynucleotide strands of nucleic acid). 2. A species of molecule which results from the joining together (usually end-to-end) of two parts obtained from different molecules. **Labelled molecule.** One incorporating a detectable atom (usually radioactive) so that the molecule can be traced through metabolic pathways, chemical reactions, etc. **Monatomic molecule.** An unusual molecule consisting of one atom only, as in the case of the elementary molecules of inert gases. **Non-polar molecule.** A molecule in which the constituent atoms have their charges evenly distributed over the outer electron shells. **Polar molecule.** One in which there is a permanent dipole due to an unevenness in the distribution of the charges on the electron shells of the atoms. **Saturated molecule.** One in which all the valency bonds are used up. **Tagged molecule.** Labelled molecule (see above). **Tetratomic molecule.** One composed of four atoms. **Triatomic molecule.** One composed of three atoms. **Unsaturated molecule.** One in which there are double or triple valency bonds capable of further combination. [dim. of L *moles* mass.]

molilalia (mol·e·lal·e·ah). Mogilalia. [Gk *molis* with difficulty, *lalein* to make an inarticulate sound.]

molimen (mo·le·men) (pl. *molimina*). The natural endeavour required for carrying out any normal function. **Molimen climacterium virile.** A condition of altered endocrine balance that occurs generally in male subjects between the ages of 45 and 55 years, caused by alteration in the internal secretion of the testis. **Menstrual molimen.** The periodical effort made by the female reproductive organs to establish menstruation. [L effort.]

Molindone (mol·in·done). BP Commission approved name for 3-ethyl-6,7-dihydro-2-methyl-5-(morpholinomethyl)indol-4(5H)-one; an antipsychotic agent.

Molisch, Hans (b. 1856). Vienna and Calcutta botanist.

Molisch's reaction, or test. General test for carbohydrates: two drops of a 15 to 20 per cent alcoholic solution of β-naphthol are added to a few millilitres of solution, and sulphuric acid poured carefully down the side of the tube so as to form a layer below the test solution. A violet ring develops at the junction of the liquids if carbohydrate is present.

molitor (mol·e·tor). The generic name of a group of viruses associated with molluscum contagiosum, myxomatosis of rabbits and some varieties of warts. [L contriver.]

Moll, Jacob Antonius (b. 1832). Utrecht ophthalmologist.

Moll's glands. Ciliary glands.

Møller, Eggert Hugo Heiberg. Copenhagen physician.

Møller, McIntosh, and Van Slyke test. Urea clearance test. *See* TEST.

Møllgaard, Holger (b. 1885). Copenhagen veterinary physiologist.

Møllgaard treatment. A method of treatment of pulmonary tuberculosis by combined gold and serum therapy. [Obsolete term].

mollities (mol·ish·e·eez). Softening or softness; malacia. **Mollities cerebri.** Encephalomalacia. **Mollities ossium.** Osteomalacia. **Mollities unguium.** Onychomalacia. [L]

mollusc (mol·usk). An animal of the phylum Mollusca.

Mollusca (mol·us·kah). A phylum of animals characterized by the bilaterally symmetrical, unsegmented body, with coelom and mantle folds which usually secrete a shell. The important classes are Gastropoda (snails), Lamellibranchiata (bivalves), and Cephalopoda (squids and octopuses). [L *molluscus* soft.]

molluscous (mol·us·kus). Resembling or pertaining to molluscum.

molluscum (mol·us·kum). A soft, round, cutaneous tumour. **Cholesterinic molluscum.** Xanthoma. **Molluscum contagiosum, Molluscum epitheliale.** Small, pearly white, infective tumours of skin with a dimple at the top. They are benign and usually multiple. They are caused by a poxvirus which is very similar in appearance to that of vaccinia but serologically distinct and extremely difficult to cultivate artificially. They may be transmitted sexually. **Molluscum fibrosum.** Skin tumours of neurofibromatosis. **Molluscum fibrosum gravidarum.** Rare multiple fibromata of the trunk which recur with each pregnancy. **Molluscum giganteum.** Large lesions of molluscum contagiosum (see above). **Molluscum lipomatodes.** Xanthoma. **Molluscum pendulum.** Pendulous lesions of molluscum fibrosum (see above). **Molluscum pseudocarcinomatosum.** Kerato-acanthoma; a small innocent tumour of the skin, usually on the face, which heals spontaneously. Histologically it resembles a squamous-celled epithelioma in certain respects and has been confused with this in the past. **Molluscum sebaceum.** 1. Molluscum contagiosum (see above). 2. Molluscum pseudocarcinomatosum (see above). **Molluscum sessile.** Molluscum contagiosum (see above). **Molluscum simplex.** Molluscum fibrosum (see above). **Molluscum varioliformis, Molluscum verrucosum.** Molluscum contagiosum (see above). [L *molluscus* soft.]

Moloney, John Bromley (b. 1924). American cancer research worker.

Moloney virus. One of the group of RNA-containing mouse leukaemia viruses.

Moloney, Paul Joseph (b. 1870). Ottawa physician.

Moloney reaction, or toxoid test. A test for hypersensitivity to diphtheria prophylactics performed by injecting diluted toxoid intracutaneously into the forearm. The toxoid reagent has been used as a substitute for, or in addition to, the Schick control fluid. A positive reaction is a characteristic local flush.

Moloy, Howard Carman (b. 1903). New York gynaecologist.

Caldwell-Moloy classification. A valuable contribution to the classification of the human female pelvis into four main types; the types are assessed by clinical and radiological examination.

molugram (**mol**·ew·gram). A name proposed as an alternative for gram-molecule. [Obsolete term.]

molybdanize (mol·**ib**·dan·ize). 1. To introduce the metal molybdenum, e.g. into an alloy. 2. To treat with molybdic acid or its salts, e.g. ammonium molybdate.

molybdate (mol·**ib**·date). A salt of molybdic acid.

molybdenous (mol·**ib**·den·us). Relating to molybdenum or its compounds.

molybdenum (mol·**ib**·den·um). An element of atomic weight 95.94, atomic number 42, and chemical symbol Mo. It is a hard white metal related to chromium and found in molybdenite, an ore which resembles graphite or black lead, whence its name. It has a high melting point, and is used to give tensile strength to tool steel. [Gk *molybdos* lead.]

molybdic (mol·**ib**·dik). 1. Pertaining to molybdenum. 2. A compound of molybdenum in which the latter is hexavalent, as in molybdic acid.

molybdous (mol·**ib**·dus). 1. Pertaining to molybdenum. 2. Term used infrequently for compounds of molybdenum in which the element displays lower valencies: such compounds mostly consist of complex ions, few true salts being known.

molysmophobia (mol·is·mo·**fo**′·be·ah). Morbid fear of infection or contamination. [Gk *molysmos* pollution, phobia.]

Momburg, Fritz August (b. 1870). Bielefeld, Germany, surgeon.

Momburg's belt. A method of compressing the abdominal aorta for the purpose of arresting post-partum haemorrhage, by encircling the waist two or three times with a rubber band or tube and making it taut.

moment (**mo**·ment). 1. In mechanics, a measure of the force tending to rotate a body; defined as the product of the force and the length of the perpendicular from the point of rotation to the direction of the force. 2. In statistics, the mean of the deviations in a frequency distribution from the means of the series, each deviation being raised to a power equal to the order of the moment, e.g. first, second, third, etc. **Moment of inertia.** In the case of a body able to rotate about an axis, the sum of each particle's mass multiplied by the square of the particle's distance from the axis. **Magnetic moment.** A characteristic parameter of a magnetic dipole, equal to the product of the pole strength and the linear separation of the poles; it is also equal to the turning couple on a dipole when perpendicular to a magnetic field of unit strength. **Product moment.** The average of the products of the deviations from a mean. [L *momentum* movement.]

monad (**mon**·ad). 1. In chemistry, an element or radical that is monovalent. 2. A unicellular protozoon. 3. A single-celled flagellate infusorian. [Gk *monas* a unit.]

monaesthetic (mon·es·**thet**·ik). Relating to or affecting one sensation or one sense. [Gk *monos* single, aesthesia.]

Monaghan respirator. An American type of cuirass respirator.

Monakow, Konstantin von (b. 1853). Zürich neurologist.

Monakow's bundle, fasciculus, or tract. The rubrospinal tract. *See* TRACT.

Monakow's nucleus. The cuneate nucleus. *See* NUCLEUS.

Monakow's theory. The theory of diaschisis: a severe injury to the central nervous system may cause temporary loss of functional continuity in certain nerve cells and fibres, giving a state of shock, or diaschisis.

Monaldi, Vincenzo (b. 1899). Rome physician.

Monaldi drainage. The insertion of a radio-opaque long flexible catheter direct into a tuberculous cavity in the lung, by means of a special trocar. Continuous suction through the catheter for some weeks reduces the cough and sputum, and often the size of the cavity. The effect is usually not lasting, and the procedure is rarely used except as an ancillary measure between two stages of a thoracoplasty to allow more complete collapse after the second stage.

monamide (**mon**·am·ide). An amide in which there is only one amido group, $CONH_2$. [Gk *monos* single, amide.]

monamine (**mon**·am·een). An amine in which there is only one amino group, NH_2. [Gk *monos* single, amine.]

monaminuria (**mon**·am·in·**ewr**′·e·ah). The presence of a monamine in the urine.

monandry (mon·**an**·dre). The rule or custom of the female having only one husband at any one time. [Gk *monos* single, *aner* man.]

monargentic (mon·ar·**jen**·tik). Denoting a compound which contains only one atom of silver in its molecule. [Gk *monos* single, L *argentum* silver.]

monarthric (mon·**ar**·thrik). Monoarticular. [Gk *monos* single, *arthron* joint.]

monarthritis (mon·ar·**thri**·tis). Inflammation in which one joint only is involved. [Gk *monos* single, *arthron* joint, *-itis* inflammation.]

monarticular (mon·ar·**tik**·ew·lar). Relating to one joint. [Gk *monos* single, L *articulus* joint.]

Monas (**mo**·nas). An obsolete generic name of a group of micro-organisms, the taxonomic position of which is now uncertain. [Gk a unit.]

monathetosis (**mon**·ath·e·**to**′·sis). An athetotic condition involving a single part of the body, e.g. a hand or a foot. [Gk *monos* single, athetosis.]

monatomic (mon·at·**om**·ik). 1. Monovalent. 2. Containing only one atom in the molecule. 3. Of a base or alcohol, possessing only one hydroxyl OH group. 4. Of an acid, having only one atom of hydrogen replaceable by a metal or basic radical. [Gk *monos* single, atom.]

monauchenos (mon·**awk**·en·os). A two-headed monster having only one neck. [Gk *monos* single, *auchen* neck.]

monaural (mon·**aw**·ral). Relating to one ear. [Gk *monos* single, L *auris* ear.]

monavitaminosis (**mon**·a·vi·tam·in·**o**′·sis). Avitaminosis caused by the lack of a single vitamin in the diet. [Gk *monos* single, vitaminosis.]

monaxial (mon·**ax**·e·al). Having a single axon. [see foll.]

monaxon (mon·**ax**·on). A neuron having a single axon. [Gk *monos* single, axon.]

Mond, Ludwig (b. 1839). British chemist.

Mond gas. Producer gas; a mixture of carbon monoxide and nitrogen formed by blowing air through red-hot coke: used for industrial heating.

Mondonesi, Filippo. Bologna physician.

Mondonesi's reflex. Bulbomimic reflex. *See* REFLEX.

Mondor, Henri (b. 1885). Paris surgeon.

Mondor's disease. Thrombophlebitis in the superficial veins of the breast, the fibrosis following which may simulate a fibrosing carcinoma.

Monge, Carlos (b. 1884). Lima pathologist.

Monge's disease. Chronic mountain sickness; an insidious disease that develops in those living at high altitudes, with features of polycythaemia, emphysema, dyspnoea, bronchitis, cyanosis, headache and mental disturbances. The condition is usually relieved by return to sea-level.

mongolism (**mon**·gol·izm). Down's syndrome. [*Mongol* an Asian race.]

mongoloid (**mong**·gol·oid). 1. Belonging to the division of the human race that inhabits North-east Asia. 2. A member of the Mongoloid race. 3. A subject with Down's syndrome. [*Mongol* an Asian race, Gk *eidos* form.]

monilated (**mon**·il·a·ted). Moniliform. [L *monile* necklace.]

monilethrix (mon·**il**·e·thrix). An affection in which the hairs are fragile and constricted at intervals, so that each hair is nodulated and resembles a string of beads. [L *monile* necklace, Gk *thrix* hair.]

Monilia (mon·**il**·e·ah). The name formerly given to a genus of fungi now known as *Candida*. **Monilia albicans.** *Candida albicans.* **Monilia pinoyi** Castellani and Chalmers 1913. *Candida albicans.* **Monilia tropicalis** Castellani and Chalmers 1913. *Candida tropicalis,* a reputed cause of bronchomoniliasis. [L *monile* necklace.]

monilial (mon·**il**·e·al). Relating or due to *Monilia.*

moniliasis (mon·il·**i**·as·is). Obsolete synonym for candidiasis, a disease caused by fungi of the genus *Candida,* especially *Candida albicans.* It affects the mucous membranes of the mouth, vagina and other parts, where it is called *thrush.* It also affects the skin, especially intertriginous areas, nails and, less frequently, the deeper organs. [L *monile* necklace, Gk *-osis* condition.]

moniliform (mon·**il**·e·form). Resembling a string of beads. [see foll.]

Moniliformis (mon·il·e·**form**·is). A genus of spiny-headed worms (*Acanthocephala*). **Moniliformis dubius** (=**moniliformis**). A not uncommon intestinal parasite of rats and field rodents; intermediate hosts are cockroaches and cellar beetles (*Blaps*). Several human infestations have occurred. [L *monile* necklace, form.]

moniliid (mon·**il**·e·id). A skin lesion associated with a *Monilia* (Candida) infection.

moniliosis (mon·il·**i**·o·sis). Candidiasis. [*Monilia,* Gk *-osis* condition.]

monilithrix (mon·**il**·e·thrix). Monilethrix.

monitor-radiation (**mon**·it·or·ra·de·**a**′·shun). An instrument for detecting, measuring, or warning of the presence of radiation which may constitute a health hazard, e.g. x- or γ-rays. [L *monere* to warn, radiation.]

monitoring (**mon**·it·or·ing). 1. The act of detection or measurement of a radioactive substance, especially detection of radioactive contamination. 2. Manual maintenance of an electrical signal at a desired value. 3. The automatic recording of pulse rate, blood pressure, respiration, etc., during an operation. **Patient monitoring.** The technique, used especially in intensive care units, of the continuous presentation of information about the patient by means of special instrumentation; the electrocardiogram is the information most commonly observed. [L *monere* to warn.]

monkey (**mung**·ke). Any member of the mammalian order Primates, except lemurs, the higher apes, and men. **Rhesus monkey.** *Macaca mulatta* (synonym *Macaca rhesus*), a smallish monkey of South-east Asia and the only one used extensively in laboratories. [etym. dub.]

monkeypox (**mung**·ke·pox). An epidemic non-fatal smallpox-like illness in monkeys, particularly in Africa. It is caused by a poxvirus related antigenically to smallpox and vaccinia viruses. The virus can infect man in whom it causes a non-fatal illness clinically similar to smallpox.

monkshood (**munx**·hud). A perennial herb, *Aconitum napellus,* of the family Ranunculaceae, cultivated in England, and a source of the alkaloid, aconitine. [Gk *monachos* solitary, AS *hod.*]

Monneret, Jules Edouard Auguste (b. 1810). Paris physician.

Monneret's pulse. A full, slow pulse occurring in some cases of jaundice.

mono-acid (mon·o·**as**·id). An alcohol or base which contains only one hydroxyl, OH, group that will combine with the hydrogen of a monobasic acid. [Gk *monos* single, acid.]

mono-acidic (**mon**·o·as·**id**′·ik). Denoting a base which has one available hydroxyl, OH, group, or a base each molecule of which will neutralize one molecule of a monobasic acid. [see prec.]

monoamine oxidase (**mon**·o·**am**·een **ox**·i·**dase**). An enzyme which degrades catecholamines to inactive forms.

mono-aminodiphosphatide (mon·o·**am**·in·o·di·**fos**′·fat·ide). Any phospholipid that contains two molecules of phosphoric acid and a single amino group.

mono-aminomonophosphatide (mon·o·**am**·in·o·mon·o·**fos**′·fat·ide). Any of the class of phospholipids that contain one molecule of phosphoric acid and a single amino group: included in this category are the lecithins and cephalins.

mono-articular (**mon**·o·ar·**tik**′·ew·lar). Monarticular.

mono-atomic (**mon**·o·at·**om**′·ik). Monatomic.

monobacillary, monobacterial (mon·o·**bas**·il·ar·e, **mon**·o·bak·**teer**′·e·al). Pertaining to or caused by one variety of micro-organism only. [Gk *monos* single, bacillus, bacterium.]

monobasic (mon·o·**ba**·sik). Term applied to an acid that has only one atom of hydrogen replaceable by a metal or basic radical. [Gk *monos* single, base.]

monoblast (**mon**·o·blast). The large basophilic-staining non-lobed precursor of the monocyte. It may be from 12 to 20 μm in diameter, and has small nucleoi. [Gk *monos* single, *blastos* germ.]

monoblastoma (**mon**·o·blas·**to**′·mah). A neoplastic growth that contains monocytes and monoblasts. [monoblast, Gk *-oma* tumour.]

monoblepsia, monoblepsis (mon·o·**blep**·se·ah, mon·o·**blep**·sis). 1. A condition in which the sight is better when one eye only is used. 2. A form of colour blindness wherein one colour only can be distinguished. [Gk *monos* single, *blepsis* sight.]

monobloc (**mon**·o·blok). An interdental splint used by Robin in 1900 for holding the mandible forward. [Gk *monos* single, Fr. *bloc* block.]

monobrachius (mon·o·**bra**·ke·us). In teratism, a one-armed monster. [Gk *monos* single, *brachion* arm.]

monobromated (mon·o·**bro**·ma·ted). Applied to a compound that contains only one atom of bromine per molecule. [Gk *monos* single, bromine.]

monobromide (mon·o·**bro**·mide). Any compound in which there is only one atom of bromine per molecule. [see prec.]

monobromisovaleryglycolurea (mon·o·**brom**·i·so·val·e·re·gli·kol·**ewr**′·e·ah). $C_3H_3N_2OCCH_2CBr(CH_3)_2$, a crystalline glycol formed from bromoisovalerianylurea; a mild hypnotic or sedative.

monobromophenol (**mon**·o·bro·mo·**fe**′·nol). OHC_6H_4Br, a violet liquid, soluble in water, obtained by the combination of bromine and phenol. It is used in ointments for the treatment of erysipelas, and in gargles and mouth-washes.

monobulia (mon·o·**bew**·le·ah). A state of the mind in which desire is concentrated on one particular object. [Gk *monos* single, *boule* will.]

monocalcic (mon·o·**kal**·sik). Any calcium compound containing only one calcium atom per molecule. [Gk *monos* single, calcium.]

monocardiogram (mon·o·**kar**·de·o·gram). Vectorcardiogram. [Gk *monos* single, cardiogram.]

monocellular (mon·o·**sel**·ew·lar). Unicellular; applied to primitive biological types. [Gk *monos* single, cell.]

monocentric (mon·o·**sen**·trik). Of a chromosome or chromatid, with only one centromere. [Gk *monos* single, *kentron* centre.]

monocephalus (mon·o·**kef**·al·us). A monster having only one head and two bodies. [Gk *monos* single, *kephale* head.]

monochloralantipyrine (**mon**·o·klor·al·an·te·**pi**′·reen). A mixture of chloral and phenazone used as an antipyretic and hypnotic.

monochlorethane (**mon**·o·klor·**e**′·thane). Ethyl chloride, C_2H_5Cl. A colourless liquid, very volatile, and used therefore as a refrigerant and as a spray for local anaesthesia. It is also employed as a general anaesthetic.

monochloride (mon·o·**klor**·ide). Any compound in which there is only one atom of chlorine per molecule. [Gk *monos* single, chlorine.]

monochlormethane (**mon**·o·klor·**me**′·thane). Methyl chloride, CH_3Cl. A gas used as a refrigerant.

monochlormethylchloroformate (**mon**·o·klor·meth·il·klor·o·**for**′·mate). Chloromethylchloroformate, $CH_2ClCOOCl$. A lacrimatory liquid used in chemical warfare.

monochlorphenol (**mon**·o·klor·**fe**′·nol). $C_6H_4Cl(OH)$, a liquid prepared by the action of chlorine on phenol and consisting of a mixture of the ortho- and para- isomers. The introduction of the chlorine atom increases the germicidal power of phenol, but the toxicity and caustic effects are also increased.

monochord (**mon**·o·kord). An instrument used in testing hearing, particularly for the higher tones. It resembles a one-stringed fiddle: the single string is usually made of steel wire, by varying the tension of which the pitch of its note may be raised or lowered. [Gk *monos* single, *chorde* cord.]

monochorea (**mon**·o·ko·**re**′·ah). A choreic condition affecting one part of the body only, e.g. head, one arm, one leg. [Gk *monos* single, chorea.]

monochorionic (**mon**·o·ko·re·**on**′·ik). Of enzygotic twins, having a single chorion. [Gk *monos* single, chorion.]

monochroic (mon·o·**kro**·ik). Having only a single colour. [Gk *monos* single, *chroa* colour of the skin.]

monochromasia, monochromasy (**mon**·o·kro·**ma**′·ze·ah, mon·o·**kro**·mas·e). Colour blindness in which all colours are perceived as a single colour. [Gk *monos* single, *chroma* colour.]

monochromat, monochromate (mon·o·**kro**·mat, mon·o·**kro**·mate). An individual affected with total colour blindness and unable to differentiate any colour of the spectrum; everything appears as black, white or grey. [see prec.]

monochromatic (**mon**·o·kro·**mat**′·ik). 1. Affected with total colour blindness. 2. Having only a single colour; monochroic. 3. A substance which will colour with a single stain at a time. [Gk *monos* single, *chroma* colour.]

monochromatism (mon·o·**kro**·mat·izm). Colour blindness. *See* BLINDNESS. [Gk *monos* single, *chroma* colour.]

monochromatophil, monochromatophile (mon·o·**kro**·mat·o·fil, mon·o·**kro**·mat·o·file). 1. Taking a single stain only. 2. Any cell or other structure that takes a single stain. [Gk *monos* single, *chroma* colour, *philein* to love.]

monochromator (**mon**·o·kro·**ma**′·tor). Any device for the selection and transmission of light of one wavelength only, e.g. the use of the spectroscope with the sodium flame as a source of monochromatic light. [Gk *monos* single, *chroma* colour.]

monochromic (mon·o·**kro**·mik). Monochroic.

monochromophil, monochromophile (mon·o·**kro**·mo·fil, mon·o·**kro**·mo·file). Monochromatophil.

monocle (**mon**·okl). 1. A single eyeglass for use when the sight of only one eye is abnormal. 2. A particular type of bandage for one eye. [Gk *monos* single, L *oculus* eye.]

monoclinic (mon·o·**klin**·ik). In crystal classification, one in which there are three axes of different lengths, two intersecting obliquely, the third at right angles to the plane of the other two. [Gk *monos* single, *klinein* to slope.]

monocorditis (**mon**·o·kord·**i**′·tis). Inflammation of one vocal cord. [Gk *monos* single, cord, Gk *-itis* inflammation.]

monocranius (mon·o·**kra**·ne·us). Monocephalus. [Gk *monos* single, *kranion* skull.]

monocrotic (mon·o·**krot**·ik). Pertaining to or marked by monocrotism.

monocrotism (mon·**ok**·rot·izm). The character of a single pulse wave which has no notch on either anacrotic or dicrotic limb. [Gk *monos* single, *krotos* beat.]

monocular (mon·**ok**·ew·lar). 1. Affecting or having a single eye. 2. Referring to vision with one eye. 3. In microscopy, provided with a single eyepiece. [Gk *monos* single, L *oculus* eye.]

monoculus (mon·**ok**·ew·lus). 1. A bandage to cover one eye. 2. A one-eyed individual; a cyclops. [see prec.]

monocyclic (mon·o·**si**·klik). In botany and zoology, consisting of one circle or whorl, or arranged in one circle or whorl. [Gk *monos* single, *kyklos* circle.]

monocyesis (**mon**·o·si·**e**′·sis). A state of pregnancy in which one fetus only is present. [Gk *monos* single, cyesis.]

monocystic (mon·o·**sist**·ik). Having, or made up of a single cyst. [Gk *monos* single, cyst.]

monocytangina (**mon**·o·site·**an**′·jin·ah). Infectious mononucleosis. [monocyte, angina.]

monocyte (**mon**·o·site). The largest, unicellular, nucleated leucocyte seen in normal blood (from 12 to 20 μm diameter). It has a hyaline or frosted-glass appearance of its bluish-staining cytoplasm, and a large, round, oval or reniform nucleus. It is capable of amoeboid movement and chemotaxis and is phagocytic. It is derived from bone marrow promonocytes and is the precursor of the motile tissue macrophage. A special type is seen in increased numbers in glandular fever. [Gk *monos* single, *kytos* cell.]

monocytic (mon·o·**sit**·ik). Pertaining to, of the nature of, or marked by monocytes.

monocytopenia (**mon**·o·si·to·**pe**′·ne·ah). A condition of the peripheral blood in which the number of monocytes is diminished. [monocyte, Gk *penes* poor.]

monocytopoiesis (**mon**·o·si·to·poi·**e**′·sis). The production of monocytes in the bone marrow. [monocyte, Gk *poiein* to make.]

monocytosis (**mon**·o·si·**to**′·sis). Mononucleosis; a condition in which there is an increase in the mononuclear cells in the circulating blood. It may occur in bacterial infections (tuberculosis, bacterial endocarditis, brucellosis, typhus), in agranulocytosis, protozoal infections (such as malaria, kala-azar, trypanosomiasis), Hodgkin's disease, Gaucher's disease, sarcoidosis, monocytic leukaemia, and tetrachloroethylene poisoning. **Leucopenic infectious monocytosis.** A special type of agranulocytosis in which there is a relative or absolute increase in monocytes. [monocyte, Gk *-osis* condition.]

monodactylism (mon·o·**dak**·til·izm). A congenital condition in which one finger or one toe only is present on the hand or the foot. [Gk *monos* single, *daktylos* finger or toe.]

monodactylous (mon·o·**dak**·til·us). Having a single toe or a single finger. [see prec.]

monoderic (mon·o·**der**·ik). Consisting of one layer only. [Gk *monos* single, *deras* skin.]

monodermoma (**mon**·o·der·**mo**′·mah). An epidermoid cyst. [Gk *monos* single, *derma* skin, *-oma* tumour.]

monodidymus (mon·o·**did**·im·us). A twin. [Gk *monos* single, *didymos* twin.]

monodiplopia (**mon**·o·dip·**lo**′·pe·ah). A diplopic condition affecting one eye only. [Gk *monos* single, *diploos* double, *opsis* sight.]

monodont (**mon**·o·dont). Having a single tooth. [Gk *monos* single, *odous* tooth.]

monodromia (mon·o·**dro**·me·ah). Conduction in one direction, especially of a nerve impulse. [Gk *monos* single, *dromos* course.]

monoecious (mon·**e**·shus). Having functional male and female reproductive organs in the same individual. [Gk *monos* single, *oikos* house.]

monoestrous (mon·**e**·strus). Having only one period of mating activity in a year. [Gk *monos* single, oestrus.]

monoethanolamine (mon·o·**eth**·an·**ol**′·am·een). Ethanolamine.

monofilm (**mon**·o·film). A monomolecular layer or section. [Gk *monos* single, film.]

monogamy (mon·**og**·am·e). The rule or custom of being married to one person at any one time; especially of a man being married to one woman only. In zoology, the habit of pairing with one mate during the mating season. [Gk *monos* single, *gamein* to marry.]

monoganglial (mon·o·**gang**·gle·al). Affecting or relating to one ganglion only. [Gk *monos* single, ganglion.]

monogastric (mon·o·**gas**·trik). Having a single stomach. [Gk *monos* single, *gaster* stomach.]

monogen (**mon**·o·jen). 1. A monovalent element. 2. An antigen which stimulates the production of a single specific antibody. [Gk *monos* single, *genein* to produce, antigen.]

monogenesis (mon·o·**jen**·es·is). 1. Asexual reproduction. 2. The theory that all organisms originate from one cell only. 3. The production of progeny of one sex only. [Gk *monos* single, genesis.]

monogenous (mon·**oj**·en·us). Developed non-sexually, as by gemmation, fission, or sporulation. [see prec.]

monogerminal (mon·o·**jer**·min·al). Produced from a single ovum; denoting twin fetuses that are contained in one yolk sac. [Gk *monos* single, germ.]

monogony (mon·**og**·on·e). Reproduction by fission, budding, or other non-sexual process. [Gk *monos* single, *gone* seed.]

monohydrate (mon·o·**hi**·drate). A compound that contains one molecule of water of crystallization. [Gk *monos* single, *hydor* water.]

monohydrated (mon·o·**hi**·dra·ted). Combined with one molecule of water of crystallization. [see prec.]

monohydric (mon·o·**hi**·drik). 1. Applied to an alcohol or base, one which contains only a single hydroxyl OH group. 2. Of any other compound, one which possesses a single atom of replaceable hydrogen. [Gk *monos* single, hydrogen.]

monohydrol (mon·o·**hi**·drol). The single molecule of water, unassociated, such as occurs in steam. [Gk *monos* single, *hydor* water.]

monohydroxyphenol (**mon**·o·hi·drox·e·**fe**'·nol). A general name for phenols which contain only one hydroxy group.

mono-infection (**mon**·o·in·**fek**'·shun). Infection with only one variety of micro-organism. [Gk *monos* single, infection.]

mono-iodide (mon·o·i·o·dide). Any compound in which there is only one atom of iodine per molecule. [Gk *monos* single, iodine.]

monoketoheptose (**mon**·o·ke·to·**hep**'·toze). 1. A heptose which contains one keto CO group. 2. $(CH_2OH)(CHOH)_4CO(CH_2OH)$, a monosaccharide produced by bacterial activity from perseitol, contained in the leaves of the Persian laurel.

monoketone (mon·o·**ke**·tone). The more usual type of ketone containing only one CO group.

monolayer (mon·o·**la**·er). A sheet of cells cultured in nutrient medium on the surface of glass bottles, test-tubes, or plastic plates. So-called because the sheet is only one cell thick, overgrowth being prevented by contact inhibition between cells. [Gk *monos* single, AS *lecgan* layer.]

monolepsis (mon·o·**lep**·sis). In breeding, transfer to the offspring of characteristics peculiar to one parent and the exclusion of the characteristics of the second parent. [Gk *monos* single, *lambanein* to take.]

monolocular (mon·o·**lok**·ew·lar). Having a single loculus. [Gk *monos* single, loculus.]

monomania (mon·o·**ma**·ne·ah). Mental derangement due to concentration of attention on one idea or subject. **Emotional monomania.** A form of monomania in which the attention is focused on a single emotion. **Intellectual monomania.** A form of monomania restricted to a small number of kindred false beliefs. [Gk *monos* single, mania.]

monomaniac (mon·o·**ma**·ne·ak). An individual suffering from monomania.

monomastigote (mon·o·**mas**·tig·ote). A mastigote having only one flagellum. [Gk *monos* single, mastigote.]

monomaxillary (mon·o·max·**il**'·ar·e). Pertaining to or affecting one jaw only. [Gk *monos* single, L *maxilla* jawbone.]

monomelic (mon·o·**mel**·ik). Pertaining to or affecting one limb only. [Gk *monos* single, *melos* limb.]

monomer (**mon**·o·mer). The molecule of a compound, such as acetylene, which by polymerization forms the unit in a polymer. [Gk *monos* single, *meros* part.]

monomercurion (**mon**·o·mer·**kewr**'·e·on). The ion of monovalent mercury, Hg^+, derived from mercurous compounds.

monomeric (mon·o·**mer**·ik). Affecting, composed of, or relating to only one segment. [Gk *monos* single, *meros* part.]

monometallic (**mon**·o·met·**al**'·ik). Denoting a compound which contains in its molecule only one atom of a metal. [Gk *monos* single, metal.]

monomethylmorphine (**mon**·o·meth·il·**mor**'·feen). Codeine.

monomethylxanthine (**mon**·o·meth·il·**zan**'·theen). Methylxanthine.

monomicrobic (**mon**·o·mi·**kro**'·bik). Denoting that one particular micro-organism is present or is responsible for certain activities in the tissues. [Gk *monos* single, microbe.]

monomoria (mon·o·**mor**·e·ah). Monomania of mild degree; the melancholic diathesis. [Gk *monos* single, *moria* silliness.]

monomorphic, monomorphous (mon·o·**morf**·ik, mon·o·**morf**·us). Of one form or structure; uniform. [Gk *monos* single, *morphe* shape.]

monomphalus (mon·**om**·fal·us). A double monstrosity, the connecting link being situated at the umbilicus. [Gk *monos* single, *omphalos* navel.]

monomyoplegia (**mon**·o·mi·o·**ple**'·je·ah). A paralytic condition that is confined to one muscle. [Gk *monos* single, *mys* muscle, *plege* stroke.]

mononephrous (mon·o·**nef**·rus). Affecting or relating to one kidney only. [Gk *monos* single, *nephros* kidney.]

mononeural, mononeuric (mon·o·**newr**·al, mon·o·**newr**·ik). Having a single neurone. Relating to or supplied by one nerve. [Gk *monos* single, *neuron* nerve.]

mononeuritis (**mon**·o·newr·**i**'·tis). Neuritis affecting one nerve. **Mononeuritis multiplex.** Neuritis occurring simultaneously in several distinct nerves, at a distance from each other. [Gk *monos* single, neuritis.]

mononoea (mon·o·**ne**·ah). The concentration of the mind upon a single matter. [Gk *monos* single, *nous* mind.]

monont (**mon**·ont). Schizont; the asexual dividing stage of the malaria parasite. [obsolete term.] [Gk *monos* single, *on* existing.]

mononuclear, mononucleate (mon·o·**new**·kle·ar, mon·o·**new**·kle·ate). 1. Having only one nucleus. 2. A cell with one nucleus; in particular, a monocyte. [Gk *monos* single, nucleus.]

mononucleosis (**mon**·o·neu·kle·**o**'·sis). **Monocytosis; Infectious mononucleosis; Infective mononucleosis; Glandular fever.** An acute febrile illness mostly in young adults. Generally mild but may be prolonged and debilitating. The main features are lymphadenopathy, fever and sore throat (which may ulcerate). Atypical lymphocytes and a monocytosis are seen in the blood, which mostly shows a rise in titre of a haemagglutinin for sheep erythrocytes (positive Paul–Bunnell test). This, in various forms, is the most commonly used diagnostic test. The disease is due to a herpes virus, EB virus. It is often transmitted from mouth to mouth. [Gk *monos* single, nucleus, Gk *-osis* condition.]

mononucleotide (mon·o·**new**·kle·o·tide). A unit in the structure of nucleic acids. It consists of a molecule of phosphoric acid combined with a molecule each of a pentose sugar, usually ribose, and a base such as adenine, cytosine, guanine, thymine, or uracil. They are usually designated as monophosphates of the nucleosides or as acids, e.g. adenosine monophosphate or adenylic acid are adenine-ribose-phosphate. Other common mononucleotides are the monophosphates of guanosine, inosine, uridine, cytidine, thymidine. [Gk *monos* single, nucleus.]

mono-osteitic (**mon**·o·os·te·**it**'·ik). Referring to inflammation occurring in only one bone. [Gk *monos* single, *osteon* bone, *-itis* inflammation.]

monoparaesthesia (**mon**·o·par·es·**the**'·ze·ah). Paraesthesia affecting one limb or one part only. [Gk *monos* single, paraesthesia.]

monoparesis (**mon**·o·par·**e**'·sis). A paretic condition affecting one part or one limb only. [Gk *monos* single, paresis.]

monopathophobia (**mon**·o·path·o·**fo**'·be·ah). Fear of a particular disease. [Gk *monos* single, pathophobia.]

monopathy (mon·**op**·ath·e). 1. A disease without any complications. 2. A disease restricted to one organ or part. [Gk *monos* single, *pathos* disease.]

monopenia (mon·o·**pe**·ne·ah). Monocytopenia.

monophagia (mon·o·**fa**·je·ah). 1. The habit of eating only one meal in the day. 2. The wish for only one kind of food. [Gk *monos* single, *phagein* to eat.]

monophasia (mon·o·**fa**·ze·ah). Extreme degree of loss of expressive language due to localized brain-disease, whereby the patient is unable to emit anything more than extremely few stereotyped utterances, either verbal or non-verbal. [Gk *monos* single, *phasis* speech.]

monophasic (mon·o·**fa**·zik). 1. Relating to or characterized by monophasia. 2. Unidirectional; displaying a single variation or phase. [see prec.]

monophobia (mon·o·**fo**·be·ah). Morbid fear of solitude. [Gk *monos* single, phobia.]

monophosphate (mon·o·**fos**·fate). A compound containing only one phosphoric-acid group. [Gk *monos* single, phosphate.]

monophthalmia (mon·of·**thal**·me·ah). The condition in which only one eye is present. This may be due to removal or destruction of its fellow but it may also occur as a congenital condition due to maldevelopment of the other eye, or to fusion of the two (cyclopia or synophthalmia). [see foll.]

monophthalmous (mon·of·**thal**·mus). One-eyed; referring to dressings, describing a bandage for application to one eye only. [Gk *monos* single, *ophthalmos* eye.]

monophthalmus (mon·of·**thal**·mus). A fetal monster with only one eye. [see prec.]

monophyletic (**mon**·o·fi·**let**′·ik). Of common ancestry. [Gk *monos* single, *phyle* race.]

monophyodont (mon·o·**fi**·o·dont). Having only one dentition, the permanent set of teeth. [Gk *monos* single, *phyein* to grow, *odous* tooth.]

monopia (mon·**o**·pe·ah). Monopsia.

monoplasmatic (**mon**·o·plaz·**mat**′·ik). Composed of only one tissue or substance. [Gk *monos* single, plasm.]

monoplast (**mon**·o·plast). A single-cell organism. [Gk *monos* single, *plassein* to mould.]

monoplastic (mon·o·**plas**·tik). 1. Relating or belonging to a monoplast. 2. Not being subject to any structural change. 3. Made up of one substance only. [see prec.]

monoplastid (mon·o·**plas**·tid). Any structural element or organism that is made up of only one cell. [Gk *monos* single, *plassein* to mould.]

monoplegia (mon·o·**ple**·je·ah). A paretic condition affecting one muscle, one group of muscles, one limb or one part of the body only. **Monoplegia masticatoria.** Paralysis in which one side of the masticatory muscles only is affected. [Gk *monos* single, *plege* stroke.]

monoplegic (mon·o·**ple**·jik). Affected with or relating to monoplegia.

monopolar (mon·o·**po**·lar). Monoterminal. [Gk *monos* single, pole.]

monops (**mon**·ops). Monophthalmus; a fetal monster with only one eye. [see foll.]

monopsia (mon·**op**·se·ah). Uni-ocular vision. [Gk *monos* single, *ops* eye.]

monopsychosis (**mon**·o·si·**ko**′·sis). Monomania. [Gk *monos* single, psychosis.]

monoptychial (mon·o·**ti**·ke·al). Disposed in one stratum only; denoting glands the cells of which are arranged in one layer on the basement membrane. [Gk *monos* single, *ptychos* layer.]

monopus (**mon**·o·pus). A fetal monster with only one leg or foot. [Gk *monos* single, *pous* foot.]

monoradicular (**mon**·o·rad·**ik**′·ew·lar). Denoting teeth which have a single root. [Gk *monos* single, L *radicula* small root.]

monorchid (mon·**or**·kid). An individual with only one testis in the scrotum. [see foll.]

monorchidic (mon·or·**kid**·ik). Relating to an individual having only one descended testis. [Gk *monos* single, *orchis* testicle.]

monorchidism, monorchism (mon·**or**·kid·izm, **mon**·or·kizm). A condition in which only one testis is apparent, the other being non-existent or undescended into the scrotum. [see prec.]

monorecidive (**mon**·o·re·**sid**′·iv). One of the manifestations of the recurrent stage of early syphilis. The lesion appears at the site of the original primary chancre and can be identified by dark-ground microscopy. [Gk *monos* single, L *recidivus* falling back.]

monorrhinic (mon·o·**ri**·nik). Relating to a single nostril. [Gk *monos* single, *rhis* nose.]

monorrhinous (mon·o·**ri**·nus). Having only one nostril situated medially. [see prec.]

monosaccharide (mon·o·**sak**·ar·ide). One of the family of simple sugars, most of which occur in nature. They are colourless crystalline compounds, soluble in water, sweet tasting, and are to be considered as polyhydric alcohols of general formula $(CH_2O)_m$, with an aldehyde CHO group (*aldoses*) or a ketone CO group (*ketoses*). Structurally they consist of a chain of carbon atoms, some of which may be asymmetric giving rise to optical activity, and are classified therefore as *dioses, trioses, tetroses, pentoses, hexoses, heptoses, octoses, nonoses* and *decoses* according to the number. Compound saccharides are produced by the union of two or more monosaccharides. [Gk *monos* single, *sakkharon* sugar.]

monosaccharose (mon·o·**sak**·ar·oze). Monosaccharide.

monoscelous (mon·o·**skel**·us). Having only one leg. [Gk *monos* single, *skelos* leg.]

monoscenism (mon·o·**se**·nizm). Living again in memory an experience in past life; the incidents are generally repeated several times in succession. [Gk *monos* single, scene.]

monose (**mon**·oze). Monosaccharide.

monoside (**mon**·o·side). Name applied to a glycoside which contains only one sugar unit. [Gk *monos* single, glycoside.]

monosodic (mon·o·**so**·dik). Any sodium compound which contains only one sodium atom per molecule. [Gk *monos* single, sodium.]

monosome (**mon**·o·some). A chromosome without a homologous partner. [Gk *monos* single, *soma* body.]

monosomian (mon·o·**so**·me·an). Applied to a double monster having a single body. [see foll.]

monosomic (mon·o·**so**·mik). Of a cell or individual, with only one member of one or more chromosome pairs. [Gk *monos* single, *soma* body.]

monosomus (mon·o·**so**·mus). A double fetus having two heads but only one body. [Gk *monos* single, *soma* body.]

monosomy (mon·o·**so**·me). The state of monosomics. [Gk *monos* single, *soma* body.]

monospasm (**mon**·o·spazm). A condition of spasm limited to one part, to one muscle or group of muscles, or to one limb. [Gk *monos* single, spasm.]

monospermy (**mon**·o·sper·me). Fertilization of an ovum by the penetration of a single spermatozoon. [Gk *monos* single, sperm.]

Monosporium (mon·o·**spo**·re·um). A genus of fungi. **Monosporium apiospermum.** A species that has been isolated from maduromycetoma and from cases of otomycosis. **Monosporium sclerotiale** Pepere 1914. A species that has been isolated from a case of mycetoma. [Gk *monos* single, *sporos* seed.]

monostearin (mon·o·**ste**·ar·in). **Self-emulsifying Monostearin BPC 1968.** Monostearin emulsificans, self-emulsifying glyceryl monostearate; a whitish waxy substance, composed chiefly of glyceryl esters of palmitic and stearic acids together with some free fatty acids, glycerin, and small amounts of other substances. It is used as an emulsifying agent for oils, fats, and waxes in the preparation of creams and ointments.

monostotic (mon·os·**tot**·ik). Pertaining to a single bone. [Gk *monos* single, *osteon* bone.]

monostratal (mon·o·**stra**·tal). Arranged in one stratum, or in a single layer. [Gk *monos* single, stratum.]

monosubstituted (mon·o·**sub**·stit·ew·ted). In organic synthesis, a compound which has had one atom or group of atoms in its molecule replaced by another. [Gk *monos* single, substitute.]

monosymptom (mon·o·**simp**·tom). One isolated symptom. [Gk *monos* single, symptom.]

monosymptomatic (**mon**·o·simp·tom·**at**′·ik). Denoting a condition in which there is manifestation of a single symptom. [see prec.]

monosynaptic (**mon**·o·sin·**ap**′·tik). Denoting a nervous pathway with only one synapse. [Gk *monos* single, *synaptein* to join.]

monosyphilid, monosyphilide (mon·o·**sif**·il·id, mon·o·**sif**·il·ide). A single syphilitic lesion of the skin or mucosa. [Gk *monos* single, syphilis.]

monoterminal (mon·o·ter·min·al). Uniterminal; the use of one terminal only in the giving of electrical treatment, the earth acting as the second terminal. This technique is employed in fulguration. [Gk *monos* single, terminal.]

monothermia (mon·o·ther·me·ah). A state in which there is no rise or fall of the bodily temperature during the day. [Gk *monos* single, *therme* heat.]

monotic (mon·ot·ik). Relating to a single ear. [Gk *monos* single, *ous* ear.]

monotocous (mon·ot·o·kus). Giving birth to one child at a time; a single birth ending pregnancy. [Gk *monos* single, *tokos* birth.]

monotonia (mon·o·to·ne·ah). Monotony of voice, resulting from a paralysed condition of the larynx. [Gk *monos* single, tone.]

Monotremata, Monotremes (mon·o·tre·mah′·tah, mon·o·treemz). A group of primitive Australasian mammals which lay eggs. They include the duck-billed platypus. [Gk *monos* single, *trema* hole.]

monotrichous (mon·ot·rik·us). Bearing a single flagellum; pertaining to Mastigophora. [Gk *monos* single, *thrix* hair.]

monoureide (mon·o·ewr·e·ide). A simple ureide derived from urea by the condensation of only one of the amino-groups with the carboxyl group of an organic acid; carbromal is an example. Monoureides are weak depressants of the central nervous system, and though safer than the diureides (e.g. barbiturates) are only moderately effective. [Gk *monos* single, ureide.]

monovalent (mon·o·va·lent). 1. Having a valency of one; applied to elements and radicals. 2. A serum antibody which is capable of combining with only one antigen or complement. [Gk *monos* single, L *valentia* strength.]

monoxenous (mon·ox·en·us). Having only a single species of host in the life cycle. [Gk *monos* single, *xenos* host.]

monoxeny (mon·ox·en·e). Parasitism in which there is only one species of host in the life cycle. [see prec.]

monozygotic (mon·o·zi·got′·ik). Resulting from or relating to a single zygote. [Gk *monos* single, *zygon* yoke.]

Monro (I), Alexander (b. 1697). Edinburgh anatomist.

Monro's abscess. A collection of neutrophils found in the epidermis in some patients with psoriasis.

Micro-abscess of Monro, Pseudo-abscess of Monro. Small accumulations of neutrophil polymorpholeucocytes in the epidermis, found in psoriasis.

Monro (II), Alexander (b. 1733). Edinburgh anatomist.

Monro's fissure, or sulcus. The hypothalamic sulcus of the third ventricle.

Foramen of Monro. Interventricular foramen; the communication between the lateral and 3rd ventricles of the brain.

Monro's line, Monro-Richter line. A line from the umbilicus to the anterior superior iliac spine.

mons (monz). An eminence or mound. **Mons pubis [NA].** The superficial cushion of fat covering the body of the pubis. **Mons veneris.** Mons pubis (see above). [L mountain.]

Monsel's solution. A solution of basic ferric subsulphate used as a styptic.

Monson's curve. The curved plane formed by the occlusal surfaces of the premolar and molar teeth.

monster (mon·ster). A grossly distorted individual, incapable of properly carrying out normal functions owing to faulty development. **Acardiac monster.** A monster without a properly developed heart and with a rudimentary circulation. **Autositic monster.** That part of a double monster that exists through its own organs as well as those of its partner which is called the parasite. **Celosomian monster.** A monster in which there is protrusion of the viscera because of defect of the thoracic or abdominal walls. **Compound monster.** Diaxial monster (see foll.). **Diaxial monster.** Symmetrical double monsters consisting of two equal or nearly equal fetuses, due to partial fusion of two originally separate embryos derived from one ovum or from the incomplete splitting of one original embryo. **Double monster.** Diaxial monster (see above). **Emmenic monster.** A menstruating infant. **Endocymic monster.** A double monster in which the parasite is contained within the body of the autositic monster. **Heterotypical monster.** A double monster in which a small parasitic twin is attached to the ventral abdominal wall of the larger twin. **Mono-axial monster.** A monster in which the original axis of one fetus is present, but some anomaly of its components has arisen. **Parasitic monster.** That part of a double monster that exists through the organs of its partner, the autositic monster. **Sirenoform monster.** A monster showing fusion of the lower extremities, the feet being absent. **Triplet monster.** A monster arising from partial or complete fusion of three fetuses. **Twin monster.** Diaxial monster (see above). [L *monstrum.*]

monstricide (mon·stris·ide). The act of destroying a monster. [monster, L *caedere* to kill.]

monstriferous (mon·strif·er·us). Producing monsters. [monster, L *ferre* to bear.]

monstriparity (mon·stre·par·it·e). The act of bringing forth a monster. [monster, L *parere* to give birth.]

monstrosity (mon·stros·it·e). 1. A monster or teratism. 2. A congenital deformity of severe degree.

monstrum (mon·strum). A monster. **Monstrum abundans.** A monster with an excess of parts. **Monstrum deficiens.** One with a deficiency of parts. **Monstrum sirenoforme.** Sirenoform monster. *See* MONSTER. [L]

Monteggia, Giovanni Battista (b. 1762). Milan physician.

Monteggia's fracture. Fracture of the shaft of the ulna with dislocation of the head of the radius.

Montenegro's test. An intradermal test for South American mucocutaneous leishmaniasis. About 0.1 ml of a flagellate suspension (*Leishmania braziliensis*) is injected.

Monteverde, Angelo (fl. 1874). Cremona physician.

Monteverde's sign. Failure to respond to an injection of ammonia as a sign of death.

Montgomery, William Fetherstone (b. 1797). Dublin gynaecologist.

Montgomery's corpuscles, glands, or tubercles. Small prominences, sebaceous glands, in the areola of the breast which become more marked in pregnancy.

Montgomery's cups, or follicles. Large, deep, mucous glands in the upper two-thirds of the endometrium of the neck of the uterus.

monticulus (mon·tik·ew·lus). In anatomy, a small mound or elevation. [L]

mood (mood). A dimension of feeling ranging from mania through elation and cheerfulness to sadness, gloom and depression. **Impure mood.** Feeling tone directed towards some object, e.g. anger. **Pure mood.** Feeling tone not directed towards an object, e.g. cheerfulness. [AS *mod* mind.]

Moon, Henry (b. 1845). London dental surgeon.

Moon's cusps. The pitted, irregular cusps of a first permanent molar tooth from a patient affected by hereditary syphilis.

Moon's molars, or teeth. Dome-shaped first permanent molar teeth due to hereditary syphilis.

Moon, Robert Charles (b. 1844). Philadelphia ophthalmologist.

Laurence-Moon-Biedl dystrophy, or syndrome. The combination of obesity, sexual under-development, retinitis pigmentosa, mental deficiency and polydactylism or syndactylism. It may be incomplete, and other abnormalities may be present. A familial congenital syndrome.

moonseed (moon·seed). Yellow sarsaparilla; the climbing plant *Menispermum canadense,* the rhizome and roots of which are used as a substitute for sarsaparilla itself. [AS *mona, seed.*]

Moor, Cresacre George (b. 1870). Exeter public analyst.

Moor's nitrogen-free agar. A medium made up from magnesium sulphate 0.2 g, potassium acid phosphate 1.0 g, glucose 10 g, agar 15 g, and distilled water to 1 litre.

Moore, Charles Hewitt (b. 1821). London surgeon.

Moore's operation. The introduction of a wire into an aneurysm to induce coagulation.

Moore-Corradi operation. The passage of a strong electric current along a wire introduced into an aneurysm.

Moore, Edward Mott (b. 1814). American surgeon.
Moore's fracture. Fracture of the lower end of the radius with luxation of the ulna.

Moore, Matthew T. (b. 1901). Philadelphia neurologist.
Moore's syndrome. Abdominal epilepsy. *See* EPILEPSY.

Moorehead, Frederick Brown (b. 1875). Chicago oral surgeon.
Moorehead's retractor. A type of dental retractor.

Mooren, Albert (b. 1828). Düsseldorf ophthalmologist.
Mooren's ulcer. A progressive chronic ulceration of the cornea, with a typical undermined and overhanging advancing edge that spreads in time across the whole cornea. It is rare and the cause is unknown.

Mooser, Hermann (b. 1891). Swiss pathologist in Mexico City.
Mooser body, Neill-Mooser body. The rickettsia of murine typhus seen in the tunica vaginalis exudate of the infected guinea-pig.
Neill-Mooser reaction, or test. A guinea-pig inoculation test for differentiating the rickettsiae. The morbid material is injected into the peritoneum; a characteristic severe inflammatory reaction of the scrotum with numerous rickettsiae in the exudate indicates that the infection is with the murine or an allied strain.

Moots, Charles William (b. 1869). Toledo, Ohio, surgeon.
Moots' formula, or rule, Moots-McKesson ratio.

$$\frac{\text{Systolic blood pressure} - \text{diastolic blood pressure}}{\text{diastolic blood pressure}} \times 100$$

should be 50 in normal persons. If it is below 25 or above 75 the subject presents a poor anaesthetic risk.

moral defective (mor·al de·**fek**·tiv). A person in whose case there exists mental defect coupled with strongly vicious or criminal tendencies and who requires control for the protection of others. [L *moralis*, defective.]

moramentia (mor·a·**men**·she·ah). A state of feeblemindedness in which the individual lacks moral sense. [moron, amentia.]

Morand, Sauveur François (b. 1697). Paris surgeon.
Morand's disease. Paresis of the extremities.
Morand's ergot, or spur. The calcar avis; a projection in the medial wall of the posterior horn of the lateral ventricle, produced by the calcarine sulcus.
Morand's foramen. The foramen caecum of the tongue.

Morat, Jean-Pierre (b. 1846). Paris physiologist.
Dastre-Morat law. Constriction of the blood vessels of the skin is usually associated with dilatation of the splanchnic blood vessels, and *vice versa.*

Morawitz, Paul Oskar (b. 1879). German physiologist.
Morawitz theory. Of blood coagulation: when blood is shed, the platelets disintegrate in contact with a water-soluble surface liberating thromboplastin (a further quantity also comes from the damaged tissues) which reacts in the presence of ionizable calcium in the blood with the plasma prothrombin to form thrombin; this thrombin then reacts with the blood fibrinogen producing fibrin.

Morax, Victor (b. 1866). Paris ophthalmologist.
Morax's diplobacillus, or diplococcus, Morax-Axenfeld bacillus, or diplococcus. *Moraxella lacunata.*

Moraxella (mor·ax·el·ah). A genus of the family Brucellaceae; short, Gram-negative, non-motile diplobacilli found as parasites and pathogens in warm-blooded animals, especially associated with diseases of the eye. **Moraxella duplex.** A species differentiated by growing in the absence of serum. **Moraxella lacunata.** The type species; short rods, from 0.4 to 2.0 μm in length, occurring in pairs or short chains. It is non-motile and Gram-negative, and is the cause of subacute infectious conjunctivitis or angular conjunctivitis in man. **Moraxella wolffi.** A cause of conjunctivitis in man. [Victor *Morax* and Karl Theodor Paul Polykarpos *Axenfeld.*]

Morazone (mor·az·one). BP Commission approved name for 2,3-dimethyl-4-(3-methyl-2-phenylmorpholinomethyl)-1-phenyl-5-pyrazolone; an analgesic.

morbid (mor·bid). 1. Belonging or relating to disease; pathological. 2. Of tissue, diseased. 3. Applied to any mental or psychic faculty that is unhealthy or that tends towards abnormality. [L *morbidus* diseased.]

morbidity (mor·**bid**·it·e). The state of being diseased or conducive to disease. [see prec.]

morbific (mor·**bif**·ik). Generating disease; pathogenic. [L *morbus* disease, *facere* to make.]

morbigenous (mor·**bij**·en·us). Morbific. [L *morbus* disease, Gk *genein* to produce.]

morbilli (mor·**bil**·e). Measles. [L little diseases.]

morbilliform (mor·**bil**·e·form). Resembling measles or the measles eruption. [morbilli, form.]

morbillous (mor·**bil**·us). Relating to measles. [morbilli.]

morbus (**mor**·bus). A disease. **Morbus anglicus.** Rickets. **Morbus apoplectiformis.** Ménière's disease. **Morbus asthenicus.** A general state of asthenia. **Morbus basedowii.** Exophthalmic goitre; Basedow's disease, Graves' disease; Parry's disease. **Morbus brightii.** Nephritis; Bright's disease. **Morbus britannicus.** Heat exhaustion and cramps in ships' firemen. **Morbus caducus.** Epilepsy; falling sickness. **Morbus cardiacus.** Morbus cordis (see below). **Morbus celsi.** Epilepsy. **Morbus coeruleus.** Congenital heart disease with cyanosis. **Morbus comitialis.** Epilepsy. **Morbus cordis.** Heart disease. **Morbus coxae senilis.** Osteo-arthritis of the hip in elderly persons. **Morbus coxarius.** Neuralgic pain felt in the coccyx; coccygodynia. **Morbus cucullaris.** Whooping-cough. **Morbus divinus.** Epilepsy. **Morbus dormitivus.** Sleeping sickness. **Morbus elephas.** Elephantiasis. **Morbus errorum.** Morbus vagabondus (see below). **Morbus gallicus.** Syphilis. **Morbus herculus.** 1. Elephantiasis. 2. Pseudohypertrophic muscular dystrophy. **Morbus maculosus neonatorum.** Haemorrhagic disease of the newborn. **Morbus maculosus werlhofii.** Thrombocytopenic purpura. *See* PURPURA. **Morbus magnus.** Epilepsy. **Morbus major.** Epilepsy. **Morbus medicorum.** An abnormal tendency to consult doctors for trifling or imaginary ailments. **Morbus miseriae.** Disease due to poverty and neglect. **Morbus moniliformis lichenoides.** A name given by Wise and Rein to an eruption of node-like masses, arranged in lines or bands, with small, flat-topped, brown papules between the nodes, hitherto called *lichen ruber moniliformis.* Wise and Rein considered that, because of the histological appearances, the malady was not a form of lichen planus. **Morbus morsus muris.** Rat-bite fever. **Morbus nauticus, Morbus naviticus.** Seasickness. **Morbus niger.** Melaena. **Morbus pedicularis, Morbus pediculosis.** Infestation with lice. **Morbus regius.** Jaundice. **Morbus sacer.** Epilepsy. **Morbus saltatorius.** Dancing mania; St. Vitus' dance. **Morbus senilis.** Arthritis deformans. **Morbus strangulatorius.** Diphtheria. **Morbus tuberculosis pedis.** Mycetoma; Madura foot. **Morbus vagabondus.** Brown pigmentation of the skin seen in tramps, and due to infestation with lice, scratching, and exposure. **Morbus vesicularis.** Pemphigus. **Morbus virginius.** Chlorosis. **Morbus vulpis.** Alopecia. [L]

mordacious (mor·**da**·she·us). Acrid, biting. [L *mordax* biting.]

mordant (**mor**·dant). Essentially a chemical reagent impregnated in a fabric, with which a dye subsequently forms an insoluble and firmly-held lake; the term is used in bacteriology and histology to mean any chemical substance (e.g. aniline, phenol, metallic salts and alkalis) which will make staining possible or easier. [L *mordere* to bite.]
See also: BUNGE.

mordanting (mor·dant·ing). The process of applying a mordant to a textile or tissue so as to facilitate subsequent dyeing or staining procedures. [see prec.]

Morel, Bénédict Augustin (b. 1809). Paris psychiatrist.
Morel ear. A congenital deformity in which the ear is flattened and the normal contours obliterated.
Morel's syndrome, Morel-Morgagni syndrome. Morgagni's syndrome.
Kraepelin-Morel disease, Morel-Kraepelin disease. Dementia praecox.
Stewart-Morel syndrome. Morgagni's syndrome.

Morestin, Hippolyte (b. 1869). Paris surgeon.

Morestin's operation. Amputation at the knee [obsolete term].

Souligoux–Morestin method. A method of lavage of the peritoneal cavity in acute peritonitis.

Morgagni, Giovanni Battista (b. 1682). Padua anatomist and pathologist.

Morgagni's appendices. Appendices vesiculosae.

Morgagni's cartilage, or tubercle. The cuneiform cartilage of the larynx.

Morgagni's caruncle. The median lobe of the prostate gland.

Columns of Morgagni. The anal columns.

Morgagni's corpuscles, globules, or spheres. Bodies found in cataractous lenses between the cortex and the capsule and produced by the coagulation of fluid breakdown products.

Crypt of Morgagni. The anal crypt.

Morgagnian cyst. A cyst of the hydatid of Morgagni (see below) attached to the testis.

Morgagni's disease. Endocranial hyperostosis.

Morgagni's foramen. 1. Foramen singulare. 2. The interval between the sternal and costal origins of the diaphragm.

Morgagni's fossa. The fossa terminalis.

frenulum of Morgagni. The prolongation of the two labia of the ileocaecal valve around the inner wall of the colon.

Morgagni's glands. Littré's glands; mucous glands in the urethra.

Morgagni's humour, or liquor. A clear fluid developing in the crystalline lens after death.

Hydrocele of the hydatid of Morgagni. Morgagnian cyst (see above).

hydatid of Morgagni. A congenital vesicle hanging by a thin stalk to the uterine tube in the female or to the epididymis in the male, and derived from the paramesonephric duct.

Morgagni's hyperostosis, or syndrome, Morel–Morgagni syndrome. Hyperostosis frontalis interna associated with obesity, headache, various endocrine abnormalities (e.g. amenorrhoea, hypertrichosis, diabetes), and various neuropsychiatric disturbances, usually occurring in middle-aged women.

Morgagni's lacunae. Lacunae urethrales.

Morgagni's nodules. A fibrocartilaginous thickening of the centre of the free margin of the cusps of the aortic and pulmonary valves.

Morgagni's prolapse. A prolapse of the mucous membrane of Morgagni's ventricle, the recess which lies between the true and false vocal cords.

Morgagni's sinus. 1. The hiatus between the base of the skull and the superior constrictor muscle of the pharynx, filled by the pharyngobasilar fascia. 2. The prostatic utricle.

Morgagni's valves. The anal valves.

Morgagni's ventricle. The sinus of the larynx.

Morgagni–Adams–Stokes disease, or syndrome. Disturbance of consciousness due to inadequate cerebral blood flow, accompanying extreme slowing of the heart or ventricular standstill; in severe cases complete loss of consciousness and even epileptiform convulsions may result. As soon as ventricular beating is resumed consciousness is rapidly regained, followed by a widespread flush (reactive hyperaemia). It occurs not infrequently when partial auriculoventricular heart block is becoming complete, and less frequently in cases of established complete heart block. Ventricular asystole may sometimes follow an episode of ventricular paroxysmal tachycardia with a similar clinical syndrome, but this is not strictly the Morgagni–Adams–Stokes syndrome. Originally described by Morgagni in 1700, it is usually called the *Stokes–Adams' syndrome.*

Morgan, Harry de Riemer (b. 1863). London physician.

Morgan's bacillus. *Proteus morgani.*

morgue (morg). Mortuary. [Fr.]

moria (mo·re·ah). An abnormal tendency to joke. [Gk folly.]

moribund (mor·e·bund). In the act of dying; almost dead. [L *moribundus* dying.]

morioplasty (mor·e·o·plas·te). The plastic restoration of parts lost through accident or disease. [Gk *morion* piece, *plassein* to mould.]

Morison, James Rutherford (b. 1853). Newcastle-upon-Tyne surgeon.

Rutherford Morison appendicectomy incision. An oblique incision in the line of the external oblique muscle which divides the deeper muscles of the abdomen in the same line; for approach to the appendix.

Rutherford Morison's method. Treatment of open infected wounds by packing them with paste of bismuth subnitrate and iodoform (BIPP); used in World War I.

Morison's paste. A mixture of exsiccated magnesium sulphate and glycerol, with a little phenol, and used as an antiseptic desiccant for boils and carbuncles.

Morison's pouch. The right subhepatic space of the peritoneum, extending from the lower surface of the right lobe of the liver and the coronary ligament above to the transverse mesocolon below.

Drummond–Morison operation. An operation for the relief of ascites in which the surfaces of the liver, spleen, and parietal peritoneum are roughened to encourage adhesions, the omentum being also roughened and sutured to the abdominal wall.

Talma–Morison operation. A combination of splenectomy, rawing of the surfaces of the viscera, and implantation of the omentum in the abdominal wall, to encourage collateral venous anastomosis in portal obstruction.

Morley, John. Manchester surgeon.

Morley's law. Referred pain law; this type of pain only arises from irritation of nerves which are sensitive to those stimuli that produce pain when applied to the surface of the body.

Moro, Ernst (b. 1874). Heidelberg paediatrician.

Moro's reaction, or test. A local tuberculin reaction produced by applying Moro's reagent to an area of skin. The original Moro test is now obsolete, but has been replaced by other percutaneous tests, e.g. the Vollmer patch test.

Moro's reagent. Percutaneous reagent; an ointment composed of equal parts of old tuberculin and lanolin, used as a tuberculin test, especially in children.

Moro reflex. 1. Embrace reflex. 2. Startle reflex. *See* REFLEX.

Moro's treatment. Pulverized carrots (or other vegetables) are made into a suspension with water in a 5 to 10 per cent concentration, and fed to babies suffering from diarrhoea or dyspepsia, for from one to two days after rehydration has been effected. No other food is given by mouth. Powdered apple, carob, or quince may be used in place of carrots.

moron (mor·on). A person with arrested or incomplete mental development of mild degree (approximate intelligence quotient 50 to 69). [Gk *moros* stupid.]

moronism, moronity, morosis (mor·on·izm, mor·on·it·e, mor·o·sis). The state of being a moron.

Moroxydine (mor·ox·id·een). BP Commission approved name for *N*-(guanidinoformimidoyl)morpholine; an antiviral agent.

morphene (mor·feen). In phonetics the smallest meaningful unit of form.

Morpheridine (mor·fer·id·een). BP Commission approved name for morpholinoethylnorpethidine; a narcotic analgesic.

morphia (mor·fe·ah). Morphine.

morphina (mor·fe·nah). Morphine.

morphine (mor·feen). 3,6-Dihydroxy-4,5-oxyphenanthrene, $C_{17}H_{19}NO_3H_2O$. A white crystalline tertiary base, occurring as the principal alkaloid in opium, to which the latter owes its characteristic pharmacological properties. It is almost insoluble in water, alcohol, or ether, and is laevorotatory. Its most important action is on the central nervous system, producing a mixture of depression and stimulation; there is marked analgesia, and the drug finds its greatest therapeutic use in the alleviation of pain. Even small doses depress the respiratory centre, and in poisoning death is the result of respiratory failure; larger doses are required to depress the motor cortex. It stimulates the spinal cord, for which reason it is never used as an anticonvulsant; it also stimulates the vomiting centre and the nucleus of the 3rd cranial nerve, the latter resulting in constriction of the pupils. Intravenous doses produce a fall in blood pressure that persists for several hours, partly due to the release of histamine from skin and muscle, which contra-indicates the use of the drug in bronchitic asthma. It frequently causes constipation by lessening peristaltic movements and inducing spasm of the intestinal musculature. It is readily absorbed when given by mouth, is destroyed in part by the liver, but is mostly stored in skeletal muscle; excretion takes place in the faeces mainly, though it may appear slightly in the urine. In addition to physiological effects, morphine produces a euphoric state with addiction that needs specialist treatment. **Ethyl morphine.** $C_{19}H_{23}O_3N$, a synthetic derivative of morphine with properties similar to codeine; when dropped into the eye it produces local irritation. **Morphine Hydrochloride BP 1973.** $C_{17}H_{19}O_3NHCl{\cdot}3H_2O$, a compound much more soluble in water than morphine itself. **Methyl morphine.** Codeine, $C_{18}H_{21}O_3N$, a compound occurring naturally to a small extent in opium, but prepared artificially. Its effects are similar to those of morphine, but less potent and not likely to cause addiction. It is commonly used in cough syrup and in analgesic tablets; the analgesia is mild in degree and increase of dose results in stimulation rather than increased narcotic effect. **Morphine Sulphate BP 1973.** $(C_{17}H_{19}O_3)_2{\cdot}H_2SO_4{\cdot}5H_2O$, a white crystalline powder soluble in water. **Morphine Tartrate BPC 1959.** $(C_{17}H_{19}O_3N)_2C_4H_6O_6{\cdot}3H_2O$, a white crystalline powder, much more soluble in water than morphine itself and used in injections. [*Morpheus*, god of sleep.]

morphinia (mor·**fin**·e·ah). Any diseased condition caused by the ingestion of an excessive amount of morphine.

morphinic (mor·**fin**·ik). Relating to morphine.

Morphinii Chloridum. *European Pharmacopoeia* name for Morphine Hydrochloride BP 1973.

morphinism (**mor**·fin·izm). A diseased condition produced by the continued absorption of morphine.

morphinomania, morphiomania (**mor**·fin·o·**ma**'·ne·ah, **mor**·fe·o·**ma**'·ne·ah). 1. An irresistible desire for morphine. 2. Mental derangement produced by the excessive intake of morphine, whether the latter be accomplished by injection or by mouth. [morphine, mania.]

morphiometry (mor·fe·**om**·et·re). The determination of the proportion or amount of morphine in a given preparation or drug. [morphine, Gk *metron* measure.]

morphodifferentiation (**mor**·fo·dif·er·en·she·**a**'·shun). The appearance of structures with a definite characteristic shape or pattern from undifferentiated precursor tissues. [Gk *morphe* form, differentiation.]

morphoea (mor·**fe**·ah). A variety of scleroderma in which there is one area of skin involvement, no visceral involvement and a good prognosis. **Acroteric morphoea.** Morphoea affecting the extremities. **Morphoea alba.** Morphoea without pigmentation. **Morphoea atrophica.** Atrophic morphoea. **Morphoea en coup de sabre, Frontoparietal morphoea.** Frontoparietal localized scleroderma with linear alopecia, sometimes accompanied by hemiatrophy of the face and unilateral defects of the skull, brain, eye or tongue. **Morphoea guttata.** Small, shiny, white maculae having a sclerodermatous structure. **Herpetiform morphoea.** Morphoea with lesions arranged as in zoster. **Morphoea linearis.** Morphoea in the form of a band. **Morphoea nigra.** 1. Brown patches which sometimes follow morphoea. 2. Large brown or black plaques of infiltration in tuberculoid leprosy. **Morphoea tuberosa.** Morphoea with thick raised lesions. [Gk *morphe* form.]

morphogenesis (mor·fo·**jen**·es·is). The production and evolution of form; growth stimulation. [Gk *morphe* shape, *genein* to produce.]

morphogenetic, morphogenic (**mor**·fo·**jen**·**et**'·ik, mor·fo·**jen**·ik). Exciting growth; evolving shape or form. [see prec.]

morphography (mor·**fog**·raf·e). Descriptive morphology. [Gk *morphe* form, *graphein* to write.]

morpholinylethylmorphine (mor·fo·**lin**·il·eth·il·**mor**'·feen). A derivative of morphine resembling codeine in its action; a sedative for coughs.

morphological (mor·fo·**loj**·ik·al). Relating to morphology.

morphology (mor·**fol**·o·je). That branch of biology dealing with the structure and form of living organisms. [Gk *morphe* form, *logos* science.]

morpholysis (mor·**fol**·is·is). The process of disintegration in which shape and form disappear. [Gk *morphe* form, *lysis* a loosing.]

morphometry (mor·**fom**·et·re). Measurement of the different forms of organism. [Gk *morphe* form, *metron* measure.]

morphon (**mor**·fon). A morphological unit. [Gk *morphoein* to give shape to.]

morphophyly (mor·**fof**·il·e). Evolution of the structure of the organs of the body. [Gk *morphe* form, *phyle* tube.]

morphosis (mor·**fo**·sis). The development of an organ or part. [Gk a forming.]

morphotic (mor·**fot**·ik). Relating to morphosis or development; concerned in the formation of the structure of an organism.

morpio, morpion (**mor**·pe·o, **mor**·pe·on) (pl. *morpiones*). An archaic name for the crab louse (*Phthirus pubis*). [Fr. *morpion*.]

Morquio, Luis (b. 1867). Montevideo physician.

Morquio's disease, Brailsford–Morquio disease. Eccentrochondrodysplasia.

Morquio's sign. In poliomyelitis the supine patient will not allow the trunk to be raised to the sitting position unless the knees are flexed.

Brailsford–Morquio syndrome. Collapse of the 1st lumbar vertebra.

Morrant Baker. *See* BAKER, WILLIAM MORRANT.

morrhua (**mor**·oo·ah). The codfish, *Gadus morrhua*. [L]

morrhuate (**mor**·oo·ate). Any salt or ester of morrhuic acid. [L *morrhua* codfish.]

morrhuine (**mor**·oo·een). $C_{19}H_{27}N_3$, a toxic alkaloid formed by decomposition in cod-liver oil, rendering it unfit for medical use. [L *morrhua* codfish.]

Morris, Sir Henry (b. 1844). London surgeon.

Morris' kidney box. The parallelogram produced on the back by two lines parallel with the midline, and 2.5 and 7 cm from it, with two transverse lines crossing them at the levels of the 11th thoracic and 3rd lumbar spinous processes. It demarcates the position of the kidney.

Morris, Robert Tuttle (b. 1857). New York surgeon.

Morris' point. A point of tenderness in chronic appendicitis about 5 cm from the umbilicus on a line from there to the right anterior superior iliac spine.

mors (morz). Death. **Mors putativa.** Apparent death. **Mors subita.** Sudden death. **Mors thymica.** A term, no longer in use, that related sudden death to an enlarged thymus gland.

morsal (**mor**·sal). Taking part in mastication, as the occlusal or masticatory surfaces of premolar and molar teeth. [L *morsus* bite.]

Morson, Albert Clifford (b. 1881). London urologist.

Morson's retractor. A three-bladed self-retaining bladder retractor with illuminated blades.

Morson's suprapubic trocar. A simple suprapubic trocar and cannula. The catheter to the bladder is inserted after withdrawal of the trocar.

morsus (**mor**·sus). A bite. **Morsus stomachi, Morsus ventriculi.** Pain over the stomach. [L]

mortality (mor·**tal**·it·e). 1. Condition or quality of liability to death. 2. Mortality rate. *See* RATE. **Actual mortality.** The number of deaths occurring per thousand insured persons. **Perinatal mortality.** Infant death occurring between the 20th week of pregnancy and the 4th week of postnatal life. Also defined as (1) death of a fetus or infant weighing 1 kg or more between the 28th week of pregnancy and the 28th day of postnatal life; (2) deaths from the 28th week of pregnancy to the 7th day after birth. **Tabular mortality.** The actual mortality as set out in a table of mortality of insured persons. [L *mortalis* mortal.]

mortamin, mortamine (mor·tam·in, mor·tam·een). A term no longer in common use; it was originally proposed for any deleterious factor or activity present in a foodstuff, in supposed contradistinction to a vitamin. [L *mors* death, amine.]

mortar (mor·tar). A vessel, often in the form of an inverted bell, made of iron, porcelain, or glass and used for crushing, grinding, or beating crude drugs by means of a pestle. [L *mortarium.*]

mortification (mor·tif·ik·a′·shun). Gangrene; necrotic death of a part. [L *mors* death, *facere* to make.]

Mortimer's disease or malady. Sarcoidosis, a case of lupus pernio described by Jonathan Hutchinson in 1894. It resembled sarcoma. [*Mrs Mortimer,* the patient after whom the disease was named.]

Morton, Samuel George (b. 1799). American craniologist.

Morton's plane. A plane including the parietal eminences and the external occipital protuberance.

Morton, Thomas George (b. 1835). Philadelphia surgeon.

Morton's disease, foot, neuralgia, or toe. A condition associated with falling of the metatarsal arch and pressure on the digital branches of the lateral plantar nerve.

Morton's metatarsalgia. Pain in the region of the heads of the metatarsal bones due to entrapment of the superficial branch of the lateral plantar nerve between the heads of the fourth and fifth metatarsal bones.

Morton's operation. Division of the plantar nerves for relief of metatarsalgia.

Morton's test. For metatarsalgia: compression of the metatarsal heads causes a sharp pain at the 2nd or 3rd metatarsal head.

mortuary (mor·tew·ar·e). 1. Relating to burial or to death. 2. A building in which the dead are placed to await identification, post-mortem examination, burial, or cremation; morgue. [L *mortuarium* tomb.]

morula (mor·ew·lah). The mass of cells formed by repeated cleavage of the ovum; mulberry mass. [L *morulus* little mulberry.]

morular (mor·ew·lar). Resembling a mulberry. [see prec.]

morulation (mor·ew·la·shun). The process in which the morula is formed.

moruloid (mor·ew·loid). Shaped like a mulberry; used to describe the colonial morphology of certain bacteria. [L *morulus* little mulberry, Gk *eidos* form.]

morulus (mor·ew·lus). The characteristic lesion of yaws. [L little mulberry.]

Morus (mor·us). A genus of trees of the family Moraceae, including the mulberry. **Morus nigra.** The species which yields the edible fruit. [L mulberry tree.]

Morvan, Augustin Marie (b. 1819). Lannilis (Finistère) physician.

Morvan's disease, or syndrome. Syringomyelia with trophic changes; these usually affect the extremities, particularly the fingers, and may give progressive painless ulceration and destruction. Similar changes may occur in leprosy.

mosaic (mo·za·ik). 1. In cytogenetics, an individual whose cells are genetically different although they have arisen from the same zygote. Sometimes used as a synonym of *chimaera.* 2. In embryology, applied to eggs or early cleavage stages in which determination is finished and presumptive areas are thus no longer influenced by their environment. 3. In clinical chromosomal anomalies, an early mitotic division, usually the first, of the zygote, undergoes loss or gain of a sex chromosome, so that two (or more) cell lines arise, one containing one chromosomal pattern and the other, or another, a different pattern. Other cells then arise by mitosis from each of these chromosomal patterns. **Developmental mosaic.** A mosaic due to mutation or mutations which have occurred during the development of the individual, for example in embryogenesis. **Gonadal mosaic.** An individual whose gonads are made up of cells with different genetic constitution. **Proliferative mosaic.** A mosaic due to a mutation occurring during the proliferation of some tissues in a fully developed individual. [Fr. *mosaïque.*]

mosaicism (mo·za·ik·izm). The condition characteristic of mosaics.

Moschcowitz, Alexis Victor (b. 1865). New York surgeon.

Moschcowitz's operation. 1. Femoral herniotomy by the inguinal route. 2. Repair of rectal prolapse by extraperitoneal encircling sutures at the level of the brim of the pelvis.

Moschcowitz, Eli (b. 1879). New York physician.

Moschcowitz's sign, or test. The lower limb is elevated, and a tourniquet applied for five minutes, after which the leg is lowered to the horizontal position and the tourniquet removed. In normal persons a hyperaemic flush extends to the toes in from 2 to 5 seconds, but when the peripheral circulation is impaired, the flush is delayed and patchy.

Mosenthal, Hermann Otto (b. 1878). New York physician.

Mosenthal's test. For renal function: the patient receives a fixed amount of diet given in the form of three meals at 8 a.m., 12 noon, and 5 p.m., with no food or fluid between meals or during the night. Urine is voided at 8 a.m. immediately before the first meal and discarded, and is then collected at two-hourly intervals until 8 p.m., and the night urine collected as a single specimen from 8 p.m. to 8 a.m. of the next day. The volume and specific gravity of all specimens are measured. In normal individuals the specific gravity varies 10 points or more between the lowest and highest; the specific gravity of the night urine is 1.018 or more; the total volume of urine passed during the day is three to four times that of the night urine. In renal failure the specific gravity is relatively low whatever the volume passed, and shows little variation between the highest and lowest values; the volume of the night urine may also equal or exceed that of the total day urine.

Moser, Paul (b. 1864). Vienna paediatrician.

Moser's serum. An antistreptococcal serum formerly used in scarlet fever.

Mosher, Harris Peyton (b. 1867). Harvard laryngologist.

Mosher's cells. Air cells sometimes present beneath the ethmoidal bulla, opening into the middle group of ethmoid cells.

Mosher drain. A copper-mesh drain for brain abscesses (obsolete).

Mosher–Toti operation. For epiphora: a method of dacryocystorrhinostomy: the bone between the lacrimal sac and nose is resected and the nasal mucosa underneath removed and also the middle turbinate. The medial wall of the sac is removed and the lateral wall pushed into the opening in the nose. No sutures are employed.

Mosler, Karl Friedrich (b. 1831). German physician.

Mosler's sign. Sternal tenderness in acute myeloblastic leukaemia.

mosquito (mos·ke·to). A fly of the family Culicidae; narrow-winged, long-legged flies with sucking mouth parts which are adapted for piercing in the females only. The presence of scales on the wing veins and elongate fringing hairs on the wing margins are diagnostic. The eggs are usually laid on the surface of water, often in rafts, and the larvae and pupae are always aquatic, though very small and temporary sources may serve; they obtain respiratory air from the surface, or occasionally from plant tissues. Mosquitoes are the normal transmitters of the causative agents of dengue, filariasis, malaria and yellow fever. The following are the most important genera: *Aëdes, Anopheles, Armigeres, Culex, Psorophora, Taeniorhynchus* and *Theobaldia.* **Anautogenous mosquito.** One whose females need a blood meal before they can lay fertile eggs. **Arygamous mosquito.** One that will not breed in confined spaces. **Autogenous mosquito.** One whose females lay fertile eggs without a blood meal. **House mosquito.** One that habitually enters human habitations; in England, *Culex pipiens* particularly. **Stenogamous mosquito.** One that will breed in confined spaces. [Sp. little fly.]

mosquitocide (mos·ke·to·side). Any agent capable of destroying mosquitos or their larvae. [mosquito, L *caedere* to kill.]

Moss, William Lorenzo (b. 1876). Baltimore haematologist.

Moss' classification. Numerical designation of the ABO blood groups I (AB), II (A), III (B), IV (O). [obsolete term.]

moss (mos). Any plant of the phylum Bryophyta, order Musci. **Bog moss.** Sphagnum moss (see below). **Ceylon moss.** The dried thallus of the alga *Gracilaria lichenoides* Agardh., from the Sri Lanka coasts; it contains much pectin and has been used as a demulcent and nutrient. **Club moss.** The spores of *Lycopodium clavatum* used as a dusting powder and also in making pills. **Iceland moss.** Cetraria. **Irish moss.** Chondrus. **Juniper moss.** Haircap; the plant *Polytrichum juniperinum.* **Muskeag moss, Peat moss.** Sphagnum. **Running moss, Snake moss.** Club moss (see above). **Sphagnum moss.** Sphagnum. [AS *mos.*]

Mosse, Max (b 1873). Berlin physician.

Mosse's syndrome. A variety of erythraemia (polycythaemia vera) associated with an enlarged cirrhotic liver, but hepatomegalia is a common finding (from 40 to 50 per cent) in polycythaemia.

Mosso, Angelo (b. 1846). Italian physiologist.

Mosso's plethysmograph. A plethysmograph composed of a glass tube containing warm water. The hand and forearm are inserted in the tube, and the variations in the level of the water induced by alterations in the volume of the limb are recorded.

Motais, Ernst (b. 1845). Angers ophthalmologist.

Motais' operation. For ptosis: a central tongue is dissected out from the superior rectus muscle of the orbit and this is brought through the levator palpebrae superioris muscle in front of the tarsal plate and stitched to the skin from 3 to 4 mm above the eyelash margin.

Motais-Parinaud operation. *See* PARINAUD'S OPERATION.

mote (mote). A dust particle. [AS *mot.*]

See also: MUELLER (J.).

moth (moth). An insect of the order Lepidoptera which is distinguished from the butterfly by not having clubbed antennae; usually nocturnal. The larvae of many moths have urticating hairs. **Clothes moth.** Any moth whose larvae feed on human clothes, woollens particularly. [AS *moththe.*]

mother (muth·er). 1. The female parent, hence, metaphorically, the source. 2. In simple vegetative reproduction, the parent cell is known as the *mother cell* and the progeny as *daughter cells.* **Expectant mother.** Correctly, a woman in her first pregnancy. A popular term for a pregnant woman whether primipara or multipara. It appears to have been first used by Sir Benjamin Ward Richardson (1828-1896). [AS *modor.*]

motile (mo·tile). Capable of spontaneous movement. [L *motare* to move frequently.]

motility (mo·til·it·e). The quality of being motile; capable of spontaneous movement. [see prec.]

motion (mo·shun). 1. The process of changing position or place. 2. Defaecation; faeces. **Active motion.** Movement produced by active muscular effort of the individual. **Passive motion.** Involuntary movement caused by external force or agency. **Vermicular motion.** Movement like that of a worm. [L *motio* movement.]

motoceptor (mo·to·sep·tor). Any sense receptor in muscle. A term not in general use. [motor, receptor.]

motofacient (mo·to·fa·shent). Producing motion; referring in particular to that phase of muscle activity after tension has risen and when movement is produced. [L *movere* to move, *facere* to make.]

motoneuron (mo·to·newr·one). A motor neuron.

motor (mo·tor). Anything that gives rise to motion. **Club motor.** Plastic motor (see below). **Motor end-plate.** The area around which a motor fibre receives its nerve fibre; the neuromuscular junction. **Motor half-centre.** Term suggested in 1914 by T. G. Brown to describe certain functional units in the nervous system. When one unit is stimulated the other member of the pair is inhibited, and *vice versa;* thus co-ordinate muscular movement is made possible. The term is not synonymous with reflex arc. **Knob motor, Loop motor.** Plastic motor (see below). **Motor march.** *See* JACKSONIAN CONVULSION (under JACKSON, J. H.). **Plastic motor.** A motor formed from muscle during a cineplastic amputation whereby the stump is designed to form a club, knob, loop, or tunnel, by which a prosthesis can be activated. **Tunnel motor.** Plastic motor (see above). [L a mover.]

motorgraphic (mo·tor·graf·ik). Having reference to the graphical recording of movements. [motor, Gk *graphein* to record.]

motorial (mo·tor·e·al). Relating to movement or to a motor centre or nerve.

motoricity (mo·tor·is·it·e). The capability of achieving movement. [L *movere* to move.]

motorium (mo·tor·e·um). The cerebral anatomical centres for motor activity.

motorogerminative (mo·tor·o·jer′·min·a·tiv). Denoting that part of the mesoderm which develops into muscular tissue. [motor, L *germinare* to sprout forth.]

Mott, Sir Frederick Walker (b. 1853). London physician and neuropathologist.

Mott's law of anticipation. Law of anticipation: the theory that when germ plasma is irritated there is often a tendency for it to continue to degenerate for a long period, thus leading to anticipation in the sense that the onset of the disease in affected individuals is earlier in every succeeding generation.

mottling (mot·ling). The appearance of a tissue that is marked with coloured blotches or spots. [etym. dub.]

Mouchet, Albert (b. 1869). French surgeon.

Mouchet's disease. Osteochondritis of the talus.

moulage (moo·lahzh). The reproduction of lesions or anatomical structures by the forming of plaster or wax models or moulds. [Fr. moulding.]

mould (mo·ld). A general term applied to describe the growth of fungi, a large group of plants belonging to the phylum Thallophyta. They are characterized by the production of septate or non-septate filaments or hyphae which branch and interlace to form a mat of growth, the mycelium. Reproduction occurs by sexual or asexual spores of different types. Numerous pathogenic and saprophytic species are recognized, e.g. *Mucor, Penicillium, Aspergillus* and the genera of the dermatophytes which commonly parasitize man and other animals. **Ear mould.** A fungus infection of the ear; otomycosis. **Radiation mould.** An individually-shaped radiation application for curietherapy. [etym. dub.]

moulding (mo·lding). The deformation of the fetal head that occurs in normal labour, caused by the pressure of the maternal tissues. [ME *molde.*]

moult (mo·lt). To cast off, or shed, and renew the hair, feathers, or skin. [ME *mouten.*]

mound (mownd). An elevation. **Anal mound.** Anal hillock; one of a pair of protuberances which develop around the anal proctodeal depression of the early embryo and contribute to the walls of the lower part of the canal. [D *mond* protection.]

mounding (mown·ding). The localized contraction of degenerating muscle in response to a sharp firm blow. [see prec.]

mount (mownt). 1. A specimen for display or examination, usually immersed in a transparent preserving medium between two glass slides. 2. To prepare a specimen in this form for examination. [OFr. *munter.*]

mounting (mown·ting). In histology, the covering of a tissue section with a transparent preserving medium such as canada balsam before applying a glass cover slip. [see prec.]

Moure's operation. 1. An approach to the upper jaw through an incision made at the side of the nose. 2. An operation for the partial resection of the upper jaw.

mouse (mows). General name for any small long-tailed rodent, particularly the house mouse, *Mus musculus.* **Joint mouse.** A cartilaginous foreign body loose in a joint. **Laboratory mouse.** *Mus musculus.* **Multimammate mouse.** Any *Mastomys* species. [AS *mus.*]

mouth [OS] (mowth). 1. Anatomically, the external orifice of the alimentary canal: a horizontal aperture (oral fissure) bounded by the lips and limited laterally by the angles of the mouth. 2. Generally and medically, as above but including the cavity of the mouth. **Angle of the mouth [angulus oris].** The lateral extremity of the oral fissure. **Ceylon mouth.** The characteristic tongue lesions of sprue. **Dry mouth.** Sjögren's syndrome. **Glassblowers' mouth.** Enlargement of the parotid glands in glassblowers. **Primitive mouth.** Blastopore. **Rubber-sore-mouth.** Soreness of the mouth due to wearing an artificial denture the base of which is made of vulcanized rubber. **Tapir mouth.** The mouth in myopathy of the facioscapulohumeral type in which the orbicularis oris muscle is wasted. The lips protrude and droop. **Trench mouth.** Vincent's angina which may affect the gums as well as the tonsils; it occurs in epidemic forms. **White mouth.** Thrush. [AS *muth.*]

mouth-wash (**mowth**·wash). An aqueous solution of a medicament or medicaments intended for gargling. **Mouth-wash of Formaldehyde BPC 1959.** A solution of formaldehyde and peppermint water. **Mouth-wash of Phenol, Alkaline, BPC 1959.** A solution of phenol, potassium hydroxide, and amaranth. **Mouth-wash of Sodium Chloride, Compound, BPC 1959.** A solution of sodium chloride, sodium carbonate, and peppermint water. **Mouth-wash of Zinc Sulphate and Zinc Chloride BPC 1959.** A solution of zinc sulphate and zinc chloride in dilute hydrochloric acid, with compound solution of tartrazine, and made up with chloroform water. [AS *muth, wascan.*]

movement (**moov**·ment). Change of position. **Active movement.** Movement by a subject's own muscular action. **Amoeboid movement.** Cellular movement similar to that of an amoeba, in which protoplasmic pseudopodia are protruded; the cytoplasm then flows into them and they swell gradually. **Angular movement.** Movement round an axis of rotation. **Associated movement.** Involuntary movement of a part of the body evoked by voluntary movement of another part. **Automatic movement.** Active movement not under control of the subject's will. **Brownian movement.** The oscillation of minute particles suspended in a liquid, e.g. the movement of non-motile bacteria in a fluid when examined microscopically. **Cardinal movements.** Rotatory movements of the eyeball from the primary position on the transverse axis, e.g. elevation and depression, and on the vertical axis, e.g. abduction and adduction. **Choreic movements, Choreiform movements.** Irregular jerky movements as seen in chorea. **Ciliary movement.** The undulatory movement of cilia of certain mammalian tissues and genera of micro-organisms. **Circus movement.** 1. A rolling type of gait with circumduction of the legs, seen in certain disorders of the basal ganglia. 2. A movement travelling continuously in a circle around a ring of muscle, said to occur in the auricles of the heart in auricular fibrillation. **Communicated movement.** Passive movement (see below). **Conjugate movements.** Movements of the two eyes together when the fixation axes remain parallel. **Contralateral associated movement.** Involuntary movement of the paralysed side in hemiplegia, resulting from voluntary movement of the corresponding part of the intact side. **Corrective fusion movements.** Reflex movements of either eye to correct any deviation of the fixation axis, and so maintain fusion. **Disjunctive movements.** Movements of the two eyes together when the fixation axes do not remain parallel, e.g. convergence and divergence. **Doll's head eye movements.** Conjugate deviation of the eyes in the opposite direction to passive head movements. It demonstrates the integrity of the pontine gaze centre and its vestibular input. **Dystonic movement.** A slow, writhing type of involuntary muscular movement, as seen in torsion spasm. **Elastic movement.** The return movement of a stretched muscle. **Fetal movements.** Muscular movements performed by the fetus *in utero*, felt by the mother usually from the fifth month onwards. **Forced movement.** 1. Passive movement. 2. Involuntary movements, e.g. somersaults, seen after section of the semicircular canals. **Gliding movement.** A sliding movement within a joint, in which there is no angulation or rotation of the components. **Hand movements.** A term used in assessing visual acuity when the sight is very poor; a degree worse than counting fingers. **Ideomotor movement.** Unconscious movement when attention is withdrawn. **Index movement.** A movement of the cephalic part of the body about the fixed caudal part. **Molecular movement.** Brownian movement (see above). **Nucleopetal movements.** Movements towards the nucleus of a cell, such as that of the male pronucleus towards the egg nucleus after fertilization. **Paradoxical movement.** Movement of the chest wall during respiration in a direction opposite to normal; usually associated with severe injuries of the chest wall. **Passive movement.** Movement imparted to an object by a force outside it. **Perverse movements.** A comprehensive term for the disorders of movement in cerebral diplegia, including ataxia, grimacing and involuntary movements. **Rapid eye movements (REMs).** Eye movements associated with dreaming and occurring during the "paradoxical" phase of sleep. **Reflex movement.** An involuntary movement caused by an external stimulus applied to some part of the afferent nervous sytem. **Rotatory movements.** Movements of the eyeball around three axes, vertical, transverse and anteroposterior. **Saccadic movements.** Jerky, rapid, forward movements of the eyes followed by a pause when reading. **Scissors movement.** 1. Scissor gait. *See* GAIT. 2. A term used in retinoscopy of the eye when the so-called shadow in the pupil moves from opposite sides of the pupil and meets in the centre; it is usually caused by mixed astigmatism. **Spontaneous movement.** A movement caused by a stimulus arising in the organism itself. **Swedish movements.** Systematized, rhythmic, gymnastic, exercises of Swedish origin for correction and treatment of deformities, especially postural, and in that, the use of apparatus. **Synkinetic movement.** An involuntary movement of one or more groups of muscles associated with, and accompanying, voluntary movement in another group. Such movement occurs particularly with maximal muscular efforts. **Translatory movements.** Movements of the eyeball forward, backward, or from side to side, with no rotatory element. **Vermicular movement.** Movement of a squirming character, resembling that of a worm. [L *movere* to move.]

See also: BROWN (R.), FRENKEL (H. S.) MAGNAN, ZSIGMONDY.

moxa (**mox**·ah). A soft combustible material employed to cauterize the skin by burning. [Jap. *moe kusa* burning herb.]

moxibustion (mox·e·**bust**·yun). The use of a moxa as a cautery upon the skin. [moxa, combustion.]

Moxipraquine (mox·e·**pra**·kween). BP Commission approved name for 8-(6-[4-(3-hydroxybutyl)piperazin-1-yl]-hexylamino)-6-methoxyquinoline; a protozoacide.

Moynihan, Berkeley George Andrew (Lord Moynihan) (b. 1865). Leeds surgeon.

Moynihan clamp. A clamp for stomach or intestine, with fenestrated (slit) blades.

Moynihan's N stitch. A seromuscular N-shaped stitch for invagination of the appendix stump after appendicectomy.

Mozer's disease. Adult myelosclerosis.

Much, Hans Christian R. (b. 1880). Hamburg physician.

Much's granules. Granules seen in some tuberculous sputa; these do not stain with the usual acid-fast stains but they do take the Gram stain; they may be degenerating tubercle bacilli.

Much-Holzmann reaction. Psychoreaction; the inhibition of the haemolytic action of cobra venom on the red blood corpuscles in schizophrenia and affective psychosis. It is now discredited.

Mucha, Victor (b. 1877). Vienna dermatologist.

Mucha's disease. Habermann's disease.

muchaematein (mews·**he**·mat·e·in). A combination of haematein and aluminium chloride, used for staining mucin.

See also: MAYER (P.).

mucicarmine (mew·se·**kar**·mine). Carmine with aluminium chloride, used for staining mucin (Mayer).

mucid (**mew**·sid). Mucilaginous, mucous, mouldy; having a slimy quality.

muciferous (mew·**sif**·er·us). Stimulating or secreting mucus. [mucus, L *ferre* to carry.]

mucification (**mew**·sif·ik·**a**′·shun). The mucous-producing changes occurring in the vaginal epithelium of many animals during pro-oestrum. First described by Stockard and Papaninolaou in 1917. [mucus, L *facere* to make.]

muciform (mew·se·form). Having the appearance of mucus. [mucus, form.]

mucigenous (mew·sij·en·us). Yielding mucus. [mucus, Gk *genein* to produce.]

mucigogue (mew·se·gog). A drug that stimulates the secretion of mucus. [mucus, Gk *agogein* to draw forth.]

mucilage (mew·sil·ij). 1. A product of the plant cell activity secreted and laid down in the cell. They are very similar in constitution to gums but are generally sulphuric esters of complex polysaccharides. 2. In pharmacy, a thick aqueous solution of a gum used for suspending insoluble substances in mixtures, or to increase the viscosity of the continuous phase of oil-in-water emulsions. They are also used as water-miscible bases for dermatological preparations, for the production of pills, as adhesives and as lubricating agents for catheters and similar surgical instruments. The most important mucilages are those of acacia, tragacanth, starch, Irish moss, the alginates of calcium and sodium and of ceratoria. Mucilages of certain cellulose derivatives are also employed. [LL *mucilago.*]

mucilaginous (mew·sil·aj·en·us). Resembling mucilage; viscid, slimy, sticky.

mucilago (mew·sil·a·go). A mucilage [LL.].

mucin (mew·sin). The glycoproteins occurring in salivary glands, skin, tendon and cartilage. They are soluble in water and dilute alkali, but are precipitated by dilute acid; the aqueous solution is extremely viscous. They are compounds of protein and the polysaccharides mucoitinsulphuric acid or chondroitinsulphuric acid. Mucin prepared from hog's stomach is used as a treatment for gastric ulcer. [mucus.]

mucinaemia (mew·sin·e·me·ah). The presence of detectable amounts of mucin in the circulating blood. [mucin, Gk *haima* blood.]

mucinase (mew·sin·aze). An enzyme which splits a mucoprotein.

mucinogen (mew·sin·o·jen). The antecedent of mucin; a glycoprotein which, in the presence of water, becomes mucin. [mucin, Gk *genein* to produce.]

mucinoid (mew·sin·oid). Resembling mucin; mucoid. [mucin, Gk *eidos* form.]

mucinosis (mew·sin·o·sis). A dermatosis with mucinous infiltrations, papular or nodular, e.g. myxoedema, either diffuse or pretibial, lichen myxoedematosus, gargoylism, mucinous degeneration in tumours, idiopathic and reticulotic mucinoses, and synovial (mucinous degeneration) cysts. **Focal mucinosis.** A flesh-coloured or white nodule in the skin caused by degeneration of connective tissue with the formation of mucin, as in a myxoid cyst. **Follicular mucinosis.** An inflammation of the skin presenting with scaling and loss of hair. Histologically there is an accumulation of acid polymucosaccharide in the sebaceous glands and in the outer root sheath of the hair follicles. Some forms are benign while others proceed to reticulosis. It may occur in lupus erythematosus and in lichen simplex. **Papular mucinosis.** Lichen myxoedematosus. [mucin, Gk *-osis* condition.]

mucinous (mew·sin·us). Of the character of mucin.

mucinuria (mew·sin·ewr·e·ah). The presence of mucin in the urine.

muciparous (mew·sip·ar·us). Secreting mucus, or giving rise to it. [mucus, L *parere* to produce.]

mucitis (mew·si·tis). Inflammation of a mucous membrane. [mucus, Gk *-itis* inflammation.]

mucivorous (mew·siv·or·us). Living on gum or mucus. [mucus, L *vorare* to devour.]

mucocartilage (mew·ko·kar·til·ij). A cartilage of soft consistency with cells contained in a mucoid matrix.

mucocele (mew·ko·seel). 1. A mucous (gelatinous) polypus. 2. A dilated cavity containing an accumulation of mucoid substance. **Mucocele of the appendix.** Distension of the appendix with mucus following a stricture at its base. **Mucocele of the gall bladder.** Distension of the gall bladder with mucus following obstruction at its neck or in the cystic duct, usually due to a gall-stone. **Suppurating mucocele.** One that contains pus. [mucus, Gk *kele* hernia.]

mucoclasis (mew·kok·las·is). The destruction or peeling-off of the mucous coat of any organ, e.g. by cauterization. [mucus, Gk *klasis* a breaking.]

mucocolitis (mew·ko·kol·i′·tis). Mucous colitis.

mucocolpos (mew·ko·kol·pos). An accumulation of mucoid material in the vagina. [mucus, Gk *kolpos* pocket.]

mucocutaneous (mew·ko·kew·ta′·ne·us). Relating to a mucous membrane and the skin. [mucus, L *cutis* skin.]

mucocyte (mew·ko·site). A mesoglial cell with mucoid degeneration of the cytoplasm. [mucus, Gk *kytos* cell.]

mucodermal (mew·ko·der·mal). Relating to the mucous membrane and skin. [mucus, Gk *derma* skin.]

muco-enteritis (mew·ko·en·ter·i′·tis). Acute catarrhal enteritis. [mucus, enteritis.]

mucofibrous (mew·ko·fi·brus). Consisting of mucous and fibrous elements and thus forming a tissue with the characteristics of both.

mucoflocculent (mew·ko·flok·ew·lent). Composed of mucoid threads. [mucus, L *floccus* tuft of wool.]

mucoid (mew·koid). Of the nature of mucus. [mucus, Gk *eidos* form.]

mucoids (mew·koidz). Glycoproteins occurring in egg white and serum, similar in nature to mucins but less viscous in aqueous solution and not so easily precipitated by acetic acid. [see prec.]

mucoitin sulphate (mew·ko·it·in· sul·fate). A constituent of salivary mucin, composed of units of glucuronic acid and acetylated glucosamine esterified with sulphuric acid.

mucolytic (mew·ko·lit·ik). Dissolving or breaking-down mucus. [mucus, Gk *lysis* a loosing.]

mucomembranous (mew·ko·mem·bran·us). Relating to or consisting of mucous membrane.

mucoperichondrium (mew·ko·per·e·kon′·dre·um). The fused mucous membrane and fibrous tissue lining the cartilages of the larynx. [mucus, Gk *peri, chondros* cartilage.]

mucoperiosteal (mew·ko·per·e·os′·te·al). Composed of mucous membrane and periosteum.

mucoperiosteum (mew·ko·per·e·os′·te·um). Periosteum which has a mucous surface, or mucous and periosteal elements combined to form a composite membrane.

mucopolysaccharide (mew·ko·pol·e·sak′·ar·ide). Polysaccharides containing hexosamine and occurring, either alone or in combination with protein, as mucins in mucoid secretions.

mucopolysaccharidoses (mew·ko·pol·e·sak·ar·id·o′·seez). A group of eponymously-named syndromes caused by inborn errors of carbohydrate metabolism (Hurler, Hunter, Sanfilippo, Morquio, Scheie, Maroteaux-Lamy). [mucopolysaccharide, Gk *-osis* condition.]

mucopolysaccharidosis (mew·ko·pol·e·sak·ar·id·o′·sis). Diseases characterized by mucopolysaccharide storage. They include: *Type I,* Hurler's syndrome or gargoylism; *Type II,* Hunter's syndrome, a sex-linked recessive form of gargoylism without corneal opacity but with deafness; *Type III,* Sanfilippo syndrome, a mild form of gargoylism; *Type IV,* Morquio's disease, eccentropolychondrodysplasia; *Type V,* Scheie's syndrome, gargoylism with normal intelligence; and *Type VI,* Maroteaux-Lamy syndrome of polydystrophic dwarfism. [mucopolysaccharide, Gk *-osis* condition.]

mucoprotein (mew·ko·pro·te·in). Glycoprotein, glucoprotein; one of the classes of conjugated proteins in which protein is combined with a polysaccharide containing hexosamine. [mucus, protein.]

mucopurulent (mew·ko·pewr·ew·lent). Composed of or containing mucus and pus.

mucopus (mew·ko·pus). Mucus that is mixed with pus.

Mucor (mew·kor). A genus of fungi belonging to the class Phycomycetes, characterized by delicate tubular filaments bearing spherical sporangia, often black in colour, and a cotton-wool-like mycelium. Several species have been known to cause infections in man and animals. *Mucor ramosissimus* was isolated from destructive lesions of the face, *Mucor pusillus* from disseminated disease, other species have been isolated from cases of phycomycosis. [L mould.]

mucoriferous (mew·kor·**if**·er·us). Coated with mould. [L *mucor* mould, *ferre* to carry.]

mucormycosis (mew·kor·mi·**ko**'·sis). A fungous disease caused by the genus *Mucor* but now generally grouped under the disease phycomycosis. [L *mucor* mould, Gk *mykes* fungus, *-osis* condition.]

mucosa (mew·**ko**·sah). Mucous membrane; the moist membrane lining the alimentary canal, glandular ducts, the respiratory, urinary and genital passages. It consists of a superficial layer of epithelium supported on a connective-tissue layer which contains nerves, blood vessels and lymphatics, and often plain muscle, glands and lymphoid tissue. The membrane may be smooth, corrugated, or provided with villous projections. **Cobblestone mucosa.** Red and swollen intestinal mucous membrane in Crohn's disease. [L mucus.]

mucosal (mew·**ko**·sal). Relating to a mucous membrane.

mucosanguineous, mucosanguinolent (mew·ko·san·**gwin**'·e·us, mew·ko·san·**gwin**'·o·lent). Composed of mucus mixed with blood. [mucus, L *sanguis* blood.]

mucosedative (mew·ko·**sed**·at·iv). Applied to a demulcent that is soothing to mucous surfaces. [mucus, sedative.]

mucoserous (mew·ko·**seer**·us). Consisting of or containing mucus and serum.

mucosin (mew·**ko**·sin). The type of mucin particular to the viscid forms of mucus, as may be found in the uterine and nasal cavities.

mucosis (mew·**ko**·sis). Mucoviscidosis.

mucositis (mew·ko·**si**·tis). Inflammation of a mucous surface. **Mucositis neuroticans agranulocytica.** Agranulocytosis with ulceration of the mucosa. [mucus, Gk *-itis* inflammation.]

mucosity (mew·**kos**·it·e). The quality of being mucous; sliminess.

mucous (**mew**·kus). Pertaining to or secreting mucus.

mucoviscidosis (mew·ko·vis·id·**o**'·sis). Fibrocystic disease of the pancreas. [mucus, L *viscidus* sticky, Gk *-osis* condition.]

mucro (**mew**·kro). A sharp end. **Mucro cordis.** The apex of the heart. [L]

mucronate (**mew**·kron·ate). Tipped with a short spine. [L *mucronatus* sharply pointed.]

mucroniform (mew·**kron**·e·form). Having the shape and characters of a spine. [L *mucro* sharp point, form.]

muculent (**mew**·kew·lent). Abundantly supplied with mucus.

mucuna (mew·**kew**·nah). The hairs from the tropical plant *Mucuna pruriens*; cowhage, cowitch. Mixed with honey or treacle it has been used as a vermifuge. [Tupi (S. Am.) name.]

mucus [NA] (**mew**·kus). The viscous secretion of mucous membrane upon which it has a protective action. Its chief constituent is mucin. [L]

Mudd, Stuart (b. 1893). Philadelphia bacteriologist.

Flosdorf-Mudd apparatus. An apparatus devised for the preservation of sera, plasma, bacteria and tissues. It consists of a manifold holding ampules of the substance which is frozen by immersion in a carbon-dioxide-acetone mixture and then dehydrated for some hours by a high-vacuum pump with primary and secondary condensers.

Mueller, Arthur (b. 1863). Munich gynaecologist.

Mueller's manoeuvre, or method. To estimate the relative size of the fetal head and maternal pelvis: two fingers are inserted into the vagina and the other hand is placed just above the pubic symphysis. The external hand pushes the head into the pelvis while the fingers of the other hand estimate the relative size of the pelvis and head.

Mueller, Friedrich von (b. 1858). Munich physician.

Mueller's sign. Capillary pulsation of the uvula in aortic incompetence without stenosis.

Mueller, Heinrich (b. 1820). Würzburg anatomist.

Mueller's fibres or cells. The sustentacular fibres of the retina.

Mueller's muscle. The plain muscle component of the palpebral muscles.

Mueller's trigone. A part of the tuber cinereum which is related to the upper surface of the optic chiasma.

Mueller, Hermann Franz (b. 1866). Vienna histologist.

Mueller's Berlin blue. A suspension of Prussian blue, used for the injection of blood vessels.

Mueller's fluid. A fixative and preserving fluid containing potassium dichromate and sodium sulphate.

Mueller, Johannes (b. 1801). Berlin physiologist.

Mueller's dust bodies, blood dust, or blood motes. Haemoconia; small round, or dumb-bell-shaped, refractile particles, showing active brownian movements, and seen in wet blood films, especially under dark-field illumination.

Mueller's canal, or duct, Muellerian duct. The paramesonephric duct. *See* DUCT.

Mueller's capsule. The glomerular capsule.

Mueller's eminence, hillock, or tubercle. A swelling on the dorsal wall of the embryonic urogenital sinus at the openings of the wolffian (mesonephric) and muellerian (paramesonephric) ducts.

Mueller's experiment. The making of a forced inspiratory effort with both nose and mouth closed to demonstrate the reverse of Valsalva's experiment.

Mueller's ganglion. A ganglion found in the prostatic plexus.

Mueller's law. 1. Biogenetic law: ontogenesis repeats phylogenesis. 2. Specific irritability law: normally each type of sensory nerve responds to its specific stimulus only, and gives rise to a specific sensation. Abnormally, it may respond to an unusual stimulus, but the induced sensation is of the same type as before.

Mueller's sarcoma. Sarcoma phyllodes; adenofibroma of the breast.

Bowman-Mueller capsule. Bowman's capsule.

Vieth-Mueller horopter. The circumference of a circle joining the fixation point and the nodal points of each eye.

Mueller, Leopold (b. 1862). Czechoslovakian ophthalmologist.

Mueller's operation. For detachment of the retina: resection of a crescent of sclera 10 mm wide and 20 mm long from the attachment of a rectus muscle to the posterior pole; the subretinal fluid is drained and the sclera sutured. Historical, 1885, and the forerunner of the scleral resection now used for detachment.

Mueller, Maurice E. Swiss surgeon in Berne.

Mueller compression technique. The use of special plates with a compression device to produce rigid fixation of fractures, osteotomies and arthrodeses.

Mueller total hip replacement. A form of arthroplasty.

Mueller, Walther. German physicist.

Geiger-Mueller counting circuit. The electrical circuit which amplifies the electrical impulses from a Geiger-Mueller tube exposed to radiation, so that they may be registered.

Geiger-Mueller counter, or tube. An instrument used for the detection of ionizing radiations. It consists of a tube filled with a gas at reduced pressure, and contains a cylindrical conducting cathode and an axial tungsten wire anode. The passage of an ionizing particle through the gas gives rise to further ionization by collision, a charge being collected on the electrodes, giving an electrical pulse of potential on the anode. The amplitude of the pulse is independent of the number of ions initially formed by the ionizing particle, so that discrimination between different types of particles is not possible.

Geiger-Mueller plateau. In a curve made by plotting the count rate of a Geiger counter against the potential applied between the electrodes, the part of the curve where the slope is minimal.

Geiger-Mueller region. The range of potential applied to an ionization chamber of Geiger counter in which the amplitude of the output pulse is independent of the number of ions formed initially by the passage of the ionizing particle through the counter.

Mueller's steatoma. Lipofibroma.

muellerian (mool·er·e·an). Applied to organs and other bodily structures associated with the name of Johannes Mueller, e.g. muellerian duct.

muellerianoma (mool·er·e·an·o′·mah). A neoplasm derived from the paramesonephric (Mueller's) duct. [muellerian duct, Gk *-oma* tumour.]

Muenchmeyer (b. 1846). Leipzig physician.

Muenchmeyer's disease. Progressive diffuse ossifying myositis.

muguet (moo·ga). Parasitic (mycotic) stomatitis; thrush. [Fr.]

muhinyo (moo·hin·yo). A term used in Uganda for continued fevers of the abortus or melitensis type of undulant fever. [local name.]

Muir, J. C. (fl. 1932).

Muir's tract, Bruce and Muir tract. Part of the septomarginal tract in cervical and thoracic regions of the spinal cord.

Muir, Sir Robert (b. 1864). Edinburgh bacteriologist.

Muir's method. For capsules: the smears are stained with strong carbol fuchsine for one minute, washed in alcohol and water, treated for thirty seconds with a mercuric chloride, tannic acid, potassium alum mordant; decolorized with 95 per cent alcohol and counterstained with methylene blue. The bacterial cells stain red and the capsules blue.

Muirhead, Archibald Laurence (b. 1863). Omaha pharmacologist.

Muirhead's treatment. Treatment of Addison's disease by adrenaline and cortex of the suprarenal gland by mouth (superseded).

mulatto (mew·lat·o). A person of mixed, black and white, parentage. [Sp. mixed-breed.]

mulberry (mul·ber·e). The fresh ripe fruits of *Morus nigra* (family Moraceae). It is cultivated in Britain. The fruit is dark purplish and globular and has a sweet but acidulous taste, containing about 10 per cent of invert sugar with malic and citric acids. It may be used to prepare a drink suitable for febrile patients, whilst the juice is slightly laxative and expectorant. Sugar is added to the juice to prepare syrup of mulberry. [L *morum* mulberry, AS *beri*.]

Mulder, Gerard Johann (b. 1802). Dutch chemist.

Mulder's test. A test for protein, depending on the formation of a yellow coloration (xanthoprotein) on the addition of nitric acid.

Mulder, Johannes (b. 1769). Dutch anatomist.

Mulder's angle. The angle between Camper's horizontal line from the spheno-occipital junction to the root of the nose.

Mules, Philip Henry (b. 1843). Manchester ophthalmologist.

Mules' operation, Mules-Dimitry operation. Evisceration followed by insertion of a glass, gold, or bone ball into the sclerotic, the sclera and conjunctiva being stitched over it.

Mules' scoop. A curette, designed for the scraping out of the entire contents of the eyeball; this leaves only the scleral shell. It is used in evisceration of the eyeball.

muliebria (mew·le·eb·re·ah). The female genitalia. [see foll.]

muliebris (mew·le·eb·ris). Belonging to or characteristic of a woman. [L relating to a woman.]

muliebrity (mew·le·eb·rit·e). 1. The state of being a woman; womanliness; the characteristics peculiar to the female sex as fully assumed at puberty. 2. Unnatural womanliness as shown by certain male types. [see prec.]

mull (mul). 1. To grind or pulverize. 2. A soft surgical muslin. **Plaster mull.** Muslin spread with gutta percha, the most common use for which is in the treatment of skin conditions. **Salve mull.** Muslin spread with ointment. [Hind. *mulmul* soft cotton cloth.]

mullein (mul·ine). The leaves of *Verbascum thapsus* Linn. (family Scrophulariaceae), sometimes used as an adulterant of digitalis. [ME *moleine*.]

multangulum (mult·ang·gew·lum). Any bone with many angles. **Multangulum majus.** The trapezium; the carpal bone on the radial side of the distal row. **Multangulum minus.** The trapezoid bone. [L *multus* many, *angulus* angle.]

multi-articular (mul·te·ar·tik′·ew·lar). Referring to or involving many joints. [L *multus* many, *articulus* joint.]

multicapsular (mul·te·kap·sew·lar). Composed of or containing many capsules. [L *multus* many, capsule.]

multicell (mul·te·sel). An organ or tissue consisting of numerous cells. [see foll.]

multicellular (mul·te·sel·ew·lar). Consisting of many cells. [L *multus* many, cell.]

Multiceps (mul·te·seps). A genus of tapeworms of which the dog is the most important determinative host. **Multiceps multiceps.** A species of which the dog and the wolf are the determinative hosts. The larval stage is usually passed in herbivora, and most commonly in the sheep in which it may cause symptoms associated with the cerebral localization of the larvae. It has been demonstrated in man several times. The larval cyst is called *Coenurus cerebralis*. [L *multus* many, *caput* head.]

multicostate (mul·te·kos·tate). Having numerous ribs. [L *multus* many, *costa* rib.]

multicuspid, multicuspidate (mul·te·kus·pid, mul·te·kus·pid·ate). Having many cusps, as in human molar teeth. [L *multus* many, cusp.]

multidentate (mul·te·den·tate). Provided with many teeth or tooth-like processes. [L *multus* many, *dens* tooth.]

multidigitate (mul·te·dij·it·ate). Having numerous fingers. [L *multus* many, digit.]

multifamilial (mul·te·fam·il′·e·al). Affecting the offspring in several generations in succession. [L *multus* many, family.]

multifetation (mul·te·fe·ta′·shun). Any gestation in which three or more fetuses are present. [L *multus* many, fetation.]

multifid (mul·te·fid). Cleft into numerous segments or parts. [L *multifidus* cloven into many parts.]

multifidus muscle [musculus multifidus (NA)] (mul·tif·id·us musl). A muscle deep to the sacrospinalis muscle whose fibres run obliquely upwards and inwards mainly from transverse to spinous processes. The deeper fibres are more oblique than the superficial.

multiflagellate (mul·te·flaj·el·ate). Having numerous flagella. [L *multus* many, *flagellum* whip.]

multiform (mul·te·form). Occurring in many forms; polymorphous. [L *multus* many, form.]

multiganglionate (mul·te·gang·gle·on·ate). Having or composed of numerous ganglia. [L *multus* many, ganglion.]

multiganglionic (mul·te·gang·gle·on′·ik). Having, referring to, or affecting numerous ganglia. [see prec.]

multigesta (mul·te·jes·tah). Multigravida. [L *multus* many, gestation.]

multiglandular (mul·te·glan·dew·lar). Referring to or derived from many glands. [L *multus* many, gland.]

multigravida (mul·te·grav·id·ah). A pregnant woman who has had two or more pregnancies. [L *multus* many, *gravidare* to impregnate.]

multi-infection (mul·te·in·fek′·shun). A mixed infection with several varieties of micro-organism; simultaneous activities of two or more such. [L *multus* many, infection.]

multikaryon (mul·te·kar·e·on). A multinucleated cell. [L *multus* many, Gk *karyon* nut.]

multilobar, multilobate, multilobed (mul·te·lo·bar, mul·te·lo·bate, mul·te·lo·bd). Having or composed of many lobes. [L *multus* many, lobe.]

multilobular (mul·te·lob·ew·lar). Provided with many lobules. [L *multus* many, lobule.]

multilocular (mul·te·lok·ew·lar). Having many loculi or compartments. [L *multus* many, *loculus* little place.]

multimammae (mul·te·mam·e). The possession of supernumerary mammary glands. [L *multus* many, *mamma* breast.]

multinodular, multinodulate (mul·te·nod·ew·lar, mul·te·nod·ew·late). Having or composed of many nodules. [L *multus* many, nodule.]

multinuclear, multinucleate, multinucleated (mul·te·new·kle·ar, mul·te·new·kle·ate, mul·te·new·kle·a·ted). Having several nuclei. [L *multus* many, nucleus.]

multipara (mul·**tip**·ar·ah). Generally, a woman who has borne two or more children; more particularly a woman who is in labour for the second time and subsequently. [see foll.]

multiparity (mul·te·**par**·it·e). 1. The state of being the mother of more than one child. 2. Birth of more than one offspring at a confinement. [L *multus* many, *parere* to give birth.]

multiparous (mul·**tip**·ar·us). 1. Having borne two or more children. 2. Having more than one child at confinement. [see prec.]

multiple (**mul**·tipl). Occurring in or affecting several parts of the body simultaneously; manifold; repeated several times. [L *multus* many, *plica* fold.]

multiplier (**mul**·te·pli·er). An instrument or apparatus used for multiplying the strength of a force. **Electron multiplier.** A vacuum tube in which electrons produced by impact of a positive ion, gamma ray, or electron with the first electrode, are accelerated down the tube striking intermediate electrodes. Multiplication of the electrons occurs by secondary emission at these electrodes, producing a very large overall multiplication of the initial number of electrons produced. **Photoelectric multiplier.** A vacuum tube containing a light-sensitive photocathode: the electron stream emitted from this under the action of light is amplified by secondary emission through striking intermediate electrodes in the tube. This electron-multiplication effect gives a high-voltage amplification without the use of an external electronic circuit. [L *multiplicare* to multiply.]

multipolar (mul·te·**po**·lar). Having more than two poles or processes, referring particularly to nerve cells. [L *multus* many, pole.]

multirooted (mul·te·**root**·ed). Having many roots, a term sometimes applied to the molar teeth. [L *multus* many, root.]

multirotation (mul·te·ro·**ta'**·shun). Mutarotation. [L *multus* many, rotation.]

multisensitivity (mul·te·sen·sit·**iv'**·it·e). Sensitivity to two or more antigens. [L *multus* many, sensitivity.]

multisynaptic (mul·te·sin·**ap'**·tik). Denoting a nervous pathway involving more than one synapse or neurone. [L *multus* many, *synaptein* to join.]

multiterminal (mul·te·**ter**·min·al). Provided with several terminals so that more than two electrodes can be employed at any one time. [L *multus* many, terminal.]

multituberculate (mul·te·tew·**ber'**·kew·late). Having a number of tubercles. [L *multus* many, tubercle.]

multivalent (mul·te·**va**·lent). 1. An element or radical that has a valency of more than two. 2. A body formed by the association of more than two chromosomes held together by chiasmata at the first division of meiosis. According to the number of chromosomes involved (3, 4, 5, 6 and so on) it is possible to distinguish *trivalent, quadrivalent, pentavalent, hexavalent,* etc. **Chain multivalent.** A multivalent forming an open configuration rather than a ring. **Ring multivalent.** A multivalent whose chromosomes are held by chiasmata to form a ring configuration. [L *multus* many, *valere* to be worth.]

muma (**moo**·mah). Myositis purulenta tropica. [Samoan name.]

Mummery, John Howard (b. 1847). London dentist.

fibres of Mummery. Fibres found in developing dentine; probably the same as Korff's fibres.

mummification (mum·if·ik·**a'**·shun). 1. Dry gangrene. 2. Concerning dead *fetus in utero*, a process of desiccation and withering. 3. Desiccation of a corpse in a dry atmosphere. [Pers. *mum* wax, L *facere* to make.]

mummying (**mum**·e·ing). A method of physical restraint in which the whole body is wrapped in a sheet so that movements of arms and legs are impossible, resembling the swathing of a mummy. [Pers. *mum* wax.]

mumps (mumps). Epidemic parotitis; an acute infectious disease caused by a virus, and spread by direct contact and droplet spray; children of school age and young adults are chiefly attacked. The incubation period is most commonly from 17 to 18 days, the extreme limits being 3 and 30 days. Painful enlargement of one or other parotid salivary gland or both is characteristic, but other salivary glands may be affected; moderate fever for from 3 to 5 days is usual. Complications include orchitis in post-pubertal males, pancreatitis and meningitis. The case mortality from mumps is very low. Treatment of an ordinary attack is symptomatic, but the use of convalescent serum and gamma globulin is under investigation for older boys who may be liable to orchitis. **Iodine mumps.** A swelling of the parotid and lacrimal glands due to iodine therapy. **Lacrimal mumps.** Mumps in which the lacrimal glands are solely or mainly involved. **Metastatic mumps.** Mumps of the testicle (orchitis), the pancreas (pancreatitis), the mammary gland (mastitis), or other organs; involvement may precede, follow, or even occur in the absence of parotitis. **Non-parotid mumps.** Mumps in which glands other than the parotid are solely involved. **Single mumps.** Swelling of one salivary gland only; unilateral parotitis. **Sublingual mumps.** Mumps in which the sublingual glands are solely or mainly involved; it is very rare for this gland only to be involved. **Submaxillary mumps.** Mumps in which the submaxillary glands are solely or mainly involved: this is one of the most common of the non-parotid types. [dial. E for lumps.]

Munchausen, Baron von. 16th century traveller and proverbial liar.

Munchausen's syndrome. A syndrome first described and named by Richard Asher in 1951. Patients with this syndrome travel from one hospital to another telling dramatic but untruthful stories, deliberately simulating acute illness, and submitting to countless unnecessary operations and investigations. A few days after admission they discharge themselves and resume their travels. Common varieties are: laparotomophilia migrans, simulating acute abdominal catastrophes; neurologica diabolica, specializing in fits, faints, and other disturbances of consciousness; and haemorrhagica histrionica, contriving spurious haematemesis or other external haemorrhage.

munity (**mew**·nit·e). The condition of being easily infected. [(incorrect) back-formation from *immunity.*]

Munk, Fritz (b. 1879). Berlin physician.

Munk's disease. Lipoid nephrosis. *See* NEPHROSIS.

Munro Kerr, John Martin (b. 1868). Glasgow gynaecologist and obstetrician.

Munro Kerr manoeuvre. A manoeuvre used to estimate the relative size of the fetal head and maternal pelvis. The procedure is the same as Mueller's manoeuvre except that the thumb of the vaginal hand is passed upwards externally towards the brim of the pelvis and the degree of overlapping can be estimated.

Munzer, Egmont (b. 1865). Prague physician.

Munzer's bundle, or tract. A bundle of fibres connecting the medial geniculate body with the reticular formation of the pons.

Muraena (mew·**re**·nah). A genus of poisonous fish. [Gk *myraina* sea eel.]

mural (**mewr**·al). Referring to or occurring in the wall of a cavity. [L *murus* wall.]

Murat, Louis (b. 1874). Paris physician.

Murat's sign, or symptom. A vibratory sensation of discomfort in one side of the chest which may occur in pulmonary tuberculosis on that side.

Murchison, Charles (b. 1830). London physician.

Murchison-Sanderson syndrome. Pel-Ebstein disease.

murder (**mer**·der). The act of unlawful killing of a human being with malice aforethought. Excusable or reduced inculpability in certain states of abnormality of mind. *See* MCNAGHTEN'S RULES and Diminished RESPONSIBILITY. [AS *mordhor.*]

Muret, Paul Louis (b. 1878). Paris surgeon.

Quénu-Muret sign. If blood is obtained from a subcutaneous puncture distal to an aneurysm after the proximal artery has been compressed, a collateral circulation can be assumed to be present.

murexide (mewr·ex·ide). Ammonium purpurate, $C_8H_4O_6N_5NH_4$. A purple-red purine derivative formed when uric acid and certain other purine compounds, e.g. caffeine, are oxidized by evaporation with nitric acid and the product is treated with ammonia. This reaction is employed as a qualitative test for these substances. [L *murex* the purple fish.]

muriate (mewr·e·ate). A chloride. [obsolete term.] [L *muria* brine.]

muriatic (mewr·e·at·ik). Relating to chlorine or hydrochloric acid. [see prec.]

Muridae (mewr·id·e). A family of the mammalian order Rodentia; mice, rats, squirrels, etc. The genera *Mus* and *Rattus*, and several genera of field rodents associated with plague, are of medical importance. [L *mus* mouse, Gk *eidos* form.]

murine (mewr·ine). Pertaining to rodents, particularly of the family Muridae. [L *mus* mouse.]

murmekiasmosis amphilaphes (mer·mek·e·as·mo'·sis am·fil·af·eez). Cutaneous warts of extremely rapid growth spreading to the face and neck; considered by some to be a tropical infection. [Gk *myrmekiasmos* warts, *amphilaphes* spreading.]

murmur (mer·mer). A continuous sound; a bruit. **Anaemic murmur.** Haemic murmur (see below). **Aortic murmur.** A murmur produced as the result of an abnormality of the left ventricular outflow tract. **Aortic diastolic murmur.** A diastolic murmur produced by regurgitation through the aortic valve; it is usually high-pitched, blowing in quality and decrescendo in form. It is audible at the upper right sternal edge and is well transmitted down the left sternal edge. **Aortic systolic murmur.** A systolic murmur produced as the result of any form of aortic stenosis or deformity of the valve. It is often harsh, has a crescendo-decrescendo form, and is audible at the upper right sternal edge with radiation up to the neck. **Apical murmur.** A murmur at the apex of the heart or lung. **Arterial murmur.** A murmur produced by blood rushing through an artery. **Blood murmur.** Haemic murmur (see below). **Brain murmur.** A murmur produced by a vascular abnormality in the brain. **Bronchial murmur.** A blowing sound produced by air rushing in and out of the bronchial tubes; breath sound. **Cardiac murmur.** A sound produced within the heart which continues through at least part of the systole or of diastole. Murmurs are produced by turbulent blood flow, and this in turn is usually the consequence of structural abnormality. **Cardiopulmonary murmur, Cardiorespiratory murmur.** The sound heard over the heart during breathing and during the heart beat, due to vibration set up by the heart striking lung tissue with every beat. It is one of the most common heart murmurs heard in childhood, particularly in thin excitable children during expiration. **Continuous murmur.** A murmur which continues from systole into diastole; such murmurs are vascular rather than cardiac in origin and their commonest cause is persistence of the ductus arteriosus. **Crescendo murmur.** A murmur steadily increasing in intensity up to a sudden termination. **Diastolic murmur.** A murmur occurring during the phase of ventricular diastole. When arising from the aortic or pulmonary valves it indicates valve incompetence, but if from the mitral or tricuspid valves, stenosis. **Displacement murmur.** A systolic murmur heard over the heart in pleurisy. **Ejection murmur.** A murmur produced by the ejection of blood from either ventricle. It is usually harsh, best heard over the base of the heart and crescendo-decrescendo in form, starting very shortly after the first heart sound (immediately after an ejection sound if one is present); the extent to which it continues up to the appropriate component of the second heart sound is related to the severity of the obstruction to the ventricular outflow from which it arises. **Endocardial murmur.** A murmur arising from within the heart. **Exocardial murmur.** A murmur arising from outside the cardiac chambers but within the mediastinum, e.g. pericardial murmur. **Expiratory murmur.** A sound heard over the lung on expiration. **Friction murmur.** The sound produced by two serous membranes rubbing together; it occurs in pericarditis, pleurisy, perisplenitis, etc.; Bright's murmur. **Full systolic murmur.** Pansystolic murmur (see below). **Functional murmur.** A murmur produced as a result of alteration of function without structural disease or damage. It is usually applied to cardiac murmurs which occur in the absence of organic heart disease, e.g. haemic murmur. **Haemic murmur.** A systolic cardiac murmur heard in patients with severe anaemia, in the absence of organic heart disease other than that attributable to long-standing anaemia. **Heart murmur.** Cardiac murmur (see above). **Holosystolic murmur.** Pansystolic murmur (see below). **Humming-top murmur.** A continuous humming sound throughout the cardiac cycle, present in normal persons and caused by the movement of blood in cervical veins. It is maximal at the base of the neck on the right side, and may be confused with the machinery murmur of a persistent ductus arteriosus. **Inorganic murmur.** A murmur arising in the absence of organic disease; usually applied to innocent murmurs in persons without disorder of cardiac structure or function. **Inspiratory murmur.** A sound heard over the lung in inspiration. **Late systolic murmur.** A murmur confined to the latter part of systole, often preceded by a systolic click and usually due to mitral regurgitation resulting from prolapse of a valve cusp as systole proceeds. **Machinery murmur.** A continuous murmur throughout systole and diastole, with systolic accentuation, heard in the 1st and 2nd intercostal spaces to the left of the sternum in patients with a persistent ductus arteriosus. It may be confused with venous hum (humming-top murmur), and is also produced by arterior-venous aneurysm or congenital aortopulmonary septal defect. **Mid-diastolic murmur.** One occurring in the middle phase of ventricular diastole. **Millwheel murmur.** A murmur sometimes heard on auscultation over the chest in the presence of air embolism. **Mitral murmur.** A murmur produced as a result of an abnormality of the mitral valve. **Mitral diastolic murmur.** A diastolic murmur produced by blood flow through the mitral valve, most commonly as a consequence of stenosis of the valve but sometimes because of abnormality of movement of the valve cusps, as may occur in aortic regurgitation (the Austin Flint murmur). It is low-pitched and rumbling in quality, starting shortly after the second sound (immediately after the opening snap if one is present); at first decrescendo in form, there is often a short presystolic crescendo immediately before the first heart sound. It is best heard at, or a little outside, the apex beat and is usually well localized. **Mitral systolic murmur.** A systolic murmur produced by regurgitation through the mitral valve. It is pansystolic in form and best heard at the apex with radiation best towards the left axilla. **Muscle murmur.** A sound produced by a muscle contracting. **Organic murmur.** A murmur produced by organic disease; usually applied to murmurs arising from cardiac valvular disease or pulmonary disease. **Pansystolic murmur.** A systolic murmur which occurs throughout the whole of systole; it usually also varies little in intensity or quality throughout its duration. **Pericardial murmur.** A harsh, grating, creaking sound during cardiac systole and diastole, due to the two layers of pericardium rubbing together. It is heard in pericarditis. **Placental murmur.** A murmur (or bruit) heard over the abdomen, due to placental blood circulating. **Pleuropericardial murmur.** A sound heard during respiration and connected with the cardiac cycle, due to a layer of pleura and pericardium striking one another. **Precardial murmur.** A murmur heard over the anterior surface of the heart, but not necessarily arising from the heart or pericardium. **Prediastolic murmur.** Systolic murmur (see below). **Presystolic murmur.** A cardiac murmur heard during the last phase of ventricular diastole leading up to the first heart sound. It occurs in mitral stenosis. **Protodiastolic murmur.** A murmur occurring in the earliest phase of ventricular diastole, as in aortic and pulmonary incompetence. **Pulmonary murmur, Pulmonic murmur.** A murmur heard over the lungs, which may be due to air moving in the bronchial tubes and alveoli, to blood moving in abnormal vascular structures (e.g. arteriovenous aneurysm), or to a sound transmitted from the heart of great vessels, e.g. transmitted murmur (see below). The term is applied to murmurs produced as a result of abnormality of the right ventricular outflow track. **Pulmonary diastolic murmur.** A diastolic murmur produced by regurgitation through the pulmonary valve. When this is secondary to pulmonary hypertension it is high-pitched and blowing in quality, mimicking an aortic diastolic murmur; this is the *Graham Steell murmur.* **Pulmonary systolic murmur.** A systolic murmur produced as the result of any form of pulmonary stenosis, deformity of the valve, or increased blood flow through a normal outflow tract, e.g. the *haemic murmur* (see above). **Regurgitant murmur.** A cardiac murmur resulting from incompetence of a valve, caused by blood regurgitating through incompletely closed valve cusps from the distal to the proximal chamber. Incompetence of the aortic and pulmonary valves causes a diastolic murmur; of the mitral and tricuspid valves, a systolic murmur. The term has also been used to indicate the type of systolic murmur, the pansystolic murmur (see above) which occurs, for example, with mitral regurgitation as distinct from the ejection type of murmur. **Respiratory murmur.** The sound produced by air moving in the bronchial tubes and alveoli of the lungs during respiration. **Short systolic murmur.** A murmur starting with the first heart sound and terminating before the second. **Stenosal murmur.** A cardiac murmur produced by obstruction of the flow of blood through a valve orifice and due to organic narrowing of the valve ring. Mitral and tricuspid stenosis both produce a diastolic murmur; aortic and pulmonary stenosis, a systolic murmur. **Systolic murmur.** A murmur occurring during cardiac systole. **To-and-fro murmur.** A murmur occurring during cardiac systole and diastole, with an interval between the two elements. It may occur as the result of valvular disease (aortic stenosis with incompetence), or in pericarditis. **Transmitted murmur.** A murmur which, arising from one organ, is transmitted along blood vessels or other structures to areas some distance from its source. **Tricuspid murmur.** A murmur produced as the result of an abnormality of the tricuspid valve. **Tricuspid diastolic murmur.** A diastolic murmur produced by blood flow through the tricuspid valve as a consequence of stenosis of the valve. It is best heard at the left lower sternal border but is otherwise similar to a *mitral diastolic murmur* (see above). **Tricuspid systolic murmur.** A systolic murmur produced by regurgitation through the tricuspid valve; it closely resembles a *mitral systolic murmur* (see above) with which it is easily confused. **Vascular murmur.** A sound produced by the passage of blood through a blood vessel. **Venous murmur.** Venous hum. **Vesicular murmur.** A soft rustling sound caused by air entering or leaving the alveoli of normal lungs. **Water-wheel murmur.** A splashing sound synchronous with cardiac systole. **Whistling murmur.** A high-pitched murmur. [L humming.]

See also: BRIGHT, DUROZIEZ, FISCHER (L.), FLINT, GIBSON, PARROT, ROGER (H. L.), SMITH (E.), STEELL, TRAUBE (L.).

Murphy, John Benjamin (b. 1857). Chicago surgeon.

Murphy's button. Two button-like hollow metal bulbs each with a central collar and stem so that the two parts may be clipped together. Formerly used in intestinal anastomosis, one open end of intestine being applied to each half of the button, the halves being clipped together, the intestine healing and the button subsequently being passed.

Murphy drip, or method. A continuous rectal drip of saline given in Fowler's position in cases of peritonitis.

Murphy's law. Jaundice due to obstruction by a gall-stone is preceded by colic, but when caused by a neoplasm or catarrh of the bile ducts there is no colic.

Murphy's kidney punch, or test. With the patient on a stool and bending forwards, the examiner's thumb is applied under the 12th rib in the renal angle. Deep-seated tenderness may be elicited in affections of the kidney or perinephric tissue.

Murphy's sign. When in cholecystitis the palpating fingers are pressed in below the rib margin in the region of the gall bladder, a deep inspiration, by causing descent of the diaphragm, will induce pain as the tender gall bladder is forced against the examiner's hand.

Murphy treatment. 1. Treatment of a patient with peritonitis in the sitting-up (Fowler) position to encourage the collection of pus in the pelvis. 2. Treatment of pulmonary tuberculosis by artificial pneumothorax, using nitrogen instead of air.

Fowler-Murphy treatment. Murphy treatment, 1st def. (see prec.).

Murphy, William Parry (b. 1892). Boston physician.

Minot-Murphy treatment. The first effective treatment introduced for pernicious anaemia, being the oral administration of raw or lightly cooked liver or of crude extracts of fresh calf liver.

Murray, John Milne (b. 1896). American psychiatrist.

Murray's test, Murray-Harvard test. Thematic apperception test. *See* TEST.

Murray, Robert Milne (b. 1855). Edinburgh obstetrician.

Milne Murray forceps. Axis-traction obstetric forceps: the axis-traction handle is attached to rods which fit on to the proximal angles of the winders in the cephalic ends of the blades, and the rods lie underneath the forceps proper.

Murri, Augusto (b. 1841). Bologna physician.

Murri's disease. Paroxysmal haemoglobinuria.

Mus (mus). A genus of small rodents, house mice. The term is used by some when *Rattus* is meant. **Mus alexandrinus.** *Rattus rattus alexandrinus.* **Mus bactrianus.** A house mouse of temperate Asia; fancy strains are known. **Mus decumanus.** *Rattus norvegicus.* **Mus frugivorus.** *Rattus rattus frug vorus.* **Mus musculus.** The house mouse of the Old World, now cosmopolitan; laboratory, white and other strains are of this species. **Mus norvegicus.** *Rattus norvegicus.* **Mus rattus.** *Rattus rattus.* [L mouse.]

Musca (**mus**·kah). A genus of flies of the family Muscidae, house flies. The mouth parts are usually adapted for sucking only, and the flies act as passive carriers of bacteria, etc. Some species can rasp the skin surface and feed on blood. **Musca autumnalis.** A species which does not normally enter houses but is an abundant European garden fly. Its larvae have occurred in intestinal myiasis. **Musca domestica.** The common house fly. It is world wide, breeding in garbage, and the larvae have occurred in cases of intestinal myiasis. **Musca nebula, Musca sorbens, Musca vicina.** Species that may act as mechanical vectors in the Orient. [L fly.]

muscacide (**mus**·kah·side). 1. Having the power to destroy flies. 2. Any agent that kills flies. [L *musca* fly, *caedere* to kill.]

muscae volitantes (**mus**·ke vol·e·**tan**·teez). The appearance in the field of vision of variously shaped figures (e.g. dots, beads, threads and the like) caused by defect of the vitreous humour or small bodies present in it. [L flying flies.]

muscarine (**mus**·kar·een). An alkaloid present in *Amanita muscaria*, a poisonous mushroom. Its pharmacological actions resemble the effects of postganglionic stimulation of parasympathetic nerves, and thus are similar to many of the actions of acetylcholine; it is not used in therapeutics. It is regarded as a choline derivative of formula $C_2H_5CHOHCH[N(CH_3)_3OH]CHO$. **Artificial muscarine, Synthetic muscarine.** Choline muscarine, a choline nitrous ester prepared by the action of nitric acid on choline. [L *musca* fly.]

muscarinism (**mus**·kar·in·izm). Muscarine poisoning; mushroom poisoning.

muscicide (**mus**·kis·ide). Muscacide.

Muscidae (**mus**·id·e). A large family of flies of the order Diptera, including the medically important genera, *Fannia, Glossina, Musca* and *Muscina.* [L *musca* fly.]

Muscina (mus·i·nah). A genus of flies of the family Muscidae.

Muscina pascuorum. A species that may act as a mechanical vector of disease. **Muscina stabulans.** A small, cosmopolitan fly whose larvae, common in garbage, have occurred in intestinal myiasis. [see prec.]

muscle [musculus (NA)] (musl). 1. Muscular tissue. 2. The organs formed of collections of muscular tissue and which by their contraction produce movement. Muscular tissue is the contractile tissue of the body and occurs in three varieties, striped or voluntary, unstriped or involuntary, and cardiac. The *striped* variety consists of long, thin, multinucleated threads which are made up of bundles of contractile fibrils, the myofibrils, showing periodic alternate dark and light striations embedded in a semifluid sarcoplasm and enclosed in a hyaline sheath, the sarcolemma. This variety is found in skeletal muscles. In the lower mammals two distinct types, the *red* and *white*, occur independently. In man they are intermingled in the one organ. The red is distinguished from the white by its colour, poor striations, the occurrence of many centrally placed nuclei, the majority of which are, however, as in the white, placed under the sarcolemma, and by its slow contraction. The difference in colour is due to the high content of the pigment myohaemoglobin. Striped or voluntary muscle receives its motor supply from the cerebrospinal nervous system. *Unstriped muscle* is mainly concerned with movements and contractions of blood vessels, alimentary canal, respiratory, urogenital systems and of glands. It often occurs in sheets, consisting of long spindle-shaped cells containing myofibrils and sarcoplasm, but devoid of cross striations. The nuclei are central. *Cardiac muscle* is found only in the heart and at the roots of the great vessels. It is cross striated and its cells are connected together in a syncytium. It displays some of the characteristics of both striped and unstriped muscle. *Unstriped* and *cardiac muscles* are supplied by the autonomic nervous system. (For specific muscles, see under qualifying adjective.) **Accessory muscle.** An additional muscle not normally present; a reinforcing muscle in a movement. **Antigravity muscle.** One of the muscles responsible for maintaining the upright posture of man or standing posture of lower animals. **Appendicular muscle.** One of the skeletal limb muscles. **Articular muscle [musculus articularis (NA)].** One attached wholly or partly into the capsule or synovial membrane of a joint. **Axial muscle.** The muscle of the trunk. **Belly of a muscle [venter (NA)].** The bulging central portion of a muscle. **Bicipital muscle.** A muscle with two heads of origin. **Bipennate muscle [musculus bipennatus (NA)].** One in which the muscle fibres converge in barb-like fashion off opposite sides of the tendon of insertion. **Cardiac muscle.** *See* MAIN DEF. (above). **Circumpennate muscle.** One in which the muscle fibres converge on all sides of the tendon of insertion. **Cutaneous muscle [musculus cutaneus (NA)].** One attached at one or both ends to the skin and responsible for moving this organ. **Dermal muscle.** The muscle of the dermis of the skin; one of the muscles inserted into and moving the hair follicle. **Eustachian muscle.** The muscle of the pharyngotympanic tube. **Extrinsic muscle.** One arising outside the part or segment, particularly of the limb. **Femoral muscle.** One of the muscles of the thigh. **Fixation muscle.** One used to fix rather than to move a part and acting as an adjustable ligament or to prevent some undesired movement during the action of another muscle. **Fusiform muscle [musculus fusiformis (NA)].** One with a spindle-shaped belly. **Hamstring muscles.** The group of muscles of the lower limb comprising the biceps femoris, the semitendinosus and the semimembranosus muscles. **Head of a muscle [caput (NA)].** A term applied to each portion of the origin of a muscle with two or more discrete origins. **Hypaxial muscles.** Muscles of the trunk supplied by the anterior primary branches of the spinal nerves and lying in front of the vertebral column. **Infrahyoid muscle.** One of the group of muscles including the sternohyoid, thyrohyoid, sternothyroid, and omohyoid. **Inspiratory muscle.** The muscle used in inspiration. **Intra-aural muscle, Intra-auricular muscle.** 1. One of the intrinsic muscles of the auricle. 2. One of the muscles of the middle ear. **Intrinsic muscle.** One lying wholly within the part or segment, particularly of a limb to be moved. **Involuntary muscle.** Unstriped muscle (*see* MAIN DEF. above). **Iridic muscle.** One of the muscles of the iris, either a dilator or sphincter of the pupil. **Joint muscle.** Articular muscle (see above). **Mimetic muscle.** A muscle used in mimicry; in man one of the facial muscles. **Multicipital muscle.** One with several heads of origin. **Multipennate muscle.** One with a branched tendon of origin or insertion from which the muscle fibres radiate like the barbs of a feather. **Non-striated muscle.** Unstriped muscle (*see* MAIN DEF. above). **Orbicular muscle [musculus orbicularis (NA)].** A muscle with circulatory disposed fibres. **Organic muscle.** Unstriped muscle (*see* MAIN DEF. above). **Pectinate muscle.** One of the muscular regions in the auricles of the heart. **Pennate muscle.** One where the muscle fibres converge on one or more sides of the tendon of origin or insertion. **Postaural muscle.** One of the extrinsic auricular muscles placed behind the auricle. **Postaxial muscle.** One placed behind the central axis of a limb. **Pre-axial muscle.** A muscle placed in front of the central axis of a limb. **Red muscle.** *See* MAIN DEF. (above). **Ribbon muscle.** A flat parallel-fibred muscle. **Riders' muscle.** One of the adductor muscles of the thigh, usually the adductor longus. **Skeletal muscles [musculi skeleti (NA)].** Muscles attached to bones. **Smooth muscle.** Unstriped muscle (*see* MAIN DEF. above). **Somatic muscle.** Striped muscle (*see* MAIN DEF. above). **Sphincter muscle [musculus sphincter (NA)].** Muscle fibres arranged as a ring around a tube or orifice. **Striated muscle.** Striped muscle (*see* MAIN DEF. above). **Striped muscle.** *See* MAIN DEF. (above). **Supernumerary muscle.** Accessory muscle (see above). **Synergic muscle, Synergistic muscle.** One which acts in conjunction with the prime mover to oppose some undesired side-effect of the latter. **Thenar muscle.** One of the intrinsic muscles of the thumb; one of the muscles of the thenar eminence. **Tricipital muscle.** A muscle with three heads of origin. **Two-joint muscle.** One which passes over and can act on two joints. **Unipennate muscle [musculus unipennatus (NA)].** One in which the muscle fibres insert on one side only of the tendon of origin or insertion. **Unstriated muscle.** Unstriped muscle (*see* MAIN DEF. above). **Unstriped muscle.** *See* MAIN DEF. (above). **Veratrinized muscle.** Isolated voluntary muscle treated with veratrine. It shows on electrical stimulation a greater height of contraction than normal, the contraction being maintained for some time and relaxation taking twenty to thirty times as long as normal. Muscles of both warm- and cold-blooded animals are affected, but the phenomenon is most easily displayed in frog muscle. **Vestigial muscle.** One which is known to have been present in a phylogenetically ancestral form and occasionally reappears. **Visceral muscle.** Unstriped muscle (*see* MAIN DEF. above). **Voluntary muscle.** Striped muscle (*see* MAIN DEF. above). **White muscle.** *See* MAIN DEF. (above). **Yolked muscle.** One heavily laden with yolk, seen only in lower vertebrates. [L *musculus.*]

See also: AEBY, ALBINUS, BELL (C.), BOWMAN, BRAUNE, BRUECKE, CASSERIO, CHASSAIGNAC, COITER, CRAMPTON (P.), DUPRÉ, DUVERNEY, ELLIS (G. V.), FALLOPIUS, FOLIUS, GANTZER, GAVARD, GUTHRIE, HILTON, HORNER (W. E.), HOUSTON, JARJAVAY, JUNG (K. G.), KLEIN, KOBELT, KOHLRAUSCH (O. L. B.), KRAUSE (K. F. T.), LANDSTRÖM, LANGER, LESSHAFT, LUSCHKA, MARCACCI, MERKEL (K. L.), MEYERHOLTZ, MUELLER (H.), OCHSNER, OEHL, PHILLIPS, PORTAL, POZZI, REISSEISEN, RIOLAN, ROUGET, ROUX (C.), RUDINGER, RUYSCH, SIBSON, SOEMMERING, SYLVIUS, THEILE, TOD, TOYNBEE, TREITZ, WILSON (J.), WOOD (J.).

muscle-bound (musl·bownd). Possessing muscles developed to excessive proportions but functionally suboptimal. [muscle, AS *bindan.*]

muscular (mus·kew·lar). 1. Of or referring to a muscle or group of muscles. 2. Provided with well-developed muscles.

muscularis (mus·kew·la·ris). The muscular layer of an organ. **Muscularis mucosae.** A layer of unstriped muscular fibres in a mucous membrane.

muscularity (mus·kew·lar·it·e). The quality of being muscular.

musculation (mus·kew·la·shun). Muscular activity.

musculature (mus·kew·la·tewr). The arrangement of the muscles in the body or in a part of it.

musculocutaneous (mus·kew·lo·kew·ta′·ne·us). Referring to muscles and to skin; denoting nerves which supply both the muscles and the skin. [muscle, L *cutis* skin.]

musculocutaneous nerve of the lower limb [nervus peroneus (fibularis) superficialis (NA)]. One of the terminal branches of the lateral popliteal nerve, supplying the peroneal muscles [rami musculares] (except the peroneus tertius), and most of the skin on the dorsum of the foot.

Lateral branch [nervus cutaneus dorsalis intermedius (NA)]. A branch of the musculocutaneous nerve supplying the skin on the adjacent sides of the third and fourth, and fourth and fifth toes.

Medial branch [nervus cutaneus dorsalis medialis (NA)]. A branch of the musculocutaneous nerve to the skin on the medial side of the big toe and in the 2nd interdigital cleft.

musculocutaneous nerve of the upper limb [nervus musculocutaneus (NA)]. A branch of the lateral cord of the brachial plexus to supply the biceps brachii, coracobrachialis and brachialis muscles [rami musculares (NA)], and the skin on the lateral side of the forearm. It also supplies the elbow and wrist joints.

musculodermic (mus·kew·lo·**der**'·mik). Musculocutaneous. [muscle, Gk *derma* skin.]

musculo-elastic (mus·kew·lo·e·**las**'·tik). Containing or made up of muscular and elastic tissue.

musculo-intestinal (mus·kew·lo·in·**tes**'·tin·al). Referring to the muscles and to the intestines.

musculomembranous (mus·kew·lo·**mem**'·bran·us). Composed of muscle an l of membranous tissue.

musculophrenic (mus·kew·lo·**fren**'·ik). Referring to or supplying the diaphragm and associated muscles. [muscle, Gk *phren* diaphragm.]

musculophrenic artery [arteria musculophrenica (NA)]. The terminal branch of the internal mammary artery, passing obliquely downwards and laterally behind the 7th, 8th, and 9th costal cartilages. It supplies the diaphragm and the lower intercostal and upper abdominal muscles and sends twigs to the pericardium.

musculophrenic veins [venae musculophrenicae (NA)]. Veins accompanying the artery of the same name and draining the diaphragm and adjacent abdominal wall into the internal mammary veins.

musculoprecipitin (mus·kew·lo·pre·**sip**'·it·in). A precipitin in serum, specifically prepared for the differentiation of meat from different animals. [muscle, precipitin.]

musculorhachidian (mus·kew·lo·rak·**id**'·e·an). Relating or belonging to the muscles of the spine. [muscle, Gk *rhachis* spine.]

musculoskeletal (mus·kew·lo·**skel**'·et·al). Relating to or composed of the muscles and the bones (skeleton).

musculospiral (mus·kew·lo·**spi**'·ral). Referring to the radial (formerly musculospiral) nerve. [muscle, spiral.]

musculotegumentary (mus·kew·lo·teg·ew·**men**'·tar·e). Referring to or affecting both the muscle and integument.

musculotendinous (mus·kew·lo·**ten**'·din·us). Referring to or made up of both muscular and tendinous tissue.

musculotonic (mus·kew·lo·**ton**'·ik). Referring to the contractility or tonicity of a muscle.

musculus (**mus**·kew·lus) (pl. *musculi*). A muscle. **Musculus incisurae helicis [NA].** A few muscle fibres occasionally to be found bridging over the fissure of Santorini. **Musculi pectinati [NA].** Muscle bundles on the inner surface of both the auricles (auricular appendages) of the heart. **Musculus uvulae [NA].** A muscle arising from the posterior nasal spine and inserted into the mucous membrane of the uvula. It elevates the uvula and palate [L].

mushbite (**mush**·bite). In dentistry, a record of the relationship between upper and lower teeth obtained by biting into a piece of softened material such as wax. [etym. dub.]

Mushin, William Woolf (b. 1910). Cardiff anaesthetist.

Coxeter-Mushin apparatus. An apparatus for closed anaesthesia, working on the "circle" principle.

mushroom (**mush**·room). Name given to both edible and poisonous fungi belonging to a sub-class of Basidiomycetes. They include the following groups: 1. Agaricaceae (mushrooms and toadstools proper), of which there are over 4600 species, some poisonous (e.g. *Amanita*), others edible (e.g. *Agaricus campestris*). 2. Polyporaceae (pore fungi), chiefly parasitic on trees and destructive to timber; some are edible. 3. Hydnaceae (spine-bearing fungi), small and woody. 4. Thelephoraceae, small mostly, the larger species being tough and leathery. 5. Clavariaceae (coral-shaped fungi), non-poisonous and including some large fungi. The most important medicinally are in the group Agaricaceae: the field or common mushroom, *Agaricus campestris* (*Psalliota campestris*) is often cultivated; *Amanita muscaria*, the fly agaric, contains the alkaloid muscarine which has pharmacological properties like those of pilocarpine and is antagonized by atropine. [ME *muscheron*.]

musicogenic (mew·zik·o·**jen**'·ik). Produced or affected by music. **Musicogenic epilepsy.** A type of epilepsy where an attack is provoked by listening to music. [Gk *mousike* music, *genein* to produce.]

musicomania (mew·zik·o·**ma**'·ne·ah). A morbid devotion to music. [Gk *mousike* music, mania.]

musicotherapy (mew·zik·o·**ther**'·ap·e). The treatment of disease by means of music. [Gk *mousike* music, therapy.]

musk (musk). The dried secretion from the preputial follicle of *Moschus moschiferus* Linn. (order Ungulata), the musk-deer. It has a strong and characteristic odour, and is used in the making of some perfumes. **Artificial musk.** A synthetic musk substitute. [Sanskrit *muska* scrotum.]

Muskens, Louis Jacob Josef (b. 1872). German neurologist.

Muskens' tonometer. An instrument for measuring the tension of the tendo calcaneus.

musophobia (mus·o·**fo**·be·ah). Unnatural dread of mice. [L *mus* mouse, phobia.]

Musset, Louis Charles Alfred de. (b. 1810). French poet who died as a result of aortic insufficiency and in whom, traditionally, the symptom was first noted.

de Musset's sign, Musset's sign. Rhythmical movement of the head and neck synchronous with each ventricular systole, seen occasionally in cases of severe free aortic incompetence and aortic aneurysm.

mussitation (mus·it·a·shun). Labial movements taking place as in speaking, but without sound being produced. [L *mussitare* to murmur to oneself.]

mustard (**mus**·tard). A plant of the genus *Brassica (Sinapis)* of the order Cruciferae. The seeds are generally used. **Bath mustard.** A mixture of black and white mustard added to the bath as a counter-irritant to increase the flow of blood through the skin and promote sweating. **Black mustard.** Sinapis nigra; the dried ripe seeds of *Brassica nigra* occurring as reddish-brown to black small spherical grains and containing a yellowish oily embryo. The chief constituent is the glucoside, sinigrin, and the enzyme, myrosin, which react in the presence of water to produce allyl isothiocyanate. There is also about 27 per cent of a fixed oil, certain proteins, and mucilage. It is used in the preparation of the expressed and volatile oils of mustard, and, mixed with white mustard, of bath mustard, mustard bran, and mustard flour. **Mustard bran.** Chiefly the seed coats of black and white mustard. **Brown mustard.** Black mustard (see above). **Mustard flour.** The powdered seeds of black and white mustard freed from the seed-coats. It increases the flow of saliva and gastric juice and is used as a condiment. It is also an emetic in cases of poisoning. Externally it is employed as a counter-irritant in the form of a poultice. **Mannitol mustard.** Mannomustine hydrochloride. **Nitrogen mustard.** Mustine hydrochloride. **White mustard.** Sinapis alba; the dried ripe seeds of *Brassica alba* Linn., occurring as small, subspherical, faintly pitted grains, yellowish-buff in colour. The chief constituent is the glucoside, sinalbin, which yields acrinyl isothiocyanate on hydrolysis by the enzyme myrosin. It is used as a rubefacient and vesicant like black mustard. **Yellow mustard.** White mustard (see prec.). [L *mustum* must.]

Mustine (**mus**·teen). BP Commission approved name for *NN*-di-(2-chloroethyl)methylamine. **Mustine Hydrochloride BP 1973.** di-(2-Chloroethyl)-methylamine hydrochloride, $CH_3N(C_2H_4Cl)_2$, HCl. A cytotoxic agent acting similarly to irradiation, but more rapid and severe in effect. In small doses its action is confined to the blood-forming organs, and, inhibiting mitotic division, it eventually destroys the precursors of the red and white blood cells in the bone marrow, and causes necrosis of the germ cells in the lymph nodes. Prolonged administration may cause agranulocytosis, severe anaemia and thrombocytopenic purpura, which may be fatal. Side-effects include venous thrombosis, nausea, vomiting, anorexia, diarrhoea, neurological disturbances and skin rashes. Antidotes are blood transfusion for anaemia, and penicillin for agranulocytosis. Its employment therapeutically should take second place to x-ray therapy, and be an alternative in cases refractory to irradiation. Best results have been obtained in Hodgkin's disease, particularly if widely disseminated; treatment of lymphosarcoma has been less consistent in results, and it is of little value in acute leukaemia as it may cause death by damaging the remaining haemopoietic tissue. In chronic myeloid leukaemia, x-ray therapy is preferred; results in carcinoma have been disappointing. The drug is given by slow intravenous saline drip, since it may cause a thrombosis if injected directly. Dosage is given in conjunction with blood counts, and may be repeated at intervals of six weeks. Combined x-ray and mustine therapy may have a dangerous effect on the bone marrow.

mutability (mew·tah·**bil**·it·e). **Nucleic acid mutability.** The tendency of a nucleic acid to vary in structure as a result of mutation. [L *mutare* to change, *sensibilis* perceptible by the senses.]

mutacism (**mew**·tah·sizm). 1. The incorrect sounding of mute letters. 2. The frequent but incorrect use of the *m* sound in speech; mimmation. [Gk *mytakismos* fondness for the letter μ.]

mutagen (**mew**·tah·jen). A physical or chemical environmental agent which induces mutation. [L *mutare* to change, Gk *genein* to produce.]

mutagenesis (mew·tah·**jen**·es·is). The process(es) by which mutations arise. [L *mutare* to change, Gk *genesis* origin.]

mutant (**mew**·tant). 1. A gene in which mutation has occurred. 2. An organism carrying a mutant gene and, usually, showing its effects. [L *mutare* to change.]

mutarotation (**mew**·tah·ro·**ta**'·shun). The change in rotation of an optically-active compound. A phenomenon exhibited by freshly prepared solutions of sugars which alter in the value of their optical activity until an equilibrium is attained: it is due to the formation of stereo-isomers. [L *mutare* to change, rotation.]

mutase (**mew**·taze). 1. An oxidoreductase or enzyme which is specifically concerned with the oxidation of aldehydes. 2. A protein food prepared from leguminous plants and used in gastro-intestinal disorders. **Aldehyde mutase.** An enzyme occurring in muscle and liver which, with coenzyme I, catalyses the conversion of aldehyde into alcohol and acid. [L *mutare* to change.]

mutation (mew·**ta**·shun). A sudden change of chromosomal material which alters the effect of this material on the physiology of the cell. Mutation of sex cells will result in the production of mutant individuals in the offspring. **Chromosomal mutations.** Relatively gross changes by inversion, polyploidy, or translocation of chromosomal material. **Gene mutation.** Mutation of an individual gene producing an allelomorph. **Somatic mutation.** Mutation in somatic cell nuclei affecting all derived cells, but not the offspring. Except in the case of certain viruses, the genetic material is universally composed of deoxyribonucleic acid (DNA). At the molecular level, mutation may result from the substitution of one DNA base by another, or by the deletion or addition of one or more bases. **Accepted point mutation.** An amino acid replacement which has occurred in related proteins as the result of the occurrence of a point mutation. **Amber mutation.** Name given to one of three types of chain-terminating mutation, due to alteration of an amino acid codon to the "nonsense" codon uracil-adenine-guanine (UAG); this results in termination of polypeptide chain synthesis at the site of the substitution. **Chain-terminating mutation.** A mutation which alters an amino acid codon to one of three types of "nonsense" codon and results in the termination of polypeptide chain synthesis at this amino acid site. **Chromosome mutation.** A change in the structure of a chromosome involving more than one gene locus. **Frame-shift mutation.** A mutation resulting from deletion or addition of a base or bases from the DNA so that the genetic information, which is translated in one direction from a fixed point in groups of three bases (a codon) at a time, is misread from the mutational site onwards—the "reading-frame" is out of phase. **Genome mutation.** A change in the chromosome number leading to heteroploidy (polyploidy and/or aneuploidy). **Induced mutation.** A mutation which has resulted from treatment with a mutagen. **Leaky mutation.** A mutation which fails to abolish function completely. **Neutral mutation.** One of a class of mutations that appear not to be involved in the process of natural selection; a mutation that is neither biologically advantageous nor deleterious. **Nonsense mutation.** The change of an amino acid codon to one of three base triplets which do not code for an amino acid; it results in termination of polypeptide chain synthesis. **Ochre mutation.** Name given to one of three types of chain-terminating mutations, due to change of an amino acid codon to the "nonsense" codon uracil-adenine-adenine (UAA). **Point mutation.** A mutation in which only a single base-pair of DNA has been changed. **Polar mutation.** A point mutation whose effects extend to other genes of the same operon located to one side only of the mutation; usually "nonsense" mutations. **Mutation rate.** The frequency of mutation per individual per generation. **Transition mutation.** A mutation due to the substitution, in one of the two strands of DNA, of a purine base by another purine, or of a pyrimidine base by another pyrimidine. **Transversion mutation.** A mutation due to the substitution of a purine base by a pyrimidine, or *vice versa*, in one of the two strands of DNA. [L *mutare* to change.]

Mutch, Joseph Raeburn (b. 1895). Aberdeen ophthalmologist.

Mutch's proptometer. A simple instrument for estimating the amount of proptosis of the eye. It rests on the upper and lower orbital margin, and a plunger is moved down until it rests on the apex of the cornea through the closed lid. The distance the plunger moves is read off on a scale.

mute (mewt). 1. Incapable of utterance. 2. An individual who does not have the faculty of speech. **Deaf mute.** A person who is dumb because he has not the faculty of hearing. [L *mutus* dumb.]

mutilation (mew·til·**a**·shun). Deliberate infliction of injuries to the body, including, at times, self-injury, often centring on the sex organs, associated with various types of psychosis. Mutilation of a victim may be a feature of sex murders, occasionally involving removal of parts of the body possibly as a form of self-gratification, or delusion of guilt. [L *mutilare* maim.]

mutism (**mewt**·izm). Dumbness; lack of the faculty of speech. In psychiatry, abnormal arrest of speaking powers. **Akinetic mutism.** A condition in which consciousness is retained but there is no movement except for the eyes and respiratory muscles, usually due to a lesion of the mid-brain. **Deaf mutism.** The state of being unable to speak because the faculty of hearing is lacking. **Hysterical mutism.** A hysterical condition in which the patient loses the power of speech. [see prec.]

mutitas (**mewt**·it·as). Dumbness. **Mutitas atonica.** Dumbness caused by disease of the lingual nerves. **Mutitas organica.** Dumbness caused by deprivation of the tongue, e.g. by operation. **Mutitas pathematica.** That due to a frightening or emotional experience. **Mutitas spasmodica.** Dumbness that occurs at spasmodic intervals. **Mutitas surdorum.** That brought on by congenital deafness. [L *mutus* dumb.]

mutualism (mew·tew·al·izm). The benefit obtained from living together, by two or more species of animals. [L *mutuus* in return.]

mutualist (**mew**·tew·al·ist). One of two or more species living together in a state of mutual advantage. [see prec.]

Myà, Giuseppe (b. 1857). Florence paediatrician.

Myà's disease. Megacolon.

myaesthesia (mi·es·**the**·ze·ah). Muscle sense. [Gk *mys* muscle, aesthesia.]

myalgia (mi·**al**·je·ah). A painful condition of a muscle or muscles. **Myalgia abdominis.** Pain in the muscles of the abdominal wall. **Myalgia capitas.** Cephalodynia. **Epidemic myalgia.** That due to Coxsackie and other viruses; epidemic pleurodynia; Bornholm disease. [Gk *mys* muscle, *algos* pain.]

myalgic (mi·**al**·jik). Affected with or referring to myalgia.

myamoeba (mi·am·**e**·bah). A muscle cell. [Gk *mys* muscle, amoeba.]

myasthenia (mi·as·**the**·ne·ah). Weakness of muscles from whatever cause. **Myasthenia cordis.** Weakness of the myocardium. **Myasthenia gastrica.** Atony of the stomach with dilatation. **Myasthenia gravis.** Muscle dysfunction and abnormal fatigability of the muscles due to impairment of conduction at the motor end-plate (or myoneural junction). Muscles innervated by the cranial nerves, especially the extrinsic ocular muscles, are usually first affected, but later the muscles of the neck, limbs, and trunk are involved. The course of the disease is variable: there may be long remissions ultimately followed by recurrence, but in some it is rapidly progressive, leading to death in a few months. **Myasthenia laryngis.** Paralysis of the internal tensor muscles of the vocal cords, usually brought about by laryngitis or vocal misuse. [Gk *mys* muscle, *astheneia* weakness.]

myasthenic (mi·as·**then**·ik). Marked by or relating to myasthenia.

myatonia, myatony (mi·a·**to**·ne·ah, mi·**at**·on·e). Amyotonia congenita. **Myatonia congenita, Myotonia dystrophica.** Myotonia atrophica; Thomsen's disease, a rare heredofamilial disease pathologically similar to muscular dystrophy. [Gk *mys* muscle, atony.]

myatrophy (mi·**at**·ro·fe). Atrophy affecting a muscle; muscular atrophy. [Gk *mys* muscle, atrophy.]

myautonomy (mi·awt·**on**·om·e). A state in which the contraction of a muscle in response to excitation is so tardy that it seems to have no connection with the latter. [Gk *mys* muscle, *autos* self, *nomos* law.]

mycelial, mycelian (mi·**se**·le·al, mi·**se**·le·an). Referring to mycelium.

mycelioid (mi·**se**·le·oid). 1. Having the appearance of a mycelium. 2. A descriptive term used of certain bacterial colonies which look like mould colonies. [mycelium, Gk *eidos* form.]

mycelium (mi·**se**·le·um). A collective term for the elements of true fungi, consisting of filaments (or hyphae) which branch and intertwine to form a dense mat of growth. **Racquet mycelium.** Hyphae in which the distal portion of each segment is swollen, producing a racquet shape. [Gk *mykes* fungus, *helos* nail.]

mycete (**mi**·seet). A fungus. [Gk *mykes* fungus.]

mycethaemia (mi·se·**the**·me·ah). Fungaemia. [Gk *mykes* fungus, *haima* blood.]

mycetism, mycetismus (**mi**·se·tizm, mi·se·**tiz**·mus). Poisoning by mushrooms. [Gk *mykes* fungus.]

mycetogenetic, mycetogenous (mi·se·to·jen·**et**'·ik, mi·se·**toj**·en·us). Caused by fungi. [Gk *mykes* fungus, *genein* to produce.]

mycetoid (**mi**·se·toid). Having the appearance of a fungus. [Gk *mykes* fungus, *eidos* form.]

mycetology (mi·se·**tol**·o·je). Mycology.

mycetoma (mi·se·**to**·mah). Name proposed by Carter (1862) for a localized mycosis of the subcutaneous and deeper tissues, most frequently affecting the exposed parts of the body, particularly the foot (Madura foot), and causing conspicuous deformity by swelling, destruction of tissue, and formation of sinuses through which pus containing granules (black, white, or red in colour) or colonies of the fungus is discharged. It may be caused by any one of a large number of fungi which fall into two main groups, *Streptomyces* and *Nocardia* causing actinomycotic mycetoma (actinomycetoma) and true filamentous fungi, e.g. *Madurella, Allescheria,* which cause maduromycetoma. Historically, this disease was known by such names as *white mycetoma* (mycetoma with white grains). The name is particularly applied to Vincent's white mycetoma caused by *Streptomyces madurae,* but there are several other white mycetomata of which, in some cases, only single examples have been described, e.g. Reynier's, Tarozzi and Raedeli's, Nicolle and Pinoy's, Brumpt's, Bouffard's, Manson's, and Musgrave and Clegg's; other mycetomata were similarly named according to the colour of the infecting colonies or to persons describing the disease or fungus. [Gk *mykes* fungus, *-oma* tumour.]

mycetozoon (mi·se·to·**zo**'·on). An organism of the class Mycetozoa, the slime fungi. [Gk *mykes* fungus, *zoon* animal.]

myco-agglutinin (mi·ko·ag·**loo**'·tin·in). A serum agglutinin having the power of agglutinating the homogenized elements of the fungus causing infection. [Gk *mykes* fungus, agglutinin.]

myco-angioneurosis (mi·ko·an·je·o·newr·**o**'·sis). A neurotic condition associated with mucous colitis. [Gk *mykes* fungus, angioneurosis.]

Mycobacteriaceae (mi·ko·bak·teer·e·**a**'·se·e). A family of the order Actinomycetales. The only genus it includes is *Mycobacterium,* the type species of which is *Mycobacterium tuberculosis.* [Gk *mykes* fungus, bacterium.]

mycobacteriosis (mi·ko·bak·teer·e·**o**'·sis). Disease caused by a species of the genus *Mycobacterium.* [*Mycobacterium,* Gk *-osis* condition.]

Mycobacterium (mi·ko·bak·**teer**'·e·um). A bacterial genus in the family Mycobacteriaceae. The organisms are slender, straight, or slightly curved rods, Gram-positive but staining with difficulty, and acid-fast by the Ziehl-Neelsen method of staining. The pathogenic species are very slow growing and require enriched media, e.g. containing egg (Dorset's egg culture medium, Loewenstein-Jensen culture medium). Two species are of particular importance in human tuberculosis: *Mycobacterium tuberculosis hominis,* the common cause of human tuberculosis, and *Mycobacterium tuberculosis bovis,* the cause of tuberculosis in cattle and other animals but sometimes infecting man, usually by drinking raw milk from infected cows. *Mycobacteria leprae,* the cause of leprosy, has not been cultivated on artificial media. The two species *Mycobacterium ulcerans* and *Mycobacterium marinum* (Balnei) are exclusively skin pathogens and grow best at a temperature of 30.32°C. In recent years, certain species of mycobacteria, provisionally called *anonymous microbacteria,* have been identified as causing mild clinical (usually respiratory) or symptomless infections in man; among the more important of these are *Mycobacterium kansasii, M. intracellulare* (formerly known as the Battey bacillus), *M. xenopi* and *M. fortuitum.* **Mycobacterium avium.** The causative organism of tuberculosis in birds. It is also known to infect pigs. **Mycobacterium balnei.** The causative organism of swimming-pool granuloma. **Mycobacterium buruli.** The organism responsible for certain forms of chronic ulceration of the skin occurring in Uganda. **Mycobacterium butyricum.** A saprophytic species found in butter. **Mycobacterium johnei.** A strongly acid-fast, Gram-positive micro-organism, morphologically like the avian form of *Mycobacterium tuberculosis.* It causes a chronic infiltration of the intestinal canal in cattle and possibly in sheep (Johne's disease). **Mycobacterium leprae.** The leprosy bacillus. **Mycobacterium muris.** The vole bacillus; the cause of a naturally occurring tuberculosis in the vole, *Microtus agrestis.* It is of low virulence for man and it has been suggested that it might be used in place of the bacillus of Calmette-Guérin, as an immunizing vaccine for humans. **Mycobacterium phlei.** The timothy-grass bacillus; a saprophytic member of the genus found on certain grains. **Mycobacterium piscium.** The cause of tuberculosis in fish and reptiles. **Mycobacterium of rat leprosy.** *Mycobacterium lepraemurium.* **Mycobacterium smegmatis.** The smegma bacillus; a saprophytic member of the genus found on the skin around the urethral orifice. **Mycobacterium stercoris.** The mist bacillus; a saprophytic member of the genus found in horse dung and manure heaps. **Mycobacterium tuberculosis.** The cause of tuberculosis in man and certain other mammals. Two varieties are differentiated on their cultural characteristics and pathogenicity for laboratory animals, *Mycobacterium tuberculosis* var. *hominis* and *Mycobacterium tuberculosis* var. *bovis.* **Mycobacterium ulcerans.** The organism responsible for certain forms of ulceration of the skin occurring in Africa and in Australia, e.g. the Burnli ulcer. [Gk *mykes* fungus, bacterium.]

Mycocandida (mi·ko·**kan**·did·ah). A generic name proposed by Langeron and Talice (1932) for a group of imperfect mycelium-forming yeast fungi which are now included in the genus *Candida.* [Gk *mykes* fungus, *Candida.*]

mycoderma (mi·ko·**der**·mah). 1. A synonym of *Geotrichum,* but it has been used loosely for other fungi. The term has now no other place in medical mycology except as a synonym of

Geotrichum. It is, however, still used in botanical mycology for certain species which reproduce by chains of cubical to oval spores. 2. Mucous membrane. **Mycoderma dermatitidis.** *Blastomyces dermatitidis.* **Mycoderma immite.** *Coccidioides immitis.* [Gk *mykes* fungus, *derma* skin.]

mycodermitis (**mi**·ko·der·**mi′**·tis). Inflammation affecting a mucous membrane. [mycoderma, Gk *-itis* inflammation.]

mycodermomycosis (**mi**·ko·der·mo·mi·**ko′**·sis). Geotrichosis. [Gk *mykes* fungus, *derma* skin, mycosis.]

mycogastritis (**mi**·ko·gas·**tri′**·tis). A fungus infection of the mucous membrane of the stomach. [Gk *mykes* fungus, gastritis.]

mycohaemia (mi·ko·**he**·me·ah). Fungaemia. [Gk *mykes* fungus, *haima* blood.]

mycoid (**mi**·koid). Fungoid. [Gk *mykes* fungus, *eidos* form.]

mycologist (mi·**kol**·o·jist). One who studies or practises the science of mycology.

mycology (mi·**kol**·o·je). The study of fungi. There is no general agreement as to the limits of the forms that should be called fungi: early mycologists included bacteria (fission fungi) and slime moulds (Mycetozoa). Though the latter are still usually included, bacteria are more often regarded as a separate group. **Medical mycology.** The study of fungi which cause disease of man and animals. [Gk *mykes* fungus, *logos* word.]

mycomyringitis (**mi**·ko·mir·in·**ji′**·tis). Myringomycosis.

mycophage (**mi**·ko·faje). A virus that destroys moulds. [Gk *mykes* fungus, *phagein* to eat.]

mycophthalmia (mi·kof·**thal**·me·ah). Ophthalmia caused by the activities of a fungus. [Gk *mykes* fungus, ophthalmia.]

mycophylaxin (**mi**·ko·fil·**ax′**·in). An old term used rather vaguely to describe any substance which protects against infection. [Gk *mykes* fungus, *phylax* guard.]

Mycoplasma (mi·ko·**plaz**·mah). A bacterial genus in the order Mycoplasmatales, associated with outbreaks of severe respiratory disease in cattle, sheep and goats (pleuropneumonia-like organisms) and of chronic respiratory infections in poultry and certain mammals. A species (*Mycoplasma pneumoniae*) has also been identified as synonymous with Eaton's agent as a cause of primary atypical pneumonia in man. There are numerous non-pathogenic species, e.g. *Mycoplasma hominis, Mycoplasma salivarium.* **F-mycoplasm.** A compound which is probably present on the anterior or middle piece of the sperms of infertile men and also in the cervical mucus of infertile women and may produce neuroaminidase-like substances. [Gk *mykes* fungus, *plassein* to mould.]

mycoprecipitin (**mi**·ko·pre·**sip′**·it·in). A precipitating antibody which produces a precipitate when mixed with bacterial or fungous fractions. Nowadays referred to simply as *precipitin.* [Gk *mykes* fungus, precipitin.]

mycoprotein (mi·ko·**pro**·te·in). Any protein elaborated by bacteria or fungi. [Gk *mykes* fungus, protein.]

mycopus (**mi**·ko·pus). Mucus mixed with pus. [Gk *mykes* fungus, pus.]

mycose (**mi**·koze). $C_{12}H_{22}O_{11}$, a disaccharide, glucose glucoside, occurring in fungi and seaweeds and also, polymerized, in ergot and moulds. [Gk *mykes* fungus.]

mycosin (**mi**·ko·sin). A nitrogenous substance found in the cell wall of fungi. [see prec.]

mycosis (mi·**ko**·sis). A disease caused by a fungus. **Mycosis favosa.** Favus. **Mycosis interdigitalis.** 1. Tinea pedis. 2. Athletes' foot. **Pulmonary mycosis.** A mycotic infection of the lung, e.g. actinomycosis, torulosis (cryptococcosis). **Water-bed mycosis.** A fungus infection of the skin following continuous use of a water bed. Terms suggesting fungal aetiology but not caused by fungi are: **Mycosis botyra.** Septic granuloma. **Mycosis cutis chronica.** Oriental sore; cutaneous leishmaniasis. **Mycosis framboesioides.** Yaws. **Mycosis fungoides.** A chronic, pruritic, pleomorphic reticulosis. It begins with lesions resembling eczema, parapsoriasis, or psoriasis, may continue as pityriasis rubra, and finally mushroom-like tumours develop. **Mycosis intestinalis.** Anthrax. **Mycosis leptothrica.** A disease of the tonsils and pharynx caused by *Leptothrix buccalis.* **Mycosis pemphigoides.** A yeast infection of the skin somewhat resembling pemphigus vulgaris. [Gk *mykes* fungus, *-osis* condition.]

See also: GILCHRIST, POSADA.

mycostasis (mi·**kos**·tas·is). Inhibition of the developmnt or reproduction of fungi. [Gk *mykes* fungus, *stasis* a standing still.]

mycotic (mi·**kot**·ik). Referring to a mycosis or, with regard to a lesion, due to fungi. [Gk *mykes* fungus.]

Mycotoruloides (**mi**·ko·tor·ew·**loi′**·deez). A generic name proposed by Langeron and Talice (1932) for a section of imperfect mycelium-forming yeast fungi which are now included in the genus *Candida.* [Gk *mykes* fungus, L *torula* roll, Gk *eidos* form.]

mycotoxin (mi·ko·**tox**·in). A toxin derived from fungi. [Gk *mykes* fungus, toxin.]

mycteric (mik·**ter**·ik). Referring to the nasal cavity. [Gk *mykter* nose.]

mycterophonia (**mik**·ter·o·**fo′**·ne·ah). A condition in which the voice is produced at the back of the nose, with characteristic nasal twang. [Gk *mykter* nose, *phone* sound.]

mycteroxerosis (**mik**·ter·o·zer·**o′**·sis). A condition of dryness affecting the nares. [Gk *mykter* nose, xerosis.]

mydaleine (mi·**da**·le·een). A ptomaine which has been isolated from putrefied viscera, e.g. liver. Alleged toxic symptoms include salivation, dilated pupils and rise of temperature followed by arrest of the heart in diastole. [Gk *mydaleos* mouldy.]

mydatoxine (mi·da·**tox**·een). $C_6H_{13}NO_2$, a poisonous ptomaine isolated from decaying fish. [Gk *mydaein* to become damp, *toxikon* poison.]

mydesis (mi·**de**·sis). 1. A putrefactive process. 2. A purulent exudation from the eyelids. [Gk *mydaein* to become damp.]

mydine (**mi**·deen). $C_9H_{11}NO_2$, a non-poisonous ptomaine isolated from the viscera of dead bodies. [Gk *mydaein* to become damp.]

mydriasine (**mi**·dre·as·een). $C_{17}H_{23}O_3NCH_3Br$, a compound used as a mydriatic, since its action is less prolonged than that of atropine.

mydriasis (mi·**dri**·as·is). Enlargement of the pupil, due to paralysis of the sphincter muscle, stimulation or spasm of the dilator muscle, or both. **Paralytic mydriasis.** Dilatation of the pupil due to paralysis of the sphincter muscle which may be due to many causes: drugs, e.g. atropine; poisons, e.g. botulism; diseases, e.g. syphilis, diphtheria. **Spasmodic mydriasis.** An early stage of spastic mydriasis. **Spastic mydriasis.** Dilatation of the pupil due to excessive contraction of the dilator muscle. It is produced artificially by cocaine drops, or in disease by irritation of the cervical sympathetic nerve, and may be an early sign of syringomyelia; it usually develops into paralytic miosis later. The condition is characterized by retention of light and convergence reflexes. **Spinal mydriasis.** Mydriasis due to a lesion in the spinal cord causing irritation of the cervical sympathetic nerve. [Gk]

mydriatic (mi·dri·**at**·ik). Any drug causing dilatation of the pupil, e.g. atropine, hyoscine, or lachesine. [see prec.]

myectomy (mi·**ek**·to·me). Excision of part or all of a muscle. [Gk *mys* muscle, *ektome* a cutting out.]

myectopia, myectopy (mi·ek·**to**·pe·ah, mi·**ek**·to·pe). Displacement of a muscle. [Gk *mys* muscle, *ektopos* out of the way.]

myelaemia (mi·el·**e**·me·ah). A word of ill-defined meaning, best avoided. 1. Myeloid leukaemia. 2. The occurrence of myelocytes in the circulating blood. [myelocyte, Gk *haima* blood.]

myelanalosis (**mi**·el·an·al·**o′**·sis). 1. A wasting condition affecting the spinal cord; myelatrophy. 2. Tabes dorsalis. [Gk *myelos* marrow, *analosis* a wasting away.]

myelapoplexy (mi·el·**ap**·o·plex·e). Haemorrhage from one of the vessels of the spinal cord; spinal apoplexy. [Gk *myelos* marrow, apoplexy.]

myelasthenia (**mi**·el·as·**the′**·ne·ah). A supposed state of exhaustion of the spinal cord [obsolete term]. [Gk *myelos* marrow, *asthenia* debility.]

myelatelia (**mi**·el·at·**e′**·le·ah). Defective development of the spinal cord. [Gk *myelos* marrow, *ateles* unaccomplished.]

myelatrophy (mi·el·**at**·ro·fe). Atrophy affecting the spinal cord. [Gk *myelos* marrow, atrophy.]

myelencephalic (mi·el·en·kef·**al**′·ik). Referring to the myelencephalon.

myelencephalitis (**mi**·el·en·kef·al·**i**′·tis). Inflammation affecting the brain and spinal cord. [Gk *myelos* marrow, encephalitis.]

myelencephalon [NA] (**mi**·el·en·**kef**′·al·on). The caudal limb of the hind-brain. It becomes the medulla oblongata when fully developed. [Gk *myelos* marrow, *egkephalos* brain.]

myelencephalospinal, myelencephalous (mi·el·en·**kef**·al·o·**spi**′·nal, mi·el·en·**kef**′·al·us). Cerebrospinal. [Gk *myelos* marrow, *egkephalos* brain, spine.]

myeleterosis (**mi**·el·et·er·**o**′·sis). Any pathological change in the spinal cord. [Gk *myelos* marrow, *heteros* other.]

myelhyperaemia (**mi**·el·hi·per·e′·me·ah). Hyperaemia affecting the spinal marrow. [Gk *myelos* marrow, hyperaemia.]

myelic (mi·**el**·ik). Referring to the spinal cord. [Gk *myelos* marrow.]

myelin (**mi**·el·in). 1. $C_{40}H_{75}NPO_{10}$, a mono-aminomono-phosphatide occurring in small amounts in the white matter of brain. 2. A fatty substance found in the sheath of medullated nerve fibres which stains black with osmic acid and blue with haematoxylin after potassium-dichromate fixation. [Gk *myelos* marrow.]

myelinated (mi·el·in·a·ted). Equipped or coated with a myelin substance (medulla).

myelination, myelinization (mi·el·in·**a**′·shun, **mi**·el·in·i·**za**′·shun). The acquisition of myelin.

myelinogenesis (**mi**·el·in·o·**jen**′·es·is). Myelination. [see foll.]

myelinogenetic (**mi**·el·in·o·jen·**et**′·ik). Developing myelin or myelination. [myelin, Gk *genein* to produce.]

myelinogeny (**mi**·el·in·**oj**′·en·e). The myelination of nerve fibres. [see prec.]

myelinolysin (**mi**·el·in·**ol**′·is·in). A lytic substance able to destroy myelin, and said to be present in the serum of patients with multiple sclerosis. [myelin, Gk *lysis* a loosing.]

myelinolysis (**mi**·el·in·**ol**′·is·is). Demyelination. **Central pontine myelinolysis.** Demyelination confined to central pontine structures, possibly due to malnutrition. [Gk *myelos* marrow, *lysis* a loosing.]

myelinoma (**mi**·el·in·**o**′·mah). A tumour formed of myelin-producing cells. [myelin, Gk *-oma* tumour.]

myelinopathy (**mi**·el·in·**op**′·ath·e). Any disease or degenerative change affecting myelin. [myelin, Gk *pathos* disease.]

myelinosis (**mi**·el·in·**o**′·sis). A variety of fat necrosis in which there is formation of myelin. [myelin, Gk *-osis* condition.]

myelitic (mi·el·**it**·ik). Referring to or characterized by myelitis.

myelitis (mi·el·**i**·tis). 1. Inflammation of bone marrow; osteomyelitis. 2. Inflammation or degeneration of the spinal cord. The symptoms are variable: local pain in the back; motor and sensory paralysis of varying degrees below the level of the lesions. **Acute myelitis.** Simple myelitis without obvious pathological causes. **Apoplectiform myelitis.** Myelitis of sudden onset. **Ascending myelitis.** Myelitis with extension upwards in the spinal cord, and corresponding interference with function of nervous tissues involved. **Bulbar myelitis.** That involving the medulla oblongata. **Cavitary myelitis.** Myelitis with formation of cavities due to the destruction of myelin. **Central myelitis.** That affecting specially the grey matter of the cord. **Myelitis cervicalis.** Myelitis affecting the cervical regions of the spinal cord and producing symptoms in the hands and arms. **Chronic myelitis.** A slowly progressing form of myelitis or the sequel of an acute myelitis. **Compression myelitis.** That due to pressure on the spinal cord by a tumour or a fracture of the spine. **Concussion myelitis.** A sequel to a concussion of the spine. **Corneal myelitis.** Myelitis affecting the grey horns of the spinal cord. **Descending myelitis.** That in which the pathological process progresses downwards in the cord. **Diffuse myelitis.** Myelitis with scattered areas of the myelitic process. **Disseminated myelitis.** Diffuse myelitis [see prec.]. **Focal myelitis.** The myelitic involvement of only a small area of the cord. **Foudroyant myelitis.** Myelitis of sudden or rapid onset. **Funicular myelitis.** Myelitis involving the posterior and lateral columns of the cord. **Haemorrhagic myelitis.** Myelitis with haemorrhagic areas, seen in specially acute cases. **Interstitial myelitis.** Myelitis in which the incidence is on the neuroglial elements of the cord. **Peri-ependymal myelitis.** Myelitis with special incidence of the morbid process in the neighbourhood of the central canal of the spinal cord. **Postvaccinal myelitis.** An acute myelitis that may, rarely, follow vaccination. **Pressure myelitis.** Compression myelitis (see above). **Transverse myelitis.** The usual type of acute myelitis involving both sides of the cord. **Traumatic myelitis.** Myelitis after injury to the cord, especially in fractures of the spine. **Myelitis vaccinia.** Part of the clinical picture of a vaccinal encephalomyelitis. [Gk *myelos* marrow, *-itis* inflammation.]

myeloblast (**mi**·el·o·blast). The most primitive precursor of the granular leucocytes; a basophilic, non-granular cell seen normally only in the bone marrow, except in certain leukaemic conditions when it may be found in the circulating blood and other organs in great or small numbers. [Gk *myelos* marrow, *blastos* germ.]

myeloblastaemia (**mi**·el·o·blas·**te**′·me·ah). The occurrence of myeloblasts in the blood. [myeloblast, Gk *haima* blood.]

myeloblastoma (**mi**·el·o·blas·**to**′·mah). A tumour consisting of myeloblasts. [myeloblast, Gk *-oma* tumour.]

myeloblastomatosis (**mi**·el·o·**blas**·to·mat·**o**′·sis). The occurrence of several myeloblastomata. [myeloblastoma, Gk *-osis* condition.]

myeloblastosis (**mi**·el·o·blas·**to**′·sis). Myeloblastic leukaemia. [myeloblast, Gk *-osis* condition.]

myelobrachium (**mi**·el·o·**bra**·ke·um). The inferior cerebellar peduncle (restiform body). [Gk *myelos* marrow, *brachion* arm.]

myelocele (**mi**·el·o·seel). Spina bifida with extrusion of the spinal cord. [Gk *myelos* marrow, *kele* hernia.]

myelocerebellar (**mi**·el·o·ser·e·**bel**′·ar). Referring to the spinal cord and to the cerebellum. [Gk *myelos* marrow, cerebellum.]

myeloclast (**mi**·el·o·klast). A cell that breaks up medullary sheaths. [Gk *myelos* marrow, *klastos* broken.]

myelocoele (**mi**·el·o·seel). The central canal of the spinal cord. [Gk *myelos* marrow, *koilia* cavity.]

myelocyst (**mi**·el·o·sist). A cyst, usually of dermoid type, arising in a medullary cavity of the spinal cord. [Gk *myelos* marrow, cyst.]

myelocystic (mi·el·o·**sist**·ik). 1. Myeloid and cystic in formation, 2. Referring to a myelocyst or characterized by its presence.

myelocystocele (**mi**·el·o·**sist**′·o·seel). A cystic tumour of the spinal cord. [Gk *myelos* marrow, *kystis* bag, *kele* hernia.]

myelocystomeningocele (**mi**·el·o·**sist**·o·men·**ing**′·go·seel). Myelocystocele associated with meningocele; a type of spina bifida, associated with hernia of the spinal cord and meninges. [Gk *myelos* marrow, *kystis* bag, *menigx* membrane, *kele* hernia.]

myelocyte (**mi**·el·o·site). An early differentiated large, granular, nucleated leucocyte (from 12 to 18 μm diameter) derived from the myeloblast, and having a round, oval, or reniform nucleus. It is normally seen in the bone marrow, but in certain leukaemic conditions appears in the circulating blood. The staining of the cytoplasmic granules differentiates these cells into *neutrophil, basophil* and *eosinophil myelocytes.* According to their degrees of maturity there are corresponding promyelocytes, myelocytes and metamyelocytes, respectively. [Gk *myelos* marrow, *kytos* cell.]

myelocythaemia (**mi**·el·o·si·**the**′·me·ah). Myelocytes in the blood; myeloid leukaemia. [myelocyte, Gk *haima* blood.]

myelocytic (**mi**·el·o·**sit**′·ik). Referring to or of the character of myelocytes.

myelocytoma (**mi**·el·o·si·**to**′·mah). Chronic myeloid leukaemia. [myelocyte, Gk *-oma* tumour.]

myelocytosis (**mi**·el·o·si·**to**′·sis). Myelocythaemia. [myelocyte, Gk *-osis* condition.]

myelodiastasis, myelodiastema (**mi**·el·o·di·**as**′·tas·is, **mi**·el·o·di·as·**te**′·mah). Destruction or necrosis of the spinal cord. [Gk *myelos* marrow, *diastasis* separation.]

myelodysplasia (**mi**·el·o·dis·**pla**′·ze·ah). Imperfect development of any portion of the spinal cord, in particular of the lower segments. [Gk *myelos* marrow, dysplasia.]

myelo-encephalic (mi·el·o·en·kef·**al**′·ik). Relating or belonging to the spinal cord and to the brain. [Gk *myelos* marrow, *egkephalos* brain.]

myelo-encephalitis (**mi**·el·o·en·kef·al·**i**′·tis). Inflammation affecting the spinal cord and the brain. **Epidemic myelo-encephalitis.** Acute poliomyelitis. [Gk *myelos* marrow, encephalitis.]

myelofibrosclerosis (**mi**·el·o·**fi**·bro·skleer·**o**′·sis). Myelofibrosis. [Gk *myelos* marrow, fibrosis.]

myelofibrosis (**mi**·el·o·fi·**bro**′·sis). A fibrotic condition of the bone marrow. [Gk *myelos* marrow, fibrosis.]

myelogenesis (**mi**·el·o·**jen**′·es·is). 1. The evolution of the nervous system; in particular, the evolution of the brain and spinal cord, 2. The process of depositing myelin around axons. [Gk *myelos* marrow, *genesis* origin.]

myelogenetic, myelogenic, myelogenous (**mi**·el·o·jen·**et**′·ik, **mi**·el·o·**jen**′·ik, mi·el·**oj**·en·us). Originating in the bone marrow. [see foll.]

myelogeny (mi·el·**oj**·en·e). The stage in the evolution of the central nervous system at which the myelin sheaths of nerve fibres reach maturity. [Gk *myelos* marrow, *genein* to produce.]

myelogone, myelogonium (**mi**·el·o·gone, **mi**·el·o·**go**′·ne·um). A primitive leucocyte of the myeloid series. [Gk *myelos* marrow, *gone* seed.]

myelogram (**mi**·el·o·gram). 1. In radiology, a radiograph of the spinal cord and subarachnoid space, made after intrathecal injection of contrast medium via the cisternal or lumbar route. 2. In haematology, a diagrammatic or tabular representation of the various cells found in the bone marrow, e.g. Schilling's haemogram. [Gk *myelos* marrow, *gramma* record.]

myelography (mi·el·**og**·raf·e). Radiography of the spinal cord and subarachnoid space by intrathecal injection of contrast medium via cisternal or lumbar route. **Air myelography.** Radiography of the spinal cord and sacral sac. Gas, including air, water-soluble or iodized oil may be used as the contrast medium injected into the subarachnoid space, usually in the lumbar region. [Gk *myelos* marrow, radiography.]

myeloid (**mi**·el·oid). 1. Similar to, originating in, or referring to bone marrow. 2. Referring to the spinal cord. 3. Resembling myelocytes. [Gk *myelos* marrow, *eidos* form.]

myeloidin (mi·el·**oid**·in). A substance similar to myelin in appearance and present in the pigmented layer of the retina. [see prec.]

myeloidosis (**mi**·el·oid·**o**′·sis). The growth of myeloid tissue, in particular hyperplasia of the tissue. [myeloid, Gk *-osis* condition.]

myelokentric (**mi**·el·o·**ken**′·trik). Producing myeloid cells. [Gk *myelos* marrow, *kentron* point.]

myelolymphangioma (**mi**·el·o·**limf**·an·je·**o**′·mah). Elephantiasis. [Gk *myelos* marrow, lymph, Gk *aggeion* small vessel, *-oma* tumour.]

myelolymphocyte (**mi**·el·o·**limf**′·o·site). An abnormal type of lymphocyte found in bone marrow. [Gk *myelos* marrow, lymphocyte.]

myelolysis (mi·el·**ol**·is·is). Disintegration of myelin. [myelin, Gk *lysis* a loosing.]

myelolytic (**mi**·el·o·**lit**′·ik). Capable of disintegrating myelin. [see prec.]

myeloma (mi·el·**o**·mah). A locally malignant tumour composed mainly of osteoclasts and found most often at the end of long bones and in the jaw or gums. As well as those referred to below, myeloid sarcoma and myeloid epulis are classed as myelomata. **Endothelial myeloma.** Diffuse endothelioma of bone in children. **Giant-cell myeloma.** A tumour of the bone marrow in which there are many giant cells. **Multiple myeloma.** Myelomatosis, a tumour arising from bone marrow and most often affecting the flat bones. It is sometimes associated with Bence-Jones proteinuria. **Osteogenetic myeloma.** Osteoclastoma. [Gk *myelos* marrow, *-oma* tumour.]

myelomalacia, myelomalacosis, myelomalaxia (**mi**·el·o·mal·**a**′·she·ah, **mi**·el·o·mal·ak·**o**′·sis, **mi**·el·o·mal·**ax**′·e·ah). Pathological softening of the spinal cord. [Gk *myelos* marrow, malacia.]

myelomatoid (mi·el·**o**·mat·oid). Having a resemblance to myeloma. [myeloma, Gk *eidos* form.]

myelomatosis (**mi**·el·o·mat·**o**′·sis). A type of malignant tumour or disease that may infiltrate the bone marrow with so-called myeloma or plasma cells which may also appear in the circulating blood. These changes are usually associated with single or multiple osteolytic lesions in the bony skeleton. The cause of the disease is unknown and the treatment unsatisfactory. Myelomatosis is associated with paraproteinaemia, the presence of large quantities of monoclonal immunoglobulin in the serum. Bence-Jones protein (free light chains) is present in the urine of a proportion of cases. [myeloma, Gk *-osis* condition.]

myelomenia (**mi**·el·o·**me**′·ne·ah). Vicarious menstruation into the spinal cord. [Gk *myelos* marrow, menses.]

myelomeningitis (**mi**·el·o·men·in·**ji**′·tis). Inflammation of the spinal cord and its membranes. [myelitis, meningitis.]

myelomeningocele (**mi**·el·o·men·**ing**′·go·seel). Spina bifida associated with herniation of the spinal cord and its membranes. [Gk *myelos* marrow, meningocele.]

myelomeninx (**mi**·el·o·**men**′·ingx). A membrane of the spinal cord. [Gk *myelos* marrow, *menigx* membrane.]

myelomyces (**mi**·el·o·**mi**′·seez). Medullary cancer. [Gk *myelos* marrow, *mykes* fungus.]

myeloneuritis (**mi**·el·o·newr·**i**′·tis). Multiple neuritis occurring in association with myelitis.

myeloparalysis (**mi**·el·o·par·**al**′·is·is). Spinal paralysis. [Gk *myelos* marrow, paralysis.]

myelopathic (**mi**·el·o·**path**′·ik). 1. Referring to or due to any disease of the spinal cord. 2. Myelogenetic. [see foll.]

myelopathy (mi·el·**op**·ath·e). Any disease affecting the spinal cord or myeloid tissues. **Cervical myelopathy.** Disease of the cervical spinal cord, especially that due to cervical spondylosis. **Radiation myelopathy.** Progressive paraplegia due to radiation damage to the spinal cord, usually after therapeutic irradiation of the neck or mediastinum. **Subacute necrotic myelopathy.** Rapidly advancing necrosis of the spinal cord with paraplegia, usually of unknown cause but sometimes associated with carcinoma. **Tropical myelopathy.** Beriberi. [Gk *myelos* marrow, *pathos* disease.]

myelopetal (mi·el·**op**·et·al). Moving in a direction towards the spinal cord; a term used in respect of nerve impulses. [Gk *myelos* marrow, L *petere* to seek.]

myelophage (**mi**·el·o·fage). A macrophage which absorbs or destroys myelin. [Gk *myelos* marrow, *phagein* to eat.]

myelophthisis (mi·el·**of**·this·is). 1. Depression and disorganization of the bone-marrow function by various space-occupying lesions and tumours in the bone-marrow cavity. It is associated with the appearance of immature red and white blood corpuscles in the circulating blood, producing a myelophthisic anaemia or leucoerythroblastosis. 2. Atrophy of the spinal cord, often with cavity formation. [Gk *myelos* marrow, *phthisis* a wasting.]

myeloplaque (**mi**·el·o·plak). Myeloplax.

myeloplasm (**mi**·el·o·plazm). The substance composing the wall of the early embryonic neural tube, supposed to be a protoplasmic syncytium derived from the neural ectodermal cells. [Gk *myelos* marrow, *plassein* to form.]

myeloplax (**mi**·el·o·plax). A multinucleated giant cell of the bone marrow. [Gk *myelos* marrow, *plax* plate.]

See also: ROBIN (C. P.).

myeloplaxoma (**mi**·el·o·plax·**o**′·mah). Endothelian myeloma. [Gk *myelos* marrow, *plax* plate, *-oma* tumour.]

myeloplegia (**mi**·el·o·**ple**′·je·ah). Spinal paralysis. [Gk *myelos* marrow, *plege* stroke.]

myelopoiesis (**mi**·el·o·poi·**e**′·sis). The development of bone marrow or of the cells that are derived from it. **Ectopic myelopoiesis, Extramedullary myelopoiesis.** The development of myeloid tissue and/or blood cells in parts of the body other than the bones. [Gk *myelos* marrow, *poiein* to form.]

myelopore (**mi**·el·o·pore). Any opening in the spinal cord. [Gk *myelos* marrow, *poros* passage.]

myeloradiculitis (mi·el·o·rad·ik·ew·**li**'·tis). Inflammation affecting the spinal cord and the posterior nerve roots. [Gk *myelos* marrow, L *radiculus* rootlet, Gk *-itis* inflammation.]

myeloradiculodysplasia (mi·el·o·rad·ik·ew·lo·dis·**pla**'·ze·ah). Imperfect development of the spinal cord and roots of the spinal nerves. [Gk *myelos* marrow, L *radiculus* rootlet, dysplasia.]

myeloradiculography (mi·el·o·rad·ik·ewl·**og**'·raf·e). Radiculography of the spinal nerve roots. [Gk *myelos* marrow, radiculography.]

myeloradiculopathy (mi·el·o·rad·ik·ew·**lop**'·ath·e). A diseased condition of the spinal cord and spinal-nerve roots. [Gk *myelos* marrow, L *radiculus* rootlet, *pathos* disease.]

myelorrhagia (mi·el·o·**ra**'·je·ah). Haemorrhage of or into the spinal cord. [Gk *myelos* marrow, *rhegnynein* to gush forth.]

myelorrhaphy (mi·el·**or**·af·e). Suture of the spinal cord which has been injured or cut. [Gk *myelos* marrow, *rhaphe* suture.]

myelosarcoma (mi·el·o·sar·**ko**'·mah). A sarcomatous tumour composed of either bone-marrow cells or myeloid substance. [Gk *myelos* marrow, sarcoma.]

myelosarcomatosis (mi·el·o·sar·ko·mat·**o**'·sis). The existence of multiple myelosarcomata throughout the body. [myelsarcoma, Gk *-osis* condition.]

myeloschisis (mi·el·**os**·kis·is). A developmental abnormality in which part of the neural canal is exposed on the surface. It is associated with spina bifida. [Gk *myelos* marrow, *schisis* a cleaving.]

myelosclerosis (mi·el·o·skler·**o**'·sis). 1. Sclerosing myelitis; spinal sclerosis. 2. A sclerotic condition affecting the bone marrow. [Gk *myelos* marrow, sclerosis.]

myelosis (mi·el·o·sis). 1. Myelomatosis or multiple myeloma. 2. Tumours of the spinal cord. 3. Hyperplasia of the myeloid elements of the bone marrow, causing changes in the circulating blood resembling chronic myeloid leukaemia, or sometimes myelophthisic anaemia. **Aleukaemic myelosis.** Myelosis in which the total white-blood-cell count is low while the differential white count may be normal. **Aleukaemic megakaryocytic myelosis.** Myelophthisic anaemia characterized by splenomegaly, polychromatophilia and, in the circulating blood, abnormal platelets, young megakaryocytes, normoblasts and often a leukaemic reaction. **Chronic myelosis.** Chronic myeloid leukaemia. **Chronic non-leukaemic myelosis.** Myelophthisic anaemia. **Funicular myelosis.** Myelosis with degenerative areas in the white matter of the spinal cord. **Leukaemic myelosis.** Myelosis with a high total white-blood-cell count and many immature myeloid cells in the blood. **Non-leukaemic myelosis.** Myelophthisic anaemia or aleukaemic myelosis. **Subleukaemic myelosis.** An aleukaemic myelosis with immature myeloid cells in the circulating blood. [Gk *myelos* marrow, *-osis* condition.]

myelospongium (mi·el·o·**spon**'·je·um). A network composed of the processes of the neuroglial cells in the embryonic neural tube. [Gk *myelos* marrow, *spoggos* sponge.]

myelosyphilis (mi·el·o·**sif**'·il·is). Any diseased condition of the spinal cord which is due to syphilis. [Gk *myelos* marrow, syphilis.]

myelosyringosis (mi·el·o·sir·in·**go**'·sis). Syringomyelia.

myelotherapy (mi·el·o·**ther**'·ap·e). Treatment with preparations made from bone marrow. [Gk *myelos* marrow, therapy.]

myelotome (mi·el·o·tome). 1. A cutting instrument used in making sections of the spinal cord. 2. An instrument for severing the spinal cord when removing the brain during a post-mortem examination. [Gk *myelos* marrow, *temnein* to cut.]

myelotomy (mi·el·**ot**·o·me). The operation for the division of nerve tracts within the spinal cord; usually division of sensory nerve tracts for the relief of intractable pain. [see prec.]

myelotoxic (mi·el·o·**tox**'·ik). 1. Having a destructive action on bone marrow. 2. Derived from diseased bone marrow. [Gk *myelos* marrow, *toxikon* poison.]

myelotoxicosis (mi·el·o·tox·ik·**o**'·sis). A disease of the bone marrow due to a chronic intoxication. [Gk *myelos* marrow, *toxikon* poison, *-osis* condition.]

myelotoxin (mi·el·o·**tox**'·in). A cytotoxin which causes disintegration of the cells of bone marrow. [Gk *myelos* marrow, toxin.]

myentasis (mi·**en**·tas·is). The stretching of a muscle. [Gk *mys* muscle, *entasis* a straining.]

myenteric (mi·en·**ter**·ik). Relating or belonging to the myenteron.

myenteron (mi·**en**·ter·on). The muscular coat of the small intestine. [Gk *mys* muscle, *enteron* bowel.]

Myers, Victor Caryl (b. 1883). Cleveland, Ohio, biochemist.

Pfiffner and Myers method. A colorimetric method: using alkaline nitroprusside ferricyanide reagent for the detection and determination of guanidine in blood.

Myers and Wardell method. For cholesterol in blood: the blood is dried on plaster of Paris, extracted with chloroform in a Soxhlet apparatus, and the cholesterol determined in the extract by the Liebermann–Burchard reaction.

myiasis (mi·i·as·is). Infestation of the body by larvae of flies; those commonly concerned are the larvae of species of *Calliphora, Chrysomyia, Cochliomyia, Drosophila, Lucilia, Musca, Oestrus, Phormia,* and *Sarcophaga.* **Creeping myiasis.** Larva migrans. **Cutaneous myiasis, Myiasis dermatosa.** Infestation of the skin by fly larvae. **Intestinal myiasis.** Infestation of the gut by fly larvae, usually through the accidental swallowing of larvae, which may survive and appear in the faeces. **Myiasis linearis.** Larva migrans. **Ocular myiasis.** Infestation of or around the eyes by fly larvae. Flies of several species lay their eggs or larvae in the eyes of sick or sleeping persons: the larvae may penetrate the cornea. **Traumatic myiasis.** Larval infestation of wounds. [Gk *myia* fly.]

myiocephalon, myiocephalum (mi·i·o·**kef**'·al·on, mi·i·o·**kef**'·al·um). Staphyloma formed by the iris through a rent in the cornea. [Gk *myia* fly, *kephale* head.]

myiodesopsia (mi·i·o·dez·**op**'·se·ah). A condition in which muscae volitantes appear before the eyes. [Gk *myia* fly, *eidos* form, *opsis* vision.]

mylacephalus (mi·la·**kef**·al·us). The lowest type of headless monstrosity. [Gk *mylax* large stone, acephalus.]

mylacris (**mil**·ak·ris). The patella. [Gk *mylakris* millstone.]

myle (**mi**·le). 1. The patella. 2. The maxilla. 3. A uterine mole. [Gk mill.]

Mylius, Franz Benno (b. 1845). Berlin chemist.

Mylius' test. For bile acids: to 5 ml of solution or of urine add three drops of 0.1 per cent aqueous solution of furfural. Layer with concentrated sulphuric acid. A red ring appears at the junction of the liquids if bile acids are present. This is a modified Pettenkofer test.

myloglossus (mi·lo·**glos**·us). That part of the superior constrictor muscle of the pharynx which arises from the mylohyoid line of the mandible. [Gk *myle* mill, *glossa* tongue.]

mylohyoid (mi·lo·**hi**·oid). Pertaining to the molar teeth of the mandible and the hyoid bone, e.g. the mylohyoid muscle of the neck. [Gk *myle* mill, *hyoid* bone.]

mylohyoid artery [ramus mylohyoideus (NA)]. *See* MAXILLARY ARTERY.

mylohyoid muscle [musculus mylohyoideus (NA)]. A flat sheet attached laterally to the mylohyoid line on the mandible and medially to the body of the hyoid bone behind and in front to a raphe, which joins it to its fellow, the two forming the floor of the mouth.

mylohyoid nerve [nervus mylohyoideus]. *See* DENTAL NERVE, INFERIOR.

myo-adenoma (mi·o·ad·en·**o**'·mah). An adenoma arising in connection with ducts of glands which contain muscle elements, such as mammary ducts. [Gk *mys* muscle, adenoma.]

myo-albumin (mi·o·al·**bew**'·min). One of the water-soluble proteins occurring in muscle. [Gk *mys* muscle, albumin.]

myo-albumose (mi·o·al·**bew**'·moze). An albumose derived from muscle protein. [Gk *mys* muscle, albumose.]

myo-architectonic (mi·o·ar·ke·tek·**ton**'·ik). Referring to the structural arrangement of muscle, or of muscle fibres. [Gk *mys* muscle, architectonic.]

myo-asthenia (mi·o·as·**the'**·ne·ah). Generalized loss of muscle power; weakness: usually a hysterical manifestation. [Gk *mys* muscle, *asthenia* lack of strength.]

myo-atrophy (mi·o·**at**·ro·fe). Muscular atrophy. [Gk *mys* muscle, atrophy.]

myoblast (**mi**·o·blast). An embryonic cell which develops into a muscle fibre. [Gk *mys* muscle, *blastos* germ.]

myoblastoma, myoblastomyoma (**mi**·o·blas·**to'**·mah, **mi**·o·blas·to·mi·**o'**·mah). Abrokosov's tumour; a rounded tumour found most frequently in the tongue, skin of the face, breasts and vulva; composed of large, pale, granular cells with eccentric nuclei and cytoplasmic granules. Formerly thought to be derived from muscle, there is now much doubt about its origin. The most recent suggestion implicates the neurolemmal cells. **Granular cell myoblastoma.** A tumour, probably of neural or nerve sheath origin, occurring on the skin or on the tongue. Its infiltration between muscle fibres has given the impression of origination from muscle cells. [myoblast, Gk *-oma* tumour.]

myobradia (mi·o·**bra**·de·ah). The slow, sluggish contraction of muscle following electrical stimulation which occurs in certain conditions. [Gk *mys* muscle, *bradys* slow.]

myocardial (mi·o·**kar**·de·al). Relating to the myocardium.

myocardiogram (mi·o·**kar**·de·o·gram). A tracing representing the cardiac muscular activity made by the use of the myocardiograph. [myocardium, Gk *gramma* a writing.]

myocardiograph (mi·o·**kar**·de·o·graf). An apparatus used in recording the action of the heart muscle. [myocardium, Gk *graphein* to record.]

myocardiopathy (mi·o·kar·de·**op'**·ath·e). An abnormal condition of the heart muscle not due to any known infective agent. The term may be applied to disorders of the heart muscle due to abnormal infiltrations (glycogen disease, amyloid disease), or to deficiency of vitamin B_1 (beriberi heart), and to Fiedler's myocarditis, and endomyocardial fibrosis. The myocardial lesion produced by diseases of the coronary arteries is best covered by the term *ischaemic heart disease*, but the designation *myocardiopathy* could be employed to differentiate the condition mentioned above from myocarditis due to specific infections or disease processes, i.e. diphtheria or rheumatic fever. [myocardium, Gk *pathos* disease.]

myocardiorrhaphy (mi·o·kar·de·**or'**·af·e). The suture of a wound of the heart. [myocardium, Gk *rhaphe* suture.]

myocardiosis (mi·o·kar·de·**o'**·sis). Myocardiopathy. [Gk *mys* muscle, *kardia* heart, *-osis* condition.]

myocardism (mi·o·**kar**·dizm). A predisposition to the development of myocardial degeneration.

myocarditic (mi·o·kar·**dit'**·ik). Referring to myocarditis.

myocarditis (mi·o·kar·**di'**·tis). Inflammation of the myocardium; it may be acute or chronic. **Acute bacterial myocarditis.** Inflammation of the myocardium due to invasion by bacteria (usually streptococci, staphylococci, or pneumococci), either locally or through the blood stream. **Acute isolated myocarditis.** An acute interstitial myocarditis characterized by widespread infiltration of the interstitial tissues with leucocytes and by some degenerative changes in the muscle fibres. Also known as *Fiedler's myocarditis*. **Chronic myocarditis.** Chronic inflammation of the myocardium as a result of previous acute inflammation. It is characterized by fibrosis following the degeneration of the muscle fibres or the infiltration of the interstitial tissue. The commonest form is rheumatic in origin. **Fibrous myocarditis.** Interstitial myocarditis (see below). **Idiopathic myocarditis.** An interstitial myocarditis characterized by infiltration with round cells, and allied to acute isolated myocarditis (Fiedler's). **Interstitial myocarditis.** Inflammation of the myocardium affecting the interstitial tissues. It is usually diffuse, but may be focal, and is characterized by infiltration with round cells and polymorphonuclear leucocytes; the muscle fibres often undergo slow degenerative changes. The condition occurs in rheumatic myocarditis and in some acute infections. **Local myocarditis.** Local areas of myocardial inflammation, parenchymatous or interstitial, or both, as a result of bacteriaemias or the direct spread of suppurative local lesions. **Parenchymatous myocarditis.** Inflammation of the myocardium involving the muscle fibres rather than the interstitial tissue. The fibres undergo cloudy swelling and degeneration, and may be destroyed and replaced by fibrous tissue. It occurs in severe diphtheric and infectious fevers, and may occur in acute fevers, scarlet fever, typhoid, meningococcal infections and diphtheria. **Rheumatic myocarditis.** Interstitial myocardial inflammation due to rheumatic fever. In the acute stage, swelling of collagen tissue and the infiltration with round cells is seen. The characteristic lesion is the Aschoff body, consisting of multinucleated giant cells, fibroblasts, and swollen collagen. In the chronic stage, the Aschoff body is transformed into a triangular area of fibrous tissue between the muscle fibres and around the blood vessels. **Suppurative myocarditis.** Suppuration of the myocardium with areas of necrosis and abscess formation, due to the action of pyogenic bacteria. **Toxic myocarditis.** Myocardial inflammation resulting from the action of toxins produced by acute infections, as in diphtheria. [myocardium, Gk *-itis* inflammation.]

See also: FIEDLER.

myocardium [NA] (mi·o·**kar**·de·um). The muscular structure of the heart; the whole mass of cardiac muscle. [Gk *mys* muscle, *kardia* heart.]

myocardosis (mi·o·kar·**do'**·sis). Myocardiopathy. [myocardium, Gk *-osis* condition.]

myocele (**mi**·o·seel). Herniation of a muscle; extrusion of a muscle through a tear in its sheath. [Gk *mys* muscle, *kele* hernia.]

myocellulitis (mi·o·sel·ew·**li'**·tis). Myositis associated with cellulitis.

myoceptor (mi·o·**sep**·tor). That part of a muscle fibre in immediate contact with the motor end-plate of the nerve, and thus the first part to receive the stimulus. The term is infrequently used. [Gk *mys* muscle, L *recipere* to receive.]

myocerosis (mi·o·ser·**o'**·sis). Waxy degeneration of muscle. **Myocerosis angiotica haemorrhagica.** Angiohyalinosis haemorrhagica. [Gk *mys* muscle, *keros* wax.]

myochorditis (mi·o·kord·**i'**·tis). Inflammation involving the muscles of the vocal cord. [Gk *mys* muscle, *chorde* cord, *-itis* inflammation.]

myochrome (**mi**·o·krome). Any one of a class of pigments obtained from muscles. [Gk *mys* muscle, *chroma* colour.]

myochronoscope (mi·o·**kron**·o·skope). A device for measuring the latent period between the arrival of a nerve impulse and the beginning of muscular contraction. [Gk *mys* muscle, *chronos* time, *skopein* to view.]

myoclonia (mi·o·**klo**·ne·ah). A condition showing clonic muscular contractions (myoclonus). **Myoclonia epileptica.** Clonic spasms seen during an epileptic attack. **Pseudoglottitic myoclonia.** Chronic spasm of the glottis as a result of coughing or laughing, sometimes terminating in momentary loss of consciousness with relief of the spasm. [Gk *mys* muscle, *klonos* contraction.]

myoclonic (mi·o·**klon**·ik). Referring to or characterized by myoclonus. **Myoclonic seizure.** An isolated epileptic seizure of unusually brief duration.

myoclonus (mi·o·**klo**·nus). 1. A sudden shock-like muscular contraction which may involve one or more muscles or a few fibres of a muscle. 2. The condition in which such contractions occur; myoclonia. **Diaphragmatic myoclonus.** Hiccup, clonic spasms of the diaphragm due to a variety of causes, such as reflex stimulation from the stomach, irritation of the phrenic nerve by pressure in the mediastinum, or from central-nervous lesions. Epidemic hiccup was a manifestation of encephalitis lethargica in certain epidemics. **Encephalitic myoclonus.** Myoclonic movements occurring during the acute stage of encephalitis lethargica; they may persist for several months. **Essential myoclonus.** Myoclonus multiplex (see below). **Facial myoclonus.** Chronic facial spasm, a disorder of adults in which there are frequent attacks of facial spasm, usually unilateral. **Myoclonus multiplex.** Paramyoclonus multiplex; a chronic disorder characterized by frequent sudden shock-like contractions of varying intensity, most frequently affecting symmetrically the proximal muscles of the limbs. There may be from 10 to 50 contractions per minute, which disappear during sleep and on voluntary movement. The mechanical excitability of the muscle is increased, but the electrical reactions are normal and there is no wasting. **Palatal myoclonus.** Unilateral or bilateral rapid rhythmic oscillation of the soft palate, often with synchronous involvement of the eyes, pharynx, larynx, and diaphragm. **Postanaesthetic myoclonus.** Temporary myoclonous sometimes seen after general anaesthesia, especially if halothane has been used. [Gk *mys* muscle, *klonos* contraction.]

See also: UNIVERRICHT.

myocoelalgia (**mi**·o·seel·**al**′·je·ah). Coeliomyalgia.

myocoele (**mi**·o·seel). The cavity of the primitive mesodermal segment, or somite, of the embryo. [Gk *mys* muscle, *koilos* hollow.]

myocolpitis (**mi**·o·kol·**pi**′·tis). Inflammation affecting the muscular coat of the vagina. [Gk *mys* muscle, *kolpos* pocket, *-itis* inflammation.]

myocomma (mi·o·**kom**·ah). One of the intersegmental connective-tissue septa between adjacent segmental myotomes of the embryo, or between the dorsal segmental muscles of lower vertebrates. [Gk *mys* muscle, comma.]

myocrismus (mi·o·**kriz**·mus). A sound heard on auscultation over a contracting muscle. [Gk *mys* muscle, *krizein* to speak.]

myoculator (mi·**ok**·ew·la·tor). An instrument for exercising the eye muscles. An image is projected on to a screen and by mechanical means is moved about in various directions. The patient, equipped with red and green glasses, has to follow it by moving the eyes and trying to keep the images superimposed. [Gk *mys* muscle, L *oculus* eye.]

myocyst (**mi**·o·sist). A cystic tumour affecting a muscle. [Gk *mys* muscle, cyst.]

myocyte (**mi**·o·site). A muscle cell. [Gk *mys* muscle, *kytos* cell.]

myocytoma (**mi**·o·si·**to**′·mah). A tumour composed of myocytes. [myocyte, Gk *-oma* tumour.]

myodegeneration (**mi**·o·de·jen·er·**a**′·shun). Muscular degeneration. [Gk *mys* muscle, degeneration.]

myodemia (mi·o·**de**·me·ah). Fatty degeneration affecting muscle tissue. [Gk *mys* muscle, *demos* fat.]

myodes (mi·**o**·deez). 1. Muscular; similar to muscle. 2. The platysma. [Gk *mys* muscle, *eidos* form.]

myodesopsia (**mi**·o·dez·**op**′·se·ah). Myiodesopsia.

myodiastasis (**mi**·o·di·**as**′·tas·is). The elevation of shortened muscle from its bony attachment. [Gk *mys* muscle, *diastasis* separation.]

myodioptre (**mi**·o·di·**op**′·ter). The contractile power of the ciliary muscle needed to increase the refractive power of the lens by one dioptre. [Gk *mys* muscle, dioptre.]

myodynamia (**mi**·o·di·**nam**′·e·ah). Muscular force, strength, or power. [see foll.]

myodynamic (**mi**·o·di·**nam**′·ik). Referring to muscular power. [Gk *mys* muscle, *dynamis* force.]

myodynamics (**mi**·o·di·**nam**′·ix). That branch of physiology which deals with the action of muscles. [see prec.]

myodynamometer (**mi**·o·di·nam·**om**′·et·er). An apparatus for determining muscular force. [Gk *mys* muscle, *dynamis* force, meter.]

myodynia (mi·o·**din**·e·ah). Pain in the muscles. [Gk *mys* muscle, *odyne* pain.]

myodystonia (**mi**·o·dis·**to**′·ne·ah). Any disorder affecting muscular tone. [Gk *mys* muscle, *dys-*, *tonos* tone.]

myodystrophia, myodystrophy (**mi**·o·dis·**tro**′·fe·ah, mi·o·**dis**·tro·fe). Muscular dystrophy. [Gk *mys* muscle, dystrophy.]

myo-elastic (**mi**·o·e·**las**′·tik). Pertaining to or composed of elastic fibres and smooth-muscle fibres. [Gk *mys* muscle, elastic.]

myo-electrical (**mi**·o·el·**ek**′·trik·al). Referring to the electrical properties of muscle. [Gk *mys* muscle, electricity.]

myo-endocarditis (**mi**·o·en·do·kar·**di**′·tis). Myocarditis associated with endocarditis.

myo-epithelial (**mi**·o·ep·e·**the**′·le·al). 1. Relating or belonging to myo-epithelium. 2. Referring to or consisting of muscle and epithelium.

myo-epithelioma (**mi**·o·ep·e·the·le·**o**′·mah). A tumour arising from the myo-epithelium of the sweat glands, closely simulating a spindle-cell sarcoma. Rarely it appears as a tumour of the breast which metastasizes to the lymph nodes. [Gk *mys* muscle, epithelium, Gk *-oma* tumour.]

myo-epithelium (**mi**·o·ep·e·**the**′·le·um). Tissue composed of smooth-muscle cells which are epithelial in origin. [Gk *mys* muscle, epithelium.]

myofascitis (**mi**·o·fas·**i**′·tis). Inflammation affecting a muscle and its fascia, especially the fascial insertion of muscle on bone. [Gk *mys* muscle, fascitis.]

myofibril, myofibrilla (mi·o·fi·bril, **mi**·o·fi·**bril**′·ah). Any of the long, thin, thread-like structures found in the cytoplasm of all types of muscle cells, but best marked in voluntary and cardiac muscle, where their presence gives rise to the longitudinal striation visible in fixed preparations. They are normally invisible in the living cell, and are composed of bundles of myofilaments. In voluntary and striated muscle they exhibit a regular alternation of dark (anisotropic) and light (isotropic) bands. [Gk *mys* muscle, fibril.]

myofibroma (**mi**·o·fi·**bro**′·mah). A tumour composed of myomatous and fibrous tissue; generally a myoma in which fibrous tissue is incorporated.

myofibrosis (**mi**·o·fi·**bro**′·sis). A degenerative lesion in which there is widespread substitution of fibrous tissue for muscle tissue. **Myofibrosis cordis.** Myofibrosis of the heart. [Gk *mys* muscle, fibrosis.]

myofibrositis (**mi**·o·fi·bro·**si**′·tis). Inflammation involving the perimysium. [Gk *mys* muscle, fibrositis.]

myofilaments (mi·o·**fil**·am·ents). Contractile filaments which are components of all types of muscle fibres. They contain actin, myosin and tropomyosin. [Gk *mys* muscle, filament.]

myofunctional (mi·o·**fungk**·shun·al). Pertaining to muscular function. [Gk *mys* muscle, function.]

myogaster (**mi**·o·gas·ter). A muscle belly. [Gk *mys* muscle, *gaster* belly.]

myogelosis (**mi**·o·jel·**o**′·sis). A hardened portion of a muscle; in particular, hardening of a gluteus muscle. [Gk *mys* muscle, L *gelare* to freeze, Gk *-osis* condition.]

myogen (**mi**·o·jen). An albumin occurring in muscle plasma. It has been separated into two fractions, A and B, which have been obtained in crystalline form. *Myogen A* is stated to possess enzymatic properties. [Gk *mys* muscle, *genein* to produce.]

myogenesis (mi·o·**jen**·es·is). The development of muscle tissue. [Gk *mys* muscle, *genesis* origin.]

myogenetic, myogenic, myogenous (**mi**·o·jen·**et**′·ik, mi·o·**jen**·ik, mi·**oj**·en·us). Derived from muscle tissue. [see prec.]

myoglia (mi·o·**gle**·ah). A fibrillary network present in muscular tissue and resembling neuroglia in appearance. [Gk *mys* muscle, *glia* glue.]

myoglobin (mi·o·**glo**·bin). Muscle haemoglobin; a respiratory pigment which occurs in the muscle cells of vertebrates and invertebrates. It is a monomeric conjugated protein containing one molecule of haem non-covalently linked to a single polypeptide chain containing 153 amino-acid residues. It is globular in shape and may exist as *reduced myoglobin* (deoxygenated myoglobin) or as *oxymyoglobin* (oxygenated myoglobin); when the iron is oxidized, *methmyoglobin* results. It functions as an oxygen carrier and store in muscle. Rarely, myoglobin variants occur in man in which one amino-acid residue is replaced by an alternative one as the result of mutation. In crush injuries, myoglobin is liberated from injured muscle and may appear in the urine (*myoglobinuria*) since it is filtered by the glomerulus and may precipitate in the renal tubules and produce anuria. **Dehaemated myoglobin.** Apomyoglobin. [Gk *mys* muscle, globin.]

myoglobinuria (**mi**·o·glo·bin·**ewr**′·e·ah). The presence of myoglobin in the urine. In horses this sometimes occurs after sharp exercise following a long period of rest, and is associated with a paralytic condition. It has been reported in man after severe exercise, and may or may not be accompanied by cramps. It also occurs in several diseases of unknown aetiology in which there is muscle necrosis and associated paralyses and cramps. **Paroxysmal idiopathic myoglobinuria.** A condition in which myoglobin is passed in the urine for from 3 to 5 days, associated with muscular pains and paralysis. The cause is not known, but attacks may be precipitated by muscular exercise or cold. The condition shows a familial pattern.

myoglobulin (mi·o·**glob**·ew·lin). A globulin present in muscle tissue. [Gk *mys* muscle, globulin.]

myognathia, myognathus (mi·og·**nath**·e·ah, mi·og·**nath**·us). A monster having a supernumerary mandible which is joined by muscular tissue and skin to the normal mandible. [Gk *mys* muscle, *gnathos* jaw.]

myogram (**mi**·o·gram). A myographic tracing. [Gk *mys* muscle, *gramma* a writing.]

myograph (**mi**·o·graf). An apparatus used in recording the degree and strength of muscular contraction. [Gk *mys* muscle, *graphein* to record.]

myographic (mi·o·**graf**·ik). Referring to a myograph, or to the records made by it.

myography (mi·**og**·raf·e). 1. The tracing of muscular movements by the myograph. 2. Description of muscles; descriptive myology.

myohaemoglobin (**mi**·o·he·mo·**glo**'·bin). The pigmented substance present in cytoplasm of the muscle fibrils, which is very similar to haemoglobin but physiologically different in having a far greater affinity for oxygen; it is spectroscopically distinct from haemoglobin, having an absorption band at about 584 nm. [Gk *mys* muscle, haemoglobin.]

myohaemoglobinaemia (**mi**·o·he·mo·glo·bin·**e**'·me·ah). Myohaemoglobin in the circulating blood. [myohaemoglobin, Gk *haima* blood.]

myohaemoglobinuria (**mi**·o·he·mo·glo·bin·**ewr**'·e·ah). Myoglobinuria. [Gk *mys* muscle, haemoglobinuria.]

myohypertrophia kymoparalytica (**mi**·o·hi·per·**tro**'·fe·ah, **ki**·mo·par·al·**it**'·ik·ah). A type of muscular dystrophy described by Oppenheim. [Gk *mys* muscle, hypertrophy, Gk *kyma* wave, paralysis.]

myohysterectomy (**mi**·o·his·ter·**ek**'·to·me). Subtotal hysterectomy; removal of the body of the uterus leaving the cervix. [Gk *mys* muscle, *hystera* uterus, *ektome* excision.]

myoid (**mi**·oid). Composed of or resembling muscle. [Gk *mys* muscle, *eidos* form.]

myoidema (mi·oid·e·mah). A localized muscular contraction produced by a light tap such as percussion over the pectoralis muscles, causing muscular contractions which result in the formation of a small lump. It is not uncommonly seen in cases of pulmonary tuberculosis, but it also occurs in other conditions of poor nutrition. [Gk *mys* muscle, *oidema* swelling.]

myoides (mi·**oid**·eez). The platysma. [see foll.]

myoideum (mi·**oid**·e·um). Muscular tissue. [Gk *mys* muscle, *eidos* form.]

myoidism (mi·**oid**·izm). The state of undue irritability of muscles to mechanical stimulation. [see prec.]

myo-ischaemia (**mi**·o·is·**ke**'·me·ah). A localized deficiency of blood supply in muscular tissue. [Gk *mys* muscle, ischaemia.]

myokinase (mi·o·**kin**·aze). An enzyme, also known as adenylate kinase, which catalyses the conversion of two molecules of adenosine diphosphate into one of adenosine triphosphate and one of adenosine monophosphate. It is important in muscle in conserving ATP concentrations in contraction and in the regulation of energy metabolism. [Gk *mys* muscle, *kinein* to move.]

myokinesimeter (**mi**·o·kin·e·**sim**'·et·er). A device for measuring the muscular contraction induced by artificial stimulation. [Gk *mys* muscle, *kinesis* movement, meter.]

myokinesis (**mi**·o·kin·**e**'·sis). Movement of muscles. [Gk *mys* muscle, *kinesis* movement.]

myokinetic (**mi**·o·kin·**et**'·ik). Pertaining to the movement of muscle, or to myokinesis.

myokymia (mi·o·**ki**·me·ah). The quivering or fibrillation of a few fasciculi of a muscle, often seen in the palpebral part of the orbicularis oculi muscle but also occurring in larger muscles. It affects debilitated persons, especially on mechanical stimulation, but may occur in normal persons on exposure to cold. Also in pathological states: continuously in facial muscles as an occasional symptom in mutiple sclerosis, and also generalized in a rare syndrome associated with sweating and muscular wasting. [Gk *mys* muscle, *kyma* wave.]

myokynine (mi·o·**ki**·neen). $C_{11}H_{30}N_2O_4$, a base, believed to be L-hexamethylornithine, occurring in human muscle.

myolemma (mi·o·**lem**·ah). Sarcolemma. [Gk *mys* muscle, *lemma* sheath.]

myolipoma (**mi**·o·lip·**o**'·mah). A myoma containing fatty tissues. [Gk *mys* muscle, *lipos* fat, *-oma* tumour.]

myological (mi·o·**loj**·ik·al). Referring to myology.

myologist (mi·**ol**·o·jist). One with especial knowledge or experience in the science of myology.

myology (mi·**ol**·o·je). That branch of science that deals with muscles and associated structures. [Gk *mys* muscle, *logos* science.]

myolysis (mi·**ol**·is·sis). Fatty degeneration or destruction of muscular tissue; adipose infiltration. **Cardiotoxic myolysis, Myolysis cardiotoxica.** Degeneration of the myocardium due to blood-borne toxins; noted in infectious diseases. **Nodular myolysis.** The formation of a nodule consisting of degenerated muscular tissue on the tongue. [Gk *mys* muscle, *lysis* a loosing.]

myoma (mi·o·mah). An innocent tumour composed of muscle elements. **Ball myoma.** A pedunculated globular myoma of the uterus. **Myoma laevicellulare.** A tumour arising from smooth, non-striated, involuntary muscle. **Myoblastic myoma.** A myoma which is sarcomatous because it is composed of embryonic muscle cells. **Myoma sarcomatodes.** A sarcoma of muscle. **Myoma striocellulare.** A tumour arising from striated voluntary muscle. **Myoma telangiectodes.** Haemangioma of muscle, a myoma rich in blood vessels, many of which are distended and spongy. [Gk *mys* muscle, *-oma* tumour.]

myomalacia (**mi**·o·mal·**a**'·she·ah). The softening of muscle due to various degenerative processes. **Myomalacia cordis.** The autolytic softening and necrosis of an area of infarction on the myocardium following coronary occlusion. It may lead to an aneurysm of the heart wall and rupture, or the area may undergo fibrosis and healing. [Gk *mys* muscle, *malakia* softening.]

myomatectomy (**mi**·o·mat·**ek**'·to·me). Extirpation of a myoma. [myoma, Gk *ektome* a cutting out.]

myomatosis (**mi**·o·mat·**o**'·sis). The formation of multiple myomata. [myoma, Gk *-osis* condition.]

myomatous (mi·**o**·mat·us). Referring to or of the character of a myoma.

myomectomy (mi·o·**mek**·to·me). 1. Extirpation of a myoma. 2. Myectomy. [Gk *mys* muscle, *-oma* tumour, *ektome* a cutting out.]

myomelanosis (**mi**·o·mel·an·**o**'·sis). Black discoloration of a part of a muscle; melanosis of muscle. [Gk *mys* muscle, *melas* black, *-osis* condition.]

myomere (**mi**·o·meer). Myotome. [Gk *mys* muscle, *meros* part.]

myometer (mi·**om**·et·er). An instrument for measuring the contractions of muscle. [Gk *mys* muscle, meter.]

myometritis (**mi**·o·me·**tri**'·tis). Inflammation involving the muscular tissue of the uterus. [Gk *mys* muscle, metritis.]

myometrium (mi·o·**me**·tre·um). The general muscular mass of the uterus. [Gk *mys* muscle, *metra* womb.]

myomohysterectomy (**mi**·o·mo·his·ter·**ek**'·to·me). Myomectomy associated with hysterectomy; extirpation of a uterus containing a myoma. [myoma, Gk *hystera* womb, *ektome* a cutting out.]

myomotomy (mi·o·**mot**·o·me). Myomectomy. [myoma, Gk *temnein* to cut.]

myonecrosis (**mi**·o·nek·**ro**'·sis). Muscle necrosis. **Clostridial**

myonecrosis. Gas gangrene. *See* GANGRENE. [Gk *mys* muscle, *necrosis* mortification.]

myoneme (**mi**·o·neem). Any of the fine contractile fibres in the ectoplasm of many protozoa. [Gk *mys* muscle, *nema* thread.]

myonephropexy (mi·o·**nef**·ro·pex·e). A form of fixation of a movable kidney by suturing the organ to muscle, usually the psoas. [Gk *mys* muscle, *nephros* kidney, *pexis* a fixation.]

myoneural (mi·o·**newr**·al). Referring to muscle and to nerve; denoting the nerve-endings in muscular tissue. [Gk *mys* muscle, *neuron* nerve.]

myoneuralgia (**mi**·o·newr·**al**'·je·ah). Neuralgic pain affecting the muscles. [Gk *mys* muscles, neuralgia.]

myoneurasthenia (**mi**·o·newr·as·**the**'·ne·ah). A state of muscular relaxation in neurasthenia; general atony and flabbiness of the muscles. [Gk *mys* muscle, neurasthenia.]

myoneure (**mi**·o·newr). A motor-nerve cell. [Gk *mys* muscle, *neuron* nerve.]

myoneurectomy (**mi**·o·newr·**ek**'·to·me). The section of the nerve supply of a muscle, sometimes used in the treatment of intermittent claudication affecting the muscles of the calf. [Gk *mys* muscle, *neuron* nerve, *ektome* a cutting out.]

myoneuroma (**mi**·o·newr·**o**'·mah). A painful tumour composed of muscle and nerves, or derivatives of these. [Gk *mys* muscle, *neuron* nerve, *-oma* tumour.]

myoneurosis (**mi**·o·newr·**o**'·sis). Any neurotic condition referring to or affecting muscles. **Colic myoneurosis, Intestinal myoneurosis.** Mucous colitis. [Gk *mys* muscle, neurosis.]

myonicity (mi·on·**is**·it·e). The ability of living muscle to relax and contract. [Gk *myon* a knot of muscle.]

myonitis (mi·on·**i**·tis). Myositis. [Gk *myon* a knot of muscle, *-itis* inflammation.]

myonosus (mi·**no**·sus). Any disease of the muscles. [Gk *mys* muscle, *nosos* disease.]

myonymy (mi·**on**·im·e). Muscle nomenclature. [Gk *mys* muscle, *onoma* name.]

myo-oedema (**mi**·o·e·**de**'·mah). 1. Muscular oedema. 2. Mounding. [Gk *mys* muscle, *oidema* a swelling.]

myopachynsis (**mi**·o·pak·**in**'·sis). A thickening of muscle fibres. [Gk *mys* muscle, *pachynsis* thickening.]

myopalmus (mi·o·**pal**·mus). Twitching of the muscles. [Gk *mys* muscle, *palmos* a quivering.]

myoparalysis (**mi**·o·par·**al**'·is·is). Muscular paralysis. [Gk *mys* muscle, paralysis.]

myoparesis (**mi**·o·par·**e**'·sis). Muscular paralysis. [Gk *mys* muscle, paresis.]

myopathia, myopathy (mi·o·**path**·e·ah, mi·**op**·ath·e). Any diseased condition of the muscles. **Acute thyrotoxic myopathy.** Myopathy occurring acutely in association with thyrotoxicosis. **Alcoholic myopathy.** Excessive alcohol intake may result in acute or chronic damage to muscle; in the acute form, severe muscle pain with myohaemoglobinuria are found. Muscle biopsy shows intracellular oedema and destruction of mitochondria. **Benign congenital myopathy.** Non-progressive muscle disease causing severe hypotonia from birth. **Carcinomatous myopathy.** Muscle disease due to remote carcinoma. **Myopathia cordis.** Myocardiopathy. **Corticosteroid myopathy.** Myopathy resulting from medication by corticosteroids. It may also be seen in Cushing's disease. **Cushing's myopathy.** Accounts for thin arms and legs due to atrophy of skeletal muscles in these regions. **Distal myopathy.** Myopathy affecting the distal parts of the limbs. **Myopathia infraspinata.** A disease characterized by the sudden onset of shoulder pain and tenderness in the infraspinatus muscle. **Megaconial myopathy.** Progressive myopathy in childhood associated with enlarged mitochondria. **Myotubular myopathy.** A probably distinct form of non-progressive congenital myopathy, possibly due to arrest of cellular development at the myotubule stage. **Nemaline myopathy.** A non-progressive congenital myopathy causing limb weakness, often associated with skeletal deformities. Rod-shaped bodies occur within muscle fibres. **Ocular myopathy.** A hereditary dystrophy affecting all the extra-ocular muscles, and producing a gradually progressive bilateral external ophthalmoplegia, going on to complete immobility of the eyes. It used to be considered nuclear in origin. It is sometimes associated with a similar condition of other muscles. **Pleoconial myopathy.** Congenital myopathy associated with an increase in abnormal mitochondria. **Myopathia rachitica.** Muscular atony in infants with rickets. **Radiation myopathy.** Following exposure to radiation, individual muscle cells show hyaline degeneration with patches of monocytic infiltration. There are associated EMG abnormalities. **Steroid myopathy.** Myopathy due to therapeutic administration of corticosteroids. [Gk *mys* muscle, *pathos* disease.]

See also: DÉJÉRINE, LANDOUZY.

myope (**mi**·ope). An individual affected with myopia. [Gk *myops* short-sighted.]

myopericarditis (**mi**·o·per·e·kar·**di**'·tis). Myocarditis associated with pericarditis.

myoperitonitis (**mi**·o·per·e·ton·**i**'·tis). Inflammation of the abdominal muscles associated with the peritoneum. [Gk *mys* muscle, peritoneum, Gk *-itis* inflammation.]

myophone (**mi**·o·fone). A device for the audible recording of the electrical potentials of muscles. Prior to the use of the cathode-ray oscillograph in electromyography, the potentials picked up from muscles were passed through an amplifier to a loud-speaker, assessment being made on the noise recorded. [Gk *mys* muscle, *phone* sound.]

myophonia (mi·o·**fo**·ne·ah). The sound caused by contraction of a muscle. [see prec.]

myopia (mi·o·pe·ah). Short sight; a condition in which the far point of the eye is inside infinity, or, expressed another way, the image of an object at infinity is in front of the retina. **Axial myopia.** Myopia in which the image falls in front of the retina because the eyeball is longer than normal. **Curvature myopia.** That due to excessive curvature of one of the refracting surfaces of the eye, usually the anterior surface of the cornea but sometimes the lens. **Empty-field myopia.** Failure to perceive objects at distances within normal visual range. When the visual field contains no perceptible details, the human eye tends to accommodate for a distance of about 2 m. **High myopia.** An arbitrary term indicating myopia exceeding a certain number of dioptres; 7 is the number chosen by some authorities, but others put it higher. **Index myopia, Indicial myopia.** That due to increase in refractive index, usually of the lens and then a prodromal sign of cataract, but it may be caused by increase in refractive index of the aqueous as in iritis. **Low myopia.** An arbitrary term indicating myopia lower than a certain number of dioptres, usually about two. **Malignant myopia.** Myopia progressing throughout life and associated with degenerative changes in the choroid and retina. **Pernicious myopia.** Malignant myopia (see prec.). **Prodromal myopia.** Myopia prodromal of cataract. **Progressive myopia.** A term applied to myopia during the time it is increasing. The majority of myopes become stabilized when growth is complete. **Space myopia.** A state of accommodation that occurs when no contours are imaged on the retina, as in high-altitude flying. Night myopia has the same mechanism. (Syn. empty-field myopia.) [Gk *myops* short-sighted.]

myopic (mi·**o**·pik). Referring to, characterized by, or affected with myopia.

myoplasm (**mi**·o·plazm). The cytoplasm of a muscle cell. [Gk *mys* muscle, *plasma* formation.]

myoplastic (mi·o·**plas**·tik). Pertaining to the use of muscle in reparative operations, or to plastic surgery of the muscles. [see foll.]

myoplasty (**mi**·o·plas·te). Reparative surgery as applied to muscle tissue. [Gk *mys* muscle, *plassein* to mould.]

myoplegia (mi·o·**ple**·je·ah). Slight paralysis of muscle or a condition in which there is decreased muscular force. [Gk *mys* muscle, *plege* stroke.]

myoporthosis (**mi**·o·por·**tho**'·sis). The correction of myopic errors and the restoration of approximately normal vision by provision of concave lenses. [Gk *myops* short-sighted, *orthos* straight.]

myoprotein (mi·o·**pro**·te·in). A protein found in muscle tissue. [Gk *mys* muscle, protein.]

myoproteose (mi·o·**pro**·te·oze). Myo-albumose. [Gk *mys* muscle, proteose.]

myopsis (mi·**op**·sis). A condition in which muscae volitantes appear before the eyes. [Gk *myia* fly, *ops* eye.]

myopsychopathy, myopsychosis (mi·o·si·**kop**·ath·e, **mi**·o·si·**ko'**·sis). Myopathies and neuromuscular affections associated with mental disturbances. [Gk *mys* muscle, pyschopathy, psychosis.]

myoreceptor (**mi**·o·re·**sep'**·tor). A proprioceptor found in skeletal muscle and excited by the contraction of muscle. [Gk *mys* muscle, receptor.]

myorrhaphy (mi·**or**·af·e). The suture of severed muscle. [Gk *mys* muscle, *rhaphe* suture.]

myorrhexis (mi·o·**rex**·is). Tearing or laceration of a muscle. [Gk *mys* muscle, *rhexis* rupture.]

myosalpingitis (**mi**·o·sal·pin·**ji'**·tis). Inflammation affecting the muscular coat of the uterine tube. [Gk *mys* muscle, salpinx, Gk *-itis* inflammation.]

myosalpinx (mi·o·**sal**·pingx). The muscular coat of the uterine tube. [Gk *mys* muscle, salpinx.]

myosan (**mi**·o·san). Denatured myosin precipitated from solutions of myosin on standing at or above room temperature.

myosarcoma (**mi**·o·sar·**ko'**·mah). A sarcoma containing non-striated muscular tissue; a combined myoma and sarcoma. [Gk *mys* muscle, sarcoma.]

myosclerosis (**mi**·o·skler·**o'**·sis). 1. Muscular sclerosis; chronic inflammation of muscle in which the interstitial tissue has become overgrown. 2. Pseudohypertrophic muscular dystrophy. [Gk *mys* muscle, *skleros* hard.]

myoscope (**mi**·o·skope). 1. An instrument used by orthoptists for training binocular vision. A moving image in red and green is thrown on a screen, and attempts at diplopia and then fusion are made by the patient who wears red and green glasses. 2. An apparatus designed for the observation of muscular contraction. [Gk *mys* muscle, *skopein* to view.]

myoseptum (mi·o·**sep**·tum). The septum of primitive connective tissue separating adjacent myotomes in the early embryo.

myoserum (mi·o·**seer**·um). The juice obtained from muscular tissue or from meat. [Gk *mys* muscle, serum.]

myosin (**mi**·o·sin). A protein found in cardiac and skeletal muscle. The thick filament which interacts with actin (thin filament) to produce muscle shortening or contraction. It contains adenosine triphosphatase which catalyses the hydrolysis of adenosine triphosphate to provide energy for the contractile process. [Gk *mys* muscle.]

myosinase (mi·o·sin·aze). The enzyme concerned in the conversion of myogen to myosin.

myosinose (mi·o·sin·oze). A proteose formed by hydrolytic action on myosin.

myosinuria (**mi**·o·sin·**ewr'**·e·ah). The presence of myosin in the urine.

myositic (mi·o·**sit**·ik). Referring to myositis.

myositis (mi·o·**si**·tis). Inflammation of voluntary muscles. **Clostridial myositis.** A myositis caused by *Clostridium welchii*; cases have been reported after sulphonamide injections. **Non-suppurative myositis.** Inflammation of muscle caused by trauma, following the intramuscular haemorrhages of scurvy or the irritation of the encapsulated larvae in trichiniasis. There may be direct spread of infection from the skin or subcutaneous tissues. **Myositis ossificans progressiva.** A progressive affection characterized by the formation of bony masses in muscles, fasciae, aponeuroses, tendons, ligaments, and bones. The muscles of the neck and back are usually first involved, but ultimately the majority of muscles are affected. **Myositis ossificans traumatica.** New bone formation in the soft tissues caused by injury, very often in association with a joint. **Myositis purulenta tropica.** Deep-seated abscesses in muscles in widely separated sites. The disease is often, but not always, associated with filariasis, and is common in Samoa, the West Indies, and West Africa. It is known in West Africa as *bungpagga*. **Suppurative myositis.** Inflammation of muscle due to infection with pyogenic organisms such as staphylococci or streptococci. It may be spreading and diffuse, or localized and forming abscesses; there are the general symptoms of a septic infection. **Tropical myositis.** Tropical pyomyositis. *See* PYOMYOSITIS. [Gk *mys* muscle, *-itis* inflammation.]

myosome (**mi**·o·some). The contractile element of muscular substance. [Gk *mys* muscle, *soma* body.]

myospasm (**mi**·o·spazm). Spasmodic contraction affecting a muscle; cramp. [Gk *mys* muscle, spasm.]

myospasmia (mi·o·**spaz**·me·ah). Any disease in which the most marked symptom is involuntary spasmodic contractions of a muscle or muscles. [see prec.]

myosteoma (**mi**·os·te·**o'**·mah). A tumour consisting of bony deposits in muscular tissue. [Gk *mys* muscle, *osteon* bone, *-oma* tumour.]

myostroma (mi·o·**stro**·mah). The stroma of muscular tissue. [Gk *mys* muscle, stroma.]

myostromin (mi·o·**stro**·min). A protein present in the framework of muscle. [see prec.]

myosuria (mi·o·**sewr**·e·ah). The presence of myosin in the urine; myosinuria. [Gk *mys* muscle, urine.]

myosuture (**mi**·o·sew·tewr). The suture of severed muscle or of separated muscle fibres. [Gk *mys* muscle, suture.]

myosynizesis (**mi**·o·sin·iz·**e'**·sis). Muscular adhesion. [Gk *mys* muscle, *synezeuxein* to hold together.]

myotactic (mi·o·**tak**·tik). Referring to the tactile sense of muscles. [Gk *mys* muscle, L *tactus* touch.]

myotamponade (mi·o·**tam**·pon·ade). The use of living muscle tissue, usually the pectoralis muscles, to compress or relax a diseased underlying lung. The muscle is isolated from its attachments, the blood supply being kept intact, and is inserted into the subpleural space between the rib and the affected lung. It is best employed as an adjunct to thoracoplasty to improve immobilization. [Gk *mys* muscle, Fr. *tampon* pack.]

myotasis (mi·**ot**·as·is). Muscular tension, as in stretching. [Gk *mys* muscle, *tasis* a straining.]

myotatic (mi·o·**tat**·ik). 1. Referring to the intrinsic or passive tension of muscle. 2. Brought about by the extension or stretching of a muscle. [see prec.]

myotenontoplasty (**mi**·o·ten·**on'**·to·plast·e). Tenomyoplasty.

myotenositis (**mi**·o·ten·o·**si'**·tis). Inflammation involving a muscle and its tendon. [Gk *mys* muscle, *tenon* tendon, *-itis* inflammation.]

myotenotomy (**mi**·o·ten·**ot'**·o·me). Surgical division of a tendon. [Gk *mys* muscle, *tenon* tendon, *temnein* to cut.]

myothermic (mi·o·**ther**·mik). Referring to alterations of muscle temperature as a result of contraction. [Gk *mys* muscle, *therme* heat.]

myotome (**mi**·o·tome). One of the series of segmental pre-muscle masses of the early embryo, derived from the somites. [Gk *mys* muscle, *temnein* to cut.]

myotomy (mi·**ot**·o·me). The dissection or division of a muscle or of muscular tissue. [see prec.]

myotonia (mi·o·**to**·ne·ah). A difficulty and slowness in relaxing muscles after effort. **Myotonia acquisita.** Tonic muscular spasm which has developed as a result of injury or secondarily to some other disease; Talma's disease. **Myotonia atrophica.** Dystrophia myontonica; a rare heredofamilial disease usually beginning between the ages of 20 and 40, and characterized by muscular atrophy most marked in the facial and sternocleidomastoid muscles but slowly progressing to the muscles of the shoulder girdle, the quadriceps, flexors of the forearm and dorsiflexors of the feet. Myotonia is present but variable in intensity and distribution, and may appear independently of the atrophy. Cataract occurs in the majority of the cases, and juvenile cataract is present in the preceding generation. **Myotonia congenita.** A rare heredofamilial disease beginning in early childhood, and characterized by prolonged muscular contraction with slow relaxation on voluntary movement or in postural muscles. It is not accompanied by muscular wasting. **Myotonia**

paradoxica. Myotonia increasing with exertion. [Gk *mys* muscle, *tonos* tone.]

myotonic (mi·o·**ton**·ik). 1. Referring to or affected with myotonia. 2. Referring to the element of tonus in muscles, in contradistinction to the myokinetic element.

myotonoid (mi·**ot**·on·oid). Applied to muscular reactions which are characterized by slow contraction and slow relaxation. [myotonia, Gk *eidos* form.]

myotonometer (**mi**·o·ton·**om**′·et·er). An apparatus used in recording the tonus of muscles. [myotonia, *metron* measure.]

myotonus (mi·o·**to**·nus). Muscle tone. *See* TONE. [Gk *mys* muscle, tone.]

myotony (mi·**ot**·on·e). Myotonia.

myotrophy (mi·**ot**·ro·fe). The nutrition of muscle tissue. [Gk *mys* muscle, *trophe* nutrition.]

myotropic (mi·o·**trop**·ik). Directed towards or drawn towards by a muscle. [Gk *mys* muscle, *trope* a turning.]

myovascular (mi·o·**vas**·kew·lar). Referring to the myocardium and the blood vessels. [Gk *mys* muscle, L *vasculum* little vessel.]

Myralact (**mir**·al·akt). BP Commission approved name for *N*-(2-hydroxyethyl)tetradecylammonium lactate; an antiseptic agent.

myrcene (**mer**·seen). A terpene which occurs in oil of bay (oleum myrciae).

myrcia (**mer**·she·ah). Bay leaves; the leaves of the plant *Pimenta acris* Kostel (family Myrtaceae) and other species. They yield an oil (oil of bay, Oleum Myrciae BPC 1949), the main constituent of which is eugenol.

myriachit (**meer**·e·ah·chit). A type of saltatory spasm, similar to lata, prevailing in Java, Borneo and parts of Russia, characterized by the patient imitating what he hears or sees. [Russian, to be epileptic.]

myriagram (**mir**·e·ah·gram). Unit of weight; ten thousand grams. [Obsolete term.] [Gk *myrioi* ten thousand, gramme.]

myrialitre (**mir**·e·ah·le·ter). Unit of volume; ten thousand litres. [Obsolete term.] [Gk *myrioi* ten thousand, litre.]

myriametre (**mir**·e·ah·me·ter). Unit of length; ten thousand metres. [Obsolete term.] [Gk *myrioi* ten thousand, metre.]

myriapoda (mir·e·**ap**·o·dah). A general term for the centipedes (Chilopoda) and millipedes (Diplopoda). [Gk *myrios* numberless, *pous* foot.]

Myrica (mir·**i**·kah). A genus of shrubs of the family Myricaceae. The dried root bark of *Myrica cerifera* Linn. has been used in the treatment of diarrhoea and as a tonic. [Gk *myrike* tamarisk.]

myricin (**mir**·is·in). $C_{15}H_{31}COOC_{30}H_{61}$, the chief constituent of beeswax (about 80 per cent).

myricyl (**mir**·is·il). The monovalent radical $C_{30}H_{61}$–, derived from myricyl alcohol.

myringa (mir·**ing**·gah). The tympanic membrane. [LL]

myringectomy (mir·in·**jek**·to·me). Tympanectomy. [myringa, Gk *ektome* a cutting out.]

myringitis (mir·in·**ji**·tis). Inflammation of the tympanic membrane. **Myringitis bullosa.** Inflammation of the tympanic membrane, with the formation of haemorrhagic bullae or blebs. [myringa, Gk *-itis* inflammation.]

myringodermatitis (mir·**ing**·go·der·mat·**i**′·tis). Inflammation of the tympanic membrane associated with an inflammation of the skin of the external ear passage. [myringa, Gk *derma* skin, *-itis* inflammation.]

myringomycosis (mir·**ing**·go·mi·**ko**′·sis). A fungus infection of the tympanic membrane. **Myringomycosis aspergillina.** Fungus infection of the tympanic membrane caused by black fungus (*Aspergillus niger*). [myringa, Gk *mykes* fungus, *-osis* condition.]

myringoplastic (mir·**ing**·go·**plas**′·tik). Relating or belonging to myringoplasty.

myringoplasty (mir·**ing**·go·plas·te). Plastic repair of the tympanic membrane. [myringa, Gk *plassein* to mould.]

myringoscope (mir·**ing**·go·skope). A speculum used in examination of the tympanic membrane; an aural speculum. [myringa, Gk *skopein* to watch.]

myringotome (mir·**ing**·go·tome). A type of knife used for incision of the tympanic membrane. [myringa, Gk *temnein* to cut.]

myringotomy (mir·ing·**got**·o·me). Incision of the tympanic membrane. [see prec.]

myrinx (**mir**·inx). The tympanic membrane. [myringa, Gk *menigx* membrane.]

Myristica (mi·**ris**·tik·ah). 1. A genus of tropical trees of the family Myristicaceae. 2. Nutmeg; the dried kernel of the seeds of *Myristica fragrans* Houtt. [L nutmeg.]

myristicene (mi·**ris**·tis·een). $C_{10}H_{14}$, an elaeoptene obtained from nutmeg oil. [see foll.]

myristicin (mi·**ris**·tis·in). 4-Allyl-6-methoxy-1,2-methylene dioxybenzene, a crystalline compound occurring in nutmeg oil. It is toxic, producing convulsions. [L *myristica* nutmeg.]

myrobalan (mi·**rob**·al·an). The dried immature fruits of *Terminalia chebula* Retz. (family Combretaceae). They contain from 20 to 30 per cent of a mixture of gallic and tannic acids, also a greenish oleoresin. The drug is used as an equivalent of gall in India, having an astringent action externally; internally, notwithstanding the large tannin content, it has a purgative action. [Gk *myron* ointment, *balanos* nut.]

myronate (**mi**·ron·ate). A salt of myronic acid. **Potassium myronate.** Sinigrin, the glucoside of black mustard.

Myrorphine (mi·**ror**·feen). BP Commission approved name for the myristoyl ester of benzylmorphine, a modified morphine with enhanced antitension activity.

myrosin (**mi**·ro·sin). An enzyme occurring in mustard seeds and horseradish root. It activates the hydrolysis of the glucosides, sinalbin and sinigrin. [Gk *myron* ointment.]

Myrrh BPC 1968 (mer). An oleo gum resin from *Commophora molmol.* Employed most frequently as the tincture, which has some antiseptic action, it is commonly used in mouth-washes and with purgatives as a carminative. The tincture consists of 20 per cent of myrrh in alcohol. [Gk *myrra.*]

myrtenol (**mir**·ten·ol). $C_{10}H_{16}O$, a terpene alcohol obtained from the Dutch myrtle, *Myrtus communis*, which also contains pinene and cineole.

myrtol (**mer**·tol). A fraction obtained from the volatile oil of the Dutch myrtle, *Myrtus communis*, distilling between 166° and 180°C. It has been recommended as an antiseptic and as a stimulant to the pulmonary and urogenital mucous membranes, and is used in bronchitis, cystitis and pyelitis.

mysophilia (mis·o·**fil**·e·ah). A pathological interest in filth or dirt, sometimes for sexual arousal. [Gk *mysos* anything that causes disgust, *philein* to love.]

mysophobia (mis·o·**fo**·be·ah). A morbid dread of faeces or any foul or dirty substance, or of coming in contact with them. [Gk *mysos* anything that causes disgust, phobia.]

mytacism (**mi**·tas·izm). The frequent but incorrect use of the *m* sound in speech. [Gk *mytakismos* fondness for the letter μ.]

mythomania (mith·o·**ma**·ne·ah). An inclination to exaggerate or to be untruthful. [Gk *mythos* legendary tale, mania.]

mythophobia (mith·o·**fo**·be·ah). An unnatural fear of making an untruthful statement. [Gk *mythos* legendary tale, phobia.]

mythoplasty (**mith**·o·plas·te). Hysteria. [Gk *mythos* legendary tale, *plassein* to fabricate.]

mytilotoxin (**mit**·il·o·**tox**′·in). $C_6H_{15}NO_2$, a poisonous substance found in mussels. [see foll.]

mytilotoxism (**mit**·il·o·**tox**′·izm). Poisoning as a result of eating mussels. [Gk *mytilos* mussel, *toxikon* poison.]

myxa (**mix**·ah). Mucus. [Gk.]

myxadenitis (**mix**·ad·en·**i**′·tis). Inflammation affecting the mucous glands. **Myxadenitis labialis.** Painless papules on the mucosa of the lip. [Gk *myxa* mucus, adenitis.]

myxadenoma (**mix**·ad·en·**o**′·mah). A tumour of mucous and glandular tissue. [Gk *myxa* mucus, adenoma.]

myxaemia (mix·e·me·ah). Mucinaemia. [Gk *myxa* mucus, *haima* blood.]

myxamoeba (mix·am·e·bah). An amoeboid cell. [Gk *myxa* mucus, amoeba.]

myxangiitis (**mix**·an·je·**i**′·tis). An inflammation of the ducts of a mucous gland. [Gk *myxa* mucus, *aggeion* vessel, *-itis* inflammation.]

myxasthenia (mix·as·the·ne·ah). Deficient secretion of mucus, causing a dryness of the mucous membrane. [Gk *myxa* mucus, asthenia.]

myxidiocy (mix·id·e·o·se). A type of myxoedema that is characterized by imperfect mental development; cretinism. [myxoedema, idiocy.]

myxiosis (mix·e·o·sis). The discharge of mucus. [Gk *myxa* mucus, *-osis* condition.]

myxo-adenoma (mix·o·ad·en·o'·mah). Myxadenoma.

Myxobacteriales (mix·o·bak·teer·e·a'·leez). A class of bacteria commonly found in soil and dung, characterized by a slimy spreading colony. [Gk *myxa* mucus, bacteria.]

myxoblastoma (mix·o·blas·to'·mah). A malignant tumour derived from cells of mucoid connective tissue. [Gk *myxa* mucus, blastoma.]

myxochondrofibrosarcoma (mix·o·kon·dro·fi·bro·sar·ko'·mah). A malignant tumour consisting of mucoid, cartilaginous, fibrous and sarcomatous tissues. [Gk *myxa* mucus, *chondros* cartilage, fibrosarcoma.]

myxochondroma (mix·o·kon·dro'·mah). A tumour containing myxomatous and chondromatous tissues.

myxochondrosarcoma (mix·o·kon·dro·sar·ko'·mah). A malignant tumour consisting of mucoid, cartilaginous and connective tissues. [Gk *myxa* mucus, chondrosarcoma.]

Myxococcus (mix·o·kok·us). A genus of saprophytic soil organisms characterized by fruiting bodies with spherical spores, the whole being enveloped in loose slime. [Gk *myxa* mucus, *kokkos* berry.]

myxocylindroma (mix·o·sil·in·dro'·mah). Cylindroma. [Gk *myxa* mucus, cylindroma.]

myxocystitis (mix·o·sist·i'·tis). Inflammation affecting the mucous coat of the urinary bladder. [Gk *myxa* mucus, cystitis.]

myxocystoma (mix·o·sist·o'·mah). A cystic tumour containing mucoid tissue. [Gk *myxa* mucus, cystoma.]

myxocyte (mix·o·site). A large stellate or polyhedral cell present in mucous tissue. [Gk *myxa* mucus, *kytos* cell.]

myxodermia (mix·o·der·me·ah). An acute condition of ecchymosis, oedematous softening of the skin and contraction of muscles. [Gk *mys* muscle, *derma* skin.]

myxodes (mix·o·deez). Similar to mucus. [Gk *myxa* mucus, *eidos* form.]

myxoedema (mix·e·de·mah). A condition due to hypothyroidism, and characterized by mucoid infiltration of the skin and subcutaneous tissue, dryness of the skin, loss of hair, sensitivity to cold, mental dullness and a low basal metabolic rate. It most often occurs in adults over forty years of age and is more common in women than in men. **Childhood myxoedema.** Juvenile myxoedema (see below). **Circumscribed myxoedema.** A localized and sharply circumscribed condition of the skin, usually over the tibia, found in thyroid disorders, commonly in hyperthyroidism. The skin is thickened, slightly reddened, often hairy, and contains an abnormal amount of mucin. **Congenital myxoedema.** Cretinism. **Infantile myxoedema.** Brissaud's infantilism. **Juvenile myxoedema.** Myxoedema occurring in children, from atrophy of the thyroid which may follow a febrile disease. **Pituitary myxoedema.** Myxoedema secondary to anterior pituitary disease. **Postoperative myxoedema.** Cachexia strumipriva; myxoedema following total ablation of the thyroid as a therapeutic measure in heart disease, or a subtotal thyroidectomy for thyrotoxicosis. **Pretibial myxoedema.** Raised irregular firm bilateral swellings of the skin of the anterolateral aspects of the legs, sometimes extending to the knees and insteps and reaching the back of the legs. The surface is usually dimpled and may be pink or brown but the colour is sometimes unchanged. Hair tends to grow on the infiltrated skin. The condition is associated with thyroid dysfunction, and hypothyroidism or hyperthyroidism. Other evidence of thyrotoxicosis is usually present. The condition may resolve spontaneously, but treatment is unsatisfactory. [Gk *myxa* mucus, *oidema* swelling.]

myxoedematoid (mix·e·deem·at·oid). Similar to myxoedema. [myxoedema, Gk *eidos* form.]

myxoedematous (mix·e·deem·at·us). Referring to or marked by myxoedema.

myxo-enchondroma (mix·o·en·kon·dro'·mah). A chondroma in which there has been degeneration of some of the mucous tissues. [Gk *myxa* mucus, enchondroma.]

myxo-endothelioma (mix·o·en·do·the·le·o'·mah). An endothelioma having some myxomatous elements. [Gk *myxa* mucus, endothelioma.]

myxofibroma (mix·o·fi·bro'·mah). An innocent tumour composed of mucoid and fibrous tissue. [Gk *myxa* mucus, fibroma.]

myxofibrosarcoma (mix·o·fi·bro·sar·ko'·mah). A mixed tumour consisting of mucoid, fibromatous and sacromatous tissues. [Gk *myxa* mucus, fibrosarcoma.]

myxoglioma (mix·o·gli·o'·mah). A glioma, the tissues of which have undergone myxomatous degeneration. [Gk *myxa* mucus, glioma.]

myxoglobulosis (mix·o·glob·ew·lo'·sis). Myxomatous degeneration with the formation of cysts in the appendix. [Gk *myxa* mucus, globule, Gk *-osis* condition.]

myxoid (mix·oid). Mucoid. [Gk *myxa* mucus, *eidos* form.]

myxoinoma (mix·o·in·o'·mah). Myxofibroma. [myxoma, inoma.]

myxolipoma (mix·o·lip·o'·mah). A tumour composed of myxomatous and lipomatous tissue.

myxoliposarcoma (mix·o·lip·o·sar·ko'·mah). A sarcoma rich in mucoid and fatty tissue. [Gk *myxa* mucus, *lipos* fat, sarcoma.]

myxoma (mix·o·mah). An innocent tumour composed of mucous tissue, most frequently found in the subcutaneous tissues of the limbs and neck. **Cardiac myxoma.** A rare jelly-like tumour, containing a large amount of mucoid substance, which develops within the heart; it occurs mostly in the left atrium, in which situation it can simulate mitral valve disease or bacterial endocarditis. **Cystic myxoma.** A myxoma in which softening and liquefaction has produced cysts. **Enchondromatous myxoma.** A myxoma arising within cartilage. **Myxoma fibrosum.** A myxoma undergoing conversion into fibrous tissue. **Infectious myxoma.** Myxomatosis. **Lipomatous myxoma.** A fatty tumour rich in mucoid tissue. **Myxoma sarcomatosum.** Myxosarcoma. **Telangiectatic myxoma.** A myxoma showing large prominent blood vessels and blood spaces. **Vascular myxoma.** A myxoma containing more than the usual number of blood vessels. [Gk *myxa* mucus, *-oma* tumour.]

myxomatosis (mix·o·mat·o'·sis). A virus disease of rabbits, not transmissible to man or other domestic animals. The virus is a poxvirus and is spread mechanically by ectoparasites. Not all rabbits are equally susceptible, *Silrilagus* species show only a mild infection whilst in *Oryctolagus* species (the wild rabbit of UK) initial spread is 99 per cent fatal. Resistant strains of rabbit soon develop, making attempts to control the rabbit population with the virus only partially successful. [myxoma, Gk *-osis* condition.]

myxomatous (mix·o·mat·us). Resembling a myxoma.

Myxomycetes (mix·o·mi·se'·teez). A genus of organisms, the slime moulds, of no medical importance. [Gk *myxa* mucus, *mykes* fungus.]

myxomyoma (mix·o·mi·o'·mah). A tumour composed of myomatous and myxomatous elements.

myxoneuroma (mix·o·newr·o'·mah). Myxoma combined with neuroma.

myxoneurosis (mix·o·newr·o'·sis). Mucous colitis; a neurosis characterized by excessive mucous secretion in the colon. [Gk *myxa* mucus, neurosis.]

myxopapilloma (mix·o·pap·il·o'·mah). A mixed tumour composed of myxomatous and papillomatous elements.

myxopoiesis (mix·o·poi·e'·sis). The production of mucus. [Gk *myxa* mucus, *poiein* to make.]

myxorrhoea (mix·o·re·ah). A discharge of mucus. **Myxorrhoea gastrica.** A condition in which the secretion of mucus in the stomach is abnormally increased. **Myxorrhoea intestinalis.** A mucoid discharge from the bowel occurring in neurotic persons suffering undue mental strain. [Gk *myxa* mucus, *rhoia* flow.]

myxosarcoma (mix·o·sar·**ko**′·mah). A malignant tumour of mucous tissue, arising either as a sarcoma from the beginning, or from malignant change in a myxoma. [Gk *myxa* mucus, sarcoma.]

myxosarcomatous (mix·o·sar·**ko**′·mat·us). Pertaining to or of the nature of a myxosarcoma.

Myxosporidia (mix·o·spo·**rid**′·e·ah). An order of Sporozoa. Most of the described forms are parasites of invertebrates; they develop intracellularly but the life histories are little known. *Encephalitozoon* is the only genus of medical interest. [Gk *myxa* mucus, spiridia.]

myxovirus (mix·o·vi·rus). Strictly, any virus which displays an affinity to the mucoprotein receptors on red cells. Originally the term was used to designate those viruses which agglutinated red blood cells readily, eluted from them through the action of the enzyme neuraminidase and failed to agglutinate red cells which had been treated previously with the enzyme. This definition has proved unsatisfactory as further knowledge has been gained. The viruses are divided into two groups, *orthomyxovirus* (which includes influenza A, B and C) and *paramyxovirus* (para-influenza types 1-4, mumps, and Newcastle disease virus). This classification leaves the position of measles, indistinguishable morphologically from the paramyxovirus group, but with a different haemagglutinin and devoid of neuraminidase, in an anomalous position which has yet to be defined. [Gk *myxa* mucus, virus.]

Myzomyia (mi·zo·**mi**·e·ah). A sub-genus of *Anopheles*. [Gk *myzein* to suck, *myia* fly.]

N

Naboth, Martin (b. 1675). Leipzig physician and anatomist.

Naboth's cyst, follicle, ovule or vesicle, Nabothian cyst. A retention cyst derived from a mucous gland of the neck of the uterus.

Naboth's glands. The mucous glands of the neck of the uterus.

nabothian (nah·**bo**·the·an). Associated with Martin *Naboth.*

nacreous (na·kre·us). Having a lustre and colour like pearl; used to describe certain bacterial colonies. [Fr. *nacre* mother of pearl.]

Nadide (nad·ide). BP Commission approved name for nicotinamide adenine dinucleotide; an antagonist to alcohol and narcotic analgesics.

Naegele, Franz Karl (b. 1778). Heidelberg obstetrician.

Naegele's obliquity. Anterior parietal presentation in which the anterior parietal line of the fetal head presents over the brim of the pelvis. It is sometimes seen in patients with a flat pelvis.

Naegele's pelvis. An obliquely contracted pelvis due to the lack, or imperfect development, of the ala of the sacrum on one side.

Naegele's rule. A rule for calculating the day that labour is due to commence: first day of the last menstrual period less 3 calendar months plus 7 days.

Naegeli, Otto (b. 1843). Zürich physician.

Naegeli's manoeuvre or method. A manoeuvre to control epistaxis in which the patient's head is pushed upwards by placing one hand under the jaw and the other under the occiput.

Naegeli, Otto (b. 1871). Zürich haematologist.

Naegeli's law. A disease in which eosinophilic polymorphonuclear leucocytes are present in numbers greater than half-normal cannot be typhoid fever; the presence of even a few eosinophils may render such a diagnosis uncertain.

Naegeli's leukaemia. A type of monocytic leukaemia said to follow a previous myelogenous leukaemia.

naevi (ne·vi). *See* NAEVUS.

naevocarcinoma (ne·vo·kar·sin·**o**'·mah). A carcinomatous growth formed in a naevus.

naevoid (ne·void). Like a naevus. [naevus, Gk *eidos* form.]

naevolipoma (ne·vo·lip·**o**'·mah). A lipomatous growth formed in a naevus. [naevus, Gk *lipos* fat, *-oma* tumour.]

naevose, naevous (ne·voze, **ne**·vus). Spotted, freckled; marked with naevi.

naevoxantho-endothelioma (ne·vo·zan·tho·en·do·the·le·**o**'·mah). Scattered, hard, yellow nodules appearing on the skin in early infancy, and sometimes familial. The face, extremities, elbows, knees and buttocks are most commonly affected and the nodules usually disappear without leaving scars. [naevus, Gk *xanthos* yellow, endothelioma.]

naevus (ne·vus) (pl. *naevi*). 1. Any birthmark. 2. A haemangioma. 3. Any localized abnormality of developmental origin. **Acanthotic naevus.** 1. A seborrhoeic wart. 2. A hard naevus in which there is hypertrophy of the prickle-cell layer. **Achromic naevus.** A local absence of pigment in flat lesions. **Naevus acneiformis unilateralis.** A band or patch containing large comedones, papules, pustules and scars; it is limited to one side of the body. **Amelanotic naevus.** A soft naevus without pigmentation. **Naevus anaemicus.** A patch of skin paler than the surrounding area, due to local vascular agenesis. **Naevus angiectodes, Angiomatous naevus.** Naevus vascularis (see below). **Naevus aplasticus.** A depressed, smooth, pigmented, hairless area of skin on the forehead or face; it is familial. **Naevus arachnoides, Naevus araneosus, Naevus araneus.** A small red, vascular dilatation from which capillaries radiate, and said to resemble a spider. **Naevus atrophicus.** A naevus with dermal and epidermal atrophy. It may be part of the focal dermal hypoplasia syndrome. **Basal-cell naevus.** A naevus with basal-cell carcinoma histology. **Blue naevus.** A well defined blue papule with pigment cells, deep in the corium. **Blue rubber-bleb naevus.** A rubbery, blue, subcutaneous, cavernous, haemangiomatous naevus, associated with haemangiomata. **Capillary naevus.** Naevus flammeus (see below). **Naevus cavernosus.** A cavernous naevus of which the superficial variety is the strawberry naevus. The deep variety may be circumscribed or diffuse, purple or bluish-black, and may be a lobulated tumour or almost flat. **Cellular naevus.** Soft naevus (see below). **Naevus cerasus.** Strawberry naevus (see below). **Cerebelliform naevus.** A soft amelanotic naevus with shape and surface resembling the cerebellum. **Cerebroid naevus.** A soft, amelanotic naevus with shape and surface resembling the cerebrum. **Comedo naevus.** A developmental abnormality of an area of skin in which the pilosebaceous follicles are filled with horny plugs. **Naevus comedonicus.** 1. Naevus acneiformis unilateralis (see above). 2. Widespread comedones with little or no sign of inflammation. **Compound naevus.** A melanocytic naevus in which the cells are both in the dermis and at the dermo-epidermal junction. **Connective-tissue naevus.** A naevus of collagenous tissue, some of which may take up elastic stains. **Cutaneous naevus.** Strawberry naevus (see below). **Dermo-epidermal naevus.** Junction naevus (see below). **Naevus elasticus.** Connective-tissue naevus (see above). **Naevus elasticus regionis mammariae.** Slightly raised, firm, whitish-yellow lesions on the chest resembling pseudoxanthoma elasticum; it occurs in Scandinavians. **Epidermal naevus, Epithelial naevus.** Hard naevus (see below). **Erectile naevus.** Strawberry naevus (see below). **Faun tail naevus.** Pony tail naevus (see below). **Naevus fibrosus.** A soft, fibrous naevus. **Naevus flammeus.** A diffuse, flat, red or purple angioma, occurring especially on the face. **Naevus flammeus nuchae.** A capillary naevus on the nape of the neck or lower part of the occiput. **Naevus foliaceus.** Naevus flammeus with bright red borders, and lines traversing it arising from a central thicker line. **Naevus follicularis.** A naevus arising from embryonic cells which are the precursors of hair follicles. **Naevus follicularis keratosus.** A band-like naevus with dilated plugged hair follicles and cavities in the corium. **Naevus fragarius.** Strawberry naevus (see below). **Giant naevus.** Any very large naevus. **Naevus gigantosus.** A large mole that may be covered with hair and mamillated; it rarely becomes malignant. **Hair follicle naevus.** Trichofolliculoma. **Hairy naevus.** A mole, usually pigmented, from which many hairs arise. **Halo naevus.** Leucoderma acquisitum centrifugum. **Hard naevus.** Raised lesions consisting of overgrowth of epidermis; it appears during the first year of life. **Hepatic naevus.** Haemorrhagic infarct of the liver. **Honeycomb naevus.** Ulerythema ophryogenes. **Naevus hypertrophicus.** A large naevus with thickening of the skin, which is thrown into folds. **Naevus ichthyosiformis systematisatus.** Naevus unius lateris (see below). **Intradermal naevus.** Cellular mole. *See* MOLE. **Junction naevus.** Usually an almost flat naevus with a deeply pigmented basal layer, and cells arising from dermo-epidermal junction. It is potentially malignant. **Keratoid naevus.** A hard naevus in which the stratum corneum is greatly thickened. **Naevus keratoticus papillomatosus.** Ichthyosis hystrix. **Naevus lichenodes.** A naevus resembling lichen planus, but paler in colour. **Linear naevus, Naevus linearis.** Naevus unius lateris in the form of a streak or band. **Naevus lipomatodes.** A soft naevus in which the infiltrate consists partly of fat cells. **Naevus lupus.** Serpiginous angioma. **Naevus lymphangiectodes, Lymphatic naevus, Naevus lymphaticus.** 1. Mixed haemangiomatous and lymphangiomatous lesions. 2. Lymphangioma circumscriptum. **Naevus maculosus.** A flat pigmented naevus. **Marginal naevus.** Junction naevus (see above). **Mast cell naevus.** An urticating naevus containing mast cells. Blistering may occur, also generalized flushing. **Naevus maternus.** Any birthmark. **Melanocytic naevus.** Any naevus of dermal melanocytes. **Mixed naevus.** 1. A mixed capillary and cavernous haemangioma. 2. A hard naevus in which both horny and prickle-cell layers are hypertrophied. **Naevus molluscum.** A soft pendulous fibroma of the skin. **Naevus morus.** Strawberry naevus (see below). **Multiplex naevus.** Sebaceous naevus (see below). **Naevus nervosus.** Naevus linearis (see above). **Neurofibromatous naevus.** A neurofibroma which is not part of a generalized neurofibromatosis; it is sometimes congenital. **Naevus neuroticus unius lateris.** Naevus linearis (see above). **Oculocutaneous naevus.** A melanocytic naevus of the skin near the eye, with melanocytosis of the iris. **Oral naevus.** A vascular, lymphangiomatous, epithelial or melanocytic naevus within the mouth. **Organoid naevus.** An epithelial naevus differentiating towards glandular, follicular or surface epithelial characteristics. **Pachydermic naevus.** A naevus with much infiltration of the corium, producing an indurated tumour. **Naevus papillaris.** Naevus linearis (see above). **Naevus papillomatosus.** A soft naevus with papillary excrescences. **Paving-stone naevus.** Connective-tissue naevus (see above). **Naevus à pernione.** Angiokeratoma. **Naevus pigmentosus.** Naevus spilus and soft naevus (see below). **Pilose naevus, Naevus pilosus.** A hard or pigmented naevus covered with hair. **Naevus planus.** A flat naevus. **Pony tail naevus.** A tuft of lumbosacral hair. It is often associated with diastematomyelia. **Porcupine naevus.** Ichthyosis hystrix. **Naevus porokeratodes.** A hyperkeratotic naevus unius lateris with punctiform depressions. **Port-wine naevus.** Naevus flammeus (see above). **Naevus profundus.** A deep type of cavernous naevus, especially of the scalp. **Raspberry naevus.** Strawberry naevus (see below). **Naevus sanguineus.** Naevus vascularis (see below). **Naevus sclerodermicus thoracis.** Naevus elasticus regionis mammariae (see above). **Sclerodermoid naevus.** A rare symmetrical disorder starting in infancy; it is characterized by thickened skin with strings of papules and some pigmentation. **Sebaceous naevus.** A naevus consisting of sebaceous-gland tissue, yellow in colour, and occurring most commonly on the scalp. Malignant changes can occur. **Seborrhoeic naevus.** Seborrhoeic wart. *See* WART. **Segmental naevus.** A soft naevus occupying 1 segment of the body. **Soft naevus.** A tumour containing pigment cells in the corium, frequently first appearing in infancy but may occur at any subsequent age; it is usually, but not necessarily, brown; also known as a *mole*. **Spider naevus.** Naevus arachnoides (see above). **Naevus spilus.** Flat brown patches on the skin, usually multiple, and frequently noticed soon after birth. **Naevus spongiosus albus mucosae.** A congenital naevus, white and spongy in appearance with many follicular openings, affecting the mouth, labia, vagina and rectum. **Stellar naevus, Stellate naevus.** Naevus arachnoides (see above). **Strawberry naevus.** A superficial type of cavernous naevus; a raised red angioma appearing in early infancy, often growing rapidly at first but frequently disappearing spontaneously by the age of 5. **Subcutaneous naevus.** A deep variety of cavernous naevus, the overlying skin being of normal colour or blue. **Naevus syringadenomatosus papilliferus.** Firm rose-red papules, some containing vesicles, arranged in groups; it is derived from the sweat glands. **Naevus syringo-adenomatosi.** A lesion clinically resembling naevus unius lateris, but histologically seen to be derived from sweat glands. **Systematized naevus.** Hard naevus (see above). **Naevus tardus.** A naevus that develops late, appearing during adolescence or adult life, but not apparent at birth. **Telangiectatic naevus.** Naevus flammeus (see above). **Naevus unilateralis comedonicus.** Naevus acneiformis unilateralis (see above). **Naevus unius lateris.** A congenital variety of hard naevus confined to one side of the person and occurring in lines or streaks; the lesions are commonly warty. **Naevus vascularis.** Congenital hypertrophy of the vessels of the skin or subcutaneous tissue, which may be capillary, cavernous or mixed. **Naevus vascularis fungosus.** A cavernous haemangioma having bluish-red tumours projecting above the skin in lobulated masses. **Naevus vasculosus.** Naevus vascularis (see above). **Venous naevus.** Naevus cavernosus (see above). **Naevus verrucosus.** 1. Naevus pigmentosus with hyperkeratosis. 2. Warty naevus unius lateris (see above). **Naevus vinosus.** Naevus flammeus (see above). **White sponge naevus.** An oral epithelial naevus. **Woolly hair naevus.** Woolly, closely-coiled hair developing early in life. **Zoniform naevus.** Segmental naevus (see above). [L birthmark.]

See also: PRINGLE (J. J.), SUTTON (R. L.), UNNA.

Nafcillin (naf·sil·in). BP Commission approved name for 6-(2-ethoxy-1-naphthamido)penicillanic acid; an antibiotic.

Nafenopin (naf·en·o·pin). BP Commission approved name for 2 - methyl - 2 - [4 - (1,2,3,4 - tetrahydro - 1 - naphthyl) - phenoxy]-propionic acid; a hypolipidaemic agent.

Naffziger, Howard Christian (b. 1884). San Francisco surgeon.

Naffziger's operation. Orbital decompression by removal of the bony roof with a transfrontal approach; it is used for thyrotropic exophthalmos and exploration.

Naffziger's syndrome. Scalenus syndrome. *See* SYNDROME.

Naffziger's test, for scalenus anticus syndrome. Pressure on the scalenus anterior muscle at the root of the neck causes tingling in the hand.

nafoxidine (naf·ox·i·dine). A diphenyldihydroxnaphthalene derivative with the formula 1 - {2[*p* - (3.4 - dihydro - 6 - methyoxy - 2 - phenyl - 1 - naphthyl) phenoxyl]ethyl} pyrrolidine hydrochloride. It is a synthetic non-steroidal anti-estrogen related structurally to clumiphene and chlorotrianisene. It combines with cytoplasmic oestrogen receptors forming a stable compound and prevents the full action of oestrogen. It has been said to have been used successfully in the treatment of post-menopausal carcinoma of the breast.

Naftazone (naf·taz·one). BP Commission approved name for 1,2-naphthaquinone 2-semicarbazone; a haemostatic agent.

Naftidrofuryl (naf·tid·ro·fewr'·il). BP Commission approved name for 2-diethylaminoethyl 2 - (1 - naphthylmethyl) - 3 - (tetrahydro - 2 - furyl)propionate; a vasodilator.

nagana (na·gah·nah). A disease of wild game and domestic cattle in Africa; caused by *Trypanosoma brucci* and transmitted by tsetse flies, *Glossina.* [Zulu.]

Nageotte, Jean (b. 1866). Paris histologist and pathologist.

Nageotte's bracelets. Transverse bands on which are circular spines found on the axons in a line with the nodes of Ranvier.

Nageotte's cell. A lymphocyte from the cerebrospinal fluid.

Nageotte's radicular nerve. The preganglionic portion of the posterior root of a spinal nerve.

syndrome of Babinski-Nageotte, syndrome of Nageotte-Babinski. Multiple medullary lesions of vascular origin, involving the pyramidal tract, medial lemniscus, restiform body and reticular structures. Clinically, hypotonia, ataxia, lateropulsion, dyssynergia and Horner's syndrome occur on the side of the lesion, and hemiplegia with loss of tactile discrimination and of proprioceptive sensation on the opposite side.

Nagler, F. P. O. 20th century Sydney bacteriologist.

Nagler's reaction. The production of opalescence in human sera by toxin of *Clostridium welchii* due to its lecithinase action. The reaction is specifically inhibited by antiserum.

Naia (nah·yah). A genus of Old World snakes, the cobras. The numerous species are all poisonous, and several frequent the vicinity of human dwellings. **Naia flava.** The Cape cobra. **Naia haie.** The Egyptian cobra or asp. **Naia hannah.** The king cobra or hamadryad, found from India to the Philippines. **Naia melanoleuca.** The black cobra of tropical Africa. **Naia naia.** The common Indian cobra. **Naia nigricollis.** The African black-necked or spitting cobra. [Hind. *nag* snake.]

nail (nale). 1. [Unguis (NA).] The flat horny plate on the dorsal surface of the terminal segment of the finger and toe. 2. A pin of metal or other material used to fix the fragments of a fractured bone. **Nail bed [matrix unguis (NA)].** The corium which underlies the nail; it shows a series of longitudinal ridges, the ridges of the nail bed. **Body of a nail [corpus unguis (NA)].** That part which is exposed on the surface. **Borders of a nail, collateral [margines laterales (NA)].** The sides of the nail. **Border of a nail, free [margo liber (NA)].** The distal projection border. **Border of a nail, hidden [margo occultus (NA)].** The border buried in the skin. **Eggshell nail** (Hyde). Upturning of the free border of the nail, associated with increased translucency of the nail. The condition is seen in erythrocyanosis and vitamin-A deficiency. **Hang nail.** *See* HANGNAIL. **Hippocratic nail.** The enlarged curved nail associated with clubbing of the finger. **Ingrowing nail, Ingrown nail.** Unguis incarnatus. If, through careless paring of a nail, a sharp corner is left at one side, the skin may be pierced, so that a painful wound, sepsis and ulceration may occur. This condition is known as ingrowing nail, and occurs usually on the great toe. **Parrot-beak nail.** A nail curved like a parrot's beak. **Primary nail field.** Anlage of the nail bed in the embryo. **Racket nail.** A short, wide thumb nail growing from a short, wide distal phalanx. **Ram's-horn nail.** Onychogryphosis or Ostlers' toe. **Nail en raquette.** Racket nail (see above). **Reedy nail.** A nail marked with furrows. **Root of a nail [radix unguis (NA)].** The proximal part which is buried in the skin. **Spoon nail.** Koilonychia, an abnormality in which the nail is thin and concave like the bowl of a spoon. The concavity is more marked transversely than longitudinally. **Turtleback nail.** A nail which is curved both laterally and longitudinally. **Nail wall [vallum unguis (NA)].** The fold of skin which borders the sides of the nail. [AS *naegel.*]

See also: KUNTSCHER, SMITH-PETERSEN, STEINMANN.

nailing (na·ling). The surgical fastening of a fractured bone by means of a nail. **Intramedullary nailing, Marrow nailing, Medullary nailing.** The fixation of the two ends of fractured long bone by means of a pin inserted into the medullary cavity of the bone. [see prec.]

naja (nah·jah). Naia.

Najjar, Victor Assad (b. 1914). American paediatrician.

Crigler–Najjar kernicterus. A form of kernicterus not associated with iso-immunization. It appears to be due to a congenital lack of enzymes responsible for the conversion of unconjugated bilirubin into its conjugated form.

Nalorphine (nal·or·feen). BP Commission approved name for *N*-allylnormorphine. **Nalorphine Hydrobromide BP 1973.** A derivative of morphine in which the *N*-methyl group has been replaced by an *N*-allyl group. It antagonizes most of the actions of morphine, and it is a most valuable and effective antidote in the treatment of overdosage with morphine, pethidine, methadone and related compounds; it does not affect depression produced by barbiturates, cyclopropane or any drug not chemically related to morphine. Administered to a normal individual it acts as a depressant of respiration and circulation; injected into a patient under the influence of an overdose of morphine, it dramatically stimulates the respiration and elevates the lowered blood pressure. It has little effect in counteracting the sedation of the patient. It is valuable in counteracting depression in the fetus induced by the administration of morphine or related drugs prior to delivery: recent reports have shown its efficacy in this respect when injected into the umbilical vein of the baby immediately after delivery and before the cord is cut. Given to morphine addicts it will not relieve the withdrawal symptoms, and when it is given after morphine the symptoms and craving immediately return. It is unlikely therefore to have addiction liability.

Naloxone (na·lox·one). BP Commission approved name for (-) - 17 - allyl - 4,5α - epoxy - 3,14 - dihydroxymorphinan - 6 - one, a powerful specific narcotic analgesic antagonist.

namangitis (nam·an·ji·tis). Lymphangitis. [Gk *nama* anything flowing, *aggeion* small vessel, *-itis* inflammation.]

Nandrolone (nan·dro·lone). BP Commission approved name for 19-norandrostenolone, a steroid hormone with tissue-building function; it shows little or no masculinizing action. **Nandrolone Decanoate BP 1973.** 17β-Decanoyloxyoestre-4-en-3-one, a synthetic androgen with actions and uses similar to those of testosterone and methandienone. It is administered intramuscularly as it is inactive when given by mouth. **Nandrolone Phenylpropionate BP 1973.** 17β-(β-Phenylpropionyloxy)oestr-4-en-3-one, an androgenic and anabolic hormone with actions and uses resembling those of testosterone and methandienone, but it is not active when given by mouth; administered by intramuscular injection.

nanism (nan·izm). A condition of abnormal smallness; dwarfism. **Senile nanism.** Progeria. **Symptomatic nanism.** Nanism associated with imperfect bone formation, sexual development and dentition. [Gk *nanos* dwarf.]

See also: PALTAUF.

Nannizzia (nan·iz·e·ah). A genus of Eurotiales. The sexual state of the genus *Microsporum*, a ringworm fungus.

nano-. A prefix indicating that the quantity which follows is to be multiplied by 10^{-9}; thus, a nanogram $= 10^{-9}$ gram. [Gk *nanos*, dwarf.]

nanocephalia (nan·o·kef·a'·le·ah). Abnormal smallness of the head. [see foll.]

nanocephalous (nan·o·kef·al·us). Having an abnormally small head. [Gk *nanos* dwarf, *kephale* head.]

nanocephalus (nan·o·kef·al·us). A fetal monster having an abnormally small or imperfectly developed head. [see prec.]

nanocephaly (nan·o·kef·al·e). Nanocephalia.

nanocormia, nanocormus (nan·o·kor·me·ah, nan·o·kor·mus). A condition in which the trunk or body is extremely small in comparison with the size of the head, arms and legs. [Gk *nanos* dwarf, *kormos* trunk.]

nanocurie (na·no·kewr·e). nCi, 10^{-9}curie. [Gk *nanos* dwarf, curie.]

nanogram (na·no·gram). 10^{-9} gram (ng).

nanoid (nan·oid). Having an undersized body; dwarfish. [Gk *nanos* dwarf, *eidos* form.]

nanomelia (nan·o·me·le·ah). A type of teratism in which the limbs are abnormally small. [see foll.]

nanomelous (nan·om·el·us). Processing abnormally small limbs. [Gk *nanos* dwarf, *melos* limb.]

nanomelus (nan·om·el·us). A fetal monster having underdeveloped or abnormally small limbs. [see prec.]

nanometre (na·no·me·ter). A unit of length, 10^{-9}m. Symbol nm. Equivalent to the obsolescent millimicron. [Gk *nanos* dwarf, *metron* measure.]

nanomol (na·no·mol). 10^{-9}mol (nmol).

nanophthalmus (nan·of·thal·mus). An eye that is congenitally small but has no other abnormality. [Gk *nanos* dwarf, *ophthalmos* eye.]

nanosecond (na·no·sek·ond). One thousand millionth part of a second. [Gk *nanos* dwarf, L *secundus* second.]

nanosomia (nan·o·so·me·ah). A dwarfish state of the body; nanism. **Nanosomia pituitaria.** Progeria. [Gk *nanos* dwarf, *soma* body.]

nanosomus (nan·o·so·mus). A dwarf. [see prec.]

nanous (nan·us). Stunted, dwarfed. [Gk *nanos* dwarf.]

nanukayami (nan·ook·ah·yah'·me). A 7-day fever due to *Leptospira hebdomadis*, occurring in Japan, China and Indonesia. There is severe headache with pains in the back and limbs and pyrexia with a saddle-back course. The field vole, *microtus montebelli*, is believed to be the main carrier. [Jap.]

nanus (nan·us). A dwarf. [Gk *nanos* dwarf.]

nape [nucha (NA)] (nape). The back of the neck. [ME.]

Naphazoline (naf·az·o·leen). BP Commission approved name for 2-(1-naphthylmethyl)-2-imidazoline. A compound used as a nasal spray in asthma and congestion of the nasal mucous membranes; it has a prolonged vasoconstrictor action. Its constant use reduces its effectiveness. The official preparation is Naphazoline Nitrate BP 1958. **Naphazoline Hydrochloride BP**

1968. The hydrochloride of Naphazoline, a vasoconstrictor as potent as adrenaline but, when injected subcutaneously or intramuscularly, it does not cause prolonged vasoconstriction. It is used almost exclusively as a topical application to relieve congestion of the nasal mucosa.

naphtha (**naf**·thah). A mixture of hydrocarbons obtained by fractionating petroleum benzine. There are 2 fractions: *mineral naphtha* (boiling range from 70° to 95°C) and *petroleum naphtha* (boiling range from 90° to 120°C). **Naphtha aceti.** Ethyl acetate. **Naphtha vitrioli.** Ether. **Wood naphtha.** Crude methyl alcohol from the destructive distillation of wood. [Gk.]

naphthalan (**naf**·thal·an). A greenish-black soft mass obtained by fractionally distilling the naphtha obtained from the Armenian highlands. It is soluble in fats and oils but not in water, and has a use in skin diseases.

naphthalene (**naf**·thal·een). $C_{10}H_8$, a white crystalline hydrocarbon obtained as a by-product in the manufacture of coal gas. It has been employed as an ointment (10 per cent) to treat scabies and pediculosis, and as a vermifuge. It is incorporated in antimoth preparations.

naphthamine (**naf**·tham·een). Hexamethylenetetramine.

naphthol (**naf**·thol). $C_{10}H_7OH$, a crystalline compound occurring in coal tar in 2 isomeric forms, α and β-naphthols. **Alpha naphthol.** A substance with phenolic character, said to have antiseptic properties greater than β-naphthol, but more irritant when given internally. It is employed in the furfural test for sugars (Molisch), for proteins containing guanidine groupings, e.g. arginine (Sakaguchi), and in the testing of urine for indoxyl. **Beta naphthol.** A more powerful antiseptic than phenol and less toxic. It has been used in ointments and lotions to treat scabies, psoriasis and eczema; it has also been used as a vermifuge in ancylostomiasis.

naphtholate (**naf**·thol·ate). Any compound formed from naphthol by the substitution of a basic atom or group for the hydrogen of the hydroxyl radical, e.g. $C_{10}H_7OK$. Naphtholates are analogous with the phenates.

naphtholism (**naf**·thol·izm). Chronic naphthol poisoning.

naphthopyrine (naf·tho·**pi**·reen). A loose compound of β-naphthol and phenazone, used as an antiseptic.

naphthoquinone (naf·tho·**kwin**·one). Dihydrodiketonaphthalene, $C_6H_4(CO)_2(CH)_2$. The α- or 1,4-isomer is the parent of the synthetic vitamin-K analogues. Vitamins K_1 and K_2 are derivatives of 2-methyl-1,4-naphthaquinone, which is itself a potent K vitamin (menaphthone).

naphthoresorcin (**naf**·tho·res·**or**′·sin). A loose compound of β-naphthol and resorcinol, used as an antiseptic.

naphthosalicin (naf·tho·**sal**·is·in). A loose compound of β-naphthol and salicin, used as an antiseptic.

naphthyl (**naf**·thil). The radical $C_{10}H_7$– which occurs in naphthol. **Naphthyl alcohol.** Naphthol. **Naphthyl benzoate.** Betanaphthol benzoate, benzonaphthol, $C_6H_5COOC_{10}H_7$, a white compound formed from β-naphthol and benzoyl chloride. **Naphthyl blue.** A safranine dyestuff. **Naphthyl ether.** One of a series of alkyl ethers used in perfumery. **Naphthyl lactate.** $CH_3CHOHCOOC_{10}H_7$, an intestinal antiseptic. **Naphthyl phenol.** Naphthol. **Naphthyl salicylate.** Betol, β-naphthyl salicylic ether, $C_{10}H_7OCOC_6H_4OH$, an intestinal antiseptic and antirheumatic.

naphthylpararosaniline (**naf**·thil·par·ah·ro·**zan**′·il·een). Isamine blue. A dye substance which has been used in the treatment of malignant growths in animals. It has also been used in human carcinoma, but without encouraging results. [naphthyl, Gk *para*, rosaniline.]

Napier, Lionel Everard (b. 1888). British physician in India.

Napier's aldehyde test. A serum test for kala-azar.

napiform (**nap**·e·form). Turnip-shaped. [L *napus* turnip, form.]

naprapath (**nap**·rah·path). One who practises naprapathy.

naprapathy (nap·**rap**·ath·e). A system of manipulative therapy based on the belief that most diseases are the result of contracted ligaments in the spine or pelvis. [Czech *napravit* to correct, Gk *pathos* disease.]

Naproxen (nap·**rox**·en). BP Commission approved name for (+)-2-(6-methoxy-2-naphthyl)propionic acid; an anti-inflammatory, analgesic and antipyretic agent.

Narath, Albert (b. 1864). Heidelberg surgeon.

Narath's hernia. Femoral hernia complicating congenital dislocation of the hip.

Narath's operation. Fixation of the omentum in the abdominal wall to encourage venous collateral circulation in portal obstruction.

narceine (**nar**·se·een). $C_{23}H_{27}O_8N$, an alkaloid related to narcotine and belonging to the isoquinoline group; it is found in opium. It has properties similar to those of papaverine but is little used in therapeutics.

narcism (**nar**·sizm). Narcissism.

narcissism (nar·**sis**·izm). 1. Love of self that is sexual in character; sexual attraction on the part of an individual to his or her own body and voluptuous excitement induced by the observation of it unclothed. 2. A state in which the individual is paramountly interested in, and considers every external happening only in its relation to, himself or herself. [*Narcissus*, in Greek mythology, a beautiful youth who fell in love with his own face mirrored in water and was changed into the flower that bears his name.]

narcissistic (nar·sis·**is**·tik). Pertaining to or characterized by narcissism.

narco-anaesthesia (**nar**·ko·an·es·**the**′·ze·ah). Basal narcosis. *See* NARCOSIS. [Gk *narke* stupor, anaesthesia.]

narco-analysis (**nar**·ko·an·**al**′·is·is). A term invented by Horsley to describe a psychotherapeutic technique, in which, by the administration (usually by intravenous injection) of a narcotic drug, the patient is put into a soporose state before being brought to discuss matters which will cause him emotional distress. [narcosis, analysis.]

narcodiagnosis (**nar**·ko·di·ag·**no**′·sis). Narco-analysis. [narcosis, diagnosis.]

narcohypnia (**nar**·ko·**hip**·ne·ah). A feeling of general bodily numbness on awakening. [Gk *narke* stupor, *hypnos* sleep.]

narcohypnosis (**nar**·ko·hip·**no**′·sis). Hypnotism in which a narcotic drug is used. [see prec.]

narcolepsy (**nar**·ko·lep·se). A condition of unknown cause characterized by a periodic uncontrollable tendency to fall asleep. Sometimes associated with cataplexy. [Gk *narke* stupor, *lambanein* to seize.]

narcoleptic (nar·ko·**lep**·tik). An individual who is subject to narcolepsy.

narcoma (nar·**ko**·mah). A condition of stupor which is the result of the administration of narcotics. [Gk *narke* stupor.]

narcomania (nar·ko·**ma**·ne·ah). 1. An ungovernable craving for narcotics. 2. Alcoholic psychosis. 3. A condition of insanity marked by symptoms of stupor. [Gk *narke* stupor, mania.]

narcomaniac (nar·ko·**ma**·ne·ak). An individual who is subject to narcomania.

narcomatous (nar·**ko**·mat·us). Referring to, characterized by, or suffering from narcoma.

narcopepsia, narcopepsis (nar·ko·**pep**·se·ah, nar·ko·**pep**·sis). A sluggish digestion. [Gk *narke* stupor, *peptein* to digest.]

narcose (**nar**·koze). In a stuporous condition. [Gk *narke* stupor.]

narcosis (nar·**ko**·sis). Stupor produced by drugs and tending to insensibility and paralysis. **Basal narcosis, Basis narcosis.** A complete unconsciousness induced as a preliminary to the establishment of surgical anaesthesia. **Electric narcosis.** Electronarcosis. **Intravenous narcosis.** Narcosis produced by intravenous injection of a drug. **Prolonged narcosis.** A therapeutic measure for neuroses in which the patient is kept under the influence of hypnotics for a long time. **Rausch narcosis.** Ether rausch. *See* RAUSCH. [Gk *narkosis* a benumbing.]

narcosomania (nar·**ko**·so·**ma**′·ne·ah). A morbid craving to be in a narcotic state. [narcosis, mania.]

narcospasm (**nar**·ko·spazm). A spasmodic condition associated with stupor. [narcosis, spasm.]

narcostimulant (nar·ko·**stim**·ew·lant). Possessing narcotic and stimulant qualities.

narcosynthesis (nar·ko·**sin**·thes·is). A form of treatment in psychiatry, in which the personality is built up again with the aid of psychotherapy during and after narcosis produced by the intravenous injection of drugs. [narcosis, synthesis.]

narcotic (nar·**kot**·ik). 1. A drug that induces a stuporous condition or sleep. 2. Having the power to induce stupor or sleep. [Gk *narke* stupor.]

narcotine (**nar**·kot·een). $C_{22}H_{23}O_7N$, an alkaloid occurring in opium as a laevorotatory isomer; the inactive form has been synthesized and named *gnoscopine.* It resembles papaverine in action, but is no longer used in therapeutics. [Gk *narke* stupor.]

narcotism (**nar**·kot·izm). 1. The stuporous condition induced by the use of a narcotic. 2. Narcotic addiction.

narcotize (**nar**·kot·ize). To subject to the influence of narcotic drugs; generally refers to laboratory animals.

narcous (**nar**·kus). Narcose.

nard (nard). Nardus root. *See* ROOT. [Gk *nardos* nard.]

Nardostachys (nar·**dos**·tak·is). 1. A genus of plants of the family Valerianaceae. 2. Nardus root. *See* ROOT. [Gk *nardos* nard, *stachys* spike.]

Naregamia (nah·re·**ga**·me·ah). 1. A genus of trees of the family Meliaceae. 2. Goanese ipecacuanha; the root of *Naregamia alata*, a tree of Western India, containing an alkaloid. It has been employed as an emetic, as a hepatic stimulant and as an expectorant. [East Ind.]

naris (**na**·ris) (pl. *nares*). A nasal opening; a nostril. **Anterior naris.** A nostril. **Posterior naris [meatus nasopharyngeus (NA)].** The opening of the nasal cavity into the nasopharynx. [L.]

narry (**nah**·re). Alcoholic gastritis in Mongolians.

nasal (**na**·zal). Referring to the nose. [L *nasus* nose.]

nasal arteries. Lateral, posterior and septal nasal arteries [arteriae nasales, posteriores, laterales, et septi (NA)]. Branches of the sphenopalatine artery to the septal and side walls of the nose. They enter the nose through the sphenopalatine foramen.

nasal bone [os nasale (NA)]. One of a pair of small bones forming the bridge of the nose and articulating with each other, and with the frontal bone, the maxilla, the ethmoid bone and the lower nasal cartilage.

nasal muscle [musculus nasalis (NA)] (**na**·zal musl). [Pars alaris] a small muscle arising from the maxilla and inserted into the alar cartilage of the nose; the dilator naris muscle. [Pars transversa] a muscle attached to the maxilla between the canine fossa and the nasal notch, and joined by an expanding aponeurosis over the cartilaginous portion of the nose.

nasal veins, external [venae nasales externae (NA)]. Tributaries of the anterior facial vein.

nasalis (na·**za**·lis). A small muscle arising from the maxilla and inserting into the skin over the bridge of the nose. [L *nasus* nose.]

nascent (**nas**·ent). 1. Being born; beginning to exist. 2. Incipient. 3. In chemistry, describing an element in an active form at the stage when it is becoming freed from a compound. [L *nascens.*]

nasiform (**na**·ze·form). Resembling a nose in shape. [L *nasus* nose, form.]

nasio-alveolar (**na**·ze·o·al·**ve**′·o·lar). In craniometry, relating to the distance between the nasion and the alveolar point.

nasiobregmatic (**na**·ze·o·breg·**mat**′·ik). In craniometry, relating to the distance between the nasion and the bregma.

nasio-inial (**na**·ze·o·**in**′·e·al). In craniometry, relating to the distance between the nasion and the inion.

nasion (**na**·ze·on). In craniometry, the midpoint of the depression where the nasal bones join the frontal bones. [L *nasus* nose.]

nasitis (na·**zi**·tis). An inflammation of the nose. [L *nasus* nose, Gk *-itis* inflammation.]

Nasmyth, Alexander (d. 1847). Scottish dental surgeon in London.

Nasmyth's cuticle or membrane. The atrophied remains of the enamel organ attached to the surface of the enamel of a newly formed tooth.

naso-antral (na·zo·**an**·tral). Relating or belonging to the nose and the maxillary sinus. [L *nasus* nose, antrum.]

naso-antritis (**na**·zo·an·**tri**′·tis). Inflammation affecting the mucous membrane of the nose and of the maxillary sinus. [L *nasus* nose, antrum, Gk *-itis* inflammation.]

naso-aural (na·zo·**aw**·ral). Relating or belonging to both the nose and ear. [L *nasus* nose, *auris* ear.]

nasobuccal (na·zo·**buk**·al). Relating or belonging to both the nose and cheek. [L *nasus* nose, *bucca* cheek.]

nasobuccopharyngeal (**na**·zo·buk·o·far·**in**′·je·al). Relating or belonging to the nose, cheek and pharynx. [L *nasus* nose, *bucca* cheek, pharynx.]

nasociliary (na·zo·**sil**·e·ar·e). Having to do with the nose and the eyelids. [L *nasus* nose, *cilium* eyelid.]

nasociliary nerve [nervus nasociliaris (NA)]. A branch of the ophthalmic nerve which runs on the medial side of the orbit and thence to the nose. It supplies the mucous membrane and skin of the nose and paranasal sinuses, and carries sensory fibres to the eye, some of which run through the ciliary ganglion.

communicating branch with the ciliary ganglion [ramus communicans cum ganglione ciliari (NA)]. A branch of the nasociliary nerve to the ciliary ganglion.

nasocular (naze·**ok**·ew·lar). Relating or belonging to the nose and eye. [L *nasus* nose, *oculus* eye.]

naso-endoscope (na·zo·**en**·do·skope). An instrument used in examination of the nasal cavity; it is equipped with its own illumination and a magnifying lens which is passed through the anterior naris. [L *nasus* nose, endoscope.]

naso-endoscopy (**na**·zo·en·**dos**′·ko·pe). A method of examining the nasal cavity and postnasal space by means of the naso-endoscope. [L *nasus* nose, endoscope.]

nasofrontal (na·zo·**frun**·tal). Relating or belonging to the nose and the frontal bones. [L *nasus* nose, frontal.]

nasofrontal vein [vena nasofrontalis (NA)]. A communicating channel linking the superior ophthalmic vein with the commencement of the angular branch of the facial vein.

nasograph (**na**·zo·graf). An instrument for determining the patency of the nose. [L *nasus* nose, Gk *graphein* to record.]

nasolabial (na·zo·**la**·be·al). Relating or belonging to the nose and lip. [L *nasus* nose, *labium* lip.]

nasolabialis (**na**·zo·la·be·**a**′·lis). The medial band of muscular fibres of the orbicularis oris muscle connecting the upper lip to the back of the nasal septum. [see prec.]

nasolacrimal (na·zo·**lak**·rim·al). 1. Relating or belonging to the nose and the lacrimal apparatus. 2. Referring to the nasal and lacrimal bones. **Nasolacrimal duct.** *See* DUCT. **Nasolacrimal groove.** *See* GROOVE. [L *nasus* nose, *lacrima* tear.]

nasology (naze·**ol**·o·je). The branch of science that deals with the study of noses. [*nasus* nose, Gk *logos* science.]

nasomalar (na·zo·**ma**·lar). Relating or belonging to the nose and the zygomatic (malar) bone. [L *nasus* nose, malar.]

nasomanometer (**na**·zo·man·**om**′·et·er). A means of measuring the changes in pressure in the nasal passages during nasal breathing. [L *nasus* nose, Gk manos rare, meter.]

naso-occipital (**na**·zo·ok·**sip**′·it·al). In craniometry, relating or belonging to the nose and the occiput. [L *nasus* nose, occiput.]

nasopalatine (na·zo·**pal**·at·ine). Belonging to the nose and the palate. [L *nasus* nose, palatine.]

nasopalpebral (na·zo·**pal**·pe·bral). Relating or belonging to the nose and the eyelids. [L *nasus* nose, *palpebra* eyelid.]

nasopharyngeal (**na**·zo·far·**in**′·je·al). Relating or belonging to the cavity of the nose and the nasal part of the pharynx. [L *nasus* nose, pharynx.]

nasopharyngitis (**na**·zo·far·in·**ji**′·tis). Inflammation involving the mucous membrane of the nasal part of the pharynx. [L *nasus* nose, pharyngitis.]

nasopharyngoscope (**na**·zo·far·**ing**′·go·skope). An instrument for inspecting the nasopharynx. [nasopharynx, Gk *skopein* to view.]

nasopharynx (na·zo·**far**·ingx). The nasal part of the pharynx.

nasorostral (na·zo·**ros**·tral). Pertaining to the nose and the rostrum of the sphenoid bone. [L *nasus* nose, rostrum.]

nasoscope (**na**·zo·skope). A rhinoscope, generally with electrically illuminated nasal speculum, used for inspection of the cavity of the nostril. [L *nasus* nose, Gk *skopein* to watch.]

nasoseptal (na·zo·**sep**·tal). Referring to the septum of the cavity of the nose. [L *nasus* nose, septum.]

nasosinusitis (na·zo·si·nus·i′·tis). Inflammation affecting the paranasal sinuses and the lining membrane of the nares. [L *nasus* nose, sinusitis.]

nasospinale (na·so·spi·**na**′·le). A point obtained by bisecting the line joining the lower margins of the nasal aperture. [L *nasus* nose, spine.]

Nasse, Christian Friedrich (b. 1778). German physician.

Nasse's law. A law formulated by Nasse (1820) on the familial inheritance of haemophilia via the female.

nastin (nas·tin). A preparation made by the ether extraction of an acid-fast streptothrix and formerly used in attempts to produce immunity to leprosy. [Gk *nastos* solid.]

nasus (na·zus). The nose. **Nasus cartilagineus.** The cartilaginous part of the nose. **Nasus incurvus.** Saddlenose. *See* NOSE. **Nasus osseus.** The bony portion of the nose. [L.]

nasute (na·zewt). 1. Having a large or long nose. 2. Having a keen sense of smell. 3. In zoology, having the nostrils prominent and sheathed. [L *nasus* nose.]

natal (na·tal). 1. Of or referring to birth. [L *natus* birth.] 2. Referring to the gluteal region. [L *nates* buttocks.]

natality (na·tal·it·e). The birth rate, i.e. the number of registered births per thousand of the population. [L *natalis* concerning birth.]

nataloin (nat·al·o·in). A name sometimes given to aloin derived from Natal aloes.

Natamycin (na·tah·**mi**·sin). BP Commission approved name for an antibiotic produced by *Streptomyces natalensis*.

nates (na·teez). 1. The buttocks. 2. The superior quadrigeminal bodies of the mid-brain. [L.]

natiform (na·te·form). Shaped like the buttocks. [L *nates* buttocks, form.]

natimortality (na·te·mor·**tal**′·it·e). The stillbirth rate. This is estimated by taking for any one year the number of stillbirths, multiplying this number by 1000 and dividing by the number of total births (live and still) for that year. This gives the proportion of stillbirths to the total birth rate. [L *natus* birth, mortality.]

National Health Service (Reorganisation) Act 1973. This Act drastically amends or repeals previous legislation and gives effect to the following policies, namely (*a*) to unify the local administration of the National Health Service under new Regional and Area Health Authorities covering the whole field of health care, (*b*) to ensure that the views of the health professions are given full weight in the planning and management of services, (*c*) to provide means in each area of representing the interests of the community, (*d*) to provide for collaboration between National Health Service and the services for which local authorities are responsible, and between the National Health Service and voluntary organisations, (*e*) to provide for the establishment of Health Service Commissioners to investigate complaints against Health Service Authorities. By virtue of the Act it is the duty of the Secretary of State to provide hospital accommodation, medical, dental and nursing services, other faculties for the care of expectant and nursing mothers and young children, facilities for the prevention of illness, the care of persons suffering from illness, the care of persons suffering from illness and their aftercare, such other services as are required for the diagnosis and treatment of illness and advice on contraception.

National Health Service (Vocational Training) Act 1976. The purpose of this Act is to tighten the entry requirement for becoming a general practitioners principal in the National Health Service by introducing a period of compulsory post-registration vocational training.

National Insurance (Industrial Injuries) Acts 1965–1974. *See* SOCIAL SECURITY ACT 1975.

Nativelle, Charles Adolph (fl. 1872). Paris chemist.

Nativelle's digitalin. A crystalline preparation of digitalis glycosides, probably chiefly digitoxin.

natraemia (nat·**re**·me·ah). The presence of excess of sodium in the blood. [L *natrium* sodium, Gk *haima* blood.]

natri (nah·tre). A popular indigenous medicine of Chile, made from the leaves and shoots of several species of *Solanum*.

natrium (nat·re·um). Sodium. **Natrii aminosalicylas.** *European Pharmacopoeia* name for Sodium Aminosalicylate BP 1973. **Natrii chloridum.** *European Pharmacopoeia* name for Sodium Chloride BP 1973. **Natrii hydrogenocarbonas.** *European Pharmacopoeia* name for Sodium Bicarbonate BP 1973. **Natrii iodidum.** *European Pharmacopoeia* name for Sodium Iodide BP 1973. **Natrii phosphas.** *European Pharmacopoeia* name for Sodium Phosphate BP 1973. **Natrii sulfas decahydricus.** *European Pharmacopoeia* name for Sodium Sulphate BP 1973. [L.]

natriuresis (nat·re·ewr·**e**′·sis). Marked sodium glomerular filtration, occasionally present with greatly increased diuresis following relief of urinary obstruction. [L *natrium* sodium, Gk *ouresis* urination.]

natron (nat·ron). A naturally occurring sodium sesquicarbonate, $Na_2CO_3NaHCO_3 \cdot 2H_2O$, found in deposits in California, Egypt and East Africa.

naturopath (na·cher·o·path). One who practises naturopathy.

naturopathic (na·cher·o·**path**′·ik). Referring to naturopathy; by means of naturopathy.

naturopathy (na·cher·**op**·ath·e). A form of therapy which excludes medicinal and surgical agents and depends entirely on natural forces, such as light, water, air, heat, massage. [L *natura* nature, Gk *pathos* disease.]

Naunyn, Bernhard (b. 1839). Strasbourg physician.

Naunyn's sign. Tenderness on deep pressure below the margin of the right ribs at the edge of the epigastrium, in cholecystitis.

nausea (naw·se·ah). A feeling of sickness with a desire to vomit. **Creatic nausea.** A dislike of the use of flesh for food. **Epidemic nausea.** A condition characterized by vomiting, giddiness, diarrhoea and nausea, and occurring in epidemic form. **Nausea gravidarum.** The morning sickness of pregnancy. **Nausea marina, Nausea navalis.** Seasickness. [Gk *nausia* seasickness.]

nauseant (naw·se·ant). 1. Producing nausea; nauseating. 2. An agent that induces nausea.

navel (na·vel). The umbilicus. **Blue navel.** Bluish discoloration around the umbilicus, considered as diagnostic of ruptured ectopic pregnancy. **Enamel navel.** A depression where the enamel septum meets the external epithelium of the enamel organ of a dental germ. [AS *nafela*.]

navicular (nav·**ik**·ew·lar). 1. Shaped like a boat; scaphoid. 2. The navicular bone of the tarsus or the scaphoid bone of the carpus. [L *navicula* small boat.]

navicular bone [os naviculare (NA)]. An irregular tarsal bone situated on the medial side of the foot, between the talus and the 3 cuneiform bones.

naviculocuboid (nav·**ik**·ew·lo·**kew**′·boid). Relating or belonging to the navicular and the cuboid bones of the foot.

naviculocuneiform (nav·**ik**·ew·lo·kew·**ne**′·e·form). Relating or belonging to the navicular and the cuneiform bones.

naviculoid (nav·**ik**·ew·loid). Scaphoid. [L *navicula* small boat, Gk *eidos* form.]

Nealbarbitone BP 1968 (ne·al·**bar**·bit·one). 5-Allyl-5-neopentylbarbituric acid; a sedative drug of the barbiturate group with actions and uses comparable with those of phenobarbitone.

near-point (neer·point). 1. The distance from the eye to the nearest point at which the eye can see minute detail clearly. This can be measured in fractions of a metre, or the reciprocal can be used, in which case the measurement is in dioptres, e.g. 10 cm, 1/10 metre or 10 D. 2. The maximum accommodative power of the eye. **Convergence near-point.** Relative near-point (see foll). **Relative near-point.** The nearest point to which the eyes can accommodate without converging. This is a hypothetical point, and represents the reciprocal of the dioptric power of concave lenses which the eyes will tolerate without blurring or doubling of the images. [AS *neah,* point.]

nearthrosis (ne·ar·**thro**·sis). False joint. [Gk *neos* new, *arthron* joint.]

nebenagglutinin (**na**·ben·ag·**loo**′·tin·in). A non-specific agglutinin. [G *neben* near, agglutinin.]

nebenkern (**na**·ben·**kern**′). An old name for the paranucleus. [G.]

nebula (**neb**·ew·lah). 1. A spray; usually a medicament in an oily, aqueous or alcoholic solution, applied to the throat or nose by means of an atomizer. Adrenaline, ephedrine and atrophine are the more usual ingredients. 2. A faint or slight corneal opacity. **Nebula frontalis.** Hyperostosis frontalis interna. [L mist.]

nebulization (**neb**·ew·li·**za**′·shun). 1. Atomization. 2. Treatment by means of a spray. [see foll.]

nebulize (**neb**·ew·lize). To reduce to a delicate spray. [L *nebula* mist.]

nebulizer (**neb**·ew·li·zer). An atomizer. [see prec.]

Necator (nek·**a**·tor). A genus of hookworms. **Necator americanus.** The American hookworm, the commonest species of hookworm throughout the tropics and probably African in origin. The adults live in the small intestine feeding on the host's blood from the mucous wall. The eggs pass out in faeces and the larvae develop in the surface layers of the soil. The larvae infect man by burrowing through the intact skin: they pass in the blood stream to the lungs, from whence they migrate subsequently to the intestine. Man is the true host but monkeys can be infected. **Necator suillus.** A species found in pigs in Africa; it may be only a form of *Necator americanus* (see above). [L murderer.]

necatoriasis (nek·a·tor·i′·as·is). Infestation with a parasite of the genus *Necator.*

neck (nek). 1. [Collum (NA)] That part of the body which connects the head with the trunk; [cervix (NA)] any narrow part of a structure which lies between and connects 2 other parts. 2. A constriction. **Bull neck.** Cervical lymphadenitis and/or cellulitis. **Derbyshire neck.** Endemic goitre. *See* GOITRE. **Limber neck.** A disease of chickens in which they droop in the neck. **Nithsdale neck.** Goitre. **Ricked neck.** A sprain of the muscles and ligaments of the neck. **Wry neck.** Torticollis. [AS *hnecca.*]

See also: MADELUNG.

neck, anterior cutaneous nerve of the [nervus transversus colli (NA)]. A sensory branch of the cervical plexus, deriving its fibres from the 2nd and 3rd cervical nerves, emerging at the posterior border of the sternomastoid muscle and passing anteriorly across the neck to supply the skin on its lateral and anterior parts [rami superiores et inferiores (NA)].

necklace (**nek**·lase). *See* CASAL. **Necklace of Venus.** Syphilitic leucoderma of the neck. [AS *hnecca,* OFr. *laz.*]

necraemia (nek·**re**·me·ah). A condition in which the blood loses its vitality, with marked erythrocytic degeneration and loss of rouleaux formation. [Gk *nekros* dead, *haima* blood.]

necrectomy (nek·**rek**·to·me). 1. Generally, excision of necrotic tissues. 2. In chronic suppuration of the middle ear, removal of necrotic elements acting as sound conductors. [Gk *nekros* dead, *ektome* a cutting out.]

necrencephalus (nek·ren·**kef**·al·us). A condition of softening of the brain. [Gk *nekros* dead, *egkephalos* brain.]

necrobacillosis (**nek**·ro·bas·il·**o**′·sis). Coagulative necrosis of animals caused by *Fusiformis necrophorus.* [Gk *nekros* dead, bacillus, Gk *-osis* condition.]

necrobiosis (**nek**·ro·bi·**o**′·sis). 1. Death of individual cells in the midst of living tissue. 2. Gradual localized death of a part or tissue as the result of retrograde processes or degeneration, e.g. atrophy of an organ. **Necrobiosis lipoidica diabeticorum.** A condition found in diabetic individuals, characterized by the presence of papular elevations on the skin, lipoid deposits and necrobiotic lesions. [Gk *nekros* dead, *biosis* life.]

necrobiotic (**nek**·ro·bi·**ot**′·ik). Referring to or produced by necrobiosis.

necrocytosis (**nek**·ro·si·**to**′·sis). Cellular decay and necrosis. [Gk *nekros* dead, *kytos* cell.]

necrocytotoxin (**nek**·ro·si·to·**tox**′·in). A toxic agent that causes cellular death. [Gk *nekros* dead, *kytos* cell, toxin.]

necrodermatitis (**nek**·ro·der·mat·i′·tis). An inflammatory lesion of the skin with cutaneous gangrene. [Gk *nekros* dead, dermatitis.]

necrogenic, necrogenous (nek·ro·**jen**·ik, nek·**roj**·en·us). Originating in dead material. [Gk *nekros* dead, *genein* to produce.]

necrological (nek·ro·**loj**·ik·al). Relating to necrology.

necrologist (nek·**rol**·o·jist). An individual who is experienced in necrology.

necrology (nek·**rol**·o·je). The science of the collation, grouping and interpretation of mortality statistics. [Gk *nekros* dead, *logos* science.]

necrolysis (nek·**rol**·is·is). Separation of a tissue as a result of its death. **Toxic epidermal necrolysis.** A bullous eruption followed by scald-like shedding of the epidermis in large sheets. It is caused by infections, drugs or other, unknown, causes and healing usually occurs in 2 weeks. [Gk *nekros* dead, *lysis* a loosing.]

necromania (nek·ro·**ma**·ne·ah). 1. An unnatural or insane delight in corpses or in death. 2. A state in which the individual has a morbid attitude towards death and thinks of it with longing. [Gk *nekros* dead, mania.]

necromimesis (**nek**·ro·mim·**e**′·sis). 1. A state of insanity in which the patient believes that he is dead. 2. Imitation of death by an individual who is mentally deranged. [Gk *nekros* dead, *mimesis* imitation.]

necronectomy (nek·ro·**nek**·to·me). Necrectomy.

necroparasite (nek·ro·**par**·ah·site). A saprophyte. [Gk *nekros* dead, parasite.]

necrophagous (nek·**rof**·ag·us). Living on or devouring dead or putrefying flesh; subsisting on carrion. [Gk *nekros* dead, *phagein* to eat.]

necrophile (**nek**·ro·file). One affected with necrophilism.

necrophilism (nek·**rof**·il·izm). 1. Unnatural pleasure in corpses and in being in their presence. 2. Sexual violation of dead bodies. [Gk *nekros* dead, *philein* to love.]

necrophilous (nek·**rof**·il·us). 1. Referring to necrophilism. 2. Feeding on dead matter; necrophagous.

necrophily (nek·**rof**·il·e). Necrophilism.

necrophobia (nek·ro·**fo**·be·ah). 1. Morbid dread of death. 2. Morbid aversion to dead bodies. [Gk *nekros* dead, phobia.]

necrophorus (nek·**rof**·or·us). *Fusiformis necrophorus.* [Gk *nekros* dead, *pherein* to carry.]

necropneumonia (**nek**·ro·new·**mo**′·ne·ah). Gangrene of the lung. [Gk *nekros* dead, *pneumon* lung.]

necropsy (nek·**rop**·se). Post-mortem examination of a body in order to establish the cause of death. [Gk *nekros* dead, *opsis* a viewing.]

necrosadism (nek·ro·**sa**·dizm). Mutilation of a corpse in order to arouse sexual feelings or to achieve sexual gratification. [Gk *nekros* dead, sadism.]

necroscopy (nek·**ros**·ko·pe). Necropsy. [Gk *nekros* dead, *skopein* to watch.]

necrose (nek·**roze**). In a necrotic condition. [Gk *nekros* dead.]

necrosin (**nek**·ro·sin). A substance present in the exudation of wounds which has a proteolytic action. [Gk *nekros* dead.]

necrosis (nek·**ro**·sis). Death of a portion of a tissue. **Anaemic necrosis.** Ischaemic necrosis (see below). **Aseptic necrosis.** The development of cystic and sclerotic degenerative changes in the heads of the femur and humerus after traumatic dislocation of the joint. **Caseous necrosis.** Necrosis in which structures or tissues are changed into a cheesy mass. **Central necrosis.** Death of the central portion of a tissue or organ. **Cheesy necrosis.** Caseous necrosis (see above). **Chemical necrosis.** Necrosis caused by a chemical agent. **Coagulation necrosis, Coagulative necrosis.** Death of a tissue with coagulation of its cells, as in infarction. **Colliquative necrosis.** Necrosis which results in liquefaction of the affected part. **Cystic medial necrosis.** Disease of large arteries in which necrosis of the media occurs with the formation of cysts; Marfan's syndrome. **Decubital necrosis.** Bedsore. **Dental necrosis.** Dental caries. *See* CARIES. **Diphtheri-**

tic necrosis. Necrosis due to infection by *Corynebacterium diphtheriae*, e.g. of the mucous membrane of the larynx which becomes white, tough and leathery, and separated from the underlying tissues. **Dry necrosis.** Necrosis which results in drying and withering of a part. **Embolic necrosis.** Infarction. **Fat necrosis.** Necrosis of adipose tissue. It occurs in the breast and the subcutaneous tissue as the result of trauma or infection, and in the abdominal cavity from the action of pancreatic enzymes released during acute pancreatitis. **Fibrinoid necrosis.** A type of necrosis found in arteries in collagen diseases. **Focal necrosis.** Necrosis that involves small circumscribed areas of tissue. **Hyaline necrosis.** Zenker's degeneration of muscle, as in typhoid fever. **Icteric necrosis.** Necrosis of the liver with jaundice. **Necrosis infantilis.** Pathological cellular disintegration occurring in marasmic infants. **Ischaemic necrosis.** Death of tissue due to the cutting-off of its blood supply. **Liquefaction necrosis, Liquefactive necrosis.** Colliquative necrosis (see above). **Mechanical necrosis.** Necrosis caused by a mechanical agent. **Medial necrosis.** Cystic necrosis of the media of the aorta, often associated with dissecting aneurysm. The aetiology is unknown, but congenital defect is postulated. It should not be confused with necrosis of the media due to syphilis. **Mercurial necrosis.** Death of tissue such as that of the colon or gum, due to mercury poisoning. **Moist necrosis.** Necrosis in which the tissues become soft and wet. **Mummification necrosis.** Dry gangrene. *See* GANGRENE. **Neonatal subcutaneous fat necrosis.** Single or multiple, rubbery or firm subcutaneous nodules or plaques in red or violaceous skin, occurring in otherwise apparently healthy neonates and usually resolving spontaneously. **Nodular subcutaneous fat necrosis.** Multiple subcutaneous nodules, sometimes ulcerative, occurring from blood-stream dissemination of lipolytic enzymes in pancreatitis or in carcinoma of the pancreas. **Peripheral necrosis.** Necrosis of the peripheral parts of the liver lobules. **Phosphorus necrosis.** Necrosis of the maxilla due to exposure to phosphorus fumes. **Physical necrosis.** Necrosis caused by a physical agent. **Pressure necrosis.** Bedsore. **Necrosis progrediens.** Progressive gangrene. *See* GANGRENE. **Progressive emphysematous necrosis.** Gas gangrene. *See* GANGRENE. **Radiation necrosis.** Necrosis caused by local overdosage of radiation. **Radium necrosis.** Death of a circumscribed volume of tissue, due to over-exposure to the rays from radium. **Simple necrosis.** Necrosis uncomplicated by infection, haemorrhage or pigmentation. **Superficial necrosis.** Death of the outer layers of any tissue. **Total necrosis.** Death of a complete structure. **Necrosis ustilaginea.** Dry gangrene caused by ergot poisoning. **X-ray necrosis.** Necrosis caused by local overdosage of x-rays. [Gk *nekros* dead, *-osis* condition.]

See also: BALSER, PAGET, ZENKER (F. A.).

necrospermia (nek·ro·**sper**·me·ah). A condition in which the seminal spermatozoa are not alive; one of the causes of male sterility. [Gk *nekros* dead, sperm.]

necrosteon (nek·**ros**·te·on). Necrosis affecting a bone. [Gk *nekros* dead, *osteon* bone.]

necrotic (nek·**rot**·ik). Marked by or referring to necrosis.

necrotomy (nek·**rot**·o·me). Dissection of a dead body. **Osteoplastic necrotomy.** Sequestrectomy. [Gk *nekros* dead, *temnein* to cut.]

necrotoxin (nek·ro·**tox**·in). A necrotizing toxin produced by certain staphylococci.

necrozoospermia (nek·ro·zo·o·**sper**′·me·ah). Necrospermia. [Gk *nekros* dead, zoospermia.]

Nectandra (nek·**tan**·drah). 1. A genus of tropical trees of the family Lauraceae. 2. Bebeeru bark; the dried trunk bark of *Nectandra rodioei* Hook. It contains the alkaloid bebeerine, and is used as a bitter stomachic and tonic. [Gk *nektar* nectar, *aner* anther.]

nectareous (nek·**ta**·re·us). Applied to any substance or liquid that has a pleasing taste. [Gk *nektareos* like nectar.]

Necturus (nek·**tewr**·us). A genus of large American salamanders. **Necturus maculatus.** The mud puppy, a species used as a laboratory animal. [Gk *nektos* swimming, *oura* tail.]

needle (ne·dl). A sharp instrument used to carry sewing material in sewing, or a sharp hollow tubular instrument along which fluid is withdrawn or injected. Also certain other similar sharply pointed apparatus. **Aneurysm needle.** A handled blunt needle used to pass a ligature round a blood vessel for ligation in continuity. **Aspirating needle.** A long hollow needle used to withdraw fluid from a cavity. **Atraumatic needle.** A round-bodied needle to which a suture is attached in direct continuity. **Boomerang needle.** A handled needle whose sewing end is curved in a half-circle or more. **Butterfly needle.** A needle used for repeated intravenous injections, so-called because of its plastic "wings" to facilitate fixation to the skin. **Cataract needle.** A needle used in removing a cataract. **Cutting needle.** A surgical needle with a cutting edge, so that it penetrates skin readily. **Differentially-loaded radium needle.** A radium needle in which the active material is not uniformly loaded along the length of the needle. **Discission needle.** A form of cataract needle. **Exploring needle.** A long, sharp, hollow needle for blindly seeking an abscess cavity. **Fascia needle.** A needle used to carry a suture of fascia lata in fascial repair of a hernia. **Harelip needle.** A tiny cannula formerly used in the harelip operation to carry sutures. **Hypodermic needle.** A needle for hypodermic injection. **Knife needle.** A slender knife with a needle point used in the cataract operation. **Ligature needle.** Aneurysm needle (see above). **Lumbar-puncture needle.** A long, straight, sharp, hollow needle used in lumbar puncture to withdraw cerebrospinal fluid, or, in spinal anaesthesia, to inject the anaesthetic into the subarachnoid space. **Radium needle.** A radium container in the form of a needle for interstitial irradiation, also used for loading surface and intracavitary applicators. **Round needle.** A needle that is circular in cross-section, and which, like an ordinary sewing needle, has no cutting edge. **Surgical needle.** Any sewing needle used in a surgical operation. **Transfusion needle.** A needle inserted into a vein for the introduction of blood in transfusion. **Ventriculopuncture needle.** A long, hollow needle for aspiration from, or injection into, the cerebellomedullary cisterna of the subarachnoid space. [AS *naedl.*]

See also: BARKER (A. E. J.), BROWNE (D.), CLOQUET (J. G.), DATTNER, EMMET, GALLIE, GORDH, GREENFIELD, HAGEDORN (W.), HOWARD-JONES, LANE (W. A.), MADDOX, OLDFIELD, PANNETT, PITKIN, REVERDIN (A.), SALAH, SAUNDERS (J. C.), SILVERMAN, SINGER, VIM, ZIEGLER.

needling (ne·dling). The puncture or discission of a cataract by a needle.

Neelsen, Friedrich Karl Adolf (b. 1854). Dresden pathologist.

Ziehl–Neelsen method or stain, for *Mycobacterium tuberculosis.* Heat-fixed smears are stained with hot strong carbolfuchsine for 5 min, decolorized with 20 per cent sulphuric acid and 95 per cent alcohol and counterstained with methylene blue or malachite green. Tubercle bacilli stain bright red, all other cells blue or green.

neencephalon (ne·en·**kef**·al·on). That part of the brain which has evolved most recently; usually applied to the cerebral hemisphere. [Obsolete term.] [Gk *neos* new, *egkephalos* brain.]

Nefopam (**nef**·o·pam). BP Commission approved name for 3,4,5,6 - tetrahydro - 5 - methyl - 1 - phenyl - 1*H* - 2,5 - benzoxazocine; a muscle relaxant.

Neftel, William Basil (b. 1830). New York physician of Russian birth.

Neftel's disease. Hysterical inability to walk, stand or sit, without the development of severe discomfort in the head and back and generalized paraesthesia; all movements are freely performed in comfort while lying down.

negative (**neg**·at·iv). 1. The opposite of positive; the absence of a particular quality. 2. The failure to react to a test. 3. In electricity, the cathode which attracts the positive current and repels the negative current. 4. In psychiatry, the attitude of opposition or resistance to suggestions. 5. A photographic image in which the bright parts of the original subject are dark, and *vice versa.* [L *negare* to deny.]

negativism (neg·at·iv·izm). An attitude of contrariness or opposition. **Active negativism.** Negativism in which the individual does the opposite of what he is asked or expected to do. **Passive negativism.** Negativism in which the individual merely fails to do what he is told or expected to do. [see prec.]

negatoscope (neg·at·o·skope). An apparatus consisting of a bright even light to demonstrate radiographs clearly. [negative, Gk *skopein* to view.]

negatron (neg·at·ron). Name given to the negatively charged electron to distinguish it from the positron.

neglect (neg·lekt). Failure to provide attentions or services for persons in need. A more serious offence than negligence may result, in the event of death, in a charge of manslaughter. [L *neglectus.*]

negligence (neg·lij·ens). An act of omission to do something which a reasonable person would ordinarily do, or the doing of something which a reasonable person would not do. [L *neglegentia* carelessness.]

Negri, Adelchi (b. 1876). Pavia pathologist.

Negri body. An intracytoplasmic inclusion body found in cerebral cells in rabies.

Negus, Victor Ewings (b. 1887). London otorhinolaryngologist.

Negus bag. A bag connected with an oesophageal tube through which water can be injected to distend the cardio-oesophageal junction in achalasia [obsolete].

Negus oesophagoscope. An instrument with proximal lighting, oval in cross-section, used for examining the oesophagus.

Neher-Harper quenching circuit. An early, simple form of quenching circuit.

neighbourhood symptoms (nabe·or·hood simp·toms). Of pituitary tumours. Headaches, visual disturbances consisting of loss of vision, bitemporal haemianopia or other signs of pressure on the optic nerves, cranial nerve palsies, hypothalamic syndromes and radiological findings.

Neill, James Maffett (b. 1894). New York bacteriologist.

Van Slyke and Neill method, for the manometric analysis of gases in blood and other solutions. The sample solution is introduced into a specially designed apparatus and the gas or gases to be determined are liberated by treating with a suitable reagent under reduced pressure. The gas volume is then adjusted to a set value and the pressure read from a manometer. The gas is removed by ejection or absorption and the pressure again read at the same gas volume. The difference between the 2 readings gives the partial pressure of the gas at the given volume, from which the gas volume at stp can be calculated.

Neill, Mather Humphrey (b. 1882). American physician.

Neill-Mooser body. The rickettsia of murine typhus seen in the tunica vaginalis exudate of the infected guinea-pig.

Neill-Mooser reaction or test. A guinea-pig inoculation test for differentiating the rickettsiae. The morbid material is injected into the peritoneum; a characteristic severe inflammatory reaction of the scrotum with numerous rickettsia in the exudate indicates that the infection is with the murine or an allied strain.

Neisser, Ernst (b. 1863). Stettin physician.

Neisser-Doering phenomenon. A phenomenon noted when an antihaemolytic substance is present in the blood capable of preventing the normal haemolysis of the red blood corpuscles.

Neisser, Max (b. 1869). Frankfort bacteriologist.

Neisser's staining method, for *Corynebacterium diphtheriae.* Smears are stained with a mixture of methylene blue in acid alcohol (sol. A) and crystal violet (sol. B) for a few seconds, and counterstained with Bismarck brown or chrysoidine for 30 s. The metachromatic (volutin) granules of *Corynebacterium diphtheriae* stain bluish-black, and protoplasm yellow or brown.

Neisser-Wechsberg phenomenon. Deviation of complement; when more specific antibody is added to a mixture of antigen and complement than can be absorbed by the antigen the excess antibody may combine with the complement. This prevents the complement from acting on the antigen-antibody complex.

Neisseria (ni·seer·e·ah). A genus of bacteria, consisting of Gram-negative cocci usually arranged in pairs. All are strict parasites and are often pathogenic; they are sensitive to penicillin. **Neisseria catarrhalis.** A species which grows singly, in pairs or in clumps. It can occur in either the normal or diseased nasopharynx, and is thus of uncertain pathogenicity. **Neisseria gonorrhoeae.** Gonococcus, the causative organisms of gonorrhoea; a Gram-negative diplococcus which is a strictly human parasite and will not produce the disease in animals. Characteristically, it is found in the cells of the urethral and cervical discharges, also in the discharge from the eyes in some cases of ophthalmia neonatorum. A small proportion of strains have become resistant to penicillin, particularly among cases of gonorrhoea in sea ports and large cities. **Neisseria meningitidis.** Meningococcus, the organism responsible for epidemic cerebrospinal meningitis (spotted fever); typically, a Gram-negative intracellular diplococcus growing slowly on enriched media such as serum agar, and ordinarily very sensitive to sulphonamides and certain antibiotics. Recently, sulphonamide-resistant strains have become prevalent in North America and in some other countries. **Neisseria pharyngis.** Non-motile Gram-negative diplococci occurring in the normal nasopharynx and very variable in colonial appearance. **Neisseria weichselbaumii.** *Neisseria meningitidis* (see above). [Albert Ludwig Siegmund *Neisser* (b. 1855), Breslau dermatologist.]

Neisseriaceae (ni·seer·e·a′·se·e). In American nomenclature, the tribe of Eubacteriales known in England as Neisserieae.

Neisserieae (ni·seer·e·e′·e). Tribal name for the bacterial genus *Neisseria.*

neisserosis (ni·seer·o·sis). Infection with the gonococcus, *Neisseria gonorrhoeae.* [neisseria, Gk *-osis* condition.]

Nélaton, Auguste (b. 1807). Paris surgeon.

Nélaton's fibre. A condensation of circular muscle of the rectum in the upper part of the ampulla said to constitute a sphincter (Nélaton's sphincter, see below).

Nélaton's line. A line joining the anterior superior iliac spine and the ischial tuberosity.

Nélaton's operation. Excision of the shoulder joint by a transverse incision.

Nélaton's sphincter. A localized thickening of circular muscle fibres in the rectal wall.

Nélaton's tumour. Desmoid tumour of the abdominal wall.

nem (nem). A unit of nutrition equal to the nutritional value of 1 gram of breast milk (von Pirquet). [G *Nahrungs Einheit Milch,* nutritional unit milk.]

nemathelminth (nem·at·hel·minth). Any member of the group Nemathelminthes; a round worm.

Nemathelminthes (nem·at·hel·min′·theez). A group of animals, sometimes considered as a phylum, containing the Acanthocephala, Gordiacea and Nematoda. These latter are more usually considered as phyla, and the group used only to separate the round worms from the flat worms (Platyhelminthes). [Gk *nema* thread, *helmins* worm.]

nemathelminthiasis (nem·at·hel·min·thi′·as·is). Nematode infestation. [nemathelminthes.]

nematization (nem·at·i·za′·shun). The process of infestation with nematodes.

nematoblast (nem·at·o·blast). A spermatid. [Gk *nema* thread, *blastos* germ.]

Nematocera (nem·at·os·er·ah). A sub-order of the Diptera. The adults are characterized by the filiform antennae; the larvae have the head well developed and, in almost all forms of medical importance, are aquatic; the pupae are free and often active. Members of the following families are of medical importance: Ceratopogonidae, Culicidae, Psychodidae, Simuliidae. [Gk *nema* thread, *keras* horn.]

nematocide (nem·at·o·side). 1. Any agent that kills nematode worms. 2. Destructive to nematodes. [nematode, L *caedere* to kill.]

Nematoda (nem·at·o·dah). A phylum of round worms. Most species are free-living or plant parasites, such forms being called *nemas*; many are, however, important parasites whose life histories may be simple, the young developing in the soil, or may involve secondary hosts. Members of the following genera are of medical importance: *Ancylostoma, Ascaris, Capillaria, Dioctophyme, Enterobius, Necator, Oesophagostomum, Strongyloides, Ternidens, Trichinella, Trichostrongylus, Trichuris.* [Gk *nema* thread, *eidos* form.]

nematode, naematoid (**nem**·at·ode, **nem**·at·oid). 1. Thread-like. 2. Referring to an endoparasitic worm of the phylum Nematoda. [see prec.]

nematology (nem·at·**ol**·o·je). The science and study of nematodes. [nematode, Gk *logos* science.]

nematosis (nem·at·**o**·sis). Infestation with nematodes. [nematode, Gk *-osis* condition.]

nematospermia (**nem**·at·o·**sper**′·me·ah). The faculty of producing spermatozoa with long thin tails, which are characteristic of the spermatozoa of man. [Gk *nema* thread, sperm.]

nemic (**nem**·ik). Referring to nematode worms. [Gk *nema* thread.]

Neoarsphenamine BPC 1963 (**ne**·o·ars·**fen**′·am·een). A complex organic arsenical derived from arsphenamine, but far more useful clinically and less toxic. It is administered intravenously for venereal diseases: solutions have to be freshly prepared as it is readily oxidized to toxic arsenoxide derivatives.

neo-arthrosis (ne·o·ar·**thro**′·sis). An artificial joint made by surgical operation. [Gk *neos* new, *arthron* joint, *-osis* condition.]

neoblast (**ne**·o·blast). That portion of the mesoderm which gives origin to the blood vessels, blood and other vascular structures. [Gk *neos* new, *blastos* germ.]

neoblastic (ne·o·**blas**·tik). Derived from or of the character of new growth. [see prec.]

neocerebellum (**ne**·o·ser·e·**bel**′·um). The most recently-evolved part of the cerebellum, i.e. the middle lobe, including the greater part of the cerebellar hemispheres. [Gk *neos* new, cerebellum.]

Neocinchophen (ne·o·**sin**·ko·fen). BP Commission approved name for ethyl 6-methyl-2-phenylquinoline-4-carboxylate, a light-yellow crystalline powder having analgesic and antipyretic properties. Like the salicylates, it increases the excretion of both exogenous and endogenous uric acid: usually the blood uric acid is lowered, but it may sometimes be raised during the increased excretion period. It is absorbed adequately from the intestinal canal and is excreted in the urine partly oxidized.

neocortex (ne·o·**kor**·tex). The most recently-evolved part of the cerebral cortex. It includes all the cerebral cortex in man, except that of the hippocampal formation and piriform areas. [Gk *neos* new, cortex.]

neocyte (**ne**·o·site). A leucocyte which has not reached maturity. [Obsolete term.] [Gk *neos* new, *kytos* cell.]

neocytosis (**ne**·o·si·**to**′·sis). The existence of neocytes in the blood. [Obsolete term.] [neocyte, Gk *-osis* condition.]

neodiathermy (**ne**·o·di·ah·**ther**′·me). Short-wave diathermy; heat generated in the tissues by a high-frequency current. It is variously known as *radiathermy* and *dialectrothermy.* [Gk *neos* new, diathermy.]

neodymium (ne·o·**dim**·e·um). A rare-earth element of atomic weight 144.2, atomic number 60 and chemical symbol Nd. It is a trivalent metal occurring in the cerite earths and gives violet salts sometimes used to colour porcelain. [Gk *neos* new, *didymos* twin.]

neofetal (ne·o·**fe**·tal). Referring to the neofetus; the state of the embryo in the ninth week of pregnancy.

neofetus (ne·o·**fe**·tus). In embryology, the organism during the ninth week; the stage of transition between the embryonic and fetal periods. [Gk *neos* new, fetus.]

neoformation (**ne**·o·for·**ma**′·shun). 1. Neoplasm. 2. Regeneration. [Gk *neos* new, formation.]

neoformative (ne·o·**for**·mat·iv). Denoting the development of new tissue. [see prec.]

neogala (ne·**og**·al·ah). Milk as first secreted after birth of the child. [Obsolete term.] [Gk *neos* new, *gala* milk.]

neogenesis (ne·o·**jen**·es·is). 1. The formation of new tissue which takes place more slowly than in the process of anagenesis. 2. Regeneration. [Gk *neos* new, genesis.]

neogenetic (**ne**·o·jen·**et**′·ik). Referring to neogenesis.

neoglycogenesis (**ne**·o·gli·ko·**jen**′·es·is). Glyconeogenesis.

neohippocratism (**ne**·o·hip·**ok**′·rat·izm). A term applied to a form of latter-day medicine which revives the principles of Hippocrates and studies the individual patient and his clinical signs and symptoms, while at the same time applying the discoveries of modern medical research in diagnosis and treatment. [Gk *neos* new, Hippocratism.]

neokinetic (**ne**·o·kin·**et**′·ik). The nervous motor mechanism regulating voluntary muscle control. [Gk *neos* new, kinetic.]

neologism (ne·**ol**·o·jism). The employment of a newly coined word. [Gk *neos* new, *logos* word.]

neomorph, neomorphism (**ne**·o·morf, ne·o·**mor**·fizm). Any new organ or part; a structure to be found in most highly developed organisms only. [Gk *neos* new, *morphe* form.]

Neomycin (ne·o·**mi**·sin). BP Commission approved name for an antibiotic obtained from a soil organism allied to *Streptomyces fradiae.* It is a mixture of 2 substances, *neomycins A and B,* and is useful against many Gram-positive and Gram-negative organisms. The official preparation is Neomycin Sulphate BP 1973.

Neomycini Sulfas (ne·o·**mi**·sin·i **sul**·fas). *European Pharmacopoeia* name for Neomycin Sulphate BP 1973.

neon (**ne**·on). A chemical element of atomic weight 20.179, atomic number 10 and chemical symbol Ne. It is a colourless inert gas occurring in the atmosphere (one part in 55 000) and used principally in neon tubes. **Neon lamp, Neon tube.** A glass tube containing neon at very low pressure: a high-voltage electric discharge through it produces a strong red glow. [Gk *neos* new.]

neonatal, neonate (ne·o·**na**·tal, **ne**·o·nate). 1. Referring to the newborn. 2. Referring to the period that succeeds delivery of a child. [see foll.]

neonatus (ne·o·**na**·tus). A newly-born child. [Gk *neos* new, L *natus* born.]

neonicotine (ne·o·**nik**·o·teen). Name given to a synthetic alkaloid prepared from pyridine and subsequently shown to be a racemic form of anabasine. [Gk *neos* new, nicotine.]

neonym (**ne**·o·nim). A new name given to any part of the organism or to any disease, injury or function. [Gk *neos* new, *onoma* name.]

neopallium (ne·o·**pal**·e·um). Neocortex. [Gk *neos* new, L *pallium* cloak.]

neopathy (ne·**op**·ath·e). 1. A disease that has been discovered recently. 2. A new condition or element arising in an already existing disease, or a complication. [Gk *neos* new, *pathos* suffering.]

neophilism (ne·**of**·il·izm). Excessive wish for or fondness of something that is novel. [Gk *neos* new, *philein* to love.]

neophobe (**ne**·o·fobe). One who dreads anything new or is strongly averse to its introduction. [Gk *neos* new, phobia.]

neophobia (ne·o·**fo**·be·ah). Abnormal fear of and morbid aversion to anything new. [see prec.]

neophrenia (ne·o·**fre**·ne·ah). A disordered mental condition occurring in the early years; the psychoses of childhood. [Gk *neos* new, *phren* mind.]

neoplasia (ne·o·**pla**·ze·ah). The growth of a neoplasm or of new tissue. [Gk *neos* new, *plassein* to form.]

neoplasm (**ne**·o·plasm). Any new and morbid formation of tissue; a tumour. **Histoid neoplasm.** One in which the tissues are similar in structure to those in which it develops. **Inflammatory fungoid neoplasm.** Mycosis fungoides. **Metastatic neoplasm.** A neoplasm which has originated from cells of a primary neoplasm that have been carried in the blood or lymph to some other tissue or organ. **Organoid neoplasm.** A neoplasm in which the tissues are similar in structure to one of the body organs. [Gk *neos* new, *plasma* something formed.]

neoplasmatase (ne·o·**plaz**·mat·aze). The filtrable matter in some particular new growths which is capable of transmitting the diseased condition to another part. [see prec.]

neoplasmatic (ne·o·plaz·**mat**'·ik). Relating to or having the character of a neoplasm.

neoplastic (ne·o·**plas**·tik). Relating or belonging to neoplasty.

neoplasty (**ne**·o·plas·te). 1. A plastic operation by which a part is restored or a new part is formed. 2. Neoplasia. [Gk *neos* new, *plassein* to mould.]

neosine (**ne**·o·seen). A nitrogenous base, one of the minor constituents of muscle.

neostigmine (ne·o·**stig**·meen). The dimethylcarbamic ester of 3-hydroxyphenyltrimethylammonium methyl sulphate, $(CH_3)_2NCOOC_6H_4N(CH_3)_3SO_4CH_3$. A synthetic alkaloid with pharmacological effects similar to physostigmine in that it inhibits cholinesterase. It thus potentiates the action of acetylcholine and stimulates the contraction of skeletal muscle; it is used therefore in myasthenia gravis. It overcomes curare block by allowing accumulation of acetylcholine at the motor end-plate and for that reason is used by anaesthetists to counteract the effect of curare-like compounds. Its parasympathetic effects, e.g. salivation and bradycardia, may be prevented by premedication with atropine. It potentiates the actions of suxamethonium and usually those of decamethonium. **Neostigmine Bromide BP 1973.** A compound employed orally in myasthenia gravis. **Neostigmine Methylsulphate BP 1973.** A compound similar to the bromide, but employed when administration by injection is required.

Neostigminii Bromidum (neo·stig·**min**·e·i **bro**·mid·um). *European Pharmacopoeia* name for Neostigmine Bromide BP 1973.

neostomy (ne·**os**·to·me). An operative procedure by which an artificial opening is made either into an organ or between 2 organs. [Gk *neos* new, *stoma* mouth.]

neostriatum (**ne**·o·stri·**a**'·tum). The most recently-evolved parts of the corpus striatum. The term is usually applied to the caudate nucleus and putamen which are said to be phylogenetically younger than the globus pallidus (the palaeostriatum). [Gk *neos* new, corpus striatum.]

Neotestudina rosatii (**ne**·o·tes·tew·**de**'·nah ro·**za**·te·i). A fungus causing white grain mycetoma in tropical Africa (Somalia, Senegal).

neothalamus (ne·o·**thal**·am·us). Term sometimes applied to the lateral and dorsomedial nuclei of the thalamus and to the pulvinar, since these structures are more highly developed in Man, and in Primates generally, than in more primitive mammals. [Gk *neos* new, thalamus.]

neo-vitamin A (**ne**·o·**vi**'·tam·in **a**). An isomer of vitamin A occurring in mammals and salt-water fish along with vitamin A. [Gk *neos* new, vitamin A.]

nephablepsia (nef·a·**blep**·se·ah). Snow blindness. *See* BLINDNESS. [Gk *nephos* cloud, ablepsia.]

nephalism (**nef**·al·izm). Abstention from all forms of alcoholic liquor. [Gk *nephalios* sober.]

nephela (**nef**·el·ah). 1. Cloudiness of the urine. 2. Leucoma. [Gk *nephele* cloud.]

nephelometer (nef·el·**om**·et·er). A photometer adapted to the measurement of the intensity of light scattered by bacteria or chemical particles suspended in a liquid. By comparing the light with that scattered by a standard suspension, an estimate of the number of bacteria or particles can be arrived at. [Gk *nephele* cloud, meter.]

nephelometry (nef·el·**om**·et·re). The estimation of bacteria or chemical particles suspended in a liquid, by use of the nephelometer.

nephelopia (nef·el·**o**·pe·ah). Dimness of vision caused by a cloudy condition of the cornea. [Gk *nephele* cloud, *ops* eye.]

nephradenoma (**nef**·rad·en·**o**'·mah). An adenoma of the kidney. [Gk *nephros* kidney, adenoma.]

nephraemia (nef·**re**·me·ah). Hyperaemia and congestion of the kidney. [Gk *nephros* kidney, *haima* blood.]

nephralgia (nef·**ral**·je·ah). Pain in the kidney. **Idiopathic nephralgia.** A pain in a kidney the cause of which cannot be determined. [Gk *nephros* kidney, *algos* pain.]

nephralgic (nef·**ral**·jik). Applied to a condition in which renal pain is a characteristic symptom. [see prec.]

nephranuria (nef·ran·**ewr**·e·ah). A condition in which the renal secretion is suppressed. [Gk *nephros* kidney, anuria.]

nephrapostasis (nef·rap·**os**·tas·is). An inflammatory suppurative state of the kidney or an abscess of the kidney. [Gk *nephros* kidney, apostasis.]

nephrasthenia (nef·ras·**the**·ne·ah). The presence of albuminuria or minor symptoms of renal disease. [Gk *nephros* kidney, asthenia.]

nephratonia, nephratony (nef·rat·**o**·ne·ah, nef·**rat**·on·e). Lessening of tone of the kidney and reduction of its output. [Gk *nephros* kidney, atony.]

nephrauxe (nef·**rawx**·e). Hypertrophy of the kidney. [Gk *nephros* kidney, *auxe* increase.]

nephrectasia (nef·rek·**ta**·ze·ah). A dilated condition of the kidney. [Gk *nephos* kidney, *ektasis* a stretching.]

nephrectasis, nephrectasy (nef·**rek**·tas·is, nef·**rek**·tas·e). A distended state of the kidney or of the pelvis of the ureter. [see prec.]

nephrectomize (nef·**rek**·to·mize). To perform the operation of nephrectomy.

nephrectomy (nef·**rek**·to·me). Extirpation of a kidney. **Abdominal nephrectomy, Anterior nephrectomy.** Removal of a kidney through abdominal incision and peritoneal cavity. **Lumbar nephrectomy.** Nephrectomy through an incision in the loin. **Posterior nephrectomy.** Lumbar nephrectomy (see above). **Radical nephrectomy.** Extirpation of the kidney with the surrounding perinephric fat and other involved tissues in cases of malignant disease. [Gk *nephros* kidney, *ektome* a cutting out.]

nephrelcosis (nef·rel·**ko**·sis). Ulceration of the mucous membrane of the pelvis or calyces of the kidney. [Gk *nephros* kidney, *helkos* ulcer.]

nephremphraxis (nef·rem·**frax**·is). Vascular obstruction in the kidneys. [Gk *nephros* kidney, *emphraxis* obstruction.]

nephresia (nef·**re**·ze·ah). Any pathological condition of a kidney. [Gk *nephros kidney.]*

nephretic (nef·**ret**·ik). Pertaining to nephresia.

nephria (**nef**·re·ah). Nephritis. [see foll.]

nephric (**nef**·rik). Referring to the kidney; renal. [Gk *nephros* kidney.]

nephridion (nef·**rid**·e·on). Nephridium.

nephridium (nef·**rid**·e·um). A type of segmental excretory tubule found in many invertebrates. Its inner end opens into the coelom, its outer end to the exterior. [Gk *nephridios* pertaining to the kidney.]

nephrism (**nef**·rizm). Chronic disease of the kidneys. [Gk *nephros* kidney.]

nephritic (nef·**rit**·ik). 1. Referring to or suffering from nephritis. 2. Referring to the kidneys. 3. Any medicament used in the treatment of renal conditions. [see prec.]

nephritides (nef·**rit**·id·eez). **See** NEPHRITIS.

nephritis (nef·**ri**·tis) (pl. *nephritides*). A bilateral disease of the kidneys of toxic origin, affecting the glomeruli, tubules and interstitial tissue in varying degree. The essential lesion is an inflammation of the glomerular capillaries, followed by degeneration of the glomerular and tubular cells and small-celled infiltration of the interstitial tissue. Clinically, it is characterized by albuminuria, haematuria, cylinduria and oedema, together with cardiovascular signs in differing combination and degree. In its complete and typical form it passes through acute, subacute and chronic stages of varying duration. **Acute focal nephritis.** A form in which comparatively few glomeruli are affected; it is characterized clinically by albuminuria and haematuria, without oedema, urea retention or hypertension. It is most common in children and the majority of cases recover completely. **Acute focal embolic nephritis.** Nephritis occurring in subacute bacterial endocarditis, caused by emboli lodging in the glomerular blood vessels. Clinically, it is revealed by transient attacks of albuminuria and haematuria without oedema or urea retention. **Azotaemic nephritis.** Chronic nephritis (see following). **Chronic**

nephritis, Chronic interstitial nephritis. Secondary contracted kidney, small white kidney, azotaemic nephritis; the third stage of nephritis, following subacute or latent nephritis or an unsuspected mild attack of nephritis (so-called "idiopathic" chronic nephritis). The kidney is small and granular with marked proliferation of interstitial tissue and thickening of arteries and arterioles. The clinical picture is varied and complex. Oedema if previously present lessens or disappears; the urine increases in volume and its specific gravity tends to be fixed at about 1010; a variable amount of albumin is present and a few casts. There is progressive urea retention and increasing hypertension and retinopathy. Cardiovascular symptoms may dominate the picture and death may occur from myocardial failure or progressive renal failure may terminate in uraemia. **Clostridial nephritis.** Nephritis due to toxins of bacteria of the genus *Clostridum*, especially those of *Clostridium welchii.* **Epidemic nephritis.** Trench nephritis, acute nephritis occurring in epidemics; besides the usual signs of nephritis, dyspnoea was usually a prominent early symptom. Epidemics occurred in the American Civil War and World War I. **Hydraemic nephritis.** Subacute nephritis (see below). **Latent nephritis.** A sequel to acute nephritis when, after apparent recovery, shown by subsidence of oedema and haematuria, there is a persistent albuminuria with some pallor and a tendency to a slight rise of blood pressure. After months or years of a slow symptomless course the condition passes into that of chronic nephritis and renal failure. **Lipomatous nephritis.** Renal lipomatosis. *See* LIPOMATOSIS. **Nephrotic nephritis.** Subacute nephritis (see below). **Radiation nephritis.** Nephritis caused by exposure to ionizing radiation. **Subacute nephritis.** Hydraemic nephritis, nephrotic nephritis, large white kidney; the second stage of nephritis in which there is increased tubular degeneration and epithelial proliferation with beginning interstitial fibrosis. Clinically, it is marked by gross oedema, albuminuria and anaemia. At first there may be no impairment of renal function or hypertension, but later these appear and progress as the condition passes into the chronic stage. **Trench nephritis.** Epidemic nephritis (see above). **Type I nephritis** (Ellis). Nephritis starting abruptly with haematuria, oedema of short duration and hypertension. It occurs mainly at the younger ages, following a recent infection, especially of the tonsils. The prognosis is favourable, as it is said that about 80 per cent recover: a few run a rapidly progressive course with death within a few months, and others after a long latent phase of symptomless albuminuria end eventually with hypertension and uraemia. **Type II nephritis.** Nephritis with an insidious onset and occurring at any age. It is characterized by a prolonged phase of general oedema and recovery is rare. [Gk *nephros* kidney, *-itis* inflammation.]

nephro-abdominal (**nef**·ro·ab·**dom**′·in·al). Referring especially to the kidney and its relation to the abdominal wall. [Gk *nephros* kidney, abdomen.]

nephrobarytosis (**nef**·ro·bar·e·**to**′·sis). A deposit of barium sulphate occurring after urethrocystography when barium sulphate has refluxed into the kidney. [Gk *nephros* kidney, barytes, Gk *-osis* condition.]

nephroblastoma (**nef**·ro·blas·**to**′·mah). Embryonal adenomyosarcoma, Wilms' tumour; a highly-malignant complex renal tumour of young children, rarely found after the tenth year, composed of a great variety of tissues suggesting abortive renal elements. [Gk *nephros* kidney, *blastos* germ, *-oma* tumour.]

nephrocalcinosis (**nef**·ro·kal·sin·**o**′·sis). The deposition of calcium in the kidneys and the formation of calculi, due to increased calcium in the blood as with hyperparathyroidism or excessive intake of vitamin D. [Gk *nephros* kidney, calcium, Gk *-osis* condition.]

nephrocapsulectomy (**nef**·ro·kap·sew·**lek**′·to·me). Removal of the renal capsule; renal decapsulation (Edebohl's operation). [Gk *nephros* kidney, capsule, Gk *ektome* a cutting out.]

nephrocapsulotomy (**nef**·ro·kap·sew·**lot**′·om·e). Incision of the renal capsule. [Gk *nephros* kidney, capsule, Gk *temnein* to cut.]

nephrocardiac (nef·ro·**kar**·de·ak). Relating or belonging to the kidney and the heart. [Gk *nephros* kidney, *kardia* heart.]

nephrocele (**nef**·ro·seel). A hernial protrusion of the kidney. [Gk *nephros* kidney, *kele* hernia.]

nephrochalazosis (**nef**·ro·kal·az·**o**′·sis). The granular kidney of chronic interstitial nephritis. [Gk *nephros kidney, chalazaein* to have tubercles.]

nephrocirrhosis (**nef**·ro·sir·**o**′·sis). Chronic interstitial nephritis. *See* NEPHRITIS. [Gk *nephros* kidney, cirrhosis.]

nephrocolic, nephrocolica (nef·ro·**kol**·ik, nef·ro·**kol**·ik·ah). 1. Referring to the kidney and the colon. 2. Renal colic. *See* COLIC. [Gk *nephros* kidney, colic.]

nephrocolopexy (**nef**·ro·ko·lo·**pex**′·e). Operative fixation, at a proper level, of the kidney and colon. [Gk *nephros* kidney, *kolon* colon, *pexis* a fixation.]

nephrocoloptosis (**nef**·ro·ko·lop·**to**′·sis). Prolapse of the kidney and colon. [Gk *nephros* kidney, colon, Gk *ptosis* a falling.]

nephrocystanastomosis (nef·ro·**sist**·an·as·to·**mo**′·sis). The establishment of an artificial passage between the kidney and the urinary bladder. [Gk *nephros* kidney, *kystis* bag, anastomosis.]

nephrocystitis (**nef**·ro·sist·**i**′·tis). Inflammation affecting the kidney and the urinary bladder. [Gk *nephros* kidney, cystitis.]

nephrocystosis (**nef**·ro·sist·**o**′·sis). Cystic formation in the kidney. [Gk *nephros* kidney, cystosis.]

nephrodystrophy (nef·ro·**dis**·tro·fe). Nephrosis. [Gk *nephros* kidney, dystrophy.]

nephroedema (nef·re·**de**·mah). 1. Hydronephrosis. 2. Oedema of the kidneys. [Gk *nephros* kidney, oedema.]

nephrogastric (nef·ro·**gas**·trik). Relating or belonging to the kidney and stomach. [Gk *nephros* kidney, *gaster* stomach.]

nephrogenetic, nephrogenic, nephrogenous (**nef**·ro·jen·**et**′·ik, nef·ro·**jen**·ik, nef·**roj**·en·us). Produced by, derived from, or originating in a kidney. [Gk *nephros* kidney, *genein* to produce.]

nephrogram (**nef**·ro·gram). The radiograph or tracing made during nephrography. [Gk *nephros* kidney, *gramma* record.]

nephrography (nef·**rog**·raf·e). Radiographic or radionuclide visualization of the kidneys. In radiological diagnosis, usually applied to a specific phase of intravenous urography, the so-called *nephrographic effect.* [Gk *nephros* kidney, *graphein* to record.]

nephrohaemia (nef·ro·**he**·me·ah). Nephraemia.

nephrohaemorrhagia (**nef**·ro·hem·or·**a**′·je·ah). A discharge of blood from the kidney. [Gk *nephros* kidney, haemorrhage.]

nephrohydrops, nephrohydrosis (nef·ro·**hi**·drops, **nef**·ro·hi·**dro**′·sis). Hydronephrosis.

nephrohypertrophy (**nef**·ro·hi·**per**′·tro·fe). Enlargement of the kidney. [Gk *nephros* kidney, hypertrophy.]

nephroid (**nef**·roid). In the shape of a kidney; like a kidney. [Gk *nephros* kidney, *eidos* form.]

nephrolith (**nef**·ro·lith). A calculus or gravel present in a kidney. [Gk *nephros* kidney, *lithos* stone.]

nephrolithiasis (**nef**·ro·lith·**i**′·as·is). A condition characterized by the presence of gravel or of renal calculi. [see prec.]

nephrolithic (nef·ro·**lith**·ik). Referring to or suffering from the presence of a nephrolith.

nephrolithotomy (**nef**·ro·lith·**ot**′·o·me). The surgical procedure of removing renal calculi by making an incision into the kidney. [Gk *nephros* kidney, lithotomy.]

nephrology (nef·**rol**·o·je). That branch of medicine which deals with the kidney and diseases affecting the kidney. [Gk *nephros* kidney, *logos* science.]

nephrolysin (nef·**rol**·is·in). A toxin which specifically affects renal cells. [Gk *nephros* kidney, *lysein* to loosen.]

nephrolysis (nef·**rol**·is·is). 1. Freeing of the kidney from inflammatory adhesions. 2. Disintegration of the kidney produced by nephrolytic agents. [Gk *nephros* kidney, *lysis* a loosing.]

nephrolytic (nef·ro·**lit**·ik). Relating, belonging or giving rise to nephrolysis.

nephroma (nef·**ro**·mah). A renal tumour or a tumour derived from renal substance. **Embryonal nephroma.** Wilms' tumour. [Gk *nephros* kidney, *-oma* tumour.]

nephromalacia (nef·ro·mal·a′·she·ah). Softening of the kidney tissues. [Gk *nephros* kidney, malacia.]

nephromegalia, nephromegaly (nef·ro·meg·a′·le·ah, nef·ro·meg′·al·e). Hypertrophy of the kidney. [Gk *nephros* kidney, *megas* great.]

nephromeiosis (nef·ro·mi·o′·sis). Shrinkage of a kidney. [Gk *nephros* kidney, *meion* less.]

nephromere (nef·ro·meer). That part of a primitive mesodermal segment which gives rise to the renal tubules. [Gk *nephros* kidney, *meros* part.]

nephron (nef·ron). The functioning unit in the kidney, composed of the renal corpuscle (the capsule of Bowman enclosing the glomerulus) and a uriniferous tubule. There are about 1 million such units in the human kidney. The glomerular filtrate passing through the tubular system is subjected to an active reabsorption of high-threshold substances, e.g. glucose, whereas the low-threshold substances, e.g. urea, are concentrated in the urine. [Gk *nephros* kidney.]

nephroncus (nef·rong·kus). A tumour of the kidney. [Gk *nephros* kidney, *ogkos* mass.]

nephronophthisis (nef·ron·of·thi·sis). Medullary cystic disease with anaemia and uraemia, often familial. [Gk *nephros* kidney, *phthisis* a wasting away.]

See also: FANCONI.

nephroparalysis, nephroparesis (nef·ro·par·al′·is·is, nef·ro·par·e′·sis). Paralysis affecting the kidney, so that the function of secretion is suspended. [Gk *nephros* kidney, paralysis, paresis.]

nephropathic (nef·ro·path·ik). Producing or caused by nephropathy.

nephropathy (nef·rop·ath·e). Disease of the kidney. **Dropsical nephropathy.** Nephritis with dropsy. **Hypo-azoturic nephropathy.** Nephritis with nitrogen retention. **Hypochloruric nephropathy.** Nephritis with retention of sodium chloride. [Gk *nephros* kidney, *pathos* disease.]

nephropexy (nef·ro·pex·e). The operation of anchoring a mobile kidney. [Gk *nephros* kidney, *pexis* fixation.]

nephropoietic (nef·ro·poi·et′·ik). Concerned with the generation or production of renal tissue. [Gk *nephros* kidney, *poiein* to make.]

nephroptosis (nef·rop·to·sis). Mobile kidney; undue mobility of the kidney found by palpation. It is usually associated with a general visceroptosis. [Gk *nephros* kidney, *ptosis* a falling.]

nephropyelitis (nef·ro·pi·el·i′·tis). Pyelonephritis; an inflammatory condition affecting the parenchyma of the kidney and the pelvis of the ureter. [Gk *nephros* kidney, pyelitis.]

nephropyelolithotomy (nef·ro·pi·el·o·lith·ot′·o·me). Removal of calculi in the pelvis of the ureter by making an incision through the substance of the kidney. [Gk *nephros* kidney, pyelolithotomy.]

nephropyeloplasty (nef·ro·pi·el·o·plas·te). A plastic resection of a portion of the pelvis of the ureter to ensure more efficient ureteral drainage in hydronephrosis. [Gk *nephros* kidney, pyeloplasty.]

nephropyosis (nef·ro·pi·o′·sis). A suppurative condition involving the kidney. [Gk *nephros* kidney, pyosis.]

nephrorrhagia (nef·ro·ra·je·ah). A discharge of blood from the kidney; renal haemorrhage. [Gk *nephros* kidney, *rhegnynein* to gush forth.]

nephrorrhaphy (nef·ror·af·e). Nephropexy. [Gk *nephros* kidney, *rhaphe* suture.]

nephrosclerosis (nef·ro·skler·o′·sis). The form of kidney disease which is due primarily to vascular lesions, the renal changes being secondary. **Arteriolar nephrosclerosis.** The kidney in benign hypertension, showing thickening of the arterioles and varying degrees of atrophy of the glomeruli and tubules, with increase of the interstitial tissue. **Benign nephrosclerosis.** The renal condition secondary to benign hypertension, in which there is thickening of the intima with hyaline and adipose degeneration of the renal arterioles and smaller arteries. There are consequent patchy areas of ischaemia and fibrotic change. In severe cases of this nature the whole kidney may become fibrotic and the name is no longer applicable. **Intercapillary nephrosclerosis.** Arteriolar nephrosclerosis (see above). **Malignant nephrosclerosis.** The condition of the kidneys associated with malignant hypertension. The essential lesion is a renal arteriolitis and arteritis with necrosis of the afferent and interlobular arterioles. In contrast with benign nephrosclerosis the disease runs a rapid and fatal course. **Nephrosclerosis without hypertension.** The condition in which arteriosclerosis affects the renal arteries as part of a general senile arteriosclerosis. There is a gradual failure of physical and mental powers; blood pressure is not raised and there are no renal symptoms. [Gk *nephros* kidney, *sklerosis* a hardening.]

nephrosis (nef·ro·sis). A syndrome caused by a primary non-inflammatory degeneration of the renal tubules and characterized by oedema, marked albuminuria, a fall in the plasma albumin and a rise in the plasma cholesterol. Hypertension and haematuria are absent and the blood urea is normal or low. Some authorities do not accept nephrosis as a distinct entity and regard it as a form of glomerulonephritis. **Acute nephrosis.** Generalized oedema with gross albuminuria, mostly seen in children; it may follow an acute pneumococcal infection or have an unknown cause. **Amyloid nephrosis.** A condition in which the nephrotic syndrome is due to amyloid degeneration of the renal blood vessels. **Chronic nephrosis.** Prolonged gross oedema with marked albuminuria; many cases are examples of the oedematous stage of subacute glomerulonephritis. **Larval nephrosis.** Albuminuria without oedema or hypertension, associated with cloudy swelling or fatty degeneration of the renal cells as in febrile albuminuria or mild toxic conditions. **Lipoid nephrosis.** Severe nephrosis with very marked lipoidal degeneration of the tubules. **Lower nephron nephrosis.** A form of nephrosis in which the distal portion of the nephron is mainly affected. **Malarial nephrosis.** A condition associated with a chronic infection with quartan malaria in children, recognized in Africa and New Guinea. It responds to prolonged antimalarial therapy. **Necrotizing nephrosis.** Severe degeneration of the epithelium of the kidney which may go on to necrosis. It is most often due to poisoning with salts of the heavy metals such as mercury, gold and bismuth, but may occur with other forms of poisoning or in certain severe infections. [Gk *nephros* kidney, *-osis* condition.]

See also: EPSTEIN (A. A.).

nephrosplenopexy (nef·ro·splen·o·pex·e). Fixation of the kidney and of the spleen by surgical methods. [Gk *nephros* kidney, spleen, Gk *pexis* fixation.]

nephrostegnosis (nef·ro·steg·no′·sis). Nephrosclerosis. [Gk *nephros* kidney, *stegnosis* a stopping.]

nephrostoma, nephrostome (nef·ro·sto·mah, nef·ro·stome). The ciliated opening of a primitive urinary tubule into the coelom; it is only found in association with the pronephros in mammalian development. [Gk *nephros* kidney, *stoma* mouth.]

nephrostomy (nef·ros·to·me). The establishment of a permanent opening into the pelvis of the ureter from the surface. [see prec.]

nephrotic (nef·rot·ik). Referring, due to, or like nephrosis.

nephrotome (nef·ro·tome). Nephromere. [see foll.]

nephrotomography (nef·ro·to·mog′·raf·e). Tomography of the kidney. [Gk *nephros* kidney, *tome* section, *graphein* to record.]

nephrotomy (nef·rot·o·me). An incision into the kidney substance. **Abdominal nephrotomy.** Nephrotomy performed through an incision into the abdomen. **Lumbar nephrotomy.** Nephrotomy performed by means of an incision in the lumbar region. [Gk *nephros* kidney, *temnein* to cut.]

nephrotoxic (nef·ro·tox·ik). Having the power to destroy or having a toxic action on the cells of the kidney. [see foll.]

nephrotoxin (nef·ro·tox·in). A cytotoxin having a destructive action specifically on the cells of the kidney. [Gk *nephros* kidney, *toxikon* poison.]

nephrotresis (nef·ro·tre·sis). Nephrostomy. [Gk *nephros* kidney, *tresis* a boring.]

nephrotrophic (nef·ro·trof·ik). Having a special affinity for, or exerting its principal effect upon, the kidney. [Gk *nephros* kidney, *trophe* nutrition.]

nephrotuberculosis (**nef**·ro·tew·ber·kew·**lo'**·sis). Disease of the kidney due to *Mycobacterium tuberculosis.* [Gk *nephros* kidney, tuberculosis.]

nephro-ureterectomy (**nef**·ro·ewr·e·ter·**ek'**·to·me). The operation of removing a kidney and its ureter either in whole or in part. [Gk *nephros* kidney, ureter, Gk *ektome* a cutting out.]

nephro-ureterocystectomy (**nef**·ro·ewr·e·ter·o·sist·**ek'**·to·me). The surgical removal of a kidney and its ureter together with a portion of the wall of the urinary bladder. [Gk *nephros* kidney, ureter, Gk *kystis* bag, *ektome* a cutting out.]

nephrozymosis (**nef**·ro·zi·**mo'**·sis). The occurrence of a local inflammation of the kidney as part of an infectious disease. [Gk *nephros* kidney, zymosis.]

neptunium (nep·**tew**·ne·um). The first of the transuranic elements to be synthesized (1940); it has an atomic weight of 237.048, atomic number 93 and chemical symbol Np. It was produced by the bomdardment of uranium 238 with fast neutrons, and has a half-life of 2.2×10^6 years. [Named after the planet *Neptune.*]

neral (**ne**·ral). β-Citral, $(CH_3)_2C{=}CH(CH_2)_2C(CH_3){=}CHCHO$. A stereo-isomer of geranial and the aldehyde corresponding to nerol, found in oils of neroli and bergamot. It is used as an aromatic and flavouring agent.

Neri, Vincenzo (b. 1882). Bologna neurologist.

Neri's sign. 1. In hemiplegia of organic origin, if the patient is supine and the affected leg is lifted the knee bends automatically. 2. In sciatica, forward bending of the trunk when the patient is standing results in flexion of the knee on the affected side. 3. The arms of a recumbent hemiplegic patient are pronated on a flat surface; the examiner's hand is placed underneath one of the arms and passive flexion at the elbow is carried out. The paralysed forearm supinates; the sound one remains pronated.

neriin (**ne**·re·in). A glycoside isolated from oleander, *Nerium oleander* (family Apocynaceae).

Nerium (**ne**·re·um). 1. A genus of trees of the family Apocynaceae. 2. Oleander, the leaves and bark of *Nerum oleander.* [Gk *nerion* oleander.]

Nernst, Hermann Walter (b. 1864). Berlin physicist.

Nernst lamp. A source of infra-red radiation, consisting of an electrically-heated filament maintained at a temperature below incandescence.

Nernst law. In order to cause a neuromuscular response the current density that must be used varies as the square root of its frequency.

Nernst's theory. The theory that tissue response to electrical stimulation depends on the ionization induced in the salts of the extracellular fluid in immediate contact with the cell membrane.

nerol (**ne**·rol). $C_{10}H_{18}O$, an isomer of geraniol found in oils of neroli and bergamot.

nerolin (**ner**·o·lin). One of the methyl-, ethyl or butyl-β-naphthyl ethers used in perfumery, instead of nerol, as an orange perfume.

nerve [nervus (NA)] (nerv). A bundle of nerve fibres along which impulses pass from one part of the body to another, each fibre being the axon of a nerve cell (neuron) surrounded by a neurilemma and often a myelin sheath. (For specific nerves, see under regional qualifying adjective or the organ or region supplied.) **Accelerator nerve.** A cardiac sympathetic nerve. **Adrenergic nerve.** An autonomic nerve that liberates an adrenal-like substance at the nerve-endings in a ganglion or muscle. **Afferent nerve.** A nerve that transmits impulses from the periphery to the centre. **Alderman's nerve.** The auricular branch of the vagus nerve; so-called because at official city dinners aldermen suffering from indigestion were reputed to rub or anoint the area of skin behind the ears as a stimulus to the vagus nerve to facilitate digestion. **Anabolic nerve.** A nerve whose stimulation promotes anabolic processes. **Nerve of arrest.** Inhibitory nerve (see below). **Articular nerve [nervus articularis (NA)].** A nerve supplying joint structures, especially the capsule. **Centrifugal nerve.** Efferent nerve (see below). **Centripetal nerve.** Afferent nerve (see above). **Cerebrospinal nerve.** A nerve originating directly from the brain or spinal cord. **Cutaneous nerve [nervus cutaneus (NA)].** A nerve entering the skin. **Depressor nerve.** A nerve that depresses the activity of an organ or a nerve centre. **Efferent nerve.** A nerve that carries impulses to the periphery. **Esodic nerve.** Afferent nerve (see above). **Excitor nerve.** A nerve whose stimulation increases the activity of an organ. **Exodic nerve.** Efferent nerve (see above). **Extrinsic nerve.** An autonomic nerve in its course external to the organ it supplies. **Gangliated nerve.** A sympathetic nerve. **Inhibitory nerve.** A nerve whose stimulation inhibits the activity of an organ. **Intrinsic nerve.** A term applied to the ultimate ramifications of autonomic nerve fibres in an organ. **Mixed nerve.** A nerve that contains both sensory and motor fibres. **Motor nerve.** A nerve that contains only or mainly motor fibres. **Pain nerve.** Sensory nerve (see below). **Parasympathetic nerves.** *See* SYSTEM, PARASYMPATHETIC NERVOUS. **Peripheral nerve.** Any of the cranial or spinal nerves. Autonomic nerves are not usually considered as peripheral nerves, but with the peripheral nerves constitute the peripheral nervous system. **Pilomotor nerve.** A motor nerve that supplies the arrectores pilorum muscles. **Pressor nerve.** A nerve whose stimulation increases vascular tension. **Secretory nerve.** An efferent nerve whose stimulation causes increased activity of the gland in which it terminates. **Sensory nerve.** An afferent nerve which conveys impulses from peripheral nerve-endings in sense organs to the cord or brain. **Somatic nerve.** Any peripheral nerve, sensory or motor, which is not part of the autonomic outflow. **Splanchnic nerve.** Any nerve supplying the abdominal viscera, and formed mainly of preganglionic sympathetic fibres. *See* SPLANCHNIC NERVES. **Sympathetic nerves.** *See* SYSTEM, SYMPATHETIC NERVOUS. **Vasoconstrictor nerve.** A nerve whose stimulation causes constriction of the arterioles. **Vasodilator nerve.** A nerve whose stimulation causes dilatation of the arterioles. **Vasomotor nerve.** Any nerve effecting constriction or dilatation of the blood vessels. **Vidian nerve.** The nerve of the pterygoid canal. [L *nervus.*]

See also: ANDERSCH, ARNOLD (F.), BELL (C.), BOCK, CASSERIO, COTUGNO (COTUNNIUS), CRUVEILHIER, CYON, EXNER, GALEN, GASKELL, GUIDI, HERING (H. E.), HIRSCHFELD (L. M.), HOFER, JACOBSON (L. L.), KRAUSE (W. J. F.), LANCISI, LANGENBECK (K. J. M.), LANGLEY, LATARGET, LUSCHKA, NAGEOTTE, RANDACIO, SAPOLINI, SCARPA, SOEMMERING, SOUSA, TIEDEMANN, VALENTIN, VOIT (M.), WALTER, WRISBERG.

nerve-ending (**nerv**·end·ing). The termination of any fibre, axonal or dendritic, arising from a nerve cell. **Annulospiral nerve-endings.** Sensory nerve-endings around the nuclear bag of muscle spindles. **Effector motor nerve-endings.** Specialized endings in the skeletal muscles; motor end-plates. **Flower-spray nerve-endings.** Receptor nerve-endings on the intrafusal fibres of muscle spindles. **Free nerve-endings [terminationes nervorum liberae (NA)].** Unencapsulated or naked nerve-endings, in which the axon, after losing its medullary sheath and neurilemma, divides into naked terminal branches often with bead-like extremities which end amongst the other tissue elements. No organized capsule or special cells are associated with these endings. **Somatic sensory nerve-endings.** Dendritic nerve-endings subserving sensation, lying in skin, muscles or tendons, as contrasted with special sense endings (in special sense organs) or visceral sensory endings (in viscera and blood vessels). The endings may be in the form of special end-organs or fine nerve nets and filaments. [nerve, AS *ende.*]

See also: DOGIEL.

nerve gases (**nerv gas**·es). Liquids that are about as volatile as kerosene, almost colourless and non-irritating: they are therefore not easily detected and act insidiously. They inhibit cholinesterase, leading to accumulation of acetylcholine, and thereby upset neuromuscular action. They produce a condition similar to acute asphyxia. [nerve, gas.]

nerve storm (**nerv** storm). An ill-defined phrase meaning any sudden attack of nervous disorder. [nerve, AS *storm.*]

nerve-stretching (**nerv**·strech·ing). Stretching of a nerve by open operation or otherwise, usually to relieve pain. [nerve, AS *streccan*.]

nervimotor (ner·ve·**mo**·tor). Referring to a motor nerve or motor activity.

nervimuscular, nervomuscular (ner·ve·**mus**·kew·lar, ner·vo·**mus**·-kew·lar). Pertaining to nerve and muscle, e.g. the nerve impulses transmitted to muscles.

nervone (**ner**·vone). A cerebroside of brain tissue.

nervotabes (ner·vo·**ta**·beez). A disorder which resembles tabes dorsalis in its symptoms but differs from it in 3 respects: the Argyll Robertson pupil is absent, tenderness is noted on muscular pressure and very often a cure can be effected. [nerve, L *tabescere* to waste.]

nervous (**ner**·vus). 1. Referring to a nerve or nerves. 2. Timid, apprehensive with little cause, easily agitated or irritable.

nervousness (**ner**·vus·nes). The state of being nervous.

nervus (**ner**·vus). Nerve. **Nervus descendens cervicalis.** A nerve formed from branches of the 2nd and 3rd cervical nerves. It joins the descending branch of the hypoglossal nerve to form the ansa hypoglossi, and helps to supply the infrahyoid group of muscles. **Nervi erigentes.** The pelvic splanchnic nerves. **Nervus spinosus [ramus meningeus (nervi mandibularis (NA))].** A small branch of the mandibular nerve which arises immediately outside the skull and enters the cerebral cavity through the foramen spinosum. It is distributed along the middle meningeal artery to the dura mater. It also sends a twig to the mastoid air cells. **Nervi terminales [NA].** A pair of small nerves composed of non-medullated fibres and bipolar and multipolar cells lying in the medial side of the olfactory tracts. They are connected centrally to the olfactory trigone and are distributed to the nasal mucous membrane. [L.]

Nesbit, Reed Miller (b. 1898). American urologist.

Reed Nesbit's intraperitoneal transplantation of ureters. Transperitoneal ureterocolic transplantation by "mucosa-to-mucosa" technique and subsequent retroperitonealization of the line of suture.

nesidiectomy (ne·sid·e·**ek**′·to·me). Excision of the inter-alveolar cell islets of the pancreas. [Gk *nesidion* islet, *ektome* a cutting out.]

nesidioblastoma (ne·**sid**·e·o·blas·**to**′·mah). A tumour of the interalveolar cell islets of the pancreas. [Gk *nesidion* islet, blastoma.]

nesidioblastosis (ne·**sid**·e·o·blas·**to**′·sis). A generalized proliferative condition affecting the interalveolar cell islets of the pancreas. [Gk *nesidion* islet, *blastos* germ, *-osis* condition.]

Nessler, A. (b. 1827). Karlsruhe chemist.

Nessler's reagent, for ammonia. 1. Dissolve 35 g of potassium iodide and 12.5 g of mercuric chloride in 800 ml of water and add cold saturated solution of mercuric chloride until after repeated shaking a slight red precipitate remains. Add 120 g of sodium hydroxide, shake until dissolved, then add a little more saturated mercuric chloride solution, followed by water to 1 litre. Shake occasionally during several days, allow to stand and decant the clear supernatant liquid for use. 2. Koch and McMeekin's method. Dissolve 22.5 g of iodine in 20 ml of water containing 30 g of potassium hydroxide. Add 30 g of mercury and shake the mixture well, keeping it in cold water as required until the supernatant liquid has lost its brown colour. Decant through glass wool into a 200 ml flask and test a drop with starch; if free iodine is absent add iodine solution of the above strength drop by drop until a faint excess is shown by starch. Dilute to 200 ml and pour the solution into 975 ml of 10 per cent sodium hydroxide. Mix and allow to clear by standing. This method is especially recommended for preparing Nessler's reagent for use in clinical analysis, e.g. blood urea, plasma proteins, etc.

nesslerization (**nes**·ler·i·**za**′·shun). The diagnostic use of Nessler's reagent.

nest (nest). Used figuratively and applied to a cluster of objects grouped like eggs in a bird's nest. **Cancer nest, Cell nest.** A concentration mass of keratin and pavement epithelium found in epitheliomata. [AS.]

See also: BRUNN.

nesteostomy, nestiostomy (nes·te·**os**·to·me). Jejunostomy [obsolete terms]. [Gk *nestis* fasting, *stoma* mouth.]

nestotherapy (nes·to·**ther**·ap·e). The treatment of disease by absolute fasting or by limitation of the quantity of food. [Gk *nestis* fasting, therapy.]

net (net). A network. **Nerve net.** A network of terminal nerve fibres, such as subserves pain sensation in the skin. Its individual fibres do not anastomose. [AS.] 1*See also:* HELD, TROLARD.

nettle (netl). Stinging nettle; the leaves and flowering tops of *Urtica dioica* (family Urticaceae). The irritant effect is due to the presence of histamine and acetylcholine in the hairs. [AS *netele*.]

Nettleship, Edward (b. 1845). London ophthalmologist.

Nettleship's punctum dilator. A blunt pointed conical instrument with a grooved handle that enables it to be twirled between the fingers. It is used for dilating the puncta lacrimalia prior to syringing or probing.

Nettleship's disease. Urticaria pigmentosa.

network [rete (NA)] (**net**·werk). Reticulum, rete or plexus: an interlacing or anastomosing system of fibres or vessels. **Acromial network [rete acromiale (NA)].** A network of arteries on the superficial surface of the acromion formed by anastomoses between acromial branches of the suprascapular and acromiothoracic arteries and the deltoid branch of the acromiothoracic artery. **Arterial network [rete arteriosum (NA)].** Any plexus of arteries or arterioles. **Network of basilar sinuses.** *See* SINUS, BASILAR. **Calcanean network [rete calcaneum (NA)].** The plexus of arteries in the subcutaneous tissues of the heel supplied by the medial and lateral calcanean branches of the peroneal artery. **Dorsal venous network of the foot [rete venosum dorsale pedis (NA)].** A network of veins on the dorsum of the foot, connected with the network on the front of the leg and with the dorsal venous arch of the foot. **Dorsal venous network of the hand [rete venosum dorsale manus (NA)].** The venous network on the dorsum of the hand, across the middle of the metacarpal bones, draining the digits and continuous with the basilic and cephalic veins at its ulnar and radial ends respectively. **Network of the elbow joint [rete articulare cubiti (NA)].** The arterial anastomosis around the elbow joint. It receives the ulnar collateral, supratrochlear, anterior and posterior ulnar recurrent, interosseous recurrent, and radial recurrent arteries and terminal branches of the profunda brachii artery. **Network of the knee [rete articulare genu (NA)].** The anastomosis around the knee joint, in which the following arteries take part: the descending genicular, medial inferior genicular, anterior tibial recurrent, circumflex fibular, lateral inferior genicular, lateral superior genicular and the descending branch of the lateral femoral circumflex artery. **Malleolar network, lateral [rete malleolare laterale (NA)].** The network of arteries around and over the lateral malleolus, receiving contributions from the anterior lateral malleolar branch of the anterior tibial artery and the malleolar branch of the peroneal artery. **Malleolar network, medial [rete malleolare mediale (NA)].** The network of arteries around and over the medial malleolus, receiving contributions from the anterior medial malleolar branch of the anterior tibial and the malleolar branch of the posterior tibial artery. **Patellar network [rete patellae (NA)].** The part of the network of the knee (see above) around the patella, sometimes referred to as the *superficial network*, as opposed to the remainder which is termed the *deep network*. **Venous network [rete venosum (NA)].** Any plexus of veins or venules. **Venous plantar network [rete venosum plantare (NA)].** A fine network of veins in the subcutaneous tissue of the sole. **Wonderful network.** Rete mirabile. [AS *net, wearc*.]

See also: HALLER, KOBELT, TEICHMANN-STAWIARSKI.

Neubauer, Johann Ernst (b. 1742). Jena anatomist and surgeon.

Neubauer's artery. The thyroidea ima artery.

Neubauer's ganglion. A ganglion formed by the junction of the inferior cervical and 1st thoracic sympathetic ganglia.

Neubauer, Otto (b. 1874). Munich physician.
Neubauer chamber. A blood-cell counting chamber. There are 2 complete sets of readings on each slide; each is divided into 9 large squares of 0.1 mm^3 each; of these the corner ones are subdivided into 16 smaller squares for white-cell counting, and the centre is divided into still smaller squares of 0.000 25 mm^3 in 16 groups of 16 squares each, for red-cell counting.
Neubauer and Fischer test. *See* TEST FOR CANCER.

Neuber, Gustav Adolf (b. 1850). Kiel surgeon.
Neuber's operation. Obliteration of a bone cavity by skin flaps turned from the side of the wound.

Neuberg, Carl (b. 1877). Berlin biochemist.
Neuberg ester. Fructofuranose monophosphate, $C_6H_{11}O_6PO(OH)_2$, which occurs with Embden ester in muscle.

Neufeld, Fred (b. 1861). German bacteriologist.
Neufeld's phenomenon. Lysis of pneumococci by bile salts.
Neufeld's reaction or test. Quellung reaction; the swelling of the capsules of pneumococci visible microscopically when a suspension of viable organisms is mixed on a microscope slide with the homologous type serum. It is a test used to identify the serological type of pneumococci.

Neumann, Ernst Franz Christian (b. 1834). Königsberg pathologist.
Neumann's cell. An immature nucleated red cell from the bone marrow.
Neumann's sheath. A differentiated layer of dentine immediately adjacent to the canal of the dentinal tubules.

Neumann, Franz Ernst (b. 1798). Königsberg physicist.
Neumann's law. The specific heats of solid compounds of similar composition are inversely proportional to the molecular weights of the compounds, i.e. the molecular heats (molecular weight multiplied by specific heat) of similar compounds are equal.

Neumann, Isidor (b. 1832). Vienna dermatologist.
Neumann's disease. Pemphigus vegetans.

neura (newr·ah). Neurone. [Gk *neuron* nerve.]

neuradynamia (newr·a·di·nam'·e·ah). Neurasthenia. [Gk *neuron* nerve, *a*, *dynamis* force.]

neuragmia (newr·ag·me·ah). Distraction of a nerve from its ganglion. [Gk *neuron* nerve, *agmos* break.]

neural (newr·al). Referring to a nerve or to the nervous system. [Gk *neuron* nerve.]

neuralgia (newr·al·je·ah). A painful affection of the nerves, due to functional disturbances or to neuritis. It is met with in a great number of morbid conditions, and varieties are frequently named from the part of the body affected, e.g. facial, brachial, supraorbital, etc. **Neuralgia amyotrophica.** Neuralgic amyotrophia. *See* AMYOTROPHIA. **Articular neuralgia.** Neuralgic pains in the neighbourhood of a joint. **Brachial neuralgia.** Aching or stabbing pains in the distribution of any of the branches of the brachial plexus, without paresis of muscle; that due to stretching or other injury of the brachial plexus. **Cardiac neuralgia.** Angina pectoris. **Cervical neuralgia.** Pain in the distribution of the sensory branches of the cervical nerves. **Cervico-occipital neuralgia.** Pain in the back of the neck and occipital regions. **Ciliary neuralgia.** A variety of neuralgia associated with migraine in which pain is felt in or behind the eye. **Cranial neuralgia.** Neuralgic pain located in various portions of the head, e.g. trigeminal neuralgia, supra-orbital neuralgia, etc. **Neuralgia facialis vera.** Geniculate neuralgia (see below). **Gastric neuralgia.** Visceral neuralgia (see below). **Geniculate neuralgia.** That due to morbid conditions of the otic ganglion of the facial nerves; pain is felt in the middle ear and auditory canal. **Glossopharyngeal neuralgia.** Paroxysmal attacks of pain in the distribution of the 9th cranial nerve. **Hepatic neuralgia.** Visceral neuralgia (see below). **Idiopathic neuralgia.** Neuralgia unaccompanied by structural nerve changes. **Intercostal neuralgia.** Neuralgic pain in intercostal spaces. **Intestinal neuralgia.** Visceral neuralgia (see below). **Mammary neuralgia.** Neuralgic pain in the breast. **Migrainous neuralgia.** Recurrent short attacks of severe unilateral pain in one eye and adjacent parts of the face and head. There may be rhinorrhoea, lacrimation and, occasionally, Horner's syndrome. More often known as *cluster headaches* or occasionally, *histaminic cephalgia.* **Otic neuralgia.** Geniculate neuralgia (see above). **Ovarian neuralgia.** Visceral neuralgia (see below). **Paratrigeminal neuralgia.** *See* RAEDER. **Postherpetic neuralgia.** Neuralgic pains in an area previously the site of a herpes zoster eruption; such pains are very intractable in treatment. **Red neuralgia.** A very painful affection of distal parts of a limb, associated with marked redness of the skin. It is obstinate to treatment, and often ends in amputation. **Sciatic neuralgia.** Sciatica. **Segmental neuralgia.** Neuralgia of a sharply defined area, e.g. of the area of supply of a single intercostal nerve. **Sphenopalatine ganglion neuralgia.** A lower-half headache, or unilateral facial pain, mainly in the orbital region and at the root of the nose. **Stump neuralgia.** Neuralgic pains in the stump of an amputated limb. **Supra-orbital neuralgia.** Neuralgia of the supra-orbital nerve. **Trifacial neuralgia, Trigeminal neuralgia.** Pain in the distribution of one or more of the sensory divisions of the 5th cranial nerve; tic douloureux. **Uterine neuralgia.** Visceral neuralgia (see following). **Visceral neuralgia.** Under this heading pains in various viscera may be described, e.g. hepatic, gastric, intestinal, ovarian, and uterine. Such pains are probably due to organic conditions in the organs named and not to a true neuralgia. [Gk *neuron* nerve, *algos* pain.]
See also: HUNT (J. R.), MORTON (T. G.), SEELIGMUELLER.

neuralgic (newr·al·jik). Referring to or of the character of neuralgia.

neuralgiform (newr·al·je·form). Resembling neuralgia. [neuralgia, form.]

neuraminidase (newr·am·in·e·daze). An enzyme (Enzyme Catalogue No. 3.2.1.18) found in broth culture filtrates from some organisms (e.g. *Vibrio cholerae*), some snake venoms (e.g. Russell's viper) and on the surface of some viruses (e.g. orthomyxovirus and paramyxovirus). Its action is to split the sialic acid residues from glycoproteins or from the surface of cells, including red blood cells.

neuranagenesis (newr·an·ah·jen'·es·is). Renewal of nervous tissue; regeneration of a nerve. [Gk *neuron* nerve, *anagenein* to regenerate.]

neurangiosis (newr·an·je·o'·sis). A neurotic condition involving the blood vessels and affecting the circulation. [Gk *neuron* nerve, *aggeion* small vessel, *-osis* condition.]

neurapophysis (newr·ap·of·is·is). One of the pair of neural arches of a vertebra, embracing the spinal cord and its membranes. [Gk *neuron* nerve, apophysis.]

neurapraxia (newr·ap·rax·e·ah). A nerve lesion attended by paralysis of short duration, but without any associated degenerative changes; recovery is usually complete (Seddon). [Gk *neuron* nerve, apraxia.]

neurarchy (newr·ar·ke). The dominating power of the cerebrospinal system over the whole body. [Gk *neuron* nerve, *arche* sovereignty.]

neurasthenia (newr·as·the·ne·ah). A neurosis in which there is marked mental and physical irritability and fatiguability. Symptoms are both physical and mental: on the mental side there is an inability to concentrate, impairment of memory, lessened control of the emotions and some depression. Physically, there is an inability to take exercise without excessive fatigue, a feeling of pressure in the head and pain in the limbs and back; the eyes are soon fatigued on reading. There may be complaint of palpitation, dyspnoea, constipation, impotence, etc. The condition may follow exhausting illnesses, prolonged lactation, insomnia or excessive consumption of tea, coffee or tobacco; in other cases the cause may be purely psychogenic. There is usually an inborn predisposition to react abnormally to mental stress. This term is at present out of favour among psychiatrists. **Abdominal neurasthenia.** Neurasthenia in which gastro-intestinal symptoms predominate. **Cardiovascular neurasthenia.** A neurasthenic condition in which submammary pain and laboured respiration are present. **Professional neurasthenia.**

Inability on the part of a patient to use movements which are commonly used in the practice of his profession, e.g. writers' cramp in a clerk. [Gk *neuron* nerve, *asthenia* debility.]

neurasthenic (newr·as·**then**·ik). 1. Referring to or suffering from neurasthenia. 2. Any person who suffers from neurasthenia.

neurataxia, neurataxy (newr·at·**ax**·e·ah, newr·at·**ax**·e). Neurasthenia. [Gk *neuron* nerve, ataxia.]

neuratrophia (newr·at·**ro**·fe·ah). Faulty nutrition of a nerve or of the central nervous system. [Gk *neuron* nerve, atrophy.]

neuratrophic (newr·at·**rof**·ik). 1. Referring to or marked by neuratrophia. 2. Any person who suffers from neuratrophia.

neuratrophy (newr·**at**·ro·fe). Neuratrophia.

neuraxial (newr·**ax**·e·al). Referring to the axon. [Gk *neuron* nerve, axis.]

neuraxis (newr·**ax**·is). The central nervous sytem [Obsolete term]. [Gk *neuron* nerve, axis.]

neuraxitis (newr·ax·**i**·tis). Encephalitis. **Epidemic neuraxitis.** Epidemic encephalitis. *See* ENCEPHALITIS. [Gk *neuron* nerve, axis, Gk *-itis* inflammation.]

neuraxon (newr·**ax**·on). The axon or axis-cylinder of a nerve cell [Obsolete term]. [Gk *neuron* nerve, axon.]

neurectasis, neurectasy (newr·**ek**·tas·is, newr·**ek**·tas·e). Nerve-stretching carried out by surgical methods. [Gk *neuron* nerve, *ektasis* a stretching.]

neurectomy (newr·**ek**·to·me). Excision of a nerve segment. **Gastric neurectomy.** Division of those branches of the vagus nerve which supply the stomach in order to reduce acid secretion. Performed in treatment of peptic ulcer. **Obturator neurectomy.** Division of the obturator nerves either in the abdomen or the groin to relieve adductor spasm in upper motor neurone paralysis. **Obturator neurectomy, anterior.** A neurectomy carried out through a thigh approach in which only the anterior branch of the obturator nerve is divided. **Opticociliary neurectomy.** Division of the optic and ciliary nerves. **Presacral neurectomy.** Removal of parasympathetic nerve fibres lying over the promontory of the sacrum. [Gk *neuron* nerve, *ektome* a cutting out.]

neurectopia, neurectopy (newr·ek·**to**·pe·ah, newr·**ek**·to·pe). 1. Nerve displacement. 2. A nerve that has an anomalous distribution. [Gk *neuron* nerve, *ektopos* out of the way.]

neurenteric (newr·en·**ter**·ik). Pertaining to the canal which exists at an early stage of development between the hind end of the neural tube and the primitive gut. [Gk *neuron* nerve, *enteron* bowel.]

neurepithelial (newr·ep·e·**the**'·le·al). Neuro-epithelial.

neurepithelium (newr·ep·e·**the**'·le·um). Neuro-epithelium.

neurergic (newr·**er**·jik). Referring to or contingent on the activity of a nerve. [Gk *neuron* nerve, *ergon* work.]

neurexeresis (newr·ex·**er**·es·is). Nerve avulsion. *See* AVULSION. [Gk *neuron* nerve, exeresis.]

neurhypnology (newr·hip·**nol**·o·je). Hypnology. [Gk *neuron* nerve, *hypnos* sleep, *logos* science.]

neuriasis (newr·i·as·is). Hypochondriasis of hysterical pattern. [Gk *neuron* nerve.]

neurilemma (newr·e·**lem**·ah). The delicate membrane investing the medullary sheath of a nerve fibre and associated with the cells of Schwann. [Gk *neuron* nerve, *lemma* sheath.]

neurilemmitis (newr·e·lem·**i**'·tis). Inflammation affecting the neurilemma. [neurilemma, Gk *-itis* inflammation.]

neurilemmoma (newr·e·lem·**o**'·mah). An innocent tumour of a nerve derived from the neurilemma. [neurilemma, Gk *-oma* tumour.]

neurilemmosarcoma (newr·e·**lem**·e·sar·**ko**'·mah). A malignant neurilemmoma. [neurilemmoma, sarcoma.]

neurimotility (newr·e·mo·**til**'·it·e). Power of movement in response to a nervous impulse. [Gk *neuron* nerve, motility.]

neurimotor (newr·e·**mo**·tor). Referring to a motor nerve or to motor activity. [Gk *neuron* nerve, motor.]

neurine (newr·een). Trimethylvinylammonium hydroxide, CH_2=$CHN(CH_3)_3OH$. An actively poisonous cadaveric alkaloid or ptomaine related to choline, produced by the bacterial decomposition of lecithin and found in brain, putrefying fish and also occurring in some fungi. Inoculation of animals causes widespread paralysis and death.

neurinoma (newr·in·o·mah). An innocent tumour of a nerve derived from the neurilemma. **Acoustic neurinoma.** Acoustic neurofibroma. *See* NEUROFIBROMA. **Malignant neurinoma.** One that has undergone malignant change. [Gk *neuron* nerve, *-oma* tumour.]

neurinomatosis (newr·in·o·mat·o'·sis). The condition of being affected with numerous neurinomata. [neurinoma, Gk *-osis* condition.]

neurit, neurite (newr·it, newr·ite). Old terms for the axon of a nerve cell. [Gk *neuron* nerve.]

neuritic (newr·**it**·ik). Relating to or suffering from neuritis.

neuritis (newr·**i**·tis). Inflammation of a nerve, with pain and tenderness and diminution or loss of function in its distribution, i.e. of sensation or motor power. It is caused by various conditions (pressure, local inflammatory conditions), numerous poisons (metallic, alcoholic), toxins of infectious diseases or lack of vitamins (beriberi). **Adventitial neuritis.** That due to changes in the sheath of the nerve. **Alcoholic neuritis.** Neuritis associated with chronic alcoholism; probably due to vitamin-B_1 deficiency. **Amyloid neuritis.** A form of peripheral neuropathy caused by local deposits of amyloid. **Arsenical neuritis.** A peripheral neuritis that may follow a large single or a repeated dose of arsenic, taken accidentally or medicinally. **Axial neuritis.** Neuritis due to changes in the parenchyma of a nerve. **Cervico-occipital neuritis.** A painful neuritis radiating over the upper branches of the cervical plexus; the great auricular nerve is usually concerned, but the supraclavicular, suprasternal and supra-acromial branches may also be involved. **Degenerative neuritis.** Neuritis due to degenerative processes in the parenchyma of a nerve. **Diabetic neuritis.** Neuritis due to metabolic disturbance in the diabetic state. **Dietetic neuritis.** Neuritis arising when the diet includes some toxic substance, e.g. alcohol, metallic poisons; also that in deficiency disease, e.g. beriberi. **Diphtheritic neuritis.** That due to the effects of toxins of diphtheria on the nerves of eye muscles or the soft palate. **Disseminated neuritis.** Peripheral neuritis (see below). **Dysenteric neuritis.** A peripheral neuritis that may follow an attack of bacillary dysentery. **Endemic neuritis.** Beriberi. **Facial neuritis.** Bell's palsy. **Neuritis fascians.** Adventitial neuritis (see above). **Influenzal neuritis.** A peripheral neuritis of the single or multiple type, a sequel to influenza. **Interstitial neuritis.** That affecting the connective tissue of a nerve. **Intra-ocular neuritis.** Optic neuritis (see below). **Ischaemic neuritis.** Neuritis resulting from impaired blood supply to a nerve as in occlusive arterial disease. **Lead neuritis.** Neuritis in lead poisoning; usually occupational. **Leprous neuritis.** A form of neuritis seen in leprosy. **Lipomatous neuritis.** A form of neuritis in which nerve fibres are destroyed and replaced by fibrous tissue with an added deposition of fat. **Lymphatic neuritis.** Inflammation of the parenchyma of a nerve. **Multiple neuritis.** Peripheral neuritis (see below). **Neuritis nodosa.** Neuritis with formation of nodules on the nerves. **Optic neuritis.** Neuritis affecting the optic disc or the optic nerve behind the eye. **Orbital optic neuritis.** Optic neuritis (see preceding). **Parenchymatous neuritis.** Neuritis with morbid changes in the nerve substance proper. **Periaxial neuritis.** Inflammation in the connective tissue surrounding the nerve. **Peripheral neuritis.** The term applied to nervous trouble caused by lesions affecting the parenchyma of peripheral motor and sensory nerves due to toxic causes, bacterial, alcoholic and metallic. **Postfebrile neuritis.** That which follows an acute infection. **Postocular neuritis.** Optic neuritis (see above). **Pressure neuritis.** Neuritis due to pressure on a nerve or nerve root, e.g. by bone or tumour. **Proliferative neuritis.** Neuritis with overgrowth of connective tissue until the nerve may appear as a fibrous cord. **Neuritis puerperalis traumatica.** Nerve lesions in the mother due to trauma during birth, e.g. sciatica. **Radicular neuritis.** Affections of nerve roots as they pass from the spinal cord through the intervertebral foramina. **Retrobulbar**

neuritis. Optic neuritis (see above). **Neuritis saturnina.** Lead neuritis (see above). **Sciatic neuritis.** Sciatica. **Segmental neuritis, Segmentary neuritis.** Inflammation occurring at several localized points of a nerve. **Shoulder-girdle neuritis.** Neuralgic amyotrophia. *See* AMYOTROPHIA. **Syphilitic neuritis, Tabetic neuritis.** Neuritis seen in cases with underlying syphilitic pathology. **Terminal neuritis.** Erythromelalgia. **Toxaemic neuritis, Toxic neuritis.** Neuritis due to some poison, bacterial or metallic. **Traumatic neuritis.** Neuritis which is the result of trauma to a nerve. [Gk *neuron* nerve, *-itis* inflammation.]

See also: EICHHORST, GOMBAULT, LEYDEN.

neuro-anastomosis (newr·o·an·as·to·**mo**'·sis). The surgical formation of an anastomosis between nerves. [Gk *neuron* nerve, anastomosis.]

neuro-anatomy (newr·o·an·**at**'·o·me). That branch of anatomical science which deals with the nervous system. [Gk *neuron* nerve, anatomy.]

neuro-arthropathy (newr·o·ar·**throp**'·ath·e). Neurogenic arthropathy. *See* ARTHROPATHY. [Gk *neuron* nerve, arthropathy.]

neuro-avitaminosis (newr·o·a·vi·tam·in·**o**'·sis). Neuritis caused by avitaminosis, usually of B_1 or aneurine.

neurobiology (newr·o·bi·**ol**'·o·je). The study of life processes in the nervous system. [Gk *neuron* nerve, biology.]

neurobiotaxis (newr·o·bi·o·**tax**'·is). The predisposition of a nerve cell to move in the direction from which it derives its stimuli. [Gk *neuron* nerve, biotaxis.]

neuroblast (newr·o·blast). Any one of the cells of the intermediate layer in the embryonic spinal cord which later gives rise to a nerve cell. [Gk *neuron* nerve, *blastos* germ.]

neuroblastoma (newr·o·blas·**to**'·mah). A highly malignant tumour of sympathoblast from the neural crest of the adrenal medulla occurring mainly in young children. The presence of HMMA or HVA in the urine confirms the diagnosis. [neuroblast, Gk *-oma* tumour.]

neurocanal (newr·o·kan·**al**'). The central canal of the spinal cord. [Gk *neuron* nerve, canal.]

neurocardiac (newr·o·**kar**·de·ak). 1. Referring to the nervous system and to the heart. 2. Concerning the nervous mechanism of the heart. 3. Referring to neurosis of cardiac type. [Gk *neuron* nerve, *kardia* heart.]

neurocele (newr·o·seel). Neurocoele.

neurocentral (newr·o·**sen**·tral). Pertaining to the sutures between the vertebral (neural) arch and centrum of an immature vertebra.

neurochemistry (newr·o·**kem**·is·tre). That branch of biochemistry concerned with the chemical changes which take place in the nervous system. [Gk *neuron* nerve, chemistry.]

neurochoroidoretinitis (newr·o·kor·**oid**·o·ret·in·**i**'·tis). An inflammatory condition involving the optic nerve, the choroid and the retina. [Gk *neuron* nerve, choroidoretinitis.]

neuroclonic (newr·o·**klon**·ik). Marked by the occurrence of clonic nervous spasms. [Gk *neuron* nerve, *klonos* any violent motion.]

neurocoele (newr·o·seel). A cavity surrounded by nervous tissue; the cavity of the embryonic nervous system, represented in the adult by the central canal of the spinal cord, ventricles of the brain, etc. [Gk *neuron* nerve, *koilos* hollow.]

neurocranial (newr·o·**kra**·ne·al). Referring to the neurocranium.

neurocranium (newr·o·**kra**·ne·um). The part of the skull enclosing and protecting the brain. [Gk *neuron* nerve, *kranion* skull.]

neurocrine (newr·o·krine). A chemical transmitter; a substance concerned in the transmission of a nerve impulse across a synapse or from the nerve to the effector organ. It is also referred to as a *local hormone.* [Gk *neuron* nerve, *krinein* to secrete.]

neurocrinia (newr·o·**krin**·e·ah). The influence of an endocrine substance on nervous tissues, [see prec.]

neurocutaneous (newr·o·kew·**ta**'·ne·us). Referring to the cutaneous nerves and to their relation to the skin. [Gk *neuron* nerve, cutaneous.]

neurocyte (newr·o·site). A nerve cell or neuron. [Gk *neuron* nerve, *kytos* cell.]

neurocytolysin (newr·o·si·**tol**'·is·in). A toxic substance that has an affinity for nerve cells which it lyses; the poison of certain colubrine snakes, e.g. the cobra, contains such a toxin. [Gk *neuron* nerve, *kytos* cell, *lysein* to loosen.]

neurocytoma (newr·o·si·**to**'·mah). A variety of glioma, found at the base of the brain, in the third or fourth ventricles, in the cerebellum, retina, abdominal sympathetic trunks, adrenals and spinal cord, which infiltrates the adjacent tissues and produces pressure symptoms early. [Gk *neuron* nerve, *kytos* cell, *-oma* tumour.]

neurodealgia (newr·o·de·**al**'·je·ah). A painful condition affecting the retina. [Gk *neuroeides* nerve-like, *algos* pain.]

neurodeatrophia (newr·o·de·at·**ro**'·fe·ah). Atrophy of the retina. [Gk *neuroeides* nerve-like, atrophia.]

neurodegenerative (newr·o·de·**jen**'·er·a·tiv). Pertaining to or characterized by degeneration of nerve tissue. [Gk *neuron* nerve, degenerate.]

neurodendrite, neurodendron (newr·o·**den**·drite, newr·o·**den**'·dron). Dendrite; the protoplasmic process (usually short) of a nerve cell which, freely branching, transmits nerve impulses to the cell and arborizes with dendrites of other nerve-cells. [Gk *neuron* nerve, *dendron* tree.]

neuroderm (newr·o·derm). That part of the primitive ectoderm which gives rise to the neural tube and crest. [Gk *neuron* nerve, *derma* skin.]

neurodermatitis (newr·o·der·mat·**i**'·tis). 1. Any skin eruption, except dermatitis artefacta, in which the principal aetiological factor is psychological. 2. Lichen simplex chronicus. **Neurodermatitis circumscripta.** Neurodermatitis affecting only a limited area. **Neurodermatitis disseminata.** Neurodermatitis affecting wide areas—sometimes the whole—of the body. [Gk *neuron* nerve, dermatitis.]

neurodermatomyositis (newr·o·**der**·mat·o·mi·o·**si**'·tis). A syndrome in which there is an inflammatory reaction of the tissues, involving the skin and subcutaneous tissue, with a clinical manifestation of nerve pain in the limb. [Gk *neuron* nerve, *derma* skin, *mys* muscle, *-itis* inflammation.]

neurodermatosis (newr·o·der·mat·**o**'·sis). A nervous condition involving the skin. [Gk *neuron* nerve, dermatosis.]

neurodermatrophia (newr·o·der·mat·**ro**'·fe·ah). Atrophy of the skin caused by a disorder of the nervous system. [Gk *neuron* nerve, *derma* skin, atrophy.]

neurodermite (newr·o·**der**·mite). Lichen simplex chronicus. [Gk *neuron* nerve, *derma* skin.]

neurodermitis (newr·o·der·**mi**'·tis). Lichen simplex chronicus. [Gk *neuron* nerve, *derma* skin, *-itis* inflammation.]

neurodes (newr·o·deez). The retina. [Gk *neuroeides* nerve-like.]

neurodiagnosis (newr·o·di·ag·**no**'·sis). Diagnosis of the disorders which affect the nervous system. [Gk *neuron* nerve, diagnosis.]

neurodiastasis (newr·o·di·**as**'·tas·is). Nerve separation. [Gk *neuron* nerve, *diastasis* a standing apart.]

neurodin (newr·o·din). Acetyl para-oxyphenylurethane, $C_6H_4(OCOCH_3)NHCOOC_2H_5$. A crystalline substance with analgesic properties.

neurodynamia (newr·o·di·**nam**'·e·ah). Nervous force. [Gk *neuron* nerve, *dynamis* force.]

neurodynamic (newr·o·di·**nam**'·ik). Relating or belonging to neurodynamia.

neurodynia (newr·o·**din**·e·ah). Neuralgia. [Gk *neuron* nerve, *odyne* pain.]

neurodystonia (newr·o·dis·**to**'·ne·ah). Dystonia associated with disordered innervation of the visceral structures. [Gk *neuron* nerve, dystonia.]

neuro-electricity (newr·o·el·ek·**tris**'·it·e). Electrical changes and phenomena in the nervous system. [Gk *neuron* nerve, electricity.]

neuro-electrotherapeutics (newr·o·el·ek·tro·ther·ap·**ew**'·tix). The treatment of affections of nerves by means of electrical apparatus. [Gk *neuron* nerve, electrotherapeutics.]

neuro-encephalomyelopathy (newr·o·en·kef·al·o·mi·el·**op**'·ath·e). A disordered condition of the nerves, brain and spinal cord. [Gk *neuron* nerve, encephalomyelopathy.]

neuro-endocrine (newr·o·**en**·do·krine). Relating or belonging to the effect produced on the organism by the nerves and the action of the ductless (endocrine) glands. [Gk *neuron* nerve, endocrine.]
neuro-enteric (**newr**·o·en·**ter**'·ik). Neurenteric.
neuro-epidermal (**newr**·o·ep·e·**der**'·mal). 1. Referring to the nerves and to the epidermis. 2. Embryonic tissue from which the above structures are formed. [Gk *neuron* nerve, epidermis.]
neuro-epithelial (**newr**·o·ep·e·**the**'·le·al). Relating or belonging to or consisting of neuro-epithelium.
neuro-epithelioma (**newr**·o·ep·e·the·le·**o**'·mah). Neurocytoma of the retina. [Gk *neuron* nerve, epithelium, Gk *-oma* tumour.]
neuro-epithelium [NA] (**newr**·o·ep·e·**the**'·le·um). Epithelial cells of ectodermal origin lining the primitive neural tube or forming part of the lining of the mucosa of the nose or of the membranous labyrinth of the internal ear, which differentiate into nerve cells. [Gk *neuron* nerve, epithelium.]
neuro-equilibrium (**newr**·o·e·kwil·**ib**'·re·um). The state of even stress or general readiness in the nervous system which permits of a prompt response to impulses. [Gk *neuron* nerve, equilibrium.]
neurofibril (newr·o·**fi**·bril). One of a large number of fine fibres within the cytoplasm and processes of nerve cells, usually only demonstrable after silver impregnation of fixed tissues. [Gk *neuron* nerve, fibril.]
neurofibrillar (newr·o·**fi**·bril·ar). Pertaining to or characterized by neurofibrils.
neurofibroma (**newr**·o·fi·**bro**'·mah). An innocent tumour composed of nerve fibres and connective tissue, arising from the sheaths of cutaneous nerves. Often multiple (von Recklinghausen's disease) and associated with congenital abnormalities of the skin, brain and blood vessels. **Acoustic neurofibroma.** A benign tumour growing from the sheath of the 8th cranial nerve. **Dumb-bell neurofibroma.** A bilobate neurofibroma arising from a spinal nerve, part of which remains within the vertebral canal and part grows through the vertebral foramen. **Plexiform neurofibroma.** A diffuse neurofibroma arising along a nerve or from several nerves. [Gk *neuron* nerve, fibroma.]
neurofibromatosis (**newr**·o·fi·bro·mat·**o**'·sis). Von Recklinghausen's disease; a familial disorder in which developmental changes occur in the skin, nervous system, bones and viscera. In the skin there is a brown pigmentation varying in size from freckles to large diffuse areas, most evident on the trunk, combined with numerous sessile or pedunculated soft pinkish swellings (mollusca fibrosa) which may reach a large size and form redundant hanging folds. Neurofibromata occur on nerve trunks, limb plexuses or spinal nerve roots where they may cause spinal compression; within the skull they most commonly occur on the 8th cranial nerve (acoustic neurofibroma). Visceral neurofibromata may also occur. Kyphosis is usually present and there may be hyperostosis of the facial bones and the long bones of the limbs. The tumours may undergo sarcomatous change and complications such as spina bifida, meningocele, epilepsy, acromegaly, infantilism, etc. are not infrequent. [Gk *neuron* nerve, fibroma, Gk *-osis* condition.]
neurofibrosarcoma (newr·o·**fi**·bro·sar·**ko**'·mah). A malignant neurofibroma. [neurofibroma, sarcoma.]
neurofibrositis (**newr**·o·fi·bro·**si**'·tis). 1. Inflammation involving the fibres of nerves; neuritis. 2. Inflammation involving nerves and fibrous tissue. [Gk *neuron* nerve, fibrositis.]
neuroganglion (newr·o·**gang**·gle·on). The ganglion of a nerve. [Gk *neuron* nerve, ganglion.]
neuroganglionitis (**newr**·o·gang·gle·on·**i**'·tis). Inflammation affecting a nerve ganglion. [Gk *neuron* nerve, ganglionitis.]
neurogastric (newr·o·**gas**·trik). Pertaining to the nerves of the stomach. [Gk *neuron* nerve, *gaster* stomach.]
neurogenesis (newr·o·**jen**·es·is). The development and growth of nerves and nervous tissue. [Gk *neuron* nerve, *genesis* production.]
neurogenetic, neurogenic, neurogenous (**newr**·o·jen·**et**'·ik, newr·o·**jen**·ik, newr·**oj**·en·us). 1. Referring to neurogenesis. 2. Producing nerve tissue. 3. Arising in a nerve. 4. Caused by some disordered condition of the nerves or nervous system. [Gk *neuron* nerve, *genein* to produce.]
neurogeny (newr·**oj**·en·e). Neurogenesis.
neuroglia (newr·**og**·le·ah). The supporting cells of the central nervous system, taking the place of the connective tissue of other systems. They are usually classified as astrocytes, oligodendroglia, ependyma (all of ectodermal origin) and microglia (of mesodermal origin). **Interfascicular neuroglia.** The oligodendroglia ranged along tracts of white matter of the central nervous system. [Gk *neuron* nerve, *glia* glue.]
neurogliacyte (newr·**og**·le·ah·site). One of the cells contained in neuroglial tissue (the so-called *spider* or *mossy cell*). [neuroglia, Gk *kytos* cell.]
neurogliacytoma (newr·**og**·le·ah·si·**to**'·mah). A growth consisting of neuroglial cells. [neurogliacyte, Gk *-oma* tumour.]
neuroglial, neurogliar (newr·**og**·le·al, newr·**og**·le·ar). Referring to the neuroglia.
neuroglioma (**newr**·o·gli·**o**'·mah). A glioma. **Neuroglioma ganglionare, Ganglionic neuroglioma.** A glioma in which are contained ganglion cells. [neuroma, glioma.]
neurogliosis (**newr**·o·gli·**o**'·sis). The occurrence of scattered formations of neurogliomata. **Neurogliosis gangliocellularis diffusa.** Epiloia. [neuroglioma, Gk *-osis* condition.]
neurohaematology (**newr**·o·he·mat·**ol**'·o·je). That division of neurology which is concerned with changes in the blood brought about by disease of nervous origin. [Gk *neuron* nerve, *haima* blood, *logos* science.]
neurohistochemistry (**newr**·o·his·to·**kem**'·is·tre). The histological examination of the nervous system using staining methods specific for certain chemicals or chemical processes. [Gk *neuron* nerve, histology, chemistry.]
neurohistology (**newr**·o·his·**tol**'·o·je). Histology in its application to nerve tissues. [Gk *neuron* nerve, histology.]
neurohumoral (newr·o·**hew**·mor·al). Relating to the impulse of a nerve and the response made by the nerve tissue. [see foll.]
neurohumoralism (newr·o·**hew**·mor·al·izm). A theory based on experimental evidence that stimulation of the nerves of the autonomic nervous system gives rise to the output of chemical substances (neurohumours) at the visceral, muscular or glandular nerve-endings. An example is the stimulation of certain sympathetic nerve fibres producing an output of adrenaline. [Gk *neuron* nerve, L *humor* fluid.]
neurohumour (newr·o·**hew**·mor). Any chemical set free by stimulation of nerve-endings. [see prec.]
neurohypnology (**newr**·o·hip·**nol**'·o·je). Hypnology. [Gk *neuron* nerve, *hypnos* sleep, *logos* science.]
neurohypophyseal (**newr**·o·hi·po·**fiz**'·e·al). Referring to the posterior lobe of the hypophysis cerebri. [see foll.]
neurohypophysis (**newr**·o·hi·**pof**'·is·is). The posterior lobe of the hypophysis cerebri. [Gk *neuron* nerve, hypophysis.]
neuroid (**newr**·oid). Nerve-like. [Gk *neuron* nerve, *eidos* form.]
neuro-induction (**newr**·o·in·**duk**'·shun). Therapy by suggestion. [Gk *neuron* nerve, L *inducere* to influence.]
neuro-inidia (**newr**·o·in·**id**'·e·ah). Faulty nutrition of a nerve cell. [Gk *neuron* nerve, L *in* not, Gk *eidar* food.]
neuro-inoma (**newr**·o·in·**o**'·mah). Neurinoma.
neurokeratin (newr·o·**ker**·at·in). A horny material forming a supporting reticulum for the myelin sheath of medullated nerve fibres. [Gk *neuron* nerve, *keras* horn.]
neurokym, neurokyme (**newr**·o·kim, **newr**·o·kime). A nervous process or action. [gk *neuron* nerve, *kyma* wave.]
neurolabyrinthitis (**newr**·o·lab·ir·in·**thi**'·tis). Inflammation affecting the nerve tissues of the labyrinth. [Gk *neuron* nerve, labyrinth, Gk *-itis* inflammation.]
neurolapine (newr·o·**lap**·een). A suspension of vaccine virus prepared by inoculation of the virus intracerebrally into rabbits; now replaced by calf lymph prepared by growing the virus in the skin of calves or sheep. [Gk *neuron* nerve, Fr. *lapin* rabbit.]
neurolemma (newr·o·**lem**·ah). Neurilemma.

neurolemmitis (**newr**·o·lem·**i**′·tis). Neurilemmitis.

neurolemmoma (**newr**·o·lem·**o**′·mah). Neurilemmoma.

neurolepsy (newr·o·**lep**·se). A state of apathy and mental detachment. (A term coined by Delay in 1959.) [Gk *neuron* nerve, *lepsis* seizure.]

neurolept (**newr**·o·lept). A butyrophenone derivative which produces neurolepsis, e.g. droperidol. [Gk *neuron* nerve, *lepsis* seizure.]

neurolipomatosis dolorosa (**newr**·o·lip·o·mat·**o**′·sis dol·or·**o**·sah). Adiposis dolorosa (Dercum's disease); a disease chiefly affecting the female sex and characterized by the presence of nerve lesions and painful local accumulations of fat. [Gk *neuron* nerve, lipomatosis, L *dolor* bodily pain.]

neurologica diabolica (newr·ol·**oj**·ik·ah di·ab·**ol**·ik·ah). *See* MUNCHAUSEN'S SYNDROME. [neurology, Gk *diabolikos* devilish.]

neurological (newr·ol·**oj**·ik·al). Pertaining to neurology.

neurologist (newr·**ol**·o·jist). One expert in the study and treatment of diseases of the nervous system. [see foll.]

neurology (newr·**ol**·o·je). The section of medicine that deals with the study and treatment of diseases of the nervous system. [Gk *neuron* nerve, *logos* science.]

neurolues (newr·o·**lew**·eez). Neurosyphilis. [Gk *neuron* nerve, L *lues* syphilis.]

neurolymph (**newr**·o·limf). The cerebrospinal fluid. [Gk *neuron* nerve, lymph.]

neurolymphomatosis (**newr**·o·limf·o·mat·**o**′·sis). Invasion of the substance of a nerve by lymphoblasts. [Gk *neuron* nerve, lymphomatosis.]

neurolysin (newr·**ol**·is·in). A cytolysin having the power to destroy nerve cells. [see foll.]

neurolysis (newr·**ol**·is·sis). 1. Destruction of nerve tissue. 2. The relief of a nerve from adhesions by operation or stretching. [Gk *neuron* nerve, *lysein* to loosen.]

neurolytic (newr·o·**lit**·ik). Referring to neurolysis.

neuroma (newr·**o**·mah). A tumour composed of nerve cells and nerve fibres. **Acoustic neuroma.** A neurofibromatous tumour on the auditory or eighth cranial nerve. **Amputation neuroma.** A tumour-like mass of proliferating nerve fibres at the site of division of a peripheral nerve. **Amyelinic neuroma.** A neuroma composed of non-medullated nerve fibres. **Appendical neuroma.** An enlargement of nerve fibres within the wall of the appendix as the result of repeated inflammation; the enlargement of nerve fibres that sometimes accompanies carcinoid of the appendix. **Cirsoid neuroma.** A congeries of elongated, irregularly thickened nerve trunks. **Neuroma cutis.** A cutaneous neuroma. **Cystic neuroma.** A neuroma or neurofibroma in which cystic degeneration has occurred, as for instance in the acoustic neurofibroma. **Digital neuroma.** Amputation neuroma occurring in the fingers; sometimes used as an alternative term to describe plantar neuroma. **False neuroma.** A tumour which is the result of proliferation of the connective tissue of a nerve trunk. **Fibrillary neuroma.** Plexiform neuroma (see below). **Ganglionar neuroma, Ganglionated neuroma, Ganglionic neuroma.** A neuroma composed of ganglion cells, occurring mainly in connection with the main sympathetic trunks and the adrenal gland. **Malignant neuroma.** A rapidly growing ganglioneuroma. **Medullated neuroma.** A neuroma which is composed of medullated nerve fibres. **Multiple neuroma.** Neurofibromatosis. **Myelinic neuroma.** Medullated neuroma (see above). **Naevoid neuroma.** The proliferation of nerve-endings which accompanies skin naevi. **Plantar neuroma.** Fibrous thickening occurring in the digital nerves to the toes, usually the second and third, causing metatarsal pain and numbness of the affected toes; always associated with dropping of the metatarsal arch. **Plexiform neuroma.** Overgrowth of nerve trunks and ganglia, in which the nerves take part in the hyperplasia. **Post-traumatic neuroma.** Proliferation of the nerve fibres that may occur within scar tissue following a wound or an amputation. **Neuroma telangiectodes.** A neuroma rich in large blood spaces. **Traumatic neuroma.** Amputation neuroma (see above). **True neuroma.** A neuroma which is composed of nerve cells and fibres. [Gk *neuron* nerve, *-oma* tumour.]

See also: VERNEUIL.

neuromalacia (**newr**·o·mal·**a**′·she·ah). Softening of nerve tissue. [Gk *neuron* nerve, malacia.]

neuromast (**newr**·o·mast). A sensory organ or area formed by a raised mass of neuro-epithelial cells. [Gk *neuron* nerve, *mastos* hill.]

neuromatosis (**newr**·o·mat·**o**′·sis). The existence of aggregations of multiple neuromata. [neuroma, Gk *-osis* condition.]

neuromatous (newr·**o**·mat·us). Relating or belonging to a neuroma or neuromatosis.

neuromechanism (newr·o·**mek**·an·izm). The general mechanism and framework associated with the function of the nervous system. [Gk *neuron* nerve, mechanism.]

neuromere (**newr**·o·meer). A spinal segment of the embryo. [see foll.]

neuromery (newr·**om**·er·e). The segmental organization of the nervous system. [Gk *neuron* nerve, *meros* part.]

neuromimesis (**newr**·o·mim·**e**′·sis). The imitation by hysterical or neurotic persons of the signs of any organic disease. [Gk *neuron* nerve, mimesis.]

neuromimetic (**newr**·o·mim·**et**′·ik). 1. Referring to neuromimesis. 2. Similar to the impulse associated with neural action; denoting those agencies that excite nervous activity.

neuromittor (new·ro·**mit**·or). That terminal part of a nerve fibril through which a stimulus is transmitted to an adjoining neurone; a word infrequently used. [Gk *neuron* nerve, L *mittere* to send.]

neuromuscular (newr·o·**mus**·kew·lar). Relating to nerves and to muscles. [Gk *neuron* nerve, muscle.]

neuromyal (newr·o·**mi**·al). Neuromuscular. [Gk *neuron* nerve, *mys* muscle.]

neuromyelitis (**newr**·o·mi·el·**i**′·tis). Myelitis associated with neuritis. **Neuromyelitis optica.** Acute myelitis associated with optic neuritis. [Gk *neuron* nerve, *myelitis.*]

neuromyic (newr·o·**mi**·ik). Neuromuscular. [Gk *neuron* nerve, *mys* muscle.]

neuromyocardium (**newr**·o·mi·o·**kar**′·de·um). A continuous tract of atypical cardiac muscle concerned with the conduction of cardiac impulse from atria to ventricles. [Gk *neuron* nerve, myocardium.]

neuromyology (**newr**·o·mi·**ol**′·o·je). Classification of muscles on the basis of nerve supply. [Gk *neuron* nerve, *mys* muscle, *logos* science.]

neuromyon (newr·o·**mi**·on). The comprehensive term for the neural mechanism of a muscle. [Gk *neuron* nerve, *mys* muscle.]

neuromyopathic (**newr**·o·mi·o·**path**′·ik). Having reference to disease that affects both muscle and nerve. [Gk *neuron* nerve, *mys* muscle, *pathos* disease.]

neuromyopathy (**newr**·o·mi·**op**′·ath·e). Disease of the nervous system and of muscles. Carcinomatous neuromyopathy, neuromyopathy due to remote carcinoma. [Gk *neuron* nerve, *mys* muscle, *pathos* disease.]

neuromyositis (newr·o·mi·o·**si**′·tis). Neuritis associated with myositis.

neuron (**newr**·on). A complete nerve cell, consisting of a cell body containing the nucleus and its processes, axonal and dendritic. The term implies that the nerve cell is structurally independent of other cells and not part of a syncytium. **Afferent neuron.** A neuron which conducts impulses towards the structure or part under consideration, usually the central nervous system as a whole. **Bipolar neuron.** A neuron with 2 processes only, a single dendrite and an axon. **Central neuron.** A neuron within the central nervous system. **Connector neuron.** Any neuron which connects 2 other neurons or groups of neurons, commonly applied to the preganglionic neuron through which cells in the central nervous system are connected with postganglionic neurons in peripheral ganglia; also to neurons which connect receptor with effector or motor neurons. **Correlation neuron.** A neuron which connects with 2 other neurons or groups of neurons and correlates their functions. **Effector neuron.** A neuron whose axon ends on muscle fibres or other effector organs; a motor neuron the stimulation of which causes movement, secretion or some other activity in a structure which is not itself nervous. **Efferent neuron.** A neuron whose axon conducts away from the particular part of the nervous system under consideration; most commonly applied to the motor neurons of the anterior grey horn of the spinal cord. **Gamma neuron.** The cell bodies giving rise to the slowly conducting gamma fibres, especially the motor supply to the muscle spindles. **Intercalary neuron, Internuncial neuron.** A neuron connecting 2 other neurons or groups of neurons. **Lower motor neuron.** A motor or effector neuron in the anterior horn of grey matter of the spinal cord. **Multipolar neuron.** A neuron with many dendritic processes arising from the cell body in addition to the axon. **Peripheral motor neuron.** An effector or motor neuron situated outside the central nervous system, usually in a sympathetic or parasympathetic ganglion. **Peripheral sensory neuron.** A neuron in a dorsal-root ganglion of a spinal nerve or in the sensory ganglion of a cranial nerve; also a receptor neuron in the olfactory mucous membrane. **Postganglionic neuron.** A neuron in a sympathetic or parasympathetic ganglion or in a peripheral autonomic plexus whose axon innervates unstriped muscle or glandular tissue directly. **Preganglionic neuron.** A neuron whose axon ends in contact with another situated in a peripheral ganglion or plexus. **Projection neuron.** A neuron situated in one of the major subdivisions of the central nervous system whose axon passes to a different major subdivision, e.g. a neuron in the cerebral cortex whose axon ends in the brain stem or spinal cord. **Pseudo-unipolar neuron.** A neuron found in sensory ganglia of the spinal and cranial nerves in which the axon and dendrite have partly fused to form a single, birfurcating process. **Pyramidal neuron.** 1. A neuron whose axon enters the pyramidal tract. 2. A neuron the cell body of which is pyramidal in shape. **Receptor neuron.** A term usually limited to neurons which receive stimuli directly from the periphery; since any neuron is capable of receiving stimuli, all are in the most general sense "receptor". **Sensory neuron.** A neuron which receives its stimulus directly from the periphery; the *primary sensory neuron.* It may be applied to neurons within the central nervous system which receive direct connections from the primary sensory neuron, such neurons being called *secondary sensory neurons,* or more generally to any neuron which appears to be concerned predominantly with sensory function. **Unipolar neuron.** A neuron with a single process. **Upper motor neuron.** A neuron in the cerebral cortex the axon of which forms one of the fibres of the pyramidal tract, and, if stimulated, causes movement. [Gk *neuron* nerve.]

neuronaevus (newr·o·**ne**·vus). A soft cellular naevus; it is so called because it is held by some that naevus cells are derived from nerve end-organs. [Gk *neuron* nerve, naevus.]

neuronal (**newr**·on·al). Characterized by or appertaining to a neuron or neurons.

neuronatrophy (newr·on·**at**·ro·fe). General term for degeneration in any neuron. [neuron, atrophy.]

neuronephric (newr·o·**nef**·rik). Relating to the nervous and renal systems, particularly the nerve supply of the kidney. [Gk *neuron* nerve, *nephros* kidney.]

neuroneuronitis (**newr**·o·newr·on·**i**′·tis). Neuronitis.

neuronic (newr·**on**·ik). Neuronal.

neuronin (**newr**·on·in). The main protein present in an axon. [neuron.]

neuronist (**newr**·on·ist). One who supports the theory that nervous tissue is made up of nerve cells (neurons) which are structurally independent and do not form a syncytium.

neuronitis (newr·on·**i**·tis). An inflammatory and degenerative condition affecting the neurons; a term used to denote neuritis of the cells and roots of spinal-cord nerves. **Infective neuronitis.** Guillain–Barré syndrome. **Vestibular neuronitis.** An acute illness considered to be due to viral infection of the vestibular nerve, and characterized by acute severe vertigo persisting for several days, followed by gradual recovery. [neurone, Gk *-itis* inflammation.]

neuronosis (newr·on·**o**·sis). Neuropathy. **Neuronosis of the skin.** Any skin affection of nervous origin. [Gk *neuron* nerve, *-osis* condition.]

neuronyxis (newr·o·**nix**·is). Nerve puncture by surgical methods. [Gk *neuron* nerve, *nyssein* to puncture.]

neuro-ophthalmology (**newr**·o·of·thal·**mol**′·o·je). The branch of ophthalmology that is concerned with the neurological aspects of the subject. [Gk *neuron* nerve, *ophthalmos* eye, *logos* science.]

neuro-otology (**newr**·o·o·**tol**′·o·je). Neurotology.

neuropapillitis (**newr**·o·pap·il·**i**′·tis). Optic neuritis. *See* NEURITIS. [Gk *neuron* nerve, papilla, Gk *-itis* inflammation.]

neuroparalysis (**newr**·o·par·**al**·is·is). Paralysis caused by a disordered condition of the nerve supplying the muscle concerned. [Gk *neuron* nerve, paralysis.]

neuroparalytic (**newr**·o·par·al·**it**′·ik). Referring to neuroparalysis.

neuropath (**newr**·o·path). An individual with a predisposition, generally hereditary, to some nervous disorder or affected with such a disease. [Gk *neuron* nerve, *pathos* disease.]

neuropathic (newr·o·**path**·ik). Referring to neuropathy.

neuropathist (newr·**op**·ath·ist). A neurologist. [Gk *neuron* nerve, *pathos* disease.]

neuropathogenesis (**newr**·o·path·o·**jen**′·es·is). The development of any disordered condition of the nervous system or the cause or origin of such a condition. [Gk *neuron* nerve, pathogenesis.]

neuropathologist (**newr**·o·path·**ol**′·o·jist). A medical practitioner, usually a trained pathologist, who specializes in the laboratory and autopsic diagnosis of diseases of the nervous sstem. [Gk *neuron* nerve, pathology.]

neuropathology (**newr**·o·path·**ol**′·o·je). The pathology of the nervous system. [Gk *neuron* nerve, pathology.]

neuropathy (newr·**op**·ath·e). A disease process, thought to be non-inflammatory, characterized by disintegration or destruction of the specialized tissues of the central or peripheral nervous system. It is generally the result of some toxic, metabolic or vascular disturbance, as for example that associated with diabetes or vitamin-B_1 deficiency. **Amyloid neuropathy.** A degeneration of peripheral nerves due to vascular deposits of amyloid. **Carcinomatous neuropathy.** A degeneration of peripheral nerves and occasionally of the cerebellum and occurring without actual malignant invasion of the nerves. Most often found in association with carcinoma of the bronchus. **Diabetic neuropathy.** A degenerative condition of sensory nerves and pathways, giving pain and absence of reflexes in the lower limbs, occurring in subjects with diabetes mellitus. **Entrapment neuropathy.** Lesions of single peripheral nerves due to pressure from surrounding tissues, especially ligaments and fascia. **Hereditary sensory neuropathy.** A rare form of sensory peripheral neuropathy transmitted by dominant inheritance and often leading to painless, mutilating lesions of the extremities. **Ischaemic neuropathy.** The degenerative changes which occur in peripheral nerves or fibres as a result of ischaemia, and occlusion of the blood vessels supplying the nerves in particular. **Progressive hypertrophic interstitial neuropathy.** A rare familial disorder characterized by the symptoms and signs of a slowly progressive peripheral neuropathy affecting both motor and sensory nerves. There is often conspicuous enlargement of peripheral nerves; pathologically, changes are most marked in the interstitial tissue of nerves and secondary degeneration of the posterior columns of the spinal cord may occur. **Subacute myelo-optic neuropathy.** A degeneration of certain long tracts of the spinal cord and of the retina, described in Japan and, occasionally elsewhere. It is attributed to chronic intoxication with clioquinol taken for diarrhoea and dysentery. **Trigeminal neuropathy.** A progressive lesion of one, or both, fifth cranial nerves, of unknown cause, usually affecting women. [Gk *neuron* nerve, *pathos* disease.]

See also: DÉJÉRINE, SOTTAS.

neurophilic (newr·o·**fil**·ik). Neurotropic. [Gk *neuron* nerve, *philein* to love.]

neurophonia (newr·o·**fo**·ne·ah). A condition in which, as a result of muscular spasm in the larynx and other structures, phonation of an abnormal type is produced, so that the patient utters involuntary cries or sounds, imitative of animals. [Gk *neurone* nerve, *phone* sound.]

neurophthisis (newr·o·**thi'**·sis). Atrophy of nervous tissue [obsolete term]. [Gk *neuron* nerve, *phthisis* a wasting away.]

neurophysin I, II and III (**new**·ro·**fi**·sin). Neurosecretory material present in the mammation hypothalamo-neurohypophyseal system concerned with the synthesis of oxytocin and vasopressin.

neurophysiologist (**newr**·o·fiz·e·**ol'**·o·jist). A scientist, sometimes a medical practitioner, who is an expert in the physiology of the nervous system. [Gk *neuron* nerve, physiology.]

neurophysiology (**newr**·o·fiz·e·**ol'**·o·je). That branch of physiology dealing with the nervous system. [Gk *neuron* nerve, physiology.]

neuropil, neuropile, neuropilem (**newr**·o·pil, **newr**·o·pile, newr·o·**pi**·lem). The complicated interlacement of dendrites and axonal terminals surrounding the nerve cell bodies of the grey matter of the central nervous system. [Gk *neuron* nerve, *pilos* felt.]

neuroplasm (**newr**·o·plazm). The protoplasm of the nerve cell body. [Gk *neuron* nerve, *plasma* formation.]

neuroplasmic (newr·o·**plaz**·mik). Pertaining to or consisting of neuroplasm.

neuroplasty (**newr**·o·plas·te). A plastic operation on a nerve or nerves. [Gk *neuron* nerve, *plassein* to mould.]

neuroplegia (newr·o·**ple**·je·ah). A paralysis of nervous activity produced by neuroplegic drugs. [Gk *neuron* nerve, *plege* stroke.]

neuroplegic (newr·o·**ple**·jik). The adjective applied to a group of substances whose action consists in the blocking of synaptic transmission in the central nervous system. [see prec.]

neuroplegics (newr·o·**ple**·jix). Neuroplegic drugs.

neuroplexus (newr·o·**plex**·us). A nerve plexus. [Gk *neuron* nerve, plexus.]

neuroploca (newr·**op**·lo·kah). A nerve ganglion. [Gk *neuron* nerve, *ploke* web.]

neuropodion, neuropodium (newr·o·**po**·de·on, newr·o·**po**·de·um). A branching set of axonal terminal fibres. [Gk *neuron* nerve, *pous* foot.]

neuropore (**newr**·o·pore). A communication between the unclosed cavity of the neural tube and the exterior, situated either at the anterior end of the brain (*anterior neuropore*) or the posterior end of the spinal cord (*posterior neuropore*) in the early embryo. [Gk *neuron* nerve, *poros* pore.]

neuropotential (**newr**·o·po·**ten'**·shal). The reserve of nervous energy. [Gk *neuron* nerve, potential.]

neuropsychiatrist (**newr**·o·si·**ki'**·at·rist). 1. A physician who specializes in neurology and psychiatry. 2. Psychiatrist. [see foll.]

neuropsychiatry (**newr**·o·si·**ki'**·at·re). That branch of medical science which deals with the study and treatment of nervous and mental disorders. [Gk *neuron* nerve, psychiatry.]

neuropsychic (newr·o·**si**·kik). Referring to the nervous and psychical functions. [Gk *neuron* nerve, *psyche* mind.]

neuropsychology (**newr**·o·si·**kol'**·o·je). Psychology founded on a neurological basis. [Gk *neuron* nerve, psychology.]

neuropsychopathic (**newr**·o·si·ko·**path'**·ik). Relating to neuropsychopathy.

neuropsychopathy, neuropsychosis (**newr**·o·si·**kop'**·ath·e, **newr**·o·si·**ko'**·sis). Any disordered condition of the nervous system and mental processes. [Gk *neuron* nerve, psychopathy, psychosis.]

neuropsychopharmacology (**newr**·o·si·ko·far·mah·**kol'**·o·je). The knowledge of drugs influencing the somatic and psychological functions of the nervous system. [Gk *neuron* nerve, *psyche* mind, *pharmakon* drug, *logos* science.]

neuropsychosis (**newr**·o·si·**ko'**·sis). Neuropsychopathy. [Gk *neuron* nerve, *psyche* mind, *-osis* condition.]

neuroradiologist (**newr**·o·ra·de·**ol'**·o·jist). A medical practitioner, usually a diagnostic radiologist, who specializes in the diagnosis of diseases of the central nervous system by radiological means. [Gk *neuron* nerve, radiology.]

neuroradiology (**newr**·o·ra·de·**ol'**·o·je). The branch of radiology concerned with the diagnosis and study of diseases of the central nervous system. [Gk *neuron* nerve, radiology.]

neurorecidive (newr·o·**re**·sid·eev). Neurorecurrence. [Gk *neuron* nerve, L *recidivare* to fall back.]

neurorecurrence (**newr**·o·re·**kur'**·ens). Usually a subacute meningitis with cranial nerve affection, developing soon after the apparently successful treatment of early syphilis. [Gk *neuron* nerve, L *recurrere* to run back.]

neuroregulation (**newr**·o·reg·ew·**la'**·shun). Control and regulation of the activity of the nervous system. [Gk *neuron* nerve, regulation.]

neurorelapse (**newr**·o·re·**laps'**). Neurorecurrence. [Gk *neuron* nerve, relapse.]

neuroretinitis (**newr**·o·ret·in·**i'**·tis). An inflammatory condition in which the optic nerve and the retina are affected. [Gk *neuron* nerve, retinitis.]

neuroretinopathy (**newr**·o·ret·in·**op'**·ath·e). Any non-inflammatory disease of the retina. [Gk *neuron* nerve, retina, Gk *pathos* disease.]

neurorrhaphy (newr·**or**·af·e). Joining by suture the 2 ends of a cut nerve; nerve anastomosis. [Gk *neuron* nerve, *rhaphe* suture.]

neurorrhexis (newr·o·**rex**·is). Interrruption of a nerve, usually the phrenic, by dividing it and forcibly withdrawing or avulsing a segment. [Gk *neuron* nerve, *rhexis* a breaking.]

neurosal (newr·**o**·sal). Of the nature of or referring to a neurosis.

neurosarcocleisis (**newr**·o·sar·ko·**kli'**·sis). Surgical withdrawal of a nerve from a bony canal which exerts pressure upon it, and replacement of the nerve in soft tissues, for the relief of certain forms of neuralgia. [Gk *neuron* nerve, *sarx* flesh, *kleisis* a closing.]

neurosarcoma (**newr**·o·sar·**ko'**·mah). A sarcoma in which nervous elements are contained. [Gk *neuron* nerve, sarcoma.]

neurosclerosis (**newr**·o·skler·**o'**·sis). A sclerotic condition affecting the tissue of a nerve or of a nerve centre, which becomes indurated by a proliferation of connective tissue. [Gk *neuron* nerve, *skleros* hard.]

neurosecretion (**newr**·o·se·**kre'**·shun). The process of elaboration and discharge of active substances by nerve cells, in a manner similar to ductless-gland cells. [Gk *neuron* nerve, L *secernere* to separate.]

neurosensory (newr·o·**sen**·sor·e). Referring to a sensory nerve. [Gk *neuron* nerve, sensory.]

neurosis (newr·**o**·sis). An illness of the personality, manifested as a functional derangement of the mind or body and differentiated in typical instances from psychosis by the retention of insight and by its less serious and less fundamental nature. **Accident neurosis.** Neurosis caused or precipitated by an accident. **Actual neurosis.** A neurosis characterized clinically by anxiety and aetiologically by disturbances of normal sex function, according to Freud. **Air neurosis.** Aeroneurosis. **Anxiety neurosis.** Neurosis characterized by anxiety, morbid fears and somatic symptoms. **Association neurosis.** Neurosis in which an associative link plays a predominant and essential part in the mechanism. **Blast neurosis.** A neurosis precipitated by the subject's experience of an explosion. **Cardiac neurosis.** Neurosis in which the symptoms are referred to the heart. **Combat neurosis.** War neurosis (see below). **Compensation neurosis.** Neurosis in which the factor of compensation is responsible for the production or prolongation of symptoms. **Compulsion neurosis.** Neurosis characterized by a repetitive compulsion to perform a certain act or acts in spite of the conscious recognition of its apparent senselessness. The act may often be shown to have a symbolic meaning. **Conversion neurosis.** A neurosis in which part of the affect or libido of the patient is thought to be converted into a physical symptom. **Craft neurosis.** Neurosis associated with a particular vocation. **Expectation neurosis.** Neurosis associated with morbid anticipation of an event. **Fatigue neurosis.** Neurosis resulting from physical fatigue. **Fixation neurosis.** Neurosis dependent on an unconscious attachment to an earlier stage of mental development; a psycho-analytic term. **Fright neurosis.** A neurosis precipitated by the subject's experience of a frightening situation. **Gastric neurosis.** Neurosis in which the symptoms are referable to the stomach. **Homosexual neurosis.** Neurosis characterized by overt or latent homosexual processes. **Intestinal neurosis.** Neurosis in which the symptoms are referable to the intestines. **Obsessional neurosis.** Neurosis characterized by the repetitive intrusion into the mind, against volition, of ideas, ruminations and phobias, often associated with compulsive actions. The ideas, apparently senseless, may often be shown to have symbolic meaning. **Obsessive-compulsive neurosis.** A neurosis characterized by the recurrent emergence into consciousness of a thought or idea, and by the recurrent performance of a certain action or actions once or repeatedly, these occurring against the will of the patient and with his recognition of their apparent meaninglessness. **Occupational neurosis.** Neurosis associated with a particular occupation. **Professional neurosis.** Neurosis associated with a particular profession. **Rectal neurosis.** Neurosis in which the symptoms are referable to the rectum. **Regression neurosis.** Fixation neurosis (see above). **Sexual neurosis.** Neurosis in which the symptoms are referable to the sexual functions. **Torsion neurosis.** Neurosis characterized by athetoid movements. [Obsolete term.] **Transference neurosis.** In treatment by psychoanalysis, the stage when tender emotion (*positive transference*), often mixed with enmity (*negative transference*), derived from old unconscious wishes of the patient, is applied to the person of the physician. In this way unconscious elements in the patient's emotional life are lived over by the patient in relation to the physician. **Traumatic neurosis.** Neurosis following trauma. **Vasomotor neurosis.** Angioneurosis. **Vegetative neurosis.** A disorder of the sympathetic or parasympathetic nervous system, associated particularly with vasomotor instability. **War neurosis.** Neurosis attributable mainly to circumstances of war. [Gk *neuron* nerve, *-osis* condition.]

See also: WESTPHAL (C. F. O.).

neurosism (**newr**·o·sizm). A condition of neurasthenia characterized by nervous activity and general irritability of the nerves. [neurosis.]

neuroskeleton (newr·o·**skel**·et·on). That part of the skeleton which surrounds and protects the central nervous system; the cranial part of the skull and the bones surrounding the vertebral (neural) canal of the vertebral column. [Gk *neuron* nerve, skeleton.]

neurosome (**newr**·o·some). 1. The cell body. 2. One of the minute granules in the protoplasm of the cell body.

neurospasm (**newr**·o·spazm). Spasmodic contractions of a muscle caused by some nervous disorder. [Gk *neuron* nerve, spasm.]

neurosplanchnic (newr·o·**splangk**·nik). Relating to the sympathetic and cerebrospinal nervous systems. [Gk *neuron* nerve, *splagchnon* seat of the feelings.]

neurospongioma (**newr**·o·spun·je·**o**′·mah). Spongioblastoma. [Gk *neuron* nerve, *spoggos* sponge, *-oma* tumour.]

neurostearic (**newr**·o·ste·**ar**′·ik). Originating in the fatty substance of nervous tissues. [Gk *neuron* nerve, *stear* fat.]

neurosthenia (newr·o·**sthe**·ne·ah). A condition in which slight stimuli excite abnormal nervous strength. [Gk *neuron* nerve, *sthenos* strength.]

neurosurgery (newr·o·**ser**·jer·e). The surgery of the nervous system. [Gk *neuron* nerve, surgery.]

neurosurgeon (**newr**·o·ser·jun). A medical practitioner, usually skilled in general surgery, who specializes in the operative treatment of diseases of the nervous system. [Gk *neuron* nerve, surgery.]

neurosuture (newr·o·**sew**·tewr). Neurorrhaphy. [Gk *neuron* nerve, suture.]

neurosyphilis (newr·o·**sif**·il·is). Any form of involvement of the nervous system by syphilis. **Asymptomatic neurosyphilis.** Persistent pathological changes of syphilitic type in the cerebrospinal fluid, without symptoms or signs of disease of the nervous system. It may precede manifest neurosyphilis by many years. **Meningeal neurosyphilis.** Acute or subacute meningitis occurring within the first few years of infection. **Meningovascular neurosyphilis.** A localized or generalized inflammation of the enclosing, supporting and nutrient tissues of the nervous system. **Parenchymatous neurosyphilis.** A primary degenerative affection of the neurons of the brain or spinal cord, e.g. tabes dorsalis, general paralysis of the insane. It occurs from 10 to 30 years after infection. **Paretic neurosyphilis.** Dementia paralytica. **Tabetic neurosyphilis.** Tabes dorsalis. [Gk *neuron* nerve, syphilis.]

neurosystemitis epidemica (**newr**·o·sis·tem·**i**′·tis ep·e·**dem**·ik·ah). The von Economo type of encephalitis; encephalitis lethargica. [Gk *neuron* nerve, system, Gk *-itis* inflammation, *epidemios* among the people.]

neurotabes (newr·o·**ta**·beez). A condition that bears a certain resemblance to locomotor ataxia. **Neurotabes diabetica.** Diabetic neuritis. *See* NEURITIS. [Gk *neuron* nerve, tabes.]

neurotendinal (newr·o·**ten**·din·al). Pertaining to nerve and tendon. [Gk *neuron* nerve, L *tendo* tendon.]

neurotension (newr·o·**ten**·shun). Nerve stretching carried out by surgical methods. [Gk *neuron* nerve, tension.]

neuroterminal (newr·o·**ter**·min·al). An end-organ. [Gk *neuron* nerve, terminal.]

neurothecitis (**newr**·o·the·**si**′·tis). Inflammation of the sheath of a nerve. [Gk *neuron* nerve, *theke* sheath, *-itis* inflammation.]

neurothele (newr·o·**the**·le). A nerve papilla. [Gk *neuron* nerve, *thele* nipple.]

neurothelion, neurothelium (newr·o·**the**·le·on, newr·o·**the**·le·um). A small-sized nerve papilla. [see prec.]

neurotherapeutics, neurotherapy (**newr**·o·ther·ap·**ewt**′·tix, newr·o·**ther**·ap·e). Treatment of diseases of the nervous system. [Gk *neuron* nerve, therapy.]

neurothlipsia, neurothlipsis (newr·o·**thlip**·se·ah, newr·o·**thlip**·sis). Compression or excitation of a nerve. [Gk *neuron* nerve, *thlipsis* pressure.]

neurotic (newr·**ot**·ik). 1. Referring to or suffering from a neurosis. 2. Relating to the nerves; useful in nerve affections. 3. One suffering from a neurosis.

neuroticism (newr·**ot**·is·izm). The state of being neurotic or of being affected with a disorder of the nervous system.

neurotization (**newr**·ot·i·**za**′·shun). 1. The implantation of a paralysed muscle by surgical means. 2. The regeneration of a nerve previously divided. [Gk *neuron* nerve.]

neurotmesis (newr·ot·**me**·sis). The total severance of a nerve caused by injury. [Gk *neuron* nerve, *tmesis* a cutting.]

neurotology (newr·ot·**ol**·o·je). A study of the function of the ear, including its cochlear and vestibular elements, in relation to the brain or nervous system. [Gk *neuron* nerve, *ous* ear, *logos* science.]

neurotome (**newr**·o·tome). 1. A fine knife having a pointed end, or a needle, used in the microdissection of nerves. 2. A neuromere. [Gk *neuron* nerve, *temnein* to cut.]

neurotomy (newr·**ot**·o·me). Cutting of a nerve. **Opticociliary neurotomy.** Division of the optic nerve together with the surrounding ciliary nerves, directly behind the eyeball. Indications are to prevent pain when enucleation is not possible, or as a prevention against sympathetic ophthalmia. This latter is of doubtful value and is rarely used today. **Retrogasserian neurotomy.** Section of the trigeminal nerve at a point between its exit from the pons and the gasserian ganglion. [Gk *neuron* nerve, *temnein* to cut.]

neurotonia (newr·o·**to**·ne·ah). 1. Lack of stability of the tonicity of the autonomic nervous system. 2. Neurotony. [Gk *neuron* nerve, tone.]

neurotonogenic (**newr**·o·to·no·**jen**′·ik). Giving rise to tonicity in a nerve. [Gk *neuron* nerve, tone, Gk *genein* to produce.]

neurotony (newr·**ot**·o·ne). Nerve-stretching. [Gk *neuron* nerve, *teinein* to stretch out.]

neurotoxia (newr·o·**tox**·e·ah). A state of intoxication affecting the nervous system; neurasthenia regarded as an auto-intoxication. [see foll.]

neurotoxic (newr·o·**tox**·ik). Having a destructive or toxic effect on nervous tissue. [Gk *neuron* nerve, *toxikon* poison.]

neurotoxin (newr·o·**tox**·in). A toxin capable of destroying nervous tissue. [see prec.]

neurotrauma (newr·o·**traw**·mah). Injury to a nerve. [Gk *neuron* nerve, *trauma* injury.]

neurotripsy (newr·o·**trip**·se). The surgical bruising or crushing of a nerve. [Gk *neuron* nerve, *tribein* to grind.]

neurotrope (newr·o·trope). Neurotropic.

neurotrophasthenia (newr·o·tro·fas·**the**′·ne·ah). A condition of nerve weakness caused by defects of nutrition. [Gk *neuron* nerve, *trophe* nourishment, asthenia.]

neurotrophic (newr·o·**trof**·ik). Relating to nutrition of the nervous system or to nutritional changes controlled by nervous influences. [Gk *neuron* nerve, *trophe* nutrition.]

neurotrophy (newr·**ot**·ro·fe). The nutrition of nervous tissue. [Gk *neuron* nerve, *trophe* nutrition.]

neurotropic (newr·o·**trop**·ik). Having a particular tendency towards nervous tissue, sometimes affinity of chemical type. [see foll.]

neurotropism, neurotropy (newr·**ot**·ro·pizm, newr·**ot**·ro·pe). A state of predilection for nervous tissue; certain chemical substances, toxins and strains of viruses are attracted. [Gk *neuron* nerve, *trepein* to turn.]

neurovaccine (newr·o·**vak**·seen). A strain of vaccinia virus prepared and maintained by cerebral passage in rabbits, with perhaps occasional testicular transfer. Viruses of this type have been much used in experimental work, especially in France, where they are said to have the advantage of freedom from secondary contamination. [Gk *neuron* nerve, vaccine.]

neurovaccinia (newr·o·vak·**sin**′·e·ah). The condition produced by inoculation with neurovaccine.

neurovaricosis, neurovaricosity (newr·o·var·ik·**o**′·sis, newr·o·var·ik·**os**′·it·e). A varicosity on the fibres of a nerve. [Gk *neuron* nerve, varicose.]

neurovariola (newr·o·var·**i**′·o·lah). Neurovaccinia. [Gk *neuron* nerve, variola.]

neurovascular (newr·o·**vas**·kew·lar). 1. Relating to the nervous and vascular systems. 2. Having reference to the vasomotor nerves. [Gk *neuron* nerve, vascular.]

neurovegetative (newr·o·**vej**·et·a·tiv). Relating to the autonomic nervous system. [Gk *neuron* nerve, L *vegere* to stir up.]

neurovirulence (newr·o·**vir**·ew·lens). The property of a strain of a parasitic organism to infect preferentially the central nervous system of the host. [Gk *neuron* nerve, L *virulentus* full of poison.]

neurovirulent (newr·o·**vir**·ew·lent). Having the property of neurovirulence. [Gk *neuron* nerve, L *virulentus* full of poison.]

neurovirus (newr·o·vi·rus). Neurovaccine. [Gk *neuron* nerve, virus.]

neurovisceral (newr·o·**vis**·er·al). Relating to the sympathetic and cerebrospinal nervous systems. [Gk *neuron* nerve, viscera.]

neurovoltometer (newr·o·volt·**om**′·et·er). An electrical instrument for estimating the degree of a patient's nervousness. [Gk *neuron* nerve, volt, meter.]

neurula (**newr**·ul·ah). The stage in the developing embryo (more particularly in amphibia) following gastrulation, in which the neural folds appear and fuse to form the neural tube. [Gk *neuron* nerve.]

neutral (**newr**·tral). 1. Being neither acid nor alkaline; having the pH value of pure water (6.9). 2. Displaying no external electric charge. [L *neutralis* neuter.]

neutralization (new·tral·i·**za**′·shun). 1. The process of neutralizing, counteracting or rendering innocuous the effect of a harmful agent. 2. In chemistry, the mixture of an acid and base in such proportions that the resultant solution displays neither acidity nor alkalinity; the union of the acid hydrogen ion with the basic hydroxyl ion to form water. 3. In bacteriology, the rendering harmless of toxin by combination with the correct amount of antitoxin. [see prec.]

neutrino (new·**tre**·no). An uncharged elementary particle that has two forms associated respectively with the electron and the muon, that is believed to be massless, and that interacts very weakly with matter after being created in the process of particle decay. [L *neuter* neither.]

neutrocclusion (new·trok·**loo**·zhun). That form of malocclusion in which the teeth are irregularly placed without any accompanying abnormal mesiodistal relationship existing between the jaws. [L *neuter* neither, occlusion.]

neutrocyte (**new**·tro·site). A neutrophil leucocyte.

neutrocytopenia (new·tro·si·to·**pe**′·ne·ah). Neutropenia. [neutrocyte, Gk *penia* poverty.]

neutrocytophilia, neutrocytosis (new·tro·si·to·**fil**′·e·ah, new·tro·si·**to**′·sis). Neutrophilia. [neutrocyte, Gk *philein* to love, *-osis* condition.]

neutroflavine (new·tro·**fla**·veen). Euflavine.

neutron (**new**·tron). One of the particles of which nuclei consist; it is of zero charge and slightly heavier than a proton. **Delayed neutron.** A neutron emitted by one of the highly excited fragments after fission of an atomic nucleus, e.g. at intervals of up to about a minute. **Epithermal neutrons.** Neutrons in the energy region of 1 eV. **Fast neutrons.** Neutrons of energy greater than an arbitrarily chosen value of, say, 1 MeV. **Prompt neutrons.** The neutrons emitted at the actual instant of fission of an atomic nucleus. **Slow neutrons.** Neutrons of energy between thermal (see following) and 100 eV. **Thermal neutrons.** Neutrons in approximately thermal equilibrium with their surroundings; at room temperature their mean energy is about 0.025 eV. Neutrons of higher energies are referred to as *fast neutrons.* [L *neuter* neither, electron.]

neutropenia (new·tro·**pe**·ne·ah). A condition in which there is a reduction below normal in the neutrophil granular leucocytes in the circulating blood. It may or may not be associated with a leucopenia and may occur after injections, associated with certain other diseases of the blood, and commonly under the influence of toxic chemical and physical agents. **Cyclic neutropenia.** A chronic neutropenia that tends to recur in a cyclic manner, with intervening normal periods of varying degree; its cause is unknown. **Idiopathic neutropenia.** Neutropenia of unknown aetiology. **Malignant neutropenia.** Agranulocytosis. **Periodic neutropenia.** Cyclic neutropenia (see above). **Primary splenic neutropenia.** A neutropenia or granulocytopenia associated with fever and painful splenomegaly, but with a normal bone marrow. [neutrophil, Gk *penia* poverty.]

neutrophil, neutrophile (**new**·tro·fil, **new**·tro·file). 1. Taking neutral stains. 2. A polymorphonuclear leucocyte which is neither predominantly acidophil nor basophil in its reaction to acid and basic dyes. **Filamented neutrophil.** A neutrophil with a nucleus consisting of 2 or more lobes connected by fine nuclear filaments. **Juvenile neutrophil.** A neutrophil precursor with undivided nucleus. **Nonfilamented neutrophil.** A neutrophil with a partially subdivided nucleus. **Rod neutrophil, Stab neutrophil.** A neutrophil with undivided nucleus. [L *neuter* neither, Gk *philein* to love.]

neutrophilia (new·tro·**fil**·e·ah). An increase in the number of neutrophil leucocytes in the blood.

neutrophilic (new·tro·**fil**·ik). Having the characteristics of a neutrophil or associated with neutrophilia.

neutrophilopenia (new·tro·fil·o·**pe**′·ne·ah). A decrease in the number of neutrophil leucocytes in the blood. [neutrophil, Gk *penia* poverty.]

neutrotaxis (new·tro·**tax**·is). The power of attraction or repulsion invested in neutrophil leucocytes. [neutrophil, Gk *taxis* a turning.]

névrodermite (na·vro·der·**meet**′). Neurodermatitis. [Fr.]

Newlands, John Alexander Reina (b. 1838). British chemist.

Newlands' law. Periodic law. *See* LAW.

Newman, David (b. 1834). Scottish surgeon.

Newman's operation. Nephropexy by suture of the renal capsule to the overlying muscles (1884).

newton (**new**·ton). The unit of force in the SI system. It is equal to the force which gives a mass of 1 kg an acceleration of 1 m s^{-2}. [Sir Isaac *Newton* English physicist.]

Newton, Sir Isaac (b. 1642). English physicist.

Newton's aberration, Newtonian aberration. Newton's rings (see below).

Newton's disc. A circle divided into 7 sectors, each painted a primary colour of the spectrum: on rapid rotation an illusion of white light is obtained.

Newton's law. The attraction between 2 bodies is directly proportional to their masses and varies inversely as the square of the distance between them.

Newton's law of colour mixtures. The spectral nature of the light resulting from the mixture of 2 other lights, of any 2 wavelengths situated between the upper end of the spectrum and green, may be determined graphically by dividing the line joining the 2 constituents inversely as the quantities of each constituent of the mixture.

Newton's law of cooling. The rate of cooling of a hot body is proportional to the difference in temperature between the body and its surroundings.

Newton's laws of motion. Laws governing motion in classical mechanics: (*a*) a body will continue in its state of rest or uniform motion in a straight line unless acted on by external forces; (*b*) the rate of change of momentum is proportional to and in the same direction as an applied force; (*c*) to every action there is an equal and opposite reaction.

Newton's rings. A series of concentric coloured rings to be seen when a convex lens is placed in contact with plane glass or another lens of different curvature; due to light-interference in the air film between the surfaces.

Newton, W. H.

Newton method, for uric acid in blood. Blood filtrate is treated with acid lithium chloride and silver nitrate solution to remove interfering substances. The filtrate is treated with urea-cyanide and a special lithium arsenotungstate reagent. After standing for 10 min at room temperature the colour is compared with standards prepared similarly.

nexus (nex·us). A link or bond; interlacing. **Nexus nervorum opticorum.** The optic chiasma. **Nexus stamineus oculi.** The ciliary body. [L a tying together.]

niacin (ni·as·in). Nicotinic acid. *See* ACID.

niacinamide (ni·as·in·am·ide). Nicotinamide.

Nialamide BP 1973 (ni·al·am·ide). *N*-(2-benzylcarbamoylethyl)-*N'*-isonicotinoylhydrazine; it is used in the treatment of angina and depression.

niamide (ni·am·ide). Nicotinamide.

Nicametate (nik·am·et·ate). BP Commission approved name for 2-diethylaminoethyl nicotinate; a peripheral vasodilator.

niccolic (nik·ol·ik). Relating to or composed of nickel. [modern L *niccolum* nickel.]

Nicergoline (ni·ser·go·leen). BP Commission approved name for 8β - (5 - bromonicotinoyloxymethyl) - 10 - methoxy - 1,6 - dimethylergoline; a vasodilator.

niche (nitch). A recess in a smooth surface. In radiology it is the direct sign of ulcer, usually gastric or duodenal. It consists of protrusion of contrast medium into the ulcer crater. The niche may be seen in profile or *en face*, depending on the incidence of the rays in relation to the organ examined. **Enamel niche.** A depression at the junction of the tooth band with the external epithelium of the dental germ. [Fr.]

See also: BARCLAY, HAUDEK.

Nichols' radiometer. A radiometer in which a vane is suspended by a quartz fibre and the action of radiation upon it is balanced by the torsion in the fibre.

nickel (nik·el). An element of atomic weight 58.71, atomic number 28 and chemical symbol Ni. It is a metal closely allied to iron, occurring naturally combined with sulphur and arsenic. It has also been found widely distributed in microscopic quantities in plants and animals, particularly in plants of the cabbage family, and in marine organisms. No compounds of nickel are used in medicine, being poisonous, but owing to the resistance of the metal to acids and oxidation it is employed in laboratory and domestic ware. Alloys of extreme hardness and non-corroding properties are used for surgical instruments, whilst the metal deposited on a carrier such as pumice or diatomite is highly efficient as a catalyser in the hydrogenation of oils and fats and other industrial processes. **Nickel carbonyl.** A gaseous industrial product arising in the hardening of steel and involving a risk of carcinoma of the nose, sinuses or bronchial tree. [abbr. from G *Kupfer-nickel* the ore from which it was first obtained.]

nicking (nik·ing). A localized constriction in retinal arteries found in arterial hypertension. [etym. dub.]

Niclosamide BP 1973 (nik·lo·sam·ide). 5-Chloro-*N*-(2-chloro-4-nitrophenyl)salicylamide; a taenicide which is effective against all tapeworms that infest man.

nicochrome (nik·o·krome). An alloy of nickel (50 per cent), chromium (14 per cent) and iron, melting at high temperature and chemically resistant; used in electric heaters and for industrial chemical-ware.

Nicocodine (nik·o·ko·deen). BP Commission approved name for 6-*O*-nicotinoylcodeine; a narcotic analgesic.

Nicodicodine (nik·o·di·ko'·deen). BP Commission approved name for 7,8-dihydro-O^3-methyl-O^6-nicotinoylmorphine; an antitussive agent.

Nicol, William (b. 1768). Edinburgh physicist.

Nicol prism. A combination of 2 prisms cut and cemented together to make a rhomb, in such a way that a ray of light passing through the rhomb is split in two, one part (*ordinary ray*) being totally reflected at the interface of the 2 prisms, and the other (*extraordinary* or *polarized ray*) passing through.

Nicola, Toufick (b. 1894). New York surgeon.

Nicola's operation. Stabilization of the shoulder in recurrent dislocation by transplantation of the long tendon of the biceps through a hole drilled in the head of the humerus.

Nicoladoni, Carl (b. 1847). German surgeon.

Nicoladoni's operation. Transplantation of a toe for the replacing of a lost finger, usually the second toe and for aesthetic reasons.

Nicoladoni tendon transference. The transfer of the peroneal muscle to replace a paralysed calf.

Nicolas, Joseph (b. 1868). Lyons dermatologist.

Durand-Nicolas-Favre disease. Lymphopathia venereum.

Nicolle, Charles Jules Henri (b. 1866). Rouen and Tunis physician.

Nicolle's method, for bacteria in tissue sections. Sections are stained in Loeffler's methylene blue, followed by tannic acid.

Novy-Nicolle-McNeal culture medium. A saline rabbit's-blood agar used for growing *Leishmania donovani*; NNN medium.

Nicolle and Pinoy white mycetoma. *See* MYCETOMA, WHITE.

Nicomorphine (nik·o·mor·feen). BP Commission approved name for 3,6-di-*O*-nicotinoylmorphine; a narcotic analgesic.

nicotiana (nik·o·she·a'·nah). Tobacco; the plant *Nicotiana tabacum* Linn. (family Solanaceae) widely cultivated, the leaves of which are dried and processed to produce tobacco as it is known in commerce. Tobacco is yellowish-brown in colour with a strong odour and a bitter acrid taste. Its chief constituent is the alkaloid nicotine and its physiological effects are due almost entirely to its nicotine content. [Jean *Nicot* de Villemain (b. 1530), French ambassador to Portugal, who first sent tobacco seed into France.]

nicotianine (nik·o·she·an·een). A volatile and fragrant crystalline principle from tobacco. [see prec.]

nicotinamidaemia (nik·o·tin·am·id·e'·me·ah). The presence of nicotinamide in the circulating blood. [nicotinamide, Gk *haima* blood.]

Nicotinamide BP 1973 (nik·o·tin·am·ide). Nicotinic-acid amide, $C_5H_4NCONH_2$. A compound isolated from heart muscle, and a component part of co-enzymes I and II which are concerned with the promotion of oxidation in the tissues, in particular the oxidation or dehydrogenation of triose phosphate formed from glucose. It can replace nicotinic acid in the treatment of pellagra and is to be preferred since it does not produce vasodilatation. It is an essential growth factor for many micro-organisms.

Nicotinamidum (nik·o·tin·am'·id·um). *European Pharmacopoeia* name for Nicotinamide BP 1973.

nicotine (nik·o·teen). β-Pyridyl-α-*N*-methylpyrrolidine, $C_{10}H_{14}N_2$. A colourless liquid alkaloid turning yellow in air and light. It has a sharp burning taste, is miscible with water and is very soluble in organic solvents such as alcohol and chloroform. It is the principal alkaloid in tobacco and may be synthesized, It has no use in medicine, and is of value chiefly as an insecticide, the soluble sulphate being employed for the purpose. [*Nicotiana.*]

nicotinism (**nik**·o·tin·izm). Tobacco or nicotine intoxication.

nicotyrine (nik·o·ti·reen). α-(β-Pyridyl)-*N*-methylpyrrole, $C_{10}H_{10}N_2$. An alkaloid obtained from tobacco. It is an intermediate in the synthesis of nicotine.

Nicoumalone BP 1973 (nik·**oo**·mal·one). 3 - [2 - Acetyl - 1 - (4 - nitrophenyl)ethyl]4-hydroxycoumarin; an anticoagulant with actions and uses similar to those of phenindione.

nictation, nictitation (nik·**ta**·shun, nik·te·**ta**·shun). The act of winking. [L *nictare* to wink.]

nidal (ni·dal). Relating to a nidus.

nidation (ni·**da**·shun). 1. Implantation; the embedding of the fertilized ovum in the uterine mucous membrane (endometrium). 2. The building up, during the intermenstrual phase, of the endometrial layers. [L *nidus* nest.]

nidulus (**nid**·ew·lus). Nerve nucleus. [L little nest.]

nidus (ni·dus) (pl. *nidi*). A nest; the focus or seat of an infection. [L.]

Niemann, Albert (b. 1880). Berlin paediatrician.

Niemann's disease, splenomegaly or syndrome, Niemann-Pick disease, Pick-Niemann disease. A rare chronic, familial condition, a disorder of lipoid metabolism, resembling Gaucher's disease, with moderate anaemia, gastro-intestinal disturbances, loss of weight, ulcerative gingivitis, an abdomen much distended by gross hepatomegalia and splenomegaly, and lymphadenopathy. The skin is pale, waxy or brownish, and there is usually retardation of mental development. There is an increase of blood cholesterol; the marrow, spleen and glands show characteristic large cells containing the phospholipide, sphingomyelin.

Niemann-Pick cells. The large reticulo-endothelial cells containing sphingomyelin characteristic of the disease.

Niewenglowski, Gaston Henri (b. 1861). Paris physicist.

Niewenglowski's rays. Phosphorescence rays emitted by certain substances after exposure to strong light.

Nifedipine (ni·**fed**·e·peen). BP Commission approved name for dimethyl 1,4 - dihydro - 2,6 - dimethyl - 4 - (2 - nitrophenyl) pyridine - 3,5 - dicarboxylate; a coronary vasodilator.

Nifenazone (nif·**en**·az·one). BP Commission approved name for 2,3 - dimethyl - 4 - nicotinamido - 1 - phenyl - 5 - pyrazolone; an anti-inflammatory analgesic agent.

Nifuratel (ni·**fewr**·at·el). BP Commission approved name for 5 - methylthiomethyl - 3 - (5 - nitrofurfurylideneamino)oxazolidin - 2 - one; it is used in the treatment of trichomoniasis.

Nifurtimox (ni·**fewr**·tim·ox). BP Commission approved name for tetrahydro - 3 - methyl - 4 - (5 - nitrofurfurylideneamino) - 1,4 - thiazine 1,1 - dioxide; it is used in the treatment of trypanosomiasis.

night-terror (nite·**ter**·er). A form of dissociated sleep occurring usually in children and consisting of a marked reaction which the child does not remember. In contrast to a child waking up from a nightmare who is unable to recall the experience. [AS *niht*, L *terror.*]

nightingale (ni·ting·gale). A sleeved scarf made of wool, very popular at one time for use by invalids. [Florence *Nightingale* (b. 1820), famous English nurse.]

nightmare (**nite**·mare). A terrifying dream. [AS *niht, mara* incubus.]

nightshade (**nite**·shade). Belladonna; deadly nightshade; a tall branching herb, *Atropa belladonna* (family Solanaceae), widely distributed in England and Europe. It has flowers with a regular pale-purple cup-shaped corolla and black berries. Its chief constituent is hyoscyamine with traces of scopolamine; atropine is the racemic form of hyoscyamine. **Deadly nightshade.** *See* MAIN DEF. (above). **Woody nightshade.** A climbing plant, *Solanum dulcamara* Linn. (family Solanaceae), with smaller flowers than belladonna and a rotate purplish corolla; its berries are bright red. It has no medicinal use. [AS *nihtscada.*]

nigral (ni·gral). Relating to the substantia nigra.

nigraniline (ni·**gran**·il·een). Nigrosin. [L *niger* black, aniline.]

nigredo (ni·**gre**·do). Nigrismus.

nigrismus (ni·**griz**·mus). Melasma. **Nigrismus linguae.** Black tongue. *See* TONGUE. [L *nigrescere* to become black.]

nigrities (ni·**grish**·e·eez). Abnormally dark pigmentation. **Nigrities linguae.** Black tongue. *See* TONGUE. [L blackness.]

nigrometer (ni·**grom**·et·er). An apparatus for comparing the densities of blacks in paint and pigment manufacture. [L *niger* black, meter.]

nigrosin (ni·gro·sin). A blue-black aniline dye used in neurological histology. [L *niger* black.]

nigua (ne·gwah). Chigger.

nihilism (ni·hil·izm). A belief that denies the existence of anything. **Therapeutic nihilism.** Disbelief in the remedial powers of drugs. [L *nihil* nothing.]

Nikethamide BP 1973 (nik·**eth**·am·ide). $C_5H_4NCON(C_2H_5)_2$, the diethylamide of nicotinic acid. It is a central nervous system stimulant, used to counteract the effects of depressants such as morphine on the respiratory centre; a convulsant in large doses.

Nikethamidum (nik·eth·**am**·id·um). *European Pharmacopoeia* name for Nikethamide BP 1973.

Nikiforoff, Mikhail Nikiforovich (b. 1858). Moscow dermatologist.

Nikiforoff's method. A method for blood-film fixation, with alcohol and ether.

Nikolsky, Pyotr Vasilyevich (b. 1855). Kiel and Warsaw dermatologist.

Nikolsky's sign. Separation of the stratum corneum from the underlying layers of the epidermis as a result of minor degrees of friction; seen typically in pemphigus foliaceus. The sign may sometimes be demonstrated in other varieties of pemphigus, but usually in these the separation occurs at the dermo-epidermal junction.

Nimorazole (ni·**mor**·az·ole). BP Commission approved name for 4-[2-(5-nitroimidazol-1-yl)ethyl]morpholine; it is used in the treatment of trichomoniasis.

ninhydrin (nin·**hi**·drin). Triketohydrindene hydrate, $C_6H_4(CO)_2C(OH)_2$. A reagent which gives a blue colour on boiling with amino acids, polypeptides and peptones.

niobium (ni·o·be·um). A rare element with atomic weight 92.9064, atomic number 41 and chemical symbol Nb. It is a grey metal resembling tantalum in properties. [Gk *Niobe* daughter of Tantalus.]

niphablepsia (nif·a·**blep**·se·ah). Snow blindness. *See* BLINDNESS. [Gk *nipha* snow, *ablepsis* blindness.]

niphotyphlosis (**nif**·o·tif·**lo**'·sis). Snow blindness. *See* BLINDNESS. [Gk *nipha* snow, *typhlosis* a making blind.]

Nippe, Martin O. H. (b. 1883). Königsberg physician.

Nippe's test. A modification of Teichmann's test: make a film of blood or stain extract upon a slide and evaporate to dryness. Add 2 drops of a reagent consisting of 0.1 g each of the chloride, bromide and iodide of potassium in 100 ml of glacial acetic acid, cover with a slip and heat gently until bubbles appear. Run in a further drop or two of reagent and examine microscopically for haemin crystals.

nipple [papilla mammae (NA)] (nipl). The conical projection from the areola of the breast on which the lactiferous ducts open. **Cracked nipple.** One showing linear abrasions in the epidermis. **Crater nipple.** A nipple which has retained an immature form, in which the lactiferous ducts open into a shallow pit rather than a conical elevation. **Retracted nipple.** One that is drawn inward by adhesions, so that it is below the skin level, as in early carcinoma of the breast. [etym. dub.]

Nirenstein, Edmund. Vienna physician.

Nirenstein and Schiff method. A modified form of Mett's method for testing for peptic activity in gastric juice.

Niridazole (ni·**rid**·az·ole). BP Commission approved name for

1-(5-nitrothiazol-2-yl)imidazolidin-2-one; it is used in the treatment of schistosomiasis.

nirls (nerlz). A type of herpes. [prob. Scot.]

nirlus (**ner**·lus). A papular eruption sometimes appearing after scarlatina or measles and which quickly subsides.

nirvanine (**ner**·van·een). Dimethylglycine-methyl-2-hydroxy-5-aminobenzoate, $(NCH_3)_2CH_2CONHC_6H_3(OH)COOCH_3$. One of many synthetic agents put out as a cocaine substitute. It was not found to be satisfactory for either local or spinal anaesthesia. [*Nirvana*, Buddhist ideal of freedom from evil.]

Nissl, Franz (b. 1860). Heidelberg neuropathologist.

Nissl acid. Fibril acid. *See* ACID.

Nissl's bodies, granules or spindles. Coarse basophilic granules surrounding the nucleus in the cytoplasm of nerve cells.

Nissl degeneration. Degeneration of a nerve cell after division of its axon.

Nissl's method, for nerve cells. A method for staining the Nissl granules of nerve cells in which, after fixation in alcohol, sections are stained in hot Nissl's methylene blue, differentiated in aniline alcohol, and cleared in cajupot oil.

Nissl's methylene blue. An aqueous solution of methylene blue containing Venetian soap.

substance of Nissl. The granular basophilic material of which Nissl's bodies or granules are composed; it stains well with toluidine blue.

nit (nit). The egg or the larva of a louse. [AS *hnitu.*]

Nitabuch, Raissa. 19th century German physician.

Nitabuch's layer or stria. A band of fibrinoid in the decidua basalis and decidua capsularis of the human placenta.

niton (**ni**·ton). The name given by Ramsay to radium emanation (radon) when discovered, because of its glowing in liquid form. [obsolete term.] [L *nitidus* shining.]

nitraemia (ni·**tre**·me·ah). The presence of an excess of nitrogen in the blood; not a generally accepted word. [nitrogen, Gk *haima* blood.]

nitramine (**ni**·tram·een). Any organic amine in which a hydrogen atom of the amino-group has been replaced by a nitro-group to form $-NHNO_2$.

nitrate (**ni**·trate). Any salt of nitric acid.

nitrated (**ni**·tra·ted). Describing any compound which has had introduced into its molecule the nitro- NO_2 group.

nitratine (**ni**·trah·teen). A naturally occurring sodium nitrate.

nitration (ni·**tra**·shun). The treatment of an organic compound with nitric or fuming nitric acid, thereby introducing into its structure the nitro- NO_2 group.

Nitrazepam BP 1973 (ni·**traz**·e·pam). 1,3-dihydro-7-nitro-5-phenyl-1,4-benzodiazepin-2-one; a tranquillizer and hypnotic.

nitre (**ni**·ter). Potassium nitrate, saltpetre, KNO_3. A white crystalline compound obtained by mixing hot strong solutions of sodium nitrate and potassium chloride, filtering off the common salt produced and allowing to crystallize. It is used internally as a diuretic and also mixed with asthma powders to make them burn well. **Chile nitre.** Sodium nitrate, $NaNO_3$, occurring in large natural deposits in Chile. **Sweet spirit of nitre.** Essentially a 2 per cent solution of ethyl nitrite (C_2H_5ONO) in alcohol. As it is often prepared by distilling a mixture of nitric acid, alcohol, sulphuric acid and copper, it usually contains traces of other substances such as acetaldehyde. It is a heart stimulant like all other nitrites. [Gk *nitron* soda.]

nitridation (ni·trid·**a**·shun). The heating of metals in nitrogen gas or ammonia to form nitrides.

nitride (**ni**·tride). A compound of 1 or more atoms of nitrogen with another element such as lithium, boron or aluminium; it evolves ammonia on treatment with water.

nitrification (**ni**·trif·ik·**a**′·shun). The chemical process in which ammonia is oxidized, usually by bacteria, into nitrous acid and thence into nitric acid. [nitric acid, L *facere* to make.]

nitrifier (**ni**·trif·i·er). A nitrifying micro-organism.

nitrifying (**ni**·trif·i·ing). Qualifying certain bacteria that convert ammonia into nitric and nitrous acids. [nitric acid, L *facere* to make.]

nitrilase (**ni**·tril·aze). A nitrile-splitting enzyme.

nitrile (**ni**·trile). Cyanide. An organic compound containing the group CN, prepared by the dehydration of an acid amide, whence it derives its name, e.g. *acetonitrile* CH_3CN, also known as *methyl cyanide.* **Acid nitrile.** A nitrile derived from an acid substitution of the CN group for the COOH. **Basic nitrile.** A tertiary amine or ammonia with its hydrogen atoms replaced by alkyl radicals.

nitrilese (**ni**·tril·eez). An enzyme which activates the formation of nitriles.

nitrite (**ni**·trite). Any salt of nitrous acid. Nitrites, particularly the organic alkyl nitrites, are vasodilator in action, with a depressor effect on the motor centres of the cord. They are used in angina pectoris, and in intestinal colic and asthma to relax smooth muscle.

nitritocobalamin (**ni**·trit·o·ko·**bal**′·am·in). Vitamin B_{12}. *See* VITAMIN B_{12}.

nitritoid (**ni**·trit·oid). Resembling the action of nitrites. [nitrite, Gk *eidos* form.]

nitrituria (ni·trit·**ewr**·e·ah). The presence of nitrites in the urine.

nitro- (**ni**·tro). In chemistry, denoting the group NO_2, derived from nitric acid. [Gk *nitron* soda.]

nitro-acid (ni·tro·**as**·id). *See* ACID, NITRO-. [nitrogen, acid.]

nitro-compound (ni·tro·**kom**·pownd). A compound containing the group NO_2. [nitrogen, compound.]

nitro-starch (ni·tro·**starch**). A compound formed by treating starch with nitric acid. It is used as a blasting explosive. [nitre, starch.]

nitro-anisole (ni·tro·**an**·is·ole). Methoxynitrobenzene, $CH_3OC_6H_4NO_2$. A substance occurring in 3 isomeric forms; it has a fragrant odour.

Nitrobacter (ni·tro·**bak**·ter). A genus of bacteria belonging to the tribe Nitrobacterieae (family Nitrobacteriaceae). They are rod-shaped non-pathogenic organisms capable of oxidizing nitrates to nitrites. The type species is *Nitrobacter winogradskyi.*

nitrobacteria (ni·tro·bak·**teer**′·e·ah). A group of bacteria occurring in soil or water, which obtain their energy by the oxidation of ammonia and other nitrogenous compounds. [nitrogen, bacterium.]

Nitrobacteriaceae (ni·tro·bak·teer·e·**a**′·se·e). A family of Gram-negative non-pathogenic bacteria, rod-shaped, ellipsoid, spherical or spiral, occurring in soil or water. Most species are non-motile. They are capable of growing without organic compounds, using carbon dioxide as the source of carbon and obtaining energy by the oxidation of ammonia, nitrite or sulphur. [see prec.]

Nitrobacterieae (ni·tro·bak·**teer**′·e·e). A tribe of bacteria of the family Nitrobacteriaceae, obtaining energy by oxidation of ammonia to nitrite or from nitrite to nitrate. Their habitat is the soil, and they are non-pathogenic.

nitrobenzene (ni·tro·**ben**·zeen). $C_6H_5NO_2$, a pale yellow poisonous liquid, not used in medicine but sometimes confused with almond oil because of its odour. It is formed by the action of nitric acid on benzene in the presence of sulphuric acid and is largely used in industry for the preparation of aniline.

nitrobenzol (ni·tro·**ben**·zol). Nitrobenzene.

nitrobenzolism (ni·tro·**ben**·zol·ism). Nitrobenzene intoxication caused by inhalation of the vapour or through absorption by the skin, or through drinking a liquid containing nitrobenzene.

nitrocellulose (ni·tro·**sel**·ew·lose). A mixture of the nitrate esters of cellulose obtained by treating cotton wool or other forms of cellulose with a mixture of nitric and sulphuric acids. Those mixtures containing about 2-3 nitro-groups per glucose residue are known as *pyroxylin* or *gun-cotton*, and solutions in a mixture of ether and alcohol are used as plastic skin under the name of *collodion.* The more highly nitrated products form the basis of the explosive cordite, and others are employed in the manufacture of celluloid and artificial silk.

nitrochloroform (ni·tro·**klor**·o·form). Trichloronitromethane, CCl_3NO_2. A dense liquid with a suffocating lacrimatory vapour that also causes vomiting; used as a choking gas in chemical warfare.

nitrodextrose (ni·tro·**dex**·troze). Nitroglucose; a little-used analogue of glyceryl trinitrate.

nitro-erythrite (**ni**·tro·er·**ith'**·rite). Diluted erythrityl tetranitrate.

nitro-erythrol (**ni**·tro·er·**ith'**·rol). Erythrityl tetranitrate, $C_4H_6(NO_3)_4$. A compound which, diluted with an equal weight of lactose, is used to reduce blood pressure in angina pectoris, asthma, etc.

nitrofural (ni·tro·**fewr**·al). Nitrofurazone.

Nitrofurantoin BP 1973 (**ni**·tro·fewr·an·**to'**·in). *N*-(5-Nitro-2-furfurylidene)-1-amino-hydantoin. A synthetic antibacterial agent indicated in the treatment of pyelonephritis, cystitis and other infections, caused by nitrofurantoin-sensitive bacteria.

Nitrofurazone (ni·tro·**fewr**·az·one). BP Commission approved name for 5-nitro-2-furfuraldehyde semicarbazone. A bacteriostatic used mainly for infections of the ear and of the vagina.

nitrogen (**ni**·tro·jen). An element of atomic weight 14.0067, atomic number 7 and chemical symbol N. It is a colourless, tasteless gas constituting 80 per cent by volume of air; combined, it forms approximately 16 per cent of the protein matter of living organisms, and occurs as sodium nitrate in vast deposits in Chile. The free gas is inert but its compounds are very active and have important biological functions; it is not poisonous but will not support life: slightly soluble in blood especially under pressure, the bubbles produced when the pressure is relieved giving rise to the symptoms associated with *caisson disease.* **Active nitrogen.** A highly reactive form of nitrogen with an after-glow, produced by an electric discharge in the gas at low pressure. **Alloxuric nitrogen.** The combined organic nitrogen of the alloxur bases. **Amide nitrogen, Amino nitrogen.** The nitrogen of protein bound up in the amido- or amino-groups. **Authentic nitrogen.** Legitimate nitrogen (see below). **Nitrogen cycle.** The circulation of nitrogen in nature in 2 ways: from the atmosphere through bacterial fixation to plant and animal tissue and thence by decay back into the atmosphere; and from inorganic nitrogen compounds of the soil through the protein of plants to that of animals and the excretion of the latter back into the soil. **Nitrogen dioxide.** NO_2, a reddish-brown vapour formed by heating the nitrates of the heavy metals. **Nitrogen distribution.** Nitrogen partition (see below). **Nitrogen equilibrium.** The condition in which an animal excretes as much nitrogen as it takes in with food. **Filtrate nitrogen.** Non-protein nitrogen (see below). **Fixed nitrogen.** Free atmospheric nitrogen converted into combined nitrogen either by purely chemical processes or, as in nature, by bacteria. **Nitrogen group.** The elements of Group Vb of the Periodic Table: nitrogen, phosphorus, arsenic, antimony and bismuth. **Illegitimate nitrogen.** Administered nitrogen which does not reappear in the excreta and the retention of which is abnormal. **Justifiable nitrogen.** Legitimate nitrogen (see below). **Nitrogen lag.** The period between the taking in of a quantity of nitrogen as protein and the excretion of the same amount in the urine, faeces and sweat. **Legitimate nitrogen.** Nitrogen which is either used in the tissues or excreted normally. **Nitrogen monoxide.** Nitrous oxide, laughing gas, N_2O, a colourless gas with a sweet taste and agreeable smell, fairly soluble in water and used as a mild anaesthetic especially in dental operations. **Nomadic nitrogen.** Free atmospheric nitrogen which takes part in the nitrogen cycle (see above). **Non-protein nitrogen.** Tissue nitrogen other than protein nitrogen. **Nitrogen partition.** The subdivision of the nitrogen of the urine under the headings of its several constituents. **Nitrogen pentoxide.** Nitric anhydride, N_2O_5, an unstable crystalline substance which forms nitric acid in water. **Nitrogen peroxide.** Nitrogen dioxide (see above). **Protein nitrogen.** The nitrogen of the tissues combined in the form of protein. **Rest nitrogen.** The tissue nitrogen unaccounted for by protein, amino acids, peptides, urea and uric acid, creatine and creatinine. **Nitrogen tetroxide.** N_2O_4, a pale-yellow solid or liquid formed by cooling nitrogen dioxide (see above). **Nitrogen trichloride.** *See* AGENE. **Nitrogen trioxide.** Nitrous anhydride, N_2O_3, a gas which behaves like a mixture of nitrogen dioxide and nitric oxide, formed by the action of nitric acid on copper. [nitre, Gk *genein* to produce.]

nitrogenase (**ni**·tro·jen·aze). An enzyme that catalyses the fixation of nitrogen in nitrogen-fixing bacteria.

Nitrogenii Oxidum (ni·tro·**jen**·e·i **ox**·id·um). *European Pharmacopoeia* name for Nitrous Oxide BP 1973.

nitrogenization (**ni**·tro·jen·i·**za'**·shun). The process of treating a substance with nitrogen or nitrogen compounds so that combination takes place.

nitrogenous (ni·**troj**·en·us). Relating to nitrogen or containing nitrogen in composition.

nitroglucose (ni·tro·**gloo**·koze). Nitrodextrose; a little-used analogue of glyceryl trinitrate.

nitroglycerin (ni·tro·**glis**·er·in). Glyceryl trinitrate, $C_3H_5(ONO_2)_3$. A dangerously explosive ester prepared by the action of nitric and sulphuric acids on glycerol. It is employed, either in a 1 per cent alcoholic solution (BPC 1959) or in tablets, as a heart stimulant, and it closely resembles erythrityl tetranitrate or ethyl nitrite in its action.

nitromannitol (ni·tro·**man**·it·ol). Mannitol hexanitrate, $C_6H_8(ONO_2)_6$. A compound similar to erythrityl tetranitrate in action but less powerful and more prolonged in effect.

nitrometer (ni·**trom**·et·er). An apparatus used for the estimation of nitrates or nitrites by liberating and measuring their nitrogen in the form of the free gas or nitric oxide. [nitrogen, meter.]

See also: LUNGE.

Nitromonas (ni·tro·**mo**·nas). *Nitrosomonas.*

nitron (**ni**·tron). 1. $C_{20}H_{16}N_4$, a triazole compound which forms a white insoluble crystalline precipitate with nitrates and is used as a reagent in the quantitative estimation of the latter. 2. An ancient Green name for natural sodium sesquicarbonate.

nitronaphthalene (ni·tro·**naf**·thal·een). $C_{10}H_7NO_2$, a crystalline compound formed by the nitration of naphthalene. It has the property of reducing fluorescence in oils; its vapour can render the cornea opaque.

nitrophenol (ni·tro·**fe**·nol). 1. Any one of a series of compounds formed by the progressive substitution of the hydrogen atoms of phenol with nitro- NO_2 groups. 2. Paranitrophenol, $C_6H_4(OH)NO_2$, a crystalline compound obtained by the nitration of phenol. It is used in the manufacture of drugs and dyestuffs and also as an indicator (pH 5-7), being colourless in acid and yellow in alkalis. 3. Picric acid.

nitropropiol (ni·tro·**pro**·pe·ol). *o*-Nitrophenylpropiolic acid, $NO_2C_6H_4C{\equiv}CCOOH$. A compound used as a distinguishing test for sugars, since it forms indigo on boiling with glucose in alkaline solution.

nitroprotein (ni·tro·**pro**·te·in). A substance produced by the action of nitric acid on certain proteins.

nitroprusside (ni·tro·**prus**·ide). A salt of nitroferricyanic acid, also called *nitroprussic acid.*

nitrosalol (ni·tro·**sal**·ol). $C_6H_4(OH)COOC_6H_4NO_2$, a yellow crystalline compound formed by the combination of nitrophenol and salicylic acid.

nitrose (**ni**·troze). Nitrososulphuric acid, nitrosulphonic acid, nitrosyl sulphuric acid, NO_2SO_3H or $NOSO_4H$. The "chamber crystals" of sulphuric-acid manufacture, formed by the solution of nitrogen dioxide in sulphuric acid.

nitrosification (ni·**tro**·sif·ik·**a'**·shun). The introduction of nitrous groups into a compound, a process of importance in the manufacture of drugs and dyes. [nitrous, L *facere* to make.]

nitrosifying (ni·**tro**·sif·i·ing). Of soil bacteria, those which oxidize the ammonia of decaying plant and animal matter into nitrous acid and nitrites. [see prec.]

nitroso (ni·**tro**·so). In organic chemistry, the group -N=O derived from nitrous acid.

Nitrosobacter (**ni**·tro·so·**bak'**·ter). *Nitrobacter.*

nitrosobacteria (ni·**tro**·so·bak·**teer'**·e·ah). A general term used to describe species belonging to the 7 genera of the tribe Nitrobacterieae.

Nitrosococcus (**ni**·tro·so·**kok'**·us). A genus of non-pathogenic soil bacteria belonging to the tribe Nitrobacterieae (family Nitrobacteriaceae). They are spherical and non-motile, and obtain their energy by the oxidation of ammonia to nitrite. The type species is *Nitrosococcus nitrosus* (Migula). [nitrogen, Gk *kokkos* berry.]

nitroso-indole (ni·**tro**·so·**in'**·dole). $C_8H_6N(NO)$, a red precipitate formed by indole with nitrous acid, which forms a very delicate test.

Nitrosomonas (**ni**·tro·so·**mo'**·nas). A genus of non-pathogenic soil bacteria belonging to the tribe Nitrobacterieae (family Nitrobacteriaceae). They are rod-shaped or spherical, motile or non-motile cells which obtain energy for growth by the oxidation of ammonia to nitrites. Their growth on media containing organic substances is poor or absent. The type species is *Nitrosomonas europaea* (Winogradsky). [nitroso, Gk *monas* unit.]

nitrosophenyldimethylpyrazol (ni·tro·so·**fe**·nil·di·meth·il·**pir'**·az·-ol). An intermediate in the preparation of amidopyrine from phenazone.

nitrososubstitution (ni·**tro**·so·sub·stit·**ew'**·shun). The replacement of any radical in a compound by the nitroso-group, -N=O. [nitroso, substitute.]

nitrosubstitution (**ni**·tro·sub·stit·**ew'**·shun). The replacement of any radical in a compound by the nitro group, NO_2. [nitro-compound, substitute.]

nitrosyl (ni·**tro**·sil). The monovalent radical NO, which forms compounds with the halogens and sulphuric acid. **Nitrosyl chloride.** NOCl, a suffocating gas formed by heating aqua regia which attacks all metals except gold and platinum.

nitrous (**ni**·trus). An oxide or oxyacid of nitrogen in which the latter is trivalent. **Nitrous anhydride.** Nitrogen trioxide, N_2O_3. **Nitrous Oxide BP 1958.** Nitrogen monoxide, N_2O.

Nitroxoline (ni·**trox**·ol·een). BP Commission approved name for 8-hydroxy-5-nitroquinoline; an antibacterial agent.

nitroxyl (ni·**trox**·il). The monovalent radical NO_2, which forms compounds with the halogens.

nitryl (**ni**·tril). The nitro-group, NO_2, which enters into nitro-substitutions, as distinguished from the nitroxyl group.

njovera (nyo·ve·rah). A non-venereal treponematosis in Africa.

no-asthenia (no·as·**the**·ne·ah). Feebleness of mind or of intellect. [Gk *nous* intellect, asthenia.]

Nobel, Alfred Bernhard (b. 1833). Swedish chemist.

Nobel prize. Monetary prizes awarded annually for outstanding contributions to chemistry, physics, physiology, medicine, literature and to the cause of world peace; the money for these prizes is derived from a fund established by *Nobel.*

nobelium (no·**bel**·e·um). The transuranic element of atomic number 102; chemical symbol No. [*Nobel* Institute, Stockholm, where the element was first reported in 1957.]

Noble, Charles Percy (b. 1863). Philadelphia gynaecologist.

Noble's position. Examination of the kidneys by palpation of the body in the upright posture; it may be of value in nephroptosis.

Nocardia (no·**kar**·de·ah). A genus of Actinomycetes. They are characterized by aerobic growths of slender filaments or rods, frequently swollen and occasionally branched, forming a mycelium. Partially acid-fast, they form no conidia, are non-motile, aerobic and Gram-positive. There are many species, some of which occur only in soil and water; others are recognized pathogens in animals and man. Species infecting man are *Nocardia asteroides* causing nocardiosis and occasionally isolated from mycetomas, *N. brasiliensis* and *N. caviae*, both agents of actinomycotic mycetoma. *Nocardia farcinica* (Trevisan 1889) was found in farcy in oxen; it is pathogenic for guinea-pig, ox and sheep, but not very pathogenic for domestic animals and other cattle. [Edmund Isidore Etienne *Nocard* (b. 1850), Paris veterinary pathologist.]

nocardial (no·**kar**·de·al). Pertaining to or due to *Nocardia.*

nocardiasis, nocardiosis (no·kar·**di**·as·is, no·**kar**·de·**o'**·sis). A term generally confined to an acute or chronic, suppurative, primary pulmonary infection due to *Nocardia asteroides* which may metastasize to the subcutaneous tissues and other organs of the body, especially the brain and meninges. Other species of *Nocardia* (*N. brasiliensis, N. caviae*) are usually grouped under the disease actinomycotic mycetoma. [*Nocardia*, Gk *-osis* condition.]

Nocht, Bernhardt Albrecht Eduard (b. 1857). Founder of Tropical Institute in Hamburg.

Nocht's method. A method of staining blood for differentiation with a mixture of 1 per cent methylene blue matured with 0.5 per cent sodium carbonate and 1 per cent eosin.

noci-association (**no**·se·as·o·se·**a'**·shun). The involuntary release of nervous energy caused by surgical and other shock. [L *nocere* to injure, association.]

nociceptive (no·se·**sep**·tiv). The action of a peripheral nerve which receives and conveys painful stimuli to the brain. [L *nocere* to injure, *capere* to receive.]

nociceptor (no·se·**sep**·tor). A nerve or nerve-ending which receives and transmits a noxious stimulus. [L *nocere* to injure, *capere* to receive.]

nocifensor (no·se·**fen**·sor). Term applied to certain groups of nerves supplying the skin and mucous membranes, which were thought by Lewis to act independently to minimize the dangers associated with trauma. [L *nocere* to injure, *defendere* to defend.]

noci-influence (no·se·**in**·floo·ens). Traumatic or other harmful effect. [L *nocere* to injure, influence.]

nociperception (**no**·se·per·**sep'**·shun). The appreciation by the nerve centres of harmful influences. [L *nocere* to injure, perception.]

noctalbuminuria (**nokt**·al·bew·min·**ewr'**·e·ah). A condition in which an abnormally large quantity of albumin is to be found in the urine secreted at night. [L *nox* night, albuminuria.]

noctambulation (**nokt**·am·bew·**la'**·shun). Somnambulism. [L *nox* night, *ambulare* to walk.]

noctiphobia (nokt·e·**fo**·be·ah). Abnormal dread of night, quietness and the darkness. [L *nox* night, phobia.]

Noctuidae (nokt·**ew**·id·e). A family of moths of which the caterpillar's hairs cause a dermatitis in man; owlet moths. [L *noctua* owl.]

nocturia (nokt·**ewr**·e·ah). The discharge of an abnormally large quantity of urine at night. [L *nox* night, urine.]

nodal (**no**·dal). Referring to a node; in particular, the atrioventricular node.

node [nodus (NA)] (node). 1. A swelling. 2. A constriction, especially if serially repeated. **Atrioventricular node [nodus atrioventricularis (NA)], Auriculoventricular node.** A mass of specialized conducting tissue under the endocardium of the right atrium near the atrioventricular valve, which is continued towards the ventricular septum as the bundle of His, and represents an important part of the conducting system of the heart. **Gouty node.** A concretion composed of sodium biurate which occurs in the neighbourhood of joints in certain sufferers with gout. It may also occur in the ears. **Lymph node.** Lymph gland. *See* GLAND. **Milkers' nodes.** Milkers' nodules. *See* NODULE. **Piedric node.** A hard sclerotium-like mass of fungus vegetating superficially on the hair shaft in the condition known as piedra. **Primitive node.** A rounded swelling of the ectoderm of a blastodermic disc at the front end of the primitive streak, from which the notochordal mesoderm is derived. **Puberty node.** A hard sub-areolar plaque occurring in about 70 per cent of pubertal boys due to oestrogen as well as androgen from the pubertal testis. It disappears spontaneously in due course. **Signal node.** A superclavicular node which is sometimes noted as the first sign of gastric cancer. **Singers' node.** The formation of a fibrous nodule on the vocal cord, usually at the junction of the anterior and middle third; commonly bilateral. It results from abuse or overuse of the vocal mechanism. **Sino-atrial node. Sino-auricular node.** Sinu-atrial node (see following). **Sinu-atrial node [nodus sinu-atrialis (NA)], Sinu-auricular node.** The pacemaker of the heart; a collection of specialized cardiac muscle fibres in the wall of the right atrium near the entrance of the superior vena cava, where the heart beat is initiated. **Syphilitic node.** A localized swelling of bone due to syphilitic periostitis. **Teachers' node.** Singers' node (see above). **Triticeous node.** Corpus triticeum. [L *nodus* knot.]

See also: ASCHOFF, BOUCHARD, FÉRÉOL, FLACK, HAYGARTH, HEBERDEN, HENSEN, HIS (W. JNR.), KEITH (A.), KOCH (W.), LE GENDRE, MEYNET, OSLER, PARROT, RAVNIER, ROSENBACH (O.), ROSENMUELLER, SCHMIDT (H. D.), SCHMORL, TAWARA, TROISIER, VIRCHOW.

nodose (**no**·dose). Having nodes or protuberances. [L *nodosus* knotty.]

nodositas (no·**dos**·it·as). Nodosity. **Nodositas crinium.** Trichorrhexis nodosa; a morbid condition in which nodular swellings form along the hair shafts, resulting in breaking of the hairs. The beard is usually affected. [L *nodosus* knotty.]

nodosity (no·**dos**·it·e). 1. The state of being nodose. 2. A node.

See also: HAYGARTH, LE GENDRE.

nodous (**no**·dus). Nodose.

nodular, nodulate, nodulated (**nod**·ew·lar, **nod**·ew·late, **nod**·ew·la·ted). 1. Of, pertaining to, or resembling a node or nodule. 2. Studded with nodules.

nodulation (nod·ew·**la**·shun). The development or existence of nodules.

nodule (**nod**·ewl). 1. A small node, or aggregation of cells. 2. [Nodulus (NA).] The most anterior part of the inferior vermis. **Accessory thymic nodules [noduli thymici accessorii (NA)].** Small isolated nodules of thymic tissue frequently found close to the thyroid gland. **Apple-jelly nodule.** The nodule of lupus vulgaris which, on diascopy, gives an apple-jelly or barley-sugar appearance. **Enamel nodule.** Enamel pearl. *See* PEARL. **Guatemala nodules.** Slowly developing fibrous nodules under the skin, usually of the scalp, caused by infection with the filarial worm *Onchocerca volvulus.* **Juxta-articular nodule.** An inflammatory nodule situated near a joint. **Lentiform nodule [processus lenticularis (NA)].** A small swelling at the end of the long process of the incus. It articulates with the head of the stapes. **Lumbar-sacral nodules.** Tender fibrotic nodules found in the lumbar-sacral region. They are due to fat herniations through the deep fascia. They may become inflamed and painful as a result of trauma. The condition responds to procaine injections. **Lymphatic nodules, aggregated [folliculi lymphatici aggregati (NA)].** Large oval aggregates of lymph nodules, mainly in the ileum but also in the lower part of the jejunum. **Lymphatic nodules, bronchial.** Small lymph nodules in the lung substance on the larger branches of the bronchi. **Lymphatic nodules, gastric [folliculi lymphatici gastrici (NA)].** Solitary lymphatic follicles in the mucous membrane of the stomach. **Lymphatic nodules of the larynx [folliculi lymphatici laryngei (NA)].** Lymphatic nodules of the mucous membrane of the larynx. **Lymphatic nodules of the rectum [folliculi lymphatici recti (NA)].** Small aggregations of lymphoid tissue in the mucous membrane. **Lymphatic nodules, solitary [folliculi lymphatici solitarii (NA)].** Small collections of lymphoid tissue found in the mucous and submucous coats of the small and large intestine. **Lymphatic nodules of the spleen [folliculi lymphatici lienales (NA)].** Localized thickenings of the white pulp around the small arteries, visible to the naked eye. **Lymphatic nodules, tubal.** Lymphoid tissue beneath the mucous membrane of the pharyngotympanic tube, especially near its pharyngeal opening. **Lymphatic nodules, vaginal.** Lymph nodules of the vagina. **Lymphatic nodules of the vermiform appendix [folliculi lymphatici aggregati appendicis vermiformis (NA)].** Masses of lymphoid tissue in the submucous coat of the vermiform appendix. **Lymphatic nodules, vesical.** Lymph nodules of the urinary bladder. **Milkers' nodules.** A *Poxvirus* infection similar to orf. Reddish, single or multiple nodules occur on the hands, having been acquired from infected udders of cows. **Pearly nodule.** A nodule found in bovine tuberculosis. **Nodules of the pulmonary valve.** *See* VALVE. **Pulp nodule.** A mass of calcified tissue found within the substance of the tooth pulp; a pulp stone. **Rheumatic nodules.** Aggregations of tissue cells of sufficient size to be detectable by the examining finger, situated in various soft tissues of the body, often over bony prominences. They occur chiefly during the course of active rheumatic fever (Aschoff's nodules) and rheumatoid arthritis, in which disease they are non-specific in structure, consisting principally of the fibroblasts and lymphoid cells. **Siderotic nodule.** Gandy-Gamna nodule; a tiny brown or yellow nodule found in the spleen in Banti's disease, composed of altered blood. **Nodule tabac.** Siderotic nodule (see above). **Typhoid nodule.** A type of nodule observed in the liver of typhoid patients, and consisting of monocytes and lymphocytes around the invading bacilli. **Typhus nodule.** Fraenkel's nodule. **Vocal nodules.** Nodules which develop on vocal cords in individuals who constantly strain the voice. [L *nodulus* a small knot.]

See also: ARANZIO, ASCHOFF, BIANCHI (G. B.), BOUCHARD, DALEN, FRAENKEL (C.), FUCHS (E.), GAMNA, HOBOKEN, KOEPPE, MORGAGNI, PEYER, SCHMORL.

nodulous (**nod**·ew·lus). Nodular; nodose.

nodulus (**nod**·ew·lus) (pl. *noduli*). A nodule. **Noduli cutanei.** Nodular subepidermal fibrosis. *See* FIBROSIS. [L a small knot.]

noegenesis (no·e·**jen**·es·is). A doctrine according to which all knowing originates in 3 fundamental laws with corresponding processes: the awareness of one's own experience, the education of relations and the eduction of correlates (Spearman). [Gk *nous* mind, *genein* to produce.]

noematachograph (**no**·e·mat·**ak**'·o·graf). A device for recording the time of a mental operation. [Gk *noema* thought, *tachys* swift, *graphein* to record.]

noematic (no·e·**mat**·ik). Relating to the understanding or to mental processes or mechanisms. [Gk *noema* thought.]

noesis (no·**e**·sis). Cognition; a psychological term for that activity of the mind by which one "knows" things, i.e. the means by which one is aware of the processes of thinking and perceiving. The faculties of understanding and reasoning are included in the term. [Gk *nous* mind.]

noetic (no·**et**·ik). Referring to noesis.

noeud vital (ner ve·**tahl**). An old physiological term, referring to the respiratory centre. [Fr. vital knot.]

Noguchi, Hideyo (b. 1876). Japanese pathologist in New York.

Noguchi's culture medium. A medium composed of rabbit blood and semisolid nutrient agar; it is employed for the cultivation of *Leptospira.*

Noguchi's luetin reaction. Luetin reaction; the appearance of a red papule following the intradermal injection of an extract (luetin) of killed cultures of several strains of *Treponema pallidum.*

Noguchi test. A qualitative test for the presence of globulin in cerebrospinal fluid in which opalescence is produced by the addition of a solution of butyric acid in normal saline and the subsequent addition of normal sodium hydroxide.

Smith-Noguchi culture medium. A medium composed of fresh rabbit kidney tissue in sterile ascitic fluid under "Vaseline" in narrow tubes; it is prepared aseptically without heat.

Noguchia (no·**goo**·che·ah). A genus of bacteria of the tribe Haemophileae (family Parvobacteriaceae). They are small, slender, Gram-negative rods, motile with flagella and encapsulated. Their optimum growth temperature is 28-30°C, but culture is difficult on ordinary media. The species are *Noguchia granulosis,* causing trachoma in man and monkeys, *N. simiae,* producing follicular conjunctivitis in rhesus monkeys, and *N. cuniculi* responsible for follicular conjunctivitis in rabbits. [Hideyo *Noguchi.*]

noise (noiz). **Thermal noise.** Electrical signals of a random nature arising in an amplifier due to the statistical behaviour of matter on an atomic scale. **White noise.** A noise purposely and simultaneously produced from frequencies throughout the auditory field. It is used for masking one ear when the auditory acuity of the other ear is being established. [etym. dub.]

noli-me-tangere (no·le·ma·**tan**'·jer·e). An old but colourful name for rodent ulcer. [L touch me not.]

noma (**no**·mah). Gangrenous stomatitis; cancrum oris. **Noma pudendi, Noma vulvae.** An ulcerative condition affecting the external genitalia of young children. [Gk *nome* distribution.]

nomadic (no·**mad**·ik). Wandering, free, loose; the term has been applied to a movable or wandering spleen, and also to spreading ulcers. In the nitrogen cycle, it is used to designate the free nitrogen of the air. [Gk *nomas* roaming.]

nomenclature (no·**men**·klat·ewr). A system of names; scientific terminology, e.g. of diseases. **Basle nomenclature.** The anatomical terminology agreed upon and incorporated in the *Basle* (*Basel*) *Nomina Anatomica.* **Nomenclature of Disease.** The title of an official publication prepared by a committee appointed by the Royal College of Physicians. **Jena nomenclature.** The anatomical terminology agreed upon and incorporated in the *Jena Nomina Anatomica.* **Paris nomenclature.** The anatomical terminology agreed upon at the Sixth International Congress of Anatomists held in Paris in July 1955. [L *nomenclatio*, a calling by name.]

Nomifensine (nom·e·**fen**·zeen). BP Commission approved name for 8 - amino - 1,2,3,4 - tetrahydro - 2 - methyl - 4 - phenylisoquinoline; a thymoleptic and CNS stimulant.

Nomina Anatomica (**nom**·in·ah an·at·**om**·ik·ah). **Basle Nomina Anatomica, NA.** The anatomical terminology adopted at Basle (Basel), Switzerland, in 1895, by the German Anatomical Society. **Jena Nomina Anatomica, JNA.** The anatomical terminology adopted at Jena, in 1933, by a committee of German anatomists. **Paris Nomina Anatomica, PNA.** The anatomical terminology agreed upon at the Sixth International Congress of Anatomists held in Paris in July 1955. The publication listing these terms is entitled *Nomina Anatomica.* [L *nomen* name, Gk *anatome* a cutting up.]

nomogenesis (no·mo·**jen**·es·is). The theory that evolution is premeditated and governed by certain inherent factors. [Gk *nomos* law, genesis.]

nomogram, nomograph (**no**·mo·gram, **no**·mo·graf). A number of scales drawn on graph paper, each denoting values of variables which are correlated by some complicated formula. By simply joining certain given values on the scales with straight lines, the values of unknown variables can quickly be read off, thus avoiding tedious calculation. [Gk *nomos* law, *gramma* a record, *graphein* to write.]

nomography (no·**mog**·raf·e). The solution of complex equations by nomograms. [Gk *nomos* law, *graphein* to write.]

nomotopic (no·mo·**top**·ik). Occurring at the customary or usual site; occurring normally. [Gk *nomos* law, *topos* place.]

non-access (non·**ak**·ses). In forensic medicine, the absence of opportunity for sexual intercourse. [L *non* not, *accedere* to approach.]

non-agglutinator (non·ag·**loo**·tin·a·tor). *See* AGGLUTINATOR, 2nd def. [L *non* not, agglutinator.]

non-antigenic (**non**·an·te·**jen**'·ik). Not giving rise to antibodies; not having the ability to produce antigenic substances. [L *non* not, antigenic.]

non compos mentis (non **kom**·pos **ment**·is). Applied to a person who is not sufficiently sound of mind to manage his own affairs. [L not in full possession of the mind.]

non-conductor (non·kon·**duk**·tor). Any substance which transmits electricity or heat only with difficulty; useful therefore as an insulator. [L *non* not, conductor.]

non-consummation (**non**·kon·sum·a·shun). A marital failure under divorce law, giving grounds for ending a marriage. A form of nullity which may arise from psychological or physical causes and applies to both male and female. Unrelated to potency. [L *non* not, *consummare* to accomplish.]

non-disjunction (non·dis·**jungk**·shun). The failure of chromosome pairs or sister chromatids to segregate regularly at cell division. **Primary non-disjunction.** A meiotic non-disjunction affecting disomic elements of the chromosome complement. **Secondary non-disjunction.** A meiotic non-disjunction involving polysomic members of the chromosome complement and presumably due to the hazards that usually accompany pairing and segregation of chromosomes present in abnormal numbers. [L *non* not, *disjunctio* a separation.]

non-electrolyte (non·el·**ek**·tro·lite). Any substance which does not yield ions in solution and which therefore does not conduct electricity. [L *non* not, electrolyte.]

non-homologous (**non**·hom·**ol**·og·us). Of chromosomes or chromosome regions which are the site of different gene loci. They do not exchange parts through pairing and crossing-over at meiosis. [L *non* not, Gk *homos* same, *logos* relation.]

non-motile (non·**mo**·tile). Incapable of voluntary movement; not motile. [L *non* not, *motilis* moving.]

non-occlusion (non·ok·**loo**·zhun). The absence of occlusion between teeth in opposite jaws. [L *non* not, occlusion.]

non-opaque (non·o·**pake**). A substance or fluid permitting the transmission of light or radiation (x-rays). [L *non* not, opaque.]

non-parous (non·**par**·us). Nulliparous. [L *non* not, *parere* to bear.]

non-phlobatannin (**non**·flo·bah·**tan**'·in). Pyrogallol tannin, any of the group of tannins which yield pyrogallol on heating, and hydrolyse to phenolic acids.

non-radiable (non·**ra**·de·abl). A substance that is completely opaque to x-rays. [L *non* not, radiation.]

non-refractive (non·re·**frak**·tiv). Not possessed of the power of deflecting light rays. [L *non* not, refraction.]

non-septate (non·**sep**·tate). Not having a septum or septa. [L *non* not, septum.]

non-specific (non·spes·**if**·ik). Applied to a disease or infection that is not due to the action of any particular micro-organism or of a drug which does not depend for its efficacy on its action on one specific micro-organism. [L *non* not, specific.]

non-union (non·**ew**·ne·on). In a case of fracture, lack of union of the 2 portions of bone. **Established non-union.** The state of affairs when it is clear that a fracture will never unite unless further active treatment is instituted. [L *non* not, union.]

non-valent (non·**va**·lent). Said of an element which has no chemical affinity and therefore does not display valency: the inert gases are such. [L *non* not, *valere* to be able.]

non-viable (non·**vi**·abl). Unable to exist independently after birth. [L *non* not, viable.]

nona (**no**·nah). A disease having certain features resembling encephalitis lethargica, an outbreak of which was recorded in southern Europe in 1889–1890. [It. ninth: because it was held to occur 9 days after the onset of influenza.]

nonacosane (non·a·**ko**·sane). $C_{29}H_{60}$, a solid hydrocarbon of the methane series, found in beeswax. [Gk *nonacosa* twenty-nine.]

nonan (**no**·nan). Having a recurrence on the ninth day. [L *nonus* ninth.]

nonane (**no**·nane). C_9H_{20}, a saturated hydrocarbon, ninth in the methane series; a colourless liquid occurring in petroleum. [see prec.]

nonigravida (no·ne·**grav**·id·ah). Denoting a woman gravid for the ninth time. [L *nonus* ninth, gravid.]

nonipara (no·**nip**·ar·ah). A woman who has given birth to 9 offspring. [L *nonus* ninth, *parere* to bear.]

Nonne, Max (b. 1861). Hamburg neurologist.

Nonne's syndrome. Cerebellar syndrome. *See* SYNDROME.

Nonne-Apelt reaction. Equal volumes of cerebrospinal fluid and saturated ammonium sulphate are shaken together and allowed to stand for at least 3 min. If globulin is present the liquid becomes opalescent, turbid or a precipitate forms, depending upon the amount present. Normal fluids remain clear or faintly opalescent.

Nonne-Milroy-Meige syndrome. Milroy's disease; chronic hereditary oedema of the legs.

nonose (**no**·noze). $C_9H_{18}O_9$, a monosaccharide composed of a chain of 9 carbon atoms: 2 such sugars have been synthesized. [L *nonus* ninth.]

nonyl (**no**·nil). The monovalent radical C_9H_{19}–, derived from the hydrocarbon nonane.

nookleptia (no·o·**klep**·te·ah). Delusion held by the mentally unsound that their thoughts are being stolen. [Gk *nous* mind, *kleptein* to steal.]

nooklopia (no·o·**klo**·pe·ah). Castrophrenia. [Gk *nous* mind, *kleptein* to steal.]

Noon, Leonard (b. 1878). London physician.

Noon's pollen unit. The amount of pollen toxin extracted from one millionth of a gram of pollen.

Noonan, Jacqueline Anne. 20th century paediatric cardiologist.

Noonan's syndrome. A condition having many of the features of Turner's syndrome. The commonest cardiovascular abnormalities, however, are pulmonary valve stenosis, left ventricular hypertrophy and cardiomyopathy. Some cases show fairly severe mental retardation. Webbing of the neck is even more common than in Turner's syndrome. The facies is typical of Turner's syndrome and short stature is characteristic. In males undescended or hypoplastic testes are common. There are no chromosomal anomalies.

noopsyche (no·o·**si**·ke). The intellectual aspect of mental activity. [Gk *nous* mind, *psyche* understanding.]

Noorden, Carl Harko von (b. 1858). Vienna physician.

von Noorden's treatment. A dietetic treatment for diabetes, now superseded.

noothymopsychic (**no**·o·thi·mo·**si'**·kik). Referring to the affective and thinking faculties of the mind. [Gk *nous* mind, *thymos* will, *psyche* understanding.]

nopalin G (**no**·pal·in **je**). A bluish eosin dye.

Noracymethadol (**nor**·as·e·**meth**·ad·ol). BP Commission approved name for 1 - ethyl - 4 - methylamino - 2,2 - diphenylpentyl acetate (α-form); a narcotic analgesic.

Noradrenaline (**nor**·ad·**ren'**·al·een). BP Commission approved name for α-(3,4-dihydroxyphenyl)-β-aminoethanol; norepinephrine. A catecholamine hormone produced with adrenaline in the suprarenal medulla. Unlike adrenaline it functions mainly as an over-all vasoconstrictor, and is sometimes used to maintain blood pressure in shock, haemorrhage, hypotension and in central vasomotor depression. It is a powerful stimulator of alpha adrenergic receptors. The official preparation is Noradrenaline Acid Tartrate BP 1973.

Noradrenalini Tartras (nor·ad·**ren**·al·in·i **tar**·tras). *European Pharmacopoeia* name for Noradrenaline Acid Tartrate BP 1973.

noratropine (nor·at·ro·peen). $C_{16}H_{21}NO_3$, a mydriatic alkaloid obtained from belladonna and other solanaceous plants. It is formed by racemizing norhyoscyamine with alkali.

Norbutrine (nor·**bew**·treen). BP Commission approved name for 2 - cyclobutylamino - 1 - (3,4 - dihydroxyphenyl)ethanol; a bronchodilator.

Norcodeine (nor·**ko**·de·een). BP Commission approved name for *N*-dimethylcodeine; a narcotic analgesic.

Nordau, Max Simon (b. 1849). Hungarian physician and sociologist in Paris.

Nordau's disease. Degeneracy.

Nordensen, Johan Wilhelm (b. 1883). Uppsala ophthalmologist.

Nordensen camera. A camera for taking photographs of the fundus of the eye.

norepinephrine (**nor**·ep·e·**nef'**·reen). Noradrenaline.

Norethandrolone BP 1973 (nor·eth·**an**·dro·lone). 17α-Ethyl-17-hydroxy-19-norandrost-4-en-3-one; used as an anabolic steroid (Nilenar). A weak androgen.

Norethisterone BP 1973 (nor·eth·**is**·ter·one). 17β - Hydroxy - 19-norpregn - 4 - en - 20 - yn - 3 - one. **Norethisterone Acetate BP 1973.** 17β - Hydroxy - acetoxy - 19 - norpregn - 4 - en - 20 - yn - 3 - one, a synthetic hormone with actions resembling those of progesterone; it has slight oestrogenic activity but no androgenic action. It is effective when given by mouth.

Norethynodrel BP 1973 (nor·eth·**in**·o·drel). 17β-Hydroxy-19-norpregn-5(10)-en-20-yn-3-one, a synthetic steroid hormone which has the actions and uses of progesterone. It may be given orally with an oestrogenic substance such as mestranol to inhibit ovulation in the practice of contraception.

Norgestrel (nor·**jes**·trel). BP Commission approved name for 13β - ethyl - 17 - hydroxy - 18,19 - dinor - 17α - pregn - 4 - en - 20 - yn - 3 - one; a progestational steroid.

norgestrienone (**nor**·jest·**ri**·en·**own**). A norsteroid which suppresses gonadotrophin secretion. It has been used together with testosterone (to maintain libido and secondary sexual characters) as a male contraceptive.

norhyoscyamine (**nor**·hi·o·**si'**·am·een). $C_{16}H_{21}NO_3$, an alkaloid present in belladonna and other solanaceous plants. It has mydriatic properties.

norleucine (nor·**lew**·seen). α-Amino-*n*-caproic acid $CH_3(CH_2)_3CH(NH_2)COOH$. An amino acid occurring in hydrolysates of certain proteins.

Norlevorphanol (nor·lev·**or**·fan·ol). BP Commission approved name for (-)-3-hydroxymorphinan; a narcotic analgesic.

norm (norm). A standard or pattern. [L *norma* rule.]

norma (**nor**·mah). In anatomy describing the particular aspect from which the skull is viewed, e.g. *norma facialis*, the skull viewed from the facial aspect, or *norma occipitalis* (*norma posterior*), the occipital or posterior aspect of the skull. [L rule.]

normal (**nor**·mal). 1. Conforming to the regular or more usual pattern. 2. In chemistry: (*a*) of a number of isomeric compounds, that one in which the carbon atoms are in a straight chain; (*b*) of a series of salts, that one in which no un-neutralized acid hydrogen or basic hydroxyl remains; (*c*) a solution used in volumetric analysis which contains 1 gram-equivalent of reagent per litre. 3. In optics, the perpendicular to a surface at any point. 4. In bacteriology, a subject who has not been immunized or treated in any way. [L *norma* rule.]

normergic (norm·er·jik). 1. Relating to normergy. 2. Having the capacity for a normal reaction. [see foll.]

normergy (norm·**er**·je). The state of being able to respond normally to stimuli. [normal, Gk *ergon* work.]

Normethadone (nor·**meth**·ad·one). BP Commission approved name for a synthetic analgesic derived theoretically from methadone by the removal of a methyl group. It is less active than either amidone or isoamidone.

normoblast (**nor**·mo·blast). A stage in the development of red blood cells when the nucleus has become condensed into a homogeneous densely staining body, normally only found in the bone marrow. In exceptional circumstances, e.g. in certain anaemias and in leukaemia, it may also appear in the circulating blood. [normal red cell, Gk *blastos* germ.]

normoblastic (nor·mo·**blas**·tik). Of the nature of, or pertaining to a normoblast.

normoblastosis (**nor**·mo·blas·**to'**·sis). Excessive proliferation of normoblasts in the marrow. [normoblast, Gk *-osis* condition.]

normocapnia (nor·mo·**kap**·ne·ah). The presence of a normal amount of carbon dioxide in the blood. [L *norma* rule, Gk *kapnos* vapour.]

normochromasia (**nor**·mo·kro·**ma'**·ze·ah). 1. A typical reaction to staining by dyes in cellular or other tissues. 2. The typical colour of the erythrocytes. [see foll.]

normochromia (nor·mo·**kro**·me·ah). The typical colour of the erythrocytes, i.e. when the haemoglobin content is normal. [normal, Gk *chroma* colour.]

normochromic (nor·mo·**kro**·mik). Of normal colour: applied to the blood picture it indicates a mean corpuscular haemoglobin concentration within the normal limits, from 33 to 35 per cent. [see prec.]

normochromocyte (nor·mo·**kro**·mo·site). An erythrocyte containing the normal amount of haemoglobin. [normal, chromocyte.]

normocrinic (nor·mo·**krin**·ik). Relating to typical secretion or to typical endocrine functions. [formal, Gk *krinein* to secrete.]

normocyte (**nor**·mo·site). An erythrocyte of typical shape, colour and size. [normal, Gk *kytos* cell.]

normocytic (nor·mo·**sit**·ik). Of the nature of, or pertaining to a normocyte.

normocytosis (**nor**·mo·si·**to'**·sis). A state of the peripheral blood in which the red blood cells are normal. [normal, Gk *kytos* cell, *-osis* condition.]

normo-erythrocyte (**nor**·mo·er·**ith'**·ro·site). Normocyte. [normal, erythrocyte.]

normoglycaemia (nor·mo·gli·se′·me·ah). A condition of the blood in which the blood sugar is within normal limits. [normal, glycaemia.]

normoglycaemic (nor·mo·gli·se′·mik). Pertaining to normoglycaemia.

normokalaemic (nor·mo·kal·e′·mik). Having a normal serum potassium level. [normal, G *Kali* potash, Gk *haima* blood.]

normolineal (nor·mo·lin·e·al). Constructed on typical lines. [normal, line.]

Normorphine (nor·mor·feen). BP Commission approved name for *N*-dimethylmorphine; a narcotic analgesic.

normosexual (nor·mo·sex·ew·al). Normal mentally and physically so far as sex is concerned.

normoskeocytosis (nor·mo·ske·o·si·to′·sis). An increase in the number of immature or young white cells, usually of the granular series (deviation or shift to the left), although the total number of white cells remains within the normal limits. *See* ARNETH CLASSIFICATION. [NORMAL, GK *skaios* left, *kytos* cell.]

normosthenuria (nor·mo·sthen·ewr′·e·ah). Normality of urinary secretion and excretion. [normal, Gk *sthenos* strength, urine.]

normotension (nor·mo·ten·shun). Normal blood pressure. [L *norma* rule, *tendere* to stretch.]

normotensive (nor·mo·ten·siv). 1. Relating to a normal blood pressure. 2. A person having a normal blood pressure. [L *norma* rule, *tendere* to stretch.]

normothermia (nor·mo·ther·me·ah). That temperature condition of the body in which the tissues function basally, being neither stimulated nor depressed. [normal, Gk *therme* heat.]

normotonic (nor·mo·ton·ik). Of normal bodily tonus.

normotopia (nor·mo·to·pe·ah). The state in which organs and other structures are normal. [normal, Gk *topos* place.]

normotopic (nor·mo·top·ik). Situated in the right place. [see prec.]

nornicotine (nor·nik·o·teen). An alkaloid present in species of *Duboisia* (family Solanaceae), and also in tobacco.

Norpipanone (nor·pip·an·one). BP Commission approved name for 4,4-diphenyl-6-piperidinohexan-3-one; an analgesic.

Norris, Richard (b. 1831). Birmingham physiologist.

Norris' corpuscles. Colourless, transparent and almost invisible disc-like corpuscles described in blood serum.

Nortriptyline (nor·trip·ti·leen). BP Commission approved name for 3 - (3 - methylaminopropylidene) - 1,2:4,5 - dibenzocyclohepta - 1,4 - diene. **Nortriptyline Hydrochloride BP 1973.** The hydrochloride of nortriptyline, an antidepressant drug with actions and uses resembling those of imipramine and amitriptyline.

norvaline (nor·val·een). α-Amino-*n*-valeric acid, $CH_3CH_2CH_2CH(NH_2)COOH$. An amino acid occurring in caseins and other proteins.

nosaetiology (nos·e·te·ol′·o·je). That section of medicine which deals with the aetiology of disease. [Gk *nosos* disease, aetiology.]

Noscapine BP 1973 (nos·kap·een). $C_{22}H_{22}NO_7$, one of the alkaloids of opium occurring in the seed capsules of *Papaver somniferum.* A respiratory stimulant and cough suppressant, it is useful in the treatment of bronchitis and whooping cough.

nose [nasus (NA)] (noze). *See* ORGAN OF SMELL. **Apex of the nose [apex nasi (NA)].** The free angle of the nose; the tip of the nose. **Bottle nose, Brandy nose.** Rhinophyma. **Bridge of the nose, Dorsum of the nose [dorsum nasi (NA)].** The region of junction of the 2 lateral surfaces of the nose; the upper part of the external surface of the nose overlying the nasal bones. **External nose [nasus externus (NA)].** The pyramidal portion of the olfactory organ projecting on the face. **Hammer nose.** Rhinophyma. **Opera-glass nose.** The nose of congenital syphilis in which the bridge is depressed and the tip tends to turn upward. **Potato nose.** Rhinophyma. **Root of the nose [radix nasi (NA)].** The upper angle of the nose, connected with the forehead. **Saddle nose, Saddleback nose.** A sunken bridge produced by injury or disease which results in damage to the nasal septum. **Strawberry nose.** Rhinophyma. **Whisky nose.** Rhinophyma. [AS *nosu.*]

nosema (no·se·mah). Any kind of disease or illness. [Gk malady.]

nosencephalus (nos·en·kef·al·us). A fetal monstrosity having an imperfect brain and lacking the frontal and temporal regions of the skull. [Gk *nosos* disease, *egkephalos* brain.]

nosepiece (noze·pees). A metal disc attached to the lower end of the tube of a microscope, bearing a number of objectives which can be rotated into position when required. [nose, piece.]

noseraesthesia (nos·er·es·the′·ze·ah). Perversion of the perceptive senses. [Gk *noseros* unwholesome, aesthesia.]

nosogenesis (nos·o·jen·es·is). Pathogenesis. [Gk *nosos* disease, *genein* to produce.]

nosogenetic, nosogenic (nos·o·jen·et′·ik, nos·o·jen·ik). Pathogenic. [see prec.]

nosogeny (nos·oj·en·e). Nosogenesis.

nosogeography (nos·o·je·og′·raf·e). The study of diseases in respect of their endemicity. [Gk *nosos* disease, geography.]

nosographic (nos·o·graf·ik). Relating or belonging to nosography.

nosography (nos·og·raf·e). A description of diseased conditions; medical literature. [Gk *nosos* disease, *graphein* to write.]

nosohaemia (nos·o·he·me·ah). A diseased state of the blood. [Gk *nosos* disease, *haima* blood.]

noso-intoxication (nos·o·in·tox·ik·a′·shun). A toxic state induced by the activity of disease process. [Gk *nosos* disease, intoxication.]

nosological (nos·ol·oj·ik·al). Referring to nosology.

nosology (nos·ol·o·je). Classification of diseases regarded as a science. [Gk *nosos* disease, *logos* science.]

nosomania (nos·o·ma·ne·ah). The erroneous belief held by an insane person that he is suffering from a particular disease; hypochondria of an extreme degree. [Gk *nosos* disease, mania.]

nosometry (nos·om·et·re). The determination of the sickness rate. [Gk *nosos* disease, *metron* measure.]

nosomycosis (nos·o·mi·ko′·sis). Any diseased condition caused by a fungus. [Gk *nosos* disease, *mykes* fungus, *-osis* condition.]

nosonomy (nos·on·o·me). Classification of diseases. [Gk *nosos* disease, *nomos* law.]

nosoparasite (nos·o·par·ah·site). A parasite to be found in association with a diseased condition; it has no aetiological relation, but has the power to alter the course of the disease [Obsolete term.] [Gk *nosos* disease, parasite.]

nosophilia (nos·o·fil·e·ah). An abnormal wish to suffer illness. [Gk *nosos* disease, *philein* to love.]

nosophobe (nos·o·fobe). One who has a morbid dread of a certain disease or of sickness generally. [Gk *nosos* disease, phobia.]

nosophobia (nos·o·fo·be·ah). An abnormal or insane fear of disease. [see prec.]

nosophthoria (nos·of·tho·re·ah). The stamping out of disease by means of prophylaxis. [Gk *nosos* disease, *phthora* destruction.]

nosophyte (nos·o·fite). A plant micro-organism that gives rise to morbid symptoms. [Gk *nosos* disease, *phyton* plant.]

nosopoietic (nos·o·poi·et′·ik). Pathogenic. [Gk *nosos* disease, *poiein* to make.]

Nosopsyllus (nos·o·sil·us). A genus of fleas. **Nosopsyllus fasciatus.** The commonest rat flea occurring in temperate and Mediterranean countries, and in ports throughout the world. It bites man and is of importance as a plague vector, particularly between rat and rat, though it does not normally become blocked with bacilli. Several closely related species occur in India, but not usually *Nosopsyllus fasciatus.* [Gk *nosos* disease, *psylla* flea.]

nosotaxy (nos·o·tax·e). Classification of diseases. [Gk *nosos* disease, *taxis* arrangement.]

nosotherapy (nos·o·ther·ap·e). The treatment of one disease by the induction of a second disease, e.g. malaria in order to modify the course of dementia paralytica. [Gk *nosos* disease, therapy.]

nosotoxic (nos·o·tox·ik). Pertaining to, or caused by, nosotoxicosis or to a nosotoxin. [Gk *nosos* disease, toxin.]

nosotoxicity (nos·o·tox·is′·it·e). The quality of being nosotoxic.

nosotoxicosis (nos·o·tox·ik·o′·sis). Any diseased condition that is caused by or combined with a state of poisoning. [Gk *nosos* disease, toxicosis.]

nosotoxin (nos·o·**tox**·in). A toxic substance that is either combined with or induces a disease. [Gk *nosos* disease, toxin.]

nosotrophy (nos·**ot**·ro·fe). The nursing and care of sick persons. [Gk *nosos* disease, *trophe* a nursing.]

nosotropic (nos·o·**trop**·ik). Applied to remedies or treatment directed against the actual disease affecting the patient. [Gk *nosos* disease, *tropos* a turning.]

nostalgia, nostalgy (nos·**tal**·je·ah, nos·**tal**·je). A strong desire to return to the birthplace or home; generally and popularly referred to as homesickness. **Cryptic nostalgia.** A condition noted amongst service recruits in which all their thoughts are centred on their homes and friends. [Gk *nostein* to return home, *algos* pain.]

nostology (nos·**tol**·o·je). Gerontology; the branch of medical science which is concerned with the physiological and pathological phenomena of senescence. [Gk *nostein* to return home, *logos* science.]

nostomania (nos·to·**ma**·ne·ah). An insane degree of homesickness. [Gk *nostein* to return home, mania.]

nostras (**nos**·tras). Indicating a disease endemic to the country of its description, as distinct from a like disease occurring in another country. [L *nostras* native.]

nostrate (**nos**·trate). Endemic. [see prec.]

nostrils [nares] (**nos**·trilz). The two elliptical external openings of the nose; external nares. [AS *nosu* nose, *thyrel* hole.]

nostrum (**nos**·trum). A patent medicine, a quack remedy or a medicine the ingredients of which are kept secret. [L *noster* our own.]

Nosworthy, Michael Denis. London anaesthetist.

Nosworthy connections. Metal devices for attaching tracheal tubes to anaesthetic circuits.

Nosworthy's record-cards. Anaesthetic record-cards on to which many variables can be transferred and retrieved by the punch-card technique.

notal (**no**·tal). Dorsal. [Gk *noton* the back.]

notalgia, notalgy (no·**tal**·je·ah, no·**tal**·je). Dorsalgia. **Notalgia paraesthetica.** Pain and paraesthesia in the area of the back supplied by posterior primary rami of the lumbar nerves and due to nerve compression. [Gk *noton* the back, *algos* pain.]

notancephalia (no·tan·kef·**a**′·le·ah). The condition in which the back of the skull is lacking. [Gk *noton* the back, *a*, *kephale* head.]

notanencephalia (no·tan·en·kef·**a**′·le·ah). A monster in which the cerebellum is absent. [Gk *noton* back, *egkephalos* brain.]

notation (no·**ta**·shun). **CDE notation.** For the Rhesus (Rh) blood group system described by Fisher and Race. Originally based on the genetic concept of 3 pairs of closely-linked alleles, C–c, D–d, E–e, determining the presence of corresponding antigens on the red cells except that the d antigen has never been identified. An alternative system of nomenclature, Rh–Hr due to Wiener, hereafter given in brackets. The common Rh antigens are as follows: $D(Rh_0)$, C(rh′), E(rh″), c(hr′), e(hr″), f, $ce(rh_i)$ and $C^W(rh^{W'})$. The gene complexes found most frequently in Caucasians are, CDe(R′), cde(r), $cDE(R^2)$, $cDe(R^0)$, $C^WDe(R'^w)$ (cdE(r″), Cde(r′) and $CDE(R^z)$. [L *notare* to mark.]

See also: FISHER, RACE, WIENER.

notch [incisura (NA)] (noch). A depression, usually on a bone, but also applied to an indentation on an organ. **Acetabular notch [incisura acetabuli (NA)].** A deficiency in the margin of the acetabulum, situated inferiorly and bridged over by the transverse ligament. **Angular notch.** Notch of the stomach, angular (see below). **Antegonial notch.** The depression in the lower border of the mandible anterior to the angle. **Anterior notch of the auricle [incisura anterior (auris) (NA)].** A notch between the supratragal tubercle and the spine of the helix. **Aortic notch.** Dicrotic notch (see below). **Cardiac notch.** Notch of the stomach, cardiac (see below). **Cerebellar notch, anterior.** A broad depression separating the cerebellar hemispheres rostral to the vermis. It lies dorsal to the mid-brain. **Cerebellar notch, posterior.** A deep notch lodging the falx cerebelli. **Clavicular notch [incisura clavicularis (NA)].** The indentation at the upper angle of the manubrium sterni for the clavicle. **Costal notch [incisura costalis (NA)].** One of the indentations on the side of the sternum for a costal cartilage. **Dicrotic notch.** The incisura on the descending limb of the normal arterial pulse tracing. It is synchronous with the closure of the aortic valve and immediately precedes the dicrotic wave. **Ethmoidal notch [incisura ethmoidalis (NA)].** The interval between the medial borders of the orbital plates of the frontal bone. **Fibular notch [incisura fibularis (NA)].** A shallow furrow on the lateral side of the lower end of the tibia, intimately related to the lower end of the fibula and giving attachment to the interosseous tibiofibular ligament. **Frontal notch [incisura (sive foramen) frontales (NA)].** A small notch or foramen in the supra-orbital margin of the frontal bone medial to the supra-orbital notch. It transmits the supratrochlear nerve. **Notch for the glossopharyngeal nerve.** *See* FORAMEN, JUGULAR. **Interarytenoid notch [incisura interarytenoidea (NA)].** The posterior part of the opening of the larynx between the arytenoid cartilages. **Intercondylar notch [fossa intercondylaris (NA)].** A non-articular depression between the condyles of the femur posteriorly and inferiorly, and giving attachment to the cruciate ligaments. **Jugular notch [incisura jugularis (NA)].** The notch on the anterior surface of the jugular process of the occipital bone, which in the articulated skull forms the posterior margin of the jugular foramen. **Lacrimal notch [incisura lacrimalis (NA)].** *See* MAXILLA, ORBITAL SURFACE. **Notch for the ligamentum teres [incisura ligamenti teretis].** A notch where the fissure for the round ligament reaches the lower border of the liver. **Notch of the lung, cardiac [incisura cardiaca pulmonis sinistri (NA)].** A notch in the anterior border of the left lung between the 4th and 6th costal cartilages, extending 4 cm or more from the mid-line. **Mandibular notch [incisura mandibulae (NA)].** A notch lying between the condyloid and coronoid processes of the mandible. **Mastoid notch [incisura mastoidea (NA)].** The groove on the deep surface of the mastoid process of the temporal bone, giving origin to the posterior belly of the digastric muscle. **Nasal notch [incisura nasalis (NA)].** The margin of the maxilla which helps to form the lower and lateral boundary of the bony external nares. **Pancreatic notch [incisura pancreatis (NA)].** The deep indentation between the uncinate process of the neck of the pancreas through which pass the superior mesenteric vessels. **Parietal notch [incisura parietalis (NA)].** The angle between the squamous and mastoid parts of the temporal bone, into which the postero-inferior angle of the parietal bone is received. **Pre-occipital notch [incisura pre-occipitalis (NA)].** A small notch occasionally present on the inferolateral border of the hemisphere of the cerebrum, close to the occipital pole. It forms the anterior limit of the occipital lobe in this region. **Pterygoid notch [incisura pterygoidea (NA)].** A gap between the anterior borders of the pterygoid plates below which lodges the tubercle of the palatine bone. **Radial notch [incisura radialis (NA)].** A concave articular area on the ulna for the articular circumference of the head of the radius. **Sciatic notch, greater [incisura ischiadica major (NA)].** A notch on the posterior border of the hip bone between the posterior inferior iliac spine and the spine of the ischium. It is converted into a foramen by the sacrotuberous and sacrospinous ligaments. **Sciatic notch, lesser [incisura ischiadica minor (NA)].** A notch on the posterior border of the ischium between the spine and the tuberosity. It is converted into the lesser sciatic foramen by the sacrotuberous and sacrospinous ligaments. **Sphenopalatine notch [incisura sphenopalatina (NA)].** *See* PERPENDICULAR PLATE OF PALATINE BONE (under PLATE). **Spinoglenoid notch.** The interval between the lateral border of the spine and the dorsal surface of the scapula. **Notch of the stomach, angular [incisura angularis (NA)].** A notch in the lesser curvature, marking the left limit of the pyloric part of the organ. **Notch of the stomach, cardiac [incisura cardiaca (NA)].** The notch at the junction of the oesophagus and the greater curvature of the stomach. **Supra-orbital notch [incisura (sive foramen) supra-orbitalis (NA)].** Supra-orbital foramen. *See* FORAMEN. **Supra-**

scapular notch [incisura scapulae (NA)]. An indentation between the root of the coracoid process and the anterolateral end of the superior border of the scapula. **Suprasternal notch [incisura jugularis (NA)].** The broad indentation on the upper border of the manubrium sterni. **Tentorial notch [incisura tentorii (NA)].** The opening enclosed by the free border of the tentorium cerebelli and the sphenoid bone, and occupied by the mid-brain. **Thyroid notch [incisura thyroidea superior (NA)].** The separation above the fused anterior borders of the laminae of the thyroid cartilage. **Thyroid notch, inferior [incisura thyroidea inferior (NA)].** The notch in the middle of the lower border of the thyroid cartilage. **Trochlear notch [incisura trochlearis (NA)].** A semilunar articular surface of the ulna for articulation with the trochlea of the humerus. **Tympanic notch [incisura tympanica (NA)].** A deficiency in the tympanic groove to which is attached the flaccid part [pars flaccida (NA)] of the tympanic membrane. **Ulnar notch [incisura ulnaris (NA)].** A smooth, concave area on the medial side of the lower end of the radius for articulation with the ulna. **Vertebral notch, inferior [incisura vertebralis inferior (NA)].** The concavity on the lower border of the pedicle of a vertebra. **Vertebral notch, superior [incisura vertebralis superior (NA)].** The concavity on the upper border of the pedicle of a vertebra. [O Fr. *enochier.*]

See also: RIVENUS, WIART.

note (note). A sound of definite pitch. **Amphoric note.** A hollow, low-pitched sound obtained by percussion over a hollow cavity. **Bell note.** Bell sound. *See* SOUND. **Cracked-pot note.** Cracked-pot sound. *See* SOUND. **Percussion note.** The sound evoked by percussion. [L *nota* a mark.]

Notechis (no·**te**·kis). A genus of poisonous snakes of the subfamily Elapinae. **Notechis scutatus.** A tiger snake found in Australia. [Gk *notos* south, *echis* snake.]

notencephalocele (no·ten·**kef**·al·o·seel). Herniation of the brain through the occipital portion of the skull. [Gk *noton* the back, *egkephalos* brain, *kele* hernia.]

notencephalus (no·ten·**kef**·al·us). A fetal monster the substance of the brain of which protrudes through an occipital defect. [Gk *noton* the back, *egkephalos* brain.]

Nothnagel, Carl Wilhelm Hermann (b. 1841). Freiburg and Vienna pharmacologist, pathologist and neurologist.

Nothnagel's bodies. Oval bodies, plain or striated and from 15 to 60 μm in diameter, sometimes found in the faeces of meat-eaters.

Nothnagel's paralysis or syndrome. Unilateral oculomotor paralysis with ipsilateral cerebellar ataxia, due to a lesion of the superior cerebellar peduncle.

Nothnagel's sign or symptom. Paralysis of emotional movement of the face with retention of willed movement, due to destruction of the centre concerned with emotional movement, which is situated centrally, in basal structures near the thalamus.

Nothnagel's type. A form of acroparaesthesia with vascular spasm and a tendency to gangrene.

nothrous (**no**·thrus). Sluggish; lifeless; stupid. [G *nothros.*]

notifiable (no·te·fi·abl). Designating infectious diseases the occurrence of which must by law be reported to health authorities. [L *nota* a mark, *facere* to make.]

notochord (**no**·to·kord). The primitive axial rod of mucoid tissue lying beneath the neural tube, about which the vertebral column and base of the skull as far forward as the sella turcica are developed. The possession of a notochord in early development is characteristic of the chordata: in lowly chordates it persists indefinitely; in higher forms it disappears, except for contributions to the nucleus pulposus of the intervertebral discs. [Gk *noton* the back, *chorde* cord.]

notochordal (no·to·**kord**·al). Relating or belonging to the notochord.

notochordoma (no·to·kord·**o**′·mah). Chordoma. 1. A neoplasm made up of notochordal tissue. 2. Specifically, a small malignant neoplasm, composed of notochordal tissue, which may occur at the union of the occipital with the sphenoid bone. 3. A term applied by Virchow to the upper portion of a persisting notochord. [notochord, Gk *-oma* tumour.]

Notoëdres (no·to·e·dreez). A genus of mites; mange mites. **Notoëdres cati.** The causative agent of mange in cats; it has been found on man, causing a scabies-like condition of short duration.

notogenesis (no·to·**jen**·es·is). Evolution of the notochord. [Gk *noton* the back, *genein* to produce.]

notomelus (no·to·**mel**·us). A fetal monster having a supplementary limb or limbs attached to the back. [Gk *noton* the back, *melos* limb.]

notomyelitis (**no**·to·mi·el·i′·tis). An inflammatory condition affecting the spinal cord. [Gk *noton* the back, myelitis.]

noumenal (**noo**·men·al). Appertaining to or concerned with the noumenon.

noumenon (**noo**·men·on). The thing-in-itself, as opposed to the phenomenon, the thing such as it appears to us (Kant). [Gk *nooumenon* thing perceived.]

nousic (**noo**·sik). Relating to or causing functional movements of the cerebrum or relating to the understanding. [Gk *nous* mind.]

novaine (no·va·een). Carnitine, $HO(CH_3)_3NCH_2CH(OH)CH_2C$-$OOH$. The betaine of β-hydroxybutyric acid, found in mammalian muscle.

novarsenobenzene, novarsenobenzol (**nov**·ar·sen·o·**ben**′·zeen, **nov**·ar·sen·o·**ben**′·zol). Neoarsphenamine.

novaurantia (nov·awr·**an**·she·ah). Orange G.

Nové-Josserand, Gabriel. 20th century French surgeon.

Nové-Josserand-McIndoe procedure. For reconstruction of the urethra: a dermo-epidermal urethral tube is used as a graft, the latter being wrapped round a bougie and introduced subcutaneously on a specially assembled trocar.

Novobiocin (no·vo·**bi**·o·sin). BP Commission approved name for the oral antibiotic obtained from *Streptomyces niveus.* It is of particular value in blood, intestinal, bone, respiratory, urinary and skin infections, with *Staphylococcus* resistant to other antibiotics, and with some strains of *Proteus.* **Novobiocin Calcium BP 1973.** The dihydrate of the calcium salt of Novobiocin, a stable preparation more stable than Novobiocin Sodium. **Novobiocin Sodium BP 1973.** The monosodium salt of Novobiocin, active against many Gram-positive organisms including *Staphylococcus aureus*; administered by mouth but it can also be given intravenously.

novovalis (no·vo·**va**·lis). A contraction of fenestra novovalis, the name given to the new window made in the semicircular canal in the fenestration operation.

Novy, Frederick George (b. 1864). Chicago bacteriologist.

Novy-Nicolle-McNeal culture medium. A saline rabbit's blood agar used for growing *Leishmania donovani*; NNN culture medium.

noxa (**nox**·ah). Any substance that has a harmful or deleterious effect. [L injury.]

noxious (**nok**·she·us). Harmful; injurious. **Noxious thing.** In law, a thing taken or administered for an unlawful purpose. It is not limited to poisonous substances, but includes anything which may be liable, under certain circumstances, to produce injury. This may depend upon the quantity as well as the nature of the substance. [see prec.]

Noxiptyline (nox·e·ti·leen). BP Commission approved name for 3 - (2 - dimethylaminoethyloxyimino) - 1,2:4,5 - dibenzocyclohepta - 1,4 - diene; an antidepressant.

Noxythiolin (nox·e·**thi**·o·lin). BP Commission approved name for *N*-hydroxymethyl-*N*-methylthiourea; an antifungal agent.

Noyes, Henry Dewey (b. 1832). American ophthalmologist.

Noyes' operation. 1. The original evisceration operation performed in 1873: the cornea was incised and the contents of the eye wiped out with a small sponge until the sclera of the eye appeared white and glistening. Historical. 2. For squint: a form of resection of the muscle.

nubecula (new·**bek**·ew·lah). 1. A faintly cloudy appearance of the urine. 2. Faint cloudiness of the cornea. [L little cloud.]

nubile (**new**·bile). Denoting a female of an age suitable for bearing children. [L *nubilis* marriageable.]

nubility (new·**bil**·it·e). Marriageableness; the condition of being of an age suitable for marriage. [see prec.]
nucha (new·kah). The nape of the neck. [Fr. *nuque*.]
nuchal (new·kal). Referring to the nape of the neck. [see prec.]
Nuck, Anton (b. 1650). Leyden physician and anatomist.
canal of Nuck, Nuck's diverticulum. The pouch of peritoneum that grows into the inguinal canal in the female; it corresponds to the vestige of the vaginal process of the male and is normally obliterated.
Nuck's hydrocele. Hydrocele of the canal of Nuck; a collection of fluid in relation to the round ligament of the female inguinal canal at a site corresponding to the vestigial canal of Nuck.
nuclear (new·kle·ar). Referring to a nucleus.
nuclease (new·kle·aze). A class of enzymes present in serum, the liver and the intestines, which hydrolyse the nucleic acids.
nucleated (new·kle·a·ted). Possessing a nucleus.
nucleide (new·kle·ide). A compound formed by nuclein with a metallic element.
nucleiform (new·**kle**·e·form). Resembling a nucleus in shape. [nucleus, form.]
nuclein (new·kle·in). An intermediate product in the hydrolysis of nucleoprotein. Further hydrolysis yields protein and nucleic acid.
nucleinase (new·kle·in·aze). Nuclease.
nucleinotherapy (new·kle·in·o·**ther**'·ap·e). The treatment of disease with nucleins: specifically, the use of sodium nucleinate in Parkinson's disease (paralysis agitans). [nuclein, therapy.]
nucleo-albumin (new·kle·o·al·**bew**'·min). Any phosphoprotein such as casein or vitellin, as distinct from a nucleoprotein. [nuclein, albumin.]
nucleo-albuminuria (new·kle·o·al·bew·min·**ewr**'·e·ah). A condition of the urine in which nucleo-albumin is present.
nucleo-analysis (new·kle·o·an·**al**'·is·is). Blood counting in respect of the nucleated leucocytes. [nucleus, analysis.]
nucleocytoplasmic (new·kle·o·si·to·**plaz**'·mik). Relating to the nucleus and to the cytoplasm of a cell.
nucleofugal (new·kle·**of**·ew·gal). Directed away from a nucleus. [nucleus, L *fugare* to avoid.]
nucleohistone (new·kle·o·**his**'·tone). A conjugated protein occurring in cell nuclei in which histone is combined with nucleic acid.
nucleoid (new·kle·oid). 1. Resembling a nucleus in shape; nucleiform. 2. A nucleiform body that is sometimes present at the centre of an erythrocyte. [nucleus, Gk *eidos* form.]
nucleolar (new·**kle**·o·lar). Relating to a nucleolus.
nucleole (new·kle·ole). Nucleolus.
nucleoliform (new·kle·**o**·le·form). Resembling a nucleolus in shape. [nucleolus, form.]
nucleolin (new·**kle**·o·lin). The substance or substances, chiefly ribose- and deoxyribose-nucleoproteins, composing the true nucleolus of all cell nuclei.
nucleolinus (new·kle·o·**li**'·nus). A concentrated or granular element in the nucleolus.
nucleoloid (new·kle·o·loid). Nucleoliform. [nucleolus, Gk *eidos* form.]
nucleolonucleus (new·kle·o·lo·**new**'·kle·us). A nucleiform body inside a nucleus.
nucleolus (new·**kle**·o·lus). Plasmosome (*true nucleolus*); a rounded body found within the nucleus of all cells. It consists of a central core containing ribosenucleic acids and a peripheral layer of deoxyribonucleic acid. **False nucleolus.** Karyosome, a small node of chromatin (deoxyribonucleic acid) liable to be confused with the true nucleolus or plasmosome. [L dim. of *nucleus*.]
nucleomicrosoma, nucleomicrosome (new·kle·o·mi·kro·**so**'·mah, new·kle·o·**mi**'·kro·some). One of the many bands of a chromosome, each possibly representing a single gene locus. [nucleus, Gk *mikros* small, *soma* body.]
nucleon (new·kle·on). A phosphorylated derivative of carnosine which occurs in muscle nucleoprotein. [nucleus.]
nucleonics (new·kle·**on**·ix). Nuclear physics.
nucleopetal (new·kle·**op**·et·al). Tending towards the nucleus of a cell. [nucleus, L *petere* to seek.]
nucleophaga (new·kle·**of**·ag·ah). A parasitic organism which destroys the nucleus of amoebae. [nucleus, Gk *phagein* to eat.]
nucleoplasm (new·kle·o·plazm). The semi-fluid protoplasm which fills the meshes of the chromatin network of the cell nucleus. [nucleus, Gk *plasma* something formed.]
nucleoprotamine (new·kle·o·**pro**'·tam·een). A conjugated protein occurring in cell nuclei in which protamine is combined with nucleic acid.
nucleoprotein (new·kle·o·**pro**'·te·in). 1. A class of conjugated proteins occurring in cell nuclei in which protein is combined with nucleic acid. 2. The form in which some viral nucleic acids are found inside the virus particles.
nucleopurine (new·kle·o·**pewr**'·een). Name given to the aminopurines, adenine and guanine, because of their occurrence in nucleoproteins.
nucleoreticulum (new·kle·o·ret·**ik**'·ew·lum). The nuclear network. [nucleus, reticulum.]
nucleosidases (new·kle·**o**·sid·á·sez). Enzymes which catalyse the hydrolysis of nucleosides into base + sugar.
nucleoside (new·kle·o·side). A compound formed by condensation of a purine or pyrimidine base with a pentose sugar. With phosphoric acid it constitutes a nucleotide unit in nucleic acid.
nucleosis (new·**kle**·o·sis). Abnormal nuclear proliferation. [nucleus, Gk *-osis* condition.]
nucleospindle (new·kle·o·**spin**'·dl). The achromatic spindle seen in mitosis. [nucleus, spindle.]
nucleotherapy (new·kle·o·**ther**'·ap·e). Nucleinotherapy.
nucleotidase (new·kle·**o**·tid·aze). Any one of a class of phosphatases which act upon nucleotides to produce nucleosides and phosphoric acid.
nucleotides (new·kle·o·ti·dz). General name for nucleoside monophosphates composed of a nitrogenous base (usually purines or pyrimidines), a pentose sugar (ribose in ribonucleotides and deoxyribose in deoxyribonucleotides) and phosphoric acid. Ribonucleotides are the components of ribonucleic acids and are important in metabolism as the nucleoside mono-, di- and triphosphates of adenosine, uridine, guanosine and cytidine. Other important ribonucleotide derivatives are NAD, NADP and coenzyme A. Deoxyribonucleotides are the components of deoxyribonucleic acids. **Diphosphopyridine nucleotide.** Coenzyme I. **Phosphopyridine nucleotides.** Co-enzymes I and II, usually referred to as diphospho- and triphosphopyridine nucleotides respectively. **Triphosphopyridine nucleotide.** Coenzyme II.
nucleotoxin (new·kle·o·**tox**'·in). 1. A toxin originating in a nucleus. 2. A toxin affecting the nucleus of a cell.
nucleus (new·kle·us). 1. A central core around which a larger structure is built in layers. 2. The positively charged central portion of an atom contributing almost the whole mass of the atom, but only a minute part of its volume. 3. A specialized part of most living cells which is enclosed in the nuclear envelope and contains genetic material in the form of DNA. 4. [NA] A collection of nerve cells within any part of the central nervous system. **Accessory nucleus [nucleus accessorius (autonomicus (NA))].** The nucleus of Edinger–Westphal. **Accessory cuneate nucleus [nucleus cuneatus accessorius (NA)].** A small mass of grey matter in the upper part of the fasciculus cuneatus dorsolateral to the main cuneate nucleus and detached from the remainder of the grey matter in this region. **Nucleus ambiguus [NA].** A group of motor-nerve cells placed deeply in the reticular formation of the medulla oblongata. It gives rise to fibres that run in the glossopharyngeal and vagus nerves, supplying branchial musculature. **Amygdaloid nucleus [corpus amygdaloideum (NA)].** One of the basal nuclei. It lies in the roof of the anterior end of the inferior horn of the lateral ventricle. **Anatomical nuclei.** *See under the respective anatomical structures.* **Arcuate nuclei [nuclei arcuati (NA)].** A flattened band on the ventral and medial surfaces of the pyramid, in which some of the anterior

external arcuate fibres relay. **Basal nuclei.** Subcortical masses of grey matter in the cerebral hemispheres, comprising the lentiform, caudate and amygdaloid nuclei, and the claustrum. **Caudal central nucleus [nucleus caudalis centralis (NA)].** A component of the oculomotor group of nuclei which sends fibres to the levator palpebrae superioris muscle. **Caudate nucleus [nucleus caudatus (NA)].** An arcuate mass of grey matter lateral to the thalamus, lying in the floor of the anterior horn and body of the lateral ventricle and in the root of the inferior horn. **Caudate nucleus, body of the [corpus nuclei caudati (NA)].** Part of the caudate nucleus lying along the floor of the lateral ventricle. **Caudate nucleus, head of the [caput nuclei caudati (NA)].** The globular anterior end of the caudate nucleus which causes a swelling in the floor of the anterior horn of the lateral ventricle. **Caudate nucleus, tail of the [cauda nuclei caudati (NA)].** The attenuated portion of the caudate nucleus, lying in the roof of the inferior horn of the lateral ventricle. **Cholane nucleus.** The cyclopentenophenanthrene skeleton, consisting of 3 six-membered rings united to 1 five-membered ring, which forms the basis of the sterols and steroids, including the sex hormones, the bile acids, the hormones of the cortex of the suprarenal glands, the toad poisons, the digitalis and strophanthus aglycones and certain carcinogenic hydrocarbons. The nucleus is so named from the hydrocarbon, cholane. **Cleavage nucleus.** The nucleus, of the egg cell or zygote, from which the other cells of the embryo are produced. **Cochlear nuclei, ventral and dorsal [nuclei cochleares, ventralis et dorsalis (NA)].** Nuclei on the dorsal and ventrolateral aspects of the inferior cerebellar peduncle, where afferent fibres from the cochlear nerve first relay. **Conjugation nucleus.** The nucleus of a fertilized ovum formed by the union of male and female pronuclei. **Nucleus of a cranial nerve [nucleus nervi cranialis (NA)].** A collection of nerve cells within the brain giving rise to the fibres of a motor cranial nerve or receiving the fibres of a sensory cranial nerve. **Cuneate nucleus [nucleus cuneatus (NA)].** The nucleus at the upper extremity of the fasciculus cuneatus, relaying proprioceptive impulses to the thalamus and cerebellum. **Daughter nucleus.** One of the 2 nuclei which ordinarily result from cell division. **Dentate nucleus [nucleus dentatus (NA)].** The main nucleus in the centre of the cerebellar hemispheres. It is flask-shaped, with crenated walls and an open mouth, the hilum. The centre contains white matter. **Dentate nucleus, hilum of the [hilus nuclei dentati (NA)].** The open mouth of the flask-shaped nucleus in the centre of the cerebellar hemispheres. **Diploid nucleus.** A nucleus having the normal double set of chromosomes, 1 set from each parent. **Dorsolateral nucleus [nucleus dorsolateralis (NA)].** One of a pair of nuclei forming part of the oculomotor group of nuclei; it is believed to be concerned with upward movement of the eye. **Dorsomedial nucleus [nucleus dorsomedialis (NA)].** A nucleus in the anterior hypothalamic area, dorsal to the ventromedial nucleus (see below) and medial to the fornix. **Nucleus emboliformis [NA].** A small centrally placed nucleus just medial to the hilum of the dentate nucleus. **Nucleus fastigii [NA].** A small centrally placed nucleus in the white matter of the vermis close to the midline. **Fertilization nucleus.** Conjugation nucleus (see above). **Free nucleus.** An isolated living cell nucleus. **Gametic nucleus.** A haploid nucleus, either male or female. **Germ nucleus, Germinal nucleus.** The male or female pronucleus of the sperm head or unfertilized ovum respectively. **Nucleus globosus [NA].** A small centrally placed nucleus medial to the nucleus emboliformis. **Gonad nucleus.** The reproductive, as opposed to the vegetative, nucleus in cells which possess both. **Gracile nucleus [nucleus gracilis (NA)].** The nucleus at the upper extremity of the fasciculus gracilis, for relay of proprioceptive impulses destined for the thalamus. **Habenular nucleus [nucleus habenulae (NA)].** Collections of neurones on the floor of the trigonum habenulae. **Haploid nucleus.** A nucleus having only half the normal somatic number of chromosomes, such as that of a germ cell after reduction division and before fertilization. **Nucleus intercalatus [NA].** A small collection of cells of unknown function lying under the hypoglossal triangle in the floor of the 4th ventricle between the hypoglossal nucleus and the dorsal nucleus of the vagus. **Intercornual nucleus, Intermediolateral nucleus.** One of the subsidiary groups of cells in the spinal medulla. **Interpeduncular nucleus [nucleus interpeduncularis (NA)].** A small collection of nerve cells between the basis pedunculi, just in front of the pons. **Interstitial nucleus [nucleus interstitialis (NA)].** An area of grey matter near the median raphe in the tegmentum of the mid-brain; it receives fibres from the ansa lenticularis. **Lateral nucleus [nucleus lateralis (NA)].** A long column of cells in the ventrolateral reticular formation, related to the spinocerebellar tract. Their axons pass to the cerebellum in the inferior cerebellar peduncle. **Lentiform nucleus [nucleus lentiformis (NA)].** One of the basal nuclei. It has biconvex surfaces, is composed of a lateral putamen and a medial globus pallidus, and medial to it is the internal capsule. **Merocyte nucleus.** A supernumerary nucleus within a fertilized ovum, the result of polyspermia or artificial introduction. **Mesoblastic nucleus.** The nucleus of a mesodermal cell. **Mother nucleus.** The nucleus which divides to give daughter nuclei. **Motion nucleus.** The micronucleus of certain protozoa, and believed to control its movements. **Nutrition nucleus.** The vegetative as opposed to the reproductive nucleus of cells which possess both. **Olivary nucleus [nucleus olivaris (NA)].** A large, crenated, hollow nucleus lying posterolateral to the pyramid, just below the level of the pons. It is a constituent of the extrapyramidal motor system. **Olivary nucleus, hilum of the [hilus nuclei olivaris (NA)].** The medial side of the olive, deficient in grey matter. **Olivary nucleus, dorsal accessory [nucleus olivaris accessorius dorsalis (NA)].** A small nucleus dorsimesal to the olive. **Olivary nucleus, medial accessory [nucleus olivaris accessorius medialis (NA)].** A curved lamina of grey matter on the ventromedian side of the olive, just dorsal to the pyramid. **Nucleus of origin [nucleus originis (NA)].** A collection of nerve cells within the central nervous system giving rise to the fibres of a nerve. **Paraventricular nucleus [nucleus paraventricularis (NA)].** One of the nuclei in the hypothalamus. **Polymorphic nucleus.** A nucleus of irregular shape, or possessing 2 or more lobes. **Polytene nucleus.** A nucleus with polytene chromosomes. **Nuclei pontis [NA].** Scattered groups of nerve cells in the basilar part of the pons, where impulses from the cerebrum to the cerebellum relay. **Posterior nucleus [nucleus posterior (NA)].** A group of cells in the side wall of the 3rd ventricle immediately dorsal to the mamillary bodies, which, when stimulated, gives rise to signs of sympathetic activity. The course of its efferent fibres is uncertain. **Pretectal nucleus [nucleus pretectalis (NA)].** A collection of nerve cells deep to the upper end of the superior quadrigeminal body, receiving afferent fibres from the optic tract and occipital cortex and sending efferents to the Edinger-Westphal nucleus. It is an important centre in the light reflex. **Nucleus pulposus [NA].** The soft pulpy centre of an intervertebral disc. It disappears in old age. **Red nucleus [nucleus ruber (NA)].** An oval-shaped collection of nerve cells in the tegmentum of the mid-brain and extending forwards into the subthalamic region. **Reproductive nucleus.** Gonad nucleus (see above). **Salivary nucleus, inferior [nucleus salivatorius inferior (NA)].** A small group of cells in the reticular formation of the medulla close to the nucleus ambiguus, giving rise to those fibres of the glossopharyngeal nerve that innervate the parotid gland. **Salivary nucleus, superior [nucleus salivatorius superior (NA)].** A small nucleus on the dorsolateral side of the motor nucleus of the facial nerve. It is the source of secretomotor fibres to the sublingual and submandibular salivary glands. **Segmentation nucleus.** Cleavage nucleus (see above). **Shadow nucleus.** A cell nucleus in process of dissolution at the stage when it has lost its chromatin and is no longer stainable. **Somatic nucleus.** The macro- as opposed to the micro-nucleus in cells which possess both. **Sperm nucleus, Spermatic nucleus.** The male pronucleus within the fertilized ovum. **Subthalamic nucleus [nucleus subthalamicus (NA)].** A small brownish nucleus lying in the forward projection of the tegmentum under the thalamus and above the base of the cerebral peduncle. **Supra-optic nucleus [nucleus supra-opticus (NA)].** One of the nuclei in the hypothalamus; it lies above the optic chiasma and sends its fibres to the posterior lobe of the hypophysis cerebri. **Tectorial nucleus.** Red nucleus (see above). **Tegmental nuclei [nuclei tegmenti (NA)].** Collections of nerve cells which lie in the reticular substance. They include the interstitial nucleus of Cajal. **Nucleus of termination [nucleus terminationis (NA)].** A nucleus into which a fibre tract discharges. **Nuclei of the thalamus.** *See* THALAMUS. **Thoracic nucleus [nucleus thoracicus (NA)].** A group of cells occupying the medial part of the base of the posterior columns in the thoracic and upper lumbar region (Clarke's column). **Trophic nucleus.** The vegetative as opposed to the reproductive nucleus of cells possessing both. **Tuberal nuclei [nuclei tuberales (NA)].** Scattered groups of cells in the tuber cinereum; some of their efferent fibres pass to the posterior lobe of the hypophysis cerebri. **Ventromedial nucleus [nucleus ventromedialis (NA)].** A nucleus situated just caudal to the anterior hypothalamic area extending back to the mamillary body and lying ventral and medial to the fornix fibres. It is part of the oculomotor group of nuclei and is believed to be concerned with the innervation of the inferior rectus muscle. **Vesicular nucleus.** A cell nucleus whose chromatin is dispersed, leaving unstained areas between the chromatin threads and granules. **Vestibular nucleus, inferior [nucleus vestibularis inferior (NA)].** An elongated nucleus between the medial nucleus and the inferior cerebellae peduncle, traversed by the fibres of the vestibulospinal tract. **Vestibular nucleus, lateral [nucleus vestibularis lateralis (NA)].** A nucleus lying lateral to the medial nucleus, containing large cells giving rise to the vestibulospinal tract; Deiters' nucleus. **Vestibular nucleus, medial [nucleus vestibularis medialis (NA)].** A large nucleus in the floor of the 4th ventricle near its lateral extremity, crossed dorsally by the auditory striae, the principal nucleus for the relay of afferent vestibular impulses. **Vestibular nucleus, superior [nucleus vestibularis superior (NA)].** A small nucleus lying above the medial and lateral vestibular nuclei. **Vitelline nucleus.** Yolk nucleus (see below). **Yolk nucleus.** A star-shaped structure within the first-formed yolk of a developing egg while it is still in the ovary. **Zygote nucleus.** The nucleus formed by the fusion of male and female pronuclei in the fertilized ovum. [L nut.]

See also: BALBIANI, BECHTEREW, BÉCLARD, BLUMENAU, BURDACH, DARKSHEVICH, DEITERS, DUVAL (M. M.), EDINGER, FUSE, GOLL, KAISER, KOELLIKER, LAURA, LUYS (J. B.), MONAKOW, PANDER, PERLIA, RAMÓN Y CAJAL, ROLLER, SCHWALBE, SCHWANN, SETCHENOV, SIEMERLING, SPITZKA (E. A.), STADERINI, STILLING, VOIT (K.), WESTPHAL (C. F. B.).

nuclide (new·klide). A species of atomic nucleus characterized by its charge, mass number and quantum state, and capable of existing for a measurable lifetime. Nuclear isomers are separate nuclides, but transient excited nuclear states and unstable intermediates in nuclear reactions are not so considered. **Daughter nuclide.** Of a given nuclide, any nuclide that originates from it by radioactive decay. [nucleus.]

nudism (new·dizm). 1. The abnormal desire of patients suffering from some mental illness to remove their clothes or to go about in the naked state. 2. A cult according to which members of particular groups do not wear clothing while they are within their own colony although they conform to conventional standards of decency when they mingle with others. [L *nudus* naked.]

nudomania (new·do·**ma**·ne·ah). Having an interest in nudism to a morbid degree. [L *nudus* naked, mania.]

nudophobia (new·do·**fo**·be·ah). A dislike or fear of being naked. [L *nudus* naked, phobia.]

Nuel, Jean Pierre (b. 1847). Ghent and Louvain ophthalmologist.

Nuel's operation, for corneoscleral rupture [obsolete].

Nuel's spaces. Intercellular spaces in the outer part of the spiral organ of the inner ear.

Nuhn, Anton (b. 1814). Heidelberg anatomist.

Nuhn's glands, Blandin and Nuhn glands. Anterior lingual glands. *See* GLAND.

cyst of Blandin and Nuhn glands. A rare cyst resulting from obstruction to the duct of one of the anterior lingual glands situated beneath the anterior part of the tongue.

nuisance (new·sans). In forensic medicine, anything that annoys or vexes or is offensive to anyone else, or to something that is of noxious character. [O Fr. from L *nocere* to harm.]

nullipara (nul·**ip**·ar·ah). A woman who has not given birth to a child. [see foll.]

nulliparity (nul·ip·**ar**·it·e). The state of not having borne any children. [L *nullus* no one, *parere* to bear.]

nulliparous (nul·**ip**·ar·us). Never having given birth to a child. [see prec.]

nullisomic (nul·e·**so**·mik). Aneuploid cell or individual lacking all members of at least 1 chromosome pair. [L *nullus* no one, Gk *soma* body.]

nullity (**nul**·it·e). Grounds for dissolution of marriage arising from unrevealed disease or unsoundness of mind at the time of marriage, of an age below consent, pregnancy by another man at the time of marriage (not disclosed) or non-consummation. [L *nullus* not any.]

numb (num). 1. Having enfeebled power of sensation or being without sensation. 2. To deaden or impair the power of sensing. [ME *nume.*]

number (**num**·ber). In chemistry, a value or index. **Acetyl number.** The oxyacids and alcohols in a fat expressed in terms of the weight (in milligrams) of potassium hydroxide required to neutralize the acetic acid produced from 1 g of fat when the latter is acetylated and then saponified. **Acid number.** The free fatty acids in a fat expressed in terms of the weight (in milligrams) of potassium hydroxide required to neutralize them. **Atomic number.** Of an element, the integer Ze, where Z is the nuclear charge and e is the charge of a proton. **Chromosome modal number.** The most common chromosome number of a cell population or of a taxonomic group (genus, family, class, order). **Dibucaine number.** Measurement of the ability of dibucaine (cinchocaine) to inhibit cholinesterase activity and assist differentiation between normal and abnormal types of cholinesterase. It is the percentage inhibition of the differential inhibitor of acetylcholine by a 10^{-5} molar concentrate of dibucaine. The normal enzyme is inhibited by about 80 per cent and the atypical variant by about 20 per cent. **Diploid number.** The number of chromosomes present in the diploid; a constant for each species. **Haploid number.** Half the number of chromosomes present in the normal somatic cell; the actual number in the gamete. **Hydrogen number.** The unsaturated fatty acids in a fat in terms of the weight of hydrogen they will absorb. **Iodine number.** The unsaturated fatty acids in a fat in terms of the weight of iodine with which they will combine. **Isotopic number.** The isotopic weight less twice the atomic number. **Mass number.** Of a nuclide, the number of protons plus neutrons in the nucleus; symbol A. **Octane number.** The percentage of octane in a mixture with normal heptane that has the same "knock" as a given sample of motor spirit. **Polar number.** The valency of an element expressed with a positive or negative sign according to its electrochemical nature. **Saponification number.** The fatty acids of a fat in terms of the weight (in milligrams) of potassium hydroxide necessary to saponify 1 g of the fat. **Thiocyanogen number.** The unsaturated fatty acids in a fat in terms of the amount of thiocyanogen they will absorb. **Transport number.** The ratio of the migration velocity of an ion to the combined velocities of anion and cation; it is of value in electrolytic work as a guide to the conductivity of the electrolyte and the concentration at the electrodes. **Wave number.** The number of electromagnetic waves per centimetre; the reciprocal of the wavelength in centimetres. [L *numerus.*]

See also: AVOGADRO, HITTORF, POLENSKÉ, REICHERT (J. S.), REYNOLDS.

numbering (**num**·ber·ing). In chemistry, the indication of the position of radicals in an organic compound by incorporating in their names the numbers of the carbon atoms to which they are attached. A carbon chain is numbered consecutively from the carbon next to the reactive radical; a ring compound begins its numbering at the heterocyclic or most fully saturated atom. **Series numbering.** The practice of numbering parts in anatomy commencing with those at the proximal or cephalic aspect. [see prec.]

numbness (**num**·nes). A condition in which there is loss or impairment of sensation in a part. **Waking numbness.** Impermanent numbness or paresis of the hands and feet experienced either after lying down for a length of time or on waking. [ME *nume.*]

nummiform (**num**·e·form). Shaped like a coin or a circular disc. [L *nummus* coin, form.]

nummular (**num**·ew·lar). 1. Shaped like a coin or circular disc. This term is commonly applied to the sputum of pulmonary tuberculosis. 2. Composed of flat, circular discs. Arranged in a rouleau as coins are stacked. [L *nummularius* of money.]

nummulation (num·ew·**la**·shun). The formation of nummular aggregations of blood corpuscles. [see prec.]

numoquin (**new**·mo·kwin). Ethylhydrocupreine.

Nunn, Thomas William (b. 1825). London surgeon.

Nunn's gorged corpuscles. Fatty epithelial cells found in ovarian cysts.

nunnation (nun·**a**·shun). 1. Stammering in which the *n* sound is used instead of other, and correct, consonants. 2. The pronouncing of words or the production of sound nasally. [Ar. *nun* letter*n.*]

nupharine (**new**·far·een). $C_{18}H_{44}O_2N_2$, an alkaloid found in species of *Nymphaea* (*Nuphar luteum* Sibth. and Sm.).

nuptiality (nup·she·**al**·it·e). The ratio of marriages to the total population. [L *nuptus* married.]

nurse (ners). 1. A person whose profession it is to care for the sick. The title is now legally confined to men and women whose names are on the State Register or State Roll of qualified nurses, with the exception of children's nurses, who are also allowed to use the title. 2. To carry out the duties of a nurse. 3. To suckle. 4. To tend, hold or clasp. **Charge nurse.** A head nurse, i.e. one who is in charge of a ward or department of a hospital. **Children's nurse.** A person who has the charge of an infant or small child. **District nurse.** A nurse whose duties consist in visiting patients in their own homes within a certain specified area. **Domiciliary nurse.** A nurse who visits patients in their own homes; a visiting nurse. **Dry nurse.** An infant's nurse who is not required to suckle it [probably obsolete]. **Factory nurse.** An industrial nurse engaged in a factory. **Graduate nurse.** A State Registered Nurse, who has completed a period of training in an approved training-school, and has passed the State examinations. **Head nurse.** A charge nurse (see above). **Hospital nurse.** A nurse whose duties are confined to the wards and departments of a hospital. **Industrial nurse.** A person engaged in caring for the physical and mental well-being of persons in industry. **Private nurse.** A nurse whose attentions are engaged and remunerated by private individuals. **Probationer nurse.** A student nurse on probation. **Public Health nurse.** A State Registered Nurse who by precept and practice assists in the teaching and maintenance of communal health, e.g. health visitors, baby clinic nurses, tuberculosis visitors, school nurses, industrial nurses. **Queen's nurse.** A State Registered Nurse or qualified midwife with an additional qualification for district work. **School nurse.** A nurse who is engaged in safeguarding the health of school children. **Special nurse.** A nurse whose duties are confined to one patient only. **State Enrolled Assistant Nurse.** A person who by training and experience during a specified period in a hospital approved by the General Nursing Council, and having passed an examination, has qualified for the State Roll of Assistant Nurses. **State Registered Nurse.** A person who by training and experience during a specified period in a hospital approved by the General Nursing Council, and having passed an examination, qualifies for the State Register of Nurses. **Student nurse.** A nurse in training. **Trained nurse.** A qualified State Registered Nurse or State Enrolled Assistant Nurse (see above). **Visiting nurse.** A domiciliary nurse. **Wet nurse.** A person who suckles a child in the place of its mother [probably obsolete]. [L *nutrix.*]

Nussbaum, Johann Nepomuk von (b. 1829). German surgeon.

Nussbaum's bracelet. A device worn around the wrist to which a pen or pencil can be attached with the object of enabling sufferers from writers' cramp to write.

Nussbaum, Moritz (b. 1850). Bonn biologist and histologist.

Nussbaum's cell. A small cell from the pyloric glands of the stomach.

Nussbaum's experiment. The ligation of the renal arteries in the frog, thus cutting off the blood supply to the glomeruli, thereby demonstrating the activity of the tubules which are supplied with blood from the renal veins.

nut (nut). A fruit characterized by being dry, indehiscent, with 1 seed coat and with a hard stony pericarp. **Bissy nuts, Gooroo nuts.** Kola. **Greek nuts.** Bitter and sweet almonds. **Kola nut.** Kola. **Monkey nut.** Peanut. **Poison nut.** Nux vomica. **Purging nut.** The seeds of *Jatropha curcas* (family Euphorbiaceae) containing about 40 per cent of fixed oil and a substance, curcin, resembling the ricin of castor oil. Both oil and seeds are strong purgatives. [AS *hnutu.*]

nutans (**new**·tans). Nodding. [L.]

nutarian (nut·a·re·an). An individual whose diet consists mainly of nuts.

nutation (new·**ta**·shun). The act of nodding habitually and involuntarily. [L *nutare* to nod.]

nutgall (**nut**·gawl). Galls; the excrescences on the twigs of the oak resulting from stimulation of the tissues by the deposition of the eggs of the gall wasp. Preparations of gall are applied externally as astringents. Nutgall is also used as a source of gallic and tannic acids. [AS *hnutu*, L *galla* gall-nut.]

Nutmeg BPC 1968 (**nut**·meg). The dried kernel of the seeds of *Myristica fragrans* Houtt., the chief constituents of which are a volatile oil consisting chiefly of terpenes and myristicin, a solid fat and amylodextrin. It has stimulant and carminative properties, but it can be toxic, producing convulsions due to the myristicin contained. The dried arillus constitutes mace. [AS *notemuge.*]

nutrient (**new**·tre·ent). 1. Supplying nourishment; for example, a nutrient artery. 2. Any drug that influences the process of metabolism or nutrition. [L *nutriens* nourishing.]

nutriment (**new**·tre·ment). Food; that which nourishes. [L *nutrimentum.*]

nutrition (new·**trish**·un). 1. Nourishment; food. *See* DIET. 2. The supply of food to the tissues and its absorption by the latter. [L *nutrire* to nourish.]

nutritional (new·**trish**·on·al). Referring to or having an effect on the process of nutrition.

nutritionist (new·**trish**·on·ist). An expert in the sciences of food and of nutrition.

nutrix (**new**·trix). A wet nurse [obsolete term]. [L female nurse.]

nutrose (**new**·troze). A compound of sodium and casein used in the preparation of culture media.

nux moschata (nux mos·**ka**·tah). Nutmeg. [L *nux* nut, Gk *moschos* musk.]

Nux Vomica BP 1973 (nux **vom**·ik·ah). The dried ripe seeds of *Strychnos nux-vomica* (family Loganiaceae), a small tree widely distributed in India. The principal constituents are the 2 alkaloids, strychnine and brucine. **Powdered nux vomica.** Nux vomica (above) finely powdered and adjusted to contain from 1.14 to 1.26 per cent of strychnine by the addition of lactose or other inert substance. [L *nux* nut, *vomere* to vomit.]

nyctalbuminuria (nikt·al·bew·min·**ewr'**·e·ah). Noctalbuminuria. [Gk *nyx* night, albuminuria.]

nyctalgia (nikt·**al**·je·ah). Pain that occurs at night; in particular, denoting the bone pains of syphilis which interrupt sleep. [Gk *nyx* nigt, *algos* pain.]

nyctalope (**nik**·tal·ope). An individual suffering from night blindness. [see foll.]

nyctalopia (nik·tal·**o**·pe·ah). Night blindness. It may be due to defective formation of visual purple such as occurs in avitaminosis especially with regard to vitamin A or defective metabolism of vitamin A (as in cirrhosis of the liver), or to scarcity of rods in the retina which may be hereditary or caused by disease, e.g. Oguchi's disease, retinitis pigmentosa or widespread choroidoretinitis. [Gk *nyx* night, *alaos* obscure, *ops* eye.]

nyctamblyopia (**nikt**·am·ble·**o'**·pe·ah). Defective vision after nightfall or in dim light. [Gk *nyx* night, *amblyopia* dim vision.]

nyctaphonia (nikt·af·**o**·ne·ah). A hysterical condition in which there is loss of voice during the night. [Gk *nyx* night, aphonia.]

nycterine (**nik**·ter·ine). 1. Nocturnal. 2. Obscure. [Gk *nykterinos* nightly.]

nycterohemeral, nyctohemeral (**nik**·ter·o·**hem'**·er·al, nik·to·**hem'**·er·al). Relating to day and to night. [Gk *nykteros* by night, *hemera* day.]

nycthemeral (nik·**them**·er·al). Nyctihemeral.

nyctihemeral (nik·te·**hem**·er·al). Referring to a measurable attribute, usually a physiological parameter, which varies in a regular manner in unison with the light-darkness daily cycle but extended to include such cyclical changes which are related to the sleep-wakefulness daily cycle. [Gk *nykteros* by night, *hemera* day.]

nyctohemeral (nik·to·**hem**·er·al). Nyctihemeral.

nyctophilia (nik·to·**fil**·e·ah). A predilection for night-time. [Gk *nyx* night, *philos* pleasing.]

nyctophobia (nik·to·**fo**·be·ah). Excessive dread of the darkness and silence of night, or of being in the dark. [Gk *nyx* night, phobia.]

nyctophonia (nik·to·**fo**·ne·ah). A condition in which there is loss of voice during the daytime. [Gk *nyx* night, *phone* voice.]

Nyctotherus (nik·**toth**·er·us). A genus of infusorian parasites, one member of which, *Nyctotherus faba*, was once thought to be a factor in the causation of trypanosomiasis. [Gk *nyktotheras* a hunter by night.]

nyctotyphlosis (**nik**·to·tif·**lo'**·sis). Night blindness. *See* BLINDNESS. [Gk *nyx* night, *typhlosis* a making blind.]

nycturia (nik·**tewr**·e·ah). 1. A condition in which the secretion of urine is more active at night and the quantity passed per hour is greater than that passed during daylight. 2. Nocturnal enuresis. *See* ENURESIS. [Gk *nyx* night, urine.]

nygma (**nig**·ma). A wound of puncture type. [Gk a prick.]

Nylander, Emmo (b. 1835). Swedish chemist.

Nylander's reagent, for sugar in urine. Dissolve 40 g of Rochelle salt and 20 g of bismuth subnitrate in 1 litre of 8 per cent sodium hydroxide solution.

Nylin's test. Of myocardial reserve: the oxygen consumption is measured after the climbing of a standard staircase at a known rate. The oxygen debt (i.e. consumption) is much greater in persons with cardiac insufficiency than in normal subjects.

nylon (**ni**·lon). A synthetic polymer of great toughness, lightness and elasticity used in many forms, including surgical suture threads. [etym. dub.]

nymph (nimf). 1. The larval form of a hemimetabolous insect. 2. The later larval form of Acarina, having 8 legs. [Gk *nymphe* maiden.]

nympha (**nimf**·ah) (pl. *nymphae*). One or other of the labia minora. [see prec.]

nymphectomy (nimf·**ek**·to·me). Removal of the nymphae, usually because of excessive size. [nympha, Gk *ektome* excision.]

nymphitis (nimf·**i**·tis). An inflammatory condition affecting the nymphae. [nympha, Gk *-itis* inflammation.]

nymphocaruncular (**nimf**·o·kar·**ung'**·kew·lar). Nymphohymeneal. [nympha, caruncula.]

nymphohymeneal (**nimf**·o·hi·**men'**·e·al). Pertaining to the labia minora and hymen, or the caruncula hymenalis. [nympha, hymen.]

nympholepsy (**nimf**·o·lep·se). 1. Ecstasy or frenzy of an erotic nature. 2. Excision of the labia minora. [Gk *nymphe* maiden, *lambanein* to seize.]

nymphomania (nimf·o·**ma**·ne·ah): Ungovernable sexual desire in women. [nympha, mania.]

nymphomaniac (nimf·o·**ma**·ne·ak). One who suffers from nymphomania.

nymphoncus (nimf·**ong**·kus). A condition of hypertrophy affecting the labia minora. [nympha, Gk *ogkas* a swelling.]

Nyssorhynchus (nis·o·**ring**·kus). A sub-genus of *Anopheles.* [Gk *nyssa* prick, *rhygchos* snout.]

nystagmic (nis·**tag**·mik). Referring to or affected with nystagmus.

nystagmiform (nis·**tag**·me·form). Similar to nystagmus. [nystagmus, form.]

nystagmograph (nis·**tag**·mo·graf). A device that registers by applied tambour and style the degree of movement of the eyeball of an individual suffering from nystagmus. [nystagmus, Gk *graphein* to record.]

nystagmography (nis·tag·**mog**·raf·e). A recording of the eye in nystagmus. [see prec.]

nystagmoid (nis·**tag**·moid). Nystagmiform. [nystagmus, Gk *eidos* form.]

nystagmus (nis·**tag**·mus). A condition in which the eyes are seen to move in a more or less rhythmical manner, from side to side, up and down, or in a rotary manner from the original point of fixation. **Amaurotic nystagmus.** That associated with blindness. **Amblyopic nystagmus.** That caused by any lesion interfering with central vision and so preventing the normal fixation reflex to develop, e.g. albinism or congenital defects or disease of the media or macula. **Ataxic nystagmus.** Nystagmus occurring on conjugate horizontal gaze, particularly affecting the abducting eye. **Aural nystagmus.** A reflex associated with hearing a loud and sudden noise. The term is sometimes loosely applied to vestibular nystagmus (see below). **Caloric nystagmus.** Nystagmus induced by irrigating the external auditory meatus with hot or cold water. It appears after a latent period of from 15 to 30 s. **Central nystagmus.** That caused by a lesion in the brain affecting the central connections of the vestibular apparatus, the cerebellum, medulla, pons or the mid-brain. **Cerebellar nystagmus.** A highly variable jerk nystagmus which may be to either side, vertical or rotatory. **Congenital nystagmus.** Nystagmus present at, or shortly after, birth and continuing throughout life. The condition may be familial and is usually of the horizontal pendular type, becoming jerky on lateral gaze. **Deviational nystagmus.** Pseudonystagmus. **Disjunctive nystagmus.** Nystagmus in which the eyes swing towards and away from each other; alternating convergence and divergence. **Dissociated nystagmus.** The movements of the two eyes are dissimilar in both amount and direction. **Downbeat nystagmus.** Vertical nystagmus with the fast phase downward. It denotes a lesion of the lower end of the brain stem or cerebellum. **Nystagmus of eccentric fixation.** A physiological form, jerky in type, which occurs when the fixation axes of the eyes are deviated laterally beyond the extent of the binocular field; it is of no pathological significance. **End-positional nystagmus, Endstellung nystagmus.** Pseudonystagmus. **Fixation nystagmus.** Nystagmus due to abnormal functioning of the fixation mechanism. It may be: 1. Experimental (optokinetic nystagmus); 2. Spontaneous: (*a*) from infancy, due to defective formation or function of the macular region, e.g. albinism; (*b*) acquired as the result of disseminated sclerosis; (*c*) latent, appearing only when one or other eye is closed; or (*d*) miners' nystagmus (see below). **Galvanic nystagmus.** That caused by electrical stimulation of the labyrinth. When the anode is applied to the labyrinth the slow movement of the nystagmus is towards the same side; when the cathode, to the opposite side. **Hereditary nystagmus.** Congenital nystagmus (see above). **Horizontal nystagmus.** Nystagmus when the eyes are moved horizontally, e.g. from side to side. **Jerk nystagmus.** Nystagmus in which the movement is quicker in one direction than in the other. The direction of the quick component is used in defining the type of nystagmus, e.g. right, left, up, down, etc. **Labyrinthine nystagmus.** That due to disturbances of the semicircular canals or their nervous connections, which may be experimental (*rotatory nystagmus*) or due to disease of the labyrinth or central nervous system. **Latent nystagmus.** Nystagmus which is only present if one eye is covered. It is often associated with squint or with alternating hyperphoria. **Lateral nystagmus.** That in which the movements of the eyes are from side to side. **Miners' nystagmus.** An acquired occupational disease of coal miners characterized by eye movements, usually pendular in the primary position, and frequently jerky in lateral gaze. The movements are regular, but may be in any direction, vertical, horizontal, rotatory or oblique. **Ocular nystagmus.** Nystagmus caused by a condition of the eye itself. **Optokinetic nystagmus.** Nystagmus caused by following moving objects, e.g. by looking out of a railway carriage window or by following vertical black marks on a rotating drum. The latter method is used extensively in experimental and clinical investigations. **Oscillating nystagmus.** Undulatory nystagmus (see below). **Palatal nystagmus.** Jerky movements occurring in the soft palate. **Paretic nystagmus.** That occurring when the eye attempts to look in the direction of action of a weakened or partly paralysed extra-ocular muscle. It may be uni-ocular. **Pendular nystagmus.** Nystagmus in which the swing of the eyes is smooth and equal in each direction. **Periodic alternating nystagmus.** Vestibular nystagmus which undergoes cyclic changes in amplitude and direction. **Positional nystagmus.** Nystagmus occurring only when the head is held in a certain position. **Resilient nystagmus.** Nystagmus in which a slow movement in one direction is followed by a rapid return movement. **Retraction nystagmus.** Nystagmus which may be horizontal, vertical or rotatory, each oscillation being associated with a jerk drawing the eyeballs back into the orbits; usually accompanied by some palsy of elevation of the eyes. **Rhythmical nystagmus.** A comparatively slow movement in one direction is followed by a rapid return in the opposite direction. **Rotatory nystagmus.** Nystagmus that occurs in 2 forms, the eyeball making rotary to-and-fro movements: (*a*) around its antero-posterior axis; or (*b*) around some other axis. **Secondary nystagmus.** After-nystagmus; that occurring on the cessation of rotation, due to the labyrinthine fluid continuing to move for a short time after the head movement has stopped. **See-saw nystagmus.** Opposed vertical movements of the eyes usually associated with chiasmal disease. **Undulatory nystagmus.** Nystagmus in which the movements have the same to-and-fro velocity. **Vertical nystagmus.** Nystagmus in which the movements are up and down. **Vestibular nystagmus.** Nystagmus due to some disorder of the semicircular canals or their nervous connections. **Vibratory nystagmus.** Nystagmus in which the movements have the same to-and-fro velocity but are of greater frequency than the undulatory form. **Visual nystagmus.** That due to defects of visual fixation, e.g. albinism. The movements are pendular. [Gk *nystagmos* a nodding.]

See also: CHEYENE (J.), STOKES (WILLIAM).

nystagmusmyoclonus (nis·tag·mus·mi·o·klo'·nus). A congenital condition of uncommon occurrence consisting of nystagmus associated with clonic muscular spasms elsewhere. [nystagmus, Gk *mys* muscle, *klonos* tumult.]

Nystatin BP 1973 (ni·stat·in). An antibiotic produced by a growth of a species of *Streptomyces.* It is used locally in the treatment of candidiasis.

nystaxis (nis·tax·is). Nystagmus. [Gk drowsiness.]

Nysten, Pierre Hubert (b. 1774). Paris physician.

Nysten's law. Rigor mortis begins in the muscles of the jaw, spreads to those of the face and neck and then to those of the trunk and arms, and lastly to the legs and feet.

nyxis (nix·is). Paracentesis. [Gk a prick.]

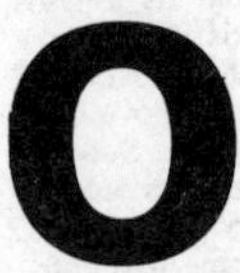

oak (oke). A tree of the genus *Quercus* (family Fagaceae). **Oak apple.** Nutgall. **Oak bark.** The dried bark obtained from the smaller branches and young stems of the British oak, collected in the spring from the trees. It contains from 15 to 20 per cent of quercitannic acid, also a phlobaphene, *oak red*, and gallic acid. It is used solely as an astringent, more especially as a wash or injection in the treatment of leucorrhoea or haemorrhoids. **Oak gall.** An excrescence on the twigs of *Quercus infectoria* resulting from the deposition of the eggs of the gall wasp. [AS *ac*.]

oakum (o·kum). A hempen material prepared from old rope; it was formerly used as a dressing material to absorb discharge from wounds and lochia. [AS *acumbe* off-combings.]

oarium (o·a·re·um). An ovary. [Gk *oarion* small egg.]

oasis (o·a·sis) (pl. *oases*). A circumscribed area of healthy tissue encircled by an area of diseased tissue. [Gk a fertile spot in the Libyan desert.]

obcaecation (ob·se·**ka**·shun). Partial blindness (a term now rarely used). [L *ob* towards, *caecitas* blindness.]

obdormition (ob·dor·**mish**·un). Anaesthesia and numbness of an extremity or a part as the result of pressure on the associated sensory nerve. [L *obdormire* to go to sleep.]

O'Beirne, James (b. 1786). Dublin surgeon.

O'Beirne's experiment. The demonstration of the mechanism of strangulated hernia by inflating a loop of bowel introduced through a hole in a sheet of cardboard or other material.

O'Beirne's sphincter or valve. A local thickening of the circular muscle fibres of the upper end of the rectum.

Obelia (o·**be**·le·ah). A genus of jelly-fish whose sting produces painful local swellings and an urticarial rash; susceptible persons may suffer from shock and collapse. [Gk *obelos* a spit.]

obeliac (o·**be**·le·ak). Referring to the obelion.

obelion (o·**be**·le·on). The point of intersection of the sagittal suture with a line joining the two parietal foramina. [Gk *obelos* a spit.]

Ober, Frank Roberts (b. 1881). Boston surgeon.

Ober's operation. Division of the tensor fasciae latae muscle for low back pain.

Ober's test. For contracture of the tensor fasciae latae muscle. With the patient on his side and the under leg flexed, if the upper leg is abducted and extended this position will be maintained without the support of the examiner's hand.

Obermayer, Friedrich (b. 1861). Vienna physician.

Obermayer's reagent. For indican. Dissolve 1 g of ferric chloride in 500 ml of concentrated hydrochloric acid.

Obermayer's test. For indican in urine. Mix 5 ml of urine with 5 ml of Obermayer's reagent; add 4 ml of chloroform and mix by repeated inversion. On separating, the chloroform is coloured blue if indican is present.

Obersteiner, Heinrich (b. 1847). Vienna neurologist.

Obersteiner-Redlich area or zone. An unmyelinated area of the lateral part of a posterior nerve root as it enters the spinal cord.

obese (o·bees). Very fat; corpulent. [L *obesus* swollen.]

obesity (o·**bees**·it·e). An excessive accumulation of fat in the body; the fat is mainly deposited in the subcutaneous tissues, the omentum, mesentery and around such organs as the heart and liver. It is essentially due to the caloric intake being in excess of the person's needs, and overeating combined with insufficient exercise is the commonest cause. In some cases there is a marked retention of water, which accounts for some of the gain in weight and size, whilst disorder of the ductless glands, especially the thyroid, pituitary and sex glands, may also be a factor. **Alimentary obesity.** That due to an excessive caloric intake. **Endocrine obesity.** Obesity due to any endocrine imbalance. **Endogenous obesity.** Obesity due to endocrine disorders. **Exogenous obesity.** Alimentary obesity (see above). **Hyperinsular obesity.** Obesity occurring in chronic hyperinsulinism. **Hypogonad obesity.** That which occurs with deficient ovarian secretion, as at the menopause, or after castration, as in eunuchs. **Hypothalamic obesity.** Obesity due to damage to or disturbance of the function of the hypothalamus. **Hypothyroid obesity.** That occurring in hypothyroidism. [L *obesitas* fatness.]

obesogenous (o·bees·**oj**·en·us). Causing or producing obesity. [obesity, Gk *genein* to produce.]

obex [NA] (o·bex). A small triangular membrane formed at the caudal angle of the roof of the 4th ventricle by the meeting of the taeniae of the ventricle. [L barrier.]

obfuscation (ob·fus·**ka**·shun). 1. The act of clouding or of rendering obscure. 2. Confusion; bewilderment. [L *obfuscare* to darken.]

object choice (**ob**·jekt chois). The object of the sexual impulses, either external (anaclitic) or internal (narcissistic). A psychoanalytical term. [L *objectum* something cast before, AS *cis*.]

objective (ob·**jek**·tiv). The lens, simple or compound, of an optical system nearest the object viewed, e.g. in a telescope or compound microscope. **Achromatic objective.** An objective having the same focal length for red and blue light. **Apochromatic objective.** An objective having the same focal length for red, green and blue light. **Fluorite objectives.** Semi-apochromatic objective (see below). **Immersion objective.** A microscope objective in which the space between objective and object is liquid-filled, usually by oil of the same refractive index as glass. **Monochromatic objective.** An objective specially designed for working with light of a single wavelength. **Semi-apochromatic objectives.** Objectives that contain some fluorite in the lenses and are intermediate in quality between achromatic and apochromatic objectives. [L *objectum* something cast before.]

oblique (ob·**leek**). 1. Deviating from a perpendicular line but not so far as to be horizontal; pointing in a slanting direction or lying in an inclined position. 2. Indirect or obscure. 3. In botany, asymmetrical, as a leaf. [L *obliquus* aslant.]

oblique muscles. External oblique muscle [musculus obliquus externus abdominis (NA)]. The most superficial of the flat muscles covering the front and lateral sides of the abdomen with its fibres directed from above downwards and medially, and ending in front and below in an aponeurosis. **Internal oblique muscle [musculus obliquus internus abdominis (NA)].** The middle layer of the flat abdominal muscles, with its fibres directed from above downwards and backwards, and its lowest free margin arching above the medial half of the inguinal ligament and over the spermatic cord.

oblique muscles of the orbit. Inferior oblique muscle of the orbit [musculus obliquus inferior (NA)]. A muscle arising from the floor of the orbit lateral to the nasolacrimal groove and passing laterally, backwards and upwards, to reach the lateral part of the sclera behind the equator. It turns the eye upwards and laterally. **Superior oblique muscle of the orbit [musculus obliquus superior (NA)].** A muscle arising above the origin of the medial rectus muscle, passing forward to end in a slender tendon which traverses a fibrocartilaginous pulley, the trochlea, is attached to the trochlear fossa of the frontal bone, and then passes backwards, downwards and laterally, to pass out into the sclera behind the equator. It turns the eye downwards and laterally.

oblique vein of the left atrium [vena obliqua atrii sinistri (NA)]. A tributary of the coronary sinus from the back of the left atrium. Of embryological significance, it is a remnant of the left duct of Cuvier.

obliquimeter (ob·le·**kwim**·et·er). An instrument used to indicate the angle of the pelvic brim in the standing patient. [L *obliquus* aslant, meter.]

obliquity (ob·**lik**·wit·e). The state of being oblique.
See also: LITZMANN, NAEGELE.

obliquus (ob·**li**·kwus). An oblique muscle. [L aslant.]

obliquus capitis inferior muscle [musculus obliquus capitis inferior (NA)] (ob·**li**·kwus **kap**·it·is in·**feer**·e·or musl). A muscle forming the inferior boundary of the suboccipital triangle, attached to the spine of the axis and the inferior aspect of the transverse process of the atlas.

obliquus capitis superior muscle [musculus obliquus capitis superior (NA)] (ob·**li**·kwus **kap**·it·is sew·**peer**·e·or musl). A muscle forming the lateral boundary of the suboccipital triangle, attached superiorly to the occipital bone between the superior and inferior nuchal line, and inferiorly to the posterior part of the transverse process of the atlas.

obliteration (ob·lit·er·**a**′·shun). Entire removal of a part of the body by operative procedure or disease. **Cortical obliteration.** A condition of the cerebral cortex in which, on microscopic examination, certain areas have failed to stain with reagents, indicating disappearance of nerve ganglion cells. [L *obliterare* to efface.]

oblitine (**ob**·lit·een). The diethyl ester of carnitine isolated from meat extract.

oblongata (ob·long·**gah**·tah). The medulla oblongata. [L *oblongus* rather long.]

obmutescence (ob·mew·**tes**·ens). Becoming or keeping dumb or silent. [L *obmutescere* to become dumb.]

obnubilation (ob·**new**·bil·**a**′·shun). A clouded condition of the mind in which thinking is not clear; a state of consciousness obstructive to normal mental processes. [L *obnubilare* to cover.]

O'Brien, Cecil Starling (b. 1889). Iowa ophthalmologist.
O'Brien method. Of facial nerve block. A method of abolishing activity in the facial nucleus by injecting the 7th cranial nerve near to the articulation of the lower jaw with anaesthetizing solution.

observerscope (ob·**zerv**·er·skope). An endoscope having 2 cylinders, thereby permitting the simultaneous inspection by 2 persons. [L *observare* to watch over, Gk *skopein* to watch.]

obsession (ob·**sesh**·un). A fixed idea or delusion that haunts the mind continually, in spite of the subject's recognition of its absurdity or irrationality. [L *obsidere* to haunt.]

obsessive (ob·**ses**·iv). Having the quality of an obsession.

obsessive-compulsive (ob·**ses**·iv·kom·**pul**′·siv). Characterized by the occurrence of thoughts and actions against the will of the subject and with his recognition of their apparent irrationality. [obsession, compulsion.]

obsolescence (ob·so·**les**·ens). Of physiological processes, the state of becoming useless because of the effects of ageing. [L *obsolescere* to decay.]

obstetric, obstetrical (ob·**stet**·rik, ob·**stet**·rik·al). Referring or belonging to obstetrics.

obstetrician (ob·stet·**rish**·un). One who is practised in obstetrics; an accoucheur.

obstetrics (ob·**stet**·rix). That branch of medicine and surgery dealing with the care of women during pregnancy, childbirth and puerperium. [L *obstetricare* to assist in delivery.]

obstetrist (ob·**stet**·rist). Obstetrician.

obstipation (ob·stip·**a**·shun). Obstinate constipation. [L *obstipare* to press.]

obstruction (ob·**struk**·shun). 1. The state of being obstructed or blocked. 2. Impediment; the object that causes the blocking. 3. The act of interrupting or clogging. **Alvine obstruction.** Constipation. **Aortic obstruction.** A condition in which the passage of blood from the left ventricle to the aorta is impeded because of adhesions or thickening of the cusps of the aortic valves. **Bladder-neck obstruction.** Conditions the symptoms of which simulate those of an enlarged prostate but without such enlargement. **False colonic obstruction.** Spastic ileus. *See* ILEUS. **Intestinal obstruction.** Any obstruction that hinders or prevents progression of the contents of the intestine. **Mitral obstruction.** A condition in which the flow of blood through the left atrioventricular opening is impeded as the result of disease of the left atrioventricular (mitral) valve. **Pyloric obstruction.** Obstruction to the pylorus from any cause, e.g. stenosis, a contracting ulcer or a malignant growth. **Ureteral obstruction.** Obstruction in the ureter. **Urinary obstruction.** Any obstruction in the passage of urine from the kidney to the meatus. [L *obstruere* to build up against.]

obstructive (ob·**struk**·tiv). Tending to block up or obstruct.

obstruent (**ob**·stroo·ent). 1. Being the cause of obstruction. 2. An astringent agent that arrests a discharge of the bowel contents or tends to cause a closure of the outlet of a canal, duct or similar structure. [L *obstruens* piling up.]

obstupefacient (ob·stew·pe·**fa**′·shent). Soporific; narcotic; applied to any agent that has a stupefying effect on a human being. [L *obstupefacere* to stupefy.]

obtund (ob·**tund**). To dull or to blunt, as, for example, sensation. [L *obtundere* to make blunt.]

obturation (ob·tewr·**a**·shun). The process of closing; a type of intestinal obstruction. Sometimes used to express the sealing of a firearm mechanism against loss of gases. [see foll.]

obturator (**ob**·tewr·a·tor). A mechanical appliance for closing or occupying a space, e.g. a dental plate to close the gap in a cleft palate; a smooth metal bulb to fit into a bronchoscope or sigmoidoscope and afford it a rounded end for insertion. **Obturator foramen.** *See* FORAMEN. **Obturator groove.** *See* GROOVE. **Obturator membrane.** *See* MEMBRANE. [L *obturare* to stop up.]

obturator artery [arteria obturatoria (NA)]. A branch of the anterior division of the internal iliac artery which, after supplying small branches to the pelvic wall and urinary bladder, escapes into the thigh through the obturator foramen and supplies the adductor muscles.

acetabular branch [ramus acetabularis (NA)]. A branch of the obturator artery which enters the hip joint through the acetabular notch and sends a nutrient twig along the ligament of the head of the femur.

anterior branch [ramus anterior (NA)]. One of the terminal branches passing along the anterior margin of the obturator foramen and supplying the adjacent muscles. It terminates by anastomosing with the posterior branch.

posterior branch [ramus posterior (NA)]. One of the terminal branches following the posterior margin of the foramen to supply the adjacent muscles and giving an acetabular branch to the hip joint. It terminates by anastomosing with the anterior branch.

pubic branch [ramus pubicus (NA)]. A small branch of the obturator artery to the back of the pubis, where it anastomoses with the pubic branch of the inferior epigastric artery. It is often enlarged, in conjunction with the pubic branch of the inferior epigastric artery, to give rise to an abnormal obturator artery which descends to the pelvis in relation to the femoral ring.

obturator externus muscle [musculus obturatorius externus (NA)] (**ob**·tewr·a·tor ex·**ter**·nus musl). A lateral rotator of the thigh, lying deeply in its upper part and arising from the obturator membrane and the adjoining bone, and inserted into the trochanteric fossa on the femur.

obturator internus muscle [musculus obturatorius internus (NA)] (**ob**·tewr·a·tor in·**ter**·nus musl). A muscle arising from the lateral wall of the true pelvis and the obturator membrane, the tendon of which passes through the lesser sciatic foramen and is inserted into the greater trochanter.

obturator internus muscle, nerve to the. A branch of the sacral plexus (root value L_5S_1,S_2).

obturator nerve [nervus obturatorius (NA)]. A large branch of the lumbar plexus (root value $L_{2, 3, 4}$), arising on the posterior abdominal wall and passing into the pelvis to emerge through the obturator foramen and supply the adductor muscles of the thigh, the skin over the upper and medial part of the thigh [ramus cutaneus] and the hip and knee joints.

anterior branch [ramus anterior (NA)]. The branch which supplies the adductor longus, gracilis and adductor brevis muscles, and the skin on the medial side of the thigh and the hip joint.

posterior branch [ramus posterior (NA)]. The branch which supplies the adductor magnus muscle, the knee joint and sometimes the adductor brevis muscle.

obturator vein [vena obturatoria (NA)]. A tributary of the internal iliac vein, draining the structures adjoining the obturator foramen.

obtuse (ob·**tews**). 1. Not acute; dull. 2. Dull of intellect, sensibility or perception; stupid. [L *obtusus* blunt.]

obtusion (ob·tew·zhun). 1. Blunted perceptibility or sensibility. 2. A state of being dulled or blunted. [L *obtundere* to dull.]

Obwegeser, Hugo. 20th century Zurich oral surgeon.

Obwegeser–Dal Pont sagittal split osteotomy. Of the mandible. Designed to separate the body from the ascending ramus with the preservation of the neurovascular bundle. This procedure can be used for advancing or retruding the mandible.

occipital (ok·**sip**·it·al). Referring to the occiput. **Occipital lobe.** The most posterior region of the cerebrum.

occipital artery [arteria occipitalis (NA)]. A large branch of the external carotid artery, running upwards and backwards with the posterior belly of the digastric muscle to reach the back of the scalp [rami occipitales (NA)]. It supplies branches to muscles, including the sternocleidomastoid [rami sternocleidomastoidei (NA)], the dura mater of the posterior cranial fossa [ramus meningeus (NA)], the mastoid air cells [ramus mastoideus (NA)], the ear [ramus auricularis (NA)] and the scalp, as far as the vertex of the skull. Its descending branch anastomoses with the vertebral, deep cervical and transverse cervical arteries.

occipital bone [os occipitale (NA)]. The composite bone at the posterior and inferior part of the skull, articulating anteriorly with the temporal, parietal and sphenoid bones, and containing the foramen magnum. It is made up of the squamous part above and behind the foramen, the basilar part in front of it and the condylar part on each side, bearing the occipital condyles.

lambdoid border [margo lambdoideus (NA)]. The superior border of the occipital bone forming the lambdoid suture with the parietal bone.

mastoid border [margo mastoideus (NA)]. The inferior border of the occipital bone articulating with the mastoid part of the temporal bone.

basilar part [pars basilaris (NA)]. The quadrilateral basal part of the occipital bone in front of the foramen magnum.

condylar part [pars lateralis (NA)]. Part of the occipital bone at the side of the foramen magnum, bearing the occipital condyle and, lateral to this, forming the posterior boundary of the jugular foramen (jugular process).

squamous part [squama occipitalis (NA)]. The part of the occipital bone above and behind the foramen magnum. Its borders are the lambdoid or superior [margo lambdoideus (NA)] and the mastoid or inferior [margo mastoideus].

occipital nerves. Greater occipital nerve [nervus occipitalis major (NA)]. A large medial branch of the posterior primary ramus of the 2nd cervical nerve, mainly cutaneous to the skin of the back of the scalp. **Lesser occipital nerve [nervus occipitalis minor (NA)].** A branch of the cervical plexus, deriving its fibres from the 2nd cervical nerve. It emerges at the posterior border of the sternocleidomastoid muscle and supplies the skin on the side of the head behind the auricle and part of the cranial surface of the auricle. **Third occipital nerve [nervus occipitalis tertius (NA)].** A branch of the medial division of the 3rd cervical nerve, to the skin of the nape of the neck.

occipital vein [vena occipitalis (NA)]. A vein lying deeply in the back of the neck, usually commencing as a plexus over the occipital bone. Commonly it receives the parietal and mastoid occipital emissary veins and the occipital diploic vein, and communicates below with the deep cervical and vertebral veins.

occipitalis (ok·**sip**·it·**a′**·lis). The occipital belly of the occipitofrontalis muscle.

occipitalization (ok·**sip**·it·al·i·**za′**·shun). A process of synostosis of the atlas with the occipital bone.

occipito-anterior (ok·**sip**·it·o·an·**teer′**·e·or). Referring to the anterior position of the occiput in the pelvis in a vertex presentation.

occipito-atloid (ok·**sip**·it·o·**at′**·loid). Referring to the occipital bone and the atlas. [occiput, atlas, Gk *eidos* form.]

occipito-axoid (ok·**sip**·it·o·**ax′**·oid). Relating to the occipital bone and the axis. [occiput, axis, Gk *eidos* form.]

occipitobasilar (ok·**sip**·it·o·**ba′**·sil·ar). Relating to the occiput and the base of the skull.

occipitobregmatic (ok·**sip**·it·o·breg·**mat′**·ik). Referring to the occiput and the bregma.

occipitocalcarine (ok·**sip**·it·o·**kal′**·kar·een). Occipital and calcarine.

occipitocervical (ok·**sip**·it·o·**ser′**·vik·al). Relating to the occiput and the neck. [occiput, L *cervix* neck.]

occipitofacial (ok·**sip**·it·o·**fa′**·shal). Relating to the occiput and the face.

occipitofrontal (ok·**sip**·it·o·**frun′**·tal). Relating to the occiput and the forehead. [occiput, L *frons* front.]

occipitofrontalis (ok·**sip**·it·o·frun·**ta′**·lis). The occipitofrontalis muscle. [see foll.]

occipitofrontalis muscle [musculus occipitofrontalis (NA)]. A muscle forming the third layer of the scalp, composed of the epicranial aponeurosis joining 2 frontal bellies [venter frontalis (NA)] inserted into the skin of the eyebrows to 2 occipital bellies [venter occipitalis (NA)] attached to the highest nuchal line.

occipitomastoid (ok·**sip**·it·o·**mas′**·toid). Relating to the occipital bone and the mastoid process of the temporal bone.

occipitomental (ok·**sip**·it·o·**men′**·tal). Relating to the occiput and the chin. [occiput, L *mentum* chin.]

occipitoparietal (ok·**sip**·it·o·par·**i′**·et·al). Referring to the occipital and parietal bones or occipital and parietal lobes of the cerebrum.

occipitoposterior (ok·**sip**·it·o·pos·**teer′**·e·or). Denoting a presentation of the fetus with the child's occiput directed towards the maternal back. [occiput, posterior.]

occipitotemporal (ok·**sip**·it·o·**tem′**·por·al). Relating to the occipital and temporal bones. **Occipitotemporal gyrus.** *See* GYRUS. **Occipitotemporal sulcus.** *See* SULCUS.

occipitothalamic (ok·**sip**·it·o·thal·**am′**·ik). Referring to the occipital lobe of the cerebrum and the thalamus.

occiput [NA] (**ok**·sip·ut). The occipital region of the head; the back part of the skull or the head. [L the back of the head.]

occlude (ok·**lood**). To close together; to shut. [L *occludere* to close up.]

occlusal (ok·**loo**·zal). 1. Pertaining to occlusion. 2. A term applied to the biting or masticatory surfaces of premolar and molar teeth. [see prec.]

occlusio (ok·**loo**·ze·o). Occlusion. **Occlusio pupillae.** Occlusion of the pupil; this and other similar terms are now seldom used. [see foll.]

occlusion (ok·**loo**·zhun). 1. The action of closing up or fact of being closed up. 2. The contact between upper and lower teeth on the closure of the jaws or during normal movements of the mandible. 3. The absorption of a gas such as hydrogen by certain solids, e.g. iron, platinum, etc. It may be attributed to chemical combination, solid solution or condensation on the surface. **Abnormal occlusion.** Occlusion in which any of the teeth do not meet normally; malocclusion. **Afunctional occlusion.** Malocclusion which is such as to prevent use of the teeth. **Anatomical occlusion.** That form of occlusion in which all the teeth are present in the arch and meet one another in a normal manner; normal occlusion. **Anterior occlusion.** That form of malocclusion in which 1 or more teeth occlude anterior to the normal position. **Buccal occlusion.** That form of malocclusion in which 1 or more teeth occlude buccal to (outside) the normal position. **Capsular occlusion.** Operative plication of the perinephric fascia for the support of a mobile kidney. **Centric occlusion.** Position of maximum interdigitation of the teeth. **Coronary occlusion.** Obstruction of the lumen of a main coronary artery or one of its branches, usually due to thrombosis associated with atherosclerosis obliterans. It occasionally results from dissecting aneurysm of the aorta, syphilis, cardiac trauma, thrombo-angiitis obliterans, periarteritis nodosa and, very rarely, from embolism. **Distal occlusion.** That form of malocclusion in which 1 or more teeth occlude posterior to the normal position. **Eccentric occlusion.** Occlusion of the teeth when the lower jaw has moved from the normal resting position. **Occlusion of the eye.** The covering of 1 eye; commonly used in amblyopia in an attempt to improve the vision of the weak eye. It is also used to obtain single vision in cases of diplopia. **Functional occlusion.** The occlusion of the teeth of opposite jaws which permits of their optimum use during the movements of the lower jaw in mastication. **Labial occlusion.** That form of malocclusion in which 1 or more teeth occlude labial (anterior) to the normal position. **Lateral occlusion.** Occlusion of the teeth when the lower jaw is moved to either side of the midline. **Lingual occlusion.** That form of malocclusion in which 1 or more teeth lie lingual (internal) to the normal position. **Mesial occlusion.** Anterior occlusion (see above). **Normal occlusion.** Anatomical occlusion (see above). **Posterior occlusion.** Distal occlusion (see above). **Post-normal occlusion.** That form of malocclusion in which the lower teeth meet the upper teeth behind the normal position. **Prenormal occlusion.** That form of malocclusion in which the lower teeth meet the upper teeth in front of the normal position. **Protrusive occlusion.** The occlusion of the teeth when the mandible is protruded. **Puerperal tubal occlusion.** Occlusion of the uterine tubes from sepsis after childbirth or abortion. **Occlusion of the pupil.** That occurring when the pupil of the eye becomes filled with exudate in iridocyclitis and the vision is obstructed; also called *occlusio pupillae.* **Occlusion of the retinal artery.** A blockage situated either in the central artery of the retina at the disc or in one of its branches, due to spasm, thrombosis or embolism. **Occlusion of the retinal vein.** A blockage situated either in the central vein of the retina at the disc or in one of its branches, due to thrombosis. **Retrusive occlusion.** The occlusion of the teeth when the mandible is retruded. **Traumatic occlusion.** An excessively forceful occlusal relationship between 2 or more teeth. [L *occludere* to close up.]

occlusive (ok·**loo**·ziv). Tending to close or shut, and bring into occlusion.

occlusocervical (ok·**loo**·so·**ser**′·vik·al). Pertaining to the occlusal surface and the neck of a tooth. [occlusal, L *cervix* neck.]

occlusometer (ok·loo·**zom**·et·er). Gnathodynamometer; an instrument with which the force necessary for closing the jaws can be measured. It consists of 2 rubber pads upon which the teeth bite, the pressure exerted being shown by the movement of a pointer along a graduated scale. [occlusion, Gk *metron* measure.]

occult (**ok**·ult). Concealed or masked; as with a disease whose signs and symptoms are obscure. [L *occultus* hidden.]

ocellus (o·**sel**·us). 1. The simple eye. 2. Rarely, an element of a compound eye of an insect. 3. A circular spot of colour like an eye. [L little eye.]

Ochlerotatus (**ok**·ler·o·**ta**′·tus). A sub-genus of *Aëdes* mosquitoes. [Gk *ochlerotatos* most troublesome.]

ochlesis (ok·**le**·sis). Any morbid condition caused or exacerbated by overcrowding. [Gk *ochlos* crowd.]

ochletic (ok·**let**·ik). Relating to, or having the characteristics of ochlesis.

ochlophobia (ok·lo·**fo**·be·ah). Abnormal fear of crowds. [Gk *ochlos* crowd, phobia.]

ochrodermatosis (**o**·kro·der·mat·**o**′·sis). The condition characterized by yellowish or sallow coloration of the skin sometimes noted in Europeans living in India and other tropical countries. [Gk *ochros* yellow, dermatosis.]

ochrodermia (o·kro·**der**·me·ah). Yellow coloration of the skin. [Gk *ochros* yellow, *derma* skin.]

Ochrogaster contraria (o·kro·**gas**·ter kon·**tra**·re·ah). A species of hairy caterpillar; contact causes urticaria followed by a papular pruritic eruption. [Gk *ochros* yellow, *gaster* belly, L *contrarius* opposite.]

ochrometer (o·**krom**·et·er). A device used in the measurement of the blood pressure in the capillary vessels; a finger is constricted by means of a rubber balloon until blanched, and the force required to induce this alteration in colour is registered in millimetres of mercury. [Gk *ochros* yellow, *metron* measure.]

ochromyia (o·kro·**mi**·e·ah). *Cordylobia.* [Gk *ochros* yellow, *myia* a fly.]

ochronosis (o·kron·**o**·sis). A metabolic disorder causing a grey or blackish pigmentation of cartilages, ligaments and other fibrous tissues, together with the excretion of urine which turns black on exposure to the air. Occasionally there is also pigmentation of the skin. It may be due to an inborn error of metabolism, alkaptonuria, in which homogentisic acid is partly excreted in the urine and partly stored in the tissues. Acquired cases are due to chronic phenol poisoning, in which hydroquinone is excreted in the urine and oxidized to pigments similar to those occurring in alkaptonuria. [Gk *ochros* yellow, *-osis* condition.]

ochronotic (o·kron·**ot**·ik). Relating to or due to ochronosis.

ochropyra (o·kro·**pi**·rah). Yellow fever. *See* FEVER. [Gk *ochros* yellow, *pyr* fire.]

Ochsner, Albert John (b. 1858). Chicago surgeon.

Ochsner method or treatment, Ochsner-Sherren method or treatment. A method of non-operative management of established peritonitis due to acute appendicitis, which involves resting the intestine completely; used also nowadays in the treatment of the appendix mass.

Ochsner's muscle or sphincter. An annular thickening of the musculature of the duodenum below the opening of the bile duct; it is doubtful if this is a normal structure.

Ochsner's ring. Circular thickening of the mucous lining of the opening of the pancreatic duct into the ampulla of the bile duct.

O'Connell, Thomas Columba James (b. 1906). Irish surgeon.

O'Connell's modification of Kehr's shoulder sign. Of rupture of the spleen. Pain in the tip of the left shoulder when the foot of the bed is raised.

O'Connor, Roderic P. (b. 1878). American ophthalmologist.

O'Connor's operation. 1. For squint; also called *cinch operation*: the muscle fibres are separated longitudinally into 4 strands. A suture consisting of a number of threads of non-absorbable material is wound twice round one strand after another and then pulled tight; this shortens the muscle by tucking. Later the suture is withdrawn. 2. For paralysis of the lateral rectus muscle of the orbit: advancement of the paralysed muscle combined with transplantation of the outer half of the superior and inferior rectus muscles, split back for 8 mm, which are sutured to the stump of the tendon of the external rectus muscle. It is usually combined with a recession of the internal rectus muscle.

Octacosactrin (**ok**·tah·ko·**sak**′·trin). BP Commission approved name for α^{1-28}_{h} corticotrophin; a synthetic corticotrophin.

octacosane (ok·tah·**ko**·sane). $C_{28}H_{58}$, a solid hydrocarbon of the methane series, found in certain plant waxes. [Gk *oktakosa* twenty-eight.]

octacosanol (ok·tah·**ko**·san·ol). $C_{28}H_{57}OH$, a solid alcohol derived from octacosane and found in wheat germ oil.

octad (**ok**·tad). Denoting an element with a valency of 8: osmium and ruthenium are the only known examples. [L *octo* eight.]

octadecanol (ok·tah·**dek**·an·ol). Octadecyl alcohol, $C_{18}H_{37}OH$. A solid alcohol which occurs as a glyceryl ether in bone marrow and fish-liver oils; it is also formed by the hydrogenation of stearic acid. [Gk *oktadeka* eighteen.]

octamethyl pyrophosphoramide (ok·tah·**meth**·il **pi**·ro·fos·**for**'·am·ide). $[(CH_3)_2N]_2POOPO[N(CH_3)_2]_2$. One of a series of phosphorus-containing systemic horticultural insecticides. It has been used in the treatment of myasthenia gravis.

octan (**ok**·tan). Having a recurrence every eighth day or at 7-day intervals. [L *octo* eight.]

octane (**ok**·tane). Dibutyl, C_8H_{18}. A saturated liquid hydrocarbon, eighth in the methane series, occurring in several isomeric forms: it is found in petroleum. Cf. OCTENE. [L *octo* eight.]

Octaphonium Chloride (ok·tah·**fo**·ne·um **klor**·ide). BP Commission approved name for benzyldiethyl-2-[4-(1,1,3,3-tetramethylbutyl)phenoxy]-ethylammonium chloride; an antiseptic.

octaploid (**ok**·tah·ploid). Octoploid.

octarius (ok·**ta**·re·us). One eighth part of a gallon; a pint. [Obsolete term.] [L *octo* eight.]

Octatropine Methylbromide (ok·tah·**tro**·peen meth·il·**bro**·mide). BP Commission approved name for 8-methyl-*O*-(2-propylvaleryl)tropinium bromide; an anticholinergic.

octavalent (ok·tah·**va**·lent). Describing an element with a valency of 8: the only known examples are osmium and ruthenium. [L *octo* eight, valency.]

octaverin (ok·**tav**·er·in). 1 - (3,4,5 - Triethoxyphenyl)6,7 dimethoxyisoquinoline, a drug possessing spasmolytic properties similar to the alkaloids of belladonna.

Octaverine (ok·**tav**·er·een). BP Commission approved name for 6,7 - dimethoxy - 1 - (3,4,5 - triethoxyphenyl)isoquinoline; an antispasmodic agent.

octene (**ok**·teen). C_8H_{16}, a liquid unsaturated olefine hydrocarbon, homologous with ethylene; its several isomers are present in the oils of bergamot and lemon. Cf. OCTANE. [L *octo* eight.]

octigravida (ok·te·**grav**·id·ah). A woman who is pregnant for the eighth time. [L *octo* eight, *gravidare* to impregnate.]

octipara (ok·**tip**·ar·ah). One who has given birth to 8 children. [L *octo* eight, *parere* to produce.]

octoferric (ok·to·**fer**·ik). Applied to a compound that has in its composition 8 atoms of iron. [L *octo* eight, *ferrum* iron.]

octoploid (**ok**·to·ploid). Having 8 times the haploid number of chromosomes in the somatic-cell nuclei. [Gk *oktoploos* eightfold, *eidos* form.]

octopoda (ok·to·**po**·dah). A sub-order of the molluscan class Cephalopoda, which contains all octopuses. [L *octo* eight, Gk *pous* foot.]

octoroon (ok·to·**roon**). An individual who is of one eighth negro blood; the child of a quadroon and a white person. [L *octo* eight, *roon* as in *quadroon*.]

octose (**ok**·toze). A monosaccharide of the general formula $C_8H_{16}O_8$; 3 isomers have been prepared synthetically. [L *octo* eight.]

octovalent (ok·to·**va**·lent). Octavalent.

octyl (**ok**·til). The radical C_8H_{17}, derived from octane. **Octyl Gallate BP 1973.** 3,4,5-Trihydroxybenzoate, an antioxidant used for preserving oils and fats. **Octyl Nitrite BPC 1968.** 2-Ethyl-*n*-hexyl nitrite, $CH_3(CH_2)_3$. $CH(C_2H_5)CH_2ONO$, a vasodilator similar to amyl nitrite, but said to be less toxic and of longer duration. [L *octo* eight.]

octylene (**ok**·te·leen). Octene.

ocular (**ok**·ew·lar). 1. Relating to the eye. 2. Eyepiece; the system of lenses in any optical instrument through which the eye views the magnified image formed by the objective. **Ocular bobbing.** Repeated downward movements of the eyes occurring with massive pontine haemorrhage. **Compensating ocular.** An eyepiece which corrects the spherical aberration due to the objective. **Huyghenian ocular.** An eyepiece composed of 2 planoconvex lenses mounted with their convex surfaces towards the objective. **Stereoscopic ocular.** A double eyepiece used to give a stereoscopic vision. **Working ocular.** An eyepiece used in microscopical working examination as distinct from any eyepiece employed in the location of the object. [L *oculus* eye.]

See also: HUYGHENS, RAMSDEN.

Oculentum (ok·ew·**len**·tum). The old BP name for an ointment prepared specially for use in the eye; Eye Ointment is the term used in the BP 1958. [see foll.]

oculist (**ok**·ew·list). A physician or surgeon who specializes in ophthalmology; an ophthalmologist. [L *oculus* eye.]

oculistics (ok·ew·**lis**·tix). The science of ophthalmology. A term not in general use. [see prec.]

oculocephalogyric (ok·ew·lo·kef·al·o·**ji**'·rik). Pertaining to the head movements carried out in association with vision. [L *oculus* eye, Gk *kephale* head, *gyros* circle.]

oculofacial (ok·ew·lo·**fa**'·shal). Referring to the eyes and the face. [*oculus* eye, face.]

oculofrontal (ok·ew·lo·**frun**'·tal). Belonging to the eyes and the forehead. [L *oculus* eye, *frons* forehead.]

oculogyration (ok·ew·lo·ji·**ra**'·shun). Ocular movement. [L *oculus* eye, gyration.]

oculogyric (ok·ew·lo·**jir**'·ik). Causing ocular movements. **Oculogyric crisis.** Involuntary contraction of the eye-muscles resulting in conjugate gaze usually though not always, in an upward direction. [see prec.]

oculometroscope (ok·ew·lo·**met**'·ro·skope). A retinoscope incorporating a mechanical device for rotating the trial lenses before the eyes. [L *oculus* eye, Gk *metron* measure, *skopein* to view.]

oculomotor (ok·ew·lo·**mo**'·tor). Causing or belonging to ocular movements. [L *oculus* eye, *motor* mover.]

oculomotor nerve [nervus oculomotorius (NA)]. The 3rd cranial nerve, arising from cells in the mid-brain, traversing the middle cranial fossa and passing through the superior orbital fissure to supply all the extrinsic muscles of the eye except the superior oblique and the lateral rectus. It also carries the nerves of supply to the sphincter of the pupil and the ciliary muscle.

inferior branch [ramus inferior (NA)]. The branch in the orbit which supplies the medial rectus, inferior rectus and inferior oblique muscles. It also sends a twig to the ciliary ganglion, through which it supplies the sphincter of the pupil and the ciliary muscle.

superior branch [ramus superior (NA)]. The branch in the orbit that supplies the superior rectus and the levator palpebrae superioris muscles.

nucleus [nucleus nervi oculomotorii (NA)]. An elongated collection of cells situated ventrally in the central grey matter of the mid-brain beside the midline at the level of the superior quadrigeminal body, and rostral to this.

oculomycosis (ok·ew·lo·mi·**ko**'·sis). Any morbid condition of the eye caused by the presence of a fungus. [L *oculus* eye, mycosis.]

oculonasal (ok·ew·lo·**na**'·zal). Referring to the eye and the nose. [L *oculus* eye, *nasus* nose.]

oculopathy (ok·ew·**lop**·ath·e). Any disease of the eye. [L *oculus* eye, Gk *pathos* disease.]

oculopupillary (ok·ew·lo·**pew**'·pil·ar·e). Designating or relating to the pupil of the eye. [L *oculus* eye, pupil.]

oculoreaction (ok·ew·lo·re·**ak**'·shun). A test devised by Calmette for the detection of tuberculosis in man; not now used on account of the severe reactions that occurred. It consisted in instilling a drop of a 1 per cent solution of tuberculin into the conjunctiva, when subsequent congestion of the conjunctival blood vessels was held to be a positive reaction. [L *oculus* eye, reaction.]

oculospinal (ok·ew·lo·**spi**'·nal). Relating to the eye and the spinal cord. [L *oculus* eye, spine.]

oculozygomatic (ok·ew·lo·zi·go·**mat**'·ik). Relating to the eye and the zygomatic process or the zygomatic bone. [L *oculus* eye, zygomatic.]

oculus (**ok**·ew·lus). The eye. **Oculus bovinus.** Buphthalmia or congenital glaucoma. [L.]

ocyodinic (o·se·o·**din**'·ik). Oxytocic. [Gk *okys* swift, *odis* pangs of labour.]

ocytocic (o·se·**to**·sik). Oxytocic. [Gk *okys* swift, *tokos* birth.]

od (od). The magnetic force supposed to produce the mesmeric or odic state. [Gk *hodos* way.]

odaxesmus (o·dax·**ez**·mus). Biting of the tongue or cheek during an epileptic seizure. [Gk *odaxein* to feel a biting pain.]

odaxetic (o·dax·**et**·ik). Arousing a sensation of itching or biting. [see prec.]

Oddi, Ruggero. 19th century Bologna surgeon.

sphincter of Oddi. Circular muscle fibres round the lower part of the common bile duct and pancreatic duct.

odditis (od·**i**·tis). Inflammation of the sphincter of Oddi situated at the termination of the common bile duct. [sphincter of *Oddi*, Gk *-itis* inflammation.]

odic (**od**·ik). Referring to the hypothetical force, od.

odogenesis (od·o·**jen**·es·is). Branching of axons. [Gk *odos* way, *genesis* origin.]

Odom, Charles Brown (b. 1909). American surgeon.

Odom's indicator. A capillary glass tube attached to the hub of a spinal needle and which contains a bubble of air that is sucked in when the point of the needle enters the extradural space. It is used by anaesthetists to locate the extradural space.

odontalgia (o·dont·**al**·je·ah). A painful condition affecting a tooth; tooth-ache. **Phantom odontalgia.** Pain at the site of an extracted tooth or a sensation that a tooth is still present after it has been extracted. [Gk *odous* tooth, *algos* pain.]

odontalgic (o·dont·**al**·jik). 1. Referring to or characterized by tooth-ache. 2. A remedy for tooth-ache. [see prec.]

odontic (o·**don**·tik). Referring to the teeth; dental. [Gk *odous* tooth.]

odontinoid (o·**don**·tin·oid). Resembling a tooth in structure or shape. [Gk *odous* tooth, *eidos* form.]

odontoblast (o·**don**·to·blast). One of a layer of columnar cells, lying on the periphery of the pulp, which form the primary and secondary dentine of a tooth. They have a peripheral process which runs along the lumen of a dentinal tube with a trophic function, a lateral or collar process and a central or pulpal process. [Gk *odous* tooth, *blastos* germ.]

odontoceramic (o·**don**·to·ser·**am**'·ik). Appertaining to porcelain teeth or to a porcelain filling in a tooth. [Gk *odous* tooth, *keramos* potter's clay.]

odontochirurgic, odontochirurgical (o·**don**·to·ki·**rer**'·jik, o·**don**·to·ki·**rer**'·jik·al). Having reference to dental surgery. [Gk *odous* tooth, *cheirourgos* surgeon.]

odontoclasis (o·**don**·to·**kla**'·sis). A dental fracture. [Gk *odous* tooth, *klasis* a breaking.]

odontogenesis (o·**don**·to·**jen**'·es·is). Odontogeny.

odontogenic (o·**don**·to·**jen**'·ik). Relating to odontogeny.

odontogeny (o·don·**toj**·en·e). The origin and formative development of the teeth. [Gk *odous* tooth, *genein* to produce.]

odontoid (o·**don**·toid). 1. Having the shape of a tooth. 2. The part of the axis (2nd cervical vertebra) articulating with the anterior arch of the atlas and tethered by the transverse ligament. [Gk *odous* tooth, *eidos* form.]

odontolith (o·**don**·to·lith). Calculus on the teeth. [Gk *odous* tooth, *lithos* stone.]

odontologist (o·don·**tol**·o·jist). A dentist. [see foll.]

odontology (o·don·**tol**·o·je). The study of the teeth and their associated structures, and of the diseases appertaining thereto. **Forensic odontology.** The study of teeth in relation to legal problems—in identification, in ageing the dead, in comparing the details of bite marks with dentition models. [Gk *odous* tooth, *logos* science.]

odontolysis (o·don·**tol**·is·is). The resorption of dental tissue. [Gk *odous* tooth, *lysis* a loosing.]

odontoma (o·don·**to**·mah). Odontome.

odontome (o·**don**·tome). A tooth-like structure in which there is abnormal arrangement of the component tissues; a solid or cystic tumour occurring in the jaws which is derived from cells concerned in tooth development. **Complex composite odontome.** An irregular rough calcified mass of dental tissue, derived from abnormal growth of the tooth germ and containing enamel, dentine, cementum and pulp. **Compound composite odontome.** A tumour which remains unerupted and which consists of a varying number of separate calcified denticles surrounded by a connective-tissue capsule. It is probably due to aberration of the enamel band and formation of additional dental germs. **Dilated composite odontome.** A tooth-like mass formed by invagination of the dentine germ by enamel-forming cells during tooth development. **Epithelial odontome.** A cyst formed by the proliferation and subsequent degeneration of the epithelial debris of Malassez in the periodontal membrane of an infected tooth in either jaw; dental cyst. **Fibrous odontome.** A rare soft tumour occurring around the root of a tooth composed mainly of fibroblasts derived from the tooth follicle; odontogenic fibroma. **Follicular odontome.** A cyst, often involving large areas of either jaw, in which the crown of an unerupted tooth projects into the cyst cavity; dentigerous cyst. **Geminated composite odontome.** A tooth-like tumour which erupts into the mouth, formed by the fusion of 2 dental germs during the process of tooth formation; true gemination. [Gk *odous* tooth, *-oma* tumour.]

odontoprisis (o·**don**·to·**pri**'·sis). Grinding of the teeth. [Gk *odous* tooth, *prisis* a sawing.]

odontotherapy (o·**don**·to·**ther**'·ap·e). Dental therapeutics, including the routine hygiene and the treatment of dental diseases. [Gk *odous* tooth, therapy.]

odontotomy (o·don·**tot**·o·me). The operation of removing a portion of a tooth, sometimes employed in the prophylactic treatment of early dental caries. [Gk *odous* tooth, *temnein* to cut.]

odor (**o**·dor). Odour. **Odor phthisicus.** The smell, said to be characteristic, of cases of advanced tuberculosis of the lungs, especially if sweating is profuse. It is different from that of other chronic febrile diseases, and is more marked if intestinal ulceration is present as a complication. [L.]

odorimeter (o·dor·**im**·et·er). A device used in carrying out odorimetry.

odorimetry (o·dor·**im**·et·re). The determination of power of the smell sense, the assessment being made by using different substances of known olfactory stimulative property. [L *odor* smell, Gk *metron* measure.]

odoriphore (**o**·dor·e·for). The name applied, out of analogy with *chromophore*, to the chemical grouping believed to be responsible for the odorous properties of a compound. [L *odor* smell, Gk *pherein* to bear.]

odorivector (o·dor·e·**vek**'·tor). A substance that carries a smell. [L *odor* smell, *vector* carrier.]

odour (**o**·dor). A smell; a perfume. Odours have been classified by Henning in the following order: fruity, flowery, spicy, resinous, scorching and putrid. **Butcher-shop odour.** The odour supposed to be characteristic of patients suffering from yellow fever. **Empyreumatic odour.** An odour associated with distillation of organic matter; a tarry smell. **Measles odour.** The musty smell that is said to be characteristic of persons with this disease. **Minimum identifiable odour, Minimum perceptible odour.** The lowest concentration of substance which will produce an olfactory stimulus. **Typhus odour.** A mousy smell that is said to be characteristic of persons with this disease. [L *odor*.]

O'Dwyer, Joseph P. (b. 1841). Cleveland physician.

O'Dwyer's operation. Intubation by means of special tubes in cases of laryngeal diphtheria.

O'Dwyer's tube. *See* INTUBATION (2nd def.).

Fell-O'Dwyer apparatus. An apparatus for performing artificial respiration and preventing collapse of the lung in operations on the chest.

odynacousis (o·din·ak·**oo**'·sis). A condition of the ear in which the hearing of noises gives rise to pain. [Gk *odyne* pain, *akouein* to hear.]

odynolysis (o·din·**ol**·is·is). Mitigation of pain. [Gk *odyne* pain, *lysis* a loosing.]

odynophagia (o·din·o·**fa**'·je·ah). A condition in which pain accompanies the act of swallowing. [Gk *odyne* pain, *phagein* to eat.]

odynophobia (o·din·o·**fo**'·be·ah). An excessive fear of pain. [Gk *odyne* pain, phobia.]

odynopoeia (o·din·o·**pe**'·ah). The induction of labour pains. [Gk *odyne* pain, *poiein* to make.]

odynuria (o·din·**ewr**·e·ah). Painful micturition. [Gk *odyne* pain, urine.]

Oeciacus (e·**si**·ak·us). A genus of bugs in the family Cimicidae. *Oeciacus hirundinis* in Europe and *O. vicarius* in America live in nests of martins and swallows, occasionally invading houses and biting man. [Gk *oikos* house.]

oeciomania (e·se·o·**ma**'·ne·ah). Oecomania.

oecoid (e·koid). The colourless stroma of an erythrocyte. [Gk *oikos* house, *eidos* form.]

oecology (e·**kol**·o·je). Var. of ECOLOGY. [Gk *oikos* house, *logos* science.]

oecomania (e·ko·**ma**·ne·ah). A disordered mental state marked by a domineering, ill-tempered and perverse attitude of the subject towards members of his or her household but by humility towards anyone in authority. [Gk *oikos* house, mania.]

oecoparasite (e·ko·**par**·ah·site). A parasitic micro-organism against which the host is protected. [Gk *oikos* house, parasite.]

oecophobia (e·ko·**fo**·be·ah). Morbid dislike or fear of the home environment. [Gk *oikos* house, *phobos* fear.]

oecosite (e·ko·site). Oecoparasite. [Gk *oikos* house, *sitos* food.]

oedema (e·**de**·mah). The presence of excessive amounts of fluid in the intercellular tissue spaces of the body, due to increased transudation of fluid from the capillaries. This may be caused by an increase of capillary blood pressure, increased permeability of the capillary wall or reduced plasma-protein osmotic pressure; all 3 factors may be present, though one usually predominates. Oedema may be localized or general. Localized oedema is seen with venous or lymphatic obstruction, around inflammatory lesions, or in some allergic conditions. **Acute circumscribed oedema, Acute essential oedema.** Angioneurotic oedema (see below). **Acute pulmonary oedema.** A paroxysmal attack of oedema of the lungs causing acute dyspnoea; so-called *cardiac asthma.* **Ambulant oedema.** Subcutaneous oedematous swellings, known as Calabar swellings, occurring in *Loa loa* infection and due to allergic response to toxins produced by this parasite. **Angioneurotic oedema.** An allergic disorder in which transient circumscribed oedematous swellings of the skin and subcutaneous tissues, and sometimes mucous membranes, occur. **Anthrax oedema.** A hard cellulitis from the invasion of the subcutaneous tissues, without any accompanying pustule. **Blue oedema.** A hysterical manifestation brought about by a muscular spasm leading to fixation of a joint or joints, followed by oedema and cyanosis of the periarticular tissues and changes within the joint. **Brown oedema.** Oedema of the lung due to venous congestion in which there is some exudation of blood from the capillaries. **Calabar oedema.** Calabar swelling. *See* SWELLING. **Cardiac oedema.** The accumulation in the interstitial tissues of a transudate of serum fluid from the blood plasma as a result of congestive heart failure. It is most evident in the dependent parts of the body, but in severe cases the oedema fluid accumulates in the serous cavities also. When oedema is generalized, involving the lower limbs and sacrum, and producing pleural effusions and ascites, the condition is known as *anasarca.* **Cerebral oedema.** Oedema of the brain, associated with such lesions as tumour, abscess, concussion or haemorrhage. **Epidemic oedema.** Epidemic dropsy. *See* DROPSY. **Famine oedema.** Oedema of the tissues due to protein deficiency from either starvation or ill-balanced diet. **Glottideal oedema.** A misnomer, as the mucosa of the vocal cords is too adherent to allow oedematous swelling. **Hepatic oedema.** Oedema due to hepatic dysfunction. **Hereditary oedema.** Milroy's disease, a familial disease characterized by a persistent oedema of both legs without obvious cause. **Hunger oedema.** Nutritional oedema (see below). **Inflammatory oedema.** Oedema occurring around an inflammatory lesion, due to exudation of protein-rich fluid from dilated capillaries whose endothelium has become more permeable from the action of toxins. **Intracellular oedema.** Retention of fluid within individual cells. **Laryngeal oedema.** Oedema of the soft tissues of the larynx which may be inflammatory, as in acute infections, or due to injury, or to the inhalation of irritant gases or foreign bodies. It occurs in some acute specific fevers. **Lymphatic oedema.** Oedema due either to congenital deficiencies or abnormalities of lymph vessel development, or to acquired obstruction, e.g. from disease or operative removal of lymph glands, or from obstruction of lymphatic vessels by inflammatory fibrosis, carcinoma or filariasis. **Malignant oedema.** Inflammatory oedema (see above) occurring after invasion by *Clostridium welchii* and associated with gas gangrene. **Menstrual oedema.** Oedema, especially around the eyes, associated with menstruation. **Oedema neonatorum.** An oedema of premature or weakly infants which develops during the first few days of life and often proves fatal. The condition may be confused with sclerema neonatorum, but is not associated with immobility of the joints. **Nephrotic oedema.** That due to lowered protein osmotic pressure caused by the loss of large amounts of albumin in the urine. There may also be retention of salt in the tissues. **Nutritional oedema.** Oedema of nephrotic type due to the low concentration of protein in the plasma following a low intake of protein. This may be widespread in time of war and famine. A similar oedema occurs in infants with gastro-intestinal disorders and marasmus. **Obstructive oedema.** Oedema due to obstruction of the efferent lymphatic channels, e.g. in filariasis, after inflammation and after surgical interference. **Physiological oedema.** Oedema of the muscles and subcutaneous tissues of the legs which may occur after much walking or standing. **Prehepatic oedema.** Oedema consequent on prehepatic hypoproteinaemia. **Pulmonary oedema.** Oedema of the lungs, as in left-sided heart failure. **Renal oedema.** That occurring in acute nephritis from increased capillary permeability through endothelium presumably damaged by a toxin. The protein content of the fluid is high (1.0 per cent or more). It also occurs in the nephrotic stage of chronic nephritis. **Senile oedema.** Swelling of the legs in old people with feeble circulation, and due to prolonged sitting. It was often seen in air-raid shelters during bombing raids. **Solid oedema.** Myxoedema. **Turban oedema.** Turban epiglottis. **Yangtze oedema.** Gnathostomiasis. *See* EPIGLOTTIS. [Gk *oidema* swelling.]

See also: BERLIN, IWANOFF, MILROY.

oedematigenous (e·de·mat·**ij**'·en·us). Producing oedema. [oedema, Gk *genein* to produce.]

oedematin (e·**de**·mat·in). The name given to the composite substance of which the microsomes of a cell are made up. [Gk *oidema* swelling.]

oedematization (e·de·mat·i·**za**'·shun). Production of oedema of the tissues.

oedematous (e·**de**·mat·us). Marked by oedema or belonging to oedema.

oedipism (e·dip·izm). The intentional infliction of injury by a subject on his own eyes. [*Oedipus*, King of Thebes, who tore out his eyes.]

Oehl, Eusebio (b. 1827). Pavia anatomist.

Oehl's layer or stratum. The clear layer of the horny zone of the epidermis.

Oehl's muscles. Muscle bundles said to occur in the chordae tendineae of the left atrioventricular valve.

Oehler, Johannes (b. 1879). German physician.

Oehler's symptom. Coldness and pallor of the lower extremities in patients with occlusive peripheral vascular disease and intermittent claudication. Coldness and pallor is increased by exercising the affected limb.

oenanthal (e·**nan**·thal). Heptyl aldehyde, heptaldehyde, $CH_3(CH_2)_5CHO$. A colourless liquid obtained by the distillation of castor oil under reduced pressure.

oenomania (e·no·**ma**·ne·ah). 1. An irresistible craving for alcohol or any other intoxicating drink, almost amounting to insanity. 2. Delirium alcoholicum. [Gk *oinos* wine, mania.]

oenoxidase (e·**nox**·id·aze). A ferment in spoiled wine which causes it to become sour. [Gk *oinos* wine, oxidase.]

oersted (er·sted). A unit of magnetic field intensity equal to

$10^3/4\pi$ A m^{-1}. [Hans Christian *Oersted* (b. 1777), Danish physicist.]

Oertel, Max Joseph (b. 1835). Munich physician.

Oertel's method or treatment. The treatment of cardiovascular disorders by dietary control, reduction of fluid intake, regulated exercises, massage and Swedish movements. Although more specific measures are now available for the treatment of the various forms of circulatory disorders, the above general management is based on sound principles, but emphasis is now laid on restriction of salt, rather than fluid, in the diet.

oese (er·zer). Öse.

oesophagalgia (e·**sof**·ag·**al**′·je·ah). A painful condition of the oesophagus. [oesophagus, Gk *algos* pain.]

oesophageal (e·**sof**·ah·**je**′·al). Relating or appertaining to the oesophagus.

oesophageal veins [venae esophageae (NA)]. Veins draining the oesophagus and ending in the left gastric vein, vena azygos, vena hemiazygos or inferior thyroid vein.

oesophagectasis (e·**sof**·ah·**jek**′·tas·is). Oesophageal dilatation. [oesophagus, Gk *ektasis* a stretching.]

oesophagectomy (e·**sof**·ah·**jek**′·to·me). Excision of a part of the oesophagus. [oesophagus, Gk *ektome* a cutting out.]

oesophagectopy (e·**sof**·ah·**jek**′·to·pe). Oesophageal displacement. [oesophagus, Gk *ektopos* out of the way.]

oesophagism, oesophagismus (e·**sof**·ah·jizm, e·**sof**·ah·**jiz**′·mus). Spasmodic contraction of the circular fibres of the muscular coat of the oesophagus. **Hiatal oesophagism, Hiatal oesophagismus.** Cardiospasm.

oesophagitis (e·**sof**·ah·**ji**′·tis). An inflammatory condition affecting the oesophagus. **Catarrhal oesophagitis.** An inflammatory condition of the mucous membrane of the oesophagus which may be *acute* or *chronic*, frequently due to reflux of gastric juice into the oesophagus. **Gangrenous oesophagitis.** A rapidly spreading destructive inflammation of the oesophagus which may occur in the terminal stages of fatal infective diseases. **Peptic oesophagitis.** Catarrhal oesophagitis (see above). **Phlegmonous oesophagitis.** Acute inflammation of the oesophageal submucosa, usually secondary to penetrating oesophageal foreign bodies, to acid poisoning or associated with cervical abscess formation. **Reflux oesophagitis.** Oesophagitis due to reflux of gastric or jejunal contents. **Ulcerative oesophagitis.** Ulceration of the oesophageal mucous membrane which may occur during the course of syphilis, tuberculosis or typhoid fever. It may be followed by stricture formation. [oesophagus, Gk *-itis* inflammation.]

oesophagocele (e·**sof**·ag·o·seel). Herniation or distension of the oesophagus, generally with breach in the muscular coat, through which the mucous and submucous coats are forced. [oesophagus, Gk *kele* hernia.]

oesophagoduodenostomy (e·**sof**·ag·o·**dew**·o·de·**nos**′·to·me). The operation of making an anastomosis between the oesophagus and the duodenum, after total gastrectomy. [oesophagus, duodenostomy.]

oesophagodynia (e·**sof**·ag·o·**din**′·e·ah). Oesophagalgia. [oesophagus, Gk *odyne* pain.]

oesophago-ectasis (e·**sof**·ag·o·**ek**′·tas·is). Dilatation of the oesophagus without demonstrable obstruction; cardiospasm. [oesophagus, Gk *ekteinein* to stretch out.]

oesophago-enterostomy (e·**sof**·ag·o·en·ter·**os**′·to·me). Surgical anastomosis of the oesophagus to the jejunum. [oesophagus, enterostomy.]

oesophagogastrectomy (e·**sof**·ag·o·gas·**trek**′·to·me). Removal of the oesophagus and the stomach. [oesophagus, gastrectomy.]

oesophagogastro-anastomosis (e·**sof**·ag·o·**gas**·tro·an·as·to·**mo**′·sis). The creation of an artificial opening between the oesophagus and the stomach. [oesophagus, Gk *gaster* stomach, anastomosis.]

oesophagogastroplasty (e·**sof**·ag·o·**gas**′·tro·plas·te). Cardioplasty; a method of relieving achalasia of the gastric cardia by a plastic operative procedure. [oesophagus, gastroplasty.]

oesophagogastroscopy (e·**sof**·ag·o·gas·**tros**′·ko·pe). Examination of the oesophagus and stomach with instruments. [oesophagus, gastroscopy.]

oesophagogastrostomy (e·**sof**·ag·o·gas·**tros**′·to·me). Oesophagogastro-anastomosis. [oesophagus, gastrostomy.]

oesophagography (e·**sof**·ah·**gog**′·raf·e). Radiographic visualization of the oesophagus after contrast filling of the lumen, usually with barium sulphate. [oesophagus, Gk *graphein* to record.]

oesophagojejunostomy (e·**sof**·ag·o·jej·oon·**os**′·to·me). The formation of an artificial communication between the oesophagus and the jejunum after total gastrectomy. [oesophagus, jejunostomy.]

oesophagology (e·**sof**·ag·**ol**′·o·je). The branch of medical science which deals with the study and treatment of disorders of the oesophagus. [oesophagus, Gk *logos* science.]

oesophagomalacia (e·**sof**·ag·o·mal·**a**′·she·ah). Pathological softening of the oesophageal walls. [oesophagus, Gk *malakia* softness.]

oesophagomycosis (e·**sof**·ag·o·mi·**ko**′·sis). Any morbid condition of the oesophagus due to the invasion of fungi. [oesophagus, mycosis.]

oesophagomyotomy (e·**sof**·ag·o·mi·**ot**′·o·me). Division of the muscle fibres of the lower end of the oesophagus. Performed at the lower end of the oesophagus in the treatment of achalasia (cardiospasm); Heller's operation. [oesophagus, Gk *mys* muscle, *temnein* to cut.]

oesophagopathy (e·**sof**·ag·**op**′·ath·e). Any morbid condition of the oesophagus. [oesophagus, Gk *pathos* disease.]

oesophagoplasty (e·**sof**·ag·o·plas·te). 1. Plastic repair of any oesophageal defect or deformity. 2. An operation to enlarge the cardio-oesophageal opening. [oesophagus, Gk *plassein* to mould.]

oesophagoplegia (e·**sof**·ag·o·**ple**′·je·ah). Oesophageal paralysis. [oesophagus, Gk *plege* stroke.]

oesophagoplication (e·**sof**·ag·o·pli·**ka**′·shun). The operation of reducing the size of an oesophageal pouch or of a dilated oesophagus by means of folds or tucks in the long axis of the wall of the oesophagus. [oesophagus, L *plicare* to double up.]

oesophagosalivation (e·**sof**·ag·o·sal·iv·**a**′·shun). An abnormal discharge of saliva associated with oesophageal carcinoma and regarded as an important sign.

oesophagoscope (e·**sof**·ag·o·skope). An endoscopic instrument used in inspection of the interior of the oesophagus. [oesophagus, Gk. *skopein* to watch.]

See also: JACKSON (C.), NEGUS.

oesophagoscopy (e·**sof**·ag·**os**′·ko·pe). Investigation of the condition of the oesophagus internally by the oesophagoscope.

oesophagospasm (e·**sof**·ag·o·spazm). Spasmodic contraction of the walls of the oesophagus.

oesophagostenosis (e·**sof**·ag·o·sten·**o**′·sis). Narrowing of the oesophagus, e.g. by a stricture. [oesophagus, stenosis.]

oesophagostoma (e·**sof**·ag·o·**sto**′·mah). Any opening into the oesophagus apart from the normal entrance and exit. [oesophagus, Gk *stoma* mouth.]

oesophagostomiasis (e·**sof**·ag·o·sto·**mi**′·as·is). A condition caused by infestation with a nematode of the genus *Oesophagostomum.*

Oesophagostomum (e·**sof**·ag·**os**′·to·mum). A genus of hookworms. The numerous species are all found in the large intestine: the young worms burrow in the intestinal epithelium, which forms conspicuous nodules around them, and the adults emerge into the lumen. **Oesophagostomum apiostomum.** A species recorded in prisoners in a Nigerian gaol; it may be the same as *Oesophagostomum bifurcum.* **Oesophagostomum bifurcum.** A species common in apes; it has been recorded rarely from man in Africa and the Far East. **Oesophagostomum stephanosoma.** A species common in apes; it has been recorded once in man in Brazil, perhaps as the cause of death. [oesophagus, Gk *stoma* mouth.]

oesophagostomy (e·**sof**·ag·**os**′·to·me). The insertion of a tube from the exterior into the oesophagus by way of a surgical wound, the tube then being passed on into the stomach for feeding purposes. [oesophagus, Gk *stoma* mouth.]

oesophagotome (e·**sof**·ag·o·tome). A scalpel of special type used for making incisions into the oesophagus. [oesophagus, Gk *temnein* to cut.]

oesophagotomy (e·sof·ag·ot'·o·me). An operation in which an incised opening into the oesophagus is made. [see prec.]

oesophagram (e·sof·ah·gram). Radiographs made during oesophagography. [oesophagus, Gk *gramma* record.]

oesophagus [esophagus (NA)] (e·sof·ag·us). The gullet, extending from the level of the cricoid cartilage to the cardiac orifice of the stomach and lying in the lower part of the neck [pars cervicalis (NA)], thorax [pars thoracica (NA)] and upper part of the abdomen [pars abdominalis (NA)], close to or in the midline. **Coat of the oesophagus, adventitious [tunica adventitia (NA)].** The loose, outer, areolar, connective-tissue coat of the oesophagus. **Coat of the oesophagus, mucous [tunica mucosa (NA)].** The innermost coat in longitudinal folds when undistended. **Coat of the oesophagus, muscular [tunica muscularis (NA)].** The main muscle layers in the wall, comparable in arrangement to the coat elsewhere in the gut, but consisting in the upper part of the tube of striped instead of unstriped muscle. **Coat of the oesophagus, submucous [tela submucosa (NA)].** The vascular and glandular coat connecting the mucous and muscular coats of the oesophagus. **Corkscrew oesophagus.** A pathological state of the oesophagus in which segmental spasms occur below the level of the aortic arch and cause alternating dilatations and contractions; radiologically, after a barium swallow, the appearance is that of a string of pearls or of a corkscrew. It has been suggested that it is produced by arteriosclerotic changes in the myenteric plexus. **Webbed oesophagus.** Rings of mucosa projecting into the lumen, usually associated with iron-deficiency anaemia. [Gk *oisophagos* gullet.]

oestradiol (e·strah·di·ol, e·strad·e·ol). Oestradiol-17β, $\Delta^{1,3,5}$-oestratriene-3,17-diol, $C_{18}H_{24}O_2$. A naturally-occurring oestrogen and the actual hormone of the ovarian follicle; a colourless steroid, slightly soluble in water and now prepared synthetically. In the female it stimulates the accessory reproductive organs and causes development of the secondary sexual characters at puberty; it also is responsible for the hypertrophy of the uterus and for the changes in the endometrium during the first half of the menstrual cycle which when acted on by progesterone prepare it for the reception of a fertilized ovum. It furthermore promotes the growth of the ducts of the mammary glands. Large doses inhibit the gonadotropic secretion of the anterior pituitary, thus influencing the normal ovarian cycle. In the male it induces atrophy of the accessory reproductive organs and inhibits spermatogenesis, hence its value in carcinoma of the prostate. Unlike the synthetic oestrogens, it is relatively inactive by mouth and has to be injected: the benzoate is used for the purpose and prolongs the action. It is of value in menstrual disorders, ovarian insufficiency, especially at the menopause, and for the treatment of infections of the vagina in children, where it promotes the growth of a cornified and more resistant epithelium; it is also used to terminate lactation, not very successfully, by inhibiting the release of prolactin. **Oestradiol Benzoate BP 1973, Oestradiol monobenzoate.** The benzoyl ester of oestradiol; it has all the physiological properties of the parent alcohol, but is the form usually employed for intramuscular injection.

Oestradioli Benzoas (e·strad·e·o'·li ben·zo·as). *European Pharmacopoeia* name for Oestradiol Benzoate BP 1973.

oestriasis (e·stri·as·is). An infection due to infestation by eggs of botflies of the genus *Oestrus.*

Oestridae (e·stri·de). A family of large hairy Diptera; botflies; warble flies. The larvae are internal parasites of mammals. The genus *Dermatobia* is of medical importance. [Gk *oistros* gadfly.]

oestrin (e·strin). A name originally applied to the oestrus-producing hormone, on the assumption that only one such hormone existed. It has now become obsolete, being replaced by the generic term *oestrogen.*

oestriol (e·stre·ol). $C_{18}H_{24}O_3$, a placental hormone with oestrogenic properties. It is $\Delta^{1,3,5}$-oestratriene - 3,16,17 - triol. **Oestriol Sodium Succinate.** BP Commision approved name for oestra - 1,3,5(10) - triene - 3,16α,17β - triol 16,17 - di(sodium succinate); it is used in the treatment of thrombocytopenic haemorrhage. **Oestriol Succinate.** BP Commission approved name for oestra - 1,3,5(10) - triene - 3,16α,17β - triol 16,17 - di(hydrogen succinate); it is used in the treatment of thrombocytopenic haemorrhage.

oestrogen (e·stro·jen). Any substance having the physiological activity of oestradiol, the follicular hormone of the ovary. [oestrum, Gk *genein* to produce.]

oestrogenic, oestrogenous (e·stro·jen·ik, e·stroj·en·us). Causing oestrus. [see prec.]

oestrone (e·strone). $C_{18}H_{22}O_2$, an oestrogen having properties similar to oestradiol, and probably formed from it during extraction, but with only 30 per cent of the potency by intramuscular injection. **Oestrone benzoate.** A compound used as an intramuscular injection in oil: its action is similar to that of oestrone. It is seldom now used.

oestrous (e·strus). Showing the characteristics of oestrus.

oestrus (e·strus). 1. The phase of intense sexual excitement in female mammals. 2. The changes in genitalia produced by injecting ovarian and hypophyseal substances into laboratory animals. [Gk *oistros* mad desire.] 3. A genus of flies, sheep warbles. **Oestrus ovis.** The common nasal fly of sheep; its larva has occasionally occurred in man, causing ocular or other myiases. [Gk *oistros* gadfly.]

Oettinger's operation. For trichiasis: the lid margin is split along the grey line in its whole length as far up as the upper border of the tarsus; the skin of the lid and lash margin is displaced upward and stitched to the upper border of the tarsus.

official (o·fish·al). Inferring that the substance (medicament) concerned is controlled by an official publication; in the UK this means the *British Pharmacopoeia* or the *British Pharmaceutical Codex.* [L *officium* office.]

Ogata, Masaki (b. 1864). Tokyo physician.

Ogata's method. A method of stimulating respiration by stroking the chest.

ogee (o·je). Ogive. [Fr. *ogive.*]

Ogilvie syndrome. Spastic ileus (obstruction by spasm) of the bowel.

ogive (o·jive). An S-shaped figure cut out of metal or any stiff material and used to measure radius of curvature. [Fr.]

ogo (o·go). Gangosa; in tertiary yaws, an ulcerative process which attacks and destroys the nasal and palatal structures. The condition may be found in any region in which yaws is endemic, particularly in the islands of the East Indies and the Pacific.

Ogston, Sir Alexander (b. 1844). Aberdeen surgeon.

Ogston's operation. 1. Removal of part of the inner femoral condyle to correct knock knee. 2. An external operation on the frontal sinus.

Ogston-Luc operation. Ogston's operation, 2nd def. (see above).

Oguchi, Chuta (b. 1875). Japanese ophthalmologist.

Oguchi's disease. A rare hereditary syndrome characterized by night blindness, marked reduction of visual fields in reduced illumination and a grey appearance of the fundus. It was first seen in Japan and later in Europe.

Ohara, Hachiro. 19th–20th century Japanese physician.

Ohara's disease. Tularaemia.

Ohm, Georg Simon (b. 1787). German physicist.

Ohm's law. The ratio between the electromotive force (E) applied to a conductor and the current it produces (C) is a constant for the particular conductor, i.e. its resistance, R, which equals E/C.

ohm (ome). The unit of electrical resistance. The ohm is the electric resistance between two points of a conductor when a constant potential difference of 1 volt, applied at these points, produces in the conductor a current of 1 ampere, the conductor not being the seat of any electromotive force. [Georg Simon *Ohm.*]

ohmammeter (ome·am·et·er). An instrument designed to measure both resistance and current in ohms and amperes respectively.

ohmmeter (ome·me·ter). An instrument which measures electrical resistance in ohms.

oidiomycosis (o·id·e·o·mi·ko′·sis). Candidosis. [oidium, mycosis.]

Oidium (o·id·e·um). The name formerly given to a genus of fungi now known as *Candida* following a period as *Monilia.* **Oidium albicans.** The former name of *Candida albicans,* the agent of thrush and other forms of candidosis. Other species are now classified as *Trichosporon.* [dim. of Gk *oon* egg.]

oikoid (oi·koid). Oecoid.

oikology (oi·kol·o·je). Oecology.

oikomania (oi·ko·ma·ne·ah). Oecomania.

oikophobia (oi·ko·fo·be·ah). Oecophobia.

oil (oil). Oils are liquids which are not miscible with water, are soluble in ether and are as a rule combustible. They may be broadly classed under 3 types: the fixed vegetable or animal oils; the volatile oils; and the mineral oils. The only difference between a fixed oil and a fat is that the former is liquid at 20°C. Oils were classified officially prior to the BP 1953 and BPC 1954 as *Oleum.* **Ajowan oil.** An antiseptic oil used for its thymol content. **Allspice oil.** Oleum pimentae. **Almond Oil BP 1973.** The fixed oil obtained by pressure from the seeds of the bitter almond, *Prunus amygdalus* Batsch. var. *amara* or var. *dulcis.* It is a pale-yellow oil consisting of the glycerides of oleic acid, with smaller amounts of linoleic, palmitic and myristic acids. It is used as a nutritive, demulcent and laxative; externally, it is applied to the skin as an emollient. It is sometimes included in cold creams and lotions for the hair. **Oil of almond, essential.** Oleum amygdalae amarae. **Oil of amber.** Oleum succini. **Oil of American wormseed.** Chenopodium oil (see below). **Oil of American wormwood.** Oleum absinthiae. **Ampule oil.** Any fixed oil suitable for suspensions in ampules. **Animal oil.** An oil containing pyridine, obtained by the distillation of bones and other animal matter. It is used only in veterinary practice for its germicidal action. **Anise Oil BP 1973, Aniseed oil.** An oil obtained by distillation from anise or from star anise, *Illicium verum* Hook. f., which is its main source. It is a colourless or pale-yellow liquid with a characteristic odour and aromatic taste. Its main constituent is anethole, and it is employed as a carminative to relieve flatulence, also in cough mixtures for its mild expectorant properties. It is also employed as a flavouring agent. **Anthos oil.** Rosemary oil (see below). **Anthracene oil.** The distillate of coal tar above 270°C, which contains carbazole and phenanthrene in addition to anthracene. **Arachis Oil BP 1973.** The fixed oil obtained by expression without heat from the seeds of *Arachis hypogaea.* It occurs as a pale-yellow liquid with a faint nut-like odour and a bland taste. It thickens slowly on exposure to air and becomes rancid. It consists of the glycerides principally of oleic and linoleic acids, and has similar properties to those of olive oil, in place of which it is sometimes used in making plasters, ointments, liniments, soaps and oily injections. It also has valuable food properties and is employed in the manufacture of margarine. **Argemone oil.** An oil obtained from the seeds of the prickly poppy, *Argemone mexicana,* used mainly in soap-making. It is used medicinally in Indian systems of medicine, and a variety of properties are claimed for it, but it is not employed in scientific medicine. Its importance from a medical point of view lies in the fact that it is a frequent contaminant of mustard oil and when present in appreciable amounts may cause peripheral vascular dilatation leading to a serious pathological syndrome, epidemic dropsy, among rice-eating peoples in India who use mustard oil with their rice. **Aromatic castor oil.** Oleum ricini aromaticum. **Oil of Australian sandal wood.** Oleum santali australiensis. **Oil of bay.** Oleum myrciae. **Ben oil, Oil of behen.** An oil obtained from the ben-nut tree. It is a bland oil used as an extractant. **Oil of benne.** Sesame oil (see below). **Oil of bergamot.** Oleum bergamottae. **Bhilawanol oil.** An oil from the nut of the tree *Semecarpus anacardium,* once used by the washerman in India (dhobie) to mark clothes. It causes marking-nut dermatitis by local irritation. The nut is also used externally and internally in Indian medicine. **Birch-tar oil.** Oleum rusci. **Oil of bitter almond.** Oleum amygdalae amarae. **Bitter Almond Oil, Volatile, BP 1958.** Purified volatile oil of bitter almond, oil of bitter almond without hydrocyanic acid; an oil prepared from the cake left after the fixed oil from bitter almonds, peach kernels or apricot kernels has been pressed out, by distillation with water and purification of the resulting distillate: this is done by shaking with lime water and ferrous sulphate, and steam distilling. It is a colourless liquid with a characteristic odour, rapidly oxidized in air and depositing benzoic acid. It is used as a flavouring agent. **Bone oil.** A tarry oily liquid obtained from bones during distillation in the preparation of animal charcoal. It is occasionally used in veterinary practice. **Bottle-nose oil.** An oil obtained from the whale, *Balaena rostrata.* It is really a wax and is used in ointment bases. **Bouchi oil.** An essential oil extracted from the leguminous weed *Psoralia corylifolia,* often used in Indian medical systems and also studied in scientific medicine. It was found to have a beneficial effect when rubbed into the decolorized skin lesions of vitiligo or leucoderma. **Buchu oil.** A volatile oil obtained from buchu. **Cade Oil BP 1958.** An oil obtained by the destructive distillation of the branches and wood of a species of *Juniperus.* It is a dark-reddish-brown to black oily liquid with an empyreumatic odour and a bitter acrid taste. Its main constituent is a sesquiterpene, cadinene, and it is used as a stimulant antiseptic in chronic skin diseases and as an ingredient of scalp preparations and medicated soaps. **Cajuput Oil BPC 1968.** An oil distilled from the fresh leaves and twigs of *Melaleuca leucadendron* and other species of *Melaleuca.* It is a colourless or yellow liquid with a camphoraceous odour and a bitter aromatic taste. It consists chiefly of cineole, together with terpineol and aldehydes, and is used chiefly as a carminative. Externally it is employed as a stimulant and counter-irritant, and is applied in combination with olive oil or turpentine liniment to rheumatic joints. **Oil of camphor, essential, Oil of camphor, light.** Rectified camphor oil (see below). **Camphor Oil, Rectified, BPC 1959.** An oil obtained as a by-product in the manufacture of camphor from the camphor laurel, *Cinnamomum camphora.* It is a colourless or yellowish liquid with the odour of camphor, its chief constituents being terpenes, safrole, acetaldehyde, camphor, terpineol, eugenol, cineole, D-pinene, phellandrene, dipentene and cadinene. It is used as a rubefacient and counter-irritant, and applied to rheumatic and inflamed joints; it is included in liniment of methyl salicylate. It also has value as a parasiticide. **Oil of camphor, white.** Rectified camphor oil (see above). **Camphorated oil.** Camphor liniment. **Caraway Oil BPC 1968.** An oil distilled from freshly crushed caraway seeds with subsequent rectification. It is a colourless or pale-yellow liquid with the odour and taste of caraway, and its main constituent is carvone. It is used as an aromatic carminative, more especially in the form of caraway water for children. **Carbolic oil.** Oleum phenolatum. **Oil of cardamom.** Oleum cardamomi. **Carron oil.** Lotio calcii hydroxidi oleosa. **Oil of cassia.** Oleum cassiae. **Castor Oil BP 1973.** A fixed oil obtained by expression from the seeds of *Ricinus communis* with subsequent bleaching. It is a colourless or pale-yellow liquid, having a faint odour and a bland, followed by a nauseating, taste. It consists chiefly of the glycerides of ricinoleic acid, together with small amounts of other glycerides, and is used as a mild purgative when, due to hydrolysis in the small intestine, the irritant alkali ricinoleate is formed. The laxative effect occurs in from 4 to 8 hours, and since there is little griping it is used in haemorrhoids and during pregnancy. Externally it may be applied as an ointment (e.g. zinc and castor oil ointment) to irritated skin. It is a valuable solvent for alkaloids to be applied to the conjunctiva. **Castor oil, aromatic.** Oleum ricini aromaticum. **Castor Oil, Sulphated, BPC 1954.** An oil prepared by the sulphonation of castor oil and subsequent neutralization. It is an emulsifying agent and detergent. **Cedar-leaf oil.** A volatile oil distilled with steam from the fresh leaves of *Thuja occidentalis.* It occurs as a colourless or yellow liquid with a distinct odour, and consists chiefly of thujone and fenchone which, in overdoses, cause convulsions due to their stimulant action on the cerebral cortex; cases of poisoning have occurred in its use as an abortifacient. It has been used internally in enuresis and menstrual disorders, but its value is questionable; externally it has a mild counter-irritant action. It is very seldom employed medicinally. **Cedarwood oil.** Oleum cedri. **Celery oil, Celery-seed oil.** An oil obtained from celery seeds and containing apiol. **Oil of chamomile.** Oleum anthemidis. **Chaulmoogra Oil BPC 1954.** An oil obtained by expression from the seeds of *Taraktogenos kurzii.* It occurs as a solid fat, or, at tropical temperatures, a brownish-yellow liquid, with a characteristic odour and an acrid taste, and consists of glycerides, principally of chaulmoogric and hydnocarpic acids. The oils from the seeds of *Hydnocarpus* species, *Carpotroche braziliensis* Endl. and *Caloncoba echinata*, have similar compositions and properties. Chaulmoogra oil has been almost entirely superseded by hydnocarpus oil (see below). **Chenopodium Oil BPC 1959.** An oil obtained by steam distillation from the fresh flowering and fruiting plants, excluding roots, of *Chenopodium ambrosiodes* Linn. var. *anthelminticum* Gray. It is a pale-yellow liquid with a penetrating camphoraceous odour and a bitter burning taste, having as its principal constituent, ascaridole. It is used as an anthelmintic, particularly for the expulsion of roundworms and for dwarf tapeworms; it should always be followed by purgation. In children it should be combined with tetrachlorethylene, especially in mixed infestation with hookworms and roundworms. Overdosage leads to toxic effects, e.g. gastro-intestinal irritation, vomiting and dizziness. It is useless against tapeworms. **Oil of cherry laurel.** A volatile oil obtained by the steam distillation of the fresh leaves of the cherry-laurel, *Prunus laurocerasus* Linn.; it resembles the oil from bitter almonds and is occasionally used as a flavouring agent. **Cinnamon Oil BP 1958.** An oil obtained by distillation from cinnamon. It is a light-yellow liquid, becoming brownish on keeping, and contains cinnamic aldehyde and eugenol. It has carminative properties; internally it is rather irritant, but is occasionally used in influenza and catarrh, though of doubtful value. It may be inhaled to stimulate bronchial secretions. It is also employed as a flavouring agent. **Oil of citron.** An oil obtained from the tree *Citrus medica.* It contains limonene. **Citronella Oil BPC 1968.** An oil obtained by distillation from *Cymbopogon citratus.* There are 2 types, the Ceylon oil and the Java oil, and the main constituents are geraniol and citronellal. It is used in perfumery and toilet preparations and is a popular insect repellent. **Clove Oil BP 1973.** An oil obtained by distillation from clove. It occurs as a colourless or pale-yellow liquid when freshly distilled, but darkens to reddish-brown on exposure to air. It has the odour and taste of clove and its chief constituent is eugenol; it also contains caryophyllin and vanillin. It has antiseptic properties and acts as a preservative; internally it is antispasmodic and carminative. Externally it is rubefacient, and is used as a counter-irritant and mild analgesic mixed with olive oil. It is also employed in dentistry as a local analgesic or obtundent, and is applied to carious cavities or freshly exposed tooth pulp. In microscopy it finds use as a clearing agent. **Clover oil.** An oil expressed from plants of species *Trifolium.* **Coconut oil.** *See* FRACTIONATED COCONUT OIL BP 1973 (below). **Cod-liver Oil BP 1973.** The fixed oil separated from the fresh liver of the cod, *Gadus callarias* (= *G. morrhua* Linn.) and other species of *Gadus*, by the application of low-pressure steam at a temperature not exceeding 85°C. The oil is cooled to about 0°C and filtered to remove the separated fat. It is a pale-yellow liquid with a fairly fishy odour and taste; its most important constituents are vitamins A and D, the oil itself consisting of the glycerides of fatty acids, mainly unsaturated palmitoleic, oleic, linoleic, gadoleic and clupadonic acids, with a lesser proportion of saturated myristic, palmitic and stearic acids. It is an important source of vitamins A and D, but the unsaturated acids present are valuable food factors as well. The *British Pharmacopoeia* requires the oil to contain not less than 600 units of vitamin-A activity and not less than 85 units of vitamin-D activity per gram. The antirachitic activity of the oil is believed to be due to vitamin D_3. Cod-liver oil is used as a dietary supplement in infants and children, as a prophylactic to improve nutrition and calcification of the bones. It may be taken plain, in an emulsion, or with extract of malt. **Colza oil.** Rape oil (see below). **Coriander Oil BP 1973.** An oil obtained by distillation from coriander. It is a pale-yellow liquid, the chief constituent of which is D-linalol, together with pinene, terpinene, geraniol and borneol. It is used internally as an aromatic stimulant and carminative. **Corn oil.** Maize oil (see below). **Cottonseed Oil BP 1968.** The refined oil obtained by expression or solvent extraction from the seeds of *Gossypium herbaceum* and other species of *Gossypium.* It is a semi-drying oil occurring as a pale-yellow liquid with a nutty taste, consisting of the glycerides chiefly of palmitic, oleic and linoleic acids, together with small amounts of myristic and stearic acids. It is used in place of olive oil in preparations for external use, and is employed for culinary purposes and in the manufacture of lard substitutes, cooking oils, margarine and soap. **Croton oil.** Oleum crotonis. **Oil of cubeb.** Oleum cubebae. **Dill Oil BP 1958.** An oil obtained by distillation from dill. It is a pale-yellow liquid with a sweet aromatic but pungent taste. Its main constituent is carvone, together with other terpenes and it is used as an aromatic carminative, especially as dill water for flatulence in infants. It may also be employed as a flavouring agent. **Doegling oil.** The oil obtained from the bottle-nose whale, *Hyperoodon rostratus.* It has similar properties to sperm oil. **Drying oil.** Any oil which thickens and hardens when exposed to air, especially when spread in a thin layer, as in paint. Poppy-seed oil and linseed oil are the principal ones and consist mainly of the esters of the unsaturated linoleic and linolenic acids which absorb oxygen from the air to form varnish-like substances. **Dwarf pine oil.** Pumilio pine oil (see below). **Empyreumatic oil.** Any oil, such as bone oil, formed by the destructive distillation of organic matter. **Essential oil.** A class of oils present in many plants and obtained by distillation in steam, by pressure or by extraction with solvents. They are oily substances which are volatile and possess a characteristic fragrance or odour. Many contain terpenes or sesquiterpenes, and owe their value chiefly to the presence of oxygenated derivatives of these which are responsible for the odours or flavours. They are used in perfumery, and medicinally as antiseptics, counter-irritants, deodorants, flavouring agents and carminatives. **Estragon oil.** Tarragon oil (see below). **Eucalyptus Oil BP 1973.** An oil obtained by rectification of the oil distilled from the fresh leaves of *Eucalyptus polybractea* R. T. Baker, *E. dumosa* A. Cunn. and other species of *Eucalyptus.* It occurs as a colourless or pale-yellow liquid, with an aromatic camphoraceous odour and a pungent taste. It contains chiefly cineole (also known as *eucalyptol*), and D-pinene together with other terpenes. It is used medicinally as an antiseptic and deodorant, is frequently employed in inhalants and is sprinkled on the handkerchief for catarrhal colds; mixed with menthol, oil of pine and tincture of benzoin, it is inhaled with steam to relieve bronchitis and asthma; it is often included in oily sprays and nasal drops, and in bougies, suppositories and pessaries as an antiseptic and deodorant. Internally it may be given in capsules or as an emulsion in the treatment of catarrhal inflammation of mucous membranes, especially of the respiratory tract and bladder. **Expressed oil.** Any oil obtained by pressure, e.g. crushing of plants between rollers, or treatment either hot or cold in hydraulic presses. The oil may be refined to remove colour, odour, colloidal matter or free fatty acid. **Oil of fennel.** Oleum foeniculi. **Fixed oil.** Any of the glyceryl esters of the higher fatty acids. They are present in plants and animals where they serve as food reserves, and are mostly obtained by expression in hydraulic presses, preferably cold for the best oils; hot expression, boiling with water, or extraction by solvents, produces inferior oils. They are non-volatile and should contain little or no free acid. They constitute important food commodities as well as medicinal agents, and are also employed in the manufacture of soap. **Fractionated Coconut Oil BP 1973.** The oil obtained from the dried solid part of the endosperm of the coconut; it is subsequently fractionated and refined and used as a basis for pharmaceutical suspensions of drugs. **Fractionated Palm Kernel Oil BP 1973.** A fat expressed from the kernels of the fruit of the palm tree. An ointment base, also used in the manufacture of soaps and margarine. **Fusel oil.** A mixture of alcohols and esters, principally amyl, isopropyl and butyl, derived from protein impurities in alcoholic fermentation processes, and present to a small extent in most alcoholic liquors. It is more toxic than ethyl alcohol, causing methaemoglobinuria and nephritis, and is never used in medicine. **Garlic oil.** An oil distilled from *Allium sativum*, containing allyl sulphide and used to stimulate bronchial secretion in the treatment of bronchitis; it should not be given to children. It is also employed as a flavouring. **Geranium Oil BPC 1959.** An oil distilled from the leaves of *Pelargonium cdoratissimum*, *P. capitatum* and *P. radula*. It is a colourless, greenish or brown liquid, with a rose-like odour, the chief constituent being geraniol. It is largely employed in perfumery, dentifrices, ointments and other preparations. **Oil of Ginger.** An essential oil obtained from ginger. It contains phellandrene and zingiberene. **Gorli oil.** An oil obtained from the plant *Caloncoba echinata*, used as an adulterant of chaulmoogra oil. **Groundnut oil.** Arachis oil (see above). **Halibut-liver Oil BP 1973.** The oil obtained from the liver of the halibut, *Hippoglossus hippoglossus*. It occurs as a pale-yellow liquid with a slight fishy odour and taste, and its most important constituents are vitamin A, of which it contains 100 times as much as cod-liver oil, and vitamin D, about 250 times as much as the latter. It is a convenient and more pleasant way of administering these vitamins than cod-liver oil. **Heavy oil.** That fraction distilled from coal tar between 230° and 270°C, and consisting chiefly of cresols, methylnaphthalenes, naphthols, xylenols, quinoline and isoquinoline. It is sold as creosote and is used for preserving wood. **Hemp-seed oil.** An oil obtained from species of the plant *Cannabis*. It is used in the manufacture of varnishes and paints. **Hydnocarpus Oil BPC 1959.** A fatty oil obtained by cold expression from the fresh ripe seeds of *Hydnocarpus wightiana* Blume. It occurs as a yellowish oil or soft fat with a slight characteristic odour and somewhat acrid taste, and contains the glycerides of chaulmoogric and hydnocarpic acids. It was largely used in the treatment of leprosy, most frequently in the form of its ethyl esters (Ethyl Esters of Hydnocarpus Oil BPC 1959). Externally the oil is a powerful rubefacient and is used as an ointment in very chronic psoriasis. **Iodised Oil BP 1958.** An iodine addition-product of poppy-seed oil obtained by treating the latter with hydriodic acid. It is a colourless or pale-yellow clear viscous oily liquid with a slightly alliaceous odour and a bland oily taste. On exposure to air and sunlight it decomposes, becoming dark brown, and as such should not be used. It is employed as a contrast medium, largely for radiological examination of the bronchus; it is non-irritant to the mucous membrane. After injection, absorption occurs in the lungs. It is also used to outline the urethra, uterus, fallopian tubes, the subarachnoid space and other body cavities. A more fluid preparation consists of the iodized esters of poppy-seed oil. **Jasmine oil.** An oil obtained from the flowers of the jasmine, *Jasminum grandiflorum*. It is used in perfumery. **Oil of juniper.** Oleum juniperi. **Juniper tar oil.** Cade oil (see above). **Kurung oil.** An oil obtained from the Indian tree *Pongamia glabra*. It is used in skin diseases. **Lavender Oil BPC 1968.** An oil obtained by distillation from the fresh flowering tops of *Lavandula officinalis* or *L. intermedia*. It occurs as a colourless, pale-yellow or yellowish-green liquid with chief constituents linalool and its acetic ester. The English oil contains cineole which is present only in traces in the French oil. It has carminative properties, but is not employed much internally, except as a flavouring agent. It is mainly used as a perfume, and sometimes as an insect repellent. **Lemon Oil BPC 1968.** An oil obtained by expression from lemon peel. It occurs as a pale-yellow or greenish-yellow liquid, with a characteristic odour and a warm, aromatic, slightly bitter taste, its main constituents being D-limonene and citral, which gives it its odour. Whilst it has carminative properties, it is chiefly used as a flavouring agent; an alcoholic solution, *prepared essence of lemon*, is used for culinary purposes. **Lemon Grass Oil BPC 1954.** An oil obtained by distillation from the entire herb of *Cymbopogon citratus* Stapf. and *C. flexuosus* Stapf. It is a reddish-yellow or brownish-red liquid with a strong odour of verbena, and contains citral with traces of geraniol, citronellal and the terpenes, limonene and dipentene. It has been used as a carminative, but is now mainly used in perfumery and as a source of citral. **Oil of lemon grass, Indian.** Lemon grass oil (see above). **Oil of linaloe.** An oil from the wood of the Mexican tree *Ocotea caudata*, used in perfumery. **Linseed Oil BP 1963.** The fixed oil obtained by cold expression from linseed, followed by clarification. It is a yellowish-brown liquid with a faint characteristic odour and a bland taste. On exposure to air it thickens to form a thin, hard, transparent film. It consists of the glycerides chiefly of linoleic and linolenic acids, with small amounts of oleic, palmitic and stearic acids. The commercial oil has a marked odour and acrid taste due to atmospheric oxidation. It may be used externally, mixed with calcium-hydroxide solution, for the treatment of burns. The purified oil has been used as a laxative. Industrially, linseed oil is employed as a drying oil in the manufacture of paints and varnishes. *Boiled linseed oil* is linseed oil which has been heated with litharge or other suitable driers to about 150°C so that metallic salts of the fatty acids are formed, which cause the oil to dry more quickly. **Lubricant oil.** Any oil with lubricant properties; fixed oils of vegetable or mineral origin may be used therapeutically for their lubricant or emollient properties to soothe inflamed and irritated mucous membranes and skin, e.g. liquid paraffin in emollient ointments or castor oil applied to the eye. They may also be used internally to soften the stools in constipation (e.g. liquid paraffin) or to retard the flow of gastric juice in gastric and duodenal ulcer (e.g. olive oil). They are mostly products of the petroleum industry, obtained in the distillation of crude petroleum. **Maize Oil BP 1973.** An oil obtained by expression from the fruits of the maize plant, *Zea mays* Linn. It consists of glycerides, mainly of oleic and linoleic acids, and has similar properties to olive oil for which it is an official substitute in Australia. It is also used in the manufacture of margarine, and as a salad oil. **Oil of male fern.** Male fern extract, an oil obtained by the extraction of the rhizome of the male fern, *Dryopteris filixmas*, with ether, and diluted with olive or other fluid vegetable oil to contain 25 per cent of filicin. It is used like male fern as an anthelminthic, particularly for tapeworm infestations; it should be administered in capsules or as an emulsion because of its unpleasant taste, and should be preceded and followed by a saline purgative. **Oil of marjoram.** An oil obtained from the herb *Origanum marjorana* and used in perfumery. **Oil of melalenca.** Oleum melalencae. **Melissa oil.** Verbena oil (see below). **Melissa oil, Indian.** Lemon grass oil (see above). **Oil of Mexican poppy.** Argemone oil (see above). **Oil of mignonette.** An oil obtained from the flowers of mignonette, *Reseda odorata*. **Mineral oil.** Any oil obtained from mineral sources, e.g. petroleum and its products; it is also applied to lubricating oils. It is commonly regarded as a synonym in medicine for liquid paraffin. **Oil of mirbane.** Nitrobenzene. **Mocaya oil.** A non-volatile oil obtained from the fruits of species of *Acrocomia* (family Palmaceae); it is identical with coconut oil (oleum cocois). **Moodooga oil.** An oil obtained from the seeds of *Butea monosperma*, used as an anthelminthic. **Mustard oil.** The term *mustard oil* is often applied to a volatile oil containing isothiocyanates. Such oils are powerful vesicants and are no longer used in medicine. **Mustard Oil, Expressed, BPC 1954.** An oil obtained by pressure from the seed of *Brassica nigra*; it is a by-product in the manufacture of the volatile oil (oleum sinapis volatile). It is a brownish-yellow or greenish-brown liquid with a mild taste, and consists chiefly of the glyceride of oleic acid. It has mild rubefacient properties, and may be applied to the chest instead of camphorated oil or as a liniment to rheumatic joints. **Oil of mustard, volatile.** Oleum sinapis volatile. **Mustard-seed oil, white.** An oil obtained from *Brassica alba*; it is used for lubricating and burning. **Oil of myrcia.** Oleum myrciae. **Oil of neroli.** Oleum neroli. **Nut oil.** Arachis oil (see above). **Nutmeg Oil BP 1958.** An oil obtained by distillation from nutmeg. It is a colourless or pale-yellow liquid, with the odour and taste of nutmeg. It consists chiefly of D-camphene and has carminative properties; it is also used as a flavouring agent. High doses of the oil induce epileptiform convulsions due to its stimulant action on the cerebral cortex. **Nutmeg oil, expressed.** A solid yellow fat containing myristicin, employed in plasters. It is obtained by hot expression from nutmeg or mace. **Olive Oil BP 1973.** The fixed oil obtained by expression from the ripe fruits of *Olea europaea* Linn. It is a pale-yellow liquid with a faint but not rancid odour and a bland taste. It consists of glycerides, mainly of oleic acid, with small amounts of palmitic, linoleic, stearic and myristic acids. It has nutritious, demulcent and mildly laxative properties, and is employed in medicine as a laxative and to inhibit secretion of gastric juice in the treatment of gastric and duodenal ulcers. It may be given per rectum to soften impacted faeces or as a vehicle for the administration of paraldehyde or ether. Externally the oil is an emollient, and is used to soothe and protect inflamed surfaces. It is frequently employed in the preparation of liniments, ointments, plasters and soaps, and as a vehicle for oily injections. It is used industrially for the manufacture of soaps. **Orange Oil BPC 1968.** An oil obtained by mechanical means from the fresh peel of the sweet orange, *Citrus sinensis* Linn., and also of the bitter orange, *C. aurantium* Linn. It occurs as a yellowish liquid with the characteristic odour of orange and a mild aromatic taste; it consists largely of the terpene, D-limonene, and is employed in perfumery and as a flavouring agent. **Oil of orange-flower water.** Oleum neroli. **Origanum oil.** An oil obtained from wild marjoram, *Origanum vulgare*, used in liniments. **Oil of orris.** A semisolid, aromatic substance obtained from orris root by steam distillation. It consists chiefly of myristic acid and small amounts of the odorous substance, irone. It is used for blending with the latter as a base for violet perfumes. **Palm-kernel oil.** *See* FRACTIONATED PALM-KERNEL OIL (above). **Patchouli oil.** An oil obtained from the plant *Pogostemon cablin*, used in perfumery. **Peanut oil.** Arachis oil (see above). **Oil of pelargonium.** Geranium oil (see above). **Peppermint Oil BP 1973.** An oil distilled from the fresh flowering tops of *Mentha piperita* and rectified if necessary. It is a colourless, pale-yellow or greenish-yellow liquid with the odour of peppermint and a pungent aromatic taste. On cooling, crystals of menthol may separate. The Japanese and Chinese oils, which are not so esteemed as the English oil, are obtained from *Mentha arvensis* var. *piperascens* and var. *glabrata*, and are richest in menthol. The oil contains, besides menthol, menthyl acetate, menthyl isovalerate and other terpenes, and is used internally as an aromatic carminative for the relief of gastric and intestinal flatulence and colic. It is also employed as a flavouring agent. Externally it has analgesic properties. It may be used as peppermint water or as peppermint spirit, and is frequently incorporated in lozenges and to flavour dentifrices and medicines. **Phenolated oil.** Oleum phenolatum. **Oil of pimento.** Oleum pimentae. **Oil of pine.** Oleum abietis. **Oil of pine, aromatic.** Pumilio pine oil (see below). **Pine-needle oil.** Oleum abietis. **Poppy-seed oil.** An oil which may be obtained by the expression of seeds of *Papaver somniferum*. It is a light-yellow odourless liquid with a faint almond flavour and a bland taste. It has no narcotic properties and is used as a substitute for olive oil for culinary and medical purposes. It contains the glycerides of stearic and palmitic acids, together with those of linoleic and oleic acids, and is used to prepare iodized oil as a drying oil in paints, for soap manufacture and for culinary purposes. **Pumilio Pine Oil BPC 1968.** An oil distilled from the fresh leaves of *Pinus mugo* var. *pumilio*. It contains chiefly L-pinene, L-phellandrene and up to 10 per cent of bornyl acetate; it has antiseptic and expectorant properties and is employed in the treatment of laryngitis and bronchitis by inhalation from hot water. Externally it is rubefacient and is used as a counter-irritant in the treatment of sprains, fibrositis and synovitis. **Rape Oil BPC 1954.** The refined oil expressed from the seeds of *Brassica napus* var. *oleifera* and certain other species of *Brassica*. It contains 50 per cent of the glycerides of erucic acid, with other glycerides, mainly of oleic and linoleic acids. It is rarely given by mouth, but is used externally in oil and liniments in place of olive oil. **Red oil.** A liquid used for colouring toilet preparations, obtained by digesting anchusa in liquid paraffin. **Oil red O.** A red fat-soluble stain used as a substitute for Sudan III in histology. It is a monoazo dye. **Oil of rose.** Oleum rosae. **Oil of rose geranium.** Geranium oil (see above). **Rosemary Oil BP 1958.** An oil distilled from the flowering tops of *Rosmarinus officinalis*. It contains borneol, bornyl acetate and other acetates. and has carminative properties, It is commonly included in hair lotions and other preparations used externally. **Sage oil.** The oil obtained from *Salvia officinalis*, garden sage. It contains cineole and pinene. **Oil of sandal wood, Oil of santal wood.** Oleum santali. **Sassafras Oil BPC 1954.** An oil obtained by distillation from the root or root bark of species of *Sassafras*. It is a pale-yellow or reddish-yellow liquid with the odour of safrole, its main constituent, and a warm aromatic taste. It has rubefacient properties and is used as an anodyne in chronic rheumatism. It is also used to destroy pediculi and their larvae, but must be applied with care to the hair in such a way that the skin is untouched. It is not used internally, large doses causing fatty degeneration of the liver. **Savory oil.** An oil obtained from species of the herb *Satureia*. It contains carvacrol. **Sesame Oil BP 1968.** The fixed oil obtained by expression from the seeds of *Sesamum indicum*. It is a pale-yellow liquid with a slight grain-like odour and a bland taste. It contains the glycerides of oleic and linoleic acids, and has similar properties to olive oil. It is used in parts of the Commonwealth in the preparation of official liniments, plasters, ointments and soaps. It is also iodated for use as an opaque medium in the x-ray examination of a directly accessible cavity of the body. Much of it goes to the manufacture of margarine. **Shale oil.** An oil distilled from bituminous shales. It contains unsaturated hydrocarbons, chiefly of the olefine series, and paraffins, and has no medicinal uses as such. **Shark oil, Shark-liver oil.** A fixed oil obtained from the livers of sharks; it closely resembles cod-liver oil to which it may be added as an adulterant. It is used in soap-making and in paint manufacture. **Oil of Siberian fir.** Oleum abietis. **Spearmint Oil BPC 1968.** An oil obtained by distillation from fresh flowering spearmint, *Mentha viridis* Linn. and *M. crispa* Roth. It is a colourless, pale-yellow or greenish-yellow liquid when freshly distilled, but becomes darker and viscid on keeping. It has a characteristic odour and a warm, slightly bitter taste; its chief constituent is carvone, together with L-limonene and L-pinene. Its uses are similar to those of peppermint oil. **Sperm oil.** An oil obtained from the head of the sperm whale, *Physeter macrocephalus* Linn. and from other species. The best quality is a pale-yellow liquid which on standing precipitates crystalline spermaceti. It consists of the glycerides of unsaturated fatty acids including palmitic acid, and is used principally in soap-making and as a burning oil and lubricant. **Spike Lavender Oil BPC 1968.** The oil obtained by distillation from the flowering herb *Lavandula latifolia* Vill. and other species of *Lavandula*. It is a pale-yellow liquid having an odour of camphor, borneol, cineole, terpineol and D-camphene. It has similar properties to lavender oil and is used in perfumery and as an insect repellent. **Sweet oil.** Olive oil (see above). **Oil of sweet birch.** Oleum betulae. **Tansy oil.** An oil obtained from the herb *Tanacetum vulgare*, tansy. It is used as an anthelminthic. **Tarragon oil.** An essential oil from the plant *Artemisia dracunculus*, tarragon. **Tea-tree oil.** Oleum melaleucae. **Oil of teaberry.** Oleum betulae. **Teel oil.** Sesame oil (see above). **Theobroma Oil BP 1973.** A solid pale-yellow fat obtained by expression from crushed and roasted theobroma seed, *Theobroma cacao*; it is a by-product in the manufacture of cocoa. It contains the glycerides of stearic, palmitic and oleic acids, and is used as a base in the preparation of suppositories, pessaries and bougies, since it melts at body temperature. It is also used in ointments and as a lubricant in the preparation of tablets. **Oil of thuja.** Cedar-leaf oil (see above). **Oil of thyme.** Oleum thymi. **Ti-tree oil.** Oleum melaleucae. **Oil of tsana.** A fixed oil containing isanic acid. **Tung oil.** An oil obtained from species of the Chinese tree *Aleurites*, used in paints and varnishes. **Tunny-liver oil.** An oil obtained from the fresh liver of the tunny fish. It contains vitamin D_3. **Turpentine Oil BP 1973, Turpentine oil, rectified.** The oil obtained by distillation and rectification from turpentine, an oleoresin from *Pinus* *palustris* and other species of *Pinus*. It is a colourless liquid with a strong odour and a bitter pungent taste. On exposure to air it becomes yellow and viscid, whilst treatment with sulphuric acid yields terebene. It contains chiefly the hydrocarbons Δ-3-carene and D- and L-pinene, together with resin acids, camphene and fenchone. It is antiseptic internally and externally. Internally it is a sialogogue and a carminative, relieving colic and giving a feeling of warmth in the stomach. Large doses may cause purging. It is absorbed unchanged into the blood, causing a leucocytosis, and is excreted through the lungs and kidneys; the skin may show eruptions and some diaphoresis. In the lungs it acts as an expectorant, assisting and softening the mucous; in the kidneys it increases the flow of urine and will lessen inflammatory exudation and retard putrefaction of the urine. Large doses, however, irritate and inflame the bladder, and there may be albuminuria and haematuria through similar action on the kidneys. It is an anthelminthic for tapeworm; given as an enema it is effective against threadworm. Applied externally to the skin it causes rubefaction and irritation, and may be employed as a counter-irritant in chronic rheumatism and in chest affections such as bronchitis and pleurisy. It relieves congestion in the bronchioles when inhaled, and is given in small doses internally in bronchitis and phthisis. **Verbena oil.** The oil obtained from species of *Verbena*. It contains citral. **Oil of verbena, Indian.** Lemon grass oil (see above). **Oil of vitriol.** Concentrated sulphuric acid. **Volatile oil.** Essential oil (see above). **Whale oil.** Sperm oil (see above). **Wheat Germ Oil BPC 1954.** An oil obtained from the embryo of wheat, *Triticum aestivum*, by expression or by solvent extraction. It is a bland yellow oil with a nutty odour and taste, and consists mainly of the glycerides of oleic, palmitic and linoleic acids. The most important constituent is, however, α-tocopherol (vitamin E) and other tocopherols. It was used in medicine at one time as a source of vitamin E, but has now been largely replaced by the synthetic tocopherol acetate. **Oil of wine, heavy.** A mixture of ethyl sulphate, ethyl sulphite and several polymeric forms of ethylene, produced by the action of sulphuric acid on ethyl alcohol followed by distillation. **Oil of wintergreen.** Oleum betulae. **Wood oil.** Gurjun balsam, an oil obtained from species of *Dipterocarpus* and used as an expectorant. **Oil of wormseed.** An oil obtained from santonica, *Artemesia maritima*, and containing cineole. [L *oleum*.]

See also: DIPPEL.

oil breakfast (oil brek·fast). An administration of olive oil, 200 ml (Volhard's), or 2 per cent oleic acid in olive oil, 100–200 ml (Boldiref's), given fasting, and drawn off from half to 1 hour later, when it contains the pancreatic juice from the duodenum. [oil, AS *brecan, faestan*.]

oinomania (oi·no·ma·ne·ah). Oenomania.

ointment (oint·ment). A semi-solid preparation of 1 or more medicaments in a suitable base, applied to the skin or mucous membrane for emollient or protective purposes or as a means of local administration. The base may be fatty or a water-in-oil emulsion where absorption is intended, or simply soft paraffin where protection is desired. For ointments listed officially before 1953 as *Unguenta*, see UNGUENTUM. **Ammoniated Mercury Ointment BP 1973.** A mixture of finely powdered ammoniated mercury and simple ointment (see below). **Ointment of Ammoniated Mercury and Coal Tar BPC 1959.** A mixture of ammoniated mercury, solution of coal tar and yellow soft paraffin. **Ointment of ammonium ichtholsulphonate.** Ointment of ichthammol. **Ointment of belladonna.** Unguentum belladonnae. **Basilicon ointment.** Ointment of colophony (see below). **Benzamine ointment.** An ointment consisting of benzamine hydrochloride, olive oil and wool fat. **Ointment of Benzocaine, Compound, BPC 1959.** An ointment consisting of benzocaine in a mixture of hamamelis and zinc oxide ointments; it is used as a surface local anaesthetic and astringent to allay irritation, as in pruritis. **Ointment of Benzoic Acid, Compound, BPC 1959.** An ointment composed of benzoic acid and salicylic acid, used in the treatment of fungous skin diseases. **Ointment of birch tar, compound.** Unguentum rusci compositum. **Blue ointment.** Ointment of mercury, dilute (see below). **Ointment of Boric Acid BPC 1959.** An ointment consisting of powdered boric acid in white paraffin ointment. **Ointment of Calamine BPC 1959.** An ointment of calamine in white soft paraffin. **Ointment of Calamine, Compound, BPC 1959.** An ointment of calamine, zinc oxide, white soft paraffin and solution of coal tar in hydrous wool fat. **Calomel ointment.** Unguentum hydrargyri subchloridi. **Ointment of camphor, hard.** Unguentum camphorae durum. **Ointment of Capsicum BPC 1959.** An ointment made of bruised capsicum in simple ointment. **Ointment of capsicum, compound.** Unguentum capsici compositum. **Cetomacrogol Emulsifying Ointment BP 1973.** A non-ionic emulsifying ointment containing Cetomacrogol Emulsifying Wax BP 1973, liquid paraffin and white soft paraffin. **Cetrimide Emulsifying Ointment BP 1973.** A cationic emulsifying ointment containing cetrimide, cetostearyl alcohol, liquid paraffin and white soft paraffin. **Ointment of chrysarobin.** Unguentum chrysarobini. **Ointment of cinchocaine, compound.** Unguentum cinchocainae compositum. **Citrine ointment.** Ointment of mercuric nitrate, strong (see below). **Coal-tar ointment.** Ointment of ammoniated mercury and coal tar (see above). **Ointment of Colophony BPC 1959.** Colophony resin in a basis of beeswax, lard and olive oil. **Danish ointment.** Unguentum potassi polysulphidi. **Dithranol Ointment BP 1973.** Dithranol in a basis of yellow soft paraffin; used in the treatment of psoriasis and chronic eczema. **Dithranol Ointment, Strong, BP 1968.** Dithranol yellow soft paraffin, applied in the treatment of psoriasis, eczema, alopecia and myotic infections of the skin. **Emulsifying Ointment BP 1973.** A mixture of emulsifying wax, white soft paraffin and liquid paraffin. **Eserine ointment.** Physostigmine ointment (see below). **Ointment of eucalyptus.** Unguentum eucalypti. **Eye ointment.** An ointment prepared specially for use in the eye. Before 1953 eye ointments were classed as *oculenta*. **Ointment of Gall BPC 1954.** An ointment containing powdered gall and lard, used in the treatment of haemorrhoids for its astringent effect. **Ointment of Gall and Opium BPC 1959.** Ointment of gall (see preceding) with powdered opium added. **Ointment of glycerin of lead subacetate.** Unguentum glycerini plumbi subacetatis. **Golden ointment.** Unguentum hydrargyri oxidi flavi. **Hamamelis Ointment BP 1958.** An ointment consisting of liquid extract of hamamelis in a wool fat and soft paraffin base; it has an astringent action and is used to treat haemorrhoids. **Hydrocortisone Ointment BP 1973.** An ointment consisting of hydrocortisone in a wool fat and white soft paraffin base. **Hydrocortisone Acetate Ointment BP 1973.** An ointment consisting of hydrocortisone acetate in a wool fat and white soft paraffin base; used in the treatment of inflammatory skin conditions. **Hydrous Ointment, Oily Cream BP 1958.** An emulsion of equal parts of ointment of wool alcohols and distilled water; used as an ointment base. **Ointment of hydrous wool fat.** Unguentum adipis lanae hydrosi. **Ointment of Ichthammol BPC 1959.** An ointment of ichthammol in wool fat and yellow soft paraffin. **Ointment of iodine.** Unguentum iodi. **Ointment of Iodine, Non-Staining, BPC 1959.** An ointment of iodine in arachis oil and yellow soft paraffin. **Ointment of Iodine with Methyl Salicylate, Non-Staining, BPC 1959.** Non-staining ointment of iodine with methyl salicylate. **Ointment of kaolin.** Unguentum kaolini. **Lanolin ointment.** Unguentum adipis lanae hydrosi. **Ointment of lead subacetate.** Unguentum plumbi subacetis. **Ointment of menthol and camphor.** An ointment consisting of menthol and camphor in soft paraffin; it is applied to the nasal passages to relieve catarrh and hay fever. **Ointment of Mercuric Nitrate, Dilute, BP 1953.** A mixture of strong ointment of mercuric nitrate (see following) with yellow soft paraffin. **Ointment of Mercuric Nitrate, Strong, BPC 1959.** An ointment consisting of mercury dissolved in nitric acid and mixed with lard and olive oil. **Mercuric oxide ointment, red.** Unguentum hydrargyri oxidi rubri. **Mercuric oxide ointment, yellow.** Unguentum hydrargyri oxidi flavi. **Mercurous chloride ointment, mild.** Unguentum hydrargyri subchloridi. **Ointment of Mercury, Compound, BPC 1959.** Strong ointment of mercury with arachis oil and camphor in beeswax. **Ointment**

of Mercury, Dilute, BPC 1959. A mixture of strong ointment of mercury and simple ointment. **Ointment of Mercury, Strong, BPC 1959.** A preparation of mercury and oleated mercury in a wool fat, white beeswax and white soft paraffin mixture; it can be used for inunction in syphilis or to destroy pediculi. **Ointment of mercury, lead and zinc.** Unguentum hydrargyri, plumbi et zinci. **Ointment of Methyl Salicylate BPC 1959.** An ointment composed of methyl salicylate in beeswax and hydrous wool fat. **Ointment of Methyl Salicylate, Compound, BPC 1959.** An ointment containing methyl salicylate, menthol, eucalyptol and cajuput oil in beeswax and hydrous wool fat. **Ointment of oil of cade.** Unguentum olei cadini. **Ointment of Oleated Mercury BP 1953.** A mixture of oleated mercury and hydrous ointment. **Paraffin Ointment BP 1968.** A mixture of beeswax, paraffin wax and white or yellow soft paraffin. **Ointment of Penicillin BPC 1959.** Benzylpenicillin in ointment of wool alcohols (see below); it may be prescribed at any strength, but if no strength is stated it is made to contain 1000 units per gram. **Physostigmine ointment.** Eserine ointment, an ointment prepared by dissolving physostigmine salicylate (0.125 per cent) in chloroform and mixing into yellow soft paraffin; it is used as a miotic in ophthalmology. **Potassium polysulphide ointment.** Unguentum potassi polysulphidi. **Ointment of resorcinol.** Unguentum resorcinolis. **Ointment of Resorcinol, Compound, BPC 1959.** An ointment containing resorcinol, bismuth subnitrate and zinc oxide. It is used in the treatment of skin diseases. **Ointment of resorcinol and bismuth.** Unguentum resorcinolis et bismuthi compositum. **Ointment of rosewater.** Unguentum aquae rosae. **Salicylic Acid Ointment BP 1973.** An ointment containing 2 per cent of salicylic acid. **Ointment of Salicylic Acid and Sulphur BPC 1959.** An ointment containing salicylic acid and sulphur in a base of hydrous ointment. **Ointment of Scarlet Red BPC 1954.** A mixture of scarlet red in simple ointment. **Simple Ointment BP 1973.** A mixture of wool fat, paraffin wax and white or yellow soft paraffin; used as an ointment base. **Sodium perborate ointment.** An antiseptic and healing ointment composed of sodium perborate in paraffin ointment base. **Ointment of spermaceti.** Unguentum cetacei. **Sulphur Ointment BP 1973.** A mixture of finely powdered sublimed sulphur in a base of simple ointment. **Ointment of tannic acid.** Unguentum acidi tannici. **Ointment of Tar BPC 1959.** A mixture of tar, lard and yellow beeswax. **Thymol ointment.** An ointment prepared by dissolving thymol in soft paraffin; used in the treatment of eczema and other skin affections. **White precipitate ointment.** Ammoniated mercury ointment (see above). **Wintergreen ointment.** Ointment of methyl salicylate (see above). **Wool Alcohols Ointment BP 1973.** A mixture of wool alcohols, hard paraffin, white or yellow soft paraffin and liquid paraffin, most frequently used as an ointment base. **Zinc Ointment BP 1973.** A preparation containing 15 per cent of zinc oxide in simple ointment. It is used as a local surface application in various skin disorders for its astringent and protective properties. **Zinc and Castor Oil Ointment BP 1973.** A mixture of zinc oxide and castor oil in benzoinated lard. It is used for its emollient, protective and healing action on irritated skin, particularly in infants. **Zinc oxide ointment.** Zinc ointment (see above). **Ointment of zinc oxide with benzoin.** Unguentum zinci oxidi cum benzoini. **Zinc Undecenoate Ointment BP 1973.** An ointment composed of zinc undecenoate and undecenoic acid in emulsifying ointment. It is used in mycotic infections. [O Fr. *oignement.*]

See also: BROOKE, CASTELLANI, HEBRA, KAPOSI, LOEWENSTEIN, LOMHOLT, MARCUSSEN, PAGENSTECHER, SCOTT, WHITFIELD.

Okazaki, R. 20th century Japanese biochemist.

Okazaki fragments. A class of deoxyribonucleic acid produced during DNA replication in *Escherichia coli.* They are some 1000–2000 nucleotide units in length and appear to be single-stranded. When joined end-to-end by a DNA ligase, they are thought to give rise to very high molecular weight daughter strands of DNA involved in replication of DNA.

Oken, Lorenz (b. 1779). German naturalist and physiologist.

Oken's body. The mesonephros.

Okra (o·krah). Bendee, gumbo; the plant *Hibiscus esculentus* (family Malvaceae), cultivated for its mucilaginous capsular fruit. It has been used for gastric ulcer. [West African name.]

Oldberg's disease. Osteochondrosis of the epiphysis of the ischiopubic junction.

Oldfield, Michael Whitaker Carlton (b. 1907). Leeds surgeon.

Oldfield needle. A type of full-circle needle for the cleft palate operation.

oleander (o·le·**an**·der). Nerium; an ornamental evergreen shrub, *Nerium oleander* (family Apocynaceae). It is highly toxic and contains a glycoside, oleandrin. [etym. dub.]

Oleandomycin (o·le·an·do·**mi**'·sin). BP Commission approved name for the antibiotic obtained from species of *Streptomyces.* It acts on Gram-positive micro-organisms but also on some Gram-negative ones and on some *Rickettsiae.* No cross-immunity has been shown between this antibiotic and most of the other more popular antibiotics.

oleandrin (o·le·**an**·drin). $C_{32}H_{48}O_9$, a cardiac glycoside obtained from oleander. On hydrolysis it yields gitoxigenin.

oleandrism (o·le·**an**·drizm). Oleander poisoning, acute or chronic; having characteristics akin to those of digitalis poisoning.

oleanol (o·**le**·an·ol). $C_{18}H_{35}OH$, an alcohol from fish-liver oils.

olease (**o**·le·aze). An oil-splitting enzyme in olive oil. [L *oleum* oil.]

oleate (**o**·le·ate). 1. Any salt or ester of oleic acid. 2. A compound obtained by interaction between the oxide or salt of a metal and olive oil. According to the method of preparation, it can be either a powder or an unctuous mass. **Lead oleate.** A compound prepared by heating litharge with olive oil and constituting the main proportion of lead plaster. **Oleate of mercury.** A soft yellow-brown substance obtained by heating mercuric oxide with oleic acid. **Zinc oleate.** A compound obtained by adding a solution of zinc sulphate to a solution of hard soap; it is used in ointments.

olecranal (o·**lek**·ran·al). Relating or belonging to the olecranon.

olecranarthritis (o·**lek**·ran·ar·**thri**'·tis). A rheumatic inflammatory condition affecting the elbow joint at the olecranon. [olecranon, arthritis.]

olecranarthrocace (o·**lek**·ran·ar·**throk**'·as·e). An inflammatory condition of the elbow joint, especially at the olecranon. [olecranon, Gk *kakia* badness.]

olecranarthropathy (o·**lek**·ran·ar·**throp**'·ath·e). Any morbid condition of the elbow joint. [olecranon, Gk *arthron* joint, *pathos* disease.]

olecranoid (o·**lek**·ran·oid). Shaped like the olecranon. [olecranon, Gk *eidos* form.]

olecranon [NA] (o·**lek**·ran·on). The prominent curved process of the ulna which lodges in the olecranon fossa. [Gk *olekranon* point of the elbow.]

olefiant (o·le·**fi**·ant). Forming or making an oil. [L *oleum* oil, *facere* to make.]

olefin (o·le·fin). Olefine.

olefine (**o**·le·feen). A member of the homologous series of unsaturated hydrocarbons having the general formula: C_nH_{2n}. The first member of the series is ethylene (originally called *olefiant gas* because of the oily ethylene chloride it forms with chlorine gas), and the members are characterized by a double bond (*olefine linkage*) which renders them very reactive. [L *oleum* oil, *facere* to make.]

olein (**o**·le·in). 1. Any glyceride of oleic acid; in particular glyceryl triolein, $(C_{17}H_{33}COO)_3C_3H_5$, a colourless oil found in olive oil and other fixed oils. 2. The mixed fatty acids resulting from the hydrolysis of fats. [L *oleum* oil.]

olenitis (o·len·**i**·tis). Inflammation affecting the elbow joint. [Gk *olene* elbow, *-itis* inflammation.]

oleochrysotherapy (o·le·o·kris·o·**ther**'·ap·e). The use of gold salts in oily suspensions in the treatment of disease. [L *oleum* oil, Gk *chrysos* gold, therapy.]

oleocreosote (o·le·o·**kre**'·o·sote). The oleate of creosote; it is used in phthisis.

oleodipalmitin (o·le·o·di·**pal′**·mit·in). $C_{17}H_{33}COOC_3H_5(OCOC_{15}H_{31})_2$, a mixed glyceride of oleic and palmitic acids which occurs in the fats of butter, cocoa and soya bean.

oleodistearin (o·le·o·di·**ste′**·ar·in). $C_{17}H_{33}COOC_3H_5(OCOC_{17}H_{35})_2$, a mixed ester of glycerol with oleic and stearic acids which occurs in the seed fats of the tropical plant *Allanblackia*, the Indian mango, *Mangifera indica* and cacao.

oleogranuloma (o·le·o·gran·ew·**lo′**·mah). A granuloma produced by continuous contact with oil or by the failure of absorption of injected oily media. It occurs particularly if such media are injected subcutaneously rather than intramuscularly. [L *oleum* oil, granuloma.]

oleoguaiacol (o·le·o·**gwi′**·ak·ol). Guaiacol oleate, $CH_3OC_6H_4OCOC_{17}H_{33}$. The ester of guaiacol and oleic acid, used as an internal antiseptic.

oleoma (o·le·o·mah). Paraffinoma; a chronic granuloma caused by constant exposure to paraffin or by the administration of paraffin by injection into the tissues. [L *oleum* oil, Gk *-oma* tumour.]

oleomargarine (o·le·o·**mar′**·jer·een, o·le·o·**mar′**·gar·een). Margarine. [Obsolete term.] [L *oleum* oil, Gk *margaron* pearl.]

oleometer (o·le·**om**·et·er). A device for testing the specific gravity and purity of oils. [L *oleum* oil, Gk *metron* measure.]

oleonucleoprotein (o·le·o·**new**·kle·o·**pro′**·te·in). The caseinogenic and fatty components of milk considered as one compound substance. [L *oleum* oil, nucleus, protein.]

oleoperitoneography (o·le·o·**per**·e·to·ne·**og′**·raf·e). Peritoneal radiography preceded by injection of iodized oil into the peritoneum. [L *oleum* oil, peritoneum, Gk *graphein* to record.]

oleoresin, oleoresina (o·le·o·**rez′**·in, o·le·o·rez·**i′**·nah). A liquid preparation obtained from natural vegetable sources by extraction with an organic solvent such as ether, acetone or alcohol, and subsequent evaporation of the solvent. As its name implies, it contains a mixture of natural oils and resins. [L *oleum* oil, resin.]

oleostearate (o·le·o·**ste**·ar·ate). A compound of a base with oleic and stearic acids. **Zinc oleostearate.** A compound prepared by treating a solution of hard soap and curd soap with zinc sulphate in water, drying and powdering the precipitate. It is used to protect the surface of the skin and absorb discharges in certain types of skin infection.

oleothorax (o·le·o·**thor′**·ax). The gradual replacement of air in an artificial pneumothorax or extrapleural pneumothorax by sterilized olive oil or liquid paraffin. [L *oleum* oil, thorax.]

oleum (o·le·um). Oil; this was classified officially prior to the BP 1953 and BPC 1954 as *Oleum.* **Oleum Abietis BPC 1949.** Oil of Siberian fir, oil of pine; an oil distilled from the fresh leaves of *Abies sibirica* (family Pinaceae). It contains esters, chiefly bornyl acetate, and has properties similar to pumilio pine oil but is not of so pleasant an odour. **Oleum absinthiae.** Oil of American wormwood, the volatile oil obtained from wormwood, *Artemesia absinthium.* It contains thujone and is a narcotic poison, causing violent epileptiform convulsions in toxic doses. It is not used medicinally nowadays. **Oleum aethereum.** A mixture of heavy oil of wine and ether. **Oleum alii essentiale.** Garlic oil. *See* OIL. **Oleum amygdalae.** Almond oil. *See* OIL. **Oleum amygdalae amarae.** Oil of bitter almond, essential oil of almond; an oil obtained by distilling moistened bitter-almond cake, and also from the cake of the seeds of the apricot or peach. The oil is produced by the interaction of amygdalin and emulsin which form benzaldehyde, benzaldehyde cyanohydrin, hydrocyanic acid and dextrose, and is adjusted to contain 4.0 per cent HCN. It is a colourless liquid with a characteristic odour, employed as a flavouring agent in confectionery, being more stable than the oil freed from hydrocyanic acid, but it should be used with caution. **Oleum amygdalae essentiale.** Oleum amygdalae amarae (see above). **Oleum amygdalae volatile purificatum.** Bitter almond oil, volatile. *See* OIL. **Oleum anethi.** Dill oil. *See* OIL. **Oleum animale aethereum.** Dippel's animal oil; an empyreumatic oil obtained during the destructive distillation of bone, ivory, hair, wool or other animal products. It consists of a mixture of amines, pyridine, pyrrole and several nitriles. It is not used in medical practice. **Oleum anisi.** Anise oil. *See* OIL. **Oleum Anthemidis BPC 1949.** Oil of chamomile, an oil obtained by distillation from recently dried flowers of *Anthemis nobilis* Linn. It occurs as a blue liquid which becomes greenish to brownish yellow in light and air. It has a pleasant aromatic odour and a burning taste, and contains esters of angelic and tiglic acids with butyl and amyl alcohols, and butyric acid. It is employed as an aromatic carminative. **Oleum arachis.** Arachis oil. *See* OIL. **Oleum aurantii.** Orange oil. *See* OIL. **Oleum aurantii florum.** Oleum neroli (see below). **Oleum Bergamottae BPC 1949.** Oil of bergamot, an oil expressed from the fresh peel of the fruit of *Citrus bergamia.* It contains the ester, linalyl acetate, which gives it its fragrance, and is used largely in perfumery, especially in hair preparations. **Oleum Betulae BPC 1949.** Oil of sweet birch, oil of wintergreen, oil of teaberry; an oil formerly obtained by distillation from the leaves of *Gaultheria procumbens,* but more so nowadays from the bark of *Betula lenta.* Its chief constituent is methyl salicylate and it is sometimes given internally in rheumatism. It is mostly applied externally, but being absorbed by the skin may give rise to eruptions; pure methyl salicylate is to be preferred. It is also incorporated in liniments and ointments for chronic rheumatism, fibrositis and lumbago. **Oleum betulae albae, Oleum betulae pyroligneum.** Oleum rusci (see below). **Oleum cadinum.** Cade oil. *See* OIL. **Oleum cajuputi.** Cajuput oil. *See* OIL. **Oleum calcis.** A thick oily liquid formed by the deliquescence of calcium chloride. **Oleum camphorae essentiale, Oleum camphorae rectificatum.** Camphor oil, rectified. *See* OIL. **Oleum carbolisatum.** Oleum phenolatum (see below). **Oleum Cardamomi BPC 1949.** Oil of cardamom, an oil obtained by distillation from the whole fruits of *Elettaria cardamomum* Maton. var. *minuscula* Burkill, cultivated in Sri Lanka and India. It is a pale-yellow liquid with a pungent odour and aromatic taste, its main constituents being esters of cineole and terpineol, together with limonene. It has carminative properties and is sometimes used as a flavouring agent. **Oleum cari, Oleum carui.** Caraway oil. *See* OIL. **Oleum caryophylli.** Clove oil. *See* OIL. **Oleum Cassiae BPC 1949.** Oil of cassia, an oil obtained by the distillation of the leaves and twigs of *Cinnamomum cassia* with subsequent rectification. In odour and taste it resembles cinnamon oil, its main constituent being cinnamic aldehyde, and it is used like that oil, but is inferior as a flavouring agent. **Oleum Cedri BPC 1949.** Cedar-wood oil, an oil obtained by distillation from the wood of various species of red cedar, the chief of which is *Juniperus virginiana.* It is a colourless or slightly yellow viscous liquid with a mild and persistent odour, consisting almost entirely of cedrene, a liquid sesquiterpene. It is used in microscopy as an immersion oil and is also employed in perfumery. **Oleum cedri folii.** Cedar-leaf oil. *See* OIL. **Oleum chaenoceti.** The oil of the whale, *Balaena rostrata.* **Oleum chaulmoograe.** Chaulmoogra oil. *See* OIL. **Oleum chenopodii.** Chenopodium oil. *See* OIL. **Oleum cinnamomi.** Cinnamon oil. *See* OIL. **Oleum citronellae.** Citronella oil. *See* OIL. **Oleum coriandri.** Coriander oil. *See* OIL. **Oleum Crotonis BPC 1949.** Croton oil, an oil expressed from the seeds of *Croton tiglium.* It is a weak drying oil, and has powerful vesicant properties due to its constituent, croton resin. Internally it is a drastic purgative, and except in very small doses is a powerful irritant to the stomach and intestines, causing vomiting, purging and collapse. Externally it is a strong counter-irritant. **Oleum Cubebae BPC 1949.** Oil of cubeb, an oil obtained by distillation from the coarsely ground fruit of *Piper cubeba.* It is a pale-yellowish to bluish-green liquid with a characteristic odour and camphoraceous taste. Its main constituents are terpenes and sesquiterpenes, and it has carminative and antiseptic properties. It was popular at one time as an antiseptic for the urogenital system in gonorrhoea and cystitis. **Oleum eucalypti.** Eucalyptus oil. *See* OIL. **Oleum fixum.** Fixed oil. *See* OIL. **Oleum Foeniculi BPC 1949.** Oil of fennel, an oil obtained by distillation from the dried ripe fruit of *Foeniculum vulgare.* It is a colourless or slightly yellow liquid with the aromatic odour of fennel and a bitter camphoraceous taste. Its chief constituents are anethole and fenchone, and it is used as an aromatic carminative, and in purgative medicines to prevent gripe. It is also used in the

oleum

treatment of intestinal colic in children. **Oleum gaultheriae.** Oleum betulae (see above). **Oleum geranii.** Geranium oil. *See* OIL. **Oleum gossypii seminis.** Cottonseed oil. *See* OIL. **Oleum graminis citrati.** Lemon grass oil. *See* OIL. **Oleum hippoglossi.** Halibut-liver oil. *See* OIL. **Oleum hydnocarpi.** Hydnocarpus oil. *See* OIL. **Oleum iodisatum.** Iodised oil. *See* OIL. **Oleum jecoris, Oleum jecoris aselli.** Cod-liver oil. *See* OIL. **Oleum Juniperi BPC 1949.** Oil of juniper; the English oil consists of the entire distillate from the dried ripe fruit of *Juniperus communis* Linn. and has the characteristic odour of the fruit; the foreign oil has a less pronounced odour and flavour. The commercial oil is obtained as a by-product in the manufacture of an alcoholic liqueur and has a powerful turpentine-like smell. It is a colourless or pale-yellow liquid with a characteristic odour and burning bitter taste, its main constituents being pinene, camphene, cadinene, terpineol and juniper camphor. It is used chiefly as a diuretic and urinary antiseptic, but should not be used where there is renal disease as it is a kidney irritant. It is also of value as a carminative in flatulence and in colic, also in lumbago. It has been employed as a reflex emmenagogue. **Oleum lavandulae.** Lavender oil. *See* OIL. **Oleum lavandulae spicatae.** Spike lavender oil. *See* OIL. **Oleum ligni santali.** Oleum santali (see below). **Oleum limonis.** Lemon oil. *See* OIL. **Oleum lini.** Linseed oil. *See* OIL. **Oleum marjoranae.** Oil of marjoram. **Oleum maydis.** Maize oil. *See* OIL. **Oleum Melaleucae BPC 1949.** Oil of melaleuca, ti-tree oil, tea-tree oil; an oil obtained by the distillation of the leaves of *Melaleuca alternifolia.* It is a colourless or pale-yellow oil with a pleasant odour, containing terpenes and cineole. It has antiseptic properties and, being used as a germicide, is a common constituent of proprietary disinfectants, especially chlorinated phenols. **Oleum menthae piperitae.** Peppermint oil. *See* OIL. **Oleum menthae viridis.** Spearmint oil. *See* OIL. **Oleum morrhuae.** Cod-liver oil. *See* OIL. **Oleum Myrciae BPC 1949.** Oil of myrcia, oil of bay; an oil obtained from the leaves of *Pimenta acris* and other close species, by distillation. It contains eugenol, myrcene, L-phellandrene, citral and other terpenes. It is not employed directly in medicine, but is included in bay rum which is used as a hair wash and as an astringent to the face after shaving. **Oleum myristicae.** Nutmeg oil. *See* OIL. **Oleum Neroli BPC 1949.** Oil of neroli, oil of orange-flower water; an oil obtained by distillation with water from the fresh blossoms of the bitter-orange tree, *Citrus aurantium* Linn. It occurs as a pale-yellow liquid, slightly fluorescent, and becoming brownish-red on exposure to light. It has an intense and characteristic odour and a bitter aromatic taste, and is used largely in perfumery. It is employed in medicine to produce concentrated orange-flower water, which is used as a flavouring agent. **Oleum nigrum.** A reddish-yellow oil obtained from the seeds of *Celastrus paniculata*; it contains formic, acetic and benzoic acids in organic combination, and is used as a diaphoretic and stimulant in rheumatism, gout and various fevers. **Oleum olivae.** Olive oil. *See* OIL. **Oleum origani.** Origanum oil. *See* OIL. **Oleum Palmae Nuclei BPC 1949.** Palm-kernel oil, a fat obtained by pressing the kernels of the fruit of the palm tree, *Eloeis guineensis.* It is a white or slightly yellow fatty substance with a pleasant odour and a nutty taste, consisting of glycerides, mainly of lauric, oleic and myristic acids, with smaller amounts of palmitic and oleic acids. It has occasionally been used as an ointment base, but is now principally confined to the manufacture of soap and margarine. **Oleum papaveris.** Poppy-seed oil, an oil which may be obtained by the expression of the seeds of *Papaver somniferum.* It is a light-yellow odourless liquid with a faint almond flavour and a bland taste. It has no narcotic properties and is used as a substitute for olive oil for medical and culinary purposes. It contains the glycerides of stearic and palmitic acids together with those of linoleic and oleic acids, and is used to prepare iodised oil, as a drying oil in paints, for soap manufacture and for culinary purposes. **Oleum percomorphum.** A mixture of the liver oils of various fishes of the order Percomorphi, containing a high proportion of vitamins A and D. **Oleum Phenolatum BPC 1949.** Phenolated oil, carbolic oil; a solution of phenol in arachis oil. Its main value lies in its emollient action and certain local anaesthetic effects on the skin; it has little bactericidal activity. **Oleum Pimentae BPC 1949.** Oil of pimento, allspice oil; an oil distilled from the dried, full-grown, unripe fruit of *Pimenta officinalis* Lindl. It is a yellow or yellowish-red liquid, having the clove-like odour of the fruit and a pungent spicy taste; it contains eugenol and a sesquiterpene. It is used as a carminative and in aperient mixtures. **Oleum pini.** Oleum abietis (see above). **Oleum Pini Aromaticum BPC 1949.** An antiseptic oil prepared by the steam distillation of weathered pine wood. **Oleum pini pumilionis.** Pumilio pine oil. *See* OIL. **Oleum pini sylvestris.** An oil from certain conifers used as an adulterant of pumilio pine oil. **Oleum rapae.** Rape oil. *See* OIL. **Oleum ricini.** Castor oil. *See* OIL. **Oleum ricini aromaticum.** Aromatic castor oil, a mixture of cinnamon and clove oils together with saccharin, vanillin and chloroform in castor oil. It is a pleasant way of administering castor oil, to which its therapeutic value is entirely due. **Oleum Rosae BPC 1949.** Oil of rose, otto of rose; an oil obtained by distillation from the fresh flowers of the damask rose, *Rosa damascena.* It occurs as a pale-yellow, semi-solid, crystalline mass, with a fragrant odour, and is chiefly employed in perfumery, also in lozenges, dentifrices, ointments and toilet preparations. **Oleum rosmarini.** Rosemary oil. *See* OIL. **Oleum Rusci BPC 1949.** Birch-tar oil, the pyroligneous oil obtained by the dry distillation of the bark and wood of *Betula pendula* and related species of *Betula.* It contains guaiacol, cresols and phenols, and is used as a local application in chronic eczema and other skin diseases. **Oleum Santali BPC 1949.** Oil of sandal wood, oil of santal wood; an oil distilled from the heartwood of *Santalum album.* It is a pale-yellow viscid liquid with a peculiar persistent odour and an unpleasant taste. It contains chiefly santalol, and is used mainly for its effect on the urogenital mucous membranes which are stimulated and disinfected; it was employed in the subacute stages of cystitis and gonorrhoea, but is now obsolete. **Oleum Santali Australiensis BPC 1949.** Oil of Australian sandal wood, an oil obtained from the wood of *Eurcarya spicata*; it has properties similar to oleum santali. **Oleum sassafras.** Sassafras oil. *See* OIL. **Oleum sesami.** Sesame oil. *See* OIL. **Oleum sinapis alba.** An oil obtained from *Brassica alba*; it is used for lubricating and burning. **Oleum sinapis expressum.** Oil of mustard, expressed. *See* OIL. **Oleum Sinapis Volatile BPC 1949.** Volatile oil of mustard, an oil which may be prepared synthetically or by distillation of the dried ripe seeds of black mustard, *Brassica nigra*, after they have been deprived of fixed oil and macerated with tepid water for several hours during which the glycoside, sinigrin, reacts hydrolytically with the ferment, myrosin, to produce mustard oil. The synthetic product is obtained by the interaction of allyl iodide and potassium thiocyanate, the allyl thiocyanate so formed being converted to the isothiocyanate on heating. It is a colourless or pale-yellow liquid with a pungent odour and an acrid taste which becomes reddish-brown on exposure to light. It contains allyl isothiocyanate, with variable amounts of allyl cyanide, carbon disulphide and allyl thiocyanate. It is strongly irritant, and applied to the skin is rapidly vesicant, causing painful blisters due to deep penetration. It is the active constituent of liniment of mustard which is used as a counter-irritant and rubefacient for application to places where plasters cannot readily be applied; it is also employed in the treatment of pneumonia and pleurisy, and to relieve deep-seated pain. **Oleum Succini BPC 1949, Oleum succini rectificatum.** Oil of amber, an oil obtained by the destructive distillation of certain resins or as the distillate of oleoresin; it was formerly obtained from amber. It is a pale-yellow liquid with a strong odour and contains retene. It has similar properties to turpentine oil and is used externally, mixed with olive oil or camphorated oil, as a mild counter-irritant. **Oleum terebinthinae, Oleum terebinthinae rectificatum.** Turpentine oil. *See* OIL. **Oleum theobromatis.** Theobroma oil. *See* OIL. **Oleum Thymi BPC 1949.** Oil of thyme, an oil distilled from the leaves and flowering tops of *Thymus vulgaris* and other species of *Thymus.* It is a reddish-brown liquid, with a strong thyme odour and a biting persistent taste; it contains thymol and the isomer, carvacrol. It has antiseptic, antispasmodic and carminative properties, and is used in the treatment of whooping-cough and bronchitis. Externally it is mixed with a vegetable oil and employed as a counter-irritant and rubefacient in the treatment of rheumatism and fibrositis. **Oleum tiglii.** Oleum crotonis (see above). **Oleum tritici germinis.** Wheat germ oil. *See* OIL. [L.]

olfact (ol·fakt). A unit measured in grams per litre to record the acuity of the sense of smell: the weakest concentration of a substance diluted in petroleum jelly of specific gravity 0.880 which can be appreciated by a group of normal people. It is known also as the *olfactory coefficient,* or the *minimal identifiable or perceptible odour.* [L *olfactus* sense of smell.]

olfactie (ol·fak·te). A unit of smell, based on the distance at which an odorous substance may be recognized in an olfactometer (Zwaardemaker). [see prec.]

olfaction (ol·**fak**·shun). 1. The sense of smell. 2. The act or process of smelling. [L *olfacere* to smell.]

olfactometer (ol·fak·**tom**·et·er). An apparatus for determining the degree of acuity of the olfactory sense. [L *olfactus* sense of smell, meter.]

olfactometry (ol·fak·**tom**·et·re). Estimation of the sensitivity of the nose to olfactory stimuli. [see prec.]

olfactophobia (ol·**fak**·to·**fo**′·be·ah). Morbid fear of odours. [L *olfacere* to smell, phobia.]

olfactory (ol·**fak**·tor·e). Associated with the sense of smell. **Olfactory hallucinatory epileptic seizure.** A variety of epilepsy characterized by hallucinations of smell, usually unpleasant in character, commonly constituting the aura. [L *olfactus* sense of smell.]

olfactory nerves [nervi olfactorii (NA)]. The nerves of smell. They arise from sensory cells in the mucous membrane of the nose and end in the olfactory bulb.

olibanum (ol·**ib**·an·um). A dried oleo-gum-resin obtained as a secretion from the bark of various species of *Boswellia* (family Burseraceae). It occurs in yellowish ovoid tears, having an agreeable balsamic odour and a somewhat bitter, spicy taste. It is used in incense and as constituent of fumigating powders. [Ar. *al-luban* frankincense.]

oligaemic (ol·ig·e·mik). Pertaining to deficiency in blood. [Gk *oligos* little, *haima* blood.]

oligaerobe (ol·ig·a·er·obe). A micro-organism which is able to grow and multiply with minimal amounts of free atmospheric oxygen as the optimum. [Gk *oligos* little, aerobe.]

oligakisuria (ol·ig·ak·is·**ewr**′·e·ah). A condition in which urine is passed at long intervals. [Gk *oligakis* seldom, urine.]

oligergasia (ol·ig·er·**ga**′·se·ah). An oligergastic condition; a mental condition caused by faulty development of the intellect or feeblemindedness.

oligergastic (ol·ig·er·**gas**′·tik). Denoting disorders of the mind founded on mental defects caused by arrested development of the brain (Adolf Meyer). [Gk *oligos* little, *ergon* work.]

olighaemia (ol·ig·**he**·me·ah). Oligohaemia.

olighidria, olighydria, oligidria (ol·ig·**hi**·dre·ah, ol·ig·**id**·re·ah). Oligohidria.

oligo-amnios (ol·ig·o·**am**′·ne·os). Oligohydramnios.

oligoblast (ol·ig·o·blast). A primitive oligodendroglial cell. [Gk *oligos* little, *blastos* germ.]

oligoblennia (ol·ig·o·**blen**′·e·ah). A condition in which there is an insufficient mucoid secretion. [Gk *oligos* little, *blenna* mucus.]

oligocardia (ol·ig·o·**kar**′·de·ah). Bradycardia. [Gk *oligos* little, *kardia* heart.]

Oligochaeta (ol·ig·o·**ke**′·tah). An order of worms including the earthworm. [Gk *oligos* little, *chaite* long hair.]

oligocholia (ol·ig·o·**ko**′·le·ah). Acholia; deficiency or lack in the secretion of bile. [Gk *oligos* little, *chole* bile.]

oligochromaemia (ol·ig·o·kro·**me**′·me·ah). Hypochromaemia; a condition in which there is an inadequate amount of haemoglobin in the blood. [Gk *oligos* little, *chroma* colour, *haima* blood.]

oligochromasia (ol·ig·o·kro·**ma**′·ze·ah). Hypochromasia. 1. A state of the nucleus of the cell body in which it contains too few chromosomes. 2. The condition of taking stain less readily and intensely than is normally the case. [Gk *oligos* little, *chroma* colour.]

oligochrosis (ol·ig·o·**kro**′·sis). Oligochromaemia. [Gk *oligos* little, *chroa* colour, *-osis* condition.]

oligochylia (ol·ig·o·**ki**′·le·ah). Hypochylia; a condition in which the secretion of chyle is deficient or in which the amount of gastric juice is lessened. [Gk *oligos* little, chyle.]

oligochymia (ol·ig·o·**ki**′·me·ah). Lack of chyme. [Gk *oligos* little, chyme.]

oligocystic (ol·ig·o·**sist**′·ik). Having only a small number of cysts. [Gk *oligos* little, cyst.]

oligocythaemia (ol·ig·o·si·**the**′·me·ah). A condition of the blood in which there is cell deficiency. [Gk *oligos* little, *kytos* cell, *haima* blood.]

oligocythaemic (ol·ig·o·si·**the**′·mik). Pertaining to or suffering from oligocythaemia.

oligocytosis (ol·ig·o·si·**to**′·sis). Oligocythaemia. [Gk *oligos* little, *kytos* cell, *-osis* condition.]

oligodacrya (ol·ig·o·**dak**′·re·ah). A condition in which there is an insufficiency of tears. [Gk *oligos* little, *dakryon* tear.]

oligodactylia (ol·ig·o·dak·**til**′·e·ah). A congenital deficiency of fingers or toes. [Gk *oligos* little, *daktylos* finger or toe.]

oligodendria (ol·ig·o·**den**′·dre·ah). Oligodendroglia.

oligodendroblastoma (ol·ig·o·**den**·dro·blas·**to**′·mah). A tumour composed of primitive oligodendroglial cells. [oligodendroglia, blastoma.]

oligodendrocyte (ol·ig·o·**den**′·dro·site). An oligodendroglial cell. [oligodendroglia, Gk *kytos* cell.]

oligodendroglia (ol·ig·o·den·**drog**′·le·ah). Neuroglial cells with small, round or oval, clear nuclei and few cell processes. They tend to form columns around the constituent medullated fibres of the white matter of the central nervous system, where possibly they play a rôle similar to that of the neurilemmal cells of Schwann in peripheral nerves. [Gk *oligos* little, *dendron* tree, neuroglia.]

oligodendroglioma (ol·ig·o·**den**·dro·gli·**o**′·mah). A tumour consisting of oligodendroglial cells. [oligodendroglia, Gk *-oma* tumour.]

oligodendrogliomatosis (ol·ig·o·**den**·dro·gli·o·mat·**o**′·sis). The diffuse occurrence of oligodendrogliomata in the meninges and ventricles. [oligodendroglioma, Gk *-osis* condition.]

oligodipsia (ol·ig·o·**dip**′·se·ah). A condition in which thirst is absent. [Gk *oligos* little, *dipsa* thirst.]

oligodontia (ol·ig·o·**don**′·she·ah). A state in which most of the teeth are lacking. [Gk *oligos* few, *odous* tooth.]

oligodynamic (ol·ig·o·di·**nam**′·ik). Powerful in exceedingly small amounts; referring for instance to the most dilute solutions of certain substances used as disinfectants. [Gk *oligos* little, *dynamis* power.]

oligo-erythrocythaemia (ol·ig·o·er·**ith**·ro·si·**the**·me·ah). Hypo-erythrocythaemia; the condition of the blood when there is a deficiency of erythrocytes. [Gk *oligos* little, *erythros* red, *kytos* cell, *haima* blood.]

oligogalactia, oligogalia (ol·ig·o·gal·**ak**′·she·ah, ol·ig·o·**ga**′·le·ah). The secretion of too small a quantity of milk. [Gk *oligos* little, *gala* milk.]

oligogenesis (ol·ig·o·**jen**′·es·is). The production of only a few offspring. [Gk *oligos* little, *genesis* birth.]

oligogenic (ol·ig·o·**jen**′·ik). Applied to inherited characters which are determined by one or a few genes. [Gk *oligos* little, *genein* to produce.]

oligogenics (ol·ig·o·**jen**′·ix). The practice and study of birth control. [see prec.]

oligoglia (ol·ig·**og**·le·ah). Oligodendroglia.

oligoglobulia (ol·ig·o·glob·**ew**′·le·ah). Oligocythaemia. [Gk *oligos* little, globule.]

oligohaemia (ol·ig·o·**he**′·me·ah). A condition in which there is an insufficient amount of blood in the body. **Oligohaemia serosa.** Hydraemia. [Gk *oligos* little, *haima* blood.]

oligohidria, oligohidrosis (ol·ig·o·**hi**′·dre·ah, ol·ig·o·hi·**dro**′·sis). A condition in which the secretion of sweat is scanty. [Gk *oligos* little, *hidros* sweat.]

oligohydramnios (**ol**·ig·o·hi·**dram**′·ne·os). A deficient secretion of liquor amnii. [Gk *oligos* little, *hydor* water, amnion.]

oligohydria (**ol**·ig·o·**hi**′·dre·ah). Oligohidria.

oligohydruria (ol·ig·o·hi·**drewr**′·e·ah). Urine that contains a relatively small percentage of water; urine of high concentration. [Gk *oligos* little, *hydor* water, urine.]

oligohypermenorrhoea (**ol**·ig·o·**hi**·per·men·o·**re**′·ah). Menstruation that occurs only rarely and in which there is an excessive discharge. [Gk *oligos* little, hypermenorrhoea.]

oligohypomenorrhoea (ol·ig·o·**hi**·po·men·o·re′·ah). Menstruation that occurs only rarely and in which there is insufficient discharge. [Gk *oligos* little, hypomenorrhoea.]

oligolecithal (**ol**·ig·o·**les**′·ith·al). Having a small yolk; denoting the yolk of a mammalian ovum in which there is an extremely small scattered quantity of deutoplasm. [Gk *oligos* little, *lekithos* yolk of egg.]

oligoleucocythaemia, oligoleucocytosis (**ol**·ig·o·**lew**·ko·si·**the**′·me·ah, **ol**·ig·o·**lew**·ko·si·**to**′·sis). Leucopenia. [Gk *oligos* little, leucocyte, Gk *haima* blood, *-osis* condition.]

oligomania (ol·ig·o·**ma**′·ne·ah). A form of insanity in which not all the mental powers are defective. [Gk *oligos* little, mania.]

oligomastigate (ol·ig·o·**mas**′·tig·ate). Possessing a small number of flagella. [Gk *oligos* little, *mastix* whip.]

oligomelus (ol·ig·o·**me**′·lus). 1. A congenital condition in which the limbs are abnormally thin. 2. A condition in which there are fewer limbs than is normal. [Gk *oligos* little, *melos* limb.]

oligomenorrhoea (**ol**·ig·o·men·o·**re**′·ah). Menstruation characterized by infrequent occurrence. [Gk *oligos* little, menorrhoea.]

oligomer (ol·ig·o·mer). Certain important biological macromolecules are composed of more than 1 identical unit or protomer and are generally referred to as *oligomers*; an example is glycogen phosphorylase of muscle which involves a combination of 2 or 4 protomers. [Gk *oligos* little, *meros* part.]

oligometallic (**ol**·ig·o·met·**al**′·ik). Applied to substances the total metallic content of which is very small. [Gk *oligos* little, metal.]

oligomorphic (ol·ig·o·**mor**′·fik). Denoting micro-organisms which pass through only a few stages during their development. [Gk *oligos* little, *morphe* form.]

oligomycin (**ol**·ig·o·**mi**′·sin). An antibiotic which inhibits oxidative phosphorylation through its action on the mitochondrial ATPase system. [Gk *oligos* little, *mykes* fungus.]

oligonatality (**ol**·ig·o·na·**tal**′·it·e). Birth rate which is below the normal. [Gk *oligos* little, L *natalis* relating to birth.]

oligonecrospermia (ol·ig·o·nek·ro·**sper**′·me·ah). A condition in which some of the spermatozoa in the semen are dead and in which the total number is less than normal. [Gk *oligos* little, *nekros* dead, sperm.]

oligopepsia (ol·ig·o·**pep**′·se·ah). Weakness of the process of digestion. [Gk *oligos* little, *peptein* to digest.]

oligophosphaturia (ol·ig·o·fos·fat·**ewr**′·e·ah). Deficiency in the amount of phosphates excreted in the urine. [Gk *oligos* little, phosphate, urine.]

oligophrenia (ol·ig·o·**fre**′·ne·ah). Mental defect. **Galactosaemic oligophrenia.** Oligophrenia found in association with the inborn error of metabolism, *galactosaemia*. **Phenylpyruvic oligophrenia.** A genetically determined disorder in which intellectual defect, commonly of severe degree, is accompanied by the urinary excretion of about 1 g daily of phenylpyruvic acid (phenylketonuria). [Gk *oligos* little, *phren* mind.]

oligoplasmia (ol·ig·o·**plaz**′·me·ah). A deficiency in the quantity of blood plasma. [Gk *oligos* little, plasma.]

oligopnoea (ol·ig·op·**ne**′·ah). Restricted breathing, the respiratory cycle being below the usual standard. [Gk *oligos* little, *pnoia* breath.]

oligopsychia (ol·ig·o·**si**′·ke·ah). Feeblemindedness. [Gk *oligos* little, *psyche* reason.]

oligoptyalism (**ol**·ig·o·**ti**′·al·izm). A lessening of the amount of saliva secreted. [Gk *oligos* little, *ptyalon* saliva.]

oligopyrene, oligopyrous (**ol**·ig·o·**pi**′·reen, **ol**·ig·o·**pi**′·rus). Lack of chromatin or nuclear constituents. [Gk *oligos* little, *pyren* kernel.]

oligoria (ol·ig·**or**·e·ah). A type of melancholia in which the patient displays abnormal aversion from or indifference to persons or things. [Gk *oligoria* contempt.]

oligosaccharide (**ol**·ig·o·**sak**′·ar·ide). A general name for di- and trisaccharides. [Gk *oligos* little, *sakcharon* sugar.]

oligosialia (**ol**·ig·o·si·**a**′·le·ah). Oligoptyalism. [Gk *oligos* little, *sialon* saliva.]

oligosideraemia (**ol**·ig·o·sid·er·**e**′·me·ah). Diminution of the iron content of the blood. [Gk *oligos* little, *sideros* iron, *haima* blood.]

oligospermatic (**ol**·ig·o·sper·**mat**′·ik). Relating or belonging to oligospermia.

oligospermia (**ol**·ig·o·**sper**′·me·ah). A condition in which too few spermatozoa are present in the semen. [Gk *oligos* little, *sperma* seed.]

Oligosporidia (**ol**·ig·o·spor·**id**′·e·ah). The name formerly given to a sub-order of Protozoa, class Sporozoa, order Sarcosporidia, characterized by the production of spores (sarcocysts) filled with sickle-shaped or oval-shaped bodies. Several species are pathogenic for animals, but very few authentic infections of man are recorded. A species of the genus, *Sarcocystis, Sarcocystis lindermannii*, infects man and is found in striated muscles, but the method of transmission is unknown, probably accidental. [Gk *oligos* little, dim. of *sporos* seed.]

oligosteatosis (**ol**·ig·o·ste·at·**o**′·sis). Insufficiency in the amount of sebum secreted. [Gk *oligos* little, *stear* fat, *-osis* condition.]

oligotrichia, oligotrichosis (**ol**·ig·o·**trik**′·e·ah, **ol**·ig·o·trik·**o**′·sis). A congenital deficiency of hair. [Gk *oligos* little, *thrix* hair, *-osis* condition.]

oligotrophia, oligotrophy (**ol**·ig·o·**tro**′·fe·ah, ol·ig·**ot**·ro·fe). Inadequate nutrition. [Gk *oligos* little, *trophe* nourishment.]

oliguria (ol·ig·**ewr**·e·ah). Daily output of urine below normal levels. [Gk *oligos* little, urine.]

olivary (**ol**·iv·a·re). 1. Relating to the olive. 2. Like an olive in shape.

olive (**ol**·iv). The evergreen tree, *Olea europaea* (family Oleaceae) and its drupaceous fruit. The latter contains a bitter glycoside and a fixed oil, *olive oil*, consisting chiefly of olein, with palmitin, linolein and arachin, used as a food, in the manufacture of soap, and in medicine as a demulcent and mild laxative. **Spurge olive.** Spurge laurel, the dried bark of *Daphne mezereum* and other species of *Daphne*. It contains a bitter glycoside, an acrid resin and a yellow colouring matter; applied to the skin it is a vesicant and is used as an epispastic. [L *oliva*.]

olive [oliva (NA)] (**ol**·iv). A smooth oval eminence on the anterolateral surface of the upper part of the medulla, overlying the olivary nucleus. [L *oliva*.]

Oliver, William Silver (b. 1836). British Army Medical Department.

Oliver's sign. Tracheal tug, a pulling of the trachea synchronous with each ventricular systole, seen in aortic aneurysm; also called *Porter's sign*. Cf. CARDARELLI'S SIGN.

olivopontocerebellar (ol·iv·o·**pon**·to·ser·e·**bel**′·ar). Pertaining to the olive, the pons and the cerebellum.

Ollier, Louis Xavier Edouard Léopold (b. 1830). Lyons surgeon.

Ollier's disease. Dyschondroplasia.

Ollier's layer. Osteoblastic layer, osteogenetic layer; the deepest layer of the periosteum, lying adjacent to the bone, and containing osteoblasts or potential osteoblasts.

Ollier-Thiersch graft. Thick split-skin graft; free grafts of large sheets of skin, usually one-half to almost full thickness, and the graft commonly employed to replace skin defects after burns.

olophonia (ol·o·**fo**·ne·ah). Imperfect speech caused by deformity or physical defect of the vocal organs. [Gk *oloos* destroying, *phone* sound.]

Olshausen, Robert von (b. 1835). German obstetrician.

Olshausen's method. An operation for the correction of uterine retroversion. The uterine ends of the round ligaments are approximated to the anterior abdominal wall by silk sutures running through peritoneum, muscle and rectal sheath.

omacephalus (o·mah·**kef**·al·us). A fetal monstrosity having an imperfectly formed head or none at all and lacking the upper extremities. [Gk *omos* shoulder, *a*, *kephale* head.]

omagra (o·**mag**·rah). A gouty condition affecting the shoulder joint. [Gk *omos* shoulder, *agra* a catching.]

omalgia (o·**mal**·je·ah). A painful condition affecting the shoulder. [Gk *omos* shoulder, *algos* pain.]

omarthralgia (o·mar·**thral**·je·ah). A painful condition affecting the shoulder joint. [Gk *omos* shoulder, *arthron* joint, *algos* pain.]

omarthritis (o·mar·**thri**·tis). An inflammatory condition affecting the shoulder joint. [Gk *omos* shoulder, arthritis.]

omarthrocace (o·mar·**throk**·as·e). Any pathological condition of the shoulder joint. [Gk *omos* shoulder, *arthron* joint, *kakos* bad.]

Ombrédanne, Louis (b. 1871). Paris surgeon.

Ombrédanne's mask. An anaesthetic mask used in Europe for ether administration.

Ombrédanne's operation. Repair of hypospadias by using the skin of the under-surface of the penis and of the scrotum to form a new urethra, and transplanting the prepuce to cover the under-surface of the penis.

Turner-Ombrédanne orchidopexy. An operation performed for undescended testicle. In this operation, after mobilization of the cord, the imperfectly descended testis is secured in the contralateral compartment of the scrotum between the septum and the inner side of the normal testis.

ombrophobia (om·bro·**fo**·be·ah). A morbid dread of rain. [Gk *ombros* rain, phobia.]

ombrophore (**om**·bro·for). A portable apparatus for applying hydrotherapy in the form of a douche or shower bath. [Gk *ombros* rain, *pherein* to bear.]

omega melancholium (o·me·gah mel·an·**ko**·le·um). A wrinkling of the skin between the eyebrows in the shape of the Greek small letter omega (ω) believed to indicate a melancholic condition.

omental (o·**ment**·al). Referring to the omentum.

omentectomy (o·ment·**ek**·to·me). The operation of excising a part of the omentum. [omentum, Gk *ektome* a cutting out.]

omentitis (o·ment·**i**·tis). An inflammatory condition affecting the omentum. [omentum, Gk *-itis* inflammation.]

omentocele (o·**ment**·o·seel). Epiplocele. [omentum, *kele* hernia.]

omentofixation (o·**ment**·o·fix·**a**′·shun). Omentopexy. [omentum, fixation.]

omentopexy (o·**ment**·o·pex·e). The operation of suturing the omentum to, or implanting it in the abdominal wall, to obtain drainage of its veins into the latter and thus relieving portal congestion in cirrhosis of the liver or other forms of portal hypertension. [omentum, Gk *pexis* a fixation.]

omentoplasty (o·**ment**·o·plas·te). The use of patches of omentum as grafts, to reinforce suture lines after anastomosis of hollow abdominal viscera or to reinforce the line of closure after repair of a perforated ulcer. [omentum, Gk *plassein* to mould.]

omentorrhaphy (o·ment·**or**·af·e). The operative procedure of suturing the omentum. [omentum, Gk *rhaphe* suture.]

omentosplenopexy (o·**ment**·o·**sple**′·no·pex·e). The combined operations of omentopexy and splenopexy.

omentotomy (o·ment·**ot**·o·me). Incision of the omentum. [omentum, Gk *temnein* to cut.]

omentovolvulus (o·**ment**·o·**vol**′·vew·lus). Omental volvulus or torsion.

omentulum (o·**ment**·ew·lum). The lesser omentum [obsolete term].

omentum (o·**ment**·um). A double layer of peritoneum connecting 2 viscera; usually applied only to those layers which connect the stomach with other viscera. **Gastrocolic omentum.** Greater omentum (see below). **Gastrosplenic omentum.** The double layer of peritoneum which connects the greater curvature of the stomach to the spleen. **Greater omentum [omentum majus (NA)].** The double layer of peritoneum which hangs down from the greater curvature of the stomach and is folded back to enclose the transverse colon. **Lesser omentum [omentum minus (NA)].** The omentum connecting the lesser curvature of the stomach to the liver. [L.]

omentumectomy (o·**ment**·um·**ek**′·to·me). Excision of the omentum. [omentum, Gk *ektome* a cutting out.]

omitis (o·**mi**·tis). Inflammation of the shoulder. [Gk *omos* shoulder, *-itis* inflammation.]

omnipotence (om·**nip**·o·tens). Infinite power. **Omnipotence of thought.** An attitude in the mental life of primitive people and of children, characterized by a belief in the magical power of thoughts and words. [L *omnis* all, *potentia* power.]

omocephalus (o·mo·**kef**·al·us). A fetal monstrosity without arms and with a head that is deficient in some of its parts. [Gk *omos* shoulder, *kephale* head.]

omoclavicular (o·mo·klav·**ik**′·ew·lar). Relating to the shoulder and the clavicle. [Gk *omos* shoulder, clavicle.]

omodynia (o·mo·**din**·e·ah). Pain in the shoulder. [Gk *omos* shoulder, *odyne* pain.]

omohyoid (o·mo·**hi**·oid). 1. Referring to the shoulder and the hyoid bone. 2. The omohyoid muscle. [Gk *omos* shoulder, hyoid.]

omohyoid muscle [musculus omohyoideus (NA)]. A muscle of 2 bellies, the superior (venter superior (NA)] attached to the body of the hyoid bone and the inferior [venter inferior (NA)] to the upper border of the scapula and the suprascapular ligaments. The intermediate tendon attaches by a fascial loop to the inner end of the clavicle and the 1st rib.

omophagia (o·mo·**fa**·je·ah). The eating of raw food, and in particular of raw flesh. [Gk *omos* unripe, *phagein* to eat.]

omosternal (o·mo·**ster**·nal). Referring to the shoulder and the sternum. [Gk *omos* shoulder, sternum.]

omosternum (o·mo·**ster**·num). The layer of fibrocartilage in the sternoclavicular joint. [see prec.]

omotocia (om·o·**to**·se·ah). Premature birth. [Gk *omos* unripe, *tokos* birth.]

omphalectomy (om·fal·**ek**·to·me). Excision of the umbilicus or of any new growth associated with it. [Gk *omphalos* navel, *ektome* a cutting out.]

omphalelcosis (om·fal·el·**ko**′·sis). A disease of the umbilicus characterized by ulceration. [Gk *omphalos* navel, *helkosis* ulceration.]

omphalic (om·**fal**·ik). Referring to the umbilicus. [Gk *omphalos* navel.]

omphalitis (om·fal·**i**·tis). General inflammatory invasion of the umbilicus. [Gk *omphalos* navel, *-itis* inflammation.]

omphalo-angiopagus (**om**·fal·o·an·je·**op**′·ag·us). Omphalosite. [Gk *omphalos* navel, *aggeion* vessel, *pagos* fixed.]

omphalocele (**om**·fal·o·seel). Umbilical hernia. [Gk *omphalos* navel, *kele* hernia.]

omphalochorion (**om**·fal·o·**kor**′·e·on). A composite fetal membrane formed by the close apposition of the yolk sac and chorion in some mammals, e.g. marsupials. [Gk *omphalos* navel, chorion.]

omphalocraniodidymus (**om**·fal·o·**kra**·ne·o·**did**′·im·us). A double monster in which the parasitic twin is joined to the skull of the autosite. [Gk *omphalos* navel, *kranion* skull, *didymos* twin.]

omphalodidymus (**om**·fal·o·**did**′·im·us). Gastrodidymus. [Gk *omphalos* navel, *didymos* twin.]

omphalo-enteric (**om**·fal·o·en·**ter**′·ik). Relating to the umbilicus and the intestine. [Gk *omphalos* navel, *enteron* bowel.]

omphalogenesis (**om**·fal·o·**jen**′·es·is). Development of the umbilicus. [Gk *omphalos* navel, *genesis* origin.]

omphaloma (om·fal·**o**·mah). An umbilical tumour. [Gk *omphalos* navel, *-oma* tumour.]

omphalomesaraic (**om**·fal·o·mes·ar·**a**′·ik). Omphalomesenteric. [Gk *omphalos* navel, *mesaraion* mesentery.]

omphalomesenteric (**om**·fal·o·mes·en·**ter**′·ik). Relating to the umbilicus and to the mesentery. [Gk *omphalos* navel, *mesos* middle, *enteron* bowel.]

omphaloncus (om·fal·**ong**·kus). An umbilical tumour. [Gk *omphalos* navel, *ogkos* a swelling.]

omphalopagus (om·fal·**op**·ag·us). A twin monster united at the umbilicus. [Gk *omphalos* navel, *pagos* fixed.]

omphalophlebitis (**om**·fal·o·fleb·**i**′·tis). A condition of inflammation affecting the umbilical veins. [Gk *omphalos* navel, phlebitis.]

omphaloproptosis (**om**·fal·o·prop·**to'**·sis). Prolapse of the umbilical cord. [Gk *omphalos* navel, proptosis.]

omphalorrhagia (**om**·fal·o·**ra'**·je·ah). Bleeding from the umbilicus. [Gk *omphalos* navel, *rhegnynein* to gush forth.]

omphalorrhexis (**om**·fal·o·**rex'**·is). Rupture of the umbilicus or of the umbilical cord. [Gk *omphalos* navel, *rhexis* rupture.]

omphalorrhoea (**om**·fal·o·**re'**·ah). An escape of lymph from the umbilicus. [Gk *omphalos* navel, *rhoia* flow.]

omphalos (**om**·fal·os). The umbilicus. [Gk navel.]

omphalosite (**om**·fal·o·site). The parasitic member of uni-ovular twins. The parasite derives its blood-supply through the autosite's umbilical cord to which it is joined. [Gk *omphalos* navel, *sitos* food.]

omphalosoter, omphalosotor (**om**·fal·o·**so'**·ter, **om**·fal·o·**so'**·tor). A device for the reinsertion of prolapsed coils of the umbilical cord during childbirth. [Gk *omphalos* navel, *soter* preserver.]

omphalospinous (**om**·fal·o·**spi'**·nus). Belonging to the umbilicus and the anterior superior iliac spine. [Gk *omphalos* navel, spine.]

omphalotaxis (**om**·fal·o·**tax'**·is). Replacement of the prolapsed coils of the umbilical cord. [Gk *omphalos* navel, *taxis* arrangement.]

omphalotome (om·**fal**·o·tome). In the second stage of labour, the instrument used in the division of the umbilical cord. [Gk *omphalos* navel, *temnein* to cut.]

omphalotomy (om·fal·**ot**·o·me). The operation of division of the umbilical cord at the end of the second stage of labour. [see prec.]

omphalotribe (om·**fal**·o·tribe). A surgical instrument for crushing the umbilical cord. [see foll.]

omphalotripsy (**om**·fal·o·**trip'**·se). The crushing of the umbilical cord after childbirth. [Gk *omphalos* navel, *tribein* to grind.]

omphalus (**om**·fal·us). The umbilicus. [Gk *omphalos* navel.]

onanism (o·nan·izm). Masturbation. [*Onan*, son of Judah.]

onanist (o·nan·ist). One who is addicted to or practises onanism.

Onanoff, Jacques (b. 1859). Paris physician.

Onanoff's reflex or sign. Bulbospongiosus reflex; reflex contraction of the bulbospongiosus muscle with retraction of the penis on the squeezing of the glans, it was alleged to occur in schizophrenia.

onaye (o·**nah**·ye). A virulent poison derived from the seeds of *Strophanthus hispidus*. [West African name.]

Onchocerca (ong·ko·**ser**·kah). A genus of filarial worms. **Onchocerca caecutiens.** A species from Central America, now usually considered the same as *Onchocerca volvulus*. **Onchocerca volvulus.** A species common in man in tropical Africa and Central America. The adult females are very long and thread-like and occur in cutaneous fibrous cysts, usually several to a cyst, which may be 25 mm (1 in) across but usually smaller, and commonly localized around joints; in America they are almost entirely confined to the head. The microfilariae migrate in the surface tissues, but not in the blood stream, their migrations causing irritation and severe damage when in the eyes. Secondary hosts are flies of the genera *Eusimulium* and *Simulium*. [Gk *ogkos* a swelling, *kerkos* tail.]

onchocerciasis, onchocercosis (**ong**·ko·ser·**ki'**·as·is, **ong**·ko·ser·**ko'**·sis). The condition caused by infestation with onchocerca.

onchocercoma (**ong**·ko·ser·**ko'**·mah). A mobile, painless nodule, usually on the scalp or on the buttocks, due to onchocerciasis. [*Onchocerca*, Gk *-oma* tumour.]

oncocyte (**ong**·ko·site). One of the cells which form the substance of any neoplasm. Most often used to describe the large pale cells (Huerthle cells) found in thyroiditis. [Gk *ogkos* a swelling, *kytos* cell.]

oncocytoma (**ong**·ko·si·**to'**·mah). An innocent oxyphil cell adenoma of the salivary glands. [Gk *ogkos* a swelling, *kytos* cell, *-oma* tumour.]

oncogenesis (ong·ko·**jen**·es·is). The origin and formation of tumours. [Gk *ogkos* a swelling, *genesis* origin.]

oncogenous (ong·**koj**·en·us). Causing or encouraging the growth of tumours. [Gk *ogkos* a swelling, *genein* to produce.]

oncograph (**ong**·ko·graf). The recording attachment of an oncometer. [Gk *ogkos* a swelling, *graphein* to record.]

oncography (ong·**kog**·raf·e). The graphic representation of the size and configuration of an organ by means of an oncometer. [see prec.]

oncoides (ong·**koid**·eez). Intumescence; turgidity. [Gk *ogkos* a swelling, *eidos* form.]

oncology (ong·**kol**·o·je). The science of new growths. [Gk *ogkos* a swelling, *logos* science.]

oncolysis (ong·**kol**·is·is). The destruction of or disposal by absorption of any neoplastic cells, particularly those of carcinoma. [Gk *ogkos* a swelling, *lysis* a loosing.]

oncolytic (ong·ko·**lit**·ik). Causing the destruction of tumour cells. [see prec.]

oncoma (ong·**ko**·mah). A tumour or intumescence. [Gk *ogkos* a swelling, *-oma* tumour.]

Oncomelania (**ong**·ko·mel·**a'**·ne·ah). A genus of snails several species of which act as intermediary hosts of *Schistosoma japonicum*, e.g. *Oncomelania formosana, O. herpensis* found in the Yangtze valley, *O. nosophora, O. nosophora slateri* and *O. quadrasi* found in the Philippines. **Oncomelania hydrobiosis.** *Oncomelania quadrasi* (see above). [Gk *ogkos* a swelling, *melas* black.]

oncometer (ong·**kom**·et·er). A device used in determining the variations in the size of the spleen, kidney or any other viscus. [Gk *ogkos* a swelling, meter.]

oncometric (ong·ko·**met**·rik). Relating to the oncometer or to oncometry.

oncometry (ong·**kom**·et·re). The determination of the size of any internal organ. [Gk *ogkos* a swelling, meter.]

oncosis (ong·**ko**·sis). The morbid state characterized by the growth of tumours. [Gk *ogkos* a swelling.]

oncosphaera, oncosphere (ong·ko·**sfeer**·ah, **ong**·ko·sfeer). The first larval form of tapeworms; it is minute and spherical, and bears 6 hooks. It develops in the secondary host into a procercoid, a cysticercus or a coenurus, according to the species. [Gk *ogkos* a swelling, *sphaira* sphere.]

oncotherapy (ong·ko·**ther**·ap·e). The treatment of tumours. [Gk *ogkos* a swelling, therapy.]

oncothlipsis (ong·ko·**thlip**·sis). Pressure which is set up in any part because of the presence of a growing tumour. [Gk *ogkos* a swelling, *thlipsis* pressure.]

oncotic (ong·**kot**·ik). Referring to or resulting from the existence of a tumour at any place in the body. [Gk *ogkos* a swelling.]

oncotomy (ong·**kot**·o·me). The procedure of incising a tumour, swelling, cyst or abscess. [Gk *ogkos* a swelling, *temnein* to cut.]

oncotropic (ong·ko·**trop**·ik). Attractive especially to neoplastic cells. [Gk *ogkos* a swelling, *trope* a turning.]

ondometer (on·**dom**·et·er). Any device with which the rate of a high-frequency oscillation may be determined. [Fr. *onde* wave, meter.]

oneiric (on·i·rik). Referring to, or like a dream. [see foll.]

oneirism (on·i·rizm). A dream-like state of consciousness. [Gk *oneiros* dream.]

oneirodynia (on·i·ro·**din'**·e·ah). Nightmare; disturbance of the sleep by abnormal dreams or painful phases. **Oneirodynia activa.** Somnambulism. [Gk *oneiros* dream, *odyne* pain.]

oneirogmus (on·i·**rog**·mus). Dreaming which is accompanied by emission of semen; nocturnal emissions. [Gk *oneiros* dream.]

oneirology (on·i·**rol**·o·je). The study or interpretation of dreams. [Gk *oneiros* dream, *logos* science.]

oneironosus (on·i·**ron**·os·us). Disordered dreaming; distress during sleep as evidence of a morbid mental state. [Gk *oneiros* dream, *nosos* disease.]

oneiroscopy (on·i·**ros**·ko·pe). Diagnosis of the patient's mental condition by investigation of his dreams; dream analysis. [Gk *oneiros* dream, *skopein* to watch.]

oniomania (**o**·ne·o·**ma'**·ne·ah). A mania for buying. [Gk *onios* for sale, mania.]

oniric (on·i·rik). Oneiric.

onirism (on·i·rizm). Oneirism.

onium (**o**·ne·um). 1. Generally, an organic grouping analogous to ammonium, in which an element such as oxygen, phosphorus or sulphur, at its highest valency, is united to a number of hydrogen atoms and to an organic radical, e.g. ROH_3. 2. In particular, the positive ion of ammonium in which the hydrogen atoms are replaced by organic radicals, forming bases of biological importance such as the betaines and cholines.

onkinocele (ong·**kin**·o·seel). A condition of swelling around the synovial sheath of a tendon. [Gk *ogkos* a swelling, *is* fibre, *kele* tumour.]

onobaio (o·no·**ba**·yo). An arrow poison, which acts as a cardiac depressant, used by the natives of Somaliland. [African name.]

onomatology (on·o·mat·**ol**′·o·je). Terminology. [Gk *onoma* name, *logos* science.]

onomatophobia (on·o·mat·o·**fo**′·be·ah). Insane fear of hearing any particular word or name. [Gk *onoma* name, phobia.]

onomatopoiesis (on·o·mat·o·poi·**e**′·sis). The formation of incorrect or senseless words by a mentally deranged person. [Gk *onoma* name, *poiein* to make.]

Ononis (o·**no**·nis). 1. A genus of plants of the family Leguminosae. 2. The root of *Ononis spinosa*. It contains saponins and has a diuretic action. [Gk rest harrow.]

Onthophagus (on·**thof**·ag·us). A genus of dung beetles. *Onthophagus bifasciatus* (from Bengal and Burma) and *O. unifasciatus* (from Sri Lanka and the East Indies) have caused intestinal canthariasis in infants in the tropical Far East. [Gk *onthos* dung, *phagein* to eat.]

ontogenesis (on·to·**jen**·es·is). The origin and evolution of the individual organism. Cf. PHYLOGENESIS. [Gk *ontos* being, *genein* to produce.]

ontogenetic, ontogenic (**on**·to·jen·**et**′·ik, on·to·**jen**·ik). Relating to ontogenesis.

ontogeny (on·**toj**·en·e). Ontogenesis.

onyalai (o·ne·a·la·e). A variety of purpura in natives of Africa. There are blood blisters in the mouth, purpuric rashes in the skin and deficiency in blood thrombocytes. [African name.]

onychalgia (on·ik·**al**·je·ah). A painful condition affecting the nails. **Onychalgia nervosa.** Painful nails without any structural changes. [Gk *onyx* nail, *algos* pain.]

onychatrophia, onychatrophy (on·ik·at·**tro**′·fe·ah, on·ik·**at**·ro·fe). A condition of atrophy affecting the nails. [Gk *onyx* nail, atrophy.]

onychauxis (on·ik·**awx**·is). Overgrowth of the nails of fingers or toes. [Gk *onyx* nail, *auxe* increase.]

onychectomy (on·ik·**ek**·to·me). The act of excising a nail or nail bed. [Gk *onyx* nail, *ektome* a cutting out.]

onychexallaxis (**on**·ik·ex·al·**ax**′·is). A condition of degeneration affecting the nails. [Gk *onyx* nail, *exallassein* to change utterly.]

onychia (on·**ik**·e·ah). Abnormality of the nail or nails, due to inflammation of the matrix. It may be produced by any of the causes which excite inflammation in other regions of the skin, e.g. infection, trauma or the presence of a foreign body. *Onychitis* is a misnomer, for the suffix *-itis* implies that inflammation can occur in the nail itself, but the nail is an avascular appendage. **Onychia craquelé.** Cracked nails. **Onychia maligna.** Destruction of the nail by ulceration of adjacent tissues: gangrene of the nail bed may supervene. **Monilial onychia.** Onychia caused by infection with *Candida albicans*, previously known as *Monilia albicans*. **Onychia parasitica.** Fungous infection of the nails. **Pianic onychia.** Secondary yaws affecting the paronychial region. **Onychia punctata.** Pitted nails. **Onychia sicca.** Literally a dry form of onychia. One form is pachyonychosis, described by Fournier, in which the nail is increased in thickness at the expense of its density so that its substance resembles the pith of a rush. **Onychia superficialis undulata.** Nails with superficial ripples across them. **Syphilitic onychia.** Changes in the nails occurring during the secondary stage of syphilis. *Dry syphilitic onychia* denotes painless nail changes produced by papular infiltrates in the nail fold or matrix. [Gk *onyx* nail.]

onychin (**on**·ik·in). A type of keratin found in the nails. [Gk *onyx* nail.]

onychitis (on·ik·**i**·tis). Onychia. [Gk *onyx* nail, *-itis* inflammation.]

onychoclasis (on·ik·**ok**·las·is). Breaking of the nails. [Gk *onyx* nail, *klasis* a breaking.]

onychocryptosis (**on**·ik·o·krip·**to**′·sis). Ingrowing toe nail. [Gk *onyx* nail, *kryptos* hidden.]

onychodynia (**on**·ik·o·**din**′·e·ah). Onychalgia. [Gk *onyx* nail, *odyne* pain.]

onychodystrophy (**on**·ik·o·**dis**′·tro·fe). Malformation of the nails from impaired nutrition. [Gk *onyx* nail, *dys-* bad, *trophe* nourishment.]

onychogenic (**on**·ik·o·**jen**′·ik). Producing nail tissue. [Gk *onyx* nail, *genein* to produce.]

onychogram (on·**ik**·o·gram). An onychographic record or tracing. [see foll.]

onychograph (on·**ik**·o·graf). An instrument which records the capillary blood pressure as found in the subungual vessels. [Gk *onyx* nail, *graphein* to record.]

onychogryphosis, onychogryposis (**on**·ik·o·grif·**o**′·sis, **on**·ik·o·grip·**o**′·sis). A condition in which the nails are bent or curved over the tips of the fingers or toes. [Gk *onyx* nail, *gryphein* to curve.]

onychohelcosis (**on**·ik·o·hel·**ko**′·sis). Ulceration affecting the nail. [Gk *onyx* nail, *helkosis* ulceration.]

onychoheterotopia (**on**·ik·o·het·er·o·**to**′·pe·ah). Abnormally placed nails. [Gk *onyx* nail, *heteros* other, *topos* place.]

onychoid (**on**·ik·oid). Resembling a finger nail in form, texture or structure. [Gk *onyx* nail, *eidos* form.]

onycholysis (on·ik·**ol**·is·is). Separation of the nail from its bed by an accumulation of cellular debris, without shedding. The condition may be symptomatic of eczema, psoriasis, syphilis, or induced by subungual corns. Idiopathic neurotic cases have been described (Debreuilh); the condition has been noted as an occupational malady in fur-fleshers. **Onycholysis partialis.** Onycholysis affecting only the distal portion of the nail. [Gk *onyx* nail, *lysein* to loosen.]

onychoma (on·ik·**o**·mah). A type of neoplasm which generally has origin in the matrix, and which is characterized by hypertrophy of the nail itself. [Gk *onyx* nail, *-oma* tumour.]

onychomadesis (**on**·ik·o·mad·**e**′·sis). Total loss of the nails, originating at the matrix. [Gk *onyx* nail, *madein* to fall off.]

onychomalacia (**on**·ik·o·mal·**a**′·she·ah). A condition of softening of the finger nails, generally associated with hapalonychia. [Gk *onyx* nail, *malakia* softness.]

onychomycosis (**on**·ik·o·mi·**ko**′·sis). Infection of a nail or nails by a fungus. **Onychomycosis favosa.** Favus of the nails. **Onychomycosis tonsurans.** Ringworm of the nails. **Onychomycosis trichophytica.** Trichophytic infection of the nails. **Onychomycosis trichophytina.** Ringworm of the nails. [Gk *onyx* nail, mycosis.]

onychonosus (on·ik·**on**·o·sus). Onychopathy. [Gk *onyx* nail, *nosos* disease.]

onycho-osteodysplasia (**on**·ik·o·os·te·o·dis·**pla**′·ze·ah). A hereditary condition which presents as a tetrad malformation of the nails, dislocating patellae, elbow dysplasia and presence of iliac horns. It is thought to have a non-sex-linked dominant inheritance. [Gk *onyx* nail, *osteon* bone, dysplasia.]

onychopacity (**on**·ik·o·**pas**′·it·e). Leuconychia. [Gk *onyx* nail, L *opacus* shaded.]

onychopathic (**on**·ik·o·**path**′·ik). Pertaining to or suffering from any diseased condition of the nails. [Gk *onyx* nail, *pathos* disease.]

onychopathology (**on**·ik·o·path·**ol**′·o·je). That branch of pathology which deals with diseases of the nails. [Gk *onyx* nail, pathology.]

onychopathy (on·ik·**op**·ath·e). Any diseased condition of the nails. [Gk *onyx* nail, *pathos* disease.]

onychophagia (**on**·ik·o·**fa**′·je·ah). The practice, of nervous origin, of biting the finger nails. [Gk *onyx* nail, *phagein* to eat.]

onychophagist (on·ik·**of**·aj·ist). An individual who is addicted to nail-biting. [see prec.]

onychophagy (on·ik·**of**·aj·e). Onychophagia.
onychophosis (**on**·ik·o·**fo'**·sis). A growth of horny epithelium underneath the toe nails. [Gk *onyx* nail, *hyphe* tissue, *-osis* condition.]
onychophyma (**on**·ik·o·**fi'**·mah). A condition of thickening or hypertrophy of the nails. [Gk *onyx* nail, *phyma* growth.]
onychoptosis (**on**·ik·op·**to'**·sis). Loosening and shedding of the nails. [Gk *onyx* nail, *ptosis* a falling.]
onychorrhexis (**on**·ik·o·**rex'**·is). Brittleness of the nails associated with splitting at the free border. [Gk *onyx* nail, *rhexis* cleft.]
onychorrhiza (**on**·ik·o·**ri'**·zah). The root of the nail. [Gk *onyx* nail, *rhiza* root.]
onychoschizia (**on**·ik·o·**skitz'**·e·ah). Onycholysis. [Gk *onyx* nail, *schizein* to split.]
onychosis (on·ik·o·sis). An atrophic or dystrophic affection of the nails. Severe dermatoses, e.g. pemphigus, pityriasis rubra pilaris, generalized exfoliative dermatitis, etc. may cause the condition. Atrophic and dystrophic affections of the nails have also been reported in tabes, general paralysis of the insane, syringomyelia and leprosy. *Favic* and *trichophytic onychosis* are due to invasion of the nails by fungi. *Staphylococcal onychosis*, which occurs after much nail-biting, is due to the formation of 1 or more tiny abscesses or pustules under the free border of the nail. *Streptococcal onychosis* is more a perionyxis than an onychosis, and the nail is affected secondarily. [Gk *onyx* nail, *-osis* condition.]
onychostroma (**on**·ik·o·**stro'**·mah). The matrix of the nail. [Gk *onyx* nail, *stroma* mattress.]
onychotillomania (**on**·ik·ot·il·o·**ma'**·ne·ah). Picking of the nails in nervous persons. [Gk *onyx* nail, *tillein* to pluck, *mania* madness.]
onychotomy (on·ik·**ot**·o·me). Incision of a nail. [Gk *onyx* nail, *temnein* to cut.]
onychotrophy (on·ik·**ot**·ro·fe). Nutrition of the nails. [Gk *onyx* nail, *trophe* nutrition.]
onychyphosis (**on**·ik·i·**fo'**·sis). Onychophosis.
onym (**on**·im). Any technical term. [Gk *onyma* name.]
o'nyong nyong (o·ne·**yong** ne·**yong**). A Central African infectious disease due to a group A arbovirus transmitted by anopheline mosquitoes. The clinical features include fever, lymphadenitis, excruciating joint pains and a maculopapular rash. [Ugandan dialect, joint breaker.]
onyx (**on**·ix). A nail of the finger or of the toe. [Gk nail.]
onyxis (on·**ix**·is). An incurving or ingrowing nail. [Gk *onyx* nail.]
onyxitis (on·ix·**i**·tis). Inflammation affecting the nail bed. [Gk *onyx* nail, *-itis* inflammation.]
oöblast (**o**·o·blast). A primitive sexual cell from which the ovum is developed. [Gk *oon* egg, *blastos* germ.]
oöcentre (o·o·sen·ter). Ovocentre; the centrosome of the ovum during the period of fertilization. [Gk *oon* egg, centre.]
oöcephalus (o·o·**kef**·al·us). A monster with an egg-shaped or triangular head. [Gk *oon* egg, *kephale* head.]
oöcyesis (**o**·o·si·**e'**·sis). Ovarian pregnancy. *See* PREGNANCY. [Gk *oon* egg, *kyesis* pregnancy.]
oöcyst (o·o·sist). The cyst which develops in the wall of the stomach of the mosquito when the oökinete comes to rest. [Gk *oon* egg, *kystis* bladder.]
oöcytase (o·o·**si**·taze). A cytase that has a destructive action on ovarian cells. [Gk *oon* egg, cytase.]
oöcyte (o·o·site). The immature ovum or egg cell, at a stage intermediate between the primordial ovum or oögonium, and the ripe ovum ready for fertilization. The primary oöcyte contains the full diploid number of chromosomes (e.g. 48 in man), and undergoes meiotic division to give rise to a secondary oöcyte and a first polar body, each with the haploid number of chromosomes (e.g. 24 in man). The secondary oöcyte in turn divides by a modified mitotic division into the mature ovum and a second polar body, each of which possesses the haploid number of chromosomes. [Gk *oon* egg, *kytos* cell.]
oödeocele (o·o·de·o·seel). Obturator hernia. *See* HERNIA. [Gk *oodes* egg-shaped, *kele* hernia.]

oögamous (o·o·gam·us). Propagating by the union of dissimilar male and female sex cells. [see foll.]
oögamy (o·o·gam·e). The process of union of dissimilar male and female sex cells. [Gk *oon* egg, *gamos* marriage.]
oögenesis (o·o·**jen**·es·is). The formation and development of the ovum. [Gk *oon* egg, *genesis* origin.]
oögenetic (**o**·o·jen·**et'**·ik). Pertaining to oögenesis.
oögenous (o·**oj**·en·us). Egg-forming. [Gk *oon* egg, *genein* to produce.]
oögonium (o·o·**go**·ne·um). 1. The primordial ovum, before maturation begins. 2. The female organ in some of the lower fungi which gives rise to one or more oöspheres (egg cells). [Gk *oon* egg, *gonos* offspring.]
oökinesis (o·o·kin·**e'**·sis). The movements of the nuclear material and achromatic spindle during maturation and fertilization of the ovum. [Gk *oon* egg, *kinesis* movement.]
oökinete (o·o·**kin**·eet). The "travelling" vermicule; the motile pear-shaped organism formed when the male microgamete of the malaria parasite fertilizes the female macrogamete. [Gk *oon* egg, *kinein* to move.]
oölemma (o·o·**lem**·ah). The zona striata. [Gk *oon* egg, *lemma* sheath.]
oöphagia, oöphagy (o·o·**fa**·je·ah, o·**of**·aj·e). The eating of eggs; the condition in which eggs make up the major portion of the food. [Gk *oon* egg, *phagein* to eat.]
oöphoralgia (**o**·of·or·**al'**·je·ah). Pain affecting the ovary. [Gk *oophoron* ovary, *algos* pain.]
oöphorauxe (**o**·of·or·**awx'**·e). Hypertrophy of the ovary. [Gk *oophoron* ovary, *auxe* increase.]
oöphorectomy (**o**·of·or·**ek'**·to·me). Excision of an ovary. [Gk *oophoron* ovary, *ektome* a cutting out.]
oöphoritis (o·of·or·**i'**·tis). Inflammation affecting an ovary. **Oöphoritis parotidea.** Oöphoritis preceding or occurring as the only evidence of epidemic parotitis. **Oöphoritis serosa.** An oedematous condition of the ovary. [Gk *oophoron* ovary, *-itis* inflammation.]
oöphorocystectomy (o·**of**·or·o·sist·**ek'**·to·me). The excision of an ovarian cyst. [Gk *oophoron* ovary, cystectomy.]
oöphorocystosis (o·**of**·or·o·sist·**o'**·sis). The formation and development of ovarian cysts. [Gk *oophoron* ovary, *kystis* bag, *-osis* condition.]
oöphoro-epilepsy (o·**of**·or·o·ep·il·**ep'**·se). Epilepsy caused by ovarian disease or disorder. [Gk *oophoron* ovary, epilepsy.]
oöphorogenous (**o**·of·or·**oj'**·en·us). Originating in the ovary. [Gk *oophoron* ovary, *genein* to produce.]
oöphorohysterectomy (**o**·of·or·o·his·ter·**ek'**·to·me). Excision of the uterus and ovaries. [Gk *oophoron* ovary, *hystera* womb, *ektome* a cutting out.]
oöphoroma (**o**·of·or·**o'**·mah). A rare ovarian tumour of middle age arising most likely from coelomic epithelial derivatives within the ovary. **Oöphoroma folliculare.** Brenner tumour. [Gk *oophoron* ovary, *-oma* tumour.]
oöphoromalacia (o·**of**·or·o·mal·**a'**·she·ah). Softening of the ovary, generally pathological in type. [Gk *oophoron* ovary, *malakia* softness.]
oöphoromania (o·**of**·or·o·**ma'**·ne·ah). Insanity arising as a sequel to some disorder of the ovary. [Gk *oophoron* ovary, mania.]
oöphoron (o·**of**·or·on). An ovary. [Gk *oon* egg, *pherein* to bear.]
oöphoropathia, oöphoropathy (o·**of**·or·o·**path'**·e·ah, o·of·or·**op'**·ath·e). Any diseased condition of an ovary or ovaries. [Gk *oophoron* ovary, *pathos* disease.]
oöphoropexy (o·**of**·or·o·pex·e). The operation in which the uterine tubes and ovaries are raised and sutured to the abdominal wall. [Gk *oophoron* ovary, *pexis* a fixation.]
oöphororrhaphy (**o**·of·or·**or'**·af·e). Suture of an ovary to the wall of the pelvis. [Gk *oophoron* ovary, *rhaphe* suture.]
oöphorosalpingectomy (o·**of**·or·o·sal·pin·**jek'**·to·me). Excision of an ovary and the uterine tube. [Gk *oophoron* ovary, salpingectomy.]
oöphorosalpingitis (o·**of**·or·o·sal·pin·**ji'**·tis). Inflammation of an ovary and the uterine tube. [Gk *oophoron* ovary, salpingitis.]

oöphorostomy (o·of·or·**os**′·to·me). The creation of an opening into an ovarian cyst in order to drain the contents. [Gk *oophoron* ovary, *stoma* mouth.]

oöphorotomy (o·of·or·**ot**′·o·me). Surgical incision of an ovary. [Gk *oophoron* ovary, *temnein* to cut.]

oöphorrhagia (o·of·or·**a**′·je·ah). Severe haemorrhage at the site of ovulation. [Gk *oophoron* ovary, *rhegnynein* to gush forth.]

oöphorrhaphy (o·of·**or**·af·e). Fixation of a prolapsed ovary by suturing the hilum to the slackened infundibulopelvic ligaments. [Gk *oophoron* ovary, *rhaphe* suture.]

oöplasm, oöplasma (o·o·plazm, o·o·**plaz**·mah). The yolk of an ovum. [Gk *oon* egg, *plasma* something formed.]

oöporphyrin (o·o·**por**·fir·in). Protoporphyrin. [Obsolete term.] [Gk *oon* egg, porphyrin.]

oösperm (o·o·sperm). A fertilized ovum; a zygote. [Gk *oon* egg, *sperma* seed.]

oösphere (o·o·sfeer). An egg cell. [Gk *oon* egg, *sphaira* sphere.]

Oöspora (o·**os**·po·rah). Generic name for several unrelated organisms [obsolete term]. **Oöspora minutissimum.** *Corynebacterium minutissimum*, the agent of erythrasma. **Oöspora tozeuri.** *Madurella mycetomi*, a cause of black-grain mycetoma. [Gk *oon* egg, *sporos* seed.]

oöspore (o·o·spore). A general term for a spore formed by the union of two sexually opposite elements. [see prec.]

oötheca (o·o·**the**·kah). An ovary. [Gk *oon* egg, *theke* case.]

oöthecalgia (o·o·the·**kal**′·je·ah). Oöphoralgia. [oötheca, Gk *algos* pain.]

oöthecitis (o·o·the·**si**′·tis). Oöphoritis. [oötheca, Gk *-itis* inflammation.]

oöthecocele (o·o·**the**·ko·seel). Ovariocele. [oötheca, Gk *kele* hernia.]

oöthecocentesis (o·o·**the**·ko·sen·**te**′·sis). Ovariocentesis. [oötheca, Gk *kentein* to stab.]

oöthecocyesis (o·o·**the**·ko·si·**e**′·sis). Ovarian pregnancy. *See* PREGNANCY. [oötheca, cyesis.]

oöthecocystosis (o·o·**the**·ko·sist·**o**′·sis). Oöphorocystosis. [oötheca, Gk *kystis* bag, *-osis* condition.]

oöthecohysterectomy (o·o·**the**·ko·his·ter·**ek**′·to·me). Oöphorohysterectomy. [oötheca, hysterectomy.]

oöthecoma (o·o·the·**ko**′·mah). An ovarian tumour. [oötheca, Gk *-oma* tumour.]

oöthecomania (o·o·the·ko·**ma**′·ne·ah). Oöphoromania. [oötheca, mania.]

oöthecopathy (o·o·the·**kop**′·ath·e). Oöphoropathy. [oötheca, Gk *pathos* disease.]

oöthecopexy (o·o·**the**·ko·pex·e). Oöphoropexy. [oötheca, Gk *pexis* fixation.]

oöthecosalpingectomy (o·o·**the**·ko·sal·ping·**jek**′·to·me). Oöphorosalpingectomy. [oötheca, salpingectomy.]

oöthectomy (o·o·**thek**·to·me). Oöphorectomy. [oötheca, Gk *ektome* a cutting out.]

oötherapy (o·o·**ther**·ap·e). The treatment of disease by means of ovarian material or extracts. [Gk *oon* egg, therapy.]

oötid (o·o·tid). The ripe ovum formed by the division of a secondary oöcyte. [Gk *oon* egg.]

oötype (o·o·tipe). A gland in flukes, concerned with the formation of shell for the fertilized egg. [Gk *oon* egg, *typos* impression.]

opacification (o·**pas**·if·ik·**a**′·shun). The process of becoming opaque; term used of the cornea or lens. [opaque, L *facere* to make.]

opacity (o·**pas**·it·e). 1. The quality or condition of being opaque. 2. An opaque or non-transparent area or spot. **Band-shaped opacity.** A degenerative condition of the cornea in which a band of opacity grows across the centre of the cornea in the position of the palpebral aperture; it is seen in long-standing iridocyclitis, and as a primary condition in old people. Also called *band keratitis.* [L *opacitas* shadiness.]

See also: CASPAR, HAAB.

opalescent (o·pal·**es**·ent). Iridescent; exhibiting a display of colours like that of an opal.

opalgia (op·**al**·je·ah). Facial neuralgia. [Gk *ops* face, *algos* pain.]

opaline (o·pal·ine). Like opal in appearance; opalescent. [L *opalus* opal.]

opaque (o·**pake**). 1. Applied to any substance that will not allow electromagnetic vibrations (e.g. light, x-rays) or other wave motion (e.g. sound) to pass through it. 2. In the case of light, non-transparent and non-translucent. [L *opacus* obscure.]

opeidoscope (op·i·do·skope). A device consisting of a tube with a delicate flexible membrane and mirror attachment, stretched across one end of the tube; by means of rays reflected from the mirror the vibrations of the voice can be demonstrated on a screen. [Gk *ops* voice, *eidos* form, *skopein* to watch.]

open (o·pen). 1. Of a wound, one exposed to the air; unprotected by skin or mucous membrane. 2. Of an infection, one in which there is a lesion that has direct access to the surface and is therefore contaminating the air with micro-organisms, e.g. in pulmonary tuberculosis. 3. Of an electrical circuit, one which is broken, so that the current is unable to pass. [AS.]

opening (o·pen·ing). An aperture. **Aortic opening.** The opening in the posterior part of the diaphragm through which the aorta passes from the thorax into the abdomen, accompanied by the vena azygos and the thoracic duct. **Openings in the diaphragm.** *See* DIAPHRAGM. **Oesophageal opening.** The opening in the diaphragm through which the oesophagus passes from the thorax into the abdomen, accompanied by the two vagi. **Orbital opening [aditus orbitae (NA)].** The roughly quadrangular opening on the bony face, which forms the base of the pyramidal orbital cavity. **Saphenous opening.** *See* FASCIA LATA. **Vena-caval opening.** The opening in the central tendon of the diaphragm through which the inferior vena cava passes from the abdomen to the thorax. [AS *open.*]

operability (op·er·ab·**il**′·it·e). The degree in which a condition is suitable for operation. [L *operari* to work.]

operable (**op**·er·abl). Term applied to a condition in which surgical intervention is justifiable; not beyond surgical relief. [see prec.]

operation (op·er·**a**·shun). 1. Surgical intervention upon a part of the body, usually performed with the use of instruments. 2. The mode of action of a drug. **Abdomino-anal operation.** An operation in which the distal colon and proximal part of the rectum are removed, the colon being anastomosed to the rectal stump to restore bowel continuity. **Banding operation.** Creation of a partial obstruction by a band around the main pulmonary artery in cases of left to right shunt. **Buttonhole operation.** A small counter-opening into an organ or cavity usually employed for the introduction of a drainage tube. **By-pass operation.** The formation of an alternative channel in the arterial system or the alimentary canal. **Celsian operation.** 1. Perineal lithotomy. 2. Excision of epithelioma of the lip by a V-shaped incision. 3. Circular amputation. **Cinch operation.** O'Connor's operation (1st def.). **Commando operation.** Excision *en bloc* of the cervical lymph nodes and the associated primary carcinoma. **Cosmetic operation.** An operation intended to improve the appearance of a feature or part of the body. **Decompression operation.** Any surgical operation on the skull that is designed to relieve pressure within the skull. **Equilibrating operation.** Tenotomy recession or myectomy of the antagonist of the paralysed muscle. **Fenestration operation.** The operation for the relief of deafness resulting from otosclerosis. A fenestra or window is made into the horizontal canal. First performed by Sourdille. **Flap operation.** Amputation with the formation of a flap so cut as to cover the stump when sutured. **Four-point operation.** Fuchs' operation (3rd def.). **Indian operation.** Rhinoplasty. **Interposition operation.** Watkins' operation. **Interval operation.** The removal of the appendix in an interval between acute attacks. **Italian operation.** The formation of an artificial nose by a skin flap from the arm. **Magnet operation.** The removal of fragments of steel or iron from the eye with a powerful magnet. **Major operation.** A surgical operation which carries risk to life. **Manchester operation.** Amputation of the cervix, anterior colporrhaphy and posterior colpoperineorrhaphy, for the treatment of uterovaginal prolapse. **Mastoid operation.** An operation on the tympanic antrum and middle ear for the relief of suppuration. Many types are described: the more limited drains the mastoid antrum and air cells; the radical operation drains the whole of the middle-ear cleft. Intermediate operations of many kinds have been described. **Minor operation.** An operation which carries no risk to life. **Open operation.** An operation performed through an open wound. **Palliative operation.** An operation to relieve symptoms without hope of cure. **Plastic operation.** An operation dependent upon the transposition of skin or other tissue. **Radical operation.** One which is intended to extirpate disease, usually malignant disease, completely. **Shelf operation.** Reconstruction arthroplasty of the hip where a shelf is turned from the ilium over the femoral head. **Subcutaneous operation.** An operation performed through a stab incision. **Surgical operation.** Any manipulation for the relief of disease or deformity, usually carrying the implication of instrumental intervention. **Tagliacotian operation.** A plastic operation on the nose. **Three-snip operation,** for epithora due to a small or closed lower punctum lacrimale. The punctum is dilated and one short snip is made with scissors vertically downwards from the punctum. The second snip is longer and made horizontally along the canaliculus towards the sac. The third snip completes the triangle, so removing part of the inner wall of the canaliculus and allowing drainage. **V-Y operation.** A method of direct advancement of soft tissues whereby after a V-shaped incision and the liberation of the tissue inside the limbs of the V, it is sewn up in the form of a Y. The amount of advancement is equal to the length of the stem of the Y. **Z-plasty operation.** A principle of rearrangement of skin tensions by making a Z-shaped incision and transposing the flaps thus formed. It is widely used in the treatment of contracted scars, webs and bands. [L *operari* to work.]

See also: ABBE, ABERNETHY, ADAMS (SIR WILLIAM), ADAMS (W.), ADELMANN, ADSON, ALBEE, ALBERT (E.), ALDRIDGE, ALLARTON, ALLINGHAM, ALOUETTE, AMMON, AMUSSAT, ANAGNOSTAKIS, ANDERSON (R.), ANDREWS, ANEL, ANNANDALE, ANTYLLUS, ARGYLL ROBERTSON, ARLT, ASCH, ASSALINI, AXENFELD, BABCOCK (W. W.), BACELLI, BACON, BALDWIN, BALDY, BALFOUR (D. C.), BALL, BALLANCE, BANKART, BARASTY, BARDENHEUER, BARKAN, BARKER (A. E. J.), BARRAQUER (I.), BARTON, BARWELL, BASSET, BASSINI, BATTLE, BAYER, BEER, BELFIELD, BENNETT (E. H.), BERENS, BERGENHEM, BERGER (P.), BERGMANN (E.), BEVAN, BIER, BIGELOW, BILLROTH, BLAIR, BLAKEMORE, BLALOCK, BLASIUS, BLASKOVICS, BLOODGOOD, BOARI, BOBBS, BOGUE, BORTHEN, BOSSALINO, BOTTINI, BOUCHERON, BOWMAN, BRAILEY, BRAQUEHAYE, BRASDOR, BRAUER, BRITTAIN, BROCK, BROCKMAN, BROPHY, BROWN (J. B.), BROWNE (D.), BRUNSCHWIG, BRYANT, BUCHANAN, BURCKHARDT, BUROW, BUTLIN, CALDWELL (G. W.), CALOT, CAMPBELL (W. C. C.), CARDEN, CARNOCHAN, CARPUE, CARTER (W. W.), CHARRIÈRE, CHAVASSE, CHEEVER, CHESELDEN, CHEYNE (W. W.), CHIARI, CHIBRET, CHIENE, CHOPART, CIVIALE, CLARK, COAKLEY, COCK, CODIVILLA, COFFEY (R. C.), COLONNA, COOPER (A. P.), CORDONNIER, CORRADI, COTTE, COTTING, COWELL, CRAFOORD, CRILE, CRITCHETT, CRUISE, CUSHING (HARVEY W.), CUTLER (N. L.), CZERMAK (W.), CZERNY (V.), DANA, DANDY, DAVAT, DAVIEL, DAVIES-COLLEY, D'AZYR, DE LAPERSONNE, DELBET (P. L. E.), DE LIMA, DÉLORME, DENIG, DENKER, DENONVILLIERS, DESAULT, DESMARRES, DICKEY (C. A.), DIEFFENBACH, DIMITRY, DIMMER, DITTEL, DOLBEAU, DONALD, DOPPLER (K.), DOYEN, DRAGSTEDT, DRUMMOND (D.), DUDLEY, DUEHRSSEN, DUNN, DUPLAY, DUPUY-DUTEMPS, DUPUYTREN, DUVAL (P.), EDEBOHLS, EKEHORN, ELLIOT (R. H.), ELY, EMMET, ESMARCH, ESTLANDER, EVERBUSCH, EWING, FARABEUF, FENTON, FERGUSSON, FINNEY, FINZI, FLAJANI, FLARER, FOERSTER (O.), FOERSTER (R.), FOLEY, FOTHERGILL (W. E.), FOWLER (G. R.), FRANCO, FRANK (R.), FREDET, FREUND, FREYER, FRICKE, FRIEDRICH, FROST, FUCHS (E.), FULLER, GABRIEL, GALEZOWSKI, GALLIE, GANT (F. J.), GAZA, GENSOUL, GERDY, GIFFORD, GIGLI, GILL, GILLESPIE, GILLIAM, GILLIES, GIRDLESTONE, GLUECK, GOLDSTEIN, GONIN, GRABER-DUVERNAY, GRAEFE, GREEN, GREEN-ARMYTAGE, GREEVES, GRIMSON, GRITTI, GROSS (R. E.), GROSS (S. W.), GUÉRIN (A. F. M.), GUYON, HACKER, HAGNER, HALSTED, HANCOCK, HANDLEY (R. S.), HARMER, HARRIS (S. H.), HARTLEY, HARTMANN (H.), HASNER, HAYNES, HEATH, HEINE (L.), HEINEKE, HELLER (E.), HERBERT, HESS (C.), HEY (W.), HEY (W. H.), HIBBS, HILTON, HIMLY, HIPPEL, HIRSCHBERG (J.), HOCHENEGG, HOFFA, HOLMES (T.), HOLTH, HORSLEY, HOTZ, HOWARTH, HUGHES (W. L.), HUGUIER, HUMMELSHEIM, HUNT (H. L.), HUNTER (J.), IMRE, JABOULAY, JACOBAEUS, JACOBSON (J.), JAEGER (E. R. J.), JAESCHE, JANEWAY (H. H.), JANSEN (A.), JARVIS, JIANU, JOBERT, JONAS (A. F.), JONES (T. W.), JONNESCO, KADER, KEEGAN, KEETLEY, KEHRER (F. ADOLPH), KELLER (W. L.), KELLY (H. A.), KELLY (J. D.), KEY (C. A.), KILLIAN, KING (B. T.), KING (J. E. J.), KIRMISSON, KNAPP, KOCHER, KOENIG (FRANZ), KOERTE, KONDOLEON, KORTZEBORN, KRASKE, KRAUSE (F. V.), KORENLEIN, KUECHLER, KUESTER, KUHNT, LAGRANGE, LAHEY, LAMBERT (V. F.), LAMBRINUDI, LANDOLT, LANE (W. A.), LANG, LANGE (F.), LANGENBECK (B. R. K.), LANNELONGUE, LANZ, LARREY, LATZKO, LAURENS, LeFORT, LEMPERT (J.), LENNANDER, LERICHE, LIMBERG, LISFRANC, LISTON, LITTLE (W. J.), LITTRÉ, LIZARS, LONGMIRE, LORD, LORENZ, LOSSEN, LOTHEISSEN, LOWSLEY, LUC, LUDLOFF, LUND, McBURNEY, McDOWELL, MacEWEN, McGILL, MACHEK, MACKENRODT, McMURRAY, McREYNOLDS, MAISONNEUVE, MAKKAS, MALGAIGNE, MARIANO, MARTIN (H. A.), MARWEDEL, MATAS, MAUNOIR, MAUNSELL, MAYDL, MAYO (C. H.), MAYO (W. J.), MEEK, MELLER, MERCIER, MIKULICZ-RADECKI, MILES, MILLIN, MIRAULT, MOORE (C. H.), MORESTIN, MORISON, MORTON (T. G.), MOSCHCOWITZ (A. V.), MOSHER, MOTAIS, MOURE, MUELLER (L.), MULES, NAFFZIGER, NARATH, NÉLATON, NEUBER, NEWMAN, NICOLA, NICOLADONI, NOYES, NUEL, OBER, O'CONNOR, O'DWYER, OETTINGER, OGSTON, OMBRÉDANNE, O'SHAUGHNESSY, OTIS, OUSILLEAU, PACI, PAGENSTECHER, PANAS, PANCOAST (J.), PARINAUD, PARKER (W.), PASSAVANT, PAUL (F. T.), PEER, PENFIELD, PÉRIER, PETER (L. C.), PETERS (G. A.), PETERSEN, PETIT (F. P.), PHELPS, PIROGOFF, POLITZER, PÓLYA, POMEROY, PONCET, PORRO, POTT, PRAUN, PRIBRAM, PRINCE, PUUSSEPP, QUÉNU, RAMSDEN, RAMSTEDT, RANSOHOFF, RECLUS, REESE, REVERDIN, RICHET, RICHTER (A. G.), RIEDEL, RIGAUD, ROBERTS (J. E. H.), ROBERTS (P. W.), ROBERTS (S. E.), RODGERS, RODMAN, ROLLET (E.), ROSE (W.), ROUGE, ROUX (C.), ROUX (J.), ROVSING, ROYLE, RYDYGIER, SAEMISCH, SAYRE, SCARPA, SCHAUTA, SCHEDE, SCHOEMAKER, SCHUCHARDT, SCHUELLER (K. H. A. L. M.), SCHWARTZE, SEMB, SENN (E. J.), SHAMBAUGH, SIMPSON (J. Y.), SIMS, SISTRUNK, SLUDER, SMITH (F.), SMITH (H.), SMITH-PETERSEN, SMITHWICK, SNELLEN, SOCIN, SOERENSEN, SOURDILLE, SPAETH, SPERINO, SPIVACK, SSABANEJEW, STACKE, STALLARD, STAMM, STEINACH, STEINDLER, STELLWAG von CARION, STEVENS (G. T.), STOFFEL, STOKES (SIR WILLIAM), STOLTZ, STREATFIELD, STROMEYER, SURMAY, SWENSON, SYME, SZYMANOWSKI, TAGLIACOZZI, TAIT, TALMA, TANSINI, TANSLEY, TAPIA, TAYLOR (C. B.), TEALE, TERSON, THIERSCH, THOMPSON (G. J.), THOMSON-WALKER, TODD (F. C.), TOREK, TORKILDSEN, TOTI, TOUROFF, TRAINOR, TRAVERS, TRENDELENBURG, TREVES, TRIPIER, TROTTER, TUFFIER, URBAN, VAN BUREN, VAN HOOK, VAN MILLIGAN, VEAU, VERHOEFF, VIDAL (A. T.), VLADIMIROFF, VOGT (A.), VOLKMANN (R.), VORONOFF, WAGNER (W.), WANGENSTEEN, WARDILL, WARDROP, WARREN, WATERS (E. G.), WATKINS (T. J.), WATSON (T. A.), WATSON (W. S.), WEBER (A.), WEBSTER, WECKER, WEIR (R. F.), WENZEL (M. J. B.), WERTHEIM, WEST (J. M.), WHEELER, WHEELHOUSE, WHIPPLE (A. O.), WHITE (J. W.), WHITEHEAD (W.), WHITMAN, WICKERKIEWICZ, WIEIVERSAVER, WILDE, WILLIAMS (H. W.), WILMS, WINIWARTER, WITZEL, WOELFLER, WOLFE, WOOD (J.), WOODMAN, WORTH, WRIGHT (J. W.), WYETH, YANKAUER, YOUNG (H. H.), ZIEGLER.

operative (op·er·at·iv). 1. Having effect; having the power of acting. 2. Pertaining to an operation. [L *operari* to work.]

operator (op·er·a·tor). 1. One who operates, e.g. one who carries out a surgical or dental operation, or one who works a machine or device. 2. In molecular genetics, indicating that proximal region of an operon to which a protein repressor specifically attaches, thus blocking the transcription and expression of the genes of the operon. [see prec.]

opercle (o·**per**·kl). Operculum.

opercular (o·**per**·kew·lar). Relating to an operculum; constructed in order to function in closing an aperture. **Opercular epilepsy.**

These seizures comprise excessive salivation with masticatory movements and clouding of consciousness, sometimes preceded by a hallucination of taste or a general somatic sensation.

operculate, operculated (o·**per**·kew·late, o·**per**·kew·la·ted). Having an operculum.

operculum (o·**per**·kew·lum) (pl. *opercula*). 1. A plug of mucus found in the cervical canal of a pregnant woman. 2. The parts of the cerebral hemisphere overlapping the insula and forming the boundaries of that region of the lateral sulcus. **Frontal operculum [operculum frontale (NA)].** The portion of the superior boundary of the lateral sulcus between the two anterior rami. **Frontoparietal operculum [operculum frontoparietale (NA)].** The portion of the superior boundary of the lateral sulcus behind the horizontal ascending ramus which overlies the insula. **Orbital operculum.** The portion of the superior boundary of the lateral sulcus in front of the anterior horizontal ramus. **Temporal operculum [operculum temporale (NA)].** The portion of the inferior boundary of the lateral sulcus which overlies the insula. **Trophoblastic operculum.** The trophoblastic cells which close the gap in the uterine epithelium after embedding of the ovum. [L cover.]

See also: ARNOLD (F.), BURDACH.

operon (**op**·er·on). A unit of genetic transcription comprising adjacent structural genes and a promotor region at one end, where the transcription of the structural genes into messenger RNA begins. In negative regulatory systems, transcription is controlled by a cytoplasmic repressor with specific affinity for an operator region lying between promotor and structural genes. [L *operari* to work.]

ophiasis (o·**fi**·as·is). Alopecia areata at the margin of the scalp, giving a serpentine hair outline. [Gk *ophis* snake.]

Ophidia (o·**fid**·e·ah). A sub-order of the reptile order Suamata. It contains all snakes. [Gk *ophidion* small snake.]

ophidiasis (o·fid·i′·as·is). Ophidism.

ophidic (o·**fid**·ik). Referring to, produced, or caused by snakes. [Gk *ophidion* small snake.]

ophidiophilia (o·**fid**·e·o·**fil**′·e·ah). A morbid affection for snakes. [Gk *ophidion* small snake, *philein* to love.]

ophidiophobia (o·**fid**·e·o·**fo**′·be·ah). An abnormal fear of snakes. [Gk *ophidion* small snake, phobia.]

ophidism (o·fid·izm). Poisoning by snake venom. [Gk *ophidion* small snake.]

Ophiophagus (o·fe·**of**·ag·us). A genus of elapine snakes. *Ophiophagus elaps* is another name for *Naia hannah* (*bungarus*), the king cobra. [Gk *ophis* snake, *phagein* to eat.]

ophiophobe (o·fe·o·phobe). One who has a morbid fear of snakes. [Gk *ophis* snake, phobia.]

ophiotoxaemia (o·fe·o·tox·**e**′·me·ah). Toxaemia caused by poisoning with snake venom. [Gk *ophis* snake, toxaemia.]

ophiotoxin (o·fe·o·**tox**′·in). The poison present in snake venom, especially the venom of the cobra. [Gk *ophis* snake, toxin.]

ophritis, ophryitis (of·**ri**·tis, of·re·i·tis). Dermatitis affecting the region of the eyebrow. [Gk *ophrys* eyebrows, *-itis* inflammation.]

ophryo-alveolo-auricular (of·re·o·al·**ve**·o·lo·aw·**rik**′·ew·lar). Term used to denote the angle formed by lines drawn between the ophryon and the alveolar and auricular points.

ophryoiniac (of·re·o·**in**′·e·ak). Relating to the ophryon and the inion.

ophryon (**of**·re·on). In craniology the juncture of the median line of the face with a line drawn from the upper margin of one orbit to another (transverse supra-orbital line). [Gk *ophrys* eyebrow.]

ophryosis (of·re·o·sis). Spasmodic contraction of the eyebrows. [Gk *ophrys* eyebrow, *-osis* condition.]

ophryphtheiriasis (**of**·rif·thi·**ri**′·as·is). Pediculosis affecting the eyelashes and eyebrows. [Gk *ophrys* eyebrow, *phtheiriosis* pediculosis.]

ophrys (**of**·ris). The eyebrow. [Gk.]

ophrytic (of·**rit**·ik). Referring to the eyebrow. [see prec.]

ophthalmagra (of·thal·**mag**·rah). Sudden pain experienced in the eye. [Gk *ophthalmos* eye, *agra* seizure.]

ophthalmalgia (of·thal·**mal**·je·ah). Neuralgic pain affecting the eyeballs. [Gk *ophthalmos* eye, *algos* pain.]

ophthalmatrophia, ophthalmatrophy (of·**thal**·mat·**ro**′·fe·ah, of·thal·**mat**·ro·fe). Atrophy of the eyeball. [Gk *ophthalmos* eye, atrophy.]

ophthalmecchymosis (**of**·thal·mek·e·**mo**′·sis). Effusion of blood into the conjunctiva. [Gk *ophthalmos* eye, ecchymosis.]

ophthalmectomy (of·thal·**mek**·to·me). Enucleation of the whole eyeball by surgical operation. [Gk *ophthalmos* eye, *ektome* a cutting out.]

ophthalmencephalon (**of**·thal·men·**kef**′·al·on). The thalamus [Obsolete term]; it may sometimes be applied to those parts of the brain surrounding the 3rd ventricle. [Gk *ophthalmos* eye, *egkephalon* brain.]

ophthalmia (of·**thal**·me·ah). A term usually applied to conjunctivitis, but sometimes used loosely for inflammation of the whole eye, e.g. sympathetic ophthalmia. **Actinic-ray ophthalmia.** Electric ophthalmia (see below). **Catarrhal ophthalmia.** Catarrhal inflammation of the conjunctiva. **Caterpillar ophthalmia, Caterpillar-hair ophthalmia.** Inflammation due to the lodgement of caterpillar hairs in the conjunctiva, characterized by the presence of a number of greyish or yellowish semitransparent nodules. **Ophthalmia eczematosa.** Phlyctenular ophthalmia (see below). **Egyptian ophthalmia.** Trachoma, but sometimes applied loosely to include all forms of conjunctivitis occurring in crowded barracks, assuming epidemic form and pursuing a more or less chronic course. **Electric ophthalmia, Flash ophthalmia.** A type of photo-ophthalmia caused by exposure of the unprotected eyes to an electric flash or to a naked arc light. It is due mainly to ultraviolet rays, though infrared and luminous rays also play a part. Characterized by hyperaemia, photophobia, blepharospasm and chemosis. **Gonorrhoeal ophthalmia.** A severe form of conjunctivitis due to gonococcal infection (60 per cent of cases of ophthalmia neonatorum are gonococcal). It was a common cause of blindness owing to corneal complications, before the antibiotics were discovered. **Granular ophthalmia.** Trachoma. **Jequirity ophthalmia.** Violent inflammation of the eye following painting of the everted lids with infusion of jequirity, a procedure which used to be employed for the treatment of trachomatous pannus. **Metastatic ophthalmia.** Ophthalmia which is usually gonorrhoeal and due to the gonococcus or its toxin being carried in the blood from the urethra to the conjunctiva. **Migratory ophthalmia.** Sympathetic ophthalmia (see below) based on Deutschmann's theory of migration of infection from the injured eye to its fellow via lymphatic channels. **Mucous ophthalmia.** Catarrhal ophthalmia (see above). **Ophthalmia neonatorum.** Purulent discharge from the eyes of an infant, commencing within 21 days of birth. Sixty per cent of cases are gonococcal, the remainder being due to streptococci, pneumococci, *Bacterium coli* and mixed infections. **Neuroparalytic ophthalmia.** A form of keratitis most commonly seen after herpes zoster ophthalmicus and after alcohol injection of the trigeminal ganglion for trigeminal neuralgia. **Ophthalmia nivialis.** A form of photo-ophthalmia due to exposure of the unprotected eyes to bright sunlight reflected from snow. **Ophthalmia nodosa.** Caterpillar ophthalmia (see above). **Phlyctenular ophthalmia.** A form of keratoconjunctivitis, occurring usually in children and characterized by the presence of small nodules at or near the limbus. Most cases are tuberculous in origin and the subjects suffer from malnutrition. **Purulent ophthalmia.** Conjunctivitis with a purulent secretion, frequently gonococcal. **Scrofulous ophthalmia.** Phlyctenular ophthalmia (see above). **Solar ophthalmia.** Glare conjunctivitis. *See* CONJUNCTIVITIS. **Spring ophthalmia.** Vernal catarrh, vernal conjunctivitis; a seasonal form of conjunctivitis characterized by flat granulations in the palpebral part of the conjunctiva and, in some forms, in the region of the limbus. The secretion contains eosinophils and the cause is probably allergic. **Strumous ophthalmia.** Phlyctenular ophthalmia (see above). **Sympathetic ophthalmia.** A specific bilateral severe inflammation of the eyes, frequently terminating in blindness. It usually appears after injury in otherwise healthy individuals, and is particularly associated with a neglected prolapse of the iris or ciliary body. **Transferred ophthalmia.** Sympathetic ophthalmia (see prec.). **Ultraviolet-ray ophthalmia.** Electric ophthalmia (see above). **Varicose ophthalmia.** Ophthalmia associated with varicosity of the conjunctival veins. **War ophthalmia.** Trachoma. [Gk *ophthalmos* eye.]

ophthalmiac (of·**thal**·me·ak). One who is afflicted with ophthalmia.

ophthalmiatric (of·**thal**·me·**at**′·rik). Relating or belonging to ophthalmic treatment. [see foll.]

ophthalmiatrics (of·**thal**·me·**at**′·rix). The treatment of diseases of the eye. [Gk *ophthalmos* eye, *iatreia* treatment.]

ophthalmic (of·**thal**·mik). Relating to the eye. [Gk *ophthalmos* eye.]

ophthalmic artery [arteria ophthalmica (NA)]. A branch of the internal carotid artery, entering the orbit through the optic foramen. After supplying numerous branches to the retina via the central artery of the retina, uveal tract and sclera via the anterior [arteriae ciliares anteriores (NA)] and long and short posterior ciliary arteries [arteriae ciliares posteriores longae et breves (NA)], the lacrimal gland via the lacrimal artery [arteria lacrimalis (NA)] and other orbital contents, it gives off anterior and posterior ethmoidal branches [arteriae ethmoidales, anterior et posterior (NA)] to the nasal cavity and terminates on the forehead as the supra-orbital [arteria supra-orbitalis (NA)] and supratrochlear [arteria supratrochlearis (NA)] arteries, and in the face as the dorsalis nasi artery [arteria dorsalis nasi (NA)]. Its other named branches are the anterior and posterior conjunctival arteries [arteriae conjunctivales anteriores et posteriores (NA)], the episcleral arteries [arteriae episclerales (NA)], the medial and lateral palpebral branches [arteriae palpebrales mediales et laterales (NA)], uniting as the superior and inferior palpebral arches [arcus palpebrales superior et inferior (NA)] and a recurrent meningeal branch [arteria meningea anterior (NA)].

ophthalmic nerve [nervus ophthalmicus (NA)]. The first division of the trigeminal nerve, supplying the eyeball, through its nasociliary branch, the lacrimal gland (lacrimal nerve), conjunctiva and eyelids, through its lacrimal and frontal and nasociliary branches, and the forehead and scalp by the frontal nerve. It also gives a twig to the dura mater (nerve to the tentorium).

ophthalmic veins. Two veins draining each orbit, the superior [vena ophthalmica superior (NA)] and inferior [vena ophthalmica inferior (NA)], communicating in front with the facial vein and usually terminating in the cavernous sinus of the dura mater and pterygoid plexus of veins respectively.

ophthalmin (of·**thal**·min). A name proposed for the causal agent of purulent ophthalmia.

ophthalmitic (of·thal·**mit**·ik). Pertaining to ophthalmitis.

ophthalmitis (of·thal·**mi**·tis). A condition of inflammation affecting the eye; ophthalmia. **Sympathetic ophthalmitis.** A severe form of bilateral uveitis of unknown aetiology, nearly always following a perforating injury of one eye. The disease starts in the injured or exciting eye, and sooner or later affects the uninjured or sympathizing eye. [Gk *ophthalmos* eye, *-itis* inflammation.]

ophthalmoblennorrhoea (of·**thal**·mo·blen·o·**re**′·ah). Gonorrhoeal ophthalmia. *See* OPHTHALMIA. [Gk *ophthalmos* eye, *blenna* mucus, *rhoia* flow.]

ophthalmocace (of·thal·**mok**·as·e). Any disease of the eye. [Gk *ophthalmos* eye, *kakos* bad.]

ophthalmocarcinoma (of·**thal**·mo·kar·sin·**o**′·mah). Carcinoma of the eye. [Gk *ophthalmos* eye, carcinoma.]

ophthalmocele (of·**thal**·mo·seel). Exophthalmos; prominence or protrusion of the eyeball, due to disease, to such an extent that the eyelid will not cover it. [Gk *ophthalmos* eye, *kele* hernia.]

ophthalmocentesis (of·**thal**·mo·sen·**te**′·sis). Puncturing of the eyeball by surgical methods. [Gk *ophthalmos* eye, *kentein* to pierce.]

ophthalmocopia (of·**thal**·mo·**kop**′·e·ah). Asthenopia. [Gk *ophthalmos* eye, *kopos* weariness.]

ophthalmodesmitis (of·**thal**·mo·dez·**mi**′·tis). Inflammation affecting the tendons or fibrotic elements of the eye. [Gk *ophthalmos* eye, *desmos* band, *-itis* inflammation.]

ophthalmodiagnosis (of·**thal**·mo·di·ag·**no**′·sis). A diagnosis based upon the oculoreaction. [Gk *ophthalmos* eye, diagnosis.]

ophthalmodiaphanoscope (of·**thal**·mo·di·af·**an**′·o·skope). An instrument employed principally for the diagnosis of intra-ocular neoplasms. [Gk *ophthalmos* eye, diaphanoscope.]

ophthalmodiastimeter (of·**thal**·mo·di·as·**tim**′·et·er). An apparatus for ascertaining the correct position in which spectacle lenses should be fixed before the eyes. [Gk *ophthalmos* eye, *diastema* interval, meter.]

ophthalmodonesis (of·**thal**·mo·don·**e**′·sis). A trembling movement or flickering of the eyes. [Gk *ophthalmos* eye, *donetos* shaken.]

ophthalmodynamometer (of·**thal**·mo·di·nam·**om**′·et·er). An instrument invented by Baillart for exercising varying amounts of pressure on the sclera while the fundus is observed with an ophthalmoscope. It is principally employed for estimation of the systolic and diastolic pressures in the ophthalmic artery. [Gk *ophthalmos* eye, dynamometer.]

ophthalmodynamometry (of·**thal**·mo·di·nam·**om**′·et·re). The determination of the ophthalmic artery pressure by direct observation of the pulsation of the central retinal artery when a known pressure is being applied to the eyeball. [see prec.]

ophthalmodynia (of·**thal**·mo·**din**′·e·ah). Pain affecting the eyeball. [Gk *ophthalmos* eye, *odyne* pain.]

ophthalmo-eikonometer (of·**thal**·mo·i·kon·**om**′·et·er). A complex instrument for measuring differences in the magnification (size and shape) of the images in the two eyes. [Gk *ophthalmos* eye, *eikon* image, meter.]

ophthalmofundoscope (of·**thal**·mo·**fun**′·do·skope). An apparatus for inspecting the fundus of the eye. [Gk *ophthalmos* eye, fundus, Gk *skopein* to view.]

ophthalmograph (of·**thal**·mo·graf). A device used in recording by photographic methods the movements of the eye of a person who is reading. [Gk *ophthalmos* eye, *graphein* to record.]

ophthalmogyric (of·**thal**·mo·**ji**′·rik). Causing ocular movements. [Gk *ophthalmos* eye, *gyros* circle.]

ophthalmoleucoscope (of·**thal**·mo·**lew**′·ko·skope). A polarizer employed in testing colour blindness. [Gk *ophthalmos* eye, *leukos* white, *skopein* to view.]

ophthalmolith (of·**thal**·mo·lith). Calculus occurring in the lacrimal apparatus. [Gk *ophthalmos* eye, *lithos* stone.]

ophthalmological (of·thal·mo·**loj**·ik·al). Pertaining to ophthalmology.

ophthalmologist (of·thal·**mol**·o·jist). A specialist in the investigation and treatment of eye diseases and defects. [see foll.]

ophthalmology (of·thal·**mol**·o·je). That branch of medical science which deals with the diseases and refractive errors of the eye. [Gk *ophthalmos* eye, *logos* science.]

ophthalmolyma (of·**thal**·mo·**li**′·mah). Destruction or mutilation of the eye so that sight is destroyed. [Gk *ophthalmos* eye, *lyme* destruction.]

ophthalmomacrosis (of·**thal**·mo·mak·**ro**′·sis). Enlargement of the eyeball. [Gk *ophthalmos* eye, *makros* large, *-osis* condition.]

ophthalmomalacia (of·**thal**·mo·mal·**a**′·she·ah). A condition of abnormal softening and shrivelling of the eyeball associated with a decrease in the globular tension. [Gk *ophthalmos* eye, *malakia softness.]*

ophthalmomelanoma (of·**thal**·mo·mel·an·**o**′·mah). A melanoma of the eye. [Gk *ophthalmos* eye, *melas* black, *-oma* tumour.]

ophthalmomelanosis (of·**thal**·mo·mel·an·**o**′·sis). A condition characterized by the formation of an ophthalmomelanoma. [Gk *ophthalmos* eye, *melas* black, *-osis* condition.]

ophthalmometer (of·thal·**mom**·et·er). An instrument with which the degrees of curvature of the corneal surface may be measured. [Gk *ophthalmos* eye, meter.]

ophthalmometroscope (of·**thal**·mo·**met**′·ro·skope). An ophthalmoscope fitted with an attachment which enables the powers and errors of refraction of the eye to be determined. [Gk *ophthalmos* eye, *metron* measure, *skopein* to view.]

ophthalmometry (of·thal·**mom**·et·re). Measurement of the refractive errors and powers of the eye by means of the ophthalmometer. [Gk *ophthalmos* eye, *metron* measure.]

ophthalmomycosis (of·**thal**·mo·mi·**ko**′·sis). Any disease process of the eye or of the accessory organs of the eye caused by fungi. [Gk *ophthalmos* eye, mycosis.]

ophthalmomyiasis (of·**thal**·mo·mi·**i**′·as·is). Infestation of the eye by fly larvae. [Gk *ophthalmos* eye, *myia* fly.]

ophthalmomyitis, ophthalmomyositis (of·**thal**·mo·mi·**i**′·tis, of·**thal**·mo·mi·o·**si**′·tis). A condition of inflammation affecting the extrinsic muscles of the eye. [Gk *ophthalmos* eye, *mys* muscle, *-itis* inflammation.]

ophthalmomyotomy (of·**thal**·mo·mi·**ot**′·o·me). Surgical division of the extrinsic muscles of the eye. [Gk *ophthalmos* eye, myotomy.]

ophthalmoncus (of·thal·**mong**·kus). A swelling or neoplasm of the eye. [Gk *ophthalmos* eye, *ogkos* a swelling.]

ophthalmoneuritis (of·**thal**·mo·newr·**i**′·tis). Inflammation affecting the ophthalmic nerve. [Gk *ophthalmos* eye, neuritis.]

ophthalmoneuromyelitis (of·**thal**·mo·**newr**·o·mi·el·**i**′·tis). Neuromyelitis optica. [Gk *ophthalmos* eye, neuromyelitis.]

ophthalmopathy (of·thal·**mop**·ath·e). Any eye disease. **Congestive ophthalmopathy.** Swelling of the eyelids which appear congested—malignant ophthalmoplegia, a dangerous complication of Graves' disease. **External ophthalmopathy.** Any morbid condition of the conjunctiva, cornea, eyelids or adnexa of the eye. **Internal ophthalmopathy.** Any morbid condition of the lens, retina or other deeper structure of the eye. [Gk *ophthalmos* eye, *pathos* disease.]

ophthalmophacometer, ophthalmophakometer (of·**thal**·mo·fak·**om**′·et·er). An instrument used to estimate the refraction of the crystalline lens by measuring the radii of curvature of its surfaces. [Gk *ophthalmos* eye, *phakos* lens, meter.]

ophthalmophantom (of·**thal**·mo·**fan**′·tom). A model of the eye used in teaching and demonstration or in practising ocular surgery. [Gk *ophthalmos* eye, phantom.]

ophthalmophlebotomy (of·**thal**·mo·fleb·**ot**′·o·me). Venesection for the purpose of relieving congestion of the veins of the conjunctiva. [Gk *ophthalmos* eye, phlebotomy.]

ophthalmophobia (of·**thal**·mo·**fo**′·be·ah). A state of hypersensitiveness in which a person has an unreasonable dislike of being stared at. [Gk *ophthalmos* eye, phobia.]

ophthalmophyma (of·**thal**·mo·**fi**′·mah). A condition of general swelling or hypertrophy of the eyeball. [Gk *ophthalmos* eye, *phyma* tumour.]

ophthalmoplastic (of·**thal**·mo·**plas**′·tik). Relating or belonging to ophthalmoplasty.

ophthalmoplasty (of·**thal**·mo·plas·te). Plastic surgery of the eye or of its adnexa. [Gk *ophthalmos* eye, *plassein* to mould.]

ophthalmoplegia (of·**thal**·mo·**ple**′·je·ah). Theoretically, the term includes all ocular-muscle palsies, but it is sometimes restricted to those caused by disease of the muscles supplied by the 3rd, 4th and 6th cranial nerves. **Acquired ophthalmoplegia.** That coming on after birth and not genetically determined. **Acute ophthalmoplegia.** Rapid paralysis of all ocular muscles, often with fever and convulsions. It can occur in many different conditions, e.g. intracranial haemorrhage in the region of the nuclei, poisoning from alcohol, lethargic encephalitis and botulism. **Basal ophthalmoplegia.** That due to disease at the base of the brain or in the meninges. **Chronic progressive external ophthalmoplegia.** A progressive hereditary paralysis of the external muscles of the eye, starting in early adult life and continuing to complete immobility of the eyes. It is now thought to be a myopathy rather than a nuclear lesion. **Complete ophthalmoplegia.** That where the muscles concerned have no movement. **Congenital ophthalmoplegia.** That where the paralysis is present in some form at birth. **Diabetic ophthalmoplegia.** That associated with diabetes. **Diphtheritic ophthalmoplegia.** That associated with diphtheria and caused by the circulating toxin. It is characterized especially by paralysis of accommodation. **Exophthalmic ophthalmoplegia.** Thyrotropic exophthalmos. *See* EXOPHTHALMOS. **Ophthalmoplegia externa.** Paralysis of the extra-ocular muscles. **Fascicular ophthalmoplegia.** That due to a lesion in the medial longitudinal bundle. **Hereditary ophthalmoplegia.** One that is genetically determined. **Hysterical ophthalmoplegia.** That found in hysterics; it is always conjugate. Also called *pseudo-ophthalmoplegia.* **Infectious ophthalmoplegia.** That due to infection, e.g. lethargic encephalitis, syphilis. **Ophthalmoplegia interna.** Palsy of some or all of the intra-ocular muscles, sphincter and dilator muscles of the iris and ciliary muscles. **Internuclear ophthalmoplegia.** Paralysis of the medial rectus muscle on lateral gaze with normal contraction on convergence. **Malignant ophthalmoplegia.** Severe and progressive ophthalmoplegia often requiring tarsorrhaphy or surgical decompression of the orbit. **Myogenic ophthalmoplegia.** That in which the paralysis is due to disease of the muscles concerned, e.g. myasthenia gravis. **Neurogenic ophthalmoplegia.** That in which the paralysis is due to a lesion of nervous origin. **Nuclear ophthalmoplegia.** That due to a lesion of one or more of the 3rd, 4th and 6th cranial-nerve nuclei. **Orbital ophthalmoplegia.** That due to orbital lesions, e.g. tumours, orbital cellulitis. **Partial ophthalmoplegia.** Palsy affecting one or more, but not all, of the ocular muscles. **Progressive ophthalmoplegia.** Ophthalmoplegia of the nuclear type, with a familial tendency; it usually starts with ptosis and gradually involves all the extra-ocular muscles. **Recurrent ophthalmoplegia.** Recurrent attacks of paralysis of the eye muscles associated with migraine. Also called *ophthalmoplegic migraine.* **Total ophthalmoplegia.** Paralysis affecting all the muscles of the eye and associated with ptosis. Unilateral cases are due to cavernous sinus or orbital affections, bilateral, to a serious intracranial lesion, or to involvement of both cavernous sinuses, as in thrombosis. **Toxic ophthalmoplegia.** That caused by circulating toxins, e.g. diphtheria, tetanus and botulism. [Gk *ophthalmos* eye, *plege* stroke.]

See also: PARINAUD.

ophthalmoplegic (of·**thal**·mo·**ple**′·jik). 1. Characterized by, referring to, or suffering from ophthalmoplegia. 2. Any agent which paralyses the ciliary muscle; a cycloplegic [see prec.]

ophthalmoptosis (of·**thal**·mop·**to**′·sis). Exophthalmos; prominence or protrusion of the eyeball, due to disease. [Gk *ophthalmos* eye, *ptosis* a falling.]

ophthalmoreaction (of·**thal**·mo·re·**ak**′·shun). Oculoreaction. [Gk *ophthalmos* eye, reaction.]

ophthalmorrhagia (of·**thal**·mo·**ra**′·je·ah). Profuse ocular haemorrhage. [Gk *ophthalmos* eye, *rhegnynein* to gush forth.]

ophthalmorrhexis (of·**thal**·mo·**rex**′·is). Rupture of the eyeball. [Gk *ophthalmos* eye, *rhexis* rupture.]

ophthalmorrhoea (of·**thal**·mo·**re**′·ah). A discharge of mucus, pus or blood from the eye. [Gk *ophthalmos* eye, *rhoia* flow.]

ophthalmoscope (of·**thal**·mo·skope). An instrument for illuminating the interior of the eye and rendering it visible through the pupil. Light is reflected from a mirror into the eye and the observer inspects through a small hole in the centre of the mirror furnished with changeable lenses, or it is refracted by a prism over the top of which the observer is able to look. Numerous varieties of ophthalmoscopes exist, usually distinguished by the name of the inventor or manufacturer, or by some special feature, e.g. polarizing, red-free, etc. **Electric ophthalmoscope.** An ophthalmoscope in which the source of light is a small bulb contained in the instrument. **Ghost ophthalmoscope.** An ophthalmoscope in which the emergent rays are reflected at right angles by a glass plate placed at 45 degrees in the beam. **Reflecting ophthalmoscope.** One in which the source of light is a lamp by the side of the patient's head. [Gk *ophthalmos* eye, *skopein* to view.]

See also: LORING, MAY (C. H.).

ophthalmoscopic (of·**thal**·mo·**skop**′·ik). Relating or belonging to the ophthalmoscope or to ophthalmoscopy.

ophthalmoscopy (of·thal·**mos**·ko·pe). Examination of the eye with an ophthalmoscope. **Direct ophthalmoscopy.** A method in which the instrument is held close to the patient's eye and the fundus is seen as a virtual, erect and magnified image. **Indirect**

ophthalmoscopy. The production of a real, inverted image of the interior of the eye by the interposition of a strong convex lens (14 to 20 D) between the patient and the observer who are seated about half a metre apart. A binocular ophthalmoscope is generally employed for this purpose. **Medical ophthalmoscopy.** Examination of the fundus for evidence of extra-ocular disease, e.g. diabetes, hyperpiesis, cerebral tumour. **Metric ophthalmoscopy.** 1. Estimation of the refraction of the patient's eye by the strength of lens required to see fundus details clearly when the observer's accommodation is relaxed. 2. Estimation in dioptres of the amount of swelling of the optic-nerve head in case of papilloedema. [Gk *ophthalmos* eye, *skopein* to view.]

ophthalmospasm (of·**thal**·mo·spazm). Spasmodic contraction of the eye. [Gk *ophthalmos* eye, spasm.]

ophthalmospintherism (of·thal·mo·**spin**′·ther·izm). An ocular condition which causes visual hallucinations to occur, these being in the form of sparks of light. [Gk *ophthalmos* eye, *spinther* spark.]

ophthalmostasia, ophthalmostasis (of·**thal**·mo·**sta**′·se·ah, of·thal·**mos**·tas·is). Fixation of the eyeball by means of the ophthalmostat. [Gk *ophthalmos* eye, *stasis* a standing still.]

ophthalmostat (of·**thal**·mo·stat). An instrument used to hold the eyeball in one particular position and so prevent involuntary movements during an operation. [Gk *ophthalmos* eye, *statos* standing.]

ophthalmostatometer (of·**thal**·mo·stat·**om**′·et·er). A device used in the measurement of the degree of protrusion of an eyeball. [Gk *ophthalmos* eye, *statos* standing, meter.]

ophthalmostatometry (of·**thal**·mo·stat·**om**′·et·re). The measurement of protrusion or retraction of the eyeballs. [see prec.]

ophthalmosteresis (of·**thal**·mo·ster·**e**′·sis). Loss or absence of an eye, or of both eyes. [Gk *ophthalmos* eye, *steresis* loss.]

ophthalmosynchysis (of·**thal**·mo·**sin**′·kis·is). Effusion of fluid into the tissues of the eyeball. [Gk *ophthalmos* eye, *sygchysis* a breaking through.]

ophthalmothermometer (of·**thal**·mo·ther·**mom**′·et·er). A thermometer used to determine the temperature of the eye. [Gk *ophthalmos* eye, thermometer.]

ophthalmotomy (of·thal·**mot**·o·me). Incision of the eyeball. [Gk *ophthalmos* eye, *temnein* to cut.]

ophthalmotonometer (of·**thal**·mo·to·**nom**′·et·er). An instrument for determining the intra-ocular tension. [Gk *ophthalmos* eye, tonometer.]

ophthalmotonometry (of·**thal**·mo·to·**nom**′·et·re). Measurement of intra-ocular tension by means of the ophthalmotonometer.

ophthalmotoxin (of·**thal**·mo·**tox**′·in). 1. Any toxin acting specifically on the eye. 2. A cytotoxin produced by injection of an emulsion prepared from the ciliary body. [Gk *ophthalmos* eye, toxin.]

ophthalmotrope (of·**thal**·mo·trope). A working model of the human eyes with the extrinsic eye muscles represented in force and direction by weighted cords. It is used to demonstrate the effect of these muscles on eye movements. [Gk *ophthalmos* eye, *trepein* to turn.]

ophthalmotropometer (of·**thal**·mo·tro·**pom**′·et·er). An instrument used in the determination of imbalance in the ocular muscles. [Gk *ophthalmos* eye, *trepein* to turn, meter.]

ophthalmotropometry (of·**thal**·mo·tro·**pom**′·et·re). The process of measuring the tension and the movements of the eyeball by means of the ophthalmotropometer.

ophthalmovascular (of·**thal**·mo·**vas**′·kew·lar). Referring to the ocular blood vessels. [Gk *ophthalmos* eye, vascular.]

ophthalmoxerosis (of·**thal**·mo·zer·**o**′·sis). A degenerative condition in which the conjunctiva becomes dry, lustreless and shrunken. It may be due to severe vitamin-A deficiency or to local disease of the eye causing cicatricial changes which close the lacrimal and accessory lacrimal-gland ducts, e.g. trachoma and pemphigus. [Gk *ophthalmos* eye, *xeros* dry.]

ophthalmoxysis (of·**thal**·mo·**zi**′·sis). Treatment of a disordered condition of the conjunctiva by means of scarification or scraping. [Gk *ophthalmos* eye, *xysis* a scraping.]

ophthalmoxyster, ophthalmoxystrum (of·**thal**·mo·**zis**′·ter, of·**thal**·mo·**zis**′·trum). An instrument used in scraping or curetting the conjunctiva. [Gk *ophthalmos* eye, *xyster* scraper.]

ophthalmula (of·**thal**·mew·lah). A scar on the eyeball. [Gk *ophthalmos* eye, *oule* scar.]

opiate (o·pe·ate). An opium preparation or sedative containing an alkaloid of opium.

opilacao (o·pil·ah·**sah**′·o). American trypanosomiasis. [Port.]

opiomania (o·pe·o·**ma**′·ne·ah). Addiction to the use of opiates. [opium, mania.]

opiomaniac (o·pe·o·**ma**′·ne·ak). One who is addicted to the use of opium. [see prec.]

opiophagia, opiophagism, opiophagy (o·pe·o·**fa**′·je·ah, o·pe·**of**·aj·izm, o·pe·**of**·aj·e). The habitual eating or using of opium. [opium, Gk *phagein* to eat.]

opiophile (o·pe·o·file). One who is devoted to the eating or smoking of opium. [opium, *philein* to love.]

Opipramol (o·**pip**·ram·ol). BP Commission approved name for 5 - {3 - [4 - (2 - hydroxyethyl)piperazin - 1 - yl]propyl} - dibenz[*b*,*f*]-azepine; an antidepressant.

Opisocrostis (o·pis·o·**kros**′·tis). A genus of fleas, some of which are vectors of plague. **Op socrostis bruneri.** A squirrel flea, a vector of plague.

opisthenar (o·**pis**·then·ar). The back of the hand. [Gk *opisthen* behind, *thenar* flat of the hand.]

opisthencephalon (o·**pis**·then·**kef**′·al·on). The cerebellum. [Gk *opisthen* behind, *kephale* head.]

opisthiobasial (o·**pis**·the·o·**ba**′·se·al). Belonging to or connecting opisthion and basion.

opisthion (o·**pis**·the·on). A craniometric point; the midpoint of the posterior margin of the foramen magnum. [Gk *opisthios* posterior.]

opisthionasial (o·**pis**·the·o·**na**′·ze·al). Belonging to or connecting the opisthion and nasion.

opisthocranion (o·**pis**·tho·**kra**′·ne·on). A craniometric point; that point on the back of the head in the midline which is most distant from the glabella. [Gk *opisthen* behind, *kranion* skull.]

opisthogenia (o·**pis**·tho·**je**′·ne·ah). Faulty development of the maxilla and mandible as a result of bony ankylosis. [Gk *opisthen* behind, *genys* lower jaw.]

opisthoglypha (o·pis·**thog**·lif·ah). A division of the snakes of the family Colubridae containing those in which 2 or more of the posterior teeth are grooved in association with the poison glands. They are all relatively harmless to man. [Gk *opisthen* behind, *glyphein* to carve.]

opisthognathism (o·pis·**thog**·nath·izm). A cranial abnormality characterized by the presence of a receding lower jaw and a gnathic index of less than 98. [Gk *opisthen* behind, *gnathos* jaw.]

opisthoporeia, opisthoporia (o·**pis**·tho·por·**i**′·ah). A condition occurring in certain patients affected by nervous disorder, the characteristic of which is walking backwards when the attempt to walk forwards is made. [Gk *opisthen* behind, *poreia* a walking.]

opisthorchiasis (o·pis·thor·**ki**′·as·is). Infection with a liver fluke of the genus *Opisthorchis.*

Opisthorchidae (o·pis·**thor**·kid·e). A family of the trematode sub-order Distomata or Fascioloidea. The genera *Clonorchis, Metorchis* and *Opisthorchis* are of medical interest. [Gk *opisthen* behind, *orchis* testicle, *eidos* form.]

Opisthorchis (o·pis·**thor**·kis). A genus of liver flukes. **Opisthorchis felineus.** A species found in man, from Central Europe to Japan. The secondary host in Europe is the fresh-water snail *Bythinia leachi.* The cercariae encyst in fish of the family Cyprinidae, and are transmitted to man when the fish is eaten raw. **Opisthorchis noverca.** A parasite of the pig and dog in India, rarely reported in man. **Opisthorchis viverrini.** A species from Taiwan, India and Thailand, found infrequently in man. The life cycle is not known, but the usual hosts are small carnivores. [Gk *opisthen* behind, *orchis* testicle.]

opisthorchosis (o·pis·thor·**ko**′·sis). Opisthorchiasis.

Opisthothalmus (o·**pis**·tho·**thal'**·mus). A genus of South African scorpions. [Gk *opisthen* behind, *thalamos* chamber.]

opisthotic (o·pis·**thot**·ik). Designating or referring to the parts situated behind the ear. [Gk *opisthen* behind, *ous* ear.]

opisthotonic (o·**pis**·tho·**ton'**·ik). Referring to opisthotonos.

opisthotonoid (o·pis·**thot**·on·oid). Resembling opisthotonos. [opisthotonos, Gk *eidos* form.]

opisthotonos (o·pis·**thot**·on·us). Tetanic spasm occurring in the muscles of the back causing the head and lower limbs to bend backward and arching of the body so that it rests on the heels and head. [Gk *opisthen* behind, *tonos* straining.]

Opitz, Hans (b. 1888). Breslau paediatrician.

Opitz disease. Thrombophlebitic splenomegaly. *See* SPLENOMEGALY.

opium (o·pe·um). Raw opium; a latex, dried or partially dried, obtained from unripe capsules of *Papaver somniferum* Linn. (family Papaveraceae). Drying of the exudate is accomplished partly by spontaneous evaporation and partly by applied heat, the product being manipulated into cakes. The principal constituent is the alkaloid morphine, together with smaller amounts of the alkaloids, narcotine, papaverine, thebaine, narceine, meconidine and numerous other minor alkaloids. Its action is primarily that of a narcotic, though preparations of opium are used as diaphoretics and sedatives in the treatment of coughs and colds (BP 1973). **Powdered Opium BP 1973.** Opium, dried, powdered and adjusted to contain 10 per cent of anhydrous morphine, by use of some suitable diluent such as lactose. **Opium Tincture BP 1973.** Laudanum, an alcoholic extract of opium adjusted to contain 1 per cent w/v of anhydrous morphine; it is a convenient preparation for the administration of opium alkaloids. **Opium Tincture, Camphorated, BP 1973.** Paregoric, an alcoholic dilution of tincture of opium with benzoic acid, camphor and anise oil. It is used in cough mixtures. **Vinegar of opium.** An extract of opium, sugar and nutmeg prepared by maceration and percolation with dilute acetic acid. It is an old preparation used for the administration of opium. [L poppy juice.]

opiumism (o·pe·um·izm). 1. The habit of taking opium. 2. The condition induced by the abuse of opium.

opocephalus (op·o·**kef**·al·us). A monstrosity without nose or mouth, united by the ears and with only 1 orbit, or alternatively with 2 eyes in very close proximity. [Gk *ops* eye, *kephale* head.]

opoclonia (op·o·**klo**·ne·ah). Rapid, irregular, jerking movements of the eyes, occurring in short bursts of diminishing intensity upon a change of fixation; attributed to a lesion of the basal ganglia. [Gk *ops* eye, *klonos* violent motion.]

opodeldoc (op·o·**del**·dok). Soap liniment. *See* LINIMENT. [etym. dub.]

opodidymus, opodymus (op·o·**did**·im·us, op·**od**·im·us). A twin monster having only 1 body, in which the 2 heads are fused together and there is partial fusion of the organs of the senses. [Gk *ops* face, *didymos* twin.]

opossum (o·**pos**·um). A marsupial of the genus *Didelphis*. Some species are potential reservoirs of infection of certain diseases of man. [Amer. Ind.]

opotherapeutic (o·po·ther·ap·**ew'**·tik). Relating to the treatment of disease by extracts of ductless glands. [Gk *opos* juice, *therapeia* treatment.]

Oppenheim, Herman (b. 1858). Berlin neurologist.

Oppenheim's disease. Myatonia congenita.

Oppenheim's gait. A gait showing large irregular oscillations of the head, extremities and trunk; a variation of the spastic gait of disseminated sclerosis.

Oppenheim's reflex or sign. 1. In spastic paraplegia, stroking the posterior edge of the medial subcutaneous surface of the tibia may give rise to contraction of the tibialis anterior, extensor hallucis longus, extensor digitorum and sometimes the peronei muscles. 2. An extensor-plantar response, indicative of pyramidal-tract disease, produced by firm downward pressure on the front of the lower part of the tibia. An elaboration of Babinski's sign.

Ziehen-Oppenheim disease. Torsion spasm; dystonia musculorum deformans.

Oppenheim, Moritz (b. 1876). Vienna dermatologist.

Urbach-Oppenheim disease. Xanthoma diabeticorum.

Oppenheimer, Isaac (b. 1855). New York physician.

Oppenheimer's treatment. A treatment for drug addiction.

oppilation (op·il·a·shun). Constipation. [L *oppilare* to stop up.]

oppilative (**op**·il·at·iv). 1. Tending to close the duct of a gland and thus cause an obstruction to outflow. 2. Causing constipation. [see prec.]

Oppler, Bruno (fl. 1903–1928). Berlin physician.

bacillus of Boas-Oppler, lactobacillus of Boas-Oppler. A species observed by Oppler in the stomach contents in gastric cancer: not cultivated and therefore not properly identified; of historical interest only. It is generally believed to be identical with *Lactobacillus acidophilus*.

Oppolzer, Johann von (b. 1808). Vienna physician.

Oppolzer's sign. In serofibrinous pericarditis the site of the apex beat alters with the position of the patient.

opponens (op·o·nenz). A name applied to certain muscles of the fingers that tend to draw these digits opposite to other digits, e.g. opponens digiti minimi. [L opposing.]

opponens digiti minimi muscle [musculus opponens digiti minimi (NA)] (op·**o**·nenz **dij**·it·i **min**·im·i musl). A deep muscle of the hypothenar eminence. It arises from the ulnar side of the wrist and is inserted along the length of the shaft of the 5th metacarpal bone. It is the main muscle of opposition of the little finger.

opponens pollicis muscle [musculus opponens pollicis (NA)] (op·**o**·nenz **pol**·is·is musl). One of the deeper muscles of the thenar eminence, and the main muscle in producing opposition of the thumb to the other fingers. It extends from the radial side of the wrist to the radial side of the shaft of the 1st metacarpal bone.

opposition (op·o·**zish**·un). In relation to the mechanics of the hand, a movement that results in the pulp surface of the thumb becoming diametrically opposed to the pulp surface of one or other of the remaining digits for the purposes of prehension. [L *opponere* to oppose.]

oppositipolar (**op**·o·zit·e·**po'**·lar). Bipolar; the state of being polarized about 2 opposite poles.

opsialgia (op·se·**al**·je·ah). Facial neuralgia. [Gk *ops* face, *algos* pain.]

opsinogen (op·**sin**·o·jen). An antigenic substance capable of causing the production of an opsonin in the blood. [opsonin, Gk *genein* to produce.]

opsinogenous (op·sin·**oj**·en·us). Capable of forming opsonins. [see prec.]

opsiometer (op·se·**om**·et·er). Optometer. [Gk *opsis* vision, meter.]

opsionosis (**op**·se·o·**no'**·sis). Any disorder of the eye or of vision. [Gk *opsis* sight, *-osis* condition.]

opsitocia (op·se·**to**·se·ah). Term for a period of pregnancy that is much longer than the normal 280 days. [Gk *opse* late, *tokos* birth.]

opsiuria (op·se·**ewr**·e·ah). A condition in which there is an excretion of larger quantities of urine while the patient is fasting than during the digestion of food. [Gk *opson* meat, urine.]

opsoclonia (op·so·**klo**·ne·ah). Opoclonia.

opsogen (**op**·so·jen). Opsinogen.

opsomania (op·so·**ma**·ne·ah). Abnormal desire for a particular article of diet, especially well-seasoned meat. [Gk *opson* meat, mania.]

opsomaniac (op·so·**ma**·ne·ak). A person affected with opsomania.

opsone (**op**·sone). Opsonin.

opsonic (op·**son**·ik). Belonging to or characterized by opsonins.

opsoniferous (op·son·**if**·er·us). Containing opsonin, and acting as a vehicle in its distribution. [opsonin, L *ferre* to carry.]

opsonification (**op**·son·if·ik·**a'**·shun). The process of making bacteria and other cellular organisms susceptible to phagocytosis. [opsonin, L *facere* to make.]

opsonify (op·son·if·i). To submit to the process of opsonification.

opsonin (op·son·in). A substance in mammalian blood having the power to render micro-organisms and blood cells more easily absorbed by phagocytes. [Gk *opsonein* to provide with food.]

opsonization (op·son·i·za'·shun). Opsonification.

opsonize (op·son·ize). Opsonify.

opsonocytophagic (op·son·o·si·to·fa'·jik). Relating to the phagocytic activity of the blood in the presence of serum opsonins.

opsonogen (op·son·o·jen). Opsinogen.

opsonoid (op·son·oid). An opsonin in which the opsonophoric substance has been inactivated. [opsonin, Gk *eidos* form.]

opsonometry (op·son·om·et·re). The estimation of the amount of opsonin present in the blood serum. [opsonin, meter.]

opsonophilia (op·son·o·fil'·e·ah). The condition in which micro-organisms are attracted to opsonins, thus rendering themselves palatable to the leucocytes. [opsonin, Gk *philein* to love.]

opsonophilic (op·son·o·fil'·ik). Belonging to, characterized by, or uniting readily with opsonins. [see prec.]

opsonophoric (op·son·o·for'·ik). 1. Opsoniferous. 2. Applied to that particular part of an opsonin which acts on micro-organisms and renders them susceptible to phagocytosis. [opsonin, Gk *pherein* to bear.]

opsonotherapy (op·son·o·ther'·ap·e). Opsonic therapy.

optaesthesia (op·tes·the·ze·ah). Visual sensibility; the power of receiving and reacting to visual influences. [optic, aesthesia.]

optic (op·tik). Optical.

optic nerve [nervus opticus (NA)]. The nerve of sight, its fibres arising from the cells in the ganglionic layer of the retina and passing in a compact bundle, approximately 25 mm (1 in) long, from the back of the eye to the optic chiasma in the cranium. It is enveloped by all 3 membranes of the brain. Developmentally it is derived from the stem of the optic cup, which is an evagination from the brain.

optical (op·tik·al). Referring or belonging to the eye or to the vision, or of use to vision. [Gk *optikos* of sight.]

optician (op·tish·an). 1. A maker or seller of spectacles or optical instruments. 2. One who makes and adjusts spectacles in accordance with the prescription of the oculist. **Dispensing optician.** An optician who sells glasses and fills prescriptions. [Gk *optikos* of sight.]

opticochiasmatic, opticochiasmic (op·tik·o·ki·az·mat'·ik, op·tik·o·ki·az'·mik). Pertaining to the optic chiasma.

opticociliary (op·tik·o·sil'·e·ar·e). Belonging to the optic and ciliary nerves.

opticocinerea (op·tik·o·sin·eer'·e·ah). The grey matter of the optic tract. [Gk *optikos* of sight, L *cinereus* ashen coloured.]

opticopupillary (op·tik·o·pew'·pil·ar·e). Belonging to the optic nerve and the pupil.

optics (op·tix). The branch of physics which deals with the laws and phenomena of light and the refraction of the eye. [Gk *optikos* of sight.]

optimal (op·tim·al). Pertaining to optimum.

optimeter (op·tim·et·er). Optometer.

optimism (op·tim·izm). 1. Predisposition to regard all that happens in the most hopeful light. 2. Term for the state of spiritual ecstasy and associated delusions of grandeur. **Therapeutic optimism.** The belief that some remedy or drug will be effective in treatment of disease. [L *optimus* best.]

optimum (op·tim·um). The best and most suitable, qualitatively and quantitatively, for the special circumstances; e.g. of food or drugs in health or disease, of temperature or other environmental condition in the growth of micro-organisms. [L *optimus* best.]

optogram (op·to·gram). The image formed on the retina by the bleaching of visual purple under the action of light. [Gk *optos* visible, *gramma* record.]

optomeninx (op·to·men·ingx). The retina. [Gk *optikos* of sight, *menigx* membrane.]

optometer (op·tom·et·er). An instrument for measuring the refraction of the eye by its limits of distant vision. Numerous varieties exist. **Coincidence optometer.** A modern accurate instrument: the image is observed through a number of prisms and divided into 2 halves which have to be properly aligned. **Hair optometer.** An instrument designed by Donders for measuring the near point of accommodation: a number of fine hairs on a white background are brought up to the eye until they blur and cannot be differentiated. [Gk *optikos* of sight, meter.]

See also: DONDERS, SCHMIDT-RIMPLER.

optometrist (op·tom·et·rist). One who practises optometry.

optometry (op·tom·et·re). The process of assessment of the visual acuity, and the correction of visual defects by the fitting of spectacles. [Gk *optikos* of sight, meter.]

optomyometer (op·to·mi·om'·et·er). An instrument for determining the strength of the ocular muscles. [Gk *optikos* of sight, myometer.]

optophone (op·to·fone). An instrument for enabling the blind to read. A beam of light is made to traverse a line of print and the light reflected from it falls on a photosensitive cell, causing variations in the current passing through the latter which are converted into audible sounds, each letter of the print thus producing a recognizable sound pattern. [Gk *optikos* of sight, *phone* voice.]

optotype (op·to·tipe). A test type, used in the assessment of visual acuity. [Gk *optikos* of sight, type.]

opzyme (op·zime). A substance extracted from ductless glands and other organs or from tumours, which contains the specific proteins of the organ from which it originates. [Gk *opson* meat, *zyme* ferment.]

ora (o·rah). Margin. **Ora serrata [NA].** The jagged edge of the retina just behind the ciliary body. [L edge.]

orad (or·ad). Towards the mouth; USA usage. [L *os* mouth, *ad* to.]

oral (or·al). 1. Belonging to the mouth. 2. Verbal; spoken by word of mouth. [see foll.]

orale (o·ra·le). The midpoint of a line drawn to form a common tangent to the inner alveolar margins of the sockets of the 2 central incisors of the maxilla. [L *oralis* relating to the mouth.]

Oram, Samuel. 20th century London cardiologist.

Holt-Oram syndrome. The association of skeletal deformities of the forearm with atrial septal defect.

orange (or·anj). 1. A colour of the visible spectrum, with wavelength 585–647 nm. 2. The yellow edible fruit of the orange tree, *Citrus aurantium* (family Rutaceae). The fresh peel of the bitter orange is used in medicine (BP 1958) as a flavouring agent and for its bitter carminative properties. It contains a volatile oil, the bitter glycoside aurantiamarin, and the glycoside hesperidin, as well as small quantities of the vitamins A, B and C. **Orange II.** A dye used as an indicator of pH. It has a range of 11.0 (yellow) to 13.0 (red). **Orange III.** Sodium dimethylaminobenzene sulphonate; a dye used as an indicator. It has a pH range of 2.8 (red) to 4.0 (yellow). **Orange IV.** A dye used as an indicator of pH. It has a range of 1.0 (red) to 2.8 (yellow). **Acridine orange.** 2,8-tetramethyldiaminoacridine, $CH[N(CH_3)_2C_6H_3]_2N$, an orange dyestuff. **Bitter orange.** The Seville orange, *Citrus aurantium amara*; the fruit is smaller than the sweet orange (see below) and its pulp more acid and bitter. The peel is largely used in medicine for flavouring. The flowers yield a fragrant oil, oil of orange-flower water (oleum neroli), and from them is also made orange-flower water. **Orange G BPC 1954.** An acid azo dye much used in histology as a counterstain. **Methyl orange.** Helianthine. **Sweet orange.** Malta orange; the fruit of *Citrus aurantium sinensis.* The fruit has a superior flavour to the bitter orange and is preferred for eating; the juice is a popular way of administering vitamin C. **Victoria orange.** The ammonium or potassium salt of dinitroparacresol, used as a dye and as a stain in histology. **Wool orange.** Orange G (see above). [Ar. *naranj.*]

Orbeli, Leon Abgarovich (b. 1882). Leningrad physiologist.

Orbeli effect or phenomenon. The improvement in the height of contraction of a fatigued muscle that occurs if its sympathetic nerve supply is stimulated at the same time as the motor nerve.

orbiculare (or·bik·ew·la′·re). The lentiform nodule of the long process of the incus. [L *orbiculus* little disc.]

orbicularis oculi muscle [musculus orbicularis oculi (NA)] (or·bik·ew·la′·ris ok·ew·li musl). A sheet of muscle in the upper and lower eyelids, composed of a palpebral, an orbital and a lacrimal portion.

lacrimal part [pars lacrimalis (NA)]. A small muscle attached to the lacrimal crest, to the fascia covering the lacrimal sac, and by 2 slips into the tarsal plates. It dilates the lacrimal sac.

orbital part [pars orbitalis (NA)]. The outer part of a sheet of muscle encircling the palpebral fissure, which extends on to the forehead, temple and cheek, and is attached medially to the frontal process of the maxilla and the medial angular process of the frontal bone.

palpebral part [pars palpebralis (NA)]. The thin inner part of the orbicularis oculi muscle lying in both eyelids, attached to the medial palpebral ligament and adjacent bone and the lateral palpebral raphe.

orbicularis oris muscle [musculus orbicularis oris (NA)] (or·bik·ew·la′·ris or·is musl). A circumoral muscle in 3 layers. The 2 superficial layers [pars marginalis, pars labialis (NA)] are attached to neither bone nor cartilage. The deep layer is attached to the incisive fossae of both jaws.

orbi-like virus (ohr·bi·like vi·rus). *See* ROTAVIRUS.

orbit [orbita (NA)] (or·bit). 1. The large bony cavity which contains the eyeball, its associated vessels, nerves, muscles and so on, formed by parts of the frontal, sphenoid, zygomatic, maxillary, ethmoid, palatine and lacrimal bones; eye socket. The roof [paries superior (NA)] is formed by the orbital plate of the frontal bone and the sphenoid bone posteriorly. The floor [paries inferior (NA)] is formed by the maxilla. The lateral wall [paries lateralis (NA)] is formed by the orbital surfaces of the zygomatic bone and the greater wing of the sphenoid bone, whilst the medial wall [paries medialis (NA)] is formed by the maxilla, the lacrimal bone, the orbital plate of the ethmoid bone, the sphenoid bone and the orbital process of the palatine bone. 2. The path of a body moving round another body. [L *orbita* wheel-track.]

orbital (or·bit·al). 1. Belonging to the orbit. 2. The motion of an electron in a field of force. There is 1 orbital for each quantized orbit. **Orbital fissure.** *See* FISSURE. **Molecular orbital.** An orbital enclosing a molecule as a whole rather than being limited to a particular constituent atom of the molecule. **Orbital opening.** *See* OPENING. **Orbital plate.** *See* PLATE. **Orbital process of the palatine bone.** *See* PROCESS. **Orbital sulcus.** *See* SULCUS.

orbitale (or·bit·a′·le). The lowest point on the orbital margin.

orbitalis muscle [musculus orbitalis (NA)] (or·bit·a′·lis musl). A thin layer of unstriped muscle bridging the inferior orbital fissure.

orbitomeatal (or·bit·o·me·a′·tal). Pertaining to the orbit and the external auditory meatus. Orbitomeatal line. *See* LINE.

orbitonasal (or·bit·o·na′·zal). Belonging to the orbit and the nasal bone or the cavity of the nose.

orbitonometer (or·bit·on·om′·et·er). An instrument for measuring the compressibility of the contents of the orbit: a contact shell is placed over the cornea and the distance the eye is pushed back into the orbit is measured for different pressures applied.

orbitonometry (or·bit·on·om′·et·re). The measurement of the compressibility of the orbital contents. It is of importance in the differential diagnosis of proptosis.

orbitopagus (or·bit·op·ag·us). A twin monster, the imperfectly developed parasite of which is in the orbit of the autosite. [orbit, Gk *pagos* joined.]

orbitostat (or·bit·o·stat). An instrument for measuring the orbital axes. [orbit, Gk *statos* placed.]

orbitotemporal (or·bit·o·tem′·por·al). Belonging to the orbital and temporal regions.

orbitotomy (or·bit·ot·o·me). The operation of incising the orbit. [orbit, Gk *temnein* to cut.]

Orbivirus (ohr·bee·vi·rus). A genus of RNA-containing viruses, 65–80 nm in diameter. The members mostly cause disease in animals (bluetongue in sheep and cattle, African horse sickness, epidemic haemorrhagic disease in deer, etc.) which is transmitted by arthropods. Only one causes disease in man, Colorado tick fever, transmitted by *Dermacentor* ticks. [L *orbis* a ring.]

orcein (or·se·in). A reddish-brown colouring material obtained from cudbear and used in the histological identification of elastic fibres. [orcin.]

orchectomy (or·kek·to·me). Orchidectomy.

orcheitis (or·ke·i·tis). Orchitis.

orcheopexy (or·ke·o·pex·e). Orchiopexy.

orcheoplasty (or·ke·o·plas·te). Orchioplasty.

orcheotomy (or·ke·ot·o·me). Orchidotomy.

orchestromania (or·kes·tro·ma′·ne·ah). Acute chorea. [Gk *orcheisthein* to leap, mania.]

orchialgia (or·ke·al·je·ah). Orchidalgia.

orchic (or·kik). Orchidic.

orchichorea (or·ke·kor·e′·ah). Involuntary twitching of the testis due to spasmodic contraction of the cremaster muscle. [Gk *orchis* testis, *choreia* a dancing.]

orchidalgia (or·kid·al·je·ah). Pain of neuralgic type affecting the testis. [Gk *orchis* testis, *algos* pain.]

orchidatrophia, orchidatrophy (or·kid·at·ro′·fe·ah, or·kid·at·ro·fe). Atrophy or shrinkage of the testis. [Gk *orchis* testis, atrophy.]

orchidauxe (or·kid·awx·e). Morbid enlargement of the testis. [Gk *orchis* testis, *auxe* increase.]

orchidectomy (or·kid·ek·to·me). Surgical removal of the testis. Male castration is the operation of bilateral orchidectomy. **Radical orchidectomy.** Removal in continuity of the testicle, spermatic cord and, after an abdominal incision, the extraperitoneal fat around the spermatic vessels up to and including the lymph nodes at the level of the renal veins. Formerly performed in the treatment of malignant tumours of the testicle. [Gk *orchis* testis, *ektome* excision.]

orchidic (or·kid·ik). Relating to the testis. [Gk *orchis* testis.]

orchidion (or·kid·e·on). A small-sized testis. [Gk little testis.]

orchiditis (or·kid·i·tis). Orchitis.

orchidocele (or·kid·o·seel). Orchiocele.

orchidocelioplasty (or·kid·o·se′·le·o·plas·te). An operation for transplanting an imperfectly descended testis in the abdominal cavity. [Gk *orchis* testis, *koilia* belly, *plassein* to mould.]

orchidodynia (or·kid·o·din′·e·ah). Orchiodynia.

orchido-epididymectomy (or·kid·o·ep·e·did·im·ek′·to·me). Excision of the testis and epididymis. [Gk *orchis* testis, epididymis, Gk *ektome* a cutting out.]

orchidometer (or·kid·o·me·ter). An instrument for measuring the volume of the testis.

orchidoncus (or·kid·ong·kus). Orchioncus.

orchidopathy (or·kid·op·ath·e). Orchiopathy.

orchidopexia, orchidopexy (or·kid·o·pex′·e·ah, or·kid·o·pex·e). Orchiopexy.

See also: OMBRÉDANNE, TURNER (P.).

orchidoplasty (or·kid·o·plas·te). Orchioplasty.

orchidoptosis (or·kid·op·to′·sis). A condition characterized by prolapse of the testis, due to the presence of a varicocele or to laxity of the scrotum. [Gk *orchis* testis, *ptosis* a falling.]

orchidorrhaphy (or·kid·or·af·e). Orchiorrhaphy.

orchidoscheocele (or·kid·os·ke·o·seel). Orchioscheocele.

orchidospongioma (or·kid·o·spon·je·o′·mah). A tuberculous tumour of the testis. [Gk *orchis* testis, *spoggos* sponge, *-oma* tumour.]

orchidotherapy (or·kid·o·ther′·ap·e). The treatment of disease by administration of testicular extracts. [Gk *orchis* testis, therapy.]

orchidotomy (or·kid·ot·o·me). Incision through the tunica albuginea of the testis for the relief of tension or for the purpose of a biopsy of the germinal epithelium. [Gk *orchis* testis, *temnein* to cut.]

orchidotyloma (or·kid·o·ti·lo′·mah). A hard, thick nodule of the testis. [Gk *orchis* testis, *tylos* callus, *-oma* tumour.]

orchiectomy (or·ke·**ek**·to·me). Surgical removal of the testis. [Gk *orchis* testis, *ektome* excision.]

orchiencephaloma (**or**·ke·en·kef·al·**o'**·mah). An encephaloma of the testis. [Gk *orchis* testis, encephaloma.]

orchiepididymitis (**or**·ke·**ep**·e·did·e·**mi'**·tis). Inflammation affecting the testis and epididymis. [Gk *orchis* testis, epididymitis.]

orchil (**or**·kil). A violet colouring matter obtained from lichens of the *Roccella* and *Lecanora* species by boiling with water, treating with ammonia and exposing to air. It contains orcein, and was at one time used as a dye; it is now employed to colour pharmaceutical preparations. The name was originally applied to the plants themselves. [O Fr. *orchel.*]

orchilytic (or·kil·**it**·ik). Destructive of testicular tissue. [Gk *orchis* testis, *lysis* a loosing.]

orchiocatabasis (**or**·ke·o·kat·**ab'**·as·is). The process of descent of the testes. [Gk *orchis* testis, *katabasis* a descending.]

orchiocele (**or**·ke·o·seel). 1. A scrotal hernia. 2. A testicular tumour. 3. Herniation of a testis. 4. A testis that is retained in the inguinal canal. [Gk *orchis* testis, *kele* hernia.]

orchiococcus (**or**·ke·o·**kok'**·us). Name formerly given to *Neisseria gonorrhoeae* when isolated from the testis. [Gk *orchis* testis, coccus.]

orchiodynia (**or**·ke·o·**din'**·e·ah). Pain affecting the testis. [Gk *orchis* testis, *odyne* pain.]

orchiomyeloma (**or**·ke·o·mi·el·**o'**·mah). A myeloma of the testis. [Gk *orchis* testis, myeloma.]

orchioncus (or·ke·**ong**·kus). A swelling or tumour of the testis. [Gk *orchis* testis, *ogkos* tumour.]

orchioneuralgia (**or**·ke·o·newr·**al'**·je·ah). Orchidalgia. [Gk *orchis* testis, neuralgia.]

orchiopathy (or·ke·**op**·ath·e). Testicular disease. [Gk *orchis* testis, *pathos* disease.]

orchiopexy (**or**·ke·o·pex·e). The surgical fixation of an undescended testis in the scrotum. [Gk *orchis* testis, *pexis* fixation.]

orchioplasty (**or**·ke·o·plas·te). A plastic operation performed on the testis. [Gk *orchis* testis, *plassein* to mould.]

orchiorrhaphy (or·ke·**or**·af·e). The operation of suturing a testis to a portion of surrounding tissue; in particular, the fixing of an imperfectly descended testis to the scrotum by stitches. [Gk *orchis* testis, *rhaphe* suture.]

orchioscheocele (or·ke·**os**·ke·o·seel). Scrotal hernia. *See* HERNIA. [Gk *orchis* testis, *oscheon* scrotum, *kele* hernia.]

orchioscirrhus (**or**·ke·o·**skir'**·us). A scirrhous tumour or sclerosis of the testis. [Gk *orchis* testis, *skirros* hard.]

orchiotomy (or·ke·**ot**·o·me). Orchidotomy.

orchis (**or**·kis). 1. Testis. 2. A genus of orchidaceous plants some of which are used for medicinal purposes; salep is made from *Orchis mascula, O. masculata* and *O. latifolia.* [Gk.]

orchitic (or·**kit**·ik). Referring to or of the nature of orchitis.

orchitis (or·**ki**·tis). Inflammation affecting the testis and characterized by hypertrophy, pain and a sensation of weight. The condition usually is caused by gonorrhoea, syphilis or tuberculosis. **Filarial orchitis.** Orchitis due to infection by *Wuchereria bancrofti.* **Metastatic orchitis.** Orchitis due to an infection circulated to the testis by the blood stream, as occurs in cases of epidemic parotitis. **Orchitis parotidea.** Testicular inflammation occurring either before the onset or, more rarely, as the only evidence of epidemic parotitis. **Orchitis variolosa.** That which occurs in a patient suffering from smallpox. **Spermatogenic granulomatous orchitis.** A granulomatous inflammation seen in the spermatic tubules. It may be due to an auto-antibody. [Gk *orchis* testis, *-itis* inflammation.]

orchitolytic (**or**·kit·o·**lit'**·ik). Destructive of testicular tissue. [Gk *orchis* testis, *lysis* a loosing.]

orchitomy, orchotomy (or·**kit**·o·me, or·**kot**·o·me). Orchidotomy.

orcin, orcinol (**or**·sin, **or**·sin·ol). 3,5-Dihydroxytoluene, $CH_3C_6H_3(OH)_2$. A compound occurring naturally as a constituent of many lichens of the species of *Roccella* and *Lecanora.* Oxidation products of orcinol are used medicinally, often in the form of lichen extracts, for their tinctorial powers.

Orciprenaline (or·se·**pren**·al·een). BP Commission approved name for (±) - 1 - (3,5 - dihydroxyphenyl) - 2 - isopropylamino-ethanol. **Orciprenaline Sulphate BP 1973.** The sulphate of Orciprenaline, a sympathomimetic amine with an action similar to that of isoprenaline sulphate but more prolonged, and it can be given by mouth.

Ord, William Miller (b. 1834). British surgeon.

Ord's operation. An operation for overcoming fresh adhesions in joints.

ordinate (**or**·din·ate). In a graph the length cut off up the vertical axis by a perpendicular to the axis from a point. [L *ordinare* to arrange in order.]

ordure (**or**·dewr). Faeces or other excremental matter. [Fr.]

oreston (or·**es**·ton). Positron. [Obsolete term.] [*Orestes,* Gk mythology.]

orexia (or·**ex**·e·ah). Appetite. [L *orexis* longing.]

orexigenic (or·**ex**·e·**jen'**·ik). Having the property of being able to improve or stimulate the appetite. [Gk *orexis* longing, *genein* to produce.]

oreximania (or·**ex**·e·**ma'**·ne·ah). Morbid urge to eat, with abnormal appetite and increase in ingestion on account of a phobia of thinness. [Gk *orexis* longing, mania.]

orexis (or·**ex**·is). Appetite. [Gk longing.]

orf (orf). Ulcerative stomatitis of sheep which may be transmitted to man by direct contact, and in whom a single vesiculo-proliferative lesion may be found on the hands or face. The disease is due to a virus of the paravaccinia group which is very similar, or identical, to that of pseudocowpox. [AS.]

organ [organum (NA)] (**or**·gan). Any differentiated part devoted to a specific function. **Absorbent organ.** A highly vascular structure containing osteoclast cells which resorb cementum and dentine of deciduous teeth, whereby their attachment to the jaw is lost. **Adipose organ.** A fat lobule, considered as an organ. **Cell organ.** A more or less permanent cell structure, such as the nucleus. **Cement organ.** The embryonic tissue which deposits cementum on the surface of a tooth. **Enamel organ.** A complex epithelial structure lying on the dental papilla, from which the enamel of a tooth is developed. **Endocrine organ.** A gland which secretes the products of its activity into the blood stream rather than into a duct; ductless gland. **Organ of generation.** Any organ that takes part in reproduction. **Genital organs [organa genitalia (NA)].** The organs of reproduction, concerned with the formation of gametes and their passage from male to female, and also, in the female, the protection and nourishment of the embryo and fetus. **Genital organs, female [organa genitalia feminina (NA)].** Internally, the ovaries, uterine tubes, uterus and vagina; externally, the pubis, labia majora et minora, clitoris, bulb of the vestibule and greater vestibular glands. **Genital organs, male [organa genitalia masculina (NA)].** The testes and epididymides, the vasa deferentia, seminal vesicles, ejaculatory ducts and the penis. The prostate and bulbo-urethral glands are accessory structures. **Gustatory organ.** Organ of taste (see below). **Organ of hearing [organum vestibulocochleare (NA)].** General term embracing the external, middle and internal ear. **Primitive fat organ.** Interscapular gland. **Rudimentary organ.** A vestigial organ whose development has been arrested. **Segmental organ.** The embryonic kidney. **Sex organ.** Any organ that is peculiar to the sex of the individual. **Organ of sight [organum visus (NA)].** *See* EYE. **Organ of smell [organum olfactus (NA)].** The external nose and nasal cavity. The former is joined to the forehead by a root which continues down the midline as the dorsum and terminates in the apex. Inferiorly, 2 apertures, the nares, are bounded by the rounded alae. The upper part of its framework is formed by the nasal bones, the frontal processes, and the maxillary and the nasal processes of the frontal bones; below this it is supplied by the upper, lower and alar cartilages on both sides. The nasal cavity is divided into two by a median septum; from the lateral walls of each half project 3 ledges, the superior, middle and inferior conchae. The upper third of the walls is covered with pale-yellowish olfactory mucous membrane; the remainder of the cavity is lined by a red, highly vascular mucoperiosteum. **Spiral organ [organum spirale (NA)].** A series of sensory and supporting cells arranged on the upper surface of the basilar membrane, from which arise auditory impulses passing to the brain along the cochlear nerve. The sensory cells consist of a single inner row of hair cells and an outer set of 3 or 4 rows, the inner and outer rods of Corti lying between. The hairs are in contact with the membrana tectoria. **Organ of taste [organum gustus (NA)].** Epithelial structures, the taste buds, situated on the tongue and adjacent parts. They are numerous on the sides of the vallate papillae and surrounding walls, on the posterior part and sides of the tongue, especially the folia linguae, and on the inferior surface of the soft palate and the posterior surface of the epiglottis. **Urinary organs [organa uropoëtica (NA)].** The kidneys, ureters, urinary bladder and urethra. **Vestigial organ.** An organ whose development has been arrested in the course of evolution. **Vomeronasal organ [organum vomeronasale (NA)].** A rudimentary organ in the lower part of the nasal septum. It is well developed in some animals. [Gk *organon* instrument.]

See also: BOJANUS, CHIEVITZ, CORTI, EIMER, GIRALDÈS, GOLGI, JACOBSON (L. L.), ROSSENMUELLER, RUFFINI, WALDEYER-HARTZ, WEBER (M. I.).

organelle (or·gan·**el**). Any cell organ or specialized part of a protozoon having some individual function such as that of movement, reproduction or metabolism. [dim. of organ.]

organic (or·**gan**·ik). 1. Relating to a body organ. 2. Having organs or an organized physical structure. 3. Relating to a substance derived from an animal or vegetable organism or to such an organism. 4. In chemistry, relating to carbon compounds. [Gk *organikos.*]

organicism (or·**gan**·is·izm). The doctrine that each individual organ of the body has a separate constitution, and that disease is an entity with regard to such organ.

organicist (or·**gan**·is·ist). One who adheres to the theory of organicism.

organification (or·**gan**·if·i·**ca**·shon). Usually applied to the conversion of iodide trapped by the thyroid cell from the blood to organic iodine which is essential before the iodine can be taken up by tyrosine to form monoiodotyrosine and diiodotyrosine.

organism (**or**·gan·izm). A single living entity whether animal or plant. **Coprozoic organism.** An organism living in excreta. **L organisms.** The pleuropneumonia group of micro-organisms that are provisionally placed in the class Schizomycetes; they are mainly associated with animal infections, but similar bodies have been demonstrated in epithelial cells in non-specific urethritis. **Nitrosifying organism.** One capable of oxidizing ammonia to nitrites. **Nitrifying organism.** One capable of oxidizing nitrates to nitrites. **Pleuropneumonia-like organisms.** *See* MYCOPLASMA. [Gk *organon* instrument.]

See also: VINCENT.

organization (or·gan·i·**za**′·shun). 1. The process by which a simple tissue is converted into a more complex tissue or organ. 2. An organized body. [see foll.]

organize (**or**·gan·ize). To convert into an organ or complex structure. [Gk *organon* instrument.]

organizer (**or**·gan·i·zer). A tissue or hormone substance which determines the line of embryonic development. Cf. ACTIVATOR. **Mesodermic organizer.** The early notochord, in its capacity as a producer of chemical substances which initiate and control the differentiation of the mesoderm into somites, etc. **Nucleolus organizer.** A chromosome region contributing to the formation of the nucleolus and containing DNA coding for ribosomal DNA. **Primary organizer.** The dorsal lip of the blastopore in lower vertebrates, or Hensen's node in higher vertebrates, in its capacity as a producer of chemical substances which bring about the differentiation of neighbouring cells of the embryo and determine their fate. [see prec.]

organofaction (or·gan·o·**fak**′·shun). The formation and evolution of a body organ. [organ, L *facere* to make.]

organogel (**or**·gan·o·jel). A gel in which the liquid forming the disperse phase is, instead of water, an organic solvent such as alcohol or benzene.

organogen (**or**·gan·o·jen). Any of the chemical elements, carbon, hydrogen, nitrogen, oxygen and phosphorus, which principally go to form the organic compounds. [organic, Gk *genein* to produce.]

organogenesis (or·gan·o·**jen**′·es·is). The origin and growth of an organ. [organ, *genesis* origin.]

organogenetic, organogenic (or·gan·o·jen·**et**′·ik, or·gan·o·**jen**′·ik). 1. Referring to organogenesis. 2. Having origin in an organ.

organogeny (or·gan·**oj**·en·e). Organogenesis.

organoid (**or**·gan·oid). 1. Resembling an organ in structure or appearance. 2. Organelle. [organ, Gk *eidos* form.]

organoleptic (or·gan·o·**lep**′·tik). The quality of being able to make an impression on the sensory receptors of a special sense organ. [organ, Gk *lambanein* to seize.]

organoma (or·gan·**o**·mah). A variety of teratoma in which parts of organs can be recognized. [organ, Gk *-oma* tumour.]

organometallic (or·gan·o·met·**al**′·ik). Denoting compounds of a metal with organic alkyl radicals, e.g. zinc methyl $Zn(CH_3)_2$ and lead tetraethyl $Pb(C_2H_5)_4$, in which the metal has replaced hydrogen atoms in the corresponding hydrocarbons: they are mostly highly volatile liquids.

organonymy (or·gan·**on**·im·e). The designation or nomenclature of the organs of the body. [organ, Gk *onyma* name.]

organopathism (or·gan·**op**·ath·izm). The view that each organ should be studied separately as far as its pathology is concerned. [see foll.]

organopathy (or·gan·**op**·ath·e). 1. Any morbid condition affecting an organ of the body. 2. The local action of drugs. [organ, Gk *pathos* disease.]

organopexia, organopexy (or·gan·o·**pex**′·e·ah, **or**·gan·o·pex·e). The operation of fixing an organ which has been misplaced or otherwise is in an abnormally mobile condition. [organ, *pexis* fixation.]

organophil, organophilic (**or**·gan·o·fil, or·gan·o·**fil**′·ik). Having an affinity for certain body organs or tissues. [organ, Gk *philein* to love.]

organophilism (or·gan·**of**·il·izm). The state of having an affinity for some particular body organs or tissues. [see prec.]

organophosphates (or·gan·o·**fos**′·fates). A series of anticholinesterase compounds causing myosis, diplopia, perspiration, lacrimation, salivation, abdominal cramps, muscular twitching and weakness. *See* DFP, DNTP, OMPA, and TEPP.

organoscopy (or·gan·**os**·ko·pe). Examination of the abdominal viscera by a surgical telescope introduced through a puncture wound in the abdominal wall. [organ, Gk *skopein* to view.]

organotherapy (or·gan·o·**ther**′·ap·e). Treatment by administration of animal organs or extracts of animal organs. [organ, therapy.]

organotrophic (or·gan·o·**trof**′·ik). Pertaining or belonging to the nutrition of the body organs. [organ, *trophe* nourishment.]

organotropism, organotropy (or·gan·**ot**·ro·pizm, or·gan·**ot**·ro·pe). The condition of bodily economy in which certain chemical substances have a special affinity for particular organs or tissues. [organ, Gk *trope* a turning.]

organule (**or**·gan·ewl). An end-organ of the sensory receptor neurones, for example a taste bud; an essential cell. [dim. of organ.]

orgasm (**or**·gazm). The climax of excitement in the sexual act. Synonymous with ejaculation in the male. [Gk *orgein* to be passionate.]

orgasmolepsy (or·gaz·mo·lep·se). A rare type of seizure precipitated by sexual intercourse and occurring at the moment of orgasm. [orgasm, Gk *lepsis* a seizing.]

orgastic (or·**gas**·tik). Referring to, or of the nature of an orgasm; characterized by orgasm.

orgeat (**or**·zhah). A French flavouring syrup prepared either with an emulsion of almonds or with a decoction of barley. [Fr. *orge* barley.]

Orgotein (or'·go·te·in). BP Commission approved name for a group of soluble metalloproteins isolated from liver, red blood cells and other mammalian tissues; anti-inflammatory.

orientation (or·e·en·ta'·shun). 1. In psychology, the determination of one's bearings in relation to the environment or to a specific aspect of it. 2. In chemistry, the disposition of the substituted elements or groups about a benzene ring, i.e. in the *ortho-*, *meta-* or *para-* positions. 3. At an interface, e.g. between water and air, the alignment of the unsymmetrical molecules of a solute like oleic acid so that the polar carboxyl groups are turned towards the water and the hydrocarbon groups to the air. Many of the phenomena of cell adsorption and enzyme action may be due to this effect. [L *oriens* the rising (sun), i.e. the East.]

orifice [orificium (NA)] (or·if·is). An opening. **Aortic orifice [ostium aortae (NA)].** The orifice through which blood from the left ventricle enters the ascending aorta. **Atrioventricular orifice, left (mitral) [ostium atrioventriculare sinistrum (NA)].** The orifice, guarded by the bicuspid (mitral) valve, through which the left atrium and ventricle communicate. **Atrioventricular orifice, right (tricuspid) [ostium atrioventriculare dextrum (NA)].** The orifice, guarded by the tricuspid valve, through which the right atrium and ventricle communicate. **Orifice of the female urethra, external [ostium urethrae externum (NA)].** The slit-like orifice directly in front of the opening of the vagina. **Ileocolic orifice [ostium ileocaecale].** The opening of the ileum into the large intestine, guarded by upper and lower folds or frenula. **Orifice of the male urethra, external [ostium urethrae externum (NA)].** The narrowed part of the urethra; a vertical slit 6 mm long. **Pulmonary orifice [ostium trunci pulmonalis (NA)].** The orifice through which blood from the right ventricle enters the pulmonary trunk. **Orifice in the stomach, cardiac [ostium cardiacum (NA)].** The junction of the oesophagus and stomach, which is devoid of an anatomical sphincter but usually resists the regurgitation of the stomach contents into the oesophagus. **Orifice in the stomach, pyloric [ostium pyloricum (NA)].** The opening from the stomach into the duodenum. **Orifice of the ureter [ostium ureteris (NA)].** The slit-like termination of a ureter; they lie 25 mm apart in the empty bladder. **Urethral orifice, internal [ostium urethrae internum (NA)].** The crescentic opening at the apex of the trigone, leading into the urethra. **Orifice of the vagina [ostium vaginae (NA)].** A median slit in the vestibule, below and behind the urethral orifice. [L *orificium.*]

orificial (or·if·ish·al). Belonging to an orifice.

orificium (or·if·ish·e·um). An opening. [L.]

oriform (or·e·form). Shaped like a mouth or opening. [L *os* mouth, form.]

Origanum (o·rij·an·um). A genus of plants of the family Labiatae. **Origanum marjorana.** Sweet marjoram, a species which yields oil of marjoram, of low phenolic content. **Origanum vulgare.** Wild marjoram, the source of origanum oil, containing up to 85 per cent of carvacrol. Other species yielding this oil are *Origanum hirtum* and *O. majoranoides.* [Gk *origanon.*]

origin (or·ij·in). The beginning; the relative fixed origin of a muscle from which it exerts its action upon its insertion, or the point on the parent stem from which a branch of a nerve or blood vessel begins. **Origin of species.** An expression that has acquired a special significance since Charles Darwin wrote his book, *On the Origin of Species by means of Natural Selection*, London, 1859, in which he propounded the theory of natural selection. [L *origo* source.]

orinasal (or·e·na·zal). Oronasal.

orinotherapy (or·in·o·ther'·ap·e). The treatment of disease by residence in mountainous areas. [Gk *oreinos* mountainous, therapy.]

orizabin (o·riz·ab·in). Scammonin; the ether-soluble portion of jalap resin. [*Orizaba*, a town in Mexico.]

Ormond, John Kelso (b. 1886). American urologist.

Ormond's disease. A form of retroperitoneal fibrosis causing ureteral obstruction.

ornithine (or·nith·een). Diaminovaleric acid. *See* ACID.

Ornithodorus (or·nith·o·dor'·us). A genus of ticks. The species are world-wide in distribution and are the most important vectors of the spirochaetes of relapsing fever. In most cases their normal hosts are not man, and consequently relapsing fever, though endemic, is sporadic in its incidence. The larvae and adults usually remain on the host for a short time only, but in some cases may remain for days; all stages can transmit spirochaetes and the females infect the eggs with them. In all species the bite is painful and may produce toxic effects. **Ornithodorus coriaceus.** A species of California and Central America which bite man painfully, but is probably not a vector. **Ornithodorus corniceps.** A species that is a potential vector of American trypanosomiasis. **Ornithodorus erraticus.** A species of Spain and North Africa, responsible for sporadic relapsing fever. The pig is a favourite host. **Ornithodorus hermsi.** A species of western North America, responsible for sporadic relapsing fever and for Q fever. Chipmunks are the usual hosts, and these invade houses in winter. **Ornithodorus lahorensis.** A species of central Asia which is a vector of relapsing fever, possibly of the exanthemic typhus, and a potential vector of American trypanosomiasis. **Ornithodorus megnini.** *Otobius megnini.* **Ornithodorus moubata.** A species of all Africa, and primarily a parasite of man, living in dwellings, a vector of Q fever and potential vector of American trypanosomiasis. It is the most important vector of relapsing fever. **Ornithodorus nereensis.** A species that is a vector of relapsing fever. **Ornithodorus nicollei.** A vector of tick-borne typhus and a potential vector of American trypanosomiasis. **Ornithodorus normandi.** A sub-species of *Ornithodorus erraticus* (see above); it transmits relapsing fever. **Ornithodorus papillipes.** *Ornithodorus tholozani* (see below). **Ornithodorus parkeri.** A species of north-western North America, which normally feeds on small rodents, but may be a sporadic vector of relapsing fever and typhus. **Ornithodorus rostratus.** A potential vector of yellow fever and of American trypanosomiasis. **Ornithodorus rudis.** A species of Central America which enters houses and feeds on man readily. It is an important vector of relapsing fever. It has been confused with *Ornithodorus talaje.* **Ornithodorus savignyi.** A vector of relapsing fever in North Africa and Asia. **Ornithodorus talaje.** A species of Central America which rarely enters houses and seldom feeds on man. **Ornithodorus tartakowskyi.** A vector of relapsing fever. **Ornithodorus tholozani.** A species of western Asia, Persia and Syria, and a sporadic vector of relapsing fever. **Ornithodorus turicatum.** A vector of relapsing fever and of Q fever and a potential vector of American trypanosomiasis. **Ornithodorus venezuelensis.** A species of Central America which may be a sporadic vector of relapsing fever and is a potential vector of American trypanosomiasis; perhaps the same as *Ornithodorus rudis.* **Ornithodorus verrucosus.** A vector of relapsing fever. [Gk *ornis* bird, *doros* a leather bag.]

ornithonyssus (or·nith·o·nis'·us). A mite infesting rats and fowls which may also infest man. [Gk *ornis* bird, *nyssein* to pierce.]

ornithosis (or·nith·o·sis). 1. A virus disease resembling psittacosis affecting pigeons, doves and probably some other birds which is conveyed to man, causing bronchitis and bronchopneumonia. 2. A generic name for all respiratory virus infections transmissible from birds to man, including psittacosis. [Gk *ornis* bird, *-osis* condition.]

ornus (or·nus). Fraxinus, the ash. [L.]

oro (o·ro). The local name (West Africa) for a poisonous decoction of a cactus.

oro-antral (or·o·an·tral). Relating to the mouth and antrum. [L *os* mouth, Gk *antron* cave.]

orolingual (or·o·ling·gwal). Belonging to, or formed by the mouth and tongue, e.g. certain sounds. [L *os* mouth, *lingua* tongue.]

oromaxillary (or·o·max·il'·ar·e). Relating to the mouth and region of the maxilla. [L *os* mouth, maxilla.]

oronasal (or·o·na·zal). Belonging to the mouth and nose. [L *os* mouth, *nasus* nose.]

oronosus (or·o·**no**·sus). Mountain sickness; anoxia. [Gk *oros* mountain, *nosos* disease.]

oropharyngeal (**or**·o·far·**in**′·je·al). Relating or belonging to the oropharynx or lying within it.

oropharynx (or·o·**far**·ingx). The part of the pharynx which lies below the soft palate and behind the mouth; the buccal part of the pharynx. [L *os* mouth, pharynx.]

Oropsylla (o·ro·**sil**·ah). A genus of fleas. *Oropsylla silantiewi* is the characteristic flea of the tarabagan (*Arctomys bobac*) and is responsible for carrying plague to man during epidemics amongst rodents in the Siberian and Mongolian steppes. Several other species are possible vectors of sylvatic plague in north-western America. [Gk *oros* mountain, *psylla* flea.]

orphenadrine (or·**fen**·ah·dreen). 2-Dimethylaminoethyl 2-methyl-diphenylmethyl ether. **Orphenadrine Citrate BP 1973.** The dihydrogen citrate of orphenadrine, used principally to relieve disability due to rigidity in Parkinsonism. It also reduces depression which accompanies advanced Parkinsonism. **Orphenadrine Hydrochloride BP 1973.** The hydrochloride of orphenadrine; action and use are those of the citrate but the hydrochloride is much more soluble in water.

orpiment (**or**·pe·ment). A naturally-occurring mineral, essentially arsenic trisulphide, As_2S_3. [L *auri pigmentum* pigment of gold.]

Orr, Hiram Winnett (b. 1877). Lincoln, Nebraska, orthopaedic surgeon.

Winnett Orr's method or treatment. The treatment of chronic osteomyelitis by opening the bone cavity, packing with petroleum jelly gauze and immobilizing the limb in closed plaster.

orrhodiagnosis (**or**·o·di·ag·**no**′·sis). Serum diagnosis. *See* DIAGNOSIS. [Gk *orrhus* serum, diagnosis.]

orrho-immunity (**or**·o·im·**ewn**′·it·e). Passive immunity. *See* IMMUNITY. [Gk *orrhos* serum, immunity.]

orrhology (or·**ol**·o·je). Serology; the science of serum and its specific powers associated with immunity. [Gk *orrhos* serum, *logos* science.]

orrhomeningitis (**or**·o·men·in·**ji**′·tis). Inflammation in which there is involvement of a serous membrane. [Gk *orrhos* serum, meningitis.]

orrhorrhoea (or·o·**re**·ah). Discharge, generally from a mucous membrane, of a serous or watery type. [Gk *orrhos* serum, *rhoia* flow.]

orrhosis (or·**o**·sis). The formation of serum. [Gk *orrhos* serum.]

orrhotherapeutic (**or**·o·ther·ap·**ew**′·tik). Relating to orrhotherapy.

orrhotherapy (or·o·**ther**·ap·e). 1. Whey cure. 2. Serum therapy. [Gk *orrhos* serum, therapy.]

Orris BPC 1949 (**or**·is). Orris root, iridis rhizoma; the rhizome of *Iris germanica* Linn., *I. pallida* Lam. and *I. florentina* Linn. (family Iridaceae). It contains about 0.2 per cent of a yellowish, buttery, aromatic substance (concrete oil of orris or butter of orris) and the ketonic substance irone. Both are used in perfumery and powdered orris root is used in toilet powder and dental preparations. [prob. corruption of *iris*.]

Orsat apparatus. An apparatus used in gas analysis for estimating carbon dioxide, oxygen and carbon monoxide in producer gases, in gases from blast furnaces and from other sources.

Orsi, Francesco (b. 1828). Pavia physician.

Orsi-Grocco method. A method of palpatory percussion of the heart.

Orth, Johannes J. (b. 1847). Berlin pathologist.

Orth's solution. A histological fixative containing formaldehyde and potassium dichromate.

orthanilamide (or·than·**il**·am·ide). Name given to the *ortho*- form of aminobenzene sulphonamide. It is inactive compared with the *para*-isomer (sulphanilamide).

orthergasia (or·ther·**ga**·ze·ah). Normal physiological action of the body. [Gk *orthos* right, *ergon* work.]

ortho- (**or**·tho). 1. Right, correct, straight. 2. In chemistry, denoting the attachment of atoms or radicals to a benzene ring in adjacent positions: the 1,2 position. [Gk *orthos* right, straight.]

ortho-arteriotony (**or**·tho·ar·teer·e·**ot**′·on·e). Arterial blood pressure normal in amount. [Gk *orthos* right, artery, tone.]

orthobiosis (**or**·tho·bi·**o**′·sis). Living of a hygienically sound life, mentally and physically. [Gk *orthos* right, *bios* life.]

Orthocaine BP 1953 (**or**·tho·kane). Methyl *m*-amino-*p*-hydroxy-benzoate, $NH_2C_6H_4(OH)COOCH_3$. A colourless, tasteless, white crystalline powder, slightly soluble in water; soluble in alcohol and ether. It is used as a local analgesic, often in the form of dusting powders, owing to its low solubility.

orthochlorophenol (**or**·tho·klor·o·**fe**′·nol). $C_6H_4(OH)Cl$. A phenolic antiseptic.

orthochlorosalol (**or**·tho·klor·o·**sal**′·ol). $C_6H_4(OH)COOC_6H_4Cl$. A compound derived from phenyl salicylate, used as an antiseptic.

orthochorea (**or**·tho·ko·**re**′·ah). A type of chorea in which the jerking movements occur only or mainly when the patient is in the erect position, standing or walking. [Gk *orthos* straight, chorea.]

orthochromatic (**or**·tho·kro·**mat**′·ik). Pertaining to a tissue or cell which stains or is coloured in the normal way. [Gk *orthos* right, *chroma* colour.]

orthochromia (or·tho·**kro**·me·ah). A condition in which the red blood cells have their full or normal amount of haemoglobin. [see prec.]

orthochromophil, orthochromophile (or·tho·**kro**·mo·fil, or·tho·**kro**·mo·file). Capable of being stained the same colour as the dye itself. [Gk *orthos* right, *chroma* colour, *philein* to love.]

orthocrasia (or·tho·**kra**·ze·ah). Physiological adjustment so that ingested matter such as certain proteins and drugs give reactions of certain fixed pattern; in contradistinction to idiosyncrasy in which the reactions are of abnormal type. [Gk *orthos* right, *krasis* a blending.]

orthocresol (or·tho·**kre**·sol). $CH_3C_6H_4OH$, a phenolic antiseptic of considerably greater disinfectant power than phenol.

orthocytosis (**or**·tho·si·**to**′·sis). The condition in which only normal mature red cells are present in the circulating blood. [Gk *orthos* right, *kytos* cell, *-osis* condition.]

orthodactylous (or·tho·**dak**·til·us). Possessing straight fingers or toes. [Gk *orthos* straight, *daktylos* finger or toe.]

orthodentine (or·tho·**den**·teen). Tubular dentine of a relatively simple pattern, as in human teeth. [Gk *orthos* straight, dentine.]

orthodiagram (or·tho·**di**·ah·gram). The x-ray radiograph of an organ recorded by the orthodiagraph.

orthodiagraph (or·tho·**di**·ah·graf). The radiograph of an organ when only a pin-point stream of parallel x-rays is used. All oblique rays are eliminated, and thus the exact size of the organ is reproduced without distortion. [Gk *orthos* straight, *dia*, *graphein* to record.]

orthodiagraphy (**or**·tho·di·**ag**′·raf·e). The production of the orthodiagraph.

orthodiascope (or·tho·**di**·ah·skope). A radiographic instrument used in performing orthodiascopy.

orthodiascopy (**or**·tho·di·**as**′·ko·pe). The visualization on the fluorescent screen of the orthodiagraphic outline of a body or organ. [Gk *orthos* straight, *dia*, *skopein* to view.]

orthodichlorobenzene (**or**·tho·di·klor·o·**ben**′·zeen). $C_6H_4Cl_2$, a colourless liquid used as a solvent and insecticide.

orthodigita (or·tho·**dij**·it·ah). The science of correcting digital deformities. [Gk *orthos* straight, L *digitus* finger or toe.]

orthodont (**or**·tho·dont). Having normal teeth. [Gk *orthos* straight, *odous* tooth.]

orthodontia (or·tho·**don**·she·ah). Orthodontics.

orthodontic (or·tho·**don**·tik). Appertaining to orthodontics.

orthodontics (or·tho·**don**·tix). That part of dental surgery which is concerned with the prevention and correction of the malocclusion of teeth. [Gk *orthos* straight, *odous* tooth.]

orthogenesis (or·tho·**jen**·es·is). 1. Evolution in which the variations are not haphazard and influenced by environment, but adopt a given direction. 2. Theory that evolution is premeditated and governed by certain intrinsic factors. [Gk *orthos* right, *genesis* origin.]

orthogenics (or·tho·**jen**·ix). Eugenics. [Gk *orthos* right, *genesis* origin.]

orthoglycaemic (**or**·tho·gli·**se**′·mik). Applicable to the state in which the amount of sugar in the blood is at normal levels. [Gk *orthos* right, *glykos* sweet, *haima* blood.]

orthognathic (or·tho·**nath**·ik). The condition in which the upper jaw is set approximately in a vertical plane when the skull is orientated on the Frankfort horizontal plane. [Gk *orthos* straight, *gnathos* jaw.]

orthograde (**or**·tho·grade). Carrying the body in the erect position, in contrast to pronograde. [Gk *orthos* straight, L *gradus* a step.]

orthokeratinization (**or**·tho·ker·at·in·i·**za**′·shun). Normal formation of keratin in skin, hair and nails. [Gk *orthos* right, *keras* horn.]

orthokinetic (**or**·tho·kin·**et**′·ik). Denoting the movement of particles in the same direction, as in sedimentation or creaming, when the effect of the brownian movement is overcome by gravity. Cf. PERIKINETIC. [Gk *orthos* straight, *kinesis* movement.]

orthometabolism (**or**·tho·met·**ab**′·ol·izm). Normal growth or normal metabolic process. [Gk *orthos* right, metabolism.]

orthometer (or·**thom**·et·er). A device for estimating the relative protrusion or retraction of the eyeballs. [Gk *orthos* right, meter.]

orthomonochlorphenol (**or**·tho·mon·o·klor·**fe**′·nol). Orthochlorophenol.

orthomorphia (**or**·tho·**mor**·fe·ah). The treatment of deformities by surgical and mechanical methods. [Gk *orthos* straight, *morphe* shape.]

orthomyxovirus (**or**·tho·mix·o·**vi**′·rus). *See* MYXOVIRUS.

orthoneutrophil, orthoneutrophile (or·tho·**new**·tro·fil, or·tho·-**new**·tro·file). Orthochromophil; staining normally with neutral dyes. [Gk *orthos* right, neutrophil.]

orthopaedia (or·tho·**pe**·de·ah). Orthopaedics.

orthopaedic (or·tho·**pe**·dik). Relating to or employed in orthopaedics.

orthopaedics (or·tho·**pe**·dix). That part of surgery which deals with the abnormalities, diseases and injuries of the locomotor system. **Dental orthopaedics.** The science and practice of the correction of malocclusion of the teeth; orthodontics. [Gk *orthos* straight, *pais* child.]

orthopaedist (or·tho·**pe**·dist). One skilled in the art of orthopaedics; an orthopaedic surgeon.

orthopercussion (**or**·tho·per·**kush**′·un). A method of percussion in which the left middle finger is flexed at a right angle and the tip of the finger applied to the chest wall. The flexed finger is then lightly struck upon the distal end of the first phalanx. [Gk *orthos* straight, percussion.]

orthophenanthroline (**or**·tho·fe·**nan**′·thro·leen). $C_{12}H_8N_2$, a heterocyclic compound which is an oxidation-reduction indicator used in volumetric analysis.

orthophony (or·**thof**·on·e). The accurate and straightforward production of sound. [Gk *orthos* straight, *phone* sound.]

orthophoria (or·tho·**for**·e·ah). The condition of muscle balance in which no deviations of the eyes occur when one or other is covered in the so-called position of rest. The presence or absence of this condition is usually determined subjectively with the Maddox rod for hypermetropia and with the Maddox wing test for myopia. [Gk *orthos* straight, *pherein* to bear.]

orthophoric (or·tho·**for**·ik). Relating to, of the nature of, or characterized by orthophoria.

orthophosphate (or·tho·**fos**·fate). A salt of orthophosphoric acid.

orthophrenia (or·tho·**fre**·ne·ah). The state in which the mind reacts normally in the ordinary circumstances of life. [Gk *orthos* right, *phren* mind.]

orthopia (or·**tho**·pe·ah). The correction or prevention of squint. [Gk *orthos* straight, *ops* eye.]

orthoplastocyte (or·tho·**plas**·to·site). A normal blood platelet. [Gk *orthos* right, plastocyte.]

orthoplessimeter (**or**·tho·ples·**im**′·et·er). A device used in orthopercussion instead of the pleximeter finger. [Gk *orthos* straight, pleximeter.]

orthopnoea (or·thop·**ne**·ah). A condition in which the patient can breathe comfortably only when he is sitting or standing erect. **Orthopnoea cardiaca.** Angina pectoris. [Gk *orthos* straight, *pnoia* breath.]

orthopnoeic (or·thop·**ne**·ik). Pertaining to orthopnoea.

orthopraxis, orthopraxy (or·tho·**prax**·is, **or**·tho·prax·e). Correction of physical deformity by surgical or other means. [Gk *orthos* straight, *praxis* a doing.]

orthopsychiatry (**or**·tho·si·**ki**′·at·re). The science and treatment of personality and behaviour disorders. [Gk *orthos* right, *psyche* mind, *iatreia* treatment.]

Orthoptera (or·**thop**·ter·ah). An order of exopterygote insects which includes cockroaches, crickets, grasshoppers and locusts. Members of the genera *Blatella*, *Blatta* and *Periplaneta* are of medical interest. [Gk *orthos* straight, *pteron* wing.]

orthoptic (or·**thop**·tik). Denoting or referring to the correction of deviation in the eyes. [see foll.]

orthoptics (or·**thop**·tix). The methods employed in the training of patients with squint. The majority of these involve the use of a modified form of stereoscope. [Gk *orthos* straight, *ops* eye.]

orthoptist (or·**thop**·tist). A specialist in the correction of squint or other results of ill-balance of ocular muscle by ocular exercises. [see prec.]

orthoptoscope (or·**thop**·to·skope). An adjustable form of reflecting stereoscope by means of which dissociated images are presented to the two eyes. The angle between the tubes can be varied and the images twisted, if necessary, so as to correspond to the type of squint in the patient and induce him to fuse them and obtain binocular vision. Many similar instruments are made with different names, e.g. synoptophore, synoptoscope, major amblyoscope. [Gk *orthos* straight, *ops* eye, *skopein* to view.]

orthorhombic (or·tho·**rom**·bik). In crystallography, a crystal system in which 3 unequal axes intersect at right angles to one another. [Gk *orthos* straight, rhomb.]

orthoroentgenography (**or**·tho·runt·yen·**og**′·raf·e). Orthodiagraphy. [Gk *orthos* straight, roentgenography.]

Orthorrhapha (or·tho·**ra**·fah). A sub-order of the insectan order Diptera. The groups Nematocera and Brachycera which are contained in it are often treated as separate sub-orders. [Gk *orthos* straight, *rhaphe* suture.]

orthoscope (**or**·tho·skope). An instrument devised by Czermak in 1851 for viewing the fundus of the eye. A glass box filled with water was fitted over the eye, the water neutralizing the corneal refraction and so allowing a view of the fundus. Of historical interest only. [Gk *orthos* straight, *skopein* to view.]

orthoscopic (or·tho·**skop**·ik). 1. Providing an image of normal and undistorted proportions. 2. Belonging to an orthoscope or relating to orthoscopy. 3. Denoting lenses which are cut from the outer part of a large-sized lens. [see prec.]

orthoscopy (or·**thos**·ko·pe). Use of the orthoscope for examining the eyes.

orthosis (or·**tho**·sis). The procedure of adjusting or otherwise correcting deformity. [Gk *orthos* straight.]

orthoskiagraph (or·tho·**ski**·ah·graf). Orthodiagraph. [Gk *orthos* straight, *skia* shadow, *graphein* to record.]

orthoskiagraphy (**or**·tho·ski·**ag**′·raf·e). Orthodiagraphy. [see prec.]

orthostatic (or·tho·**stat**·ik). Referring to or due to the maintenance of an upright position. [Gk *orthos* straight, *statikos* causing to stand.]

orthostatism (or·tho·**stat**·izm). An upright standing posture of the body. [see prec.]

orthostereoscope (or·tho·**steer**·e·o·skope). An apparatus used for producing stereoscopic radiographs. [Gk *orthos* straight, stereoscope.]

orthosympathetic (**or**·tho·sim·path·**et**′·ik). An epithet applied to the sympathetic nervous system proper, in distinction from the parasympathetic. [Gk *orthos* straight, sympathetic.]

orthoterion, orthoterium (or·tho·**teer**·e·on, or·tho·**teer**·e·um). A device used to straighten abnormally curved limbs. [Gk *orthoter* straightener.]

orthotherapy (or·tho·**ther**·ap·e). Treatment of diseases or disorders by correcting the posture of the patient. [Gk *orthos* straight, therapy.]

orthotic (or·**thot**·ik). 1. Relating to orthosis. 2. Orthostatic.

orthotonos, orthotonus (or·**thot**·on·os, or·**thot**·on·us). A tetanic spasm in which the head, body and limbs are held fixedly and rigidly in a straight line. [Gk *orthos* straight, *tonos* tension.]

orthotopic (or·tho·**top**·ik). In the correct place. [Gk *orthos* right, *topos* place.]

orthotrophy (or·**thot**·ro·fe). 1. A state of normal or proper nourishment. 2. The ordinary physiological process of assimilating food. [Gk *orthos* right, *trophe* nourishment.]

orthotropic (or·tho·**trop**·ik). Growing vertically in an upward or downward extension; said of roots, stems and abdominal, pelvic or thoracic neoplasms. [Gk *orthos* straight, *trepein* to turn.]

orthotropism (or·**thot**·ro·pizm). Vertical growth. [see prec.]

orthropsia (or·**throp**·se·ah). The ability to see better in twilight and early dawn than at mid-day when the sun is bright. [Gk *orthros* dawn, *ops* eye.]

orthuria (orth·**ewr**·e·ah). Micturition occurring at normal intervals. [Gk *orthos* right, urine.]

Ortolani, Marius. 20th century Italian orthopaedic surgeon.

Ortolani's sign (sometimes referred to as Ortolani's *jerk* or *click*). The snapping sensation which can be produced by reducing a congenital dislocation of the hip in the newborn.

Oryza (o·**ri**·zah). A genus of cereals (family Gramineae), including *Oryza sativa* Linn. from which rice is obtained. [Gk rice.]

oryzamin (o·**ri**·zam·in). Vitamin B_1. [Gk *oryza* rice.]

os (os) (pl. *ossa*). Bone. **Os acetabuli.** A scale of bone formed in the triradiate acetabular cartilage and fusing with the 3 main bones about the age of puberty. **Os calcis.** Calcaneum. **Os centrale [NA].** An occasional additional bone found between the scaphoid, trapezoid and capitate bones in the carpus. It is constant in many mammals. **Os costale [NA].** The bony part of a rib. **Os epitympanicum.** Part of the squamous temporal roofing in the middle ear which has a separate centre of ossification in early fetal life. **Os magnum.** The capitate bone. **Os novum.** Newly formed bone. **Os purum.** The name for bone freed from fat and connective tissue, used for grafting. **Os sepiae.** Cuttle-fish bone; the internal shell of the cuttle fish, used when crushed in tooth powder. **Os trigonum [NA].** An ossicle in the position of and replacing the posterior tubercle of the talus. [L.]

os (os) (pl. *ora*). A mouth. **Pinhole os.** Extreme atresia of the os uteri in under-developed women. **Os uteri, external [ostium uteri (NA)].** The opening in the vaginal part of the neck of the uterus. **Os uteri, internal.** The isthmus of the uterus. [L.]

osazone (o·**sa**·zone). A condensation compound of phenylhydrazine with reducing sugars. They are sparingly soluble in water and crystallize well in characteristic forms that serve to identify the sugars.

Osborne, Thomas Burr (b. 1859). New Haven, Connecticut, biochemist.

Osborne and Folin method, for total sulphur in biological material. Organic matter is destroyed and sulphur converted to sulphate by fusing with sodium peroxide. The sulphate is determined by precipitation as $BaSO_4$.

Osborne and Mendel salt mixture. Calcium carbonate, magnesium carbonate, sodium carbonate, potassium carbonate, phosphoric acid, hydrochloric acid, manganese sulphate, citric acid and iron citrate, with sodium fluoride and potassium aluminium sulphate. It is used as a tonic salt mixture to supply mineral salts.

oscedo (os·**se**·do). 1. The act of yawning. 2. Aphthous stomatitis. [L *oscitare* to gape.]

oschea (os·ke·ah). The scrotum. [Gk *oscheon.*]

oscheal (os·ke·al). Of or relating to the scrotum. [see prec.]

oscheitis (os·ke·i·tis). Inflammatory invasion of the scrotal tissues. [Gk *oscheon* scrotum, *-itis* inflammation.]

oschelephantiasis (os·kel·e·fan·**ti**′·as·is). Elephantiasis of the scrotum. [Gk *oscheon* scrotum, elephantiasis.]

oscheocele (os·ke·o·seel). 1. A scrotal tumour or swelling. 2. A scrotal hernia. [Gk *oscheon* scrotum, *kele* hernia.]

oscheohydrocele (os·ke·o·**hi**′·dro·seel). Scrotal hydrocele. [Gk *oscheon* scrotum, hydrocele.]

oscheolith (os·ke·o·lith). A calculus in the sebaceous glands of the scrotum, sometimes referred to as scrotal calculus. [Gk *oscheon* scrotum, *lithos* stone.]

oscheoma, oscheoncus (os·ke·**o**·mah, os·ke·**ong**·kus). A neoplastic tumour of the scrotum. [Gk *oscheon* scrotum, *-oma* tumour.]

oscheoplasty (os·ke·o·plas·te). A plastic or reparative operation performed on the scrotum. [Gk *oscheon* scrotum, *plassein* to mould.]

oschitis (os·**ki**·tis). Oscheitis.

Oscillaria malariae (os·il·a·re·ah mal·a·re·e). The name originally suggested by Laveran for the malaria parasite discovered by him. [L *oscillare* to swing, malaria.]

oscillation (os·il·**a**·shun). 1. The act or motion of swinging to and fro, as of a pendulum. 2. Vibration. **Bradykinetic oscillation.** Slow, choreiform movements which recur at intervals in cases of epidemic encephalitis. [L *oscillare* to swing.]

oscillator (os·il·a·tor). 1. An apparatus used in mechanical therapeutics, similar to a vibrator. 2. A means of sustaining oscillations in an electrical circuit. [see prec.]

oscillogram (os·il·o·gram). The tracing made by an oscillograph.

oscillograph (os·il·o·graf). An instrument for recording oscillations produced by changes in electrical potential. **Cathode-ray oscillograph.** An instrument used for the presentation of phenomena which can be represented by an electric potential varying with time, often regularly recurring. The value of the potential is given by the vertical deflection of a spot of light caused by the impingement of an electron beam on a fluorescent screen. Auxiliary electronic circuits can cause uniform horizontal motion of the spot, leading to the presentation of a wave trace on the screen representing the variation of the applied potential with time. [L *oscillare* to swing, Gk *graphein* to record.]

oscillometer (os·il·**om**·et·er). An instrument used in the measurement of various kinds of oscillation, and in particular those of the blood stream, in which the disappearance and return of the pulse are marked by a vibrating needle. A fairly accurate method of estimating systolic and diastolic blood pressure. [L *oscillare* to swing, Gk *metron* measure.]

oscillometric (os·il·o·**met**′·rik). Relating to the oscillometer or to oscillometry.

oscillometry (os·il·**om**·et·re). The process of making observations with the oscillometer.

oscillopsia (os·il·**op**·se·ah). Oscillating vision. [L *oscillare* to swing, Gk *opsis* vision.]

oscilloscope (os·**il**·o·skope). 1. Oscillograph. 2. An apparatus used in electrical work to identify alternating currents. 3. A cathode-ray tube adapted to demonstrate the shape of the wave curve of high-frequency oscillations. [L *oscillare* to swing, Gk *skopein* to watch.]

Oscinidae (os·in·i·de). A family of the dipteran sub-order Cyclorrhapha. The genera *Hippelates, Oscinis* and *Siphunculina* are of medical interest. [L *oscen* singing bird.]

Oscinis (os·in·is). A genus of small flies. *Oscinis pallipes* from the West Indies may be a vector of yaws. [see prec.]

oscitancy (os·it·an·se). The tendency to yawn; drowsiness; dullness. [see foll.]

oscitate (os·it·ate). To yawn. [L *oscitare* to yawn.]

oscitation (os·it·**a**·shun). Yawning. [see prec.]

osculum (os·kew·lum). A pore or small opening. [L little mouth.]

Öse (er·zer). The German name, now obsolete, for a platinum wire looped at one end, the other being fixed into a glass or aluminium rod; used in bacteriological and virus work for sampling colonies, making sub-cultures and other techniques. [G loop.]

Osgood, Edwin Eugene (b. 1899). Portland, Oregon, physician.

Osgood-Haskins test, for urinary proteins. Mix 5 ml of urine with 1 ml of 50 per cent acetic acid and 3 ml of saturated sodium chloride solution. Proteins are precipitated immediately in the cold. If the precipitation dissolves upon boiling and reappears on cooling it is Bence-Jones protein. This test is particularly useful for the detection of Bence-Jones proteinuria, especially where the results of other tests are inconclusive.

Osgood, Robert Bayley (b. 1873). Boston orthopaedic surgeon.

Osgood disease, Osgood-Schlatter disease. Osteochondritis of the epiphysis of the tibial tuberosity.

O'Shaughnessy, Laurence (b. 1900). British surgeon.

O'Shaughnessy's operation. Cardiomentopexy.

Osiander, Johann Friedrich (b. 1787). Göttingen obstetrician.

Osiander's sign. The pulsation of the uterine arteries felt through the vaginal fornices in pregnancy.

oside (o·zide). The compound saccharides which split into simple sugars on hydrolysis.

Osler, Sir William (b. 1849). Montreal, Philadelphia, Baltimore and Oxford physician.

Osler's disease, Osler-Vaquez disease, Vaquez-Osler disease. Polycythaemia vera.

Osler's node or sign. A small, raised, red, tender patch found on the pads of the fingers, and occasionally toes, in bacterial endocarditis. It is transient, and due to infected cutaneous embolus.

Osler's phenomenon. The immediate agglutination of blood platelets after the withdrawal of the blood from the circulatory system.

Osler's triad. Telangiectasis, capillary fragility and hereditary haemorrhagic diathesis.

Osler-Libman-Sacks syndrome. Non-bacterial verrucose endocarditis associated with systemic lupus erythematosus.

Rendu-Osler-Weber disease. Hereditary haemorrhagic telangiectasia. *See* TELANGIECTASIA.

osmaesthesia (os·mes·**the**·ze·ah). The sensibility of the olfactory apparatus to recognize and differentiate odours. [Gk *osme* odour, aesthesia.]

osmate (**oz**·mate). Any salt of the hypothetical osmic acid: formed by the combination of osmium tetroxide with strong alkalis, they have the general formula $OsO_4 \cdot 2MOH$.

osmatic (oz·**mat**·ik). 1. Pertaining to the sense of smell. 2. Characterized by a normal sense of smell. [Gk *osme* odour.]

osmesis (oz·**me**·sis). Olfaction; the act of smelling. [Gk.]

osmic (**oz**·mik). 1. Related to or containing osmium. 2. Applied to any compound formed by tetravalent osmium.

osmicate (**oz**·mik·ate). To stain with osmium tetroxide (osmic acid).

osmics (**oz**·mix). The science of smells and smelling. [Gk *osme* odour.]

osmidrosis (oz·mid·**ro**·sis). Bromhidrosis; a condition in which the perspiration is foul-smelling. [Gk *osme* odour, *hidros* sweat.]

osmification (**oz**·mif·ik·**a**'·shun). The process of staining or impregnating with osmium tetroxide. [osmium, L *facere* to make.]

osmiophilic (oz·me·o·**fil**'·ik). Having an affinity for osmium tetroxide. [osmium, Gk *philein* to love.]

osmiophobic (**oz**·me·o·**fo**'·bik). Showing a tendency to resist staining with osmic acid. [osmic acid, Gk *phobein* to fear.]

osmiridium (oz·mir·**id**·e·um). An alloy of osmium and iridium which occurs naturally and is used for tipping instruments.

osmium (**oz**·me·um). An element of atomic weight 190.2, atomic number 76 and chemical symbol Os. It is a hard, very dense metal, found alloyed with iridium in the platiniferous sands of South America, Australia and Russia. It has a high melting-point (2700°C) and is used in electric-light filaments. **Osmium tetroxide.** OsO_4, an oxide of osmium, often referred to as *osmic acid* and used in the histological staining of fats. [Gk *osme* smell.]

osmoceptor (**oz**·mo·sep·tor). Osmoreceptor; receptor of smell stimuli. [Gk *osme* smell, L *recipere* to receive.]

osmodysphoria (**oz**·mo·dis·**for**'·e·ah). A morbid detestation of certain odours. [Gk *osme* odour, *dysphoros* hard to bear.]

osmogen (**oz**·mo·jen). An embryo substance, or one from which an active ferment is produced. [Gk *osmos* impulse, *genein* to produce.]

osmolagnia, osmolagny (oz·mo·**lag**·ne·ah, oz·mo·**lag**·ne). Sexual desire aroused by odour. [Gk *osme* odour, *lagneia* lust.]

osmolality (os·mo·lal·it·e). The osmotic concentration of a fluid expressed as the number of osmols of solute per kilogram of solution. [Gk *osmos* impulse.]

osmolar (oz·**mo**·lar). Osmotic.

osmology (oz·**mol**·o·je). 1. Osphresiology. 2. The branch of science concerned with osmoses. [Gk *osme* odour, *osmos* impulse, *logos* science.]

osmometer (oz·**mom**·et·er). 1. An apparatus for determining osmotic pressure. [Gk *osmos* impulse.] 2. Olfactometer; an apparatus for determining the degree of acuity of the olfactory sense. [Gk *osme* odour, *metron* measure.]

osmonosology (**oz**·mo·nos·**ol**'·o·je). The science which deals with olfactory disorders. [Gk *osme* odour, *nosos* disease, *logos* science.]

osmophilic (oz·mo·**fil**·ik). Of a type or quality that favours and leads to osmosis. [Gk *osmos* impulse, *philein* to love.]

osmophobia (oz·mo·**fo**·be·ah). Morbid fear of strong odours. [Gk *osme* odour, phobia.]

osmophore (**oz**·mo·fore). The elements of a chemical formula that are responsible for the smell. [Gk *osme* odour, *pherein* to bear.]

osmoreceptor (**oz**·mo·re·**sep**'·tor). One of the postulated centres in the hypothalamus which are sensitive to the osmolality of the plasma and which regulate the secretion of antidiuretic hormone. [Gk *osmos* impulse, L *recipere* to receive.]

osmoregulator (oz·mo·**reg**·ew·la·tor). Any device employed to control the penetration of x-rays. [Gk *osmos* impulse, regulator.]

osmoregulatory (**oz**·mo·reg·ew·**la**'·tor·e). Influencing or controlling the extent and speed of the process of osmosis. [osmosis, regulator.]

osmosis (oz·**mo**·sis). The movement of solvent molecules across a membrane to an area where there is a higher concentration of solute to which the membrane is impermeable. [Gk *osmos* impulse.]

osmotic (oz·**mot**·ik). Relating to or having the property of osmosis.

osmyl (**oz**·mil). Any variety of strong smell, either distasteful or pleasing. [Gk *osme* odour, *hyle* matter.]

osology (o·**sol**·o·je). The science concerning the body fluids. [Gk *ozein* to have a smell, *logos* science.]

osone (**o**·sone). A ketonic aldehyde resulting from the hydrolysis of an osazone: an intermediary compound formed in the synthesis of a ketose from the isomeric aldose.

osphrasia (os·**fra**·ze·ah). Olfaction; the sense of smell. [Gk *osphresis* smell.]

osphresiolagnic (os·fre·ze·o·**lag**'·nik). An individual who experiences sexual satisfaction from the inhalation of odours. [Gk *osphresis* smell, *lagneia* lust.]

osphresiological (os·**fre**·ze·o·**loj**'·ik·al). Relating or belonging to osphresiology.

osphresiology (os·**fre**·ze·**ol**'·o·je). The study and science which deals with the sense of smell and with the nature and production of odours. [Gk *osphresis* smell, *logos* science.]

osphresiometer (os·**fre**·ze·**om**'·et·er). Olfactometer; an apparatus for determining the degree of acuity of the olfactory sense. [Gk *osphresis* smell, *metron* measure.]

osphresiophilia (os·**fre**·ze·o·**fil**'·e·ah). A morbid interest in odours. [Gk *osphresis* smell, *philein* to love.]

osphresiophobia (os·**fre**·ze·o·**fo**'·be·ah). A morbid dislike of odours. [Gk *osphresis* smell, *phobein* to fear.]

osphresis (os·**fre**·zis). The sense of smell. [Gk smell.]

osphretic (os·**fret**·ik). Olfactory; referring to the sense of smell. [see prec.]

osphyalgia (os·fe·**al**·je·ah). Myalgic pain in the lumbar region, hip and flanks. [Gk *osphys* hip, *algos* pain.]

osphyarthrosis (os·fe·ar·**thro**'·sis). Coxitis; inflammatory affection of the hip joint. [Gk *osphys* hip, arthrosis.]

osphyitis (os·fe·i·tis). Inflammation affecting the lumbar region. [Gk *osphys* hip, *-itis* inflammation.]
osphyomyelitis (os·fe·o·mi·el·i′·tis). Inflammation affecting the spinal cord in the lumbar region. [Gk *osphys* hip, myelitis.]
ossein, osseine (os·e·in, os·e·een). 1. The organic matrix of bone. 2. The collagenous material extractable from bone. [L *os* bone.]
osseo-albumoid (os·e·o·al·bew′·moid). An albuminous protein extractable from bone. [L *os* bone, albumoid.]
osseo-aponeurotic (os·e·o·ap·on·ewr·ot′·ik). Referring to bone and an aponeurosis. [L *os* bone, aponeurosis.]
osseocartilaginous (os·e·o·kar·til·aj′·in·us). Osteochondrous. [L *os* bone, cartilage.]
osseofibrous (os·e·o·fi′·brus). Composed of or having the quality of bone and fibrous tissue. [L *os* bone, fibre.]
osseomucin (os·e·o·mew′·sin). A mucinous material, possibly chondroitin sulphate, extractable from bone. [L *os* bone, mucin.]
osseomucoid (os·e·o·mew′·koid). A mucoid substance forming part of the structure of bone. [L *os* bone, mucoid.]
osseosonometer (os·e·o·son·om′·et·er). An apparatus employed in the measurement of the conduction of sound through bony tissue. [L *os* bone, *sonus* sound, meter.]
osseosonometry (os·e·o·son·om′·et·re). Determination of the strength of the conduction of sound through bony tissue by means of the osseosonometer.
osseous (os·e·us). Consisting of or like bone. [L *os* bone.]
ossicle (os·ikl). A small bone. **Auditory ossicles [ossicula auditus (NA)].** The malleus, incus and stapes in the middle ear. **Mental ossicles.** Small ossicles appearing at the symphysis mandibulae in the fetus about the seventh month. After birth they fuse with the mandible and are responsible for the formation of the mental protuberance. **Pterion ossicle.** A cranial sutural bone found in the region of the pterion. [L *ossiculum* little bone.]
See also: ANDERNACH, BERTIN, KERCKRING, RIOLAN, SPIX.
ossiculectomy (os·ik·ewl·ek′·to·me). Operative removal of an ossicle, or of the auditory ossicles. [L *ossiculum* little bone, Gk *ektome* a cutting out.]
ossiculotomy (os·ik·ewl·ot′·o·me). Any operation involving incision of the auditory ossicles. [L *ossiculum* little bone, Gk *temnein* to cut.]
ossiculum (os·ik·ew·lum) (pl. *ossicula*). An ossicle. **Ossicula mentalia.** Mental ossicles. *See* OSSICLE. [dim. of L *os* bone.]
ossidesmosis (os·e·dez·mo′·sis). Osteodesmosis. [L *os* bone, Gk *desmos* band.]
ossiferous (os·if·er·us). 1. Bone-producing. 2. Containing bony tissue. [L *os* bone, *ferre* to bear.]
ossific (os·if·ik). Producing or developing into bone. [L *os* bone, *facere* to make.]
ossification (os·if·ik·a′·shun). The process by which bone is formed, consisting essentially of 3 phases: the deposition of a meshwork of collagenous fibres, the deposition of a cementing mucopolysaccharide around these fibres, and the impregnation of the cement with microcrystals of calcium phosphate and calcium carbonate. It is believed that specialized cells, osteoblasts, are responsible for the formation of bone; many of these are trapped within the calcified matrix as bone cells or osteocytes. **Cartilaginous ossification, Endochondral ossification.** The replacement of cartilage by bone, whereby most of the cartilage is removed and bone deposited on spicules of residual calcified cartilage. **Heterotopic ossification.** The development of bone in tissues other than skeletal. **Intramembranous ossification.** The formation of bone within a connective-tissue membrane without the appearance of cartilage. **Metaplastic ossification.** The conversion of soft tissue into bone. [L *os* bone, *facere* to make.]
ossifluence (os·if·loo·ens). A process of softening affecting bone substance. [L *os* bone, *fluere* to become weak.]
ossifluent (os·if·loo·ent). Derived from the breaking-down of bone. [see prec.]
ossiform (os·e·form). Like bone. [L *os* bone, form.]
ossify (os·e·fi). To convert or develop into bone. [L *os* bone, *facere* to make.]
ossiphone (os·e·fone). An instrument which utilizes hearing by bone condition; it is used as an aid for the deaf. [L *os* bone, Gk *phone* sound.]
ostaemia (os·te·me·ah). Abnormal amount of blood in a bone, causing congestion. [Gk *osteon* bone, *haima* blood.]
osteal (os·te·al). Having reference to bone. [Gk *osteon* bone.]
ostealgia (os·te·al·je·ah). Pain affecting a bone. [Gk *osteon* bone, *algos* pain.]
ostealgic (os·te·al·jik). Relating or belonging to, or characterized by pain in the bones. [see prec.]
ostealloeosis (os·te·al·e·o′·sis). A morbid change which occurs in the bone tissue, for example in the formation of an osteosarcoma. [Gk *osteon* bone, *alloioein* to be changed for the worse.]
osteamoeba (os·te·am·e′·bah). Osteoblast. [Gk *osteon* bone, amoeba.]
ostein, osteine (os·te·in, os·te·een). Ossein. [Gk *osteon* bone.]
osteite (os·te·ite). A discrete element of bony tissue or centre of ossification. [Gk *osteon* bone.]
osteitic (os·te·it·ik). Relating to or suffering from osteitis.
osteitis (os·te·i·tis). Inflammation of bone due to infection or injury. **Acute osteitis.** Acute osteomyelitis; a fulminating infection of bone generally due to infection by pyogenic cocci. **Apical osteitis.** Osteitis around the apex of a tooth, usually due to infection. **Chronic osteitis.** The late stage of the above type of infection, or a low-grade infection of bone of long duration. **Chronic non-suppurative osteitis.** Garre's osteitis, sclerosing osteitis; a chronic inflammatory condition of bone, associated with sclerosis and thickening and due to infection by pyogenic cocci. **Osteitis cystica multiplex.** Sarcoidosis involving the bone marrow; the term has also been applied to other conditions producing multiple cystic growths in the bone marrow. **Osteitis deformans.** Paget's disease, a chronic disease of the skeleton, in which there is softening of the bone followed by thickening of the cortex. The condition when generalized leads to marked deformity. **Osteitis fibrosa cystica.** Parathyroid osteitis, a generalized rarefaction of bone, associated with cyst formation and replacement of bone by fibrous tissue due to excessive parathyroid secretion, the result of enlargement of one or more of the parathyroid glands. The condition results in marked weakness and gross deformity of the bones. **Osteitis fibrosa localisata.** A localized change, usually in a long bone, where bone is replaced by fibrous tissue with cyst formation. The condition is not associated with disturbance of the parathyroid glands. **Gummatous osteitis.** Inflammation of bone secondary to infection by the specific organism, i.e. spirochaeta of syphilis or bacillus of tuberculosis. **Parathyroid osteitis.** Osteitis fibrosa cystica (see above). **Osteitis pubis.** Inflammation of the pubic symphysis which occurs after certain pelvic operations such as prostatectomy. **Radiation osteitis.** Osteitis that results from injudicious dosage with x-rays or radium. **Residual osteitis.** Osteitis remaining in the jaw after an infected tooth has been removed. **Sclerosing osteitis.** Chronic non-suppurative osteitis (see above). **Tuberculous osteitis.** Gummatous osteitis (see above). [Gk *osteon* bone, *-itis* inflammation.]
See also: GARRÉ.
ostembryon (ost·em·bre·on). A process of ossification of a fetus. [Gk *osteon* bone, embryo.]
ostempyesis (ost·em·pi·e′·sis). Suppuration in a bone. [Gk *osteon* bone, empyesis.]
osteo-acousia (os·te·o·ak·oo′·se·ah). Bone conduction. [Gk *osteon* bone, *akouein* to hear.]
osteo-anabrosis (os·te·o·an·ah·bro′·sis). Atrophy or rarefaction of bone. [Gk *osteon* bone, anabrosis.]
osteo-anaesthesia (os·te·o·an·es·the′·ze·ah). A condition in which a bone is insensitive to the touch. [Gk *osteon* bone, anaesthesia.]
osteo-anagenesis (os·te·o·an·a·jen′·es·is). Bone regeneration. [Gk *osteon* bone, anagenesis.]
osteo-aneurysm (os·te·o·an′·ewr·izm). A bone aneurysm. [Gk *osteon* bone, aneurysm.]
osteo-arthritis (os·te·o·ar·thri′·tis). Osteo-arthrosis. Chronic arthritis of a degenerative type, usually but not invariably

associated with increasing age. It is not accompanied by a generalized constitutional disorder and affects particularly the hips, spine, thumb bases and distal interphalangeal joints of the hands. Osteo-arthritis of the knees may be associated with obesity and at any site may follow severe or repeated trauma. **Hyperplastic osteo-arthritis.** Osteo-arthritis in which there is an associated proliferation of the synovial membrane of the joints. [Gk *osteon* bone, arthritis.]

osteo-arthropathy (os·te·o·ar·**throp**′·ath·e). Pseudohypertrophic pulmonary osteo-arthropathy (see below). **Pseudohypertrophic pulmonary osteo-arthropathy.** A joint condition affecting particularly the ankles, knees and wrists, associated usually with carcinoma of the bronchus but sometimes with other conditions, usually of the lung, and accompanied by clubbing of the fingers. [Gk *osteon* bone, *arthron* joint, *pathos* disease.]

osteo-arthrosis (os·te·o·ar·**thro**′·sis). Osteo-arthritis. **Osteo-arthrosis juvenilis.** Koehler's disease. [Gk *osteon* bone, arthrosis.]

osteo-arthrotomy (os·te·o·ar·**throt**′·o·me). Operative removal of the articular end of a bone. [Gk *osteon* bone, *arthron* joint, *temnein* to cut.]

osteo-articular (os·te·o·ar·**tik**′·ew·lar). Of the nature of or belonging to the bones and joints. [Gk *osteon* bone, L *articulus* joint.]

osteoblast (**os**·te·o·blast). A large pyriform or ovoid cell with an eccentric hypochromatic nucleus containing from 1 to 3 large nucleoli, basophilic cytoplasm, a large Golgi element and numerous mitochondria. It is thought to play a major role in the deposition of bone matrix. [Gk *osteon* bone, *blastos* germ.]

osteoblastic (os·te·o·**blas**′·tik). Referring to, of the nature of, or consisting of osteoblasts.

osteoblastoma (os·te·o·blas·**to**′·mah). A benign tumour found in children and young people. It occurs most frequently in the vertebral column or in the short bones of the hand or foot, and consists of osteoblasts which may produce a patchy osteoid matrix. [osteoblast, Gk *-oma* tumour.]

osteocampsia, osteocampsis (os·te·o·**kamp**′·se·ah, os·te·o·**kamp**′·sis). Curvature of a bone as occurs in cases of osteomalacia and rickets. [Gk *osteon* bone, *kampsis* a curving.]

osteocarcinoma (os·te·o·kar·sin·**o**′·mah). 1. Carcinoma of a bone. 2. A tumour composed of osteomatous and carcinomatous tissue. [Gk *osteon* bone, carcinoma.]

osteocartilaginous (os·te·o·kar·til·**aj**′·in·us). Osteochondrous; made up of bone and cartilage. [Gk *osteon* bone, cartilage.]

osteocele (**os**·te·o·seel). A testicular or scrotal tumour composed of bone tissue. [Gk *osteon* bone, *kele* hernia.]

osteocephaloma (os·te·o·kef·al·**o**′·mah). A soft encephaloid sarcoma of bone. [Gk *osteon* bone, encephaloma.]

osteochondral (os·te·o·**kon**′·dral). Of or relating to bone and cartilage, especially a bone and its articular cartilage. [Gk *osteon* bone, *chondros* cartilage.]

osteochondritis (os·te·o·kon·**dri**′·tis). A degenerative change in 1 or more epiphyses, commencing with necrosis and fragmentation followed by repair and regeneration. **Osteochondritis deformans juvenilis.** Osteochondritis of the spine in adolescents resulting in kyphosis. **Osteochondritis dissecans.** A disease of unknown aetiology in which fragments of articular cartilage of a joint, most commonly of the knee, are detached from the joint surface. Clinically there is pain and swelling with intermittent locking of the joint. **Osteochondritis of the hip.** Osteochondritis of the epiphysis of the head of the femur. **Osteochondritis of the lunate.** Kienboeck's atrophy. **Osteochondritis of the tarsal navicular.** Koehler's disease. **Osteochondritis of the tuberosity of the tibia.** Osgood-Schlatter disease. **Vertebral osteochondritis.** Osteochondritis deformans juvenilis (see above). [Gk *osteon* bone, *chondros* cartilage, *-itis* inflammation.]

osteochondrodysplasia (os·te·o·kon·dro·dis·**pla**′·ze·ah). Disease or abnormal development of bony-cartilaginous junctions. [Gk *osteon* bone, chondrodysplasia.]

osteochondrodystrophia deformans (os·te·o·kon·dro·dis·**tro**′·fe·ah de·**form**·anz). Eccentrochondrodysplasia. [Gk *osteon* bone, chondrodystrophia, L deforming.]

osteochondrodystrophy (os·te·o·kon·dro·**dis**′·tro·fe). 1. Eccentrochondrodysplasia. 2. Lipochondrodystrophy. [Gk *osteon* bone, chondrodystrophy.]

osteochondrolysis (os·te·o·kon·**drol**′·is·is). Osteochondritis dissecans. [Gk *osteon* bone, *chondros* cartilage, lysis.]

osteochondroma (os·te·o·kon·**dro**′·mah). A tumour composed of both bony and cartilaginous tissues. [Gk *osteon* bone, *chondros* cartilage, *-oma* tumour.]

osteochondromatosis (os·te·o·kon·dro·mat·**o**′·sis). A disease characterized by the occurrence of multiple osteochondromata. **Synovial osteochondromatosis.** The development of osteochondromata in the synovial membranes of joints, with subsequent detachment to become pedunculated or loose bodies in the joints. [osteochondroma, Gk *-osis* condition.]

osteochondrophyte (os·te·o·**kon**′·dro·fite). A tumour composed of bony and cartilaginous elements. [Gk *osteon* bone, *chondros* cartilage, *phyton* plant.]

osteochondrosarcoma (os·te·o·kon·dro·sar·**ko**′·mah). A tumour composed of bony, cartilaginous and sarcomatous tissues. [Gk *osteon* bone, chondrosarcoma.]

osteochondrosis (os·te·o·kon·**dro**′·sis). Osteochondritis. **Osteochondrosis deformans.** Osteochondritis deformans juvenilis. **Osteochondrosis dissecans.** Osteochondritis dissecans. **Juvenile osteochondrosis.** Osteochondritis deformans juvenilis. [Gk *osteon* bone, chondrosis.]

osteochondrous (os·te·o·**kon**′·drus). Relating to, having the characteristics, or made up of bone and cartilage. [Gk *osteon* bone, *chondros* cartilage.]

osteoclasia, osteoclasis (os·te·o·**kla**′·ze·ah, os·te·**ok**·las·is). 1. The fracture or refracture of a bone by surgical means for the purpose of correcting a deformity. 2. The breaking-down and absorption of bone tissue by osteoclasts. [Gk *osteon* bone, *klasis* a breaking.]

osteoclast (**os**·te·o·klast). 1. An instrument for breaking a bone. 2. A large multinuclear cell which produces physiological or pathological resorption of bone; especially one of the cells which help in the physiological resorption of the roots of deciduous teeth. In disease they may also help to resorb the root of a permanent tooth. [Gk *osteon* bone, *klasis* a breaking.]

osteoclastic (os·te·o·**klas**′·tik). Relating to or having the characteristics of an osteoclast or of osteoclasia.

osteoclastoma (os·te·o·klas·**to**′·mah). A tumour occurring at the ends of long bones in young adults. It consists of giant-celled osteoclasts scattered throughout a spindle-cell stroma. Usually benign, but an occasional tumour metastasizes. Multiple osteoclastomata, particularly in unusual sites, suggest the possibility of hyperparathyroidism. [osteoclast, Gk *-oma* tumour.]

osteocomma (os·te·o·**kom**′·ah). One of the segments, e.g. a vertebra, in a series of skeletal structures. [Gk *osteon* bone, *komma* fragment.]

osteocope (**os**·te·o·kope). Severe pain in a bone or in several bones, generally occurring in spasms and mostly associated with syphilitic infection. [Gk *osteon* bone, *kopos* pain.]

osteocopic (os·te·o·**kop**′·ik). Pertaining to osteocope.

osteocranium (os·te·o·**kra**′·ne·um). The cranium of a fetus after ossification has occurred. [Gk *osteon* bone, cranium.]

osteocystoma (os·te·o·sist·**o**′·mah). A cystic tumour occurring in a bone. [Gk *osteon* bone, *kystis* bag, *-oma* tumour.]

osteocyte (**os**·te·o·site). A bone cell. [Gk *osteon* bone, *kytos* cell.]

osteodentoma (os·te·o·den·**to**′·mah). An odontome consisting of bony and dentinal elements. [Gk *osteon* bone, L *dens* tooth, Gk *-oma* tumour.]

osteodermatoplastic (os·te·o·der·mat·o·**plas**′·tik). Relating to the growth of bony elements in cutaneous tissues. [Gk *osteon* bone, *derma* skin, *plassein* to mould.]

osteodermatous (os·te·o·**der**′·mat·us). Relating to osteodermia.

osteodermia (os·te·o·**der**′·me·ah). A condition in which bony changes have occurred in the skin. [Gk *osteon* bone, *derma* skin.]

osteodesmosis (os·te·o·dez·**mo**′·sis). 1. The growth of bone and tendinous tissues. 2. The formation of bone in a tendon. [Gk *osteon* bone, *desmos* band.]

osteodiastasis (os·te·o·di·**as'**·tas·is). The separation of a bone or of 2 contiguous bones. [Gk *osteon* bone, diastasis.]

osteodynia (os·te·o·**din'**·e·ah). Ostealgia. [Gk *osteon* bone, *odyne* pain.]

osteodysmetamorphosis (os·te·o·dis·met·ah·**mor'**·fo·sis). Hypophosphatasia. [Gk *osteon* bone, *dys-*, metamorphosis.]

osteodystrophia, osteodystrophy (os·te·o·dis·**tro'**·fe·ah, os·te·o·**dis'**·tro·fe). A disorder of bone, especially a metabolic disorder. **Osteodystrophia cystica.** Cystic disorder of bone, such as that seen in hyperparathyroidism. **Osteodystrophia deformans.** Osteitis deformans; Paget's disease of bone. **Osteodystrophia fibrosa.** Fibrous disorder of bone, such as that seen in Albright's disease and in hyperparathyroidism. **Osteodystrophia juvenilis.** Osteitis fibrosa cystica in a child. **Renal osteodystrophy.** Osteodystrophy due to renal disease; renal rickets. [Gk *osteon* bone, dystrophia.]

osteo-ectomy (os·te·o·**ek'**·to·me). The operation of removing a bone or segment of bone. [Gk *osteon* bone, *ektome* a cutting out.]

osteo-ectopia (os·te·o·ek·**to'**·pe·ah). Bone displacement. [Gk *osteon* bone, ectopia.]

osteo-encephaloma (os·te·o·en·kef·al·**o'**·mah). Osteocephaloma.

osteo-enchondroma (os·te·o·en·kon·**dro'**·mah). Osteochondroma. [Gk *osteon* bone, enchondroma.]

osteo-epiphysis (os·te·o·ep·**if'**·is·is). Any epiphysis of bone. [Gk *osteon* bone, epiphysis.]

osteofibrochondrosarcoma (os·te·o·fi·bro·**kon**·dro·sar·**ko'**·mah). A tumour composed of bony, fibrous, cartilaginous and muscular elements. [Gk *osteon* bone, fibre, chondrosarcoma.]

osteofibrolipoma (os·te·o·fi·bro·lip·**o'**·mah). A tumour containing bony, fibrous and fatty tissue. [Gk *osteon* bone, fibrolipoma.]

osteofibroma (os·te·o·fi·**bro'**·mah). A tumour made up of bone and fibrous tissue. [Gk *osteon* bone, fibroma.]

osteofibromatosis (os·te·o·fi·bro·mat·**o'**·sis). The development of multiple osteofibromata. **Cystic osteofibromatosis.** Jaffe-Lichtenstein disease. [osteofibroma, Gk *-osis* condition.]

osteofibrosis (os·te·o·fi·**bro'**·sis). Osteosclerosis; Albers-Schoenberg or marble-bone disease. [Gk *osteon* bone, fibrosis.]

osteogenesis (os·te·o·**jen'**·es·is). The formation of bone. **Osteogenesis imperfecta, fragilitas ossium.** A congenital abnormality of the skeleton, due to imperfect bone formation and associated with a peculiar blue colour of the sclerotic coat of the eye. The bones are brittle and fracture with trivial violence. [Gk *osteon* bone, *genein* to produce.]

osteogenetic (os·te·o·jen·**et'**·ik). Pertaining to osteogenesis.

osteogenic (os·te·o·**jen'**·ik). Applied to any structure that has its origin in or is made up of tissue from which bone grows or is repaired. [see foll.]

osteogenin (os·te·**oj**·en·in). A substance extractable with alcohol from fresh bony tissues, which is thought to be capable of inducing heterotopic bone formation when injected into muscles or connective tissues. [Gk *osteon* bone, *genein* to produce.]

osteogenous (os·te·**oj**·en·us). Osteogenic.

osteogeny (os·te·**oj**·en·e). Osteogenesis.

osteohalisteresis (os·te·o·**hal**·is·ter·**e'**·sis). Deprivation or lack of the mineral portions of a bone, so that there is general softening. [Gk *osteon* bone, *hals* salt, *steresis* privation.]

osteohydatidosis (os·te·o·hi·dat·id·**o'**·sis). Hydatid disease of the bones. [Gk *osteon* bone, *hydatis* vesicle, *-osis* condition.]

osteohypertrophic (os·te·o·hi·per·**tro'**·fik). Associated with overgrowth of bones. [Gk *osteon* bone, *hyper, trophe* nourishment.]

osteoid (os·te·oid). 1. Like bone. 2. The basic tissue of bone before calcification takes place. [Gk *osteon* bone, *eidos* form.]

osteolipochondroma (os·te·o·**lip**·o·kon·**dro'**·mah). A chondroma containing also bony and fatty tissue. [Gk *osteon* bone, *lipos* fat, chondroma.]

osteolipoma (os·te·o·lip·**o'**·mah). A lipoma with bony constituents. [Gk *osteon* bone, lipoma.]

osteolith (os·te·o·lith). A bone which has undergone petrifaction. [Gk *osteon* bone, *lithos* stone.]

osteology [osteologia (NA)] (os·te·**ol**·o·je). That branch of medicine which is concerned with the study and structure of the bones. [Gk *osteon* bone, *logos* science.]

osteolysis (os·te·**ol**·is·is). 1. The absorption and breaking-down of bone tissue by osteoclasts. 2. Deprivation or removal of bone calcium. [Gk *osteon* bone, *lysis* a loosing.]

osteolytic (os·te·o·**lit'**·ik). Pertaining to or undergoing the process of osteolysis.

osteoma (os·te·**o**·mah). An innocent tumour of bone. **Cancellous osteoma.** An osteoma mainly composed of cancellous bone. **Cavalryman's osteoma.** Rider's bone, exostosis; a tumour-like mass of bone which may form in the adductor muscles of riders as the result of continuous mild injury. **Compact osteoma.** An osteoma of compact bone. **Osteoma cutis.** A bony tumour of the skin. **Osteoma dentale.** A mass of hyperplastic bone or a true osteoma, arising in connection with displaced and inflamed teeth. **Osteoma durum, Osteoma eburneum.** A very hard osteoma with ivory-like bone. **Heteroplastic osteoma.** An osteoma which arises within tissues other than bone, as the result of metaplasia. **Homoplastic osteoma.** A true osteoma, i.e. one which arises within bone. **Ivory osteoma.** An osteoma mainly composed of hard eburnated bone. **Osteoma medullare.** An osteoma which is rich in marrow spaces. **Osteoid osteoma.** A curiously localized, painful innocent tumour of long and short bones, situated within the substance of the bone and composed of osteoid tissue. **Osteoma sarcomatosum.** Osteosarcoma; either an osteoma which has become sarcomatous or a sarcoma which forms much bony tissue. **Osteoma spongiosum.** An osteoma of cancellous spongy bone. [Gk *osteon* bone, *-oma* tumour.]

osteomalacia (os·te·o·mal·**a'**·she·ah). Mollities ossium; adult rickets; softening of the bones. A general disease of the bones due to a deficiency of vitamin D, which may be caused by a diet deficient in the vitamin, or a deficient absorption of vitamin D and calcium as in steatorrhoea. It is most commonly found in women, often associated with pregnancy, and occurs endemically among the underfed populations of parts of India, China, Japan and some of the poorer countries of Europe. It is essentially rickets occurring in adults, and shows the same pathological changes, giving rise to severe deformities especially of the spine, pelvis and thorax. The bones are soft and flexible so that they bend, whilst deformities of the pelvis cause diffulty in labour and necessitate Caesarean section. Untreated cases eventually become bedridden, anaemic and cachectic. [Gk *osteon* bone, *malakia* softness.]

osteomatoid (os·te·**o**·mat·oid). Like an osteoma. [osteoma, Gk *eidos* form.]

osteomatosis (os·te·o·mat·**o'**·sis). A condition in which multiple osteomata occur. [osteoma, Gk *-osis* condition.]

osteomere (os·te·o·meer). One of the units or segments of a skeletal structure composed of a number of such units, e.g. a vertebra. [Gk *osteon* bone, *meros* part.]

osteometry (os·te·**om**·et·re). That branch of anthropometry which deals with the size and measurement of bones. [Gk *osteon* bone, *metron* measure.]

osteomiosis (os·te·o·mi·**o'**·sis). Wasting of bone. [Gk *osteon* bone, *meioein* to diminish.]

osteomucoid (os·te·o·**mew'**·koid). Osseomucoid. [Gk *osteon* bone, mucoid.]

osteomyelitic (os·te·o·mi·el·**it'**·ik). Pertaining to, having the nature of, or characterized by osteomyelitis.

osteomyelitis (os·te·o·mi·el·**i'**·tis). Inflammation of the interior of a bone, especially affecting the marrow spaces. **Acute osteomyelitis.** Osteomyelitis of rapid onset and progression. **Chronic osteomyelitis.** Continuing suppuration of a bone the seat of acute osteomyelitis; Brodie's circumscribed abscess of bone. **Haemorrhagic osteomyelitis.** An osteomyelitis with which is associated much local haemorrhage. **Juvenile osteomyelitis.** Osteomyelitis of the epiphyseal regions of long bones in young children. **Sclerosing osteomyelitis.** Garré's osteomyelitis. **Typhoid osteomyelitis.** Osteomyelitis, usually of ribs or spine, occurring during typhoid fever. **Osteomyelitis variolosa.** Osteomyelitis occurring as a complication of smallpox. [Gk *osteon* bone, myelitis.]

See also: GARRÉ.

osteomyelodysplasia (os·te·o·mi·el·o·dis·**pla**′·ze·ah). Rarefaction of bone associated with leucopenia. The condition is often associated with irregular fever. [Gk *osteon* bone, *myelos* marrow, dysplasia.]

osteomyelography (os·te·o·mi·el·**og**′·raf·e). The visualization of the bone marrow by x-rays and also by radioactive isotopes. [Gk *osteon* bone, *myelos* marrow, *graphein* to record.]

osteon (os·te·on). A cylindrical unit of compact bone structure built around a central, vascular canal and composed of concentric bony lamellae. [Gk bone.]

osteoncus (os·te·**ong**·kus). 1. An osteoma. 2. An exostosis. [Gk *osteon* bone, *ogkos* a swelling.]

osteonecrosis (os·te·o·nek·**ro**′·sis). 1. Bone necrosis. 2. Ischaemic change developing in bone as a feature of decompression sickness. [Gk *osteon* bone, necrosis.]

osteoneuralgia (os·te·o·newr·**al**′·je·ah). Neuralgia affecting a bone. [Gk *osteon* bone, neuralgia.]

osteonosus (os·te·o·**no**′·sus). Any disease of bone. [Gk *osteon* bone, *nosos* disease.]

osteo-odontoma (os·te·o·o·don·**to**′·mah). A tumour arising from structures which normally give origin to teeth. [Gk *osteon* bone, *odous* tooth, *-oma* tumour.]

osteo-onychodysplasia (os·te·o·**on**·ik·o·dis·**pla**′·ze·ah). Hereditary osteo-onychodysplasia. Nail-patella syndrome. *See* SYNDROME. [Gk *osteon* bone, *onyx* nail, dys-, *plasis* a forming.]

osteopaedion (os·te·o·**pe**′·de·on). A dead fetus which has undergone calcification. [Gk *osteon* bone, *paidion* young child.]

osteoparectasis (os·te·o·par·**ek**′·tas·is). 1. Excessive lengthening of a bone. 2. Production of over-extension in the treatment of a fractured bone or limb. [Gk *osteon* bone, *parekteinein* to stretch out along.]

osteopath (ós·te·o·path). One who is expert in the practice of osteopathy.

osteopathia (os·te·o·**path**′·e·ah). Any pathological change in bone; disease of bone. [Gk *osteon* bone, *pathos* disease.]

osteopathic (os·te·o·**path**′·ik). Relating to osteopathy.

osteopathist (os·te·**op**·ath·ist). Osteopath.

osteopathology (os·te·o·path·**ol**′·o·je). Any disease of bone. [Gk *osteon* bone, pathology.]

osteopathy (os·te·**op**·ath·e). 1. Disease of bone. 2. A system of treatment of disease by manipulation. **Alimentary osteopathy, Hunger osteopathy, War osteopathy.** Changes in the skeleton produced by deficiency of food, producing weakness and bone pains often with multiple fractures. [Gk *osteon* bone, *pathos* disease.]

osteoperiosteal (os·te·o·per·e·**os**′·te·al). Relating to bone and the periosteum overlying it. [Gk *osteon* bone, periosteum.]

osteoperiostitis (os·te·o·per·e·os·**ti**′·tis). A condition of inflammation affecting a bone and its overlying periosteum. **Alveodental osteoperiostitis.** Periodontitis. [Gk *osteon* bone, periostitis.]

osteopetrosis (os·te·o·pet·**ro**′·sis). A condition in which the bones undergo a process of condensation: the borders of the smaller bones condense and bandlike areas of compact bone form at the epiphyseal lines of the long bones. *See* ALBERS-SCHOENBERG DISEASE. [Gk *osteon* bone, *petra* stone, *-osis* condition.]

osteophage (os·te·o·faje). Osteoclast, 2nd def. [Gk *osteon* bone, *phagein* to eat.]

osteophagia (os·te·o·**fa**′·je·ah). The eating of bone in order to satisfy a craving for phosphorus or calcium. [see prec.]

osteophlebitis (os·te·o·fleb·**i**′·tis). Inflammation affecting the blood vessels of a bone. [Gk *osteon* bone, phlebitis.]

osteophony (os·te·**of**·o·ne). Bone conduction. [Gk *osteon* bone, *phone* sound.]

osteophore (os·te·o·for). A forceps having strong teeth and curved blades, used in the crushing of bone. [Gk *osteon* bone, *pherein* to carry away.]

osteophyma (os·te·o·**fi**′·mah). Applied generally to swellings or tumours of bone. [Gk *osteon* bone, *phyma* a growth.]

osteophyte (os·te·o·fite). Exostosis or dendriform outgrowth on a bone. [Gk *osteon* bone, *phyton* that which has grown.]

osteophytosis (os·te·o·fi·**to**′·sis). A morbid state marked by the presence of osteophytes. [osteophyte, Gk *-osis* condition.]

osteoplaque (os·te·o·plak). A plate, stratum or layer of bone. [Gk *osteon* bone, *plax* something flat.]

osteoplast (os·te·o·plast). An osteoblast; a formative cell which is derived from the layer of osteogenetic mesenchyme and forms one of the bone cells of a developing bone. [see foll.]

osteoplastic (os·te·o·**plas**′·tik). 1. Osteogenetic. 2. Relating to osteoplasty. [Gk *osteon* bone, *plassein* to form.]

osteoplasty (os·te·o·plas·te). A plastic operation performed on the bones. [see prec.]

osteopoikilosis, osteopoikily (os·te·o·poi·kil·**o**′·sis, os·te·o·**poi**′·kil·e). A congenital disease of bone characterized by dense areas scattered throughout the skeleton. [Gk *osteon* bone, *poikilos* mottled.]

osteoporosis (os·te·o·por·**o**′·sis). Rarefaction of bone. **Osteoporosis circumscripta cranii.** Localized rarefaction of the bones of the skull; Schueller's disease. **Neurogenic osteoporosis.** Decalcification of bone following damage or disease of the nervous system. **Senile osteoporosis.** Osteoporosis developing in old age. [Gk *osteon* bone, *poros* passage, *-osis* condition.]

osteoporotic (os·te·o·por·**ot**′·ik). Pertaining to osteoporosis.

osteopsathyrosis (os·te·op·sath·e·**ro**′·sis). A condition of abnormal fragility of bones leading to multiple fractures. [Gk *osteon* bone, *psathyros* crumbling.]

osteoradionecrosis (os·te·o·**ra**·de·o·nek·**ro**′·sis). Bony necrosis occurring after treatment by irradiation. [Gk *osteon* bone, radionecrosis.]

osteorrhagia (os·te·o·**ra**′·je·ah). Haemorrhage from a bone. [Gk *osteon* bone, *rhegnynein* to gush forth.]

osteorrhaphy (os·te·**or**·af·e). The operation of suturing or wiring together the fragments of a fractured bone. [Gk *osteon* bone, *rhaphe* suture.]

osteosarcoma (os·te·o·sar·**ko**′·mah). Osteogenic sarcoma; a malignant neoplasm of bone cells. [Gk *osteon* bone, sarcoma.]

osteosarcomatous (os·te·o·sar·**ko**′·mat·us). Having the properties of an osteosarcoma.

osteoscirrhus (os·te·o·**skir**′·us). Scirrhous carcinoma of bone. [Gk *osteon* bone, *skirrhos* hard.]

osteosclerosis (os·te·o·skler·**o**′·sis). Hardening of the bony spaces as the result of chronic inflammation or stimulation of bone cells. **Osteosclerosis fragilis, Osteosclerosis generalisata.** Excessive calcification of the bony skeleton. **Osteosclerosis myelofibrosis.** A widely-distributed osteosclerosis associated with reduction in the bone marrow as the result of leukaemia or chronic anaemia. [Gk *osteon* bone, sclerosis.]

osteosclerotic (os·te·o·skler·**ot**′·ik). Relating to, of the nature of, or characterized by osteosclerosis.

osteoscope (os·te·o·skope). An instrument for testing an x-ray apparatus using a standard absorption bone medium. [Gk *osteon* bone, *skopein* to view.]

osteoseptum (os·te·o·**sep**′·tum). The bony part of the septum of the nose. [Gk *osteon* bone, septum.]

osteosis (os·te·o·sis). Bone formation, and in particular the process by which connective tissue is invaded by bone. **Osteosis cutis.** The occurrence of bone-containing nodules in the skin. **Parathyroid osteosis.** Generalized osteitis fibrosa cystica. [Gk *osteon* bone, *-osis* condition.]

osteospongioma (os·te·o·spon·je·**o**′·mah). An osteoma composed of cancellous or spongy bone. [Gk *osteon* bone, *spoggia* sponge, *-oma* tumour.]

osteosteatoma (os·te·o·ste·at·**o**′·mah). A sebaceous cyst containing some bone tissue. [Gk *osteon* bone, steatoma.]

osteostixis (os·te·o·**stix**′·is). Puncture of a bone by surgical methods. [Gk *osteon* bone, *stizein* to puncture.]

osteosuture (os·te·o·**sew**′·tewr). The operation of suturing or wiring together the fragments of a fractured bone. [Gk *osteon* bone, suture.]

osteosynovitis (os·te·o·si·no·**vi'**·tis). Synovitis which is associated with osteitis of the surrounding bones. [Gk *osteon* bone, synovitis.]

osteosynthesis (**os**·te·o·**sin'**·thes·is). Fixation and apposition of pieces of a fractured bone by means of plates, wire or sutures. [Gk *osteon* bone, synthesis.]

osteotabes (**os**·te·o·**ta'**·beez). A morbid condition which mainly affects infants, in whom there is destruction of the bone-marrow cells. [Gk *osteon* bone, tabes.]

osteotelangiectasia, osteotelangiectasis (**os**·te·o·tel·an·je·ek·**ta'**·ze·ah, **os**·te·o·tel·an·je·**ek'**·tas·is). An osteosarcoma infiltrated with dilated capillary vessels. [Gk *osteon* bone, telangiectasia.]

osteothrombosis (**os**·te·o·throm·**bo'**·sis). Thrombosis in the blood vessels of a bone. [Gk *osteon* bone, thrombosis.]

osteotome (**os**·te·o·tome). A chisel used in incising a bone. [Gk *osteon* bone, *temnein* to cut.]

osteotomy (os·te·**ot**·o·me). The operation of cutting through a bone. **Cuneiform osteotomy.** Removal of a wedge of bone. **Cup-and-ball osteotomy.** Division of a bone so that the divided ends are shaped to fit as a cup-and-ball. **External (or lateral) rotation osteotomy.** That used in congenital dislocation of the hip. **Hinge osteotomy.** Division of a bone with angulation of one fragment upon the other. **Intertrochanteric osteotomy.** Division of the upper end of the femur between the trochanters. **Linear osteotomy.** Division of a bone by a straight cut. **Subtrochanteric osteotomy.** Division of the shaft of the femur immediately below the greater trochanter. **Transtrochanteric osteotomy.** Division of the upper shaft of the femur through the region of the trochanters. **Triplane osteotomy.** A subtrochanteric osteotomy of the femur designed to correct the 3 deformities of slipped upper femoral epiphysis (external rotation, adduction and extension). [Gk *osteon* bone, *temnein* to cut.]

See also: WARD, WASSMUND.

osteotribe, osteotrite (**os**·te·o·tribe, **os**·te·o·trite). A rasp for scraping away decayed bone tissue. [Gk *osteon* bone, *tribein* to wear away.]

osteotrophy (os·te·**ot**·ro·fe). The nutrition of bone tissue. [Gk *osteon* bone, *trophe* nutrition.]

osteotylus (os·te·**ot**·il·us). The callus which surrounds the ends of a fractured bone. [Gk *osteon* bone, *tylos* callus.]

osteotympanic (**os**·te·o·tim·**pan'**·ik). Referring to the skull and the middle ear (tympanic cavity). [Gk *osteon* bone, tympanic cavity.]

Osterberg, Arnold Edwin (b. 1894). Rochester, Minnesota, biochemist.

Benedict and Osterberg method, for sugar in urine. The urine is treated with activated charcoal and filtered. To the filtrate is added saturated picric-acid solution, sodium-carbonate solution and a few drops of acetone. The red colour is matched against standards.

osthexia, osthexy (os·**thex**·e·ah, os·**thex**·e). A morbid state in which ossification takes place in abnormal or unusual places. [Gk *osteon* bone, *hexis* condition of body.]

ostial, ostiary (**os**·te·al, **os**·te·ar·e). Relating to an orifice or ostium. [L *ostium* entrance.]

ostitis (os·**ti**·tis). Osteitis.

ostium [NA] (**os**·te·um) (pl. *ostia*). A mouth or opening, e.g. *ostium abdominale*, the opening at the fimbriated end of the uterine tube into the abdominal cavity. **Ostium primum.** In the fetal heart, an opening in the lower part of the atrial septum which normally closes at or soon after birth. **Ostium secundum.** In the fetal heart, an opening (the foramen ovale) in the upper part of the atrial septum which normally closes at or soon after birth. [L.]

ostoclasty (**os**·to·klas·te). Osteoclasia.

ostoid (**os**·toid). Osteoid.

ostosis (os·**to**·sis). Osteogenesis. [Gk *osteon* bone.]

ostraceous (os·**tra**·shus). Resembling the shell of an oyster. [Gk *ostrakon* oyster shell.]

ostracosis (os·trah·**ko**·sis). A morbid change that occurs in a bone in which it acquires the texture of an oyster shell. [Gk *ostrakon* oyster shell, *-osis* condition.]

ostreasterol (**os**·tre·ah·**steer'**·ol). $C_{29}H_{47}OH$, a natural sterol occurring in molluscs. [Gk *ostreon* oyster, sterol.]

Ostreogrycin (**os**·tre·o·**gri'**·sin). BP Commission approved name for the antibiotic obtained from *Streptomyces ostreogriseus.*

ostreotoxism, ostreotoxismus (**os**·tre·o·**tox'**·izm, **os**·tre·o·tox·**iz'**·mus). A form of poisoning that is caused by the eating of infected or contaminated oysters. [Gk *ostreon* oyster, *toxikon* poison.]

Ostwald-Folin pipette. A combined bulb-capillary pipette devised for measuring blood or other viscous fluid.

otacoustic (o·tak·**oos**·tik). 1. Aiding the sense of hearing. 2. Relating to the sense of hearing. [Gk *otakoustein* to listen surreptitiously.]

otacousticon (o·tak·**oos**·tik·on). An ear trumpet. [see prec.]

otagra (o·**tag**·rah). Otalgia. [Gk *ous* ear, *agra* seizure.]

otalgia (o·**tal**·je·ah). Pain in the ear. **Otalgia dentalis.** Pain reflected to the ear as a result of dental disease. **Geniculate otalgia.** Pain arising in the ear from an inflammation of the ganglion of the facial nerve. **Otalgia intermittens.** Intermittent earache from any cause. **Reflex otalgia.** Pain referred to the ear as a result of a lesion elsewhere, most commonly in the tongue, larynx, pharynx or teeth. **Secondary otalgia.** An otalgia dependent upon a lesion at a distance; similar to reflex otalgia (see above). **Tabetic otalgia.** Otalgia in tabes dorsalis. [Gk *ous* ear, *algos* pain.]

otalgic (o·**tal**·jik). 1. Relating or belonging to earache. 2. A remedy for earache. [see prec.]

otantritis (o·tan·**tri**·tis). Oto-antritis.

otaphone (**o**·tah·fone). Otophone.

otectomy (o·**tek**·to·me). Excision of the contents of the ear. [Gk *ous* ear, *ektome* excision.]

othaematoma (**ote**·he·mat·**o'**·mah). Haematoma auris. [Gk *ous* ear, haematoma.]

othaemorrhagia (**ote**·hem·o·**ra'**·je·ah). A discharge of blood from the ear. [Gk *ous* ear, haemorrhage.]

othaemorrhoea (**ote**·hem·o·**re'**·ah). Discharge of blood or of haemorrhagic fluid from the ear. [Gk *ous* ear, *haima* blood, *rhoia* flow.]

othelcosis (ote·hel·**ko**·sis). Ulceration or suppuration affecting the ear, generally any involvement of auricle, auditory canal or middle ear. [Gk *ous* ear, *helkosis* ulceration.]

othygroma (ote·hi·**gro**·mah). Distension of the lobule of the auricle due to the presence of fluid. **Othygroma nephriticum.** A condition in which the lobule of the auricle becomes elongated on account of facial oedema. [Gk *ous* ear, hygroma.]

otiatric (o·te·**at**·rik). Relating to the therapeutics of aural diseases. [Gk *ous* ear, *iatros* surgeon.]

otic (**o**·tik). Aural. [Gk *ous* ear.]

oticodinia, oticodinosis (**o**·tik·o·**di'**·ne·ah, **o**·tik·o·di·**no'**·sis). Vertigo due to the existence of disease in the ear. [Gk *ous* ear, *dine* a whirling.]

Otis, Fessenden Nott (b. 1825). American urologist.

Otis' operation. An operation for internal urethrotomy, in which the stricture was divided from within, using a specially constructed urethrotome, with the blade concealed in the bulb.

otitic (o·**tit**·ik). Pertaining to otitis.

otitis (o·**ti**·tis). Inflammation of the ear. **Aviation otitis.** Inflammation of the ear as a result of flying, now usually called otitic barotrauma. **Otitis crouposa.** That associated with the formation of a fibrinous membrane. **Otitis desquamativa.** Desquamative inflammation of the external ear and the tympanic membrane. **Otitis diphtheritica.** Otitis crouposa (see above). **Otitis externa.** Any form of inflammation of the outer ear passage. **Otitis externa circumscripta.** Otitis externa furunculosa (see below). **Otitis externa diffusa.** Diffuse inflammation of the external auditory meatus. **Otitis externa furunculosa, Furuncular otitis.** Inflammation of the outer ear passage which produces localized boils, usually associated with the hair follicles of the meatus.

Otitis haemorrhagica. Haemorrhagic inflammation of the tympanic cavity and tympanic membrane, the latter having haemorrhagic bullae on it; a condition often found in influenzal affections of the ear. **Otitis interna.** Inflammation of the internal ear, more correctly called labyrinthitis. **Otitis labyrinthica.** Otitis interna (see prec.). **Otitis mastoidea.** Inflammation of the middle ear, associated with a mastoid infection. **Otitis media.** Inflammation of the middle ear. **Otitis media catarrhalis acuta.** Acute inflammation of the middle-ear cleft, associated with the formation of catarrhal exudate. **Otitis media catarrhalis chronica.** A chronic form of catarrhal inflammation of the middle-ear cleft. **Otitis media purulenta acuta.** Acute inflammation of the middle-ear cleft, with pus formation. **Otitis media purulenta chronica.** A chronic inflammatory condition of the middle ear, often the only symptom of which is otorrhoea. **Otitis media sclerotica.** A sclerosing or dry type of catarrhal inflammation of the middle ear. **Otitis media serosa.** Inflammation of the middle ear, associated with exudate formation which may not be of an inflammatory origin. **Otitis media suppurativa.** Otitis media purulenta chronica (see above). **Mucosis otitis, Mucosus otitis.** A form of catarrhal otitis. **Otitis mycotica.** Otitis associated with fungus infection. **Otitis parasiticus.** 1. An inflammatory condition of the ear associated with any parasitic infection. 2. Oto-acariasis. **Otitis purulenta chronica.** Chronic purulent inflammation of the middle-ear cleft. **Otitis sclerotica.** A form of otosclerosis. [Gk *ous* ear, *-itis* inflammation.]

oto-acariasis (o·to·ak·ar·**i**'·as·is). Mite infection of the ear. [Gk *ous* ear, acariasis.]

oto-antritis (o·to·an·**tri**'·tis). Inflammation affecting the tympanic antrum and the epitympanic recess. [Gk *ous* ear, antritis.]

otobiosis (o·to·bi·**o**'·sis). The presence of a tick in the ear, most commonly *Otobius megnini*. [*Otobius*, Gk *-osis* condition.]

Otobius (o·**to**·be·us). A genus of ticks. **Otobius megnini.** The ear tick of southern North America, the larvae of which live in the ears of domestic animals and sometimes man, particularly children. The adults are free living. [Gk *ous* ear, *bios* life.]

otoblennorrhoea (o·to·blen·o·**re**'·ah). Mucous discharge from the ear. [Gk *ous* ear, blennorrhoea.]

otocariasis (o·to·kar·**i**'·as·is). Oto-acariasis.

otocatarrh (o·to·kat·**ar**'). A catarrhal infection of the ear. [Gk *ous* ear, catarrh.]

otocephalus (o·to·**kef**·al·us). A monster in which the nose and mandible are absent, the ears are either joined or are set near each other below the skull and there is either 1 fused eye or 2 contained in a single orbit. [Gk *ous* ear, *kephale* head.]

otocerebritis (o·to·ser·e·**bri**'·tis). Oto-encephalitis. [Gk *ous* ear, cerebrum, Gk *-itis* inflammation.]

otocleisis (o·to·**kli**·sis). Occlusion of the auditory canals, e.g. by new growth or waxy plug. [Gk *ous* ear, *kleisis* closure.]

otoconia (o·to·**ko**·ne·ah) (pl. *otoconiae*). Otolith. [Gk *ous* ear, *konia* dust.]

otocrane (o·to·krane). Otocranium.

otocranial (o·to·**kra**·ne·al). Pertaining to the otocranium.

otocranium (o·to·**kra**·ne·um). That part of the skull in which the inner ear (membranous labyrinth) is embedded; the petromastoid part of the temporal bone. [Gk *ous* ear, *kranion* skull.]

otocyst (o·to·sist). The embryonic auditory vesicle. [Gk *ous* ear, *kystis* bag.]

otodynia (o·to·**din**·e·ah). Earache. [Gk *ous* ear, *odyne* pain.]

oto-encephalitis (o·to·en·kef·al·**i**'·tis). Inflammation affecting the brain, the result of spread of an inflammatory process from the middle ear. [Gk *ous* ear, encephalitis.]

otoganglion (o·to·**gang**·gle·on). The otic ganglion. [Gk *ous* ear, ganglion.]

otogenic, otogenous (o·to·**jen**·ik, o·**toj**·en·us). Arising from within the ear, especially with reference to inflammatory processes. [Gk *ous* ear, *genein* to produce.]

otohemineurasthenia (o·to·**hem**·e·newr·as·**the**'·ne·ah). Defective hearing on one side, of neurasthenic origin. [Gk *ous* ear, *hemi* half, neurasthenia.]

otolaryngology (o·to·lar·in·**gol**'·o·je). The sciences of otology and laryngology considered together.

otolite (o·to·lite). Otolith.

otolith (o·to·lith). 1. [Statocona (NA).] Minute crystals of calcium carbonate adhering to the hair cells of the maculae of the utricle and saccule in the inner ear; it subserves the function of orientation to gravity and comparable forces. 2. A calculus in the middle ear. [Gk *ous* ear, *lithos* stone.]

otolithiasis (o·to·lith·**i**'·as·is). A state in which calculi (otoliths) develop in the middle ear.

otological (o·to·**loj**·ik·al). Pertaining to otology.

otologist (o·**tol**·o·jist). An ear specialist (aurist). [see foll.]

otology (o·**tol**·o·je). That branch of medicine which deals with the science and treatment of aural diseases. [Gk *ous* ear, *logos* science.]

otomassage (o·to·mas·**ahzh**). Massage of the tympanic membrane and auditory ossicles, carried out at regular intervals, the methods being those of using sound waves and puffs of air in the auditory canal or vibratory percussion of the tympanic membrane itself. [Gk *ous* ear, massage.]

otomastoiditis (o·to·mas·toid·**i**'·tis). A morbid condition in which there is simultaneous occurrence of otitis and mastoiditis.

otomicroscope (o·to·**mi**·kro·skope). A microscope used in examination of the ear. [Gk *ous* ear, microscope.]

otomucormycosis (o·to·**mew**·kor·mi·**ko**'·sis). A fungus disease of the ear caused by a parasite of the genus *Mucor*; mucormycosis of the ear. [Gk *ous* ear, mucormycosis.]

otomyasthenia (o·to·mi·as·**the**'·ne·ah). 1. Debility of the muscles of the ear which prevents the normal amplification and selection of sounds. 2. Imperfect hearing caused by paresis of the stapedius and tensor tympani muscles. [Gk *ous* ear, myasthenia.]

Otomyces (o·to·**mi**·seez). The genus *Aspergillus*. [Obsolete term.] [Gk *ous* ear, *mykes* fungus.]

otomycosis (o·to·mi·**ko**'·sis). Myringomycosis; any lesion of the external ear due to the presence of a fungus. Hyphal elements and/or sporing heads must be demonstrated in debris obtained from the ear, culture alone is insufficient. Commonly caused by *Aspergillus* species and also by dermatophytes, *Mucor, Allescheria, Penicillium, Absidia, Rhizopus* and *Candida* species. [Gk *ous* ear, *mykes* fungus, *-osis* condition.]

otomyiasis (o·to·mi·**i**'·as·is). Infestation of the ear with arthropod larvae. [Gk *ous* ear, myiasis.]

otoncus (o·**tong**·kus). Any tumour of the ear. [Gk *ous* ear, *ogkos* a swelling.]

otonecrectomy, otonecronectomy (o·to·nek·**rek**'·to·me, **o**·to·-nek·ro·**nek**'·to·me). Excision of necrosed aural tissues in the middle ear. [Gk *ous* ear, *nekros* dead, *ektome* a cutting out.]

otoneuralgia (o·to·newr·**al**'·je·ah). Pain in the ear of neuralgic type. [Gk *ous* ear, neuralgia.]

otoneurology (o·to·newr·**ol**'·o·je). Neurotology.

otopathy (o·**top**·ath·e). Any morbid condition of the ear. [Gk *ous* ear, *pathos* disease.]

otopharyngeal (o·to·far·**in**'·je·al). Belonging to the middle ear and the pharynx. [Gk *ous* ear, pharynx.]

otophone (o·to·fone). 1. An external instrument to assist hearing. 2. A tube used in auscultation of the ear. [Gk *ous* ear, *phone* sound.]

otophthalmic (o·tof·**thal**·mik). Belonging to or relating to the ear and the eye. [Gk *ous* ear, *ophthalmos* eye.]

otophyma (o·to·**fi**·mah). Hyperplasia of connective tissue and sebaceous glands of the ear, similar to that in rhinophyma. [Gk *ous* ear, *phyma* tumour.]

otopiesis (o·to·**pi**·e·sis). Indrawing of the tympanic membrane. [Gk *ous* ear, *piesis* a pressing.]

otoplasty (o·to·plas·te). Plastic surgery of the external ear performed in order to rectify defects or deformities. [Gk *ous* ear, *plassein* to mould.]

otopolypus (o·to·**pol**·ip·us). Polypus of the external auditory meatus. [Gk *ous* ear, polypus.]

otopyorrhoea (o·to·pi·or·**re**'·ah). A discharge of purulent substance from the ear, commonly flowing from the middle ear through a perforated tympanic membrane. [Gk *ous* ear, pyorrhoea.]

otopyosis (o·to·pi·o′·sis). Suppuration of the ear, occurring either in the tympanic cavity or in the external auditory meatus. [Gk *ous* ear, pyosis.]

otor (o·tor). Aural. [Gk *ous* ear.]

otorhinolaryngology (o·to·ri·no·lar·in·gol′·o·je). That branch of medical science which deals with the structure, functions and diseases of the ear, nose and larynx; considered as one speciality. [Gk *ous* ear, *rhis* nose, larynx, Gk *logos* science.]

otorhinology (o·to·ri·nol′·o·je). The branches of medical science which deal with the study and treatment of disease of the ear and nose. [Gk *ous* ear, *rhis* nose, *logos* science.]

otorrhagia (o·to·ra·je·ah). Haemorrhage from the external ear. [Gk *ous* ear, *rhegnynein* to gush forth.]

otorrhoea (o·to·re·ah). An escape of fluid, in particular purulent or mucopurulent fluid, from the ear. **Cerebrospinal otorrhoea.** The flow of cerebrospinal fluid from the ear as a result of congenital malformation, injury or disease. It is frequently concomitant of fractures involving the base of the skull. [Gk *ous* ear, *rhoia* flow.]

otosalpinx (o·to·sal·pingx). The pharyngotympanic tube. [Gk *ous* ear, *salpigx* trumpet.]

otosclerectomy, otoscleronectomy (o·to·skler·ek′·to·me, o·to·skler·o·nek′·to·me). Excision of the auditory ossicles in order to remove bones which have become ankylosed. [Gk *ous* ear, *skleros* hard, *ektome* a cutting out.]

otosclerosis (o·to·skler·o′·sis). A pathological change in the middle and internal ear resulting from a thickening of the bone of the periotic capsule, which produces deafness, most commonly of the obstructive or middle-ear type, but often associated with inner-ear deafness as well. There appears to be a familial tendency to the condition, and it is commoner in the female; it may be precipitated or made worse by child-bearing. [Gk *ous* ear, *skleros* hard, *-osis* condition.]

otoscope (o·to·skope). A tube or funnel used for the examination of ears. [Gk *ous* ear, *skopein* to view.]

See also: BRUNTON, SIEGLE.

otoscopic (o·to·skop·ik). Relating to otoscopy.

otoscopy (o·tos·ko·pe). Inspection of the ear and particularly of the tympanic membrane with the aid of the otoscope.

otosis (o·to·sis). Mishearing of sounds or words uttered, and the resultant errors of comprehension. [Gk *ous* ear, *-osis* condition.]

otosteal (o·tos·te·al). Belonging to the auditory ossicles. [Gk *ous* ear, *osteon* bone.]

otosteon (o·tos·te·on). 1. An otolith. 2. One of the auditory ossicles. [see prec.]

ototomy (o·tot·o·me). 1. Dissection of the ear. 2. Anatomy of the ear. 3. Puncture or incision of the tympanic membrane. [Gk *ous* ear, *temnein* to cut.]

Ott, Adolf (b. 1835). Prague physician.

Ott's test, for nucleoprotein in urine. Mix equal volumes of urine and saturated sodium-chloride solution and add Almén's reagent slowly. A bulky precipitate indicates nucleoprotein.

ottar (ot·ar). Otto.

Otten, Max (b. 1877). Magdeburg physician.

Otten vaccine. An antiplague vaccine used in Java; it is composed of living avirulent *Pasteurella pestis.*

Otto, Adolf Wilhelm (b. 1786). Breslau surgeon and anatomist.

Otto's disease. An osteo-arthritic protrusion of the acetabulum into the pelvic cavity. The resulting deformity when bilateral is known as *Otto's pelvis.*

Otto, Friedrich Wilhelm Robert (b. 1837). Brunswick chemist.

Stas-Otto method. A method used in toxicological analysis for the isolation of non-volatile organic poisons from viscera and other biological material. The material is thoroughly minced, acidified with tartaric acid and extracted several times with alcohol. The alcohol is removed from the extract and the residue dissolved in dilute acid. The acid solution is extracted with a non-miscible solvent, usually chloroform, which removes acidic and neutral substances, and is then made alkaline and re-extracted to remove basic substances. The latter include the alkaloids with the exception of morphine. Morphine is finally removed by adding an equal volume of alcohol to the alkaline aqueous solution and extracting with chloroform.

otto (ot·o). Attar; a general name for any volatile oil. **Otto of rose.** A volatile oil distilled with steam from the fresh flowers of *Rosa gallica, R. damascena, R. alba* and *R. centifolia*; also from varieties of these species (family Rosaceae). It contains the alcohols, geraniol and citronellol, the sesquiterpene alcohol, nerol, and also phenylethyl alcohol. Other compounds present are linalool, eugenol, nonyl aldehyde, traces of citral and 2 solid hydrocarbons of the paraffin series. [Ar. *atar* perfume.]

Ouabain BP 1958 (wah·ba·in). Strophanthin-G, $C_{29}H_{44}O_{12}{\cdot}8H_2O$. A crystalline glycoside obtained from the seeds of *Strophanthus gratus* French (family Apocynaceae) and the wood of *Acocanthera schimperi* Schwenf. It is similar in physiological action to strophanthin-K but is excreted more rapidly and is twice as active; it is used in congestive cardiac failure.

ouabaio (wah·ba·yo). The wood or root of the tree *Acocanthera schimperi* from which Arnaud in 1888 obtained a crystalline glycoside identical with strophanthin of *Strophanthus gratus* and named it ouabain. It is used as an arrow poison in parts of Africa.

Oudin, Paul (b. 1851). Paris radiologist and physiotherapist.

Oudin resonator. Apparatus for producing *Oudin current*, which is a high-frequency current from only one pole or terminal at one time used in electrotherapy.

oudinization (oo·dahn·i·za′·shun). Treatment by the high-frequency effluve. [Paul *Oudin.*]

oula (oo·lah). Gum or gingiva. [Gk *oulon.*]

oulectomy (oo·lek·to·me). 1. Ulectomy; removal of scar tissue. [Gk *oule* scar, *ektome* a cutting out.] 2. Gingivectomy. [Gk *oulon* gum, *ektome* a cutting out.]

oulhaemorrhagia (ool·hem·o·ra′·je·ah). A discharge of blood from the gums. [Gk *oulon* gum, haemorrhage.]

oulitis (oo·li·tis). Gingivitis. [Gk *oulon* gum, *-itis* inflammation.]

ouloid (oo·loid). 1. Shaped like a scar but not caused by a cutaneous lesion. 2. A cicatricial spot caused by degeneration of the subcutaneous tissues and observed in cases of dermal syphilis and lupus. [Gk *oule* scar, *eidos* form.]

oulorrhagia (oo·lo·ra·je·ah). Oulhaemorrhagia. [Gk *oulon* gum, *rhegnynein* to gush forth.]

oulotomy (oo·lot·o·me). 1. Incision of scar tissue. [Gk *oule* scar, *temnein* to cut.] 2. Incision of the gums. [Gk *oulon* gum, *temnein* to cut.]

ounce (owns). A unit of weight equal to 28.349 g. **Apothecary ounce** (℥), by weight 31.103 g, or 480 grains, or approximately $\frac{11}{10}$ of an Imperial ounce. **Ounce avoirdupois.** Imperial ounce (see below). **Fluid ounce** (℥ fl), 28.416 cc, or $\frac{1}{20}$ part of an Imperial pint, or 480 minims; the volume occupied at 16.7°C by one ounce (437.5 grains) of distilled water. **Imperial ounce** (1 oz), by weight $\frac{1}{16}$ part of a pound, or 437.5 grains, or 28.349 grams. [L *uncia.*]

ourari (oo·rah·re). Curare.

Ousilleau's operation. For lymphoedema: excision of redundant scrotal tissues in filarial lymphoedema of the scrotum.

outbreeding (owt·breeding). Genetic. Producing a greater difference in progeny than would be determined by random breeding. [ME *out*, AS *brédan.*]

outflow (owt·flo). Any emergence analogous to the flowing out of water. **Craniosacral outflow.** Nerve fibres linking the parasympathetic and central nervous systems, running in certain cranial and sacral nerves. **Thoracolumbar outflow.** Nerve fibres linking the sympathetic and central nervous systems, running in the thoracic and lumbar nerves. [ME *out*, AS *flowan.*]

outlay (owt·la). A surface graft. **Epithelial outlay.** A form of split-skin graft in which the graft is smaller than the area which it covers, leaving a rim to be epithelialized from its edges. [ME *out*, AS *leegan.*]

outlet (owt·let). An opening permitting egress; usually taken to mean the pelvic outlet. **Outlet of the pelvis.** *See* PELVIS. **Outlet of the thorax.** *See* THORAX. [ME *out, leten.*]

outlimb (owt·lim). The distal portion of an extremity. [ME *out,* limb.]

outpocketing (owt·pok·et·ing). The procedure of inserting the stump of an excised pedunculated tumour or other pedicle between the edges of the external wound before they are sutured. [ME *out, poket.*]

output (owt·put). The quantity produced. **Cardiac output.** The volume of blood expelled from the left ventricle in 1 minute. [ME *out,* AS *putian.*]

ovalbumin (ov·al·bew·min). The principal protein of egg white, in which it constitutes about 70 per cent of the total protein. It is a crystalline albumin with a molecular weight of about 40 000. [L *ovum* egg, albumin.]

ovalocyte (o·val·o·site). An elliptical erythrocyte. [L *ovum* egg, erythrocyte.]

ovalocytosis (o·val·o·si·to'·sis). A condition in which numerous elliptical erythrocytes are found in the blood. [L *ovum* egg, erythrocytosis.]

ovaralgia, ovarialgia (o·var·al·je·ah, o·var·e·al'·je·ah). Pain affecting the ovary. [ovary, Gk *algos* pain.]

ovarian (o·va·re·an). Belonging to an ovary.

ovarian artery [arteria ovarica (NA)]. A paired ventrolateral branch from the abdominal aorta, passing obliquely downwards and laterally across the psoas major muscle and the ureter to which it sends twigs [rami ureterici (NA)]. It enters the pelvic cavity, runs medially within the infundibulopelvic ligament and supplies the ovary, uterine tube, the round ligament of the uterus and the side of the uterus itself, where it anastomoses with the uterine artery.

ovarian veins. *See* TESTICULAR (OVARIAN) VEINS.

ovariectomy (o·var·e·ek'·to·me). Excision of an ovary. [ovary, Gk *ektome* a cutting out.]

ovariocele (o·va·re·o·seel). Hernia of an ovary. **Vaginal ovariocele.** Protrusion of an ovary through the wall of the vagina. [ovary, Gk *kele* hernia.]

ovariocentesis (o·va·re·o·sen·te'·sis). Puncture of an ovary or of an ovarian cyst by surgical means. [ovary, Gk *kentein* to puncture.]

ovariocyesis (o·va·re·o·si·e'·sis). Ovarian pregnancy. *See* PREGNANCY. [ovary, Gk *kyesis* pregnancy.]

ovariodysneuria (o·va·re·o·dis·newr'·e·ah). Pain affecting the ovary. [ovary, dysneuria.]

ovario-epilepsy (o·va·re·o·ep'·il·ep·se). Convulsive hysteria. [ovary, epilepsy.]

ovariogenic (o·va·re·o·jen'·ik). Originating in the ovary. [ovary, Gk *genein* to produce.]

ovariohysterectomy (o·va·re·o·his·ter·ek'·to·me). Excision of the uterus and ovaries. [ovary, Gk *hystera* womb, *ektome* a cutting out.]

ovariolytic (o·va·re·o·lit'·ik). Having the power to destroy ovarian cells or other ovarian tissue. [ovary, lysis.]

ovarioncus (o·va·re·ong'·kus). A tumour of the ovary. [ovary, Gk *ogkos* a swelling.]

ovariopathy (o·va·re·op'·ath·e). Disease of the ovary. [ovary, Gk *pathos* disease.]

ovariorrhexis (o·va·re·o·rex'·is). Rupture of an ovary. [ovary, Gk *rhexis* rupture.]

ovariosalpingectomy (o·va·re·o·sal·pin·jek'·to·me). Excision of ovary and uterine tube. [ovary, Gk *salpigx* trumpet, *ektome* a cutting out.]

ovariosteresis (o·va·re·o·ster·e'·sis). Excision of an ovary. [ovary, Gk *steresis* loss.]

ovariostomy (o·va·re·os'·to·me). The creation of an opening into an ovarian cyst in order to drain the contents. [ovary, Gk *stoma* mouth.]

ovariotestis (o·va·re·o·tes'·tis). Ovotestis.

ovariotherapy (o·va·re·o·ther'·ap·e). The treatment of disease by means of ovarian material or extracts. [ovary, therapy.]

ovariotomy (o·va·re·ot'·o·me). 1. Excision of an ovary. 2. Excision of a tumour of the ovary. **Abdominal ovariotomy.** Removal of an ovary by the abdominal route. **Normal ovariotomy.** Excision of an uninfected ovary. **Vaginal ovariotomy.** Removal of an ovary by the vaginal route. [ovary, Gk *temnein* to cut.]

ovariotubal (o·va·re·o·tew'·bal). Belonging to an ovary and the uterine tube.

ovariprival (o·var·e·pri'·val). Caused by, or on account of lack of ovaries. [ovary, L *privare* to deprive.]

ovaritis (o·var·i·tis). An inflammatory condition of an ovary or of both ovaries. [ovary, Gk *-itis* inflammation.]

ovarotherapy (o·var·o·ther'·ap·e). The treatment of disease by means of ovarian material or extracts. [ovary, therapy.]

ovary [ovarium (NA)] (o·var·e). The female gonad, one of a pair of organs attached to the posterior surface of the broad ligament by a mesovarium. The smooth pinkish surface becomes increasingly pitted with scars after ovulation begins. It has 2 ends, the tubal [extremitas tubaria (NA)] and the uterine [extremitas uterina (NA)]. [L *ovum* egg.]

free border [margo liber (NA)]. The curved border opposite to the mesovarian border separating the medial and lateral surfaces [facies medialis et facies lateralis (NA)].

mesovarian border [margo mesovaricus (NA)]. The short, straight border to which is attached the ovarian mesentery.

hilum [hilus ovarii (NA)]. The attached border where the vessels and nerves enter and leave.

ovaserum (o·vah·seer·um). The antiserum produced by immunization of an animal with egg albumin. [L *ovum* egg, serum.]

ovatherapy (o·vah·ther·ap·e). Ovarotherapy.

overbite (o·ver·bite). The vertical overlap of upper over the lower teeth. [AS *ofer,* bite.]

over-compensation (o·ver·kom·pen·sa'·shun). A compensatory procedure or reaction that goes beyond the immediate requirements to effect compensation. [AS *ofer,* compensation.]

over-correction (o·ver·kor·ek'·shun). 1. In ophthalmology, referring to the prescribing of a lens of too high a power in refraction work. 2. The presence of deformity of the fragments opposite to that of the original deformity as a result of manipulation. [AS *ofer,* correction.]

over-determination (o·ver·de·ter·min·a'·shun). In psycho-analysis, a process by which a single symbol represents 2 or more objects. [AS *ofer,* determination.]

over-exposure (o·ver·ex·po'·zewr). A radiographic term used to describe a radiograph that has been made with too large a quantity of x-rays, usually milliampere-seconds. [AS *ofer,* exposure.]

overflow (o·ver·flo). Flooding or uninterrupted discharge of fluid, e.g. bile, saliva, urine, tears. [AS *ofer, flowan.*]

overhang (o·ver·hang). The shoulder or ledge produced at the neck of a tooth by an imperfect filling or crown. [AS *ofer, hangian.*]

Overholt, R. H. 20th century American surgeon.

Overholt position. A position on the operating table during thoracotomy in which the patient is prone and the head-end of the table tilted down, in order to localize secretions in the diseased upper lobe. Described in 1946.

overjet (o·ver·jet). The horizontal overlap of upper over the lower teeth. [AS *ofer,* Fr. *jeter* to throw.]

over-maturity (o·ver·mat·ewr'·it·e). Beyond the normal date of maturity. [AS *ofer,* maturity.]

over-maximal (o·ver·max·im·al). Beyond the normal maximum. [AS *ofer,* maximum.]

over-penetration (o·ver·pen·e·tra'·shun). A radiographic term denoting the use of too great a kilovoltage, so that the radiograph lacks contrast. [AS *ofer,* penetration.]

over-productivity (o·ver·prod·uk·tiv'·it·e). A mental condition the signs of which are constant and incoherent talking, glancing from one subject to another, extreme cerebral and physical activity and destructive and noisy behaviour. [AS *ofer,* product.]

over-riding (o·ver·ri·ding). 1. The overlapping of one fragment of a fractured bone over the other portion. 2. Overlapping fetal skull bones shown on the radiographs, indicating intra-uterine death. 3. Dextroposition of the aorta with complete transposition of the great vessels. [AS *ofer, ridan.*]

overstain (o·ver·stane). In histology, to stain a preparation very densely prior to differentiation. [AS *ofer,* stain.]

overstrain (o·ver·strane). Excessive strain caused by overexertion. [AS *ofer,* L *stringere* to pull tight.]

overstress (o·ver·stres). Overactivity which brings on overstrain. [AS *ofer,* stress.]

overt (o·**vert**). Open; evident; uncovered; patent. **Overt infection.** An obvious infection with symptoms and/or the demonstrable presence of the causal organism; not latent. [O Fr. *ovrir* to open.]

overtoe (o·ver·to). A form of hallux varus in which the big toe lies above the rest. [AS *ofer,* toe.]

Overton, Charles Ernst (b. 1865). German anaesthetist.

Meyer-Overton theory. A theory referring to the action of anaesthetic agents. It is suggested that this depends on the difference in affinities between the anaesthetic and the lipoid on the one hand and other constituents of the nerve cell on the other.

overtone (o·ver·tone). Harmonic. Any of the fainter (secondary) notes of higher pitch which are created by and accompany the sounding of any particular note (fundamental). They are characteristic of the note-producing instrument and give what is known as quality. **Psychic overtone.** In psychiatry, the sum of associated mental feelings which accompany a thought process. [AS *ofer,* tone.]

over-transfusion (o·ver·trans·**few**′·zhun). The signs and symptoms which may follow the transfusion of an excess of fluid into the blood stream. [AS *ofer,* L *transfundere* to pour through.]

over-ventilation (o·ver·ven·til·**a**′·shun). Hyperventilation. [AS *ofer,* ventilation.]

ovi (o·vi). Of an egg. **Ovi albumen.** The white of a domestic fowl's egg. **Ovi vitellus.** Yolk of egg, containing about 20 per cent of oil, 15 per cent of protein, 7 per cent of lecithin, in the form of an emulsion in about 50 per cent of water. It is a natural source of vitamins A and B, and is used in pharmacy as an emulsifying agent, especially for cod-liver oil and turpentine oil. [L *ovum* egg.]

ovicapsule (o·ve·kap·sewl). The inner coat of a vesicular ovarian follicle. [L *ovum* egg, capsule.]

oviducal, oviducent (o·ve·**dew**·kal, o·ve·**dew**·sent). Pertaining to the uterine tubes. [L *ovum* egg, *ducere* to pass.]

oviduct (o·ve·dukt). A uterine tube. *See* TUBE. [L *ovum* egg, duct.]

oviferous (o·**vif**·er·us). Bearing or containing ova. [L *ovum* egg, *ferre* to bear.]

ovification (o·vif·ik·**a**′·shun). Ovulation. [L *ovum* egg, *facere* to make.]

oviform (o·ve·form). Shaped like an egg; bearing resemblance to an ovum. [L *ovum* egg, form.]

ovigenesis (o·ve·**jen**·es·is). The formation and development of the ovum. [see foll.]

ovigenetic, ovigenic, ovigenous (o·ve·jen·**et**′·ik, o·ve·**jen**·ik, o·**vij**·en·us). Capable of producing ova. [L *ovum* egg, Gk *genein* to produce.]

ovigerm (o·ve·jerm). An oöblast; a primitive sex cell from which the ovum is developed. [L *ovum* egg, germ.]

ovigerous (o·**vij**·er·us). Oviferous. [L *ovum* egg, *gerere* to bear.]

oviparous (o·**vip**·ar·us). Producing offspring in the form of eggs. [L *ovum* egg, *parere* to bring forth.]

oviposit (o·ve·**poz**·it). To lay eggs; a term applied especially to insects. [see foll.]

oviposition (o·ve·po·**zish**′·un). The act of laying eggs. [L *ovum* egg, *ponere* to place.]

ovipositor (o·ve·**poz**·it·or). An appendicular structure found in many insects, by means of which the eggs are inserted in places suitable for their development. In higher Diptera the ovipositor is formed from the posterior body segments, which are telescopic. [see prec.]

ovisac (o·ve·sak). A vesicular ovarian follicle. [L *ovum* egg, *saccus* bag.]

ovium (o·ve·um). A mature ovum (Waldeyer).

ovo-albumin (o·vo·**al**·bew·min). The albumin in the white of egg. [L *ovum* egg, albumin.]

ovoblast (o·vo·blast). The primitive ovum. [L *ovum* egg, Gk *blastos* germ.]

ovocentre (o·vo·sen·ter). The centrosome of the ovum, which appears after the entry of the sperm during fertilization. [L *ovum* egg, centre.]

ovocyte (o·vo·site). Oöcyte. [L *ovum* egg, Gk *kytos* cell.]

ovoflavin (o·vo·**fla**·vin). A flavin present in egg white. [L *ovum* egg, *flavus* yellow.]

ovogenesis (o·vo·**jen**·es·is). Oögenesis. [L *ovum* egg, Gk *genesis* origin.]

ovoglobulin (o·vo·**glob**·ew·lin). The globulin of egg white. [L *ovum* egg, globulin.]

ovogonium (o·vo·**go**·ne·um). Oögonium. [L *ovum* egg, Gk *gone* seed.]

ovoid (o·void). 1. An isotope applicator for intravaginal use in radiotherapy. 2. Egg-shaped. [L *ovum* egg, Gk *eidos,* form.]

ovolysin (o·**vol**·is·in). A serum antibody acting on egg white. [L *ovum* egg, Gk *lysein* to loosen.]

ovolytic (o·vo·**lit**·ik). Having the power to split up egg albumin. [see prec.]

ovomucin (o·vo·**mew**·sin). A glycoprotein present in egg white in which it constitutes about 2 per cent of the total protein. [L *ovum* egg, mucin.]

ovomucoid (o·vo·**mew**·koid). A glycoprotein present in egg white, constituting about 13 per cent of the total protein. [L *ovum* egg, mucoid.]

ovoplasm (o·vo·plazm). The yolk of an ovum. [L *ovum* egg, plasma.]

Ovoplasma orientale (o·vo·**plaz**·mah or·e·en·**ta**·le). A name formerly given to *Leishmania tropica.* [L *ovum* egg, plasma, *oriens* rising (sun), i.e. the east.]

ovoprecipitin (o·vo·pre·**sip**′·it·in). A precipitin in serum, specific for egg albumin. [L *ovum* egg, precipitin.]

ovoserum (o·vo·**se**·rum). The serum from an animal which has been injected with egg albumin. The serum contains a precipitin specific for the egg albumin of the species with which the animal has been inoculated. [L *ovum* egg, serum.]

ovotestis (o·vo·**tes**·tis). A hermaphrodite gonad consisting of ovarian and testicular substance.

ovotherapy (o·vo·**ther**·ap·e). The treatment of disease by means of ovarian substance or extracts. [L *ovum* egg, therapy.]

ovotid (o·vo·tid). Oöcyte. [L *ovum* egg.]

ovovitellin (o·vo·vit·**el**′·in). The vitellin (nucleo-albumin) contained in egg yolk. [L *ovum* egg, vitellin.]

ovoviviparous (o·vo·viv·**ip**′·ar·us). Producing eggs which are hatched within the body. [L *ovum* egg, *vivus* living, *parere* to give birth.]

ovular (o·vew·lar). Belonging to an ovum or ovule.

ovulation (o·vew·**la**·shun). The development and discharge of an ovum from the vesicular ovarian follicle. **Amenstrual ovulation.** Ovulation occurring in the absence of menstruation, as during lactation.

ovulatory (o·vew·**la**·tor·e). Relating to ovulation.

ovule (o·vewl). 1. Ovum. 2. Small cyst. [L *ovulum* small egg.] *See also:* NABOTH.

ovulogenous (o·vew·**loj**·en·us). Capable of producing ovules. [ovule, Gk *genein* to produce.]

ovulum (o·vew·lum). An ovum. [L small egg.]

ovum [NA] (o·vum). A female germ cell or egg. Strictly speaking, the term is only applied to unfertilized eggs, but it is commonly used to denote the early embryo and its membranes derived from the growth of the fertilized ovum. **Alecithal ovum.** An egg without microscopically demonstrable yolk. **Blighted ovum.** An abortus in which the chorion is present but the embryo has disappeared. **Centrolecithal ovum.** An egg with centrally placed yolk surrounded by a thin shell of cytoplasm, as in insects. **Dropsical ovum.** The name applied to a small, relatively hydramniotic conception sac in which the fetus is absent. **Holoblastic ovum.** An egg in which cleavage involves the whole cell and not merely the non-yolky cytoplasm. **Lecithal ovum.** An egg with microscopically demonstrable yolk. **Megalecithal ovum.** Telolecithal ovum (see below). **Meroblastic ovum.** An egg in which cleavage is partial, involving only the cap of non-yolky cytoplasm. **Primordial ovum.** The female germ cell in the cortex of the ovary, before maturation and follicle ripening. **Telolecithal ovum.** An egg with much yolk, having the cytoplasm confined to one pole. [L.]

See also: BRYCE, HERTIG, MILLER (J. W.), PETERS (H.), ROCK, TEACHER.

Owen, Sir Richard (b. 1804). London anatomist and palaeontologist.

line of Owen. Contour line; one of the microscopic markings in dentine produced by the superimposition of interglobular spaces.

Owren, Paul A. (b. 1905). Oslo haematologist.

Owren's disease. A haemorrhagic disease resembling haemophilia that Owren has described as being due to a deficiency of Factor V, an accelerating factor for the conversion of prothrombin to thrombin.

ox bot, ox warble (**ox** bot, **ox** waw·bl). The larvae of warble flies, *Hypoderma bovis.* [AS *oxa,* Irish *boiteag* maggot, Swedish *varbulde* boil.]

oxacid (ox·**as**·id). Oxyacid: any acid that has oxygen in its composition.

Oxacillin (ox·ah·**sil**·in). BP Commission approved name for 6-(5-methyl-3-phenyl-4-isoxazolecarboxamido)penicillanic acid; an antibiotic.

oxalaemia (ox·al·**e**·me·ah). The presence of an abnormal quantity of oxalates in the blood. [Gk *oxalis* sorrel, *haima* blood.]

oxalate (**ox**·al·ate). A salt or ester of oxalic acid.

oxalated (**ox**·al·a·ted). Subjected to treatment with sodium-oxalate solution, e.g. blood.

oxalation (ox·al·**a**·shun). Treatment with sodium oxalate, e.g. blood which is being made non-coagulable.

oxalism (**ox**·al·izm). Poisoning by any salt of oxalic acid or by oxalic acid.

oxalium (ox·**a**·le·um). A name for potassium hydrogen oxalate, potassium binoxalate, COOHCOOK.

oxaloacetate (ox·al·o·**as**′·et·ate). $COOHCH_2COCOOH$, an intermediate of the citric-acid cycle. Formed from malate by malate dehydrogenase, it condenses with acetyl CoA under the agency of citrate synthase to yield citrate.

oxaluria (ox·al·**ewr**·e·ah). The presence of an abnormally large amount of oxalic acid or of oxalates (chiefly calcium oxalate) in the urine. [oxalate, urine.]

oxalyl (**ox**·al·il). The divalent acyl radical -OCCO-, derived from oxalic acid.

oxalylurea (ox·al·il·ewr·**e**′·ah). Parabanic acid.

oxamide (ox·**am**·ide). 1. Diamide, oxalic acid amide, $(CONH_2)_2$. A white crystalline substance which, like biuret, gives a violet coloration with copper sulphate. 2. Any of the derivatives of diamide (above) formed by replacing hydrogen atoms of the amino-groups by alkyl radicals.

oxamidine (ox·**am**·id·een). Amidoxime.

Oxamniquine (ox·**am**·ne·kween). BP Commission approved name for 6 - hydroxymethyl - 2 - isopropylaminomethyl - 7 - nitro-1,2,3,4-tetrahydroquinoline; it is used in the treatment of schistosomiasis.

Oxandrolone (ox·**an**·dro·lone). BP Commission approved name for 17β-hydroxy-17α-methyl-2-oxa-5α-androstan-3-one; an anabolic steroid.

Oxantel (**ox**·an·tel). BP Commission approved name for 1,4,5,6-tetrahydro-1-methyl-2-(*trans*-3-hydroxystyryl)pyrimidine; an anthelminthic.

Oxaprozin (ox·ah·**pro**·zin). BP Commission approved name for 3-(4,5-diphenyloxazol-2-yl)propionic acid; an anti-inflammatory agent.

oxatyl (**ox**·at·il). The carboxyl group, COOH.

Oxazepam (ox·**az**·e·pam). BP Commission approved name for 7 - chloro - 1,3 - dihydro - 3 - hydroxy - 5 - phenyl - 1,4 - benzodiazepin - 2 - one; a tranquillizer.

oxeladin (ox·**el**·ad·in). BP Commission approved name for diethylaminoethoxyethyl α:α-diethylphenyl acetate. It acts on the cough centre of the central nervous system.

Oxethazaine (ox·**eth**·az·ane). BP Commission approved name for 2-di-[($\alpha\alpha N$-trimethylphenethylcarbamoyl)methyl]-aminoethanol; a local anaesthetic.

oxidant (**ox**·id·ant). Oxidizing agent.

oxidase (**ox**·id·aze). An enzyme which brings about biological oxidation by activating the oxygen of molecular oxygen, hydrogen peroxide, etc. **Amine oxidase.** Monamine oxidase (see below). **Amino-acid oxidase.** An enzyme occurring in the liver and kidneys, which oxidizes the α-amino acids to the corresponding keto acids. **Ascorbic-acid oxidase.** An enzyme contained in fresh fruits and vegetables which catalyses the oxidation of ascorbic acid to dehydroascorbic acid. It is a copper-protein complex. **Cytochrome oxidase.** An enzyme present in most cells, which oxidizes reduced cytochrome back to cytochrome. **Diamine oxidase.** Histaminase, an enzyme present in many tissues, notably the kidney and placenta, which catalyses the oxidation of diamines. **Dopa oxidase.** An enzyme present in the skin, which converts 3,4-dihydroxyphenylalanine to melanin. **Histamine oxidase.** Diamine oxidase (see above). **Monoamine oxidase.** A widely distributed mitochondrial flavoprotein enzyme which oxidizes a variety of monoamines to the corresponding aldehyde; these amines include the catecholamines and dietary amines such as tyramine and phenylethylamine. **Monophenol oxidase.** Tyrosinase, an enzyme present in various animal and plant tissues, which converts tyrosine into a red indole compound and thence to melanin, or monohydroxyphenols generally into catechols and thence to quinones. **Phenol oxidase.** Phenolase. **Polyphenol oxidase.** A copper-protein enzyme which catalyses the oxidation of such phenolic compounds as catechol. **Tyramine oxidase.** Tyrosinase. **Xanthine oxidase.** An enzyme present in milk and in liver which catalyses the oxidation of xanthine and hypoxanthine to uric acid. It is a yellow enzyme. [oxidation.]

oxidasic (ox·id·**a**·zik). Belonging to or having the characteristics of an oxidase.

oxidasis (ox·id·**a**·sis). The process of oxidation activated by an oxidase.

oxidation (ox·id·**a**·shun). 1. The process of burning or rusting in air. 2. The combination of a substance with oxygen. 3. The addition to a compound, of oxygen or other electronegative element. 4. The removal from a compound, of hydrogen or other electropositive element. 5. The increase of an element's valency. 6. The increase of an element's positive charge by removal of negatively-charged electrons. **Aerobic oxidation.** Oxidation in the tissues by means of molecular oxygen activated by an aerobic oxidase. **Anaerobic oxidation.** Oxidation in the tissues that does not involve molecular oxygen, but is effected by the removal of hydrogen activated by a dehydrogenase. **Beta oxidation.** The breaking-down in the body of the long carbon chains of the saturated fatty acids by successive oxidations of the atom at the β-position, next but one to the terminal COOH group. **Mixed function oxidation.** The process in liver whereby many drugs and steroids are metabolized. Both molecular oxygen and NADPH are involved, together with the extramitochondrial electron transport system containing the cytochromes b_5 and P-450. [oxide.]

oxidation-reduction (ox·id·a·shun·re·**duk**′·shun). The simultaneous process of oxidation and reduction regarded as a transfer of electrons from reducing agent to oxidizing agent.

oxide (**ox**·ide). A compound of an element or radical with oxygen. **Acid oxide.** An oxide which combines with bases or dissolves in water to form an acid: usually the oxides of non-metals, e.g. SO_3. **Amphoteric oxide.** An oxide which may act as both a weak base and a weak acid, e.g. Al_2O_3. **Basic oxide.** An oxide that forms salts with acids or dissolves in water to yield a base: certain metallic oxides, e.g. Na_2O. **Compound oxide.** An oxide that acts as if it were a mixture of 2 oxides, e.g. Fe_3O_4. **Indifferent oxide, Neutral oxide.** An oxide which behaves as neither a base nor an acid, e.g. H_2O. **Nitrous oxide.** N_2O, a sweet-smelling, non-irritating, colourless gas in common use, possessing anaesthetic properties. First described in 1772 by Joseph Priestley and used as an anaesthetic by Horace Wells in Boston in 1844. It is neither flammable nor explosive, but supports the combustion of other agents even in the absence of oxygen. The boiling point is $-89°C$, the molecular weight is 44 and the specific gravity is 1.5. In anaesthesia it acts as an excellent analgesic when given with at least 20 per cent of oxygen. **Saline oxide.** A term for a salt produced by a basic oxide. [Gk *oxys* sharp, acid.]

oxidization (**ox**·id·i·**za'**·shun). Oxidation.

oxidize (**ox**·id·ize). To bring about the process of oxidation.

oxidoreductase (**ox**·id·o·re·**duk'**·taze). General term including any enzyme that is involved in an oxidation-reduction system.

oxidoreduction (**ox**·id·o·re·**duk'**·shun). Oxidation-reduction.

oxidosis (ox·id·**o**·sis). Acidosis. [oxide, Gk *-osis* condition.]

oxigram (**ox**·e·gram). A record of the oxygen content of the blood over a period. [oxygen, Gk *gramma* record.]

oxime (**ox**·ime). Any of the compounds resulting from the condensation of hydroxylamine with aldehydes or ketones: they have the general formula RCH=NOH or R_2C=NOH.

oximeter (ox·**im**·et·er). An apparatus for determining the oxygen content of the blood. **Ear oximeter.** An oximeter modified for determining the oxygen content of the blood flowing through the ear. [oxygen, Gk *metron* measure.]

oximetry (ox·**im**·et·re). The measurement of the oxygen content of the blood. [see prec.]

oximide (ox·**im**·ide). $(CO)_2NH$, the internal anhydride of oxamic acid.

oxk (o·**ex**·ka). A strain of *Proteus* agglutinated by the blood of patients with mite-borne typhus.

oxoglutarate (ox·o·**gloo**·tar·ate). An intermediate of the citric-acid cycle, formed from isocitrate by the action of isocitrate dehydrogenase.

oxonaemia (ox·on·e·me·ah). Acetonaemia; the presence of acetone bodies in the blood.

oxonium (ox·o·ne·um). Term applied to salts formed from ethers in which the oxygen atom, behaving quadrivalently, combines with acids in a manner similar to the nitrogen atom in ammonium compounds.

oxonuria (ox·o·**newr**·e·ah). Acetonuria; the presence of an excess quantity of acetone bodies in the urine.

oxophenarsine (ox·o·**fen**·ar·seen). 3-Amino-4-hydroxyphenylarsine oxide, $(NH_2)C_6H_3(OH)AsO$. A logical successor to the arsenobenzene derivatives used in the treatment of syphilis, yaws and relapsing fever, and effective in much smaller doses. The hydrochloride and tartrate are administered by injection, the tartrate being regarded as giving fewer side-reactions than the hydrochloride. **Oxophenarsine Hydrochloride BP 1953.** $C_6H_6O_2NAs,HCl$. **Oxophenarsine Tartrate BP 1953.** $C_6H_6O_2NAsC_4H_6O_6{\cdot}2H_2O$.

oxosteroid (ox·o·**steer**·oid). A steroid compound with an oxygen radicle in the steroid skeleton.

Δ5-4 3, oxosteroid isomerase (ox·o·**steer**·oid i·so·**mer**·ase). An enzyme which converts a steroid oxygenated at the C_3 position in which the double bond is between the 5 and 6 positioned carbon atoms in Ring B, to a steroid with a double bond between C_5 and C_4 in Ring A.

oxozone (**ox**·o·zone). O_4, a form of oxygen shown to occur with ozone: it combines with unsaturated hydrocarbons.

Oxpentifylline (ox·pen·**tif**·il·een). BP Commission approved name for 3,7-dimethyl-1-(5-oxohexyl)xanthine; a vasodilator.

Oxprenolol (ox·**pren**·o·lol). BP Commission approved name for 1-(*o*-allyloxyphenoxy)-3-isopropylaminopropan-2-ol; a beta-adrenergic receptor blocking agent.

oxyacetone (ox·e·**as**·et·one). Acetol, acetyl carbinol, CH_3COCH_2OH. A compound obtained from cane-sugar manufacture and used in organic synthesis.

oxyachrestia (**ox**·e·a·**kres'**·te·ah). A defective supply of glucose to the neurones of the central nervous system, responsible for the nervous symptoms and signs of hypoglycaemia. [Gk *oxys* sharp, *a-*, *chresis* use.]

oxyacid (**ox**·e·as·id). Oxacid: any acid that has oxygen in its composition.

oxyacoa, oxyacoia (**ox**·e·ah·**ko'**·ah, **ox**·e·ah·**koi'**·ah). Oxyecoia; abnormal acuity of hearing. [Gk *oxys* sharp, *akoe* the sense of hearing.]

oxyaesthesia (**ox**·e·es·**the'**·ze·ah). Hyperaesthesia. [Gk *oxys* sharp, aesthesia.]

oxyaphia (ox·e·**af**·e·ah). 1. Extreme sensitiveness to touch. 2. Marked acuteness of the sense of touch. [Gk *oxys* sharp, *haphe* touch.]

oxyarthritis (**ox**·e·ar·**thri'**·tis). Arthritis of acute type. [Gk *oxys* sharp, arthritis.]

oxybiontic (**ox**·e·bi·**on'**·tik). Aerobic. [oxygen, Gk *bios* life.]

oxyblepsia (ox·e·**blep**·se·ah). Abnormal sharpness of vision. [Gk *oxys* sharp, *blepsis* sight.]

oxybromide (ox·e·**bro**·mide). Any oxy- or hydroxy- compound that also contains a bromine atom.

Oxybuprocaine (ox·e·**bew**·pro·kane). BP Commission approved name for 2-diethylaminoethyl 4-amino-3-butoxybenzoate; a local anaesthetic.

oxybutyria, oxybutyricacidaemia (ox·e·bew·**tir'**·e·ah, ox·e·bew·**tir**·ik·as·id·**e'**·me·ah). The presence of oxybutyric acid in the blood.

oxycalorimeter (**ox**·e·kal·or·**im'**·et·er). An apparatus for the determination of the heat of combustion of organic materials by measurement of the volume of oxygen consumed when known weights of the substances are burnt in oxygen, each litre of oxygen being equivalent to approximately 5 kilocalories. [oxygen, calorimeter.]

oxycamphor (ox·e·**kam**·for). $C_{10}H_{15}O(OH)$, an oxidation product of camphor, said to be of use in dyspnoea.

oxycephalia (**ox**·e·kef·**a'**·le·ah). Oxycephaly.

oxycephalic (**ox**·e·kef·**al'**·ik). Pertaining to oxycephaly.

oxycephalous (ox·e·**kef**·al·us). Denoting a skull which has a cranial-height index of more than 77. [oxycephaly.]

oxycephalus (ox·e·**kef**·al·us). Oxycephaly.

oxycephaly (ox·e·**kef**·al·e). A cranial deformity characterized by abnormal height and sloping of the skull so that the crown is peaked, the cranial-height index being more than 77, exophthalmos and defective sight, probably caused by too early union of the sagittal and coronal sutures resulting in limited development of the vault of the skull. [Gk *oxys* sharp, *kephale* head.]

oxychinolin (ox·e·**kin**·o·lin). Potassium hydroxyquinoline sulphate. An antiseptic employed in skin affections, and active against *Staphylococcus aureus.* It is used as a perspiration deodorant and as the active constituent of numerous chemical contraceptives.

oxychloride (ox·e·**klor**·ide). 1. Any oxy- or hydroxy- compound that also contains a chlorine atom. 2. A basic chloride, such as bismuth oxychloride, BiOCl.

oxycholine (ox·e·**ko**·leen). Muscarine, $C_8H_{19}O_3N$. A poisonous alkaloid found in certain toadstools, especially *Agaricus muscarius.* Its pharmacological actions are very similar to pilocarpine, stimulating the parasympathetic-nerve receptors, and it is antagonized by atropine. It promotes secretions, slows the heart and stimulates unstriped muscle such as that of the gastro-intestinal tract; also, the pupil is contracted. It is not used medicinally.

oxychromatic (**ox**·e·kro·**mat'**·ik). Acidophilic: 1. Applied to a substance capable of absorbing acid stains or having an affinity for them, e.g. an acid-staining cell of the anterior lobe of the hypophysis cerebri. 2. Applied to any organism that flourishes in a medium of strongly acid reaction. [Gk *oxys* sharp, *chroma* colour.]

oxychromatin (ox·e·**kro**·mat·in). That portion of the chromatin which stains readily with acid aniline dyes. [see prec.]

Oxycinchophen (ox·e·**sin**·ko·fen). BP Commission approved name for hydroxyphenylcinchonic acid. One of a series of hydroxylated cinchophen compounds having an antidiuretic action and decreasing tubular reabsorption. It has an antipyretic action and has been tried in the treatment of acute rheumatic fever and other collagen diseases, but it does not appear to be superior to the salicylates. It is not well tolerated, showing undesirable side effects, especially during prolonged administration, such as diarrhoea, vomiting, skin rashes and tinnitus.

oxycinesia, oxycinesis (ox·e·sin·e′·ze·ah, ox·e·sin·e′·sis). Oxykinesis.

Oxycodone (ox·e·**ko**·done). BP Commission approved name for dihydrohydroxycodeinone, an analgesic and narcotic similar to morphine in activity.

oxydesis (ox·e·**de**·sis). The acid-binding power of blood and other tissues. In the case of blood it is measured by the amount of M/100 hydrochloric acid required to be added to blood without causing agglutination of red cells. [Gk *oxys* sharp, *desis* a binding.]

oxydetic (ox·e·**det**·ik). Referring to the acid-binding power oxydesis.

oxydimorphine (ox·e·di·**mor**′·feen). Dehydromorphine, $C_{34}H_{36}N_2O_6{\cdot}3H_2O$. One of the less important alkaloids of opium; also prepared by oxidizing morphine.

oxydoreductase (ox·e·do·re·**duk**′·taze). Oxidoreductase.

oxyecoia (ox·e·ek·**oi**′·ah). A condition in which there is abnormal acuteness of hearing. [Gk *oxys* sharp, *akoe* the sense of hearing.]

Oxyfedrine (ox·e·**fed**·reen). BP Commission approved name for L - 3 - [(β - hydroxy - α - methylphenethyl)amino] - 3′ - methoxypropiophenone; a coronary vasodilator.

Oxygen BP 1973 (ox·e·jen). An element of atomic weight 15.9994, atomic number 8 and chemical symbol O. A colourless, odourless and tasteless gas, slightly soluble in water, constituting approximately one-fifth of the atmosphere, half of the earth's crust and two-thirds of plant and animal tissue. It is essential for all forms of life, either free or combined oxygen being utilized to provide energy and for combustion. It combines with most elements to form oxides which in turn yield acids and bases. There are 2 isotopes, O^{17} and O^{18}. For medical purposes it is manufactured by the fractional distillation of liquid air and stored in the gaseous state in metal cylinders under pressure. **Atomic oxygen.** O, a highly active form of oxygen prepared by passing electric discharges through the gas at low pressures. **Hyperbaric oxygen.** Oxygen under increased atmospheric pressure. Its use is mostly indicated for relief of temporary arterial insufficiency, e.g. after fractures, in ergot poisoning and also in gas gangrene. [Gk *oxys* sharp, *genein* to produce.]

oxygenase (ox·e·jen·aze). An enzyme system that activates oxidation in the tissues by molecular oxygen: it consists of an enzyme peroxidase and an auto-oxidation substance. **Haem oxygenase.** An enzyme that catalyses the removal of a specific methane carbon atom, as carbon monoxide, from haemoglobin which is thereby converted to choleglobin. **α-Methyl oxygenase.** Haem oxygenase (see above).

oxygenate (ox·e·jen·ate). To treat with oxygen or impregnate with the gas.

oxygenation (ox·e·jen·**a**′·shun). The impregnation of a substance with oxygen gas. **Diffusion oxygenation.** Oxygenation of the blood from alveolar oxygen in the absence of respiratory movement, due to the high affinity of haemoglobin for oxygen.

oxygenator (ox·e·jen·a·tor). An artificial device for the oxygenation of blood during cardiopulmonary by-pass. Varieties include *thin film oxygenators* (either screen or rotating disc), *membrane oxygenators* and *bubble oxygenators.* **Membrane oxygenator.** A silicone-rubber membrane used for oxygenation and carbon dioxide elimination during cardiopulmonary by-pass. **Pump oxygenator.** An apparatus which pumps oxygenated blood through the body during cardiopulmonary by-pass. **Rotating disc oxygenator.** A device for oxygenating blood during cardiopulmonary by-pass in which a thin film of blood adheres to a disc dipping into a channel of blood and rotating in an atmosphere of oxygen.

oxygenic (ox·e·**jen**·ik). 1. Possessing the characteristics of oxygen. 2. Constituted of, or containing, oxygen.

Oxygenium (ox·e·**jen**·e·um). *European Pharmacopoeia* name for Oxygen BP 1973.

oxygenize (ox·e·jen·ize). 1. Oxygenate. 2. Oxidize.

oxygeusia (ox·e·**gews**·e·ah). More than normal acuteness or too great acuteness of the sense of taste. [Gk *oxys* sharp, *geusis* taste.]

oxyhaem (ox·e·heem). The compound formed by co-ordination of haem with oxygen, which is present in combination with globin in oxyhaemoglobin.

oxyhaemoglobin (ox·e·he·mo·**glo**′·bin). *See* HAEMOGLOBIN.

oxyhaemoglobinometer (ox·e·he·mo·glo·bin·**om**′·et·er). An apparatus for measuring the amount of oxygen which is present in the blood. [oxygen, haemoglobin, meter.]

oxyhaemograph (ox·e·**he**·mo·graf). An apparatus for measuring blood-oxygen continuously. [oxygen, Gk *haima* blood, *graphein* to record.]

oxyhaemotherapy (ox·e·he·mo·**ther**′·ap·e). Any method which increases the oxygenation of the lung, either by high altitude, inducing polycythaemia, or increasing the depth of respiration by exercise, or by the administration of extra oxygen. [oxygen, Gk *haima* blood, *therapeia* treatment.]

oxyhaloid (ox·e·**hal**·oid). Any oxy- or hydroxy- compound that also contains a halogen atom.

oxyhydrocephalus (ox·e·hi·dro·**kef**′·al·us). Hydrocephalus in which the top of the head slopes to a peak. [Gk *oxys* sharp, hydrocephalus.]

oxyiodide (ox·e·**i**·o·dide). Any oxy- or hydroxy- compound that also contains an atom of iodine.

oxykinesia, oxykinesis (ox·e·kin·e′·ze·ah, ox·e·kin·e′·sis). A condition in which pain is felt when movement is carried out. [Gk *oxys* sharp, *kinesis* movement.]

oxykrinin (ox·e·**krin**·in). Secretin, the secretory hormone of the pancreas. [Obsolete term.] [Gk *oxys* sharp, *krinein* to separate.]

oxylalia (ox·e·**la**·le·ah). Abnormal rapidity of speech. [Gk *oxys* sharp, *lalia* talking.]

oxyleucotin (ox·e·**lew**·ko·tin). $C_{34}H_{32}O_{12}$, a constituent of coto bark.

oxylith (ox·e·lith). Sodium peroxide, Na_2O_2. A yellowish powder which evolves oxygen on warming with water and is used in bleaching teeth, wool, sponges, bone, etc. [oxygen, Gk *lithos* stone.]

oxyluciferin (ox·e·lew·**sif**′·er·in). *See* LUCIFERIN.

Oxymel (ox·e·mel). A mixture of honey and diluted acetic acid (BPC 1954). **Oxymel of Squill BPC 1959.** An acetic-acid extract of squill to which honey has been added; used in coughs. [Gk *oxys* sharp, *meli* honey.]

Oxymesterone (ox·e·**mes**·ter·one). BP Commission approved name for 4-hydroxy-17α-methyltestosterone; an anabolic agent.

Oxymetholone (ox·e·**meth**·o·lone). BP Commission approved name for 4,5α-dihydro-2-hydroxymethylene-17α-methyltestosterone; an anabolic agent.

oxymetry (ox·**im**·et·re). Oximetry.

oxymorphine (ox·e·**mor**·feen). Oxydimorphine.

Oxymorphone (ox·e·**mor**·fone). BP Commission approved name for dihydrohydroxymorphinone, an analgesic and narcotic with morphine-like activity.

oxymyoglobin (ox·e·mi·o·**glo**′·bin). *See* MYOGLOBIN. [oxygen, myoglobin.]

oxymyohaemoglobin (ox·e·mi·o·he·mo·**glo**′·bin). Oxidized myohaemoglobin.

oxynarcotine (ox·e·**nar**·kot·een). $C_{22}H_{23}O_8N$, an alkaloid occurring in opium and closely related to narcotine. Like narcotine, it yields cotarnine upon oxidation with ferric chloride.

oxyneurine (ox·e·**newr**·een). Betaine.

oxynitrilase (ox·e·**ni**·tril·aze). An enzyme that activates the conversion of oxynitriles into aldehydes.

oxynitrile (ox·e·ni·trile). An organic compound which contains both an OH group and a CN– radical, e.g. glycollic nitrile, $OHCH_2CN$.

oxyntic (ox·in·tik). Secreting matter of acidic character. [Gk *oxynein* to make sour.]

oxyopia (ox·e·o·pe·ah). Abnormal visual acuity. [Gk *oxys* sharp, *opsis* vision.]

oxyosis (ox·e·o·sis). Acidosis. [Gk *oxys* sharp, *-osis* condition.]

oxyosmia (ox·e·oz·me·ah). Hyperosmia: 1. Abnormal acuteness of the sense of smell. 2. Sensitiveness to odour of such degree that it amounts to morbidity. [Gk *oxys* sharp, *osme* odour.]

oxyosphresia (ox·e·os·fre′·ze·ah). Oxyosmia. [Gk *oxys* sharp, *osphresis* sense of smell.]

oxypathia (ox·e·path·e·ah). Any condition marked by acuteness of sensation. [Gk *oxys* sharp, *pathos* disease.]

oxypathic (ox·e·path·ik). Relating to or marked by oxypathia.

oxypathy (ox·ip·ath·e). 1. A condition presumed to be due to inability to eliminate unoxidized acids, the latter combining with the fixed alkalies of the body; the gouty diathesis. 2. Oxypathia. [Gk *oxys* sharp, *pathos* disease.]

Oxypertine (ox·e·per·teen). BP Commission approved name for 1 - [2 - (5,6 - dimethoxy - 2 - methylindol - 3 - yl)ethyl]-4-phenylpiperazine; a psychotropic agent.

Oxyphenbutazone BP 1973 (ox·e·fen·bew′·tah·zone). The monohydrate of 4-butyl-2-(4-hydroxyphenyl)-1-phenylpyrazolidine-3,5-dione. It has the same actions, uses and side-effects as phenylbutazone in the symptomatic treatment of acute gout and in rheumatoid arthritis when these diseases have failed to respond to less toxic drugs. It has no obvious therapeutic advantages over phenylbutazone.

Oxyphencyclimine (ox·e·fen·si′·klim·een). BP Commission approved name for 1,4,5,6 - tetrahydro - 1 - methylpyrimidin - 2 - methyl - α - cyclohexylmandelate. **Oxyphencyclimine Hydrochloride BP 1973.** The hydrochloride of Oxyphencyclimine, an anticholinergic drug with the peripheral, but not the central, actions of atropine.

Oxyphenisatin (ox·e·fen·i′·sat·in). BP Commission approved name for 3,3-di-(4-hydroxyphenyl)oxindole. **Oxyphenisatin Acetate BPC 1968.** 3,3-di(*p*-acetoxyphenyl)oxindole; its actions and uses are those of bisacodyl, a laxative acting almost exclusively on the colon. It is given by mouth as tablets.

Oxyphenonium Bromide (ox·e·fen·o′·ne·um bro·mide). BP Commission aproved name for 2-diethylaminoethyl-α-cyclohexyl-α-phenylglycollate methobromide, an anticholinergic agent employed for adjunctive therapy in peptic ulcer and spasm of the gastro-intestinal tract.

oxyphil, oxyphile (ox·e·fil, ox·e·file). Acidophil: 1. A substance capable of absorbing acid stains or having an affinity for them. 2. An acid-staining cell of the anterior lobe of the hypophysis cerebri. 3. Any organism that flourishes in a medium of strongly acid reaction. **Amphophilic oxyphil.** A cell which has greater affinity for acid dyes but which takes the stain also of basic dyes; amphophilic acidophil. [Gk *oxys* sharp, *philein* to love.]

oxyphilic, oxyphilous (ox·e·fil·ik, ox·if·il·us). Acidophilic. [see prec.]

oxyphonia (ox·e·fo·ne·ah). Shrillness or an abnormally high pitch of the voice. [Gk *oxyphonos* with a clear shrill voice.]

oxyphor (ox·e·for). Oxycamphor.

oxyplasm (ox·e·plazm). That part of the cytoplasm which is readily stained with acid dyes. [Gk *oxys* sharp, plasma.]

oxypolygelatin (ox·e·pol·e·jel′·at·in). An oxidized product of polymerized gelatin that has been used as a transfusion substitute for blood plasma.

oxyproline (ox·e·pro·leen). Hydroxyproline.

oxypurine (ox·e·pewr·een). A generic name for the hydroxyl derivatives of purine. Of these the most important are uric acid (2,6,8-trioxypurine) and xanthine (2,6-dioxypurine).

Oxypurinol (ox·e·pewr·in·ol). BP Commission approved name for 1*H*-pyrazolo[3,4-*d*]pyrimidin-4,6-diol; a xanthine oxidase inhibitor.

oxyqua (ox·e·kwah). Oxygenated water used in nausea and vomiting. [oxygen, L *aqua* water.]

oxyquinoline (ox·e·kwin·o·leen). Hydroxyquinoline, C_9H_7ON. A compound of which there are 8 isomers, one of which, 8-oxyquinoline, is used in medicine. It is a powerful bacteriostatic, and is usually employed as a mixture of the sulphate with potassium sulphate dissolved in water.

oxyrhine (ox·e·rine). 1. Possessing a sharply pointed nose or snout. 2. Possessing an abnormally acute sense of smell. [Gk *oxys* sharp, *rhis* nose.]

oxysalt (ox·e·sawlt). Any salt formed by an oxyacid.

oxysparteine (ox·e·spar·te·een). $C_{15}H_{24}ON_2$, a compound obtained by the oxidation of sparteine; it does not possess the curare-like effect of the latter on motor nerves.

11-oxysteroids (ox·e·steer·oids). Any compound in which an oxygen atom is attached to the steroid nucleus in position 11, as in cortisone.

17-oxysteroids (ox·e·steer·oidz). 17-Ketosteroids. *See* KETOSTEROID.

Oxytetracycline (ox·e·tet·rah·si′·kleen). BP Commission approved name for 4 - dimethylamino - 1,4,4*a*,5,5*a*,6,11,12*a*-octahydro - 3,5,6,10,12,12*a*-hexahydroxy - 6 - methyl-1,11,dioxonaphthacene -2 - carboxyamide, a crystalline antibiotic isolated from the culture medium of *Streptomyces rimosus.* It is a bactericide with a wide range of activity similar to that of aureomycin, but has no value in tuberculosis, leprosy or diseases caused by filamentous fungi. The dihydrate and the hydrochloride have been officially recognized in the BP 1973.

Oxytetracyclini Dihydras (ox·e·tet·rah·si′·klin·i di·hi·dras). *European Pharmacopoeia* name for Oxytetracycline Dihydrate BP 1973.

Oxytetracyclini Hydrochloridum (ox·e·tet·rah·si′·klin·i hi·dro·klor·id·um). *European Pharmacopoeia* name for Oxytetracycline Hydrochloride BP 1973.

oxytocia (ox·e·to·se·ah). Rapid childbirth. [see foll.]

oxytocic (ox·e·to·sik). 1. Promoting childbirth. 2. An agent which hastens parturition. [Gk *oxys* quick, *tokos* birth.]

oxytocin (ox·e·to·sin). The fraction of the extract of the posterior lobe of the hypophysis cerebri which causes contraction of uterine muscle and of plain muscle generally, except that of the bronchi. [see prec.]

oxytoxin (ox·e·tox·in). Any substance that is produced by the process of oxidizing a toxin.

oxytropism (ox·e·tro·pizm). The response of living organisms to oxygen. [oxygen, Gk *trope* a turning.]

oxytuberculin (ox·e·tew·ber′·kew·lin). A tuberculin prepared from highly virulent strains of tubercle bacilli and modified by oxidation. It is no longer used.

oxyuria, oxyuriasis (ox·e·ewr·e·ah, ox·e·ewr·i′·as·is). Infestation with a nematode worm of the genus *Enterobius,* previously named *Oxyuris.*

oxyuricide (ox·e·ewr·e·side). Any agent which destroys nematode worms of the genus *Enterobius* (*Oxyuris*). [oxyuris, L *caedere* to kill.]

oxyurid (ox·e·ewr·id). A pinworm. [oxyuris.]

Oxyuridae (ox·e·ewr·id·e). A family of the nematode super-family or sub-order Oxyuroidea. The genus *Enterobius* is of medical interest. [Gk *oxys* sharp, *oura* tail, *eidos* form.]

oxyurifuge (ox·e·ewr·e·fewj). Oxyuricide. [oxyuris, L *fugare* to put to flight.]

oxyuriosis (ox·e·ewr·e·o′·sis). Oxyuria. [oxyuria, Gk *-osis* condition.]

Oxyuris (ox·e·ewr·is). 1. A superseded generic name for the human threadworm *Enterobius vermicularis.* 2. A genus of threadworm whose members are not of medical importance. [Gk *oxys* sharp, *oura* tail.]

Oxyuroidea (ox·e·ewr·oid′·e·ah). A super-family or sub-order of the nematode sub-order or order Ascaridata. The family Oxyuridae is of medical interest. [Gk *oxys* sharp, *oura* tail, *eidos* form.]

oxyzymol (ox·e·zi·mol). Carvacrol, methyl isopropyl phenol, $CH_3C_6H_3(OH)CH(CH_3)_2$. An isomer of thymol occurring in savory oil, caraway oil and origanum oil. It is an oily liquid, similar to creosote, and with germicidal and local anaesthetic properties.

ozaena (o·ze·nah). 1. Probably a constitutional condition associated with dyspituitarism which causes a vasoconstriction and obliterates arteritis of the nasal mucosa; this results in atrophy and rhinitis, and, clinically, an offensive odour. 2. Any offensive nasal discharge. [Gk *ozein* to have a smell.]

ozaenous (o·ze·nus). Suffering from ozaena; relating or belonging to or having the characteristics of ozaena.

ozamin (o·zam·in). Benzopurpurine.

ozocerite (o·zo·ser·ite). A crude ceresin wax occurring as a natural paraffin in Galicia and the Caucasus. When bleached it constitutes ceresine, a substitute for beeswax. [Gk *ozein* to have a smell, *keros* wax.]

ozochrotia (o·zo·kro·she·ah). A condition in which the skin has an offensive smell. [Gk *ozein* to have a smell, *chroa* skin.]

ozochrotous (o·zok·ro·tus). Having a fetid odour of the skin. [see prec.]

ozoena (o·ze·nah). Ozaean.

ozokerite (o·zo·ker·ite). Ozacerite.

ozonator (o·zo·na·tor). An apparatus for producing ozone.

ozone (o·zone). O_3, an allotrope of oxygen formed by the action of ultraviolet light or an electrical discharge on oxygen or air: it does not occur naturally in air. When pure it is a blue gas with a peculiar smell, highly unstable and very reactive. It is used to sterilize drinking water, to purify air in ventilation and as a powerful oxidizing and bleaching agent. [Gk *ozein* to have a smell.]

ozone-ether (o·zone·e'·ther). A mixture of ethyl ether, hydrogen peroxide and alcohol. It is used as an antiseptic and in the treatment of whooping-cough, being more stable than an aqueous solution of hydrogen peroxide. [ozone, ether.]

ozonide (o·zo·nide). An unstable additive compound formed by ozone with unsaturated hydrocarbons: the absorption of ozone by the pinene of turpentine to form pinene ozonide, $C_{10}H_{16}O_3$, is used in the quantitative estimation of the gas.

ozonization (o·zo·ni·za'·shun). Saturation with ozone.

ozonize (o·zo·nize). To saturate with ozone.

ozonizer (o·zo·ni·zer). A device used in the application of ozone to sinuses, wounds and so on.

ozonometer (o·zone·om·et·er). An apparatus for measuring the amount of ozone in the atmosphere.

ozonometry (o·zone·om·et·re). The measurement of the amount of ozone present in the air.

ozonophore (o·zo·no·for). 1. An erythrocyte. 2. A granule of the cytoplasm. [ozone, Gk *phoros* bearer.]

ozonoscope (o·zo·no·skope). Any device for demonstrating the presence of ozone: a test paper impregnated with an indicator such as starch-iodide that is sensitive to ozone. [ozone, Gk *skopein* to watch.]

ozostomia (o·zo·sto·me·ah). Halitosis. [Gk *ozostomos* with bad breath.]

Ozzard's filariasis. Infection with *Mansonella ozzardi.*

P

paaj (pah·aj). A contact dermatitis from the leaves of red quebracho, *Schinopsis lorentzii*, which grows in Argentina.

pabular (pab·ew·lar). Pertaining to food. [pabulum.]

pabulin (pab·ew·lin). The protein and fatty substances which are found in the blood after food has been digested. [L *pabulum* food.]

pabulum (pab·ew·lum). Food. [L.]

Pacchioni, Antonio (b. 1665). Rome anatomist.

Pacchionian bodies, or corpuscles. Enlarged arachnoid villi; they consist of protrusions of the arachnoid membrane through the dura into the venous lacunae on either side of the superior sagittal sinus and, to a less extent, into the sinus itself. They become enlarged by proliferation of fibrous tissue and of arachnoid mesothelial cells, and are usually calcified in old age. It is thought that cerebrospinal fluid drains through the arachnoid villi into the venous blood stream. The name is applied only to the villi when they become enlarged by fibrosis and mesothelial proliferation, and when this has occurred it is doubtful if the original function is preserved.

Pacchionian depressions. Depressions on the inner surface of the cranial vault which mark the position of large, often calcified, arachnoid villi; they are usually present only in old age.

Pacchionian glands, Pacchionian granulations. Pacchionian bodies (see above).

pacemaker (pase·ma·ker). The sinu-atrial node of Keith and Flack; a small collection of specialized nervous tissue which lies at the junction of the superior vena cava and the right atrium in the mammalian heart. It originates and controls the rate and rhythm of the atria and ventricles, causing the atria to contract and pass the impulse to the atrioventricular node which initiates ventricular contraction. Rarely, the atrioventricular node takes over the rôle of pacemaker if the rate of impulse formation at the sinu-atrial node is depressed below the natural frequency of the former; the sinu-atrial node is then activated retrogradely. **Cardiac pacemaker.** *See* MAIN DEF. (prec.). **Ectopic pacemaker.** An abnormal focus in the heart which usurps the function of the sinu-atrial node in initiating cardiac contraction. It may lie in the atrium, atrioventricular node, or in the ventricle. **External pacemaker.** 1. A device used to stimulate the heart electrically by the discharge of impulses from outside the chest wall, used as emergency treatment for cardiac standstill or in heart block with severe bradycardia. 2. A cardiac pacemaker system with electrodes in contact with the heart but the connecting wires brought out through the skin to an external electrical impulse generator. **Idioventricular pacemaker.** The taking over of the function of the pacemaker by the atrioventricular node. **Sequential pacemaker.** A device used to stimulate the atria and then, after an appropriate interval, the ventricles; used in patients with heart block when it is desired to preserve atrial transport function. **Shifting pacemaker.** The term applied to describe the association of abrupt changes in heart rate with similarly abrupt alterations in the P-wave morphology in the electrocardiogram, usually initiated by a premature impulse. **Ventricular inhibited pacemaker.** A demand pacemaker (see above) which is inhibited from discharging an impulse for a preselected period after each detected QRS complex, used in patients with intermittent heart block. **Ventricular-triggered pacemaker.** A demand pacemaker (see above) which discharges an impulse as soon as a QRS complex is detected and also spontaneously after a preselected interval following the preceding impulse if triggering does not occur first; the triggered impulses permit identification of continuing pacemaker function in patients with intermittent heart block during periods of normal conduction. **Wandering pacemaker.** The term applied to describe the association of a heart rate variation as in sinus arrhythmia with varying P-wave morphology and P-R interval in the electrocardiogram. [L *passus* step, ME *maken*.]

pachaemia (pak·e·me·ah). Pachyhaemia.

pachismus (pak·iz·mus). Thickening. [Gk *pachys* thick.]

pachometer (pak·om·et·er). Pachymeter.

Pachon, Michel Victor (b. 1867). Bordeaux physiologist.

Pachon method, or test. Oscillometry test: the oscillometer (devised by Pachon) is an instrument which measures the degree of pulsation of the extremities, and is a rough guide to the patency of large arteries. Two cuffs are placed round the extremity, one of which is filled with air at a known pressure. The difference in pressure between this collecting cuff and the arterial pressure is recorded on a dial. If no major arteries are patent, no pulsation will be recorded, and no movement of the needle will occur.

pachulosis (pak·ew·lo·sis). Pachylosis.

pachyacria (pak·e·ak·re·ah). 1. Acromegaly. 2. A morbid condition marked by thickening of the soft tissues of the ends of the fingers or toes. [Gk *pachys* thick, *akron* end.]

pachyblepharon, pachyblepharosis (pak·e·blef·ar·on, pak·e·blef·ar·o'·sis). A condition in which the eyelid becomes thickened, noticeably near the tarsal margins. [Gk *pachys* thick, *blepharon* eyelid, *-osis* condition.]

pachycarpine (pak·e·kar·peen). Sparteine, $C_{15}H_{26}N_2$. An alkaloid occurring in broom, *Cytisus scoparius.* Its salts are used in the treatment of cardiac disease.

pachycephalia (pak·e·kef·a'·le·ah). Pachycephaly.

pachycephalic, pachycephalous (pak·e·kef·al'·ik, pak·e·kef·al·us). Pertaining to or characterized by pachycephaly.

pachycephaly (pak·e·kef·al·e). Morbid thickening of the skull. [Gk *pachys* thick, *kephale* head.]

pachycheilia, pachychilia (pak·e·kih·le·ah). Abnormal thickness or swelling of the lips. [Gk *pachys* thick, *cheilos* lip.]

pachycholia (pak·e·ko·le·ah). Thickness of the bile. [Gk *pachys* thick, *chole* bile.]

pachychromatic (pak·e·kro·mat'·ik). Having, or characterized by, coarse chromatin filaments. [Gk *pachys* thick, *chroma* colour.]

pachycolpismus (pak·e·kol·piz'·mus). Pachyvaginitis. [Gk *pachys* thick, *kolpos* vagina.]

pachydactylia (pak·e·dak·til'·e·ah). Pachydactyly.

pachydactylous (pak·e·dak·til·us). Pertaining to pachydactyly.

pachydactyly (pak·e·dak·til·e). Abnormal thickening of a finger or toe, particularly at the tip. [Gk *pachys* thick, *daktylos* finger or toe.]

pachyderma (pak·e·der·mah). Pachydermia.

pachydermatocele (pak·e·der·mat·o·seel). 1. Tumours occurring in some cases of dermatolysis (Valentine Mott). 2. Filarial elephantiasis. [Gk *pachys* thick, *derma* skin, *kele* tumour.]

pachydermatosis (pak·e·der·mat·o'·sis). Chronic pachydermia. [pachydermia, Gk *-osis* condition.]

pachydermatous (pak·e·der·mat·us). Pertaining to pachydermia.

pachydermia (pak·e·der·me·ah). Hypertrophy of the skin and subcutaneous tissue, due to blockage of lymph channels; the surface of the affected integument often becomes verrucose. The condition may be noted in Milroy's disease, filariasis, and other maladies. **Pachydermia circumscripta, Pachydermia laryngis.** A heaping-up of the epithelium over the vocal cords, but particularly over the vocal processes. **Pachydermia lymphangiectatica.** Pachydermia arising in association with diffuse lymphangioma. **Occipital pachydermia.** Pachydermia confined to the occipital area on which site the skin develops into folds. **Pachydermia verrucosa.** Papillomatous growths on the vocal cords. **Pachydermia vesicae.** Leucoplakia vesicae. [Gk *pachys* thick, *derma* skin.]

pachydermic (pak·e·**der**·mik). Pachydermatous.

pachydermoperiostosis (pak·e·**der**·mo·per·e·os·**to**′·sis). A rare clinical syndrome characterized by the thickening and excessive folding of the skin, especially over the face, and peripheral changes resembling hypertrophic pulmonary osteo-arthropathy. The incidence is sometimes familial. [Gk *pachys* thick, *derma* skin, periostosis.]

pachyglossal, pachyglossate (pak·e·**glos**·al, pak·e·**glos**·ate). Having a tongue of abnormal thickness. [see foll.]

pachyglossia (pak·e·**glos**·e·ah). Excessive thickening of the tongue. [Gk *pachys* thick, *glossa* tongue.]

pachygnathous (pak·ig·**nath**·us). Pertaining to or marked by a large or thick jaw. [Gk *pachys* thick, *gnathos* jaw.]

pachygyria (pak·e·**ji**·re·ah). Broadening and flattening of the gyri of the cerebral hemispheres. [Gk *pachys* thick, gyrus.]

pachyhaematous (pak·e·**he**·mat·us). Relating to pachyhaemia.

pachyhaemia (pak·e·**he**·me·ah). A condition characterized by concentration and thickening of the blood. [Gk *pachys* thick, *haima* blood.]

pachyhymenic (**pak**·e·hi·**men**′·ik). Pachymenic.

pachyleptomeningitis (**pak**·e·lep·to·men·in·**ji**′·tis). Inflammation affecting the dura mater and the pia mater simultaneously. [Gk *pachys* thick, *leptos* thin, meningitis.]

pachylosis (pak·e·**lo**·sis). A chronic dermatosis, especially of the legs, with thickening of the skin which becomes harsh and dry. [Gk *pachylos* thick.]

pachymenia (pak·e·**me**·ne·ah). Abnormal thickness of the skin or other membranes. [Gk *pachys* thick, *hymen* membrane.]

pachymenic (pak·e·**men**·ik). Pertaining to pachymenia.

pachymeningitis (**pak**·e·men·in·**ji**′·tis). Inflammation of the dura mater. **Cerebral pachymeningitis.** Inflammation of the dura mater of the brain. **Pachymeningitis cervicalis hypertrophica.** A condition in which the space between the cord and dura in the cervical region is occupied by a firm fibrous growth, ultimately showing signs of pressure on the nerve roots and cord in the region, i.e. pain and paralysis of muscle. It is pathologically identical with haemorrhagic internal pachymeningitis of the brain (see below). **Circumscribed pachymeningitis.** Localized pachymeningitis in various regions. **Epidural pachymeningitis.** Inflammation or suppuration in the extradural tissues of the spinal canal. **External pachymeningitis.** Inflammation of the outer layers of the dura. **Haemorrhagic pachymeningitis.** An obsolete synonym for chronic subdural haematoma. **Haemorrhagic internal pachymeningitis, Pachymeningitis haemorrhagica interna.** That due to localized thickening between the dura and the brain with possible haemorrhages into the new tissue. Pachymeningitis cervicalis hypertrophica (see above) is a similar condition within the cervical dura. **Internal pachymeningitis.** Inflammation of the inner layer of the dura mater. **Pachymeningitis intralamellaris.** Intradural inflammation or abscess. **Purulent pachymeningitis.** Pachymeningitis associated with infection by pyogenic organisms. **Pyogenic pachymeningitis.** Infection of the dura by pyogenic bacteria, usually secondary to cranial or vertebral osteitis. **Serous internal pachymeningitis.** Pachymeningitis cervicalis hypertrophica (see above). **Syphilitic pachymeningitis.** That in which the basal pathology is syphilitic. [Gk *pachys* thick, *menigx* membrane, *-itis* inflammation.]

pachymeningopathy (**pak**·e·men·in·**gop**′·ath·e). Disease of the dura mater apart from that caused by inflammation. [Gk *pachys* thick, *menigx* membrane, *pathos* disease.]

pachymeninx (pak·e·**men**·ingx). The dura mater. [Gk *pachys* thick, *menigx* membrane.]

pachymeter (pak·**im**·et·er). An instrument used to determine the thickness of any object, especially those of slender construction or of thinness; the measurements can be made to 0.025 mm. [Gk *pachys* thick, *metron* measure.]

pachynsis (pak·**in**·sis). Thickening; thickening due to pathological causes. [Gk.]

pachyntic (pak·**in**·tik). 1. Pertaining to pachynsis. 2. Showing abnormal thickening.

pachyonychia (**pak**·e·on·**ik**′·e·ah). Excessive thickening of the nails. **Pachyonychia congenita.** A congenital defect of the nails, characterized by much thickening, and sometimes associated with defects in other structures of ectodermal origin. [Gk *pachys* thick, *onyx* nail.]

pachyonychosis (**pak**·e·on·ik·**o**′·sis). Onychia sicca. [Gk *pachys* thick, *onyx* nail, *-osis*, conditon.]

pachyonyxis (**pak**·e·on·**ix**′·is). Pachyonychia.

pachyotia (pak·e·**o**·she·ah). Abnormal thickness of the ears; boxers' ear; cauliflower ear. [Gk *pachys* thick, *ous* ear.]

pachypelviperitonitis (**pak**·e·pel·ve·per·it·on·**i**′·tis). Pelvic peritonitis characterized by thickening of the affected tissues. [Gk *pachys* thick, pelviperitonitis.]

pachyperiosteitis (**pak**·e·per·e·os·te·**i**′·tis). Pachyperiostitis.

pachyperiosteoderma (**pak**·e·per·e·**os**·te·o·**der**′·mah). A rare syndrome, consisting of periostitis with enlargement of the fingers and toes and furrowing of the skin of the forehead. [Gk *pachys* thick, *peri*, *osteon* bone, *derma* skin.]

pachyperiostitis (**pak**·e·per·e·os·**ti**′·tis). Inflammation of the periosteum of long bones, causing morbid thickening of the bones. [Gk *pachys* thick, periostitis.]

pachyperiostosis (**pak**·e·per·e·os·**to**′·sis). A condition in which there is a great thickening of the periosteum of the long bones. [Gk *pachys* thick, periosteum, Gk *-osis* condition.]

pachyperitonitis (**pak**·e·per·it·on·**i**′·tis). Inflammation affecting the peritoneum associated with thickening. [Gk *pachys* thick, peritonitis.]

pachypleuritis (**pak**·e·ploor·**i**′·tis). Inflammation affecting the pleura associated with thickening of the involved membrane. [Gk *pachys* thick, pleuritis.]

pachypodous (pak·**ip**·od·us). Possessing feet large in size and of more than normal thickness. [Gk *pachys* thick, *pous* foot.]

pachyrhinic (pak·e·**rin**·ik). Characterized by or possessing a thick or abnormally flat and broad nose. [Gk *pachys* thick, *rhis* nose.]

pachysalpingitis (**pak**·e·sal·pin·**ji**′·tis). Chronic parenchymatous salpingitis. [Gk *pachys* thick, salpingitis.]

pachysalpingo-oöthecitis, pachysalpingo-ovaritis (**pak**·e·sal·-ping·go·o·o·the·**si**′·tis, **pak**·e·**sal**·ping·go·o·var·**i**′·tis). An inflammatory condition of the ovary and uterine tube associated with induration of the affected parts. [Gk *pachys* thick, *salpigx* trumpet, oöthecitis, ovaritis.]

pachysomia (pak·e·**so**·me·ah). Morbid thickening of the soft tissues of the body such as occurs in acromegaly. [Gk *pachys* thick, *soma* body.]

pachytene (**pak**·e·teen). That stage in meiosis when the paired homologous chromosomes contract owing to spiralization, and become much thicker than in the preceding leptotene and zygotene stages. [Gk *pachys* thick, *tainia* ribbon.]

pachytes (pak·i·teez). 1. Thickening. 2. Pachyblepharon. [Gk *pachytes* thickness.]

pachytic (pak·it·ik). 1. Characterized by thickness or obesity. 2. Capable of inspissating the body fluids. [see prec.]

pachytrichous (pak·it·rik·us). A term applied to growth of hair, each strand of which is thicker than normal. [Gk *pachys* thick, *thrix* hair.]

pachyvaginalitis (**pak**·e·vaj·in·al·**i**′·tis). Chronic inflammation and thickening of the tunica vaginalis testis. [Gk *pachys* thick, vaginalitis.]

pachyvaginitis (**pak**·e·vaj·in·**i**′·tis). A chronic inflammatory condition of the vagina associated with thickening of its walls. **Cystic pachyvaginitis, Pachyvaginitis cystica.** Emphysematous vaginitis. [Gk *pachys* thick, vaginitis.]

Paci, Agostino. Pisa surgeon.

Paci's operation. Manipulative reduction of a congenital dislocation of the hip.

pacing (pa·sing). The technique of artificial stimulation of the heart used in failure of the normal impulse formation, excessive bradycardia, or heart block (*see also* PACEMAKER). **Atrial pacing.** The technique of electrically stimulating the atria, used in failure of normal impulse formation or excessive bradycardia, or when it is desired to drive the heart at a rate faster than the physiological one. **Coupled pacing.** The technique of pacing the ventricles by two impulses close together, used to enhance ventricular contractility. **Endocardial pacing.** Artificial pacing of the heart using electrodes, in contact with the endocardium, which have been introduced pervenously. **Epicardial pacing.** Artificial pacing of the heart using electrodes placed on the epicardial surface of the heart by open operation. **Overdrive pacing.** The technique of pacing the heart faster than its natural rate so as to capture control of the heart beat, used in attempts to terminate certain abnormal rhythms or paroxysms of tachycardia. **Paired pacing.** Coupled pacing (see above). **Programmed pacing.** The technique of pacing the heart at preselected intervals after the naturally occurring P waves or QRS complexes in a preselected proportion of beats, e.g. 1 in 7. The method is used in the study of naturally occurring arrhythmias in an attempt to initiate a paroxysm of tachycardia so as to define its mechanism. **Sequential pacing.** The technique of pacing using a sequential pacemaker. **Ventricular pacing.** The technique of electrically stimulating the ventricle, used in failure of normal impulse formation, excessive bradycardia, or heart block. [L *passus* step.]

Pacini, Filippo (b. 1812). Florence anatomist.

Pacini's corpuscles, Vater-Pacini corpuscles. Lamellated corpuscles, subserving pressure sense.

Pacini's fluid, or diluting solution. A solution used as a diluent in the enumeration of red blood corpuscles; it contains mercuric chloride 2 g, sodium chloride 4 g, glycerin 26 g, distilled water 226 g.

Pacini's foramen. The tentorial notch. *See* NOTCH.

pacinitis (pas·in·i·tis). Inflammation of the corpuscles of Pacini. [*Pacini*, Gk *-itis* inflammation.]

pack (pak). 1. A method of treatment where a blanket or sheet is used to envelope a patient either wholly or partially. 2. A tampon or plug of gauze or cotton-wool, used for packing an orifice such as the vagina or the nose. **Cold pack.** A method of temperature reduction now almost obsolete, by which the patient is wrapped in a sheet wrung out of cold water. **Hot pack.** Hot blankets, wet or dry, used to promote sweating. **Ice pack.** A poultice of crushed ice, used for local cooling, or, in larger quantities, for refrigeration anaesthesia. **Partial pack.** A large hot fomentation, used locally for the reduction of inflammation or the easement of pain. **Wet pack.** Treatment by wrapping the patient in wet sheets and enveloping the whole in dry blankets. [ME *pakke.*]

packer (pak·er). An instrument for introducing a gauze pack into the vagina or into a wound.

packing (pak·ing). 1. The act of filling a wound or other cavity to obliterate it, or to prevent bleeding from its walls. 2. The material used in filling a wound or cavity. [ME *pakken.*]

pad (pad). 1. A flat cushion, or an arrangement of several thicknesses of resilient, soft, and possibly absorbent, material: used to localize or distribute pressure, to protect from friction, or to absorb discharges. 2. A localized thickening. **Abdominal pad.** A gauze and cotton-wool pad, used to absorb discharges from an abdominal wound. **Buccal pad of fat [corpus adiposum buccae].** A large mass of fat which separates the buccinator muscle from the overlying part of the masseter muscle and mandible. **Pad of the corpus callosum.** The splenium of the corpus callosum. **Fat pad.** A mass of adipose tissue, e.g. synovial fat pad, sucking pad. **Infrapatellar pad of fat [corpus adiposum infrapatellare (NA)].** The collection of fat in the synovial membrane deep to the ligamentum patellae. **Ischiorectal pad of fat [corpus adiposum fossae ischiorectalis (NA)].** Fatty tissue filling the ischiorectal fossa, traversed by many bands of fibrous tissue. **Knuckle pads.** Fibrous nodules which develop on the dorsal surfaces of the fingers. **Periarterial pad.** The juxtaglomerular apparatus of the nephron, in the form of a collection of specialized granular cells around the afferent arteriole to the glomerulus. **Retropubic pad of fat.** The pad of fat which normally occupies the retropubic space. **Ring pad.** A gauze and cotton-wool pad, made in the form of a ring; used to protect the bony prominences of a patient confined to bed. **Sucking pad, Suctorial pad.** A mass of fat on the surface of the buccinator muscle, most marked in infants. **Synovial fat pad.** A localized collection of fat in the synovial membrane of joints. [etym. dub.]

See also: BICHAT, MALGAIGNE.

Padgett, Earl C. (b. 1893). American surgeon.

Padgett's dermatome. A calibrated instrument consisting of a drum and cutting blade for the cutting of free split skin grafts of the desired thickness.

paedarthrocace (pe·dar·**throk**·as·e). Suppuration of the joints affecting children. [Gk *pais* child, arthrocace.]

paedatrophia (pe·dat·**ro**·fe·ah). Paedatrophy.

paedatrophy (pe·**dat**·ro·fe). 1. Marasmus. 2. Tabes mesenterica. [Gk *pais* child, atrophy.]

paederast (**pe**·der·ast). One addicted to the practice of paederasty.

paederasty (**pe**·der·as·te). Sodomy practised by adults with boys. [Gk *pais* boy, *erastes* lover.]

paederosis (pe·der·**o**·sis). An abnormal state in which adults show sexual passion for children. [Gk *pais* child, *eros* love.]

Paederus (**pe**·der·us). A genus of staphylinid beetles. **Paederus columbinus.** A species producing anal secretions which cause a blistered dermatitis, in tropical South America. **Paederus fuscipes.** A species of western Asia which causes a blistered dermatitis if squashed. **Paederus sabaeus.** A beetle with blister-producing properties. [Gk *paideros* rouge.]

paediatric (pe·de·**at**·rik). Relating to the medical care and treatment of children, and in general to the study of children's diseases. [see foll.]

paediatrician (pe·de·at·**rish**'·un). One skilled in the treatment of diseases of childhood. [Gk *pais* child, *iatreia* treatment.]

paediatrics (pe·de·**at**·rix). The section of medical science that deals with the care and development of children, with the diseases that affect them, and with the treatment of such diseases. [see prec.]

paediatrist (pe·de·**at**·rist). Paediatrician.

paediatry (pe·de·**at**·re). Paediatrics.

paedication (pe·dik·**a**·shun). Paederasty. [Gk *pais* boy.]

paedicterus (pe·**dik**·ter·us). Icterus neonatorum. [Gk *pais* child, icterus.]

paedion (**pe**·de·on). 1. A child. 2. A fetus. [Gk *paidion* young child.]

paedodontia (pe·do·**don**·she·ah). Paedodontics.

paedodontics (pe·do·**don**·tix). The department of the science of dentistry that deals with the correction and abnormalities of the teeth of children. [Gk *pais* child, *odous* tooth.]

paedodontology (pe·do·don·**tol**'·o·je). Paedodontics.

paedogenesis (pe·do·**jen**·es·is). The reproduction of young by parents who are in the pre-adult or larval stage. [Gk *pais* child, *genesis* birth.]

paedology (pe·**dol**·o·je). The science which is concerned with the systematic study of child life and development. [Gk *pais* child, *logos* science.]

paedometer (pe·**dom**·et·er). A device used to measure the length of an infant. [Gk *pais* child, *metron* measure.]

paedometry (pe·**dom**·et·re). Measurement of the length of an infant by means of the paedometer.

paedomorphism (pe·do·**mor**·fizm). The retaining of infantile traits by an organism after reaching maturity. [Gk *pais* child, *morphe* form.]

paedonosology (pe·do·nos·**ol**'·o·je). Paediatrics. [Gk *pais* child, *nosos* disease, *logos* science.]

paedonosos, paedonosus (pe·do·**nos**·os, pe·do·**nos**·us). Any disease which occurs in childhood. [Gk *pais* child, *nosos* disease.]

paedontology (pe·don·**tol**·o·je). Paedodontics. [Gk *pais* child, *odous* tooth, *logos* science.]

paedopathy (pe·**dop**·ath·e). Paediatrics. [Gk *pais* child, *pathos* disease.]

paedophilia (pe·do·**fil**·e·ah). An exaggerated affection for children. **Paedophilia erotica.** A type of sexual perversion directed to children. [Gk *pais* child, *philein* to love.]

paedophobia (pe·do·**fo**·be·ah). Extreme fear aroused by the sight of infants or dolls. [Gk *pais* child, phobia.]

paedotrophy (pe·do·**tro**·fe). Application of the principles of hygiene in the management of children. [Gk *pais* child, *trophe* nourishment.]

Paessler, Heinrich (b. 1860). German physician.

Romberg–Paessler syndrome. Tachycardia, low blood pressure, shock, and abdominal distension, caused by dilation of the splanchnic blood vessels.

Pagano, Giacomo (fl. 1883). Palermo physiologist.

Pagano's reaction. A local reaction to tuberculin applied to the urinary meatus. This test is obsolete.

Page, Herbert William (b. 1845). London surgeon.

Page's disease. Railway spine. *See* SPINE.

Pagenstecher, Alexander (b. 1828). Wiesbaden ophthalmologist.

Pagenstecher's ointment. Unguentum hydrargyri oxidi flavi.

Pagenstecher's operation. 1. For ptosis: the passage of double-armed silk braided sutures subcutaneously from the free border of the eyelid to just above the eyebrow. They are left in for from 2 to 4 weeks, so forming fibrous bands connecting the lid to the occipitofrontalis muscle. 2. For cataract: extraction of the lens within its capsule by passing a special scoop behind the lens and lifting it out against counter-pressure on the cornea with a hook.

Pagenstecher's suture. For ptosis. *See* PAGENSTECHER'S OPERATION (above).

Paget, Sir James (b. 1814). London surgeon.

Paget's abscess. Residual abscess; one occurring near the site of an earlier abscess and due to pyrogenic organisms remaining from the latter.

Paget's cells. Cells with hyperchromatic nuclei and vacuolated cytoplasm found in Paget's disease of the nipple.

Paget's disease. 1. Osteitis deformans. 2. A pseudo-eczematous condition of the nipple and areola, sometimes spreading to the surrounding skin, due to intra-epithelial spread of carcinoma cells from the underlying breast ducts.

extramammary Paget's disease. A plaque resembling Paget's disease both clinically and histologically, but occurring in the axilla, on the penis or scrotum, vulva or perianal skin.

Paget's recurrent fibroid. A spindle-cell sarcoma of low malignancy found in the subcutaneous tissue of the abdominal wall or thighs, with a special tendency to recur after removal, but not to disseminate.

Paget's quiet necrosis. A condition in which a small portion of the articular surface of a bone separates as a sequestrum. The condition usually occurs in the lower end of the femur.

Paget's test. A solid tumour feels hardest in the centre, whereas a cystic tumour is least hard in the centre.

pagetoid (**paj**·et·oid). Like Paget's disease. [Sir James *Paget*, Gk *eidos* form.]

Pagniello, R. (fl. 1920). Italian physician.

Pagniello's point. A point painful to light pressure when a finger is drawn over the 9th left costal interspace in patients suffering from malaria.

pagoplexia (pa·go·**plex**·e·ah). Frostbite, or chilblains. [Gk *pagos* frost, *plege* stroke.]

pain (pane). 1. The distressing sensation excited by noxious stimuli of sufficient intensity acting on nerve-endings in the skin, viscera, muscles, bones, joints, etc. The pain sensation has different qualities according to the tissue affected and the producing agent. It is variously described as cutting, stabbing, burning, boring, throbbing, gripping, shooting, spasmodic. Pain arising in the skin may be excited by injury, inflammation, pressure, great heat or cold; in muscles by ischaemia; and in hollow organs by tension. It may be of central nervous origin or psychogenic. 2. Used in the plural, generally indicating the contractions of labour. **After pains.** Pains caused by uterine contraction in the puerperium, especially common in multiparae. **Bearing-down pains.** Contractions of the uterus accompanied by a desire to strain as at stool. **Boring pain.** The pain occurring deep in the tissues as if produced by a boring instrument. **Central pain.** Pain resulting from a lesion of centrally situated nervous tissues. **Excentric pain.** Pain due to irritation of posterior nerve roots, but felt in peripheral tissues. **Expulsive pains.** Bearing-down pains (see above). **False pains.** Pains similar to those of labour but less severe and always ineffective. **Fulgurant pain, Fulgurating pain.** Lightning pain (see below). **Functional pain.** Pain which occurs without any organic cause, and is due to a disorder of the mind. **Girdle pain.** Pain in girdle distribution, usually following the course of a thoracic spinal nerve and resulting from disease in the spinal cord or in the spinal canal or exit foramina. **Growing pains.** Vague pains in the legs of children, difficult to localize but usually referred to the muscles or tendons. At one time they were regarded as a definite sign of rheumatism; although doubt is now thrown upon this, the pains should be regarded with suspicion and other signs of rheumatism sought for. **Heterotopic pain.** Referred pain (see below). **Homotopic pain.** Pain felt at the point of injury. **Hunger pain.** Pain referred to the epigastrium, occurring some hours after a meal, and relieved by food. It is characteristic of a peptic ulcer. **Ideogenous pain.** Pain arising in the mind. **Intermenstrual pain.** Pain between the menses. **Jumping pain.** Sudden sharp pain in joint disease when the articular cartilage is destroyed. The pain is produced by muscle spasm. **Labour pains.** The contraction of the uterus in labour. **Lancinating pain.** A sharp, stabbing pain. **Lightning pain.** A pain of short duration like a flash of lightning, repeated after intervals of a few seconds and occurring in bouts which may last for days. It is most often felt in the legs but may occur in any part. It is characteristic of tabes dorsalis. **Middle pain.** Pain in the mid-cycle, usually occurring at the time of ovulation. **Niggling pains.** Irregular or ineffective bowel or uterine contractions. **Night pain.** Jumping pain (see above). **Parenchymatous pain.** Pain arising in the parenchyma of an organ. **Phantom-limb pain.** Pain which appears to be localized in a limb that has been amputated. **Postprandial pain.** Pain occurring immediately after a meal. **Psychogenic pain.** Functional pain (see above). **Referred pain.** A pain arising in a viscus and referred to an area of skin that is connected through its sensory nerves to the same segment of the nervous system as the afferent autonomic fibres from the viscus. Thus, pain arising in the gall bladder may be felt at the angle of the right scapula and at the right shoulder, and the pain of angina pectoris is felt over the sternum and radiates to the left shoulder and down the left arm or maybe to the epigastrium. **Root pain.** Pain in the area of supply of a spinal root, usually due to disease of, or pressure upon, the root concerned. **Shooting pain.** Lightning pain (see above). **Starting pain.** Muscular spasms, generally in the legs, occurring in the early stages of sleep. **Terebrant pain, Terebrating pain.** A boring pain. **Visceral pain.** Pain which is caused by a lesion or disturbance of function of a viscus. It may be felt in the viscus itself, as with intestinal colic or the pains of childbirth, and tends to be diffuse and difficult to localize. In hollow viscera the stimulus is the stretching of unstriped-muscle fibres. The pain may also be referred through autonomic fibres to an area of the surface that is innervated by somatic fibres from the same spinal segment. **Wandering pain.** A pain which wanders from site to site. [L *poena* penalty.]

See also: CHARCOT.

painful (**pane**·ful). 1. Causing pain. 2. Having the characteristics of pain.

painless (**pane**·les). Free from pain. [pain, AS *leas*.]

paint (pa·nt). In pharmacy, a liquid preparation for application to the skin or mucous membrane; such preparations usually contain substances with antiseptic, analgesic, astringent, or caustic properties and are often coloured. [OFr. *peindre.*]

See also: CASTELLANI, MANDL.

pair production (pare pro·**duk**·shun). The phenomenon of the production of positive and negative electrons in pairs by the interaction of high energy photons with matter; in the process the photon disappears, and an electron pair is produced. The process commences at 1.2 MeV and increases in importance at higher energies. [L *par* equal, *producere* to lead forth.]

Pajot, Charles (b. 1816). Paris obstetrician.

Pajot's hook. A decapitating hook.

Pajot's manoeuvre, or method. Tangential pressure exerted on obstetric forceps to give a resultant force in the direction of the birth canal. The left hand usually pulls the handles downwards and the right hand pulls them upwards and outwards. The procedure was first suggested by Saxtorph.

Pal, Jacob (b. 1863). Vienna physician.

Pal's crisis. A tabetic ocular crisis, consisting of a stabbing pain in the eye, lacrimation, and photophobia.

Pal's modification of Weigert's myelin-sheath stain, Weigert-Pal method. After fixation in formalin, followed by mordanting in a mixture of potassium dichromate and chrome alum, sections are stained in Weigert's haematoxylin, blued with lithium carbonate, and differentiated with potassium permanganate followed by oxalic acid. Myelin sheaths are stained blue-black against a clear background.

palaeo- (pal·e·o). A prefix most commonly used in relation to parts of particular structures in the central nervous system, denoting that the part in question is older in an evolutionary sense than the rest of the structure under consideration. Since the evolutionary history of structures in the central nervous system is usually uncertain, at least in detail, the term lacks precision and is sometimes used differently by different authors. [Gk *palaios* old.]

palaeocerebellar (pal·e·o·ser·e·**bel**′·ar). Belonging to the palaeocerebellum.

palaeocerebellum (pal·e·o·ser·e·**bel**′·um). Those parts of the cerebellum which are older in an evolutionary sense. It may be applied to that part of the cerebellum which receives direct vestibular connections, i.e. the nodule, flocculus and lingula, or, more usually, to the anterior and posterior lobes as a whole, but excluding the middle lobe (the neocerebellum). [Gk *palaios* old, cerebellum.]

palaeocinetic (pal·e·o·sin·**et**′·ik). Palaeokinetic.

palaeocortex (pal·e·o·**kor**′·tex). Those parts of the cortex of the cerebral hemisphere which are thought to be oldest in an evolutionary sense. The term may be applied to the cortex of the hippocampal formation and the pyriform lobe (uncus), but is more usually limited to the latter. [Gk *palaios* old, cortex.]

palaeo-encephalon (pal·e·o·en·**kef**′·al·on). Those parts of the whole brain that are phylogenetically older than the rest; this excludes the cerebral cortex. [Gk *palaios* old, encephalon.]

palaeogenesis (pal·e·o·**jen**·e·sis). Palingenesis, 1st def. [Gk *palaios* old, *genesis* origin.]

palaeokinetic (pal·e·o·kin·**et**′·ik). A term applied, in mammals, to the extrapyramidal nervous pathways which are concerned with postural and associated automatic movement. These pathways are the representatives of the more primitive ones found in submammals. [Gk *palaios* old, *kinetikos* of motion.]

palaeontology (pal·e·on·**tol**′·o·je). The study of the now extinct forms of organized life in past geological periods, demonstrable in fossilized remains. [Gk *palaios* old, *logos* science.]

palaeopallium (pal·e·o·**pal**′·e·um). Palaeocortex. [Gk *palaios* old, pallium.]

palaeopathology (pal·e·o·path·**ol**′·o·je). The science of the diseases occurring in ancient times, as revealed by the study of fossilized remains, bones, mummies. [Gk *palaios* old, pathology.]

palaeophrenia (pal·e·o·**fre**′·ne·ah). 1. Primitive thought. 2. (Secondarily to 1.) Schizophrenia, which is thought to be accompanied by a return to primitive modes of thought. [Gk *palaios* old, *phren* mind.]

palaeopsychology (pal·e·o·si·**kol**′·o·je). The investigation of primitive modes of thought. [Gk *palaios* old, psychology.]

palaeosensation (pal·e·o·sen·**sa**′·shun). Primordial sensation of acute pain and definite alterations in temperature, as distinct from later sensations, e.g. the epicritic sensations. [Gk *palaios* old, sensation.]

palaeostriatal (pal·e·o·stri·**a**′·tal). Belonging to the palaeostriatum.

palaeostriatum (pal·e·o·stri·**a**′·tum). That part of the corpus striatum which is thought to be oldest in an evolutionary sense, i.e. the globus pallidus. [Gk *palaios* old, corpus striatum.]

palaeothalamus (pal·e·o·**thal**′·am·us). A term of doubtful validity which has been applied to the anterior thalamic nuclei and to the intralaminar and midline nuclei of the thalamus. It implies that these parts of the thalamus are older in an evolutionary sense than others. [Gk *palaios* old, thalamus.]

palatal (**pal**·at·al). Belonging to the palate or to the palatine bone.

palate [palatum (NA)] (**pal**·at). The roof of the mouth, consisting of an anterior part, the hard palate, supported by the palatine processes of the maxilla and the palatine bone, and a mobile posterior part, the soft palate, projecting into the pharynx. **Artificial palate.** A plate inserted into the mouth to cover the gap of a cleft palate. **Bony palate [palatum osseum (NA)].** Hard palate (see below). **Cleft palate.** A congenital fissure in the midline of the hard palate. **Falling palate.** An elongated uvula. **Gothic palate.** A high arched palate. **Hard palate [palatum durum].** The anterior part of the roof of the mouth, made up by the palatine processes of the maxillae and the horizontal plates of the palatine bone. **Premaxillary palate, Primary palate, Primitive palate.** The early partition between nasal cavities and mouth, formed from the frontonasal process. It represents the premaxillary element of the palate. **Secondary palate.** The definitive palate of mammals, which includes large contributions from the maxillary arches of the embryo, in addition to the early contribution from the frontonasal process. **Soft palate [palatum molle velum palatinum (NA)].** The fold from the posterior border of the hard palate (see above) extending into the pharynx. [L *palatum.*]

palatic (pal·**at**·ik). Palatal.

palatiform (pal·**at**·e·form). Like a palate. [palate, form.]

palatine (**pal**·at·ine). Belonging or relating to the palate.

palatine arteries. The arteries that supply the palate. **Palatine artery, ascending [arteria palatina ascendens (NA)].** A branch of the facial artery lying on the superior constrictor muscle of the pharynx; it is the principal artery to the soft palate. **Palatine artery, descending [arteria palatina descendens (NA)].** The branch of the maxillary artery which descends in the greater palatine canal and there gives off the lesser palatine arteries and is then continued as the greater palatine artery. **Palatine artery, greater [arteria palatina major (NA)].** *See* MAXILLARY ARTERY. **Palatine arteries, lesser [arteriae palatinae minores (NA)].** *See* MAXILLARY ARTERY.

palatine bone [os palatinum (NA)]. A bone situated between the maxilla and the pterygoid plate and forming a large part of the palate and side wall of the nose.

palatine nerves. **Greater palatine nerve [nervus palatinus major (NA)].** A nerve to the hard palate from the sphenopalatine ganglion. **Nasal branches of the greater palatine nerve [rami nasales posteriores inferiores (laterales) (NA)].** Branches to the side wall of the posterior part of the nose. **Lesser palatine nerves [nervi palatini minores (NA)].** Branches from the sphenopalatine ganglion to the soft palate and nasopharynx.

palatine veins. Veins which follow the greater or lesser palatine arteries from the palate to the pterygoid plexus. **External palatine vein [vena palatina externa (NA)].** One of the veins draining the tonsil into the anterior or common facial vein.

palatitis (pal·at·**i**·tis). Inflammation of the palate. [palate, Gk *-itis* inflammation.]

palatoglossal (pal·at·o·**glos**′·al). Belonging or relating to the palate and the tongue. [palate, Gk *glossa* tongue.]

palatoglossus (**pal**·at·o·**glos**′·us). The palatoglossus muscle. [see prec.]

palatoglossus muscle [musculus palatoglossus (NA)]. A small muscle extending from the soft palate to the tongue in the palatoglossal arch (anterior pillar of the fauces). It elevates the back of the tongue, and approximates the palatoglossal arch to the midline.

palatognathous (pal·at·og·nath·us). Having a cleft palate. [palate, Gk *gnathos* jaw.]

palatognathus (pal·at·og·nath·us). Cleft palate. *See* PALATE. [see prec.]

palatograph (**pal**·at·o·graf). Palatomyograph.

palatography (pal·at·og·raf·e). The process of recording by means of the palatomyograph the palatal movements while the subject is speaking. [palate, Gk *graphein* to record.]

palatolabial (**pal**·at·o·**la**′·be·al). Belonging to the palate and the lips. [palate, L *labium* lip.]

palatomaxillary (**pal**·at·o·max·**il**′·ar·e). Belonging to the palate and the maxilla.

palatomyograph (**pal**·at·o·**mi**′·o·graf). A myograph with which the movements of the palate while the subject is speaking can be recorded.

palatonasal (**pal**·at·o·**na**′·zal). Relating to the palate and the nose. [palate, L *nasus* nose.]

palatopagus parasiticus (pal·at·**op**·a·gus par·ah·**sit**·ik·us). A condition in which a teratoma, or remnants of a parasitic twin fetus, is attached to the hard palate. [palate, Gk *pagos* that which is fixed, parasite.]

palatopharyngeal (**pal**·at·o·far·**in**′·je·al). Belonging to the palate and the pharynx.

palatopharyngeus (**pal**·at·o·far·**in**′·je·us). The palatopharyngeus muscle.

palatopharyngeus muscle [musculus palatopharyngeus (NA)]. A muscle arising from the back of the hard palate and the soft palate and running in the palatopharyngeal fold (posterior pillar of the fauces) to the posterior border of the thyroid cartilage and wall of the pharynx. It is an elevator of the pharynx.

palatoplasty (**pal**·at·o·plas·te). Plastic surgery of the palate. [palate, Gk *plassein* to mould.]

palatoplegia (**pal**·at·o·**ple**′·je·ah). Paralysis affecting the soft palate. [palate, Gk *plege* stroke.]

palatopterygoid (**pal**·at·o·**ter**′·ig·oid). Pertaining to the palate and the pterygoid process of the sphenoid bone.

palatorrhaphy (pal·at·**or**·af·e). Suture of a cleft palate. [palate, Gk *rhaphe* suture.]

palatosalpingeus (**pal**·at·o·sal·**pin**′·je·us). The tensor palati muscle. [palate, Gk *salpigx* trumpet.]

palatoschisis (pal·at·**os**·kis·is). Cleft palate. [palate, Gk *schisis* a cleaving.]

palato-uvularis (**pal**·at·o·ew·vew·**la**′·ris). The musculus uvulae. [palate, uvula.]

palatum (pal·a·tum). The palate. **Palatum fissum.** Cleft palate. *See* PALATE. **Palatum mobile.** The soft palate. *See* PALATE. **Palatum ogivale.** An unusually pointed palate. **Palatum pendulum.** The soft palate. *See* PALATE. [L.]

Palfyn, Jean (b. 1650). Paris and Ghent anatomist and surgeon.
Palfyn's sinus. A space, which is not generally recognized, within the crista galli, said to communicate with frontal and ethmoidal air sinuses.

palicinesia, palicinesis (**pal**·e·sin·**e**′·ze·ah, **pal**·e·sin·**e**′·sis). Palikinesia.

paligraphia (**pal**·e·graf·ia). A phenomenon whereby an aphasic patient continues to write a word or phrase which he has already written.

palikinesia, palikinesis (**pal**·e·kin·**e**′·ze·ah, **pal**·e·kin·**e**′·sis). A pathological condition in which involuntary movements are repeated constantly. [Gk *palin* again, *kinesis* movement.]

palilalia (pal·e·**la**·le·ah). A symptom whereby the patient repeats the last word or two of a verbal statement, the words tailing off in a diminuendo fashion, and with increasing rapidity. **Aphonic palilalia.** Silent articulatory movements of the lips at the end of a word or phrase that has just been uttered. [Gk *palin* again, *lalein* to babble.]

palinal (**pal**·in·al). Pertaining to a motion backwards; moving backwards. [Gk *palin* backwards.]

palindromia (pal·in·**dro**·me·ah). The recrudescence of a disease or a relapse. [Gk, a running back.]

palindromic (pal·in·**dro**·mik). Recurring or relapsing. [see prec.]

palingenesis (pal·in·**jen**·es·is). 1. The hereditary transmission, in man and in animals, through successive generations, of a tendency to develop certain characteristics which have not been apparent in intermediate generations; this may explain certain abnormalities occurring in man. 2. Renewal or restoration of a lost part. 3. In entomology, metamorphosis. [Gk *palin* again, *genesis* origin.]

palingraphia (pal·in·**graf**·e·ah). Involuntary repetition of letters, whole words, or parts of words, in writing. [Gk *palin* again, *graphein* to write.]

palinmnesis (pal·in·**ne**·sis). Recollection of earlier experiences and events. [Gk *palin* backwards, *mnesis* memory.]

palinodia (pal·in·**o**·de·ah). A recrudescence of a disease; a relapse. [Gk *palin* again, *odos* approach.]

palinphrasia (pal·in·**fra**·ze·ah). Paliphrasia.

paliphrasia (pal·e·**fra**·ze·ah). Involuntary and needless repetition of words or phrases. [Gk *palin* again, *phrasein* to utter.]

palirrhoea (pal·e·**re**·ah). 1. Regurgitation. 2. Recrudescence of a discharge of mucoid character. [Gk *palirroia* reflux of water.]

palite (**pal**·ite). Chloromethylchloroformate, $CH_2ClCOOCl$. A lacrimatory liquid, the vapour of which is used in chemical warfare as a choking gas.

palladium (pal·**a**·de·um). An element of atomic weight 106.4, atomic number 46, and chemical symbol Pd. It is a white metal, found in native crude platinum and osmiridium: employed pure or alloyed with gold for dental work, and generally as a substitute for platinum. **Palladium black.** A catalyst in hydrogenation processes, consisting of finely divided metallic palladium. **Palladium chloride.** $PdCl_2$, a soluble crystalline substance of value as a reagent in analysis, and as an antiseptic. **Palladium sponge.** A spongy form of palladium that has the ability to absorb large volumes of hydrogen gas; it is also used as a catalyst. [*Pallus*, goddess in Gk mythology.]

pallaesthesia (pal·es·**the**·ze·ah). Appreciation of vibrations; that sensation noticed when the handle of a vibrating tuning-fork is placed over bony surfaces lying beneath the skin. [Gk *pallein* to quiver, aesthesis.]

pallaesthetic (pal·es·**thet**·ik). Characterized by pallaesthesia.

pallamine (**pal**·am·een). A colloidal form of palladium.

pallanaesthesia (**pal**·an·es·**the**′·ze·ah). A condition in which the power to receive vibrations is lacking or has been lost, or in which the vibrations of a tuning-fork cannot be appreciated. [Gk *pallein* to quiver, anaesthesia.]

pallescence (pal·**es**·ens). Pallor; a pallid appearance. [L *palescere* to lose colour.]

pallhypaesthesia (**pal**·hi·pes·**the**′·ze·ah). Hypopallaesthesia.

pallial (**pal**·e·al). Belonging to the pallium.

palliate (**pal**·e·ate). To alleviate; to mitigate the severity of a disease. [see foll.]

palliation (pal·e·a·shun). Alleviation of suffering or symptoms. [L *palliare* to cloak.]

palliative (**pal**·e·at·iv). 1. Serving to mitigate pain or the severity of a disease. 2. A medicine which alleviates but does not cure. [see prec.]

pallidectomy (pal·id·**ek**·to·me). Surgical destruction of part of the thalamus in the treatment of Parkinson's disease by chemical means (*chemopallidectomy*) or freezing (*cryopallidectomy*). [L *pallidus* pale, Gk *ektome* a cutting out.]

pallidum (**pal**·id·um). The globus pallidus of the lentiform nucleus. [L *pallidus* pale.]

pallium [NA] (**pal**·e·um). Literally a mantle; applied to that part of the wall of the embryonic hemisphere vesicle in which the cerebral cortex is developed. It is sometimes used as a synonym for the cerebral cortex. [L.]

pallor (pal·or). Paleness. **Pallor chloroticus.** The pallor peculiar to individuals suffering from chlorosis. **Pallor eximus.** Abnormal pallor, as a rule caused by a condition of anaemia. **Pallor luteus.** Chlorosis. **Pallor pathematicus.** That caused by experiencing fright or terror. **Pallor virginum.** Chlorosis. [L.]

pallypaesthesia (pal·ip·es·**the**′·ze·ah). Hypopallaesthesia.

palm [palma manus (NA)] (pahm). The palmar surface of the hand. **Handball palm.** Contusion and swelling of the palm in handball players. **Liver palm.** The intense bluish-red, or liver-coloured appearance of the hands in pink disease. [L *palma*.]

palm (pahm). A tree of the family Palmae, including the date and coconut. **Coconut palm.** The tree *Cocos nucifera* yielding the fruit known as the *coconut*, a valuable food and the source of the vegetable oil used in soap and margarine manufacture. The dried, white, fleshy endosperm is *copra*. **Date palm.** The tree *Phoenix dactylifera;* its fruit, the date, is a valuable food containing a high percentage of sugar. [L *palma*.]

palma (**pal**·mah). 1. The palm of the hand [palma manus.] 2. The palm tree. [L.]

palmae plicatae (**pal**·me pli·**ka**·te). Rugae of the vagina. [L, palm branches folded together.]

palmaesthesia (pal·mes·**the**·ze·ah). Pallaesthesia. [Gk *palmos* a quivering, aesthesia.]

palmaesthetic (pal·mes·**thet**·ik). Belonging to the sense of vibration. [see prec.]

palmanaesthesia (pal·man·es·**the**′·ze·ah). Pallanaesthesia. [Gk *palmos* a quivering, anaesthesia.]

palmar [palmaris (NA)] (**pah**·mar, **pal**·mar). Belonging to the palm of the hand. **Palmar arch.** *See* ARCH. [L *palma* palm.]

palmaris brevis muscle [musculus palmaris brevis (NA)] (pal·**ma**·ris **brev**·is musl). A small muscle on the medial side of the hand arising from the flexor retinaculum and inserted into the skin over the hypothenar eminence, which it wrinkles when the palm is cupped.

palmaris longus muscle [musculus palmaris longus (NA)] (pal·**ma**·ris **long**·gus musl). A slender flexor muscle extending approximately along the midline of the forearm from the medial epicondyle to the palmar aponeurosis. It is frequently absent.

palmatine (**pal**·mat·een). $C_{21}H_{23}O_5N$, an alkaloid found in calumba root *Jateorrhiza palmata,* and a strong respiratory depressant.

palmature (**pal**·mat·ewr). An abnormal condition of the hand in which there is union or webbing of the fingers. [L *palma* palm.]

palmic (**pal**·mik). 1. Belonging to or characterized by saltatory spasm (palmus). 2. Belonging to the pulse. [Gk *palmos* a quivering.]

palmin (**pal**·min). Palmitin.

palmiped (**pal**·mip·ed). Web footed. [L *palma* palm, *pes* foot.]

palmital (**pal**·mit·al). Palmitic aldehyde. *See* ALDEHYDE.

palmitate (**pal**·mit·ate). Any salt or ester of palmitic acid.

palmitin (**pal**·mit·in). 1. Tripalmitin, glycerol tripalmitate, $(C_{15}H_{31}COO)_3C_3H_5$, a solid ester, one of the principal constituents of palm oil, mutton suet, and other animal and vegetable fats and oils. 2. Any of the glycerol esters of palmitic acid which occur in natural fats and oils.

palmitone (**pal**·mit·one). $C_{15}H_{31}COC_{15}H_{31}$, a ketone derived from palmitic acid.

palmityl (**pal**·mit·il). The acyl group, $C_{15}H_{31}CO$-, which occurs in compounds formed by palmitic acid.

palmodic (pal·**mod**·ik). Belonging to or suffering from saltatory spasm (palmus). [Gk *palmodes* quivering.]

palmoplantar (pahm·o·**plan**·tar). Pertaining to the palmar surface of the hand and the plantar aspect of the foot. [palm, L *planta* the sole of the foot.]

palmoscopy (pal·**mos**·ko·pe). Observation of the beat of the heart or pulse. [Gk *palmos* a quivering, *skopein* to watch.]

palmprints (**pahm**·printz). Prints similar to fingerprints giving detail sufficient to establish identity, used in crime investigation. [L *palma* palm, ME *prent*.]

palmus (**pal**·mus). 1. Saltatory spasm. 2. A throbbing or leaping movement. 3. The heart beat. [Gk *palmos* a quivering.]

palograph (**pal**·o·graf). An instrument for recording pulse tracings, in which the impulses are transmitted to a column of fluid in a U-shaped tube, the movements of the surface of the fluid in the open limb of the tube being traced on moving smoked paper. [Gk *pallesthein* to vibrate, *graphein* to record.]

palography (pal·**og**·raf·e). Sphygmography by means of the palograph.

palp (palp). A chemoreceptory appendage in the region of the mouth in many animals, especially molluscs and arthropods. **Labial palp.** That of the third pair of mouth parts of insects. **Maxillary palp.** That of the second pair of mouth parts of insects. [L *palpare* to touch gently.]

palpable (**pal**·pah·bl). That can be appreciated by the sense of touch; capable of being palpated. [see prec.]

palpate (**pal**·pate). To examine or explore by feeling or pressing with the palms and fingers. [see foll.]

palpation (pal·**pa**·shun). The method of physical examination in which the hands are applied to the surface of the body, so that by the sense of touch information is obtained about the condition of the skin, the underlying tissues, and organs. In the examination of the skin, its texture, temperature, thickness, disturbances of sensation, localized or general swellings, etc., are noted. Palpation of the chest determines the range and any irregularity of expansion on respiration, also the sites of pulsations, thrills, friction, and vocal fremitus. Examination of the abdomen reveals any areas of tenderness or rigidity, enlargement or undue mobility of such organs as the liver, spleen, or kidneys, and the presence of abnormal swellings or free fluid. Palpation of the neck, axillae, and groins may reveal enlarged lymphatic glands, and palpation of the limbs is used to determine the tone of muscles, the mobility of joints, the presence of joint crepitus, and the presence of tenderness in muscles, nerves, or joints. **Bimanual palpation.** Palpation in which one hand is placed posteriorly in the loin and is pushed forwards towards the other hand placed on the front of the abdomen; deep-seated organs such as the kidneys and liver may be more easily felt. Bimanual palpation of pelvic organs is practised by inserting one finger in the vagina or rectum and the opposite hand on the abdominal wall. **Fingertip palpation.** The method in which only the tips of the fingers are used to appreciate the sense of resistance, which varies according to the nature of the underlying tissues, whether air-containing, solid, or fluid. [L *palpare* to touch gently.]

palpatometer (pal·pat·**om**·et·er). An instrument for determining the degree of arterial pressure. [palpation, Gk *metron* measure.]

palpatometry (pal·pat·**om**·et·re). The determination of the degree of pressure which can be exerted without producing pain. [see prec.]

palpatopercussion (**pal**·pat·o·per·**kush**′·un). Physical examination in which combined palpation and percussion are used.

palpatorium (pal·pa·**tor**·e·um). An instrument used in abdominal palpation for the purpose of detecting tender areas during examination with a fluoroscope.

palpebral (**pal**·peb·ral). Of or belonging to an eyelid or the eyelids. **Palpebral fissure.** *See* FISSURE. [L *palpebra* eyelid.]

palpebral arteries. **Lateral palpebral arteries [arteriae palpebrales laterales].** *See* OPHTHALMIC ARTERY. **Medial palpebral arteries [arteriae palpebrales mediales].** *See* OPHTHALMIC ARTERY.

palpebral veins. Veins of the eyelids; the upper [vena palpebralis superioris (NA)] is a tributary of the supraorbital vein, and the lower [vena palpebralis inferioris (NA)] is a tributary of the anterior facial vein.

palpebralis (pal·peb·**ra**·lis). The levator palpebrae superioris muscle of the orbit. [L *palpebra* eyelid.]

palpebrate (**pal**·peb·rate). 1. To wink. 2. In zoology, having eyelids. [L *palpebra* eyelid.]

palpebration (pal·peb·**ra**·shun). 1. The act of winking. 2. Excessive frequency of winking. [see prec.]

palpebritis (pal·peb·ri·tis). Blepharitis. [L *palpebra* eyelid, Gk *-itis* inflammation.]

palpebrofrontal (pal·peb·ro·frun′·tal). Belonging to the eyelid and the brow. [L *palpebra* eyelid, *frons* forehead.]

palpitate (pal·pit·ate). To beat rapidly; to throb or flutter. A term generally used with reference to the abnormally fast rate of the heart. [see foll.]

palpitation (pal·pit·a·shun). Undue awareness of the heart beat, occasioned by anxiety, rapid heart action, premature contractions, or paroxysms of abnormal rhythm. [L *palpitare* to flutter.]

palpus (pal·pus). Palp.

palsy (pawl·ze). Loss of function, motor or sensory, in some part of the body; a term applied, by convention, to certain forms of paralysis. In many instances the words *paralysis* and *palsy* are used alternatively. **Birth palsy.** Palsy which is the result of injury to the brain during the birth (hemiplegia or diplegia) or to the brachial plexus. **Brachial birth palsy.** Birth palsy (see prec.). **Bulbar palsy.** Palsy due to degeneration of the nuclear cells of the lower cranial nerves; it is associated with progressive muscular atrophy. **Congenital cerebral palsy.** Congenital spastic paraplegia. **Craft palsy.** Occupational palsy (see below). **Creeping palsy.** A vague term applied to several forms of paralysis, especially tabes dorsalis and paralysis agitans. **Crossed-leg palsy.** Paralysis caused by sitting with one leg crossed over the other; this causes pressure on the peroneal nerve. **Crutch palsy.** Palsy due to pressure by a crutch on nerves in the axilla. **Divers' palsy.** Caisson disease. *See* DISEASE. **Drummers' palsy.** Palsy of the ungual phalanx of the thumb by rupture of the tendon of the extensor pollicis longus muscle. **Epidemic infantile palsy.** Acute anterior poliomyelitis. *See* POLIOMYELITIS. **Gaze palsy.** A supranuclear ophthalmoplegia resulting in a defect of conjugate eye movements. **Hammer palsy.** Spasmodic affection of the muscles of the upper limb due to over-use. **Hod-carriers' palsy.** Paralysis due to pressure on the long or posterior thoracic nerve causing paralysis of the serratus magnus muscle and unilateral winged scapula. **Infantile palsy.** Acute anterior poliomyelitis. *See* POLIOMYELITIS. **Infantile cerebral palsy.** Spastic or athetotic paralysis of cerebral origin occurring in infancy, including diplegia and hemiplegia. It is usually due to a birth injury. **Ischaemic palsy.** Paralysis due to interference with the blood supply from any cause, e.g. Volkmann's ischaemic paralysis. **Lead palsy.** A paralysis due to lead poisoning, of which wrist drop is a common example. **Night palsy.** A condition which is not a true palsy. **Occupational palsy.** Palsy associated with a specific occupation. **Painters' palsy.** Lead palsy (see above). **Pressure palsy.** That due to pressure on nerves by various causes, e.g. crutch palsy (see above). **Printers' palsy.** Nervous effects on groups of muscles in constant employment, analogous to writers' cramp. **Progressive bulbar palsy.** Progressive bulbar paralysis. *See* PARALYSIS. **Progressive supranuclear palsy.** A chronic progressive degenerative disease of the central nervous system beginning in middle age and characterized by conjugate ocular palsies, dystonia of the neck, and eventually widespread rigidity. The cause is unknown. **Pseudobulbar palsy.** Bulbar symptoms due to supranuclear lesions. **Saturday-night palsy.** Radial nerve palsy caused by pressure from the hard arm of a chair during a drunken sleep. **Scriveners' palsy.** Writers' cramp. **Shaking palsy.** Paralysis agitans; parkinsonism. **Wasting palsy.** Progressive muscular atrophy. *See* ATROPHY. [Corruption of Gk *paralysis.*]

See also: BELL (C.), DUCHENNE, ERB, FÉRÉOL, LANDRY.

Paltauf, Arnold (b. 1860). Prague physician.

Paltauf's dwarf. Pituitary dwarf. *See* DWARF.

Paltauf's dwarfism, Paltauf's nanism. A type of dwarfism in which sexual retardation and short stature are associated with status lymphaticus. The last is probably an erroneous observation, the condition being identical with pituitary infantilism.

Paltauf-Sternberg disease. Lymphadenoma.

paludal (pal·ew·dal). 1. Malarial. 2. Marshy. [see foll.]

paludide (pal·ew·dide). A skin eruption believed to be malarial in origin. [L *palus* stagnant water.]

paludism (pal·ew·dizm). Malaria. [see prec.]

palustral (pal·us·tral). 1. Marshy. 2. Malarial. [L *paluster* marshy.]

palustrine (pal·us·treen). $C_{12}H_{24}O_2N_2$, a poisonous alkaloid found in *Equisetum palustre.*

Pamaquin BP 1953 (pam·ah·kwin). The 8-(4-diethylamino-1-methylbutylamino)-6-methoxyquinoline salt of 2,2′-dihydroxy-1,1′-dinaphthylmethane-3,3′-dicarboxylic acid, $C_{42}H_{45}O_7N_3$. It is a relatively toxic drug and, although it has some action on all the blood forms of the malaria parasites, it is too dangerous for general use in the treatment of malaria. It acts, however, on the gametocytes, especially those of *Plasmodium falciparum,* in small and non-toxic doses, and in slightly larger doses (15 mg t.d.s.) it eradicates the exo-erythrocytic stages of *P. vivax, P. malariae* and *P. ovale* from the liver, thus preventing late relapses. The patient should be under strict medical observation while taking pamaquin. The first sign of toxicity is cyanosis due to methaemoglobinaemia, but a more important adverse effect is the precipitation of acute haemolysis in patients whose erythrocytes are deficient in the enzyme glucose-6-phosphate dehydrogenase.

pamaquine (pam·ah·kween). Pamaquin.

pambotano (pam·bo·tah·no). The root bark of *Calliandra houstoni* (family Leguminosae), a tree of Mexico. The only active constituent is a saponin which is a cardiac depressant. The root has been used as a vermifuge and antiperiodic. [Sp.]

pampiniform (pam·pin·e·form). Tendril-shaped, e.g. a plexus of veins. **Pampiniform plexus.** *See* PLEXUS. [L *pampinus* vine tendril, form.]

pampinocele (pam·pin·o·seel). Varicocele. [L *pampinus* vine tendril, Gk *kele* hernia.]

pan (pahn). Betel.

panacea (pan·ah·se·ah). A universal remedy; a cure-all. [Gk *panakeia.*]

panaesthesia (pan·es·the·ze·ah). The normal undifferentiated conscious state of awareness of being alive and of general organic sensation; vital sense. The state comprises the ordinary rise and fall of spirits, including normal mental function, within physiological limits. [Gk *pan* all, aesthesia.]

panaesthetic (pan·es·thet·ik). Referring or belonging to panaesthesia.

panagglutinable (pan·ag·loo·tin·abl). Describing red blood cells which are agglutinable by every group of blood serum of the same species. [see foll.]

panagglutination (pan·ag·loo·tin·a′·shun). The agglutination of red blood cells by sera of all blood groups of the same species. [Gk *pan* all, agglutination.]

panagglutinin (pan·ag·loo·tin·in). An agglutinin in blood serum which agglutinates the red blood cells belonging to all blood groups in the same species. [see prec.]

panaris, panaritium (pan·ar·is, pan·ar·ish·e·um). Inflammation in the finger pulp or nail fold. **Analgesic panaris, Panaris analgicum.** Painless ulceration of the fingers in syringomyelia; also called *Morvan's disease.* [L.]

panarteritis (pan·ar·ter·i′·tis). An inflammatory condition in which all the coats of an artery are affected simultaneously. [Gk *pan* all, artery, Gk *-itis* inflammation.]

panarthritis (pan·ar·thri·tis). Inflammation in which all the joints of the body or all the tissues of any particular joint are involved. [Gk *pan* all, arthritis.]

Panas, Photinos (b. 1832). Greek ophthalmologist in Paris.

Panas' operation. 1. For ptosis: a tongue of skin and orbicularis fibres is fashioned from the upper eyelid and passed subcutaneously to be sutured to the occipitofrontalis muscle in the centre of the eyebrow. Now modified by Hunt, Tansley, and Machek. 2. For trichiasis and entropion: a horizontal incision is made in the skin of the upper eyelid 4 mm above the lid margin right through all the structures, including the conjunctiva. The skin and orbicularis are dissected up and down and the lash margin sutured to the upper border of the tarsus, so turning the lower flap outward. 3. Linear proctotomy. *See* PROCTOTOMY.

panatrophy (pan·at·ro·fe). 1. Atrophy affecting all the tissues or parts of an organ or body structure. 2. Atrophy affecting all the structures of the body. [Gk *pan* all, atrophy.]

Panax (pa·nax). A genus of araliaceous plants. **Panax quinquefolium.** Chinese ginseng; a species to the root of which the Chinese have attributed magic healing properties. It contains a glucosidal principle, together with a saponin and a bitter principle. [Gk *pan* all, *akos* cure.]

pancarditis (pan·kar·di·tis). Inflammation affecting the heart in all its tissues. [Gk *pan* all, *kardia* heart, *-itis* inflammation.]

panchontee (pan·shon·te). A gum from the Indian tree, *Bassia elliptica* (family Sapotaceae); it resembles gutta percha. [Tamil name.]

Pancoast, Henry Khunrath (b. 1875). Philadelphia radiologist.

Pancoast's syndrome. Horner's syndrome due to involvement of the cervical sympathetic, and brachial neuralgia due to involvement of the brachial plexus by a peripherally situated bronchogenic carcinoma in the lung apex (superior pulmonary sulcus tumour).

Pancoast's tumour. Superior sulcus tumour; a tumour at the apex of the lung which involves the brachial plexus and cervical sympathetic chain and so produces a characteristic syndrome comprising ptosis, enophthalmia, meiosis, with motor and sensory changes in the arm of the same side. The growth may also destroy the neighbouring bony structures.

Pancoast, Joseph (b. 1805). New Jersey surgeon.

Pancoast's operation. For trigeminal neuralgia: section of the trigeminal nerve at the foramen ovale.

pancolectomy (pan·kol·ek·to·me). Removal of the whole colon. Often necessary in the treatment of ulcerative colitis. [Gk *pan* all, colon, Gk *ektome* a cutting out.]

pancolpohysterectomy (pan·kol·po·his·ter·ek'·to·me). The complete surgical removal of the uterus and vagina. [Gk *pan* all, *kolpos* vagina, *hystera* uterus, *ektome* excision.]

pancrealgia (pan·kre·al·je·ah). Pancreatalgia.

pancreas [NA] (pan·kre·as). A large compound racemose gland lying transversely on the posterior abdominal wall in the epigastric and left hypochondriac regions of the abdomen. It consists of a head [caput pancreatis (NA)], lying in the loop of the duodenum, and a body [corpus pancreatis (NA)], both retroperitoneal, and a tail [cauda pancreatis (NA)], which turns forward in the lienorenal ligament to reach the hilum of the spleen. Its external secretion, containing proteolytic, lipolytic, and other enzymes, is discharged by main and accessory ducts into the second part of the duodenum. It contains also the pancreatic islets (of Langerhans) which produce both insulin and glucagon, secreting these substances directly into the blood stream. The neck of the pancreas is the part between the head and the body, corresponding to a groove on the posterior surface of the pancreas, lodging in the end of the superior mesenteric vein and the beginning of the portal vein. There are three surfaces of the body of the pancreas. The anterior surface [facies anterior (NA)] is the surface between the superior [margo superior (NA)] and anterior [margo anterior (NA)] borders. It lies behind the lesser sac of the peritoneum, which intervenes between it and the posterior surface of the stomach. The posterior surface [facies posterior (NA)] is the non-peritoneal surface in contact with the aorta, left renal vessels, left crus of the diaphragm, and the anterior surface of the left suprarenal gland and the upper pole of the left kidney. The splenic vein runs between the surface of these structures. The inferior surface [facies inferior (NA)] is the peritoneal-covered surface, narrow on the right, broadening towards the left, which lies between the anterior [margo anterior (NA)] and inferior [margo inferior (NA)] borders. It is in contact with the duodenojejunal flexure, the coils of the small intestine, and the splenic flexure. **Accessory pancreas [pancreas accessorium (NA)].** Small collections of pancreatic tissue sometimes found in the wall of the stomach, duodenum, or jejunum. **Annular pancreas.** A congenital abnormality in which a ring of pancreatic tissue partly, or completely, surrounds the second part of the duodenum. It may cause vomiting in the newborn. **Dorsal pancreas.** The pancreatic rudiment which grows from the dorsal border of the duodenum in the embryo, and from which part of the head and the body and tail of the pancreas are formed. **Lesser pancreas.** A term applied to the uncinate process of the head of the pancreas when it is separate from the rest of the organ. **Ventral pancreas.** The pancreatic rudiment which grows from the ventral border of the duodenum in common with the hepatic diverticulum in the embryo, and from which the uncinate process of the head of the pancreas is formed. [Gk *pan* all, *kreas* flesh.]

See also: ASELLI, WINSLOW.

pancreatalgia (pan·kre·at·al'·je·ah). Sensation of pain in the pancreas. [pancreas, Gk *algos* pain.]

pancreatectomy (pan·kre·at·ek'·to·me). Excision of a part of or the entire pancreas. [pancreas, Gk *ektome* a cutting out.]

pancreatemphraxis (pan·kre·at·em·frax'·is). Hypertrophy or congestion of the pancreas caused by blockage of the pancreatic duct. [pancreas, emphraxis.]

pancreatic (pan·kre·at·ik). Belonging to the pancreas.

pancreatic veins [venae pancreaticae (NA)]. Tributaries of the splenic vein.

pancreaticocholecystostomy (pan·kre·at·ik·o·ko·le·sist·os'·to·me). The surgical implantation of a pancreatic fistula into the gall bladder. [pancreas, Gk *chole* bile, *kystis* bladder, *stoma* mouth.]

pancreaticoduodenal (pan·kre·at·ik·o·dew·o·de'·nal). Belonging to the pancreas and the duodenum.

pancreaticoduodenal arteries. Inferior pancreaticoduodenal artery [arteria pancreaticoduodenalis inferior (NA)]. *See* MESENTERIC ARTERY, SUPERIOR. **Superior pancreaticoduodenal artery [arteria pancreaticoduodenalis superior (NA)].** *See* HEPATIC ARTERY, COMMON.

pancreaticoduodenal veins [venae pancreaticoduodenales (NA)]. Tributaries of the superior mesenteric vein, draining the pancreas and duodenum and accompanying the corresponding arteries.

pancreaticoduodenectomy (pan·kre·at·ik·o·dew·o·de·nek'·to·me). Surgical removal of the pancreas and duodenum; Whipple's operation. [pancreas, duodenum, Gk *ektome* excision.]

pancreaticoduodenostomy (pan·kre·at·ik·o·dew·o·de·nos'·to·me). The surgical implantation of a pancreatic fistula, or of the pancreatic duct, or of the cut surface of pancreas, into the duodenum. [pancreas, duodenum, Gk *stoma* mouth.]

pancreatico-enterostomy (pan·kre·at·ik·o·en·ter·os'·to·me). The surgical implantation of a pancreatic fistula, or of the pancreatic duct, or of the cut surface of pancreas, into the jejunum. [pancreas, Gk *enteron* intestine, *stoma* mouth.]

pancreaticogastrostomy (pan·kre·at·ik·o·gas·tros'·to·me). The surgical implantation of a pancreatic fistula, or of the pancreatic duct, or of the cut surface of pancreas, into the stomach. [pancreas, Gk *gaster* stomach, *stoma* mouth.]

pancreaticojejunostomy (pan·kre·at·ik·o·jej·oon·os'·to·me). The surgical implantation of a pancreatic fistula, or of the pancreatic duct, or of the cut surface of pancreas, into the jejunum. [pancreas, jejunum, Gk *stoma* mouth.]

pancreaticosplenic (pan·kre·at·ik·o·splen'·ik). Relating or belonging to the pancreas and the spleen.

Pancreatin BP 1973 (pan·kre·at·in). The dried alcoholic extract of the pancreas of certain animals, e.g. hog, ox. It contains the enzymes trypsin, amylase and lipase, and is administered orally to assist digestive weakness, or is added to foods such as milk, oatmeal, gruel, beef tea, etc., in order to predigest fat, protein, and carbohydrates before consumption.

pancreatism (pan·kre·at·izm). A term comprising all the activities of the pancreas.

pancreatitic (pan·kre·at·it'·ik). Of the nature of or relating to pancreatitis.

pancreatitis (pan·kre·at·i'·tis). Inflammation of the pancreas. **Acute pancreatitis.** Inflammation following the escape of pancreatic enzymes into the pancreas, usually due to biliary disease or alcoholism, and causing symptoms of an acute abdomen. **Acute haemorrhagic pancreatitis.** Severe pancreatitis with haemorrhagic necrosis producing shock and paralysis of the gut; it is often fatal. **Acute parenchymatous pancreatitis.** A complication of mumps and possibly other virus infections. **Chronic pancreatitis.** Chronic inflammation usually following repeated attacks of acute pancreatitis with developing fibrosis and calcification of the gland; it may lead to diabetes and steatorrhoea. [pancreas, Gk *-itis* inflammation.]

pancreatoduodenectomy (pan·kre·at·o·dew·o·de·**nek**′·to·me). Surgical removal of the head of the pancreas together with the duodenum. [pancreas, duodenum, Gk *ektome* excision.]

pancreatoduodenostomy (pan·kre·at·o·dew·o·de·**nos**′·to·me). Pancreaticoduodenostomy.

pancreato-enterostomy (pan·kre·at·o·en·ter·**os**′·to·me). Pancreatico-enterostomy.

pancreatogenic, pancreatogenous (pan·kre·at·o·**jen**′·ik, pan·kre·at·**oj**′·en·us). Having origin in the pancreas. [pancreas, Gk *genein* to produce.]

pancreatogram (pan·kre·**at**·o·gram). The radiograph made during pancreatography. [pancreas, Gk *gamma* record.]

pancreatograph (pan·kre·**at**·o·graf). Pancreatogram. [pancreas, Gk *graphein* to record.]

pancreatography (pan·kre·at·**og**′·raf·e). Radiographic or radionuclide visualization of the pancreas, covering retroperitoneal gas insufflation, contrast filling of the pancreatic duct, angiography and scanning. [pancreas, Gk *graphein* to record.]

pancreatoid (pan·kre·at·oid). Like the pancreas. [pancreas, Gk *eidos* form.]

pancreatolith (pan·kre·**at**·o·lith). A calculus or concretion present in the pancreas. [pancreas, Gk *lithos* stone.]

pancreatolithectomy (pan·kre·**at**·o·lith·**ek**′·to·me). The surgical removal of a pancreatolith. [pancreas, lithectomy.]

pancreatolysis (pan·kre·at·**ol**′·is·is). Destruction of the pancreatic substance. [pancreas, Gk *lysis* a loosing.]

pancreatolytic (pan·kre·at·o·**lit**′·ik). Pertaining to pancreatolysis.

pancreatomy (pan·kre·**at**·o·me). Pancreatotomy.

pancreatoncus (pan·kre·at·**ong**′·kus). A pancreatic tumour. [pancreas, Gk *ogkos* a swelling.]

pancreatopathy (pan·kre·at·**op**′·ath·e). Any disordered condition of the pancreas. [pancreas, Gk *pathos* disease.]

pancreatotomy (pan·kre·at·**ot**′·o·me). Incision of the pancreas, generally with a view to removing neoplasm or calculus. [pancreas, Gk *temnein* to cut.]

pancre-ectomy (pan·kre·**ek**·to·me). Pancreatectomy.

pancreolith (pan·kre·o·lith). Pancreatolith.

pancreolysis (pan·kre·**ol**·is·is). Pancreatolysis.

pancreolytic (pan·kre·o·**lit**′·ik). Pancreatolytic.

pancreopathia, pancreopathy (pan·kre·o·**path**′·e·ah, pan·kre·**op**′·ath·e). Any disordered condition of the pancreas. [pancreas, Gk *pathos* disease.]

pancreotherapy (pan·kre·o·**ther**′·ap·e). Treatment by the utilization of pancreatic tissue. [pancreas, therapy.]

pancreozymin (pan·kre·o·**zi**′·min). *See* CHOLECYSTOKININ-PANCREOZYMIN.

Pancuronium Bromide (pan·kewr·o·ne·um **bro**·mide). BP Commission approved name for $3\alpha,17\beta$-diacetoxy-$2\beta,16\beta$-dipiperidino-5α-androstane dimethobromide; a neuromuscular blocking agent introduced into anaesthetic practice as a non-depolarizing relaxant in 1967.

pancytopenia (pan·si·to·**pe**′·neah). A reduction in all the cellular elements (red cells, white cells, platelets) of the blood, and usually due to a marrow dyscrasia. This cellular depression is seen in aplastic and refractory anaemias, myelophthisic anaemias, and acute leukaemias. **Hypersplenic pancytopenia.** Pancytopenia due to overaction of hypertrophied spleen (hypersplenism). [Gk *pan* all, *kytos* cell, *penia* poverty.]

pandemia (pan·**de**·me·ah). An epidemic that affects the major proportion or all of the inhabitants of a region or a country. [see foll.]

pandemic (pan·**dem**·ik). 1. Said of a disease that extends over a large area, possibly the whole world. 2. A pandemic disease. 3. More rarely, implying involvement of all or a large majority of the people in a limited area. [Gk *pan* all, *demos* the people.]

pandemicity (pan·dem·**is**·it·e). The quality of being pandemic.

pandemy (pan·dem·e). Pandemia.

Pander, Heinrich Christian von (b. 1794). Würzburg embryologist.

Pander's false amnion. The chorionic membrane.

island of Pander. Blood island; a small localized area of blood formation found on the wall of the yolk sac in the early embryo.

Pander's layer. Splanchnopleure.

Pander's nucleus. A small mass of grey matter found in the subthalamic region of the brain.

pandiculation (pan·**dik**·ew·**la**′·shun). A stretching of the trunk, arms and legs, attended by yawning, after waking from sleep or when fatigued. [L *pandiculari* to stretch oneself.]

Pandy, Kálmán (b. 1868). Budapest psychiatrist.

Pandy's test. For globulin in cerebrospinal fluid: to 0.5 ml of reagent in a very small test-tube add 1 drop of fluid. A turbidity or precipitate, depending upon the amount present, indicates globulin. The reagent consists of 7 g of phenol dissolved in 100 ml of water.

Pane, Nicola. Naples physician.

Pane's serum. An antipneumococcal serum.

panel (pan·el). 1. A list of names; in Law, the list of persons summoned on a jury, and hence applied to the whole jury. 2. A list of names of registered medical practitioners, who were willing to receive insured patients for treatment under the National Health Insurance Scheme (Great Britain). The name was also applied to the list of insured patients assigned to such a medical practitioner. [L *pannus* list.]

panencephalitis (pan·en·kef·al·**i**′·tis). **Sclerosing panencephalitis, Subacute sclerosing panencephalitis, SSPE.** A chronic progressive and fatal degeneration in the brain cells of children as a late sequel of measles. It is a rare complication and appears to be due to a reactivation of latent measles virus within the central nervous system. The mechanism of this reactivation is not understood but virus-like structures and inclusions are widespread in the brain at post-mortem, and, using co-cultivation techniques, an atypical measles virus has been recovered. *Dawson's inclusion body panencephalitis.* *See* LEUCO-ENCEPHALITIS. [Gk *pan* all, encephalitis.]

panendoscope (pan·**en**·do·skope). A foreoblique cystoscope which gives a wide view of the bladder (McCarthy). The objective system of the telescope has a double-acting prism which deflects the angle of the optical axis about 25 degrees. The telescope is slender, and accordingly the sheath has ample accommodation for a wide range of endovesical operating instruments. [Gk *pan* all, *endon* within, *skopein* to view.]

Paneth, Josef (b. 1857). Vienna physiologist.

Paneth's cell, or granule. An eosinophil granular epithelial cell from the intestinal crypts of Lieberkühn, probably secreting digestive enzymes; also known as *Davidoff's cell.*

pang (pang). A sudden, transitory and extreme pain. **Breast pang.** Angina pectoris. **Brow pang.** Supraorbital neuralgia. [etym. dub.]

pangenesis (pan·**jen**·es·is). The theory that each cell of the adult body is represented by a particle in the gametes. Now of historical interest only. [Gk *pan* all, *genein* to produce.]

pangenetic (pan·jen·**et**·ik). Belonging to pangenesis.

panglossia (pan·**glos**·e·ah). Excessive or insane talkativeness. [Gk *pagglossia* wordiness.]

Pangonia (pan·**go**·ne·ah). A genus of African flies of the family Tabanidae, with very elongate proboscis. Their bites are painful to man and they carry trypanosomes, especially to camels.

panhaematopenia (pan·he·mat·o·**pe**′·ne·ah). A deficiency of all of the various blood cells. **Primary splenic panhaematopenia.** Hypersplenism. [Gk *pan* all, *haima* blood, *penia* poverty.]

panhaematopoiesis (pan·**he**·mat·o·poi·**e**′·sis). Production and development of all of the cellular elements of the blood. [Gk *pan* all, *haima* blood, *poiesis* production.]

panhaematopoietic (pan·**he**·mat·o·poi·**et**′·ik). Pertaining to panhaematopoiesis.

panhaemocytophthisis (pan·**he**·mo·si·to·**thi**′·sis). Deficiency of all cellular elements of the blood, resulting from failure in the formative tissue or from other causes. [Gk *pan* all, *haima* blood, *kytos* cell, *phthisis* a wasting.]

panhidrosis (pan·hid·**ro**·sis). Perspiration over the entire body surface. [Gk *pan* all, *hidros* sweat.]

panhydrometer (pan·hi·**drom**·et·er). A form of hydrometer suitable for the determination of the specific gravity of any liquid. [Gk *pan* all, hydrometer.]

panhygrous (pan·**hi**·grus). Moist in every part. [Gk *pan* all, *hygros* moist.]

panhyperaemia (**pan**·hi·per·**e**′·me·ah). Widespread plethora. [Gk *pan* all, hyperaemia.]

panhypopancreatism (**pan**·hi·po·**pan**′·kre·at·izm). The condition in which there is depression of both the external and internal secretions of the pancreas. [Gk *pan* all, *hypo*, pancreas.]

panhypopituitarism (pan·**hi**·po·pit·**ew**′·it·ar·izm). Defective function of the whole of the pituitary gland, as in Simmonds' disease. [Gk *pan* whole, *hypo*, pituitary gland.]

panhysterectomy (**pan**·his·ter·**ek**′·to·me). The complete surgical removal of the uterus. [Gk *pan* all, *hystera* uterus, *ektome* excision.]

panhystero-oöphorectomy (pan·**his**·ter·o·o·of·or·**ek**′·to·me). Surgical excision of the whole uterus with one or both ovaries. [Gk *pan* all, *hystera* uterus, *oon* egg, *pherein* to bear, *ektome* excision.]

panhysterosalpingectomy (pan·**his**·ter·o·sal·pin·**jek**′·to·me). Surgical excision of the whole uterus and the uterine tubes. [Gk *pan* all, *hystera* uterus, *salpigx* tube, *ektome* excision.]

panhysterosalpingo-oöphorectomy (pan·**his**·ter·o·sal·ping·go·o·of·or·**ek**′·to·me). Surgical excision of the whole uterus, ovaries, and uterine tubes. [Gk *pan* all, *hystera* uterus, *salpigx* tube, *oon* egg, *pherein* to bear, *ektome* excision.]

panic (**pan**·ik). A sudden unreasonable feeling or expression of alarm or fear that may lead to unreasonable and precipitate acts; the state of mind is rapidly conveyed to other persons all of whom may behave similarly. [Gk *panikos* of the god Pan.]

panicula (pan·**ik**·ew·lah). A tumour or other swelling. [L, little swelling.]

Panidazole (pan·id·**a**·zole). BP Commission approved name for 2-methyl-5-nitro-1-[2-(4-pyridyl)ethyl]-imidazole; an amoebacide.

panidrosis (pan·id·**ro**·sis). Panhidrosis.

panimmunity (pan·im·**ewn**·it·e). Immunity to several bacterial or viral infections. [Gk *pan* all, immunity.]

panivorous (pan·**iv**·or·us). Referring to persons or groups who are essentially bread eaters; existing on bread. [L *panis* bread, *vorare* to devour.]

Panizza, Bartolomeo (b. 1785). Pavia anatomist and surgeon.

Panizza's foramen. A congenital lesion of the interventricular septum of the heart.

Panizza's plexuses. Lymphatic plexuses in the lateral fossae of the frenulum of the prepuce.

panleucopenia (**pan**·lew·ko·**pe**′·ne·ah). 1. A deficiency of all the white-cell elements in the blood. 2. A virus disease in cats. Also called *cat distemper* or *cat plague.* [Gk *pan* all, *leukos* white, *penia* poverty.]

panmixia (pan·**mix**·e·ah). 1. In biology, indiscriminate and unselective crossing. 2. Sexual association of individuals of different races. [Gk *pan* all, *mixis* intercourse.]

panmnesia (pan·**ne**·ze·ah). A latent recollection of every impression made upon the mind or sensibilities. [Gk *pan* all, *mnesis* remembrance.]

panmyeloid (pan·**mi**·el·oid). Relating to all the cellular elements of the bone marrow. [Gk *pan* all, *myelos* marrow, *eidos* form.]

panmyelopathy (**pan**·mi·el·**op**′·ath·e). A disease affecting all the blood-forming elements in the bone marrow. [Gk *pan* all, *myelos* marrow, *pathos* disease.]

panmyelophthisis (**pan**·mi·el·**of**′·this·is). A general wasting or atrophy of the bone marrow. [Gk *pan* all, *myelos* marrow, *phthisis* a wasting.]

panmyelosis (**pan**·mi·el·**o**′·sis). A condition in which there is proliferation of all the constituent cells of the bone marrow. [Gk *pan* all, *myelos* marrow.]

panmyelotoxicosis (**pan**·mi·el·o·tox·ik·**o**′·sis). A state in which all the various elements of the bone marrow are subject to toxic effects. [Gk *pan* all, *myelos* marrow, *toxikon* poison.]

panners' disease. Koehler's disease; osteochondrosis of the navicular bone.

Pannett, Charles Aubrey. London surgeon.

Pannett's needle. A relatively fine needle, about 100 mm in length, for lumbar puncture.

panneuritis (pan·newr·**i**·tis). Multiple neuritis. **Panneuritis epidemica.** Beriberi. [Gk *pan* all, neuritis.]

panniculalgia (**pan**·ik·ewl·**al**′·je·ah). A neurosis in which there is a sensation of pain in areas of the subcutaneous fat. [panniculus, Gk *algos* pain.]

panniculitis (pan·**ik**·ewl·**i**′·tis). A condition of chronic inflammation of the superficial fascia, in which the skin is hardened, and small subcutaneous masses of induration are found over the abdomen and upper part of the thorax and on the inner aspects of the thighs and arms. **Mesenteric panniculitis.** Inflammation of the mesenteric fat, mainly in males. **Nodular non-suppurative panniculitis, Relapsing febrile non-suppurative panniculitis.** A rare condition of unknown causation, characterized by the presence of nodular formations in the subcutaneous tissues, and prolonged, intermittent relapsing pyrexia. [panniculus, Gk *-itis* inflammation.]

panniculus (pan·**ik**·ewl·us). A sheet of membranous tissue. **Panniculus adiposus.** The superficial fascia which contains fatty pellicles. **Panniculus carnosus.** A thin sheet of muscle found in the superficial fascia of hairy-coated animals, but which in human beings is found principally in the platysma muscle. **Panniculus hymeneus.** The hymen of the vagina. **Panniculus subtilis.** The pia mater of the brain. **Panniculus transversus.** The diaphragm. **Panniculus virginis.** The hymen of the vagina. [L, small piece of cloth.]

pannus (**pan**·us). Superficial vascularization of the cornea associated with a cellular infiltration, finally becoming granulation tissue. **Pannus carateus.** Pinta. **Pannus crassus.** A type of trachomatous pannus which is particularly thick with dense opacification of the cornea. **Pannus degeneraticus.** Superficial corneal opacification and vascularization found in degenerate blind eyes, often associated with corneal bullae in the early stages. **Eczematous pannus.** Phlyctenular pannus (see below). **Leprotic pannus.** Superficial vascularization and cellular infiltration of the cornea occurring in cases of leprosy. It usually follows limbal nodules or superficial punctate keratitis. **Phlyctenular pannus.** A superficial vascularization of the cornea, with some loss of epithelium and opacity; usually situated around the periphery and extending centrally, not particularly above, as in trachoma. **Pannus sarcomatosus.** A type of trachomatous pannus which shows extreme thickness and very marked opacification of the cornea. **Scrofulous pannus.** Phlyctenular pannus (see above). **Pannus siccus.** The scarring or late stage of trachomatous pannus. **Pannus tenuis.** A type of trachomatous pannus which is very thin, with only slight corneal opacification. **Rheumatoid pannus.** The thickened and chronically inflamed synovium which is found over the articular surfaces of joints affected by rheumatoid arthritis. **Trachomatous pannus.** A superficial vascularization and cellular infiltration of the cornea coming on in the second and third stages of trachoma. It always starts at the upper limbus and extends downwards, and is of great diagnostic importance. **Pannus vasculosus.** A type of trachomatous pannus showing very marked vascularization. [L, cloth.]

panodic (pan·od·ik). Panthodic. [Gk *pan* all, *hodos* way.]

panophobia (pan·o·fo·be·ah). Pantophobia.

panophthalmia, panophthalmitis (pan·of·thal·me·ah, pan·of·thal·mi′·tis). Inflammation affecting all parts of the eye. **Panophthalmia purulenta.** An acute form of panophthalmia characterized by suppuration and protrusion of the eyeball, leading as a rule to blindness. [Gk *pan* all, *ophthalmos* eye, *-itis* inflammation.]

panoptic (pan·op·tik). Rendering everything microscopically visible; applied to certain stains used for histological sections and for protozoa. [Gk *pan* all, *opsis* vision.]

panoptosis (pan·op·to·sis). A condition in which all the viscera are prolapsed. [Gk *pan* all, *ptosis* a falling.]

panosteitis, panostitis (pan·os·te·i′·tis, pan·os·ti·tis). Inflammation in which the whole of a bone is affected. [Gk *pan* all, *osteon* bone, *-itis* inflammation.]

panotitis (pan·o·ti·tis). Inflammation affecting every part of the ear, but particularly the middle ear. [Gk *pan* all, otitis.]

panphobia (pan·fo·be·ah). Pantophobia.

panplegia (pan·ple·je·ah). Total paraplegia. [Gk *pan* all, *plege* stroke.]

Pansch, Adolf (b. 1841). Kiel anatomist.

Pansch's fissure, or sulcus. The intraparietal sulcus of the parietal lobe of the cerebrum.

pansclerosis (pan·skler·o·sis). General hardening of a part or tissue. [Gk *pan* all, sclerosis.]

panseptum (pan·sep·tum). The nasal septum in its entirety. [Gk *pan* all, septum.]

pansinuitis (pan·si·new·i′·tis). Pansinusitis.

pansinusitis (pan·si·nus·i′·tis). Inflammation in which there is involvement of all the sinuses. [Gk *pan* all, sinusitis.]

pansphygmograph (pan·sfig·mo·graf). An instrument used for the simultaneous recording of the pulse, and cardiac and respiratory thoracic movements. [Gk *pan* all, sphygmograph.]

Panstrongylus (pan·stron·jil·us). A genus of bugs, sometimes regarded as a subgenus of *Triatoma*. **Panstrongylus geniculatus.** A species from tropical South America which normally lives in burrows of armadilloes, but may bite man and act as a vector for *Trypanosoma cruzi*. **Panstrongylus megistus.** The barbiero bug of northern Brazil, the Guianas, and Peru. It is a normal inhabitant of dwellings and its bites are painful. It is an important vector of *Trypanosoma cruzi*. [Gk *pan* all, *stroggylos* round.]

pantachromatic (pant·a·kro·mat′·ik). Completely achromatic. [Gk *pan* all, achromatic.]

pantalar (pan·ta·lar). Around the talus. [Gk *pan* all, talus.]

pantalgia (pant·al·je·ah). Pain affecting all parts of the body. [Gk *pan* all, *algos* pain.]

pantamorphia (pant·a·mor·fe·ah). A condition in which there is malformation of all the parts or structures. [Gk *pan* all, *amorphia* ill shape.]

pantamorphic (pant·a·mor·fik). Having no shape or form. [Gk *pan* all, *a*, *morphe* shape.]

pantanencephalia (pant·an·en·kef·a′·le·ah). Total anencephalia; complete congenital lack of cerebrum as found in certain monsters. [see foll.]

pantanencephalic (pant·an·en·kef·al′·ik). Pertaining to total anencephalia. [Gk *pan* all, anencephalia.]

pantanencephalus (pant·an·en·kef′·al·us). A fetal monster in which there is total absence of brain substance. [see prec.]

pantankyloblepharon (pant·ang·ki·lo·blef′·ar·on). Complete union of the eyelid margins. [Gk *pan* all, *agkyle* noose, *blepharon* eyelid.]

pantaphobia (pant·a·fo·be·ah). Complete fearlessness. [Gk *pan* all, *a*, *phobos* fear.]

pantatrophia (pant·at·ro·fe·ah). Pantatrophy.

pantatrophous (pant·at·ro·fus). Lacking all nutrition. [see foll.]

pantatrophy (pant·at·ro·fe). General atrophy; an advanced state of malnutrition. [Gk *pan* all, atrophy.]

Panthenol (pan·then·ol). BP Commission approved name for (±)-2,4-dihydroxy-*N*-(3-hydroxypropyl)-3,3-dimethylbutyramide; it is used in the treatment of paralytic ileus and postoperative distension.

pantherapist (pan·ther·ap·ist). A practitioner who employs any suitable means of treatment, irrespective of whether it is obtained from his own or other systems of medicine. [Gk *pan* all, therapy.]

panthodic (pan·thod·ik). Radiating from one centre, referring to nerve stimuli. [Gk *pan* all, *odos* way.]

panting (pant·ing). Breathing quickly, spasmodically or with difficulty, with heaving of the chest. [OFr. *pantaisier* to be breathless.]

pantochromism (pant·o·kro·mizm). The property of a substance that is capable of existence in two or more dissimilarly coloured varieties. [Gk *pan* all, *chroma* colour.]

pantograph (pant·o·graf). 1. An apparatus used in tracing the outlines of the thorax. 2. A device composed of a system of levers which can be adjusted, connecting a pencil with a tracing stylet, used in the reproduction of diagrams, plans, and other drawings to any required scale. [Gk *pan* all, *graphein* to write.]

pantography (pant·og·raf·e). The art of using the pantograph.

pantomime (pant·o·mime). Movements carried out in silence and with strict deliberation in order to express an idea or feeling.

pantomorph (pant·o·morf). That which is capable of assuming all shapes. [see foll.]

pantomorphia (pant·o·mor·fe·ah). 1. The state of being symmetrical. 2. The condition of being able to assume or take any shape at all. [Gk *pan* all, *morphe* form.]

pantomorphic (pant·o·mor·fik). Relating or belonging to pantomorphia. Term applied to something that can assume any shape, or that can appear in any form. [see prec.]

pantophobia (pant·o·fo·be·ah). 1. A condition of morbid apprehension in regard to all things. 2. An indeterminate fear of an unknown harmful thing. [Gk *pan* all, phobia.]

pantoplethora (pant·o·pleth·or·ah). A state of general hyperaemia. [Gk *pan* all, plethora.]

pantoptosis (pant·op·to·sis). Generalized visceroptosis. [Gk *pan* all, ptosis.]

pantoscopic (pant·o·skop·ik). A term applied to reading glasses, the top half of which, being cut away, allows the wearer to see clearly in the distance. [Gk *pan* all, *skopein* to view.]

pantostat (pant·o·stat). Polystat; an instrument which, when connected to the electric mains, supplies direct (galvanic), low frequency (faradic) and sinusoidal currents. [obsolete term.] [Gk *pan* all, *statos* standing.]

pantothermia (pant·o·ther·me·ah). A condition in which there are variations of body temperature, the cause of which cannot be determined. [Gk *pan* all, *therme* heat.]

pantotropic (pant·o·trop·ik). With the property of being attracted to many tissues. [Gk *pan* all, *tropos* a turning.]

pantoyl taurine (pant·o·il taw·reen). $CH_2OHC(CH_3)_2CHOHCO NHCH_2CH_2SO_3H$, a substance capable of inhibiting the growth of many bacterial cultures on account of the competitive antagonism it exhibits for the essential pantothenic acid.

pantropic (pan·trop·ik). Pantotropic.

panturbinate (pan·ter·bin·ate). The whole structure comprised by the inferior, middle and superior nasal conchae, together with the bony and soft tissue. [Gk *pan* all, turbinate.]

Panum, Peter Ludvig (b. 1820). Copenhagen physiologist.

Panum's area. A zone around the horopter within which images of points are seen singly although they fall on non-corresponding areas of the retina.

panus (pa·nus). An inflamed lymph gland in which there is no pus formation. **Panus faucium.** An inflamed lymph gland in the throat. **Panus inguinalis.** A bulbo. [L, a swelling.]

panzootic (pan·zo·ot·ik). A disease of animals that is widespread. Cf. PANDEMIC. The word is also used adjectivally. [Gk *pan* all, *zoon* animal.]

pap (pap). 1. A nipple. 2. Any food of soft, pulpy consistency. [etym. dub.]

Papain BPC 1954 (pap·a·in). A proteolytic enzyme, or mixture of enzymes, obtained from the unripe fruit of *Carica papaya*. It is a white or light-brown powder, used as an aid to protein digestion when the natural ferments are deficient as in pancreatic disease, and also in the manufacture of proteolysed liver preparations. Used in blood group serology to treat red cells, after which they can be agglutinated in saline suspensions by blocking antibodies.

papainase (pap·a·in·aze). Catheptic enzyme. A group of proteolytic enzymes which includes cathepsin, papain and bromelin.

papainum (pap·a·in·um). Papain.

Papanicolaou, George N. (b. 1883). Greek physician in America. **Papanicolaou's stain or smear.** A method of staining smears of various body secretions (from bronchi, bladder, vagina and gastro-intestinal tract) to detect the presence of a malignant process.

Papaver (pap·a·ver). A genus of plants of the family Papaveraceae; the poppies. **Papaver rhoeas.** Corn poppy, red poppy; a species the leaves of which are used for their red colouring matter. **Papaver somniferum.** The poppy from the capsules of which opium is obtained. [L, poppy.]

Papaveretum BPC 1968 (pap·av·er·e'·tum). A mixture of the hydrochlorides of the total alkaloids of opium, 20 mg are said to contain 13.3 mg of morphine. It is used for analgesia and as a pre-operative sedative, often with hyoscine.

papaverine (pap·av·er·een). $C_{20}N_{21}NO_4$, an optically inactive alkaloid derived from opium. It is a spasmolytic, relaxing the smooth muscle of the intestinal tract, biliary tract, bronchioles, ureters and the blood vessels, especially during spasms; it tends also to relax the coronary arteries. It has little action on the central nervous system and does not cause sleep or analgesia. Its chief value is in peripheral or pulmonary arterial embolism for increasing the collateral circulation and for producing vasodilatation in peripheral vascular diseases. **Papaverine Hydrochloride BP 1973.** The most commonly employed water-soluble salt of papaverine, administered orally, subcutaneously, or (for asthma) as a spray. **Papaverine Sulphate BPC 1963.** A preparation more soluble in water than papaverine hydrochloride; its action and uses are similar to those of the hydrochloride. [L *papaver* poppy.]

Papaverinii Chloridum. *European Pharmacopoeia* name for Papaverine Hydrochloride BP 1973.

papaveris capsula (pap·a·ver·is **kap**·sew·lah). Poppy capsule. [L *papaver* poppy, capsule.]

Papaveroline (pap·ah·**ver**·o·leen). BP Commission approved name for 1-(3,4-dihydroxybenzyl)-6,7-dihydroxyisoquinoline; a vasodilator.

papaw (pap·aw). 1. The seed of *Asimina triloba*, a small tree of the family Anonaceae, the fruits of which have a high nutritive value. The bark is used as a bitter and contains the alkaloid, anolobine. 2. Pawpaw. [Sp. *papaya.*]

papaya (pap·a·yah). The juice from the fruit of the tree *Carica papaya;* it contains the proteolytic enzyme, papain.

papayotin (pap·a·yo·tin). A proteolytic enzyme obtained from the pawpaw, *Carica papaya.* It is a protein digestant in acid, alkaline or neutral media, and is chiefly used in chronic dyspepsia and gastric fermentation.

paper (pa·per). A material manufactured in sheets from wood pulp, esparto and other cellulose materials, such as cloth rags, and impregnated with fillers to render it non-absorbent, or treated in other special ways for particular purposes. **Amboceptor paper.** Paper used in a test for syphilis; now obsolete. **Aniline-acetate paper.** A test paper for detecting oxidizing agents, e.g. hypochlorite. **Antigen paper.** Amboceptor paper (see above). **Articulating paper.** A carbon paper which when bitten upon marks the points of contact between the upper and lower teeth. **Blue-litmus paper.** Paper for testing for acidity (acid turns it red), being impregnated with blue litmus. **Congo-red paper.** A paper impregnated with Congo red; it is turned blue by acids, red by alkalis. **Filter paper.** A porous paper used to separate a solution from suspended particles. **Helianthin paper.** Methyl-orange paper (see below). **Litmus paper.** A paper impregnated with litmus; acids turn it red, alkalis blue. **Methyl-orange paper.** A paper impregnated with methyl orange; acids turn it pink, alkalis orange. **Red-litmus paper.** A paper impregnated with red litmus; alkalis turn it blue. **Test paper.** Non-glazed paper soaked in solutions of various reagents, dried, and cut into strips suitable for certain chemical tests. **Turmeric paper.** A paper impregnated with turmeric; soaked in solutions of boric acid and dried, it turns pink; the colour is changed to green by alkali. **Wax paper.** Paper impregnated with paraffin wax to render it waterproof. [Gk *papyros* papyrus.]

papilla [NA] (pap·il·ah). Any small elevation shaped like a nipple. **Alpine papillae.** Elongated dermal papillae seen in several skin diseases, characteristically in psoriasis. **Circumvallate papilla.** A type of papilla on the tongue, surrounded by a walled depression. **Conical papillae [papillae conicae (NA)].** Small papillae found in the anterior ridge-like projections of the corium of the skin towards the surface. The epidermis is moulded over these. **Dental papilla [papilla dentis (NA)].** The mesodermal core of the bell-shaped tooth germ or enamel organ. **Duodenal papilla, greater [papilla duodeni major (NA)].** A small projection on the medial wall of the second part of the duodenum, on the apex of which the ampulla of the bile duct opens. **Duodenal papilla, smaller [papilla duodeni minor (NA)].** A small rounded elevation on to which the accessory pancreatic duct opens. **Engorged papilla.** Choked disc. *See* DISC. **Filiform papillae [papillae filiformes (NA)].** Numerous pointed projections of the mucous membrane of the dorsal surface of the anterior two-thirds of the tongue, giving this part its characteristic roughness. **Foliate papillae [papillae foliatae (NA)].** Rudimentary papillae in folds on the sides of the tongue. **Fungiform papillae [papillae fungiformes (NA)].** Rounded and somewhat club-shaped projections of the mucous membrane of the tongue, mainly situated on the tip and sides of the organ. **Genital papilla.** The midline swelling at the ventral end of the cloacal membrane in early embryos which gives rise to the distal end of the penis or clitoris; genital tubercle. **Hair papilla [papilla pili (NA)].** The central part of a hair bulb. **Incisive papilla [papilla incisiva (NA)].** A small median eminence at the extreme anterior part of the palate, behind the interval between the median incisor teeth. **Interdental papilla.** The papilla of gum between adjacent teeth. **Lacrimal papilla [papilla lacrimalis (NA)].** A small conical elevation on the margin of each eyelid at its medial end, pierced by the lacrimal canaliculus. **Lingual papillae [papillae linguales (NA)].** The papillae found on the tongue; they are the filiform, conical, fungiform, vallate and foliate. **Optic papilla.** Optic disc. *See* DISC. **Parotid papilla [papilla parotidea (NA)].** The elevation in the mucous membrane of the cheek upon which lies the orifice of the parotid duct. **Renal papillae [papillae renales (NA)].** Conical apices of the renal pyramids, projecting into the minor calyces. **Sublingual papilla [caruncula sublingualis (NA)].** A small eminence on which the submandibular duct opens, situated on either side of the tongue. **Tactile papilla.** A papilla occurring in the corium; it contains tactile corpuscles. **Vallate papillae [papillae vallatae (NA)].** About 10 large button-like projections of the mucous membrane of the tongue, rich in taste buds and parallel with and in front of the sulcus terminalis. Each projection is surrounded by a circular depression. [L, nipple.]

See also: BERGMEISTER.

papillary (pap·il·ar·e). Belonging to or like a papilla.

papillary muscles [musculi papillares (NA)]. Special portions of the columnae carneae forming conical projections into the ventricular cavities. The chordae tendineae are attached to their apices. **Anterior papillary muscle of the right ventricle [musculus papillaris anterior (NA)].** A cone-shaped bundle arising from the anterior ventricular wall and attached by its chordae tendineae to the anterior and inferior cusps of the right atrioventicular (tricuspid) valve. **Inferior papillary muscle of the left ventricle [musculus papillaris posterior (NA)].** A large, cone-shaped muscle bundle arising from the left ventricular wall, from the apex of which chordae tendineae run to the right-hand portion of both cusps of the left atrioventricular (mitral) valve. **Inferior**

papillary muscle of the right ventricle [musculus papillaris posterior (NA)]. A muscle composed of two or three bundles arising from the inferior wall, from which chordae tendineae pass to the inferior and medial cusps of the right atrioventricular (tricuspid) valve. **Septal papillary muscles [musculi papillares septales (NA)].** Small cone-shaped bundles arising from the interventricular septum from which chordae tendineae pass to the anterior and medial cusps of the right atrioventricular (tricuspid) valve. **Superior papillary muscle of the left ventricle [musculus papillaris anterior (NA)].** A large, cone-shaped muscle bundle arising from the left ventricular wall, from the apex of which chordae tendineae run to the left-hand portion of both cusps of the left atrioventricular (mitral) valve.

papillate (**pap**·il·ate). 1. Covered with papillae. 2. Characterized by papillary projections, e.g. in bacterial plate cultures.

papillectomy (pap·il·**ek**·to·me). 1. Surgical removal of a papilloma. 2. Removal of congested or bleeding papillae from the kidney, pelvis, or bladder. [papilla, Gk *ektome* excision.]

papilliferous (pap·il·**if**·er·us). Papillate; bearing papillae. [papilla, L *ferre* to bear.]

papilliform (pap·il·e·form). Formed like or resembling a papilla.

papillitis (pap·il·i·tis). Inflammation of the optic disc or nerve head. **Chronic lingual papillitis.** Enlargement of the filiform papillae of the tongue; hairy tongue. **Necrotizing papillitis.** Necrosis of the tips of the renal pyramids occurring in diabetes and in chronic phenacetin poisoning. **Renal papillitis.** Inflammation of a renal papilla often progressing to necrosis, occurring in diabetes, after drug administration, and uricacidaemia. [papilla, Gk *-itis* inflammation.]

papillo-adenocystoma (**pap**·il·o·ad·en·o·sist·**o'**·mah). An innocent cystic glandular tumour in which the lining membrane is thrown into numerous fine folds. [papilla, adenocystoma.]

papillocarcinoma (**pap**·il·o·kar·sin·**o'**·mah). A cancer which grows outwards from a surface or projects into a hollow cavity, imitating a wart in its structure. [papilla, carcinoma.]

papilloedema (pap·il·e·**de**·mah). Oedema of the optic nerve head, as opposed to papillitis which is inflammatory. The commonest cause is raised intracranial pressure from cerebral tumour. [papilla, oedema.]

papilloma (pap·il·o·mah). An innocent stalked tumour of surface or lining epithelium. **Papilloma acuminatum.** Condyloma acuminatum, a papilloma with moist sharply defined projections, found chiefly about the genitals and usually venereal. **Papilloma choroideum.** A papilloma or papillary outgrowth derived from the living cells of the choroid plexus. **Cylindrical-cell papilloma.** A papilloma lined by tall columnar cells, as in the rectum. **Papilloma diffusum.** A papilloma which spreads over an extensive region of tissue; multiple papillomata on the legs and buttock. **Papilloma durum, Hard papilloma.** A papilloma which feels hards because of the large amount of fibrous tissue in its core. **Intracanalicular papilloma.** A papilloma of the ducts of the breast in which the duct epithelium is compressed by the growth of fibrous tissue around the ducts, giving bizarre-shaped clefts. **Intracystic papilloma.** Papillo-adenocystoma. **Papilloma molle.** Soft papilloma (see below). **Papilloma neuropathicum, Papilloma neuroticum.** Neurofibroma; von Recklinghausen's disease. **Soft papilloma.** A papilloma of soft consistency resulting either from limited keratin formation or from maceration due to being situated in a fold from which evaporation is difficult. **Squamous-cell papilloma.** A papilloma lined by squamous cells, as in the skin. **Papilloma venereum.** Papilloma acuminatum (see above). **Villous papilloma.** A papilloma with very thin and multiple excrescences, common in the urinary bladder. [L *papilla* nipple, Gk *-oma* tumour.]

papillomatosis (**pap**·il·o·mat·**o'**·sis). 1. The condition of being affected with papillomata. 2. The condition of diffuse formation of papillomata, e.g. in the bladder. [papilloma, Gk *-osis* condition.]

papillomatous (pap·il·o·mat·us). Having the characteristics of or relating to a papilloma.

Papillomavirus (pap·il·o·mah·**vi'**·rus). One of the two genera of viruses that make up the Papovaviruses. The viruses of the genus are DNA-containing spherical viruses about 50 nm in diameter. The members include the viruses of human warts and those of papillomatosis in various animal species including cows, dogs, rabbits, deer, horses and monkeys. The viruses cause single or multiple benign tumours. [L *papilla* nipple, Gk *-oma* tumour, L *virus* poison.]

papilloretinitis (**pap**·il·o·ret·in·**i'**·tis). Inflammation involving the optic disc (papilla) and the retina; usually employed in connection with sympathetic ophthalmitis and with renal disease. The term retinitis is now obsolete, retinopathy being used in its place. [papilla, retina, Gk *-itis* inflammation.]

papillosarcoma (**pap**·il·o·sar·**ko'**·mah). A sarcoma which forms excrescences, and projects from a body surface. [papilla, sarcoma.]

papillose (**pap**·il·oze). Bearing papillae.

papillous (**pap**·il·us). Papillary.

papillula (pap·**il**·ew·lah). 1. A small-sized papilla. 2. A nipple.

Papio (pap·e·o). A genus of West African monkeys that are often infected with the trematode *Pseudodiscus watsoni* which also infects man. [Fr. *papion* baboon.]

papoid (**pap**·oid). A proteolytic enzyme from pawpaw fruit. [papaya, Gk *eidos* form.]

Papovavirus (pap·o·vah·vi·rus). A family of viruses comprising the genera *Papillomavirus* and *Polyomavirus.* The properties of the Papovaviruses include the possession of DNA and the ability to initiate tumours, usually benign with the large (50 nm) Papillomaviruses and frequently malignant with the smaller (40 nm) Polyomaviruses. [*pa*pilloma, *po*lyoma, *va*cuolating agent, L *virus* poison.]

Pappenheim, Artur (b. 1870). Berlin physician.

Pappenheim's stain. A mixture of methyl green and pyronine, used to differentiate between ribonucleic and deoxyribonucleic acids: the former stains red, the latter greenish-blue. **Unna–Pappenheim stain.** A stain containing methyl green and pyronine, used especially for demonstrating plasma cells.

Pappenheimer, Alwin Max (b. 1877). New York biochemist.

Pappenheimer's bodies, Pappenheimer's inclusion bodies. Iron-containing granules which are Feulgen-negative, seen in mature and immature red blood corpuscles, and in normoblasts and other red-cell precursors in the bone marrow, usually in patients with haemolytic anaemia, but also after splenectomy in certain haemolytic anaemias; they are said to indicate haemoglobin anabolism and to be related to punctate basophilia, apparently being formed in the bone marrow and removed by the spleen.

pappose, pappous (**pap**·oze, **pap**·us). Covered with fine down. [pappus.]

pappus (**pap**·us). 1. The first downy hair which grows on the chin of the male at puberty. 2. The lanugo. [Gk *pappos* down.]

paprika (pap·re·kah). Green pepper, sweet pepper; the dried fruits of *Capsicum annum* L. (family Solanaceae), used as a condiment. It is rich in vitamin C. [Hungarian.]

papula (pap·ew·lah). Papule.

papular (pap·ew·lar). Relating to, composed of, marked by, or having the nature of a papule.

papulation (pap·ew·la·shun). The development of papules, as occurs in certain eruptive lesions.

papule (**pap**·ewl). A small, superficial, circumscribed, solid elevation of the skin, not larger than a few millimetres in diameter. Papulae may be acuminate, flat, or obtuse. **Moist papule, Mucous papule.** Lesions of secondary syphilis occurring on contiguous or opposing surfaces of the skin, or on the mucosae, particularly in the mouth. **Pearly penile papules.** Physiological, pearly, wart-like or hair-like papules at the corona glandis. **Squamous papule.** A papula having a scaly surface. [L *papula* pimple.]

See also: CELSUS.

papuliferous (pap·ew·**lif**·er·us). Bearing or covered with papules. [papule, L *ferre* to bear.]

papulo-erythematous (pap·ew·lo·er·e·**the**'·mat·us). Characterized by an eruption of papules on an erythematous surface.

papuloid (pap·ew·loid). Shaped like a papule. [papule, Gk *eidos* form.]

papulopustular (pap·ew·lo·**pus**'·tew·lar). Descriptive of an eruption of papules and pustules.

papulopustule (pap·ew·lo·**pus**'·tewl). A papule which is altering its characteristics to those of a pustule.

papulosquamous (pap·ew·lo·**skwa**'·mus). Papular and squamous; said of an eruption. [papule, L *squama* scale.]

papulovesicular (pap·ew·lo·ves·**ik**'·ew·lar). A term applied to skin rashes possessing both papules (small solid elevations) and vesicles (small blisters).

papyraceous (pap·ir·a·shus). Papery. [Gk *papyros* paper.]

Paquelin, Claude André (b. 1836). Paris physician.

Paquelin's cautery. A cautery carrying a platinum point with a content of platinum mesh heated by the passage of a volatile hydrocarbon.

para- (par·ah). 1. A prefix, from the Greek preposition *para*, meaning *beside, beyond, near, wrong*. 2. In organic chemistry, a prefix given to compounds of benzene in which the substituted radicals occupy positions opposite to one another in the ring. Cf. ORTHO, META. 3. Generally, a prefix applied to anything that bears a similarity or relationship to something else.

para-acetphenetidin (par·ah·as·et·fen·**et**'·id·in). Acetophenetidin, phenacetin, $CH_3CONHC_6H_4OC_2H_5$. A white crystalline compound, only sparingly soluble in water, used as an analgesic. It is a safer antipyretic than acetanilide.

para-actinomycosis (par·ah·ak·tin·o·mi·**ko**'·sis). Pseudo-actinomycosis. [Gk *para*, actinomycosis.]

para-agglutinin (par·ah·ag·**loo**'·tin·in). A partial agglutinin. [Gk *para*, agglutinin.]

para-amidophenetol (par·ah·**am**·id·o·**fen**'·et·ol). *p*-Aminophenetole, *p*-aminophenylethyl ether, phenetidin, $NH_2C_6H_4OC_2H_5$. A base used in the manufacture of dyestuffs, and also in the preparation of phenacetin and allied antipyretic drugs.

para-aminobenzoate (par·ah·**am**·in·o·**ben**'·zo·ate). Any salt or ester of para-aminobenzoic acid.

para-aminohippurate (par·ah·**am**·in·o·**hip**'·ewr·ate). A salt of para-aminohippuric acid.

para-amnesia (par·ah·am·**ne**'·ze·ah). 1. Distortion of memory with confabulation. 2. In a more restricted sense, *déja vu* phenomena. *See* DÉJA VU. [Gk *para*, amnesia.]

para-anaesthesia (par·ah·an·es·**the**'·ze·ah). Anaesthesia of the lower half of the body, including the legs. [Gk *para*, anaesthesia.]

para-analgesia (par·ah·an·al·**je**'·ze·ah). A condition of analgesia affecting the lower extremities and the lower part of the body. [Gk *para*, analgesia.]

para-appendicitis (par·ah·ap·en·dis·**i**'·tis). Inflammation of the vermiform appendix with extension to the adnexa. [Gk *para*, appendicitis.]

Parabelminus carioca (par·ah·**bel**·min·us kar·i·**o**·kah). A reduviid bug; a potential vector of American trypanosomiasis.

parabion, parabiont (par·**ab**·e·on, par·**ab**·e·ont). One of two or more individual organisms living in a state of parabiosis. [Gk *para*, *bion* a living thing.]

parabiosis (par·ah·bi·**o**'·sis). The experimental joining together of two individuals, whether adult or embryo. **Vascular parabiosis.** The experimental joining together of the circulations of two individuals; sometimes called *cross-circulation*. [Gk *para*, *bios* life.]

parabiotic (par·ah·bi·**ot**'·ik). Belonging to or having the nature of parabiosis.

parablast (par·ah·blast). That portion of the mesoderm which gives origin to the blood vessels, blood and other vascular structures. [Gk *para*, *blastos* germ.]

parablastic (par·ah·**blas**·tik). Belonging to or originating in the parablast.

parablastoma (par·ah·blas·**to**'·mah). A tumour formed from parablastic substance. [parablast, Gk *-oma* tumour.]

parablepsia, parablepsis (par·ah·**blep**·se·ah, par·ah·**blep**·sis). False or defective vision. [Gk *para*, *blepsis* sight.]

parabulia (par·ah·**bew**·le·ah). Abnormality of will power. [Gk *para*, *boule* will.]

Parabuthus (par·ah·**bew**·thus). A genus of South African scorpions.

paracaecitis (par·ah·se·**si**'·tis). Paratyphlitis. [Gk *para*, caecum, Gk *-itis* inflammation.]

paracaine (par·ah·kane). Procaine hydrochloride.

paracanthoma (par·ak·an·**tho**'·mah). A tumour occurring in the prickle-cell layer of the skin. [Gk *para*, *akantha* prickle, *-oma* tumour.]

paracanthosis (par·ak·an·**tho**'·sis). A condition in which a new growth of the skin or other developmental abnormality arises in the prickle-cell layer of the skin. [Gk *para*, *akantha* prickle, *-osis* condition.]

paracardiac (par·ah·**kar**·de·ak). Close to the heart. [Gk *para*, *kardia* heart.]

paracarmine (par·ah·**kar**·mine). An alcoholic solution of carminic acid, also containing calcium chloride; it is used as a histological stain: Mayer's paracarmine. [Gk *para*, carmine.]

See also: MAYER (P.).

paracasein (par·ah·**ka**·se·in). A term not included in British nomenclature, denoting the insoluble form of casein produced by the action of rennin. In the British system of nomenclature the soluble form is caseinogen and the insoluble form is casein. [Gk *para*, casein.]

paracentesis (par·ah·sen·**te**'·sis). Surgical puncture, tapping, or needling of a cavity for evacuation of harmful content, or for removal of fluid material for diagnosis. **Paracentesis abdominis.** Tapping of the abdomen by needle, usually for the removal of ascitic fluid. **Paracentesis auris.** Incision of the tympanic membrane in order to drain fluid from the middle-ear cavity. **Paracentesis bulbi.** Puncture of the eyeball. **Paracentesis capitis.** Removal of the fluid from the ventricle of the brain by needle for the treatment of hydrocephalus. **Paracentesis oculi.** Paracentesis bulbi (see above). **Paracentesis pericardii.** Aspiration of the pericardial sac for diagnosis or treatment of pericarditis. **Paracentesis pulmonis.** Puncture of the lung by needle. **Paracentesis thoracis.** Aspiration by needle of the fluid, or air, or both, from the pleural cavity. **Paracentesis tunica vaginalis.** Paracentesis of the tunica vaginalis testes for the relief of hydrocele. **Paracentesis tympani.** Puncture of the tympanic membrane for the drainage of an infected middle ear. **Paracentesis vesicae.** Withdrawal of fluid from the bladder by needle puncture for the relief of urinary obstruction. [Gk *para*, *kentesis* a puncturing.]

paracentetic (par·ah·sen·**tet**'·ik). Pertaining to paracentesis.

paracentral (par·ah·**sen**·tral). Lying close to a centre or central part. [Gk *para*, centre.]

paracephalus (par·ah·**kef**·al·us). A monster with an underdeveloped and malformed head, imperfect limbs and trunk, and undeveloped organs of the senses. [Gk *para*, *kephale* head.]

paracerebellar (par·ah·ser·e·**bel**'·ar). Belonging to the lateral part of the cerebellum. [Gk *para*, cerebellum.]

paracetaldehyde (par·as·et·**al**'·de·hide). Paraldehyde.

Paracetamol BP 1973 (par·**as**·et·am·ol). *p*-Acetamidophenol; an analgesic.

parachloralose (par·ah·**klor**·al·oze). $CCl_3C_7H_{11}O_6$, a compound isomeric with glucochloral and produced similarly by the action of chloral on glucose, but without the hypnotic properties of the former.

parachlorometacresol (par·ah·klor·o·met·ah·**kre**'·sol). Chlorocresol.

parachlorometaxylenol (par·ah·klor·o·met·ah·**zi**'·len·ol). Chloroxylenol, $OHC_6H_2(CH_3)_2Cl$. A powerful bacteriostatic used in the well-known "pine" disinfectants.

parachlorophenol (par·ah·klor·o·**fe**'·nol). HOC_6H_4Cl, a bacteriostatic used in lupus, phthisis, and in dental fillings.

parachlorphenol (par·ah·klor·**fe**'·nol). Parachlorophenol.

paracholera (par·ah·**kol**·er·ah). A condition resembling cholera clinically, but not due to the true cholera vibrio. The term is sometimes used for infection with *Vibrio cholerae El Tor.* [Gk *para,* cholera.]

paracholia (par·ah·**ko**·le·ah). Disorder of bile secretion. [Gk *para, chole* bile.]

parachordal (par·ah·**kord**·al). Pertaining to the paired cartilaginous plates flanking the anterior end of the notochord, from which the hind part of the base of the skull is derived. [Gk *para, chorde* cord.]

Parachordodes (par·ah·kor·**do**'·deez). A genus of Gordiacea. The adults, horse-hair worms, are free-living in fresh water; the larvae are parasitic in insects. In western Europe individuals of three species, *P. tolosanus, P. violaceus,* and *P. pustulosus,* are said to have been ingested and subsequently vomited. [Gk *para, chorde* cord, *eidos* form.]

parachroia (par·ah·**kroi**·ah). Abnormal complexion or colouring of the skin. [Gk *para, chroia* colour of skin.]

parachroma (par·ah·**kro**·mah). An alteration in the colour of the skin. [Gk *para, chroma* colour.]

parachromatin (par·ah·**kro**·mat·in). 1. The achromatic material which is believed to produce spindle fibres. 2. In contraposition to orthochromatin; that part of the chromatin which is thought to be unstable and particularly sensitive to the action of genetic and environmental factors. [Gk *para, chroma* colour.]

parachromatism (par·ah·**kro**·mat·izm). Faulty assessment of colour values, not amounting to true colour blindness. [see prec.]

parachromatoblepsia (par·ah·kro·mat·o·**blep**'·se·ah). Parachromatism. [Gk *para, chroma* colour, *blepsis* sight.]

parachromatopsia (par·ah·kro·mat·**op**'·se·ah). Colour blindness. [Gk *para, chroma* colour, *opsis* sight.]

parachromatosis (par·ah·kro·mat·**o**'·sis). Parachroma. [parachroma, Gk *-osis* condition.]

parachrosis (par·ah·**kro**·sis). The occurrence of a cutaneous disease which is characterized by pigmentation. [Gk *para, chros* colour.]

parachymosis (par·ah·ki·**mo**'·sis). A pathological condition affecting a secreting organ or a secretion. [Gk *para, chymos* juice.]

paracinesia, paracinesis (par·ah·sin·**e**'·se·ah, par·ah·sin·**e**'·sis). Parakinesia.

paracinetic (par·ah·sin·**et**'·ik). Parakinetic.

paraclonus (par·ah·**klo**·nus). Paramyoclonus multiplex. [Gk *para,* clonus.]

paracmastic (par·ak·**mas**·tik). 1. Abating. 2. Having a period of decline. 3. Pertaining to the paracme. [see foll.]

paracme (par·**ak**·me). 1. The phase of subsidence of a fever or disease. 2. In biology, the period of decline of life, the involutional stage. [Gk *para, akme* highest point.]

Paracoccidioides brasiliensis (par·ah·kok·sid·e·**oi**'·deez bras·il'·e·**en**·sis). The causative organism of paracoccidioidomycosis, appearing in tissue as large, spherical or oval cells bearing single or multiple buds. In culture at elevated temperatures the yeast form is reproduced; at room temperature the fungus grows slowly as a membranous, wrinkled colony which may form short, aerial mycelium. Occasionally a few sessile microconidia are produced. [Gk *para, kokkos* berry, *eidos* form, Sp. *brasil* Brazil.]

paracoccidioidomycosis (par·ah·kok·sid·e·oi·do·mi·**ko**'·sis). South American blastomycosis; a primary pulmonary disease which may disseminate to chronic granulomatous disease of skin, mucous membranes, lymph nodes and internal organs. It is due to infection by *Paracoccidioides brasiliensis.* [Gk *para, kokkos* berry, *eidos* form, *mykes* fungus, *-osis* condition.]

paracoele (par·ah·seel). One of the lateral ventricles of the brain. [Gk *para, koilos* hollow.]

paracoenaesthesia (par·ah·se·nes·**the**'·ze·ah). Any deviation from the normal functioning and state of well-being of the body. [Gk *para,* coenaesthesia.]

paracolic (par·ah·**kol**·ik). By the side of the colon. [Gk *para,* colon.]

paracolon (par·ah·**ko**·lon). An ill-defined group of Gram-negative bacilli belonging to the family Enterobacteriaceae. They ferment glucose with gas formation; lactic fermentation is delayed or negative. Certain species are regarded as pathogenic for man, causing gastroenteritis. [Gk *para,* colon.]

paracolpitis (par·ah·kol·**pi**'·tis). A condition of inflammation affecting the cellular tissues adjacent to the vagina. [Gk *para,* colpitis.]

paracolpium (par·ah·**kol**·pe·um). The tissues around the vagina. [Gk *para, kolpos* vagina.]

paracone (par·ah·kone). In the tritubercular theory of evolution, the name given to the anteroexternal cusp of an upper molar tooth. [Gk *para, konos* cone.]

paraconid (par·ah·**ko**·nid). The anteroexternal cusp of a lower molar tooth. [Gk *para, konos* cone.]

paraconiine, paraconin (par·ah·**ko**·ne·een, par·ah·**ko**·nin). $C_5H_8N(C_3H_7)$, a synthetic alkaloid related to coniine and prepared from butyric aldehyde; a poisonous liquid with a peculiar odour.

paracoto (par·ah·**ko**·to). A South American bark having a similarity to coto, obtained from an unidentified tree believed to be a laurel, *Ocotea pseudocoto* Rusby. It yields the crystalline substance, paracotoin. [Gk *para,* coto.]

paracotoin (par·ah·ko·**to**'·in). A crystalline principle obtained from paracoto, and used in the treatment of night-sweats.

paracousia, paracousis (par·ak·**oo**·se·ah, par·ak·**oo**·sis). Any abnormal condition of the hearing sense. **Paracousia duplicata.** Diplacusis. **Paracousia perversa, Paracousia willisii.** Increased acuity of hearing when a deaf subject is surrounded by noise. [Gk *para, akouein* to hear.]

See also: WILLIS.

paracoxalgia (par·ah·kox·**al**'·je·ah). Pain resembling that caused by inflammation of the hip joint (coxitis). [Gk *para,* coxalgia.]

paracresalol (par·ah·**kres**·al·ol). Salicylic ester of cresol, used mainly as an external antiseptic.

paracresol (par·ah·**kre**·sol). $HOC_6H_4CH_3$, one of the three isomers of cresol, used either alone or in the crude mixture, as a disinfectant.

paracrisis (par·ah·**kri**·sis). Any secretory disorder. [Gk *para, krisis* separation.]

paracrystals (par·ah·**kris**·talz). Crystals having two-dimensional symmetry, instead of three-dimensional; regarded as imperfect crystals. The description is applied to certain plant viruses in pure form, e.g. tobacco mosaic. [Gk *para,* crystal.]

paracusia, paracusis (par·ak·**ew**·se·ah, par·ak·**ew**·sis). Paracousia.

paracyesis (par·ah·si·**e**'·sis). Ectopic pregnancy. *See* PREGNANCY. [Gk *para, kyesis* pregnancy.]

paracynanche (par·ah·si·**nang**'·ke). Inflammation of the muscles and cellular tissue of the throat. [Gk *para,* cynanche.]

paracystic (par·ah·**sist**·ik). Surrounding or alongside of the bladder. [Gk *para, kystis* bag.]

paracystitis (par·ah·sist·**i**'·tis). A condition of inflammation affecting the connective and other tissues which adjoin or are near the bladder. [Gk *para,* cystitis.]

paracystium (par·ah·**sist**·e·um). The tissues adjoining the urinary bladder. [Gk *para, kystis* bag.]

paracytic (par·ah·**si**·tik). Denoting abnormal or extraneous cells found in the blood, body organs, or tissues. [Gk *para, kytos* cell.]

paradenitis (par·ad·en·**i**'·tis). Inflammation affecting the tissues which surround a gland. [Gk *para,* adenitis.]

paradental (par·ah·**den**·tal). Periodontic. [see foll.]

paradentium (par·ah·**den**'·she·um). Periodontium. [Gk *para,* L *dens* tooth.]

paradichlorobenzene (par·ah·di·klor·o·**ben**'·zeen). $C_6H_4Cl_2$, an insecticide of great value for the destruction of moths and furniture beetles.

paradidymal (par·ah·**did**·im·al). 1. Belonging to the paradidymis. 2. Situated beside or alongside the epididymis.

paradidymis [NA] (par·ah·**did**·im·is). A vestige of the mesonephros found anteriorly in the spermatic cord, a little above the head of the epididymis, and consisting of a few convoluted tubules. [Gk *para,* epididymis.]

paradimethylaminobenzaldehyde (par·ah·di·**meth**·il·am·in·o·ben·**zal'**·de·hide). $(CH_3)_2NC_6H_4CHO$, a reagent used for the detection and determination of the therapeutically active alkaloids of ergot, with which it gives a blue coloration.

paradioxybenzene (par·ah·di·ox·e·**ben'**·zeen). Hydroquinone, or quinol.

paradiphtherial, paradiphtheritic (par·ah·dif·**theer'**·e·al, par·ah·dif·ther·**it'**·ik). Having some resemblance to diphtheria. [Gk *para*, diphtheria.]

paradox (par·ah·dox). **Post-hypoxia paradox.** Usually the lowering of consciousness caused by hypoxia clears quickly when oxygen is given. Rarely there may be a transient deterioration of the level of consciousness after correcting the oxygen deficit in the inspired air, which may be accompanied by a convulsion; this is the *post-hypoxia paradox*. [Gk *paradoxos* strange.]

See also: WEBER (E. H.).

paradoxia (par·ah·**dox**·e·ah). Term applied to a scheme or statement that is apparently contrary to fact. **Paradoxia sexualis.** Sexual activity outside the appropriate age of corresponding physiological activity, i.e. before puberty, and in old age. [Gk *paradoxos* strange.]

paradysentery (par·ah·**dis**·en·ter·e). 1. A diarrhoeal condition which is like a mild type of dysenteric infection. 2. Dysentery due to *Shigella flexneri* and other organisms of the genus *Shigella* that have been included under the species *Shigella paradysenteriae* by American bacteriologists. [Gk *para*, dysentery.]

para-eccrisis (par·ah·**ek**·ris·is). Any disorder of excretion or secretion. [Gk *para*, eccrisis.]

para-enteric (par·ah·en·**ter'**·ik). 1. Paratyphoid. 2. Outside the intestinal tract. [Gk *para*, enteric.]

para-epilepsy (par·ah·ep·il·**ep'**·se). A non-convulsive type of epilepsy in which the attack consists of the aura only and consciousness is not lost. [Gk *para*, epilepsy.]

para-eponychia (par·ah·ep·o·**nik'**·e·ah). A paronychial and eponychial infection occurring simultaneously. [Gk *para*, eponychium.]

para-equilibrium (par·ah·e·kwil·**ib'**·re·um). Vertigo caused by a disordered condition of the vestibular apparatus of the ear, and sometimes accompanied by nausea, nystagmus and other reactions. [Gk *para*, equilibrium.]

paraesthesia (par·es·**the**·ze·ah). Numbness and tingling. [Gk *para*, *aisthesis* sensation.]

See also: BERGER (O.), BERNHARDT (M.).

paraesthetic (par·es·**thet**·ik). Of the nature of or affected with paraesthesia.

paraffin (par·ah·fin). The name given to any hydrocarbon or mixture of hydrocarbons of the paraffin series which can be represented by the chemical formula, $C_nH_{(2n+2)}$, and which constitute the most inactive of all organic compounds. Physically they show a gradation from the lower members (e.g. methane, ethane, propane) which are gases used as illuminants, through the liquid members, mixtures of which are sold as fuel (petrol, gasoline, kerosene, paraffin oil), or *liquid paraffin*, to the semisolids, petroleum jelly, employed as lubricants, and finally to the solid mixtures such as *paraffin wax*, or *hard paraffin* (*solid paraffin*) used for candles, polishes, for sealing vessels and for immobilizing limbs. **Surgical paraffin.** Liquid paraffin of a certain viscosity and suitably purified for medicinal purposes. [L *parum* little, *affinis* related.]

paraffinoma (par·ah·fin·**o'**·mah). 1. A chronic granuloma caused by constant exposure to paraffin or by the administration of paraffin by injection into the tissues. 2. A granulomatous condition of the pelvic colon, occurring in patients with diverticulosis of the pelvic colon who have been taking liquid paraffin as an aperient for a long time. [paraffin, Gk *-oma* tumour.]

paraffinum (par·ah·fi·num). The Latin name for paraffin, so called because of the chemical inertness of the group of hydrocarbons. [L *parum* little, *affinis* related.]

parafibrinogen (par·ah·fi·**brin'**·o·jen). A substance like fibrin which results from repeated salting-out of fibrinogen. [Gk *para*, fibrinogen.]

paraflagellate (par·ah·**flaj**·el·ate). Bearing one or more paraflagella.

paraflagellum (par·ah·flaj·**el'**·um). A small supernumerary flagellum. [Gk *para*, flagellum.]

paraflocculus (par·ah·**flok**·ew·lus). A small mass of grey matter sometimes present in the cerebellum and adjoining the flocculus. [Gk *para*, flocculus.]

parafollicular cell (par·ah·fol·**ik'**·u·lar sel). Of the thyroid gland, derived from the fourth branchial pouch. Sometimes referred to as C-cells because they secrete calcitonin.

paraform (par·ah·form). Paraformaldehyde.

Paraformaldehyde BPC 1968 (par·ah·for·**mal'**·de·hide). Trioxymethylene, $(CH_2O)_3$. A white solid polymer of formaldehyde, used as an antiseptic.

Parafossarulus (par·ah·fos·**ar'**·ew·lus). A genus of operculate fresh-water snails. **Parafossarulus striatulus.** A species found from India to Japan; the main secondary host of the fluke *Clonorchis sinensis*.

parafuchsine (par·ah·**fook**·seen). Pararosaniline chloride.

parafunction (par·ah·**fungk**·shun). An abnormality of function. [Gk *para*, function.]

parafunctional (par·ah·**fungk**·shun·al). Pertaining to perversion of function. [see prec.]

paragammacism, paragammacismus (par·ah·**gam**·ah·sizm, par·ah·gam·ah·**siz'**·mus). 1. The incorrect utterance of *g*, *k*, and *ch* sounds. 2. Substitution of other letters, e.g. *d*, *e*, for the letters *g* and *k*. [Gk *para*, *gamma* Gk letter G.]

paraganglioma (par·ah·gang·gle·**o'**·mah). A benign or malignant tumour of chromaffin cells found in the adrenal gland, and other derivatives of the sympathetic nervous system. [Gk *para*, ganglioma.]

paraganglion (par·ah·**gang**·gle·on). A small mass of chromaffin tissue found in close relationship with a sympathetic ganglion or in a sympathetic plexus. They are largest in the infant at birth, and tend subsequently to atrophy. **Paraganglion caroticum.** The carotid body, a mass of epithelioid cells with a few chromaffin cells, situated behind the common carotid artery at its bifurcation. It has a large nerve supply from the glossopharyngeal nerve, and is probably a chemoreceptor concerned in the regulation of blood pressure. [Gk *para*, ganglion.]

See also: WIESEL, WIESNER.

paraganglionoma (par·ah·gang·gle·on·**o'**·mah). Paraganglioma.

paragenitalis (par·ah·jen·it·**a'**·lis). That part of the embryonic mesonephros which persists as the paradidymis in the male and the paroöphoron in the female. [Gk *para*, L *genitalis* genital.]

parageusia (par·ah·**gew**·se·ah). 1. Abnormality of the sense of taste. 2. An offensive taste in the mouth. [Gk *para*, *geusis* a taste of a thing.]

paragglutination (par·ag·loo·tin·**a'**·shun). Group agglutination; the agglutination of several members of serologically related bacteria by a serum prepared specifically for one of the group, due to the presence in the serum of an agglutinin specific for one or more antigens common to other members of the group. It is well marked in the Salmonella group of organisms. Monospecific sera may be obtained by absorption of group agglutinins. [Gk *para*, agglutination.]

paraglobulin (par·ah·**glob**·ew·lin). Fibrinoplastin, serum globulin; a globulin present in blood serum, blood cells and in many connective tissues. [Gk *para*, globulin.]

paraglobulinuria (par·ah·**glob**·ew·lin·**ewr'**·e·ah). The passage of serum globulin in the urine. [Gk *para*, globulinuria.]

paraglossa (para·ah·**glos**·ah). Swelling or hypertrophy of the tongue. [Gk *para*, *glossa* tongue.]

paraglossia, paraglossitis (par·ah·**glos**·e·ah, par·ah·glos·**i'**·tis). An inflammatory condition of the sublingual tissues. [see prec.]

paragnathous (par·**ag**·nath·us). Characterized by the existence of an accessory jaw, e.g. in certain monsters. [Gk *para*, *gnathos* jaw.]

paragnathus (par·ag·**nath**·us). A monster with an accessory mandible, generally on one side of the face. [see prec.]

paragnosis (par·ag·**no**·sis). Posthumous diagnosis based on historical descriptions of the symptoms of famous personages. [Gk *para, gnosis* knowledge.]

paragonimiasis (par·ah·gon·im·**i**′·as·is). The state of being infected by the lung fluke, genus *Paragonimus.*

Paragonimus (par·ah·**gon**·im·us). A genus of lung flukes. Three species are generally recognized, *P. kellicotti* from mink in North America, *P. ringeri* from man in Taiwan and *P. westermani* from a tiger from Bengal; a fourth, *P. compactus,* has also been described as possibly infecting man, but it is not clear whether these are good species or, if so, where exactly they occur. Infestations in man occur throughout the tropical Far East, Japan, Korea, North and Central Americas and eastern regions of Nigeria. The adults are surrounded by cysts of host tissue in the bronchi; these burst to liberate eggs which reach the exterior in the sputum. Secondary hosts are operculate freshwater snails, particularly *Melania* species in the Far East, *Pomatopsis lapidaria* in North America, and *Ampullaria luteostoma* in Central America. The cercariae encyst in crustacea, particularly crabs (*Eriocheir* and *Potamon* species) and crayfish (*Astacus* species) in the Far East, crayfish (*Cambarus* species) in North America, and crabs (*Pseudothelphusa iturbei*) in Central America. [Gk *para, gonimos,* generative.]

Paragordius (par·ah·**gor**·de·us). A genus of Gordiacea. The adults, horse-hair worms, are free-living; the larvae are parasitic in insects. In western Europe and North America individuals of two species, *P. tricuspedatus* and *P. varius,* are said to have been ingested and subsequently vomited. [Gk *para,* Gordiacea.]

paragrammatism (par·ah·**gram**·at·izm). A defect of speech in which the patient uses wrong words and is incapable of arranging words in their correct grammatical sequence, as well as the certain incorrect use of words by schizophrenics. Cf. APHASIA. [Gk *para, gramma* letter.]

paragranuloma (par·ah·gran·ew·**lo**′·mah). A benign form of Hodgkin's disease affecting lymph glands only. [Gk *para,* granuloma.]

paragraphia (par·ah·**graf**·e·ah). 1. A condition noted in persons suffering from certain mental diseases, characterized by spelling errors and the use of an incorrect word instead of the intended one. 2. A disorder marked by absence of the power to write from dictation. [Gk *para, graphein* to write.]

parahaematin (par·ah·**he**·mat·in). A compound of haematin with denatured globin. Reduced in alkaline solution, it forms haemochromogen. [Gk *para,* haematin.]

parahaemoglobin (par·ah·he·mo·**glo**′·bin). A form of crystalline haemoglobin found in tissues where there has been severe haemolysis. [Gk *para,* haemoglobin.]

parahaemophilia (par·ah·he·mo·**fil**′·e·ah). Congenital haemorrhagic diathesis: a congenital haemorrhagic disease resembling haemophilia but having a prolonged clotting time of venous blood, and a prolonged one-stage prothrombin time; it is associated with deficiency of Factor V (Owren). [Gk *para,* haemophilia.]

parahepatic (par·ah·hep·**at**′·ik). Lying alongside or adjacent to the liver. [GK *para, hepar* liver.]

parahepatitis (par·ah·hep·at·**i**′·tis). Inflammation affecting the structures beside or around the liver. [Gk *para,* hepatitis.]

parahidrosis (par·ah·hid·**ro**′·sis). Any abnormal condition of the sweat secretion. [Gk *para, hidros* sweat.]

parahypnosis (par·ah·hip·**no**′·sis). Disordered sleep as occurs in hypnosis or narcosis. [Gk *para, hypnos* sleep.]

para-infection (par·ah·in·**fek**′·shun). A disease which in all respects resembles an infectious disease, but in which the micro-organisms typical of that disease are not present. [Gk *para,* infection.]

para-infectious (par·ah·in·**fek**′·shus). 1. Connected with or coming after infection. 2. Caused by the state induced by infection and not by the infection itself. [see prec.]

para-influenza (par·ah·in·floo·**en**′·zah). Strictly, an infection due to a para-influenza virus which may cause any syndrome from inapparent infection to a severe upper respiratory tract infection with or without croup. The diagnosis depends on laboratory rather than clinical evidence. [Gk *para,* influenza.]

para-influenza virus (par·ah·in·floo·**en**′·zah **vi**·rus). An enveloped RNA-containing virus associated with upper respiratory tract infections in man and morphologically identical with other paramyxoviruses and measles virus. The virus is pleomorphic in appearance and there are four genetically stable serological types: 1. (*syn* haemadsorption virus type 2, newborn pneumonitis virus, haemagglutinating virus of Japan (HVJ, Sendai)); 2. (*syn.* croup-associated virus); 3. (*syn.* haemadsorption virus type 1, bovine shipping fever virus); and 4. (with two subtypes 4a and 4b). Simian virus type 5 (SV5), found as an apparent commensal in monkey tissues, is closely related to para-influenza type 2, and may be identical with it. Para-influenza viruses have surface haemagglutinin and neuraminidase antigens, and most can fuse cells in culture even when inactivated with formalin.

para-influenzal (par·ah·in·floo·**en**′·zal). 1. Indirectly connected with influenza. 2. Consequent upon an attack of influenza.

parakeratosis (par·ah·ker·at·**o**′·sis). Imperfect formation of horn cells of the epidermis characterized by the persistence of nuclei, incomplete formation of keratin, and moistness and swelling of the horn cells. **Parakeratosis brillante** (Gougerot). Pseudo-atrophoderma colli. **Parakeratosis gonorrhoeica.** Keratoderma blenorrhagica. **Parakeratosis ostracea.** Parakeratosis scutularis (see below). **Parakeratosis pityriasiformis, Parakeratosis pityroides.** A variety of eczematid with fine scaling. **Parakeratosis psoriasiformis.** A variety of eczematid resembling psoriasis. **Parakeratosis pustulosa.** A chronic scaly condition around the nails of the fingers and toes of children. **Parakeratosis scutularis.** A very rare dermatosis with livid red patches containing horny balls and large shield-shaped scales, with adherent horny frills enclosing bundles of hairs on the scalp. **Parakeratosis variegata.** A rare chronic dermatosis, resistant to treatment, consisting of yellowish-red lichenoid network with a little fine scaling; probably closely related to parapsoriasis en plaques. [Gk *para, keras* horn, *-osis* condition.]

parakinesis (par·ah·kin·**e**′·sis). Any abnormality of movement in the muscles due to a nervous affection; in ophthalmology, irregularity of action of one of the ocular muscles. [Gk *para, kinesis* motion.]

parakinetic (par·ah·kin·**et**′·ik). Suffering from or pertaining to parakinesia.

parakrine (par·ah·krine). Applied to hormones which act solely on the cells immediately neighbouring those which secrete them. Mainly applied to gastro-intestinal hormones.

paralactate (par·ah·**lak**·tate). Any salt of paralactic acid.

paralalia (par·ah·**la**·le·ah). An abnormality of speech characterized particularly by the habitual substitution of one letter for another or the utterance of a sound other than the one intended. **Paralalia literalis.** Loss of the ability to utter the sounds of specific letters. [Gk *para, lalia* talking.]

paralambdacism (par·ah·**lam**·dah·sizm). A condition in which the letter *l* is mispronounced or in which another consonant is substituted for it. [Gk *para, lambda* Gk letter L.]

Paraldehyde BP 1973 (par·**al**·de·hide). 1. $(CH_3CHO)_n$, a mixture of polymers of acetaldehyde obtained by treating the latter with a drop of concentrated sulphuric acid followed by purification. It is a hypnotic and can be administered orally, intravenously, or per rectum, being dissolved in water, normal saline, or olive oil respectively. 2. The trimeric compound $(CH_3CHO)_3$ produced by the polymerization of acetaldehyde.

paraldehydism (par·**al**·de·hi·dizm). The toxic state caused by abuse of paraldehyde.

Paraldehydum. *European Pharmacopoeia* name for Paraldehyde BP 1973.

paraleipsis (par·ah·**li**·psis). Any abnormality of the sebaceous outflow. [Gk *para, aleipsein* to anoint.]

paraleprosis, paraleprosy (par·ah·lep·**ro**′·sis, par·ah·**lep**·ro·se). Ill-conceived words that are said to mean a mild type of leprosy. [Gk *para,* leprosy.]

paralepsy (par·ah·lep·se). Psycholepsy. [Gk *para*, epilepsy.]

paralerema (par·ah·ler·e′·mah). Delirium or the utterances of delirious individuals. [see foll.]

paraleresis (par·ah·ler·e′·sis). Delirium or a mild type of mental defect. [Gk *paralereein* to talk great nonsense.]

paralexia (par·ah·lex·e·ah). Inability to read correctly, characterized by the substitution or transference of words or syllables. [Gk *para, lexis* diction.]

paralexic (par·ah·lex·ik). Belonging to or suffering from paralexia.

paralgesia (par·al·je·ze·ah). 1. Paraesthesia marked by the occurrence of pain. 2. A condition in which sensation in the skin is abnormal and unpleasant, e.g. there is a sensation of cold or of heat or of formication. [Gk *para, algos* pain.]

paralgesic (par·al·je·zik). Suffering from or characterized by paralgesia.

paralgia (par·al·je·ah). Paralgesia.

paralgic (par·al·jik). Paralgesic.

paralipophobia (par·ah·li·po·fo′·be·ah). Abnormal dread of being neglectful of something, even of trivial nature. [Gk *paraleipein* to neglect, phobia.]

parallactic (par·al·ak·tik). Relating to a parallax.

parallagma (par·al·ag·mah). Displacement of a bone or overlapping of the ends of a fractured bone. [Gk, exchange.]

parallax (par·al·ax). The apparent movement, relative to each other, of two objects at different distances from the eye, when the observer's head is moved. **Binocular parallax.** The basis of stereoscopic vision and depth perception: when the eyes alter fixation from a distant object to one nearer, the former becomes double, the image on the right belonging to the right eye, that on the left to the left eye. **Crossed parallax.** Heteronymous parallax (see below). **Direct parallax.** Homonymous parallax (see below). **Entopic parallax.** A method by which the position of opacities in the eye can be estimated from their movement, relative to the pupil or to the reflection by the cornea of the source of light, when the patient moves his eye. **Heteronymous parallax.** A form of parallax in which, when one eye is covered, an object viewed by the open eye seems to move towards the former. **Homonymous parallax.** A phenomenon in stereoscopic parallax: when fixation is changed from a near to a distant object, the near object becomes double, the right image belonging to the left eye and the left one to the right eye. **Stereoscopic parallax,** the phenomena of parallax in relation to stereoscopic vision. [Gk, in turn.]

parallelism (par·al·el·izm). The state of being parallel or similar. Automatism. **Parallelism of disease.** The tendency of some diseased conditions to resemble other diseases. [Gk *parallelos* side by side.]

parallelometer (par·al·el·om′·et·er). An instrument used in dentistry for ensuring that planes or surfaces are parallel to one another. [parallel, meter.]

parallergia (par·al·er·je·ah). Parallergy.

parallergic (par·al·er·jik). Relating to or characterized by an allergic state in which the body acquires a susceptibility to non-specific stimuli after it has first been sensitized with a specific allergen. [Gk *para*, allergy.]

parallergin (par·al·er·jin). An antigenic substance which is capable of causing a parallergic reaction.

parallergy (par·al·er·je). A state in which an allergic condition caused by sensitization with a special allergen creates a tendency in the body to react to non-specific stimuli. [Gk *para*, allergy.]

paralodion (par·ah·lo·de·on). Partially dried and shredded nitrocellulose used in the preparation of histological embedding media. [Gk *para*, collodion.]

paralogia (par·ah·lo·je·ah). False reasoning. **Thematic paralogia.** Mental disorder in which the patient dwells unduly on one subject. [Gk *para, logos* reason.]

paralogism (par·al·o·jizm). 1. False or illogical reasoning. 2. The utterance of nonsensical or illogical words by insane individuals. [see prec.]

paralogy (par·al·o·je). Paralogia.

paralyse (par·al·ize). To affect with paralysis; to produce paralysis in the body or in any part or structure of it. [Gk *paralyein* to be palsied.]

paralyser (par·al·i·zer). 1. Any substance or action that is able to bring about paralysis. 2. Any substance which, by its poisoning effect upon the catalyst, slows down or prevents a chemical action. [Gk *paralyein* to be palsied.]

paralysis (par·al·is·is). Loss of motor power due to a functional or organic disorder of neural or neuromuscular mechanisms; also called *palsy.* **Abducens paralysis.** Paralysis of the external rectus muscle of the orbit due to a lesion involving the 6th cranial nerve or its nucleus. The eye will be convergent, and diplopia will be present on looking to the side of the lesion. **Abductor paralysis.** Paralysis of abduction, especially of the vocal cords. **Absolute pupillary paralysis.** Complete paralysis of the pupil with dilatation, which is unaffected by light or accommodation reflexes, direct or consensual. It is caused by a lesion of the 3rd cranial nerve nucleus or its efferent pathway. **Paralysis of accommodation.** Paralysis of the ciliary muscle, causing inability to focus near objects. It may be due to a lesion of the 3rd cranial nerve or Edinger–Westphal nucleus (affecting the parasympathetic fibres), or the local effect of a cycloplegic drug, e.g. atropine. **Acoustic paralysis.** Nerve deafness. *See* DEAFNESS. **Acute amyotrophic paralysis.** Any acute illness with rapid muscular wasting owing to disease of anterior horn cells or motor nerves. One form, neuralgic amyotrophy or shoulder-girdle neuritis, is believed to be a virus infection and commonly follows trauma or a febrile illness. It is characterized by severe pain and rapid wasting of shoulder-girdle muscles. The term can also be applied to acute anterior poliomyelitis. **Acute ascending paralysis.** A condition of multiple aetiology, characterized by successive flaccid paralysis of legs, trunk, arms and muscles of respiration. Some cases are due to poliomyelitis, others to acute infectious polyneuritis; others are perhaps of biochemical origin. Also called *Landry's paralysis.* **Acute atrophic paralysis.** Acute anterior poliomyelitis. *See* POLIOMYELITIS. **Acute infectious paralysis.** This unsatisfactory term usually refers to acute anterior poliomyelitis, but can be applied to infectious polyneuritis. **Acute progressive paralysis.** Acute ascending paralysis (see above). **Acute spreading paralysis.** A spreading paralysis of which there are several forms; Landry's paralysis is a good example, though not all forms are reversible. **Acute wasting paralysis.** Acute paralysis owing to muscular wasting. **Paralysis agitans.** Parkinsonism, the shaking palsy: a condition of late middle life, characterized by mask-like facies, rigidity of the limbs with tremor of the hands of the "pill-rolling" type, a festinant gait and a general clumsiness of muscular movements. It is due to degenerative changes in the corpus striatum. **Paralysis agitans, juvenile.** The parkinsonian syndrome developing in early life, due to degeneration of the globus pallidus. **Alcoholic paralysis.** Paralysis due to alcoholic peripheral neuropathy. **Alternate paralysis, Alternating paralysis.** Paralysis which affects cranial nerves on one side of the body and the opposite limbs; due to a lesion in or near the brain stem. **Amaurotic pupillary paralysis.** Loss of the direct pupil reaction to light, associated with blindness on the same side, caused by damage to the retina or optic nerve. The consensual reaction from the stimulation of the normal pupil on the good side is retained. **Ambiguo-accessorius paralysis.** Schmidt's syndrome; paralysis of the soft palate, larynx, neck muscles, sternocleidomastoid muscle and trapezius muscle. **Ambiguo-accessorius-hypoglossal paralysis.** Jackson's syndrome; hemilateral associated paralysis of the larynx, soft palate, tongue and muscles of the neck. **Ambiguohypoglossal paralysis.** Tapia's syndrome; paralysis of the tongue and larynx. **Ambiguospino-accessorius paralysis.** Palatolaryngeal hemiparesis. **Ambiguospinothalamic paralysis.** Avellis' syndrome. **Amyotrophic paralysis.** Paralysis due to muscular wasting of neuropathic origin. **Anaesthesia paralysis.** Paralysis after administration of an anaesthetic; it can be of various types, including lesions of the brachial plexus after general anaesthesia in Trendelenburg's position, and a variety of

paralysis

complications, affecting the lower limbs particularly, after spinal anaesthesia. **Anapeiratic paralysis.** Occupational paralysis (see below). **Anterior spinal paralysis.** Acute anterior poliomyelitis. *See* POLIOMYELITIS. **Arsenical paralysis.** Peripheral neuropathy due to disease of the spinal cord or motor roots, which spreads in a cephalic direction. **Ascending tick paralysis.** Progressive spinal paralysis which extends upwards towards the brain, due to the bite and continued attachment to the body of certain ticks. It has been reported mainly from the USA and is chiefly of importance in children and small domestic animals. In treatment it is essential to remove the tick. **Association paralysis.** Progressive bulbar paralysis (see below). **Asthenic bulbar paralysis.** Myasthenia gravis affecting bulbar muscles. **Asthenobulbospinal paralysis.** Myasthenia gravis. **Atrophic muscular paralysis.** Paralysis due to muscular atrophy; applied particularly to progressive muscular atrophy (motor neuron disease). **Atrophic spinal paralysis.** Muscular wasting of spinal origin due to disease of anterior horn cells; either inflammatory (acute anterior poliomyelitis) or degenerative (motor neuron disease). **Atrophospastic paralysis.** Amyotrophic lateral sclerosis; a form of motor neuron disease giving muscular wasting in the upper limbs and spasticity of the lower extremities. **Axillary paralysis.** Paralysis of the deltoid muscle due to a lesion of the circumflex nerve. **Basal-ganglionic paralysis.** Weakness due to a lesion of the basal ganglia, as in paralysis agitans. **Bifacial paralysis.** Paralysis of both sides of the face. **Birth paralysis.** Paralysis, usually of an upper limb due to a brachial plexus lesion; due to an injury during delivery. **Brachial paralysis.** Paralysis of an arm. **Brachiofacial paralysis.** Paralysis affecting the face and an arm. **Bulbar paralysis.** Progressive bulbar paralysis (see below). **Bulbospinal paralysis.** Progressive bulbar paralysis with disease of the pyramidal tracts. **Capsular paralysis.** Paralysis due to a lesion of the pyramidal fibres in the internal capsule. **Central paralysis.** Paralysis due to a lesion of the spinal cord or brain. **Centrocapsular paralysis.** Paralysis resulting from a lesion of the internal capsule. **Centrocortical paralysis.** Paralysis due to disease of the cerebral cortex. **Cerebral paralysis.** Paralysis of cerebral origin. **Cerebral infantile ataxic paralysis.** One form of congenital diplegia, probably due to cerebral maldevelopment, giving spasticity of the lower limbs, ataxia, and perhaps mental defect. **Cerebral spastic infantile paralysis.** Congenital spastic paraplegia. **Cerebrocerebellar infantile diplegic paralysis.** A term covering the wide variety of types of infantile diplegia in which spasticity, involuntary movements, mental defect and severe ataxia may occur, suggesting disease of cerebral hemispheres, cerebellum and basal ganglia. **Cerebrospinal hereditary paralysis.** A rare hereditary condition, often beginning in adolescence, and usually giving a spastic paraplegia, although hemiplegia or quadriplegia may occur. It is usually called *congenital spastic paraplegia,* or *diplegia.* **Cervical sympathetic paralysis.** Horner's syndrome. **Chlorotic paralysis.** Paralysis occurring in patients with chlorosis. **Circumflex paralysis.** Paralysis of the circumflex nerve. **Complete paralysis.** Total loss of motility. **Compression paralysis.** Paralysis resulting from nerve compression. **Conjugate paralysis.** Paralysis of the conjugate movements of the two eyes together, either upwards or downwards, to right or left. The fixation axes remain parallel, and there is absence of diplopia. The lesion is situated above the 3rd, 4th and 6th cranial nerve nuclei. **Convergence paralysis.** A paralysis of the convergence of the eyes, with full movement of the internal rectus muscles in all conjugate movements, due to a lesion of the convergence centre in the mid-brain or its afferent or efferent connections. It is common in postencephalitis. **Cortical paralysis.** That resulting from a lesion of the cerebral cortex. **Creeping paralysis.** A vague term applied to several forms of paralysis, especially tabes dorsalis and paralysis agitans. **Crossed paralysis, Cruciate paralysis.** Unilateral cranial-nerve paralysis with contralateral hemiplegia, due to a brain-stem lesion involving cranial-nerve nuclei and the pyramidal tract. **Crural paralysis.** Paralysis of the leg, and particularly the thigh. **Crutch paralysis.** Paralysis of one or both upper limbs due to compression of the brachial plexus by the pressure of a crutch in the axilla. **Decubitus paralysis.** Paralysis from nerve compression due to lying in one position for a prolonged period. **Dental paralysis.** Acute anterior poliomyelitis of bulbar type, occurring after teeth extraction or in teething children. **Diphtheric paralysis, Diphtheritic paralysis.** An important sequela of diphtheria, occurring in the second or third week of convalesence, and affecting the palate, eye, limbs, trunk, diaphragm and intercostals. It may be arrested at any stage and is due to a toxin produced by the diphtheria bacilli at the site of the lesion. **Divergence paralysis.** A paralysis of divergence of the eyes with full movement of the external rectus muscles in all conjugate movements. It is due to a lesion of the brain stem. **Divers' paralysis.** Caisson disease. *See* DISEASE. **Drummers' paralysis.** A paralysis of extension of the terminal phalanx of the left thumb, occurring in drummers. **Drunkards'-arm paralysis.** Paralysis of the radial nerve due to falling asleep after a drinking bout, with the arm hanging over the back of a chair; also called *Sunday-morning paralysis, Saturday-night paralysis.* **Emotional paralysis.** Hysterical paralysis (see below), consequent upon emotional stress. **Epidemic infantile paralysis.** Acute anterior poliomyelitis. *See* POLIOMYELITIS. **Epidural ascending spinal paralysis.** A syndrome of transient root pains, ascending paralysis, sensory loss, sphincter disorder and amyotrophy, due to spinal pachymeningitis with thrombophlebitis of dural veins. **Essential paralysis.** Paralysis of unknown aetiology. **Exhaustion paralysis.** Paralysis owing to exhaustion or overwork; usually hysterical as in battle exhaustion. **External ocular paralysis.** Paralysis of the external ocular muscles, including the levator palpebrae superioris. **Extra-ocular paralysis.** Paralysis of the extrinsic muscles of the eye. **Facial paralysis.** Any paralysis of the facial musculature. The peripheral, nuclear, or infranuclear types causes paralysis of all muscles of the affected side of the face; the supranuclear or upper motor neuron type affects only the lower half of the face. **Familial periodic paralysis.** A rare familial disorder characterized by attacks of generalized flaccid paralysis, often on waking; the attacks, which may be precipitated by the administration of glucose, are due to hypokalaemia and may be relieved by the administration of a potassium salt. In some forms the serum potassium is increased. **Familial recurrent paralysis.** Attacks of familial periodic paralysis (see prec.) which are unduly prolonged. **Fascicular paralysis.** A paralysis of individual eye muscles due to a lesion situated in the course of the 3rd, 4th or 6th cranial nerves between the nuclei and point of emergence from the brain stem. It is characterized by simultaneous paralysis of opposite extremities. Also called *stem paralysis.* **Paralysis festinans.** The festinant gait of paralysis agitans; the patient walks with the body thrown forward as if chasing his own centre of gravity. **Flaccid paralysis.** The type of paralysis in which the affected muscles lose their tone completely, and tendon reflexes depending upon the muscles concerned for their activity are diminished or lost. **Functional paralysis.** Paralysis not due to organic disease; hysterical paralysis (see below). **Galloping paralysis.** A form of general paralysis with very rapid progression of the disease. **General paralysis, General paralysis of the insane.** Dementia paralytica found in late stages of syphilis; a condition characterized by progressive dementia, often with delusions of grandeur. Tremor of the lips and tongue is common and there may be progressive spastic paralysis of the extremities. Pathologically there is severe atrophy of the anterior two-thirds of the brain. **Ginger paralysis.** A polyneuropathy, affecting particularly motor nerves to the distal portions of the extremities, caused by contamination of liquor with tricresyl phosphate. It was first recognized in Jamaica, and called *Jamaica ginger* or *Jamaica jake paralysis.* **Glossolabial paralysis.** Glossopharyngeal paralysis (see below). **Glossolabiolaryngeal paralysis.** Progressive bulbar paralysis affecting the muscles of the lips, tongue and larynx. **Glossopharyngeal paralysis.** Progressive bulbar paralysis, affecting the muscles of the tongue, lip and pharynx. **Hemianopic pupillary paralysis.** Loss of the direct reaction to light of both pupils in cases of hemianopia, when a thin beam of light is directed from the blind side. The lesion must be situated distal to the point where the pupillary pathways leave the optic tract. *See* WERNICKE'S HEMIANOPIC PUPIL REACTION. **Hemiplegic paralysis.** Loss of power and function on one side of the body, including the face, head, trunk, and upper and lower limbs. **Histrionic paralysis.** Name given to facial paralysis (Bell's palsy) since the facial expression is altered radically. **Hypoglossal paralysis.** Paralysis of one-half of the tongue due to injury or disease of the hypoglossal nerve or its nucleus. **Hypokalaemic paralysis.** Periodic paralysis associated with low serum potassium levels. **Hysterical paralysis.** Paralysis or muscular weakness of hysterical origin. **Immunological paralysis.** Immunological tolerance. *See* TOLERANCE. **Incomplete paralysis.** Paresis; partial paralysis. **Indian-bow paralysis.** Paralysis of the extrinsic muscles of the larynx. **Infantile paralysis.** Acute anterior poliomyelitis. *See* POLIOMYELITIS. **Infantile spastic paralysis.** Cerebral diplegia; Little's disease. **Infantile spinal paralysis.** Acute anterior poliomyelitis. *See* POLIOMYELITIS. **Infranuclear paralysis.** A paralysis of individual eye muscles due to a lesion situated in the course of the 3rd, 4th or 6th cranial nerves below the nuclei. It is characterized by diplopia and involvement of the pupil and ciliary muscle. **Internal ocular paralysis.** Paralysis of the ciliary muscle and the contractor muscle of the pupil, causing loss of accommodation and a dilated pupil. **Ischaemic paralysis.** Paralysis due to muscular infarction or nerve ischaemia, e.g. Volkmann's ischaemic contracture. **Jake paralysis, Jamaica ginger paralysis, Jamaica jake paralysis.** Ginger paralysis (see above). **Juvenile paralysis.** General paralysis of the insane in young people, usually due to congenital syphilis. **Juvenile paralysis agitans.** Paralysis agitans, juvenile (see above). **Labial paralysis, Labioglossolaryngeal paralysis.** Progressive bulbar paralysis, affecting muscles of the lips or of the lips, tongue and larynx. **Laryngeal paralysis.** Paralysis of the intrinsic muscles of the larynx. **Lateral-gaze paralysis.** Paralysis of the external rectus muscle of the orbit contralaterally. It is found with a lesion of the pons, and is sometimes accompanied by paralysis of lateral rotation of the head. **Lead paralysis.** Paralysis due to myopathy caused by lead poisoning; once thought to be due to a lead neuritis. **Lenticular paralysis.** Paralysis due to disease of the lenticular nucleus. **Lingual paralysis.** Paralysis of the tongue. **Local paralysis.** Paralysis which is confined to a single muscle or to a group of muscles, or to one part of a member. **Lumbosacral-cord paralysis.** Paralysis following parturition, resulting from pressure of the fetal head on the lumbosacral cord. **Masticatory paralysis.** Paralysis of the muscles innervated by the trigeminal nerve, the masticatory muscles. **Medullary tegmental paralysis.** Several types of paralysis produced by lesions of the tegmentum of the medulla, including Cestan–Chenais syndrome, Tapia's syndrome, and the Babinski–Nageotte syndrome. **Mesencephalic paralysis.** Crossed hemiplegia due to a mid-brain lesion. **Mimetic paralysis.** Paralysis of the facial musculature. **Mixed paralysis.** Combined motor and sensory defects. **Morning paralysis.** 1. Familial periodic paralysis; attacks are often worse in the early morning. 2. Drunkard's-arm paralysis; Sunday-morning paralysis. **Motor paralysis.** Paralysis of motor nerves or pathways and hence of voluntary muscles. **Multiple paralysis.** Paralysis affecting several limbs. **Musculospiral paralysis.** Paralysis of muscles supplied by the radial nerve, chiefly the wrist and finger extensors, giving rise to a dropped wrist. **Myogenic paralysis, Myopathic paralysis.** Paralysis owing to primary disease of muscle, as in muscular dystrophy. **Myosclerotic paralysis.** Pseudohypertrophic muscular dystrophy; the term can also be applied to cases of chronic dermatomyositis. **Narcosis paralysis.** Anaesthesia paralysis (see above); postanaesthetic paralysis. **Neural paralysis.** Neuropathic muscular weakness; paralysis due to disease of nerves. **Night nurses' paralysis.** Affective hypotonia; a form of temporary immobility provoked by startle. **Notariorum paralysis.** Writers' cramp, an occupational neurosis. **Nuclear paralysis.** Paralysis due to a lesion of a nerve nucleus in the central nervous system; usually applied to lesions of the nuclei of motor cranial nerves, and especially to the 3rd, 4th and 6th cranial nerves in the mid-brain. **Obstetric paralysis.** Birth palsy; paralysis due to injury to the infant during parturition. **Occupational paralysis.** Weakness due to excessive use of certain muscles, to nerve compression in the course of an occupation, or to any other cause incidental to a specific occupation. **Oculomotor paralysis.** Paralysis of either all or some of the ocular muscles supplied by the 3rd cranial nerve (superior, inferior and internal rectus; inferior oblique and levator palpebrae superioris). In complete paralysis there is ptosis, the eye being rotated outwards and slightly downwards, the pupil dilated and accommodation paralysed. It is caused by a lesion involving the 3rd cranial nerve or its nucleus. **Oculophrenicorecurrent paralysis.** A combination of Horner's syndrome and phrenic and recurrent laryngeal nerve paralysis, due to an upper mediastinal lesion. **Organic paralysis.** Paralysis due to an organic, as distinct from a functional, lesion of the neuromuscular system. **Parotitic paralysis.** Paralysis complicating mumps; usually due to an allergic encephalopathy, as is the case with paralytic complications of most infectious fevers. **Periodic paralysis.** Recurrent attacks of muscular weakness. **Peripheral paralysis.** That due to a lesion somewhere between the nerve cells of origin of a motor nerve within the central nervous system and the motor end-plate in the muscle. **Peroneal paralysis.** Crossed-leg palsy. *See* PALSY. **Phonetic paralysis.** Paralysis of the laryngeal muscles concerned with phonation, and hence of the vocal cords. **Postdiphtheritic paralysis.** Diphtheritic paralysis (see above). **Posthemiplegic paralysis.** A residual hemiplegia. **Posticus paralysis.** Paralysis of abduction of the vocal cords as may occur in a laryngeal crisis of tabes dorsalis; a very unsatisfactory term, rarely used in the UK. **Pressure paralysis.** Paralysis caused by pressure upon a nerve. **Progressive bulbar paralysis.** The bulbar form of motor neuron disease in which wasting, weakness and fasciculation of laryngeal, pharyngeal, tongue and facial muscles occur, giving rise to progressive dysarthria and dysphagia. There may also be evidence of pyramidal-tract disease in the extremities. **Pseudobulbar paralysis.** A condition resembling progressive bulbar paralysis, in which dysarthria and dysphagia occur but may be associated with gross emotional lability. In this case the weakness of bulbar muscles is of upper motor neuron type; the condition results from multiple bilateral infarcts of the cerebral cortex in an artherosclerotic individual. **Pseudohypertrophic muscular paralysis.** Pseudohypertrophic muscular dystrophy. *See* DYSTROPHY. **Psychic paralysis.** Hysterical paralysis (see above). **Reflex paralysis.** Paralysis of muscles supplied by a motor nerve resulting from sensory irritation in the distribution of the corresponding sensory nerve. **Reflex pupillary paralysis.** A loss of the direct and consensual pupil reaction to light, with normal vision and near reflex, e.g. Argyll Robertson pupil. The lesion is situated somewhere between the 3rd cranial-nerve nucleus and the point where the pupillary motor fibres decussate centrally after leaving the optic tract. **Root paralysis.** Paralysis of ocular muscles due to a lesion involving the 3rd, 4th and 6th cranial nerves at their exit from the brain. It is characterized by the involvement of all muscles supplied by the nerve concerned. **Saturday-night paralysis.** Drunkards'-arm paralysis (see above). **Segmental paralysis.** Paralysis of muscles supplied by the anterior horn cells of one segment of the spinal cord. **Sensory paralysis.** Loss of sensation. **Serum paralysis.** A paralysis which may follow the injection of serum. Single nerves (e.g. the nerve to the serratus anterior muscle) may sometimes be involved; on other occasions there is extensive motor root involvement, affecting particularly muscles of the shoulder girdle. **Sleep paralysis.** A state experienced by a person while going to sleep (predormitial) or on waking (postdormitial); consciousness is present but muscular movement is lost as well as the ability to speak. Usually seen in patients otherwise normal but may be associated with narcolepsy or other forms of sleep disturbance (*syn.* waking paralysis). **Spastic paralysis.** Paralysis with increased muscular tone and exaggerated deep reflexes, owing to liberation of the muscles from pyramidal control. **Spastic spinal paralysis.** Disease of the lateral columns of the spinal cord, giving spasticity of the extremities. **Spinomuscular paralysis.** Paralysis owing to disease of anterior cells of the spinal cord, producing muscular wasting. **Spinoneural paralysis.**

Paralysis due to disease of the anterior horn cells of the cord and hence of efferent nerves; essentially the same as spinomuscular paralysis (see prec.) **Stem paralysis.** Fascicular paralysis (see above). **Sunday-morning paralysis.** Drunkards'-arm paralysis (see above). **Supranuclear paralysis.** Paralysis of the conjugate or disjunctive movements of the two eyes together. It is characterized by lack of diplopia. The lesion is situated above the 3rd, 4th and 6th cranial-nerve nuclei. **Syphilitic spastic spinal paralysis.** Syphilitic spastic paraplegia. *See* PARAPLEGIA. **Temporary paralysis.** Transient or short-lived paralysis; due perhaps to a drug, to brief pressure upon a nerve, or to hysteria. **Tic paralysis.** Tic; habit spasm. An unsatisfactory term that is rarely used. **Tick paralysis.** Ascending tick paralysis (see above). **Thyrotoxic periodic paralysis.** Paralysis associated with thyrotoxicosis. **Tourniquet paralysis.** Paralysis due to pressure of a tourniquet which has been applied too tightly, e.g. around the arm. **Trigeminal paralysis.** Paralysis of the muscles of mastication (masseter, pterygoids, temporals). **Trochlear paralysis.** Paralysis of the superior oblique muscle of the orbit due to a lesion involving the 4th cranial nerve or its nucleus. There will be a manifest vertical squint with diplopia on looking down and to the side opposite to that of the lesion; the head tilts to the normal side. **Trunk paralysis.** Paralysis of the ocular muscles due to a lesion involving the 3rd, 4th and 6th cranial nerves after they have left the brain. It is characterized by involvement of all muscles supplied by the nerve concerned. **Uveoparotitic paralysis.** Sarcoidosis with neurological involvement. **Paralysis vacillans.** Chorea. **Vasomotor paralysis.** Paralysis of vasomotor nerves, giving rise to vascular dilatation. **Waking paralysis.** Temporary inability to move on waking; one form of the hypnogogic state. **Wasting paralysis.** The progressive muscular atrophy form of motor neuron disease. **Writers' paralysis.** Writers' cramp; notariorum paralysis. [Gk.]

See also: BELL (C.), BERNHARDT (M.), BROWN-SÉQUARD, CESTAN, CHENAIS, CLARK, CRUVEILHIER, DÉJÉRINE-KLUMPKE, DUCHENNE, ERB, FOVILLE, GUBLER, HEINE (J.), JACKSON (J. H.), KUSSMAUL, LANDRY, LISSAUER, LITTLE (W. J.), MILLARD, NOTHNAGEL, POTT, TODD (R. B.), VOLKMAN (R.), WEBER (H. D.), ZENKER (F. A.).

paralyssa (par·ah·**li**·sah). A disease like, or identical with, rabies, transmitted by the bite of vampire bats, especially *Desmodus rotundus.* Epizootics of the disease occur among these bats, which can also act as long-term carriers of the virus. It is suggested that the virus of paralyssa may be identical with that causing a cattle disease *mal de caderas* in South America. [Gk *para, lyssa* rabies.]

paralytic (par·al·**it**·ik). 1. Having the characteristics of or suffering from paralysis. 2. An individual afflicted with paralysis.

paramagenta (**par**·ah·maj·**en'**·tah). Pararosaniline chloride. [Gk *para,* magenta.]

paramagnetic (**par**·ah·mag·**net'**·ik). Attracted to the poles of a magnet; describing any substance that takes up a position in a magnetic field parallel to the lines of force. [Gk *para,* magnetic.]

paramania (par·ah·**ma**·ne·ah). A disordered condition of the emotions in which the patient has pleasure or delight in complaining. [Gk *para,* mania.]

paramastigote (par·ah·**mas**·tig·ote). A mastigote furnished with a small supernumerary flagellum alongside the large flagellum. [Gk *para,* mastigote.]

paramastitis (par·ah·mas·**ti'**·tis). Inflammation affecting the tissues in the neighbourhood of the mammary gland. [Gk *para,* mastitis.]

paramastoid (par·ah·**mas**·toid). Near or alongside the mastoid process of the temporal bone. [Gk *para,* mastoid.]

paramastoiditis (**par**·ah·mas·toid·**i'**·tis). In cases of mastoiditis, inflammation involving the temporal bone. [Gk *para,* mastoiditis.]

paramecium (par·a·**me**·se·um). Paramoecium.

paramedian (par·ah·**me**·de·an). Located near the median line. [Gk *para,* median.]

paramedical (par·ah·**med**·ik·al). Having some association with medicine. [Gk *para,* medicine.]

paramenia (par·ah·**me**·ne·ah). Menstrual disorder or irregularity. **Paramenia obstructionis.** Amenorrhoea. [Gk *para,* menses.]

parameningococcus (**par**·ah·men·ing·go·**kok'**·us). A Gram-negative diplococcus belonging to the genus *Neisseria* and closely related to *Neisseria meningitidis.* It occurs in the nasopharynx of man, and may be a cause of cerebrospinal fever. [Gk *para,* meningococcus.]

parameniscitis (**par**·ah·men·is·**i'**·tis). Inflammation of a parameniscus. [parameniscus, Gk *-itis* inflammation.]

parameniscus (**par**·ah·men·**is'**·kus). The tissue around the meniscus of the knee. [Gk *para,* meniscus.]

paramesial (par·ah·**me**·ze·al). Paramedian. [Gk *para, mesos* middle.]

parameter (par·**am**·et·er). An attribute in terms of which it is convenient to express other related attributes so that they can be regarded as being dependent upon the selected attribute. [Gk *para, metron* measure.]

Paramethadione BP 1973 (**par**·ah·meth·ah·**di'**·one). 5-Ethyl-3,5-dimethyloxazolidine-2,4-dione. An anticonvulsant that has proved useful in controlling petit mal when other drugs have failed. Patients should be kept under strict observation, as it sometimes acts as a marrow depressant.

Paramethasone (par·ah·**meth**·az·one). BP Commission approved name for 6α-fluoro-16α-methylprednisolone; it is used in corticosteroid therapy.

parametric (par·ah·**me**·trik). Pertaining to the parametrium.

parametritic (**par**·ah·me·**trit'**·ik). Characterized by or pertaining to parametritis.

parametritis (**par**·ah·me·**tri'**·tis). A cellulitis of the tissues of the parametrium. [parametrium, Gk *-itis* inflammation.]

parametrium [NA] (par·ah·**me**·tre·um). Cellular tissue lying anteriorly between the supravaginal portion of the cervix and the bladder, along the sides of the cervix itself and laterally between the layers of the broad ligaments. [Gk *para, metra* womb.]

parametropathy (**par**·ah·met·**rop'**·ath·e). Any disease of the parametrium. [parametrium, Gk *pathos* disease.]

paramido-acetophenone (par·**am**·id·o·as·et·o·**fen'**·one). $NH_2C_6H_4COCH_3$, a compound which has been used in Ehrlich's diazo test for certain aromatic substances in the urine.

paramimia (par·ah·**mim**·e·ah). A morbid state marked by the use of gestures which are inappropriate to the words spoken. [Gk *para, mimos* actor.]

paramnesia (par·am·**ne**·ze·ah). The recall of events which have not occurred but which the person believes have happened; this may be due to confusion of fact and phantasy or dream contents. It may occur in normal as well as in pathological states. [Gk *para,* amnesia.]

Paramoecium (par·ah·**me**·se·um). An oval, ciliated protozoon parasite belonging to the class Ciliata (Infusoria). The only species pathogenic for man is *Balantidium coli* (syn. *Paramoecium coli*), the cause of balantidial dysentery, which occurs in the large intestine. The vegetative form is 60–100 μm long and 50–70 μm broad, and is actively motile. The encysted forms are 45–65 μm long. [Gk *paramekos* oblong.]

paramonochlorophenol (**par**·ah·mon·o·klor·o·**fe'**·nol). $C_6H_4(OH)Cl$, a chlorophenol used as an antiseptic and bacteriostatic. It is a stronger germicide than phenol but more toxic.

paramorphane (par·ah·**mor**·fane). Paramorphine.

paramorphia (par·ah·**mor**·fe·ah). Abnormality of form or structure. [Gk *para, morphe* shape.]

paramorphic (par·ah·**mor**·fik). Characterized by paramorphia.

paramorphine (par·ah·**mor**·feen). Thebaine, $C_{19}H_{21}NO_3$. A highly toxic opium alkaloid with very little narcotic action. It is a dimethylmorphine.

paramorphism, paramorphosis (par·ah·**mor**·fizm, par·ah·**mor**·fo·sis). The phenomenon of a substance changing its crystalline form or physical properties without any accompanying alteration of chemical structure: it is due to a rearrangement of molecules. [Gk *para, morphe* form, *-osis* condition.]

Paramphistomatidae (par·**am**·fe·sto·**mat'**·id·e). A family of the trematode suborder Amphistomata. The genus *Watsonius* is of medical interest. [Gk *para, amphi* double, *stoma* mouth, *eidos* form.]

paramphistomiasis (par·am·fe·sto·mi'·as·is). A parasitic disease due to *Watsonius watsoni* or *Gastrodiscoides hominis*, trematodes of the family *Paramphistomatidae*. It occurs in Egypt and the United States.

Paramphistomoidea (par·am·fe·sto·moi'·de·ah). Amphistomata; a suborder of the trematode order Prosostomata. The families Gastrodiscidae and Paramphistomatidae are of medical interest. [Gk *para, amphi* double, *stoma* mouth, *eidos* form.]

paramucin (par·ah·mew·sin). The gummy material found within ovarian cysts and related chemically to mucin. [Gk *para*, mucin.]

paramusia (par·ah·mew·se·ah). Deterioration or partial loss of the ability to play or read music correctly. [Gk *para, a, mousike* music.]

paramyelin (par·ah·mi·el·in). A mono-aminomonophosphatide present in the white matter of brain. [Gk *para*, myelin.]

paramyoclonus multiplex (par·ah·mi·ok'·lo·nus mul·te·plex). Myoclonus multiplex; a chronic disorder of the muscles characterized by frequent sudden shock-like contractions of varying intensity, most frequently affecting symmetrically the proximal muscles of the limbs. There may be from 10 to 50 contractions per minute, which disappear during sleep and on voluntary movement. The mechanical excitability of the muscles is increased, but the electrical reactions are normal and there is no wasting. [Gk *para*, myoclonus, L, multiple.]

paramyotone (par·ah·mi·o·tone). Atypical myotonus.

paramyotonia, paramyotonus (par·ah·mi·o·to'·ne·ah, par·ah·mi·ot'·on·us). Any condition in which muscular relaxation is abnormal. **Paramyotonia congenita.** A form of congenital myotonia in which the sudden prolonged tonic muscular contractions occur only after exposure to cold. [Gk *para*, myotonia.]

Paramyxovirus (par·ah·mix'·o·vi·rus). A genus of RNA-containing enveloped viruses, very pleomorphic in the electron microscope, which have haemagglutinin and neuraminidase surface antigens. The average size of the virus particles is about 200 nm. The members of the genus which infect man are para-influenza viruses types 1–4, mumps virus and Newcastle disease virus. Measles virus, which is indistinguishable morphologically, differs antigenically and functionally and is not a true member of the genus. [Gk *para, myxa* mucus, L *virus* poison.]

paranaesthesia (par·an·es·the'·ze·ah). Para-anaesthesia.

paranalgesia (par·an·al·je'·ze·ah). Para-analgesia.

paranaphthalene (par·ah·naf·thal·een). Anthracene.

paranasal (par·ah·na·zal). By the side of the nose. [Gk *para*, L *nasus* nose.]

paranephric (par·ah·nef·rik). 1. Situated adjacent to the kidney. 2. Relating to the suprarenal glands. [Gk *para, nephros* kidney.]

paranephritis (par·ah·nef·ri'·tis). 1. A condition of inflammation affecting the suprarenal glands. 2. An inflammatory condition involving the connective tissue adjacent to and about the kidney. **Lipomatous paranephritis.** Renal lipomatosis. *See* LIPOMATOSIS. [Gk *para*, nephritis.]

paranephros, paranephrus (par·ah·nef·ros, par·ah·nef·rus). A suprarenal gland. [Gk *para, nephros* kidney.]

paraneural (par·ah·newr·al). Near or beside a nerve. [Gk *para, neuron* nerve.]

paraneurismus (par·ah·newr·iz'·mus). Any disordered condition of the nerves or abnormality of their function. [Gk *para, neuron* nerve.]

parangi (pah·ran·je). Sri Lankan name for yaws.

paranoia (par·ah·noi·ah). A mental disorder, originally described by Kraepelin as a distinctive syndrome, characterized by slow insidious onset, and the gradual development of delusional ideas of a superficially not grossly bizarre or irrational kind, while the personality remains fairly well preserved; hallucinations should be rare and unimportant, or not seen at all. This condition is not now generally considered to be a syndrome in its own right, but merely a chronic but otherwise benign form of paranoid schizophrenia. All subclasses of paranoia, such as those mentioned below, are now obsolete in psychiatric terminology. **Acute hallucinatory paranoia.** Any acute psychosis of whatever causation, with florid delusions and hallucinations. **Alcoholic paranoia.** A chronic paranoid psychosis seen not infrequently in confirmed drinkers, in which delusional ideas are prominent. The aetiology is doubtful, and is often considered as due to the combination of chronic alcoholic intoxication and a schizoid predisposition. **Paranoia hallucinatoria.** A psychosis showing both delusions and hallucinations. **Heboid paranoia.** An obsolete term for hebephrenic schizophrenia. **Litigious paranoia.** A paranoid psychosis leading the sufferer, who feels himself to be persecuted, to seek obstinately for legal redress. **Querulous paranoia.** A paranoid psychosis leading the patient to make constant complaint, e.g. to medical men or men of law. **Paranoia simplex.** Paranoia of a typical kind, not classifiable as a subtype. [Gk *para, nous* mind.]

paranoic (par·ah·no·ik). Of, characterized by, or suffering from paranoia.

paranoid (par·ah·noid). Like paranoia. [paranoia, Gk *eidos* form.]

paranoidism (par·ah·noid·izm). The character or condition of one afflicted with paranoia. [see prec.]

paranomia (par·ah·no·me·ah). A form of aphasia characterized by the incorrect naming of objects. **Myotactic paranomia.** Aphasia in which the names of objects touched cannot be remembered and are therefore called by incorrect titles. **Visual paranomia.** Aphasia in which the names of objects seen cannot be recalled and are therefore named incorrectly. [Gk *para, onoma* name.]

paranormal (par·ah·nor·mal). Lying outside the range of normal scientific investigations. [Gk *para*, normal.]

paranuclear (par·ah·new·kle·ar). Relating to or containing a paranucleus. [Gk *para*, nucleus.]

paranucleate (par·ah·new·kle·ate). 1. Possessing a paranucleus. 2. Any salt or ester of paranucleic acid.

paranucleolus (par·ah·new·kle'·o·lus). A minute basophil body in the enveloping sac of the nucleus. [Gk *para*, nucleolus.]

paranucleus (par·ah·new·kle·us). A small body similar to a nucleus occasionally found in the cytoplasm adjacent to the nucleus of a cell. [Gk *para*, nucleus.]

para-oesophageal (par·ah·e·sof·ah·je'·al). By the side of the oesophagus. [Gk *para*, oesophagus.]

para-omphalic (par·ah·om·fal'·ik). Para-umbilical. [Gk *para, omphalos* navel.]

para-oral (par·ah·or·al). Parenteral. [Gk *para*, L *os* mouth.]

para-osmia (par·ah·oz·me·ah). Parosmia.

para-osteoarthropathy (par·ah·os·te·o·ar·throp'·ath·e). Paraplegia associated with a morbid condition of the bones and joints. [Gk *para*, osteoarthropathy.]

para-otitis interna (par·ah·o·ti'·tis in·ter·nah). Circumscribed labyrinthitis, occurring in acute or chronic suppurative otitis media, in which the endosteum is exposed through destruction of the bony wall of the labyrinth. There is vertigo, but no inner-ear deafness. [Gk *para*, otitis, L, inside.]

paraoxymethylacetanilide (par·ah·ox·e·meth·il·as·et·an'·il·ide). Acetophenetidin.

parapancreatic (par·ah·pan·kre·at'·ik). Lying near or alongside the pancreas. [Gk *para*, pancreas.]

paraparesis (par·ah·par·e'·sis). An incomplete paralysis affecting the lower extremities. [Gk *para, paresis* paralysis.]

paraparetic (par·ah·par·et'·ik). Relating to or suffering from paraparesis.

parapathia (par·ah·path·e·ah). Psychoneurosis; emotional imbalance. [Gk *para, pathos* disease.]

parapedesis (par·ah·ped·e'·sis). Secretion or excretion through an abnormal channel. [Gk *para, pedesis* an oozing.]

parapemphigus (par·ah·pem·fig·us). Pemphigoid. [Gk *para, pemphix* bubble.]

paraperitoneal (par·ah·per·it·on·e'·al). Lying near or beside the peritoneum. [Gk *para*, peritoneum.]

parapertussis (par·ah·per·tus'·is). Mild pertussis caused by *Bordetella parapertussis*. [Gk *para*, pertussis.]

parapestis (par·ah·**pes**·tis). Pestis minor. [Gk *para*, L *pestis* plague.]

paraphasia (par·ah·**fa**·ze·ah). The evocation of an inappropriate sound in place of a desired word or phrase. Cf. APHASIA. **Central paraphasia.** Incomplete aphasia caused by a lesion of the cerebral cortex. **Choreic paraphasia.** Incomplete aphasia in which a number of words are combined to form a nonsensical phrase or sentence. [Gk *para*, aphasia.]

paraphasic (par·ah·**fa**·zik). Having the qualities of or affected with paraphasia.

paraphemia (par·ah·**fe**·me·ah). A type of aphasia in which the wrong words are constantly used. [Gk *para*, *pheme* any word.]

paraphenetolcarbamide (par·ah·**fen**·et·ol·**kar'**·bam·ide). Dulcin, phenetidinurea, $C_2H_5OC_6H_4NHCONH_2$. A derivative of urea, some two hundred times sweeter than sugar and used as a sweetening agent.

paraphenylenediamine (par·ah·**fen**·il·een·**di'**·am·een). $C_6H_4(NH_2)_2$, a compound derived from aniline, used chiefly for dyeing the hair and in photographic processing. It is liable to cause dermatitis, especially in sensitive individuals.

paraphia (par·**af**·e·ah). An abnormal state of the tactile sense. [Gk *para*, *aphe* the sense of touch.]

paraphilia (par·ah·**fil**·e·ah). Sexual perversion. [Gk *para*, *philein* to love.]

paraphiliac (par·ah·**fil**·e·ak). 1. A sexual pervert. 2. Marked by sexual perversion. [see prec.]

paraphimosis (par·ah·fi·**mo'**·sis). 1. A condition in which a phimosed prepuce is forcibly retracted behind the glans penis with the result that the fold of prepuce distal to the phimotic constriction becomes grossly oedematous owing to obstruction of its venous and lymphatic drainage. 2. In ophthalmology, a rare condition seen in infants in the presence of orbicularis oculi muscle spasm. This prevents the lids returning to their normal position and finally causes congestion, oedema and strangulation of the lids, when anaesthesia may be necessary to return them to their normal postition. [Gk *para*, *phimoein* to muzzle.]

paraphobia (par·ah·**fo**·be·ah). A mild degree of phobia in which the patient is hesitant or reluctant in the performance of certain acts or about remaining in a particular place, although he is not entirely inhibited from doing so. [Gk *para*, phobia.]

paraphonemia (par·ah·fon·**em'**·ia). An inability to distinguish between phonemes which are somewhat similar in their acoustic properties.

paraphonia (par·ah·**fo**·ne·ah). Morbid change of the tone or other disorder of the voice. **Paraphonia puberum, Paraphonia pubescentium.** The alteration in a boy's voice when he reaches puberty. [Gk *para*, *phone* voice.]

paraphora (par·**af**·or·ah). 1. A mild degree of mental derangement. 2. Unstable equilibrium caused by intoxication. [Gk, distraction.]

paraphrasia (par·ah·**fra**·ze·ah). A type of aphasia in which the individual is unable to speak in a coherent manner. **Paraphrasia praeceps.** Paraphrasia in which the patient speaks in a hasty and incoherent manner. **Paraphrasia tarda.** A condition characterized by slowness in expressing one's thoughts. **Paraphrasia verbalis.** The interjection of an unsuitable word. **Paraphrasia vesana.** Confusion of thoughts and words. [Gk *para*, *phrasein* to utter.]

paraphrenesis (par·ah·fren·**e'**·sis). 1. Amentia. 2. Delirium. [see foll.]

paraphrenia (par·ah·**fre**·ne·ah). A paranoid psychosis, i.e. involving the gradual development of delusional ideas of increasing absurdity, of hallucinations, and slow and progressive deterioration of personality, in the absence of any known organic cause. Though the term is in general use, it is clinically equivalent to a chronic and insidious paranoid schizophrenia, usually with late age of onset. All subclasses, such as those mentioned below, are now obsolete in psychiatric terminology. **Paraphrenia confabulans.** A paraphrenic psychosis in which the patient confabulates, i.e. he does not merely misinterpret the experience he undergoes but seems also to be inventing the experiences themselves. **Paraphrenia expansiva.** A paraphrenic psychosis in which the delusions take a grandiose form, and the predominant mood is one of euphoria. **Paraphrenia phantastica.** A paraphrenic psychosis in which the delusions are of a fantastic kind, e.g. involve supernatural experiences and agencies. **Paraphrenia systematica.** A paraphrenic psychosis in which the delusions are closely knit, mutually interdependent, and form one or more related wholes. [Gk *para*, *phren* mind.]

paraphrenic (par·ah·**fre**·nik). 1. Suffering from paraphrenia, or pertaining to it. 2. In the neighbourhood of the diaphragm. [Gk *para*, *phren* mind, *phren* diaphragm.]

paraphrenitis (par·ah·fren·**i'**·tis). A condition of inflammation affecting the tissues in the neighbourhood of the diaphragm. [Gk *para*, *phren* diaphragm, *-itis* inflammation.]

paraphronesis (par·ah·fron·**e'**·sis). Paraphrenesis.

paraphronia (par·ah·**fro**·ne·ah). A mental condition in which there is an alteration in character and disposition. [Gk *para*, *aphron* silly.]

paraphysial (par·ah·**fiz**·e·al). Belonging to the paraphysis.

paraphysis (par·**af**·is·is). 1. A derivative of the roof plate in the development of the forebrain. 2. In botany, a sterile filament occurring in mosses and algae, accompanying the sexual organs. [Gk, attachment.]

paraphyte (par·ah·fite). Applied to vegetations, denoting that they are proliferating in the form of excrescences. [Gk *para*, *phyton* plant.]

paraphyton (par·ah·**fi**·ton). A vegetable parasite. [see prec.]

paraplasm (par·ah·plazm). 1. Hyaloplasm; the fluid-like constituent of the cytoreticulum of the cell body. 2. Any unusual conformation of the protoplasm. [Gk *para*, plasma.]

paraplasma flavigenum (par·ah·**plaz**·mah flav·e·**je**·num). The name given by Harold Seidelin to bodies that he observed in the red blood cells and thought were the cause of yellow fever. [Gk *para*, plasma, L *flavus* yellow, Gk *genein* to produce.]

paraplasmic (par·ah·**plaz**·mik). Belonging to the paraplasm.

paraplastic (par·ah·**plas**·tik). 1. Paraplasmic. 2. Having abnormal formative powers. 3. Deformed; misshapen. [Gk *para*, *plassein* to mould.]

paraplastin (par·ah·**plas**·tin). A chromatophilic substance other than chromatin that occurs in both nucleus and cytoplasm of a cell. [see prec.]

paraplectic (par·ah·**plek**·tik). Paraplegic. [Gk *paraplektos* striken aside.]

paraplegia (par·ah·**ple**·je·ah). Paralysis of the lower part of the body and limbs, due to numerous causes, e.g. fractured spine and damage to the cord, various tract degenerations in the cord, and polyneuritis. **Alcoholic paraplegia.** Paraplegia due to peripheral neuritis caused by alcohol. **Ataxic paraplegia.** That due to posterior and lateral sclerosis of the cord with subacute combined degeneration. **Cerebral paraplegia.** Paraplegia due to a bilateral lesion of the brain. **Cervical paraplegia.** Paraplegia due to a lesion in the cervical part of the cord and showing weakness in the arms in addition to the legs. **Congenital spastic paraplegia.** One of the types of birth palsy showing bilateral spasticity of limbs. **Paraplegia dolorosa.** Paraplegia associated with pain, and due to pressure on the spinal nerves. **Paraplegia in extension.** Paraplegia due to an incomplete spinal-cord lesion, with spasticity of the extensor muscles of the legs. **Flaccid paraplegia.** Paraplegia with loss of tone in the paralysed muscles. **Paraplegia in flexion.** Paraplegia due to a complete spinal-cord lesion, with spasticity of the flexor muscles of the legs. **Hysterical paraplegia.** Paraplegia that is a hysterical manifestation and is unassociated with any organic lesion. **Infantile spasmodic paraplegia, Infantile spastic paraplegia.** Congenital spastic paraplegia (see above). **Primary spastic paraplegia.** That due to degeneration in the pyramidal tracts. **Progressive spastic paraplegia.** Any progressive, spastic weakness of the legs; often used as a synonym for hereditary *spastic paraplegia.* **Spastic paraplegia.** Paraplegia depending on disturbed nutrition of the cortex in aged people. **Spastic cerebral paraplegia.** Cerebral paraplegia (see above). **Paraplegia superior.** Paraplegia of both arms. **Syphilitic spastic paraplegia.** A progressive paralysis of the lower limbs of spastic type, associated with early bladder defect and minimal sensory changes; it is syphilitic in aetiology. **Toxic paraplegia.** The effect on the peripheral nerves of some poison, e.g. alcohol. [Gk *para, plege* stroke.]

See also: ERB, GOWERS, POTT.

paraplegic (par·ah·**ple**·jik). Having the characteristics of paraplegia, or suffering from paraplegia.

paraplegiform (par·ah·**ple**·je·form). Resembling paraplegia. [paraplegia, form.]

paraplegy (par·ah·**ple**·je). Paraplegia.

parapleuritis (par·ah·ploor·**i**′·tis). An inflammatory condition of the chest wall. [Gk *para*, pleuritis.]

parapneumonia (par·ah·new·**mo**·ne·ah). A condition which resembles pneumonia in its clinical symptoms but in which the *Streptococcus pneumoniae* or other specific organism cannot be found. [Gk *para*, pneumonia.]

parapoplexy (par·**ap**·o·plex·e). 1. A mild type of apoplexy; pseudo-apoplexy. 2. An attack similar to that of apoplexy but with a different cause. [Gk *para*, apoplexy.]

parapraxia, parapraxis (par·ah·**prax**·e·ah, par·ah·**prax**·is). The faulty performance of purposive actions, another movement being substituted for the one intended. [Gk *para, praxis* a doing.]

paraproctitis (par·ah·prok·**ti**′·tis). Inflammation affecting the paraproctium. [paraproctium, Gk *-itis* inflammation.]

paraproctium (par·ah·**prok**·te·um). The connective tissues around the rectum and anus. [Gk *para, proktos* the hinder parts.]

paraprostatitis (par·ah·pros·tat·**i**′·tis). Inflammation affecting the tissues about the prostate gland. [Gk *para*, prostatitis.]

paraproteinaemia (par·ah·pro·te·in·**e**′·me·ah). A condition in which serum proteins that are normally absent, or present only in minimal amounts, are present, or present in larger amounts; these proteins include macroglobulin, and cryoglobulin. [Gk *para*, protein, *haima* blood.]

paraproteins (par·ah·**pro**·teenz). Proteins which appear in large quantities in the serum as a result of some pathological disturbance, and which are the inactive equivalent of some biologically active protein. [Gk *para, proteios* of first rank.]

parapsia, parapsis (par·**ap**·se·ah, par·**ap**·sis). Paraphia.

parapsoriasis (par·ah·sor·**i**′·as·is). A group of doubtfully related dermatoses characterized by chronicity, resistance to treatment and a supposed resemblance to psoriasis. **Parapsoriasis acuta.** Pityriasis lichenoides et varioliformis acuta. **Parapsoriasis atrophicans.** An eruption consisting of recurrent crops of minute vesiculopustules on an erythematous base which leave atrophy on healing. **Parapsoriasis guttata.** Pityriasis lichenoides chronica. **Parapsoriasis herpetiformis.** A very rare chronic dermatosis characterized by widespread vesicular eruption, sterile on culture. **Parapsoriasis lichenoides.** Retiform parapsoriasis (see below). **Parapsoriasis maculata.** Parapsoriasis en plaques (see below). **Parapsoriasis papulata.** Retiform parapsoriasis (see below). **Parapsoriasis en plaques.** Flat, slightly scaly, red or reddish-yellow, very chronic patches on the skin, with very little or no thickening; it may be a precursor of mycosis fungoides. **Retiform parapsoriasis.** Parakeratosis variegata (Unna); lichen variegatus (Crocker): a variety of parapsoriasis that forms a widespread network over the limbs and trunk; it is red or bluish in colour, sometimes resembling psoriasis, at other times lichen planus, and is resistant to treatment. **Parapsoriasis varioliformis.** Pityriasis lichenoides et varioliformis acuta. [Gk *para*, psoriasis.]

parapsychology (par·ah·si·**kol**′·o·je). The study of extrasensory phenomena such as telepathy and thought-reading. [Gk *para*, psychology.]

parapsychosis (par·ah·si·**ko**′·sis). Temporary abnormality of the thought processes causing irrational thinking. [Gk *para*, psychosis.]

Parapsyllus (par·ah·**sil**·us). A genus of fleas, some of which are vectors of plague. [Gk *para, psylla* flea.]

parapyramidal (par·ah·pir·**am**′·id·al). Situated alongside or adjacent to a pyramid. [Gk *para*, pyramid.]

parapyruvate (par·ah·pi·**roo**′·vate). A pyruvate condensation product which is a potent inhibitor of pyruvate dehydrogenase. [Gk *para*, pyruvate.]

parareaction (par·ah·re·**ak**′·shun). A term employed in the system of psychiatry devised by Adolf Meyer, to include parergasia and all other psychoses in which delusional and hallucinatory experiences occur in clear consciousness, and logical thinking is undisturbed, e.g. the paranoid state which may develop with deafness. [GK *para*, reaction.]

pararectal (par·ah·**rek**·tal). 1. Near or alongside the rectum. 2. Near or beside a rectus muscle. [Gk *para*, rectum.]

parareflexia (par·ah·re·**flex**′·e·ah). Any abnormal condition or disturbance of the reflexes. [Gk *para*, reflex.]

pararenal (par·ah·re·nal). Situated beside the kidney. [Gk *para*, L *ren* kidney.]

pararhotacism (par·ah·**ro**·tah·sizm). Wrong pronunciation of the letter *r*. [Gk *para, rho* letter *r*.]

pararosaniline (pah·ah·ro·**zan**′·il·een). The base $OHC(C_6H_4NH_2)_3$, from which are derived the magenta dyes. **Pararosaniline chloride.** Parafuchsine, $(C_6H_4NH_2)_2C{=}C_6H_4NH_2Cl$. A basic dye and an effective germicide against Gram-positive organisms. It is particularly effective against staphylococci, *Corynebacterium diphtheriae* and *Pseudomonas aeruginosa* and in Vincent's angina. It forms a precipitate with necrotic tissue and is used therefore in burns.

pararrhythmia (par·ah·**rith**·me·ah). Cardiac arrhythmia in which two distinct rhythms are working simultaneously. [Gk *para*, arrhythmia.]

pararrhythmus (par·ah·**rith**·mus). Disordered rhythm. [Gk *para*, rhythm.]

pararthrema, pararthresis (par·ar·**thre**·mah, par·ar·**thre**·sis). Subluxation of a joint. [Gk *para, arthron* joint.]

pararthria (par·**ar**·thre·ah). A disorder of speech marked by difficult utterance. [Gk *para, arthroein* to utter distinctly.]

parasacral (par·ah·**sa**·kral). Near or alongside the sacrum. [Gk *para*, sacrum.]

parasagittal (par·ah·**saj**·it·al). Parallel with the median plane. [Gk *para*, L *sagitta* arrow.]

parasalpingitis (par·ah·sal·pin·**ji**′·tis). Inflammation of the tissues around or alongside a uterine tube. [Gk *para*, salpingitis.]

parascarlatina, parascarlet (par·ah·skar·lat·**e**′·nah, par·ah·**skar**·let). Fourth disease. *See* DISEASE. [Gk *para*, scarlatina.]

parasecretion (par·ah·se·**kre**′·shun). 1. Paracrisis; any secreting disorder. 2. Hypersecretion. [Gk *para*, secretion.]

parasellar (par·ah·**sel**·ar). Adjacent to the pituitary fossa. [Gk *para*, sellar.]

parasigmatism (par·ah·**sig**·mat·izm). A defect of speech characterized by the substitution of some other sound for that of the letter *s* or *z*; lisping. [Gk *para, sigma* letter *s*.]

parasinusoidal (par·ah·si·nus·**oid**′·al). Near or along the track of a cerebral or other sinus. [Gk *para*, sinusoidal.]

parasitaemia (par·ah·sit·**e**′·me·ah). Parasites in the blood. [parasite, Gk *haima* blood.]

parasite (par·ah·site). An organism which lives on another living organism (the host), at the expense of the latter, and is often specially modified for that existence. **Accidental parasite.** One that is normally not parasitic, but under particular circumstances can lead a parasitic existence. **Aestivo-autumnal parasite.** *Plasmodium falciparum*, the cause of malignant tertian malaria. **Auxiliary parasite.** One which acts in combination with another parasite. **Coelozoic parasite.** A parasite living in the coelomic cavity. **Commensal parasite.** One which lives by sharing the food of the host, but does not injure the host. **Cytozoic parasite.** An intracellular parasite. **Diheteroxenic parasite.** A parasite which requires two hosts to complete its cycle. **Ectophytic parasite.** A plant parasite; epiphytic parasite (see below). **Ectozoic parasite.** An ectoparasite. **Endophytic parasite.** One which lives in the interior of the plant host. **Entozoic parasite.** One which lives in the gut lumen. **Epiphytic parasite.** One which lives on the external surface of the plant host. **Erratic parasite.** One that is encountered in an organ or tissue other than that in which it normally lives. **Facultative parasite.** One which is capable of a saprophytic existence apart from the host for a period. **Haematozoic parasite.** One which lives in the blood. **Half parasite.** One which is not entirely dependent on its host. **Incidental parasite.** A parasite on an alien host. **Inquiline parasite.** An organism deriving protection but not nourishment from another organism. **Intermittent parasite.** One which appears periodically in the host. **Karyozoic parasite.** An intranuclear parasite. **Malaria parasite.** One of the four known species of *Plasmodium* which on injection into the body by anopheline mosquitoes produce malaria. **Obligatory parasite.** One which is incapable of existence apart from its host. **Occasional parasite.** One which is only occasionally parasitic. **Optimal parasite.** Facultative parasite (see above). **Partial parasite.** Half parasite (see above). **Pathogenic parasite.** One which causes disease of the host. **Periodic parasite.** One to which occasional parasitic life is necessary. **Placental parasite.** Omphalosite. **Quartan parasite.** *Plasmodium malariae,* the cause of quartan malaria. **Specific parasite.** One which is confined to a particular type of host. **Sporadic parasite.** An organism that is only rarely parasitic in the species in which it is found. **Stenotrophic parasite.** A parasite that lives in one species only. **Temporary parasite.** One which is parasitic during only a part of its life cycle. **Tertian parasite.** *Plasmodium vivax,* the cause of benign tertian malaria. **True parasite.** One entirely dependent on the host. [Gk *parasitos* guest.]

parasitic (par·ah·**sit**·ik). Belonging to or having the characteristics of a parasite; living in or on, and subsisting on another organism, e.g. bacteria peculiar to human beings.

parasiticidal (par·ah·sit·is·**i**′·dal). Pertaining to parasiticide.

parasiticide (par·ah·**sit**·is·ide). A substance destructive to parasites. [parasite, L *caedere* to kill.]

parasitifer (par·ah·**sit**·if·er). 1. The host of a parasitic organism. 2. Of teratisms, the autosite. [parasite, L *ferre* to bear.]

parasitiferism (par·ah·si·**tif**′·er·izm). The condition of delusions affecting certain persons who believe that they are infested with parasites. [see prec.]

parasitism (**par**·ah·si·tizm). 1. Infestation with parasites. 2. The general state of parasitic existence. 3. The relation of a parasite to its host.

parasitization (par·ah·sit·i·**za**′·shun). Infestation or infection with a parasite.

parasitogenesis (par·ah·si·to·**jen**′·es·is). 1. The growth of parasites. 2. A state of the body which facilitates invasion by parasites. [parasite, Gk *genein* to produce.]

parasitogenetic, parasitogenic (par·ah·si·to·jen·**et**′·ik, par·ah·si·to·**jen**′·ik). 1. Relating to conditions which facilitate infestation by parasitic organisms. 2. Caused or produced by parasites. [see prec.]

parasitoid (**par**·ah·si·toid). Like a parasite. [parasite, Gk *eidos* form.]

Parasitoidea (par·ah·sit·**oi**′·de·ah). A super-family of the acarine order Parasitiformes. The family Dermanyssidae is of medical interest. [see prec.]

parasitologist (par·ah·sit·**ol**′·o·jist). One who makes a special study of parasitology.

parasitology (par·ah·sit·**ol**′·o·je). The section of zoology which deals with the science and study of parasites. **Medical parasitology.** The branch of the science of medicine that deals with parasites in their relation to man, especially the disease-producing or carrying parasites; it is usually understood that bacteria and other fungi, and viruses are excluded. [parasite, Gk *logos* science.]

parasitophobia (par·ah·si·to·**fo**′·be·ah). 1. Abnormally great fear of parasites. 2. The morbid belief held by an individual that he is suffering from infestation with parasitic organisms. [parasite, phobia.]

parasitosis (par·ah·si·**to**′·sis). Any disease characterized by infestation with parasites. The development of a morbid condition characterized by parasitic infestation. [parasite, Gk *-osis* condition.]

parasmallpox (par·ah·**smawl**·pox). Alastrim. [Gk *para,* smallpox.]

parasoma, parasome (par·ah·**so**·mah, **par**·ah·some). An irregular structure found in the cytoplasm adjacent to the nucleus. [Gk *para, soma* body.]

parasomnia (par·ah·**som**·ne·ah). A mild degree of insomnia. [Gk *para,* insomnia.]

paraspadia, paraspadias (par·ah·**spa**·de·ah, par·ah·**spa**·de·as). A condition in which the external urethral orifice is on one side of the penis. [Gk *paraspaein* to draw away from.]

paraspasm (**par**·ah·spazm). Muscular spasm affecting both legs; spastic paraplegia. [Gk *para,* spasm.]

paraspecific (par·ah·spes·**if**′·ik). Applied to remedies, having other therapeutic actions in addition to the specific one. [Gk *para,* specific.]

parasplenic (par·ah·**splen**·ik). Situated beside the spleen. [Gk *para,* spleen.]

parasteatosis (par·ah·ste·at·**o**′·sis). Any abnormal state of the sebaceous secretion. [Gk *para,* steatosis.]

parasternal (par·ah·**ster**·nal). Near or alongside the sternum. [Gk *para,* sternum.]

parastramnia, parastremma (par·ah·**stram**·ne·ah, par·ah·**strem**·ah). Twisting of the face and mouth. [Gk *parastrephein* to twist aside.]

parastruma (par·ah·**stroo**·mah). Hypertrophy of the parathyroid gland, simulating goitre. [Gk *para,* L *struma* scrofulous tumour.]

parasympathetic (par·ah·sim·path·**et**′·ik). The craniosacral subdivision of the autonomic nervous system, functionally antagonistic to the sympathetic division. Parasympathetic preganglionic fibres emerge in the 3rd, 7th, 9th and 10th cranial nerves, and in the 2nd, 3rd and 4th sacral-nerve roots. Functionally they are, in general, vasodilators to the abdominal viscera, and secretomotor, also causing slowing of the heart beat, peristalsis in the alimentary canal, etc. **Spinal parasympathetic.** Parasympathetic fibres which emerge in the 2nd, 3rd and 4th sacral-nerve roots, and form the *nervi erigentes.* [Gk *para,* sympathetic.]

parasympathicotonia (par·ah·sim·path·ik·o·**to**′·ne·ah). A syndrome in which the vagus (or parasympathetic nervous system) is supposed to predominate functionally over the sympathetic nervous system. The hyperexcitability is shown by constricted pupils, narrow palpebral fissures, low blood pressure, slow pulse, a tendency to excessive sweating, and sensitiveness to atropine and pilocarpine. It may play a part in allergic conditions, such as urticaria, hay fever, asthma, etc. It is a theoretical conception which oversimplifies the clinical facts. [parasympathetic, Gk *tonos* tone.]

parasympatholytic (par·ah·sim·path·o·**lit**′·ik). Antiparasympathomimetic; anticholinergic. [Gk *para, sympathein* to feel with, *lysis* a loosing.]

parasympathomimetic (par·ah·sim·path·o·mim·**et**′·ik). Relating to or simulating the actions of the parasympathetic nervous system. [Gk *para, sympathein* to feel with, *mimesis* imitation.]

parasympathotonia (par·ah·sim·path·o·**to**′·ne·ah). Parasympathicotonia.

parasynanche (par·ah·**sin**·an·ke). An imprecise term for inflammation of the throat muscles or the parotid gland [obsolete term]. [Gk *para,* synanche.]

parasynapsis (par·ah·sin·**ap**′·sis). The pairing of homologous chromosomes in meiosis. [Gk *para, synapsis* conjugation.]

parasynovitis (par·ah·si·no·**vi**′·tis). Inflammation affecting the tissues associated with a synovial sac. [Gk *para,* synovitis.]

parasyphilis (par·ah·**sif**·il·is). Quaternary syphilis [obsolete term]. [Gk *para,* syphilis.]

parasyphilitic (par·ah·sif·il·**it**′·ik). Pertaining to parasyphilis.

parasystole (par·ah·**sis**·to·le). The phenomenon of the heart beat being controlled at the same time by two independent foci, each discharging at its own rate. In this situation the focus which discharges more rapidly dominates, but the other focus will capture the heart when its discharge occurs between those of the fast focus if the heart is non-refractory. (*See* Parasystolic RHYTHM.) [Gk *para,* systole.]

paratarsium (par·ah·tar·se·um). General term for the tissues in close association with the tarsus—ligaments and connective tissue. [Gk *para*, tarsus.]

paratenon (par·ah·ten·on). The tissue (areolar and adipose) of a tendon sheath, which fills up vacant spaces and surrounds the tendon. [Gk *para*, *tenon* tendon.]

paratereseomania (par·ah·ter·e·se·o·ma′·ne·ah). A manic condition characterized by abnormal desire to observe fresh sights; insane inquisitiveness. [Gk *parateresis* observation, mania.]

parathelioma (par·a·the·le·o′·mah). A tumour in the vicinity of the nipple. [Gk *para*, *thele* nipple, *-oma* tumour.]

parathermy (par·ah·ther·me). Through-heating of the tissues by long- or short-wave diathermy. [Gk *para*, diathermy.]

parathion (par·ah·thi·on). Dinitrothiophosphate (DNTP). *See* ORGANOPHOSPHATES.

parathormone (par·ah·thor·mone). The hormone secreted by the parathyroid glands, the function of which is the control of the calcium level in the blood. This name is seldom now used and *parathyroid hormone* is preferred. [parathyroid, hormone.]

parathymia (par·ah·thi·me·ah). A disturbance of the affective state, in which emotions are felt which are inappropriate to the circumstances or to the actions which accompany them. [Gk *para*, *thymos* mind.]

parathyroid glands (par·ah·thi·roid glandz). These consist of an upper and lower pair of small flattened reddish discs of glandular tissue about 5 mm in diameter, though one or both of the lower pair may be found in the mediastinum. They are concerned with calcium metabolism, mobilizing calcium from the bone into the blood and thence into the urine and diminishing the output of phosphate from bone. Both they and the thyroid gland also secrete (thyro-) calcitonin.

parathyroidal (par·ah·thi·roid′·al). Belonging to the parathyroid glands.

parathyroidectomize (par·ah·thi·roid·ek′·to·mize). To remove a parathyroid gland in a patient or an experimental animal. [parathyroid, Gk *ektome* a cutting out.]

parathyroidectomy (par·ah·thi·roid·ek′·to·me). The operation for removal of a parathyroid gland. [see prec.]

parathyroidoma (par·ah·thi·roid·o′·mah). A tumour derived from a parathyroid gland or consisting of tissue which resembles that of a parathyroid gland. [parathyroid, Gk *-oma* tumour.]

parathyropathy (par·ah·thi·rop′·ath·e). Parathyroid disease. [parathyroid, Gk *pathos* disease.]

parathyrotoxicosis (par·a·thi·ro·tox·ik·o′·sis). Any condition due to overaction of the parathyroid hormones: hyperparathyroidism. [parathyroid, toxicosis.]

parathyrotrophic (par·ah·thi·ro·trof′·ik). Applied to anything that increases the growth of the parathyroid glands and induces greater activity in them. [parathyroid, Gk *trophe* nourishment.]

parathyrotrophin (par·ah·thi·ro·trof′·in). Parathyrotrophic hormone. Its existence is in doubt.

parathyrotropic (par·ah·thi·ro·trop′·ik). Having affinity for the parathyroid glands. [parathyroid, Gk *trepein* to turn.]

paratonia (par·ah·to·ne·ah). 1. Hyperextension. 2. A type of paralysis characterized by a hypertonic state of one set of muscles and a hypotonic state of the antagonist group. [Gk *para*, *tonos* tension.]

paratonsillar (par·ah·ton·sil·ah). Near the tonsils. [Gk *para*, tonsil.]

paratony (par·at·on·e). Paratonia.

paratopia (par·ah·to·pe·ah). Displacement. [Gk *para*, *topos* place.]

paratrachoma (par·ah·trak·o′·mah). Conjunctivitis caused by genital inclusion virus, usually in the newborn. Also called *inclusion blennorrhoea*. [Gk *para*, trachoma.]

Paratriatoma hirsuta (par·ah·tri·at·o′·mah hir·sew·tah). A reduviid bug; a potential vector of American trypanosomiasis. [Gk *para*, *tri-* three, *atomos* uncut, L, hairy.]

paratrichosis (par·ah·trik·o′·sis). Abnormality in the character or distribution of hair. [Gk *para*, trichosis.]

paratrimma (par·ah·trim·ah). 1. Intertrigo. 2. Chafing. [see foll.]

paratripsis (par·ah·trip·sis). 1. Irritation. 2. Chafing. 3. Reduction of catabolic activity with consequent reduction of protoplasmic waste. [Gk *paratribein* to rub beside.]

paratriptic (par·ah·trip·tik). 1. Produced by or causing chafing. 2. Retarding bodily wasting. [see prec.]

paratrope (par·at·ro·pe). Wrenching of a limb. [Gk, a turning away.]

paratrophic (par·ah·trof·ik). Deriving or needing sustenance from living organic material; parasitic. [Gk *paratrephein* to live at the expense of another.]

paratrophy (par·at·ro·fe). 1. The deriving of nutrition by a parasite from its host's tissues. 2. Atrophy through nutritional defect. [Gk *para*, atrophy.]

paratuberculosis (par·ah·tew·ber·kew·lo′·sis). A morbid condition characterized by symptoms of tuberculosis but in which *Mycobacterium tuberculosis* cannot be discovered [obsolete term]. [Gk *para*, tuberculosis.]

paratuberculous (par·ah·tew·ber′·kew·lus). 1. Relating or belonging to paratuberculosis. 2. Being connected indirectly with tuberculosis.

paratyphlitis (par·ah·tif·li′·tis). Perityphlitis. [Gk *para*, *typhlos* blind, *-itis* inflammation.]

paratyphoid (par·ah·ti·foid). 1. Paratyphoid fever. *See* FEVER. 2. Pertaining to paratyphoid fever. [Gk *para*, typhoid fever.]

paratyphus (par·ah·ti·fus). Paratyphoid fever. *See* FEVER.

paratypical (par·ah·tip·ik·al). Deviating from the normal type. [Gk *para*, type.]

para-umbilical (par·ah·um·bil·i′·kal). Situated near or beside the umbilicus. [Gk *para*, umbilicus.]

para-umbilical veins [venae para-umbilicales (NA)]. Small veins along the ligamentum teres, connecting with the veins of the abdominal wall (systemic system) on the one hand, and with the left branch of the portal vein (hepatic portal system) on the other.

para-ungual (par·ah·ung·gwal). Near, or next to, a nail. [Gk *para*, *unguis* nail.]

para-urethra (par·ah·ewr·e′·thrah). A supernumerary urethra. [Gk *para*, urethra.]

para-urethral (par·ah·ewr·e′·thral). Lying beside or near to the urethra. [see prec.]

para-urethritis (par·ah·ewr·e·thri′·tis). An infective or inflammatory condition in which the tissues alongside or near the urethra are involved. [para-urethra, Gk *-itis* inflammation.]

para-uterine (par·ah·ew·ter·ine). Near or beside the uterus. [Gk *para*, uterus.]

paravaccinia (par·ah·vak·sin′·e·ah). A subgroup of the poxviruses differing in morphology from the smallpox-vaccinia-cowpox group. The virus particles are large (250 nm), oval and contain DNA. The members of the subgroup are the viruses of pseudocowpox (milkers' nodule virus), orf (contagious pustular dermatitis) and stomatitis papulosa of cattle. The viruses of pseudocowpox and orf are closely related, difficult to grow in cell culture and may occasionally infect man by direct contact with infected cows or sheep respectively. [Gk *para*, L *vaccinus* of a cow.]

paravaginal (par·ah·vaj·in·al). Situated close to or beside the vagina. [Gk *para*, vagina.]

paravaginitis (par·ah·vaj·in·i′·tis). An inflammatory condition affecting the cellular tissues adjacent to the vagina. [Gk *para*, vaginitis.]

paravariola (par·ah·var·e′·o·lah). Alastrim. [Gk *para*, variola.]

paravenin (par·ah·ven·in). A product obtained by collecting the venoms of certain poisonous snakes, mixing them and then rendering the mixture partly inactive. It has been used in treating nerve exhaustion, hysteria and functional nervous disorders. [Gk *para*, L *venenum* poison.]

paravenous (par·ah·ve·nus). Beside or situated near a vein. [Gk *para*, vein.]

paravertebral (par·ah·ver·te·bral). Situated alongside of the spinal column, or a vertebra. [Gk *para*, vertebra.]

paravesical (par·ah·**ves**·ik·al). Near the urinary bladder. [Gk *para,* L *vesica* bladder.]

paravitaminosis (par·ah·vi·tam·in·**o′**·sis). A syndrome that is similar to an avitaminosis, but not due to lack of vitamins. [Gk *para,* vitaminosis.]

paraxanthine (par·ah·**zan**·theen). 1,7-Dimethylxanthine, $C_7H_8N_4O_2$. A purine derivative, isomeric with theophylline and theobromine, which occurs in minute quantity in normal urine, and in many animal organs. Its chief physiological significance appears to be as inhibitor of thyroid hormone.

paraxial (par·**ax**·e·al). By the side of or close to an axis of any part or body. [Gk *para,* axis.]

paraxon (par·**ax**·on). A collateral branch from the axon of a nerve cell; an obsolescent term. [Gk *para,* axon.]

Parazoa (par·ah·**zo**·ah). A subkingdom of the animal kingdom containing only the phylum Porifera; the sponges. [see foll.]

parazoon (par·ah·**zo**·on). Any one member of the subkingdom Parazoa. [Gk *para, zoon* animal.]

parchment crackling (**parch**·ment **krak**·ling). The abnormal sensation and sound produced by pressure on cranial bones which are affected by craniotabes. This localized thinning of the cranial bones is usually due to rickets, but also occurs in the group of chondrodysplasias and cranial dysostoses. [Fr. *parchemin,* AS *cracian.*]

parectasia (par·ek·**ta**·ze·ah). Parectasis.

parectasis (par·**ek**·tas·is). Overstretching or overdistension of an organ or part. [Gk *para,* ectasia.]

parectropia (par·ek·**tro**·pe·ah). Apraxia. [Gk *para, ektrope* digression.]

paregoric (par·e·**gor**·ik). The popular name for camphorated tincture of opium, containing 5 per cent of tincture of opium (≡ 0.05 per cent morphine) as well as benzoic acid, camphor and anise oil; used in cough mixtures. [Gk *paregorikos* consoling.]

paregorism (par·**e**·gor·izm). Addiction to opium caused by constant dosage with paregoric.

pareira (par·**a**·rah). The dried root of *Chondrodendron tomentosum* of the family Menispermaceae, a plant of Brazil. It contains several alkaloids, including bebeerine, isobebeerine and β-chondrodendrine. It is thought to be the source of tube curare, and *d*-tubocurarine has been prepared from it, according to report. [Port. *parreira brava* wild vine.]

pareleidin (par·el·**e**·id·in). Keratin. [Gk *para,* eleidin.]

parencephalia (par·en·kef·**a′**·le·ah). A congenital abnormality of the brain. [Gk *para, egkephalos* brain.]

parencephalitis (par·en·kef·al·**i′**·tis). An inflammatory condition affecting the cerebellum. [Gk *para,* encephalitis.]

parencephalocele (par·en·**kef**·al·o·seel). Cerebellar hernia. [parencephalon, Gk *kele* hernia.]

parencephalon (par·en·**kef**·al·on). The cerebellum. [Gk *para, egkephalos* brain.]

parencephalous (par·en·**kef**·al·us). 1. Having a congenital deformity of the brain. 2. Relating to a parencephalus. [see foll.]

parencephalus (par·en·**kef**·al·us). A monster with a congenital cerebral deformity. [Gk *para, egkephalos* brain.]

parenchyma [NA] (par·**en**·ki·mah). The specific or functional constituent of a gland or organ, in contradistinction to its supporting framework. **Parenchyma testis [NA].** The glandular part of the testis; it consists of the seminiferous tubules. [Gk *para,* enchyma.]

parenchymal, parenchymatic (par·**en**·ki·mal, par·en·ki·**mat′**·ik). Belonging to or having the characteristics of parenchyma.

parenchymatitis (par·en·ki·mat·**i′**·tis). An inflammatory state of the parenchyma or organs, glands and other structures. [parenchyma, Gk *-itis* inflammation.]

parenchymatous (par·**en**·ki·mat·us). Parenchymal.

parenol (**par**·en·ol). An emulsion of water, wool fat and soft paraffin; used as an ointment base.

parent (**pa**·rent). Of a nuclide, that radioactive nuclide from which it is formed by decay. [L *parens.*]

parental (par·**en**·tal). Belonging to or originating in the parents. [L *parens* parent.]

parentalism (par·**en**·tal·izm). In psychiatry, the characteristics of possessiveness and power of ownership displayed by a parent towards his or her child. [see prec.]

parenteral (par·**en**·ter·al). Introduced subcutaneously, intravenously, or by any route other than by way of the digestive tract. [Gk *para, enteron* bowel.]

parepididymal (par·ep·e·**did′**·e·mal). Belonging to the paradidymis.

parepididymis (par·ep·e·**did′**·e·miz). Paradidymis.

parepigastric (par·ep·e·**gas′**·trik). Close to the epigastric region. [Gk *para,* epigastrium.]

parepithymia (par·ep·e·**thi′**·me·ah). A condition marked by perverted craving or appetite; morbid longing. [Gk *para, epithymia* longing.]

parerethisis, parerethism (par·er·**eth**·is·is, par·**er**·eth·izm). Over-excitation or over-stimulation. [Gk *para, erethizein* to excite.]

parergasia (par·er·**ga**·ze·ah). A term invented by Adolf Meyer to include all forms of schizophrenia, which are regarded in Meyerian psychopathology as a reaction of the personality to past and present experience, rather than as endogenous psychoses. [Gk *para, ergein* to work.]

parergasic, parergastic (par·er·**ga**·zik, par·er·**gas**·tik). Of or pertaining to parergasia.

paresis (par·**e**·sis, **par**·es·is). 1. Partial paralysis. 2. Frequently used as a synonym of paralysis. **Canal paresis.** Failure of the semicircular canal to react to caloric stimulation. **Galloping paresis.** A rapidly progressive form of general paralysis. **General paresis.** That due to cerebral syphilis; also called *dementia paralytica* and *general paralysis of the insane.* **Juvenile paresis.** A juvenile form of general paresis (see above). **Paresis sine paresei.** An early stage in neurosyphilis when symptoms are minimal but the cerebrospinal fluid shows a picture suggestive of the disease. [Gk, paralysis.]

pareso-analgesia (par·e·so·an·al·**je′**·ze·ah). Partial paralysis with loss of sensation. [paresis, analgesia.]

paretic (par·**et**·ik). Relating to, characterized by, or affected with paresis.

parfocal (par·**fo**·kal). Literally of equal focus, but applied in practice to instruments, e.g. the modern form of corneal microscope, in which changes of magnification can be obtained without having to re-focus. [L *par* equal, focus.]

Pargyline (**par**·ji·leen). BP Commission approved name for *N*-benzyl-*N*-methylprop-2-ynylamine; a hypotensive agent.

parhaemoglobin (par·he·mo·**glo′**·bin). A form of haemoglobin; not a specific word. [Gk *para,* haemoglobin.]

Parham, Frederick William (b. 1856). American surgeon.

Parham band. A metal strip used for the internal fixation of spiral fractures of the long bones.

parhedonia (par·he·**do**·ne·ah). A Freudian term for abnormalities of sexuality, such as the obsessive desire to see, to exhibit, or to touch the sexual organs of oneself or another. [Gk *para, hedonia* pleasure.]

parhidrosis (par·hid·**ro**·sis). Any abnormal condition of the sweat secretion. [Gk *para, hidros* sweat.]

paricine (**par**·is·een). $C_{16}H_{18}ON_2·\frac{1}{2}H_2O$, one of the less important alkaloids of cinchona.

paries [NA] (**par**·e·eez) (pl. *parietes*). The wall or boundary of a cavity; the most superficial parts of a structure or organ. [L.]

parietal (par·**i**·et·al). Of or relating to the walls of any cavity or organ. [L *paries* wall.]

parietal bone [os parietale (NA)]. A quadrilateral skull bone meeting its fellow along its medial border and lying between the frontal and occipital bones and above the temporal bone. It forms a large part of the cranial vault [facies externa (NA)], and its point of great convexity near the centre constitutes the parietal eminence. A longitudinal groove on its inner surface [facies interna (NA)], along its median border, forms part of the sulcus for the sagittal sinus in the articulated skull. **Frontal angle [angulus frontalis (NA)].** The anterosuperior angle of the parietal bone; it occurs at the bregma where the sagittal and coronal sutures meet.

Mastoid angle [angulus mastoideus (NA)]. The postero-inferior angle of the parietal bone; it meets the occipital bone and the mastoid part of the temporal bone at the asterion.
Occipital angle [angulus occipitalis (NA)]. The posterosuperior angle of the parietal bone; it occurs at the lambda where the sagittal and lambdoid sutures meet.
Sphenoidal angle [angulus sphenoidalis (NA)]. The antero-inferior angle of the parietal bone; it fits between the frontal bone and the greater wing of the sphenoid bone.
Frontal border [margo frontalis (NA)]. The border that articulates with the frontal bone.
Occipital border [margo occipitalis (NA)]. The border that articulates with the occipital bone.
Sagittal border [margo sagittalis (NA)]. The border that articulates with its fellow of the opposite side.
Squamous border [margo squamosus (NA)]. The border that articulates with the squamous part of the temporal bone.

parietalia (par·i·et·**a**'·le·ah). Those bones which taken together comprise the cranial vault. [L *paries* wall.]

parietaria (par·i·et·**a**'·re·ah). Wall pellitory; the herb of *Parietaria officinalis* (family Urticaceae), formerly employed as a diuretic in urinary complaints and dropsy. [L *paries* wall.]

parietes (par·i·et·eez). *See* PARIES.

parietitis (par·i·et·**i**'·tis). Inflammation affecting the wall or walls of an organ. [L *paries* wall, Gk *-itis* inflammation.]

parietofrontal (par·i·et·o·**frun**'·tal). Of or belonging to the parietal and frontal bones or to the gyri or fissures similarly named.

parietomastoid (par·i·et·o·**mas**'·toid). Relating or belonging to the parietal bone and the mastoid part of the temporal bone.

parieto-occipital (par·i·et·o·ok·**sip**'·it·al). Relating or belonging to the parietal and occipital bones, or to the cerebral gyri similarly named.

parietosphenoid (par·i·et·o·**sfe**'·noid). Relating to the parietal and sphenoid bones.

parietosplanchnic (par·i·et·o·**splangk**'·nik). Parietovisceral. [L *paries* wall, Gk *splanchnon* viscus.]

parietosquamosal (par·i·et·o·skwa·**mo**'·sal). Belonging to the parietal bone and the squamous part of the temporal bone.

parietotemporal (par·i·et·o·**tem**'·por·al). Belonging to the parietal bones and temporal bones or to the cerebral gyri of similar name.

parietovisceral (par·i·et·o·**vis**'·er·al). 1. Relating to the walls of a cavity and the viscera contained therein. 2. Both parietal and visceral. [L *paries* wall, viscus.]

parigenin (par·ij·en·in). $C_{27}H_{44}O_3$, a genin obtained by the hydrolysis of the saponin parillic acid.

Parinaud, Henri (b. 1844). Paris ophthalmologist.
Parinaud's conjunctivitis, or oculoglandular syndrome. Unilateral chronic granulomatous conjunctivitis with marked enlargement of the regional lymph glands, going on to suppuration, and associated with a fever. Some of the cases turn out to be tuberculous, others have been attributed to a *Leptothrix, Sporotrichum schencki,* or a filter-passing virus.
Parinaud's operation, Motais–Parinaud operation. For ptosis: a method very similar to Motais' operation of using the superior rectus muscle of the orbit.
Parinaud's ophthalmoplegia, or syndrome. Paralysis of conjugate upward deviation of the eyes, due to a lesion in the mid-brain at the level of the anterior corpora quadrigemina; a form of supranuclear ocular paralysis.

Paris, M. (fl. 1791). French surgeon.
Paris's disease. Coarctation of the aorta.

Paris Nomenclature (**par**·is no·**men**·klah·tcher). The anatomical terminology agreed upon at the Sixth International Congress of Anatomists held in Paris in July 1955.

Paris Nomina Anatomica (**par**·is **nom**·in·ah an·at·**om**·ik·ah). PNA, the anatomical terminology agreed upon at the Sixth International Congress of Anatomists held in Paris in July 1955. [L *nomen* name, Gk *anatome* dissection.]

paristhmic (par·is·mik). Belonging to the tonsils. [see foll.]

paristhmion (par·**is**·me·on). A tonsil. [Gk *para, isthmos* neck.]

paristhmitis (par·is·**mi**·tis). Tonsillitis. [paristhmion, Gk *-itis* inflammation.]

paritol (**par**·it·ol). A synthetic substitute for heparin, being a polysylphonic acid ester of polyanhydromannuronic acid.

parity (**par**·it·e). The condition or fact of having borne children. [L *parere* to give birth.]

Parker, H. M. 20th century British-American physicist.
Paterson and Parker method or system of radium dosage. The Manchester system; a scheme of radium distribution for interstitial, intracavitary and surface application, designed to provide homogeneity of tumour dose and simplify the necessary calculations.

Parker, Ralph R. (b. 1888). American zoologist.
Spencer–Parker vaccine. A vaccine of Rocky Mountain spotted fever made from ground-up ticks.

Parker, Willard (b. 1800). New York surgeon.
Parker's operation. An operation for lateral perineal lithotomy, early 19th century. He performed the first cystotomy for repair of rupture of the bladder.
Bard–Parker knife. A knife with a metal handle, and detachable renewable blades.

Parker, William Kitchen (b. 1823). London anatomist.
Parker's arches. Occipital arches of the developing vertebrate skull.

Parkes' syndrome. Vomiting, sleepiness, irregularity of breathing and bowel action; the signs consist of cyanosis, acetonuria, enlargement of the liver and signs of meningeal irritation. These symptoms and signs, occurring as they may in various epidemics amongst children, are due to a bacteriological or virus infection, and their specific aetiology should be determined, and this term avoided.

Parkinson, James (b. 1755). English physician.
Parkinson's disease. Paralysis agitans.
Parkinson's facies, mask, or sign. The mask-like facial expression of parkinsonism.
Parkinson's syndrome, Parkinsonian syndrome. Parkinsonism; mask-like facies, excessive salivation, loss of emotional and associated movements, static tremor inhibited by movement, and a festinant gait, due to a lesion of the globus pallidus and often the substantia nigra (the palaeostriatum). If due to degeneration it is called *paralysis agitans,* if to chronic encephalitis lethargica, *postencephalitic parkinsonism.* Also caused by certain drugs and by manganese poisoning.

Parkinson, Sir John (b. 1885). London cardiologist.
Wolff–Parkinson–White syndrome. This consists of physiological bundle-branch block with short P–R interval, probably as a result of an abnormal short conducting pathway between atria and ventricles. This results in premature excitation of one ventricle (usually the right), and gives rise to functional block of the left bundle. It occurs as a congenital anomaly in an otherwise normal heart, and is associated with a liability to repeated paroxysms of tachycardia. A similar electrocardiographic appearance may sometimes be seen as a result of nodal rhythm resulting from acquired cardiac lesions.

parkinsonism (**par**·kin·son·izm). Parkinson's syndrome. *See* PARKINSON, JAMES. **Arteriosclerotic parkinsonism.** A condition with some resemblance to Parkinson's disease, resulting from cerebral arteriosclerosis, but not associated with tremor. More accurately termed *arteriosclerotic pseudoparkinsonism.* **Idiopathic parkinsonism.** Parkinson's disease; paralysis agitans. **Postencephalitic parkinsonism.** Parkinsonism following encephalitis lethargica.

parkinsonism–dementia complex. A specific disease of unknown cause occurring on the island of Guam and causing dementia and a parkinsonian-like state, and possibly progressive muscle wasting.

Parks, Alan Guyatt. London surgeon.
Parks' operation. For anorectal fistulae. An operation, the essential feature of which is the excision of the infected anal

gland and associated abscess which, it is postulated, is the primary cause of the fistula.

Parks' operation. For haemorrhoids. Submucous removal of the haemorrhoidal plexus of veins and arteries, preserving the mucous membrane.

paroccipital (par·ok·**sip**·it·al). Close to the occipital bone. [Gk *para*, occiput.]

parodontal (par·o·**don**·tal). Periodontic. [Gk *para*, *odous* tooth.]

parodontitis (par·o·don·**ti'**·tis). Periodontitis. [Gk *para*, *odous* tooth, *-itis* inflammation.]

parodontosis (par·o·don·**to'**·sis). Periodontosis; periodontitis complex. [Gk *para*, *odous* tooth, *-osis* condition.]

parodynia (par·o·**din**·e·ah). Difficult labour; dystocia. [L *parere* to bring forth, *odyne* pain.]

paroecius (par·e·she·us). In biology, denoting male and female organs which develop side by side. [Gk *para*, *oikos* a single house.]

parogen (**par**·o·jen). A vasoliment.

parolivary (par·**ol**·iv·ar·e). Situated beside or close to the olivary body. [Gk *para*, olivary.]

Paromomycin (par·o·mo·**mi'**·sin). BP Commission approved name for an antibiotic produced by *Streptomyces rimosus* forma *paromomycinus*. **Paromomycin Sulphate BP 1968.** The sulphates of paromomycin, effective against a wide range of pathogenic bacteria in the intestinal tract. It is also effective in infections with *Entamoeba histolytica*.

paromphalocele (par·**om**·fal·o·seel). A hernial protrusion near the umbilicus. [Gk *para*, *omphalos* navel, *kele* hernia.]

Parona, Francesco. Milan surgeon.

space of Parona. A fascial plane between the superficial and deep groups of the muscles of the forearm.

paroniria (par·on·i·re·ah). Dreaming which has a frightening or morbid character. **Paroniria ambulans.** Somnambulism. **Paroniria salax.** Unrestful sleep associated with lustful dreams and nocturnal emissions. [Gk *para*, *oneiros* dream.]

paronychia (par·on·**ik**·e·ah). Pyogenic inflammation in the tissue around the nail or around the bone of the distal phalanx of a toe or finger; whitlow. **Mycotic paronychia.** Paronychia caused by a mycotic infection, commonly *Candida albicans*. **Paronychia tendinosa.** Pyogenic infection of the synovial sheath of a finger. [Gk *para*, *onyx* nail.]

paronychial (par·on·**ik**·e·al). Relating or belonging to, or of the nature of a paronychia.

paronychomycosis (par·**on**·ik·o·mi·**ko'**·sis). Mycotic paronychia.

paronychosis (par·**on**·ik·**o'**·sis). 1. A pathological state of the tissues surrounding the nails. 2. The development of a nail in an abnormal situation. [Gk *para*, *onyx* nail, *-osis* condition.]

paroöphoric (par·o·**of**·or·ik). Belonging to the paroöphoron.

paroöphoritis (par·o·**of**·or·**i'**·tis). 1. Inflammation affecting the paroöphoron. 2. Inflammation affecting the structures around the ovary. [paroöphoron, Gk *-itis* inflammation.]

paroöphoron [NA] (par·o·**of**·or·on). A group of vestigial mesonephric tubules situated in the broad ligament of the uterus medial to the ovaries. [Gk *para*, *oon* egg, *pherein* to bear.]

parophthalmia (par·of·**thal**·me·ah). Inflammation of the cellular and connective tissue in the neighbourhood of the eye. [Gk *para*, *ophthalmos* eye.]

parophthalmoncus (par·of·thal·**mon'**·kus). A tumour situated close to the eye. [Gk *para*, *ophthalmos* eye, *ogkos* a swelling.]

paropion (par·o·pe·on). An eye shade. [Gk *para*, *ops* eye.]

paropsis (par·**op**·sis). Disorder of sight. [Gk *para*, *opsis* vision.]

paroptic (par·**op**·tik). Relating to the coloured fringes around an image due to diffraction of light at the sharp edges of the object. [see prec.]

paroral (par·**or**·al). In biology, beside the mouth. [Gk *para*, L *os* mouth.]

parorasis (par·or·**a**·sis). Any abnormality of the visual sense or of colour vision, generally hallucinatory. [Gk *para*, *horaein* to see.]

parorchidium (par·or·**kid**·e·um). 1. Displacement of a testis. 2. Non-descent of a testis. [Gk *para*, *orchis* testicle.]

parorexia (par·o·**rex**·e·ah). A nervous state characterized by perversion of appetite and a strong desire for certain foods or for substances which are unsuitable as food. [Gk *para*, *orexia* desire for a thing.]

parosmia (par·**oz**·me·ah). Perversion of the sense of smell, even to a stage at which odours not in existence are perceived. [Gk *para*, *osme* smell.]

parosphresis (par·os·**fre**·sis). Parosmia. [Gk *para*, *osphresis* smell.]

parosteal (par·**os**·te·al). Belonging to the outer layer of the periosteum. [Gk *para*, periosteum.]

parosteitis (par·**os**·te·i'·tis). Inflammation of the structures closely associated with a bone. [Gk *para*, *osteon* bone, *-itis* inflammation.]

parosteosis (par·**os**·te·**o'**·sis). Ossification in the soft tissues adjacent to the periosteum. [Gk *para*, *osteon* bone, *-osis* condition.]

parostia (par·**os**·te·ah). Any abnormal ossification. [Gk *para*, *osteon* bone.]

parostitis (par·os·**ti**·tis). Parosteitis.

parostosis (par·os·**to**·sis). Parosteosis.

parotic (par·**ot**·ik). Beside or close to the ear. [Gk *para*, *ous* ear.]

parotid (par·**ot**·id). 1. Occurring near the ear. 2. The parotid gland. *See* GLAND. [see prec.]

parotid veins [venae parotideae (NA)]. Veins draining the parotid gland into the posterior facial vein or its superficial temporal or maxillary tributaries.

parotidean (par·**ot**·id·**e'**·an). Belonging to the parotid gland.

parotidectomy (par·**ot**·id·**ek'**·to·me). Surgical removal of the parotid gland. **Conservative parotidectomy.** Surgical removal of the parotid gland, partially or completely, with preservation of the facial nerve; commonly performed for pleomorphic adenomas. **Radical parotidectomy.** Surgical removal of the parotid gland with sacrifice of the facial nerve and sometimes of involved surrounding tissues; performed for carcinoma and other malignant tumours of the parotid. **Subfacial parotidectomy.** Surgical removal of that part of the parotid gland which lies deep to the facial nerve. **Superfacial parotidectomy, Superficial parotidectomy.** Surgical removal of that part of the parotid gland which lies superficial to the facial nerve. [parotid gland, Gk *ektome* a cutting out.]

parotiditis (par·**ot**·id·**i'**·tis). Parotitis.

parotidoscirrhus (par·**ot**·id·o·**skir'**·us). 1. Parotidosclerosis. 2. A scirrhous tumour of the parotid gland. [parotid, Gk *skirrhos* hard.]

parotidosclerosis (par·**ot**·id·o·skler·**o'**·sis). A sclerosed state of the parotid gland.

parotis (par·**o**·tis). The parotid gland. *See* GLAND. **Parotis accessoria.** The accessory parotid gland. *See* GLAND. [Gk *para*, *ous* ear.]

parotitic (par·o·**tit**·ik). Relating to or suffering from parotitis.

parotitis (par·o·**ti**·tis). An inflammatory state of the parotid glands. **Chronic parotitis.** Persistent enlargement of the parotid gland as a result of chronic infection. **Coeliac parotitis.** Parotitis which is consequent upon abdominal injury or disease. **Epidemic parotitis.** Mumps, an infectious disease due to a paramyxovirus, characterized by swelling of the salivary glands, especially the parotids, with occasional involvement of the testes, ovaries, or pancreas. Meningitis is a relatively common complication. **Metastatic parotitis.** Symptomatic parotitis (see below). **Parotitis phlegmonosa.** That in which the swelling is succeeded by suppuration. **Postoperative parotitis.** Inflammation of the parotid gland after operation, due to organisms ascending along the duct from the mouth; predisposed to by poor oral hygiene and dehydration. Now rare. **Recurrent parotitis.** Recurrent inflammation of the parotid gland, usually secondary to obstruction of the duct as by a calculus or to deficiency of secretion. **Symptomatic parotitis.** Parotitis which occurs as a secondary lesion following an injury or disease. [parotid gland, Gk *-itis* inflammation.]

parotomegaly (par·ot·o·**meg'**·al·e). Enlargement of the parotid gland without pathology. [parotid gland, Gk *megas* large.]

parous (pa·rus). Of a woman, one who has borne one or more children. [L *parere* to bear.]

parovarian (par·o·va·re·an). 1. Relating to the epoöphoron (parovarium). 2. Occurring beside or close to the ovary. [Gk *para*, ovary.]

parovariotomy (par·o·va·re·ot'·o·me). The operation of incising or removing a cyst of the epoöphoron. [parovarium, Gk *temnein* to cut.]

parovaritis (par·o·var·i'·tis). Inflammation affecting the epoöphoron (parovarium). [parovarium, Gk *-itis* inflammation.]

parovarium (par·o·va·re·um). The epoöphoron. [Gk *para*, ovary.]

paroxia (par·ox·e·ah). Pica. [Gk *para*, *oxetes* pungency of taste.]

paroxyntic (par·ox·in·tik). Paroxysmal. [Gk *paroxyntikos* exciting.]

paroxysm (par·ox·izm). 1. A sudden attack or exacerbation of a disease or of symptoms, particularly recurrent symptoms. 2. A convulsion. [Gk *paroxysmos* irritation.]

paroxysmal (par·ox·iz·mal). Having the characteristics of a paroxysm.

Parrish, Edward (b. 1822). Philadelphia pharmacist.

Parrish's camphor mixture. Aromatic camphor mixture; tincture of lavender, sugar and camphor water, used as a carminative.

Parrish's syrup. A tonic syrup intended especially for children and containing the phosphates of iron, calcium, potassium and sodium, flavoured with orange-flower water and coloured with cochineal.

Parrot, Joseph Marie Jules (b. 1839). Paris physician.

Parrot's atrophy of the newborn. A primary atrophy or marasmus of newborn infants.

Parrot's disease, or pseudoparalysis. Epiphyseal osteochondritis of syphilitic origin, producing pseudoparalysis.

Parrot's murmur. A soft sound heard during cardiac asystole.

Parrot's node. A syphilitic node on the outer table of the skull.

Parrot's sign. 1. The ciliospinal reflex. *See* REFLEX. 2. Parrot's node (see above).

Parrot's ulcer. Small ulcerated areas on the mucous membrane of the mouth, pharynx, and less commonly throughout the gastrointestinal tract, caused by *Candida albicans;* thrush.

parru (par·oo). Yaws.

Parry, Caleb Hillier (b. 1755). Bath physician.

Parry's disease. Exophthalmic goitre. (Parry gave an excellent description of this disease as early as 1786.)

Parry-Romberg syndrome. Progressive wasting of the tissues, starting in one side of the brow and spreading so as to involve the face and perhaps the homolateral upper limb and mamma.

pars [NA] (parz). A part. **Pars anterior hypophyseos.** The anterior lobe of the hypophysis cerebri (pituitary gland). It produces hormones which influence growth and the activity and development of the sexual glands and other ductless glands. **Pars basalis.** That part of the endometrium that remains after menstruation and from which the endometrium regenerates. **Pars buccalis, Pars buccalis hypophyseos.** The anterior lobe and middle part of the hypophysis cerebri, both of which are developed from the ectoderm of the embryonic mouth, or stomatodaeum. **Pars functionalis.** That part of the endometrium which is shed during menstruation. **Pars intermedia hypophyseos.** The middle part of the hypophysis cerebri. **Pars nervosa hypophyseos.** The posterior lobe of the hypophysis cerebri which develops from the floor of the 3rd ventricle of the brain. It forms hormones which raise blood pressure, cause uterine muscle to contract and regulate the excretion of water by the kidney, etc. **Pars optica hypothalami.** That part of the hypothalamus which lies above the optic chiasma. **Pars plana.** The posterior part of the ciliary body of the eye lying between the ora serrata and ciliary processes. **Pars posterior hypophyseos.** Pars nervosa hypophyseos (see above). **Pars squamosa.** A squamous or flattened part; usually applied to certain bones of the skull, e.g. pars squamosa of the temporal bone. **Pars tuberalis hypophyseos.** An extension of the anterior lobe of the hypophysis cerebri along its stalk and around the tuber cinereum of the hypothalamus. [L, a part.]

parsley (par·sle). The herb *Carum petroselinum* (family Umbelliferae) which is used for culinary purposes; the root and fruit are employed medicinally. [ME *persely.*]

partal (par·tal). Relating to parturition.

parthenicine (par·then·is·een). One of the antipyretic alkaloids obtained from the plant *Parthenium hysterophorus.*

parthenine (par·then·een). An alkaloid with antipyretic properties derived from the plant *Parthenium hysterophorus.*

parthenium (par·the·ne·um). Feverfew; the herb *Chrysanthemum parthenium* (family Compositae). The flower heads are very similar to chamomile in appearance and odour. [Gk *parthenos* virgin.]

parthenogenesis (par·then·o·jen'·es·is). Non-sexual reproduction by means of an egg independent of fertilization by the male. **Artificial parthenogenesis.** The growth of an unfecundated ovum by such means as mechanical or chemical stimuli. [Gk *parthenos* virgin, *genesis* origin.]

parthenogenetic (par·then·o·jen·et'·ik). Reproducing without union of the male and female organisms. [see prec.]

parthenology (par·then·ol·o·je). The branch of gynaecology which is concerned with virgins. [Gk *parthenos* virgin, *logos* science.]

parthenoplasty (par·then·o·plas·te). The production of a faked virginal state by suture of the ruptured hymen. [Gk *parthenos* virgin, *plassein* to mould.]

parthogenesis (par·tho·jen·es·is). Parthenogenesis.

particle (par·tikl). A minute fragment or speck; now usually understood to mean any of the fundamental units of matter studied by atomic physics. **Alpha particle.** A particle consisting of two neutrons and two protons (the nucleus of the helium atom) emitted by certain radioactive elements. **Attraction particle.** The centriole, a minute darkly staining granule at the centre of the centrosome in resting cells and the aster in dividing cells. **Beta particle.** An electron, of positive or negative charge, emitted during the beta decay of a radionuclide. **Colloid particle.** A solid particle in the disperse phase of a colloidal system, having an average diameter of from 5 nm to 100 nm. **Dane particles.** Particles about 42 nm in diameter found in the serum of some Australia-antigen-positive patients with serum hepatitis. By electron microscopy they are seen in association with Australia antigen particles and may be mature virus particles. **Disperse particles.** The particles of the internal phase of a colloidal system. **Elementary particle.** In nuclear physics, a subatomic particle such as an electron, proton, neutron, etc., forming part of atomic structure. **Fast-charged particle.** A charged atomic particle moving at a velocity that is an appreciable proportion of the velocity of light, e.g. one-fifth. **Gamma particle.** Gamma ray. *See* RAY. **Nuclear particles.** Howell-Jolly bodies; nuclear remnants occasionally seen in red blood corpuscles. They are spherical, eccentrically placed granules, about 1 μm diameter. **Virus particle.** The smallest complete unit of a virus; the virion. [L *particula* small part.]

See also: ZIMMERMANN (G. H. E.).

particulate (par·tik·ew·late). Pertaining to or existing in the form of, or made up of, discrete particles.

partigen (par·te·jen). Partial antigen. *See* ANTIGEN.

partinium (par·tin·e·um). An aluminium-tungsten alloy employed for its lightness and hardness.

partition (par·tish·un). When a substance is soluble to some extent in two or more immiscible liquids, the distribution of that substance between the liquids on the latter being shaken together and allowed to separate again. [L *partitio* a dividing.]

parturient (par·tewr·e·ent). 1. In the process of bringing forth young. 2. Relating to parturition. 3. A parturient woman. [L *parturire* to have the pains of labour.]

parturifacient (par·tewr·e·fa'·shent). 1. Inducing or accelerating delivery. 2. Giving relief during the process of child-bearing. 3. A drug that induces, accelerates, or gives relief during parturition. [L *parturire* to have the pains of labour, *facere* to cause.]

parturiometer (par·tewr·e·om′·et·er). An instrument determining the expulsive force of the uterus. [parturition, meter.]

parturition (par·tewr·ish·un). The process of childbirth. [L *parturire* to have the pains of labour.]

partus (par·tus). Labour, delivery, childbirth, or parturition. [L, a bringing forth.]

parulis (par·ew·lis). Abscess on a tooth which points on the gum; a gumboil. [Gk *para, oulon* the gums.]

parumbilical (par·um·bil·i′·kal). Para-umbilical.

parungual (par·ung·gwal). Occurring by the side of the nail. [Gk *para,* L *unguis* nail.]

paruria (par·ewr·e·ah). 1. Any defect of micturition. 2. Any disordered state of the urine. [Gk *para,* urine.]

parurocystis (par·ewr·o·sist′·is). A supplementary urinary bladder. [Gk *para, ouron* urine, *kystis* bag.]

parvicellular (par·ve·sel·ew·lar). Relating to or made up of small cells. [L *parvus* small, cellular.]

Parvobacteriaceae (par·vo·bak·teer·e·a′·se·e). A family of bacteria belonging to the order Eubacteriales in Rahn's classification (1937): it includes three genera, *Brucella, Pasteurella,* and *Haemophilus.* [L *parvus* small, bacterium.]

parvoline (par·vo·leen). 2-Ethyl-3,5-dimethylpyridine, $C_2H_5C_5H_2N(CH_3)_2$. An oily ptomaine produced in decaying fish and horse flesh.

parvule (par·vewl). A pilule, or small pill or pellet. [L *parvulus* very small.]

Paryphostomum (par·e·fos·to·mum). A genus of flukes. **Paryphostomum safrartefex,** a rare parasite of man; a specimen was recovered from a child in Assam with the symptoms similar to those of fasciolopsiasis. [Gk *paryphe* border, *stoma* mouth.]

Pascal, Blaise (b. 1623). French scientist.

Pascal's law. The pressure exerted at a point on a confined fluid is transmitted unchanged throughout the whole fluid.

pascal (pas·cal). The unit of pressure being equal to 1 newton per square metre. Symbol Pa. [Blaise *Pascal.*]

paschachurda (pas·kah·koor·dah). A crusted ulcer which is part of an endemic dermatosis, occurring in Central Asia.

Paschen, Enrique (b. 1860). Hamburg bacteriologist.

Paschen body, or granule, Buist-Paschen body. The elementary body in skin lesions in smallpox and vaccinia.

Paschutin, Victor Vasilyevich (b. 1845). St Petersburg pathologist.

Paschutin's degeneration. Hydrocarbonaceous degeneration.

pasimology (pas·im·ol′·o·je). Sign-language.

paspalism (pas·pal·izm). A form of poisoning attributed to the seeds of the Indian grass *Paspalum scorbiculatum.* [Gk *paspalos* millet.]

passage (pas·ij). 1. An opening, meatus, or channel. 2. The act of moving from one place to another. 3. The introduction into a cavity of an instrument such as a sound, catheter, or probe. 4. An evacuation of the bowels. **Alveolar passage.** Infundibulum of the lung. **False passage.** A passage made through the walls of a canal, usually as the result of inept introduction of a catheter. [L *passus* step.]

See also: BOLL.

Passavant, Philip Gustav (b. 1815). Frankfort surgeon.

Passavant's bar. A small sphincter-like ring of muscle which runs horizontally round the pharynx at the level of the hard palate. It is now regarded as a muscle of the soft palate which remained in its original position after the larynx migrated lower into the neck in man.

Passavant's cushion, or ridge. The prominence formed on the pharyngeal wall by Passavant's bar.

Passavant's operation. For synechia: by breaking down the adhesions; obsolete.

Passiflora (pas·e·flor·ah). A genus of twining plants; the passion flowers. **Passiflora incarnata.** A species the fluid extract of the leaves of which is used as an antispasmodic and sedative. [L *passio* passion, *flos* flower.]

passion (pash·un). 1. Enduring of pain or suffering. 2. A specific intense emotion. 3. Sexual love. **Ileac passion.** Ileus. [L *passio.*]

passional (pash·un·al). Pertaining to one of the passions, exhibiting or influenced by any of the passions.

passive (pas·iv). Not spontaneous, or not produced by the active effort of the individual. [L *passivus.*]

passivism (pas·iv·izm). A type of sexual perversion characterized by submission of one partner (usually the male) to unnatural sexual practices desired by the other partner, who may be of either sex. [L *passivus* passive.]

passivist (pas·iv·ist). Anyone who is the subject of passivism.

passivity (pas·iv·it·e). The mental state of being inactive or submissive. [L *passivus* passive.]

pasta (pas·tah). Paste. [L.]

paste (pa·st). An unctuous or gelatinous mass intended for external application. The basis of most pastes is soft paraffin (e.g. Lassar's paste), but glycogelatin is used for some (e.g. Unna's paste), whereas others contain no extraneous pasty material but owe their unctuous nature to the principal ingredient, as in almond paste. **Almond paste.** A confection of crushed almonds, sugar, etc. **Arsenical paste.** An arsenical paste used as a caustic in dentistry. **Bismuth paste.** A mixture of bismuth carbonate and white soft paraffin. **Chillie paste.** Unguentum capsici compositum. **Guarana paste.** A paste of crushed seeds of guarana, and containing theobromine and tannin. **Phosphorus paste.** Phosphorus mixed with flour; used as a rat poison. **Vienna paste.** Vienna powder. *See* POWDER. **XYZ paste.** A paste of equal parts of bismuth picrate and ammoniated mercury in liquid paraffin; a wound dressing. [L *pasta.*]

See also: ABBOT, BECK (E. G.). BOUGARD, BROOKE, BUCKLEY, DUPUYTREN, ESMARCH, IHLE, LANDOLFI, LASSAR, MORISON, UNNA.

paster (pas·ter). The reading segment of a bifocal spectacle lens.

Pasteur, Louis (b. 1822). Paris chemist, bacteriologist and immunologist. An early protagonist of the "germ" theory of infection, introduced live attenuated vaccines against anthrax and rabies.

Pasteur effect. The inhibiting effect of oxygen upon the fermentation of carbohydrates by living cells.

Pasteur's solution, or yeast water. A culture medium containing yeast ash, ammonium carbonate and glucose.

Pasteur's theory. The obsolete theory that immunity to an infection was the result of the exhaustion of foodstuffs necessary for reproduction and growth of the causal microorganisms.

Torula of Pasteur. The name *Torula* was used in a general sense for yeasts by Pasteur.

Pasteur's vaccine. Rabies vaccine. *See* VACCINE.

Pasteur-Chamberland filter. A bacterial filter similar to the Coors or Kitasato filter.

Pasteurella (pas·ter·el·ah). A bacterial genus in the family Brucellaceae; different species within the genus are associated with widespread infections among wild and domestic mammals. The pasteurellae are small, ovoid, Gram-negative bacilli showing bipolar staining with non-motile and motile species, aerobic or facultatively anaerobic with a tendency to involution forms in older cultures. Man may become secondarily infected from the animal reservoir as in plague, ordinarily transmitted from rats to man by the rat flea, and in tularaemia transmitted to man during handling of infected hares, rabbits, etc., and possibly also by ticks. Two other species occasionally infect man: *Pasteurella multocida (P. septica),* which causes acute haemorrhagic septicaemia among many animal species and may cause local septic lesions in man following cat or dog bites; and *P. pseudotuberculosis,* naturally associated with a chronic granulomatous infection in guinea-pigs, which may cause mesenteric lymphadenitis, mostly in children. Fowl cholera, due to a pasteurella, was originally studied by Pasteur in the development of live attenuated vaccines. [Louis *Pasteur.*]

pasteurelleae (pas·ter·el·e·e). A tribe of bacteria of the family Parvobacteriaceae, containing three genera—*Pasteurella, Malleomyces* and *Actinobacilius.* [Louis *Pasteur.*]

pasteurellosis (pas·ter·el·o′·sis). A term usually applied to infections with organisms of the genus *Pasteurella* in animals;

strictly it could be applied to similar infections in man, e.g. plague and tularaemia. [*Pasteurella*, Gk *-osis* condition.]

Pasteuria (pas·ter·e·ah). A genus of the family Pasteuriaceae. **Pasteuria ramosa.** A micro-organism parasitic in the body cavities of species of *Daphnia*. [Louis *Pasteur*.]

pasteurism (pas·ter·izm). The method of active immunization with attenuated cultures introduced by Louis Pasteur.

pasteurization (pas·ter·i·za′·shun). A process by which foods and food products, e.g. milk, fruit juices, wine, etc., are protected from putrefaction or fermentation. It involves a short exposure to heat at a lower temperature than that employed in ordinary sterilization, commonly for milk to 72°C for 20 seconds or 63°C for 30 minutes, followed by rapid cooling. The employment of the process in dairying has been an important factor in the elimination of tuberculosis and other infections conveyed by milk. [Louis *Pasteur*.]

pasteurizer (pas·ter·i·zer). A machine used in the pasteurization of fluids.

Pastia, C. Rumanian physician.

Pastia's lines, or sign. Transverse lines in the creases of the skin at the bend of the elbow, which are observed in scarlet fever after the rash has faded elsewhere. They are of some diagnostic value in late cases.

pastille (pas·teel). 1. A gelatin base impregnated with medicament and poured into moulds of a size suitable for sweetmeats. They may be sugar-coated to prevent them from adhering to one another, and are intended to be sucked. 2. In radiotherapy, a small paper disc covered with barium platinocyanide which undergoes colour changes when exposed to radiation. Formerly used for estimations of dose. [L *pastillus* little roll.]

Patau, Klaus. American geneticist.

Patau's syndrome. A syndrome of small head and often cleft lip and palate, deformed nose, micrognathia and scalp defect. It is usually fatal and is due to trisomy 13–15.

patch (pach). 1. A piece of material, especially plaster, applied to the skin, either to assist a healing process or for cosmetic purposes. 2. An area of tissue, particularly skin or mucous membrane, which is abnormal in appearance. **Butterfly patch.** The term applied to certain skin lesions when they affect both cheeks and the nose, especially lupus erythematosus but also erysipelas; a distribution which simulates a butterfly with extended wings. **Café-au-lait patches.** Brown skin patches seen in normal people but especially associated with epiloia, neurofibromatosis and Albright's syndrome; smaller moles are found in large numbers in Turner's (Albright's) syndrome. **Cotton-wool patch.** A soft, white patch of exudate, with ill-defined edges, seen in the retina, usually in cases of renal or malignant hypertensive retinopathy. **Herald patch.** The first visible lesion of pityriasis rosea. **Milk patch.** Macula albida. **Moth patch.** An area of chloasma. **Mucous patch.** The homologue of the roseola on mucous membranes (Gougerot). A greyish-white, or pearly, slightly raised lesion, with red edges, often seen on mucosae (particularly in the mouth) in secondary syphilis. Mucous patches are highly infective, usually multiple, and often from 5 to 10 mm in diameter. **Opaline patch.** Mucous patch (see above). **Salmon patches** (of Hutchinson) 1. A pinkish area seen in the cornea during the course of specific interstitial keratitis. One of the diagnostic features of Hutchinson's disease. 2. Pink telangiectases present at birth on the forehead, eyelids or nape of the neck, most of which fade spontaneously. **Sandy patches.** Ulcers in the bladder in schistosomiasis; the deposits of urates give them the sandy quality. **Smokers' patch.** Leucoplakia of the mouth. **White patch.** Milk spots; irregular, whitish, patches of fibrous tissue on the surface of the heart, most frequently over the ventricles, and considered to be caused by constant friction. [ME *pacche*.]

See also: BITOT, FOURNIER, HUTCHINSON, PEYER.

patefaction (pat·e·fak·shun). The process of laying open or exposing. [L *patefacere* to lay open.]

patella [NA] (pat·el·ah). The knee cap: a sesamoid bone lying in front of the knee joint and situated in the tendon of the quadriceps femoris muscle. It has two surfaces, the anterior [facies anterior (NA)] and the posterior [facies articularis (NA)]. **Apex of the patella [apex patellae (NA)].** The blunted inferior extremity formed by the meeting of the medial and lateral borders, to which the patellar tendon is attached. **Base of the patella [basis patellae (NA)].** The superior border of the patella, to which is attached the part of the quadriceps femoris muscle derived from the rectus femoris and the vastus intermedius muscles. **Patella bipartita.** A patella ossified in two parts. **Patella cubiti.** An occasional sesamoid bone in the triceps tendon of the arm. **Floating patella.** A patella which is forced away from the femoral condyle by a large effusion into the knee joint. **Patella partita.** A patella subdivided into several parts. **Slipping patella.** Recurrent dislocation of the patella. [L, small disc.]

patellapexy (pat·el·ah·pex·e). Fixation by suture of the patella to the lower end of the femur. [patella, Gk *pexis* fixation.]

patellar (pat·el·ar). Belonging to the patella.

patellectomy (pat·el·ek·to·me). The operation of removing the patella. [patella, Gk *ektome* a cutting out.]

patelliform (pat·el·e·form). In the shape of a patella.

patellofemoral (pat·el·o·fem′·or·al). Relating to the patella and to the femur.

patelloid (pat·el·oid). Patelliform. [patella, Gk *eidos* form.]

patency (pa·ten·se). The state of being freely exposed or open. [L *patens* open.]

patent (pa·tent). Open or exposed. [see prec.]

Paterson, Donald Gildersleeve (b. 1892). Minnesota psychologist.

Pintner-Paterson test. A series of non-verbal tests (including form-boards, cube tests and assembly tests) designed to test the intelligence of subjects who are deaf or who do not speak English.

Paterson, Donald Ross (b. 1863). Cardiff otolaryngologist.

Paterson's forceps. A bronchoscopic forceps with a distally controlled cupped hinged beak for the removal of foreign bodies or tissues for biopsy from the trachea or bronchi.

Paterson syndrome, Paterson-Kelly syndrome, Kelly-Paterson syndrome. Plummer-Vinson syndrome.

Paterson, James Ralston Kennedy. Manchester radiotherapist.

Paterson and Parker method or system of radium dosage. The Manchester system; a scheme of radium distribution for interstitial, intracavitary and surface application, designed to provide homogeneity of tumour dose and simplify the necessary calculations.

Paterson, Robert (b. 1814). Edinburgh physician.

Paterson corpuscle, Henderson-Paterson body. The inclusion body of molluscum contagiosum.

Patey, David Howard. London surgeon.

Patey's operation. A modified radical operation for carcinoma of the breast in which the breast and axillary lymph nodes are removed in continuity, as in the Halsted operation but without removal of the pectoralis major muscle.

path (pahth). In physiology, the chain of nerve cells and their processes along which a nerve impulse travels, whether the chain is motor or sensory. **Incisor path.** The path taken by the incisal edges of the lower teeth as they move from the position of centric occlusion to edge-to-edge contact with the upper teeth. [AS *paeth*.]

pathema (path·e·mah). Any pathological condition. [Gk, misfortune.]

pathergasia (path·er·ga·ze·ah). Term devised by Adolf Meyer to connote all forms of mental reaction of an abnormal (pathological) kind. [Gk *pathos* suffering, *ergein* to work.]

pathergia (path·er·je·ah). Pathergy.

pathergic (path·er·jik). Pertaining to or marked by pathergy.

pathergization (path·er·ji·za′·shun). The act of assuming the pathergic state.

parthergy (path·er·je). An abnormal response to an allergen. [Gk *pathos* suffering, *ergein* to work.]

pathetic (path·et·ik). 1. Affecting or stirring the emotions; belonging to the feelings. 2. Rare name for the 4th cranial nerve. [Gk *pathetos* subject to suffering.]

patheticus (path·et·ik·us). The 4th, or trochlear, cranial nerve, supplying the superior oblique muscle of the orbit. [see prec.]

pathetism (**path**·et·izm). Hypnotism or mesmerism. [Gk *pathetos* subject to suffering.]

pathetist (**path**·et·ist). A hypnotist. [see prec.]

pathfinder (**pahth**·fi·nder). A device for locating strictures of the urethra, when a series of delicate filiform guides are passed to the face of the stricture until one negotiates the channel. [AS *paeth, findan.*]

pathic (**path**·ik). 1. The passive partner in perverted sexual practices. 2. Pathological. [Gk *pathein* to suffer.]

patho-amine (path·o·**am**·een). A name sometimes applied to the ptomaines, or toxic amines produced by the bacterial decomposition of protein.

patho-anatomy (**path**·o·an·**at**′·o·me). Pathological anatomy.

pathobiology (**path**·o·bi·**ol**′·o·je). Pathology. [pathology, biology.]

pathobolism (path·**ob**·ol·izm). A state of disordered metabolism. [Gk *pathos* disease, metabolism.]

pathoclisis (path·o·**klis**·is). 1. A specific fundamental sensitivity for certain toxic substances. 2. A specific attraction of certain toxins for particular groups of organs. [Gk *pathos* suffering, *klisis* inclination.]

pathocrine (**path**·o·krine). Relating to or characterized by pathocrinia.

pathocrinia (path·o·**krin**·e·ah). Any derangement of endocrine function. [Gk *pathos* disease, endocrine.]

pathodixia (path·o·**dix**·e·ah). An exaggerated tendency to exhibit injuries or morbid lesions. [Gk *pathos* suffering, *deiknymein* to display.]

pathogen (**path**·o·jen). Any living organism or other agent which is the cause of disease. [Gk *pathos* disease, *genein* to produce.]

pathogenesis (path·o·**jen**·es·is). The generation and production, or the mode of origin and development, of morbid or diseased conditions. **Drug pathogenesis.** The production of morbid symptoms by means of drugs. [see prec.]

pathogenetic (**path**·o·jen·**et**′·ik). Pathogenic.

pathogenic (path·o·**jen**·ik). Causing or producing disease. [Gk *pathos* disease, *genein* to produce.]

pathogenicity (**path**·o·jen·**is**′·it·e). The quality of being capable of causing disease, a quality that varies in degree. [see prec.]

pathogeny (path·**oj**·en·e). Pathogenesis.

pathognomonic (**path**·og·no·**mon**′·ik). Descriptive of a sign or symptom which is typical or characteristic and by which a disease can be recognized. [Gk *pathos* disease, *gnomon* index.]

pathognomy (path·**og**·no·me). 1. Diagnosis of disease by recognition of typical symptoms and signs. 2. The psychological diagnosis of a diseased state by study of the patient's subjective sensations. [Gk *pathos* disease, *gnome* opinion.]

pathognostic (path·og·**nos**·tik). Pathognomonic. [Gk *pathos* disease, *gnosis* knowledge.]

patholesia (path·o·le·ze·ah). Any hysterical state. [pathological, Gk *laien* to wish.]

pathological (path·o·**loj**·ik·al). 1. Relating to pathology. 2. Caused by or causing disease. 3. Indicating a diseased state or condition. [Gk *pathos* disease, *logos* science.]

pathologist (path·**ol**·o·jist). An expert in pathology; any person who specializes in the study of morbid anatomy.

pathology (path·**ol**·o·je). 1. By derivation, the science of disease; that branch of medical science that deals with the causes of disease and with their effect on the structure and functions of the body tissues. In the UK the word has a wide application and includes studies of the causal agents of disease, but in the USA the meaning is more restricted, and—unqualified—the word is confined to morbid anatomical and histopathological studies. 2. The sum of the morbid processes and changes that occur in the body tissues in a specific disease. **Cellular pathology.** Pathology considered from the point of view of the cell. **Chemical pathology.** Biochemistry. **Clinical pathology.** The application of pathology to clinical work, particularly with regard to the diagnosis of disease by laboratory methods. **Comparative pathology.** Pathology which treats of the diseases of animals and man, comparatively. **Dental pathology.** That branch of pathology which deals with diseases of the teeth and jaws and surrounding soft tissues. **Dermal pathology.** Pathology of the skin. **Exotic pathology.** A system of pathology foreign to the country or school in which it has become engrafted. **Experimental pathology.** The science of artificially induced disease. **External pathology.** Surgical pathology (see below). **Forensic pathology.** 1. The study of trauma and disease in relation to the needs of the law. 2. The practice of autopsy and laboratory techniques in the investigation of deaths of medicolegal interest. **Functional pathology.** The functional changes engendered by structural alterations in tissues. **General pathology.** The general laws associated with disease. **Geographical pathology.** The pathology which deals with the geographical distribution of diseases and their characteristics. **Gynaecological pathology.** The pathology of diseases peculiar to women. **Humoral pathology.** Pathology of the body fluids and their constituents. **Internal pathology, Medical pathology.** The pathology of diseases not easily accessible to operative procedures. **Mental pathology.** The pathology of mental processes. **Ophthalmic pathology.** Pathology of the eye. **Oral pathology.** Dental pathology (see above). **Plant pathology.** The pathology of plant life. **Special pathology.** The pathology of particular organs or tissues. **Surgical pathology.** The pathology of diseases accessible to surgical procedures. **Vegetable pathology.** Plant pathology (see above). [Gk *pathos* disease, *logos* science.]

patholysis (path·**ol**·is·is). Disintegration of diseased tissues. [Gk *pathos* suffering, *lysis* a loosing.]

pathomaine (**path**·o·mane). Any one of the cadaveric alkaloids considered to be pathogenic. [pathogenic, ptomaine.]

pathomania (path·o·**ma**·ne·ah). Moral insanity; compulsive urge to do wrong. [Gk *pathos* disease, mania.]

pathomeiosis (**path**·o·mi·**o**′·sis). The condition of mind of a patient in which he is disposed to underestimate the gravity of his disease. [Gk *pathos* disease, *meioein* to make smaller.]

pathometabolism (**path**·o·met·**ab**′·ol·izm). Metabolism in diseased conditions. [Gk *pathos* disease, metabolism.]

pathometric (path·o·**met**·rik). Relating to pathometry.

pathometry (path·**om**·et·re). 1. Determination of the number of persons suffering from a specific disease at any given time and of the conditions which make for a diminution or increase in that number. 2. A term used by Sir Ronald Ross to denote the quantitative estimation of parasitic infection in individuals or classes of individuals. [Gk *pathos* disease, *metron* measure.]

pathomimesis, pathomimia, pathomimicry (**path**·o·mim·**e**′·sis, path·o·**mim**·e·ah, path·o·**mim**·ik·re). Malingering. [Gk *pathos* disease, mimesis.]

pathomorphism, pathomorphology (path·o·**mor**·fizm, **path**·o·mor·**fol**′·o·je). Abnormal morphology. [Gk *pathos* disease, morphology.]

pathoneurosis (**path**·o·newr·**o**′·sis). A type of neurosis which influences the functioning of the body. [Gk *pathos* disease, neurosis.]

pathonomia, pathonomy (path·o·**no**·me·ah, path·**on**·o·me). The study of the laws of morbid processes. [Gk *pathos* disease, *nomos* law.]

patho-occlusion (**path**·o·ok·**loo**′·zhun). Malocclusion. [Gk *pathos* disease, occlusion.]

pathophilia (path·o·**fil**·e·ah). The state in which a patient with some form of chronic ill-health accommodates himself to circumstances. [Gk *pathos* disease, *philein* to love.]

pathophobia (path·o·**fo**·be·ah). An abnormal fear of disease. [Gk *pathos* disease, phobia.]

pathophoresis (**path**·o·for·**e**′·sis). The carrying or transmitting of disease. [Gk *pathos* disease, *pherein* to carry.]

pathophoric, pathophorous (path·o·**for**·ik, path·**of**·or·us). Conveying disease; sometimes applied to certain insects. [see prec.]

pathophysiology (**path**·o·fiz·e·**ol**′·o·je). The study of the effect of pathological changes in structure on the normal physiological processes. [Gk *pathos* disease, physiology.]

pathopleiosis (**path**·o·pli·**o**′·sis). A condition in which the patient tends to exaggerate the seriousness of his disease. [Gk *pathos* disease, *pleion* greater than.]

pathopoiesia, pathopoiesis (**path**·o·poi·**e**′·se·ah, **path**·o·poi·**e**′·sis). 1. The aetiology of disease. 2. The predisposition of a subject to become affected with disease. [Gk *pathos* disease, *poiein* to cause.]

pathopsychology (**path**·o·si·**kol**′·o·je). The psychology of mental disorder. [Gk *pathos* disease, psychology.]

pathopsychosis (**path**·o·si·**ko**′·sis). A psychotic disorder which has detrimental effect on the functions of the body. [Gk *pathos* disease, psychosis.]

pathoradiography (**path**·o·ra·de·**og**′·raf·e). The examination of morbid lesions by means of x-ray photography. [Gk *pathos* disease, radiography.]

pathoroentgenography (**path**·o·runt·yen·**og**′·raf·e). Pathoradiography. [Gk *pathos* disease, roentgenography.]

pathosis (path·o·sis). A pathological condition. [Gk *pathos* disease.]

pathotropism (path·o·**tro**·pizm). The affinity of drugs for morbid structures. [Gk *pathos* disease, *trope* a turning.]

pathway (pahth·way). A course, track or way; specifically, the linked neurones through whose cells and along whose processes a nervous impulse travels either from the periphery to the centre *(afferent pathway)* or from the centre to the effector organ *(efferent pathway)*. **Internuncial pathways.** Neurones which link together other neurones in a nervous pathway. **Pentose phosphate pathway.** The pathway of carbohydrate metabolism whereby glucose 6-phosphate may give rise to pentose sugars. In fatty-acid synthesis it is important as a source of NADPH. [AS *paeth, weg.*]

patient (pa·shent). Strictly a person who suffers patiently; from the physician's point of view one who is sick and requires treatment. [L *pati* to suffer.]

Patrick, James. Glasgow surgeon.

Patrick's solution. A solution of cocaine muriate and alcohol for injection into the trigeminal nerve.

Patrick's brachial-plexus block technique. A method of injecting anaesthetic solutions in the region of the brachial nerves at the root of the neck.

patrilineal (pat·re·**lin**·e·al). Relating to descent through the male line. [L *pater* father, *linea* line.]

patroclinous (pat·ro·**kli**·nus). Having characteristics which are inherited from the male parent. [Gk *patros* father, *klinein* to lean.]

patten (pat·en). A metal support worn on the shoe of the sound foot to prevent weight-bearing in disease of the opposite leg. When wearing a patten the patient can use crutches, swinging the diseased leg. [Fr. *patin.*]

pattern (pat·ern). A model, example, instance; hence, an arrangement or plan. **Action pattern.** The more or less constant manner in which an individual responds to certain stimuli. The manner may be congenital or acquired. **Behaviour pattern.** The characteristic arrangement of behavioural response. **Muscle pattern.** Muscles that are grouped together and respond as a group to stimulation. **Occlusal pattern.** In dentistry, the shape, size and relationship of the crowns of the teeth in upper and lower dental arches. **Skeletal pattern.** In dentistry, the shape, size and relationship of the basal part of the maxilla and the mandible. **Startle pattern.** The manner, typical of an individual, in which he responds to an unexpected stimulus. **Stimulus pattern.** Grouped stimuli that constantly arise in a given situation. [ME *patron.*]

patulin (pat·ew·lin). An antibiotic produced by the mould *Penicillium patulum.* It is active against Gram-positive and Gram-negative organisms as well as fungi, but is toxic to animals. It has been shown to be identical with the clavacin of *Aspergillus clavatus,* and with the claviformin of *Penicillium claviforme,* once believed to have possibilities in the treatment of the common cold. [see foll.]

patulous (pat·ew·lus). Freely expanded; patent. [L *patulus* standing open.]

Pauchet, Victor (b. 1869). Paris surgeon.

Pauchet's manoeuvre, Lardennois-Pauchet method. In gastrectomy a vascular separation of greater omentum by its division close to its attachment to the transverse colon.

Paul, Frank Thomas (b. 1851). English surgeon.

Paul's operation. Stage resection of colon, which is withdrawn as a loop on the surface of the abdomen and removed some days later to leave a double colostomy, the colostomy being finally closed after crushing of the spur which forms between the two ends of the extruded loop. Also called *Mikulicz operation.*

Paul's tube. A glass tube flanged at one end, used in intestinal surgery for drainage.

Paul, Gustav (b. 1859). Vienna physician.

Paul's test. A laboratory test for the diagnosis of smallpox, involving the inoculation of the contents of the patient's pustules into rabbits or guinea-pigs, through the cornea. A positive reaction is the development of a keratitis.

Paul, John Rodman (b. 1893). New Haven physician.

Paul-Bunnell reaction, or test. A laboratory test used to confirm a clinical diagnosis of infectious mononucleosis (glandular fever): dilutions of the patient's serum are mixed with a suspension of washed sheep's corpuscles and incubated, and the degree of agglutination is noted. The test depends on the presence of sheep heterophil antibodies (agglutinins) in the blood in glandular fever, and is almost specific.

Paul, Robert William. London engineer.

Bragg-Paul pulsator. An apparatus consisting of a rubber bag wrapped round the chest wall; by means of a pump the air pressure within the bag is increased and released at a given frequency. It is used to provide artificial respiration in cases of respiratory failure.

paulocardia (paw·lo·**kar**·de·ah). An uncommon term, originally intended to describe (*a*) unusual prolongation of cardiac diastole, or (*b*) a sensation that the heart has ceased to beat. [Gk *paula* a stopping, *kardia* heart.]

pause (pawz). An interval of inaction, or rest. **Compensatory pause.** In cardiology the protracted interval after an extra-systole which counterbalances the extra beat, thereby causing the total rate of the beat to remain unchanged. [Gk *pausis* a stopping.]

pausimenia (paw·se·**me**·ne·ah). Menopause. [Gk *pausis* a stopping, *men* month.]

Pautrier, Lucien M.A. (b. 1876). Strasbourg dermatologist.

Pautrier's giant lichenification. Thickened plaques of lichenification with a warty surface as sometimes seen in the genitofemoral region.

Angiolupoid of Brocq and Pautrier. A cutaneous sarcoid of the Boeck type, characterized by bluish-red, round or oval nodules and plaques about 5–20 mm in diameter. The lesions are few in number and occur especially on the upper parts of the sides of the nose, near the inner canthi of the eyes and on the cheeks adjacent to these parts.

pavaex (pa·va·ex). Pavex.

pavement (pa·vment). Any structure that has a pattern like a pavement or a tiled floor. [L *pavimentum* pavement of tiles.]

pavementing (pa·vment·ing). A condition of the blood vessels in which the walls are covered with a layer of leucocytes. [see prec.]

pavex (pa·vex). An apparatus used in the treatment of peripheral vascular disease by alternating pressure for the purpose of passive exercise. [passive, vascular, exercise.]

pavilion (pav·**il**·e·on). Any flared end of a canal; the term is largely obsolete. **Pavilion of the ear.** The auricle. **Pavilion of the oviduct.** The fimbriated end of the oviduct. **Pavilion of the pelvis.** The upper flaring part of the pelvis. [L *papilio* tent.]

pavitation (pav·it·a·shun). Fright and trembling amounting to demoralization. [L *pavere* to quake with fear.]

Pavlov, Ivan Petrovich (b. 1849). Russian physiologist.
Pavlov's method. A method for the study of the conditioned reflexes.
Pavlov's pouch, or stomach. A surgically isolated cul-de-sac of the stomach, with intact blood and nerve supply, from which gastric juice can be collected free from contamination with food; it opens to the exterior.

pavor (pa·vor). Terror. **Pavor diurnus.** A fit of screaming on awakening during the day. **Pavor nocturnus.** A condition similar to nightmare occurring in children. [L, fear by night.]

Pavy, Frederick William (b. 1829). London physician.
Pavy's disease. Recurrent albuminuria.

Pawlik, Karl (b. 1849). Prague gynaecologist.
Pawlik's grip. A method of abdominal palpation with the palm of the right hand on the pubic symphysis and the fingers parallel to one inguinal ligament and the thumb to the other. By pressing downwards and inwards the presenting part may be felt.
Pawlik's triangle, or trigone. An area on the anterior wall of the vagina in contact with the base (trigone) of the bladder.

pawpaw (paw·paw). 1. The melon tree, *Carica papaya* (family Caricaceae); the dried and purified latex of the fruit furnishes the proteolytic enzyme, papain. 2. Sometimes applied to papaw, the seed of *Asimina triloba*. [Sp. *papaya*.]

Paxton, Francis Valentine (b. 1840). Chichester physician.
Paxton's disease. Trichorrhexis nodosa.

Payr, Erwin (b. 1871). Leipzig surgeon.
Payr's clamp. A heavy crushing clamp.
Payr's disease. Adhesions and kinking between the transverse and descending parts of the colon.
Payr's membrane. The presplenic fold of the peritoneum, passing from the gastrosplenic ligament to blend with the phrenico-colic ligament.
Payr's sign. Tenderness on pressure along the inner side of the foot, found in venous thrombosis.

Péan, Jules Emile (b. 1830). Paris surgeon.
Péan's forceps. The earliest French artery forceps.

peanut (pe·nut). The edible fruit of *Arachis hypogaea* Linn. (family Leguminosae); from it is expressed a fixed oil, peanut or arachis oil, used in place of olive oil, and in the manufacture of margarine. [AS *pise, hnutu*.]

pear (pa·er). *See* ARZBERGER. [AS *pere*.]

pearl (perl). 1. Small pellets of mucoid material. 2. A native calcium carbonate. 3. A common type of pill coating, consisting of french chalk and mucilage. **Enamel pearl.** A type of odontome; a small nodule of enamel which is formed on the root of a molar tooth near the neck. Also called *enamel nodule, enameloma.* **Epidermic pearls, Epithelial pearls.** Whorls of epithelial cells arranged in a concentric manner, found in sections of malignant skin tumours. **Gouty pearl.** A colloquial term for the gouty tophus, a concretion of sodium biurate, often deposited around the joints or in the ears of sufferers with gout. [LL *perla*.]
See also: BOHN, ELSCHNIG, EPSTEIN (A.), LAËNNEC.

pearlash (perl·ash). Potassium carbonate, K_2CO_3. An alkali obtained by lixiviating the ashes of wood and purifying the solution. [pearl, ash.]

Pearson, George (b. 1751). London physician and chemist.
Pearson's solution. A solution of sodium arsenate, Na_3AsO_4, about 0.17 per cent w/v.

Pearson, Karl (b. 1857). British mathematician and anthropologist.
Pearson's formula. A formula for estimating the stature from certain long bones. Now superseded by the more accurate *Trotter and Gleser formulae* owing to underestimates from the use of Pearson's formula.
Poisson-Pearson formula. A statistical formula based on pure mathematics for calculating percentage of error. It has been used *inter alia* in malariology.

peau d'orange (po·daw·rahnzh). A condition caused by lymphatic oedema and characterized by the existence of dimples on the skin; typical of established scirrhous carcinoma of the breast and of elephantiasis. [Fr., orange rind.]

pebble (pebl). The name given to the variety of rock crystal which is the basis from which optical lenses may be cut. [etym. dub.]

Pecazine (pek·ah·zeen). BP Commission approved name for 10-(1-methyl-3-piperidylmethyl) phenothiazine; used in the treatment of anxiety states.

peccant (pek·ant). 1. Inducing disease. 2. Morbid. [L *peccare* to go wrong.]

peccatiphobia (pek·at·e·fo'·be·ah). Exaggerated fear of doing wrong. [L *peccatum* sin, phobia.]

Pechlin, Johannes Nicolaus (b. 1644). Kiel and Stockholm anatomist.
Pechlin's glands. The lymphatic nodules of the intestine.

pechyagra (pek·e·ag·rah). A gouty condition affecting the elbow joint. [Gk *pechys* forearm, *agra* a catching.]

Pecilocin (pe·sil·o·sin). BP Commission approved name for an antibiotic produced by *Paecilomyces varioti banier* var. *antibioticus;* it is used in the treatment of fungal infections of the skin.

Peck, Samuel Mortimer (b. 1900). New York dermatologist.
Peck's test. A test for purpura haemorrhagica, in which moccasin-snake venom (0.1 ml) injected intradermally produces a purpuric effect within an hour, whereas a control injection of normal saline at another site does not do so.

Pecquet, Jean (b. 1622). Montpellier and Paris physician.
Pecquet's cisterna, or reservoir. The cisterna or receptaculum chyli; the dilatation at the beginning of the thoracic duct anterior to the bodies of the 1st and 2nd lumbar vertebrae.
duct of Pecquet. The thoracic duct. *See* DUCT.

pectase (pek·taze). An enzyme occurring in ripening fruits which is concerned with the transformation of insoluble pectin (pectose) into soluble pectin. [Gk *pektos* congealed.]

pecten (pek·ten). 1. A vascular pleated membrane which extends from the optic disc for a variable distance into the vitreous. It is best developed in birds, but a comparable structure is present in some reptiles and fishes. 2. A sharp ridge extending laterally from the pubic tubercle and giving attachment to the pectineal part of the inguinal ligament. 3. The junction of stratified squamous and columnar epithelium in the wall of the anal canal. 4. The outer margins of the lamina cribrosa sclerae. [L, comb.]
See also: STROUD.

pectenitis (pek·ten·i·tis). A condition of inflammation affecting the middle third of the anal canal, generally causing interference with the action of the sphincter ani muscle. [pecten, Gk *-itis* inflammation.]

pectenosis (pek·ten·o·sis). Hardening and fibroid degeneration of the middle third of the anal canal, characterized by the development of a ring-like formation of fibrous tissue (the pecten band). [pecten, Gk *-osis* condition.]

pectenotomy (pek·ten·ot·o·me). The act of cutting into the pecten band of the anal canal. [pecten, Gk *temnein* to cut.]

pectic (pek·tik). Relating to or composed of pectin.

pectin (pek·tin). Any of the vegetable mucilages found in fruits such as ripe oranges, lemons and apples, in roots such as beet and turnip, and generally in plant tissues. They are hydrolysed on boiling with the weak fruit acids, or by pectase. into a pentosan and pectic acid: it is the gelation of the latter in a high concentration of sugar that brings about the setting of jams and fruit jellies. **Apple pectin.** A pectin obtained from apple pomace, containing also starches and colouring matter. It is a coarse or fine powder which forms a viscous colloidal solution in water; it is probably the most important component in the apple treatment for diarrhoea. It may be used as an emulsifying agent, and solutions of purified pectin have also been employed intravenously as a substitute for plasma after haemorrhage and shock. [Gk *pektos* congealed.]

pectinase (pek·tin·aze). An enzyme found in plant tissues which hydrolyses pectins and causes them to form gels. [Gk *pektos* congealed.]

pectinate (pek·tin·ate). Comb-shaped. [L *pecten* comb.]

pectineal (pek·tin·e·al). Belonging to the pubis; relating to any structure resembling a comb. Ridged. [L *pecten* comb.]

pectineus (pek·tin·e·us). The pectineus muscle. [see prec.]

pectineus muscle [musculus pectineus (NA)]. A small muscle in the groin, so called because it arises from the pectineal line of the pubis. It is inserted just below the lesser trochanter of the femur, and is an adductor and flexor of the hip.

pectiniform (pek·tin·e·form). Shaped like a comb. [L *pecten* comb, form.]

pectinose (pek·tin·oze). Arabinose. [Gk *pektos* congealed.]

pectization (pek·ti·za·shun). The process of gel formation; gelation. [Gk *pektos* congealed.]

pectoral (pek·tor·al). 1. Belonging to the thorax. 2. Applied to therapeutic agents which have good effect in respiratory diseases. [L *pectus* breast.]

pectoral nerves. Lateral pectoral nerve [nervus pectoralis lateralis (NA)]. A branch of the lateral cord of the brachial plexus to the pectoralis major muscle; it also supplies the shoulder joint. **Medial pectoral nerve [nervus pectoralis anterior medialis (NA)].** A branch of the medial cord of the brachial plexus to the pectoralis muscles. It carries fibres from the 7th cervical and 1st thoracic roots of the brachial plexus.

pectoral veins [venae pectorales (NA)]. Small veins which drain the structures of the pectoral region into the subclavian or axillary veins.

pectoralgia (pek·tor·al·je·ah). A sensation of pain in the thorax. [L *pectus* breast, Gk *algos* pain.]

pectoralis (pek·tor·a·lis). A pectoralis muscle. [L *pectus* breast.]

pectoralis major muscle [musculus pectoralis major (NA)] (pek·tor·a·lis ma·jor musl). A large muscle on the front of the upper part of the chest arising from the clavicle [pars clavicularis (NA)], sternum, costal cartilages [pars sternocostalis (NA)], and aponeuroses of the external oblique muscle [pars abdominalis (NA)], and inserted by tendon into the lateral lip of the bicipital groove. It underlies the breast, and forms the anterior wall of the axilla.

pectoralis minor muscle [musculus pectoralis minor (NA)] (pek·tor·a·lis mi·nor musl). A triangular muscle lying deep to the pectoralis major muscle and running from the 3rd, 4th and 5th ribs to the coracoid process.

pectoriloquy (pek·tor·il·o·kwe). In auscultation the clear transmission of articulate voice sounds through the thoracic wall in an area where it should not normally be heard. It may, for example, be heard over a cavity or a consolidated lobe of the lung. **Aphonic pectoriloquy.** Transmission of widespread sounds through a serous, non-purulent pleuritic effusion. **Whispering pectoriloquy.** In which the whispered voice is conducted directly to the ear through the stethoscope in an area of the chest where it should not normally be heard. A more delicate sign than bronchophony but heard under the same physical conditions. [L *pectus* breast, *loqui* to speak.]

pectorophony (pek·tor·of·on·e). Increase of vocal resonance noted on auscultation of the chest. [L *pectus* breast, Gk *phone* sound.]

pectose (pek·toze). A polysaccharide precursor of pectin, existing in unripe fruits and vegetables. [Gk *pektos* congealed.]

pectosinase (pek·to·sin·aze). An enzyme present in unripe fruits and vegetables which activates the conversion of pectose into pectin as the ripening proceeds. [see prec.]

pectous (pek·tus). 1. Gelatinous. 2. Relating to or composed of pectin. [Gk *pektos* congealed.]

pectus (pek·tus). The anterior part of the thorax or breast. **Pectus carinatum.** Pigeon breast. *See* BREAST. **Pectus excavatum.** Cobblers' chest. *See* CHEST. **Pectus gallinatum.** Pigeon breast. *See* BREAST. [L.]

ped-. For words beginning with **ped-**, *see also* PAED-.

pedal (ped·al). 1. Belonging to the foot. 2. Belonging to the pes hippocampi, or any other structure by the name of pes. [L *pes* foot.]

pedesis (ped·e·sis). 1. Leaping. 2. The brownian movement. [Gk.]

Pedetes caffer (ped·e·teez kaf·er). A giant jerboa that is a reservoir of plague infection in South Africa. [Gk *pedetes* leaper, Kaffir.]

pedialgia (ped·e·al·je·ah). Neuralgic pain affecting the foot. [Gk *pedion* sole of the foot, *algos* pain.]

pedicel (ped·e·sel). Foot process; one of the many processes of a podocyte which is applied to the surface of the basal lamina of the glomerular capillaries, interdigitating with the pedicles of adjacent podocytes. [L *pediculus* little foot, Gk *kytos* cell.]

pedicellate, pedicellated (ped·is·el·ate, ped·is·el·a·ted). Pediculate.

pedicellation (ped·is·el·a′·shun). The formation of a pedicle.

pedicle (ped·ikl). 1. The narrowing stem of a tumour, organ, or skin flap. 2. Pedicle of the vertebral arch (see below). **Tube pedicle.** A tube of skin anchored at each end, and designed for transference, often in several stages, to make good a full-thickness skin loss at some distant site. **Vascular pedicle.** The attachment of a viscus or of a tumour, which contains its main blood vessels. **Pedicle of the vertebral arch [pediculus arcus vertebrae (NA)].** The bridge which connects the lamina of a vertebra with the body. [L *pediculus* little foot.]

pedicled (ped·ikld). Pediculate.

pedicular (ped·ik·ew·lar). 1. Relating to a pedicle. [pedicle.] 2. Relating to or due to the presence of lice. [L *pediculus* louse.]

pediculate (ped·ik·ew·late). Provided with a pedicle.

pediculation (ped·ik·ew·la′·shun). 1. Infestation with lice. [L *pediculus* louse.] 2. The process of developing a pedicle. [L *pediculus* little foot.]

pediculicide (ped·ik·ew·le·side). An agent which destroys lice. [L *pediculus* louse, *caedere* to kill.]

Pediculidae (ped·ik·ew·lid·e). A family of the insectan order Anoplura. The genera *Pediculus* and *Phthirus* contain the lice that infest man. [L *pediculus* louse, Gk *eidos* form.]

Pediculoides (ped·ik·ew·loi′·deez). A genus of mites. **Pediculoides ventricosus.** The louse mite, a common species in stored products, straw, etc. The gravid females show an enormous enlargement of the body into a spherical sac; they are normally parasitic on insects but commonly attack man, causing great irritation, rash and fever (grain itch, grocers' itch, or bakers' itch). Distribution is mostly holarctic but they are widely distributed by commerce. [see foll.]

Pediculoididae (ped·ik·ew·loi′·did·e). A family of the acarine superfamily Tarsonematoidea. The genus *Pediculoides* is of medical interest. [L *pediculus* louse, Gk *eidos* form.]

pediculophobia (ped·ik·ew·lo·fo′·be·ah). Extreme fear of infestation with lice. [L *pediculus* louse, phobia.]

pediculosis (ped·ik·ew·lo′·sis). A disease of the skin characterized by infestation with lice. **Pediculosis capillitii, Pediculosis capitis.** An affection marked by the presence of *Pediculus humanus* var. *capitis* in the hair. **Pediculosis corporis.** Pediculosis vestimenti (see below). **Pediculosis inguinalis.** Pediculosis pubis (see below). **Pediculosis palpebrarum.** Infestation of the eyelashes with the crab louse, *Phthirus pubis.* **Pediculosis pubis.** An affection characterized by infestation of the hair of the pubic region with *Phthirus pubis* usually sexually transmitted. **Pediculosis vestimenti, Pediculosis vestimentorum.** The presence of *Pediculus humanis* var. *corporis* on the clothes which subsequently transfer to the body of the affected individual. [L *pediculus* louse, Gk *-osis* condition.]

pediculous (ped·ik·ew·lus). Infested with pediculi.

Pediculus (ped·ik·ew·lus). A genus of sucking lice, Anoplura, whose species infest man, the higher apes and South American monkeys. They are vectors of typhus and relapsing fever in man. *P. humanus humanus (P. humanus* var. *capitis),* the head louse, and *P. humanis corporis (P. corporis),* the body or clothes louse, are both world-wide in distribution and recognized as subspecies which have almost achieved specific rank. They will cross, but the offspring are abnormal. The former lives solely on the fine hairs of the head, the latter on clothing near the skin of the body. **Pediculus capitis.** *P. humanus humanus* (see above).

Pediculus vestimenti. *P. humanus corporis* (see above). [L, louse.]

pedicure (ped·e·kewr). 1. Chiropody. 2. A chiropodist. [L *pes* foot, *cura* healing.]

Pediococcus (ped·e·o·kok′·us). A genus of bacteria belonging to the family Micrococcaceae. They are non-motile cocci occurring singly, in pairs, or in tetrads, and produce acidification and clouding of wort and beer; non-pathogenic. **Pediococcus acidilactici.** A species from spoiled malt mash, which produces lactic acid. **Pediococcus albus.** A species from spoiled beer and water. **Pediococcus aurantiacus,** (syn. *P. maggiorae*), a species found in the human nasal passages and on the skin of the human foot. **Pediococcus cerevisiae.** A species from sarcina-sick wort, yeast and beer. There are many other species described from wort, yeast, beer, horse urine and anchovy pickle. [L *pes* foot, Gk *kokkos* berry.]

pedion (pe·de·on). The plantar surface of the foot. [Gk, sole of the foot.]

pedionalgia (pe·de·on·al′·je·ah). Pain in the sole of the foot. **Pedionalgia epidemica.** Erythroedema polyneuropathy (pink disease). [Gk *pedion* sole of the foot, *algos* pain.]

pediphalanx (ped·e·fa·langx). A phalanx of the foot. [L *pes* foot, phalanx.]

pedistibulum (ped·e·stib·ew·lum). The stapes. [L *pes* foot, *stabulum* stall.]

pedium (pe·de·um). Pedion.

Pedley, F. G. American biochemist.

Shohl and Pedley method. For calcium in urine: urine is oxidized with sulphuric acid and ammonium persulphate, calcium is precipitated as oxalate, the calcium oxalate is filtered, washed and titrated with standard permanganate solution.

pedodynamometer (ped·o·di·nam·om′·et·er). A device for determining the muscular power of a leg. [L *pes* foot, dynamometer.]

pedograph (ped·o·graf). An imprint of the weight-bearing surface of the foot; it is usually made on paper. [L *pes* foot, Gk *graphein* to record.]

pedometer (ped·om·et·er). An instrument used to count the number of steps taken by an individual and so to register the distance walked. [L *pes* foot, Gk *metron* measure.]

pedometry (ped·om·et·re). Measurement by means of the pedometer of the distance travelled on foot.

peduncle [pedunculus (pediculus) (NA)]. (ped·ungkl). 1. A small foot. 2. A stalk, or stem (in anatomy, the commoner meaning). **Cerebellar peduncle, inferior [pedunculus cerebellaris inferior (NA)].** Restiform body, a prominent band of fibres which appears to be a continuation cranially of the posterolateral regions of the spinal cord; it forms the lateral boundary of the lower part of the 4th ventricle, and disappears in the cerebellum. It consists mainly of fibres afferent to the cerebellum, notably the dorsal spinocerebellar tract, but has many other components. **Cerebellar peduncle, middle [pedunculus cerebellaris medius (NA)].** The lateral extension of the transverse fibres of the pons, which disappears into the cerebellum. It consists almost entirely of fibres from the pontine nuclei to the middle lobe of the cerebellum (neocerebellum). **Cerebellar peduncle, posterior.** Inferior cerebellar peduncle (see above). **Cerebellar peduncle, superior [pedunculus cerebellaris superior (NA)].** Flattened bands of the fibres which emerge from the cerebellum and pass cranially on either side of the superior medullary velum. They consist almost entirely of fibres from the dentate nucleus to the red nucleus of the mid-brain, and to the thalamus. **Cerebral peduncle [pedunculus cerebri (NA)].** Literally the stalk of the cerebral hemisphere; there are two, right and left, which appear as prominent, more or less cylindrical masses of nerve fibres at the upper border of the pons and diverge on the ventral (anterior) aspect of the mid-brain to disappear into their respective hemispheres. They consist mainly of corticopontine and pyramidal-tract fibres which, after passing through the internal capsule, descend in the cerebral peduncles. **Peduncle of the flocculus [pedunculus flocculi (NA)].** An attenuated strand of nervous tissue which joins the flocculus to the nodule of the vermis of the cerebellum. **Peduncle of the mamillary body [pedunculus corporis mamillaris (NA)].** A bundle of nerve fibres passing from the mamillary body to the tegmentum of the mid-brain. Many end in the cells of the reticular formation of the brain stem. **Olfactory peduncle.** The elongated stalk of the olfactory bulb; it lies on the orbital surface of the frontal lobe and joins the olfactory bulb to the brain a little in front of the anterior perforated space. It consists of secondary olfactory fibres which pass back into the olfactory tracts. **Pineal peduncle.** The stalk of the pineal body. **Thalamic peduncle, inferior [pedunculus thalami inferior (NA)].** Fibres passing from the hypothalamus to the thalamus. [L dim. of *pes* foot.]

peduncular (ped·ung·kew·lar). Belonging to a peduncle.

pedunculate, pedunculated (ped·ung·kew·late, ped·ung·kew·la·ted). Having a peduncle; stalked.

pedunculotomy (ped·ung·kew·lot·o·me). The operation of incision of a cerebral peduncle formerly used in the treatment of Parkinson's disease. [peduncle, Gk *temnein* to cut.]

peenash (pe·nash). Rhinitis caused by infestation of the nose with insect larvae. [E. Indian name.]

Peer, Arthur Lyndon (b. 1899). Newark surgeon.

Lyndon Peer operation, or technique. Diced autogenous cartilage is used in this method of reconstruction of the pinna. A preformed mould is established to match the normal ear and is buried under the postauricular skin. Further skin grafting is necessary to form the helix and the postauricular sulcus.

peg (peg). A shaped piece of metal, wood, or bone, or other material, which is driven into similar or dissimilar material to hold it in position. **Bone peg.** A piece of bone or metal which is inserted into the pieces of bone at the site of a fracture to hold them in the normal position. **Chelsea peg.** The old type of peg leg used to replace a leg amputated below the knee. It is made so that the wearer kneels on a pad that is fixed to the top of the peg. The peg is held in position by a wooden extension that passes along the lateral side of the thigh and is fixed by a belt around the waist. **Peg leg.** An artificial leg incorporating a wooden shin with a peg end instead of an articulated foot and ankle. [ME *pegge*.]

peganine (peg·an·een). $C_{11}H_{12}ON_2$, an alkaloid, obtained from the plant, *Adhatoda vasica,* which is found in South Asia. It has been used in pulmonary disease.

pegology (pe·gol·o·je). The study of springs, especially of those which supply mineral and medicinal waters. [Gk *pege* spring, *logos* science.]

peinotherapy (pi·no·ther·ap·e). Hunger cure. *See* CURE. [Gk *peina* hunger, therapy.]

pejorative (pe·jor·at·iv). Becoming worse; adverse; unfavourable. [L *pejor* worse.]

Pekelharing, Cornelis Adrianus (b. 1848). Utrecht physiologist.

Pekelharing's theory. Blood coagulation occurs when calcium is liberated from thrombin, and forms fibrin by combining with fibrinogen.

Pel, Pieter Klazes (b. 1852). Amsterdam physician.

Pel-Ebstein disease, fever, or syndrome. The characteristic undulant fever of Hodgkin's disease, a remittent pyrexia that occurs daily and reaches its highest point (40°C, or so) after about 5 days, then gradually subsides to recur after a period of from 10 to 14 days, is referred to as *Pel-Ebstein fever* or *Pel-Ebstein syndrome.* The term *Pel-Ebstein disease* is only rarely and unjustifiably used for the whole disease.

pelade (pel·ade). 1. Alopecia areata. 2. A disease which resembles pellagra. **Achromic pelade.** A condition characterized by atrophy and whitening of the skin. **Pelade décalvante.** Alopecia totalis. [Fr.]

peladic (pel·ad·ik). Of the nature of, or relating to, pelade.

peladophobia (pel·ad·o·fo′·be·ah). Extreme dread of becoming bald. [pelade, phobia.]

pelage (pel·ij). A comprehensive term for the hair covering of the body of man or of the lower mammals. [Fr., hair.]

pelagism (pel·ij·izm). Seasickness. [Gk *pelagos* sea.]

pelentan (pel·en·tan). Ethyl biscoumacetate.

Pelger, Karel (b. 1885). Amsterdam physician.

Pelger's nuclear anomaly, Pelger–Hüet anomaly. Of the granulocytes: an anomaly inherited as a mendelian dominant in otherwise apparently well persons. It is characterized by an increase in the numbers of juvenile or band forms of granulocytes or polymorphonuclear leucocytes which have dumb-bell, kidney-shaped or bilobed nuclei. These cells may sometimes exceed the numbers of ordinary segmented granulocytes, and may be associated with certain infections or with very active cell-formation in the marrow.

Pelger's cell. A neutrophil with a bilobal nucleus.

pelicometer (pel·ik·om·et·er). Pelvimeter. [Gk *pelyx* bowl, *metron* measure.]

pelidisi (pel·e·de·ze). A unit employed in von Pirquet's index for the measurement of the nutritional status of children. It is the cube root of 10 times the weight in grams, divided by the sitting height in centimetres. The normal value is taken as 100; values under 95 are considered to represent under-nutrition, and over 100, over-nutrition. The unit is not in use in the UK. [L *pondus decies linearis divisus sidentis (altitudo)*, weight, ten, line divided, sitting (height).]

pelidnoma (pel·id·no·mah). A circumscribed dark-coloured patch or spot on the skin. [Gk *pelidnos* livid, *-oma* tumour.]

pelioma (pel·e·o·mah). Purpura. **Pelioma typhosum.** A purpuric rash which sometimes occurs in typhoid fever. [Gk *pelios* livid, *-oma* tumour.]

peliosis (pel·e·o·sis). Purpura. **Peliosis rheumatica.** Purpura rheumatica. [Gk *pelios* livid.]

Pelizaeus, Friedrich (b. 1850). Cassel neurologist.

Merzbacher–Pelizaeus disease, Pelizaeus–Merzbacher disease. Familial centrolobar sclerosis, also called *aplasia axialis extracorticalis congenita;* a progressive disorder of infancy with dementia, spasticity, cerebellar disturbances and involuntary movements of the head and eyes. It is related to Schilder's disease, Krabbe's disease and Scholz's disease.

Pelkan, K. F. Californian biochemist.

Bloor, Pelkan and Allen method. For cholesterol in blood: the blood is treated with alcohol-ether to precipitate proteins and extract the cholesterol. The filtrate is evaporated, the residue is dissolved in chloroform, and the cholesterol determined by the Liebermann–Burchard reaction.

pellagra (pel·ag·rah). An endemic deficiency disease prevalent among the poor in countries where maize is the staple article of diet. It is due to a deficiency of certain factors of the vitamin-B_2 complex (nicotinic acid, riboflavine and pyridoxine). It is characterized by a loss of weight and general weakness, together with distinctive signs affecting the skin, and alimentary and nervous systems. An erythema occurs on parts of the skin exposed to light, accompanied by itching and burning sensations, going on to a severe dermatitis with desquamation and exfoliation. Pigmentation and atrophy of the skin may follow. Glossitis and stomatitis appear early, and the tongue becomes a fiery red (beet tongue). Anorexia, nausea and vomiting are present, and a persistent diarrhoea occurs in the late stages. Mental symptoms such as depression, irritability, headache and burning sensations occur early, and later there may be rigidity combined with coarse tremors. Numbness and paralysis of the extremities are common, and in untreated cases insanity may result. **Monkey pellagra.** A deficiency disease of caged monkeys in which they lose condition and weight, and may die. It is curable by nicotinic acid. **Pellagra sine pellagra.** Pellagra without the skin signs. **Typhoid pellagra.** A severe fulminating form marked by severe prostration, tremor, muscular rigidity, convulsions and death. [It. *pelle* skin, *agra* rough.]

pellagragenic (pel·ag·rah·jen'·ik). Giving rise to pellagra. [pellagra, Gk *genein* to produce.]

pellagral (pel·ag·ral). Characterized by or belonging to pellagra.

pellagramin (pel·ag·ram·in). The antipellagra vitamin, now identified with nicotinamide, or nicotinic acid [obsolete term].

pellagraphobia (pel·ag·rah·fo'·be·ah). A morbid fear of becoming affected with pellagra. [pellagra, phobia.]

pellagrazein (pel·ah·gra·ze·in). A hypothetical toxin of damaged maize, suggested as a possible cause of pellagra. [pellagra, L *zea* maize.]

pellagrin (pel·ag·rin). One suffering from pellagra.

pellagroid (pel·ag·roid). A morbid state which is like that of pellagra but in which the symptoms are of mild type. [pellagra, Gk *eidos* form.]

pellagrose (pel·ag·rose). Pellagrous.

pellagrous (pel·ag·rus). Suffering from or having the characteristics of pellagra.

pellant (pel·ant). Cleansing; tending to purify. [L *pellere* to drive out.]

Pellegrini, Augusto. Florence surgeon.

Pellegrini–Stieda disease. Ossification in the upper part of the medial collateral ligament of the knee as a result of injury.

pellentia (pel·en·she·ah). Abortifacient drug [obsolete term]. [L *pellere* to drive.]

pellet (pel·et). A preparation of steroid hormone, principally confined to oestrogen (stilboestrol and oestradiol) and testosterone, rather than testosterone propionate which tends to extrude. Progesterone also tends to extrude and must be implanted deeply. This method of administration prolongs the hormonal effect. Stilboestrol pellets last about 2 months, oestradiol 9 months, and testosterone 4–6 months.

pelletierine (pel·et·i·er·een). $C_8H_{15}ON$, an akaloid closely related to coniine and found as a racemic isomer in the root bark of the pomegranate, *Punica granatum* Linn. (family Punicaceae). It is chiefly used as the tannate, which invariably consists of a mixture of the tannates of the several pomegranate alkaloids. It is employed as a vermifuge. [Joseph *Pelletier* (b. 1782), French chemist.]

pellicle (pel·ikl). 1. A thin film or skin. 2. A scum, as occurs on the surface of a bacterial growth, or a crust formed on the surface of a saturated solution during evaporation. [L *pellicula* little skin.]

pellicula (pel·ik·ew·lah). Epidermis. [L, little skin.]

pellicular, pelliculous (pel·ik·ew·lar, pel·ik·ew·lus). Pertaining to or having the characteristics of a pellicle.

pellitorine (pel·it·or·een). A crystalline substance occurring in pyrethrum. [see foll.]

pellitory (pel·it·or·e). 1. Name given to plants of the genera *Pyrethrum* and *parietania* (family Compositae). 2. Pyrethrum root; the dried root of *Anacyclus pyrethrum* DC, containing pellitorine, is used in lozenges and pastilles to promote salivation. [Gk *pyrethron* feverfew.]

Pellizzi, G. B.

Pellizzi's syndrome. Macrogenitosomia praecox.

pellucid (pel·ew·sid). Translucent; clear. [L *pellucidus* transparent.]

pelma (pel·mah). The sole of the foot. [Gk.]

pelmatic (pel·mat·ik). Belonging to the sole of the foot. [see prec.]

pelmatogram (pel·mat·o·gram). An impression of the sole of the foot; such footprints may be made by covering the plantar surface with black pigment and pressing the foot on white paper, or by using a smooth plaque of moist plaster of Paris. [Gk *pelma* sole of the foot, *gramma* mark.]

pelohaemia (pel·lo·he·me·ah). A condition in which the blood is thicker than normal. [Gk *pelos* clay, *haima* blood.]

pelopathist (pe·lop·ath·ist). One who practises pelotherapy. [see foll.]

pelopathy (pe·lop·ath·e). Pelotherapy. [Gk *pelos* clay, *pathos* disease.]

pelotherapy (pe·lo·ther·ap·e). Treatment of diseased conditions by the use of mud, peat, or earth baths or packs. [Gk *pelos* clay, therapy.]

peltate (pel·tate). 1. Like a shield in shape. 2. In botany, applied to a leaf the stalk of which is attached to the lower surface. [L *pelta* shield.]

Peltier, Jean Charles Athanase (b. 1785). French physicist.
Peltier effect. The liberation or absorption of heat which takes place at the junction where a current passes from one material to another.

peludo (pel·**ew**·do). *Euphractus sexcinctus*, a species of armadillo that acts as a reservoir of *Trypanosoma cruzi.* [Sp., hairy.]

pelvic (**pel**·vik). Relating to the pelvis.

pelvicellulitis (pel·ve·sel·ew·**li**'·tis). Pelvic cellulitis.

pelvicephalography (pel·ve·kef·al·**og**'·raf·e). Determination of the size of the head of the fetus and of the birth canal by means of x-ray examination. [pelvis, Gk *kephale* head, *graphein* to record.]

pelvicephalometry (pel·ve·kef·al·**om**'·et·re). Measurement of the diameters of the fetal head in proportion to the diameters of the maternal pelvis. [pelvis, Gk *kephale* head, *metron* measure.]

pelvicliseometer (pel·ve·kli·se·**om**'·et·er). An apparatus used to ascertain the degree of pelvic inclination, as well as to measure the various diameters of the pelvis. [pelvis, cliseometer.]

pelvifixation (pel·ve·fix·**a**'·shun). Fixation of a floating or displaced pelvic organ by surgical methods to the wall of the pelvic cavity.

pelvigraph (**pel**·ve·graf). A device which records graphically the contour and dimensions of the pelvis. [pelvis, Gk *graphein* to record.]

pelvigraphy (pel·**vig**·raf·e). Radiography of the uterus, tubes and pelvic organs, after injection of a water-soluble contrast medium into the uterus. In addition to the uterine cavity and tubes, the broad ligament and the peritoneal pouches can be demonstrated. [see prec.]

pelvilithotomy (pel·ve·lith·**ot**'·o·me). Pelviolithotomy.

pelvimeter (pel·**vim**·et·er). A caliper-like instrument used to determine the diameters and capacity of the pelvis. [pelvis, Gk *metron* measure.]
See also: MARTIN (A.).

pelvimetry (pel·**vim**·et·re). Measurement of the pelvic shape or dimensions. **Combined pelvimetry.** Pelvimetry from observations made on abdominal and vaginal examination. **Digital pelvimetry.** Pelvimetry made with the fingers; usually vaginal. **External pelvimetry.** Pelvimetry by means of external measurements. **Instrumental pelvimetry.** External pelvimetry (see above) made with a pelvimeter. **Internal pelvimetry.** Digital pelvimetry (see above). **Manual pelvimetry.** Pelvimetry made with the hands. **X-ray pelvimetry.** Pelvimetry by means of x-rays. [see prec.]

pelviography (pel·ve·**og**·raf·e). Pelvioradiography.

pelviolithotomy (pel·ve·o·lith·**ot**'·o·me). Removal by surgical methods of stone from the pelvis of the ureter. [pelvis, lithotomy.]

pelvioneostomy (pel·ve·o·ne·**os**'·to·me). The operation of excising the constricted segment of a ureter and transplanting the upper end of the lower part into a new opening into the pelvis of the ureter. [pelvis, neostomy.]

pelvioperitonitis (pel·ve·o·**per**·it·on·**i**'·tis). Pelvic peritonitis. *See* PERITONITIS.

pelvioplasty (**pel**·ve·o·plas·te). A plastic operation performed on the pelvis for the purpose of enlarging the outlet; generally pubiotomy. [pelvis, Gk *plassein* to mould.]

pelvioradiography (pel·ve·o·ra·de·**og**'·raf·e). Radiographical inspection of the pelvis.

pelviostomy (pel·ve·**os**·to·me). 1. Resection of the pelvis of the ureter with implantation of the ureter into the lower end of the pelvis. 2. Simple drainage of the pelvis of the ureter by a tube. More specific terms are used in the surgery of hydronephrosis, e.g. ureteropyeloplasty, ureteroneopyelostomy, etc. [pelvis, Gk *stoma* mouth.]

pelviotomy (pel·ve·**ot**·o·me). 1. Section of the pelvic bones. 2. Pyelotomy. [pelvis, Gk *temnein* to cut.]

pelviperitonitis (pel·ve·per·it·on·**i**'·tis). Pelvic peritonitis. *See* PERITONITIS.

pelviradiography (pel·ve·ra·de·**og**'·raf·e). Pelvioradiography.

pelvirectal (pel·ve·**rek**·tal). Belonging to the pelvis and to the rectum.

pelvis [NA] (**pel**·vis). 1. The basin-shaped ring of bone at the lower end of the trunk, composed of the two innominate bones and the sacrum and coccyx. It is differentiated into a sacral part, a pubic part and an iliac part. 2. (Of the ureter): a funnel-shaped dilatation at the upper end of the ureter. **Pelvis aequabiliter justo major.** An unusually large gynaecoid pelvis. **Pelvis aequabiliter justo minor.** A gynaecoid pelvis of below average dimensions. **Android pelvis.** A female pelvis resembling that of the male in configuration. **Anthropoid pelvis.** A female pelvis with its greatest dimensions in the anteroposterior plane. It is more correctly termed *pithecoid pelvis.* **Assimilation pelvis.** *High assimilation:* the condition where the last lumbar vertebra is united to the sacrum, making the sacrum a long narrow unit of six segments instead of the usual five. *Low assimilation:* in this condition there are only four sacral segments, making it a short broad unit. **Beaked pelvis.** A condition occurring in osteomalacia where the inward pressure of the femurs produces a distortion of the horizontal pubic rami. **Brachypellic pelvis.** A term, now largely obsolete, for the normal female pelvis. **Caoutchouc pelvis.** The light, soft, decalcified, and hence unusually flexible pelvis seen in advanced osteomalacia. **Contracted pelvis.** 1. A pelvis sufficiently reduced in any dimension as to cause difficulty in the passage of a normal-sized fetus. 2. A pelvis in which there is a diminution of more than 15 mm below the average, in any important dimension. **Coxalgic pelvis.** A deformed pelvis resulting from hip-joint disease. **Dolichopellic pelvis.** Anthropoid pelvis (see above). **Dwarf pelvis.** A rare type of pelvis retaining the infantile shape, with the bones united by cartilage. **Elastic pelvis.** Caoutchouc pelvis (see above). **Extrarenal pelvis.** A manifestation of hydronephrosis, where most of the pelvis of the ureter is forced outside the kidney. **False pelvis [pelvis major (NA)].** That portion of the pelvis above the pelvic inlet, bounded behind by the 5th and part of the 4th lumbar vertebrae and the sacrum, and laterally by the alae of the ilium. **Fissured pelvis.** A rachitic pelvis grossly flattened in the anteroposterior plane. **Flat pelvis.** A pelvis contracted in the anteroposterior diameter. The contraction is usually chiefly of the inlet. **Floor of the pelvis.** The muscular sling forming the lower boundary of the pelvis. **Frozen pelvis.** The result of chronic inflammation, tumour, or endometriosis: the pelvic viscera are "frozen" together and immobile. **Funnel pelvis.** A pelvis gradually narrowing from the inlet to the outlet. The inlet may or may not be reduced. **Generally contracted pelvis.** A pelvis reduced in all its dimensions below the average. **Giant pelvis.** Pelvis aequabiliter justo major (see above). **Greater pelvis.** False pelvis (see above). **Gynaecoid pelvis.** The average or normal female pelvis. **India-rubber pelvis.** Caoutchouc pelvis (see above). **Inlet of the pelvis [apertura pelvis superior (NA)].** The upper opening into the pelvis, bounded by the brim of the pelvis. **Pelvis justo major.** Pelvis aequabiliter justo major (see above). **Pelvis justo minor.** Pelvis aequabiliter justo minor (see above). **Kyphorachitic pelvis.** The pelvis associated with true rachitic kyphosis. It may be virtually normal, or present the changes of the ordinary rachitic pelvis. **Kyphoscoliorachitic pelvis.** The pelvis of rachitic kyphoscoliosis, which usually shows a reduced anteroposterior diameter and an oblique deformity of the brim. **Kyphotic pelvis.** The pelvis associated with kyphosis. The deformity varies with the situation of the kyphosis, but a funnel type of pelvis tends to be produced. **Lesser pelvis.** True pelvis (see below). **Malacosteon pelvis.** Osteomalacic pelvis (see below). **Masculine pelvis.** Android pelvis (see above). **Pelvis nana.** The true dwarf pelvis (see above). **Obliquely contracted pelvis.** Naegele's pelvis. **Pelvis obtecta.** The pelvis associated with severe kyphosis. **Osteomalacic pelvis.** The pelvis in osteomalacia. The changes vary from mild anteroposterior flattening to gross compression in all diameters, producing the charactistic "beaked" appearance. **Outlet of the pelvis [apertura pelvis inferior (NA)].** The diamond-shaped lower circumference of the pelvis bounded by the pubic arch, ischial tuberosities and coccyx, and the sacrotuberous ligaments. **Pelvis ovalis.** A funnel-shaped depression of the tympanic membrane, at the bottom of which is the fenestra vestibuli. **Pithecoid pelvis.** Anthropoid pelvis (see above). **Pelvis plana.** Flat pelvis (see above). **Platypelloid pelvis.** Flat pelvis (see above). **Prague**

pelvis. Spondylolisthetic pelvis (see below). **Pseudo-osteomalacic pelvis.** A rachitic pelvis with changes simulating those characteristic of osteomalacia. **Rachitic pelvis.** The pelvis in rickets. A wide range of changes is found, but the most characteristic is a flattened inlet and a flared, increased outlet. **Renal pelvis.** Pelvis of the ureter (see below). **Reniform pelvis.** A kidney-shaped pelvic brim. **Rostrate pelvis.** The beaked pelvis of osteomalacia. **Pelvis rotunda.** A funnel-shaped depression of the tympanum, at the bottom of which is the fenestra cochleae. **Round pelvis.** A pelvis with a brim that is almost circular. **Rubber pelvis.** Caoutchouc pelvis (see above). **Scoliotic pelvis.** The pelvis in severe scoliosis, where the sacrum assumes an abnormal position leading to slight asymmetry of the pelvis. **Simple flat pelvis.** The flat pelvis unassociated with rickets. **Spider pelvis.** An anomaly of the renal pelvis showing on the pyelogram as long, string-like lines. **Split pelvis.** One showing a separation of the pubic symphysis. **Spondylolisthetic pelvis.** A pelvis where the last lumbar vertebra is dislocated forwards on the sacrum. **Stove-in pelvis.** A driving inwards of part of the pelvis as a result of a severe compression injury. **Transversely contracted pelvis.** Robert's pelvis. **Triradiate pelvis.** The pelvis in severe osteomalacia. **True pelvis [pelvis minor (NA)].** That part of the pelvis below the pelvic inlet, containing the pelvic colon, rectum, urinary bladder and some of the generative organs. **Pelvis of the ureter [pelvis renalis (NA)].** The funnel-shaped dilatation at the upper end of the ureter. [L, basin.]

See also: NAEGELE, OTTO (A. W.), ROBERT.

pelvisacral (pel·ve·**sa**·kral). Belonging to the pelvis and the sacrum.

pelvisacrum (pel·ve·**sa**·krum). The pelvis and the sacrum considered together as one unit.

pelviscope (**pel**·ve·skope). An x-ray apparatus with a fluorescent screen, used to visualize the bony pelvis. [pelvis, Gk *skopein* to view.]

pelvisection (pel·ve·**sek**·shun). Surgical section of any part of the pelvis, e.g. pubiotomy, symphyseotomy.

pelvisternum (pel·ve·**ster**·num). The cartilage of the symphysis pubis.

pelvitomy (pel·**vit**·o·me). Pelviotomy.

pelvitrochanterian (**pel**·ve·tro·kan·**teer**'·e·an). Pertaining to the pelvis and to the greater trochanter of the femur.

pelviureterography (**pel**·ve·ewr·e·ter·**og**'·raf·e). The radiography of the pelvis of the ureter, calcyces and ureter, when they are filled with a radio-opaque fluid.

pelviureteroradiography (**pel**·ve·ewr·e·ter·o·ra·de·**og**'·raf·e). Pelviureterography.

pelvoscopy (pel·**vos**·ko·pe). Generally, examination of a pelvis, but chiefly used for the examination of the pelvis of the ureter. [pelvis, Gk *skopein* to examine.]

pelvospondylitis (**pel**·vo·spon·dil·**i**'·tis). Inflammation of the pelvic portion of the spine. [pelvis, Gk *sphondylos* vertebra, *-itis* inflammation.]

pelycalgia (pel·ik·**al**·je·ah). Pelvic pain. [Gk *pelyx* bowl, *algos* pain.]

pelycephalometry (**pel**·e·kef·al·**om**'·et·re). Pelvicephalometry. [Gk *pelyx* bowl, *kephale* head, *metron* measure.]

pelycogram (**pel**·ik·o·gram). A radiograph of the pelvis. [Gk *pelyx* bowl, *gramma* a writing.]

pelycograph (**pel**·ik·o·graf). A radiograph of the pelvis. [Gk *pelyx* bowl, *graphein* to record.]

pelycography (pel·ik·**og**·raf·e). X-ray examination of the pelvic viscera, with air or carbon dioxide as a contrast medium. [see prec.]

pelycometer (pel·ik·**om**·et·er). Pelvimeter. [Gk *pelyx* bowl, *metron* measure.]

pelycometresis (**pel**·ik·o·met·**re**'·sis). Pelvimetry. [Gk *pelyx* bowl, *metresis* measurement.]

pelycometry (pel·ik·**om**·et·re). Pelvimetry. [Gk *pelyx* bowl, *metron* measure.]

pelycotomy (pel·ik·**ot**·o·me). Pelviotomy. [Gk *pelyx* bowl, *temnein* to cut.]

pelyometer (pel·e·**om**·et·er). Pelvimeter. [Gk *pelyx* bowl, *metron* measure.]

pelyometresis (**pel**·e·o·met·**re**'·sis). Pelvimetry. [Gk *pelyx* bowl, *metresis* measurement.]

Pemoline (**pem**·o·leen). BP Commission approved name for 2-imino-5-phenyloxazolidin-4-one; a central nervous stimulant.

pemphigoid (**pem**·fig·oid). 1. Pertaining to, resembling, characterized by, or of the nature of pemphigus. 2. An idiopathic bullous disease mostly affecting the elderly, with subepidermal bullae and no acanthosis. Remissions occur in about one-half and may be permanent. **Benign mucosal pemphigoid.** A subepidermal bullous disease of the aged, affecting skin, mucosae and conjunctivae, causing shrinkage, scarring, adhesions, ectropion and severe loss of vision. **Cicatricial pemphigoid.** Benign mucosal pemphigoid (see above). [Gk *pemphix* bubble, *eidos* form.]

pemphigus (**pem**·fig·us). An eruption characterized by the formation of bullae in successive crops, usually without antecedent lesions. **Pemphigus acutus, Pemphigus acutus febrilis gravis.** An acute, general, infectious disease with a bullous eruption. **Pemphigus arthriticus.** Dermatitis herpetiformis. **Pemphigus benignus.** 1. A mild type of pemphigus chronicus (see below). 2. Familial benign chronic pemphigus (see below). 3. Pemphigus erythematosus (see below). **Pemphigus chloroticus.** Pemphigus virginum (see below). **Pemphigus chronicus.** A chronic, progressive, often fatal disease, characterized by the formation of bullae upon apparently normal skin. **Pemphigus circinatus.** Dermatitis herpetiformis. **Pemphigus congenitalis.** Epidermolysis bullosa. **Pemphigus contagiosus.** Impetigo contagiosa bullosa. **Pemphigus diphtheriticus.** Pemphigus chronicus (see above) in which the contents of the bullae are yellow, and fibrin is deposited on their base. **Pemphigus disseminatus, Pemphigus diutinus.** Pemphigus chronicus (see above) in which very large numbers of bullae form a widespread eruption. **Pemphigus epidemicus neonatorum.** A bullous form of impetigo contagiosa. **Pemphigus erythematosus.** A variety of pemphigus characterized by bullous eruption on the trunk with eruption resembling lupus erythematosus on the face; sometimes lesions resembling seborrhoeic dermatitis may be present. **Familial benign chronic pemphigus.** A chronic, benign, familial disorder, characterized by bullae and dyskeratosis. **Febrile pemphigus.** Pemphigus acutus (see above). **Pemphigus foliaceus.** A chronic variety of pemphigus, characterized by flaccid bullae and exfoliation. **Pemphigus gangraenosus.** Dermatitis gangraenosa infantum. **Pemphigus haemorrhagicus.** Pemphigus chronicus (see above) with haemorrhage into the bullae. **Pemphigus hystericus.** A bullous variety of dermatitis artefacta. **Juvenile pemphigus.** Juvenile dermatitis herpetiformis, a bullous disease of childhood mostly affecting the face, lower abdomen, buttocks and external genitalia. The bullae are subepidermal. **Pemphigus leprosus.** Bullous eruption in leprosy. **Pemphigus localis.** Pemphigus solitarius (see below). **Pemphigus malignus.** A severe, rapidly progressive type of pemphigus chronicus (see above). **Pemphigus neonatorum.** Impetigo neonatorum. **Pemphigus neuroticus.** Pemphigus hystericus (see above). **Ocular pemphigus.** Benign mucosal pemphigoid. *See* PEMPHIGOID. **Pemphigus prurigineus, Pemphigus pruriginosus.** Dermatitis herpetiformis. **Pemphigus solitarius.** A single bulla which may be coccal in origin, or may be a manifestation of pemphigus chronicus (see above). **Pemphigus syphiliticus.** A bullous syphilid. **Pemphigus traumaticus hereditarius.** Epidermolysis bullosa. **Pemphigus vegetans.** A rare, chronic variety of pemphigus, in which vegetations form rapidly at the base of the bullae. **Pemphigus virginum.** A benign, bullous, or vesicular eruption of anaemic girls. **Pemphigus vulgaris.** Pemphigus chronicus (see above). [Gk *pemphix* bubble.]

Pempidine (**pem**·pid·een). BP Commission approved name for 1,2,2,6,6-pentamethylpiperidine.

Pempidine Tartrate BP 1968. The hydrogen tartrate of pempidine, a ganglion-blocking agent acting on both sympathetic and parasympathetic ganglia. Its use in the treatment of arterial hypertension depends on producing adequate block at the sympathetic ganglia and consequent peripheral vasodilatation.

penalgesia (pen·al·je·ze·ah). A reduction in the number of pain spots in an area of skin. [Gk *penia* poverty, *algos* pain.]

Penamecillin (pen·am·e·sil'·in). BP Commission approved name for acetoxymethyl 6-phenylacetamidopenicillanate; an antibiotic.

penatin (pen·at·in). An antibiotic, toxic for man and animals, produced by *Penicillium notatum.*

Penbutolol (pen·bew·to·lol). BP Commission approved name for (−)-1-*tert*-butylamino-3-(2-cyclopentylphenoxy)propan-2-ol; a β-adrenergic blocking agent.

pencil (pen·sil). 1. A stick or roll of caustic having a pointed end like that of a pencil. 2. A cylindrical roll of lint or other material; a tent. [L *penicillum* paintbrush.]

Pende, Nicolo (b. 1880). Genoa and Bari physician.

Pende's metabolic body type. Pende described three biotypes, hyperanabolic, orthometabolic, hypercatabolic. He introduced the term "endocrinology".

Pendecamaine (pen·dek·am·ane). BP Commission approved name for *N,N*-dimethyl-(3-palmitamidopropyl)aminoacetic acid betaine; a surface-active agent.

Pendred, Vaughan (b. 1869). London physician.

Pendred's syndrome. A familial disease with goitre developing in childhood or later and nerve deafness developing at birth or early childhood and occurring in non-iodine-deficient areas. It is due to deficient iodination of inorganic iodide taken up by the thyroid cells. There are raised circulating levels of triiodothyronical (T-3) and exaggerated response of thyroid-stimulating hormone (TSH) to thyrotrophin-releasing hormone (TRH).

pendular (pen·dew·lar). Pertaining to or moving like a pendulum. [see foll.]

pendulous (pen·dew·lus). 1. Swinging. 2. Hanging freely. [L *pendulus* swinging.]

Penethamate Hydriodide (pen·eth·am·ate hi·dri·o·dide). BP Commission approved name for benzylpenicillin 2-diethylaminoethyl-ester hydriodide; a compound which is used in all cases where penicillin is indicated, but appears to have a special affinity for lung tissue. It is also of value when subjects show special sensitivity to other penicillin preparations.

penetrance (pen·e·trance). The frequency with which a dominant, or double recessive gene, or gene association, manifests itself. This depends on other genes or on non-genetic factors. [L *penetrare* to penetrate.]

penetration (pen·e·tra·shun). 1. The act of entry into, of piercing or penetrating. 2. Medicolegally, penetration of the penis into the vagina, which alone constitutes rape. Seminal emission is not necessary, nor is injury to the hymen essential. Proof of penetration of the vulva is sufficient. 3. The depth of focus of a lens [obsolete term]. **X-ray penetration.** The degree to which rays are able to penetrate matter; hard rays show a high degree of penetration and soft rays a low degree. [L *penetrare* to penetrate.]

penetrometer (pen·e·trom·et·er). An apparatus once used for measuring the penetrating power (quality, hardness) and intensity of x-rays. Usually associated with the name of Benoist. *See* BENOIST'S SCALE.

Penfield, Wilder Graves (b. 1891). Montreal neurological surgeon.

Foerster-Penfield operation. Cortical scar excision for epilepsy.

Penfluridol (pen·floo·rid·ol). BP Commission approved name for 4-(4-chloro-3-trifluoromethylphenyl)-1-[4,4-di(4-fluorophenyl) butyl] piperidin-4-ol; a neuroleptic agent.

penial (pe·ne·al). Penile; relating or belonging to the penis.

penicidin (pen·e·si·din). Patulin.

Penicillamine BP 1973 (pen·e·sil·am·een). (−)-3,3-dimethylcysteine, a chelating agent used to facilitate elimination of certain toxic metallic ions from the body tissues. It is mainly used in the treatment of hepatolenticular degeneration (Wilson's disease) where it increases the output of copper; it is also used in the treatment of poisoning by lead and iron, and cystinuria. **Pencillamine Hydrochloride BP 1973.** The hydrochloride of pencillamine, with the same actions and uses.

penicillase (pen·e·sil·aze). Penicillinase.

penicillate (pen·e·sil·ate). Provided with a tuft of fine hairs. [L *penicillum* paintbrush.]

penicilli [NA] (pen·e·sil·i). The terminal arterioles of the splenic branches of the splenic artery. They arise as a tuft of straight vessels immediately after the arterial branches emerge from the lymphatic nodules of the spleen (malpighian bodies) and terminate in the splenic capillaries. [L *penicillum* paintbrush.]

penicilliform (pen·e·sil·e·form). Shaped like a pencil. [L *penicillum* paintbrush, form.]

penicillin (pen·e·sil·in). An antibiotic produced by *Penicillium notatum,* first described by Fleming in 1929 and purified and adapted for therapeutic use by Florey and Chain in 1941. It is now produced by surface culture of *Penicillium notatum* or submerged culture of *Penicillium chrysogenum.* The purified product is a yellow powder, issued in the form of the calcium or sodium salt in sealed airtight containers. There are four principal penicillins, F, G, K and X; fraction G is benzyl-penicillin, the most active and stable, and forming the greater part of commercial products. Penicillin is bactericidal to many bacteria pathogenic for man, and is usually given intramuscularly or subcutaneously for the treatment of infections caused by staphylococcus, streptococcus, pneumococcus, meningococcus, gonococcus, *Leptospira icterohaemorrhagiae* and *Clostridium;* it has also been used with success in the treatment of anthrax, actinomycosis and syphilis. **Benethamine penicillin.** BP Commission approved name for a salt of penicillin G with an organic base. It is the *N*-benzyl-*p*-phenylethylamine salt of penicillin G, a substance relatively insoluble in water, and producing prolonged effective blood levels when given by intramuscular injection as an aqueous suspension. It is less toxic than procaine penicillin, and is well tolerated and stable at room temperatures, but is not suitable for intravenous injection. Effective serum levels of penicillin are maintained for 3 days or more following a single intramuscular injection of 300 000 units. It is indicated in the treatment of infections caused by bacteria fully sensitive to penicillin, but not where a quick effect is required, when sodium penicillin is indicated. **Benzathine Penicillin BP 1973.** *N,N'*-dibenzylethylenediamine dipenicillin G, used in the treatment of infections caused by all penicillin-sensitive organisms. **Benzethamine penicillin.** Benethamine penicillin (see above). **Clemizole Penicillin.** BP Commission approved name for benzylpenicillin combined with 1-*p*-chlorobenzyl-2-pyrrolidino-methylbenzimidazole; an antibiotic with anti-allergic properties. **Crystalline penicillin G.** Benzylpenicillin. **Depot penicillin.** Any preparation which liberates penicillin slowly from the site of injection, thus enabling the frequency of dosage to be markedly reduced. Earlier means of ensuring this included the injection of oily suspensions of penicillin, but procaine benzylpenicillin is now used, by means of which therapeutic levels of penicillin can be maintained in the blood stream after one injection of 300 000 units. Another method of depot therapy is the use of procaine benzylpenicillin in oil with aluminium stearate, which maintains a reasonable blood level for seven days after one injection. ***N,N',*-Dibenzylethylenediamine penicillin.** A sparingly-soluble complex prepared by coupling *N,N'*-dibenzylethylenediamine with penicillin; it shows promise as a depot-therapy form of the antibiotic. **Penicillin G.** Benzylpenicillin. **Penicillin O.** Allylmercaptomethyl penicillin produced by growing the mould in a medium containing allylmercaptomethylacetic acid. **Procaine Penicillin BP 1973.** The monohydrate of the procaine salt of benzylpenicillin. It is only slightly soluble in water, and penicillin is slowly liberated from it at the site of injection. It is administered as an aqueous suspension, and injection is less painful than is the case with the other penicillin salts. **Repository penicillin.** Depot penicillin (see above). **Penicillin V.** Phenoxymethylpenicillin. [L *penicillum* paintbrush.]

penicillin-fast (pen·e·sil·in·fahst'). Of a micro-organism, resistant to the action of penicillin. [penicillin, AS *faest.*]

penicillinase (pen·e·sil·in·aze). 1. An enzyme secreted by penicillin-fast bacteria. It inactivates penicillin, hence such an organism must be absent from penicillin injections. 2. BP Commission approved name for an enzyme obtained from cultures of *Bacillus cereus* which hydrolyses benzylpenicillin to penicilloic acid.

penicilliosis (pen·e·sil·e·o'·sis). A rare mycosis in some animals, but doubtful in man. It is difficult to diagnose unequivocably owing to ubiquity of *Penicillium* spores in the environment, thus penicillia may occur in patients with various diseases almost certainly without harmful effects. [L *penicillum* paintbrush, Gk *-osis* condition.]

Penicillium (pen·e·sil·e·um). A genus of fungi belonging to the group Ascomycetes, many species of which possess antibiotic activity due to the penicillins produced during their metabolism. Certain species are pathogenic to man. **Penicillium charlesii.** A species that produces carlic acid. **Penicillium chrysogenum.** A species from which penicillin is produced by submerged culture. **Penicillium citrinum.** A species that produces the antibiotic citrinin. **Penicillium claviforme.** A species that produces the antibiotic claviformin, identical with clavacin. **Penicillium crustaceum, Penicillium glaucum.** The common blue-green mould; it has been found in chronic catarrh of the eustachian tube. **Penicillium griseofulvum.** The species that produces the antibiotic griseofulvin. **Penicillium luteum.** A species that produces luteic acid. **Penicillium montoyai.** A species once thought to be responsible for pinta, of tropical America, now recognized as a treponematosis. **Penicillium notatum.** A species employed in surface culture, the penicillin being extracted from the filtrate. **Penicillium patulum.** A species that produces the antibiotic patulin, identical with clavacin. **Penicillium puberulum.** A species that produces penicillic acid. **Penicillium purpurogenum.** A species that produces gluconic acid in glucose. **Penicillium spinulosum.** A species that produces the antibiotic spinulosin. **Penicillium terrestre.** A species that produces terrestric acid. [L *penicillum* paintbrush.]

penicillus (pen·e·sil·us). Any one of the small straight vessels into which the arterioles divide when they enter the red pulp of the spleen. [L *penicillum* paintbrush.]

penile (pe·nile). Relating or belonging to the penis.

penis [NA] (pe·nis). The male organ of copulation, cylindrical in form and capable of enlargement and erection as a result of the engorgement of the cavernous spaces within its substance. **Body of the penis [corpus penis (NA)].** The main free portion of the penis, anterior to the pubic symphysis. **Penis captivus.** Retention of the penis within the vagina as a result of vaginismus. **Chordeic penis.** A painful curved erection of the penis with the concavity downwards, associated with the extension of gonorrheal inflammation to the corpus spongiosum urethrae. **Clubbed penis.** A curvature which may include torsion of the penis, frequently associated with hypospadias or epispadias. **Dorsum of the penis [dorsum penis (NA)].** The upper surface of the penis. **Hairy penis.** Pearly penile papules. *See* PAPULE. **Neck of the penis [collum glandis (NA)].** The constriction proximal to the glans penis. **Penis plastica.** Peyronie's disease; a condition in which the corpora cavernosa penis contain plaques of acellular fibrous tissue which form actual nodules and interfere with erection. **Root of the penis [radix penis (NA)].** The attached portion of the penis in the perineum. **Urethral surface of the penis [facies urethralis (NA)].** The undersurface of the body of the penis. **Webbed penis.** A penis which is concealed in whole or part beneath the skin of the scrotum or the perineum. [L.]

penis, arteries of the (or of the clitoris). Deep artery of the penis (or of the clitoris) [arteria profunda penis (clitoridis) (NA)]. A branch of the internal pudendal artery. **Dorsal artery of the penis (or of the clitoris) [arteria dorsalis penis (clitoridis) (NA)].** A branch of the internal pudendal artery.

penis, artery of the bulb of the, or of the vestibule [arteria bulbi penis et arteria bulbi vestibuli (vaginae) (NA)]. A branch of the internal pudendal artery.

penis, nerves of the (or of the clitoris). Cavernous nerves of the penis (or of the clitoris) [nervi cavernosi penis (clitoridis) (NA)]. Two branches, greater and lesser, from the prostatic plexus to the cavernous tissues of the penis, or, in the female, from the uterovaginal plexus to the clitoris. **Dorsal nerve of the penis (or of the clitoris) [nervus dorsalis penis (clitoridis) (NA)].** A branch of the perineal nerve.

penis, veins of the (or of the clitoris). Cavernous veins of the penis [venae cavernosae (NA)]. Cavernous spaces: large cavernous spaces filling the corpora cavernosa penis and the corpus spongiosum penis, into which the helicine arteries open. **Deep veins of the penis (or of the clitoris) [venae profundae penis (clitoridis) (NA)].** Tributaries of the prostatic venous plexus in the male, or of the vesical plexus in the female. They enter the pelvis beneath the pubic symphysis. **Dorsal vein of the penis, deep [vena dorsalis penis profunda (NA)].** A tributary of the prostatic plexus, entering the pelvis beneath the pubic symphysis. **Dorsal veins of the penis (or of the clitoris), superficial [venae dorsales penis (clitoridis) superficiales (NA)].** Tributaries of the superficial external pudendal veins.

penis, vein of the bulb of the, or of the vestibule [vena bulbi penis et vena bulbi vestibuli (NA)]. A tributary of the internal pudendal vein draining the erectile tissue of the bulb.

penitis (pe·ni·tis). Any inflammatory condition of the penis. [penis, Gk *-itis* inflammation.]

pennate (pen·ate). 1. Winged or feathered. 2. Penniform. [L *penna* feather.]

penniform (pen·e·form). Having the appearance of a feather; shaped like a feather. [L *penna* feather, form.]

pennyroyal (pen·e·roi·al). The common name for the perennial herb, *Mentha pulegium* Linn., which yields a volatile oil containing the ketone, pulegone. The plant is used as a carminative, stimulant and emmenagogue; the oil is a powerful but dangerous ecbolic and intestinal irritant, now rarely used in medicine. **American pennyroyal.** The dried leaves and flowering tops of the plant, *Hedeoma pulegioides,* which yields a volatile oil similar in composition and properties to that from *Mentha pulegium.* [OFr. *poliol* thyme, *roial.*]

pennyweight (pen·e·wate). A unit of weight equal to 1.56 g (24 grains or $\frac{1}{20}$ part of a troy ounce) not used in pharmacy. [AS *pening, gewiht.*]

penology (pe·nol·o·je). The science and study which deals with punishment of crime, especially that section of criminology which treats of corrective and reformative measures. [Gk *poine* penalty, *logos* science.]

penoplasty (pe·no·plas·te). Any plastic operation on the penis. [penis, Gk *plassein* to mould.]

penoscrotal (pe·no·skro·tal). Pertaining to the penis and the scrotum.

Penrose, Charles Bingham (b. 1862). Philadelphia surgeon.

Penrose drain. Cigarette drain; a drain of gauze surrounded by waterproof material, rubber, or gutta percha.

pentabasic (pen·tah·ba·sik). 1. Denoting an acid that has five atoms of hydrogen replaceable by a metal or radical. 2. Of an alcohol, one containing 5 hydroxyl groups. [Gk *pente* five, basic.]

pentachromic (pen·tah·kro·mik). Designating an individual who is partially colour blind and can identify 5 colours only of the 6 spectral colours of Edridge-Green's classification of colour blindness. [Gk *pente* five, *chroma* colour.]

Pentacosactride (pen·tak·o·sak'·tride). BP Commission approved name for D-Ser^{1}-Nle^{4}-(Val-NH$_2$)^{25}-$\beta^{1\text{-}25}$-corticotrophin; a synthetic corticotrophin.

pentacyclic (pen·tah·si·klik). In organic chemistry, describing a ring composed of 5 atoms. [Gk *pente* five, *kyklos* circle.]

Pentacynium Methylsulphate (pen·tah·si·ne·um meth·il·sul'·fate). BP Commission approved name for 4-[2-(5-cyano-5,5-diphenylpentyldimethylammonio)ethyl]-4-methylmorpholonium di(methyl sulphate); a ganglion blocking agent used in treatment of hypertension.

pentad (pen·tad). General term denoting an element or radical with a valency of 5. [Gk *pente* five.]

pentadactyl, pentadactyle (pen·tah·**dak**·til, pen·tah·**dak**·tile). Having 5 toes or 5 fingers on the hand or foot. [Gk *pente* five, *daktylos* finger or toe.]

Pentaerythritol Tetranitrate (**pen**·tah·er·**ith**'·rit·ol tet·rah·**ni**·trate). BP Commission approved name for pentaerythrityl tetranitrate. A vasodilator with a prolonged action. It is more stable than glyceryl trinitrate, and is useful in anginal pain, its effect lasting up to 4 hours.

pentaerythrityl tetranitrate (**pen**·tah·er·**ith**'·rit·il tet·ra·**ni**·trate). Pentaerythritol tetranitrate.

Pentagastrin BP 1973 (pen·tah·**gas**·trin). *N*-t-butyloxycarbonyl-β-alanyl-L-tryptophyl-L-methionyl-L-aspartyl-L-phenylalanine amide; a gastrin-like polypeptide used to stimulate gastric secretion.

pentahydric (pen·tah·**hi**·drik). Describing the presence of 5 hydrogen atoms.

pental (**pen**·tal). Trimethyl-ethylene, β-iso-amylene, $(CH_3)_2CCHCH_3$. A colourless oily liquid once tried as a general anaesthetic but found to be unduly toxic.

Pentalamide (pen·**tal**·am·ide). BP Commission approved name for 2-pentyloxybenzamide; it is used in the treatment of fungal infections.

Pentamethonium (**pen**·tah·meth·**o**'·ne·um). An organic radical derived by substitution from ammonium. It is the pentamethylene member of a series of polymethylene bis[trimethylammonium] radicals of general formula $(CH_3)_3\,N^+(CH_3)_nN^+(CH_3)_3$ known as *methonium* bases, *n* in this case being 5. The simple salts act like the homologue hexamethonium by paralysing transmission across the ganglionic synapse, and are used to lower blood pressure. Hexamethonium, however, is more commonly employed for the purpose, being more active. **Pentamethonium Bromide.** BP Commission approved name for the bromide. Its action is similar to the iodide, which is also approved. **Pentamethonium Iodide.** BP Commission approved name for the iodide of pentamethonium, used like hexamethonium iodide to block the sympathetic and parasympathetic ganglia, and of value in the treatment of hypertension.

pentamethyl violet (**pen**·tah·meth·il **vi**·o·let). Methyl violet, methylrosaniline. A mixture of pararosanilines, mostly the pentamethyl pararosaniline chloride, closely related to gentian violet. It is used as a bactericide against staphylococci, *Corynebacterium diphtheriae, Pseudomonas aeruginosa* and other Gram-positive organisms; also used in Vincent's angina and against moulds, e.g. *Candida, Torula, Epidermophyton* and *Trichophyton.* It is also employed as an anthelminthic and in the treatment of burns. [Gk *pente* five, methyl, L *viola.*]

pentamethylenediamine (pen·tah·**meth**·il·een·**di**'·am·een). Cadaverine, $H_2N(CH_2)_5NH_2$. A nitrogenous base (ptomaine) occurring as a product of bacterial decomposition of protein and formerly believed to be a cause of food poisoning.

pentamethylenetetrazole (pen·tah·**meth**·il·een·**tet**'·rah·zole). Leptazol.

Pentamidine (pent·**am**·id·een). BP Commission approved name for 4,4'-diamidino-α,ω-diphenoxypentane. One of a series of amidines used in the treatment of African trypanosomiasis, especially against arsenic-resistant strains. They are effective in early cases, but are of little use once the central nervous system is involved. They are also employed in kala-azar, appearing relatively more active in the Sudanese form which tends to be resistant to antimony. **Pentamidine Isethionate BP 1973.** $[NH_2C(=NH)C_6H_4O]_2(CH_2)_5(C_2H_6SO_4)_2$, the usual form in which the drug is employed.

pentane (**pen**·tane). C_5H_{12}, a highly inflammable liquid hydrocarbon, fifth of the methane series, which occurs in petroleum: it is very volatile, and is used as an anaesthetic and refrigerant. [Gk *pente* five.]

pentanone (**pen**·tan·one). Diethylketone.

pentanucleotide (pen·tah·**new**·kle·o·tide). A breakdown product of a nucleic acid, comprising 5 nucleotide residues per molecule. [Gk *pente* five, nucleotide.]

Pentapiperide (pen·tah·**pip**·er·ide). BP Commission approved name for 1-methyl-4-(3-methyl-2-phenylvaleryloxy)piperidine; an anticholinergic agent.

pentaploid (**pen**·tah·ploid). Having five times the haploid number of chromosomes in the somatic cell nuclei. [Gk *pentaploos* fivefold, *eidos* form.]

pentapyrrolidinium tartrate (**pen**·tah·pir·ol·id·**in**'·e·um **tar**·trate). Pentolinium tartrate.

Pentaquine (**pen**·tah·kween). BP Commission approved name for 6-methoxy-8-(5-isopropylamino-amylamino)quinoline, an antimalarial drug. There is a tendency towards its replacement by primaquine.

pentasomic (pen·tah·**so**·mik). Of polysomic cells or individuals, with five replicas of the same chromosome. [Gk *pente* five, *soma* body.]

Pentastoma (pen·tah·**sto**·mah). A name erroneously used for Pentastomida. [Gk *pente* five, *stoma* mouth.]

pentastomes (**pen**·tah·sto·mz). A general name for the tongue worms of several genera. [see prec.]

pentastomiasis (**pen**·tah·sto·**mi**'·as·is). Infestation with endoparasitic arthropods, known as *tongue worms,* which suck blood. Genera infesting man are *Pentastomida, Linguatula* and *Armillifer.* [Gk *pente* five, *stoma* mouth.]

Pentastomida (pen·tah·**sto**·**mid**·ah). A class of worm-like arthropods, perhaps related to mites; sometimes considered as a phylum. The adults bear 4 claws anteriorly; they are parasites of vertebrates, particularly reptiles. Secondary hosts of the young are also vertebrates. Members of the genera *Armillifer, Linguatula* and *Porocephalus* are of medical importance. [see prec.]

pentatomic (pent·at·**om**·ik). 1. Pentavalent (*see* MULTIVALENT). 2. Describing a molecule composed of 5 atoms. 3. Of an alcohol, one containing 5 hydroxyl groups. [Gk *pente* five, atom.]

Pentatrichomonas (**pen**·tah·trik·o·**mo**'·nas). A genus of flagellate protozoa. *Pentatrichomonas ardin delteili* is a form of *Trichomonas hominis* with 5 flagella. [Gk *pente* five, *thrix* hair, *monas* unit.]

pentavaccine (pen·tah·**vak**·seen). A general term used to describe a vaccine made from 5 species of bacteria; applied to a vaccine containing the bacilli causing typhoid, paratyphoid A, paratyphoid B, cholera and Malta fever. [Gk *pente* five, vaccine.]

pentavalent (pen·tah·**va**·lent). *See* MULTIVALENT. [Gk *pente* five, valent.]

Pentazocine (pent·**az**·o·seen). BP Commission approved name for 1,2,3,4,5,6-hexahydro-8-hydroxy-6,11-dimethyl-3-(3-methylbut-2-enyl)-2,6-methano-3-benzazocine; a morphine-like analgesic but with less tendency of producing dependence than morphine.

pentene (**pen**·teen). Any hydrocarbon of the formula C_5H_{10}; amylene.

Penthienate (pen·**thi**·en·ate). BP Commission approved name for 2-diethylaminoethyl α-cyclopentyl-2-thiopheneglycolate, an anticholinergic agent that inhibits gastric activity and secretion. It has also been used in hyperhidrosis.

Penthrichloral (pen·thri·**klor**·al). BP Commission approved name for 5,5-di(hydroxymethyl)-2-trichloromethyl-1,3-dioxane; a hypnotic and sedative.

Pentifylline (pen·**tif**·il·een). BP Commission approved name for 1-hexyl-3,7-dimethylxanthine; a vasodilator.

pentobarbital sodium (pen·to·**bar**·bit·al **so**·de·um). Pentobarbitone sodium.

Pentobarbitone Sodium BP 1973 (pen·to·**bar**·bit·one **so**·de·um). Monosodium ethyl-methylbutyl barbiturate, $C_{11}H_{17}O_3N_2Na$. One of many variants of the barbiturate complex. It is sedative, antispasmodic and hypnotic.

Pentolinium Tartrate BP 1973 (pen·to·**lin**·e·um **tar**·trate). A hypotensive agent used for the treatment of malignant hypertension, arteriosclerosis with hypertension, etc., and to induce hypotension during anaesthesia.

pentosaemia (pen·to·se·me·ah). The presence of pentose in the blood. [pentose, Gk *haima* blood.]

pentosan (**pen**·to·san). Any of the polysaccharides formed from pentose units. They have the general formula $(C_5H_8O_4)_n$, and are represented principally by araban from gum arabic, and xylan from straw. **Methyl pentosan.** A gum such as fucosan which, on hydrolysis, produces a methyl pentose.

pentosazone (pen·**to**·sa·zone). General term for an osazone formed by phenylhydrazine with a pentose.

pentose (**pen**·toze). Any of a class of sugars containing 5 carbon atoms in a chain and having the general formula $C_5H_{10}O_5$. They occur in nature in complex form as pentosans, glycosides, and in the nucleic acids. Free pentoses, chiefly L-xyloketose, occur in the urine in the condition pentosuria. [Gk *pente* five.]

pentosidase (pen·**to**·sid·aze). An enzyme which attacks the oxygen linkage in compound saccharides composed of pentose units.

pentoside (**pen**·to·side). A compound which contains a pentose unit: the most important are the nucleosides which are composed of a pentose united to a purine or pyrimidine base.

pentosuria (pen·to·**sewr**·e·ah). The presence of pentose in the urine. **Essential pentosuria, Idiopathic pentosuria.** An inborn error of metabolism, the chemical importance of which is that it may be mistaken for diabetes mellitus or renal glycosuria.

pentosuric (pen·to·**sewr**·ik). Pertaining to or suffering from pentosuria.

pentoxide (pent·**ox**·ide). Any oxide which contains 5 atoms of oxygen in its molecule, e.g. phosphorus pentoxide, P_2O_5. [Gk *pente* five, oxide.]

pentyl (**pen**·til). Amyl; the monovalent group C_5H_{11}, which occurs in normal amyl alcohol. **Pentyl hydride.** Pentane. [Gk *pente* five.]

pentylenetetrazole (**pen**·til·een·**tet**'·rah·zole). Leptazol.

penumbra (pen·**um**·brah). A half-shadow formed round the deep shadow or umbra when a source of light is large and placed near the object casting the shadow. [L *paene* almost, *umbra* shadow.]

peonin (pe·o·nin). $O{=}C_6H_4{=}C(C_6H_4OH)(C_6H_4NH_2)$, the amino derivative of aurin; a pararosaniline dye used as a pH indicator.

peotillomania (pe·o·til·o·ma'·ne·ah). A nervous tic consisting in continual pulling of the penis. [Gk *peos* penis, *tillein* to pull, mania.]

peotomy (pe·**ot**·o·me). Amputation of the penis. [Gk *peos* penis, *temnein* to cut.]

pepo (**pe**·po). The dried ripe seeds of the pumpkin, *Cucurbita pepo*, used as a non-toxic vermifuge. [L, pumpkin.]

Pepper, William (b. 1874). Philadelphia physician.

Pepper syndrome, or type. Primary sarcoma of the suprarenals in young infants, with metastases in the liver, with resultant liver failure.

pepper (**pep**·er). 1. The dried fruits of various plants of the genus *Piper* (family Piperaceae). 2. Black pepper (see foll.). **Black pepper.** The dried, fully grown, but unripe fruit of *Piper nigram* Linn.; it contains 2 per cent of volatile oil, consisting mostly of the terpenes, phellandrene and dipentene, an alkaloid, piperine and a resin, chavicine. **Cayenne pepper.** Capsicum; the dried ripe fruits of *Capsicum minimum* Roxb. (family Solanaceae), used as a condiment. Externally it is applied in the form of a plaster or medicated wool for counter-irritation; a tincture is given as a carminative in dyspepsia and flatulence. **Red pepper.** Cayenne pepper (see prec.). **Tailed pepper.** Cubeb; the dried fruits of *Piper cubeba* Linn. **Water pepper.** The leaves of *Polygonum hydropiper.* **White pepper.** The fruits of *Piper nigrum* Linn. which have ripened and from which the pericarp has been separated after soaking in salt or lime water. It is less pungent and aromatic than black pepper and has a more delicate flavour. [L *piper.*]

peppermint (**pep**·er·mint). The dried leaf and flowering tops of the herb *Mentha piperita* Linn. (family Labiatae), largely cultivated for the volatile oil distilled from the fresh plant. **Japanese peppermint.** The species *Mentha arvensis* var. *piperascens,* from which is distilled an oil containing up to 90 per cent of menthol but inferior in flavour to that of *Mentha piperita.* [pepper, Gk *mintha* mint.]

pepsic (**pep**·sik). Peptic.

pepsigogue (**pep**·se·gog). A substance that stimulates the secretion of pepsin. [pepsin, Gk *agogein* to lead.]

pepsin (**pep**·sin). The proteolytic enzyme of the stomach, secreted by the gastric mucosa in an inactive form, pepsinogen, which requires acid for activation to pepsin. It is a protein of the albumin class, with a molecular weight of about 35 000, and shows optimal activity at pH 1.8 converting proteins mainly into peptones. It is used medicinally (BPC 1959) to aid digestion, chiefly in cases of hypochlorhydria, commercial preparations being assayed by their ability to digest several thousand times their own weight of coagulated egg albumen to soluble digestion products. **Elixir of pepsin.** A solution of pepsin in alcohol and aromatic elixir containing 5.5 per cent w/v of pepsin. **Glycerin of pepsin.** A solution of pepsin in acidified glycerin and water containing 15 per cent w/v of pepsin. [Gk *pepsis* digestion.]

pepsinase (**pep**·sin·aze). A member of a group of protein-splitting enzymes which occur in gastric juice and, acting in acid medium, hydrolyse proteins into polypeptides. [see prec.]

pepsinate (**pep**·sin·ate). To treat or mix with pepsin; to impregnate with pepsin.

pepsinia (pep·**sin**·e·ah). The secretion of pepsin.

pepsiniferous (pep·sin·**if**·er·us). Yielding, secreting or producing pepsin. [pepsin, L *ferre* to bear.]

pepsinogen (pep·**sin**·o·jen). The inactive precursor of pepsin secreted by the stomach, which is activated by acid to pepsin. [see foll.]

pepsinogenous (pep·sin·**oj**·en·us). Producing pepsin. [pepsin, Gk *genein* to produce.]

pepsinum (pep·**si**·num). Pepsin.

peptic (**pep**·tik). 1. Promoting or relating to digestion. 2. Pertaining to, resembling or containing pepsin. [see foll.]

pepticity (pep·**tis**·it·e). A good state of digestion. [Gk *peptein* to digest.]

peptid (**pep**·tid). Peptide.

peptidase (**pep**·tid·aze). A member of a group of protein-splitting enzymes which attack peptides, converting them into amino acids. They occur as a mixture of specific peptidases in the erepsin of intestinal juice, and in plants, yeasts and certain micro-organisms.

peptide (**pep**·tide). A unit in the structure of proteins, consisting of 2 or more amino acids linked by their respective carboxyl and amino groups into a molecular chain: they are known as di-, tri-, tetra-, octa-, deca- or polypeptides according to the number of amino acids involved. **Cyanogen bromide peptide.** A peptide derived by treatment of a larger polypeptide with cyanogen bromide in formic acid, which reacts with the side chain of methionine and breaks the peptide bond involving the carboxyl group of this residue. **Peptide link.** The group -CONH-, which unites amino acids into polypeptides. **Non-coded peptide.** One of a class of peptides that are not assembled in living cells on a specific messenger RNA as template. **Peptide map.** A fingerprint of a partial digest of a protein. **Peptide map analysis.** The examination of fingerprints of a protein digest by staining reactions for specific amino acids (e.g. reactions for tryptophan, methionine, tyrosine, histidine and arginine). [Gk *peptein* to digest.]

peptidolytic (pep·tid·o·**lit**'·ik). Having the power to break up peptides and digest them. [peptide, Gk *lysis* a loosing.]

peptidyl transferase (**pep**·tid·il **trans**·fer·aze). An enzyme that catalyses the formation of peptide bonds during the assembling of amino-acid residues into polypeptides on ribosomes. It is a protein that forms part of the 50S subunit of the ribosome. [Gk *peptein* to digest, L *transferre* to bring across.]

peptinotoxin (pep·tin·o·**tox**'·in). A poisonous intestinal product supposed to be due to imperfect digestion of proteins by pepsin. [pepsin, toxin.]

peptization (pep·ti·za·shun). 1. The conversion of a gel into a liquid state (sol), especially when brought about by enzymes. 2. The dispersion by mechanical means of fine insoluble particles through a liquid to form a colloidal solution. [Gk *peptein* to digest.]

peptogaster (pep·to·gas·ter). The alimentary canal. [Gk *peptein* to digest, *gaster* stomach.]

peptogastric (pep·to·gas·trik). 1. Peptic. 2. Belonging to the alimentary canal. [see prec.]

peptogen (pep·to·jen). Any substance that promotes the secretion of pepsin, e.g. meat extract. [pepsin, Gk *genein* to produce.]

peptogenic, peptogenous (pep·to·jen·ik, pep·toj·en·us). 1. Able to assist digestion. 2. Having the characteristics of a peptogen. 3. In physiological chemistry, capable of yielding peptone, or of being converted into it. [peptone, Gk *peptein* to digest, *genein* to produce.]

peptolysis (pep·tol·is·sis). The hydrolysis of peptone. [peptone, Gk *lysis* a loosing.]

peptolytic (pep·to·lit·ik). Capable of causing the hydrolysis of peptone. [see prec.]

peptonaemia (pep·to·ne·me·ah). The presence of peptone in the blood. [peptone, Gk *haima* blood.]

peptone (pep·tone). A product of the partial hydrolysis of proteins, e.g. by the action of pepsin. Peptones are soluble in water, acids and alkalis, and are not precipitated by complete saturation with ammonium sulphate or sodium sulphate. Commercial peptones are prepared from meat fibrin or casein, by digestion either with pepsin alone or with pepsin followed by trypsin, the composition of the final product being thus varied to provide a range of peptones suitable to general and special bacteriological purposes. **Beef peptone.** Peptone prepared by digestion of beef with pancreatin. **Casein peptone.** Peptone prepared by digestion of casein with pepsin or trypsin. **Gelatin peptone.** Peptone prepared by peptic digestion of gelatin. [Gk *pepton* digesting.]

See also: DUNHAM (E. K.).

peptonic (pep·ton·ik). Relating or belonging to, secreting, or containing peptone.

peptonization (pep·to·ni·za′·shun). The enzymic process whereby proteins are converted into peptones.

peptonize (pep·to·nize). To change protein to peptone by enzymic action.

peptonoid (pep·to·noid). Any substance that has some resemblance to peptone. [peptone, Gk *eidos* form.]

peptonolysis (pep·to·nol·is·is). The hydrolysis of peptone.

peptonuria (pep·to·newr·e·ah). A condition in which peptones are found in the urine. **Enterogenous peptonuria.** Peptonuria caused by intestinal disease. **Hepatogenous peptonuria.** That which is caused by a diseased condition of the liver. **Nephrogenic peptonuria.** Peptonuria which is caused by renal disease. **Puerperal peptonuria.** That which occurs during the puerperium. **Pyogenic peptonuria.** Peptonuria caused by suppuration.

peptophilic (pep·to·fil·ik). Growing well in peptone solution, e.g. certain bacteria. [peptone, Gk *philein* to love.]

peptotoxin (pep·to·tox·in). Any toxic substance produced in the peptone stage of protein breakdown.

per-. 1. A prefix, from the Latin preposition *per*, meaning *through, all over, very, completely.* 2. In chemistry, a prefix meaning *more than,* with reference to the highest valence of a series.

peracephalus (per·a·kef·al·us). In teratology, an acephalous monster without arms, and with malformed thorax. [L *per*, Gk *a*, *kephale* head.]

peracetate (per·as·et·ate). 1. Any salt or ester of peracetic acid. 2. Of several acetates of an element or radical, that one which contains the highest proportion of acetic radical.

peracid (per·as·id). 1. An acid formed by an element displaying its highest valency, e.g. persulphuric acid, $H_2S_2O_8$. 2. Any organic acid containing the group -COOOH. [L *per*, acid.]

peracidity (per·as·id·it·e). Hyperacidity. [see prec.]

peracute (per·ak·ewt). Hyperacute. [L *peracutus* very acute.]

perarticulation (per·ar·tik·ew·la′·shun). Diarthrosis. [L *per*, *articulus* joint.]

Peratizole (per·at·i·zole). BP Commission approved name for 1-[4-(2,4-dimethylthiazol-5-yl)butyl]-4-(methylthiazol-2-yl)piperazine; an antihypertensive agent.

peratodynia (per·at·o·din′·e·ah). Cardiodynia; heartburn. [Gk *peraein* to pierce right through, *odyne* pain.]

perborate (per·bor·ate). A salt of perboric acid.

perborax (per·bor·ax). Sodium perborate, $NaBO_3·4H_2O$, which in solution yields free hydrogen peroxide. It is used as an oxidizing agent and in dentrifrices.

percept (per·sept). The mental image, or product of perception, of any object in space. [see foll.]

perception (per·sep·shun). The interpretation by the cerebrum of the afferent nervous impulses produced by sensory stimuli. **Depth perception.** The impression of depth and distance and the position of objects relative to each other. It is mainly due to stereoscopic vision, but a certain degree is present in monocular vision. **Extrasensory perception.** Perception or communication not mediated by known receptors; also includes *precognition* (knowledge of future events). **Parapsychological perception.** Clairvoyance. **Simultaneous macular perception.** A low grade of binocular vision when the images, falling on the maculae of the two eyes are both appreciated by the cerebrum instead of one or the other being suppressed. Although these two images may be superimposed to form one, no proper fusion with amplitude exists at this stage of binocular vision. A term commonly used in orthoptics. **Subliminal perception.** Measurable responses to stimuli below the threshold of conscious perception. **Visual perception.** The interpretation by the cerebrum of the afferent nervous impulses produced by light stimuli on the retinal elements of the eye. [L *percipere* to perceive.]

perceptive (per·sep·tiv). 1. Endowed with perceptive power. 2. Relating or belonging to perception.

perceptivity (per·sep·tiv·it·e). The power or faculty of perception.

perceptorium (per·sep·tor·e·um). Any sensory nerve centre. [L *percipere* to perceive.]

perchlorate (per·klor·ate). Any salt of perchloric acid. **Perchlorate discharge test.** *See* TEST.

perchlorethylene (per·klor·eth·il·een). Tetrachloroethylene.

perchlorhydria (per·klor·hi·dre·ah). Hyperchlorhydria. [L *per*, chlorhydria.]

perchloride (per·klor·ide). Of the several chlorides of an element or radical, that one which contains the largest proportion of chlorine. **Perchloride of mercury.** Mercuric chloride.

perchlormethane (per·klor·me·thane). Carbon tetrachloride.

perchlormethylformate (per·klor·meth·il·for′·mate). Diphosgene, trichloromethylchloroformate, $ClCOOCCl_3$. A polymer of phosgene used in chemical warfare as a choking gas under the names *perstoff* and *superpalite.*

perclusion (per·kloo·zhun). Incapability of carrying out any movement. [L *per*, *claudere* to halt.]

percolate (per·kol·ate). 1. To undergo percolation. 2. The liquid issuing from the base of a percolator, and containing the soluble matter of the drug.

percolation (per·kol·a·shun). The subjection of a substance, in a suitable state of subdivision, to the solvent action of a gravitating liquid. Percolation is the most efficient method of extracting the soluble matter of a drug of vegetable origin, as by this means it is possible to exhaust the drug completely. The powdered drug is packed into a vertical cylinder fitted with a tap at the bottom, and the solvent poured over; when the liquid commences to drip from the base the tap is usually closed for some hours in order to allow the soluble matter to pass into solution, after which the tap is opened and percolation allowed to continue, either until the drug is exhausted (i.e. pure solvent only is obtained) or until the solution becomes too weak to make further percolation worth while. [L *percolare* to filter through.]

percolator (per·kol·a·tor). In pharmacy, a long, funnel-shaped glass vessel with a tubular extremity used to extract the soluble constituents of a solid drug. [see prec.]

percuss (per·**kus**). To perform percussion. [L *percutere* to strike through.]

percussible (per·**kus**·ibl). Detectable on percussion.

percussion (per·**kush**·un). The art of striking the thoracic or abdominal wall in order to produce sound vibrations from which the nature of the underlying structures can be deduced; it is based on the fact that when an elastic body capable of vibrating is struck, a sound will be produced. The sounds vary in intensity, pitch and quality or timbre: percussion over a normal chest gives a characteristic resonant note; in pathological conditions the note may become more or less resonant, varying from hyperresonance, or tympany, to complete dullness. Originally percussion was practised with a small rubber-tipped hammer called a *plexor* with which a small piece of bone or ivory called the *pleximeter*, placed flat against the chest, was struck; nowadays the fingers are invariably used, and have the advantage that the tactile sense of resistance can add to the information obtained by percussion. **Auditory percussion.** That in which the character of the sound produced is noted. **Auscultatory percussion.** A method of determining the boundaries of a solid- or gas-containing organ by listening to the sound vibrations set up by light percussion. The stethoscope is placed over the centre of the organ and percussion is practised from outside the boundaries towards the centre. When the margin is reached, the sounds increase in intensity. **Coin percussion.** A method of auscultatory percussion in which a coin is placed on one part of the chest and struck with another coin while the observer listens with a stethoscope at a different part of the chest: a ringing bell-like sound is sometimes heard over a pneumothorax or large cavity. **Comparative percussion.** Percussion over corresponding parts of the two lungs to compare, for instance, the resonance of a healthy lung with the other which may be the seat of disease. **Deep percussion.** Percussion with firm blows in order to obtain vibrations from deep tissues. **Definitive percussion.** Percussion to define the outline of an organ. **Direct percussion.** Immediate percussion (see below). **Drop-stroke percussion.** Percussion in which the percussion hammer is allowed to fall by its own weight on to the pleximeter. **Immediate percussion.** Percussion in which no pleximeter is used and the percussion finger strikes directly on the chest wall. **Indirect percussion.** That in which a finger, or some substance used as a pleximeter, intervenes between the percussing finger and the area percussed. **Mediate percussion.** Indirect percussion by the use of plexor and pleximeter, fingers, or instruments. **Palpatory percussion.** Percussion in which the fingers are pressed successively over various parts of the chest but no blow is struck. It is a method of palpation and not percussion. **Piano percussion.** Immediate percussion with the four fingers successively, beginning with the little finger. **Respiratory percussion.** Percussion during respiration to detect differences between the sounds during inspiration and expiration. **Strip percussion.** Percussion of the chest from above downward over a narrow strip of the chest wall. **Tangential percussion.** Percussion in which the pleximeter is held vertically on the chest wall and the strokes are applied to the pleximeter in a direction parallel with the surface of the skin. **Threshold percussion.** Goldscheider's percussion; percussion performed by tapping lightly with the finger upon a glass-rod pleximeter, one end of which is covered with a rubber cap and rests upon an intercostal space. The method confines the vibrations to a very small area, and has been used to delimit the boundaries of organs such as the heart. [L *percutere* to strike through.]

See also: GOLDSCHEIDER, KROENIG.

percussopunctator (per·**kus**·o·**pungk**'·ta·tor). A hammer-like instrument studded with short needles which is employed in multiple acupuncture, a sharp knock driving their points into the tissues. [percussion, puncture.]

percussor (per·**kus**·or). A type of hammer used in percussion. [L, striker.]

percutaneous (per·kew·**ta**·ne·us). Effected through the skin; referring in particular to inunction in which the skin is whole. [L *per, cutis* skin.]

Percy, James Fulton (b. 1864). Galesburg, Illinois, surgeon.

Percy treatment. Cautery of the carcinomatous cervis with a hot iron to control bleeding before the radium is inserted (obsolete).

perectomy (per·**ek**·to·me). Peritectomy.

perencephaly (per·en·**kef**·al·e). A condition characterized by the presence of multiple cysts in the brain. [Gk *pera* pouch, *egkephalos* brain.]

Perényi, Josef. Budapest histologist.

Perényi's solution. A histological fixative containing nitric acid, alcohol and chromic acid.

Perethynol (per·**eth**·in·ol). A preparation of dried or fresh heart muscle of a horse in the form of a colloidal suspension with chloroethylene and alcohol.

perezone (per·e·zone). Pipitzahoic acid.

perfectionism (per·**fek**·shun·izm). A mental state in which the subject has as his aim an impossibly high standard of behaviour; he attributes the failure to reach it to his own shortcomings and consequently feels baffled and defeated. [L *perficere* to complete.]

perflation (per·**fla**·shun). 1. The act of blowing a current of air through or into a cavity or channel so that the walls are forced apart and the accumulated discharges expelled. 2. A system of natural ventilation by which air is introduced into a room as the result of movement of natural air currents. [L *perflare* to blow through.]

perforans (per·for·anz). A term used to designate certain nerves and muscles which penetrate other structures. **Perforans gasseri.** The musculocutaneous nerves. **Perforans manus.** The flexor digitorum profundus muscle. [L, piercing through.]

perforating arteries [arteriae perforantes (NA)] (**per**·for·a·ting **ar**·ter·iz). Branches, usually three in number of the profunda femoris artery, which pierce the adductor magnus muscle and supply the muscles in the back of the thigh and the vastus lateralis muscle. **Perforating arteries of the kidney.** Interlobular arteries which continue their course right through the cortex and emerge onto the surface of the kidney where they anastomose with the capsular arteries.

perforating veins [venae perforantes (NA)] (**per**·for·a·ting **va**·nz). 1. Tributaries of the profunda femoris vein which pierce the adductor muscles with the arteries of the same name. 2. Veins accompanying the corresponding arteries through the upper five or six intercostal spaces lateral to the sternum. The second, third and fourth help to drain the breast.

perforation (per·for·a·shun). A hole made through the whole thickness of a membrane or similar tissue, or through any substance. [L *perforare* to pierce through.]

See also: BEZOLD (F.).

perforator (**per**·for·a·tor). A sharp instrument for making holes in bone, particularly for perforating the fetal head to facilitate labour. [see foll.]

perforatorium (**per**·for·a·**tor**'·e·um). The head cap (acrosome) of a spermatozoon. [L *perforare* to pierce through.]

perfrication (per·frik·a·shun). Massage with an embrocation or ointment; inunction. [L *perfricare* to rub over.]

perfrigeration (**per**·frij·er·a'·shun). Frostbite. [L *perfrigere* to be very cold.]

Perfringens (per·**frin**·jenz). *Clostridium welchii* [obsolete term]. [L *perfringere* to shatter.]

perfusate (per·**few**·zate). The liquid used in a perfusion.

perfuse (per·**fewz**). To pass a liquid through or over an organ or other tissue. [see foll.]

perfusion (per·**few**·zhun). The passage of fluid through an organ or tissue. **Extracorporeal perfusion.** The use of an extracorporeal system, consisting usually of a pump and an oxygenator, to perfuse the whole body. **Organ perfusion.** The perfusion of an organ to maintain its viability. [L *perfundere* to pour over.]

perhalation (per·hal·a·shun). A method of anaesthetic administration in which the patient breaths through the meshes of a pad of cotton gauze onto which is dropped a volatile liquid anaesthetic agent; the so-called "open" method. [L *per*, *halare* to breathe.]

Perhexiline (per·**hex**·il·een). BP Commission approved name for 2-(2,2-dicyclohexylethyl)piperidine; it is used in the treatment of angina pectoris.

perhydride (per·**hi**·dride). Hydrogen peroxide.

peri-. A prefix, from the Greek preposition *peri*, meaning *around, enclosing, near.*

periacinal, periacinous (per·e·**as**·in·al, per·e·**as**·in·us). Located around an acinus. [Gk *peri*, L *acinus* berry.]

periadenitis (per·e·ad·en·**i**′·tis). Inflammation affecting the structures surrounding a gland. **Periadenitis mucosa necrotica recurrens.** Major aphthae; deep painful ulcers which tend to persist and leave a scar on healing. Occasionally a feature of Behçet's syndrome. [Gk *peri*, adenitis.]

periadventitial (per·e·ad·ven·**tish**′·al). Situated around the external (adventitial) coat of an artery. [Gk *peri*, adventitia.]

perialgia (per·e·**al**·je·ah). Pain of great intensity. [Gk *peri*, *algos* pain.]

perialienitis (per·e·a·le·en·**i**′·tis). Inflammation in which the structures surrounding a foreign body are affected. [Gk *peri* around, L *alienus* foreign, Gk *-itis* inflammation.]

periampullary (per·e·am·**pul**′·ar·e). Around the ampulla, e.g. Vater's ampulla. [Gk *peri*, L *ampulla* jug.]

periamygdalar (per·e·am·**ig**′·dal·ar). Peritonsillar. [Gk *peri*, *amygdale* almond.]

periamygdalitis (per·e·am·ig·dal·**i**′·tis). Peritonsillitis. [Gk *peri*, *amygdale* almond, *-itis* inflammation.]

perianal (per·e·**a**·nal). Surrounding the anus. [Gk *peri*, anus.]

periangeitis, periangiitis (per·e·an·je·**i**′·tis). Inflammation affecting the tissues surrounding a blood or lymph vessel. [Gk *peri*, *aggeion* small vessel, *-itis* inflammation.]

periangiocholitis (per·e·an·je·o·ko·**li**′·tis). Inflammation of the structures lying around the bile ducts or interlobular bile capillaries. [Gk *peri*, *aggeion* small vessel, *chole* bile, *-itis* inflammation.]

periangioma (per·e·an·je·**o**′·mah). A tumour which is located around a blood vessel. [Gk *peri*, *aggeion* small vessel, *-oma* tumour.]

periangitis (per·e·an·**ji**′·tis). Periangeitis.

perianth (**per**·e·anth). The calyx and corolla of a flower together, if both be present, or either, if the other be absent. [Gk *peri*, *anthos* flower.]

periaortic (per·e·a·**or**′·tik). Situated around the aorta. [Gk *peri*, aorta.]

periaortitis (per·e·a·or·**ti**′·tis). An inflammatory condition affecting the connective tissues which surround the aorta. [Gk *peri*, aorta, Gk *-itis* inflammation.]

periapical (per·e·**a**·pik·al). Lying around the apex of the root of a tooth. [Gk *peri*, apex.]

periappendicitis (per·e·ap·en·dis·**i**′·tis). Local peritonitis around an inflamed appendix. **Periappendicitis decidualis.** Decidual cells in the peritoneum of the appendix in cases of tubal pregnancy, due to adhesions between the ovum and the appendix. [Gk *peri*, appendicitis.]

periappendicular (per·e·ap·en·**dik**′·ew·lar). Situated around the vermiform or other appendix. [Gk *peri*, appendix.]

periapt (**per**·e·apt). An amulet worn against disease. [Gk *periaptein* to put round oneself.]

periarterial (per·e·ar·**teer**′·e·al). Situated around an artery. [Gk *peri*, artery.]

periarteritis (per·e·ar·ter·**i**′·tis). Inflammation of the outer coat of arteries and of the surrounding tissues. **Periarteritis gummosa.** Gummatous involvement of the outer arterial wall and surrounding tissue in the late stages of syphilitic arteritis. The early lesion consists of an infiltration of mononuclear cells into the adventitia, with endarteritis of the vasa vasorum, and spread into the media, producing necrosis. **Periarteritis nodosa.** Polyarteritis nodosa, an inflammatory disease of the smaller arteries which involves, in different stages, all the coats of the vessel which are infiltrated with lymphocytes, granulocytes and eosinophils. Exudation and necrosis occur, which result in thrombosis, aneurysm formation and haemorrhage; there is also a perivascular inflammatory reaction. The disease may follow almost any course, and is usually fatal. The cause is unknown, but cases have been reported following the administration of certain drugs, e.g. sulphonamides. **Syphilitic periarteritis.** Periarteritis gummosa (see above). [Gk *peri*, artery, Gk *-itis* inflammation.]

periarthric (per·e·**ar**·thrik). Periarticular. [Gk *peri*, *arthron* joint.]

periarthritis (per·e·ar·**thri**′·tis). Inflammation in which the parts surrounding a joint are involved. **Acute calcific periarthritis.** An inflammatory condition associated with the deposition of calcific material in periarticular soft tissues, particularly of the shoulder joint. **Scapulohumeral periarthritis.** An inflammatory condition of the muscles surrounding the shoulder joint, and leading to limitation of movement of the joint. [Gk *peri*, arthritis.]

periarticular (per·e·ar·**tik**′·ew·lar). Around a joint; in the cellular and fibrous tissues surrounding a joint. [Gk *peri*, L *articulus* joint.]

periatrial (per·e·**a**·tre·al). Surrounding the atrium of the heart. [Gk *peri*, atrium.]

periauricular (per·e·aw·**rik**′·ew·lar). 1. Surrounding an atrium of the heart. 2. Surrounding the concha of the auricle. [Gk *peri*, auricle.]

periaxial (per·e·**ax**·e·al). Around an axis. [Gk *peri*, axis.]

periaxillary (per·e·ax·**il**′·ar·e). Around the axilla. [Gk *peri*, axilla.]

periaxonal (per·e·**ax**·on·al). Surrounding an axon. [Gk *peri*, axon.]

periblast (**per**·e·blast). The cytoplasm. [Gk *peri*, *blastos* germ.]

periblastic (per·e·**blas**·tik). 1. Belonging to the cytoplasm. 2. Developing from the surface of the ovum. [see prec.]

periblepsia, periblepsis (per·e·**blep**·se·ah, per·e·**blep**·sis). The insane-like stare of an individual who is delirious. [Gk *peri*, *blepein* to look.]

peribronchial (per·e·**brong**·ke·al). Located about a bronchus or its subdivisions. [Gk *peri*, bronchus.]

peribronchiolar (per·e·brong·ke·**o**′·lar). Lying around the bronchioles. [Gk *peri*, bronchiolus.]

peribronchiolitis (per·e·brong·ke·o·**li**′·tis). Inflammation affecting the structures surrounding the bronchioles. [Gk *peri*, bronchiolus, Gk *-itis* inflammation.]

peribronchitis (per·e·brong·**ki**′·tis). A severe bronchitis in all parts of the lobe and thickening of the connective tissue around the bronchus, in most cases amounting to bronchopneumonia of subacute type. [Gk *peri*, bronchitis.]

peribrosis (per·e·**bro**·sis). An ulcerative state of either the medial or lateral angle of the eye. [Gk *peri*, *brosis* an eating into.]

peribulbar (per·e·**bul**·bar). Situated around any bulb, especially the eyeball. [Gk *peri*, bulb.]

peribursal (per·e·**ber**·sal). Situated around a bursa. [Gk *peri*, bursa.]

pericaecal (per·e·**se**·kal). Lying around the caecum. [Gk *peri*, caecum.]

pericaecitis (per·e·se·**si**′·tis). Inflammatory involvement of the structures surrounding the caecum. [Gk *peri*, caecum, Gk *-itis* inflammation.]

perical (**per**·ik·al). Mycetoma.

pericanalicular (per·e·kan·al·**ik**′·ew·lar). Referring to structures or reactions around a canaliculus. [Gk *peri*, canaliculus.]

pericapillary (per·e·kap·**il**′·ar·e). Surrounding a capillary. [Gk *peri*, capillary.]

pericapsular (per·e·**kap**·sew·lar). Occurring around a capsule. [Gk *peri*, capsule.]

pericardectomy (per·e·kar·**dek**′·to·me). Pericardiectomy.

pericardiac (per·e·**kar**·de·ak). Pericardial.

pericardiacophrenic artery [arteria pericardiacophrenica (NA)] (per·e·**kar**·de·ak·o·**fren**′·ik **ar**·ter·e). A branch of the internal mammary artery accompanying the phrenic nerve.

pericardiacophrenic veins [venae pericardiacophrenicae (NA)] (per·e·**kar**·de·ak·o·**fren**′·ik **va**·nz). Venous drainage of the pericardium and adjacent part of the diaphragm; they are tributaries of the internal mammary veins.

pericardial (per·e·**kar**·de·al). 1. Relating to the pericardium. 2. Situated around or surrounding the heart. [Gk *peri, kardia* heart.]

pericardial veins [venae pericardiacae (NA)]. Tributaries of the vena azygos and the internal mammary veins.

pericardiectomy (per·e·kar·de·**ek**'·to·me). Surgical removal of the pericardium when it is thick, tough and hard as a result of chronic pericarditis, and thus embarrassing the action of the heart. [pericardium, Gk *ektome* excision.]

pericardiocentesis (per·e·**kar**·de·o·sen·**te**'·sis). Puncture of the pericardium for aspiration. [pericardium, Gk *kentein* to pierce.]

pericardiolysis (per·e·kar·de·**ol**'·is·is). Removal of a portion of sternum, ribs and pericardium, to slacken adhesions of the heart to other intrathoracic organs. [pericardium, Gk *lysis* a loosing.]

pericardiomediastinitis (per·e·**kar**·de·o·**me**·de·as·tin·**i**'·tis). Inflammation of the pericardium and of the mediastinum; indurative mediastinitis. [pericardium, mediastinitis.]

pericardiophrenic (per·e·**kar**·de·o·**fren**'·ik). Relating to the pericardium and the diaphragm. [pericardium, Gk *phren* diaphragm.]

pericardiopleural (per·e·**kar**·de·o·**ploor**'·al). Belonging to the pericardium and the pleura.

pericardiorrhaphy (per·e·kar·de·**or**'·af·e). Suture of a pericardial wound. [pericardium, Gk *rhaphe* suture.]

pericardiostomy (per·e·kar·de·**os**'·to·me). The making of an opening into the pericardium through the wall of the thorax for the purpose of draining an effusion. [pericardium, Gk *stoma* mouth.]

pericardiosymphysis (per·e·**kar**·de·o·**sim**'·fis·is). A condition characterized by the formation of adhesions between the parietal and visceral serous layers of the pericardium. [pericardium, Gk *symphyein* to grow into one.]

pericardiotomy (per·e·kar·de·**ot**'·o·me). The operation of making an incision into the pericardium. [pericardium, Gk *temnein* to cut.]

pericarditic (per·e·kar·**dit**'·ik). Relating to pericarditis.

pericarditis (per·e·kar·**di**'·tis). Inflammation of the pericardium, visceral, parietal, or both. **Acute benign pericarditis.** Acute pericarditis, with or without effusion, which typically resolves in a short time without complications; occasionally there may be some associated myocarditis and sometimes constrictive pericarditis develops later. The aetiology is generally not evident but it is thought that most cases are due to viral infection. **Acute fibrinous pericarditis.** Acute inflammation of the pericardium attended by fibrinous exudation into the sac and also inflammatory changes in the endothelial cells of the pericardium. **Adherent pericarditis, Adhesive pericarditis.** Obliteration of the pericardial sac by dense fibrous adhesions resulting from previous inflammation. It may be localized or generalized, and calcification may occur. *Internal adhesive pericarditis* (concretio cordis) denotes adhesion between the two pericardial layers and may produce obliteration of the sac. *External adhesive pericarditis* (accretio cordis) denotes adhesion between the pericardium and neighbouring structures. The heart is often damaged as a result of the associated carditis, but is not compressed by constrictive pericarditis. **Bacterial pericarditis.** Inflammation of the pericardium due to infection with bacteria, usually staphylococci, pneumococci or streptococci, but many other organisms may be responsible. Infection occurs through the blood stream, local extension in the chest, from the abdomen via the diaphragm, or from external wounds. **Bread-and-butter pericarditis.** Inflammation of the pericardium which produces thick fibrinous tenacious deposits on the pericardial surfaces. **Pericarditis calculosa.** *See* CONSTRICTIVE PERICARDITIS (below). **Carcinomatous pericarditis.** Pericardial inflammation due to involvement by malignant disease, usually secondary to primary neoplasm within the thorax. **Constrictive pericarditis.** Widespread generalized adhesive pericarditis with dense fibrous thickening of the pericardium, often incorporating calcified plaques, which encloses the heart in a rigid case, impeding the filling of the heart. Previously most commonly the result of tuberculous infection, it now most frequently appears to be a consequence of previous overt or silent viral infection; it may also follow pyogenic infection or haemopericardium, but it does not follow rheumatic pericarditis. **Dry pericarditis.** Inflammation of the pericardium without development of an effusion. It results from infections, uraemia, rheumatic fever, trauma, malignant disease, myocardial infarction, infection with yeasts, parasites, etc., and certain collagen diseases. **Pericarditis with effusion.** A collection of fluid in the pericardial sac as the result of inflammation. **Pericarditis externa et interna.** Inflammation of the internal (serous) and external (fibrous) pericardial sacs. **External pericarditis.** Inflammation of the external pericardial sac (fibrous pericardium). **Fibrinous pericarditis.** That in which the pericardium is covered with a lymph exudate that coagulates on the surface and may assume a considerable thickness, and lead to the characteristic bread-and-butter appearance. **Fibrous pericarditis.** Inflammation of the pericardium resulting from the formation of fibrous adhesions. **Haemorrhagic pericarditis.** Inflammation of the pericardium with production of a blood-stained effusion. It is usually, but not always, due to malignant or tuberculous invasion. **Localized pericarditis.** Local areas of pericardial inflammation which may give rise to the fibrous flat white epicardial patches known as *milk spots.* **Mediastinal pericarditis.** An extensive form of external adhesive pericarditis in which the pericardium is adherent to the surrounding mediastinal structures. It may be associated with constriction of the heart. **Pericarditis due to myocardial infarction.** Localized or extensive dry pericarditis as a result of myocardial infarction which extends to the epicardial surface of the heart. **Pericarditis obliterans, Obliterating pericarditis.** Internal adhesive pericarditis which obliterates the pericardial sac. **Purulent pericarditis.** Bacterial pericarditis (see above). **Rheumatic pericarditis.** Inflammation of the pericardium due to rheumatic fever. **Serofibrinous pericarditis.** Fibrinous pericarditis which progresses to the formation of a serous pericardial effusion. **Pericarditis sicca.** Dry pericarditis (see above). **Suppurative pericarditis.** Bacterial pericarditis (see above). **Syphilitic pericarditis.** Pericarditis due to syphilis infection with the spirochaete *Treponema pallidum.* **Traumatic pericarditis.** Pericarditis resulting from injuries of the chest wall which produce rupture of small vessels and the oozing of blood into the pericardial sac. The small amount of blood organizes into a fibrinous exudate. Extensive haemorrhage may occur, producing haemopericardium, and such trauma may activate quiescent tuberculous pericarditis. **Tuberculous pericarditis.** Pericarditis due to infection with *Mycobacterium.* **Typhoid pericarditis.** Pericarditis due to typhoid fever. **Uraemic pericarditis.** Dry pericarditis, or pericarditis with effusion, occurring in the terminal stages of chronic renal insufficiency with uraemia; sometimes secondary bacterial infection is present. **Pericarditis villosa.** Pericarditis with an exudate which forms villous shaggy masses. [pericardium, Gk *-itis* inflammation.]

See also: CONCATO.

pericardium [NA] (per·e·**kar**·de·um). A membrane enveloping the heart and formed of two parts, a fibrous investing sac, the *fibrous pericardium* [pericardium fibrosum (NA)], and a *serous pericardium* [pericardium serosum (NA)] lining the sac, and a visceral layer [lamina visceralis (epicardium) (NA)] covering the surface of the heart. **Adherent pericardium.** A pericardium in which the parietal layer is adherent to the epicardium. **Bread-and-butter pericardium.** *See* PERICARDITIS, BREAD-AND-BUTTER. **Calcified pericardium.** A pericardium in which there are plaques of calcification. **Cardiac pericardium.** Visceral pericardium (see below). **Parietal pericardium.** The outer layer of the serous pericardium which is not in direct contact with the heart muscle. **Shaggy pericardium.** Bread-and-butter pericardium. *See* PERICARDITIS, BREAD-AND-BUTTER. **Visceral pericardium.** That surface of the pericardium which is in direct contact with the heart muscle; the epicardium. [Gk *peri, kardia* heart.]

pericardosis (per·e·kar·**do**′·sis). Involvement of the pericardium by any disease process other than infection. [pericardium, Gk *-osis* condition.]

pericardotomy (per·e·kar·**dot**′·o·me). Pericardiotomy.

pericarp (per·e·karp). The fruit of a plant, with the exception of the seeds and pulp. [Gk *peri, karpos* fruit.]

pericellular (per·e·**sel**·ew·lar). Situated around a cell. [Gk *peri,* cell.]

pericemental (per·e·se·**men**′·tal). Periodontal. [Gk *peri,* cementum.]

pericementitis (per·e·se·men·**ti**′·tis). Periodontitis. [pericementum, Gk *-itis* inflammation.]

pericementum (per·e·se·**men**′·tum). The connective tissue between the root of a tooth and the alveolar bone; the periodontal membrane. [Gk *peri,* cementum.]

pericephalic (per·e·kef·**al**′·ik). Around the head. [Gk *peri, kephale* head.]

pericerebral (per·e·**ser**·e·bral). Surrounding the cerebrum. [Gk *peri,* cerebrum.]

perichareia (per·e·kar·**i**′·ah). Violent and delirious exultation or rejoicing. [Gk, exceeding great joy.]

pericholangeitis, pericholangitis (per·e·ko·lan·je·**i**′·tis, per·e·ko·lan·**ji**′·tis). Inflammation of the structures lying around the bile ducts or interlobular bile capillaries. [Gk *peri, chole* bile, *aggeion* small vessel, *-itis* inflammation.]

pericholecystitis (per·e·ko·le·sist·**i**′·tis). Inflammation involving the peritoneal tissues which surround the gall bladder. [Gk *peri, chole* bile, *kystis* bag, *-itis* inflammation.]

perichondral, perichondrial (per·e·**kon**·dral, per·e·**kon**·dre·al). Belonging or relating to, or made up of perichondrium.

perichondritic (per·e·kon·**drit**′·ik). Relating to or suffering from perichondritis.

perichondritis (per·e·kon·**dri**′·tis). An inflammatory state of the perichondrium. [perichondrium, Gk *-itis* inflammation.]

perichondrium [NA] (per·e·**kon**·dre·um). The fibrotic connective tissue of a cartilage, springing from adjacent parts and generally consisting of white fibrous tissue. [Gk *peri, chondros* cartilage.]

perichondroma (per·e·kon·**dro**′·mah). A tumour derived from the perichondrium. [perichondrium, Gk *-oma* tumour.]

perichord (per·e·kord). The stout membranous sheath surrounding the notochord. [Gk *peri, chorde* cord.]

perichordal (per·e·**kord**·al). Relating or belonging to, or situated around the notochord. [see prec.]

perichoroidal (per·e·kor·**oid**′·al). Pertaining to or situated around the choroid coat of the eye. [Gk *peri,* choroid.]

perichrome (per·e·krome). A nerve cell in which the tigroid (Nissl's) bodies are dispersed throughout the cytoplasm. [Gk *peri, chroma* colour.]

periclaustral (per·e·**klaw**·stral). Situated around the claustrum of the brain. [Gk *peri,* claustrum.]

pericolic (per·e·**ko**·lik). Situated around the colon. [Gk *peri,* colon.]

pericolitis, pericolonitis (per·e·ko·**li**′·tis, per·e·ko·lon·**i**′·tis). Inflammation of the peritoneal and subperitoneal coats of the colon. It is usually caused by spread of infection from the mucous membrane, and may lead to adhesions between portions of the bowel, local abscesses, or peritonitis. **Pericolitis dextra.** Inflammation around the ascending colon. **Pericolitis sinistra.** Inflammation around the descending colon or the sigmoid flexure; the symptoms may resemble those of appendicitis, but on the left side. It may complicate diverticulosis. [Gk *peri,* colon, Gk *-itis* inflammation.]

pericolpitis (per·e·kol·**pi**′·tis). An inflammatory condition affecting the connective tissue which surrounds the vagina. [Gk *peri, kolpos* vagina, *-itis* inflammation.]

Pericoma (per·**ik**·o·mah). A genus of sand flies of the family Psychodidae. **Pericoma townsvillensis.** A species found in Queensland; a serious pest whose painful bites cause small lesions which heal slowly.

periconchal (per·e·**kong**·kal). Surrounding any concha, particularly the concha of the auricle. [Gk *peri, kogche* shell.]

periconchitis (per·e·kong·**ki**′·tis). Inflammation affecting the periosteum of the orbit. [Gk *peri, kogche* shell, *-itis* inflammation.]

pericorneal (per·e·**kor**·ne·al). Around the cornea. [Gk *peri,* cornea.]

pericoronal (per·e·**kor**·on·al). Around the crown of a tooth. [Gk *peri, L corona* crown.]

pericoronitis (per·e·kor·on·**i**′·tis). Inflammation of the soft tissues surrounding the crown of an erupting tooth. [Gk *peri,* L *corona* crown, Gk *-itis* inflammation.]

pericoxitis (per·e·kox·**i**′·tis). Inflammation of the periarticular parts around the hip joint. [Gk *peri,* L *coxa* hip, Gk *-itis* inflammation.]

pericranial (per·e·**kra**·ne·al). 1. Belonging or relating to the pericranium. 2. Situated around the skull.

pericranitis (per·e·kra·**ni**′·tis). Pericranial inflammation [pericranium, Gk *-itis* inflammation.]

pericranium (per·e·**kra**·ne·um). The periosteum on the outer surface of the skull bones. **Pericranium interum.** The endocranium. [Gk *peri,* cranium.]

Pericyazine (per·e·si·az·een). BP Commission approved name for 2-cyano-10-[3-(4-hydroxypiperidino)propyl] phenothiazine; a tranquillizer.

pericystic (per·e·**sist**·ik). 1. Lying around a cyst. 2. Surrounding either the gall bladder or the urinary bladder. [Gk *peri, kystis* bag.]

pericystitis (per·e·sist·**i**′·tis). Inflammation in which the structures around a bladder are affected, particularly those around the urinary bladder. [Gk *peri,* cystitis.]

pericystium (per·e·**sist**·e·um). 1. The vascular tissues which surround certain types of cyst. 2. A comprehensive term for the structures situated around the urinary bladder or the gall bladder. [Gk *peri, kystis* bag.]

pericyte (per·e·site). A perivascular cell. [Gk *peri, kytos* cell.]

pericytial (per·e·**sish**·al). Pericellular. [see prec.]

peridectomy (per·e·**dek**·to·me). Peritectomy.

perideferentitis (per·e·def·er·en·**ti**′·tis). Inflammation affecting the parts situated around the vas deferens. [Gk *peri,* vas deferens, Gk *-itis* inflammation.]

peridentine (per·e·**den**·teen). The calcified tissue which immediately surrounds the dentine of the root of a tooth; cement, cementum. [Gk *peri,* dentine.]

peridentitis (per·e·den·**ti**′·tis). Periodontitis. [Gk *peri,* L dens tooth, Gk *-itis* inflammation.]

periderm (per·e·derm). The outer layer of flattened cells from the early embryonic skin. [Gk *peri, derma* skin.]

peridermal, peridermic (per·e·**der**·mal, per·e·**der**·mik). Relating to the periderm; cuticular.

peridesmic (per·e·**dez**·mik). Belonging or relating to the peridesmium; surrounding a ligament. [Gk *peri, desmos* band.]

peridesmitis (per·e·dez·**mi**′·tis). Inflammation affecting the peridesmium. [peredesmium, Gk *-itis* inflammation.]

peridesmium (per·e·**dez**·me·um). The areolar layer covering a ligament. [Gk *peri, desmos* band.]

peridiastole (per·e·di·**as**′·to·le). Prediastole. [Gk *peri,* diastole.]

peridiastolic (per·e·di·as·**tol**′·ik). Prediastolic. [see prec.]

perididymis (per·e·**did**·im·is). The coats of the testis, the tunica vaginalis and the tunica albuginea. [Gk *peri, didymos testicle.]*

perididymitis (per·e·did·im·**i**′·tis). Inflammation of the perididymis. [perididymis, Gk *-itis* inflammation.]

peridiverticulitis (per·e·**di**·ver·tik·ew·**li**′·tis). Inflammation affecting the tissues surrounding an intestinal diverticulum. [Gk *peri,* diverticulum, Gk *-itis* inflammation.]

periductal, periductile (per·e·**duk**·tal, per·e·**duk**·tile). Around a duct, particularly a mammary duct. [Gk *peri,* duct.]

periduodenitis (per·e·dew·o·de·**ni**′·tis). Inflammation around the duodenum that may lead to deformity of the latter which becomes surrounded and fixed by adhesions. [Gk *peri,* duodenum, Gk *-itis* inflammation.]

periencephalitis (per·e·en·kef·al·i′·tis). Inflammation of the membranes and surface of the brain involving the cortex. [Gk *peri*, encephalitis.]

periencephalomeningitis (per·e·en·kef·al·o·men·in·ji′·tis). Chronic inflammation of the cerebral cortex and meninges. [Gk *peri*, *egkephalos* brain, meningitis.]

periendothelioma (per·e·en·do·the·le·o′·mah). A combined perithelioma and endothelioma.

periendymal (per·e·en·dim·al). Periependymal.

perienteric (per·e·en·ter′·ik). Occurring around the intestine. [Gk *peri*, *enteron* bowel.]

perienteritis (per·e·en·ter·i′·tis). Inflammation in which the peritoneal coat of the intestine is involved. [perienteron, Gk *-itis* inflammation.]

perienteron (per·e·en·ter·on). The visceral peritoneum or the peritoneal cavity in the embryo. [Gk *peri*, *enteron* intestine.]

periependymal (per·e·ep·en′·dim·al). Surrounding the ependyma. [Gk *peri*, ependyma.]

periepithelioma (per·e·ep·e·the·le·o′·mah). A variety of endothelioma. [Gk *peri*, epithelioma.]

Périer, Charles (b. 1836). Paris surgeon.

Périer method, or operation. For laryngeal carcinoma: total laryngectomy, the operation commencing at the trachea and the larynx being removed from below upwards.

perifascicular (per·e·fas·ik′·ew·lar). Situated around a fasciculus. [Gk *peri*, fasciculus.]

perifibral, perifibrous (per·e·fi·bral, per·e·fi·brous). Situated around a fibre. [Gk *peri*, fibre.]

perifistular (per·e·fis·tew·lar). Occurring around a fistula. [Gk *peri*, fistula.]

perifocal (per·e·fo·kal). Situated around a focus of infection. [Gk *peri*, focus.]

perifollicular (per·e·fol·ik′·ew·lar). Situated around a follicle. [Gk *peri*, follicle.]

perifolliculitis (per·e·fol·ik·ew·li′·tis). Inflammation around a pilosebaceous follicle. **Perifolliculitis capitis abscedens et suffodiens.** An inflammatory disease of the scalp resembling acne conglobata, with the formation of abscesses and sinuses. **Conglomerative pustular perifolliculitis.** Acute pustular ringworm of the glabrous skin. **Granulomatous perifolliculitis.** An infiltrated nodular eruption with scaling of the legs, mostly of women, caused by *Trychophyton rubrum* infection. **Superficial pustular perifolliculitis.** Bockhart's impetigo. [Gk *peri*, follicle, Gk *-itis* inflammation.]

perigangliitis (per·e·gang·gle·i′·tis). Inflammation in which the tissues around a ganglion are affected. [Gk *peri*, ganglion, Gk *-itis* inflammation.]

periganglionic (per·e·gang·gle·on′·ik). Surrounding a ganglion. [Gk *peri*, ganglion.]

perigastric (per·e·gas·trik). Around the stomach; relating to the portion of visceral peritoneum which lies over the stomach. [Gk *peri*, *gaster* stomach.]

perigastritis (per·e·gas·tri′·tis). Inflammation affecting the portion of visceral peritoneum which lies over the stomach. [Gk *peri*, gastritis.]

perigemmal (per·e·jem·al). Situated around one of the taste buds; denoting a certain type of nerve-ending in which fibrils surround an end-bulb. [Gk *peri*, L *gemma* bud.]

periglandular (per·e·glan·dew·lar). Situated around a gland or a collection of glands. [Gk *peri*, gland.]

periglandulitis (per·e·glan·dew·li′·tis). Inflammation affecting the tissues which surround a small gland. [Gk *peri*, gland, Gk *-itis* inflammation.]

periglial (per·e·gli·al). Around the neuroglia cells of the brain. [Gk *peri*, neuroglia.]

periglossitis (per·e·glos·i′·tis). Inflammation affecting the structures about the tongue. [Gk *peri*, *glossa* tongue, *-itis* inflammation.]

periglottic (per·e·glot·ik). Situated about the tongue, more especially at the base. [see foll.]

periglottis (per·e·glot·is). The mucous membrane of the tongue. [Gk *peri*, *glotta* tongue.]

perignathic (per·e·nath·ik). Occurring about the jaws. [Gk *peri*, *gnathos* jaw.]

perihepatic (per·e·hep·at′·ik). 1. Surrounding the liver. 2. Pertaining to the tissues situated around the liver. [Gk *peri*, *hepar* liver.]

perihepatitis (per·e·hep·at·i′·tis). Inflammation of the peritoneal capsule of the liver. **Acute perihepatitis.** That occurring secondarily to acute infections of the liver. **Chronic perihepatitis.** Local thickenings of the capsule of the liver which may be found in many conditions, such as cirrhosis of the liver, heart failure, tuberculosis or cancer of the peritoneum, irritation of an infected gall bladder, or gastric ulcer. **Perihepatitis chronica hyperplastica.** A disease in which the peritoneal coat of the liver is greatly thickened and converted into a white mass resembling the sugar icing of a cake. The contraction of the fibrous mass may cause atrophy of the underlying liver substance. A similar thickening of the capsule of the spleen and other parts of the peritoneum may be associated. It also occurs in polyserositis in which there is thickening of the pericardium and pleura with obliteration of the sacs. [Gk *peri*, *hepar* liver, *-itis* inflammation.]

perihernial, periherniary (per·e·her·ne·al, per·e·her·ne·ar·e). 1. Surrounding a hernia. 2. Pertaining to the tissues around a hernia. [Gk *peri*, hernia.]

peri-insular (per·e·in·sew·lar). Situated around an insula, particularly the cerebral insula (island of Reil). [Gk *peri*, L *insula* island.]

perijejunitis (per·e·jej·oon·i′·tis). Inflammation of the structure situated about the jejunum. [Gk *peri*, jejunum, Gk *-itis* inflammation.]

perikaryon (per·e·kar·e·on). The cytoplasm; the general mass of protoplasm forming the cell contents, as distinct from the nucleus and associated structures. [Gk *peri*, *karyon* nut.]

perikeratic (per·e·ker·at′·ik). Pericorneal. [Gk *peri*, *keras* horn.]

perikinetic (per·e·kin·et′·ik). Denoting the movement of particles indiscriminately in all directions, as in the brownian movement. [Gk *peri*, *kinesis* movement.]

perilabyrinth (per·e·lab·ir·inth). The tissues by which the labyrinth of the ear is surrounded. [Gk *peri*, labyrinth.]

perilabyrinthitis (per·e·lab·ir·in·thi′·tis). Inflammation of the structures which are situated around the labyrinth. [Gk *peri*, labyrinth, Gk *-itis* inflammation.]

perilaryngeal (per·e·lar·in′·je·al). Surrounding or occurring about the larynx. [Gk *peri*, larynx.]

perilaryngitis (per·e·lar·in·ji′·tis). Inflammation in which the areolar connective tissue surrounding the larynx is involved. [Gk *peri*, laryngitis.]

perilenticular (per·e·len·tik′·ew·lar). Pertaining to the tissues surrounding the lens. [Gk *peri*, lens.]

periligamentous (per·e·lig·am·en′·tus). Surrounding a ligament. [Gk *peri*, ligament.]

perilobar (per·e·lo·bar). Situated around a lobe. [Gk *peri*, lobe.]

perilobulitis (per·e·lob·ew·li′·tis). Inflammation of the connective tissue which invests the lobules of the lung. [Gk *peri*, lobule, Gk *-itis* inflammation.]

perilymph [perilympha (NA)] (per·e·limf). In anatomy, the fluid identical in substance with the cerebrospinal fluid, which fills the bony labyrinth separating the latter from the membranous labyrinth of the ear. [Gk *peri*, lymph.]

perilymphadenitis (per·e·limf·ad·en·i′·tis). Inflammation affecting the tissues surrounding a lymph gland. [Gk *peri*, lymphadenitis.]

perilymphangeal, perilymphangial (per·e·limf·an′·je·al). Surrounding a lymph vessel. [Gk *peri*, lymph, Gk *aggeion* small vessel.]

perilymphangitis (per·e·limf·an·ji′·tis). Inflammation of the tissues situated around a lymph vessel. [Gk *peri*, lymphangitis.]

perilymphatic (per·e·limf·at′·ik). 1. Relating to the perilymph. 2. Perilymphangeal.

perimadarous (per·e·mad·ar·us). Describing a spreading ulcer where the epidermis peels away from the areas to which the ulcer is about to extend. [Gk *peri*, *madaros* bald.]

perimandibular (per·e·man·**dib**'·ew·lar). Relating or belonging to, surrounding, or in the region of the mandible. [Gk *peri*, mandible.]

perimastitis (per·e·mas·**ti**'·tis). Inflammation of the areolar tissue which surrounds the mammary gland. [Gk *peri*, mastitis.]

perimedullary (per·e·med·**ul**'·ar·e). Situated around the medulla oblongata or any bone marrow. [Gk *peri*, L *medulla* marrow.]

perimeningitis (per·e·men·in·**ji**'·tis). Inflammation of the dura mater; pachymeningitis. [Gk *peri*, meningitis.]

perimeter (per·**im**·et·er). 1. Circumference. 2. An instrument for measuring circular outlines, e.g. the extent of the visual fields. **Dental perimeter.** An instrument used in conservative dentistry for measuring the circumference of a tooth. **Projection perimeter.** An instrument for recording the visual fields, using a projected circle of light as the target. **Recording perimeter, Self-recording perimeter.** An instrument which automatically records the visual fields on a special chart. Lister's model is in common use. [Gk *peri*, *metron* measure.]

See also: LISTER (W.).

perimetric (per·e·**met**·rik). 1. Relating to a perimeter or perimetry. 2. Periuterine; relating to the perimetrium. [Gk *peri*, *metron* measure, *metra* womb.]

perimetritic (per·e·me·**trit**'·ik). Relating to perimetritis.

perimetritis (per·e·me·**tri**'·tis). Inflammation affecting the perimetrium. [perimetrium, Gk *-itis* inflammation.]

perimetrium (per·e·**me**·tre·um). The peritoneal investment of the uterus. [Gk *peri*, *metra* womb.]

perimetrosalpingitis (per·e·**me**·tro·sal·pin·**ji**'·tis). A term which covers parametritis, perisalpingitis, perimetritis and other forms of pelvic inflammation.

perimetry (per·**im**·et·re). The making of measurements with a perimeter, e.g. measuring the acuity of perception throughout the entire visual field.

perimyelis (per·e·**mi**·el·is). 1. Endosteum; the membrane of highly vascular areolar tissue which lines the medullary cavity of the long bones. 2. The pia mater of the spinal cord. [Gk *peri*, *myelos* marrow.]

perimyelitis (per·e·mi·el·**i**'·tis). 1. Inflammation of the perimyelis; endosteitis. 2. Spinal meningitis. [perimyelis, Gk *-itis* inflammation.]

perimyelography (per·e·mi·el·**og**'·raf·e). The x-ray visualization, by means of an opaque or non-opaque contrast medium, of the subarachnoid space of the spinal cord. [perimyelis, *graphein* to record.]

perimyo-endocarditis (per·e·**mi**·o·en·do·kar·**di**'·tis). Inflammation affecting simultaneously the pericardium, myocardium, and endocardium. [Gk *peri*, *mys* muscle, endocardium, Gk *-itis* inflammation.]

perimyositis (per·e·mi·o·**si**'·tis). A condition characterized by inflammation of the connective tissue investing a muscle. [Gk *peri*, *mys* muscle, *-itis* inflammation.]

perimysial (per·e·**mi**·se·al). Belonging to the perimysium.

perimysiitis, perimysitis (per·e·mi·se·**i**'·tis, per·e·mi·**si**'·tis). Inflammation of the perimysium. [perimysium, Gk *-itis* inflammation.]

perimysium [NA] (per·e·**mi**·se·um). The connective tissue sheath of a muscle composed of an enveloping layer, *perimysium externum*, from which arise septa, the *perimysium internum*, dividing the organ into bundles. [Gk *peri*, *mys* muscle.]

perinatal (per·e·**na**·tal). At about the time of birth. The term incorporates pre- and postnatal periods. [Gk *peri*, L *natus* birth.]

perineal (per·in·**e**·al). Belonging to the perineum.

perineal artery, transverse [arteria perinealis (NA)]. A branch of the internal pudendal artery.

perineal nerve [nervus perinei (NA)]. A branch of the pudendal nerve to supply the skin of the scrotum in the male (or the skin of the labium majus in the female), and the muscles in the perineum in front of the anus, including the sphincter urethrae. **Scrotal (labial) branches [nervi scrotales posteriores, nervi labiales posteriores (NA)].** Branches of the perineal nerve to the scrotum (or labium majus).

perineauxesis (per·in·e·awx·**e**'·sis). Repair of a perineal tear by plastic surgery and suturing of the torn edges so that the integrity of the part is restored. [perineum, Gk *auxesis* increase.]

perineocele (per·in·**e**·o·seel). Perineal hernia, which in position may be ischiorectal, between the bladder and rectum, or between the vagina and rectum. [perineum, Gk *kele* hernia.]

perineocolporectomyomectomy (per·in·e·o·kol·po·**rek**·to·mi·o·**mek**'·to·me). Extirpation of a myoma by incising the perineum, vagina and rectum. [perineum, Gk *kolpos* vagina, rectum, myoma, Gk *ektome* a cutting out.]

perineoplasty (per·in·**e**·o·plas·te). A plastic operation performed on the perineum. [perineum, *plassein* to mould.]

perineorrhaphy (per·in·e·**or**·af·e). Suture of the perineum, usually carried out for the repair of laceration. [perineum, *rhaphe* suture.]

perineoscrotal (per·in·e·o·**skro**'·tal). Belonging to the perineum and the scrotum.

perineostomy (per·in·e·**os**·to·me). Perineal urethrostomy. [perineum, Gk *stoma* a mouth.]

perineosynthesis (per·in·e·o·**sin**'·thes·is). The repair by operation of a perineum which has been lacerated completely. [perineum, synthesis.]

perineotomy (per·in·e·**ot**·o·me). An incision through the perineum by the anteroposterior route. [perineum, Gk *temnein* to cut.]

perineovaginal (per·in·e·o·**vaj**'·in·al). Belonging to the perineum and to the vagina.

perineovaginorectal (per·in·e·o·vaj·i·no·**rek**'·tal). Belonging to the perineum, vagina and rectum.

perineovulvar (per·in·e·o·**vul**'·var). Belonging to the perineum and the vulva.

perinephrial (per·e·**nef**·re·al). Relating or belonging to the perinephrium.

perinephric (per·e·**nef**·rik). Situated around the kidney. [Gk *peri*, *nephros* kidney.]

perinephritic (per·e·nef·**rit**'·ik). Relating to or having the characteristics of perinephritis.

perinephritis (per·e·nef·**ri**'·tis). Inflammation affecting the perinephrium, associated with thickening of the renal capsule and adherence to the perirenal tissues. [Gk *peri*, nephritis.]

perinephrium, perinephros (per·e·**nef**'·re·um, per·e·**nef**·ros). The connective and fatty tissues surrounding the kidney. [Gk *peri*, *nephros* kidney.]

perineum [NA] (per·in·**e**·um). The area between the medial sides of the thighs laterally, the scrotum anteriorly, and the buttocks posteriorly. Its deep boundaries are the pubic arch anteriorly, the inferior pubic ramus and the ischial ramus laterally, and the sacrotuberous ligament and coccyx posteriorly. **Shot-gun perineum.** A name suggested by Denis Browne for the congenital abnormality in which the anal and vaginal openings are side by side. **Watering-can perineum, Watering-pot perineum.** The multiple fistulae subsequent to uncontrolled strictures of the urethra. There has usually been a sequence of attacks of periurethral inflammation with abscess formation. [Gk *perineos.*]

perineural (per·e·**newr**·al). Situated around a nerve. [Gk *peri*, *neuron* nerve.]

perineurial (per·e·**newr**·e·al). Relating or belonging to the perineurium.

perineuritic (per·e·newr·**it**'·ik). Relating to or affected with perineuritis.

perineuritis (per·e·newr·**i**'·tis). Inflammation affecting the perineurium. **Retrobulbar perineuritis.** Inflammation of the sheath of the optic nerve behind the eyeball. [perineurium, Gk *-itis* inflammation.]

perineurium (per·e·**newr**·e·um). A delicate smooth transparent membrane forming a sheath round a bundle of nerve fibres. [Gk *peri*, *neuron* a nerve.]

perinuclear (per·e·**new**·kle·ar). Surrounding a nucleus. [Gk *peri*, nucleus.]

periocular (per·e·**ok**·ew·lar). Periophthalmic; occurring or situated around the eye. [Gk *peri*, L *oculus* eye.]

period (peer·e·od). 1. Interval of time. 2. The menses. **Absolute refractory period.** Refractory period (see below). **Childbearing period.** The years between the menarche and the menopause. **Eclipse period.** 1. In bacteriophage infection, the period that elapses between entry of the virus genetic material into the bacterial cell and the time at which mature, infective virus particles can first be found when the infected cells are broken down. 2. In bacterial transformation, the period during which the donor DNA, taken up by recipient bacteria, cannot be re-extracted from them as transforming DNA. This is because, following uptake, the DNA is stripped to a single-stranded state which is itself non-transforming. **Ejection period.** Ejection time. See TIME. **Gestation period.** The period between conception and parturition; about 40 weeks in man. **Half-life period, Half-value period.** The time required for one-half of the atoms of any sample of a radioactive isotope of an element to disintegrate. Each radioactive isotope has a characteristic half-life period: these vary from microseconds to many thousands of years. **Incubation period.** The latent stage or interval between the time of infection and the development of the first symptoms, which varies greatly for different diseases. **Intersystolic period.** A–C interval [obsolete term]. **Iso-electric period.** A period in the heart's cycle when the potentials at two electrodes are exactly balanced, so that no deflexion is shown by the galvanometer. **Period of isometric contraction.** *See* CONTRACTION. **Period of isometric relaxation.** *See* RELAXATION. **Lag period.** The interval of time which elapses after inoculation of a medium with a micro-organism, before multiplication begins. **Latency period, Latent period.** 1. Incubation period (see above). 2. The time elapsing between the application of a stimulus and the resulting effect. 3. In psycho-analysis, the period between the ages of about 4 or 5 and puberty during which there is little manifest interest in sexual matters. 4. In physiology, a term used in estimating the integrity of muscle fibres. **Menstrual period, Monthly period.** The menses. **Patent period.** Of a micro-organismal infection, the period during which it can be demonstrated in the blood or tissues. **Prepatent period.** Of a micro-organismal infection, the period between infection and the demonstration of the micro-organism in the blood or other tissues. **Postsphygmic period.** Isometric relaxation [obsolete term]. *See* RELAXATION. **Presphygmic period.** Isometric contraction [obsolete term]. *See* CONTRACTION. **Pulse period.** The duration of the arterial or venous pulse, determined by the sum of the lengths of the various phases of the cardiac cycle. **Quarantine period.** The time required for the detention or isolation of contacts of an infectious disease, such as smallpox. It is equivalent to the maximum incubation period. **Reaction period.** The stage of recovery after shock; the hyperaemia which occurs within a few seconds after the circulation of a limb has been completely obstructed for a few mintues due to the accumulation of dilator substances. **Refractory period.** A phase at, and immediately following, the maximal activity in a muscle or nerve, when no response to another stimulus is possible. This is the *absolute refractory period.* **Relative refractory period.** The period after activation of nerve or muscle, during recovery, when it can only be excited again by a stimulus greater than that normally required. **Respiratory period,** a pause in breathing, or apnoea, which follows voluntary overbreathing or occurs as Cheyne-Stokes respiration in pathological conditions such as increased intracranial pressure, uraemia, or heart failure. **Safe period.** A period during the menstrual cycle when conception is least likely to take place. Intercourse should not take place less than 5 days before, or until 5 days after, ovulation; a form of contraception dependent upon normal health, a normal cycle, and an accurate calculation of the time of ovulation. **Sphygmic period.** Ejection time [obsolete term]. *See* TIME. **Vulnerable period.** A brief period during the recovery phase of the ventricle, after contraction, corresponding approximately to the time of the peak of the T wave on the electrocardiogram when a stimulus applied to the ventricle may precipitate ventricular fibrillation. [Gk *peri, hodos* way.]

periodate (per·i·o·date). Any salt of periodic acid.

periodic (peer·e·**od**·ik). Characterized by periodicity. **Periodic law.** *See* LAW. **Periodic paralysis.** Recurrent attacks of muscular weakness. **Periodic table.** *See* TABLE.

periodic acid–Schiff, PAS (peer·e·**od**·ik **a**·sid shif). Positive or negative reaction. A staining reaction characteristic of glycoprotein compounds as in the basophil cells of the pituitary.

periodicity (peer·e·od·**is**′·it·e). Repeating at regular intervals of time. **Filarial periodicity.** The regular diurnal or nocturnal appearance of the larvae of filarial worms in the peripheral blood. In certain species, e.g. *Wuchereria bancrofti* in Asia, the larvae are found in the blood of the skin at night but not in the daytime. In *Loa loa* infection of Africa the larvae are found in the surface circulation in the daytime only. **Malarial periodicity.** The regular occurrence of paroxysms of malaria, the intervals depending on the species of parasite concerned. [Gk *periodikos* periodical.]

periodontal (per·e·o·**don**′·tal). Periodontic.

periodontia (per·e·o·**don**′·she·ah). In dentistry, the study and treatment of morbid conditions of the periodontal membrane.

periodontic (per·e·o·**don**′·tik). Lying around a tooth, as the periodontal membrane which attaches a tooth to the alveolar bone. [Gk *peri, odous* tooth.]

periodontics (per·e·o·**don**′·tix). Periodontia.

periodontitis (per·e·o·don·**ti**′·tis). Inflammation of the periodontal membrane. **Acute local periodontitis.** An acute inflammation of the periodontal membrane of a single tooth; an acute periapical abscess. **Chronic local periodontitis.** A chronic inflammation of the periodontal membrane of a single tooth; a chronic periapical granuloma or an abscess. Chronic suppurative periodontitis. Pyorrhoea. **Periodontitis complex.** A condition in which there is rapid irregular resorption of alveolar bone and loss of periodontal membrane without obvious cause; periodontosis, diffuse alveolar atrophy. **Periapical periodontitis.** Inflammation around the apex of the root of a tooth. **Periodontitis simplex.** Destruction of the periodontal membrane and alveolar bone surrounding the teeth, mainly local in origin. [Gk *peri, odous* tooth, *-itis* inflammation.]

periodontium [NA] (per·e·o·**don**′·she·um). The periodontal membrane; the term may also include the alveolar bone and gum surrounding the root of a tooth. [Gk *peri, odous* tooth.]

periodontoclasia (per·e·o·don·to·**kla**′·ze·ah). The destruction and loss of the tissues investing a tooth. [Gk *peri, odous* tooth, *klasis* a breaking off.]

periodontosis (per·e·o·don·**to**′·sis). Any degenerative change occurring in alveolar periosteum (periodontium). [periodontium, Gk *-osis* condition.]

periodoscope (peer·e·**od**·o·skope). A contrivance in the form of a chart for calculating the probable date of labour, calculated from the date of the last menstrual period. [period, Gk *skopein* to watch.]

periodynia (per·e·o·**din**′·e·ah). Acute pain affecting the entire body. [Gk *peri, odyne* pain.]

perioesophageal (per·e·e·**sof**·ah·**je**′·al). Occurring around the oesophagus. [Gk *peri,* oesophageal.]

perioesophagitis (per·e·e·**sof**·ah·**ji**′·tis). Inflammation affecting the structures surrounding the oesophagus. [Gk *peri,* oesophagus, Gk *-itis* inflammation.]

periomphalic (per·e·om·**fal**′·ik). Periumbilical. [Gk *peri, omphalos* navel.]

perionychia (per·e·on·**ik**′·e·ah). Perionyxis. [see foll.]

perionychium (per·e·on·**ik**′·e·um). The epidermis of the bed and sides of the nail. [Gk *peri, onyx* nail.]

perionyx [NA] (per·e·**on**·ix). A remnant of the eponychium which is perpetuated in the narrow fold overlapping the proximal portion of the lunule. [Gk *peri, onyx* nail.]

perionyxis (per·e·on·**ix**′·is). Inflammation around a nail or the nails. [see prec.]

perioöphoritis (per·e·o·of·or·**i**′·tis). Inflammation of the portion of peritoneum which lies over the ovary. [Gk *peri,* oöphoron, Gk *-itis* inflammation.]

perioöphorosalpingitis (per·e·o·of·or·o·sal·pin·ji′·tis). Inflammation affecting the tissues around the ovary and uterine tube. [Gk *peri,* oöphoron, salpingitis.]

perioöthecitis (per·e·o·o·the·si′·tis). Perioöphoritis. [Gk *peri, oon* egg, *theke* sheath, *-itis* inflammation.]

perioöthecosalpingitis (per·e·o·o·the·ko·sal·pin·ji′·tis). Perioöphorosalpingitis. [Gk *peri, oon* egg, *theke* sheath, salpingitis.]

periophthalmia (per·e·of·thal′·me·a). Periophthalmitis.

periophthalmic (per·e·of·thal′·mik). Occurring or situated around the eye: circumocular. [Gk *peri, ophthalmos* eye.]

periophthalmitis (per·e·of·thal·mi′·tis). Inflammation affecting the parts which surround the eye. [Gk *peri, ophthalmos* eye, *-itis* inflammation.]

perioptic (per·e·op·tik). Periophthalmic. [Gk *peri, optikos* of sight.]

perioptometry (per·e·op·tom′·et·re). The estimation of the limit of the field of vision or of the acuity of peripheral vision. [Gk *peri, optos* visible, meter.]

perioral (per·e·or·al). Around or surrounding the mouth. [Gk *peri,* L *os* mouth.]

periorbit [periorbita (NA)] (per·e·or·bit). The periosteum lining the orbit. It is continuous with that on the surface of the facial bones in front and with the outer layer of the dura mater through the superior orbital fissure and optic tract. [Gk *peri,* orbit.]

periorbital (per·e·or·bit·al). 1. Belonging to the periorbit. 2. Occurring around the orbit; circumorbital. [see prec.]

periorbitis, periorbititis (per·e·or·bi′·tis, per·e·or·bit·i′·tis). Inflammation of the periorbit; orbital periostitis. [periorbit, Gk *-itis* inflammation.]

periorchitis (per·e·or·ki′·tis). Inflammation of the tunica vaginalis testis following orchitis or epididymitis. **Periorchitis adhaesiva.** Periorchitis causing adhesion of the two layers of the sac. **Periorchitis haemorrhagica.** Periorchitis which occurs in severe inflammation with haemorrhagic effusion into the sac. The sac may become lined with fibrinous deposit, resulting in thickening of the membrane. **Periorchitis prolifera.** A condition in which the tunica vaginalis undergoes hyperplasia and much thickening. Small wart-like projections may form, become separate and remain as free bodies in the sac. **Periorchitis purulenta.** Periorchitis in which the inflammation goes on to suppuration due to septic infection. [Gk *peri, orchis* testis, *-itis* inflammation.]

periorchium (per·e·or·ke·um). The parietal layer of the tunica vaginalis testis. [Gk *peri, orchis* testis.]

periosteal (per·e·os·te·al). Relating or belonging to the periosteum. [Gk *peri, osteon* bone.]

periosteitis (per·e·os·te·i′·tis). Periostitis.

periosteoma (per·e·os·te·o′·mah). 1. A tumour of the periosteum. 2. A bony outgrowth from the tissues surrounding a bone. [periosteum, Gk *-oma* tumour.]

periosteomatosis (per·e·os·te·o·mat·o′·sis). Periosteosis. [periosteoma, Gk *-osis* condition.]

periosteomedullitis (per·e·os·te·o·med·ul·i′·tis). Inflammation affecting the periosteum and the marrow of a bone. [periosteum, medullitis.]

periosteomyelitis (per·e·os·te·o·mi·el·i′·tis). Inflammation in which the entire bone, including marrow and periosteum, is affected. [periosteum, myelitis.]

periosteo-oedema (per·e·os·te·o·e·de′·mah). Oedema affecting the periosteum.

periosteophyma (per·e·os·te·o·fi′·mah). 1. Hypertrophy of the periosteum. 2. Periosteophyte. [periosteum, Gk *phyma* a growth.]

periosteophyte (per·e·os·te·o·fite). A bony tumour growing outwards from the periosteum. [periosteum, Gk *phyton* that which has grown.]

periosteorrhaphy (per·e·os·te·or′·af·e). The operation suturing the edges of divided periosteum. [periosteum, Gk *rhaphe* suture.]

periosteosis (per·e·os·te·o′·sis). The morbid state characterized by the development of multiple periosteomata. [periosteoma, Gk *-osis* condition.]

periosteosteitis (per·e·os·te·os·te·i′·tis). Periostitis and osteitis occurring simultaneously.

periosteotome (per·e·os·te·o·tome). A knife used in incising the periosteum in the separation of the periosteum from a bone. [Periosteum, Gk *temnein* to cut.]

periosteotomy (per·e·os·te·ot′·o·me). The operation of making an incision into the periosteum and down to the bone. [see prec.]

periosteous (per·e·os·te·us). Relating or belonging to periosteum, or having the character of periosteum.

periosteum [NA] (per·e·os·te·um). A dense membrane of connective tissue which covers all but the articular surfaces of bones. It consists mainly of collagenous fibres, but contains some elastic tissue. It is vascular, and the blood vessels are found chiefly in its superficial layer; the deeper layer is less vascular and contains many fibroblasts. It is in the deeper layer that osteoblasts are found in developing bones and in pathological conditions (e.g. repair of fracture) in adult bones. Collagenous fibres extend from the deeper layers directly into the bone as Sharpey's fibres. **Alveolar periosteum [periodontium (NA)]** The periodontal membrane; the periosteum lining the alveolar cavities of the mandible and maxilla and joining the bone to the cementum of the teeth. [Gk *peri, osteon* bone.]

periostitic (per·e·os·tit′·ik). Relating to, of the natue of, or suffering from periostitis.

periostitis (per·e·os·ti′·tis). Inflammation of the periosteum. **Periostitis albuminosa, Albuminous periostitis.** Periostitis associated with a collection of clear serous fluid beneath the periosteum. **Dental periostitis.** Inflammation of the dental periosteum. **Diffuse periostitis.** Periostitis affecting a large area of bone. **Haemorrhagic periostitis.** Periostitis associated with an accumulation of blood beneath the periosteum, usually due to direct injury. **Periostitis hyperplastica.** Chronic thickening of the periosteum. **Periostitis interna cranii.** Inflammation of the periosteum on the inner surface of the skull. **Orbital periostitis.** Inflammation of the periosteum of the orbit: usually an extension from an acute frontal, maxillary, or ethmoidal sinusitis. **Precocious periostitis.** Syphilitic periostitis occurring early in the disease. [periosteum, Gk *-itis* inflammation.]

periostoma (per·e·os·to′·mah). Periosteoma.

periostomedullitis (per·e·os·to·med·ul·i′· tis). Periosteomedullitis. [periosteum, medullitis.]

periostosis (per·e·os·to′·sis). A bony growth from the surface of a bone. [Gk *peri, osteon* bone.]

periostosteitis (per·e·ost·os·te·i′·tis). Inflammation affecting simultaneously the bone and its periosteum. [periosteum, *osteon* bone, *-itis* inflammation.]

periostotome (per·e·os·to·tome). Periosteotome.

periostotomy (per·e·os·tot′·o·me). Periosteotomy.

periotic (per·e·o·tik). 1. Surrounding the ear. 2. Occurring around the internal ear. 3. referring to the mastoid and petrous parts of the temporal bone. [Gk *peri, ous* ear.]

periovaritis (per·e·o·var·i′·tis). Perioöphoritis. [Gk *peri,* ovary, Gk *-itis* inflammation.]

periovular (per·e·o·vew·lar). Surrounding the ovum. [Gk *peri,* ovum.]

peripachymeningitis (per·e·pak·e·men·in·ji′·tis). Inflammation involving the parietal layer of the dura mater. [Gk *peri, pachys* thick, meningitis.]

peripancreatic (per·e·pan·kre·at′·ik). Occurring about the pancreas. [Gk *peri,* pancreas.]

peripancreatitis (per·e·pan·kre·at·i′·tis). Inflammation affecting the peritoneal tissues which surround the pancreas. [Gk *peri,* pancreatitis.]

peripapillary (per·e·pap·il′·ar·e). Occurring around a papilla, and especially around the optic disc. [Gk *peri,* papilla.]

peripatetic (per·e·pat·et′·ik). Walking about; applied to cases of fever, e.g. typhoid fever, in which the patient remains up and about. Ambulatory is the more usual term. [Gk *peripatein* to walk about.]

peripenial (per·e·pe·ne·al). Situated about the penis. [Gk *peri,* penis.]

peripericarditis (per·e·per·e·kar·di′·tis). Pericarditis with adherence of the pericardium to the pleura and wall of the thorax. [Gk *peri,* pericarditis.]

periphacitis (per·e·fas·i'·tis). Inflammation of the periphacus. [periphacus, Gk *-itis* inflammation.]

periphacus (per·e·fak·us). The capsule of the lens of the eye. [Gk *peri, phakos* lens.]

periphakitis (per·e·fak·i'·tis). Periphacitis.

peripharyngeal (per·e·far·in'·je·al). Occurring or situated about the pharynx. [Gk *peri,* pharynx.]

peripheral (per·if·er·al). Relating or belonging to the periphery; occurring at or near the periphery, or on the surface of an organ or of the body.

peripheraphose (per·if·er·af·oze). An aphose which originates in the peripheral part of the visual mechanism.

peripherocentral (per·if·er·o·sen'·tral). Pertaining to the periphery and to the centre of a part or of the body.

peripheroceptor (per·if·er·o·sep'·tor). A receptor at the peripheral termination of a peripheral sensory neuron which receives the stimulus.

peripheromittor (per·if·er·o·mit'·or). That part of a neuron which is in contact with the effector organ and is responsible for transmitting the stimulus. [periphery, L *mittere* to send.]

peripheroneural (per·if·er·o·newr'·al). Relating to those nerves which are to be found on the surface of the body. [periphery, Gk *neuron* nerve.]

peripherophose (per·if·er·o·foze). A subjective sensation of light due to stimulation of the retina or optic nerve. [periphery, phose.]

periphery (per·if·er·e). The outer boundary or surface, away from the centre. [Gk *periphereia* a circumference.]

periphlebitic (per·e·fleb·it'·ik). 1. Pertaining to or having the characteristics of periphlebitis. 2. Suffering from periphlebitis.

periphlebitis (per·e·fleb·i'·tis). 1. Inflammation affecting the external coat of a vein, resulting from injury or from an inflammatory process in its neighbourhood. 2. Inflammation affecting the connective tissues which surround a vein. **Sclerosing periphlebitis of the chest wall.** Mondor's disease. [Gk *peri,* phlebitis.]

periphoria (per·e·for·e·ah). Cyclophoria. [Gk *peri, pherein* to carry.]

periphrastic (per·e·fras·tik). Characterized by the use of more words than are necessary and circumlocutory ways of giving expression to thoughts. [Gk *peri, phrasein* to utter.]

periphrenitis (per·e·fren·i'·tis). Inflammation of the parts which are situated around the diaphragm. [Gk *peri, phren* diaphragm, *-itis* inflammation.]

Periplaneta (per·e·plan·e'·tah). A genus of large, pale brown cockroaches. **Periplaneta americana.** The American cockroach, a cosmopolitan commensal of man; it is an intermediate host of *Moniliformis dubius.* **Periplaneta australasiae.** The Australian cockroach, a less common, but cosmopolitan commensal of man. [Gk *periplanein* to wander about.]

periplasm (per·e·plazm). A thin layer of hyaline substance surrounding an animal cell. [Gk *peri, plasma* something formed.]

periplastic (per·e·plas·tik). 1. Pertaining to the matrix of an organ or part. 2. Surrounding the nucleus of an animal cell. [Gk *peri, plassein* to form.]

peripleural (per·e·ploor·al). Occurring or situated about the pleura. [Gk *peri,* pleura.]

peripleuritis (per·e·ploor·i'·tis). Inflammation affecting the structures lying between the pleura and the chest wall. [Gk *peri,* pleura, Gk *-itis* inflammation.]

Periploca (per·ip·lo·kah). A genus of plants including the climbing dog's bane, *Periploca graeca.* They contain the cardiac glycosides, periplocin and periplocymarin. [Gk *periplokos* entwined.]

periplocin (per·ip·lo·sin). $C_{36}H_{56}O_{13}$, a little-used cardiac glycoside obtained from *Periploca graeca.*

periplocymarin (per·ip·lo·si'·mar·in). $C_{30}H_{46}O_8$, a cardiac glycoside found in the bark of *Periploca graeca.*

periplogenin (per·ip·lo·jen'·in). $C_{23}H_{34}O_5$, a heart poison of steroid structure occurring as an aglycone in the glycoside, periplocin.

peripneumonia, peripneumonitis (per·e·new·mo'·ne·ah, per·e·new·mon·i'·tis). 1. Pneumonia. 2. Pleurisy affecting the surface of the lung (visceral pleurisy). [Gk *peri,* pneumonia, pneumonitis.]

peripolar (per·e·po·lar). Surrounding a pole. [Gk *peri,* pole.]

periporitis (per·e·po·ri'·tis). Multiple abscesses of sweat glands, especially in infants. [Gk *peri, poros* passage, *-itis* inflammation.]

periportal (per·e·por·tal). Surrounding the portal vein, especially in the liver. [Gk *peri,* L *porta* gate.]

periproctic (per·e·prok·tik). Perianal. [Gk *peri, proktos* anus.]

periproctitis (per·e·prok·ti'·tis). Inflammation affecting the connective tissue surrounding the rectum and anus. [Gk *peri, proktos* anus, *-itis* inflammation.]

periprostatic (per·e·pros·tat'·ik). Surrounding the prostate. [Gk *peri,* prostate.]

periprostatitis (per·e·pros·tat·i'·tis). Inflammation of the tissues which are situated around the prostate. [L *peri,* prostatitis.]

peripyema, peripyemia (per·e·pi·e'·mah, per·e·pi·e'·me·ah). Suppuration occurring around an organ or part. [Gk *peri, pyon* pus.]

peripylephlebitis (per·e·pi·le·fleb·i'·tis). Inflammation affecting the structures surrounding the portal veins. [Gk *peri, pyle* gate, phlebitis.]

peripylic (per·e·pi·lik). Periportal. [Gk *peri, pyle* gate.]

peripyloric (per·e·pi·lor'·ik). Occurring or situated in the neighbourhood of the pylorus. [Gk *peri,* pylorus.]

periradicular (per·e·rad·ik'·ew·lar). Situated around a root, particularly around the root of a tooth. [Gk *peri, radicula* rootlet.]

perirectal (per·e·rek·tal). Round the rectum. [Gk *peri,* rectum.]

perirectitis (per·e·rek·ti'·tis). Periproctitis. [Gk *peri,* rectum, Gk *-itis* inflammation.]

perirenal (per·e·re·nal). Situated around a kidney. **Perirenal insufflation.** Insufflation of oxygen in the tissues surrounding the kidney with subsequent radiological visualization to determine the size and position of the tumour or structure lying above the kidney. [Gk *peri,* L *ren* kidney.]

perirhinal (per·e·ri·nal). Occurring about the nose. [Gk *peri, rhis* nose.]

perisalpingitis (per·e·sal·pin·ji'·tis). Inflammation affecting the peritoneum and other structures surrounding a uterine tube. [Gk *peri,* salpingitis.]

perisalpingo-ovaritis (per·e·sal·ping·go·o·var·i'·tis). Perioöphorosalpingitis. Inflammation of the ovaries and uterine tubes, with adhesions. [Gk *peri, salpigx* trumpet, ovary, Gk *-itis* inflammation.]

perisalpinx (per·e·sal·pingx). The coat, formed of the peritoneum, which covers the superior aspect of the uterine tube. [Gk *peri, salpigx* trumpet.]

periscleritis (per·e·skler·i'·tis). Episcleritis. [Gk *peri, skleros* hard, *-itis* inflammation.]

perisclerium (per·e·skler·e·um). Fibrous tissue situated around the cartilage which is undergoing a process of ossification. [Gk *peri, skleros* hard.]

periscopic (per·e·skop·ik). Applied in optics to a curved form of spectacle lens (meniscus) which allows clear vision when the eye looking through it is moved over a relatively wide field. [Gk *peri, skopein* to view.]

perisigmoiditis (per·e·sig·moid·i'·tis). Pericolitis of the sigmoid flexure. [Gk *peri,* sigmoid, Gk *-itis* inflammation.]

perisinuitis (per·e·si·new·i'·tis). Perisinusitis.

perisinuous (per·e·sin·ew·us). Occurring or situated about a sinus. [see foll.]

perisinusitis (per·e·si·nus·i'·tis). Inflammation of the structures which are situated around a sinus. [Gk *peri,* sinus.]

perispermatitis (per·e·sper·mat·i'·tis). Inflammation affecting the parts around the spermatic cord. **Perispermatitis serosa.** Encysted hydrocele of the spermatic cord. [Gk *peri,* spermatic cord, Gk *-itis* inflammation.]

perisplanchnic (per·e·**splangk**·nik). Situated around any viscus. [Gk *peri, splagchnon* viscus.]

perisplanchnitis (**per**·e·splangk·**ni**′·tis). Inflammation affecting the tissues around a viscus; perivisceral peritonitis. [Gk *peri, splagchnon* visucs, *-itis* inflammation.]

perisplenic (per·e·**splen**·ik). Situated around or occurring in the immediate neighbourhood of the spleen. [Gk *peri,* spleen.]

perisplenitis (per·e·splen·**i**′·tis). Inflammation of the peritoneum which invests the spleen and of the parts surrounding that organ. **Perisplenitis cartilaginea.** Inflammatory hyperplasia of the splenic capsule, resulting in such thickening of the tissue that it resembles cartilage in its hardness. [Gk *peri,* spleen, Gk *-itis* inflammation.]

perispondylic (**per**·e·spon·**dil**′·ik). Occurring around a vertebra. [Gk *peri, spondylos* vertebra.]

perispondylitis (**per**·e·spon·dil·**i**′·tis). Periarthritis or fibrositis of the spine. [Gk *peri, spondylos* vertebra, *-itis* inflammation.]

See also: GIBNEY.

Perisporiaceae (**per**·e·spo·re·**a**′·se·e). Obligate plant pathogens, dark mildews. [Gk *peri, sporos* seed.]

perissad (per·is·ad). In chemistry, applied to an element or radical with a valency that is an odd number. [obsolete term.] [Gk *perissos* uneven.]

perissodactylous (per·is·o·**dak**′·til·us). Referring to an individual who has an uneven number of fingers or toes. [Gk *perissos* uneven, *daktylos* finger or toe.]

peristalsis (per·e·**stal**·sis). The vermiform movement of the intestine and other tubes, produced by a wave of alternate contraction and relaxation of the tube, which impels the contents forward. **Mass peristalsis.** Forcible peristaltic movements lasting only a very short time, which propel the contents of the intestine from one part of the colon to the next. **Reversed peristalsis.** A wave of contraction which propels the contents of the tube in the reverse direction. [Gk *peristellein* to clasp.]

peristaltic (per·e·**stal**·tik). Relating to or having the characteristics of peristalsis.

peristaltin (per·e·**stal**·tin). A glycoside, $C_{14}H_{18}O_8$, derived from cascara bark.

peristaphyline (per·e·**staf**·il·ine). Periuvular. [Gk *peri, staphyle* uvula.]

peristaphylitis (**per**·e·staf·il·**i**′·tis). Inflammation affecting the soft palate and the tissues which surround the uvula. [Gk *peri, staphyle* uvula, *-itis* inflammation.]

peristerna (per·e·**ster**·nah). The lateral parts of the thorax. [Gk *peri,* sternum.]

peristole (per·is·to·le). The ability of the wall of the stomach to contract around its contents after food has been ingested. [Gk *peristellein* to clasp.]

peristolic (per·is·**tol**·ik). Pertaining to or characterized by peristole.

peristoma (per·e·**sto**·mah). Peristome.

peristomal, peristomatous (per·e·**sto**·mal, per·e·**sto**·mat·us). Situated or occurring about a mouth. [see foll.]

peristome (per·e·stome). A depression lined with cilia leading to the cytostome in certain types of protozoa. [Gk *peri, stoma* mouth.]

peristroma (per·e·**stro**·mah). 1. The inner coat of any tubular structure. 2. The membrane on which the intestinal villi are based. [Gk *peri, stroma* mattress.]

peristrumitis (**per**·e·stroo·**mi**′·tis). Inflammation of the structures surrounding a goitre. [Gk *peri,* L *struma* scrofulous tumour, Gk *-itis* inflammation.]

peristrumous (per·e·**stroo**·mus). Situated around or close to a goitre. [Gk *peri,* L *sturma* scrofulous tumour.]

perisynovial (**per**·e·si·**no**′·ve·al). Situated or occurring about a synovial structure. [Gk *peri,* synovial membrane.]

perisyringitis chronica nasi (**per**·e·sir·in·**ji**′·tis **kron**·ik·ah **na**·zi). Granulosis rubra nasi. [Gk *peri, syrigx* pipe, *-itis* inflammation, *chronos* time, L *nasus* nose.]

perisystole (per·e·**sis**·to·le). The pause in the cardiac rhythm that occurs between the diastole and the systole. [Gk *peri,* systole.]

perisystolic (**per**·e·sis·**tol**′·ik). Relating or belonging to the perisystole; preceding the systole. [see prec.]

peritalar (per·e·ta·lar). Around the talus. [Gk *peri,* L *talus* ankle.]

peritectomy (per·e·**tek**·to·me). The removal of a ring of conjunctival tissue surrounding the cornea. [Gk *peri, ektome* excision.]

peritendineum [NA] (**per**·e·ten·**din**′·e·um). The sheath-like process which invests a tendon and maintains the lubrication of the fibres. [Gk *peri,* L *tendo* tendon.]

peritendinitis (**per**·e·ten·din·**i**′·tis). Inflammation of a tendon sheath. **Peritendinitis calcarea.** Peritendinitis associated with calcareous deposits in the inflamed sheath. **Peritendinitis crepitans.** Peritendinitis associated with marked grating felt on movement of the tendon. **Peritendinitis serosa.** Peritendinitis with effusion of fluid into the sheath. [Gk *peri,* L *tendo* tendon, Gk *-itis* inflammation.]

peritendonitis (**per**·e·ten·don·**i**′·tis). Peritendinitis.

peritenon (per·e·**ten**·on). A tendon sheath. [Gk *peri, tenon* tendon.]

peritenonitis (**per**·e·ten·on·**i**′·tis). Peritendinitis. [peritenon, Gk *-itis* inflammation.]

perithecium (per·e·**the**·se·um). The subglobose or flask-like ascocarp of certain fungi and angiocarpic lichens. [Gk *peri, theke* case.]

perithelial (per·e·**the**·le·al). Relating to the perithelium.

perithelioma (**per**·e·the·le·**o**′·mah). A tumour derived from the perithelium. [perithelium, Gk *-oma* tumour.]

perithelium (per·e·**the**·le·um). The system of cells and connective-tissue fibres forming a sheath around small blood vessels. [Gk *peri, thele* nipple.]

perithoracic (**per**·e·thor·**as**′·ik). 1. Surrounding the thorax. 2. Pertaining to the tissues around the thorax. [Gk *peri,* thorax.]

perithyreoiditis (**per**·e·**thi**·re·oid·**i**′·tis). Perithyroiditis.

perithyroiditis (**per**·e·**thi**·roid·**i**′·tis). Inflammation affecting the capsule of the thyroid gland. [Gk *peri,* thyroid gland, Gk *-itis* inflammation.]

peritomy (per·it·o·me). 1. The operation of removing a circular strip of the conjunctiva for the relief of pannus. 2. Circumcision. [Gk *peri, temnein* to cut.]

peritoneal (**per**·it·o·**ne**′·al). Belonging to the peritoneum.

peritonealgia (**per**·it·o·ne·**al**′·je·ah). Sensation of pain in the peritoneum. [peritoneum, Gk *algos* pain.]

peritoneocentesis (**per**·it·o·**ne**·o·sen·**te**′·sis). Paracentesis of the cavity of the peritoneum for the purpose of withdrawing fluid. [peritoneum, Gk *kentein* to stab.]

peritoneoclysis (**per**·it·o·**ne**·o·**kli**′·sis). Peritoneal irrigation. [peritoneum, Gk *klysis* a washing out.]

peritoneography (**per**·it·o·ne·**og**′·raf·e). Radiography within the peritoneal cavity.

peritoneomuscular (**per**·it·o·**ne**·o·**mus**′·kew·lar). Pertaining to peritoneal and muscular tissue.

peritoneopathy (**per**·it·o·ne·**op**′·ath·e). Any diseased state of the peritoneum. [peritoneum, Gk *pathos* disease.]

peritoneopericardial (**per**·it·o·**ne**·o·per·e·**kar**′·de·al). Belonging to the peritoneum and the pericardium.

peritoneopexy (per·it·o·**ne**·o·pex·e). The surgical fixation of the uterus by the vaginal route, carried out in order to relieve retroflexion. [peritoneum, Gk *pexis* fixation.]

peritoneoplasty (per·it·o·**ne**·o·plas·te). Surgical covering, by flaps of peritoneum, of raw areas on the surface of an abdominal organ. [peritoneum, Gk *plassein* to mould.]

peritoneorrhexis (per·it·o·ne·o·**rex**′·is). Peritoneal rupture. [peritoneum, Gk *rhexis* a breaking.]

peritoneoscope (**per**·it·o·**ne**′·o·skope). An endoscope, or surgical periscope, for inspection of the contents of the abdomen through a stab incision in the abdominal wall. [peritoneum, Gk *skopein* to view.]

peritoneoscopy (**per**·it·o·ne·**os**′·ko·pe). Inspection of the peritoneum by passing the peritoneoscope through the wall of the abdomen.

peritoneotome (**per**·it·o·**ne**′·o·tome). The peritoneal analogue of the dermatome, being the area of peritoneum supplied by a posterior nerve root. [peritoneum, Gk *tomos* a cutting.]

peritoneotomy (**per**·it·o·ne·**ot**′·o·me). Incision of the peritoneum. [peritoneum, Gk *temnein* to cut.]

peritoneum [NA] (**per**·it·o·**ne**′·um). The serous membrane which lines the whole abdominal cavity, covers the abdominal viscera and forms the outer layers of the mesenteries, omenta and peritoneal ligaments which are associated with the abdominal and pelvic viscera. It consists of a single layer of flattened mesothelial cells [tunica serosa]. In the male it is a closed cavity, and a small part is separated to form the lining of the tunica vaginalis testis. In the female the uterine tubes open into the peritoneal cavity. **Parietal peritoneum [peritoneum parietale].** The serous membrane lining the inner aspect of the abdominal wall. **Visceral peritoneum [peritoneum viscerale].** The serous membrane covering an abdominal or pelvic viscus. [Gk *peri*, *teinein* to stretch.]

peritonism (**per**·it·on·izm). A state of shock characterized by symptoms similar to those occurring in cases of peritonitis but in which inflammation is not present. [peritoneum.]

peritonitic (**per**·it·on·**it**′·ik). Belonging to or characterized by peritonitis.

peritonitis (**per**·it·on·**i**′·tis). Inflammation of the peritoneum caused by bacterial infection. **Acute generalized peritonitis.** Peritonitis secondary to infection from a neighbouring organ, as from the bursting of an appendical abscess or the perforation of an ulcer of the stomach or bowel. Symptoms are very acute and severe, and death may occur in 24 hours in fulminating cases. **Acute spreading peritonitis.** Peritonitis in which the infection spreads more gradually from the primary focus (e.g. appendix) and eventually becomes general; coils of intestines become adherent and pockets of pus form. It may follow unrelieved intestinal obstruction. **Adhesive peritonitis.** Peritonitis in which adhesions may form as a sequel to a mild acute peritonitis. In tuberculosis, extensive adhesions may form after absorption of the fluid and the cavity of the peritoneum be obliterated, with the intestines bound in a confused mass. **Aseptic peritonitis.** Any form of peritonitis other than that caused by infection, e.g. by irritant chemicals, or biological substance such as bile, by trauma during an operation, or by radioactive material or x-rays. **Biliary peritonitis.** Peritonitis complicated by the entrance of bile into the cavity, as in rupture of the gall bladder or bile duct. **Chronic peritonitis.** A form of peritonitis in which the peritoneum becomes much thickened and ascites is the prominent symptom. It occurs as part of a polyserositis, or in connection with perihepatitis, perisplenitis, or adherent pericardium. **Diaphragmatic peritonitis.** Inflammation of the lower surface of the diaphragm. **Encysted peritonitis.** Collections of pus localized by peritoneal adhesions. **Fibrocaseous peritonitis.** Tuberculous peritonitis (see below). **Gonococcal peritonitis.** An acute form of peritonitis occurring in the course of gonococcal infection. **Haemorrhagic peritonis.** Peritonitis in which the ascitic fluid contains much blood. **Malignant peritonitis.** Cancer of the peritoneum usually occurring secondarily to a primary source in the abdomen. The primary source may also be the breast or other distant organ. **Meconium peritonitis.** Inflammation of peritoneum by meconium which has escaped from ruptured intestine *in utero* or soon after birth; it may be secondary to meconium ileus. **Pelvic peritonitis.** Peritonitis in which the inflammation is limited to the pelvic peritoneum. **Pneumococcal peritonitis.** Peritonitis due to infection with pneumococci *(Streptococcus pneumoniae)*. **Primary peritonitis.** That caused by direct infection from outside, or via the blood or lymph. **Puerperal peritonitis.** Part of a general or localized puerperal infection. **Secondary peritonitis.** That caused by infection from an adjoining viscus or infected tissue. **Septic peritonitis.** Peritonitis due to pyogenic organisms causing suppuration and abscess formation. **Peritonitis serosa.** One in which a copious serous ascitic fluid is present. **Streptococcal peritonitis.** Peritonitis due to infection with streptococci. **Tuberculous peritonitis.** A peritonitis most often secondary to tuberculous mesenteric glands or some other abdominal focus such as tuberculosis of the uterine tubes or tuberculous intestinal ulcers. [peritoneum, Gk *-itis* inflammation.]

peritonization (**per**·it·on·i·**za**′·shun). Peritoneoplasty. [peritoneum.]

peritonsillar (per·e·**ton**·sil·ar). Occurring about a tonsil. [Gk *peri*, tonsil.]

peritonsillitis (**per**·e·ton·sil·**i**′·tis). Inflammation affecting the tissues about a tonsil or both tonsils. [Gk *peri*, tonsilitis.]

peritracheal (**per**·e·trak·**e**′·al). Occurring or situated about the trachea. [Gk *peri*, trachea.]

peritracheitis (**per**·e·trak·e·**i**′·tis). Inflammation in which the tissues around the trachea are affected. [Gk *peri*, tracheitis.]

peritricha (per·e·trik·ah). Bacteria provided with flagella arranged indiscriminately over the bacterial cell. [Gk *peri*, *thrix* hair.]

peritrichal (per·e·**trik**·al). Peritrichous.

peritrichial (per·e·**trik**·e·al). Surrounding a hair follicle. [see foll.]

peritrichous (per·e·**trik**·us). 1. Applied to infusoria in which the cilia are limited to the region around the mouth. 2. Applied to bacteria which have flagella projecting over the entire surface. [Gk *peri*, *thrix* hair.]

peritrochanteric (**per**·e·tro·kan·**ter**′·ik). Occurring or in a position about a trochanter. [Gk *peri*, trochanter.]

perityphlic (per·e·**tif**·lik). Pericaecal. [Gk *peri*, *typhlos* blind.]

perityphlitic (**per**·e·tif·**lit**′·ik). Characterized by or affected with perityphlitis.

perityphlitis (**per**·e·tif·**li**′·tis). Inflammation which affects the peritoneal tissue around the caecum and vermiform appendix, a term widely used before the word *appendicitis* was introduced. **Perityphlitis actinomycotica.** A form of actinomycosis which occurs in the pericaecal area. [Gk *peri*, *typhlos* blind, *-itis* inflammation.]

periumbilical (**per**·e·um·**bil**′·ik·al). Situated or occurring around the umbilicus. [Gk *peri*, umbilicus.]

periungual (per·e·**ung**·gwal). Occurring or situated around a nail. [Gk *peri*, L *unguis* nail.]

periureteric (**per**·e·ewr·e·**ter**′·ik). Surrounding a ureter. [Gk *peri*, ureter.]

periureteritis (**per**·e·ewr·e·ter·**i**′·tis). Inflammation affecting the structures about a ureter. [Gk *peri*, ureter, Gk *-itis* inflammation.]

periurethral (**per**·e·ewr·**e**′·thral). Situated or occurring about the urethra. [Gk *peri*, urethra.]

periurethritis (**per**·e·ewr·e·**thri**′·tis). Inflammation of the periurethral tissues. [Gk *peri*, urethra, Gk *-itis* inflammation.]

periuterine (per·e·**ew**·ter·ine). Situated or occurring around the uterus. [Gk *peri*, uterus.]

periuvular (per·e·**ew**·vew·lar). Situated or occurring around the uvula. [Gk *peri*, uvula.]

perivaginal (per·e·**vaj**·in·al). Situated or occurring about the vagina. [Gk *peri*, vagina.]

perivaginitis (**per**·e·vaj·in·**i**′·tis). Inflammation of the tissues surrounding the vagina. [Gk *peri*, vaginitis.]

perivascular (per·e·**vas**·kew·lar). Surrounding or occurring around a vessel. [Gk *peri*, L *vasculum* little vessel.]

perivasculitis (**per**·e·vas·kew·**li**′·tis). Inflammation affecting the perivascular sheath of a blood or lymph vessel. [Gk *peri*, L *vasculum* little vessel, Gk *-itis* inflammation.]

perivaterian (**per**·e·vat·**er**′·e·an). Around the ampulla of Vater. [Gk *peri*, Vater's ampulla.]

perivenitis (**per**·e·ven·**i**′·tis). Inflammation affecting the parts around a vein. [Gk *peri*, L *vena* vein, Gk *-itis* inflammation.]

perivenous (per·e·**ve**·nus). Situated around a vein. [Gk *peri*, L *vena* vein.]

perivertebral (per·e·**ver**·te·bral). Situated or occurring around a vertebra. [Gk *peri*, vertebra.]

perivesical (per·e·**ves**·ik·al). Situated or occurring around the urinary bladder. [Gk *peri*, L *vesica* bladder.]

perivesicular (**per**·e·ves·**ik**′·ew·lar). Situated around or occurring around a seminal vesicle. [Gk *peri*, vesicle.]

perivesiculitis (per·e·ves·ik·ew·li'·tis). Inflammation involving the investing tissues of a seminal vesicle. [Gk *peri*, vesicle, Gk *-itis* inflammation.]

perivisceral (per·e·vis·er·al). Situated or occurring in the immediate neighbourhood of a viscus or viscera. [Gk *peri*, viscera.]

pervisceritis (per·e·vis·er·i'·tis). Inflammation of the tissues which surround a viscus or viscera. [Gk *peri*, viscera, Gk *-itis* inflammation.]

perivitelline (per·e·vit·el'·ine). Occurring or situated around a yolk. [Gk *peri*, L *vitellus* yolk.]

perixenitis (per·e·zen·i'·tis). An inflammatory reaction which affects the structures surrounding a foreign body. [Gk *peri*, *xenos* strange, *-itis* inflammation.]

perkinism (per·kin·izm). An empirical method of treatment in which disease is purported to be treated by applying metals with magnetic and magic properties. It had a considerable vogue in America and a Perkins' Institute was established in London. In 1796 Perkins patented his tractors, two metallic rods which were drawn over the skin of the affected part. [Elisha *Perkins*].

Perkins, Elisha (b. 1740). A quack of Norwich, Connecticut.

Perkins' tractor. *See* PERKINISM.

Perlapine (per·lap·een). BP Commission approved name for 6-(4-methylpiperazin-1-yl)-11*H*-dibenz [*b*,*e*]-azepine; a hypnotic drug.

perle (perl). A soft capsule made and filled by mass-production methods. [Fr. pearl.]

perlèche (per·lesh). 1. A disease, often due to riboflavine deficiency, occurring amongst children, in which the epithelium at the angle of the mouth becomes thickened and desquamatous, forming painful fissures. 2. Candidiasis. [Fr. *perlècher* to lick thoroughly with the tongue.]

Perlia, Richard (fl. 1889). Krefeld ophthalmologist.

Perlia's nucleus. A single convergence centre situated between the two nuclei of the medial recti muscles of the orbit in the medial part of the 3rd cranial-nerve nuclei in the mid-brain.

perlingual (per·ling·gwal). Through the tongue; referring to the giving of drugs which are reabsorbed from the tongue's surface. [L *per*, *lingua* tongue.]

Perls, Max (b. 1843). Giessen pathologist.

Perls' anaemia bodies. Small, mobile, club-shaped bodies seen in the blood in some patients with pernicious anaemia.

Perlsucht (perl·sookt). Tuberculosis of cattle. **Perlsucht bacillen-emulsion (BPE).** German tuberculin derived from bovine tubercle bacilli; no longer used. **Perlsucht-tuberculin original (PTO).** Early German tuberculin, no longer used. **Perlsucht-tuberculin rest (PTR).** Early German tuberculin; no longer used. [G.]

permanganate (per·mang·gan·ate). Any of the salts formed by the unstable permanganic acid: they possess strong oxidizing properties.

permeability (per·me·ab·il'·it·e). The degree to which a body is permeable to another substance, i.e. allows that substance to pass through it. **Capillary permeability.** The extent to which the capillary walls allow the fluid elements of the blood to pass through them; this permeability is increased, for example, by the injection of non-specific protein. **Magnetic permeability.** μ, the ratio of the magnetism induced in a body to the strength of the field which induces it. Where μ is greater than 1, the body is said to be *paramagnetic;* if less than 1 it is *diagmagnetic.* [L *permeare* to pass through.]

permeable (per·me·abl). Allowing the passage or penetration of liquids. [see prec.]

permease (per·me·aze). An enzyme or carrier which acts specifically to transport a compound from one side of a membrane to the other. [L *permeare* to pass through.]

permeation (per·me·a·shun). Penetration into and diffusion throughout an organ or tissue, e.g. of a chemical substance, physical rays, an infection, or a malignant growth. [L *permeare* to pass through.]

permixion (per·mik·shun). In chemistry, a mixture. [L *permiscere* to mix.]

Permutit (per·mew·tit). 1. Proprietary name for a silicate prepared by the fusion of kaolin, felspar, pearl ash and sodium hydrate. Powdered, it acts as a water-softener, removing calcium and magnesium ions from water in which it is placed and giving out sodium ions in exchange. 2. The process used in water-softening. [L *permutare* to exchange.]

perna (per·nah). Chlorinated naphthalenes which give rise to chlorine acne or perna disease when handled incautiously. [*per*chlor*na*phthalene.]

pernasal (per·na·zal). Through the nose. [L *per*, nose.]

perniciosiform (per·nish·e·o'·se·form). Apparently pernicious; denoting a diseased condition which resembles, but is not, a malignant or pernicious process. [pernicious, form.]

pernicious (per·nish·us). 1. Destructive. 2. Injurious. 3. Denoting a disease of abnormal severity which is apt to end fatally, e.g. pernicious anaemia before the introduction of liver treatment. [L *perniciosus* dangerous.]

pernio (per·ne·o) (pl. *perniones*). Chilblain. [L.]

perniosis (per·ne·o·sis). A term used to denote those cutaneous conditions which are caused by exposure to cold; a chronic state characterized by the presence of chilblains on many parts of the body. [pernio, Gk *-osis* condition.]

pernoctation (per·nok·ta·shun). Insomnia. [L *pernoctatio* wakefulness.]

perobrachius (pe·ro·bra·ke·us). A congenital abnormality affecting the arms. [Gk *peros* maimed, *brachion* arm.]

perocephalus (pe·ro·kef·al·us). In teratism, a monster having an imperfectly formed head. [Gk *peros* maimed, *kephale* head.]

perocheirus, perochirus (pe·ro·ki·rus). A monster with deformed hands. [Gk *peros* maimed, *cheir* hand.]

perocormus (pe·ro·kor·mus). In teratology, a monster the body of which is very defective or greatly deformed. [Gk *peros* maimed, *kormos* trunk.]

perodactylia (pe·ro·dak·til'·e·ah). Imperfect growth of either fingers or toes. [Gk *peros* maimed, *daktylos* finger or toe.]

perodactylus (pe·ro·dak·til·us). A fetus having imperfectly developed or defective fingers or toes, one or more of which may be lacking. [see prec.]

peromelia (pe·ro·me·le·ah). In teratism, the condition in which development of the limbs is defective. [Gk *peros* maimed, *melos* limb.]

peromelus (pe·rom·el·us). A monster having defective limbs. [see prec.]

peromoplasty (pe·rom·o·plas·te). The creation of a fresh stump after an amputation when there is projection of the end of the bone. [Gk *peroma* a maiming, *plassein* to mould.]

peronarthrosis (per·on·ar·thro'·sis). Saddle joint. *See* JOINT. [Gk *perone* brooch, *arthron* joint.]

perone (per·o·ne). The fibula. [Gk, brooch.]

peroneal (per·o·ne·al). Pertaining to the fibula, or to the lateral or fibular aspect of the leg. [see prec.]

peroneal artery [arteria peronea (fibularis)(NA)]. A branch of the posterior tibial artery which arises in the upper part of the leg and descends in close relation to the fibula to the ankle joint, where it takes part in the arterial anastomosis there. **Calcanean branches [rami calcanei (NA)].** Branches to the side of the heel. **Communicating branch [ramus communicans (NA)].** A branch which joins the posterior tibial artery. **Lateral malleolar branches [rami malleolares laterales (NA)].** Branches to the lateral malleolus. **Perforating branch [ramus perforans (NA)].** A branch which perforates the interosseous membrane near the ankle to gain the front of the ankle joint.

peroneal nerves. Common peroneal nerve. Lateral popliteal nerve. **Deep peroneal nerve.** Anterior tibial nerve. **Superficial peroneal nerve.** Musculocutaneous nerve of the lower limb.

peroneal veins [venae peroneae (fibulares) (NA)]. The venae comitantes of the peroneal artery. They are tributaries of the posterior tibial veins.

peroneotibial (per·o·ne·o·tib'·e·al). Relating or belonging to the fibula and tibia. [*perone*, tibia.]

peroneus brevis muscle [musculus peroneus (fibularis) brevis (NA)] (per·o·**ne**·us **brev**·is musl). A muscle arising from the lower two-thirds of the lateral surface of the fibula and inserted into the base of the 5th metatarsal bone. It is an evertor of the foot.

peroneus longus muscle [musculus peroneus (fibularis) (NA) longus] (per·o·**ne**·us **long**·gus musl). A muscle arising from the upper two-thirds of the lateral surface of the fibula and passing obliquely across the sole of the foot to be inserted into the medial cuneiform bone and the base of the 1st metatarsal bone. It is an evertor of the foot.

peroneus tertius muscle [musculus peroneus (fibularis) tertius (NA)] (per·o·**ne**·us **ter**·shus musl). A small muscle in the extensor compartment of the leg, arising at the lower third of the fibula and inserted into the base of the 5th metatarsal bone. Sometimes it is missing.

pero-olfactorius (pe·ro·ol·fak·**tor**'·e·us). The layer of olfactory nerve fibres forming the superficial layer of the olfactory bulb. [L *pero* boot of rough leather, olfactory bulb.]

peroplasia (pe·ro·**pla**·ze·ah). A deformity resulting from imperfect growth. [Gk *peros* maimed, *plassein* to form.]

peropus (pe·**ro**·pus). A monster having badly formed or defective feet. [Gk *peros* maimed, *pous* foot.]

peroral (per·**or**·al). Through the mouth. [L *per*, mouth.]

perosomus (pe·ro·**so**·mus). In teratology, a monster the body of which is greatly deformed. [Gk *peros* maimed, *soma* body.]

perosplanchnica (pe·ro·**splangk**·nik·ah). Defective development of the viscera. [Gk *peros* maimed, *splagchnon* viscus.]

perosseous (per·**os**·e·us). Through bone. [L *per*, *os* bone.]

peroxidase (per·**ox**·id·aze). One of a group of enzymes composed of protein combined with haem which occur in lung, liver and spleen tissue, in seedlings and in root vegetables such as horse-radish and potatoes. They catalyse the transfer of active oxygen from hydrogen peroxide or organic peroxides to an oxygen acceptor in tissue respiration.

peroxidate (per·**ox**·e·date). To oxidize to the fullest extent. [L *per*, oxidize.]

peroxide (per·**ox**·ide). 1. In a series of oxides formed by an element, commonly applied to that oxide which has the largest proportion of oxygen. 2. More accurately, an oxide containing the group -O-O, which yields hydrogen peroxide with dilute acids. **Peroxide of hydrogen.** Hydrogen peroxide.

peroxidize (per·**ox**·id·ize). 1. To peroxidate. 2. To treat with hydrogen peroxide.

peroxisomes (per·**ox**·e·so·mz). Components of the lysosome fraction, in liver and kidney only in mammals. Of unknown function, they contain certain enzymes such as catalase and urate oxidase. [L *per*, Gk *oxys* sharp, *soma* body.]

peroxydase (per·**ox**·id·aze). Peroxidase.

peroxydasis (per·ox·id·**a**·sis). The process of oxygen transfer activated by peroxidase.

peroxydate (per·**ox**·id·ate). Peroxidate.

peroxydol (per·**ox**·id·ol). Sodium perborate.

Perphenazine 1973 (per·**fen**·ah·zeen). 2-Chloro-10-[3-{4-(2-hydroxyethyl)piperazin-1-yl}-propyl]phenothiazine; used in the treatment of anxiety states and to prevent and treat nausea and vomiting.

perplication (per·plik·**a**·shun). The operation of drawing the free end of a divided artery through an incision made in its wall immediately above the cut, for the purpose of arresting haemorrhage. [L *per*, *plicare* to double up.]

Perroncito, Aldo (b. 1882). Pavia histologist.

Perroncito's apparatus, phenomenon, or spirals. A skein-like form assumed by the abortive axons in the proximal stump of a regenerating peripheral nerve.

persalt (**per**·sawlt). Of a series of salts formed by an oxyacid with a base, that one which contains the highest proportion of oxygen.

perseitol (**per**·se·tol). The alcohol, $CH_2OH(CHOH)_5CH_2OH$, found in the tropical plant *Laurus persea.*

perseulose (**per**·sew·loze). $(CH_2OH)(CHOH)_4CO(CH_2OH)$, a monosaccharide produced by bacterial activity from perseitol.

perseveration (per·sev·er·**a**'·shun). The continuation or recurrence of an experience or activity, without the appropriate exciting stimulus. **Clonic perseveration.** Recurrence of a movement. **Tonic perseveration.** Continuation of a posture. **Verbal perseveration.** A meaningless persistence of verbal activity. [L *perseverare* to persist.]

persimmon (per·**sim**·on). An edible fruit, *Diospyros virginiana*, said to be useful in diarrhoea because of its astringent properties when unripe. [Amer. Ind. (Algonquian) name.]

Persio BPC 1949 (**per**·se·o). Cudbear, red indigo; a red colouring matter obtained from certain lichens and used for colouring acid solutions; it turns blue with alkali.

persona (per·**so**·nah). The outer attitude adopted by a person towards others and towards his environment. [L, a mask.]

personality (per·son·**al**·it·e). The conscious living human being in his mental aspects (contrast with physique), especially as a unique individual distinct and differentiable from his fellows; more narrowly, the temperamental, conative and emotional aspects of the individual, his intellectual qualities being disregarded. **Alternating personality.** A personality which conspicuously varies between two states, e.g. of emotional tone; it has also been used as equivalent to double personality [obsolete term]. **Cycloid personality.** An abnormal personality type reflecting the fundamental psychological symptoms of the manic-depressive psychosis in the form of minor personality traits (Kretschmer). **Dissociated personality.** A personality type abnormally likely to show evidence of dissociation into two or more independent streams of mental activity. **Double personality.** A state of hysterical dissociation in which the individual presents himself to his associates at different times as two distinct persons, perhaps styling himself on separate occasions with two different names, and showing markedly different, even contrasting, personality traits. The memories of the two personalities may be supplementary to one another and mutually exclusive, or the memory of one may exclude but be included in that of the other. This condition has sometimes apparently arisen spontaneously, but has more often been the product of suggestion, e.g. by the psychotherapist. **Dual personality.** A personality which in opposing sets of circumstances may appear in two markedly contrasting aspects; more narrowly, equivalent to *double personality* (see prec.). **Extraverted personality.** A personality type which is distinguished by a striving towards identification with and dependence on the object (Jung). **Feeling-type personality.** A personality type characterized by the orientation of the personality by feeling, i.e. by a subjective value judgement with appropriate affect (Jung). **Introverted personality.** A personality type which is distinguished by self-assertion in the presence of the object struggling against dependence on it. **Intuition-type personality.** A personality type characterized by the orientation of the personality by intuition, i.e. by transmission and interpretation of perceptions in an unconscious way (Jung). **Personality inventory.** A self-completion questionnaire concerning personal characteristics and behaviour. **Multiple personality.** A state analogous to that of double personality (see above). **Neurotic personality.** A personality type with major or minor neurotic symptoms, and likely to develop or to have developed a neurotic illness. **Psychopathic personality.** A personality with one or more traits developed to such an inadequate or excessive degree as to cause suffering or damage either to the individual himself or the society in which he lives; more narrowly, an individual whose traits of personality lead him persistently into asocial or antisocial paths. As a psychiatric diagnostic category, some clinicians would use the term to include only those whose abnormality of personality has arisen in the course of development, and to exclude those whose abnormality has arisen in later life, e.g. from disease of trauma of the brain. **Schizoid personality.** Having qualities resembling those found in greater degree in schizophrenics, or qualities which may be found by catamnesis in schizophrenics before the onset of the illness, or found in the relatives of schizophrenics, i.e. coldness, eccentricity, reserve, etc. (Note: this term is not generally used in any very precise way; different clinicians tend to have their own usage.) **Seclusive personality.** A personality with a tendency to seclusiveness; an individual who tends to shut himself off from his fellows. **Sensation-type personality.** A personality type characterized by the orientation of the personality by sensation, i.e. by conscious sense perception (Jung). **Shut-in personality.** A personality shut in on itself, insufficiently attentive to and insufficiently reactive to the psychological environment. **Split personality.** 1. Dissociated personality (see above). 2. A common lay synonym for schizophrenia. **Syntonic personality.** A personality with the quality of reacting to the environment with spontaneity, directness and immediacy, and with warm emotional tone (contrast schizoid personality). The syntonic personality is frequently used to include all forms of the cyclothyme, but especially denotes the more balanced type. **Thinking-type personality.** A personality type characterized by the orientation of the personality by thinking, i.e. the active directed connection of presentations (Jung). [L *personalis* of a person.]

personology (per·son·**ol**·o·je). The study of personality. [personality, Gk *logos* discourse.]

perspiration (per·spir·**a**·shun). 1. The act or process of sweating; the excretion of sweat. 2. Sweat. **Foetid perspiration.** Bromhidrosis. **Insensible perspiration.** The evaporation of water which diffuses through the epidermis from the deepest layers of the skin, and which does not wet the skin. **Sensible perspiration.** The evaporation of water from the fluid actively secreted by the sweat glands; the sweat appears as droplets at the mouths of the glands. [L *per, spirare* to breathe.]

perstoff (**per**·shtoff). The choking gas, diphosgene, used in chemical warfare: also known as *superpalite.* [hyper, G *Stoff* substance.]

perstriction (per·**strik**·shun). Control of haemorrage by compressing or ligating the blood vessel. [L *per, stringere* to draw tight together.]

persulphate (per·**sul**·fate). Any salt formed by persulphuric acid: all are powerful oxidizing agents.

persulphide (per·**sul**·fide). A sulphide, analogous to a peroxide, which contains a greater proportion of sulphur than any other sulphide of the particular element.

pertechnate (per·**tek**·nate). The ion formed by the combination of the elements oxygen and technetium TcO_4. This is used as a label for a variety of radiopharmaceuticals employing the isotope of technetium ^{99m}Tc. [L *per* more than, technetium.]

Perthes, Georg Clemens (b. 1869). Leipzig surgeon.

Perthes' disease, Calvé–Perthes disease, Legg–Calvé–Perthes disease. Coxa plana; osteochondritis of the upper femoral epiphysis.

Perthes' incision. For exposure of the gall bladder: a vertical incision from the xiphoid process to the umbilicus with a horizontal angled extension from its lower end to the costal margin.

Perthes' method. A method of continuous drainage of a pleural effusion into an airtight receiver exhausted by water suction.

Pertik, Otto (b. 1852). Budapest pathologist.

Pertik's diverticulum. A lateral extension of the pharyngeal recess, not always present.

pertubation (per·tew·**ba**·shun). The blowing of air into the uterine tubes in order that they may be rendered patent. [L *per*, tube.]

pertussal (per·**tus**·al). Relating or belonging to pertussis.

pertussis (per·**tus**·is). Whooping-cough. [L *per, tussis* cough.]

pertussoid (per·**tus**·oid). In certain aspects, like whooping-cough. [pertussis, Gk *eidos* form.]

peruanum (per·oo·**a**·num). An element reported in a Peruvian mineral, the claim for which was unfounded.

peruol (**per**·oo·ol). Benzyl benzoate, a compound which occurs in balsam of Peru, and also prepared synthetically; it is used in the treatment of scabies.

peruscabine (per·oo·**ska**·been). Benzyl benzoate, a compound occurring in balsam of Peru, and also prepared synthetically; it is used in the treatment of scabies.

Peruvian bark (per·**oo**·ve·an bark). Cinchona.

peruvin (per·**oo**·vin). Name applied to cinnamic alcohol which is obtained from balsam of Peru.

pervenous (per·**ve**·nus). Literally, through a vein; the term is often used to describe the route used to reach the heart when catheters or electrodes are passed to it along a vein. [L *per, vena* vein.]

perversion (per·**ver**·shun). The turning aside of a function from its proper use. **Sexual perversion.** Abnormality of the sexual instinct. [L *pervertere* to turn about.]

pervert (**per**·vert). One who is perverted. **Sexual pervert.** One addicted to abnormal sexual practices. [see prec.]

pervigilium (per·vij·**il**·e·um). Insomnia. [L, a watching throughout the night.]

pervious (**per**·ve·us). Permeable. [L *pervius* passable.]

pes (paze) (pl. *pedes*). The foot. **Pes abductus.** A deformity in which the anterior part of the foot is turned away from the midline of the body. **Pes adductus.** A deformity in which the anterior part of the foot is turned towards the midline of the body. **Pes anserinus.** The conjoint insertion into the tibia of the sartorius, gracilis and semitendinosus muscles. **Pes arcuatus.** Pes cavus (see below). **Pes calcaneus.** Talipes calcaneus. **Pes cavus.** 1. A foot with an abnormally high arch. 2. Claw foot. **Pes corvinus.** Crow's feet; skin wrinkles radiating from the outer canthi of the eyes. **Pes equinovarus.** Talipes equinovarus. **Pes equinus.** Talipes equinus. **Pes excavatus.** Pes cavus (see above). **Pes febricitans.** Elephantiasis. **Pes gigas.** Macropodia. **Pes hippocampi [NA].** The expanding extremity of the hippocampus in the anterior end of the floor of the inferior horn of the lateral ventricle. Its surface is marked by several ridges. **Pes malleus valgus.** Hammer toe. *See* TOE. **Pes olfactorius.** The root of the olfactory bulb. **Pes planus.** Flat foot. **Pes pronatus.** Talipes valgus. **Pes supinatus.** Talipes varus; pes adductus (see above). **Pes valgoplanus.** Flat foot. **Pes valgus.** Deviation of the foot outward at the talocalcanean joint. **Pes varus.** Talipes varus. [L.]

pessary (**pes**·ar·e). 1. A device worn in the vagina to support the uterus in its correct position or vaginal walls. 2. A contraceptive device worn in the vagina to prevent the entry of spermatozoa into the cervical canal. 3. A medicament that is inserted into the vagina; it is usually made of glycogelatin or cocoa butter in which is dissolved a spermicide, e.g. quinine, or some other antiseptic. It is used either as a contraceptive or for the treatment of a vaginal infection. **Air-ball pessary.** An inflatable rubber balloon sometimes useful in cases of complete prolapse. **Check pessary, Contraceptive pessary.** An occlusive rubber pessary which prevents the entry of spermatozoa into the cervical canal. **Cup pessary.** A pessary about 75 mm long, having a cup at one end to support the cervix. **Diaphragm pessary.** A shallow cup-shaped pessary used to prevent conception. **Doughnut pessary.** A ring-shaped pessary for correcting prolapse. **Electric pessary.** A vaginal pessary carrying electrodes to stimulate the muscles of the pelvic floor and around the urethrovesical junction in cases of stress or urgency incontinence of urine. **Pessary forms.** Erythrocytes in which the central colourless area of the hypochromic red corpuscle encroaches on the peripheral coloured zone so that only a narrow rim of coloured cytoplasm remains, giving the impression of a pessary. **Prolapse pessary.** Any pessary to correct prolapse. **Retroversion pessary.** Any pessary designed to correct retroversion. **Ring pessary.** A circular rubber pessary. **Stem pessary.** A pessary having a stem which fits into the cervical canal. [L *pessarium.*]

See also: HODGE, SMITH (A. J.), THOMAS (T. G.).

pessima (**pes**·im·ah). A dermatosis characterized by firm pustules which spread all over the body and are surrounded by inflammation. [L, worst.]

pessimism (**pes**·im·izm). A tendency to take a dark or the most hopeless view of things; in extreme cases, the exhibition of such a disposition may amount to a psychosis. **Therapeutic pessimism.**

A disposition to underestimate the curative value of drugs. [L *pessimus* worst.]

pessulum, pessum, pessus (pes·ew·lum, pes·um, pes·us). A pessary. [Gk *pessos* oval-shaped stone.]

pest (pest). Plague. **Siberian pest.** Anthrax. [L *pestis.*]

pesticaemia (pes·tis·e·me·ah). 1. *Pasteurella pestis* in the blood. 2. Septicaemic plague. [L *pestis* plague, Gk *haima* blood.]

pesticide (pes·tis·ide). A comprehensive word to include substances that will kill any form of pest, e.g. insects, rodents and bacteria. [L *pestis* plague, *caedere* to kill.]

pestiferous (pes·tif·er·us). Pestilential; plague-bearing. [L *pestiferus* pestilential.]

pestilence (pes·til·ens). Any infectious or contagious disease occurring in epidemic and virulent form. [L *pestilentia* infectious disease.]

pestilential (pes·til·en·shal). Pertaining to, having the nature of, or producing pestilence.

pestis (pes·tis). Plague; a febrile disease caused in human beings by a bacillus, *Pasteurella pestis,* usually carried by rat fleas. Glandular swellings (buboes) are a common feature, and the death rate is high. **Pestis ambulans.** Subclinical plague or plague with few symptoms. **Pestis bubonica.** Typical plague with buboes in the groin. **Pestis fulminans.** Rapidly fatal plague. **Pestis inguinaria.** Pestis bubonica (see above). **Pestis major.** Typical bubonic plague. **Pestis minor.** A mild form of plague. **Pestis orientalis.** The plague; pest. **Pestis siderans.** Rapidly fatal plague. [L.]

pestle (pesl). An implement shaped like a club used for pulverizing, crushing, or breaking substances in a mortar. [L *pistillum.*]

pestology (pes·tol·o·je). The science and study of pests. [L *pestis* plague, Gk *logos* science.]

petalobacteria (pet·al·o·bak·teer′·e·ah). Bacterial micro-organisms so clustered together that they form a pellicle. [Gk *petalon* leaf, bacteria.]

petalococcus (pet·al·o·kok′·us). Any coccus which belongs to an aggregated group of cocci constituting a pellicle. [Gk *petalon* leaf, *kokkos* berry.]

petechia (pet·e·ke·ah). A small spot, generally reddish or purple and ranging in size from a pinpoint to a pinhead, appearing under the epidermis and caused by extravasation of blood. **Petechiae tardieu.** Minute spots of bleeding from venules and capillaries engorged and distended by venous stasis or obstruction, and thus rendered penetrable to whole blood. The feature described by *Auguste Tardieu* as characteristic of asphyxia; commonly seen in the scalp, face, eyelids or conjunctiva following strangling, but not confined to cases of violence. [It. *petecchia.*]

petechial (pet·e·ke·al). Belonging to or having the characteristics of petechiae.

petechiasis (pet·e·ki·as·is). 1. A morbid state characterized by the presence of petachiae. 2. A predisposition to the development of petechiae.

Peter, Charles Félix Michel (b. 1824). Paris physician.

Peter's law. Atheroma most commonly affects blood vessels where they change their direction.

Peter, Luther Crouse (b. 1869). Philadelphia ophthalmologist.

Peter's operation. For oculomotor paralysis: transplantation of the superior oblique tendon to the insertion of the internal rectus muscle of the orbit, with advancement of the latter.

Peters, George Armstrong (b. 1859). Canadian surgeon.

Peters' operation. A method of transplantation of the ureters to the rectum by the extraperitoneal route for exstrophy of the bladder.

Peters, Hubert (b. 1859). Budapest and Vienna gynaecologist.

Peters' ovum. One of the classical early human embryos.

Petersen, Ferdinand (b. 1845). Kiel surgeon.

Petersen's bag. An inflatable rubber bag for insertion into the rectum to raise the bladder during the operation of suprapubic cystotomy.

Petersen's operation. A modification of high lithotomy.

pethidine (peth·id·een). Ethyl-1-methyl-4-phenylpiperidine 4-carboxylate, $(C_2H_5COO)(C_6H_5)C_5H_8N(CH_3)$. A synthetic analgesic, usually used in the form of the hydrochloride (BP 1973) which is a colourless, almost odourless crystalline solid with a bitter taste, and very soluble in water. It is mostly administered intramuscularly, and has approximately one-half the activity of codeine and one-tenth that of morphine. It has a sedative action, but is not a potent hypnotic. It also exhibits powerful spasmolytic action, being more effective than papaverine but less so than atropine. Its use may be accompanied by unpleasant side reactions, such as dizziness and nausea, and may lead to addiction.

petiolate, petiolated (pet·e·o·late, pet·e·o·la·ted). Having a stalk, stem, or peduncle. [petiole.]

petiole (pet·e·ole). A peduncle, stalk or stem. [L *petiolus* little foot.]

Petit, Alexis Thérèse (b. 1791). Paris physician.

Dulong and Petit law. The atomic heats (i.e. atomic weight multipled by specific heat) of almost all solid elements are constant, approximately equal to 6.3. Exceptions are elements of low atomic weight and high melting point.

Petit, Antoine (b. 1718 or 1722). Paris anatomist and surgeon.

Petit's ligaments. The uterosacral ligaments. *See* LIGAMENT.

Petit, François Pourfour du (b. 1664). Paris ophthalmologist and anatomist.

Petit's canal. The space between the anterior and posterior suspensory fibres of the lens.

Petit's operation. For stricture of the lacrimal sac (obsolete).

Petit's sinuses. Sinuses of the aorta.

Petit, Jean Louis (b. 1664). Paris anatomist and surgeon.

Petit's disease. Eventration of the diaphragm.

Petit's hernia. Lumbar hernia; hernia through the lumbar triangle of Petit in the loin.

Petit's triangle. The lumbar triangle, formed by the iliac crest, the latissimus dorsi muscle, and the external oblique muscle of the abdomen.

Petit, Paul (b. 1889). French anatomist.

Petit's aponeurosis. That part of the broad ligament of the uterus below and behind the ligament of the ovary.

petit mal (pet·e mal). A form of epileptic fit beginning in childhood and characterized by abrupt loss of consiousness without falling or convulsion, with rapid recovery. **Petit mal status.** *See* STATUS. [Fr., little illness.]

petits maux (pet·e mo). The mild pains which herald the onset of labour. [Fr., little pains.]

Petragnani, Giovanni (b. 1893). Italian bacteriologist.

Petragnani culture medium. A medium prepared from fresh milk, peptone, potato meal, fresh potato, glycerol, hen egg and malachite green, for the culture of *Mycobacterium tuberculosis.*

Petren, Karel (b. 1868). Uppsala physician.

Petren's treatment. Treatment of diabetes by a high-fat diet, now superseded.

Petri, Richard Julius (b. 1852). Berlin bacteriologist.

Petri dish, or plate. A shallow circular glass dish and cover of varying diameter, used for solid culture media.

petrifaction (pet·re·fak·shun). The process of converting organic matter into stone or into a stony substance; calcification. [L *petra* stone, *facere* to make.]

pétrissage (pa·tre·sahj). A manipulation employed in massage, the tissues being picked up and kneaded between the operator's hands. [Fr., kneading.]

petrobasilar (pet·ro·ba·sil·ar). Belonging to the petrous part of the temporal bone and the basilar part of the occipital bone.

Petroff, Strashimis Alburtus (1882). Chicago bacteriologist.

Petroff's culture medium. An egg medium for growing *Mycobacterium tuberculosis.*

Petroff's method. A method for concentrating tubercle bacillus material.

petrogenous (pet·roj·en·us). Produced from rocks; in the petrogenous hypothesis of endemic goitre, the latter is believed to be caused by water containing deposits or impregnations derived from certain rocks. [Gk *petros* stone, *genein* to produce.]

petrolatoma (pet·rol·a·to'·mah). A tumour that may devlop after the injection of liquid petrolatum. [petrolatum, Gk *-oma* tumour.]

petrolatum (pet·rol·a·tum). Soft paraffin, petroleum jelly; a mixture of semisolid hydrocarbons produced during the distillation of petroleum. *See also* PARAFFIN. **Petrolatum album.** White soft paraffin. **Liquid petrolatum, Petrolatum liquidum.** Liquid paraffin for medicinal use. **Petrolatum molle album.** White soft paraffin. **Petrolatum molle flavum.** Yellow soft paraffin. **Petrolatum saponatum liquidum, Petrolatum saponatum spissum.** Liquid paraffin or soft paraffin respectively, mixed with ammonia and oleic acid, and used as vehicles for iodine or phenol; known as liquid or solid *Petrox*. **Petrolatum spissum.** Soft paraffin. [L *petra* rock, *oleum* oil.]

petrolene (pet·rol·een). 1. Asphalt. 2. A mixture of hydrocarbons obtained from bitumen; soluble in petrol or benzene. [see prec.]

petroleum (pet·ro·le·um). 1. Mineral oil, a mixture of paraffin and other hydrocarbons occurring naturally as a thick oil in the USA, Russia, Iran, Borneo, and elsewhere. It is obtained by drilling so-called wells, and the crude oil undergoes several stages of fractionation. 2. Light petroleum, petroleum ether, a solvent consisting of mixtures of liquid paraffin hydrocarbons and marketed in various boiling ranges, e.g. 40-60°C (principally pentane and hexane), 60-80°C, 80-100°C, 100-120°C, etc., according to the requirements. **Petroleum benzine.** The fraction of petrol distilling between 35° and 80°C. **Petroleum ether.** *See* MAIN DEF. 2 (above). **Petroleum jelly.** Soft paraffin; a semisolid mixture of paraffin hydrocarbons, naturally yellow in colour, but often bleached. It is used as a lubricant, an ointment base and as a protective. **Light petroleum.** *See* MAIN DEF. 2 (above). [L *petra* rock, *oleum* oil.]

petrolization (pet·rol·i·za'·shun). A process in which paraffin in fine spray is spread on the surface of water in lakes, streams, swamps, and so on, the object being to destroy the larvae of mosquitoes. [see prec.]

petromastoid (pet·ro·mas·toid). 1. Belonging to the petrous and mastoid parts of the temporal bone. 2. The otocranium.

petro-occipital (pet·ro·ok·sip'·it·al). Belonging to the petrous part of the temporal bone and to the occipital bone.

petrosa (pet·ro·sah). The petrous part of the temporal bone. [Gk *petros* stone.]

petrosal (pet·ro·sal). Relating to the petrous part of the temporal bone. **Petrosal sinus.** *See* SINUS OF THE DURA MATER.

petrosal nerves. Deep petrosal nerve [nervus petrosus profundus (NA)]. A twig from the carotid sympathetic plexus in the foramen lacerum, joining the greater superficial petrosal nerve to form the nerve of the pterygoid canal. Its fibres run through the sphenopalatine ganglion to be distributed to the orbit, nose, palate and pharynx. **Greater superficial petrosal nerve [nervus petrosus major (NA)].** A branch of the ganglion of the facial nerve which emerges through a small slit on the anterior surface of the petrous part of the temporal bone and travels in a narrow groove on this surface (groove for the greater superficial petrosal nerve) to the foramen lacerum where it joins the deep petrosal nerve to form the nerve of the pterygoid canal. It probably carries parasympathetic fibres. **Lesser superficial petrosal nerve [nervus petrosus minor (NA)].** A branch formed in the petrous part of the temporal bone by the union of two roots, one from the glossopharyngeal nerve via the tympanic plexus and one from the facial nerve. It emerges into the middle temporal fossa where it lies in a narrow groove (groove for the lesser petrosal nerve) lateral to the greater superficial petrosal nerve, and leaves usually through the foramen ovale to join the otic ganglion. It probably carries parasympathetic fibres.

petrosalpingostaphylinus (pet·ro·sal·ping·go·staf·il·i'·nus). The levator muscle of the soft palate. [Gk *petros* stone, *salpigx* tube, *staphyle* uvula.]

petroselinum (pe·tro·sel·i'·num). A genus of umbelliferous plants. **Petroselinum crispum.** Parsley *(Carum petroselinum)*. [Gk *petros* stone, *selinon* parsley.]

petrositis (pet·ro·si·tis). Inflammation affecting the petrous part of the temporal bone. [petrous, Gk *-itis* inflammation.]

petrosomastoid (pet·ro·so·mas'·toid). Petromastoid.

petrosphenoid (pet·ro·sfe·noid). Belonging to the petrous part of the temporal bone and to the sphenoid bone.

petrosquamosal, petrosquamous (pet·ro·skwa·mo'·sal, pet·ro·skwa·mus). Belonging to the petrous and squamous parts of the temporal bone.

petrostaphylinus (pet·ro·staf·il·i'·nus). The levator muscle of the soft palate. [Gk *petros* stone, *staphyle* uvula.]

petrous (pet·rus). 1. Like a rock or stone. 2. Petrosal. [Gk *petros* stone.]

petrox (pet·rox). Liquid paraffin or soft paraffin, mixed with ammonia and oleic acid; it is used as a vehicle for medicaments such as iodine or phenol, and is denoted *liquid* or *solid* according to the type of paraffin used. [Gk *petros* stone.]

petroxolin (pet·rox·o·lin). A solution or suspension of a drug in solid or liquid petrox.

Petruschky, Johannes (b. 1863). Danzig bacteriologist.

Petruschky's spinalgia. Pain and/or tenderness over the interscapular region induced by inflamed tuberculous parabronchial or paratracheal glands.

Pettenkofer, Max Joseph von (b. 1818). Munich chemist and hygienist.

Pettenkofer's reaction, or test. For bile acids in urine: to 5 ml of urine add 5 drops of 5 per cent sucrose and layer with concentrated sulphuric acid. A red ring appears at the junction of the liquids if bile acids are present.

Pettenkofer's theory. The obsolete theory that a low level of ground water is necessary for the occurrence of epidemics, and that the bacteria of typhoid fever, cholera, etc., must ripen in dry soil before they cause disease in healthy subjects.

Pettit, A. French bacteriologist.

Pettit's serum. A serum for the treatment of poliomyelitis.

Petz, Alador de. Hungarian surgeon.

Petz clamp. A crushing clamp by which metal clips may be inserted to close the crushed end of stomach or bowel.

peucine (pew·seen). A resinous pitch obtained from crude turpentine. [Gk *peuke* fir.]

peucinous (pew·sin·us). Resinous. [Gk *peukinos* fir gum.]

peucyl (pew·sil). A hemiterpene liquid hydrocarbon, C_5H_8, prepared from turpentine oil. [Gk *peuke* fir.]

Peutz, J. L. A. Dutch physician.

Peutz-Jeghers syndrome. A rare condition in childhood, although more frequent in later life, said to be inherited through a Mendelian dominant gene of high penetration. A child with brown pigmented spots on the circumoral skin and on the intra-oral mucous membrane presents with abdominal pain associated with marked borborygmi. The pigmented spots show melanin deposits in the basal-cell layer. Intestinal intussusception caused by polyposis is found at operation, sometimes in multiple areas; polypi are not found in other areas common to their development.

pexia (pex·e·ah). Pexis.

pexic (pex·ik). Having the ability to fix substances in the tissues. [see foll.]

pexin (pex·in). Rennet, or the enzyme contained in rennet; it causes milk to coagulate. [Gk *pexis* fixation.]

pexis (pex·is). The making fast of substances in the tissues; surgical fixation, as a rule effected by means of sutures. [Gk *pexis* fixation.]

Peyer, Johann Conrad (b. 1653). Swiss anatomist.

Peyer's glands, or nodules. The lymphatic nodules, both solitary and aggregated, of the intestine.

Peyer's patches, or plaques. The aggregated lymphatic nodules of the intestines.

peyote (pa·o·ta). Mescaline.

Peyronie, François de la (b. 1678). Paris surgeon.

Peyronie's disease. Chordee due to induration of the corpora cavernosa.

Peyrot, Jean Joseph (b. 1843). Paris surgeon.

Peyrot's thorax. A chest obliquely oval in section; it is seen in large pleural effusions.

Pfahler's method. A saturation method of irradiation, based on work done by Kingery: uneven fractionation of dose, with large initial dose followed by smaller doses designed to keep the radiation effect at its maximum.

Pfannenstiel, Hermann Johann (b. 1862). Breslau gynaecologist.

Pfannenstiel's incision. A curved incision convex downwards just above the pubis, with transverse division of both rectus abdominis sheaths and separation of the rectus abdominis muscles in the midline.

Pfeiffer, Emil (b. 1846). Wiesbaden physician.

Pfeiffer's disease, or glandular fever. Infectious mononucleosis.

Pfeiffer, Richard Friedrich Johannes (b. 1858). Breslau bacteriologist.

Pfeiffer's bacillus. *Haemophilus influenzae.*

Pfeiffer's phenomenon. Intraperitoneal lysis of *Vibrio cholerae* in immunized guinea-pigs.

Pfeiffer's reaction. The loss of motility, swelling and lysis of *Vibrio cholerae* caused by addition of complement and antiserum to the organisms.

Pfeiffer apparatus. An apparatus designed for the analysis of coal gas. Also known as *Pfeiffer's explosion pipette.*

Pfeifferella (fi·fer·el·ah). A former genus of bacteria belonging to the family Parvobacteriaceae. The type species was *P. mallei*, the cause of glanders in horses, man, sheep, and goats; *P. whitmori* was the causal organism of melioidosis. [Richard Friedrich Johannes *Pfeiffer*.]

Pfiffner, Joseph John (b. 1903). American biochemist.

Pfiffner and Myers method. A colorimetric method using alkaline nitroprusside ferricyanide reagent for the detection and determination of guanidine in blood.

Pflueger, Eduard Friedrich Wilhelm von (b. 1829). Bonn physiologist.

Pflueger's cord, or tube. Ovarian tube; an ingrowth of germinal epithelium from the surface of the ovary in the form of a cord or tube, from which primitive ovarian follicles are derived.

Pflueger's law. A nerve fibre is stimulated when catelectrotonus develops, or anelectrotonus disappears, but not when the reverse occurs.

pfropfhebephrenia (fropf·he·be·fre′·ne·ah). A hebephrenic psychosis occurring in a mental defective. [G *Pfropf* graft, hebephrenia.]

pfropfschizophrenia (fropf·skitz·o·fre′·ne·ah). A schizophrenic psychosis occurring in a mental defective. [G *Pfropf* graft, schizophrenia.]

Pfuhl, Adolph (b. 1842). German physician.

Pfuhl's sign. On aspiration the flow from a subphrenic abscess increases on inspiration but lessens with pyopneumothorax.

Pfund's gold-plated glass. A very thin layer of gold placed between a lens of crown glass and one of Crookes-A tint; this excludes the infrared and ultraviolet rays.

phacentocele (fas·en·to·seel). Phacocele. [Gk *phakos* lens, *entos* within, *kele* hernia.]

phacitis (fas·i·tis). Suppurative infiltration of the lens; not a true inflammation. [Gk *phakos* lens, *-itis* inflammation.]

phaco-anaphylaxis (fak·o·an·ah·fil·ax′·is). An allergic reaction to lens protein. [Gk *phakos* lens, anaphylaxis.]

phacocele (fak·o·seel). Dislocation of the crystalline lens of the eye, usually through a wound of the sclera into the subconjunctival space. [Gk *phakos* lens, *kele* hernia.]

phacocyst (fak·o·sist). The capsule of the lens. [Gk *phakos* lens, *kystis* bag.]

phacocystectomy (fak·o·sist·ek′·to·me). Removal of part of the lens capsule; an alternative procedure to needling or discission for cataract. [Gk *phakos* lens, *kystis* bladder, *ektome* excision.]

phacocystitis (fak·o·sist·i′·tis). Inflammation affecting the capsule of the lens of the eye. [phacocyst, Gk *-itis* inflammation.]

phaco-emulsification (fak·o·e·mul·sif·ik·a′·shun). A method of cataract extraction performed by washing out lens matter emulsified by an ultrasonic probe. Only a small limbal incision is needed. [Gk *phakos* lens, L *emulgere* to mix out, *facere* to make.]

phaco-erisis, phaco-erysis (fak·o·er·e′·sis). Removal of the crystalline lens by means of a small cup which is made to attach itself to the lens capsule by suction. [Gk *phakos* lens, *erysis* removal.]

phacoglaucoma (fak·o·glaw·ko′·mah). The sum of the alterations in the structure of the crystalline lens caused by glaucoma. [Gk *phakos* lens, glaucoma.]

phacohymenitis (fak·o·hi·men·i′·tis). Phacocystitis. [Gk *phakos* lens, *hymen* membrane, *-itis* inflammation.]

phacoid (fak·oid). Shaped like a lentil; lenticular. [Gk *phakos* lentil, *eidos* form.]

phacoiditis (fak·oi·di·tis). Phacitis; inflammation affecting the lens of the eye. [Gk *phakos* lens, *eidos* form, *-itis* inflammation.]

phacoidoscope (fak·oi·do·skope). Phacoscope. [Gk *phakos* lens, *eidos* form, *skopein* to watch.]

phacolysin (fak·ol·is·in). A protein derived from the lens, subcutaneous injection of which was at one time thought to bring about cure of early cataract (lens antigen treatment). [Gk *phakos* lens, *lysein* to loosen.]

phacolysis (fak·ol·is·is). Solution of the crystalline lens, usually brought about by dividing the anterior capsule (needling or discission) or by removing part of it with forceps (capsulectomy). It was performed at one time for high myopia, but abandoned because of the liability to subsequent retinal detachment. [Gk *phakos* lens, *lysein* to loosen.]

phacolytic (fak·o·lit·ik). Relating or belonging to phacolysis.

phacoma (fak·o·mah). A tumour of the lens of the eye. **Retinal phacoma.** Phacomatoses. [Gk *phakos* lens, *-oma* tumour.]

phacomalacia (fak·o·mal·a′·she·ah). A morbid condition characterized by softening of the lens; soft cataract. [Gk *phakos* lens, *malakia* softness.]

phacomatoses (fak·o·mat·o′·sees). A generic name suggested by Van der Hoeve for the following syndromes: neurofibromatosis (von Recklinghausen's disease), tuberous sclerosis (Bourneville's disease), angiomatosis (von Hippel–Lindau disease), and the Sturge–Weber syndrome. They are characterized by being genetically determined, congenital neuro-ectodermal lesions, often minimal at birth but becoming multiple tumours or cysts, sometimes malignant, situated most frequently in the central nervous system and the retina. [phacoma, Gk *-osis* condition.]

phacometachoresis (fak·o·met·ah·kor·e′·sis). Displacement of the lens of the eye. [Gk *phakos* lens, *metachoresis* change of place.]

phacometer (fak·om·et·er). 1. An apparatus used to estimate the refractive power of a lens. 2. Phacoscope. [Gk *phakos* lens, *metron* measure.]

phacopalingenesis (fak·o·pal·in·jen′·es·is). Regeneration of the lens of the eye. [Gk *phakos* lens, *palin* again, *genein* to produce.]

phacoplanesis (fak·o·plan·e′·sis). Dislocation of the crystalline lens; wandering lens. [Gk *phakos* lens, *planesis* a wandering.]

phacosclerosis (fak·o·skler·o′·sis). Hard cataract; induration of the lens. [Gk *phakos* lens, *skleros* hard.]

phacoscope (fak·o·skope). An instrument in the form of a dark chamber by means of which variations occurring during accommodation of the lens may be observed. [Gk *phakos* lens, *skopein* to watch.]

phacoscopy (fak·os·ko·pe). Inspection of the lens with the aid of a phacoscope.

phacoscotasmus (fak·o·skot·az′·mus). Opacification of the eye lens. [Gk *phakos* lens, *skotasmos* a clouding.]

phacotherapy (fak·o·ther·ap·e). The concentration through a lens of the sun's rays as a means of cauterizing superficial skin lesions. [Gk *phakos* lens, therapy.]

phaenakistoscope (fe·nah·kis·to·skope). Stroboscope. [Gk *phenakistes* imposter, *skopein* to watch.]

phaeochrome (**fe**·o·krome). Chromaffin; pertaining to cells which have an affinity for chromium salts owing to the presence of adrenaline or some of its derivatives. [Gk *phaios* dark, *chroma* colour.]

phaeochromoblast (fe·o·**kro**·mo·blast). The precursor cells of those medullary and paraganglionic cells which exhibit a chromaffin reaction. [phaeochrome, Gk *blastos* germ.]

phaeochromoblastoma (fe·o·**kro**·mo·blas·**to**'·mah). A malignant tumour composed of embryonic chromaffin cells. [phaeochromoblast, Gk *-oma* tumour.]

phaeochromocyte (fe·o·**kro**·mo·site). A cell which stains densely with chromium salts owing to the presence of adrenaline or its derivatives. It is found in the adrenal medulla and the paraganglia. [phaeochrome, Gk *kytos* cell.]

phaeochromocytoma (fe·o·**kro**·mo·si·**to**'·mah). Chromaffinoma, occurring chiefly in the adrenal medulla and staining brown with dichromate resulting from oxidation products of catecholamine and giving rise to hypertension, hypermetabolism and hyperglycaemia with excessive production of catecholamines. Provocative tests with histamine or tyramine are dangerous in the presence of severe hypertension. The α-adrenergic blocking agent phentolamine causes an increased fall in blood pressure. [phaeochrome, Gk *kytos* cell, *-oma* tumour.]

phaeosporotrichosis (**fe**·o·spo·ro·trik·**o**'·sis). Inflammatory infection with subcutaneous abscesses caused by pigmented (brown) fungi, e.g. *Phialophora gougerottii, P. richardsiae, P. spinifera.* Tissue preparations show dark, branching hyphae in abscess contents. The disease must not be confused with chromomycosis which, in tissue, produces only single or clustered, round, thick-walled bodies which divide by fission not budding. [Gk *phaios* dark, *Sporotrichum,* Gk *-osis* condition.]

phage (faje). Bacteriophage. (Gk *phagein* to eat.]

phage-typing (**faje**·ti'·ping). The identification of particular strains of different bacteria by the use of strain-specific bacteriophages which will lyse only that particular strain. Applied to many bacteria but particularly to salmonellae and staphylococci. [Gk *phagein* to eat, *typos* mark.]

phagedaena, phagedena (faj·e·**de**·nah). An obstinate ulcerative condition of the skin and subcutaneous tissues, characterized by sloughing and quick extension to surrounding tissues. **Phagedaena geometrica.** A chronic destructive ulceration of soft tissue, showing burrows and circular and trefoil ulcers. It is a gangrenous pyoderma, seen in the late stages of syphilis, oriental sore and tuberculosis, but is rare nowadays. **Sloughing phagedaena.** Hospital gangrene. *See* GANGRENE. **Phagedaena tropica, Tropical phagedaena.** Ulcus tropicum. [Gk phagedaina canker.]

phagelysis (**faje**·li·sis). Phagocytolysis. [phage, lysis.]

phagocytable (fag·o·**si**·tabl). Capable of submission to phagocytic action.

phagocyte (**fag**·o·site). A cell that has the power of ingesting, and usually digesting, micro-organisms, protozoa, tissue and blood cells, particulate matter and foreign substances. They may be free (motile) like the microphages or polymorphonuclear leucocytes and macrophages or monocytes; or fixed (non-motile) as in the case of the reticuloendothelial cells. **Alveolar phagocyte.** Phagocytic cells present in the pulmonary alveoli having the power of ingesting foreign substances inhaled into the lungs from the air. **Endothelial phagocyte.** Endotheliocyte. **Globuliferous phagocyte.** A phagocyte that has the power to ingest erythrocytes. **Melaniferous phagocyte.** A phagocyte with the power of taking up blood pigments. **Mobile phagocyte.** Leucocyte. **Sessile phagocyte.** A non-motile or fixed phagocyte. [Gk *phagein* to eat, *kytos* cell.]

phagocytic (fag·o·**sit**·ik). Produced, characterized by, or relating to phagocytes or phagocytosis.

phagocytize (**fag**·o·sit·ize). Phagocytose.

phagocytoblast (fag·o·**si**·to·blast). A primitive cell which develops into a phagocyte. [phagocyte, Gk *blastos* germ.]

phagocytolysis (**fag**·o·si·**tol**'·is·is). The splitting-up or disintegration of phagocytic cells. [phagocyte, Gk *lysis* loosing.]

phagocytolytic (**fag**·o·si·to·**lit**'·ik). Relating or belonging to phagocytolysis.

phagocytose (fag·o·**si**·toze). To engulf and digest bacteria and other foreign substances.

phagocytosis (**fag**·o·si·**to**'·sis). The ingestion of micro-organisms, cells and foreign particles by cells of the reticuloendothelial system known as *phagocytes.* Phagocytosis may be *induced* by the action of serum opsonins on bacterial cells, or *spontaneous,* e.g. the ingestion of dyestuffs and other non-antigenic particles. [phagocyte, Gk *-osis* condition.]

phagodynamometer (**fag**·o·di·nam·**om**'·et·er). A device used to determine the degree of force expended in masticating various kinds of food. [Gk *phagein* to eat, dynamometer.]

phagokaryosis (**fag**·o·kar·e·**o**'·sis). Phagocytic action carried on by the cell nucleus. [Gk *phagein* to eat, *karyon* nucleus, *-osis* condition.]

phagological (fag·o·**loj**·ik·al). 1. Relating to phagology. 2. Bacteriophagic.

phagology (fag·**ol**·je). The science which deals with feeding or eating. [Gk *phagein* to eat, *logos* science.]

phagolysis (fag·**ol**·is·is). Phagocytolysis. [phage, *lysis* a loosing.]

phagolytic (fag·o·**lit**·ik). Phagocytolytic.

phagomania (fag·o·**ma**·ne·ah). 1. Hyperorexia occurring in insane subjects. 2. An obsession in which the topic of eating is the predominant idea. [Gk *phagein* to eat, mania.]

phagophobia (fag·o·**fo**·be·ah). Fear of eating. [Gk *phagein* to eat, phobia.]

phagopyrism, phagopyrismus (fag·o·**pi**·rizm, **fag**·o·pi·**riz**'·mus). Undue sensitiveness to articles of diet, e.g. oysters, cheese and pork resulting in the appearance of symptoms of slight poisoning. [Gk *phagein* to eat, *pyr* fire.]

phagopyrosis (**fag**·o·pi·**ro**'·sis). Heartburn after the ingestion of food. [Gk *phagein* to eat, pyrosis.]

phagosome (**fag**·o·some). Heterophagosome. [Gk *phagein* to eat.]

phagotherapy (fag·o·**ther**·ap·e). Treatment by overfeeding or superalimentation. [Gk *phagein* to eat, *therapeia* treatment.]

Phagus (**fa**·gus). A genus of viruses which includes the bacteriophages. [Gk *phagein* to eat.]

phak-. For words beginning with **phak-**, *see* PHAC-.

phalacrosis (fal·ak·**ro**·sis). Alopecia. [Gk *phalakros* bald-headed.]

phalacrotic, phalacrous (fal·ak·**rot**·ik, fal·**ak**·rus). Relating to baldness. [see prec.]

phalangeal (fal·**an**·je·al). Relating or belonging to a phalanx.

phalangectomy (fal·an·**jek**·to me). 1. Removal of a phalanx of hand or foot. 2. Amputation of a finger. [phalanx, Gk *ektome* a cutting out.]

phalanges (of the hand and foot) [ossa digitorum manus et ossa digitorum pedis (NA)] (fal·**an**·geeze, fa·**lan**·geez) (sing. *phalanx*). The main bones of the digits of both the hand and foot. There are three, the proximal [phalanx proximalis (NA)], middle [phalanx media (NA)] and distal [phalanx distalis (NA)] in each digit except the thumb and big toe where there are two phalanges, the proximal and distal only. Each phalanx possesses a base [basis phalangis (NA)] with an articular surface for the corresponding metacarpal or metatarsal bone in the case of the 1st phalanx and for the more proximal member in the case of the middle and distal phalanges, a cylindrical or somewhat flattened shaft [corpus phalangis (NA)], and a distal end or head [caput phalangis (NA)] which, in the case of the middle and proximal phalanges articulates with the more distal member of the digit. The head of the distal phalanx is non-articular. The phalanges afford attachment for the tendons of the digits and their fibrous sheaths. [Gk *phalagx* a line of soldiers.]

See also: DEITERS.

phalangette (fal·an·**jet**). The distal phalanx. **Drop phalangette.** Falling of the distal phalanx and loss of the power to extend it when the hand is prone, because of rupture or overstretching of the extensor tendons close to the point of their insertion into the phalanx. [Fr., small phalanx.]

phalangitis (fal·an·**ji**·tis). Inflammation affecting a phalanx.

Phalangitis syphilitica. Dactylitis syphilitica. [phalanx, Gk *-itis* inflammation.]

phalangization (fal·an·ji·za′·shun). The creation by plastic surgery of a stump for use as a finger. [phalanx.]

phalangophalangeal (fal·an·go·fal·an′·je·al). Relating to two adjacent phalanges.

phalangosis (fal·an·go·sis). 1. The development of the eyelashes in rows. 2. Ptosis. [Gk *phalagx* a line of soldiers, *-osis* condition.]

phalanx (fal·angx, fa·langx). *See* PHALANGES.

phallalgia (fal·al·je·ah). Pain affecting the penis. [Gk *phallos* penis, *algos* pain.]

phallanastrophe (fal·an·as·tro·fe). An upward twisting of the penis. [Gk *phallos* penis, *anastrophe* a turning back.]

phallaneurysm (fal·an·ewr·izm). An aneurysm of one of the blood vessels of the penis. [Gk *phallos* penis, aneurysm.]

phallectomy (fal·ek·to·me). The operation of amputation of the penis. [Gk *phallos* penis, *ektome* a cutting out.]

phallic (fal·ik). Relating or belonging to the penis. **Phallic worship.** Worship of the phallus as an emblem of the generative or creative power of nature. [Gk *phallos* penis.]

phallicism (fal·is·izm). The cult of phallic worship.

phalliform (fal·e·form). Shaped like the penis. [Gk *phallos* penis, form.]

phallin (fal·in). A toxalbumin derived from *Amanita phalloides,* the death-cup fungus. [Gk *phallos* penis.]

phallitis (fal·i·tis). Inflammation of the penis. [Gk *phallos* penis, *-itis* inflammation.]

phallocampsis (fal·o·kamp·sis). Chordee. [Gk *phallos* penis, *kampsis* a curving.]

phallocrypsis (fal·o·krip·sis). A condition in which the penis is retracted, so that it is almost invisible. [Gk *phallos* penis, *krypsis* concealment.]

phallodynia (fal·o·din·e·ah). Pain in the penis. [Gk *phallos* penis, *odyne* pain.]

phalloid (fal·oid). Like a penis in shape. [Gk *phallos* penis, *eidos* form.]

phalloncus (fal·ong·kus). A penile swelling or tumour. [Gk *phallos* penis, *ogkos* a swelling.]

phalloplasty (fal·o·plas·te). Plastic or reparative surgery of the penis. [Gk *phallos* penis, *plassein* to mould.]

phallorrhagia (fal·o·ra·je·ah). Penile haemorrhage. [Gk *phallos* penis, *rhegnynein* to gush forth.]

phallorrhoea (fal·o·re·ah). Gonorrhoea in a male subject. [Gk *phallos* penis, *rhoia* flow.]

phallotomy (fal·ot·o·me). Incision of the penis. [Gk *phallos* penis, *temnein* to cut.]

phallus (fal·us). The penis. [Gk *phallos.*]

phanerogam (fan·er·o·gam). In botany, a flowering plant which produces seeds. [Gk *phaneros* visible, *gamos* marriage.]

phanerogenetic, phanerogenic (fan·er·o·jen·et′·ik, fan·er·o·jen′·ik). Denoting a disease of known aetiology. [Gk *phaneros* visible, genesis.]

phaneromania (fan·er·o·ma′·ne·ah). A morbid habit marked by preoccupation with some external growth or part, such as picking at a pimple or wart, pulling the moustache or biting the nails. [Gk *phaneros* visible, mania.]

phaneroscope (fan·er·o·skope). An instrument consisting of a lens which concentrates the light from a lamp on the skin, making it semitransparent and facilitating the examination of cutaneous structures. [Gk *phaneros* visible, *skopein* to watch.]

phaneroscopy (fan·er·os·ko·pe). Examination of the skin by means of the phaneroscope.

phanerosis (fan·er·o·sis). 1. The act or process of becoming visible. 2. The liberation of a substance which hitherto has not been apparent as it has been held in combination. **Fat phanerosis.** A morbid state in which fat previously not evident in the tissues has become liberated on account of disease and therefore capable of being seen and stained. [Gk *phaneros* visible.]

phanerosterol (fan·er·os·ter·ol). A sterol occurring in certain higher plants. [Gk *phaneros* visible, sterol.]

phanerous (fan·er·us). Phanic. [Gk *phaneros* visible.]

phanerozoite (fan·er·o·zo′·ite). An exo-erythrocytic form of the malaria parasite that appears concomitantly with, or later than, the earliest parasite of the erythrocytic phase. [Gk *phaneros* visible, *zoon* animal.]

phanic (fan·ik). Evident; visible. [Gk *phanikos.*]

Phanquone BP 1973 (fan·kwone). 4,7-Phenanthroline-5, 6-quinone; an anti-amoebic.

phantasia (fan·ta·ze·ah). The occurrence of an illusion or hallucination. [Gk, appearance.]

phantasm (fan·tazm). 1. An optical illusion; a phantom; an illusory image. 2. A manifestation of distorted mentality in delirium. [Gk *phantasma* vision.]

phantasmatomoria (fan·taz·mat·o·mor′·e·ah). Dementia or childish behaviour associated with delusions. [phantasm, Gk *moria* folly.]

phantasmoscopia (fan·taz·mo·sko′·pe·ah). The experience of hallucinations of ghosts. [Gk *phantasma* vision, *skopein* to view.]

phantasy (fan·tas·e). A quality of the imagination, leading to the development of thought or imagery from conventional paths into ones lacking one or more of the prerequisites of reality; concretely, a mental picture or invented story having such a dream-like quality. The term has no precise usage in medicine. [Gk *phantasia* appearance.]

phantom (fan·tom). 1. An apparition; a phantasm. 2. A model of the whole or of a part of the body used to practise or demonstrate operative methods. 3. A mass of absorbing material roughly equivalent in radiation absorbing and scattering properties to human tissues *(water phantom, wax phantom),* sometimes of a complicated structure to imitate varying densities of structures in the human body. [Gk *phantasma* vision.]
See also: SCHULTZE.

pharbitin, pharbitisin (far·bit·in, far·bit·is·in). Names given to the resin obtained from kaladana.

pharcidous (far·sid·us). Wrinkled or rugose. [Gk *pharkis* a wrinkle.]

pharmaceutical (far·mah·sew·tik·al). Relating or belonging to drugs or pharmacy; or engaged in pharmacy. [Gk *pharmakeuein* to administer a drug.]

pharmaceutics (far·mah·sew·tix). 1. Pharmacy. 2. Pharmaceutical remedies.

pharmaceutist (far·mah·sew·tist). A pharmacist.

pharmacist (far·mah·sist). Pharmaceutical chemist, pharmaceutist, chemist and druggist, dispensing chemist. Titles restricted by law to Fellows or Members of the Pharmaceutical Society of Great Britain (FPS or MPS); the title *chemist* is similarly restricted when used in connection with a retail shop. Membership of the Society may be obtained by any person of 21 years of age and over who has satisfied certain conditions as to training, etc., and passed the Society's examinations. A holder of a degree in pharmacy of a British university is normally exempted from the examinations, except in the subject of forensic pharmacy, upon the passing of which he may be admitted to membership provided he has complied with certain conditions of training. [Gk *pharmakeuein* to administer a drug.]

pharmacochemistry (far·mah·ko·kem′·is·tre). Pharmaceutical chemistry. *See* CHEMISTRY. [Gk *pharmakon* drug, chemistry.]

pharmacodiagnosis (far·mah·ko·di·ag·no′·sis). The use of drugs in diagnosis. [Gk *pharmakon* drug, diagnosis.]

pharmacodynamic (far·mah·ko·di·nam′·ik). Relating to the action and effects of drugs. [Gk *pharmakon* drug, *dynamis* power.]

pharmacodynamics (far·mah·ko·di·nam′·ix). The science of drugs especially with regard to their physiological effects and therapeutic action. [see prec.]

pharmaco-endocrinology (far·mah·ko·en·do·krin·ol′·o·je). The study of the effect of drugs on the function of the ductless glands. [Gk *pharmakon* drug, endocrinology.]

pharmacogenetics (far·mah·ko·jen·et′·ix). The study of inherited differences of reactions of individuals to certain drugs. [Gk *pharmakon* drug, *genesis* origin.]

pharmacognosist (far·mah·**kog**·no·sist). One who is experienced in pharmacognosy.

pharmacognosy (far·mah·**kog**·no·se). The study of crude drugs of vegetable and animal origin. [Gk *pharmakon* drug, *gnosis* knowledge.]

pharmacologist (far·mah·**kol**·o·jist). One who is expert in the science of pharmacology.

pharmacology (far·mah·**kol**·o·je). That branch of medical science which deals especially with the action, but also of the properties and characteristics, of drugs. [Gk *pharmakon* drug, *logos* science.]

pharmacomania (far·mah·ko·**ma**'·ne·ah). 1. An insane craving for drugs or for self-drugging. 2. Morbid preoccupation with administration of medicines. [Gk *pharmakon* drug, mania.]

pharmacon (far·mah·kon). A drug or a medicine. [Gk *pharmakon.*]

pharmaco-oryctology (far·mah·ko·or·ik·**tol**'·o·je). The sum of knowledge regarding mineral drugs. [Gk *pharmakon* drug, *oryktos* dug out, *logos* science.]

pharmacopaedia, pharmacopaedics (far·mah·ko·**pe**'·de·ah, far·mah·ko·**pe**'·dix). The study and science of drugs and their preparation. [Gk *pharmakon* drug, *paideia* education.]

pharmacophilia (far·mah·ko·**fil**'·e·ah). An abnormal fondness for medicines or drugs. [Gk *pharmakon* drug, *philein* to love.]

pharmacophobia (far·mah·ko·**fo**'·be·ah). Morbid fear of taking drugs or medicines. [Gk *pharmakon* drug, *phobos* fear.]

pharmacopoeia (far·mah·ko·**pe**'·ah). 1. A work, especially one published authoritatively, containing descriptions of drugs which are used in the practice of medicine, with methods of their preparation, their formulae and dosages, and directions for determining purity and strength; most countries have their national pharmacopoeia. 2. In the abstract, the whole range of drugs used in medicine. **British Pharmacopoeia.** A book published periodically under the auspices of the General Medical Council. All drugs included in this book are said to be "official". **Extra Pharmacopoeia.** A periodic (every 4 or 5 years) publication, under the auspices of the Pharmaceutical Society of Great Britain, giving technical information about official and non-official drugs, for the use of doctors, pharmacists and others. Also called *Martindale's Extra Pharmacopoeia.* **Pharmacopoeia Internationalis, International Pharmacopoeia.** A pharmacopoeia published under the auspices of the World Health Organization with the object of establishing an international nomenclature and internationally agreed standards for the preparation of drugs. [Gk *pharmakon* drug, *poiein* to make.]

pharmacopoeial (far·mah·ko·**pe**'·al). Relating to the pharmacopoeia; denoting a drug listed in the pharmacopoeia, therefore official.

pharmacopsychosis (far·mah·ko·si·**ko**'·sis). Any of the mental disorders caused by addiction to drugs, alcohol or poisons. [Gk *pharmakon* drug, psychosis.]

pharmacotherapeutic (far·mah·ko·ther·ap·**ew**'·tik). Relating to pharmacotherapy.

pharmacotherapeutics (far·mah·ko·ther·ap·**ew**'·tix). That branch of therapeutics associated with the use of drugs. [see foll.]

pharmacotherapy (far·mah·ko·**ther**'·ap·e). The treatment of disease with drugs. [Gk *pharmakon* drug, therapy.]

pharmacy (far·mas·e). 1. The art or practice of preparing and dispensing drugs. 2. A druggist's shop. **Chemical pharmacy.** Pharmaceutical chemistry. *See* CHEMISTRY. **Galenic pharmacy.** The pharmacy of drugs which are derived from plants or animals. [Gk *pharmakon* drug.]

Pharmacy and Poisons Act 1933. 1. Provided that every person registered as a pharmacist becomes a member of the Pharmaceutical Society which registers pharmacists and supervises pharmaceutical practice. 2. Provided for the establishment of a Poisons Board to advise the Home Secretary. The Poisons Board prepares the Poisons List. Part I specifies certain poisons required to be sold only by an authorized seller of poisons, i.e. a pharmacist, or one who is under the direct supervision of a pharmacist, on registered premises. Part II specifies other poisons in common use for other purposes than the treatment of human ailments which the public may obtain, and these may be sold by anybody whose name is on the local authority's list. Part II includes such substances as spirit of salt, disinfectants, etc. Normally Part I poisons may only be sold upon a prescription of a duly qualified medical practitioner, dentist or veterinary surgeon, but (except certain poisons in Schedule IV) may be sold without prescription provided that the purchaser is known to the vendor and that the purchaser signs an entry in the poisons register.

See also: MISUSE OF DRUGS ACT 1971; POISONS ACT 1972.

pharyngalgia (far·in·**gal**·je·ah). Pain in the pharynx. [pharynx, Gk *algos* pain.]

pharyngeal (far·**in**·je·al). Belonging or relating to the pharynx.

pharyngeal artery, ascending [arteria pharyngea ascendens (NA)]. The smallest branch of the external carotid artery, arising on its medial side. It runs upwards on the wall of the pharynx, which it supplies [rami pharyngei (NA)], and gives branches also to the middle ear [arteria tympanica inferior (NA)] and to the dura mater of the middle and posterior cranial fossae [arteria meningea posterior (NA)].

pharyngeal nerve [ramus pharyngeus (NA)]. A branch which passes back from the pterygopalatine nerves through the palatinovaginal canal to the mucous membrane of the nasopharynx.

pharyngeal veins [venae pharyngeae (NA)]. Veins which arise in a venous plexus around the pharynx and end in the internal jugular vein or its tributary.

pharyngectasia (far·in·jek·**ta**'·se·ah). Pharyngocele. [pharynx, Gk *ektasis* a stretching.]

pharyngectomy (far·in·**jek**'·to·me). An operation in which a portion of the pharynx is removed. [pharynx, Gk *ektome* a cutting out.]

pharyngemphraxis (far·in·jem·**frax**'·is). Pharyngeal obstruction. [pharynx, Gk *emphrassein* to block up.]

pharyngism, pharyngismus (far·in·jizm, far·in·**jiz**·mus). Pharyngospasm. [pharynx.]

pharyngitic (far·in·**jit**·ik). Relating or belonging to, having the characteristics of, or suffering from pharyngitis.

pharyngitis (far·in·**ji**·tis). Inflammation of the pharynx; it may be due to organismal infection, or to reflex disturbance from another part of the body, such as the gastrointestinal tract, or the pelvis, particular in the female. **Acute pharyngitis.** An acute inflammation of the pharynx. **Atrophic pharyngitis.** Inflammation of the pharynx associated with dryness and atrophy of the mucosa. **Catarrhal pharyngitis.** A catarrhal inflammation of the pharynx, as found in the common cold. **Chronic pharyngitis.** Chronic inflammation of the pharynx, often associated with the formation of lymphoid granules in the pharyngeal mucosa. **Croupous pharyngitis.** Pharyngitis associated with the formation of a false membrane. **Diphtheritic pharyngitis.** Pharyngitis due to invasion with the bacillus of diphtheria, and associated with the formation of a false membrane. **Follicular pharyngitis.** A pharyngitis associated with inflammation of the lymphatic follicles of the region. **Gangrenous pharyngitis.** A rapidly acute and most commonly fatal pharyngitis with gangrenous patches and the formation of sloughs in the lining. **Granular pharyngitis.** Chronic inflammation of the pharynx associated with hypertrophy of the isolated lymphatic follicles of the region and particularly the lateral pharyngeal bands. **Pharyngitis herpetica.** Herpetic inflammation of the pharynx. **Hypertrophic pharyngitis.** Pharyngitis associated with the thickening of the lining in general, and the lymphoid bands in particular. **Pharyngitis keratosa.** A condition where the formation of stalactite-like, horny outgrowths of cornified epithelial cells appear on the lymphoid tissue of the pharynx. **Lithaemic pharyngitis.** An inflammation of the pharynx resulting from a disturbance in the metabolism of the nitrogenous elements in the blood. **Membranous pharyngitis.** Inflammation of the pharynx associated with the formation of false membrane, usually due to diphtheritic infection. **Phlegmonous pharyngitis.** Acute parenchymatous inflammation of the pharynx, with the formation of abscesses. **Pharyngitis sicca.** A form of atrophic pharyngitis, with excessive drying and crusting. **Ulcerative pharyngitis.** A septic ulcerative condition of the pharynx. It used to be found fairly commonly in old-fashioned, badly ventilated hospital wards. [pharynx, Gk *-itis* inflammation.]

pharyngo-amygdalitis (far·ing·go·am·ig·dal·**i**′·tis). Pharyngotonsillitis. [pharynx, Gk *amygdale* almond, *-itis* inflammation.]

pharyngocele (far·**ing**·go·seel). 1. Herniation of a portion of the pharynx. 2. A diverticulum or cystic malformation of the pharynx. [pharynx, Gk *kele* hernia.]

pharyngodynia (far·**ing**·go·**din**′·e·ah). Pain affecting the pharynx. [pharynx, Gk *odyne* pain.]

pharyngo-epiglottic, pharyngo-epiglottidean (far·**ing**·go·ep·e·glot′·ik, far·ing·go·ep·e·glot·**id**′·e·an). Relating or belonging to the pharynx and the epiglottis.

pharyngoglossal (far·**ing**·go·**glos**′·al). Belonging or relating to the pharynx and the tongue. [pharynx, Gk *glossa* tongue.]

pharyngoglossus (far·**ing**·go·**glos**′·us). Those fibres of the superior constrictor muscle of the pharynx which are attached to the tongue. [see prec.]

pharyngokeratosis (far·**ing**·go·ker·at·**o**′·sis). Keratosis pharyngis.

pharyngolaryngeal (far·**ing**·go·lar·in·**je**′·al). Relating to both pharynx and larynx.

pharyngolaryngectomy (far·**ing**·go·lar·in·**jek**′·to·me). Surgical removal of the hypopharynx and larynx. [pharynx, larynx, Gk *ektome* excision.]

pharyngolaryngitis (far·**ing**·go·lar·in·**ji**′·tis). Inflammation affecting the pharynx and the larynx together. [pharynx, larynx, Gk *-itis* inflammation.]

pharyngolith (far·**ing**·go·lith). A calculus or concretion in the walls of the pharynx. [pharynx, Gk *lithos* stone.]

pharyngology (far·ing·**gol**·o·je). That branch of medical science which is concerned with the pharynx and the diseases and disorders to which it is subject. [pharynx, Gk *logos* science.]

pharyngolysis (far·ing·**gol**·is·is). Pharyngoparalysis. [pharynx, Gk *lysis* a loosing.]

pharyngomaxillary (far·**ing**·go·max·**il**′·a·re). Relating or belonging to both the pharynx and jaw. [pharynx, maxilla.]

pharyngomycosis (far·**ing**·go·mi·**ko**′·sis). Any lesion of the pharyngeal mucous membrane which is due to invasion by fungi. [pharynx, mycosis.]

pharyngonasal (far·**ing**·go·**na**′·zal). Belonging or relating to both the pharynx and the nose. [pharynx, L *nasus* nose.]

pharyngo-oesophageal (far·**ing**·go·e·sof·ah·**je**′·al). Relating or belonging to the pharynx and the oesophagus.

pharyngo-oesophagus (far·**ing**·go·e·**sof**′·ag·us). The pharynx and oesophagus considered as a single structure.

pharyngo-oral (far·**ing**·go·**or**′·al). Belonging to the pharynx and the mouth. [pharynx, L *os* mouth.]

pharyngopalatine (far·**ing**·go·**pal**′·at·ine). Belonging to the pharynx and the palate.

pharyngoparalysis (far·**ing**·go·par·**al**′·is·is). Paralysis affecting the muscles of the pharynx.

pharyngoperistole (far·**ing**·go·per·**is**′·to·le). Pharyngostenosis. [pharynx, Gk *peristellein* to contract.]

pharyngoplasty (far·**ing**·go·plas·te). Plastic or reparative surgery of the pharynx. [pharynx, Gk *plassein* to mould.]

pharyngoplegia (far·**ing**·go·**ple**′·je·ah). Pharyngoparalysis. [pharynx, Gk *plege* stroke.]

pharyngorhinitis (far·**ing**·go·ri·**ni**′·tis). Inflammation affecting the nasal part of the pharynx. [pharynx, rhinitis.]

pharyngorhinoscopy (far·**ing**·go·ri·**nos**′·ko·pe). Examination of the nasal part of the pharynx and posterior nares with the rhinoscope.

pharyngorrhagia (far·**ing**·go·**ra**′·je·ah). Bleeding from the pharynx. [pharynx, Gk *rhegnynein* to gush forth.]

pharyngorrhoea (far·**ing**·go·re′·ah). A mucoid discharge from the pharynx. [pharynx, Gk *rhoia* flow.]

pharyngosalpingitis (far·**ing**·go·sal·pin·**ji**′·tis). Inflammation of the pharynx and the pharyngotympanic tube. [pharynx, salpingitis.]

pharyngoscleroma (far·**ing**·go·skler·**o**′·mah). A pharyngeal scleroma, the induration affecting the mucous membrane.

pharyngoscope (far·**ing**·go·skope). An instrument used in inspection of the pharyngeal mucosa. [pharynx, *skopein* to watch.]

pharyngoscopy (far·ing·**gos**·ko·pe). Inspection of the pharynx by means of the pharyngoscope.

pharyngospasm (far·**ing**·go·spazm). Spasmodic contraction of the muscles of the pharynx.

pharyngospasmodic (far·**ing**·go·spaz·**mod**′·ik). Pertaining to spasm of the constrictor muscles of the pharynx.

pharyngostaphylinus (far·**ing**·go·staf·il·**i**′·nus). The palatopharyngeus muscle. [pharynx, Gk *staphyle* uvula.]

pharyngostenosis (far·**ing**·go·sten·**o**′·sis). Stenosis of the pharyngeal lumen.

pharyngostenous (far·**ing**·go·**ste**′·nus). Pertaining to stricture or narrowing of the lumen of the pharynx. [pharynx, Gk *stenos* narrow.]

pharyngotherapy (far·**ing**·go·**ther**′·ap·e). Treatment of any disease of the pharynx. [pharynx, therapy.]

pharyngotomy (far·ing·**got**·o·me). An operation for the exposure and exploration of the pharynx or pharyngeal tube. **Anterior pharyngotomy.** The operative approach to the pharynx through its anterior wall. **External pharyngotomy.** Any operation where an external approach is made to the pharynx. **Lateral pharyngotomy.** An approach to the pharynx and hypopharynx from the side of the neck, as opposed to a midline approach. **Lateral transhyoid pharyngotomy.** An approach to the pharynx from the side, with removal of part of the hyoid bone. **Subhyoid pharyngotomy, Subhyoidean pharyngotomy.** An approach to the pharynx through the thyrohyoid membrane. [pharynx, Gk *temnein* to cut.]

pharyngotonsillitis (far·**ing**·go·ton·sil·**i**′·tis). Inflammation affecting the pharynx and the tonsil. [pharynx, tonsillitis.]

pharyngoxerosis (far·**ing**·go·zer·**o**′·sis). Xerosis of the pharynx. [pharynx, Gk *xeros* dry.]

pharynx [NA] (**far**·ingx). The part of the foregut which extends from the base of the skull above to the beginning of the oesophagus at the level of the 6th cervical vertebra. It lies anterior to the upper six cervical vertebrae and prevertebral muscles and behind the nasal cavities, mouth and larynx. Its walls are formed of fibrous tissue reinforced with muscles. It is subdivided into *(a)* the nasopharynx [pars nasalis (NA)], the most superior part, receiving the openings of the posterior nares anteriorly and the pharyngotympanic tubes laterally, and purely respiratory in function; *(b)* the oral part [pars oralis (NA)] which lies behind the mouth and is both respiratory and alimentary in fuction, and *(c)* the laryngeal part [pars laryngea (NA)] lying behind the larynx which opens into its anterior wall. The latter part is alimentary and respiratory in function, except below the opening of the larynx where it is only alimentary. [Gk, throat.]

pharynx, constrictor muscles of the. Three muscles on either side of the pharynx, the superior [musculus constrictor pharyngis superior (NA)], the middle [musculus constrictor pharyngis medius (NA)] and the inferior [musculus constrictor pharyngis inferior (NA)], inserted mainly into the median raphe. The superior arises from the medial pterygoid lamina [pars pterygopharyngeal (NA)], buccopharyngeal part [pars buccopharyngea (NA)], the mandible [pars mylopharyngea (NA)] and the tongue [pars glossopharyngea (NA)]; the middle arises from the stylohyoid ligament [pars chondropharyngea (NA)] and the cornua of the hyoid bone [pars ceratopharyngea (NA)]; the inferior arises from the thyroid [pars thyreopharyngea (NA)] and cricoid cartilages [pars cricopharyngea (NA)].

phase (faze). 1. The appearance at any one moment of a thing which undergoes change, usually a cyclic change. 2. The stage which any pathological condition or physiological process has reached at any given moment. 3. Term applied to each of the homogeneous parts separated from each other by surfaces which go to make up a heterogeneous system, e.g. ice, water and water vapour. 4. In a wave motion, the displacement of any point from the central position, e.g. points at the tops of successive crests are said to be in equal phase. **Bacterial phase.** Phases of growth: when a medium is inoculated there is first a lag phase when the organisms enlarge but do not divide; this is followed by a phase of active division, the *logarithmic phase.* Later, division ceases and the stationary phase occurs. Finally, the cells begin to die; this is referred to as the *phase of decline.* Certain bacteria, in particular the *Salmonella,* are subject to diphasic variation in their flagellar antigens; the specific phase is known as *phase I* and the group phase as *phase II.* **Continuous phase.** Disperse medium. *See* MEDIUM. **Phase of decline.** That period in the growth of a bacterial culture when the viable count is falling. **Discontinuous phase.** Disperse phase (see foll.). **Disperse phase.** The phase of a colloidal solution corresponding to the solute of a true solution. **Ejection phase.** Ejection time. *See* TIME. **Erythrocytic phase.** With reference to the life cycle of the plasmodium, the period when it lies within the erythrocyte. **External phase.** Disperse medium. *See* MEDIUM. **Group phase.** Bacterial phase (see above). **Internal phase.** Disperse phase (see above). **Isometric relaxation phase.** Isometric relaxation. *See* RELAXATION. **Lag phase.** An early phase after inoculation of medium when the organisms enlarge but do not multiply. **Logarithmic phase.** The phase of active division of bacteria in a culture medium. **Maximal ejection phase.** The period early during ventricular systole when blood is being rapidly ejected. **Phase of meditation.** The latent interval between the causative stimulus and the appearance of a psychogenic state. **Meiotic phase.** That phase of oögenesis and spermatogenesis in which the number of chromosomes per cell is halved. **Motofacient phase.** That phase of muscular activity during which movement occurs. **Negative phase.** That part of the cycle of an artifical ventilating machine when the pressure is subatmospheric. **Non-motofacient phase.** That phase of muscular activity during which tension alters but no movement occurs. **Positive phase.** A rise in antibody after booster doses of antigen. **Post-meiotic phase.** The phase after the meiotic phase (see above). **Premeiotic phase.** The phase before the meiotic phase (see above). **Premenstrual phase.** The secretory phase of the endometrium. **Prereduction phase.** Premeiotic phase (see above). **Proliferative phase.** The building up of the uterine mucosa which follows menstruation and precedes ovulation. **Protodiastolic phase.** Protodiastole. **Reduced ejection phase.** The period late during ventricular systole when the ejection of the blood is slackening. **Reduction phase.** Meiotic phase (see above). **Specific phase.** Bacterial phase (see above). **Stationary phase.** That period in the growth of a bacterial culture when the viable count is neither increasing nor decreasing. **Synaptic phase.** The meiotic phase in which homologous chromosomes unite in pairs. [Gk *phasis* appearance.]

phase reversal (faze re·ver·sal). Deflections of similar form but opposite sign in two contiguous electro-encephalographic channels linked by the bipolar method: indicative of a focus beneath the common electrode. [phase, L *reversus* turned back.]

phaseolunatin (fa·se·o·loon′·a·tin). $C_{10}H_{17}O_6N$, a glycoside obtained from the lima bean, *Phaseolus lunatus.*

phasin, phasine (fa·sin, fa·seen). A type of vegetable protein that agglutinates erythrocytes.

phasmid (faz·mid). A causal chemoceptor of certain nematodes. [Gk *phasma* apparition.]

Phasmidia (faz·mid·e·ah). A class of the phylum Nematoda, or subclass when Nematoda is treated as a class; characterized by the presence of phasmids. [see prec.]

phasmophobia (faz·mo·fo·be·ah). Fear of ghosts. [Gk *phasma* apparition, *phobein* to fear.]

phatnorrhagia (fat·no·ra·je·ah). Haemorrhage from a dental alveolus. [Gk *phatne* manger, *rhegnynein* to gush forth.]

phatnorrhoea (fat·no·re·ah). Pyorrhoea alveolaris. [Gk *phatne* manger, *rhoia* flow.]

phellandral (fel·an·dral). $C_{10}H_{16}O$, an aldehydic terpene occurring in water-fennel oil.

phellandrene (fel·an·dreen). One of a group of isomers of formula $C_{10}H_{16}$ occurring as constituents of volatile oils (fennel, cinnamon, eucalyptus, etc.), and classified as monocyclic terpenes. They are of little medical importance.

phellandrium (fel·an·dre·um). The fruits of the water fennel, *Phellandrium aquaticum* Linn. (= *Oenanthe phellandrium* Lamk.) of the family Umbelliferae. They have been used in chronic bronchial affections. [Gk *phellandrion.*]

Phelps, Abel Mix (b. 1851). New York surgeon.

Phelps' operation. Operative correction of talipes by division of the tight structures in the sole and removal of a wedge of bone.

Phelps' splint. A metal splint used in the treatment of talipes equinovarus.

Phemister, Dallas Burton (b. 1882). Chicago orthopaedic surgeon.

Phemister graft. A technique of sliver onlay bone grafting of ununited fractures without disturbing the pseudo-arthrosis.

phemitone (fem·e·tone). Methylphenobarbitone.

phenacaine (fen·ah·kane). Ethenyl-*p*-diethoxy-diphenyl-amidine, $(C_2H_5OC_6H_4N)C(CH_3){=}(NHC_6H_4OC_2H_5)$. A colourless synthetic compound employed as a local anaesthetic. **Phenacaine hydrochloride.** A soluble derivative of value in the production of anaesthesia of the eye.

Phenacemide (fen·as·em·ide). BP Commission approved name for (phenylacetyl)urea, $C_6H_5CH_2CONHCONH_2$. A drug used in the treatment of epilepsy; it is most useful in the psychomotor types of seizure which are difficult to control with anticonvulsants. It should not be used in persons with liver dysfunction or in those who are liable to personality disorders. Nausea and vomiting are common symptoms, and fever, rashes and jaundice may be caused.

Phenacetin BP 1973 (fen·as·et·in). Aceto phenetidin, $CH_3CONHC_6H_4OC_2H_5$. A compound used medicinally as an analgesic. It is a safer antipyretic than acetanilide.

Phenacetinum. *European Pharmacopoeia* name for Phenacetin BP 1973.

phenacetolin (fen·as·et·o·lin). $C_{16}H_{12}O_2$, a compound employed as an indicator for pH (5.5–6.5), being brown in acid and red in alkaline solutions.

phenacite (fen·as·ite). A naturally occurring silicate of beryllium.

Phenactropinium Chloride (fen·ak·tro·pin′·e·um klor·ide). BP Commission approved name for *N*-phenacyl-homotropinium chloride; used in the production of controlled hypotension.

Phenadoxone (fen·ah·dox·one). BP Commission approved name for 6-morpholino-4,4-diphenylheptan-3-one, $O(CH_2CH_2)NCH(CH_3)CH_2C(C_6H_5)_2COC_2H_5$, a potent analgesic which, so far, has not shown much tendency to become a drug of addiction. It has only a slight hypnotic action, and does not cause constipation; it is replacing morphine as the drug of choice for the treatment of chronic pain.

Phenaglycodol (fen·ah·gli·ko·dol). BP Commission approved name for 2-*p*-chlorophenyl-3-methylbutane-2,3-diol; a sedative.

phenakistoscope (fen·ak·is·to·skope). A stroboscope. [Gk *phenakistes* imposter, *skopein* to watch.]

phenamidine (fen·am·id·een). 4,4′-Diamidino-diphenyl ether. One of the less successful diamidines used in leishmaniasis and trypanosomiasis; it is also used as an antiseptic.

Phenampromide (fen·am·pro·mide). BP Commission approved name for *N*-(1-methyl-2-piperidinoethyl)propionanilide; a narcotic analgesic.

phenanthrene (fen·an·threen). $C_{14}H_{10}$, a colourless crystalline hydrocarbon isomeric with anthracene and found likewise in coal tar. It dissolves in alcohol with a blue fluorescence. Its peculiar structure of three benzene rings forms the basis of the cyclopentenophenanthrene skeleton from which the sterols, bile acids and sex hormones are built up. [phenol, Gk *anthrax* coal.]

phenarsone sulphoxylate (fen·ar·sone sulf·ox·il·ate). $C_7H_8AsNNa_2O_6S$, the sodium formaldehyde sulphoxylate derivative of 3-amino-4-hydroxybenzene arsonic acid. It is an organic arsenical used for infections of the cervix and vagina by *Trichomonas vaginalis.*

phenate (**fe**·nate). Any salt formed by a phenol as a weak acid with a base, e.g. potassium phenate, C_6H_5OK: they correspond with the alcoholates.

Phenazocine (fen·**az**·o·seen). BP Commission approved name for 1,2,3,4,5,6-hexahydro-8-hydroxy-6,11-dimethyl-3-phenethyl-2,6-methano-3-benzazocine. **Phenazocine Hydrobromide BP 1973.** The hemihydrate of the hydrobromide of phenazocine; an analgesic more powerful, weight for weight, than morphine and, in therapeutic doses, less liable than morphine to cause unpleasant side effects. It is a drug of addiction.

Phenazone BPC 1968 (**fen**·ah·zone). 1-Phenyl-2,3-dimethyl-5-pyrazolone, a colourless, odourless, crystalline solid, having a slightly bitter taste, and soluble in water or alcohol. It is a rapidly acting antipyretic, reducing temperature in fever by depression of the heat centre in the hypothalamus. Its mild and safe analgesic action makes it valuable in the relief of headache and neuralgia. It also has a local haemostatic action. **Phenazone salicylate.** Obtained by heating phenazone and salicylic acid in equimolecular proportions; it is used as an antipyretic and mild analgesic for the treatment of rheumatic ailments and sciatica.

Phenazopyridine (**fen**·az·o·**pi**′·rid·een). BP Commission approved name for 2,6-diamino-3-phenylazopyridine; an analgesic.

Phenbenicillin (**fen**·ben·e·**sil**′·in). BP Commission approved name for α-phenoxybenzylpenicillin; an antibiotic.

Phenbutrazate (fen·**bew**·traz·ate). BP Commission approved name for 2-(3-methyl-2-phenylmorpholino)ethyl 2-phenylbutyrate; an appetite suppressant.

Phencyclidine (fen·**si**·klid·een). BP Commission approved name for 1-(1-phenylcyclohexyl)piperidine); an analgesic.

Phendimetrazine (fen·di·**met**·raz·een). BP Commission approved name for (+)-3,4-dimethyl-2-phenylmorpholine; it is used in the treatment of obesity.

phene (feen). The six-membered benzene ring. [Gk *phainein* to appear.]

Phenelzine (fen·**el**·zeen). BP Commission approved name for phenethylhydrazine; used in anxiety states.

Phenelzine Sulphate BP 1973. Phenethylhydrazine hydrogen sulphate, a white powder with a pungent odour and characteristic taste. A monoamine oxidase inhibitor, it is an effective anti-depressant and is used in the treatment of certain neurotic depressive states.

Phenethicillin (fen·**eth**·is·**il**′·in). BP Commission approved name for 6-(α-phenoxypropionamido)penicillanic acid.

Phenethicillin Potassium BP 1973. A mixture of the potassium salts of 6-D(+)- and 6-L(-)-(α-phenoxypropionamido)penicillanic acid; an antibiotic with many of the actions and uses of penicillin. Like phenoxymethylpenicillin, it can be given by mouth as it is not inactivated by the gastric hydrochloride.

phenetidin (fen·**et**·id·in). *p*-Amino-ethoxybenzene, *p*-ethoxy-aniline, $C_2H_5OC_6H_4NH_2$. The ethyl ether of *p*-aminophenol; upon acetylation it yields phenacetin. **Phenetidin amygdalate.** Amygdophenin.

phenetidinurea (fen·et·id·in·ewr·**e**′·ah). Dulcine.

phenetidinuria (fen·**et**·id·in·**ewr**′·e·ah). Phenetidin in the urine, sometimes as a result of administration of phenacetin.

phenetol, phenetole (**fen**·et·ol, fen·et·**ole**). $C_6H_5OC_2H_5$, an ethereal liquid formed from phenol and ethyl sulphate. Its amino derivative is the starting point of the phenacetin drugs.

Pheneturide (fen·**et**·ewr·ide). BP Commission approved name for (2-phenylbutyryl)urea; an anticonvulsant.

Phenformin (fen·**for**·min). BP Commission approved name for *N*-phenethyldiguanide.

Phenformin Hydrochloride BP 1973. The hydrochloride of *N*-phenethyldiguanide; an oral hypoglycaemic agent used in the treatment of diabetes mellitus.

Phenglutarimide BP 1963 (fen·gloo·**tar**·im·ide). α-2-Diethyl-aminoethyl-α-phenyl glutarimide. The hydrochloride (BPC 1963), a synthetic preparation with atropine-like actions, was formerly used in the treatment of Parkinsonism.

phengophobia (fen·go·**fo**·be·ah). Abnormal dread of daylight; photophobia. [Gk *pheggos* daylight, phobia.]

phenicate (**fen**·e·kate). 1. A phenate or salt of phenol. 2. To treat with phenol for disinfecting purposes.

Phenindamine (fen·**in**·dam·een). BP Commission approved name for 1,2,3,4-tetrahydro-2-methyl-9-phenyl-2-azafluorene, an anti-histaminic, usually administered orally as the hydrogen tartrate. **Phenindamine Tartrate BP 1973.** The form in which the drug is most usually administered.

Phenindione BP 1973 (fen·in·**di**·one). 2-Phenyl indane-1,3-dione, an anticoagulant that has been used in several conditions, including coronary thrombosis. A high initial dose and relatively low maintenance doses are used, and haemorrhage can be controlled with vitamin K.

Pheniodol BP 1958 (fen·**i**·o·dol). β-(4-Hydroxy-3,5-di-iodo-phenyl)-α phenylpropionic acid. An opaque contrast medium used in cholecystography. It is given by mouth only. It has largely superseded iodophthalein, since it is more palatable and less likely to cause vomiting and diarrhoea.

Pheniprazine (fen·**ip**·raz·een). BP Commission approved name for α-methylphenethylhydrazine; it is used in the treatment of depressive conditions.

Pheniramine (fen·**ir**·am·een). BP Commission approved name for 3-dimethylamino-1-phenyl-1-2′-pyridylpropane; an antihistamine.

phenmethylol (fen·**meth**·il·ol). Benzyl alcohol, $C_6H_5CH_2OH$. An aromatic liquid occurring in Peru and tolu balsams; used in perfumery and as a local anaesthetic and anodyne.

Phenmetrazine (fen·**met**·rah·zeen). BP Commission approved name for tetrahydro-3-methyl-2-phenyl-1,4-oxazine. **Phenmetrazine Hydrochloride BP 1973.** 3-Methyl-2-phenylmorpholine hydrochloride, an anorexic agent which has been used in conjunction with dieting in the treatment of obesity.

phenobarbital (fe·no·**bar**·bit·al). Phenobarbitone.

Phenobarbitalum. *European Pharmacopoeia* name for Phenobarbitone BP 1973.

Phenobarbitone BP 1973 (fe·no·**bar**·bit·one). Phenyl ethyl-malonylurea, 5-phenyl-5-ethyl barbituric acid, $(C_6H_5)(C_2H_5)C(CONH)_2{=}CO$. A slow and long-lasting barbiturate; a sedative and hypnotic having a particularly strong action on the motor cortex. It is particularly valuable in the treatment of epilepsy, especially grand mal, but its use is limited owing to the development of a progressive tolerance to the drug. As a sedative it is employed in neurasthenia, hysteria, hyperthyroidism, and chorea, and it is also used in the vomiting of pregnancy and in insomnia. Idiosyncrasy occasionally occurs, urticarial skin eruptions being the commonest reaction, whilst habituation and dependence may result from continuous treatment. Toxic doses cause respiratory depression, for which picrotoxin is the best analeptic. **Phenobarbitone Sodium BP 1973. Soluble phenobarbitone.** The water-soluble sodium derivative of phenobarbitone. Orally, its action is slightly more rapid than that of phenobarbitone, and the aqueous solutions may be administered by injection, but the solutions are unstable.

Phenobutiodil (**fen**·o·bewt·**i**′·o·dil). BP Commission approved name for α-(2,4,6-tri-iodophenoxy) butyric acid; a contrast medium for oral cholecystography and cholangiography.

phenocoll (**fen**·o·kol). *p*-Aminoacetophenetidin, $C_2H_5OC_6H_4NHCOCH_2NH_2$. An analgesic usually used in the form of the hydrochloride, a colourless crystalline solid with a saline taste, and fairly soluble in water. It is employed in the treatment of rheumatic ailments, and also for the relief of neuralgia and headaches.

phenocopy (**fen**·o·kop·e). An organism with features resembling those possessed by a mutation, but resulting from abnormal environmental conditions. [Gk *phainein* to appear, copy.]

phenol (**fe**·nol). 1. Name given to any member of a series of hydroxybenzenes in which one or more hydroxyl groups are linked directly to the benzene nucleus. 2. Carbolic acid, C_6H_5OH, a colourless crystalline compound, slightly soluble in water but more so in alcohol or ether. It is obtained from coal tar and is widely used in industry in the manufacture of plastics, drugs and dyes. It is a weak disinfectant, not greatly affected by the presence of organic matter, and, because of the absence of marked selective action, provides a convenient standard for other disinfectants (Rideal–Walker coefficient). Though the first disinfectant to be extensively used, it is seldom employed now since it is toxic to tissue cells in the concentrations that will kill bacteria. It is chiefly used for sanitary purposes, though still prescribed in mouth-washes and gargles, and because of its local anaesthetic properties is of value in the treatment of urticarial skin conditions. It may also be used locally as a cauterizing agent (BP 1973). **Phenol bismuth.** Bismuth phenolate, $C_6H_5OBi(OH)_2$, an insoluble white powder containing a variable amount of phenol combined with bismuth oxide. It is used as an internal disinfectant, as it slowly liberates phenol in the intestine. **Phenol camphor.** Carbolic camphor, a fungistatic and local anaesthetic, used to relieve itching of the skin and in epidermophytosis, though it may cause tissue damage. **Iodized phenol.** 10 per cent iodine in liquefied phenol, used in ringworm of the scalp and in chronic hydrocele. **Liquefied Phenol BP 1973.** 80 per cent phenol made by adding water to phenol. It is more easily handled than phenol and is used in lotions, gargles and mouth-washes. **Phenol red.** Phenolsulphonphthalein. **Phenol salicylate.** Salol, $OHC_6H_4COOC_6H_5$, a compound of phenol and salicylic acid which, given by mouth, is hydrolysed in the intestine, liberating phenol. It has been used as an intestinal antiseptic in the treatment of enteritis, but it is impossible to administer a sufficiently high dose without toxic effects. It has also been used in rheumatism. **Phenol sulphoricinate.** A solution of phenol in sulphoricinic acid; a 20 per cent solution is used in tuberculosis of the throat. [Gk *phainein* to appear, L *oleum* oil.]

phenolaemia (fe·nol·e·me·ah). A condition marked by the existence of phenols in the blood. [phenol, Gk *haima* blood.]

phenolase (fe·nol·aze). Phenol oxidase, an enzyme which activates the oxidation of phenolic compounds in the metabolism.

phenolate (fe·nol·ate). 1. A salt of phenol corresponding with an alcoholate. 2. To treat with phenol for disinfecting purposes; to phenicate.

phenolated (fe·nol·a·ted). 1. Having phenol as a main constituent. 2. Disinfected with phenol.

phenolic (fe·nol·ik). Relating to or obtained from phenol.

phenolipoid (fe·no·lip·oid). Phenololipoid.

phenolization (fe·nol·i·za′·shun). The method of treating contaminated wounds with a strong solution of phenol (carbolic acid).

phenologist (fen·ol·o·jist). One who has made a special study of the science of phenology.

phenology (fen·ol·o·je). The study of climatic effects on living things. [Gk *phainein* to appear, *logos* discourse.]

phenoloid (fe·nol·oid). Substances of phenolic character such as cresols and xylenols. [Obsolete term.] [phenol, Gk *eidos* form.]

phenololipoid (fe·nol·o·lip′·oid). A compound of phenol and camphor with a sterol such as cholesterol, employed therapeutically for its bactericidal properties.

Phenolphthalein BP 1973 (fe·nol·thal·e·in). Dihydroxyphthalophenone, dihydroxytriphenylmethane 2-carboxylic acid anhydride; a triphenylmethane derivative obtained by heating phenol with phthalic anhydride in the presence of concentrated sulphuric acid. It is a colourless compound, slightly soluble in water, used as an indicator (pH 8.2–10.0). It is tasteless and odourless, and is a powerful cathartic acting directly on the wall of the bowel causing a copious watery secretion within 6–8 hours of administration.

phenolphthaline (fe·nol·thal·een). $(C_6H_4OH)_2CHC_6H_4COOH$, a reduction product of phenolphthalein.

phenolquinine (fe·nol·kwin·een). Quinine carbolate, QuC_6H_5OH, a slightly soluble compound chiefly used as an antiseptic.

phenolsulphonate (fe·nol·sul·fon·ate). A salt or ester of phenosulphonic acid.

Phenolsulphonphthalein BP 1968 (fe·nol·sul·fon·thal′·e·in). A triphenylmethane dye derived from phenol and *o*-sulphobenzoic acid anhydride. It is a bright red crystalline compound, soluble in water, and used as an indicator (pH 6.8–8.4). Its sodium salt is injected intravenously and its rate of appearance in the urine noted as a test of renal function.

phenoltetrachlorphthalein (fe·nol·tet·rah·klor·thal′·e·in). $[NaOOCC_6H_4C(C_6H_2Cl_2ONa){=}(C_6H_2Cl_2{=}O)]\cdot 3H_2O$, a triphenylmethane dye obtained by condensing phenol with tetrachlorphthalic anhydride. It is a deep purple compound used in a test for hepatic function, since it is removed from the blood stream almost exclusively by the liver.

phenoltetraiodophthalein (fe·nol·tet·rah·i·o·do·thal′·e·in). Iodophthalein, $[NaOOCC_6H_4C(C_6H_2I_2ONa){=}(C_6H_2I_2O)]\cdot 3H_2O$. The disodium salt of tetraiodophenolphthalein; a dark blue crystalline solid, soluble in water to give a deep blue solution which exhibits the phenomenon of dichroism. It is used in radiography of the biliary tract on account of its being opaque to x-rays and its secretion by the liver in the bile. It may be administered orally or intravenously.

phenoluria (fe·nol·ewr·e·ah). A condition marked by the existence of phenols in the urine.

phenome (fen·ome). The outward visible expression of a genetically determined characteristic. [Gk *phainein* to appear.]

phenomenon (fen·om·en·on). An observed fact or event; an objective sign; a remarkable occurrence. **Abstinence phenomenon.** Unpleasant symptoms such as insomnia, restlessness, occurring after withdrawal of a drug from an addict. **Anaphylactoid phenomenon.** Anaphylactoid reaction. *See* REACTION. **Arm phenomenon.** Pool's phenomenon. **Autokinetic phenomenon.** The illusion of apparent movement in an object seen, the impression being not quite the same as real movement, and somewhat different for various observers. **Blanching phenomenon.** *See* SCHULTZ-CHARLTON PHENOMENON. **Brake phenomenon.** The tendency of muscle to be maintained in its resting position owing to the activity of antagonistic muscles. **Break-off phenomenon.** A sensation of being separated from the earth sometimes described as being poised on a knife-edge, which may be felt at altitudes above 9000 m (30 000 ft). This symptom may cause apprehension. At these heights the horizon is below the pilot's gaze; the absence of orientating cues may be the cause of the phenomenon. **Cervicolumbar phenomenon.** Sensations which may occur in the neck when a lesion exists in the lower part of the spinal cord or alternatively weakness and sensory phenomena in the lower limbs occurring on neck movement in cervical-cord disease. **Cheek phenomenon.** Pressure on the cheeks below the zygoma, in cases of meningitis, may result in flexion of both arms with upward jerking. **Cogwheel phenomenon.** 1. The discontinuous and therefore jerky resistance offered to passive stretching by a hypertonic muscle; negro phenomenon. 2. The type of muscular rigidity which may be noted in advanced cases of paralysis agitans; the muscles show a plastic rigidity on passive stretching, which progresses in an intermittent, jerky manner. **Conglutinin phenomenon.** Conglutination reaction. *See* REACTION. **Dental phenomenon.** Faradic stimulation of hyperaesthetic areas on the body surface gives rise, in the presence of toothache, to sensations in the gums. **Diaphragm phenomenon.** Litten's sign; using oblique illumination, changes in the contour of the thorax may be seen to accompany respiration, and to be related to movements of the diaphragm. **Doll's head phenomenon.** Contralateral deviation of the eyes on rapid passive movement of the head; a normal reflex. **Entopic phenomena.** The perception, under certain conditions, of opacities or opaque bodies situated in the eye in front of the perceptive layer of the retina, either in the media, retinal circulation, or deeper layers of the retina. Also the perception of halos caused by the diffraction of light by the cornea, or lens, and the perception of variegated forms of light seen in the dark; the latter also called *intrinsic light of the retina, light chaos,* or *luminous dust.* **Face phenomenon, Facialis phenomenon.** A condition, present in hypoparathyroidism, in which a twitch of the facial muscles occurs when the skin of the face is tapped over the facial nerve. Obsolete term; the sign is now known as *Chvostek's sign.*

Finger phenomenon. Involuntary extension and separation of the fingers on raising the arm in case of hemiparesis; also called *Souques' phenomenon.* **Flicker phenomenon.** The rate at which objects can be merged before the eyes. **Foot phenomenon.** Ankle clonus. *See* CLONUS. **Great-toe phenomenon.** Babinski's sign. **Hip-flexion phenomenon.** If a patient with spastic paralysis of one or both lower limbs attempts to sit up from the supine position the movement begins with flexion at the affected hip joint or joints; a similar movement occurs on lying down. **Interference phenomenon.** 1. The prevention or alteration of the pharmacological or therapeutic action of one drug by another. 2. A protective mechanism against viruses, in which a less harmful virus (the interfering virus) enters and multiplies in living host cells, or is adsorbed on to them. When a second more virulent virus comes along, entry to the cell is blocked. **Isomorphic phenomenon.** Koebner's phenomenon. **Jaw-winking phenomenon.** Jaw-winking syndrome. *See* SYNDROME. **Knee phenomenon.** The knee jerk; the reflex of the patellar tendon. **LE phenomenon.** The formation of LE cells in the blood of a patient with systemic lupus erythematosus. **Leg phenomenon.** Schlesinger's sign; flexion of the hip joint with a bent knee causes an extensor spasm of the knee and supination of the foot (present in tetany). **Lip phenomenon.** Reflex movements of the lips in sleeping babies when the angle of the mouth is tapped. **Lupus erythematosus cell phenomenon.** Antinuclear factor (antibodies) in the blood of patients with lupus erythematosus which react with the nuclei of dead or damaged leucocytes, the resultant distorted nuclei subsequently being ingested by phagocytic leucocytes to form lupus erythematosus (LE) cells. **Metallic phenomenon.** The metallic coin sound or bell note heard over a pneumothorax. **Muscle phenomenon.** Myotatic irritability. *See* IRRITABILITY. **Neck phenomenon.** Brudzinski's sign. **Negro phenomenon.** Cogwheel phenomenon 1st def. (see above). **Orbicularis phenomenon.** Pilcz-Westphal phenomenon. **Overflow phenomenon.** The spread of a reflex from one side of the body to the other. **Palmoplantar phenomenon.** Filipovitch's sign; yellow coloration of the prominent parts of the palms and soles in typhoid fever. **Paradoxical diaphragm phenomenon.** The paralysed side of the diaphragm moves upwards on inspiration and downwards on expiration, the reverse of the movement on the sound side. **Paradoxical phenomenon of dystonia.** Hunt's paradoxical phenomenon. **Peroneal-nerve phenomenon.** Lust's phenomenon. **Phrenic phenomenon.** Diaphragm phenomenon (see above). **Platysma phenomenon.** Strong contraction of the platysma of the unaffected side when the mouth is opened wide in hemiplegia. **Pronation phenomenon.** Immediate involuntary pronation of the forearm on the affected side in hemiplegia after both forearms have been passively supinated. **Prozone phenomenon.** The existence of a region of the dilution range among the low dilutions in which an antiserum fails to agglutinate the homologous bacteria, although it agglutinates it in higher dilutions. This phenomenon also occurs in tests for titres of bacteriolytic and precipitating sera. **Puppet-head phenomenon.** Sudden elevation of the eyes after forward flexion of the head in postencephalitic patients. **Radial phenomenon.** Dorsal extension of the wrist occurring when the fingers are flexed. **Rash extinction phenomenon.** Schultz-Charlton phenomenon. **Rebound phenomenon.** The tendency for antagonistic muscles to contract spontaneously as soon as stimulation of a group of muscles ceases. When the examiner grasps the patient's wrist and attempts to draw the arm into extension against the patient's resistance and then suddenly releases the wrist the patient's hand rebounds towards his body. The phenomenon indicates motor disorder due to cerebellar lesion. **Release phenomenon.** Unmasking of the activity of a lower nervous centre when a higher controlling centre is inhibited or destroyed. **Second set phenomenon.** The increased rapidity of rejection of a second transplant of skin or other tissue from the same donor to the same recipient. **Spring-like phenomenon.** Rebound phenomenon (see above). **Staircase phenomenon.** Treppe; increase in force of muscular contraction in response to the first few of a series of constant stimuli. The phenomenon is due to the beneficial accumulation of products of contraction, until finally a steady state is reached. **Phenomenon of successive contrast.** The seeing of an after-image of an opposite kind to the original image, when the stimulus is replaced by one of similar or of a different type. Thus, after a circular area of white light has been looked at for a period, if a larger and square area of similar light is then stared at, there will be a dark patch in the centre of the square of the same size and shape as the original stimulus. Again, if a red book is looked at and then the gaze shifted to a square area of white light, there will be a green patch (the complementary colour) in the centre, the same size as the red book. **Super-cooling phenomenon.** The cooling of living cytoplasm to much lower degrees than would be expected, in order to produce solidification and death of the tissue. **Tibial phenomenon.** Struempell's sign. **Toe phenomenon.** Babinski's sign. **Tongue phenomenon.** Contraction of the tongue produced by tapping it (present in tetany). **Ulnar phenomenon.** Analgesia of the ulnar nerve observed in some psychoses. **Zone phenomenon.** Inhibition of agglutination or other antigen-antibody reaction by excess of either reagent. [Gk *phainomenon* anything seen.]

See also: ARTHUS, ASCHNER, AUBERT, BABINSKI, BELL (C.), BORDET, BRANHAM, BRAY, BROWN (R.), CHARLTON, CHEYNE (J.), CUSHING (HARVEY W.), DALE, DANYSZ, DEBRÉ, DÉJÉRINE, D'HERELLE, DOERING, DONATH, DOPPLER (C. J.), DUCKWORTH, DU NOÜY, DUPUY-DUTEMPS, ERB, ERBEN, FÅHRAEUS, FILIPOVITCH, FLINT, FRIEDREICH, GAERTNER (G.), GAUSSEL, GENGOU, GERHARDT (C. C. A. J.), GERSUNY, GOWERS, GRAEFE, GRASSET, GUNN, HAMMERSCHLAG, HATA, HECHT, HEIDENHAIN, HERING (H. E.), HIRST, HOCHSINGER, HOFFMANN (J.), HOLMES (G. M.), HOUSSAY, HUNT (J. R.), KIENBOECK, KOCH (R.), KOEBNER, KOHNSTAMM, KUEHNE (W.), LANDSTEINER, LEEDE, LEICHTENSTERN, LICHTHEIM, LIESEGANG, LITTEN, LUST, NEISSER (E.), NEISSER (M.), NEUFELD, ORBELI, OSLER, PERRONCITO, PFEIFFER (R. F. J.), PILCZ (A.), POOL, PORRET, PURKINJE, QUECKENSTEDT, QUINQUAUD, RAYNAUD, RIEGER, RITTER (J. W.), ROLLET (A.), RUMPEL, RUST, SCHRAMM, SCHUELLER (A.), SCHULTZ, SCHWARTZMANN, SHERRINGTON, SINKLER, SOLOVIEFF, SOUQUES, STOKES (WILLIAM), STRAUS, STRUEMPELL, TRAUBE (L.), TROUSSEAU, TULLIO, TWORT, TYNDALL, VON STOCKERT, VULPIAN, WARTENBERG, WECHSBERG, WEDENSKY, WESTPHAL (A. K. O.), WESTPHAL (C. F. O.), WEVER, WILLIAMS (C. J. B.).

Phenomorphan (fe·no·mor·fan). BP Commission approved name for 3-hydroxy-*N*-(2-phenylethyl)morphinan; a potential drug of addiction.

phenone (fe·none). One of a family of mixed ketones which incorporate a phenyl group with a methyl radical or its homologue, e.g. acetophenone, $C_6H_5COCH_3$.

Phenoperidine (fe·no·per·id·een). BP Commission approved name for ethyl 1-(3-hydroxy-3-phenylpropyl)-4-phenylpiperidine-4-carboxylate; a narcotic analgesic with actions similar to those of morphine. It has been used with a major tranquillizer or sedative, e.g. droperidol to produce neuroleptanalgesia.

Phenoprobamate (fe·no·pro·bam·ate). BP Commission approved name for 3-phenylpropyl carbamate; a skeletal muscle relaxant.

Phenothiazine (fe·no·thi·az·een). Thiodiphenylamine, C_6H_4=S NH)=C_6H_4. A light yellow crystalline compound which is the parent of a number of important dyes. It is insoluble in water but soluble in organic solvents such as alcohol or acetone. It is toxic to both threadworm and roundworm in man, but owing to its toxicity is restricted as an anthelminthic to veterinary practice.

phenotype (fen·o·tipe). The organism itself as opposed to its genetic constitution, the genotype. The same phenotype may appear even when the genotype is different, e.g. homozygotes, and heterozygotes where an allelomorph is dominant. Different phenotypes may appear even when the genotype is the same, as a result of differences of environment during development. **Rh phenotypes.** The antigenic properties of individuals which result from the action of different alleles at the Rh locus. [Gk *phainein* to appear, *typos* type.]

phenotypical (fen·o·tip·ik·al). Relating or belonging to phenotypes.

phenoxin (fe·nox·in). Carbon tetrachloride.

Phenoxybenzamine (fen·ox·e·ben′·zam·een). BP Commission approved name for 2-(*N*-benzyl-2-chloroethylamino)-1-phenoxypropane. **Phenoxybenzamine Hydrochloride BP 1973.** The hydrochloride of phenoxybenzamine; it combats the vasoconstrictor effects of adrenaline and noradrenaline. Its action is similar to that of phentolamine mesylate but more prolonged.

Phenoxyethanol BPC 1968 (fen·ox·e·eth′·an·ol). $C_6H_5OCH_2CH_2OH$, a bactericide effective against *Pseudomonas aeruginosa* even in the presence of serum.

Phenoxymethylpenicillin BP 1973 (fen·ox·e·meth·il·pen·e·sil′·in). 6-Phenoxyacetamidopenicillanic acid, an antibiotic formed by strains of *Pencillium notatum* or related organisms. **Phenoxymethylpenicillin Calcium BP 1973.** The dihydrate of the calcium salt of phenoxymethylpenicillin; an antibiotic with actions similar to those of phenoxymethylpenicillin but it is absorbed more readily from the alimentary tract. **Phenoxymethylpenicillin Potassium BP 1973.** The potassium salt of phenoxymethylpenicillin; an antibiotic with actions similar to those of benzylpenicillin, but it can be taken by mouth as it is not destroyed by the gastric juice.

Phenoxymethylpenicillinum (fen·ox·e·meth·il·pen·e·sil′·in·um). *European Pharmacopoeia* name for Phenoxymethylpenicillin BP 1973.

phenoxypropandiol (fen·ox·e·pro·pan′·di·ol). $C_6H_5OCH_2CHOHCH_2OH$, a phenyl ester of glycerol, formerly used as an analgesic.

Phenoxypropazine (fen·ox·e·pro′·paz·een). BP Commission approved name for (1-methyl-2-phenoxyethyl)hydrazine; a monoamine oxidase inhibitor.

phenozygous (fen·oz·ig·us). Denoting a skull which is narrower than the face, so that the zygomatic arches are apparent when the head is looked at from above. [Gk *phainein* to appear, *zygoma* cheekbone.]

Phenprocoumon (fen·pro·koo·mon). BP Commission approved name for 4-hydroxy-3-(1-phenylpropyl) coumarin; used in anticoagulant therapy.

Phensuximide (fen·sux·im·ide). BP Commission approved name for *N*-methyl-α-phenylsuccinimide; used in the treatment of epilepsy and petit mal.

Phentermine (fen·ter·meen). BP Commission approved name for $\alpha\alpha$-dimethylphenethylamine; it is used in the treatment of obesity.

phentetiophthalein sodium (fen·tet·i·o·thal′·e·in so·de·um). The disodium salt of phenoltetraiodophthalein. It is used as a contrast medium in x-ray work, and in tests of liver function.

Phentolamine (fen·tol·am·een). BP Commission approved name for 2-*N*-(3-hydroxyphenyl)-*p*-toluidinomethyl-2-imidazoline; usually the mesylate (BP 1968). An α-adrenergic blocking drug suppressing or reducing the pressor activity of circulating adrenaline and noradrenaline; in high doses it is also a sympathicolytic drug blocking the pressor effects produced by stimulation. It is used clinically for its almost specific adrenolytic action; principally in the diagnosis and treatment of phaeochromocytoma, when it is sometimes referred to as rogitine. The diagnostic test is based on the fact that phentolamine causes an immediate and marked drop in blood pressure when this is raised, as in phaeochromocytoma, due to the secretion of excessive amounts of adrenaline and/or noradrenaline (*see* TEST). The drug is also used during the surgical removal of the adrenal tumour to counteract adrenaline and/or noradrenaline which may be discharged in large quantities into the circulation as a result of emotional stress, anaesthesia, or surgical manipulation of the tumour. It is given pre-operatively or during the operation. It has also been used successfully in the treatment of peripheral vascular disorders such as peripheral arteriosclerosis, Buerger's disease, varicose ulcer and frostbite. It has been tried for the treatment of essential hypertension, and is suitable for short-term treatment such as between courses of other agents and for the treatment of hypertensive crises. Side effects, however, may develop, necessitating cessation of treatment, and tolerance may be produced in 3 months. The side effects include tachycardia, diarrhoea, nausea, vomiting and syncope.

phenyl (fe·nil). The monovalent organical radical, C_6H_5, derived from phenol. **Phenyl alcohol.** Phenol. **Phenyl aminosalicylate.** BP Commission approved name for phenyl-4-aminosalicylate, used in the treatment of tuberculosis. **Phenyl carbinol.** Benzyl alcohol, a compound occasionally used to produce local anaesthesia by application or subcutaneous injection in a 1–4 per cent solution in saline; it may, however, be irritant. It is sometimes placed on the exposed nerve for toothache, and may also be used in ointments and lotions as an antipruritic. **Phenyl hydrate.** Phenol. **Phenyl salicylate.** Salol, $OHC_6H_4COOC_6H_5$, a compound which is slowly hydrolysed in the intestine when given by mouth, and has been used therefore as an intestinal antiseptic in the treatment of enteritis; it is impossible, however, to give sufficietly high doses without toxic effects. It is also employed in rheumatic conditions, but sodium salicylate is safer.

phenylacetamide (fe·nil·as·et·am·ide). Acetanilide, $C_6H_5NHCOCH_3$. An acetyl derivative of aniline; lustrous white scales, easily sublimating, odourless, and soluble in water. It is used as an antipyretic, but continued administration is likely to produce methaemoglobinaemia.

phenylacetylurea (fe·nil·as·et·il·ewr·e′·ah). Phenacemide.

phenylalanine (fe·nil·al·an·een). Phenylaminopropionic acid, $C_6H_5CH_2CH(NH_2)COOH$. An essential amino acid formed during the breakdown of protein; it provides the benzene nucleus for the metabolism.

phenylamine (fe·nil·am·een). Aniline.

phenylaminoethanol (fe·nil·am·in·o·eth′·an·ol). Phenylethanolamine, $C_6H_5CHOHCH_2NH_2$. A compound related chemically to ephedrine and similar in physiological action.

phenylaniline (fe·nil·an·il·een). Diphenylamine, $NH(C_6H_5)_2$. A colourless compound derived from aniline and of importance in the manufacture of dyestuffs. A solution in sulphuric acid affords a delicate test for nitric acid with which it gives an intense blue coloration. It is also used as an indicator in the volumetric analysis of ferrous salts.

phenylarsine oxide (fe·nil·ar·seen ox·ide). C_6H_5AsO, an arsenical compound used in the treatment of syphilis.

phenylate (fe·nil·ate). Phenolate

phenylbromoacetonitrile (fe·nil·bro·mo·as·et·o·ni′·trile). Bromobenzylcyanide, $C_6H_4BrCH_2CN$. A colourless liquid used in chemical warfare as a tear gas.

Phenylbutazone BPC 1973 (fe·nil·bew·tah·zone). 4-*n*-Butyl-1,2-diphenylpyrazolidine-3,5-dione; it is used in the treatment of rheumatic disorders.

Phenylbutazonum (fe·nil·bew·tah·zo·num). *European Pharmacopoeia* name for Phenylbutazone BP 1973.

phenylcarbylamine chloride (fe·nil·kar·bil·am·een klor·ide). $C_6H_5NCCl_2$, a lacrimatory gas used in chemical warfare.

phenylchinoline (fe·nil·kin·o·leen). Phenylquinoline.

phenyldichlorarsine (fe·nil·di·klor·ar′·seen). $C_6H_5AsCl_2$, a vesicant liquid used in the manufacture of blister gases employed in chemical warfare.

phenyldimethylpyrazolone (fe·nil·di·meth·il·pi·raz′·o·lone). Phenazone.

phenylene (fe·nil·een). The divalent radical C_6H_4 which occurs in derivatives of benzene. **Phenylene blue.** Indamine, $NH_2C_6H_4N{=}C_6H_4NH_2Cl$; a synthetic dye prepared from aniline and paraphenylene diamine. **Phenylene brown.** Bismarck brown, $C_6H_4[N_2C_6H_3(NH_2)_2]_2$; a basic dye used for staining mucin, cartilage matrix and other basophilic substances.

phenylenediamine (fe·nil·een·di′·am·een). $C_6H_4(NH_2)_2$, three isomeric compounds: the ortho-form is used as a test for ferric compounds, the meta-form is a delicate reagent for nitrites with which it gives a brown coloration, and the para-form is employed as a hair dye.

Phenylephrine Hydrochloride BP 1973 (fe·nil·ef·reen hi·dro·klor·ide). $C_9H_{13}NO_2HCl$, a fairly non-toxic vasoconstrictor, used to reduce nasal congestion in sinusitis, rhinitis, hay fever, etc., and locally in the eye as a mydriatic. It is also used with local analgesics to prolong the action by vasoconstriction and to treat hypotension.

phenylethanolamine (**fe**·nil·eth·an·**ol**'·am·een). Phenylamino-ethanol, $C_6H_5CHOHCH_2NH_2$. A compound related chemically to ephedrine and similar in physiological action.

phenylethene (fe·nil·**eth**·een). Styrene, cinnamene, $C_6H_5CH=CH_2$. An unsaturated hydrocarbon obtained from storax and also occurring in coal tar. It polymerizes to form compounds which are used in the manufacture of plastics.

phenylethylaceto-urea (**fe**·nil·eth·il·as·et·o·ewr·**e**'·ah). Phenylethylhydantoin.

phenylethylalcohol (**fe**·nil·eth·il·**al**'·ko·hol). Benzyl carbinol, $C_6H_5CH_2CH_2OH$. A compound which occurs naturally in rose and geranium oils, and is employed in perfume manufacture. It has certain anaesthetic properties.

phenylethylamine (**fe**·nil·eth·il·**am**'·een). $C_6H_5CH_2CH_2NH_2$, a toxic amine formed during the putrefaction of meat by the breaking down of phenylalanine.

phenylethylhydantoin (**fe**·nil·eth·il·hi·**dan**'·to·in). $(C_6H_5)(C_2H_5)C_3H_2O_2N_2$, a compound which is used as a hypnotic in chorea, but its side reactions, especially capillary injury, restrict its value.

phenylethylmalonylurea (**fe**·nil·eth·il·mal·on·il·ewr·**e**'·ah). Phenobarbitone.

phenylgalactosazone (**fe**·nil·gal·ak·**to**'·sa·zone). $CH_2OH(CHOH)_3C=(NNHC_6H_5)CH=(NNHC_6H_5)$, a compound derived from galactose with phenylhydrazine. It forms characteristic crystals which serve to distinguish galactose from the other hexoses.

phenylglucosazone (**fe**·nil·gloo·**ko**'·sa·zone). $CH_2OH(CHOH)_3C=(NNHC_6H_5)CH=(NNHC_6H_5)$, a compound of glucose with phenylhydrazine which forms characteristic yellow crystals. It is identical with the osazones formed by fructose and mannose, but clearly distinguishable from phenylgalactosazone.

phenylglycolphenetidin (fe·nil·**gli**·kol·fen·**et**'·id·in). Phenetidin amygdalate, amygdophenin, $C_2H_5OC_6H_4NHCOCH(OH)C_6H_5$. A phenetidin derivative employed as an analgesic.

phenylhydrazine (fe·nil·**hi**·draz·een). $C_6H_5NHNH_2$, a colourless crystalline compound which combines with aldehydes and ketones to form hydrazones and osazones, and is used therefore for the identification of monosaccharides. It is also important as the starting point for many drugs and dyes. Mixed with blood it produces methaemoglobin, and reduces the number of red cells; it is used in polycythaemia, but caution is necessary as it may have serious toxic effects on the liver and kidneys. **Phenylhydrazine hydrochloride.** $C_6H_5NHNH_2HCl$, the water-soluble salt of phenylhydrazine; administered in capsules whenever the drug is indicated. It is also used as a reagent for the detection of aldehydes, ketones and reducing sugars.

phenylhydrazone (fe·nil·**hi**·draz·one). A compound of the type $RCH=NNHC_6H_5$, formed by the interaction of phenylhydrazine with an aldehyde. It is the formation of such compounds, and the derived osazones, with the aldehyde groups of certain sugars, that serves to identify the latter.

phenylhydroxylamine (**fe**·nil·hi·drox·il·**am**'·een). C_6H_5NHOH, colourless, acicular crystals, soluble in hot water, alcohol and ether; met with the organic chemical industry. Absorbed through the skin, inhaled, or swallowed, it causes livid cyanosis, dyspnoea, irritation of the central nervous system with trismus, twitchings and nystagmus, respiratory and circulatory disturbances, and unconsciousness.

phenylic (fe·**nil**·ik). Relating to phenol.

phenylindanedione (**fe**·nil·in·dane·**di**'·one). Phenindione.

phenylketonuria (**fe**·nil·ke·to·**newr**'·e·ah). A hereditary disorder of phenylalanine metabolism characterized by the presence of phenylpyruvic acid in the urine, and accumulation of phenylalanine metabolites that produce brain damage resulting in severe mental retardation. Brain damage can be prevented by a low phenylalanine diet. [phenyl, ketonuria.]

phenyl-lactosazone (**fe**·nil·lak·**to**'·sa·zone). The osazone derived from lactose with phenylhydrazine; yellow crystals of characteristic appearance which serve to identify lactose.

phenylmercuric (**fe**·nil·mer·**kewr**'·ik). Describing a compound of mercury which contains the phenyl radical, C_6H_5-; many of these compounds are important bacteriostatic agents. **Phenylmercuric Acetate BPC 1968.** $C_6H_5HgOOCCH_3$, a crystalline solid, slowly soluble in water, the solution having a bactericidal or bacteriostatic value depending upon concentration. It is used as a chemical contraceptive, though its spermicidal action is much reduced at pH greater than 7.2. **Phenylmercuric Nitrate BP 1973,** $C_6H_5HgOHC_6H_5HgNO_3$, a colourless crystalline compound, slightly soluble in water but an efficient bacteriostatic even in high dilution. It is used for the direct medication of wounds and for disinfection of the skin; also, at concentration 0.1 per cent, as a bacteriostatic in the routine preparation of solutions for injection.

phenylmethylacetone (**fe**·nil·meth·il·**as**'·et·one). Acetophenone, phenylmethyl ketone, $C_6H_5COCH_3$. A colourless liquid with the odour of bitter almonds; insoluble in water but soluble in alcohol and oils. It is used in perfumery, and medicinally as a hypnotic.

phenylmethylcarbinol (**fe**·nil·meth·il·**kar**'·bin·ol). $C_6H_5CH(OH)CH_3$, a compound prepared from acetophenone, and employed as a local anaesthetic.

Phenylpropanolamine (**fe**·nil·pro·pan·**ol**'·am·een). 2-Amino-1-phenylpropan-1-ol. **Phenylpropanolamine Hydrochloride BP 1973.** The hydrochloride of phenylpropanolamine; a sympathomimetic agent with actions similar to those of ephedrine.

phenylpropylmethylamine hydrochloride (fe·nil·**pro**·pil·meth·il·**am**'·een hi·dro·**klor**·ide). $C_6H_5CH(CH_3)CH_2NHCH_3HCl$, a synthetic nasal vasoconstrictor of the amphetamine type.

phenylquinoline (fe·nil·**kwin**·o·leen). $C_6H_5C_9H_6N$, a compound derived from quinoline which resembles quinine in action.

phenylthiourea (**fe**·nil·thi·o·ewr·**e**'·ah). A compound which is tasteless to some persons and bitter to others. It contains the group =N-C=S, the ability to taste which is inherited and is dependent on a single gene pair. People who can taste it are either homozygous or heterozygous for the dominant allele. Thiourea and thiouracil also contain the significant group.

Phenyltoloxamine (**fe**·nil·tol·**ox**'·am·een). BP Commission approved name for *N*-2-(2-benzylphenoxy)ethyldimethylamine; an antihistamine.

Phenyramidol (fe·nir·**am**·id·ol). BP Commission approved name for 1-phenyl-2-(2-pyridylamino)ethanol; an analgesic.

Phenytoin (fen·it·**o**·in). 5,5-Diphenylhydantoin. **Phenytoin Sodium BP 1973.** Soluble phenytoin, diphenylhydantoin sodium. The monosodium derivative of 5,5-diphenylhydantoin, a colourless hygroscopic compound giving an alkaline solution in water. It is an anticonvulsant used in epilepsy, having the advantage that its hypnotic action is negligible. Toxic side reactions (nausea, dizziness, skin rashes) have been observed in some cases. It is administered in capsules or tablets with copious draughts of water because of its alkalinity.

pheo-. For words beginning with **pheo-**, *see* PHAEO-.

pheromone (**fer**·o·mone). This is not, strictly speaking, a hormone which affects only the organism that produces it. Pheromones affect the development, reproduction and behaviour of other members of the same species, but usually of the opposite sex. The path of communication is usually olfactory, and they may, in fact, be odours given off by, say, male rodents which modify or regulate the sexual cycle of females, inducing regular ovulation leading to pregnancy or, on the other hand, blocking pregnancy. The presence or absence of the male parent at a critical postnatal phase may affect the sexual behaviour of the offspring when they become mature.

phial (**fi**·al). A small glass vessel or bottle for holding or administering medicine. [Gk *phiale* bowl.]

phialide (**fi**·al·ide). Sterigma; a specialized spore-bearing cell, usually flask-shaped, from the narrow tubular neck of which spores arise in chains by a process of successive apical growth and abstriction cutting off the terminal segment. [Gk *phiale* bowl, *eidos* form.]

Phialophora (fi·al·**of**·or·ah). A genus of hyphomycetous fungi, several species of which are agents of chromomycosis, e.g. *Phialophora compacta, P. dermatitidis, P. pedrosoi, P. verrucosa. P. jeanselmei* has been isolated from black-grain mycetoma, and *P. gougerottii, P. richardsiae* and *P. spinifera* have been isolated from subcutaneous abscesses in phaeosporotrichosis. [Gk *phiale* bowl, *phoros* bearing.]

Philip, Sir Robert William (b. 1857). Edinburgh physician.

Philip's gland. An enlarged gland above the clavicle in children, regarded as indicative of intrathoracic tuberculosis.

Philippe, Claudien (b. 1866). Paris pathologist.

Gombault-Philippe triangular bundle, triangular tract of Gombault-Philippe. The triangular strand of the fasciculus gracilis in the conus medullaris; a part of the septomarginal tract.

Philipson's reflex. On passive lengthening of the quadriceps femoris muscle on one side a reflex shortening of the opposite quadriceps, with extension at the knee joint, ensues.

Phillips' muscle. An uncommon slip of muscle arising from the lateral ligament of the wrist and the styloid process of the radius, and having insertion into the phalanges of the thumb.

Philometridae (fil·o·**met**·rid·e). The name of a family of nematodes, said by some authorities to contain *Dracunculus* within the superfamily Filarioidea.

philoneism (fil·o·**ne**·izm). Excessive interest in or fondness of something that is novel. [Gk *philein* to love, *neos* new.]

philopatridomania (fil·o·pat·rid·o·**ma**'·ne·ah). A desire, bordering on insanity, of a person to return to his homeland; extreme degree of homesickness. [Gk *philopatria* love of one's country, mania.]

philtre (**fil**·ter). Any drug that is held to be able to excite sexual passion or love. [Gk *philtron* love potion.]

philtrum [NA] (**fil**·trum). 1. The medial shallow depression on the outer surface of the upper lip. 2. Philtre. [Gk *philtron* love potion.]

phimosiectomy (fi·mo·se·**ek**'·to·me). Circumcision for the treatment of phimosis. [phimosis, *ektome* a cutting out.]

phimosientomy, phimosiotomy (fi·mo·se·**en**'·to·me, fi·mo·se·**ot**'·o·me). The operation of incising a constricted prepuce. [phimosis, Gk *entemnein* to cut in.]

phimosis (fi·**mo**·sis). Narrowing of the preputial orifice so that the foreskin cannot be readily retracted. Usually congenital but may be acquired as a result of inflammatory fibrosis. **Labial phimosis, Oral phimosis, Phimosis oris.** Atresia of the oral orifice. **Phimosis palpebrarum.** A general diminution of the palpebral fissure, a rare developmental anomaly, more commonly called *congenital blepharophimosis.* **Phimosis vaginalis.** Narrowness of the vaginal orifice. [Gk, a stopping up.]

phimotic (fi·**mot**·ik). Relating to or characterized by phimosis.

phlebalgia (fleb·**al**·je·ah). Pain in venules or varices in connection with a nerve. [Gk *phleps* vein, *algos* pain.]

phlebangioma (**fleb**·an·je·o'·mah). Venous aneurysm. [Gk *phleps* vein, *aggeion* small vessel, *-oma* tumour.]

phlebarteriectasia (**fleb**·ar·teer·e·ek·ta'·ze·ah). A general dilatation of the veins and arteries. [Gk *phleps* vein, artery, Gk *ektasis* a stretching.]

phlebarteriodialysis (**fleb**·ar·teer·e·o·di·**al**'·is·is). Arteriovenous aneurysm. [Gk *phleps* vein, artery, Gk *dialysis* a destroying.]

phlebasthenia (fleb·as·**the**·ne·ah). A condition marked by general loss of tone and vitality of the walls of the arteries and veins. [Gk *phleps* vein, asthenia.]

phlebectasia, phlebectasis (fleb·ek·**ta**·ze·ah, fleb·**ek**·tas·is). A varicosity; a dilated condition of the veins. **Phlebectasia laryngis.** A condition characterized by chronic dilatation of the laryngeal veins, and in particular of those of the vocal folds. [Gk *phleps* vein, *ektasis* a stretching.]

phlebectomy (fleb·**ek**·to·me). The operation of excising a segment of or the whole of a vein, as may be done in cases of varicose veins. [Gk *phleps* vein, *ektome* a cutting out.]

phlebectopia, phlebectopy (fleb·ek·**to**·pe·ah, fleb·**ek**·to·pe). Displacement or abnormal course of a vein. [Gk *phleps* vein, *ektopos* out of the way.]

phlebemphraxis (fleb·em·**frax**·is). Obstruction of a vein by a clot of blood. [Gk *phleps* vein, *emphrassein* to block up.]

phlebexeresis (fleb·ex·**er**·e·sis). The withdrawal of a varicose vein by traction through a small incision at one of its extremities. [Gk *phleps* vein, exeresis.]

phlebhepatitis (**fleb**·hep·at·i'·tis). Inflammation of the hepatic veins. [Gk *phleps* vein, *hepar* liver, *-itis* inflammation.]

phlebismus (fleb·**iz**·mus). Plugging and overdistention of a vein, with resultant congestion. [Gk *phleps* vein.]

phlebitic (fleb·**it**·ik). Relating to or characterized by the presence of phlebitis.

phlebitis (fleb·**i**·tis). Inflammation of a vein: *endophlebitis,* inflammation of the internal coat of the vein; *periphlebitis,* inflammation of the external coat from inflammation invading from without. **Adhesive phlebitis.** Inflammation of the endothelium followed by the formation of a thrombus which adheres to the wall and obliterates the vein. The clot may organize and the vein become a fibrous cord, but in some cases the clot may soften and break down so that the circulation is restored. **Gouty phlebitis.** Phlebitis occurring with the gouty diathesis. **Plastic phlebitis.** Adhesive phlebitis (see above). **Puerperal phlebitis.** Phlebitis occurring after childbirth in the uterine veins and spreading to neighbouring veins such as the iliac and femoral. **Sinus phlebitis.** Phlebitis and thrombosis of a cerebral sinus, e.g. the lateral sinus in middle-ear disease. The longitudinal sinus and the cavernous sinus are other common sites. **Suppurative phlebitis.** The result of infection with a pyogenic organism, either from a neighbouring septic focus or in septicaemia. **Syphilitic phlebitis.** Phlebitis which may occur in syphilis as a result of syphilitic endophlebitis or gummatous infiltration. In congenital syphilis it may affect the umbilical vein. **Toxic phlebitis.** Acute infective phlebitis with toxic symptoms. **Tuberculous phlebitis.** Phlebitis due to the spread of infection to a vein from a neighbouring tuberculous focus. It may result in tubercle bacilli entering the blood stream and causing a general infection. Phlebitis of veins in the extremities, most often the femoral, is not uncommon in advanced phthisis, as in other exhausting diseases. **Typhoid phlebitis.** A sequel to typhoid fever. [Gk *phleps* vein, *-itis* inflammation.]

See also: TIDY.

phlebocarcinoma (**fleb**·o·kar·sin·**o**'·mah). Carcinoma affecting a vein. [Gk *phleps* vein, carcinoma.]

phlebocholosis (**fleb**·o·ko·**lo**'·sis). Any diseased condition of the veins. [Gk *phleps* vein, *cholos* defective.]

phleboclysis (**fleb**·o·**kli**·sis). The intravenous injection in quantity of saline or other fluid. **Drip phleboclysis.** Intravenous drip. [Gk *phleps* vein, *klysis* a washing out.]

phlebogenous (fleb·**oj**·en·us). Having origin in the veins. [Gk *phleps* vein, *genein* to produce.]

phlebogram (**fleb**·o·gram). 1. The radiograph made during phlebography. 2. A tracing of the venous pulse made by the phlebograph. [Gk *phleps* vein, *gramma* a writing.]

phlebograph (**fleb**·o·graf). An instrument for recording venous pulsations. [Gk *phleps* vein, *graphein* to record.]

See also: MACKENZIE (J.).

phlebography (fleb·**og**·raf·e). 1. Radiographic visualization of veins after the injection of a radio-opaque contrast medium into the lumen of the vessel. 2. The tracing of the venous pulse by means of a plebograph. 3. Venography. [see prec.]

phleboid (**fleb**·oid). 1. Having resemblance to a vein. 2. Containing many veins or composed of veins. 3. Venous. [Gk *phleps* vein, *eidos* form.]

phlebolite (**fleb**·o·lite). Phlebolith.

phlebolith (**fleb**·o·lith). A calcareous concretion in a vein produced by calcification of an old thrombus. [Gk *phleps* vein, *lithos* stone.]

phlebolithiasis (**fleb**·o·lith·i'·as·is). A condition in which there is a tendency to formation of phleboliths. [Gk *phleps* vein, lithiasis.]

phlebolitic (fleb·o·**lit**·ik). Relating to or of the nature of a phlebolith.

phlebology (fleb·**ol**·o·je). That branch of medical science which deals with the anatomy and diseases of the veins. [Gk *phleps* vein, *logos* science.]

phlebomanometer (**fleb**·o·man·**om**′·et·er). An instrument for measuring venous blood pressure. [Gk *phleps* vein, manometer.]

phlebometritis (**fleb**·o·met·**ri**′·tis). Inflammation in which the uterine veins are affected. [Gk *phleps* vein, *metra* womb, *-itis* inflammation.]

phlebomyomatosis (**fleb**·o·mi·o·mat·**o**′·sis). A morbid condition characterized by induration of the walls of a vein due to overgrowth of irregularly arranged muscle fibres. [Gk *phleps* vein, myoma, Gk *-osis* condition.]

phlebopexy (fleb·o·**pex**·e). Extraserous transplantation of the testicle, with preservation of the reticulum of veins; it was formerly done for varicocele. [Gk *phleps* vein, *pexis* a fixation.]

phlebophlebostomy (**fleb**·o·fleb·**os**′·to·me). An operation whereby a communication is made between two veins. [Gk *phleps* vein, *stroma* mouth.]

phlebophlogosis (**fleb**·o·flo·**go**′·sis). Phlebitis. [Gk *phleps* vein, phlogosis.]

phlebophthalmotomy (**fleb**·of·thal·**mot**′·o·me). Venesection for the purpose of relieving congestion of the veins of the conjunctiva. [Gk *phleps* vein, *ophthalmos* eye, *temnein* to cut.]

phlebopiezometry (**fleb**·o·pi·e·**zom**′·et·re). Estimation of the venous blood pressure. [Gk *phleps* vein, *plezein* to squeeze, *metron* measure.]

phleboplasty (**fleb**·o·plas·te). Plastic repair of a vein in case of defect or wound. [Gk *phleps* vein, *plassein* to mould.]

phleboplerosis (**fleb**·o·pler·**o**′·sis). A morbid condition in which the veins are distended. [Gk *phleps* vein, *plerosis* a filling up.]

phleborrhagia (fleb·o·**ra**·je·ah). A profuse discharge of blood from a vein; venous haemorrhage. [Gk *phleps* vein, *rhegnynein* to gush forth.]

phleborrhaphy (fleb·**or**·af·e). Suture of a vein. [Gk *phleps* vein, *rhaphe* seam.]

phleborrhexis (fleb·o·**rex**·is). Rupture of a vein. [Gk *phleps* vein, *rhexis* rupture.]

phlebosation (fleb·o·za·shun). Phlebosclerosation.

phlebosclerosation (**fleb**·o·skler·o·**za**′·shun). The production of an artificial sclerotic condition in the treatment of varicose veins. [see foll.]

phlebosclerosis (**fleb**·o·skler·**o**′·sis). Sclerosis of a vein, and in particular induration of the tunica intima of a vein; chronic phlebitis. [Gk *phleps* vein, sclerosis.]

phlebosis (fleb·**o**·sis). A condition characterized by simple (abacterial) inflammation of a vein. [Gk *phleps* vein, *-osis* condition.]

phlebostasis (fleb·**os**·tas·is). 1. Venostasis. 2. Compression of the veins of an arm or leg in order to shut off some of the blood from the circulation. [Gk *phleps* vein, *stasis* a standing still.]

phlebostenosis (**fleb**·o·sten·**o**′·sis). Stenosis of a vein. [Gk *phleps* vein, stenosis.]

phlebostrepsis (fleb·o·**strep**·sis). Torsion of the cut or torn end of a vein for the purpose of arresting haemorrhage. [Gk *phleps* vein, *strephein* to twist.]

phlebothrombosis (**fleb**·o·throm·**bo**′·sis). Thrombosis in the veins. [Gk *phleps* vein, thrombosis.]

phlebotome (**fleb**·o·tome). A lancet used especially in venesection. [see foll.]

phlebotomist (fleb·**ot**·om·ist). One who practises venesection. [Gk *phleps* vein, *temnein* to cut.]

phlebotomize (fleb·**ot**·om·ize). To perform venesection. [see prec.]

Phlebotomus (fleb·**ot**·o·mus). A genus of small flies of the family Psychodidae, sand flies. The numerous species are world-wide and almost sole vectors of the various diseases caused by species of Leishmania. The adults are sluggish fliers, mostly nocturnal; the females alone suck blood in almost all species. The larvae develop in cracks in walls, rubble and rubbish heaps. The names *Adlerius, Brumptius, Brumptomyia, Larroussius, Lutzia, Prophlebotomus, Sergentomyia (= Newsteadia)* and *Sintonius* have been used as subgeneric, or as generic, in certain groups of species here considered in *Phlebotomus*. **Phlebotomus argentipes.** An important vector of kala-azar in India. **Phlebotomus caucasicus.** A transmitter of cutaneous leishmaniasis in South Russia. **Phlebotomus chinensis.** A vector of kala-azar in China. **Phlebotomus fischeri.** A probable vector of American leishmaniasis. **Phlebotomus intermedius.** Probably a principal vector of espundia (American leishmaniasis) in South and Central America, and possibly of kala-azar. **Phlebotomus japatasi.** A vector of cutaneous ulcerative leishmaniasis. **Phlebotomus langeroni.** A probable vector of kala-azar. **Phlebotomus langeroni orientalis.** A probable vector of kala-azar. **Phlebotomus longicuspis.** A probable vector of kala-azar. **Phlebotomus longipalpis.** A suspected vector of kala-azar. **Phlebotomus macedonicus.** *Phlebotomus perfiliewi* (see below). **Phlebotomus major.** A vector of infantile kala-azar in the Mediterranean area. **Phlebotomus martini.** The vector of East African kala-azar. **Phlebotomus migonei.** Probably a vector of espundia in South and Central America. **Phlebotomus noguchii.** An unimportant vector of oroya fever (bartonellosis) in the Peruvian Andes. **Phlebotomus papatasii.** The principal vector of oriental sore in North Africa, and the principal (and perhaps sole) vector of sand-fly fever in southern Europe and North Africa. The virus is transmitted to the eggs. **Phlebotomus perfiliewi.** A vector of oriental sore in Italy. **Phlebotomus perniciosus.** A vector of infantile kala-azar in the Mediterranean area. **Phlebotomus peruensis.** A vector of bartonellosis. **Phlebotomus pessoai.** A probable vector of espundia in South and Central America. **Phlebotomus roubaudi.** A probable vector of oriental sore. **Phlebotomus sergenti.** The most important vector of oriental sore in the Middle East and India. **Phlebotomus sergenti mongolensis.** A probable vector of kala-azar in China. **Phlebotomus squamipes.** A transmitter of mucocutaneous leishmaniasis in Surinam and Brazil. **Phlebotomus taianensis.** A probable vector of kala-azar in China. **Phlebotomus verrucarum.** The principal vector of oroya fever in the Peruvian Andes. **Phlebotomus whitmani.** A probable vector of American leishmaniasis. [Gk *phleps* vein, *tomos* a cutting.]

phlebotomy (fleb·**ot**·o·me). Venesection. **Bloodless phlebotomy, Medical phlebotomy.** The technique of trapping blood in the veins of the limbs by the application of tourniquets at a tension below that required to obstruct the arterial flow; used, in the emergency treatment of acute pulmonary congestion or oedema, to reduce the central blood volume. [Gk *phleps* vein, *temnein* to cut.]

phlebotropism (fleb·**ot**·ro·pizm). Attraction to the veins. [Gk *phleps* vein, *trope* a turning.]

phledonia (fle·**do**·ne·ah). Delirium or delirious speech. [Gk *phledon* a babbler.]

phlegm (flem). 1. Mucus, especially that secreted in the respiratory passages. 2. One of the four humours of ancient physiology, indicating coolness or sluggishness of temperament; self-restraint. [Gk *phlegma.]*

phlegmasia (fleg·**ma**·ze·ah). An inflammation. **Phlegmasia alba dolens.** Typically an acute oedema of the leg occurring in recently delivered women due to lymphatic obstruction. This is often secondary to a deep femoral thrombosis. It is a term which has unfortunately been used to describe deep femoral thrombosis also. **Cellulitic phlegmasia.** Septic inflammation of connective tissue of the leg following parturition. **Thrombotic phlegmasia.** Acute oedema of the leg from venous obstruction due to thrombosis of veins. [Gk, turgescence.]

phlegmatic (fleg·**mat**·ik). 1. Relating to phlegm. 2. Not excitable; dull or apathetic in humour.

phlegmon (**fleg**·mon). Inflammation of connective tissue without pus formation. **Bronze phlegmon.** A gas-producing infection of subcutaneous tissues associated with bronze discoloration of the skin. **Diffuse phlegmon.** Spreading cellulitis without localization. **Emphysematous phlegmon, Gas phlegmon.** Cellulitis or gangrene due to gas-producing organisms. **Ligneous phlegmon.** Chronic, painless, low-grade cellulitis of the neck without suppuration or systemic disturbance. **Woody phlegmon.** Ligneous phlegmon (see prec.). [Gk *phlegmone* inflammation.]

See also: DUPUYTREN.

phlegmona diffusa (fleg·**mo**·nah dif·**ew**·sah). Diffuse phlegmon. [Gk *phlegmone* inflammation, L *diffusus* spread out.]

phlegmonodoea (**fleg**·mon·o·**de**′·ah). A form of enteritis [obsolete term]. [see foll.]

phlegmonoid (**fleg**·mon·oid). Having resemblance to phlegmon. [Gk *phlegmone* inflammation, *eidos* form.]

phlegmonosis (fleg·mon·**o**·sis). 1. Fever. 2. Inflammation. [Gk *phlegmone* inflammation, *-osis* condition.]

phlegmonous (**fleg**·mon·us). Relating or belonging to or characterized by a phlegmon; descriptive of cellulitis.

phlobaphene (**flo**·bah·feen). A reddish resinous substance obtained by boiling a phlobatannin with dilute hydrochloric acid; phlobaphenes occur in nature associated with the tannins of fruit rinds. [Gk *phloios* bark, *baphe* dye.]

phlobatannin (flo·bah·**tan**·in). Catechol tannin. Any member of the group of tannins which form the colouring of certain fruit rinds: on heating they are converted into catechol. [Gk *phloios* bark, *baphe* dye, tannin.]

phloem (**flo**·em). In plant anatomy, that part of the vascular structure which consists of sieve-tubes and associated tissues, and carries synthesized sugars and proteins through the plant. It is differentiated into *primary phloem,* formed from procambium, and *secondary phloem* which is produced by the cambium. [Gk *phloios* bark.]

phlogistic (flo·**jis**·tik). Inflammatory; relating to inflammation or fever. [Gk *phlogistos* set on fire.]

phlogocyte (**flo**·go·site). One of the cells found in inflamed tissue; a plasma cell. [Gk *phlogosis* burning heat, *kytos* cell.]

phlogocytosis (**flo**·go·si·**to**′·sis). The state of the blood when phlogocytes are present in it. [phlogocyte, Gk *-osis* condition.]

phlogogen (**flo**·go·jen). Any substance which is capable of giving rise to inflammation. [Gk *phlox* flame, *genein* to produce.]

phlogogenic, phlogogenous (flo·go·**jen**·ik, flo·**goj**·en·us). Exciting or producing inflammation. [see prec.]

phlogosis (flo·**go**·sis). 1. Superficial inflammation. 2. Specific term for erysipelas. [Gk, burning heat.]

phlogotic (flo·**got**·ik). Having reference to inflammatory processes. [see prec.]

phloretin (flor·e·tin). A polyhydroxyketone, $C_6H_4(OH)CH_2CH_2COC_6H_2(OH)_3$, produced by the partial hydrolysis of the glycoside phloridzin. Like the latter, it is capable of inducing glycosuria in animals.

phlorhizin (flo·ri·zin). Phloridzin.

phloridzin (flo·**rid**·zin). $C_6H_4(OH)CH_2CH_2COC_6H(OH)_2OC_6H_{11}O_5$, a bitter glucoside occurring in the root bark of apple, pear, plum, and other rosaceous trees. It is a powerful inhibitor of specific transport systems for glucose and other sugars in a variety of animal cells and micro-organisms. Its action on glucose transport by the renal tubule leads to failure of glucose reabsorption and thus to *phloridzin diabetes.* [Gk *phloios* bark, *rhiza* root.]

phlorizin (flo·ri·zin). Phloridzin.

phloroglucin, phloroglucinol (flor·o·**gloo**·sin, flor·o·**gloo**·sin·ol). 1,3,5-Trihydroxybenzene, $C_6H_3(OH)_3$. A compound which occurs widely in plants as a constituent of flavone and anthocyanin pigments, and in phloridzin, quercetrin, hesperidin, etc. It is used as a reagent, serving as a test for lignin in woody substances (red coloration), with vanillin for the detection of hydrochloric acid in the stomach, and in the detection of pentoses where it gives an insoluble compound with the furfural formed. **Phloroglucin vanillin.** Test solutions of phloroglucin and vanillin in dehydrated alcohol; they are mixed immediately prior to use and yield a cherry-red coloration with the hydrochloric acid of gastric juice drawn from the stomach.

phlorol (**flor**·ol). $C_6H_4(OH)C_2H_5$, a colourless oil occurring in creosote.

phlorose (**flor**·oze). The sugar obtained by the hydrolysis of the glucoside, phloridzin: it is identical with glucose.

phlorrhizin (flo·ri·zin). Phloridzin.

phloryl (**flor**·il). A phenolic compound occurring in creosote.

phloxine (**flox**·een). A bright-red acid stain included in the xanthene series. With blue staining of cell nuclei it can be used as a counterstain.

phlyctena (flik·**te**·nah). 1. A small blister, particularly that produced by a superficial degree burn. 2. A raised nodule forming in the conjunctiva or cornea of the eye at or near the limbus, usually going to ulceration. It is composed mainly of lymphocytes, but leucocytes appear after ulceration. It is an allergic response by the conjunctival and corneal epithelium to a specific allergen, most commonly the tubercle bacillus, but other organisms and allergens can be responsible. [Gk *phlyktaina* blister.]

phlyctenar (**flik**·ten·ar). Relating to a phlyctena; characterized by the presence of phlyctenae.

phlyctenoid (**flik**·ten·oid). 1. Having resemblance to a phlyctena or vesicle. 2. Phlyctenular. [phlyctena, Gk *eidos* form.]

phlyctenosis (flik·ten·**o**·sis). An eruption of blisters or phlyctenae. **Phlyctenosis aggregata.** A herpetic condition characterized by a close grouping of the vesicles. **Phlyctenosis labialis.** Herpes labialis. **Phlyctenosis sparsa.** Phlyctenosis marked by the presence of only a small number of vesicles which are not in close contact with each other. **Phlyctenosis streptogenes.** A cutaneous condition caused by infection with streptococci. [phlyctena, Gk *-osis* condition.]

phlyctenotherapy (**flik**·ten·o·**ther**′·ap·e). A method of treatment in which the serum from a blister produced by cantharides is removed and injected subcutaneously. [Gk *phlyktaina* blister, *therapeia* treatment.]

phlyctenula (flik·**ten**·ew·lah). Phlyctenule.

phlyctenular (flik·**ten**·ew·lar). Relating or belonging to a phlyctenule, or characterized by an eruption of phlyctenules or phlyctenule-like lesions.

phlyctenule (**flik**·ten·ewl). 1. A very small vesicle of the cornea or conjunctiva. 2. A phlyctena. [L dim. of Gk *phlyktaina* blister.]

phlyctenulosis (**flik**·ten·ew·**lo**′·sis). Phlyctenular conjunctivitis. **Allergic phlyctenulosis.** A condition characterized by the presence of phlyctenules, due to some allergic idiosyncrasy. **Tuberculous phlyctenulosis.** Occurrence of phlyctenules as indicating the tuberculous diathesis. [phlyctenule, Gk *-osis* condition.]

phlysis (**fli**·sis). 1. A phlyctenule. 2. A type of whitlow. [Gk *phlyein* to rise up.]

phlyzacium (fli·**za**·se·um). 1. A small pustule. 2. Ecthyma. **Phlyzacium acutum.** Ecthyma. [Gk *phlyzakion* pustule.]

phobia (fo·be·ah). 1. Fear. 2. Used as a suffix it is preceded by the thing or condition which is the object of fear or aversion. There is a tendency to manufacture such words unnecessarily as phobias are seldom specific. The two in most common use are claustrophobia and agoraphobia, fear of closed and open spaces respectively, but others are in current use and are defined in the appropriate place. [Gk *phobos* fear.]

phobic (**fo**·bik). Relating to or characterized by a phobia.

phobodipsia (fo·bo·**dip**·se·ah). Hydrophobia. [Gk *phobos* fear, *dipsa* thirst.]

phobophobia (fo·bo·**fo**·be·ah). An abnormal fear of developing a phobia, generally a symptom of mental strain. [Gk *phobos* fear.]

phocenine (**fo**·sen·een). $C_3H_5(OCOC_4H_9)_3$, a liquid fat found in the oil of the porpoise. [Gk *phokaina* porpoise.]

phocomelia, phocomely (fo·ko·**me**·le·ah, fo·**kom**·el·e). 1. Absence of central elements of limbs with foreshortening. 2. A deformity in which the legs are developed, but the arms are absent or undeveloped. [Gk *phoke* seal, *melos* limb.]

phoenixin (fe·**nix**·in). Carbon tetrachloride.

Pholcodine BP 1973 (**fol**·ko·deen). The 3-(2-morpholinoethyl) ether of morphine. It is used for the relief of cough. **Pholcodine Tartrate BPC 1963.** Pholcodine di(hydrogen tartrate) trihydrate; it is more soluble in water than pholcodine.

Pholedrine (**fol**·ed·reen). BP Commission approved name for *p*-(2-methylaminopropyl)phenol, a sympathomimetic drug, which acts as a vasopressor by constricting the peripheral vessels directly; it is prescribed in the form of the sulphate.

phon (fon). A unit of the objective loudness of sounds. [Gk *phone* sound.]

phonacoscope (fo·**nak**·o·skope). The bell-shaped resonance chamber employed in phonacoscopy.

phonacoscopy (fo·nak·**os**·ko·pe). Combined auscultation and percussion with a bell-shaped resonating chamber incorporating a percussion hammer which is applied to the front of the chest while the examiner listens at the back. [Gk *phone* sound, *akouein* to hear, *skopein* to examine.]

phonal (**fo**·nal). Relating to the voice. [Gk *phone* voice.]

phonasthenia (fo·nas·**the**·ne·ah). A weakness or difficulty in the act of phonation. It occurs in professional voice users as a result of overstrain or misuse of the vocal mechanism. [Gk *phone* voice, asthenia.]

phonation (fo·**na**·shun). The act of producing purposive sound by means of the larynx. [Gk *phone* voice.]

phonatory (**fo**·nat·or·e). Relating to or promoting phonation. **Vocal phonatory.** Vocal cord. *See* CORD.

phonautogram (fo·**naw**·to·gram). The record traced by the phonautograph. [Gk *phone* sound, *autos* self, *gramma* a writing.]

phonautograph (fo·**naw**·to·graf). An instrument for recording the vibrations of the air arising as a result of sound, including that of the voice. [Gk *phone* sound, *autos* self, *graphein* to record.]

phone (fone). The minimum distinctive sound-feature into which any given flow of speech can be analyzed. [Gk *phone* sound.]

phoneme (**fo**·neem). A minimum unit of distinctive sound-feature. [Gk *phonema* voice.]

phonendoscope (fo·**nen**·do·skope). A stethoscope in which the chest piece consists of a flat shallow metal cup about 30 mm diameter closed by a diaphragm. [Gk *phone* sound, *endon* within, *skopein* to examine.]

phonendoskiascope (fo·**nen**·do·**ski**′·ah·skope). A phonendoscope combined with a fluorescent screen so that the heart movements can be observed at the same time as the heart sounds are heard. [Gk *phone* sound, *endon* within, *skid* shadow, *skopein* to examine.]

phonetic (fo·**net**·ik). 1. Relating to speech sounds. 2. Relating to the voice. [Gk *phone* voice.]

phonetics (fo·**net**·ix). 1. That department of phonology which is concerned with analysis and classification of actual speech sounds. 2. The science of the vocal sounds used in language-systems. [see prec.]

phoniatrics, phoniatry (fo·ne·**at**·rix, fo·ne·**at**·re). The treatment of disorders and defects of speech; speech therapy. [Gk *phone* voice, *iatrikos* the art of healing.]

phonic (**fo**·nik). Phonetic.

phonism (**fo**·nizm). A complex type of synaesthesia in which the feeling, seeing, smelling, tasting, or even thinking of some particular thing gives rise to a sensation of hearing. [Gk *phone* sound.]

phono-auscultation (fo·no·aws·**kul**·**ta**′·shun). Auscultation by means of a tuning-fork laid over the organ to be examined; a stethoscope is laid over the organ and the vibrations from the tuning fork are heard through the stethoscope. [Gk *phone* sound, auscultation.]

phonocardiogram (fo·no·**kar**·de·o·gram). The record produced by the phonocardiograph. [Gk *phone* sound, *kardia* heart, *gramma* a writing.]

phonocardiograph (fo·no·**kar**·de·o·graf). An instrument for recording heart sounds and murmurs graphically. [Gk *phone* sound, *kardia* heart, *graphein* to record.]

phonocardiography (**fo**·no·kar·de·**og**′·raf·e). The mechanical registration of the sounds of the heart by means of the phonocardiograph. **Spectral phonocardiography.** The technique of analysing the recorded heart sounds according to their frequency content as well as their time of occurrence.

phonocatheter (**fo**·no·kath·et·er). A catheter having a microphone in its tip. [Gk *phone* sound, catheter.]

phono-electrocardioscope (**fo**·no·el·ek·tro·**kar**′·de·o·skope). A double-beam cathode-ray oscilloscope with which two phenomena such as the phonocardiogram and the electrocardiogram, or the electrocardiogram and the sphygmogram, may be seen simultaneously. [Gk *phone* sound, electrocardiogram, *skopein* to watch.]

phono-electrocardioscopy (**fo**·no·el·ek·kar·de·**os**′·ko·pe). Simultaneous direct visual recording of two circulatory phenomena, such as by the phonocardiogram and the sphygmogram, or the phonocardiogram and the electrocardiogram, by means of a double-beam cathode-ray oscilloscope (phono-electrocardioscope).

phonogram (**fo**·no·gram). A graphic curve of the duration and intensity of sounds such as those of the heart. [Gk *phone* sound, *gramma* a writing.]

phonology (fo·**nol**·o·je). The science of vocal sounds and their changes. [Gk *phone* voice, *logos* science.]

phonomania (fon·o·**ma**·ne·ah). A form of insanity characterized by homicidal tendencies. [Gk *phonos* murder, mania.]

phonometer (fo·**nom**·et·er). Phon meter; an instrument for measuring the loudness of sounds. [Gk *phone* sound, meter.]

phonomyoclonus (**fo**·no·mi·o·**klo**′·nus). A condition in which sound is noted on auscultation over a myoclonic muscle, demonstrating that fibrillary contractions are present although they cannot be seen. [Gk *phone* sound, myoclonus.]

phonomyogram (fo·no·**mi**·o·gram). The graphic record of the sound caused by the action of a muscle. [Gk *phone* sound, *mys* muscle, *gramma* a writing.]

phonomyography (**fo**·no·mi·**og**′·raf·e). The registration of the various sounds caused by contraction of muscle tissue. An oscillograph receives the sounds from a microphone situated over the muscle. [Gk *phone* sound, *mys* muscle, *graphein* to record.]

phonopathy (fo·**nop**·ath·e). Any diseased state of the vocal organs that affects speech. [Gk *phone* voice, *pathos* disease.]

phonophobia (fo·no·**fo**·be·ah). 1. In cases of laryngeal paralysis, aversion to speaking on account of the pain caused. 2. Exaggerated and morbid fear of speaking above a whisper. 3. Morbid fear of any noise or sound. [Gk *phone* voice, phobia.]

phonophore (**fo**·no·for). 1. The small bones of the ear. 2. A funnel-shaped stethoscope. 3. An electrical instrument for the conveying of laryngeal sounds to the ear of a deaf person. [Gk *phone* sound, *pherein* to bear.]

phonopneumomassage (**fo**·no·**new**·mo·mas·**ahzh**′). Massage of the ligaments, muscles and articulating surfaces of the middle ear by means of a jet of air forced into the external auditory meatus. [Gk *phone* sound, *pneuma* air, *massein* to knead.]

phonopsia (fo·**nop**·se·ah). A condition in which there is perception of colour when particular sounds are heard. [Gk *phone* sound, *opsis* sight.]

phonoreceptor (**fo**·no·re·**sep**′·tor). A receptor for sound impulses. [Gk *phone* sound, receptor.]

phonorenography (**fo**·no·re·**nog**′·raf·e). A phonocatheter is placed retrogradely in the renal pelvis connected to a pre-amplifier; pulse and sound recordings are made at different levels. [Gk *phone* sound, L *ren* kidney, Gk *graphein* to record.]

phonoscope (**fo**·no·skope). An instrument for obtaining a photographic record of the heart sounds, as in phonocardiography. [Gk *phone* sound, *skopein* to view.]

phonoscopy (fo·**nos**·ko·pe). 1. The photographic recording of the sounds of the heart by means of the phonoscope. 2. Determination of the boundaries of organs by means of a stethoscope, while percussion is performed on the adjoining parts.

phonoselectoscope (fo·no·sel·**ek**′·to·skope). An instrument which eliminates the lower or normal range of chest sounds enabling the higher-pitched pathological sounds to be more clearly heard in auscultation. [Gk *phone* sound, L *seligere* to separate, Gk *skopein* to watch.]

phonostethograph (fo·no·**steth**·o·graf). An arrangement for the amplification and recording on a disc of the chest sounds. [Gk *phone* sound, *stethos* chest, *graphein* to record.]

phoorsa (**foor**·sah). The name used in India for *Echis carinatus*, a poisonous viper.

phoresis (for·e·sis). The driving of chemical ions into the tissues by means of an electric current. [Gk *pherein* to bear.]

phoria (for·e·ah). Heterophoria. **Monofixational phoria.** A microtropia with an associated heterophoria. [Gk *phora* orbit.]

phoriascope (for·e·ah·skope). A modified stereoscope employed in orthoptic exercises. [Gk *pherein* to bear, *skopein* to view.]

Phoridae (for·id·e). A family of the dipteran suborder Cyclorrhapha. The genus *Apiochaeta* is of medical interest. [Gk *phor* robber bee.]

Phormia (**for**·me·ah). A genus of sheep blow flies. **Phormia regina.** A species whose larvae have been found in intestinal myiasis in man.

phoroblast (**for**·o·blast). Connective tissue. [Gk *phoros* bearer, *blastos* germ.]

phorocyte (**for**·o·site). One of the cells found in connective tissue. [Gk *phoros* bearer, *kytos* cell.]

phorocytosis (**for**·o·si·**to'**·sis). General increase of the cells in connective tissue. [phorocyte, Gk *-osis* condition.]

phorology (for·**ol**·o·je). The science dealing with the study of carriers of disease. [Gk *phoros* bearer, *logos* science.]

phorometer (for·**om**·et·er). An instrument for measuring the type and amount of heterophoria, consisting of two Maddox rods with double rotating prisms. [Gk *phora* movement, meter.]

phorometry (for·**om**·et·re). Determination of the variety and degree of heterophoria by means of the phorometer.

phorone (**for**·one). Di-isopropylidene acetone, $(CH_3)_2C{=}CHCO\,CH{=}(CH_3)_2$. A compound derived from acetone, of value in organic synthesis.

phoroplast (**for**·o·plast). Connective tissue. [Gk *phoros* bearer, *plastos* formed.]

phose (foze). Any sensation of bright light or colour in the line of vision. [Gk *phos* light.]

phosgene (**fos**·jeen). Carbon oxychloride, carbonyl chloride, $COCl_2$. A colourless gas with a suffocating odour prepared by the oxidation of chloroform. It is used in chemical warfare as a choking gas.

phosgenic (fos·**jen**·ik). Producing light; photogenic. [Gk *phos* light, *genein* to produce.]

phosis (**fo**·sis). The establishment and maintenance of a phose.

phosphagen (**fos**·fah·jen). The name given to creatine phosphate (in vertebrate tissues) and to arginine phosphate (in invertebrate tissues) which act as energy stores in tissues. Phosphagens may be metabolized in muscle during contraction and in nerve during conduction of a nerve impulse. Thus, creatine phosphate can react with adenosine diphosphate to give creatine and adenosine triphosphate which supplies the energy for muscle contraction and nerve conduction; it can be regenerated from adenosine triphosphate and creatine during recovery. [phosphate, Gk *genein* to produce.]

phosphamidase (fos·**fam**·id·aze). An enzyme occurring in the cytoplasm of cells of the liver, adrenal cortex, pancreatic islets and certain other tissues; it also occurs in higher concentration in malignant tumours and in the grey matter of the central nervous system. It is stated to attack an N = P bond.

phosphataemia (fos·fat·**e**·me·ah). A condition marked by excess of phosphates in the blood. [phosphate, Gk *haima* blood.]

phosphatase (**fos**·fat·aze). General term for those specific enzymes which attack phosphoric esters. They occur widely in fermenting organisms and in the tissues, especially in the blood, in which they play an important part in the cycle of muscle contraction, and also in the ossifying zone of bones, in which they are concerned in calcification (bone enzyme). **Acid phosphatase.** Increase in the serum values occurring in prostatic neoplasms. **Alkaline phosphatase.** An enzyme particularly associated with bone formation; the serum level is raised in certain bone-forming tumours. **Serum phosphatase,** the particular phosphatase in blood serum.

phosphate (**fos**·fate). Any salt formed by orthophosphoric acid, H_3PO_4. Phosphates occur naturally in minerals and in the deposits of sea-birds' excreta. They also constitute a proportion of tissue, tissue fluids and bone. They are used in medicine as tonics and in deficiency diseases of bone. **Acid phosphate.** A phosphate in which one (secondary) or two (primary) hydrogen atoms of the original acid remain unreplaced by the base, e.g. disodium hydrogen phosphate. Na_2HPO_4, and sodium dihydrogen phosphate, NaH_2PO_4. **Alkali phosphate.** A phosphate of an alkali metal such as sodium. **Bone phosphate.** Calcium phosphate, $Ca_3(PO_4)_2$, the principal inorganic constituent of bone. **Dibasic phosphate.** A phosphate such as Na_2HPO_4. **Earthy phosphate.** A phosphate of a metal of the alkaline earths such as calcium or magnesium. **Hexose phosphate.** Any ester of a sugar and phosphoric acid which is involved in sugar metabolism and the cycle of muscle contraction. **Monobasic phosphate.** A primary phosphate such as NaH_2PO_4. **Normal phosphate.** A tertiary phosphate. **Primary phosphate.** A phosphate which still contains two of the hydrogen atoms of the original acid, e.g. NaH_2PO_4. **Secondary phosphate.** A phosphate which contains one of the hydrogen atoms of the original acid, e.g. Na_2HPO_4. **Stellar phosphate.** The star-shaped crystals of calcium hydrogen phosphate, $CaHPO_4{\cdot}2H_2O$, appearing in urinary deposits and calculi. **Tertiary phosphate.** A phosphate in which all the hydrogen atoms of the original acid have been replaced by a base, e.g. Na_3PO_4. **Triose phosphate.** The general name given to the two compounds, glyceraldehyde phosphate and dihydroxyacetone phosphate, which play a part in muscle glycogenolysis, sugar fermentation and photosynthesis. Also known as *phosphotrioses*. **Triple phosphate.** The phosphate of ammonium and magnesium excreted in the urine as "coffin-lid" crystals or in feathery form, according to alkalinity.

phosphatese (**fos**·fat·eez). An enzyme system believed to activate the synthesis of hexose phosphates in the formation of lactic acid from glycogen in muscle.

phosphatic (fos·**fat**·ik). Relating to or characterized by phosphates.

phosphatides (fos·fat·i·dz). Phosphatidic acids; esters of glycerol containing two fatty acids and one phosphoric acid and, hence, are diacyl-L-α-glycerophosphoric acids. They are intermediates in the biosynthesis of triglycerides and phospholipids.

phosphatidosis (fos·fat·id·**o'**·sis). Niemann-Pick disease; a generalized disease of the reticulo-endothelial system in which the cells are filled with a complex lipoid material mainly composed of phospholipids. [phosphatide, Gk *-osis* condition.]

phosphatometer (fos·fat·**om**·et·er). An apparatus used to determine the amount of phosphates present in a specimen of urine. [phosphate, Gk *metron* measure.]

phosphatoptosis (**fos**·fat·op·**to'**·sis). A spontaneous and abnormally large deposit of phosphates in the urine. [phosphate, Gk *ptosis* a falling.]

phosphaturia (fos·fat·**ewr**·e·ah). 1. An excess of phosphates in the urine. 2. Phosphatoptosis.

phosphene (**fos**·feen). A subjective sensation of light due to non-luminous stimulation of the retina. **Accommodation phosphene.** A sensation produced by sudden accommodation causing traction on the retina and seen if the patient is in the dark. **Detachment phosphene.** One due to the movements of a detached retina. **Movement phosphene.** One due to sudden eye movements in the dark. **Pressure phosphene.** One in which the stimulus is provided by pressure on the eyeball; "seeing stars". [Gk *phos* light, *phainein* to manifest.]

phosphide (**fos**·fide). A compound of the element phosphorus with another element, e.g. calcium phosphide, Ca_3P_2. The action of water on metallic phosphides is to generate phosphine. Used medicinally instead of phosphorus.

phosphine (**fos**·feen). 1. Hydrogen phosphide, PH_3. A colourless gas with a garlic odour, extremely poisonous and spontaneously inflammable. 2. Any of the organic compounds such as triethylphosphine, $(C_2H_5)_3P$, formed by replacing the hydrogen atoms of hydrogen phosphide with alkyl radicals. 3. Leather yellow, a dye used in the treatment of trypanosomiasis and as a bacteriological stain.

phosphite (**fos**·fite). Any salt formed by orthophosphorous acid, H_3PO_3.

phosphoadenosine phosphosulphate (**fos**·fo·ad·**en**'·o·seen fos·fo·**sul**·fate). PAPS; a nucleotide important in sulphur metabolism.

phospho-aminolipid (**fos**·fo·am·in·o·**lip**'·id). Any phospholipid of the cephalin or lecithin type, where an amine base is incorporated into the structure.

phospho-arginine (fos·fo·**ar**·jin·een). The phosphagen of the muscle of invertebrates, its function being analogous to that of creatine phosphate in the muscle metabolism of vertebrates.

phosphocreatine (fos·fo·**kre**·at·een). Phosphagen.

phosphodiesterase (**fos**·fo·di·**es**'·ter·aze). A type of phosphatase catalysing the hydrolysis of a phosphate ester bond in compounds containing two such bonds. Of particular importance in this class is cyclic 3'5'-AMP phosphodiesterase which inactivates cyclic 3'5'-AMP by hydrolysis to 5'-AMP.

phosphoenolpyruvate (fos·fo·**e**·nol·pi·**roo**'·vate). CH_2=C $(OPO_3H_2)COOH$, an intermediate in glycolysis and gluconeogenesis; a precursor of neuraminic acid. **Phosphoenolpyruvate carboxykinase.** The gluconeogenic enzyme which catalyses the conversion of oxaloacetate into phosphoenolpyruvate, with GTP as phosphate donor.

phosphofructokinase (**fos**·fo·fruk·to·**ki**'·naze). The glycolytic enzyme catalysing the phosphorylation of fructose-6-phosphate by ATP. Frequently pinpointed as a regulatory step; inhibited by ATP and citrate; activated by AMP, ADP, phosphate and fructose diphosphate.

phosphoglobulin (fos·fo·**glob**·ew·lin). A phosphoprotein, the protein moiety of which is of the globulin class. Examples are vitellin and livetin of egg yolk.

phosphoglyceraldehyde (**fos**·fo·glis·er·**al**'·de·hide). CHOCH $(OH)CH_2OPO(OH)_2$. An intermediate compound formed from fructose-1,6-diphosphate in the biological conversion of glycogen or glucose to pyruvic acid.

phosphoglycerate (fos·fo·**glis**·er·ate). **Phosphoglycerate 2- and 3-**, glycolytic intermediates. Interconverted by *phosphoglycerate mutase.* **Phosphoglycerate kinase.** The enzyme which catalyses the reversible phosphorylation of 3-phosphoglycerate by ATP.

phosphohexoisomerase (**fos**·fo·hex·o·i·**som**'·er·aze). An enzyme occurring in animal and plant tissues which catalyses the conversion of glucose-6-phosphate to fructose-6-phosphate, a reaction that forms one of the steps in the biological conversion of glycogen or glucose to pyruvic acid.

phospholipid, phospholipine (fos·fo·**lip**·id, fos·fo·**lip**·een). Any of the compound lipids, mainly lecithins, cephalins and sphingomyelins, which occur in brain and cell tissue. They contain phosphoric acid and a nitrogenous base united to aliphatic acids and glycerol or sphingosine.

phospholipidaemia (**fos**·fo·lip·id·**e**'·me·ah). An increase of phospholipid in the blood. [phospholipide, Gk *haima* blood.]

phosphomonoesterase (**fos**·fo·mon·o·**es**'·ter·aze). A type of phosphatase that activates the hydrolysis of phosphoric esters which contain only one phosphate group.

phosphonecrosis (**fos**·fo·nek·**ro**'·sis). A necrotic condition of the alveolar process of the jaw that may affect those who work with phosphorus.

phosphonium (fos·**fo**·ne·um). A family of compounds formed by the feebly basic phosphine containing the radical PH_4, analogous to ammonium NH_4. The hydrogen atoms may in turn be replaced by alkyl radicals giving rise to a series of organic compounds such as tetramethyl phosphonium hydroxide, P $(CH_3)_4OH$.

phosphopenia (fos·fo·**pe**·ne·ah). A condition characterized by inadequate quantities of phosphorus in the body. [phosphorus, Gk *penes* poor.]

phosphoprotein (fos·fo·**pro**·te·in). A member of a class of proteins in which protein is combined with phosphoric acid, either by peptide or ester linkage. The chief members of this class are casein in milk, and vitellin and livetin in egg yolk. The phosphoric acid is readily removed from the compound molecule by alkaline hydrolysis, or by the action of enzymes such as phosphatase or trypsin.

phosphor (**fos**·for). Any material which emits light when it absorbs ionizing radiation. The general term used to designate the sensitive volume of a scintillation counter whether this be a crystal, a plastic, or a liquid. [Gk *phos* light, *pherein* to bear.]

phosphorated (**fos**·for·a·ted). Phosphoretted.

phosphorenesis (fos·for·**en**·es·is). Disease due to the presence of an excessive amount of calcium phosphate in the body.

phosphorescence (fos·for·**es**·ens). 1. The glow of yellow phosphorus in air, produced by slow oxidation. 2. The emission of visible light without appreciable accompanying heat by substances which have been exposed to radiation of any kind, after such radiation has ceased. 3. The luminosity produced by certain creatures, e.g. glow worms. [Gk *phos* light, *pherein* to bear.]

phosphorescent (fos·for·**es**·ent). Luminous without appreciable heat. [see prec.]

phosphoretted (fos·for·**et**·ed). Phosphorated; impregnated with, or forming a compound with phosphorus. **Phosphoretted hydrogen.** Phosphine, hydrogen phosphide, PH_3.

phosphorhidrosis, phosphoridrosis (**fos**·for·hid·**ro**'·sis, **fos**·for·id·**ro**'·sis). The secretion of sweat which has a luminous or phosphorescent character. [phosphorus, Gk *hidros* sweat.]

phosphoribosyl transferase (fos·for·**ib**·o·sil **trans**'·fer·aze). The enzyme which converts hypoxanthine and guanine to inosinic and guanylic acids, a stage in the degradation of purines to uric acid. This enzyme is deficient in the Lesch–Nyhan syndrome.

phosphorism (**fos**·for·izm). Chronic phosphorus poisoning.

phosphornecrosis (**fos**·for·nek·**ro**'·sis). Phosphonecrosis.

phosphorolysis (fos·for·**ol**·is·is). The splitting-off of phosphoric acid from its esters by an enzyme (phosphorylase). Reversal of the action leads to the production of esters of phosphoric acid. [phosphorus, Gk *lysis* a loosing.]

phosphoroscope (**fos**·for·o·skope). An apparatus by the use of which the amount of phosphorescence may be determined. [phosphorus, Gk *skopein* to watch.]

phosphorous (**fos**·for·us). Of the nature of phosphorus or containing phosphorus; particularly applied to compounds of phosphorus in which the element is trivalent, e.g. phosphorous acid.

phosphorpenia (fos·for·**pe**·ne·ah). Phosphopenia.

phosphoruria (fos·for·**ewr**·e·ah). 1. A condition marked by the secretion of phosphorescent urine. 2. A condition in which free phosphorus exists in the urine.

phosphorus (**fos**·for·us). An element of atomic weight 30.974, atomic number 15, and chemical symbol P. It occurs widely in nature in the combined state in the form of minerals (e.g. apatite) and is an essential constituent of all plants and animals. As phosphates, it enters into body structure (phytates, bone salts), is a constituent of nerve tissue and bone marrow (nucleoproteins, lecithins, cephalins, sphingomyelins), and plays an important part in the metabolism (carbohydrate, lipid, calcium, etc.). It is a non-metal, having several allotropic forms. *Ordinary, or yellow phosphorus* is a white waxy solid, extremely poisonous, and on exposure to air may ignite spontaneously with the formation of oxides. *Red phosphorus, amorphous phosphorus,* a dark-red powder obtained by heating yellow phosphorus out of contact with air, is non-poisonous, is not oxidized in air, and unlike yellow phosphorus, is insoluble in organic solvents such as carbon disulphide. It has replaced yellow phosphorus in match manufacture. Other forms include β- and γ- varieties of yellow phosphorus, *metallic (black) phosphorus,* and *violet phosphorus.* The element is tri- and pentavalent, giving rise to a wide range of oxides, acids and halogen derivatives. **Labelled phosphorus, Radioactive phosphorus.** ${}_{15}P^{32}$, the radioactive isotope of phosphorus produced by the bombardment of ordinary phosphorus with deuterons. It has a half-life of approximately 15 days, and has been used in the investigation of the part played by phosphorus in metabolism. [Gk *phos* light, *pherein* to bear, because of the glow of the element (yellow allotrope) in air.]

phosphoryl (**fos**·for·il). The trivalent radical ≡PO.

phosphorylases (fos·**for**·il·a·zez). Enzymes in plant tissues and micro-organisms which catalyse reaction between glycogen or the components of starch and phosphate to give glucose-1-phosphate. These enzymes are physiologically important in the breakdown of glycogen and starch, and in animal tissues are under hormonal control being activated by cyclic 3′5′AMP through phosphorylation by ATP catalysed by protein kinase.

phosphorylation (**fos**·for·il·**a**′·shun). A general term for the formation of an organic phosphate in a biological system, for example as the result of enzyme-catalysed transfer of the terminal or γ-phosphate of ATP. Thus, the phosphorylation of glucose by hexokinase is given by glucose + ATP → glucose-6-phosphate + ADP. The term is also used to describe the formation of ATP in metabolism by *substrate level phosphorylation* in which, for example, phosphoenol pyruvate formed in glycolysis can react with ADP to give ATP and pyruvate and by *respiratory chain or oxidative phosphorylation,* the process whereby electron flow in the respiratory chain drives the formation of ATP from ADP and phosphate by an, as yet, unknown mechanism.

phosphorylcholine (**fos**·for·il·**ko**′·leen). The phosphoric ester of choline which occurs, combined with glycerol and aliphatic acids, in lecithins.

phosphosugar (fos·fo·**shug**·er). A descriptive general term for the combinations of sugars with phosphoric acid which play so important a part in biological systems, e.g. hexosephosphate.

phosphotidate (fos·**fot**·id·ate). Any ester of glycerophosphoric acid and an aliphatic acid which is found in the cytoplasm of the plant cell.

phosphotriose (fos·fo·**tri**·oze). Name applied to either glyceraldehyde phosphate or dihydroxyacetone phosphate, both of which occur in muscle glycogenolysis, photosynthesis and sugar fermentation. Also known as *triose phosphate.*

phosphuria (fos·**fewr**·e·ah). Phosphaturia.

phot (fot). A unit of intensity of illumination, being defined as the intensity produced by one lumen per square centimetre. [Gk *phos* light.]

photalgia (fo·**tal**·je·ah). Ocular pain set up by light rays; severe photophobia. [Gk *phos* light, *algos* pain.]

photechy (**fo**·tek·e). The radioactive property acquired by objects as a result of previous irradiation. [Gk *phos* light, *echein* to have.]

photic (**fo**·tik). Relating or belonging to light. [Gk *phos* light.]

photism (**fo**·tizm). A visual form or feeling, either of light or colour, evoked by some sensation (taste, smell, touch, hearing, heat, or cold) or thought. [Gk *photismos* illumination.]

photo-actinic (**fo**·to·ak·**tin**′·ik). Sending out luminous rays and rays of the spectrum (actinic). [Gk *phos* light, *aktis* ray.]

photo-aesthesia, photo-aesthesis (**fo**·to·es·**the**′·ze·ah, **fo**·to·es·**the**′·sis). 1. Response to stimulation of light. 2. Photophobia. [Gk *phos* light, aethesia.]

photo-aesthetic (**fo**·to·es·**thet**′·ik). 1. Sensitive to light. 2. Relating to photo-aesthesia. [see prec.]

photo-allergy (fo·to·**al**·er·je). Sensitiveness to light as an allergic manifestation. [Gk *phos* light, allergy.]

photobacterium (**fo**·to·bak·**teer**′·e·um). A bacterium possessing a photosynthetic mechanism. [Gk *phos* light, bacterium.]

photobiology (**fo**·to·bi·**ol**′·o·je). The study of the action of light on living organisms. [Gk *phos* light, biology.]

photobiotic (**fo**·to·bi·**ot**′·ik). Pertaining to organisms which require light for existence and vigorous growth. [Gk *phos* light, *bios* life.]

photocatalyst, photocatalyser (fo·to·**kat**·al·ist, fo·to·**kat**·al·i·zer). A catalyst which depends for its action on the effect of light of a particular wavelength. [GK *phos* light, catalyst.]

photocauterization (**fo**·to·kaw·ter·i·**za**′·shun). Cauterization by means of x-rays, radium or other radioactive agent. [Gk *phos* light, cautery.]

photocautery (fo·to·**kaw**·ter·e). 1. An instrument used in photocauterization. 2. Photocauterization.

photoceptor (**fo**·to·sep·tor). Photoreceptor.

photochemical (fo·to·**kem**·ik·al). Relating to chemical action under the influence of light. [Gk *phos* light, chemistry.]

photochemistry (fo·to·**kem**·is·tre). The study of chemical actions brought about by light or other forms of radiant energy. [see prec.]

photochromatic (fo·to·kro·**mat**′·ik). 1. Relating to coloured light. 2. Belonging to or produced by colour photography. [Gk *phos* light, *chroma* colour.]

photocinetic (**fo**·to·sin·**et**′·ik). Photokinetic.

photocoagulation (**fo**·to·ko·ag·ew·**la**′·shun). Coagulation of tissue produced by an intense beam of light, used in the treatment of retinal disease. [Gk *phos* light, L *coagulare* to curdle.]

photocolorimeter (**fo**·to·kol·or·**im**′·et·er). An instrument for measuring the depth of colour; it includes colour filters and photo-electric cells. [Gk *phos* light, colorimeter.]

photodensitometer (**fo**·to·den·sit·**om**′·et·er). An apparatus for translating strip chromatograms, which have been obtained by electrophoresis, into graphs. [Gk *phos* light, densitometer.]

photodermatism (fo·to·**der**·mat·ism). The quality of sensitivity of the epithelium of the skin to light. [Gk *phos* light, *derma* skin.]

photodermatosis (**fo**·to·der·mat·**o**′·sis). A skin lesion resulting from exposure to light. [Gk *phos* light, *derma* skin, *-osis* condition.]

photodermia (fo·to·**der**·me·ah). Cutaneous lesions caused by exposure to light. [Gk *phos* light, *derma* skin.]

photodromy (fo·**tod**·ro·me). The directional movement exhibited by certain particles in suspension under the influence of light either positively (towards) or negatively (away from) the source. [Gk *phos* light, *dromos* a running.]

photodynamic (**fo**·to·di·**nam**′·ik). Fluorescent; having the ability to emit light of a certain wavelength when radiated with light of another wavelength. [Gk *phos* light, *dynamis* power.]

photodynamics (**fo**·to·di·**nam**′·ix). The science which deals with the force exerted by light, and with its relation to plant movement. [see prec.]

photodynia (fo·to·**din**·e·ah). Sensation of pain induced by rays of light. [Gk *phos* light, *odyne* pain.]

photodysphoria (**fo**·to·dis·**for**′·e·ah). Photophobia. [Gk *phos* light, *dysphoros* hard to bear.]

photo-electric (**fo**·to·el·**ek**′·trik). Pertaining to the release of electrons by the action of light. [Gk *phos* light, electron.]

photo-electricity (**fo**·to·el·ek·**tris**′·it·e). Electricity produced by the action of light. [see prec.]

photo-electrometer (**fo**·to·el·ek·**trom**′·et·er). An apparatus containing a photo-electric cell, used for estimating small quantities of substances in solution by measuring the amount of light absorbed by the solution and comparing it against a standard solution of the same substance. It is of great value where substances have to be measured in very small concentrations, or where quantities of material such as blood constituents are small, or where there are no satisfactory chemical methods of estimation. [Gk *phos* light, electrometer.]

photo-electron (**fo**·to·el·**ek**′·tron). Any electron which is discharged from the surface of a metal when light impinges upon it. [Gk *phos* light, electron.]

photo-element (fo·to·**el**·em·ent). 1. Any element, metallic or otherwise, employed to convert variations in light intensity into equivalent variations of an electric current, e.g. selenium. 2. Any element which emits electrons when light falls upon its surface thereby setting up a photo-electric current. [Gk *phos* light, element.]

photo-erythema (**fo**·to·er·e·**the**′·mah). An erythematous condition caused by light rays. [Gk *phos* light, erythema.]

photofluorogram (**fo**·to·floo·**or**′·o·gram). The photographic record produced in photofluorography.

photofluorography (fo·to·floo·or·**og'**·raf·e). The production of photographs of the fluorescent screen image, used chiefly in mass miniature radiographs. [Gk *phos* light, fluorescence, Gk *graphein* to write.]

photofluoroscope (**fo**·to·floo·**or'**·o·skope). An apparatus used to photograph the fluorescent x-ray screen. [Gk *phos* light, fluorescence, Gk *skopein* to watch.]

photofluoroscopy (fo·to·floo·or·**os'**·ko·pe). Photofluorography. [see prec.]

photogastroscope (fo·to·**gas**·tro·skope). An instrument used in photography of the interior of the stomach. [Gk *phos* light, gastroscope.]

photogen (**fo**·to·jen). The substance which is the potential source of phosphorescence in certain photogenic micro-organisms. [see foll.]

photogene (**fo**·to·jeen). After-image; the visual impression which remains after the stimulation of the retina has ceased. [Gk *phos* light, *genein* to produce.]

photogenesis (fo·to·**jen**·es·is). 1. Phosphorescence. 2. State of bacteria in which they give out light. [see prec.]

photogenic, photogenous (fo·to·**jen**·ik, fo·**toj**·en·us). 1. Emitting or producing light; phosphorescent. 2. Produced by the action of light. [Gk *phos* light, *genein* to produce.]

photohaematachometer (**fo**·to·he·mah·tak·**om'**·et·er). An instrument for making a photographic record of the rate of blood flow. [Gk *phos* light, *haima* blood, *tachys* swift, meter.]

photo-inactivation (**fo**·to·in·ak·tiv·**a'**·shun). The use of light, usually in conjunction with suitable sensitizing dyes, to inactivate viruses, complement, etc. [Gk *phos* light, L *activus* active.]

photokinesis (**fo**·to·kin·**e'**·sis). Movement which is set up by stimulation of light rays. [Gk *phos* light, *kinesis* movement.]

photokymograph (fo·to·**ki**·mo·graf). An apparatus in which the movements of a beam of light (or of a shadow) are recorded by the use of photography. [Gk *phos* light, *kyme* wave, *graphein* to record.]

photology (fo·**tol**·o·je). The science of light. [Gk *phos* light, *logos* science.]

photoluminescence (**fo**·to·loo·min·**es'**·ens). The property of becoming luminescent by exposure to the action of light waves. [Gk *phos* light, luminescence.]

photolysis (fo·**tol**·is·is). 1. Chemical change in a solution brought about by light. 2. The dissolution of cells by the action of light. [Gk *phos* light, *lysis* a loosing.]

photolyte (**fo**·to·lite). 1. Any substance that undergoes photolysis. 2. The product resulting from photolysis.

photolytic (fo·to·**lit**·ik). Relating to photolysis; exhibiting a tendency to photolysis in light.

photomagnetism (fo·to·**mag**·net·izm). Magnetism resulting from the atomic absorption of circularly polarized light. [Gk *phos* light, magnetism.]

photomania (fo·to·**ma**·ne·ah). 1. The development of symptoms of insanity because of long exposure to intense light. 2. A morbid craving, amounting to insanity, for light. [GK *phos* light, mania.]

photometer (fo·**tom**·et·er). An instrument with which the intensities of two sources of light may be compared. **Flame photometer.** An instrument used to measure the concentration of certain inorganic elements in solution from the intensity of the characteristic colour they produce when introduced into a flame. **Flicker photometer.** A device by means of which the eye is exposed alternately to the two surfaces to be compared; the the frequency of this alteration can be adjusted to where the colour difference disappears whilst the flicker due to the difference in brightness remains. [Gk *phos* light, meter.]

See also: FOERSTER (R.), PULFRICH.

photometry (fo·**tom**·et·re). 1. The science of measurement of light intensity. 2. The measurement of the reaction to light of an organism. **Flame photometry.** Chemical analysis by means of the flame photometer. **Flicker photometry.** Flicker test. See TEST. [see prec.]

photomicrograph (fo·to·**mi**·kro·graf). A photograph of a microscopical object, taken through a compound microscope.

photomicrography (fo·to·mi·**krog'**·raf·e). The process of making a photomicrograph.

photomicroscope (fo·to·**mi**·kro·skope). A combination of a camera and microscope used to take photographs of microscopic objects.

photomicroscopy (**fo**·to·mi·**kros'**·ko·pe). The photography of microscopic objects by the aid of the photomicroscope.

photomorphism, photomorphosis (fo·to·**mor**·fizm, fo·to·**mor**·fo·sis). The alterations in structure made in organisms by their exposure to light. [Gk *phos* light, *morphe* shape.]

photomotor (fo·to·**mo**·tor). Pertaining to the muscular reaction to light that causes pupillary contraction. [Gk *phos* light, L *movere* to move.]

photomultiplier (fo·to·**mul**·tip·li·er). A vacuum tube containing a cathode emitting electrons under the action of light. These are accelerated to strike intermediate electrodes, thereby producing larger numbers of electrons by secondary emission. The final multiplied electron output is collected, furnishing a potential pulse on the collector. The light sensitivity of the photomultiplier in thus very high. [Gk *phos* light, L *multiplex* many-folded.]

photon (**fo**·ton). A quantum of electromagnetic radiation. [Gk *phos* light.]

photone (**fo**·tone). 1. A hallucination of light. 2. Visualization of light. [Gk *phos* light.]

photonosus (fo·to·**no**·sus). Any morbid condition due to prolonged exposure to intense light. [Gk *phos* light, *nosos* disease.]

photo-ophthalmia (**fo**·to·of·**thal'**·me·ah). Ophthalmia produced by intense light. [Gk *phos* light, ophthalmia.]

photoparaesthesia (**fo**·to·par·es·**the'**·ze·ah). A condition in which the sensitiveness of the retina is perverted or defective. [Gk *phos* light, paraesthesia.]

photopathological (**fo**·to·path·o·**loj'**·ik·al). Pertaining to the detrimental effect of light on the organism. [Gk *phos* light, pathology.]

photopathy (fo·**top**·ath·e). 1. Any morbid condition due to prolonged exposure to intense light. 2. The attractive or repellent effect of light upon living organisms. [Gk *phos* light, *pathos* disease.]

photoperceptive (**fo**·to·per·**sep'**·tiv). Able to see light. [Gk *phos* light, perception.]

photoperiodism (fo·to·**peer**·e·od·izm). The physiological changes in animals and plants brought about by the variations in the alternations of light and darkness. [Gk *phos* light, *periodos* cycle.]

photophilic (fo·to·**fil**·ik). 1. Light-loving; denoting plants which require strong light in order to flourish, or which are able to grow in strong light. 2. Seeking light. [GK *phos* light, *philein* to love.]

photophobia (fo·to·**fo**·be·ah). 1. Morbid dread of, or aversion to being in well-lit places. 2. Abnormal intolerance of, or sensitiveness to light; term used particularly of the eyes. [Gk *phos* light, *phobos* fear.]

photophobic (fo·to·**fo**·bik). Relating or belonging to, characterized by, or affected with photophobia.

photophore (**fo**·to·for). A lamp for rhinoscopy or laryngoscopy. [Gk *phos* light, *pherein* to bear.]

photopia (fo·**to**·pe·ah). Light adaptation; the adjustment by which the eye accommodates itself to bright light. [Gk *phos* light, *ops* eye.]

photopic (fo·**top**·ik). Applied to light of moderate or high intensity, sufficient to allow of colour perception. [see prec.]

photopsia, photopsy (fo·**top**·se·ah, fo·**top**·se). A sensation of light, as of flashes or sparks, associated with disease of the retina. [Gk *phos* light, *opsis* vision.]

photoptic (fo·**top**·tik). Relating or belonging to or affected with photopsia.

photoptometer (fo·top·**tom**·et·er). An instrument for measuring the smallest amount of light which allows an object to be seen. [see foll.]

photoptometry (fo·top·**tom**·et·re). Measurement of light perception. [Gk *phos* light, *optein* to see, *metron* measure.]

photoradiometer (**fo**·to·ra·de·**om**′·et·er). An apparatus for measuring the intensity of x-rays (now obsolete). [Gk *phos* light, radiometer.]

photoreaction (fo·to·re·**ak**′·shun). Any chemical reaction that takes place through the influence of light. [Gk *phos* light, reaction.]

photoreactivation (**fo**·to·re·ak·tiv·**a**′·shun). Enzymatic repair of DNA lesions produced by ultraviolet radiations, which takes place only in the presence of light. In contraposition to dark DNA repair. [Gk *phos* light, L *re-*, *activus* active.]

photoreceptive (**fo**·to·re·**sep**′·tiv). Able to receive light rays. [Gk *phos* light, reception.]

photoreceptor (**fo**·to·re·**sep**′·tor). A nerve-ending that receives light stimuli. [Gk *phos* light, receptor.]

photoscan (**fo**·to·skan). A scan composed of a series of marks obtained by a photographic process; a scintiscan obtained by this means in contrast to one obtained by a mechanical printer. [Gk *phos* light, L *scandere* to climb.]

photoscope (**fo**·to·skope). 1. Any instrument for observing light or the effects of light. 2. A special device for recording the movements of the mouth in speech and used for the instruction of deaf mutes. [Gk *phos* light, *skopein* to view.]

photosensitive (fo·to·**sen**·sit·iv). Relating to an organism or substance which is capable of being stimulated by the influence of light. [Gk *phos* light, sensitive.]

photosensitivity (**fo**·to·sen·sit·**iv**′·it·e). Sensitivity to light. [see prec.]

photosensitization (**fo**·to·sen·sit·i·**za**′·shun). The act of rendering an organism or substance sensitive to the action of light. **Cross-photosensitization.** That occurring between immunochemically related light substances, e.g. sulphonamides and phenothiazines. [see foll.]

photosensitize (fo·to·**sen**·sit·ize). To render an organism or substance sensitive to the action of light. [Gk *phos* light, sensitize.]

photostable (**fo**·to·sta·bl). Unaltered by the action of light. [Gk *phos* light, stable.]

photostethoscope (fo·to·**steth**·o·skope). A lamp which converts sounds magnified by a microphone into flashes of light and is used for recording the beats, or for continuous observation of the fetal heart. [Gk *phos* light, *stethos* chest. *skopein* to watch.]

photosynthesis (fo·to·**sin**·the·sis). In plant physiology, the combining or building up of chemical substances which occurs by means of the action of light, especially the process by which carbohydrates are compounded from carbon dioxide and water in the chlorophyll-containing tissues of plants when under exposure to light. [Gk *phos* light, synthesis.]

phototactic (fo·to·**tak**·tik). Relating or belonging to phototaxis.

phototaxis (fo·to·**tax**·is). The reaction of micro-organisms and cells to light stimulus in which they migrate either towards (*positive phototaxis*) or away from (*negative phototaxis*) the light or a luminous body. [Gk *phos* light, *taxis* arrangement.]

phototherapy (fo·to·**ther**·ap·e). The employment of light in the treatment of disease. [Gk *phos* light, *therapeia* treatment.]

phototonus (fo·**tot**·o·nus). Sensitivity in an organism produced by exposure to light. [Gk *phos* light, *tonos* tension.]

phototoxis (fo·to·**tox**·is). The condition resulting from excessive exposure to light or other form of radiant energy. [Gk *phos* light, *toxikon* poison.]

phototrophic (fo·to·**trof**·ik). Pertaining to the use of light in metabolism. [Gk *phos* light, *trophe* nourishment.]

phototropic (fo·to·**trop**·ik). Pertaining to phototropism.

phototropism (fo·to·**trop**·izm). 1. The movement of plants or other living organisms either towards (*positive phototropism*) or away from (*negative phototropism*) the light. 2. Alteration of colour effected in an organism under the influence of light. [Gk *phos* light, *trope* a turning.]

photuria (fo·tewr·e·ah). Micturition in which the urine has phosphorescent characters. [Gk *phos* light, urine.]

Phoxinus (**fox**·in·us). A genus of fresh-water fish. *Phoxinus laevis* is the minnow, which is used as a laboratory animal. [Gk *phoxinos* a river fish.]

Phragmidiothrix (frag·**mid**·e·o·thrix). A generic name suggested by Engler (1882) for a single species of non-branching, filamentous bacteria, enclosed in a sheath, now known as *Crenothrix*, a genus of the family Crenothrichaceae. They are non-pathogenic, and have their habitat in water. [Gk *phragmos* enclosure, *thrix* hair.]

phragmoplast (**frag**·mo·plast). The equatorial element of the spindle in plant cells, from which new cellulose walls are generated after cell division. [Gk *phragmos* enclosure, *plassein* to form.]

phren (fren). 1. The diaphragm. 2. Old-fashioned term for the mind. [Gk.]

phrenalgia (fren·**al**·je·ah). 1. Psychalgia; mental distress or pain associated with mental effort, the state occurring particularly in melancholia. 2. A condition of pain occurring in the diaphragm. [Gk *phren* mind, diaphragm, *algos* pain.]

phrenasthenia (fren·as·**the**·ne·ah). 1. Feeble-mindedness. 2. A condition marked by loss of tone in the diaphragm. [Gk *phren* mind, diaphragm, asthenia.]

phrenasthenic (fren·as·**then**·ik). 1. A feeble-minded individual. 2. Relating or belonging to phrenasthenia. [see prec.]

phrenasthesia (fren·as·**the**·ze·ah). Idiocy. [Gk *phren* mind, *a*, *sthenos* strength.]

phrenatrophia (fren·at·**ro**·fe·ah). 1. The state of idiocy. 2. Cerebral atrophy. [Gk *phren* mind, atrophy.]

phrenauxe (fren·**awx**·e). Cerebral hypertrophy. [Gk *phren* mind, *auxe* increase.]

phrenectomy (fren·**ek**·to·me). Phrenicectomy.

phrenemphraxis (fren·em·**frax**·is). The operation of crushing the phrenic nerve, [phrenic nerve, Gk *emphrassein* to block up.]

phrenesia (fren·e·ze·ah). Encephalitis. [Gk *phren* mind.]

phrenesiac (fren·e·ze·ak). A person affected with phrenesis.

phrenesis (fren·e·sis). Insanity, frenzy, delirium. [Gk.]

phrenetic (fren·**et**·ik). 1. Insane; frenzied; delirious. 2. A maniac. [see prec.]

phrenic (**fren**·ik). 1. Relating to the mind or intellect. 2. Relating to the diaphragm. [Gk *phren* mind, diaphragm.]

phrenic arteries [arteriae phrenicae inferiores (NA)]. Branches of the abdominal aorta, given off as the aorta passes between the diaphragmatic crura. They are on the underside of the diaphragm, and supply the superior suprarenal branches to the suprarenal glands.

phrenic nerve [nervus phrenicus (NA)]. A paired nerve; one of the branches of the cervical plexus, deriving its fibres from the 3rd, 4th and 5th cervical nerves and descending through the neck and thorax to supply the diaphragm [rami phrenico-abdominales (NA)], pericardium [ramus pericardiacus (NA)] and pleura. It may receive fibres from the 5th cervical nerve through the nerve to the subclavius muscle. **Accessory phrenic neves [nervi phrenici accessorii (NA)].** The fibres of the 5th cervical nerve to the phrenic nerve when these fibres take an independent course in the neck, usually travelling in the nerve to the subclavius muscle and joining the main phrenic nerve in the thorax.

phrenic veins [venae phrenicae inferiores et superiores (NA)]. Veins draining both surfaces of the diaphragm, generally terminating on the right in the inferior vena cava and on the left in one or more of the following veins: renal, suprarenal or inferior vena cava.

phrenicectomize (fren·e·**sek**·tom·ize). To excise either a part or the whole of the phrenic nerve. [see foll.]

phrenicectomy (fren·e·**sek**·to·me). The operation of excising a portion of a phrenic nerve. [phrenic nerve, Gk *ektome* a cutting out.]

phreniclasia, phreniclasis (fren·e·**kla**·ze·ah, fren·e·**kla**·sis). The operation of clamping a phrenic nerve. [phrenic nerve, Gk *klasis* a breaking.]

phrenicocolic (**fren**·ik·o·**kol**′·ik). Pertaining to the diaphragm and the colon. [Gk *phren* diaphragm, colon.]

phrenico-exeresis (**fren**·ik·o·ex·**er**′·e·sis). Phrenic avulsion; phrenicectomy. [phrenic nerve, exeresis.]

phrenicogastric (**fren**·ik·o·**gas**′·trik). Relating or belonging to diaphragm and the stomach. [Gk *phren* diaphragm, *gaster* stomach.]

phreniconeurectomy (**fren**·ik·o·newr·**ek**′·to·me). The operation of excising a part or the whole of a phrenic nerve. [phrenic, Gk *neuron* nerve, *ektome* a cutting out.]

phrenicosplenic (**fren**·ik·o·**splen**′·ik). Relating or belonging to the diaphragm and the spleen. [Gk *phren* diaphragm, spleen.]

phrenicotomy (fren·ik·**ot**·o·me). Division of a phrenic nerve. This results in paralysis of that part of the diaphragm supplied by the nerve. [phrenic nerve, Gk *temnein* to cut.]

phrenicotripsy (**fren**·ik·o·**trip**′·se). Phreniclasia. [phrenic nerve, Gk *tripsis* a rubbing away.]

phrenitis (fren·**i**·tis). 1. Encephalitis. 2. Delirium. 3. Inflammation affecting the diaphragm. [Gk *phren* mind, diaphragm, *-itis* inflammation.]

phrenoblabia (fren·o·**bla**·be·ah). Mental derangement. [Gk *phren* mind, *blabe* damage.]

phrenocardia (fren·o·**kar**·de·ah). A neurasthenic condition in which submammary pain and laboured respiration are present. [Gk *phren* mind, *kardia* heart.]

phrenocolic (fren·o·**kol**·ik). Pertaining to the diaphragm and the colon. [Gk *phren* diaphragm, colon.]

phrenocolopexy (fren·o·**ko**·lo·pex·e). The operation of suturing to the diaphragm a displaced or prolapsed transverse colon. [Gk *phren* diaphragm, colon, Gk *pexis* fixation.]

phrenocostal (fren·o·**kos**·tal). Relating or belonging to the diaphragm and the ribs. [Gk *phren* diaphragm, L *costa* rib.]

phrenodynia (fren·o·**din**·e·ah). Pain in the diaphragm. [Gk *phren* diaphragm, *odyne* pain.]

phrenogastric (fren·o·**gas**·trik). Relating or belonging to the diaphragm and the stomach. [Gk *phren* diaphragm, *gaster* stomach.]

phrenoglottic (fren·o·**glot**·ik). Relating to the diaphragm and the glottis. [Gk *phren* diaphragm, glottis.]

phrenoglottismus (**fren**·o·glot·**iz**′·mus). Glottic spasm caused by some affection of the diaphragm. [see prec.]

phrenograph (**fren**·o·graf). An instrument used for recording graphically movements of the diaphragm. [Gk *phren* diaphragm, *graphein* to record.]

phrenohepatic (**fren**·o·hep·**at**′·ik). Relating or belonging to the diaphragm and the liver. [Gk *phren* diaphragm, *hepar* liver.]

phrenolepsia (fren·o·**lep**·se·ah). Insanity. [Gk *phren* mind, *lepsis* a carrying off.]

phrenology (fren·**ol**·o·je). The study of the mind, character and faculties of an individual by the shape of his head. The theory on which it is based is not accepted. [Gk *phren* mind, *logos* science.]

phrenoparalysis (**fren**·o·par·**al**′·is·is). Phrenoplegia. [Gk *phren* mind, diaphragm, paralysis.]

phrenopathic (**fren**·o·path·ik). Psychopathic. [see foll.]

phrenopathy (fren·**op**·ath·e). Any morbid mental state. [Gk *phren* mind, *pathos* disease.]

phrenopericarditis (**fren**·o·per·e·kar·**di**′·tis). A condition marked by attachment of the apex of the heart to the diaphragm as a result of adhesions. [Gk *phren* diaphragm, pericarditis.]

phrenoplegia, phrenoplegy (fren·o·**ple**·je·ah, fren·o·**ple**·je). 1. Sudden failing of mental power, or the onset of psychosis. 2. Diaphragmatic paralysis. [Gk *phren* mind, diaphragm, *plege* stroke.]

phrenoptosis (fren·op·**to**·sis). A condition in which there is abnormal displacement downwards of the diaphragm. [Gk *phren* diaphragm, *ptosis* fall.]

phrenosin (**fren**·o·sin). $C_{48}H_{91}NO_8$, a glycolipid occurring in brain tissue. It is a white crystalline substance, insoluble in ether but soluble in warm alcohol, and hydrolysed by acids to give galactose, sphingosine and phrenosinic acid.

phrenospasm (**fren**·o·spazm). 1. Spasmodic contraction of the diaphragm. 2. Achalasia of the cardia of the stomach. [Gk *phren* diaphragm, spasm.]

phrenosplenic (fren·o·**splen**·ik). Relating or belonging to the diaphragm and the spleen. [Gk *phren* daphragm, spleen.]

phrenosterol (fren·**os**·ter·ol). An isomeric form of cholesterol which has been isolated from extracts of brain. [Gk *phren* mind, sterol.]

phricasmus (frik·**az**·mus). Cutis anserina. [Gk *phrike* a shivering.]

phrictopathic (frik·to·**path**·ik). A peculiar form of shudder or sensation of shuddering observed in certain functional disorders. [Gk *phriktos* to be shuddered at, *pathos* disease.]

phronemophobia (**fron**·e·mo·**fo**′·be·ah). Fear of or aversion to thinking. [Gk *phronema* thought, phobia.]

phronesis (fron·**e**·sis). Stability of mind and critical faculty. [Gk *phronein* to have understanding.]

phronetal (fron·**e**·tal). Concerning the process of thought. [see prec.]

phrynoderma (frin·o·**der**·mah). Toad skin; a sign of avitaminosis A. The whole skin becomes dry, and on various areas at the pilosebaceous orifices there are closely set dome-shaped papules resembling the skin of a toad. The most affected parts are usually the outer surfaces of the arms and the anterior and external aspects of the thighs. [Gk *phrynos* toad, *derma* skin.]

phrynolysin (fri·**nol**·i·sin). A lysin or toxin found in *Bombinator igneus*, the fire-toad; it haemolyses the blood of certain animals. [Gk *phrynos* toad, *lysis* a loosening.]

phthalate (**thal**·ate). Any salt or ester formed by phthalic acid.

phthalein (**thal**·e·in). Name applied to any of the dyes prepared from phthalic anhydride and a phenol: some are used as indicators and also are employed in medicine for their purgative action. **Alphanaphthol phthalein.** An indicator used for pH determination (7.3–8.4), changing from pink (acid) to green (alkali). **Orthocresol phthalein.** A pH indicator (8.2–9.2), which is colourless in acid and red in alkali.

phthalic anhydride (**thal**·ik an·**hi**·dride). $C_6H_4(CO)_2O$, a crystalline substance prepared from phthalic acid and used in the manufacture of drugs and dyestuffs. [na*phthal*ene.]

phthaline (**thal**·een). A colourless compound formed from the corresponding phthalein by reduction; easily reoxidized to the phthalein.

phthalocyanine (thal·o·**si**·an·een). One of a family of intense pigments synthesized from phthalonitrile. Structurally phthalocyanines consist of a porphyrin ring with a metallic atom at the centre and are therefore related to chlorophyll and haemoglobin. The copper compound is a vivid persistent blue dye. [phthalic, Gk *kyanos* blue.]

phthalonitrile (thal·o·**ni**·trile). $C_6H_4(CN)_2$, a compound used in the preparation of the phthalocyanine dyes.

phthalylsulphacetamide (**thal**·il·sul·fas·**et**′·am·ide). $C_6H_4(COOH)CONHC_6H_4SO_2NHCOCH_3$. A sulphonamide drug used in the treatment of gastrointestinal infections on account of its extremely slow absorption from the gut.

Phthalylsulphathiazole BP 1973 (**thal**·il·sul·fah·**thi**′·az·ole). $C_6H_4(COOH)CONHC_6H_4SO_2NHC_3H_2NS$. Like succinylsulphathiazole and phthalylsulphacetamide, a drug that is only slowly absorbed, and is therefore used in the treatment of infections of the gut.

phtheiriophobia (**thi**·re·o·**fo**′·be·ah). Unnatural fear of lice. [Gk *phtheiriaein* to be lousy, phobia.]

phthersigenic (ther·se·**jen**·ik). Pertaining to that type of mental disorder which is marked by a degradation or deterioration. [Gk *phthersigenes* destroying the race or family.]

phthiocerol (thi·o·**se**·rol). $C_{35}H_{72}O_3$, a crystalline alcohol isolated from the lipoid fraction of *Mycobacterium tuberculosis* (var. *hominis*).

phthiocol (**thi**·o·kol). 3-Hydroxy-2-methyl-1,4-naphthoquinone, $C_{10}H_4O_2(CH_3)(OH)$. A yellow crystalline pigment which can be extracted from cultures of *Mycobacterium tuberculosis* (var. *hominis*). It is related to vitamin K and has antihaemolytic properties. It is a growth factor for Johne's bacillus.

phthiriasis (thir·**i**·as·is). Infestation with lice of the genus *Phthirus*. [Gk *phtheir* louse.]

phthiriophobia (thi·re·o·**fo′**·be· ah). Phtheiriophobia.

phthirus (thir·us). The sucking louse, *Phthirus pubis*, a specific parasite of man, and confined to areas of coarse hair, particularly in the pubic region, but also of the chest, axillae, and eyebrows and lashes. It causes irritation and purple patches at hair bases, but is not apparently a disease vector. [Gk *phtheir* louse.]

phthisic, phthisical (**thi**·zik, **thi**·zik·al). Belonging to, suffering from, or having the characteristics of phthisis.

phthisiogenesis (**thi**·ze·o·**jen′**·es·is). The rise and establishment of the active phthisical state in any person. [phthisis, Gk *genein* to produce.]

phthisiogenetic, phthisiogenic (**thi**·ze·o·jen·**et′**·ik, **thi**·ze·o·**jen′**·ik). 1. Causing phthisis. 2. Relating to the origin of phthisis. [see prec.]

phthisiomania (**thi**·ze·o·**ma′**·ne·ah). An erroneous idea amounting almost to an insane conviction on the part of an individual that he is suffering from pulmonary tuberculosis. [phthisis, mania.]

phthisiophobia (**thi**·ze·o·**fo′**·be·ah). An unnatural fear of pulmonary tuberculosis or of tuberculous persons. [phthisis, phobia.]

phthisis (**thi**·sis). 1. Any wasting disease in which the whole body is involved or only a part of the body. 2. Pulmonary tuberculosis. A reference to phthisis without qualification nowadays invariably means the latter disease. **Abdominal phthisis.** Tabes mesenterica; tuberculosis of the intestines and mesenteric glands. **Apicocaudal phthisis.** Tuberculosis affecting the upper segment of the lower or dorsal lobe of the lung. **Bacillary phthisis.** Pulmonary tuberculosis in which tubercle bacilli have been found [obsolete term]. **Basal phthisis.** Tuberculosis of the lower or dorsal lobes of one or both lungs. **Black phthisis.** Anthracosis. **Bronchial phthisis.** Inflammatory or ulcerative tuberculous lesions of the larger bronchi in cases of tuberculosis of the lungs. It may give rise to stenosis and areas of alveolar collapse or even atelectasis of a lobe if blockage is complete. **Phthisis bulbi.** A soft and shrunken eye usually following severe inflammation or injury. **Phthisis corneae.** A shrunken and contracted cornea following severe injury or inflammation of the cornea, associated with shrinking and softening of the globe. **Phthisis desperata.** Progressive incurable tuberculosis of the lungs. **Diabetic phthisis.** Acute caseous pulmonary tuberculosis in diabetics. **Dorsal phthisis.** Pott's disease; tuberculosis of the spine. **Essentia phthisis of the eye.** The term originally used by von Graefe for the condition of hypotension of the eye. Also called *ophthalmomalacia*. **Fibroid phthisis.** Chronic pulmonary tuberculosis in which fibrotic changes have taken place in the diseased parenchyma or pleura to such an extent that it is the predominant clinical feature, causing loss of elasticity of the lung and often deformity of the thoracic wall, displacement of the heart, mediastinum and diaphragm. **Flax-dressers' phthisis.** A fibroid pneumonic condition due to inhalation of fine particles of flax by those employed in dressing flax. **Phthisis florida.** Acute febrile pulmonary tuberculosis with widespread bronchopneumonic lesions which may become confluent and necrotic or caseous. **Galloping phthisis.** Phthisis florida (see above). **Glandular phthisis.** Tuberculosis of lymph glands. **Grinders' phthisis.** The association of pneumoconiosis with chronic pulmonary tuberculosis, occurring in knife grinders. The primary cause of the pneumoconiosis is the inhalation of grindstone dust. **Hepatic phthisis.** Wasting caused by chronic hepatic disease. **Phthisis incipiens.** The earliest stage of pulmonary tuberculosis in which it can be diagnosed, either by clinical, radiological or bacteriological means. The term does not necessarily imply a good prognosis. **Knife-grinders' phthisis.** Grinders' phthisis (see above). **Laryngeal phthisis.** Tuberculosis of the larynx. **Marble-cutters' phthisis.** Calcicosis. **Mediterranean phthisis.** Malta fever. *See* FEVER. **Miners' phthisis.** Silicosis. **Phthisis nodosa.** Miliary tuberculosis. *See* TUBERCULOSIS. **Non-bacillary phthisis.** Disease of the lungs simulating tuberculosis but due to other causes. **Pancreatic phthisis.** Wasting caused by chronic pancreatic disease. **Phthisis phlegmatica.** Tuberculosis occurring without loss of weight. **Pneumonic phthisis.** *See* PNEUMONIA, TUBERCULOUS. **Potters' phthisis.** The association of pneumoconiosis with chronic pulmonary tuberculosis, occurring in potters. The primary cause of the pneumoconiosis is the inhalation of the silicious dust in the manufacture of pottery. **Rand miners' phthisis.** Silicosis. **Phthisis renalis.** Tuberculosis of the kidneys. **Stone-cutters' phthisis.** The association of pneumoconiosis with chronic pulmonary tuberculosis, occurring in stone cutters. The primary cause of the pneumoconiosis is the inhalation of silica dust in the course of the worker's occupation. **Phthisis ventriculi.** Wasting of the mucous membrane of the stomach. [Gk, a wasting away.]

phycochromoprotein (fi·ko·kro·mo·**pro′**·te·in). A term used to designate the chromoproteins of seaweeds. [Gk *phykos* seaweed, chromoprotein.]

phycocyan (fi·ko·**si**·an). A blue pigment occurring in seaweeds. It is one of the phytochrome class of chromoproteins. [Gk *phykos* seaweed, *kyanos* blue.]

phycocyanin (**fi**·ko·si·**an′**·in). A blue colouring matter present in the *Cyanophyceae*, an order of blue-green algae found in water reservoirs. [see prec.]

phyco-erythrin (fi·ko·**er**·ith·rin). A red pigment occurring in seaweeds. It is one of the phytochrome class of chromoproteins. [Gk *phykos* seaweed, *erythros* red.]

phycology (fi·**kol**·o·je). The study of algae. [Gk *phykos* seaweed, *logos* science.]

phycomycetes (**fi**·ko·mi·**se′**·teez). Fungi having typically aseptate mycelium; some are pathogenic for man and animals, e.g. *Mucor* species in otomycosis and *Absidia corymbifera* in phycomycosis. [Gk *phykos* seaweed, *mykes* fungus.]

phycomycosis (**fi**·ko·mi·**ko′**·sis). An acute fungus infection of lungs, central nervous system or other organs, characterized by inflammation and vascular thrombosis in patients with debilitating or underlying disease (e.g. diabetes), and those due to filamentous fungi (e.g. *Mucor, Rhizopus, Absidia*). **Phycomycosis entomophthorae.** A subcutaneous infection in man and horses due to *Entomophthora coronata*, which has a predeliction for nasal tissue. **Subcutaneous phycomycosis.** Chronic infection of subcutaneous tissues with elephantiasis of affected part due to *Basidiobolus haptosporus* (*B. meristrosporus*)—originally thought to be caused by *B. ranarum*. [Gk *phykos* seaweed, *mykes* fungus, *-osis* condition.]

phycogalactic (**fi**·go·gal·**ak′**·tik). Lactifuge; any agent that arrests or diminishes lactation. [Gk *phygein* to be banished, *gala* milk.]

phylacagogic (fi·**lak**·ah·**goj′**·ik). Capable of inducing the formation of protective antibodies (phylaxins). [phylaxin, Gk *agogos* leading forth.]

phylactic (fi·**lak**·tik). Pertaining to the production of protective antibodies. [Gk *phylax* guard.]

phylactotransfusion (fi·**lak**·to·trans·**few′**·zhun). Immunotransfusion; the transfusion of blood from a donor who has been immunized with a vaccine made from the organism causing the infection in the recipient. [Gk *phylax* guard, transfusion.]

phylaxin (fi·**lax**·in). Antibody; any of the substances present, or induced by bacterial antigens, in body tissues and fluids, which are protective against infection, e.g. bactericidins, bacteriolysins, opsonins, complement-fixing antibodies. [Gk *phylax* guard.]

phylaxiology (fi·**lax**·e·**ol′**·o·je). The science which treats of protection against infection. [Gk *phylax* guard, *logos* science.]

phylaxis (fi·**lax**·is). Activity against infection, on the part of the organism. [Gk, a guarding.]

phyletic (fi·**let**·ik). Of or pertaining to a phylum.

Phyllanthus (fil·**an**·thus). A genus of tropical and subtropical trees of the family Euphorbiaceae. Preparations of *Phyllanthus niruri* Linn. and of several other species are used in India and Malaysia as external applications and as diuretics. The root bark of *Phyllanthus engleri* Max., a Zambian species, is reported to be extremely toxic. [Gk *phyllon* leaf, *anthos* flower.]

phyllode (**fil**·ode). Leaf-like; applied to tumours which have a leaf-like, lobular appearance when cut. [Gk *phyllon* leaf, *eidos* form.]

phylloporphyrin (fil·o·**por**·fir·in). $C_{31}H_{35}N_4COOH$, a porphyrin which constitutes part of the molecule of chlorophyll. [Gk *phyllon* leaf, porphyrin.]

phyllopyrrole (fil·o·**pir**·ole). 2,3,5-Trimethyl-4-ethylpyrrole, one of the basic fission products of haem, chlorophyll and bilirubin. [Gk *phyllon* leaf, pyrrole.]

phylloquinone (fil·o·**kwin**·one). Vitamin K_1.

phylogenesis (fi·lo·**jen**·es·is). The race history or evolution of a species, family, or order of animals or plants; the ancestral history of an individual organism. [Gk *phylon* tribe, *genesis* origin.]

phylogenetic, phylogenic (fi·lo·jen·**et**'·ik, fi·lo·**jen**·ik). Relating to phylogenesis.

phylogeny (fi·**loj**·en·e). Phylogenesis.

phylum (**fi**·lum). A major classificatory division of the animal kingdom, containing one or more classes. Sometimes also used in plant systematics. [Gk *phylon* tribe.]

phyma (**fi**·mah). A circumscribed swelling of the skin. [Gk, growth.]

Physalia (fiz·a·le·ah). A genus of Coelenterata. **Physalia arethusa.** The Portuguese man-of-war of tropical and subtropical oceans; it has a large blue float and long tentacles which can give painful stings. [Gk *physallis* bubble.]

physaliphore (fiz·**al**·e·for). A highly vacuolated cell met with especially in the rare tumour of the notochord, the chordoma. [Gk *physallis* bubble, *pherein* to bear.]

physalis (fiz·al·is). A giant epithelial cell found in certain forms of carcinoma. [Gk *physallis* bubble.]

Physaloptera (fiz·al·**op**·ter·ah). A genus of large round worms. **Physaloptera caucasica.** A species which occurs in the stomach and small intestine, where it does considerable damage. The secondary hosts are not known. It has been found once in man in eastern Europe. **Physaloptera mordens.** A species which has been found in man, not uncommonly, in tropical Africa. The usual hosts are monkeys. It is probably the same species as the preceding. [Gk *physallis* bubble, *pteron* wing.]

physalopteriasis (fiz·al·op·ter·**i**'·as·is). Infestation with nematode worms of the genus *Physaloptera.*

Physalopteridae (fiz·al·op·**ter**'·id·e). A family of the nematode super-family Spiruroidea. [*Physaloptera,* Gk *eidos* form.]

physconia, physcony (fis·**ko**·ne·ah, **fis**·ko·ne). Any enlargement of the abdomen. **Physconia adiposa.** An adipose state of the abdomen. **Physconia aquosa.** Ascites. **Physconia biliosa.** A distended state of the gall bladder. **Physconia mesenterica.** Tabes mesenterica. [Gk *physke* sausage.]

physic (**fiz**·ik). 1. The science of healing diseases. 2. A drug; in particular, a cathartic. 3. To treat with medicines or to purge. [Gk *physikos* natural.]

See also: CULVER.

physical (**fiz**·ik·al). 1. Relating to the body. 2. Relating to material or matter. 3. Relating to physics. [see prec.]

physician (fiz·**ish**·un). 1. One who practises the healing art; a doctor. 2. One who practises medicine as distinct from surgery. 3. A Fellow or Member of a College of Physicians. **House physician.** A physician resident in a hospital who acts under the orders of the attending physician and during his absence. [Gk *physikos* natural.]

physicist (**fiz**·is·ist). 1. A specialist in physics. 2. One who holds the belief that the vital phenomena can be explained solely on chemical and physical principles. [see prec.]

Physick, Philip Syng (b. 1768). Philadelphia surgeon.

Physick's pouch. Proctitis confined to the rectal pouches which are distended.

physicochemical (fiz·ik·o·**kem**'·ik·al). Pertaining to physical chemistry.

physicogenic (fiz·ik·o·**jen**'·ik). 1. Of physical origin. 2. Produced by physical means. [physical, Gk *genein* to produce.]

physicopyrexia (fiz·ik·o·pi·**rex**'·e·ah). Pyrexia produced by physical means, usually as a therapeutic measure.

physicotherapeutics, physicotherapy (fiz·ik·o·ther·ap·**ew**'·tix, fiz·ik·o·**ther**'·ap·e). Physiotherapy.

physics (**fiz**·ix). The branch of science dealing with the phenomena and laws of nature and with the structure of matter, comprising the nature of fundamental particles and the laws governing their motions and general behaviour. **Atomic physics.** The study of the physical properties of the atom, its structure, energy and internal changes. **Molecular physics.** The study of molecules in motion, particularly the phenomena of temperature, aggregation and diffusion. **Nuclear physics.** The study of the atomic nucleus, its structure, energy and disintegration, and of the subatomic particles. [Gk *physikos* natural.]

physinosis (fiz·in·o·sis). Any disease caused by physical agents. [physical, Gk *nosos* disease.]

physiochemical (fiz·e·o·**kem**'·ik·al). Biochemical. [Gk *physis* nature, chemistry.]

physiochemistry (fiz·e·o·**kem**'·is·tre). Biochemistry. [see prec.]

physiogenesis (fiz·e·o·**jen**'·es·is). Embryology. [see foll.]

physiogeny (fiz·e·**oj**·en·e). The origin of vital function. [Gk *physis* nature, genesis.]

physiognomy (fiz·e·**og**·no·me). 1. The art of judging the dominant temper and other mental characteristics by studying the face and the general carriage of the body. 2. The expression and appearance of the face used as an aid to diagnosis. 3. The face. [Gk *physis* nature, *gnomon* guide.]

physiognosis (fiz·e·og·**no**'·sis). A method of diagnosis of which the general appearance and expression of the face is the basis. [Gk *physis* nature, *gnosis* knowledge.]

physiological (fiz·e·o·**loj**'·ik·al). 1. Relating to physiology. 2. Normal, in contrast to pathological or morbid; term used of the vital processes. [Gk *physis* nature, *logos* science.]

physiologist (fiz·e·**ol**·o·jist). One expert in the science of physiology.

physiology (fiz·e·**ol**·o·je). The study of the phenomena presented by living organisms, the classification of these phenomena, and the recognition of their sequence and significance. **Animal physiology.** The physiology of animal species. **Applied physiology.** Practical physiology; physiological knowledge applied directly to practical medical problems. **Aviation physiology.** Physiology with special reference to conditions during flying. **Cellular physiology.** The physiology of cells. **Comparative physiology.** The study of the physiology of different animal species. **General physiology.** The general scientific basis of physiology. **Hominal physiology, Human physiology.** The physiology of human beings. **Morbid physiology, Pathogenetic physiology, Pathological physiology.** The physiological interpretation of pathological phenomena. **Vegetable physiology.** The physiology of plants. [Gk *physis* nature, *logos* science.]

physiolysis (fiz·e·**ol**·is·is). The decay and disintegration of tissues as a natural process. [Gk *physis* nature, *lysis* a loosing.]

physiomedicalism (fiz·e·o·**med**·ik·al·izm). A system of medical treatment in which only bland natural remedies are used. [Gk *physis* nature, medicine.]

physioneurosis (fiz·e·o·newr·**o**'·sis). A true neurosis, in contrast to a psychoneurosis. [Gk *physis* nature, neurosis.]

physionomy (fiz·e·**on**·o·me). The science which treats of the laws of nature. [Gk *physis* nature, *nomos* law.]

physiopathic (fiz·e·o·**path**'·ik). Denoting the functional nervous affections which do not have a psychopathic basis. [Gk *physis* nature, *pathos* disease.]

physiopathological (fiz·e·o·path·o·**loj**'·ik·al). 1. Relating or belonging to physiopathology. 2. Belonging to the physiological and pathological states.

physiopathology (fiz·e·o·path·**ol**'·o·je). Pathological physiology; the physiological interpretation of pathological phenomena.

physiophyly (fiz·e·o·**fi**'·le). That branch of phylogenesis which is concerned with the evolution and development of physical function. [Gk *physis* nature, *phyle* tribe.]

physiopsychic (fiz·e·o·**si**'·kik). Relating or belonging to body as well as to mind; psychosomatic. [Gk *physis* nature, *psyche* mind.]

physiopyrexia (fiz·e·o·pi·**rex**'·e·ah). Any form of therapeutic pyrexia. [Gk *physis* nature, pyrexia.]

physiotherapy (fiz·e·o·**ther**·ap·e). The employment of physical measures in building up the physique, correcting deformities and restoring function after disease or injury. [Gk *physis* nature, *therapeia* treatment.]

physique (fiz·**eek**). The structural bodily organization and development or constitution, or appearance. [Fr.]

physocele (**fi**·so·seel). 1. A circumscribed tumour containing air or gas. 2. A hernial sac distended with flatus. 3. Distension of the scrotum caused by an accumulation in it of gas or air. [Gk *physa* air, *kele* tumour.]

physocephalus, physocephaly (fi·so·**kef**·al·us, fi·so·**kef**·al·e). Emphysematous swelling of the head. [Gk *physa* air, *kephale* head.]

physohaematometra (**fi**·so·he·mat·o·**met**'·rah). An accumulation of air or gas with blood in the uterus and consequent distension of the organ. [Gk *physa* air, *haima* blood, *metra* womb.]

physohydrometra (**fi**·so·hi·dro·**met**'·rah). A collection of air and serous fluid in, and consequent distension of, the cavity of the uterus. [Gk *physa* air, *hydor* water, *metra* womb.]

physometra (**fi**·so·met·rah). The presence in the cavity of the uterus of gas or air. [Gk *physa* air, *metra* womb.]

physoncus (fi·**song**·kus). A tumour caused by an accumulation of air. [Gk *physa* air, *ogkos* a swelling.]

Physopsis (fi·**sop**·sis). A subgenus of snails of the genus *Bulinus*, some species of which are intermediary hosts of *Schistosoma*. **Physopsis africana.** An African snail, an intermediary host of *Schistosoma haematobium, S. intercalatum* and *S. mattheei*. **Physopsis globosa.** Differs only slightly from *Physopsis africana*. **Physopsis nasuta** var. **martens.** Probably identical with *Physopsis africana*. **Physopsis ovoidea.** A subspecies of *Physopsis africana*. **Physopsis tchadiensis.** An intermediary host of *Schistosoma haematobium*. [Gk *physis* growth, *ops* eye.]

physopyosalpinx (**fi**·so·pi·o·**sal**'·pingx). The presence of gas and pus in the uterine tube. [Gk *physa* air, *pyon* pus, *salpigx* trumpet.]

physoscheocele (fi·**sos**·ke·o·seel). Distension of the scrotum caused by an accumulation in it of gas or air. [Gk *physa* air, *oscheon* scrotum, *kele* hernia.]

physospasmus (fi·so·**spaz**·mus). Spasmodic colic, with flatulence. [Gk *physa* air, spasm.]

physostigma (fi·so·**stig**·mah). The ripe seeds of the West African plant, *Physostigma venenosum* Balf. (family Leguminoseae). They contain about 0.2 per cent of myotic alkaloids, the most important of which is physostigmine. [Gk *physa* air, *stigma* mark.]

Physostigmine BPC 1968 (fi·so·**stig**·meen). Eserine, $C_{15}H_{21}N_3O_2$. An alkaloid obtained from Calabar beans, the dried seeds of *Physostigma venenosum*. It inhibits the action of cholinesterase, the enzyme which destroys acetylcholine in the body. It potentiates all the muscarinic effects of acetylcholine, but its influence on the nicotinic properties is more complex. Physostigmine increases the cholinergic response at neuromuscular junctions in skeletal muscle so that close arterial injection of acetylcholine to such a junction, which would normally produce a single twitch of the muscle, causes a tetanic response. Similarly, if the muscle has been curarized, physostigmine will tend to restore conduction. In sympathetic ganglia, physostigmine potentiates inhibitor effects rather than excitor. It is sometimes used to reduce intra-ocular pressure by the instilling of a few drops of solution into the eye: the pupil is constricted, thus opening the canal of Schlemm in the filtration angle of the eye. It is also used in a similar way to reverse the effect of homatropine when the latter has been administered for diagnostic purposes. Together with posterior pituitary extract, it has been employed to restore intestinal tone after operations, but is less effective than carbachol in this respect. Because of its action at neuromuscular junctions in skeletal muscle, it has also been tried in myasthenia gravis, but neostigmine has proved more effective in doses that do not produce circulatory disturbance. **Physostigmine Salicylate BP 1973.** $C_6H_5(OH)COOC_{15}H_{21}N_3O_2$, the form most commonly used; it consists of colourless crystals which gradually turn red on exposure to air, and is moderately soluble in water. **Physostigmine Sulphate BPC 1968.** $(C_{15}H_{21}N_3O_2)_2H_2SO_4$, a deliquescent salt soluble in water or alcohol. [see prec.]

Physostigminii Salicylas. *European Pharmacopoeia* name for Physostigmine Salicylate BP 1973.

physostigminism (fi·so·**stig**·min·izm). Physostigmine poisoning.

physovenine (fi·so·**ven**·een). $C_{14}H_{18}N_2O_3$, a minor alkaloid which occurs together with physostigmine in the Calabar bean. It has myotic properties similar to those of physostigmine. [physostigmine, L *venenum* poison.]

phytagglutinin (fi·tag·**loo**·tin·in). A phytotoxin with the power of agglutinating red blood corpuscles.

phytase (**fi**·taze). An enzyme which hydrolyses phytin (inositol hexaphosphoric ester), yielding inositol and phosphoric acid. It occurs in liver and in certain cereals.

phytate (**fi**·tate). 1. Phytin. 2. Any salt or ester formed by phytic acid.

phytid (**fi**·tid). A cutaneous, hypersensitivity response to a dermatophyte infection. [Gk *phyton* plant.]

phytin (**fi**·tin). The calcium-magnesium salt of inositol phosphoric acid (phytic acid), obtained from various plants, in particular from the seeds. It has been recommended for neurasthenia, and in cases of anaemia, but its efficacy seems to be somewhat uncertain.

phyto-albumin (**fi**·to·al·**bew**'·min). An albumin of plant origin. [Gk *phyton* plant, albumin.]

phytobezoar (fi·to·**be**·zo·ar). A concretion formed of vegetable fibres and other matter such as the skins and seeds of fruit, and on occasion starch granules and globules of fat, which may be present in the stomach. [Gk *phyton* plant, bezoar.]

phytochemistry (fi·to·**kem**·is·tre). That branch of science which deals with the chemical changes that take place in vegetable organisms. [Gk *phyton* plant, chemistry.]

phytochrome (**fi**·to·krome). A plant chromoprotein. [Gk *phyton* plant, *chroma* colour.]

phytogenesis (fi·to·**jen**·es·is). The origin or formation and evolution of plant organisms. [Gk *phyton* plant, *genesis* origin.]

phytogenetic, phytogenic (fi·to·jen·**et**·ik, fi·to·**jen**·ik). Phytogenous.

phytogenous (fi·**toj**·en·us). 1. Relating to phytogenesis. 2. Originating from a plant; produced by a plant growth. [Gk *phyton* plant, *genein* to produce.]

phytogeny (fi·**toj**·en·e). Phytogenesis.

phytohormone (fi·to·**hor**·mone). A plant hormone that takes part in the repair of damaged vegetable tissues. [Gk *phyton* plant, hormone.]

phytoid (**fi**·toid). Having resemblance to a plant; term applied to an animal having many biological characteristics belonging to a vegetable. [Gk *phyton* plant, *eidos* form.]

phytol (**fi**·tol). Phytyl alcohol, tetramethylhydroxy hexadecane, $CH_3[(CH_3)CH(CH_2)_3]_3CCH_3{=}CHCH_2OH$. An alcohol obtained by the hydrolysis of chlorophyll which is a phytyl ester. It is the precursor of the carotenoids and a unit in the structure of vitamin K_1.

phytolacca (fi·to·**lak**·ah). Poke root; the root of a North American plant, *Phytolacca americana* Linn. (family Phytolaccaceae). It contains a bitter resin, also a saponin, and has purgative and emetic properties. **Phytolacca berries.** The ripe fruits of the above plant, which have similar properties to those of the root but are milder in action. [Gk *phyton* plant, L *lacca* lac.]

phytolaccin (fi·to·**lak**·sin). A crystalline neutral principle said to be present in phytolacca.

phytomelin (fi·**tom**·el·in). Rutin, $C_{27}H_{30}O_{16}$. A glycoside occurring in the leaves of rue.

Phytomenadione BP 1973 (**fi**·to·men·ah·**di**'·one). 2-Methyl-3-phytyl-1,4-naphthaquinone; an antidote to anticoagulants of the dicoumarol type.

Phytomonas (fi·**tom**·on·as). A generic term formerly applied to bacteria causing necrosis in plants; now known as *Xanthomonas*, because they produce a yellow water-insoluble pigment. About 50 species have been identified. [Gk *phyton* plant, *monos* single.]

phytonosis (fi·to·**no**·sis). Any disease caused by a plant. [Gk *phyton* plant, *nosos* disease.]

phytoparasite (fi·to·**par**·ah·site). Any plant which lives parasitically. [Gk *phyton* plant, parasite.]

phytopathogenic (fi·to·path·o·**jen**′·ik). Giving rise to a morbid process in a plant. [Gk *phyton* plant, pathogenic.]

phytopathology (fi·to·path·**ol**′·o·je). 1. Plant pathology. 2. The pathology of those diseases which are due to vegetable parasites. [Gk *phyton* plant, pathology.]

phytopathy (fi·**top**·ath·e). Any morbid condition occurring in plants. [Gk *phyton* plant, *pathos* disease.]

phytophagous (fi·**tof**·ag·us). Vegetarian; herbivorous. [Gk *phyton* plant, *phagein* to eat.]

phytopharmacology (fi·to·far·mah·**kol**′·o·je). The science which deals with the influence of drugs on the growth and development of plants. [Gk *phyton* plant, *pharmakon* drug, *logos* science.]

phytoplasm (fi·to·plazm). The protoplasm of plant cells. [Gk *phyton* plant, *plasma* something formed.]

phytopneumonoconiosis (fi·to·new·mon·o·kon·e·**o**′·sis). A lung condition comparable to pneumoconiosis, produced by vegetable dust particles. [Gk *phyton* plant, pneumoconiosis.]

phytoprecipitin (fi·to·pre·**sip**′·it·in). A precipitin produced as the result of immunization with vegetable protein. [Gk *phyton* plant, L *praecipitare* to precipitate.]

phytosis (fi·to·sis). Any disease (e.g. skin lesion) produced by a vegetable parasite. [Gk *phyton* plant, *-osis* condition.]

phytosterin (fi·to·**steer**·in). Phytosterol.

phytosterol (fi·to·**steer**·ol). 1. The characteristic sterols occurring in the higher plants and derived from the vegetable oils. 2. The mixture of sitosterol isomers with formula $C_{29}H_{50}O$, obtained from wheat germ. [Gk *phyton* plant, sterol.]

phytosterolin (fi·to·**steer**·ol·in). The glucoside of phytosterol.

phytosyntax (fi·to·**sin**·tax). The synthesis of complex organic compounds from simpler substances which takes place in a plant in the presence of sunlight. [Gk *phyton* plant, *syntassein* to assemble.]

phytotherapy (fi·to·**ther**·ap·e). The system of therapy in which plants are utilized. [Gk *phyton* plant, therapy.]

phytothromboplastin (fi·to·throm·bo·**plas**′·tin). A thromboplastin of vegetable origin. [Gk *phyton* plant, thromboplastin.]

phytotoxic (fi·to·**tox**·ik). Having a poisonous effect on plants. [Gk *phyton* plant, toxic.]

phytotoxin (fi·to·**tox**·in). Any toxin derived from a plant, e.g. abrin, ricin, crotin. [Gk *phyton* plant, toxin.]

phytotrichobezoar (fi·to·tri·ko·**be**′·zo·ar). A bezoar composed of vegetable fibres and animal hair. [Gk *phyton* plant, *thrix* hair, bezoar.]

phytovitellin (fi·to·vi·**tel**′·in). A vegetable protein similar to vitellin found in rye, wheat, maize and certain other seeds. [Gk *phyton* plant, vitellus.]

phytoxanthin (fi·to·**zan**·thin). Xanthin. [Gk *phyton* plant, xanthin.]

phytyl (fi·til). The organic radical $CH_3[(CH_2)CH(CH_2)_3]_3CCH_3{=}CHCH_2$ derived from phytol.

pia mater (pi·ah **ma**·ter). A delicate, highly vascular membrane of connective tissue which is in intimate contact with the central nervous system (both brain [pia mater encephali] and spinal cord [pia mater spinalis]) and dips into all fissures and sulci, following every irregularity of the surface. It is connected by fine trabeculae with the arachnoid membrane, and forms a sheath round the larger blood vessels as they enter the nervous system. [L, tender mother.]

pia-arachnitis (pi·ah·ar·ak·**ni**′·tis). Leptomeningitis. [pia mater, arachnitis.]

pia-arachnoid (pi·ah·ar·**ak**′·noid). The pia mater and the arachnoid mater considered as one membrane.

pial (pi·al). Relating to the pia mater.

pian (pe·**ahn**). Yaws. **Pian bois.** Espundia, mucocutaneous leishmaniasis, forest yaws; it is not related to pian or yaws, which is a spirochaetal disease. **Pian cayenne.** Mucocutaneous leishmaniasis. **Pian datre.** Lichen framboesianus, a secondary manifestation of yaws. **Haemorrhagic pian.** A haemorrhagic eruption in verruga peruana (cutaneous bartonellosis) of South America, not related to yaws. [Fr.]

pianides (pe·**ahn**·i·dz). Hypochromic macules of secondary yaws. [Fr. *pian* yaws.]

pianoma (pe·ahn·o·mah). Raspberry-like exudative papillomatosis in secondary yaws (daughter yaws). [Fr. *pian* yaws, Gk *-oma* tumour.]

piarachnitis (pi·ar·ak·**ni**′·tis). Leptomeningitis. [pia mater, arachnitis.]

piarhaemia (pi·ar·**he**·me·ah). Lipaemia. [Gk *piar* fat, *haima* blood.]

piastrenaemia (pi·as·tren·**e**′·me·ah). Megakaryocytic leukaemia; a leukaemic condition associated with a megakaryocytic hyperplasia of bone marrow, and sometimes with an increase of megakaryocytes in the blood. It is usually seen in chronic myeloid leukaemia or myelophthisic anaemias.

Piazza's fluid or solution. A solution containing sodium chloride 1 g, ferric chloride 1 g, in 4 ml distilled water, used to coagulate blood.

piblokto (pib·**lok**·to). A type of hysteria occurring in women in Greenland. [Eskimo.]

Pic, Adrien (b. 1863). Lyons physician.

Bard-Pic syndrome. Progressive jaundice with enlargement of the gall bladder and cachexia, due to carcinoma of the head of the pancreas.

pica (pi·kah). An abnormal craving to eat substances not fit for food (e.g. wood, lead pencils, chalk), to which children and pregnant women may be subject. The state may be found in patients with anaemia and in certain types of hysteria and insanity. [L, magpie.]

Picea (pi·se·ah). A genus of coniferous trees of the family Pinaceae. **Picea abies** Linn. (= *Picea excelsa* Link). The Norway spruce fir and the source of Burgundy pitch. [L, pitch pine.]

picene (pi·seen). $C_{22}H_{14}$, a hydrocarbon which occurs in coal tar.

piceous (pi·se·us). 1. Relating or having resemblance to, or containing pitch. 2. In zoology, pitch-black in colour. [L *piceus* pitchy.]

pichi (pe·che). A South American shrub, *Fabiana imbricata* Ruiz and Pavon, of the family Solanaceae. A tincture prepared from the resinous leaves and twigs is used in hepatic and urinary disorders. [Araucan, small thing.]

Pick, Arnold (b. 1851). Prague neurologist and psychiatrist.

Pick's convolutional atrophy. Lobar sclerosis. *See* SCLEROSIS.

Pick's bundle. Fibres of the pyramidal tract which take an aberrant course through the medulla oblongata.

Pick's dementia, or disease. A form of dementia presenilis characterized by focal cerebral atrophy of the frontal and temporal lobes, often with aphasia and agnosia.

Pick's disease of the brain. A localized atrophy of the brain in which the outer laminae of the cortex are replaced by an intense gliosis, often giving rise to a status spongiosus.

Pick's pseudo-apraxia. Apraxia arising from motor perserveration.

Pick's vision. A condition occurring in lesions of the pons which affect the posterior longitudinal bundle. In consequence of this, objects appear disorientated and not in their correct position.

Pick, Filipp Josef (b. 1834). Prague dermatologist.

Pick's disease. Erythromelia of arms and legs.

Pick, Friedel (b. 1867). Prague physician.

Pick's disease, or syndrome. Constrictive mediastinopericarditis giving rise to chronic venous congestion and cirrhosis of the liver, a condition allied to polyorrhomenitis.

Pick, Ludwig (b. 1868). Berlin pathologist and paediatrician.

Pick's cells, Niemann-Pick cells. The large reticulo-endothelial cells characteristic of Pick's disease.

Pick's disease, Niemann-Pick disease, Pick-Niemann disease. A rare, chronic, familial condition, a disorder of lipoid metabolism, resembling Gaucher's disease, with moderate anaemia, gastrointestinal disturbances, loss of weight, ulcerated gingivitis, an abdomen much distended by gross hepatomegaly and splenomegaly and lymphadenopathy. The skin is pale, waxy or brownish, and there is usually retardation of mental development. There is an increase of blood cholesterol; the marrow, spleen and glands show characteristic large cells containing the phospholipid, sphingomyelin.

Pick-Herxheimer disease. Acrodermatitis chronica atrophicans.

pick (pik). A dental instrument for removing debris from between the teeth. [AS *piken.*]

Pickerill's line. Imbrication line; any of the minute parallel lines occurring on the surface of the enamel of a tooth due to the outcropping of the enamel prisms.

Pickering, George White (b. 1904). British physician.

Lewis and Pickering test. Reactive hyperaemia test; a test to detect organic arterial occlusion in a limb. Full vasodilatation in the limb is obtained by immersion in hot water, the limb is elevated to drain venous blood, and a sphygmomanometer cuff is then applied and inflated to above the systolic blood pressure. After 5 minutes the cuff is removed. In a normal limb a flush spreads distally, reaching the digits in 2–5 seconds, but when organic vascular disease is present, the flush spreads slowly, and is patchy in distribution.

pickwickian (pik·**wik**·e·an). Obese. **Pickwickian syndrome.** *See* SYNDROME. [After the fat boy "Joe" in *Pickwick Papers* by Charles Dickens.]

Pickworth's method or test. *See* BENZIDINE AND NITROPRUSSIDE PEROXIDASE TEST.

Picloxydine (pik·**lox**·id·een). BP Commission approved name for 1,4-di-(4-chlorophenylguanidinoformimidoyl)piperazine; a bactericide and fungicide.

pico-. A prefix indicating that the quantity which follows is to be multiplied by 10^{-12}; thus, a picogram = 10^{-12} gram [It. *pico* small.]

picofarad (pi·ko·**far**·ad). 10^{-12} farad (pF). [It. *pico* small, farad.]

picogram (**pi**·ko·gram). 10^{-12} gram (pg).

picoline (**pik**·o·leen). Methylpyridine, $C_5H_4N(CH_3)$. A compound homologous with pyridine which occurs in three isomeric forms, all pungent liquids extracted from bone oil and coal tar. The α-compound is employed in medicine as a sedative. [L *pix* pitch, *oleum* oil.]

picomole (**pi**·ko·mole). 10^{-12} mole (pmol).

Picornavirus (pi·**korn**'·ah·**vi**·rus). A family name for small (20–30 nm) RNA-containing viruses without envelopes. Included are enteroviruses, rhinoviruses and some small animal RNA viruses. [It. *pico* small, RNA, L *virus* poison.]

picraconitine (pik·rak·**on**·it·een). $C_{32}H_{45}O_{10}N$, one of the alkaloids present in aconite leaves.

picramin (**pik**·ram·in). Amarine; a poisonous substance found in bitter almonds.

Picramnia (pik·**ram**·ne·ah). A genus of shrubs and small trees of the family Simarubaceae. The bark of *Picramnia antidesma* Sw. is known as *cascara amarga* and is used as a bitter tonic. [Gk *pikros* bitter, *thamnos* shrub.]

picrasma (pik·**raz**·mah). Quassia. **Picrasma excelsa.** Picroena excelsa. [Gk *pikrasmos* bitterness.]

picrasmin (pik·**raz**·min). A bitter principle isomeric with quassin. [see prec.]

picrate (**pik**·rate). Any salt formed by picric acid.

picrocarmine (pik·ro·**kar**·mine). A double stain (carmine with picric acid), used for staining nerve tissue.

See also: RANVIER, WEIGERT.

picrocrocin (pik·ro·**kro**·sin). Saffron bitter, $C_{38}H_{66}O_{17}$. A glucosidic principle found in saffron.

Picroena (pik·**re**·nah). A genus of trees of the family Simarubaceae. **Picroena excelsa.** A species which is the source of quassia wood. [Gk *pikros* bitter.]

picroformol (pik·ro·**for**·mol). Bouin's fluid; an aqueous solution of picric acid and formaldehyde used as a histological fixative.

picrogeusia (pik·ro·**gew**·se·ah). Bitterness of taste. [Gk *pikros* bitter, *geuma* a taste of a thing.]

picrol (**pik**·rol). $(OH)_2C_6HI_2SO_2OK$, a colourless antiseptic used for the same purpose as iodoform.

picronigrosin (pik·ro·**ni**·gro·sin). A combination of picric acid and nigrosin in alcohol, sometimes used as a stain for chromatin.

picropodophyllin (pik·ro·pod·**of**'·il·in). A lactone of podophyllic acid which occurs in podophyllum.

picropyrine (pik·ro·**pi**·reen). A compound formed by antipyrin with picric acid. It is a yellow crystalline substance.

picrorhiza (pik·ro·**ri**·zah). The rhizome and root of a Himalayan plant, *Picrorhiza kurroa* Royle, of the family Scrophulariaceae. Known as *Indian gentian,* it is used in India as an aperient and bitter tonic. [Gk *pikros* bitter, *rhiza* root.]

picrosclerotine (pik·ro·**skle**·ro·teen). The name given by Dragendorff and Podwyssozki in 1877 to ergotinine, $C_{35}H_{39}O_5N_5$, a crystalline alkaloid of ergot first obtained by Tanret in 1875; Jakoby named the same substance *secaline.* It was regarded as inert but is readily transformed into ergotoxine, $C_{35}H_{41}O_6N_5$, which contains an additional molecule of water.

Picrotoxin BP 1968 (pik·ro·**tox**·in). $C_{30}H_{34}O_{13}$, the active principle obtained from the seeds of *Anamirta cocculus;* a powerful respiratory stimulant and convulsive agent. It stimulates the cerebrospinal axis from above downward, affecting chiefly the cerebral cortex, mid-brain and medulla; only affecting the spinal cord in large doses. In the unanaesthetized person it causes convulsions, at first tonic and then clonic. Stimulation of the central nervous system is eventually followed by depression, and death results from respiratory failure. Its main use is in antagonizing the central depression following overdoses of the narcotic drugs, particularly the barbiturates. It has little effect against alcohol and the ureides. While convulsive doses need to be given to stimulate the respiratory centres in the unanaesthetized animal, this is more readily stimulated in the anaesthetized animal. [Gk *pikros* bitter, *toxikon* poison.]

picrotoxinism (pik·ro·**tox**·in·izm). Picrotoxin poisoning.

picrotoxinum (**pik**·ro·tox·**i**'·num). Picrotoxin.

Pictet, R. Swiss chemist.

Pictet liquid. A mixture of liquefied sulphur dioxide and carbon dioxide: used as a refrigerant.

pictograph (**pik**·to·graf). Name given to a set of test types in the form of pictures, used for children and illiterates. [L *pictus* painted, Gk *graphein* to write.]

picture (**pik**·tcher, **pik**·tewr). **Blood picture.** The overall results and interpretation revealed through an examination of the blood by the usual haematological techniques which determine red cells, white cells, platelets, haemoglobin, differential white-cell count, and sometimes reticulocytes, red-cell volume, or corpuscular haemoglobin values. [L *pictus* painted.]

See also: VAUBAN.

pidan (**pe**·dan). The Chinese name for preserved eggs.

piedra (pi·a·drah). Piedra nostras, chignon disease, Beigel's disease, tinea nodosa, trichomycosis nodosa, trichomycosis nodularis; a fungus disease of the hair shaft characterized by the formation of hard nodules giving a metallic quality to the hair when combed. Two forms occur: *black piedra* commonly in subtropical and tropical areas and due to infection by *Piedraia hortae,* and *white piedra* more common in temperate areas and caused by *Trichosporon beigelii.* [Sp., stone.]

Piedraia (pi·ed·**ri**·ah). Generic name proposed by Fonseca and Arêa Leão (1928) for the fungus that causes black piedra (trichosporosis), a hair affection occurring in tropical climates. The only recognized species is *Piedraia hortae.*

piesaesthesia (pi·e·zes·**the**'·ze·ah). Pressure sense. [Gk *piezein* to press upon, aesthesia.]

piesimeter, piesometer (pi·e·**zim**·et·er, pi·e·**zom**·et·er). An instrument for the measurement of pressure by piezo-electric effect, i.e. the production of a charge on a crystal surface proportional to the pressure applied to it. [Gk *piezein* to press upon, *metron* measure.]

See also: HALES.

piezaesthesia (pi·e·zes·**the**′·ze·ah). Piesaesthesia.

piezochemistry (pi·e·zo·**kem**′·is·tre). The chemistry of reactions that take place under pressure. [Gk *piezein* to press upon, chemistry.]

piezo-electricity (pi·e·zo·el·ek·**tris**′·e·te). The development of electric charges by certain crystals when subjected to strain. [Gk *piezein* to press upon, electricity.]

piezometer (pi·e·**zom**·et·er). Piesimeter.

Pifenate (pi·**fen**·ate). BP Commission approved name for ethyl 2,2-diphenyl-3-(2-piperidyl)propionate; an analgesic.

pigment (**pig**·ment). 1. A dyestuff, or stain. 2. A paint; in pharmacy, a paint to be applied to the throat or nose. 3. Any coloured substance occurring in animal or plant tissue. **Bile pigment.** Any of the colouring matters characteristic of bile, the most important being bilirubin and biliverdin. **Blood pigment.** A term applied to haemoglobin and various of its derivatives. The more important blood pigments are oxyhaemoglobin, methaemoglobin, sulphmethaemoglobin, haematin, haemochromogen and haematoporphyrin. **Ceroid pigment.** A waxy, insoluble, acid-fast, yellow pigment found within or close to the liver cells in some cases of cirrhosis, and sometimes in muscle and ganglion cells. **Cholera-red pigment.** A colour base found in cultures of the cholera vibrio. When sulphuric acid is added to a culture of the vibrio in peptone water the characteristic cholera-red reaction is obtained. **Endogenous pigment.** Any pigment produced within the body. **Exogenous pigment, Extraneous pigment.** Any pigment introduced into the body from external sources, e.g. colouring matter in food. **Lipochrome pigment.** A carotenoid. **Malarial pigment.** Pigment formed by the malaria parasites from the haemoglobin of the red blood cells. It is seen in the parasite itself, especially in the older forms, but is eventually deposited in the liver and spleen. **Melanotic pigment.** Any of a group of pigments, including and related to melanin, which produce colour in hair and fur and in the skin, as well as in melanotic sarcoma. **Respiratory pigment.** Any pigment, such as ferroporphyrin, cytochrome or flavine, which has an essential function in the oxidative processes of respiration. [L *pigmentum* paint.]

pigmentation (pig·men·**ta**·shun). Deposition of pigment. **Addisonian pigmentation.** Due to lack of ACTH and melanocyte-stimulating hormone-inhibiting hormone. **Carotinoid pigmentation.** Pigmentation due to carotene. **Cervicofacial pigmentation.** Riehl's melanosis. **Exogenous pigmentation, Extraneous pigmentation.** Pigmentation of skin or mucosae due to pigment or pigments of exogenous origin. **Haematogenous pigmentation.** Pigmentation due to a blood-borne pigment. **Malarial pigmentation.** The accumulation in the liver and spleen of dark-brown pigment derived from the break-down of the red blood cells by the malaria parasite. **Vagabonds' pigmentation.** Cutaneous pigmentation due to long-standing infection with *Pediculi.* The pigmentation is most pronounced on the upper part of the back, but in exceptional cases it is generalized and of a dark hue.

pigmented (**pig**·men·ted). Coloured by a deposit of pigment.

pigmentodermia (pig·men·to·**der**′·me·ah). Chromatodermatosis; any disease of the skin in which pigmentation is one of the main features. [pigment, Gk *derma* skin.]

pigmentogenesis (pig·men·to·**jen**′·es·is). The production of pigment. [pigment, Gk *genein* to produce.]

pigmentolysin (pig·men·**tol**·is·in). A lysin that destroys pigment. [pigment, lysin.]

pigmentolysis (pig·men·**tol**·is·is). 1. The disappearance of the tigroid (Nissl's) bodies in the protoplasm of a nerve cell when the nerve fibre connected with the cell is severed, or during fatigue. 2. The breaking-up and the destruction by lysis of the chromatin of cell substance. [pigment, Gk *lysis* a loosing.]

pigmentophage (pig·**men**·to·faje). A phagocytic cell, in particular in the hair, which destroys pigment. [pigment, Gk *phagein* to eat.]

pigmentophore (pig·**men**·to·for). A pigment-carrying cell. [pigment, Gk *phorein* to bear.]

pigmentum (pig·**men**·tum). 1. In pharmacy, a paint. *See* PAINT. 2. Pigment; coloured matter. **Pigmentum nigrum.** Literally, black pigment; it could be applied to the black pigment (melanin) in any pigmented cell or chromatophore, e.g. in the choroid coat of the eye. [L.]

Pignet, Maurice Charles Joseph (b. 1871). Paris physician.

Pignet's formula, or standard. The length of the body in centimetres minus the sum of the body weight in kilograms and the circumference of the chest at greatest expansion in centimetres. When the sum is less than 10 the person is regarded as very strong; between 10 and 15, strong; 15 to 20, good; 20 to 25, medium; 25 to 30, weak; above 30, very weak. It is an index used in the selection of army recruits.

pigweed (**pig**·weed). A plant of the genus *Chenopodium;* a common allergen. [ME *pigge,* AS *weod.*]

piitis (pi·i·tis). Inflammation affecting the pia mater. [pia mater, Gk *-itis* inflammation.]

pikrococin (pik·ro·**kos**·in). Saffronal glucoside, $CHO(CH_3)_3C_6H_5C_6H_{10}O_5$. A compound found in saffron.

pila (**pi**·lah). Any one of the large spaces found in the spongy substance of bone. [L, pillar.]

pilar, pilary (**pi**·lar, **pil**·ar·e). Relating or belonging to the hair; hairy; downy. [L *pilus* hair.]

pilaster (pi·**las**·ter). An anomalous ridge that may be present on the femur. [Fr. *pilastre* column.]

pilastered (pi·**las**·terd). Arranged in columns. [see prec.]

pilatio (pi·**la**·she·o). A fissure in the cranium. [see foll.]

pilation (pi·**la**·shun). A fracture of hair-like dimensions such as may be found in the skull. [L *pilus* hair.]

Pilcher, Lewis Stephen (b. 1845). Brooklyn surgeon.

Pilcher bag. An inflatable rubber bag, now seldom used, designed to control bleeding from the prostatic bed following operation.

Pilcz, Alexander (b. 1871). Austrian neurologist.

Pilcz's sign, Pilcz-Westphal phenomena, or reaction, Westphal-Pilcz phenomenon, reaction or pupillary reflex. Contraction of the pupil of the eye on reflex or voluntary closure, or attempted closure, of the lids; unilateral.

Pilcz, Jan (b. 1870). Polish neurologist.

Pilcz's reflex. Constriction of the pupil when the attention is drawn to an object, analogous to pupillary constriction on convergence; also called the *attention reflex.*

Pilcz's treatment. The treatment of dementia paralytica by the induction of fever through the injection of the erysipelas toxin.

pile (pile). 1. An assemblage of similar objects heaped upon one another. 2. A haemorrhoid; a dilatation of a branch or branches of the haemorrhoidal veins. The term is also loosely applied to other anal swellings. **Acute pile.** Subcutaneous haematoma beside the anus. **Atomic pile.** An assembly of nuclear fissile material and a moderator, in which a self-sustaining controllable chain reaction involving nuclear fission can take place. An obsolete term replaced by *nuclear reactor.* **External pile.** A tag of skin at the anus. **First-degree pile.** Internal pile (see following). **Internal pile.** Dilatation of veins of the rectal (venous) plexus just inside the anus. **Intero-external pile.** An internal pile which has grown down into the subcutaneous tissue round the anus. **Muscular pile.** Layers of muscle tissue arranged in a manner similar to the plates in a battery so that an electrical current is produced. **Nuclear pile.** An assembly of one material whose atomic nuclei are capable of undergoing fission, e.g. uranium, and a second material whose nuclei absorb neutrons to a negligible extent, but which slow down neutrons in collisions, e.g. graphite or heavy water. Beyond a certain critical size the rate of formation of neutrons by fission exceeds the rate of removal of neutrons by absorption and diffusion outwards: a chain reaction for the neutrons can then proceed at an ever-increasing rate. In practice a steady limited rate is maintained by introducing some neutron-absorbing material (e.g. cadmium) into the pile as "control rods". **Oesophageal pile.** Dilatation of a submucous vein of the oesophagus in portal hypertension. **Prolapsed pile.** An internal pile which has protruded through the anus. **Prostatic pile.** The dilated varicose veins seen cystoscopically in the intravesical lobes of a congested prostate; not a good term. **Second-degree pile.** An internal pile which protrudes at stool but returns or can be returned subsequently. **Sentinel pile.** A tag of indurated skin at the lower end of an anal fissure. **Thermo-electric pile.** An instrument used for the detection of radiant heat, consisting of a large number of thermocouples joined in series to obtain the maximum sensitivity. **Third-degree pile.** Prolapsed pile (see above). **Thrombosed pile.** A pile whose main vein has solidified by clot. **Voltaic pile.** An assembly of primary electric cells in series in one container, producing a high potential. [L *pila* pillar, ball.]

pileous (pi·le·us). Hairy. [L *pilus* hair.]

piles (pi·lz). Haemorrhoids. [L *pila* ball.]

pileum (pi·le·um). A cerebellar hemisphere. [L, felt skull-cap.]

pili (pi·li). Hairs. **Pili annulati.** Leucotrichia annularis, ringed hair. **Pili incarnati.** Ingrowing hairs. **Pili torti.** Twisted hairs. [L.]

piliation (pi·le·a·shun). The process of development and growth of hair. [L *pilus* hair.]

piliform (pi·le·form). With the appearance of hair. [L *pilus* hair.]

pilimictio, pilimiction (pi·le·**mik**·she·o, pi·le·**mik**·shun). 1. The passage of urine containing hairs such as may occur in cases of dermoid cyst. 2. The passage of urine containing hair-like filaments of mucus. [L *pilus* hair, micturition.]

pill (pil). A spherical or ovoid body containing medicament and intended to be swallowed whole. Most pills are machine-made and are coated, partly to disguise the taste of the medicament and partly to preserve them from the deleterious effects of storage and transport; pills ordered in small quantities to an individual prescription are made by hand. The most common coatings are sugar and pearl, but varnishing, gilding and silvering are still employed. Except when it is more economical to make pills by hand for small quantities of any special formula, pills have no advantages and many disadvantages compared with tablets and are rapidly becoming obsolete. Proprietary pills, however, still have wide popularity, mainly as purgatives and for kidney disturbances. **The pill.** *See* ORAL CONTRACEPTION. **Blue pill.** A pill of metallic mercury finely dispersed in syrup, glucose, glycerin and liquorice; used as an aperient. **Bulk pill.** A mass ready to be rolled and cut to form pills of any required size. **Dinner pill.** A pill containing quinine, belladonna, aloe and podophyllum resin; it is intended to be taken with meals. **Pill of Ferrous Carbonate BPC 1959.** Blaud's Pill, a pill containing ferrous carbonate; formerly used in anaemia but now replaced by ferrous-sulphate tablets. **Guy's pill.** Compound pill of digitalis; a pill containing equal parts of squill, digitalis and blue pill; used in cardiac oedema. This is often attributed to W. A. Guy, but incorrectly. He has no reference to it. It appears that the pill was used at Guy's Hospital, London, founded by Thomas Guy (1644–1724). **Iron pill.** Pill of ferrous carbonate (see above). [L *pila* ball.]

See also: ADDISON (T.), BAILLIE, BLAUD, GREGORY, HUTCHINSON.

pillar (pil·ar). An elongated structure which appears to support another structure; usually arranged in pairs beneath either end of an arch-like structure, e.g. pillars of fauces, the folds of mucous membrane covering the palatoglossal and palatopharyngeus muscles on either side of the passage from mouth to pharynx beneath the arch-like palate. **Pillar of a microscope.** The metal upright mounted on the base, carrying the stage and arm. [L *pila* pillar.]

See also: USKOW.

pilleum (pil·e·um). Pilleus.

pilleus (pil·e·us). The membrane sometimes covering a child's head at birth; a caul or lucky cap. **Pilleus ventriculi.** The first part of the duodenum; duodenal cap. [L, felt skull-cap.]

pilocarpine (pi·lo·**kar**·peen). $C_{11}H_{16}O_2N_2$, an alkaloid occurring in jaborandi leaves and other species of *Pilocarpus*. It increases the secretion of salivary, pancreatic, intestinal and gastric glands when injected; it also reduces the heart beat and contracts the bronchioles. It is used in eye drops to contract the pupil, solutions of the nitrate being generally employed. **Pilocarpine Hydrochloride BPC 1968.** $C_{11}H_{16}O_2N_2HCl$, a salt of pilocarpine used for the same purposes. **Pilocarpine Nitrate BP 1973.** $C_{11}H_{16}O_2N_2HNO_3$, the water-soluble nitrate of pilocarpine and the salt of preference whenever aqueous solutions of the drug are indicated.

Pilocarpinii Nitras. *European Pharmacopoeia* name for Pilocarpine Nitrate BP 1973.

Pilocarpus (pi·lo·**kar**·pus). A genus of shrubs of the family Rutaceae. **Pilocarpus microphyllus.** A species which is the source of jaborandi. [Gk *pilos* cap, *karpos* fruit.]

pilocystic (pi·lo·**sist**·ik). Denoting those encysted dermoid tumours which are hollow and contain hair. [L *pilus* hair, cyst.]

pilocytic (pi·lo·**si**·tik). Consisting of hair-shaped cells. [L *pilus* hair, Gk *kytos* cell.]

pilo-erection (pi·lo·e·**rek'**·shun). Erection of the hair. [L *pilus* hair, erection.]

pilogenic (pi·lo·**jen**·ik). A lesion produced by hairs. [L *pilus* hair, Gk *genein* to produce.]

pilology (pi·**lol**·o·je). The science which deals with the hair, its diseases and their treament. [L *pilus* hair, *logos* science.]

pilomatrixoma (pi·lo·ma·trix·o'·mah). Calcifying epithelioma (of Malherbe). [L *pilus* hair, matrix, Gk *-oma* tumour.]

pilomotor (pi·lo·**mo**·tor). Moving the hair, applied to certain muscles of the skin. [L *pilus* hair, motor.]

pilonidal (pi·lo·**ni**·dal). Having a growth of hair in a cyst, nidus, or other internal part. [L *pilus* hair, *nidus* nest.]

pilose (pi·loze). Hairy; downy; having a covering of hair. [L *pilus* hair.]

pilosebaceous (pi·lo·se·**ba'**·shus). Relating to the hair follicles and sebaceous glands. [L *pilus* hair, *sebum* fat.]

pilosis, pilosism (pi·**lo**·sis, **pi**·lo·sizm). A condition in which the growth of hair is excessive or is present in an unusual place. [L *pilus* hair, Gk *-osis* condition.]

pilosity (pi·**los**·it·e). Hairiness. [see prec.]

pilous (pi·lus). Pilose.

pilula (pil·ew·lah) (pl. *pilulae*). A pill. [L, little ball.]

pilular (pil·ew·lar). Relating to or like a pill. [see prec.]

pilule (pil·ewl). A small pill, generally of pellet type, although there are no official limitations in size. [L *pilula* little ball.]

pilus (pi·lus). A hair-like protein appendage, of much smaller diameter than flagellum, often present in large numbers at surface of Gram-negative intestinal bacilli and associated with pellicle formation in fluid culture. **Sex pilus.** A special pilus, produced by donor bacteria and determined by sex factor genes, which is required for conjugation with recipient bacteria; these pili are the site of adsorption of "male-specific" bacteriophages. [L.]

pimelecchysis (pim·el·**ek**·is·is). An abnormal discharge of fatty or sebaceous material. [Gk *pimele* fat, *ekcheein* to pour out.]

pimelitis (pim·el·i·tis). Inflammation of the fatty tissue. [Gk *pimele* fat, *-itis* inflammation.]

pimeloma (pim·el·o·mah). Lipoma. [Gk *pimele* fat, *-oma* tumour.]

pimelopterygium (pim·el·o·ter·ij'·e·um). A collection of fat in the conjunctiva. [Gk *pimele* fat, *pteryx* wing.]

pimelorrhoea (pim·el·o·re'·ah). A state of diarrhoea in which the stools contain fatty elements. [Gk *pimele* fat, *rhoia* flow.]

pimelorthopnoea (pim·el·or·thop·ne'·ah). A condition in which, because of obesity, the patient experiences discomfort and difficulty in breathing when he is lying down. [Gk *pimele* fat, *orthos* straight, *pnoiein* to breathe.]

pimelosis (pim·el·o·sis). 1. Transformation of tissue into fat, usually as a degenerative process. 2. Obesity. 3. Lipomatosis. [Gk *pimele* fat, *-osis* condition.]

pimelotic (pim·el·**ot**·ik). 1. Relating to or having the characteristics of pimelosis. 2. Suffering from pimelosis.

pimeluria (pim·el·ewr·e·ah). Lipuria. [Gk *pimele* fat, urine.]

Pimenta (pim·**en**·tah). A genus of tropical American trees of the family Myrtaceae. The leaves of *Pimenta acris* Kostel yield oil of bay, and *Pimenta officinalis* Lindl. is the source of allspice. The fruits of *Pimenta officinalis* Lindl. yield a volatile oil, oleum pimentae, which contains eugenol, and is used as a carminative and flavouring agent. [Sp. *pimienta.*]

pimento (pim·**en**·to). Pimenta.

Piminodine (pim·**in**·o·deen). BP Commission approved name for ethyl-4-phenyl-1-(3-phenylaminopropyl)piperidine-4-carboxylate; a narcotic analgesic.

Pimozide (**pim**·o·zide). BP Commission approved name for 1-{1-[4,4-bis(4-fluorophenyl)butyl]-4-piperidyl}-benzimidazolin-2-one; a tranquillizer.

Pimpinella (pim·pin·**el**·ah). A genus of herbs of the family Umbelliferae, widely distributed. **Pimpinella anisum.** The species which is the source of aniseed. **Pimpinella saxifraga.** The lesser or salad burnet; a species reported as having carminative and diaphoretic properties. [It., pimpernel.]

pimple (**pim**·pl). Popular term for a papule or pustule of small size. [etym. dub.]

pin (pin). 1. A long, sharp, metal skewer or nail for transfixion or fixation of a bone or bones. 2. A post or peg used in the fixation of an artificial crown to the root of a tooth. **Pin and arc.** A technique used in radiotherapy for beam location. [AS *pinn.*]

See also: SMITH-PETERSEN, STEINMANN.

pinacoid (**pin**·ah·koid). Describing molecular arrangements in layers, with parallel faces. [Gk *pinax* tablet, *eidos* form.]

pinacyanole (pin·ah·**si**·an·ole). A carbocyanine dye used for staining frozen sections, and for mitochondria supravitally. It is also employed in the red-sensitization of photographic plates.

pinang (**pe**·nang). A Malayan name for the areca-nut tree, *Areca catechu* Linn.

Pinard, Adolphe (b. 1844). Paris obstetrician.

Pinard's manoeuvre. A method of bringing down the extended leg in breech presentation by pressure with the finger behind the knee, thus enabling the ankle to be grasped.

pince-ciseaux (pahns·se·**zo**). Scissors in which the blades are held apart by a spring and approximated by pressure on the handle. The best known type is the de Wecker's iris scissors. [Fr.]

pincement (pahns·**mahn**). In massage, a manipulation in which the flesh is nipped or pinched. [Fr., pinching.]

Pindolol (**pin**·do·lol). BP Commission approved name for 1-(indol-4-yloxy)-3-isopropylaminopropan-2-ol; a β-adrenergic receptor blocking agent.

pine (pine). A general name for coniferous trees, mostly members of the genus *Pinus.* They yield turpentine and various essential oils and resins. **Scotch pine.** *Pinus sylvestris* Linn. **White pine.** *Pinus strobus.* [L *pinus.*]

pineal (**pin**·e·al). 1. Belonging or relating to the pineal body. *See* BODY. 2. Resembling a pine cone in shape. **Pineal tumour.** May cause precocious puberty by pressure on the hypothalamus. [L *pineus* pine cone.]

pinealectomy (**pin**·e·al·**ek**'·to·me). Extirpation of the pineal body. [pineal body, Gk *ektome* a cutting out.]

pinealoblastoma (**pin**·e·al·o·blas·**to**'·mah). An invasive tumour of the pineal body. [pineal body, blastoma.]

pinealoma (**pin**·e·al·**o**'·mah). A benign tumour of the pineal body. [pineal body, Gk *-oma* tumour.]

pinealopathy (**pin**·e·al·**op**'·ath·e). Any morbid condition affecting the pineal body. [pineal body, Gk *pathos* disease.]

pineapple (**pine**·apl). The fruit of *Ananas sativus* Schult. (family Bromeliaceae). It contains bromelin, a proteolytic enzyme, and acts as a diuretic. The unripe fruit has an irritant action. [pine, AS *aeppel.*]

Pinel, Philippe (b. 1745). Paris physician.

Pinel's system. The treatment of mental disorder without the use of any form of restraint.

pinene (**pi**·neen). The terpene hydrocarbon, $C_{10}H_{16}$, that is the main constituent of turpentine oil, and also occurs in the oils of sage, juniper, eucalyptus and peppermint. It exists in two optically active isomeric forms, both liquids with characteristic odours, and is used as a solvent.

pineoblastoma (**pin**·e·o·blas·**to**'·mah). A tumour composed of rudimentary pineal cells. [pineal, blastoma.]

pineocytoma (**pin**·e·o·cy·**to**'·mah). A tumour of mature pineal cells.

pinguecula, pinguicula (pin·**gwek**·ew·lah, pin·**gwick**·ew·lah). A small yellowish elevation of the conjunctiva near the corneal margin, usually on the nasal side, due to hyaline degeneration of subconjunctival connective tissue. Formerly thought to be fatty. [L *pinguiculus* rather fat.]

pinguid (**pin**·gwid). 1. Fat. 2. Soapy. [L *pinguis* fat.]

piniform (**pin**·e·form). Resembling a pine cone in shape; conical. [L *pineus* pine cone, form.]

pinite, pinitol (**pin**·ite, **pin**·it·ol). Inositol monomethyl ether, $C_6H_6(OH)_5.OCH_3$. A substance which occurs in rubber latex from species of *Hevea.*

Pinkerton, Herbert Harvey. Glasgow anaesthetist.

Pinkerton's catheter. A rubber or plastic catheter with a curve near the tip to facilitate its introduction into one or other of the main-stem bronchi, for purposes of suction.

Pinkus, Felix (b. 1868). Berlin dermatologist.

Pinkus' disease. Lichen nitidus.

Pinkus' fibro-epithelial tumour. A benign but premalignant tumour of the skin resembling a seborrheic keratosis but with the histology of a basal cell carcinoma with fibrous overgrowth.

pinna (**pin**·ah). The auricle of the ear; the external part of the auditory apparatus. **Pinna nasi.** Ala of the nose. [L, wing.]

pinnal (**pin**·al). Relating or belonging to a pinna; auricular.

pinocarveol (pi·no·**kar**·ve·ol). $C_{10}H_{16}O$, a terpene alcohol which is a constituent of the oil of *Eucalyptus globulus.*

pinocyte (**pi**·no·site). A type of macrophage which imbibes and assimilates tissue fluids. [Gk *pinein* to drink, *kytos* cell.]

pinocytosis (**pi**·no·si·**to**'·sis). The process whereby a cell engulfs fluid to form an intracellular vesicle. Minute invaginations occur in the cell membrane and then close to trap the fluid vesicle. [Gk *pinein* to drink, *kytos* cell, *-osis* condition.]

pinole (**pi**·nole). $C_{10}H_{16}O$, a terpene compound present in pine needles or prepared from pinene. Its hydrate is sobrerole.

pinosylvine (pi·no·**sil**·veen). 3,5-Dihydroxystilbene, $C_{14}H_{12}O_2$. So called because it occurs in the heartwood of pine.

Pinoy, E. French mycologist.

Nicolle and Pinoy white mycetoma. *See* MYCETOMA, WHITE.

Pins, Emil (b.1845). Vienna physician.

Pins' sign. Relief of precordial pain or discomfort connected with acute pericarditis or effusion, by leaning forward and drawing the knees up to the chest. The pericardium itself (except the lower third) is insensitive to pain; pain in pericarditis is either due to coincident pleural involvement, or to irritation of the phrenic nerve which supplies its lower third. Leaning forward perhaps tends to separate the inflamed surfaces and so lessen the pain.

pins-and-needles (pinz·and·**ne**·dlz). A popular term; a form of paraesthesia; a sensation of pricking as produced by release of a tourniquet after temporary constriction. [AS *pinn, naedl.*]

pinselhaare (pin·sel·**har**·ah). Trichostasis spinulosa. [G, paint-brush hairs.]

pint (**pi**·nt). A unit of capacity for liquids equal to 568.26 ml, being one-eighth of a gallon, or 20 fluid oz. The American pint equals 473 ml, being 16 fluid oz. [OFr. *pinte.*]

pinta (**peen**·tah). Mal del pinto; a disease which is chiefly troublesome in the tropical parts of the Western hemisphere, and caused by *Treponema carateum* (Brumpt) (or *T. herrejoni*); possibly it is transmitted by flies or biting insects. The primary lesion is a plaque which may persist for from 5 to 12 months. The secondary stage is characterized by an eruption of various types of lesions (psoriasiform, lichenoid, eczematoid, etc.), and is followed after a long period by a tertiary stage which is manifest in the skin by the appearance of areas of hyper- and hypo-pigmentation. Systemic manifestations, including cardiovascular lesions, may occur. In some 60 per cent of cases the Wassermann reaction is positive. [Sp., spot.]

pintado (pin·**tah**·do). A patient with pinta.

pintid (**pin**·tid). The symptomatic dermal lesion of pinta.

Pintner, Rudolf. American psychologist.

Pintner–Paterson test. A series of non-verbal tests (including form-boards, cube tests and assembly tests) designed to test the intelligence of subjects who are deaf or who do not speak English.

pinto (**peen**·to). Pinta.

Pinus (**pi**·nus). A genus of coniferous trees of the family Pinaceae. **Pinus mugo.** A species a variety of which yields pumilio pine oil. **Pinus palustris.** Brown pine; a species which is a source of colophony. **Pinus strobus.** White pine; a species the bark of which is used in the treatment of coughs. **Pinus sylvestris.** A species which is the source of Stockholm tar. **Pinus taeda.** A species which yields colophony. [L.]

pinus (**pi**·nus). The pineal body. [L, pine.]

pinworm (**pin**·werm). Threadworm. *Enterobius vermicularis,* probably the commonest internal parasite of the white man and the causal agent of oxyuriasis. The adults (females 15 mm, males 5 mm) live in the caecum and colon from which the females migrate to lay eggs perianally, or may disintegrate after passing through the anus: eggs are therefore infrequent in faeces, but may be widely disseminated in dust. The word is not current in the United Kingdom. [AS *pinn, wyrm.*]

pio-epithelium (**pi**·o·ep·e·**the′**·le·um). Epithelium in which there are deposits of fat globules, a degenerative manifestation. [Gk *pion* fat, epithelium.]

pionaemia (pi·on·e·me·ah). Lipaemia. [Gk *pion* fat, *haima* blood.]

Piophila (pi·**of**·il·ah). A genus of small flies. **Piophila casei.** A common commensal fly which normally breeds in decaying refuse. It also breeds in cheese and the larvae, cheese skippers, are one of the commonest causes of intestinal myiasis. [Gk *pion* fat, *philein* to love.]

Piorkowski, Max (b. 1859). Berlin bacteriologist.

Piorkowski's staining method. To demonstrate metachromatic granules: alkaline methylene blue is followed by acid differentiation and eosin counterstaining.

piorthopnoea (**pi**·or·thop·**ne′**·ah). Shortness of breath, markedly increased when the supine position is adopted, resulting from general adiposity. [Gk *pion* fat, *orthos* straight, *pnoia* breath.]

pioscope (**pi**·o·skope). An instrument used at one time for the rough estimation of the fat content of milk by comparing the colour of the sample with a graded series of known content. [Gk *pion* fat, *skopein* to view.]

Piotrowski, Alexander (b. 1878). Berlin neurologist.

Piotrowski's sign. Dorsiflexion of the foot as a result of percussion of the tibialis anterior muscle; an excessive response indicates pyramidal-tract disease.

Pipamazine (pip·**am**·ah·zeen). BP Commission approved name for 10-[3-(4-carbamoylpiperidino)propyl]-2-chlorophenothiazine; used in the treatment of pregnancy sickness.

Pipamperone (pip·**am**·per·one). BP Commission approved name for 1-[3-(4-fluorobenzoyl)propyl]-4-piperidinopiperidine-4-carboxamide; a tranquillizer.

Pipazethate (pip·**az**·eth·ate). BP Commission approved name for 2-(2-piperidino-ethoxy)ethyl 10-thia-1,9-diaza-anthracene-9-carboxylate; a cough suppressant.

Pipenzolate (pi·**pen**·zo·late). BP Commission approved name for *N*-ethyl-3-piperidyl benzilate; used in the treatment of peptic ulcers.

Pipenzolate Bromide. BP Commission approved name for 3-benziloyloxy-1-ethyl-1-methylpiperidinium bromide; an antispasmodic.

Piper (**pi**·per). 1. A genus of tropical and subtropical climbing herbs and shrubs of the family Piperaceae; the peppers. 2. Piper nigrum (see below). **Piper album.** White pepper; the fruits, more completely ripe, of *Piper nigrum* Linn. stripped of the pericarp and dried. **Piper angustifolium.** The leaves of the plant are reported to have astringent and styptic properties. **Piper betel.** The source of betel leaves, said to have carminative properties. Mixed with lime and areca nut, the leaves are largely used in India as a masticatory. **Piper cubeba.** A species the fruits of which are known as cubebs. The oil was formerly administered in genito-urinary infections. **Piper methysticum.** The source of kava rhizome; in the form of an extract it has been used as a urinary antiseptic. **Piper nigrum.** Black pepper; the dried unripe fruits of *Piper nigrum* Linn. They contain a volatile oil, the alkaloid piperine, and the resin chavicine. In addition to its use as a condiment, it is employed medicinally as a diaphoretic and stimulant. [L, pepper.]

piperazine (pi·**per**·az·een). Hexahydropyrazine, diethylenediamine, a heterocyclic compound which is a uric-acid solvent. Various salts have been recommended for gout. **Piperazine Adipate BP 1973.** A compound used similarly to the hydrate. **Piperazine calcium edetate.** A chelate produced by treating ethylenediamine-*N,N,N′,N′*-tetra-acetic acid with calcium carbonate and piperazine; an anthelmintic. **Piperazine Citrate BP 1973.** A compound used similarly to the hydrate. **Piperazine Hydrate BPC 1968.** The hexahydrate of piperazine, used in the treatment of threadworm and roundworm infestation. **Piperazine Phosphate BP 1973.** A compound used similarly to the hydrate. **Triclofenol Piperazine.** BP Commission approved name for piperazine di-(2,4,5-trichlorophenoxide); an anthelmintic.

piperic (pi·**per**·ik). Relating to or containing pepper. [L *piper* pepper.]

piperidine (pi·**per**·id·een). $CH_2(CH_2.CH_2)_2NH$, a strong organic base which occurs in pepper as the alkaloid, piperine. Both the base itself and its salts are uric-acid solvents.

Piperidolate (pip·**er**·id·o·late). BP Commission approved name for 1-ethyl-3-piperidyl diphenyl acetate; a parasympatholytic drug.

piperine (**pi**·per·een). $C_{17}H_{19}O_3N$, a colourless crystalline alkaloid occurring to the extent of 9 per cent in black pepper. It has no particular pharmaceutical properties.

piperism (**pi**·per·izm). Poisoning by means of pepper, generally demonstrated by an attack of acute gastritis. [L *piper* pepper.]

piperitone (pi·**per**·it·one). $C_{10}H_{16}O$, a terpene ketone occurring mainly in the leaves of species of *Eucalyptus.*

Piperocaine (pi·**per**·o·kane). BP Commission approved name for 3-(2-methylpiperidino)propyl benzoate. It is used in the form of the hydrochloride (BP 1963) as a synthetic local analgesic.

piperonal (pi·**per**·o·nal). Heliotropin, $CH_2{=}O_2{=}C_6H_3CHO$. An aldehyde which can be prepared from piperine or from safrole, and occurring naturally in species of *Spiraea.* It has the odour of heliotrope and is used mainly in perfumery; it has a slight bacteriostatic action.

Piperoxan (pip·er·**ox**·an). BP Commission approved name for 2-piperidinomethylbenzo-1,4-dioxan. It is an α-adrenergic blocking agent.

pipette (pip·**et**). 1. A specially constructed glass tube used in the measurement and transference of definite amounts of liquids or gases. 2. To employ the pipette. [Fr., little pipe.]

See also: FOLIN, OSTWALD, PFEIFFER.

Pipothiazine (pip·o·**thi**·az·een). BP Commission approved name for 2-dimethylsulphamoyl-10-(3-[4-(2-hydroxyethyl)piperidino]-propyl)phenothiazine; a neuroleptic agent.

Pipoxolan (pip·**ox**·o·lan). BP Commission approved name for 5,5-diphenyl-2-(2-piperidinoethyl)-1,3-dioxolan-4-one; an antispasmodic.

Pipradrol (**pip**·rad·rol). BP Commission approved name for α-2-piperidylbenzhydrol, a central nervous stimulant with actions and uses similar to those of amphetamine; it is usually used in the form of the hydrochloride.

Piprinhydrinate (pip·rin·**hi**·drin·ate). BP Commission approved name for diphenylpyraline salt of 8-chlorotheophylline; an antihistamine.

pipsissewa (pip·**sis**·se·wah). Chimaphila, the dried leaves of the evergreen plant *Chimaphila umbellata* (Linn.) Nutt. (family Pyrolaceae), containing a crystalline substance arbutin, tannin, resin and gum. It is diuretic and astringent and has been used in renal disease. [Amer. Ind.]

piptonychia (pip·ton·**ik**·e·ah). Loosening and shedding of the nails. [Gk *piptein* to fall, *onyx* nail.]

piqûre (pe·kewr). Puncture. **Piqûre diabétique.** Claude Bernard's experimental puncture of the floor of the 3rd ventricle which causes glycosuria. [Fr.]

Piracetam (pi·ras·et·am). BP Commission approved name for 2-oxopyrrolidin-1-ylacetamide; a cerebral stimulant.

Piria, Raffaele (b. 1815). Turin chemist.

Piria's test. For tyrosine: add a few drops of concentrated sulphuric acid to a little of the substance on a watch glass and warm on a boiling-water bath for 20 minutes. Neutralize with solid calcium carbonate, filter, concentrate the filtrate and add a few drops of very dilute neutral ferric-chloride solution. A violet colour indicates tyrosine.

Piridoxilate (pi·rid·ox·e·late). BP Commission approved name for the reciprocal salt ot (5-hydroxy-4-hydroxymethyl-6-methyl-3-pyridyl)methoxyglycolic acid with [4,5-bis-(hydroxymethyl)-2-methyl-3-pyridyl]oxyglycolic acid (1:1); it is used in the treatment of angina.

Pirie, George Alexander (b. 1864). Dundee radiologist.

Pirie's bone. A rare accessory bone in the tarsus, between the dorsal parts of the talus and the navicular bone.

piriform (pir·e·form). Pear-shaped. [L *pirum* pear, form.]

piriformis (pir·e·for·mis). The piriformis muscle. [see prec.]

piriformis muscle [musculus piriformis (NA)]. A muscle lying on the back of the hip joint, arising from the pelvic surface of the middle pieces of the sacrum and inserted into the top of the greater trochanter.

Piritramide (pi·rit·ram·ide). BP Commission approved name for 4-(4-carbamoyl-4-piperidinopiperidino)-2,2-diphenylbutyronitrile; an analgesic.

Pirogoff, Nikolai Ivanovich (b. 1810). Russian surgeon.

Pirogoff's amputation, or operation. An osteoplastic variant of Syme's operation, the posterior process of the calcaneum being retained in the flap and apposed to the cut end of the tibia.

Pirogoff's angle. The venous angle demarcated by the subclavian and internal jugular veins.

Pirogoff's triangle. A triangular area in the submandibular region bounded by the posterior belly of the digastric muscle, the hypoglossal nerve and the posterior border of the mylohyoid muscle.

Pironella conica (pir·o·nel·ah kon·ik·ah). A snail that acts as an intermediary host of *Heterophyes heterophyes* in Egypt.

piroplasm (pi·ro·plazm) (pl. *piroplasms*). Piroplasma (an accepted anglicism).

piroplasma (pi·ro·plaz·mah) (pl. *piroplasmata*). Name applied to certain parasites which inhabit the red blood corpuscles of mammals; they do not form the pigment so characteristic of the genera, *Haemoproteus* and *Plasmodium.* Each parasite consists of a minute portion of cytoplasm and a nucleus: when a vacuole is present it may be difficult to distinguish it from a young ring form of a malarial parasite. Included under this designation are *Theileria (Babesia) parva,* the cause of African Coast fever of cattle, *Babesia bigemina,* the cause of Texas fever of cattle, and other species of *Babesia* which attack dogs, sheep, and horses. [L *pirum* pear, Gk *plasma* anything formed.]

piroplasmosis (pi·ro·plaz·mo'·sis). A group of very fatal diseases occurring chiefly in cattle and horses, caused by infection with one of a group of the pathogenic protozoa, piroplasma, which attack the red blood corpuscles. The organisms are transmitted by ticks. No case of human piroplasmosis has so far been reported. **Bovine piroplasmosis.** 1. Texas or red-water fever, a widespread disease in South America, the southern states of North America, North and South Africa, and Australia. It is associated with haemoglobinuria, and is caused by infection with *Babesia bigemina.* 2. African Coast fever, a variety characterized by fever and enlargement of lymph glands but without haemoglobinuria; the organism concerned is *Theileria (Babesia) parva.* **Canine piroplasmosis.** A disease caused by *Babesia canis.* **Equine piroplasmosis.** A variety occurring in horses, mules and donkeys in South Africa and caused by *Babesia equi* which is conveyed by ticks. **Ovine piroplasmosis.** A disease in sheep caused by *Babesia ovis.* [piroplasma, Gk *-osis* condition.]

Pirquet, Clemens Peter von (b. 1874). Vienna immunologist.

von Pirquet's reaction, or test. The reaction produced by scarifying an area of skin through a drop of tuberculin. A positive reading of the test indicates sensitization to tuberculin, but does not differentiate between tuberculous infection and clinical disease.

Piscidia (pis·id·e·ah). A genus of tropical trees of the family Leguminoseae. The bark of *Piscidia erythrina* Linn. has sedative and narcotic properties and has been employed to relieve pain and induce sleep. It is used by the natives of the West Indies as a fish poison. [L *piscis* fish, *caedere* to kill.]

pisco (pis·ko). A type of brandy made in the neighbourhood of Pisco in Peru.

pisiform (pi·se·form). 1. Like a pea. 2. The pisiform bone. [L *pisum* pea, form.]

pisiform bone [os pisiforme (NA)]. A small bone of the carpus articulating with, and in front of, the triquetral bone.

Piskacek, Ludwig (b. 1854). Vienna obstetrician.

Piskacek's sign. Deviation of the pregnant uterus to the right or left, simulating a cystic tumour of the adnexa.

Pistacia (pis·ta·she·ah). A genus of trees of the family Anacardiaceae and widely distributed. **Pistacia lentiscus.** A Mediterranean species which is the source of mastic. [Gk *pistake,* pistachio tree.]

Pistia stratiotes (pis·te·ah stra·te·o·teez). A tropical water plant of Asia (family Araceae). It is used in native medicine as an external application and the root is said to be laxative. This plant is associated with the aetiology of Malayan filariasis; the larvae of the insect transmitter, *Taeniorhyncus,* of the causal organism, *Wuchereria malayi,* obtain air by piercing the hollow underwater stems of this plant. [Gk *pistos* watery, *stratiotes* soldier.]

pistil (pis·til). The ovule-bearing organ of a plant, comprising the ovary and stigma, sometimes the style also. [L *pistillum* pestle.]

pit (pit). 1. Any indentation of a surface. 2. Any small but moderately deep depression on the external surface of an embryo. **Anal pit.** An ectoderm-lined depression in the early embryo which gives rise to the cavity of the lower half of the anal canal; proctodaeum. **Auditory pit.** An ectoderm-lined depression lateral to the hind-brain of an early embryo which sinks deeper, becomes separated from the surface, and gives rise to the cavity of the otic or auditory vesicle from which the epithelial lining of the internal ear is derived. **Basilar pit.** A pit in the palatal surface of an incisor tooth which is frequently the site of dental caries. **Chrome pits.** Skin ulcers caused by chromium. **Ear pit.** A familial depression occasionally occurring on the anterior aspect of the helix. **Gastric pits.** Gastric foveolae; the minute orifices of the ducts of the gastric glands opening on the surface of the mucous membrane of the stomach. **Granular pits [foveolae granulares (NA)].** The irregular depressions on the interior of the skull caused by the arachnoid granulations. **Pit on the head of the femur [fovea capitis femoris (NA)].** A small depression just below the centre of the head of the femur for the ligament of the head (ligamentum teres). **Lens pit.** An ectoderm-lined depression adjacent to the optic cup, from which the transient cavity of the crystalline lens of the eye is derived. **Olfactory pit.** An ectoderm-lined depression of the frontonasal process of the early embryo which represents the future nasal cavity on one side. **Optic pit.** A depression which forms in the optic area of the anterior part of the neural ectoderm in the embryo. This deepens to form the optic vesicle. **Primitive pit.** A small depression at the centre of Hensen's node at the anterior end of the primitive streak of an early embryo. It may represent part of the blastopore of lower vertebrates. **Pterygoid pit [fovea pterygoidea (NA)].** The depression on the anterior surface of the neck of the mandible. **Tonsillar pits [fossulae tonsillares (NA)].** Small tubes of the covering mucous membrane which ramify into the substance of the tonsil. [AS *pytt.*]

See also: HOWSHIP.

pitch (pich). 1. In acoustics, the character of a note, depending upon the frequency of vibration of the body producing the sound. [ME *picchen.*] 2. The residue remaining in a still after the destructive distillation of such substances as coal or wood. The name is also given to natural asphalts of various kinds. [L *pix.*] **Black pitch.** Tar; an inflammable substance obtained by the destructive distillation of various species of pine, mainly *Pinus sylvestris.* It is a blackish semi-liquid, and contains many phenols and cresols which give it disinfectant properties. **Burgundy pitch.** A semi-solid oleoresin obtained from the stem of the spruce, *Picea excelsa* Link. It occurs as an opaque yellowish-brown substance, brittle at ordinary temperatures, and contains pimarolic acid and a volatile oil. **Canada pitch.** The resinous exudation of the hemlock spruce of the USA and Canada, *Tsuga canadensis.* It is a brittle, hard, opaque substance, dark reddish-brown in colour, and containing resin and a volatile oil. It has been used as a gentle rubefacient. **Hard pitch.** A pitch obtained from the distillation of coal. **Jew's pitch.** Bitumen. **Liquid pitch.** Black pitch (see above). **Mineral pitch.** Bitumen. **Naval pitch.** Black pitch (see above). **Soft pitch.** A type of pitch obtained from coal tar.

pitchblende (pich·blend). A natural form of uranium oxide, U_3O_8, which occurs as a black mineral in Bohemia, Saxony, Colorado and Africa. It is the chief source of radium. [G *Pechblende.*]

Pitfield, Robert Lucas (b. 1870). Philadelphia physician.

Pitfield's fluid, or solution. A diluent solution containing acacia gum 20 g, in 50 ml of distilled water, to which is added 50 g glacial acetic acid and 0.1 g gentian violet; for use in the enumeration of white blood corpuscles.

pith (pith). 1. To destroy a part or the whole of the central nervous system in an animal, as in preparing it for physiological experiments. The nervous tissue is broken up, and thus rendered inactive, by movement of a blunt probe inserted through a foramen; or more or less of the upper part of the nervous system is removed through an opening made in the skull. 2. Bone marrow. 3. The soft cellular material to be found in stalks of plants. 4. The internal constituents of a hair. 5. Generally, the contents of the spinal canal—medulla and cord. [AS *pitha.*]

pithecoid (pith·e·koid). Resembling an ape. [Gk *pithekos* ape, *eidos* form.]

Pithecolobium lobatum (pith·e·ko·**lo**·be·um lo·**ba**·tum). A tree that grows in Indonesia and produces a fruit, djengkol, which is sometimes eaten and causes poisoning.

pithiatic (pith·i·**at**·ik). Pithiatric.

pithiatism (pith·i·at·izm). A method of influencing the mind by the use of persuasion. [Gk *peithein* to persuade, *iatos* curable.]

pithiatric (pith·i·**at**·rik). 1. Pertaining to pithiatism. 2. Curable by suggestion and persuasion.

pithiatry (pith·i·at·re). The treatment of disease by suggestion and persuasion. [Gk *peithein* to persuade, *iatreia* healing.]

Pitkin, George Philo (b. 1885). New Jersey surgeon.

Pitkin menstruum. A preparation of gelatin, dextrose, acetic acid and distilled water, used as a vehicle for certain drugs administered parenterally, to delay their diffusion and hence retard their action.

Pitkin spinal needle. A fine flexible needle with stilette, used for spinal puncture.

pitometer (pe·**tom**·et·er). An apparatus used in the measurement of variations of speed of water flowing through pipes, and for checking waste. [Henri *Pitot* (b. 1695), French physicist and engineer.]

Pitres, Jean Albert (b. 1848). Bordeaux physician.

Pitres' areas. Areas of the cerebral cortex.

Pitres' sections. Six planes of coronal section made through the brain at post-mortem examination. These were first used in a study of the cortical motor centres in 1895 and are rarely used today.

Pitres' sign. Hyperaesthesia of the skin of the scrotum and hyperalgesia of the testis on pressure in a case of tabes dorsalis.

pitting (pit·ing). 1. Indentation of tissue after the skin has been pressed with the finger; an indication of the presence of oedema. 2. Formation of pits or depressions. [AS *pytt.*]

pituicyte (pit·**ew**·is·ite). A cell in the pars nervosa hypophyseos, which is essentially a modified neuroglia cell. [pituitary, Gk *kytos* cell.]

pituita (pit·**ew**·it·ah). Glue-like mucus; phlegm. [L, phlegm.]

pituitary (pit·**ew**·it·ar·e). An endocrine gland situated in the pituitary fossa of the sphenoid bone; the hypophysis cerebri. The anterior part consists of three types of cells, basophil, eosinophil and chromophobe; the last are thought to have no secretory function, the others secrete the various anterior pituitary hormones. The posterior part, or pars nervosa stores oxytocin and vasopressin. The intermediate part is not present in all species and is not thought to have any function in the human being. **Powdered Pituitary (Posterior Lobe) BP 1973.** A powder prepared from the posterior lobe of mammalian pituitary bodies. It has oxytocic, pressor, antidiuretic and hyperglycaemic actions, but it is used mainly for its antidiuretic effect in the control of diabetes insipidus. It is administered by subcutaenous injection or as a snuff by nasal insufflation. **Pituitary stalk.** The nerve fibres running down from the hypothalamus to the posterior lobe. [L *pituita* phlegm.]

pituitectomy (pit·**ew**·it·**ek'**·to·me). Surgical removal of the hypophysis cerebri. The term "hypophysectomy" is preferred. [pituitary gland, Gk *ektome* a cutting out.]

pituitous (pit·**ew**·it·us). Pertaining to pituita or the secretion of pituita.

pituri (pit·ew·re). The leaf of *Duboisia hopwoodii* F. Muell. (family Solanaceae), known as *Australian tobacco.* It contains piturine, an alkaloid similar to nicotine.

piturine (pit·ew·reen). A very uncommon name for nicotine; it is usually applied in the form of the alkaloid derived from *Duboisia hopwoodii.*

pityriasic (pit·e·ri·as·ik). 1. Relating to or characterized by pityriasis. 2. Affected with pityriasis.

pityriasis (pit·e·**ri**·as·is). A name used somewhat indiscriminately for several cutaneous maladies marked by the formation of scales resembling bran. The word was applied originally by Robert Willan to a group of cutaneous affections, the lesions of which are characterized by delicate pellucid scales, like small flakes of mica, and by the absence of any obvious sign of inflammation. **Pityriasis alba.** Furfuraceous scaling occurring on limited oval or round areas as seen on the cheeks of children. The lesions are not erythematous. **Pityriasis amiantacea.** Asbestos-like, sticky, adherent scaling of the scalp as seen in severe psoriasis, lichen simplex and pityriasis sicca. The scales extend up the hair shafts. It is not a fungal condition, hence the synonym *tinea amiantacea* is best abandoned. **Pityriasis capitis.** Dandruff. **Pityriasis circinata.** 1. Pityriasis rosea (see below). 2. A seborrhoeic eruption seen only on bald scalps (Sabouraud). **Pityriasis circinata et marginata** (Vidal). Petalloid seborrhoeic dermatitis as seen on the chest or elsewhere. **Pityriasis disséminé.** Pityriasis rosea (see below). **Pityriasis folliculorum** (Ayres). Dryness, roughness and scaling of the skin of the face, associated with sensations of irritation or burning. *Demodex folliculorum* is present in the affected areas. **Pityriasis lichenoides chronica.** A form of parapsoriasis. **Pityriasis lichenoides et varioliformis acuta.** A form of guttate parapsoriasis having an acute onset, polymorphic lesions and a variable duration from a few weeks to several months. In some cases the initial lesions resemble those of varicella, but scaling papules and nodules may also be noted. **Pityriasis linguae.** Transitory benign plaques of the tongue. **Pityriasis maculata et circinata** (Duhring). Pityriasis rosea (see below). **Pityriasis nigricans.** Black sweating; the melanhidrotic variety of chromhidrosis. **Pityriasis pilaris.** Keratosis pilaris. **Pityriasis rosea.** Gilbert's pityriasis; an eruption of unknown cause, often preceded by the appearance of a herald patch, usually but not invariably affecting only those parts of the trunk and limbs covered by a high-necked short-sleeved vest, and characterized by the appearance of oval or round, rosy or fawn-coloured superficial medallions covered with furfuraceous scales. The long axes of the oval lesions tend to follow the lines of cleavage of the skin. Macular, urticarial, papular and vesicular varieties of the eruption are recognized. The disease is self-limited and runs a course of from 6 to 10 weeks; recurrences are uncommon. **Pityriasis rotunda.** Circular, well-defined patches of scaling, mostly on the trunk or proximal parts of the limbs, occurring in the Far East and elsewhere; it is non-fungal but of undetermined cause. **Pityriasis rubra.** Exfoliative dermatitis, usually generalized. The variety known as pityriasis rubra (Hebra) is characterized by small scales, some degree of atrophy, and often has a fatal termination. **Pityriasis rubra pilaris.** An intractable malady of unknown cause characterized by small reddish-brown, acuminate, horny, follicular papules, and red scaly patches widely distributed over the cutaneous surface. **Pityriasis sicca.** Dandruff associated with diminished secretion of the sebaceous glands of the scalp. **Pityriasis simplex.** Pityriasis alba (see above). **Pityriasis simplex capitis** (Sabouraud). Dandruff. **Pityriasis steatoides.** Dandruff in which the scales are greasy and less easily detached than in pityriasis simplex capitis. Sabouraud stated that the condition occurs diffusely on the vertex and temples as far as the retro-auricular regions, where it often forms isolated patches. The malady usually develops about the age of 15 or 16 years, and is associated with loss of hair. Localized areas of petalloid seborrhoeic dermatitis, as commonly seen on the central area of the front of the chest in men as well as elsewhere, has been regarded as a form of steatoid pityriasis. **Pityriasis streptogenes.** Dry, discrete, oval or circular, slightly pink or whitish scaly patches on the cheeks or chin, not infrequently seen in children. Despite the title there is little evidence that the lesions are caused by streptococci. **Pityriasis versicolor.** Chromophytosis, dermatomycosis furfuracea, hodi-potsy, parasitic achromia of Jeanselme, pityriasis versicolor tropica, tinea versicolor; a superficial fungus infection of the skin, caused by *Malassezia furfur,* and characterized by brownish maculae over the trunk. In dark-skinned persons the infection causes pseudo-achromia. **Pityriasis vulgaris.** Dandruff. [Gk *pityron* bran.]

See also: GIBERT, HEBRA.

pityroid (**pit**·e·roid). Furfuraceous, scaly; branny. [Gk *pityron* bran, *eidos* form.]

pityrosporon (pit·e·**ros**·por·on). *Pityrosporum.*

pityrosporum (pit·e·**ros**·por·um). A yeast-like organism having globose to ellipsoidal cells which bud on a more or less broad base. Budding occurs at one pole and leaves a collarette from which younger buds emerge; they are released by fission of a septum. Mycelium or pseudomycelium is rarely produced in culture. Three species are recognized: *Pityrosporum orbiculare* associated with the disease pityriasis versicolor; *P. ovale,* a commensal on the skin of man and implicated in pityriasis capitis; and *P. pachydermatis (P. canis),* a commensal on the skin of animals and sometimes associated with disease, e.g. otitis externa in dogs. *Pityrosporum orbiculare* is considered by some as synonymous with *Malassezia furfur;* others prefer the name *Pityrosporum furfur.* [Gk *pityron* bran, *sporos* seed.]

Pivampicillin (piv·am·pe·**sil**'·in). BP Commission approved name for 6-[D(−)-α-aminophenylacetamido]penicillanate; an antibiotic.

Pivhydrazine (piv·**hi**·draz·een). BP Commission approved name for *N*-benzyl-*N'*-pivaloylhydrazine; a monoamine oxidase inhibitor.

pivot (**piv**·ot). In dentistry, a post used for attaching an artificial crown to the root of a natural tooth. [Fr.]

pivoting (**piv**·ot·ing). The attaching of an artificial crown to the root of a natural tooth by means of a post, or pivot.

pix (pix) (gen. *picis*). Pitch. **Pix abietinarum.** Black pitch. *See* PITCH. **Pix betula.** Birch tar; an oil obtained from *Betula alba* Linn., used in skin diseases. **Pix burgundica.** Burgundy pitch. *See* PITCH. **Pix carbonis.** Coal tar. *See* TAR. **Pix carbonis praeparata.** Prepared coal tar. **Pix liquida, Pix pini.** Black pitch. *See* PITCH. [L.]

Pizotifen (pi·**zot**·e·fen). BP Commission approved name for 4-(9,10-dihydrobenzo-[4,5]-cyclohepta-[1,2-*b*]-thien-4-ylidene)-1-methylpiperidine; a migraine prophylactic.

placebo (plas·**e**·bo). A pharmacologically inactive substance which is administered as a drug either to satisfy a patient's desire for medication or in the course of drug trials. [L, I shall please.]

placenta [NA] (plas·**en**·tah). A complex structure, peculiar to pregnancy. It is attached to the uterine wall of the mother and connected to the child by the umbilical cord. Through the vessels of this cord is provided all the material for the metabolism and growth of the fetus. **Abruption of placenta.** Premature separation of the normal placenta. **Accessory placenta.** Succenturiate placenta (see below). **Placenta accreta.** A placenta in which the chorionic villi have invaded the uterine musculature, as there is no dividing line between the stratum compactum and stratum spongiosum and no line of cleavage can be found by the operator. **Adherent placenta.** One which remains attached to the uterine wall beyond the normal time allowed for separation. **Battledore placenta.** One in which the cord is inserted into the periphery. **Bilobed placenta, Placenta bipartita.** A placenta with two lobes which are not separated from one another. **Placenta circumvallata.** A placenta with a central depression which is surrounded by a raised rim. **Cirsoid placenta.** One in which the vessels on the fetal surface appear varicose. **Placenta diffusa.** A villous placenta. **Discoid placenta, Placenta discoidea.** A round placenta. **Placenta duplex.** A placenta having two separate lobes. **Placenta fenestra.** One in which there is a deficiency of placental tissue in one area of the placenta which is covered by membrane. **Fetal part of the placenta [pars fetalis (NA)].** That portion formed from the chorion rondosum, the villi of which invade the decidua basalis. **Fundal placenta.** One which is implanted in the fundus of the uterus. **Haemochorial placenta.** A type of placenta found in higher primates, including man, and in some other mammals in which fetal chorionic villi are bathed directly by the maternal blood stream, no maternal tissues intervening. **Horse-shoe placenta.** One having a horse-shoe shape; it occurs sometimes with twins. **Incarcerated placenta.** One which has separated from the uterine wall but is trapped in the uterus. **Placenta increta.** A type of placenta accreta where the placenta has penetrated into the uterine muscle. **Placenta marginata.** One which has a large amount of tissue at its edge. **Placenta membranacea.** A placenta in which the whole of the chorion frondosum has developed into placental tissue. **Multilobed placenta, Placenta multipartita.** One having many lobes. **Placenta praevia.** A placenta situated in or encroaching upon the lower uterine segment. **Placenta praevia, central.** Placenta praevia, fourth degree (see below). **Placenta praevia, first degree.** A placenta in which the greater part is attached to the upper uterine segment, and only the lower margin dips into the lower segment. **Placenta praevia, fourth degree.** A placenta so low that its centre corresponds roughly with the centre of the internal os uteri and therefore covers the os even when this is fully dilated. **Placenta praevia, lateral.** A placenta attached to the side of the lower uterine segment so that its edge does not reach the internal os uteri. **Placenta praevia, marginal.** A placenta the edge of which at its junction with the membranes crosses the internal os uteri. **Placenta praevia, second degree.** A placenta the edge of which reaches the internal os uteri. **Placenta praevia, third degree.** A placenta overlapping the internal os uteri when closed but not covering it entirely when it is fully dilated. **Retained placenta.** Non-delivery of the placenta from the genital canal after waiting an appropriate time after the birth of the child. **Placenta succenturiata, Succenturiate placenta.** A smaller placenta united to the main placenta by a leash of the umbilical vessels bridging the gap of amnion and chorion. **Trilobed placenta, Placenta tripartita.** A placenta having three lobes. **Uterine part of the placenta [pars uterina (NA)].** Most of the endometrium forming the decidua basalis, except the deeper portion of the stratum spongiosum. **Zonary placenta.** One which forms a ring round part of the ovum. [L, flat cake.]

placental (plas·en·tal). Belonging or relating to the placenta. **Placental hormones.** Hormones produced by the placenta.

Placentalia (plas·en·ta·le·ah). A subclass of the Mammalia, containing all living forms except the Marsupialia and the Monotremata. The young are attached to the uterine wall by a placenta.

placentation (plas·en·ta·shun). The process whereby a placenta is formed. It involves the formation of the chorion, its vascularization from adjacent fetal membranes such as the allantois or yolk sac, its association with the uterine wall by means of interlocking processes or active erosion in certain regions, and the subsequent development of an organ composed partly of fetal and partly of maternal tissue, whereby exchange of respiratory gases, nutritive materials and waste products between fetus and mother is achieved.

placentin (plas·en·tin). A vague term applied to any extract of placenta.

placentitis (plas·en·ti·tis). Inflammation affecting the placenta. [placenta, Gk *-itis* inflammation.]

placentography (plas·en·tog·raf·e). The x-ray visualization of the placenta, either by straight partly filtered x-rays or by means of a radio-opaque contrast medium or an appropriate radiopharmaceutical concentrating in the vascular placenta. **Indirect placentography.** The radiographic demonstration of the relationship between the presenting fetal part and the bladder and the soft tissues between it and the rectum. In placenta praevia there is an appreciable gap between these parts. Opaque contrast medium or air is injected into the bladder, and air into the rectum. **Radioisotope placentography.** The determining of the site of the placenta by injecting radioactive materials into the maternal blood stream and thereafter identifying maximum radioactivity over the placental bed. **Ultrasonic placentography.** Visualization of the placental site by ultrasonic scanning of the pregnant uterus. [placenta, radiography.]

placentoid (plas·en·toid). Having resemblance to a placenta. [placenta, Gk *eidos* form.]

placentolysin (plas·en·tol·is·in). A lysin formed in the serum of an animal in response to injections of placental cells and destructive to the placentae of animals from which the cells originated. [placenta, Gk *lysis* a loosing.]

placentoma (plas·en·to·mah). A tumour originating in and developing from remnants of retained placenta. [placenta, Gk *-oma* tumour.]

placentopathy (plas·en·top·ath·e). Any morbid condition of the placenta. [placenta, Gk *pathos* disease.]

placentotherapy (plas·en·to·ther′·ap·e). Treatment by administration of preparations derived from the placenta. [placenta, therapy.]

placentotoxin (plas·en·to·tox′·in). A supposed toxin formed by the placenta and thought to cause some of the toxaemias of pregnancy.

placentula (plas·en·tew·lah). A small-sized placenta. [L, little cake.]

Placido, A. (fl. 1882). Portuguese oculist.

Placido's disc. A large disc with concentric black and white circles, used for diagnosing conical cornea and irregular astigmatism. The disc is held in front of the patient and the shape of the image reflected by the cornea is examined through a hole in the centre of the instrument.

Placobdella (plak·o·del·ah). A genus of leeches. **Placobdella catenigra.** A small Mediterranean form which bites man readily. [Gk *plax* flat round plate, *bdella* leech.]

placode (plak·ode). An ectodermal thickening, especially one which presages the formation of a sensory organ in the head region of the embryo, e.g. nasal, otic or lens placode. **Auditory placode.** A thickened region of the surface ectoderm lateral to the hind-brain, from which the otic vesicle and part of the acousticofacial ganglia are derived. **Dorsolateral placode.** A thickened line of ectoderm along the side of an embryo of a fish or amphibian which gives rise to the lateralline organ. Its most anterior part represents the auditory placode. **Epibranchial placode.** A thickened region of the surface ectoderm above the root of a branchial arch of an embryo, which may be partly incorporated in the neighbouring cranial-nerve ganglion. **Lens placode.** A thickened region of the surface ectoderm adjacent to the optic cup, from which the crystalline lens of the eye is derived. **Olfactory placode.** A thickened region of the surface ectoderm of the frontonasal process of an embryo, from which the lining of the nasal cavity is derived. [Gk *plax* flat round plate, *eidos* form.]

pladaroma, pladarosis (plad·ar·o·mah, plad·ar·o·sis). A soft tumour occurring on the eyelid. [Gk *pladaros* moist, *-oma* tumour.]

plaga ignis (pla·gah ig·nis). Anthrax. [L *plaga* a stroke, *ignis* fire.]

plagiocephalic (pla·je·o·kef·al′·ik). Relating or belonging to, or showing the characteristic shape of head of plagiocephaly.

plagiocephalism (pla·je·o·kef′·al·izm). Plagiocephaly.

plagiocephaly (pla·je·o·kef′·al·e). A deformity of the head marked by a greater development anteriorly of one side of the skull and of the other side posteriorly, resulting in an asymmetrical and twisted appearance due to closure of half of the coronal suture. [Gk *plagios* aslant, *kephale* head.]

plague (pla·g). 1. A word at one time applied to any severe pestilence, but, since many of the historical plagues can be recognized as having been due to *Pasteurella pestis* infection, the word has come to be applied specifically to the disease caused by this infection. It is characterized by high fever, with rigors, great prostration, and usually lymphadenitis. It is often fatal, but the newer antibiotics have reduced the death rate. When the lungs are mainly affected it is known as *pneumonic plague;* in this form it is particularly severe and usually fatal, and secondary cases arising are likely to run true to type. The term *bubonic* is applied when the lymph glands are affected, and *septicaemic* when the constitutional symptoms outweigh the local ones; actually all cases of bubonic plague are septicaemic at some stage of the infection. The term "pestis minor" is applied to very mild infections when only one group of glands is affected and the constitutional symptoms are minimal. The infection is transmitted to man from rodents by the agency of rodent fleas; *pneumonic plague* may also be transmitted by droplets. 2. The term plague is still applied to a variety of serious outbreaks of a variety of diseases in animals, e.g. *cattle* plague—rinderpest, *fowl* plague—a virus infection. **Ambulant plague, Ambulatory plague.** A mild form, symptomless or almost symptomless. **Black plague.** A severe haemorrhagic form: the name usually applied to the classical plagues. **Bubonic plague.** *See* MAIN DEF. 1 (above). **Cellulocutaneous plague.** A severe form with cutaneous complications. **Domestic plague.** Urban plague (see below). **Glandular plague.** Bubonic plague. **Larval plague, Minor plague.** Pestis minor. **Pneumonic plague.** *See* MAIN DEF. 1 (above). **Septicaemic plague.** *See* MAIN DEF. 1 (above). **Sylvatic plague.** *Pasteurella pestis* infection among wild rodents in rural areas, especially in North America and South Africa; it may be transmitted to man sporadically. **Urban plague.** The form of plague transmitted from domestic rats to man by the rat flea; severe outbreaks of epidemic proportions may develop. [L *plaga* stroke.]

plakins (pla·kinz). Substances that are lytic to organisms and said to be extractable from blood platelets. [Gk *plax* flat round plate.]

Planck, Max (b. 1858). German physicist.

Planck's constant. The fundamental constant of proportionality between energy and the frequency of quanta of electromagnetic radiation. It is equal to 6.6256×10^{-34}Js, symbol *h*.

Planck's quantum hypothesis. Electromagnetic energy is emitted from a source in discrete quanta, the energy of which is equal to $h\nu$, where ν is the frequency of the radiation and *h* Planck's constant.

plane (plane). A flat surface. Mathematically, a surface that contains a straight line and all other straight lines which intersect the latter from a point in space. **Alveolocondylean plane.** A plane through the alveolar point and the line tangential to the lower surfaces of the occipital condyles; the alveolocondyloid plane of Broca, used in anthropometry. **Planes of anaesthesia.** The four levels into which A. E. Guedel divided the third stage of surgical anaesthesia. **Auriculoinfra-orbital plane.** The plane passing through the centres of the external auditory meatuses and the lowest points on the margins of the orbits, used in anthropometry. **Axiobuccolingual plane.** The plane which passes through a molar or premolar tooth, parallel to the long axis in a buccolingual direction. **Axiolabiolingual plane.** The plane which passes through an incisor or canine tooth, parallel to the long axis of the tooth, in a labiolingual direction. **Axiomesiodistal plane.** The plane which passes through a tooth, parallel to the axis, in a mesiodistal direction. **Bite plane.** The plane occupied by the biting surfaces of teeth. **Cleavage plane.** The plane at which division of a cell occurs. **Coronal plane.** A vertical plane at right angles to the median plane. **Cove plane.** A term used to describe the shape of the T wave of the electrocardiogram in a lead facing a muscle damaged by myocardial infarction: the S-T segment is elevated above the iso-electric level and the T wave sharply and deeply inverted and pointed. **Datum plane.** A plane of reference for craniometric measurements. **Equatorial plane of the eye.** The plane dividing the eyeball into anterior and posterior halves. **Facial plane.** The plane joining the pogonion and nasion. **Plane of fixation.** The plane in which the fixation axes of the two eyes lie. **Focal planes.** The planes which lie at right angles to the common optical axis of a system of lenses and pass through the focal points; used in the schematic eye. **Frankfort horizontal plane.** The plane passing through the lower margins of the orbits (the orbitale) and the upper margins of the external auditory orifices (the porion), used in anthropometry when comparing skulls. **Frontal plane.** Coronal plane (see above). **Horizontal plane.** 1. Any plane of the erect body parallel to the horizon. 2. A plane passing through a tooth at right angles to its longitudinal axis. **Plane of incidence.** The plane in which lie the incident ray of light, the normal to the surface at the point of incidence, and the reflected or refracted ray. **Plane of the inlet of the pelvis.** The plane passing through the promontory of the sacrum behind and the arcuate line on either side. **Intercristal plane, Intertubercular plane.** The horizontal plane passing through the tubercles of the iliac crests. **Labiolingual plane.** A plane passing through the labial and lingual surfaces of a tooth parallel to its long axis. **Mandibular plane.** The plane represented by a line drawn to touch the two most dependent points of the mandible. **Median plane.** The anteroposterior plane dividing the body into right and left halves. **Mesiodistal plane.** A plane passing through the mesial and distal surfaces of a tooth. **Midclavicular plane.** A vertical plane passing through the middle of the clavicle. **Midsagittal plane.** Median plane (see above). **Narrow pelvic plane.** Plane of the outlet of the pelvis (see below). **Nodal planes.** The planes lying at right angles to the common optical axis of a system of lenses and passing through the nodal points. **Nuchal plane.** The outer surface of the squamous part of the occipital bone below the superior curved lines. **Occipital plane.** The surface of the occipital bone above the superior nuchal lines. **Occlusal plane.** A plane passing through the occlusal surfaces of the teeth. **Orbital plane.** The plane dropped from the orbitale at right angles to the Frankfort horizontal plane. **Plane of the outlet of the pelvis.** A flat surface bounded in front by the lower border of the pubic symphysis, laterally by the tips of the ischial spines, and posteriorly by the lower border of the last sacral vertebra. **Parasagittal plane.** A plane parallel to the sagittal plane. **Principal planes.** The planes which lie at right angles to the common optic axis of a system of lenses and pass through the principal points; used in the schematic eye. **Plane of regard.** Plane of fixation (see above). **Sagittal plane.** An anteroposterior plane. **S-N plane.** The plane drawn from the midpoint of the sella turcica to the nasion. **Spinous plane.** The horizontal plane, drawn with the body erect, through the anterior superior iliac spine. **Subcostal plane.** The horizontal plane, with the body erect, at the level of the lowest parts of the 10th costal cartilages. **Transpyloric plane** (of Addison). An imaginary horizontal plane, with the body erect, placed midway between the suprasternal notch and the pubic symphysis. Posteriorly it cuts the lower border of the body of the 1st lumbar vertebra. **Transtubercular plane.** Intertubercular plane (see above). **Transverse plane.** Horizontal plane (see above). **Umbilical plane.** The horizontal plane through the umbilicus. [L *planum* level ground.]

See also: ADDISON (C.), AEBY, BAER (K. E.), BLUMENBACH, BOLTON, BROCA, DAUBENTON, HENSEN, HODGE, LISTING, MECKEL, MORTON (S. G.).

planiceps (pla·ne·seps). Having a flat head, or marked tendency towards flat-headedness. [L *planus* flat, *caput* head.]

planigram (pla·ne·gram). A radiograph of a layer or section of the body made by body-section radiography. [L *planus* flat, Gk *gramma* a writing.]

planigraphy (pla·**nig**·raf·e). Body-section radiography.

See RADIOGRAPHY. [L *planus* flat, Gk *graphein* to record.]

planimeter (pla·**nim**·et·er). An apparatus with jointed levers and a recording index for measuring the area of a plane figure or surface by passing a tracer around the boundaries. [L *planus* flat, Gk *metron* measure.]

planiography (pla·ne·**og**·raf·e). Planigraphy.

planipes (**pla**·nip·eez). Flat foot. [L *planus* flat, *pes* foot.]

planithorax (pla·ne·**thor**·ax). A diagram of the thorax illustrating in plan the front and the back. [L *planus* flat, thorax.]

planocellular (pla·no·**sel**·ew·lar). Belonging or relating to or composed of flat cells. [L *planus* flat, cell.]

planococcus (plan·o·**kok**·us). A former generic term for motile coccal cells dividing in two planes [obsolete term]. [Gk *plane* wandering, *kokkos* berry.]

planoconcave (pla·no·**kon**·kave). Applied to a lens that is flat on one surface, concave on the other. [L *planus* flat, concave.]

planoconical (pla·no·**kon**·ik·al). With one side flat and the other conical. [L *planus* flat, conical.]

planoconvex (pla·no·**kon**·vex). Applied to a lens that is flat on one surface, convex on the other. [L *planus* flat, convex.]

planocyte (**plan**·o·site). A wandering cell. [Gk *plane* wandering, *kytos* cell.]

planography (plan·**og**·raf·e). Body-section radiography.

See RADIOGRAPHY. [L *planus* flat, radiography.]

planomania (plan·o·**ma**·ne·ah). A form of insanity marked by a craving to wander from place to place. [Gk *plane* wandering, mania.]

Planorbis (plan·**or**·bis). A genus of pulmonate fresh-water molluscs. The species are usually small, with the shell in the form of a flattened coil. *Planorbis dufouri*, an intermediary host of *Schistosoma haematobium*, and *Planorbis metidjensis* are at present the only snails of this genus recognized as a host of flukes pathogenic to man; other species have now been reclassified in different genera. **Planorbis adowensis.** *Biomphalaria alexandrina pfeifferi.* **Planorbis alexandrinus.** *Biomphalaria alexandrina.* **Planorbis boissyii.** *Biomphalaria alexandrina.* **Planorbis bridouxianus.** *Biomphalaria alexandrina tanganyicensis.* **Planorbis centrimetalis.** *Tropicorbis centrimetalis.* **Planorbis choanomphalus.** *Biomphalaria alexandrina choanomphala.* **Planorbis coenosus.** An intermediary host of *Fasciolopsis buski.* **Planorbis corneus** var. **metidjensis.** *Planorbis dufouri.* **Planorbis dufouri.** *See* MAIN DEF. (above). **Planorbis glabratus.** *Australorbis glabratus.* **Planorbis guadeloupensis.** *Australorbis glabratus.* **Planorbis herbini.** *Biomphalaria alexandrina pfeifferi.* **Planorbis metidjensis.** An intermediary host of *Schistosoma haematobium* in Portugal. **Planorbis metidjensis var. dufouri.** *Planorbis dufouri.* **Planorbis olivaceus.** *Australorbis centrimetalis olivaceus.* **Planorbis pfeifferi.** *Biomphalaria alexandrina pfeifferi.* **Planorbis rupelli.** *Biomphalaria alexandrina pfeifferi.* **Planorbis stanleyi.** *Biomphalaria alexandrina stanleyi.* **Planorbis sudanicus.** *Biomphalaria alexandrina tanganyicensis.* **Planorbis tanganikanus.** *Biomphalaria alexandrina tanganyicensis.* **Planorbis tanganyicensis.** *Biomphalaria alexandrina tanganyicensis.* [L *planus* flat, *orbis* circle.]

planorheumatism (plan·o·**roo**·mat·izm). Rheumatism that flits about from joint to joint or focus to focus. [Gk *plane* wandering, rheumatism.]

planosarcina (plan·o·**sar**·sin·ah). A former generic term for motile coccal cells dividing in three planes [obsolete term]. [Gk *plane* wandering, L *sarcina* pack.]

planotopokinesia (**plan**·o·**to**·po·kin·e′·ze·ah). Spatial disorientation. *See* DISORIENTATION. [Gk *plane* wandering, *topos* place, *kinesis* movement.]

planovalgus (pla·no·**val**·gus). Flat foot with valgus or everted heel. [L *planus* flat, *valgus* bowlegged.]

Plantago (plan·**ta**·go). A genus of herbs of the family Plantaginaceae; the plantains. **Plantago major.** The common plantain or ripple grass; the seeds once formed a popular remedy for diarrhoea and dysentery and a decoction made from the leaves was said to have diuretic and cooling properties. **Plantago ovata.** A species that is the source of spaghula. **Plantago psyllium.** The species that yields psyllium. [L.]

plantain (**plan**·tane). 1. The common name for all plants belonging to the genus *Plantago*, but particularly applied to the common plantain, *Plantago major*, whose seeds were at one time used medicinally. The seeds of *Plantago psyllium* are used as a mild laxative. 2. A tropical fruit, *Musa sapientum*, an important source of food in some tropical countries. [L *plantago*.]

plantalgia (plan·**tal**·je·ah). Pain affecting the plantar surface of the foot due to general weakness of the foot, especially flat foot. [L *planta* sole of the foot, Gk *algos* pain.]

plantar [plantaris (NA)] (**plan**·tar). Relating or belonging to the sole of the foot. [L *planta* sole of the foot.]

plantar arteries. Lateral plantar artery [arteria plantaris lateralis (NA)]. One of the terminal branches of the posterior tibial artery, arising behind the medial malleolus and passing first laterally across the sole of the foot and then turning medially to the base of the 1st intermetatarsal space where it anastomoses with the dorsalis pedis artery to form the plantar arterial arch. Superficial branches go to the skin and subcutaneous tissues of the sole of the foot. **Medial plantar artery [arteria plantaris medialis (NA)].** One of the terminal branches of the posterior tibial artery, arising behind the medial malleolus and supplying the medial side of the foot and big toe [ramus superficialis (NA)]. The deep branch [ramus profundus (NA)] joins the 1st plantar metatarsal artery.

plantar nerves. Lateral plantar nerve [nervus plantaris lateralis (NA)]. One of the terminal branches of the posterior tibial nerve. It passes to the lateral side of the foot and supplies the muscles and skin of this region [ramus superficialis (NA)], the skin of the lateral one and a half toes and all the interosseous muscles of the foot, the lateral three lumbricals and the adductor hallucis [rami profundi (NA)]. **Medial plantar nerve [nervus plantaris medialis (NA)].** One of the terminal branches of the posterior tibial nerve, arising at the ankle and passing along the medial side of the sole of the foot. It supplies the small muscles and skin in this region and on the skin on the plantar surfaces of the medial three and a half toes.

plantar veins. Lateral and medial plantar veins. The venae comitantes of the lateral and medial plantar arteries. They are tributaries of the posterior tibial veins.

plantaris (plan·ta·ris). The plantaris muscle. [L *planta* sole of the foot.]

plantaris muscle [musculus plantaris (NA)]. A slender muscle deep to the gastrocnemius, arising from the lateral supracondylar line on the femur and inserted to the calcaneum on the medial side of the tendo calcaneus. Sometimes absent.

plantation (plan·**ta**·shun). The insertion of a tooth, either by replantation, i.e. the replacement of a tooth into the bony socket from which it has been removed by accident or design, or by transplantation, i.e. the insertion of a similar tooth from another mouth into a bony socket from which a tooth has just been removed. [L *planta* a shoot for setting.]

plantigrade (**plan**·te·grade). In zoology, applied to animals that place the whole of the plantar surface of the foot on the ground in walking, man as well as most of the bears. [L *planta* sole of the foot, *gradi* to walk.]

plantose (**plan**·toze). An edible protein obtained from rape seed.

planula (**plan**·ew·lah). The larval stage of a coelenterate. [dim. of L *planus* flat.]

planum (**pla**·num). A plane or flat surface; in anatomy, a surface which is more or less flat and reasonably extensive. **Planum supracochleare.** The upper surface of the developing petrous part of the temporal bone on which the facial nerve lies; later the nerve becomes enclosed in a bony canal. [L *planus* flat.]

planuria (plan·**ewr**·e·ah). Extravasation of urine by an abnormal channel, e.g. a fistula. [Gk *plane* wandering, urine.]

plaque (plahk). A flat area; a patch. **Bacterial plaque.** A film of living and dead micro-organisms, food debris, desquamated degenerated cells and mucus, lying on the enamel surface of a tooth and thought to induce the commencement of dental caries. **Bacteriophage plaque.** A small visible area of clearing in confluent bacterial growth on solid media, due to localized phage infection; when a diluted phage suspension is plated with an excess of sensitive bacteria, isolated plaques represent phage clones derived from multiplication of single particles and analogous to bacterial colonies. **β-ray plaque.** A container for phosphorus, radium or strontium for surface application of β-rays. **Blood plaque.** Blood platelet. *See* PLATELET. **Dental plaque.** Bacterial plaque (see above). **Fibromyelinic plaques.** Areas of proliferation of medullated nerve fibres at the sites of arteriosclerotic necrosis in the brain. **Gelatinoid plaque.** Bacterial plaque (see above). **Mucinous plaque.** Bacterial plaque (see above). **Mucous plaque.** Mucous patch; a whitish superficial ulcer on mucous membranes, occurring in secondary syphilis. **Opaline plaque.** Opaline patch; a lesion of secondary syphilis. **Radium plaque.** A radium container for surface application, sometimes thin-walled on one side to permit transmission of β-rays (β-ray plaque). **Senile plaques.** Areas of partial or complete necrosis found in the cerebral cortex of the aged. **Talc plaque.** A dense opaque line or ragged mass seen radiographically in a small proportion of talc workers and miners; an opaque deposit on the pleural surface at the periphery of lung fields. [Fr.]

See also: LICHTHEIM, PEYER, REDLICH-FISCHER.

plasm (plazm). Plasma.

plasma (**plaz**·mah). 1. The fluid portion of the blood in which the blood corpuscles are suspended. *See* BLOOD PLASMA (below). 2. Corpuscle-free lymph. 3. Sometimes used to mean cytoplasm or protoplasm. 4. May refer to Starch Glycerin BP 1958, a starch glyceride used in pharmacy for ointments and emulsion. 5. May refer to the concentration of some compound in the plasma, e.g. plasma testosterone concentration, as opposed to serum, e.g. serum globulin. **Blood plasma.** The yellow fluid portion of blood in which the blood cells are suspended; when whole blood is treated with an anticoagulant to prevent clotting, it is the clear supernatant liquid than can be separated after sedimentation or centrifugation from the thick sedimented layer of blood cells. It will clot when treated appropriately, producing a clear liquid resembling or identical with blood serum. **Citrated plasma.** Plasma prepared from blood, containing added citrate to prevent clotting. **Dried Human Plasma BP 1973.** A dried preparation of Whole Human Blood BP 1973. **Germ plasma.** The substance which represents the physical basis of heredity and is transmitted from generation to generation by the germ cells. **Lymph plasma.** Corpuscle-free lymphatic fluid. **Plasma marinum.** Sea water diluted to make it isotonic with blood serum. **Muscle plasma.** The spontaneously coagulable juice expressed from muscle tissue. **Oxalate plasma.** Blood plasma containing ammonium oxalate (1 per cent) to prevent clotting. **Plasma removal.** The separation of plasma from blood cells after their sedimentation on standing or after centrifugation. **Salt plasma.** Blood plasma containing an added neutral salt to prevent clotting. **Plasma skimming.** A phenomenon said to occur in small capillaries whereby contraction prevents the blood corpuscles from passing through, although the plasma flows through freely. **True plasma.**

Blood plasma prepared out of contact with air so that the gas content remains unchanged. [Gk *plassein* to mould.]

plasma-albumin (plaz·mah·al·bew′·min). Albumin normally present in the plasma.

plasmablast (plaz·mah·blast). A very primitive cell with the characteristic nucleus of the plasma-cell series; seen in bone marrow, rarely in the blood, in myelomatosis and glandular fever. [plasma, Gk *blastos* germ.]

plasmacule (plaz·mah·kewl). One of numerous tiny granules believed to exist in the blood plasma. [dim. of plasma.]

plasmacyte (plaz·mah·site). A plasma cell. [plasma, Gk *kytos* cell.]

plasmacytoma (plaz·mah·si·to′·mah). A malignant tumour composed of plasma cells, most often found in lymph nodes and bone marrow. [plasmacyte, Gk *-oma* tumour.]

plasmacytosis (plaz·mah·si·to′·sis). A condition characterized by the existence of plasmacytes in the blood. [plasmacyte, Gk *-osis* condition.]

plasmagene (plaz·mah·jeen). A self-reproducing particle in cells, having the characteristics of a gene but not situated on a chromosome. [plasma, gene.]

plasma-globulin (plaz·mah·glob·ew·lin). Globulin normally present in the plasma.

plasmaphaeresis (plaz·mah·fe·re·sis). The process of removing by venesection a large volume of blood to which is added an anticoagulant (sodium citrate), separating the red blood cells from the plasma by centrifugation or sedimentation under sterile conditions, washing them free from plasma with a selected isotonic saline solution, and then transferring them into the patient as a suspension in fresh isotonic solution. [plasma, Gk *aphairesis* a taking away.]

plasmarrhexis (plaz·mah·rex·is). Disintegration of cell protoplasm. [plasma, Gk *rhexis* rupture.]

plasmase (plaz·maze). Thrombin. [plasma.]

plasmasome (plaz·mah·some). A granule in a granular leucocyte. [plasma, Gk *soma* body.]

plasmatherapy (plaz·mah·ther·ap·e). Therapeutic transfusion of blood plasma.

plasmatic (plaz·mat·ik). 1. Relating to or having the characteristics of plasma. 2. Plastic. [Gk *plassein* to mould.]

plasmatogamy (plaz·mah·tog·am·e). Fusion of two or more cells, the individual nuclei being preserved. [plasma, Gk *gamos* marriage.]

plasmatorrhexis (plaz·mah·to·rex′·is). Rupture and herniation of cell contents because of the internal pressure exercised by the protoplasm. [plasma, Gk *rhexis* rupture.]

plasmatosis (plaz·mah·to·sis). The conversion of cell protoplasm into liquid form. [plasma, Gk *-osis* condition.]

plasmexhidrosis, plasmexidrosis (plaz·mex·hid·ro′·sis, plaz·mex·id·ro′·sis). The extravasation of plasma from the blood vessels. [plasma, Gk *ex*, hidrosis.]

plasmic (plaz·mik). 1. Amply provided with protoplasm. 2. Plasmatic.

plasmid (plaz·mid). A genetic element of bacteria, additional to the normal genome, which replicates independently of the chromosome but co-ordinately with the cell; it includes sex factors (= transmissible plasmids) and often carries genetic determinants of resistance to antibiotics and metal ions. [plasma.]

Plasmin (plaz·min). BP Commission approved name for the proteolytic enzyme derived from the activation of plasminogen. [plasma.]

See also: DENIS (P. S.).

Plasminogen (plaz·min·o·jen). BP Commission approved name for the specific substance derived from plasma which, when activated, has the property of lysing fibrinogen, fibrin and some other proteins.

plasmocyte (plaz·mo·site). Plasmacyte.

plasmocytoma (plaz·mo·si·to′·mah). Plasmacytoma.

plasmodesma, plasmodesmus (plaz·mo·dez·mah, plaz·mo·dez·mus). Cement substance binding adjacent cells. [plasma, Gk *desmos* band.]

plasmodial (plaz·mo·de·al). Relating or belonging to a plasmodium.

plasmodiblast (plaz·mo·de·blast). Trophoblast. [plasmodium, Gk *blastos* germ.]

plasmodicidal (plaz·mo·de·si′·dal). Capable of destroying plasmodia. [plasmodium, L *caedere* to kill.]

plasmodicide (plaz·mo·de·side). A substance that is able to destroy plasmodia; an antimalarial drug. [see prec.]

Plasmodiidae (plaz·mo·de·e·de). A family of the sporozoan order Haemosporidia. It contains the genus *Plasmodium.*

plasmoditrophoblast (plaz·mo·de·tro′·fo·blast). The syncytiotrophoblast; that part of the trophoblast which covers the chorionic villi and in which no cell boundaries are visible. It actively erodes the decidua in early pregnancy, and later becomes the most important constituent of the placental barrier separating the maternal and fetal blood streams. [plasmodium, trophoblast.]

Plasmodium (plaz·mo·de·um). 1. The name of a genus of sporozoa of the order Haemosporidia. There are numerous species that infect man, monkeys and other animals, and birds, respectively. The plasmodia that infect man cause malaria, and those of other species cause varying degrees of morbidity in their hosts. Several plasmodial species of monkeys and birds have been used extensively in the study of malaria and especially for screening antimalarial drugs. The important species that infect man are: *Plasmodium falciparum,* which causes malignant tertian, subtertian or aestivo-autumnal malaria, a dangerous form of malaria that is sometimes fatal, especially in children, but shows a low rate of relapse; *P. malariae,* which causes quartan malaria; *P. ovale,* which causes a mild form of malaria with little tendency to relapse; *P. tenue,* possibly a subspecies of *P. falciparum;* and *P. vivax,* which causes benign tertian malaria, an infection that is seldom fatal but shows a marked tendency to relapse. The important species infecting monkeys are: *P. cynomolgi, P. gonderi, P. (Hepatocytis) kochi, P. inui, P. knowlesi, P. reichenowi, P. rodhaini,* and *P. schwetzi.* The important species that infect birds are: *P. cathemerium, P. elongatum* and *P. relictum* of the canary, *P. lophurae* of the duck and *P. gallinaceum* of fowls. *P. bergei,* an infection of the rat, is a recent important addition to the plasmodia used in chemotherapeutic assays. 2. A multinucleated mass of protoplasm formed by the union of two or more cells with loss of cell boundaries. **Exo-erythrocytic plasmodium.** A malarial plasmodium of the exo-erythrocytic stage, i.e. in the liver parenchyma cells. **Plasmodium wilsoni.** A species name of doubtful validity. [Gk *plasma* anything formed, *eidos* type.]

Plasmodroma (plaz·mo·dro·mah) (pl. *plasmodromata*). A subphylum of the Protozoa. It contains the classes Mastigophora, Sarcodina and Sporozoa. The nucleus is usually single and movement, when present, is by flagella or pseudopodia. [Gk *plasma* anything formed, *dromos* running.]

plasmogamy (plaz·mog·am·e). Reproduction by cell fusion. [Gk *plasma* anything formed, *gamos* marriage.]

plasmology (plaz·mol·o·je). The science dealing with the microscopical granules or ultimate corpuscles of living structure. [plasma, Gk *logos* science.]

plasmolyse (plaz·mo·lize). To induce plasmolysis in a cell.

plasmolysis (plaz·mol·is·is). Dissolution or contraction of cell protoplasm, the result of dehydration by osmotic action, with shrinkage from the surrounding cell wall. [plasma, Gk *lysis* a loosing.]

plasmolytic (plaz·mo·lit·ik). Relating or belonging to or distinguished by plasmolysis.

plasmoma (plaz·mo·mah). 1. A collection of plasma cells which resembles a tumour. 2. Plasmocytoma. [plasma, Gk *-oma* tumour.]

plasmophagocytosis (plaz·mo·fag·o·si·to′·sis). The disposal of plasma by phagocytes. [plasma, phagocyte, Gk *-osis* condition.]

plasmophagous (plaz·mof·ag·us). Denoting certain organisms which cause decomposition of organic matter. [plasma, Gk *phagein* to eat.]

plasmoptysis (plaz·**mop**·tis·is). Expression of protoplasm from a cell as a result of rupture of the wall of the cell. [plasma, Gk *ptyein* to disgorge.]

plasmorrhexis (plaz·mo·**rex**·is). Bursting of a cell due to internal pressure, with extrusion of the plasma. [plasma, Gk *rhexis* rupture.]

plasmoschisis (plaz·**mos**·kis·is). Disintegration of cell plasma. [plasma, Gk *schisis* a cleaving.]

plasmosin (**plaz**·mo·sin). A cytoplasmic nucleoprotein. [plasma.]

plasmosome (**plaz**·mo·some). The true nucleolus of the cell nucleus; a rounded body containing both ribo- and deoxyribonucleic acids, and thought to be involved in the initial stages of protein manufacture by the cell. [Gk *plasma* anything formed, *soma* body.]

plasmotherapy (plaz·mo·**ther**·ap·e). The use of blood plasma in treatment. [plasma, Gk *therapeia* treatment.]

plasmotropic (plaz·mo·**trop**·ik). Relating to or effecting plasmotropism.

plasmotropism (plaz·**mot**·rop·izm). Degeneration and disintegration of erythrocytes in the bone marrow, spleen or liver as a result of haemolytic action there, the cells in the general circulation, however, not undergoing any change. [plasma, Gk *tropos* a turning.]

plasmozyme (**plaz**·mo·zime). Prothrombin. [plasma, Gk *zyme* leaven.]

plasome (**plas**·ome). Hypothetically, the smallest amount of protoplasm which retains all the characteristics. [plasma, Gk *soma* body.]

plassomyxineae (plas·o·mix·**in**'·e·e). The acidophilic inclusion bodies found in the lesions of molluscum contagiosum [obsolete term]. [Gk *plassein* to form, *myxa* slime.]

plasson (**plas**·on). Protoplasm, generally in a non-nucleated, non-differentiated state. [Gk, that which forms.]

plastein (**plas**·te·in). Proteins synthesized by proteolytic enzymes such as pepsin and trypsin from the products of peptic digestion of proteins. Plasteins appear to be high molecular polypeptides which differ from the proteins originally digested. [Gk *plassein* to form.]

plaster (**plah**·ster). Any preparation of a medicament in a resinous, plastic, rubber or unctuous base spread on calico or linen and maintained in close contact with the skin for a considerable time. They may be used to exclude dirt and hold the edges of a wound together or to enable certain medicaments to permeate the subdermal tissues. **Adhesive plaster.** A rubber basis spread on calico, linen or plastic, and used in strips for closing small wounds or holding dressings in position. **Barium plaster.** Plaster containing a high proportion of barytes (barium sulphate), used as a protective building material. **Belladonna plaster.** A plaster impregnated with the alkaloids of belladonna root and used for lumbago. **Blistering plaster, Cantharides plaster.** A plaster containing cantharidin, used to produce blisters on the skin. **Corn plaster.** A resin plaster containing from 5 to 25 per cent of salicylic acid, sometimes with Indian hemp or other anodyne, and used to destroy corns, warts and hard skin. **Court plaster.** An isinglass plaster used to protect small cuts. **Diachylon plaster.** Lead plaster (see below). **Elastic plaster.** A rubber plaster spread on an elastic backing and suitable for movable parts of the body. **Lead plaster, Litharge plaster.** The basis of many medicated plasters, made by boiling lead monoxide (litharge) with olive oil for some hours followed by kneading under hot water to remove the glycerol produced. **Plaster of Paris.** A white powder, calcium sulphate hemihydrate, $Ca SO_4 \cdot \frac{1}{2}H_2O$, which is mixed to a paste with water and sets slowly with slight expansion to a hard mass; used for plaster bandages and jackets. **Plaster of pitch.** A plaster of burgundy pitch, frankincense or olibanum, resin, yellow beeswax, olive oil and distilled water. It is an old preparation used in chronic bronchitis, rheumatism and lumbago, and is now obsolete. **Poor man's plaster.** Plaster of pitch (see prec.). **Resin plaster.** A plaster base made from turpentine resin (colophony) and used as an adhesive plaster with or without added medicament. **Tobruk plaster.** Tobruk splint. *See* SPLINT. **ZO plaster, Zinc oxide plaster.** A resin plaster containing zinc oxide and used for cuts. [Gk *emplastron.*]

See also: WHITMAN.

plaster-mass (**plah**·ster·**mas**'). A resinous or plaster mass medicated or unmedicated that is used to make plaster by spreading it on some supporting material. [plaster, L *massa.*]

plastic (**plas**·tik). 1. Formative. 2. Able to be moulded or formed; pliable. 3. Capable of restoring structures or repairing structural deficiencies. 4. In dentistry, applied to any material (e.g. amalgam) that can be readily moulded and used as a filling. [Gk *plassein* to mould.]

plasticity (plas·**tis**·it·e). The state or quality of being plastic.

plastics (**plas**·tix). 1. Plastic surgery. 2. Any of the numerous organic synthetic or processed materials that are mostly thermoplastic or thermosetting polymers of high molecular weight and that can be moulded, cast, extruded, drawn, or laminated into objects, films or filaments.

plastid (**plas**·tid). A round or oval body within the cytoplasm of a plant cell, containing a pigment such as chlorophyll or storage material such as oil or starch. [Gk *plastos* formed.]

plastidogenetic (plas·tid·o·jen·**et**'·ik). Producing plastids. [plastid, Gk *genein* to produce.]

plastidule (**plas**·tid·ewl). A molecular unit of protoplasm. [dim. of plastid.]

plastiosome (**plas**·te·o·some). Mitochondria. [Gk *plassein* to form, *soma* body.]

plastochondria (plas·to·**kon**·dre·ah). Mitochondria of granular type. [Gk *plastos* formed, *chondros* granule.]

plastocont (**plas**·to·kont). A rod-shaped chondriosome. [Gk *plastos* formed, *kontos* pole.]

plastocytaemia (plas·to·si·**te**'·me·ah). Plastocytosis. [plastocyte, Gk *haima* blood.]

plastocyte (**plas**·to·site). Blood platelet. *See* PLATELET. [Gk *plastos* formed, *kytos* cell.]

plastocytopenia (plas·to·si·to·**pe**'·ne·ah). A condition marked by a lessening in the number of blood platelets to below the normal range. [plastocyte, Gk *penes* poor.]

plastocytosis (plas·to·si·**to**'·sis). A condition characterized by an increase in the number of blood platelets well above normal range. [plastocyte, Gk *-osis* condition.]

plastodynamia (plas·to·di·**nam**'·e·ah). The physiological property or potential for development, active or passive. [Gk *plastos* formed, *dynamis* power.]

plastogamy (plas·**tog**·am·e). Protozoan union in which the protoplasm of several individuals is fused but without union of the nuclei taking place. [Gk *plastos* formed, *gamos* marriage.]

plastogel (**plas**·to·jel). A colloidal gel that has a considerable amount of plasticity.

plastosome (**plas**·to·some). Any granule or filament of the protoplasm which is readily stained with dyes. [Gk *plastos* formed, *soma* body.]

plastron (**plas**·tron). The sternum and attached costal cartilages. [Fr., breastplate.]

plate (plate). 1. Any flattened structure. 2. In dentistry, an artificial denture. 3. A glass culture plate (Petri dish). 4. In bacteriology, to inoculate culture media contained in glass plates (Petri dishes) with bacteria or other micro-organisms or with material suspected as containing them. 5. To fix metal plates to fractured bones in order to maintain fragments in apposition. **Alar plate.** One of the paired dorsolateral thickenings of the embryonic neural tube from which sensory or afferent neurones arise, and in which the processes of the dorsal root neurones end. **Anal plate.** A temporary membrane in the embryo, separating the hind-gut and the proctodaeal derivatives of the anal canal. **Approximation plate.** A plate of bone used in the 19th century in bowel anastomosis. **Axial plate.** The primitive streak of the embryo. **Basal plate.** One of the paired ventrolateral thickenings of the embryonic neural tube from which the motor neurones are derived. **Base plate.** That portion of a prosthetic appliance which rests on the mucosa and supports either artificial teeth or a bite block. **Bite plate.** In prosthetic dentistry, a plate made of wax or other plastic material and used to record the normal relationship between the upper and the lower jaw. **Blood plate.** Blood platelet. *See* PLATELET. **Bone plate.** 1. Approximation plate (see above). 2. A metal plate used for approximating bones. *See* MAIN DEF. 5 (above). **Cardiogenic plate.** A plate of mesodermal cells at the anterior end of the early embryo, from which the paired endothelial heart tubes are derived. **Cell plate.** A thickening which appears across the centre of the spindle towards the end of cell division, along the line of separation into daughter cells. **Chorionic plate.** That part of the chorion from which the placental villi arise; it forms the inner wall of the placenta. **Cloacal plate.** The cloacal membrane of the early embryo, separating the hind-gut from the ectodermal cloaca. **Closing plate.** One of the epithelial membranes separating the ectodermal clefts from the underlying pharyngeal pouches in the embryo. **Collecting plate.** The negative plate of an electric cell; a plate electrode in an ionization chamber, connected to the instrument used to measure the charge carried by the ions that fall on it. **Cough plate.** A Petri dish, containing a suitable medium (e.g. Bordet–Gengou for whooping-cough), over which the patient coughs; used for the isolation of *Haemophilus pertussis.* **Cribriform plate [lamina cribrosa (NA)].** A horizontal bony plate which joins the ethmoidal labyrinth to the perpendicular plate and has perforations in it to transmit olfactory nerves. **Cutis plate.** A dermatome; that part of a somite from which a segmental area of skin dermis is derived. **Deck plate.** The roof plate of the embryonic neural tube, connecting the alar laminae. **Dental plate.** A prosthesis constructed of metal, acrylic resin or vulcanized rubber, made to the shape of the mouth to support artificial teeth; an artificial denture. **Dorsal plate.** Deck plate (see above). **Dorsolateral plate.** Alar plate (see above). **Equatorial plate.** The plate-like mass of chromosomes across the equator of the spindle at metaphase in mitotic cell division. **Ethmovomerine plate.** The back part of the cartilaginous nasal septum of the embryo, from which the ethmoidal septum and the vomer are derived. **Facial plate.** One of the swellings around the primitive mouth of the embryo, viz. frontonasal, maxillary and mandibular processes, from which the facial region is developed. **Floor plate.** The floor of the neural tube of the embryo. **Frontal plate.** A cartilaginous plate at the side of the back of the nose in the embryo, between the sphenoid and ethmoid cartilages. **Frontonasal plate.** Frontonasal process. *See* PROCESS. **Generating plate.** The positive plate of a voltaic cell. **Horizontal plate of the palatine bone [lamina horizontalis (NA)].** The flattened horizontal part of the palatine bone which forms the back of the hard palate. Its upper surface [facies nasalis (NA)] forms part of the floor of the nasal cavity, and its lower surface [facies palatina (NA)] forms the posterior part of the hard palate. **Lateral mesoblastic plate.** The most lateral part of the early embryonic mesoderm in which the coelom develops; it forms the basis of the body wall and the muscular and serous coats of the alimentary canal. **Location plate.** A dental plate in which pieces of metal are buried; when inserted in the mouth it localizes under x-rays the position of fragments of tooth retained in the jaws. **Meatal plate.** A solid strand of ectodermal cells which later hollows out to become the lining of the external auditory meatus in the embryo. **Medial plate.** Mesial plate (see below). **Medullary plate.** The middle ectodermal thickening of the embryonic disc, which later enfolds to become the neural tube. **Mesial plate.** The intermediate cell mass between the somites and the lateral mesoblastic plate of the embryo, from which the urogenital organs are formed. **Metaphase plate.** The equatorial plate of the spindle where the chromosomes come to equilibrium at metaphase of meiosis or mitosis. **Muscle plate.** Myotome; that part of the somite from which the segmented striated muscles are formed. **Neural plate.** Medullary plate (see above). **Notochordal plate.** A narrow band of cells in the mid-dorsal line of the early embryonic gut, which later constricts to become the notochord. **Nuclear plate.** Equatorial plate (see above). **Optic plate.** A thickened area of the wall of the front end of the neural tube from which the optic outgrowths are derived in the early embryo. **Oral plate.** The buccopharyngeal membrane of the early embryo, separating the stomatodaeum from the pharynx. **Orbital plate of the ethmoid bone [lamina orbitalis (NA)].** A flat plate of bone forming the lateral wall of the ethmoidal labyrinth, and part of the medial wall of the orbit. **Orbital plate of the frontal bone [pars orbitalis (NA)].** That part of the frontal bone which forms the roof of the orbit, except for a small portion posteriorly. **Parachordal plate.** One of the two plates of condensed mesoderm, later cartilage, lying on either side of the frontal end of the notochord and developing into the basi-occipital and basisphenoidal portions of the skull. **Parietal plate.** The outer layer of the intermediate cell mass, as compared with the visceral plate (see below). **Perpendicular plate of the ethmoid bone [lamina perpendicularis (NA)].** A thin, flat, bony plate which lies in the midsagittal plane, forming the upper third of the nasal septum. **Perpendicular plate of the palatine bone [lamina perpendicularis (NA)].** The ascending portion of the palatine bone which presents mainly in the lateral wall of the nose. Above, it supports the orbital and sphenoidal processes which are separated by a notch (the sphenopalatine notch). It forms part of the lateral nasal wall [facies nasalis (NA)], and its lateral surface [facies maxillaris (NA)] articulates with the nasal surface of the maxilla. **Polar plate, Pole plate.** A flattened body seen in some cells at the end of the spindle during mitosis. **Pour plate.** A term used to describe a plate of culture medium to which the material under examination has been added before the agar or gelatin has set. **Primitive plate.** Primitive streak. *See* STREAK. **Primitive-joint plate.** A plate of condensed mesenchyme lying between the cartilaginous precursors of the bones at the site of future joints. It disappears in synovial joints, with the formation of the synovial cavity, but persists in less movable joints. **Prochordal plate.** A thickening of the roof of the yolk sac in front of the notochord in the situation of the future buccopharyngeal membrane. **Pterygoid plate, lateral [lamina lateralis processus pterygoidei (NA)].** The lateral of the two plates forming the pterygoid process. **Pterygoid plate, medial [lamina medialis processus pterygoidei (NA)].** The medial of the two plates forming the pterygoid process. **Retaining plate.** An appliance used in orthodontics to keep teeth that have moved in their new position. **Reticular plate.** A specialized form of nerve-ending in the ciliary body of the eye in the form of fine nerve terminals. **Roof plate.** The roof of the neural tube. **Segmental plate.** The paraxial mesoderm before it has become subdivided into somites. **Sinus plate.** A rod of ectodermal cells traversing the glans penis, which later hollows out to become the lining of the terminal portion of the urethra. **Stomatodaeal plate.** Oral plate (see above). **Streak plate.** A Petri dish containing some suitable solid nutrient medium which has been inoculated in such a way as to produce discrete bacterial colonies. **Subgerminal plate.** A sheet of cells delaminated from the blastoderm of large-yolked eggs, forming the floor of the subgerminal cavity. **Suction plate.** A dental plate held in place by suction. **Tarsal plate.** A plate of dense fibrous tissue incorporated in and supporting either eyelid; the larger superior [tarsus superior (NA)] plate is semi-ovoid in form and the smaller inferior [tarsus inferior (NA)] one is long and narrow. **Trial plate.** A plate of wax, shellac or other base-plate material, used as a temporary support for artificial teeth during the construction of an artificial denture. **Tympanic plate.** The plate of bone forming the floor and sides of the external auditory meatus. **Urethral plate.** A sagittally placed plate of cells in the embryonic phallus which breaks down to form part of the male urethra. **Vascular foot plate.** A flattened foot-like process at the ends of some of the branches of astroglial cells in the central nervous system, attached to the wall of a capillary. **Ventral plate.** The floor plate of the neural tube, between the basal laminae. **Ventrolateral plate.** Basal plate (see above). **Visceral plate.** The inner stratum of the intermediate cell mass after that structure has been divided by the coelom in lower vertebrates. **Wing plate.** Alar plate (see above). [OFr.]

See also: KUEHNE (W.), LANE (W. A.), PETRI, SENN (N.), STRASBURGER.

Plateau, Joseph Antoine Ferdinand (b. 1801). Belgian physicist.

Talbot-Plateau law. In periodic light stimuli, the speed of which is rapid enough to produce a sensation of uniform brightness, this resultant impression is the mean of the periodic impression.

plateau (plat·o). 1. An elevated tract of flat country; hence any elevated flat portion of a plotted graph or curve. 2. In psychology, the flattening out of the curve of learning. **Ventricular plateau.** The flattening of the summit of the intraventricular pressure curve during the latter portion of the ejection phase of ventricular systole. [Fr.]

See also: GEIGER, MUELLER (W.).

platelet (plate·let). A blood platelet. **Blood platelet.** A very small cell in the blood, originating from the megakaryocytes in the marrow, and liberating thromboplastin, essential for the clotting of blood, when damaged or shed extravascularly. **Giant platelet.** Large blood platelets with a staining capacity similar to that of normal blood platelets, and found in some cases of chronic myeloid leukaemia, polycythaemia, and very occasionally in thrombocytopenic purpura. [dim. of plate.]

platinic (plat·**in**·ik). 1. Relating to platinum. 2. Denoting a compound of platinum in which the latter is quadrivalent.

platinite (**plat**·in·ite). An alloy with a coefficient of expansion approximately that of glass and employed therefore instead of platinum for the sealing of electrodes into electric lamps and vacuum tubes. It consists of iron (56 per cent) and nickel (44 per cent).

platinode (**plat**·in·ode). Platinum electrode; the platinum pole of an electrolytic apparatus such as that employed in conductivity determinations. [platinum, Gk *hodos* way.]

platinoid (**plat**·in·oid). A German-silver type of alloy used in electrical resistances; it consists of copper (60 per cent), zinc (24 per cent), nickel (14 per cent), and tungsten (2 per cent). [platinum, Gk *eidos* form.]

platinous (**plat**·in·us). 1. Relating to platinum. 2. Denoting a compound of platinum in which the latter is divalent.

platinum (**plat**·in·um). An element of atomic weight 195.09, atomic number 78, and chemical symbol Pt. It is a hard white metal which occurs in alluvial sands and gravels in the Urals, California, Australia and elsewhere. Of high melting point, and chemically resistant, it is used in laboratory ware, in electrical apparatus as electrodes and electrical contacts (same coefficient of expansion as glass), as an industrial catalyst, and in jewellery. It is employed in dentistry, and in surgery where other metals would be corroded by body fluids. **Platinum chloride.** $PtCl_4$, usually in solution as chloroplatinic acid, used as a reagent for alkaloids. [Sp. *plata* silver.]

platode, platoid (**plat**·ode, **plat**·oid). In biology, applied to anything flat or broad, e.g. a worm. [Gk *platys* broad, *eidos* form.]

platonychia (plat·on·**ik**·e·ah). A dystrophy of the nail. **Platonychia acuta abrata.** Round, white, thickened spots on the finger nails, thought to be a manifestation of psoriasis; a very rare condition. [Gk *platys* broad, *onyx* nail.]

Platt, Sir Harry. 20th century British orthopaedic surgeon.

Putti-Platt operation. A reconstructive procedure for the repair of recurrent dislocation of the shoulder, using the tendon of the subscapularis muscle as an anterior ligament.

platybasia (plat·e·**ba**·se·ah). A developmental abnormality of the basi-occiput and upper cervical spine. [Gk *platys* flat, basis.]

plactycephalic, platycephalous (plat·e·kef·**al**′·ik, plat·e·**kef**·al·us). Relating or belonging to platycephaly.

platycephaly (plat·e·**kef**·al·e). Broadness of the skull, the vertical index being less than 70. [Gk *platys* broad, *kephale* head.]

platycnemia (plat·e·**ne**·me·ah). A condition marked by abnormal lateral flatness of the upper end of the tibia. [Gk *platys* flat, *kneme* leg.]

platycnemic (plat·e·**ne**·mik). Relating or belonging to platycnemia.

platycoelous (plat·e·**se**·lus). Describing the body of a vertebra that is flat on one surface and concave on the others; such vertebrae are not found in man. [Gk *platys* flat, *koilos* hollow.]

platycoria (plat·e·**kor**·e·ah). Mydriasis. [Gk *platys* broad, *kore* pupil.]

platycrania (plat·e·**kra**·ne·ah). Platycephaly produced by artificial means. [Gk *platys* broad, *kranion* skull.]

platycyte (**plat**·e·site). An epithelioid cell [obsolete term]. [Gk *platys* broad, *kytos* cell.]

platyglossal (plat·e·**glos**·al). Having a flattened and broad tongue. [Gk *platys* broad, *glossa* tongue.]

platyhelminth (plat·e·**hel**·minth). A member of the phylum Platyhelminthes, a flat worm.

Platyhelminthes (**plat**·e·hel·**min**′·theez). A phylum which includes the classes Trematoda (flukes) and Cestoidea (tapeworms); they are triploblastic acoelomate animals, without blood system and with the gut closed posteriorly. Life cycles of parasitic forms are complex, and usually include secondary hosts. [Gk *platys* flat, *helmins* worm.]

platyhieric (**plat**·e·hi·**er**′·ik). Having a broad sacrum, with a sacral index over 100. [Gk *platys* broad, *hieron* sacrum.]

platymeria (plat·e·**me**·re·ah). A condition marked by lateral compression of the femur; unusual broadness of the femur. [Gk *platys* broad, *meros* part.]

platymeric (plat·e·**me**·rik). Relating or belonging to platymeria.

platymorphia (plat·e·**mor**·fe·ah). A flattening of the structure of the eyeballs so that the anteroposterior diameter is short, with the result that hypermetropia is developed. [Gk *platys* flat, *morphe* shape.]

platymorphic (plat·e·**mor**·fik). Relating or belonging to platymorphia; shallow-eyed.

platyonychia (**plat**·e·on·**ik**′·e·ah). Excessive flatness of the nails. [Gk *platys* flat, *onyx* nail.]

platyopia (plat·e·**o**·pe·ah). Broadness of the face, with the nasomalar index below 107.5. [Gk *platys* broad, *ops* face.]

platyopic (plat·e·**o**·pik). 1. Relating or belonging to platyopia. 2. Applied to a face of abnormally great breadth.

platypellic, platypelloid (plat·e·**pel**·ik, plat·e·**pel**·oid). Applied to a pelvis, which has an index of less than 90. [Gk *platys* wide, *pella* bowl, *eidos* form.]

platypodia (plat·e·**po**·de·ah). Flat foot. [Gk *platys* flat, *pous* foot.]

platyrhine (**plat**·e·rine). Having a short broad nose. Applied to a skull the nasal index of which is more than 53. [Gk *platys* broad, *rhis* nose.]

platyrhiny (plat·e·**ri**·ne). The condition of having a nose broad in proportion to its height or length. [see prec.]

platysma [NA] (plat·**iz**·mah). A thin sheet of muscle in the superficial fascia of the neck. It is attached below to the skin over the upper two intercostal spaces; above it blends with the superficial muscles around the mouth, and has some attachment to the lower border of the mandible. [Gk *platys* flat.]

platysmal (plat·**iz**·mal). Relating or belonging to the platysma.

platyspondylia, platyspondylisis (**plat**·e·spon·**dil**′·e·ah, **plat**·e·spon·**dil**′·is·is). A congenital condition characterized by flattening of the bodies of the vertebra. [Gk *platys* flat, *spondylos* vertebra.]

platystaphyline (plat·e·**staf**·il·ine). Denoting a palate which is flat and broad. [Gk *platys* broad, *staphyle* palate.]

platystencephalia (**plat**·is·ten·kef·**a**′·le·ah). The state of having a skull that is wide at the back, associated with prognathism. [Gk *platystos* broadest, *egkephalon* brain.]

platystencephalic (**plat**·is·ten·kef·**al**′·ik). Relating or belonging to platystencephalia.

platytrope (**plat**·e·trope). Concerning the body, either of two lateral homologues. [Gk *platys* broad, *trope* turn.]

Plaut, Hugo Karl (b. 1858). Leipzig physician.

Plaut's angina, or ulcer. Vincent's angina.

Playfair, William Smoult (b. 1836). London physician.

Playfair's treatment. A treatment by systematic rest and feeding.

Plecoglossus altivelis (ple·ko·glos·us al·te·ve·lis). A fish that acts as an intermediary host of *Metagonimus yokogawai*. [Gk *plekein* to weave, *glossa* tongue, L *altus* high, *velum* covering.]

Plectranthus (plek·tran·thus). A genus of tropical herbs (family Labiatae); several species are used in African native medicine. **Plectranthus secundus.** A species used in India. [Gk *plektron* hammer, *anthos* flower.]

Plectridium (plek·trid·e·um). A generic term for certain species of the genus *Clostridium* proposed by Fischer in 1895 [obsolete term]. [Gk *plektron* hammer.]

plectrum (plek·trum). 1. The uvula. 2. The malleus bone of the ear. 3. The styloid process of the temporal bone. [Gk *plektron* hammer.]

pledget (plej·et). A small piece of cotton wool, used chiefly as a swab for mopping up exudates, effusions or discharge from wounds. [etym. dub.]

plegaphonia (ple·jaf·o·ne·ah). A substitute method of auscultation in cases in which the patient cannot or is not allowed to speak. By percussion over the larynx or trachea, vibrations are produced similar to those normally set up in the larynx by speech. [Gk *plege* stroke, *a*, *phone* voice.]

Plehn, Albert (b. 1861). Berlin physician.

Plehn's granules. Basophil granules in the gametocytes of malaria parasites.

pleiades (pli·ah·deez). A group of hypertrophied or swollen lymph glands. [*Pleiades*, cluster of small stars in the constellation Taurus.]

pleiochromia (pli·o·kro·me·ah). 1. Generally, an increase in pigment. 2. Particularly, an increase in the secretion of bile pigment so that the bile is of a deeper tint than normally. [Gk *pleion* more, *chroma* colour.]

pleiotropia (pli·o·tro·pe·ah). In genetics, the appearance of two or more characters which are controlled by a single gene; if one such character is present and controlled by such a gene the others will also be present. [Gk *pleion* more, *trepein* to turn.]

pleniloquence (plen·il·o·kwens). Excessive talkativeness. [L *plenus* full, *loqui* to speak.]

pleocholia (ple·o·ko·le·ah). Excessive flow of bile. [Gk *pleon* more, *chole* bile.]

pleochroic (ple·o·kro·ik). Exhibiting the phenomenon of pleochroism; relating to pleochroism. **Pleochroic halo.** The concentric coloured rings round a speck of radioactive material in a mineral; they are due to α-rays and afford evidence of the age of the mineral. [Gk *pleon* more, *chroa* colour.]

pleochroism (ple·o·kro·izm). General term for the phenomenon displayed by certain crystals which affect light differently in different directions, and consequently vary in colour according to the axis along which they are viewed. Di- and tri-chroism are particular cases, being variations along two and three axes respectively. The term is sometimes applied erroneously to fluorescence. [see prec.]

pleochromatic (ple·o·kro·mat'·ik). Pleochroic. [see foll.]

pleochromatism (ple·o·kro·mat·izm). Pleochroism. [Gk *pleon* more, *chroma* colour.]

pleochromocytoma (ple·o·kro·mo·si·to'·mah). A tumour made up of cells of different colours. [Gk *pleon* more, *chroma* colour, cytoma.]

pleocytosis (ple·o·si·to'·sis). The condition in which, as in some diseases of the central nervous system, there is an increase in leucocytes in the cerebrospinal fluid. [Gk *pleon* more, *kytos* cell, *-osis* condition.]

pleodermatitis (ple·o·der·mat·i'·tis). Eruptions with a wide range of morphological variation on different individuals but having the same drug cause. [Gk *pleon* more, *derma* skin, *-itis* inflammation.]

pleomastia (ple·o·mas·te·ah). A condition characterized by the presence of three or more mammary glands or nipples. [Gk *pleon* more, *mastos* breast.]

pleomastic (ple·o·mas·tik). Relating to, or marked by pleomastia.

pleomorphic (ple·o·mor·fik). Relating to or characterized by pleomorphism.

pleomorphism (ple·o·mor·fizm). 1. Occurrence in more than one form. 2. The existence of several distinct types in the same species or group; polymorphism. 3. The capacity of some crystals to crystallize in two or more crystal forms. [Gk *pleon* more, *morphe* form.]

pleomorphous (ple·o·mor·fus). Pleomorphic.

pleonasm (ple·on·azm). A condition characterized by the presence of supernumerary parts or organs. [Gk *pleonazein* to be more than enough.]

pleonectic (ple·on·ek·tik). 1. Characterized by or relating to pleonexia. 2. Denoting blood which has an abnormally great saturation of oxygen, i.e. more than 79 per cent. [see foll.]

pleonexia, pleonexy (ple·on·ex·e·ah, ple·on·ex·e). 1. A psychotic condition in which there is abnormal desire for possession or acquisition; morbid greed. 2. A pathological state of the blood in which the haemoglobin in the circulation retains more than the normal amount of oxygen and so gives up to the tissues a smaller quantity of oxygen than in normal circumstances. [Gk *pleonexia* greediness.]

pleonosteosis (ple·on·os·te·o'sis). A condition distinguished by an excessive degree of ossification, abnormally increased and premature ossification. [Gk *pleon* more, *osteon* bone, *-osis* condition.]

pleoptics (ple·op·tix). An orthoptic technique in which central vision is not attempted. [Gk *pleon* more, *ops* eye.]

plerocercoid (ple·ro·ser·koid). A solid vermiform larva of tapeworms of the order Pseudophyllidea, the scolex of which is invaginated. They develop in the secondary hosts where they are known by the pseudogeneric name of *Sparganum*. Species of *Diphyllobothrium* have plerocercoid larvae. [Gk *pleroun* to complete, *kerkos* tail, *eidos* form.]

plerosis (pler·o·sis). 1. The replacement of tissue which has been lost during a spell of ill-health. 2. Plethora. [Gk, a filling up.]

Plesch, Johann (b. 1878). Berlin physician.

Plesch's test. The blood in the pulmonary arteries in cases of patent ductus arteriosus contains more oxygen than that in the right ventricle, owing to passage of oxygenated blood from the aorta via the ductus. This increase in pulmonary-artery oxygen saturation can be detected by obtaining blood samples from the pulmonary artery and right side of the heart with the cardiac catheter, and analysing their oxygen content.

plesiomorphism (ple·ze·o·mor'·fizm). Resemblance in shape. [Gk *plesios* near, *morphe* form.]

plesiopia (ple·ze·o·pe·ah). A condition of myopia caused by long-standing strain on the accommodation in which the convexity of the lens is increased. [Gk *plesios* near, *ops* eye.]

plessaesthesia (ples·es·the'·ze·ah). A form of palpatory percussion [obsolete term]. [Gk *plessein* to strike, *aisthesis* sensation.]

plessigraph (ples·e·graf). A type of pleximeter constructed to indicate any minute differences in the nature of the sounds produced on percussion; there is a pencil holder on the stem and a coloured crayon with which the surface anatomy may be traced, or areas delineated. [Gk *plessein* to strike, *graphein* to record.]

plessimeter (ples·im·e·ter). Pleximeter. [Gk *plessein* to strike, *metron* measure.]

plessor (ples·or). A small hammer with a rubber tip, used in percussion of the chest or for testing tendon reflexes; plexor. [Gk *plessein* to strike.]

plethora (pleth·or·ah, ple·thor·ah). A name formerly given to a supposed condition due to an excessive volume of blood. A so-called plethoric person was red-faced and of full-blooded appearance; we now know that is is due to dilatation of superficial blood vessels and not to an increase in the blood volume. It is doubtful whether an increase in the volume of blood ever occurs without alteration in its composition. Temporary increase may occur after excessive water drinking, in some anaemias, congestive cardiac failure and uraemia. In polycythaemia vera the increased volume is due to the excessive number of red corpuscles without increase of the plasma. [Gk *plethore* fullness.]

plethysmogram (pleth·**iz**·mo·gram). The tracing made by the plethysmograph. [Gk *plethynein* to increase, *gramma* a writing.]

plethysmograph (pleth·**iz**·mo·graf). An apparatus used to determine and register the alterations in size of an organ or limb. **Finger plethysmograph.** One which records the variation in the volume of blood in one finger. **Impedance plethysmograph.** A device which observes the change in volume by measuring the concurrent changes of electrical impedance. [see foll.]

See also: FRANCK, MOSSO.

plethysmography (pleth·iz·**mog**·raf·e). A method of assessing changes in the volume of organs, mainly used for measuring blood flow in limbs or digits. **Venous-occlusion plethysmography.** The method in which the limb to be tested is inserted and sealed into a rigid box containing air or water: a cuff is placed round the limb proximal to the box and suddenly inflated to a pressure below diastolic but above venous pressure. This traps arterial blood in the tissue within the box, causing an increase in volume, which in turn produces an increase of pressure in the box that is recorded by a sensitive device, thus measuring the amount and rate of increase in volume resulting from the arterial inflow. [Gk *plethynein* to increase, *graphein* to record.]

plethysmometer (pleth·iz·**mom**·et·er). An apparatus used in measurement of the degree of swelling of a blood vessel. [Gk *plethynein* to increase, *metron* measure.]

plethysmometry (pleth·iz·**mom**·et·re). Estimation of the swelling of a blood vessel by means of the plethysmometer.

pleura [NA] (ploor·ah). The serous membrane which covers the lungs, *pulmonary (visceral) pleura* [pleura pulmonalis (NA)], and the inner aspect of the thoracic cavity, *parietal pleura* [pleura parietalis], on each side of the thoracic cavity. The mediastinal space containing the heart, pericardium, great vessels and oesophagus lies between the right and left pleura. The visceral and parietal layers are continuous round the root of the lung and in the pulmonary ligament; elsewhere, while the two layers are normally in contact, there is a potential space between them, the cavity of the pleura, which becomes actual when filled with effusion, air, etc., such a condition being accompanied of necessity by a greater or lesser degree of collapse of the lung. **Cervical pleura [cupula pleurae (NA)].** The part of the parietal pleura ascending into the neck above the apex of the lung. **Costal pleura [pleura costalis (NA)].** The part of the parietal pleura lining the chest wall. **Diaphragmatic pleura [pleura diaphragmatica (NA)].** The part of the parietal pleura clothing the upper surface of the diaphragm. **Mediastinal pleura [pleura mediastinalis (NA)].** The part of the parietal pleura forming the surface layer of the mediastinum. That part of it covering the fibrous pericardium is called the *pericardial pleura.* **Parietal pleura.** *See* MAIN DEF. (above). **Pericardial pleura.** *See* MEDIASTINAL PLEURA (above). **Pulmonary pleura.** *See* MAIN DEF. (above). **Visceral pleura.** *See* MAIN DEF. (above). [Gk, rib.]

pleuracentesis (**ploor**·ah·sen·**te**′·sis). Pleurocentesis.

pleuracotomy (ploor·ah·**kot**·o·me). The act of making an incision through the chest wall and inserting a drainage tube into the pleura. [pleura, Gk *temnein* to cut.]

pleuragraphy (ploor·**ag**·raf·e). Pleurography.

pleural (ploor·al). Relating or belonging to the pleura.

pleuralgia (ploor·**al**·je·ah). Pain affecting the pleura or the region of the ribs. [Gk *pleura* rib, *algos* pain.]

pleuralgic (ploor·**al**·jik). Relating or belonging to, or suffering from pleuralgia.

pleurapophyseal (ploor·ap·of·iz·**e**′·al). Relating to a pleurapophysis.

pleurapophysis (ploor·ap·**of**·is·is). A rib or the structure that takes its place in the cervical or lumbar region of the vertebral column, e.g. the lateral process of a vertebra. [Gk *pleura* rib, apophysis.]

pleurarthrocace (ploor·ar·**throk**·as·e). 1. Any morbid condition affecting the costovertebral joints. 2. Costal caries. [Gk *pleura* rib, arthrocace.]

pleurectomy (ploor·**ek**·to·me). Surgical excision of pleura, e.g. one thickened and stiffened from chronic empyema. [pleura, Gk *ektome* excision.]

pleurisy (ploor·is·e). Inflammation of the pleura; this may be due to mechanical or chemical irritation, but most usually to infection secondary to disease of the lung or chest wall. So-called *idiopathic* or *primary pleurisy* is in reality secondary to an unrecognized lesion in the lung. The initial change is hyperaemia, with serous exudation into the subpleural tissues and on the pleural surface, followed by deposition of fibrin. The lesion may then completely resolve or lead to pleural adhesions and thickening. Often the fluid exudate increases and may go on to a considerable effusion with collapse of the lung, while if pyogenic organisms are responsible the fluid becomes purulent and an empyema forms. **Acute dry pleurisy.** Pleurisy without recognizable effusion. A localized pleurisy may be due to trauma, but is usually secondary to disease of the lung such as bronchiectasis, abscess, infarction or neoplasm, and especially pneumonia; tuberculosis is a common cause and a dry pleurisy may be the first sign of a tuberculous lesion of the lung. **Basal pleurisy.** Pleurisy at the base of the lung. **Cholesterol pleurisy.** Pleurisy in which the milky appearance of the effusion is due to the presence of cholesterol crystals. **Chronic dry pleurisy.** A sequel to an acute dry pleurisy in which organization of the fibrinous exudate has led to adhesions between the two layers of the pleura. **Chylous pleurisy.** Pleurisy in which the fluid is milky in appearance from emulsified fat. It may be present with tuberculosis or carcinoma of the pleura. **Diaphragmatic pleurisy.** Inflammation of the pleural covering of the diaphragm, revealed by very severe pain in the epigastric and hypochondrial regions of the abdomen and by referred pain via the phrenic nerve to the shoulder; pleural friction is not usually heard. **Pleurisy with effusion.** Pleurisy in which the inflammation has proceeded to effusion. The fluid has a high specific gravity (1018 to 1020) and, owing to the large amount of fibrin, clots on standing. Usually the cytology shows a preponderance of lymphocytes. The majority of cases are due to tuberculosis; they may occur during the secondary or allergic stage of pulmonary tuberculosis before the lung lesion has been recognized, or at later stages with obvious disease. A serofibrinous effusion may be present in the early stage of a pleurisy which later becomes purulent, as with pneumonia. **Encapsulated pleurisy.** A localized collection of pleural exudate shut off by adhesions. **Fibrinous pleurisy.** Acute dry pleurisy (see above). **Foetid pleurisy.** A suppurative pleurisy in which the pus has a foetid odour due to the presence of *Escherichia coli* or anaerobic organisms. **Plastic pleurisy.** Acute dry pleurisy (see above). **Pulsating pleurisy.** A pulsating swelling on the chest wall, usually near the nipple, due to pus tracking from the pleural space between the ribs into the subcutaneous tissues where it forms a localized abscess; when on the left side pulsations are transmitted from the heart and the swelling simulates an aneurysm. **Purulent pleurisy.** Empyema, a condition most commonly secondary to inflammation of the lung, especially to pneumonia and bronchopneumonia; in other cases bronchiectasis, abscess or gangrene of the lung, phthisis, osteomyelitis of a rib, or a subdiaphragmatic abscess may be the cause. The epyema may be localized and encysted by adhesions cutting off the rest of the pleural cavity; this is usually between the lung and the chest wall but may be interlobar or between the lung and the diaphragm or mediastinum. The encysted empyema is characteristic of a pneumococcal infection and is a sequel to lobar pneumonia; the pus is thick and yellowish. A total empyema is not confined by adhesions but occupies the whole pleural space; it is found with streptococcal infection and usually accompanies a bronchopneumonia of varying origin. The pus is thin and greenish. **Serofibrinous pleurisy.** Pleurisy with effusion (see above). **Pleurisy sicca.** Acute dry pleurisy (see above). **Suppurative pleurisy.** Purulent pleurisy (see above). [Gk *pleuritis.*]

pleuritic (ploor·**it**·ik). 1. Relating or belonging to, or suffering from pleurisy. 2. A person suffering from pleurisy.

pleuritis (ploor·i·tis). Pleurisy. [Gk.]
pleuritogenous (ploor·e·**toj**·en·us). Producing pleurisy. [pleurisy, Gk *genein* to produce.]
pleurobronchitis (**ploor**·o·brong·**ki**'·tis). Pleurisy and bronchitis occurring simultaneously.
pleurocele (**ploor**·o·seel). 1. Herniation of the lung or pleura; pneumocele. 2. The presence of serous fluid in the cavity of the pleura. [pleura, Gk *kele* hernia.]
pleurocentesis (**ploor**·o·sen·**te**'·sis). The operation of puncturing the chest so as to tap the cavity of the pleura. [pleura, Gk *kentein* to prick.]
pleurocentral (ploor·o·**sen**·tral). Relating to a pleurocentrum.
pleurocentrum (ploor·o·**sen**·trum). The lateral half of a vertebral centrum. [Gk *pleura* rib, centrum.]
pleurocholecystitis (**ploor**·o·ko·le·sist·**i**'·tis). Inflammation affecting the pleura and gall bladder simultaneously. [pleura, cholecystitis.]
pleuroclysis (ploor·**ok**·lis·is). Washing out of the cavity of the pleura by injection of a fluid. [pleura, Gk *klysis* a washing out.]
pleurocollesis (**ploor**·o·kol·**e**'·sis). Adhesion of the visceral to the parietal pleura. [pleura, Gk *kollesis* a gluing.]
pleurocutaneous (**ploor**·o·kew·**ta**'·ne·us). Relating to the pleura and the skin. [pleura, L *cutis* skin.]
pleurodynia (ploor·o·**din**·e·ah). Rheumatic inflammation of the intercostal muscles of one side, usually attended by severe pain and tenderness. **Epidemic pleurodynia, Epidemic diaphragmatic pleurodynia.** An epidemic virus disease affecting the intercostal muscles on one or both sides of the chest, characterized by acute pain and a short febrile period, with the possibility of recurrence of the symptoms. Bornholm disease. [Gk *pleura* rib, *odyne* pain.]
pleurogenic, pleurogenous (ploor·o·**jen**·ik, ploor·**oj**·en·us). Of pleural origin. [pleura, Gk *genein* to produce.]
pleurogram (**ploor**·o·gram). A radiograph of the cavity of the pleura into which has been injected a contrast medium, usually a radio-opaque oil. [pleura, Gk *gramma* record.]
pleurography (ploor·**og**·raf·e). Radiographical examination of the cavity of the pleura. [pleura, Gk *graphein* to record.]
pleurohepatitis (**ploor**·o·hep·at·**i**'·tis). Hepatitis with associated inflammation of the pleura in the neighbourhood. [pleura, Gk *hepar* liver, *-itis* inflammation.]
pleurolith (**ploor**·o·lith). A calculus existing in the pleura. [pleura, Gk *lithos* stone.]
pleurolysis (ploor·**ol**·is·is). Pneumolysis; the operation of separating the lung and parietal pleura from the endothoracic fascia for the purpose of collapsing the lung. [pleura, Gk *lysis* a loosing.]
pleuro-oesophageal muscle [musculus pleuro-esophageus (NA)] (**ploor**·o·e·sof·ah·**je**'·al musl). Slips of the muscle coat of the oesophagus which pass to the left pleura.
pleuroparietopexy (**ploor**·o·par·**i**'·et·o·pex·e). The operation of suturing the pulmonary pleura to the parietal pleura, so fixing the lung to the wall of the thorax. [pleura, L *paries* wall, Gk *pexis* fixation.]
pleuropericardial (**ploor**·o·per·e·**kar**'·de·al). Relating to the pleura and the pericardium.
pleuropericarditis (**ploor**·o·per·e·kar·**di**'·tis). Inflammation of the pleura and pericardium occurring simultaneously. [pleura, pericardium, Gk *-itis* inflammation.]
pleuroperitoneal (**ploor**·o·per·it·on·**e**'·al). Belonging to the pleura and the peritoneum.
pleuroperitoneum (**ploor**·o·per·it·on·**e**'·um). The pleura and peritoneum regarded as one membrane.
pleuroperitonitis (**ploor**·o·per·it·on·**i**'·tis). Inflammation of the pleura and peritoneum occurring simultaneously. [pleura, peritoneum, Gk *-itis* inflammation.]
pleurophorous (ploor·**of**·or·us). Provided with a membrane. [Gk *pleura* side, *pherein* to bear.]
pleuropneumonia (**ploor**·o·new·**mo**'·ne·ah). Acute lobar pneumonia. *See* PNEUMONIA. [pleurisy, pneumonia.]
pleuropneumonolysis (**ploor**·o·new·mon·**ol**'·is·is). An obsolete term for thoracoplasty. [pleura, Gk *pneumon* lung, *lysis* a loosing.]
pleuropulmonary (ploor·o·**pul**·mon·ar·e). Relating to the pleura and the lungs. [pleura, L *pulmo* lung.]
pleuropyesis (**ploor**·o·pi·**e**'·sis). Pleurisy with septic type of effusion; empyema. [pleura, Gk *pyein* to suppurate.]
pleurorrhagia (ploor·o·**ra**·je·ah). Pleural haemorrhage. [pleura, Gk *rhegnynein* to gush forth.]
pleuroscopy (ploor·**os**·ko·pe). Examination of the cavity of the pleura through an incision in the wall of the thorax. [pleura, Gk *skopein* to watch.]
pleurosoma, pleurosomus (ploor·o·**so**·mah, ploor·o·**so**·mus). A monster with eventration in the upper abdominal and thoracic areas, associated with under-development of the arm on the side of the intestinal protrusion. [Gk *pleura* rib, *soma* body.]
pleurospasm (**ploor**·o·spazm). Muscular cramp generally affecting the lateral thoracic region. [Gk *pleura* rib, spasm.]
pleurothoracopleurectomy (**ploor**·o·thor·ak·o·ploor·**ek**'·to·me). Surgical excision of parietal pleura and ribs to permit the soft tissues of the chest wall to sink in and obliterate a chronic empyema cavity. [pleura, thorax, pleurectomy.]
pleurothotonos, pleurothotonus (ploor·o·**thot**·on·os, ploor·o·**thot**·on·us). Tetanus in which the body is bent laterally in spasm. [Gk *pleurothen* from the side, *tonos* tension.]
pleurotin (ploor·**o**·tin). $C_{20}H_{22}O_5$, an antibiotic prepared from culture filtrates from *Pleurotus griseus.*
pleurotome (**ploor**·o·tome). A guarded knife for incising the outer layer of the pleural membrane. [pleura, Gk *temnein* to cut.]
pleurotomy (ploor·**ot**·o·me). The operation of incising the pleura, and gaining entrance to the cavity of the pleura, so as to allow effusions to escape. [see prec.]
Pleurotus griseus (ploo·**ro**·tus **griz**·e·us). A species of Basidiomycetes which produces the antibiotic, pleurotin.
pleurovisceral (ploor·o·**vis**·er·al). Referring to the visceral pleura.
plexal (plex·al). Relating to or characterized by a plexus.
plexalgia (plex·**al**·je·ah). A condition characterized by insomnia, general fatigue, pains in several parts of the body and excitability noted in troops who have undergone prolonged exposure to wet and cold. [Gk *plessein* to strike, *algos* pain.]
plexiform (**plex**·e·form). Like or forming a plexus. [plexus, form.]
pleximeter (plex·**im**·et·er). 1. A flat disc of ivory or bone placed in contact with the chest; on this disc the examiner strikes his finger in mediate percussion. 2. A glass disc which when applied to the surface of the skin indicates the state of the skin when subjected to pressure. [Gk *plessein* to strike, *metron* measure.]
pleximetric (plex·e·**met**·rik). Relating to a pleximeter; referring to mediate percussion.
pleximetry (plex·**im**·et·re). The employment of the pleximeter in diagnosis.
plexitis (plex·**i**·tis). Inflammation involving a nerve plexus. [plexus, Gk *-itis* inflammation.]
plexometer (plex·**om**·et·er). Pleximeter.
plexor (**plex**·or). A small hammer with a rubber-tipped head, used in percussion of the chest and for testing for deep reflexes. [Gk *plessein* to strike.]
plexus [NA] (**plex**·us). An interwoven network of blood vessels, nerves or lymphatics. **Aortic plexus, abdominal [plexus aorticus abdominalis (NA)].** A plexus of sympathetic nerve fibres around, but mainly in front of, the abdominal aorta. It receives branches from the lumbar part of the sympathetic trunk and communicates with the coeliac plexus. **Aortic plexus, thoracic [plexus aorticus thoracicus (NA)].** A fine sympathetic nerve plexus along the thoracic aorta and its branches. It receives its fibres from the upper ganglia on the thoracic part of the sympathetic trunk. **Areolar (venous) plexus [plexus venosus areolaris (NA)].** The venous plexus deep to the areola of the mammary gland. It is drained into the lateral thoracic and adjacent tributaries of the intercostal veins. **Brachial plexus [plexus brachialis (NA)].** A plexus situated in the posterior triangle of the neck (supraclavicular part [pars supraclavicularis (NA)]), and in the axilla (infraclavicular part [pars infraclavicularis (NA)]), formed from the anterior primary rami of the lower four cervical and the upper two thoracic spinal nerves. Its branches supply the

muscles and skin of the upper limb. The three trunks [trunci plexus brachialis (NA)] emerge at the lateral border of the scalenus anterior muscle. The upper trunk [truncus superior (NA)] is formed by the anterior primary rami of the 5th and 6th cervical nerves, the middle [truncus medius (NA)] by that of the 7th cervical nerve, and the lower [truncus inferior (NA)] by the union of the anterior primary rami of the 8th cervical and 1st thoracic nerves. **Cardiac plexus [plexus cardiacus** (NA)]. A large autonomic nerve plexus placed partly behind the bifurcation of the pulmonary artery (deep part), and partly in front of the right pulmonary artery (superficial part). **Carotid plexus, common [plexus caroticus communis** (NA)]. The plexus of sympathetic fibres around the common carotid artery; it consists of postganglionic fibres which descend from the superior cervical ganglion. **Carotid plexus, external [plexus caroticus externus** (NA)]. Branches, mostly postganglionic, from the superior cervical ganglion which twine around the external carotid artery and its branches. They supply the skin and blood vessels of the face and scalp, the submaxillary (submandibular) gland and the carotid sinus. **Carotid plexus, internal [plexus caroticus internus** (NA)]. A plexus of sympathetic fibres around the internal carotid artery, consisting mostly of postganglionic fibres with cells of origin in the superior cervical ganglion. The plexus is disposed in two main parts, internal and external, along corresponding sides of the artery. Besides furnishing filaments to several cranial nerves, the plexus supplies the deep petrosal nerve to the sphenopalatine ganglion and the sympathetic root to the ciliary ganglion. **Cavernous plexus of the conchae [plexus cavernosi concharum** (NA)]. A plexus of submucous veins, especially thick over the lower part of the septum and the lower two conchae; it also contains the arteriovenous anastomosis. **Cavernous plexus of the penis (or of the clitoris).** An autonomic nerve plexus in the cavernous tissue of the penis or clitoris. **Cervical plexus [plexus cervicalis** (NA)]. A plexus in the neck, formed from the anterior primary rami of the upper four cervical nerves. Its branches supply the muscles and skin of the neck and also the diaphragm. The cutaneous branches all emerge at the posterior border of the sternocleidomastoid muscle. **Choroid plexus of the fourth ventricle [plexus choroideus ventriculi quarti** (NA)]. Two vascular invaginations of the lower part of the roof of the 4th ventricle. The lateral portion of each passes out of the lateral aperture of the ventricle immediately above the glossopharyngeal nerve. **Choroid plexus of the lateral ventricle [plexus choroideus ventriculi lateralis** (NA)]. A vascular fringe of pia mater, covered by ependyma, projecting into the choroidal fissure of each cerebral hemisphere and lying within the body (central part) of the lateral ventricle, the collateral trigone and the inferior horn. It is supplied by the anterior and posterior choroid arteries and drains into the internal cerebral vein. **Choroid plexus of the third ventricle [plexus choroideus ventriculi tertii** (NA)]. A paired vascular fold of pia mater, covered by ependyma, projecting into the roof of the 3rd ventricle. **Ciliary ganglionic plexus.** A plexus derived from the long and short ciliary nerves and situated around the iris. It supplies the dilator and sphincter muscles of the pupil. **Coccygeal plexus [plexus coccygeus** (NA)]. A small trunk formed by branches of the 4th and 5th lumbar nerves and the coccygeal nerve. It supplies the skin in the region of the coccyx. **Coeliac plexus [plexus celiacus** (NA)]. A large sympathetic plexus around the origin of the coeliac artery, receiving the greater and lesser splanchnic nerves and some twigs from the vagus nerve, and giving off twigs along the branches of the coeliac and superior mesenteric, renal and suprarenal arteries. **Dental plexus, inferior [plexus dentalis inferior** (NA)]. A plexus formed by communications between the dental branches of the inferior dental nerve. The alveolar part supplies the molars and premolars and the incisor part supplies the incisors. The canines may be supplied from either part. **Dental plexus, superior [plexus dentalis superior** (NA)]. Communications between the anterior, middle and posterior superior dental nerves just superior to the teeth of the maxilla. They give branches to the teeth and gums [rami dentales superiores, rami gingivales superiores (NA)]. **Enteric plexus [plexus entericus].** The autonomic plexus in the wall of the gut. **Femoral plexus [plexus femoralis** (NA)]. The plexus of sympathetic fibres around the femoral artery. **Gastric plexus.** A nerve plexus derived from the gastric branches of the vagus nerve to the anterior and posterior surfaces of the stomach. **Gastric plexus, left [plexus gastricus** (NA)]. An extension of the coeliac plexus along the left gastric artery and its branches. It receives accessions from the vagus nerve and sends fibres to the pyloric sphincter. **Haemorrhoidal plexus.** Rectal (venous) plexus (see below). **Hepatic plexus [plexus hepaticus** (NA)]. An extension of the coeliac plexus along the hepatic artery and its branches. It receives accessions from the vagus and phrenic nerves. **Hypogastric plexus [plexus hypogastricus superior (nervus presacralis)** NA]. A plexus of nerve fibres which descends into the pelvis in front of the termination of the aorta and the commencement of the common iliac vessels. Its fibres join the aortic plexus and lower lumbar ganglia with the pelvic plexuses. **Iliac plexus [plexus iliacus** (NA)]. The sympathetic plexus around the iliac arteries. **Intermesenteric plexus [plexus intermesentericus** (NA)]. The plexus which unites the coeliac and superior mesenteric plexuses. **Laryngeal plexus.** An extension of the pharyngeal plexus onto the inferior constrictor muscle. It receives trunk fibres from the sympathetic and the external laryngeal nerve. **Lumbar plexus [plexus lumbalis** (NA)]. A nerve plexus formed by the anterior primary rami of the upper four lumbar nerves; it lies in the psoas major muscle. **Lumbosacral plexus [plexus lumbosacralis** (NA)]. An inclusive name for the combined lumbar and sacral plexus. **Lymphatic plexus [plexus lymphaticus** (NA)]. Any plexus of lymphatic vessels. **Mesenteric plexus, inferior [plexus mesentericus inferior** (NA)]. The plexus of autonomic nerve fibres around the inferior mesenteric artery and its branches. It is an extension of the aortic plexus. **Mesenteric plexus, superior [plexus mesentericus superior** (NA)]. An autonomic nerve plexus along the superior mesenteric artery and its branches. It receives fibres from the coeliac plexus and the vagus nerve. **Myenteric plexus [plexus myentericus** (NA)]. A plexus of autonomic nerve fibres interspersed with ganglion cells, situated in the muscular coat of the gut; Auerbach's plexus. **Oesophageal plexus [plexus esophageus** (NA)]. A nerve plexus between the muscle layers and in the submucous coat of the oesophagus, derived from the branches of the vagus and sympathetic nerves and supplying the mucous membrane and muscle of the oesophagus. **Ovarian plexus [plexus ovaricus** (NA)]. An autonomic nerve plexus along the ovarian artery. It receives twigs from the renal and aortic plexuses and extends to the ovary. **Pampiniform plexus [plexus pampiniformis** (NA)]. A plexus of veins in the spermatic cord, draining the testes and terminating in the lower abdomen in the testicular vein. **Pancreatic plexus [plexus pancreaticus** (NA)]. Extensions of the coeliac plexus along the arteries to the pancreas. **Parotid plexus [plexus parotideus** (NA)]. A plexus formed by the facial nerve in the parotid gland. **Pelvic plexus [plexus hypogastricus inferior (plexus pelvinus** NA)]. An autonomic nerve plexus, interspersed with ganglia, on both sides of the posterior part of the pelvic splanchnic nerves and distributed to the pelvic viscera. **Periarterial plexus [plexus periarterialis** (NA)]. The plexus of nerve fibres in the adventitial coat of arteries, consisting mainly but not exclusively of non-medullated postganglionic sympathetic fibres. **Pharyngeal plexus [plexus pharyngeus** (NA)]. A plexus of nerves in the wall of the pharynx formed by branches of the glossopharyngeal, vagus and sympathetic nerves, and supplying motor fibres to the muscles of the soft palate, also sensory fibres to the mucous membrane of the pharynx. **Pharyngeal (venous) plexus [plexus pharyngeus** (NA)]. The plexus of veins on the surface of the pharynx draining into the pterygoid plexus and thence into the internal jugular and common facial veins. **Prostatic plexus [plexus prostaticus** (NA)]. An autonomic nerve plexus alongside the prostate; it is a continuation of the pelvic plexus to supply the prostate, seminal vesicles, and erectile tissue of the penis. **Prostatic (venous) plexus [plexus venosus prostaticus** (NA)]. A plexus partly within and partly around the fascial capsule of the prostate. It communicates with the vesical plexus, and drains into the internal iliac veins. **Pterygoid (venous) plexus [plexus pterygoideus (NA)].** A large venous plexus in the pterygoid region, receiving veins from the nose, palate, jaws, cavernous sinus of the dura mater and orbit. It is drained by the maxillary vein into the posterior facial vein. **Pulmonary plexus [plexus pulmonalis (NA)].** 1. A plexus formed mainly from branches of the vagus and sympathetic nerves, placed in front and behind the roots of the lungs respectively, and supplying motor fibres to the muscles, with sensory fibres to the mucous membrane of the bronchi. 2. Fibres of the vagus nerve conveying parasympathetic fibres to the pulmonary plexus (see prec.). **Rectal plexus, inferior [plexus rectalis inferior (NA)].** The lowermost part of the plexus of autonomic nerves around the rectum and the upper part of the anal canal. **Rectal plexus, middle [plexus rectalis medius (NA)].** An extension of the pelvic plexus around the wall of the rectum. Its branches join those of the superior rectal plexus. **Rectal plexus, superior [plexus rectalis superior (NA)].** The extension of the inferior mesenteric plexus around the superior rectal artery and rectum. It receives accessions from the pelvic splanchnic nerves and supplies the wall of the rectum. **Rectal (venous) plexus [plexus venosus rectalis (hemorrhoidalis) (NA)].** The plexus of veins surrounding the rectum. **Renal plexus [plexus renalis (NA)].** A plexus along the renal artery. It receives branches from the coeliac plexus, aorticorenal ganglion, aortic plexus, the lowest splanchnic nerve and the vagus. It accompanies the arteries to the kidney and also sends filaments to the testicular plexus and ureter. **Sacral plexus [plexus sacralis (NA)].** The plexus formed by the lumbosacral trunk and the anterior primary rami of the 1st, 2nd, 3rd, and part of the 4th, sacral nerves. It lies on the posterior wall of the pelvis and supplies the buttock, back of the thigh and leg, sole of the foot and perineum, and gives branches to the pelvic viscera. **Sacral (venous) plexus, anterior [plexus venosus sacralis (NA)].** A plexus in front of the sacrum, draining the internal iliac veins. **Solar plexus.** Coeliac plexus (see above). **Spinal nerve plexuses [plexus nervorum spinalium (NA)].** Any of the plexuses of spinal nerves, e.g. the cervical, brachial, lumbar or sacral. **Splenic plexus [plexus lienalis (NA)].** An extension of the coeliac plexus along the splenic artery and its branches. **Subclavian plexus [plexus subclavius (NA)].** A plexus of postganglionic fibres from the inferior cervical ganglion on the subclavian artery. **Submucous plexus [plexus submucosus (NA)].** A plexus of autonomic nerve fibres interspersed with ganglion cells, situated in the submucous coat of the gut; Meissner's plexus. **Suboccipital plexus [plexus venosus suboccipitalis (NA)].** A plexus of veins over the suboccipital triangle, draining mainly into the vertebral and deep cervical veins. **Subpapillary plexus.** A plexus of arterial branches beneath the corium from which fine capillaries pass into the papillae. **Subserous plexus [plexus subserosus (NA)].** An autonomic plexus under the peritoneal coat of the gut. **Suprarenal plexus [plexus suprarenalis (NA)].** Extensions of the coeliac plexus together with branches from the greater splanchnic nerve close to the suprarenal gland. It contains preganglionic fibres which are distributed to the medulla of the suprarenal gland. **Sympathetic plexuses [plexus autonomici (NA)].** Nerve plexuses, mainly prevertebral in position, in connection with the sympathetic nervous system; the principal ones are the cardiac, solar (coeliac), and hypogastric. They consist of a mixture of nerve fibres and nerve cells, and furnish branches to the viscera. **Testicular plexus [plexus testicularis (NA)].** An autonomic nerve plexus along the testicular artery. It receives twigs from the renal and aortic plexuses and extends to the testis. **Thyroid plexus [plexus thyroideus impar (NA)].** The venous network on the front of the trachea formed by communications between the right and left thyroid veins. **Tympanic plexus [plexus tympanicus (NA)].** A plexus of nerve fibres on the promontory of the tympanic membrane, which receives fibres from the glossopharyngeal nerve and the carotid plexus of the sympathetic system. The plexus supplies the mucous membrane of the middle ear, tympanic antrum, mastoid air cells and pharyngotympanic tube. **Ureteric plexus [plexus uretericus (NA)].** A sympathetic plexus along the ureter. It receives fibres from the renal plexus and aorticorenal ganglion and the aortic plexus. **Uterine (venous) plexus [plexus venosus uterinus (NA)].** A venous plexus at the attachment of the broad ligament, draining the uterus and emptying into the internal iliac vein. **Uterovaginal plexus [plexus uterovaginalis (NA)].** An autonomic plexus, interspersed with ganglia cells, around the vagina and neck of the uterus; it is a continuation of the pelvic plexus to supply these organs and the erectile tissue of the vestibule. **Vaginal (venous) plexus [plexus venosus vaginalis (NA)].** A venous plexus around the vagina, draining this organ and emptying into the internal iliac vein. **Plexus of the vas deferens [plexus deferentialis (NA)].** A peripheral portion of the pelvic plexus supplying the vas deferens. **Vascular plexus [plexus vasculosus (NA)].** Any network of blood vessels. **Venous plexus [plexus venosus (NA)].** A network of interconnecting veins. **Vertebral plexus of the inferior cervical ganglion [plexus vertebralis (NA)].** A plexus of postganglionic fibres from the inferior cervical ganglion on the vertebral artery. **Vertebral (venous) plexus [plexus venosi vertebrales internus et externus (anterior et posterior) (NA)].** Venous plexus along the vertebral column, lying outside (external vertebral plexus) and inside the vertebral canal (internal vertebral plexus). Each main subdivision is further distinguished into an anterior or posterior plexus according to position in front of or behind the vertebral column or spinal cord. These plexuses drain the muscles around and the structures within the vertebral column, and drain eventually into the vertebral, posterior intercostal, lumbar and sacral veins. At the foramen magnum they communicate with the venous sinuses of the dura mater. **Vesical plexus [plexus vesicalis (NA)].** An autonomic nerve plexus, a continuation of the pelvic plexus, lying alongside the bladder. It supplies the bladder, vas deferens and seminal vesicle. **Vesical (venous) plexus [plexus venosus vesicalis (NA)].** A venous plexus around the base of the bladder, continuous below with the prostatic plexus in the male and vaginal plexus in the female. It drains into the internal iliac vein. [L, plaited.]

See also: AUERBACH, CRUVEILHIER, EXNER, HALLER, HELLER (J. F.), HOVIUS, JACQUES, LEBER, MEISSNER, PANIZZA, RANVIER, REMAK (R.), SANTORINI, SAPPEY, STENSEN, TROLARD, WALTHER.

plica [NA] (**pli**·kah). A fold or plait. **Caecal plica.** Caecal fold; a fold of peritoneum behind the caecum which forms the right boundary of the retrocaecal recess. **Genital plica.** The genital fold or ridge on the medial side of the mesonephros of the embryo, overlying the developing gonad. **Plica polonica.** Matted and infested hair. **Plica semilunaris conjunctivae [NA].** A semilunar fold of conjunctiva lateral to the lacrimal caruncle. **Septal plica.** One of the transient ridges seen at the back of the nasal septum in the embryo. **Plicae tubariae** [NA]. Longitudinal folds of the mucous coat of the uterine tube. **Urorectal plica.** A fold of peritoneum on each lateral wall of the embryonic cavity, containing the mesonephric and paramesonephric ducts as they pass towards the urogenital sinus. In the male they fuse to become the urorectal septum, in the female the broad ligaments and uterus. [L *plicare* to fold.]

plicadentin (pli·kah·**den**·tin). A condition in which the dentine of a tooth is folded in a complex manner in relation to a complex pulp chamber; it is found only in certain animals, and never in man. [L *plicare* to fold, dentine.]

plicate (**pli**·kate). Folded; tucked. [L *plicatus.*]

plication (pli·**ka**·shun). 1. The act of folding. 2. A fold. 3. An operation for shortening a muscle or for decreasing the size of a hollow viscus by taking tucks in its walls. [L *plicare* to fold.]

plicotomy (pli·**kot**·o·me). The operation of dividing the posterior malleolar fold of the tympanic membrane. [L *plicare* to fold, Gk *temnein* to cut.]

pliers (**pli**·erz). An instrument with a pincer movement, used for holding small objects; also used for bending and cutting metal. Many and various forms are used in dentistry. [Fr. *pli* fold.]

Plimmer, Henry George (b. 1856). London protozoologist.

Plimmer's body. An intracellular body found in cancer cells and degenerative in origin.

Plimmer's salt. Sodium antimony tartrate.

plint, plinth (plint, plinth). An apparatus on which the patient lies or sits in remedial gymnastics. [Gk *plinthos* tile.]

pliophite (**pli**·o·fite). Denoting a cell which is amply provided with reserves of nutriment. [Gk *pleion* more, *phyein* to make to grow.]

ploidy (**ploid**·e). The number of chromosome sets in a cell; e.g. 1,2,3 sets equals haploidy, diploidy, triploidy, and so on. [Gk *eidos* form.]

plombage (plom·**bahzh**). 1. The packing of bone cavities with antiseptic preparations. 2. The packing of lung or pleural cavities with inert material. [Fr., stopping.]

plombe (plom). A word introduced by Professor Custodis of Dusseldorf to describe the implants he used to produce infolding of the sclera in cases of detachment of the retina. The implants now usually consist of silicon rubber.

plot (plot). *See* KURIE.

plug (plug). 1. An occluding pack usually introduced firmly to control bleeding, e.g. into the nasal cavity in epistaxis. 2. To insert such a plug. 3. In dentistry, to use a plugger to condense a filling into a cavity prepared in a tooth. **Cervical plug.** Mucous plug (see below). **Epithelial plug.** Any mass of epithelial cells temporarily occluding the lumen of an embryonic tubular structure or opening, e.g. the oesophageal and duodenal plugs. **Kite-tailed plug.** A plug consisting of several balls of gauze or wool strung together so as to facilitate their removal. **Meconium plugs.** Anorectal plugs of meconium, causing temporary obstruction. **Mucous plug.** The hypothetical plug of mucus which blocks the canal of the cervix during pregnancy. It is probably a constant outpouring of mucus. **Yolk plug.** The mass of yolk-laden cells temporarily occluding the blastopore at the end of amphibian gastrulation. [etym. dub.]

See also: CORNER (E. M.), DITTRICH, ECKER, IMLACH, TRAUBE (L.).

plugger (**plug**·er). An instrument used to condense and consolidate a filling material in a cavity in a tooth. **Amalgam plugger.** An instrument for condensing and consolidating amalgam. **Automatic plugger.** A spring-loaded plugger operated by hand pressure or a dental engine for consolidating gold foil or amalgam. **Back-action plugger.** A plugger with a reverse action used for condensing a filling in a tooth. **Electromagnetic plugger.** A plugger operated by an electromagnet. **Foil plugger.** An instrument used for condensing cohesive gold foil, piece by piece, into a solid mass in a cavity in a tooth. **Foot plugger.** A plugger with a foot-shaped end. **Gold plugger.** A plugger for compressing and consolidating gold foil. **Hand plugger.** A plugger that is hand operated. **Reverse plugger.** Back-action plugger (see above). [see prec.]

plumbagin (plum·**ba**·jin). 2-Methyl-5-hydroxy-1,4-naphthaquinone, $C_6H_4(CO)_2C(CH_3)COH$. A yellow compound derived from various shrubs of the family Plumbaginaceae; it has very slight vitamin-K activity.

plumbago (plum·**ba**·go). 1. Graphite, black lead. An allotropic form of carbon found naturally in Siberia, Sri Lanka and the USA; a soft dark-grey chemically inert crystalline substance used for lead pencils, electrodes, crucibles, and as a lubricant. 2. A genus of tropical herbs of the family Plumbaginaceae; leadworts. [L *plumbum* lead.]

plumbic (**plum**·bik). 1. Of, relating to, like, or containing lead. 2. Applied to a compound of trivalent lead. [L *plumbum* lead.]

plumbism (**plum**·bizm). Lead poisoning. [see prec.]

plumbite (**plum**·bite). Any compound formed by the solution of lead monoxide, PbO, in alkali hydroxides; it may be regarded as derived from a hypothetical plumbous acid, H_2PbO_2. [L *plumbum* lead.]

plumbotherapy (plum·bo·**ther**·ap·e). The treatment of disease by means of lead preparations. [L *plumbum* lead, therapy.]

plumbous (**plum**·bus). Applied to a compound of divalent lead.

plumbum (**plum**·bum) (gen. *plumbi*). Lead. **Plumbi acetas.** Lead acetate. **Plumbi carbonas.** Lead carbonate, white lead, $2PbCO_3$ $Pb(OH)_2$, a white amorphous compound used in ointment form as an astringent. **Plumbi monoxidum, Plumbi oxidum.** Lead monoxide. [L.]

Plummer, Henry Stanley (b. 1874). Rochester, Minnesota, physician.

Plummer's sign. Inability to step onto a chair, occurring in thyrotoxic myasthenia.

Plummer-Vinson anaemia, or syndrome, Vinson-Plummer syndrome. Chronic hypochromic microcytic anaemia with dysphagia, glossitis and achylia gastrica, due to iron deficiency.

plumose, plumous (**ploom**·oze, **ploom**·us). 1. Like a feather. 2. Provided with feathers. [L *pluma* small soft feather.]

plumper (**plum**·per). The labial flange of an artificial denture, or of an obturator worn in the mouth, which has been built up in order to hold the soft tissues of the lips and cheeks in their natural position. [ME *plumpe*.]

Plunket's caustic. A paste made by incorporating arsenic, and sulphur, with the bruised plants *Ranunculus acris* and *Ranunculus flammula.*

pluricytopenia (ploor·e·si·to·**pe**'·ne·ah). Pancytopenia. [L *plus* more, Gk *kytos* cell, *penia* poverty.]

pluridyscrinia (**ploor**·e·dis·**krin**'·e·ah). The simultaneous occurrence of dysfunction in more than one endocrine organ. [L *plus* more, Gk *dys*, *krinein* to separate.]

plurifetation (**ploor**·e·fe·**ta**'·shun). The conception of more than one child. [L *plus* more, fetus.]

pluriglandular (ploor·e·**glan**·dew·lar). Of several glands. [L *plus* more, gland.]

plurigravida (ploor·e·**grav**·id·ah). A woman who has had at least two children and who is again pregnant; multigravida. [L *plus* more, *gravida* pregnant.]

plurilocular (ploor·e·**lok**·ew·lar). Multilocular. [L *plus* more, *loculus* little place.]

plurimenorrhoea (**ploor**·e·men·o·**re**'·ah). Abnormally frequent recurrence of the menstrual period. [L *plus* more, menorrhoea.]

plurinuclear (ploor·e·**new**·kle·ar). Having a number of nuclei. [L *plus* more, nucleus.]

pluri-orificialis (**ploor**·e·or·if·is·e·**a**'·lis). Pertaining to several orifices. [L *plus* more, *orificium* opening.]

pluripara (ploor·**ip**·ar·ah). One who has had several children; multipara. [L *plus* more, *parere* to bear.]

pluriparity (ploor·e·**par**·it·e). The condition or fact of having borne several children; multiparity. [see prec.]

pluripolar (ploor·e·**po**·lar). Referring to a cell with several poles. [L *plus* more, pole.]

pluripotent, pluripotential (ploor·**ip**·o·tent, **ploor**·e·po·**ten**'·shal). 1. Having more than one way of action. 2. Having more than a single effect. [L *plus* more, *potens* powerful.]

pluriresistant (**ploor**·e·riz·**is**'·tant). Resistant to several drugs of different types. [L *plus* more, resistant.]

pluriseptate (ploor·e·**sep**·tate). Consisting of or provided with more than a single septum. [L *plus* more, septum.]

plutomania (ploo·to·**ma**·ne·ah). 1. A delusion amounting to insanity of being possessed of riches. 2. An obsession with the idea of great wealth. [Gk *ploutos* riches, mania.]

plutonism (ploo·**to**·nizm). A condition caused by over-exposure to plutonium; degenerative changes occur. [Obsolete term.]

plutonium (ploo·**to**·ne·um). A radioactive metallic element of atomic number 94 and chemical symbol Pu. It was obtained in 1940 by the bombardment of uranium 238 with neutrons, neptunium being produced as an intermediate, and has a half-life of 2.4×10^4 years. Thermal neutrons produce fission, and the element has been used in an atomic bomb (Nagasaki 1945) and in nuclear power plants. [Named after the planet *Pluto.*]

pnein (**ne**·in). A hypothetical respiratory stimulant once believed to be present in the blood; now discredited. [Gk, to breathe.]

pneodynamics (**ne**·o·di·**nam**'·ix). Pneumodynamics. [Gk *pnoe* breath, *dynamis* force.]

pneograph (**ne**·o·graf). Pneumograph. [Gk *pnoe* breath, *graphein* to record.]

pneometer (ne·**om**·et·er). Pneumatometer. [Gk *pnoe* breath, *metron* measure.]

pneophore (**ne**·o·fore). An instrument used in the performance of artificial respiration. [Gk *pnoe* breath, *phoros* bearer.]

pneoscope (**ne**·o·skope). Pneumograph. [Gk *pnoe* breath, *skopein* to watch.]

pneuma (**new**·mah). 1. A breath. 2. The vital principle; the primordial substance. **Perivascular pneuma.** Cumbo's sign. [Gk, air.]

pneumal (**new**·mal). Belonging to the lungs. [Gk *pneumon* lung.]

pneumameter (new·**mam**·et·er). A device to which is attached a scale which demonstrates the air capacity of the lungs, used to exercise the lungs as part of the after-treatment in empyema. [Gk *pneuma* air, *metron* measure.]

pneumarthrography (new·mar·**throg**·raf·e). Pneumoarthrography.

pneumarthrosis (new·mar·**thro**·sis). 1. The presence of gas or air in a joint. 2. Distension of a joint with oxygen in order to assist radiographical inspection. [Gk *pneuma* air, *arthron* joint, *-osis* condition.]

pneumascope (**new**·mah·skope). Pneumograph. [Gk *pneuma* air, *skopein* to watch.]

pneumascos (new·**mas**·kos). Pneumoperitoneum. [Gk *pneuma* air, *askos* leather bag.]

pneumatelectasis (**new**·mat·el·**ek**'·tas·is). Pulmonary atelectasis. [Gk *pneumon* lung, atelectasis.]

pneumathaemia (new·mah·**the**·me·ah). The presence of bubbles of gas or air in the blood. [Gk *pneuma* air, *haima* blood.]

pneumatic (new·**mat**·ik). 1. Relating to air or gas. 2. Containing air; having cavities filled with air. 3. Relating to respiration. 4. Worked by means of compressed air, e.g. an instrument. [Gk *pneuma* air.]

pneumatics (new·**mat**·ix). That branch of physics which deals with the mechanical properties of air and gases. [Gk *pneuma* air.]

pneumatinuria (**new**·mat·in·**ewr**'·e·ah). Pneumaturia.

pneumatism (**new**·mat·izm). Medicine as practised by the pneumatists.

pneumatists (**new**·mat·ists). A school of medicine of the 1st century B.C., members of which based their teaching and practice on the function and make-up of the vital air passing from the lungs to the heart and arteries, from there dispersing through the whole body. [see foll.]

pneumatization (**new**·mat·i·**za**'·shun). The development of air cells or air-filled cavities within a structure; in particular, their development within the bones of the skull, e.g. paranasal sinuses. [Gk *pneuma* air.]

pneumatized (**new**·mat·i·zd). 1. Containing air. 2. Containing air cells. [see prec.]

pneumatocardia (**new**·mat·o·**kar**'·de·ah). The existence of bubbles of air or gas in the blood of the chambers of the heart. [Gk *pneuma* air, *kardia* heart.]

pneumatocele (new·**mat**·o·seel). 1. Herniation of the lung. 2. A sac or tumour filled with gas. **Pneumatocele cranii.** An air-filled tumour under the scalp, after an accident in which the nasal sinuses were involved. [Gk *pneuma* air, *kele* hernia.]

pneumatochemical (**new**·mat·o·**kem**'·ik·al). 1. Pertaining to the treatment of diseases of the lungs by means of inhalations. 2. Relating or belonging to the chemistry of gases. [Gk *pneuma* air, chemistry.]

pneumatodyspnoea (**new**·mat·o·**disp**'·ne·ah). Laboured breathing or shortness of breath caused by emphysema of the lungs. [Gk *pneuma* air, dyspnoea.]

pneumatogeny (new·mat·**oj**·en·e). Artificial respiration. [Gk *pneuma* air, *genein* to produce.]

pneumatogram (new·**mat**·o·gram). Pneumogram.

pneumatograph (new·**mat**·o·graf). Pneumograph.

pneumatology (new·mat·**ol**·o·je). 1. The science of gases and their use in various kinds of treatment. 2. The science of respiration. [Gk *pneuma* air, *logos* science.]

pneumatometer (new·mat·**om**·et·er). A type of spirometer used in determining the amount of air inhaled and exhaled. [Gk *pneuma* air, *metron* measure.]

pneumatometry (new·mat·**om**·et·re). Measurement by means of the pneumatometer, of the air inhaled and exhaled.

pneumatomphalocele (new·mat·**om**·fal·o·seel). An umbilical hernia which is filled with gas. [Gk *pneuma* air, *omphalos* navel, *kele* hernia.]

pneumatophore (**new**·mat·o·fore). An oxygen breathing apparatus used in rescuing mine workers; it generally consists of a bag filled with oxygen, a tube and mouthpiece. [Gk *pneuma* air, *phoros* bearer.]

pneumatorrhachis (new·mat·**or**·ak·is). The presence of gas in the spinal canal. [Gk *pneuma* air, *rhachis* backbone.]

pneumatoscope (**new**·mat·o·skope). An instrument for auscultatory percussion of the chest. [Gk *pneumon* lung, *skopein* to view.]

pneumatosis (new·mat·**o**·sis). The presence of gas in an abnormal situation such as the pleural or peritoneal cavity. **Pneumatosis abdominis.** Pneumoperitoneum. **Pneumatosis cystoides intestinalis.** A rare disorder (of obscure origin) of the intestinal wall in which gas-filled bullae are found, usually without symptoms; it may be congenital or associated with pyloric stenosis. **Pneumatosis intestinalis.** Tympanites. **Pneumatosis pulmonum.** Either pneumothorax or pulmonary emphysema [obsolete term]. [Gk *pneuma* air, *-osis* condition.]

pneumatotherapy (**new**·mat·o·**ther**'·ap·e). 1. The treatment of disease by the use of condensed or rarefied air. 2. The administration of gases in order to control pain, in the treatment of pneumonia, for the induction of an anaesthetic state and for resuscitation purposes. [Gk *pneuma* air, therapy.]

pneumatothorax (**new**·mat·o·**thor**'·ax). Pneumothorax.

pneumaturia (new·mat·**ewr**·e·ah). The passing of air or gas with urine; the cause is either urinary decomposition or a vesicointestinal fistula. [Gk *pneuma* air, urine.]

pneumatype (**new**·mah·tipe). The pattern formed by the deposit of air exhaled through the nose onto a glass surface. It is used for comparison of the permeability of the two nasal passages. [Gk *pneuma* air, *typos* impression.]

pneumectomy (new·**mek**·to·me). Pneumonectomy.

pneumo-alveolography (**new**·mo·al·ve·o·**log**'·raf·e). Radiography of the pulmonary alveoli, a preliminary injection of radio-opaque substance having been made into the veins. [Gk *pneumon* lung, alveolus, Gk *graphein* to record.]

pneumo-arctia (new·mo·**ark**·she·ah). Pulmonary stenosis. *See* STENOSIS. [Gk *pneumon* lung, L *arctare* to contract.]

pneumo-arthrogram (new·mo·**ar**·thro·gram). The radiograph made during pneumo-arthrography. [Gk *pneuma* air, arthrogram.]

pneumo-arthrography (**new**·mo·ar·**throg**'·raf·e). X-ray examination of joints which have been injected with air. [Gk *pneuma* air, arthrography.]

pneumobacillus (**new**·mo·bas·**il**'·us). *Streptococcus pneumoniae.* [Gk *pneumon* lung, bacillus.]

pneumobronchotomy (**new**·mo·brong·**kot**'·o·me). The operation of incising the lungs and bronchi. [Gk *pneumon* lung, bronchotomy.]

pneumobulbar, pneumobulbous (new·mo·**bul**·bar, new·mo·**bul**·bus). Relating to the lungs and the respiratory centre of the medulla oblongata. [Gk *pneumon* lung, bulb.]

pneumocace (new·**mok**·as·e). Gangrene of the lung. [Gk *pneumon* lung, *kakos* bad.]

pneumocardial (new·mo·**kar**·de·al). Relating to the lungs and the heart. [Gk *pneumon* lung, *kardia* heart.]

pneumocele (**new**·mo·seel). Pneumatocele.

pneumocentesis (**new**·mo·sen·**te**'·sis). Lung puncture in order to aspirate the contents of a cavity. [Gk *pneumon* lung, *kentesis* a pricking.]

pneumocephalon (new·mo·**kef**·al·on). Pneumocephalus. **Pneumocephalon artificiale.** Treatment by means of air introduced inside the cranium. [see foll.]

pneumocephalus (new·mo·**kef**·al·us). The presence of air or gas in the ventricles of the brain. [Gk *pneuma* air, *kephale* head.]

pneumochemical (new·mo·**kem**·ik·al). Pneumatochemical.

pneumocholecystitis (new·mo·ko·le·sist·**i**′·tis). Cholecystitis caused by gas-producing organisms, so that air forms in the gall bladder. [Gk *pneuma* air, cholecystitis.]

pneumochysis (new·**mok**·is·is). Oedema of the lungs. [Gk *pneumon* lung, *chysis* a pouring.]

pneumocirrhosis (new·mo·sir·**o**′·sis). Pulmonary fibrosis. [Gk *pneumon* lung, cirrhosis.]

pneumococcaemia (new·mo·kox·**e**′·me·ah). The presence of pneumococci *(Streptococcus pneumoniae)* in the blood. [pneumococcus, Gk *haima* blood.]

pneumococcal, pneumococcic (new·mo·**kok**·al, new·mo·**kox**·ik). Relating to or caused by the pneumococcus *(Streptococcus pneumoniae).*

pneumococcidal, pneumococcocidal (new·mo·kox·**i**′·dal, new·mo·kok·o·**si**′·dal). Having the power to destroy pneumococci *(Streptococcus pneumoniae).* [pneumococcus, L *caedere* to kill.]

pneumococcolysis (new·mo·kok·**ol**′·is·is). The process of destroying pneumococci *(Streptococcus pneumoniae).* [pneumococcus, Gk *lysis* a loosing.]

pneumococcosis (new·mo·kok·**o**′·sis). A morbid condition marked by pneumococcal invasion of the tissues. [pneumococcus, Gk *-osis* condition.]

pneumococcosuria (new·mo·kok·o·**sewr**′·e·ah). The excretion of pneumococci *(Streptococcus pneumoniae)* in the urine.

Pneumococcus (new·mo·**kok**·us). A bacterial genus in the family Lactobacillaceae; the generic name is *Streptococcus pneumoniae* but is sometimes called *Diplococcus pneumoniae.* It is a Gram-positive ovoid capsulated diplococcus, facultative anaerobe, bile-soluble and sensitive to optochin. It is associated with a wide range of upper and lower respiratory tract infections, including lobar and bronchopneumonia. [Gk *pneumon* lung, coccus.]

See also: FRAENKEL (A.), WEICHSELBAUM.

pneumocolon (new·mo·**ko**·lon). 1. A condition marked by the existence of air in the colon. 2. Distension of the colon with air for diagnostic purposes. [Gk *pneuma* air, colon.]

pneumoconiosis (new·mo·kon·e·**o**′·sis). An industrial disease of the respiratory system caused by the inhalation of microscopical metallic or mineral particles. The diagnosis is made radiologically and the x-ray appearances vary from miliary mottling to gross opacities, as in advanced silicosis. The symptoms depend, as does the radiological picture, on the degree of fibrosis caused in the lung by the presence of the foreign particles which depends on their nature. There may accordingly be no symptoms at one end of the spectrum or the most distressing dyspnoea at the other. Cf. ANTHRACOSIS, ASBESTOSIS, BAGASSOSIS, BYSSINOSIS, SIDEROSIS, SILICOSIS. **Pneumoconiosis siderotica.** Siderosis. **Talc pneumoconiosis.** Pneumoconiosis caused by the inhalation of talc, e.g. in a rubber factory. [Gk *pneumon* lung, *konis* dust, *-osis* condition.]

pneumocrania, pneumocranium (new·mo·**kra**·ne·ah, new·mo·**kra**·ne·um). The presence of gas or air beneath the dura mater. [Gk *pneuma* air, cranium.]

pneumocyst (new·mo·sist). A cyst, generally found in the lungs or the intestinal wall, containing air or other gases. [Gk *pneuma* air, cyst.]

Pneumocystis carinii (new·mo·**sist**·is kar·**in**·e·i). A micro-organism of uncertain position in classification which causes pneumonia in animals and has been reported as a pathogen in children. It is a major cause of pneumonia in children with agammaglobulinaemia. [see prec.]

pneumocystogram (new·mo·**sist**·o·gram). A radiographic film of the bladder after intravesical injection of air as contrast medium. [Gk *pneuma* air, *kystis* bladder, *gramma* record.]

pneumocystography (new·mo·sist·**og**′·raf·e). Radiography of the bladder after the latter has been insufflated with air. [Gk *pneuma* air, *kystis* bladder, *graphein* to record.]

pneumoderma, pneumodermia (new·mo·**der**·mah, new·mo·**der**′·me·ah). The presence of air in the tissues so that the skin becomes swollen; subcutaneous emphysema. [Gk *pneuma* air, *derma* skin.]

pneumodograph (new·**mod**·o·graf). An apparatus used to record the degree of efficiency of nasal respiration. [Gk *pneuma* air, *hodos* way, *graphein* to record.]

pneumodynamics (new·mo·di·**nam**′·ix). The mechanics of respiration. [Gk *pneuma* air, *dynamis* force.]

pneumodynia (new·mo·**din**·e·ah). Sensation of pain in the lung. [Gk *pneumon* lung, *odyne* pain.]

pneumo-empyema (new·mo·em·pi·**e**′·mah). The presence of pus and gas within the pleural space. [Gk *pneuma* air, empyema.]

pneumo-encephalitis (new·mo·en·kef·al·**i**′·tis). Newcastle disease of fowls. [Gk *pneuma* air, *egkephalos* brain, *-itis* inflammation.]

pneumo-encephalogram (new·mo·en·**kef**′·al·o·gram). The radiograph made during pneumo-encephalography. [Gk *pneuma* air, *egkephalos* brain, *gramma* record.]

pneumo-encephalography (new·mo·en·kef·al·**og**′·raf·e). Encephalography carried out after gas or air has been introduced into the intracranial cerebrospinal fluid space. [Gk *pneuma* air, *egkephalos* brain, *graphein* to record.]

pneumo-encephalomyelography (new·mo·en·**kef**·al·o·mi·el·**og**′·raf·e). Radiological examination of the cerebrospinal spaces after they have been filled with air. [Gk *pneuma* air, *egkephalos* brain, myelography.]

pneumo-encephalos (new·mo·en·**kef**′·al·os). Gas in the brain substance. [Gk *pneuma* air, *egkephalos* brain.]

pneumogalactocele (new·mo·gal·**ak**′·to·seel). A galactocele containing gas. [Gk *pneuma* air, *gala* milk, *kele* tumour.]

pneumogastric (new·mo·**gas**·trik). Relating to the lungs and the stomach. **Pneumogastric nerve.** The vagus nerve. [Gk *pneumon* lung, *gaster* stomach.]

pneumogastrography (new·mo·gas·**trog**′·raf·e). Radiography of the stomach which has previously been filled with air. [Gk *pneuma* air, *gaster* stomach, *graphein* to record.]

pneumogram (new·mo·gram). 1. The tracing made by a pneumograph. 2. The radiograph made during pneumography. [Gk *pneuma* air, *gramma* record.]

pneumograph (new·mo·graf). An instrument for recording chest movements during respiration. [Gk *pneumon* lung, *graphein* to record.]

pneumography (new·**mog**·raf·e). 1. Tracing of the movements of respiration by means of the pneumograph. 2. Pneumoradiography. **Cerebral pneumography.** Pneumoventriculography.

pneumohaemia (new·mo·**he**·me·ah). The presence of air in the arteries or veins. [Gk *pneuma* air, *haima* blood.]

pneumohaemopericardium (new·mo·**he**·mo·per·e·**kar**′·de·um). An accumulation of air and blood in the pericardium. [Gk *pneuma* air, *haima* blood, pericardium.]

pneumohaemothorax (new·mo·he·mo·**thor**′·ax). An accumulation of gas or air and blood in the cavity of the thorax. [Gk *pneuma* air, *haima* blood, thorax.]

pneumohydrometra (new·mo·hi·dro·**me**′·trah). A condition in which fluid and gas or air have collected in the uterus. [Gk *pneuma* air, *hydor* water, *metra* womb.]

pneumohydropericardium (new·mo·**hi**·dro·per·e·**kar**′·de·um). The presence of fluid and gas or air in the cavity of the pericardium. [Gk *pneuma* air, *hydor* water, pericardium.]

pneumohydrothorax (new·mo·hi·dro·**thor**′·ax). The presence of serous fluid and air or gas in the cavity of the pleura. [Gk *pneuma* air, *hydor* water, thorax.]

pneumohypoderma, pneumohypodermia (new·mo·hi·po·**der**′·mah, new·mo·hi·po·**der**′·me·ah). Infiltration of air into the subcutaneous tissues; subcutaneous emphysema. [Gk *pneuma* air, *hypo*, *derma* skin.]

pneumokoniosis (new·mo·kon·e·**o**′·sis). Pneumoconiosis.

pneumolipoidosis (new·mo·lip·oid·**o**′·sis). Bronchopneumonia caused by inhalation of fatty particles. [Gk *pneumon* lung, lipoidosis.]

pneumolith (**new**·mo·lith). 1. Small calcified concretions found in the lung. 2. One of the hardened patches present in the lungs in chronic pulmonary tuberculosis. [Gk *pneumon* lung, *lithos* stone.]

pneumolithiasis (**new**·mo·lith·**i**′·as·is). The presence of areas of calcification in the lungs. [see prec.]

pneumology (new·**mol**·o·je). The branch of medical science which is concerned with the lungs and other respiratory organs. [Gk *pneumon* lung, *logos* science.]

pneumolysis (new·**mol**·is·is). The operation of separating the lung and parietal pleura from the endothoracic fascia for the purpose of collapsing the lung. **Extrapleural pneumolysis.** Apicolysis. **Intrapleural pneumolysis.** The operation of collapsing the lung by stripping the pulmonary from the visceral pleura. [Gk *pneumon* lung, *lysis* a loosing.]

pneumomalacia (**new**·mo·mal·**a**′·she·ah). Pathological softening of the lung tissue. [Gk *pneumon* lung, malacia.]

pneumomassage (**new**·mo·mas·**ahzh**′). Massage of the tympanic membrane by air; an old-fashioned treatment for deafness. [Gk *pneuma* air, massage.]

pneumomediastinum (**new**·mo·me·de·as·**ti**′·num). 1. The presence of air in the mediastinum. 2. Insufflation of air into the mediastinum as an aid to x-ray diagnosis. [Gk *pneuma* air, mediastinum.]

pneumomelanosis (**new**·mo·mel·an·**o**′·sis). Darkening of the lung tissue resulting from inhalation of black particles such as those of coal dust. [Gk *pneumon* lung, *melas* black, *-osis* condition.]

pneumometer (new·**mom**·et·er). Pneumatometer.

pneumometry (new·**mom**·et·re). Pneumatometry.

pneumomoniliasis (**new**·mo·mon·il·**i**′·as·is). Pulmonary candidiasis. [Gk *pneumon* lung, moniliasis.]

pneumomycosis (new·mo·mi·**ko**′·sis). Disease of the lungs resulting from the presence of fungi. [Gk *pneumon* lung, *mykes* fungus, *-osis* condition.]

pneumomyelography (**new**·mo·mi·el·**og**′·raf·e). Radiography of the vertebral canal after its injection with air or oxygen. [Gk *pneuma* air, *myelos* marrow, *graphein* to record.]

pneumonaemia (new·mon·e·**me**·ah). Hyperaemia of the lungs. [Gk *pneumon* lung, *haima* blood.]

pneumonalgia (new·mon·**al**·je·ah). Pain affecting the lung. [Gk *pneumon* lung, *algos* pain.]

pneumonectasia, pneumonectasis (**new**·mon·ek·**ta**′·ze·ah, new·mon·**ek**·tas·is). Pulmonary emphysema. [Gk *pneumon* lung, ectasia.]

pneumonectomy (new·mon·**ek**·to·me). Total or partial surgical removal of diseased lung tissue. **Partial pneumonectomy.** Lobectomy. **Radical pneumonectomy.** Removal of the lung together with the lymph nodes at the root of the lung. **Total pneumonectomy.** Excision of the complete lung. [Gk *pneumon* lung, *ektome* a cutting out.]

pneumonere (**new**·mo·neer). The splanchnic mesenchyme of the embryonic lung buds. [Gk *pneumon* lung.]

pneumonia (new·**mo**·ne·ah). A general disease in which the essential lesion is an inflammation of the spongy tissue of the lung with consolidation of the alveolar exudate; the term is often applied to the local pathological lesion only. Classically two varieties were described, *lobar pneumonia* and *bronchopneumonia*, but several causes and varieties are now recognized. **Abortive pneumonia.** A name given to cases which after an abrupt onset and all the symptoms of pneumonia, terminate in from 1 to 3 days before definite signs of consolidation have developed. **Acute lobar pneumonia.** Pleuropneumonia, the classical type of pneumonia in which the consolidation has a lobar distribution. It is an acute specific infectious disease caused by a virulent type of pneumococcus. Pathologically four stages of the pulmonary lesion are described: *congestion*, in which the blood vessels are engorged and a serofibrinous exudate appears in the alveoli and increases in amount; *red hepatization*, in which the lung becomes solid and the alveoli are filled with fibrinous clot containing many red blood corpuscles; *grey hepatization*, in which the capillaries are obliterated by the pressure of the exudate and the alveoli are packed with polymorphonuclear cells and distintegrating red cells; and finally, *resolution*, in which liquefaction and absorption of the exudate takes place through the action of intracellular ferments and the lung is restored to normal. These stages are the result of post-mortem studies of fatal cases and are not necessarily present in every case. There are many degrees of severity both pathologically and clinically. The disease typically has an abrupt onset with a rigor in adults and convulsions or vomiting in children. The temperature rises rapidly and remains at a high level with slight remissions for several days. The stabbing pain in the side, the short, dry cough ending in a grunt, the sticky, rusty sputum, rapid respirations, hot dry skin, excitement or delirium, make an unmistakable picture. The fever usually ends by crisis, and in a few hours the temperature, respirations and pulse drop to normal and convalescence begins. In about one-third the temperature falls by lysis over 2 or 3 days. **Apical pneumonia.** Pneumonia in which the consolidation is limited to the upper lobe of one lung. High temperatures and cerebral symptoms may be marked. **Aspiration pneumonia.** Acute bronchopneumonia caused by the aspiration of infected material into the lungs. This may be due to accident or occur during anaesthesia or coma. The infected material may be food particles, or septic material from ulcerating growths of the upper air passages, or be aspirated from suppurative lesions in other parts of the lung. There is widespread bronchitis and bronchopneumonia, which may go on to abscess, gangrene or empyema. **Asthenic pneumonia.** Pneumonia associated with severe prostration, seen in enfeebled elderly persons. The symptoms and signs in the lung may be slight. **Atypical pneumonia.** Primary atypical pneumonia (see below). **Central pneumonia.** Pneumonia in which the lesion is deep-seated, and physical signs are absent or slight until the disease has extended to the periphery. **Chronic pneumonia, Chronic interstitial pneumonia.** Bronchopneumonia in which complete resolution has not taken place and pulmonary fibrosis occurs. It may be complicated by suppurative processes such as abscess or bronchiectasis. **Contusional pneumonia.** Traumatic pneumonia (see below). **Creeping pneumonia.** Acute lobar pneumonia in which consolidation appears successively in other lobes of the same or opposite lung before clearing up in the first. With each extension there is an exacerbation of the fever. **Croupous pneumonia.** Acute lobar pneumonia (see above). **Double pneumonia.** Acute lobar pneumonia affecting both lungs. **Epidemic pneumonia.** Pneumonia occasionally occurring in small epidemics, mainly in institutions such as barracks, mental hospitals and jails. **Fibrinous pneumonia.** Acute lobar pneumonia (see above). **Giant cell pneumonia.** An interstitial pneumonia of children with inclusion bodies in multinucleated giant cells. It may be due to measles virus. *Hecht's pneumonia.* **Haemorrhagic pneumonia.** Pneumonia in which the alveolar exudate and sputum are markedly haemorrhagic, as in infection with haemolytic streptococci and the influenza bacillus. **Hypostatic pneumonia.** A low-grade pneumonia occurring with passive congestion of the posterior bases of the lungs in bedridden patients with enfeebled hearts. **Larval penumonia.** Abortive pneumonia (see above). **Lipoid pneumonia.** A chronic proliferative lesion caused by the entry of oil globules into the alveoli. It may follow the use of oily nasal drops, forcible feeding with milk, or the aspiration of oil-contaminated water when swimming. **Lobar pneumonia.** Acute lobar pneumonia (see above). **Lobular pneumonia.** Bronchopneumonia, pneumonia in which the consolidation has a patchy lobular distribution. Beginning in the bronchi, the disease spreads to the lobular bronchioles (bronchiolitis) and the corresponding air sacs and alveoli, and also to neighbouring alveoli and the interalveolar interstitial tissue. Between the patches of consolidation are areas of collapse, oedema and emphysema, in varying degree. The alveolar exudate contains desquamated epithelial cells, large numbers of white blood corpuscles but only a few red corpuscles, and little, if any, fibrin.

Although a pure pneumococcal infection can cause a lobular pneumonia in infants, the infection is usually a mixed one due to a variety of micro-organisms, several of which may be associated although one usually predominates. Common organisms are pneumococci of less virulent types, streptococci, staphylococci, *Haemophilus influenzae*, but occasionally it may be due to the organisms of typhoid, plague, diphtheria, and other specific infectious diseases. In children it is a common complication of measles or whooping-cough, and at all ages of epidemic influenza. In the elderly it may terminate a chronic bronchitis especially when associated with debilitating diseases such as chronic renal disease, cardiovascular degeneration, chronic nervous diseases, diabetes, etc. Clinically the onset is more gradual than in lobar pneumonia, the temperature is more remittent, dyspnoea and cyanosis are early and prominent symptoms, and defervescence is by lysis. The course may be measured by weeks rather than by days; convalescence is slow, and fibrosis with bronchiectasis is a not uncommon sequel. **Louisiana pneumonia.** A virus pneumonia. **Massive pneumonia.** A form of pneumonia in which the bronchi are also filled with consolidated exudate. The combination of dullness with absent or feeble breath sounds may suggest a pleural effusion, but the heart is not displaced. **Migratory pneumonia.** Creeping pneumonia (see above). **Oil-aspiration pneumonia.** Lipoid pneumonia (see above). **Plague pneumonia.** The pneumonic form of oriental plague in which the plague bacilli are inhaled directly into the lungs from the droplets sprayed into the air by infected persons when coughing. It is extremely infectious and fatal. An intense haemorrhagic confluent bronchopneumonia is produced. An extensive epidemic occurred in Manchuria in 1911, and it accounted for the majority of the deaths in the "Black Death". **Pneumococcal lobular pneumonia.** Primary bronchopneumonia, a pneumonia occurring mainly in children under 2 years of age, and due to a pure pneumococcal infection. In its onset and course it resembles lobar pneumonia. High temperatures and cerebral symptoms are common. **Postoperative pneumonia.** Pneumonia following operations especially upon the abdomen. Although the anaesthetic and restriction of diaphragmatic movement may be factors, most of the cases so diagnosed are cases of either massive collapse, aspiration bronchopneumonia or pyogen infarction. **Primary atypical pneumonia.** A term denoting a group of relatively mild allied conditions of non-bacterial origin which have an insidious onset with malaise, shivering, headache and muscular pains, followed by moderate fever and an irritating cough. Physical signs may be marked without severe symptoms, but chest x-ray reveals extensive diffuse mottling particularly at the bases. The disease is rarely complicated or fatal; it is often accompanied by an increase in serum antibodies to *Mycoplasma pneumoniae*, which is the most common causative organism. **Secondary pneumonia.** Pneumonia occurring in the course of a specific infectious disease such as typhoid, plague, diphtheria, tularaemia, etc. **Suppurative pneumonia.** Septic bronchopneumonia, bronchopneumonia which goes on to suppuration and abscess formation, especially after the inhalation of infected material. In other cases it may be due to staphylococci, β-haemolytic streptococci or *Haemophilus influenzae* which have gained entrance to the lung. **Terminal pneumonia.** Pneumonia occurring as a terminal infection, especially in elderly and debilitated patients. It is of the asthenic type. **Traumatic pneumonia.** Pneumonia occurring after a blow on the chest wall. Cases so described in reality have haemorrhagic infiltration into the lung and pleura, but a bronchopneumonic consolidation may sometimes follow as the result of secondary infections. **Tuberculous pneumonia.** Pneumonia due to the inhalation of caseous material into the bronchi. It may take a lobar form (pneumonic phthisis), but a bronchopneumonia is more common. In either case the diagnosis from acute lobar pneumonia or bronchopneumonia may be difficult at first, but after a time the failure of resolution, the signs of breaking-down of the lung, and the appearance of tubercle bacilli in the sputum enable the diagnosis to be made. **Pneumonia types.** In the classification of the pneumococci in presulphonamide drugs, there were three main specific serological types and a fourth omnibus group which included many non-pathogenic strains. The pneumonias were correspondingly grouped and treated with the corresponding antiserum. Type III was the most severe. **Unresolved pneumonia.** The apparent failure of the consolidation to resolve after 3 or 4 weeks which may be due to the exudate becoming organized into fibrous tissue, or the presence of a lung abscess or localized empyema. **Virus pneumonia.** Inflammation of the lung which may occur in the course of some virus diseases, including infection with the following viruses: adenovirus, chickenpox (varicella), cytomegalovirus, infectious mononucleosis (glandular fever), influenza A and B, measles, para-influenza, respiratory syncytial virus. The extent and severity of lung involvement will depend on the virus, the age of the patient (more severe at the extremes of life) and the severity of the initial virus infection. Most of the viruses listed do not infect the lungs initially or specifically but by extension usually from the upper respiratory tract. Secondary bacterial infection often occurs and complicates the clinical picture. **White pneumonia.** A congenital syphilitic condition found in still-born children or those dying shortly after birth. There is a cellular infiltration of the interalveolar tissue, with degeneration and desquamation of the epithelium. On section, the lung is firm, smooth, and has a greyish-white colour. [Gk *pneumon* lung.]

See also: FRIEDLAENDER, HECHT, LOEFFLER (W.).

pneumonic (new·**mon**·ik). 1. Pertaining to pneumonia, e.g. pneumonic crisis, pneumonic consolidation. 2. A term used to describe any consolidation of the lung which resembles that of pneumonia.

pneumonitis (new·mon·i·tis). Inflammation of the lung: the present use of the term is imprecise, covering as it does a heterogeneous group of lesions ranging from the radiological opacities in mild catarrhal infections, through atypical pneumonia and virus pneumonia, to grave suppurative diseases. [Gk *pneumon* lung, *-itis* inflammation.]

pneumonocele (**new**·mon·o·seel). Pneumatocele.

pneumonocentesis (**new**·mon·o·sen·**te'**·sis). Pneumocentesis.

pneumonocirrhosis (**new**·mon·o·sir·**o'**·sis). Pneumocirrhosis.

pneumonococcus (**new**·mon·o·**kok'**·us). *Streptococcus pneumoniae.*

pneumonoconiosis (**new**·mon·o·kon·e·**o'**·sis). Pneumoconiosis.

pneumonograph (**new**·mon·o·graph). Pneumograph.

pneumonography (**new**·mon·**og**·raf·e). Pneumography.

pneumonolipoidosis (new·mon·o·lip·oid·**o'**·sis). Pneumolipoidosis.

pneumonolysis (new·mon·**ol**·is·is). Pneumolysis.

pneumonomelanosis (**new**·mon·o·mel·an·**o'**·sis). Pneumomelanosis.

pneumonometer (new·mon·**om**·et·er). Pneumatometer.

pneumonomoniliasis (**new**·mon·o·mon·il·**i'**·as·is). Pulmonary candidiasis.

pneumonomycosis (**new**·mon·o·mi·**ko'**·sis). Pneumomycosis.

pneumonoparesis (**new**·mon·o·par·**e'**·sis). Pneumoparesis.

pneumonopathy (new·mon·**op**·ath·e). Pneumopathy.

pneumonopexy (**new**·mon·o·pex·e). Pneumopexy.

pneumonopleuritis (**new**·mon·o·ploor·**i'**·tis). Pneumopleuritis.

pneumonorrhagia (**new**·mon·o·**ra'**·je·ah). Pneumorrhagia.

pneumonorrhaphy (new·mon·**or**·af·e). Pneumorrhaphy.

pneumonosis (new·mon·o·sis). Pneumopathy; any diseased or morbid condition of the lungs. **Traumatic pneumonosis.** A condition of acute emphysema and damage to lung structure, sometimes resulting in aero-embolism or pneumothorax, due usually to the effects of explosive decompression, but occasionally to direct impact. [Gk *pneumon* lung, *-osis* condition.]

pneumonotherapy (**new**·mon·o·**ther'**·ap·e). Pneumotherapy.

pneumonotomy (new·mon·**ot**·o·me). Pneumotomy.

pneumo-oxygenator (new·mo·**ox**·e·jen·a·tor). An apparatus used for the inhalation of large amounts of oxygen. [Gk *pneuma* air, oxygen.]

pneumoparesis (**new**·mo·par·**e'**·sis). An inelastic condition of lung tissue allowing infiltration of passive exudate into the air cells. [Gk *pneumon* lung, *paresis* a letting go.]

pneumopathy (new·**mop**·ath·e). Any morbid condition affecting the lungs. **Eosinophilic pneumopathy.** Loeffler's eosinophilia. [Gk *pneumon* lung, *pathos* disease.]

pneumopericarditis (**new**·mo·per·e·kar·**di**'·tis). Pericarditis associated with the presence of air or gas in the pericardial sac. [Gk *pneuma* air, pericarditis.]

pneumopericardium (**new**·mo·per·e·**kar**'·de·um). The presence of air or gas in the pericardial sac; the condition may be the result of trauma through the wall of the thorax or of communication with a cavity or organ in which air has accumulated. [Gk *pneuma* air, pericardium.]

pneumoperitoneal (**new**·mo·per·it·o·**ne**'·al). Relating or belonging to pneumoperitoneum.

pneumoperitoneum (**new**·mo·per·it·o·**ne**'·um). Air or gas within the peritoneal cavity. It may be due to a perforating ulcer or wound, or may be induced therapeutically to cause partial collapse of the lung in pulmonary tuberculosis. It is also induced to aid radioscopy of the abdominal organs. **Artificial pneumoperitoneum.** The deliberate introduction of air into the peritoneal cavity through the abdominal wall with the object of raising the diaphragm; this decreases the size of the thoracic cavity and produces relaxation of the lung. It is used in selected cases of pulmonary tuberculosis to rest the affected parts. With predominantly unilateral disease it may be used in conjunction with crushing the phrenic nerve. The air is introduced into the peritoneal cavity through a needle attached to the standard artificial pneumothorax apparatus, and refills must usually be given once a week. **Diagnostic pneumoperitoneum.** That achieved by either direct injection through the abdominal wall or by per-uterine inflation if one of the uterine tubes is patent. By its aid radiographs will show pelvic and abdominal soft tissues against a translucent background. **Indirect pneumoperitoneum.** A leakage of air from an established artificial pneumothorax through a defect in the diaphragm into the peritoneal cavity. Rare. **Therapeutic pneumoperitoneum.** Artificial pneumoperitoneum (see above). [Gk *pneuma* air, peritoneum.]

pneumoperitonitis (**new**·mo·per·it·on·**i**'·tis). Acute peritonitis complicated by the presence of gas or air in the peritoneal cavity. [pneumoperitoneum, Gk *-itis* inflammation.]

pneumopexy (**new**·mo·pex·e). Suture of the lung to the wall of the thorax. [Gk *pneumon* lung, *pexis* fixation.]

pneumophone (**new**·mo·fone). An instrument for measuring the pressure in the middle ear. [Gk *pneuma* air, *phone* sound.]

pneumophonia (new·mo·**fo**·ne·ah). A form of vocal disability characterized by phonatory waste in speaking, producing a breathy quality of the voice. [see prec.]

pneumopleuritis (**new**·mo·ploor·**i**'·tis). Combined pneumonia and pleurisy. [Gk *pneumon* lung, pleuritis.]

pneumopleuroparietopexy (new·mo·**ploor**·o·par·i·et·o·**pex**'·e). Surgical or chemical fixation of the lung to the parietal pleura as a preliminary to opening a pulmonary abcess. [Gk *pneumon* lung, pleura, L *paries* wall, Gk *pexis* fixation.]

pneumoprecordium (new·mo·pre·**kord**'·e·um). An accumulation of air in the precordial space. [Gk *pneuma* air, precordium.]

pneumopreperitoneum (**new**·mo·**pre**·per·it·o·**ne**'·um). 1. An accumulation of air in the space between the transversalis fascia and the parietal peritoneum. 2. In radiographical diagnosis, insufflation of air between the transversalis fascia and the parietal peritoneum. [Gk *pneuma* air, peritoneum.]

pneumoprotein (new·mo·**pro**·te·in). Any of the proteins elaborated by *Streptococcus pneumoniae.*

pneumopyelogram (new·mo·**pi**·el·o·gram). A radiographic film of a kidney after injection of oxygen as contrast medium into its pelvis through a ureteric catheter. Such films sometimes demonstrate calculi of low density, and papillomata of the pelvis of the ureter. [Gk *pneuma* air, pyelogram.]

pneumopyelography (**new**·mo·pi·el·**og**'·raf·e). Pyelography in which, instead of an opaque medium, oxygen is used as an insufflated gas in the pelvis of the ureter. [Gk *pneuma* air, pyelography.]

pneumopyopericardium (**new**·mo·**pi**·o·per·e·**kar**'·de·um). The presence of air and pus in the pericardial cavity. [Gk *pneuma* air, *pyon* pus, pericardium.]

pneumopyothorax (**new**·mo·pi·o·**thor**'·ax). Pyopneumothorax.

pneumoradiography (**new**·mo·ra·de·**og**'·raf·e). Injection of a part with air or oxygen and subsequent examination by x-rays. [Gk *pneuma* air, radiography.]

pneumoresection (**new**·mo·re·**sek**'·shun). Partial resection of a lung. [Gk *pneumon* lung, resection.]

pneumoretroperitoneum (**new**·mo·re·tro·per·it·o·**ne**'·um). The presence of air in the retroperitoneal space. [Gk *pneuma* air, retroperitoneum.]

pneumoroentgenography (**new**·mo·runt·yen·**og**'·raf·e). Pneumoradiography. [Gk *pneumon* lung, roentgenography.]

pneumorrhachis (new·mo·**rak**·is). 1. The presence of gas or air in the vertebral canal. 2. In radiographical examination, the instillation of air or gas into the vertebral canal. [Gk *pneuma* air, *rhachis* spine.]

pneumorrhagia (new·mo·**ra**·je·ah). 1. The occurrence of haemorrhage from the lung; haemoptysis. 2. Infarction of the lungs. [Gk *pneumon* lung, *rhegnynein* to gush forth.]

pneumorrhaphy (new·**mor**·af·e). The operation of suturing a wound of the lung. [Gk *pneumon* lung, *raphe* suture.]

pneumosclerosis (**new**·mo·skler·**o**'·sis). Pulmonary fibrosis. [Gk *pneumon* lung, *sklerosis* hardening.]

pneumoscrotum (new·mo·**skro**·tum). Emphysema of the scrotal tissues. [Gk *pneuma* air, scrotum.]

pneumosepticaemia (**new**·mo·sep·te·**se**'·me·ah). A fulminating fatal type of influenzal pneumonia. [Gk *pneumon* lung, sepsis, Gk *haima* blood.]

pneumoserosa (**new**·mo·ser·**o**'·sah). Insufflation of air into a joint cavity as a preliminary to x-ray examination.

pneumoserothorax (**new**·mo·seer·o·**thor**'·ax). The presence of gas or air and serous fluid in the cavity of the thorax. [Gk *pneuma* air, serum, thorax.]

pneumosilicosis (**new**·mo·sil·ik·**o**'·sis). Invasion of the lung tissue by minute dust particles, these carrying a certain amount of silica. [Gk *pneumon* lung, silicosis.]

pneumostratigraphy (**new**·mo·strah·**tig**'·raf·e). A radiological method of demonstrating the pancreas by a combination of retroperitoneal insufflation of oxygen and gaseous distension of the stomach. [Gk *pneuma* air, L *stratum* layer, Gk *graphein* to record.]

pneumotachograph (new·mo·**tak**·o·graf). An instrument which measures the volume of pulmonary ventilation. [Gk *pneuma* air, *tachos* swiftness, *graphein* to record.]

pneumotherapy (new·mo·**ther**·ap·e). 1. Pneumatotherapy; treatment of disease by the use of condensed or rarefied air. 2. The treatment of pulmonary disorders. [Gk *pneuma* air, *pneumon* lung, therapy.]

pneumothermomassage (new·mo·**ther**·mo·mas·**ahzh**'). The use of hot medicated air in physiotherapy. [Gk *pneuma* air, *therme* heat, massage.]

pneumothorax (new·mo·**thor**·ax). The presence of air or gas within the thorax, resulting in partial or complete collapse of the lung. **Artificial pneumothorax.** The intentional introduction of air between the visceral and parietal layers of the pleura, producing relaxation and consequent partial collapse of the underlying lung. Its therapeutic use was confined to selected cases of tuberculosis of the lung but it was much used before the introduction of effective chemotherapy. **Clicking pneumothorax.** Pneumothorax in which a clicking noise is heard by the patient; this is usually synchronous with the heart beat. **Closed pneumothorax.** The presence of air between the intact layers of pleural membrane, resulting in partial or complete collapse of the lung. **Diagnostic pneumothorax.** The induction of an artificial pneumothorax (see above) to determine the position of an intrathoracic lesion in relation to the lung. **Extrapleural pneumothorax.** A pneumothorax produced surgically by the separation of both layers of the pleura from the endothoracic fascia of the mediastinum and chest wall, used in the treatment of tuberculosis of the upper parts of the lungs. **Idiopathic pneumothorax.** The escape of alveolar air into the pleural space without any clinically apparent lesion in the lung. Most commonly, however, this is due to the rupture of an emphysematous bulla or a tuberculous focus too small to be discovered except by thoracoscopy. **Induced pneumothorax.** Artificial pneumothorax (see above). **Insatiable pneumothorax.** Artificial pneumothorax requiring frequent large refills owing to rapid absorption of gas from the intrapleural space. **Open pneumothorax.** A pneumothorax which communicates with the atmosphere through an open wound in the chest wall. **Spontaneous pneumothorax.** A pneumothorax arising of its own accord from rupture of some abnormality of the pleural surface of the lung. **Sucking pneumothorax.** A pneumothorax with a fistulous opening. **Tension pneumothorax.** A pneumothorax in which the rupture of the pleura forms a valvular opening through which air is forced during coughing but cannot escape, and the intrapleural pressure becomes positive. **Therapeutic pneumothorax.** Artificial pneumothorax (see above). **Traumatic pneumothorax.** Pneumothorax resulting from damage to the chest wall or lung surface, or both, causing leakage of air into the intrapleural space. **Valvular pneumothorax.** A traumatic or spontaneous pneumothorax (see above) wherein air can enter, but cannot leave, the intrapleural space during respiration. [Gk *pneuma* air, thorax.]

pneumotomy (new·**mot**·o·me). The making of an incision into the lung, e.g. for the purpose of drainage. [Gk *pneumon* lung, *temnein* to cut.]

pneumotoxin (new·mo·**tox**·in). A toxin produced by the pneumococcus (*Streptococcus pneumoniae*) and presumed to be the cause of symptoms. Attempts to separate specific soluble toxins from pneumococci have failed, and active immunity is antibacterial and not antitoxic. [Gk *pneumon* lung, toxin.]

pneumotropic (new·mo·**trop**·ik). 1. Having a disposition or preference for the lungs. 2. Having a predilection for pneumococci. [Gk *pneumon* lung, *trope* a turning.]

pneumotyphoid, pneumotyphus (new·mo·**ti**·foid, **new**·mo·**ti**·fus). Typhopneumonia.

pneumo-uria (new·mo·**ewr**·e·ah). Pneumaturia.

pneumoventricle (new·mo·**vent**·rikl). An accumulation of air in the ventricles of the brain. [Gk *pneuma* air, ventricle.]

pneumoventriculography (**new**·mo·ven·**trik**·ew·**log**′·raf·e). X-ray examination of the ventricles of the brain after the cerebrospinal fluid has been removed and replaced with oxygen or air. [Gk *pneuma* air, ventricle, Gk *graphein* to record.]

pneusis (**new**·sis). 1. Respiration. 2. Anhelation; panting in association with dyspnoea. **Pneusis pertussis.** Whooping- cough. [Gk *pneein* to breathe.]

pnigma (**nig**·mah). Strangulation [obsolete term]. [Gk, a choking.]

pnigophobia (ni·go·**fo**·be·ah). A morbid apprehension on the part of an individual that he will choke; a state that may be present in cases of angina pectoris. [Gk *pnigoeis* choking, phobia.]

pock (pok). 1. A localized skin lesion, especially one due to small-pox or chickenpox. 2. A discrete infective focus on the chorio-allantoic membrane of a fertile egg due to a virus, though not all viruses infect this membrane or produce discrete lesions. **Stone pock.** Acne. [AS *pocc*.]

pock-mark (**pok**·mark). A pitted scar that may remain on the skin after a smallpox pustule has healed. [AS pocc, *meark.]*

pocket (**pok**·et). A cavity, usually a patent cavity, e.g. a pathological space between a tooth and the gum. **Accessory pocket.** The term applied to a perigastric cavity as seen at a barium meal in the erect position. Three layers are visible in the cavity: from above downward, air, fluid and barium. **False pocket.** A space between the enamel of a tooth and the gum when the latter has undergone hypertrophic or hyperplastic changes. **Gingival pocket.** Periodontal pocket (see below). **Haem pocket.** The region of a polypeptide chain of a haemoprotein molecule in which the haem prosthetic group is lodged. **Intra-oral pocket.** A pocket or slot made artificially in the mouth to retain a prosthesis, in plastic surgery of the face. **Periodontal pocket.** A pathological increase in the depth of the gingival crevice surrounding a tooth at the gum margin, often extending on to the root surface. **True pocket.** Periodontal pocket (see above). [Fr. *pochette.*]

See also: RATHKE, SEESSEL, TROELTSCH.

pocketing (**pok**·et·ing). 1. The occurrence of closed, or nearly closed, pockets of pus anywhere in the body. 2. The enclosing of the stump of the pedicle of an excised ovarian or other tumour in the edges of the closed incision. [Obsolete term.] [see prec.]

podagra (pod·**ag**·rah). Gout, particularly that which affects the big toe. [Gk, gout in the feet.]

podagral, podagric, podagrous (pod·**ag**·ral, pod·**ag**·rik, pod·**ag**·rus). 1. Gouty; relating or belonging to gout. 2. Afflicted with gout. [see prec.]

podalgia (pod·**al**·je·ah). Sensation of pain in the foot. [Gk *pous* foot, *algos* pain.]

podalic (pod·**al**·ik). 1. Relating or belonging to the feet. 2. Effected by means of the feet, used in obstetrics to describe a method of turning the fetus *in utero* (podalic version). [Gk *pous* foot.]

podarthral (pod·**ar**·thral). Relating or belonging to the metatarsophalangeal joint of the foot (podarthrum). [Gk *pous* foot, *arthron* joint.]

podarthritis (pod·ar·**thri**·tis). Inflammation affecting any of the joints of the foot. [Gk *pous* foot, arthritis.]

podarthrocace (pod·ar·**throk**·as·e). Caries of the joints of the foot. [Gk *pous* foot, arthrocace.]

podarthrum (pod·**ar**·thrum). A metatarsophalangeal joint. [Gk *pous* foot, *arthron* joint.]

podelkoma (pod·el·**ko**·mah). Mycetoma. [Gk *pous* foot, *helkos* ulcer, *-oma* tumour.]

podencephalus (pod·en·**kef**·al·us). A monster the major portion of whose brain is outside the cranium, only a pedicle attaching it to the top of the head. [Gk *pous* foot, *egkephalos* brain.]

podiatrist (po·**di**·at·rist). A chiropodist. [Gk *pous* a foot, *iatros* surgeon.]

podiatry (po·**di**·at·re). Chiropody. [see prec.]

podobromhidrosis (**pod**·o·brom·**hid**·**ro**′·sis). Sweating of the feet, with very offensive smell. [Gk *pous* foot, bromhidrosis.]

podocyte (**pod**·o·site). One of the complex epithelial cells which form an incomplete covering for the capillaries of the glomeruli of the kidney. [Gk *pous* foot, *kytos* cell.]

pododynamometer (**pod**·o·di·nam·**om**′·et·er). A dynamometer for measuring the strength of the leg or foot muscles. [Gk *pous* foot, dynamometer.]

pododynia (pod·o·**din**·e·ah). Pain of burning character affecting the sole of the foot, e.g. in those who sit in cramped positions, such as tailors; physical or other signs are absent. [Gk *pous* foot, *odyne* pain.]

podoedema (pod·e·**de**·mah). Oedema of the feet. [Gk *pous* foot, oedema.]

podogram (**pod**·o·gram). 1. An imprint of the sole of the foot. 2. A traced outline of the sole of the foot. [Gk *pous* foot, *gramma* a writing.]

podograph (**pod**·o·graf). The apparatus with which a podogram is made. [Gk *pous* foot, *graphein* to record.]

podology (pod·**ol**·o·je). The branch of medical science which deals with the feet. [Gk *pous* foot, *logos* science.]

podometer (pod·**om**·et·er). Pedometer. [Gk *pous* foot, *metron* measure.]

podophyllin (pod·o·**fil**·in). Podophyllum resin.

podophyllotoxin (pod·o·**fil**·o·**tox**′·in). $C_{15}H_{16}O_6$, a crystalline purgative substance occurring in podophyllum. Podophyllum resin contains from 20 to 40 per cent according to source.

Podophyllum (pod·o·**fil**·um). A genus of plants of the family Berberidaceae. The root and rhizome (BPC 1968) of *Podophyllum peltatum* Linn., also known as *may-apple,* and *wild* or *American mandrake,* found in eastern Canada and the USA, yields from 2 to 8 per cent of the podophyllum resin which has strong purgative properties. **Indian Podophyllum BPC 1968.** The dried roots and rhizome of a Himalayan species, *Podophyllum hexandrum* Royle (*Podophyllum emodi* Wall.). It yields from 6 to 12 per cent of a resin similar in properties to that obtained from *Podophyllum peltatum* but differs slightly in composition. **Podophyllum Resin BP 1968.** A mixture of resins obtained from *Podophyllum peltatum* and also from *Podophyllum hexandrum.* It is a purgative. [Gk *pous* foot, *phyllon* leaf.]

podopompholyx (pod·o·**pom**·fol·ix). A pompholyx eruption of the feet. [Gk *pous* foot, *pompholyx* bubble.]

poecil-. For words beginning with **poecil-**, see POIKIL-.

Poehl, Alexander Vasilyevich (b. 1850). Russian biochemist.

Poehl's test. The cholera-red reaction. *See* REACTION.

poenology (pe·**nol**·o·je). Penology; the science and study which deals with the correction and punishment of crime. [Gk *poine* penalty, *logos* science.]

Poggendorf, Johann Christian (b. 1796). German physicist.

Poggendorf cell. Bichromate cell. *See* CELL.

poganiasis (po·go·**ni**·as·is). 1. An excessively heavy growth of beard. 2. A growth of beard on the face of a woman. [Gk *pogonias* bearded.]

pogonion (po·**go**·ne·on). In craniometry, the most anterior point of the chin, the mental point. [Gk, little beard.]

pogonium (po·go·ne·um). 1. Pogonion. 2. A small beard. [see prec.]

Pogostemon (po·go·**ste**·mon). A genus of herbs of the family Labiatae. **Pogostemon cablin.** The source of patchouli oil, used in perfumery. [Gk *pogon* beard, *stemma* wreath.]

poikilergasia (**poi**·kil·er·**ga**′·ze·ah). A psychopathic constitution (Adolf Meyer). [Gk *poikilos* varied, ergasia.]

poikilionia (poi·kil·i·**o**′·ne·ah). Variations in the concentration of electrolytes in the blood. [Gk *poikilos* varied, ion.]

poikiloblast (**poi**·kil·i·**o**′·blast). An irregularly shaped nucleated erythrocyte. [Gk *poikilos* varied, *blastos* germ.]

poikilocyte (**poi**·kil·o·site). An erythrocyte, usually bigger than normal and irregularly shaped, associated with the condition of pernicious anaemia and other anaemias. [Gk *poikilos* varied, *kytos* cell.]

poikilocythaemia (**poi**·kil·o·si·**the**′·me·ah). Poikilocytosis. [poikilocyte, Gk *haima* blood.]

poikilocytosis (**poi**·kil·o·si·**to**′·sis). A condition of the blood in which there are large numbers of poikilocytes, as in pernicious and certain other anaemias. [poikilocyte, Gk *-osis* condition.]

poikilodentosis (**poi**·kil·o·den·**to**′·sis). Mottled enamel. [Gk *poikilos* varied, L *dens* tooth, Gk *-osis* condition.]

poikiloderma (**poi**·kil·o·**der**′·mah). Variegated skin. **Poikiloderma atrophicans vasculare.** Poikiloderma vascularis atrophicans (see below). **Poikiloderma congenitale.** A congenital defect of the skin, first described by M.S. Thomson, which begins in infancy and is characterized by telangiectasia, pigmentation and fine atrophy. The eruption develops on the buttocks and cheeks, and spreads to involve other areas. Abnormalities of the bones may be noted. **Reticulated pigmented poikiloderma.** Poikiloderma of Civatte; a reticulated pigmentation of the face, neck and upper part of the chest, occurring in middle-aged women. It is thought to be the same condition as Riehl's melanosis. **Poikiloderma vascularis atrophicans** (Jacobi). Atrophia cutis reticularis cum pigmentatione (Zinsser), atrophoderma erythematodes reticularis (Muller), dermatitis atrophicans reticularis (Glück); a generalized dermatosis of unknown cause, almost invariably occurring in adult life, approximately symmetrical in distribution, and characterized by widespread telangiectasia, pigmentation and cutaneous atrophy. The buccal mucosae may be affected. [Gk *poikilos* varied, *derma* skin.]

See also: CIVATTE.

poikilodermatomyositis (**poi**·kil·o·**der**·mat·o·mi·o·**si**′·tis). A variety of dermatomyositis with poikilodermatous changes. [Gk *poikilos* varied, dermatomyositis.]

poikilodermia (**poi**·kil·o·**der**′·me·ah). Poikiloderma.

poikilodermie et poikilodermatomyosite (**poi**·kil·o·**der**′·me et **poi**·kil·o·der·**mat**′·o·mi·o·site). The poikilodermatous skin changes which follow some cases of dermatomyositis; this French term was once widely used.

poikilonymy (poi·kil·**on**·im·e). The use of terms from several nomenclatures to denote the same organ or part. [Gk *poikilos* varied, *onoma* name.]

poikilopicria (**poi**·kil·o·**pik**′·re·ah). Changes in the acid-base balance of the blood due to alterations in the anion concentrations. [Gk *poikilos* varied, *pikros* bitter.]

poikiloplastocyte (**poi**·kil·o·**plas**′·to·site). A blood platelet of abnormal shape. [Gk *poikilos* varied, plastocyte.]

poikilotherm (**poi**·kil·o·therm). An animal whose temperature varies with that of its surroundings. [see foll.]

poikilothermal, poikilothermic (**poi**·kil·o·**ther**′·mal, **poi**·kil·o·**ther**′·mik). 1. Relating or belonging to poikilothermism. 2. Denoting certain cold-blooded animals or plants the temperatures of which vary with the temperature of their surroundings. 3. Having the capacity to exist in media of varying temperature. [Gk *poikilos* varied, *therme* heat.]

poikilothermism, poikilothermy (**poi**·kil·o·**ther**′·mizm, **poi**·kil·o·**ther**′·me). The capacity of living organisms, including cold-blooded animals, to adapt themselves to changes of environmental temperature. [see prec.]

poikilothrombocyte (**poi**·kil·o·**throm**′·bo·site). A blood platelet of distorted shape. [Gk *poikilos* varied, thrombocyte.]

poikilothymia (**poi**·kil·o·**thi**′·me·ah). A condition characterized by abnormal swings of mood from depression to elation. [Gk *poikilos* varied, *thymos* mind.]

point (point). 1. A minute spot; [punctum (NA)] a small designated area, especially on the skin surface; the sharp end of an object. 2. To approach and to be about to reach the surface; applied especially to an abscess which works its way towards the skin or into a hollow organ such as the vagina or rectum. **Point of an abscess.** The part of an abscess where its rupture seems imminent; its summit. **Achromic point.** The stage during the hydrolysis of starch by amylases when the iodine indicator no longer gives a colour reaction, signifying the completion of the breakdown of erythrodextrin. **Alveolar point.** The prosthion. **Apophyseal point.** A point midway between the lower borders of the nostrils. **Auricular point.** The centre of the orifice of the external auditory meatus. **Boiling point.** The temperature at which liquid boils or at which the vapour pressure of the liquid is equal to the atmospheric pressure. **Cardinal points.** Three pairs of points, the two nodal points, the two principal points, and the two principal foci, of a system of lenses centred in the same optical axis. By Gauss' theorem, if the combined points are known the image can be easily constructed. They are used in ophthalmology in the schematic eye. **Cold point.** A spot on the skin which gives a vivid sense of cold when touched with the end of a cold metal rod and does not give a sensation of heat when touched with a warm instrument. **Cold rigor point.** The level of cold temperature at which cell activity ceases. **Conjugate points.** The positions, which can be reversed, of image and object when rays of light are deflected to form an image. **Contact point.** The point on the interproximal surface of a tooth abutting on an adjoining tooth. **Point of convergence.** 1. The point to which rays of light converge. 2. Near point; far point (see below). **Corresponding retinal points.** Paired points in the retinae of the two eyes which are stimulated by the same object and so give rise to a binocular sensation of a single fused image, e.g. the maculae. **Critical point.** 1. The temperature above which it is impossible to liquefy a gas by application of pressure alone. 2. The highest possible temperature at which a liquid condition is possible; above it the substance can exist only as a gas. 3. The temperature at which a change in the physical properties of a substance occurs. **Deaf point.** Deaf field. *See* FIELD. **Dew point.** 1. The temperature at which moisture actually in the atmosphere is sufficient to saturate it. 2. The temperature to which air must be cooled to produce saturation, or to cause dew to form. **Point of direction.** That portion of the presenting part of a fetus which temporarily approaches or ultimately comes to pass under the pubic arch. **Point of divergence.** The point in an optical system from which rays of light diverge. **Dorsal point.** A point between the spinous processes of the vertebrae at the level of the 4th and 5th intercostal spaces 20 or 30 mm from the middle line. It is tender in cases of biliary colic. **Points douloureux.** Tender points on the course of a nerve with neuralgia. **Point of election.** Site of election; the optimum level at which to carry out an operative procedure, applied especially to amputation and to bowel resection. **Far point.** 1. Of accommodation: the furthest distance from the eye at which an object can be clearly seen, i.e. when accommodation is fully relaxed. 2. Of convergence: the point at which the visual axes of the two eyes meet when at rest, usually at infinity as axes are often slightly divergent. **Fixation point.** The point or object at which the gaze is directed and through which the visual axis and fixation axes pass. **Flash point.** A specific constant for volatile liquids whose vapours are inflammable; the lowest temperature at which the vapour will ignite. **Focal point.** The point at which rays of light, or their prolongation, meet when deflected either by refraction or reflection; the focus. **Freezing point.** The temperature at which a substance changes from the liquid to the solid state. **Fusing point.** Melting point (see below). **Gaussian points.** Geometrical points introduced by Gauss, used in the theory of compound lenses for ray-tracing through the system. **Homologous point.** In radiology, identical points in stereometric or stereoscopic films. **Hot point.** A spot on the skin which gives a sensation of warmth when touched with a hot instrument but does not respond to cold. **Hystero-epileptogenic point, Hysterogenous point.** A point which, when pressed upon, may provoke a hysterical or hystero-epileptic seizure; a very unsatisfactory term. **Identical retinal points.** Corresponding retinal points (see above). **Point of incidence.** The point at which a ray of light falls on a surface. **Iso-electric point.** The particular pH value of solution (true or colloidal) of an amphoteric electrolyte such as an amino acid or protein at which the molecules of the latter are electrically neutral owing to equality of ionization. At this point the molecules will not migrate ionically and the substance has minimum solubility, a fact made use of in precipitating proteins. **Jugal point.** The point of meeting of the zygomatic arch and the frontal process of the zygomatic bone. **Point of maximum impulse.** The point at which the apex beat of the heart is felt most intensely. **Melting point.** The characteristic and constant temperature at which a solid changes into a liquid state. **Mental point.** The pogonion. **Motor point.** That point on the skin over a muscle at which electrical stimulation causes contraction of the muscle. **Nasal point.** The nasion. **Near point.** 1. Of accommodation: the nearest distance from the eye at which small print can be seen clearly, using maximum accommodation. 2. Of convergence: the nearest distance from the eyes to which an object can be brought without becoming double. *See also* NEAR-POINT. **Neutral point.** In titration, the point at which the indicator changes, denoting neutralization of the reactant solutions. **Nodal points.** Of the eye, the optical centre; of any system of lenses, two points situated on the common optical axis corresponding to the optical centre of a single lens. An incident ray passing through the first nodal point will emerge from the system through the second nodal point, and parallel to the original incident ray. In the schematic eye of Gullstrand they are situated close together in the posterior part of the crystalline lens. **Occipital point.** The point in the median plane upon the occipital bone that lies farthest from the glabella. **Ossification point.** Centre of ossification. **Painful point.** In cases of neuralgia in the distribution of a particular nerve, exquisitely tender points along the course of the nerve; these are also known as *puncta dolorosa* or *Valleix's points.* **Phrenic pressure point.** A point on the right phrenic nerve between the sternocleidomastoid and scalenus anterior muscles which is tender in disease of the gall bladder. **Pre-auricular point.** A point immediately in front of the auricular point on Reid's base line. **Pressure point.** 1. A point at which pain is felt on deep pressure. 2. A small area where on account of the prominence of a bone near the surface, and of continual external pressure on the skin that may result from the unchanged position of a patient lying in bed, or from pressure of some appliance on such areas, the skin becomes red and sore, and may break down and form a bedsore. 3. A point at which pressure should be exerted to control haemorrhage from an underlying artery. **Pressure-arresting point.** A point, pressure upon which arrests spasm. **Pressure-exciting point.** A point, pressure upon which excites spasm. **Principal points.** Two points situated on the common optical axis of a system of lenses and corresponding to the conjugate foci of a single lens. In the schematic eye of Gullstrand they are situated close together in the anterior chamber. **Reflection point.** The point on the surface of a body at which a ray of light is reflected. **Refraction point.** The point on the surface of a body at which a ray of light is refracted. **Point of regard.** Fixation point (see above). **Registration point.** In craniometry, the midpoint of the perpendicular dropped from the midpoint of the sella turcica to the Bolton nasion plane. It is used to orientate lateral skull x-rays. **Retromandibular tender point.** A point of tenderness situated behind the ramus of the lower jaw, below the lobe of the ear and in front of the mastoid process. In cases of meningitis, pressure on this point causes severe pain. **Point of reversal.** During retinoscopy of the eye, the point where the so-called shadow in the pupil changes its movement from with to against that of the mirror, or *vice versa.* **S point.** The centre of the sella turcica. **Saturation point.** 1. In hygrometry: the temperature to which the atmosphere must be lowered so that the moisture it contains saturates it, and dew is deposited. 2. Of a solution: the particular concentration of solute at which the solvent will take up no more for the given temperature. **Scapular point.** A tender zone at the inferior angle of the scapula in brachial neuritis. **Spinal point, Subnasal point.** The midpoint of the lower border of the nasal orifice. **Supra-auricular point.** A point on the posterior root of the zygomatic arch directly above the auricular point. **Supranasal point.** The ophryon. **Supra-orbital point.** 1. The midpoint of the transverse supra-orbital line; ophryon. 2. In cases of supra-orbital neuralgia, a tender point in the region of the supra-orbital notch; a Valleix's point. **Thermal death point.** The degree of heat necessary to kill all the organisms in a culture in a given time (usually 10 minutes). **Trigger point.** A point, the stimulation of which may initiate changes in neighbouring or distant parts of the organism. **Triple point.** If a substance can exist in three phases, e.g. liquid, solid, vapour, a pressure–temperature equilibrium line can be found for each phase pair, liquid/solid, solid/vapour, liquid/vapour. The triple point is the point of intersection of the three equilibrium lines, and is defined by a temperature and a pressure. **Vital point.** An area in the floor of the 4th ventricle, overlying the respiratory centre, puncture of which causes death. [L *punctus* pricked.]

See also: ADAMSON, ADDISON (C.), BARKER (A. E. J.), BEARD, BOAS, BOLTON, BREWER (G. E.), BROCA, CAPURON, CHAUFFARD, CLADO, COPE (V. Z.), COVA, DESJARDIN, ERB, GUÉNEAU DE MUSSY, HALLÉ, HARTMANN (H.), HUETER, KANAVAL, KEEN, KIENBOECK, KOCHER, KUEMMELL, LANZ, LENZMANN, LIAN, LOTHEISSEN, MCBURNEY, MACKENZIE, MAYO-ROBSON, MÉGLIN, MORRIS (R. T.), PAGNIELLO, RAMOND (F.), ROLANDO, SUDECK, TROUSSEAU, VALLEIX, VOGT (P. F. E.), VOILLEMIER, WEBER (W. E.), ZIEMSSEN.

pointillage (point·il·ahzh). Massage with the tips of the fingers. [Fr., stippling.]

pointing (point·ing). The process of reaching a point. **Pointing of an abscess.** The process by which pus from a deep-seated abscess tracks to and inflames the skin or the epithelium of a hollow viscus, which it may eventually penetrate. **Past pointing.** Incoordination of voluntary movements seen in disseminated sclerosis. [L *punctus* pricked.]

Poirier, Paul (b. 1853). Paris surgeon.

Poirier's gland. A lymph node lying on the uterine artery in the base of the broad ligament.

Poirier's line. A line from the nasion, passing 5 mm above the external auditory meatus, extending to the lambda.

poise (poiz). A unit of viscosity equal to 0.1 Pa.s (pascal second) defined as the tangential shearing force over 10^{-4}m^2 area of liquid which is moving with a velocity gradient of 0.01 m/s. [J. L. M. *Poiseuille.]*

Poiseuille, Jean Léonard Marie (b. 1799). Paris physiologist. **Poiseuille's law.** The rate of flow of a liquid in a tube is given by the formula (*Poiseuille's formula*)

$$\frac{\pi pr^4}{8l\eta}$$

where p is the pressure of the liquid, r the radius of the tube, l its length, and η the coefficient of viscosity.
Poiseuille's space. In a cross-section of a blood vessel, the space at the periphery in which the movement of the red blood cells is reduced to a minimum.

poison (poi·zn). A noxious substance which, by its action on organs or tissues of the body, can impair function or destroy life. **Acrid poison.** An irritant poison. **Acronarcotic poison, Acrosedative poison.** A poison having both irritant and depressive actions, e.g. chloroform, aconite. **Arrow poison.** A poison used for tipping arrows, e.g. curare. **Cellular poison.** One causing damage to cells. **Corrosive poison.** One that burns or otherwise destroys tissue. **Fatigue poison.** A toxic substance formed in muscle action and limiting further activity. **Fugu poison.** Toxic matter in the flesh of fish of the genus *Tetrodon,* found in Eastern waters. **Haemotropic poison.** A toxin acting especially on erythrocytes, e.g. cobra venom. **Irritant poison.** One causing irritation of surfaces with which it comes into contact, e.g. arsenic. **Mitotic poison.** One that acts by preventing mitosis. **Muscle poison.** One impairing the function of muscle, e.g. lead. **Narcotic poison.** A poison which depresses the brain centres, causing unconsciousness, e.g. opium. **Ordeal poison.** A noxious substance administered to a suspected person as a method of deciding guilt or innocence, e.g. a toxic bark used by savages. **Primrose poison.** The sap of *Primula obconica,* a cause of contact dermatitis. **Sedative poison.** One causing depression of the vital centres, e.g. bromide; under certain circumstances, alcohol. **Toot poison.** *See* CORIARIA SARMENTOSA. **Vascular poison.** A poison that damages blood vessels and affects vasomotor activities. [L *potio* drink.]

Poisons Act 1972. This Act consolidates certain enactments relating to poisons. It retains the Poison Board, an advisory committee, and the Poison List, both established by the Pharmacy and Poisons Act 1933. The List consists of non-medicinal poisons which are prohibited from being sold except by a person lawfully conducting a retail pharmacy business or by a person whose name is on a local authority list. The regulation of sale of poisons extends to a prescribed manner of labelling of poison containers, including the name of the poison, the proportion it bears to the ingredients of the container and the name and address of the seller. The Secretary of State is empowered to make rules for (a) regulating, restricting or prohibiting the sale of poisons and (b) the storage, transport and labelling of poisons.

poisoning (poi·zning). The condition brought about by a poison. **Acetosalicylic-acid poisoning, Acetylsalicylic-acid poisoning.** That due either to ingestion of a large quantity of aspirin (suicidal) or idiosyncrasy to the drug (accidental). With large quantities death may be rapid or delayed. The symptoms are sweating, air hunger and vomiting. **Ackee poisoning.** A frequently fatal illness, occurring especially in children in the West Indies, due to the eating of unripe fruit of the ackee tree, *Blighia sapida;* this fruit is not normally poisonous and malnutrition is probably an essential factor. Gastrointestinal irritation is followed after a calm interval by cerebral vomiting, convulsions and coma. The toxic factors are hypoglycins A and B, which cause profound hypoglycaemia; the effect is more marked in malnourished children. **Aconite poisoning.** Poisoning by the active principle of *Aconitum napellus* (monkshood, wolfsbane), causing especially pressure on the chest, numbness and paralysis. **Alcohol poisoning.** 1. Ethyl alcohol (acute); symptoms will vary according to the individual, the form and conditions under which the alcohol is taken (e.g. full or empty stomach). It acts first as an excitant, and then as a depressant of the nervous system, the various stages being irritability, excitability, inco-ordination, delayed reaction time, slurring of speech, coma, respiratory failure and death. Blood and urine analysis show the ratio to be 1:1.3 and in most cases with a blood level of 0.2 per cent there will be some symptoms, whilst with 0.5 per cent coma and death may occur. There may, however, be a wide individual variation. 2. Methyl alcohol; symptoms are headaches, nausea, abdominal cramps, muscular weakness, dyspnoea and cyanosis, and coma. It has a special toxic effect in some cases, causing blindness. Fatal dose is 120-240 g. **Amidopyrine poisoning, Aminopyrine poisoning.** Poisoning which may be due to deliberate overdose of amidopyrine (aminopyrine), but more commonly to idiosyncrasy resulting in agranulocytosis (agranulocytic angina), for which reason the drug is in the fourth Schedule of the Pharmacy and Poisons Act. **Amphetamine poisoning.** Poisoning by amphetamine; cases have been described with definite mental symptoms of paranoic character. It is suggested that it can become a drug of addiction. **Aniline poisoning.** Poisoning in industry from inhalation or absorption through the skin of aniline; also from absorption of shoestains, and, in babies, from marked napkins inadequately washed. Acute symptoms are headache, weakness, difficulty in breathing, cyanosis, and occasionally death in coma; chronic symptoms are slight cyanosis, headache, abdominal discomfort and anaemia. **Antimony poisoning.** A poisoning similar to that of arsenic (see foll). **Arsenic poisoning.** The poisoning most commonly associated with homicide, but also frequently used for suicide. There are signs of irritation of the intestine, vomiting, colic pains, diarrhoea, tremors and collapse, usually associated with burning of the mouth a short while after ingestion. **Arsphenamine poisoning.** Poisoning by diaminodihydroxyarsenobenzene dihydrochloride, the original Ehrlich–Hata antisyphilitic of 1910, or any of its derivatives. The toxic symptoms may be similar to those of neoarsphenamine after therapeutic injection, and are related to idiosyncrasy. Oxidation occurs if the compound is exposed to air, greatly increasing toxicity (e.g. cracked ampules). **Aspirin poisoning.** Acetosalicylic-acid poisoning (see above). **Barbital poisoning.** Barbiturate poisoning (see foll.). **Barbiturate poisoning.** Poisoning by barbituric acid or its derivatives which may be suicidal or accidental. Barbiturates are respiratory depressants, the rapidity of death and course of coma being dependent upon such things as whether the barbiturate belongs to the rapid, intermediate or slow groups, and renal or liver damage. **Benzene poisoning.** Poisoning by benzene produced in the distillation of coal tar. It may result in granulocytopenia and aplastic anaemia. **Beryllium poisoning.** Poisoning by the inhalation from the coating of strip-lighting tubes. Of slow development; the symptoms may appear as late as 3 years, with chronic pneumonia (granuloma of the lungs). **Blood poisoning.** A vague non-medical term for septicaemia, and/or toxaemia. **Brass poisoning.** Metal-fume fever. *See* FEVER. **Bromide poisoning.** The condition arising from the cumulative action of bromides taken over too long a period. It causes acne, diminished skin sensibility and sexual power, mental depression and confusion, and may lead to delirium and death. A concentration in the blood of more than 200 mg/100 ml produces definite intoxication. **Broom poisoning.** The symptoms following eating the tops of the common broom plant, *Cytisus scoparius,* due to the contained alkaloids, sparteine and cysticine. They produce paralysis of the peripheral nerve-endings and autonomic ganglia, and cardiac depression. **Cadmium poisoning.** Poisoning by cadmium, used in plating metallic objects and in various metallurgic processes. Poisoning has occurred from the storage of acid foods in plated containers, giving rise to symptoms of gastrointestinal irritation. **Calor-gas poisoning.** This is an inert gas with very small CO content, but poisoning can occur from partial combustion in a confined space, when carbon monoxide will be formed. **Camphor poisoning.** Poisoning by camphor, used in the manufacture of moth repellents and in liniments. It can cause gastrointestinal and neurological symptoms. **Can poisoning.** An American term for poisoning associated with the consumption of tinned (canned) foods.

Cannabis-indica poisoning. Poisoning by hashish, marihuana or Indian hemp, commonly smoked in cigarettes (reefers) which has a depressant action on the brain and produces a sense of lightness with a feeling of power, accompanied by a distortion of time and space. There is a release of inhibition with increased suggestibility and pleasant intoxication. There are no withdrawal symptoms. **Carbon-disulphide poisoning.** An illness marked by weakness, giddiness and insomnia, and by visual and auditory symptoms. It may produce a picture of parkinsonism, thalamic syndrome or choreo-athetosis. It is caused through inhalation of the vapour of carbon disulphide which is used as a solvent. **Carbon-monoxide poisoning.** Asphyxia produced by the inhalation of carbon monoxide and due to its combination with haemoglobin for which it has over 200 times the affinity that oxygen has. Oxygen carriage to the tissues is thus prevented. **Carbon-tetrachloride poisoning.** Poisoning by carbon tetrachloride, used as a fat solvent and also as an anthelminthic; it may cause liver and renal damage. **Cheese poisoning.** Poisoning from toxic substances in the milk of cows that have fed on noxious vegetables. This occurs in some North American provinces at certain seasons. **Chlorate poisoning.** Poisoning commonly by potassium chlorate, causing methaemoglobinaemia and sometimes acute nephritis. The symptoms that follow may include abdominal pain, vomiting, diarrhoea, dyspnoea with a feeling of suffocation, and bluish coloration of the lips. **Chlorine poisoning.** Poisoning by chlorine, an irritant gas producing pulmonary oedema. **Chromium poisoning.** Poisoning by chromic acid and its salts used in tanning, plating, and in the chemical industry. It can produce skin lesions and cancer. **Cryolite poisoning.** Poisoning occurring among aluminium workers from the mineral, cryolite, used in the manufacture of the metal. **Cyanide poisoning.** Poisoning from the action of hydrocyanic acid, either inhaled (fumigation), or ingested, or formed by hydrolysis of cyanides by free hydrochloric acid in the stomach. It is a rapidly absorbed protoplasmatic poison with toxic effects on the tissue enzymes, causing death from anoxia. Common sources are industrial (sodium cyanide), or domestic (potassium or sodium cyanide in killing beetles, or for the destruction of wasps' nests). **Delayed chloroform poisoning.** Toxic hepatitis sometimes seen after chloroform anaesthesia. **Dinitrobenzene poisoning.** Poisoning by any of the three isomeric nitrobenzenes of which the *meta*-compound is the most important. Moderate occupational exposure (from 2 to 4 weeks) causes anaemia with stippled red cells, moderate cyanosis and fatigue. Severe exposure causes marked cyanosis, headache, vertigo, nausea and vomiting. **Dinitrocresol poisoning.** Poisoning by the sodium salt of dinitro-orthocresol, used as a fungicide and insecticide. It causes disorder of the carbohydrate metabolism by interfering with the synthesis of bonded phosphates, the available energy being dissipated as heat; hence this substance, or dinitrophenol, which has a similar action, was used for the treatment of obesity previous to 1939. It causes symptoms akin to heatstroke, sweating, high temperature, dyspnoea and death with indefinite autopsy findings. **Dinitrophenol poisoning.** Poisoning similar to dinitrocresol poisoning. Subacute poisoning causes anorexia, nausea, pyrexia, vomiting, occasionally agranulocytosis, cataract formation and hepatitis; acute poisoning gives symptoms similar to dinitrocresol. **Dioxane poisoning.** Poisoning by dioxane used as solvent for resins, waxes, and in laboratories. Inhalation causes anorexia, vomiting, oliguria, anuria and uraemia, enlarged liver and jaundice. Death occurs from haemorrhagic nephritis and necrosis of the liver. **Dural poisoning.** Poisoning from magnesium in the alloy duralumin used in aircraft construction. **Ethylene poisoning.** Poisoning by ethylene, a colourless gas which when inhaled in sufficiently high concentrations can cause nausea, sometimes preceded by excitement. **Fluoride poisoning.** Poisoning by fluorides used as vermin killers and for moth-proofing. In the acute form it causes nausea, thirst, burning in the mouth and oesophagus, fascicular twitchings and epileptiform convulsions. In the chronic form loss of appetite, nausea and vomiting, osteosclerosis and mottling of the teeth. **Food poisoning.** Poisoning resulting from consumption of harmful foods. These may be articles ordinarily poisonous, such as toadstools eaten in mistake for mushrooms, or articles harmless to most persons but which produce allergic symptoms in individuals sensitive to them. More commonly, the food is wholesome in itself but rendered poisonous from outside sources. Salmonella-group organisms conveyed in food cause infective gastroenteritis. Some types of *Staphylococcus* and *Clostridium botulinum* produce toxins which are not destroyed by cooking. The former is a fairly common cause of severe gastrointestinal upset; the latter is rare, but its action on the central nervous system is often lethal. Rye contaminated by ergot may cause abortion, gangrene and a type of mania. Foods may be contaminated with chemical substances such as arsenic, by faulty manufacture or storage, or rendered toxic by excessive or ill-chosen preservatives. **Fugu poisoning.** Poisoning the result of eating the roe and other parts of certain fish of the species *Diodon, Triodon,* and *Tetradon,* which inhabit eastern Asiatic waters. **Garage poisoning.** Carbon monoxide asphyxia from the exhaust gases of motor-car engines allowed to run in closed spaces. **Gossypol poisoning.** Poisoning from cotton-seed cake. **Hydrogen-fluoride poisoning.** Poisoning by hydrofluoric acid which will cause severe if not fatal burns on the skin which do not look very obvious on examination. It is a respiratory irritant. **Hydrogen-sulphide poisoning.** Poisoning by hydrogen sulphide, a gas with an offensive odour in low concentration but which may not be recognized by smell in high concentration. It is an irritant and a depressant of the central nervous system. It is a constituent of sewer gas and is also used as a laboratory reagent. In industry it is found in petrol distillation, glue and artificial silk manufacture. If inhaled in high concentration (1 in 1000) it causes rapid collapse, convulsions and death; in low concentration, amnesia, delirium and hallucinations, with sleepiness. **Iron poisoning.** Poisoning by iron salts. Ferrous-sulphate tablets mistaken for sweets by children cause vomiting, collapse and, later, liver necrosis. Ferric chloride is a corrosive when taken by mouth, causing vomiting, diarrhoea with collapse, and haemorrhages. Iron encephalopathy, sometimes fatal, has been recorded from therapeutic administration of iron preparations. **Lead poisoning.** Plumbism; acute, or more often chronic, intoxication by lead or its salts. Acute lead poisoning causes severe gastroenteritis. The chronic form is characterized by intestinal colic, anaemia with blue stippling of a proportion of the erythrocytes, and muscular paralysis first affecting the long extensors of the middle and ring fingers, then the long extensors of the wrists (wrist drop). Encephalopathy may occur, also laryngeal paralysis. A blue line may appear on the gums, but indicates absorption not poisoning. Tetra-ethyl-lead, added to petrol, is readily absorbed through the skin. It may cause muscular weakness, tremors, restlessness, delirium and violent mania. **Lewisite poisoning.** Poisoning by the irritant war gas, causing vesication and lung irritation. **Loco poisoning.** Locoism; selenium poisoning in domestic animals from eating vegetables growing in soil containing this element. **Meat poisoning.** Food poisoning from meat. **Methyl-bromide poisoning.** Poisoning by methyl bromide causing local irritation of the eyes, headache, giddiness, vomiting and double vision; there may be a symptom-free period followed by muscular cramps and twitchings, incoordination and diplopia. Sources are refrigeration fluid and some fire extinguishers. **Methyl-chloride poisoning.** Poisoning similar to methyl bromide poisoning, caused by methyl chloride used in the chemical industry and in refrigerators. **Methyl-iodide poisoning.** Poisoning similar to methyl-bromide and methyl-chloride poisoning, caused by methyl iodide used in the chemical industry. **Mushroom poisoning.** The true edible mushroom does not cause poisoning and most fungi are edible. Those particularly poisonous are *Amanita phalloides* in which there is a phosphorus-like action leading to death from hepatic necrosis, and *Amanita muscaria* which has an acetylcholine-like action with salivation, sweating, blurred vision and contracted pupils. Recovery is usual. **Mussel poisoning.** Mytilotoxism; poisoning attributed to eating mussels. The effects are said to be due to mytilotoxin, and the symptoms described include unconsciousness, lividity, stertorous breathing, dilated pupils and diminished reflexes. **Mustard-gas poisoning.** Exposure to low concentrations of mustard gas causes erythema after several hours. More severe exposure produces vesication and ulceration (3rd to 4th day), laryngitis, tracheitis and bronchitis. **Neoarsphenamine poisoning.** Poisoning by the sodium salt of the methylene-sulphoxylate derivative of 3,3-diamino-4,4-dihydroxyarsenobenzene. Toxic symptoms may follow its therapeutic use: 1. Immediate (nitritoid) reaction; flushing of the face, burning taste, oedema of the tongue and eyelids, nausea, vomiting, perspiration, dyspnoea, cyanosis and precordial pain. 2. Herxheimer reaction (1-4 hours); pyrexia, exacerbation of symptoms of syphilis and intensification of secondary rash. 3. Dermatitis (1-14 days); usually subsiding, but exfoliative dermatitis may occur. Purpura, aplastic anaemia and nephritis have been recorded. Hepatitis, previously attributed to the drug, is now believed to be due to virus infection from syringes or apparatus. **Nicotine poisoning.** Poisoning by nicotine insecticide, very rapid and fatal in adequate dosage. It has been used criminally, usually in the form of snuff added to beer or other liquids. There is burning in the mouth, nausea, vomiting, diarrhoea, palpitation, pulmonary oedema and death, sometimes with convulsions and twitchings. **Nitrobenzene poisoning.** Poisoning by nitrobenzene which is more toxic than dinitrobenzene, being absorbed through the skin (shoe dyes), with cyanosis, rapid irregular pulse, nausea, vomiting, epigastric pain and headaches. **Phenytoin poisoning.** Poisoning by soluble phenytoin (sodium diphenylhydantoin) used in epilepsy where the effective dose is near the toxic dose. It causes dizziness, diplopia, fever, dermatitis, purpura, and sometimes greatly increased incidence of fits. Hyperplasia of the gums follows prolonged administration. **Phosphorus poisoning.** Poisoning by yellow phosphorus which is very toxic. There are three stages, acute with nausea, vomiting, and collapse in a matter of hours, a latent period, and death from liver failure. **Potato poisoning.** Poisoning from solanine, found beneath the skin of shrivelled, germinating potatoes. Headaches, vomiting, and muscle cramps are caused. **Sausage poisoning.** Botulism; a rare but often fatal variety of food poisoning due to the action on the nervous system of preformed toxin of *Clostridium botulinum.* **Sewer-gas poisoning.** Poisoning by sewer gases consisting mostly of hydrogen sulphide, but it should be borne in mind that other gases such as carbon monoxide can get into sewers. **Shellfish poisoning.** 1. Enteric infection from shellfish gathered in waters contaminated by sewage. 2. Allergic symptoms in persons sensitive to certain shellfish. 3. Mytilotoxism. **Shoe-dye poisoning.** That which occurs as a result of wearing shoes or clothing dyed with liquids containing aniline or nitrobenzene. Absorption takes place through the skin, causing headache, giddiness, vomiting and extreme cyanosis which is due to conversion of haemoglobin into a pigment of doubtful constitution. Coma and death are readily caused by these substances, but are uncommon in persons whose only exposure is through wearing shoes thus dyed. **Spider poisoning.** Systematic poisoning from the bites of certain spiders. That of the black-widow spider, *Latrodectus mactans,* causes dilatation of the pupils, cyanosis, oedema of the face and extremities, and neurotoxic and peritoneal signs. **Tetrachlorethane poisoning.** Poisoning from a chlorinated hydrocarbon, tetrachlorethane, used as a solvent for cellulose acetate in the manufacture of the dope used for waterproofing aeroplane wings in World War I and in the making of non-inflammable cinema films. It causes severe gastrointestinal symptoms and toxic hepatitis progressing to acute yellow atrophy. **Tetrachloroethylene poisoning.** Poisoning by tetrachloroethylene used as a solvent in industry and also as an anthelminthic. Toxic doses may cause giddiness and vertigo with excessive perspiration. **Thiouracil poisoning.** Poisoning by thiouracil used for the treatment of hyperthyroidism; toxic reactions are produced in about 13 per cent of people, with agranulocytosis, purpura, giddiness and abdominal pain. **Tobacco poisoning.** That due to the alkaloid, nicotine (see above). **Trichlorethylene poisoning.** Poisoning by trichlorethylene used as a solvent in dry-cleaning and as an anaesthetic. It causes unconsciousness and prolonged exposure may be fatal. Optic neuritis followed by atrophy and sensory paralysis of the 5th cranial nerve has been reported from chronic exposure. Taken by mouth it causes salivation and vomiting with liver failure. **Trinitrotoluene poisoning.** Poisoning from the absorption, chiefly through the skin, of trinitrotoluene, a coal-tar derivative handled mainly in the filling of shells by munition workers. The toxic effects include dermatitis, headache, severe gastrointestinal upset, drowsiness, staggering gait, hepatic necrosis and aplastic anaemia.

Poisson, Francis (b. 1871). Lille surgeon and anatomist.

Poisson's fossa. The inferior duodenal peritoneal fossa which is occasionally found and which extends behind the third part of the duodenum.

Poisson, Simeon Denis (b. 1781). French mathematician.

Poisson distribution curve. A curve whose ordinates represent the probability of occurrence of the various possible discrete numbers of events represented by the abscissae when the Poisson law applies.

Poisson law. This is a particular case of the binominal distribution when the probability of an event is very small but when the number of trials is very large so that the mean is finite. The probability of η events $P(\eta)$, when the mean number is μ, is

$$P(\eta) = \frac{e^{-\mu}\mu^{\eta}}{\eta!}$$

The variance of η is μ. This law describes the fluctuations in the numbers of atoms of a radioactive substance which disintegrate in successive time intervals.

Poisson's ratio. The ratio of the lateral strain to the longitudinal strain for a bar acted on by a stress parallel to its length.

Poisson-Pearson formula. A formula used for finding the percentage of error in calculating the endemic index of malaria in a district or locality.

poitrinaire (pwah·treen·a·er). One affected with pulmonary tuberculosis or other chronic thoracic disease. [Fr., a consumptive.]

poke, pokeweed (poke, **poke**·weed). Common names for *Phytolacca.* **Poke berries.** Phytolacca berries. **Poke root.** Phytolacca. [ME *poke,* AS *weod.]*

Poland, Alfred (b. 1920). London surgeon.

Poland's syndrome. Microsyndactyly of one hand with absence of the costal part of the pectoralis major muscle on the same side.

polar (po·lar). 1. Relating or belonging to a pole. 2. Provided with poles, applied to those nerve cells which have one process or more.

polarimeter (po·lar·**im**·et·er). An apparatus for measuring the angle through which the plane of a beam of polarized light is rotated by any interposed substance. An adaptation for liquids is used as a saccharimeter in the analysis of sugars. [see foll.]

polarimetry (po·lar·**im**·et·re). The measurement of the rotation of the plane of a beam of polarized light when passed through certain substances. [polarization, meter.]

polariscope (po·**lar**·e·skope). 1. Polarimeter. 2. An apparatus for the study of phenomena due to polarized light. It consists normally of a polarizer and analyser, both Nicol prisms or polarizing films, between which is placed the substance to be examined. [polarization. Gk *skopein* to watch.]

polariscopic (po·lar·e·**skop**·ik). Referring to the polariscope or to polarimetry.

polariscopy (po·lar·**is**·ko·pe). 1. Polarimetry. 2. The study of the phenomena associated with polarized light. [polarization, Gk *skopein* to watch.]

polaristrobometer (po·lar·is·tro·**bom'**·et·er). A particular form of polarimeter or saccharimeter in which the field is divided vertically into zones. The zero point is reached when the zones appear equally dark, thus enabling a high degree of accuracy to be attained. [polarization, Gk *strobos* a twisting, meter.]

polarity (po·**lar**·it·e). 1. The quality of being polar or of having two points of opposite tendencies. 2. The positivity or negativity of terminals in an electrical circuit. **Dynamic polarity.** That polarity shown in regard to the passage of impulses through nerve cells.

polarization (**po**·lar·i·**za**′·shun). 1. Radiation, which is of a wave nature and in which the vibration occurs in a plane at right angles to the direction of propagation of the wave, is polarized when the vibration in that plane occurs only in certain directions and not at random. The phenomenon of polarization can therefore be observed in electromagnetic radiation, such as light, x-rays or radio waves, which are stated to be plane-polarized if vibration occurs in one direction only in the vibration plane. Plane polarization of light may be produced by passage through a Nicol prism or a sheet of Polaroid. Light may also be circularly or elliptically polarized, and the polarization may be partial or complete. 2. The phenomenon of production of a back e.m.f. in an electrolytic cell by the decomposition products of the electrolyte of the cell. **Cellular polarization.** The condition of muscle and nerve cells in the resting phase; there is a positive charge on the external surface of the cell membrane as compared to the interior of the cell. **Circular polarization.** Light polarized in such a way that the electric vector of the wave motion rotates around the axis of the direction in which the light is propagated. **Electric polarization.** The creation of an electric dipole in an atom as the result of application of an electric field. **Polarization of electrodes.** The accumulation of a charge derived from ions at the electrodes of a cell. **Electrolytic polarization.** The accumulation of the products of ionic dissociation, e.g. gas molecules, at the electrodes, producing increased resistance and eventual stoppage. **Elliptical polarization.** Light polarized in such a way that the electric vector of the wave motion rotates in an ellipse about the direction in which the light is propagated. **Plane polarization.** Light polarized in such a way that the electric vector of the wave motion is in one plane only, the magnetic vector being in the plane at right angles to this, the plane of polarization. **Rotatory polarization.** The rotation of the plane of a beam of plane-polarized light when passed through certain media, e.g. a solution of an optically active isomer. [L *polus* pole.]

polarize (**po**·lar·ize). To produce polarization.

polarizer (**po**·lar·i·zer). The part of a polariscope which causes polarization of light.

polarogram (po·**lar**·o·gram). The curve produced in polarography.

polarography (po·lar·**og**·raf·e). Polarographic analysis; a method of chemical analysis depending upon variations in the potential curve observed when the given substance is electrolysed, employing a dropping mercury electrode. [pole, Gk *graphein* to record.]

Polaroid (**po**·lar·oid). The trade name for a synthetic plastic which has the property of polarizing light.

Poldine Methylsulphate BP 1973 (**pol**·deen meth·il·**sul**′·fate). 2-Benziloyloxymethyl-1,1-dimethylpyrrolidinium methylsulphate; an anticholinergic drug. A selective action on the alimentary canal is claimed. It is used in gastrointestinal disorders for its sustained atropine-like effects.

pole (pole). 1. Either end of any axis. 2. The middle point of the reflecting surface of a mirror. 3. The positive or negative plate of a primary or secondary cell. 4. A point which may be taken as the origin of the magnetic forces of a magnet. On a bar magnet the poles are normally near the ends of the bar. 5. [Polus (NA).] The extremity of a rounded organ, or the highest point on a convex surface. **Animal pole.** That end of the early ovum which shows, or is destined to show, greatest proliferation and metabolic activity, and which eventually forms the head end of the embryo. **Antigerminal pole.** The end of a large-yolked egg, opposite to the germinal disc. **Cephalic pole.** The head of the fetal ovoid. **Pole of the eyeball, anterior [polus anterior** (NA)**].** The central, most anterior, point of the cornea, situated at the anterior end of the geometrical axis. **Pole of the eyeball, posterior [polus posterior** (NA)**].** The central, most posterior, point of the sclera, situated at the posterior end of the geometrical axis. **Frontal pole [polus frontalis** (NA)**].** The anterior extremity of the frontal lobe. **Germinal pole.** The end of a large-yolked egg which contains the germinal disc. **Pole of the lens of the eye, anterior [polus anterior lentis** (NA)**].** The central and most anterior point on the anterior curved surface of the lens, being the anterior end of the axis. **Pole of the lens of the eye, posterior [polus posterior lentis** (NA)**].** The central and most posterior point on the posterior curved surface of the lens, being the posterior end of the axis. **Lower pole.** Antigerminal pole (see above). **Negative pole.** The pole of a primary or secondary cell to which current flows through the external circuit. **Nutritive pole.** Antigerminal pole (see above). **Occipital pole [polus occipitalis** (NA)**].** The rounded posterior extremity of the occipital lobe. **Pelvic pole.** The breech of the fetal ovoid. **Placental pole.** The part of the uterus containing the placenta. **Positive pole.** The pole of a primary or secondary cell from which current flows through the external circuit. **Temporal pole [polus temporalis** (NA)**].** The rounded anterior extremity of the temporal lobe of the cerebrum. **Upper pole.** Germinal pole (see above). **Vegetal pole, Vegetative pole.** Antigerminal pole (see above). **Vitelline pole.** Antigerminal pole (see above). [L *polus.*]

Polemonium (pol·e·**mo**·ne·um). A genus of herbs of the family Polemoniaceae. **Polemonium caereuleum.** Jacob's ladder; a British species used as a diaphoretic and expectorant. **Polemonium reptans.** Abscess root; an American species used for the same purposes as *Polemonium caeruleum.* [Gk *polemonion.*]

Polenské number or value. The number of millilitres of 0.1 M alkali required to neutralize the volatile water-insoluble fatty acids obtained from 5 g of fat.

polianite (**pol**·e·an·ite). Pyrolusite.

Polidexide (pol·e·**dex**·ide). BP Commission approved name for dextran cross-linked with epichlorhydrin and *O*-substituted with 2-diethylaminoethyl groups, some of them quaternized with diethylaminoethyl chloride; it is an anticholesterolaemic agent.

poliheteroxenous (pol·e·het·er·**ox**′·en·us). With numerous intermediate hosts. [Gk *polys* many, *heteros* different, *xenos* host.]

poliocidal (pol·e·o·**si**′·dal). Having the capacity to destroy the virus of acute anterior poliomyelitis. [Gk *polios* grey, L *caedere* to kill.]

polioclastic (pol·e·o·**klas**′·tik). Denoting the viruses of rabies, encephalitis lethargica and poliomyelitis which tend to break down the grey matter of the brain and/or spinal cord. [Gk *polios* grey, *klastos* broken in pieces.]

polio-encephalitis (pol·e·o·en·kef·al·**i**′·tis). Acute inflammation of the grey matter of the brain. The varieties noted have all the same basal pathology, and differ only in the acuteness of the attack and the varying special localization in the brain grey matter. In some cases there are implications of the cord (polio-encephalomyelitis). **Polio-encephalitis acuta infantum.** A febrile type seen in small children, liable to be followed by paralysis. **Acute bulbar polio-encephalitis.** A type affecting specially the grey matter of the bulb. **Anterior superior polio-encephalitis.** Wernicke's encephalopathy; a disorder due to aneurine deficiency and characterized by petechiae and congestion of the mid-brain and diencephalon with vomiting, ophthalmoplegia, nystagmus, disorder of consciousness and sometimes ataxia. **Polio-encephalitis haemorrhagica superior.** Polio-encephalitis affecting the grey matter in the neighbourhood of the 3rd and 4th ventricles. [Gk *polios* grey, encephalitis.]

polio-encephalomeningomyelitis (pol·e·o·en·**kef**·al·o·men·**ing**·go·mi·el·**i**′·tis). Inflammation affecting the grey matter of the spinal cord and brain as well as the meninges. [Gk *polios* grey, *egkephalos* brain, meninges, myelitis.]

polio-encephalomyelitis (pol·e·o·en·**kef**·al·o·mi·el·**i**′·tis). Polio-encephalitis in which the cord is also involved. [Gk *polios* grey, *egkephalos* brain, myelitis.]

polio-encephalopathy (pol·e·o·en·kef·al·**op**′·ath·e). Any pathological condition of the grey matter of the brain. [Gk *polios* grey, *egkephalos* brain, *pathos* disease.]

polio-encephalotropic (pol·e·o·en·kef·al·o·trop'·ik). Having a marked affinity for the grey matter of the brain. [Gk *polios* grey, *egkephalos* brain, *trope* a turning.]

poliomyelencephalitis (pol·e·o·mi·el·en·kef·al·i'·tis). Polio-encephalomyelitis.

poliomyeliticidal (pol·e·o·mi·el·it·is·i'·dal). Having a destructive action on the virus of poliomyelitis. [poliomyelitis, L *caedere* to kill.]

poliomyelitis (pol·e·o·mi·el·i'·tis). An acute inflammation of the anterior horn cells of the spinal cord due to an enterovirus infection. The great majority of cases in an unprotected population are due to polioviruses (Syn. acute anterior poliomyelitis, infantile paralysis). A flaccid paralysis of the limbs served by the damaged lower motor neurons may result, though paralysis is an uncommon sequel of infection with the virus which often does not progress beyond the cells of the gut. There is no specific treatment, other than supportive, and there is some recovery of function following reduction in the reactive oedema in the central nervous system. Adequate protection can be provided by immunization. There are two forms of vaccine: live attenuated virus (Sabin type) and formalized inactivated virus (Salk type). **Bulbar poliomyelitis.** Poliomyelitis with involvement of the brain-stem nuclei giving rise to progressive bulbar paralysis, respiratory and vasomotor failure. [Gk *polios* grey, *myelos* marrow, *-itis* inflammation.]

poliomyelo-encephalitis (pol·e·o·mi·el·o·en·kef·al·i'·tis). Polio-encephalomyelitis. [Gk *polios* grey, *myelos* marrow, encephalitis.]

poliomyelopathy (pol·e·o·mi·el·op'·ath·e). Any disease affecting the grey matter of the spinal cord and medulla oblongata. [Gk *polios* grey, *myelos* marrow, *pathos* disease.]

polioneuromere (pol·e·o·newr·o·meer). A segment of the grey matter of the spinal cord in the embryo. [Gk *polios* grey, *neuron* nerve, *meros* part.]

polioplasm (pol·e·o·plazm). The granular protoplasm of a cell. [Gk *polios* grey, plasma.]

poliosis (pol·e·o·sis). 1. Greying of the hair resulting from lack of pigment. 2. Premature canities. **Poliosis eccentrica.** Irregular patches of white hair; partial albinism. [Gk *polios* grey.]

poliothrix (pol·e·o·thrix). Canities; the process of turning grey-haired. [Gk *polios* grey, *thrix* hair.]

poliovirus (pol·e·o·vi·rus). The most frequent cause of human poliomyelitis. A small 25 nm RNA virus of the enterovirus genus. There are three serological types of which type I is most likely to cause a paralytic infection. Attenuated strains have been produced by repeated passage in monkey kidney cells in culture, and have been used in oral vaccines (Sabin-type vaccine). Type III has proved to be the most difficult type to attenuate and often provokes the least response to a trivalent vaccine containing all three serotypes. A vaccine using virus inactivated with formalin (Salk-type vaccine) and given by intramuscular injection was developed before the Sabin vaccine. This gives good individual protection but does little to hinder spread of the wild virus in the community. [Gk *polios* grey, L *virus* poison.]

Polish plait (po·lish plat). Plica polonica; a condition seldom seen and once thought to be peculiar to Poles, but also reported from many parts of the world. The "plait" is a matted mass of hair, lice, dirt, serum and pus developing on the crown of the head and due to parasitic invasion, infection and neglect. [*Poland*, OFr. *pleit.*]

polisography (pol·is·og·raf·e). The making of more than one exposure on a radiographic film. [Gk *polys* many, *isos* equally divided, *graphein* to record.]

Politzer, Adam (b. 1835). Vienna otologist.

Politzer's abscess. An abscess occurring rarely in the internal auditory meatus as a complication of suppurative labyrinthitis.

Politzer's acoumeter. For testing hearing: a standard sound simulating a watch tick is produced by the fall of a percussion hammer on to a steel cylinder. The distance at which this acoumeter can be heard when horizontally in line with each external auditory meatus is measured, the opposite ear being occluded by a moistened finger.

Politzer's bag. A bag of flexible rubber, used for inflating the middle ear.

Politzer's cone. A triangle area of light, the apex of which is at the tip of the malleus with the general direction downwards and forwards, the base of the triangle being formed at the junction of the drum with the tympanic annulus. It is an optical effect resulting from the convexity of the drum head.

Politzer's operation. For the treatment of chronic middle-ear deafness: by making an artificial opening into the ear-drum, or by dividing the ligament of the malleus.

Politzer's hearing test. A vibrating tuning fork in front of the nostrils is normally heard more clearly on deglutition. In a unilateral middle-ear disease, with an impermeable pharyngotympanic tube, vibrations will be perceived only in the normal ear. In middle-ear disease with a patent tube, the tuning fork will appear louder on the affected side. In unilateral internal-ear types of deafness, the vibrations are heard only in the normal ear. In cases of inactive otitis media with perforation or cicatrices of the tympanic membrane, the sound heard through an auscultatory tube may appear much increased.

Politzer's treatment. The forcing of air along the pharyngotympanic tube by the sudden increase of the pressure in the postnasal space. A rubber bag (Politzer's bag) is introduced into one nostril, the opposite nostril is blocked, and the patient blows out his cheeks. The sudden compression of the bulb produces a sudden rise in postnasal pressure, and some of this air tends to escape along the pharyngotympanic tube.

politzerization (pol·it·zer·i·za'·shun). Inflation of the middle ear and pharyngotympanic tube by the Politzer bag. **Negative politzerization.** The withdrawal of secretions contained in a cavity by a sucking action produced by the Politzer bag attached to a tube introduced into the cavity. [Adam *Politzer.*]

pollakiuria (pol·ak·e·ewr'·e·a). Frequent micturition. [Gk *pollache* often, *ouron* urine.]

pollantin (pol·an·tin). An antitoxic horse-blood serum obtained by inoculating the horse with pollen extracts. It was formerly used in the treatment of hay fever, but is now discredited. [pollen, Gk *anti.*]

pollen (pol·en). The fine powdery dust expelled from the anthers of seed plants; each granule is a male fecundating agent or microspore. [L, dust.]

pollenogenic (pol·en·o·jen'·ik). Producing or produced by pollen. [pollen, Gk *genein* to produce.]

pollenosis (pol·en·o·sis). Hay fever. *See* FEVER. [pollen, Gk *-osis* condition.]

pollex (pol·ex) (pl. *pollices*). The thumb. **Pollex extensus.** The permanent backward deviation of the thumb. **Pollex flexus.** Fixed flexion of the thumb. **Pollix pedis.** The big toe. **Pollex valgus.** Fixed deviation of the thumb towards the fingers. **Pollex varus.** Fixed deviation of the thumb away from the fingers. [L.]

pollicial (pol·is·e·al). Relating or belonging to the thumb. [L *pollex* thumb.]

pollicization (pol·is·i·za'·shun). A plastic surgical procedure in which an artificial thumb is constructed from neighbouring tissue. [L *pollex* thumb.]

pollination (pol·in·a·shun). In botany, the process by which pollen is dusted on the stigma of a seed plant so that fertilization takes place.

pollinosis (pol·in·o·sis). Hay fever. *See* FEVER. [pollen, Gk *-osis* condition.]

Pollitzer, Sigmund (b. 1859). New York dermatologist.

Pollitzer's disease. Folliclis.

pollodic (pol·od·ik). Panthodic; denoting nerve stimuli which radiate from one centre. [Gk *polys* many, *hodos* way.]

pollopas (pol·o·pas). A type of glass whose power of absorbing ultraviolet and infrared radiation is less than that of flint glass.

pollution (pol·ew·shun). 1. The act of polluting. 2. Defilement. 3. The voluntary or involuntary emission of semen at other times than during coitus. **Diurnal pollution, Pollution nimiae.** Spermatorrhoea. **Nocturnal pollution.** Involuntary emission of semen during sleep. [L *polluere* to defile.]

polocyte (**po**·lo·site). Polar body; one of the small cells which are cast off from the ovum during its maturation divisions. [Gk *polos* pole, *kytos* cell.]

polonium (po·**lo**·ne·um). A radioactive element of atomic number 84, and chemical symbol Po. It is one of the disintegration products of uranium and its longest-lived isotope ^{210}Po has a half-life of 138.4 days. [*Poland*, native land of the discoverer, Mme Curie.]

Poloxalkol (pol·**ox**·al·kol). BP Commission approved name for a polymer of ethylene oxide, propylene oxide and propylene glycol; a surface-active agent.

Polphila (pol·**fi**·lah). A genus of Australian finches that may be infected with ornithosis.

poltophagy (pol·**tof**·aj·e). Thorough mastication so that the food is reduced to a pulpy mass; Fletcherism. [Gk *poltos* porridge, *phagein* to eat.]

polus (**po**·lus). A pole; the extremity of a rounded organ, or the highest point of a convex surface, e.g. the frontal pole of the brain. [L.]

Pólya, Eugene Jenö Alexander (b. 1876). Budapest surgeon.

Pólya's gastrectomy, or operation. Gastrectomy with reconstitution by implantation of the stomach end-to-side in the jejunum.

polyacid (pol·e·**as**·id). An alcohol or base which contains two or more hydroxyl OH groups that will combine with the hydrogen atoms of acids. [Gk *polys* many, acid.]

polyacoustic (**pol**·e·ak·**oos**'·tik). 1. Magnifying or multiplying sound. 2. A device for magnifying sound. [Gk *polys* much, *akoustos* audible.]

polyacrylonitrile (**pol**·e·ak·ril·o·**ni**'·trile). Polyvinyl cyanide, a polymer of vinyl cyanide used as the synthetic fibre.

polyadenia (**pol**·e·ad·**e**'·ne·ah). Lymphadenoma. [Gk *polys* many, *aden* gland.]

polyadenitis (**pol**·e·ad·en·**i**'·tis). Inflammation affecting several glands simultaneously, more especially in the neck. **Malignant polyadenitis.** Bubonic plague. *See* PLAGUE. [Gk *polys* many, adenitis.]

polyadenoma (**pol**·e·ad·en·**o**'·mah). Multiple adenomata. [Gk *polys* many, adenoma.]

polyadenomatosis (**pol**·e·ad·en·o·mat·**o**'·sis). A morbid condition marked by the presence of multiple adenomata. [polyadenoma, Gk *-osis* condition.]

polyadenopathy (**pol**·e·ad·en·**op**'·ath·e). Any morbid condition in which many glands are involved simultaneously. [Gk *polys* many, *aden* gland, *pathos* disease.]

polyadenosis (**pol**·e·ad·en·**o**'·sis). A disordered condition of several glands; an unsatisfactory word. [Gk *polys* many, *aden* gland, *-osis* condition.]

polyadenous (pol·e·**ad**·en·us). Relating to, bearing or involving many glands. [Gk *polys* many, *aden* gland.]

polyaemia (pol·e·e·me·ah). An increase in the volume of the blood; such increase of volume with a normal composition of the blood probably does not occur. The volume of plasma is very constant and depends upon the balance between the fluid in the vessels and in the tissue spaces; any tendency for the volume to increase leads to fluid passing from the vessels to the tissues and urine. Drinking a considerable volume of water causes only a slight dilution of the blood. The increase in volume after intravenous injection of normal saline is only temporary, whilst hypertonic saline injected intravenously or *per rectum* causes a flow of fluid from tissue spaces to the blood and has a longer effect. The corpuscular volume can vary considerably and so alter the total volume of blood, which volume is also increased temporarily by contraction and emptying of the spleen. An increased volume occurs during pregnancy and with exposure to high external temperatures. Pathologically it is moderately increased in congestive heart failure, cirrhosis of the liver, chlorosis, splenomegaly, leukaemia and erythrocytosis, and greatly increased in polycythaemia vera. [Gk *polys* much, *haima* blood.]

polyaesthesia (**pol**·e·es·**the**'·ze·ah). A disorder of sensation in which a stimulus such as that of a single touch is felt in several places. [Gk *polys* many, aesthesia.]

polyaesthetic (**pol**·e·es·**thet**'·ik). Relating or belonging to polyaesthesia.

polyalgesia (**pol**·e·al·**je**'·ze·ah). A disorder of sensation in which a single painful stimulus, e.g. the pricking of a pin, gives the feeling that several have been made. [Gk *polys* many, algesia.]

polyamine (pol·e·**am**·een). An amine that contains two or more NH_2 groups. [Gk *polys* many, amine.]

polyaminostyrene (**pol**·e·am·in·o·**sti**'·reen). A polymerized derivative of styrene used as an ion-exchange resin.

polyandrous (pol·e·**an**·drus). Referring to polyandry.

polyandry (pol·e·**an**·dre). 1. The mating of a female with more than one male during the same period. 2. The result of fertilization of an egg by more than one sperm. [Gk *polys* many, *aner* man.]

Polyangium (pol·e·**an**·je·um). A genus of the order Myxobacteriales, characterized by rounded or coiled cysts surrounded by a well-developed membrane either free or embedded in a slimy layer. They are found in soil, rabbit dung and on wet wood. [Gk *polys* many, *aggeion* vessel.]

polyarteritis (**pol**·e·ar·ter·**i**'·tis). Inflammation affecting a number of arteries simultaneously. **Cutaneous polyarteritis nodosa.** Livedo with painful nodulation, mainly affecting the legs; the nodules occur in crops and there may also be myalgia. Other organs are seldom affected and the prognosis is fair. **Polyarteritis nodosa.** A collagen disease characterized pathologically by inflammatory changes and fibrinoid necrosis in the walls of medium-sized and small arteries. Clinically there is a generalized constitutional illness with manifestations in most systems but particularly skin lesions, hypertension, renal failure, ischaemic cerebral lesions, peripheral neuropathy, a variety of pulmonary conditions and arthralgia. The disease affects males most commonly and carries a serious prognosis. [Gk *polys* many, *arteria* artery, *-itis* inflammation.]

polyarthralgia (**pol**·e·ar·**thral**'·je·ah). Pain affecting several joints. [Gk *polys* many, *arthron* joint, *algos* pain.]

polyarthric (pol·e·**ar**·thrik). Pertaining to or involving many joints. [Gk *polys* many, Gk *arthron*.]

polyarthritis (**pol**·e·ar·**thri**'·tis). An inflammatory condition affecting more than one joint. Rheumatoid arthritis is an example. **Polyarthritis rheumatica acuta.** Rheumatic fever. *See* FEVER. **Seronegative polyarthritis.** A group of conditions in which there is inflammation of many joints but negative serological tests for rheumatoid arthritis. It includes some cases of rheumatoid arthritis and other conditions which resemble it, including Reiter's disease and arthritis associated with other diseases, e.g. psoriasis and ulcerative colitis. **Tuberculous polyarthritis.** Polyarthritis associated with tuberculosis as a primary factor. [Gk *polys* many, *arthron* joint, *-itis* inflammation.]

polyarthropathy (**pol**·e·ar·**throp**'·ath·e). A pathological condition involving many joints. [Gk *polys* many, *arthron* joint, *pathos* disease.]

polyarticular (**pol**·e·ar·**tik**'·ew·lar). Polyarthric. [Gk *polys* many, L *articulus* joint.]

polyatomic (**pol**·e·at·**om**'·ik). 1. Describing a compound composed of several atoms. 2. Applied to an acid which has several replaceable hydrogen atoms, or to an alcohol or base which has several replaceable hydroxyl groups. [Gk *polys* many, atom.]

polyauxotroph (pol·e·**awx**·o·trofe). An organism which needs to be provided with many food substances before it will grow and reproduce. Used particularly in genetics of lower plants. [Gk *polys* many, *auxanein* to grow, *trophe* nutrition.]

polyauxotrophic (**pol**·e·awx·o·**trof**·ik). Having the properties of a polyauxotroph.

polyavitaminosis (**pol**·e·a·vit·am·in·**o**'·sis). A morbid condition caused by deficiency of several vitamins in the diet. [Gk *polys* many, avitaminosis.]

polyaxon (pol·e·**ax**·on). A nerve cell with more than one axon. [Gk *polys* many, axon.]

polyaxonic (**pol**·e·ax·**on**′·ik). Relating to or indicating a polyaxon.

polybasic (pol·e·**ba**·sik). 1. Applied to an acid that has two or more atoms of hydrogen replaceable by a metal or basic radical. 2. Sometimes applied to the salt formed by the replacement of such hydrogen atoms. [Gk *polys* many, base.]

polyblast (**pol**·e·blast). A wandering macrophage of connective tissue, especially numerous in inflammation. [Gk *polys* many, *blastos* germ.]

polyblennia (pol·e·**blen**·e·ah). The secretion of an abnormally large amount of mucus. [Gk *polys* much, *blenna* mucus.]

polycardia (pol·e·**kar**·de·ah). Tachycardia. [Gk *polys* many, *kardia* heart.]

polycellular (pol·e·**sel**·ew·lar). Consisting of many cells; multicellular. [Gk *polys* many, cell.]

polycentric (pol·e·**sen**·trik). Provided with a number of centres; multinuclear. [Gk *polys* many, centre.]

polyceptor (pol·e·**sep**·tor). A term in Ehrlich's side-chain theory, no longer used but meaning an amboceptor able to fix several complements. [Gk *polys* many, L *recipere* to receive.]

polycheiria (pol·e·**ki**·re·ah). A developmental abnormality in which a supernumerary hand is present. [Gk *polys* many, *cheir* hand.]

polychemotherapy (**pol**·e·kem·o·**ther**′·ap·e). Treatment by the administration of a number of different chemotherapeutic agents at the same time without attempting to decide which is likely to be the effective one. [Gk *polys* many, chemotherapy.]

polychloral (pol·e·**klor**·al). A polymer of chloral and pyridine having hypnotic properties.

polycholia (pol·e·**ko**·le·ah). Excessive production and flow of bile. [Gk *polys* much, *chole* bile.]

polychondritis (**pol**·e·kon·**dri**′·tis). A disease mostly of the middle-aged, sometimes associated with rheumatoid arthritis, lupus erythematosus or Hashimoto's disease. The cartilages most affected are those of the nose and ears, the larynx and trachea, and the costal and joint cartilages. [Gk *polys* many, *chondros* cartilage, *-itis* inflammation.]

polychrest, polychrestus (**pol**·e·krest, pol·e·**krest**·us). A homoeopathic term. 1. Efficacious and often used in treatment of many diseases. 2. A drug applicable in the treatment of many diseases. [Gk *polys* much, *chrestos* useful.]

polychroism (pol·e·**kro**·izm). The phenomenon displayed by certain crystals which affect light differently in different directions and consequently appear to vary in colour according to the axis along which they are viewed. [Gk *polys* many, *chroa* colour.]

polychromaemia (**pol**·e·kro·**me**′·me·ah). A condition marked by an increase in the quantity of haemoglobin present in the blood. [Gk *polys* many, *chroma* colour, *haima* blood.]

polychromasia (**pol**·e·kro·**ma**′·ze·ah). 1. Polychromatophilia. 2. Variation in the haemoglobin content of the erythrocytes or the haemoglobinated normoblasts. [Gk *polys* many, *chroma* colour.]

polychromate (pol·e·**kro**·mate). A person who is able to distinguish many colours. **Abnormal polychromate.** Anyone who confuses one colour with another. [see prec.]

polychromatia (**pol**·e·kro·**ma**′·she·ah). Polychromatophilia. [see foll.]

polychromatic (**pol**·e·kro·**mat**′·ik). Showing or having many colours; multicoloured. [Gk *polys* many, *chroma* colour.]

polychromatocyte (pol·e·**kro**·mat·o·site). A cellular tissue cell, usually an erythrocyte or normoblast, capable of taking up different stains or dyes. [Gk *polys* many, *chroma* colour, *kytos* cell.]

polychromatocytosis (**pol**·e·kro·mat·o·si·**to**′·sis). An increased number of polychromatocytes in the blood. [polychromatocyte, Gk *-osis* condition.]

polychromatophil (pol·e·**kro**·mat·o·fil). 1. A cellular tissue cell, usually an erythrocyte or normoblast, capable of taking up different stains or dyes. 2. Capable of taking up stains or dyes of different colours. [see foll.]

polychromatophilia (**pol**·e·kro·mat·o·**fil**′·e·ah). 1. An increased number of polychromatophils in the blood. 2. The ability to take up different stains or dyes or to develop different staining reactions, commonly exhibited by the red blood cells (erythrocytes, normoblasts) in certain blood diseases such as pernicious anaemia, haemolytic anaemias, etc. [Gk *polys* many, *chroma* colour, *philein* to love.]

polychromatophilic (**pol**·e·kro·mat·o·**fil**′·ik). Taking up different stains or colours. [see prec.]

polychromatosis (**pol**·e·kro·mat·**o**′·sis). Polychromatocytosis.

polychromia (pol·e·**kro**·me·ah). Increased or unnatural pigmentation in any part of the body. [Gk *polys* many, *chroma* colour.]

polychromic (pol·e·**kro**·mik). Polychromatic.

polychromophil (pol·e·**kro**·mo·fil). Polychromatophil.

polychromophilia (**pol**·e·kro·mo·**fil**′·e·ah). Polychromatophilia.

polychylia (pol·e·**ki**·le·ah). Production of an excessive quantity of chyle. [Gk *polys* much, chyle.]

polychylic (pol·e·**ki**·lik). Relating or belonging to polychylia.

polycistronic (**pol**·e·sis·**tron**′·ik). Pertaining to more than one cistron or gene; e.g. polycistronic messenger RNA carries, on a single molecule, the genetic information from several adjacent structural genes of an operon. [Gk *polys* many, L *cis* on this side, *trans* on the other side, referring to a complementation test.]

polyclinic (pol·e·**klin**·ik). 1. Not restricted to the treatment of certain diseases only. 2. A hospital providing clinical treatment of and instruction in all forms of disease. [Gk *polys* many, *kline* bed.]

polyclonia (pol·e·**klo**·ne·ah). Clonic spasms. [Gk *polys* many, clonus.]

polycoria (pol·e·**kor**·e·ah). The existence of a supernumerary pupil in one eye. **Polycoria spuria.** Polycoria marked by the presence of a number of openings on the iris. **Polycoria vera.** The presence of several pupils, each having a sphincter. [Gk *polys* many, *kore* pupil.]

polycrotic (pol·e·**krot**·ik). Relating or belonging to, or characterized by polycrotism.

polycrotism (pol·e·**krot**·izm). A condition in which there are several subsidiary waves to each stroke of the pulse, noted in the sphygmograph as minor peaks in the descending phase. [Gk *polys* many, *kroteein* to beat.]

polycyclic (pol·e·**si**·klik). Pertaining to or having many rings or whorls. [Gk *polys* many, *kyklos* circle.]

polycyesia, polycyesis (**pol**·e·si·**e**′·se·ah, **pol**·e·si·**e**′·sis). Multiple pregnancy. [Gk *polys* many, *kyesis* pregnancy.]

polycystic (pol·e·**sist**·ik). Composed of or containing many cysts, e.g. a hydatid cyst. [Gk *polys* many, cyst.]

polycystoma (**pol**·e·sist·**o**′·mah). Polycystic disease, a condition in which many congenital cysts are found in such organs as the kidneys, liver and pancreas. [Gk *polys* many, cystoma.]

polycyte (**pol**·e·site). A normal-sized polymorphonuclear neutrophil leucocyte having a hypersegmental or complex nucleus, usually associated with acute or chronic infections. [Gk *polys* many, *kytos* cell.]

polycythaemia (**pol**·e·si·**the**′·me·ah). A condition in which there is an abnormal increase in the number of red cells in the circulating blood; there is usually an associated increase in the amount of cellular haemoglobin, in the volume of packed red cells and in blood viscosity. These increases, which may be relative or absolute, may arise from different causes, e.g. it is physiological in newborn infants and among those living at high altitudes with lowered oxygen tension of the blood, and occurs in cardiac and pulmonary diseases, after haemoconcentration, and after exposure to certain chemical and physical agents, besides arising from unknown causes (polycythaemia vera). The patient has a characteristic plum-coloured skin and mucous membranes. Polycythaemia arising from a known stimulus is usually referred to as *erythrocytosis,* while the term *erythraemia* is applied to the polycythaemia vera of unknown aetiology. **Absolute polycythaemia.** An absolute increase in the total amount of red blood cells, packed-cell volume and haemoglobin, e.g. in polycythaemia vera. **Chronic splenomegalic polycythaemia.** Polycythaemia vera (see below). **Cryptogenic polycythaemia** (Cabot). Polycythaemia vera (see below). **Polycythaemia cyanotica.** Polycythaemia vera (see below). **Polycythaemia hypertonica.** Gaisboeck's syndrome; a condition with polycythaemia, hypertension, arteriosclerosis and cardiac enlargement, but without splenomegaly. **Polycythaemia megalosplenica, Polycythaemia myelopathica.** Polycythaemia vera (see below). **Myelopathic polycythaemia** (Weber). Polycythaemia vera (see below). **Primary polycythaemia.** Polycythaemia vera (see below). **Relative polycythaemia.** An apparent increase in the number of red blood cells, the packed-cell volume and cellular haemoglobin, as a result of a loss of blood plasma or body fluids, or an abnormally lowered fluid intake, causing haemoconcentration with lowered total blood volume. **Polycythaemia rubra.** Polycythaemia vera (see below). **Secondary polycythaemia.** Polycythaemia arising as a secondary result of some other condition, e.g. chronic or pulmonary conditions, Ayerza's syndrome, etc. **Splenomegalic polycythaemia.** Polycythaemia vera (see foll.). **Polycythaemia vera.** A polycythaemia of unknown aetiology and relative chronic duration, characterized by marked increases in the red cell count (7 000 000–14 000 000/mm^3), packed-cell volume (up to 92 per cent), and cellular haemoglobin (140–200 per cent; 20.7–29.6 g), with similar increases in numbers of leucocytes (20 000–30 000/mm^3), platelets (may be as high as 3 000 000/mm^3), and total blood volume. Clinically there is a typical plum or maroon colour of the skin and mucous membranes, splenomegaly, hyperpiesis and various vasomotor and neurological features, with occasionally hepatomegalia, duodenal ulcer or haemorrhagic manifestations. A deletion of one arm of an F chromosome (presumably No. 20) has been found in the bone marrow cells of patients with this condition. **Polycythaemia vera cum splenomegalia.** Polycythaemia vera (see prec.). [Gk *polys* many, *kytos* cell, *haima* blood.]

polycytosis (pol·e·si·to'·sis). A morbid condition characterized by a marked increase in the number of leucocytes and erythrocytes without increase in the volume of the plasma. [Gk *polys* many, *kytos* cell.]

polydactylia (pol·e·dak·til'·e·ah). Polydactylism.

polydactylism (pol·e·dak·til·izm). The presence of more than the normal number of fingers or toes on a hand or a foot. [Gk *polys* many, *daktylos* finger or toe.]

polydactyly (pol·e·dak·til·e). Polydactylism.

polydeficiency (pol·e·de·fish'·en·se). A deficiency of several different food factors, especially vitamins. [Gk *polys* many, deficiency.]

polydipsia (pol·e·dip·se·ah). An excessive degree of thirst often associated with diabetes insipidus. **Polydipsia ebrioria.** A morbid longing for intoxicating liquors. [Gk *polys* much, *dipsa* thirst.]

polydisperse (pol·e·dis·pers). A term applied to a colloidal sol in which the colloid is dispersed in particles of varying size. Most colloidal sols are of this nature, probably the commonest example being a solution of gelatin. [Gk *polys* many, disperse.]

polydontia (pol·e·don·she·ah). The presence of more than the usual number of teeth. [Gk *polys* many, *odous* tooth.]

polydyscrinia (pol·e·dis·krin'·e·ah). The simultaneous occurrence of disorder in more than one endocrine organ. [Gk *polys* much, *dys-*, *krinein* to secrete.]

polydysplasia (pol·e·dis·pla·ze·ah). The condition of possessing multiple developmental abnormalities. **Hereditary ectodermal polydysplasia.** Hereditary ectodermal dysplasia. *See* DYSPLASIA. [Gk *polys* many, *dys-*, *plassein* to form.]

polyelectrolyte (pol·e·el·ek'·tro·lite). Any polymerized substance such as a polysaccharide or rubber, or any compound of high molecular weight such as a protein, which is capable of acting as an electrolyte. [Gk *polys* many, electrolyte.]

polyembryony (pol·e·em·bre·on·e). In embryology, the production of two or more embryos from a single egg. [Gk *polys* many, embryo.]

polyene (pol·e·een). An organic compound containing two or more double bonds. When the double bonds alternate with single bonds as in butadiene, CH_2=CHCH=CH_2, they are said to be *conjugate*, and as such have a tendency to polymerize forming rubber-like substances: the natural yellow colouring matters, carotenes, are of this type.

polyergic (pol·e·er·jik). Capable of acting in a number of different ways. [Gk *polys* many, *ergon* work.]

polyethylene (pol·e·eth·il·een). A synthetic resin of the formula $(CH_2CH_2)_n$, produced by the polymerization of ethylene under high pressure. It is tough and flexible, is a good electrical insulator and is not affected by water. It has been used in surgery.

Polygala (po·lig·al·ah). A genus of plants, milkworts (family Polygalaceae) with many species. **Polygala polygama.** Bitter milkwort, a perennial shrub containing a saponin and used as a bitter tonic, also, in larger doses, as a laxative. **Polygala senega.** Senega, the dried root of the milkwort containing the saponins, senegin, and polygalic acid. [Gk *polys* many, *gala* milk.]

polygalactia (pol·e·gal·ak'·she·ah). An over-abundant secretion of milk. [see prec.]

polygalin (pol·ig·al·in). Polygalic acid, one of the two glycosidal saponins (the other being senegin) present in senega root, *Polygala senega,* and to which the drug owes its properties.

polygamous (pol·ig·am·us). Pertaining to polygamy.

polygamy (pol·ig·am·e). The mating of one male with more than one female, or, used more loosely, the mating of an individual of either sex with more than one spouse. [Gk *polys* many, *gamos* marriage.]

polyganglionic (pol·e·gang·gle·on'·ik). 1. Relating or belonging to a number of ganglia. 2. Provided with many ganglia. [Gk *polys* many, ganglion.]

polygastria (pol·e·gas·tre·ah). Abnormally large secretion of gastric juice. [Gk *polys* much, gastric juice.]

Polygeline (pol·e·jel·een). BP Commission approved name for a polymer of urea and polypeptides derived from denatured gelatin; it is used for the restoration of blood volume.

polygen (pol·e·jen). 1. An element that has more than one valency and is thus able to form more than one series of compounds. 2. A complex antigen which, on inoculation into the animal body, gives rise to two or more specific antigens, e.g. *Salmonella typhi* (Vi antigen; O antigens; specific H antigen). [Gk *polys* many, *genein* to produce, antigen.]

polygenesis (pol·e·jen·es·is). The process of producing numerous offspring. [Gk *polys* many, *genein* to produce.]

polygenic (pol·e·je·nik). Applied to characters whose expression is controlled by a number of genes. Often used in connection with characters which are largely genetic, but in whose expression non-genetic factors also play a part. [Gk *polys* many, gene.]

Polyglactin (pol·e·glak·tin). BP Commission approved name for lactic acid polyester with glycolic acid; used as a synthetic absorbable suture.

polyglandular (pol·e·glan·dew·lar). 1. Relating to or originating in several glands. 2. Pertaining to the secretions of a number of glands. [Gk *polys* many, gland.]

polyglobulism (pol·e·glob·ew·lizm). Polycythaemia. [Gk *polys* many, globule.]

polygnathus (pol·e·nath·us). In teratism, a double monster the parasite of which is united with the autosite at the jaw. [Gk *polys* many, *gnathos* jaw.]

Polygonatum (pol·e·go·na'·tum). Solomon's seal; a perennial herbaceous plant, *Polygonatum officinale* (family Liliaceae), said to be emetic. The root was used in bruises and skin eruptions. [Gk *polys* many, *gony* knee.]

Polygonum (po·lig·o·num). A genus of plants (family Polygonaceae) many species of which are astringent, diuretic and stimulant. **Polygonum bistorta.** Snakeweed, adder's wort; the rhizome contains tannin and is used as an astringent. **Polygonum cuspidatum.** A wild plant from Japan; it has purgative properties. **Polygonum hydropiper.** Water pepper, smartweed; a plant used domestically, also as a diuretic and in amenorrhoea. [Gk *polys* many, *gonia* angle.]

polygram (pol·e·gram). The tracing recorded by a polygraph. [Gk *polys* many, *gramma* a writing.]

polygraph (pol·e·graf). An instrument for making two or more simultaneous records of the jugular pulse, the arterial pulse, the apex beat or the respiratory movements. The pulsations are transmitted through air-containing tubes to tambours which move levers recording on smoked paper fastened to a revolving drum. Sometimes referred to as the "lie detector". [Gk *polys* many, *graphein* to record.]

See also: MACKENZIE (J.).

polygyria (pol·e·**ji**·re·ah). The existence of an abnormally large number of cerebral gyri. [Gk *polys* many, gyrus.]

polyhaemia (pol·e·**he**·me·ah). Polyaemia.

polyhexoside (pol·e·**hex**·o·side). Polysaccharide. [Gk *polys* many, hexoside.]

polyhidria (pol·e·**hid**·re·ah). Polyhidrosis.

polyhidrosis (**pol**·e·hid·**ro**′·sis). Excessive sweating, the sweat glands being stimulated by sympathetic nerves. It is often a prominent symptom in thyrotoxicosis, but may occur in syringomyelia, especially over the face and arms; more often it is a neurosis and excited by emotional disturbances. Complete division of the spinal cord is followed by excessive sweating of the lower part of the body which is cut off from the control of higher centres. Localized polyhidrosis is common in the axillae, palms and soles; the skin becomes moist and macerated and is liable to become infected. [Gk *polys* much, *hidros* sweat.]

polyhydramnion, polyhydramnios (**pol**·e·hi·**dram**′·ne·on, **pol**·e·hi·**dram**′·ne·os). An abnormality of pregnancy in which liquor amnii exists in an excessive quantity. [Gk *polys* much, hydramnion.]

polyhydric (pol·e·**hi**·drik). 1. Applied to an alcohol or base which contains several hydroxyl OH groups. 2. Any compound which possesses two or more replaceable atoms of hydrogen. [Gk *polys* many, hydrogen.]

polyhydruria (**pol**·e·hi·**droor**′·e·ah). Abnormal increase in the watery constituent of the urine. [Gk *polys* much, hydruria.]

polyhypermenorrhoea (**pol**·e·hi·per·men·o·**re**′·ah). Frequent menstruation associated with an excessive flow. [Gk *polys* much, hypermenorrhoea.]

polyhypomenorrhoea (**pol**·e·hi·po·men·o·**re**′·ah). Frequent menstruation associated with a scanty flow. [Gk *polys* much, hypomenorrhoea.]

polyidrosis (**pol**·e·id·**ro**′·sis). Polyhidrosis.

polyinfection (**pol**·e·in·**fek**′·shun). A mixed infection with several varieties of organism. [Gk *polys* many, infection.]

polykaryocyte (pol·e·**kar**·e·o·site). A giant cell in which there are several nuclei. [Gk *polys* many, karyocyte.]

polykaryon (pol·e·**kar**·e·on). A cell with more than two nuclei. [Gk *polys* many, *karyon* nut.]

polylecithal (pol·e·**les**·ith·al). Megalecithal. [Gk *polys* many, lecithal.]

polyleptic (pol·e·**lep**·tik). Denoting a disease in which there are many relapsing and exacerbating phases, with abatements as well as paroxysmal increases in the severity of the symptoms. [Gk *polys* many, *lambanein* to seize.]

polylogia (pol·e·**lo**·je·ah). Garrulity caused by mental disturbance. [Gk *polys* much, *logos* discourse.]

polymastia (pol·e·**mas**·te·ah). The state in which in human beings there are more than two distinct mammary glands. [Gk *polys* many, *mastos* breast.]

polymastigate (pol·e·**mas**·tig·ate). Having more than one flagellum. [see foll.]

Polymastigida, Polymastigina (pol·e·mas·**tig**·id·ah, pol·e·mas·-tig·in·ah). An order of the Mastigophora which includes the more complex flagellates associated with man. More than three flagella are present. It includes *Chilomastix, Giardia* and *Trichomonas.* [Gk *polys* many, *mastix* lash.]

polymastigote (pol·e·**mas**·tig·ote). A micro-organism having more than one flagellum. [see prec.]

polymazia (pol·e·**ma**·ze·ah). Polymastia. [Gk *polys* many, *mazos* breast.]

polymelia (pol·e·**me**·le·ah). In teratism, the condition of having more than the normal number of limbs or parts of limbs, as in polydactylism. [Gk *polys* many, *melos* limb.]

polymelus (pol·**im**·el·us). A monster with supernumerary limbs or parts of limbs. [see prec.]

polymenia, polymenorrhoea (pol·e·**me**·ne·ah, **pol**·e·men·o·**re**′·ah). Abnormally frequent recurrence of menstruation. [Gk *polys* many, menorrhoea.]

polymer (**pol**·e·mer). Any organic compound which has the same percentage composition as another, but a molecular weight a multiple of the latter; polymeride. [Gk *polys* many, *meros* part.]

polymerase (**pol**·e·mer·ase). **DNA polymerase.** A class of enzymes which catalyse synthesis of DNA from a mixture of deoxyribonucleoside triphosphates. They only function in the presence of a nucleic acid primer which also acts as a template for the assembling of new DNA and, thus, determines its base composition and sequence. There are three types: *(a)* DNA polymerase I, believed to function in the repair of DNA; *(b)* DNA polymerase II, probably the enzyme responsible for DNA replication; *(c)* RNA-dependent DNA polymerase, thought to be responsible for neoplastic transformation in cells. **DNA-dependent RNA polymerase, DNA-directed RNA polymerase.** Transcriptase.

polymeria (pol·e·**me**·re·ah). The existence of more than the normal number of body organs or parts. [Gk *polys* many, *meros* part.]

polymeric (pol·e·**mer**·ik). 1. Pertaining to a structure which is derived from two or more somites, such as certain striated muscles. 2. Denoting similar chemical constitution but different molecular size; exhibiting polymerism. [see prec.]

polymeride (pol·**im**·er·ide). Polymer.

polymerism (pol·**im**·er·izm). 1. The chemical phenomenon in which several molecules of a compound unite, without elimination of any simpler substance, to form a new compound with new properties the molecular weight of which is a whole number multiple of that of the original compound. 2. Polymeria. [Gk *polys* many, *meros* part.]

polymerization (pol·**im**·er·i·**za**′·shun). The combination of two or more molecules of a compound to form a polymer.

polymerize (pol·**im**·er·ize). To undergo the process of conversion into a polymer, or to bring about such a conversion.

polymetameric (**pol**·e·met·am·**er**′·ik). Possessing or derived from numerous segments. [Gk *polys* many, metamere.]

polymicrobial, polymicrobic (**pol**·e·mi·**kro**′·be·al, **pol**·e·mi·**kro**′·bik). Pertaining or due to a number of species of micro-organism. [Gk *polys* many, microbe.]

polymicrolipomatosis (**pol**·e·**mi**·kro·lip·o·mat·**o**′·sis). A morbid condition marked by the presence of a number of small nodular lipomata in the subcutaneous connective tissue. [Gk *polys* many, *mikros* small, lipoma, Gk *-osis* condition.]

polymicrotome (pol·e·**mi**·kro·tome). A microtome for cutting a number of histological sections at one time. [Gk *polys* many, microtome.]

polymitus (pol·e·**mi**·tus). Name applied by early observers to the exflagellated microgametocyte of the malarial parasite, owing to its resemblance to a protozoon of the same name which has no medical significance. [Gk *polys* many, *mitos* thread.]

Polymnia (po·**lim**·ne·ah). A genus of composite-flowered plants. **Polymnia uvedalia.** Leafcup, bearsfoot; the root is used as a stimulant, laxative and anodyne. [Gk, one of the Muses.]

polymorph (**pol**·e·morf). A polymorphonuclear leucocyte. *See* LEUCOCYTE.

polymorphic (pol·e·**mor**·fik). Polymorphous.

polymorphism (pol·e·**mor**·fizm). The ability to assume several distinct forms; the condition of being polymorphous. **Chromosome polymorphism.** The presence in the population of two or more alternative forms of one or more chromosomes which are maintained in the population in frequencies too high to be accounted for by recurrent mutations. **Haemoglobin polymorphism.** The existence in a population of two or more forms of haemoglobin.

polymorphocellular (pol·e·mor·fo·sel′·ew·lar). Relating to or composed of cells of a number of distinct shapes or varieties. [Gk *polys* many, *morphe* form, cell.]

polymorphocyte (pol·e·**mor**·fo·site). Myelocyte. [GK *polys* many, *morphe* form, *kytos* cell.]

polymorphonuclear (**pol**·e·mor·fo·**new**′·kle·ar). 1. Having a nucleus that may take one of several different shapes. 2. A polymorphonuclear leucocyte. *See* LEUCOCYTE. **Filament polymorphonuclear.** A polymorphonuclear in which the nuclei are joined by the fine filaments of nuclear materials. **Non-filament polymorphonuclear.** A polymorphonuclear in which the nuclei are joined by broad bands of nuclear material. [Gk *polys* many, *morphe* form, nucleus.]

polymorphous (pol·e·**mor**·fus). Relating or belonging to or existing in a number of distinct forms. **Polymorphous perverse.** Relating to the stage in development of the libido when it has the potentialities for various, even perverse, modes of expression. [Gk *polys* many, *morphe* form.]

polymyalgia (**pol**·e·mi·**al**′·je·ah). Myalgia affecting a number of muscles. **Polymyalgia rheumatica.** A syndrome in which elderly people complain of pain and morning stiffness in the muscles of the shoulder and pelvic girdles. The condition is probably due to inflammation of joint capsules, tendons and ligaments, is associated with giant-cell arteritis in many cases, and responds to steroids. [Gk *polys* many, *mys* muscle, *algos* pain.]

polymyarian (**pol**·e·mi·a′·re·an). Polymyerial.

polymyerial (**pol**·e·mi·**e**′·re·al). Of nematode worms, having many flask-shaped muscle cells attached to the body wall. At one time of classificatory importance. [Gk *polys* many, *mys* muscle.]

polymyoclonus (**pol**·e·mi·o·**klo**′·nus). Multiple clonic spasms as seen in encephalitis. [Gk *polys* many, *mys* muscle, clonus.]

polymyositis (**pol**·e·mi·o·**si**′·tis). A collagen disease in which there is diffuse inflammation of striated muscle. It may be acute or chronic and associated with skin changes (dermatomyositis), evidence of other collagen diseases, e.g. scleroderma, and sometimes with malignant tumours, especially of the bowel. **Polymyositis haemorrhagica.** A type of dermatomyositis characterized by the occurrence of haemorrhages in and between the muscles and sometimes into the skin and mucous membranes. **Trichinous polymyositis.** Myositis in trichiniasis. [Gk *polys* many, myositis.]

Polymyxin (pol·e·**mix**·in). BP Commission approved name for an antibiotic produced by strains of *Bacillus polymyxa*. The several types are designated A, B, C, D and E, e.g. polymyxin A. **Polymyxin B Sulphate BP 1973.** The sulphate of polymyxin B, used against Gram-negative bacteria.

Polymyxini B Sulfas (pol·e·**mix**·in·i be **sul**·fas). *European Pharmacopoeia* name for Polymyxin B Sulphate BP 1973.

polynesic (pol·e·**ne**·sik). Occurring in various foci, e.g. certain infections and inflammations. [Gk *polys* many, *nesos* island.]

polyneural (pol·e·**newr**·al). 1. Relating to or receiving branches from a number of nerves. 2. Affecting several nerves. [Gk *polys* many, *neuron* nerve.]

polyneuralgia (pol·e·newr·**al**′·je·ah). A neuralgic condition affecting several nerves at the same time. [Gk *polys* many, neuralgia.]

polyneuramin (pol·e·**newr**·am·in). The polyneuritic vitamin (vitamin B_1) [obsolete term].

polyneuritic (**pol**·e·newr·**it**′·ik). Relating or belonging to or affected with polyneuritis.

polyneuritis (**pol**·e·newr·**i**′·tis). Inflammation of many nerves; multiple and peripheral neuritis. **Acute febrile polyneuritis.** One associated with fever and widespread paresis of muscles of the neck, trunk and limbs. **Acute infective polyneuritis.** Guillain-Barré syndrome. **Polyneuritis cerebralis menieriformis.** Multiple neuritis involving the auditory, vestibular, and 5th and 7th cranial nerves; an early syphilitic manifestation; Frankl-Hochwart's disease. **Polyneuritis cranialis.** A polyneuritis of the cranial nerves, including the oculomotor. This may occur with a generalized polyneuritis, but may be unassociated with neuritis of the limbs. **Diabetic polyneuritis.** Polyneuritis occurring as a complication in long-standing cases of diabetes mellitus. **Endemic polyneuritis.** Beri-beri. **Jamaica ginger polyneuritis.** A form seen in the USA in 1932, due to the use of an alcoholic extract of ginger, but adulterated with triorthocresyl phosphate, the actual cause of the neuritis. **Polyneuritis potatorum.** Alcoholic neuritis. **Progressive hypertrophic polyneuritis.** A rare heredofamilial polyneuritis, caused by hypertrophy of the sheaths of Schwann and the nerve trunks. **Uraemic polyneuritis.** Polyneuritis in renal failure. [Gk *polys* many, neuritis.]

polyneuromyositis (pol·e·**newr**·o·mi·o·**si**′·tis). Inflammation of tendon sheaths and bursae in several parts of the body. [Gk *polys* many, *neuron* nerve, myositis.]

polyneuropathy (**pol**·e·newr·**op**′·ath·e). A morbid state in which a number of nerves are affected at the same time. **Erythroedema polyneuropathy.** Pink disease. [Gk *polys* many, *neuron* nerve, *pathos* disease.]

polyneuroradiculitis (**pol**·e·**newr**·o·**rad**·**ik**·**ew**·**li**′·tis). Inflammation involving the nerve roots, the peripheral nerve and the spinal ganglia. [Gk *polys* many, *neuron* nerve, radiculitis.]

Polynoxylin (pol·e·**nox**·e·lin). BP Commission approved name for poly[methylenedi(hydroxymethyl)urea]; it is used in the treatment of skin disorders.

polynuclear (pol·e·**new**·kle·ar). Multinuclear; having several nuclei. [Gk *polys* many, nucleus.]

polynucleate, polynucleated (pol·e·**new**·kle·ate, pol·e·**new**·kle·a·ted). Multinuclear. [see prec.]

polynucleolar (**pol**·e·new·**kle**′·o·lar). Pertaining to or containing several nucleoli. [Gk *polys* many, nucleolus.]

polynucleosis (**pol**·e·new·kle·**o**′·sis). A morbid state characterized by the presence of many polynuclear cells in the blood or in an exudation. [Gk *polys* many, nucleus, Gk *-osis* condition.]

polyodontia (**pol**·e·o·**don**′·she·ah). The presence of more than the normal number of teeth. [Gk *polys* many, *odous* tooth.]

polyoestrous (pol·e·**e**·strus). Exhibiting two or more oestrous periods in a year. [Gk *polys* many, oestrous.]

polyoma (pol·e·**o**·mah). Normally an inapparent virus infection of some strains of laboratory mice and also of wild mice. Stocks of the virus grown in susceptible cells can be used to induce tumours of multiple histological types in suckling mice, guinea-pigs and hamsters. The tumours are transplantable but virus may not be recoverable from the transplanted tumours. The tumours are generally malignant, but the virus is not known to affect man. [Gk *polys* many, *-oma* tumour.]

Polyomavirus (pol·e·o·mah·**vi**′·rus). One of the two genera of viruses that make up the Papovaviruses. The viruses are DNA-containing spherical viruses about 40 nm in diameter, and they include the viruses of polyoma, simian vacuolating virus and rabbit vacuolating virus. Morphologically similar viruses have been isolated from man and one has shown a slight antigenic cross-reaction with the simian vacuolating virus (SV40). Their role, if any, in human disease has yet to be established. Polyoma, SV40 and rabbit vacuolating virus either do not grow in man or cause an inapparent infection. [Gk *polys* many, *-oma* tumour, L *virus* poison.]

polyonychia (**pol**·e·on·**ik**′·e·ah). The presence of more than one nail on a finger or toe. [Gk *polys* many, *onyx* nail.]

polyopia, polyopsia, polyopy (pol·e·**o**·pe·ah, pol·e·**op**·se·ah, pol·e·o·pe). Perception of more than one image of the object looked at. **Binocular polyopia.** Polyopia present only when both eyes are open and due to some form of squint. In this case only two images are seen and the condition is usually called *diplopia*. **Polyopia monophthalmica.** Polyopia present monocularly; there are many causes for this, e.g. irregularities of the surface of the cornea, early cataract, partial dislocation of the lens or high uncorrected astigmatism. [Gk *polys* many, *ops* eye.]

polyorchidism (pol·e·**or**·kid·izm). The state of having supernumerary testes. [Gk *polys* many, *orchis* testis.]

polyorchis (pol·e·**or**·kis). One who has one or more supernumerary testes. [see prec.]

polyorchism (pol·e·**or**·kizm). Polyorchidism.

polyorexia (**pol**·e·o·**rex**′·e·ah). Bulimia; a diseased condition characterized by perpetual and voracious appetite for food. [Gk *polys* much, *orexis* appetite.]

polyorrhymenitis, polyorrhymenosis (pol·e·or·hi·men·i′·tis, pol·e·or·hi·men·o′·sis). Polyserositis, Concato's disease; a widespread inflammation of the serous membranes, accompanied by effusion and thickening of the membranes themselves. There may be peritonitis, bilateral pleurisy and pericarditis. The peritoneum is much thickened, especially over the liver and spleen, the capsules of which are converted into glistening white fibrous layers resembling iced sugar, and the organs become shrunken. The pleural sacs may become obliterated, the pericardium adherent and often calcified, and there is an associated mediastinitis. Some cases have been regarded as tuberculous, but in most the cause is unknown. [Gk *polys* many, *orrhos* serum, *hymen* membrane, *-itis* inflammation, *-osis* condition.]

polyostotic (pol·e·os′·tot·ic). Fibrous dysplasia. *See* ALBRIGHT'S SYNDROME.

polyotia (pol·e·o·she·ah). The presence of a supernumerary auricle on either or both sides of the head. [Gk *polys* many, *ous* ear.]

polyoxyls (pol·e·ox·ilz). Non-ionic emulsifying surface-active agents. They are a mixture of the monostearate and distearate esters of a condensation polymer of ethylene oxide. BP Commission approved names are: **Polyoxyl 8 Stearate,** polyoxyethylene 8 stearate, having a polymer length equivalent to 8 oxyethylene units; and **Polyoxyl 40 Stearate,** polyoxyethylene 40 stearate, having a polymer length equivalent to 40 oxyethylene units. [Gk *polys* many, *oxys* sharp.]

polyp (pol·ip). Polypus; a tumour with a stalk, arising from mucous membranes or the body surface. **Fibro-epithelial polyp.** A soft, pedunculated protrusion on the skin, usually of a flexure and often multiple. **Lipoid polyp.** A cholesterol polyp of a strawberry gall bladder. **Umbilical polyp.** A polypoid mass of granulation tissue at the umbilicus. [Gk *polys* many, *pous* foot.]

polypapilloma (pol·e·pap·il·o′·mah). Multiple papillomata. **Polypapilloma tropicum.** Yaws. [Gk *polys* many, papilloma.]

polyparasitism (pol·e·par·ah·sit·izm). A condition characterized by infestation with several kinds of parasite. [Gk *polys* many, parasite.]

polyparesis (pol·e·par·e′·sis). General paralysis of the insane. [Gk *polys* much, paresis.]

polypathia (pol·e·path·e·ah). 1. The presence of two or more diseases at the same time. 2. The frequent return of symptoms after a remission. [Gk *polys* many, *pathos* disease.]

polypectomy (pol·ip·ek·to·me). The operation of removal of a polyp. [polyp, Gk *ektome* a cutting out.]

polypeptidaemia (pol·e·pep·tid·e′·me·ah). A condition characterized by the existence of polypeptides in the blood. [polypeptide, Gk *haima* blood.]

polypeptides (pol·e·pep·ti·dz). Proteins which are composed of several amino acids linked to one another by the peptide grouping, =CH–CO–NH–CH=. **Nascent polypeptide.** A polypeptide chain at various stages of its product at the ribosomes. **Primary structure of a polypeptide.** Amino-acid sequence. *See* SEQUENCE. [Gk *polys* many, peptide.]

polypeptidorrhachia (pol·e·pep·tid·o·rak′·e·ah). Polypeptides in the cerebrospinal fluid, or the toxic meningitis which may result therefrom. [polypeptide, Gk *rhachis* backbone.]

polyperiostitis hyperaesthetica (pol·e·per·e·os·ti′·tis hi·per·es·thet′·ik·ah). A chronic inflammatory state of the periosteum, characterized by excessive sensitiveness of the skin and soft tissues in the neighbourhood. [Gk *polys* much, *peri, osteon* bone, *-itis* inflammation, hyperaesthesia.]

polyphagia (pol·e·fa·je·ah). 1. Gluttony. 2. Bulimia; a morbid desire for every kind of food. [Gk *polys* much, *phagein* to eat.]

polyphalangism (pol·e·fal·an′·jizm). The condition of having more than the usual number of phalanges in a finger or toe. [Gk *polys* many, phalanx.]

polyphany (pol·if·an·e). Changes produced in several structures or properties of an organism by a single genetic change. [Gk *polys* many, *phainein* to show.]

polyphase (pol·e·faze). Possessing or constituted of several phases, as when several alternating currents are superimposed to give approximate uniformity. [Gk *polys* many, phase.]

polyphenoloxidase (pol·e·fe·nol·ox′·id·aze). An enzyme occurring in bacteria, fungi and higher plants which activates the oxidation of polyphenolic compounds in metabolism. It does not affect the monophenols, such as tyrosine.

polyphenols (pol·e·fe·nolz). General term applied to di- and trihydroxyl phenols, e.g. catechol, $C_6H_4(OH)_2$, pyrogallol, $C_6H_3(OH)_3$.

polyphobia (pol·e·fo·be·ah). Excessive fear of many things. [Gk *polys* many, phobia.]

polyphrasia (pol·e·fra·ze·ah). Insane or morbid garrulity; extreme volubility. [Gk *polys* much, *phrasein* to utter.]

polyphyletic (pol·e·fi·let′·ik). Relating to or derived from more than one source; derived from more than one ancestral type. [Gk *polys* many, *phyle* tribe.]

polyphyletism (pol·e·fi·let·izm). The view that the blood cells are formed from more than one stem cell. [see prec.]

polyphyodont (pol·e·fi·o·dont). Having many sets of teeth which replace one another. [Gk *polys* many, *phyein* to produce, *odous* tooth.]

polypi (pol·e·pi). *See* POLYPUS.

polypiferous (pol·ip·if·er·us). Bearing or producing a polypus. [polypus, L *ferre* to bear.]

polypiform (pol·ip·e·form). Polypoid. [polypus, form.]

polyplasmia (pol·e·plaz·me·ah). A condition of the blood in which there is either extreme fluidity or excess of plasma. [Gk *polys* much, plasma.]

polyplastic (pol·e·plas·tik). 1. Composed of several different structural elements. 2. Polymorphous. [Gk *polys* many, *plastos* formed.]

polyplastocytosis (pol·e·plas·to·si·to′·sis). A condition characterized by an increase in the number of blood platelets. [Gk *polys* many, plastocyte, Gk *-osis* condition.]

Polyplax (pol·e·plax). A genus of lice. **Polyplax spinulosa.** The common rat louse which is capable of transmitting murine typhus from rat to rat. It is not known to attack man. [Gk *polys* many, *plax* flat round plate.]

polyplegia (pol·e·ple·je·ah). Paralysis affecting a number of muscles at the same time. [Gk *polys* many, *plege* stroke.]

polypleurodiaphragmotomy (pol·e·ploor·o·di·ah·frag·mot′·o·me). Transthoracic surgical approach to the upper abdomen by removal of several ribs and incision of the diaphragm from above. [Gk *polys* many, *pleura* rib, diaphragm, Gk *temnein* to cut.]

polyploid (pol·e·ploid). Having three or more sets of the haploid number of chromosomes in somatic cell nuclei. Polyploids, as a rule, are sterile when mated with normal diploids, and are thus rare in forms without asexual reproductive mechanisms. They are common in flowering plants where polyploidy is an important mechanism of speciation. [Gk *polyplous* many times.]

polyploidization (pol·e·ploid·i·za′·shun). The process converting haploid or diploid cells or individuals into polyploids. [Gk *polyplous* many times.]

polyploidy (pol·e·ploi·de). The state of being polyploid.

polypnoea (pol·ip·ne·ah). A condition in which the respiration is abnormally rapid and shallow or is panting. [Gk *polys* many, *pnoiein* to breathe.]

polypodia (pol·e·po·de·ah). In teratism, the condition of having supernumerary feet. [Gk *polys* many, *pous* foot.]

Polypodium (pol·e·po·de·um). Fern root; a genus of ferns several species of which are claimed to have medicinal properties. **Polypodium vulgare.** Brakeroot, rockbrake; a species the slender rhizome of which is knotty, has a sweet taste and faintly acrid odour, and is used with the leaves as an expectorant, tonic and alterative. [Gk *polys* many, *pous* foot.]

polypoid (pol·e·poid). Like a polypus. [polypus, Gk *eidos* form.]

polypoidosis (pol·e·poid·o′·sis). Polyposis.

polyporous (pol·ip·or·us). Containing a large number of pores. [see foll.]

Polyporus (pol·ip·or·us). A genus of fungi, including the species *Polyporus officinalis* which is the source of agaric acid. [Gk *polys* many, *poros* pore.]

polyposis (pol·e·po·sis). A rare condition, sometimes familial, in which the colon is studded with polypi growing from the mucous membrane. It is marked by frequent passage of bright red blood from the bowel which may lead to severe anaemia; secondary inflammatory lesions may be caused by secondary infections, and diarrhoea then develops. Sometimes polypi like small grapes are passed from the bowel. They may cause chronic intussusception, and there is a considerable tendency for the polypi to become malignant. Multiple polypi also occur in the stomach, bladder and nose, usually secondary to infections. **Polyposis coli, Familial polyposis.** *See* MAIN DEF. (above). **Polyposis gastrica.** Multiple polypi of the gastric mucosa. **Polyposis intestinalis.** Multiple polypi of the intestinal mucous membrane. **Polyposis ventriculi.** Polyposis gastrica (see above). [polypus, Gk *-osis* condition.]

polypotome (pol·ip·o·tome). An instrument used for excising a polypus. [polypus, Gk *temnein* to cut.]

polypotrite (pol·ip·o·trite). An instrument used to crush polypi. [polypus, L *terere* to grind.]

polypous (pol·e·pus). Relating to or having the characteristics of a polypus.

polyptychial (pol·e·tik·e·al). Arranged in several layers; applied to those glands in which the cells on the basement membrane are arranged in a series of layers. [Gk *polys* many, *ptyx* layer.]

polypus (pol·e·pus) (pl. *polypi*). A tumour with a stalk, arising from mucous membranes or the body surface. **Polypus angiomatodes.** A highly vascular polypus which resembles a pedunculated angioma, especially common in the nasal cavities. **Antrochoanal polypus.** A unilateral polypoid condition of the maxillary antrum, the affected mucosa being continuous by means of a pedicle through an accessory ostium with a polypus extending into the posterior choana of the nose. **Bleeding polypus.** A vascular polypus which bleeds easily when touched. **Blood polypus.** A mass of fibrin deposited on a piece of retained placenta. **Bronchial polypus.** A pedunculated mass, usually inflammatory, arising from the mucous membrane of a bronchus. **Cardiac polypus.** A post-mortem clot in the heart cavities, especially the right. **Cellular polypus.** A papilloma. **Choanal polypus.** A polypus occupying the posterior choana of the nose, often extending into the postnasal space and visible on posterior rhinoscopy. **Polypus cysticus.** A polypus rich in cystic spaces. **Fibrinous polypus.** A mass of fibrin attached to a bleeding site or necrotic tissue. **Fibrous polypus.** A pedunculated fibroma. **Fleshy polypus.** A soft fibroma or sarcoma. **Gelatinous polypus.** A pedunculated myxoma; a polypus of the nose which secretes mucus. **Gum polypus.** Localized hyperplasia of the gingival margin; a soft, fairly sensitive tumour caused by chronic irritation, attached to the gingival margin. **Hydatid polypus, Polypus hydatidosus.** Hydatidiform mole. **Lipomatous polypus.** A pedunculated lipoma. **Malignant polypus.** A pedunculated sarcoma or carcinoma. **Mucous polypus.** Gelatinous polypus (see above). **Nasal polypus.** An inflammatory or tumour mass protruding into the nasal cavities, often caused by enlarged lymphatic follicles. **Osseous polypus.** An osteophyte or an osteoma. **Placental polypus.** Blood polypus (see above). **Pulp polypus.** Hyperplasia of the pulp of a tooth, occurring when the roof of the pulp chamber has been lost owing to caries, allowing a pink insensitive mass of tissue connected with the pulp to occupy a carious cavity. **Raspberry cellular polypus.** A small angioma, especially of the lip. **Schistosomal polypus.** A colonic polypus due to the presence of ova of *Schistosoma mansoni* in the submucosa of the colon or rectum. **Soft polypus.** Fleshy polypus (see above). **Spongy polypus.** Polypus cysticus (see above). **Polypus telangiectodes.** Polypus angiomatodes (see above). **Vascular polypus.** Polypus angiomatodes (see above). [Gk *polys* many, *pous* foot.]

polyradiculitis (pol·e·rad·ik·ew·li′·tis). Inflammation affecting roots of nerves, particularly the roots of the spinal nerves. [Gk *polys* many, radiculitis.]

polyradiculoneuropathy (pol·e·rad·ik·ew·lo·newr·op′·ath·e). Generalized disease of the peripheral nerves and spinal roots. **Acute polyradiculoneuropathy.** Guillain-Barré syndrome. [Gk *polys* many, L *radix* root, Gk *neuron* nerve, *pathos* disease.]

polyradiotherapy (pol·e·ra·de·o·ther′·ap·e). The use of several types of radiant energy in the treatment of disease. [Gk *polys* many, radiotherapy.]

polyribosomes (pol·e·ri·bo·somes). A cluster of ribosomes held together by a strand of messenger RNA. [Gk *polys* many, ribosomes.]

polyrrhoea (pol·e·re·ah). A copious flow or discharge of thin watery fluid. [Gk *polys* much, *rhoia* flow.]

polysaccharase, polysaccharidase (pol·e·sak·ar·aze, pol·e·sak·ar·id·aze). A class of enzyme which splits up polysaccharides. Examples are amylases which act on starch and glycogen, and cellulases capable of breaking down cellulose.

polysaccharide (pol·e·sak·ar·ide). A class of complex carbohydrates in which the molecule is built up by combination of five or more monosaccharide residues. The latter may be derived from the same sugar or from different sugars, whilst the more complex polysaccharides, such as those of bacterial origin, are built up from uronic-acid residues as well as different parent sugar units. The best-known polysaccharides are those derived from one parent sugar; starch, glycogen and cellulose, for example, are derived entirely from glucose units. **Bacterial polysaccharide.** A polysaccharide derived from bacteria, or their capsules, by extraction. **Capsular polysaccharide.** Polysaccharide material which can be extracted from the capsules of bacteria. The capsular polysaccharide of the pneumococci is a hapten, and is used in the serological typing of this species. **Immune polysaccharides.** Polysaccharides present in micro-organisms that are capable of acting as antigens and stimulating specific immunity response. **Pneumococcus polysaccharide.** Capsular polysaccharide (see above). **Specific polysaccharide.** A polysaccharide obtained from micro-organisms, usually by extraction, which will react by precipitation with the specific antiserum prepared from the homologous organism. [Gk *polys* many, saccharide.]

polysarcia (pol·e·sar·se·ah). Obesity. **Polysarcia cordis.** Fatty infiltration of the heart; cor adiposum. [Gk *polys* much, *sarx* flesh.]

polysarcous (pol·e·sar·kus). Relating or belonging to polysarcia; obese. [see prec.]

polyscelia (pol·e·se·le·ah). A type of polymelia, in which there are more than two legs. [Gk *polys* many, *skelos* leg.]

polyscelus (pol·is·el·us). A monster having more than two legs. [see prec.]

polyscope (pol·e·skope). An illuminating instrument with which a body cavity may be lighted up, the interior examined and its limits defined. [Gk *polys* much, *skopein* to watch.]

polyserositis (pol·e·seer·o·si′·tis). Inflammation affecting the serous membranes in association with effusion of serous fluid. [Gk *polys* much, serositis.]

polysialia (pol·e·si·a′·le·ah). A condition in which there is increased secretion or flow of saliva. [Gk *polys* much, *sialon* saliva.]

polysinuitis (pol·e·si·new·i′·tis). Polysinusitis.

polysinusitis (pol·e·si·nus·i′·tis). Inflammation affecting two or more sinuses at the same time. [Gk *polys* many, sinusitis.]

polysome (pol·e·some). A group of ribosomes attached to a single molecule of messenger RNA. They can be seen in electron micrographs of preparations from both prokaryotic and eukaryotic cells. [Gk *polys* many, *soma* body.]

polysomia (pol·e·so·me·ah). The state of being a polysomus.

polysomic (pol·e·so·mik). Describing an essentially diploid organism or nucleus in which one or more chromosomes are present at least in triplicate (that is trisomic, tetrasomic, double trisomic, and so on). [Gk *polys* many, *soma* body.]

polysomus (pol·e·**so**·mus). A monster with one head and two or three bodies joined together. [see prec.]

polysomy (pol·e·**so**·me). The state characteristic of polysomics. [Gk *polys* many, *soma* body.]

polysorbates (pol·e·**sor**·ba·tz). Non-ionic emulsifying surface-active agents consisting of polyoxyethylene esters or ethers of sorbitol. They are yellow to brown liquids of varying viscosity, stable to pH changes and to high concentrations of electrolytes. They are given different numbers according to their composition, viscosity, etc. BP Commission approved names are: **Polysorbate 20,** polyoxyethylene 20 sorbitan monolaurate; **Polysorbate 40,** polyoxyethylene 20 sorbitan monopalmitate; **Polysorbate 60,** polyoxyethylene 20 sorbitan monostearate; **Polysorbate 65,** polyoxyethylene 20 sorbitan tristearate; **Polysorbate 80,** polyoxyethylene 20 sorbitan mono-oleate; **Polysorbate 85,** polyoxyethylene 20 sorbitan trioleate.

polyspermia, polyspermism, polyspermy (pol·e·**sper**·me·ah, pol·e·**sper**·mizm, pol·e·**sper**·me). 1. An excessively profuse seminal secretion. 2. Penetration of the ovum by more than one spermatozoon. [Gk *polys* many, sperm.]

polystat (**pol**·e·stat). An instrument which, when connected to the electric mains, supplies galvanic, faradic and sinusoidal currents. [Gk *polys* many, *statos* standing.]

polystichia (pol·e·**stik**·e·ah). The presence of more than one row of lashes on an eyelid. [Gk *polys* many, *stichos* row.]

polystomatous (pol·e·**sto**·mat·us). Characterized by the presence of, or provided with, a number of apertures or mouths. [Gk *polys* many, *stoma* mouth.]

polystyrene (pol·e·**sti**·reen). A synthetic resin of formula $(CH_2=CHC_6H_5)_n$, produced by the polymerization of styrene from ethylene and benzene. It is glass-like in clarity, of high tensile strength and impervious to moisture; used for laboratory ware and for optical purposes.

polysuspensoid (**pol**·e·sus·**pen**'·soid). A colloidal solution in which the disperse phase consists of particles in various states of suspension. [Gk *polys* many, suspensoid.]

polysynovitis (**pol**·e·si·no·**vi**'·tis). Inflammation of a number of synovial membranes. [Gk *polys* many, synovitis.]

polytendinitis (**pol**·e·ten·din·**i**'·tis). Inflammation in which a number of tendons are affected simultaneously. [Gk *polys* many, L *tendo* tendon, Gk *-itis* inflammation.]

polytendinobursitis (**pol**·e·ten·din·o·ber·**si**'·tis). Inflammation of tendon sheaths and bursae in several parts of the body. [Gk *polys* many, L *tendo* tendon, bursitis.]

polyteny (pol·e·**ten**·e). The result of multiple lateral duplication of the chromosome as it occurs, for example, in some tissues of Diptera where it leads to the formation of giant chromosomes. [Gk *polys* many, *tainia* band.]

polythelia, polythelism (pol·e·**the**·le·ah, pol·e·**the**·lizm). A condition in which supernumerary nipples are present on either the mammary gland or another part of the body. [Gk *polys* many, *thele* nipple.]

polythene (**pol**·e·theen). Polyethylene; a general name for the several synthetic resins produced by the polymerization of ethylene. They have been used in surgery.

Polythiazide (pol·e·**thi**·az·ide). BP Commission approved name for 6-chloro-3,4-dihydro-2-methyl-3-(2,2,2-trifluoroethylthiomethyl)-1,2,4-benzothiadiazine-7-sulphonamide 1,1-dioxide; a diuretic.

polytocous (pol·**it**·o·kus). In zoology, producing several young at a time. [Gk *polys* many, *tokos* birth.]

polytrichia, polytrichosis (pol·e·**trik**·e·ah, **pol**·e·trik·**o**'·sis). Hirsuties. [Gk *polys* many, *thrix* hair, *-osis* condition.]

Polytrichum (pol·e·**trik**·um). A genus of mosses (family Musci). **Polytrichum juniperinum.** Haircap, juniper moss; the whole plant is used as a diuretic. [Gk *polys* many, *thrix* hair.]

polytrophia (pol·e·**tro**·fe·ah). Over-feeding with its resultant effect on the tissues and the mechanism of the body generally. [Gk *polys* much, *trophe* nourishment.]

polytrophic (pol·e·**trof**·ik). 1. Denoting a micro-organism which produces two or more different varieties of fermentation. 2. Relating or belonging to polytrophia. [see prec.]

polytrophy (pol·e·**tro**·fe). Polytrophia.

polytropic, polytropous (pol·e·**trop**·ik, pol·**it**·ro·pus). Denoting those substances which affect two or more kinds of tissue. [Gk *polys* many, *trope* a turning.]

polyunguia (pol·e·**ung**·gwe·ah). The presence of more than one nail on a finger or toe. [Gk *polys* many, L *unguis* nail.]

polyuria (pol·e·**ewr**·e·ah). Increase in the amount of the urine excreted, usually due to diabetes insipidus. **Polyuria spastica.** Polyuria occurring intermittently, associated with neurotic symptoms and convulsions. [Gk *polys* much, urine.]

polyuric (pol·e·**ewr**·ik). Pertaining to or characterized by polyuria.

polyvalent (pol·e·**va**·lent). Having several valencies, as applied to a chemical element; by analogy, used in immunology. [Gk *polys* many, valency.]

Polyvinox (pol·e·**vi**·nox). BP Commission approved name for poly(butylvinyl ether); it is used in the treatment of skin diseases, wounds and burns.

polyvinyl cyanide (pol·e·**vi**·nil **si**·an·ide). A polymer of vinyl cyanide, also known as *polyacrylonitrile.* It is used in a synthetic fibre.

polyvinylpyrrolidone (pol·e·**vi**·nil·pir·**ol**'·id·one). Povidone.

Pomatopsis lapidaria (po·mat·**op**·sis lap·id·**a**·re·ah). A species of fresh-water snail in North America; it acts as secondary host to *Paragonimus.* [Gk *poma* a cover, *opsis* sight, L *lapis* stone.]

pomegranate (**pom**·gran·ate). Pomegranate root bark, the dried root and stem bark of *Punica granatum* Linn. (family Punicaceae). It contains the alkaloid pelletierine together with tannins, and is used as a taenicide. **Pomegranate rind.** The dried pericarp of the fruit. It contains tannins but no alkaloids, and is used as an astringent. [L *pomum* apple, *granatus* many seeded.]

Pomeroy, R. H. 20th century American gynaecologist.

Pomeroy's operation. An abdominal method of sterilization: a loop of the central portion of the uterine tube is crushed, ligated with catgut, and the loop excised.

pomphoid (**pom**·foid). Having the characteristics of and resembling a blister. [Gk *pomphos* blister, *eidos* form.]

pompholygometer (**pom**·fo·le·**gom**'·et·er). An instrument for counting bubbles. [Gk *pompholyx* bubble, *metron* measure.]

pompholyhaemia (**pom**·fo·le·**he**'·me·ah). Bubbles in the blood, as in caisson disease. [Gk *pompholyx* bubble, *haima* blood.]

pompholyx (**pom**·fo·lix). 1. Any morbid cutaneous condition characterized by the presence of bullous eruptions. 2. Dyshidrosis; an acute vesicular type of eczema (sometimes called *cheiropompholyx*) which attacks the palms and sides of the fingers and the soles of the feet, particularly in individuals who perspire freely. [Gk, bubble.]

pomphus (**pom**·fus). A blister. [Gk *pomphos.*]

pomum adami (**po**·mum ad·**am**·i). The laryngeal prominence on the front of the neck. [L, Adam's apple.]

ponceau (pon·**so**). **Ponceau B.** Biebrich scarlet; a red dye used as a counterstain in histology. **Ponceau 2R.** Scarlet red. *See* RED. **Ponceau 3R.** Cumidine red. *See* RED.

Poncet, Antonin (b. 1849). Lyons surgeon.

Poncet's disease, or rheumatism. An inflammatory condition of the joints or periarticular structures resulting from the presence of a tuberculous focus elsewhere in the body; tuberculous rheumatism.

Poncet's operation. Lengthening of the tendo calcaneus for talipes.

pond lily (pond **lil**·e). The yellow pond lily, *Nuphar (Nymphaea) advena,* and the white pond lily, *Nymphaea odorata* (family Nymphaeaceae), the roots of which have astringent, antiseptic and demulcent properties. The powdered root is often used as a poultice. [AS *pund,* L *lilium.*]

Ponder, Eric (b. 1898). American physiologist.

Cooke and Ponder classification, formula, or method. A simplification of Arneth's count or index in which polymorphonuclear leucocytes are divided into five groups according to the number of their nuclear lobes united by fine filaments. The nucleus is considered to be undivided if parts of it are still united by even a small band of nuclear material.

ponderal (**pon**·der·al). Relating or belonging to weight. [L *pondus* weight.]

pondostatural (pon·do·**stat**·ewr·al). Relating to weight and height. [L *pondus* weight, stature.]

Ponfick, Emil (b. 1844). Breslau pathologist.

Ponfick's shadows. Ghost or phantom blood cells.

Pongamia (pon·**ga**·me·ah). A genus of leguminous East Indian trees. **Pongamia glabra.** A species which gives a fixed oil, kurung oil, when pressed. The oil is used in skin diseases, especially in pityriasis versicolor and other parasitic skin diseases. [Malay *pongam.*]

Ponndorf, Wilhelm Hermann Friedrich (b. 1864). Weimar physician.

Ponndorf's vaccination. An obsolete method of vaccination with concentrated tuberculin, drops of which were placed on scarified skin.

ponograph (**po**·no·graf). An instrument designed to estimate, and record visually, sensitiveness to pain. [Gk *ponos* pain, *graphein* to record.]

ponopalmosis (po·no·pal·**mo**'·sis). Palpitation on effort; a term used for *effort syndrome.* [Gk *ponos* pain, *palmos* palpitation, *-osis* condition.]

ponophobia (po·no·**fo**·be·ah). 1. Morbid fear of pain. 2. Morbid aversion to work or other exertion, or of becoming fatigued. [Gk *ponos* pain, phobia.]

ponos (**po**·nos). The name given in Greece to the Mediterranean form of kala-azar. [Gk *ponos* pain.]

pons [NA] (ponz). A bridge; any tissue which bridges across some space or structure. Specifically, the bridge-like mass of nerve cells and fibres on the anterior aspect of the brain stem, between the cerebral peduncles and mid-brain cranially and the medulla oblongata caudally *(pons varolii).* **Dorsal part of the pons [pars dorsalis pontis (NA)].** The part of the pons lying dorsal to the transverse fibres of the pons and directly continuous with the medulla oblongata. **Ventral part of the pons [pars ventralis pontis (NA)].** The ventral part of the pons, containing the nuclei pontis and many longitudinal and tranverse fibres.

See also: VAROLIO (VAROLIUS).

pontibrachium (pon·te·**bra**·ke·um). The middle cerebellar peduncle. [L *pons* bridge, *bracchium* arm.]

pontic (**pon**·tik). 1. An artificial tooth on a bridge which replaces a natural tooth. 2. Pontile. [L *pons* bridge.]

ponticular (pon·**tik**·ew·lar). Pertaining to the transverse fibres of the pons. [see foll.]

ponticulus (pon·**tik**·ew·lus). A little bridge. An old anatomical word that has fallen into disuse. [dim. of L *pons* bridge.]

pontile (**pon**·tile). Relating to or occurring in the pons.

pontimeter (pon·**tim**·et·er). An instrument for measuring the depth of the "bridge" (posterior meatal wall) before its removal in the radical mastoid operation. [L *pons* bridge, meter.]

pontine (**pon**·tine). Pontile.

pontobulbar (pon·to·**bul**·bar). Relating or belonging to the pons and the medulla oblongata. [pons, bulb.]

pontobulbia (pon·to·**bul**·be·ah). A condition in which the pons and medulla oblongata contain cavities. [see prec.]

pontocerebellar (pon·to·ser·e·**bel**'·ar). Relating or belonging to the pons and the cerebellum.

pontocrural (pon·to·**kroo**·ral). Relating or belonging to the pons and the cerebral peduncles. [pons, L *crus* leg.]

pontoon (pon·**toon**). A loop of the small intestine. [L *ponto* ferry-boat.]

Pool, Eugene Hillhouse (b. 1874). New York surgeon.

Pool's phenomenon. Contraction of the arm muscles on the stretching of the brachial plexus (present in tetany).

Pool-Schlesinger sign. *See* SCHLESINGER'S SIGN.

pool (pool). Any collection of substances in one place for future distribution, especially an accumulation of blood in the blood vessels of any region of the body caused by delaying of the venous flow; this may be physiological or pathological. **Abdominal pool.** The blood present in the splanchnic vessels which is increased in volume in cases of shock, thus depriving peripheral regions of blood. **Blood pool.** The storage of donors' blood at a blood transfusion centre. **Metabolic pool.** The whole of absorbable substances in the body. [AS *pol.*]

poplar (**pop**·lar). Populus.

poples [NA] (**pop**·lees). The posterior surface of the knee. [L, the ham.]

poplitaeus (pop·le·**te**·us). Popliteus.

popliteal (pop·le·**te**·al). Relating or belonging to the space behind the knee joint. [L *poples* the ham.]

popliteal artery [arteria poplitea (NA)]. A continuation of the femoral artery in the popliteal fossa. Branches, the sural arteries [arteriae surales (NA)], are supplied to the muscle bellies at the back of the knee joint; five other branches, the lateral superior genicular artery [arteria genu superior lateralis (NA)], the medial superior genicular artery [arteria genu superior medialis (NA)], the middle genicular artery [arteria genu media (NA)], the lateral inferior genicular artery [arteria genu inferior lateralis (NA)], and the medial inferior genicular artery [arteria genu inferior medialis (NA)], form the arterial anastomosis around the knee joint, supplying the joint structures and soft tissues around the joint and the patella.

popliteal nerves. The two terminal branches of the sciatic nerve. **Lateral popliteal nerve [nervus peroneus (fibularis) communis (NA)].** A smaller terminal branch of the sciatic nerve. It arises on the back of the thigh, winds round to the front of the leg, and supplies directly or through its branches the short head of the biceps femoris muscle, the extensor muscles of the foot, the peroneal muscles and the skin on the lateral side of the leg and most of the dorsum of the foot. The sural communicating branch [ramus communicans peroneus (fibularis) (NA)] runs from the lateral popliteal nerve to join the sural nerve. **Medial popliteal nerve [nervus tibialis (NA)].** The larger of the two terminal branches of the sciatic nerve. It arises on the back of the thigh and descends to the lower border of the popliteus muscle; it is continued in the leg as the posterior tibial nerve. It supplies most of the hamstring muscles, the popliteus, soleus and gastrocnemius muscles [rami musculares (NA)], articular branches to the knee [nervus interosseus cruris (NA)], and the sural nerve to the skin on the outer and posterior sides of the lower part of the leg.

popliteal vein [vena poplitea (NA)]. A large vessel formed in the popliteal fossa by the union of the anterior and posterior tibial veins. It leaves the fossa through the adductor magnus muscle to become the femoral vein in the thigh.

popliteus (pop·le·**te**·us). The popliteus muscle. [L *poples* the ham.]

popliteus muscle [musculus popliteus (NA)]. A flat, triangular muscle in the floor of the popliteal fossa, stretching from the lateral condyle of the femur to the upper part of the posterior surface of the tibia. It medially rotates the tibia and helps to flex the knee.

poppy (**pop**·e). Red poppy, *Papaver rhoeas* (family Papaveraceae), a common herb in England. The scarlet petals contain a colouring agent for which they are chiefly used. The opium poppy, *Papaver somniferum,* is grown mainly in Macedonia, Bulgaria, Turkey, Iran and India; the latex obtained from the capsule is dried to give opium which contains the important alkaloids morphine, codeine, narcotine, papaverine and thebaine. The seeds yield a pale-yellow fixed oil consisting of the glycerides of linolenic, linoleic, oleic and palmitic acids, and is used as a drying oil by artists as well as for culinary and technical purposes. **Poppy capsule, Poppy heads.** The dried fruit of *Papaver somniferum* Linn. Traces of opium alkaloids, especially morphine (up to about 0.3 per cent), cause the capsules to possess a mildly sedative action. They are used for the preparation of poultices for boils, etc., and for syrup of poppy, a sedative incorporated in cough mixtures. [AS *popig.*]

population (pop·ew·**la**·shun). A group of individuals defined by a common characteristic (e.g. area of residence). [LL *populatus* to inhabit.]

populin (pop·ew·lin). $C_{20}H_{22}O_8$, a glycoside occurring in the bark and leaves of species of poplar. It is the benzoyl derivative of salicin.

Populus (pop·ew·lus). A genus of trees of the family Salicaceae, including the poplars and aspens. **Populus candicans.** A species yielding balm of Gilead, used as a stimulant, tonic and diuretic. **Populus tremula.** The aspen; the bark contains the glycosides salicin and populin. [L, poplar.]

poradenia (po·rad·e·ne·ah). Poradenitis.

poradenitis (po·rad·en·i′·tis). Inflammatory disease of lymphatic glands, characterized by the formation of small abscesses. **Poradenitis nostras, Subacute inguinal poradenitis, Poradenitis venerea.** Lymphopathia venereum. [Gk *poros* passage, *aden* gland, *-itis* inflammation.]

pore [porus (NA)] (pore). A small opening on an epithelial surface, or a small communication between adjacent cavities. **Interalveolar pore.** One of the openings supposed to exist between adjacent alveoli in the lung. **Nuclear pore.** A region where the two layers of the nuclear envelope come together to form a thin membrane, the site of a potential communication between nucleus and cytoplasm. **Slit pore.** Filtration slit, the narrow winding space between the bases of adjacent pedicles in the renal glomerulus, through which the glomerular filtrate has to pass to reach the urinary space. **Sweat pore [porus sudoriferus (NA)].** The superficial opening of the duct, lying on the palm and soles on the summits of the curved ridges of the epidermis. **Taste pore [porus gustatorius (NA)].** The external opening of a taste bud. [Gk *poros* passage.]

See also: KOHN (H.).

porencephalia, porencephalus, porencephaly (po·ren·kef·a′·le·ah, po·ren·kef·al·us, po·ren·kef·al·e). Cystic formations in the cerebral cortex due to defective development. [Gk *poros* passage, *egkephalos* brain.]

Porfiromycin (por·fir·o·mi′·sin). BP Commission approved name for 6-amino-8-carbamoyloxymethyl-1-1a,2,8,8a,8b-hexa-hydro-8a-methoxy-1,5-dimethylazirino[2′,3′,3,4]-pyrrolo[1,2-α]indole-4,7-dione; an antibiotic.

Porifera (por·if·er·ah). A phylum of the animal kingdom; the sponges. [Gk *poros* passage, L *ferre* to bear.]

poriomania (por·e·o·ma′·ne·ah). A form of mental disorder characterized by wandering, usually in a state of impaired consciousness. [Gk *poreia* journey, mania.]

porion (po·re·on). The midpoint on the upper margin of the external auditory meatus which, together with a point on the inferior margin of the orbital aperture, is used to define the Frankfort horizontal plane. [Gk *poros* passage.]

pork (pork). The flesh of swine used as an article for diet. **Measly pork.** Pork which is infested with so-called cysticercus cellulosae (the larval form of *Taenia solium*); if it is insufficiently cooked it may cause infection in human beings. [L *porcus* hog.]

pornographomania (por·no·graf·o·ma′·ne·ah). A morbid interest in obscene writing. [Gk *porne* prostitute, *graphein* to write, mania.]

pornography (por·nog·raf·e). Explicit description or exhibition of sexual activity in literature, films, etc., intended to stimulate erotic rather than aesthetic feelings. [Gk *porne* prostitute, *graphein* to write.]

pornolagnia (por·no·lag·ne·ah). Sexual attraction towards prostitutes. [Gk *porne* prostitute, *lagneia* lust.]

porocele (po·ro·seel). Herniation into the scrotum associated with hardening and thickening of the essential structures of the hernial sac. [Gk *poroein* to become hardened, *kele* hernia.]

porocephaliasis (po·ro·kef·al·i′·as·is). Infection with a species of the genus *Porocephalus;* it is rare in man.

Porocephalida (po·ro·kef·al′·id·ah). An order of the phylum or arthropod class Pentastomida. The families Linguatulidae and Porocephalidae are of medical interest. [Gk *poros* passage, *kephale* head.]

Porocephalidae (po·ro·kef·al′·id·e). A family of the arthropod class Pentastomida. The genera *Armillifer* and *Porocephalus* are of medical interest. [see prec.]

porocephalosis (po·ro·kef·al·o′·sis). Porocephaliasis.

Porocephalus (po·ro·kef·al·us). A genus of Pentastomida. **Porocephalus crotali.** The lung worm of rattlesnakes in tropical and subtropical America. The larvae have been found rarely in human viscera. **Porocephalus subulifer.** A lung worm of various snakes in tropical Africa. The larva has been found rarely in human viscera. [Gk *poros* passage, *kephale* head.]

porofolliculitis (po·ro·fol·ik·ew·li′·tis). An acute superficial pustular folliculitis due to staphylococci. Also known as *Bockhart's impetigo.* [Gk *poros* passage, folliculitis.]

porokeratosis (po·ro·ker·at·o′·sis). A name suggested by Vittorio Mibelli in 1893 for a malady which he considered was essentially a hyperkeratosis occurring about the sweat pores; other observers have disputed this view. This rare malady can occur on any part of the skin, but is usually seen on the hands. The primary lesion is an acuminate horny papule which becomes surrounded by a horny raised collar. The latter spreads centrifugally and assumes the pattern of a festooned seam enclosing an area of flat, somewhat atrophic skin. The cause is unknown; the lesion is indolent and treatment is unsatisfactory. [Gk *poros* passage, *keras* horn, -osis condition.]

poroma (po·ro·mah). 1. Hardening of the tissues supervening on an inflammatory condition. 2. Callosity. 3. Exostosis. **Eccrine poroma.** A benign tumour of the palm or sole, arising from the intra-epidermal portion of a sweat duct. [Gk, callus.]

poroplastic (por·o·plas·tik). Referring to a substance which is porous and plastic, e.g. felt, in the making of splints.

porosis (por·o·sis). Abnormal rarefaction of a bone by thinning of its trabeculae; osteoporosis. **Cerebral porosis.** The occurrence of cyst-like cavities in brain substance. **Porosis palpebrae.** Chalazion. [Gk *poros* passage.]

porosity (por·os·it·e). 1. The quality of being porous. 2. A pore; a perforation.

porotic (por·ot·ik). 1. Aiding or influencing the growth of connective or fibrous tissue and thus of callus. 2. Like callus. [Gk *poroein* to become hardened.]

porotomy (por·ot·o·me). Meatotomy; incision of the urethral meatus. [Gk *poros* passage, *temnein* to cut.]

porous (po·rus). 1. Containing pores. 2. Allowing liquid to pass through. [Gk *poros* passage.]

porphin (por·fin). $C_{20}H_{14}N_4$, a 16-membered ring compound consisting of 4 pyrrole units linked by -CH= groups. The molecule is believed to exhibit resonance due to the shifting of the double bonds, the conjugate arrangement of which is responsible for the colour of its derivatives. It gives rise to the porphyrins, and may therefore be regarded as the parent of haemoglobin and chlorophyll.

porphobilinogen (por·fo·bi·lin′·o·jen). 2-Aminomethyl-4-2′-carboxyethyl-3-carboxymethylpyrrole, a chromogen sometimes present in the urine in porphyrinuria. It is converted to porphyrin by the action of light, heating at 100°C for 30 minutes, or by dilute hydrochloric acid.

porphyran (por·fir·an). A metalloporphyrin; a porphyrin combined with a metal such as iron, copper, magnesium or manganese. Such compounds have biological catalytic properties and include the haemochromes, cytochromes and chlorophylls. **Protein porphyran.** A compound of a protein and a porphyran, such as haemoglobin and other oxygen-transfer and respiratory pigments. [Gk *porphyros* purple.]

porphyria (por·fi·re·ah). A metabolic disorder in which porphyrin is retained in the tissues; it is always associated with an excess of porphyrin in the blood (porphyrinaemia) and in the urine (porphyrinuria). There is probably a constitutional predisposition to porphyria. It may be precipitated by certain drugs, the sulphonamides. **Acquired porphyria.** Porphyria resulting from liver damage due to alchohol or drugs (barbiturates, sulphonamides, griseofulvin, oestrogens or chloroquine). There is a bullous light-sensitivity rash with scarring, increased fragility of the skin, defective healing of wounds and hirsutism. **Acute idiopathic porphyria.** An inborn error of metabolism transmitted by dominant inheritance and characterized by attacks of abdominal pain, polyneuritis and psychotic symptoms. Porphobilinogen is present in the urine. **Acute intermittent porphyria.** Hepatic porphyria (see below). **Bantu porphyria.** Darkening of the skin, bullous eruptions, neurological syndromes, passage of urine which turns pink on standing, and hypertrichosis of the forehead in women. Excessive consumption of millet beer and crude spirits is a constant factor. The liver and spleen are usually enlarged and liver function tests are abnormal; uroporphyrin excretion is excessive; porphobilinogen and faecal porphyrins are normal. **Congenital porphyria.** A rare, genetic, erythropoietic porphyria in which there is a defect of haem synthesis in erythrocytes and release of porphyrin from normoblasts in the marrow with its excretion in the urine. Severe photosensitivity develops in infancy, with hypertrichosis, redness and oedema, and blistering, sometimes haemorrhagic. Mutilations result, including scars, ulcers, ectropion, milia, scarring alopecia, destruction of nasal and aural cartilages and even of the terminal phalanges. There is often a haemolytic anaemia, sometimes relieved by splenectomy. **Porphyria cutanea tarda.** Acquired porphyria (see above). **Erythropoietic porphyria.** 1. Congenital porphyria (see above). 2. Erythropoietic protoporphyria. *See* PROTOPORPHYRIA. **Hepatic porphyria.** 1. *Acute intermittent porphyria,* genetically determined but induced by drugs, e.g. barbiturates, sulphonamides and oestrogens. It causes abdominal pain, dark urine and neuropsychiatric symptoms. 2. *Porphyria variegata;* light sensitivity, skin fragility and attacks of acute intermittent porphyria, but genetically distinct from the acute intermittent porphyria described above. **Symptomatic cutaneous porphyria.** Acquired porphyria (see above). **Turkish porphyria.** An outbreak of porphyria due to consumption of seed grain dressed with benzene hexachloride. **Porphyria variegata.** Hepatic porphyria (see above). [Gk *porphyros* purple.]

porphyrin (**por**·fir·in). 1. One of a family of biological pigments derived from porphin by substitution of methyl and other alkyl groups for hydrogen atoms around the ring. They contain no metallic atom, and occur widely in plant and animal tissue, and in oil shales and coal, as the result of the breakdown of porphyrans. By combination with atoms of iron or magnesium they give rise to the pigments of oxygen-transfer and respiration in animals or plants respectively. 2. Porphyrine. [see prec.]

porphyrinaemia (**por**·fir·in·e′·me·ah). A condition characterized by the presence of porphyrin in the blood. [porphyrin, Gk *haima* blood.]

porphyrine (**por**·fir·een). $C_{21}H_{25}O_2N_3$, a minor alkaloid of alstonia bark.

porphyrinogen (por·fir·**in**·o·jen). Porphobilinogen. [porphyrin, Gk *genein* to produce.]

porphyrinuria (**por**·fir·in·**ewr**′·e·ah). The secretion of an excessive quantity of porphyrin in the urine.

porphyrism (**por**·fir·izm). Porphyria.

porphyruria (por·fir·**ewr**·e·ah). Porphyrinuria.

porphyryl (**por**·fir·il). Iron-free haemin. [Gk *porphyros* purple.]

Porret's phenomenon. Kuehne's phenomenon; on passing a continuous current through a muscle fibre, a wave of contraction arises at the positive pole and passes towards the negative pole.

porriginous (por·**ij**·in·us). Relating or belonging to porrigo; scurfy.

porrigo (por·**i**·go). Scurf or scales in the head, brows or beard [obsolete term]. **Porrigo contagiosa.** Impetigo contagiosa. **Porrigo decalvans.** Alopecia areata. **Porrigo favosa.** Favus. **Porrigo furfurans.** Tinea capitis. **Porrigo lavalis, Porrigo lupinosa, Porrigo scutulata.** Favus. [L, dandruff.]

Porro, Eduardo (b. 1842). Milan obstetrician.

Porro's hysterectomy, or operation. Caesarean section followed by subtotal hysterectomy with marsupialization of the cervical stump. The name of Porro is often incorrectly applied to the modern caesarean subtotal hysterectomy.

porta (**por**·tah). Gateway; the entrance into an organ through which pass the main vessels. **Porta hepatis** [L.]. The gateway of the liver through which enter the portal vein and the hepatic arteries and from which the hepatic ducts leave. [L.]

portacaval (por·tah·**ka**·val). Relating to the inferior vena cava and the portal vein, e.g. portacaval anastomosis.

Portal, Baron Antoine (b. 1742). French anatomist.

Portal's muscle. The deep portion of the brachialis muscle inserted into the articular capsule of the elbow joint.

portal (**por**·tal). Relating or belonging to a porta or hilum, and particularly to the porta hepatis. **Entry portal.** The area of body surface through which a beam of radiation is applied to a patient; the field. **Exit portal.** The area of body surface through which a beam of radiation leaves the patient; the emergent ray.

portal vein [vena portae (NA)]. The main vein draining the abdominal part of the alimentary canal, the spleen, pancreas and gall bladder to the liver. It is formed behind the neck of the pancreas by the union of the superior mesenteric and splenic veins, and terminates at the porta hepatis by dividing into right and left branches. The right branch [ramus dexter (NA)] divides into anterior and posterior segmental veins [ramus anterior et posterior (NA)]. The left branch [ramus sinister (NA)] passes to the left [pars transversa (NA)] and then bends downwards to lie in the depths of the umbilical fossa [pars umbilicalis (NA)]. The pars transversa gives branches to the caudate lobe [rami caudati (NA)] and the pars umbilicalis gives lateral branches [rami laterales (NA)] to the left lobe, and medial branches [rami mediales (NA)] to the quadrate lobe.

porte-aiguille (port·a·**gwe**). A needle-holder. [Fr.]

porte-cordon (port·kor·**don**). An instrument used in the replacement of a prolapsed umbilical cord. [Fr. *porter* to carry, *cordon* cord.]

porte-ligature (port·**lig**·at·ewr). An instrument used to convey a ligature into a deep wound or part. [Fr. *porter* to carry, ligature.]

porte-mèche (port·**mesh**). A packer in the form of a metal probe with a fork at one end, for packing a wound with gauze or other material. [Fr. *porter* to carry, *mèche* wick.]

porte-moxa (port·**mox**·ah). An appliance for retaining the combustible material, moxa, against the skin, for counter-irritation by heat. [Fr. *porter* to carry, moxa.]

porte-noeud (port·**nerd**). A forked instrument for carrying a ligature around the tip of a forceps controlling a deeply placed bleeding vessel. [Fr. *porter* to carry, *noeud* knot.]

Porteous, Stanley David (1883). Hawaiian psychiatrist.

Porteous maze test. A series of mazes, printed on paper, which the subject is required to trace in pencil from entrance to exit; the score (based on success and time) is supposed to provide an estimate of one aspect of intelligence.

Porter, William Henry (b. 1790). Dublin surgeon.

Porter's fascia. The pretracheal fascia.

Porter's sign. Tracheal tug. *See* TUG.

porter (**por**·ter). A dark, bitter beer, brewed from partly charred malt. [etym. dub.]

portio [NA] (**por**·she·o). A part; the term has been used in compounds such as *portio vaginalis cervicis,* but is rare in present-day English anatomy. [L.]

Portuguese man-of-war (port·ew·**geez** man·ov·**wor**). A jelly fish of the genus *Physalia* that inhabits tropical and subtropical waters; its sting is very painful and even dangerous.

porus [NA] (**po**·rus). An orifice; an opening; a pore. **Porus acusticus externus [NA].** The lateral orifice of the external auditory meatus. **Porus acusticus internus [NA].** The medial orifice of the internal auditory meatus. **Porus opticus.** The opening in the sclera which admits the optic nerve. **Porus sudoriferus [NA].** The surface opening of a sweat gland. [L].

Posada, Alejandro (b. 1870). Argentine protozoologist.

Posada's disease, or mycosis, Posada-Wernicke disease. Coccidioidomycosis.

Posadasia spheriforme (pos·ah·**da**·se·ah sfer·e· **for**·me). A former name for the fungus *Coccidioides immitis,* the cause of coccidioidomycosis [obsolete term]. [Alejandro *Posada.]*

posed (po·zd). In dentistry, describing the position of a tooth. Thus, normally posed, regularly posed, denotes a tooth in normal position, as distinct from malposed, a tooth in abnormal position. [L *ponere* to place.]

posiomania (po·se·o·**ma'**·ne·ah). Dipsomania. [Gk *posis* drink, mania.]

position (poz·**ish**·un). 1. The site occupied by an object in relation to other objects. 2. Attitude or posture of a person. 3. A state, condition or situation in relation to other conditions; a mental attitude towards a proposition. 4. In organic chemistry, the system of denoting the carbon atom in a chain or a ring to which a radical is attached. Thus, in an unbranched chain, the 1-, 2- or 3-position, or the α-, β- or γ- position; in a ring, the ortho-, meta- or para-position. **Alpha position.** *See* ALPHA. **Amino-acid position.** The numbered location of an amino-acid residue in a polypeptide proceeding from the amino to the carboxyl end of the chain. **Anatomical position.** The position of the body to which reference is made when using descriptive anatomical terms. The body is imagined as standing erect with the feet together and the palms of the hands facing forwards. **Apparent position.** The point in space where the object seen appears to the viewer to be. **Beta position.** *See* BETA. **Cadaveric position.** The semi-abducted position of the vocal cords which is seen when the laryngeal muscles are paralysed on both sides. **Coiled position.** A position in which the patient lies on his side with the legs well drawn up. **Delta position.** *See* DELTA. **Dorsal position.** The supine position with the patient lying on his back. **Dorsal elevated position.** The supine position with the head and shoulders raised. **Dorsal recumbent position.** A position in which the patient lies on the head, back and shoulders. **Dorsal rigid position.** The supine position with the legs drawn up to the body. **Dorsosacral position.** A position in which the patient lies on his back with the legs flexed at the knees and the thighs flexed on to the abdomen with the legs abducted. **Emprosthotonos position.** General spasm of the body with the head and feet forward and the abdominal muscles tightly contracted. **English position.** Left lateral recumbent position (see below). **Equinus position.** The position of the foot in talipes equinus. **First position.** Left occipito-anterior position of the vertex presentation. **Flipper position.** A position of decerebrate rigidity, due to a mid-brain lesion, with extension of arms and legs, pronation of forearms, flexion of wrists, and plantar flexion of feet, resembling the posture of a seal. **Positions of the fetus.** *See* PRESENTATION. **Fourth position.** Left occipitoposterior position of the vertex presentation. **Frog position.** The position of full abduction of both hips used in the treatment of congenital dislocation of the hip. **Gamma position.** *See* GAMMA. **Genucubital position.** Knee-elbow position; the patient rests on knees and elbows with his head supported on his hands. **Genupectoral position.** Knee-chest position; the patient rests on the knees and chest with his arms crossed beyond his head. **High pelvic position.** Trendelenburg's position; a position with the table tilted head down, the patient being prevented from slipping off by shoulder or pelvic supports, and by having the legs hanging over the end of the table. It is very commonly used in gynaecological operations. **Horizontal position.** One in which the patient lies on his back with legs extended. **Jack-knife position.** A position of the patient on the urological couch when the shoulders are elevated and the thighs are at right angles to the abdomen. The position is comfortable and facilitates urethral instrumentation. **Kidney position.** A position in which approach to the kidney is facilitated by having the patient lying on his side, the uppermost arm being drawn forwards and secured to a vertical support. **Knee-chest position.** Genupectoral position (see above). **Knee-elbow position.** Genucubital position (see above). **Kneeling-squatting position.** One in which the patient squats with his legs pressed against the abdomen and the body erect. **Lateral recumbent position.** One in which the patient lies on one or other side with the upper knee and thigh drawn upwards. **Latero-abdominal position.** Sims' position; semiprone position (see below). **Leap-frog position.** A position in which the patient rests on his knees and hands with arms straight. **Lithotomy position.** A position in which the patient lies on his back with legs flexed and his thighs on his abdomen and abducted. **Meta position.** *See* META-. **Obstetrical position.** Left lateral recumbent position (see above). **Occipito-anterior position.** The position of the fetus *in utero* when the head presents and is flexed and the occiput lies to the front. **Occipitoposterior position.** That in which the fetal occiput lies in or above the posterior half of the pelvis. **Opisthotonos position.** One in which the patient is arched backwards and rests on the back of his head and his heels. **Ortho position.** *See* ORTHO-. **Orthopnoeic position.** One in which the patient sits up and slightly forwards, with the arms supported on the arms of a chair or a small table. **Orthotonos position.** One in which the patient is rigid, with head, body and legs extended. **Para position.** *See* PARA-. **Prone position.** Face downwards. **Second position.** Right occipito-anterior position of the occiput. **Semiprone position.** Sims' position; the patient lies on the left side with the right knee and thigh drawn well up above the left. The left arm is put behind the back and allowed to hang over the edge of the couch. The chest and abdomen are allowed to fall forwards, thus creating a negative pressure in the abdomen and allowing the vagina to fill with air. **Semireclining position.** One in which the patient is partially upright, with the back supported on pillows or a bed rest. **Shoe-and-stocking position.** Lying with one leg crossed over the other. **Sitting position.** Orthopnoeic position (see above). **Supine position.** Lying on the back. **Third position.** Right occipitoposterior position of the vertex presentation. **Unilateral position.** Lying on one side. [L *positio.]*

See also: ADAMS, ALBERT, BOYCE, BOZEMAN, CASSELBERRY, DEPAGE, DUNCAN (J. M.), EDEBOHLS, ELLIOT (J. W.), FOWLER (G. R.), GRANGER, KRASKE, MAYO-ROBSON, NOBLE, PROETZ, ROSE (E.), SCHULTES (SCULTETUS), SIMON (G.), SIMS, STERN, TRENDELENBURG, VALENTINE, WALCHER, WATERS (C. A.), WOLFENDEN.

positive (**poz**·it·iv). 1. The opposite of negative; a quantity in excess of one. 2. A response to a test, usually disclosing some abnormality. 3. In electricity, the anode which attracts the negative current and repels the positive current. 4. In psychiatry, the complete agreement to suggestions. 5. A photographic image. [L, *positivus.*]

positron (**poz**·it·ron). *See* ELECTRON.

Poskine (**pos**·keen). BP Commission approved name for *O*-propionylhyoscine; a central nervous system depressant, used in the treatment of travel sickness.

Posner, Adolph (b. 1906). New York ophthalmologist.

Posner-Schlossman syndrome. Glaucomatocyclitic crises; recurrent unilateral non-congestive glaucoma characterized by an open angle and keratic precipitates.

posological (po·so·**loj**·ik·al). Relating or belonging to posology.

posology (po·**sol**·o·je). That branch of medical science which deals with dosage. [Gk *posos* of any size or number, *logos* science.]

posset (**pos**·et). A beverage made of hot milk curdled with wine or ale, and flavoured with sugar and spices. It was at one time recommended for colds and other ailments. [ME *poshote.*]

post. Prefix, from the Latin preposition and adverb, meaning *after, behind.*

post mortem (post **mor**·tem). After death. 1. Carried out or occurring after death. 2. A colloquial term for a post mortem examination; an autopsy. [L.]

See also: HUMAN TISSUE ACT 1961.

post natal (post **na**·tal). 1. Relating or belonging to the period immediately following birth. 2. Occurring after birth. [L *post, natus* birth.]

post partum (post **par**·tum). After childbirth. [L.]

postabortal (post·ab·**or**·tal). Taking place after an abortion. [L *post,* abortion.]

postacetabular (post·as·et·**ab'**·ew·lar). Occurring or situated behind the acetabulum. [L *post,* acetabulum.]

postacidotic (post·as·id·**o'**·tik). After acidosis. [L *post,* acidosis.]

postanaesthetic (**post**·an·es·**thet**′·ik). Occurring after or resulting from general anaesthesia. [L *post*, anaesthesia.]
postanal (post·**a**·nal). Behind the anus. [L *post*, anus.]
postapoplectic (**post**·ap·o·**plek**′·tik). Occurring after an apoplectic attack. [L *post*, apoplexy.]
postauditory (post·**aw**·dit·or·e). Occurring behind the auditory nerve. [L *post*, auditory.]
postauricular (post·aw·**rik**·ew·lar). Referring to the ear, occurring behind one of the auricles. [L *post*, auricle.]
postaxial (post·**ax**·e·al). Behind an axis, for example, the postaxial border of the upper extremity. [L *post*, axis.]
postbrachial (post·**bra**·ke·al). Occurring or situated on the posterior portion of the upper arm. [L *post*, Gk *brachion* arm.]
postbuccal (post·**buk**·al). Situated behind the buccal region. [L *post*, *bucca* cheek.]
postbulbar (post·**bul**·bar). Occurring behind the medulla oblongata. [L *post*, bulb.]
postcaecal (post·**se**·kal). Relating or belonging to the area behind the caecum. [L *post*, caecum.]
postcaesarean (post·se·**zare**·e·an). Occurring after caesarean section. [L *post*, caesarean.]
postcardinal (post·**kar**·din·al). Pertaining to the paired veins which drain the posterior part of the early embryo into the common cardinal veins or ducts of Cuvier. [L *post*, cardinal vein.]
postcava (post·**ka**·vah). The inferior vena cava. [L *post*, vena cava.]
postcaval (post·**ka**·val). Relating to the inferior vena cava. [see prec.]
postcentral (post·**sen**·tral). Behind a centre, e.g. the postcentral gyrus of the cerebral hemisphere. [L *post*, centre.]
postcerebellar (**post**·ser·e·**bel**′·ar). Situated or occurring in the posterior cerebellar region. [L *post*, cerebellum.]
postcerebral (post·**ser**·e·bral). Occurring or located behind the cerebrum. [see prec.]
postcibal (post·**si**·bal). Occurring after the taking of food. [L *post*, *cibus* food.]
postclavicular (post·klav·**ik**·ew·lar). Behind the clavicle. [L *post*, clavicle.]
postclimacteric (**post**·kli·mak·**ter**′·ik). Occurring after the climacteric. [L *post*, climacteric.]
postcoital (post·**ko**·it·al). After sexual intercourse. **Postcoital test.** The examination of the cervical mucus within 5 hours of coitus to see whether there are adequate, progressively moving sperms to enable fertilization to take place, provided the test is carried out around the time of ovulation, other fertility factors being excluded. [L *post*, coitus.]
postcommissure (post·**kom**·is·ewr). The posterior commissure of the cerebellum. [L *post*, commissure.]
postcondylar (post·kon·**di**·lar). Situated behind a condyle. [L *post*, condyle.]
postconnubial (post·kon·**ew**·be·al). Occurring after marriage. [L *post*, *connubium* marriage.]
postconvulsive (post·kon·**vul**·siv). Occurring after a convulsion. [L *post*, convulsion.]
postcordial (post·**kord**·e·al). Occurring or situated behind the heart. [L *post*, *cor* heart.]
postcornu (post·**kor**·new). The posterior horn of the lateral ventricle of the cerebral hemisphere. [L *post*, *cornu* horn.]
postcribrum (post·**kri**·brum). The posterior perforated substance of the mid-brain. [L *post*, *cribrum* sieve.]
postcricoid (post·**kri**·koid). Behind the cricoid cartilage. [L *post*, Gk *krikos* ring, *eidos* form.]
postcubital (post·**kew**·bit·al). Occurring on the dorsal aspect of the forearm. [L *post*, *cubitus* length of forearm.]
postdevelopmental (**post**·de·vel·op·**men**′·tal). After the developmental phase. [L *post*, development.]
postdiastolic (**post**·di·as·**tol**′·ik). Following the diastole, or occurring after it. [L *post*, diastole.]
postdicrotic (post·di·**krot**·ik). Occurring after the dicrotic pulse wave. [L *post*, dicrotic.]
postdigestive (post·di·**jes**·tiv). After digestion. [L *post*, digestion.]
postdiphtheritic (**post**·dif·ther·**it**′·ik). After diphtheria. [L *post*, diphtheria.]
postdivision (**post**·div·**izh**′·un). *See* PREDIVISION. [L *post*, division.]
postdormitum (post·**dor**·mit·um). The period of increasing wakefulness immediately succeeding sleep. [L *post*, *dormire* to sleep.]
postductal (post·**duk**·tal). A term applied to coarctation of the aorta of the adult type, indicating that the narrowing is below the opening of the ductus arteriosus. Cf. PREDUCTAL. [L *post*, duct.]
postdural (post·**dewr**·al). Situated or occurring behind the dura mater. [L *post*, dura mater.]
postembryonic (**post**·em·bre·**on**′·ik). Happening after embryonic life. [L *post*, embryo.]
postencephalitic (**post**·en·kef·al·**it**′·ik). 1. Happening after or occurring as a sequel to encephalitis. 2. Relating or belonging to postencephalitis. [see foll.]
postencephalitis (**post**·en·kef·al·**i**′·tis). A condition, characterized by abnormal and capricious behaviour, which may be observed in patients who have not long recovered from encephalitis lethargica. [L *post*, encephalitis.]
postepileptic (**post**·ep·il·**ep**′·tik). Following an epileptic seizure. [L *post*, epilepsy.]
posterior [NA] (pos·**teer**·e·or). Behind a part; the back of a part; dorsal. [L, behind.]
posterior vein of the left ventricle [vena posterior ventriculi sinistri (NA)]. A vein draining the diaphragmatic surface of the left ventricle and ending in the coronary sinus or the great cardiac vein.
postero-anterior (**pos**·ter·o·an·**teer**′·e·or). From the back to the front. [L *posterus* coming after, *anterior* before.]
posterocclusion (**pos**·ter·ok·**lew**′·zhun). Disto-occlusion. [L *posterus* coming after, occlusion.]
postero-external (**pos**·ter·o·ex·**ter**′·nal). Situated on the lateral side posteriorly. [L *posterus* coming after, external.]
postero-inferior (**pos**·ter·o·in·**feer**′·e·or). Situated in a posterior and inferior position.
postero-internal (**pos**·ter·o·in·**ter**′·nal). Situated on the medial side of a posterior aspect. [L *posterus* coming after, internal.]
posterolateral (**pos**·ter·o·**lat**′·er·al). Behind and to the lateral side. [L *posterus* coming after, *latus* side.]
posteromedial (**pos**·ter·o·**me**′·de·al). Behind and to the medial side. [L *posterus* coming after, *medius* middle.]
posteromedian (**pos**·ter·o·**me**′·de·an). Occupying the central position posteriorly. [see prec.]
postero-occlusion (**pos**·ter·o·ok·**lew**′·zhun). Disto-occlusion. [L *posterus* coming after, occlusion.]
posteroparietal (**pos**·ter·o·par·**i**′·et·al). Relating or belonging to the posterior portion of the parietal bone.
posterosuperior (**pos**·ter·o·sew·**peer**′·e·or). Situated behind and above. [L *posterus* coming after, *superior* above.]
posterotemporal (**pos**·ter·o·**tem**′·por·al). Occurring or situated in the posterior portion of the temporal bone.
posteruptive (post·e·**rup**·tiv). After eruption. [L *post*, eruption.]
postethmoid (post·**eth**·moid). Situated behind the ethmoid bone. [L *post*, ethmoid.]
postfebrile (post·**feb**·rile). Following or occurring as a sequel to a febrile condition. [L *post*, febrile.]
postganglionic (**post**·gang·gle·**on**′·ik). Literally, posterior to a ganglion. More usually interpreted as beyond or distal to a ganglion; e.g. a postganglionic fibre is the axon of a nerve cell situated in a ganglion, and therefore proceeds beyond or distally from the ganglion. [L *post*, ganglion.]
postgeniculatum, postgeniculum (**post**·jen·ik·ew·**la**′·tum, post·-jen·ik·ew·lum). The medial geniculate body of the metathalamus. [L *post*, geniculate.]
postglenoid (post·**gle**·noid). In a position posterior to a glenoid fossa. [L *post*, glenoid.]

postgrippal (post·**grip**·al). Postinfluenzal. [L *post*, Fr. *grippe* influenza.]

posthaemorrhage (post·**hem**·or·ij). Secondary haemorrhage. [L *post*, haemorrhage.]

posthaemorrhagic (**post**·hem·or·**ah'**·jik). Occurring as a sequel to, or following, haemorrhage. [see prec.]

posthalgia (pos·**thal**·je·ah). General term for pain affecting the penis. [Gk *posthe* foreskin, *algos* pain.]

posthemiplegic (**post**·hem·e·**ple'**·jik). Resulting from or occurring after hemiplegia. [L *post*, hemiplegia.]

posthepatic (post·hep·**at**·ik). Occurring or situated behind the liver. [L *post*, Gk *hepar* liver.]

posthetomy (pos·**thet**·o·me). Circumcision. [Gk *posthe* foreskin, *temnein* to cut.]

posthioplastic (**pos**·the·o·**plas'**·tik). Relating or belonging to posthioplasty.

posthioplasty (**pos**·the·o·plas·te). Plastic repair of the prepuce. [Gk *posthe* foreskin, *plassein* to mould.]

posthippocampal (**post**·hip·o·**kam'**·pal). Situated or occurring behind the hippocampus. [L *post*, hippocampus.]

posthitis (pos·**thi**·tis). Inflammation involving the prepuce. [Gk *posthe* foreskin, *-itis* inflammation.]

postholith (**pos**·tho·lith). A preputial concretion. [Gk *posthe* foreskin, *lithos* stone.]

posthoncus (pos·**thong**·kus). Any preputial tumour or swelling. [Gk *posthe* foreskin, *ogkos* a swelling.]

posthumeral (post·**hew**·mer·al). Occurring behind the humerus. [L *post*, humerus.]

posthumous (**post**·hew·mus). Occurring after death of the originator, e.g. publication of a book, birth of a child or granting an award. [L *post*, *humare* to bury.]

posthyoid (post·**hi**·oid). Pertaining to or occurring in the area behind the hyoid bone. [L *post*, hyoid.]

posthypnotic (post·hip·**not**·ik). Occurring after hypnosis. [L *post*, hypnosis.]

posthypophysis (post·hi·**pof**·is·is). The posterior lobe of the hypophysis cerebri. [L *post*, hypophysis.]

postictal (post·**ik**·tal). After a stroke or attack. [L *post*, *ictus* blow.]

posticteral (post·**ik**·ter·al). After jaundice has cleared. [L *post*, *ikteros* jaundice.]

posticus (post·i·kus). Another name for posterior, used in old anatomical nomenclature. [L, behind.]

postinfluenzal (**post**·in·floo·**en'**·zal). Occurring as a result of, or succeeding, influenza. [L *post*, influenza.]

postinsula (post·**in**·sew·lah). The posterior portion of the insula. [L *post*, insula.]

postischial (post·**is**·ke·al). Relating or belonging to the region behind the ischium. [L *post*, ischium.]

postmalarial (post·mal·a·re·al). Occurring as a result of an attack of malaria, or following malaria. [L *post*, malaria.]

postmastoid (post·**mas**·toid). Relating to the part behind the mastoid process of the temporal bone, or situated in that part. [L *post*, mastoid.]

postmaturity (post·mat·**ewr**·it·e). Overmaturity; beyond the normal date of maturity. [L *post*, maturity.]

postmaximal (post·**max**·im·al). Occurring after the maximum has been attained. [L *post*, maximum.]

postmeatal (post·me·a·tal). Situated or occurring behind a meatus. [L *post*, meatus.]

postmedian (post·**me**·de·an). Posterior to a median plane or line. [L *post*, median.]

postmediastinal (**post**·me·de·as·**ti'**·nal). 1. Posterior to the mediastinum. 2. Relating or belonging to the posterior mediastinum. [see foll.]

postmediastinum (**post**·me·de·as·**ti'**·num). The posterior mediastinum. [L *post*, mediastinum.]

postmeiotic (post·mi·**ot**·ik). Pertaining to a cell following meiosis or reduction division. [L *post*, meiosis.]

postmenopausal (**post**·men·o·**pawz'**·al). Taking place after the menopausal epoch. [L *post*, menopause.]

postmenstrua (post·**men**·stroo·ah). The phase which succeeds the end of a menstrual period. [L *post*, menstruation.]

postmesenteric (**post**·mes·en·**ter'**·ik). Occurring behind or situated posteriorly to the mesentery. [L *post*, mesentery.]

post-mortem (post·**mor**·tem). After death. Also loosely used to describe an examination of the body after death (autopsy) by a pathologist (sectio cadaveris). **Post-mortem lividity.** *See* LIVIDITY. **Post-mortem rigidity.** *See* RIGIDITY.

postnarial (post·**na**·re·al). Relating to the posterior nasal apertures. [see foll.]

postnaris (post·**na**·ris). A posterior nasal aperture; the posterior naris. [L *post*, *naris* nostril.]

postnasal (post·**na**·zal). 1. Pertaining to the region behind the nose. 2. Referring to the posterior part of the nasal fossae. [L *post*, *nasus* nose.]

postnatal (post·**na**·tal). 1. Relating or belonging to the period immediately following birth. 2. Occurring after birth. [L *post*, *natus* birth.]

postnecrotic (post·nek·**rot**·ik). Taking place after necrosis of tissue or of a part of the body. [L *post*, necrosis.]

postneuritic (post·newr·**it**·ik). Referring to any disease which arises as a sequel to neuritis. [L *post*, neuritis.]

postnodular (post·**nod**·ew·lar). Relating to or situated in the part behind the middle (nodular) lobe of the cerebellum. [L *post*, nodule.]

postocular (post·**ok**·ew·lar). Situated behind the eyeball. [L *post*, *oculus* eye.]

postoesophageal (**post**·e·sof·ah·**je'**·al). Behind the oesophagus. [L *post*, oesophagus.]

postolivary (post·**ol**·iv·ar·e). Situated behind the olivary nucleus. [L *post*, olivary.]

postoncolytic (**post**·ong·ko·**lit'**·ik). After the destruction of a tumour or tumour cells. [L *post*, oncolysis.]

postoperative (post·**op**·er·a·tiv). Pertaining to or occurring in the period succeeding a surgical operation. [L *post*, operation.]

postopticus (post·**op**·tik·us). Any one of the quadrigeminal bodies (optic lobes). [L *post*, optic.]

postoral (post·**or**·al). 1. Occurring in the posterior portion of the mouth. 2. Situated behind the mouth. [L *post*, *os* mouth.]

postorbital (post·**or**·bit·al). Behind the orbit. [L *post*, orbit.]

postpalatal, postpalatine (post·**pal**·at·al, post·**pal**·at·ine). Pertaining to the part behind, or the posterior part of, the palate or the palatine bone. [L *post*, palate.]

postpallium (post·**pal**·e·um). The part of the cerebral cortex which lies behind the central sulcus. [L *post*, *pallium* coverlet.]

postpaludal (post·**pal**·ew·dal). Postmalarial. [L *post*, *palus* swamp.]

postparalytic (**post**·par·al·**it'**·ik). Succeeding, or resulting from, paralysis. [L *post*, paralysis.]

postpartum (post·**par**·tum). Relating to the period immediately following childbirth. [L *post*, *parturire* to have the pains of labour.]

postpharyngeal (post·far·**in**·je·al). Pertaining to the part behind the pharynx; occurring behind the pharynx. [L *post*, pharynx.]

postpituitary (post·pit·**ew**·it·ar·e). 1. Occurring behind the hypophysis cerebri (pituitary body). 2. Relating to the posterior lobe of the hypophysis cerebri. [L *post*, pituitary.]

postpleuritic (post·ploor·**it**·ik). Succeeding, or occurring as a sequel to, pleurisy. [L *post*, pleurisy.]

postpneumonic (post·new·**mon**·ik). Succeeding, or resulting from, pneumonia. [L *post*, pneumonia.]

postpontile (post·**pon**·tile). Below or behind the pons. [L *post*, pons.]

postprandial (post·**pran**·de·al). After dinner or after a meal. [L *post*, *prandere* to lunch.]

postpuberal, postpubescent (post·**pew**·ber·al, post·pew·**bes**·ent). Occurring after the period of puberty. [L *post*, puberty.]

postpyknotic (post·pik·**not**·ik). Pertaining to the stage following pyknosis; in the dissolution of the nucleus after cell death. [L *post,* pyknosis.]
postpyramidal (post·pir·**am**·id·al). Pertaining to or situated behind the pyramidal tract. [L *post,* pyramid.]
postradiation (**post**·ra·de·**a**'·shun). After radiation, after excessive radiation, e.g. with x-rays or radioactive isotopes. [L *post,* radiation.]
postrhinal (post·**ri**·nal). Postnasal. [L *post,* Gk *rhis* nose.]
postrolandic (post·ro·**lan**·dik). Occurring behind the central sulcus of the cerebrum (fissure of Rolando). [L *post,* fissure of Rolando.]
postrotatory (post·ro·**ta**·tor·e). After rotation. [L *post,* rotation.]
postsacral (post·**sa**·kral). Pertaining to the part situated behind or below the sacrum. [L *post,* sacrum.]
postscapular (post·**skap**·ew·lar). Posterior to the scapula, or behind it. [L *post,* scapula.]
postscarlatinal (post·skar·**lat**·in·al). Succeeding scarlatina. [L *post,* scarlatina.]
postsinusoidal (**post**·si·nus·**oid**'·al). After the sinusoids, e.g. postsinusoidal obstruction of the liver. [L *post, sinus* curve, Gk *eidos* form.]
postsphenoid (post·**sfe**·noid). The posterior portion of the body of the sphenoid bone in the embryo. Its centre of ossification is distinct from that of the anterior portion (presphenoid). [L *post,* sphenoid.]
postsphygmic (post·**sfig**·mik). Following the arterial pulse wave. [L *post,* Gk *sphygmos* pulse.]
postsplenic (post·**splen**·ik). Pertaining to or situtated in the part posterior to the spleen; lying behind the spleen. [L *post,* spleen.]
poststenotic (post·**sten**·ot·ik). Situated after a stenosis. [L *post,* Gk *stenos* narrow, *-osis* condition.]
postsylvian (post·**sil**·ve·an). Occurring or situated behind the lateral sulcus (fissure of Sylvius) in the cerebrum. [L *post,* fissure of Sylvius.]
postsyphilitic (**post**·sif·il·**it**'·ik). Occurring after an infection with syphilis. [L *post,* syphilis.]
postsystolic (post·sis·**tol**·ik). In the cardiac cycle, occurring at the end of the systole. [L *post,* systole.]
post-tarsal (post·**tar**·sal). 1. Posterior to the tarsus. 2. Relating or belonging to the posterior portion of the tarsus. [L *post,* tarsus.]
post-tibial (post·**tib**·e·al). Relating or belonging to the part of the leg posterior to the tibia. [L *post,* tibia.]
post-traumatic (post·traw·**mat**·ik). Taking place after or as the result of trauma. **Post-traumatic epilepsy.** An organic epilepsy secondary to brain lesions due to injury. [L *post,* trauma.]
post-tussis (post·**tus**·is). After coughing. [L *post, tussis* a cough.]
post-typhoid (post·**ti**·phoid). Succeeding typhoid fever; occurring as a result of an attack of typhoid fever. [L *post,* typhoid.]
postulate (**pos**·tew·late). 1. A proposition whose acceptance is demanded. 2. A hypothesis put forward as a basis for argument. [L *postulare* to demand.]
See also: AVOGADRO, EHRLICH, EWING, KOCH (R.).
postural (**pos**·tewr·al). 1. Relating to or caused by position or posture. 2. Effected by posture, as treatment of fracture. [see foll.]
posture (**pos**·tewr). Position, attitude or carriage of the body. An attitude of body or mind, often used in a derogatory sense. **Active alerted posture.** Posture in which each mobile part is firmly locked to its corresponding fixed part. **Inactive slumping posture.** Posture in which the dead weight of the mobile parts exerts a strain on muscles and ligaments of joints. **Incompetent lip posture.** In dentistry, the position of the lips in resting tonus, where there is no lip seal possible without active conscious contraction of the surrounding muscles. **Passive supported posture.** Posture when sitting or lying without strain on mobile parts. [L *ponere* to place.]
postuterine (post·**ew**·ter·ine). Behind the uterus. [L *post,* uterus.]
postvaccinal (post·**vax**·in·al). Occurring after or as a sequel to vaccination. [L *post,* vaccine.]
postvaccinial (post·vax·**in**·e·al). Occurring after and/or arising from vaccinia. [L *post,* vaccinia.]
postvital (post·**vi**·tal). A term used in connection with the staining of recently killed cells. [L *post, vita* life.]
potable (**po**·tabl). Drinkable; fit for drinking. [L *potare* to drink.]
Potain, Pierre Charles Edouard (b. 1825). Paris physician.
Potain's apparatus, or aspirator. An apparatus which enables fluid to be withdrawn through a cannula, attached by tubing to a bottle in which negative pressure is produced by means of a pump.
Potain's congestion. Pleuropulmonary congestion; congestion of the lungs, either passive, as in heart failure, or active, as in inflammation.
Potain's disease. Pulmonary oedema. *See* OEDEMA.
Potain's sign. Dullness to the right of the sternum in the upper two intercostal spaces, in cases of dilatation of the ascending aorta.
Potain's syndrome. Dilatation of the right ventricle and increase of the second pulmonary sound in cases of gastric dilatation.
Potamon (**pot**·a·mon). A genus of fresh-water crabs, of which some species are capable of acting as intermediary hosts of the fluke *Paragonimus westermani.* [Gk *potamos* river.]
potamophobia (**pot**·am·o·**fo**'·be·ah). Morbid dread of rivers or any expanse of water. [Gk *potamos* river, phobia.]
potash (**pot**·ash). 1. Term applied generally to potassium compounds. 2. Pot-ashes; wood-ash lixiviated with water and the solution concentrated in iron pots to yield a crude potassium carbonate, K_2CO_3. 3. Caustic potash, potassium hydroxide, KOH. **Potash alum.** Potassium alum. *See* ALUM. **Caustic potash.** Potassium hydroxide. **Sulphurated Potash BPC 1968.** Liver of sulphur; a mixture of sulphite and thiosulphate, and other compounds of potassium obtained by the fusion of sublimed sulphur with potassium carbonate. It is used in the form of a lotion in aqueous media for external application to the skin in the treatment of scabies and acne. **Sulphuretted potash.** Potassium sulphide. [Dutch *potasschen.*]
potassa (pot·**as**·ah). Potash. **Potassa caustica.** Potassium hydroxide. **Potassa sulphurata.** Sulphurated potash. [L.]
potassaemia (pot·as·**e**·me·ah). The presence of abnormally large quantities of potassium in the blood. [potassium, Gk *haima* blood.]
potassic (pot·**as**·ik). Relating to potassium, or having potassium in its composition.
potassiocupric (pot·as·e·o·**kew**'·prik). Applied to a compound that contains both potassium and divalent copper, e.g. potassiocupric carbonate, $K_2CO_3CuCO_3$. [potassium, L *cuprum* copper.]
potassiocuprous (pot·as·e·o·**kew**'·prus). Applied to a compound that contains both potassium and monovalent copper, as in potassium cuprocyanide, $KCu(CN)_2$, used in electroplating. [see prec.]
potassiomercuric (pot·as·e·o·mer·**kewr**'·ik). Applied to a compound that contains potassium and divalent mercury. **Potassiomercuric iodide.** K_2HgI_4, a germicide and antiseptic more soluble than mercuric iodide; also a reagent for alkaloids.
potassium (pot·**as**·e·um). An element of atomic weight 39.098, atomic number 19, and chemical symbol K (*kalium*). It is a soft white metal, related to sodium and even more highly reactive. It occurs naturally in sea water, as the silicate in primary rocks and granites, and in vast deposits as the chloride in Saxony, Galicia, California and elsewhere. It is a constituent of all plants and animals, exceeding sodium in amount, but, unlike the latter, is to be found in the tissues rather than the fluids. In plants it is concerned in photosynthesis and growth; in animals the ion is essential for tissue excitability. It has a depressant action, however, on voluntary and unstriped muscle, and on the central nervous system and the heart; the ion is excreted rapidly by the kidneys when taken orally, and is of value as a diuretic. The element as it occurs in nature is slightly radioactive, due to the presence of the isotope ${}_{19}K^{40}$, but no biological significance has

been traced to this. **Potassium acetate.** CH_3COOK, a compound employed as a diuretic and diaphoretic and to reduce the pain and frequency of micturition caused by highly acid urine. It is also used in pathology for hardening and preserving tissues to retain their colour (Kaiserling's method). **Potassium acid phosphate.** KH_2PO_4, a soluble compound used in buffer solutions; it renders the urine acid and is of value as a diuretic. Administered in small frequent doses, it is claimed to be more effective than the sodium salt. **Potassium acid tartrate.** Purified cream of tartar, $HOOC(CHOH)_2COOK$, a compound used as a saline purgative; it has also been used for dusting surgical gloves in place of starch. **Potassium ammonium antimonyl tartrate.** Antiluctin, $K(NH_4)_2(SbO)(C_6H_4O_6)_2$, an antisyphilitic. **Potassium antimonyl tartrate.** Antimony potassium tartrate. **Potassium arsenate.** K_2HAsO_4, a compound used like sodium arsenate therapeutically. **Potassium arsenite.** A solution of arsenic trioxide in potassium hydroxide and neutralized with hydrochloric acid; arsenical solution (Fowler's solution), used as a convenient way of administering arsenic. **Potassium aurobromide.** $KAuBr_4$, a double salt of potassium and gold bromides used as a convenient way of administering gold. **Potassium aurocyanide.** $KAu(CN)_2$, a soluble gold compound which has been occasionally administered internally and locally in lupus and syphilitic ulcerations. **Potassium Bicarbonate BP 1968.** $KHCO_3$, a compound more soluble than sodium bicarbonate, but with similar properties and used in the treatment of gastric hyperacidity, acidosis and to reduce the acidity of the urine. It is also used with expectorants in the treatment of bronchitis. **Potassium bichromate.** Potassium dichromate (see below). **Potassium binoxalate.** HOOCCOOK, a soluble compound used in dyeing and to remove stains. **Potassium biphosphate.** Potassium acid phosphate (see above). **Potassium bismuth tartrate.** $K(BiO)(C_4H_4O_6)$, a compound used in the treatment of syphilis, and, in higher doses, as an emetic. **Potassium bisulphate.** $KHSO_4$, a compound occasionally used in conjunction with sodium bicarbonate as a saline laxative. **Potassium bisulphite.** Potassium metabisulphite (see below). **Potassium bitartrate.** Potassium acid tartrate (see above). **Potassium Bromide BP 1973.** KBr, a compound with a sedative action on the central nervous system, depressing psychical function, the motor area, the medulla and the cord. It has a direct action on the nerve cells and is used in controlling epilepsy and allaying cerebral excitement; by depression of the medulla and cord it diminishes reflexes and promotes sleep. In conjunction with chloral formamide it is of value in seasickness and the sickness of pregnancy. Continued administration of large doses results in accumulation and symptoms of brominism. **Potassium bromortho-oxybenzoate, Potassium bromsalicylate.** $OHC_6H_3BrCOOK$, a compound used as an antirheumatic. **Potassium carbolate.** C_6H_5OK, a compound with antiseptic properties, used occasionally in diarrhoea and dysentery. **Potassium carbonate.** $K_2CO_3 \cdot 1\frac{1}{2} H_2O$, a compound more caustic and irritant than potassium bicarbonate and seldom given internally; externally it has been employed as a lotion in eczema and urticaria. **Potassium Chlorate BPC 1968.** $KClO_3$, a mild astringent used in stomatitis, tonsilitis and other inflammatory conditions of the mouth and pharynx, usually as a mouth-wash or gargle, but sometimes in the form of lozenges. Internally it is rapidly absorbed and only slowly eliminated by the kidneys, hence administration may be attended with toxic effects. **Potassium Chloride BP 1973.** KCl, a salt commonly used for administering the potassium ion; since the ion is rapidly excreted by the kidneys it is an efficient diuretic, and in cardiac oedema may replace common salt in the diet. It is an important constituent of Ringer's solution. Injected subcutaneously or intravenously it has a depressant action on cardiac muscle and nerve tissues. It has been employed to improve conduction at the nerve-endings in myasthenia gravis and in familial periodic paralysis, also in the treatment of Ménière's disease. Toxic effects may be produced where excretion is delayed, as in renal insufficiency. **Potassium Citrate BP 1973.** $C_3H_4OH(COOK)_3 \cdot H_2O$, a compound with diaphoretic, diuretic, and febrifugal properties. It is excreted as the carbonate, rendering the urine alkaline, and is given in cystitis, gout and enuresis when this is due to over-acid urine; it is also used to prevent crystalluria in sulphonamide treatment. Large doses are given in acidosis. **Potassium dichromate.** $K_2Cr_2O_7$, an actively astringent and mildly antiseptic orange-red compound; in concentrated solution it is vigorously caustic. By mouth an irritant corrosive poison, it is little used in medicine, but is a valuable oxidizing agent used for laboratory purposes and in industry. **Potassium dihydrogen phosphate.** Potassium acid phosphate (see above). **Potassium di-iodoresorcinmonosulphate.** $C_6HI_2(OH)_2SO_3K$, a compound used as a wound antiseptic. **Potassium dithiocarbonate.** K_2COS_2, a compound which has been used in skin diseases. **Effervescent potassium citrate.** An effervescent preparation of potassium citrate, containing also sodium bicarbonate, and citric and tartaric acids. **Potassium ferricyanide.** $K_3Fe(CN)_6$, a soluble red compound used as a reducing agent in the laboratory and in photographic processes. **Potassium ferrocyanide.** $K_4Fe(CN)_6$, a soluble yellow compound used as a laboratory reagent and in photography; it has diaphoretic properties and has been used in the night sweats of phthisis. **Potassium fluoresceinate.** The potassium salt of fluorescein, used to detect corneal injury and ulceration. **Potassium Gluconate BPC 1968.** $C_6H_{11}KO_7$, the potassium salt of gluconic acid; given by mouth for the prevention and treatment of potassium deficiency in patients on diuretic therapy. **Potassium glycerophosphate.** A compound used like other glycerophosphates for nervous diseases and debilitated conditions, but of doubtful value. **Potassium guaiacolsulphonate.** A soluble compound used as a substitute for guaiacol and employed as an expectorant and antiseptic in the treatment of bronchitis, but of doubtful value. **Potassium hydrate, Potassium Hydroxide BP 1973.** KOH, a white compound, highly soluble in water; it is a powerful caustic and in solution may be used as a potent escharotic. Small doses freely diluted may be employed as an antacid internally, but other antacids are to be preferred. **Potassium Hydroxyquinoline Sulphate BPC 1968.** A mixture of potassium sulphate and hydroxyquinoline sulphate. It has bactericidal and deodorant properties, is rarely used internally, but externally is employed as a lotion in mycosis and eczema; it is also of value as a spermicide. **Potassium hypochlorite.** KOCl, a soluble compound with bleaching and disinfectant properties. **Potassium Hypophosphite BPC 1963.** KH_2PO_2, a compound used as a "nerve tonic" but there is no evidence of its effectiveness. **Potassium iodate.** KIO_3, a soluble deliquescent compound used in solution as a reagent, and occasionally employed like potassium chlorate in diseases of mucous surfaces. **Potassium Iodide BP 1973.** KI, a soluble white crystalline compound with diuretic and expectorant properties. Being partly excreted by the bronchial glands it renders the bronchial mucus less viscid and hence is of value in chronic catarrhs and bronchitis. It promotes the resolution or absorption of recently formed fibrous tissue and is for this reason used in the later stages of syphilis to aid the action of antisyphilitic drugs. In large doses it is employed in the treatment of actinomycosis, sporotrichosis and blastomycosis. Tending to reduce pain, it is of some help in cases of circulatory disease. It is used for the prophylaxis and treatment of simple goitre and also in the early treatment of exophthalmic goitre prior to operation. Externally it may be applied locally to enlarged glands as a liniment with soap. Idiosyncrasy exists in certain people, and side-effects such as mental depression and nervousness may result from prolonged administration. **Potassium Menaphthosulphate.** BP Commission approved name for dipotassium 2-methyl-1,4-disulphatonaphthalene dihydrate. It is the potassium salt of the disulphuric acid ester of reduced menaphthone, and resembles acetomenaphthone and the corresponding phosphoric acid ester more closely than it does menaphthone. It reduces the coagulation time of the blood. **Potassium mercuric iodide.** $KIHgI_2$, a yellow compound insoluble in water but soluble in potassium-iodide solution; it is a powerful germicide and is used externally as a skin disinfectant, for irrigation, and for the disinfection of instruments. It is also employed in Mayer's reagent for alkaloids, and in Nessler's reagent for the estimation of ammonia. **Potassium metabisulphite.** $K_2S_2O_5$, a compound used as an antiseptic and antifermentative in thrush, ringworm and other skin diseases. It is also employed as a food preservative, and in pharmacy as an anti-oxidant. **Potassium Nitrate BP 1973.** KNO_3, saltpetre; a colourless crystalline compound, soluble in water. By mouth it acts as a saline diuretic, but in larger doses may cause irritation of the kidneys and gastrointestinal tract. It is occasionally used in gargles for sore throats, and saltpetre balls (sal prunella) were sucked for this purpose at one time. **Potassium nitrite.** KNO_2, a compound which exhibits the physiological effects of nitrites, but the sodium salt is to be preferred. **Normal potassium tartrate.** Potassium tartrate (see below). **Potassium osmate.** K_2OsO_4, a salt which has been used in rheumatic affections and sciatica; it has been suggested for injection along the nerve trunk. **Potassium oxyquinoline sulphate.** Potassium Hydroxyquinoline Sulphate (see above). **Potassium penicillin G.** The crystalline potassium salt of benzylpenicillin. **Potassium Perchlorate BP 1963.** $KClO_3$, it interferes with the iodine-binding mechanism of the thyroid gland and was formerly used in the treatment of thyrotoxicosis. **Potassium Permanganate BP 1973.** $KMnO_4$, a soluble, dark-purple compound with disinfectant and deodorant properties owing to its oxidizing action. It is employed as a solution for cleansing foul ulcers or abscesses, as a gargle, mouth-wash and also for vaginal and urethral irrigation. A strong solution has a powerful styptic action. It is a valuable antidote in morphine poisoning, and is of use in snake bite. **Potassium phenate, Potassium phenolate.** Potassium carbolate (see above). **Potassium phosphate.** K_2HPO_4, a soluble compound used as a saline purgative and mild diuretic. **Potassium salicylate.** $C_6H_4(OH)COOK$, a soluble compound of value in certain rheumatic conditions. **Potassium sodium cyanide.** The commerical potassium cyanide; really a mixture of sodium and potassium cyanide. It is used mainly in entomology for destroying insects. **Potassium sodium tartrate.** Rochelle salt, $NaOOC(CHOH)_2COOK$, a saline cathartic with a diuretic action, turning the urine alkaline. It is employed as a mild purgative, and is a constituent of Seidlitz powder. **Potassium Sorbate BPC 1968.** The potassium salt of 2,4-hexadienoic acid, it has anti-fungal and antibacterial properties and is used pharmaceutically as a preservative. **Potassium sulphate.** K_2SO_4, a soluble compound used as a saline purgative; it may also potentiate the action of local anaesthetic solutions. **Potassium sulphide.** K_2S, a compound little used in medicine. **Potassium sulphite.** K_2SO_3, an antiseptic and antizymotic compound. **Potassium sulphocyanide.** Potassium Thiocyanate (see below). **Potassium tartrate.** $KOOCH(CHOH)_2COOK$, a compound used as a laxative and diuretic; sal vegetabile. **Potassium Thiocyanate BPC 1954.** KCNS, a compound used as a reagent in analysis; it is also employed in medicine by mouth to relax unstriped muscle, and it is of value in arterial hypertension. [potash.]

potency (po·ten·se). 1. The inherent quality of having power or strength. 2. The capacity of the male to perform the sexual act. 3. In homoeopathy, the increased efficacy of a drug produced by dilution or attenuation. 4. The homoeopathic preparation of a medicine above the thirtieth dilution. **Reactive potency.** The power to react. [L *potentia* power.]

See also: BIOLOGICAL STANDARDS ACT 1976.

potentia (po·ten·she·ah). Power. **Potentia coeundi.** The capacity to have sexual intercourse. **Potentia concepiendi.** The capacity to conceive. **Potentia generandi.** The power to beget children. [L.]

potential (po·ten·shal). 1. Capable of coming into action. 2. The power to do work. 3. An unrealized capacity, an unused force or source of energy. 4. In electricity, voltage, the electromotive force which drives a current from one point to another; the work required to bring a unit positive charge to a certain point from infinity. **Action potential.** The voltage changes occurring inside a cell (heart, nerve) when it is depolarized, due to ionic movements into and out of the cell. **After potential.** The smaller wave which follows the main action potential wave (spike) in an oscillograph tracing. **Autonomous potentials.** Potentials arising spontaneously in neurones, i.e. without extraneous stimulation. **Bio-electric potential.** That which is manifested in biological phenomena. **Constant potential.** In radiological practice, a unidirectional potential that has small periodic variations. The periodic component is called a *ripple potential.* **Critical potential.** The particular ionic potential at which the addition of charged ions to a colloidal system brings about the precipitation of the colloid. **Demarcation potential.** The difference in electrical potential between the parts of a muscle or nerve that has been severed. **Difference of potential.** The electrical potential difference between two points, numerically equal to the work done in moving unit positive charge from the point at lower potential to that of higher potential. **Earth potential.** The electric potential of the earth, taken as zero, and the standard of reference. **Electrical potential.** The voltage between two points. **Electrochemical potential.** The potential drop across all of the ionic layers from the surface of the particle to the solution. Also called *epsilon potential.* **Electrocortical potentials.** Potentials arising in the cerebral cortex and observed by means of leads placed either on the exposed cortex or outside the intact skull. **Electrode potential.** The potential set up between a metal (electrode) and a solution of one of its salts (electrolyte) in which it is immersed. It is due either to the emission of cations from the metal into the solution (*negative electrode potential*) or to the deposition of cations on the metal from the solution (*positive electrode potential*). **Electrokinetic potential.** A potential at the interface between the semipermeable membrane and a solution on either side. Also called *zeta potential.* **Electrotonic potential.** That potential led off from either side of bipolar electrodes when a nerve is stimulated by direct current. **Epsilon potential.** Electrochemical potential (see above). **Evoked potential.** Potential occurring as a result of stimulation applied to a nerve. **Ground potential.** Earth potential (see above). **Injury potential.** The potential developed between injured and uninjured parts of a nerve, due to the fact that at the injured site the negatively charged inner surface of the polarized membrane is exposed. Also called *demarcation potential.* **Ionization potential.** The work which must be done to remove an electron completely from an atom. **Magnetic potential.** The work required to bring up a unit magnetic (north-seeking) pole from infinity to a defined point. **Membrane potential.** The difference in potential between the two sides of a membrane or cell wall. **Monophasic action potential.** The type of record of the electrical activity that is associated with stimulation of the atrium of the heart, which is obtained by means of a small suction electrode applied to the inner surface of the atrium after pervenous introduction; the record has close similarity to that obtained of the membrane potential by the use of intracellular micro-electrodes. **Oxidation-reduction potential.** The relative potential exerted by a non-reacting electrode in a solution, as measured against that exerted by a normal hydrogen electrode; the potential difference between a non-reacting electrode and a reversible oxidation–reduction system in which it is immersed. **Pulsating potential.** A unidirectional potential which undergoes periodic variations in magnitude at a frequency related to that of the mains supply. **Radiation potential.** The energy required to transfer an electron from one position in the atom to another position where its energy level would be greater. **Redox potential.** Oxidation-reduction potential (see above). **Resonance potential.** Radiation potential (see above). **Ripple potential.** *See* CONSTANT POTENTIAL (above). **Saturation potential.** The potential applied to an ionization chamber or two-electrode valve which is sufficient to remove ions or electrons to the electrodes at the rate at which they are produced. Increase of potential above saturation does not produce an increase in current. **Spike potential.** That demarcation potential which, as it passes the uninjured part of a nerve, and as recorded by means of a cathode-ray or other oscillograph, gives rise to a large brief monophasic wave. **Streaming potential.** Potential due to the movement of fluids, as of the blood in the blood vessels. **Zeta potential.** Electrokinetic potential (see above). [L *potentia* power.]

potentialization (po·ten·shal·i·za′·shun). Potentiation.

potentiation (po·ten·she·a′·shun). A word usually applied to the action of drugs which together exert an effect greater than the total effect if the drugs were taken separately. Classification of the interaction of two drugs is determined most simply by the administration of half the dose of one drug necessary for a given effect with half the corresponding dose of the other. If the combination does not produce the effect, the drugs are antagonists; if it just causes the effect, their actions are additive; if it causes more than the given effect, there is *potentiation.* **Postextrasystolic potentiation.** In cardiology, the increase in the forcefulness of the ventricular contraction which occurs in the beat which follows an extrasystole and which is independent of any effect secondary to altered filling of the ventricle because of the interruption of the normal rhythm. [L *potentia* power.]

potentiometer (po·ten·she·om′·et·er). A graduated and variable resistance used in the accurate comparison of electrical voltages. [potential, meter.]

potentiometric (po·ten·she·o·met′·rik). Relating to or involving the use of a potentiometer.

potentize (po·ten·tize). 1. To produce potency in a drug. 2. In homoeopathy, to produce potency in a drug by dilution.

potentor (po·ten·tor). A mechanical device used in the treatment of impotence in a male subject, particularly that due to loss or deficiency of erectile power. [L *potentia* power.]

potocytosis (po·to·si·to′·sis). The assumed capacity of cells to convey fluid substances from one to another location in themselves. [Gk *potos* drink, *kytos* cell.]

potomania (po·to·ma·ne·ah). An uncontrollable urge to drink alcoholic beverages, often ending in alcoholism. [Gk *potos* drink, mania.]

Pott, Percival (b. 1714). London surgeon.

Pott's anastomosis, or operation. An anastomosis between the anterior aspect of the descending aorta and the posterior aspect of the left pulmonary artery, used for the palliation of various forms of cyanotic congenital heart disease in which the blood flow to the lungs is diminished.

Pott's aneurysm. An aneurysmal varix.

Pott's boss, or curvature. The abnormal curvature of the spine which is the result of disease of the vertebrae.

Pott's caries, or disease. Tuberculosis of the spine.

Pott's clamp. A clamp devised to shut off the edge of a large vessel while not interrupting the flow through the vessel, so that the edge may be used for anastomosis.

Pott's fracture. Fracture of the lower end of the fibula with outward displacement of the ankle and foot, and with or without fracture of the medial malleolus of the tibia.

Pott's gangrene. Senile gangrene; that due to arterial changes in elderly patients.

Pott's paralysis, or paraplegia. Paralysis resulting from tuberculous disease of the spine (Pott's disease).

Pott's puffy tumour. A collection of pus beneath the scalp, associated with osteomyelitis of a bone of the skull.

Pottenger, Frances Marion (b. 1869). St Louis physician.

Pottenger's sign. Palpation with light touch to detect different degrees of resistance according to the underlying structures.

Potter, Caryl Ashby (b. 1886). St Joseph, Minnesota, physician.

Potter treatment. The administration of decinormal hydrochloric acid to prevent tryptic activity in the treatment of intestinal fistulae.

Potter, Hollis Elmer (b. 1880). Chicago radiologist.

Potter-Bucky diaphragm, Bucky-Potter diaphragm. Bucky diaphragm.

Potter, Irving White (b. 1868). Buffalo, New York, obstetrician.

Potter version. The performance of podalic version as a routine procedure at the conclusion of the first stage of labour.

Potts, Willis John (b. 1895). Chicago paediatric surgeon.

Potts' clamp. A clamp which allows a lumen to be preserved in the aorta and blood to continue to flow through it while an anastomosis is being made between it and other vessels.

Potus Imperialis BPC 1949 (po·tus im·pe·re·a·lis). Imperial drink, haustus imperialis; a mixture prepared from potassium acid tartrate, citric acid, sucrose, lemon oil, tincture of lemon and water. [L, imperial drink.]

pouch (powch). A small sac-like appendage or pocket whose cavity communicates with that of a larger parent structure. **Abdominovesical pouch.** The peritoneal pouch between the abdominal wall and the distended bladder. **Branchial pouch.** One of the series of 4 or 5 saccular diverticulae of the lateral wall of the embryonic pharynx. **Craniobuccal pouch, Craniopharyngeal pouch.** Rathke's pouch; a diverticulum from the roof of the primitive mouth cavity from whose walls the glandular anterior part of the pituitary gland is developed. **Enterocoelic pouch.** One of the series of paired dorsolateral pouches of the archenteron or primitive gut of Amphioxus, from which the mesodermal segments are formed. **Neurobuccal pouch.** Craniobuccal pouch (see above). **Pharyngeal pouch.** Branchial pouch (see above). **Recto-uterine pouch [excavatio recto-uterina (NA)].** A peritoneal pouch, open upwards, lying between the vagina and the rectum, bounded laterally by the recto-uterine folds; Douglas' pouch. **Rectovaginal pouch.** Recto-uterine pouch (see prec.). **Rectovesical pouch [excavatio rectovesicalis (NA)].** A peritoneal pocket with its mouth directed upwards, between the bladder and the rectum in the male. **Suprapatellar synovial pouch.** Suprapatellar bursa. *See* BURSA. **Uterovesical pouch [excavatio vesico-uterina (NA)].** A peritoneal pouch lying between the uterus and the bladder and bounded laterally by the round ligaments of the uterus. **Visceral pouch.** Branchial pouch (see above). [OFr. *pouche.]*

See also: BROCA, DOUGLAS (J.), HARTMANN (H.), MORISON, PAVLOV, PHYSICK, RATHKE, SEESSEL, TROELTSCH, WILLIS.

poudrage (poo·drahzh). Powdering. **Pleural poudrage.** The act of covering pleural surfaces with a powder for the purpose of stimulating the formation of adhesions. [Fr.]

Poulet, Alfred (b. 1848). Paris physician.

Poulet's disease. Rheumatic osteoperiostitis.

poultice (pole·tis). A soft, moist mass made of some cohesive substance, e.g. bread, linseed, bran, to which water has been added. It is usually used hot, for surface application in order to encourage local circulation and to relieve pain. **Kaolin poultice.** *See* KAOLIN. **Mustard poultice.** A poultice made with dry mustard and linseed. The term is sometimes applied to a mustard plaster which is made of equal parts of mustard and flour, moistened to a suitable consistency. [L *puls* pap.]

pounce (powns). Powdered sandarac. [Fr. *ponce* pumice.]

pound (pownd). A unit of weight equal to 0.45359 kg, defined as the weight *in vacuo* of the Imperial Standard Pound. It is the avoirdupois pound, equivalent to 16 oz av., or 7000 grains. **Apothecaries' pound.** 12 oz, 5760 grains, 340 grams. **Troy pound.** Used for gold and silver, 12 oz, 5760 grains, 340 grams. [L *pondus* weight.]

Poupart, François (b. 1616). Paris surgeon.

Poupart's ligament. Inguinal ligament; the thickened lower edge of the aponeurosis of the external oblique muscle, which spans the gap between the anterior superior iliac spine and the pubic tubercle.

Poupart's line. A line drawn on the abdomen passing perpendicularly upwards from the centre of Poupart's ligament.

poverty (pov·er·te). 1. The quality of being poor in substance or elements. 2. Deficiency or absence of necessary material to maintain existence. 3. Of bodily condition, poor, lean, or feeble. **Emotional poverty.** A lessening of the capacity to feel and exhibit, e.g. sympathy, love. [L *paupertas.]*

Povidone (po·vi·done). BP Commission approved name for poly(vinylpyrrolidone), a white, slightly hygroscopic powder, very soluble in water, giving a clear and somewhat viscous solution. It is a polymerized form of vinylpyrrolidone, the average molecular weight ranging between 30 000 and 60 000. A preparation is used as a blood substitute in pathological conditions associated with diminished blood volume, such as shock and haemorrhage, in the form of a 3.5 per cent solution containing potassium chloride, calcium chloride, magnesium chloride and sodium bicarbonate, being isotonic with blood and having a viscosity almost identical with blood plasma proteins; it is given by slow intravenous infusion, and permits a filling of the blood vessels persisting for about 18 hours. It is well tolerated, there is a freedom from risk of anaphylactic reactions, and it does not affect kidney and liver functions. A hypertonic solution has also been used in the preparation of depot injections to retard the absorption of the medicament.

Povidone-iodine (po·vid·one·i·o·deen). BP Commission approved name for a complex produced by reacting iodine with poly-(vinylpyrrolidone); a topical antiseptic.

powder (pow·der). A mixture of two or more dry substances, usually intended for internal use. They are prepared by mixing the smaller ingredient or ingredients with gradually increasing quantities of the larger, then sieving, usually through a No. 60 sieve, and lightly triturating. If the quantity of an ingredient is less than 65 mg (1 grain), trituration is made with a diluent such as lactose; if a potent ingredient is ordered by itself in a powder, the weight of each powder should be made up to 130 mg (2 grains) by the addition of an inert substance such as lactose. The degree of coarseness or fineness of a powder is specified by the size of the mesh of the sieve through which the powder is able to pass. *Coarse Powder* (10/44) is defined by the *British Pharmacopoeia* as one which passes through a No. 10 sieve completely, and not more than 40 per cent through a No. 44 sieve; *Moderately Coarse Powder* (22/60) passes through a No. 22 sieve, and not more than 40 per cent through a No. 60; *Moderately Fine Powder* (44/85) passes through a No. 44 sieve, but not more than 40 per cent through a No. 85; *Fine Powder* (85) passes completely through a No. 85 sieve; *Very Fine Powder* passes completely through a silk sieve in which not less than 45 meshes go to 10 mm in each transverse direction parallel to the threads. Describing the fineness of a powder by a number means that the particles of the powder will all pass through the sieve distinguished by that number. **Aluminium powder.** A powder consisting mainly of the powdered metal, but containing appreciable amounts of oxide. Streak acid, used as a lubricant during the manufacture, protects the metal from excessive oxidation. It is employed as a dusting powder to prevent irritation by discharges. **Aluminium hydrate powder, Aluminium hydroxide powder.** Dried aluminium hydroxide gel. *See* GEL. **Antimonial powder.** Antimonious oxide diluted with calcium phosphate. It is used as an expectorant and diaphoretic. **Apple powder.** The dried pomace of the apple (*Pyrus malus*); it is a source of pectin, and may be used in the treatment of diarrhoea. **Aromatic powder.** A mixture of cinnamon, ginger and cardamom powders. It is used as a carminative and as a flavouring agent. **Bitter apple powder.** Colocynth powder; the powdered dry pulp of the unripe fruit of *Citrullus colocynthis* (family Cucurbitaceae). It is used as a drastic hydragogue cathartic, and is normally prescribed with hyoscyamus to prevent griping. **Bleaching powder.** Chlorinated lime, calx chlorinata, chloride of lime; a preparation obtained by exposing slaked lime to chlorine gas until absorption ceases. It contains not less than 30 per cent of available chlorine, and is used as a powerful and rapid deodorant. **Blood-plasma powder.** A sterile, completely water-soluble plasma powder obtained by separating plasma from whole blood by sedimentation or centrifugation of the blood cells, and drying it under sterile conditions by a freeze-drying technique or a spray dryer. It can be reconstituted by solution in sterile water for venous infusion. **Borosalicylic powder.** A mixture of boric acid and salicylic acid which is used as a dusting powder in the treatment of wounds. **Chiniofon powder.** A mixture of 7-iodo-8-hydroxy-quinoline-5-sulphonic acid with sodium bicarbonate. It is used in the treatment and prevention of amoebiasis. **Colocynth powder.** Bitter apple powder (see above). **Composition powder.** A mixture of powdered bayberry, ginger, capsicum and clove, used as a domestic remedy for colds. **Compound chalk powder.** A mixture of powdered chalk with acacia and sugar, used as an antacid and in the treatment of diarrhoea. It is sometimes regarded as a mixture of calcium carbonate, magnesium carbonate and sodium bicarbonate. **Compound powder of jalap.** Prepared jalap with ginger and potassium tartrate. It is a powerful purgative. **Compound powder of morphine.** A powder composed of morphine sulphate, camphor, liquorice and chalk; Tully's powder. **Dusting powder.** Any fine powder prepared for application by dusting to the skin. **Effervescent powder.** Sodium potassium tartrate and sodium bicarbonate wrapped in blue paper separately from tartaric-acid powder in white paper. When the two are mixed in water they form an effervescent saline cathartic and diuretic. **Goa powder.** A substance found in cavities in the trunk of the tree *Andira araroba* Aguiar. (family Leguminosae). It occurs as a coarse, amber-brown powder containing fragments of wood. It is applied, in the form of an ointment, as a stimulant and parasiticide in psoriasis, acne rosacea and ringworm, the action being due to its content of chrysarobin. **Grey powder.** Mercury with chalk; a mixture of mercury with chalk, the mercury having been triturated with the chalk until the mixture has a uniform grey colour and no metallic globules are visible under an average magnifying glass. It is used as a laxative and antisyphilitic; also in small doses as a mild purgative, but may be toxic for children. **Impalpable powder.** A very fine powder, the particles of which cannot be felt as distinct bodies. **Insect powder.** A powder destructive to insects, e.g. pyrethrum. **Jesuit's powder.** Cinchona. **Karaya gum powder.** A powder used prophylactically to prevent ileostomy dermatitis. **NCI powder.** A mixture of naphthalene, creosote and iodoform, used as an insecticide and delousant. **Persian insect powder.** Pyrethrum. **Portland powder.** A mixture of equal parts of the roots of *Aristolochia rotunda* and *Gentiana lutea*, the tops and leaves of *Teucrium chamaedrys* and *Erythraea centaurium*, and the leaves of *Ajuja chamaepitys*, used as a remedy for gout in former days. **Seidlitz powder.** Effervescent powder (see above). **Serum powder.** Zinc oxide treated with freshly prepared serum, then dried and sterilized. It is used as an antiseptic dressing powder. **Styptic powder.** A powder consisting of alum, acacia, gum, colophony and tragacanth, used as a haemostatic powder. **Talcum powder.** Talc, a native hydrous magnesium silicate freed from limestone, marble and other impurities, and finally powdered until it is elevated by a current of air. It may be medicated for application of medicaments to the skin to prevent drying or to allay irritation, or perfumed for toilet purposes. Pharmaceutically, it is used as a filtering aid and as a dispersing agent. It was formerly employed to facilitate the putting on of rubber gloves, but even small amounts were found to cause granuloma and a specially prepared starch powder is now used for this purpose. **Vienna powder.** Vienna paste; a mixture of potassium hydroxide and slaked lime with alcohol or glycerin, it is used as an escharotic. [L *pulvis* dust.]

See also: CASTILLON, DOVER, DUPUYTREN, GOULARD, GREGORY, HUFELAND, JAMES (R.), JEPHSON, SCHULTZE (B. S.), SIPPY, TULLY, VIGO, VINCENT.

Power, Marschelle Harnly (b. 1894). Nebraska biochemist at the Mayo Clinic.

Cutler, Power and Wilder test. A chemical test for Addison's disease which depended upon the induction of an exacerbation of the disease by the withholding of salt. It is now obsolete because of its danger.

Robinson-Power-Kepler test. For Addison's or Simmonds' disease: on the day before the test the patient has three ordinary meals without added salt, but does not eat or drink anything after 6 p.m. At 10.30 p.m. the bladder is emptied and the urine discarded. Urine is collected between 10.30 p.m. and 7.30 a.m. (night specimen). Breakfast is omitted. At 8.30 a.m. the bladder is emptied and the patient then drinks within the next 45 minutes 20 ml of water per kg body weight. Urine is collected separately at 9.30, 10.30, 11.30 and 12.30. The volumes of all specimens are measured. If the volume of any single hourly day specimen is larger than the volume of the night urine, the test is negative and Addison's or Simmonds' disease is presumed to be excluded. If positive, however, further evidence is obtained. Blood is taken and the urea and chlorides determined in the plasma, and the same substances are determined in the night urine. The factor *A* is then calculated as follows: (urea in urine ÷ urea in plasma) × (chloride in plasma ÷ chloride in urine) × (volume of largest single hourly day urine ÷ volume of night urine), concentrations being in mg per 100 ml and volumes in ml. If *A* is greater than 30 the test is negative and Addison's disease is presumed excluded. If it is less than 25 the patient probably has Addison's or Simmond's disease, provided that nephritis has been excluded.

power (pow·er). Capacity or ability to perform an act or to produce an effect. **Aligning power.** The capacity of the eye to recognize the smallest alterations in lateral deviations in the situation of a line. **Back vertex power.** The reciprocal of the posterior focal length of a lens or number of lenses. It is important in spectacle lenses and those in the trial frame during refraction, as it indicates the exact effect of these on the rays of light entering the eye. **Candle power.** Luminous intensity expressed in candles. **Converging power.** Refractive power (see below). **Focal power.** Refractive power (see below). **Fusion duction power.** The ability to maintain fusion of the two images from the two eyes when disjunctive ocular movements are taking place. Measured by an amblyoscope or synoptophore in degrees of arc, or by prisms in prism dioptres. Also called *vergence power.* **Phylactic power.** Ability of an organism to protect itself from infection. **Refractive power.** The amount that an optical system bends the rays of light which pass through it. It is measured in dioptres, as the reciprocal of the focal length of that system. **Resolving power.** The ability of the eye to see two closely approximated objects as separate objects. **Vergence power.** Fusion duction power (see above). [Fr. *pouvoir.]*

pox (pox). 1. Any eruptive disease with vesicles or pustules (pocks); specifically, an eruptive disease due to a virus of the smallpox group, and affecting man or animals. 2. An old term for syphilis. **Crystal pox.** Varicella. **Fowl pox.** *See* FOWL-POX. **Glass pox.** An old synonym for both varicella and mild smallpox (alastrim). **Great pox.** An old term for syphilis. **Horse pox.** Equine variola. *See* VARIOLA. **Kaffir pox.** Mild smallpox. **Milk pox.** A variety of smallpox similar to mild smallpox (alastrim). **Mouse pox.** Infectious ectromelia; a virus disease of mice, related to vaccinia and other pock diseases. **Rickettsial pox.** *See* RICKETTSIALPOX. **Samoa pox.** Mild smallpox. **Sanaga pox.** Alastrim. **Sheep pox.** Ovine variola. *See* VARIOLA. **Wart pox.** Variola verrucosa. **Water pox.** Ground itch; a rash caused by the entry of ancylostome larvae into the skin. **White pox.** Mild smallpox. [ME *pokkes.*]

poxvirus (pox·vi·rus). A genus of large DNA-containing viruses with a predilection for epithelial surfaces. The members of the group show a considerable heterogeneity of characters. A common nucleoprotein antigen has been reported to be present in most members of the group but this needs to be confirmed. By morphology the group can be divided into two subgroups: the majority, including the viruses of smallpox, vaccinia and cowpox, fall into one group whose virions are brick-shaped (about 250 × 200 nm) with thread-like structures arranged apparently at random over the surface; the other, paravaccinia, subgroup, including the viruses of pseudocowpox and orf, has virions which are more oval and elongated (250 × 150 nm) with surface threads arranged in a regular spiral. Individual members of the poxvirus group can be identified serologically or through the following characteristics: 1. Pock morphology and/or ceiling temperature when grown on the chorio-allantoic membrane of fertile eggs. 2. Host range in animals or cell culture. Members of the group pathogenic for man include the viruses of smallpox (including alastrim), cowpox, monkeypox, molluscum contagiosum, pseudocowpox and orf. Vaccinia is closely related antigenically to smallpox and is used as a vaccine against it. [ME *pokkes,* L *virus* poison.]

Pozzi, Samuel Jean (b. 1846). Paris anatomist and gynaecologist.

Pozzi's muscle. The extensor digitorum brevis muscle of the hand; a rare anomaly in man.

practice (prak·tis). 1. The regular application of medical knowledge and skill in the diagnosis and treatment of disease by a medical practitioner. 2. A collective term for the patients of a medical practitioner. **Contract practice.** An arrangement made with a practitioner by an organization, society or benefit club, for the medical care of its members, either by a stipend paid at regular intervals or at so much a head. **Group practice.** The co-operation of several medical practitioners, usually in partnership, for the diagnosis and treatment of patients. Frequently, one partner specializes in medicine, another in surgery, etc. **Panel practice.** A term formerly used for the practice of a medical practitioner receiving insured patients under the National Health Insurance Scheme (Great Britain). [Gk *praktikos* fit for action or business.]

practitioner (prak·tish·un·er). One engaged in the practice of medicine.

Practolol BP 1973 (prak·to·lol). (±)-4-(2-Hydroxy-3-isopropylaminopropoxy)acetanilide. Used to inhibit β-adrenergic stimulation in the heart; it controls supraventricular arrhythmias and improves exercise tolerance in patients with angina pectoris.

prae-. For words beginning **prae-**, see also PRE-.

praecoid (pre·koid). Like dementia praecox. [dementia praecox, Gk *eidos* form.]

praecox (pre·kox). Occurring in early life or at an early stage. [L, premature.]

praevia, praevius (pre·ve·ah, pre·ve·us). Going before in time or place. [L.]

pragmatagnosia (prag·mat·ag·no'·se·ah). A condition in which there is failure to distinguish objects which hitherto have been readily recognized. **Visual pragmatagnosia.** Term used by some to indicate object blindness. [Gk *pragma* object, *agnosia* obscurity.]

pragmatamnesia (prag·mat·am·ne'·ze·ah). A condition in which the ability to recall the appearance of objects is lost. **Visual pragmatamnesia.** Term used by some to describe the mental state which is characterized by failure to recall the visual image of an object. [Gk *pragma* object, *amnesia* forgetfulness.]

pragmatic (prag·mat·ik). Relating to pragmatism.

pragmatics (prag·mat·iks). The branch of semantics which concerns signs and their relation to users.

pragmatism (prag·mat·izm). In philosophy, the belief that the meaning of any assertion or conception is to be found in its practical results, and that the sole object of thinking is to evolve conceptions which shall form the basic tenets of behaviour. [Gk *pragma* deed.]

Prajmalium Bitartrate (praj·ma·le·um bi·tar·trate). BP Commission approved name for *N*-propylajmalinium hydrogen tartrate; it is used in the treatment of heart arrhythmias.

Pralidoxime Iodide (pral·id·ox·eem i·o·dide). BP Commission approved name for picolinaldoxime methiodide; an anticholinergic, used especially in poisoning with organic phosphorus.

Pramiverine (pram·iv·er·een). BP Commission approved name for 4,4-diphenyl-*N*-isopropylcyclohexylamine; a spasmolytic.

Pramoxine (pram·ox·een). BP Commission approved name for 4-[3-(4-butoxyphenoxy)propyl] morpholine; a local anaesthetic.

Prampine (pram·peen). BP Commission approved name for *O*-propionylatropine; an anticholinergic, and ganglion blocking agent.

prana apparatus. A wooden tube equipped with a wooden rammer for compressing carbon-dioxide snow into sticks.

prandial (pran·de·al). Relating or referring to a meal. [L *prandium* lunch.]

praseodymium (pra·se·o·dim'·e·um). An element of the rare earths with atomic weight 140.92, atomic number 59, and chemical symbol Pr. It is a yellowish trivalent highly reactive metal which is found with neodymium in cerite. It forms light-green salts, whence its name. [Gk *prasaios* leek-green, *didymos* twin.]

Praun, Eduard (b. 1866). Wiesbaden otolaryngologist.
Nebinger-Praun operation. An external operation on the frontal sinus.

Prausnitz, Otto Carl Willy (b. 1876). Breslau bacteriologist.
Prausnitz-Kuestner reaction, or test. Production of local passive sensitization by an intracutaneous injection of serum from a hypersensitive subject. Kuestner himself was hypersensitive to certain fish and the reaction was first demonstrated with his serum.
reversed Prausnitz-Kuestner reaction, or test. The reaction, a weal, that appears when the antibody is given after the administration of the antigen, instead of before, as in the Prausnitz-Kuestner reaction.

praxiology (prax·e·**ol**·o·je). The science that is concerned with behaviour. [Gk *praxis* action, *logos* science.]

praxis (**prax**·is). The performance of a purposive act. [Gk, action.]

Prazepam (**pra**·ze·pam). BP Commission approved name for 7-chloro-1-(cyclopropylmethyl)-1,3-dihydro-5-phenyl-1,4-benzodiazepin-2-one; a muscle relaxant.

Prazitone (**praz**·it·one). BP Commission approved name for 5-phenyl-5-(2-piperidyl)methylbarbituric acid; an antidepressant.

Prazosin (**pra**·zo·sin). BP Commission approved name for 1-(4-amino-6,7-dimethoxyquinazolin-2-yl)-4-(2-furoyl)piperazine; an antihypertensive agent.

pre-. A prefix from the Latin preposition *prae*, meaning *before*.

pre-adult (pre·**ad**·ult). Preceding adult life. [L *prae*, adult.]

pre-agonal, pre-agonic (pre·**ag**·on·al, pre·ag·**on**·ik). Immediately preceding death. [L *prae*, Gk *agon* struggle.]

pre-albuminuric (pre·al·bew·min·**ewr**'·ik). Taking place before the onset of albuminuria. [L *prae*, albuminuria.]

pre-anaesthesia (pre·an·es·**the**'·ze·ah). Premedication or basal narcosis. [L *prae*, anaesthesia.]

pre-anaesthetic (pre·an·es·**thet**'·ik). Referring to premedication and to basal narcosis. [see prec.]

pre-anal (pre·**a**·nal). Situated anterior to the anus. [L *prae*, anus.]

pre-antiseptic (pre·an·te·**sep**'·tik). Belonging to the era before antiseptic methods were introduced, particularly in surgical practice. [L *prae*, antiseptic.]

pre-aortic (pre·a·**or**·tik). Occurring or situated anterior to the aorta. [L *prae*, aorta.]

pre-aseptic (pre·a·**sep**·tik). Belonging to the period preceding the adoption of aseptic principles in surgical operations. [L *prae*, aseptic.]

pre-atactic, pre-ataxic (pre·at·**ak**·tik, pre·at·**ax**·ik). Pertaining to the period that immediately precedes the onset of ataxia. [L *prae*, ataxia.]

pre-auditory (pre·**aw**·dit·or·e). Occurring in front of the auditory nerve. [L *prae*, auditory.]

pre-auricular (pre·aw·**rik**·ew·lar). Referring to the ear, occurring in front of one of the auricles. [L *prae*, auricle.]

pre-auricular veins. Anterior auricular veins.

pre-axal (pre·**ax**·al). Occurring anteriorly to an axon. [L *prae*, axon.]

pre-axial (pre·**ax**·e·al). In front of an axis of the body or of a limb, as for example of the lateral border of the upper extremity. [L *prae*, axis.]

prebacillary (pre·**bas**·il·ar·e). Referring to a stage in a disease before bacilli *(sensu lato)* are discoverable. [L *prae*, bacillus.]

prebase (**pre**·base). The posterior surface (base) of the pharyngeal part of the tongue. [L *prae*, base.]

prebasilar (pre·**ba**·sil·ar). In front of the basilar part of the occipital bone. [L *prae*, basilar.]

prebasophilic (pre·ba·so·**fil**'·ik). Applied to premyelocytes that are precursors of basophils before they develop their characteristic basophilic quality. [L *prae*, basophil.]

prebladder (pre·**blad**·er). A large cavity developed anterior to the internal urethral orifice of the urinary bladder within the capsule which envelops the prostate gland. [L *prae*, bladder.]

Prebluda, Harry Jacob (b. 1911). Baltimore biochemist.
Prebluda and McCollum test. For vitamin B_1: diazotized *p*-aminoacetophenone is added to the test solution and the red colour produced is extracted with xylene and compared with standards obtained with pure aneurine hydrochloride treated similarly.

prebrachial (pre·**bra**·ke·al). Antebrachial. [see foll.]

prebrachium (pre·**bra**·ke·um). A superior brachium of one of the quadrigeminal bodies. [L *prae*, *brachium* arm.]

precancer (pre·**kan**·ser). A growth, not actually cancerous, that will probably develop into a malignant tumour. [L *prae*, cancer.]

precancerosis (pre·kan·ser·**o**'·sis). Any condition which leads to or is the forerunner of cancer. [L *prae*, cancer, Gk *-osis* condition.]

precancerous (pre·**kan**·ser·us). Relating or belonging to the stage in which a precancer develops, before the growth has become malignant. [L *prae*, cancer.]

precapillary (pre·**kap**·**il**·ar·e). A tiny vein or arterial branch. [L *prae*, capillary.]

precarcinomatous (pre·kar·sin·o'·mat·us). Relating or belonging to the period before the formation of a carcinoma. [L *prae*, carcinoma.]

precardiac (pre·**kar**·de·ak). Situated in front of the heart; precordial. [L *prae*, Gk *kardia* heart.]

precardinal (pre·**kar**·din·al). Pertaining to the paired veins which drain the head end of the early embryo into the common cardinal veins. In part, the precardinals persist as the internal jugular veins. [L *prae*, cardinal.]

precartilage (pre·**kar**·til·ij). Temporary cartilage in the embryo. [L *prae*, cartilage.]

precava (pre·**ka**·vah). The superior vena cava. [L *prae*, vena cava.]

precentral (pre·**sen**·tral). 1. In front of a centre or the centre. 2. Anterior to the central sulcus of the cerebrum. [L *prae*, centre.]

prechordal (pre·**kord**·al). Situated anterior to the notochord. [L *prae*, chord.]

precipitable (pre·**sip**·it·abl). Being in a state favourable to precipitation; the condition of an ion that will be thrown out of solution if another ion is added.

precipitant (pre·**sip**·it·ant). Any substance which brings about the precipitation of another substance from solution. **Group precipitant.** A reagent employed in qualitative analysis which precipitates the metals of a particular group.

precipitate (pre·**sip**·it·ate). 1. A substance, previously in solution, which has been made to settle out, e.g. the deposit formed as the result of the interaction of a bacterial polysaccharide with its specific antiserum, or the insoluble compound produced by the addition of a reagent to a solution. 2. To cause a precipitate to form, e.g. the deposition of silver chloride when a solution of silver nitrate is added to a solution of sodium chloride. **Black precipitate.** Mercurous oxide, Hg_2O. **Green precipitate.** Basic copper acetate (of variable composition). **Keratic precipitates, Keratitic precipitates.** An important diagnostic sign of inflammation of the uveal tissues of the eye: small greyish-white spots formed by cells and protein matter free in the anterior chamber, adhering to the back of the cornea in clumps. Also called *keratitis punctata*. **Red precipitate.** Red mercuric oxide, HgO. **White precipitate.** Ammoniated mercury, NH_2HgCl. **Yellow precipitate.** Yellow mercuric oxide, HgO. [L *praecipitare* to throw down.]

precipitation (pre·sip·it·**a**'·shun). 1. The formation of fine solid particles in a solution and their subsequent separation and settlement. 2. The formation of fine particles in a biological fluid as a result of the reaction of a precipitin with an antigen. **Group precipitation.** 1. In bacteriology, precipitation by a specific antiserum of an antigen common to a group of closely related organisms, e.g. haemolytic streptococci. 2. In qualitative chemical analysis, the precipitation of all the metals of a particular group by the addition of a single group reagent. [L *praecipitare* to throw down.]

precipitin (pre·**sip**·it·in). An antibody which, when mixed with its specific antigen in a soluble form, causes precipitation. **Heat precipitin.** A precipitin prepared by the injection of heated antigen; the antibody reacts with both heated and unheated antigen.

precipitinogen (pre·sip·it·in'·o·jen). An antigen which is capable of giving rise to the production of precipitating antibodies when injected into an animal. [precipitin, Gk *genein* to produce.]

precipitinoid (pre·sip·it·in·oid). A partial antibody which, while unable to produce precipitation when mixed with its antigen, retains its affinity to the latter. [precipitin, Gk *eidos* form.]

precipitum (pre·sip·it·um). The precipitate produced by the activity of a precipitin.

precirrhosis (pre·sir·o·sis). Splenic and hepatic enlargement that precedes the development of cirrhotic changes. [L *prae*, cirrhosis.]

precision (pre·sizh·un). The precision of a measurement is given by an estimate of the variance of the measurement-response parameter divided by the slope of the response curve at the point where the measurement is made. [L *praecaedere* cut short.]

preclavicular (pre·klav·ik·ew·lar). Anterior to the clavicle. [L *prae*, clavicle.]

preclinical (pre·klin·ik·al). Referring to the stage of a disease before the clinical symptoms can be recognized and a diagnosis made. [L *prae*, clinical.]

preclival (pre·kli·val). Occurring in front of the lobulus clivi of the cerebellum. [L *prae*, lobulus clivi.]

precocious (pre·ko·shus). Developed before the normal time; more developed either physically or mentally than is natural or normal at any particular age. [L *praecoquere* to ripen beforehand.]

precocity (pre·kos·it·e). The state of premature development of faculties and mental powers; forwardness. **Heterosexual precocity.** Development at an early age of the secondary sex characters of the opposite sex, e.g. virilism in a female child due to an adrenal cortical tumour. **Isosexual precocity.** Development of the sexual characteristics of the same sex, e.g. granulosa-cell tumour in a female infant due to the oestrogen secreted by the tumour. **Sexual precocity.** As opposed to precocious puberty, due to oestrogen or androgen produced at an early age but not in response to LH/FSH.SH, e.g. granulosa cell of the ovary producing oestrogen or interstitial-cell tumour producing androgen. *Precocious puberty* is normal puberty accompanied by ovulation in girls and production of mature sperms in boys.

precognition (pre·kog·nish·un). Awareness of an event before it has happened, sometimes taking the form of a detailed vision of the event. [L *prae* before, *cognitio* to know.]

precommissure (pre·kom·is·ewr). The anterior horn of the lateral ventricle of the brain. [L *prae*, *commissura* a joining together].

preconscious (pre·kon·shus). A term used by adherents of the Freudian doctrine to denote any mental impression that is forgotten for the time being but needs only slight effort to bring it back to mind. [L *prae*, conscious.]

preconvulsant (pre·kon·vul·sant). Occurring in the stage in epilepsy before the onset of a convulsive attack. [see foll.]

preconvulsive (pre·kon·vul·siv). Occurring before a convulsive seizure. [L *prae*, convulsion.]

precordia (pre·kord·e·ah). Precordium.

precordial (pre·kord·e·al). Belonging to the precordium.

precordialgia (pre·kord·e·al'·je·ah). Pain affecting the precordium. [precordium, Gk *algos* pain.]

precordium (pre·kord·e·um). The part of the anterior aspect of the thorax which overlies the heart. [L *prae*, *cor* heart.]

precornu (pre·kor·new). The anterior horn of the lateral ventricle of the brain. [L *prae*, *cornu* horn.]

precostal (pre·kos·tal). Situated or occurring in front of the ribs. [L *prae*, *costa* rib.]

precranial (pre·kra·ne·al). Situated or occurring in the anterior portion of the skull. [L *prae*, cranium.]

precribrum (pre·krib·rum). The anterior perforated substance of the brain. [L *prae*, *cribrum* sieve.]

precritical (pre·krit·ik·al). Occurring before the crisis in a disease. [L *prae*, crisis.]

precuneal (pre·kew·ne·al). Anterior to the cuneus. [L *prae*, *cuneus* wedge.]

precuneate (pre·kew·ne·ate). Relating or belonging to the precuneus.

precuneus [NA] (pre·kew·ne·us). A lobule on the medial surface of the cerebral hemisphere, bounded anteriorly by the upturned portion of the sulcus cinguli, posteriorly by the parieto-occipital sulcus, inferiorly by the callosal sulcus, and superiorly by the superomedial margin of the hemisphere. [L *prae*, *cuneus* wedge.]

predentine (pre·den·teen). A soft collagenous material secreted by the odontoblasts of the developing tooth; it is later calcified to become dentine. [L *prae*, dentine.]

prediastole (pre·di·as·to·le). A part of the early diastolic phase or late systolic phase of the cardiac cycle and represented by the momentary pause before diastole actually begins. [L *prae*, diastole.]

prediastolic (pre·di·as·tol'·ik). Relating or belonging to the prediastole.

predicrotic (pre·di·krot·ik). In a sphygmogram, coming before the dicrotic notch, denoting an interruption in the wave. [L *prae*, dicrotic.]

predigested (pre·di·jes·ted). Applied to food that has undergone the process of predigestion.

predigestion (pre·di·jes·chun). The artificially produced initiation of the digestive process in starch and protein before they are used as food. [L *prae*, digestion.]

predispose (pre·dis·poze). To induce bodily susceptibility or vulnerability to disease. [see foll.]

predisposition (pre·dis·po·zish'·un). The state of being particularly susceptible to a certain disease; diathesis favourable to the development of disease. [L *prae*, *disponere* to arrange.]

predivision (pre·div·izh'·un). In cytogenetics, the segregation to opposite poles of the chromatids of a univalent at the first, rather than the second meiotic division *(postdivision)*. [L *prae*, division.]

Prednisolamate (pred·nis·ol·am·ate). BP Commission approved name for prednisolone 21-diethylaminoacetate. **Prednisolamate Hydrochloride BPC 1963.** $C_{27}H_{40}ClNO_6$, a white, odourless crystalline powder; it is employed in the treatment of inflammatory skin conditions.

Prednisolone BP 1973 (pred·nis·o·lone). 1,2-Dehydrohydrocortisone, 11β,17α,21-trihydroxypregna-1,4-diene-3,20-dione. It is used similarly to cortisone, and is administered by mouth in the form of tablets. **Prednisolone Acetate BP 1963.** The acetyl derivative of prednisolone, used for the same purposes. **Prednisolone Pivalate BP 1973.** A white, odourless crystalline powder which may be prepared by partial synthesis. It is used in the treatment of rheumatic diseases and inflammatory conditions of the skin. **Prednisolone Sodium Phosphate BP 1973.** The disodium salt of the 21-phosphate ester of prednisolone; an adrenocortical steroid administered intravenously.

Prednisolonum (pred·nis·o·lo'·num). *European Pharmacopoeia* name for Prednisolone BP 1973.

Prednisone BP 1973 (pred·ne·sone). 1,2-Dehydrocortisone, 17α,21-dehydroxypregna-1,4-diene-3,11,20-trione. A drug used similarly to cortisone but in smaller doses and given by mouth. **Prednisone Acetate BP 1968.** The acetate of prednisone, and the method of choice for administration of the drug.

Prednisonum (pred·nis·o·num). *European Pharmacopoeia* name for Prednisone BP 1973.

Prednylidene (pred·ni·le·deen). BP Commission approved name for 11β,17α,21-trihydroxy-16-methylenepregna-1,4-diene-3,20-dione; a corticosteroid.

predormition, predormitium (pre·dor·mish·un, pre·dor·mish·e·um). The state of disordered consciousness which precedes sound sleep. [L *prae*, *dormire* to sleep.]

preductal (pre·duk·tal). A term applied to coarctation of the aorta of the infantile type, indicating that the narrowing is above the entrance of the ductus arteriosus. [L *prae*, duct.]

pre-eclampsia (pre·ek·lamp·se·ah). A condition arising in pregnancy and characterized by the presence of any two of the following: hypertension, oedema, proteinuria. It is a precursor of eclampsia. [L *prae*, eclampsia.]

pre-elacin (pre·el·as·in). A precursor of elacin, arising from degenerated elastic tissue. [L *prae*, elacin.]

pre-eosinic (pre·e·o·sin'·ik). Referring to the eosinophilic promyelocyte. [L *prae*, eosin.]

pre-epiglottic (pre·ep·e·glot'·ik). Situated anterior to the epiglottis. [L *prae*, epiglottis.]

pre-eruptive (pre·e·rup·tiv). Preceding eruption. [L *prae*, eruption.]

pre-erythrocyte (pre·er·ith·ro·site). An imprecise term best avoided. 1. A pre-erythrocytic malaria parasite. 2. An early stage of the red blood cell, e.g. an erythroblast. [L *prae*, erythrocyte.]

pre-erythrocytic (pre·er·ith·ro·si'·tik). Before the erythrocytic phase; said of a malarial parasite. [see prec.]

pre-excitation (pre·ek·si·ta'·shun). In cardiology, excitation of part of the ventricular myocardium before the remainder is excited by the impulse conducted normally through the His bundle system; the Wolff-Parkinson-White syndrome. [L *prae*, *excitare* to rouse.]

preflagellate (pre·flaj·el·ate). Denoting a protozoon in the stage which precedes the formation of flagella. [L *prae*, flagellum.]

preformation (pre·for·ma·shun). An old theory that the germ cell contains in minute form the complete organism, which unfolds in development. [L *prae*, formation.]

prefrontal (pre·frun·tal). 1. Pertaining to or occurring in the anterior portion of the frontal lobe of the brain. 2. The middle portion of the ethmoid bone. [L *prae*, frontal.]

preganglionic (pre·gang·gle·on'·ik). Of autonomic nerve fibres, those that have not synapsed in an autonomic ganglion. [L *prae*, ganglion.]

pregeminal (pre·jem·in·al). Belonging to a pregeminum.

pregeminum (pre·jem·in·um). Either one of the superior quadrigeminal bodies. [L *prae*, *geminus* twin.]

pregeniculatum, pregeniculum (pre·jen·ik·ew·la'·tum, pre·jen·ik·-ew·lum). The lateral geniculate body. [L *prae*, geniculate.]

pregnancy (preg·nan·se). The state of being with child; the condition from conception to delivery of the conceptus. **Abdominal pregnancy.** Implantation of the fertilized ovum in the abdominal cavity. **Ampullary pregnancy.** Development of the conceptus in the ampullary portion of the uterine tube. **Angular pregnancy.** Implantation of the conceptus in the uterine angle. **Bigeminal pregnancy.** Twin pregnancy (see below). **Broad-ligament pregnancy.** Development of the conceptus in the broad ligament of the uterus. **Cervical pregnancy.** Pregnancy occurring in the cervix. **Cornual pregnancy.** Lodgement of the fertilized ovum in a rudimentary uterine horn. **Ectopic pregnancy.** Pregnancy in which the fertilized ovum is implanted at some site other than the usual one in the uterine cavity. **Exochorial pregnancy.** Pregnancy in which the fetus lies outside the membranes and is in direct contact with the uterus. **Extra-uterine pregnancy.** Ectopic pregnancy (see above). **Fallopian pregnancy.** Pregnancy in a uterine (fallopian) tube. **False pregnancy.** Phantom pregnancy (see below). **Heterotopic pregnancy.** Combined intra- and extra-uterine pregnancies. **Hydatid pregnancy.** Pregnancy which develops into a hydatidiform mole. **Hysterical pregnancy.** Phantom pregnancy (see below). **Interstitial pregnancy.** Lodgement of the fertilized ovum in the interstitial segment of the uterine tube. **Intraligamentary pregnancy.** Broad-ligament pregnancy (see above). **Intramural pregnancy.** Interstitial pregnancy (see above). **Intraperitoneal pregnancy.** Abdominal pregnancy (see above). **Intra-uterine pregnancy.** A pregnancy in which the fertilized ovum is implanted in the normal way in the uterine cavity. **Membranous pregnancy.** Exochorial pregnancy (see above). **Mesenteric pregnancy.** Tuboligamentary pregnancy (see below). **Molar pregnancy.** Degeneration of the conceptus into a hydatidiform or carneous mole. **Multiple pregnancy.** Simultaneous development of two or more fetuses. **Mural pregnancy.** Interstitial pregnancy (see above). **Nervous pregnancy.** Phantom pregnancy (see below). **Ovarian pregnancy.** Pregnancy developing in the ovary. **Ovario-abdominal pregnancy.** The type in which an ovarian pregnancy becomes secondarily implanted in the abdomen. **Parietal pregnancy.** Interstitial pregnancy (see above). **Phantom pregnancy.** Pseudocyesis; the occurrence of subjective symptoms of pregnancy with increase in size of the abdomen but without the presence of a fertilized ovum or true pregnancy. **Plural pregnancy.** Multiple pregnancy (see above). **Prolonged pregnancy.** That which extends beyond the average period: in the human the usual length is 266 days between fertilization and expulsion of the ovum, or, as is calculated, 280 days from the first day of the last normal menstrual period. **Sarcofetal pregnancy.** The concurrent development of both a hydatidiform mole and fetus. **Spurious pregnancy.** Phantom pregnancy (see above). **Stump pregnancy.** Development of the conceptus in the residual medial end of the tube after partial salpingectomy. **Tubal pregnancy.** Fallopian pregnancy (see above). **Tubo-abdominal pregnancy.** A tubal pregnancy which extends during development into the abdominal cavity. **Tuboligamentary pregnancy.** Tubal pregnancy which extends between the layers of the broad ligament. **Tubo-ovarian pregnancy.** A pregnancy where the implantation site includes both the tube and ovary. **Tubo-uterine pregnancy.** Interstitial pregnancy (see above). **Twin pregnancy.** The simultaneous development of two fetuses. **Uterine pregnancy.** The normal implantation and subsequent development of the fertilized ovum in the uterus. **Utero-abdominal pregnancy.** Twin pregnancy with one conceptus in the uterus and the other in the abdominal cavity. **Utero-ovarian pregnancy.** Twin pregnancy with one fetus in the uterus and the other in the ovary. **Uterotubal pregnancy.** Interstitial pregnancy (see above). [L *praegnans* bearing child.]

pregnanediol (preg·nane·di·ol). 17(β)-[1(α)-Hydroxyethyl]-etiocholane-3(α)-ol, $C_{21}H_{33}O_2$. An inactive end-product in the metabolism of progesterone, found in the urine after ovulation and during pregnancy in the form of pregnanediol sodium glucuronidate. In the follicular phase the urinary pregnanediol is less than 1 mg/24 h. In the luteal phase the concentration is 2-5 mg. Any value over 2 mg indicates that ovulation has taken place.

pregnane-3α,20α-diol (preg·nane·di·ol). A compound used as a standard in the determination of urinary pregnanediol.

pregnanetriol (preg·nane·tri·ol). A metabolite of progesterone found in congenital adrenal hyperplasia.

pregnant (preg·nant). Gravid; being with child. [L *praegnans.*]

pregnene (preg·neen). Δ^4-Pregnene, $C_{21}H_{34}$. A crystalline steroid; it forms the nucleus of progesterone, the hormone of the corpus luteum.

pregneninolone (preg·nen·in·o·lone). Alternative name for Ethisterone BP 1968. 17(β)-ethinyl-Δ^4-androstene-3-one-17(α)-ol. $C_{21}H_{28}O_2$. A synthetic preparation, not found in the animal body, with pharmacological action similar to that of progesterone, though weaker; unlike the latter it is almost as active by mouth as when injected.

Pregnenolone (preg·nen·o·lone). BP Commission approved name for 3β-hydroxypregn-5-en-20-one; a synthetic steroid produced from the naturally occurring steroid, progesterone. It is used in the treatment of rheumatoid arthritis.

prehabilitation (pre·hab·il·it·a'·shun). The early stages of the rehabilitation of injured persons to take their place in industry or in other activities. [L *prae*, habilitation.]

prehallux (pre·hal·ux). An accessory bone found occasionally on the lateral border of the navicular bone. [L *prae*, hallux.]

prehemiplegic (pre·hem·e·ple'·jik). Preceding hemiplegia. [L *prae*, hemiplegia.]

prehensile (pre·hen·sile). Capable of or adapted to grasping. [see foll.]

prehension (pre·hen·shun). The act of seizing or grasping. [L *prehendere* to seize.]

prehepaticus (pre·hep·at·ik·us). The segment of the inferior vena cava anterior to the liver. [L *prae*, Gk *hepar* liver.]

prehyoid (pre·hi·oid). Anterior to the hyoid bone; usually referring to an accessory thyroid gland. [L *prae*, hyoid.]

pre-ictal (pre·ik·tal). Prior to a stroke or attack. [L *prae, ictus* blow.]

pre-icteral (pre·ik·ter·al). Prior to the development of jaundice. [L *prae*, Gk *ikteros* jaundice.]

pre-insula (pre·in·sew·lah). The anterior part of the insula. [L *prae*, insula.]

prelacrimal (pre·lak·rim·al). Anterior to the lacrimal sac. [L *prae*, lacrimal.]

prelacteal (pre·lak·te·al). Prior to the beginning of full lactation and before the secretion of breast milk is adequate. [L *prae*, lactation.]

prelaryngeal (pre·lar·in·je·al). In front of the larynx. [L *prae*, larynx.]

preleproma (pre·lep·ro·mah). A macular leprotic lesion which histologically resembles an inflammatory lesion and in which lepra bacilli are scanty. [L *prae*, Gk *lepra* leprosy, *-oma* tumour.]

prelimbic (pre·lim·bik). Anterior to the limbus laminae spiralis. [L *prae*, limbus.]

prelocalization (pre·lo·kal·i·za′·shun). A term used with reference to the segregation at definite sites within the egg of formative materials which later become distributed within specific cells, tissues or organs of the embryo. [L *prae*, *locus* place.]

prelocomotion (pre·lo·ko·mo′·shun). The early attempts at walking made by a child, in which it shows its purpose but cannot fulfil it on account of lack of muscular co-ordination. [L *prae*, *locus* place, *motio* movement.]

prelum (pre·lum). A press. **Prelum abdominale.** Compression of the abdominal viscera between the diaphragm and wall of the abdomen such as occurs in micturition, defaecation and labour by the act of straining down. **Prelum arteriale.** A tourniquet. [L.]

prelumbar (pre·lum·bar). Situated in front of the loins or the lumbar vertebrae. [L *prae*, lumbar.]

premalignant (pre·mal·ig·nant). Preceding the development of overt malignant changes; precancerous. [L *prae*, malignant.]

premaniacal (pre·man·i·ak·al). Preceding an attack of mania or a maniacal outbreak. [L *prae*, mania.]

premature (prem·ah·tewr). Happening before the normal or usual time; referring to an infant born before the appointed time but capable of independent existence. [L *praematurus* too early.]

premaxilla (pre·max·il·ah). The incisive bone of the maxilla. [L *prae*, maxilla.]

premaxillary (pre·max·il·ar·e). Anterior to the maxilla. [see prec.]

premedicant (pre·med·ik·ant). A general term describing any one drug used in conjunction with, but administered prior to, a second. It has been used largely in connection with the administration of basal anaesthetics which are often supplemented by one of the more usual gaseous anaesthetics immediately prior to and during the course of the operation. Hence *premedication.* [L *prae*, *medicare* to drug.]

premedication (pre·med·ik·a′·shun). A term first used in the 1920s for drugs designed to facilitate the induction, maintenance and recovery from anaesthesia. [L *prae*, *medicare* to drug.]

premenstrual (pre·men·stroo·al). Occurring in the stage before a menstrual period begins. [see foll.]

premenstruum (pre·men·stroo·um) (pl. *premenstrua*). The stage immediately before the start of a menstrual period. [L *prae*, menstruum.]

premolar (pre·mo·lar). 1. Anterior to the molar teeth. 2. Any one of the two teeth situated directly in front of the molars on each side of the upper and lower jaws. [L *prae*, molar.]

premonition (pre·mon·ish·un). A sense of foreboding of an event, usually of a disagreeable nature. [L *prae*, *monere* to warn.]

premonocyte (pre·mon·o·site). Promonocyte. [L *prae*, monocyte.]

premorbid (pre·mor·bid). Occurring before the appearance of morbid signs and symptoms. [L *prae*, morbid.]

premortal (pre·mor·tal). Referring to the period just before death. [L *prae*, *mors* death.]

premunition (pre·mew·nish·un). A state of active immunity that is dependent on the presence of an inactive infection with the same species in the host, e.g. in malaria in Africans from hyperendemic or holo-endemic areas. [L *praemunitio* a fortifying in advance.]

premycosic (pre·mi·ko·sik). A nonce-word, now accepted as an adjective which may probably be used in relation to any eruption or phenomenon that precedes the appearance of the characteristic tumour or mycosic stage of mycosis fungoides. [L *prae*, mycosis.]

premyeloblast (pre·mi·el·o·blast). A precursor cell of the myeloblast, intermediate between the non-differentiated haemocytoblast and the differentiated myeloblast. [L *prae*, myeloblast.]

premyelocyte (pre·mi·el·o·site). Promyelocyte. [L *prae*, myelocyte.]

prenarcosis (pre·nar·ko·sis). The state brought about by the administration of sedatives, narcotics or anaesthetics as a preliminary to the induction of full anaesthesia. [L *prae*, Gk *narke* numbness.]

prenarcotic (pre·nar·kot·ik). Occurring before the induction of full narcosis. [see prec.]

prenaris (pre·na·ris) (pl. *prenares*). An anterior nasal aperture. [L *prae*, *naris* nostril.]

prenasal (pre·na·zal). Anterior to the nasal cavity or the nose. [L *prae*, *nasus* nose.]

prenatal (pre·na·tal). Preceding birth; antenatal. [L *prae*, *natus* birth.]

preneoplastic (pre·ne·o·plas′·tik). Pertaining to the period preceding the establishment of a tumour in the tissues. [L *prae*, neoplasm.]

preneutrophilic (pre·new·tro·fil′·ik). Referring to the neutrophilic promyelocyte. [L *prae*, neutrophil.]

prenidatory (pre·ni·da·tor·e). Existing before nidation occurs. [L *prae*, *nidus* nest.]

Prentice's law. For each 10 mm of decentralization, a spherical lens displaces an object by the same number of prism dioptres as the dioptric strength of the lens.

Prenylamine (pren·il·am·een). BP Commission approved name for *N*-(3,3-diphenylpropyl)-α-methylphenethylamine; it is used in the treatment of angina pectoris.

pre-occipital (pre·ok·sip·it·al). Occurring in front of the occipital bone. [L *prae*, occiput.]

pre-operative (pre·op·er·a·tiv). Occurring before an operation. [L *prae*, operation.]

pre-operculum (pre·o·per·kew·lum). The frontal operculum of the brain. [L *prae*, operculum.]

pre-optic (pre·op·tik). In front of one of the superior quadrigeminal bodies. [see foll.]

pre-opticus (pre·op·tik·us). One of the superior quadrigeminal bodies (anterior optic lobes). [L *prae*, optic.]

pre-oral (pre·or·al). Occurring in front of the mouth. [L *prae*, *os* mouth.]

pre-oxygenation (pre·ox·e·jen·a′·shun). Breathing oxygen to reduce tissue nitrogen before take-off, with a view to lessening the risk of aero-embolism. [L *prae*, Gk *oxys* sharp, *genein* to produce.]

prepalatal, prepalatine (pre·pal·at·al, pre·pal·at·ine). Anterior to the hard palate. [L *prae*, palate.]

prepallium (pre·pal·e·um). The anterior portion of the cerebral hemisphere (the frontal lobe) which is situated in front of the central sulcus. [L *prae*, *pallium* coverlet.]

preparalytic (pre·par·al·it′·ik). Referring to the state or stage before paralysis has set in. [L *prae*, paralysis.]

preparation (prep·ar·a·shun). 1. A making ready. 2. A specimen set up for demonstration in anatomy or pathology. 3. A medicament. **Cavity preparation.** The removal of decay, the shaping, and the toilet of a cavity in a tooth, before inserting a filling material. **Corrosion preparation.** A specimen made by filling hollow organs or tubes with a substance which is left intact after the tissues have been dissolved in caustic or acid. **Cover-glass preparation.** A cytological preparation in which a cover-glass is used to protect the matter, or one in which a drop of blood or other matter is placed between two cover-glasses that are subsequently drawn apart. **Hanging-drop preparation.** A preparation in which a drop of fluid is placed on a cover-glass which is inverted over a hollow-ground slide or over a ring of petroleum jelly on a slide, so that the drop remains suspended. **Heart-lung preparation.** A preparation designed originally for analysis of the mechanical and physical factors influencing cardiac muscle in warm-blooded animals. Blood passes in the normal way through the heart and lungs, but the rest of the animal's circulation is replaced by an artificial circulation in which factors such as pressure, temperature, etc., are completely under control of the observer. The preparation may also be used as a pump and oxidizing agent for the perfusion of isolated organs. **Impression preparation.** A microscopical preparation of a young bacterial culture in the stage of active multiplication on a solid medium; prepared by impressing a coverslip lightly on the colony to be examined. [L *praeparare* to make ready.]

prepartal (pre·**par**·tal). Referring to the period which immediately precedes the onset of labour. [L *prae*, *partus* time of bearing.]

prepatellar (pre·pat·el·ar). Occurring in front of the patella. [L *prae*, patella.]

prepatent (pre·**pa**·tent). Before becoming manifest. Of infections, before the parasite appears. [L *prae*, *patere* to lie open.]

prepeduncle (pre·**ped**·ungkl). The superior cerebellar peduncle. [L *prae*, peduncle.]

prepenile (pre·**pe**·nile). In front of the penis. [L *prae*, penis.]

preperception (pre·per·**sep**·shun). The anticipatory set or readiness for a perception which, when it comes, is thereby intensified. [L *prae*, perception.]

preperforatum, preperforatus (pre·per·for·**a**′·tum, **pre**·per·for·**a**′·tus). The anterior perforated substance of the rhinencephalon. [L *prae*, perforation.]

preperitoneal (pre·per·it·o·**ne**′·al). Situated in front of the peritoneum. [L *prae*, peritoneum.]

prephthisis (pre·**thi**·sis). The incipient stage of pulmonary tuberculosis. [L *prae*, phthisis.]

preplacental (pre·plas·**en**·tal). Occurring before the development of the placenta. [L *prae*, placenta.]

prepollex (pre·**pol**·ex). A supernumerary thumb. [L *prae*, *pollex* thumb.]

preponderance (pre·**pon**·der·ans). The condition of exceeding some related thing in size, weight or function. **Directional preponderance.** A term used when nystagmus produced by caloric stimulation of the vestibular mechanism may show excessive reaction in one direction. **Ventricular preponderance.** A term used to denote cardiac enlargement due to preponderant hypertrophy of one or other ventricle. It is generally used as an electrocardiographic term, *right ventricular preponderance* arising out of right ventricular hypertrophy, and *left ventricular preponderance* out of hypertrophy of the left ventricle. The latter is, however, normally preponderant over the right ventricle owing to the increased thickness of its musculature. [L *praeponderare* to outweigh.]

prepontile (pre·**pon**·tile). Occurring or situated in front of or above the pons. [L *prae*, *pons* bridge.]

prepotency (pre·**po**·ten·se). The greater capacity possessed by one parent than the other of passing on to the offspring hereditable characters peculiar to himself or herself. [L *praepotens* very powerful.]

prepotent (pre·**po**·tent). Pertaining to, possessing, or characterized by prepotency.

preprotein (pre·**pro**·te·in). A presumed ancestral precursor of proteins which was not synthesized on information coded in nucleic acids. [L *prae*, Gk *proteios* of first rank.]

prepsychotic (pre·si·**kot**·ik). Pertaining to a mental state preceding the development of a psychosis. [L *prae*, psychosis.]

prepubertal (pre·**pew**·bert·al). Existing in or happening in the period before puberty. **Prepubertal testicular failure.** *See* AGENESIS, TESTICULAR. [see foll.]

prepuberty (pre·**pew**·ber·te). The phase which immediately precedes puberty. [L *prae*, puberty.]

prepubescent (pre·pew·**bes**·ent). Prepubertal.

prepuce [preputium (NA)] (**pre**·pews). The fold of thin skin covering the neck of the penis which overhangs the glans penis for varying distances. **Prepuce of the clitoris [preputium clitoridis (NA)].** A fold formed by the conjunction anteriorly of each labium minus, overlapping the glans of the clitoris. **Redundant prepuce.** An excessive amount of preputial skin. [L *praeputium* foreskin.]

prepucectomy (pre·pew·**sek**·to·me). Circumcision. [prepuce, Gk *ektome* a cutting out.]

prepucotomy (pre·pew·**kot**·o·me). Preputiotomy.

preputial (pre·**pew**·shal). Relating or belonging to the prepuce.

preputiotomy (pre·pew·she·**ot**′·o·me). Any operation of incising the prepuce other than complete circumcision; e.g. incising the dorsal surface of the prepuce in cases of phimosis. [prepuce, Gk *temnein* to cut.]

prepyloric (pre·pi·**lor**·ik). Anterior to the pylorus. [L *prae*, pylorus.]

prepyloric vein [vena prepylorica (NA)]. A tributary of the right gastric or the portal vein, from the front of the pylorus. At operation it indicates the site of the pyloric junction.

prepyramidal (pre·pir·**am**·id·al). Occurring in front of the pyramid of the medulla oblongata. [L *prae*, pyramid.]

prerectal (pre·**rek**·tal). Anterior to the rectum. [L *prae*, rectum.]

prerenal (pre·**re**·nal). Occurring or situated in front of the kidney or occurring before reaching the kidneys, e.g. of blood changes. [L *prae*, *ren* kidney.]

preretinal (pre·**ret**·in·al). Anterior to the retina. [L *prae*, retina.]

presbyatrics, presbyatry (pres·be·**at**·rix, **pres**·be·at·re). Geriatrics. [Gk *presbys* old man, *iatreia* treatment.]

presbycousis (pres·be·**koo**·sis). The natural failure of hearing with advancing years, caused by degenerative changes in the internal ear. [Gk *presbys* old man, *akousis* hearing.]

presbyonosus (pres·be·o·**no**′·sus). Any disease that affects old people only. [Gk *presbys* old man, *nosos* disease.]

presbyope (**pres**·be·ope). An individual affected with presbyopia.

presbyophrenia (pres·be·o·**fre**′·ne·ah). Dementia, comprising intellectual impairment and disorders of behaviour arising in old age: especially the type characterized by overactivity and by gross memory impairment. [Gk *presbys* old man, *phren* mind.]

presbyopia (pres·be·**o**·pe·ah). Gradual diminution in the focusing power of the eye due to hardening of the lens rendering it less flexible. It continues uniformly throughout life; thus at the age of 8 years the focusing power is about 14 D, at 60, 0.75 D. **Premature presbyopia.** Presbyopia in which the loss of focusing power is greater than it should be for the age of the patient. Common causes are early glaucoma, prolonged residence in the tropics and states of exhaustion. [Gk *presbys* old man, *ops* eye.]

presbyopic (pres·be·**o**·pik). 1. Relating or belonging to presbyopia. 2. A person affected with presbyopia.

presbysphacelus (pres·bis·**fas**·el·us). Gangrene as a lesion associated with senile changes. [Gk *presbys* old man, *sphakelos* gangrene.]

presbytia (pres·**bish**·e·ah). Presbyopia.

presbytiatrics (pres·bit·e·**at**′·rix). Geriatrics. [Gk *presbys* old man, *iatreia* treatment.]

presbytic (pres·**bit**·ik). Presbyopic.

presbytism (**pres**·bit·izm). Presbyopia.

prescapula (pre·**skap**·ew·lah). The suprascapular part of the scapula. [L *prae*, scapula.]

prescapular (pre·**skap**·ew·lar). 1. Anterior to the scapula. 2. Relating to the suprascapular part of the scapula. [see prec.]

preschizophrenic (pre·skits·o·**fren**′·ik). Pertaining to the mental state before the full development of schizophrenia. [L *prae*, schizophrenia.]

presclerosis (pre·skler·**o**·sis). The condition of arterial hypertension generally the forerunner of arteriosclerosis. [L *prae*, sclerosis.]

presclerotic (pre·skler·**ot**′·ik). Relating or belonging to the stage before sclerosis occurs. [see prec.]

Prescoting (**pres**·kot·ing). A proprietary process of presscoating tablets. The advantages are the simplicity of the procedure, the fact that it can be applied to hygroscopic substances so that they are unaffected by moisture and that it produces a practically tasteless tablet which is unlikely to have an attraction for children.

prescribe (pre·**skribe**). The act of writing out or otherwise giving directions for the preparation and administration of a medicament. [L *prae, scribere* to write.]

prescription (pre·**skrip**·shun). The written direction from a doctor to a pharmacist for the preparation of medicaments in a suitable form for administration to a patient. Traditionally the prescription commences with the letter ℞ which signifies the Latin, *recipe*, "take". There follows the body of the prescription with details of the medicaments, their quantities and the manner in which they are to be supplied, i.e. whether mixture, tablets, pills, injection, etc. Finally the "signature" gives directions to the patient for taking the medicine. [see prec.]

presecretin (pre·se·**kre**·tin). The precursor of secretin, present in the mucous membrane of the duodenum. [L *prae*, secretin.]

presegmenter (pre·seg·**men**·ter). A mature schizont of any species of *Plasmodium* just prior to the development of the intracellular merozoites called *segmenters.* [L *prae*, segmenter.]

presenile (pre·**se**·nile). Relating to a condition affecting persons in early or middle life of which the characteristics are those of old age; prematurely old. [L *prae, senex* aged.]

presenility (pre·sen·**il**·it·e). Premature old age. [see prec.]

presenium (pre·**se**·ne·um). The stage which precedes the beginning of old age. [L *prae, senex* aged.]

present (pre·**zent**). To appear first at the external os uteri, a term used to describe the action of a fetal part as it moves to occupy the neck of the uterus. [L *praesentare* to show.]

presentation (prez·en·**ta**·shun). In obstetrics, that part of the fetus which occupies the centre of the pelvic canal and the part which the examining finger feels on vaginal examination. The types of presentation are usually described by prefixing the name of the part of the fetus that presents. The following classical presentations of the fetus *in utero*, for each of which there are several positions, are recognized. *Vertex Presentation:* the occiput the point of direction. Positions: left occipito-anterior (LOA); right occipito-anterior (ROA); left occipitoposterior (LOP); right occipitoposterior (ROP); left occipitolateral (LOL); right occipitolateral (ROL); persistent occipitoposterior (POP). *Face Presentation:* the chin the point of direction. Positions: left mento-anterior (LMA), also called mentolaevo anterior (MLA); right mento-anterior (RMA); left mentoposterior (LMP); right mentoposterior (RMP); persistent mentoposterior (PMP); left mentolateral (LML); right mentolateral (RML). *Breech Presentation:* the sacrum the point of direction. Positions: left sacro-anterior (LSA), also called left dorso-anterior (LDA) and sacrolaevo anterior (SLA); right sacro-anterior (RSA), also called right dorso-anterior (RDA); left sacroposterior (LSP), also called left dorsoposterior (LDP); right sacroposterior (RSP), also called right dorsoposterior (RDP); left sacrolateral (LSL); right sacrolateral (RSL). *Brow Presentation:* Positions: left fronto-anterior (LFA), also called frontolaeva anterior (FLA); right fronto-anterior (RFA); left frontoposterior (LFP); right frontoposterior (RFP); left frontolateral (LFL); right frontolateral (RFL). Other, less common, presentations are referred to below. **Arm presentation.** As for shoulder presentation (see below) when an arm has prolapsed. **Complete breech presentation.** Presentation of the fetus with both thighs and both knees fully flexed, and the feet present alongside the buttocks. **Compound presentation.** That in which a limb has prolapsed and is lying by the side of the main presenting part. **Presentation of the cord.** That in which the umbilical cord is lying before the main presenting part. **Footling presentation.** A variety of breech presentation; one or both feet present in advance of the buttocks. **Frank breech presentation.** A type in which both legs are extended along the fetal abdomen. **Hand and head presentation.** *See* COMPOUND PRESENTATION (above). **Incomplete breech presentation.** Any departure from the complete breech presentation, such as footling, or knee presentation. **Knee presentation.** *See* INCOMPLETE BREECH PRESENTATION (above). **Parietal presentation.** The condition when the fetal head presents in the pelvic brim, with the occiput lying laterally; obliquity of the head causes one or other parietal bone to be the leading part. **Placental presentation.** Placenta praevia. **Polar presentation.** Presentation of the cephalic or pelvic end of the fetus. **Shoulder presentation.** The presentation associated with transverse or oblique lie of the fetus. **Torso presentation, Transverse presentation.** Presentation of the fetal trunk such as occurs when the fetal lie is oblique or transverse. **Undetermined presentation.** Of the fetus, a term used for statistical purposes when a woman has delivered unattended. [L *praesentare* to show.]

preservative (pre·**zer**·vat·iv). Any substance added to a medicinal preparation or foodstuff to increase its keeping properties; it may act by reducing decomposition by moulds or bacteria, or by suppressing more definite chemical reactions, e.g. oxidation reduction. The most common preservatives include sugar, ethyl alcohol, sulphur dioxide and benzoic acid. Special regulations issued by the Department of Health and Social Security exist to control the use of preservatives in food. [L *praeservare* to keep.]

presphenoid (pre·**sfe**·noid). The anterior part of the body of the sphenoid bone. [L *prae*, sphenoid.]

presphygmic (pre·**sfig**·mik). Preceding the arterial pulse. The presphygmic period of the heart is that period between the onset of ventricular systole and the opening of the semilunar valves. [L *prae*, Gk *sphygmos* pulse.]

prespinal (pre·**spi**·nal). Occurring or located in front of the spine. [L *prae*, spine.]

prespondylolisthesis (pre·**spon**·di·lo·lis·**the**′·sis). A congenital condition characterized by a defect of both pedicles of the 5th lumbar vertebra, without displacement of the body of the vertebra, and predisposing to spondylolisthesis. [L *prae*, spondylolisthesis.]

pressinervoscopy (pres·e·ner·**vos**′·ko·pe). A method of diagnosing by noting the results of pressure upon the sympathetic and parasympathetic nerves. [pressure, nerve, Gk *skopein* to examine.]

pressor (**pres**·or). A substance which has the action of raising blood pressure. **Pressor amine, Pressor base.** Amines or nitrogenous bases of plant or animal origin, which have the ability to raise blood pressure (sympatheticomimetic). **Pressor-X.** A substance believed to have been extracted from the kidney and other animal tissues which experimentally produces a rise of blood pressure. [L *premere* to press.]

pressoreceptive (**pres**·o·re·**sep**′·tiv). The property of being sensitive to rises in blood pressure as shown for instance by receptor nerve-endings in the aorta and carotid sinus: stimulation of these by a rise of blood pressure produces a lowering of the pressure. [see foll.]

pressoreceptor (**pres**·o·re·**sep**′·tor). A nerve-ending affected by change of pressure, notably present in the carotid sinus and aorta. [pressure, L *recipere* to receive.]

pressosensitive (pres·o·**sen**·sit·iv). Pressoreceptive. [pressure, L *sentire* to feel.]

pressure (**presh**·er). 1. The force exerted by one body on another, e.g. by weight or muscular thrust. 2. The force exerted by a liquid or gas on its surroundings, e.g. blood pressure, atmospheric pressure. 3. A state of physical or mental stress caused by compelling circumstances, e.g. working at high pressure, or the pressure of business. **Abdominal pressure.** That within the abdomen caused by coincident contractions of the diaphragm and abdominal muscles. **Atmospheric pressure.** The pressure exerted by the atmosphere, which is about 101 kPa (15lb/in^2) at sea level. **Blood pressure.** *See* BLOOD PRESSURE. **Brain pressure.** The pressure within the capillaries of the brain. **Cardiac back pressure.** The pressure in the atria or veins supposed to result from failure of the ventricles to expel their contents adequately; it is the basis of the concept of backward cardiac failure. The concept is valid in so far as the pressure reflects the end-systolic volume of the ventricles and the compliance of the ventricular walls, but it ignores the importance of the fact that the filling is due to the pumping of the ventricle at the other end of the circulation and that the pressure is also dependent on the tone (compliance) of the venous system and atria. **Central venous pressure.** The pressure of blood in the right atrium which is at the level of the manubriosternal angle; it is estimated by means of a manometer attached to a cannula running into the inferior or superior vena cava, represented by the height above the manubriosternal angle of the column of fluid in the manometer measured, if possible, with the patient recumbent. *High central venous pressure* indicates cardiac failure, *low central venous pressure* indicates low blood pressure. **Cerebrospinal pressure.** The pressure of the cerebrospinal fluid; normally, with the patient lying on one side, it is from 100 to 150 mm of fluid. **Critical pressure.** The pressure corresponding to the critical point. **Critical closing pressure.** The intraluminal pressure in a terminal arteriole which is just low enough for the natural tension of the arteriolar wall to cause the vessel to collapse and close. **Diastolic pressure.** In an artery, the level of the pressure immediately prior to the upstroke of the next pulse; in a ventricle, the pressure during diastole, especially the end-diastolic pressure, either just before the transmitted rise in pressure due to atrial systole (the "a" wave) or the level to which the pressure falls after the "a" wave, prior to the onset of ventricular systole. **End-diastolic pressure.** The pressure of the blood in the ventricles at the end of diastole prior to the next ventricular systole. This is usually measured after the "a" wave due to atrial contraction, but before the "a" wave when it is desired to study ventricular function unaffected by the effects of atrial function. **Endocardial pressure.** The pressure exerted on the endocardium by the pressure of blood within the cavities of the heart. **Hydrostatic pressure.** Pressure within a closed fluid system. **Imbibition pressure.** Pressure in a gel caused by absorption of liquid. **Intra-abdominal pressure.** The intraperitoneal pressure. **Intra-atrial pressure.** The pressure of blood within the atria of the heart. **Intracranial pressure.** The pressure in the subarachnoid space between the skull and the brain; if there is free circulation of the fluid and the patient is recumbent this is the same as the cerebrospinal pressure as measured by lumbar puncture. **Intra-ocular pressure.** The pressure maintained by the ocular contents as measured by a manometer: normally from 2.7 to 3.3 kPa (20 to 25 mmHg). **Intraperitoneal pressure.** The pressure within the peritoneal cavity. **Intrapleural pressure.** The pressure within the pleural cavity. **Intrapulmonic pressure.** The pressure of the air inside the lungs. **Intrathecal pressure.** The pressure of the cerebrospinal fluid within the theca, as measured by lumbar puncture. **Intrathoracic pressure.** The pressure within the thoracic cage, usually, but not necessarily, within the pleural cavity. **Intraventricular pressure.** The pressure of blood within the ventricles of the heart, which varies with the phase of the cardiac cycle. **Jugular venous pressure.** The pressure of blood within the jugular veins, which reflects the systemic venous pressure and the pressure within the right atrium. In normal individuals the upper level of mean venous pressure does not rise above the sternal angle when the subject is lying at an angle of 45 degrees, but is elevated in congestive heart failure and in certain other forms of cardiac and circulatory disorders. **Negative pressure.** Any pressure below that of the atmosphere measured as the difference between the atmospheric pressure and a lower pressure. **Osmotic pressure.** The tendency for solvent molecules to pass across a membrane from a low concentration of solute to a higher concentration may be completely prevented by applying a pressure. This pressure is the *effective osmotic pressure.* It is dependent on the number of particles in solution and is independent of the type. **Partial pressure.** The pressure exerted by any particular constituent of a mixture of gases. **Portal venous pressure.** The pressure, normally about 6–12 ml of saline, within the portal venous system; it is raised in cirrhosis and certain other conditions in which there is intra- or extrahepatic obstruction. **Positive pressure.** Any pressure above that of the atmosphere, measured as the difference between the atmospheric pressure and a higher pressure. **Positive end-expiratory pressure.** The use of slight positive pressure towards the end of expiration during intermittent positive pressure ventilation. It increases the functional residual capacity above the closure volume of the lungs. **Pulse pressure.** The difference between the systolic and diastolic arterial pressures. **Solution pressure.** 1. The force which tends to bring into solution the molecules of a solid immersed in a solvent. 2. The pressure which drives the ions of a metal from itself into the surrounding solution. **Systolic pressure.** In an artery or a ventricle, the highest pressure of the blood attained during systole. **Vapour pressure.** The pressure exerted by the molecules of a liquid or solid given off as a vapour. In an enclosed space the vapour pressure will attain a maximum dependent on the temperature. **Wedge pressure.** Usually the pressure which can be measured by a manometer attached to one end of a fluid-filled catheter when the other end of the catheter is wedged into a distal branch of the pulmonary artery; in these circumstances, provided there is no important pulmonary vascular disease distal to the point of wedging, the pressure recorded is that in the pulmonary veins and, thus, that in the left atrium. Less commonly the catheter may be wedged in a distal pulmonary vein when it will register the pulmonary arterial pressure. [L *premere* to press.]

See also: DONDERS.

presternum (pre·**ster**·num). The manubrium sterni. [L *prae,* sternum.]

Preston's salt. Smelling salt; aromatized ammonium carbonate, with or without addition of ammonia, used as a stimulant and restorative, especially in fainting.

presuppurative (pre·sup·ewr·a·tiv). Denoting an early phase in an inflammatory process which precedes the collection or formation of pus. [L *prae,* suppuration.]

presylvian (pre·**sil**·ve·an). Relating to the horizontal anterior ramus of the lateral sulcus (fissure of Sylvius). [L *prae,* fissure of Sylvius.]

presymptom (pre·**simp**·tom). Prodromal symptom. [L *prae,* symptom.]

presymptomatic (pre·simp·tom·**at**′·ik). Referring to presymptom.

presystole (pre·**sis**·to·le). The interval in the cardiac cycle immediately preceding systole. [L *prae,* systole.]

presystolic (pre·sis·**tol**·ik). Relating or belonging to the presystole.

Pretamazium Iodide (pret·am·a·ze·um i·o·dide). BP Commission approved name for 4-(biphenyl-4-yl)-3-ethyl-2-[4-(pyrrolidin-1-yl)styryl]thiazolium iodide; it is used in the treatment of enterobiasis.

pretarsal (pre·**tar**·sal). Anterior to the tarsus. [L *prae,* tarsus.]

pretibial (pre·**tib**·e·al). Situated or occurring in front of the tibia. [L *prae,* tibia.]

pretracheal (pre·**trak**·e·al). Anterior to the trachea. [L *prae,* trachea.]

pretuberculosis (pre·tew·ber·kew·**lo**′·sis). A stage in which tuberculosis is established but in which the characteristic symptoms or lesions are not obvious. [L *prae,* tuberculosis.]

pretuberculous (pre·tew·**ber**·kew·lus). Relating or belonging to the stage before the signs of tuberculosis may be recognized, or to the period during which tuberculosis was not established. [see prec.]

pretympanic (pre·tim·**pan**·ik). Occurring in front of the middle ear (tympanic cavity). [L *prae,* tympanum.]

pre-urethritis (pre·ewr·eth·**ri**′·tis). Inflammation affecting the lesser vestibular glands about the external urethral orifice. [L *prae,* urethritis.]

prevalence (**prev**·al·ens). **Point prevalence.** The proportion of cases (or manifestations) in a defined population at a particular point of time (*see also* INCIDENCE). **Period prevalence.** The proportion of cases (or manifestations) occurring during a specified period of time in a defined population. [L *praevalentia* superior force.]

Prevel's sign. Acceleration of the heart on assuming the upright position from the horizontal position.

preventive (pre·**ven**·tiv). Prophylactic. [L *praevenire* to anticipate.]

preventriculosis (pre·ven·trik·ew·**lo**′·sis). Achalasia of the cardia. [L *prae, ventriculus* stomach, Gk *-osis* condition.]

preventriculus (pre·ven·**trik**·ew·lus). The cardiac orifice of the stomach. [L *prae, ventriculus* stomach.]

preverbitum (pre·**ver**·bit·um). Those processes of thought which take place immediately prior to speech evocation.

prevermis (pre·**ver**·mis). The superior vermis of the cerebellum. [L *prae*, vermis.]

prevertebral (pre·**ver**·te·bral). Anterior to the body of a vertebra or to the vertebral column. [L *prae*, vertebra.]

prevertiginous (pre·ver·**tij**·in·us). Pertaining to a condition of vertigo in which the individual tends to fall forward, having the sensation that he has been pushed in the back. [L *prae*, vertigo.]

prevesical (pre·**ves**·ik·al). Anterior to or occurring in front of the urinary bladder. [L *prae, vesica* urinary bladder.]

previable (pre·**vi**·abl). Before the point at which extra-uterine existence is possible. [L *prae*, viable.]

previtamin (pre·**vi**·tam·in). The precursor of a vitamin as it occurs in nature; a provitamin. [L *prae*, vitamin.]

Prevost, Jean Louis (b. 1838). Swiss physician.

Prevost's law, or sign. Conjugate deviation of the head and eyes towards the side of the affected hemisphere and away from the paralysed limbs; seen in hemiplegia due to frontal lobe damage.

Preyer, Wilhelm Thierry (b. 1841). Jena physiologist and chemist.

Preyer's reflex. A reflex movement of the ears resulting from stimulation of the auditory mechanism.

prezone (**pre**·zone). Prozone. [L *prae*, zone.]

prezonular (pre·**zon**·ew·lar). Pertaining to that part of the eye lying in front of the zonular fibres, supporting the lens, and behind the iris. [L *prae*, zonular.]

prezygapophysis (pre·zi·gah·**pof**′·is·is). Anterior zygapophysis; the superior articular process of a vertebra. [L *prae*, zygapophysis.]

priapism (**pri**·ap·izm). A distressing condition in which there is more or less persistent erection of the penis, as a rule not due to sexual desire but caused by penile injuries, stone in the urinary bladder, or lesions of the spinal cord. It also occurs in leukaemia. [Gk *priapos* phallus.]

priapitis (pri·ap·**i**·tis). Inflammation affecting the penis. [Gk *priapos* phallus, *-itis* inflammation.]

priapus (**pri**·ap·us). The penis. [Gk *priapos* phallus.]

Pribram, Bruno Oskar (b. 1887). Berlin surgeon.

Pribram's operation. Cholecystectomy by thermocoagulation.

Price, Ernest Arthur (b. 1882). London chemist.

Carr–Price test. For vitamin A: a transient blue colour is given by vitamin A when 0.2 ml of a chloroform solution containing the vitamin is mixed with 2 ml of chloroform saturated with antimony trichloride.

Carr–Price unit. A colour equal to 1 Lovibond blue unit given by 0.04 g of sample in 0.2 ml of solvent when mixed with 2 ml of antimony trichloride reagent shows unit vitamin-A potency.

Price, Ivor Noble Orpwood. 20th century London venereologist.

Price precipitation reaction. A serological test for syphilis.

Price-Jones, Cecil (b. 1863). London haematologist.

Price-Jones curve. The curve obtained by the somewhat laborious Price-Jones method; the diameters (in μm) of from 200 to 500 erythrocytes are plotted on a graph as the abscissa against their frequency (i.e. the number of cells in each size group) as the ordinate. The curve so produced lies approximately symmetrically about the mean of 7.2 μm; diameters greater than 7.718 μm and less than 6.686 μm are definitely abnormal.

Price-Jones method. A method for the direct measurement of the diameters of red cells from images of the cells in a stained film magnified to an optimum size by the microscope and conveniently projected by a prism on to a flat horizontal plane (see above).

Priestley, Joseph (b. 1733). English scientist.

Priestley's mass. A green or brown stain occurring in a young person on those parts of Nasmyth's membrane which have not been worn off the surface of the enamel of a tooth.

Prilocaine (**pril**·o·kane). BP Commission approved name for *N*-(2-propylaminopropionyl)-*o*-toluidine. **Prilocaine Hydrochloride BP 1973.** The hydrochloride of the basic substance; a local analgesic with actions similar to those of lignocaine but with a tendency to produce methaemoglobin by its metabolites.

Primaquine (**prim**·ah·kween). BP Commission approved name for 8-(4-amino-1-methylbutylamino)-6-methoxyquinoline; an antimalarial drug given in succession to chloroquine, amodiaquine or quinine in order to eliminate the persistent exo-erythrocyte phase of the parasite in infections with *Plasmodium vivax, P. malariae* or *P. ovale.* **Primaquine Phosphate BP 1973.** The phosphate of primaquine, used similarly to the base.

primary (**pri**·mar·e). First, or of first importance. [L *primus* first.]

primate (**pri**·mate). A member of the order Primates.

Primates (pri·**ma**·teez). An order of the chordate class Mammalia, which includes Lemuroidea, lemurs, and Anthropoidea, monkeys, apes and man. Characterized by the large brain, well-developed eyes set forward, giving, in many, stereoscopic vision, and the limbs developed for climbing by grasping with hands and feet. [L *primus* first.]

prime mover (prime **moo**·ver). A muscle which produces a movement by shortening, thus approximating its attachments.

primer (**pri**·mer). A class of molecule required to initiate the synthetic reactions catalysed by certain enzymes (e.g. a glucose oligosaccharide for glucagen synthetase, appropriate nucleic acids for RNA and DNA polymerases). [L *primus* first.]

primeverose (**pri**·me·ver·oze). 6-[-β-D-xylosido]-D-glucose. A disaccharide occurring as a constituent of various natural glycosides such as gaultherin.

Primidone BP 1973 (**prim**·e·done). 5-Phenyl-5-ethylhexahydropyrimidine-4,6-dione. An anticonvulsant drug which appears to be of use in the treatment of epilepsy, probably more so in major epilepsy than in minor epilepsy.

primigravida (pri·me·**grav**·id·ah). One who is pregnant for the first time. [L *primus* first, *gravidus* pregnant.]

primipara (pri·**mip**·ar·ah). A woman who has had one child. [see foll.]

primiparity (pri·me·**par**·it·e). The condition of having had one child. [L *primus* first, *parere* to bear.]

primiparous (pri·**mip**·ar·us). Referring to a woman who is giving or has given birth to her first child. [see prec.]

primitiae (pri·**mish**·e·e). Name given to that portion of the liquor amnii which is expelled before the child is born. [L *primus* first.]

primitive (**prim**·it·iv). 1. Rudimentary; earliest or early in the process of development. 2. Of people, uncivilized; simple. 3. Crude. [L *primitus* for the first time.]

primordial (pri·**mor**·de·al). In biology, existing in the simplest form; primitive, early or undeveloped. **Primordial sex cells.** These are differentiated early in embryonic development and migrate to the genital ridge forming the fetal ovary, acting as stem cells for the primordial ova present at birth.

primordium (pri·**mor**·de·um). Anlage; in embryology, the first undifferentiated grouping of cells from which any organ or part will develop. [L, origin.]

primula (**prim**·ew·lah). Primrose, *Primula vulgaris* (family Primulaceae); the root and herb contain saponin and bitter principles but are seldom used. **Primula obconica.** A primula with powerful skin-sensitizing properties, derived from glandular hairs on its flowers, stems and leaves. [dim. of L *primus* first.]

primulin (**prim**·ew·lin). A crystalline compound found in the root of the cowslip, *Primula veris.*

primuline (prim·ew·**leen**). $C_6H_3CH_3(SNC)C_6H_3(SNC)C_6H_4NH_2$, a thiazole base prepared from *p*-toluidine which gives a number of yellow ingrain dyes. It is also used in a process of fabric printing.

Prince, Arthur E. (b. 1853). Illinois ophthalmologist.

Prince's muscle clamp, or forceps. A light muscle clamp with small teeth on each blade, designed to hold the extra-ocular muscle in squint operations.

Prince's operation. For squint: resection and advancement of the muscle, using a special clamp *(Prince's muscle clamp)* with teeth. A pulley suture is placed vertically near the limbus through the sclera and the resected muscle sutured to this.

Prince's rule. A steel tape calibrated in both centimetres and dioptres for measuring the distance of the near point and also giving the amount of accommodation in dioptres.

princeps (prin·seps). Literally, principal; usually applied to an artery, e.g. princeps pollicis artery. [L.]

princeps pollicis artery [arteria princeps pollicis] (**prin**·seps **pol**·is·is **ar**·ter·e). *See* RADIAL ARTERY.

Princeteau's tubercle. A tubercle at the apex of the temporal bone.

principle (**prin**·sipl). 1. In science, a rule or theory. 2. Active principle; the ingredient, or ingredients, of a drug or other substance to which its pharmaceutical activity is due. **Anterior pituitary-like principle.** Gonadotrophin [obsolete term]. **Anti-anaemia principle.** A principle present in liver extracts which effects remission of symptoms in pernicious anaemia. It has been shown that the disease is the immediate result of folic-acid deficiency, but the fundamental principle is now believed to be vitamin B_{12}. **Anti-insulin principle.** A hormone present in the anterior part of the pituitary, the action of which is antagonistic to that of insulin and tends to produce a rise in the level of the blood sugar. **Displacement principle.** A method of introducing fluids into the nasal air sinuses through their natural ostium, devised by A. W. Proetz of St Louis, USA. It is based on the fact that if a liquid is placed near the ostium joining two air-containing cavities, one of which is a closed cavity, suction applied to the non-closed cavity will result in air escaping from the closed cavity, its place being taken by the fluid in contact with the ostium. **Glucotrophic principle.** Anti-insulin principle (see above). **Haematinic principle.** Anti-anaemia principle (see above). **Pleasure principle.** In psycho-analysis, the principle which determines that unconscious mental processes strive towards gaining pleasure, drawing back from any operation which might arouse unpleasantness. **Reality principle.** In psycho-analysis, the principle which determines that unconscious mental processes, in addition to being guided by the pleasure principle, take into account also the conditions imposed by the outer world. **Transforming principle.** The agent responsible for bacterial transformation. Discovered to be highly polymerized deoxyribonucleic acid (DNA) by O. T. Avery *et al.* (1944), the first direct evidence that genetic material is composed of DNA. [L *principium.*]

See also: ARCHIMEDES, BRAGG, DOPPLER (C. J.), LE CHATELIER.

Pringle, John James (b. 1855). London dermatologist.

Pringle's disease, or naevus. A red vascular type of sebaceous adenoma.

Pringle, Seton Sidney (b. 1879). Dublin surgeon.

Pringle's band. A fold of peritoneum which extends from the mesocolon to the antimesenteric border of the proximal part of the jejunum.

Seton Pringle clamp. A fine crushing-clamp, used in aseptic excision of the colon.

Prinos (**pri**·nos). A genus or subgenus of aquifoliaceous shrubs assigned to the genus *Ilex* (holly). *Prinos verticillatus,* winterberry, feverbush, the American black alder, has a bark which is astringent and is used in diarrhoea. [Gk, oak.]

print (print). **Radiographic print.** A photographic print on paper, made from either a positive or negative x-ray film. [ME *prent.*]

Prinzmetal, Myron (b. 1908). American cardiologist.

Prinzmetal's angina. Anginal variant; an uncommon form of angina pectoris in which the pain is experienced at rest, often nocturnally, rather than in relation to effort, and during the attacks there is S–T segment elevation in the electrocardiogram instead of depression as usually occurs with angina. Reported cases have often had a bad prognosis.

Prionurus citrinus (pri·**on**·ew·rus sit·**ri**·nus). A poisonous scorpion. [Gk *prion* saw, *oura* tail, L, lemon-coloured.]

prisilidene hydrochloride (pris·**il**·id·een hi·dro·**klor**·ide). Alphaprodine.

prism (prizm). 1. A solid figure which is triangular or polygonal in cross-section, and is bounded by parallelograms. 2. In optics, a solid triangular refracting medium which breaks up white light into its constituent spectral colours and alters the direction of the rays of light, so moving the apparent position of an object viewed through it towards the apex. It is incorporated in spectacle lenses to overcome ocular muscle imbalance or paresis, and is also a component of spectroscopes, binoculars, etc. **Adverse prisms.** Those used in treating ocular muscle imbalance by making the weak muscle work hard by the apparent movement of the object in the same direction as the action of the muscle. **Prism dioptre.** A scale for measuring the deviating power of prisms: a one-dioptre prism will deviate a ray of light a distance of 10 mm when measured on a plane situated at right angles to the base of the prism, at a distance of 1 m. **Enamel prisms [prismata adamantina (NA)].** Calcified rods or prisms that are surrounded by organic prism cuticle and joined together by interprismatic substance to form the hard enamel on the surface of a tooth; an enamel rod. **Relieving prisms.** Those used in treating ocular muscle imbalance by resting the weak muscle with the apparent movement of the fixation object in the opposite direction to the action of the muscle. **Verger prism.** A prism used to test or train the ability of the eyes to converge, diverge or supraverge whilst still maintaining fusion, e.g. Maddox prism verger. [Gk *prisma* that which is sawn through.]

See also: GOLDMANN, MADDOX, NICOL.

prismatic (priz·**mat**·ik). 1. Like a prism in shape. 2. Relating to or produced by a prism.

prismoid, prismoidal (**priz**·moid, priz·**moid**·al). Having resemblance to a prism. [prism, Gk *eidos* form.]

prismoptometer (priz·mop·**tom**·et·er). A revolving prism for testing the duction power of the eyes. [prism, Gk *optos* seen, meter.]

prismosphere (**priz**·mo·sfeer). A spectacle lens in which a prism is combined with a sphere.

Pristinamycin (**pris**·tin·ah·**mi**′·sin). BP Commission approved name for an antibiotic produced by *Streptomyces pristina spiralis.*

Pritchard, Urban (b. 1845). London aural surgeon.

Pritchard's reticulated membrane. Intercellular membrane found in the bony ampullae in mammals.

Pritchett, Ida W. (b. 1891). New York pathologist.

Bull and Pritchett serum. A serum used for gas gangrene.

Privey, Paul (b. 1885). French physician.

Lesieur-Privey sign. The presence of albumin in sputum. It is positive in tuberculosis and acute or subacute congestive conditions of the lungs, such as pneumonia, but it is not specific.

Lesieur-Privey test. For albumin in sputum in cases of suspected tuberculosis, emphysema with cardiac dilatation and pneumonia. An equal quantity of 3 per cent acetic acid is well shaken up with the sputum and allowed to stand for some time, then filtered. If albumin is present, this clear filtrate becomes cloudy on boiling.

pro-. A prefix, from the Greek and Latin prepositions *pro,* meaning *before, in front of, in place of, forward.*

pro-accelerin (pro·ak·**sel**·er·in). *See* CONVERTIN.

pro-actinium (pro·ak·**tin**·e·um). Protactinium.

pro-actinomyces (pro·ak·tin·o·**mi**′·seez). The name proposed by Jensen for those Actinomyces which reproduce aerobically by fragmentation of the mycelial filaments. The generic name *Nocardia* Trevisan 1889 has precedence for these organisms. [Gk *pro,* actinomyces.]

pro-actinomycin (pro·**ak**·tin·o·**mi**′·sin). A chemically undefined antibiotic substance produced by certain species of *Nocardia.* It is more active against Gram-positive than Gram-negative micro-organisms. [see prec.]

proal (pro·al). Pertaining to or having a forward movement. [Gk *pro.*]

pro-amnion (pro·am·ne·on). A membrane in front of the definitive embryonic area in the early development of certain embryos, where ectoderm and entoderm are in contact. [Gk *pro,* amnion.]

pro-antithrombin (pro·an·te·throm′·bin). A precursor of antithrombin. [Gk *pro,* antithrombin.]

pro-arrhythmic (pro·a·rith·mik). The property of a drug which produces cardiac arrythmia. [Gk *pro, a, rhythmos* rhythm.]

pro-atlantal artery (pro·at·lan·tal). An embryonic artery, the first of the intersegmental arteries, which lies cranial to the first cervical somite. [Gk *pro,* atlas.]

pro-atlas (pro·at·las). An anomalous vertebral element occasionally found between the atlas and the occipital bone. [Gk *pro,* atlas.]

proband (pro·band). A propositus; the person with a certain malady or condition whose family history or pedigree is being constructed in order to discover whether or not any relatives of this person, either in the existing or previous generations, are suffering or have suffered from the same condition. [L *probare* to test.]

probang (pro·bang). A flexible rod which was formerly introduced into the oesophagus for testing and localizing strictures, and the displacing of foreign bodies towards the stomach. It is not much used now, since the introduction of x-ray diagnosis and peroral endoscopy. The type of end attached to the rod varies. **Ball probang.** A probang with a bulbous end. **Bristle probang, Horse probang.** One possessing an end with expansile tuft of horsehair. **Sponge probang.** One fitted with a sponge at the end.

probe (probe). 1. An instrument for exploring the depths of a wound or a sinus. 2. Any device inserted into a medium to obtain information about the nature of the medium. **Blunt probe.** A probe with a blunt leading end. **Bullet probe.** A slender probe, commonly malleable, used in searching for a bullet in a wound. **Drum probe.** A probe with a sounding device to help in the detection of metallic foreign bodies in wounds. **Electric probe.** Telephonic probe (see below). **Eyed probe.** A probe with an eye at one end, used to introduce a guiding thread along a fistula. **Lacrimal probe.** A small probe designed for passing down the lacrimal passages. Liebreich's or Bowman's are commonly used. **Scissors probe.** Scissors with a probe fused to one blade, used in exploring and laying open a fistula. **Space probe.** An instrumental rocket which attains an altitude above 4000 miles (one earth's radius), designed to gather information about the environment. **Telephonic probe.** A probe attached to a telephone headphone in which a sound is recorded when the probe touches metal. **Uterine probe.** An instrument to determine the length and direction of the uterine cavity. **Vertebrated probe.** A flexible probe consisting of several articulated metal segments. **Wire probe.** A soft malleable probe, often of silver. [L *probare* to test.]

See also: ANEL, BOWMAN, BRACKETT, DESJARDIN, FLUHRER, GIRDNER, LIEBREICH, LUCAE, MAYO (C. H.).

Probenecid BP 1973 (pro·ben·es·id). *p*-(di-*n*-Propylsulphamoyl) benzoic acid. A compound used in the treatment of gout; it is administered over long periods.

proboscis (pro·bos·is). The elongate, often retractile, structure at the anterior end of many animals, often associated with feeding; especially elongate mouth-parts of insects, e.g. Diptera, Hemiptera and Hymenoptera. [Gk *proboskis* elephant's trunk.]

Probucol (pro·bew·kol). BP Commission approved name for 4,4′-(isopropylidenedithio)bis(2,6-di-*tert*-butylphenol); an antihypercholesterolaemic agent.

Procainamide (pro·ka·nam·ide). BP Commission approved name for *p*-amino-*N*-(2-diethylaminoethyl)benzamide. It depresses irritability of the thyro-epiglottic muscle; the effect is more prolonged than that of procaine hydrochloride, and it is better tolerated. The hydrochloride (BP 1973) is useful in the treatment of ventricular and atrial arrhythmias and extrasystoles. Administered intravenously it causes less hypotension than does procaine hydrochloride. Repeated administration has given rise to granulocytopenia.

procaine (pro·kane). Ethocaine, diethylaminoethyl-*p*-aminobenzoate, $NH_2C_6H_4COOCH_2CH_2N(C_2H_5)_2$. A colourless crystalline synthetic base, usually administered as the hydrochloride (BP 1973). It is soluble in water and is used in place of cocaine on account of its lower toxicity. Its action is rapid in onset, especially when injected, and is prolonged by administration with adrenaline which constricts the blood vessels around the site of injection. **Procaine benzylpenicillin.** Procaine Penicillin. *See* PENICILLIN. **Procaine borate.** A salt considered more active and less toxic than the hydrochloride, used as a surface analgesic in ophthalmic and dental practice. **Procaine penicillin.** *See* PENICILLIN.

Procainii Chloridum. *European Pharmacopoeia* name for Procaine Hydrochloride BP 1973.

procallus (pro·kal·us). The organized blood clot between the separated parts of a fractured bone, which is eventually replaced by callus. [Gk *pro,* callus.]

procambium (pro·kam·be·um). The long slender cells in the growing points and root tips of a plant; they develop into vascular tissue. [Gk *pro,* LL *cambium* nutriment.]

Procarbazine (pro·kar·baz·een). BP Commission approved name for *N*-4-isopropylcarbamoylbenzyl-*N*′-methylhydrazine; it is used in the treatment of Hodgkin's disease.

procarboxypeptidase (pro·kar·box·e·pep′·tid·aze). The zymogen of carboxypeptidase. [Gk *pro,* carboxypeptidase.]

procaryote (pro·kar·e·ote). Prokaryote.

procatarctic (pro·kat·ark·tik). Applied to the predisposing cause of a disease, or to the primary or the exciting cause. [Gk *prokatarktikos* beginning beforehand.]

procatarxis (pro·kat·arx·is). 1. The initial or exciting cause. 2. Predisposition. 3. The onset of a disease, the predisposition being already present. [Gk *prokatarchomaein* to begin first.]

procedure (pro·seed·yer). *See* ELSBERG, HUMBY, MCINDOE, NOVÉ-JOSSERAND. [L *procedere* to proceed.]

procephalic (pro·kef·al·ik). In biology, relating or belonging to the anterior portion of the head. [Gk *pro, kephale* head.]

procercoid (pro·ser·koid). A larval stage of tapeworms, occurring in the intermediary host. [Gk *pro, kerkos* tail, *eidos* form.]

procerus muscle [musculus procerus (NA)] (pro·se·rus musl). A small skin muscle at the root of the nose, continuous above with the frontal belly of the occipitofrontalis muscle. [L *procerus* stretched.]

process (pro·ses). 1. A course of action or of events. 2. [Processus (NA)]. An outgrowth of tissue. 3. In chemistry, any method of preparing a particular compound. **ABC (alum, blood, clay) process.** A rough method of treating crude sewage by adding alum, blood, clay, charcoal or other substances to it. These precipitate the sludge and deodorize the sewage. It has been superseded by modern methods of sewage purification. **Accessory process.** Process of a lumbar vertebra, accessory (see below). **Acromial process, Acromion process.** Acromion. **Alveolar process.** 1. Process of the mandible, alveolar (see below). 2. Process of the maxilla, alveolar (see below). **Ameloblastic process.** The process from one of the ameloblast cells of the enamel organ which goes to form the matrix upon which calcium salts are deposited to form enamel; a Tomes' process. **Articular process.** 1. Process of the sacrum, superior articular (see below). 2. [Zygapophysis (NA)] Process of a vertebra, inferior articular, superior articular (see below). **Process of the arytenoid cartilage, muscular [processus muscularis (NA)].** The lateral angle of the arytenoid cartilage, to which the lateral and posterior crico-arytenoid muscles are attached. **Process of the arytenoid cartilage, vocal [processus vocalis (NA)].** The anterior angle of the arytenoid cartilage, giving attachment to the vocal ligament. **Process of the atlas, transverse.** The long bony process projecting laterally from the atlas. **Process of the axis, odontoid [dens (NA)].** A toothlike, bony, upward projection from process

the body of the axis. **Axis-cylinder process.** A branch of an axis-cylinder. **Bremsstrahlung process.** *See* BREMSSTRAHLUNG. **Caudate process [processus caudatus (NA)].** A tongue of liver tissue joining the caudate lobe to the remainder of the right lobe. **Process of a cervical vertebra, costal [processus costarius (NA)].** The anterior bar of the transverse process of a cervical vertebra in front of and lateral to the canal for the vertebral artery. **Ciliary processes [processus ciliares (NA)].** Foldings of the choroid of the eye in the ciliary body, arranged circularly and giving attachment to the suspensory ligament of the lens. **Clinoid processes.** Processes of the sphenoid bone, anterior clinoid, middle clinoid, posterior clinoid (see below). **Condyloid process.** Process of the mandible, condyloid (see below). **Coracoid process [processus coracoideus (NA)].** A strong, curved process arising from the upper surface of the neck of the scapula. **Coronoid process.** 1. Process of the mandible, coronoid (see below). 2. Process of the ulna, coronoid (see below). **Costal process.** 1. Process of a cervical vertebra, costal (see above). 2. The mesenchymal primordium of a rib in the early embryo, which arises as an outgrowth from the sclerotome. **Dendritic process.** A branching process, such as the dendrite of a nerve cell. **Process of the ethmoid bone, uncinate [processus uncinatus (NA)].** A bony bar springing from the labyrinth of the ethmoid bone and curving downward to articulate with the inferior nasal concha to form the medial boundary of the hiatus semilunaris. **Ethmoidal process.** Process of the inferior nasal concha, ethmoidal (see below). **Falciform process.** Process of the sacro-tuberous ligament, falciform (see below). **Process of the fibula, styloid [apex capitis fibulae (NA)].** An eminence on the posterolateral aspect of the head of the fibula which gives attachment to the tendon of the biceps femoris muscle. **Foot process.** A pedicel. **Frontal process.** 1. Process of the maxilla, frontal (see below). 2. Process of the zygomatic bone, frontal (see below). **Frontonasal process.** The embryonic anlage of the nose, upper lip and front part of the palate, first appearing as a median swelling rostral to the stomatodaeum or primitive mouth. **Globular process.** One of two rounded swellings of the median nasal process bounding the inner margin of the olfactory pits. **Head process.** A sagittal rod of mesoderm in front of and derived from the primitive node of the early embryo and destined to give rise to the notochord. Its cells are responsible for the axial organization of the embryo during its early development. **Process of the incus, long [crus longum (NA)].** A slender process projecting downward parallel, medial and posterior to the handle of the malleus. It terminates in a small swelling, the lentiform nodule, which articulates with the head of the stapes. **Process of the incus, short [crus breve (NA)].** A blunt process, covered with cartilage at the tip, which projects horizontally backward into a fossa in the posterior wall of the tympanic cavity. **Process of the inferior nasal concha, ethmoidal [processus ethmoidalis (NA)].** A bony plate projecting upward to articulate with the uncinate process of the ethmoid bone. **Intrajugular process.** 1. Process of the occipital bone, intrajugular (see below). 2. Process of the temporal bone, intrajugular (see below). **Jugular process.** Process of the occipital bone, jugular (see below). **Lacrimal process [processus lacrimalis (NA)].** A process on the superior border of the inferior nasal concha forming part of the nasolacrimal canal. **Process of a lumbar vertebra, accessory [processus accessorius (vertebrarum lumbalium) (NA)].** A rough elevation on the posterior aspect of the transverse process of a lumbar vertebra, near its root. **Lyophil process.** Drying *in vacuo* from the frozen state; a method of preserving bacteria and sera. **Processes of the malleus.** *See* MALLEUS. **Mamillary process.** Process of a vertebra, mamillary (see below). **Process of the mandible, alveolar.** The upper part of the body of the mandible; the alveolar part of the mandible. **Process of the mandible, condyloid [processus condylaris (NA)].** The projection from the upper posterior part of the ramus of the mandible bearing the condyle. **Process of the mandible, coronoid [processus coronoideus (NA)].** The flattened triangular projection from the upper anterior part of the ramus of the mandible to which the temporal muscle is attached. **Mastoid process.** Process of the temporal bone, mastoid (see below). **Process of the maxilla, alveolar [processus alveolaris (NA)].** The part of the maxilla which bears the tooth sockets. **Process of the maxilla, frontal [processus frontalis (NA)].** A process extending upward to articulate with the frontal and nasal bones. **Process of the maxilla, palatine [processus palatinus (NA)].** The medially directed process of the maxilla which helps to form the hard palate and articulates behind with the palatine bone. **Process of the maxilla, zygomatic [processus zygomaticus (NA).** A part of the anterior surface of the maxilla articulating above with the zygomatic bone. **Maxillary process [processus maxillaris (NA)].** A flat plate from the inferior nasal concha forming part of the medial wall of the maxillary sinus. **Maxillary process of the embryo.** That part of the 1st pharyngeal arch which lies above the mouth in an early embryo, and in which the upper jaw and associated structures are developed. **Medial angular process.** The termination of the supra-orbital margin of the nasal part of the frontal bone. **Muscular process.** Process of the arytenoid cartilage, muscular (see above). **Nasal process, lateral.** That part of the frontonasal process of the early embryo which lies lateral to the olfactory pit, and from which the ala of the nose is derived. **Nasal process, median.** That part of the frontonasal process of the early embryo which lies between the olfactory pits. **Notochordal process.** Head process (see above). **Process of the occipital bone, intrajugular [processus intrajugularis (NA)].** A bony spicule which projects into the jugular notch. **Process of the occipital bone, jugular [processus jugularis (NA)].** The quadrilateral plate of bone projecting laterally from the condylar part and forming the posterior border of the jugular foramen. **Process of the occipital bone, paramastoid [processus paramastoideus (NA)].** A bony eminence on the inferior surface of the jugular process of the occipital bone. **Odontoblastic process.** The peripheral process from one of the odontoblast cells of the tooth pulp which provides nutrition to the dentine. **Odontoid process.** Process of the axis, odontoid (see above). **Opercular process.** A projection from the hinder edge of the 2nd pharyngeal arch, which helps to bridge over and close the precervical sinus. **Orbital process.** Process of the palatine bone, orbital (see below). **Palatal process.** Palatine process, lateral (see below). **Palatine process.** Process of the maxilla, palatine (see above). **Palatine process, lateral.** A shelf-like inward projection from the maxillary process of the embryo, from which one-half of the palate is derived. **Process of the palatine bone, orbital [processus orbitalis (NA)].** An upward and laterally directed projection from the perpendicular plate of the palatine bone, articulating with the ethmoid and sphenoid bones at the back of the orbit. **Process of the palatine bone, sphenoidal [processus sphenoidalis (NA)].** A projection directed upward and medially from the perpendicular plate of the palatine bone to articulate with the sphenoid bone and vomer. **Process of the pancreas, uncinate [processus uncinatus (NA)].** A prolongation from the lower and left part of the head upward and to the left behind the superior mesenteric vessels. **Papillary process [processus papillaris (NA)].** A rounded projection from the inferior left portion of the caudate lobe of the liver. **Paramastoid process.** Process of the occipital bone, paramastoid (see above). **Protoplasmic process.** A thick, as opposed to a thin, fibrous process of the cell body of a neuron or neuroglial cell. **Pterygoid process.** Process of the sphenoid bone, pterygoid (see below). **Pterygospinous process [processus pterygospinosus (NA)].** Occasional backward projection from the lower end of the lateral pterygoid plate connected by a ligament, sometimes ossified, to the spine of the sphenoid. **Process of the radius, styloid [processus styloideus (NA)].** A downward-directed projection on the lateral side of the lower end of the radius. **Process of the sacrotuberous ligament, falciform [processus falciformis (NA)].** That portion of the ligament attaching to the inferior ramus of the ischium; it has a crescentic margin. **Process of the sacrum, superior articular [processus articularis superior (NA)].** The upwardly directed bony projection from the base of the sacrum, bearing the joint surfaces for articulation with the 5th vertebra. **Septal process** [crus mediale (NA)]. The part of the lower nasal cartilage that joins its neighbour in the lower part of the nasal septum. **Process of the sphenoid bone, anterior clinoid [processus clinoideus anterior (NA)].** A process on the medial end of the posterior border of the lesser wing. **Process of the sphenoid bone, middle clinoid [processus clinoideus medius (NA)].** One of a pair at the lateral ends of the tuberculum sellae. **Process of the sphenoid bone, posterior clinoid [processus clinoideus posterior (NA)].** One of a pair situated at the ends of the anterosuperior border of the dorsum sellae. **Process of the sphenoid bone, pterygoid [processus pterygoideus (NA)].** A process projecting downward from the junction of the body and the greater wing, and composed of the two pterygoid plates. **Process of the sphenoid bone, vaginal [processus vaginalis (NA)].** A thin scale on the inferior surface of the body, which articulates with the ala of the vomer. **Sphenoidal process.** Process of the palatine bone, sphenoidal (see above). **Sphenoidal process of the nasal septum [processus posterior (sphenoidalis) (NA)].** The extension posteriorly of the cartilage of the nasal septum. **Spinous process of a vertebra.** *See* SPINE OF A VERTEBRA. **Styloid process.** 1. Process of the fibula, styloid (see above). 2. Process of the radius, styloid (see above). 3. Process of the temporal bone, styloid (see below). 4. Process of the third metacarpal bone, styloid (see below). 5. Process of the ulna, styloid (see below). **Subgerminal process.** A cellular mass derived from the deep layer of the blastoderm in a large-yolked egg. **Sucker process.** A process from an astrocyte which is attached to the wall of a small blood vessel. **Supracondylar process [processus supracondylaris (NA)].** A hook-shaped process sometimes found projecting from the anteromedial surface of the shaft of the humerus, about 50 mm above the medial epicondyle. It is usually converted by a fibrous band into a foramen transmitting the median nerve and brachial artery; this foramen occurs normally in many animals. **Process of the talus, posterior.** The process that receives the attachment of the talofibular ligament. **Temporal process.** Process of the zygomatic bone, temporal (see below). **Process of the temporal bone, intrajugular [processus intrajugularis (NA)].** A bony spicule which projects into the jugular notch. **Process of the temporal bone, mastoid [processus mastoideus (NA)].** A blunted process projecting from the mastoid part downward and forward below the external auditory meatus. **Process of the temporal bone, styloid [processus styloideus (NA)].** A slender tapering process of variable length, projecting downward and forward from the inferior surface of the temporal bone. The sheath [vagina processus styloidei (NA)] forms part of the inferior border of the tympanic plate. **Process of the temporal bone, zygomatic [processus zygomaticus (NA)].** The zygoma; a process which projects forward from the external surface of the squamous temporal bone to form the posterior part of the zygomatic arch. **Process of the third metacarpal bone, styloid [processus styloideus (NA)].** A bone process projecting proximally from the base of the bone. **Transverse process.** Process of a vertebra, transverse (see below). **Process of the ulna, coronoid [processus coronoideus (NA)].** A bracket-like projection from the front of the ulna just below the olecranon. It forms the lower part of the trochlear notch. **Process of the ulna, styloid [processus styloideus (NA)].** A short, rounded projection at the lower end of the ulna. **Uncinate process.** 1. Process of the ethmoid bone, uncinate (see above). 2. Process of the pancreas, uncinate (see above). **Vaginal process.** Process of the sphenoid bone, vaginal (see above). **Process of a vertebra, inferior articular [processus articularis inferior (zygapophysis) (NA)].** The bony projection from the lamina of a vertebra, bearing the articular surface for the vertebra below. **Process of a vertebra, mamillary [processus mamillaris (NA)].** A rough elevation on the superior articular process of a vertebra for muscle attachment. **Process of a vertebra, superior articular [processus articularis superior (zygapophysis) (NA)].** An upward projection from the junction of the pedicle and lamina, bearing the articular surface for the vertebra above. **Process of a vertebra, transverse [processus transversus (NA)].** The bony process projecting laterally from the vertebral arch. **Vocal process.** Process of the arytenoid cartilage, vocal (see above). **Xiphoid process [processus xiphoideus (NA)].** The lowest piece of the sternum, so called because of its sword-shape. **Zygomatic process [processus zygomaticus (NA)].** 1. A projection of the frontal bone forming the lateral boundary of the superciliary arch. 2. Process of the maxilla, zygomatic (see above). 3. Process of the temporal bone, zygomatic (see above). **Process of the zygomatic bone, frontal [processus frontalis (NA)].** The upwardly directed process of the zygomatic bone articulating with the frontal bone and the greater wing of the sphenoid bone. **Process of the zygomatic bone, temporal [processus temporalis (NA)].** The backwardly directed prolongation of the zygomatic bone which articulates with the zygomatic process of the temporal bone. [L *processus.*]

See also: BLUMENBACH, CIVININI, DEITERS, FOLIUS, GOTTSTEIN, GOWERS, INGRASSIA, LENHOSSÉK, RAU, RIEDEL, STIEDA (L.), TODD (R. B.), TOMES (C. S.).

processus [NA] (pro·ses·us). Process. **Processus cochleariformis [NA].** A curved part of the bony septum over which passes the tendon of the tensor tympani muscle. **Processus vaginalis of the peritoneum [processus vaginalis peritonei (NA)].** A peritoneal process in the fetus, traversing the inguinal canal and reaching the scrotum. The testis invaginates the posterior wall. Its proximal portion is obliterated, and the distal portion becomes the tunica vaginalis testis. [L.]

procheilon (pro·**ki**·lon). The slight prominence formed by the termination of the philtrum in the central part of the outer surface of the upper lip. [Gk *pro, cheilos* lip.]

Prochlorperazine (pro·klor·**per**·az·een). BP Commission approved name for 2-chloro-10-[3-(4-methylpiperazin-1-yl)propyl] phenothiazine. **Prochlorperazine Maleate BP 1973.** The di(hydrogen maleate) of the base; it is used effectively as an anti-emetic in the control of nausea, vomiting and motion sickness. **Prochlorperazine Mesylate BP 1973.** The dimethanesulphate of prochlorperazine; its actions and uses are similar to those of chlorpromazine. It is particularly effective in the management of nausea and vomiting and in the treatment of migraine.

prochondral (pro·**kon**·dral). Pertaining to the stage which precedes the development of cartilage. [Gk *pro, chondros* cartilage.]

prochordal (pro·**kord**·al). Prechordal. [Gk *pro,* chord.]

prochoresis (pro·kor·e·sis). The movement downward of partly digested food as it is propelled through the pylorus and down the alimentary canal. [Gk *prochoreein* to advance.]

prochorion (pro·**ko**·re·on). Part of the ectodermal covering of a blastocyst, which will later form part of the chorion. [Gk *pro,* chorion.]

prochromosome (pro·**kro**·mo·some). Chromocenter formed by positively heterochromatic chromosome regions situated near the centromere. [Gk *pro,* chromosome.]

prochymosin (pro·ki·mo·sin). Renninogen; the precursor of the enzyme, chymosin (rennin). [Gk *pro,* chymosin.]

procident (**pro**·sid·ent). 1. Relating to procidentia. 2. In a prolapsed state. [see foll.]

procidentia (pro·sid·**en**·she·ah). Prolapse of any part or organ; denoting especially prolapse of the uterus to such degree that the neck of the uterus protrudes beyond the vulva. [L *procidere* to fall down forward.]

Proclonol (pro·**klo**·nol). BP Commission approved name for 4,4′-dichloro-α-cyclopropylbenzhydrol; an acaricide and fungicide.

procoelia (pro·**se**·le·ah). The lateral ventricle of the cerebral hemisphere. [Gk *pro, koilia* cavity.]

procoelous (pro·**se**·lus). Hollowed out on the anterior surface, as the body of a vertebra. [see prec.]

proconceptive (pro·kon·**sep**·tiv). 1. Facilitating conception. 2. A drug which facilitates conception by adjusting the hydrogen-ion concentration of the vaginal secretion. [L *pro,* conception.]

proconvertin (pro·kon·**ver**·tin). A factor (factor VII) concerned in the clotting of blood, which under the influence of calcium and thromboplastin is converted into convertin (stable component) according to Owren. [L *pro,* convertin.]

procreate (pro·kre·ate). To beget or to produce offspring. [see foll.]

procreation (pro·kre·a·shun). The action of procreating. [L *procreare* to beget.]

procreative (**pro**·kre·at·iv). Pertaining to procreation.

proctagra (prok·**tag**·rah). Pain affecting the anus or the parts surrounding that organ. [Gk *proktos* anus, *agra* a catching.]

proctalgia (prok·**tal**·je·ah). Neuralgic pain in the anus or lower part of the rectum. **Proctalgia fugax, Nocturnal proctalgia.** A pain that occurs periodically in the rectum; its occurrence follows a definite pattern and is possibly muscular in origin. It is usually relieved by the taking of food or drink. It is not associated with any organic lesion. [Gk *proktos* anus, *algos* pain.]

proctatresia (prok·tat·re·ze·ah). Imperforate anus. [Gk *proktos* anus, atresia.]

proctectasia, proctectasis (prok·tek·**ta**·ze·ah, prok·**tek**·tas·is). A dilated condition of the anus or rectum. [Gk *proktos* anus, ectasia.]

proctectomy (prok·**tek**·to·me). Surgical removal of the rectum. [Gk *proktos* anus, *ektome* excision.]

proctencleisis (prok·ten·**kli**·sis). Proctostenosis. [Gk *proktos* anus, *egkleiein* to shut fast.]

procteurynter (prok·tewr·**in**·ter). A hydrostatic or pneumatic rectal dilator. [Gk *proktos* anus, *eurynein* to widen.]

procteurysis (prok·**tewr**·is·is). Dilatation of the rectum with a procteurynter.

proctitis (prok·**ti**·tis). Inflammation of the rectum. This may be a simple catarrhal inflammation from the irritation of a faecal mass or a foreign body, or due to a specific infection such as amoebic dysentery, syphilis, gonorrhoea, schistosomiasis, etc. **Amoebic proctitis.** Proctitis associated with *Entamoeba histolytica* infection. **Epidemic gangrenous proctitis.** A fatal disease attacking natives of Guyana, Surinam, French Guiana, Venezuela, Fiji and neighbouring countries and islands; it is most frequent in children. It begins as a severe inflammation of the rectum which rapidly spreads, ulcerates and becomes gangrenous. [Gk *proktos* anus, *-itis* inflammation.]

proctocele (**prok**·to·seel). Prolapse of a portion of the rectum. **Vaginal proctocele.** Hernial protrusion of the rectum into the vagina. [Gk *proktos* anus, *kele* hernia.]

proctoclysis (prok·**tok**·lis·is). The method of introducing large quantities of fluid into the rectum by slow injection. [Gk *proktos* anus, *klysis* a drenching.]

proctococcypexy (prok·to·**kok**·se·pex·e). The fixation of the rectum to the coccyx to prevent prolapse. [Gk *proktos* anus, coccyx, Gk *pexis* fixation.]

proctocolitis (**prok**·to·kol·**i**′·tis). Inflammation involving the rectum and part of the colon. [Gk *proktos* anus, colitis.]

proctocolonoscopy (**prok**·to·ko·lon·**os**′·ko·pe). Examination of the interior of the rectum and pelvic colon. [Gk *proktos* anus, colon, Gk *skopein* to watch.]

proctocolpoplasty (prok·to·**kol**·po·plas·te). The closing of a rectovaginal fistula by surgical means. [Gk *proktos* anus, *kolpos* vagina, *plassein* to mould.]

proctocystoplasty (prok·to·**sist**·ɔ·plas·te). An operation on the rectum and bladder in order to close a rectovesical fistula. [Gk *proktos* anus, *kystis* bag, *plassein* to mould.]

proctocystotome (prok·to·**sist**·o·tome). A guarded knife for the incision of the base of the bladder, or of a vesical diverticulum, through a rectal wall (obsolete). [Gk *proktos* anus, *kystis* bladder, *temnein* to cut.]

proctocystotomy (**prok**·to·sist·**ot**′·o·me). The operation of incising the urinary bladder from the rectum in order to remove a stone from the bladder. [see prec.]

proctodaeum (prok·**to**·de·um). The primitive anus, consisting of an ectoderm-lined depression separated from the entodermal cloaca by an anal membrane. It later forms the lower half of the definitive anal canal. [Gk *proktos* anus, *hodaios* concerning a way.]

proctodynia (prok·to·**din**·e·ah). Sensation of pain in the anus and the anal region. [Gk *proktos* anus, *odyne* pain.]

procto-elytroplasty (**prok**·to·el·**it**′·ro·plas·te). Proctocolpoplasty. [Gk *proktos* anus, *elytron* sheath, *plassein* to mould.]

proctogenic (prok·to·**jen**·ik). Developing from the anus or rectum. [Gk *proktos* anus, *genein* to produce.]

proctological (prok·to·**loj**·ik·al). Relating or belonging to proctology.

proctologist (prok·**tol**·o·jist). One who makes a special study of diseases of the anus and rectum and their treatment. [see foll.]

proctology (prok·**tol**·o·je). That branch of medical science which is concerned with the anus and rectum and the diseases to which they are subject. [Gk *proktos* anus, *logos* science.]

proctoparalysis (**prok**·to·par·**al**′·is·is). Paralysis affecting the muscles of the anus and rectum, associated generally with a condition of incontinence. [Gk *proktos* anus, paralysis.]

proctoperineoplasty (**prok**·to·per·in·**e**′·o·plas·te). Reparative surgery of the anus and perineum. [Gk *proktos* anus, perineum, Gk *plassein* to mould.]

proctoperineorrhaphy (**prok**·to·per·in·e·**or**′·af·e). Suture of the anus and perineum. [Gk *proktos* anus, perineum, Gk *rhaphe* suture.]

proctopexy (**prok**·to·pex·e). The operation of suturing the rectum to a neighbouring part. [Gk *proktos* anus, *pexis* fixation.]

proctophobia (prok·to·**fo**·be·ah). A peculiar state of apprehension or fear that affects many sufferers with rectal disease. [Gk *proktos* anus, phobia.]

proctoplasty (**prok**·to·plas·te). A plastic operation on the anus and rectum. [Gk *proktos* anus, *plassein* to mould.]

proctoplegia (prok·to·**ple**·je·ah). Proctoparalysis. [Gk *proktos* anus, *plege* stroke.]

proctopolypus (prok·to·**pol**·e·pus). A polypus of the rectum. [Gk *proktos* anus, polypus.]

proctoptoma (prok·top·**to**·mah). Proctoptosia.

proctoptosia, proctoptosis (prok·top·**to**·se·ah, prok·top·**to**·sis). A prolapsed condition of the anus and rectum. [Gk *proktos* anus, *ptosis* a falling.]

proctorrhagia (prok·to·**ra**·je·ah). Haemorrhage from the rectum. [Gk *proktos* anus, *haima* blood.]

proctorrhaphy (prok·**tor**·af·e). The operation of suturing lacerations of the anus or rectum. [Gk *proktos* anus, *rhaphe* suture.]

proctorrhoea (prok·to·**re**·ah). A discharge of mucus from the anus. [Gk *proktos* anus, *rhoia* flow.]

proctoscope (**prok**·to·scope). A speculum for inspecting the rectum. **Fenestrated proctoscope.** A proctoscope with a slit at one part of its circumference through which a pile mass protrudes for injection. **Slotted proctoscope.** Fenestrated proctoscope (see prec.). **St Mark's proctoscope.** A special proctoscope carrying an electric bulb developed at St Mark's Hospital for Diseases of the Rectum, London. [Gk *proktos* anus, *skopein* to view.]

See also: GABRIEL, TUTTLE.

proctoscopy (prok·**tos**·ko·pe). Examination of the rectum by means of a proctoscope.

proctosigmoidectomy (**prok**·to·sig·moid·**ek**′·to·me). Surgical excision of the rectum together with the pelvic colon. [Gk *proktos* anus, sigmoid, Gk *ektome* excision.]

proctosigmoiditis (**prok**·to·sig·moid·**i**′·tis). Inflammation affecting the rectum and pelvic colon. [Gk *proktos* anus, sigmoid, Gk *-itis* inflammation.]

proctosigmoidoscopy (**prok**·to·sig·moid·**os**′·ko·pe). Inspection of the rectum and pelvic colon with the sigmoidoscope. [Gk *proktos* anus, sigmoid, Gk *skopein* to watch.]

proctospasm (**prok**·to·spazm). Spasmodic contraction of the rectum, sometimes extending to the anus and causing anal tenesmus. [Gk *proktos* anus, spasm.]

proctostasis (prok·**tos**·tas·is). Constipation caused by the lack of power of the rectum to respond to the stimulus causing defaecation. [Gk *proktos* anus, *stasis* a standing still.]

proctostenosis (**prok**·to·sten·**o**′·sis). Stenosis of the anus or rectum. [Gk *proktos* anus, stenosis.]

proctostomy (prok·**tos**·to·me). The operation of establishing a permanent opening into the rectum. [Gk *proktos* anus, *stoma* mouth.]

proctotome (**prok**·to·tome). A proctotomy knife.

proctotomy (prok·**tot**·o·me). The surgical division of a rectal or anal structure, or the opening of an imperforate anus. **External proctotomy.** Division of a stricture of the anus by a cut through skin. **Internal proctotomy.** The blind division of a rectal stricture from within the cavity of the rectum. **Linear proctotomy.** Proctotomy by vertical incisions. [Gk *proktos* anus, *temnein* to cut.]

proctovalvotomy (**prok**·to·val·**vot**′·o·me). Incision of the anal valves. [Gk *proktos* anus, valve, Gk *temnein* to cut.]

procumbent (pro·**kum**·bent). Lying with the face downwards; prone. [L *procumbere* to fall forward.]

procuration (prok·ewr·**a**·shun). In law, broadly to procure or attempt to procure any woman to become a prostitute. It applies equally to procuring a woman to practice prostitution herself or to enter a brothel either in the United Kingdom or abroad. [L *procurare* to take charge of.]

Procurator Fiscal (**prok**·ewr·a·tor **fis**·kal). The Scottish equivalent to the Coroner, responsible for enquiry into sudden deaths of obscure, traumatic or suspicious character.

procursive (pro·**ker**·siv). The type of epilepsy in which the sufferer runs aimlessly just before the first phase of the fit is established. [L *procursus* a running forward.]

procurvation (pro·ker·**va**·shun). The condition of the body, of being inclined or bent forward. [L *procurvare* to bend forward.]

Procyclidine (pro·**si**·klid·een). BP Commission approved name for 1-cyclohexyl-1-phenyl-3-pyrrolidinopropan-1-ol. One of a group of synthetic substances with a peripheral antispasmodic action and other parasympatholytic effects. In high doses it stimulates the central nervous system, and has been suggested for use in parkinsonism. **Procyclidine Hydrochloride BP 1973.** The hydrochloride of procyclidine; it is used in the symptomatic treatment of paralysis agitans.

Procyon lotor (**pro**·se·on **lo**·tor). The racoon, subject to guinea-worm infection in North America.

prodigiosin (**pro**·dij·e·**o**′·sin). $C_{20}H_{25}ON_3$, a red pigment produced by cultures of *Serratia marcescens (Bacillus prodigiosus).*

prodromal (pro·**dro**·mal). Relating or belonging to a prodrome; premonitory, as symptoms.

prodrome (**pro**·drome) (pl. *prodromes*). An early premonitory symptom which is not infrequently of a different nature from the symptoms of the true onset of the disease. [Gk *prodromos* running before.]

prodromic, prodromous (pro·**dro**·mik, pro·**dro**·mus). Prodromal.

product (**prod**·ukt). 1. An effect or result of a natural process. 2. Any substance produced by a chemical reaction, or by a manufacturing process. 3. The result of multiplying two or more numbers together. **Addition product.** Any substance formed by the direct union of two compounds without the elimination of any part. **Cleavage product.** Split product (see below). **Fission products.** The stable and unstable nuclides resulting from fission. **Gene product.** The molecule that is produced as a result of the expression (or transcription) of a gene in a living cell. The *primary* gene product is a ribonucleic acid molecule (usually a messenger RNA). The *secondary* gene product is a specific polypeptide chain. **Reaction product.** Any compound formed by a chemical reaction. **Solubility product.** The product of the concentrations of the respective ions of an electrolyte in saturated solution, i.e. in contact with undissolved electrolyte. This is a constant for any given temperature: if therefore more of one ion is added, some of the other ion will be precipitated, a fact of importance biologically, e.g. in bone formation. **Spallation product.** An isotope formed by bombardment of an element with very-high-energy particles, leading to a complete disintegration of the parent nucleus with formation of a daughter element very different from the parent element in atomic mass and number. **Split product.** Any compound formed by the splitting of another, e.g. by hydrolysis. **Substitution product.** Any compound obtained by substituting other elements or radicals for those in the molecule of the original compound. **Volatility product.** The product of the concentrations of vapours when in equilibrium with their liquids. [L *producere* to produce.]

production rate (pro·**duk**·shun rate). The rate at which a compound, such as a hormone, is produced by its gland or organ of secretion.

productive (pro·**duk**·tiv). Of a lesion, one that forms fresh tissue. [L *producere* to produce.]

proemial (pro·**e**·me·al). Prodromal. [L *prooemium* prelude.]

pro-encephalus (pro·en·**kef**·al·us). A monster a large portion of the brain of which protrudes through a fissure in the frontal area of the skull. [Gk *pro*, *egkephalos* brain.]

pro-erythroblast (pro·er·**ith**·ro·blast). The earliest stage in the development of the erythrocyte, before the erythroblast. [Gk *pro*, erythroblast.]

pro-erythrocyte (pro·er·**ith**·ro·site). Reticulocyte. [Gk *pro*, erythrocyte.]

Proetz, Arthur Walter (b. 1888). St Louis otolaryngologist.

Proetz position. Extreme extension of the head used by Proetz in his replacement treatment of sinus disease.

Proetz test. For olfactory acuity: the sense of smell in each nostril is tested by the application of 10 easily recognizable odorous substances of varying dilutions in bottles constituting an olfactometer. In normal people, the weakest solution of each of the test substances which can be recognized by the sense of smell is known as an olfact, the minimal identifiable or perceptive odour or the coefficient of olfaction.

Proetz treatment. Displacement principle; a method of introducing fluids into the nasal air sinuses through their natural ostia. It is based on the fact that if a liquid is placed near the ostium joining two air-containing cavities one of which is a closed cavity, suction applied to the non-closed cavity will result in air escaping from the closed cavity, its place being taken by the fluid in contact with the ostium.

Profadol (**pro**·fad·ol). BP Commission approved name for 1-methyl-3-propyl-3-(3-hydroxyphenyl)pyrrolidine; an analgesic and antitussive.

professional secrecy (pro·**fesh**·un·al **se**·kre·se). The maintenance of secrecy about matters which come to the knowledge of a medical practitioner through private or confidential communications from patients. In a court of law, this knowledge is not privileged, but no person is bound to answer any question without being ordered to do so by the court; he must first protest. [L *professio* profession, *secretus* secret.]

Profeta, Giuseppe (b. 1840). Genoa dermatologist.

Profeta's immunity. The so-called immunity to syphilis said to be possessed by the healthy children of syphilitic parents.

Profeta's law. The apparently healthy infant born of a syphilitic mother will not become infected by its mother. (These infants have already been infected *in utero* and are in the latent stage of syphilis; their Wassermann reactions are positive.)

profibrinolysin (**pro**·fi·brin·**ol**′·is·in). The inactive precursor of the proteolytic enzyme fibrinolysin, carried in the globulin fraction of the blood. [Gk *pro*, fribrinolysin.]

Profichet, Georges Charles (b. 1873). French physician.

Profichet's syndrome. Calcinosis; the deposition of calcium salts in the skin and subcutaneous tissues.

Proflavine (pro·**fla**·veen). 2,8-Diamino-acridine, $NH_2C_6H_3(CHN)C_6H_3NH_2$. A compound which is an effective germicide against Gram-positive micro-organisms in alkaline media, and at one time used as a trypanocide. It is excreted unchanged in the urine and acts as an effective urinary antiseptic. A 0.1 per cent solution is employed as a germicide for mucous membranes and for washing out wounds; it is also incorporated as an oleate in ointments and emulsions for application to open wounds. It has a weaker antiseptic action than acriflavine, but is more rapid and less toxic. **Proflavine Hemisulphate BP 1968.** Neutral proflavine sulphate, a neutral sulphate of proflavine.

profluvium (pro·**floo**·ve·um). A discharge of ordinary or excessive amount. **Profluvium alvi.** Diarrhoea. **Profluvium lactis.** Flow of milk in excessive quantity. **Profluvium muliebre.** Leucorrhoea. **Profluvium sanguinis.** Haemorrhage. **Profluvium seminis.** 1. Spermatorrhoea. 2. Expulsion of seminal fluid from the vagina after coitus. [L, a flowing forth.]

profondometer (pro·fond·**om**·et·er). An apparatus used for accurately locating foreign bodies or abnormal areas by means of the fluorescent screen: site lines are taken at right angles to each other. [L *profundus* deep, meter.]

profunda (pro·**fun**·dah). Applied to blood vessels that are deeply embedded in the tissues. **Profunda cervicis.** The deep cervical artery. [L *profundus* deep.]

profunda artery of the tongue [arteria profunda linguae (NA)]. *See* LINGUAL ARTERY.

profunda brachii artery [arteria profunda brachii (NA)]. (pro·**fun**·dah **bra**·ke·i ar·ter·e). The main branch of the brachial artery, accompanying the radial nerve to the back of the arm, entering the spiral groove and usually ending by dividing into anterior [arteria collateralis radialis (NA)] and posterior [arteria collateralis media (NA)] descending branches which run in front of and behind the lateral epicondyle to take part in the anastomosis around the elbow. It usually gives off an ascending branch [ramus deltoideus (NA)] which runs up between the long and lateral heads of the triceps, anastomosing with the posterior circumflex humeral artery and supplying the deltoid muscle. **Nutrient branches to the humerus [arteriae nutriciae humeri (NA)].** An occasional branch entering the humerus behind the deltoid tuberosity.

profunda femoris artery [arteria profunda femoris (NA)]. (pro·**fun**·dah **fem**·or·is **ar**·ter·e). A large branch of the femoral artery to the muscles of the thigh.

profunda femoris vein [vena profunda femoris] (pro·**fun**·dah **fem**·or·is vane). A large tributary of the femoral vein, just below the inguinal ligament. It accompanies the correspondingly named artery and drains the thigh muscles.

profunda vein of the tongue [vena profunda linguae (NA)]. The vein draining the tip and deep parts of the tongue joining the sublingual vein to form the vena comitans of the hypoglossal nerve.

progaster (pro·**gas**·ter). The archenteron. [Gk *pro*, *gaster* belly.]

progenesis (pro·**jen**·es·is). The development of germ cells prior to and during fertilization. [Gk *pro*, *genein* to produce.]

progenia (pro·je·ne·ah). Prognathism. [Gk *pro*, *genus* chin.]

progenital, progenitalis (pro·**jen**·it·al, pro·**jen**·it·a′·lis). On the surface of the external genitalia. [L *pro*, genitalia.]

progenitor (pro·**jen**·it·or). Ancestor. [Gk *pro*, *genein* to produce.]

progeny (**proj**·en·e). Offspring. [L *progenies* offspring.]

progeria (pro·je·re·ah). Hutchinson-Gilford syndrome. Premature senility; a rare condition in which the changes of senility occur in childhood. The children are stunted, the sex organs are infantile, the face is old-looking and wizened, the cranial hair is absent or scanty and white, the skin parchment-like, and the arteries atheromatous. It is an endocrine disorder of uncertain pathology. *See* DWARFISM. [Gk *pro*, *geras* old age.]

progestasert (pro·jes·**ta**·sert). A system built on the principle of an intrauterine, T-shaped contraceptive device designed to deliver 65 mg of progesterone regularly each day for a year so that the endometrium is under the influence of 25 mg daily, thus producing a high percentage rate of locally induced contraception for at least 1 year.

progestational (pro·jes·**ta**·shun·al). Denoting the phase in the menstrual cycle which immediately precedes the onset of menstruation, during the functional activity of the corpus luteum and secretory activity of the endometrium. [L *pro*, gestation.]

Progesterone BP 1973 (pro·**jes**·ter·one). A C21 steroid produced by the corpus luteum and the placenta. Luteinizing hormone causes release of progesterone during the luteal phase of the menstrual cycle. It is responsible for the endometrial changes during the secretory or progestational phase of the menstrual cycle, and for the cyclic, cervical and vaginal changes.

Progesteronum (pro·jes·ter·o′·num). *European Pharmacopoeia* name for Progesterone BP 1973.

progestogen (pro·**jes**·to·jen). Any substance having an action identical with that of progesterone.

proglossis (pro·**glos**·is). The tip of the tongue. [Gk *pro*, *glossa* tongue.]

proglottid (pro·**glot**·id). Proglottis.

proglottis (pro·**glot**·is) (pl. *proglottides*). A sexual segment of adult tapeworms. Each proglottis contains a full set of reproductive organs, and when mature is shed from the posterior end of the worm. [Gk *pro*, *glossa* tongue.]

prognathic (prog·**nath**·ik). Prognathous.

prognathism (**prog**·nath·izm). A condition in which there is abnormal projection of one or both jaws. **Alveolosubnasal prognathism.** In craniometry the degree of prognathism calculated by the angle created by the line connecting the alveolocondylean plane and the alveolar and subnasal points. [Gk *pro*, *gnathos* jaw.]

prognathometer (prog·nath·**om**·et·er). An instrument used in determining the type and extent of prognathism. [prognathism, Gk *metron* measure.]

prognathous (prog·**nath**·us). Having a gnathic index of above 103: characterized by prognathism. [Gk *pro*, *gnathos* jaw.]

prognose (prog·**noze**). Prognosticate; to make a prognosis. A slovenly word that is not generally accepted, but is being used with increasing frequency and may in time oust the longer word. [see foll.]

prognosis (prog·**no**·sis). The considered opinion of the probable course and outcome of an illness based upon all the relevant attainable facts of the case. **Prognosis anceps.** An uncertain prognosis. **Prognosis fausta.** A good prognosis. **Prognosis infausta.** An unfavourable prognosis. **Prognosis quoad restitutio ad integrum.** The prognosis as to whether the patient will be restored to normal or be left with damaged organs. **Prognosis quoad vita.** An opinion as to whether the patient will live. [Gk *pro*, *gnosis* knowledge.]

prognostic (prog·**nos**·tik). 1. Relating or belonging to prognosis. 2. Applied to any symptom or sign on which prognosis may be founded.

prognosticate (prog·**nos**·tik·ate). To forecast the course which a disease may take and the outcome that may be expected. [Gk *pro*, *gnosis* knowledge.]

progonism (**pro**·gon·izm). The occurrence of a triad in which the characteristic appearances of kidneys, spleen and appendix at birth are exceptionally well defined.

progonoma (pro·gon·o·mah). A tumour in which lost ancestral characters are revived. [Gk *pro*, *gonos* seed, *-oma* tumour.]

progranulocyte (pro·**gran**·ew·lo·site). Promyelocyte. **Progranulocyte A.** A leucoblast. **Progranulocyte S.** A promyelocyte. [Gk *pro*, granulocyte.]

progression (pro·**gresh**·un). 1. Onward movement. 2. The act of moving forward; the act of walking. **Backward progression.** The act of walking backward peculiar to certain diseases of the nervous system. **Crosslegged progression.** Walking with the toes turned inward and the feet put down one in front of the other. **Metadromic progression.** The ability to run although almost unable to walk noted in persons who have survived an attack of encephalitis lethargica. [L *progredi* to advance.]

progressive (pro·**gres**·iv). 1. Advancing, moving forward. 2. Applied to a condition or to the course of a disease, used particularly in an unfavourable sense. [see prec.]

Proguanil Hydrochloride BP 1973 (pro·**gwan**·il hi·dro·**klor**·ide). Chlorguanide hydrochloride, the hydrochloride of N^1-*p*-chlorophenyl-N^5-isopropyldiguanide, $C_{11}H_{16}N_5ClHCl$. An antimalarial drug that acts on the asexual forms of all plasmodial species producing at least a clinical remission; in adequate dosage it produces a radical cure in *Plasmodium falciparum* infection, and it is a valuable malarial suppressive. It also renders gametocytes non-viable. Its toxicity is very low, and it can be taken in therapeutic doses indefinitely. Its limitation is that its prolonged administration, especially in small doses, is liable to lead to the development of drug resistance in a plasmodial strain, and that there are strains of *Plasmodium falciparum* that apparently enjoy a natural resistance to the drug.

Prohemistomum (**pro**·hem·is·**to**·mum). A genus of trematodes. *Prohemistomum vivax,* known from the intestines of cats and dogs, is said to have occurred in man once.

Proheptazine (pro·**hep**·taz·een). BP Commission approved name for hexahydro-1,3-dimethyl-4-phenylazepin-4-yl propionate; a narcotic analgesic.

prohistiocyte (pro·**his**·te·o·site). The precursor of a histiocyte, a large reticular cell of irregular outline, chromatic nucleus, and eosinophilic cytoplasm. [Gk *pro,* histiocyte.]

pro-insulin (pro·**in**·sew·lin). A single-chain protein precursor of insulin in its biosynthesis which is converted to insulin (containing two chains) by proteolytic enzymes which remove a central peptide (the C or connecting peptide). [Gk *pro,* insulin.]

proiosystole (**pro**·e·o·**sis**'·to·le). A premature contraction of the heart, a type of extrasystole. [Gk *proios* early, systole.]

proiosystolia (**pro**·e·o·sis·**to**'·le·ah). A condition characterized by the occurrence of proiosystoles.

proiotia (pro·e·o·she·ah). Premature development of the sexual organs. [Gk *proios* early.]

projectile (pro·**jek**·tile). Impelling or throwing forward; descriptive of a certain type of vomiting. [L *projectio* a throwing forward.]

projection (pro·**jek**·shun). 1. The throwing of anything in a forward direction. 2. The extension of a part forwards. 3. The reference of a sensation to the object which is considered to arouse it. 4. The process of interpretation of objects and events in the light of the subject's thoughts and experiences, as in projection tests. 5. The ascription of mental processes not recognized to be of personal origin to persons or situations in the outer world. **Eccentric projection.** More commonly called *referred sensation,* that is, one which is felt at a place other than that at which the stimulus is actually applied. **Erroneous projection.** False projection (see foll.). **False projection.** False positioning of an object in space from the image received by an eye with paresis of an external ocular muscle. The object is falsely moved in the direction of the normal action of the paresed muscle. **Projection of light.** A rough test used in opthalmology for the normality of the posterior segment of the eye, when this cannot be seen owing to opacities of the media. The patient points towards a light held in various positions. **Radiographic projection.** A defined position of the patient in relation to the x-ray tube used in diagnostic radiography. [see prec.]

projectoscope (pro·**jek**·to·skope). An apparatus in which reflected light is used to throw pictures on a screen [projection, Gk *skopein* to watch.]

prokaryoblast (pro·**kar**·e·o·blast). Pro-erythroblast. [Gk *pro,* karyoblast.]

prokaryocyte (pro·**kar**·e·o·site). An immature nucleated erythrocyte intermediate between a karyoblast and a karyocyte. [Gk *pro,* karyocyte.]

prokaryote (pro·**kar**·e·ote). An organism whose cells contain no membrane-bound nucleus or other membranous organelles (such as mitochondria, endoplasmic reticulum, Golgi body). Their cells are simpler in structure and smaller than eukaryotic cells. Such cells are characteristic of bacteria, blue-green algae and some other micro-organisms. [Gk *protos* first, Gk *karyon* nut.]

prokaryotic (**pro**·kar·e·**ot**'·ik). Appertaining to the cells of bacteria and a few other unicellular organisms which are characterized by naked DNA (unassociated with protein) as genetic material, no nuclear membrane, and absence of a mitotic or meiotic cycle. [Gk *pro, karyon* nut.]

See also: EUKARYOTIC, GENOPHORE.

prolabium (pro·la·be·um). 1. The exposed carmine margin of the lip. 2. The slight elevation in which the philtrum of the lip terminates; the procheilon. [L *pro, labium* lip.]

prolactin (pro·**lak**·tin). A polypeptide hormone produced by the anterior pituitary and responsible for the stimulation of milk production. **Prolactin-inhibiting hormone, PIH.** A peptide hormone elatorated by the hypothalumus which inhibits the release of prolactin from the pituitary. **Prolactin, PRL.** Regulates luteal function on some species — it is structurally similar to human growth hormone. It may be released by suckling or ACTH. It initiates and maintains lactation in suitably prepared breasts. Excessive production may lead to galactorrhoea in either sex. [L *pro, lac* milk.]

prolamin (**pro**·lam·in). Gliadin; a type of protein occurring in the seeds of cereals. They are insoluble in water, but soluble in aqueous alcohol (50–80 per cent), and are not coagulated by heat. They contain a high proportion of proline, whence the name, and include the gliadin of wheat, zein of maize and hordein of barley.

prolapse (pro·**laps**). The sinking down or protrusion of a part or viscus. **Prolapse of the cord.** Expulsion of the umbilical cord past the presenting part. **Prolapse of the gastric mucosa.** Folds of gastric mucosa prolapsed through the pylorus, which may simulate a peptic ulcer. **Prolapse of the iris.** Extrusion of any part of the iris tissue through a perforating wound of the eyeball following injury, operation or perforating ulcer. **Prolapse of the rectum.** A protrusion of the mucous membrane of the rectum through the anal orifice; it is especially common in infants with diarrhoea. **Urethral prolapse.** Prolapse of urethral mucosa in women, seen in acute form in childhood and old age. **Prolapse of the uterus.** *First degreee:* descent of the cervix uteri to the vaginae introitus. *Second degree:* descent of the cervix uteri outside the introitus vaginae, but part of the uterus still in the vagina. *Third degree:* descent of the whole uterus outside the introitus vaginae. *Complete prolapse or procidentia:* third degree prolapse (see above). **Prolapse of the vagina.** Laxity and descent of the vaginal walls (cystocele, enterocele, rectocele), often associated with uterine prolapse. [L *prolapsus* a falling.]

See also: MORGAGNI.

prolapsus (pro·**laps**·us). Prolapse. **Prolapsus ani.** Anal prolapse. **Prolapsus recti.** Rectal prolapse. **Prolapsus uteri.** Uterine prolapse. [L, a falling.]

prolepsis (pro·**lep**·sis). The recurrence of the paroxysm of a periodical disease at regularly shortening intervals. [Gk *pro, lambanein* to seize.]

proleptic (pro·**lep**·tik). Relating or belonging to prolepsis; anticipating.

proleucocyte (pro·**lew**·ko·site). Leucoblast. [Gk *pro,* leucocyte.]

proleukaemia (pro·lew·**ke**·me·ah). Leuco-erythroblastic anaemia. *See* ANAEMIA. [Gk *pro,* leukaemia.]

proliferate (pro·**lif**·er·ate). To produce by the multiplication of similar cells or parts, and thus to grow; hence proliferating. [L *proles* offspring, *ferre* to bear.]

proliferation (pro·**lif**·er·**a**'·shun). The process of proliferating. **Atrophic proliferation.** The reproduction of cells in atrophic tissues. **Fibroblastic proliferation, Fibroplastic proliferation.** The formation of reparative connective-tissue cells, fibroblasts, during the healing of wounds. [see foll.]

proliferative, proliferous (pro·**lif**·er·a·tiv, pro·**lif**·er·us). Multiplying; reproductive. [L *proles* offspring, *ferre* to bear.]

proligerous (pro·**lij**·er·us). 1. Bearing an ovum or offspring. 2. Germinating. [L *proles* offspring, *gerere* to produce.]

prolinaemia (pro·lin·e·me·ah). Excess of proline, hydroxyproline and glycine in blood and urine, with mild mental retardation. [proline, Gk *haima* blood.]

prolinase (**pro**·lin·aze). An enzyme of the peptidase class occurring in the intestine and other animal tissues and in yeast. It catalyses the breakdown of polypeptides containing proline, to yield proline and simpler polypeptides.

proline (**pro**·leen). α-Pyrrolidine carboxylic acid, an amino acid which occurs as a product of hydrolysis of proteins, and is classed physiologically as a non-essential amino acid. It is found in high concentration in collagen.

Prolintane (pro·**lin**·tane). BP Commission approved name for 1-(α-propylphenethyl)pyrrolidine; it is used as a tonic.

prolinuria (pro·lin·**ewr**·e·ah). Amino-aciduria of proline, hydroxyproline and glycine, due to renal tubular defect. Autosomal recessive.

prolymphocyte (pro·**limf**·o·site). A large immature cell (12–18 μm) intermediate between the lymphoblast and lymphocyte. [Gk *pro*, lymphocyte.]

prolysine (pro·**li**·seen). α-Amino-δ-hydantoin-valeric acid, $C_8H_{13}N_3O_4$. An amino acid which has been isolated from protein hydrolysates.

Promazine (**pro**·maz·een). BP Commission approved name for 10-(3-dimethylaminopropyl)phenothiazine. **Promazine Hydrochloride BP 1973.** The hydrochloride of promazine, a tranquillizing agent used in the treatment of psychotic illnesses; it potentiates the action of analgesics.

promegakaryocyte (**pro**·meg·ah·**kar**′·e·o·site). An immature megakaryocyte, varying in histological appearance according to its stage of maturity, from its formation from the megakaryoblast to its final conversion into the megakaryocyte. [Gk *pro*, megakaryocyte.]

promegaloblast (pro·**meg**·al·o·blast). Erythrogone (Dameshek); a large, early, primitive non-haemoglobinated erythroblast or nucleated red cell (16–27 μm in diameter) having evenly distributed nuclear chromatin with from 3 to 5 nucleoli. There is a proportionally greater amount of cytoplasm (usually basophilic) than in the pronormoblast. It is the cell intermediate between the haemohistioblast, or haemocytoblast, and the basophilic or early megaloblast. It is not normally seen in the circulating blood, but is found in the bone marrow in megaloblastic anaemias. [Gk *pro*, megaloblast.]

promegalokaryocyte (pro·**meg**·al·o·**kar**′·e·o·site). Promegakaryocyte.

prometaphase (pro·**met**·ah·faze). The stage of cell division during which the spindle is formed and the chromosomes move towards the equatorial plate. [Gk *pro*, metaphase.]

Promethazine (pro·**meth**·az·een). BP Commission approved name for *N*-(2-dimethyl-amino-*n*-propyl)-phenothiazine. **Promethazine Hydrochloride BP 1973.** $C_{17}H_{20}N_2SHCl$: a highly active antihistaminic with long-lasting effects, especially useful in urticaria and because it causes drowsiness. **Promethazine Theoclate BP 1973.** The 8-chlorotheophyllinate of promethazine. A useful drug for the treatment of motion sickness, not contra-indicated in pregnancy.

promethium (pro·**me**·the·um). A radioactive element of the rare-earth series, produced by the bombardment of neo- and praseodymium with deuterons, or of uranium with neutrons. It has an atomic number of 61 and chemical symbol Pm. It is very unstable, the most stable isotope being that of mass 145 with a half-life of 30 years. It was originally named *illinium*. [*Prometheus*, who brought fire to Earth.]

Promethoestrol (pro·meth·e·strol). BP Commission approved name for 3,4-di(4-hydroxy-3-methylphenyl)hexane. It has oestrogenic properties similar to those of stilboestrol, and is used to control menopausal symptoms and to suppress lactation. It is used as the dipropionate.

promille (pro·**mil**). The expression of the percentage concentration or proportion, often used for alcohol concentration in mg/100 ml, but also used for weight/weight or volume/volume percentages.

prominence [prominentia (NA)] (**prom**·in·ens). An elevation or projection. **Prominence of the facial nerve canal [prominentia canalis facialis (NA)].** An elevation of the medial wall of the epitympanic recess, above the fenestra vestibuli, produced by the underlying facial canal. **Genital prominence.** The genital eminence of the embryo. **Laryngeal prominence [prominentia laryngea (NA)].** The subcutaneous projection formed by the angle of junction of the two laminae of the thyroid cartilage. **Prominence of the lateral semicircular canal [prominentia canalis semicircularis lateralis (NA)].** A prominence on the medial wall of the epitympanic recess, above and parallel to that caused by the canal for the facial nerve. **Prominence of the malleus [prominentia mallearis (NA)].** An elevation on the tympanic membrane visible on otoscopic examination, and produced by the underlying lateral process of the malleus. **Spiral prominence [prominentia spiralis (NA)].** An elevation in the lateral wall of the duct of the cochlea which forms the lower limit of the stria vascularis. The vas prominens lies beneath it. **Styloid prominence [prominentia styloidea (NA)].** An elevation in the posterior wall of the tympanic cavity produced by the upper end of the styloid process of the temporal bone. [L *prominentia* a jutting out.]

See also: AMMON.

prominentia (prom·in·**en**·she·ah). A prominence. [L, a jutting out.]

promnesia (pro·**ne**·ze·ah). The impression of recalling events that have never taken place. [Gk *pro*, *mnesis* remembrance.]

promonocyte (pro·**mon**·o·site). A large young cell (12–20 μm in diameter) with fewer neutral red bodies than a monocyte, and intermediate between the monoblast and monocyte. [Gk *pro*, monocyte.]

promontory [promontorium (NA)] (**prom**·on·tor·e). A projection. **Double promontory.** An anomalous condition in which the second sacral segment is angulated backwards so that the upper border of its body forms a second or *false promontory*. **Promontory of the sacrum [promontorium (NA)].** The prominent anterior border of the upper surface of the first sacral segment. **Promontory of the tympanic cavity [promontorium (NA)].** An elevation on the medial wall of the tympanic cavity produced by the first coil of the cochlea. [L *promontorium* headland.]

See also: TERRIER.

promoter (pro·**mo**·ter). 1. That portion of the operator gene which is responsible for the binding of the repressor protein. 2. Any substance which, though possessing no catalytic properties itself, assists the activity of catalysts in specific reactions. [L *promovere* to move forward.]

Promoxolan (pro·**mox**·o·lan). BP Commission approved name for 4-hydroxymethyl-2,2-di-isopropyl-1,3-dioxolan; a sedative.

promyeloblast (pro·**mi**·el·o·blast). Premyeloblast.

promyelocyte (pro·**mi**·el·o·site). The most primitive or earliest undifferentiated granular white cell of the granulocytic leucocytes, normally only seen in the bone marrow, but appearing in the blood in certain leukaemias. [Gk *pro*, myelocyte.]

pronaeus (pro·**ne**·us). The vagina, or the vestibule of the vagina. [Gk *pronaios* the court before a temple.]

pronate (**pro**·nate). 1. To place in a prone position. 2. Lying prone. 3. With reference to the hand and forearm, to carry out the action of pronation. [L *pronare* to bend forward.]

pronation (pro·**na**·shun). The movement by which the hand is rotated, normally through 180 degrees, from a position in which the palm is facing directly upward to one where it is facing directly downward. **Pure pronation.** Pronation when the elbow is flexed to 90 degrees [see prec.]

pronatoflexor (pro·**na**·to·**flex**′·or). Pertaining to the pronator and flexor muscles.

pronator (pro·**na**·tor). A muscle producing the movement of pronation, i.e. rotating the forearm so that the palm of the hand faces downwards. [L *pronare* to bend forward.]

pronator quadratus muscle [musculus pronator quadratus (NA)]. (pro·**na**·tor kwod·**ra**·tus musl). A deep muscle on the front of the forearm, lying across and attached to the lower fifth of the radius and ulna. It pronates the forearm and hand.

pronator teres muscle [musculus pronator teres (NA)] (pro·**na**·tor **ter**·eez musl). The most radially placed of the superficial forearm muscles. It arises from the medial epicondyle [caput humerale (NA)] and coronoid process of the ulna [caput ulnare (NA)] and is inserted into the lateral side of the middle of the shaft of the radius. It pronates the forearm and hand.

pronaus (pro·**na**·us). Pronaeus.

prone (prone). 1. Lying flat with the face downward. 2. Of the hand, when rotated so that the palm faces downward. [L *pronus* stooping forward.]

pronephric (pro·**nef**·rik). Pertaining to the pronephros.

pronephron (pro·**nef**·ron). A tubule of the pronephros.

pronephros (pro·**nef**·ros). The first type of kidney to appear both in phylogenesis and ontogenesis. It remains the permanent kidney of the most primitive vertebrates, but is replaced by a mesonephros in fish and amphibia and by a metanephros in birds, reptiles and mammals. It consists of segmental tubules each associated with a glomerulus at its medial end and opening laterally into a longitudinally running pronephric duct. [Gk *pro*, *nephros* kidney.]

Pronethalol (pro·**neth**·al·ol). BP Commission approved name for 2-isopropylamino-1-(2-naphthyl)ethanol; an adrenaline antagonist.

prong (prong). A colloquial term applied to the root of a tooth. [etym. dub.]

pronograde (pro·no·grade). Denoting the posture of those animals which stand or move with their bodies in a horizontal posture. [L *pronus* stooping forward, *gradi* to walk.]

pronometer (pro·**nom**·et·er). An instrument for measuring rotation of the forearm. [pronation, meter.]

pronormoblast (pro·**nor**·mo·blast). The intermediate precursor of the normoblast in the maturation of the red cell in the bone marrow. [Gk *pro*, normoblast.]

prontosil (**pron**·to·sil). 2,4-Diaminoazobenzene-4′-sulphonamide, $(NH_2)_2C_6H_3NNC_6H_4SO_2NH_2$. The first sulphonamide, now only of historical interest, originally prepared by Domagk. It has been replaced in medical practice by the more effective and often more readily accessible sulphonamides such as sulphanilamide, sulphathiazole, sulphacetamide, sulphadiazine, etc.

pronucleus (pro·**new**·kle·us). In embryology, either of the two nuclei after maturation of the ovum but before fusion occurs and the cleavage nucleus is formed. **Female pronucleus.** The nucleus of the ovum. **Male pronucleus.** The nucleus of the spermatozoon. [Gk *pro*, nucleus.]

pro-otic (pro·**o**·tik). Occurring in front of the internal ear (periotic capsule). [Gk *pro*, *ous* ear.]

pro-ovarium (pro·o·**va**·re·um). The epoöphoron; a rudimentary structure situated between the ovary and the uterine tube. It consists of several short tubules which, with the paroöphoron, are all that remains of the mesonephros. [Gk *pro*, ovary.]

prop (prop). A support. **Dental prop.** Mouth prop, a device for separating the teeth and propping open the mouth. [etym. dub.]

propagation (prop·ag·**a**·shun). Multiplication; increasing or causing to increase. [L *propagare* to generate.]

propalinal (pro·**pal**·in·al). Having a forward and backward movement. [Gk *pro*, *palin* back.]

Propamidine (pro·**pam**·id·een). BP Commission approved name for one of a series of amidines used mainly as a bacteriostatic in burns and wounds, being effective against staphylococci, streptococci and clostridia. It is usually administered in the form of the isethionate.

propancreatitis (pro·pan·kre·at·**i**′·tis). Acute suppurative pancreatitis. [Gk *pro*, pancreatitis.]

propandiolal (pro·pan·**di**·ol·al). Glyceraldehyde.

propandiolone (pro·pan·**di**·ol·one). Dihydroxyacetone.

propane (**pro**·pane). C_3H_8, a gaseous hydrocarbon, third in the methane series, which is found in the natural gas of oil wells. It is used as a refrigerant.

Propanidid BP 1973 (pro·**pan**·e·did). Propyl 4-diethylcarbamoylmethoxy-3-methoxyphenylacetate, a very short-acting anaesthetic injected intravenously. Induction is rapid and general anaesthesia lasts for about 5 minutes.

propanol (**pro**·pan·ol). Propyl alcohol. *See* ALCOHOL.

Propantheline Bromide BP 1973 (pro·**pan**·thel·een **bro**·mide). β-Di-isopropylaminoethylxanthene-9-carboxylate methobromide; an anticholinergic for the treatment of gastritis, peptic ulcer, hyperhidrosis and hyperemesis gravidarum.

propargyl (pro·**par**·jil). Propinyl, protyl. The radical $CH{\equiv}CCH_2-$ which is derived from propargyl alcohol: so called because of the compound it forms with silver. [Gk *protos* first, *argyros* silver.]

Propatylnitrate (pro·pat·il·**ni**′·trate). BP Commission approved name for 1,1,1-trisnitratomethylpropane; a coronary vasodilator.

propene (**pro**·peen). Propylene, CH_3CHCH_2. An unsaturated olefine hydrocarbon gas formed as a by-product in the cracking of high molecular weight petroleum hydrocarbons for petrol fractions. It has been used as an inhalant anaesthetic, mainly in the USA, but safer and more potent gaseous anaesthetics have displaced it.

propenol (**pro**·pen·ol). Allyl alcohol. *See* ALCOHOL.

propenyl (**pro**·pen·il). 1. The monovalent group, $CH_3{=}CH{=}CH-$, from propylene. 2. Glyceryl, $C_3H_5{\equiv}$, the trivalent radical of glycerin.

propeptone (pro·**pep**·tone). Hemialbumose.

propeptonuria (pro·pep·ton·**ewr**′·re·ah). Hemialbumosuria; a condition in which propeptone (hemialbumose) is present in the urine.

properdin (pro·**per**·din). A term, originally coined by Pillemer, for a protein component of a system responsible for the non-specific killing of Gram-negative bacteria and neutralization of viruses, and now confirmed as β-globulin which acts in conjunction with complement and magnesium ions in the lysis of Gram-negative bacteria.

Properidine (pro·**per**·id·een). BP Commission approved name for isopropyl 1-methyl-4-phenylpiperidine-4-carboxylate; a narcotic analgesic.

properitoneal (pro·per·e·ton·**e**′·al). 1. Occurring between the parietal portion of the peritoneum and the abdominal wall, as a hernia. 2. Occurring in front of the peritoneum. [Gk *pro*, peritoneum.]

prophage (**pro**·faje). The inert form in which the genetic material of temperate bacteriophage is propagated by lysogenic bacteria. [Gk *pro*, *phagein* to eat.]

prophase (**pro**·faze). The first stage in mitosis in which the chomosomes become visible as long, thin, double threads. [Gk *pro*, *phasis* appearance.]

prophenpyridamine (pro·fen·pir·**id**′·am·een). $C_6H_5CH(C_5H_4N)CH_2CH_2N(CH_3)_2$, a synthetic antihistaminic.

Prophlebotomus (pro·fleb·**ot**·om·us). A subgenus of *Phlebotomus*. [Gk *pro*, *Phlebotomus*.]

prophylactic (pro·fil·**ak**·tik). 1. Pertaining to the prevention of the development of disease. 2. A preventive agent or remedy used to ward off an infection. **Scarlet Fever Prophylactic BP 1963.** A sterile filtrate or a culture of *Streptococcus pyogenes* for immunizing against scarlet fever. It is injected intracutaneously or subcutaneously in increasing doses at weekly intervals. *See* ANTITOXIN, SERUM, TOXOID and VACCINE, all of which are used as prophylactics. [Gk *prophylax* advance guard.]

See also: HAFFKINE.

prophylaxis (pro·fil·**ax**·is). 1. The art of preventing disease. 2. Preventive treatment. 3. In dentistry, the science and practice of using measures to prevent the onset of diseases of the teeth and neighbouring soft tissues: *oral prophylaxis; dental prophylaxis.* **Causal prophylaxis.** Eradication of the causal factor of the disease. **Chemical prophylaxis.** Prevention by chemical means, by the use of chemical antiseptics. **Clinical prophylaxis.** The prevention of the development of signs and symptoms of the disease without necessarily eradicating the causal factor, e.g. in malaria, by schizonticidal drugs. **Collective prophylaxis.** The guarding of the public from disease. **Drug prophylaxis.** The administration of drugs as protection against infection, in particular malarial infection. **Gametocidal prophylaxis.** The administration of drugs in order to kill malarial gametocytes in individuals. **Individual prophylaxis.** The guarding of an individual against disease by measures that will protect him alone, e.g. vaccination. **Mechanical prophylaxis.** Prevention by mechanical means, by protecting the part from the source of infection, e.g. by gloves or condom. **Serum prophylaxis.** Prophylaxis afforded by the administration of immune serum. **Suppressive prophylaxis.** Drug prophylaxis in malaria which prevents the development of clinical symptoms but does not necessarily eradicate the infection. [see prec.]

Propicillin (pro·pe·**sil**·in). BP Commission approved name for 6-(α-phenoxybutyramido)penicillanic acid. **Propicillin Potassium**

BP 1973. A mixture of the potassium salts of propicillin; an antibiotic with uses similar to those of phenoxymethylpenicillin but it is less readily inactivated by penicillinase.

propinyl (pro·pin·il). Propargyl.

Propiolactone (pro·pe·o·lak′·tone). BP Commission approved name for *β*-propiolactone; an antiseptic substance which may be used as the inactivating agent in the preparation of certain bacterial and viral vaccines.

Propiomazine (pro·pe·o·maz·een). BP Commission approved name for 10-(2-dimethylaminopropyl)-2-propionyl-phenothiazine; a hypnotic.

propionate (pro·pe·on·ate). Any salt or ester of propionic acid.

Propionibacterium (pro·pe·on·e·bak·teer′·e·um). A genus of the family Lactobacteriaceae. The micro-organisms that constitute this genus consist of Gram-positive, non-motile, non-sporing rods, anaerobic or micro-aerophilic, which ferment carbohydrates with the production of propionic and acetic acids and carbon dioxide. They are found in dairy products, especially in hard cheeses, and are non-pathogenic. **Propionibacterium acnes.** An organism which is resident on the skin, particularly in sebaceous follicles. It is likely that in the obstructed follicles of acne vulgaris it plays an aggravating role. [Gk *pro, pion* fat, bacterium.]

Propiram Fumarate (pro·pir·am few·mar·ate). BP Commission approved name for *N*-(1-methyl-2-piperidinoethyl-*N*-(2-pyridyl)-propionamide fumarate; an analgesic.

proplasmacyte (pro·plaz·mah·site). A Tuerk cell. [Gk *pro,* plasmacyte.]

propolycyte (pro·pol·e·site). A young polycyte. [Gk *pro,* polycyte.]

propositus (pro·pos·it·us). Proband. [L *pro, ponere* to place.]

propoxyphene (pro·pox·e·feen). Dextropropoxyphene, 4-dimethylamino-1,2-diphenyl-3-methyl-2-propionyl-oxybutane; an analgesic.

Propranolol (pro·pran·o·lol). BP Commission approved name for (±)-1-isopropylamino-3-(1-naphthyloxy)propan-2-ol. **Propranolol Hydrochloride BP 1973.** The hydrochloride of propranolol, a specific blocker acting on *β*-receptors and used to abolish cardiac arrhythmias due to heart disease, digitalis or anaesthetics.

proprioceptive (pro·pre·o·sep′·tiv). Pertaining to those sensory impulses arising mainly in the joints, tendons and muscles. [L *proprius* one's own, *capere* to take.]

proprioceptor (pro·pre·o·sep′·tor). Any termination of a sensory nerve which is to be found, for example, in muscles, joints, tendons. [see prec.]

propriospinal (pro·pre·o·spi′·nal). Relating exclusively to the spine or spinal cord. [L *proprius* one's own, spine.]

proprius (pro·pre·us). Exclusive; individual; applied to certain muscles. [L, one's own.]

proptometer (prop·tom·et·er). An apparatus for measuring proptosis.

See also: MUTCH.

proptosis (prop·to·sis). Forward displacement of the eyeball. In some cases the eyeball comes straight forward; in others, the displacement is combined with a lateral, vertical or oblique component. [Gk *pro, ptosis* a falling.]

propulsion (pro·pul·shun). 1. The process of driving or pushing forward. 2. Displacement of the centre of gravity caused by stumbling on uneven ground or being pushed, causing the patient to lean or fall forward; a tendency noted in those suffering from paralysis agitans and other nervous disorders. 3. Festination. [L *propellere* to drive forward.]

propyl (pro·pil). The organic radical, $CH_3CH_2CH_2$–, which is derived from normal propyl alcohol. **Propyl docetrizoate.** BP Commission approved name for propyl 3-diacetylamino-2,4,6-tri-iodobenzoate; it is used in bronchography. **Propyl Gallate BP 1973.** 3,4,5-Trihydroxybenzoate; it is an anti-oxidant in fats and fixed oils. **Propyl Hydroxybenzoate BP 1973.** $HOC_6H_4COOC_3H_7$, the normal propyl ester of *p*-hydroxybenzoic acid, used as a bacteriostatic and fungistatic in pharmaceutical preparations. It is also useful as an anti-oxidant in fats and oils.

propylamine (pro·pil·am·een). An aliphatic amine with ammoniacal odour. It occurs in two isomeric forms, normal propylamine, $CH_3CH_2CH_2NH_2$, and isopropylamine, $CH_3CHNH_2CH_3$. Derivatives of the latter are used as sympathomimetic drugs, e.g. ephedrine, amphetamine, etc.

propylene (pro·pil·een). 1. The divalent radical, $-CH(CH_3)CH_2=CH_2CH_2CH_2-$. 2. Propene, methylethylene, CH_3CHCH_2, of the olefine series; an unsaturated hydrocarbon gas formed as a by-product in the cracking of high molecular weight petroleum hydrocarbons for petrol fractions. It has been used as an inhalant anaesthetic, mainly in the USA, but safer and more potent gaseous anaesthetics have displaced it. **Propylene Glycol BP 1973.** $CH_3CHOHCH_2OH$, a solvent finding increasing use in the extraction and presentation of drugs. It has been used to replace glycerin as a solvent, as solutions are less viscous and the solvent itself will inhibit the growth of fungi and micro-organisms as efficiently as ethyl alcohol.

Propylhexedrine (pro·pil·hex·ed·reen). BP Commission approved name for 1-cyclohexyl-2-methylaminopropane. It is a volatile sympathomimetic, having a similar action to that of amphetamine; it is used for the relief of nasal congestion.

Propyliodone BP 1973 (pro·pil·i·o·done). The *n*-propyl ester of 3,5-di-iodo-4-pyridone-*N*-acetic acid. Prepared as a 50 per cent w/v suspension in water, which has an iodine content of about 30 per cent, it is a radiographic agent of special advantage in bronchography. It is isotonic with body fluids, is less irritant than other aqueous contrast media, is less likely to produce alveolar filling, and provides well-defined shadows persisting for at least 30 minutes. It is rapidly absorbed, and eliminated via the urine in a few days. It is used in the diagnosis of bronchiectasis, to investigate conditions such as bronchogenic carcinoma and lung tumours, cysts and abcesses, also in certain cases of tuberculosis. It is administered by the usual routes used in bronchography; intubation by the cricothyroid routes is preferred.

propylparaben (pro·pil·par·ah·ben). Propyl hydroxybenzoate.

Propylthiouracil BP 1973 (pro·pil·thi·o·ewr′·as·il). $C_7H_{10}ON_2S$, an antithyroid drug of the thiouracil type. It is more active and less toxic than the parent compound.

propyphenazone (pro·pe·fen·az·one). BP Commission approved name for 4-isopropyl-2,3-dimethyl-1-phenyl-5-pyrazolone; an analgesic.

proquamezine (pro·kwam·ez·een). BP Commission approved name for 10-(2,3-bisdimethylaminopropyl)phenothiazine; a spasmolytic.

prorrhaphy (pro·raf·e). Advancement; the operation of detaching at the point of its insertion a muscle or tendon and reattaching it at a point farther forward; in the case of muscles this procedure is carried out in order to correct the action of the muscle, e.g. in squint, or uterine retroversion. [Gk *pro, rhaphe* suture.]

prorubriblast (pro·roo·bre·blast). Pro-erythroblast. [Gk *pro,* rubriblast.]

Proscillaridin (pro·sil·ar·id·in). BP Commission approved name for 3*β*,14*β*-dihydroxybufa-4,20,22-trienolide 3-rhamnoside; a cardiac glycoside.

proscolex (pro·sko·lex). A larval form of tapeworm; the oncosphere within its membranous envelope. [Gk *pro, skolex* worm.]

prosecretin (pro·se·kre·tin). Said to be the precursor of secretin, and contained in epithelial cells. [L *pro,* secretin.]

prosect (pro·sekt). To dissect a cadaver or any part of it for the purpose of anatomical demonstration. [L *prosecare* to cut off.]

prosector (pro·sek·tor). One who dissects anatomical subjects for demonstration purposes. [see prec.]

prosectorium (pro·sek·tor·e·um). Dissecting-room or room in which anatomical specimens are prepared. [L *prosecare* to cut off.]

prosencephalon (pros·en·kef·al·on). The forebrain. [Gk *pro, egkephalos* brain.]

Proskauer, Bernhard (b. 1851). Berlin hygienist.

Voges-Proskauer reaction. A reaction involving the production of acetyl methyl carbinol by the typhoid group, and not by the coliform group. A culture of the organism in glucose broth is made alkaline with potassium hydroxide; a red colour slowly develops when positive.

proso (**pro**·so). A table cereal prepared from a variety of Russian millet.

prosodemes (pros·o·**dem**·ez). A variation of a phoneme due to quality of tone and pitch.

prosodemic (pros·o·**dem**·ik). Used of contact infection, the passage of disease from one individual to another; an outbreak of disease arising in this way. [Gk *proso* forward, *demos* people.]

prosodic (**pros**·od·ik). Chromatic accent, or melody of speech. **Prosodic units.** Prosodemes.

prosody (**pros**·od·ah). The fluctuations in pitch and tempo of articulated speech.

prosopagnosia (**pros**·o·pag·**no**′·se·ah). A variety of visual agnosia in which the patient is unable to recognize faces or even his own reflection in a mirror. [Gk *prosopon* face, agnosia.]

prosopagus (pros·**op**·ag·us). A twin monster of which the tumour-like mass which constitutes the parasite is attached to the cheek or the orbit of the autosite. [Gk *prosopon* face, *pagos* fixed.]

prosopalgia (pros·o·**pal**·je·ah). Trigeminal neuralgia; tic douloureux. [Gk *prosopon* face, *algos* pain.]

prosopalgic (pros·o·**pal**·jik). Pertaining to or affected with trigeminal neuralgia. [see prec.]

prosopantritis (**pros**·o·pan·**tri**′·tis). Inflammation affecting one or both frontal sinuses. [Gk *prosopon* face, *antron* cave, *-itis* inflammation.]

prosopantrum (pros·o·**pan**·trum). A frontal sinus. [Gk *prosopon* face, *antron* cave.]

prosopic (pro·**so**·pik). Facial. [Gk *prosopon* face.]

prosoplasia (pros·o·**pla**·ze·ah). 1. Differentiation beyond the physiological limits of the cells forming certain tissues. 2. The process of growth of cells or other tissue so that they become possessed of higher functions. [Gk *pros* in addition to, *plassein* to form.]

prosopoanoschisis (**pros**·o·po·an·**os**′·kis·is). Oblique facial cleft. [Gk *prosopon* face, *ano*, *schisis* a splitting.]

prosopodiaschisis (**pros**·o·po·di·**as**′·kis·is). An elaborate operation in the evisceration of the nasal sinuses. [Gk *prosopon* face, *dia*, *schisis* a splitting.]

prosopodiplegia (**pros**·o·po·di·**ple**′·je·ah). Paralysis of the face and both lower limbs. [Gk *prosopon* face, *di-*, *plege* stroke.]

prosopodynia (**pros**·o·po·**din**′·e·ah). Sensation of pain in the face. [Gk *prosopon* face, *odyne* pain.]

prosopodysmorphia (**pros**·o·po·dis·**mor**′·fe·ah). Hemiatrophy of the face. [Gk *prosopon* face, *dys*, *morphe* form.]

prosopolepsy (**pros**·o·po·**lep**′·se). Estimation of the character of an individual based on facial expression and features. [Gk *prosopon* face, *lambanein* to take.]

prosoponeuralgia (**pros**·o·po·newr·**al**′·je·ah). Neuralgic pain affecting the face; trigeminal neuralgia. [Gk *prosopon* face, neuralgia.]

prosopopagus (pros·o·**pop**·ag·us). Conjoined twins with the parasitic twin attachment to the facial region. [Gk *prosopon* face, *pagos* fixed.]

prosopopilar, prosopopilary (**pros**·o·po·**pi**′·lar, **pros**·o·po·**pi**′·lar·e). Characterized by a heavy growth of hair on the face. [Gk *prosopon* face, L *pilus* hair.]

prosopoplegia (**pros**·o·po·**ple**′·je·ah). Paralysis of the facial nerve; Bell's palsy. [Gk *prosopon* face, *plege* stroke.]

prosopoplegic (**pros**·o·po·**ple**′·jik). Relating or belonging to or suffering from prosopoplegia. [see prec.]

prosoposchisis (pros·o·**pos**·kis·is). Any facial fissure of congenital origin, e.g. hare-lip. [Gk *prosopon* face, *schisis* a splitting.]

prosoposcopy (pros·o·**pos**·ko·pe). Examination of the face, and in particular studying the alterations in features and expression caused by certain diseases. [Gk *prosopon* face, *skopein* to watch.]

prosopospasm (pros·**o**·po·spazm). Spasm of the facial muscles, e.g. in tetanus. [Gk *prosopon* face, spasm.]

prosoposternodymia (**pros**·o·po·ster·no·**dim**′·e·ah). A type of teratism in which the twin fetuses are joined together at the face and sternum. [Gk *prosopon* face, sternum, Gk *didymos* twin.]

prosopothoracopagus (**pros**·o·po·thor·ah·**kop**′·ag·us). A double monster in which the fetuses are attached to each other by the thorax, neck and face. [Gk *prosopon* face, thorax, Gk *pagos* fixed.]

prosopotocia (**pros**·o·po·**to**′·se·ah). Face presentation in childbirth. [Gk *prosopon* face, *tokos* birth.]

prosopus varus (**pros**·o·pus **va**·rus). Congenital oblique facial deformity due to hemiatrophy of the head. [Gk *prosopon* face, L *varus* crooked.]

prososthenia quadrasi (pros·os·**the**·ne·ah **kwad**·ra·si). *Oncomelania quadrasi.*

prosostomata (pros·o·**sto**·mat·ah). Prostomata.

prospermia (pro·**sper**·me·ah). Premature ejaculation of semen. [Gk *pro*, sperm.]

prostaglandins (pros·tah·**glan**·dinz). A series of fatty acids found in many body tissues, especially in semen, lungs and brain. A tissue extract prepared from the prostate gland. There are three main groups — PGA, PGE and PGF — distinguished by the configuration of the ring. They have a wide variety of actions, including cardiovascular and gastric effects, dilatation of the bronchi, and metabolic actions. They cause uterine contractions and may be responsible for some of the local effects of inflammation. They are produced by the testis as well as by androgen. Both are increased under the influence of gonadotrophin, and prostaglandin synthesis is maintained by adrenocortical activity.

prostatalgia (pros·tat·**al**·je·ah). Pain involving the prostate gland. [prostate gland, Gk *algos* pain.]

prostatauxe (pros·tat·**awx**·e). Hypertrophy of the prostate gland; prostatic enlargement. [prostate gland, Gk *auxe* increase.]

prostate [prostata (NA)] (**pros**·tate). A gland, confined to the male, which surrounds and is continuous with the neck of the bladder. It may be divided into a median and two lateral lobes, and consists of muscular [substantia muscularis (NA)] and glandular [substantia glandularis] tissue. It is traversed by the first part of the urethra and the ejaculatory ducts. **Apex of the prostate [apex prostatae (NA)].** The inferior aspect of the gland in contact with the fascia covering the sphincter urethrae muscle. **Base of the prostate [basis prostatae (NA)].** The superior surface of the gland in contact with the neck of the urinary bladder. The urethra traverses it nearer its anterior border than the posterior. **Funnel-neck prostate.** A dilatation of the proximal urethra due to relaxation of the internal sphincter, so that the posterior urethra becomes cone-shaped, the base of the cone directed towards the bladder and the apex to the triangular ligament. The condition is seen cystoscopically in cases of spinal syphilis and certain other diseases of the central nervous system. It may be demonstrated by the cysto-urethrogram. **Lobe of the prostate, median [lobus medius (NA)].** The small portion, sometimes devoid of glandular tissue, between the urethra and ejaculatory ducts. **Lobe of the prostate, right and left [lobus (dexter et sinister) (NA)].** The main portion of the gland on either side of the midline below the ejaculatory ducts. **Surface of the prostate, anterior [facies anterior) (NA)].** A narrow surface between base and apex, separated from the lower part of the pubic symphysis by a plexus of veins and fat. The urethra emerges from it near the apex. **Surface of the prostate, inferolateral (right and left) [facies inferolateralis (NA)].** Convex surfaces separated from the superior surfaces of the levator ani muscle by a plexus of veins embedded in the fibrous tissue capsule of the organ. **Surface of the prostate, posterior [facies posterior (NA)].** A triangular surface between the base and apex, separated from the ampulla of the rectum by connective tissue. Near the upper border the ejaculatory ducts enter at a depression, below which the surface is partially divided by a vertical median groove. [Gk *prostates* one standing before.]

prostatectomy (pros·tat·**ek**·to·me). Excision of a part or of the whole of the prostate gland. **Perineal prostatectomy.** Removal of the prostate by the perineal route. **Retropubic prevesical**

prostatectomy. Removal of the prostate through a suprapubic abdominal incision and by incising the capsule of the prostate to expose the adenoma. The bladder wall is not incised. **Suprapubic transvesical prostatectomy.** Removal of the prostate by an abdominal suprapubic incision and by enucleating the prostate transvesically. **Transurethral prostatectomy.** Transurethral resection. *See* RESECTION. [prostate gland, Gk *ektome* a cutting out.]

prostathelcosis (pros·tat·hel·**ko**′·sis). Ulceration of the prostate gland. [prostate gland, Gk *helkosis* ulceration.]

prostatic (pros·**tat**·ik). Relating or belonging to the prostate gland.

prostaticovesical (pros·**tat**·ik·o·**ves**′·ik·al). Relating to the prostate gland and the urinary bladder. [prostate gland, vesicle.]

prostatism (**pros**·tat·izm). The abnormal mental and physical condition associated with disease of the prostate gland, and in particular that state which is consequent upon urinary obstruction caused by enlargement of the gland. **Vesical prostatism.** Urinary retention similar to that existing in disease of the prostate gland but occurring without any other evidence of prostatic disorder.

prostatitic (pros·tat·**it**·ik). Relating to or affected with prostatitis.

prostatitis (pros·tat·**i**·tis). Any inflammatory condition of the prostate gland. [prostate gland, Gk *-itis* inflammation.]

prostatocystitis (**pros**·tat·o·sist·**i**′·tis). Inflammation affecting the prostatic part of the urethra, with spread to the urinary bladder. [prostate gland, cystitis.]

prostatocystotomy (**pros**·tat·o·sist·**ot**′·o·me). An incision made through the prostate and the bladder by perineal or retropubic dissection. [prostate gland, Gk *kystis* bladder, *temnein* to cut.]

prostatodynia (**pros**·tat·o·**din**′·e·ah). Painful condition of the prostate gland. [prostate gland, Gk *odyne* pain.]

prostatography (pros·tat·**og**·raf·e). Radiography of the prostate gland. [prostate gland, Gk *graphein* to record.]

prostatolith (pros·**tat**·o·lith). A prostatic calculus. [prostate gland, Gk *lithos* stone.]

prostatolithotomy (**pros**·tat·o·lith·**ot**′·o·me). The operation of incising the prostate gland in order to remove a calculus. [prostatolith, Gk *temnein* to cut.]

prostatomegaly (**pros**·tat·o·**meg**′·a·le). Enlargement of the prostate gland. [prostate gland, *megas* great.]

prostatometer (pros·tat·**om**·et·er). An instrument for gauging the size of the enlarged prostate (obsolete). [prostate gland, meter.]

prostatomy (pros·**tat**·o·me). Prostatotomy.

prostatomyomectomy (**pros**·tat·o·mi·o·**mek**′·to·me). Excision of a myoma in the prostate gland. [prostate gland, myomectomy.]

prostatoncus (pros·tat·**ong**·kus). A prostatic tumour. [prostate gland, Gk *ogkos* a swelling.]

prostatorrhoea (**pros**·tat·o·**re**′·ah). A gonorrhoeal or catarrhal exudation from the prostate gland. [prostate gland, Gk *rhoia* flow.]

prostatotomy (pros·tat·**ot**·o·me). The operation of incising the prostate gland. [prostate gland, Gk *temnein* to cut.]

prostatovesiculectomy (**pros**·tat·o·ves·ik·ew·**lek**′·to·me). Surgical removal of the prostate gland and the seminal vesicles. [prostate gland, vesicle, Gk *ektome* a cutting out.]

prostatovesiculitis (**pros**·tat·o·ves·ik·ew·**li**′·tis). An inflammatory condition in which there is involvement of the prostate gland and the seminal vesicles. [prostate gland, vesicle, Gk *-itis* inflammation.]

prosternation (pro·ster·**na**·shun). A hysterical condition in which the back is habitually inclined forwards although the spine remains flexible; there is always compensatory extension of the head. [L *prosternare* to throw down in front.]

prosthesis (**pros**·the·sis). 1. An artificial part, e.g. a leg or arm. 2. Artificial restoration of some part which has been lost. **Acrylic prosthesis.** A portion of inert acrylic material suitably fashioned and introduced into the tissues to make good a deficiency, usually in the skeleton. **Cosmetic prosthesis.** Prosthesis undertaken to make appearance more acceptable. **Dental prosthesis.** A fixed or removable appliance to replace lost teeth. **Functional prosthesis.** Prosthesis undertaken to provide or supplement useful activity. **Maxillofacial prosthesis.** An artificial restoration of the contour of the face and jaw by means of an appliance, following injury or surgery. **Ocular prosthesis.** Artificial eye. **Paraffin prosthesis.** Remoulding of a part by the subcutaneous injection of paraffin. **Total joint prosthesis.** A prosthetic replacement of a joint where both joint surfaces are replaced by artificial components. **Valve prosthesis.** A mechanical substitute for a diseased cardiac valve, used for aortic and mitral valve replacement. [Gk, addition.]

See also: GERSUNY, JUDET, SAUERBRUCH, VANGHETTI.

prosthetic (pros·**thet**·ik). Relating to prosthesis or to prosthetics.

prosthetics (pros·**thet**·ix). That section of surgical science which deals with the replacement of an absent limb, part or organ by an artificial one. **Dental prosthetics.** The science and practice of replacing teeth and adjacent hard and soft tissues which have been lost, by an artificial substitute. [Gk *prosthesis* addition.]

prosthion (**pros**·the·on). The lowest point on the alveolar process of the maxilla between the two central incisor teeth; the alveolar point. [Gk *prostheos* foremost.]

prostholytic (pros·tho·**lit**·ik). Successively changing. [Gk *prosthen* further, *lyein* to release.]

Prostomata (pro·**sto**·mat·ah). An order of the trematode subclass Digenea. The suborders Amphistomata and Strigeata are of medical interest. [Gk *pro*, *stoma* mouth.]

prostrate (**pros**·trate). 1. Lying flat at full length. 2. Greatly reduced in or deprived of strength. [L *prostratus* thrown down.]

prostrated (**pros**·tra·ted). Exhausted; deprived of strength, unable to move. [see prec.]

prostration (pros·**tra**·shun). The condition of extreme exhaustion of body or mind. **Electric prostration.** Prostration due to lightning stroke or severe electric shock. The patient becomes unconscious, pale, pulseless, and respirations stop; there may be a state of suspended animation requiring artificial respiration. **Heat prostration.** Heat exhaustion, a condition of prostration due to heat, in which the patient is faint or unconscious, pale and sweating; blood pressure is low and the pulse feeble and quick. Deficiency of salts in the body from excessive sweating is an important factor. **Nervous prostration.** Neurasthenia; a state of irritable weakness and depression which may follow severe infections, prolonged illness, exhausting experiences, or it may be psychogenic in origin. [L *prosternere* to throw down.]

protactinium (pro·tak·**tin**·e·um). A radioactive element of atomic number 91, and chemical symbol Pa. It occurs in pitchblende, and is formed by the disintegration of uranium-235; it has a half life of 34 000 years, forming actinium with the emission of an α-particle. [Gk *protos* first, actinium.]

protagon (**pro**·tag·on). A term for certain lipoid materials extractable from nerve tissue [obsolete term]. [Gk *protos* first, *agon* leading.]

protal (**pro**·tal). Existing at or before birth; hereditary. [Gk *protos* first.]

protaminase (pro·**tam**·in·aze). An enzyme of the proteinase class occurring in the intestine, which hydrolyses protamines to peptides.

protamine (**pro**·tam·een). A class of proteins occurring solely in the sperm of fish. They are the simplest of the natural proteins, are soluble in water, and strongly basic by reason of their high proportion of the basic amino acids histidine, arginine and lysine, especially arginine. Examples are salmine from salmon, and sturine from sturgeon. [Gk *protos* first, amine.]

Protaminobacter (pro·**tam**·in·o·**bak**′·ter). A genus of non-pathogenic bacteria belonging to the family Pseudomonadaceae, with habitat in soil and water. Two species are described, *Protaminobacter alboflavum* and *Protaminobacter rubrum.* [protamine, bacterium.]

protandry (pro·**tan**·dre). In hermaphrodite animals, the development of mature sperms by the male organs before the ova of the female organs are ripe; it prevents self-fertilization. [Gk *protos* first, *aner* man.]

protanomalopia, protanomalopsia (pro·tan·om·al·**o**′·pe·ah, pro·tan·om·al·**op**′·se·ah). Partial colour blindness of the anomalous trichromatic type, in which the red portion of the spectrum is imperfectly perceived. [Gk *protos* first (red is the first primary colour), *anomalos* irregular, *ops* eye.]

protanomaly (pro·tan·**om**·al·e). Protanomalopia.

protanope (pro·tan·ope). One afflicted with protanopia.

protanopia, protanopsia (pro·tan·o·pe·ah, pro·tan·**op**·se·ah). A form of partial colour blindness in which the red portion of the spectrum is not perceived; red blindness. [Gk *protos* first (red is the first primary colour), *a, ops* eye.]

Protea (pro·te·ah). A genus of trees of the family Proteaceae found in wet and warm regions, many species of which have medicinal properties. **Protea juice.** A pectoral honey obtained from the flowers of various species of *Protea.* **Protea mellifera.** Sugar bush, a large bush indigenous to South Africa. An infusion of the leaves has been used in dysentery. [Gk *Proteus* sea-god who could change shape.]

protean (pro·te·an). Proteiform.

protease (pro·te·aze). Any proteolytic enzyme which breaks down protein by splitting the peptide linkage, -CONH-. **Fig-tree protease.** The active principle of leche de higueron from the latex of certain species of figs, used in the treatment of worm infections, especially ascariasis and trichuriasis; the worms are digested.

protectin (pro·tek·tin). 1. A substance which forms when blood serum is allowed to stand. According to Noguchi it delays or prevents haemolysis of erythrocytes. 2. A fine adhesive paper to cover a small wound and draw its edges together. [L *protegere* to cover in front.]

protection (pro·**tek**·shun). In radiology, provisions designed to reduce exposure of personnel to ionizing radiation. [see prec.]

protective (pro·**tek**·tiv). 1. Guarding against infection or disease; prophylactic; providing protection or conferring immunity. 2. Thin oiled silk tissue used in surgical dressings. [L *protegere* to cover in front.]

protector (pro·**tek**·tor). Any substance which protects a catalyser from inhibition or poisoning. **Lead protector.** A lead-impregnated shield to protect the body or part of the body (e.g. gonads) during diagnostic x-ray procedures. [see prec.]

proteic (pro·**te**·ik). Referring to or characterized by the presence of protein.

proteid (pro·te·id). Protein.

proteidic (pro·te·**id**·ik). Proteic.

proteidin (pro·te·id·in). A bacteriolytic substance [obsolete term]. **Pyocyanase proteidin.** A bacteriolytic substance derived from *Pseudomonas aeruginosa,* used at one time for protective inoculation against diphtheria.

proteidogenous (pro·te·id·**oj**′·en·us). Proteinogenous.

proteiform (pro·te·e·form). Changing form; taking different shapes. [Gk *Proteus,* sea-god who could change shape, form.]

protein (pro·te·in). Any of a class of organic nitrogenous compounds formed by condensation of various α-amino acids, occurring in every living cell and forming an essential constituent of it. Most proteins form colloidal solutions which are precipitated by strong salt solutions, alcohol, heavy metals and complex reagents such as those used for precipitating alkaloids. They also give certain characteristic colour reactions such as the biuret, xanthoproteic and Millon's reactions. Hydrolysis of proteins, as the result of acid, alkali or enzymatic action, yields products with successively smaller molecules (derived proteins) and, when complete, the constituent amino acids. The proteins are classified according to three main groups, namely, *simple, conjugated* and *derived proteins.* **Acute phase protein.** C-reactive protein (see below). **Alcohol-soluble protein.** A term which has been applied to the prolamins. **Autogenic protein.** A self-generating protein which can reproduce itself within the living cell. An example is chromatin of cell nuclei. **Protein binding, Protein bound.** A hormone or other compound bound to protein in the blood stream. **C-reactive protein.** A protein appearing in the blood in various human inflammatory conditions; originally discovered by its ability to precipitate with the polysaccharide C-substance of pneumococcal cell walls. **Complete protein.** Any protein which contains all of the amino acids essential for maintenance of health. **Compound protein, Conjugated protein.** Any compound formed by union of a protein with a non-protein group; the latter is termed *prosthetic group.* Subdivision of this group is made into the following classes: phosphoproteins; chromoproteins; nucleoproteins; and glycoproteins. **Denatured protein.** Protein which has undergone a change, other than by proteolysis, so that the specific character is lost. **Derived protein.** Any of a group of protein derivatives formed by hydrolytic breakdown of proteins. The classes in this group are metaproteins, proteoses, peptones and polypeptides. **Early protein.** Those bacteriophage proteins which are synthesized early, after infection of sensitive bacteria, and are usually concerned with replication of the phage genetic material. **Foreign protein.** A protein derived from some animal or plant other than that into which it is introduced. **Haem protein.** Haemoprotein. **Immune protein.** Those antibodies or antitoxins responsible for, or helpful in, the immunity of a host to invasion by foreign toxic materials. **Internal protein.** In bacteriophage infection, the small fraction of protein which is injected, in association with the phage DNA, into the host cell. **Iron-porphyrin protein.** One containing iron and porphyrin, e.g. haemoglobin, but there are many others. **Late proteins.** Those bacteriophage proteins which are synthesized late, following infection of sensitive bacteria, and usually comprise structural components of the progeny phage particles. **Mild Silver Protein BPC 1968.** Argentoproteinum mite; dark brown granules containing approximately 20 per cent Ag, but less bactericidal and less irritant than silver protein. **Myeloma protein.** A structurally homogeneous paraprotein (immunoglobulin) produced by neoplastic plasma cells in myelomatosis. The term *M component* is used to denote the occurrence of the *m*onoclonal immunoglobulins in *m*yelomatosis and *m*acroglobulinaemia (*see also* BENCE-JONES PROTEIN). **Native protein.** Any protein in its undenatured and undegraded form. **Plasma protein.** Protein substances present in blood plasma, including albumin, globulins of various types (such as α- and β-globulins), immune bodies or γ-globulin, antihaemophilic globulin and fibrinogen, among others. **Prophylactic measles protein.** The γ-globulin fraction of serum that contains antibodies active against the measles virus. This is given in the form of convalescent serum, placental concentrated extract (rarely used now) or as the purified concentrated γ-globulin. **Related protein.** One of a group of proteins which appear to have been derived from a common ancestral gene, either through chromosome or gene doubling or through divergence of species. **Serum protein.** Any of the proteins of blood serum. **Silver Protein BP 1968.** Argentoproteinum, strong silver protein; a yellowish powder containing approximately 8 per cent Ag, but highly bactericidal. **Simple protein.** Any protein which yields amino acids only upon hydrolysis. The classes of simple proteins are protamines, histones, gliadins (prolamines), glutelins, scleroproteins, albumins and globulins. **Specific protein.** One capable of calling forth a specific allergic reaction. [Gk *proteios* of first rank.]

See also: BENCE-JONES.

proteinaemia (pro·te·in·e′·me·ah). A misleading word, best avoided, since protein is a normal constituent of blood. It is, however, sometimes used to imply an increase in the protein content of the blood, for which the correct word is hyperproteinaemia. [protein, Gk *haima* blood.]

proteinase (pro·te·in·aze). Endopeptidase, a class of proteolytic enzymes which sever central linkages of proteins rather than terminal ones, thus producing peptones and peptides. Various proteinases have optimal activity at acid, alkaline or neutral pH, and are further classified as pepsinases, tryptases and papainases respectively.

protein-binding (pro·te·in **bind**′·ing). The attachment of molecules of a drug to serum proteins, with a consequent alteration of their effect. [Gk *proteios* of first rank, AS *bindan.*]

proteinic (pro·te·in·ik). Proteic.

proteinivorous (pro·te·in·iv'·or·us). Subsisting on protein foodstuffs. [protein, L *vorare* to devour.]

proteinochrome (pro·te·in·o·krome). The rose-red coloration given by tryptophan with bromine. [protein, Gk *chroma* colour.]

proteinochromogen (pro·te·in·o·kro'·mo·jen). Tryptophan, so called because of the rose-red coloration it gives with bromine. [protein, Gk *chroma* colour, *genein* to produce.]

proteinogenous (pro·te·in·oj'·en·ous). 1. Derived from protein. 2. Favouring the formation of, or producing, proteins. [protein, Gk *genein* to produce.]

proteinosis (pro·te·in·o'·sis). The accumulation of protein in excess in the tissues. In myxoedema a mucoid-like protein accumulates extracellularly and extravascularly. **Lipoid proteinosis.** A condition in which yellow deposits of a mixture of a lipoid and protein occur, especially on the mucous surface of the lips, beneath the tongue and on the fauces. Nodules may also occur on the face and limbs. **Pulmonary alveolar proteinosis.** A disease in which alveoli become filled with protein and lipid, with consequent respiratory failure; the cause is unknown. [protein, Gk *-osis* condition.]

proteinotherapy (pro·te·in·o·ther'·ap·e). Parenteral administration of a foreign protein in treatment of disease; protein therapy.

proteinphobia (pro·te·in·fo'·be·ah). Excessive distaste for foods containing protein. [protein, phobia.]

proteinuria (pro·te·in·ewr'·e·ah). A condition marked by the presence of protein in the urine. Cf. ALBUMINURIA.

See also: BENCE-JONES.

proteinuric (pro·te·in·ewr'·ik). Relating or belonging to proteinuria.

proteoclastic (pro·te·o·klas'·tik). Proteolytic. [protein, Gk *klasis* a breaking.]

proteolysis (pro·te·ol·is·is). The process of hydrolysis of proteins to soluble degradation products. [protein, Gk *lysis* a loosing.]

proteolytic (pro·te·o·lit'·ik). Pertaining to proteolysis; capable of splitting or absorbing protein.

proteometabolic (pro·te·o·met·ab·ol'·ik). Relating to protein metabolism.

proteometabolism (pro·te·o·met·ab'·ol·izm). The absorption and use of proteins by physiological processes; protein metabolism.

Proteomyces infestans (pro·te·o·mi·seez in·fes·tanz). *Trichosporon cutaneum.* [Gk *protos* first, *mykes* fungus, L *infestare* to make hostile.]

proteopepsis (pro·te·o·pep'·sis). Protein digestion. [protein, Gk *pepsis* digestion.]

proteopeptic (pro·te·o·pep'·tik). 1. Relating or belonging to proteopepsis. 2. Capable of digesting protein.

proteopexic (pro·te·o·pex'·ik). Relating or belonging to proteopexy.

proteopexis (pro·te·o·pex'·is). Proteopexy.

proteopexy (pro·te·o·pex·se). The fixation of proteins in the tissues or organs. [protein, Gk *pexis* fixation.]

proteophilic (pro·te·o·fil'·ik). With a preference for a medium rich in protein. [protein, Gk *philein* to love.]

proteose (pro·te·oze). A product of the partial hydrolysis of protein which is less complex in composition than metaprotein but more so than peptone. Proteoses are soluble in water, dilute salt solutions, dilute acids and akalis, but are precipitated by saturation with sodium sulphate or with ammonium sulphate. They are not coagulable by heat.

See also: BENCE-JONES.

proteosotherapy (pro·te·o·so·ther'·ap·e). The administration by subcutaneous or intravenous injection of foreign proteose in treatment of disease; proteose therapy.

proteosuria (pro·te·o·zewr'·e·ah). The presence of proteose in the urine.

proteotherapy (pro·te·o·ther'·ap·e). Proteinotherapy.

proteotoxin (pro·te·o·tox'·in). The foreign protein which causes the phenomenon of anaphylaxis when injected into an animal. [protein, toxin.]

Proteroglypha (pro·ter·og·lif·ah). A division of the snakes of the family Colubridae; it includes those that have grooved anterior maxillary teeth in association with poison glands. Some of the most highly poisonous species, e.g. the cobras, are Proteroglypha. [Gk *proteros* earlier, *glyphein* to carve.]

protest (pro·test). **Masculine protest.** The mechanisms which result from a person's drive to escape from a rôle actually or supposedly inferior (Adler). [L *protestari* to aver.]

proteuria (pro·te·ewr·e·ah). Proteinuria.

Proteus (pro·te·us). A bacterial genus in the family Enterobacteriaceae, widely distributed in the environment and in the intestines of man and animals. Gram-negative, actively motile bacilli which swarm on suitable culture media, they are associated with infections of wounds, pressure sores, urinary tract, etc. (*Proteus vulgaris, P. mirabilis, P. rettgeri* species); *Proteus morganii* may be causally related to infantile gastroenteritis. Urea is decomposed and trimethylamine oxide reduced by all species. **Proteus mirabilis.** A species whose habitat is in putrefying matter and water; it is found in putrid meat, in abscesses and in cases of gastroenteritis. It has no action on mannitol, produces acid and gas from sucrose but not from maltose, and does not form indole. **Proteus morganii.** A species found in the human intestinal canal and occurring in gastroenteritis and cystitis. It has no action on mannitol, sucrose or maltose; it forms indole. **Proteus rettgeri.** A species whose habitat is the intestinal canal of poultry and birds, and occurring in the faeces from sporadic and epidemic cases of gastroenteritis. It produces acid from mannitol and sucrose but not maltose, and forms indole. **Proteus vulgaris.** A species occurring in putrefying materials and found in putrid meat, in abscesses, in cases of otitis media and cystitis, and in faeces. It has no action on mannitol, produces acid and gas from sucrose and maltose, and forms indole. Suspensions of "X" strains of this species (X19, X2 and XK) are used for diagnosis by agglutination of the serum from typhus patients. [Gk *Proteus*, sea-god who could change shape.]

prothesis (pro·the·sis). Prosthesis. [Gk *pro, thesis* a placing.]

prothetic (pro·thet·ik). Relating or belonging to prothesis; prosthetic.

Prothionamide (pro·thi·on·am·ide). BP Commission approved name for 2-propylisonicotinthioamide; it is used in the treatment of tuberculosis.

Prothipendyl (pro·thi·pen·dil). BP Commission approved name for 10-(3-dimethylaminopropyl)-9-thia-1,10-diaza-anthracene; a tranquillizer.

prothrombase (pro·throm·baze). Prothrombin.

prothrombin (pro·throm·bin). A constituent of normal blood plasma that, in the presence of thromboplastin, calcium and a factor V, forms thrombin, and is essential for the normal clotting of blood. When present in reduced amounts, as in congenital hypoprothrombinaemia, vitamin-K deficiency, obstructive jaundice, or after dicoumarol and other anticoagulant therapy, a haemorrhagic condition may develop. **Fraction A prothrombin** (component A prothrombin). The labile factor of the prothrombin complex, which disappears from stored blood or plasma, but is not diminished by dicoumarol or by vitamin-K deficiency; it is probably identical with Owren's factor V, and with thrombogen (Nolf). **Fraction B prothrombin** (component B prothrombin). The second non-labile factor present with component A in the prothrombin complex, and is probably the true or classical prothrombin which is reduced by dicoumarol and by vitamin-K deficiency; it may exist in the blood in a free and an inactive form (presurcor). [L *pro*, thrombin.]

prothrombinaemia (pro·throm·bin·e'·me·ah). Prothrombin in the blood in normal or excessive amounts. [prothrombin, Gk *haima* blood.]

prothrombinopenia (pro·throm·bin·o·pe'·ne·ah). Hypoprothrombinaemia; a congenital or acquired condition in which there is a deficiency of prothrombin in the blood, causing haemorrhagic manifestations. It may follow excessive treatment with dicoumarol, or similar anticoagulants, or a deficient intake or absorption of vitamin K, while disease of the liver and bile ducts may be causal factors. It is relieved by treatment with vitamin K or its analogues. [prothrombin, Gk *penes* poor.]

prothrombokinase (pro·**throm**·bo·**kin**'·aze). A blood plasma globulin which is the precursor of the clotting enzyme, thrombokinase (thromboplastin), necessary for the conversion of prothrombin into thrombin during the initial stages of the blood-clotting mechanism. [Gk *pro*, thrombokinase.]

prothyl (pro·thil). Protyl.

prothymia (pro·**thi**·me·ah). A state in which the mentality is advanced in degree and the will well developed. [Gk *pro, thymos* mind.]

protidaemia (pro·tid·e·me·ah). Proteinaemia.

protidolytic (pro·tid·o·**lit**'·ik). Proteolytic.

protinium (pro·**tin**·e·um). Protium.

protiodide (prot·i·o·dide). Proto-iodide.

Protirelin (pro·**ti**·rel·in). BP Commission approved name for 1-[*N*-(5-oxo-L-prolyl)-L-histidyl]-L-prolinamide; a thyrotrophin-releasing hormone.

Protista (pro·**tis**·tah). A classificatory grouping, sometimes given the status of a Kingdom, which contains all single-celled organisms, both animals and plants. [Gk, the very first.]

protistology (pro·tis·**tol**·o·je). Microbiology. [Gk *protistos* the very first, *logos* science.]

protium (**pro**·te·um). Name given to hydrogen of atomic weight 1 to differentiate it from the isotopes *deuterium* and *tritium*. [Gk *protos* first.]

protoactinium (pro·to·ak·**tin**'·e·um). Protactinium.

Protobactereae (pro·to·bak·**teer**'·e·e). A tribe of bacteria described by Rahn (1937) but no longer accepted. The two genera in the tribe, *Carboxydomonas* and *Methanomonas*, obtain their energy by oxidizing CO to CO_2, or in the latter case methane to CO_2 and water; they are now included in the families Streptomycetaceae and Pseudomonadaceae, respectively. [Gk *protos* first, bacterium.]

protobiology (pro·to·bi·**ol**'·o·je). The science which is concerned with micro-organisms of smaller size than bacteria, e.g. bacteriophages. [Gk *protos* first, biology.]

Protobios (pro·to·**bi**·os). A generic name proposed for the bacteriophages. The type species, *Protobios bacteriophagus* (d'Herelle), is no longer identifiable and the genus is not therefore recognized nowadays. [Gk *protos* first, *bios* life.]

protoblast (pro·to·blast). A blastomere that gives rise to an organ or part. [Gk *protos* first, *blastos* germ.]

protoblastic (pro·to·**blas**·tik). Relating or belonging to a protoblast.

protobrochal (pro·to·**bro**·kal). Denoting the first phase in the formation of an ovary. [Gk *protos* first, *brochos* mesh of a net.]

protochloride (pro·to·**klor**·ide). Of the several chlorides of an element or radical, that one which contains the lowest proportion of chlorine. [Gk *protos* first, chloride.]

protochlorophylline (pro·to·klor·o·**fil**'·een). A colourless compound formed by the reduction of the plant pigment, chlorophyll. [Gk *protos* first, chlorophyll.]

protocone (pro·to·kone). In the tritubercular theory of evolution, the name given to the anterior-internal cusp of an upper molar tooth. [Gk *protos* first, *konos* cone.]

protoconid (pro·to·**ko**·nid). In the tritubercular theory of evolution, the name given to the anterior-external cusp of a lower molar tooth. [Gk *protos* first, *konos* cone.]

protocurarine (pro·to·kew·**rah**'·reen). $C_{19}H_{23}O_2N$, one of the most active of the curare alkaloids, derived from pot curare.

protocurine (pro·to·**kewr**·een). $C_{20}H_{22}NO_3$, one of the curare alkaloids, obtained from pot curare.

protodiastole (pro·to·di·**as**'·to·le). Protodiastolic phase, or interval; the period in the heart cycle immediately following the reduced ejection phase of ventricular systole. It constitutes the earliest phase of diastole, or relaxation, of the ventricles of the heart. [Gk *protos* first, diastole.]

protodiastolic (pro·to·di·as·**tol**'·ik). Relating to the pause that immediately succeeds the diastole. [see prec.]

protoduodenitis (pro·to·dew·o·de·**ni**'·tis). An inflammatory state of the protoduodenum. [protoduodenum, Gk *-itis* inflammation.]

protoduodenum (pro·to·dew·o·**de**'·num). The upper half of the duodenum, derived from the embryonic foregut. [Gk *protos* first, duodenum.]

proto-erythrocyte (pro·to·er·**ith**'·ro·site). A nucleated red cell, or erythroblast, having a very deeply staining nucleus. [Gk *protos* first, erythrocyte.]

protogala (pro·to·**gah**·lah). Colostrum. [Gk *protos* first, *gala* milk.]

protogaster (pro·to·gas·ter). The foregut. [Gk *protos* first, *gaster* stomach.]

protogonoplasm (pro·to·**go**·no·plazm). The protoplasm of the primordial sexual cells of the early embryo [obsolete term]. [Gk *protos* first, *gonos* offspring, plasm.]

protohaemin (pro·to·**he**·min). Haemin, haematin chloride, $C_{34}H_{32}O_4N_4FeCl$. A dark-brown crystalline porphyrin derivative which forms in old blood clots. [Gk *protos* first, haemin.]

protohaemocytoblast (pro·to·he·mo·**si**'·to·blast). A cell that develops from a bone marrow cell and becomes an erythrocyte. [Gk *protos* first, haemocytoblast.]

protohydrogen (pro·to·**hi**·dro·jen). 1. Protium. 2. An element with atomic weight 0.081, believed at one time to exist in certain nebulae and stars. [Gk *protos* first, hydrogen.]

proto-iodide (pro·to·i·o·dide). Of the several iodides of an element or radical, that one which contains the least proportion of iodine. [Gk *protos* first, iodide.]

protokaryote (pro·to·**kar**·e·ote). Prokaryote. [Gk *protos* first, *karyon* nut.]

Protokylol (pro·to·**ki**·lol). BP Commission approved name for 1-(3,4-dihydroxyphenyl)-2-(α-methyl-3,4-methylene-dioxyphenethylamino)ethanol; a sympathomimetic drug.

protoleucocyte (pro·to·**lew**·ko·site). A small lymphoid cell, or lymphocyte, seen in the spleen and marrow. [Gk *protos* first, leucocyte.]

protomer (**pro**·to·mer). The fundamental structural unit of certain oligomeric proteins which are formed by the combination of two or more protomers. [Gk *protos* first, *meros* part.]

protometrocyte (pro·to·**me**·tro·site). A common precursor or mother-cell in the bone marrow, giving rise to the red and white blood-cell series. [Gk *protos* first, *meter* mother, *kytos* cell.]

Protomonadina (pro·to·mon·ad·**i**'·nah). An order of mastigophoran Protozoa which contains forms of simple structure and with only one or two flagella. The order includes the haemoflagellates *Trypanosoma* and *Leishmania*, as well as *Embadomonas* and various coprozoic forms. [Gk *protos* first, *monas* unit.]

proton (**pro**·ton). A nuclear particle of mass number 1, having a charge equal and opposite to that of an electron and a mass of 1.672×10^{-24} g. [Gk *protos* first.]

protonephron (pro·to·**nef**·ron). A tubule of the pronephros. [Gk *protos* first, *nephros* kidney.]

protonephros (pro·to·**nef**·ros). The pronephros. [see prec.]

protonic (pro·**ton**·ik). Relating or belonging to a proton.

protonitrate (pro·to·**ni**·trate). The lowest nitrate formed by any element or radical, in that it contains the least proportion of the nitro group, NO_2. [Gk *protos* first, nitrate.]

protopathic (pro·to·**path**·ik). 1. Relating or belonging to the first symptom or lesion; primary. 2. Denoting the initial sign of the partial restoration of function in an injured nerve. 3. Relating to a certain type of nerve which is affected only by the coarser type of stimulus (pain, and high or low temperatures) and not by localization stimuli or the more refined sensory influences. [Gk *protos* first, *pathos* disease.]

protopecten (pro·to·**pek**·ten). Pectose. [Gk *protos* first, pecten.]

protopepsia (pro·to·**pep**·se·ah). One of the initial digestive processes which is in action high up in the digestive system, e.g. the action of saliva on starch, which takes place in the mouth. [Gk *protos* first, *peptein* to digest.]

protophylline (pro·to·**fil**·een). Protochlorophylline. [Gk *protos* first, *phyllon* leaf.]

protophyte (pro·to·fite). Any single-celled vegetable organism, e.g. a bacterium. [Gk *protos* first, *phyton* that which has grown.]

protopine (pro·to·peen). Fumarine, $C_{20}H_{19}O_5N$. An alkaloid occurring in opium and other papaveraceous plants.

protoplasia, protoplasis (pro·to·pla·ze·ah, pro·to·pla·sis). The initial building up of cells into a tissue. [Gk *protos* first, *plassein* to form.]

protoplasm (pro·to·plazm). The essential material basis of living matter, consisting of proteins, fats, carbohydrates, inorganic salts and water, in a labile colloidal state. **Functional protoplasm.** That part of the protoplasm which is essential to life, as opposed to the temporary storage components. **Totipotential protoplasm.** Undetermined protoplasm which possesses the potentiality for differentiating into any of the various types of protoplasm found in the organism. [Gk *protos* first, *plasma* something formed.]

protoplasmatic (pro·to·plaz·mat'·ik). Protoplasmic.

protoplasmic (pro·to·plaz·mik). Relating to or composed of protoplasm.

protoplast (pro·to·plast). Rounded, osmotically fragile forms of bacteria from which the cell wall has been removed, leaving only the cytoplasmic membrane bounding the cytoplasm; spheroplast. [Gk *protos* first, *plassein* to mould.]

protoporphyria (pro·to·por·fir'·e·ah). The presence of protoporphyrin in the blood. **Erythropoietic protoporphyria.** An inherited condition with light sensitivity, a bizarre eruption of tingling urticarioid or eczematoid lesions, sometimes with vesiculation, crusting and scarring. The erythrocyte protoporphyrin levels and, sometimes, the plasma protoporphyrin levels are raised. [Gk *protos* first, porphyrin, Gk *haima* blood.]

protoporphyrin (pro·to·por·fir·in). $C_{34}H_{34}O_4N_4$, the porphyrin which, combined with iron, forms the haem moiety of the haemoglobin molecule. It is also the porphyrin constituent of myoglobin, haemoprotein enzymes and respiratory pigments of certain other species. [Gk *protos* first, porphyrin.]

protoporphyrinuria (pro·to·por·fir·in·ewr'·e·ah). The presence of protoporphyrin in the urine.

protoproteose (pro·to·pro·te·oze). In the USA classification this corresponds to the primary proteose of British nomenclature. This term is applied to proteoses which are precipitated by half-saturation with ammonium sulphate. [Gk *protos* first, proteose.]

protoribosome (pro·to·ri·bo·some). A presumed ancestral precursor of present-day ribosomes, thought to have existed before the appearance of cellular organisms. [Gk *protos* first, ribose, Gk *stoma* body.]

protosalt (pro·to·sawlt). Of the several salts formed by a base with a particular acid, that one which contains the lowest proportion of the acid radical. [Gk *protos* first, salt.]

protospasm (pro·to·spazm). A spasm which, beginning in one limb or muscle, later becomes generalized. [Gk *protos* first, spasm.]

protostoma (pro·to·sto·mah). Blastopore. [Gk *protos* first, *stoma* mouth.]

protosulphate (pro·to·sul·fate). Of the several sulphates formed by an element or radical, that one which contains the lowest proportion of the sulphate radical, SO_4. [Gk *protos* first, sulphate.]

Prototheca (pro·to·the·kah). An achloric mutant of the green alga, *Chlorella*. Several species have been described, e.g. *Prototheca segbwema* (an achloritic alga capable of invading the epidermis of the foot to produce many granulomatous lesions; reported from Sierra Leone), *P. wickerhamii* and *P. portoricensis*. Strains have been isolated from diseased tissues in animals. [Gk *protos* first, *theke* sheath.]

protothecosis (pro·to·the·kos'·sis). A rare infection of the skin, occurring in man or animals, by an alga, Prototheca. There is often a heavy infiltration of eosinophil leucocytes. [Gk *protos* first, *theke* sheath, *-osis* condition.]

Prototheria (pro·to·the·re·ah). A subclass of the class Mammalia that contains only the Monotremata. [Gk *protos* first, *ther* beast.]

proto-tRNA (pro·to·tee·ar·en·a). A class of presumed ancestral precursors of present-day tRNA. It is thought to have existed prior to the development of cellular organisms. [Gk *protos* first, transfer ribonucleic acid.]

prototrophic (pro·to·trof·ik). Denoting those organisms which obtain sustenance from inorganic material, e.g. most plants. [Gk *protos* first, *trophe* nutrition.]

prototype (pro·to·tipe). The primary or original form from which all other types or forms arise. [Gk *protos* first, type.]

protoveratrine (pro·to·ver·at'·reen). $C_{39}H_{61}O_{13}N$, an alkaloid recently used for hypertension, but it causes sinus bradycardia.

protovertebra (pro·to·ver·te·brah). The mesenchymal primordium of a vertebra, resulting from the fusion of a pair of segmental sclerotomes. [Gk *protos* first, vertebra.]

protovertebral (pro·to·ver·te·bral). Belonging to or relating to a protovertebra.

protoxide (pro·tox·ide). Of the several oxides of an element or radical, that one which contains the lowest proportion of oxygen. [Gk *protos* first, oxide.]

protoxylem (pro·to·zi·lem). The elements which differentiate from the procambium in a plant and become xylem. [Gk *protos* first, xylem.]

protozoa (pro·to·zo·ah). A subkingdom or phylum of animals which includes all non-cellular forms; they are often placed with non-cellular plant forms in the group Protista. Members of the subphyla Ciliophora, Mastigophora, Sarcodina and Sporozoa are of medical importance. [Gk *protos* first, *zoon* animal.]

protozoacide (pro·to·zo·as·ide). 1. Capable of destroying protozoa. 2. An agent used to destroy protozoa. [protozoa, L *caedere* to kill.]

protozo-agglutinin (pro·to·zo·ag·loo'·tin·in). An agglutinin in the blood of man and animals suffering from protozoal infections; it agglutinates the infecting protozoon. It has been described in leishmaniasis and trypanosomiasis.

protozoal, protozoan (pro·to·zo·al, pro·to·zo·an). Pertaining to or caused by protozoa.

protozoiasis (pro·to·zo·i'·as·is). Any morbid condition caused by protozoa.

protozoology (pro·to·zo·ol'·o·je). That branch of zoological science which is concerned with the protozoa. [protozoa, Gk *logos* science.]

protozoon (pro·to·zo·on). An organism consisting of one cell and belonging to the protozoa. [Gk *protos* first, *zoon* animal.]

protozoophage (pro·to·zo·o·faje). A phagocytic cell which is capable of ingesting protozoa. [protozoon, *phagein* to eat.]

protraction (pro·trak·shun). A drawing forward, as that of the shoulder caused when the serratus anterior muscle draws the scapula forward, or of the jaw caused by the pterygoid muscles. [L *pro*, *trahere* to draw.]

protractor (pro·trak·tor). An instrument for the surgical removal of foreign bodies, especially bullets and dead bone from wounds. [see prec.]

Protriptyline (pro·trip·ti·leen). BP Commission approved name for 7-(3-methylaminopropyl)-1,2,5,6-dibenzocycloheptatriene. **Protriptyline Hydrochloride BP 1973.** The hydrochloride of protriptyline, an antidepressant.

protrusio acetabuli (pro·troo·se·o as·et·ab·ew·li). An acetabulum of abnormal depth, giving the appearance of protrusion of the femoral head into the pelvis. [L, protrusion of the acetabulum.]

protuberance (pro·tew·ber·ans). A blunt projection or swelling. **Frontal protuberance.** The frontal eminence; the convex forward bulge of the frontal bone above the eyebrow. **Laryngeal protuberance.** The prominence of the thyroid cartilage of the larynx. **Mental protuberance [protuberantia mentalis (NA)].** The prominence of the chin formed at the lower border of the body of the mandible. **Natiform protuberance.** The buttock. **Occipital protuberance, external [protuberantia occipitalis externa (var. crista occipitalis externa) NA].** A blunt projection about the middle of the outer aspect of the squama of the occipital bone to which the ligamentum nuchae is attached. **Occipital protuberance, internal [protuberantia occipitalis**

interna (var. crista occipitalis interna) NA]. A blunt projection about the middle of the inner aspect of the squama of the occipital bone. **Parietal protuberance.** The prominent convexity of the parietal bone which overlies the parietal lobe of the cerebrum. [L *pro, tuberare* to swell.]

See also: AMMON.

protyl (**pro**·til). 1. Propargyl, the radical $CH \equiv CCH_2$–. 2. Protyle.

protyle (**pro**·tile). Archyle; the postulated fundamental form of matter from which all the chemical elements are believed to have been built up. [Gk *protos* first, *hyle* raw material.]

protyrosinase (pro·ti·**ro**·sin·aze). Precursor of tyrosinase. [Gk *pro,* tyrosinase.]

Proust, Louis Joseph (b. 1755). French chemist.

Proust's law. Law of constant composition.

Proust, P. T. (fl. 1822). Paris physician.

Proust's space. The rectrovesical pouch.

Proust-Lichtheim manoeuvre. The technique whereby an aphasic patient, though unable to evolve the appropriate term, can nevertheless indicate how many syllables are entailed, by squeezing the examiner's hand, or by tapping the table the appropriate number of times.

provertebra (pro·**ver**·te·brah). Protovertebra.

Providentia (pro·vid·**en**·she·ah). A bacterial genus closely related to *Proteus.*

provisional (pro·**vizh**·on·al). Temporary; carried out or applied for the time being only. [L *providere* to make preparation for.]

provitamin (pro·**vi**·tam·in). A substance which is converted into a vitamin in the animal organism and hence shares the activity of the vitamin. **Provitamin A.** Carotene. **Provitamin D.** Ergosterol. [Gk *pro,* vitamin.]

provocation (prov·o·**ka**·shun). A defence in law on a charge of homicide, usually murder, which reduces the offence to manslaughter. Provocation by taunting or some act by the deceased which might cause a reasonable person temporary loss of self-control. [L *provocare* to call forth.]

provocative (pro·**vok**·at·iv). Serving to provoke or stimulate, e.g. reaction, reflex or response to treatment. [L *provocare* to call forth.]

Prowazek, Stanislaus Josef Mathias von (b. 1875). Hamburg protozoologist.

Prowazek body. The *Rickettsia prowazekii;* the causal organism of typhus fever.

Prowazek-Greeff bodies, Prowazek-Halberstaedter bodies, or corpuscles. Intracellular bodies found in trachomatous secretions and believed to represent a stage in the life history of the causal virus.

proximal [proximalis (NA)] (**prox**·im·al). 1. Nearest to the centre of the body, or to the point of origin or attachment; in contrast to distal. 2. In dentistry, applied to the surface of a tooth nearest to the front of the mouth (the mesial surface). [L *proximus* nearest.]

proximate (**prox**·im·ate). Nearest; approximate. [see prec.]

proximo-ataxia (**prox**·im·o·at·**ax**′·e·ah). Ataxia in which the proximal parts of the extremities are involved.

proximobuccal (**prox**·im·o·**buk**′·al). Relating to the proximal and labial (buccal) surfaces of a tooth.

proximolabial (**prox**·im·o·**la**′·be·al). Relating to the proximal and labial surfaces of a tooth.

proximolingual (**prox**·im·o·**ling**′·gwal). Relating to the proximal and lingual surfaces of a tooth.

Proxymetacaine (prox·e·**met**·ah·kane). BP Commission approved name for 2-diethylaminoethyl 3-amino-4-propoxybenzoate. The hydrochloride (BPC 1968) is a local anaesthetic suitable for use in the eye as a 0.5 per cent solution.

Proxyphylline (prox·e·**fi**·leen). BP Commission approved name for 7-(2-hydroxypropyl)-1,3-dimethylxanthine; used in the treatment of asthma, and bronchitis.

prozonal (pro·**zo**·nal). Describing the position of a nerve or other structure which passes into a limb anterior or cranial to the limb girdle. [see foll.]

prozone (**pro**·zone). That region of the dilution range among the low dilutions in which an antiserum fails to agglutinate the homologous bacteria, although it agglutinates it in higher dilutions. The phenomenon also occurs in tests for titres of bacteriolytic and precipitating sera. [Gk *pro,* zone.]

prozygosis (pro·zi·**go**·sis). In teratism, the state in which the two heads of a twin monster are fused into one. [Gk *pro, zygon,* yoke, *-osis* condition.]

pruinate (**proo**·in·ate). Covered with whitish dusty substance which resembles hoar-frost. [L *pruina* hoar-frost.]

prunase (**proo**·naze). An enzyme occurring in cherry-laurel leaves and bitter almonds. It is concerned with the hydrolysis of the glycosides of species of *Prunus* and is a constituent of the mixture of enzymes known as *emulsin.*

prunasin (proo·**na**·sin). One of the products brought about by the hydrolysis of the enzyme amygdalase on amygdalin.

Prune BPC 1959 (proon). The dried ripe fruit of the plum, *Prunus domesticus* Linn. It contains from 12 to 25 per cent of sugar as well as malic acid and other organic acids; used medicinally as a mild laxative, usually in conjunction with stronger laxatives such as senna. [L *prunum* plum.]

Prunella (proo·**nel**·ah). A genus of labiate plants. **Prunella vulgaris.** Self-heal, heal-all, carpenter weed; a herb with purplish flowers in a dense terminal spike. It has an astringent action and is used in internal haemorrhage and diarrhoea. [dim. of L *prunus* plum-tree.]

Prunus (**proo**·nus). 1. A genus of rosaceous trees and shrubs. 2. *See* PRUNE. **Prunus amygdala.** 1. The sweet almond, *Prunus communis* Arcang. var. *dulcis* Schneider, the seeds of which contain from 45 to 50 per cent of a bland fixed oil (oil of almonds) and about 20 per cent of proteins amongst which is included a mixture of enzymes known as *emulsin.* They are used as a demulcent and for food purposes, especially as a non-starchy food in diabetes. 2. The bitter almond, *Prunus communis* Arcang. var. *amara* Schneider, indistinguishable botanically from the sweet almond except that the seeds contain in addition amygdalin which gives them a bitter taste and liberates, when decomposed by the enzyme emulsin, dextrose, hydrocyanic acid and benzaldehyde. They are used as a sedative and for flavouring purposes, but caution is necessary because of the hydrocyanic acid content. **Prunus domestica.** A species the dried ripe fruits of which (prunes) contain 40 per cent of dextrose and are used for food purposes. The seeds contain fixed oil and amygdalin. **Prunus laurocerasus.** Cherry-laurel, a species the leaves of which contain a glycoside, which is decomposed by an enzyme also present, prunase, into dextrose, benzaldehyde and hydrocyanic acid. Cherry-laurel water (aqua laurocerasi) is prepared from the leaves and is used as a gastric sedative on account of the hydrocyanic acid content, and also in eye lotions. **Prunus serotina.** A species the bark of which (wild cherry bark, Virginian prune bark) yields hydrocyanic acid and benzaldehyde when moistened with water, owing to the glycoside prunasin being hydrolysed by the enzyme prunase also present. A syrup prepared from it is used for coughs. **Prunus spinosa.** The common blackthorn, wounds from which may cause persistent foreign-body granulomatous lesions in the skin. **Prunus virginiana.** *Prunus serotina* (see above). [L, plum-tree.]

pruriginous (proo·**rij**·in·us). Pertaining to, causing, or affected with prurigo.

prurigo (proo·**ri**·go). An itching papular eruption. The name is usually reserved for certain syndromes in which an idiopathic pruritus is the main feature. **Prurigo aestivalis.** Hydroa aestivale, recurrent summer eruption (Hutchinson), hydroa vacciniforme (Bazin), hydroa puerorum (Unna); a vesicular eruption occurring every summer on exposed areas: the sites are marked by scarring when the rash subsides. The malady usually develops in childhood, lessens at puberty and ceases in adult life. Sunlight is the exciting cause. Porphyrins may be present in the urine. **Prurigo agria.** Prurigo ferox (see below). **Circumscribed prurigo.** Lichen simplex chronicus. **Dermographic prurigo.** Prurigo with urtication and excoriations, mostly affecting sites of friction from clothing. **Diathetic prurigo.** Besnier's prurigo, a chronic eruption affecting particularly the flexor surfaces of the knees, elbows and wrists, also the back of the neck; it develops usually in early childhood and may be associated with xeroderma. From time to time eczematous reactions occur, which may be widespread. This form of prurigo is often associated with asthma, and is one of the more characteristic manifestations of the atopic state. **Prurigo ferox.** The severe type of Hebra's prurigo, a generalized prurigo, commencing in infancy and often persisting throughout adult life. During the first year of life the malady commences as an urticarial rash, but soon the typical papules appear. Itching is severe, and secondary lesions such as excoriations, pustules, boils and abscesses may be noted. The skin becomes pigmented and thickened. In some cases the symptoms are severe (*prurigo ferox*), in others they are less troublesome (*prurigo mitis*). **Flexual prurigo.** Besnier's prurigo; flexure eczema. **Prurigo gestationis.** A pruriginous eruption occurring in the last 3 months of pregnancy. **Prurigo hiemalis.** Pruritus hiemalis. **Prurigo lymphatica.** Prurigo occurring as a leading symptom in Hodgkin's disease. **Prurigo mitis.** The milder type of Hebra's prurigo (*see* PRURIGO FEROX, above). **Prurigo nodularis.** A rare eruption, usually in women, characterized by the appearance of indurated, itching papules and nodules on the extremities. **Postscabietic prurigo.** A prurigo that follows an attack of scabies; it is largely psychological. **Prurigo simplex** (Brocq). Papular urticaria. **Summer prurigo.** Any irritating papular eruption occurring on the exposed surfaces of the skin each summer, and regressing in winter, of which the cause is exposure to sunlight. **Prurigo uratica.** A crusted papular eruption associated with urticaria and due to gout. **Prurigo vulgaris.** Lichen simplex chronicus. **Winter prurigo.** Pruritus hiemalis. [L, an itching.]

See also: BESNIER, HEBRA, HUTCHINSON.

pruritic (proo·rit·ik). 1. Relating to or causing pruritus. 2. Irritating, itching.

pruritus (proo·ri·tus). Itching; a cutaneous subjective symptom producing a desire to scratch (MacLeod). **Pruritus aestivalis.** Troublesome itching which recurs whenever the weather is hot. **Pruritus ani.** Itching at the anal orifice. **Autotoxic pruritus.** Itching due to endogenous toxins occurring, for example, in jaundice, uraemia, gout and chronic cholecystitis. **Bath pruritus.** Itching which develops immediately after a bath, and usually involves the lower part of the trunk, the thighs and legs. **Essential pruritus.** Localized or generalized pruritus not preceded by any obvious skin disease. **Pruritus hiemalis.** Winter prurigo, frost itch, prurigo hiemalis; a malady of northern climates: the itching occurs only during cold weather when the patient undresses. The legs are usually affected, but other areas may be involved. **Pruritus punctata, Punctate pruritus.** Itching points in the skin, occurring without any visible lesion or cause. **Pruritus senilis.** Generalized pruritus occurring in old age, believed to be due to atrophic and degenerative changes in the skin. **Symptomatic pruritus.** Localized or generalized itching due to disease, infection or infestation of the skin. Symptomatic pruritus may also be due to some systemic malady, e.g. Hodgkin's disease. **Pruritus vulvae.** Itching of the vulva. [L *prurire* to itch.]

See also: DUHRING.

Prussak, Alexander (b. 1839). Russian otologist.

Prussak's fibres, or striae. Fibres bounding the flaccid part of the tympanic membrane.

Prussak's space. A small recess, formed by the folding of the mucous membrane, situated between the neck of the malleus and the tympanic membrane and communicating with the tympanic cavity via the posterior pockets of the tympanic membrane.

prussiate (**prus**·e·ate, **prush**·e·ate). Name applied loosely to cyanides, ferrocyanides and ferricyanides, because of their derivation from prussic (hydrocyanic) acid.

psalis (**sa**·lis). The fornix cerebri. [Gk, vault.]

psalterial (sal·**teer**·e·al). Relating or belonging to the psalterium.

psalterium (sal·**teer**·e·um). 1. The hippocampal commissure. 2. A collection of fibres running longitudinally along the floor of the aqueduct of the mid-brain. [L, stringed instrument.]

psamma (**sam**·ah). A deposit of sandy substance in the urine. [Gk *psammos* sand.]

psammism (**sam**·izm). The use of the sand bath in physical treatment. [see prec.]

psammocarcinoma (**sam**·o·kar·sin·**o'**·mah). A carcinoma rich in small calcifying concretions. [Gk *psammos* sand, carcinoma.]

Psammolestes (sam·o·**les**·teez). A genus of reduviid bugs. **Psammolestes arthuri, Psammolestes coreodes.** Species that are a potential vector of American trypanosomiasis (Chagas' disease). [Gk *psammos* sand, *lestes* robber.]

psammoma (sam·**o**·mah). A hard tumour, usually a meningioma, found in the brain membranes, choroid plexus, and even in the brain substance; it is rich in calcareous particles. [Gk *psammos* sand, *-oma* tumour.]

Psammomys rondairei (sam·**o**·mis ron·da·i·re·i). A North African rodent subject to plague infection. [Gk *psammos* sand, *mys* mouse.]

psammosarcoma (**sam**·o·sar·**ko'**·mah). A sarcoma in process of calcification. [Gk *psammos* sand, sarcoma.]

psammotherapy (sam·o·**ther**·ap·e). The use of sand baths as a form of treatment, e.g. in diseases of rheumatic type. [Gk *psammos* sand, therapy.]

psammous (**sam**·us). Sandy. [Gk *psammos* sand.]

psanoscopy (san·**os**·ko·pe). The method of determining the limits of a superficial pathological area by passing the tip of the index finger lightly over the skin to note the change in resistance or tenseness which occurs in passing from the normal to the abnormal area. [Gk *psanein* to touch, *skopein* to view.]

pselaphesia, pselaphesis (sel·af·e·ze·ah, sel·af·e·sis). The tactile sense. [Gk *pselaphesis* a touching.]

pselaphia (sel·**af**·e·ah). Palpation; digital examination. [see prec.]

psellism, psellismus (**sel**·izm, sel·**iz**·mus). 1. Stuttering or stammering. 2. A faulty mode of speech caused by a defect such as cleft palate or hare-lip. 3. The substitution of one letter sound for another; the mispronunciation of letters. **Psellismus mercurialis.** The incomprehensible, jerky, quick speech of those suffering from the tremor which is associated with mercurial intoxication. [Gk *psellos* indistinctly uttered.]

pseudaesthesia (sewd·es·**the**·ze·ah). 1. Sensation of a subjective type unrelated to any objective stimulus. 2. Sensation of a kind completely unrelated to that which should have been the result of the particular stimulus. 3. Imaginary perception of a sense referred to a part that has been amputated. 4. Imaginary sensation of any kind. [Gk *pseudes* false, aesthesia.]

Pseudamphistomum (sewd·am·**fis**·to·mum). A genus of liver flukes. **Pseudamphistomum truncatum.** A species, common in carnivores, which has occasionally occurred in man in eastern Europe and Asia. [Gk *pseudes* false, *amphi, stoma* mouth.]

pseudaphe, pseudaphia (sewd·**af**·e, sewd·**af**·e·ah). Pseudaesthesia. [Gk *pseudes* false, *haphe* touch.]

pseudarthrosis (sewd·ar·**thro**·sis). A false joint formed between the fragments of a fractured bone which have failed to unite. [Gk *pseudes* false, arthrosis.]

Pseudechis (sewd·**ek**·is). A genus of snakes of the subfamily Elapinae. **Pseudechis porphyriacus.** The poisonous black snake. **Pseudechis scutellatus.** A large poisonous snake of Australasia. [Gk *pseudes* false, *echis* snake.]

pseudelminth (sewd·**el**·minth). An artefact or foreign body which resembles a parasitic worm. [Gk *pseudes* false, *helmins* worm.]

pseudinoma (sewd·in·o·mah). A false tumour generally hard and imitative of a fibroma. [Gk *pseudes* false, *is* fibre, *-oma* tumour.]

pseudo-acanthosis (**sew**·do·ak·an·**tho'**·sis). **Pseudo-acanthosis nigricans.** A pigmented velvety thickening of the flexural skin, often with skin tags, occurring in obese, dark-complexioned individuals. [Gk *pseudes* false, *akantha* thorn, *-osis* condition.]

pseudo-acephalus (sew·do·a·**kef'**·al·us). A parasitic twin that is apparently headless but has cranial rudiments. [Gk *pseudes* false, *a, kephale* head.]

pseudo-achondroplasia (**sew**·do·a·kon·dro·**pla**′·ze·ah). A condition resembling achondroplasia but developing after birth; spondylo-epiphyseal dysplasia. Autosomal recessive. [Gk *pseudes* false, *a* without, *chondros* cartilage, *plassein* to form.]

pseudo-achromia (**sew**·do·a·**kro**′·me·ah). A partial hypopigmentation of the skin caused by pityriasis versicolor or tinea versicolor, an infection by the fungus *Malassezia furfur.* [Gk *pseudes* false, *a, chroma* colour.]

pseudo-acid (sew·do·**as**·id). A neutral organic compound which forms salts like a true acid owing to tautomeric molecular rearrangement. [Gk *pseudes* false, acid.]

pseudo-aconitine (**sew**·do·ak·**on**′·it·een). Acraconitine. [Gk *pseudes* false, aconitine.]

pseudo-acousia, pseudo-acousis, pseudo-acousma (**sew**·do·ak·**oo**′·se·ah, **sew**·do·ak·**oo**′·sis, **sew**·do·ak·**oos**′·mah). A defective hearing of sounds as if the quality and pitch were altered. [Gk *pseudes* false, *akoue* hearing.]

pseudo-actinomycosis (**sew**·do·ak·tin·o·mi·**ko**′·sis). A chronic granulomatous disease resembling actinomycosis, but caused by mycelial organisms other than the typical *Actinomyces bovis.* The term includes streptothrichosis, cladothricosis, pseudotuberculosis, nocardiasis, etc. [Gk *pseudes* false, actinomycosis.]

pseudo-aesthesia (**sew**·do·es·**the**′·ze·ah). Pseudaesthesia.

pseudo-agglutination (**sew**·do·ag·loo·tin·**a**′·shun). 1. Pseudohaemagglutination: the arrangement of erythrocytes in rouleaux, simulating agglutination. 2. Any other form of false agglutination. [Gk *pseudes* false, agglutination.]

pseudo-agraphia (**sew**·do·a·**graf**′·e·ah). Partial agraphia characterized by inability of the individual to write legibly or intelligibly although he can make a correct copy of writing. [Gk *pseudes* false, agraphia.]

pseudo-ainhum (sew·do·**ine**·hum). A term sometimes applied to ainhum when it is secondary to some congenital deformity, scleroderma, leprosy, syringomyelia or mutilating palmaplantar keratoderma. [Gk *pseudes* false, ainhum.]

pseudo-albuminuria (**sew**·do·al·**bew**·min·**ewr**′·e·ah). A condition, found mainly in young people, in which a small quantity of albumin is present in the urine at particular times of the day. [Gk *pseudes* false, albuminuria.]

pseudo-alveolar (**sew**·do·al·**ve**′·o·lar). Having the semblance of the structure of alveolar tissue. [Gk *pseudes* false, alveolus.]

pseudo-amenorrhoea (**sew**·do·am·en·or·**e**′·ah). Menstruation taking place with retention of the menses in the uterus or vagina. [Gk *pseudes* false, amenorrhoea.]

pseudo-anaemia (**sew**·do·an·**e**′·me·ah). Paleness of the complexion without the clinical or blood signs which are peculiar to anaemia. **Pseudo-anaemia angiospastica.** Pseudo-anaemia produced by vasoconstriction. [Gk *pseudes* false, anaemia.]

pseudo-anaphylactic (**sew**·do·an·ah·fil·**ak**′·tik). Relating or belonging to pseudo-anaphylaxis.

pseudo-anaphylaxis (**sew**·do·an·ah·fil·**ax**′·is). Anaphylactoid shock; a reaction with symptoms resembling those of anaphylaxis, produced by intravenous injection into normal animals of substances such as tissue extracts, snake venom, kaolin, charcoal, foreign sera, suspensions of bacteria, foreign red blood corpuscles, agar, starch and peptone. [Gk *pseudes* false, anaphylaxis.]

pseudo-angina (sew·do·an·**ji**′·nah). A condition found in nervous subjects, in which the predominant symptom is precordial pain; the attack is succeeded by fatigue and exhaustion, but is not as a rule associated with cardiac disease. [Gk *pseudes* false, angina.]

pseudo-angioma (**sew**·do·an·je·**o**′·mah). 1. The formation of a new canal through a thrombus in the portal vein, i.e. restoration of former lumen. 2. The angioma of transitory type such as that which sometimes forms on an amputation stump during the healing process. **Urethral pseudo-angioma.** A urethral carbuncle. [Gk *pseudes* false, angioma.]

pseudo-ankylosis (**sew**·do·an·kil·**o**′·sis). False or fibrous ankylosis. [Gk *pseudes* false, ankylosis.]

pseudo-anodontia (**sew**·do·an·o·**don**′·she·ah). A state in which the teeth are formed but eruption does not take place. [Gk *pseudes* false, anodontia.]

pseudo-anorexia (**sew**·do·an·or·**ex**′·e·ah). Refusal of food owing to fear of the pain caused by swallowing or resultant indigestion. [Gk *pseudes* false, anorexia.]

pseudo-antagonist (**sew**·do·an·**tag**′·on·ist). A muscle which, by flexing a given joint, diminishes the power of contraction of another flexor of the joint which acts also on a second joint. [Gk *pseudes* false, antagonist.]

pseudo-aphacia (**sew**·do·af·**a**′·se·ah). A word little used now, signifying apparent absence of the lens, as opposed to its dislocation, e.g. into the vitreous. In this condition, although the cortex of the lens has disappeared by absorption and shrinkage, the capsule and adventitious fibrous tissue are still present. [Gk *pseudes* false, aphacia.]

pseudo-apoplexy (sew·do·**ap**·o·plex·e). A state which simulates that of apoplexy but is not the result of cerebral haemorrhage. [Gk *pseudes* false, apoplexy.]

pseudo-appendicitis (**sew**·do·ap·en·dis·**i**′·tis). A condition characterized by symptoms of appendicitis but in which the appendix is healthy. **Pseudo-appendicitis zooparasitica.** The presence of parasites, e.g. worms, in the appendix. [Gk *pseudes* false, appendicitis.]

pseudo-apraxia (**sew**·do·ap·**rax**′·e·ah). A condition marked by extreme clumsiness and inco-ordination, with wrong use of everything handled. [Gk *pseudes* false, apraxia.]

See also: PICK (A.).

pseudo-arrhenia (**sew**·do·ar·**e**′·ne·ah). Pseudohermaphroditism in the female. [Gk *pseudes* false, *arrhen* male.]

pseudo-arteriosclerosis (**sew**·do·ar·**teer**·e·o·skler·**o**′·sis). A condition in which the arteries are tortuous, signs thus being produced which simulate those occurring in cases of true arteriosclerosis. [Gk *pseudes* false, arteriosclerosis.]

pseudo-asthma (sew·do·**as**·mah). Dyspnoea. [Gk *pseudes* false, asthma.]

pseudo-ataxia (**sew**·do·at·**ax**′·e·ah). A state of ataxia which is not caused by tabes dorsalis or other organic spinal lesion. [Gk *pseudes* false, ataxia.]

pseudo-athetosis (**sew**·do·ath·e·**to**′·sis). A derangement observed in those affected with tabes dorsalis and posterolateral sclerosis, characterized by athetosic movements of the fingers when the eyes are closed and the arms stretched out. [Gk *pseudes* false, athetosis.]

pseudo-atrophoderma colli (**sew**·do·at·ro·fo·**der**′·mah **kol**·li). An abnormality of the skin of the neck in which glossy, apparently atrophic, white areas of skin are surrounded by zones of darker colour, the deeper hue being due to minute folds in the skin. On microscopical examination, histological evidence of atrophy is not found. Spontaneous involution of the lesions may occur. Areas other than the neck may be affected. [Gk *pseudes* false, atrophoderma, L, of the neck.]

pseudobacillus (**sew**·do·bas·**il**′·us). Any object seen under the microscope that resembles a bacillus though it is not one, e.g. a very small rod-shaped red blood cell resembling a micro-organism. [Gk *pseudes* false, bacillus.]

pseudobacterium (**sew**·do·bak·**teer**′·e·um). Any object seen under the microscope which has the appearance of a bacterium though it is not one. [Gk *pseudes* false, bacterium.]

pseudobase (**sew**·do·base). A neutral organic compound which forms salts like a true base owing to tautomeral molecular rearrangement. [Gk *pseudes* false, base.]

pseudoblepsia, pseudoblepsis (sew·do·**blep**·se·ah, sew·do·**blep**·sis). False or defective vision. [Gk *pseudes* false, *blepein* to look.]

pseudobulbar (sew·do·**bul**·bar). Seemingly, but not in fact, caused by a lesion of the medulla oblongata. [Gk *pseudes* false, bulb.]

pseudocartilage (sew·do·**kar**·til·ij). Any tissue which resembles cartilage. [Gk *pseudes* false, cartilage.]

pseudocartilaginous (**sew**·do·kar·til·**aj**′·in·us). Relating or belonging to, or made up of tissue which is like cartilage in appearance and texture. [see prec.]

pseudocast (**sew**·do·kahst). A false cast occurring in urine deposits. [Gk *pseudes* false, cast.]

pseudocephalocele (sew·do·**kef**·al·o·seel). Non-congenital cerebellar hernia resulting from injury to or disease of the skull. [Gk *pseudes* false, cephalocele.]

pseudocerebrin (sew·do·**ser**·e·brin). $C_{44}H_{92}NO_8$, a substance formed by the hydrolysis of the protagon derived from brain tissue. [Gk *pseudes* false, cerebrin.]

pseudochalazion (sew·do·kal·**az**'·e·on). A tumour on the eyelid generally of the nature of a sarcoma or syphilitic lesion and having the appearance of a chalazion. [Gk *pseudes* false, chalazion.]

pseudochiasma (sew·do·ki·**az**'·mah). A chiasma-like configuration resulting from chromatid adhesion at homologous or non-homologous points during meiotic or mitotic cell division. [Gk *pseudes* false, chiasma.]

pseudocholecystitis (sew·do·ko·le·sist·**i**'·tis). A condition which is like inflammation of the gall bladder but not in fact inflammatory; in most cases the reaction is an allergic one, caused by eating certain kinds of food, to which the patient is susceptible. [Gk *pseudes* false, cholecystitis.]

pseudocholera (sew·do·**kol**·er·ah). A rare synonym for melioidosis. [Gk *pseudes* false, cholera.]

pseudocholesteatoma (sew·do·ko·le·ste·at·**o**'·mah). Horny epithelium found in a conglomerated mass in the tympanic cavity in chronic inflammation of the middle ear and having a strong resemblance to cholesteatoma. [Gk *pseudes* false, cholesteatoma.]

pseudocholinesterase (sew·do·ko·lin·**es**'·ter·aze). Applied to enzymes of the cholinesterase type which are most active in splitting choline esters, as distinct from acetylcholinesterase (also called *true cholinesterase*) which is most active in splitting acetylcholine. One person in 3000 is deficient in pseudocholinesterase and cannot adequately destroy the muscle relaxant, succinylcholine. [Gk *pseudes* false, cholinesterase.]

pseudochorea (sew·do·kor·**e**'·ah). Muscular inco-ordination, simulating true chorea. [Gk *pseudes* false, chorea.]

pseudochromaesthesia (sew·do·kro·mes·**the**'·ze·ah). An incomplete type of chromaesthesia in which there is perception of colour during the experience of hearing sounds. [Gk *pseudes* false, chromaesthesia.]

pseudochromhidrosis (sew·do·krome·hid·**ro**'·sis). Sweating distinguished by a local pigmentation on the skin caused by bacterial activity there. [Gk *pseudes* false, chromhidrosis.]

pseudochromia (sew·do·**kro**·me·ah). A condition in which the impression of colour is incorrect or at fault. [Gk *pseudes* false, *chroma* colour.]

pseudochromidrosis (sew·do·kro·mid·**ro**'·sis). Pseudochromhidrosis.

pseudochromosome (sew·do·**kro**·mo·some). A rod-like Golgi body of spermatocytes [obsolete term]. [Gk *pseudes* false, *chroma* colour, *soma* body.]

pseudochylous (sew·do·**ki**·lus). Like chyle but lacking the fatty or milky element. [Gk *pseudes* false, chyle.]

pseudocirrhosis (sew·do·sir·**o**'·sis). A disease which resembles cirrhosis of the liver, and is sometimes caused by inflammation of the pericardium; cardiac liver; Pick's disease. **Pericarditic pseudocirrhosis.** Pick's disease; Pick's syndrome. [Gk *pseudes* false, cirrhosis.]

pseudoclonus (sew·do·**klo**·nus). A clonic spasm which lasts for only a short time. [Gk *pseudes* false, clonus.]

pseudocoarctation (sew·do·ko·ark·**ta**'·shun). Kinking of the aorta just distal to the origin of the left subclavian artery, mimicking coarctation of the aorta but without true obstruction of the lumen. [Gk *pseudes* false, L *coarctare* to press together.]

pseudocodeine (sew·do·**ko**·de·een). $C_{18}H_{21}O_3N$, an isomer of codeine formed by the methylation of γ-isomorphine. It is a hypnotic resembling but less effective than codeine. [Gk *pseudes* false, codeine.]

pseudocoele (sew·do·seel). The cavity of the septum lucidum. [Gk *pseudes* false, *koilia* cavity.]

pseudocolloid (sew·do·**kol**·oid). A mucoid or colloid-like substance found on occasion in ovarian cysts and elsewhere. **Pseudocolloid of the lips.** Fox-Fordyce disease. [Gk *pseudes* false, colloid.]

pseudocoloboma (sew·do·kol·o·**bo**'·mah). A cicatrix or minute fissure on the iris which resembles a coloboma. [Gk *pseudes* false, coloboma.]

pseudocolonies (sew·do·**kol**·on·iz). Aggregations on the surface of a bacterial culture plate which are due to a physical change in the medium and not to micro-organismal growth. [Gk *pseudes* false, colony.]

peudoconjugation (sew·do·kon·jew·**ga**'·shun). The coming together and joining of individuals of a species without the interchange of nuclear material. [Gk *pseudes* false, L *conjugare* to yoke together.]

pseudoconstipation (sew·do·kon·stip·**a**'·shun). A condition observed in young infants on a diet of milk in which, after a period of regular (reflex) opening of the bowels, motions are passed only at relatively long intervals. There is no organic lesion to account for this, and change to a mixed diet usually effects a cure. [Gk *pseudes* false, constipation.]

pseudocorpus luteum (sew·do·kor·pus **loo**·te·um). A ripening vesicular ovarian follicle which does not break apart and discharge its ovum, and subsequently undergoes luteinization. [Gk *pseudes* false, corpus luteum.]

pseudocowpox (sew·do·**cow**·pox). A virus disease primarily of the teats and udders of cows which may be transmitted mechanically to cow-workers, etc., on whom milker's nodules (hard reddish nodules) then develop. The causative virus is a poxvirus of the paravaccinia subgroup. The disease is benign though the lesions may be indolent. [Gk *pseudes* false, AS *cu*, ME *pokkes*.]

pseudocoxalgia (sew·do·kox·**al**'·je·ah). Osteochondrosis of the capitular epiphysis (head) of the femur. [Gk *pseudes* false, coxalgia.]

pseudocrisis (sew·do·**kri**·sis). A sudden temporary lowering of the temperature occurring in pneumonia and some other diseases, which is succeeded by a heightened temperature; a false crisis. [Gk *pseudes* false, crisis.]

pseudocroup (sew·do·**kroop**). 1. Laryngismus stridulus. 2. Thymic asthma. [Gk *pseudes* false, croup.]

pseudocyesis (sew·do·si·**e**'·sis). Phantom pregnancy. *See* PREGNANCY. [Gk *pseudes* false, *kyesis* pregnancy.]

pseudocylindroid (sew·do·**sil**·in·droid). A small fragment of substance such as mucus present in the urine. It has resemblance to a cylindroid or other renal cast and may be of seminal origin. [Gk *pseudes* false, cylindroid.]

pseudocyst (sew·do·sist). False cyst; a cyst-like space which develops in a tissue as the result of softening or necrosis of the tissue. **Pseudocyst of the pancreas.** A cyst formed by distension of the lesser sac of the peritoneum as the result of leakage of pancreatic juice and consequent peritoneal irritation. [Gk *pseudes* false, cyst.]

pseudodecidual (sew·do·de·**sid**'·ew·al). The structure of the endometrium when the patient is treated with an oral contraceptive. It is so abnormal as to prevent implantation of a fertilized ovum.

pseudodementia (sew·do·de·**men**'·she·ah). A condition of extreme general apathy found in hysterical persons whose behaviour corresponds with their conception of insanity although they do not exhibit any signs of true dementia. [Gk *pseudes* false, dementia.]

pseudodextrocardia (sew·do·dex·tro·**kar**'·de·ah). Pathological displacement of the heart to the right side of the thorax, the concomitant physical signs simulating dextrocardia. [Gk *pseudes* false, dextrocardia.]

pseudodiarrhoea (sew·do·di·ar·**e**'·ah). Paradoxical diarrhoea. [Gk *pseudes* false, diarrhoea.]

pseudodiascope (sew·do·**di**·ah·skope). An instrument for demonstrating that visual sensations can last longer than the duration of the stimuli producing them. [Gk *pseudes* false, *dia*, *skopein* to view.]

pseudodiastolic (sew·do·di·as·**tol**'·ik). Seemingly, but not actually, diastolic. [Gk *pseudes* false, diastole.]

pseudodiphtheria (sew·do·dif·**theer**′·e·ah). Any disease with membranous formation resembling that of diphtheria. [Gk *pseudes* false, diphtheria.]

pseudodiphtheritic (sew·do·dif·ther·**it**′·ik). Relating or belonging to pseudodiphtheria.

pseudodiploidy (sew·do·dip·**loid**′·e). The presence of a diploid chromosome number without a true diploid complement of genes. This may result from duplication, deficiency, or both. [Gk *pseudes* false, *diploos* double, *eidos* form.]

Pseudodiscus watsoni (sew·do·**dis**·kus **wat**·son·i). A trematode that rarely affects man; it is normally a parasite of certain monkeys of the genera *Cercopithecus* and *Papio.* [Gk *pseudes* false, *diskos* disc.]

pseudodysentery (sew·do·**dis**·en·ter·e). A condition in which dysenteric symptoms are observed but which are due to causes other than infection with specific dysentery micro-organisms. It is, however, an ill-conceived word in view of the fact that the definition of dysentery includes many conditions other than that caused by specific micro-organisms. [Gk *pseudes* false, dysentery.]

pseudodyspepsia (sew·do·dis·**pep**′·se·ah). Gastric disorder of neurasthenic origin. [Gk *pseudes* false, dyspepsia.]

pseudo-embryonic (sew·do·em·bre·**on**′·ik). Seemingly, but not in fact, embryonic. [Gk *pseudes* false, embryonic.]

pseudo-emphysema (sew·do·em·fi·**se**′·mah). A morbid state which is like emphysema but caused by an obstructive condition of the bronchi which is transient. [Gk *pseudes* false, emphysema.]

pseudo-encephalitis (sew·do·en·kef·al·**i**′·tis). A morbid condition which resembles encephalitis but is caused by profuse, dehydrating diarrhoea. [Gk *pseudes* false, encephalitis.]

pseudo-encephalus (sew·do·en·**kef**′·al·us). A monster the brain of which is lacking, as well as the main bones of the skull; the latter is occupied by a vascular growth of mixed elements. [Gk *pseudes* false, *egkephalos* brain.]

pseudo-endometritis (sew·do·en·do·met·**ri**′·tis). A morbid state which resembles endometritis, characterized by overgrowth of the glands and stroma, circulatory abnormalities and atrophy of endothelial and other structures. [Gk *pseudes* false, endometritis.]

Pseudoephedrine (sew·do·**ef**·ed·reen). BP Commission approved name for (+)-2-methylamino-1-phenylpropan-1-ol, a stereoisomer of ephedrine; it is used as an antihistaminic and a cough suppressant.

pseudo-epilepsy (sew·do·ep·il·**ep**′·se). A condition which resembles epilepsy but which is, in part or entirely, due to rickets. [Gk *pseudes* false, epilepsy.]

pseudo-epiphysis (sew·do·ep·**if**′·is·is). The extremity of a bone, especially of a metacarpal, which superficially appears to have been ossified independently of the shaft but is in reality continuous with it, the mistake arising from the presence of a region of defective ossification near the end of the bone. [Gk *pseudes* false, epiphysis.]

pseudo-epithelioma (sew·do·ep·e·the·le·**o**′·mah). A cutaneous lesion which resembles an epithelioma. [Gk *pseudes* false, epithelioma.]

pseudo-erysipelas (sew·do·er·e·**sip**′·el·as). Inflammation affecting the subcutaneous tissues and simulating erysipelas. [Gk *pseudes* false, erysipelas.]

pseudo-exfoliation (sew·do·ex·fo·le·**a**′·shun). **Pseudo-exfoliation of the lens.** A condition affecting the elderly in which a white flaky material of unknown origin is deposited on the anterior surface of the lens and pupil margin. Simple glaucoma eventually supervenes. [Gk *pseudes* false, L *ex, folium* leaf.]

pseudo-exophoria (sew·do·ex·o·**for**′·e·ah). Exophoria due not to imbalance of the extra-ocular muscles but to diminished activity of the centre for accommodation. [Gk *pseudes* false, exophoria.]

pseudofever (sew·do·**fe**·ver). A questionable word used to indicate a state of high temperature without any discoverable exciting cause, and in many cases a hysterical manifestation. [Gk *pseudes* false, fever.]

pseudofibrin (sew·do·**fi**·brin). Parafibrinogen. [Gk *pseudes* false, fibrin.]

pseudoflagellata (sew·do·flaj·el·**a**′·tah). The microgametes of species of *Plasmodium;* they are produced in the mosquito gut from microgametocytes (the flagellated bodies). [Gk *pseudes* false, L *flagellum* whip.]

pseudofluctuation (sew·do·fluk·tew·**a**′·shun). Fluctuation elicited from soft solid swellings such as lipomata [obsolete term]. [Gk *pseudes* false, fluctuation.]

pseudofolliculitis (sew·do·fol·ik·ew·**li**′·tis). A papulopustular condition of the beard areas caused by ingrowing hairs. [Gk *pseudes* false, folliculitis.]

pseudofracture (sew·do·**frak**·tewr). A linear area of rarefaction of bone seen in x-rays, particularly of the scapula and pelvis in patients with osteomalacia. [Gk *pseudes* false, fracture.]

pseudofructose (sew·do·**fruk**·tose). Psicose, $CH_2OHCO(CHOH)_2CH_2OH$. A stereo-isomer of fructose.

pseudoganglion (sew·do·**gang**·gle·on). Local thickening or nodulation of a nerve simulating a ganglion. [Gk *pseudes* false, ganglion.]

pseudogastralgia (sew·do·gas·**tral**′·je·ah). A condition of pain simulating gastralgia which is not evoked by any disorder of the stomach and not in fact affecting the stomach but probably some contiguous organ such as the heart. [Gk *pseudes* false, gastralgia.]

pseudogenus (sew·do·je·nus). Having similar structural characteristics of a particular genus but not actually belonging to the genus in binominal nomenclature. [Gk *pseudes* false, genus.]

pseudogeusaesthesia (sew·do·gews·es·**the**′·ze·ah). A type of synaesthesia in which sensation of colour is evoked by the sensation of taste. [Gk *pseudes* false, *geusis* taste, aesthesia.]

pseudogeusia (sew·do·**gew**·se·ah). A condition in which there is a sensation of taste independent of any afferent stimuli. [Gk *pseudes* false, *geusis* taste.]

pseudoglaucoma (sew·do·glaw·**ko**′·mah). A condition of progressive atrophy and cupping of the optic disc, associated with field loss, simulating true glaucoma. The intra-ocular tension is never raised. [Gk *pseudes* false, glaucoma.]

pseudoglioma (sew·do·gli·**o**′·mah). A white reflex in the pupil caused by exudate in the vitreous and not by the presence of a new growth of the retina. It may follow meningitis and pyaemia, and is also seen in retrolental fibroplasia. [Gk *pseudes* false, glioma.]

pseudoglobulin (sew·do·**glob**·ew·lin). Water-soluble globulin which is not precipitated from salt solutions by dialysis against distilled water. Pseudoglobulin fractions occur in blood serum, in animal tissues and in milk, and may be separated from the euglobulin fractions by dialysis, which precipitates the latter, followed by precipitation by half-saturation with ammonium sulphate. [Gk *pseudes* false, globulin.]

pseudoglottis (sew·do·**glot**·is). False glottis. [Gk *pseudes* false, glottis.]

pseudogonococcus (sew·do·gon·o·**kok**′·us). Name given to a micrococcus isolated from urethral pus, now known as *Sarcina pseudogonorrhoeae* in the family Micrococcaceae. [Gk *pseudes* false, gonococcus.]

pseudogonorrhoea (sew·do·gon·o·**re**′·ah). Non-specific urethritis with urethral discharge. [Gk *pseudes* false, gonorrhoea.]

pseudogout (sew·do·**gowt**). Arthritis of large joints, characterized by calcification of articular cartilage and menisci with calcium pyrophosphate crystals in the synovial fluid. [Gk *pseudes* false, gout.]

pseudographia (sew·do·**graf**·e·ah). The writing of hieroglyphs that are without meaning. [Gk *pseudes* false, *graphein* to record.]

pseudogynaecomastia (sew·do·gi·ne·ko·**mas**′·te·ah). Mammary enlargement due to fat, in the male. [Gk *pseudes* false, *gyne* woman, *mastos* breast.]

pseudohaemagglutination (sew·do·he·mag·loo·tin·a′·shun). Aggregation of erythrocytes in rouleaux, simulating haemagglutination. [Gk *pseudes* false, haemagglutination.]

pseudohaemophilia (sew·do·he·mo·**fil**′·e·ah). One of several types of haemorrhagic condition occurring in either sex and resembling in many ways haemophilia (haemophilia in the female; hereditary haemophilia; afibrinogenopenia; prothrombinopenia). Features of haemophilia and of purpura may be noted. **Pseudohaemophilia hepatica.** A condition occurring in persons suffering from cirrhosis of the liver marked by the abnormal duration of the clotting time of the blood. **Hereditary pseudohaemophilia.** A familial haemorrhagic disease, occurring in either sex, and having normal platelet count and clotting time, but prolonged bleeding time, delayed clot retraction and increased capillary fragility. [Gk *pseudes* false, haemophilia.]

pseudohaemoptysis (sew·do·he·**mop**′·tis·is). A condition in which blood in the sputum is not from the lungs or bronchi. [Gk *pseudes* false, haemoptysis.]

Pseudohaje (sew·do·**ha**·je). A genus of snakes of the subfamily Elapinae; they are highly poisonous. [Gk *pseudes* false, Ar. *hayyah* snake.]

pseudohallucination (sew·do·hal·ew·sin·**a**′·shun). A hallucination recognized by the subject to have no external correlate. [Gk *pseudes* false, hallucination.]

pseudohemiacardius (sew·do·hem·e·a·**kar**′·de·us). A parasitic twin with no thorax. [Gk *pseudes* false, *hemi-* half, *a*, *kardia* heart.]

pseudohermaphrodism (sew·do·her·**maf**′·ro·dizm). Pseudohermaphroditism.

pseudohermaphrodite (sew·do·her·**maf**·ro·dite). One affected with pseudohermaphroditism.

pseudohermaphroditism (sew·do·her·**maf**′·ro·dit·izm). A congenital condition in which the gonads are either testes or ovaries but the external genitals are characteristic of the opposite sex or are a mixture of both male and female characters. It is classified into *testicular* or *male*, or *ovarian* or *female*, according to whether the gonads present are testes or ovaries, irrespective of the condition of the external genitals. [Gk *pseudes* false, hermaphroditism.]

pseudohernia (sew·do·**her**·ne·ah). Inflammation affecting an inguinal lymph gland or a hernial sac giving rise to symptoms and signs of strangulated hernia. [Gk *pseudes* false, hernia.]

pseudoheterotopia (sew·do·het·er·o·**to**′·pe·ah). The apparent occurrence of cells or tissues in abnormal situations due to their displacement by manipulation at autopsy, especially displaced grey and white matter in the central nervous system. [Gk *pseudes* false, heterotopia.]

pseudohydronephrosis (sew·do·hi·**dro**·nef·**ro**′·sis). A condition which is the result of the occurrence of a paranephric cyst; the signs and symptoms simulate those of hydronephrosis. [Gk *pseudes* false, hydronephrosis.]

pseudohydrophobia (sew·do·hi·dro·**fo**′·be·ah). Pseudorabies; a neurosis that may simulate rabies, in which there is irritability and mental depression and, in some cases, paroxysms. The condition may be observed in people who have been bitten by a dog supposedly rabid. [Gk *pseudes* false, hydrophobia.]

pseudohypertrophic (sew·do·hi·per·**trof**′·ik). Relating to or of the nature of pseudohypertrophy.

pseudohypertrophy (sew·do·hi·**per**′·tro·fe). Enlargement of an organ or part caused by overgrowth of fatty or fibrous tissue and not by overgrowth of the functioning elements. **Muscular pseudohypertrophy.** Pseudohypertrophic muscular dystrophy. *See* DYSTROPHY. [Gk *pseudes* false, hypertrophy.]

pseudohypha (sew·do·**hi**·fah). A filament resembling a hypha from the terminal cells of which are produced chlamydospores. [Gk *pseudes* false, hypha.]

pseudohypo-aldosteronism (sew·do·**hi**·po·al·do·**steer**′·on·izm). A salt-losing condition of infancy in which renal tubules are insensitive to salt-retaining hormones. [Gk *pseudes* false, *hypo* deficient, aldosteronism.]

pseudohypoparathyroidism (sew·do·**hi**·po·par·ah·**thi**′·roid·izm). A condition of end-organ resistance (Seabright bantam syndrome) to parathormone, characterized by hypocalcaemia, growth failure, short fingers and other skeletal disorders, ectopic calcification and often mental retardation. (The Seabright bantam cock's comb is like the hen's because of resistance to androgen.) **Pseudo-pseudohypoparathyroidism.** A condition with physical signs of pseudohypoparathyroidism but with normal levels of calcium and phosphorus in the blood. [Gk *pseudes* false, *hypo* deficient, parathyroid gland.]

pseudo-icterus (sew·do·**ik**·ter·us). Pseudojaundice. [Gk *pseudes* false, *ikteros* jaundice.]

pseudo-ileus (sew·do·**i**·le·us). Adynamic ileus; paralysis of the muscular wall of a segment of the bowel so that no movement takes place and a condition resembling intestinal obstruction occurs. It is seen with infarcts of the intestines due to obstruction of mesenteric arteries, and may also follow operations on the abdomen or injuries. [Gk *pseudes* false, ileus.]

pseudo-influenza (sew·do·in·floo·**en**′·zah). A vague term for any influenza-like infection, epidemic or sporadic, which is distinct from true virus influenza. [Gk *pseudes* false, influenza.]

pseudo-ion (sew·do·**i**·on). Name given to a charged particle in the disperse phase of a colloidal solution, owing to its migratory behaviour under an electrical potential. [Gk *pseudes* false, ion.]

pseudo-isochromatic (sew·do·i·so·kro·**mat**′·ik). Commonly applied to diagrams for testing colour discrimination (e.g. Isihara's test), in which dots, though differing in colour, appear similar to the colour-blind individual. [Gk *pseudes* false, *isos* equal, *chroma* colour.]

pseudo-isochromosome (sew·do·i·so·**kro**′·mo·some). A metacentric chromosome with homologous ends but non-homologous proximal segments. This chromosome cannot be the direct result of misdivision of the centromere. [Gk *pseudes* false, *isos* equal, chromosome.]

pseudojaundice (sew·do·**jawn**·dis). Discoloration of the skin produced by alterations in the blood, e.g. in Addison's disease, or by ingestion of coloured drugs and other substances, and not caused by hyperbilirubinaemia. [Gk *pseudes* false, jaundice.]

pseudokeratin (sew·do·**ker**·at·in). A keratin-like substance found in the skin and tissues of the nervous system. [Gk *pseudes* false, keratin.]

pseudoleprosy (sew·do·**lep**·ro·se). Punudos. [Gk *pseudes* false, leprosy.]

pseudoleukaemia (sew·do·lew·**ke**′·me·ah). Pseudosplenic leukaemia; a term applied to a variety of conditions with glandular enlargement, but without leukaemic changes in the blood. **Pseudoleukaemia cutis.** A pseudoleukaemic condition with cutaneous skin lesions. **Pseudoleukaemia gastrointestinalis.** A condition in which there is extensive infiltration of the mucous membrane of the gastrointestinal tract by lymphocytes, but without clinical or haematological evidence of leukaemia. **Infantile pseudoleukaemia.** Anaemia pseudoleukaemica infantum (von Jaksch), splenic anaemia of infants; a non-leukaemic condition described by von Jaksch in children under 3 years of age, showing a severe, often haemolytic type of anaemia, with erythroblasts in the blood, leucocytosis, a relative lymphocytosis, splenomegaly, hepatomegalia and enlarged lymphatic glands. Many patients recover and it is now considered to be a symptom complex and not a specific disease, associated with many conditions such as malnutrition, gastrointestinal disorders, rickets, syphilis, tuberculosis and other infections. **Pseudoleukaemia lymphatica.** A pseudoleukaemic condition without splenomegaly but showing involvement of lymphatic glands, as may be seen in Hodgkin's disease and certain lymphoid conditions of the intestines and kidneys. **Myelogenous pseudoleukaemia.** Myelomatosis. [Gk *pseudes* false, leukaemia.]

Pseudolimax (sew·do·**li**·max). *Iodamoeba.* [Gk *pseudes* false, *limax* slug.]

pseudolipoma (sew·do·lip·**o**′·mah). Neuropathic oedema, pseudo-oedema; a subcutaneous swelling occurring in hysterical patients simulating oedema, but without pitting on pressure. It is due to a fatty infiltration. [Gk *pseudes* false, lipoma.]

pseudolithiasis (sew·do·lith·**i**′·as·is). A condition in which there are symptoms such as those to be found in biliary colic, especially with spasmodic seizures in the region of the gall bladder. [Gk *pseudes* false, lithiasis.]

pseudologia, pseudology (sew·do·**lo**·je·ah, sew·**dol**·o·je). Falsehood in speech. **Pseudologia fantastica.** 1. Pathological lying. 2.

A state in which an extensive series of untruths is recounted, the subject believing it to be true. [Gk *pseudes* false, *logos* word.]

pseudoluxation (sew·do·lux·**a**′·shun). Partial dislocation of a joint. [Gk *pseudes* false, luxation.]

pseudolymphocyte (sew·do·**limf**·o·site). A leucocyte resembling a small lymphocyte, having neutrophil granules in the cytoplasm surrounding the deeply staining nucleus. [Gk *pseudes* false, lymphocyte.]

pseudolyssa (sew·do·**lis**·ah). Pseudorabies. [Gk *pseudes* false, lyssa.]

pseudomalaria (**sew**·do·mal·**a**′·re·ah). A febrile condition with frequent rigors, resembling malaria but due to other toxic causes. [Gk *pseudes* false, malaria.]

pseudomamma (sew·do·**mam**·ah). A glandular structure having the appearance of a nipple or of an entire mammary gland, found on occasion in dermoid cysts of the ovary. [Gk *pseudes* false, mamma.]

pseudomania (sew·do·**ma**·ne·ah). 1. Feigned insanity. 2. Speaking untruthfully as a manifestation of mental disease. [Gk *pseudes* false, mania.]

pseudomasturbation (**sew**·do·mas·ter·**ba**′·shun). A nervous tic consisting in continual pulling of the penis. [Gk *pseudes* false, masturbation.]

pseudomegacolon (sew·do·**meg**·ah·ko·lon). Dilatation of the colon occurring in the adult. [Gk *pseudes* false, megacolon.]

pseudomelanosis (**sew**·do·mel·an·**o**′·sis). A dark-coloured greenish or blackish pigmentation particularly of the surface of the abdominal viscera observed after death. It is caused by ferrous sulphide, the result of the action of sulphuretted hydrogen on the iron of broken-down haemoglobin. [Gk *pseudes* false, melanosis.]

pseudomembrane (sew·do·**mem**·brane). A false membrane such as is found in diphtheria. [Gk *pseudes* false, membrane.]

pseudomembranous (sew·do·**mem**·bran·us). Relating to or of the nature of a false membrane. [see prec.]

pseudomeningitis (sew·do·men·in·**ji**′·tis). A condition with symptoms like meningitis, with recovery. **Dental pseudomeningitis.** Symptoms suggesting meningitis in children with difficult dentition. [Gk *pseudes* false, meningitis.]

pseudomeningocele (**sew**·do·men·**ing**′·go·seel). A spurious meningocele arising from the skull with a fistula into one of the cerebral ventricles, as described by Billroth in 1862. [Gk *pseudes* false, meningocele.]

pseudomeninx (sew·do·**men**·ingx). A false membrane. [Gk *pseudes* false, *menigx* membrane.]

pseudomenstruation (**sew**·do·men·stroo·**a**′·shun). Haemorrhage from the uterus giving the appearance of menstruation but not associated with the basic changes in the endometrial tissues. [Gk *pseudes* false, menstruation.]

pseudometaplasia (**sew**·do·met·ah·**pla**′·ze·ah). An alteration in the form of a cell, resulting from external pressure or tension, and liable to be mistaken for true metaplasia. [Gk *pseudes* false, metaplasia.]

pseudomethaemoglobin (**sew**·do·met·he·mo·**glo**′·bin). A pigment derived from haemoglobin, observed in the serum of patients with haemolytic diseases, particularly blackwater fever, and after incompatible blood transfusions. It was formerly regarded as haematin, and later as methaemoglobin, but has been distinguished from the latter pigment by spectroscopic tests, its α band being situated between that of methaemoglobin and sulphmethaemoglobin and disappearing when the serum is treated with sodium hydrosulphite or strong ammonium sulphide, but not affected by dilute ammonium sulphide, ammonia or Stokes reagent. It may also be detected by Schumm's test. [Gk *pseudes* false, methaemoglobin.]

pseudomnesia (sew·do·**ne**·ze·ah). A condition in which the memory is perverted so that there is an impression of remembering events which in fact have not taken place. [Gk *pseudes* false, *mnesis* remembrance.]

Pseudomonadaceae (**sew**·do·mo·nad·**a**′·se·e). In systematic bacteriology, a family characterized as Gram-negative, straight or spirally curved rods, aerobic, non-sporing, and usually motile by polar flagella. The family comprises two tribes, Pseudomonadeae and Spirilleae. [see foll.]

pseudomonas (sew·do·**mo**·nas). A bacterial genus in the family Pseudomonadaceae; Gram-negative, non-sporing, motile bacilli, many producing pigments (greenish and fluorescent). They are widely distributed in the environment. **Pseudomonas aeruginosa.** *Pseudomonas pyocyanea* (see below). **Pseudomonas fluorescens.** A non-pathogenic strain; probably a saprophytic variant of *Pseudomonas pyocyanea.* **Pseudomonas pyocyanea.** The species associated with the term "blue pus" because of the bluish-green colour; it is causally related to human infections, often acquired in hospitals, e.g. wounds, eyes, urinary tract and, occasionally, meninges (purulent meningitis). [Gk *pseudes* false, *monas* unity.]

pseudomotor (sew·do·**mo**·tor). Productive of abnormal movements. [Gk *pseudes* false, L *motor* mover.]

pseudomycelium (**sew**·do·mi·**se**′·le·um). A form of mycelium-like growth characteristic of certain fungi such as *Candida.* [Gk *pseudes* false, mycelium.]

pseudomycosis sarcinia (**sew**·do·mi·**ko**′·sis sar·**sin**·e·ah). A disease of the lung at one time considered to be due to infection with *Sarcina virchowii.* [Gk *pseudes* false, mycosis, *Sarcina.*]

pseudomyopia (**sew**·do·mi·**o**′·pe·ah). A state in which patients with defective sight, not due to myopia, hold objects close to the eyes in order to see them. [Gk *pseudes* false, myopia.]

pseudomyxoma (**sew**·do·mix·**o**′·mah). A tumour or tumour-like condition that is rich in mucus. **Pseudomyxoma peritonei.** Mucinous infiltration of the peritoneum as the result of rupture of an ovarian cyst or of a mucocele of the appendix. [Gk *pseudes* false, *myxa* mucus, *-oma* tumour.]

pseudonarcotic (**sew**·do·nar·**kot**′·ik). Having a sedative effect but not producing narcosis. [Gk *pseudes* false, narcosis.]

pseudonarcotism (**sew**·do·**nar**·kot·izm). A stuporous state, of hysterical origin, resembling narcotism but not induced by the taking of drugs. [see prec.]

pseudoneoplasm (sew·do·**ne**·o·plasm). 1. A swelling of non-neoplastic character which may be diagnosed as neoplasm on account of the similarity of the clinical signs. 2. A phantom tumour. 3. Any circumscribed fibrous exudate of temporary duration resulting from an inflammatory condition. [Gk *pseudes* false, neoplasm.]

pseudoneuralgia (**sew**·do·newr·**al**′·je·ah). The pains which are peculiar to rickets (Charcot). [Gk *pseudes* false, neuralgia.]

pseudoneuritis (**sew**·do·newr·**i**′·tis). The blurring and apparent (sometimes actual) swelling of the optic disc which is seen in some cases of high hypermetropia and astigmatism as a physiological condition. Before papilloedema was differentiated from optic neuritis, all cases of swelling of the nerve head were designated optic neuritis, but it is usual nowadays to term the first-mentioned conditions *pseudopapilloedema.* [Gk *pseudes* false, neuritis.]

pseudoneuroma (**sew**·do·newr·**o**′·mah). A tumour present in a nerve trunk, but not composed of nerve substance; a false neuroma. [Gk *pseudes* false, neuroma.]

pseudonucleolus (**sew**·do·new·**kle**′·o·lus). A karyosome, or particle of chromatin within a cell nucleus, liable to be confused with the true nucleolus, or plasmosome. [Gk *pseudes* false, nucleolus.]

pseudonucleus (sew·do·**new**·kle·us). A swelling on a fibrous process of a cell, superficially resembling a nucleus. [Gk *pseudes* false, nucleus.]

pseudonystagmus (**sew**·do·nis·**tag**′·mus). Nystagmus of eccentric fixation, deviational nystagmus, Endstellung nystagmus, end-positional nystagmus: a horizontal nystagmoid movement of the eyes on extreme lateral gaze. It is physiological and of common occurrence, and is due to the fixation point being outside the binocular field. [Gk *pseudes* false, nystagmus.]

pseudo-ochronosis (**sew**·do·ok·ron·**o**′·sis). The condition of ochronosis when produced by artificial means. [Gk *pseudes* false, ochronosis.]

pseudo-ophthalmoplegia (**sew**·do·of·thal·mo·**ple**′·je·ah). 1. Hysterical ophthalmoplegia. 2. Conjugate paralysis of the eyes in which the voluntary movement is lost but reflex movement retained, e.g. inability to look to the left but ability to adduct the right eye in convergence. [Gk *pseudes* false, ophthalmoplegia.]

pseudo-optogram (sew·do·**op**·to·gram). In the preparation of an optogram, the rods may be stripped off the retina, leaving only the cones; this produces a false image. [Gk *pseudes* false, optogram.]

pseudo-osteomalacia (**sew**·do·os·te·o·mal·**a**'·she·ah). Rachitic softening of bones. [Gk *pseudes* false, osteomalacia.]

pseudopapilloedema (**sew**·do·pap·il·e·**de**'·mah). A congenitally swollen optic disc simulating papilloedema. Usually seen in hypermetropes and may also be due to buried drüsen. [Gk *pseudes* false, papilla, oedema.]

pseudoparalysis (**sew**·do·par·**al**'·is·is). The inability to move a limb or limbs. The loss of muscular power is only apparent, and there is no true paralysis. In infants it may be due to a painful condition of joints or bones as a result of syphilis, scurvy, rickets, etc. **Congenital atonic pseudoparalysis.** Amyotonia congenita. **Pseudoparalysis myasthenica.** Name applied to the muscular fatigue and weakness of myasthenia gravis. **Syphilitic pseudoparalysis.** Parrot's pseudoparalysis, that due to osteochondritis in congenital syphilis of infants. [Gk *pseudes* false, paralysis.]

See also: PARROT.

pseudoparaphrasia (**sew**·do·par·ah·**fra**'·ze·ah). A condition marked by disconnected and totally inconsequent speech and the constant use of incorrect names and words. [Gk *pseudes* false, paraphrasia.]

pseudoparaplegia (**sew**·do·par·ah·**ple**'·je·ah). Hysterical paraplegia. *See* PARAPLEGIA. [Gk *pseudes* false, paraplegia.]

pseudoparapsoriasis (**sew**·do·par·ah·sor·**i**'·as·is). Chronic superficial dermatitis. [Gk *pseudes* false, parapsoriasis.]

pseudoparasite (sew·do·**par**·ah·site). An object that resembles a parasite, but is not one. [Gk *pseudes* false, parasite.]

pseudoparesis (**sew**·do·par·e'·sis). Hysterical paralysis. *See* PARALYSIS. [Gk *pseudes* false, paresis.]

pseudoparkinsonism (sew·do·**par**·kin·son·izm). Any condition in which the developing muscular rigidity simulates parkinsonism. A well-known one is due to cerebral atheroma. **Arteriosclerotic pseudoparkinsonism.** A condition with some resemblance to Parkinson's disease resulting from cerebral arteriosclerosis. [Gk *pseudes* false, parkinsonism.]

pseudopelade (sew·do·**pe**·lade). A type of cicatricial alopecia in which one or several areas of baldness develop, extend peripherally, and may become confluent. The skin of the affected zones is white, smooth and slightly depressed. The cause is unknown. [Gk *pseudes* false, pelade.]

pseudopellagra (**sew**·do·pel·**ag**'·rah). Symptoms resembling those found in true pellagra which may occur in alcohol addicts. [Gk *pseudes* false, pellagra.]

pseudopelletierine (**sew**·do·pel·e·**ti**'·er·een). $C_9H_{15}NO$, one of the alkaloids of the pomegranate. Its derivatives have certain value as local anaesthetics.

pseudopericardial (**sew**·do·per·e·**kar**'·de·al). Apparently, but not in fact, derived from or related to the pericardium. [Gk *pseudes* false, pericardium.]

pseudoperitonitis (**sew**·do·per·it·on·**i**'·tis). A state of shock or acute neurosis characterized by symptoms similar to those occurring in cases of peritonitis but in which the characteristic peritoneal inflammation is not present. [Gk *pseudes* false, peritonitis.]

pseudophacia fibrosa (sew·do·**fak**·e·ah fi·**bro**·sah). Replacement of the lens by fibrous tissue. [Gk *pseudes* false, *phakos* lens, L, fibrous.]

pseudophlegmon (sew·do·**fleg**·mon). The local redness and swelling of the skin which is not inflammatory, but a vasomotor phenomenon. [Gk *pseudes* false, phlegmon.]

See also: HAMILTON.

pseudophoto-aesthesia (**sew**·do·fo·to·es·**the**'·ze·ah). A type of synaesthesia in which a sensation of light is perceived when any of the other organs of sense is stimulated. [Gk *pseudes* false, photo-aesthesia.]

Pseudophyllidea (**sew**·do·fil·**id**'·e·ah). An order of Cestoidea. The species have lateral or terminal slits or bothria on the scolex. The genus *Diphyllobothrium* is of medical interest. [Gk *pseudes* false, *phyllon* leaf.]

pseudoplasm (**sew**·do·plazm). A neoplasm-like swelling that does not involve any structural change and disappears spontaneously; a phantom tumour. [Gk *pseudes* false, *plasma* something formed.]

pseudoplegia (sew·do·**ple**·je·ah). 1. Pseudoparalysis. 2. Hysterical paralysis. [Gk *pseudes* false, *plege* stroke.]

pseudopneumonia (**sew**·do·new·**mo**'·ne·ah). A disease in which there are many symptoms characteristic of pneumonia but in which the pulmonary lesions are not to be found. [Gk *pseudes* false, pneumonia.]

pseudopod (**sew**·do·pod). Pseudopodium.

pseuopodiospore (sew·do·**po**·de·o·spore). Amoebula. [Gk *pseudes* false, *pous* foot, spore.]

pseudopodium (sew·do·**po**·de·um). A protoplasmic process extruded by an amoeba to facilitate movement or to ingest food. [Gk *pseudes* false, *pous* foot.]

pseudopolymelia paraesthetica (**sew**·do·pol·e·**me**'·le·ah par·es·**thet**·ik·ah). A paraesthesia in which there is the subjective and illusory sensation of movements in parts of the body. [Gk *pseudes* false, *polys* many, *melos* limb, paraesthesia.]

pseudopolyposis (**sew**·do·pol·e·**po**'·sis). Widely scattered polypi in the intestine; often a result of previous inflammation. [Gk *pseudes* false, polypus, *-osis* condition.]

pseudoporencephalia (**sew**·do·po·ren·kef·**a**'·le·ah). The existence of a condition simulating porencephalia but lacking the mental symptoms peculiar to this defect. [Gk *pseudes* false, porencephalia.]

pseudopregnancy (sew·do·**preg**·nan·se). Phantom pregnancy; any abdominal condition resembling pregnancy. [Gk *pseudes* false, pregnancy.]

pseudo-pseudohypoparathyroidism (sew·do·**sew**·do·hi·po·par·ah·**thi**'·roid·izm). A syndrome that demonstrates many of the clinical signs but none of the biochemical features of pseudohypoparathyroidism, the serum calcium level being normal.

pseudopsia (sewd·**op**·se·ah). False or defective vision. [Gk *pseudes* false, *opsis* vision.]

pseudopterygium (**sew**·do·ter·**ij**'·e·um). A fold of conjunctiva that has become attached to the cornea following an injury or ulcer near the limbus. It is differentiated from a true pterygium by the passing of a probe under the neck at the limbus. [Gk *pseudes* false, *pterygion* wing.]

pseudoptosis (sewd·op·**to**·sis). Abnormally small palpebral fissure. [Gk *pseudes* false, *ptosis* fall.]

pseudoptyalism (sew·do·**ti**·al·izm). Dribbling of saliva, due to excessive accumulation resulting from failure to swallow it for any reason, e.g. dysphagia. [Gk *pseudes* false, *ptyalon* saliva.]

pseudopunicine (sew·do·**pew**·nis·een). Pseudopelletierine.

pseudopus (**sew**·do·pus). A fluid substance that has the appearance of, but is not, pus, [Gk *pseudes* false, pus.]

pseudorabies (sew·do·**ra**·beez). A virus disease of animals due to a herpesvirus and showing a wide range of severity from an almost inapparent infection in pigs to a severe pruritis in cattle, sheep and carnivores (mad itch). It is not easily transmitted to man in whom only a mild pruritus occurs. [Gk *pseudes* false, L *rabere* to rave.]

pseudorachitis (**sew**·do·rak·**i**'·tis). Osteitis deformans. [Gk *pseudes* false, rachitis.]

pseudoreaction (**sew**·do·re·**ak**'·shun). A false reaction. [Gk *pseudes* false, reaction.]

pseudoreduction (**sew**·do·re·**duk**'·shun). The pairing of homologous chromosomes in meiosis, resulting in the apparent halving of their number. [Gk *pseudes* false, reduction.]

pseudoreminiscence (**sew**·do·rem·in·**is**'·ens). Confabulation; the recital of experiences that have no foundation in fact, usually in compensation for a gap in memory. [Gk *pseudes* false, reminiscence.]

pseudorheumatism (sew·do·**roo**·mat·izm). Any form of multiple arthritis not of the same aetiology as that of acute rheumatism.

Infectious pseudorheumatism. Infectious polyarthritis and/or synovitis that is not due to the streptococci which cause acute rheumatism. [Gk *pseudes* false, rheumatism.]

pseudorhonchus (sew·do·**rong**·kus). A false râle; an adventitious sound heard on auscultation of the lungs and resembling one associated with pulmonary disease. [Gk *pseudes* false, *rhogchos* snore.]

pseudorickets (sew·do·**rik**·etz). Renal rickets; osteodystrophy. [Gk *pseudes* false, rickets.]

pseudorubella (**sew**·do·roo·**bel**′·ah). Exanthema subitum; roseola infantilis; roseola infantum; sixth disease. [Gk *pseudes* false, rubella.]

pseudosarcoma (**sew**·do·sar·**ko**′·mah). A spindle cell epithelioma in x-irradiated skin, histologically resembling fibrosarcoma. [Gk *pseudes* false, sarcoma.]

pseudoscarlatina (**sew**·do·skar·lat·**e**′·nah). A condition in which there is an erythematous rash resembling that of scarlet fever but without the other signs of that disease. It may be due to certain drugs such as copaiba, to the injection of serum, or to septic poisoning. [Gk *pseudes* false, scarlatina.]

pseudosclerema (**sew**·do·skler·**e**′·mah). Adiponecrosis subcutanea neonatorum. [Gk *pseudes* false, *skleros* hard.]

pseudoscleroderma (**sew**·do·skler·o·**der**′·mah). The pigmented, oedematous indurated skin of the lower third of the leg in the post-thrombotic syndrome. [Gk *pseudes* false, scleroderma.]

pseudosclerosis (**sew**·do·skler·**o**′·sis). A disease with symptoms of disseminated sclerosis but without the lesions, and due to a neurosis; Westphal's pseudosclerosis. **Pseudosclerosis spastica.** 1. Inflammatory induration simulating fibrosis. 2. Westphal's pseudosclerosis; hysteria with symptoms of disseminated sclerosis. [Gk *pseudes* false, sclerosis.]

See also: STRUEMPELL, WESTPHAL (C. F. O.).

pseudosmallpox (sew·do·**smawl**·pox). Variola minor. [Gk *pseudes* false, smallpox.]

pseudosmia (sew·**doz**·me·ah). A condition in which the subject perceives odours that do not exist. [Gk *pseudes* false, *osme* odour.]

pseudosolution (**sew**·do·sol·**ew**′·shun). Name applied to a colloidal solution to differentiate it from a true solution. [Gk *pseudes* false, solution.]

pseudospleen (**sew**·do·spleen). An accessory spleen. [Gk *pseudes* false, spleen.]

pseudostoma (sew·do·**sto**·mah). An artificial gap between the cells of an epithelium, resulting from shrinkage in the preparation of sections. [Gk *pseudes* false, *stoma* mouth.]

pseudostratified (sew·do·**strat**·e·fide). Describing a type of columnar epithelium in which the nuclei of adjacent cells lie at different levels, so that the epithelium appears stratified to superficial observation. [Gk *pseudes* false, stratum.]

pseudosyphilis (sew·do·**sif**·il·is). A condition in which the skin manifestations resemble those of syphilis, but clear up with non-specific treatment. [Gk *pseudes* false, syphilis.]

pseudosyringomyelia (**sew**·do·sir·**ing**·go·mi·**e**′·le·ah). A disorder of the spinal cord characterized by cavitation, due to cysts, injuries or imperfect development. [Gk *pseudes* false, syringomyelia.]

pseutotabes (sew·do·**ta**·beez). A general wasting of the muscles with recovery in the absence of any syphilitic pathology. It is possibly associated with polyneuritis, with symptoms suggesting tabes dorsalis. **Alcoholic pseudotabes.** Peripheral neuritis due to alcohol. **Pseudotabes arsenicosa.** Arsenical neuritis. **Diabetic pseudotabes.** Peripheral neuritis due to diabetes. **Pseudotabes mesenterica.** Tuberculosis of mesenteric glands. **Pseudotabes peripherica.** The pseudotabes of peripheral neuritis. **Pseudotabes pituitaria.** Simmonds' disease; gross general wasting, atrophy of skin and bones, and premature senility. **Pupillotonic pseudotabes.** Tonic pupil; Adie's syndrome. [Gk *pseudes* false, tabes.]

pseudotetanus (sew·do·**tet**·an·us). Long-continued tonic spasm of the muscles which simulates tetanus but where *Clostridium tetani* cannot be isolated. **Hysterical pseudotetanus.** Tonic spasm of the muscles of hysterical origin. [Gk *pseudes* false, tetanus.]

Pseudothelphusa (**sew**·do·thel·**few**′·sah). A genus of crayfish, a possible intermediary host of *Paragonimus westermani.* [Gk *pseudes* false, *Thelphousa* town in Arcadia.]

pseudothrill (**sew**·do·thril). A false thrill. [Gk *pseudes* false, thrill.]

pseudotrachoma (**sew**·do·trak·**o**′·mah). A condition affecting the eyes and eyelids, simulating trachoma. [Gk *pseudes* false, trachoma.]

pseudotrichiniasis, pseudotrichinosis (sew·do·trik·in·**i**′·as·is, **sew**·do·trik·in·**o**′·sis). Acute disseminated dermatomyositis which superficially resembles trichiniasis. [Gk *pseudes* false, trichiniasis.]

pseudotropine (sew·do·**tro**·peen). $C_8H_{15}NO$, an optically inactive sterero-isomer of tropine produced by the hydrolysis of certain species of coca. [Gk *pseudes* false, tropine.]

pseudotruncus arteriosus (sew·do·**trung**·kus **ar**·teer·e·**o**′·sus). A term sometimes applied to pulmonary atresia with a ventricular septal defect. The pulmonary blood flow is carried to the pulmonary arteries by collateral vessels from the aorta. [Gk *pseudes* false, L *truncus* trunk, artery.]

pseudotuberculoma (**sew**·do·tew·ber·kew·**lo**′·mah). A granulomatous mass resembling tuberculosis but not caused by the tubercle bacillus. **Pseutotuberculoma silicoticum.** A granulomatous mass caused by the impaction of siliceous material, especially gravel, in the subcutaneous tissues. [Gk *pseudes* false, tubercle, Gk *-oma* tumour.]

pseudotuberculosis (**sew**·do·tew·ber·kew·**lo**′·sis). A collective term for certain diseases of the lungs in man or animals which are due to micro-organisms other than the tubercle bacillus. **Pseudotuberculosis hominis streptothrica.** Any streptothrix infection in man in which the lesions resemble tuberculosis. [Gk *pseudes* false, tuberculosis.]

pseudotumour (**sew**·do·tew·mor). A phantom tumour. *See* TUMOUR. **Pseudotumour cerebri.** Papilloedema and perhaps headache and abducent-nerve palsy with various causes, especially corticosteroid medication and sinus thrombosis. **Orbital pseudotumour.** A chronic inflammatory condition of the tissues of the orbit, presenting with symptoms of a new growth.

pseudotympanites, pseudotympany (**sew**·do·tim·pan·**i**′·teez, sew·do·**tim**·pan·e). Distension of the abdomen due to such causes as air swallowing or hysterical spasm of the diaphragm. [Gk *pseudes* false, tympanites.]

pseudotyphoid (sew·do·**ti**·foid). Any of a number of diseases with symptoms resembling those of typhoid fever which are not produced by the *Salmonella typhi* and in which the lesions characteristic of that disease are absent. [Gk *pseudes* false, typhoid.]

pseudotyphus (sew·do·**ti**·fus). Any disease, other than a rickettsiosis, resembling typhus. [Gk *pseudes* false, typhus.]

pseudovacuole (sew·do·**vak**·ew·ole). A vacuole-like structure in a cell that is not in fact a vacuole; occurring in a blood or fixed tissue cell, it may be a parasite. [Gk *pseudes* false, vacuole.]

pseudovalves (**sew**·do·valvz). False valves; tiny endocardial pockets which develop in the wall of the left ventricle when the aortic valve is incompetent. [Gk *pseudes* false, valves.]

pseudovariola (**sew**·do·var·**i**′·o·lah). Variola minor. [Gk *pseudes* false, variola.]

pseudovermicule, pseudovermiculus (sew·do·**ver**·mik·ewl, sew·do·ver·**mik**′·ew·lus). A term used by Danilewski (1889) for a stage in the developing gregarine in the mosquito, and subsequently applied to the corresponding stage in the plasmodium; this stage is now called the *oökinete.* [Gk *pseudes* false, L *vermiculus* little worm.]

pseudovoice (**sew**·do·vois). A voice produced by artificial means in an individual who has lost his natural voice following the removal of the larynx. It may be accomplished by means of an instrument or by the use of the pharynx to produce a pharyngeal voice. This latter usually requires special training. [Gk *pseudes* false, voice.]

pseudovomiting (sew·do·**vom**·it·ing). Regurgitation of food and other matter from the oesophagus or stomach without any attempt to expel it. [Gk *pseudes* false, vomiting.]

pseudoxanthoma elasticum (sew·do·zan·**tho**′·mah e·**las**·tik·um). A papular eruption affecting the sides of the neck and other areas, particularly the skin folds on the trunk and the flexor surfaces of the larger joints. The papules are discrete, from 2 to 5 mm in diameter, irregular in size and outline, arranged in rows, and the colour of old ivory; occasionally plaques are formed by their coalescence. The lesions tend to be symmetric in distribution and they do not itch. Oral lesions have been described. Frequently angioid streaks are found in the retinae. [Gk *pseudes* false, xanthoma, elastic tissue.]

pseudozooglea (sew·do·zo·**og**′·le·ah). Bacterial clumps which do not readily break up into their components in a watery menstruum, but which are not embedded in a jelly-like mass. [Gk *pseudes* false, zooglea.]

pseudulcus (sewd·**ul**·kus). A sore which has the appearance of, but is not, an ulcer. **Pseudulcus ventriculi.** A type of neurosis in which sensations in the stomach simulate the symptoms of gastric ulcer. [Gk *pseudes* false, L *ulcus* ulcer.]

psi (si). A term coined to designate any phenomenon inexplicable by recourse to scientific knowledge; a paranormal phenomenon. [Greek letter.]

psicose (si·koze). $CH_2OH(CHOH)_3COCH_2OH$, a ketohexose, stereo-isomeric with fructose and corresponding in structure with ribose.

Psilocybin (si·lo·si·bin). BP Commission approved name for 3-(2-dimethylaminoethyl)indol-4-yl dihydrogen phosphate; a psychotomimetic drug.

psilosis (si·**lo**·sis). 1. Loss or falling of the hair. 2. Sprue. **Psilosis pigmentosa.** Pellagra. [Gk *psilos* bald.]

psilothron (**si**·lo·thron). A depilatory agent. [Gk *psiloein* to strip bare.]

psilotic (si·**lot**·ik). 1. Depilatory. 2. Characterized by psilosis. [see prec.]

psittacosis (sit·ah·**ko**·sis). An acute infectious avian disease especially affecting parrots caused by a filtrable virus, and transmitted to human beings. In man the condition closely resembles typhoid fever but signs of primary atypical pneumonia are also present; slight abdominal distension, fever and diarrhoea are characteristic symptoms. [Gk *psittakos* parrot.]

psoas (so·as). A psoas muscle. [Gk *psoa* muscle of the loin.]

psoas major muscle [musculus psoas major (NA)] (so·as **ma**·jor musl). A long muscle extending from the sides of the vertebral column in the lumbar region to the lesser trochanter of the femur. It is a strong flexor of the hip joint.

psoas minor muscle [musculus psoas minor (NA)] (so·as **mi**·nor musl). A slender muscle running from the 12th thoracic and 1st lumbar vertebrae to the arcuate line on the ilium. It is frequently absent.

psodymus (**sod**·im·us). A twin monster having separate heads and thoraces and united from the lumbar region downwards. [Gk *psoa* muscle of the loin, *didymos* twin.]

psoitis (so·i·tis). Inflammation affecting one of the psoas muscles or its sheath. [Gk *psoa* muscle of the loin, *-itis* inflammation.]

psomophagia, psomophagy (so·mo·**fa**·je·ah, so·**mof**·aj·e). The habit of swallowing food which has not been thoroughly masticated. [Gk *psomos* gobbet, *phagein* to eat.]

psora (**so**·rah). A name which in the past has been applied to scabies, impetigo *(ulcerated psora)* and various forms of pityriasis and scaly eczematous conditions (*rough* or *leprous psora*). [Gk, itch.]

psorelcosis (so·rel·**ko**·sis). Ulceration of the skin due to scabies or other itching conditions [obsolete term]. [Gk *psora* itch, *helkos* ulcer, *-osis* condition.]

psorenteria (so·ren·**teer**·e·ah). A pathological condition of the intestines in which the closed follicles are unduly prominent. [Gk *psora* itch, *enteron* intestine.]

psorenteritis (so·ren·ter·i′·tis). An inflammation of the intestines, characteristic of Asiatic cholera. [Gk *psora* itch, enteritis.]

psoriasic (so·re·**as**·ik). Pertaining to, characterized by, or suffering from psoriasis.

psoriasiform (so·**ri**·as·e·form). Having the appearance of psoriasis. [psoriasis, form.]

psoriasis (so·**ri**·as·is). A chronic inflammatory disease of the skin, characterized by the appearance, usually on certain sites of election (knees, elbows, scalp), of whitish or silvery laminated scales, aggregated in greater or less profusion on slightly raised, well-marginated, reddish patches. Widespread efflorescences of the eruption may occur. The lesions are dry, and have a predilection for extensor surfaces. Psoriasis is neither infectious nor contagious. **Psoriasis annularis.** Circular or oval ring-like lesions of psoriasis. **Psoriasis arthropathica.** Psoriatic arthropathy. *See* ARTHROPATHY. **Psoriasis buccalis.** Leucoplakia of the mouth. **Psoriasis circinata.** A form of psoriasis in which the lesions are small coin-like discs. **Psoriasis diffusa.** 1. The term now used to denote a severe efflorescence in which large areas are completely covered with the eruption. 2. Employed by Willan to denote psoriasis pistorum (see below). **Psoriasis discoides.** Psoriasis nummularis (see below). **Erythrodermic psoriasis.** Psoriasis universalis (see below). **Exfoliative psoriasis.** Psoriasis universalis (see below). **Psoriasis figurata.** A figurate or patterned form of the eruption. **Psoriasis follicularis.** A form of psoriasis punctata (see below), in which the lesions appear to be follicular. **Psoriasis geographica.** Psoriasis in which lesions spread peripherally and may run into one another, so that they form gyrate figures that resemble the map of a group of islands. **Psoriasis guttata.** A form of the eruption in which the numerous lesions resemble drops of wax on the skin. **Psoriasis gyrata.** A type in which the eruption is arranged in rings. **Psoriasis inveterata.** Psoriasis in which the lesions are remarkably resistant to treatment. **Psoriasis linguae.** Leucoplakia of the tongue. **Napkin psoriasis.** Psoriasiform lesions mostly in the napkin area and sometimes associated with *Candida albicans* infection. **Psoriasis nummularis.** Psoriasis in which the eruption consists of coin-shaped discs. **Psoriasis ostreacea.** Psoriasis in which the scales accumulate until the lesions resemble small oyster-shells. **Psoriasis palmaris et plantaris.** Involvement of the palms and soles with psoriasis. **Psoriasis pistorum.** Bateman's name for scaly occupational eruptions occurring among persons, particularly bakers, who work among dusty substances; bakers' itch. **Psoriasis punctata.** A psoriasis eruption, usually widespread, of tiny maculopapules covered with scales. **Pustular psoriasis.** A symmetrical eruption of small sterile pustules which dry up to form a brownish scab; crops of pustules keep appearing. The malady undergoes periods of exacerbation and quiescence. **Psoriasis rupioides.** Psoriasis ostreacea (see above), particularly if, as sometimes happens, the scales are stuck together with a gum-like exudation. **Psoriasis spondylitica.** Ankylosing spondylitis associated with psoriasis. This is a variety of psoriatic arthropathy which may occur with changes in other joints. **Psoriasis of the tongue.** Leucoplakia of the tongue. **Psoriasis universalis.** A severe generalized eruption of psoriasis in which almost the whole of the skin surface is involved. [Gk, itch.]

psoriatic (so·ri·**at**·ik). Pertaining to, characterized by, or suffering from psoriasis.

psoric (**so**·rik). Relating to or characterized by psora or scabies.

psoroid (**so**·roid). Like psora or scabies. [psora, Gk *eidos* form.]

Psorophora (so·**rof**·or·ah). A genus of large mosquitoes, not generally associated with disease (except see below). **Psorophora ferox.** A mosquito that is a potential vector of yellow fever. [Gk *psora* itch, *pherein* to bear.]

psorophthalmia (so·rof·**thal**·me·ah). An ulcerative type of marginal blepharitis. [Gk *psora* itch, ophthalmia.]

Psoroptes (so·**rop**·teez). A genus of mites parasitic in domestic animals, but seldom attacking man. **Psoroptes communis.** The species that causes psoroptosis in domestic animals. [Gk *psora* itch, *Sarcoptes*.]

psoroptosis (so·rop·**to**·sis). A form of scabies which affects sheep, horses and cattle, but which is almost unknown in man.

Psoroptes communis is the mite responsible, and the lesions it produces are characterized by thick scabs and severe pruritus, but burrows are not found. [psoroptes, Gk *-osis* condition.]

psorosperm (**so**·ro·sperm). The encysted stage in Sporozoa; the term is now archaic. [Gk *psoros* rough, *sperma* seed.]

psorospermiasis, psorospermosis (**so**·ro·sper·**mi**'·as·is, so·ro·sper·**mo**'·sis). Proliferative follicular psorospermosis; psorospermose folliculaire végétante; Darier's disease; keratosis follicularis (White and Brown); keratosis vegetans (Crocker): a chronic eruption, often familial, characterized by the appearance of small, firm, follicular, reddish papules, which enlarge and may coalesce to form papilliferous, confluent, crusted excrescences. The mucosae may be involved. The eruption usually begins in childhood on the face and head; later the front of the chest, the loins, the groins and the genital regions are involved. [Gk *psoros* rough, *sperma* seed, *-osis* condition.]

psorous (**so**·rus). Psoric.

psychagogia, psychagogy (si·kah·**go**·je·ah, si·kah·**go**·je). A state in which the mental processes are excited or stimulated to greater activity. [Gk *psyche* mind, *agogos* eliciting.]

psychalgalia (si·kal·**ga**·le·ah). Psycho-algalia.

psychalgia (si·**kal**·je·ah). 1. Pain of mental causation. 2. The pain of mental distress. [Gk *psyche* mind, *algos* pain.]

psychalia (si·**ka**·le·ah). An abnormal mental condition characterized by the imaginary hearing of voices and visual hallucinations. [Gk *psyche* mind.]

psychanopsia (si·kan·**op**·se·ah). Mind blindness. *See* BLINDNESS. [Gk *psyche* mind, anopsia.]

psychasthenia (si·kas·**the**·ne·ah). 1. All psychoneuroses other than hysteria (Janet). 2. Those psychoneuroses characterized especially by fears and phobias. [Gk *psyche* mind, *astheneia* lack of strength.]

psychasthenic (si·kas·**then**·ik). Pertaining to or having the characteristics of psychasthenia.

psyche (**si**·ke). Mind, as opposed to body. [Gk, mind.]

psycheclampsia (si·ke·**klamp**·se·ah). Psychlampsia.

psychedelic (**si**·ki·de·lik). 1. Mind-opening. 2. Pertaining to drugs whose immediate action seems to expand the consciousness and enlarge the vision. [Gk *psyche* mind, *deloun* manifest.]

psycheism (**si**·ke·izm). Hypnotism. [Gk *psyche* mind.]

psychentonia (si·ken·**to**·ne·ah). Fatigue or over-exercise of the mind. [Gk *psyche* mind, *entonos* strained.]

psychiatric (si·ki·**at**·rik). Belonging or relating to psychiatry.

psychiatrics (si·ki·**at**·rix). The science of psychiatry.

psychiatrist (si·**ki**·at·rist). A medically qualified person who has undergone postgraduate training extending over many years in psychiatry.

psychiatry (si·**ki**·at·re). The branch of medicine dealing with disorders involving mental life and behaviour. [Gk *psyche* mind, *iatreia* medical treatment.]

psychic (**si**·kik). Pertaining to a class of alleged phenomena belonging to that branch of learning known as parapsychology. [Gk *psyche* mind.]

psychical (si·kik·al). Psychic. [Gk *psyche* mind.]

psychinosis (si·kin·**o**·sis). Any disordered state of the mind; psychopathy. [Gk *psyche* mind, *nosos* disease.]

psychism (**si**·kizm). The theory that all forms of life are animated by a universal fluid. [Gk *psyche* spirit.]

psychlampsia (si·**klamp**·se·ah). Acute mania. [Gk *psyche* mind, *lampsis* shining.]

psycho-algalia (si·ko·al·**ga**'·le·ah). A melancholic state which on occasion leads to suicide, characterized by distorted visual and auditory sensations and producing fear or hopelessness. [Gk *psyche* mind, *algos* pain.]

psycho-allergy (si·ko·**al**·er·je). Acquired sensitization to a mental concept. [Gk *psyche* mind, allergy.]

psycho-analysis (si·ko·an·**al**'·is·is). 1. A procedure developed by Freud for the investigation of unconscious mental processes, in particular by the use of free association and the study of dreams. 2. A method based upon that investigation, for the treatment of mental disorders. 3. A system of psychological development based on information obtained along these lines. [Gk *psyche* mind, analysis.]

psycho-analyst (si·ko·**an**·al·ist). One who practises psycho-analysis.

psycho-analytic (si·ko·an·al·**it**'·ik). Relating to psycho-analysis.

psycho-asthenia (si·ko·as·**the**'·ne·ah). Mental deficiency. [Obsolete term.] [Gk *psyche* mind, asthenia.]

psycho-asthenics (si·ko·as·**then**'·ix). That branch of medicine which deals with the study and treatment of feeble-minded persons. [Obsolete term.] [see prec.]

psycho-ataxia (si·ko·at·**ax**'·e·ah). A state of disordered mentality in which the individual is confused, lacks the ability to concentrate, and is easily excited. [Gk *psyche* mind, ataxia.]

psycho-auditory (si·ko·**aw**·dit·or·e). Relating or belonging to consciousness and perception of sound and to the intelligent interpretation of it. [Gk *psyche* mind, auditory.]

psychobiology (si·ko·bi·**ol**'·o·je). 1. The study of man as an integrated person, within the general framework of biology. 2. The name given to the school of psychiatry of Adolf Meyer. [Gk *psyche* mind, biology.]

psychocatharsis (si·ko·kath·**ar**'·sis). Catharsis 2nd def. [Gk *psyche* mind, catharsis.]

psychochemistry (si·ko·**kem**·is·tre). The employment of chemical science in the study of psychology and in the treatment of psychological and behaviour disorders. [Gk *psyche* mind, chemistry.]

psychochromaesthesia (si·ko·kro·mes·**the**'·ze·ah). Sensations of colour associated with auditory or other non-visual stimuli. [Gk *psyche* mind, *chroma* colour, *aisthesis* sensation.]

psychochrome (si·ko·krome). In synaesthesia, the mental association that causes any particular sensory stimulus to give rise to perception of a particular colour. [Gk *psyche* mind, *chroma* colour.]

psychocinesia (si·ko·sin·**e**'·se·ah). Psychokinesia.

psychocoma (si·ko·**ko**·mah). Stupor associated with melancholia. [Gk *psyche* mind, coma.]

psychocortical (si·ko·**kor**·tik·al). Belonging to the mind and to the cerebral cortex. [Gk *psyche* mind, cortex.]

psychocutaneous (si·ko·kew·**ta**'·ne·us). Applied to a cutaneous phenomenon induced by psychological mechanisms. [Gk *psyche* mind, L *cutis* skin.]

Psychoda (si·**ko**·dah). A genus of Diptera; moth flies. The larvae, which are normally saprophagous, have caused accidental intestinal myiasis. [Gk *psyche* butterfly.]

psychodiagnostics (si·ko·di·ag·**nos**'·tix). The study of personality by means of the Rorschach test (a standardized and modified ink-blot projection test), in which the subject reports what objects he sees in a series of designs. [Gk *psyche* mind, diagnosis.]

Psychodidae (si·**ko**·did·e). A family of the dipteran suborder Nematocera. The genus *Phlebotomus* is of medical interest. [Gk *psyche* butterfly, *eidos* form.]

psychodometer (si·ko·**dom**·et·er). An instrument for measuring the stimulus–response reaction time: a tuning fork set into vibration and marking a smoked drum provides the stimulus; the response to the sound disconnects the fork from the drum and interrupts the record. [Gk *psyche* mind, *hodos* way, meter.]

psychodometry (si·ko·**dom**·et·re). The measurement of stimulus-response time. [see prec.]

psychodrama (si·ko·**drah**·mah). The use of drama in the diagnosis and treatment of psychiatric disorders: the patients act out a theme of their own choosing, and in this procedure have an opportunity to express and resolve their own personal conflicts. [Gk *psyche* mind, *drama* act.]

psychodynamic (si·ko·di·**nam**'·ik). Relating or belonging to psychodynamics. [see foll.]

psychodynamics (si·ko·di·**nam**'·ix). The science dealing with mental powers and processes. [Gk *psyche* mind, *dynamis* power.]

psycho-epilepsy (si·ko·ep·il·**ep**'·se). A condition due to hysterical neurosis, but with movements resembling those of epilepsy. [Gk *psyche* mind, epilepsy.]

psychogalvanometer (si·ko·gal·van·**om**′·et·er). An instrument giving galvanometric readings indicating apparent changes in the electrical resistance of the skin resulting from emotional activity. The phenomenon is actually due to changes in the rate of sweating, and the instrument can be designed to furnish a permanent photographic record, as in the "lie detector". [Gk *psyche* mind, galvanometer.]

psychogenesis (si·ko·**jen**·es·is). The development of the mind or of its powers and faculties. [Gk *psyche* mind, *genein* to produce.]

psychogenetic, psychogenic, psychogenous (si·ko·jen·**et**′·ik, si·ko·**jen**·ik, si·**koj**·en·us). 1. Relating or belonging to psychogenesis. 2. Developing or originating in the mind; of mental causation. [see prec.]

psychogeny (si·**koj**·en·e). Psychogenesis.

psychogeusic (si·ko·**gew**·sik). Relating or belonging to the perception of taste. [Gk *psyche* mind, *geusis* taste.]

psychognosis (si·kog·**no**·sis). The process of psychiatric diagnosis, more especially through hypnosis. [Gk *psyche* mind, *gnosis* knowledge.]

psychognostic (si·kog·**nos**·tik). Relating or belonging to psychognosis.

psychogram (**si**·ko·gram). 1. A chart depicting a subject's personality traits. 2. The visualization of the subject of a thought. [Gk *psyche* mind, *gramma* record.]

psychograph (**si**·ko·graf). A written description of a subject's personality traits. [Gk *psyche* mind, *graphein* to record.]

psychokinesia, psychokinesis (si·ko·kin·e′·ze·ah, **si**·ko·kin·**e**′·sis). Outbursts of uncontrolled cerebral activity resulting in explosive action. [Obsolete term.] [Gk *psyche* mind, *kinesis* movement.]

psychokym (**si**·ko·kime). The hypothetical physical and physiological bases of mental activity. [Gk *psyche* mind, *kyma* wave.]

psycholagny (**si**·ko·lag·ne). Sexual excitement and gratification obtained by mental visualization of, or imaginary participation in, the sexual act. [Gk *psyche* mind, *lagneia* lust.]

psycholepsy (**si**·ko·lep·se). 1. A mild type of psychotic or psychasthenic seizure in which the mood suddenly swings towards melancholy and there may be temporary confusion or blindness. 2. Psychic epilepsy; latent epilepsy.

psycholeptic (si·ko·**lep**·tik). Pertaining to an emotion reaction, postulated by Janet to be caused by a fall in emotional tension. [Gk *psyche* mind, *lepsis* seizure.]

psycholexia (si·ko·**lex**·e·ah). A form of alexia in which the patient can read quite correctly, but has no comprehension. [Obsolete term.]

psycholinguistics (si·ko·ling·**gwis**′·tix). The study of linguistics as connected with human behaviour. [Gk *psyche* mind, L *lingua* tongue.]

psychological (si·ko·**loj**·ik·al). Relating or belonging to psychology.

psychologist (si·**kol**·o·jist). One who has made a special study of psychology.

psychology (si·**kol**·o·je). That branch of science which deals with the mind and mental processes. **Abnormal psychology.** The branch of psychology dealing with abnormal mental processes. **Analytical psychology.** The school of psychology founded by Jung as a departure from that of Freud, widening the concept of the libido and extending the contents of the unconscious mind. **Applied psychology.** The science of psychology, as applied to everyday life with its family, social and industrial relations. **Atomic psychology.** The branch of psychology which holds that mental processes can be satisfactorily explained by an analysis of their component parts. **Behaviouristic psychology.** The school of psychology concerned with objective responses and behaviour to the exclusion of introspection and conscious processes and associated with the name of Watson. **Child psychology.** The branch of psychology dealing with the special problems of childhood and children. **Cognitive psychology.** The branch of psychology concerned with knowing and intellection. **Collective psychology.** The branch of psychology concerned with the behaviour of organisms in groups and as groups. **Comparative psychology.** The branch of psychology concerned with the differences and resemblances between the mental processes of various species. **Constitutional psychology.** The branch of psychology concerned with the relation between mind and constitution. **Criminal psychology.** The branch of psychology concerned with crime and the criminal. **Crowd psychology.** The branch of psychology concerned with crowd behaviour. **Depth psychology.** The branch of psychology concerned with unconscious processes. **Differential psychology.** The branch of psychology concerned with differences between individuals and between groups. **Dynamic psychology.** The study of the mind considered with respect to mental processes and the energy directing them, in particular from the psycho-analytic viewpoint. **Educational psychology.** The branch of psychology concerned with the problems of education. **Empirical psychology.** A method of studying mental processes based on the examination of facts and on practice, rather than on general principles. **Employment psychology.** The branch of psychology concerned with the study of employment problems. **Existential psychology.** A psychological system based on introspection. **Experimental psychology.** The branch of psychology using experimental methods for the study of psychological problems. **Folk psychology.** The branch of psychology concerned with the study of primitive peoples. **Functional psychology.** The branch of psychology concerned with the interpretation and meaning of mental phenomena, rather than with their description. **General psychology.** The branch of psychology concerned with the study of the principles of mental functioning. **Gestalt psychology.** The school of psychology emphasizing that mental processes cannot be analysed into their component parts without a loss of their essential features, because these processes are unitary in their nature. **Group psychology.** The branch of psychology concerned with the study of the mental processes of individuals as members of a group, and of the groups themselves. **Hormic psychology.** The school of psychology emphasizing the importance of instinctive and purposive striving towards a goal. **Individual psychology.** The branch of psychology emphasizing individual differences, in particular the school of psychology associated with the work of Adler. **Industrial psychology.** The branch of psychology concerned with the practical problems presented in industry. **Infant psychology.** The branch of psychology concerned with the mental processes of infants. **Objective psychology.** The branch of psychology concerned with the study of mental processes from without. **Occupational psychology.** The branch of psychology concerned with the special problems arising in different occupations. **Organismic psychology.** The branch of psychology concerned with the study of organisms as such. **Physiological psychology.** The study of the physiological bases of mental processes. **Social psychology.** The branch of psychology concerned with mental processes operating in social groups. **Statistical psychology.** The branch of psychology having as its chief method and technique the use of statistics. **Subjective psychology.** The branch of psychology concerned with the study of mental processes from within, by introspection. **Topological psychology.** The system of psychology developed by Kurt Lewin, attempting to describe and analyse the total environment or "life-space" of the individual. **Vocational psychology.** The branch of psychology concerned with the selection of occupations for persons, and of persons for occupations. [Gk *psyche* mind, *logos* science.]

psychomathematics (si·ko·math·em·**at**′·ix). The application of mathematics to the science of psychology. [Gk *psyche* mind, mathematics.]

psychometer (si·**kom**·et·er). An instrument for measuring reaction time. [Gk *psyche* mind, meter.]

psychometrics (si·ko·**met**·rix). The quantitative estimation of personality; the measurement of intelligence. [see prec.]

psychometry (si·**kom**·et·re). 1. Measurement of the reaction time by means of a psychometer. 2. Psychometrics. 3. In psychical research, the apparent derivation of facts related to the past history of an object by handling the object.

psychomotor (si·ko·**mo**·tor). 1. Concerned with the motor effects of mental activity. 2. A term applied to a form of epilepsy in which mental phenomena and motor activity coexisted. [Gk *psyche* mind, motor.]

psychoneurological (si·ko·newr·o·**loj**'·ik·al). Pertaining to the study of psychoneuroses. [Gk *psyche* mind, neurology.]

psychoneurosis (si·ko·newr·**o**'·sis). A group of mental disorders characterized by a faulty emotional response to the stresses of life, and consisting of anxiety state, hysteria, reactive depression and obsessive-compulsive neurosis. **Defence psychoneurosis.** A psychoneurosis in which the characteristic mental mechanism is the protection of the ego against instinctual demands (psychoanalysis). **Psychoneurosis maidica.** A term applied to the nervous manifestations of pellagra. **Paranoid psychoneurosis.** A psychoneurosis in which undue suspicion is a predominant characteristic. [Gk *psyche* mind, neurosis.]

psychoneurotic (si·ko·newr·**ot**'·ik). 1. One affected by a psychoneurosis. 2. Pertaining to a psychoneurosis.

psychonomics, psychonomy (si·kon·**om**·ix, si·**kon**·o·me). That section of psychological medicine which deals with the laws of mental activities in general. [Gk *psyche* mind, *nomos* law.]

psychonosema (si·ko·no·**se**'·mah). Any unspecified mental disorder. [Gk *psyche* mind, *nosema* disease.]

psychonosis (si·ko·**no**·sis). A disorder or disease that is of mental origin. [Gk *psyche* mind, *nosos* disease.]

psycho-optic (si·ko·**op**·tik). Pertaining to the psychic part of the process of visual perception. [Gk *psyche* mind, *optikos* of sight.]

psychoparesis (si·ko·par·**e**'·sis). Feebleness of mind. [Gk *psyche* mind, *paresis* a letting go.]

psychopath (**si**·ko·path). One whose behaviour is abnormal and may be antisocial; generally one with a psychopathic personality, outwardly normal but with a potential for abnormal conduct. [Gk *psyche* mind, *pathos* disease.]

psychopathia (si·ko·**path**·e·ah). Psychopathy. **Psychopathia chirurgicalis.** An insane urge to have a surgical operation. **Psychopathia martialis.** War neurosis. *See* NEUROSIS. **Psychopathia sexualis.** A disease of the mind in which abnormal sexual feelings are experienced. [see prec.]

psychopathic (si·ko·**path**·ik). Relating to psychopathy.

psychopathist (si·**kop**·ath·ist). A specialist in mental diseases. [Gk *psyche* mind, *pathos* disease.]

psychopathologist (si·ko·path·**ol**'·o·jist). A person who has made a special study of the pathology of abnormal mental states. [see foll.]

psychopathology (si·ko·path·**ol**'·o·je). The pathology of mental diseases and disorders, especially of the mental mechanisms and thought processes. [Gk *psyche* mind, pathology.]

psychopathosis (si·ko·path·**o**'·sis). The mental disorder exhibited by a psychopathic personality. [psychopath, Gk *-osis* condition.]

psychopathy (si·**kop**·ath·e). Any congenital or acquired disorder or disease of the mind; insanity. [Gk *psyche* mind, *pathos* disease.]

psychopharmacology (si·ko·far·mah·**kol**'·o·je). The science which deals with the actions and application of drugs which exert powerful actions on the higher parts of the central nervous system and on mental state and behaviour. Such drugs are referred to as *psychotropic drugs.* [Gk *psyche* mind, pharmacology.]

psychophonasthenia (si·ko·fo·nas·**the**'·ne·ah). A disorder of speech due to mental defect. [Gk *psyche* mind, phonasthenia.]

psychophylaxis (si·ko·fil·**ax**'·is). Generally, the maintenance of mental health; otherwise the application of specific hygienic methods in order to prevent the onset of mental disease. [Gk *psyche* mind, *phylax* protector.]

psychophysical (si·ko·**fiz**·ik·al). Pertaining to the relationship between body and mind. [Gk *psyche* mind, *physikos* natural.]

psychophysics (si·ko·**fiz**·ix). The branch of psychology concerned with the relationship between physical stimuli and mental responses. [see prec.]

psychophysiology (si·ko·fiz·e·**ol**'·o·je). That section of physiology which treats of the mind and its functions. [Gk *psyche* mind, physiology.]

psychoplasm (si·ko·plazm). Protyle. [Gk *psyche* mind, *plassein* to mould.]

psychoplegia (si·ko·**ple**·je·ah). A sudden and generally unexpected attack of mental illness. [Gk *psyche* mind, *plege* stroke.]

psychoplegic (si·ko·**ple**·jik). 1. Relating or belonging to psychoplegia. 2. A drug or other agent which by controlling afferent stimuli diminishes mental activity or the severity of a physical disturbance. [see prec.]

psychopneumatology (si·ko·new·mat·**ol**'·o·je). The science of the inter-relationship between the mind and the body. [Gk *psyche* mind, *pneuma* breath, *logos* science.]

psychoprophylaxis (si·ko·pro·fil·**ax**'·is). 1. Psychological techniques applied to the prevention of emotional maladjustment and the fostering of healthy psychological developments. 2. A system of relaxation and other exercises designed to minimize pain during childbirth. [Gk *psyche* mind, *prophylax* advance guard.]

psychoreaction (si·ko·re·**ak**'·shun). The inhibition of the haemolytic action of cobra venom on the red blood corpuscles in schizophrenia and affective psychosis (Much–Holzmann reaction): obsolete. [psychosis, reaction.]

psychorrhagia (si·ko·**ra**·je·ah). The apparent conflict associated with the separation of body and mind at death. [Gk *psyche* mind, *rhegnynein* to gush forth.]

psychorrhexis (si·ko·**rex**·is). A severe type of anxiety neurosis which may be the result of shock. [Gk *psyche* mind, *rhexis* rupture.]

psychorrhoea (si·ko·**re**·ah). A profuse, incoherent stream of mental activity. [Gk *psyche* mind, *rhoia* flow.]

psychorrhythmia (si·ko·**rith**·me·ah). A condition in which the mind involuntarily repeats previous voluntary action. [Gk *psyche* mind, rhythm.]

psychosensorial, psychosensory (si·ko·sen·**sor**'·e·al, si·ko·**sen**·sor·e). Pertaining to the perception of sensory stimuli. [Gk *psyche* mind, sense.]

psychosexual (si·ko·**sex**·ew·al). Pertaining to the mental aspects of sex. [Gk *psyche* mind, sex.]

psychosin (si·**ko**·sin). $C_{24}H_{47}NO_7$, a basic substance in which sphingosine is combined with galactose, which remains after removal of the acid moiety of the phrenosin molecule.

psychosis (si·**ko**·sis). A term applied generally to any kind of mental disorder, especially to those groups in which the disorder is more serious, more fundamental, and characterized by lack of insight, as distinct from psychoneurosis. **Affective psychosis.** Psychosis characterized by a primary disturbance in mood, especially manic-depressive psychosis. **Alcoholic psychosis.** Psychosis attributable to acute or chronic alcoholism. **Alternating psychosis.** Manic-depressive psychosis (see below). **Arteriosclerotic psychosis.** A psychosis caused by arteriosclerotic changes in the brain. **Circular psychosis.** Psychosis characterized by an alternation of mania and depression. **Climacteric psychosis.** A psychosis associated with the menopause. **Degenerative psychosis.** A psychosis characterized by deterioration in conduct and behaviour. **Depressive psychosis.** A psychosis in which the patient is in a state of melancholia, depression and despondency. **Drug psychosis.** Psychosis attributable to the taking of drugs. **Epileptic psychosis.** Psychosis attributable to epilepsy. **Exhaustion psychosis.** That due to physical exhaustion. **Famine psychosis.** Psychosis attributable to famine. **Febrile psychosis.** That caused by fever. **Functional psychosis.** Psychosis due to a disturbance of function, not of structure, of the central nervous system: especially schizophrenia and affective psychosis. **Gestational psychosis.** Psychosis attributable to or occurring during pregnancy. **Idiophrenic psychosis.** Psychosis originating in the mind or brain alone. **Infection-exhaustion psychosis.** Psychosis occurring during and attributable to an infection and physical exhaustion. **Involutional psychosis.** Psychosis occurring usually at the involutional period of life and characterized by agitation and morbid concern with health. **Manic psychosis.** A psychosis in which the patient is in an excited and elated emotional state. **Manic-depressive psychosis.** Psychosis characterized by an attack or attacks of both mania and depression. **Organic psychosis.** Psychosis attributable to organic disease of the brain. **Paranoic psychosis, Paranoid psychosis.** Paranoia. **Psychosis polyneuritica.** Psychosis associated with polyneuritis; more especially when both are due to vitamin-B deficiency. **Post-infectious psychosis.** Psychosis following an acute infectious disease. **Presenile psychosis.** Any psychosis associated with degenerative lesions of the brain substance with or without cerebral arteriosclerosis. **Prison psychosis.** Psychosis attributable to imprisonment. **Puerperal psychosis.** A psychosis associated with childbirth. **Purpose psychosis.** A mental state in which the symptoms can be seen to be fulfilling some purpose. **Reactive psychosis.** A psychosis considered to be a reaction to some environmental event. **Senile psychosis.** That due to old age. **Situational psychosis.** Psychosis due to mental stress arising in the environment. **Toxic psychosis.** Psychosis due to toxins either introduced into the body or formed there. **Traumatic psychosis.** A mental disorder following an injury to the head in which it may be assumed that the symptoms are due to the cerebral injury; psychic trauma is not associated with this term. **Zoophil psychosis.** Psychosis characterized by attraction to animals. [Gk *psyche* mind, *-osis* condition.]

See also: CHEYNE (J.), KORSAKOFF, STOKES (WILLIAM).

psychosomatic (si·ko·so·**mat'**·ik). Pertaining to the body-mind relationship. [Gk *psyche* mind, *soma* body.]

psychosurgery (si·ko·**ser**·jer·e). The treatment of mental disorder by operation on the brain. [Gk *psyche* mind, surgery.]

psychotechnics (si·ko·**tek**·nix). The application of psychological knowledge to practical problems. [Gk *psyche* mind, *technikos* skilful.]

psychotherapeutics (si·ko·ther·ap·**ew'**·tix). Psychotherapy.

psychotherapist (si·ko·**ther**·ap·ist). One who practises psychotherapy.

psychotherapy (si·ko·**ther**·ap·e). The treatment of mental disease by psychological methods. [Gk *psyche* mind, *therapeia* treatment.]

psychotic (si·**kot**·ik). 1. Relating or belonging to a psychosis. 2. Characterized by mental disorder. [Gk *psyche* mind, *-osis* condition.]

psychotomimetic (si·**kot**·o·mim·**et'**·ik). Circumstances, especially medication with certain drugs or the presence of toxins, which produce mental disturbances resembling those that are characteristic of psychoses, especially changes in mood and emotional state, and disordered perception with hallucinations or delusions. [psychosis, Gk *mimetikos* imitative.]

psychotrine (si·ko·treen). $C_{28}H_{36}O_4N_2$, an alkaloid which occurs with cephaeline and emetine in the root of *Psychotria ipecacuanha.*

psychovisual (si·ko·**viz**·ew·al). Of or pertaining to vision not associated with retinal stimuli. [Gk *psyche* mind, vision.]

psychro-aesthesia (si·kro·es·**the'**·ze·ah). A state of abnormal sensory receptivity in which cold is felt in a part of the body that in reality is warm. [Gk *psychros* cold, aesthesis.]

psychro-algia (si·kro·**al**·je·ah). Pain caused by sensation of cold. [Gk *psychros* cold, *algos* pain.]

psychro-apostema (si·kro·ap·**os'**·te·mah). Cold abscess. [Gk *psychros* cold, *apostema* abscess.]

psychrolusia (si·kro·**loo**·se·ah). The habitual taking of baths, or of bathing, in cold water. [Gk *psychros* cold, *louein* to bathe.]

psychrometer (si·**krom**·et·er). The wet-and-dry-bulb hygrometer, used to determine the relative humidity of the air. **Sling psychrometer.** One in which the evaporation from the wet bulb is accelerated by whirling the instrument at the end of a leather strap. [Gk *psychros* cold, meter.]

See also: ASSMANN.

psychrophilic (si·kro·**fil**·ik). Describing bacteria which grow and multiply best at temperatures below that of the human body, usually from 15 to 20°C. [Gk *psychros* cold, *philein* to love.]

psychrophobia (si·kro·**fo**·be·ah). Morbid aversion to cold, or undue sensitivity to cold. [Gk *psychros* cold, phobia.]

psychrotherapy (si·kro·**ther**·ap·e). A method of treatment by the application of cold, e.g. cold baths, ice packs, etc. [Gk *psychros* cold, *therapeia* treatment.]

psyctic (**sik**·tik). Cooling. [Gk *psyxis* a cooling.]

Psyllium BPC 1968 (**sil**·e·um). The seeds of the herb *Plantago psyllium* Linn. and *P. indica* (*P. arenaria*) (family Plantaginaceae) which contain mucilage in the cells of the epidermis which swells and dissolves when the seeds are immersed in water. They are taken dry or after being soaked in water, and are used as a demulcent in intestinal irritation; as a bulk-producing medium in chronic constipation since they absorb and retain water. They may also be used as a poultice. [Gk *psyllion* flea-wort.]

ptarmic (**tar**·mik). Causing sneezing, or an agent that causes sneezing, e.g. snuff. [see foll.]

ptarmus (**tar**·mus). An attack of sneezing spasmodic in character. [Gk *ptarmos* a sneezing.]

pteric (**ter**·ik). Of or relating to the pterion.

pteridine (**ter**·id·een). A hypothetical ring structure, $C_4H_2N_2N_2C_2H_2$, which constitutes a unit in the wing-pigments of butterflies, and in the vitamin compound, folic acid. [Gk *pteron* wing.]

Pteridophyta (ter·id·**of**·it·ah). A division of the plant kingdom including the ferns, club mosses and horsetails; fern-like plants with root, stem and leaves, and a multicellular female organ which does not give rise to a seed. [Gk *pteron* wing, *phyton* plant.]

pteridophyte (**ter**·id·o·fite). Any of the Pteridophyta.

pterin (**ter**·in). One of a family of biological pigments found in the wings of butterflies, e.g. xanthopterin, $C_6H_5O_2N_5$, a heterocyclic ring compound. [Gk *pteron* wing.]

pterion (**teer**·e·on, **ter**·e·on). A point on the skull where the greater wing of the sphenoid bone, the parietal bone and the squamous part of the temporal bone meet. [Gk *pteron* wing.]

pternalgia (tern·**al**·je·ah). Pain affecting the heel. [Gk *pterna* heel, *algos* pain.]

Pterocarpus BPC 1949 (ter·o·**kar**·pus). Pterocarpus ligni; the heartwood of *Pterocarpus santalinus* Linn. which yields a red colouring matter. It was used as a colouring agent in pharmacy. [Gk *pteron* wing, *karpos* fruit.]

pteroylglutamate (ter·o·il·**gloo'**·tam·ate). A salt of folic acid.

pterygial (ter·**ij**·e·al). Relating or belonging to a pterygium.

pterygium (ter·**ij**·e·um). A degenerative condition in which a triangular area of fleshy conjunctiva extends on to the cornea, with the apex towards the pupil, usually situated on the nasal side. It is common in windy dusty climates. **Cicatricial pterygium.** Pseudopterygium. **Pterygium colli.** A congenital band of fascia stretching from the mastoid process of the temporal bone to the clavicle. **Congenital pterygium.** A pterygium present at birth. **Pterygium unguis.** Abnormal adhesion of the cuticle to the finger nail. [Gk *pterygion* wing.]

pterygoid (**ter**·e·goid). 1. In anatomy, like a wing in shape, applied to various structures in the region of the sphenoid bone. 2. A pseudopterygium. **Pterygoid canal.** *See* CANAL. [Gk *pteryx* wing, *eidos* form.]

pterygoid canal, artery of the [arteria canalis pterygoidei (NA)]. A branch of the maxillary artery or of the greater palatine artery to the upper part of the pharynx and the pharyngotympanic tube.

pterygoid canal, nerve of the [nervus canalis pterygoidei (radix facialis) (NA)]. A nerve lying in the canal of the same name, formed by the union of the greater superficial petrosal and deep petrosal (sympathetic) nerves. It ends in the sphenopalatine ganglion.

pterygoid canal, veins of the [venae canalis pterygoidei (NA)]. Veins accompanying the artery of the pterygoid canal.

pterygoid muscles. Lateral pterygoid muscle [musculus pterygoideus lateralis (NA)]. A masticatory muscle attached anteriorly by two heads to the lateral surface of the lateral pterygoid lamina and the inferior surface of the greater wing of the sphenoid bone, and posteriorly to a notch below the head of the mandible, the capsule and disc of the temporomandibular joint. **Medial pterygoid muscle [musculus pterygoideus medialis (NA)].** A masticatory muscle attached above by two heads to the medial surface of the lateral pterygoid lamina, the tubercle of the palatine bone and the maxillary tuberosity, and below to the medial aspect of the mandible from the angle to the mandibular foramen.

pterygoid muscles, nerves to the. *See* MANDIBULAR NERVE.

pterygoma (ter·e·go·mah). 1. A persistent enlargement of the labia minora which hinders sexual intercourse. 2. The lobule of the auricle. [Gk *pteryx* wing, *-oma* tumour.]

pterygomandibular (ter·e·go·man·**dib**′·ew·lar). Relating or belonging to the pterygoid process of the sphenoid bone and the mandible.

pterygomaxillary (ter·e·go·max·**il**′·ar·e). Relating or belonging to the pterygoid process of the sphenoid bone and the maxilla.

pterygopalatine (ter·e·go·**pal**′·at·ine). Relating or belonging to the pterygoid process of the sphenoid bone and the palatine bone.

pterygopalatine nerves. *See* MAXILLARY NERVE, GANGLIONIC BRANCHES.

pterygopharyngeus (ter·e·go·far·**in**′·je·us). 1. The palatopharyngeus muscle. 2. That portion of the superior constrictor muscle of the pharynx which originates in the medial pterygoid plate.

pterygospinous (ter·e·go·**spi**′·nus). Relating or belonging to the pterygoid process of the sphenoid bone and the spine of the sphenoid bone.

pterygotemporal (ter·e·go·**tem**′·por·al). Relating or belonging to the pterygoid process of the sphenoid bone and to the temporal bone.

ptiloma (ti·lo·mah). That portion of the eyelid which is stripped of its eyelashes in ptilosis. [Gk *ptilon* down.]

ptilosis (ti·**lo**·sis). 1. Falling of the eyelashes. 2. A type of pneumoconiosis produced by inhaling the dust of ostrich feathers. [Gk *ptilon* down.]

ptisan (tiz·an). Tisane; a medicinal decoction. [Gk *ptisane* barley.]

ptomainaemia (to·ma·**ne**·me·ah). The toxic condition resulting from the presence of a harmful ptomaine in the blood. [ptomaine, Gk *haima* blood.]

ptomaine (to·mane, to·ma·een). A collective term first applied by Franz Selmi in 1878 to a group of basic nitrogenous compounds formed in the putrefaction of proteins. The term has now no precise meaning. A number of those produced in decomposing animal matter cause toxic symptoms when injected and were formerly regarded as important in the aetiology of food poisoning, but amines of identical composition are formed in the breakdown of protein in the normal intestine. Amounts necessary to produce symptoms when taken by mouth are not produced in food until it is obviously rotten and unlikely to be consumed. Only two ptomaines cause active poisoning of inoculated animals, neurine and mydaleine. [Gk *ptoma* corpse.]

ptomainotoxism (to·ma·no·**tox**′·izm). The state of poisoning caused by the presence of a harmful ptomaine. [ptomaine, toxin.]

ptomatine (to·mat·een). Ptomaine.

ptomatinuria (to·mat·in·**ewr**′·e·ah). A condition marked by the existence of ptomaines in the urine.

ptomatropine (to·**mat**·ro·peen). Substances formed in protein decomposition which cause mydriasis and other symptoms, simulating in some degree those due to atropine. Clinically they do not give the reactions of atropine. [ptomaine, atropine.]

ptomatropinism, ptomatropism (to·mat·**ro**·pin·izm, to·**mat**·ro·pizm). Symptoms simulating belladonna poisoning, due to ptomatropines.

ptosed (to·zd). 1. Affected with ptosis. 2. Prolapsed. [see foll.]

ptosis (to·sis). The prolapse or dropping of an organ; drooping of the upper eyelid, e.g. from paralysis of the 3rd cranial nerve. **Abdominal ptosis.** Enteroptosis. **Ptosis adiposa.** Drooping of the upper eyelid caused by orbital fat coming forward into the lid owing to its atrophic condition. **Bilateral ptosis.** Ptosis involving both eyes. **Congenital ptosis.** Ptosis from birth, often hereditary. It is due to malformation or defective innervation of the levator palpebrae superioris muscle. **Hysterical ptosis.** A drooping of the upper eyelid caused by spasm of the orbicularis oculi muscle. **Mechanical ptosis.** Ptosis due to thickening and increase of weight of the upper eyelid, e.g. in trachoma. **Morning ptosis.** Waking ptosis (see below). **Myogenic ptosis.** Drooping of the upper eyelid caused by diseases of the levator palpebrae superioris muscle, usually myasthenia gravis or muscular dystrophy. **Neurogenic ptosis.** Ptosis due to paralysis of the 3rd cranial nerve. **Paralytic ptosis.** A drooping of the upper eyelid caused by a lesion of the 3rd cranial nerve or its connections. **Senile ptosis.** Drooping of the upper eyelid seen in the aged, due to loss of orbital fat and lack of tone of the levator palpebrae superioris muscle. **Sympathetic ptosis, Ptosis sympathetica.** A slight drooping of the upper eyelid due to paralysis of Mueller's muscle, and not of the levator palpebrae superioris muscle; part of Horner's syndrome. **Traumatic ptosis.** Ptosis following injury to the levator muscles, e.g. in fractures of the skull including the frontal bone. **Visceral ptosis.** Abdominal ptosis (see above). **Waking ptosis.** Difficulty in raising the upper eyelid on waking. It is not uncommon and is sometimes due to an early stage of keratoconjunctivitis sicca. [Gk, a falling.]

See also: HORNER (J. F.).

ptotic (to·tik). Relating to, characterized by, or affected with ptosis.

ptyalagogue (ti·al·ag·og). Ptyalogogue.

ptyalectasis (ti·al·**ek**·tas·is). The operation of dilating one of the salivary ducts. [Gk *ptyalon* spittle, *ektasis* a stretching.]

ptyalin (ti·al·in). An amylase secreted in saliva, which is similar to if not identical with pancreatic amylase. It converts starch to dextrins and ultimately to maltose, but is inactivated by gastric secretion of acid and is not therefore regarded as an essential factor in digestion. Its action is optimal at pH 6. [Gk *ptyalon* spittle.]

ptyalinogen (ti·al·**in**·o·jen). The precursor of ptyalin, the amylase of the salivary glands. [ptyaline, Gk *genein* to produce.]

ptyalism (ti·al·izm). A condition in which there is increased secretion or flow of saliva. **Mercurial ptyalism.** Salivation due to mercurial poisoning. [Gk *ptyalon* spittle.]

ptyalith (ti·ah·lith). A salivary calculus. [Gk *ptyalon* spittle, *lithos* stone.]

ptyalocele (ti·al·o·seel). A salivary cyst, the result of stenosis of a salivary duct. **Sublingual ptyalocele.** Ranula. [Gk *ptyalon* spittle, *kele* hernia.]

ptyalogenic (ti·al·o·**jen**′·ik). 1. Produced by saliva or by salivation. 2. Formed from saliva. [Gk *ptyalon* spittle, *genein* to produce.]

ptyalogogue (ti·al·o·gog). 1. Producing an increased discharge of saliva. 2. An agent that increases the flow of saliva. [Gk *ptyalon* spittle, *agogos* eliciting.]

ptyalography (ti·al·**og**·raf·e). Injection of an opaque medium into the ducts of the salivary glands and subsequent x-ray examination of the ducts. [Gk *ptyalon* spittle, *graphein* to record.]

ptyalolith (ti·al·o·lith). A salivary calculus. [Gk *ptyalon* spittle, *lithos* stone.]

ptyalolithiasis (ti·al·o·lith·**i**′·as·is). A condition characterized by the production or presence of salivary calculi. [see prec.]

ptyalolithotomy (ti·al·o·lith·**ot**′·o·me). The surgical operation of incising a salivary gland or duct for the purpose of removing a calculus. [ptyalolith, Gk *temnein* to cut.]

ptyalorrhoea (ti·al·o·**re**′·ah). An excessive flow of saliva. [Gk *ptyalon* saliva, *rhoia* flow.]

ptyalosis (ti·al·**o**·sis). Ptyalism. [Gk *ptyalon* saliva, *-osis* condition.]

ptysis (ti·sis). Spitting of saliva. [Gk *ptyein* to spit.]

ptysma (tiz·mah). Saliva. [Gk, spittle.]

ptysmagogue (tiz·mah·gog). A drug which increases the secretion of saliva, e.g. pilocarpine. [Gk *ptysma* spittle, *agogos* eliciting.]

pubarche (pew·**bar**·ke). The first appearance of pubic hair. [L *puber* youth, Gk *arch* beginning.]

puberal, pubertal (**pew**·ber·al, **pew**·ber·tal). Relating or belonging to puberty. [L *puber* youth.]

pubertas (pew·ber·tas). Puberty. **Pubertas plena.** The attainment of full sexual maturity. **Pubertas praecox.** Puberty occurring at an abnormally early age. [L.]

puberty (**pew**·ber·te). The epoch in a person's life at which the sex glands become active. In the male the testes enlarge and spermatocytogenesis begins. The external genitalia increase in size, hair develops on the face, trunk, the axillae and the pubic region; the larynx grows and the voice becomes deeper. There is considerable muscular development and body growth, associated with important psychological changes. In the female the ovaries, uterus and vagina enlarge, menstruation begins, the breasts increase in size and hair appears in the axillae and the pubic region. Psychological changes occur as the girl matures towards adolescence and womanhood. **Delayed puberty.** Puberty occurring at a later age than normal; arbitrarily, puberty occurring later than 17 years of age. **Precocious puberty.** Puberty occurring at an earlier age than normal; arbitrarily, puberty occurring earlier than 9 years of age. True precocious puberty is brought about by early production of LH/FSH-RH, luteinizing hormone/follicle-stimulating hormone, by the hypothalamus. Most cases of precocious puberty in girls are "idiopathic" whereas in boys there is nearly always a tumour of the hypothalamus or pineal gland. [L *pubertas*.]

pubes (**pew**·beez). The pubic hair or the area covered by this hair. [L.]

pubescence (pew·**bes**·ens). 1. The state of being pubescent. 2. Lanugo. [L *pubescere* to arrive at the age of puberty, to be covered with hair.]

pubescent (pew·**bes**·ent). 1. Reaching puberty. 2. Hairy. [see prec.]

pubic (**pew**·bik). Relating or belonging to the pubic region or to the pubis.

pubioplasty (**pew**·be·o·plas·te). Plastic surgery of the pubic region. [pubis, Gk *plassein* to mould.]

pubiotomy (pew·be·**ot**·o·me). The surgical division of the pubis to one side of the midline, to enlarge the pelvic diameter in labour. [pubis, Gk *temnein* to cut.]

pubis [os pubis (NA)**]** (**pew**·bis). The anterior portion of the hip bone, joining its fellow to form the pubic symphysis in the median plane. **Body [corpus ossis pubis** (NA)**].** In the Birmingham Revision of the BNA Terminology, that portion of the pubis which meets its fellow at the pubic symphysis and forms the anterior part of the bone; in the BNA terminology, that part of the pubis which takes part in the formation of the acetabulum. **Symphyseal surface [facies symphysialis** (NA)**].** The oval surface of the pubic bone which articulates with its fellow through the pubis symphysis.

Public Health Act 1936. *See:* HEALTH AND SAFETY AT WORK ACT 1974, HEALTH SERVICES ACT 1976, HEALTH SERVICES AND PUBLIC HEALTH ACT 1968, NATIONAL HEALTH SERVICES ACTS, NATIONAL HEALTH SERVICE (VOCATIONAL TRAINING) ACT 1976.

pubocapsular (pew·bo·**kap**·sew·lar). Of or relating to the pubis and articular capsule of the hip joint.

pubococcygeal (**pew**·bo·kok·**sij**′·e·al). Belonging or related to the pubis and the coccyx.

pubococcygeus muscle [musculus pubococcygeus (NA)**]** (**pew**·bo·kok·**sij**′·e·us musl). That portion of the levator ani muscle arising from the pubis and sweeping back around the anal canal to be attached to the coccyx.

pubofemoral (pew·bo·**fem**·or·al). Relating or belonging to the pubis and the femur.

puboprostatic (**pew**·bo·pros·**tat**′·ik). Belonging to the pubis and the prostate gland.

puboprostatic muscle [musculus puboprostaticus (NA)**].** The muscular tissue of the puboprostatic ligaments.

puborectalis muscle [musculus puborectalis (NA)**]** (**pew**·bo·rek·**ra**′·lis musl). The fibres of the levator ani muscle which arise from the pubis and become continuous as a sling with those of the opposite side around the anorectal junction.

pubotibial (pew·bo·**tib**·e·al). Relating or belonging to the pubis and the tibia.

pubovesical (pew·bo·**ves**·ik·al). Belonging to the pubis and the urinary bladder. [pubis, L *vesicula* small bladder.]

pubovesical muscle [musculus pubovesicalis (NA)**].** Fibres of the external longitudinal coat of muscle which pierce the median puboprostatic ligament and then attach to the body of the pubis.

puddling (**pud**·ling). A condition when radio-opaque contrast media collect in puddles. If an opaque contrast medium is used for hysterosalpingography when peritoneal adhesions are present, the medium on escaping from the tubes may collect in puddles instead of spreading out as a free smear over the pelvic peritoneum. [ME *podel*.]

pudenda (pew·**den**·dah). *See* PUDENDUM.

pudendagra (pew·den·**dag**·rah). Pain affecting the genital organs, in particular those of the female. **Pudendagra pruriens.** Pruritus vulvae. [pudenda, Gk *agra* a catching.]

pudendal (pew·**den**·dal). Relating or belonging to the pudendum.

pudendal arteries. External pudendal arteries [arteriae pudendae externae (NA)**].** The superficial and deep branches of the femoral artery to the skin and superficial fascia of the scrotum and penis in the male and of the labium majus in the female [rami scrotales anteriores et rami labiales anteriores (NA)]. The inguinal branches [rami inguinales (NA)] go to the spermatic cord and its coverings. **Internal pudendal artery [arteria pudenda interna** (NA)**].** A branch of the anterior division of the internal iliac artery which leaves the pelvis through the greater sciatic foramen and then enters the perineum through the lesser sciatic foramen. It supplies all the structures in the perineum, and scrotal (labial) branches [rami scrotales posteriores et rami labiales posteriores (NA)] to the scrotum or labia.

pudendal nerve [nervus pudendus (NA)**].** A branch of the sacral plexus (root value S2, 3, and 4), emerging through the greater sciatic foramen and passing into the perineum through the lesser sciatic foramen. It gives branches to the muscle and skin of the perineum.

pudendal veins. External pudendal veins [venae pudendae externae (NA)**].** Tributaries of the saphenous vein near its termination, from the external genitalia, including scrotal (labial) tributaries [venae scrotales (vel labiales) anteriores (NA)]. **Internal pudendal veins [venae pudendae internae** (NA)**].** Tributaries of the internal iliac vein, draining the perineum and intimately connected with the prostatic plexus; receives also scrotal (labial) tributaries [venae scrotales (vel labiales) posteriores (NA)]. They accompany the arteries of the same name.

pudendum (pew·**den**·dum) (pl. *pudenda*). The external genitalia. **Pudendum muliebre [pudendum femininum** (NA)**].** The mons pubis, labia majora and minora, the clitoris, the vestibule of the vagina, the bulb of the vestibule and the greater vestibular glands, considered together. [L *pudens* modest.]

pudic (**pew**·dik). Pudendal. [L *pudicus* modest.]

puerilism (**pew**·er·il·izm). Childishness; the abnormal condition of an adult when his mind reverts to its childhood state. [L *puerilis* childish.]

pueritia (pew·er·**ish**·e·ah). The state of second childhood. [L, boyhood.]

puerpera (pew·**er**·per·ah). A woman who has just been delivered or is being delivered of a child. [L *puerperus* relating to childbirth.]

puerperal (pew·**er**·per·al). Relating to the puerperium; relating, belonging, or due to childbirth; occurring after childbirth. **Puerperal eclampsia.** Seizures due to an endogenous intoxication during pregnancy or labour. [see prec.]

puerperalism (pew·**er**·per·al·izm). Any morbid state resulting from or associated with childbirth. **Infantile puerperalism.** Any diseased condition affecting the newborn child. **Infectious puerperalism.** Infection as the cause of disease in childbirth. [L *puerperus* relating to childbirth.]

puerperant (pew·**er**·per·ant). Puerpera.

puerperium (pew·er·**peer**·e·um). The period during which the reproductive organs are returning to their normal condition following labour. The duration is about 6 weeks. [L *puerperus* relating to childbirth.]

puff (puf). A short, soft blowing murmur. **Veiled puff (of Skoda).** A faint inspiratory murmur which becomes suddenly loud and bronchial on deep inspiration. It is probably due to the sudden removal of an obstruction in a bronchial tube communicating with a cavity. [ME *puf.*]

See also: SKODA.

puffball (**puf**·bawl). Lycoperdon; a fungus, *Lycoperdon bovista,* forming a globose or depressed ball varying from 100 to 300 mm in diameter. It is whitish when young, the internal white mass consisting of spores and fine thread-like fibres. The lower spongy portion is used as a haemostatic. [ME *puf, bal.*]

puffiness (**puf**·e·nes). A term applied to swollen tissues, especially the skin, and indicative of a slightly oedematous state. [ME *puf.*]

Pugh, William Thomas Gordon (b. 1872). British orthopaedic surgeon.

Pugh's traction. Traction applied to the lower limbs by tying extension tapes to the end of the bed after elevating the lower end. Originally used to correct deformity in tuberculosis of the hip.

pugil, pugillus (**pew**·jil, pew·**jil**·us). A pinch or handful [obsolete term]. [L *pugillus* handful.]

pujos blancos (**poo**·hos **blank**·os). A form of diarrhoea in which the motions are pale; it occurs in Chile. [Sp. white straining.]

pukeweed (**pewk**·weed). Lobelia, Indian tobacco; the herb *Lobelia inflata* (family Campanulaceae), the leaves and tops of which are used as an expectorant, emetic, diaphoretic and anti-asthmatic. [ME *puken,* weed.]

Pulex (**pew**·lex) (pl. *pulices*). A genus of fleas. **Pulex brasiliensis.** *Xenopsylla brasiliensis.* **Pulex cheopis.** *Xenopsylla cheopis.* **Pulex irritans.** The flea that commonly parasitizes man, very widely distributed, though absent from some desert areas; the pig and probably cattle are also true hosts, as well as some wild mammals, e.g. badger and fox. It is now a relatively uncommon insect in most civilized cities where the chief forms biting man are cat and dog fleas (*Ctenocephalides*) but it may be sometimes abundant on pig farms. It is of little importance in plague transmission because it does not normally occur on rats, nor does it become blocked when plague bacteria are ingested. It can act as secondary host to the tapeworm *Dipylidium caninum,* and as an arthropod host of *Hymenolepis diminuta.* In earlier literature almost all species of flea were placed in *Pulex.* **Pulex penetrans.** *Tunga.* **Pulex serraticeps.** *Ctenocephalides canis.* [L.]

Pulfrich, C. 20th century German physicist.

Pulfrich photometer. An abridged spectrophotometer in which two beams of light are passed successively through colour filters, absorption cells and variable apertures, and are then brought together by means of prisms. Colours of liquids in the cells are matched by adjusting the apertures, using rotating drums calibrated directly in optical densities.

Pulfrich refractometer. An instrument for the rapid determination of the refractive index of a solid or liquid.

PULHEEMS (**pul**·heemz). A system of mental and physical classification used in recruitment for the fighting services in the United Kingdom: P = Physical capacity, U = Upper limbs, L = Locomotion, H = Hearing, $\left.\begin{matrix}E\\E\end{matrix}\right\}$ = Vision in right and left eyes, M = Mental capacity, S = Emotional stability.

pulicaris (pew·lik·**a**·ris). Covered with macular spots resembling flea bites. **Pulicaris morbus.** Typhus, on account of the petechial rash to be seen on patients with this disease. [L *pulex* flea.]

pulicatio (pew·le·**ka**·she·o). A condition in which the body is infested with fleas. [L *pulex* flea.]

pulices (**pew**·le·seez). *See* PULEX.

pulicicide (pew·**lis**·is·ide). Pulicide.

Pulicidae (pew·**lis**·id·e). A family of Siphonaptera. The genera *Ctenocephalides, Pulex* and *Xenopsylla* contain species of medical importance. [L *pulex* flea.]

pulicide (**pew**·lis·ide). Any agent which kills fleas. [L *pulex* flea, *caedere* to kill.]

pulicosis (pew·lik·**o**·sis). An irritated condition of the skin as the result of bites of *Pulex irritans.* [L *pulex* flea, Gk *-osis* condition.]

pull (pul). To draw or drag. **Mesenteric pull.** A subjective feeling of pulling when the patient lies on the left side, due to the dragging effect of the mesentery. It has been regarded as a sign of appendicitis. [AS *pullian.*]

pulley (**pul**·e). 1. A mechanical device, usually in the form of a wheel or drum, for altering direction. 2. A trochlea. **Muscular pulley [trochlea muscularis].** A connective-tissue loop through which a tendon passes, by which it alters its direction. [ME *polie.*]

pullulate (**pul**·ew·late). To germinate. [see foll.]

pullulation (pul·ew·**la**·shun). The act of budding, as a form of reproduction; it is commonly seen in yeasts. [L *pullulare* to sprout.]

pulmo-aortic (**pul**·mo·a·**or**′·tik). 1. Relating or belonging to the lungs and the aorta. 2. Belonging to one of the pulmonary arteries and the aorta. [L *pulmo* lung, aorta.]

pulmolith (**pul**·mo·lith). A lung calculus. [L *pulmo* lung, Gk *lithos* stone.]

pulmometer (pul·**mom**·et·er). A type of spirometer used in determining the amount of air inhaled and exhaled. [L *pulmo* lung, meter.]

pulmometry (pul·**mom**·et·re). Measurement by means of the pulmometer of the air inhaled and exhaled.

pulmonary (**pul**·mon·ar·e). Belonging to, connected with, or affecting the lungs. [L *pulmoneus* relating to the lungs.]

pulmonary arteries. Left pulmonary artery [arteria pulmonalis sinistra (NA)]. The shorter and narrower of the two branches of the pulmonary trunk. It is distributed to the left lung. The lobar branches of the left pulmonary artery are named according to the lobe which they supply, thus: apical [ramus apicalis (NA)]; anterior descending [ramus anterior descendens (NA)]; posterior [ramus posterior (NA)]; anterior ascending [ramus anterior ascendens (NA)]; lingular [ramus lingularis (NA)], dividing into superior [ramus lingularis superior (NA)] and inferior [ramus lingularis inferior (NA)]; apical of the inferior lobe [ramus apicalis (superior) lobi inferioris (NA)]; subapical [ramus subapicalis (sub-superior) NA]; medial basal [ramus basalis medialis (NA)]; anterior basal [ramus basalis anterior (NA)]; lateral basal [ramus basalis lateralis (NA)]; and posterior basal [ramus basalis posterior (NA)]. The basal part [pars basalis] is that part of the artery to the left lower lobe between the origin of the branch to the apical lobe and the other branches to the lower lobe. **Right pulmonary artery [arteria pulmonalis dextra (NA)].** The longer and wider of the two branches of the pulmonary trunk. It is distributed to the right lung. The lobar branches of the right pulmonary artery are named according to the lobe which they supply, thus: apical [ramus apicalis (NA)]; anterior [rami anterior ascendens et descendens (NA)]; posterior [rami posterior ascendens et descendens (NA)] of the middle lobe [ramus lobi medii (NA)], branching into lateral [ramus lateralis (NA)] and medial [ramus medialis (NA)] parts; apical of the inferior lobe [ramus apicalis (superior) lobi inferioris (NA)]; subapical [ramus subapicalis (sub-superior) NA]; medial basal [ramus basalis medialis (cardiacus) (NA)]; anterior basal [ramus basalis anterior (NA)]; posterior basal [ramus basalis posterior]; and lateral basal [ramus basalis lateralis (NA)]. The basal part [pars basalis (NA)] is that part of the artery to the right lower lobe between the origin of the branch to the apical lobe and the other branches to the lower lobe.

pulmonary veins [venae pulmonales (NA)]. Left pulmonary veins [venae pulmonales sinistrae (NA)]. Veins returning blood from the left lung to the left atrium, usually two in number, the superior and inferior veins [venae pulmonales superior sinistra et inferior sinistra (NA)]. Within the lung, their distribution corresponds approximately to the segmental bronchi but most of their tributaries have two components, one of which [pars intrasegmentalis (NA)] drains a segment but the other of which [pars infrasegmentalis (intersegmentalis) NA] is intersegmental in position and drains more than one segment. The main tributaries of the superior vein are the apicoposterior [ramus apicoposterior (NA)], anterior [ramus anterior (NA)] and lingular [ramus lingularis (NA)], while those of the inferior vein are the apical [ramus apicalis (NA)], a common basal vein [vena basalis communis (NA)] and an inferior basal vein [vena basalis inferior (NA)]. **Right pulmonary veins [venae pulmonales dextrae (NA)].** Veins returning blood from the right lung to the right atrium, usually two in number, the superior and inferior veins. Most of the tributaries of these have intra- and infrasegmental components [pars intrasegmentalis et pars infrasegmentalis (intersegmentalis) NA]. The main tributaries of the superior vein [vena pulmonalis superior dextra (NA)] are the apical [ramus apicalis (NA)], anterior [ramus anterior (NA)], posterior [ramus posterior (NA)] and, from the middle lobe, the middle lobe veins [ramus lobi medii (NA)]. The latter has lateral and medial branches [pars lateralis et medialis (NA)]. The inferior vein [vena pulmonalis inferior dextra (NA)] tributaries are the apical vein [ramus apicalis (NA)] and the common basal vein [vena basalis communis (NA)] which is formed by the junction of the anterior and inferior basal veins [ramus basalis anterior et vena basalis inferior (NA)].

pulmonectomy (pul·mon·**ek**·to·me). Pneumonectomy. [L *pulmo* lung, Gk *ektome* a cutting out.]

pulmonic (pul·**mon**·ik). Pulmonary.

pulmonitis (pul·mon·i·tis). Pneumonia. [L *pulmo* lung, Gk *-itis* inflammation.]

pulmonohepatic (**pul**·mon·o·hep·**at**'·ik). Pertaining to the lungs and the liver, or situated between the lungs and the liver. [L *pulmo* lung, Gk *hepar* liver.]

pulmonoperitoneal (**pul**·mon·o·per·it·o·**ne**'·al). Pertaining to the lungs and the peritoneum. [L *pulmo* lung, peritoneum.]

pulmotor (**pul**·mo·tor). An apparatus used in artificial respiration of asphyxiated persons by which oxygen is pumped into and out of the lungs. [L *pulmo* lung, *motor* mover.]

pulp (pulp). 1. Any soft, flaccid, juicy tissue, especially when surrounded by harder material. 2. In dentistry, the pulp of a tooth. *See* TOOTH. **Coronal pulp [pulpa coronale (NA)].** That part of the tooth pulp which lies in the crown of a tooth. **Dead pulp.** A pulp which is non-vital. **Dental pulp.** Pulp of a tooth. *See* TOOTH. **Devitalized pulp.** A pulp which has been rendered non-vital. **Digital pulp.** The soft but firm cushion of flesh on the plantar and palmar aspects of the distal phalanges of the fingers and toes, respectively. **Enamel pulp.** That part of the enamel organ of a developing tooth which consists of a mass of stellate-shaped cells; the stellate reticulum. **Pulp of an intervertebral disc.** The nucleus pulposus; a soft gelatinous structure at the centre of an intervertebral disc. **Mummified pulp.** Tooth pulp which has been affected by dry gangrene. **Non-vital pulp.** Tooth pulp which is dead. **Parchment pulps.** Dry, cracked finger pulps persistently depressed after pressuure. **Putrescent pulp.** Tooth pulp which has undergone necrosis, producing a foul odour. **Radicular pulp [pulpa radicularis (NA)].** That part of the pulp which occupies the root canal of a tooth. **Splenic pulp [pulpa lienis (NA)].** Splenic tissue divided into white pulp composed of typical lymphoid tissue associated with the arteries, and atypical lymphoid tissue, the red pulp, arranged in cords forming a spongy framework between the terminal venous blood vessels. **Pulp of a tooth.** *See* TOOTH. **Vaccine pulp.** 1. The epithelium and underlying vesicular pulp which is scraped from the skin of the vaccinated sheep or calf in the preparation of smallpox vaccine (vaccine lymph). 2. A term sometimes used in laboratories for a sand-and-paper-pulp filter for removing larger particles from cultures, tissue emulsions, exudates, etc. **Vertebral pulp.** Pulp of an intervertebral disc (see above). **Vital pulp.** A tooth pulp which is alive. **White pulp.** The lymphoid, as opposed to the blood-filled reticular tissue of the spleen. **Wood pulp.** A cellulose obtained by the delignification of shredded wood. It is used as a cheap substitute for cotton wool. [L *pulpa* flesh.]

pulpa (**pul**·pah). Pulp. [L, flesh.]

pulpal, pulpar (**pul**·pal, **pul**·par). Relating to pulp.

pulpation (pul·**pa**·shun). 1. The act of pulping or reducing to pulp. 2. The state of having been reduced to pulp. [pulp, *facere* to make.]

pulpectomy (pul·**pek**·to·me). The removal of the pulp from a tooth. [pulp, Gk *ektome* excision.]

pulpefaction, pulpifaction (pul·pe·**fak**·shun). Pulpation. [pulp, L *facere* to make.]

pulpiform (**pul**·pe·form). Pulpy; having resemblance to pulp.

pulpify (**pul**·pe·fi). To make pulp of; to reduce to pulp. [pulp, L *facere* to make.]

pulpitis (**pul**·pi·tis). 1. Inflammation of the pulp of a tooth. 2. Inflammation of the pulp of a finger or toe. **Acute pulpitis.** Acute inflammation of the pulp of a tooth, due to bacterial, traumatic, chemical, thermal or electrical causes. **Acute closed pulpitis.** Acute inflammation of the tooth pulp not associated with a breach in continuity of the surrounding dentine, accompanied by considerable pain. Resolution may sometimes occur; alternatively a local pulp abscess may form, or mass gangrene of the pulp tissue occur. **Acute open pulpitis.** Acute inflammation of the tooth pulp resulting from breach in continuity of the surrounding dentine by caries or trauma. Suppuration may occur, or the condition may become chronic. **Chronic pulpitis.** A low-grade inflammation of the tooth pulp, generally due to infection by the organisms of dental caries, or occurring subsequent to acute open pulpitis. **Chronic closed pulpitis.** Chronic inflammation of the tooth pulp not associated with breach in continuity of the surrounding dentine, as in slowly advancing dental caries. **Chronic open pulpitis.** Usually an acute open pulpitis upon which a chronic state has supervened. **Chronic open hyperplastic pulpitis.** A condition in which hyperplasia of the pulp tissue occurs, pushing its way through an aperture in the wall of the pulp cavity to form a soft, insensitive, pink mass at the base of a carious cavity; pulp polypus. **Chronic open ulcerative pulpitis.** A relatively painless condition in which an ulcer is present on the exposed surface of the tooth pulp. [pulp, Gk *-itis* inflammation.]

pulpless (**pulp**·les). Having had the pulp removed, as a tooth; a dead tooth.

pulpotomy (pul·**pot**·o·me). The removal of part of the pulp of a tooth. [pulp, Gk *temnein* to cut.]

pulpy (**pul**·pe). The condition of a solid when it is soft and moist; pulpiform. [L *pulpa* flesh.]

pulque (**pool**·ke). A fermented liquid from species of *Agave*, used as a beverage in Mexico. [Sp.]

pulsate (**pul**·sate). To expand and contract rhythmically as in the rhythm of the heart. [L *pulsare* to beat.]

pulsatile (**pul**·sat·ile). Beating in rhythmic fashion. [L *pulsatio* a beating.]

pulsatilla (pul·sat·il·ah). Pasque flower, passe flower, wind flower, meadow anemone, Easter flower; the herb *Anemone pulsatilla* Linn. (family Ranunculaceae), used as an antispasmodic and alterative, especially in menstrual disorders. [dim. from L *pulsare* to beat.]

pulsation (pul·**sa**·shun). A regular beating or throbbing, as of the heart or an artery. **Expansile pulsation.** That in which the area affected can be felt or seen to be becoming greater in dimensions with the occurrence of each pulse. **Suprasternal pulsation.** Arterial pulsation near the suprasternal notch, due either to the presence of an aneurysm or to other dilated condition of the arch of the aorta. [L *pulsatio* a beating.]

pulsator (pul·**sa**·tor). A machine for providing artificial respiration in cases of respiratory failure. [see prec.]

See also: BRAGG, PAUL (R. W.).

pulse (puls). 1. The wave of increased pressure within an artery caused by the systole of the left ventricle; the arterial pulse (see below). 2. A regularly recurring variation in quantity, usually referring to the change of arterial tension caused by the heart beat. There are also radar pulses, light pulses, etc. **Abdominal pulse.** Pulsus abdominalis; the pulse of the abdominal aorta seen or felt in persons with a thin abdominal wall. **Abrupt pulse.** One that strikes the finger sharply or rapidly. **Allorrhythmic pulse.** A regularly intermittent pulse. **Alternating pulse.** Pulsus alternans;

regular alternation of the volume of the pulse produced by alternation of the strength of the ventricular contraction; it is only rarely detectable by palpation and is usually observed on sphygmomanometry. It is usually a sign of grave prognosis. **Anacrotic pulse.** One which shows a small wave on the ascending limb. **Anadicrotic pulse.** One with two notches on the ascending limb. **Arachnoid pulse.** A small, feeble, thread-like pulse. **Arterial pulse.** The rhythmic expansion and collapse of arteries, produced by the pressure variations at the root of the aorta which are propagated throughout the arterial system. The peripheral arterial pulse curve, usually recorded from the radial artery at the wrist, consists of a sharp upstroke (anacrotic limb) during ventricular systole, a rounded peak and a slower downstroke (catacrotic limb) which is interrupted by a notch oscillation (dicrotic notch). The initial portion of the upstroke of the pulse is produced by rapid early ejection of blood from the ventricle. As ejection slows, the upstroke becomes less steep, the peak of the pulse wave is reached and then the pulse wave begins to fall to the dicrotic notch; the last signals aortic valve closure and the end of systole. **Auriculovenous pulse.** The venous pulse wave due to atrial (auricular) contraction, which precedes that due to ventricular contraction [obsolete term]. **Bigeminal pulse.** Pulsus bigeminus; a pulse in which the beats occur in pairs. This is nearly always due to coupled ectopic beats but may also occur with the Wenckebach phenomenon when the cycle is repeated over three beats. **Bisferiens pulse.** Pulsus bisferiens; a pulse with two beats, and a tracing shows two waves at the apex. It is not uncommon with aortic stenosis associated with incompetence. **Brachial pulse.** The pulse felt in the brachial artery. **Capillary pulse.** Quincke's pulse; pulsation seen in the capillaries. It may be observed in the nail bed, or by pressing on the lips with a glass slide when the margin between the red and the blanched part can be seen to ebb and flow. It occurs with aortic incompetence, but not exclusively so. **Caprizant pulse.** Pulsus capricans; an old term given by Rufus of Ephesus in the 2nd century to an irregular "leaping" pulse. It was probably due to extrasystoles. **Carotid pulse.** The pulse felt in the carotid artery. **Catacrotic pulse.** A pulse with three waves, including the dicrotic wave, on the descending limb. **Catadicrotic pulse.** A pulse with a dicrotic wave on the descending or catacrotic limb. **Collapsing pulse.** Water-hammer pulse; a large-amplitude pulse with rapid upstroke and downstroke nearly always due to aortic regurgitation. **Cordy pulse.** A hard, high-tension pulse. **Coupled pulse.** Bigeminal pulse (see above). **Decurtate pulse.** A pulse which gradually tapers away. **Deficient pulse.** Dropped-beat pulse (see below). **Dicrotic pulse.** Pulsus dicroticus; a pulse with an exaggerated dicrotic wave. It is best marked in pulses of low tensions. **Digitalate pulse.** Bigeminal pulse (see above). **Dropped-beat pulse.** Pulsus deficiens, pulsus intermittens; a pulse in which an occasional beat is absent. It may occur with extrasystole, or heart block. **Entoptic pulse.** One in which each pulse beat is accompanied by the subjective sensation of flashes of light in the eyes. **Epigastric pulse.** Pulsation in the epigastrium conducted from the abdominal aorta. It may also be due to pulsation of the liver or an enlarged right ventricle. **Febrile pulse.** A full bounding pulse, later becoming quick and feeble. **Filiform pulse.** Thready pulse (see below). **Full pulse.** Pulsus magnus; a large-volume pulse with light pulse pressure. **Funic pulse.** Pulsation in the umbilical cord. **Hard pulse.** Cordy pulse (see above). **Hepatic pulse.** Pulsation of the liver, as in tricuspid incompetence. **High-tension pulse.** Cordy pulse (see above). **Hyperdicrotic pulse.** One in which the dicrotic notch on the pulse tracing falls lower than the commencement of the systolic rise. It is due to instrumental inertia and a rapid pulse. **Intermittent pulse.** Dropped-beat pulse (see above). **Irregular pulse.** Any pulse that is irregular in force or rhythm. **Jugular pulse.** Pulsation in the jugular vein. **Mouse-tail pulse.** Decurtate pulse (see above). **Negative venous pulse.** A term used under the theory that the venous pulsation was due to a wave of negative pressure or suction caused by the dilatation of the atrium. **Normal venous pulse.** Venous pulse (see below). **Paradoxical pulse.** Pulsus paradoxus; a pulse which becomes smaller during inspiration. It is an exaggeration of the normal respiratory variation of the pulse and occurs with cardiac tamponade and constrictive pericarditis. **Positive venous pulse.** A pulse in which the tracing shows an absence of the "a" wave and a prominent "v" wave due to ventricular contraction. **Pulse pressure.** *See* PRESSURE. **Quadrigeminal pulse.** A pulse with four beats followed by a pause. **Quick-rising pulse.** Collapsing pulse (see above). **Radial pulse.** The pulse felt in the radial artery. **Respiratory pulse.** Pulsation in the jugular veins in health, seen after exercise. **Retrosternal pulse.** Pulsation visible in the suprasternal notch. **Running pulse.** A small, quick, irregular pulse. **Sixty-six pulse.** A pulse with a rate of 66 which was supposed to be characteristic of vagotonia. **Tense pulse.** Cordy pulse (see above). **Thready pulse.** Pulsus filiformis; a thin, barely perceptible pulse. **Trigeminal pulse.** Pulsus trigeminus; a pulse with three beats followed by a pause. **Unequal pulse.** A pulse in which the beats vary in size. **Vaginal pulse.** Pulsation sometimes observed in the vagina during pregnancy. **Vagus pulse.** A slow regular pulse due to overaction of the vagus nerve. **Venous pulse.** The central venous pulse formed by pressure changes in the great veins and right atrium occurring during the cardiac cycle. Similar changes occur in the left atrium but these are not available for clinical examination. The venous pulse can be observed in the neck if the subject is made to recline at the correct angle. Two positive waves, the "a" and "v", can normally be seen but a third, smaller, "c" wave can be detected with suitable instruments. The "a" wave is produced by atrial systole; when the atrium relaxes the pressure falls, the "x" descent. The fall is quickly interrupted by the "c" wave produced by the billowing of the tricuspid valve cusps into the atrium at the commencement of ventricular systole. After this, the fall in pressure is resumed to reach the "x" point. Venous return to the atrium whilst the tricuspid valve is still closed then causes the pressure to rise again to the "v" wave. With the onset of ventricular relaxation the tricuspid valve cusps sink down and then the valve opens, allowing blood to enter the ventricle; this results in a fall in the atrial pressure, the "y" descent. If diastole persists for long enough, venous return will fill the combined atrioventricular cavity until equilibrium is reached and the pressure becomes stable before the onset of the next atrial systole, the "z" point. **Ventricular venous pulse.** A venous pulse showing only the "v" wave. **Water-hammer pulse.** Collapsing pulse (see above). The name derives from an old children's toy consisting of an evacuated glass cylinder containing some water; the pulse is likened to the sensation produced by the slapping of the water on the end of the cylinder when it is inverted. **Wiry pulse.** Thready pulse (see above). [L *pulsare* to beat.]

See also: BAMBERGER (H.), CORRIGAN, KUSSMAUL, MONNERET, QUINCKE, RIEGEL.

pulse (puls). The edible seed of a leguminous plant. [L *puls* porridge.]

pulseless (**puls**·les). Having no pulse or pulsation.

pulsellum (pul·**sel**·um). A flagellum which propels from behind. [L *pulsus* a striking.]

pulsimeter (pul·**sim**·et·er). An apparatus used to determine the rapidity and force of the pulse. [pulse, meter.]

pulsion (**pul**·shun). Any act of driving or propelling in any direction. **Lateral pulsion.** Movement of involuntary kind to one side, e.g. in walking. [L *pulsare* to drive away.]

pulsometer (pul·**som**·et·er). Pulsimeter.

pulsus (**pul**·sus). The pulse. **Pulsus abdominalis.** Abdominal pulse. *See* PULSE. **Pulsus alternans.** Alternating pulse. *See* PULSE. **Pulsus bigeminus.** Bigeminal pulse. *See* PULSE. **Pulsus bisferiens.** Bisferiens pulse. *See* PULSE. **Pulsus capricans.** Caprizant pulse. *See* PULSE. **Pulsus celer.** A pulse which rises and falls quickly. It does not refer to the pulse rate. **Pulsus cordis.** The cardiac apex beat. **Pulsus deficiens.** Dropped-beat pulse. *See* PULSE. **Pulsus dicroticus.** Dicrotic pulse. *See* PULSE. **Pulsus durus.** A hard, high-tension pulse. **Pulsus filiformis.** Thready pulse. *See* PULSE. **Pulsus frequens.** A very rapid pulse. **Pulsus intermittens.** Dropped-beat pulse. *See* PULSE. **Pulsus**

irregularis perpetuus. The pulse of atrial fibrillation which is completely irregular in force and rhythm. **Pulsus magnus.** Full pulse. *See* PULSE. **Pulsus magnus et celer.** A full pulse with high pulse pressure that rises and falls abruptly as in cases of aortic incompetence. **Pulsus paradoxus.** Paradoxical pulse. *See* PULSE. **Pulsus parvus.** A small pulse. **Pulsus parvus et tardus.** A small pulse with low pulse pressure that rises and falls slowly as in cases of aortic stenosis. **Pulsus plenus.** A large, full pulse. **Pulsus rarus.** A very slow pulse, as with heart block. **Pulsus tardus.** A pulse with a gradual rise and fall. **Pulsus trigeminus.** Trigeminal pulse. *See* PULSE. [L.]

pultaceous (pul·ta·shus). Pulpy; macerated; nearly fluid or having the qualities of a poultice. [L *puls* porridge.]

pulver (**pul**·ver). A powder; a word used in prescription writing. [L *pulvis* dust.]

pulverin (**pul**·ver·in). Barilla; impure sodium carbonate obtained by burning seaweeds and kelps. [see prec.]

pulverization (pul·ver·i·**za'**·shun). 1. The act of reducing to powder or dust. 2. The condition of having been reduced to dust. [L *pulvis* dust.]

pulverize (**pul**·ver·ize). To reduce to a fine powder. [see prec.]

pulverulent (pul·**ver**·ew·lent). Like powder or dust. [L *pulverulentus* dusty.]

pulvinar [nucleus posterior (pulvinar thalami) (NA)] (pul·**vi**·nar). The posterolateral part of the thalamus which overlaps the superior quadrigeminal body and the medial geniculate body. It is particularly well developed in the human thalamus and is connected to the para- and peristriate areas of the cortex (the visuopsychic area). [L *pulvinus* cushion.]

pulvinate (**pul**·vin·ate). Shaped like a cushion. [see prec.]

pulvis (**pul**·vis) (pl. *pulveres*). A powder. All powders were listed officially as *Pulveres* before 1953. [L, dust.]

pumiline (**pew**·mil·een). Dwarf pine oil, pine-needle oil, oleum pini pumilionis, pumilio pine oil; the oil from the young branches of *Pinus pumilio* (family Pinaceae). It is a colourless or yellowish liquid with a pleasant aromatic odour, containing L-pinene, L-phellandrene, sylvestrine, bornyl acetate, and cadinene. It is used like turpentine.

pump (pump). An instrument for removing or forcing liquids or gases. **Air pump.** A pump for removing air from, or forcing air into, an enclosure. **Balloon pump.** An instrument used to provide assistance to the circulation when this is acutely insufficient; it consists of a balloon passed into the aorta from the femoral artery which is automatically inflated during cardiac diastole and deflated during cardiac systole by an external machine triggered from the electocardiogram. **Breast pump.** An apparatus used to remove milk from the breast. **Dental pump.** An apparatus for removing secretions from the mouth during dental operations. **Diffusion pump.** A vacuum pump charged with mercury or with oil, depending for its action on the rapid motion of mercury or oil vapour through a jet. **Filter pump.** Water pump (see below). **Force pump.** A pump for raising water or other liquid to a higher level, or for compressing air or other gases. **Molecular pump.** A vacuum pump depending for its action on the dragging force, due to viscosity, exerted on gas molecules by a rapidly rotating surface close to a stationary one. **Pump oxygenator.** An apparatus which takes over the functions of the heart and lungs; cardiopulmonary by-pass. **Rotary pump.** A vacuum pump depending for its action on the rotation of a metal cylinder set eccentrically inside another cylinder. **Saliva pump.** Dental pump (see above). **Sodium pump.** A complex transport system in the cell membrane of animals which maintains the high intracellular concentration of potassium and the low intracellular sodium in animal cells. It is a complex lipoprotein which catalyses the coupled movements of sodium and potassium against concentration gradients, the energy required being derived from the breakdown of ATP. **Stomach pump.** An apparatus for removing the contents of the stomach by means of suction through a flexible tube. **Vacuum pump.** A pump for producing low pressures in a vessel by removal of air or other gases. **Water pump.** A pump for producing low pressures, depending for its action on the rapid motion of a jet of water. [ME *pumpe.]*

See also: ALVERGNIAT, LINDBERG, WOODYATT.

pumpkin (**pump**·kin). *Cucurbita maxima* (family Cucurbitaceae), a native of the Levant, but cultivated also on the shores of the Mediterranean and elsewhere. The seeds should be deprived of their seed coats when not more than a month old; they contain an acrid resin and about 30 per cent of a reddish fixed oil, neither of which has therapeutic activity. The seeds are used as a taenicide. [OFr. *pompon.*]

puna (**poo**·nah). Altitude sickness. *See* SICKNESS. [Sp., Andean tableland.]

punch (punsh) 1. An instrument for making a small circular hole in a sheet of material. 2. An alcoholic liquor consisting of hot wine or spirit with fruits, or their juices, and sugar. **Pin punch.** An instrument used for making holes in a piece of metal through which the pins of an artificial tooth pass to secure retention. **Plate punch.** An instrument for making circular holes in a dental plate made of metal. [L *pungere* to prick.]

See also: AINSWORTH, CAULK, MURPHY (J. B.), THOMPSON (G. J.).

punch drunk (**punsh** drunk). A condition occurring in pugilists caused by repeated cerebral concussion as the result of blows; it may be marked by uncertain gait with dragging of the feet, slow muscular movement, hesitant speech, tremor and impairment of the intellect. [punch, AS *drincon.*]

puncta (**pungk**·tah). *See* PUNCTUM.

punctate, punctated (**pungk**·tate, pungk·**ta**·ted). Marked with minute coloured or elevated dots, points or punctures. [L *punctum* point.]

punctation (pungk·**ta**·shun). The fine granules in the red-cell cytoplasm which stain red with Romanovsky stains. They are associated with the benign tertian malaria parasite, *Plasmodium vivax,* and also with *Plasmodium ovale.* [L *punctum* point.]

puncticulum (pungk·**tik**·ew·lum). A minute spot or point, generally of petechial type. [L, little point.]

punctiform (**pungk**·te·form). Of the size and shape of a point; used to describe minute colonies of bacteria growing on solid media. [L *punctum* point, form.]

punctograph (**pungk**·to·graf). A metallic pointer used to help in the localization of foreign bodies. [L *punctum* point, Gk *graphein* to record.]

punctum [NA] (**pungk**·tum) (pl. *puncta*). Point. **Punctum caecum.** Blind spot; the physiological blind area, temporal to the fixation point, found in examination of the uniocular visual field. It is due to the absence of retina where the optic nerve passes through the coats of the eye. **Puncta dolorosa.** Valleix's points. **Puncta lacrimalia [NA].** The orifices of the lacrimal canaliculi on the lacrimal papillae. **Punctum proximum.** Near point. *See* POINT. **Puncta pruritica.** Itching spots. **Punctum remotum.** Far point. *See* POINT. [L.]

punctumeter (pungk·**tum**·et·er). One of the many instruments used for measuring accommodation range. [L *punctum* point, meter.]

punctura (pungk·**tewr**·ah). Puncture. **Punctura exploratoria.** Exploratory puncture. *See* PUNCTURE. [L.]

puncture (**pungk**·tcher). 1. The operation of piercing a viscus or a swelling either to establish the nature of its content or to empty it. 2. The wound made by such a piercing. **Cistern puncture, Cisternal puncture.** The introduction of a needle into the cerebellomedullary cisterna via the suboccipital tissue. **Cranial puncture.** 1. The passage of a brain needle into cerebral substance for diagnostic purpose; ill-defined usage: obsolete. 2. Ventricular puncture (see below). **Cricothyroid puncture.** The insertion of a needle and the injection of a solution of a local analgesic through the cricothyroid membrane to depress the cough reflex. **Diabetic puncture.** Needling of a point in the floor of the 3rd ventricle of the brain in experimental animals which causes glycosuria; piqûre diabetes. **Epigastric puncture.** Marfan's method. **Exploratory puncture.** Investigation of the nature of a swelling or the content of a cavity by piercing it with a sharp instrument, often a hollow needle. **Gland puncture.** The puncture of a gland with a hypodermic needle in order to obtain some material for diagnostic purposes; it is a procedure used in the diagnosis of enlarged inguinal lymph glands in venereal disease, in plague, in trypanosomiasis and in Sudanese kala-azar. **Heat puncture.** Punctate injury to the base of the brain in the region of the hypothalamus which causes a rise in body temperature. **Intra-atrial puncture.** Puncture of the right atrium with a long needle for the purpose of making an intracardiac injection in the treatment of cardiac asystole; the ventricular route is more commonly employed. **Intracisternal puncture.** Cisternal puncture (see above). **Intraventricular puncture.** Puncture of the ventricle for the purpose of making an intracardiac injection. **Lumbar puncture.** Insertion of a hollow needle into the intradural (subarachnoid) or the extradural space. **Spinal puncture.** Lumbar puncture (see above). **Splenic puncture.** Puncture of the spleen through the abdominal wall as a diagnostic measure in certain diseases. **Sternal puncture.** Removal of marrow from the sternum through a stout needle as a diagnostic measure, especially in blood diseases. **Suboccipital puncture.** Cisternal puncture (see above). **Suprapubic puncture.** An emergency method of relieving acute retention of urine by passing a needle into the bladder immediately above the pubes. **Thecal puncture.** Lumbar puncture (see above). **Tibial puncture.** A puncture of the tibia in mid-shaft with a sternal puncture needle, to obtain marrow fluid or blood for diagnostic purposes, or to give small transfusions, in young children. **Tonsil puncture.** An exploratory puncture of the tonsil, usually carried out for the establishment of the diagnosis of abscess formation, or as a means of obtaining tissue for microscopic examination. **Ventricular puncture.** The introduction of a brain needle into the ventricles of the brain (usually the lateral) and removal of cerebrospinal fluid for diagnosis and therapy. [L *punctura.*]

See also: BERNARD (C.), CORNING, MARFAN, QUINCKE.

pungent (pun·jent). Of a taste or an odour, one that is sharp, biting, penetrating or stinging. [L *pungens* pricking.]

Punica (pew·nik·ah). A genus of plants of the family Punicaceae. The important medical species is *Punica granatum* Linn., the pomegranate, the root bark of which is the source of pelletierine, isopelletierine and pseudopelletierine. A mixture of the tannates of these alkaloids is used as a taenicide. [L *punicum malum* pomegranate.]

puniceous (pew·**nis**·e·us). Carmine or purple in colour. [L *puniceus* pomegranate red.]

punicine (pew·nis·een). Pelletierine; one of the alkaloids obtained from the bark and root of the pomegranate, *Punica granatum* Linn., and used as an anthelminthic. [see prec.]

Puntius javanicus (**pun**·she·us jah·**van**·ik·us). A freshwater fish used in antimalarial work.

punudos (poo·**noo**·dos). A disease resembling leprosy occurring in Guatemala. [Sp.]

pupa (pew·pah). A stage in the life cycle of endopterygote insects between larva and adult. It is a quiescent form showing the external characters of the adult though with unexpanded wings, as a mould on to which the adult musculature is developed. **Coarctate pupa.** An exarate pupa within the last larval skin which forms a puparium, e.g. *Musca.* **Exarate pupa.** One with the limb and wing rudiments free, e.g. *Culex.* [L, doll.]

pupal (pew·pal). Relating to or of the nature of a pupa.

puparium (pew·**pa**·re·um). The last larval skin of higher Diptera, retained and hardened as protective covering for pupa.

pupil [pupilla (NA)] (pew·pil). The aperture in the iris through which light enters the eye. **Artificial pupil.** An opening made surgically in the iris when the central part of the cornea or lens is not transparent, or when the pupil has become displaced, usually as the result of iris prolapse. **Cat's-eye pupil.** A white reflex present in the pupil due to intra-ocular neoplasm, to inflammatory changes behind the lens, or to retrolental fibroplasia. **Fixed pupil.** A condition in which the pupil fails to dilate or contract to light or convergence, owing to the iris being bound down by adhesions to the lens capsule, or to interference with the nerve supply of the iris as in acute glaucoma. **Keyhole pupil.** A pupil with keyhole shape, due to absence of a part of the iris (coloboma) as a result of iridectomy or of congenital malformation. **Multiple pupil.** One in which more than one opening is present in the iris. **Myotonic pupil.** Tonic pupil (see below). **Pinhole pupil.** A very small pupil; this may be congenital, due to the use of miotics (e.g. eserine) or to inflammatory iritis. **Tonic pupil.** A condition of which three types are described, though they are probably variations of the same condition: delayed reaction to light; delayed reaction to convergence; and delayed or absent reaction to both, with absence of tendon reflexes (Adie's syndrome). [L *pupilla* little girl.]

See also: ADIE, ARGYLL ROBERTSON, HUTCHINSON.

pupillary (pew·pil·ar·e). Relating or belonging to the pupil.

pupillatonia (pew·pil·at·**o**′·ne·ah). A condition in which the pupil does not respond to the stimulus of light. [pupil, atony.]

pupillometer (pew·pil·**om**·et·er). An instrument with which the pupil of the eye may be measured. [pupil Gk *metron* measure.]

pupillomotor (pew·pil·o·**mo**′·tor). Belonging to pupillary movement.

pupilloplegia (pew·pil·o·**ple**′·je·ah). Paralysis of the pupil. [pupil, Gk *plege* stroke.]

pupilloscope (pew·pil·o·skope). An instrument for measuring pupil reactions. [pupil, Gk *skopein* to view.]

pupilloscopy (pew·pil·**os**·ko·pe). Retinoscopy. [see prec.]

pupillostatometer (pew·pil·o·stat·**om**′·et·er). An instrument for estimating pupillary or interpupillary distance. [pupil, Gk *statos* placed, meter.]

pupillotonia (pew·pil·o·**to**′·ne·ah). Tonic pupil. *See* PUPIL.

Pupipara (pew·**pip**·ar·ah). A division of the dipteran suborder Cyclorrhapha. The members are all larviparous parasites. The family Hippoboscidae is of medical interest. [pupa, L *parere* to bring forth.]

pure (pewr). Unmixed; unadulterated. Biologically, free from admixture with any other strain. The ideal state, chemically, in which a substance consists of that substance and nothing else. Of science, the theoretical study as distinct from the practical application. **Bacteriologically pure.** 1. Sterile; free from living bacteria. 2. Consisting of a single strain of bacteria only. [L *purus.*]

purgatin (per·gat·in). Purgatol, anthrapurpurin diacetate, $C_6H_4(CO)_2C_6H(OH)(OOCCH_3)_2$. A compound which is used as a laxative.

purgation (per·ga·shun). Evacuation of the rectum by means of purgatives; catharsis. [L *purgatio* a cleansing.]

purgative (**per**·gat·iv). 1. Cathartic; promoting evacuation. 2. Any substance which promotes evacuation of the bowel. They can be divided into two classes, those which cause purgation by irritating the mucous membrane of the alimentary canal, and those which have a mechanical action increasing the bulk of the gut contents, or lubricating their passage through the alimentary canal. The irritant group increase the rate of peristalsis and thus shorten the time taken for the faeces to traverse the alimentary canal. In consequence of this, absorption is limited and the faeces reach the rectum in a more fluid state than is usual. In this group are calomel, rhubarb, cascara, senna, aloes, phenolphthalein and castor oil. The group having a mechanical action are the saline purgatives, agar-agar and liquid paraffin. [L *purgare* to purge.]

purgatol (**per**·gat·ol). Purgatin.

purge (perj). 1. To induce evacuation of the lower bowel. 2. A cathartic. [L *purgare* to purge.]

puric (pewr·ik). 1. Of the nature of or characterized by the presence of pus. 2. Relating to purine. [L *pus* corrupt matter; purine.]

puriform (pewr·e·form). Having resemblance to pus. [pus, form.]

purify (pewr·e·fi). To free completely, or as nearly as possible, from associated but unwanted substances. [L *purus* pure, *facere* to make.]

purinaemia (pewr·in·e·me·ah). The presence of purine or xanthine bases in the blood. [purine, Gk *haima* blood.]

purinaemic (pewr·in·e·mik). Relating or belonging to, or suffering from purinaemia.

purine (pewr·een). $C_5H_4N_4$, a complex cyclic diureide which does not occur free in nature but is distributed widely in the form of hydroxy-, amino- or methyl- derivatives. **Amino purine.** Nucleopurine, one of the purines containing an amino group, such as adenine or guanine, which appear in the decomposition products of the nucleic acids. **Purine base, Purine body.** Any of the purine derivatives which are found as animal waste products; they include xanthine, hypoxanthine and uric acid. **Endogenous purine.** Any purine in the body derived from the breakdown of the nucleotides of nucleic acids. **Exogenous purine.** Any purine in the body derived from foodstuffs taken in. **Methyl purine.** Any of the purines in which one or more methyl groups have been substituted; examples are the alkaloids, theobromine, theophylline and caffeine. **Purine nuclease.** An enzyme occurring in the intestinal mucosa, which breaks down nucleosides into the purine base and sugar. [pus, urine.]

purinolytic (pewr·in·o·lit'·ik). Splitting purines. [purine, Gk *lysis* a loosing.]

purinometer (pewr·in·om·et·er). An instrument used to measure the amount of purine or xanthine bases in the urine. [purine, Gk *metron* measure.]

purity (pewr·it·e). **Radiochemical purity.** Of a radioactive material, the proportion of the total activity that is present in the stated chemical form. **Radionuclidic purity.** Of a radioactive material, the proportion of the total activity which is in the form of the stated radionuclide. [L *purus* pure.]

Purkinje, Johannes Evangelista (b. 1787). Prague and Breslau physiologist.

Purkinje cells, or corpuscles. Large nerve cells in the cerebellar cortex, with dendrites which branch in the molecular layer and axons which pass into the white matter of the cerebellum.

Purkinje's fibres. Specialized subendocardial muscle fibres forming part of the conducting system of the heart.

Purkinje's figure, or image. An entoptic image produced by the shadow of the retinal vessels.

Purkinje layer. The middle zone of the cerebellar cortex.

Purkinje's phenomenon, or shift. Red colours become less luminous and blue more luminous, when the intensity of light becomes low (e.g. twilight), and the eye changes from photopic to scotopic vision and becomes dark-adapted; that is to say there is a shift of the region of maximum sensitivity of the human eye from yellow towards the blue end of the spectrum.

pupillomotor Purkinje phenomenon. When the adaptation of the eye is changed from photopic to scotopic, the maximum pupillary reaction takes place with green light instead of yellow.

Purkinje's vesicle. Germinal vesicle. *See* VESICLE.

Purkinje-Sanson images. The three images formed by the anterior surface of the cornea and the anterior and posterior surfaces of the lens, respectively, when a light source is held in front of the eye. They are of historical interest, as the alteration in the size and position of the latter two on accommodation proved that this was due to alteration in curvature of the lens.

purohepatitis (pewr·o·hep·at·i'·tis). An inflammatory condition of the liver which has progressed to the stage of suppuration. [pus, hepatitis.]

puromucous (pewr·o·mew·kus). Mucopurulent. [pus, mucus.]

Puromycin (pewr·o·mi·sin). BP Commission approved name for 3-(2-amino-*p*-methoxyhydrocinnamido)-3'-deoxy-*N,N*-dimethyladenosine; an antibiotic.

purone (pewr·one). $C_5H_8O_2N_4$, a purine compound formed by the reduction of uric acid.

purple (per·pl). A colour formed by mixing red and blue rays. **Aniline purple.** Mauveine. **Purple hearts.** A lay description of dexamphetamine and aminobarbitone tablets tinted blue, in use among drug addicts. **Retinal purple.** Visual purple (see below). **Royal purple.** Tyrian purple (see following). **Tyrian purple.** The Purple of the Ancients; 6,6'-dibromoindigo, the pigment of the snail *Murex brandaris,* native to the Eastern Mediterranean and exported as a dye from Tyre. **Visual purple.** Rhodopsin; a light-sensitive substance found only in the rods of the retina of the eye. It is bleached by the action of light, when it breaks down into visual yellow, and a protein. Vitamin A is necessary for its resynthesization. [L *purpura.*]

purpura (per·pewr·ah). A disease or condition of known or unknown aetiology, characterized by haemorrhagic manifestations mainly as petechiae or ecchymoses in the skin, or haemorrhages in or from mucous membranes and other tissues. **Purpura abdominalis.** A purpura due to urticarial, serous or haemorrhagic effusions into the intestinal mucosa; Henoch's purpura. **Allergic purpura, Anaphylactoid purpura.** A non-thrombocytopenic purpura, often of great chronicity and showing poor response to treatment. It is usually associated with other allergic manifestations such as urticaria, erythema, serous effusions into organs and tissues, asthma and rheumatic swellings of joints. The bleeding time, platelet count, clot retractability and blood coagulation are all normal, while splenomegaly is unusual; abdominal colic is often noted. **Purpura angioneurotica.** Allergic purpura (see above). **Purpura annularis telangiectodes.** A malady, chiefly affecting young males, which commences on the legs and feet and is characterized by telangiectatic, purpuric and atrophic lesions. The condition may be symptomatic of polycythaemia. **Purpura arthritica.** Purpura rheumatica (see below). **Athrombocytopenic purpura.** Non-thrombocytopenic purpura (see below). **Brain purpura.** Multiple pericapillary cerebral haemorrhages of toxic origin. **Cachectic purpura.** Symptomatic or secondary purpura occurring in cachectic states. **Dysproteinaemic purpura.** Purpura due to hyperglobulinaemia or to cryoglobulinaemia, the latter occurring mostly on parts exposed to cold. **Purpura fulminans.** A rare, severe, fulminating, usually fatal non-thrombocytopenic purpura resembling allergic purpura and often secondary to severe infections in children. **Haemogenic purpura, Purpura haemorrhagica.** Thrombocytopenic purpura (see below). **Hereditary familial purpura simplex.** A purpura simplex (see below) occurring as a familial condition, usually in women (Davis). **Purpura hyperglobulinaemia.** A chronic purpura of unknown aetiology, associated with hyperglobulinaemia (Waldenström). **Idiopathic purpura.** Purpura of unknown aetiology. **Idiopathic thrombocytopenic purpura.** A purpuric disease of unknown aetiology associated with petechiae or ecchymoses in the skin, or bleeding from mucous membranes and into body tissues, due to a severe thrombocytopenia in the blood. There is usually prolonged bleeding time, a positive capillary fragility test, normal blood clotting time and variable anaemia, and the condition is nearly always cured by splenectomy. **Purpura iodica.** A purpuric condition sometimes following iodide therapy. **Itching purpura.** Pruritic angiodermatitis; purpura, mainly on the legs, of orange-brown colour in which mild eczematous changes are seen histologically in the overlying epidermis. Varieties include clothing dermatitis (at sites of friction), carbromal sensitivity and Schamberg's disease. **Purpura maculosa.** 1. Purpura characterized by small macular cutaneous lesions. 2. Idiopathic thrombocytopenic purpura (see above). **Malignant purpura.** Acute meningococcal septicaemia. **Purpura neonatorum.** A condition at one time thought to be mainly due to syphilis but undoubtedly associated with the haemorrhagic state in the newborn; in this syndrome hypoprothrombinaemia is due to the exhaustion of the vitamin K absorbed *in utero* from the mother before the bacterial content of the intestinal canal of the infant has reached a condition in which it is able to synthesize vitamin K in sufficient amounts. **Purpura nervosa.** Allergic purpura (see above). **Non-thrombocytopenic purpura, Non-thrombopenic purpura.** A purpuric condition without any reduction in the number of platelets in the blood. **Orthostatic purpura.** A purpura occurring in the lower limbs, due to capillary weakness in certain people after prolonged standing. **Purpura pulicosa.** Purpuric spots caused by insect bites, usually fleas. **Purpura rheumatica.** A condition associated with acute arthritis in which localized haemorrhages occur in the skin, mucous membranes and elsewhere. The cause is unknown. **Purpura senilis.** A simple purpura seen in old people, due to senile changes in the vessel walls without any serological changes in blood coagulation. **Purpura simplex.** A mild purpuric condition without abnormalities of blood coagulation, commonly seen in women. **Stasis purpura.** Purpura of the ankles and feet, usually yellowish brown, resulting from venous insufficiency in the legs. **Symptomatic or secondary thrombocytopenic purpura.** Thombocytopenic purpura (see below) secondary to known primary causes such as leucocytotoxic drugs, radioactive agents and other toxic factors. **Purpura symptomatica.** Purpura occurring in acute infectious diseases. **Purpura telangiectatica arciformis** (Touraine). Purpura annularis telangiectodes (see above). **Thombocytolytic purpura.** Thrombocytopenic purpura (see foll.) **Thrombocytopenic purpura, Thrombopenic purpura.** Any purpura associated with marked thrombocytopenia, prolonged bleeding time, non-retractile clot, normal clotting time and slight to moderate splenomegaly. **Thrombotic thrombocytopenic purpura.** A rare, fatal, acute thrombocytopenic purpura with widespread plate thrombi in the capillaries and usually seen in females. **Toxic purpura.** A symptomatic or secondary thrombocytopenic purpura (see above) that has been caused by exposure to, or ingestion of, some toxic substance or agent. **Purpura urticans.** Lesions of urticaria with some haemorrhage into their substance. **Purpura variolosa.** A form of haemorrhagic smallpox in which the prodromal stage is intensely severe, with haemorrhages into the skin generally and from all the mucous membranes. Death invariably occurs. **Vascular purpura.** Non-thrombocytopenic purpura (see above). [L, purple.]

See also: HENOCH, MAJOCCHI, MINOT, SCHOENLEIN, WALDENSTRÖM (J. G.).

purpuraceous (per·pewr·a·shus). Purple-coloured. [L *purpura* purple.]

purpurate (per·pewr·ate). Any salt or ester of purpuric acid, such as murexide, ammonium purpurate, $C_8H_4O_6N_5NH_4$.

purpureaglucoside (per·pewr·e·ah·gloo′·ko·side). A true glucoside occurring in the fresh leaves of the foxglove, *Digitalis purpurea.* They are *purpureaglucoside* A, $C_{47}H_{74}O_{18}$, which hydrolyses to digitoxin and glucose, and *purpureaglucoside* B, $C_{47}H_{74}O_{19}$, which yields gitoxin and glucose. Hydrolysis by enzymes in this way occurs so rapidly after collection of the leaves that the true glucosides do not exist in digitalis preparations.

purpuric (per·pewr·ik). Pertaining to, or having the characteristics of, or marked by the presence of purpura.

purpuriferous, purpurigenous (per·pewr·if·er·us, per·pewr·ij·en·us). 1. Forming or yielding a purple-coloured pigment. 2. Forming visual purple. [L *purpura* purple, *ferre* to bear, Gk *genein* to produce.]

purpurin (per·pewr·in). 1. 1,2,4-Trihydroxyanthraquinone, $C_6H_4(CO)_2C_6H(OH)_3$. A natural dye occurring in madder; also obtained synthetically by the oxidation of alizarin. It is responsible for the red staining of newly deposited bone in animals fed with madder. 2. Uroerythrin. [L *purpura* purple.]

purpurinuria (per·pewr·in·ewr′·e·ah). An excess of uroerythrin (purpurin) in the urine.

purpuriparous (per·pewr·ip·ar·us). Purpuriferous.

purpurogenous (per·pewr·oj·en·us). Producing rhodopsin (visual purple). [L *purpura* purple, Gk *genein* to produce.]

purring (per·ing). Having a low vibrating murmur like the purring of a cat. [onomat.]

Purtscher, Otmar (b. 1852). Innsbruck ophthalmologist.

Purtscher's disease, or retinopathy. Large, pale, exudate-like areas in the fundus with haemorrhages, following crushing injuries or fractures in any part of the body.

purulence, purulency (pewr·ew·lens, pewr·ew·lens·e). 1. The quality of being purulent. 2. Suppuration; the process of pus formation. [pus.]

purulent (pewr·ew·lent). 1. Characterized by the presence of pus. 2. Producing or containing pus; suppurative.

puruloid (pewr·ew·loid). Having resemblance to, or having the characters of pus; puriform. [pus, Gk *eidos* form.]

Purves Stewart. *See* STEWART, SIR JAMES PURVES.

pus (pus). A liquid product of inflammation, containing dead and digested tissue fragments, dead cells including leucocytes, and sometimes bacteria, all suspended in serum. **Anchovy-sauce pus.** The brown pus of an amoebic abscess of the liver. **Blue pus.** The pigmented pus produced by *Pseudomonas pyocyanea.* **Cheesy pus.** The thick semisolid pus of a tuberculous abscess. **Chocolate-sauce pus.** Sometimes a better description of pus from an amoebic liver abscess, than the classical one, anchovy-sauce (see above). **Curdy pus.** Pus containing protein coagulum. **Ichorous pus.** A thin, watery, but often malodorous pus secreted by an ulcerating surface. **Laudable pus.** A term applied, before the use of antiseptic technique, to a thick, yellowish, odourless pus which, when secreted from a wound, was considered to be a natural forerunner of healthy granulation. **Sterile pus.** Pus from which organisms cannot be cultured, as from an abscess sterilized by chemotherapy, or from some tuberculous abscesses. [L.]

pustula (pus·tew·lah). Pustule. [L, blister.]

pustulant (pus·tew·lant). 1. Forming or producing pustules. 2. A substance that causes a pustular eruption, e.g. croton oil.

pustular (pus·tew·lar). 1. Pertaining to or having the characteristics of a pustule. 2. Covered with or composed of pustules.

pustulation (pus·tew·la·shun). The presence or production of pustules.

pustule (pus·tewl). A small well-defined elevation on the skin containing pus. **Compound pustule.** A pustule composed of two or more enclosed spaces. **Malignant pustule.** Anthrax of the skin. **Post-mortem pustule.** One caused by infection during dissection of a cadaver. **Primary pustule.** A pustule produced although no earlier papular or vesicular lesion could be found. **Secondary pustule.** A pustule formed after the appearance of papular or vesicular eruptions. **Simple pustule.** A pustule consisting of only one chamber. [L *pustula.*]

pustuliform (pus·tew·le·form). Having the shape and appearance of a pustule. [pustule, form.]

pustulocrustaceous (pus·tew·lo·krus·ta′·shus). Characterized by the presence of pustular eruptions over which a scabbed covering or crust has formed. [pustule, crust.]

pustuloderma (pus·tew·lo·der′·mah). Any skin lesion in which pustular elevations are formed. [pustule, Gk *derma* skin.]

pustulose (pus·tew·loze). Pustular.

pustulosis (pus·tew·lo·sis). A pustular eruption. **Palmoplantar pustulosis.** Pustular inflammation of the palms and soles. **Persistent pustulosis.** Palmoplantar pustulosis (see above). **Pustulosis vacciniformis acuta.** Kaposi's varicelliform eruption. [pustule, Gk *-osis* condition.]

pustulous (pus·tew·lus). Pustular.

putamen [NA] (pew·ta·men). The part of the lentiform nucleus which lies lateral to the globus pallidus and medial to the external capsule, claustrum and cortex of the insula. It receives connections from the suppressor areas of the cortex. [L, a paring.]

Putnam, James Jackson (b. 1846). Boston neurologist.

Putman-Dana symptom complex. Putnam–Dana syndrome.

Putman-Dana syndrome, Dana-Putnam syndrome. Sclerosis of the lateral columns of the spinal cord, with variable dorsal column involvement. The description can be applied to many cases of disseminated sclerosis, and it is doubtful if the syndrome is a separate entity.

putrefaction (pew·tre·fak·shun). The process of decomposition of animal and vegetable matter by living organisms, usually bacteria, resulting in the formation of products characterized by nauseating odours, and of toxins bringing about poisoning upon ingestion. The more characteristic products of putrefaction are formed by decomposition of proteins, and include cadaverine, putrescine, trimethyl amine, ammonia, sulphuretted hydrogen and mercaptans. [L *puter* rotten, *facere* to make.]

putrefactive (pew·tre·fak·tiv). 1. Relating or belonging to putrefaction. 2. Of the nature of, or causing or promoting putrefaction.

putrefy (pew·tre·fi). To become or to cause to become putrid; to make gangrenous. [L *puter* rotten, *facere* to make.]

putrescence (pew·**tres**·ens). Incomplete or total decay; a state of rapidly progressing rotting. [L *putrescere* to become rotten.]

putrescent (pew·**tres**·ent). In a state of active rotting. [see foll.]

putrescentia (pew·tre·**sen**·she·ah). Putrefaction. **Putrescentia uteri.** A severe form of acute endometritis in which there is blood-stained discharge resulting from ulceration of the uterine wall. [L *putrescere* to become rotten.]

putrescine (**pew**·tres·een). Tetramethylenediamine, $NH_2CH_2CH_2CH_2CH_2NH_2$. A ptomaine with an unpleasant semen-like odour obtained by Brieger in 1888 from decomposing flesh and also from cultures of *Vibrio cholerae.*

putrid (**pew**·trid). Decomposed; in a state of advanced rot. [L *putridus.*]

Putti, Vittorio (b. 1880). Bologna orthopaedic surgeon.

Putti's mattress. A divaricator pillow used in the treatment of congenital dislocation of the hip.

Putti-Platt operation. A reconstructive procedure for the repair of recurrent dislocation of the shoulder, using the tendon of the subscapularis muscle as an anterior ligament.

putty (**put**·e). *See* HORSLEY. [Fr. *potée* potful.]

Puussepp, Lyudvig Martinovich (b. 1875). Leningrad and Dorpat neurosurgeon.

Puussepp's operation. Incision of the cystic spinal cord for syringomyelia.

Puussepp's reflex. Pressure upon the posterolateral aspect of the sole of the foot produces abduction of the little toe; said to occur in disorders of both pyramidal and extrapyramidal pathways.

pyaemia (pi·**e**·me·ah). The invasion of and multiplication in the blood of pyogenic organisms, giving rise to multiple abscesses in various parts of the body. **Arterial pyaemia.** Pyaemia in which the focus of infection is a bacterial endocarditis that produces septic emboli in the arteries and so gives rise to metastatic abscesses. **Cryptogenic pyaemia.** Pyaemia in which the original focus of infection is not discovered. **Otogenic pyaemia.** Pyaemia resulting from suppurative ear disease. **Portal pyaemia.** Suppurating pyelophlebitis. **Systemic venous pyaemia.** A pyaemia secondary to a septic wound or to other localized suppurative infection. Invasion of a vein leads to septic thrombi and emboli which produce multiple abscesses in internal organs. [Gk *pyon* pus, *haima* blood.]

pyaemic (pi·**e**·mik). Characterized by the presence of, or relating to pyaemia.

pyaemid (pi·**e**·mid). A pustular lesion of the skin in pyaemia due to metastatic spread.

pyapostasis (pi·ap·**os**·tas·is). Metastasis of pus from an inflammatory area to another part. [Gk *pyon* pus, apostasis.]

pyarthrosis (pi·ar·**thro**·sis). Acute suppurative arthritis. [Gk *pyon* pus, arthrosis.]

pyecchysis (pi·**ek**·is·is). Escape of pus as a stream. [Gk *pyon* pus, *ek*, *chysis* stream.]

pyelectasia, pyelectasis (pi·el·ek·**ta**′·ze·ah, pi·el·**ek**·tas·is). A dilated condition of the pelvis of the ureter. [Gk *pyelos* pelvis, *ektasis* a stretching.]

pyelic (pi·**el**·ik). Belonging to the pelvis of the ureter. [Gk *pyelos* pelvis.]

pyelitic (pi·el·**it**·ik). 1. Relating to pyelitis. 2. Suffering from pyelitis.

pyelitis (pi·el·**i**·tis). Inflammation of the pelvis of the kidney due to blood-borne infection from the renal parenchyma, or ascending infection when there is obstruction of the lower urinary channels. **Acute pyelitis.** That associated with severe pain and tenderness in the loins, high fever and pyuria. **Calculous pyelitis.** Infection associated with a calculus which has led to obstruction at the pelvi-ureteric junction. **Chronic pyelitis.** Repeated attacks of pyelitis associated with obstruction of the pelvi-ureteric junction or persistent foci of infection in the renal parenchyma. **Pyelitis cystica.** A low-grade form of chronic irritation of the pelvis of the ureter leading to the formation of minute cysts. **Haematogenous pyelitis.** A pyelonephritis in which the organisms have reached the renal parenchyma and pelvis from the blood stream; resolution may occur, or the disease may become suppurative. **Haemorrhagic pyelitis.** An acute form of pyelitis occurring in the debilitated, or when the causal organism is virulent. **Suppurative pyelitis.** That occurring when there is obstruction to the free drainage of urine from an infected renal pelvis, or when infection complicates hydronephrosis or renal calculus. **Urogenous pyelitis.** A term employed when ascending infection has occurred from the bladder to the kidney, usually associated with obstruction in the lower urinary tract. [Gk *pyelos* pelvis, *-itis* inflammation.]

pyelocaliectasis (pi·el·o·kal·e·**ek**′·tas·is). Enlargement of both the renal pelvis and calyces of a kidney. [Gk *pyelo* pelvis, *kalyx* shell, *ektasis* a stretching.]

pyelocystitis (pi·el·o·sist·**i**′·tis). Inflammation affecting the pelvis of the ureter and the urinary bladder. [Gk *pyelos* pelvis, *kystis* bag, *-itis* inflammation.]

pyelocystostomosis (pi·el·o·sist·o·sto·**mo**′·sis). The creation of a passage between the pelvis of the ureter and the urinary bladder. [Gk *pyelos* pelvis, *kystis* bag, *stoma* mouth, *-osis* condition.]

pyelofluoroscopy (pi·el·o·floo·or·**os**′·ko·pe). Inspection of the pelvis of the ureter by fluoroscopic methods. [Gk *pyelos* pelvis, fluoroscopy.]

pyelogram (pi·el·o·gram). A radiograph of the urinary tract, visualizing the calyces and pelves of both kidneys with the aid of a radio-opaque fluid. The latter is given intravenously and concentrates in the calyces. **Dragon pyelogram.** A pyelogram in which the isthmuses of the calyces are greatly lengthened in congenital polycystic kidneys. [Gk *pyelos* pelvis, *gramma* mark.]

pyelograph (pi·el·o·graf). Pyelogram. [Gk *pyelos* pelvis, *graphein* to record.]

pyelography (pi·el·**og**·raf·e). X-ray examination of the kidneys and ureters after the structures have been filled with contrast medium. **Air pyelography.** Pneumopyelography. **Ascending pyelography.** Pyelography in which the radio-opaque medium is introduced through ureteric catheters and a cystoscope. **Excretion pyelography, Intravenous pyelography.** Pyelography in which the radio-opaque medium is administered as an intravenous injection; it is concentrated in the renal tubules, and visualized in the calyces and pelves. **Infusion pyelography.** Urography carried out by means of slow intravenous infusion of a large volume of dilute radio-opaque contrast medium. **Respiration pyelography.** Pyelography with radiographs taken in different degrees of respiration, showing the movement of the kidneys in relation to the respiratory cycle. **Retrograde pyelography.** Ascending pyelography (see above). [Gk *pyelos* pelvis, *graphein* to record.]

pyelo-interstitial (pi·el·o·in·ter·**stish**′·al). Pertaining to the interstices of the renal pelvis. [Gk *pyelos* pelvis, L *interstitium* a space between.]

pyelolithotomy (pi·et·o·lith·**ot**′·o·me). Removal by surgical methods of stone from the pelvis of the ureter. [Gk *pyelos* pelvis, *lithos* stone, *temnein* to cut.]

pyelolymphatic (pi·el·o·limf·**at**′·ik). Pertaining to the renal pelvis and lymphatic drainage of the renal pyramids, e.g. pyelolymphatic backflow occurring during retrograde pyelography due to back pressure. [Gk *pyelos* pelvis, L *lympha* water.]

pyelometry (pi·el·**om**·et·re). 1. Pelvimetry; the measurement of the diameters of the pelvis. 2. The measurement of the contractions of the pelvis of the ureter as recorded through an indwelling ureteric catheter, especially adapted for the purpose. [Gk *pyelos* pelvis, *metron* measure.]

pyelonephritic (pi·el·o·nef·**rit**′·ik). Suffering from or of the nature of pyelonephritis.

pyelonephritis (pi·el·o·nef·**ri**′·tis). Inflammation affecting the kidney and the pelvis of the ureter. [Gk *pyelos* pelvis, nephritis.]

pyelonephrosis (pi·el·o·nef·**ro**′·sis). Any disease of the kidney and the pelvis of the ureter other than an acute inflammation. [Gk *pyelos* pelvis, *nephros* kidney.]

pyeloparenchymal (**pi**·el·o·par·**en'**·ki·mal). Pertaining to the renal pelvis and parenchyma, e.g. pyeloparenchymal backflow occurring during retrograde pyelography due to back pressure. [Gk *pyelos* pelvis, *para, egchyma* infusion.]

pyelopathy (pi·el·**op**·ath·e). Any disease of the pelvis of the ureter. [Gk *pyelos* pelvis, *pathos* disease.]

pyelophlebitis (**pi**·el·o·fleb·**i'**·tis). Inflammation of the veins of the pelvis of the ureter. [Gk *pyelos* pelvis, phlebitis.]

pyeloplasty (**pi**·el·o·plas·te). Any plastic operation performed on the pelvis of the ureter. [Gk *pyelos* pelvis, *plassein* to mould.]

pyeloplication (**pi**·el·o·pli·**ka'**·shun). The plastic reduction in size of a pelvis of the ureter that is dilated, or a hydronephrosis, by suitably planned resection and resuture of the pelvic wall. [Gk *pyelos* pelvis, L *plicare* to fold.]

pyelorenal (**pi**·el·o·**re'**·nal). Pertaining to the renal pelvis and the tubules of the kidney. [Gk *pyelos* pelvis, L *ren* kidney.]

pyeloscopy (pi·el·**os**·ko·pe). X-ray investigation of the pelvis of the ureter and neighbouring renal tissues. [Gk *pyelos* pelvis, *skopein* to watch.]

pyelostomy (pi·el·**os**·to·me). Cutting an opening in the pelvis of the ureter so that flow of urine may be diverted for a certain period of time, and the ureter thus kept free of urine. [Gk *pyelos* pelvis, *stoma* mouth.]

pyelotomy (pi·el·**ot**·o·me). The operation of incising the pelvis of the ureter. [Gk *pyelos* pelvis, *temnein* to cut.]

pyelotubular (**pi**·el·o·**tew'**·bew·lar). Pertaining to the renal pelvis and tubules of the kidney, e.g. pyelotubular backflow occurring during retrograde pyelography due to back pressure. [Gk *pyelos* pelvis, L *tubulus* a small tube.]

pyelo-ureterectasis (**pi**·el·o·ewr·e·ter·**ek'**·tas·is). Dilatation of the ureter and pelvis of the ureter. [Gk *pyelos* pelvis, ureter, Gk *ektasis* extension.]

pyelo-ureterography (**pi**·el·o·ewr·e·ter·**og'**·raf·e). Pyelography. [Gk *pyelos* pelvis, ureter, Gk *graphein* to record.]

pyelo-ureteroplasty (**pi**·el·o·ewr·**e'**·ter·o·plas·te). A plastic operation involving the ureter and pelvis of the ureter. [Gk *pyelos* pelvis, ureter, Gk *plassein* to mould.]

pyelovenous (**pi**·el·o·**ve'**·nus). Pertaining to the renal pelvis and the venous circulation of the kidney, e.g. pyelovenous backflow occurring during retrograde pyelography due to back pressure. [Gk *pyelos* pelvis, L *venosus* veiny.]

pyemesis (pi·**em**·es·is). The act of vomiting purulent material. [Gk *pyon* pus, *emeein* to vomit.]

Pyemotes (pi·em·o·teez). A genus of mites.

pyencephalus (pi·en·**kef**·al·us). A cerebral abscess. [Gk *pyon* pus, *egkephalos* brain.]

pyesis (pi·e·sis). Pyosis.

pygal (pi·gal). Relating or belonging to the buttocks. [Gk *pyge* buttocks.]

pygalgia (pi·**gal**·je·ah). Painful buttocks. [Gk *pyge* buttocks, *algos* pain.]

pygalopubic (**pi**·gal·o·**pew'**·bik). Relating or pertaining to the buttocks and the pubic region. [Gk *pyge* buttocks, pubis.]

Pygiopsylla (pi·je·**op**·sil·ah). A genus of fleas. **Pygiopsylla ahalae.** A common flea of commensal rats in China, Japan and Indonesia; it carries plague from rat to rat. [Gk *pyge* buttocks, *psylla* flea.]

pygmalionism (pig·**ma**·le·on·izm). A type of erotomania in which the subject falls in love with a statue or an object which he has created. [*Pygmalion,* in classical mythology, a sculptor who fell in love with a maiden he had carved out of marble.]

pygodidymus (pi·go·**did**·im·us). A monster with one body but double pelvis and hips. [Gk *pyge* buttocks, *didymos* twin.]

pygomelus (pi·**gom**·el·us). A double monster of which the parasite, consisting of a limb or limbs, is attached to or in the region of the buttock. [Gk *pyge* buttocks, *melos* limb.]

pygopagus (pi·**gop**·ag·us). A fully developed twin monster joined together at the buttocks, usually back-to-back with fused sacrum and coccyx. [Gk *pyge* buttocks, *pegos* fixed.]

pyic (**pi**·ik). Relating to pus; of the nature of pus. [Gk *pyon* pus.]

pyknaemia (pik·**ne**·me·ah). Thickening of the blood, as with haemoconcentration, polycythaemia or plethora. [Gk *pyknos* thick, *haima* blood.]

pyknic (**pik**·nik). A bodily constitution characterized by a stocky build, a broad face, short massive neck, a large chest and abdomen, and a tendency to obesity. The face is red with prominent venules on the cheeks. Subjects are supposed to have a predisposition to arteriosclerosis, gout, diabetes, osteo-arthritis and affective mental disorders. [Gk *pyknos* thick.]

pyknocytes (**pik**·no·si·tz). Contracted red blood corpuscles with projecting spikes. They may be 5 per cent of a premature baby's corpuscles. [Gk *pyknos* thick, *kytos* cell.]

pyknocytosis (**pik**·no·si·**to'**·sis). Infantile pyknocytosis, an acute, self-limiting haemolytic anaemia of unknown cause, with pyknocytes in the blood. [Gk *pyknos* thick, *kytos* cell, *-osis* condition.]

pyknodysostosis (**pik**·no·dis·os·**to'**·sis). 1. Of Maroteaux and Lamy: short stature, osteosclerosis, dental anomalies, small face, delayed fontanelle closure; autosomal recessive. 2. Of Stanesco: short stature, osteosclerosis, thin cranium and facial bone, brachycephaly; autosomal dominant. [Gk *pyknos* thick, *dys-* difficult, *osteon* bone.]

pykno-epilepsy (**pik**·no·ep·il·**ep'**·se). A variety of minor epileptiform attack, seen in children. [Gk *pyknos* frequent, epilepsy.]

pyknohaemia (pik·no·**he**·me·ah). Pyknaemia.

pyknolepsy (pik·no·**lep**·se). The occurrence of very frequent attacks of petit mal epilepsy. The prognosis is regarded (Gélineau) as exceptionally favourable. [Gk *pyknos* frequent, *epilepsia* seizure.]

pyknometer (pik·**nom**·et·er). A form of accurately graduated pipette or glass-stoppered density bottle used in the determination of the specific gravities of liquids. [Gk *pyknos* thick, meter.]

pyknometry (pik·**nom**·et·re). The determination of the specific gravities of liquids by the use of a pyknometer.

pyknomorphic, pyknomorphous (pik·no·**mor**·fik, pik·no·**mor**·fus). Denoting especially a nerve cell in which the stainable parts are packed closely together. [Gk *pyknos* thick, *morphe* form.]

pyknophrasia (pik·no·**fra**·ze·ah). The thick, coarse type of enunciation to be noted in certain neuromuscular conditions of the face. [Gk *pyknos* thick, *phrasis* speech.]

pyknoplasson (**pik**·no·plas·on). Plasson in its unexpanded form. Cf. CHASMATOPLASSON. [Gk *pyknos* thick, plasson.]

pyknosis (pik·**no**·sis). The process of condensation of nuclear material into a homogenous deeply staining body following death of the cell. [Gk *pyknos* thick, *-osis* condition.]

pyknosomatic (**pik**·no·so·**mat'**·ik). A bodily constitution characterized by a pronounced development of the body cavities, with a tendency to the distribution of fat about the trunk, but with a more slender construction of the motor apparatus. [Gk *pyknos* thick, *soma* body.]

pyknotic (pik·**not**·ik). Of or relating to pyknosis; thick set. [Gk *pyknos* thick.]

Pyle, Edwin (b. 1891). American orthopaedic surgeon.

Pyle's syndrome. An autosomal recessive syndrome with flat nasal bridge and cranial-nerve compression by bone overgrowth; metaphyses widened.

pylephlebitis (**pi**·le·fle·**bi'**·tis). Thrombosis of the portal vein; a rare complication of cirrhosis of the liver or malignant disease of the liver, pancreas or stomach. **Adhesive pylephlebitis.** Non-suppurative pylephlebitis (see foll.) **Non-suppurative pylephlebitis.** Thrombosis of the portal vein as a complication of liver disease, but in which there is no preceding or succeeding suppuration. **Suppurative pylephlebitis.** Thombosis of the portal vein secondary to a septic intra-abdominal infection, especially appendicitis. It results in the formation of numerous abscesses. [Gk *pyle* gate, phlebitis.]

pylethrombophlebitis (**pi**·le·throm·bo·fleb·**i'**·tis). Thrombosis of the portal vein in association with pylephlebitis. [Gk *pyle* gate, thrombosis, phlebitis.]

pylethrombosis (pi·le·throm·**bo′**·sis). A condition characterized by the presence of thrombi in the portal vein or in any branch of it. [Gk *pyle* gate, thrombosis.]

pylic (py·lik). Of or belonging to the portal vein; portal. [Gk *pyle* gate.]

pylometer (pi·**lom**·et·er). An instrument used in the bladder to determine the degree of obstruction at the orifice of the ureter. [Gk *pyle* gate, *metron* measure.]

pylon (**pi**·lon). A simplified artificial (lower) limb sometimes issued as a temporary measure, consisting of a socket to which is attached two ash side supports terminating in a peg end shod in rubber. [Gk, gate.]

pyloralgia (pi·lor·**al**·je·ah). Any type of pyloric pain. [pylorus, Gk *algos* pain.]

pylorectomy (pi·lor·**ek**·to·me). Excision of the pylorus and antrum of the stomach. [pylorus, Gk *ektome* excision.]

pyloric (pi·**lor**·ik). Relating or belonging to the pylorus.

pyloristenosis (pi·**lor**·e·sten·**o′**·sis). Pylorostenosis.

pyloritis (pi·lor·**i**·tis). Inflammation affecting the pylorus. [pylorus, Gk *-itis* inflammation.]

pylorochesis (pi·**lor**·o·**ke′**·sis). Pyloric obstruction. [pylorus, Gk *ochesis* a holding.]

pylorodilator (pi·**lor**·o·di·**la′**·tor). An instrument used to dilate the pylorus in cases of stenosis or of spasm.

pylorodiosis (pi·**lor**·o·di·**o′**·sis). The operation of dilatation of the pylorus by a finger either invaginating the stomach wall or introduced through an incision in the wall. [pylorus, Gk *diosis* pushing apart.]

pyloroduodenitis (pi·**lor**·o·dew·o·de·**ni′**·tis). An inflammatory condition of the mucous membranes of the pylorus and duodenum. [pylorus, duodenum, Gk *-itis* inflammation.]

pylorogastrectomy (pi·**lor**·o·gas·**trek′**·to·me). Excision of the pylorus with the adjacent portion of the stomach. [pylorus, Gk *gaster* stomach, *ektome* excision.]

pylorojejunostomy (pi·**lor**·o·jej·oon·**os′**·to·me). Anastomosis of the jejunum to the pyloric end of the stomach, usually performed after excision of the pancreas and duodenum. [pylorus, jejunum, Gk *stoma* mouth.]

pyloromyotomy (pi·**lor**·o·mi·**ot′**·o·me). Division of the pyloric sphincter. [pylorus, Gk *mys* muscle, *temnein* to cut.]

pyloroplasty (pi·**lor**·o·plas·te). Plastic surgical enlargement of a pathologically narrow or spastic pyloric channel, usually by a longitudinal incision which is sewn up transversely; it is sometimes combined with excision of an ulcer. [pylorus, Gk *plassein* to mould.]

pyloroptosis (pi·**lor**·op·**to′**·sis). Dropping of the pyloric end of the stomach. [pylorus, Gk *ptosis* a falling.]

pyloroschesis (pi·lor·**os**·ke·sis). Pyloric obstruction. [pylorus, Gk *schesis* a checking.]

pyloroscirrhus (pi·lor·o·**skir′**·us). A scirrhous tumour of the pylorus. [pylorus, Gk *skirros* hard.]

pyloroscopy (pi·lor·**os**·ko·pe). General inspection of the pylorus and adjacent structures. [pylorus, Gk *skopein* to watch.]

pylorospasm (pi·**lor**·o·spazm). Spasmodic contraction of the pylorus or of the pyloric portion of the stomach. **Congenital pylorospasm.** Infantile spasmodic contraction of the pylorus caused by antenatal conditions. **Reflex pylorospasm.** That which is induced by a morbid condition outside the stomach.

pylorostenosis (pi·**lor**·o·sten·**o′**·sis). Pyloric stricture. [pylorus, Gk *stenosis* a narrowing.]

pylorostomy (pi·lor·**os**·to·me). The operative insertion of a feeding tube into the pyloric antrum; a type of gastrostomy. [pylorus, Gk *stoma* mouth.]

pylorotomy (pi·lor·**ot**·o·me). The operation of incising the pylorus. [pylorus, Gk *temnein* to cut.]

pylorus [NA] (pi·**lor**·us). The distal end of the stomach which opens into the first part of the duodenum. It is defined by the great development of circular muscle fibres which form the pyloric sphincter. [Gk *pyle* gate, *ouros* guard.]

Pym, Sir William (b. 1772). Military surgeon in the West Indies. **Pym's fever.** A fever that occurred in a small island, Bulama (possible the modern Bolama), off the coast of Portuguese Guinea and was accurately described by Pym: it was probably yellow fever, but he thought it might not be the same and called it *Bulam fever.*

pyoarthrosis (pi·o·ar·**thro′**·sis). Pyarthrosis.

pyoblenna (pi·o·**blen**·ah). Mucus mixed with pus cells. [Gk *pyon* pus, *blenna* mucus.]

pyoblennorrhoea (pi·o·blen·o·re′·ah). Suppurative blennorrhoea. [Gk *pyon* pus, *blenna* mucus, *rhoia flow.]*

pyocalyx (pi·o·**ka**·lix). Pus in one or more of the kidney calyces, almost of necessity associated with suppurative pyelonephritis. [Gk *pyon* pus, calyx.]

pyocele (**pi**·o·seel). Enlargement of a tube or cavity, e.g. a hernial sac, due to retention of accumulated pus. [Gk *pyon* pus, *kele* hernia.]

pyocenosis (pi·o·sen·**o′**·sis). The process of removing the purulent contents of a cavity. [Gk *pyon* pus, *kenoein* to drain.]

pyocephalus (pi·o·**kef**·al·us). The presence of pus in the ventricles. **Circumscribed pyocephalus.** Cerebral abscess. [Gk *pyon* pus, *kephale* head.]

pyochezia (pi·o·**ke**·ze·ah). The presence of pus in the stools. [Gk *pyon* pus, *chezein* to go to stool.]

pyocine (**pi**·o·seen). An antibacterial substance derived from the genus *Pseudomonas pyocyanea* and used, epidemiologically, for the subdivision of this species into types. [Gk *pyon* pus.]

pyococcic (pi·o·**kok**·sik). Characterized by the existence of cocci which give rise to pus. [Gk *pyon* pus, coccus.]

pyococcus (pi·o·**kok**·us). Any coccus which produces or forms pus. [see prec.]

pyocoelia (pi·o·**se**·le·ah). A condition characterized by the presence of pus in the abdominal cavity. [Gk *pyon* pus, *koilia* cavity.]

pyocolpocele (pi·o·**kol**·po·seel). A vaginal tumour which contains purulent matter. [Gk *pyon* pus, colpocele.]

pyocolpos (pi·o·**kol**·pos). An accumulation of purulent matter in the vagina. [Gk *pyon* pus, *kolpos* vagina.]

pyoculture (pi·o·**kul**·tcher). The culture of pus from suppurative lesions on bacteriological nutrient media. [Gk *pyon* pus, culture.]

pyocyanase (pi·o·si·an·aze). A proteolytic enzyme produced in cultures by *Pseudomonas pyocyanea.* It is exceedingly thermostabile and possesses bactericidal and bacteriolytic properties. It is not related to the pigments also produced by this organism. [Gk *pyon* pus, cyanase.]

pyocyanic (pi·o·si·**an′**·ik). Relating or belonging to, or characterized by the presence of *Pseudomonas pyocyanea* (blue pus). [Gk *pyon* pus, *kyanos* blue.]

pyocyanin (pi·o·si·an·in). A blue-green pigment, soluble in chloroform and water, produced during growth by *Pseudomonas pyocyanea.* It is a complex phenazone compound and can be crystallized. [see prec.]

pyocyanobacterin (pi·o·si·an·o·**bak′**·ter·in). A vaccine consisting of a killed suspension in physiological salt solution of *Pseudomonas pyocyanea.* [Gk *pyon* pus, *kyanos* blue, bacterium.]

pyocyanogenic (pi·o·si·an·o·**jen′**·ik). Yielding pyocyanin. [pyocyanin, Gk *genein* to produce.]

pyocyanolysin (pi·o·si·an·**ol′**·is·in). A substance found in filtrates of old cultures of *Pseudomonas pyocyanea.* It haemolyses the red blood corpuscles of dogs, rabbits, sheep and man. [Gk *pyon* pus, *kyanos* blue, lysin.]

pyocyanosis (pi·o·si·an·**o′**·sis). Infection with *Pseudomonas pyocyanea.* [Gk *pyon* pus, *kyanos* blue, *-osis* condition.]

pyocyst (**pi**·o·sist). A cyst filled with purulent matter. [Gk *pyon* pus, cyst.]

pyocystogram (pi·o·**sist**·o·gram). The radiograph made during pyocystography. [Gk *pyon* pus, cystogram.]

pyocystography (pi·o·sist·**og′**·raf·e). Radiographic examination of the evacuated cystic cavity after injection of a contrast medium, usually gas. [Gk *pyon* pus, cystography.]

pyocyte (**pi**·o·site). A pus cell. [Gk *pyon* pus, *kytos* cell.]

pyoderma (pi·o·**der**·mah). Any eruption characterized by the presence of pus in the skin. **Pyoderma chancriforme.** Necrosis with ulceration, apparently due to infection in a debilitated individual. **Pyoderma faciale.** An acneiform eruption limited to the face, and characterized by cyanotic erythema, superficial and deep abscesses, and cysts; sinus tracts may link the cystic lesions. The onset is rapid, and the course fulminating. Comedones are not seen. The condition occurs in girls after adolescence. **Pyoderma gangraenosum.** An eruption, usually associated with ulcerative colitis, in which lesions like furuncles develop, undergo necrosis and produce ulcers which spread peripherally. Vegetations may develop during healing. Staphylococci, streptococci and other bacteria have been cultured from the lesions. **Pyoderma superficialis.** Impetigo. **Pyoderma ulcerosum tropicalum.** An infective ulcerative disease of the skin preceded by vesiculation. It is found in northern Australia. [Gk *pyon* pus, *derma* skin.]

pyodermatitis vegetans (**pi**·o·der·mat·**i**′·tis **vej**·e·tans). A malady in which numerous small pustules surrounded by areas of hyperaemia appear in crops, coalesce, and become covered with crusts. Under the crusts vegetations proliferate. The sites of election are the groins and axillae, but the scalp or lips may be affected. The buccal mucosa may be involved, in which case there is no crusting, but superficial ulcers form. [Gk *pyon* pus, dermatitis, L *vegetare* to enliven.]

pyodermatosis (pi·o·der·mat·**o**′·sis). Any disease of the skin caused by infection with pyogenic matter. [Gk *pyon* pus, dermatosis.]

pyodermia (pi·o·**der**·me·ah). Pyoderma.

pyoedema (pi·e·**de**·mah). Purulent oedema. [Gk *pyon* pus, oedema.]

pyofaecia (pi·o·**fe**·se·ah). The presence of pus in the stools. [Gk *pyon* pus, faeces.]

pyogenes (pi·**oj**·en·eez). Pyogenic.

pyogenesis (pi·o·**jen**·es·is). The mechanism of pus production. [Gk *pyon* pus, *genein* to produce.]

pyogenetic (pi·o·jen·**et**′·ik). Pyogenic.

pyogenic (pi·o·**jen**·ik). Forming or producing pus. [see foll.]

pyogenin (pi·**oj**·en·in). Any substance, whether from bacterial growth or not, that produces a local acute inflammatory reaction on injection. [Gk *pyon* pus, *genein* to produce.]

pyogenous (pi·**oj**·en·us). Pyogenic.

pyohaemia (pi·o·**he**·me·ah). Pyaemia.

pyohaemothorax (**pi**·o·he·mo·**thor**′·ax). An accumulation of pus and blood in the cavity of the pleura. [Gk *pyon* pus, *haima* blood, thorax.]

pyoid (**pi**·oid). Having resemblance to pus. [Gk *pyon* pus, *eidos* form.]

pyolabyrinthitis (**pi**·o·lab·ir·in·**thi**′·tis). Inflammation and suppuration of the aural labyrinth. [Gk *pyon* pus, labyrinth, Gk *-itis* inflammation.]

pyolymph (**pi**·o·limf). Lymph contaminated by pus. [Gk *pyon* pus, lymph.]

pyometra (pi·o·**me**·trah). A collection of pus in the uterus. [Gk *pyon* pus, *metra* womb.]

pyometritis (**pi**·o·me·**tri**′·tis). Inflammation and suppuration of the uterus. [Gk *pyon* pus, *metra* womb, *-itis* inflammation.]

pyometrium (pi·o·**me**·tre·um). Pyometra.

pyomyositis (**pi**·o·mi·o·**si**′·tis). Suppurative myositis. **Tropical pyomyositis.** The occurrence of deep intramuscular abscesses associated with pyrexia in tropical countries, but most commonly in Africa; its aetiology is still a matter for discussion, but frequently there is a streptococcus or staphylococcus in the pus. [Gk *pyon* pus, *mys* muscle, *-itis* inflammation.]

pyonephritis (**pi**·o·nef·**ri**′·tis). Inflammation and suppuration of the kidney. [Gk *pyon* pus, nephritis.]

pyonephrolithiasis (**pi**·o·nef·ro·lith·**i**′·as·is). A collection of calculi and of pus in the kidney. [Gk *pyon* pus, *nephros* kidney, *lithos* stone.]

pyonephrosis (**pi**·o·nef·**ro**′·sis). Distension of the pelvis and calyces of the kidney with pus. [Gk *pyon* pus, *nephros* kidney.]

pyonephrotic (**pi**·o·nef·**rot**′·ik). Relating or belonging to, of the nature of, or characterized by pyonephrosis.

pyo-ovarium (**pi**·o·o·**va**′·re·um). An accumulation of pus in an ovary; an ovarian abscess. [Gk *pyon* pus, ovary.]

pyopericarditis (**pi**·o·per·e·kar·**di**′·tis). Purulent pericarditis. [Gk *pyon* pus, pericarditis.]

pyopericardium (**pi**·o·per·e·**kar**′·de·um). A collection of pus in the pericardium. [Gk *pyon* pus, pericardium.]

pyoperitoneum (**pi**·o·per·it·o·**ne**′·um). A collection of pus in the cavity of the peritoneum. [Gk *pyon* pus, peritoneum.]

pyoperitonitis (**pi**·o·per·it·on·**i**′·tis). Purulent peritonitis. [Gk *pyon* pus, peritonitis.]

pyophagia (pi·o·**fa**·je·ah). The swallowing of purulent material. [Gk *pyon* pus, *phagein* to eat.]

pyophthalmia, pyophthalmitis (pi·of·**thal**·me·ah, **pi**·of·thal·**mi**′·tis). Purulent ophthalmia. [Gk *pyon* pus, opthalmia, ophthalmitis.]

pyophylactic (**pi**·o·fil·**ak**′·tik). Affording protection against pyogenic infection. [Gk *pyon* pus, *phylax* protector.]

pyophysometra (**pi**·o·fi·so·**me**′·trah). An accumulation of pus and gas in the uterus. [Gk *pyon* pus, *physa* wind, *metra* womb.]

pyoplania (pi·o·**pla**·ne·ah). Seeping of pus from one tissue into another or into the tissues in general. [Gk *pyon* pus, *plane* a wandering about.]

pyopneumocholecystitis (pi·o·new·mo·ko·le·sist·**i**′·tis). Inflammation in association with enlargement of the gall bladder resulting from the presence in it of pus and gas. [Gk *pyon* pus, *pneuma* air, cholecystitis.]

pyopneumocyst (pi·o·**new**·mo·sist). A cyst filled with pus and gas. [Gk *pyon* pus, *pneuma* air, cyst.]

pyopneumohepatitis (pi·o·**new**·mo·hep·at·**i**′·tis). Liver abscess containing gas as a result of the action of gas-producing organisms. [Gk *pyon* pus, *pneuma* air, *hepar* liver, *-itis* inflammation.]

pyopneumopericardium (pi·o·**new**·mo·per·e·**kar**′·de·um). A condition marked by a purulent effusion into the pericardial cavity, as well as the presence of air and gas. [Gk *pyon* pus, *pneuma* air, pericardium.]

pyopneumoperitoneum (pi·o·**new**·mo·per·e·ton·e′·um). A collection of pus and gas in the cavity of the peritoneum. [Gk *pyon* pus, *pneuma* air, peritoneum.]

pyopneumoperitonitis (pi·o·**new**·mo·per·it·on·i′·tis). Peritonitis associated with an accumulation of pus and air in the cavity of the peritoneum. [Gk *pyon* pus, *pneuma* air, peritonitis.]

pyopneumothorax (**pi**·o·new·mo·**thor**′·ax). An inflammatory condition characterized by the presence of purulent fluid and gas in a pleural cavity. It may be tuberculous or non-tuberculous, and is associated with partial or complete collapse of the underlying lung. **Subphrenic pyopneumothorax.** A subphrenic abscess. [Obsolete term.] [Gk *pyon* pus, *pneuma* air, *thorax* chest.]

pyopoiesis (pi·o·poi·**e**′·sis). Formation of pus. [Gk *pyon* pus, *poiein* to produce.]

pyopoietic (**pi**·o·poi·**et**′·ik). Relating or belonging to pyopoiesis.

pyoptysis (pi·**op**·tis·is). Expectoration of purulent matter or of pus. [Gk *pyon* pus, *ptyein* to spit.]

pyopyelectasis (**pi**·o·pi·el·**ek**′·tas·is). A distended condition of the pelvis of the ureter because of accumulation of pus or purulent fluid. [Gk *pyon* pus, *pyelos* pelvis, *ektasis* a stretching.]

pyorrhagia (pi·o·**ra**·je·ah). A copious discharge of pus. [Gk *pyon* pus, *rhegnynein* to gush forth.]

pyorrhoea (pi·o·**re**·ah). A discharge of pus. **Pyorrhoea alveolaris.** A suppurative process occurring in the supporting tissues of the teeth, accompanied by loosening of those teeth which are involved; chronic suppurative periodontitis. **Pyorrhoea profunda.** Pyorrhoea alveolaris with deep pockets that persistently exude pus. [Gk *pyon* pus, *rhoia* flow.]

pyorrhoeal (pi·o·**re**·al). Relating or belonging to pyorrhoea, particularly pyorrhoea alveolaris.

pyorubin (pi·o·**roo**·bin). A red, water-soluble pigment, produced by *Pseudomonas aeruginosa.* [Gk *pyon* pus, L *ruber* red.]

pyosalpingitis (**pi**·o·sal·pin·**ji**′·tis). Purulent inflammation of the uterine tube. [Gk *pyon* pus, salpingitis.]

pysosalpingo-oöphoritis, pyosalpingo-oöthecitis (pi·o·sal·-ping·go·o·of·or·i′·tis, pi·o·sal·ping·go·o·o·the·si′·tis). Inflammation affecting the ovary and uterine tube, associated with an accumulation of purulent matter. [Gk *pyon* pus, *salpigx* trumpet, oöphoron, oötheca, Gk *-itis* inflammation.]

pyosalpinx (pi·o·sal·pingx). Inflammation of the uterine tube which has progressed to pus formation. [Gk *pyon* pus, *salpigx* trumpet.]

pyosapraemia (pi·o·sap·re′·me·ah). Pyaemia. [Gk *pyon* pus, *sapros* diseased, *haima* blood.]

pyosclerosis (pi·o·skler·o′·sis). Sclerosis of a part attended by inflammation and suppuration. [Gk *pyon* pus, sclerosis.]

pyosepticaemia (pi·o·sep·te·se′·me·ah). Pyaemia associated with septicaemia.

pyoseroculture (pi·o·seer·o·kul·tcher). A culture made by the implantation of pus into blood serum. [Gk *pyon* pus, serum, culture.]

pyosis (pi·o·sis). Suppuration; pus formation. **Pyosis palmaris.** A pustular infection of the palms occurring particularly in Indian children. **Pyosis tropica.** A pustular impetiginoid infection of the skin, capped by a crust. It occurs in Sri Lanka, China, and in other hot countries. [Gk *pyon* pus, *-osis* condition.]

See also: CASTELLANI, CORLETT, MANSON.

pyospermia (pi·o·sper·me·ah). The occurrence of pus in the seminal fluid. [Gk *pyon* pus, sperm.]

pyostatic (pi·o·stat·ik). 1. Checking a suppurative process. 2. An agent capable of checking the formation of pus. [Gk *pyon* pus, *statikos* causing to stand.]

pyothorax (pi·o·thor·ax). Purulent pleurisy; empyema. **Subphrenic pyothorax.** A subphrenic abscess. [Gk *pyon* pus, thorax.]

pyotorrhoea (pi·o·to·re′·ah). A purulent discharge from the ear. [Gk *pyon* pus, *ous* ear, *rhoia* flow.]

pyotoxaemia (pi·o·tox·e′·me·ah). The existence in the blood of toxins of pyogenic micro-organisms. [Gk *pyon* pus, toxaemia.]

pyoturia (pi·o·tewr·e·ah). Pyuria.

pyo-umbilicus (pi·o·um·bil′·ik·us). Infection of the umbilicus with purulent discharge. [Gk *pyon* pus, umbilicus.]

pyo-urachus (pi·o·ewr·a·kus). An accumulation of pus in the urachus. [Gk *pyon* pus, urachus.]

pyo-ureter (pi·o·ewr·e′·ter). The presence of pus in a ureter, to the point of distension or obstruction. [Gk *pyon* pus, ureter.]

pyovesiculosis (pi·o·ves·ik·ew·lo′·sis). A collection of pus confined in the seminal vesicles. [Gk *pyon* pus, vesicle, Gk *-osis* condition.]

pyoxanthine (pi·o·zan·theen). A brownish-red or yellow pigment obtained by the oxidation of pyocyanin exposed to air. [Gk *pyon* pus, *xanthos* yellow.]

pyoxanthose (pi·o·zan·those). Pyoxanthine.

pyraconitine (pi·rak·on·it·een). $C_{32}H_{43}O_9N$, an alkaloid obtained by heating aconitine at its melting point; it resembles aconitine in action. [Gk *pyr* fire, aconitine.]

pyraloxin (pi·ral·ox·in). A product of the oxidation of pyrogallol, which has been used in skin diseases.

pyramid (pir·am·id). An eminence rising to an apex and resting on a polygonal base; in anatomy, an eminence or mass of tissue shaped more or less like a cone. **Pyramid of the cerebellum.** Pyramid of the vermis (see below). **Pyramids of the kidney.** Renal pyramids (see below). **Pyramid of light.** A bright reflection from the tympanic membrane which extends downwards and forwards from the handle of the malleus; the cone of light. **Pyramid of the medulla oblongata [pyramis (medullae oblongatae) (NA)].** Either of the two elevations formed by the pyramidal (corticospinal) tracts on the ventral aspect of the medulla oblongata. **Pyramid of the middle ear.** Pyramid of the tympanum (see below). **Olfactory pyramid [trigonum olfactorium (NA)].** The expanded end of the olfactory peduncle which is attached to the brain. **Renal pyramids [pyramides renales (NA)].** Conical masses of tissue which form the medulla of the kidney, the apices of which project into the minor calyces. The base [basis pyramidis] of each conical pyramid abuts on the cortex. **Pyramid of the tympanum [eminentia pyramidalis (NA)].** A small bony conical eminence on the posterior wall of the tympanic cavity, containing the stapedius muscle, the tendon of which emerges from its apex. **Pyramid of the vermis [pyramis (vermis)].** The most dorsal part of the inferior vermis between the uvula and the lobulus tuberis. **Pyramid of the vestibule [pyramis vestibuli (NA)].** The anterior end of a vestibular crest of the bony labyrinth. [Gk *pyramis.*]

See also: FERREIN, LALOUETTE, MALACARNE, MALPIGHI.

pyramidal (pir·am·id·al). 1. In the shape of a pyramid. 2. In anatomy, relating or belonging to any structure in association with which the name, pyramid, is used.

pyramidale (pir·am·id·a′·le). The triquetral bone. [Gk *pyramis* pyramid.]

pyramidalis muscle [musculus pyramidalis (NA)] (pir·am·id·-a′·lis musl). A small muscle, triangular in shape, arising from the pubic crest and inserted into the linea alba.

pyramidalis muscle of the auricle [musculus pyramidalis auriculae (NA)]. Fibres of the tragicus muscle which reach the spine of the helix.

pyramidotomy (pir·am·id·ot′·o·me). An operation for cutting pyramidal tracts in the brain stem for the relief of certain involuntary movements. [pyramid, Gk *temnein* to cut.]

pyran (pi·ran). A six-membered heterocyclic compound which exists only in derivatives, and in two isomeric forms, α- and γ-. In the modern system of sugar nomenclature the monosaccharides are regarded as related to the γ-compound.

pyranose (pi·ran·oze). In sugar nomenclature, the form in which a monosaccharide is regarded structurally as consisting of a six-membered ring; so called from the relation of this structure to the cyclic compound, pyran.

Pyrantel (pi·ran·tel). BP Commission approved name for 1,4,5,6-tetrahydro-1-methyl-2-[*trans*-2-(2-thienyl)vinyl]pyrimidine; an anthelmintic.

pyranyl (pi·ran·il). The heterocyclic group C_5H_5O–, which occurs in compounds of pyran.

Pyrazinamide BP 1973 (pi·raz·in·am·ide). Pyrazinoic acid amide, a bacteriostatic drug used in the treatment of tuberculosis.

pyrazine (pi·raz·een). $C_4H_4N_2$, a crystalline diazine compound isomeric with pyrimidine; it has a heliotrope smell, and is the parent of a number of important drugs.

pyrazole (pi·raz·ole). A group of five-membered ring compounds, and in particular the compound CH=CHNHN=CH, from which the others are derived.

pyrazoline (pi·raz·ol·een). $NHCH_2CH_2CH{=}N$, a heterocyclic compound produced by the reduction of pyrazole.

pyrazolone (pi·raz·ol·one). Any member of a group of isomeric ketopyrazolines of the formula C_3H_4NO, or derivative of such. They form the basis of several useful analgesics and antipyretics, the most important being phenazone (phenyldimethylpyrazolone).

pyrectic (pi·rek·tik). Pyretic.

pyrene (pi·reen). $C_{16}H_{10}$, an aromatic hydrocarbon consisting structurally of four condensed benzene rings. It is a yellow solid which occurs in coal tar, and possesses carcinogenic properties.

Pyrenochaeta (pi·ren·o·ke′·tah). A genus of fungi widely distributed in soil and on vegetation. **Pyrenochaeta romeroi.** A species causing black-grain mycetoma. [Gk *pyren* fruit stone, *chaite* hair.]

pyrenolysis (pi·reen·ol·is·is). The disintegration of the nucleolus of a cell. [Gk *pyren* fruit stone, *lysis* a loosing.]

Pyrenomycetes (pi·re·no·mi·se′·teez). A class of fungi. [Gk *pyren* fruit stone, *mykes* fungus.]

pyretherapy (pi·re·ther·ap·e). Pyretotherapy.

pyrethrin (pi·re·thrin). Any of the esters which occur in pyrethrum flower.

pyrethrine (pi·re·threen). Pellitorine, a crystalline substance occurring in pyrethrum.

pyrethrolone (pi·re·thro·lone). A mixture of keto alcohols occurring in pyrethrum flowers as the esters of chrysanthemum mono- and dicarboxylic acids (pyrethrins) to which the plant owes its insecticidal properties.

pyrethrum (pi·re·thrum). Pellitory. **Pyrethrum Flower BPC 1954.** Dalmatian insect flowers; the flower of *Chrysanthemum cinerariaefolium* Vis. (family Compositae). They owe their insecticidal properties to pyrethrins I and II which occur together to the extent of from 0.4 to 2 per cent of the dry drug. Kerosene or petroleum extracts, or solutions of the drugs themselves, are used as fly sprays; aircraft are sprayed with pyrethrum extracts to destroy insect vectors of disease (e.g. *Aëdes aegypti*). **Pyrethrum root.** The dried root of *Anacyclus pyrethrum,* used as a sialogogue. [Gk *pyrethron.*]

pyretic (pi·ret·ik). 1. Relating or belonging to fever. 2. Characterized by the presence of fever; febrile. [Gk *pyretos* fever.]

pyreticosis (pi·ret·e·ko'·sis). Any condition characterized by elevation of body temperatures. [Gk *pyretos* fever, *-osis* condition.]

pyretogen (pi·ret·o·jen). An agent which produces fever. [see foll.]

pyretogenesis (pi·ret·o·jen'·es·is). The origin or method of production of fever. [Gk *pyretos* fever, *genein* to produce.]

pyretogenetic, pyretogenic, pyretogenous (pi·ret·o·jen·et'·ik, pi·ret·o·jen'·ik, pi·ret·oj·en·us). 1. Inducing or causing fever. 2. Resulting from fever. [see prec.]

pyretolysis (pi·ret·ol·is·is). 1. Diminution of an attack of fever. 2. A lysinogenic process which is accelerated by rise in temperature. [Gk *pyretos* fever, *lysis* a loosing.]

pyretotherapy (pi·ret·o·ther'·ap·e). 1. The treatment of fever. 2. The method of treatment by raising the patient's temperature either by external heat or by such means as the intravenous injection of protein substances (protein shock) or the production of malaria. [Gk *pyretos* fever, *therapeia* treatment.]

pyrexia (pi·rex·e·ah). A fever; a condition characterized by fever. [Gk *pyressein* to be feverish.]

pyrexial, pyrexic (pi·rex·e·al, pi·rex·ik). Relating or belonging to pyrexia; febrile.

pyrexin (pi·rex·in). A substance present in the exudation of wounds which causes fever. [Gk *pyressein* to be feverish.]

pyrexiophobia (pi·rex·e·o·fo'·be·ah). A dread of fever. [pyrexia, phobia.]

pyrexy (pi·rex·e). Pyrexia.

pyrheliometer (pire·he·le·om'·et·er). An instrument designed to measure the heating of any surface by the sun. It consists of either a sensitive thermocouple or a strip of blackened platinum; from the rise in temperature due to absorption of the sun's rays the energy received per second per unit area of surface can be calculated. [Gk *pyr* fire, *helios* sun, meter.]

pyridazine (pi·rid·az·een). $C_4H_4N_2$, a liquid isomeric with pyrimidine and pyrazine.

pyridina (pir·id·e·nah). Pyridine.

pyridine (pir·id·een). C_5H_5N, a heterocyclic compound obtained by the distillation of organic matter (coal, bone). It is a colourless liquid with an unpleasant characteristic smell, used to render methylated spirit unfit for drinking. It has a local irritant action, and has been used in medicine in the treatment of asthma by inhalation.

pyridostigmine (pir·id·o·stig'·meen). BP Commission approved name for 3-dimethylcarbamoyloxy-1-methylpyridinum. **Pyridostigmine Bromide BP 1973.** The bromide of the base, used in the treatment of myasthenia gravis and to reverse the effects of curare and its congeners.

pyridoxal (pir·id·ox·al). $(CH_3)(OH)C_5HN(CHO)(CH_2OH)$, a naturally occurring derivative of pyridoxine. It is the precursor of pyridoxal 5′-phosphate which is an essential factor for a number of metabolic reactions of amino acids such as transamination and decarboxylation catalysed by aminotransferases (transaminases) and decarboxylases.

pyridoxamine (pir·id·ox·am·een). Pyridoxine.

pyridoxine (pir·id·ox·een). Adermin, 3-hydroxy-4,5-bis(hydroxymethyl)-2-methylpyridine, $(CH_2OH)_2C_5HN(OH)(CH_3)$, vitamin B_6. A factor, deficiency of which causes in rats a florid symmetrical dermatitis of the extremities, epileptiform seizures and haematuria. Similar deficiency effects are seen in pigs and chicks, but little is known about its relation to human nutrition. **Pyridoxine Hydrochloride BP 1973.** $C_8H_{11}O_3NHCl$, a pure form of pyridoxine usually prepared by synthesis and used therapeutically. It has been employed in the treatment of radiation sickness, muscular dystrophy, agranulocytosis, and nausea and vomiting of pregnancy.

Pyridoxinii Chloridum. *European Pharmacopoeia* name for Pyridoxine Hydrochloride BP 1973.

β-pyridyl carbinol (be·tah·pir'·id·il kar·bin·ol). Nicotinyl alcohol, 3-pyridyl methanol, $C_5H_4NCH_2OH$. The alcohol corresponding to nicotinic acid; a vasodilator, used for disorders of peripheral and cerebral vessels. In addition it is useful for disorders of the coronary vessels, e.g. angina pectoris.

pyriform (pir·e·form). Having the shape of a pear. [L *pirum* pear, form.]

pyriformis (pir·e·for·mis). Piriformis; the piriformis muscle.

Pyrimethamine BP 1973 (pi·re·meth·am·een). 2,4-Diamino-5-4′-chlorophenyl-6-ethylpyrimidine, an antimalarial drug used widely for the prophylaxis of malaria. It has no place in the treatment of the acute disease.

pyrimidine (pi·rim·id·een). 1. $C_4H_4N_2$, a crystalline cyclic compound not found in nature as such. Its many derivatives are of great biological importance, entering as they do into the structure of vitamins B_1 and B_2, and the nucleic acids. 2. Name applied to any derivative of 1. **Amino pyrimidine.** One of the pyrimidines occurring as nucleosides: cytosine and methylcytosine. **Pyrimidine base.** Any of the pyrimidines occurring in the nucleic acids: uracil, thymine, cytosine and methylcytosine.

pyrithiamine (pi·rith·i·am·een). $C_{14}H_{19}ON_3$, a compound related structurally to aneurine (thiamine), the -S- group in the thiazole ring of the latter being replaced by -CH=CH-. Feeding to mice produces symptoms of thiamine deficiency which are cured by thiamine.

Pyritinol (pi·rit·in·ol). BP Commission approved name for di-(5-hydroxy-4-hydroxymethyl-6-methyl-3-pyridylmethyl)disulphide; a sedative.

pyroborate (pi·ro·bor·ate). Any salt or ester of pyroboric acid.

pyrocatechin (pi·ro·kat·e·kin). $C_6H_4(OH)_2$, an isomer of resorcinol which occurs in various plants and was originally obtained from catechu but is now mainly synthesized. It has properties rather similar to resorcinol and has a germicidal activity, but is only used to a limited extent in medicine.

pyrocatechinuria (pi·ro·kat·e·kin·ewr'·e·ah). The excretion in the urine of pyrocatechin (catechol), a dihydroxybenzene used in medicine as an antipyretic.

pyrocatechol (pi·ro·kat·e·kol). Pyrocatechin.

pyrodextrin (pi·ro·dex·trin). A tasteless brown substance of uncertain composition obtained by heating starch. [Gk *pyr* fire, dextrin.]

pyrodine (pir·o·deen). An impure form of acetylphenylhydrazine. It has powerful antipyretic properties, but is dangerous to use because of its destructive action on red cells. It has been employed in the treatment of polycythaemia.

pyrogallol (pi·ro·gal·ol). Pyrogallic acid, $C_6H_3(OH)_3$. A trihydric phenol obtained from extract of gall or by decomposing gallic acid by heat. It has powerful reducing properties and hence is used as a photographic developer and for the absorption of oxygen in gas analysis. Medicinally it has germicidal properties inferior to phenol; it is irritant and, in concentrated solutions, caustic. Internally it is poisonous, irritating the gastrointestinal tract and acting like phenol on the central nervous system. It is used only to a limited extent in medicine, mostly for application to the skin in certain diseases such as psoriasis and lupus.

pyrogen (pi·ro·gen). 1. A fever-producing substance; any toxic substance formed by micro-organisms which causes a rise of temperature when injected into the human or animal body. 2. Any foreign protein producing a rise of temperature when injected. Pyrogen may be used to test the capacity of the pituitary to secrete ACTH. **Distilled-water pyrogen.** Any filtrable, thermostabile substance produced by water-borne bacteria; it may be present in distilled water, unless distillation is immediately followed by sterilization. It causes severe rigors and rise in temperature when the water is injected into man and animals. [Gk *pyr* fire, *genein* to produce.]

pyrogenetic, pyrogenic, pyrogenous (pi·ro·jen·**et'**·ik, pi·ro·**jen**·ik, pi·**roj**·en·us). 1. Inducing or causing fever. 2. Resulting from fever. [see prec.]

pyrolagnia (pi·ro·**lag**·ne·ah). A type of sexual perversion in which excitement and satisfaction are obtained by means of incendiarism or by witnessing the spectacle of a large fire. [Gk *pyr* fire, *lagneia* lust.]

pyroligneous, pyrolignic (pi·ro·**lig**·ne·us, pi·ro·**lig**·nik). Concerned with or produced by the destructive distillation of wood. [Gk *pyr* fire, L *lignum* wood.]

pyrolusite (pi·ro·**lew**·site). The principal ore of manganese: a black crystalline form of manganese dioxide, MnO_2, found in Russia, Japan and Canada; so called from its use as a decolorizer in glass manufacture. [Gk *pyr* fire, *lysis* a loosing.]

pyrolysis (pi·**rol**·is·is). In chemistry, the splitting up of compounds by heating. [Gk *pyr* fire, *lysis* a loosing.]

pyrolytic (pi·ro·**lit**·ik). Prepared by, or having a tendency to pyrolysis.

pyromania (pi·ro·**ma**·ne·ah). Morbid domination of the mind by the subject of fires; insane disposition to incendiarism. [Gk *pyr* fire, mania.]

pyromaniac (pi·ro·**ma**·ne·ak). A person affected with pyromania.

pyrometer (pi·**rom**·et·er). An instrument for measuring high temperatures such as those in furnaces, usually by the effects of the radiation emitted upon thermocouples or electrical resistances, or optically by comparing the glow with an incandescent standard of known temperature. [Gk *pyr* fire, meter.]

pyrone (**pi**·rone). Two isomeric heterocyclic compounds, α-pyrone and γ-pyrone, both of which form the basis of many natural products such as pyrocatechol tannins, meconic acid, plant pigments (flavones).

pyronine (**pi**·ron·een). Any one of a family of dyestuffs derived from diphenylmethane, used in the dyeing of cotton and silk, and employed as bacteriological and histological stains. **Pyronine B.** Tetraethyldiaminoxanthene chloride; has a blue shade. **Pyronine G.** Tetramethyldiaminoxanthene chloride; dyes silk and mordanted cotton red.

pyronyxis (pi·ro·**nix**·is). Ignipuncture; the cauterization of tissues by the insertion of needles at red heat. [Gk *pyr* fire, *nyssein* to pierce.]

pyrophobia (pi·ro·**fo**·be·ah). Morbid fear of fire. [Gk *pyr* fire, phobia.]

pyrophoric (pi·ro·**for**·ik). Having the property of glowing or igniting spontaneously in air. [Gk *pyr* fire, *pherein* to carry.]

pyrophorus (pi·ro·**for**·us). Any substance which, when exposed to air, glows intensely and bursts into flame; usually a metal or mixture of a metal and its oxide in such a finely divided state that it is oxidized rapidly. [Gk *pyr* fire, *pherein* to carry.]

pyrophosphate (pi·ro·**fos**·fate). Any salt or ester of pyrophosphoric acid.

pyroplasma (pi·ro·**plaz**·mah). *Piroplasma.*

pyroptothymia (pi·**rop**·to·**thi'**·me·ah). Insanity characterized by the delusion on the part of the subject that he is wrapped in flames. [Gk *pyr* fire, *ptoeein* to be distracted, *thymos* mind.]

pyropuncture (pi·ro·**pungk**·tcher). Ignipuncture. [Gk *pyr* fire, puncture.]

pyroscope (**pi**·ro·skope). A form of differential thermometer used to indicate the intensity of heat or cold due to any body. [Gk *pyr* fire, *skopein* to watch.]

pyrosis (pi·**ro**·sis). Heartburn; gastric hyperacidity and burning pain in the epigastrium. [Gk *pyrosis* burning.]

pyrotic (pi·**rot**·ik). 1. Relating or belonging to pyrosis. 2. Burning; caustic. 3. Any caustic agent used in medical treatment. [see prec.]

Pyroxylin BP 1973. (pi·**rox**·i·lin). Nitrocellulose. In composition it approximates to a cellulose tetranitrate, $C_6H_6O_5(NO_3)_4$, and is made by the action of nitric and sulphuric acids on cotton-wool. Dissolved in a mixture of ether and alcohol it forms a protective film when painted over small wounds and the solvent allowed to evaporate. When colophony and castor oil is added to the solution, there is less tendency for the film to crack. [Gk *pyr* fire, *xylon* wood.]

pyrro-aetioporphyrin (**pir**·o·e·te·o·**por'**·fir·in). $C_{30}H_{34}N_4$, a red crystalline porphyrin obtained from chlorophyll and closely related to the aetioporphyrin derived from haemin.

Pyrrobutamine (pir·o·**bewt**·am·een). BP Commission approved name for 1-(4-*p*-chlorophenyl-3-phenylbut-2-enyl)pyrrolidine; an antihistamine.

Pyrrocaine (**pir**·o·kane). BP Commission approved name for *N*-(pyrrolidin-1-ylacetyl)-2,6-xylidine; a local anaesthetic.

pyrrole (**pir**·ole). A heterocyclic compound which is the parent substance of a large number of important natural compounds among which the following are notable: blood and bile pigments, chlorophyll, indican, certain alkaloids such as nicotine, and some of the amino acids contained in proteins. It is a colourless liquid with the odour of chloroform, occurring in coal tar and bone oil.

pyrrolidine (pir·**ol**·id·een). 1. Tetramethylene imine, $(CH_2CH_2)_2NH$, a colourless base derived from pyrrole, which occurs in tobacco: it is the parent of certain nicotine alkaloids and of the amino acid, proline. 2. $C_{11}H_{18}N_2$, an alkaloid from the wild carrot, *Daucus carota.*

pyrroline (**pir**·ol·een). $(CHCH_2)_2NH$, a colourless base formed by the reduction of pyrrole.

pyrroporphyrin (pir·o·**por**·fir·in). $C_{30}H_{33}N_4COOH$, one of a series of porphyrins derived from chlorophyll-a by treatment with alkali at comparatively high temperature.

Pyrus (**pi**·rus). A genus of trees of the Pomoideae division of the family Rosaceae, including the apple, pear, quince and medlar. The only important medical species is *Pyrus cydonia* Linn., the quince, used for its mucilage. [L, pear.]

pyruvaemia (pi·roo·ve·me·ah). The presence of an abnormally increased quantity of pyruvic acid in the blood. [pyruvic acid, Gk *haima* blood.]

pyruvate (pi·**roo**·vate). $CH_3COCOOH$, an intermediate of carbohydrate oxidation.

pyuria (pi·**ewr**·e·ah). A condition in which pus is present in the urine. **Abacterial pyuria.** A virus infection of the bladder and urethra which may be characterized by an acute phase of considerable severity: a more chronic form may be accompanied by a urethral discharge. In the absence of bacilli, the acute phase may be mistaken for tuberculosis. Resolution may be hastened by arsphenamine therapy. **Miliary pyuria.** The presence of miliary bodies, composed of blood cells, pus cells, and epithelium in the urine. [Gk *pyon* pus, urine.]

Q

qcepo (ksa·po). A form of dermal leishmaniasis with tubercles on the skin.
quack (kwak). A fraudulent empiric; one who claims medical skill that he does not possess. [Du. *kwakzalven* to peddle salves.]
quadrant (kwod·rant). One quarter of a circle. A division of any anatomical area that can be divided by the imaginary bisecting lines, one vertical and the other horizontal, e.g. abdomen, tympanic cavity, retina. These are referred to as the right upper, left upper, etc. [L *quadrans* a fourth part.]
quadrantanopia, quadrantanopsia (kwod·rant·an·o'·pe·ah, kwod·rant·an·op'·se·ah). Loss of a quadrant of visual field. [quadrant, Gk *opsis* vision.]
quadratipronator (kwod·ra·te·pro·na'·tor). The pronator quadratus muscle [obsolete term].
quadratus (kwod·ra·tus). Quadrate or four-sided; used as a descriptive term for four-sided muscles, e.g. quadratus femoris, quadratus lumborum. [L square.]
quadratus femoris muscle [musculus quadratus femoris (NA)] (kwod·ra·tus fem·or·is musl). A quadrilateral muscle stretching from the ischial tuberosity to the trochanteric crest on the femur.
quadratus femoris muscle, nerve to the. A branch of the sacral plexus (root value L4, 5, S1).
quadratus lumborum muscle [musculus quadratus lumborum (NA)] (kwod·ra·tus lum·bor·um musl). A quadrilateral muscle on the posterior wall of the abdomen, stretching from the iliac crest to the last rib, and attached medially to the transverse processes of the lumbar vertebrae.
quadribasic (kwod·re·ba·sik). 1. Of an acid, one that has 4 atoms of hydrogen replaceable by a metal or radical. 2. Of an alcohol, one containing 4 hydroxyl groups. [L *quattuor* four, base.]
quadriceps femoris muscle [musculus quadriceps femoris (NA)] (kwod·re·seps fem·or·is musl). The mass of muscles on the front of the thigh which have a common insertion into the patella; the vasti lateralis, intermedius and medialis, and the rectus femoris muscles. They are all extensors of the knee joint. **Quadriceps lag.** See LAG. [L *quattuor* four, *caput* head.]
quadriceps surae (kwod·re·seps sewr·e). The muscles inserted through the tendo calcaneus into the calcaneus: the 2 heads of the gastrocnemius and the soleus muscles. [see prec.]
quadricepsplasty (kwod·re·seps·plas·te). The division of scars and adhesions around the quadriceps to restore movement to the knee. [L *quattuor* four, *caput* head, Gk *plassein* to mould.]
quadricuspid (kwod·re·kus·pid). 1. Of a tooth, having 4 cusps. 2. Denoting an aortic valve which consists of 4 semilunar segments. [L *quattuor* four, cusp.]
quadridigitate (kwod·re·dij·it·ate). Having only 4 digits on a hand or a foot. [L *quattuor* four, digit.]
quadrigeminal (kwod·re·jem·in·al). Fourfold; composed of 4 parts. **Quadrigeminal bodies.** *See* BODY. [see foll.]
quadrigeminum (kwod·re·jem·in·um) (pl. *quadrigemina*). One of the quadrigeminal bodies. [L fourfold.]
quadrilateral (kwod·re·lat·er·al). *See* CELSUS. [L *quattuor* four, *latus* side.]
quadrilocular (kwod·re·lok·ew·lar). Having 4 chambers, cavities, spacies or cells. [L *quattuor* four, *loculus* small space.]
quadripara (kwod·rip·ar·ah). A woman who is giving birth to her fourth child or who has given birth to 4 children. [see foll.]
quadriparity (kwod·re·par·it·e). The state of having given birth to 4 children. [L *quattuor* four, *parere* to bear.]
quadriparous (kwod·rip·ar·us). Having given birth to 4 children. [see prec.]
quadripartite (kwod·re·par·tite). Consisting of or split into 4 parts. [L *quattuor* four, part.]
quadriplegia (kwod·re·ple·je·ah). A condition in which both arms and both legs are paralysed. [L *quattuor* four, Gk *plege* stroke.]
quadripolar (kwod·re·po·lar). Denoting a cell which has 4 poles. [L *quattuor* four, pole.]
quadrisect (kwod·re·sekt). To divide into 4 equal parts. [L *quattuor* four, *secare* to cut.]
quadrisection (kwod·re·sek·shun). The process of dividing into 4 equal parts. [see prec.]
quadritubercular (kwod·re·tew·ber'·kew·lar). Possessing 4 tubercles or cusps. [L *quattuor* four, tubercle.]
quadrivalent (kwad·re·va·lent). 1. Applied to an element or radical that has a valency of 4. 2. A body formed at the first meiotic division by the association of 4 chromosomes which are held together by chiasmata.[L *quattuor* four, valency.]
quadroon (kwod·roon). 1. The offspring of a mulatto and a white person, i.e. having one quarter Negro blood. 2. In biology, an analogous hybrid. [Sp. *cuarteron.*]
quadruplet (kwod·roo·plet). 1. Any one of 4 children born in the same labour. 2. Denoting such a birth. [L *quadruplus* fourfold.]
quadruplochromosome (kwod·roo·plo·kro'·mo·some). A chromosome consisting of 8 chromatids and resulting from 3 successive replications not followed by chromatid segregation (double endoreduplication). [L *quadruplus* fourfold, Gk *chroma* colour, *soma* body.]
Quain, Sir Richard (b. 1816). London physician.
Quain's degeneration. Myocardial fibrosis.
qualimeter (kwol·im·et·er). A device incorporating materials of different radiation opacity for measuring the quality or hardness of a beam of ionizing radiation. [L *qualis* what kind, meter.]
quality (kwol·it·e). 1. The harmonic content of a musical note. 2. The spectral content of a radiation beam, e.g. "hard", having a short wavelength and high penetration. It is usually measured in terms of half-value thickness of suitable material. [L *qualis* what kind.]
quantimeter (kwon·tim·et·er). An apparatus for measuring the total amount of x-rays in an x-ray field. [L *quantus* how much, meter.]
quantivalence (kwon·te·va·lens). Valency; the number of atoms of hydrogen an element or radical will combine with or displace from combination, [L *quantus* how much, valency.]
quantivalent (kwon·te·va·lent). Having the attribute of quantivalence.
Quant's sign. A T-shaped depression in the occipital bone sometimes occurring in rickets.
quantum (kwon·tum). 1. The unit in which the energy associated with radiation is emitted or absorbed; it varies with the frequency of the radiation ν and equals $h\nu$ where h is Planck's constant. 2. The legal term for the amount of damages claimed or awarded in actions at law for compensation. [L as much as.]
quarantine (kwor·an·teen). 1. The detention, enforced by international law, of persons coming by sea, land or air, or of ships coming from ports where infectious disease is either present or suspected. 2. The period of such detention which is usually that of the incubation period of the disease in question. 3. The place where persons are detained and medically inspected. 4. Prohibition of entrance and departure from a place of detention for suspected or declared infections. 5. To detain or segregate for

suspected infectious disease. **Land quarantine.** Detention or prohibition of persons coming by land from a region where infectious disease is present or suspected. **Shot-gun quarantine.** Illegal enforcement of quarantine, as occurred in some yellow-fever epidemics when persons coming from an infected region were fired on by rifles or cannon. [It. *quarantina* from L *quadraginta* forty, the period of quarantine being formerly often 40 days.]

quart (kwort). A unit of capacity, equal to 1.136 litres, being one-fourth of a gallon; 2 pints, equivalent to 40 fluid ounces. **Imperial quart.** The British standard quart (1.136 litres). **American quart.** For liquid measure equals 0.946 litres and for dry measure equals 1.101 litres. [L *quartus* a fourth.]

quartan (kwor·tan). 1. Recurring at roughly 72-hour intervals, that is on the fourth day. 2. A malarial fever showing such periodicity, that due to infection with *Plasmodium malariae.* **Double quartan.** Infection with 2 broods of *Plasmodium malariae* with resulting fever on 2 successive days with 1 day free from fever. **Triple quartan.** Fever occurring every day from infection with 3 broods of *Plasmodium malariae.* [L *quartanus* concerning the fourth.]

quartana (kwor·**ta**·nah). A quartan fever. **Quartana duplex.** Double quartan. *See* QUARTAN. **Quartana triplex.** Triple quartan. *See* QUARTAN. [see prec.]

quartipara (kwor·**tip**·**ar**·ah). Quadripara. [L *quartus* fourth, *parere* to bear.]

quartiparous (kwor·**tip**·**ar**·us). Quadriparous. [see prec.]

quartz (kwortz). Silica, rock crystal. A natural form of silicon dioxide, SiO_2, found widely in rocks and sand. It occurs in crystals of the hexagonal system ranging from white to smoky brown. It forms the basis of granite and the porphyrins, and also appears in rare forms used as precious stones, e.g. amethyst. It is employed in optical instruments for lenses and prisms, being transparent to ultraviolet light or, when fused, in the manufacture of acid- and heat-resistant chemical ware. [G *quarz.*]

quassia (kwosh·e·ah). Quassia wood, quassiae lignum; the dried stemwood of *Picroena excelsa* (Sw.) Lindl. (family Simarubaceae), known in commerce as *Jamaica quassia.* It usually occurs in chips or raspings which break readily; it contains a bitter principle, quassin, and extracts or infusions are used as bitter tonics and in horticultural insect repellents (BPC 1968). **Surinam quassia.** The wood of *Quassia amara* Linn., used as an adulterant for quassia but easily distinguished microscopically from the true drug. [*Quassi*, a Surinam negro, 18th century.]

quassia cup (kwosh·e·ah kup). A cup made from quassia wood which contains a very bitter substance, quassin. When water is placed in the cup a very small quantity of quassin dissolves, rendering the water bitter. Drinks from such cups used to be taken as a tonic to stimulate jaded appetites.

quassin (kwos·in). A mixture of the 2 crystalline bitter principles, α- and β-picrasmin, obtainable from quassia wood. It has an extremely bitter and persistent taste.

quaternary (kwot·**ern**·ar·e). 1. Fourth. 2. In chemistry, a compound constituted of 4 elements. **Quaternary amine.** An organic compound derived from ammonium hydroxide, NH_4OH, by replacing the hydrogen atoms with alkyl radicals. **Quaternary base.** Quaternary amine (see prec.). **Quaternary structure.** *See* STRUCTURE.[L *quattuor* four.]

Quatrefages, Jean Louis Armand de Bréau (b. 1810). French naturalist.

Quatrefages' angle. The parietal angle. *See* ANGLE.

quebrachamine (ke·**brah**·kam·een). $C_{19}H_{26}N_2$, an alkaloid which occurs in quebracho bark. It is much less potent than yohimbine.

quebrachine (ke·**brah**·keen). Yohimbine, $C_{21}H_{26}O_3N_2$. One of the alkaloids present in the bark of *Aspidosperma quebracho*, used as a bitter tonic and aphrodisiac. It is also found in yohimbé bark.

quebrachite, quebrachitol (ke·**brah**·kite, ke·**brah**·kit·ol). Inositol methyl ether, $C_6H_6(OH)_5(OCH_3)$. A compound derived from quebracho, used as a sugar substitute in diabetes.

quebracho (ke·**brah**·ko, ke·**brah**·cho). The dried bark of *Aspidosperma quebracho* Schlecht. (family Apocyanaceae). It contains the alkaloids aspidospermine, yohimbine (quebrachine) and quebrachamine. It is used as a bitter tonic. [Sp axebreaker.]

Queckenstedt, Hans Heinrich Georg (b. 1876). Rostock physician.

Queckenstedt's phenomenon, sign or test. The pressure of the cerebrospinal fluid is measured with a manometer; if during the process either, or both, jugular veins are compressed, the pressure in a normal person rises rapidly and rapidly returns to the normal 10–15 kPa(80–120 mm Hg) when the veins are released. If there is a block in the spinal subarachnoid space or interference with escape of fluid from the cerebral cavity, the rise will be absent or slight. Also, if withdrawal of fluid causes a persistent fall of 50 per cent, obstruction to the normal flow of fluid is probable.

quenching (kwen·shing). Stoppage of an electrical discharge; in a Geiger counter, by an external electronic circuit. [etym. dub.]

Quénu, André Victor Alfred (b. 1852). Paris surgeon.

Quénu's operation. A sacral form of excision of the rectum.

Quénu-Muret sign. If blood is obtained from a subcutaneous puncture distal to an aneurysm after the proximal artery has been compressed, a collateral circulation can be assumed to be present.

quercetrin (kwer·set·rin). A hypertensive agent. Where vitamin-C deficiency is associated with capillary dysfunction, tablets of quercetrin and ascorbic acid are used.

quercitol (kwer·sit·ol). $CH_2{=}(CHOH)_4{=}CHOH$, a sweet compound occurring in oak bark.

Quercus (kwer·kus). The oak genus of the family Fagaceae. **Quercus infectoria.** The species on which galls are formed as a result of the deposition of the eggs of the gall wasp; the galls are a source of tannic acid. **Quercus robur.** The oak; the bark is used as an astringent and as a tanning material. [L.]

Quervain, Fritz de (b. 1868). Berne surgeon.

Quervain's disease. Chronic tenosynovitis of the abductor pollicis longus and extensor pollicis brevis muscles.

Quetelet, Lambert Adolphe Jacques (b. 1796). Brussels mathematician and astronomer.

Quetelet's rule. In adults the weight of the body should be as many kilograms as the length expressed in centimetres exceeds 100.

Quevenne, Théodore Auguste (b. 1805). French physician.

Quevenne's iron. Reduced iron. *See* IRON.

Queyrat, Auguste (b. 1872). Paris dermatologist.

Queyrat's erythroplasia. Erythematous, circumscribed, papular eruption of the glans penis, coronal sulcus or prepuce.

Quick, Armand James (b. 1894). Milwaukee biochemist.

Quick's test, for haemophilia and jaundice. 1. *Hippuric acid synthesis test.* A biochemical test of liver function in which, after a dose of sodium benzoate (6 g) given orally, the liver conjugates the benzoic acid with glycine to form hippuric acid which is excreted in the urine in quantities inversely proportional to the degree of liver damage; normally not less than 3 g hippuric acid is excreted in 4 h. 2. A test for the amount of prothrombin present in the blood plasma, and used as a test in the diagnosis of haemophilia. An excess quantity of a solution of thromboplastin (from tissue or brain extract) is added to the oxalated blood plasma; after the addition of a fixed amount of M/40 calcium chloride, the time required for the formation of a firm clot is the plasma prothrombin time and is inversely proportional to the amount of prothrombin present in the plasma. The normal plasma prothrombin time is from 12 to 20 s.

quick (kwik). 1. A part sensitive to touch, specifically that part of a finger or toe which bears the nail; vital living flesh. 2. Pregnant and conscious of the movements of the fetus. [ME *quic* living.]

quicken (kwik·en). To show signs of life, e.g. a fetus *in utero.* [see prec.]

quickening (kwik·en·ing). The moment in pregnancy at which the first movements of the fetus are felt by the mother, usually in the fourth or fifth month. [ME *quic* living.]

quicklime (**kwik**·lime). Burnt lime, caustic lime, calcium oxide, CaO. A white substance manufactured by calcining limestone in kilns; it forms calcium hydroxide when slaked with water. [ME *quic* living, lime.]

quicksilver (**kwik**·sil·ver). The old name for mercury. [ME *quic* living, silver.]

quickwater (**kwik**·wor·ter). Mercuric nitrate solution. [ME *quic* living, water.]

Quillaia BP 1973 (kwil·a·ah). Quillaiae cortex, quillaia bark, soap bark; the dried inner part of the bark of *Quillaja saponaria* Molina (family Rosaceae) and of other species of *Quillaja*. It occurs in large flat pieces and contains about 10 per cent of saponins. Extracts are used as emulsifying agents for tars, etc. [Chilean *quillái*.]

quillain (**kwil**·ane). Saponin.

quina (ke·nah). An old name for cinchona bark. [Sp. bark.]

Quinacillin (kwin·as·**il**·in). BP Commission approved name for 3-carboxyquinoxalin-2-ylpenicillin; an antibiotic.

Quinalbarbitone Sodium BP 1973 (kwin·al·**bar**·bit·one **so**·de·-um). The monosodium derivative of 5-allyl-5-(1-methyl-butyl) barbituric acid, a short-acting barbiturate more active than barbitone itself. It is employed in insomnia and anxiety states.

quinamine (**kwin**·am·een). $C_{19}H_{24}O_2N_2$, one of the minor alkaloids of cinchona bark.

quinaphenin (kwin·ah·**fen**·in). A white powder obtained by the action of quinine on the hydrochlorate of eloxyphenylcarbamic acid. It has been used in whooping-cough.

quinaquina (ke·nah·**ke**'·nah). An old name for cinchona bark. [Sp. *quina* bark.]

quinate (**kwin**·ate). Any salt or ester of quinic acid.

quince (kwins). The fruit of *Pyrus cydonia* (family Rosaceae). The seeds contain about 20 per cent of mucilage in the testa with a fixed oil and protein. Preparations are used in lotions and creams, and as suspending agents. [ME *coyns*.]

Quincke, Heinrich Irenaeus (b. 1842). Kiel physician.

Quincke's disease. Angioneurotic oedema. *See* OEDEMA.

Quincke's meningitis. Pseudotumour cerebri.

Quinke's pulse or sign. Capillary pulse, pulsation seen in the capillaries. It may be observed in the nail bed or by pressing on the lips with a glass slide when the margin between the red and blanched part can be seen to ebb and flow. It occurs with aortic incompetence, patent ductus arteriosus and other conditions in which there is a high pulse pressure.

Quincke's puncture. Lumbar puncture; the withdrawal of cerebrospinal fluid through a needle introduced into the spinal subarachnoid space: for diagnostic or therapeutic purposes.

Quinestradol (kwin·e·strad·ol). BP Commission approved name for 3 - cyclopentyloxyoestra - 1,3,5(10) - triene - 16α,17β-diol; an oestrogen.

Quinestrol (kwin·e·strol). BP Commission approved name for 3 - cyclopentyloxy - 19 - nor - 17α-pregna - 1,3,5,(10) - trien - 20 - yn - 17 - ol; an oestrogen.

Quinethazone (kwin·**eth**·az·one). BP Commission approved name for 7 - chloro - 2 - ethyl - 1,2 - dihydro - 6 - sulphamoyl - quinazolin - 4 - one; a diuretic.

quinetum (kwin·e·tum). Defined by the Malaria Commission of the League of Nations as a mixture of equal parts of quinine, cinchonine and cinchonidine. It provides a remedy for malaria in a cheaper form than quinine by itself.

Quingestanol (kwin·jes·tan·ol). BP Commission approved name for 3 - cyclopentyloxy - 19 - nor - 17α-pregna - 3,5 - diene - 20 - yn - 17 - ol; a progestational steroid.

quinia (kwin·e·ah). Quinine.

quinicine (**kwin**·is·een). Quinotoxine, $C_{20}H_{24}O_2N_2$. An alkaloid of cinchona; it is also derived from quinine by heating in dilute acetic acid. It is an isomer of quinine.

quinidine (**kwin**·id·een). $C_{20}H_{24}N_2O_2$, a stereo-isomer of quinine, its pharmacological actions being similar and of equal effect in malaria; it is used in people showing an idiosyncrasy to quinine. It is readily absorbed by mouth and the sulphate (BP 1973) is the form generally employed. Its most important use is in the treatment of auricular fibrillation, as it prolongs the refractory period of heart muscle and decreases its excitability and the rate of conduction of the impulse. It is effective in the prevention of paroxysmal fibrillation and in early persistent fibrillation, as in Graves' disease or in toxic or infective diseases, e.g. rheumatic fever; it is not so effective when the disease is of long standing, and there is also the danger that intramural thrombi present may become dislodged with a return to normal sinus rhythm. The drug may be of value in auricular flutter and in paroxysmal tachycardia. Occasional idiosyncrasies have been known to occur. **Quinidine tannate.** A compound administered occasionally in diarrhoea.

quinine (**kwin**·een). $C_{20}H_{24}O_2N_2$, an alkaloid obtained from cinchona bark. In high concentrations it is a general protoplasmic poison and bacteriostatic, depressing phagocytosis and ciliary action, It has a specific effect on the malaria parasite, particularly the erythrocytic forms, against which it is active in the body in concentrations which have no deleterious effects on the body cells themselves. It is readily absorbed by mouth and is excreted in the urine or destroyed in the liver so that there are no cumulative results. It has no significant effect on blood pressure, respiration or the central nervous system at normal therapeutic doses, but in high doses it causes a marked fall in the blood pressure due to a depressant action on the heart muscle and also by arterial dilatation, The effects on the heart are similar to those produced by quinidine. Quinine weakens the contraction of voluntary muscle, the excitability of the motor end-plate being depressed; it accentuates the weakness of the muscles in myasthenia gravis for which it has been used as a diagnostic. It stimulates smooth muscle, particularly the uterus, and may be employed as an abortifacient and as an oxytocic. High doses depress the central nervous system, leading to confusion and ataxia. This may be observed in people who show an idiosyncrasy to the drug. Effects may also be observed on the special senses and the drug may produce deafness and disturbance of vision. Sensitive persons may also develop skin rashes and urticarial eruptions. Because of its exceedingly bitter taste, it is used to stimulate the gastric secretions and to improve the appetite. Its toxic effect on the nerves causes a local anaesthesia of long duration when it is injected, preceded by a brief stimulation of the sensory nerve-endings. The chloride is generally used for this purpose. It is a valuable sclerosing agent and can be used, chiefly as quinine and urethane, in the treatment of varicose veins, haemorrhoids and hydrocele. While it has antipyretic properties apart from its specific effects in malaria, it is inferior in this respect to the salicylates. The most important use of quinine is in the treatment of malaria, but its mode of action is not clear. It is chiefly active on the dividing stages of the parasite, the merozoites quickly disappearing from the blood; it should be given a few hours before a paroxysm is expected. It does not destroy the sporozoites or the tissue forms in *Plasmodium vivax.* Although it eradicates the gametocytes of *P. vivax* and *P. malariae* (quartan fever), and injures those of *P. falciparum* (malignant tertian malaria), its main usefulness is due to its action on the sporulating stage. While it has a suppressive action in persons exposed to infected mosquitoes, it is not a true causal prophylactic because it has no action on the sporozoites or the tissue parasites. After quinine treatment relapses are prone to occur in benign tertian and quartan malaria. These may be reduced by combining quinine with pamaquin or pentaquine. **Quinine BPC 1963.** A preparation of the alkaloid. **Quinine acetate.** $QuCH_3COOH$, where Qu represents the quinine molecule, $C_{20}H_{24}N_2O_2$; a slightly soluble compound acting like the sulphate. **Quinine acetylsalicylate.** $QuCH_3COOC_6H_4COOH$, a compound resembling quinine salicylate in action and used as an analgesic in neuralgia and sciatica; it is sometimes used at the onset of influenza or the common cold. **Quinine acid hydrochloride, Acid quinine hydrochloride.** Quinine dihydrochloride (see below). **Quinine acid sulphate.** Quinine bisulphate (see below). **Quinine albuminate.** A yellow compound used chiefly as a tonic. **Quinine arsenate.** $Qu_2H_3AsO_4$, a compound used as an antiperiodic in malarial conditions, but its action is chiefly due to its arsenic content. **Quinine arsenite.** $Qu_2H_2AsO_3$, a compound used like the arsenate. **Quinine benzoate.** QuC_6H_5COOH, a compound with the properties of quinine salts but little used. **Quinine bismuth iodide.** Quinine and bismuth iodide, proposed for the systemic effect of bismuth in the treatment of syphilis. **Quinine Bisulphate BP 1973.** QuH_2SO_4, a compound preferred to the sulphate for tablets, though its solutions are not stable to heat. It is used in eye lotions for interstitial keratitis, trachoma, purulent ophthalmia and in ophthalmic diphtheria; a solution is employed for irrigation in cystitis. **Quinine borate.** QuH_3BO_3, of value as an antiseptic and antipyretic. **Quinine bromate.** $QuHBrO_3$, a compound used occasionally as an antiseptic and antipyretic. **Quinine camphorate.** $QuC_8H_{14}(COOH)_2$, an insoluble compound used as an antiseptic and antipyretic. **Quinine carbolate.** Phenolquinine, QuC_6H_5OH, a slightly soluble compound chiefly used as an antiseptic, **Quinine carbonate.** Qu_2CO, aristoquinine, an insoluble, almost tasteless, compound used in malaria and whooping-cough. **Quinine chlorocarbonic ester.** $QuCOCl$, an antipyretic. **Quinine chlorophosphate.** $QuHCl{\cdot}2H_3PO_4$, a compound used in the treatment of malaria. **Quinine chocolate.** A pastille containing quinine hydrochloride in a chocolate base to conceal the taste. **Quinine cinnamate.** $QuC_9H_8O_2$, an antiseptic and antipyretic. **Quinine citrate.** $Qu_2C_3H_4(OH)(COOH)_3$, a compound with little taste and the general properties of quinine. **Quinine Dihydrochloride BP 1973.** $Qu{\cdot}2HCl$, a salt of quinine recommended for intravenous or intramuscular injection when administration of quinine by mouth is contra-indicated. **Quinine dihydrochloride carbonate.** A double salt of quinine. **Quinine eosolate.** A derivative of quinine and creosote, used like the sulphate. **Quinine ethyl carbonate.** $QuCO_2C_2H_5$, a compound with slight taste, used in quinine therapy. **Quinine ethyl sulphate.** $Qu(C_2H_5)SO_4$, a compound used occasionally for injections. **Quinine ferrichloride.** A brown scaly compound used as a haemostatic. **Quinine ferrocyanide.** $QuH_4Fe(CN)_6$, an antipyretic. **Quinine formate.** $QuHCOOH$, quinoform, said to be less irritant than other quinine salts and recommended for injection. **Quinine glycerophosphate.** $Qu_2H_2PO_4C_3H_7O_2$, a compound used as a general tonic, especially in compound syrup preparations. **Quinine hydriodide.** $QuHI$, a pale-yellow compound used in chronic rheumatism. **Quinine hydrobromide.** $QuHBr$, a compound which is less likely to produce cinchonism and is used in neuralgia and acute rheumatism for its sedative action, and in the treatment of exophthalmic goitre. **Quinine Hydrochloride BP 1973.** $QuHCl$, a compound more soluble than the sulphate, more readily absorbed and less irritating. It is used in malaria and also in the form of pessaries in leucorrhoea and as a contraceptive. With urethane, it is employed as a sclerosing agent in varicose veins and as a lotion in corneal ulcers. **Quinine hydrochlorocarbamide.** Quinine and urea hydrochloride (see below). **Quinine hydrochlorosulphate.** $QuHClH_2SO_4$, a very soluble compound and highly acid. **Quinine hydroquinone hydrochloride.** A compound used as an antipyretic. **Quinine iodobismuthate.** A double salt of variable composition, approximating to the formula $(BiI_3)_2QuHI$. It is a means of administering bismuth in the treatment of syphilis. It acts more slowly than other preparations of bismuth, and is useful for patients who cannot tolerate, or who are resistant to, arsenic and mercury. **Quinine iodohydroiodate.** $QuIHI$, a brown compound which has been tried in the treatment of syphilis. **Quinine lactate.** $QuCH_3CHOHCOOH$, a soluble form of quinine suitable for injections. **Quinine methochloride.** A compound produced by the methylation of quinine; it blocks transmission at the myoneural junction. **Quinine muriate.** Quinine hydrochloride (see above). **Quinine nucleinate.** A preparation which has been used intramuscularly in syphilis. **Quinine oleate.** A mixture of quinine and oleic acid used in ointments. **Quinine peptonate.** A powder containing quinine and peptone, used as a tonic. **Quinine phenate, Quinine phenolate.** Quinine carbolate (see above). **Quinine phosphate.** A compound chiefly included in iron-quinine and strychnine-phosphate syrups (e.g. Easton's syrup). **Quinine phosphohydrochloride.** $QuHCl{\cdot}2H_2PO_4$, a compound used as an antiperiodic and for the relief of headaches. **Quinine phthalate.** $Qu_2C_6H_4(COOH)_2$, a compound used like the sulphate. **Quinine saccharate.** A compound of quinine and sucrose used as an antipyretic. **Quinine salicylate.** $QuC_6H_4(OH)COOH$, a sparingly soluble compound used in neuralgia and rheumatic conditions, also in the common cold and influenza. **Quinine silicofluoride.** An antiseptic and antipyretic. **Quinine stearate.** $QuC_{17}H_{35}COOH$, a compound used in ointments. **Quinine Sulphate BP 1973.** $Qu_2H_2SO_4$, the most widely used salt of quinine; a white crystalline compound, slightly soluble in water, more so in acid solution, and not suitable for injection, **Quinine sulphochloride.** Quinine hydrochlorosulphate (see above). **Quinine sulphocresolate.** An intestinal antiseptic, **Quinine sulpho-ethylate.** Quinine ethyl sulphate (see above). **Quinine sulphotartrate.** A combination of quinine sulphate and tartaric acid, used as an antipyretic and antiseptic. **Quinine sulphovinate.** Quinine ethyl sulphate (see above). **Quinine tannate.** An amorphous yellow powder which is inefficient for quinine therapy as its absorption is slow, but it can be given to young children as it is tasteless. **Quinine and urea hydrochloride.** A mixture of urea and quinine hydrochloride used as a sclerosing agent in varicose veins; it is also employed as a long-lasting local anaesthetic when injected, and to produce nerve block. By the parenteral route in weak solutions, it is of value in quinine therapy. **Quinine urethane.** A compound of quinine and urethane which is non-irritant and is employed for intravenous injection purposes (varicose veins). **Quinine valerate, Quinine valerianate.** QuC_4H_9COOH, a compound used in the treatment of headaches and nervous debility. [Sp. *quina* bark.]

quininephytine (kwin·in·ef·it·een). Quinine anhydroxymethylene diphosphate. A compound used as a tonic and antiperiodic.

quininism (kwin·in·izm). Cinchonism; chronic poisoning with cinchona or any of the alkaloids of cinchona bark. Various toxic symptoms are produced, e.g. cerebral congestion, giddiness, tinnitus, rash, nausea, mental and cardiac disturbances, and circulatory or respiratory failure.

quininize (kwin·in·ize). To treat with quinine or cinchona alkaloids.

quininurethane (kwin·in·ewr·e·thane). Quinine and urethane hydrochloride. A non-irritating compound of quinine and urethane injected hypodermically as a sclerosing agent in the treatment of varicose veins.

quiniometry (kwin·e·om·et·re). The determination of the cinchona alkaloids in cinchona barks. [quinine, meter.]

quinism (kwin·izm). Quininism.

quinizarin (kwin·iz·ar·in). 1,4-Dihydroxy-anthroquinone, $C_6H_4(CO)_2C_6H_2(OH)_2$. A colourless solid; it is used as a powder in neurological investigations (*see* SWEATING TEST).

quinoform (kwin·o·form). Chinoform, quinine formate, $C_{20}H_{24}O_2N_2HCOOH$. A soluble white crystalline compound used subcutaneously in quinine therapy.

quinoid (kwin·oid). In organic chemistry, a cyclic aromatic compound containing the six-membered carbon ring characteristic of quinone as distinct from the benzenoid ring. This is a powerful chromophoric structure and enters into the composition of many important dyestuffs.

quinol (kwin·ol). Hydroquinone, $C_6H_4(OH)_2$. A dihydriphenol prepared by reducing quinone with sulphur dioxide; it occurs naturally as the glycoside, arbutin, in bearberry leaves. It is used mainly as a photographic developer but it has also certain antiseptic properties.

quinoline (kwin·ol·een). $C_6H_4{=}CH(N)(CH)_2$, a heterocyclic base constituted of a benzene ring fused with pyridine nucleus. It is to be found in coal tar and bone oil, and may be prepared from certain alkaloids such as quinine and cinchonine. It is a colourless liquid with characteristic odour, having an antipyretic effect but too toxic for therapeutic use. Chiniofon sodium is a derivative used in amoebic dysentery.

quinone (**kwin**·one). 1. Para-benzoquinone, $O=C_6H_4=O$, a yellow crystalline compound with a penetrating odour, prepared from aniline by oxidation, It is used in the manufacture of hydroquinone for drugs and dyestuffs. 2. Any one of a family of cyclic diketones containing the quinone structure. **Quinone monoxime.** Quinoxime.

quinonoid (**kwin**·on·oid). Quinoid.

quinophan (**quin**·o·fan). Cinchophen, $C_6H_5C_9H_5NCOOH$. A compound which causes an increase in excretion of uric acid by the kidneys and is used in the treatment of gout and rheumatism. It may produce untoward reactions in susceptible individuals, particularly in the liver.

quinosol (**kwin**·o·sol). 8-Hydroxyquinoline sulphate, $C_9H_6(OH)N_2H_2SO_4$. A yellow crystalline powder used as an antiseptic and deodorizer, also as a contraceptive. **Quinosol benzoate.** A derivative used as a germicide and fungicide in the treatment of skin diseases.

quinotoxine (kwin·o·**tox**·een). Quinicine.

quinovatine (kwin·o·vat·een). $C_{23}H_{26}O_4N_2$, an alkaloid of cinchona bark.

quinovin (kwin·**o**·vin). $C_{30}H_{48}O_8$, a glycoside present in cinchona bark.

quinoxime (kwin·**ox**·ime). Quinone monoxime, $O=C_6H_4=NOH$. A stable tautomeric form of *p*-nitrosophenol obtained from quinone and hydroxylamine.

Quinquaud, Charles Emile (b. 1841). Paris physician.

Quinquaud's disease. Sycosis of the scalp causing loss of hair with scarring; folliculitis decalvans.

Quinquaud's phenomenon or sign. A propulsive fine tremor noted when the patient's outstretched fingers are placed against the vertical palm of the examiner's hand. It is due to tremors of the interossei muscles and is said to occur in alcoholics.

quinquecuspid (kwin·kwe·**kus**·pid). Denoting a molar tooth that has 5 cusps or tubercles. [L *quinque* five, cusp.]

quinquetubercular (**kwin**·kwe·tew·**ber**'kew·lar). Provided with 5 tubercles or cusps, as a molar tooth. [L *quinque* five, tubercle.]

quinquina (kin·**ke**·nah). An old name for cinchona. [Sp. *quina* bark.]

quinquivalent (kwin·kwe·**va**·lent). Applied to an element or radical that has a valency of 5. [L *quinque* five, valency.]

quinsy (**kwin**·ze). Peritonsillar abscess. *See* ABSCESS. **Lingual quinsy.** Suppuration and inflammation of the lingual tonsil and structures in its neighbourhood. [Gk *kynagche* a bad kind of sore throat.]

quinsy opener (**kwin**·se **o**·pen·er). *See* THOMSON (ST. CLAIR). [quinsy, ME *openen.*]

quintan (**kwin**·tan). 1. Occurring every fifth day. 2. Fever occurring at such intervals. [L *quintanus* concerning the fifth.]

quintessence (kwin·**tes**·ens). A pure or highly concentrated extract. [LL *quinta essentia* the fifth essence (ether) of the Pythagoreans.]

Quintin, René (fl. 1912). French physician.

Quintin treatment. Subcutaneous injection of sea water as a treatment for various states of malnutrition.

quintipara (kwin·**tip**·ar·ah). A woman who is giving birth to her fifth child or who has given birth to 5 children. [L *quintus* fifth, *parere* to bear.]

quintisternal (kwin·te·**ster**·nal). Relating or belonging to the sternebra. [L *quintus* fifth, sternum.]

quintuplet (**kwin**·tew·plet). 1. One of 5 children born in the same labour. 2. Denoting such a birth. [L *quintuplex* fivefold.]

quinuclidine (kwin·**ew** klid·een). The bridged ring in the quinine molecule which is characteristic of all the cinchona alkaloids.

quionine (**kwe**·o·neen). A mixture of cinchona alkaloids, chiefly cinchonidine, used in place of quinine, being relatively tasteless.

quotidian (kwo·**tid**·e·an). 1. Recurring daily. 2. Applied to a variety of malarial fever in which the attacks recur every day. **Double quotidian.** Applied to a fever to which there are 2 attacks a day. [L *quotidianus* daily.]

quotient (**kwo**·shent). The number obtained by dividing one number by another. **Accomplishment quotient.** Achievement quotient (see following). **Achievement quotient.** A term used in the educational assessment of children by educational psychologists. It represents the ratio between the achievement age, as shown by certain tests, and the mental age. **Albumin quotient.** The amount of albumin in blood plasma related to the total albumin content of the blood. **Blood quotient.** The value obtained by dividing the amount of haemoglobin in the blood by the erythrocyte count, both expressed as percentages of their normal values. **Caloric quotient.** The amount of heat formed per unit weight of oxygen consumed in oxidative processes. In gram-calories (gram-joules) per milligram of oxygen, it varies from 3.2 to 3.5 (13.4–14.7) according to the material consumed. Closely related to it is the *calorific value* of oxygen, used in metabolic calculations and assessed at about 5 kilocalories (21kJ) per litre. **Developmental quotient.** A mathematical term for the relationship between developmental age (i.e. a figure based on the recognized criteria for development of the epiphyses, growth, height, weight, mental and physical capacities, etc. at a certain age), and the chronological or actual age. Sometimes denoted by

$$\frac{\text{Developmental age}}{\text{Actual (chronological) age}}$$

D:N quotient. D:N ratio. *See* RATIO. **Intelligence quotient.** 1. The figure, multiplied by 100, obtained by dividing the score expressed in years and months on a standardized intelligence test, by the chronological age (with a variable ceiling) of the person obtaining the score. 2. A figure with a similar range and significance to that given in 1, but obtained indirectly without the use of tests scored in terms of age. **Non-protein respiratory quotient.** The respiratory quotient applicable to the metabolism of a mixed food containing particular proportions of fat and carbohydrate only. **Protein quotient.** The relative amounts of globulin and albumin in blood plasma, represented as a fraction. **Rachidian quotient.** Ayala's index or quotient. **Respiratory quotient.** The ratio of the volume of carbon dioxide produced in respiration during a given time to the volume of oxygen consumed during the same time, the volumes of the 2 gases being measured at the same temperature, pressure and humidity. Its value varies according to the nature of the material being combusted and to the variations of respiratory volume. When respiration is in a steady state and the body at rest its value ranges from 1.0 for carbohydrate combustion to 0.72 for fat combustion; usually the value is about 0.8. [L *quotiens* how often.]

See also: AYALA.

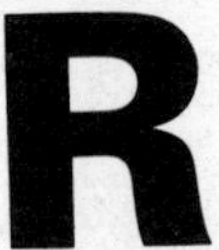

rabiate (ra·be·ate). Rabid. [L *rabere* to rave.]

rabic (ra·bik). Relating or belonging to rabies; rabid.

rabicidal (ra·be·si·dal). Capable of destroying the virus of rabies. [rabies, L *caedere* to kill.]

rabid (rab·id). Relating to rabies; suffering from rabies. [L *rabidus* raving.]

rabies (ra·beez). Hydrophobia; a virus disease of warm-blooded animals, particularly foxes, wolves and bats. Other species including domestic animals are infected through contact with these species. The disease can be communicated to man by the bite of a rabid animal in whose saliva the virus is present. Though potentially possible, person to person transmission does not occur. Once endemic throughout the world, the disease is still widespread in Asia and America. In Europe it is spreading westwards from Poland towards W. France. Scandinavia and Great Britain are rabies-free due to careful control measures and quarantine, respectively. The incubation period is 2–6 weeks and, infrequently, even longer. In man and most animals the disease, once it develops, is fatal though the long incubation period allows post-exposure immunization to be effective. In animals the symptoms include a change in behaviour pattern and the diagnosis can be suspected in wild animals which lose their fear of man. In dogs the symptoms are a moodiness and restlessness followed by fits of rage with excess salivation and a two-toned bark ("furious rabies"). Paralysis and death follow after 3 or 4 days. Post mortem, Negri bodies in the brain, particularly the hippocampus, are diagnostic, as is a positive fluorescent antibody test on the brain tissue. Vaccines are available, mostly using virus inactivated by phenol. Due to side-effects, poor antigenicity and discomfort to the patient, they are not suitable for general prophylaxis but are reserved for post-exposure immunization of persons bitten by animals suspected of being rabid. Such a course of immunization should be given as soon as possible. **Rabies canina.** Rabies of the canine species; canine madness. **Dumb rabies.** Rabies in which the furious stage does not develop. Though the dog is less aggressive it is just as infectious if it bites. Paralysis is an early symptom; as the lower jaw is partially paralysed the animal has difficulty in feeding. **False rabies.** Pseudorabies, mad itch; an infection of the central nervous system of many animal species. Unlike rabies, it is not transmissible to man and the infected animals are not aggressive. Itching of the hindquarters is a point of differentiation from rabies. It is due to a herpesvirus. The name is also given to the symptoms sometimes displayed by those who think they have contracted rabies. **Rabies felina.** Cat rabies. **Furious rabies.** The "furious" stage of rabies, in which the dog runs long distances and is aggressive to man as well as to another of his own species. Exhaustion may alternate with paroxysms of fury. **Paralytic rabies.** An atypical form of rabies, reported in cattle and human beings in Trinidad and South America, in which the virus causes an acute ascending myelitis. Transmission is by the bites of vampire bats. The term is also used as a synonym for dumb rabies (see above). **Street rabies.** Furious rabies in dogs. **Sullen rabies.** The paralytic or dumb rabies of dogs. **Tanacetic rabies.** A rabies-like condition produced in rabbits by injection of tansy oil (*Tanacetum vulgare*). **Wolf rabies.** Rabies in the wolf. [L *rabere* to rave.]

rabies virus (ra·beez vi·rus). The causative agent of rabies. It is an RNA-containing virus of the family Rhabdoviridae, probably bullet-shaped (though more pleomorphic than other members of the group), about 150 nm long and 100 nm wide. Only one antigenic type has been described though marked differences in virulence are found between wild ("street") strains and strains passed in the laboratory ("fixed strains"). Phenolized vaccines have been made from infected rabbit brain (Semple), duck embryos and after passage in eggs. None of these vaccines are suitable (because of side-effects, poor antigenicity and discomfort to the recipient) for routine prophylaxis but they have been used for post-exposure immunization. A new vaccine prepared in human diploid cells has shown itself to be free of these disadvantages though its high cost may mean that it is used only to protect selected high risk groups and those bitten by animals suspected of being rabid.

rabietic (ra·be·et·ik). Rabid.

rabific (ra·bif·ik). Causing rabies. [rabies, L *facere* to make.]

rabiform (ra·be·form). Having resemblance to rabies. [rabies, form.]

rabigenic (ra·be·jen·ik). Causing rabies. [rabies, Gk *genein* to produce.]

Rable, Carl (b. 1853). Vienna anatomist.

Rable's chromoformic acid solution. A mixture of chromic and formic acids used as a fixative, especially for invertebrate tissues.

Race, Robert Russell (b. 1907). London haematologist.

Fisher and Race notation. *See* NOTATION.

race (rase). 1. A distinct ethnic stock marked by unaltering traits transmitted through the offspring. 2. A group of individuals having like characteristics, as if they had originated from a common ancestor. 3. A breed or strain of a species. 4. A root, especially a root of ginger. [It. *razza*.]

racemation (ras·e·ma·shun). Racemization.

raceme (ras·eem). 1. A type of inflorescence in which the flowers are arranged alternately on opposite sides of the stem, the oldest flower being at the base. 2. In chemistry, a racemic compound; an equimolecular mixture of the dextro- and laevo-rotatory isomers of an optically-active compound, which displays no optical activity. It is said to be *externally compensated* and is denoted by the prefix DL-. **Compound raceme.** A raceme in which each single flower is replaced by a raceme of flowers. **False raceme.** A scorpoid cyme, distinguishable from a true raceme by the positions of the bracts which occur at the base of each pedicel but on the opposite side of what appears to be the main stem; in the true raceme the pedicels occur in the axis of the bracts and the main stem. [L *racemus* bunch of grapes.]

Racemethorphan (ras·e·meth·or′·fan). BP Commission approved name for DL-3-methoxy-*N*-methylmorphinan. The racemic isomer of Levomethorphan with very similar action.

racemic (ras·e·mik). Optically inactive but resolvable in the way of all racemic compounds. **Racemic compound, racemic form.** An isomer of an optically-active compound which displays no optical rotation by reason of its being a mixture or loose molecular association in equal parts of the mutually compensating dextro- and laevo-rotatory isomers; it can be separated into the latter by physical or chemical methods. Usually denoted by the prefix DL-, it derives its name from the racemic acid in grape juice. [L *racemus* bunch of grapes.]

racemization (ras·e·mi·za′·shun). The production of the racemic form of an optically-active compound, either by mixing the dextro- and laevo-rotatory isomers in equal proportions, or by bringing about the chemical conversion of one of the latter into half of the opposite isomer.

Racemoramide (ras·e·**mor**·am·ide). BP Commission approved name for (±) - 1 - (β - methyl - γ - morpholino - $\alpha\alpha$ - diphenylbutyryl) - pyrrolidine; used in the treatment of hypertension.

Racemorphan (ras·e·**mor**·fan). BP Commission approved name for DL - 3 - hydroxy - *N* - methylmorphinan. The best known of the morphinan group of analgesic drugs, said to be free from the disadvantages of morphine.

racemose (**ras**·e·moze). 1. Pertaining to a raceme. 2. Growing in the form of a bunch of grapes, i.e. with nodular terminations. [L *racemus* bunch of grapes.]

racephedrine (ras·**ef**·ed·reen). Racemic ephedrine, DL - ephedrine, $C_{10}H_{15}ON$. A synthetic form of ephedrine, similar to but less active than the naturally occurring laevorotatory form.

rachial (**ra**·ke·al). Rachidial.

rachialgia (ra·ke·**al**·je·ah). 1. Any painful affection of the vertebral column, particularly Pott's disease. 2. Lead colic. [Gk *rhachis* backbone, *algos* pain.]

rachialgitis (ra·ke·al·**ji**'·tis). A condition marked by pain and inflammation of the vertebral column. [Gk *rhachis* backbone, *algos* pain, *-itis* inflammation.]

rachianaesthesia (ra·ke·an·es·**the**'·ze·ah). Spinal anaesthesia. *See* ANAESTHESIA. [Gk *rhachis* backbone, anaesthesia.]

rachiasmus (ra·ke·**az**·mus). Spasmodic twitching of the muscles at the back of the neck, often noted in the first stage of an epileptic attack. [Gk *rhachis* backbone.]

rachicele (**ra**·ke·seel). The hernial protrusion in spina bifida. [Gk *rhachis* backbone, *kele* hernia.]

rachicentesis (ra·ke·sen·**te**'·sis). Lumbar puncture. *See* PUNCTURE. [Gk *rhachis* backbone, *kenteein* to puncture.]

rachidial, rachidian (ra·**kid**·e·al, ra·**kid**·e·an). Relating or belonging to the vertebral column; spinal. [Gk *rhachis* backbone.]

rachilysis (ra·**kil**·is·is). A method of correction of curvatures of the spine by traction and pressure. [Gk *rhachis* backbone, *lysis* a loosing.]

rachiocampsis (ra·ke·o·**kamp**'·sis). Spinal curvature. *See* CURVATURE. [Gk *rhachis* backbone, *kampsis* a curving.]

rachiocentesis (ra·ke·o·sen·**te**'·sis). Lumbar puncture. *See* PUNCTURE. [Gk *rhachis* backbone, *kenteein* to puncture.]

rachiochysis (ra·ke·**ok**·is·is). A collection of fluid in the vertebral canal. [Gk *rhachis* backbone, *chysis* a pouring.]

rachiodynia (ra·ke·o·**din**'·e·ah). Pain arising from the vertebral column. [Gk *rhachis* backbone, *odyne* pain.]

rachiokyphosis (ra·ke·o·ki·**fo**'·sis). Kyphosis. [Gk *rhachis* backbone, kyphosis.]

rachiometer (ra·ke·**om**·et·er). An instrument used to determine the degree of spinal curvature, natural or pathological. [Gk *rhachis* backbone, *metron* measure.]

rachiomyelitis (ra·ke·o·mi·el·**i**'·tis). Inflammation of the spinal cord. [Gk *rhachis* backbone, myelitis.]

rachioparalysis (ra·ke·o·par·**al**'·is·is). Paralysis affecting the muscles of the spine. [Gk *rhachis* backbone, paralysis.]

rachiopathy (ra·ke·**op**·ath·e). Any diseased condition of the vertebral column. [Gk *rhachis* backbone, *pathos* disease.]

rachiophyma (ra·ke·o·**fi**'·mah). A tumour of the vertebral column. [Gk *rhachis* backbone, *phyma* a growth.]

rachioplegia (ra·ke·o·**ple**'·je·ah). Spinal paralysis. [Gk *rhachis* backbone, *plege* stroke.]

rachioscoliosis (ra·ke·o·sko·le·**o**'·sis). Lateral curvature of the spine. [Gk *rhachis* backbone, scoliosis.]

rachiostrophosis (ra·ke·o·strof·**o**'·sis). Spinal curvature. *See* CURVATURE. [Gk *rhachis* backbone, *strophos* twisted band.]

rachiotome (**ra**·ke·o·tome). An instrument especially designed for dividing vertebral laminae. [Gk *rhachis* backbone, *temnein* to cut.]

rachiotomy (ra·ke·**ot**·o·me). An operation which involves section of a portion of the vertebral column. [see prec.]

rachipagus (ra·**kip**·ag·us). A double monster the two individuals of which are fused along the vertebral column. [Gk *rhachis* backbone, *pagos* fixed.]

rachis (**ra**·kis). The vertebral column. **Rachis nasi.** The line connecting the root with the apex of the nose. [Gk *rhachis* backbone.]

rachischisis (ra·**kis**·kis·is). Spina bifida; a congenital developmental defect of the vertebral column and spinal cord resulting from a failure of the neural tube in the embryo to close and separate from the ectodermal tissue forming the skin; this prevents the mesodermal tissues, which should form the vertebral arches, from meeting and closing over the developing cord. The fissure is usually posterior and median and in 90 per cent of cases affects the lumbosacral region. In severe cases a sac protrudes through the opening; this may contain meninges only (meningocele) or include also the cord (meningomyelocele). In milder cases there is no protrusion, but a pigmented dimple or tuft of hair may suggest the fault which can be confirmed by X-rays. There may be no neurological symptoms, or weakness of the legs may be present at birth or be first noticed as the child grows up, especially at puberty. The paralysis is flaccid with absent reflexes. Sensation is impaired over the area of the root distribution and there is usually enuresis. Associated malformations such as cleft palate, hare-lip, and hydrocephalus are frequent. Severe forms are incompatible with life, and the child is stillborn or lives for a very short time. Milder cases may improve with medical treatment, and in carefully selected cases benefit may result from operation. **Rachischisis partialis.** The defect in only one portion of the vertebral column. **Rachischisis totalis.** Rare cases in which the whole vertebral column is affected. [Gk *rhachis* backbone, *schizein* to split.]

rachitamin (ra·**kit**·am·in). An obsolete name for the antirachitic vitamin, vitamin D.

rachitasterol (ra·kit·ah·**steer**'·ol). An obsolete name for the sterol which prevents rickets, i.e. vitamin D. [Gk *rhachis* backbone, sterol.]

rachitic (ra·**kit**·ik). Relating to, characterized by, or affected with rickets. [see foll.]

rachitis (ra·**ki**·tis). Rickets. **Rachitis adultorum.** Adult rickets; osteomalacia. **Rachitis fetalis annularis.** Congenital enlargement of the epiphyses of long bones. **Rachitis fetalis micromelica.** Congenital shortness of the bones. **Rachitis senilis.** Osteomalacia. **Rachitis tarda.** Late rickets occurring in adolescents. [Gk *rhachis* backbone, *-itis* inflammation.]

rachitism (**ra**·kit·izm). Rickets. [see prec.]

rachitogenic (ra·kit·o·**jen**'·ik). Giving rise to rickets. [rachitis, Gk *genein* to produce.]

rachitome (**ra**·kit·ome). An instrument especially designed for dividing vertebral laminae. [Gk *rhachis* backbone, *temnein* to cut.]

rachitomy (ra·**kit**·o·me). 1. Incision for the purpose of laying bare the spinal cord; laminectomy. 2. Division of the vertebral column of the fetus in order to make delivery easier. [see prec.]

rack (rak). A framework. **Retinoscopy rack.** A number of convex and concave lenses arranged in a line, suitably mounted in instrument form, so that the lenses can be placed in turn in front of the pupil during retinoscopy. [D *rek.*]

raclage, raclement (rah·**klahzh**, rahkl·**mahn**). Removal of granulations or of soft tissue by friction, as with a hard brush. [Fr. scraping.]

rad (rad). Radiation absorbed dose, the unit of absorbed dose of ionizing radiation. One rad is equal to 0.01 J/kg. Symbol rad.

radal (**ra**·dal). A 20 per cent solution of silver protein.

raddle (radl). Reddle, red-ochre. A natural sesquioxide of iron, Fe_2O_3; a form of haematite and clay which occurs widely as a red earth. So-called from its use in marking sheep and as a colouring matter. [AS *read* red.]

Rademacher, Johann Gottfried (b. 1772). German physician.

Rademacher's system. The contention that each form of disease has its appropriate remedy.

Radford, E. P. 20th century American physician.

Radford nomogram. A nomogram which relates body weight to the tidal volume and respiratory rate necessary for the maintenance of a normal alveolar carbon dioxide tension. Described in 1954.

radial [radialis (NA)] (ra·de·al). 1. Belonging or referring to the radius of the forearm or to any radius. 2. Radiating. **Goose-neck radial.** A radial artery which has become calcified and curved, and on palpation gives the impression of a goose neck. **Radial notch.** *See* NOTCH.

radial artery [arteria radialis (NA)]. The smaller of the two terminal branches of the brachial artery. It passes along the radial side of the forearm, under cover of the brachioradialis muscle, as far as the front of the wrist; then winds backwards across the floor of the anatomical snuffbox to the back of the hand, and terminates by passing forwards between the two heads of the first dorsal interosseous artery to become the deep palmar arch with perforating branches [rami perforantes (NA)] to the interosseous spaces. In the forearm it gives off the radial recurrent branch [arteria recurrens radialis (NA)], taking part in the anastomosis around the elbow, and muscular branches. It supplies multiple carpal [ramus carpeus palmaris, ramus carpeus dorsalis (NA)], palmar metacarpal [ramus palmaris superficialis, arteriae metacarpeae palmares (NA)] and digital branches to the hand and fingers, and the princeps pollicis artery [arteria princeps pollicis (NA)] to the thumb.

radial nerve [nervus radialis (NA)]. The largest branch of the posterior cord of the brachial plexus (root value C5, 6, 7, 8, and possibly T1). It supplies, through its branches, the extensor muscle [rami musculares (NA)] and most of the skin [ramus superficialis (NA)] of the extensor surface of the arm and forearm and the skin over the radial half of the dorsum of the hand and the dorsal surfaces of the lateral three and half digits. There is also a communicating branch with the ulnar nerve [ramus communicans ulnaris (NA)].

radial veins [venae radiales (NA)]. Vessels accompanying the radial artery; they join with the ulnar veins to form the brachial veins.

radiale (ra·de·a·le). An anthropometric point; the upper border of the head of the radius.

radialis (ra·de·a·lis). Belonging or referring to the radius, e.g. flexor carpi radialis muscle.

radialis indicis artery [arteria radialis indicis (NA)]. *See* PALMAR ARCH, SUPERFICIAL (under ARCH).

radian (ra·de·an). A unit of angular measurement; the angle subtended at the centre of a circle by an arc equal in length to the radius. It is equivalent to approximately 57.3°. An ophthalmic lens of one radian would have one plane surface whose length equalled the radius of curvature of the other surface.

radiant (ra·de·ant). 1. Proceeding outwards in all directions from a given point. 2. Issuing rays. 3. Applied to any object which issues energy in the form of rays. [L *radiare* to shine.]

radiate (ra·de·ate). 1. To spread out like spokes of a wheel from a given centre. 2. To give out rays of energy such as heat, light, x-rays, etc. 3. Having radial parts. 4. Of structures, characterized by radial symmetry. [see prec.]

radiathermy (ra·di·ah·ther′·me). Short-wave diathermy. *See* DIATHERMY. [radiation, diathermy.]

radiation (ra·de·a·shun). 1. Electromagnetic energy existing in space. 2. The emission of energy in the form of electromagnetic waves, or of particles charged or uncharged with electricity. 3. In medicine, ionizing radiation used for therapeutic or diagnostic purposes. 4. The divergence of anything from a central point, e.g. in anatomy, a spreading of fibres from a central origin. **Actinic radiation.** Ultraviolet radiation (see below). **Annihilation radiation.** The electromagnetic radiation resulting from the mutual annihilation of two particles of opposite charge. In the case of a collision between a positive and a negative electron, the annihilation radiation consists of two photons, each of energy about 0.51 MeV, emitted in directions opposite to each other. **Auditory radiation (radiatio acustica (NA)].** Fibres from the medial geniculate body which pass into the internal capsule and then sweep laterally, beneath the lentiform nucleus, to the auditosensory area. **Background radiation.** The radiation detected in the absence of the source of interest. In the case of ionizing radiation, the background is derived from traces of radioactive materials which occur widely, from irrelevant sources of radioactivity in the neighbourhood, and from cosmic radiation. **Back-scattered radiation.** Radiation which is scattered in directions approximately opposite to the direction of the primary beam. In clinical medicine this term is often loosely—and inaccurately—used to indicate any scattered radiation, back-, forward- or side-scattered. **Broad-beam radiation.** The condition in which there is no collimation of a beam of x- or γ-rays which penetrate material and in which there is an admixture of scattered radiation with the emergent beam. *See* NARROW-BEAM RADIATION (below). **Radiation of the corpus callosum [radiatio corporis callosi (NA)].** The spread of the fibres of the corpus callosum above the lateral ventricles to reach different regions of the cerebral cortex. **Corpuscular radiation.** Radiation, the physical properties of which are explicable by the hypothesis of its emission as discrete corpuscles, e.g. α-radiation from radioactive bodies. **Direct radiation.** In the case of x-rays all radiation except the useful beam, coming from within the x-ray tube and tube housing. *See* PRIMARY RADIATION (below). **Electromagnetic radiation.** Waves moving with the velocity of light and exhibiting properties partly electrical and partly magnetic, the oscillating electrical displacements being accompanied by oscillating magnetic fields at right angles, whilst the direction of propagation is at right angles to both. **Fluorescent radiation.** Radiation emitted by a fluorescent substance under the action of some type of excitation, the radiation emitted being characteristic of the substance and not the excitation, e.g. visible light emitted by a fluorescent substance under ultraviolet excitation. **Forward-scattered radiation.** Radiation which is scattered in a direction approximately that of the primary beam. **Fractionated radiation.** Radiotherapy by means of repeated applications, so that the total dose is given in fractions. **Gamma radiation.** Electromagnetic radiation emitted by atomic nuclei. Also called *gamma rays.* **Hard radiation.** Rays of relatively short wavelength. In radiotherapy, the range is from 100 kV to several million volts; in diagnostic radiology, rays from 80 to 150 kV are considered hard. **Infrared radiation.** Invisible radiation beyond the red end of the spectrum, which exhibits a heating effect. **Interstitial radiation.** Interstitial irradiation. *See* IRRADIATION. **Ionizing radiation.** Electromagnetic or corpuscular radiation capable of producing ionization. **Irritative radiation.** Radiation with ultraviolet light to the point of erythema. **Mitogenetic radiation, Mitogenic radiation.** A hypothetical emanation from dividing cells, supposed to induce a similar state in neighbouring cells. **Narrow-beam radiation.** The condition in which the collimation of a beam of x- or γ-rays which penetrates material is designed to prevent the scattered electromagnetic radiation, produced during the Compton process of absorption of the radiation in the material penetrated, from reaching the measuring equipment. **Optic radiation [radiatio optica (NA)].** Fibres from the lateral geniculate body which pass in the retrolentiform portion of the internal capsule to the striate area. **Photochemical radiation.** Radiation which produces chemical changes. **Primary radiation.** 1. X-rays, radiation coming directly from the target of the x-ray tube. Except for the useful beam, the bulk of this radiation is absorbed in the tube housing. 2. β- and γ-rays, radiation coming directly from the radioactive source. **Protracted radiation.** Radiotherapy given at a low dose rate; also used for fractionated radiation (see above) spread over a long period of time. **Quantity of radiation.** Time integral of intensity. It is the total energy which has passed through unit area perpendicular to the beam, and is expressed in watt-seconds per square metre. **Radioactive radiation.** Radiation of any type arising from a radioactive substance. **Scattered radiation.** Radiation which, during passage through a substance, has been deviated in direction. It may also have been modified by an increase in wavelength (Compton effect). It is one form of secondary radiation. **Secondary radiation.** Radiation, other than the primary radiation, emitted by any matter irradiated with x-rays, γ-rays, etc. It may consist either of x-rays, electrons, or ultraviolet radiation. **Side-scattered radiation.** Radiation which is scattered in directions approximately at right angles to the direction of the primary beam. **Soft radiation.** Rays of relatively long wavelength. In radiotherapy, soft rays include Grenz rays (from 1 to 15 kV) and x-rays up to about 100 kV; in diagnostic radiology, rays from 40 to 60 kV are considered soft. **Solar radiation.** Radiation from the sun. **Stray radiation.** Radiation not serving any useful purpose. It includes direct radiation, and secondary radiation from irradiated objects, and represents the portion of the radiation against which special protective measures have to be taken. **Thalamic radiation.** The fibre tracts from the thalamus radiating into the cortex of the hemispheres and passing through the internal capsule. **Ultraviolet radiation.** Electromagnetic radiation having shorter wavelengths than those of visible light and longer wavelengths than those of x-rays. **Useful-beam radiation.** That part of the primary radiation which passes through the aperture, cone, or other device for collimating the x-ray beam. [L *radiare* to shine.]

See also: CERENKOV, GRATIOLET, HULDSCHINSKY, ROLLER.

radiator (ra·de·a·tor). Anything which radiates light or heat. **Hydrogenous radiators.** For neutron counters: fast neutrons may not be directly detected, being non-ionizing particles. If they are allowed to fall on a radiator containing hydrogen atoms, protons are produced by recoil and may be detected. The hydrogenous radiator may be a layer of polythene of known thickness and hydrogen content. [see prec.]

radical (rad·ik·al). 1. Appertaining to a root, or springing from a root. 2. Metaphorically, going to the root of anything, e.g. radical cure; fundamental or basal. 3. In chemistry, a group of atoms, e.g. CH_3, NH_2, which enters into combination in the same way as a single atom, and which may be substituted intact for an element or for another radical in a compound. **Acid radical.** The electronegative group, e.g. SO_4^{2-}, remaining when the acid hydrogen is subtracted from the molecule of an acid. **Acyl radical.** The group remaining when the acid hydroxyl is subtracted from the molecule of an organic acid, e.g. CH_3CO. **Alcohol radical.** The group remaining when the alcoholic hydroxyl is subtracted from the molecule of an alcohol. **Alkyl radical.** The monovalent radical remaining when a hydrogen atom is subtracted from an aliphatic or aromatic hydrocarbon. **Alphyl radical.** An alkyl radical (see prec.) derived from an aliphatic hydrocarbon. **Aryl radical.** An alkyl radical (see above) derived from an aromatic hydrocarbon. **Colour radical.** A chromophore; any group, e.g. N=N, which, introduced into an organic compound, confers upon it colour. **Electronegative radical.** A group of atoms above hydrogen in the electrochemical series, i.e. having a more negative electrode potential. **Electropositive radical.** A group of atoms below hydrogen in the electrochemical series, i.e. having a more positive electrode potential. **Free radical.** The highly reactive and short-lived state in which a radical can exist freely. Thus methylene, CH_2, produced by the decomposition of diazomethane at low pressure, can be demonstrated, though it lasts a mere fraction of a second. **Organic radical.** Any group which gives an organic compound its specific character, e.g. COOH, conferring acidity, or any alkyl radical (see above) entering into combination like a single atom. [L *radix* root.]

radiciform (rad·is·e·form). 1. Having the appearance or the characters of a root. 2. Like the root of a tooth in shape. [L *radix* root, form.]

radicle (rad·ikl). 1. A rootlet; a small root. [L *radicula.*] 2. Radical.

radicotomy (rad·ik·ot·o·me). Section of the roots of the spinal nerves. [L *radix* root, Gk *temnein* to cut.]

radiculalgia (rad·ik·ew·lal′·je·ah). Pain due to disease of the sensory nerve roots. [radicle, Gk *algos* pain.]

radicular (rad·ik·ew·lar). Having the character of or relating to a radicle or root, particularly those of the spinal nerves.

radiculectomy (rad·ik·ew·lek′·to·me). Removal of a nerve root or rootlet; especially removal of posterior spinal nerve roots. [radicle, Gk *ektome* a cutting out.]

radiculitis (rad·ik·ew·li′·tis). Inflammation affecting the root of a spinal nerve, in particular that part of the root between the spinal cord and the intervertebral foramen of the vertebrae. [radicle, Gk *-itis* inflammation.]

radiculoganglionitis (rad·ik·ew·lo·gang·gle·on·i′·tis). Inflammation affecting the posterior roots of the spinal nerves and their ganglia. [radicle, ganglion, Gk *-itis* inflammation.]

radiculogram (rad·ik·ew·lo·gram). The radiograph made during radiculography. [radicle, Gk *gramma* record.]

radiculography (rad·ik·ew·log·raf·e). The x-ray study of the spinal nerve roots and their sheaths after the injection of a radio-opaque contrast medium, e.g. *water-soluble lumbar radiculography.* [radicle, Gk *graphein* to record.]

radiculomedullary (rad·ik·ew·lo·med·ul′·ar·e). Pertaining to the nerve roots and the spinal cord. [radicle, medulla.]

radiculomeningomyelitis (rad·ik·ew·lo·men·ing·go·mi·el·i′·tis). Inflammation of the nerve roots, the meninges, and the spinal cord. [radicle, meninges, myelitis.]

radiculomyelopathy (rad·ik·ew·lo·mi·el·op′·ath·e). Disease of the spinal cord and spinal nerve roots. [radicle, Gk *myelos* marrow, *pathos* disease.]

radiculoneuritis (rad·ik·ew·lo·newr·i′·tis). Acute febrile polyneuritis. [radicle, neuritis.]

radiculoneuropathy (rad·ik·ew·lo·newr·op′·ath·e). A morbid condition of spinal nerve roots between the spinal cord and intervertebral foramen of the vertebrae. [radicle, Gk *neuron* nerve, *pathos* disease.]

radiculopathy (rad·ik·ew·lop′·ath·e). Any diseased condition of the roots of nerves. [radicle, Gk *pathos* disease.]

radiferous (ra·dif·er·us). Applied to any mineral or chemical mixture that contains radium or radioactive elements. [radium, L *ferre* to bear.]

radio-. Prefixed to a noun, indicating that the named material is in a radioactive form; for example, radiocobalt is the radioactive form of cobalt. [L *radius* ray.]

radioactinium (ra·de·o·ak·tin′·e·um). Thorium-227 a radioactive isotope which is produced by the emission of a β-particle from actinium. It has a half-life of approximately 19 days, and disintegrates into actinium X (radium-223).

radioactive (ra·de·o·ak′·tiv). Having the attribute of radioactivity.

radioactivity (ra·de·o·ak·tiv′·it·e). The property of certain nuclides of emitting radiation by the spontaneous transformation of their nuclei. **Artificial radioactivity, Induced radioactivity.** The production of radioactivity by an interference with the nuclei of atoms whereby the normal equilibrium between protons and neutrons is upset. It is usually effected by bombardment with neutrons. [radiation, activity.]

radioarsenic (ra·de·o·ar′·sen·ik). Radioactive arsenic; ^{74}As is the radioactive isotope of arsenic most commonly used.

radio-autograph (ra·de·o·aw′·to·graf). Autoradiograph.

radio-autography (ra·de·o·aw·tog′·raf·e). Autoradiography.

radiobicipital (ra·de·o·bi·sip′·it·al). Relating or belonging to the radius and the biceps muscle.

radiobiology (ra·de·o·bi·ol′·o·je). The section of medical science which studies the effect of radiation on living tissue, including tissue cultures, and on single cells. [radiation, biology.]

radiobismuth (ra·de·o·biz′·muth). Radioactive bismuth. ^{206}Bi is the principal radioactive isotope of bismuth of medical importance.

radiobromine (ra·de·o·bro′·meen). Radioactive bromine. ^{82}Br is a commonly used radioactive isotope of bromine.

radiocaesium (ra·de·o·se′·se·um). Radioactive caesium. The radioactive isotope of caesium ^{132}Cs has a restricted diagnostic use but ^{137}Cs is widely used as a source of gamma rays in teleradiotherapy.

radiocalcium (ra·de·o·kal′·se·um). Radioactive calcium. The radioactive isotopes of medical importance are ^{45}Ca and ^{47}Ca.

radiocarbon (ra·de·o·kar′·bon). Radioactive carbon. Only one radioactive isotope of carbon occurs naturally, ^{14}C; this isotope and also ^{11}C are the two carbon isotopes most commonly used in nuclear medicine.

radiocardiography (ra·de·o·kar·de·**og**′·raf·e). If a radioactive substance is injected into a vein, its passage through the heart and great vessels can be followed by measuring the radioactivity with a suitable radiation detector, usually a scintillation counter. The variations in radioactivity in various parts of the heart can be graphically recorded, and a time-concentration curve can thus be derived from which the cardiac output and circulation time can be ascertained. [radioactivity, Gk *kardia* heart, *graphein* to record.]

radiocarpal (ra·de·o·**kar**′·pal). 1. Relating or belonging to the radius and the carpal bones. 2. On the lateral (radial) side of the carpus.

radiochemical (ra·de·o·**kem**′·ik·al). 1. Of radiochemistry. 2. A compound containing a radioactive atom or atoms. [radiation, Gk *chemeia* alchemy.]

radiochemistry (ra·de·o·**kem**′·is·tre). The preparation, purification, and study of the properties of the radioactive elements and of chemical compounds incorporating them. [radiation, Gk *chemeia* alchemy.]

radiochroism (ra·de·o·**kro**′·izm). The degree of filtration or absorption of x-rays and other radiation which takes place in a substance. [radiation, Gk *chroma* colour.]

radiochromium (ra·de·o·**kro**′·me·um). Radioactive chromium. A commonly used radioactive isotope of chromium is ^{51}Cr. [radiation, Gk *chroma* colour.]

radiocinematograph (ra·de·o·sin·em·**at**′·o·graf). An apparatus consisting of a ciné camera attached to an x-ray apparatus to record the moving image on the fluorescent x-ray screen. [radiation, cinematograph.]

radiocobalt (ra·de·o·**ko**′·bawlt). Radioactive cobalt. The radioactive isotopes of cobalt ^{57}Co and ^{58}Co are commonly used in medical investigation, while ^{60}Co is used as a source of gamma rays in teleradiotherapy. [radiation, G *Kobold* goblin found in mines.]

radiocolloid (ra·de·o·**kol**′·oid). Radioactive material in a colloidal condition. [radiation, Gk *kolla* glue, *eidos* form.]

radiocopper (ra·de·o·**kop**′·er). Radioactive copper. ^{64}Cu and ^{67}Cu are commonly used radioactive isotopes of copper. [radiation, L *cuprum* copper.]

radiocystitis (ra·de·o·sis·**i**′·tis). A chronic inflammation of the bladder due to radiotherapeutic treatment of the urinary tract. [radiation, Gk *kystis* bladder, *-itis* inflammation.]

radiodermatitis (ra·de·o·der·mat·**i**′·tis). Dermatitis caused by exposure to ionizing radiation. **Acute radiodermatitis.** Erythema and oedema occurring within 48 h after exposure, proceeding to vesiculation and extravasation of blood with defective healing in the most severe examples. It is usually due to some error in technique. **Chronic radiodermatitis.** Atrophy or poikiloderma following repeated small exposures to x-rays. It becomes apparent some years after the exposures. The skin is dry and atrophic, with depigmentation and patchy hyperpigmentation, telangiectasia and, later, dyskeratoses or squamous epitheliomata. Cicatricial alopecia or brittle, deformed nails may result, depending on the area exposed. [radiation, Gk *derma* skin, *-itis*, inflammation.]

radiodiagnosis (ra·de·o·di·ag·**no**′·sis). The clinical science which involves the use of x-rays in the diagnosis of disease. [radiation, Gk *dia, gnosis* knowledge.]

radiodiaphane (ra·de·o·**di**′·ah·fane). An instrument for visualizing an object, with radium as the source of energy. Of historical interest only. [radium, Gk *dia, phanein* to appear.]

radiodigital (ra·de·o·**dij**′·it·al). 1. Belonging to the radius and the fingers. 2. Referring to the fingers on the lateral (radial) side of the hand. [radius, digit.]

radio-element (ra·de·o·**el**′·e·ment). Radioactive element. An element that exhibits radioactivity; this may be natural, as in elements of atomic weight greater than that of lead and in certain isotopes of a few light elements, or produced artificially by any one or more of a large variety of nuclear reactions. [radiation, L *elementum* element.]

radio-epidermitis (ra·de·o·ep·e·der·**mi**′·tis). A general term for the reaction of the skin to radiation, comprising erythema, dry desquamation and moist desquamation, either subsiding or going on to healing with epilation, loss of secretion, telangiectasis, and scarring, or to necrosis, according to the severity of the reaction produced. [radiation, epidermitis.]

radio-epithelitis (ra·de·o·ep·e·the·**li**′·tis). A condition similar to radio-epidermitis, but applying to mucous membranes as well as to the skin; otherwise known as *mucositis.* [radiation, epithelitis.]

radiofluorine (ra·de·o·**floo**′·or·een). Radioactive fluorine. A commonly used radioactive isotope of fluorine is ^{18}F. [radiation, fluorine.]

radiofrequency (ra·de·o·**fre**′·kwen·se). A frequency of electromagnetic radiation in the range used for radio communications.

radiogallium (ra·de·o·**gal**′·e·um). Radioactive gallium. The radioactive isotope ^{67}Ga has been used as a tumour localizing agent. [radiation, L *Gallia* Gaul.]

radiogen (ra·de·o·jen). Any radioactive material. [radiation, Gk *genein* to produce.]

radiogenic (ra·de·o·**jen**′·ik). Caused by treatment with ionizing radiation. [see prec.]

radiogold (ra·de·o·**go**′·ld). Radioactive gold. ^{198}Au is the principal radioactive isotope of gold of medical importance. In colloidal form it is used both as a diagnostic and as a therapeutic agent. [radiation, gold.]

radiogram (ra·de·o·gram). Radiograph. Radiogram is a word that should be avoided since it is also used popularly for a combined wireless receiver and gramophone. [radiation, Gk *gramma* record.]

radiograph (ra·de·o·graf). The recorded image of an object on an x-ray film. [radiation, Gk *graphein* to record.]

radiographer (ra·de·og·raf·er). A qualified x-ray technician, one skilled in the art and practice of making x-ray examinations. [see prec.]

radiography (ra·de·**og**·raf·e). The making of x-ray photographic records. **Body-section radiography.** Tomography; a special technique that shows images of structures lying in a predetermined plane of tissue, while blurring out by movement the images of the structures in other planes, above or below. **Cinematographic radiography.** The recording of movements in radiography by means of a motion-picture camera. **Double-contrast radiography.** Radiography of a hollow organ into which has been introduced two contrast media of different densities. If air is injected into a colon immediately after evacuation of a barium enema, the opacity of residual barium adhering to the mucous membrane will be accentuated by the translucent medium within the lumen. **Mass miniature radiography.** The x-raying of large numbers of people in a short time, carried out with a mass miniature x-ray apparatus. The size of the film image in England is usually 35 mm while in America 5 × 4 cm films are used. **Miniature-film radiography.** Radiography on small films, obtained by photographing the screen image of the part under examination; it is largely used in mass miniature radiography of the chest. **Mucosal-relief radiography.** Radiography of a hollow organ lined by mucous membrane, after the mucosa has been coated with a thin layer of opaque contrast medium. By this technique small mucosal lesions, which would be obscured by larger quantities of contrast medium, can be revealed. It is used extensively in gastro-intestinal radiography. **Serial radiography.** The taking of several radiographs of selected areas at specially timed intervals. **Spot-film radiography.** The making of localized spot films during the course of a barium-meal examination. [radiation, Gk *graphein* to record.]

radiohumeral (ra·de·o·**hew**′·mer·al). Belonging to the radius and the humerus, e.g. the radiohumeral articulation.

radio-immunoassay (ra·de·o·**im**·ewn·o·**as**′·a). A method developed by Berson and Yalow for the microassay of peptide hormones and other molecules that are antigenic. The method is based on competition between radioactively labelled antigen and unlabelled standard or unknown solutions of antigen for a fixed quantity of antibody and assay of the radioactivity of the antigen–antibody complex. The method has been widely used to assay hormones in blood and can assay concentrations down to 10^{-9} molar with ease. [radiation, immunity, assay.]

radio-indium (ra·de·o·**in**′·de·um). Radioactive indium. The radioactive isotope of indium ^{113m}In is widely used as a scanning agent. [radiation, indium.]

radio-iodine (ra·de·o·i′·o·deen). Radioactive iodine. Naturally-occurring iodine is mono-isotopic (^{127}I), all other isotopes of iodine, of which there are many, are radioactive. The medically most familiar of these are ^{123}I, ^{125}I, ^{131}I and ^{132}I. [radiation, iodine.]

radio-iridium (ra·de·o·ir·**id**′·e·um). Radioactive iridium. The radioactive isotope of iridium ^{192}Ir is used as a radiotherapeutic agent in a form suitable for insertion into the region to be treated. [radiation, iridium.]

radio-iron (ra·de·o·i′·on). Radioactive iron. ^{55}Fe and ^{59}Fe are commonly used radioactive isotopes of iron. [radiation, iron.]

radio-isotope (ra·de·o·i′·so·tope). An unstable isotope which decays to a stable state by emitting characteristic radiation. Usually the substance is an element which has been rendered radioactive by artificial means. Such an isotope can be incorporated in the molecule of a substance normally present in the body of man or animal. This "tagged" or "labelled" substance can be given orally or parenterally, and its distribution in the body determined by means of an apparatus sensitive to its radiations, such as the scintillation counter. Breakdown products of the tagged substance can also be traced and isolated and information thus obtained about its intermediary metabolism.

radiokrypton (ra·de·o·**krip**′·ton). Radioactive krypton. The radioactive isotope ^{85}Kr is commonly used where radioxenon is not available. [radiation, krypton.]

radiokymography (ra·de·o·ki·**mog**′·raf·e). A method of recording radiographically on a single film the movements of an organ by means of an x-ray kymograph. [radiation, kymograph.]

radiolesion (ra·de·o·**le**′·zhun). A lesion due to exposure to radium or x-rays.

radiological (ra·de·o·**loj**′·ik·al). Relating or belonging to radiology.

Radiological Protection Act 1970. This Act provides for the establishment of a National Radiological Protection Board and an Advisory Committee, with functions concerning the protection of people from radiation hazards and for connected purposes.

radiologist (ra·de·**ol**·o·jist). A medical practitioner who is a specialist in the application of ionizing radiation in the diagnosis and treatment of disease. [see foll.]

radiology (ra·de·**ol**·o·je). The science of x-ray technique applied both to diagnostic and therapeutic x-rays. [radiation, Gk *logos* science.]

radiolucency (ra·de·o·**lew**′·sen·se). The varying degree of permeability of an object to x-rays, ranging from being almost completely radioparent to being radio-opaque. [see foll.]

radiolucent (ra·de·o·**lew**′·sent). Allowing x-rays to pass through with little filtration. Cf. RADIOPARENT. [radiation, L *lucere* to shine.]

radioluminescence (ra·de·o·lew·min·**es**′·ens). The fluorescence of certain substances, e.g. zinc sulphide, barium platinocyanide, in x-rays, or in the radiation from radioactive materials. [radiation, luminescence.]

radiolus (ra·**de**·o·lus). A sound; a probe. [L small rod.]

radiomercury (ra·de·o·**mer**′·kewr·e). Radioactive mercury. Two radioactive isotopes of mercury are of medical interest, ^{197}Hg and ^{203}Hg. [radiation, mercury.]

radiometal (ra·de·o·**met**′·al). An alloy of iron (50 per cent), nickel (45 per cent), and copper (5 per cent), which has a high magnetic permeability and is used in cables and transformers. [radiation, metal.]

radiometallography (ra·de·o·met·al·**og**′·raf·e). The use of x-rays or the penetrating rays of radioactive substances for the examination of metal castings, welded joints, and alloys. [radiation, metal, Gk *graphein* to record.]

radiometer (ra·de·**om**·et·er). An instrument for measuring intensity of radiation. **Pastille radiometer.** An obsolete apparatus for measuring the intensity of x-rays by colour changes taking place in a barium platinocyanide disc. **Photographic radiometer.** A radiometer in which strips of photographic paper, after exposure and processing, are compared with a standard of reference.

See also: CROOKES, NICHOLS.

radiomicrometer (ra·de·o·mi·**krom**′·et·er). An apparatus used for measuring very small changes in radiation. [radiation, Gk *mikros* small, meter.]

radiomimetic (ra·de·o·mim·**et**′·ik). A term applied to cytotoxic (antimitotic) drugs which, by interfering with mitosis, have actions comparable to ionizing radiation. [radiation, Gk *mimetikos* imitative.]

radiomutation (ra·de·o·mew·**ta**′·shun). Changes effected in the character of a cell by exposure to ionizing radiation. [radiation, L *mutare* to change.]

radion (ra·de·on). Name applied formerly to the α- and β-particles emitted by radioactive elements.

radionecrosis (ra·de·o·nek·**ro**′·sis). Necrosis or ulceration of the tissues which may be a consequence of exposure to ionizing radiation.

radioneuritis (ra·de·o·newr·**i**′·tis). Neuritis occurring in those who have been exposed to ionizing radiation, usually only evident following massive exposure. [radiation, neuritis.]

radionuclide (ra·de·o·**new**′·klide). A nuclide which is radioactive. [radiation, nucleus.]

radio-opacity (ra·de·o·o·**pas**′·it·e). The state, quality, or property of being radio-opaque.

radio-opaque (ra·de·o·o·**pake**′). Radio density of higher degree than that of the surrounding structures. This can be absolute in the case of thick heavy metals, but the term is commonly used in a relative sense when one structure, or contrast medium, is denser than another. [radiation, opaque.]

radiopalmar (ra·de·o·**pal**′·mar). 1. Belonging to the radius and the palm. 2. Belonging to the radial (lateral) side of the palm.

radiopaque (ra·de·o·**pake**). Radio-opaque.

radioparency (ra·de·o·**pa**′·ren·se). Radiolucency. [radiation, L *parere* to appear.]

radioparent (ra·de·o·**pa**′·rent). Permitting the passage of x-rays without filtration; radiotransparent. Cf. RADIOLUCENT. [see prec.]

radiopathology (ra·de·o·path·**ol**′·o·je). The section of pathology which is concerned with the effects of radiation on cells and tissues.

radiopelvimetry (ra·de·o·pel·**vim**′·et·re). X-ray examination of the pelvis in order to determine its measurements. [radiation, pelvis, meter.]

radiopharmaceutical (ra·de·o·far·mah·**sew**′·tik·al). A radioactive pharmaceutical preparation used either as a diagnostic agent or as a radiotherapeutic agent. [radiation, Gk *pharmakeuein* to administer a drug.]

radiophobia (ra·de·o·**fo**·be·ah). Pathological fear of x-rays and radiation. [radiation, phobia.]

radiophosphorus (ra·de·o·**fos**′·for·us). Radioactive phosphorus. ^{32}P is the only radioactive isotope of phosphorus of medical importance. [radiation, Gk *phos* light, *pherein* to bear.]

radiophotography (ra·de·o·fo·**tog**′·raf·e). The process of recording photographically an image produced by x-rays on a fluorescent screen. [radiation, photography.]

radioplastic (ra·de·o·**plas**′·tik). Describing a method of constructing an artifical model of an organ or diseased area from measurements obtained radiologically. [radiation, Gk *plassein* to mould.]

radiopotassium (ra·de·o·pot·**as**′·e·um). Radioactive potassium. Only one radioactive isotope of potassium occurs naturally, ^{40}K; the medically most commonly used is ^{42}K. [radiation, potassium.]

radioreaction (ra·de·o·re·**ak**′·shun). A reaction shown by any part of the body, in particular the skin, to radiation.

radioreceptor (ra·de·o·re·**sep**′·tor). A device which responds in a detectable manner to incident radiant energy. [radiation, L *recipere* to receive.]

radioresistance (ra·de·o·re·**zis'**·tans). The property of relative resistance of living matter to irradiation.

radioresistant (ra·de·o·re·**zis'**·tant). Describing living matter which is relatively resistant to irradiation.

radioresponsive (ra·de·o·res·**pon'**·siv). Radiosensitive.

radioscope (ra·de·o·skope). An obsolete apparatus used for detecting and measuring x-radiation. [radiation, Gk *skopein* to view.]

radioscopy (ra·de·**os**·ko·pe). Visualization with the human eye of the image on a fluorescent screen during x-ray examination. [see prec.]

radioselenium (ra·de·o·sel·**e'**·ne·um). Radioactive selenium. ^{75}Se is medically the most important radioactive isotope of selenium. [radiation, selenium.]

radiosensitive (ra·de·o·**sen'**·sit·iv). Capable of being readily acted upon, either beneficially or harmfully, by radiant energy of any kind, e.g. from ionizing radiation. [radiation, sensitive.]

radiosensitivity (ra·de·o·sen·sit·**iv'**·it·e). The state of being radiosensitive.

radiosodium (ra·de·o·**so'**·de·um). Radioactive sodium. ^{22}Na and ^{24}Na are commonly used radioactive isotopes of sodium. [radiation, sodium.]

radiostereoscopy (ra·de·o·steer·e·**os'**·ko·pe). The stereoscopic viewing of the fluorescent screen image produced by x-rays. [radiation, stereoscopy.]

radiostrontium (ra·de·o·**stron'**·she·um). Radioactive strontium. ^{85}Sr and ^{87m}Sr are both used in diagnosis, while ^{90}Sr is a dangerous constituent of the fall-out from nuclear explosions. [radiation, strontium.]

radiosulphur (ra·de·o·**sul'**·fer). Radioactive sulphur. ^{35}S is the only radioactive isotope of sulphur of medical importance. [radiation, sulphur.]

radiotantalum (ra·de·o·**tan'**·tal·um). Radioactive tantalum. The radioactive isotope of tantalum ^{182}Ta is used as a radiotherapeutic agent in a form suitable for insertion into the region to be treated. [radiation, tantalum.]

radiotellurium (ra·de·o·tel·**ew'**·re·um). Polonium. Radium F. A radioactive element produced as a step in the disintegration of radium. It has a half-life of 136 days. So-called because it occurs in the tellurium obtained from pitchblende. [radiation, tellurium.]

radiotherapeutics (ra·de·o·ther·ap·**ew'**·tix). Radiotherapy.

radiotherapist (ra·de·o·**ther**·ap·ist). A specialist in radiotherapy.

radiotherapy (ra·de·o·**ther'**·ap·e). The treatment of patients with ionizing radiations. [radiation, Gk *therapeia* treatment.]

radiothermy (ra·de·o·**ther**·me). The therapeutic use of radiant heat or short-wave diathermy. [radiation, Gk *therme* heat.]

radiothorium (ra·de·o·**thor'**·e·um). A radioactive element produced during the disintegration of thorium. It has a half-life of 1.9 years, and emits an α-particle passing into thorium X. It occurs in pitchblende and is inseparable from thorium.

radiotomy (ra·de·**ot**·o·me). Tomography; body-section radiography. [radiation, Gk *tome* section.]

radiotoxaemia (ra·de·o·tox·**e'**·me·ah). An obsolete term describing the side-effects of exposure to ionizing radiation. [radiation, toxaemia.]

radiotransparent (ra·de·o·trans·**pa'**·rent). Radioparent. [radiation, L *trans, parere* to appear.]

radiotropic (ra·de·o·**trop'**·ik). Responsive to radiation. [radiation, Gk *trepein* to turn.]

radiotropism (ra·de·o·**trop'**·izm). A tendency to respond in a particular way to irradiation. [see prec.]

radio-ulnar (ra·de·o·**ul'**·nar). Relating or belonging to the radius and the ulna. **Radio-ulnar joint.** *See* JOINT.

radioxenon (ra·de·o·**ze'**·non). Radioactive xenon. ^{133}Xe is the only radioactive isotope of xenon of medical importance. [radiation, xenon.]

radioyttrium (ra·de·o·**it'**·re·um). Radioactive yttrium. ^{90}Y is the radioactive isotope of yttrium of medical importance. It is used as a radiotherapeutic agent as a colloid or adsorbed onto microspheres. [radiation, yttrium.]

radium (ra·de·um). A radioactive element of atomic number 88, and chemical symbol Ra. It is a white metal, occurring naturally in pitchblende, carnotite and other uranium ores, and resembles barium in chemical properties. It is a member of the uranium radioactive series with a half-life of 1580 years, transforming into radon with the emission of an α-particle and thence through the remaining decay products in the series to stable lead. It used to be widely used in radiotherapy and industrial radiography chiefly for the γ-rays emitted by its decay products which have a quantum energy varying from 0.2 to 2.2 MeV; the α- and β-emissions of its decay products also have applications in radiotherapy. Its importance has been greatly diminished by the use of artificial radio-elements both in radiotherapy and in industrial radiography. The salts are extremely toxic and are employed in luminous paints. **Radium A, B, C, D, E, and F.** A series of radioactive elements which occur in the disintegration of uranium through the uranium series to end in lead. **Radium G.** Stable lead (^{206}Pb), the final decay product of the uranium-radium series. [L *radius* ray.]

radius (ra·de·us) (pl. *radii*). The line joining the centre of a circle or sphere to the circumference or surface. **Radius fixus.** The line from the hormion to the inion. **Radii of the lens of the eye [radii lentis (NA)].** Faint lines of suture radiating from the poles to the equator; three are present in the fetus, six or more in the adult. **Nuclear radius.** The radius of the atomic nucleus, determined by an experimental method based on a theoretical hypothesis of nuclear structure. The experimental methods include measurement of fast neutron scattering, and α-particle emission from radioactive nuclei. Agreement between different methods is good, and values range from 2×10^{-13} to 10^{-12} cm with increasing atomic weight. [L ray.]

radius [NA] (ra·de·us). The lateral bone of the forearm, articulating above with the capitulum of the humerus, below with the scaphoid and lunate bones, and medially with the ulna. [see prec.]

Articular circumference [circumferentia articularis (NA)]. The smooth circumference of the head of the radius that articulates with the ulna.

Head [caput radii (NA)]. The uppermost part of the radius, articulating above with the capitulum of the humerus and medially with the ulna.

Neck [collum radii (NA)]. The constriction immediately below the head of the radius.

Shaft [corpus radii (NA)]. The main part of the bone connecting the upper and lower ends. It is slightly curved, triangular in cross-section, and widens towards the lower end. Its medial or interosseous border [margo interossea (NA)] is sharp and adjacent to the ulna and gives attachment to the interosseous membrane; its remaining borders are ill-defined and placed anteriorly [margo anterior (NA)] and posteriorly [margo posterior (NA)]. The anterior border curves medially above towards the tuberosity where it is known as the anterior oblique line. Between the interosseous and anterior borders is the anterior surface [facies anterior (NA)] which gives attachment to the flexor pollicis longus and pronator quadratus muscles. The lateral surface [facies lateralis (NA)] is bounded by the anterior and posterior borders and gives insertion in its middle part to the pronator teres muscle whilst the posterior surface [facies posterior (NA)] is bounded by the posterior and interosseous borders and gives attachment to the deep extensor muscles of the hand.

Carpal articular surface [facies articularis carpea (NA)]. The smooth, concave, lower surface of the radius for articulation with the proximal row of carpal bones.

radix [NA] (ra·dix) (pl. *radices*). A root. **Radix cochlearis nervi acustici.** The cochlear division of the 8th cranial nerve. **Radices parietales venae cavae inferiores.** The tributaries of the inferior vena cava which arise in the walls of the abdomen, such as the lumbar and diaphragmatic veins. **Radix sympathici gangli ciliaris.** Sympathetic postganglionic fibres from the carotid plexus which pass through the ciliary ganglion to the eyeball.

Radix vestibularis nervi acustici. The vestibular division of the 8th cranial nerve. **Radices viscerales venae cavae inferiores.** The tributaries of the inferior vena cava which arise in viscera, such as the hepatic, renal, and suprarenal veins. [L.]

radon (ra·don). Niton, radium emanation. A radioactive element of atomic number 86, and chemical symbol Rn. It is a colourless gas belonging to the inert-gas family, produced by the disintegration of radium with emission of an α-particle. It emits in turn an α-particle and becomes radium A. It has a half-life of approximately 4 days. **Radon seed.** A small bead containing radon formerly used in radiotherapy for insertion into the region to be irradiated. [radiation.]

Radovici, Jean G. (b. 1868). Paris physician.

Radovici's sign. The palmomental reflex; exaggeration suggests pyramidal-tract disease. When the response occurs on the side opposite to that of the thenar eminence which is stimulated, facial weakness on the silent side is likely.

raffinase (raf·in·aze). An enzyme found in yeast which hydrolyses raffinose into fructose and melibiose.

raffinose (raf·in·oze). Melitose, $C_{18}H_{32}O_{16}$. A dextrorotatory trisaccharide, fructose-β- glucose-6-α-galactoside, found in sugar beet, beetroot, molasses, eucalyptus manna, cotton seeds, and in certain cereals and fungi. Hydrolysis by dilute acids or the enzyme, raffinase, yields fructose and melibiose.

rage (raje). Violent anger. **La rage.** Rabies. **Sham rage.** A phenomenon seen in decorticated animals, when motor and autonomic reactions similar to those occurring in rage in a normal animal appear in response to mild stimuli. [Fr.]

ragle (rahgl). Hallucinations of oases experienced in the desert. [Fr.]

ragocyte (rag·o·site). A leucocyte with cytoplasmic inclusions containing gamma globulin, found in synovial effusions of patients with rheumatoid arthritis and other forms of arthritis. Also called *RA cells.*

ragweed (rag·weed). Ambrosia, the American ragweed, the airborne pollen of which can cause chronic dermatitis of exposed parts and where clothing is in close contact with the skin.

Raillietina (ri·le·et·e′·nah). A genus of tapeworms. The numerous species are parasites of birds and mammals, secondary hosts, where known, being arthropods. There are a number of records from man in various parts of the tropics, but all are casual. Old World forms were once described under the name of *Raillietina madagascariensis,* but several species were probably involved.

Raimist, J. M. 20th century Berlin psychiatrist.

Raimist's sign. The hand is held by the examiner so that the forearm is vertical, and is then suddenly let go. A sound hand remains upright, a paretic one flexes abruptly at the wrist.

Rainey, George (b. 1801). London anatomist.

Rainey's corpuscle. The spore of *Sarcocystis lindemanni.*

raised (ra·zd). Describing colonies of bacteria that are elevated above the surface of the medium. [AS *risan.*]

raisin (ra·zin). A grape partially dried in the sun, or artificially. **Corinthian raisin.** A small raisin, or currant, prepared from a variety of seedless grapes grown in the eastern Mediterranean; it is used in cooking. [OFr. *raizin.*]

râle (rahl). An abnormal adventitious sound accompanying the breath sounds heard on auscultation. In old classifications râles were divided into dry and moist. *Dry râles* are now called *rhonchi* and the old term is no longer used. Râles (moist) are the sounds produced by air bubbling through secretions or fluid in the trachea or bronchi, the sound depending on the size of the tube in which it is produced and varies from the coarsest in the trachea (*death rattle*) to the finest in the terminal bronchioles (*crepitations*). The quality of the sound depends on the nature of the tissue through which it is conducted to the ear, and the râles (coarse, medium or fine) are further subdivided into *consonating* or *crackling* and *non-consonating* or *bubbling—crackling* if they are conducted through solid lung or a cavity, and *non-consonating* if the lung is not consolidated as, for example, in bronchitis. **Sibilant râle.** A high-pitched rhonchus. *See* RHONCHUS. **Sonorous râle.** A low-pitched rhonchus. *See* RHONCHUS. [Fr rattle.]

ramal (ra·mal). Belonging to a ramus or branch.

Raman, Sir Chandrasekhara Venkata (b. 1888). Indian physicist.

Raman effect. An effect discovered by Raman in 1928, and similar to the Compton effect, but observed in the optical part of the spectrum. A monochromatic beam of light of high intensity concentrated on certain materials (solids, liquids, or gases) will produce a faint scattered light in which is found the original wavelength and also certain new wavelengths which are sharp and definite. These are caused by collision between quanta of radiation and molecules of matter. The energy of incident quanta is much smaller than in the Compton effect; the quanta cannot remove electrons from the atom, they can only excite each atom into one of its stationary states.

ramenta (ra·men·tah). Shreds or filings. **Ramenta ferri.** Iron filings. [L.]

rami (ra·mi). *See* RAMUS.

ramicotomy (ram·ik·ot·o·me). Ramisection. [L *ramus* branch, Gk *temnein* to cut.]

ramification (ram·if·ik·a′·shun). 1. The act or the process of branching. 2. A small branch from a main nerve or blood vessel. [L *ramus* branch, *facere* to make.]

ramify (ram·if·i). 1. To form or spread out into branches. 2. To branch out in several directions. [see prec.]

ramisection (ram·e·sek·shun). The operation of cutting communicating branches connecting the spinal cord with sympathetic ganglia; done for relief of spasm of blood vessels whose sympathetic (vasoconstrictor) supply is thus interrupted. It is part of the operation of sympathectomy. [L *ramus* branch, *secare* to cut.]

ramisectomy (ram·e·sek·to·me). Ramisection.

ramitis (ram·i·tis). Inflammation affecting a nerve root. [L *ramus* branch, Gk *-itis* inflammation.]

Ramon, Gaston Leon (b. 1886). French veterinary pathologist.

Ramon's flocculation test. An *in vitro* method of standardizing diphtheria antitoxin. Falling amounts of antitoxic serum are mixed with a constant amount of toxin in a series of tubes. The tube first showing flocculation contains a neutralized mixture of toxin and antitoxin, and this affords a basis for assessing potency. The method has also been applied to certain other antitoxic sera.

Ramón y Cajal, Santiago (b. 1852). Madrid histologist.

Cajal cells. 1. Astrocytes. 2. Multipolar nerve cells in the cerebral cortex giving branched processes parallel to the surface.

Cajal method. The impregnation of neuroglial cells by means of a mixture of mercuric and gold chlorides after formalin-ammonium bromide fixation.

Cajal's double method. A repetition of the osmium-bichromate stage, after the silver bath, in Golgi's quick method for the impregnation of nervous tissue, in order to intensify the latter.

Interstitial nucleus of Cajal. A small nucleus in the lateral wall of the third ventricle just above the oculomotor nucleus, at the upper limit of the medial longitudinal bundle, to which it contributes. Afferent fibres to the nucleus arise in the globus pallidus, substantia nigra, superior quadrigeminal bodies, and the vestibular nuclei.

Ramond, F. 20th century French physician.

Ramond's point. Tenderness between the heads of the right sternocleidomastoid muscle that may be found in gall-bladder disease.

Ramond, Louis (b. 1879). Paris physician.

Ramond's sign. Rigidity of the sacrospinalis muscle with a serous pleural effusion, which relaxes when the fluid becomes purulent.

ramose, ramous (ra·moze, ra·mus). 1. Branched. 2. Composed of or having branches or lateral divisions. 3. Having resemblance or belonging to, or having the character of a branch. [L *ramus* branch.]

Ramsay Hunt. *See* HUNT, JAMES RAMSAY.

Ramsbotham, John (b. 1767). London obstetrician.

Ramsbotham's hook. An instrument for decapitating the fetus.

Ramsden, Jesse (b. 1735). British optician.

Ramsden ocular. An eyepiece composed of two planoconvex lenses mounted with their convex surfaces towards one another.

Ramsden's operation. Ligation of the subclavian artery through an incision above the clavicle.

Ramstedt, Wilhelm Conrad (b. 1867). Münster surgeon.

Ramstedt's operation, Fredet-Ramstedt operation. Division by a longitudinal incision of the hypertrophied pyloric muscle for the relief of congenital hypertrophic stenosis.

ramulus (ram·ew·lus). A small branch or ramus. [L.]

ramus [NA] (ra·mus) (pl. *rami*). A branch; most commonly used for branches of nerves, but applied also to other structures. **Horizontal anterior ramus [ramus anterior (NA)].** A short fissure of the cerebral hemisphere extending horizontally forward from the stem of the lateral fissure into the lower part of the frontal lobe from the stem. **Horizontal ascending ramus [ramus ascendens (NA)].** A short fissure of the cerebral hemisphere extending vertically from the stem of the lateral fissure into the frontal lobe. It sometimes has a common origin with the horizontal anterior ramus. **Ischiopubic ramus.** The bar of bone formed by the ramus of the ischium and the inferior ramus of the pubis. **Ramus of the ischium [ramus ossis ischii (NA)].** The bone which extends forwards from the body of the ischium to join the inferior ramus of the pubis. **Ramus of the mandible [ramus mandibulae (NA)].** The broad quadrilateral portion of the mandible projecting upwards from the posterior end of the body, behind the lower teeth. It is flattened from without inward and presents two surfaces, lateral and medial, and an anterior and posterior border. It gives insertion to the bulk of the muscles of mastication. **Posterior ramus [ramus posterior (NA)].** The longest ramus of the lateral fissure of the cerebral hemisphere, extending backwards with a terminal upward curve. **Pubic ramus, inferior [ramus inferior ossis pubis (NA)].** The bone which extends from near the symphysis to join the ramus of the ischium. **Pubic ramus, superior [ramus superior ossis pubis (NA)].** The bone which extends from near the symphysis to the acetabulum, cranial to the obturator foramen. It has three surfaces, a smooth one towards the pelvic cavity (pelvic surface), a triangular pectineal surface above, and an obturator surface directed downwards and backwards and grooved for the obturator nerve. [L.]

Rana (ra·nah). A genus of frogs. **Rana esculenta.** The edible frog. **Rana nigromacula.** A species in which the plerocercoid stage of the tapeworm *Diphyllobothrium mansoni* occurs in nature. Man is rarely a host. **Rana pipiens.** A North American frog. **Rana temporaria.** The common European frog. *See also:* FROG. [L.]

rancid (ran·sid). Having an offensive, sour, or sharp taste or odour; applied especially to fats and oils which have become rank and sour owing to chemical decomposition and the production of fatty acids. [L *rancidus* stinking.]

rancidity (ran·sid·it·e). The condition of being rancid. **Chemical rancidity.** The estimation of the decomposition of fats and oils into free fatty acids in terms of the peroxide value.

Randacio, Francesco (b. 1821). Palermo anatomist.

Randacio's nerves. Branches of the sphenopalatine ganglion.

Randolph, Nathaniel Archer (b. 1858). American physician.

Randolph's diluting fluid, or solution. A diluting fluid used in the enumeration of and permitting the staining of white blood corpuscles; it is prepared by freshly mixing equal quantities of stock solutions of methylene blue (0.1 per cent) and phloxine (0.1 per cent) in 50 per cent propylene glycol and diluting this with an equal volume of distilled water.

Raney, Rupert B. Los Angeles neurosurgeon.

Raney's ganglionectomy and trunk section. Division of the thoracic communicating branches and sympathetic trunk, without excision.

range (ra·nj). 1. The interval between the lowest and highest values of a series of data, e.g. in statistics, deviations from a mean. 2. The distance travelled by an ionizing particle, usually expressed in centimetres of air at standard temperature and pressure. The range of the particle is dependent on the initial energy of the particle and the absorber through which the particle is travelling. **Range of accommodation.** The distance between the far point, the farthest distance that an object can be clearly seen with accommodation fully relaxed, and the near point, the nearest distance that an object can be seen clearly with maximum accommodation. Range of accommodation is measured in distance, inches or centimetres. Amplitude of accommodation is measured in dioptres. **Range of audibility.** The auditory field enclosed within the upper and lower limits of audibility. **Range of convergence.** The distance between the far point, i.e. where the visual axes meet when the eyes are at rest, and the near point, i.e. the nearest distance to the eyes that an object can be brought without becoming double. **Range of sensibility.** The intensity of a sensation is proportional to the logarithm of the stimulus which evokes it; also called *Fechner's law.* [OFr.]

ranine (ra·nine). 1. Relating to a ranula. 2. Relating to the inferior surface of the tip of the tongue, in particular to the branches of the artery and vein supplying that region. [L *rana* frog.]

Ranke, Johannes (b. 1836). Munich physician and anthropologist.

Ranke's angle. An angle between the horizontal plane of the skull and a line joining the nasion and prosthion. Ranke described this angle prior to the general adoption of the Frankfort horizontal plane.

Ranke, Karl Ernst (b. 1870). Munich physician.

Ranke's stages. Ranke described three stages for tuberculosis. 1. The primary infection. 2. The stage of generalized infection. 3. The stage of chronic infection.

rankenangioma (rang·ken·an·je·o′·mah). Cirsoid aneurysm. *See* ANEURYSM.

Rankin, Fred Wharton (b. 1886). Rochester, Minnesota, surgeon.

Rankin clamp. A three-bladed clamp used extensively before the introduction of antibiotics in extraperitoneal colon resection.

Ransohoff, Joseph Louis (b. 1853). Cincinnati surgeon.

Ransohoff's operation. For chronic empyema: the multiple division of thickened pleura, grid-iron fashion, over the lung.

ranula (ran·ew·lah). A cystic swelling of the floor of the mouth, immediately to one or other side of the middle line, caused by extravasation into the interstitial tissues of mucus from one of the mucous glands. **Burrowing ranula.** A rare condition in which, in addition to the swelling in the floor of the mouth, there is a swelling in the neck due to the mucous extravasation spreading interstitially between the muscles of the floor of the mouth. [dim. of L *rana* frog.]

ranular (ran·ew·lar). Pertaining to or having the characters of ranula.

Ranunculaceae (ran·ung·kew·la′·se·e). A family of plants, including the crowfoots and buttercups, characterized by having a flower with five sepals, five petals, many stamens, and few to many pistils. A few drugs of medicinal importance (aconite, black hellebore, cimicifuga, and stavesacre seeds) are derived from genera of this family. [L *ranunculus* small frog.]

Ranvier, Louis Antoine (b. 1835). Paris pathologist.

Ranvier's one-third alcohol. A 30 per cent solution of alcohol in water, used to soften tough tissues.

Ranvier's node. A regularly repeated constriction of a medullated nerve fibre.

Ranvier's cross. A cruciate figure, seen at Ranvier's nodes, of nerve fibres stained with silver nitrate.

Ranvier's disc. A thin, transverse plate seen at Ranvier's nodes after staining with silver nitrate. It corresponds to the transverse limb of a Ranvier's cross.

Ranvier's membrane. Renaut's layer.

Ranvier's formic acid method. Tissues are impregnated in a mixture of gold chloride and formic acid in the dark, and later reduced in formic acid in the light. Nerve cells and processes are impregnated.

Ranvier's picrocarmine. A mixture of carmine, picric acid, and ammonia, used as a histological stain. Nuclei are stained red, cytoplasm yellow.

Ranvier's plexus. A nerve plexus derived from the stroma immediately underlying the anterior elastic lamina of the cornea.

Ranvier's segment. The internodal portion of a nerve fibre.

Merkel-Ranvier cell. A melanoblast of the skin.

Raoult, François Marie (b. 1830). French physicist.

Raoult's laws. Laws relating to dilute solutions: (*a*) the ratio of the lowering of the vapour pressure produced by dissolving a given quantity of solute in a given weight of solvent, to the original vapour pressure of the solvent, is equal to the ratio of the respective numbers of molecules of solute and solvent present; (*b*) the elevation of the boiling point of the solution above that of the pure solvent, and the depression of the freezing point, are both proportional to the same molecular ratio.

rape (rape). The unlawful sexual intercourse of a woman without her consent, by force, fear, or fraud. Full penetration by the penis is not necessary nor is seminal emission; a mere entry into the vulva is sufficient. **Feigned rape.** Falsely alleged in attempts at extortion or for revenge, sometimes by those suffering delusions but most frequently deliberate. Fabricated rape injuries may also be committed on the dead, as in necrophilism. **Statutory rape.** In the UK, sexual intercourse of a girl under the age of consent, with or without her acquiescence. Certain persons, e.g. female idiots and imbeciles, and girls under the age of 16, are, in law, unable to give consent. Therefore, sexual intercourse or attempted sexual intercourse of a girl under the age of 13 years is always unlawful, as it is also of a girl between the ages of 13 and 16; in the former case the offence is more serious, but in the latter case it will be a defence if the accused had reasonable cause to believe the girl to be over 16, provided that (1) he is under the age of 23 at the time, and (2) he has not been charged before with a similar offence. The term *statutory rape* is of USA origin, but is understood in this country. [L *rapere* to seize.]

raphania (raf·a·ne·ah). Rhaphania.

raphe [NA] (ra·fe). A seam; often used in anatomy for the line or plane of junction of the two halves of a structure which is formed in the embryo from bilateral rudiments. **Amniotic raphe.** The line of thickened amnion marking the site of fusion of the amniotic folds in reptiles, birds, and many mammals. **Anococcygeal raphe.** A fibrous band which passes from the anus to the coccyx and to which the posterior parts of the levator ani muscles are attached. **Buccal raphe.** A ridge of the buccal epithelium of the embryo, marking the site of fusion of the mandibular and maxillary components of the cheek. **Lateral palpebral raphe [raphe palpebralis lateralis (NA)].** A weak ligament formed by the fibrous tissue of the orbital septum reinforced by fibres of the orbicularis oculi muscle; it is superficial to the lateral palpebral ligament. **Median raphe of the medulla oblongata [raphe (NA)].** The median seam which separates the right and left halves of the medulla oblongata. **Median raphe of the pons [raphe (NA)].** The median seam separating the right and left halves of the pons. **Raphe of the mid-brain.** The median seam separating the right and left halves of the tegmentum of the mid-brain. **Palatine raphe [raphe palati (NA)].** The line in the median saggital plane along which the two halves of the palate are joined in the embryo. **Raphe of the penis [raphe penis (NA)].** An anterior continuation of the raphe of the scrotum along the under-surface of the penis. **Raphe of the perineum [raphe perinei (NA)].** A posterior continuation of the raphe of the scrotum to the anus. **Raphe of the pharynx [raphe pharyngis (NA)].** The fibrous seam in the midline of the posterior aspect of the pharynx separating the constrictor muscles of the two sides. **Raphe of the scrotum [raphe scroti (NA)].** A cutaneous ridge in the midline separating the two halves of the scrotum. **Raphe of the tongue.** The fibrous septum which separates the right and left halves of the tongue and to which some of the intrinsic muscles are attached. [Gk *rhaphe.*]

See also: STILLING.

raphidiospore (raf·id·e·o·spor). Rhaphidiospore.

rapport (rap·ort). A relationship of mutual sympathy and understanding. [Fr.]

raptus (rap·tus). 1. A seizure or violent attack. 2. Rape. **Raptus haemorrhagicus.** Haemorrhage of sudden onset. **Raptus maniacus.** An attack of frenzy which lasts only a short time. **Raptus melancholicus.** A sudden attack of violent excitement occurring in a melancholiac. **Raptus nervorum.** Spasm or cramp. [L *rapere* to seize.]

rarefaction (ra·re·fak·shun). 1. The reduction of the density of a substance. 2. The attenuation of a gas, either by increasing the volume of the vessel in which it is contained or by pumping out some of the gas. **Rarefaction of bone.** The increasing of the porosity of bone. [L *rarus* thin, *facere* to make.]

rarefy (ra·re·fi). 1. To reduce the density or increase the porosity of a substance. 2. To become less dense. [see prec.]

Rasbora donicornicus (raz·bo·rah do·ni·kor·nik·us). A barbel fish that eats cyclops and is therefore used in the prophylaxis of guinea-worm infection.

rasceta (ras·se·tah). The wrinkles or lines which traverse the skin on the palmar aspect of the wrist. [LL *rasare* to scrape often.]

Rasch, Hermann (b. 1873). Berlin obstetrician.

Rasch's sign of pregnancy. The altered consistency of the uterus in pregnancy.

rash (rash). A cutaneous eruption. **Amygdalotomy rash.** Tonsillectomy rash (see below). **Aniline rash.** A dermatosis attributed to exposure to aniline. **Antitoxin rash.** A skin eruption following the injection of antitoxic serum, possibly occurring as part of the syndrome of serum sickness. **Astacoid rash.** Lobster rash (see below). **Cable rash.** A cutaneous eruption caused by exposure to the fumes of chlorinated naphthalene, used for insulating cables. **Canker rash.** Scarlet fever. **Caterpillar rash.** A somewhat urticarial, itching eruption, caused by contact with the hairs of a caterpillar. Many caterpillars belonging to some eight different families of *Lepidoptera* can cause the eruption. **Detergent rash.** A contact dermatitis of the face and hands occurring after contact with certain detergent fluids; it may also occur after contact with clothes that have been washed with detergents. **Diaper rash.** Jacquet's erythema; an erythematous eruption on the napkin area of infants. If hygienic care is poor the affected area may extend as high as the axillae and as low as the heels and calves; secondary infection may produce ulceration in the affected area. It is caused by a persistent damp condition of the skin which is the more easily affected by the free ammonia liberated through the interaction of acid urine and badly washed napkins. Treatment consists of allowing the skin to regain normal texture by frequent washing and careful drying after bladder and bowel action. The use of washing powders for napkins has also been a cause. **Drug rash.** An eruption caused by the ingestion or injection of drugs. There are four aetiological varieties: (*a*) an immediate allergic eruption; (*b*) a rash caused by overdosage or cumulative effect; (*c*) an allergic reaction developing after prolonged administration; amd (*d*) a rash caused by release of toxins due to the action of the drug on pathogenic organisms in a septic focus. **Enema rash.** An erythematous rash caused by a soap enema. **Flannel rash.** Seborrhoeic dermatitis, particularly of the petaloid variety. **Gum rash.** An erythematous eruption which occurs on the cheeks and chin, and sometimes on the anterior aspect of the chest, of infants during the teething period, when there is an unusual flow of saliva whose pH becomes slightly more acid. This predisposes towards multiplication of the normal saprophytes which may act as pathogens and set up an allergic reaction, the rash; the sodden condition of the skin may add further complication through infection with micro-organisms. **Heat rash.** A term usually indicating miliaria (prickly heat). **Hop rash.** Contact dermatitis caused by exposure to hops. **Hydatid rash.** An urticarial or erythematous rash with pruritus following the internal rupture of a hydatid cyst. **Lily rash.** Contact dermatitis usually due to daffodils or jonquils. **Lobster rash.** A reddish eruption sometimes observed in smallpox, which has been likened to the shell of a boiled lobster. It occurs only in grave haemorrhagic cases. **Medicinal rash.** Drug rash (see above). **Mulberry rash.** The blotchy rash of typhus fever, consisting of irregular dusky mottling. **Napkin rash.** Diaper rash (see above). **Nettle rash.** Urticaria. **Nickel rash.** Dermatitis due to intimate contact with nickel-plated articles. **Plant rash.** A rash produced by contact with certain plants, e.g. primula. **Rose rash.** Roseola; 1. Any rose-coloured eruption. 2. Epidemic roseola, rubella, rubeola, or German measles. **Scarlet rash.** Any scarlatiniform eruption, including scarlet fever. **Serum rash.** A skin eruption following the injection of an antitoxic or other serum into a person sensitive to serum protein. **Tonsillectomy rash.** A rash which sometimes occurs after tonsillectomy. **Tooth rash.** Gum rash (see above). **Vaccine rash.** A rash which occurs after an injection of vaccine or a vaccination. **Wandering rash.** Geographical tongue. *See* TONGUE. [OFr. *rasche* scurf.]

Rashkind, William Jacobson (b. 1922). American paediatric cardiologist.

Rashkind procedure. The creation of an enlarged atrial septal defect in patients with transposition of the great arteries (vessels) who have insufficient mixing of the two circulations. The technique involves the passage of a balloon catheter, introduced pervenously through an existing patent foramen ovale or small septal defect, into the left atrium; the balloon is then inflated and the catheter withdrawn so as to rupture the atrial septum.

Rasmussen, Fritz Waldemar (b. 1834). Copenhagen physician.

Rasmussen's aneurysm. An erosion aneurysm of a branch of the pulmonary artery in a tuberculous cavity in the lung, often rupturing and causing haemoptysis.

Rasori, Giovanni (b. 1766). Italian physician.

Doctrine of Rasori. Some substances are contrastimulating in application and lessen excitability by an antagonistic effect to that produced by the stimulating substance.

Method of Rasori. Repeated blood-letting.

rasorianism, rasorism (ra·zor·e·an·izm, ra·zor·izm). Doctrine of Rasori.

raspatory (ras·pat·o·re). An instrument used to scrape the periosteum from bone. [OFr. *rasper.*]

raspberry (rahz·ber·e). The fruit of *Rubus idaeus* Linn. (family Rosaceae), used only as a flavouring, but the leaves are said to contain a water-soluble principle which relieves uterine pains. [etym. dub.]

Rastelli, Gian Carlo (b. 1933). American thoracic surgeon.

Rastelli's operation. The procedure used for the correction of suitable forms of transposition of the great arteries (vessels) by means of a conduit within the venous ventricle conducting oxygenated blood from the arterial ventricle to the aorta and the attachment of a prosthesis with a valve at its base to the venous ventricle to conduct blood to the distal part of the pulmonary artery which is detached from its origin; the proximal part of the artery is closed as a blind-end.

rat (rat). 1. A rodent of the genus *Rattus.* The species are particularly numerous in the tropical Far East where many wild and agricultural species (and sub-species of *R. rattus*) are important as plague reservoirs and normal hosts of the mite vectors of scrub typhus. There are two species which are world-wide commensals of man, in both of which plague is an endemic disease. The names *brown, common, Hanoverian, Norway,* and *sewer* refer to *R. norvegicus.* The names *alexandrine, black, house, old English, roof, ship,* and *tree* refer to *R. rattus* and its three commensal races or colour forms, *rattus, alexandrinus,* and *frugivorus. Cane rat* is *R. culmorum* of Queensland. *Laboratory rat, albino, hooded, pied,* and all other laboratory stocks are *R. norvegicus.* 2. A general term for a rodent of medium size belonging to many different groups, but not rats in sense 1. *Cotton rat* is *Sigmodon hispidus,* a New World rodent used as a laboratory animal; *Egyptian rat* is *Arvicanthus niloticus,* an important house rat of Mediterranean Africa; *wood rat* is a species of the genus *Neotoma,* rodents of North America which may act as plague reservoirs. [AS *raet.*]

ratafia (rat·ah·fe·ah). 1. A liqueur flavoured with essence of almonds, or with the kernels of cherry, peach, or apricot. Also a biscuit so flavoured. 2. A variety of cherry. [Malay *arag* arrack, *tafia* a distilled spirit.]

ratanhia, ratany (rat·an·e·ah, rat·an·e). Rhatany.

rate (rate). A velocity; a frequency; a numerical proportion between two things. **Basal metabolic rate.** Measure of the energy expenditure of the body in the resting state, a few hours after the absorption of the last meal and under comfortable environmental and subjective conditions. It is expressed in various terms, e.g. as joules (kilocalories) per m^2 body surface per hour (usually about 40), or as ml oxygen consumed per minute per m^2 body surface. It is proportional to body surface, not to body weight. **Birth rate.** The number of live births in a year divided by the estimated total population of the area at the middle of that year; it is usually expressed per 1000 of population. **Blood sedimentation rate.** Erythrocyte sedimentation rate (see below). **Case rate.** Morbidity rate; the number of cases of a specified disease occurring in a year, calculated per 100 or other unit of the total population living at all ages. It may be computed on the entire population or for specific age groups or classes. **Case fatality rate.** The number of registered or notified deaths per 100 notified cases of a specified disease. **Circulation rate.** The velocity of the blood flow, an expression of the volume of blood discharged by the heart per minute (minute volume). Cardiac output normally refers to the minute volume of the left ventricle, except when there is an abnormal communication between the right and left sides of the heart or between the pulmonary artery and the aorta. Unless the blood volume is diminished, reduction in cardiac output entails a decrease in circulation time. **Counting rate.** 1. Mortality rate; the ratio between the number of registered deaths and the population of a country or a rural or urban area during a given period, usually one year. The number of deaths is calculated per 1000 of the population during the given period. 2. The rate at which a detector of ionizing radiation is recording photons or ionizing particles. **Death rate.** The total deaths occurring in a year divided by the estimated total population of the area at the middle of that year; it is usually expressed per 1000 of population. Often known as the *crude death rate.* **Death rate, standardized.** The death rate at all ages calculated to allow for the different age and sex compositions of the population involved. **Dose rate.** In radiology, the radiation dose received per unit time. **Erythrocyte sedimentation rate.** A measure of the speed (in mm per hour) of sedimentation or settling of the erythrocytes in citrated plasma when it is allowed to stand under standard conditions in a vertical glass column. The rate varies considerably in various physiological and pathological conditions. **Fatality rate.** Lethality rate; the number of deaths from a specified disease per 100 cases of that disease. **Fertility rate.** The number of live births in a year divided by the female population of child-bearing age (usually 15–44 years); it is usually expressed per 1000. **Heart rate.** The number of contractions made by the ventricles per minute. Usually the atria beat at the same speed as the ventricles, unless complete or incomplete dissociation has occurred, when the atrial rate is usually faster (atrioventricular block), but they may even be slower (ventricular escape). In atrial fibrillation the atria contract rapidly, irregularly, and ineffectively, a high degree of atrioventricular block being present. Many of the ventricular contractions are weak because the diastolic pause following the previous beat has not been long enough to allow adequate ventricular filling. Such weak beats may not be transmitted to the radial pulse, thus producing a pulse deficit. This also sometimes occurs when a ventricular ectopic contraction follows close upon the preceding sinus beat. **Infant mortality rate.** The number of deaths in any one year of childen under the age of one year per 1000 live births in that year. **Lethality rate.** Fatality rate (see above). **Maternal mortality rate.** The number of deaths associated with childbirth in any one year per 1000 live births in the same period. **Morbidity rate.** Case rate (see above). **Mortality rate.** The number of deaths under one year of age occurring in one year divided by the total live births in that year; it is usually expressed per 1000. *Maternal mortality rate* is the number of deaths ascribed to puerperal causes divided by the total of live births and (usually) stillbirths; it is usually expressed per 1000. *Neonatal mortality rate* is the number of deaths in the first 28 days of life, occurring in one year, divided by the total live births in that year; it is usually expressed per 1000. *Perinatal mortality rate*, the number of stillbirths plus the deaths in the first week of life per 1000 total births. **Mutation rate.** The frequency of mutation per individual per generation. **Neonatal mortality rate.** The number of deaths in infants under one month per 1000 living births. **Oöcyst rate.** The percentage of female anopheles caught in nature that on dissection show the presence of plasmodial oöcysts in the mid-gut. **Parasite rate.** The percentage of persons harbouring malarial or other specified parasites in a particular country or district, or in a certain age group. A term sometimes used in malarial investigation. **Pulse rate.** The number of beats per minute of the radial or other superfical arterial pulse. Usually this is the same as the heart rate, but they may differ (pulse deficit). The venous pulse rate reflects the speed of the atria, and may be measured by examination of the jugular veins; normally the rate is the same as the radial pulse, but it is more rapid in the case of complete or partial atrioventricular block. **Reproduction rate.** A method of estimating the fertility of the population which indicates whether a population is or is not reproducing itself. *Gross reproduction rate* is the number of female infants born to each woman of child-bearing age; from this the *net reproduction rate* is calculated by application of the female mortality rates. If the net reproduction rate is less than one, the population will diminish. **Respiration rate.** The number of inspirations per minute. **Respiratory rate.** The rate of interchange of gases between the tissues and the blood. **Sedimentation rate.** Erythrocyte sedimentation rate (see above). **Sickness rate.** Case rate (see above). **Spleen rate.** The percentage of persons with palpable enlarged spleens in a particular district or in a certain age group. A term used in malarial investigation. **Sporozoite rate.** The percentage of female anopheles caught in nature that on dissection show the presence of plasmodial sporozoites in the salivary glands. **Standardized death rate.** The death rate at all ages calculated for purposes of comparison, and corrected either by the *direct* or *indirect* method for the age and sex composition of the population concerned. **Stillbirth rate.** Natimortality; this rate is obtained by taking the number of stillbirths (i.e. infants born dead) in a year, multiplying by 1000, and dividing by the number of total births (live and still) in that year. It is therefore the proportion of stillbirths to the general birth rate. [L *ratum* from *reri* to calculate.]

ratemeter (rate·me·ter). An instrument which performs the function of integrating the electrical pulses produced by a radiation detector in a period of time and indicates the mean counting rate on a suitable meter. [L *ratum* from *reri* to calculate, Gk *metron* measure.]

Rathke, Martin Heinrich (b. 1793). Königsberg anatomist.

Rathke's cyst. A simple cyst derived from distension of Rathke's pouch.

Rathke's duct. A persistent portion of the paramesonephric duct in the male, opening into the prostatic urethra.

Rathke's pouch. A depression or diverticulum in the roof of the embryonic mouth just anterior to the buccopharyngeal membrane, the walls of which give rise to the anterior lobe of the pituitary gland.

Rathke's trabecula. The trabeculae cranii constituting the front portion of a pair of longitudinal cartilaginous bars which flank the hypophysis cerebri and form part of the developing neurocranium.

Rathke's tumour. A tumour of the craniopharyngeal pouch or hypophyseal duct.

ratin (rat·in). A strain of *Salmonella enteritidis*, pathogenic to rats, and used formerly as an exterminator. It is no longer employed for this purpose as it was shown to be the cause occasionally of gastro-enteritis in humans.

ratio (ra·she·o). The relation or proportion that one thing bears to another of the same kind in respect of magnitude or quantity; the numerical quotient. **Absorption ratio.** The ratio of the amount of energy absorbed by a surface to the amount of energy falling upon it; the absorptive power of a surface. **A-G ratio, Albumin-globulin ratio.** The relation of the serum albumin to the serum globulin, which is normally over 1; in nephritis, kala-azar, lymphopathia venereum, and many other diseases it is much below 1, even as low as 0.25. **Anthropophilic ratio.** Human blood ratio (see below). **Aperture ratio.** The ratio of the diameter of the aperture of a photographic lens to its focal length (*f*), usually specified as the fraction *f/n* where *n* is called the *f*-number, the exposure needed being proportional to the square of this number. It is customary to mark the apertures in a series such that the exposure needed is doubled in passing from one to the next, hence the series *f*/1, *f*/1.4, *f*/2, *f*/2.8, *f*/4, etc., to *f*/22.6. **Birth-death ratio.** Vital index; the proportion of births to deaths in a population during a certain period of time, usually one year. **Body-weight ratio.** The weight in grams divided by the height in centimetres. **Cardiothoracic ratio.** The ratio, expressed as a percentage, of the overall diameter of the heart to the maximum transverse diameter of the chest, from the inner surfaces of the ribs, as measured on a teleradiograph of the chest. Normal hearts have ratios less than 50. **Chromosome-arm ratio.** The ratio of the longer to the shorter arm of a chromosome. **Coding ratio.** The number of nucleotide bases in DNA or RNA whose sequence specifies a single amino acid; now known to be three. **Curative ratio.** The ratio of the effective dose to the toxic dose. **D:N ratio, G:N ratio.** The ratio of glucose (dextrose) to nitrogen in the urine of fasting phloridzinized dogs, which forms the basis for calculation of glucose derived from protein in metabolism experiments. The value 3.6 is generally used. **Hand ratio.** The ratio of the length of the hand to its width. **Human blood ratio.** The ratio of the number of mosquitoes (or other blood-sucking insects) that have fed on human blood, to the number that have fed on blood of other species. **Karyoplasmic ratio.** Nucleocytoplasmic ratio (see below). **Lymphocyte-monocyte ratio.** Lymphocyte-monocyte index. *See* INDEX. **Mendelian ratio.** The ratio in which the offspring, or later generations, show the characters of their parents. In the simplest case, the F_2 offspring of parents showing two expressions of an allelomorphic pair of genes will show these expressions in the ratio 3 dominant to 1 recessive. **Monocyte-leucocyte ratio.** Monocyte-leucocyte index. *See* INDEX. **Monocyte-lymphocyte ratio.** The ratio of monocytes to lymphocytes in the circulating blood; it has been used as a measure of tuberculous conditions, improvement being associated with a fall in the number of monocytes and a rise in lymphocytes. **Nucleocytoplasmic ratio, Nucleoplasmic ratio.** The ratio of the volumes of nucleus and cytoplasm within a given cell. **Ocular micrometer ratio.** In microscopy, the value of a unit on the eyepiece micrometer scale expressed in the units of the stage micrometer scale, usually mm. **Oxygen enhancement ratio.** The ratio of isoeffect doses of radiation in oxic and anoxic conditions. **Polymorphonuclear lymphocyte ratio.** Polymorphonuclear lymphocyte index. *See* INDEX. **Sex ratio.** The ratio of males to females, usually expressed as a percentage. *Primary sex ratio* is the ratio of male to female zygotes. *Secondary sex ratio* is the ratio of male to female births. *Tertiary sex ratio* is the ratio of males to females at sexual maturity. **Standardized mortality ratio (SMR).** The ratio of deaths in a defined population to the deaths that would have been expected in that population if each group (usually defined by sex and age) had been exposed to some selected standard rates. **T ratio.** The ratio which a statistical constant has to its standard error. **Therapeutic ratio.** The ratio of the median lethal dose to the median effective dose; the higher the ratio the safer the drug. [L, proportion.]

See also: MCKESSON, MOOTS, POISSON (S. D.), VIETH.

ration (**rash**·un). The set allowance of food and drink apportioned to a man or animal for a given period. **Basal ration.** A ration which provides ample energy but which does not have certain requisite vitamins. [L *ratio* proportion.]

rational (**rash**·un·al). 1. Applied to a person who is in possession of his reasoning faculties, e.g. neither delirious nor comatose; reasonable. 2. Founded on reason; not empirical. 3. Having understanding; sensible. [see foll.]

rationale (rash·un·a·le). 1. A reasoned explanation of principles, e.g. of a hypothesis or an action, 2. The fundamental principle or all the principles involved in carrying out a certain procedure. [L *rationalis* reasonable.]

rationalization (**rash**·un·al·i·**za**'·shun). The provision of a reason to justify an act which is in fact determined by some process other than reason. [see prec.]

ratsbane (**rats**·bane). 1. Any poison used to kill rats, particularly one containing arsenic. 2. White arsenic, arsenic trioxide, As_2O_3, so-called from its use as a rat poison. [rat, AS *bana* murder.]

rattle (ratl). A râle. **Death rattle.** The sound produced in a dying person by air passing through a collection of mucus in the trachea and large bronchi. [ME *ratelen.*]

rattlesnake (**ratl**·snake). A crotaline snake of the New World of the genus *Crotalus.* All the species, which are very poisonous, have the horny epidermal layer of the skin of the tail formed as a "rattle". [rattle, AS *snaca.*]

Rattus (rat·us). A very large genus of rodents, the rats. *Rattus norvegicus,* the brown, common, sewer, Hanoverian, or Norway rat, is now world-wide; introduced to the British Isles in the 18th century, characteristic of temperate areas, though present in tropical ports and towns. *R. rattus,* the old English, black, house, or ship rat, now world-wide, introduced in the Middle Ages, characteristic of warmer areas and ports in temperate areas. It exists in three colour forms, *R. rattus rattus* which is black, and *R. rattus alexandrinus* and *R. rattus frugivorus* which are grey-brown with fawn or white bellies. Both species are important reservoirs of the organisms of plague (*pasteurella pestis*), Weil's disease, rat-bite fever, as well as being of general public health importance. *R. norvegicus* is a reservoir for *Trichinella spiralis.* Wild species in the tropical Far East may be reservoirs of rickettsias. [L rat.]

Rau (Ravius), Johannes Jacobus (b. 1668). Amsterdam anatomist.

Rau's apophysis, or process. The anterior process of the malleus.

Rauber, August Antinous (b. 1841). Dorpat anatomist.

Rauber's layer. The part of the trophoblast in some embryos which disappears to expose the underlying embryonic area.

raucedo, raucetas (raw·se·do, **raw**·sit·as). Hoarseness caused by an inflammatory condition of the mucous membranes of the larynx and pharynx. **Raucedo catarrhalis.** Hoarseness caused by inflammation of the larynx. **Raucedo potatorum.** Hoarseness due to the drinking of whisky or other distilled spirits. **Raucedo syphilitica.** Persisting hoarseness resulting from secondary syphilis of the larynx. [L *raucitas* hoarseness.]

Rauchfuss, Charles Andreyevich (b. 1835). Russian physician.

Rauchfuss' triangle. Grocco's triangle.

rausch (rowsh). Literally, intoxication. **Ether rausch.** Ether intoxication; but also used to denote light ether anaesthesia. [G.]

Rauscher, Frank Joseph (b. 1931). American virologist.

Rauscher virus. A viral agent associated with mouse leukaemia. Like Friend virus it may be a complex of two viruses and may not actually cause the disease. It is RNA-containing and does not affect man.

Rauwolfia Serpentina BPC 1968 (raw·**wol**·fe·ah ser·pen·**te**'·nah). The dried root of *Rauwolfia serpentina* Benth. (family Apocynaceae). It is a sedative and hypnotic widely used in India for insomnia and certain types of insanity. Cases of depression in rauwolfia therapy in hypertension have been reported, and it is advisable to suspend the drug where these symptoms appear. **Rauwolfia Vomitoria BPC 1968.** The dried roots of *Rauwolfia vomitoria* Afz. (family Apocynaceae); it is employed in the production of reserpine. [Leonhard *Rauwolf,* 16th century German botanist.]

Rauzier, Georges (b. 1862). Montpellier physician.

Rauzier's disease. Oedema with cyanosis.

ravius. *See* RAU.

ray (ra). 1. A straight-line beam of electromagnetic radiation such as light or heat. 2. The term has come to be extended to a stream of particles, e.g. helium nuclei, at high velocity and behaving like a radiation. **Abiotic rays.** Ultraviolet rays with wavelengths extending from 290 to 20 nm. **Actinic rays.** Light which promotes chemical action, e.g. decomposition of photographic emulsion, especially the sun's rays rich in ultraviolet frequencies. **Alpha rays.** α-Rays, a stream of positively charged helium nuclei projected from the atom of a radioactive element at high velocity but with low penetration power. **Astral rays.** Cytoplasmic fibrils forming the aster in the metaphase of mitosis. **Beta rays, β-rays.** A stream of negatively-charged beta particles, or electrons, ejected at high velocity from the atoms of disintegrating radioactive elements. **Biotic rays.** Ultraviolet rays with wavelengths extending from 390 to 290 nm. **Border rays, Bordering rays.** Very soft x-rays of low penetration and of wavelength around 0.3 nm; Grenz rays. **Canal rays.** Positive rays (see below), so-called because they were produced by J. J. Thompson in 1910 through a canal drilled in the cathode of a discharge tube. **Cathode rays.** A stream of electrons emitted in a straight line from the surface of the cathode in a discharge tube; impinging on a target they give rise to x-rays. **Characteristic rays.** Secondary rays emitted from a metallic surface bombarded by x-rays. Their wavelength is virtually proportional to the reciprocal of the square of the metal's atomic weight. **Chemical rays.** Actinic rays (see above). **Convergent rays.** Light rays brought to a focus by a convex lens or concave mirror. **Cosmic rays.** A very penetrating radiation of uncertain origin arriving from outer space and detected on Earth by its ionizing effects. It consists of charged particles (protons and electrons) producing mesons in the upper atmosphere which in turn create showers of high-energy electrons and subsequently photons and positrons. **Direct ray.** Primary ray (see below). **Direction ray.** Light ray (see below). **Divergent rays.** Light rays apparently proceeding from a focus after passing through a concave lens or after reflection from a convex mirror. **Extraordinary ray.** *See* NICOL PRISM. **Gamma rays, γ-rays.** The photons of gamma radiation. **Glass rays.** Rays produced at the glass walls of an x-ray tube by the impact of cathode rays. **Grenz rays.** Very soft x-rays of wavelength around 0.3 nm and of low penetration, produced by low-voltage tubes. **H-rays.** A proton beam (obsolete term). **Hard rays.** X-rays of short wavelength (3 pm) and high penetration, produced by high-voltage tubes. **Heat rays.** Radiation of the infrared region of the spectrum, producing the phenomena of radiant heat. **Hertzian rays.** Radio waves; electromagnetic waves produced by an oscillating circuit and demonstrated by Hertz in 1886. They have a wavelength longer than those of the infrared region of the spectrum. **Homocentric rays.** All rays of a pencil converging to or diverging from a point. **I-ray.** A radiation said to emanate from the brain during various thought processes; its existence is very much in doubt. **Incident ray.** A ray of light meeting a surface at a point; the angle between it and the normal to the surface at the point is known as the *angle of incidence.* **Indirect rays.** Glass rays (see above). **Infrared rays.** Electromagnetic radiations of wavelengths greater than those of the visible spectrum but less than those of radio waves. They give rise to the phenomenon of radiant heat. As they have the power of penetrating fog better than visible light rays they have been used in infrared photography. **Intermediate rays.** Rays which are longer than x-rays but shorter than ultraviolet rays. **Light ray.** A straight line drawn to represent the direction of light. A collection of rays is called a beam or pencil. **Luminous rays.** The visible spectrum; light rays having a wavelength longer than the ultraviolet range and shorter than the infrared. **Mitogenetic rays.** Rays said to be produced by dividing cells and having an effect on photographic plates. They are probably not rays but emanations of volatile chemical substances. **Monochromatic ray.** A ray of light composed of radiation of the one wavelength, or as near to it as possible. **N-ray.** A form of wave said to emanate from the ether, and first described by Blondlot. The rays are said to be of shorter wavelength than light rays and to have the property of rendering bodies luminous; they are also said to have the effect of diminishing luminosity. [Obsolete.] **Neutron ray.** A stream of neutrons produced, e.g., by bombarding a beryllium target with deuterons from a cyclotron and collimating the beam. **Ordinary ray.** *See* NICOL PRISM. **Parallel rays.** Light rays from a source which can be considered at infinity, e.g. from the sun. Such rays may be focused at the exact focal point of a concave mirror or a convex lens. **Photographic rays.** Ultraviolet rays, so-called because of their strongly actinic effect on a photographic emulsion. **Polar ray.** Astral ray (see above). **Polarized ray.** *See* NICOL PRISM. **Positive rays.** A stream of positively-charged ions produced by cathode rays in a gas at low pressure and passing, under the influence of the potential, towards the cathode itself. **Primary ray.** Term applied to the x-ray as it emerges from the tube; also the radiation of a radioactive substance. **Reflected ray.** The ray of light reflected from a surface at the point where the incident ray (see above) strikes it; the angle between it and the normal to the surface at the point is known as the *angle of reflection.* **Refracted ray.** The ray entering the second medium after refraction at the surface of junction in the case of light passing obliquely from one to another. The angle between it and the normal to the surface at the point of incidence is known as the *angle of refraction.* **Secondary rays.** A stream of electrons emitted by a metallic surface when x-rays impinge upon it. **Soft rays.** X-rays of long wavelength (about 0.3 nm) and low penetration produced by a tube at a low voltage. **Supersonic rays.** Pressure waves in air or any other medium, similar to sound waves but of frequencies higher than those of audible sound. **Transition rays.** Very soft x-rays, so-called because they lie in the region between x-rays and ultraviolet light. **Ultraviolet rays.** Electromagnetic waves of lengths between those of soft rays and visible light, the longest being just below the wavelength of violet light. They may be reflected, refracted, and polarized like visible light, and will affect a photographic plate, but they are stopped by most media transparent to visible light, e.g. ordinary glass. Sunlight is rich in such rays to which it owes its properties as a bactericide and its ability to produce vitamin D in the skin by irradiation. **Visible light rays.** Light rays of the range of wavelength covered by the visible portion of the spectrum. **W rays.** Grenz rays (see above). **X-rays.** *See* X-RAYS. [L *radius.*]

See also: BECQUEREL, BLONDLOT, BUCKY, FERREIN, FINSEN (N. R.), GOLDSTEIN (E.), GURVICH, LENARD, MILLIKAN, NIEWENGLOWSKI, ROENTGEN, SAGNAC, WOOD (R. W.).

rayage (ra·ij). The dosage of ionizing radiations (obsolete term). [ray.]

Rayer, Pierre François Olive (b. 1793). Paris dermatologist.

Rayer's disease. Xanthoma.

Rayleigh, John William Strutt, Lord (b. 1842). English physicist.

Rayleigh's refractometer. An instrument for measuring the refractive index of a gas by the interference of two beams produced by two narrow slits placed close together.

Raymond, Fulgence (b. 1844). Paris neurologist.

Raymond's syndrome. Ipsilateral 6th cranial nerve paresis with contralateral hemiplegia.

Raymond type of apoplexy. Premonitory paraesthesiae in the hand which is about to be paralysed in an attack of apoplexy.

Cestan–Raymond syndrome, Raymond–Cestan syndrome. Cestan–Chenais syndrome.

Raynaud, Maurice (b. 1834). Paris physician.

Raynaud's disease, or syndrome. Intermittent pallor and cyanosis of the extremities precipitated by a degree of coldness that would not affect a normal person.

Raynaud's phenomenon, or sign. Attacks of pallor and cyanosis of the extremities on exposure to moderate degrees of cold; such attacks are the main features of Raynaud's disease.

Razoxane (raz·ox·ane). BP Commission approved name for 1,2-bis(3,5-dioxopiperazin-1-yl)propane; an antineoplastic agent.

re-. Latin prefix meaning *again.*

reaching (**reech**·ing). The act of straining to vomit; retching. [AS *hraecan* to spit.]

react (re·**akt**). 1. To respond to stimulation. 2. To show chemical activity; to take part in a chemical reaction. [L *re-*, *agere* to act.]

reactance (re·**akt**·ans). A factor in an electric circuit which contributes to its impedance to an alternating current. It is defined as 2π times the self-inductance of the circuit multiplied by the frequency of the current. [see prec.]

reactant (re·**akt**·ant). Any substance which takes part in a chemical reaction to form a new product known as the *product.*

reaction (re·**ak**·shun). 1. Any effect produced by a stimulus. 2. In mechanics, a force set up by and opposing an acting force. 3. In chemistry, the interaction between chemical compounds producing other chemical compounds; the term is often applied to any observable colour change produced by indicators or reagents in chemical analysis. **Abortin reaction.** A diagnostic symptom complex in animals suffering from infection by *Brucella abortus*; marked by loss of appetite, rise in temperature, and diarrhoea, when given an injection of the extract. **Accelerated reaction.** *See* VACCINOID REACTION, 1st def. (below). **Accommodation reaction.** Accommodation reflex. *See* REFLEX. **Accommodation convergence reaction.** Near reflex. *See* REFLEX. **Addition reaction.** Chemical reaction between two compounds which combine to form a new compound. **Affective reaction.** A mental reaction characterized by a primary change in mood towards depression, elation, or, less characteristically, anxiety. **Agglutinoid reaction.** That in which an antiserum fails to agglutinate the homologous bacteria in low dilutions, although it does so in higher dilutions. *See* PROZONE. **Alarm reaction.** The first stage of the response of an animal to a violent stimulation or stress to which it is unadapted. There are, amongst other things, loss of muscle tone, fatigue, and fall in body temperature. **Aldehyde reaction.** *See* ALDEHYDE TEST. **Allergic reaction.** The response of cells to contact with a substance to which they are sensitized or allergic. Basically the reaction comprises in varying measure contraction of unstriped muscle and increased exudate, hence such manifestations as asthma, hay fever, urticaria, diarrhoea, and vomiting, contraction of the colon, etc. **Amphicrotic reaction, Amphoteric reaction.** The reaction of a compound which is capable of behaving as an acid or alkali according to the circumstances. **Analytic reaction.** *See* CHEMICAL REACTION (below). **Anamnestic reaction.** The renewed production of antibody in response to an antigenic stimulus. The term is correctly used if the second stimulating antigen is identical with the original sensitizing antigen. **Anaphylactic reaction.** The hypersensitive condition induced in some animals and humans by parenteral contact with certain antigens. If the initial contact is followed several weeks later by a second contact with the same substance, especially if the second contact is by intravenous injection, there may result severe convulsion, and shock, possibly severe enough to cause death. **Anaphylactoid reaction.** One in which the signs may appear similar to those in anaphylactoid shock. **Anatoxin reaction.** The treatment of diphtheria toxin with formalin, showing its toxicity without affecting its antigenicity. **Anergastic reaction.** A behaviour abnormality dependent on the permanent loss of the brain substance from a disease process or from trauma. **Annihilation reaction.** The reaction between a positive and negative electron in which the particles are annihilated and their energy (including that corresponding to their rest masses) appears in the form of two gamma-ray quanta. **Anserine reaction.** Goose flesh. *See* FLESH. **Antalgesic**

reaction, **Antalgic reaction.** That reaction which is an attempt to avoid pain. **Antigen–antibody reaction.** The reaction of an antigen with its specific antibody to form a complex which *in vitro* may manifest itself by agglutination, precipitation, etc. **Associative reaction.** A reaction depending on associative mental processes. **Axon reaction, Axonal reaction.** Chromatolysis; the series of morphological changes in a nerve cell body following severance of its axon. **Bacteriolytic reaction.** A type of antigen–antibody reaction in which the bacterium (antigen) is lysed by the action of complement and specific antibody, which in this case is known as a *bacteriolysin.* **Biological false positive reaction.** A positive Wassermann reaction that is not due to *Treponema pallidum* or related *Treponema* species, but due to antibodies against antigens present in many body tissues and present in man auto-immune diseases; it may also occur in pregnancy and in some acute and chronic infections. **Biphasic reaction.** A reaction that occurs in two stages, or has two parts. **Biuret reaction.** *See* BIURET TEST. **Blanching reaction.** Schultz–Charlton phenomenon. **Cadaveric reaction.** The complete lack of response to electrical stimulation of affected muscles in familial periodic paralysis. **Caloric vestibular reaction.** The response of the semicircular canals to stimulation with hot and cold water; water at 30 and 44°C is run into each ear in turn for 40 s with the head flexed to 30°. Nystagmus is normally induced for 2 min. **Chain reaction.** A reaction that proceeds in stages, each stage being initiated by the one preceding; uranium fission by neutrons in a nuclear reactor with the production of further neutrons, and so on, is an example. **Chemical reaction.** *See* MAIN DEF. 3 (above). **Cholera reaction, Cholera-red reaction.** A test dependent on the production of indole and nitrites in peptone water. Four to eight drops of pure sulphuric acid are added to a 24-h vibrio culture in peptone broth. The reaction is positive, indicated by the development of a pink coloration, with cultures of vibrios of group A (Heiberg) which include the true cholera vibrios. The reaction is of value for screening, but is not specific. **Citochol reaction.** *See* LENTOCHOL REACTION (below). **Complement fixation reaction.** The demonstration of a positive antigen–antibody reaction by the removal of added complement. The removal of complement is then demonstrated by the inability of the solution to lyse sensitized red cells. **Conglutination reaction.** A modified agglutination test in which higher specificity is obtained by first removing the agglutinins from the specific immune sera, which is then allowed to react with fresh complement and the bacteria together with a protein isolated from seeds of leguminous plants. **Consensual reaction.** A consensual reflex; commonly applied to contraction of the pupil on stimulation of the contralateral retina. **Consensual light reaction.** The contraction of the pupil of one eye when its fellow is exposed to a light stimulus. **Constitutional reaction.** A generalized reaction, one that is neither focal nor local. **Convergence reaction.** Convergence reflex. *See* REFLEX. **Coupled reactions.** Reactions that are linked together. **Cross reaction.** An antigen–antibody reaction which takes place between an antibody and antigenic material of a type other than that used to stimulate the production of the antibody, e.g. agglutination of bacteria by serum prepared against a related species. **Cutaneous reaction.** 1. A local reaction to an antigen that is applied to or injected into the skin. It is usually a manifestation of either allergy (hypersensitivity), e.g. to pollens, or insufficiency of circulating antitoxin, as in positive Schick or Dick tests. 2. A reaction to a scratch test, e.g. the Pirquet test for tuberculin sensitivity. This usage differentiates it from a tuberculin intradermal test (Mantoux), and from a percutaneous test (Moro). **Cutituberculin reaction.** Moro's reaction. **Decidual reaction.** A change occurring in the endometrium in early pregnancy, to facilitate the embedding and nourishment of the fertilized ovum; a similar change may be seen on the surface of the ovaries and in the cervix. The hormone progesterone is thought to play an important part in producing this reaction. **Defence reaction.** A mental response in defence of the psyche. **Degeneration reaction.** The reaction of muscle to electrical stimulation after degeneration of its motor nerve. At such a time it is usually inexcitable to a brief faradic shock. **Delayed reaction.** One in which the reaction reaches its fastigium after a considerable interval. (Cf. EARLY REACTION, below.) **Desmoplastic reaction.** The formation of fibrous tissue in response to an irritant. **Diazo reaction.** A specific reaction of primary aromatic amines in which a diazo salt is formed by the action of cold nitrous acid upon the amine in dilute mineral acid solution. This salt may be coupled in alkaline solution with a phenol or another amine to give an azo dye. *See also* EHRLICH'S DIAZO REACTION. **Disergastic reaction.** A behaviour abnormality directly dependent on a disorder of the brain through poor support of its functioning from toxic, infectious, metabolic, and traumatic causes. **Distant reaction.** A localized reaction that occurs at some distance from the point of application of the excitant. **Early reaction.** A reaction that reaches fastigium within a very short time, minutes or hours, as opposed to a delayed reaction that may take some days to appear; not infrequently the same excitant will cause both an early and delayed reaction. **Electric reaction.** That reaction which occurs in response to an electrical stimulation. **Electrotonic reaction.** A fall of blood pressure and dilatation of the splanchnic blood vessels following stimulation of the depressor nerve. **Endothermal reaction, Endothermic reaction.** Any chemical reaction in which heat is absorbed. **Energonic reaction.** Any chemical reaction which absorbs energy. **Epidermotropic reaction.** A reaction to infection or other stimulus that occurs in the epidermal tissues only. **Erythraematoid reaction.** Erythrocytosis or increase in the number of red blood corpuscles in the circulating blood, usually from stimulation of the bone marrow. **Exergonic reaction.** Any chemical reaction which liberates energy. **Reaction of exhaustion.** The change produced in living tissues by exhaustion, whereby the threshold to electrical stimulation is raised. **Exothermal reaction, Exothermic reaction.** Any chemical reaction in which heat is liberated. **False-negative reaction.** A negative reaction that does not indicate the true state of affairs, e.g. through non-specificity of the test, or a fault in technique. Cf. FALSE-POSITIVE REACTION (foll.). **False-positive reaction.** A positive reaction that does not indicate the true state of affairs. Cf. FALSE-NEGATIVE REACTION (prec.). **Flaginac reaction.** A series of tests used to show the presence of *Bacterium coli* in water: fluorescein in glucose neutral broth—*FL*, acid and gas production in lactose medium—*AG*, positive indole production—*IN*, and production of acid and clotting in milk—*AC*. **Focal reaction.** A reaction that occurs at the focus of infection, or at the site of a previous injection. **Fuchsinophil reaction.** Having an affinity for acid fuchsine which is not removed by picric acid. **Furfural reaction.** The production of a bright-red colour when furfural comes into contact with aniline acetate. The reaction is used as a test for laevulose, furfural being one of the products of decomposition by boiling with acid. **Guaiacum reaction.** *See* GUAIACUM TEST. **Haemolytic reaction.** A severe haemolytic destruction of red blood corpuscles as occurs in acute haemolytic anaemias. **Hemianopic pupillary reaction.** That found in certain cases of homonymous hemianopia when the lesion is situated in the region of the optic tract; the pupils of both eyes fail to react to a thin beam of light projected from the blind side. They react normally to a light from the opposite side. Described by Wernicke. **Hyperthymergastic reaction.** Hyperthymergasia. **Hypothymergastic reaction.** Hypothymergasia. **Immune reaction.** The slight local reaction, without pustule formation, following the inoculation of smallpox lymph into an immune person. **Indirect-light reaction.** Consensual-light reaction (see above). **Intracutaneous reaction.** A local reaction obtained in non-immune people following an intradermal injection of a minute amount of specific toxin, e.g. diphtheria toxin in the Schick test. **Intracuti reaction.** Intracutaneous reaction, especially applied to the Frei test. **Irreversible reaction.** A chemical reaction which, once started, must proceed to its end in one direction only; usually by reason of the removal by precipitation or volatilization of one or more of the products. **K.H. reaction.** A combined complement fixation and haemagglutination reaction useful in the diagnosis of glanders in mules, asses, and pregnant mares, the blood of which may be anticomplementary. **Lentochol reaction.** Name given to one of two procedures for carrying out the Sachs-Georgi precipitation test for syphilis. Cholesterolized alcoholic extract of human or bullock heart, a solution of normal saline, and the patient's serum are used; positive serum gives a flocculent precipitate. The *lentochol reaction* is a slow reaction, whilst the *citochol reaction,* in which a more concentrated extract of heart is used, is rapid. Many modifications of the test are now in common use. **Lepra reaction.** An acute febrile condition which occurs in lepromatous leprosy, with high pyrexia due to the rapid multiplication of the specific bacilli and their dissemination throughout the reticulo-endothelial system. It is an ineffective defence reaction against the invading bacilli. **Leucocytic reaction.** An increase or diminution in the number of leucocytes in the circulating blood under the influence of various toxic agents, drugs, and medicines. **Leukaemic reaction, Leukaemoid reaction.** Changes in the circulating blood in which there appear immature white blood corpuscles in varying stages of immaturity producing a blood picture closely resembling leukaemia. **Light reaction.** Direct-light reflex. *See* REFLEX. **Lignin reaction.** The red colour given by lignin with phloroglucin and concentrated hydrochloric acid. **Local reaction.** A reaction that occurs at the site of injection. Cf. FOCAL REACTION (above). **Longitudinal reaction.** The displacement, due to degeneration of motor nerves, of the cutaneous points for electrical stimulation of muscle. **Luetin reaction.** Noguchi's luetin reaction; the appearance of a red papule following the intradermal injection of an extract (luetin) of killed cultures of several strains of *Treponema pallidum.* **Lymphatic reaction.** 1. Glandular fever; infectious mononucleosis. 2. A reaction occurring in lymphatism or status lymphaticus, in which all the lymphatic tissues are in excess. An unsatisfactory term to be avoided. **Magnetic reaction.** Extension of the leg induced reflexly by pressure on the sole of the foot. **Mitsuda reaction.** A specific test for the actual or potential capacity of the body to put up a successful defence against leprosy. It consists in observing the skin reaction to the injection of lepromin; a positive reaction, read about the 30th day after injection, is indicative of leprosy. The test is analogous to the Mantoux test in tuberculosis, and can be positive only in the presence of a primary focus. **Moccasin-venom reaction.** A skin test (Peck, Rosenthal, and Erf) for the determination of abnormal capillary-vessel fragility; the test consists in the intradermal injection of 0.1 ml of a standard (1 unit) moccasin-snake-venom solution (1:3000) which is compared with a control intradermal injection of normal saline (0.1 ml) after one hour; a haemorrhagic area greater than 1 cm diameter at the site of the venom injection indicates abnormally fragile capillaries and is positive in thrombocytopenic purpura and purpura secondary to benzene poisoning, aplastic anaemia, leukaemia, and subacute bacterial endocarditis. The test is also used for prognosis, which is considered to be good if a positive becomes a negative reaction. **Mouse-tail reaction.** 1. Straub-Herrman reaction; the raising and stiffening of the mouse tail produced by an analgesic drug such as morphine, due to a spasm of the anal sphincter. 2. The reaction of the mouse tail to an applied heat or electrical stimulus which is used in evaluating analgesic drugs. **Myasthenic reaction.** On applying repeated electrical stimulation to a myasthenic muscle the induced contraction steadily decreases in strength and duration, and complete exhaustion appears much more quickly than in normal muscle. **Myotonic reaction.** Erb's reaction; a prolonged contraction with slow relaxation when a muscle is stimulated electrically with a galvanic or faradic current. **Myotonic pupillary reaction.** A delayed and slow contraction of the pupil of the eye both to light and convergence followed by a delayed dilatation. It is usually unilateral and is found commonly in young women, often associated with loss of tendon reflexes and known as *Adie's syndrome.* **(n, α) reaction.** A nuclear reaction in which a neutron enters the nucleus and an α-particle is emitted. **(n,γ) reaction.** A nuclear reaction in which a neutron enters the nucleus of an atom to form an isotope of one higher atomic weight, surplus energy being emitted as a γ-ray. **(n, p) reaction.** A nuclear reaction in which a neutron enters the nucleus and a proton is emitted. **Nadi reaction.** Indophenol test. *See* TEST. **Neurotonic reaction.** Persistence of the effect (muscular contraction) of stimulation after the stimulus has ceased. **Neurotonic pupillary reaction.** A delayed and slow contraction of the pupil of the eye to light, followed by delayed dilatation. **Ninhydrin reaction.** The production of a blue colour by proteins and all amino acids, except proline and hydroxyproline, upon boiling with ninhydrin. **Nitritoid reaction.** Nitritoid crisis. *See* CRISIS. **Nuclear reaction.** A physical process occurring within the atomic nucleus. **Oxidase reaction.** The demonstration of oxidase enzymes in leucocytes by means of alphanaphthol and dimethylparaphenylenediamine. **Pain reaction.** Dilatation of the pupil when pain is felt. **Panblastotropic reaction.** One that occurs in the tissues of all three embryonic layers. **Paradoxical pupillary reaction.** Three phenomena have been described under this name: 1. The mydriatic action of adrenaline on the denervated iris. 2. Dilatation of the pupil in response to light. 3. Dilatation of the pupil in response to pain in the contralateral leg. **Parallergic reaction.** An allergic state towards one specific substance predisposes to sensitiveness to other allergens which may have different kinds of reaction. **Paternity reaction.** Paternity test. *See* TEST. **Percutaneous reaction.** The reaction produced by the application of a reagent, e.g. tuberculin, in ointment form. The advantage of the method is that the needle-prick is obviated. The disadvantage is variable absorption in successive tests. *See* MORO'S REACTION. **Periodic acid-Schiff reaction.** A histochemical reaction in which sections are treated with periodic acid to oxidize 1,2-glycol groups to dialdehydes which are then identified by treatment with Schiff's reagent. The method is used to study mucosubstances and is useful for staining basement membranes. **Ponceau-fuchsine reaction.** In cases of virilism of adrenal origin the cortical cells contain granules which stain a vivid red with a ponceau-fuchsine stain. **Precipitin reaction.** The demonstration of antigen-antibody combination by formation of a precipitate of the complex. **Protein-tyrosine reaction.** Devised by Proske and Watson: a simple colorimetric test based on the fact that proteins possess chromogenic properties which can be measured quantitively against the colour produced by pure tyrosine in the presence of a phenol reagent. The chromogenic value is constant for a given protein and the intensity of colour produced is an indication of the amount of protein present. The test is non-specific, but its high sensitivity in malaria has given rise to claims that it is a useful adjunct to the laboratory diagnosis of this disease. **Psychogalvanic reaction.** The change in electrical resistance of the skin following on emotional activity. **Quellung (G swelling) reaction.** A term used by Neufeld to describe the swelling of the pneumococcus capsule when specific antibody is added to material (sputum, culture) containing the pneumococcus. The apparent swelling is due to the deposition of antibody around the capsule, making it more visible. **Radiation reaction.** Response of tissues or patient to the effects of radiation. **Rash extinction reaction.** Schultz-Charlton phenomenon. **Recurrent reaction.** The reappearance or exacerbation (revivescence) of a positive tuberculin reaction in response to a subcutaneous injection of tuberculin. **Reversible reaction.** A chemical reaction that may proceed in either direction according to circumstances, the products of the reaction combining to reform the original substances. **Rosindole reaction.** A test for indole production in peptone water by *Bacterium coli*: after 2 days' growth, 1 ml of ether is added to the culture and the mixture shaken. After separation, 0.5 ml of Ehrlich's reagent is added and the solution gently agitated. A rose colour appears in the ether layer if indole is present. **Serum-formalin reaction.** Aldehyde test. *See* TEST. **Specific reaction.** An antigen-antibody reaction which takes place only with the type of antigen used to stimulate the production of the antibody. **Tendon reaction.** The tendon reflex. **Toxin-antitoxin reaction.** A manifestation of the antigen-antibody reaction in which the antigen is toxic; this is usually demonstrated by precipitation *in vitro.* **Transfer reaction.** A delayed cutaneous inflammatory reaction obtained when sensitized lymphocytes from the recipient of a skin graft are injected into the graft donor; a graft-versus-host reaction. **Transfusion reaction.** A reaction following transfusion, due to incompatibility or other causes. **Traumatic reaction.** The psychological reaction to a traumatic mental experience. **Uniphasic reaction.** A reaction occurring in one stage only. **Vaccinoid reaction.** 1. A reaction to smallpox vaccination, which is associated with partial immunity: all the stages (papule, vesicle, pustule) are of shorter duration (*accelerated reaction*), and milder than in the typical primary reaction. 2. Any reaction resembling vaccinia. **Vestibular pupillary reaction.** Dilatation of the pupil induced by stimulation of the semicircular canals. **White graft reaction.** Very rapid rejection of a skin graft before it becomes vascularized in an animal highly immune to the antigens of the graft. **Xanthoproteic reaction.** Xanthoproteic test. *See* TEST. **Xanthydrol reaction.** The precipitation of xanthydrol crystals from an acetic acid solution of xanthydrol by tissues combining urea, as in uraemia. [L *re-*, *agere* to act.]

See also: ADAMKIEWICZ, ALLWORDEN, APELT, ARTHUS, AVERY, BECHTEREW, BEIJERINCK, BENCE-JONES, BERGH, BITTORF, BORCHARDT, BRIEGER, BRODIE (T. G.), BUNNELL (W. W.), CALMETTE, CANNIZZARO, CHANTEMESSE, CHARLTON, CUSHING (HARVEY W.), DALE, DICK, DOCHEZ, EHRLICH, ERB, FELIX, FEULGEN, FICKER, GHILARDUCCI, GMELIN, GRAEFE, GRIGNARD, GRUBER (M.), GRÜNBAUM, HENLE, HENRY (A. F. G.), HERXHEIMER, HOFMANN (H.), HOLZMANN, JAFFÉ (M.), JARISCH, JOLLY (F.), KOCH (R.), KRAUSS, KUESTNER (H.), LEWIS (T.), LIEBERMANN-BURCHARD, LOEWI, LOHMANN, MACHADO-GUERREIRO, MANOILOFF, MARCHI, MIDDLEBROOK, MILIAN, MILLON, MOELLER (A.), MOLISCH, MOLONEY, MOOSER, MORO, MUCH, NAGLER, NEILL (M. H.), NEUFELD, NOGUCHI, NONNE, PAGANO, PAUL (J. R.), PETTENKOFER, PFEIFFER (R. F. J.), PILCZ (A.), PIRQUET, PRAUSNITZ, PRICE (I. N. O.), PROSKAUER, RIVALTA (F.), RUBINO, RUMPF, RUSSO, RUTTIN, SAENGER (A.), SCHARDINGER, SCHICK, SCHULTZ, SCHWARTZMANN, SELIVANOFF, SNELLING, SOLERA, TOURNAY, TRAMBUSTI, VITALI, VOGES, VOISENET-RHODE, VULPIAN, WASSERMANN, WEIDEL, WEIL (E.), WERNICKE (K.), WESTPHAL (A. K. O.), WIDAL, WILDBOLZ.

reactivate (re·ak·tiv·ate). To make active again; particularly applied to an old or heated serum to which fresh complement is added. [see foll.]

reactivation (re·ak·tiv·a′·shun). The rendering of anything active again. **Multiplicity reactivation.** *See* VIRUS REACTIVATION (below). **Reactivation of serum.** The restoration of immune activity to serum by the addition of fresh complement. **Virus reactivation.** A latent virus may be stimulated to produce complete infectious virus by reactivating procedures such as ultraviolet light or cell fusion. Incomplete or defective virus particles may be rescued by other virions whose defect lies elsewhere in the viral genome (*multiplicity reactivation*). [L *re-*, activity.]

reactivity (re·ak·tiv·it·e). Of any medium, the intrinsic power of reaction. [see prec.]

reactor (re·**ak**·tor). 1. An electric circuit element which stores energy. 2. A nuclear reactor (see below). **Nuclear reactor.** A large and complex installation for the production of controlled nuclear fission, used as a source of energy as in electrical power stations. Its medical importance is as a source of radionuclides and, to a lesser extent, as a source of neutrons and of other radiation for radiotherapy. [L *re-*, *agere* to act.]

reagent (re·a·jent). Any compound taking part in a chemical reaction. The term has come to be applied in particular to any chemical compound or mixture of compounds, usually in solution, employed in chemical analysis or for the detection of biological constituents. **Acid-molybdate reagent.** For phosphates: dissolve 16 g of ammonium molybdate in a mixture of 100 ml of 0.88 ammonia and 100 ml of water. Allow to stand until clear, filter, and pour into 800 ml of concentrated nitric acid. **Arsenophosphotungstic acid reagent** (Benedict). For uric acid: dissolve 100 g of sodium tungstate in 600 ml of water, add 50 g of arsenic pentoxide and 25 ml of 85% phosphoric acid and then 20 ml of concentrated hydrochloric acid. Boil for 20 min, cool, and make up to 1 l with water. **Benzidine reagent.** For the detection of blood: mix 2 ml of a 3% solution of benzidine in cold glacial acetic acid with 1 ml of 10 volume (3%) hydrogen peroxide. **Biuret reagent.** For proteins. *Gies*: 10% potassium hydroxide solution, 1 l; 3% copper sulphate solution, 25 ml. *Welker*: to 40% sodium hydroxide solution add 1% copper sulphate solution drop by drop with stirring until the solution is a deep blue colour. **Diazo reagent.** For van den Bergh reaction: A. Dissolve 1 g of sulphanilic acid in 250 ml of M/10 hydrochloric acid and dilute to 1 l with water. B. Dissolve 0.5 g of sodium nitrite in 100 ml of water. For use, add 0.3 ml of B to 10 ml of A. For Ehrlich's diazo reaction: A. Dissolve 5 g of sodium nitrite in 1 l of distilled water. B. Dissolve 5 g of sulphanilic acid in 50 ml of hydrochloric acid and 1 l of water. For use, mix 1 of A with 50 or 100 of B. **Dinitrosalicylic acid reagent.** For glucose in urine: to 10 g of crystallized phenol add 22 ml of 10% sodium hydroxide, dissolve in a little water and dilute to 100 ml. To 6.9 g of sodium bisulphite add 69 ml of the alkaline phenol solution and then 300 ml of 4.5% sodium hydroxide solution, 255 g of sodium potassium tartrate, and 880 ml of 1% dinitrosalicylic acid. **Formalin-sulphuric acid reagent.** For the detection of opium alkaloids, apomorphine, and diamorphine: 1 volume of formalin mixed with 5 volumes of concentrated sulphuric acid. **General reagent.** Any reagent employed in chemical analysis to determine the general class to which a substance belongs. **Group reagent.** A reagent employed in systematic qualitative analysis to determine the group to which a compound belongs. **Nadi reagent.** For oxidases. 1. 1% β-naphthol in 95% alcohol. 2. 1% aqueous *p*-phenylenediamine hydrochloride. Add equal volumes of the reagents to the test solution. **Percutaneous reagent.** An ointment composed of equal parts of old tuberculin and lanolin used as a tuberculin test, especially in children. **Special reagent.** Any reagent employed to identify a particular substance in chemical analysis, as distinct from a general reagent (see above). **Thiocyanogen reagent.** A special reagent containing thiocyanogen, used in the assay of fats to determine the thiocyanogen value. **Uric acid reagent** (Folin 1934). To 100 g of molybdate-free sodium tungstate add slowly, with mixing, 30 ml of syrupy phosphoric acid in 150 ml of water. Boil gently for one hour under a reflux, decolorize with a drop of bromine, boil to expel excess of bromine, cool and dilute with water to 500 ml. [L *re-*, *agere* to act.]

See also: ALMÉN, BACH, BARFOED, BERTRAND, BIAL, BLACK (O. F.), COOMBS, CROSS, DENIGÈS, DRAGENDORFF, EHRLICH, ESBACH, EXTON, FEHLING, FLORENCE, FOLIN, FOUCHET, FROEHDE, GIES, GRIGNARD, GUENZBERG, ILOSVAY, KASTLE, MAYER (F. F.), MILLON, MOERNER, MORO, NESSLER, NYLANDER, OBERMAYER, ROBERTS (W.), SAHLI, SALKOWSKI, SCHEIBLER, SCHIFF (H.), SCHWEITZER, SONNENSCHEIN, STOKES (W. R.), SULKOWITCH, SUMNER, TAKATA, TAKAYAMA, TANRET, TOEPFER, TRIBOULET, UFFELMANN, WELKER, WINKLER (A. C.), WU.

reagin (re·a·jin). 1. A term used by some writers to cover the antibody-like substances responsible for allergic phenomena. 2. Part of the gamma-globulin fraction of serum. **Atopic reagin.** Antibodies present in the serum of naturally hypersensitive persons, which can produce passive hypersensitivity when injected into normal subjects. [see prec.]

realgar (re·al·gar). A natural form of arsenic disulphide, As_2S_2, found as a red mineral, and one of the sources of arsenic. [Ar. *rahj al-ghar* powder of the mine.]

reamer (reem·er). A small instrument used in dentistry for enlarging the size of the root canal of a tooth. [AS *ryman* to make room.]

reamination (re·am·in·a′·shun). The restoration of an amino group to a compound which has already undergone deamination. [L *re-*, amino.]

reamputation (re·am·pew·ta′·shun). Amputation performed on a part or limb which has previously undergone amputation. [L *re-*, amputate.]

reanimate (re·an·im·ate). 1. To revive. 2. To reinvigorate. [L *re-*, *animus* mind.]

rearrangement (re·ar·a·nj·ment). In cytogenetics, a chromosome structural change; this may occur within the same chromosome (intrachange) and involve only one arm (intraradial or intrabrachial) or both arms (extraradial or heterobrachial). The rearrangement may also occur between two or more chromosomes (interchange); this may involve homologous or non-homologous chromosomes and may or may not be unbalanced, thus leading or not to duplication and/or deficiency. [L *re-*, OFr. *à* to, *rangier* rank.]

reattachment (re·at·**ach**·ment). The process whereby the fibres of the periodontal membrane are reattached to the alveolar bone and to the cementum of a tooth which has become loosened or has been replanted. [L *re-*, OFr. *attachier.*]

Réaumur, René Antoine Ferchault (b. 1683). French natural philosopher.

Réaumur scale and thermometer. A thermometer calibrated on the Réamur scale, a scale of temperature having the melting point of ice at 0°R, and the boiling point of water at 80°R. Obsolete.

rebasing (re·**ba**·sing). The process of remodelling the fitting surface of an artificial denture to secure perfect adaptation to the tissues of the mouth. [L *re-*, Gk *basis* base.]

rebound (re·bownd). The renewal of reflex activity after the stimulus which evoked the original action has been removed. [OFr. *rebondir.*]

rebreathing (re·**bre**·thing). In anaesthetic administration, the partial or total breathing-in by a patient of his expired gases and vapours. The method conserves and concentrates the agents used and conserves the patient's heat and water vapour. If the method is total, then the oxygen naturally used up must be replaced and the carbon dioxide produced, removed. [L *re-*, breath.]

recalcification (re·kal·sif·ik·a'·shun). The replacement of lost calcium salts in the tissues of the body. [L *re-*, calcium, L *facere* to make.]

recapitulation (re·kap·it·ew·**la**'·shun). The occurrence in ontogenesis of characters or stages which are characteristic of the adults of ancestral forms, e.g. a developing bird or mammal shows traces of gill slits which are present in adult fish. Such characters are not in fact like those of the adult of the ancestor but like its embryo. [L *re-*, *capitulum* small head.]

receiver (re·se·ver). 1. A receptacle for the collection of a gas or the products of a distillation. 2. The jar in an air pump in which the vacuum is created. 3. A menstrual pad or napkin. **Manchester receiver.** A small metal trough with a handle; the edge opposite the handle is shaped concavely to fit the curve of the cheek, so that it can be applied closely under the eye to catch the fluid during irrigation. [L *recipere* to receive.]

receptacular (re·sep·**tak**·ew·lar). Of the nature of or relating to a receptaculum.

receptaculum (re·sep·**tak**·ew·lum) (pl. *receptacula*). A receptacle. **Receptaculum chyli.** The cisterna chyli, or Pecquet's cistern; the dilatation at the beginning of the thoracic duct anterior to the bodies of the 1st and 2nd lumbar vertebrae. **Receptacula lactis.** The dilatations of the ducts of the mammary gland near their openings on the nipple; the lactiferous sinuses. **Receptaculum seminis.** The seminal vesicle. *See* VESICLE. [L.]

receptive (re·**sep**·tiv). Of the mind, having the ability to receive, take in, and absorb ideas or impressions. [see foll.]

receptor (re·**sep**·tor). 1. A specialized sensory nerve-ending, often of characteristic structure, by which stimuli are transmuted into nerve impulses. 2. The name commonly applied to the molecular groupings on cell surfaces which react with hormones and drugs and through which their effects on cells are initiated. Such combination has been detected by the binding of radioactively labelled molecules to cell membrane preparations. 3. A postulate of the Ehrlich side-chain theory, now obsolete, e.g. free receptor, sessile receptor, receptor of the first order, etc. **Contact receptor.** A receptor appreciating contact with the stimulating source, e.g. touch. **Distance receptor.** A receptor which appreciates stimuli from a distant source, e.g. of light or sound. **Gustatory receptor.** A taste receptor, located in the taste buds. **Pressure receptor.** 1. A receptor responding to the stimulus of pressure, e.g. in the skin. 2. A receptor responding to internal pressure changes, e.g. in the vascular system, as in aortic receptors. They really respond to stretching of the walls and should be classed as stretch receptors. Often called *pressoreceptor* or *baroceptor.* **Stretch receptors.** Receptors which are stimulated by stretching, e.g. the muscle spindles. **Tension receptor.** A sensory nerve-ending specialized to respond to a change of tension in the tissue in which it is situated. **Visual receptors.** The percipient end-organs of the retina, i.e. the rods and cones. [L *recipere* to receive.]

recess [recessus (NA)] (re·**ses**, **re**·ses). A depression or fossa. **Aortic recess.** A space enclosed by the reflection of the parietal layer of the serous pericardium on to the ascending aorta. **Attic recess.** Epitympanic recess (see below). **Auditory recess.** Auditory pit, a depression on the side of the head of an embryo at the site of invagination of the auditory placode to form the auditory vesicle. **Cochlear recess.** Recess of the vestibule, cochlear (see below). **Costodiaphragmatic recess [recessus costodiaphragmaticus (NA)].** A recess between the costal and diaphragmatic pleurae, about 5 cm in vertical extent. **Costomediastinal recess [recessus costomediastinalis (NA)].** A recess anteriorly placed between the costal and mediastinal pleurae. **Duodenal recess, inferior [recessus duodenalis inferior (NA)].** A peritoneal pocket to the left of the third part of the duodenum and opening upwards. It lies behind a peritoneal fold running from the duodenum to the peritoneum of the posterior abdominal wall. **Duodenal recess, superior [recessus duodenalis superior (NA)].** A small peritoneal pocket to the left of the third part of the duodenum and opening downwards, lying behind a peritoneal fold running from the duodenum to the parietal peritoneum of the posterior abdominal wall. **Elliptical recess.** Recess of the vestibule, elliptical (see below). **Epitympanic recess [recessus epitympanicus (NA)].** The portion of the tympanic cavity lying above the level of the tympanic membrane. It contains most of the incus and the upper half of the malleus. The cupolar part [pars cupularis (NA)] constitutes the superior portion. **Recess of the fourth ventricle, lateral [recessus lateralis ventriculi quarti (NA)].** A long, narrow prolongation from the widest part of the ventricle curving around the dorsum of the inferior cerebellar peduncle. **Hepatorenal recess [recessus hepatorenalis (NA)].** A pouch of peritoneum lying behind and below the right lobe of the liver and in front of the right suprarenal gland, upper part of the right kidney, second part of the duodenum, the hepatic flexure of the colon, the transverse mesocolon, and the head of the pancreas. It is bounded above by the inferior layer of the coronary ligament and the right triangular ligament. Also known as *Morison's pouch.* **Ileocaecal recess, inferior [recessus ileocaecalis inferior (NA)].** A peritoneal recess with its mouth directed downwards and to the left. It lies between the ileocaecal fold (bloodless fold of Treves) and the mesentery of the vermiform appendix. **Ileocaecal recess, superior [recessus ileocaecalis superior (NA)].** A peritoneal diverticulum between the vascular fold of the caecum, and the mesentery of the terminal ileum. Its mouth is directed downwards and to the left. **Infundibular recess.** Recess of the third ventricle, infundibular (see below). **Recess of the lesser sac of the peritoneum, lower [recessus inferior omentalis (NA)].** An inferiorly placed diverticulum between the stomach and the pancreas. **Recess of the lesser sac of the peritoneum, upper [recessus superior omentalis (NA)].** A superiorly directed diverticulum lying between the caudate lobe of the liver and the diaphragm. **Lienal recess [recessus lienalis (NA)].** That part of the omental bursa which extends into the dorsal mesogastrium and is bounded on the left by the gastrosplenic and lienorenal ligaments. **Optic recess.** Recess of the third ventricle, optic (see below). **Paraduodenal recess [recessus paraduodenalis (NA)].** A peritoneal pocket open to the right, lying behind the termination of the inferior mesenteric vein. **Recess of the pelvic mesocolon [recessus intersigmoideus (NA)].** A small diverticulum of peritoneum with its mouth directed downwards and to the left, and lying at the apex of the angulated attachment of the pelvic mesocolon. The left ureter lies behind it. **Recess of the pharynx [recessus pharyngeus (NA)].** The lateral extension of the pharynx behind the tubal elevation; recess of Rosenmueller. **Pineal recess.** Recess of the third ventricle, pineal (see below). **Recesses of the pleura [recessi pleurales (NA)].** Slit-like extensions at the periphery of the pleural cavities into which the lungs extend only in forced inspiration. **Pneumato-enteric recess.** The upper recess of the lower sac of the embryonic peritoneal cavity. **Retrocaecal recess [recessus retrocaecalis (NA)].** A wide-mouthed peritoneal pocket between the caecum and the peritoneum of the iliac fossa. **Retroduodenal recess [recessus retroduodenalis (NA)].** A small pocket of peritoneum passing behind the fourth part of the duodenum from its left margin. **Spheno-ethmoidal recess [recessus spheno-ethmoidalis (NA)].** A narrow interval, bounded above by the cribriform plate of the ethmoid and the body of the sphenoid and below by the superior nasal concha, into which opens the sphenoidal air sinus. **Spherical recess.** Recess of the vestibule, spherical (see below). **Subhepatic recess [recessus subhepatici (NA)].** The lower part of the supracolic division of the peritoneal cavity. It lies between the liver and the upper surface of the transverse mesocolon. **Subphrenic recess [recessus subphrenici (NA)].** The recess between the diaphragm and the upper surface of the right lobe of the liver. It is limited behind by the right triangular ligament. **Suprapineal recess.** Recess of the third ventricle, suprapineal (see below). **Recess of the third ventricle, infundibular [recessus infundibuli (NA)].** A recess into the base of the infundibulum of the hypophysis. **Recess of the third ventricle, optic [recessus opticus (NA)].** A prolongation of the cavity of the ventricle into the interval between the commencing optic tracts. **Recess of the third ventricle, pineal [recessus pinealis (NA)].** A recess into the stalk of the pineal body. **Recess of the third ventricle, suprapineal [recessus suprapinealis (NA)].** A recess of the ependymal roof passing backwards above the stalk of the pineal body. **Triangular recess.** An occasionally occurring evagination of the lamina terminalis of the 3rd ventricle between the anterior commissure and the anterior pillars of the fauces. **Recesses of the tympanic membrane.** Anterior, posterior, and superior recesses formed by the folding of the mucous membrane on the internal surface of the tympanic membrane. **Recess of the vestibule, cochlear [recessus cochlearis (NA)].** A recess in the lower part of the vestibule, lodging the base of the cochlea. **Recess of the vestibule, elliptical [recessus ellipticus (NA)].** A recess in the posterior part of the vestibule, lodging the utricle. **Recess of the vestibule, spherical [recessus sphericus (NA)].** A recess in the anterior part of the vestibule, lodging the saccule. [L *recedere* to retreat.]

See also: ARLT, HYRTL, JACQUEMET, KUHNT, REICHERT (K. B.), ROSENMUELLER, TARIN, TROELTSCH.

recession (re·**sesh**·un). 1. The act of drawing back. 2. In dentistry, the condition in which the supporting tissues recede and expose the roots of the teeth. **Systolic recession.** Recession or retraction of the left lower ribs and intercostal spaces in the axillary region and left posterior chest wall during ventricular systole, due to adhesions between the heart and the diaphragm as the result of adhesive pericarditis (adherent pericardium). It was first described by Broadbent in 1895, and the sign should not be confused with recession or retraction of the anterolateral chest wall, subcostal angle, or epigastrium, which may occur when the heart is greatly enlarged in the absence of pericardial adhesions. [see foll.]

recessive (re·**ses**·iv). 1. A gene which will only produce its characters when present in a homozygous state. The converse of dominant. 2. By extension, the organism or character itself. **Double recessive.** An organism which is homozygous for a recessive gene, so that it shows the characters of that gene. **Partial recessive.** A gene whose ability to produce its characters is only partly eliminated by the presence of its dominant. [L *recedere* to retreat.]

recessus [NA] (re·**ses**·us). A recess. **Recessus sacciformis [NA].** The synovial pouch projecting upwards in front of the lower end of the interosseous membrane from the main cavity of the inferior radio-ulnar joint. [see prec.]

rechloridation (re·klor·id·**a**′·shun). The giving of chlorides, e.g. by adding table salt to the drinking water. [L *re-*, chloride.]

recidivation (re·sid·iv·**a**′·shun). Of a disease, a relapse; also applied to relapses by criminals. [see foll.]

recidivism (re·**sid**·iv·izm). Tendency to relapse into bad behaviour. [L *recidivus* falling back.]

recidivist (re·**sid**·iv·ist). 1. Any patient who when ill is liable to relapse. 2. A patient who shows a tendency to re-enter hospital for treatment, particularly one who takes undue advantage of the voluntary system in mental hospitals. 3. In forensic medicine, an incorrigible criminal who, although antisocial in behaviour, does not fall into the category of the legally insane. [see prec.]

recidivity (re·sid·**iv**·it·e). The tendency to relapse in illness or to return to hospital or to gaol. [L *recidivus* falling back.]

recipe (**res**·ip·e). A formula for a compounded preparation, either for medicinal or culinary purposes. The name is not used for a prescription written for a particular individual but is usually confined to formulae intended for laymen. [see foll.]

recipient (re·**sip**·e·ent). The receiver of the blood in blood transfusion. **Universal recipient.** A person to whom any type of human blood can be given without the occurrence of agglutination or precipitation. [L *recipere* to receive.]

recipiomotor (re·**sip**·e·o·**mo**′·tor). Referring to reception of motor stimuli. [L *recipere* to receive, *motor* mover.]

Recklinghausen, Friedrich Daniel von (b. 1833). Strasbourg pathologist.

Recklinghausen's canals. Lymph or tissue spaces.

Recklinghausen's disease. 1. Multiple neurofibromatosis. 2. Osteitis fibrosa cystica.

Recklinghausen's tonometer. A tonometer for deriving the arterial blood pressure from measurement of the tension on the arterial wall produced by the column of blood within the artery.

Recklinghausen's tumour. Adenomyosis of the uterus.

Recklinghausen-Appelbaum disease. Haemochromatosis.

reclination (rek·lin·**a**·shun). Couching; an operation in which the lens is dislocated out of the pupil and turned down into the vitreous. [L *reclinare* to bend back.]

Reclus, Paul (b. 1847). Paris surgeon.

Reclus' disease. Cystic enlargement of the breast.

Reclus' operation. Iliac colostomy.

recoil (re·**koil**). The motion acquired by a particle through ejecting another particle or photon. [OFr. *reculer.*]

recombination (re·kom·bin·**a**′·shun). 1. Joining together again. 2. In genetics, the coming together of gene combinations in the offspring which were not present in either parent. It is due to independent assortment of allelomorphs during gametogenesis and to random fertilization. 3. The reunion of chemical compounds formed by a chemical reaction to reproduce the original substances. **Ionic recombination.** Combination of positive ions with electrons or negative ions, resulting in the formation of neutral atoms. This process takes place after ionization of a gas, due to random contact between ions and electrons. [L *re-*, combination.]

recomposition (re·kom·po·**zish**′·un). The recombination of parts after a period of temporary separation. [L *recomponere* to rearrange.]

recompression (re·kom·**presh**·un). The method of treatment adopted for compressed-air illness (caisson disease). On the appearance of symptoms, the man is placed in a recompressing apparatus or room and the pressure is increased to the level at which he had been working. After this recompression the reduction of pressure to that of the atmosphere is carried out very slowly, and may take several hours. The whole process is more usually defined as *decompression.* [L *re-*, *compremere* to press together.]

reconstituted (re·**kon**·stit·ew·ted). Referring to the solution in sterile distilled water of "freeze-dried" or desiccated blood plasma or serum, used for transfusion purposes when whole blood is not required. [L *re-*, *constituere* to set up.]

recovery (re·**kuv**·er·e). The process of being restored to health and strength after illness or enfeeblement or disablement from any cause. [ME *recoveren*.]

recrement (**rek**·re·ment). A secretory product, e.g. bile, which is ultimately reabsorbed rather than excreted. [L *recrementum* refuse.]

recrementitious (**rek**·re·men·**tish**'·us). Relating to or composed of a recrement.

recrudescence (re·kroo·**des**·ens). A return of symptoms of disease after a period of abatement. [L *recrudescere* to break out again.]

recrudescent (re·kroo·**des**·ent). Relating or belonging to recrudescence.

recruitment (re·**kroot**·ment). In voluntary muscle contraction, the process of bringing more and more motor units into action when additional voluntary effort is required. **Loudness recruitment.** In unilateral deafness due to cochlea disease, the difference in sensitivity to a sound stimulus between the deaf and normal ear decreases as the intensity of the sound increases. In other words, the loudness-level difference is reduced as intensity is increased. [Fr. *recroître* to grow again.]

rectal (**rek**·tal). Relating or belonging to the rectum.

rectal arteries. The arterial supply to the rectum and anal canal, consisting of an unpaired superior rectal and paired middle and inferior rectal arteries. **Inferior rectal artery [arteria rectalis inferior (NA)].** A branch of the internal pudendal artery. **Middle rectal artery [arteria rectalis media (NA)].** A small branch from the anterior division of the internal iliac artery. **Superior rectal artery [arteria rectalis superior (NA)].** *See* INFERIOR MESENTERIC ARTERY.

rectal veins. Veins which drain the rectum and anal canal into both the portal and systemic systems, the anastomosis between which lies at the junction of the upper and lower half of the anal canal. **Inferior rectal veins [venae rectales inferiores (NA)].** Tributaries of the internal pudendal veins. They form part of the drainage of the rectal plexuses, and through these communicate with the superior rectal veins, thus forming an important portacaval anastomosis. **Middle rectal vein [vena rectalis media (NA)].** An inconstant vein draining the rectal plexuses into the internal iliac veins. **Superior rectal vein [vena rectalis superior (NA)].** The main venous drainage of the rectum, draining both the internal and external rectal plexuses, and continued upward above the pelvis as the inferior mesenteric vein.

rectalgia (rek·**tal**·je·ah). Pain in the anus or lower part of the rectum. [rectum, Gk *algos* pain.]

rectectomy (rek·**tek**·to·me). Proctectomy. [rectum, Gk *ektome* a cutting out.]

rectification (**rek**·tif·ik·**a**'·shun). 1. The process of straightening anything that is curved or out of alignment; the purification of a substance; the correction of error or aberration. 2. In chemistry, the distillation of a liquid to separate impurities. [Obsolete term.] 3. In electricity, the transformation of an alternating current into a direct one. 4. In mathematics or statistics, the measurement of the length of a curve. [Obsolete term.] **Full-wave rectification.** Rectification in which both half-cycles of the alternating current wave-form are used to produce the direct current. **Half-wave rectification.** Rectification in which only one half-cycle of the alternating current wave-form is used to produce the direct current. [L *rectus* straight, *facere* to make.]

rectified (**rek**·te·fide). 1. Purified; refined, e.g. a liquid. 2. Straightened. 3. Of electricity, a direct current obtained from an alternating current. [see foll.]

rectifier (**rek**·te·fi·er). A device for converting an alternating current into a direct current by inversion or suppression of alternate half-waves. [L *rectus* straight, *facere* to make.]

recti-ischial (rek·ti·is·ke·al). Pertaining to the rectum and the ischium.

rectitis (rek·ti·tis). Proctitis. **Epidemic gangrenous rectitis.** Epidemic gangrenous proctitis. **Granular rectitis.** A granular excoriation of the lower end of the rectum. [rectum, Gk *-itis* inflammation.]

recto-abdominal (rek·to·ab·**dom**'·in·al). Relating or belonging to the rectum amd the abdomen.

rectocele (**rek**·to·seel). Protrusion of the wall of the rectum into the perineum or vagina. [rectum, Gk *kele* hernia.]

rectoclysis (rek·**tok**·lis·is). Proctoclysis. [rectum, Gk *klysis* a washing out.]

rectococcygeal (**rek**·to·kok·**sij**'·e·al). Belonging to the rectum and the coccyx.

rectococcygeal muscle [musculus rectococcygeus (NA)]. A band of muscle fibres usually found connecting the longitudinal coat of the rectum to the front of the coccyx in the median plane.

rectococcypexy (rek·to·**kok**·se·pex·e). Proctococcypexy. [rectum, coccyx, Gk *pexis* fixation.]

rectocoele (**rek**·to·seel). Rectocele. [rectum, Gk *koilos* hollow.]

rectocolitis (**rek**·to·kol·**i**'·tis). An inflammatory condition involving the rectum and part of the colon. [rectum, colitis.]

rectocolonic (**rek**·to·ko·**lon**'·ik). Belonging or referring to the rectum and the colon.

rectocystotomy (**rek**·to·sist·**ot**'·o·me). The operation of incising the urinary bladder from the rectum in order to remove a stone from the bladder. [rectum, Gk *kystis* bag, *temnein* to cut.]

rectofistula (rek·to·**fis**·tew·lah). A fistula in the rectum.

rectogenital (rek·to·**jen**·it·al). Relating or belonging to the rectum and the genitalia.

rectolabial (rek·to·**la**·be·al). Relating to the rectum and the labia majora and minora.

rectoperineorrhaphy (**rek**·to·per·in·e·**or**'·af·e). Reparative surgery of the anus and perineum. [rectum, perineum, Gk *rhaphe* suture.]

rectopexy (**rek**·to·pex·e). The operation of suturing the rectum to a neighbouring part. [rectum, Gk *pexis* fixation.]

rectophobia (rek·to·**fo**·be·ah). A peculiar state of apprehension or fear that affects many sufferers with rectal disease. [rectum, phobia.]

rectoplasty (**rek**·to·plas·te). A plastic operation on the anus and rectum. [rectum, Gk *plassein* to mould.]

rectorectostomy (**rek**·to·rek·**tos**'·to·me). Anastomosis between two portions of the rectum [rectum, Gk *stoma* mouth.]

rectoromanoscope (**rek**·to·ro·**man**'·o·skope). Sigmoidoscope. [rectum, romanoscope.]

rectorrhaphy (rek·**tor**·af·e). The operation of suturing lacerations of the rectum or anus. [rectum, Gk *rhaphe* suture.]

rectoscope (**rek**·to·skope). Proctoscope. [rectum, Gk *skopein* to watch.]

rectosigmoid (rek·to·**sig**·moid). A term applied to the region of junction between the rectum and the pelvic (sigmoid) colon.

rectosigmoidectomy (**rek**·to·sig·moid·**ek**'·to·me). Removal of the rectum and sigmoid colon as a treatment of prolapse of the rectum. [rectosigmoid, Gk *ektome* excision.]

rectosigmoidoscopy (**rek**·to·sig·moid·**os**'·ko·pe). Inspection of the rectum and pelvic colon by means of special instruments, e.g. a sigmoidoscope. [rectosigmoid, Gk *skopein* to watch.]

rectostenosis (**rek**·to·sten·**o**'·sis). Stenosis of the anus or rectum.

rectostomy (rek·**tos**·to·me). The operation of establishing a permanent opening into the rectum. [rectum, Gk *stoma* mouth.]

rectotomy (rek·**tot**·o·me). Proctotomy. [rectum, Gk *temnein* to cut.]

recto-urethral (**rek**·to·ewr·**e**'·thral). Belonging to the rectum and the urethra.

recto-urethral muscle [musculus recto-urethralis (NA)]. Some anterior fibres of the longitudinal muscle coat of the rectum which are attached to the perineal body. [rectum, urethra.]

recto-uterine (rek·to·**ew**·ter·ine). Relating or belonging to the rectum and the uterus.

recto-uterine muscle [musculus recto-uterinus (NA)]. Bands of muscle fibres in the uterosacral ligament.

rectovaginal (**rek**·to·vaj·**i**'·nal). Relating or belonging to the rectum and the vagina.

rectovagino-abdominal (rek·to·vaj·i·no·ab·**dom'**·in·al). Pertaining to the rectum, vagina, and abdomen: used with reference to an obstetric examination with the fingers of one hand in the rectum and vagina and the other hand on the abdominal wall.

rectovesical (rek·to·**ves**·ik·al). Belonging to the rectum and the urinary bladder. [rectum, L *vesica* urinary bladder.]

rectovesical muscle [musculus rectovesicalis (NA)]. Fibres of the external longitudinal coat which are carried on to the front of the rectum.

rectum [NA] (rek·tum). The part of the large bowel between the pelvic colon and the anal canal extending from the third piece of the sacrum to a point 3.5 cm in front of and below the tip of the coccyx. It is curved in the sagittal plane to fit the sacrococcygeal hollow; in the coronal plane it is sinuous, with curves to the right above and below an intermediate curve to the left; opposite these are three horizontal folds in the wall. Its upper two-thirds are retroperitoneal, and its lower third below the level of the peritoneum. Its lower end, or ampulla, is in contact anteriorly with the prostate in the male and the lower part of the vagina in the female. **Mucous coat of the rectum [tunica mucosa (NA)].** A coat covered with columnar epithelium which dips down into the deeper layers as simple tubular glands containing numerous goblet cells. Solitary lymphoid nodules are also present. **Muscular coat of the rectum [tunica muscularis (NA)].** A coat much thicker than the rest of the large intestine and consisting of an inner circular [stratum circulare (NA)] and an outer longitudinal [stratum longitudinale (NA)] layer. The latter, while completely investing the organ, is disposed mainly as a broad band on the anterior and posterior surfaces. **Submucous coat of the rectum [tela submucosa (NA)].** A coat composed of loose areolar tissue allowing free movement of the mucous membrane on the muscular coat. [L *rectus* straight.]

rectus (rek·tus). Straight; denoting any structure with a straight course, e.g. rectus capitis lateralis muscle. [L.]

rectus abdominis muscle [musculus rectus abdominis (NA)] (**rek**·tus ab·**dom**·in·is musl). A long flat muscle on the front of the abdomen, separated from its fellow by the linea alba and attached to the body of the pubis below and the 5th, 6th, and 7th costal cartilages above.

rectus capitis muscles (**rek**·tus **kap**·it·is muslz). Four paired muscles attached to the base of the skull above and to the atlas or axis below. **Rectus capitis anterior muscle [musculus rectus capitis anterior (NA)].** A paired muscle attached below to the lateral mass of the atlas and above to the basilar part of the occipital bone in front of the condyle. **Rectus capitis lateralis muscle [musculus rectus capitis lateralis (NA)].** A paired muscle attached superiorly to the jugular process of the occipital bone and inferiorly to the transverse process of the atlas. **Rectus capitis posterior major muscle [musculus rectus capitis posterior major (NA)].** One of a pair of muscles forming the medial boundaries of the suboccipital triangles, attached inferiorly to the spine of the axis and superiorly to the lateral part of the inferior nuchal line and the subjacent bone. **Rectus capitis posterior minor muscle [musculus rectus capitis posterior minor (NA)].** One of a pair of small muscles attached inferiorly to the tubercle of the atlas and superiorly to the medial third of the inferior nuchal line and the subjacent bone.

rectus femoris muscle [musculus rectus femoris (NA)] (**rek**·tus **fem**·or·is musl). One of the quadriceps mass of muscle, arising from the front of the ilium and inserted into the base of the patella. It is a weak flexor of the hip and extensor of the knee.

rectus muscles of the orbit. Muscles arising from the common tendinous ring and controlling the movements of the orbit. **External rectus muscle of the orbit.** Lateral rectus muscle of the orbit (see below). **Inferior rectus muscle of the orbit [musculus rectus inferior (NA)].** A muscle arising from the lower part of the common tendinous ring and inserted into the sclera anterior to the equator of the eyeball via a tendinous expansion. It turns the eye downwards and slightly medially. **Internal rectus muscle of the orbit.** Medial rectus muscle of the orbit (see below). **Lateral rectus muscle of the orbit [musculus rectus lateralis (NA)].** A muscle arising from the lateral part of the common tendinous ring and from the orbital surface of the greater wing of the sphenoid bone. It turns the eye laterally. **Medial rectus muscle of the orbit [musculus rectus medialis (NA)].** A muscle arising from the medial part of the common tendinous ring and inserted into the sclera anterior to the equator of the eyeball via a tendinous expansion. It turns the eye medially. **Superior rectus muscle of the orbit [musculus rectus superior (NA)].** A muscle arising from the upper part of the common tendinous ring and inserted into the sclera anterior to the equator of the eyeball via a tendinous expansion. It turns the eye upwards and slightly medially.

recumbent (re·**kum**·bent). 1. Lying down; reclining. 2. In biology, leaning; applied to structures that appear to lean against the surface of the part from which they extend. [L *recumbere* to lie down.]

recuperate (re·**kew**·per·ate). To recover in health and strength, as in convalescence. [L *recuperare* to regain.]

recuperation (re·kew·per·**a'**·shun). The process of recuperating.

recuperative (re·**kew**·per·a·tiv). 1. Relating or belonging to recuperation. 2. Having the power of recovery from illness. 3. Tending to restore to health.

recur (re·**ker**). To return or reappear; hence *recurring.* [see foll.]

recurarization (re·kew·rah·ri·**za'**·shun). The return of non-depolarizing neuromuscular block following its apparent reversal by an anticholinesterase agent. [L *re-*, curare.]

recurrence (re·**ker**·ens). 1. The reappearance of symptoms of a disease after a period of abeyance or remission. 2. In malariology, according to James' classification a return of fever and the reappearance of parasites in the peripheral blood later than 24 weeks after recovery from the primary attack, that is, usually later than 26 weeks after the primary infection. [L *recurrere* to run back.]

recurrent (re·**kur**·ent). 1. Of disease or a lesion, returning or showing a tendency to return from time to time. 2. In anatomy, a structure which turns back in the opposite direction to that of its previous course, e.g. certain nerves and branches of vessels. **Recurrent utterance.** Monophasia. [see prec.]

recurrent arteries. Branches, anterior and posterior, from the anterior tibial artery, which ascend to the arterial anastomosis around the knee joint. **Interosseous recurrent arteries, Ulnar recurrent arteries.** *See* ULNAR ARTERY.

recurvation (re·ker·**va**·shun). Curvature or bending in a backward direction; backward flexure. [L *recurvare* to bend back.]

recurvatum (re·ker·**va**·tum). A recurvation. **Tibial recurvatum.** A backward deformity at the knee or in the lower leg due to malformation or malunion of the tibia. [L *recurvare* to bend back.]

red (red). That colour of the visible spectrum which has the longest wavelength (approximately 650 nm). **Aniline red.** Magenta. **Bordeaux red.** Cerasine. **Bromphenol red.** An indicator with a pH range from 6.0 (yellow) to 7.0 (red). **Caesar red.** Eosin B. **Carmine red.** $C_{11}H_{12}O_7$, a red stain derived from carmine. **Cerasine red.** Sudan III. **Chinese red.** Mercuric sulphide. **Chlorophenol red.** Sodium dichlorphenolsulphonephthalein, $(C_6H_2Cl_2OH)_2CC_6H_4SO_3Na$, an indicator with a pH range from 5.5 to 6.5. **Congo red.** *See* CONGO RED. **Corallin red.** A derivative of pararosaniline. **Cotton red 4B.** Benzopurpurine 4B. **Cresol red.** Orthocresol sulphonephthalein, a compound used as a pH indicator (7.2–8.8). **Cumidine red.** A red dye used as a food colouring. **Direct red.** Congo red. **Direct red 4B.** Benzopurpurine 4B. **Fast red B, or P.** Cerasine. **Kino red.** An insoluble phlobaphene resulting from the decomposition of kinotannic acid. **Magdala red, Naphthalene red.** A naphrosafranin dye occasionally used as a nuclear stain. **Naphthol red.** Amaranth. **Neutral red.** Dimethyldiaminotoluphenazine hydrochloride, $(CH_3)_2NC_6H_3N_2C_6H_2(CH_3)NH_2{\cdot}HCl$, a dye used as an indicator, having a pH value 7.5, and also employed in the flaginac reaction for *Bacterium coli.* **Oil red.** General name for a series of fat stains: oil red AS, O, B, and 3B are synonyms for

Sudan III; oil red O and oil red 4B are of the Sudan type. **Orange red.** Sandix, a natural form of red-lead oxide, Pb_3O_4, a little lighter in colour than the latter and used as a pigment. **Paris red.** 1. Red ferric oxide, Fe_2O_3, employed in medicine as a styptic and industrially as a polishing abrasive in lens manufacture. 2. Red lead. *See* LEAD. **Phenol red.** Sodium phenosulphonephthalein, $(C_6H_4OH)_2CC_6H_4SO_3Na$, a bright red dye used as an indicator (pH 7.7), and as a test for kidney function. **Provisional red.** A coloured substance which can be obtained from rhodopsin. **Scarlet Red BPC 1959.** Sudan IV, Biebrich scarlet red; the azo dye, *o*-toluene azo-*o*-toluene azo-*β*-naphthol, $C_7H_7N_2C_7H_6N_2C_{10}H_6OH$. It is employed therapeutically in the treatment of burns and ulcers since it has the power of stimulating the growth of epithelial cells. It is usually applied in the form of an ointment. **Scarlet red sulphonate.** The sodium salt of azobenzene disulphonic acid azo-*β*-naphthol, used like scarlet red. **Sensitol red.** A carbocyanine dye, $C_2H_5C_9H_6NCH{=}CH{-}CH{=}C_9H_6NIC_2H_5$, with a germicidal action on staphylococci; it is also used as a red sensitizer in photography. **Sudan red.** Magdala red (see above). **Toluylene red.** A base prepared by the oxidation of indamine; the parent of neutral red. **Tony red.** Sudan III. **Trypan red.** An acid azo dye, $(NaSO_3)_2C_{10}H_4(NH_2)N_2C_6H_4C_6H_3(SO_2OH)N_2C_{10}H_4(SO_3Na)_2(NH_2)$, used as a vital stain, and the first chemotherapeutic agent employed against trypanosomes (Ehrlich). **Turkey red.** A red dye obtained from the roots of species of *Rubia.* **Venetian red.** Red ferric oxide. **Vital red.** A dye used in the estimation of blood volume by directly injecting intravenously and determining the concentration of the dye in the blood plasma. **Wool red.** Amaranth. [AS *read.*]

red-ochre (red·o·ker). Raddle. [red, Gk *ochros* yellow.]

red-out (red·owt). Under negative *G* force, objects in the visual field appear redder than normal; the cause is uncertain, possibly venous engorgement of the retina. [red, AS *ut.*]

red tide (red tide). A phenomenon due to an abnormal multiplication in the sea of dinoflagellates: *Gonyaulax* and *Gymnodinium* spp. produce a heat-stable neurotoxin which may kill fish and seabirds, and the flesh of the former may be lethal to man. Water-filtering molluscs, which retain and concentrate the toxin to which they are immune, constitute the greatest danger to man. Death occurs through respiratory paralysis. The toxin is a small molecule and is not antigenic; therefore no antitoxin exists. Treatment is symptomatic. [AS *read* MLG *getide.*]

Reddish's malt-extract bouillon. Malt-extract bouillon; a medium prepared from malt extract 100 g, water to 1 l.

reddle (redl). Raddle. [AS *read* red.]

Redecker's frühinfiltrat. Assmann's focus.

redecussate (re·de·kus·ate). To decussate for the second time. [L *re-*, *decussare* to cross like an X.]

redia (re·de·ah). The third stage in the life histories of trematode flukes; a stationary form developed from a sporocyst in the snail host. They produce, asexually, either further rediae or cercariae. [Francesco *Redi*, 1626–1697, Italian naturalist.]

redifferentiation (re·dif·er·en·she·a′·shun). The reassumption of mature characteristics by anaplastic cells. [L *re-*, differentiation.]

redintegration (red·in·teg·ra′·shun). The arousal of a response by a fraction of the stimulus originally arousing it. [L *redintegrare* to make whole again.]

redislocation (re·dis·lo·ka′·shun). The recurrence of a dislocation after its correction. [L *re-*, dislocate.]

Redlich, Emil (b. 1866). Vienna neurologist.

Obersteiner-Redlich area, or zone. An unmyelinated area of the lateral part of a posterior nerve root as it enters the spinal cord.

Redlich-Fischer miliary plaques. Small pigmented glial plaques found in the brain in cases of senile psychosis.

redox (re·dox). Oxidation-reduction. In chemistry, the simultaneous processes of oxidation and reduction regarded as a transfer of electrons from reducing agent to oxidizing agent. **Redox indicator.** A dyestuff used to detect the oxidative tendencies of a system, or to compare redox potentials. **Redox potential.** A measurement of the intensity of an oxidation-reduction system in terms of the readiness with which electrons are exchanged.

redresser (re·dres·er). An instrument used in the correction of a deformity or in the restoration of a part to its normal position. [Fr. *redresser* to set right.]

redressment (re·dres·ment). 1. Restoration of a dislocated part to its normal position or the rectification of a deformity. 2. A second or renewed dressing. **Redressment forcé.** The rectification by force of a deformity, in particular genu valgum. [Fr., straightening.]

reduce (re·dews). 1. To restore any part to its normal situation, e.g. reduce a hernia. 2. In chemistry, to remove oxygen or to add hydrogen; to convert a compound of an element into a compound in which the element has a lower valency, e.g. ferric to ferrous chloride. 3. To slim; to lower one's weight by dieting. [L *reducere* to lead back.]

reducible (re·dew·sible). Able to be reduced; replaceable in proper position as, for example, a hernia.

reducine (re·dew·seen). $C_{12}H_{24}N_6O_9$, a toxic alkaloid derived from urochrome, the pigment of urine.

reductant (re·duk·tant). A reducing agent.

reductase (re·duk·taze). Any enzyme that activates the reduction of a compound. As every reduction is necessarily accompanied by oxidation, they are more correctly termed *oxidoreductases.* **Aldehyde reductase.** An enzyme in muscle and liver which converts aldehydes into alcohols and acids. **Cytochrome reductase.** A yellow enzyme occurring in yeast and liver which catalyses the reduction of cytochrome C. **Methaemoglobin reductase.** An enzyme in red blood cells which reduces methaemoglobin; its activity requires the co-enzyme NADH (reduced nicotinamide adenine dinucleotide).

See also: SCHARDINGER.

reduction (re·duk·shun). 1. The restoration of displaced tissues to their natural position as, for example, in fracture or hernia. 2. In chemistry, the removal of oxygen from, or the addition of hydrogen to, a compound. This involves the reduction of the valency of one of the elements concerned, and the process may be regarded as an electronic interchange, the reduced element gaining one or more electrons. 3. Reduction of chromosomes, the halving of the number of chromosomes which occurs as a result of the first maturation division of primary spermatocytes and oöcytes. **Reduction en bloc.** The dangerous disappearance of a hernial swelling, usually following manipulation, but only by the displacement of the hernia sac with its contents unreduced. **Closed reduction.** Manual reduction of a fracture or dislocation without exposing the parts. **Delayed reduction.** Reduction of a fracture which has been deferred for some time, e.g. until severe swelling has subsided. **Hydrostatic reduction.** A method of reducing intussusception using fluid (usually a thin, soft barium) run into the rectum under slight pressure. **Immediate reduction.** Reduction of a fracture as soon as the patient comes for treatment, as against delayed reduction (see above) or slow reduction by continuous sustained traction to a limb for some days. **Reduction en masse.** Reduction en bloc (see above). **Open reduction.** The operative procedure of reduction of a fracture or dislocation by exposing the displaced bones. **Tetrathionate reduction.** The reduction of a salt of tetrathionic acid to a thiosulphate. This reaction is employed in certain enrichment media for the growth of typhoid, paratyphoid, and other *Salmonella* bacilli in faeces. [L *reducere* to lead back.]

See also: HIPPOCRATES.

reductone (re·duk·tone). OHCH=C(OH)CHO, an enolic form of hydroxymethylglyoxal obtained by the disintegration of glucose. It has reducing properties similar to ascorbic acid but no antiscorbutic effect: it appears to take part in the growth of bacteria and is competed for by sulphonamides.

reductor (re·duk·tor). 1. Any apparatus used in reducing a part. 2. Any muscle which has the action of retraction. [L, one who brings back.]

redundancy (re·**dun**·dan·se). The state of being superfluous, excessive, can be omitted without loss of significance. **Gratuitous redundancy.** The interpolation by a patient with mild asphasia, of verbiage, comparatively low in reference function, although not wholly beside the point.

reduplicated (re·**dew**·plik·a·ted). Of sounds, repeated, especially one of the heart sounds. [L *re-*, *duplicare* to repeat.]

reduplication (re·dew·plik·**a**'·shun). 1. A doubling, e.g. of heart sounds, when the first or second sound is repeated. 2. The state of a part when it is folded back on itself. [see prec.]

reduviid (re·**dew**·vi·id). Belonging to the family of bugs, Reduviidae. [see foll.]

Reduviidae (re·dew·**vi**·id·e). A family of Hemiptera, assassin bugs. All the species are carnivorous, and members of the genera *Reduvius, Rhodnius,* and *Triatoma* (including *Panstrongylus*) are of medical importance. Many others bite man painfully. [L *reduvia* hangnail.]

Reduvius (re·**dew**·vi·us). A genus of bugs of the family Reduviidae. **Reduvius personatus.** The big bed bug, a common commensal of man which feeds on bed bugs and other insects. It bites man rarely, but painfully. [see prec.]

Reed, Dorothy Mendenhall (b. 1874). Baltimore pathologist.

Dorothy Reed cells, Sternberg-Reed cells. The typical giant cells of Hodgkin's disease.

Reed-Hodgkin disease (a term confined to the USA). Lymphadenoma.

re-education (re·ed·ew·**ka**'·shun). Instruction of incapacitated individuals or of those affected with some mental disorder, so that some or all of their lost ability may be regained. The term is also applied to structures, e.g. muscle, subjected to exercises so that they regain their normal function. [L *re-*, *educere* to lead out.]

Reenstierna, John (fl. 1913). Swedish dermatologist.

Ito-Reenstierna test. A test for chancroid infection by intradermal injection of a suspension of killed *Haemophilus ducreyi.* An inflammatory papule developing within 48 hours indicates present or past infection. The skin does not react until about 14 days after infection, and the test is believed to remain positive for the remainder of the patient's life.

re-entry (re·**en**·tre). In cardiology, the phenomenon in which a depolarization front may be able to advance down one pathway whilst being blocked along another and then, while the first pathway is refractory, pass back up the second, now conductive, and thereby return towards its origin to find the first pathway again conducting. In this way, a circulatory movement may be established and tachycardia be produced. This is the mechanism of the paroxysmal tachycardia in the Wolff-Parkinson-White and the Lown-Ganong-Levine syndromes, and probably also many other examples of paroxysmal tachycardia. [L *re-*, Fr. *entrée* entry.]

Reese, Robert Grigg (b. 1866). New York ophthalmologist.

Reese's operation. 1. For orbital exploration: a transconjunctival route is adopted, usually from the temporal side, using a canthotomy and, if necessary, dividing the external rectus muscle. 2. For squint: resection of a portion of the muscle, the end of which is sutured to the stump with one mattress suture in the centre and two single sutures at each border.

re-evolution (re·e·vol·**ew**'·shun). John Hughlings Jackson's term for the symptoms which follow an epileptic fit during the return to consciousness. [L *re-*, *evolvere* to unroll.]

refection (re·**fek**·shun). Restoration; recovery. [L *re-*, *facere* to make.]

refectious (re·**fek**·shus). Denoting agents that are able to induce refection.

reference (**ref**·er·ens). The act of referring to some person or thing. **Idea of reference.** *See* IDEA. **Peripheral reference.** The reference of touch, pain, and thermal stimuli to the boundary zone of an anaesthetic area when such stimuli are applied within the area: a transient phenomenon occurring during the regeneration of a peripheral sensory nerve after section. [L *referre* to bring back.]

refine (re·**fine**). To reduce to a pure state; to purify. [L *re-*, *finire* to finish.]

reflected (re·**flek**·ted). 1. Rebounded; thrown back, as rays of light from a mirror. 2. Effected by the sending of a nervous impulse to a nerve centre, when it is conveyed by a motor nerve to a peripheral part. 3. In anatomy, a structure that is folded back on itself. [see foll.]

reflection (re·**flek**·shun). 1. The turning back of a beam of radiation (heat, light, sound) by a polished surface which it does not penetrate. The ray before reflection is known as the *incident ray,* and after reflection the *reflected ray.* 2. Where a membrane covers an organ and is then folded back. 3. The casting of the mind over past thoughts in the light of some present situation. [L *reflectere* to bend back.]

See also: BRAGG.

reflector (re·**flek**·tor). A device which throws back rays of light or heat or waves of sound. **Dental reflector.** Dental mirror. *See* MIRROR. [see prec.]

reflectoscope (re·**flek**·to·skope). A type of lantern in which the light is reflected. [reflection, Gk *skopein* to view.]

reflex (**re**·flex). 1. Reflected light or colour; an image; an effect coming back to the origin. 2. The immediate and involuntary response (e.g. of muscle or gland) to stimulus from a receptor (e.g. sense organ). **Abdominal reflex.** Reflex contraction of the muscles of the abdominal wall on stroking the overlying skin; clinically the most important of the cutaneous reflexes, the abdominal reflexes, are diminished or lost in disease of the pyramidal tract. **Abdominocardiac reflex.** Reflex slowing of the heart mediated through the vagus nerve in response to stimulation of abdominal viscera. **Accommodation reflex.** The reflex contraction of the pupils of the eyes on accommodation. **Achilles tendon reflex.** Contraction of the calf muscles, with consequent plantar flexion of the foot, on striking the Achilles tendon sharply; the ankle jerk, a normal tendon reflex. **Acquired reflex.** Conditioned reflex (see below). **Acromial reflex.** On tapping the acromion sharply, flexion of the forearm and slight internal rotation of the hand occur. **Adductor reflex.** Contraction of the adductors of the thigh, evoked by tapping the tendon of the adductor magnus muscle, or its lowest point of insertion into the medial condyle of the femur, with the thigh in adduction. **Allied reflex.** Two separate reflexes arising on stimuli in widely separated regions of the body, producing common or even antagonistic effects. **Anal reflex.** A scratch on the skin of the perianal region producing contraction of the sphincter ani externus muscle. **Ankle reflex.** Achilles tendon reflex (see above). **Antagonistic reflex.** Two reflexes antagonistic in effect and so, when acting together, producing no resultant. **Anticus reflex.** Piotrowski's sign. **Arterial light reflex.** Reflex streak. *See* STREAK. **Attention reflex.** Constriction of the pupil when the attention is drawn to an object, analogous to pupillary constriction on convergence. **Attitudinal reflexes.** Reflexes which automatically control the action of the skeletal musculature in the adoption of the various attitudes of the body. **Auditory reflex.** Any reflex effect resulting from stimulation of the auditory nerve, such as jumping as a result of loud noises, or the closing of the eyes. **Aural reflex.** Any form of reflex resulting from stimulation of any part of the aural mechanism. **Auricle reflex.** Involuntary movements carried out by the auricle or pinna in response to sound. **Auriculocervical nerve reflex.** Snellen's reflex. **Auriculopalpebral reflex.** Kehrer's reflex; Kirsch's reflex. **Auriculopressor reflex.** Reflex vasoconstriction due to a rise in pressure in the right auricle and great veins. **Aurosensory pupillary reflex.** Reflex dilatation of the pupil occurring on tactile or thermal stimulation of the middle ear, or by rapidly altering the air pressures. **Axon reflex.** A reflex in which an afferent impulse travels along a nerve fibre to a point of branching and then centrifugally to an effector end-organ, without entering a nerve cell body. It is possible that reflexes of this type play a part in vasomotor activity. **Basal joint reflex.**

Finger–thumb reflex (see below). **Behaviour reflex.** Conditioned reflex (see below). **Biceps reflex.** The normal contraction of the biceps brachii muscle on percussing its tendon of insertion. **Bladder reflex.** The desire to urinate which arises when the bladder contains a certain quantity of urine. **Blinking reflex.** Closure of the eye when an object approaches the eye rapidly. **Body-righting reflex.** A righting reflex induced by asymmetric stimulation of the body wall by external pressure. **Bone reflex.** It used to be considered that certain reflex muscular contractions were evoked by stimulation of bone, and they were called bone reflexes; it is now known that they result from stretching of muscle tendons as they are inserted into the bone. **Bulbocavernous reflex.** Bulbospongiosus reflex (see below). **Bulbomimic reflex.** Pressure upon the eyeball which produces contraction of muscles of both sides of the face in patients who are in coma as a result of toxaemia; in coma due to cerebral haemorrhage, contraction occurs only on the side opposite to the lesion. **Bulbospongiosus reflex.** Tapping upon the dorsum of the penis causing retraction of the bulbocavernous portion, owing to contraction of the bulbospongiosus muscle. **Cardiorespiratory reflex.** A reflex present at birth in full-term infants, and initiated by change of pressure in intracranial blood vessels, as a result of change from intra-uterine to atmospheric pressure; less easily elicited in the premature and immature baby. **Cardiovascular reflexes.** Changes in cardiovascular function resulting from stimulation of heart or blood vessels by changes of intravascular tension, heart rate, blood gases, or blood hydrogen-ion concentration (pH): e.g. Bainbridge reflex. **Carotid sinus reflex.** Increase of pressure within the carotid sinus at the bifurcation of the common carotid artery causing a reflex fall in blood pressure, vasodilatation, and slowing of the heart. These effects are the result of vagal stimulation, the afferent fibres of the reflex being contained in the sinus nerve, a branch of the glossopharyngeal nerve, which ramifies within the carotid sinus and has central connections with the cardio-inhibitory and vasomotor centres. The efferent limb of the cardiac portion of the reflex is the vagus nerve. A fall in pressure in the carotid sinus causes a rise in blood pressure, cardiac acceleration, and vasoconstriction, the afferent limb being formed by sympathetic fibres. **Carpophalangeal reflex.** Bechterew's reflex; tapping of the extensor tendons of the wrist when it is flexed, giving reflex extension. **Chain reflex.** An integrated action produced as the resultant of several separate reflexes, each of which is activated by the preceding one. **Chin reflex, Chin-jerk reflex.** The jaw jerk; reflex contraction of the masseter muscle following a brisk downward tap on the point of the jaw as the mouth hangs loosely open. **Choroidal reflex.** Red reflex (see below). **Ciliospinal reflex.** Pinching of the skin of the neck which produces dilatation of the ipsilateral pupil. **Cochlear pupillary reflex.** Dilatation of the pupil, preceded by a slight temporary contraction, following intense cochleal stimulation; it is bilateral but is more marked on the same side. **Cochleo-orbicular reflex, Cochleopalpebral reflex.** Contraction of the orbicularis oculi muscle resulting from the stimulus of the auditory mechanism. **Cochleopupillary reflex.** Cochlear pupillary reflex (see above). **Cochleostapedial reflex.** Contraction of the stapedius muscle after a loud noise. **Coeliac-plexus reflex.** A fall in blood pressure observed when the upper viscera are handled during abdominal operations. **Concealed reflex.** A reflex whose activity is masked by that of a more dominant reflex resulting from the same stimulus. **Conditional reflex, Conditioned reflex.** An acquired reflex built upon an inborn one by the association of a new or conditioned stimulus with an unconditioned one. Thus, the secretion of saliva when food is placed in the mouth is an unconditioned reflex, the contact of food with the mouth being an unconditioned stimulus; if the placing of food is repeatedly accompanied by another stimulus, such as the sounding of a given note (the conditional stimulus) then ultimately that stimulus, without the unconditioned one, will cause the reflex of salivary secretion. A more appropriate term is conditioned response rather than reflex. **Conjunctival reflex.** Approximation and closure of the eyelids on the touching of the conjunctiva. **Consensual reflex.** A reflex response occurring on one side of the body as a result of stimulation of the opposite side; a crossed reflex. **Consensual light reflex.** The simultaneous contraction of the opposite pupil when one only is exposed to light. **Contact reflex.** Flexion at the hip and knee induced by a light touch on the dorsum of the foot. **Contralateral reflex.** When a reflex is elicited on one side of the body a response may sometimes occur on the opposite side as an overflow phenomenon; the term is also applied to the flexion of the leg which may occur on passive flexion of the opposite leg in cases of meningitis. **Convergence reflex.** The reflex contraction of the pupils of the two eyes when convergence takes place. **Convulsive reflex.** A reflex response consisting of inco-ordinated and convulsive muscular contractions. **Co-ordinated reflex.** A reflex resulting in an integrated, co-ordinated movement of several muscles. **Corneal reflex.** 1. Reflex blinking on touching the cornea; part of the protective mechanism of the eye and one of the last reflexes to disappear during induction of anaesthesia. 2. The reflection by the anterior corneal surface of any source of light in front of the eye. **Corneomandibular reflex, Corneopterygoid reflex.** With the subject's mouth open, one cornea is touched lightly; the lower jaw moves towards the opposite side. **Coronary reflex, Coronary artery reflex.** Alteration in the calibre of the coronary arteries as a result of nervous influences. Stimulation of the sympathetic nervous system is thought to dilate them, and of the parasympathetic to constrict them. **Corrective fusion reflex.** The reflex movement of one or other eye that takes place in heterophoria in order to maintain fusion. **Cough reflex.** That caused by irritation in the larynx. **Cranial reflex.** Any reflex whose pathway is mediated via cranial nerves. **Cremasteric reflex.** Stimulation of the skin on the anteromedial aspect of the male thigh causes retraction of the testis on the same side; the reflex is diminished or lost in pyramidal-tract disease. **Crossed reflex.** Consensual reflex (see above). **Crossed-extension reflex.** Extension of the opposite leg with plantar flexion during elicitation of an extensor-plantar response. **Cry reflex.** 1. A reflex present at birth in full-term infants, and absent in premature and immature infants, until maturity asserts itself. It is used in assessment of maturity in relation to the feeding of premature babies. 2. Spontaneous cry, during sleep, made by children suffering from tuberculous diseases of the joints, usually of the lower limbs, due to relaxation of muscle spasm, which exists during consciousness, so that areas of bone, denuded by disease of their protective cartilaginous covering, contact each other and a painful message is sent to the brain. **Cuboidodigital reflex.** Bechterew-Mendel reflex. **Cutaneous reflex.** Stimulation of the skin which causes wrinkling or goose flesh. **Cutaneous pupillary reflex.** Ciliospinal reflex (see above). **Dark reflex.** Dilatation of the pupil caused by alteration of the illumination from bright to one of low intensity or darkness; direct or consensual as in light reflex of which it is the converse. **Dartos reflex.** Application of cold to the perineum resulting in wormlike contraction of the dartos muscle. **Deep reflex, Deeper reflex.** Any reflex evoked by stimulation of a deeply situated structure; the term *deep reflex* is usually applied to the tendon reflexes to distinguish them from the superficial or cutaneous reflexes. **Defence reflex.** A protective reflex, e.g. withdrawal on painful stimulation. **Deflator reflexes.** Pulmonary receptors which on forcible deflation of the lungs result in stimulation of the inspiratory centre. They probably play no part in the regulation of normal quiet breathing. **Delayed reflex.** A reflex in which the response occurs an abnormally long time after the stimulus has been applied. **Depressor reflex.** 1. A reflex vasodilatation or fall in the arterial blood pressure; such a response can result from a variety of stimuli, particularly stimulation of the carotid sinus. 2. Reflex depression of motor activity. **Determinate reflex.** One in which response occurs at the site of stimulation. **Digital reflex.** 1. Tapping of the palmar aspect of the terminal phalanges of the fingers, when held slightly flexed, evoking reflex finger flexion; the finger jerk. 2. On snapping the terminal phalanx of the patient's middle finger, or on eliciting the finger jerk, sudden flexion of the terminal phalanx of the thumb occurs; also called

Hoffmann's reflex. Both the finger jerk and Hoffmann's reflex are evidence of increased neuromuscular excitability and if greatly exaggerated, or present on one side only, indicate pyramidal-tract disease. **Direct reflex.** A response occurring on the same side of the body as the stimulus. **Direct light reflex.** Light falling upon the retina which produces reflex contraction of the homolateral sphincter of the pupil and constriction of the pupil. **Doll's-head reflex.** In conjugate paralysis of the eyes, if the head is moved suddenly in the opposite direction to that of the paralysis, the eyes will rotate towards the paralysed side and then swing back again to their original position. **Dorsal reflex.** Contraction of the sacrospinalis and other muscles of the back, produced by stimulation of the overlying skin. **Dorsocuboidal reflex.** Bechterew-Mendel reflex. **Duodenal reflex.** Reflex tenderness produced by pinching the abdominal muscles directly above the umbilicus. **Elbow reflex, Elbow-jerk reflex.** Triceps reflex (see below). **Embrace reflex.** If an infant is laid on a table, striking the table on either side will cause the arms to be thrown out in an embracing attitude; also called *Moro's embrace reflex.* **Emergency light reflex.** When an excessive amount of light reaches the retina, in addition to constriction of the pupil, closure of the eyelids and lowering of the brow occurs. **Enterogastric reflex.** Inhibition of the vagus nerve by stimulation of receptors in the duodenum. **Epigastric reflex.** A movement simulating withdrawal which occurs in the epigastrium on stimulation of the skin of this region or in the area supplied by the 5th and 6th dorsal nerves in the axilla. **Erector-spinae reflex.** Dorsal reflex (see above). **Eyeball-compression reflex, Eyeball-heart reflex.** Oculocardiac reflex (see below). **Eyelash reflex.** Contraction of the eyelids caused by gentle touching of the eyelashes; the reflex disappears on entering the second stage of anaesthesia. **Eyelid reflex.** Contraction of the eyelids caused by gentle raising of the upper eyelid; the reflex disappears on entering the third stage of anaesthesia. **Eyelid-closure reflex.** The conjunctival reflex and the corneal reflex (see above). **Facial reflex.** Bulbomimic reflex (see above). **Fascial reflex.** A muscular contraction produced by tapping the fascia overlying the muscle. **Faucial reflex.** Gagging as a result of stimulation of the fauces. **Femoral reflex.** Extension of the knee and plantar flexion of the toes on stimulating the skin of the upper and anterior part of the thigh. **Finger-thumb reflex.** Flexion of the basal joint and extension of the terminal joint of the thumb caused by passive flexion of the metacarpophalangeal joint of one of the fingers; also called the *basal-joint reflex,* or *Meyer's reflex.* **Fixation reflex.** The reflex movement of the eyes that takes place when a light stimulus falls on the periphery of the retina, in order to bring this stimulus on to the fovea. **Fixation head-turning reflex.** In conjugate paralysis of the eyes, if the head is moved in the opposite direction to the paralysis, while an object straight ahead is fixated, the eyes will move towards the paralysed side. **Flexion reflex of leg.** Flexion of the leg induced by tapping the medial hamstring tendons. **Fontanelle reflex.** Gruenfelder's reflex. **Foot reflex.** If the foot is held in the dorsiflexed position, a sharp tap on the ball of the foot will produce reflex plantar flexion; this is simply another way of demonstrating the Achilles tendon reflex. **Foveolar reflex.** The spot of light which is seen in the centre of the macula on ophthalmoscopy, due to light reflection from the fovea centralis. **Front-tap reflex.** Contraction of the calf muscles when the stretched muscles over the front of the extended leg are percussed. **Gag reflex.** The closing of the glottis and the cessation of respiration evoked by stimulation of the sensory nerves of the mouth, pharynx, or larynx, either by the introduction of a solid or liquid or by the inspiration of irritating vapour. **Gastrocolic reflex.** Powerful contractions of the colon which propel its contents forwards when food enters the stomach. **Gastro-ileac reflex, Gastro-ileal reflex.** Contractions of the ileum together with opening of the ileocolic valve when food enters the stomach. **Genital reflex.** Reflex stimulation of the genital organs or their accessories by physiological or pathological processes. **Gluteal reflex.** Contraction of the gluteus muscles on stroking the overlying skin. **Grasp reflex, Grasping reflex.** Reflex grasping on stimulation of the palm of the hand, e.g. a finger which is touching the palm may be grasped firmly; seen in disease or injury of the prefrontal lobe. An analogous response may occur on stroking the sole of the foot. It is not only a pathological sign but is present at birth in all babies, whether mature or immature; it should disappear about 6 weeks after birth. **Great-toe reflex.** A generic term for all manoeuvres which produce reflex upward movement of the big toe in pyramidal lesions. **Gustatolacrimal reflex.** Lacrimation, in addition to salivation, on taking food, often seen after a damaged facial nerve has regenerated and probably due to crossed reinnervation; also called *the syndrome of crocodile tears.* **Heel-tap reflex.** An extensor-plantar response produced by tapping the heel; a method of evoking the Babinski response in a case of pyramidal-tract disease. **Hepatojugular reflex.** Pressure on the liver causing a rise in the cervical venous pressure in persons with congestive failure of the right ventricle. **Humoral reflex.** Symptoms produced by the transmission of chemical substances such as hormones in the blood, and not through nervous channels. **Hypochondrial reflex.** A sudden inspiration caused by a quick thrust beneath the costal margin. **Hypogastric reflex.** Bechterew's reflex. **Hypothenar reflex.** Pressure on the pisiform bone produces contraction of the palmaris brevis muscle. **Ileogastric reflex.** Gastro-ileal reflex (see above). **Inborn reflex.** A reflex that is an essential property of the untrained nervous system and is common to all members of a species; an unconditioned reflex. **Indirect reflex.** A consensual or crossed reflex (see above). **Indirect light reflex.** Consensual light reflex (see above). **Infraspinatus reflex.** Tapping of the tendon of the infraspinatus muscle produces lateral rotation of the arm and extension at the elbow joint. **Inguinal reflex.** Geigel's reflex. **Intercoronary reflex.** Alteration in the lumen of coronary arteries as a result of reflexes arising within the heart or coronary vessels. Clear-cut evidence of the existence of these reflexes is wanting. **Interscapular reflex.** A stimulus applied to the back in the midline between the scapulae may cause contraction of the rhomboids and approximation of the scapulae. **Intestinal reflex.** Myenteric reflex (see below). **Inverted radial reflex.** No contraction of the brachioradialis muscle occurs on tapping its tendon, but finger flexion is produced. This reflex is due to disease of the 5th cervical segment of the spinal cord, affecting the anterior horn cells and so causing absence of the normal radial reflex, but also affecting the pyramidal tract to give abnormal activity of reflexes mediated by lower segments. **Iris-contraction reflex.** Pupillary reflex (see below). **Irritant vapour reflex.** Slowing of the heart produced by inhalation of an irritant vapour, through stimulation of the nasal branches of the 5th cranial nerve. Respiration may be inhibited similarly. **Jaw-jerk reflex.** Chin reflex (see above). **Knee-jerk reflex.** Patellar reflex (see below). **Labyrinthine reflex.** Any reflex response to stimulation of the vestibular apparatus. **Landau reflex.** With the infant prone, neck and hips extended, the body forms a convex arc; gentle pressure on the head or neck flexes it, the lower extremities drop and the arc is reversed. **Laryngeal cough reflex.** A cough produced by irritation of the fauces and larynx; a protective mechanism. **Laughter reflex.** That resulting from tickling. **Lid reflex.** Westphal-Pilcz reaction. **Light reflex.** 1. Of the tympanic membrane; the triangular cone of light that in the normal drum has its apex at the lower tip of the malleus (or umbo) and its base at the periphery of the drum about 5 o'clock; it is an optical phenomenon resulting from the concave nature of the drum head. 2. Of the retina; the circular area of light reflected from the retina during ophthalmoscopy. 3. Of the pupil; contraction of the pupil when the eye is exposed to a bright light. *See also* CONSENSUAL LIGHT REFLEX, DIRECT LIGHT REFLEX (above). **Lip reflex.** Movement of the lips in sleeping infants, which may be spontaneous or elicited by a sudden tap over the angle of the mouth. **Long-circuit reflex.** A long reflex arc with its centre in the brain or brain stem. **Lumbar reflex.** Dorsal reflex (see above). **Lung reflex.** Dilatation of the underlying lung tissue caused by irritation of the skin by percussion or cold. **Macular reflex.** The circle of reflected light seen around the edge of the macula on ophthalmoscopy. **Mandibular reflex.** Chin reflex (see above). **Mass reflex.** In a patient with complete transection of the spinal cord, whether due to trauma or to disease, stimulation below the level of the lesion produces a complex reflex response, including flexion of the legs, evacuation of the bladder and bowels, and profuse sweating below the level of the lesion. **Middle-ear-disease reflex.** The reaction of adults and children (as manifested by a rise in temperature) seems to vary in the less virulent forms of inflammation of the middle-ear cleft. This is thought to be a reflex disturbance reflecting the individual differences in the stability of the central nervous system. **Motor reflex.** A reflex produced by direct stimulation of the peripheral effector nerve-endings; e.g. contraction of a muscle evoked by irritation or stimulation of the muscle. **Muscle-tendon reflex, Muscular reflex.** Stretch reflex (see below). **Myenteric reflex.** On stimulation of an intestinal segment, the segment above contracts and that below relaxes. **Myotatic reflex.** Stretch reflex (see below). **Nasal reflex.** Irritation of the nasal lining producing sneezing. **Nasomental reflex.** Tapping of the side of the nose causing contraction of the mentalis muscle. **Naso-ocular reflex.** Flushing of the conjunctiva on stimulation of the nasal mucous membrane. **Near reflex.** One consisting of three synergic reflex actions taking place on myopia and equally in both eyes. These are contraction of the pupil, accommodation, and convergence. **Nociceptive reflex.** A reflex elicited by a pain stimulus. **Nostril reflex.** In pulmonary disease the anterior naris on the side of the disease is reduced in size. **Obliquus reflex.** Stroking the skin below the inguinal ligament, particularly its lateral portion, induces contraction of the homolateral external oblique muscle. **Oculocardiac reflex.** Aschner's phenomenon; a reflex slowing of the heart due to pressure on the eyball. It is mediated through the connection of the sensory nucleus of the trigeminal nerve with the nucleus of the vagus nerve, stimulation of which slows the heart, and is sometimes deliberately induced to terminate attacks of paroxysmal supraventricular tachycardia. **Oculocephalogyric reflex.** The physiological reflex whereby the head, body, and eyes are directed towards the point which is engaging the subject's attention. **Oculopharyngeal reflex.** Spontaneous closing of the eyes and rapid movements of deglutition produced by stimulation of the conjunctiva of the bulb. **Oculopupillary reflex, Oculosensory reflex.** On tactile or thermal stimulation of the eyelids, cornea, or conjunctiva, the pupil dilates slightly at first and then contracts. **Oesophagosalivary reflex.** Salivation following irritation of the oesophagus. **Ophthalmic reflex.** McCarthy's reflex. **Optical-blinking reflex.** Reflex blinking caused by a bright light or by some object being brought close to the eye. **Opticofacial winking reflex.** The protective closure of the eyelids when an object is brought suddenly into the field of vision; also called *winking reflex.* **Orbicularis reflex.** Westphal-Pilcz reaction. **Orthocardiac reflex.** A compensatory reflex to ensure an adequate venous return to the heart in the erect position: the blood pressure rises slightly owing to reflex vasoconstriction and prevents pooling of blood in the lower limbs. In spite of this, the cardiac output falls slightly in the erect position. **Palatal reflex, Palatine reflex.** 1. Swallowing on stimulation of the palate. 2. Elevation of the soft palate when it is touched. **Palmar reflex.** Stimulation of the palm of the hand causing flexion of the fingers. **Palm-chin reflex, Palmomental reflex.** Vigorous stroking or scratching of the thenar eminence producing contraction of chin and lower lip muscles on the same side, often with dimpling; said to be exaggerated in pyramidal-tract disease. **Paradoxical ankle reflex.** Plantar flexion of the foot upon percussion of the dorsal surface of the ankle joint. **Paradoxical flexor reflex.** Gordon's reflex. **Paradoxical patellar reflex.** 1. With the patient supine and the knee extended, a tap on the patellar tendon may cause contraction of the adductor muscles. 2. Sudden forcible flexion of the knee may cause reflex extension, owing to stretching of the patellar tendon; this is an elaboration of the knee jerk. **Paradoxical pupillary reflex.** Dilatation of the pupil when light falls on the retina, occasionally seen in early cases of tabes or GPI; also called *Bechterew's reflex.* **Patellar reflex.** On tapping the patellar tendon which is stretched passively, contraction of the quadriceps femoris muscle and extension at the knee joint occur; the knee jerk. **Patellar tendon reflex.** Patellar reflex (see above). **Patello-adductor reflex.** Contraction of the contralateral adductor muscles on eliciting the knee jerk; also called *MacCormac's reflex.* **Pathic reflex.** Reflex muscular action in response to stimulation of a sensory nerve. [obsolete term.] **Pathological reflex.** A reflex resulting from organic disease of the nervous system. **Pectoral reflex.** Adduction and internal rotation of the arm due to contraction of the pectoralis muscles on percussion over the humerus at the point of insertion of the pectoralis major muscle. **Penile reflex, Penis reflex.** Bulbospongiosus reflex (see above). **Perception reflex.** Reflex motor activity resulting from conscious perception. **Periosteal reflex.** Many of the muscle tendon reflexes (e.g. the knee jerk) were once considered to result from stimulation of the periosteum, but it is now realized that they are due to stretching of muscle tendons as they become inserted into the periosteum and bone. **Peroneal reflex.** When the peroneal muscles are stretched, by passive inversion of the foot, a blow over the muscles will produce reflex contraction and eversion of the foot. **Pharyngeal reflex.** Contraction of the pharyngeal muscles associated with gagging, due to stimulation of the pharyngeal mucosa. **Phasic reflex.** Co-ordinated reflex (see above). **Pilomotor reflex.** Erection of the dermal papillae (goose flesh) on stroking the skin or on exposure to cold or emotional stimuli. **Placing reflex.** If the dorsum of the foot of a young infant is drawn against the underside of a table top, the foot is placed on top of the table. **Plantar reflex.** In normal subjects over the age of one year, stroking the lateral aspect of the sole of the foot will induce flexion of all toes, the flexor-plantar response. In pyramidal-tract disease an extensor response (the Babinski reflex) ensues. **Plasticity reflex.** The reflex maintenance by a rigid limb of passively imposed posture. **Platysmal reflex.** Constriction of the ipselateral pupil on nipping the platysma; the effect is opposite to that observed in the ciliospinal reflex (see above). **Pneocardiac reflex.** Irritant vapour reflex (see above). **Pneopneic reflex.** Alteration of the respiratory rhythm on introducing an irritating gas into the air passages. **Postural reflex.** Any of the numerous reflexes concerned in the maintenance of posture. **Pressor reflex.** An increase in the arterial blood pressure occurring as a reflex response to a variety of stimuli and mediated via vasomotor nerves. **Proprioceptive reflex.** Reflex muscular activity occurring in response to afferent stimuli of proprioceptive type; one form of postural reflex, concerned with maintenance or alteration of position. **Protective reflex.** Any physiological reflex that results in protection from immediate threatened danger, e.g. blinking reflex. **Psychic reflex.** A reflex of which the afferent part is mentally initiated. **Psychocardiac reflex.** The quickening of the heart beat from emotional cause. **Psychogalvanic reflex.** The change in electrical resistance of the skin following on emotional activity. **Pterygocorneal reflex.** Corneomandibular reflex (see above). **Pulmonary reflex.** Hering-Breuer reflex. **Pupillary reflex.** 1. Pupillary constriction when light falls on the retina of the same eye; the light reflex. 2. Constriction of the pupil when light falls on the opposite retina; the consensual light reflex. 3. Constriction on convergence and dilatation on divergence of the eyes; usually called the *near reflex.* 4. Constriction of the pupil when the patient attempts to close the eyes; also called *Westphal's pupillary reaction, Westphal-Pilcz reaction.* **Purposive reflex.** One designed to protect the individual generally, e.g. the curling up of the hedgehog. **Quadriceps reflex.** Patellar reflex (see above). **Quadripedal extensor reflex.** Brain's reflex; when a patient with a hemiplegia assumes the "all fours" position, the flexed arm extends reflexly. **Radial reflex.** Contraction of the brachioradialis muscle, causing flexion of the elbow joint, on tapping the point of insertion of the muscle into the lateral aspect of the lower end of the radius. **Red reflex.** The red light seen in the pupil of the eye during ophthalmoscopy or retinoscopy, caused by the reflection of light by the vascular choroid. **Regional reflex.** Segmental reflex (see below).

Renorenal reflex. A disturbance of the contralateral or sound kidney in unilateral renal disease, which may be accompanied by severe contralateral renal pain or anuria. **Resistance reflex.** Babinski reflex. **Retrobulbar pupillary reflex.** The unsustained light reaction of the semi-dilated pupil of retrobulbar (optic) neuritis. **Righting reflexes.** Reflexes by which correct posture is restored. **Rooting reflex.** Stimulating an infant's cheek causes turning of the head to that side. **Scapular reflex.** Interscapular reflex (see above). **Scapulohumeral reflex, Scapuloperiosteal reflex.** Adduction and lateral rotation of the arm due to contraction of the subscapularis muscle, when the medial border of the scapular is percussed. **Scratch reflex.** The action of scratching that is precipitated by tickling or touching the skin. **Scrotal reflex.** Dartos reflex (see above). **Segmental reflex.** A reflex whose pathway involves a single segment of the spinal cord. **Sensory blinking reflex.** Reflex blinking taking place on any irritative stimulation of the cornea, conjunctiva, or lashes, e.g. corneal reflex (see above). **Sexual reflex.** Erection of the genitalia and subsequent orgasm and/or ejaculation as a result of erotic stimulation. **Simple reflex.** A reflex whose motor component may involve only a single muscle. **Skin reflex.** Platysmal reflex (see above). **Skin pupillary reflex.** Ciliospinal reflex (see above). **Sneezing reflex.** Nasal reflex (see above). **Sole reflex.** Plantar reflex (see above). **Spinal reflex.** Any reflex whose pathway involves the spinal cord but not the brain. **Startle reflex.** Movements of the head and limbs as a result of sudden noise or bright light affecting a full-term infant. Premature and immature infants may show no such response. **Static reflex.** Reflex maintenance of stance. **Statokinetic reflex.** Any reflex that controls the posture of the body in movement. **Stepping reflex.** If the soles of a young infant's feet are placed on a table with the infant upright, he steps in primitive walking. **Stretch reflex.** Reflex contraction of a muscle when it is stretched due to stimulation of proprioceptive receptors in the muscle; tendon reflexes are due to this mechanism. **Sucking reflex.** Stroking the lips of an infant produces sucking. **Summation reflex.** A reflex produced by the combined or summated effect of several nerve impulses. **Superficial reflex.** Any reflex produced by superficial stimulation, e.g. the abdominal and cremasteric reflexes (see above). **Supinator jerk reflex, Supinator longus reflex.** Radial reflex (see above). **Supra-orbital reflex.** McCarthy's reflex. **Suprapatellar reflex.** When a finger is placed along the upper border of the patella and is percussed sharply, reflex contraction of the quadriceps femoris muscle results; a variation of the patellar reflex. **Suprapubic reflex.** Stroking the abdominal wall in a lower and outer quadrant causing deviation of the linea alba to the stimulated side; the lower abdominal reflex. **Supra-umbilical reflex.** Epigastric reflex (see above); the upper abdominal reflex. **Swallowing reflex.** The successive reflexes concerned in the mechanism of swallowing; the sequence is initiated when food reaches the palate or the pharynx. **Tactile reflex.** Any reflex caused by stimulation of the tactile end-organs. **Tarsophalangeal reflex.** Plantar flexion of the toes as a result of a tap on the dorsum of the foot. **Tendon reflex.** Any reflex muscular contraction in response to lengthening of the muscle as a result of a tap upon the tendon of insertion; *see* STRETCH REFLEX (above). **Testicular-compression reflex.** Kocher's reflex. **Threat reflex.** Involuntary closure of the eyes upon a threatening gesture towards the face. **Tibio-abductor reflex.** A tap on the medial aspect of the tibia causing either abduction of the stimulated leg or adduction of the contralateral leg. **Toe reflex.** In spastic paralysis forceful plantar flexion of the big toes causing spontaneous flexion of all other joints in the lower extremity concerned. **Tonic reflex.** A sustained reflex. **Tonic neck reflex.** The head of a young infant, or of an older child with cerebral damage, is turned to one side with the trunk lying supine; the limbs on that side may flex while the limbs on the opposite side may extend. **Traction reflexes.** Reflex contraction of the muscles of the anterior abdominal wall and of the larynx in response to traction on the mesentery, peritoneum or other viscus; seen during anaesthesia. **Triceps reflex.** Extension at the elbow joint induced by tapping the triceps tendon near its insertion into the olecranon, with the elbow held semiflexed. **Trigeminal reflex.** Oculopupillary reflex (see above). **Trigeminocervical reflex.** Reflex contraction of the neck muscles on tapping the skin in the distribution of the homolateral trigeminal nerve. **Ulnar reflex.** Pronation of the forearm and adduction of the hand induced by percussion over the distal end of the ulna. **Unconditioned reflex.** An inborn reflex common to all members of a species. **Urinary reflex.** Bladder reflex (see above). **Vagal reflex.** The nerve reflex that ensues upon stimulation of any of the receptor areas serving the vagal tone control of heart beat and respiration. Stimulation causes slowing, or arrest, of the heart beat or respiration. A cause of sudden death during operative or anaesthetic, or other, procedures in the sensitive areas—throat, glottis, vagal sheath, pleura, peritoneum, cervix uteri. **Vagotonic pupillary reflex.** Dilatation of the pupil occurring on deep inspiration, and contraction with deep expiration. **Vagus reflex.** Increased sensitivity to pressure over the vagus nerve when the lung is tuberculous. **Vascular reflex, Vasomotor reflex.** A reflex response of the vascular system. **Vasopressor reflex.** Reflex rise of blood pressure, usually associated with vasoconstriction. **Vasovagal reflex.** A stimulation of the vagus nerve through one of its many receptors, causing slowing or arrest of heart and respiratory rhythm. Sensitive areas are throat, glottis, vagal sheath, pleural or peritoneal membranes, visceral form or tension, urethra, cervix uteri. A cause of sudden death without trace. **Vesical reflex.** The urge to urinate set up by distension of the bladder. **Vestibulo-ocular reflex.** Reflex movement of the eyes induced by stimulation of the semicircular canals. **Virile reflex.** Contraction of the bulbospongiosus muscle in response to stimulation of the glans penis (Hughes' reflex). **Visceral reflex.** A reflex of a viscus. **Viscerocardiac reflex.** Reflex slowing of the heart mediated through the vagus nerve, resulting from visceral stimulation. **Visceromotor reflex.** Muscular contraction of the abdominal wall resulting from visceral pain. **Viscerosensory reflex.** Referred tenderness of an area of skin due to disease of an internal organ. **Viscerotrophic reflex.** Referred trophic changes in the skin due to disease of an internal organ. **Visuocortical reflex.** Focusing attention on a bright surface causes contraction of the pupil, while a dark surface causes dilatation. It is carried out in a dark room, but even then it is difficult to exclude the effect of the light and near reflex. Described by Haab. **Vomiting reflex.** Vomiting induced by the touching of the mucous membrane of the throat. **Winking reflex.** Opticofacial winking reflex (see above). **Wrist clonus reflex.** Clonus produced by hyperextension at the wrist joint. **Zygomatic reflex.** Percussion over the zygoma may produce lateral movement of the lower jaw to the same side. [L *reflectere* to bend back.]

See also: ABRAMS, ARGYLL ROBERTSON, ASCHNER, BABINSKI, BAINBRIDGE, BARKMAN, BECHTEREW, BRAIN, BREUER, BRISSAUD, BUZZARD, CAPPS, CHADDOCK, DAVIDSOHN, ERBEN, ESCHERICH, GAULT, GEIGEL, GIFFORD, GONDA, GORDON (A.), GOWERS, GRUENFELDER, HENNEBERG, HERING (K. E. K.), HIRSCHBERG (L. K.), HOFFMANN (J.), HUGHES (C. H.), JACOBSOHN, JOFFROY, JUSTER, KEHRER (F. A.), KISCH, KOCHER, LIDDELL, LOVÉN, LUST, MCCARTHY (D. J.), MacCORMAC, MAGNUS, MAREY, MAYER (K.), MENDEL (K.), MONDONESI, MORO, ONANOFF, OPPENHEIM (H.), PHILIPSON, PILCZ (A.), PILCZ (J.), PREYER, PUUSSEPP, REMAK (E. J.), RIDDOCH, ROGER (G. H.), ROSSOLIMO, RUGGERI, SCHAEFFER, SHERRINGTON, SNELLEN, SOMAGYI, STOOKEY, STRUEMPELL, THROCKMORTON, WEISS (L.), WERNICKE (K.), WESTPHAL (A. K. O.), WHYTT.

reflexogenic (re·flex·o·**jen**'·ik). Producing, causing, or intensifying reflex action. [reflex, Gk *genein* to produce.]

reflexograph (re·**flex**·o·graf). An apparatus designed to time and record reflexes such as knee jerks. [reflex, Gk *graphein* to write.]

reflexometer (re·flex·**om**·et·er). An apparatus for measuring the stretching force required to produce a muscular contraction, or any device which measures the force necessary to evoke a reflex.

reflexophil, reflexophile (re·**flex**·o·fil, re·**flex**·o·file). Having exaggerated reflex activity. [reflex, Gk *philein* to love.]

reflux (re·flux). A backward flow; regurgitation. **Biliary reflux.** Reflux of bile from the common bile duct into the pancreatic duct. **Chylous reflux.** Retrograde flow of chyle from lacteals of mesentery into serous cavities with production of chyloperitoneum and chylothorax, into internal organs such as the bladder, or into the skin with the production of chylous blisters and fistulae. **Ureteric reflux.** Reflux of urine from the bladder into the ureters during micturition. **Urethrovesiculodifferential reflux.** The movement of an injected or liquid substance or seminal fluid from the prostatic part of the urethra into the genital canal. **Vesico-ureteric reflux.** Reflux of urine from the bladder up a ureter during the act of micturition. [L *refluere* to flow back.]

refract (re·**frakt**). 1. To deflect or deviate, e.g. a ray of light. 2. To determine refractive errors of the eye. [see foll.]

refraction (re·**frak**·shun). 1. The bending or deviation of electromagnetic radiation in passing obliquely from one transparent medium to another of different density; the ray before refraction is called the *incident ray,* and after refraction, the *refracted ray.* 2. In ophthalmology, the process of testing the eyes by various methods, both objective and subjective, in an attempt to estimate the refractive errors present and with a view to the correction of these with glasses if necessary. **Atmospheric refraction.** Rays of light are bent when they pass through areas of gas of different densities. This may cause apparent elevation (*superior mirage*) or lowering (*inferior mirage*) of the object; *looming, towering* and *stooping* are other terms used to describe these mirages. **Atomic refraction.** The product of the specific refraction and the atomic weight. **Double refraction.** The splitting of the incident ray (*see* MAIN DEF. 1 above) by refraction into two rays, thus producing two images. Light passed through Iceland spar shows double refraction. **Dynamic refraction.** That carried out when the eyes are in a state of active accommodation and convergence. Retinoscopy, with the patient fixing an object on the instrument, is the usual method employed. **Index of refraction.** Refractive index. *See* INDEX. **Refraction of light.** The alteration in the velocity of light when it passes from one transparent medium into another; this causes the rays to become bent, the amount of bending depending upon the difference in refractive indices. **Molecular refraction.** The product of the specific refraction and the molecular weight; the molecular refraction of a substance can be obtained roughly by adding the atomic refractions of the atoms composing the molecule. **Specific refraction.** For a gas of density ρ and refractive index μ, the ratio $(\mu-1)/\rho$, or more accurately $(\mu^2-1)/(\mu^2+2)\rho$, which is a constant for any particular substance at a given temperature. **Static refraction.** That carried out when the accommodation of the eyes is in a state of relaxation, either by the use of cycloplegics, or by the patient fixing a distant object. This is the method in common use. [L *refringere* to break apart.]

refractionist (re·**frak**·shun·ist). One who is expert in measuring the power of ocular refraction and in correcting any refractive errors.

refractionometer (re·frak·shun·**om**′·et·er). Refractometer.

refractive (re·**frak**·tiv). 1. Relating or belonging to refraction. 2. Having the capacity to refract, or instrumental in the process of refraction.

refractivity (re·frak·**tiv**·it·e). In optics, the quality of being refractive, power of refraction; the ability to refract.

refractometer (re·frak·**tom**·et·er). An instrument for measuring the refractive index of different substances in the form of a solid, liquid, or gas.

See also: JAMIN, PULFRICH, RAYLEIGH.

refractometry (re·frak·**tom**·et·re). Determination of the power of refraction by means of the refractometer.

refractory (re·**frak**·tor·e). 1. Obstinately resistant to the effects of treatment. 2. Indicating a slow or negative reaction to any physical, chemical, or other force or stimulus. [L *refringere* to break apart.]

refractoscope (re·**frak**·to·skope). An instrument used in auscultation by which a sound can be focused and localized. [refraction, Gk *skopein* to watch.]

refracture (re·**frak**·tewr). The surgical rebreaking of a formerly fractured bone in which there is faulty union and deformity, the aim being to correct the deformity. [L *refringere* to break apart.]

refrangibility (re·fran·jib·**il**′·it·e). The quality or capability of being refrangible.

refrangible (re·**fran**·jibl). Having the capacity to be refracted.

refresh (re·**fresh**). To remove the granulations and ingrowing epithelium of the edges of a wound, thus making them raw again for resuture. [OFr. *refrescher.*]

refrigerant (re·**frij**·er·ant). A medium which cools, particularly as applied to liquids which are usually circulated through the heat exchanger of a cold store, domestic refrigerator, etc. [L *refrigerare* to make cool.]

refrigeration (re·frij·er·**a**′·shun). 1. Cooling. 2. The act of lowering the temperature as a form of treatment, e.g. by immersion in cold water. 2. The production of cold in a body by reducing the temperature and conveying away its heat. [L *refrigerare* to make cool.]

refringent (re·**frin**·jent). Refractive.

Refsum, Sigvald. 20th century Norwegian physician.

Refsum's disease. A heredodegenerative disorder characterized by progressive nerve deafness, cerebellar ataxia, peripheral neuropathy, and often pigmentary changes in the retina.

refusion (re·**few**·zhun). The act of withdrawing blood and subsequently returning it to the circulation. [L *refundere* to pour back.]

regard (re·**gard**). Gaze; a directed look, with attention. **Plane of regard.** The plane which passes through the point of regard and the centre of rotation of the eye. **Point of regard.** The point towards which the eye is looking. [Fr. *regarder* to look at.]

Regaud, Claude (b. 1870). French radiologist.

Regaud's fixing fluid. A solution of potassium bichromate and formalin in water; used for the preservation of mitochondria in cells.

Regaud and Lacassagne technique for cancer of the cervix uteri. The treatment of carcinoma of the neck of the uterus by means of uterine radium tubes and vaginal cork containers retained by a colpostat, using relatively small quantities of radium and continuous irradiation for 5 days. Also known as *Paris technique.*

regenerate (re·**jen**·er·ate). 1. To generate again; to reproduce. 2. To renew; to reinvigorate. [L *re-*, *generare* to produce.]

regeneration (re·jen·er·**a**′·shun). The repair or reproduction of tissue or of a part which has been damaged. [see prec.]

regimen (**rej**·im·en). Prescribed rules regulating the mode of life, especially as regards diet, rest, exercise, sleep, etc. **Regimen sanitatis salernitanum.** A famous medical work written in verse, the product of the Salerno school in the 12th century. [L, rule.]

region (**re**·jun). 1. [Regio (NA)] A part or division of the body, either well- or ill-defined, usually named after some prominent anatomical feature within the region. 2. A geographical region. **Abdominal region [regio abdominalis (NA)].** Any one of the nine regions into which the abdomen may be divided by the two midclavicular planes and the subcostal (or, sometimes, transpyloric) and intercristal planes. From above down they are the left hypochondriac, epigastric, and right hypochondriac regions; the left lumbar, umbilical, and right lumbar regions; the left inguinal, pubic, and right inguinal regions. **Abdominal region, lateral [regio lateralis (dextra et sinistra) NA].** The side of the trunk. **Anal region [regio analis (NA)].** The part of the perineum posterior to a line joining the front of the two ischial tuberosities. **Antebrachial region, anterior [regio antebrachii anterior (NA)].** The front of the forearm. **Antebrachial region, posterior [regio antebrachii posterior (NA)].** The inner aspect of the forearm. **Antebrachial ulnar region.** Antebrachial region, posterior (see above). **Antebrachial volar region.** Antebrachial region, anterior (see above). **Axillary region [regio axillaris (NA)].** The region of the armpit. **Basilar region.** The part of the base of the skull anterior to the foramen magnum. **Brachial**

region, anterior **[regio brachii anterior (NA)].** The front of the arm. **Brachial region, posterior [regio brachii posterior (NA)].** The back of the arm. **Buccal region [regio buccalis (NA)].** The cheek area of the face. **Calcanean region [regio calcanea (NA)].** The heel. **Cervical region, anterior [regio colli anterior (NA)].** The front of the neck. **Cervical region, lateral [regio colli lateralis (NA)].** The lateral part of the neck behind the sternocleidomastoid muscle. **Ciliary region.** The part of the eye occupied by the ciliary body and muscle. **Crural region, anterior [regio cruris anterior (NA)].** The front of the leg. **Crural region, posterior [regio cruris posterior (NA)].** The back of the leg. **Cubital region, anterior [regio cubiti anterior (NA)].** The front of the elbow. **Cubital region, posterior [regio cubiti posterior (NA)].** The back of the elbow. **Deltoid region [regio deltoidea (NA)].** The area over and deep to the deltoid muscle. **Digital volar region.** The palmar aspect of the fingers. **Epencephalic region.** The alar plate of the developing neural tube. **Epigastric region [regio epigastrica (NA)].** The region of the abdomen between the right and left lateral planes and above the transpyloric plane. **Extrapolar region.** That part of the body not affected by the current from the electrodes during electrical treatment. **Femoral region.** The thigh. **Femoral region, anterior [regio femoris anterior (NA)].** The front of the thigh. **Femoral region, posterior [regio femoris posterior (NA)].** The back of the thigh. **Frontal region [regio frontalis (NA)].** The region of the forehead. **Genito-urinary region.** Urogenital triangle. *See* TRIANGLE. **Gluteal region [regio glutea (NA)].** The buttock. **Hypencephalic region.** The basal plate of the developing neural tube. **Hypochondriac regions, right and left [regio hypochondriaca (dextra et sinistra) NA].** The regions of the front of the trunk and abdominal cavity below the mammary region, lateral to the lateral planes and above the transpyloric plane. They lie in front of the axillary lines. **Hypogastric region.** Pubic region (see below). **Iliac regions.** Inguinal regions (see below). **Infraclavicular region [regio infraclavicularis (NA)].** The hollow below the clavicle. **Inframammary region.** The part of the chest wall directly below the breast. **Infra-orbital region [regio infraorbitalis (NA)].** The region of the face immediately below the eye. **Infrared region.** The region of the spectrum of radiation between the visible red and microwave regions of the electromagnetic spectrum, covering a wavelength range of approximately 1000 nm to 1 mm. **Infrascapular region [regio infrascapularis (NA)].** The part of the chest wall below the inferior angle of the scapula. **Infraspinous region.** The area below the spine of the scapula. **Infratemporal region [regio infratemporalis (NA)]. Inguinal regions, right and left [regio inguinalis (dextra et sinistra) NA].** The groin. **Ischiorectal region.** The area overlying the ischiorectal fossa. **Region of the knee, anterior [regio genus anterior (NA)].** The front of the knee. **Region of the knee, posterior [regio genus posterior (NA)].** The back of the knee. **Lumbar regions, right and left [regio lumbalis (NA)].** The loins; the regions between the costal margin and iliac crests and extending from the lateral borders of the vertebral column to the axillary lines. **Mammary region [regio mammaria (NA)].** The part of the chest occupied by the breast. **Mental region [regio mentalis (NA)].** The area between the lower lip and the chin margin. **Motor region.** The posterior part of the precentral area of the brain, controlling volitional movements. **Nasal region [regio nasalis (NA)].** The front of the face, the nose and its immediate surroundings. **Nuchal region [regio colli posterior (NA)].** The region of the neck behind the posterior triangle and related to the trapezius muscle. **Occipital region [regio occipitalis (NA)].** The part of the scalp overlying the occipital bone. **Olecranal region.** The point of the elbow. **Olfactory region of the mucous membrane of the nose [regio olfactoria tunicae mucosae nasi (NA)].** The thickened portion of mucous membrane, lying in the olfactory region of the nose, which is concerned with the perception of odours. It is innervated by the first cranial (olfactory) nerve. **Oral region [regio oralis (NA)].** The region round the mouth. **Orbital region [regio orbitalis (NA)].** The region of the face round the eye. **Parietal region [regio parietalis (NA)].** The region of the head overlying the parietal bone. **Parotideomasseteric region [regio parotideomasseterica (NA)].** The posterior part of the face, over the masseter muscle and the parotid gland. **Popliteal region.** The back of the knee. **Precordial region.** The part of the anterior chest wall overlying the heart. **Prefrontal region.** The part of the frontal lobe of the cerebrum anterior to the motor and premotor cortex; sometimes restricted to the rostral extremity of the lobe. **Pretectal region.** Part of the mid-brain deep to the upper part of the superior quadrigeminal body. **Pterygoid region.** The region of the face over the pterygoid muscles. **Pubic region [regio pubica (NA)].** The region of the abdomen between the right and left lateral planes and below the intertubercular plane. **Respiratory region [regio respiratoria (NA)].** The greater part of the nasal cavity, excluding only the olfactory region. **Rolandic region.** Motor region (see above). **Sacral region [regio sacralis (NA)].** The region of the trunk related to the sacrum. **Sacrococcygeal region.** Sacral region (see prec.). **Satellite region.** The satellite and the secondary constriction which separate it from the rest of the chromosome. **Scapular region [regio scapularis (NA)].** The region of the trunk related to the scapula. **Sensory region.** Postcentral area. *See* AREA. **Regions of the spinal cord.** The five divisions (cervical, thoracic, lumbar, sacral, and coccygeal) corresponding to the nerves given off. **Sternocleidomastoid region [regio sternocleidomastoidea (NA)].** The part of the neck over and under the sternocleidomastoid muscle. **Subicular region.** The subiculum. **Submandibular region.** The region immediately beneath the jaw on either side. **Submaxillary region.** The undersurface of the chin lateral to the mental and submental regions. **Submental region.** The area of the chin overlying the submental triangle. **Subthalamic region.** The forward extension of the tegmentum beneath the posterior part of the thalamus. **Superior maxillary region.** The part of the face between the upper lip and the orbits. **Supraclavicular region.** The hollow above the clavicle on each side. **Suprapubic region.** Pubic region (see above). **Supraspinous region.** The area of the back overlying the upper part of the scapula, above the spine. **Suprasternal region.** The hollow in the midline of the neck above the suprasternal notch. **Tegmental region.** The part of the mid-brain dorsal to the paired substantia nigra, ventral to the aqueduct of the mid-brain. **Temporal region [regio temporalis (NA)].** The region of the temples. **Trabecular region.** The longitudinal strip of mesenchyme and cartilage giving rise to the body of the sphenoid bone. **Umbilical region [regio umbilicalis (NA)].** The region of the abdomen bounded by the right and left lateral planes, the transpyloric plane, and the intertubercular plane. **Vertebral region [regio vertebralis (NA)].** The region of the trunk related to the vertebral column. **Volar region of the hand.** The palmar aspect of the hand. **Zygomatic region [regio zygomatica (NA)].** The part of the face over the zygomatic bone. [L *regio*.]

See also: BROCA, GEIGER, MUELLER (W.).

regional (re·jun·al). Relating or belonging to a region.

regression (re·gresh·un). 1. A turning back, reverting to a former condition; the disappearance of the symptoms or signs of a disease. 2. Reversion to an earlier stage; in psycho-analysis, the return of the libido to infantile aims. 3. The tendency of the offspring of extreme parents to be less extreme. *See* GALTON'S LAW. 4. In statistics, the trend for a group, reduced as regards a particular quality to a common standard of comparison or to a mean, to have a mean value approximating to the general mean in a related quality. [L *regredi* to go back.]

regressive (re·gres·iv). 1. Pertaining to regression, or characterized by it. 2. Relapsing. 3. Of symptoms, abating. [see prec.]

regular (reg·ew·lar). 1. Orderly. 2. Constant or habitual. 3. Typical. 4. Having menstrual periods at normal intervals. [see foll.]

regulation (reg·ew·la·shun). 1. The process of adjustment to an accepted level or standard. 2. The adjustment of behaviour or the physical arrangement of an organism to altered conditions. [L *regula* rule.]

regulator (reg·ew·la·tor). 1. A device for regulating the passage or flow of air, blood, water, etc. 2. In genetics, a gene that codes for the production of a regulatory macromolecule which is often a repressor protein and is functional when it binds to an operator gene. **Regulator sites.** A name given to the chemical groups on enzymes through which cell metabolites and other molecules regulate the catalytic activity of enzymes. *Regulator* sites are to be distinguished from *catalytic* or *active* sites, which are the chemical groups which effect catalysis. [L *regula* rule.]

See also: KEKWICK, MARRIOTT (H. L.).

regulus (reg·ew·lus). 1. The metal or metallic alloy obtained when an ore is reduced. 2. A metallic-like compound of sulphur which arises in the smelting of certain metals. The name is alchemical in origin and was originally applied to antimony which alloyed with gold. **Regulus of antimony.** Crude metallic antimony. **Regulus of Venus.** An alloy of copper and antimony. [L *regulus* little king.]

regurgitant (re·ger·jit·ant). Flowing or throwing backwards or in a direction opposite to the normal direction. [L *re-*, *gurgitare* to flow.]

regurgitation (re·ger·jit·a'·shun). 1. The return of swallowed food into the mouth as occurs with oesophageal obstruction and pharyngeal diverticula. It may also occur in certain forms of dyspepsia and be associated with flatulence due to air swallowing. 2. The passive flow of liquid from the stomach or oesophagus into the pharynx in the absence of vomiting. 3. The return of blood through a heart valve. **Aortic regurgitation.** Aortic incompetence. *See* INCOMPETENCE. **Duodenal regurgitation.** Return of the alkaline duodenal contents into the stomach. **Mitral regurgitation.** Mitral incompetence. *See* INCOMPETENCE. **Paravalvular regurgitation.** Paravalvular incompetence. *See* INCOMPETENCE. **Pulmonary regurgitation.** Pulmonary incompetence. *See* INCOMPETENCE. **Tricuspid regurgitation.** Tricuspid incompetence. *See* INCOMPETENCE. [see prec.]

Reh's test. A cutaneous test for the diagnosis of diphtheria, in which toxin is introduced by punctate scarification. It is now obsolete, as it is less reliable than the Schick test, in which a measured volume of diluted toxin is injected intradermally.

rehabilitate (re·hab·il·it·ate). To re-educate a person who has been sick or injured to take his place in the world; this often necessitates training in some occupation to suit the handicapped condition. [L *re-*, *habilitas* ability.]

rehabilitation (re·hab·il·it·a'·shun). The process of rehabilitating.

rehalation (re·hal·a·shun). Rebreathing. [L *re-*, *halare* to breathe.]

Rehfuss, Martin Emil (b. 1887). Philadelphia physician.

Rehfuss' method. A technique for fractional removal of the stomach contents after the Ewald test-meal by a special tube (see foll.).

Rehfuss' tube. A stomach tube designed for the removal of samples of gastric contents at intervals during a fractional test-meal. It consists of a narrow-bore rubber tube with a metal tip having slotted perforations.

rehydration (re·hi·dra·shun). In a subject who has been dehydrated, the adjustment of the water balance by the giving of fluids by mouth or other ways. [L *re-*, hydrate.]

Reich, Ferdinand (b. 1799). German engineer.

Reich-Lunge apparatus. An absorption apparatus where the non-absorbed gaseous remainder is measured after each absorption treatment; used in gas analysis.

Reichel, Friedrich Paul (b. 1858). Chemnitz gynaecologist and surgeon.

Reichel's chondromatosis. A condition in which multiple cartilaginous neoplasms are present within the articular capsule of the knee joint. Unilateral chondrodysplasia.

Reichel's duct. Cloacal duct. *See* DUCT.

Reichel, John (b. 1886). American bacteriologist.

Reichel's filter. A porcelain bacterial filter similar to the Kitasato filter.

Reichert, Joseph Seraphim (b. 1889). American chemist.

Reichert number, or value. The number of ml of 0.1 N alkali required to neutralize the water-soluble, volatile, fatty acids obtained from 5 g of fat.

Reichert, Karl Bogislaus (b. 1811). Berlin anatomist.

Reichert's canal. Part of the membranous labyrinth connecting the duct of the cochlea to the saccule.

Reichert's cartilage. The cartilage of the hyoid arch of the embryo; it is represented in the adult by the stapes styloid process of the temporal bone, stylohyoid ligament, and the lesser cornu of the hyoid bone.

Reichert's membrane. The anterior elastic lamina of the cornea; Bowman's membrane.

Reichert's recess. A small depression enclosed by the two limbs of the vestibular crest of the bony labyrinth; the cochlear recess of the vestibule.

Reichert's scar. A fibrinous area on the fertilized embedded ovum in place of the decidual tissue which is present over the rest of the conceptus.

Reichmann, Mikola (b. 1851). Warsaw physician.

Reichmann's disease, or syndrome. Excessive and continuous secretion of gastric juice.

Reichmann's rod. A short ivory rod with a grooved handle, used for auscultatory percussion of the stomach. The stethoscope was placed over the stomach and the rod pressed vertically down over the stomach area and scratched with the finger whilst being moved centrifugally towards the periphery of the organ. A change in pitch of the sound took place when the margin of the stomach was passed.

Reichmann's sign. The presence of acid food residues in the fasting stomach on waking in the morning.

Reichstein, Tadeus (b. 1897). Zürich biochemist.

Reichstein's substance M. 17-Hydroxycorticosterone.

Reichstein's substance S. 17-Hydroxy-11-deoxycorticosterone.

Reid, Robert William (b. 1851). Aberdeen anatomist.

Reid's base line. A line joining the infra-orbital point to the superior border of the external auditory meatus. Also known as the *anthropological base line* and the *Frankfurt line.* Accepted by the Munich Congress of 1877 as the base line of the skull.

Reil, Johann Christian (b. 1759). Dutch anatomist in Halle.

Reil's ansa. A bundle of fibres running in the inferior thalamic peduncle.

Band of Reil. Moderator band. *See* BAND.

Island of Reil. The insula; an area of cerebral cortex bounded by the circular sulcus and lying at the bottom of the lateral (sylvian) fissure.

Reil's ribbon. Medial lemniscus. *See* LEMNISCUS.

Reil's sulcus. The sulcus bounding the insula.

Reil's triangle. The trigone of the lateral lemniscus; a triangle bounded by the superior cerebellar peduncle, the inferior quadrigeminal body, and the midline.

Reimann, Hobart Ansteth (b. 1897). Philadelphia physician.

Reimann's epidemic diarrhoea. A mild epidemic diarrhoea in infants, probably of virus origin.

reimplantation (re·im·plan·ta'·shun). 1. The reinsertion in its original situation of an organ or part which has been removed. 2. In dental surgery, the replacing in its socket of a tooth that has been removed. [L *re-*, implant.]

Reinecke acid. Tetrathiocyanodiammono-chromic acid, $H[Cr(CHS)_4(NH_3)_2]$. It is used as a reagent for proline, histidine, and choline.

Reinecke salt. $NH_4[Cr(CNS)_4(NH_3)_2]$, the ammonium salt of tetrathiocyanodiammono-chromic acid. It is a specific reagent for proline and hydroxyproline, both of which it precipitates.

reinfection (re·in·fek·shun). A second infection with the same or a similar micro-organism. [L *re-*, infect.]

reinforcement (re·in·fors·ment). Added strength or force; augmentation. In dentistry, the strengthening of a denture by means of a metal strip or wire. **Reinforcement of reflex.** The increased reflex irritability seen when the subject performs mental or muscular work whilst a reflex is being elicited, or when certain selected stimuli are applied to parts of the body other than that concerned in the reflex itself. [Fr. *renforcement.*]

Reinhold, John Gunther (b. 1900). Philadelphia biochemist.

Reinhold and Shiels method. For blood cholesterol: a similar method to that of Myers and Wardell, anhydrous sodium sulphate being used instead of plaster of Paris for drying the serum prior to extraction.

reinnervation (re·in·er·va'·shun). The attempt at restoration of function in a paralysed muscle by grafting a live nerve. [L *re-*, innervate.]

reinoculation (re·in·ok·ew·la'·shun). A new inoculation from an exogenous source which succeeds an earlier inoculation with the type of micro-organism used on the first occasion. [L *re-*, inoculate.]

Reinsch, Adolf (b. 1862). German physician.

Reinsch's test. For the detection of arsenic, antimony, and mercury: liquids such as urine are acidified with one-fifth of their volume of pure arsenic-free hydrochloric acid; solid materials are mixed to a thin paste with distilled water and then similarly acidified. A strip of pure copper foil previously tested and found free from contaminants is placed in the solution and the latter is heated to gentle boiling for five minutes. If a black stain is formed upon the copper the latter is removed and washed gently with water, alcohol, and ether, and dried by slight warming. It is then folded and placed in a narrow glass tube, the upper part of the tube is first warmed and the foil is then carefully heated to obtain a sublimate in the upper part of the tube. When cool the sublimate is examined under the microscope. Arsenic gives characteristic octahedral crystals of arsenious oxide; antimony, an amorphous deposit; mercury, globules of metallic mercury. Bismuth gives a black stain in the first part of the test but no sublimate.

reintegration (re·in·teg·ra'·shun). In its psychiatric connotation, the building-up of the mind into a unified whole once more. [L *re-*, *integrare* to make whole.]

reintubation (re·in·tew·ba'·shun). Reinsertion of a tube. [L *re-*, intubation.]

Reisseisen, Franz Daniel (b. 1773). Strasbourg anatomist.

Reisseisen's muscle. Smooth muscle fibres in the walls of the bronchioles.

Reissner, Ernst (b. 1824). Dorpat anatomist.

Reissner's canal. The duct of the cochlea.

Reissner's fibre. A cylindrical fibre said to run the whole length of the central canal of the spinal cord: a very questionable entity in man though it has been found in lower mammals.

Reissner's membrane. The vestibular membrane of the cochlea.

Reiter, Hans (b. 1881). Berlin bacteriologist.

Reiter's arthritis, disease, or syndrome. A clinical syndrome consisting of abacterial urethritis, bilateral conjunctivitis, and polyarthritis. Balanitis and keratoderma blennorrhagica may also occur. Pericarditis with electrocardiographic changes has been reported in a few cases. The aetiology is unknown. In some cases, as in Reiter's original description, enteritis without urethritis may be present.

Reiter protein. A protein extract of the non-pathogenic Reiter strain of *Treponema pallidum* used in the complement fixation test for the serological diagnosis of syphilis.

rejoining (re·join·ing). In cytogenetics, the fusion of broken chromatid or chromosome ends to restore the normal structure (restitution) or to produce rearrangements (reunion). [L *re-*, *jungere* to join.]

rejuvenescence (re·joo·ven·es'·ens). Enhancement of bodily and mental health as a result of renewed vitality. [L *re-*, *juvenis* youth.]

Rekoss. 19th century Königsberg instrument maker.

Rekoss disc. The original rotating disc designed to change the lenses in the ophthalmoscope.

relapse (re·laps). The recurrence of a disease after seeming recovery. Cf. RECRUDESCENCE. **Intercurrent relapse.** A relapse which takes place before the fever has completely subsided. **Rebound relapse.** The return of symptoms in a severe, or even more severe, form, after the cessation of certain special treatment which has temporarily caused a remission. [L *relabi* to fall back.]

relation (re·la·shun). 1. Affinity, interdependence, or connection between parts or organs. 2. In anatomy, the situation of a part of the body in respect of other parts. **Centric relation.** The most horizontally retruded relationship of the mandible to the maxilla at the physiologically appropriate vertical separation of the jaws. *See also:* CENTRIC OCCLUSION. **Range-energy relation.** An experimental or theoretical relation between the range of an ionizing particle in matter and its initial energy. [L *relatio* a bringing back.]

See also: GEIGER.

relax (re·lax). 1. To become weak, to slacken, as tension. 2. To become less severe. 3. To provoke movement of the bowels. [L *relaxare* to ease.]

relaxant (re·lax·ant). 1. Causing relaxation; relieving strain. 2. An agent which diminishes strain or tension. 3. A laxative. 4. Muscle relaxant; a myoneural blocking agent. **Anti-depolarizing relaxants.** A group of myoneural blocking agents which act by competitive inhibition of acetylcholine, e.g. tubocurarine. **Muscle relaxants.** A group of drugs, many of which act by interfering with the passage of nervous impulses from fibres into muscle, used in anaesthesia. **Non-depolarizing relaxants.** Myoneural blocking agents which prevent the access of acetylcholine to the receptor protein of the myoneural junction so that no depolarization, no resting potential of the motor end-plate and no muscular contraction takes place, e.g. tubocurarine chloride. [see foll.]

relaxation (re·lax·a·shun). 1. A slackening of tension or strain, especially of the muscles. 2. Alleviation of pain. 3. Abatement of severity. **Cardio-oesophageal relaxation.** Persistent relaxation of the gastrocardiac junction during infancy, usually associated with intermittent oesophageal hiatus hernia. **Isometric relaxation.** A loss of tone of a muscle without any shortening of the muscle fibrils. In cardiology, the phase of ventricular systole during ventricular relaxation when both the atrioventricular and semilunar valves are closed. **Isovolumic relaxation.** In cardiology, the phase at the end of ventricular systole when the ventricular muscle is relaxing whilst both the atrioventricular and semilunar valves are closed. [L *relaxare* to ease.]

relaxin (re·lax·in). A hormone obtained from the serum of pregnant animals and from the corpora lutea of sows; it relaxes the pelvic ligaments during pregnancy.

relief (re·leef). Alleviation of pain or suffering. [L *relevare* to lighten.]

relieve (re·leev). To alleviate pain or to free from physical or mental discomfort. [see prec.]

religiosus (rel·ij·e·o'·sus). A name sometimes applied to the superior rectus muscle of the eyeball. [L religious.]

reluxation (re·lux·a·shun). Redislocation; the recurrence of a dislocation after it has been reduced. [L *re-*, *luxare* to dislocate.]

rem (rem). Unit of biological dose given by the product of the absorbed dose in rads and the relative biological efficiency of the radiation. [*R*oentgen *e*quivalent *m*an.]

Remak, Ernst Julius (b. 1849). Berlin neurologist.

Remak's reflex. On stroking the upper anterior surface of the thigh, if extension of the knee occurs with plantar flexion of the first three toes and possibly of the foot, this indicates pyramidal-tract disease.

Remak's sign, or symptom. 1. Polyaesthesia; a single stimulus may be perceived as if it were more than one applied in several different places. 2. Delay in the perception of a painful stimulus. Both may be observed in cases of tabes dorsalis.

Remak's type. Paralysis of wrist and finger extensor muscles, giving rise to wrist drop; this may be due to a radial nerve lesion.

Remak, Robert (b. 1815). Berlin neurologist.

Band of Remak. An obsolete term for the axis-cylinder.

Remak's fibre. A non-medullated nerve fibre.

Remak's ganglion. Numerous ganglia of the autonomic nervous system bear the name of this neurologist.

Remak's plexus. Meissner's plexus.

remedial (rem·e·de·al). Designed to correct or cure. [see foll.]

remedy (rem·ed·e). Any agent used for the cure or alleviation of the symptoms of a disease. **Specific remedy.** A drug or method of treatment which is capable of arresting or eliminating a disease process, in contrast to a symptomatic remedy which, though it ameliorates some of the manifestations, does not alter the underlying pathology. [L *remediare* to cure.]

Remijia (re·mij·e·ah). A genus of plants (family Rubiaceae) which contain alkaloids allied to quinine. The bark of *Remijia pedunculata* Flueck (cuprea bark) contains quinine and cupreine, but it is too scarce to be used as a source of these alkaloids. [*Remijo*, a 19th century Colombian physician.]

remineralization (re·min·er·al·i·za′·shun). Re-establishment in the body of mineral constituents of which it has been deprived by illness or by errors of diet. [L *re-*, mineral.]

remission (re·mish·un). A period in which symptoms are absent or greatly diminished. A disease may show alternate remissions and recurrences over a period. [see foll.]

remittence (re·mit·ens). Temporary remission, but not entire cessation, of symptoms. [L *remittere* to abate.]

remittent (re·mit·ent). Characterized by spells of amelioration and aggravation; said of a febrile disease which is characterized by periods of abatement. [see prec.]

Remlinger, R. (b. 1871). French physician.

Remlinger's sign. In typhus, difficulty in protruding the tongue and tremulousness of the tongue.

remnant (rem·nant). That which remains; a fragment. **Acroblastic remnant.** That part of the Golgi apparatus and associated cytoplasm of the spermatid which is cast off and not used in making a spermatozoon. **Allantoic remnant.** The vestigial entodermal allantoic diverticulum found in the umbilical cord of the human fetus near the umbilicus, and connected through the umbilicus with the urachus and bladder. [OFr. *remenant* remaining.]

ren (ren). The kidneys. **Ren amyloideus.** Lardaceous disease of the kidneys. **Ren mobilis.** Movable kidney. *See* KIDNEY. **Ren unguliformis.** Horseshoe kidney. *See* KIDNEY. [L.]

renal (re·nal). Of or relating to the kidney or the kidneys. [see prec.]

renal artery [arteria renalis (NA)]. Either of two large arteries from the side of the abdominal aorta, passing across the corresponding crura of the diaphragm to enter the hila of the kidneys. They supply twigs to the ureter [rami ureterici (NA)] and a small inferior suprarenal artery [arteria suprarenalis inferior (NA)]. Capsular branches [rami capsulares (NA)] are fine branches supplying the capsule of the kidney. On reaching the kidney (or sometimes before) the renal artery divides into a large anterior branch and a smaller posterior branch [rami anterior et posterior (NA)], although this mode of branching is subject to considerable variation. These then give rise to a total of five segmental arteries which are named as follows: apical [arteria segmenti superioris (NA)], upper (anterior) [arteria segmenti anterioris superioris (NA)], lower (anterior) [arteria segmenti anterioris inferioris (NA)], lower [arteria segmenti inferioris (NA)], and posterior [arteria segmenti posterioris (NA)]. There is only a negligible anastomosis between the segmental arteries.

renal veins [venae renales (NA)]. Tributaries of the inferior vena cava, the left vein draining the testicle or ovary and the corresponding suprarenal gland, as well as the kidney.

Renaut, Joseph Louis (b. 1844). Lyons anatomist.

Renaut's body. Pale granules seen in degenerating nerve fibres in cases of muscular dystrophy.

Renaut's layer. The malpighian layer of the skin.

Rendu, Henri Jules Louis Marie (b. 1844). Paris physician.

Rendu's tremor. An intention tremor of hysterical origin.

Rendu-Osler-Weber disease. Hereditary haemorrhagic telangiectasia. *See* TELANGIECTASIA.

renghas (reng·gas). The plant *Gluta renghas* of the family Anacardiaceae. Its sap causes a dermatitis.

renicardiac (ren·e·kar·de·ak). Relating or belonging to the kidney and heart. [L *ren* kidney, Gk *kardia* heart.]

reniculus (ren·ik·ew·lus). A lobule of the kidney. [dim. of L *ren* kidney.]

reniform (ren·e·form). Kidney-shaped. [L *ren* kidney, form.]

renin (re·nin). A proteolytic enzyme secreted by the juxtaglomerula cells of the kidney. It catalyses the conversion of circulating angiotensinogen to angiotensin I, which is then converted to angiotensin II causing release of aldosterone from the kidney. Renin secretion is controlled in three ways: (a) blood pressure within the arteriole supplying the juxtamedullary cells, (b) supply of Na^+ ions reaching the distal tubule, (c) sympathetic nervous system. [L *ren* kidney.]

reniportal (ren·e·por·tal). 1. Relating to the hilum of the kidney. 2. Pertaining to the renal and portal circulations. [L *ren* kidney, *porta* gate.]

renipuncture (ren·e·pungk·tcher). Surgical incision or puncture of the capsule of the kidney; sometimes carried out for renal pain due to capsular tension in some forms of cystic disease. [L *ren* kidney, *punctura* a pricking.]

renitis (ren·i·tis). Nephritis. [L *ren* kidney, Gk *-itis* inflammation.]

rennet (ren·et). A preparation used for curdling milk, generally obtained from the stomach of a calf. It contains the enzyme rennin, and is used in cheesemaking. [ME *rennen* to run.]

rennin (ren·in). Rennet, chymosin; an enzyme present in gastric juice, and prepared from the fourth stomach of the calf. It coagulates milk by converting caseinogen into casein. Cf. RENIN. [see prec.]

renninogen (ren·in·o·jen). The precursor of rennin (chymosin) present in peptic cells. Now called *chymosinogen.* [rennin, Gk *genein* to produce.]

renninum (ren·i·num). Rennin. [L.]

rennogen (ren·o·jen). Renninogen.

renocutaneous (re·no·kew·ta′·ne·us). Of or relating to the kidneys and the skin. [L *ren* kidney, *cutis* skin.]

renocyte (re·no·site). A kidney cell. [L *ren* kidney, Gk *kytos* cell.]

renogastric (re·no·gas·trik). Relating to the kidneys and the stomach. [L *ren* kidney, Gk *gaster* stomach.]

renography (re·nog·raf·e). The dynamic study of the functional state of the kidneys by means of continuous measurements of radioactivity made external to the body. **Computer-assisted blood background subtraction renography (CABBS).** A method by which the radioactivity recorded during renography is corrected for non-renal radioactivity by means of an analogue or a digital computer. **Radioisotope renography.** Renography (see above). [L *ren* kidney, Gk *graphein* to record.]

reno-intestinal (re·no·in·tes′·tin·al). Relating or belonging to the kidneys and the intestine. [L *ren* kidney, intestine.]

renopathy (ren·op·ath·e). Nephropathy. [L *ren* kidney, Gk *pathos* disease.]

renoprival (re·no·pri·val). Resulting from removal or loss of function of the kidneys. [L *ren* kidney, *privare* to deprive.]

renopulmonary (re·no·pul·mon·ar·e). Relating or belonging to the kidneys and the lungs. [L *ren* kidney, *pulmo* lung.]

renotrophic (re·no·trof·ik). Having a special affinity for, or exerting its principal effect upon, kidney tissue. [L *ren* kidney, Gk *trophe* nourishment.]

renunculus (re·nung·kew·lus). Reniculus.

reo-like virus (ree·o·like vi·rus). *See* ROTAVIRUS.

reorganization (re·or·gan·i·za′·shun). Healing by growth of any tissue identical with that of the part which was injured. [L *re-*, Gk *organon* member.]

reovirus (re·o·vi′·rus). A group of spherical viruses (75 nm in diameter), unusual in containing double-stranded RNA. Originally thought to be an echovirus serotype (10), they are a distinct group with three antigenic types. Though isolated from children with respiratory or gut infections, it is not clear whether they do in fact cause disease. Distribution in man is widespread. [*R*espiratory *e*nteric *o*rphan *viruses.*]

re-oxidation (re·ox·e·**da'**·shun). The process of reabsorbing oxygen, as does the haemoglobin of the blood. [L *re-*, oxidation.]

repair (re·**pa**·er). Anaplerosis; restoration of the structure of an injured part. **DNA repair.** Enzymatic repair of DNA lesions induced by ultraviolet, x- and gamma-rays, radiomimetic drugs and other physical and chemical agents. Different repair mechanisms are known, either dependent on light (photoreactivation) or occurring in the dark (excision and recombinational repair): *photoreactivation* acts only on ultraviolet-induced lesions and relies on an enzyme which is stimulated by light; the *excision* repair degrades a segment of the damaged strand and then resynthesizes it, using the normal strand as a template; *recombinational* repair tends to achieve the production of undamaged DNA strands by genetic recombination between the damaged DNA strands and their newly synthesized replicas. **Filigree repair.** A method of hernial repair involving the insertion in the parietes at the point of weakness of a mesh of (silver) wire. *See also* FICKLING. [L *reparare* to restore.]

repatency (re·**pa**·ten·se). 1. The state of being opened or patent after having been closed for a time, said of a part or vessel. 2. Of a ligated vessel, reopening of the lumen because either the knot of the ligature has slipped or absorption of the ligature has occurred too rapidly. [L *re-*, *patens* open.]

repeatability. The extent to which repeated measurements agree.

repellent (re·**pel**·ent). 1. Causing subsidence of a swelling. 2. Any agent that keeps insect pests away or prevents irritation of the skin by their attacks. [L *repellere* to drive away.]

repercolation (re·**per**·ko·la·shun). Percolation of a drug for a second or third time by a liquor previously used to extract the same drug. [L *re-*, percolate.]

repercussion (re·per·**kush**·un). In obstetrics, ballottement. [L *repercussio* a rebounding.]

repercussive (re·per·**kus**·iv). 1. Dispersing or driving in. 2. A repellent agent. [see prec.]

repercutient (re·per·**kew**·shent). In obstetrics, pertaining to or causing a repercussion. [L *repercutere* to cause to rebound.]

replacement (re·**plase**·ment). The process of replacing. [Fr.]

replantation (re·plan·**ta**·shun). 1. The planting of anything again; reimplantation. 2. The replacement of a tooth in its socket. [L *re-*, *plantare* to set.]

repletion (re·**ple**·shun). Plethora; a condition of surfeit, as of eating. [Fr.]

replica plating (**rep**·lik·ah **pla**·ting). A technique for obtaining clonal replicas of bacterial cultures growing on the surface of agar plates. The pile of a velveteen pad is pressed against the growth to pick up a topographically oriented sample of it, replicas being made by superimposing the pad on the surface of uninoculated plates which are then incubated. [L *replicare* to fold back, OFr. plate.]

replicase (**rep**·lik·aze). **DNA replicase.** A DNA-dependent DNA polymerase so far isolated only from bacteria but which is thought to be the enzyme responsible for replication of DNA in living cells; DNA polymerase II. **RNA replicase.** The class of RNA polymerases which are dependent for their activity on the presence of RNA as primer and template. They are responsible for the replication of viral RNA in infected bacteria; RNA-dependent (-directed) RNA polymerase. [L *replicare* to fold back, *-ase* enzyme.]

replication (rep·lik·a·shun). 1. A doubling-back of tissue. 2. The performance of an experiment repeatedly or for a second time in similar conditions in order that the probability of error may be reduced to the minimum. 3. The process whereby the genetic material (chromosomal DNA or viral RNA) is duplicated. **Semi-conservative replication.** Of double-stranded DNA, means that each of the two parental strands is conserved in the daughter double-helical molecules, the other two daughter strands being newly synthesized using the parental strands as templates. [L *replicare* to fold back.]

replicator (**rep**·lik·a·tor). In molecular biology, the postulated site on chromosomal DNA on which a protein 'initiator' acts to start replication. [L *replicare* to fold back.]

replicon (**rep**·lik·on). A unit of replication of the genome of a cell or organism. This, in viruses and bacteria, may represent the whole genome while in higher organisms it corresponds to only a relatively small segment of a chromosome. [L *replicare* to fold back.]

repolarization (re·po·lar·i·**za'**·shun). The recovery of muscle or nerve membrane to a polarized state after the passage of an excitation. [L *re-*, polarization.]

reposing (re·**po**·zing). Restoring a displaced part to its normal position; reducing. [L *reponere* to put back.]

reposition (re·po·**zish**·un). Restoration of an organ or part to its normal position; commonly used for the inverted uterus. [see prec.]

repositor (re·**poz**·it·or). An instrument used for replacing displaced organs to their normal site; an instrument used in the treatment of a prolapsed umbilical cord, or for the replacement of an inverted uterus from below. [L *reponere* to put back.]
See also: AVELING.

representation (**rep**·re·zen·**ta'**·shun). The act of representing. **Mental representation.** Perceptual experience of the external world. The term implies that perception is not a passive mirroring process. **Object representation.** Internalized, non-linguistic sensorimotor *schema* acquired from manipulation of an external object. Important in the early intellectual development of a child. **Sensorimotor representation.** The order of representation of different parts of the body in the motor and somatosensory cortex. **Symbolic representation.** In psychoanalysis, the disguised conscious expression of repressed wishes or impulses in the form of symptoms, manifest dream content, slips of tongue and similar manifestations. [L *re-*, *praesentare* to be at hand.]

repressibility (re·**pres**·ib·**il'**·it·e). In genetics, the property of some structural genes by virtue of which they can be repressed and their activity switched off. [L *reprimere* to press back.]

repression (re·**presh**·un). 1. The active rejection by the superego of unacceptable instinctual impulses and their associated ideas so that they are forced from consciousness into the unconscious. 2. In genetics, the process by which the activity of a structural gene is stopped or switched off; it involves the combination of a functional repressor molecule to an operator gene. **Reactive repression.** Repression as a result of an external stimulus. [L *reprimere* to press back.]

repressor (re·**pres**·or). A protein synthesized under the direction of a regulator gene; such a protein may be able to bind to an operator gene and in that way repress its activity, or it may require that it be bound by one or more small molecular weight molecules (called *corepressors*) to do this, in which case it is called an *aporepressor*. [L *reprimere* to press back.]

reproduction (re·pro·**duk**·shun). Production by an individual or a cell of other individuals or cells which are like, or potentially able to become like, the individual or cells producing them. **Asexual reproduction.** Reproduction by any means other than the production of gametes; production of spores, fission, gemmation, and vegetative reproduction are the principal means. **Bisexual reproduction.** Sexual reproduction with two gametes. **Sexual reproduction.** Reproduction by the formation of gametes. In its normal form microgametes (spermatozoa) are produced by the male, and macrogametes (ovules) by the female. These fuse to form the zygote. Parthenogenesis is, however, a form of sexual reproduction. **Somatic reproduction.** Asexual reproduction by budding-off of multicellular fragments. **Unisexual reproduction.** Sexual reproduction with one gamete. [L *re-*, *producere* to produce.]

reproductive (re·pro·**duk**·tiv). Relating or belonging to, or instrumental in reproduction.

Reptilia (rep·**til**·e·ah). A class of the phylum Chordata; reptiles. Living forms have dry, scaled skins, are poikilothermal and reproduce by laying eggs. The orders Crocodilia and Squamata may be of medical interest. [L *reptilis* creeping.]

repullulation (re·pul·ew·**la'**·shun). 1. A renewal of growth by the process of budding or sprouting. 2. The renewed growth of a morbid process; recurrence. [L *repullulare* to sprout out again.]

repulsion (re·**pul**·shun). 1. The opposite of attraction; repugnance. 2. The action which two bodies exert upon one another when they tend to increase their mutual distance from one another; hence the force which drives them apart. **Capillary repulsion.** The force between two floating bodies when brought near, if one is wetted by the liquid and the other is not. [L *repellere* to drive away.]

resazurin (rez·**az**·ewr·in). A red dye used as a histological stain.

Rescinnamine (res·**in**·am·een). BP Commission approved name for methyl-*O*-(3,4,5-trimethoxycinnamoyl)reserpate; a tranquillizer and hypotensive.

research (re·**serch**). Scientific investigation: the establishment of facts and their significance by experiment; the scientific collection and analysis of data. **Clinical research.** The collection and analysis of data and experimentation at the bedside, rather than in the laboratory. **Medical research.** Research in any kind of medical science. **Psychic research, Psychical research.** The science of phenomena beyond the domain of ordinary or physiological psychology and having relation, for example, to telepathic or clairvoyant processes. [OFr. *recercher.*]

resect (re·**sekt**). 1. To cut out a portion of tissue or an organ, e.g. the intestine. 2. With regard to a joint, to remove the articular surfaces. [L *re-*, *secare* to cut.]

resectable (re·**sekt**·abl). Able to be resected; generally used in reference to diseased joints.

resection (re·**sek**·shun). 1. Surgical removal of a part, usually of some magnitude, e.g. jaw, stomach, colon, etc. 2. Removal of a portion of one of the extra-ocular muscles, usually followed by uniting the cut end with sutures, so as to shorten the muscle. **Gastric resection.** Surgical removal of the stomach, partially or totally. It is commonly practised in the treatment of peptic ulcer and cancer of the stomach. **Resection of a joint.** Removal of the articulating portions of the bones in a joint. **Rib resection.** An operation which involves removal of a rib, either a long length in order to improve access, or a short length to establish drainage in infection of the pleural space. **Root resection.** The operation of resection of the apex of a dead tooth to eradicate infection; it is usually accompanied by curettage of surrounding infected alveolar bone. **Scleral resection.** Removal of a crescentic portion of sclera, an operation usually performed for the cure of retinal detachment. **Submucous resection.** Of the nasal septum; the classical operation for the removal of a deflexion of the cartilaginous or bony nasal septum, leaving the mucous membrane of the septum intact and complete at the end of the operation. The term is often contracted to SMR. **Transurethral resection.** Resection of the prostate gland under endoscopic visual control by a resectoscope passed through the urethra. **Window resection.** Of the nasal septum: the old-fashioned operation for the removal of the bony or cartilaginous nasal septum. [L *re-*, *secare* to cut.]

See also: BALFOUR (D. C.), SCHEDE.

resectoscope (re·**sekt**·o·skope). An instrument for transurethral prostatic resection. The operation is done under visual control, either directly or through a foroblique telescope. [resection, Gk *skopein* to view.]

resectoscopy (re·sekt·**os**·ko·pe). Transurethral resection of the prostate. [see prec.]

resene (rez·een). Any member of a family of oxygenated compounds which constitute certain resins such as copal, dammar, olibanum, and mastic. They are of indeterminate composition and, being insoluble in alkalis, their resins are employed in varnish making.

Reserpine BP 1973 (res·er·peen). One of the crystalline alkaloids of *Rauwolfia serpentina*, $C_{33}H_{40}O_9N_2$; it has also been obtained from the Australian species *constricta*. It is indicated in neuropsychiatric disorders and hypertension. Cases of depression in rauwolfia therapy in hypertension have been reported, and it is advisable to suspend the drug where these symptoms appear.

reserve (re·**zerv**). Remainder; potentiality; anything stored against a future contingency. **Alkali reserve.** The volume of carbon dioxide measured at standard temperature and pressure held by 100 ml of blood plasma in either the free or combined state which can be liberated by acid. The alkali reserve normally lies between 53 and 77 ml per 100 ml plasma, but is increased in alkalosis and decreased in acidosis. **Cardiac reserve.** The reserve energy of the heart muscle which permits it to perform more work in response to physiological stimuli. When the reserve of the heart is exhausted, cardiac insufficiency occurs. **Diminished cardiac reserve.** Reduction of the ability of the heart to meet increased demands upon it. The normal heart has a considerable reserve which enables it to adapt itself to a greatly increased work load without becoming insufficient, whereas the damaged heart has an impaired reserve, may fail to meet the increased load, and will develop insufficiency. **Myocardial reserve.** The ability of the myocardium to perform extra work when the need arises. [L *reservare* to save up.]

reservoir (rez·er·vwahr). A source of supply; a store or collection. **Reservoir of infection, Reservoir of virus.** Epidemiological terms applied to any natural source of repeated infection, e.g. in central Asia the gerbil constitutes a reservoir of infection for *Leishmania tropica* from which the parasite is carried by sand flies to man who then develops cutaneous leishmaniasis; there is an implication that the source is static, as in the above case where the gerbils suffer very little from the infection and do not usually die. Man, as well as animals, and insects also, may act as a reservoir of infection. The word *virus* may be applied in a special sense to mean filtrable virus, or in a general sense to mean any pathogen. [see prec.]

See also: PECQUET.

reshaping (re·**sha**·ping). Modifying the shape, e.g. in a filling, crown, bridge, or artificial denture. [L *re-*, AS *scieppan.*]

residue (rez·id·ew). That which remains when something else has been removed, e.g. ash, precipitate. **Amino-acid residue.** *External*: an amino acid which is located on the surface of a globular polypeptide and is usually hydrophilic. *Internal*: an amino acid which is located away from the surface of a globular polypeptide and is usually a hydrophobic residue. **Day residue.** In psychoanalysis, those remnants of the waking activity of the mind from which it has not been possible to withdraw all cathexis, and which are therefore connected with a wish that is expressed in a dream. [L *residuum.*]

residuum (rez·**id**·ew·um). Remainder, residue; that which remains after the removal of other substances from a mixture by such means as filtration, centrifugalization, etc. **Sporal residuum.** In protozoology, the residual substance after sporulation. [L.]

resilience (re·**zil**·e·ens). 1. The capability of a body to assume its original form after it has been stretched or compressed; rebound; elasticity. 2. Power of recuperation. [L *resilire* to spring back.]

resilient (re·**zil**·e·ent). Relating to or exhibiting resilience.

resin (**rez**·in). The name given to a group of solid or semi-solid amorphous substances of complex nature. They have no definite melting points, and are insoluble in water, but usually soluble in alcohol, chloroform, or ether. They are mixtures of resin acids (e.g. abietic acid), alcohols, phenols, esters, and inert substances. **Anionic exchange resin.** *See* ION-EXCHANGE RESINS (below). **Cationic exchange resin.** *See* ION-EXCHANGE RESINS (below). **Colophony resin.** Colophony. **Guaiacum resin.** A resin obtained from the stem of *Guaiacum officinale* Linn. or *G. sanctum* Linn. It is a dark-greenish substance, used as a local stimulant or as an irritant in gout and rheumatism. **Gum resin.** A class of resin associated with gum; as a volatile oil is usually present they are often known as *oleo gum resins*, e.g. myrrh, frankincense, gamboge, etc. **Ion-exchange resins.** Synthetic ionizable resins which may be acidic or basic. The labile ions may be exchanged for other ions of similar charge in solution; in this way inorganic salts can be completely removed from solution, a property utilized in the preparation of drinking water from sea water without distillation. Resins which absorb the negative acid radicals from solution are known as *anionic exchange resins*;

these, for example, can bind the hydrochloric acid and pepsin in the stomach and release them again in the alkaline medium of the small intestine, a fact used in the treatment of hyperpacidity. *Cationic exchange resins* remove metallic ions and positive radicals from solution due to the presence of free COOH or SO_2OH groups on the surface of the resin. Carboxylic resins bind cations at all pH levels above 5, but sulphonic resins will bind cations down to pH levels of 3. **Ipomoea Resin BPC 1959.** That obtained from *Ipomoea orizabensis* and known also as *scammony resin*. **Jalap Resin BPC 1959.** The resin from *Ipomoea purga* (jalap) the root of which contains up to 20 per cent; it is a powerful irritant purgative. **Oleo resin.** A resin containing oil and resin but no gum, as differing from the oleo gum resin; examples are Canada turpentine, balsam of copaiba, and sandarac. **Oleo gum resin.** Gum resin (see above). **Podophyllum Resin BP 1973.** That obtained from *Podophyllum peltatum* or *P. hexandrum* (Indian podophyllum), known as *podophyllin*; it is a drastic but slow-acting purgative. **Polyacrylic carboxylic acid resin.** A mixture of the potassium and ammonium salts of a polyacrylic resin. It is used to eliminate sodium ions from the body, and is hence of value in the treatment of oedema. **Polyvinyl resins.** A group of synthetic resins made by the polymerization of vinyl compounds. They are used in the plastics industry, and also as ion-exchange resins. **Scammony resin.** Ipomoea resin (see above). **Sodium sulphonic ion-exchange resin.** A cationic exchange resin which has been found of value in the treatment of anuria. Potassium ions are removed and replaced by sodium ions: ammonium ion resins are contra-indicated in such cases as they increase acidity and the already high urea level. **Sulphonated polystyrene resin.** A cationic exchange resin capable of removing potassium, sodium and other metallic ions from solution. Clinical trials indicate that it might be valuable for controlling sodium and potassium concentration in the intestine. **Turpentine resin.** Colophony, the residue left after distillation of turpentine oil from the crude oleo resin of various species of *Pinus*. [L *resina*.]

resin-uptake (rez·in up·take). Denoting the proportion of a radioactive material adsorbed onto an ion-exchange resin when the resin is competing with some other binding agent. In general medical literature it is most usually applied in connection with a particular index of thyroid function where the distribution of radioactive tri-iodothyronine between thyroxine-binding globulin and a resin is estimated by measuring the *resin-uptake* of radioactivity. [L *resina*, uptake.]

resina (rez·i·nah). Resin; when not qualified, turpentine resin or colophony is inferred. [L.]

resinate (rez·in·ate). Any compound formed by the acids of resins with alkalis or metallic bases. They are used in soap manufacture and also in printing inks, polishes, and paint driers.

resinotannol (rez·in·o·tan'·ol). A member of a group of alcohols derived from resin esters which are coloured and give a tannin reaction with iron salts.

resinous (rez·in·us). 1. Relating to, having the characteristics of, or containing resin. 2. Derived from resin.

res ipsa loquitur. A doctrine used in law in respect of acts of negligence, especially in medicine. [L the thing speaks for itself.]

resistance (re·zis·tans). 1. Opposition to force, or a force in opposition. 2. In electricity, the opposition encountered by a current in a conductor; it is defined as the ratio between the electromotive force and the current, and is expressed in ohms. 3. In psycho-analysis, active opposition, preventing unconscious and repressed material from manifesting in the conscious. **Acid resistance.** The property possessed by some bacteria, after staining, of resisting decolorization with acid. **Acid-alcohol resistance.** The property possessed by the tubercle bacillus and allied species of resisting the decolorizing action of alcohol or strong mineral acids; it is made use of in diagnosis. **Acquired resistance.** Acquisition by a bacterial population of the ability to grow in the presence of an antibacterial agent either by the selection of mutants or by inducing production of an enzyme destroying the agent. It can occur *in vitro* or in the course of therapy. **Airway resistance.** The resistance offered by the airways to flow of respiratory gas in and out of the lungs. **Bacterial resistance.** 1. The general ability of a bacterial species to resist physical or chemical agencies. 2. The lack of susceptibility of a strain of a bacterial species (normally included in the spectrum of an antibacterial agent) to such a degree as to render therapy with the agent ineffectual. **Cross resistance.** Acquired resistance of a bacterial strain conferring simultaneous resistance to another antibacterial agent. It is an indication that the two agents are related and have basically similar action. **Essential resistance.** Internal resistance (see below). **External resistance, Extraordinary resistance.** The resistance of the external electrical circuit, i.e. the resistance of the circuit outside the cell, battery, or generator producing the current. **Haemolytic resistance.** Osmotic fragility of erythrocytes. **Inductive resistance.** Reactance; a component of the impedance of a circuit carrying an alternating current. **Internal resistance.** The resistance of the cell, battery, or generator producing a current in an external circuit. **Natural resistance.** 1. The ability of a bacterial species to grow in the presence of an antibacterial agent. 2. The existence in a normally susceptible species of such a strain before the introduction into general use of that particular antibacterial agent. **Peripheral resistance.** The resistance offered by the systemic arterioles, and to a lesser extent by the capillaries, to the flow of blood. It is measured as the mean blood pressure divided by the cardiac output and is expressed as units (mm Hg/l/min or Pa/l/min). Maintenance of an adequate peripheral resistance is the essential peripheral mechanism for maintaining the arterial blood pressure. Increase in peripheral resistance, due to organic or functional narrowing of the arterioles, causes an increase in diastolic arterial pressure, and decrease in peripheral resistance, due to dilatation of the arterioles, causes pooling of blood and a fall in blood pressure. **Resistance transfer factor.** *See* FACTOR. **Vascular resistance.** The quantitative expresssion of the peripheral resistance (see above) in a vascular bed. It is usually derived by analogy with Ohm's law from the mean minute flow of blood and the mean pressure drop across the vascular bed under examination. Although a useful clinical concept, it ignores the reality of pulsatile flow and is not scientifically valid. **Vital resistance.** The natural resistance of an individual to the effects of overwork, fatigue, infections, and diseases generally. [L *resistere* to withstand.]

resistivity (re·zis·tiv·it·e). The specific resistance of a substance to an electric current. It is defined as the resistance in ohms across opposite faces of a cube of the material with sides of length 1 cm.

resolution (rez·o·lew·shun). 1. The abatement of any pathological process, and the process of return of the affected tissues to normal structure and function. 2. Expressing the degree to which detail can be distinguished, e.g. in a microscope image. **Resolution of autoradiographs.** No generally applicable quantitative index of resolution exists for autoradiographs. Qualitative estimates are used in terms of particular structures of tissues or cells which can be distinguished. [see foll.]

resolve (re·zolv). 1. In inflammation, to return to the normal condition without suppuration. 2. To divide a substance into constituent parts. [L *resolvere* to loosen.]

resolvent (re·zolv·ent). 1. Causing resolution of a tumour or swelling. 2. An agent that checks an inflammation or effects absorption of a new growth. [see prec.]

resonance (rez·on·ans). 1. The amplification of a sound by sympathetic vibrations in another medium, e.g. a contained volume of air, the natural vibration frequency of which is synchronous with one of the tones of the sound. Percussion of the chest produces resonance in the underlying structures and the tone varies according to whether the lungs are normal, emphysematous, pneumonic, or displaced by air as in a pneumothorax; the breath sounds produced by air passing through the glottis are reinforced by the vibration of the air in the trachea, bronchi, and lungs, and so become modified into the various kinds of vesicular or bronchial breathing. The larger the volume of air in vibration the lower the pitch of the sound. 2. In chemistry, mesomerism. **Amphoric resonance.** The sound heard over large smooth-walled cavities which has an echoing character; a low fundamental tone is combined with high-pitched overtones which die out more slowly. **Bandbox resonance.** The hyper-resonant note heard over an emphysematous lung. **Bell-metal resonance.** A resonance which has the same significance as amphoric resonance. **Boxy resonance.** A high-pitched tympanitic note heard over a relaxed lobe of a lung, e.g. above a pleural effusion. **Cracked-pot resonance.** The sound sometimes heard on percussion over a cavity communicating with a small bronchus; it is due to air being forced out of a cavity through a small opening. It is heard on percussion of the chest of a crying child, and can be imitated by clasping the hands together so as to enclose some air and striking them sharply on the knee. **Electron spin resonance, ESR.** Measurement over a range of frequency of electromagnetic radiation of the power absorbed by a substance when placed in a magnetic field. This is essentially a method of measuring unpaired electrons and has been applied to the detection of free radicals in cancer research. **Hydatid resonance.** A peculiar tone sometimes heard on auscultatory percussion over the lung containing a hydatid cyst. **Nuclear magnetic resonance, NMR.** A method for defining the character of covalent bonds by measuring the magnetic moment of the atomic nuclei involved. **Osteal resonance.** A characteristic tone obtained on percussion over superficial bones. **Shoulder-strap resonance.** Resonance in the lung in the area above the clavicle. **Skodaic resonance.** A high-pitched tympanitic note heard over relaxed lung, e.g. the lung above a moderate pleural effusion. **Supraclavicular resonance.** Shoulder-strap resonance (see above). **Tympanitic resonance.** The drum-like, low-pitched resonance heard over a large, air-containing space such as a pneumothorax or over the abdomen. **Vesicular resonance.** The characteristic resonance obtained over normal lung. It has been likened to the note produced by percussion of a loaf of bread where similarly the air is contained in a multitude of tiny spaces. **Vesicular-tympanitic resonance.** A resonance midway between normal (vesicular) and tympanitic resonance. **Vocal resonance.** The sounds heard over the chest whilst a patient is speaking. A marked increase in the sound is called *bronchophony.* **Whispering resonance.** The sound heard on auscultation of the whispering voice. **Wooden resonance.** A dull note with some tympanitic quality. [see foll.]

resonant (rez·on·ant). Producing a vibrating sound on percussion; resounding. [L *resonare* to sound again.]

resonator (rez·on·a·tor). 1. Any object, such as a stretched string, which may be caused to vibrate in unison with another vibrating object. 2. An open-ended box or cylinder so designed that it will vibrate with, and amplify the sound of, a tuning fork brought near it. 3. An electrical circuit in which an oscillating current may be induced by oscillations in another circuit. [see prec.]
See also: OUDIN.

resorcin (rez·or·sin). Resorcinol.

resorcinism (rez·or·sin·ism). A state of chronic poisoning caused by resorcinol.

resorcinol (rez·or·sin·ol). *m*-Dihydroxybenzene, $C_6H_4(OH)_2$. An isomer of catechol and hydroquinone; a soluble white compound with antiseptic properties, used in ointments and hair lotions (BP 1973). It was also used in ear drops but is no longer administered internally owing to its toxic properties. **Resorcinol monacetate.** $C_6H_4(OH)OCOCH_3$, a viscous oil used for acne, seborrhoea, dandruff, etc. **Resorcinol phthalein.** Fluorescein, $C_{20}H_{12}O_5$, a compound, the sodium salt of which is used in solution for detecting damage to the cornea, the damaged parts staining green. [resin, orcin.]

resorption (re·sorp·shun). 1. The removal, by absorption, of anything already produced. 2. In dentistry, the removal of the calcified parts of the teeth and jaws. **Pathological resorption.** The resorption of cement, dentine, and bone as a result of disease. **Physiological resorption.** The normal process of resorption of the cement and dentine of the roots of a deciduous tooth. [L *resorbere* to suck back.]

respirable (res·pir·abl). 1. Adapted for or capable of respiration. 2. Fit to be breathed.

respiration (res·pir·a·shun). The complex process by which the gaseous interchange between the tissues and the external atmosphere is effected. This includes the mechanism for the entrance of air into the lungs by the respiratory movements, the diffusion of oxygen from the alveolar air into the blood, the transport of oxygen in the circulation to the tissues by means of haemoglobin, its absorption by the tissues, the oxidation processes in the living cells and the production of carbon dioxide, and conversely the conveyance of carbon dioxide from the tissues to the lungs, and its elimination. **Abdominal respiration.** Breathing carried out mainly by the abdominal muscles. **Accelerated respiration.** A respiratory rate of more than 25 a minute. **Aerobic respiration.** The biochemical processes concerned with the use of oxygen to conserve energy as adenosine triphosphate. **Anaerobic respiration.** The biochemical processes which lead to the formation of adenosine triphosphate without the use of oxygen; Embden–Meyerhoff pathway. Conversion of glucose to pyruvate and lactic acid. **Artificial respiration.** A technique by which the respiratory movements are carried out artificially in the absence of the natural movements, now usually carried out by intermittent positive pressure. *Eve method:* the patient lies prone upon a plank or stretcher to which he is lashed. He is tilted head downwards at an angle of 45 degrees and is then tilted feet down through the same angle. The movements are repeated 12 times a minute. The weight of the abdominal contents pushes and pulls the diaphragm alternatively by gravity. *Holger Nielsen method:* the patient is prone and the chest is alternately compressed below the scapulae and then raised off the ground by pulling up the upper arms. *Howard method:* the patient is in a supine position with a roll of clothes beneath the thorax and the head lower than the abdomen. Pressure is applied to the lower ribs and upper abdomen 16 times a minute. *Mouth-to-mouth method:* the patient is supine; the operator grips the nose and inflates the lungs by breathing into the patient's mouth. *Schafer method:* the patient is prone; the operator kneels astride the patient, places his hands over the lower ribs on each side, and alternately throws his weight forward on to his hands and leans back, taking the weight off the hands about 12 times a minute. *Sylvester method:* the patient is supine and the tongue is held out; the operator grasps the arms at the elbows and presses them firmly against the sides of the chest for 2 s and then pulls the arms upwards so that they lie in the long axis of the body on each side of the head. The two movements are repeated 15 times a minute. **Assisted respiration.** Assisting shallow respiration through a face-piece or tracheotomy tube either manually, using a compressible bag, or with the aid of an apparatus working automatically. **Asthmatoid respiration.** Expiratory dyspnoea accompanied by wheezing. **Cerebral respiration.** Slow and deep respirations with raised intracranial pressure. **Clavicular respiration.** Respiration with excessive movements of the clavicles. **Cog-wheel respiration.** Respiration in which the breath sounds, especially the inspiratory phase, are interrupted and jerky. **Controlled respiration.** Control of a patient's breathing by manual or mechanical means after deliberately abolishing spontaneous respiration; a widely practised anaesthetic technique. **Controlled diaphragmatic respiration.** Deliberate use of diaphragmatic breathing with the idea of limiting the movements at the apices. **Costal respiration.** Breathing mainly carried out by the thoracic movements. **Divided respiration.** Respiration with a distinct pause between the inspiratory and expiratory movements. **Dyspnoeic respiration.** Dyspnoea. **Electrophrenic respiration.** Respiration induced by stimulation of the phrenic nerve. **External respiration.** The part of respiration concerned with the interchange of gases between the atmosphere and the alveolar air, and between the alveolar air and the lung capillaries. **Extrinsic respiration.** Breathing of air from a bag in such a way that the expired air is not rebreathed. **Fetal respiration.** The gaseous interchange between the maternal and fetal bloods. **Forced respiration.** Respiration in which the accessory muscles of respiration are brought into play. **Hissing respiration.** Dyspnoea with a hissing sound, encountered in uraemia. **Intermittent positive pressure respiration (IPPR).** Intermittent positive pressure ventilation. *See* VENTILATION. **Internal respiration.** The passage of oxygen from the blood to the tissues and of carbon dioxide from the tissues to the blood. **Intrinsic respiration.** Breathing the same volume of air over and over again. **Laboured respiration.** Difficult respiration in which the accessory muscles are brought into use. **Meningitic respiration.** Biot's respiration; a form of periodical breathing in which a phase of rapid breathing is followed abruptly by a pause of from 10-30 seconds; it may occur with meningitis affecting the medullary region. **Nasal respiration.** Breathing through the nose. **Paradoxical respiration.** The type of respiration which may be seen in a patient with a flail or an open chest, when the handicapped lung becomes inflated during expiration and deflated during inspiration by gases from the sound lung. **Pendel-Luft type of respiration.** The movement of air from one lung to the other during inspiration when an open pneumothorax is present; it can be at once controlled by sealing the chest wall opening. It is accompanied by a pendulum movement of the heart and mediastinum, unless the latter is fixed by inflammatory changes. **Periodic respiration.** Breathing of the Biot or Cheyne-Stokes types in which periods of rapid respiration are followed by slow breathing or complete cessation for a time. **Placental respiration.** The gaseous exchange between the maternal and fetal bloods in the placenta. **Pneumotoxic respiration.** Short, shallow, rapid, irregular respiration occurring in acute inflammatory conditions of the lung or pleural membranes, e.g. acute lobar pneumonia, bronchopneumonia, pleurisy, and acute tuberculous conditions, owing to reflex disturbance from pleural or hilar nerve impulses. *See* HERING-BREUER REFLEX. **Prenatal respiration.** Fetal respiration (see above). **Senile respiration.** The feeble breathing of old age. **Slow respiration.** Respiration the rate of which is below 12 a minute. **Stertorous respiration.** Loud, noisy breathing with a snoring and rattling character, heard in comatose patients. **Thoracic respiration.** Costal respiration (see above). **Tissue respiration.** The oxidation of metabolites in the tissue cells and the production of carbon dioxide. **Uraemic respiration.** Dyspnoeic breathing with a hissing character. **Vicarious respiration.** Increased breathing of one lung when the other is out of action. [L *respirare* to breathe.]

See also: BIOT, BOUCHUT, CHEYNE (J.), KUSSMAUL, STOKES (WILLIAM).

respirator (res·pir·a·tor). An apparatus placed over the nose and mouth to enable medicated vapours to be inhaled, or to prevent the inhalation of dangerous dusts or gases, e.g. the gas mask used during the war. **Respirator cabinet.** A closed small, bare room in which a patient breathes air strongly charged with an antiseptic such as creosote in the treatment of bronchiectasis. **Cuirass respirator.** A device surrounding the chest and abdomen to produce artificial respiration by means of intermittent air pressure mechanically supplied. **Intermittent negative-pressure respirator.** A respirator in which the air is sucked in by application of negative pressure to the chest wall, as in the case of the iron lung. **Intermittent positive-pressure respirator.** An apparatus for the mechanical maintenance of artificial respiration by the intermittent direct insufflation of air, or of oxygen containing mixtures of gases, into the respiratory system. The apparatus differs radically from the *intermittent negative-pressure respirators*, e.g. the iron lung, in that the air is blown in and not sucked in by the application of negative pressure to the chest wall as in the case of the latter. **Radcliffe respirator.** A pressure-pre-set, time-cycled artificial ventilating machine driven by electricity, batteries, or by hand. [L *respirare* to breathe.]

See also: BOTH, CLEVEDON, DRINKER, MONAGHAN, YEO.

respiratory (res·**pir**·at·or·e). Relating or belonging to respiration.

respire (res·**pire**). To breathe. [L *respirare*.]

respirometer (res·pir·**om**·et·er). An instrument used to ascertain the nature or quality of the respiratory movements. [respiration, meter.]

response (res·**pons**). The reaction of an organism or part of an organism to a stimulus. **Extensor-plantar response.** In the Babinski phenomenon, the big toe is dorsiflexed (extended) when the sole of the foot, especially at the lateral margin, is stimulated by having a blunt object drawn along it. **Flexor-plantar response.** Flexion of all the toes on stimulation of the lateral aspect of the sole of the foot. **Immune response.** The total immunological reaction to a stimulus; it includes not only antibody formation but also the development of hypersensitivity and various cellular phenomena, and even immunological tolerance. *Primary immune response* is the response to second or subsequent exposure to a given antigen; it may be slight or undetectable but the individual is said to be primed or sensitized. *Secondary immune response* is the response to second or subsequent exposure to a given antigen. The classical secondary response involves the rapid production of high titres of circulating antibody; other possible responses are the elicitation of immediate or delayed hypersensitivity reactions. **Inverse response.** A response which is in the opposite sense to that which is expected. **Reticulocyte response.** An increase in the rate of formation of reticulocytes in the bone marrow as shown by an increased number in the blood; this occurs in pernicious anaemia following treatment with active anti-anaemic preparations, the reticulocyte count reaching a maximum about 4-8 days later and then falling to normal levels of less than 1.0 % of the erythrocytes; a similar reticulocyte response also follows iron treatment for hypochromic anaemias, and a smaller one after severe haemorrhage. **Thalamic response.** A raised threshold of somatic sensations combined with an exaggerated reaction to stimuli above the threshold: a feature of thalamic damage. **Triple response.** The phenomenon seen in the skin after injection of histamine or heavy stroking: a red line due to capillary dilatation, a widespread flare due to arteriolar dilatation, and finally a weal at the site of the red line due to exudation from capillaries. It was first described by Sir Thomas Lewis. **Visually-evoked response.** Electrical changes recorded from the surface of the occipital cortex or from scalp electrodes in response to retinal stimulation by repeated flashes of light. [L *respondere* to reply.]

responsibility (res·**pons**·ib·il'·it·e). Diminished responsibility, a term used in criminal proceedings on charges of murder, to excuse or reduce the culpability on the grounds of a disturbance of mind sufficient to remove the real intent. *See* MENS REA. [L *respondere* to reply.]

rest (rest). 1. Repose; the refraining from volitional muscular or mental effort; a remission of muscular or mental effort. 2. An island of embryonic tissue retained into adult life. It is supposed to be the site of origin of certain types of tumour. **Adrenal rests.** Small masses, identical with the suprarenal cortex, in the region of the gland and elsewhere. **Bed rest.** 1. A contrivance for supporting a bed patient in a sitting or semisupine position. 2. Rest in bed. **Carbon rest.** The residual amount of carbon present in the substances left in the filtrate after deproteinizing blood. **Embryonal rest, Epithelial rest, Fetal rest.** A minute collection of cells, embryonic or partly differentiated, which persists from the early days of development of the human being throughout life in a dormant state, but sometimes assumes the features of growing tissue and even becomes malignant. **Occlusal rest.** A metal spur extending from a partial denture, which rests on the biting surface of a tooth. **Suprarenal rests.** Aberrant suprarenal tissue sometimes found above the kidney. [AS.]

See also: COHNHEIM, MALASSEZ, WALTHARD.

restbite (rest·bite). The occlusion of the teeth of the natural dentition or of artificial dentures when the jaws are at rest, leaving a free-way space between upper and lower teeth. [rest, bite.]

restibrachium (res·te·**bra**·ke·um) (pl. *restibrachia*). An inferior cerebellar peduncle. [L *restis* rope, brachium.]

restiform (res·te·form). Shaped like a rope; ropelike. **Restiform body.** *See* BODY. [L *restis* rope, form.]

restis (res·tis). Restibrachium.

restitution (res·te·**tew**·shun). 1. The restoring of anything to its original shape or position. 2. In obstetrics, the turning of the fetal head usually through 45 degrees to the right or the left after it has emerged from the vulva. [L *restituere* to restore.]

restocythaemia (res·to·si·**the**′·me·ah). Fragments of broken-up erythrocytes in the circulating blood. [L *restare* to remain, Gk *kytos* cell, *haima* blood.]

restoration (res·tor·a·shun). The action of being restored to a normal position or state; the fact of being thus restored. **Buccal restoration.** A filling placed on the buccal side of a tooth. [L *restaurare* to restore.]

restorative (re·**stor**·at·iv). 1. Having the power to restore or renew health, vigour, or consciousness. 2. An agent that promotes the restoration or renewal of health or consciousness. [see prec.]

restraint (re·**stra**·nt). 1. The act or process of checking or controlling a physical or mental action. 2. The enforced confinement of persons affected with a violent type of insanity, e.g. acute mania. **Chemical restraint.** Medicinal restraint (see below). **Mechanical restraint.** Controlling a violently insane person by mechanical means, e.g. in a strait jacket or a special chair or bed. **Medicinal restraint.** Control of a maniacal person by drugs, e.g. hypnotics. [L *restringere* to confine.]

restriction (re·**strik**·shun). In bacteria, the process whereby foreign DNA which enters the cell is recognized and broken down by endonuclease enzymes. [L *restringere* to confine.]

restringent (re·**strin**·jent). Astringent. [see prec.]

restropin (res·tro·pin). A factor, said to be present in blood, and supposed to have the power of stimulating the reticulo-endothelial system. [*re*ticulo-endothelial *s*ystem, Gk *trepein* to turn.]

resublimation (re·sub·lim·**a**′·shun). In chemistry, a method of purification based on successive sublimations. [L *re-*, *sublimare* to raise up.]

resublimed (re·sub·li·md). Having undergone several successive sublimations. [see prec.]

resultant (re·**zul**·tant). 1. Any substance produced by a chemical action between so-called *reactants.* 2. In mechanics, the net single force in size and direction that is the equivalent of several forces acting together at various angles. [L *resultare* to rebound.]

resupinate (re·sew·pin·ate). 1. Inverted in position. 2. To turn over on the back. [L *resupinare* to bend backwards.]

resupination (re·sew·pin·**a**′·shun). 1. The act of turning or the state of lying on the back. 2. The act of turning to an inverted position. [see prec.]

resuscitate (re·**sus**·it·ate). 1. To restore to life or consciousness after death apparently has occurred. 2. To revive. [see foll.]

resuscitation (re·sus·it·**a**′·shun). 1. The act or process of restoring to life or consciousness anyone who is gravely collapsed or apparently dead. 2. The state of being resuscitated. 3. Revival. **Emergency resuscitation.** Resuscitation following cardiac arrest; it requires external cardiac massage and artificial ventilation followed by after-care and treatment of complications. It is instituted as soon as cardiac arrest is recognized, as delay of more than 3 min results in brain damage and low cardiac output, both irreversible if the patient survives. **Expired air resuscitation.** A technique of treatment of apnoea in which the operator forces his expired air under pressure into the lungs of the subject, so giving him about 16 per cent of oxygen. [L *resuscitare* to revive.]

See also: DRINKER.

resuscitator (re·**sus**·it·a·tor). An apparatus by means of which breathing is restarted in asphyxiated persons. [see prec.]

resuture (re·**sew**·tewr). Secondary suture. [L *re-*, suture.]

RET (ret). A unit of absorbed dose used for comparative purposes allowing for differences in fractionation. (Not accepted as an international unit.) [*R*ad *E*quivalent *T*herapy.]

retainer (re·**ta**·ner). An apparatus used in dentistry for retaining in their correct position teeth whose malposition has been corrected. [L *retinere* to hold.]

Retan, George Matthew (b. 1889). Syracuse paediatrician.

Retan's treatment. The treatment of intussusception by distending the colon with a barium enema, and following with manipulation.

retardation (re·tar·**da**·shun). 1. Mental backwardness. 2. A slowing of thought or action. **Executive retardation of thought.** A slowing of the action dictated by a thought. **Initial retardation of thought.** A slowing of a thought leading to an action. **Psychomotor retardation.** A slowing of thought and action. **Retardation of thought.** A slowing of thought. [L *retardare* to check.]

retardin (re·**tar**·din). A substance obtained from the pancreas which has been stated to regulate fat metabolism. [see foll.]

retarding (re·**tar**·ding). Delaying or slowing; hindering. [L *retardare* to check.]

retch (retch). To make a straining ineffective effort to vomit; hence *retching.* [AS *hraecan* to spit.]

rete [NA] (re·te) (pl. *retia*). A net or network; in anatomy, of nerves, blood vessels, or tubules. The term has been applied in many parts of the body to anastomosing networks of arteries or veins, but this use is largely obsolete. **Rete malpighii.** Rete mucosum (see below). **Rete mirabile [NA].** A plexus formed by the splitting of an artery into many branches which again unite to form a single vessel; it is found in many animals, but in man only in the glomerulus of the kidney where the afferent arteriole breaks up into a number of capillaries which then join to form the efferent arteriole. **Rete mucosum.** The layers of the epidermis of the skin, deep to the granular layer. **Rete testis [NA].** An anastomosing network of tubules in the mediastinum testis into which the seminiferous tubules open; the tubules of the rete testis end in the efferent ducts of the testis. [L.]

retene (ret·een). Methylisopropylphenanthrene, $CH_3C_{14}H_8CH(CH_3)_2$. A crystalline hydrocarbon found with pyrene in coal tar and in the tars of some pines. It is used as a starting point for certain dyestuffs.

retentio mensium (re·**ten**·she·o **men**·se·um). Cryptomenorrhoea; retention of the menstrual flow due to congenital or acquired genital-canal stenosis. [L.]

retention (re·**ten**·shun). The holding back in the body of substances which are normally excreted. **Heat retention.** A condition occurring in normally anhydrous persons, in which the temperature rises several degrees with accompanying vertigo, headache, and restlessness. **Retention of urine.** The retention of urine in the bladder owing to obstruction of the outflow or muscular weakness of the bladder wall. [L *retinere* to hold.]

retethelioma (re·te·the·le·**o**′·mah). Reticulo-endothelial sarcoma.

retial (re·te·al). Belonging to or having the characters of a rete.

reticular, reticulated (re·**tik**·ew·lar, re·**tik**·ew·la·ted). Relating or belonging to a reticulum or reticula.

reticulation (re·**tik**·ew·**la**′·shun). 1. The quality or state of being reticulated or netlike. 2. The formation or the presence of a reticulum or network, as in erythrocytes while blood regeneration is actively proceeding. **Dust reticulation.** A preliminary stage of pneumoconiosis, occurring predominantly in coal miners, which may progress in anthracosis. [L *reticulum* little net.]

reticulin (re·**tik**·ew·lin). The protein derived from reticular fibres of connective tissue.

reticulocyte (re·**tik**·ew·lo·site). A non-nucleated young red cell intermediate between the nucleated normoblast and normal red cell; it contains strands of nuclear material which take up supravital stains such as brilliant cresyl blue and show a basket-like or reticulated appearance. Normally, they are seen in peripheral blood to the extent of 0.5–2.0 per cent of the red cells, but may be much increased in numbers (5.0–70 per cent) in certain diseases such as haemolytic anaemia, after severe haemorrhages, or for a short time (3–24 days) following commencement of active therapy in pernicious or iron-deficiency anaemias. **Myocardial reticulocyte.** A muscle tissue cell with a peculiar structure of its nucleus, usually seen in normal cardiac muscle and cells. [reticulum, Gk *kytos* cell.]

reticulocytogenic (re·**tik**·ew·lo·si·to·**jen**′·ik). Producing or causing production of reticulocytes. [reticulocyte, Gk *genein* to produce.]

reticulocytoma (re·**tik**·ew·lo·si·**to**′·mah). A misleading term for a variety of net-cell sarcoma. [reticulum, Gk *kytos* cell, *-oma* tumour.]

reticulocytopenia (re·**tik**·ew·lo·si·to·**pe**′·ne·ah). Diminution in the number of reticulocytes in the blood. [reticulocytes, Gk *penes* poor.]

reticulocytosis (re·**tik**·ew·lo·si·**to**′·sis). The presence of an excessive number of reticulocytes in the blood. **Leukaemic reticulocytosis.** Monocytic leukaemia. [reticulocyte, Gk *-osis* condition.]

reticulo-endothelial (re·**tik**·ew·lo·en·do·**the**′·le·al). Pertaining to reticulo-endothelium.

reticulo-endothelioma (re·**tik**·ew·lo·en·do·the·le·**o**′·mah). A reticulo-endothelial tumour. [reticulo-endothelium, Gk *-oma* tumour.]

reticulo-endotheliosis (re·**tik**·ew·lo·en·do·the·le·**o**′·sis). 1. Reticulosis; an abnormal increase in the reticulo-endothelial cells in certain diseases, but exact classification is difficult as there are close similarities to chronic monocytic leukaemia, Hodgkin's disease, and diseases of the reticulo-endothelial system. 2. Monocytic leukaemia. **Leukaemic reticulo-endotheliosis.** Monocytic leukaemia, a severe leukaemic condition characterized by a disturbance of the monocytic series of white cells, usually causing a rapidly fatal acute monocytic leukaemia. **Non-lipoid reticulo-endotheliosis, Systemic aleukaemic reticulo-endotheliosis.** Letterer–Siwe disease; a non-familial condition occurring in young children with hyperplasia of the reticulo-endothelial cells, splenomegaly, hepatomegalia, haemorrhagic manifestations, and anaemia. [reticulo-endothelium, Gk *-osis* condition.]

reticulo-endothelium (re·**tik**·ew·lo·en·do·**the**′·le·um). The basic substance which forms the reticulo-endothelial system. [reticulum, endothelium.]

reticulogranuloma (re·**tik**·ew·lo·gran·ew·**lo**′·mah). Histiocytosis X (Letterer-Christian disease). [reticulum, granule, Gk *-oma* tumour.]

reticulohistiocytary (re·**tik**·ew·lo·his·te·o·**si**′·tar·e). Relating to or consisting of histiocytes of the reticulo-endothelial system.

reticulohistiocytoma (re·**tik**·ew·lo·**his**·te·o·si·**to**′·mah). A giant-cell xanthomatous granulomatosis affecting the skin and mucous membranes and the synovial membranes, particularly of the long bones of the hands and feet in which crippling deformity may result. [reticulum, histiocyte, Gk *-oma* tumour.]

reticuloma (re·**tik**·ew·**lo**′·mah). A tumour made up of reticulo-endothelial cells (monocytes). [reticulum, Gk *-oma* tumour.]

reticulopenia (re·**tik**·ew·lo·**pe**′·ne·ah). Reticulocytopenia.

reticuloplasmocytoma (re·**tik**·ew·lo·**plaz**·mo·si·**to**′·mah). A tumour composed of reticulocytes and plasma cells (plasmocytes). [reticulocyte, plasmocyte, Gk *-oma* tumour.]

reticulosarcoma (re·**tik**·ew·lo·sar·**ko**′·mah). Clasmatocytic lymphoma; a malignant tumour composed of large monocytic cells derived from the reticulo-endothelium of lymph glands and spleen chiefly. **Dicytocytic reticulosarcoma.** A reticulin-forming reticulo-endothelial tumour. **Dicytosyncytial reticulosarcoma.** A highly cellular dicytocytic reticulosarcoma. **Lymphoblastic reticulosarcoma, Lymphocytic reticulosarcoma, Lymphoid reticulosarcoma.** Lymphocytic lymphoma. **Myeloblastic reticulosarcoma, Polymorphic reticulosarcoma, Syncytial reticulosarcoma.** Lymph-gland tumours of the reticulosarcoma type; a classification not universally recognized. [reticulum, Gk *sarx* flesh, *-oma* tumour.]

reticulosis (re·**tik**·ew·**lo**′·sis). 1. An increase in reticulo-endothelial cells in bone marrow and blood; reticulo-endotheliosis. 2. Reticulocytosis. **Giant follicular reticulosis.** A non-invasive type of reticulosis characterized by a prolonged and very benign clinical course. Unlike the other reticuloses, the neoplastic process tends to remain localized to a single group of nodes for many months. The organs most commonly involved are the lymph glands and spleen. **Histiocytic reticulosis.** Histiocytosis X. **Histiomonocytic reticulosis.** Net-cell sarcoma. *See* SARCOMA. **Leukaemic reticulosis.** Monocytic leukaemia. **Lipomelanic reticulosis.** Dermatopathic lymphadenitis; the histological changes seen in the rubbery enlarged lymph nodes in non-reticulotic and in pre-reticulotic erythroderma. They include a normal architecture with an increase of reticulum cells containing melanin or fat. In some cases the histological appearances of a true reticulosis may become apparent after months or several years. **Lymphoid medullary reticulosis.** A generalized diffuse proliferation of small lymphocytes, as observed in lymphatic leukaemia. **Lymphoreticular reticulosis.** An increase in lymphoid tissue in the lymph glands, with severe generalized reticular proliferation. **Myeloid reticulosis.** A fatal acute disease of the blood, characterized by splenomegaly and infiltration of the bone marrow with abnormal types of reticular cells. [reticulo-endothelium, Gk *-osis* condition.]

See also: SÉZARY.

reticulothelioma (re·**tik**·ew·lo·the·le·**o**′·mah). Reticulo-endothelioma.

reticulum (re·**tik**·ew·lum). A mesh, or network. **Endoplasmic reticulum.** A network of membrane-bound flattened vesicles whose inner compartments, called *cisternae*, interconnect to form channels that penetrate the whole of the cytoplasm of eukaryotic cells. It may be *rough* (its outer surface being studded with ribosomes) or *smooth* (having no attached ribosomes). Its main function is to serve as an intracellular transport system to the periphery of the cell. **Nuclear reticulum.** The network of precipitated chromatin within the nucleus of a fixed and stained cell. **Sarcoplasmic reticulum.** The network of fine tubules, resembling smooth endoplasmic reticulum, which is found in the sarcoplasm of muscle fibres. **Stellate reticulum.** The network of stellate cells within the early enamel organ of a developing tooth. [L little net.]

See also: CHIARI, EBNER.

retiform (re·te·form). Reticular; like network. [L *rete* net, form.]

retina [NA] (ret·in·ah). The innermost coat of the eyeball, consisting of a pigmented layer which is adherent to the choroid coat, the optic part [pars optica retinae (NA)], and extends forwards to line the back of the ciliary processes and iris, the ciliary [pars ciliaris retinae (NA)] and iridial [pars iridica retinae (NA)] parts of the retina, and the sensitive nervous layer (the retina proper) continuous posteriorly with the optic nerve and ending in front at an irregular margin, the ora serrata, just behind the ciliary body. The retina proper is a thin membrane, containing visual purple (rhodopsin) which bleaches rapidly when exposed to light. Where the optical axis of the lens meets it the retina shows a yellow pigmentation, the macula lutea, in the centre of which is a depression, the fovea centralis. A circular pale area to the medial side of the macula indicates the site of entry of the optic nerve (the optic disc) and corresponds to the blind spot. The retina proper consists of nine layers, from within out: 1, the membrana limitans interna; 2, the stratum opticum or nerve-fibre layer; 3, the ganglionic layer; 4, the inner plexiform layer; 5, the inner nuclear layer; 6, the outer plexiform layer; 7, the outer nuclear layer; 8, the membrana limitans externa; and 9, the neuro-epithelial layer, the true photoreceptors. **Fleck retina.** Retina with multiple small white or yellow spots. Fundus flavimaculatus, fundus albipunctatus, multiple drüsen of the fundus, and Doyne's honeycomb choroiditis are all conditions which can be called fleck retina. **Leopard retina.** The variegated retina of retinitis pigmentosa. **Shot-silk retina.** One that gives a shimmering effect on examination, caused by moving light reflexes from the ophthalmoscope, most commonly seen in hypermetropes and children. It is a physiological condition. **Tigroid retina.** One often seen in persons with much pigment. The dark choroidal pigment stands out between the choroid vessels as darkish patches all over the fundus. It is not pathological. **Watered-silk retina.** Shot-silk retina (see above). [L *rete* net.]

retina, central artery of the [arteria centralis retinae (NA)]. The sole artery of the retina, entering the eyeball along the optic nerve, and dividing into superior and inferior branches immediately after entering the retina, each of which divides further into nasal [arteriolae nasales retinae, superior et inferior (NA)] and temporal [arteriolae temporales retinae, superior et inferior (NA)] branches. The temporal branches supply twigs to the macula [arteriola macularis, superior et inferior (NA)]. The medial retinal branch [arteriola medialis retinae (NA)] is a small artery arising in the nasal side of the optic disc and distributed to the adjacent retina.

retina, central vein of the [vena centralis retinae (NA)]. The sole vein of the retina, formed by the junction of the superior and inferior tributaries which in turn receive blood from the nasal [venulae nasales retinae, superior et inferior (NA)], the temporal [venulae temporales retinae, superior et inferior (NA)], and the macular [venula macularis, superior et inferior (NA)] branches. The medial retinal branch [venula medialis retinae] accompanies the medial retinal branch of the central artery of the retina. It leaves the eyeball along the optic nerve.

retinaculum (ret·in·**ak**·ew·lum) (pl. *retinacula*). 1. [NA] A tie or fascial band holding a structure in position. 2. A sharp, hooked instrument used for pulling tissues aside at operation. **Retinaculum of the ankle, flexor [retinaculum musculorum flexorum (NA)].** A thickening of fascia passing back from the medial malleolus to the calcaneum over the long flexor tendons and the posterior tibial vessels and nerves. **Retinaculum of the ankle, inferior extensor [retinaculum musculorum extensorum inferius (NA)].** A Y-shaped band of deep fascia passing medially from the lateral side of the upper surface of the calcaneum, and dividing medially into two bands, the upper of which goes to the medial malleolus and the lower to the plantar aponeurosis. **Retinaculum of the ankle, inferior peroneal [retinaculum musculorum peroneorum (fibularium) inferius (NA)], Retinaculum of the ankle, superior peroneal [retinaculum musculorum peroneorum (fibularium) superius (NA)].** Fibrous slings over the peroneal tendons on the lateral side of the tarsus. **Retinaculum of the ankle, superior extensor [retinaculum musculorum extensorum superius (NA)].** A thickening of deep fascia attached to the lower ends of the shafts of the tibia and fibula and extending over the tendons of the extensor muscles. **Retinaculum of the arcuate ligament.** The diverging bundles of fibres arising from the head of the fibula and blending with either end of the arcuate ligament; the anterior band is sometimes called the *short lateral ligament of the knee.* **Caudal retinaculum [retinaculum caudale (NA)].** The fibrous tissue attaching the skin to the coccyx. **Retinacula cutis [NA].** Bands of fibrous tissue linking the corium to the underlying tissue, especially in the neighbourhood of a joint. **Retinaculum of the patella, lateral [retinaculum patellae laterale (NA)].** An accessory ligament superficial to the capsule, lying between the patella, its tendon, and the lateral ligament. It is formed by a blending of deep fascia strengthened by the iliotibial tract and the tendinous expansion of the vastus lateralis muscle. **Retinaculum of the patella, medial [retinaculum patellae mediale (NA)].** An accessory ligament superficial to the capsule, lying between the patella, its tendon, and the medial ligament. It is formed by a blending of deep fascia and the tendinous expansion of the vastus medialis muscle. **Ungual retinacula [retinacula unguis (NA)].** Bands of connective-tissue fibres which ascend from the periosteum over the ungual phalanx and expand in a brush-like fashion under the nail. **Retinaculum of the wrist, extensor [retinaculum extensorum (NA)].** A broad thickening of the deep fascia over the back of the wrist, over the extensor tendons. **Retinaculum of the wrist, flexor [retinaculum flexorum (NA)].** A strong ligament across the front of the hollow of the carpus, over the flexor tendons of the fingers and median nerve. A slip, or superficial part, crosses the ulnar vessels and nerve. [L halter.]

See also: BARRY, WEITBRECHT.

retinal (**ret**·in·al). Pertaining to the retina.

retinene (**ret**·in·een). A yellow carotenoid which is formed in the retina of the eye by decomposition of a pigment termed *visual yellow* produced from rhodopsin by the action of light. The rhodopsin cycle is completed by the conversion of retinene into vitamin A which combines with protein to regenerate rhodopsin.

retinitis (ret·in·**i**·tis). Inflammation of the retina. Since the important part of the retina is the nervous tissue, which shows only slight inflammatory changes, this term has been largely abandoned and *retinopathy*, which is non-committal, substituted for it. **Retinitis albuminurica.** An obsolete term for renal retinopathy. **Central punctate retinitis.** An old name for a common form of diabetic retinopathy, characterized by small, well-defined spots of hard, yellowish-white exudate, with a few small, round haemorrhages situated mainly around the macular region. **Retinitis disciformans.** Now commonly known as *disciform degeneration of the macula* or *senile macular exudative choroiditis,* the latter being the old name. **Retinitis pigmentosa.** A genetically determined, bilateral, primary degeneration of the retina, becoming clinically diagnosable in childhood and gradually progressing to blindness at about middle age. Characterized by poor night vision, constricted visual fields, bone-corpuscle pigmentation of the retina, alternation of the retinal vessels, and waxy atrophy of the optic discs. **Retinitis punctata albescens.** Albipunctate dystrophy. *See* DYSTROPHY. **Septic retinitis.** A benign inflammatory condition of the retina associated with a general systemic infection, most commonly endocarditis. It is characterized by white spots, usually surrounded by a haemorrhage, seen in the region of the disc, and called *Roth's spots.* [retina, Gk *-itis* inflammation.]

See also: ROTH (M.).

retinoblastoma (**ret**·in·o·blas·**to**′·mah). A malignant glioma of the retina which occurs almost exclusively in infants. It is congenital in origin and embryonic in structure. [retina, blastoma.]

retinochoroid (**ret**·in·o·**kor**′·oid). Relating or belonging to the retina and the choroid.

retinochoroiditis (**ret**·in·o·kor·oid·**i**′·tis). Choroidoretinitis. **Retinochoroiditis juxtapapillaris.** Jensen's retinopathy; choroidoretinitis near the disc margin. It is associated with the production of vitreous opacities and of a scotoma. [retinochoroid, Gk *-itis* inflammation.]

retinocystoma (**ret**·in·o·sist·**o**′·mah). A retinal glioma. [retina, cyst, Gk *-oma* tumour.]

retinodialysis (**ret**·in·o·di·**al**′·is·is). Disinsertion; a term applied to a tear in the retina in its anterior part, at or near the ora serrata. [retina, Gk *dialysis* a separation.]

retinograph (**ret**·in·o·graf). A photograph of the retina.

retinography (ret·in·**og**·raf·e). Retinal photography.

retinoid (**ret**·in·oid). 1. Having resemblance to the retina. [retina, Gk *eidos* form.] 2. Having resemblance to a resin; resinlike. [Gk *rhetine* resin, *eidos* form.]

retinol (**ret**·in·ol). 1. $C_{32}H_{16}$, a liquid hydrocarbon from pitch or resin, formerly in use as a urinary antiseptic and in gonorrhoea. 2. BP Commission approved name for vitamin A alcohol.

retinomalacia (**ret**·in·o·mal·**a**′·she·ah). Softening of the retina. [retina, Gk *malakia* softness.]

retinomeningo-encephalitis (**ret**·in·o·men·**ing**·go·en·kef·al·**i**′·tis). Inflammation of the brain and meninges with retinal haemorrhages, lasting for 2 to 6 weeks but usually ending in recovery. [retina, Gk *menigx* membrane, encephalitis.]

retinopapillitis (**ret**·in·o·pap·il·**i**′·tis). Inflammation of the optic disc and retina. [retina, papilla, Gk *-itis* inflammation.]

retinopathia (**ret**·in·o·**path**′·e·ah). Retinopathy.

retinopathy (ret·in·**op**·ath·e). Any diseased condition of the retina, usually associated with impairment of vision, distortion of objects, and oedema and sometimes haemorrhages into the substance of the retina. It has now largely replaced the term *retinitis.* **Actinic retinopathy.** The changes occurring after exposure to excessive actinic light. **Angiopathic retinopathy.** A retinopathy in which the blood vessels of the retina are affected. **Apoplectic retinopathy.** The presence of numerous retinal haemorrhages, usually caused by thrombosis of the central vein. **Arteriosclerotic retinopathy.** The fundal appearances associated with arteriosclerosis and benign hypertension; the vessels show differing calibre, increase in the streak reflex, and nipping at the arteriovenous crossings. Small scattered haemorrhages and small spots of hard white exudate are seen, mostly at the posterior pole. There is no oedema of the disc or retina. **Central angiospastic retinopathy.** Central serous retinopathy (see below). **Central disc-shaped retinopathy.** Disciform degeneration of the macula. **Central recurrent retinopathy.** A rare form of central retinopathy associated with syphilis and characterized by a corresponding scotoma. The attacks last for a few days and tend to recur with increasing frequency. **Central relapsing retinopathy.** A syphilitic affection of the macular region, characterized by the development of a grey or yellowish area. **Central serous retinopathy.** A generally benign macular retinal detachment affecting young adults, self-limiting but often recurrent, caused by focal leakage of serous fluid through the pigment epithelium. **Cerebral retinopathy.** Damage to the retina associated with intracranial inflammation. **Circinate retinopathy.** A condition occurring usually in the aged and characterized by a ring of brilliant white spots around the macula which itself undergoes degenerative changes; it is frequently associated with arteriosclerosis. **Circumpapillary retinopathy.** Retinopathy occurring in the region round the optic disc. **Diabetic retinopathy.** The changes occurring in the retina as a result of diabetes. These include changes in the blood vessels, formation of minute aneurysms and of exudate, haemorrhages, and retinal detachment. **Diffuse retinopathy.** Widespread disease in the superficial layers of the retina. **Diffuse parenchymatous retinopathy.** Diffuse retinopathy in which the deeper layers of the retina are also involved. **Exudate retinopathy.** Coats' disease; sometimes applied to central senile exudative choroiditis or disciform degeneration of the macula due to haemorrhage from the choriocapillaries. **Glycosuric retinopathy.** Diabetic retinopathy (see above). **Gravidic retinopathy.** Retinal changes in association with the toxaemia of pregnancy, resembling those of renal retinopathy but prognosis is much better and serous exudate tends to be greater, sometimes producing temporary retinal detachment. It is an indication for the termination of pregnancy. **Haemorrhagic retinopathy.** Retinopathy characterized by profuse haemorrhages. **Hepatic retinopathy.** Retinal changes occurring in association with hepatitis. **Hypertensive retinopathy.** Retinal changes occurring in association with arterial hypertension. These include alterations in the vessels, haemorrhages, exudates, retinal oedema, and sometimes papilloedema. **Leukaemic retinopathy.** Retinal changes found in leukaemia: the retinal vessels are dilated, the arteries and veins being almost of the same colour; the whole fundus is pale, haemorrhages may have a pale centre, and the disc is often blurred. **Macular retinopathy.** 1. Central relapsing retinopathy (see above). 2. A generic term applicable to any form of retinal changes affecting the central region. **Metastatic retinopathy.** Pyaemic infection of the retina by way of the vessels. **Nephritic retinopathy.** Renal retinopathy (see below). **Pigmented retinopathy.** More accurately termed *pigmentary degeneration of the retina*, a primary degeneration of the outer layers of the retina, particularly the rods. It is bilateral, progressive, and hereditary; consanguinity of parents may be a factor. It is associated with progressive contraction of the retinal vessels and fields of vision, night blindness, and the aggregation of pigment into masses shaped like bone corpuscles. **Proliferating retinopathy.** Formation of fibrous bands in the retina following intra-ocular haemorrhage, and in some cases a low-grade infection; they cause retinal detachment by their contraction. **Punctate retinopathy.** Primary retinal degeneration, sometimes familial, associated with contraction of fields, night blindness, formation of numerous small white spots, and optic atrophy. It may be applied to widespread development of small colloid excrescences of Bruch's membrane. **Purulent retinopathy.** A condition which may be exogenous when it is part of the panophthalmitis which follows the introduction of pyogenic organisms through an infected wound, or endogenous when the organisms arrive via the blood stream. In the latter the emboli are usually multiple and panophthalmitis follows. **Renal retinopathy.** A condition formerly regarded as a clinical entity, characterized by formation of a star figure at the macula, soft white patches, haemorrhages in the retina, and sclerotic changes in the vessels; these latter are now considered as the important feature and renal retinopathy as part of the hypertensive variety. **Septic retinopathy.** Purulent retinopathy (see above). **Solar retinopathy.** Retinal changes following excessive exposure to sunlight, usually when the patient has been looking directly at the sun, e.g. eclipse blindness. **Splenic retinopathy.** Leukaemic retinopathy (see above). **Stellate retinopathy.** A generic term applied to the presence of white lines radiating from the macula, due to retinal oedema. **Striate retinopathy.** The presence of brown or dark red striae in the retina (angioid streaks), usually occurring in connection with haemorrhages. They are due to ruptures in Bruch's membrane in which calcium has been deposited. **Suppurative retinopathy.** Purulent retinopathy (see above). **Syphilitic retinopathy.** Syphilis may affect the retina and optic nerve in a variety of different ways, the commonest being that due to infection of the underlying choroid. Primary retinal lesions are associated with the blood vessels and several types are described, according to their distribution. In most, the retina becomes oedematous, grey, cloudy, and opaque, either locally or generally, and there may be occlusion of vessels. **Uraemic retinopathy.** The retinal changes occurring in uraemia; these may be of the renal type, but in some cases may be surprisingly slight. **Vascular retinopathy.** Any vascular disease affecting the retina. **Venous stasis retinopathy.** Dilated veins, peripheral deep retinal haemorrhages, and micro-aneurysms, due to chronically reduced retinal blood flow for whatever cause. [retina, Gk *pathos* disease.]

See also: COATS, JACOBSON (J.), JENSEN (E. Z.), PURTSCHER.

retinophotoscopy (ret·in·o·fo·**tos**'·ko·pe). Retinoscopy. [retina, photoscopy.]

retinoschisis (ret·in·**os**·kis·is). Splitting of the retina into two layers, the dehiscence usually being between the receptors and the bipolar cells. Senile degenerative and juvenile hereditary forms occur. Also known as *giant retinal cyst.* [retina, Gk *schisis* division.]

retinoscope (**ret**·in·o·skope). The instrument used in retinoscopy. **Electric retinoscope.** One that incorporates its own source of light for reflection through the pupil in the form of a small electric bulb supplied from the mains or a battery in the handle of the instrument. **Streak retinoscope.** One that produces a linear light in the pupil instead of the more usual circular one. In self-illuminating instruments this is achieved by the use of a linear source of light, but in the simple mirror, a round source of light is employed and reflected by a planocylindrical mirror. It makes the determination of the astigmatic error simpler and more accurate.

retinoscopy (ret·in·**os**·ko·pe). The procedure employed for objective determination of errors of refraction. Light is shone into the patient's eyes from a mirror, plane or concave, with a hole in the middle of it through which the observer notes the movements of the reflex from the patient's fundus: the nature of these indicates the type of refractive error and the lenses required to neutralize them. The word *retinoscopy* is unsatisfactory since the retina is invisible, and alternatives have been suggested, e.g. *shadow test, skiascopy.* **Dynamic retinoscopy.** An objective method of measuring the accommodation by retinoscopy of the eye in a state of active accommodation and convergence. Sometimes (in USA) called *dynamic skiametry.* [retina, Gk *skopein* to view.]

retinosis (ret·in·**o**·sis). Any pathological condition of the retina which is characterized by a process of degeneration but in which inflammation is not present. [retina, Gk *-osis* condition.]

retinoskiascopy (**ret**·in·o·ski·**as**'·ko·pe). Retinoscopy. [retina, skiascopy.]

retort (re·**tort**). 1. A vessel used in distillation; made of glass or metal it is bulbous in shape and is provided with a long tapering neck that inclines laterally. 2. A heated chamber designed for the distillation of coal, tar, petroleum, or metals such as zinc and mercury. 3. An autoclave used in industry for cooking sealed cans by superheated steam. [L *retortus* bent back.]

retothelial (re·to·**the**·le·al). Pertaining to or composed of reticulo-endothelial cells.

retothelioma (re·to·the·le·**o**′·mah). A reticulo-endothelial tumour. [reticulothelium, Gk *-oma* tumour.]

retothelium (re·to·**the**·le·um). Reticulo-endothelium.

retract (re·**trakt**). 1. To shrink back. 2. To draw or pull back or in. 3. To become shorter. [L *retractare* to draw back.]

retractile (re·**trak**·tile). Capable of being retracted or drawn back; hence *retractility.*

retraction (re·**trak**·shun). 1. The act of pulling back. 2. A shrinking; a condition of being drawn back. 3. In dentistry, the pulling backwards of a tooth or a group of teeth. **Clot retraction.** Contraction of clotted normal blood on standing, with expression of serum, being completed in 24 hours. This contraction depends on a plentiful supply of platelets, otherwise the clot is soft, friable, and does not contract, as may occur in thrombocytopenic purpura, or also sometimes in fibrinogenopenia or hypoprothrombinaemia. **Systolic retraction.** Systolic depression; recession of the sternum or ribs overlying the heart during systole, due to adherence of the pericardium to the chest wall. [see foll.]

retractor (re·**trak**·tor). An instrument designed for pulling aside tissues to improve exposure at operation. **Abdominal retractor.** An instrument for holding apart the edges of an abdominal wound. **Hook retractor.** A metal handle which carries at one end a hook (or hooks), blunt or sharp, large or small; widely used in surgical dissections. **Malleable copper retractor.** A flat strip of copper which can be bent into different curves and used as a retractor in a variety of shapes. **Nerve retractor.** A small, curved instrument of metal or glass for holding a nerve trunk or root. **Periosteal retractor.** An instrument used for lifting periosteum off bone. **Rib retractor.** An instrument consisting of two strong metal retractors which can be made to separate by a thumbscrew ratchet; used to separate the ribs in chest operations. **Self-retaining retractor.** Any retractor designed to remain in position and to maintain continuous retraction, even when unsupported, e.g. in goitre, bladder, mastoid, and abdominal operations. **Tonsil pillar retractor.** A handle carrying a shallow lip at one end which pulls the pillar aside in improving access to the nasopharyngeal tonsil. **Toothed retractor.** A retractor with a finely-toothed blade for holding skin flaps in plastic surgery. [L *retractare* to draw back.]

See also: DESMARRES, MOOREHEAD, MORSON, SIMON (GUSTAV).

retrahens aurem (re·tra·henz **aw**·rem). The auricularis posterior muscle. [L, drawing back the ear.]

retrenchment (re·**trench**·ment). A plastic procedure for the removal of redundant tissue. [Fr. *retrancher* to cut back.]

retro-. Prefix, from the Latin adverb *retro,* meaning *backward.*

retro-action (ret·ro·**ak**·shun). 1. Operation in a backward direction. 2. Reaction. [L *retro, agere* to act.]

retro-auricular (ret·ro·aw·**rik**′·ew·lar). Occurring behind or in a position at the back of the auricle. [L *retro,* auricle.]

retrobronchial (ret·ro·**brong**·ke·al). Situated or occurring behind a bronchus. [L *retro,* bronchus.]

retrobuccal (ret·ro·**buk**·al). Relating to the back portion of the mouth, or behind the mouth. [L *retro, bucca* cheek.]

retrobulbar (ret·ro·**bul**·bar). 1. Posterior to the eyeball. 2. Behind the pons. [L *retro,* bulb.]

retrocaecal (ret·ro·**se**·kal). Situated behind the caecum. **Retrocaecal recess.** *See* RECESS. [L *retro,* caecum.]

retrocalcaneobursitis (ret·ro·kal·**ka**·ne·o·ber·**si**′·tis). Inflammation or thickening of the bursae associated with, and especially the bursa of the tendo calcaneus, the bursa between the tendo calcaneus and the posterior surface of the calcaneum. [L *retro,* calcaneum, bursitis.]

retrocardiac (ret·ro·**kar**·de·ak). Situated or occurring behind the heart. [L *retro,* Gk *kardia* heart.]

retrocatheterism (ret·ro·**kath**·et·er·izm). The passing of a catheter through a suprapubic opening downward through the urethra to the external orifice. [L *retro,* catheter.]

retrocedent (ret·ro·**se**·dent). 1. Moving back; returning. 2. Striking inwards from the surface and involving an interior organ. [L *retrocedere* to go back.]

retrocervical (ret·ro·**ser**·vik·al). Occurring behind the neck of the uterus. [L *retro,* cervix.]

retrocession (ret·ro·**sesh**·un). 1. Backward movement. 2. Displacement backward, e.g. position of an organ. 3. Reorientation of a tumour or other disease process so that it leaves a superficial area to become established in an internal organ, with characteristic changes of symptoms and signs. 4. Relapse. [L *retrocedere* to go back.]

retroclavicular (ret·ro·klav·**ik**′·ew·lar). Situated or occurring behind the clavicle. [l *retro,* clavicle.]

retroclusion (ret·ro·**kloo**·zhun). A type of acupressure in which the needle is passed just above the cut end of the artery and after being turned round is passed again below the vessel so that it emerges from the tissues close to the point of entrance. [L *retro, claudere* to shut.]

retrocolic (ret·ro·**kol**·ik). Occurring or situated behind the colon. [L *retro,* colon.]

retrocollic (ret·ro·**kol**·ik). Relating or belonging to the back of the neck. [L *retro, collum* neck.]

retrocollis (ret·ro·**kol**·is). Retrocollic spasm, a type of torticollis in which the head is extended.

retrocursive (ret·ro·**ker**·siv). Characterized by the action of stepping backwards, as in retrocursive epilepsy. [L *retro, currere* to run.]

retrodeviation (ret·ro·de·ve·**a**′·shun). Backward displacement, e.g. retroflexion, retroversion. [L *retro,* deviation.]

retrodisplacement (ret·ro·dis·**plase**′·ment). Any backward displacement of an organ or part. [L *retro,* displacement.]

retrodural (ret·ro·**dewr**·al). Behind the dura mater. [L *retro,* dura mater.]

retroflexed (ret·ro·flext). Turned or bent backwards abruptly; in a state of retroflexion. [L *retro, flectere* to bend.]

retroflexion (ret·ro·**flek**·shun). The bending backward upon itself of an organ, e.g. the uterus when the body is bent so that it forms an angle with the neck. [see prec.]

retrogasserian (ret·ro·gas·**eer**′·e·an). Relating to the sensory root of the trigeminal (gasserian) ganglion. [L *retro,* gasserian.]

retrognathia (ret·ro·**nath**·e·ah). A condition in which the jaws are receded in relation to the frontal plane of the forehead. [L *retro,* Gk *gnathos* jaw.]

retrograde (ret·ro·grade). Of movement, backwards, in a direction opposite to that of the previous motion, or of the normal motion; degenerative. [L *retro, gradus* step.]

retrography (ret·**rog**·raf·e). Mirror writing. *See* WRITING. [L *retro,* Gk *graphein* to write.]

retrogression (ret·ro·**gresh**·un). 1. Catabolism. 2. Any process of degeneration. [L *retrogradi* to move backward.]

retro-ileal (ret·ro·i·le·al). Behind the ileum. [L *retro, ilia* intestines.]

retro-infection (ret·ro·in·**fek**′·shun). An infectious condition transmitted by the fetus to the mother. [L *retro,* infection.]

retro-insular (ret·ro·**in**·sew·lar). Behind the insula. [L *retro,* insula.]

retro-iridian (ret·ro·i·**rid**′·e·an). Posterior to the iris. [L *retro,* iris.]

retrojection (re·tro·**jek**·shun). The lavage of a cavity by the injection of a fluid. [L *retro,* injection.]

retrolabyrinthine (ret·ro·lab·ir·**in**′·thine). Situated or occurring behind the aural labyrinth. [L *retro,* labyrinth.]

retrolental (ret·ro·**len**·tal). Behind the lens of the eye. [L *retro,* lens.]

retrolingual (ret·ro·**ling**·gwal). 1. Relating to the posterior part of the tongue. 2. Behind the tongue. [L *retro, lingua* tongue.]

retromalleolar (ret·ro·mal·**e**′·o·lar). Behind a malleolus. [L *retro,* malleolus.]

retromammary (ret·ro·**mam**·ar·e). Behind the mammary gland. [L *retro,* mammary.]

retromandibular (ret·ro·man·**dib**′·ew·lar). Behind the mandible, e.g. relating to a certain point below the mastoid process, tender in mastoid inflammation. [L *retro,* mandible.]
retromastoid (ret·ro·**mas**·toid). Behind the mastoid process of the temporal bone. [L *retro,* mastoid.]
retromaxillary (ret·ro·max·**il**′·ar·e). Behind the maxilla. [L *retro,* maxilla.]
retromolar (ret·ro·**mo**·lar). Behind the last molar tooth. [L *retro,* molar.]
retromorphosis (ret·ro·mor·**fo**′·sis). 1. Retrograde metamorphosis; a degeneration. 2. Catabolism.
retronasal (ret·ro·**na**·zal). 1. Behind the nose. 2. Relating or belonging to the posterior nares. [L *retro, nasus* nose.]
retro-ocular (ret·ro·**ok**·ew·lar). Posterior to the eyeball; retrobulbar. [L *retro, oculus* eye.]
retro-oesophageal (ret·ro·e·sof·ah·**je**′·al). Behind the oesophagus. [L *retro,* oesophagus.]
retropatellar (ret·ro·pat·**el**′·ar). Behind the patella. [L *retro,* patella.]
retroperitoneal (ret·ro·per·it·o·**ne**′·al). Occurring or situated behind the peritoneum. [L *retro,* peritoneum.]
retroperitoneum (ret·ro·per·it·o·**ne**′·um). The retroperitoneal space.
retroperitonitis (ret·ro·per·it·on·**i**′·tis). An inflammatory condition affecting the cellular structures behind the peritoneum. [retroperitoneum, Gk *-itis* inflammation.]
retropharyngeal (ret·ro·far·**in**′·je·al). Behind the pharynx. [L *retro,* pharynx.]
retropharyngitis (ret·ro·far·in·**ji**′·tis). Inflammation involving the posterior part of the pharynx. [retropharynx, Gk *-itis* inflammation.]
retropharynx (ret·ro·**far**·ingx). The posterior part of the pharynx. [L *retro,* pharynx.]
retroplacental (ret·ro·plas·**en**′·tal). Behind the placenta. [L *retro,* placenta.]
retroplasia (ret·ro·**pla**·ze·ah). Degeneration of a cell or tissue to a lower type. [L *retro,* Gk *plassein* to form.]
retroposed (ret·ro·**po**·zd). Displaced backwards, but not retroflexed or retroverted. [L *retro, ponere* to place.]
retroposition (ret·ro·po·**zish**′·un). 1. Backward displacement. 2. Reposition. [see prec.]
retropubic (ret·ro·**pew**·bik). Behind the pubis. **Retropubic pad.** *See* PAD. **Retropubic space.** *See* SPACE. [L *retro,* pubis.]
retropulsion (ret·ro·**pul**·shun). 1. The pushing or forcing back of a part such as the presenting head of the fetus in labour. 2. An involuntary backward walking or running which sometimes occurs in tabes dorsalis or paralysis agitans. 3. An abnormal mode of walking characterized by bending of the body backwards. [L *retro, pellere* to move.]
retrorectal (ret·ro·**rek**·tal). Situated or occurring behind the rectum. [L *retro,* rectum.]
retrorsine (ret·**ror**·seen). $C_{18}H_{25}O_6N$, a poisonous alkaloid obtained from certain plants of the genus *Senecio* which includes many common weeds like ragwort and groundsel. It has caused fatal necrosis of the liver and kidney damage in livestock. It forms the toxic factor in "bush teas" or herbal infusions in tropical areas and is well known as causing veno-occlusive disease of the liver in Jamaica.
retrospection (ret·ro·**spek**·shun). The action of recalling past events. [L *retro, spicere* to look.]
retrospondylolisthesis (ret·ro·**spon**·dil·o·lis·**the**′·sis). A deformity in which the sacrum lies in front of the 5th lumbar vertebra. [L *retro,* spondylolisthesis.]
retrostalsis (ret·ro·**stal**·sis). Reverse peristalsis; antiperistalsis. [L *retro, stellein* to place.]
retrosternal (ret·ro·**ster**·nal). Posterior to the sternum. [L *retro,* sternum.]
retrosymphysial (ret·ro·sim·**fiz**′·e·al). Situated behind the pubic symphysis. [L *retro,* symphysis.]
retrotarsal (ret·ro·**tar**·sal). Behind the tarsus of the eyelid. [L *retro,* tarsus.]
retrotracheal (ret·ro·trak·**e**′·al). Behind the trachea. [L *retro,* trachea.]
retro-uterine (ret·ro·**ew**·ter·ine). Behind the uterus. [L *retro,* uterus.]
retrovaccination (ret·ro·vak·sin·**a**′·shun). The vaccination of a cow or calf with vaccine virus obtained from a human subject. [L *retro,* vaccination.]
retrovaccine (ret·ro·**vak**·seen). The vaccine virus obtained after retrovaccination.
retrovagal (ret·ro·**va**·gal). Behind the vena cava, usually inferior. [L *retro,* vagus nerve.]
retroversioflexion (ret·ro·ver·se·o·**flek**′·shun). Retroversion in association with retroflexion.
retroversion (ret·ro·**ver**·shun). Inclination of an organ in a backward direction. **Retroversion of the neck of the femur.** Backward tilting of the head and neck of the femur. **Retroversion of the uterus.** A condition where the uterus is tipped backwards on its axis. [L *retro, vertere* to turn.]
retroverted (ret·ro·ver·ted). Inclined or turned backwards. [see prec.]
retrusion (re·**troo**·zhun). Malposition of a tooth, or of a group of teeth, lying behind the normal position. [L *re-, trudere* to thrust.]
Retzius, Anders Adolf (b. 1796). Stockholm anatomist.
Retzius' cave, cavity, or space. Loose areolar tissue between the anterior surface of the bladder and the posterior surface of the pubic bones, constituting a potential space. Ascribed in error to Retzius who actually described a collection of fatty areolar tissue in front of the bladder.
Retzius' fibres. Axial filaments of the outer phalangeal cells (Deiters') of the organ of Corti.
Gyri of Retzius. Small elevations of cortex frequently found on the posterior surface of the splenial gyrus.
Retzius' ligament. The stem of the Y-shaped inferior extensor retinaculum of the ankle, forming loops for the extensor digitorum longus and peroneus tertius muscles.
Retzius' veins. Veins connecting the portal and systemic systems on the posterior abdominal wall; the portacaval anastomosis. Cf. SCHMIEDEL'S ANASTOMOSIS.
Retzius, Magnus Gustaf (b. 1842). Stockholm anatomist.
Body of Retzius. A pigmented mass of protoplasm at the lower end of an outer hair cell of the cochlea.
Retzius foramen, Key–Retzius foramen. The lateral aperture of the 4th ventricle: also called *Luschka's foramen.*
Gyrus of Retzius. A gyrus within the hippocampus.
Lines, or striae of Retzius. Concentric lines seen running through the enamel in a cross-section of the crown of a tooth. They are brown in transmitted light and colourless in reflected light.
Key and Retzius corpuscles. Sensory nerve-endings in the skin.
Key and Retzius sheath. A single layer of cuboidal cells in the inner layer of the hair follicle; Henle's sheath.
reunient (re·**ewn**·e·ent). Connecting separated parts. [L *re-, unire* to unite.]
reunion (re·**ewn**·e·on). The uniting again of parts in which continuity has been lost, such as takes place in the healing of a wound. [see prec.]
Reuss, August Ritter von (b. 1841). Vienna ophthalmologist.
Reuss' colour charts. Pseudo-isochromatic diagrams for testing colour vision, in which coloured letters are printed on a background of different colour which, to the colour-blind patient, looks the same.
revaccination (re·vak·sin·**a**′·shun). Repeated vaccination. [L *re-,* vaccination.]
revascularize (re·**vas**·kew·lar·ize). To restore a vascular supply to an organ or tissue. [L *re-, vasculum* small vessel.]
revellent (re·**vel**·ent). 1. Causing revulsion. 2. A counter-irritant by means of which revulsion may be effected. [L *revellere* to be separated from.]
reverberation (re·ver·ber·**a**′·shun). Continuous self-propagated nervous activity due to repetitive transmission of a nerve impulse

through a closed circuit of neurons. [L *reverberare* to strike back.]

Reverdin, Albert (b. 1881). Geneva surgeon.

Reverdin's needle. A long, sharp, handled needle whose eye is mechanically opened and closed by a trigger at the handle.

Reverdin, Jacques Louis (b.1842). Geneva surgeon.

Reverdin's graft, method, or operation. Pinch grafts; small circular deep grafts a few millimetres in diameter sliced off so that the centre is of whole skin and the periphery of epidermis only.

reverie (rev·er·e). 1. A state of deep or abstracted musing; idle imagining. 2. Disconnected or loosely woven trail of ideas through the mind such as occurs in day-dreaming. [Fr., idle fancy.]

reverse (re·vers). In bandaging, the name given to the half-turn used when a conical part of a limb, e.g. the calf, is being bandaged, the lower borders of the overlapping turns being thus kept parallel. [see foll.]

reversible (re·ver·sibl). Having the ability to return to the original state. [L *revertere* to turn back.]

reversion (re·ver·shun). The appearance in offspring of characters present in much earlier generations but not in the immediate ancestors. Apparent reversion is usually due to the appearance of a rare recessive, or to mutation. [see prec.]

See also: MANTOUX.

revertose (re·ver·toze). $C_{12}H_{22}O_{11}$, a disaccharide produced by the action of the enzyme maltase on D-glucose; it is an isomer of maltose.

Revilliod, Léon (b. 1835). Swiss physician.

Revilliod's sign. In facial paralysis of lower motor neuron type, there is inability to close the affected eye.

Revision (re·vizh·un). **Birmingham revision.** BR: the non-official name applied by anatomists to the nomenclature approved by the Anatomical Society of Great Britain and Ireland at a meeting in Birmingham in 1933. Cf. BASLE NOMINA ANATOMICA. [L *revisere* to visit again.]

revitalization (re·vi·tal·i·za'·shun). The act of giving life to, reanimating, reactivating, or refreshing a living cell or tissue which is tending to die. [L *re-*, *vitalis* living.]

revival (re·vi·val). The act of restoring to a state of consciousness. **Visuo-auditory revival.** The recall to the mind of things seen and heard in the past. [L *re-*, *vivus* alive.]

revivescence (re·viv·es·ens). A focal hypersensitivity reaction whereby an injection of tuberculoprotein into the tissues produces a reaction about distant tuberculous lesions or at the site of a previous skin tuberculin test. [L *revivescere* to revive.]

revivification (re·viv·if·ik·a'·shun). 1. Revivescence. 2. The refreshing or scraping of the surfaces of a wound in order that union may take place. [L *re-*, *vivus* alive, *facere* to make.]

revolute (rev·o·lewt). Rolled or turned backwards. [L *revolvere* to roll back.]

revulsant (re·vul·sant). Revulsive.

revulseur (re·vul·ser). An instrument consisting of many fine needle points which are dipped in an irritant liquid and used in Baunscheidt's air-puncture treatment of "chronic rheumatism", thus providing a drastic form of counter-irritation. [L *revellere* to draw back.]

revulsion (re·vul·shun). 1. The drawing away of blood from a pathological area to another area. 2. The diversion of a disease from one part to another. [L *revulsio* a plucking away.]

revulsive (re·vul·siv). 1. Causing revulsion. 2. A counter-irritant by means of which revulsion may be effected.

Reye, Ralph Douglas Kenneth. 20th century Sydney pathologist.

Reye's disease. Encephalohepatitis.

Reyn, Axel (b. 1872). Copenhagen dermatologist.

Finsen-Reyn lamp. A modification of the Finsen lamp.

Reynier's white mycetoma. *See* MYCETOMA, WHITE.

Reynolds, Osborn. 19th century British physicist.

Reynolds' number. Defined as vl/ν where v is a velocity of fluid flow, l a dimension of the apparatus in which flow occurs, and ν the kinematic viscosity = viscosity η/ρ where ρ is the density of the fluid and η the viscosity. Flow is similar in geometrically similar conditions, when the Reynolds' number is the same. For example, the onset of turbulence occurs in tubes at a Reynolds' number of approximately 1200.

rhababerone, rhabarberone (rah·bab·er·one, rah·bar·ber·one). Trihydroxymethylanthraquinone, $C_6H_2(OH)_2(CO)_2C_6H_2(OH)(CH_3)$. An alcoholic compound found in rhubarb, aloe, and senna; it is isomeric with emodin. [Gk *rha* rhubarb, *barbaros* foreign.]

Rhabditata (rab·de·ta·tah). A sub-order of roundworms, whose members are small and mostly free living. It includes *Strongyloides* and *Rhabditis*. [Gk *rhabdos* rod.]

rhabditic (rab·dit·ik). Relating to the genus, *Rhabditis*.

Rhabditidae (rab·dit·id·e). A family of the nematode suborder Rhabditata. The genera *Diploscapter* and *Rhabditis* are of medical interest. [Gk *rhabdos* rod, *eidos* form.]

rhabditiform (rab·dit·e·form). Of larval nematodes, having resemblance to *Rhabditis*, with a posterior bulb in the oesophagus, as in first larvae of *Ancyclostoma* and *Necator*. [*Rhabditis*, form.]

Rhabditis (rab·di·tis). A genus of nematode worms. The very small adults are normally free living but often coprophagous. **Rhabditis donbass.** Species which have been recorded from human faeces in Russia. **Rhabditis hominis.** A species which has been recorded frequently in human faeces; they are probably not true parasites, but may live perianally. **Rhabditis niellyi.** A species recorded from human skin once in France. **Rhabditis pellio.** A species recorded once from the human vagina in Hungary. **Rhabditis schachtielli.** *Rhabditis donbass* (see above). [Gk *rhabdos* rod.]

rhabdium (rab·de·um). The fibre of a striped muscle. [Gk *rhabdos* rod.]

rhabdocyte (rab·do·site). Polymorphonuclear leucocyte. *See* LEUCOCYTE. [Gk *rhabdos* rod, *kytos* cell.]

rhabdoid (rab·doid). Rod-shaped. [Gk *rhabdos* rod, *eidos* form.]

Rhabdomonas (rab·do·mo·nas). A genus of the family Thiorhodaceae (the purple sulphur bacteria). They are found in mud and water, and the type species is *Rhabdomonas roseus*. [Gk *rhabdos* rod, *monas* unit.]

rhabdomyeloblastoma (rab·do·mi·el·o·blas·to'·mah). A rare malignant tumour composed of embryonic striped-muscle cells, arising chiefly in the skeletal muscles and the tongue. [Gk *rhabdos* rod, myeloblastoma.]

rhabdomyochondroma (rab·do·mi·o·kon·dro'·mah). A tumour composed of elements of rhabdomyoma and chondroma.

rhabdomyolysis (rab·do·mi·ol'·is·is). Paroxysmal idiopathic myoglobulinuria. [Gk *rhabdos* rod, *mys* muscle, *lysis* a loosing.]

rhabdomyoma (rab·do·mi·o'·mah). A tumour of striped-muscle tissue which may be innocent or malignant. **Congenital rhabdomyoma of the heart.** A congenital abnormality that resembles a tumour of the heart in infants and young children, composed of striped-muscle fibres. **Rhabdomyoma uteri.** A malignant mixed tumour of the uterus containing striped-muscle fibres amongst its cells. [Gk *rhabdos* rod, myoma.]

rhabdomyomyxoma (rab·do·mi·o·mix·o'·mah). A combined myxoma and rhabdomyoma.

rhabdomyosarcoma (rab·do·mi·o·sar·ko'·mah). A mixed tumour with the characters of rhabdomyoma and sarcoma.

Rhabdomys pumilio (rab·do·mis pew·mil·e·o). A bush mouse, a host of *Pasteurella pestis*. [Gk *rhabdos* rod, *mys* mouse, L *pumilio* pygmy.]

Rhabdonema (rab·do·ne·mah). *Strongyloides*. [Gk *rhabdos* rod, *nema* thread.]

rhabdophobia (rab·do·fo·be·ah). Morbid dread aroused by the sight of a stick; morbid fear of a whipping or beating. [Gk *rhabdos* rod, phobia.]

rhabdosarcoma (rab·do·sar·ko'·mah). A malignant rhabdomyoma. **Renal rhabdosarcoma.** Wilms' tumour of infants. [rhabdomyoma, sarcoma.]

Rhabdovirus (**rab**·do·vi′·rus). A genus of RNA-containing viruses with a bullet- or rod-shaped appearance. The only attribute common to all the members is the morphology of the virions, and not all are regular; rabies, for example, shows considerable pleomorphism. Most rhabdoviruses affect only animals or plants, but those that affect man include rabies, Marburg virus and, following accidental laboratory exposure, vesicular stomatitis virus. [Gk *rhabdos* rod, L *virus* poison.]

rhachi-. For words beginning with *rhachi, see* RACHI-. The former is more correct but the latter is more usual.

rhacoma (rak·o·mah) (pl. *rhacomata*). 1. An excoriation. 2. A pendulous scrotum. [Gk *rhakoma* rag.]

rhacous (**rak**·us). Wrinkled; lacerated. [Gk *rhakos* tattered.]

rhaebocrania (re·bo·**kra**·ne·ah). Torticollis. [Gk *rhaibokranos* crook-headed.]

rhaeboscelia (re·bo·se·le·ah). A deformed state of the legs, e.g. bow leg, knock knee. [Gk *rhaibos* crooked, *skelos* leg.]

rhaebosis (re·**bo**·sis). Crookedness of any part that normally is straight, e.g. the leg. [Gk *rhaibos* crooked.]

rhaestocythaemia (res·to·si·**the**′·me·ah). The presence of disintegrated erythrocytes in the blood. [Gk *rhaiein* to destroy, *kytos* cell, *haima* blood.]

rhagades, rhagadia (rag·ad·eez, rag·a·de·ah). Fissures, chaps, or cracks in the skin, in particular those occurring at the anus and at the angle of the mouth in syphilis. [Gk, chinks.]

rhagadiform (rag·**ad**·e·form). Fissured; cracked. [Gk *rhagas* chink, form.]

rhagoid (**rag**·oid). Having resemblance to a grape. [Gk *rhax* grape, *eidos* form.]

rhamma (**ram**·ah). A suture. [Gk *rhamnos* thorn.]

rhamnetin (**ram**·net·in). Quercetin-7-methyl ether, $C_{16}H_{12}O_7$. A colouring matter present as a glucoside in the ripe fruit of the buckthorn, *Rhamnus cathartica.*

rhamni (**ram**·ni). **Rhamni Purshianae Cortex.** *European Pharmacopoeia* name for Cascara BP 1973.

rhamninose (**ram**·nin·oze). $C_{18}H_{32}O_{14}$, a trisaccharide constituted of two units of rhamnose and one of glucose, which is found in the Persian berry and species of *Rhamnus*; it is an isomer of robinose.

rhamnitol (**ram**·nit·ol). $CH_3(CHOH)_4CH_2OH$, a pentahydric alcohol obtained by the reduction of rhamnose.

rhamnocathartin (**ram**·no·kath·**ar**′·tin). A purgative glucoside present in the fruit of the buckthorn, *Rhamnus cathartica.*

rhamnose (**ram**·noze). Isodulcite, $CH_3(CHOH)_4CHO$. A methylpentose found in quercetrin, xanthorhamnin, and other glycosides from species of *Rhamnus.* It has been observed in the urine in cases of pentosuria.

rhamnoside (**ram**·no·side). 1. Any glycoside which contains units of rhamnose, such as xanthorhamnin. 2. $C_{21}H_{20}O_9$, a compound obtained from species of *Rhamnus.*

rhamnoxanthin (ram·no·**zan**·thin). $C_{20}H_{20}O_9$, a glucoside present in the bark of *Rhamnus frangula.*

Rhamnus (**ram**·nus). A genus of trees and shrubs of the family Rhamnaceae, including *Rhamnus purshiana* DC. (cascara), *R. frangula* Linn. (alder buckthorn), and *R. cathartica* Linn. (buckthorn). The barks of cascara and frangula are used as purgatives; the berries of buckthorn are a veterinary cathartic. [Gk *rhamnos* buckthorn.]

rhaphania (raf·a·ne·ah). A disorder characterized by spasms of the limbs, attributed to poisoning by the seeds of *Rhaphanus rhaphanistrum.* Poisoning occurs from continued consumption of seed accidentally admixed with grain. [Gk *rhaphanos* cabbage.]

Rhaphanus (**raf**·a·nus). A genus of cruciferous plants which includes *Rhaphanus sativus*, the common radish. [see prec.]

rhaphe (ra·fe). Raphe.

rhaphidiospore (raf·**id**·e·o·spore). The needle-shaped sporozoite injected by the mosquito in transmitting malaria. [Gk *rhaphidion* little needle, spore.]

rhapontic (rap·**on**·tik). A variety of rhubarb grown in Siberia and England but not admitted recognition in the *British Pharmacopoeia.* It does not contain the aloe-emodin derivatives found in Chinese rhubarb, but a specific glycoside, rhaponticin. [Gk *rha* rhubarb, *Pontikos* of the Black Sea.]

rhaponticin (rap·**on**·tis·in). A crystalline glycoside which occurs in rhapontic rhubarb.

rhatany (**rat**·en·e). Krameria; the dried root of *Krameria triandra* Ruiz. et Pav. (family Leguminosae). It contains about 10 per cent of tannin and is used as an astringent, usually in lozenges with cocaine. [Port. *ratanhia.*]

rhegma (**reg**·mah). 1. A fracture. 2. A rupture. 3. A fissure. [Gk, breakage.]

Rhei rhizoma (ri ri·**zo**·mah). Rhubarb.

rheic (re·ik). Relating or belonging to rhubarb. [Gk *rheon* rhubarb.]

rhein (re·in). Rheinic acid, dihydroxyanthraquinonecarboxylic acid, $(OH)C_6H_3(CO)_2C_6H_2(OH)COOH$. A yellow compound found in senna leaves and rhubarb. [Gk *rheon* rhubarb.]

rhembasmus (rem·**baz**·mus). Mental uncertainty or indecision; state of distraction. [Gk *rhembomein* to act at random.]

rhenium (**re**·ne·um). A very rare element of atomic weight 186.2, atomic number 75, and chemical symbol Re, which occurs in certain molybdenites. It is a metal resembling manganese in properties and is used in minute quantities to increase the electrical resistance of tungsten. [L *Rhenus* Rhine.]

rheobase (**re**·o·base). Rheobasis.

rheobasic (re·o·**ba**·sik). Relating or belonging to rheobasis.

rheobasis (re·o·**ba**·sis). In physiology, the least amount of electrical current that will produce a stimulated response. [Gk *rheos* current, *basis* step.]

rheochord (**re**·o·kord). A rheostat. [Obsolete term.] [Gk *rheos* current, *chorde* chord.]

rheology (re·**ol**·o·je). The study of flow and deformation of matter. [Gk *rheos* stream, *logos* science.]

rheometer (re·**om**·et·er). 1. A galvanometer. [Obsolete term.] 2. An instrument used for the measurement of the velocity of blood flow. [Gk *rheos* current, meter.]

rheonome (**re**·o·nome). An instrument by which electrical currents of varying strength can be used to stimulate nerves or muscles. [Gk *rheos* current, *nemein* to distribute.]

rheophore (**re**·o·fore). A high-voltage circuit connection in which a wire or tape is kept taut by a spring-worked drum. [Gk *rheos* current, *pherein* to bear.]

rheoscope (**re**·o·skope). A galvanoscope; an electrical apparatus which indicates the strength and direction of an electrical current passing through it. [Gk *rheos* current, *skopein* to watch.]

rheostat (**re**·o·stat). A variable resistance which, incorporated into an electrical circuit, can be adjusted to provide any desired strength of current. [Gk *rheos* current, *statikos* causing to stand.]

rheostosis (re·**os**·to·sis). A condition of hyperostosis marked by the presence of streaks in the bones. [Gk *rheos* current, *osteon* bone, *-osis* condition.]

rheotachygraphy (re·o·tak·**ig**′·raf·e). The recording of the curve of variation in the electromotive state of muscles. [Gk *rheos* current, *tachys* swift, *graphein* to record.]

rheotaxis (re·o·**tax**·is). The movement of a body in a fluid in response to the flow. [Gk *rheos* current, *taxis* arrangement.]

rheotome (**re**·o·tome). An interrupter; any appliance designed to make and break an electrical current at required intervals. **Differential rheotome.** One used in physiology to demonstrate muscle currents. [Gk *rheos* current, *temnein* to cut.]

rheotrope (**re**·o·trope). A reversing switch; a device used to reverse the direction of an electrical current. [Obsolete term.] [Gk *rheos* current, *trepein* to turn.]

rheotropism (re·**ot**·rop·izm). Rheotaxis. [see above.]

rhesus (**re**·sus). A blood group system, discovered by Landsteiner and Wiener in 1940, clinically important because incompatibilities between mother and child can result in the immunization of the mother to produce antibodies that react against the fetal red cells. The child may consequently suffer from haemolytic disease of the newborn, which is treated by transfusions. The disease can be prevented by treating parturient women, at risk for production of antibodies in subsequent pregnancies, with powerful Rh antibodies to obviate the immunizing potential of transplacentally leaked Rh-incompatible fetal cells. *See* MONKEY. [Gk *Rhesos* legendary king of Thrace.]

rheum (re·um). Rhubarb. [Gk *rheon* rhubarb.]

rheum, rheuma (room, roo·mah). A catarrhal or watery discharge from the skin or mucous membranes. **Epidemic rheum.** Influenza. **Salt rheum.** Eczema. [Gk *rheuma* flow.]

rheumatic (roo·**mat**·ik). 1. Relating or belonging to rheumatism or arthritis. 2. A person suffering from rheumatism or arthritis.

rheumatid (roo·**mat**·id). A lesion of the skin seen in rheumatic persons.

rheumatin (**roo**·mat·in). Saloquinine salicylate; the salicylate of a salicylic acid ester of quinine. A white tasteless powder, slightly soluble in water, which has been used in neuralgia, rheumatism, etc.

rheumatism (**roo**·mat·izm). A non-specific term usually used by lay persons for any painful condition arising in musculoskeletal tissues. **Acute rheumatism.** Acute rheumatic fever; a disease following infection with haemolytic streptococcus characterized by fever, arthropathy and often carditis, nodules and rashes. **Acute articular rheumatism.** The characteristic form of acute rheumatism in adults in which fever and arthritis are prominent features. It may be due to pyogenic infection of joints. **Cerebral rheumatism.** Acute rheumatic fever associated with cerebral symptoms; chorea. **Chronic rheumatism.** Rheumatoid arthritis; osteo-arthritis and arthritis; also applied to chronic non-articular forms of rheumatism. **Chronic articular rheumatism.** The chronic form of rheumatoid arthritis, osteo-arthritis, or gout. **Desert rheumatism.** Transient arthralgia due to systematic infection with coccidioidomycosis. **Gonorrhoeal rheumatism.** Arthritis, often affecting many joints, occurring as the sequel to a systemic infection with the gonococcus. This often results in ankylosis of the affected joints. **Rheumatism of the heart.** Endocarditis, myocarditis, or pericarditis due to rheumatic fever; it often results in permanent valvular deformity. **Lumbar rheumatism.** Lumbago. **Muscular rheumatism.** A painful affection of unknown causation affecting the voluntary muscles and their fascial coverings. **Non-articular rheumatism.** Pain arising in musculoskeletal tissues but not in the joints themselves. A modern synonym of fibrositis. **Osseous rheumatism.** Osteo-arthritis. **Palindromic rheumatism.** Recurrent attacks of acute arthritis which may be the initial manifestations of rheumatoid arthritis. **Soft-tissue rheumatism.** Fibrositis. **Subacute rheumatism.** A mild, but often protracted, type of rheumatic fever which may originate in this form, or result from an initial acute attack. It may lead to cardiac complications. **Synovial rheumatism.** Rheumatism affecting principally the synovial sheaths of certain muscle groups. **Trench rheumatism.** Pain affecting the lumbar region of soldiers in the course of trench warfare. **Tuberculous rheumatism.** Arthritis due to infection of the synovium or the subchondral cartilage with *Mycobacterium tuberculosis.* It commonly affects children or elderly people, and is generally monarticular. **Visceral rheumatism.** Rheumatic changes occurring in an internal organ such as the heart. [Gk *rheumatismos* that which flows.]

See also: BESNIER, HEBERDEN, PONCET.

rheumatismal (roo·mat·**iz**·mal). Rheumatic; relating or belonging to rheumatism.

rheumatocelis (**roo**·mat·o·**ke**′·lis). Purpura rheumatica. [Gk *rheuma* flux, *kelis* spot.]

rheumatodynia (**roo**·mat·o·**din**′·e·ah). Pain of a dull, gnawing type, generally associated with rheumatic conditions, and reactive to weather conditions. [rheumatism, Gk *odyne* pain.]

rheumatoid (**roo**·mat·oid). Having resemblance to rheumatism in one or several characters. **Rheumatoid arthritis.** *See* ARTHRITIS. **Rheumatoid factors.** *See* FACTOR. [rheumatism, Gk *eidos* form.]

rheumatology (roo·mat·**ol**·o·je). That branch of medicine which is concerned with the diagnosis and treatment of rheumatic disorders. [rheumatism, Gk *logos* science.]

rheumic (**roo**·mik). Catarrhal discharge or watery flow from a membrane. [rheum.]

rhexis (**rex**·is). Rupture or bursting of an organ or vessel. [Gk, a breaking.]

rhicnosis (rik·**no**·sis). Wrinkling of the skin caused by atrophy of the underlying muscles. [Gk *rhiknos* shrivelled.]

rhigolene (**rig**·o·leen). A petroleum distillate (mostly butane and pentane, 18 to 21°C), used like ethyl chloride as a local anaesthetic for minor surgical procedures.

rhigos (**ri**·gos). Rigor. [Gk, cold.]

rhigosis (rig·o·sis). The sense of cold. [Gk *rhigos* cold.]

rhigotic (rig·**ot**·ik). Relating or belonging to rhigosis.

rhinaesthesia (ri·nes·**the**·ze·ah). The sense of smell. [Gk *rhis* nose, aesthesia.]

rhinal (**ri**·nal). Relating or belonging to the nose; nasal. [Gk *rhis* nose.]

rhinalgia (ri·**nal**·je·ah). Pain involving the nose. [Gk *rhis* nose, *algos* pain.]

rhinallergosis (ri·nal·er·**go**′·sis). Hay fever. [Gk *rhis* nose, allergy, Gk *-osis* condition.]

rhinantralgia (ri·nan·**tral**·je·ah). Pain arising within the nasal chambers. [Gk *rhis* nose, *antron* cavity, *algos* pain.]

rhinelcos (ri·**nel**·kos). An ulceration in the nose. [Gk *rhis* nose, *elkos* ulcer.]

rhinencephalic (ri·nen·kef·**al**′·ik). Relating or belonging to the rhinencephalon.

rhinencephalon [NA] (ri·nen·**kef**·al·on). The parts of the forebrain which are concerned in the functions of olfaction, namely the olfactory bulbs, peduncles, anterior perforated substance, piriform area, and amygdaloid nuclei. The septum, hippocampus, fornix, the gyrus fornicatus, mamillary bodies, and anterior thalamic nuclei are commonly included under this term, but their relationship to olfactory function is uncertain. [Gk *rhis* nose, *egkephalos* brain.]

rhinencephalus (ri·nen·**kef**·al·us). A monster with a tube-like nose or fold of skin instead of a nose, and a cyclopean eye below it. [see prec.]

rhinenchysis (ri·**nen**·kis·is). Douching of the nasal cavities. [Gk *rhis* nose, *egcheein* to pour in.]

rhineurynter (ri·newr·**in**·ter). A rubber bag which is dilatable, and may be used for checking haemorrhage in the nose. [Gk *rhis*nose, *eurynein* to dilate.]

rhiniatry (ri·**ni**·at·re). The treatment of diseases and affections of the nose. [Gk *rhis* nose, *iatreia* healing.]

rhinic (**ri**·nik). Relating or belonging to the nose; nasal. [Gk *rhis* nose.]

rhinion (**ri**·ne·on). In craniometry, the lower and most prominent point of the internasal suture. [Gk *rhinion* nostril.]

rhinism, rhinismus (ri·nizm, ri·**niz**·mus). Of the voice, characterized by a nasal timbre. [Gk *rhis* nose.]

rhinitis (ri·**ni**·tis). An inflammation of the nasal mucous membrane. **Acute catarrhal rhinitis.** The mildest form of inflammation of the nasal mucous membrane, most commonly seen in the common cold. **Allergic rhinitis.** Rhinitis of an allergic origin, the best recognized type of this condition being hay fever. **Anaphylactic rhinitis.** Loosely used as part of allergic rhinitis. **Aseptic rhinitis.** An inflammatory response of the nasal mucous membrane induced by the local application of mechanical irritants, or by the ingestion of certain drugs. **Atrophic rhinitis.** A nasal condition characterized by atrophy of the mucous membrane of the nose and interference with its ciliary mechanism, resulting in a drying and crusting of the nasal passages. **Rhinitis caseosa.** An accumulation of foul-smelling, cheesy material in the nose. **Chronic rhinitis.** A chronic form of inflammation of the nasal passages, often associated with excessive discharge and congestion, and thickening of the nasal lining. **Chronic catarrhal rhinitis.** Inflammation of the nasal mucosa, producing a chronic excess of secretion. **Croupous rhinitis.** Inflammation of the nasal mucosa, associated with a false membrane. **Dyscrinic rhinitis.** Rhinitis thought to result from a disturbance of the endocrine organs. **Fibrinous rhinitis.** A rhinitis associated with the formation of a false membrane of diphtheritic origin. **Gangrenous rhinitis.** An acute gangrenous destruction of the nasal lining resulting from severe diphtheria, or a severe streptococcal infection. Rarely seen nowadays. **Hypertrophic rhinitis.** Hypertrophy or enlargement of the nasal mucous membrane, usually resulting from a chronic or low-grade inflammation. **Infective rhinitis.** An inflammatory response of the nasal mucous membrane to certain bacterial or virus infections. **Membranous rhinitis.** Fibrinous rhinitis (see above). **Polypoid rhinitis.** A chronic inflammatory response of the nasal mucous membrane associated with the formation of polypi. **Pseudomembranous rhinitis.** A fibrinous rhinitis not resulting from the diphtheria bacillus. **Purulent rhinitis.** An acute septic infection of the nasal mucosa as seen particularly in measles, but less commonly in scarlet fever; believed by some to be the starting point for atrophic rhinitis (see above). **Scrofulous rhinitis.** Rhinitis resulting from malnutrition, now rarely seen; probably resulting from vitamin deficiency. **Rhinitis sicca.** Excessive dryness of the nasal mucosa; probably related to atrophic rhinitis (see above), but without the typical crust formation. **Simple rhinitis.** A chronic inflammatory condition of the nasal mucous membrane. **Syphilitic rhinitis.** A chronic rhinitis, usually accompanied by scanty, foul-smelling discharge, with ulceration and necrosis of the bony part of the nasal septum. In the late stage, it is followed by perforation of the bony nasal septum. **Tuberculous rhinitis.** Rhinitis of tuberculous origin. It may be a lupoid type of destructive ulceration, or a solitary tuberculoma of the nasal septum. **Vasomotor rhinitis.** Rhinorrhoea resulting from over-secretion of mucus from the nasal lining resulting from allergy or sometimes from a neurovascular imbalance. [Gk *rhis* nose, *-itis* inflammation.]

rhino-anemometer (ri·no·an·e·**mom**'·et·er). An instrument for measuring the air which passes through the nose during the act of respiration. [Gk *rhis* nose, *anemos* wind, meter.]

rhino-antritis (ri·no·an·**tri**'·tis). Inflammation affecting the nasal cavity and maxillary sinus on one or both sides. [Gk *rhis* nose, antrum, Gk *-itis* inflammation.]

rhinoblennorrhoea (ri·no·blen·o·**re**'·ah). Rhinorrhoea; profuse discharge of thin mucus from the nose. [Gk *rhis* nose, *blenna* mucus, *rhoia* flow.]

rhinobyon (ri·no·be·on). Any form of nasal plug. [Gk *rhis* nose, *byein* to plug.]

rhinocanthectomy (ri·no·kan·**thek**'·to·me). Excision of the inner canthus. [Gk *rhis* nose, canthus, Gk *ektome* excision.]

rhinocaul (ri·no·kawl). The olfactory peduncle. [Gk *rhis* nose, caul.]

rhinocephalia, rhinocephaly (ri·no·kef·**a**'·le·ah, ri·no·**kef**·al·e). A congenital abnormality associated with cyclopia, in which the nose is replaced by a tubular proboscis projecting from the forehead above the fused eyes. [Gk *rhis* nose, *kephale* head.]

rhinocheiloplasty (ri·no·**ki**·lo·plas·te). A plastic surgical procedure for modifying or restoring the nose and lip. [Gk *rhis* nose, *cheilos* lip, *plassein* to form.]

rhinocleisis (ri·no·**kli**·sis). Nasal obstruction. [Gk *rhis* nose, *kleisis* a closing.]

rhinocnesmus (ri·no·**nez**·mus). Irritability or itching of the nose. [Gk *rhis* nose, *knesmos* itching.]

rhinodacryolith (ri·no·**dak**·re·o·lith). A lacrimal stone occurring in the nasolacrimal duct. [Gk *rhis* nose, *dakryon* tear, *lithos* stone.]

rhinodynia (ri·no·**din**·e·ah). Pain in the nose. [Gk *rhis* nose, *odyne* pain.]

rhinoedema (ri·ne·**de**·mah). Nasal oedema. [Gk *rhis* nose, oedema.]

Rhinoestrus (ri·**ne**·strus). A genus of botflies of the family Oestridae. **Rhinoestrus purpureus.** A species of eastern Europe, Asia and North Africa that deposits larvae in the noses and eyes of mammals, including man. [Gk *rhis* nose, *oistros* desire.]

rhinogenous (ri·**noj**·en·us). Originating in the nose. [Gk *rhis* nose, *genein* to produce.]

rhinokyphectomy (ri·no·ki·**fek**'·to·me). An operation for the removal of a hump on the nose. [Gk *rhis* nose, *kyphos* ridge, *ektome* excision.]

rhinokyphosis (ri·no·ki·**fo**'·sis). Abnormal height and protuberance of the bridge of the nose. [Gk *rhis* nose, *kyphosis* hump-back.]

rhinolalia (ri·no·**lal**·e·ah). A voice that is nasal in quality owing to disease or abnormality of the nasal passages; rhinism. **Rhinolalia aperta.** That which is due to abnormally great size of the posterior nasal apertures. **Rhinolalia clausa.** That which is caused by partial or complete closure of the posterior nasal apertures. **Open rhinolalia.** Rhinolalia. Rhinolalia aperta (see above). [Gk *rhis* nose, *lalein* to talk.]

rhinolaryngitis (ri·no·lar·in·**ji**'·tis). Inflammation of the mucous membrane of the larynx and the nose. [Gk *rhis* nose, laryngitis.]

rhinolaryngology (ri·no·lar·in·**gol**'·o·je). That branch of medical science which deals with the nose and the larynx. [Gk *rhis* nose, larynx, Gk *logos* science.]

rhinolerema, rhinoleresis (ri·no·ler·**e**'·mah, ri·no·ler·**e**'·sis). A perverted sense of smell. [Gk *rhis* nose, *leros* nonsense.]

rhinolith (ri·no·lith). A concretion in the cavity of the nose; nasal calculus. [Gk *rhis* nose, *lithos* stone.]

rhinolithiasis (ri·no·lith·**i**'·as·is). Formation of rhinoliths.

rhinological (ri·no·**loj**·ik·al). Relating or belonging to rhinology.

rhinologist (ri·**nol**·o·jist). A nose specialist; one who has made a special study of diseases of the nose. [see foll.]

rhinology (ri·**nol**·o·je). The branch of medical science concerned with the nose and the diseases affecting it. [Gk *rhis* nose, *logos* science.]

rhinomanometer (ri·no·man·**om**'·et·er). An instrument for measuring the air pressure inside the nose and therefore for assessing the degree of nasal obstruction. [Gk *rhis* nose, *manos* thin, meter.]

rhinomeiosis (ri·no·mi·**o**'·sis). Shortening or other reduction of the size of the nose by operative means. [Gk *rhis* nose, *meioein* to make smaller.]

rhinometaplasty (ri·no·**met**·ah·plas·te). Rhinoplasty. [Gk *rhis* nose, *meta, plassein* to mould.]

rhinometer (ri·**nom**·et·er). An instrument used to measure the width of the nose or of its cavities. [Gk *rhis* nose, meter.]

rhinomiosis (ri·no·mi·**o**'·sis). Rhinomeiosis.

rhinommectomy (ri·nom·**ek**·to·me). Rhinocanthectomy. [Gk *rhis* nose, *omma* eye, *ektome* excision.]

rhinomycosis (ri·no·mi·**ko**'·sis). A fungal infection of the mucous membrane of the nose. [Gk *rhis* nose, mycosis.]

rhinonecrosis (ri·no·nek·**ro**'·sis). Necrosis of the bony framework of the nose. [Gk *rhis* nose, necrosis.]

rhinoneurosis (ri·no·newr·**o**'·sis). 1. A psychoneurotic condition which is characterized by various nasal symptoms. 2. Any functional nervous disease of the nose. [Gk *rhis* nose, neurosis.]

rhinopathia, rhinopathy (ri·no·**path**·e·ah, ri·**nop**·ath·e). Any morbid condition of the nose. **Rhinopathia vasomotoria.** Hay fever. [Gk *rhis* nose, *pathos* disease.]

rhinopharyngeal (ri·no·far·**in**'·je·al). Relating or belonging to the cavity of the nose and the nasal part of the pharynx. [Gk *rhis* nose, pharynx.]

rhinopharyngitis (ri·no·far·in·**ji**'·tis). Inflammation affecting the mucous membrane of the nasal part of the pharynx. **Rhinopharyngitis mutilans.** In tertiary yaws, an ulcerative process which attacks the nasal and palatal structures and destroys them. [rhinopharynx, Gk *-itis* inflammation.]

rhinopharyngocele (ri·no·far·**ing**'·go·seel). An air-containing cyst arising either from the pharynx or the nose. [Gk *rhis* nose, pharynx, Gk *kele* tumour.]

rhinopharyngolith (ri·no·far·**ing**'·go·lith). A calcareous concretion in the rhinopharynx. [rhinopharynx, Gk *lithos* stone.]

rhinopharynx (ri·no·**far**·inx). The nasal part of the pharynx. [Gk *rhis* nose, pharynx.]

rhinophonia (ri·no·**fo**·ne·ah). The condition of the voice when it has a nasal timbre. [Gk *rhis* nose, *phone* sound.]

rhinophore (ri·no·for). A cannula which, when it is inserted into the nostrils, promotes easier respiration. [Gk *rhis* nose, *pherein* to carry.]

rhinophycomycosis (ri·no·fi·ko·mi·**ko′**·sis). Phycomycosis entomophthorae; an infection in man and animals (especially horses) involving, preferentially, nasal and paranasal sinuses, which may disseminate eventually to the brain and other tissues. It is caused by the phycomycete *Entomophthora coronata.* [Gk *rhis* nose, *phykos* seaweed, *mykes* fungus, *-osis* condition.]

rhinophyma (ri·no·**fi**·mah). A severe type of acne rosacea found in association with hypertrophy of the skin and congestion of the subcutaneous tissue, so that the nose assumes the appearance of a lobulated tumour. [Gk *rhis* nose, *phyma* tumour.]

rhinoplastic (ri·no·**plas**·tik). Relating or belonging to rhinoplasty.

rhinoplasty (**ri**·no·plas·te). The operative correction of a deformity of the nose resulting from injury, disease, or congenital defect. [Gk *rhis* nose, *plassein* to form.]

rhinopolypus (ri·no·**pol**·e·pus). A nasal polypus. [Gk *rhis* nose, polypus.]

rhinopsia (ri·**nop**·se·ah). Convergent squint. *See* SQUINT. [Gk *rhis* nose, *opsis* sight.]

rhinoreaction (ri·no·re·**ak′**·shun). Moeller's reaction. [Gk *rhis* nose, reaction.]

rhinorrhagia (ri·no·**ra**·je·ah). Profuse epistaxis. [Gk *rhis* nose, *rhegnynein* to gush forth.]

rhinorrhaphy (ri·**nor**·af·e). An operation performed for the correction of epicanthus, in which an oval portion of skin is removed from the bridge of the nose and the edges of the wound are drawn together and sutured so that the slack portion is taken up. [Gk *rhis* nose, *rhaphe* suture.]

rhinorrhoea (ri·no·**re**·ah). Profuse discharge of thin mucus from the nose. **Cerebrospinal rhinorrhoea.** A discharge of cerebrospinal fluid from the nose. **Paroxysmal rhinorrhoea, Spasmodic rhinorrhoea.** Allergic rhinitis; attacks of swelling of the nasal mucous membrane associated with severe sneezing and profuse watery discharge. It is a common allergic manifestation caused by sensitization of the mucous membrane to some substance, usually of a protein nature, which has entered by inhalation. Pollen, animal dusts such as dandruff, particles of hair or feathers, or house dust are the most common, but sometimes sensitization to some infested substance, e.g. a food or drug, may occur. [Gk *rhis* nose, *rhoia* flow.]

rhinosalpingitis (ri·no·sal·pin·**ji′**·tis). Inflammation affecting the mucous membrane of the nose and the lining of the pharyngotympanic tube. [Gk *rhis* nose, salpingitis.]

rhinoscleroma (ri·no·skler·**o′**·mah). A chronic inflammatory process found most commonly as a primary lesion in the nose, tending to spread and involve the larynx and pharynx. It is due to infection with *Klebsiella rhinoscleromatis,* resembling *Bacterium friedländeri.* Microscopically, it may resemble the chronic inflammation of syphilis and tuberculosis, but the structure in its typical form contains Mikulicz's cells and Russell's bodies. Formerly it was most commonly found amongst the inhabitants of middle Europe, but it now has a world-wide distribution. [Gk *rhis* nose, *skleros* hard, *-oma* tumour.]

rhinoscope (**ri**·no·skope). A nasal speculum with a mirror used in posterior rhinoscopy. [Gk *rhis* nose, *skopein* to watch.]

rhinoscopic (ri·no·**skop**·ik). Relating or belonging to rhinoscopy or to the rhinoscope.

rhinoscopy (ri·**nos**·ko·pe). Examination of the nasal cavities. **Anterior rhinoscopy.** Examination of the nasal cavity through the anterior nares. **Median rhinoscopy.** Inspection of the nasal cavity and the openings of the ethmoidal and other sinuses with the aid of a long nasal speculum. **Posterior rhinoscopy.** Inspection of the nasal cavity through the nasal part of the pharynx. [Gk *rhis* nose, *skopein* to watch.]

rhinosinusopathia (ri·no·si·nus·o·**path′**·e·ah). Any disease of the nasal and accessory sinuses. [Gk *rhis* nose, sinus, *pathos* disease.]

rhinosporidiosis (ri·no·spor·id·e·**o′**·sis). An infection of the mucosae of the nose, larynx, eyes, ears, and sometimes of the vagina and skin, caused by *Rhinosporidium seeberi* and characterized by the development of polypoid growths which contain large numbers of the parasite. It occurs in man, the cow, and the horse, and is found chiefly in India but also in other countries. This disease must not be confused with *rhinophycomycosis* in which the organism is present in subcutaneous tissues as wide, sparsely septate mycelium. [*Rhinosporidium,* Gk *-osis* condition.]

Rhinosporidium (ri·no·spor·**id′**·e·um). A fungus which has not been isolated in culture but reproduces in the tissues of the host by a cycle of single to multispored sporangia. No mycelium has been observed. **Rhinosporidium kinealyi** Minchin and Fantham 1905. *Rhinosporidium seeberi.* **Rhinosporidium seeberi** (Wernicke) Seeber 1912. The cause of rhinosporidiosis. This name has priority, the species being originally described by Wernicke in 1900 as *Coccidium seeberi.* [Gk *rhis* nose, *spora* seed.]

rhinostenosis (ri·no·sten·**o′**·sis). Pathological narrowing of a nasal passage. [Gk *rhis* nose, stenosis.]

rhinothrix (**ri**·no·thrix). A hair growing within the nostril. [Gk *rhis* nose, *thrix* hair.]

rhinotomy (ri·**not**·o·me). Any incisive operation on the nose. [Gk *rhis* nose, *temnein* to cut.]

rhinovaccination (ri·no·vak·sin·**a′**·shun). The application of vaccines or vaccine toxoids to the mucous membrane of the nose. [Gk *rhis* nose, vaccine.]

Rhinovirus (ri·no·**vi′**·rus). A genus of small spherical RNA-containing viruses (25 nm in diameter) forming part of the Picornavirus family. They are one of the major causes of the common cold syndrome and normally infect only the nose and throat, with spread by droplets. There are about 100 serotypes which makes the production of an adequate vaccine virtually impossible. [Gk *rhis* nose, L *virus* poison.]

Rhipicephalus (ri·pe·**kef**·al·us). A genus of ixodic ticks which are vectors of the rickettsiae of tick-borne typhus and Q fever, of tick-borne relapsing fever, and probable vectors of Rift Valley fever; they are potential vectors of *Trypanosoma cruzi* and *Brucella tularensis* and they cause ascending tick paralysis. **Rhipicephalus appendiculatus.** A vector of tick-borne typhus and probably of the virus of Rift Valley fever, and the spirochaete of relapsing fever. **Rhipicephalus sanguineus.** The European dog tick, a vector of tick-borne typhus (boutonneuse fever) and of Q fever; a potential vector of American trypanosomiasis (*Trypanosoma cruzi*). **Rhipicephalus simus.** A vector of tick-borne typhus and a cause of ascending tick paralysis. [Gk *rhipis* fan, *kephale* head.]

rhiptasmus (rip·**taz**·mus). Choreic movements of jerking or twitching type which may be exemplified in chorea or paralysis agitans. [Gk *rhiptazein* to throw oneself about.]

rhitidectomy (rit·id·**ek**·to·me). Rhytidectomy.

rhitidosis (rit·id·**o**·sis). Rhytidosis.

rhizanaesthesia (ri·zan·es·**theez′**·e·ah). Subarachnoid anaesthesia produced by the injection of an anaesthetic solution into the subarachnoid space in which lie the spinal nerve roots. [Gk *rhiza* root, anaesthesia.]

Rhizobium (ri·**zo**·be·um). A genus of the family Rhizobiaceae. They are minute Gram-negative aerobic organisms which are able to fix atmospheric nitrogen when living symbiotically in the root nodules of leguminous plants. The type species is *Rhizobium leguminosarum.* [Gk *rhiza* root, *bios* life.]

rhizodontropy (ri·zo·**don**·tro·pe). The attachment of an artificial crown to the root of a tooth. [Gk *rhiza* root, *odous* tooth, *trope* a turning.]

rhizodontrypy (ri·zo·**don**·trip·e). The drilling of a hole through the root into the pulp chamber of a tooth in order to provide drainage for pus formed as a result of pulp necrosis. [Gk *rhiza* root, *odous* tooth, *trype* hole.]

Rhizoglyphus (ri·**zog**·lif·us). A genus of mites. *Rhizoglyphus parasiticus* causes dermatitis of the feet in India. [Gk *rhiza* root, *glyphein* to carve.]

rhizoid, rhizoidal (**ri**·zoid, ri·**zoid**·al). Having resemblance to a root; branching irregularly, like a root, as in certain bacteriological plate cultures. [Gk *rhiza* root, *eidos* form.]

rhizoma (ri·**zo**·mah). Rhizome.

rhizome (**ri**·zome) (pl. *rhizomata, rhizomes*). A rootlike stem growing underground or along the surface which gives off subterranean roots and sends out leafy shoots or buds from its upper side. [Gk *rhizoma* root.]

rhizomelic (ri·zo·**mel**·ik). Relating or belonging to, or affecting the hip and shoulder joints, i.e. the "roots" of the limbs. [Gk *rhiza* root, *melos* limb.]

rhizomeningomyelitis (ri·zo·men·**ing**·go·mi·el·**i**′·tis). Inflammation of the nerve roots, the membranes, and the spinal cord. [Gk *rhiza* root, meninges, myelitis.]

rhizomorphoid (ri·zo·**mor**·foid). Shaped like a root. [Gk *rhizoma* root, *morphe* shape, *eidos* form.]

rhizoneuron (ri·zo·**newr**·on). A motor nerve cell. [Gk *rhiza* root, *neuron* nerve.]

rhizonychia, rhizonychium (ri·zon·**ik**·e·ah, ri·zon·**ik**·e·um). The root of the nail. [Gk *rhiza* root, *onyx* nail.]

rhizopod (**ri**·zo·pod). A member of the class Rhizopoda.

Rhizopoda (ri·**zop**·od·ah). A class or sub-class of Protozoa, characterized by the absence of cuticle and, as a rule, flagella or cilia, movement being by pseudopodial flow. Many species are naked, but most bear a shell, often of very complex form. Most medically important forms are naked amoebae. [Gk *rhiza* root, *pous* foot.]

Rhizopus (**ri**·zo·pus). A genus of the Mucoraceae. Some species cause destruction of soft fruits and bulbs and a few are potentially but feebly pathogenic for man. **Rhizopus arrhizus.** A species isolated from cases of phycomycosis in man. **Rhizopus equinus** Lucet and Costantin 1903. A species isolated from a horse and later from swine. It is pathogenic for rabbits. **Rhizopus microsporus** van Tieghem 1875. A pathogenic species which has been isolated from horses and is also pathogenic for guinea-pigs. **Rhizopus niger** (Ciaglinski and Hewelke) Barthelat 1903. A fungus which has been isolated from cases of black tongue. It is not pathogenic for rabbits or guinea-pigs. **Rhizopus oryzae.** A species isolated from cases of phycomycosis in man. **Rhizopus parasiticus** (Lucet and Costantin) Lendner 1908. A species isolated from a human lung. [Gk *rhiza* root, *pous* foot.]

rhizotomy (ri·**zot**·o·me). The cutting of a nerve root, commonly a posterior (or sensory) root, for the relief of intractable pain limited to the area of distribution of one or more roots: hence, *posterior spinal rhizotomy* for pain in limbs and trunk, or (most commonly) *trigeminal rhizotomy* for persistent tic douloureux. More rarely an anterior root section is done for relief of persistent spasm or involuntary movement of limited root distribution. Apart from trigeminal root section, to be effective the operation has to deal with more than one adjacent root. [Gk *rhiza* root, *temnein* to cut.]

rhodalline (ro·**dal**·een). Thiosinamine.

rhodamine (**ro**·dam·een). Any member of a family of dyestuffs related to fluorescein: they are amino phthaleins containing substituted amino groups, and form salts which are fast dyes. **Rhodamine B.** Tetraethylrhodamine chloride, a violet-red dye for mordanted cotton. **Rhodamine S.** A succinic derivative of dimethylrhodamine chloride. [Gk *rhodon* rose, amine.]

rhodanate (**ro**·dan·ate). Any salt or ester of rhodanic (thiocyanic) acid.

rhodeorrhetin (ro·de·o·**ret**′·in). Convolvulin, the glycosidal resin obtained from jalap.

rhodeose (**ro**·de·oze). $CH_3(CHOH)_4CHO$, an isomer of fucose, occurring in convolvulin and jalapin.

rhodium (**ro**·de·um). An element of atomic weight 102.9055, atomic number 45, and chemical symbol Rh. It is a hard metal closely resembling platinum, and found with the latter in platiniferous alluvial sands. It is used in electroplating and in thermocouples. [Gk *rhodon* rose.]

Rhodnius (**rod**·ne·us). A genus of reduviid bugs. *Rhodnius brumpti, R. domesticus, R. pallescens, R. pictipes* and *R. prolixus*, human parasites living in houses in northern South America, are important secondary hosts of *Trypanosoma cruzi. R. prolixus* has been used extensively as a laboratory animal.

Rhodobacillus (ro·do·bas·**il**′·us). An obsolete genus: the organisms so described are now included in the genus *Rhodopseudomonas.* [Gk *rhodon* rose, bacillus.]

Rhodobacterium (ro·do·bak·**teer**′·e·um). An obsolete genus now included in the genus *Rhodopseudomonas.* [Gk *rhodon* rose, bacterium.]

Rhodocapsa (ro·do·**kap**·sah). An obsolete genus now included in part under the genus *Rhabdomonas.* [Gk *rhodon* rose, *kapsa* basket.]

Rhodococcus (ro·do·**kok**·us). **Rhodococcus Molisch** 1907. An obsolete genus now part of the genus *Rhodopseudomonas.* **Rhodococcus Zopf** 1891. An obsolete genus of cocci now included in the genus *Micrococcus.* [Gk *rhodon* rose, coccus.]

rhodocyte (**ro**·do·site). An erythrocyte. [Gk *rhodon* rose, *kytos* cell.]

rhodogenesis (ro·do·**jen**·es·is). The reconstitution of the visual purple in the retina after it has been bleached by exposure to bright light. [rhodopsin, Gk *genein* to produce.]

rhodophylactic (ro·do·fil·**ak**′·tik). 1. Relating or belonging to rhodophylaxis. 2. Capable of restoring or maintaining rhodopsin.

rhodophylaxis (ro·do·fil·**ax**′·is). Regeneration of the visual purple. [rhodopsin, Gk *phylaxis* a guarding.]

rhodoporphyrin (ro·do·**por**·fir·in). $C_{30}H_{32}N_4(COOH)_2$, a red crystalline porphyrin obtained by the action of alkalis on chlorophyll. [Gk *rhodon* rose, porphyrin.]

Rhodopseudomonas (ro·do·sew·do·**mo**′·nas). A genus of unicellular rod-shaped or spherical bacteria, producing a pigment system composed of chlorophyll and carotenoids. [Gk *rhodon* rose, *pseudes* false, *monas* unit.]

rhodopsin (ro·**dop**·sin). Visual purple; a deep-red pigment formed in the outer sections of the rods. It is bleached by light to visual yellow, retinene, and is synthesized from a protein and vitamin A, probably by the retinal pigment epithelium. [Gk *rhodon* rose, *opsis* vision.]

rhodopterin (ro·**dop**·ter·in). A bluish-red compound obtained by the oxidation of the wing pigment, pterin. [Gk *rhodon* rose, pterin.]

Rhodotorula (ro·do·**tor**·ew·lah). A genus of fungi, species of which (e.g. *Rhodotorula rubra* (*mucilaginosa*)) have been implicated in cases of septicaemia and endocarditis in compromised individuals. [Gk *rhodon* rose, L *torulus* small swelling.]

rhodoxanthin (ro·do·**zan**·thin). $C_{40}H_{50}O_2$, a carotenoid pigment found in the red berries of the yew, *Taxus baccata*, and rose fruits. [Gk *rhodon* rose, xanthin.]

rhoeadine (**re**·ad·een). $C_{21}H_{21}O_6N$, a crystalline non-poisonous alkaloid occurring in opium and in rose petals. It is found particularly in *Papaver rhoeas.*

rhoebdesis (reb·**de**·sis). Resorption. [Gk *rhoibdeein* to swallow greedily down.]

rhomb (romb). An oblique, equilateral parallelogram. [Gk *rhombos.]*

rhombencephalitis (rom·ben·kef·al·**i**′·tis). Encephalitis of the brain stem, with disturbance of consciousness and ocular paralysis as salient features. [rhombencephalon, Gk *-itis* inflammation.]

rhombencephalon [NA] (rom·ben·**kef**·al·on). The hind-brain. [rhomb, Gk *egkephalos* brain.]

rhombocoele (**rom**·bo·seel). The 4th ventricle of the brain, situated in the hind-brain. The term has also been applied to the terminal ventricle in the conus medullaris of the spinal cord. [Gk *rhombus* rhomb, *koilos* hollow.]

rhomboid (**rom**·boid). Being similar in outline to a rhomb. [rhomb, Gk *eidos* form.]

See also: MICHAELIS (G. A.).

rhomboid major muscle [musculus rhomboideus major (NA)]. A quadrilaterally-shaped muscle running from the upper thoracic spinous processes to the lower two-thirds of the vertebral border of the scapula.

rhomboid minor muscle [musculus rhomboideus minor (NA)]. A quadrilaterally-shaped muscle running from the ligamentum nuchae and the spines of the 7th cervical and 1st thoracic vertebrae to the vertebral border of the scapula at the apex of the spine.

rhomboids, nerve to the [nervus dorsalis scapulae (NA)]. A branch of the 5th cervical root of the brachial plexus.

Rhombomys opimus (**rom**·bo·mis op·i·mus). A gerbil, a reservoir of infection of *Leishmania tropica* in Turkmenistan. [Gk *rhembein* to turn around, *mys* mouse, L *opimus* fat.]

rhonchal, rhonchial (**rong**·kal, **rong**·ke·al). Relating to, caused by, or having the character of a rhoncus.

rhonchus (**rong**·kus) (pl. *rhonchi*). The sound produced as air passes in and out with respiration in bronchi which are partially obstructed. The obstruction may be due to tenacious mucus, swollen mucous membrane, muscular spasm, a neoplasm, or external pressure. This follows the physical law that a sound is produced by vibrations set up when air passes through a narrow constriction into a wider space; the sound is amplified by resonance of the air in the tube. The larger the volume of air the lower the pitch of the sound. Rhonchi produced in the trachea or large bronchi are low-pitched and are called *sonorous*, as in tracheobronchitis. In the smaller bronchi the rhonchi are of higher pitch or *sibilant*, as in asthma. Various descriptive terms are also used such as *snoring, groaning, whistling, squeaking, wheezing*. Rhonchi are also termed *dry râles* in the older classifications of adventitious sounds. [Gk *rhogchos* snore.]

Rhopalopsyllus cavicola (ro·pal·**op**·sil·us ka·ve·**ko**·lah). A species of flea that is a potential transmitter of plague in South America. [Gk *rhopalon* club, *psylla* flea, L *cavicolus* cave-dweller.]

rhotacism (**ro**·tah·sizm). 1. The excessive use or incorrect pronunciation of the letter *r*. 2. Stammering over the letter *r*. [Gk *rho* letter *r*.]

rhotanium (ro·**ta**·ne·um). A non-oxidizing alloy of gold and palladium, used instead of platinum in laboratory ware.

Rhubarb BP 1973 (**roo**·barb). The rhizome of *Rheum palmatum* Linn., and possibly other species and hybrids of *Rheum* excepting *R. rhaponticum* Linn., cultivated in China and Tibet; it is deprived of most of its bark and dried. It contains water-soluble glycosides of derivatives of anthraquinone, and is used as a purgative. The stem of the rhubarb contains little purgative glycoside and is not used in medicine. [Gk *rha* rhubarb, L *barbarus* wild.]

Rhus (roos). A genus of plants of the family Anacardiaceae. **Rhus cotinus.** Venetian sumach. *See* SUMACH. **Rhus javanica.** The species which is the source of Chinese and Japanese galls. **Rhus toxicodendron.** The poison ivy, a North American tree which is said to cause dermatitis. A preparation of the leaves has been employed externally as an irritant. [Gk *rhous* sumac.]

rhynchota (rin·**ko**·tah). Hemiptera, the bugs. [Gk *rhynchos* snout, *ous* ear.]

rhypophobia (ri·po·**fo**·be·ah). Pathological fear of dirt and filth. [Gk *rhypos* dirt.]

Rhypus (**ri**·pus). A genus of Diptera. Larvae, which are normally saprophagous, have caused accidental intestinal myiasis. [Gk *rhypos* dirt.]

rhysema (ri·**se**·mah). Wrinkle. [Gk *rhysema* wrinkle.]

rhysis (**ri**·sis). Any type of watery effusion, particularly from the nasal mucous membrane. [Gk *rhysis* a flowing.]

rhythm (rithm). The regular recurrence of an action or function. **Alpha rhythm.** In electro-encephalography, the normal dominant activity of the postcentral cortex. It is a regular wave form with a frequency varying between 8 and 13 Hz (c/s); it is seen most clearly in the occipital regions and varies greatly in amount in different individuals. In some normal subjects alpha activity is almost continuous and of high amplitude; in others it is extremely scanty. As a rule, the rhythm is inhibited by visual or mental attention. **Atrial rhythm.** The cardiac rhythm resulting from a focus in the atria which is discharging regularly, either at a rate in excess of that of the sinus node or in the presence of sinus arrest or exit block. **Atrioventricular (auriculoventricular) nodal rhythm.** The cardiac rhythm which results when the atrioventricular node assumes control of the heart beat, either because the sinu-atrial node is suppressed altogether or is discharging more slowly than the intrinsic rate of the atrioventricular node which then "escapes" (nodal bradycardia) or when the atrioventricular node develops an intrinsic rate of impulse formation faster than the sinus node (nodal tachycardia). **Beta rhythm.** In electro-encephalography, fast activity with a frequency between 14 and 24 Hz (c/s). A certain amount of beta activity is often recorded, particularly from the frontal lobes, in normal individuals, but this activity may be particularly profuse in anxious subjects, during the onset of sleep, and in patients taking barbiturates. **Bigeminal rhythm.** Coupled rhythm (see below). **Cantering rhythm.** Gallop rhythm (see below). **Cardiac rhythm.** The regularly recurring beating of the heart. In the normal heart excitation begins at the sinu-atrial node, producing atrial contraction. Activation of the atrioventricular node follows and produces ventricular contraction. Each atrial and ventricular systole constitutes a regularly recurring cardiac cycle. **Circadian rhythm.** Regular changes in certain physiological functions which recur approximately at 24-h intervals. Body temperature and urinary excretion rate are two examples. **Circus rhythm.** A regular rapid cardiac rhythm resulting from the continuing passage of a stimulating wavefront round a pathway which results in its re-entry to the beginning of the pathway with each circuit. It is the basis of most forms of tachycardia. **Coronary sinus rhythm.** The term sometimes used to describe the cardiac rhythm which is represented on the electrocardiogram by a supraventricular rhythm with negative P waves in leads II, III and aVF, suggesting that the focus initiating atrial depolarization is low in the atrium, possibly in the region of the coronary sinus. **Coupled rhythm.** Ventricular ectopic beats alternating with sinus beats and followed by a compensatory pause before the next sinus beat, producing coupling of the heart beats. **Delta rhythm.** In electro-encephalography, any activity at a frequency of 3.5 Hz (c/s) or less. Such activity is normal during deep sleep or in very young infants, but when seen in the waking record of an adult it is definitely abnormal. If paroxysmal it may indicate epilepsy; if focal it suggests the presence of a localized cortical lesion. **Dual rhythm.** The cadence produced by the first and second heart sounds, without added sounds. **Ectopic rhythm.** The abnormal rhythm in which the site of impulse formation lies in some ectopic focus outside the usual pacemaker. Such a focus may be anywhere in the atrial, atrioventricular nodal, or ventricular tissue. Ectopic rhythms arise when the natural pacemaker is depressed or when ectopic foci become irritable. **Fetal rhythm.** Embryocardia, tic-tac rhythm; equal spacing of the two heart sounds, with alteration in the quality of the first heart sound which resembles that of the second; it occurs in severe circulatory failure. **Gallop rhythm.** The cadence produced by three heart sounds in each cycle (gallop rhythm) in the presence of a tachycardia. This cadence resembles the galloping or cantering of a horse. *Presystolic gallop rhythm* (atrial gallop) is due to the presence of an added sound in presystole, usually the atrial sound, and occurs in left ventricular failure, atrial hypertrophy, and in the presence of a prolonged P-R interval. *Protodiastolic gallop rhythm* is due to the presence of an audible third sound, and is found in left ventricular failure, constrictive pericarditis, and frequently in mitral regurgitation. *Summation gallop rhythm* is due to the summation of the atrial and third sounds in mid-diastole when there is a considerable degree of tachycardia or when the P-R interval is markedly prolonged. **Gamma rhythm.** Ultra-fast activity (25 Hz (c/s) and over) in the electro-encephalogram. Its significance is obscure, but a certain amount of this activity may be seen in normal individuals. **Idioventricular rhythm.** A slow cardiac rhythm due to the repeated discharge of a focus within the ventricle, seen with sinus arrest or complete heart block. **Junctional rhythm.** The cardiac rhythm resulting from the regular discharge of impulses from a focus in tissue in the region of the atrioventricular node. This term is sometimes used in preference to *atrioventricular nodal rhythm* (see above) as commonly precise location of the focus to the atrioventricular node is not possible. **Nodal rhythm.** Atrioventricular nodal rhythm (see above). **Parasystolic rhythm.** The cardiac rhythm which occurs when two independent foci are driving the heart. This most commonly results from a regular discharging ventricular ectopic focus in the presence of sinus rhythm; in the electrocardiogram this is manifested by ventricular ectopic beats which are not coupled by identical time intervals to the preceding sinus beat but which have time intervals between them which are multiples of the period of the parasystolic focus and by fusion beats, due to coincident occurrence of ventricular excitation by normally conducted impulses and by the parasystolic focus. **Pendulum rhythm.** Fetal rhythm (see above). **Quadruple rhythm.** The cadence produced by four heart sounds in each cycle; it is not heard in normal hearts. **Reciprocal rhythm.** A type of nodal rhythm in which retrograde block between the atrioventricular and sinu-atrial nodes becomes so great that the impulse from the former, having activated the atrium, spreads down and activates the ventricle which has by that time ceased to be refractory. **Reversed rhythm.** Nodal rhythm with retrograde conduction to the atria, causing the latter to contract later than the ventricles. **Sinus rhythm.** The normal heart rhythm due to conduction of impulses from the sinu-atrial node to the atrioventricular node; the ventricles contract after each beat of the atria. **Supranodal rhythm.** A cardiac rhythm resulting from impulses arising at a site close to, but above, the atrioventricular node. **Theta rhythm.** In electro-encephalography, activity of a frequency between 4 and 7 Hz (c/s). Waves of this frequency normally occur in the electro-encephalogram of a child below the age of 12 years. In an adult record they are definitely abnormal and may indicate immaturity, dysrhythmia, or deep-seated pathology. **Tic-tac rhythm.** Fetal rhythm (see above). **Triple rhythm.** The cadence produced by the first and second heart sounds, with the addition in each cycle of an extra sound which may be in early diastole (*protodiastolic triple rhythm*), late diastole (*presystolic triple rhythm*), or in systole (*systolic triple rhythm*). In the protodiastolic type the added sound is usually a third heart sound which is not heard in normal adults though frequently present in children; in the presystolic type it is an exaggerated atrial sound not normally heard but which may be present if the atrium is enlarged or the P-R interval prolonged; an added sound in early systole is usually an ejection sound arising from the aorta or pulmonary artery at the time of the opening of the corresponding valve occurring in the presence of dilatation of the vessel; an added sound later in systole most commonly arises from the mitral valve apparatus and is often followed by a late systolic murmur due to mitral regurgitation. **Ventricular rhythm.** Nodal rhythm (see above). [Gk *rhythmos*.]

See also: BERGER (H.).

rhythmeur (**rith**·mer). A device which makes rhythmic interruption in the current of an X-ray apparatus.

rhythmicity (rith·**mis**·it·e). Regular periodicity. Of muscle, having rhythmic contractions.

rhythmotherapy (rith·mo·**ther**·ap·e). Treatment of disorders by the use of rhythm, e.g. the beating of time in cases of stammering. [rhythm, therapy.]

rhytidectomy (rit·id·**ek**·to·me). The plastic operation, carried out mainly for cosmetic reasons, of excising wrinkles and stretching and joining the cut edges of skin so that a smooth surface may be produced. [Gk *rhytis* wrinkle, *ektome* a cutting out.]

rhytidosis (rit·id·**o**·sis). Shrivelling and sinking in of the cornea, a sign of impending death. [Gk *rhytis* wrinkle, *-osis* condition.]

rib (rib). **Rib notching.** A radiological sign of coarctation of the aorta in which the lower borders of the upper ribs show irregular indentations due to the enlargement and tortuosity of the intercostal arteries forming part of the anastomotic circulation around the coarctation. *See* RIBS. [AS.]

Ribbert, Moritz Wilhelm Hugo (b. 1855). Zürich pathologist.

Ribbert's method. Alcohol-fixed material is mordanted in phosphomolybdic acid and stained with phosphomolybdic acid haematoxylin. Connective-tissue fibres are stained blue.

Ribbert's theory. The theory that tumours develop when cells are released from the control of associated tissue, especially connective tissue, because of reduced tension in those tissues.

Ribbert's thrombosis. Coagulation of blood within the vascular system just before or at the moment of death. It occurs in the right side of the heart and in the pulmonary artery; the thrombi are tough and stringy and do not adhere to the endothelium.

ribbon (**rib**·on). *See* REIL. [Fr. *riban*.]

Ribes, François (b. 1765). Paris and Rome physician.

Ribes' ganglion. A collection of ganglion cells in the cranial part of the sympathetic nervous system. It is situated on the anterior communicating artery.

ribodesose (rib·o·des·oze). 2-Desoxy-D-ribose, $CH_2OH(CHOH)_2CH_2CHO$. The pentose sugar which is found in animal nucleic acid combined with a purine or pyrimidine in the form of a nucleoside.

Riboflavine BP 1973 (ri·bo·**fla**·veen). Lactoflavine, 6,7-dimethyl-9-(D-1′-ribityl)-isoalloxazine, $C_{17}H_{20}N_4O_6$. A water-soluble heat-stabile vitamin of the B group; also known as *vitamin* B_2. It is a yellow pigment found in milk, grasses and malt, some algae, yeast and meat, including liver and kidney, and can also be synthesized. It is an essential part of the enzyme system in the carbohydrate metabolism of cells; deficiency in man produces cheilosis and other changes in skin and mucous membranes. [ribose, flavin.]

Riboflavinum. *European Pharmacopoeia* name for Riboflavine BP 1973.

ribofuranose (ri·bo·**fewr**·an·oze). In sugar nomenclature, the furanose form of ribose containing the five-membered furane ring.

ribonuclease (ri·bo·**new**·kle·aze). The class of endonucleases which only hydrolyse ribonucleic acids.

ribonucleoprotein (ri·bo·new·kle·o·**pro**′·te·in). A class of conjugated proteins that contain ribonucleic acid. The protein fraction is usually very basic, and is usually a protamine or a histone.

ribonucleotide (ri·bo·**new**·kle·o·tide). A class of nucleotides in which the pentose is D-ribose.

ribopyranose (ri·bo·**pi**·ran·oze). In sugar nomenclature the pyranose form of ribose containing the six-membered pyran ring.

ribose (**ri**·boze). D-ribose, $CH_2OH(CHOH)_3CHO$. An aldopentose, stereoisomeric with arabinose, which occurs in yeast-nucleic acid, riboflavine, and co-enzymes I and II; also in the glycoside from croton seeds. L-ribose can be synthesized from L-arabinose.

ribosome (**ri**·bo·some). One of a class of minute RNA-containing particles present mainly in the cytoplasm of living cells and visible in electron micrographs. They are the intracellular site for protein synthesis by providing a surface for the localized interaction of the participating molecules. Those from *Escherichia coli* have a molecular weight of 2.6×10^6 daltons and can be dissociated into two subunits of which one, the *30S subunit* (S = Svedberg unit) contains a single 16S RNA molecule, some 20 different species of protein and can bind a single strand of messenger RNA, while the other, the *50S subunit*, contains two different RNA molecules (one 5S, the other 23S), some 35 different species of protein molecule and two binding sites for transfer RNA molecules (one is called the A or aminoacyl-tRNA site and the other the P or peptidyl-tRNA site). Those from eukaryotes are larger, have a molecular weight of 4.2×10^6 daltons and contain a *40S subunit* (in which the RNA is 18S), and a *60S subunit* (in which the RNA is 5S and 28S). Their subunit protein composition, as well as functions, appear to be similar to those of the corresponding *E. coli* subunits. In the cytoplasm they may occur as free subunits, in clusters aligned on a single strand of messenger RNA (when they are called *polysomes* or *polyribosomes*) or as individual ribosomes attached to the outer surface of the endoplasmic reticulum. Ribosomes may be found in nuclei and especially in nucleoli, where they appear to be produced. Mitochondrial and chloroplast ribosomes occur in mitochondria and chloroplasts respectively, and are similar in size to those from prokaryotes. [ribose, Gk *soma* body.]

ribs [costae (NA)] (ribz). Slender, curved bars of bone articulating with the bodies of the thoracic vertebrae posteriorly and slightly expanded in front to receive the costal cartilages. They partly encircle the thorax or upper part of the abdomen. **Angle of a rib, anterior.** A ridge on the outer surface of the shaft of the 4th to the 8th ribs, near their anterior ends, to which the lower digitations of the serratus anterior muscle are attached. **Angle of a rib, posterior [angulus costae (NA)].** The ridge on the outer aspect of the shaft of a rib, not far from the tubercle, where the curvature is greatest. It gives attachment to the iliocostocervical muscle. **Cervical rib.** A supernumerary rib connected with the 7th cervical vertebra. It may vary from an exaggerated costal process prolonged as a fibrous band attached to the 1st rib, to a long rib articulated at its origin and also distally to the 1st rib. It may in some cases interfere with the nerve supply to the arm and give rise to sensory, motor and vasomotor symptoms. **False rib [costa spuria (NA)].** A rib which does not articulate through its costal cartilage directly with the sternum: one of the last five pairs of ribs. **Floating rib.** Either of the 11th or 12th ribs. **Head of a rib [caput costae (NA)].** The posterior extremity of a rib which articulates with the body of a thoracic vertebra at the articular facet [facies articularis capitis costae.] **Neck of a rib [collum costae (NA)].** The flattened part of a rib which succeeds the head; its sharp, upper border is the crest. **Shaft of a rib [corpus costae (NA)].** The main body of a rib, anterior to the tubercle. **Slipping rib.** Recurrent dislocation of a costal cartilage. **Stove-in ribs.** A driving inwards of part of the ribs as a result of a severe compression injury. **Supernumerary rib.** Cervical rib (see above). **True rib [costa vera (NA)].** A rib which articulates with a thoracic vertebra behind, and with the sternum in front through a costal cartilage: one of the first seven pairs of ribs. **Typhoid rib.** Osteomyelitis of a rib due to an infection with *Salmonella typhi*, usually a sequel of typhoid fever. [AS.]

See also: ZAHN.

Ricard, Alfred Louis (b. 1858). French surgeon.

Ricard's amputation. Intertibiocalcaneal disarticulation, a variant of the Syme amputation; the foot is removed, the talus being enucleated and the calcaneum wedged between the tibia and fibula.

rice (ri·s). The seeds of *Oryza sativa* (family Gramineae). The edible part of the grain consists of the endosperm, the pericarp, the aleuron layer, and the germ. In order to prepare rice for food, some degree of polishing is necessary. The degree of polishing varies, but a high degree, which is necessary to produce the white rice that is sold in the UK and other Western countries, entails the removal of all but the endosperm. Almost the whole of the vitamin B_1 is contained in the polishings, and the consumption of polished rice exclusively has led to beriberi. Rice is a staple food in many Eastern countries, consisting mostly of carbohydrate, and finds favour elsewhere in the preparation of cakes, puddings, etc. **Parboiled rice.** Rice that has been subjected to steaming while still in the husk; by this means some of the vitamin B_1 is adsorbed by the endosperm and therefore not lost in subsequent milling or polishing. **Polished rice.** Rice that has been polished and consists of the endosperm only. **Rice polishings.** The discarded residue, containing the outer layers and the germ, separated in the milling of rice. It is rich in vitamin B_1. **White rice.** The rice grain ordinarily on sale; polished rice (see above). [Gk *oryza*.]

Rich, Arnold Rice (b. 1893). Baltimore pathologist.

Hamman-Rich syndrome. Idiopathic diffuse interstitial fibrosis of the lungs, usually fatal.

Richard, Felix Adolphe (b. 1822). Paris surgeon.

Richard's fringe. The fimbriated extremity of the uterine tube.

Richardson, Sir Benjamin Ward (b. 1828). London physician.

Richardson's method, or sign. A test of death: a tight ligature is applied to the arm, and if life is present the veins on the distal side become more distended.

Riches, Eric William (b. 1897). London surgeon.

Riches' apparatus. The introduction of a self-retaining catheter (size 16 F) to the bladder at a point midway between the umbilicus and the pubis. The catheter is mounted on a special introducer in the end of which there is incorporated a small knife blade.

Riches' suprapubic catheter introducer. *See* RICHES' APPARATUS (above).

Richet, Louis Dominique Alfred (b. 1816). Paris surgeon.

Richet's canal. A canal in the anterior abdominal wall which surrounds the round ligament as it pierces the fibres of the transversus abdominis muscle.

Richet's fascia. The fascial covering of Richet's canal.

Richet's operation. For cicatricial ectropion and canthoplasty, when the outer canthus is involved only: a crescentic area of skin is excised at the outer canthus, including the scar tissue; this frees the outer canthus. The remaining raw area is filled by a form of Z-plasty operation.

Richter, August Gottlieb (b. 1742). Göttingen surgeon.

Richter's hernia. Protrusion of a small portion of the wall of the intestine into a hernia, the main portion of its circumference remaining within the abdomen.

Richter's operation. 1. For iridotomy. 2. For stricture of the nasolacrimal duct. Both procedures are obsolete.

Monro-Richter line. A line from the umbilicus to the anterior superior iliac spine.

Richter, Ina May (b. 1885). Santa Barbara, California, physician.

Clough and Richter syndrome. An anaemia associated with marked auto-agglutination of erythrocytes, usually indicative of myelomatosis.

ricin (ri·sin). An albumin obtained from castor-oil seeds (*Ricinus communis*). It is highly toxic, producing agglutination of the red blood cells when injected.

ricinine (ris·in·een). $C_8H_8O_2N_2$, an alkaloid occurring in castor oil, but not contributing to the therapeutic properties of the latter.

ricinism (ris·in·izm). Gastro-enteritis with bleeding, accompanied by hepatic congestion and jaundice, the result of ingestion of seeds of *Ricinus communis*.

ricinoleate (ri·sin·o·le·ate). Any salt of ricinoleic acid.

Ricinus (ris·in·us). A genus of plants of the family Euphorbiaceae. The seeds of *Ricinus communis* Linn. are the source of castor oil, of which they contain about 50 per cent; they also contain a very poisonous toxin, ricin, which makes the exhausted seeds unfit for cattle food. [L.]

rickets (rik·etz). A disturbance of the calcium/phosphorus metabolism which occurs in the growing child as a result of vitamin-D deficiency. Predisposing factors include active skeletal growth, prematurity, grossly defective maternal diet in breast-fed babies, sole use of unfortified winter-fed-cows' milk, irregular exposure of the skin to radiation from ultraviolet light, and too early addition of starch so that inositol phosphoric acid prevents absorption of vitamin D from the intestines. Classical symptoms relate to generalized hypotonicity and retarded development, so that respiratory, gastro-intestinal, dental, nervous, and skin disorders occur before the classical signs of skeletal deformity. These depend on the degree of softening of the bones and on the amount of weight-bearing to which they have been subjected. Treatment consists of administration of vitamin D combined with exposure to sunlight or ultraviolet irradiation. Prophylaxis consists of regular administration of vitamin D to the premature and to the artificially-fed infant from the end of the first month of life, and to the breast-fed from the end of the second month. Vitamin D should be continued throughout the growth period of childhood. **Acrobatic rickets.** A term applied to rickets in which there is extreme muscular laxity so that the joints can be bent into almost any position. **Adult rickets.** Osteomalacia. **Congenital rickets.** An ambiguous term loosely applied to several conditions, e.g. achondroplasia and osteogenesis imperfecta. **Fetal rickets.** True rickets developing in intra-uterine life, when the mother has osteomalacia. It is also used for several other congenital deficiencies associated with defective bone formation. It is a vague term best avoided. **Late rickets.** Rachitic changes in bone due to long-standing renal impairment. **Recrudescent rickets.** Late or adolescent rickets. **Renal rickets.** Typical bony changes occurring in older children, associated with severe impairment of renal function. Radiologically there are two types: classical infantile type, and woolly stippled appearance of long bones and skull. **Resistant rickets.** A condition when enormous daily doses of vitamin D fail to produce improvement. Further investigations may show renal impairment, or abnormality of the cystine metabolism. [prob. corruption of rachitis.]

Rickettsia (rik·et·se·ah). A genus of micro-organisms in the family Rickettsiaceae, occupying an intermediate position between the smaller bacteria and the larger viruses. They resemble bacteria in being visible by the light microscope, dividing by binary fission, and being susceptible to the action of certain antibiotics. They are, however, obligate intracellular parasites, like viruses. The rickettsiae live under natural conditions in the intestines of certain blood-sucking insects—lice, fleas, mites and ticks. Man, if infected by lice, develops epidemic typhus due to *Rickettsia prowazeki.* **Rickettsia akari.** The causal organism of rickettsialpox. **Rickettsia australis.** The causal organism of Queensland tick typhus. **Rickettsia burneti, Coxiella burneti.** The cause of Q fever. **Rickettsia conori.** The cause of boutonneuse fever. **Rickettsia mooseri.** The cause of flea-borne typhus. **Rickettsia muricola.** *Rickettsia mooseri.* **Rickettsia orientalis.** The cause of scrub typhus. **Rickettsia pediculi.** An extracellular rickettsia, a normal inhabitant of the louse, which causes no disease. **Rickettsia prowazeki.** The cause of classical typhus. **Rickettsia prowazeki var. mooseri.** *Rickettsia mooseri* (see above). **Rickettsia quintana.** The cause of trench fever. **Rickettsia Rickettsii.** The cause of Rocky Mountain spotted fever. **Rickettsia tsutsugamushi.** *Rickettsia orientalis* (see above), the cause of scrub typhus. **Rickettsia typhi.** *Rickettsia mooseri* (see above). [Howard Taylor *Ricketts,* 1871-1910, American pathologist.]

Rickettsiaceae (rik·et·se·a'·se·e). A family of micro-organisms that contains the genera *Rickettsia* and *Coxiella.*

rickettsial (rik·et·se·al). Due to the presence of a species of *Rickettsia.*

rickettsialpox (rik·et·se·al·pox). A mild febrile disease with a vesiculopapular rash, first observed in New York in 1946 and caused by *Rickettsia akari.* It occurs in the house mouse *Mus musculus,* and may be transmitted by the mite *Allodermanyssus sanguineus.* [*Rickettsia,* pox.]

rickettsiosis (rik·et·se·o'·sis). General term for diseases caused by rickettsial infection. [*Rickettsia,* Gk *-osis* condition.]

rickettsiostatic (rik·et·se·o·stat'·ik). Inhibiting the growth of *Rickettsia.* [*Rickettsia,* Gk *statos* standing.]

rickety (rik·et·e). Rachitic.

Ricord, Philippe (b. 1800). Paris physician.

Ricord's chancre. A rare, parchment-like, initial lesion of syphilis.

rictal (rik·tal). Relating or referring to a cleft or fissure. [see foll.]

rictus (rik·tus). 1. A cleft or fissure. 2. Any gaping condition, e.g. of the beak in birds. **Rictus lupinus.** Cleft palate. [L, the opening of the mouth.]

Riddoch, George (b. 1888). London neurologist.

Riddoch's reflex. Mass reflex. *See* REFLEX.

Rideal, Samuel (b. 1863). English chemist.

Rideal-Walker coefficient. A number intended to represent the ratio of bactericidal effectiveness of a substance compared to phenol as a standard.

Rideal-Walker method. A method of assessing efficiency of disinfectants, in relation to phenol as a standard.

ridge (rij). A crest; a raised border. **Alveolar ridge.** The ridge in the edentulous jaw that is left after the alveolar processes have been absorbed. **Basal ridge.** A ridge of enamel on the inner surface of an incisor or canine tooth near its neck; the cingulum. **Buccocervical ridge, Buccogingival ridge.** The ridge on the buccal surface of a deciduous molar tooth near the neck. **Dental ridge.** The tooth-bearing part of the jaw which supports an artificial denture when the natural teeth have been lost. **Genital ridge, Germ ridge, Gonadal ridge.** A longitudinal ridge on the ventromedial side of the mesonephros from which the gonads are derived. **Interureteric ridge.** A ridge caused by a thickened bar of muscle fibres joining the two ureteric orifices. **Linguogingival ridge.** A ridge on the lingual surface of incisor and canine teeth near the gingival margins. **Mandibular ridge.** The ridge on the mandibular arch homologous with the maxillary ridge. **Marginal ridges [cristae marginalis (NA)].** Ridges of enamel which join the inner and outer cusps of molar and premolar teeth on the mesial and distal aspects of the occlusal surfaces of the crown. **Maxillary ridge.** The line of thickened ectoderm on the alveolar portions of the maxillary processes of the embryo from which the enamel organs of the upper teeth are derived. **Medullary ridge.** One of the two raised margins of the neural groove. **Mesonephric ridge.** A longitudinal elevation in the posterolateral wall of the coelom of the fetus, overlying the mesonephros. **Milk ridge.** A line of thickened ectoderm on the ventral thoraco-abdominal wall from which the mammary glands are derived. **Ridges of the nail bed [cristae matricis unguis (NA)].** The series of longitudinal ridges on the corium beneath the nail. **Neural ridge.** The margin of the neural groove. **Oblique ridge.** A ridge of enamel joining the antero-internal to the postero-external cusp on the occlusal surface of an upper second deciduous and first permanent molar tooth. **Palatine ridge.** One of the lines of thickened mucous membrane on the front part of the hard palate. **Pulmonary ridge.** A ridge of mesenchyme, found in the embryo, connecting the dorsal end of the septum transversum with the wolffian body and is the anlage of both the pleuropericardial and pleuroperitoneal membranes; Mall's ridge. **Ridges of the sacrum, transverse [linea transversae (NA)].** The low bony crests which mark the lines of fusion of adjacent sacral vertebrae. **Ridges of the skin [cristae cutis (NA)].** Ridges on the epidermis, corresponding to the papillae of the dermis. They have a constant pattern for each individual, and these patterns are used in criminological work. **Supplemental ridge.** An additional or abnormal enamel ridge on the crown of a tooth. **Supracondylar ridge, lateral.** The sharp lateral border of the lower end of the shaft of the humerus, terminating at the lateral epicondyle. **Supracondylar ridge, medial.** The sharp medial border of the lower end of the shaft of the humerus, terminating at the medial epicondyle. **Supra-orbital ridge.** Superciliary arch. *See* ARCH. **Temporal ridge.** The ridge that runs across the frontal and parietal bones to the zygomatic process. **Transverse ridges [cristae transversalis (NA)].** 1. Ridges which run across the occlusal surface of a tooth in a transverse direction. 2. Ridges of the sacrum, transverse (see above). **Triangular ridge [crista triangularis (NA)].** The triangular surface which descends from the cusp of a tooth towards the centre of its occlusal surface. **Urethral ridge of the vagina [carina urethralis vaginae (NA)].** The median longitudinal prominence in the lower part of the anterior vaginal wall caused by the urethra. **Urogenital ridge.** Wolffian ridge (see foll.). **Wolffian ridge.** A longitudinal ridge on either side of the embryonic mesentery in which the mesonephros and associated structures are developed. [AS *hyrcg.*]

See also: MALL, PASSAVANT, WOLFF (K. F.).

ridgel, ridgeling (rij·el, rij·ling). A man or animal lacking one testis, either because of congenital defect or because of surgical operation. [English dialect.]

Ridley, Humphrey (b. 1653). English anatomist.

Ridley's bay, or sinus. A venous sinus encompassing the pituitary body.

Riedel, Bernhard Moritz Carl Ludwig (b. 1846). Jena surgeon.

Riedel's disease, struma, or thyroiditis. Chronic fibrous or ligneous thyroiditis of unknown aetiology associated clinically with dyspnoea, dysphagia, and hoarseness of voice, and usually with the slow onset of thyroidism.

Riedel's lobe, or process. A tongue-like downward projection of liver substance from the right lobe of the liver; a relatively common congenital abnormality.

Riedel's radical frontal-sinus operation. For chronic frontal sinusitis: through an external incision the frontal sinus floor is removed, the sinus mucosa completely curetted away, the frontonasal ethmoidal cells and the nasal process of the superior maxilla removed, and an osteoplastic flap of the anterior sinus wall and soft tissues made and allowed to fall back in contact with the posterior wall of the sinus.

Rieder, Hermann (b. 1858). Munich physician.

Rieder cell. A large primitive cell, probably a myeloblast, with bi- or multi-lobed and twisted nucleus. It is found in the blood in myeloblastic leukaemia and is looked upon by some workers as a lymphoblast and by others as an obsolescent and degenerating lymphocyte.

Rieder-cell leukaemia. A form of myeloblastic leukaemia in which many Rieder cells are present.

Riegel, Franz (b. 1843). Cologne and Giessen physician.

Riegel's pulse. Diminution of the arterial pulse during expiration.

Leube-Riegel test-dinner. A test-meal sometimes used to study gastric function. It consists of beef soup, beef steak, white bread, and water.

Rieger, Herwigh (b. 1898). Austrian ophthalmologist.

Rieger's syndrome. Dystrophia myotonica with dysplasia of iris and of teeth.

Rieger's phenomenon. Brake phenomenon. *See* PHENOMENON.

Riehl, Gustav (b. 1855). Vienna dermatologist.

Riehl's melanosis. A facial melanosis, mostly affecting women and thought to be due to some ingredient of a cosmetic, sometimes with an additional factor of malnutrition.

Riesman, David (b. 1867). Philadelphia physician.

Riesman's sign. 1. In hyperthyroidism, a murmur can be heard on auscultating over the eyeball. 2. Softening of the eyeball with diabetic coma.

Rietti, Fernando (b. 1890). Italian pathologist.

Rietti-Greppi-Micheli disease. Thalassaemia.

Rieux, Léon. 19th century French surgeon.

Rieux's hernia. Internal hernia at the site of the retrocaecal recess.

Rifamide (ri·fah·mide). BP Commission approved name for rifamycin B diethylamide; an antibiotic.

Rifampicin (rif·**am**·pe·sin). BP Commission approved name for 3-(4-methylpiperazin-1-yliminomethyl)-rifamycin, $C_{43}H_{58}N_4O_{12}$, an antibiotic compound which has been found to inhibit the replication of a number of viruses in cell cultures *in vitro*, but it has not been shown to be of therapeutic use in viral infections. It is used in bacterial infections.

Rifamycin (ri·fah·**mi**·sin). BP Commission approved name for antibiotics isolated from a strain of *Streptomyces mediterranei.* Specific substances are designated by a terminal letter; thus Rifamycin B.

rifling (ri·fling). A forensic term used to describe the spiral grooving of the interior of the barrel of bullet-firing weapons designed to impart a gyroscopic stability to the projectile, and leaving scoring marks on the bullet. [O Fr. *riffle* a stick.]

Riga, Antonio (fl. 1900). Naples physician.

Riga's aphthae, or disease. Cachectic aphthae; aphthous ulcers which occur on the tongue, inner cheeks, palates, oesophagus, and gastro-intestinal tract in a rare syndrome seen among children who are severely undernourished and whose oral hygiene is bad. Antibiotic therapy is sometimes successful, but the outcome is usually fatal.

Fede-Riga disease, Riga-Fede disease. Traumatic ulceration, with induration, of the frenulum of the tongue, caused by trauma from the lower incisor teeth during the process of sucking, and occurring therefore only during the suckling period after the eruption of the lower incisors.

Rigaud's operation. An operation for urethral fistula: a square flap is taken from below the fistula, turned over it, and reinforced by flaps from each side.

Riggs, John Mankey (b. 1810). Baltimore dentist.

Riggs' disease. Chronic suppurative periodontitis; pyorrhoea alveolaris.

right [dexter (NA)] (rite). Dextral; relating, or belonging, to the right as opposed to the left. [AS *riht.*]

right-brained (rite·**bra**·nd). Referring to a person in whom the speech centre is in the right instead of, as normally, in the left cerebral hemisphere. [AS *riht*, brain.]

right-eared (rite·**eerd**). Using the right ear more than the left. [AS *riht*, ear.]

right-eyed (rite·**ide**). Using the right eye more than the left. [AS *riht*, eye.]

right-footed (rite·**fut**·ed). Using the right foot, when there is a choice, in preference to the left, as in hopping. [AS *riht* foot.]

right-handed (rite·**hand**·ed). Tending, when there is a choice, to use the right hand rather than the left. [AS *riht*, hand.]

rigid (**rij**·id). Stiff, unbending; hard, not pliant. [L *rigidus.*]

rigiditas (rij·**id**·it·as). 1. Stiffness. 2. Rigidity; rigor. **Rigiditas articulorum.** Extracapsular ankylosis. *See* ANKYLOSIS. **Rigiditas cadaverica.** Rigor mortis. [L.]

rigidity (rij·**id**·it·e). The state of stiffness and inflexibility. **Anatomical rigidity.** Rigidity of the neck of the uterus in labour without local disease. **Cadaveric rigidity.** Rigor mortis. **Cerebellar rigidity.** Rigidity of the trunk muscles in a patient with a midline cerebellar lesion. There is arching of the back and head retraction, and the limbs may also be rigid; the position resembles that of opisthotonos. The rigidity is probably due to a secondary effect upon the brain stem rather than to the cerebellar lesion. **Clasp-knife rigidity.** The type of rigidity seen in spastic paralysis; on attempting passive movement the muscles are at first stiff, but then give suddenly. **Cogwheel rigidity.** A type of muscular rigidity seen in parkinsonian and other extrapyramidal disorders; on passive stretching of a muscle it relaxes and stiffens intermittently, giving a jerky movement. **Decerebrate rigidity.** The exaggerated extensor muscle tone due to interruption of extrapyramidal pathways at a level between the red nucleus above and the vestibular nuclei below. It is concluded that normally the higher centres prevent overaction of the vestibular nuclei. **Hemiplegic rigidity.** Clasp-knife or spastic rigidity in the paralysed limbs. **Lead-pipe rigidity.** Rigidity which remains uniform throughout the full range of passive movement, as in bending a lead pipe; seen in diseases of the basal ganglia, such as parkinsonism. **Muscle rigidity.** The stiffness and fixity of muscles as seen in parkinsonism and catatonia. **Mydriatic rigidity.** An unsatisfactory name for Westphal's pupillary reflex. **Pathological rigidity.** Rigidity of the neck of the uterus in late pregnancy or labour due to local disease. **Post-mortem rigidity.** The progressive stiffening of muscle after death, due to chemical changes, developing during the first 24 h, later passing off. **Spastic rigidity.** Clasp-knife rigidity (see above). [L *rigiditas.*]

rigor (**ri**·gor). 1. A shivering fit associated with a sensation of chilliness of the skin, although the internal temperature may be rising; also called, more popularly, *chill* or *chills.* 2. Stiffness, rigidity. **Acid rigor.** Coagulation of muscle proteins by acids, particularly lactic acid. **Heat rigor.** Muscular cramps due to excessive sweating and consequent loss of sodium chloride. **Rigor mortis.** Stiffening of the muscles that occurs at varying times after death in a specified manner, commencing in the head (eyelids) and passing down to the lower limbs. **Rigor nervorum.** Tetanus. **Rigor tremens.** Paralysis agitans. [L.]

Riley, Conrad Milton (b. 1913). American paediatrician.

Riley-Day syndrome. Familial dysautonomia. *See* DYSAUTONOMIA.

rima[NA] (**ri**·mah). A cleft or fissure. **Rima glottidis [NA].** The cleft between the vocal folds in the larynx. The intermembranous part [pars intermembranacea (NA)] lies between the vocal folds; the intercartilaginous part [pars intercartilaginea (NA)] lies between the arytenoid cartilages. **Rima respiratoria.** Rima vestibuli (see foll.). **Rima vestibuli [NA].** The cleft between the vestibular folds of the larynx. **Rima vocalis.** Rima glottidis (see above). [L.]

rimal (**ri**·mal). Belonging to a rima.

rimantidine (rim·**an**·te·deen). α-Methyl-1-adamantane-methylamine hydrochloride, $C_{21}H_{21}N{\cdot}HCl$. Similar in structure and activity to amantidine hydrochloride, it has been used in the prophylaxis against influenza A virus.

Rimiterol (rim·it·er·ol). BP Commission approved name for *erythro* - 3,4 - dihydroxy - α - (2 - piperidyl) - benzyl alcohol; a bronchodilator.

rimose, rimous (ri·moze, ri·mus). Characterized by the presence of many chinks, cracks, or fissures. [L *rima* cleft.]

rimula (rim·ew·lah). A very small fissure, particularly of the brain or spinal cord. [L, small chink.]

Rindfleisch, Georg Eduard (b. 1836). Würzburg pathologist.

Rindfleisch's cell. An eosinophil granular leucocyte.

Rindfleisch's folds. Semilunar reflections of the serous pericardium around the beginning of the ascending aorta.

ring (ring). 1. [Anulus (NA).] An annulus; any circular organ, or the structure surrounding a circular opening. 2. In chemistry, a linkage of atoms by valency bonds into a closed chain. The term has been extended to a system of such rings, e.g. cyclopentenophenanthrene ring. **Androstane ring.** Cholane ring (see below). **Annular ring.** A radiographically opaque ring shadow with translucent centre, due to a small encysted pneumothorax. It may simulate a tuberculous cavity. **Anorectal ring.** A complex fibromuscular ring which is made up of the sphincter ani internus muscle, the puborectalis muscle, and the deep part of the sphincter ani externus muscle. **Atrial ring.** The circle of muscle surrounding the orifice of the atrioventricular canal between the atrium and ventricle in the embryo mammalian heart. The sinu-atrial node develops at this site. **Benzene ring.** A hexagonal closed chain of six carbon atoms linked alternately by single and double bonds, and forming the basis of a great family of aromatic compounds. **Carbocyclic ring.** Any ring in which all the atoms of the closed chain are carbon atoms. **Cholane ring.** The androstane ring; the cyclopentenophenanthrene ring structure (steroid ring) with methyl substitutions at the 10 and 13 positions, and an OH group at position 3. It is present in cholesterol and cholic acid. **Ciliary ring [orbiculus ciliaris (NA)].** A forward continuation of the choroid of the eye behind the iris; part of the ciliary body. **Common tendinous ring [anulus tendineus communis (NA)].** A fibrous ring enclosing the optic foramen and the medial end of the superior orbital fissure. **Constriction ring, Contraction ring.** A localized annular spasm of the uterus occurring in labour. It is usually a manifestation of inco-ordinate uterine activity. **Cyclopentenophenanthrene ring.** A saturated ring system consisting of three six-membered carbon rings joined to a five-membered carbon ring. It forms the basis of the sterols and steroids, including the bile acids and sex hormones. **Femoral ring [anulus femoralis (NA)].** The opening leading into the medial compartment of the femoral sheath; a potential source of hernia. **Fibrous rings of the heart [anuli fibrosi (NA)].** Rings surrounding the atrioventricular orifices and forming part of the skeleton of the heart. **Heterocyclic ring.** Any ring in which the closed chain includes atoms of other elements besides carbon. **Homocyclic ring.** Any ring in which the closed chain is composed entirely of atoms of the same element. **Inguinal ring, deep [anulus inguinalis profundus (NA)].** The site where the spermatic cord in the male, or the round ligament of the uterus in the female, passes through the transversalis fascia. It is marked by an oval depression on the deep aspect of the anterior abdominal wall, halfway between the anterior superior iliac spine and the pubic symphysis and just above the inguinal ligament. **Inguinal ring, superficial [anulus inguinalis superficialis (NA)].** The triangularly-shaped opening in the aponeurosis of the external oblique muscle, just above and lateral to the pubic tubercle, which transmits the spermatic cord in the male, or the round ligament of the uterus in the female. **Ring of the iris, inner [anulus iridis minor (NA)].** The inner circular zone at the inner margin of the iris. **Ring of the iris, outer [anulus iridis major (NA)].** The outer circular zone at the periphery of the iris. **Isocyclic ring.** Homocyclic ring (see above). **Neonatal ring.** A microscopic marking seen in the enamel and the dentine of all deciduous teeth and first permanent molar teeth at the junction of those parts of the tissues formed before birth with those formed after birth. **Pleural ring.** Annular ring (see above). **Retraction ring.** A palpable ridge formed in obstructed labour in the uterus at the junction of the upper and lower uterine segments. It marks the lower border of the active uterine muscle. Also known as *Bandl's ring.* **Steroid ring, Sterol ring.** Cyclopentenophenanthrene ring (see above). **Tympanic ring [anulus tympanicus (NA)].** An incomplete ampulla of bone supporting the tympanic membrane in the fetus and newborn. From it is developed the bony external auditory meatus of the adult. **Umbilical ring [anulus umbilicalis (NA)].** The deficiency in the fetal linea alba which transmits the umbilical arteries and vein and the allantois. It is replaced by a scar after birth. **Vascular ring.** A condition in which, due to a developmental anomaly of the system of embryonic aortic arches, the oesophagus and trachea are completely encircled by major blood vessels, pressure from which may require treatment. A number of varieties of the condition can occur, such as double aortic arch. **White rings.** Tiny white rings seen in Bowman's membrane of the cornea, about 0.5 mm in diameter and made up of minute white spots. First described by Coats. [AS *hring.*]

See also: ALBL, BANDL, BICKEL, CABOT, CANNON, DOELLINGER, FLEISCHER, GRAEFENBERG, KAYSER (B.), LANDOLT, LIESEGANG, LOEWE, LOWER, LUSK, MAXWELL (P. W.), MERKEL (F. S.), NEWTON (I.), OCHSNER, SCHROEDER, SOEMMERING, STRUEMPELL, VOSSIUS, WALDEYER-HARTZ.

Ringer, Sydney (b. 1835). London physician.

Ringer mixture, or solution. An aqueous solution of the following percentage composition: sodium chloride 0.65, potassium chloride 0.014, calcium chloride 0.012, sodium bicarbonate 0.02, disodium hydrogen phosphate 0.001, glucose 0.2, water to 100. This solution was designed for use with the tissues of frogs.

Ringer mixture, or solution, for injection. Compound injection of sodium chloride; an isotonic solution of sodium chloride (0.85 per cent) with potassium chloride (0.03 per cent) and calcium chloride (0.048 per cent), used for intravenous injections for fluid replacement.

Ringer lactate solution for injection. Compound sodium lactate injection; a sterile, aqueous, isotonic solution of sodium chloride (0.6 per cent) and lactic acid (0.24 per cent), with potassium chloride and calcium chloride.

Ringer–Locke solution. An aqueous solution of sodium chloride, potassium chloride, calcium chloride, dextrose, and sodium bicarbonate, used in physiological experiments.

Ringer–Tyrode solution. An aqueous solution of sodium chloride, potassium chloride, calcium chloride, magnesium chloride, dextrose, sodium acid phosphate, and sodium bicarbonate, used in physiological experiments.

ringworm (ring·werm). Tinea; invasion of the skin or its appendages (hair or nails) by fungi which do not invade the deeper organs. **Ringworm of the axillae.** Tinea axillaris; a form usually caused by *Epidermophyton floccosum, Trichophyton mentagrophytes* or *T. rubrum.* **Ringworm of the beard.** Tinea barbae; a form usually caused by an ectothrix variety of *Trichophyton*, e.g. *T. verrucosum*, or occasionally by an endothrix variety, e.g. *T. violaceum* or *T. sulphureum.* Sometimes the eruption is very superficial, but usually the parasite causes much inflammation and brawny, granulomatous swellings appear; the follicles on the affected areas ooze pus, and the hairs are loosened and are easily extracted. **Black-dot ringworm.** A ringworm of the scalp, usually caused by fungi of the genus *Trichophyton*, in which the patient appears to be suffering from alopecia areata, but on close examination it is seen that the hairs are still present but are broken off at their points of exit from the follicles. **Ringworm of the body.** Tinea circinata. **Bowditch island ringworm, Burmese ringworm, Chinese ringworm.** Tinea imbricata. **Cattle ringworm,** Ringworm caused by *Trichophyton verrucosum* and transmitted from cattle. **Crusted ringworm.** Tinea favosa; favus. **Ectothrix ringworm.** Infection of the hair, characterized by the formation of a sheath of spores around the hair shaft. It may be due to *Microsporum* or *Trichophyton* spp; infections of hair by the former species usually fluoresce under Wood's light. **Endothrix ringworm.** Infection of the hair by *Trichophyton* spp, characterized by the formation of interpilary spores. **Ringworm of the feet.** Tinea pedis. **Ringworm of the glabrous skin.** Tinea circinata. **Ringworm of the groins.** Tinea cruris. **Ringworm of the hairless skin.** Tinea circinata. **Honeycomb ringworm.** Tinea favosa; favus. **Indian ringworm.** Tinea imbricata. **Ringworm of the nails.** Tinea unguium; infections caused by *Trichophyton* spp, particularly *T. rubrum*, and by *Epidermophyton floccosum*, but only rarely by *Microsporum* species. **Oriental ringworm.** Tinea imbricata. **Ringworm of the scalp.** Tinea capitis, an affection in children caused by *Microspora*, usually *Microsporum audouinii* and often *M. canis*; less commonly by endothrix *Trichophytons*, e.g. *T. sulphureum* or *T. violaceum.* In adults, infection from animals, particularly with *T. mentagrophytes*, may occur. **Tokelau ringworm.** Tinea imbricata. [ring, AS *wyrm.*]

Rinne, Heinrich Adolf (b. 1819). Hildesheim otologist.

Rinne's test. In the diagnosis of deafness: a vibrating tuning fork is placed over the mastoid process; when it ceases to be heard, the prongs are held close to the external auditory meatus. A normal person should hear it for as long again. This is termed a *positive Rinne* response. If the sound is not heard when transferred to the meatus, the test is repeated, with the fork held first at the meatus and then over the mastoid process. If now the vibrations are heard by bone conduction, after hearing by aerial conduction has ceased, the result is known as a *negative Rinne* response. A diminished positive Rinne response occurs in early cases of middle-ear deafness, and is distinguished by a slight diminution in the hearing by aerial conduction and a correspondingly slight increase in the hearing by bone conduction. A negative Rinne response is characteristic of conductive types of deafness. In cases of perceptive, internal-ear types of deafness, a positive Rinne response usually occurs, but hearing by both air and bone conduction is reduced. A false negative Rinne response is found in cases of unilateral sensorineural hearing loss.

Riolan, Jean (b. 1577). French physician.

Riolan's arcades. Arterial arches formed by anastomoses between adjacent branches of the mesenteric vessels.

Riolan's bones, or ossicles. Small bones sometimes found in the thin layer of fibrocartilage which separates the occipital bone from the petrous part of the temporal bone.

Riolan's bouquet. A group of muscles and ligaments attached to the styloid process of the temporal bone.

Riolan's muscles. A bundle of muscle fibres belonging to the palpebral part of the orbicularis oculi muscle; it runs along the lip margins.

ripa (ri·pah). A line of reflection of ependyma from the ventricular wall onto the choroid plexus. [L river bank.]

riparian (ri·pa·re·an). 1. Relating or belonging to the ripa. 2. Marginal. [see prec.]

Ripart and Petit solution. An indifferent mounting medium containing copper salts, camphor, and acetic acid.

Risley, Samuel D. (b. 1845). American ophthalmologist.

Risley's prisms. Two prisms which can rotate in opposite directions by means of a set screw on their frame, thereby varying their combined prismatic power; used in a trial frame for testing ocular muscle balance.

risorius muscle [musculus risorius (NA)] (ri·sor·e·us musl). A muscle arising from the fascia over the parotid gland and inserted into the skin at the angle of the mouth. [L *ridere* to laugh.]

Risser, Joseph Charles (b. 1892). New York surgeon.

Risser plaster jacket. For scoliosis: a special divided plaster jacket with turnbuckles, used for the gradual correction of spinal curvature.

ristin (ris·tin). Ethylene glycol monobenzoate, $C_6H_5CO_2CH_2CH_2OH$. A compound used like benzyl benzoate as a cure for scabies.

Ristocetin (ris·to·se·tin). BP Commission approved name for the antimicrobial substances produced by a species of *Nocardia*; it is used in antibiotic therapy.

risus (ri·sus). Laughter. **Risus caninus, Risus sardonicus.** A grinning distortion of the face caused by tension in the frontal belly of the occipitofrontalis muscle and in the muscles at the angles of the mouth, which occurs particularly in cases of tetanus. [L.]

Ritodrine (ri·to·dreen). BP Commission approved name for *erythro* - 1 - (4 - hydroxyphenyl) - 2 - (4 - hydroxyphenethylamino)propan - 1 - ol; a uterine relaxant.

Ritter, Johann Wilhelm (b. 1776). German physiologist.

Ritter's fibres. Retinal fibres lying between the rods and cones. It was supposed by Ritter that they were the outer prolongations of optic-nerve fibres, but their existence has not been confirmed and they are probably only artifacts.

Ritter's law. A nerve can be stimulated both by the opening and the closing of an electric current.

Ritter's tetanus. Tetanic contractions occurring in muscle at the opening of an electric circuit which has been closed for some time.

Ritter-Rollet phenomenon, or sign. On mild electrical stimulation, the foot flexes; on vigorous stimulation, it extends.

Ritter-Valli law. When section separates a portion of a nerve from its parent nerve cell, irritability is first increased and later lost; both changes progress centrifugally.

Ritter Von Rittershain, Gottfried (b. 1820). Prague paediatrician.

Ritter's disease. Dermatitis exfoliativa neonatorum.

rivalry (ri·val·re). **Binocular rivalry, Retinal rivalry.** A phenomenon that occurs when different figures of equal potency are received by the two eyes, e.g. in a stereoscope, when first one is seen and then the other. Fusion is impossible; instead, first one image then the other is seen, or a pattern made up from bits of each. The choice of image depends mainly on interest and the intensity of the impression. [L *rivalis* rival.]

Rivalta, Fabio (b. 1863). Bologna pathologist.

Rivalta's reaction. The formation of a white cloud in the wake of a drop of fluid falling through dilute acetic acid (0.1 ml glacial acetic acid in 150 ml water). Positive reactions are given mainly by exudates, presumably due to the presence of seromucoid. The test is not completely specific.

Rivalta, Sebastiano (b. 1852). Italian veterinary surgeon.

Rivalta's disease. Actinomycosis.

river (riv·er). *See* DURET. [L *rivus* brook.]

Rivinus, Augustus Quirinus (b. 1652). Leipzig anatomist and botanist.

Rivinus' canals, or ducts. The ducts of the sublingual glands: they open into the floor of the mouth.

Rivinus' gland. The sublingual gland. *See* GLAND.

Rivinus' incisura, incisure, or notch. The tympanic notch. *See* NOTCH.

Rivinus' membrane. The flaccid part of the tympanic membrane.

rivulose (riv·ew·loze). Of colonies of bacteria, marked by irregular wavy lines. [L *rivulus* rivulet.]

rivus lacrimalis [NA] (ri·vus lak·rim·a·lis). The channel between the eyelids and the eyeball when the eyes are closed. [L brook of tears.]

riziform (riz·e·form). Having the appearance of an aggregation of rice grains. [Fr. *riz* rice, form.]

roach (ro·ch). USA term for cockroach, by abbreviation.

Roaf, Herbert Eldon (b. 1881). London physiologist.

Roaf's theory. A modification of the trichromatic theory of colour vision. Roaf suggests three types of receptor, one stimulated by all light waves, a second by only the long and medium waves, and a third by the long waves only. This is achieved by filters of coloured globules in front of the receptors.

Robert, Heinrich Ludwig Ferdinand (b. 1814). German gynaecologist.

Robert's pelvis. A transversely contracted pelvis due to imperfect development of the alae of the sacrum.

Roberts, James Ernest Helme (b. 1881). London surgeon.

Roberts' operation. Obliteration of a chronic empyema cavity by a rectangular flap of whole thickness of chest wall.

Roberts, Percy Willard (b. 1867). New York surgeon.

Roberts' operation. An operation for recurrent dislocation of the shoulder.

Roberts, Sam Earl (b. 1887). Kansas otolaryngologist.

Roberts' operation. For the correction of a deflected nasal septum: obsolete.

Roberts, Sir William (b. 1830). London physician.

Roberts' reagent. For protein: a mixture of 1 volume concentrated nitric acid and 5 volumes saturated aqueous magnesium sulphate.

Roberts' test. For protein in urine: the urine is layered upon Roberts' reagent in a test-tube. A white turbidity or precipitate at the junction of the liquids indicates protein.

Robertshaw, Frank Leonard. 20th century Manchester anaesthetist.

Robertshaw low-resistance double-lumen tube. An endobronchial tube for the control of each lung independently during thoracic anaesthesia. Described in 1962.

Robertson, Muriel. 20th century London bacteriologist.

Robertson's cooked-meat culture medium. Used for the culture of anaerobic organisms, prepared from 500 g minced fresh meat cooked in 500 ml N/20 sodium hydroxide. The meat is added to tubes of 1 per cent peptone infusion broth in proportion of three parts of broth to one of cooked meat.

robin (**rob**·in). A poisonous principle from the bark of the common locust, *Robinia pseudacacia.* It is used as a purgative. [Jean *Robin*, 1550-1629, French botanist.]

Robin, Charles Phillippe (b. 1821). Paris anatomist.

Robin's myeloplaxes. Large multinucleated cells in bone; the osteoclasts.

Robin's spaces. Originally a term used to describe adventitial lymph spaces within the walls of the cerebral blood vessels; such lymph spaces have been shown by Weed not to exist.

Virchow-Robin space. The space that surrounds blood vessels as they enter the brain substance and that communicates with the subarachnoid space. The cerebral vessels carry with them into the brain double sleeves of meninges, the outer walls of which are formed of pia, and the inner walls of arachnoid mater. The spaces that lie between the two layers are the *Virchow-Robin spaces*; they are also called the *perivascular spaces.*

Robin, Edouard Charles Robert (b. 1847). Paris physician.

Gubler-Robin typhus. Typhus fever with renal complications.

Robin, Pierre (b. 1867). French histologist and stomatologist.

Pierre Robin syndrome. Congenital small chin, cleft palate and glossoptosis—falling back of the tongue so that swallowing and breathing are obstructed.

Robinia (rob·**in**·e·ah). A genus of plants including the common or black locust, *Robinia pseudacacia.* [Jean *Robin*, 1550-1629, French botanist.]

robinin (**rob**·in·in). A glycoside occurring in the common locust, *Robinia pseudacacia.* [see prec.]

robinose (**rob**·in·oze). $C_{18}H_{32}O_{14}$, a hygroscopic trisaccharide isomeric with rhamninose and found in species of *Robinia* as the glycoside, robinin.

Robinow, C. F. 20th century bacteriologist in Canada.

Robinow's method. For chromatinic bodies of bacteria: smears are fixed with osmic acid. After treatment with hot hydrochloric acid they are stained by Giemsa's method. The chromatinic bodies can be seen as purplish structures within the cells.

Robinson, Andrew Rose (b. 1845). New York dermatologist.

Robinson's disease. Hydrocystoma.

Robinson, Fred Byron (b. 1857). Chicago anatomist.

Robinson's abdominal brain. The coeliac ganglion. *See* GANGLION.

Robinson's circle. The anastomoses of the uterine and ovarian arteries with the common iliac artery and the abdominal aorta.

Robinson, F. J. 20th century American physician.

Robinson-Power-Kepler test. For Addison's or Simmonds' disease: on the day before the test the patient has three ordinary meals without added salt, but does not eat or drink anything after 6 pm. At 10.30 pm the bladder is emptied and the urine discarded. Urine is collected between 10.30 pm and 7.30 am (night specimen). Breakfast is omitted. At 8.30 am the bladder is emptied and the patient then drinks within the next 45 minutes 20 ml of water per kg body weight (9 ml per lb). Urine is collected separately at 9.30, 10.30, 11.30 and 12.30. The volumes of all specimens are measured. If the volume of any single hourly day specimen is larger than the volume of the night urine the test is negative and Addison's or Simmond's disease is presumed to be excluded. If positive, however, further evidence is obtained. Blood is taken and the urea and chlorides determined in the plasma, and the same substances are determined in the night urine. The factor *A* is then calculated as follows: (urea in urine ÷ urea in plasma) × (chloride in plasma ÷ chloride in urine) × (volume of largest single hourly day urine ÷ volume of night urine), concentrations being in mg per 100 ml and volumes in ml. If *A* is greater than 30 the test is negative and Addison's disease is presumed excluded. If it is less than 25 the patient probably has Addison's or Simmonds' disease, provided that nephritis has been excluded.

Robison, Robert (b. 1883). British biochemist.

Robison ester. Crude glucopyranose monophosphate, obtained during the action of yeast on glucose or fructose; it contains Embden and Neuberg esters.

Robison ester dehydrogenase. An enzyme which, in the presence of co-enzyme II, activates the conversion of the ester into phosphoric gluconic acid.

Robles, Rodolphe. 20th century Guatemalan physician.

Robles' disease. Pseudoleprosy or punudos, an unclassed disease of Guatemala.

roborating (ro·bor·a·ting). Strengthening, tonic. [L *roborare* to strengthen.]

Roccella (rok·**sel**·ah). A genus of lichens (family Parmeliaceae).

Roccella tinctoria. The species which is the source of litmus. [It. *rocca* rock.]

Rock, John (b. 1890). Boston gynaecologist.

Hertig-Rock embryo. One of a number of beautifully-preserved and accurately-dated early human embryos, acquired and described by Hertig and Rock in 1952.

Hertig-Rock ovum. A fertilized human ovum, 7-7½ days old, described in 1945.

Rockley's sign. A straight edge is placed at the outer edge of each orbit from the corresponding malar prominences. If either malar bone is depressed, the difference in the angle of the edges is obvious.

rod (rod). Any thin, straight, slender structure. **Enamel rods.** Enamel prisms. *See* PRISM. **Muscle rod.** A myofibril. **Retinal rod.** One of the two visual end-organs of the retina, responsible for scotopic vision and situated mainly at the periphery and decreasing towards the centre; thin cylindrical structures in the outermost layer of the retina up against the pigment epithelium, containing visual purple. [AS *rodd.*]

See also: CORTI, HEIDENHAIN, KOENIG (C. J.), MADDOX, MECKEL, REICHMANN.

rodent (ro·dent). A member of the mammalian order Rodentia.

Rodentia (ro·**den**·she·ah). An order of the class Mammalia, small medium-sized animals characterized by the single pair of perpetually growing incisors in each jaw, and grinding molars; rats, mice, marmots, squirrels, suslik, moles, etc. *Arctomys,*

Citellus, Marmota, Microtus, Mus, Rattus, and *Spermophilus* are the genera of medical interest. [L *rodere* to gnaw.]

Rodgers, John Kearny (b. 1793). New York surgeon.

Rodgers' operation. An operation for lateral perineal lithotomy, early 19th century.

Rodman, William Louis (b. 1858). Philadelphia surgeon.

Rodman's operation. Radical excision of the breast with axillary lymph glands.

rodonalgia (ro·don·al·je·ah). Erythromelalgia. [Gk *rhodon* rose, *algos* pain.]

Rodriguez' test. A method of testing the skin in leprosy: a drop of histamine (1 in 1000) is placed near the margin of the affected skin area and another drop on the normal skin; the skin is pricked by a needle through each drop, and a red flare at the site indicates that the skin is normal.

Roe, Joseph Hyram (b. 1892). Washington biochemist.

Roe-Kahn method. For calcium in serum: calcium is precipitated as phosphate from a protein-free serum filtrate; the phosphate in the precipitate is determined by the method of Fiske and Subbarow to give an indirect measure of calcium.

Roeder's treatment. Aspiration of debris from the tonsil bed by means of suction.

Roemer, Paul (b. 1873). German ophthalmologist.

Roemer's serum. An antipneumococcal serum.

Roemer's theory. Cataract formation is due to toxins, entering the lens from the aqueous humour and caused by a derangement of the ciliary epithelium.

Roentgen, Wilhelm Konrad von (b. 1845). Würzburg physicist.

Roentgen irradiation. The application of roentgen rays (x-rays) to a substance; usually meaning x-ray treatment.

Roentgen rays. X-rays.

roentgen (**runt**·yen). The unit of dose of x- and gamma-rays but not other ionizing radiation. It is the quantity of x- or gamma-radiation such that the associated corpuscular emission per 0.001293 g of air produces, in air, ions carrying one electrostatic unit of quantity of electricity of either sign. ($1R = 2.58 \times 10^{-4}$ coulombs per kg.) **Roentgen per hour at one metre.** A measure of the x-ray output of a therapy machine. [W. K. von *Roentgen*.]

roentgen-equivalent (**runt**·yen·e·**kwiv'**·al·ent). A unit for expressing the dose of some ionizing radiation other than x- or gamma-rays in terms comparable to the roentgen. **Roentgen-equivalent man.** *See* REM. **Roentgen-equivalent physical.** *See* REP. [roentgen, equivalent.]

roentgenism (**runt**·yen·izm). 1. The application of x-rays (roentgen rays) in the treatment of disease. 2. Deleterious effects produced by excessive application of x-rays. [Obsolescent term.]

roentgenkymography (**runt**·yen·ki·**mog'**·raf·e). The recording of moving images on a single x-ray film. [Obsolescent term.] [roentgen, kymograph.]

roentgenocardiogram (**runt**·yen·o·**kar'**·de·o·gram). A polygraphic tracing of the pulsations of the heart by means of x-rays (roentgen rays). [roentgen, cardiogram.]

roentgenocinematography (**runt**·yen·o·sin·e·mat·**og'**·raf·e). Cinematographic radiography. *See* RADIOGRAPHY. [roentgen, Gk *kinema* motion, *graphein* to record.]

roentgenogram (**runt**·yen·o·gram). X-ray radiograph. [roentgen, Gk *gramma* a writing.]

roentgenograph (**runt**·yen·o·graf). X-ray radiograph. [see foll.]

roentgenography (runt·yen·**og**·raf·e). Radiography. **Section roentgenography.** Tomography; body-section radiography. [roentgen, Gk *graphein* to record.]

roentgenokymograph (**runt**·yen·o·**ki'**·mo·graf). A kymograph which traces the movements of inner structures shown by means of x-rays (roentgen rays).

roentgenology (runt·yen·**ol**·o·je). The branch of radiology which is concerned with the use of x-rays (roentgen rays) in diagnosis and treatment. [roentgen, Gk *logos* science.]

roentgenolucent (**runt**·yen·o·**lew'**·sent). Radiolucent. [roentgen, L *lucere* to shine.]

roentgenometer (runt·yen·**om**·et·er). Radiometer. [see foll.]

roentgenometry (runt·yen·**om**·et·re). The accurate measurement of an object by x-rays: the direct measurement of structures shown on the x-ray radiograph after multiplication by the correction factor, the correction factor being a tube-object distance divided by a tube-image distance. [Obsolescent term.] [roentgen, meter.]

roeteln, roetheln (**ret**·eln). Rubella. [G *roteln* roseola.]

Roffo, Angel H. (b. 1882). Buenos Aires pathologist.

Roffo's test. *See* TEST FOR CANCER.

Roger, Georges Henri (b. 1860). French physiologist.

Roger's reflex, or syndrome. Excessive secretion of saliva from oesophageal irritation, e.g. by a growth.

Roger, Henri Louis (b. 1811). French physician.

Bruit de Roger, Roger's murmur. A harsh, systolic murmur, usually accompanied by a thrill, heard in the 3rd and 4th intercostal spaces to the left of the sternum in patients with patency of the ventricular septum.

Roger's disease, maladie de Roger. A congenital cardiac malformation consisting of an isolated small defect in the membranous portion of the ventricular septum, unassociated with other lesions.

Roger's sign. A subnormal temperature in the late stages of tuberculous meningitis.

Rogers, Sir Leonard (b. 1868). Calcutta and London physician.

Rogers' treatment. The treatment of cholera by intravenous injections of hypertonic salines to counteract dehydration and loss of salts; pyrogen-free distilled water containing 140 g sodium chloride to the pint.

rogitine (roj·i·tene).*See* PHENTOLAMINE.

rogue (ro·g). Of laboratory stock animals, an individual that departs from the normal behaviour patterns expected of that stock, to the detriment of the stock or experimental work. In botanical genetics, an individual variant within a stock. [etym. dub.]

Rohr, Karl (b. 1863). Berne embryologist and gynaecologist.

Rohr's layer, or stria. A band of fibrinoid lining the intervillous space of the placenta on the decidual surface and spreading to cover some of the villi themselves.

Rokitansky, Carl Freiherr von (b. 1804). Vienna pathologist.

Aschoff-Rokitansky sinuses. A radiological sign seen in the wall of the gall bladder at cholecystography. The appearance is of multiple small diverticula.

Rokitansky's disease. Acute yellow atrophy. *See* ATROPHY.

Rokitansky's diverticulum. A traction diverticulum of the oesophagus.

Rokitansky's hernia. Mucosal hernia; protrusion of the gastro-intestinal mucosa through a wound in the seromuscular coat.

Rokitansky's kidney. Amyloid kidney; a pathological condition in which the blood vessels of the kidney, the tunica of the tubules, and the interstitial tissue, have undergone waxy degeneration.

Rolandic (ro·**lan**·dik). Pertaining to Luigi Rolando; describing any structure named after Rolando.

Rolando, Luigi (b. 1773). Turin anatomist.

Rolando's area, or zone. The precentral gyrus.

Rolando's cell. A neurone from the gelatinous matter of the posterior horn of grey matter of the spinal cord.

Rolando's column. An elevation on the lateral aspect of the medulla oblongata, possibly caused by the descending tract and nucleus of the trigeminal nerve.

Rolando's fasciculus, or substance. The gelatinous matter of the posterior horn of grey matter of the spinal cord; substantia gelatinosa.

Fissure of Rolando, Rolando's sulcus. The central sulcus of the cerebrum.

Funiculus of Rolando. The funiculus cuneatus of the medulla oblongata.

Rolando's line. A line drawn between Rolando's points which marks the position of the central sulcus of the cerebrum.

Rolando's points. The points at the upper and lower ends of Rolando's line. The upper point is about 10 mm behind the mid-point between the glabella and the external occipital protuberance: the lower point is about 50 mm above the pre-auricular point.

Rolando's tubercle. Part of the funiculus cuneatus of the medulla oblongata.

Rolicypram (rol·e·si·pram). BP Commission approved name for (+) - 5 - oxo - *N* - (*trans* - 2 - phenylcyclopropyl) - L - pyrrolidine - 2 - carboxamide; an antidepressant.

Rolitetracycline (ro·le·tet·rah·si'·kleen). BP Commission approved name for *N*-(pyrrolidin-1-ylmethyl)tetracycline; an antibiotic.

roll (role). **Cotton-wool roll.** A roll made of cotton wool, used to maintain dryness of a tooth during operations of conservative dentistry. **Iliac roll.** Sigmoid sausage; a sausage-shaped mass felt in the left iliac fossa, caused by a collection of faeces or induration of the sigmoid. [OFr. *rolle.*]

Roller, Christian Friedrich Wilhelm (b. 1802). German neurologist.

Roller's nucleus. A collection of small cells in the anterior part of the nucleus of the hypoglossal nerve.

Rolleston, Sir Humphry Davy (b. 1862). London physician.

Rolleston's rule. A method of predicting the effect of age on the average and maximum normal values of the systolic blood pressure in adults: it should be 100 mm mercury plus half the age in years, and should not exceed 100 mm plus the age in years. The rule can no longer be regarded as valid; the higher levels of systolic pressure found in middle-aged and elderly persons is probably due to atherosclerosis and rigidity of the aorta.

Rollet, Alexander (b. 1834). Austrian physiologist.

Rollet's delomorphous cell. Parietal cell. *See* CELL.

Rollet's stroma. Stroma of the erythrocytes.

Rollet's secondary substance. The isotropic portions of a striated muscle fibre.

Ritter-Rollet phenomenon, or sign. On mild electrical stimulation, the foot flexes; on vigorous stimulation, it extends.

Rollet, E. 20th century French ophthalmologist.

Rollet's operation. 1. Blepharoplasty for upper lid defects, by Z flaps (*Rollet incision*). 2. For enucleation: implantation of skin and fat taken from the deltoid region within Tenon's capsule following enucleation. Of historical interest.

Rollier, Auguste (b. 1874). Swiss physician.

Rollier's formula, radiation, or treatment. A system of treatment of surgical tuberculosis by gradually increasing exposures to sunlight.

rolling (ro·ling). A term applied to assault and robbery on premises to which access has been obtained by agreement to sexual intercourse, often homosexual. A beating-up to which there may be no complaint owing to the risk of ill-repute. [O Fr. *rolle.*]

Romaña, Cecilio. 20th century Brazilian physician.

Romaña's sign. Unilateral oedema of the eyelids and inflammation of the lacrimal gland in American trypanosomiasis.

romanopexy (ro·man·o·pex·e). Sigmoidopexy. [L *Romanus* Roman, Gk *pexis* fixation.]

romanoscope (ro·man·o·skope). A sigmoidoscope. [L *Romanus* Roman, Gk *skopein* to watch.]

Romanovsky, Dmitri Leonidovich (b. 1861). Russian physician.

Romanovsky's stain, and method. One of the earliest of the contrast stains for malaria and other protozoal parasites on which many other staining methods (Leishman's, Giemsa's, etc.) are based so that the term has become generic; it shows up the chromatin particles deep red and the cytoplasm of the parasites blue. The original Romanovsky stain was a watery stain so that prior fixation of blood films with methyl alcohol was necessary, but some others are made with methyl alcohol and this obviates prior fixation of blood films.

Romberg, Moritz Heinrich (b. 1795). Berlin physician.

Romberg's disease, or trophoneurosis. Facial trophoneurosis; facial hemiatrophy.

Romberg's sign, or test. With the feet together the patient closes his eyes: swaying or falling is indicative of sensory ataxia due to loss of appreciation of position sense in the lower limbs. It is seen in tabes dorsalis and subacute combined degeneration of the cord.

Romberg's spasm. Spasm of the muscles of mastication during the act of chewing.

Romberg station. The position of the body in which Romberg's sign is elicited; the patient stands upright with the feet together.

Howship-Romberg sign, Romberg-Howship sign. Pain due to an obturator hernia may be referred along the obturator nerve into the medial part of the thigh; often accompanied by tenderness in the adductor region.

Romberg-Paessler syndrome. Tachycardia, low blood pressure, shock, and abdominal distensions, caused by dilatation of the splanchnic blood vessels.

Parry-Romberg syndrome. Progressive wasting of the tissues starting in one side of the brow and spreading so as to involve the face and perhaps the homolateral upper limb and mamma.

Rombergism (rom·berg·izm). The state of exhibiting a positive Romberg's sign. [Moritz Heinrich *Romberg.*]

rongeur (rawn·zher). Forceps used to gouge away or nip out portions of bone. [Fr. *ronger* to gnaw.]

Rönne, Henning Kristian Trappaud (b. 1878). Copenhagen ophthalmologist.

Rönne's nasal step. A nasal visual-field loss which terminates at the horizontal meridian either above or below, so giving the appearance of a step. It is found typically in chronic glaucoma and is due to the affected band of nerve fibres not extending over the horizontal raphe of the retina.

room (room, rum). **Low-background room.** A heavily radiation-shielded room in which is usually installed a whole body counter. [AS *rúm.*]

root (root). 1. That part of the plant axis which is developed from the radicle of the embryo and grows directly downwards. Roots usually possess a certain arrangement of the vascular tissues. In medicine the name is often applied to all subaerial parts. 2. [Radix (NA).] The origination of a structure, e.g. of a nerve, or the part of a structure embedded in another tissue, e.g. of a tooth. **Anatomical root.** That part of a tooth which is covered by cementum. **Root of the aorta.** The origin of the ascending aorta from the left ventricle. **Belladonna Root BPC 1959.** The root of the plant *Atropa belladonna*; extracts are used in liniments. **Clinical root [radix clinica (NA)].** The portion of a tooth which does not project into the mouth cavity. **Congo root.** A bitter tonic derived from the root of *Psoralea*, used in the treatment of chronic diarrhoea. **Cube root.** Lonchocarpus. **Dandelion root.** Taraxacum. **Deadly nightshade root.** Belladonna root (see above). **Kut root, Kuth root.** A name given to the root of *Saussurea lappa* C. B. Clarke. **Liquorice root.** The root and stolons of *Glycyrrhiza glabra* Linn. **Mexican scammony root.** Ipomoea. **Nardus root.** The rhizome and roots of *Nardostachys jatamansi* (family Valerianaceae). It resembles valerian. **Root of the neck.** The base of the neck. **Roots of the olfactory tract.** *See* TRACT. **Orris root.** *See* ORRIS. **Papoose root.** The blue cohosh; the dried rhizome and roots of *Caulophyllum thalictroides* Linn. (family Berberidaceae). It contains the alkaloid, caulophylline, and several glycosides. **Pink root.** Spigelia. **Pleurisy root.** Common name for the root of *Asclepias tuberosa* Linn. (family Asclepiadaceae) which has diaphoretic and expectorant properties. **Senega root.** Senega. **Texan snake root.** Serpentaria. **Virginian snake root.** Serpentaria. [AS *rot.*]

See also: CULVER.

rootlets [fila radicularia (NA)] (root·lets). Small bundles of nerve fibres which emerge from the spinal cord and unite in each segment to form the anterior or posterior roots. [dim. of AS *rot.*]

ropy (ro·pe). Stringy and glutinous; generally applied to sputa and precipitates. [AS *rap* rope.]

Roque's syndrome. Originally related to mydriasis with ptosis and enophthalmia occurring in some cases of ulcerative endocarditis: in tuberculous cases it is also called *Horner's* or

Horner-Bernard syndrome, and results from a unilateral irritating or destructing lesion of the cervical sympathetic chain from pressure of diseased tracheobronchial lymph glands, chronic apical pleurisy, or from surgical trauma incurred in thoracoplasty or extrapleural pneumothorax operations, or in operations on the phrenic nerve. It is characterized by slight ptosis, miosis or mydriasis, enophthalmia, and sometimes dryness of the skin of the face on the same side. The state of the pupil depends on the lesion being irritative or destructive.

Rorschach, Hermann (b. 1884). Swiss psychiatrist.

Rorschach test. An ink-blot projection test in which the subject is presented with a series of bisymmetrical cards (some in colour) and is asked "What does it look like? What could this be?". The responses depend on the personality of the subject, and are scored for location determinants, content, and originality, thus yielding an estimate of various personality traits.

Rosa (ro·zah). A genus of plants of the family Rosaceae; various species are the sources of the flowers from which oil of rose (oleum rosae) is prepared. **Rosa canina.** Dog rose, the source of the rose hips of commerce; an excellent source of vitamin C. [L rose.]

rosacea (ro·za·se·ah). A chronic condition of the nose and central portion of the face characterized by flushing, dilatation of the vessels, and scattered red papules at the openings of the follicles. In severe cases there is overgrowth of the skin and subcutaneous tissue which converts the nose into a rhinophyma; acne rosacea. **Rosacea hypertrophica.** Chronic pachydermia. **Lupoid rosacea.** Yellowish-brown nodules, lupoid on diascopy and with a tuberculoid histology but non-tuberculous; probably a foreign-body reaction to rosacea. **Ocular rosacea.** Blepharitis, conjunctivitis or keratitis occurring with rosacea. [L *rosaceus* rosy.]

rosaceiform (ro·za·se·e·form). Like acne rosacea. [acne rosacea, form.]

rosalia (ro·za·le·ah). 1. Scarlatina. 2. Measles. 3. Erythema. [L *rosa* rose.]

rosaniline (ro·zan·il·een). 1. Any one of the family of dyes derived from rosaniline base. 2. Rosaniline base, triaminodiphenyltolyl carbinol, $NH_2(CH_3)C_6H_3C(OH)(C_6H_4NH_2)_2$, prepared from aniline, gives a series of salts which are important magenta-red mordantless dyes for wool and sik. **Rosaniline acetate.** A red dye for wool and silk. **Rosaniline hydrochloride.** Fuchsine. **Rosaniline trisulphonic acid.** A dye, the salts of which are mixed in acid fuchsine.

rosary (ro·zar·e). **Rachitic rosary, Rickety rosary.** Rows of knobs which are found on the epiphyses of the ribs of children suffering from rickets. [LL *rosarium* chaplet.]

Rose, Edmund (b. 1836). Berlin and Zürich surgeon.

Rose's position. A position with the head extended over the end of the table to obviate aspiration of blood during operations on the mouth and throat.

Rose's tamponade. Heart tamponade. *See* TAMPONADE.

Rose's tetanus. Head tetanus; tetanus following a wound of the head, especially of the eyebrow region. It is characterized by trismus, facial paralysis on one side, and marked dysphagia. The symptoms superficially resemble those of rabies.

Rose, William (b. 1847). English surgeon.

Rose's operation. 1. An operation for the repair of hare-lip. 2. Removal of the trigeminal ganglion for trigeminal neuralgia.

rose (roze). The wild or cultivated flowers of various species of *Rosa* (family Rosaceae) esteemed for their use in perfumery. **Attar of rose.** The volatile oil of the damask rose, used in perfumery. **Damask rose.** The flowers of *Rosa damascena* Mill., one of the sources of attar of rose. **Rose Fruit BPC 1954.** The fresh ripe fruits of various species of *Rosa*, especially *R. canina* Linn. (the dog rose) and *R. arvensis* Huds. (the field rose). The fruits contain malic and citric acids, sugar, tannin and about 1 per cent of ascorbic acid. They form one of the richest sources of natural vitamin C, and are used in the preparation of rose-hip syrup. **Otto of rose.** Attar of rose (see above). [L *rosa.*]

rose bengal (roze beng·gawl). Dichlortetraiodofluorescein, $C_{20}H_4I_4Cl_2O_5K_2$. A dye used as a bacterial stain and also as a test of liver function. In nuclear medicine it is often labelled with radio-iodine, both as an agent for investigating the functional state of the liver and as a scanning agent.

rosein, roseine (ro·ze·in, ro·ze·een). Names applied to magenta (fuchsine) and rosaniline acetate alike. [L *rosa* rose.]

rosella (ro·zel·ah). Rubella. [dim. of L *rosa* rose.]

rosemary (roze·mar·e). The flowering tops of an evergreen shrub, *Rosmarinus officinalis* Linn. (family Labiatae). They contain the volatile oil, rosemary oil. **Marsh rosemary.** The root of the American sea-lavender, *Statice caroliniana* (family Plumbaginaceae). It is used as an astringent. [L *ros* dew, *marinus* of the sea.]

Rosenbach, Anton Julius Friedrich (b. 1842). Göttingen surgeon.

Rosenbach's disease, or erysipeloid, Baker-Rosenbach disease. An infective dermatitis due to infection with *Erysipelothrix rhusiopathiae*; erysipeloid: also known as *erythema serpens.*

Rosenbach, Ottomar (b. 1851). Berlin physician.

Rosenbach's law. In neuropathic lesions of anterior horn cells or nerve trunks, paralysis affects the extensor muscles before the flexors.

Rosenbach's sign. 1. Absence of the abdominal reflexes in intra-abdominal disease which gives protective or reflex rigidity of the abdominal wall. 2. Unilateral absence of the abdominal reflexes in hemiplegia. 3. The fine tremor of the closed eyelids in exophthalmos with thyrotoxicosis. 4. Hysterical inability to close the eyes on command.

Rosenbach's syndrome. Paroxysmal tachycardia leading to cardiac failure with dyspnoea and pulmonary congestion, and precordial pain with vomiting due to acute coronary artery insufficiency.

Rosenbach-Gmelin test. For bile pigments: filter 10-20 ml of urine acidified with a few drops of dilute hydrochloric acid through a small heavy filter paper. Add a drop of nitric acid to the filter and note the colour changes, as in Gmelin's test.

Heberden-Rosenbach nodes. The small osseous nodes which occur around the distal interphalangeal joints in certain cases of arthritis. A benign form of the disease, which is probably inherited.

Semon-Rosenbach law. In progressive organic diseases of the recurrent laryngeal nerve, the abductor element of the vocal cord movement is impaired before that of the adductor element.

Rosenberg, Edward Frank (b. 1908). Chicago physician.

Hench-Rosenberg syndrome. Palindromic rheumatism. *See* RHEUMATISM.

Rosenheim, Otto (b. 1871). London biochemist.

Rosenheim and Drummond method. For total and ethereal sulphates in urine: inorganic sulphates are precipitated with benzidine, and the benzidine sulphate titrated with standard alkali. Total sulphates are determined similarly after hydrolysis with hydrochloric acid.

Rosenheim-Drummond test. A colour test used for detecting vitamin A in cod-liver oil. It is based on the violet colour which is formed when one drop of concentrated sulphuric acid is added to one or two drops of cod-liver oil previously dissolved in anhydrous fat solvent.

Rosenheim, Theodor (b. 1860). Berlin physician.

Rosenheim's sign. A friction sound heard in the left epigastrium in perigastritis.

Rosenmueller, Johann Christian (b. 1771). Leipzig anatomist.

Rosenmueller's body, organ of Rosenmueller. The epoöphoron of the broad ligament of the uterus.

Rosenmueller's cavity, fossa, or recess. Pharyngeal recess; a recess in the lateral wall of the nasopharynx posterior to the opening of the pharyngotympanic tube.

Rosenmueller's gland, or node. 1. The palpebral process of the lacrimal gland. 2. The lymph gland which occupies the femoral ring. French authors generally call it the *gland of Cloquet*, while the Germans call it the *gland of Rosenmueller*.

Rosenmueller's valve. A fold of mucous membrane guarding the common opening of the lacrimal canaliculi into the lacrimal sac.

Rosenow, Edward Carl (b. 1875). American bacteriologist.

Rosenow's serum. An antistreptococcal serum prepared from organisms isolated from cases of poliomyelitis. [obsolete term.]

Rosenthal, Friedrich Christian (b. 1780). Greifswald anatomist.

Rosenthal's vein. The basal vein of the cerebral hemispheres.

Rosenthal, Isidor (b. 1836). Greifswald physiologist.

Rosenthal's canal. The spiral canal of the modiolus; it lodges the spiral ganglion of the cochlea.

roseola (ro·ze·o·lah). Any rose-coloured eruption; rose rash. **Epidemic roseola.** Epidemic rose rash, rubella, rubeola, or German measles. **Roseola febrilis.** A non-pathognomic rash sometimes seen in malaria and other febrile conditions. **Idiopathic roseola.** A rose-coloured eruption occurring independently of any obvious infection. **Roseola infantilis, Roseola infantum.** Exanthema subitum; pseudorubella; sixth disease. **Roseola scarlatiniforme.** An erythematous rash similar to that of scarlet fever. **Symptomatic roseola.** A rose-coloured eruption appearing as a manifestation of an eruptive fever. **Syphilitic roseola.** An eruption of rose-coloured spots early in the secondary stage of syphilis. **Roseola typhosa.** The rose spots or rash of typhoid fever which may appear about the 7th day. **Roseola urticata.** The rash of the secondary stage of syphilis that has assumed an urticarial character. **Roseola vaccinia.** A red rash after vacciniation. [L *roseus* rosy.]

roseolous (ro·ze·o·lus). 1. Pertaining to roseola. 2. Having the appearance of, or resembling, roseola or rash.

Roser, Wilhelm (b. 1817). German surgeon.

Roser's line. A line drawn from the anterior superior iliac spine to the ischial tuberosity. It is more often called *Nélaton's line* and it is of value in the clinical examination of the hip joint.

Roser's sign, Roser-Braun sign. Absence of pulsation of the dura mater; a sign of underlying tumour, abscess, or cyst.

rosette (ro·zet). Any structure resembling a heraldic rose. **Malarial rosette.** The sporulating body of the malarial parasite, representing the stage of complete schizogony. In the benign tertian form it consists of 14–24 spores or merozoites; in the quartan from 6–12; in the subtertian they are more numerous, the maximum being 32. [dim. of L *rosa* rose.]

rosin (roz·in). Colophony; an oleo resin obtained from various species of pine. It is distilled to extract the turpentine: the glassy amber mass left, consisting mainly of abietic acid and resene, is used to a limited extent in pharmacy to prepare plasters and ointments, but it is important in the manufacture of varnishes, soaps, waxes, and linoleum. [L *resina*.]

rosin-weed (roz·in·weed). The herb and root of *Silphium laciniatum* (family Compositae). It secretes an oleo resin used as a chewing gum. [rosin, AS *weod*.]

rosinol (roz·in·ol). $C_{32}H_{16}$, a liquid hydrocarbon from pitch or resin, formerly in use as a urinary antiseptic and in gonorrhoea.

rosmarinus (roz·mar·i·nus). Rosemary.

rosolene (roz·o·leen). An oily fraction in the distillation of pine pitch. [L *resina* resin, *oleum* oil.]

Ross, Sir George William (b. 1841). Toronto physician.

Ross–Jones test. A test similar to the Nonne–Apelt reaction.

Ross, Sir Ronald (b. 1857). British protozoologist in India.

Ross's cycle. The cycle of development of the malaria parasite in man and the *Anopheles* mosquito, in the first demonstration of which Ross played a major rôle.

Black spore of Ross. A degenerated oöcyst showing chitin in the infected mosquito.

Rossbach, Michael Josef (b. 1842). Jena physician.

Rossbach's disease. Hyperchlorhydria.

Rossolimo, Gregory Ivanovich (b. 1860). Moscow neurologist.

Rossolimo's reflex, or sign. The reflex in the foot which corresponds to the digital reflex; on tapping the plantar surfaces of the toes, reflex plantar flexion occurs. This reflex is exaggerated in pyramidal-tract disease or in increased neuromuscular excitability from whatever cause.

Rost, Ernest Reinhold (b. 1872). British physician in India.

Mitsudd-Rost test. Lepromin test. *See* TEST.

Rostan, Léon (b. 1790). Paris physician.

Rostan's asthma. Cardiac asthma; paroxysmal cardiac dyspnoea.

rostellum (ros·tel·um). The anterior region of the scolex of a tapeworm which often bears hooks. [L, dim. of *rostrum* beak.]

rostral (ros·tral). 1. Relating or having resemblance to a rostrum or any anatomical beak-like structure. 2. Having a rostrum or beak. 3. Cephalic.

rostrate (ros·trate). Having a beak or hook-like process. [rostrum.]

rostriform (ros·tre·form). Resembling a beak in shape. [rostrum, form.]

rostrum (ros·trum). A beak. **Rostrum of the corpus callosum [rostrum corporis callosi (NA)].** The anterior part of the corpus callosum which bends back below the septum lucidum to join the lamina terminalis. **Rostrum of the sphenoid bone [rostrum sphenoidale (NA)].** The beak-like projection in the midline of the anterior surface of the body of the sphenoid bone which fits between the alae of the vomer. [L.]

rot (rot). 1. Decomposition; decay. 2. To become decomposed. **Barcoo rot.** A pyodermatous ulcer; desert sore. **Grinders' rot.** Grinders' phthisis, knife-grinders' phthisis; the association of pneumoconiosis with chronic pulmonary tuberculosis occurring in knife grinders. The primary cause of the pneumoconiosis is the inhalation of silica dust from stone grinding wheels. The pneumoconiosis makes the lungs more vulnerable to infection from tuberculosis. **Jungle rot.** An ill-defined lay term for any ulceration or skin disease acquired in a tropical rural environment. **Knife-grinders' rot.** Grinders' rot (see above). **Liver rot.** *Fasciola hepatica* infection in sheep; the infection is relatively common in sheep but also occurs in man. **Potters' rot.** Potters' phthisis; the association of pneumoconiosis with chronic pulmonary tuberculosis occurring in potters. The primary cause of the pneumoconiosis is the inhalation of the silicious dust in the mixing of the dried china clay or kaolin for use in the pottery industry. **Sheep rot.** Liver rot (see above). [AS *rotian*.]

rotameter (ro·tam·et·er). A flowmeter used for measuring anaesthetic gases. It consists of a conical glass tube inside which a vaned metal float rotates, indicating the amount of gas flowing by its height. Described in 1908 by Kueppers. [L *rota* wheel, Gk *metron* measure.]

rotation (ro·ta·shun). 1. The act of turning round an axis; the motion of a solid body about an axis, called the axis of rotation. 2. In dentistry, malposition of a tooth due to turning around its longitudinal axis. The movement of a misplaced tooth around its longitudinal axis into a normal position by an orthodontic appliance. **Anterior rotation.** A rotation forwards. **Forceps rotation.** Rotation of the fetal head with forceps. **Manual rotation.** Rotation of the fetal head with the hand. **Molecular rotation.** The product of the specific rotation of an optically-active compound and its molecular weight divided by 100. **Optical rotation.** The rotation of the plane of a beam of polarized light when passed through solutions of certain optically-active substances. **Specific rotation.** The rotation of the plane of polarization produced by a 10-cm length of a solution containing 1 g per ml of solute, at the given temperature and for the particular light used. It is a constant for the substance in question for the given temperature and wavelength. **Wheel rotation** (of Helmholtz). The rotation of the eyeball about the fixation axis; rolling, torsion. [L *rotare* to rotate.]

See also: HELMHOLTZ.

rotatores muscles [musculi rotatores (NA)] (ro·ta·to·reez muslz). Small, deeply placed dorsal muscles, they are attached to the transverse process of the vertebra below, and to the spine of the vertebra immediately above. They are subdivided into the cervical [musculi rotatores cervicis (NA)], the thoracic [musculi rotatores thoracis (NA)], and the lumbar [musculi rotatores lumborum (NA)]. [L rotators.]

Rotavirus (roh·ta·vi·rus). An RNA-containing cubic virus 55 or 70 nm in diameter depending on whether the outer surface layer is present. Frequently associated with enteritis in children under the age of 5 years and with a worldwide distribution, it has yet to be grown in routine cell cultures. It resembles both the reoviruses and orbiviruses, with whom it makes up the family of Reoviridae, but is distinct from both. Morphologically and antigenically similar viruses are implicated in enteritis of the newborn of many animal species, including calves, piglets, mice and lambs. Also known as duovirus, orbi-like virus and reo-like virus. [L *rota* a wheel.]

Rotch, Thomas Morgan (b. 1848). Boston paediatrician.

Rotch's sign. Dullness to percussion in the right cardiohepatic angle in pericardial effusion. It may also be found in enlargement of the right atrium in tricuspid-valve disease.

rotenone (ro·ten·one). $C_{23}H_{22}O_6$, a crystalline substance occurring to the extent of 16 per cent in derris rhizome, and 3–10 per cent in the root of *Lonchocarpus nicou* (cube root). It is of value as an insecticide, especially for the control of warble fly.

Roth, Moritz (b. 1839). Basle pathologist.

Roth's disease, or retinitis. A mild form of septic retinitis occurring in patients with systemic infections, especially endocarditis, and characterized by transient yellowish-white spots (*Roth's spots*), often surrounded by a ring of blood.

Roth's spots. Any white-centred retinal haemorrhage. Originally described in bacterial endocarditis but also seen in collagen diseases, dysproteinaemias, leukaemias, and pernicious anaemia.

Roth, Paul (b. 1871). Battle Creek, Michigan, physiologist.

Benedict-Roth apparatus. An apparatus for determining the metabolic rate. It consists of a tank filled with oxygen and suspended in water: the patient breathes through a tube from the tank, carbon dioxide is removed by soda lime and the decrease in volume of the gas in the tank gives a direct measure of the oxygen consumed.

Roth, Vladimir Karlovich (b. 1848). Russian neurologist.

Roth's disease, symptom complex, or syndrome, Bernhardt-Roth symptom complex, or syndrome, Roth-Bernhardt disease. Meralgia paraesthetica; Bernhardt's disease.

Rothberg-Evans sugar tube. A tube used in the determination of blood sugar.

Rothera, Arthur Cecil Hamel (b. 1880). Melbourne biochemist.

Rothera's test. For acetone and aceto-acetic acid in urine: a powdered mixture of ammonium sulphate (100 parts) and sodium nitroprusside (1 part) is used. 5 ml of urine are saturated with the powder in a test-tube and 1 to 2 ml of concentrated ammonia added with mixing. A purple colour which fades rapidly on standing should be regarded as negative; a purple colour which persists and deepens on standing is positive. Acetone in urine indicates ketosis.

Rothmund, August (b. 1830). Munich ophthalmologist.

Rothmund-Thomson syndrome. Poikiloderma congenitale.

Rotter, Helmut. 20th century Budapest physician.

Rotter's test. A clinical test for vitamin-C deficiency: about 0.05 ml of 2,6-dichlorphenolindophenol is injected intracutaneously with a tuberculin syringe. If the dye is decolorized in 10 min, the subject is absorbing an adequate amount of vitamin C. The test is a useful one, but not entirely reliable.

rottlera (rot·ler·ah). The gland and hairs of the capsules of *Mallotus philippinensis* (family Euphorbiaceae), an East Indian shrub.

rottlerin (rot·ler·in). Mallotoxin, $C_{22}H_{20}O_6$. A bitter yellowish-pink crystalline compound occurring in rottlera, and used as an anthelminthic against tapeworm.

rotula (rot·ew·lah). 1. The patella. 2. A disc-shaped bony process. 3. A lozenge. [L, little wheel.]

rotular (rot·ew·lar). Patellar. [see prec.]

Rouge, Louis Philippe (b. 1833). Lausanne surgeon.

Rouge's operation. A sublabial approach to the nasal passages.

rouge (roozh). Red ferric oxide, Fe_2O_3, employed in medicine as a styptic and in industry as a polishing abrasive in lens manufacture. [Fr., red.]

Rouget, Antoine D. (fl. 1867). French physiologist.

Rouget cell. A flattened cell with numerous processes wrapped around the capillaries of frogs and other amphibia and thought to contract and constrict the vessels when stimulated by the sympathetic nervous system.

Rouget's muscle. A circular bundle of fibres in the inner part of the ciliary muscle.

rough (ruf). A term used to describe the colonial morphology of bacteria (the colonies are rough with a spreading edge). Specifically of a type of variation to which many bacterial species are liable (smooth to rough variation): the *rough* variant usually shows rough colonies and is deficient in a surface antigen associated with virulence. [AS *ruh.*]

roughage (ruf·ij). Any coarse substance in the diet, e.g. bran, cellulose, potato skins, which acts as an intestinal stimulant and promotes peristaltic action. [see prec.]

rouleau (rool·o). Erythrocytes found in shed blood which have formed rolls by adhering to each other. [Fr., cylinder.]

round-head (rownd·hed). A deformed skull attributed to synostosis of the frontal and parietal bones. [OFr. *rund,* head.]

roundworm (rownd·werm). A member of the Nemathelminthes, particularly the Nematoda. [OFr. *rund, AS wyrm.*]

Rous, Francis Peyton (b. 1879). New York virologist.

Rous' sarcoma. Transplantable fowl sarcoma caused by a virus complex.

Rous' sarcoma virus. A complex of two or more interacting RNA viruses which can cause, in fowls, a transplantable sarcoma. Tumours are also produced in other animal species but not in man.

Rous' test. For haemosiderin in urine: examine a portion of the centrifuged deposit for cells containing brown granules; suspend the rest of the deposit in a mixture of equal parts of 2 per cent potassium ferrocyanide and 1 per cent hydrochloric acid. After standing for 10 min centrifuge, and examine the deposit microscopically. Haemosiderin granules will have become blue. Positive results may occur in haemosiderosis of the kidney.

Rousseau, Louis François Emanuel (b. 1788). Paris anatomist.

Rousseau's bone. An accessory bone situated anterior to the lacrimal bone in the medial wall of the orbit. (The lacrimal bone is occasionally represented by several ossicles.)

Rousselot, Charles (b. 1880). Paris physician.

Rousselot's caustic. A caustic composed of mercuric sulphide, arsenic trioxide, and burnt sponge.

Roussy, Gustave (b. 1874). French neurologist.

Darier-Roussy sarcoid. Subcutaneous lesions similar to those of erythema induratum, but not necessarily confined to the lower limbs; probably of tuberculous origin.

Syndrome of Déjérine-Roussy, Roussy-Déjérine syndrome. Thalamic syndrome. *See* SYNDROME.

Roussy-Lévy disease, or syndrome. Peroneal muscular atrophy associated with cerebellar ataxia and scoliosis: it is familial.

Routier, Daniel (b. 1887). French physician.

Laubry, Routier, and van Bogaert sign. Presystolic gallop rhythm (atrial gallop). *See* RHYTHM, GALLOP.

Roux, César (b. 1857). Swiss surgeon.

Roux' muscle. The recto-urethral muscle.

Roux' operation. 1. A form of intestinal anastomosis in the shape of a Y, the intestine being divided and its proximal end anastomosed end-to-side to the distal loop, so that a portion of the distal loop remains for anastomosis to another viscus, e.g. gall bladder or oesophagus. 2. Excision of the tongue by dividing the mandible in the middle line. 3. One of the early operations for cancer of the oesophagus.

Roux, Jules (b. 1807). French surgeon.

Roux' operation. For exstrophy of the bladder: closure by means of two flaps, dissected from the abdomen and the scrotum respectively.

Roux, Pierre Paul Emile (b. 1853). Paris bacteriologist.

Roux' bottle, or flask. A large flat bottle holding approximately 1 litre with an eccentrically placed neck, for use in microbiological cell culture.

Roux' serum. Diphtheria antitoxic serum.

Roux' spatula. A metal spatula for inoculating culture media.

Roux' stain. A double stain, gentian violet and methyl green.

Roux' syringe. A glass and metal syringe with composition plunger; it can be sterilized in boiling oil.

Rovida, Carlo Leopoldo (b. 1844). Italian physician.

Rovida's hyaline substance. A material produced when pus is treated with 10 per cent sodium chloride.

Rovighi, Alberto (b. 1856). Bologna physician.

Rovighi's sign. Fremitus felt over a superficial hepatic hydatid cyst.

Rovsing, Nils Thorkild (b. 1862). Copenhagen surgeon.

Rovsing's operation. Plication of the anterior wall of the stomach and fixation of the stomach high on the anterior abdominal wall to relieve gastroptosis.

Rovsing's sign. Pressure in the left iliac fossa will often, in acute appendicitis, cause pain in the right iliac fossa at the site of the appendix.

Rowland, Russell Sturgis (b. 1874). Detroit physician.

Rowland's disease. Xanthomatosis.

Rowntree, Leonard George (b. 1883). Rochester, Minnesota, physician.

Rowntree and Geraghty test. Phenolsulphonephthalein test. *See* TEST.

Royle, Norman Dawson (d. 1944). Australian surgeon.

Royle's operation. Lumbar ganglionectomy.

rub (rub). The rough sound audible by auscultation, which is produced by the rubbing together of inflamed membranes. **Pericardial rub.** The rub which may occur with pericarditis. **Pleural rub.** The rub which may occur with pleurisy. [etym. dub.]

rubber (**rub**·er). An elastic substance prepared from the juice, or latex, of species of the Euphorbiaceae (particularly *Hevea*), grown in South America, India, Malaya, and elsewhere. It consists of a polymerized hydrocarbon, polyisoprene, $[CH_2CHC(CH_3)=CH_2]_n$, in a colloidal solution of protein, resins, and mineral salts. It is soluble in chloroform, and carbon disulphide; mixed with sulphur and in the presence of accelerators it may be converted into *vulcanized rubber.* **Antistatic rubber.** Rubber to which has been added substances, such as carbon, to make it a conductor of static electricity; used to reduce the incidence of the build-up of static charges and hence sparks in, for example, anaesthetic circuits. **Lead rubber.** Rubber containing a high proportion of lead compounds. It is used as a flexible material protective against x-rays. [etym. dub.]

rubber-dam (rub·er·**dam**). A sheet of thin rubber which is used by dentists in order to protect an area, e.g. a tooth socket, from contamination by saliva. [rubber, AS *dam.*]

rubedo (roo·**be**·do). A temporary redness of the skin; blushing. [L *ruber* red.]

rubefacient (roo·be·**fa**·shent). Causing reddening of the skin. [L *ruber* red, *facere* to make.]

rubefaction (roo·be·**fak**·shun). Redness of the skin produced by the application of a counter-irritant substance. [see prec.]

rubella (roo·**bel**·ah). German measles; a mild acute virus disease, occurring most frequently between 5 and 15 years of age, although adults are often attacked. After an incubation period of about 18 days there is slight temperature and headache, a rose-pink papular or macular rash, and enlarged glands in the neck. The mortality is negligible and no specific treatment is necessary. Congenital defects (cataract, deaf-mutism, cardiac lesions, etc.) in the child are correlated with rubella in the mother in the early months of pregnancy. **Rubella scarlatinosa.** Another name for so-called *fourth disease,* a mild infection different from rubella, scarlet fever, and measles. The existence of this condition is not generally accepted. The name is also given to the scarlatiniform type of rubella. [L *ruber* red.]

rubella virus (roo·**bel**·ah **vi**·rus). A pleomorphic enveloped RNA-containing virus of the family Togaviridae about 75 nm in size. The cause of rubella, it has marked teratogenic properties in pregnancy, particularly in the first 3 months. Only one antigenic type is known and live vaccines with minimum post-vaccination excretion of the virus are available. Protection following immunization is adequate but its duration is not yet known. Vaccination is usually offered to girls before puberty or post-partum to adult women, but with women of child-bearing age vaccination should normally only be given under adequate contraceptive cover.

rubellin (roo·**bel**·in). A cardiac stimulant extracted from the liliaceous plant *Urginea rubella.* Its action is similar to that of digoxin. [see prec.]

Ruben, Henning. 20th century Copenhagen anaesthetist.

Ruben valve. A plastic valve which closes automatically during the expiratory phase of intermittent positive pressure ventilation and prevents rebreathing.

rubeola (roo·**be**·o·lah). This term has been used as a synonym for two different virus diseases, measles and rubella. Presently it is often used as a synonym for measles, but the term should be avoided because of the confusion which exists. [L *ruber* red.]

rubeosis (roo·be·**o**·sis). Redness of the skin, in particular red discoloration of the skin. **Rubeosis iridis.** New vessel formation on the anterior surface of the iris, most commonly seen in thrombotic glaucoma and diabetes. **Rubeosis iridis diabetica.** Diabetic congestion of the eyeball. [L *ruber* red, Gk *-osis* condition.]

ruber (**roo**·ber). Red; the red nucleus of the mid-brain. [L.]

rubescence (roo·**bes**·ens). 1. A reddening of the skin. 2. Blushing. 3. A ruddy complexion. [L *rubescere* to become red.]

rubescent (roo·**bes**·ent). 1. Of a reddish colour. 2. Becoming red. [see prec.]

Rubia (**roo**·be·ah). A genus of plants (family Rubiaceae). *Rubia tinctoria* Linn., a European species, and *R. cordifolia* Linn., indigenous to India, are reputed to be medicinally active and have been employed as tonics and astringents. Both these plants yield a red dye known as *Turkey red.* [L *ruber* red.]

rubidium (roo·**bid**·e·um). An element of atomic weight 85.4678, atomic number 37, and chemical symbol Rb. It is a soft white alkaline metal resembling sodium and potassium and extremely reactive. It occurs in certain mineral waters and in sea water, and is a microconstituent of human tissue. Its salts have been used in medicine in the same way as potassium salts but they do not appear to have any special merits though stated to be better tolerated. **Rubidium and ammonium bromide.** $RbBr{\cdot}3(NH_4)Br$, a compound used like potassium bromide. [L *rubidus* red, from the red line in its spectrum.]

rubiginose, rubiginous (roo·**bij**·in·oze, roo·**bij**·in·us). Rust-coloured; term applied to sputum. [L *rubigo* rust.]

rubijervine (roo·be·**jer**·veen). $C_{26}H_{43}O_2N$, an inactive alkaloid obtained from species of *Veratrum,* white and green hellebore, so called from the purple colour of its solution in sulphuric acid. [L *rubeus* red, *jerva* green hellebore.]

Rubin, Isador Clinton (b. 1883). New York gynaecologist.

Rubin's test. For patency of the uterine tubes: carbon dioxide under pressure is injected into the uterus with an air-tight cannula, and by means of a kymograph, patency of the tubes and their peristalsis can be demonstrated.

rubin, rubine (**roo**·bin, **roo**·been). Fuchsine. [L *ruber* red.]

Rubini's essence. Essence of camphor.

Rubino's reaction. In leprosy, an agglutination-sedimentation test with sheep's corpuscles: the serum is reputed to contain a specific substance which causes agglutination and sedimentation of these corpuscles.

Rubner, Max (b. 1854). Berlin physiologist.

Rubner's law. 1. The law of constant energy consumption; the rapidity of growth is proportional to the intensity of the metabolic process. 2. The law of constant growth quotient; the same fractional part of the entire energy is used for growth.

This growth quotient, as might be expected, is many times greater in young than in adult organisms.

Rubner's test. 1. For carbon monoxide in blood: take a solution of lead acetate, add 5 volumes of it to the blood and shake well. If CO is present the blood remains pink, while normal blood becomes dark brown. 2. For lactose in urine: to 10 ml of urine add about 3 g of lead acetate, shake well and filter. Boil the filtrate. If lactose is present the solution turns brick red and a red precipitate forms. Glucose gives a red solution and a yellow precipitate.

rubor (roo·bor). Redness due to the existence of an inflammatory process. **Regional rubor.** A condition noted after the occurrence of cyanosis locally and marked by isolated reddening spots. [L, redness.]

rubrescin (roo·bres·in). An indicator consisting of a mixture of resorcinol and chloral hydrate. [L *ruber* red.]

rubreserine (roo·bres·er·een). $C_{13}H_{16}N_2O_2$, a deep-red crystalline colouring matter derived from eseroline and physostigmine (eserine).

rubriblast (roo·bre·blast). Haemocytoblast. [L *ruber* red, Gk *blastos* germ.]

rubric (roo·brik). 1. Red. 2. Relating to the red nucleus. [L *ruber* red.]

rubricyte (roo·bre·site). An early or intermediate normoblast; a term introduced by Osgood and not universally accepted. [L *ruber* red, Gk *kytos* cell.]

rubrin (roo·brin). Haematin. [L *ruber* red.]

rubrum congoensis (roo·brum kong·go·en·sis). Congo red. *See* RED.

rubrum scarlatinum (roo·brum skar·lat·in·um). Scarlet red. *See* RED.

Rubus (roo·bus). A genus of rosaceous plants including the blackberry (*Rubus fructicosus*), raspberry (*R. idaeus* Linn.), dewberries (*R. caesius*) and cloudberries (*R. chaemaemorus*). [L bramble.]

Ruck, Karl von (b. 1849). North Carolina physician.

von Ruck's vaccine. An obsolete vaccine prepared from killed tubercle bacilli.

ructation (ruk·ta·shun). Eructation. [see foll.]

ructus (ruk·tus). Eructation. **Ructus hystericus.** Eructation associated with a hysterical condition, wind being released with a pronounced bubbling, belching sound. [L, belching.]

Rudbeckia (rud·bek·e·ah). A genus of composite-flowered herbs of North America, including the cone flower, *Rudbeckia laciniata*, thimble weed, which has diuretic properties, and *R. hirta*. [Olof *Rudbeck*, 1630–1702, Upsala physician, and his son of the same name, 1660–1740.]

rudiment [rudimentum (NA)] (rood·e·ment). In embryology, the earliest stage in the differentiation of an organ; primordium; anlage. **Amnio-embryonic rudiment.** The inner cell mass; a knot of cells at one pole of a blastocyst from which the embryo proper and the amnion are derived. **Lens rudiment.** The lens vesicle of the early embryonic eye. [L *rudimentum* beginning.]

rudimentary (rood·e·ment·ar·e). 1. Relating or belonging to a rudiment. 2. Vestigial.

Rudinger, Nicolaus (b. 1832). Munich anatomist.

Rudinger's muscle. The muscularis mucosae of the rectum.

rue (roo). The herb *Ruta graveolens* Linn., garden rue, of the family Rutaceae. It is used as an emmenagogue and antispasmodic. **Goat's rue.** The herb *Galega officinalis* (family Leguminoseae), used as a diuretic and vermifuge. [Gk *rhyte*.]

Ruffini, Angelo (b. 1864). Bologna histologist.

Ruffini's bodies, brushes, corpuscles, cylinders, or organs. Organized sensory nerve-endings in the dermis having a brush-like terminal formation and thought to be the receptors for the modality of warmth. It is, however, possible that they are artefacts.

Ruffini's sheath. The continuation of the perineurium on the finest branches of peripheral nerves.

rufiopin (roo·fe·o·pin). Tetrahydroxyanthraquinone, $C_6H_2(OH)_2(CO)_2C_6H_2(OH)_2$. One of the isomeric compounds derived by the catalytic hydroxylation of anthraquinone.

Rufocromomycin (roo·fo·kro·mo·mi'·sin). BP Commission approved name for an antibiotic produced by *Streptomyces rufochromogenus*.

ruga (roo·gah) (pl. *rugae*). A ridge. **Rugae gastricae.** Folds of the mucous membrane in the contracted stomach which disappear on distension; they are mostly longitudinal in direction. **Rugae palatinae.** Ridges in the mucous membrane of the hard palate. **Rugae of the scrotum.** Irregular ridges in the skin of the scrotum produced by contraction of the dartos muscle. **Rugae of the stomach.** Rugae gastricae (see above). **Rugae of the urinary bladder.** Folds appearing in the mucous coat, except over the trigone. **Rugae of the vagina [rugae vaginales (NA)].** Transverse ridges in the mucous membrane of the vagina. [L.]

Ruge, Reinhold (b. 1862). Kiel hygienist.

Ruge's solution. A fixative containing formaldehyde and glacial acetic acid.

Ruggeri, Ruggero (d. 1905). Bologna physician.

Ruggeri's reflex, or sign. In extreme convergence of the eyes in order to fix a very near object, there may be tachycardia due to reflex sympathetic stimulation.

rugine (roo·zheen). Raspatory. [Fr., rasp.]

rugitus (roo·jit·us). The rumbling or gurgling sound made by movement of flatus in the intestines. [L roaring.]

rugose (roo·goze). 1. Bearing rugae. 2. Wrinkled; corrugated. [L *ruga* ridge.]

rugosity (roo·gos·it·e). 1. The state of being rugose. 2. A wrinkle, fold or ruga. 3. The natural condition of the skin of the fully developed scrotum. The skin of the scrotum of the patient with undescended testicles is undeveloped and does not show rugae.

rugous (roo·gus). Rugose.

Ruhmkorff, Heinrich Daniel (b. 1823). German instrument maker.

Ruhmkorff coil. An induction coil with a fixed secondary winding, and fitted with a condenser to produce space discharges.

rule (rool). 1. A guiding principle usually based upon experiment or observation. It may have the validity of a law in some cases, or be merely an empirical rule-of-thumb in others. 2. A rigid rod for measuring length. **Milk rule.** In healthy babies, after the neonatal period, the required quantity of milk in 24 hours should be one-tenth of the body weight. This quantity should not exceed 600 g. **Phase rule.** In the case of several phases of equilibrium, the degrees of freedom plus the number of phases equals the number of components plus two. [L *regula* model.]

See also: ABEGG, BUDIN, CLARK, FRIED, GIBBS, GIBSON, HARDY, HOFF, HUDSON (C. S.), JACKSON (J. H.), LIEBERMEISTER, LOSSEN, MCNAGHTEN, MOOTS, NAEGELE, PRINCE, QUETELET, ROLLESTON, SCHULTZE (E.), SPIVACK, TRAUBE (M.).

rum (rum). A spirit distilled from the fermented products of sugar manufacture, particularly molasses. There are two main varieties, Jamaica and Demerara, and it may contain 51–59 per cent of alcohol by volume. **Bay rum.** An alcoholic solution of oleum myrciae, used in cosmetics and as hair lotion. **Cherry rum.** Rum in which cherries have been steeped. [etym. dub.]

rumbling (rum·bling). The rumbling or gurgling sound made by movement of flatus in the intestines. [ME *romblen*.]

Rumex (roo·mex). A genus of plants of the order Polygonaceae, including sorrel (*Rumex acetosa*), sheep sorrel (*R. acetosella*), water dock (*R. aquaticus*), and yellow dock (*R. crispus*). Popularly reputed to be a cholagogue. [L sorrel.]

rumicin (roo·mis·in). $C_{15}H_{10}O_4$, a compound obtained from dock root, *Rumex crispus*, used in the treatment of skin diseases. It is an isomer of chrysophanic acid.

rumination (roo·min·a·shun). A condition observed in infants marked by the regurgitation of food after most feeds, a portion of which is vomited and the remainder swallowed. [L *ruminare* to chew over again.]

rump (rump). The gluteal region; the buttocks. [Dan. *rumpe*.]

Rumpel, Theodor (b. 1862). Hamburg surgeon.

Rumpel-Leede phenomenon, or sign, Leede-Rumpel phenomenon. The production of minute subcutaneous haemorrhages or petechiae by applying a tourniquet for 10-15 min to the upper arm of a patient with a scarlatinal rash on the forearm. The test is positive in scarlet fever, purpura, and certain other blood diseases.

Rumpf, Heinrich Theodor Maria (b. 1851). German physician.

Rumpf's reaction, or sign. 1. Tachycardia in response to a painful stimulus, in neurasthenia: it does not occur when pain is simulated. 2. Contractions of muscle after cessation of faradization, in traumatic neurosis.

Mannkopf-Rumpf sign. Rumpf's reaction, or sign, 1st def. (above).

runaround (run·ar·ownd). A superficial paronychia round the edge of the nail, leaving the bone unaffected. [ME *rinnen*, OFr. *rund.*]

Runeberg, Johan Wilhelm (b. 1843). Helsinki physician.

Runeberg's disease. Pernicious anaemia. *See* ANAEMIA.

runround (run·rownd). Runaround.

rupia (roo·pe·ah). A pustular eruption seen occasionally in secondary syphilis, characterized by the formation of encrusted ulcers. The bases of the lesions are infiltrated, their edges clear-cut; the adjacent skin is pigmented, and the ulcers are covered with conical or oval, dark-brown laminated crusts. **Rupia escharotica.** Dermatitis gangraenosa infantum. [Gk *rhypos* filth.]

rupial (roo·pe·al). Pertaining to, caused by, or having resemblance to rupia.

rupioid (roo·pe·oid). Having resemblance to rupia. [rupia, Gk *eidos* form.]

rupture (rup·tcher). 1. Hernia. 2. The breaking or forcible disruption of continuity of a part. 3. To break, usually applied to an organ or soft part, or to cause a hernia. **Defence rupture.** A failing of the natural resistance of the body to infection; for example, in miners the failing of the protective powers of the body to ward off tuberculosis when silica dust is inhaled. **Tubal rupture.** Rupture of tubal ectopic pregnancy. [L *rumpere* to break.]

Rusconi, Mauro (b. 1776). Pavia physician and biologist. **Anus of Rusconi.** The blastopore.

rush (rush). **Peristaltic rush.** Any one of the waves of contraction which run from one end of the intestine to the other and promote the passage downwards of the intestinal contents. [AS *risc.*]

Rush, Leslie V. 20th century Mississippi orthopaedic surgeon.

Rush nail. A solid intramedullary nail used in the internal fixation of fractures of long bones.

Russell, Frederick Fuller (b. 1870). Auburn, New York, pathologist.

Russell's double-sugar agar. A medium containing peptone 20 g, sodium chloride 5 g, lactose 10 g, glucose 1 g, agar 20 g, Andrade's indicator 10 ml, and water to 1 litre.

Russell's double-sugar agar with lead acetate. Russell's double-sugar agar with the addition of basic lead acetate 0.05 per cent.

Hiss and Russell bacillus. *Shigella flexneri.*

Russell, Patrick (b. 1727). Irish physician in India.

Russell's viper. *Vipera russelli* of India, Burma, and Thailand.

Russell, R. Hamilton. 20th century Melbourne surgeon.

Russell traction. A method of traction on the leg by weights and pulleys.

Russell, William (b. 1852). Edinburgh physician.

Russell's bodies. Acidophilic inclusions set free by the disintegration of plasma cells, often found in the wall of the alimentary canal.

Russell, William James (b. 1830). London chemist.

Russell effect. The effect which certain substances have on the emulsion of a photographic plate when in close proximity to it, and detected when the plate is developed in the ordinary way.

Russo, Mario (b. 1866). Italian physician.

Russo reaction. An obsolete test made by adding methylene blue to the urine of typhoid patients.

Rust, Johann Nepomuk (b. 1775). Berlin surgeon.

Rust's phenomenon, or syndrome. Stiff neck and the necessity of supporting the head with both hands in moving from the horizontal to the upright position, or vice versa. It is characteristic of a lesion (caries or new growth) of the cervical vertebrae.

rust (rust). 1. The hydrated ferric oxide, $2Fe_2O_3{\cdot}3H_2O$, which results from the exposure of iron to air and water. The term has been extended to the corrosive coating formed in a similar manner upon other metals exposed to the atmosphere. 2. A parasitic fungus forming coloured spores on the leaves and stems of higher plants. [AS *rust.*]

ruta (roo·tah). Rue. **Ruta graveolens.** Garden rue; used as an emmenagogue and antispasmodic.

ruthenium (roo·the·ne·um). An element of atomic weight 101.07, atomic number 44, and chemical symbol Ru. It is a hard brittle metal resembling platinum and occurring in platiniferous sands and gravels and in the mineral, laurite. It melts at a higher temperature than does platinum. [*Ruthenia* a Russian province.]

Rutherford, Ernest (Lord Rutherford) (b. 1871). British physicist.

Rutherford atom. The original idea of the atom as a miniature solar system in which electrons revolve like planets about a central sun or positive nucleus of concentrated mass.

Rutherford scattering. Scattering of a charged particle by matter, due only to coulomb forces between the particle and the nuclear charge and not to specifically nuclear forces.

Rutherford's theory. Telephone theory; the theory of central analysis. This explanation of the cochlear mechanism implies that the cochlea merely picks up the sound waves and transfers them to the nerve of hearing and thence to the brain, where they are analysed for pitch. In this theory the cochlea plays a passive rôle.

Rutherford (ruth·er·ford). A unit of radioactivity; that quantity of a radioactive substance which decays at the rate of 10^6 disintegrations/s. [Obsolete term.] [Ernest *Rutherford.*]

rutidosis (roo·tid·o·sis). Rhytidosis. [Gk *rhytis* wrinkle.]

rutilism (roo·til·izm). Having red or auburn hair. [L *rutilus* auburn.]

rutin (roo·tin). $C_{27}H_{30}O_{16}$, a crystalline alcohol occurring in tomato, tobacco, and rue leaves.

rutinose (roo·tin·oze). A disaccharide composed of units of rhamnose and glucose, which occurs in rue, tomatoes, and tobacco.

Ruttan, Robert Fulford (b. 1856). Montreal physician.

Ruttan and Hardisty test. For blood: to 1 ml of test solution add 1 ml of 4 per cent *o*-toluidine in glacial acetic acid and 1 ml of 10 volumes hydrogen peroxide. A blue colour develops if blood is present.

Ruttin, Erich (b. 1880). Prussian otologist working in Vienna.

Ruttin's reaction. Found in the compensatory or latent stage of labyrinthitis: rotational responses appear to be normal, and caloric and auditory tests are negative.

rutting (rut·ing). The phase of intense sexual excitement in female mammals. [Fr. *rut.*]

Ruysch, Frederik (b. 1638). Dutch anatomist.

Ruysch's disease. Megacolon.

Ruysch's muscle. A muscle of the fundus of the uterus.

Ruysch's tube. A small vestigial structure in the nasal septum.

Tunic of Ruysch, tunica of Ruysch. The capillary layer of the tunica vasculosa of the eye; the choriocapillary lamina.

Ruysch's veins. Retzius' veins.

Ruzicka, Vladimir (b. 1870). Prague biologist.

Ruzicka's stain. A mixture of methylene blue and neutral red, used to distinguish living and dead cells, the former staining blue, the latter red.

Rydygier, Ludwig Ritter von (b. 1850). Lemberg surgeon.

Rydgier's operation. Removal of cancer of the rectum by a sacral route.

rye (ri). The food grain obtained from the plant *Secale cereale* Linn. It is grown extensively in northern Europe and elsewhere, and is used in breadmaking. **Rye smut, Spurred rye.** Ergot; the diseased seed of rye. [AS *ryge.*]

Ryle, John Alfred (b. 1882). London, Cambridge and Oxford physician.

Ryle's tube. A stomach tube designed for removal of samples of gastric contents at intervals during a fractional test meal and also for keeping the stomach empty. It consists of a narrow-bore rubber or plastic tube having a blind end in which an oval lead weight is inserted with holes punched in the tube just above the weight.

rytidosis (ri·tid·o·sis). Rhytidosis.

S

sabadilla (sab·ah·**dil**·ah). The ripe seeds of *Schoenocaulon officinale* A. Gray (family Liliaceae). It contains alkaloids, the most important being cevadine (crystallized veratrine) which is highly toxic and sternutatory. The mixture of alkaloids constitutes amorphous commercial veratrine. Sabadilla has been used as a parasiticide, particularly for head pediculi. [Sp. *cebadilla* barley.]

sabadilline (sab·ah·**dil**·een). An alkaloid obtained from sabadilla. [see prec.]

sabadine (**sab**·ad·een). An alkaloid occurring in sabadilla and related to veratrine.

sabadinine (sab·**ad**·in·een). An alkaloid found in sabadilla.

Sabbatia (sab·a·she·ah). A genus of American herbs of the family Gentianaceae, including American centaury (*Sabbatia angularis*) and quinine flower (*S. elliotti*). [L. *Sabbati*, 18th century Italian botanist.]

Sabin, Albert Bruce (b. 1906). New York bacteriologist.

Sabin's syndrome. Internal hydrocephalus, or microcephaly, choroidoretinitis, convulsions and cerebral calcification in toxoplasmosis.

Sabin and Feldmann's slide neutralization test. In toxoplasmosis; equal parts of peritoneal exudate from infected mice and the subject's serum are incubated at 37°C for 1 h; a drop of methylene blue is added and the mixture is examined microscopically. In the absence of antimony, 90 per cent of toxoplasma take the stain; if antimony is present, less than 50 per cent.

Sabin vaccine. Live attenuated (by passage through monkey kidney cell culture) poliovirus of types 1, 2 and 3 given as an oral vaccine for protection against poliomyelitis. It is effective both in protecting the vaccinee and in limiting spread of wild virus in the community.

sabina (sab·i·nah). The fresh or dried young shoots of *Juniperus sabina* Linn. (family Pinaceae), a small evergreen shrub indigenous to southern Europe and cultivated in England. [L (*herba*) *Sabina* a juniper.]

sabinene (**sab**·in·een). $C_{10}H_{16}$, a terpene found in wormwood.

Sabouraud, Raymond Jacques Adrien (b. 1864). Paris dermatologist.

impetigo sicca of Sabouraud. Pityriasis alba.

Sabouraud's culture medium. A medium for pathogenic fungi, made from peptone 10 g, maltose 40 g, agar 18 g and water 1 litre.

Sabouraudites (sab·oo·ro·**di**'·teez). A generic name proposed by Ota and Langeron 1923, for those ringworm fungi which, in culture, produce microconidia isolated or in clusters, macroconidia or pluriseptate spindles, spiral hyphae, nodular organs and pectinate bodies. The species included belong chiefly to the genera *Microsporum* and the small-spore ectothrix group of *Trichophyton*, as well as some other species of *Trichophyton* which are chiefly parasites of the lower animals. [R. J. A. *Sabouraud*.]

Sabrazés, Jean Emile (b. 1867). French physician.

Sabrazés breath-holding test. For anaesthetic risk. Resting on a couch, the patient takes a deep breath, closes his nose and mouth and holds his breath as long as he can. 25 s and over constitutes a normal; less than 15 s indicates severe impairment of function.

sabulous (**sab**·ew·lus). Sandy; gritty. [L *sabulum* sand.]

sabulum (**sab**·ew·lum). Acervulus. [L sand.]

saburra (sab·**ewr**·ah). A foul state of the mouth or stomach resulting from decomposition of food. [L sand used as ballast.]

saburral (sab·**ewr**·al). Pertaining to or having the character of saburra.

sac [saccus (NA)] (sak). A bag-like structure. **Abdominal sac.** That part of the fetal coelom which becomes the peritoneal cavity. **Air sac.** The small terminal cavities opening into the atria. **Allantoic sac.** The entodermal portion of the allantois attached to the apex of the embryonic bladder. **Alveolar sac.** Air sac (see above). **Amniotic sac.** The fluid-filled sac which surrounds the embryo of higher vertebrates. **Aneurysmal sac.** A localized dilatation of the diseased wall of an artery, so that a bag-like projection results; a saccular aneurysm. **Conjunctival sac [saccus conjunctivae (NA)].** The space enclosed by the conjunctiva; it is open in the front when the eyelids are separated. **Dental sac, Dentinal sac.** The connective tissue which surrounds the developing dental germ, from which the periodontal membrane and the cementum are formed; the tooth follicle. **Embryonic sac.** The embryonic blastodermic vesicle. **Endolymphatic sac [saccus endolymphaticus (NA)].** The blind end of the endolymphatic duct. **Fetal sac, Gestational sac.** The sac containing the fetus in extra-uterine gestation. **Hernial sac.** The pouch of peritoneum (or of modified peritoneum), congenital or acquired, into which organs and tissues pass to cause the hernial swelling. **Lacrimal sac [saccus lacrimalis (NA)].** An expanded sac at the upper end of the nasolacrimal duct, receiving the lacrimal canaliculi on its lateral aspect. It is lodged in the fossa formed by the lacrimal bone and the frontal process of the maxilla, to which it is bound by the lacrimal fascia. **Nasal sac.** Invagination of ectoderm in the embryo which forms the primitive nasal cavity. **Pericardial sac.** Pericardium. **Sac of the peritoneum, greater.** The major portion of the peritoneal cavity, bounded anteriorly by the parietal peritoneum of the anterior abdominal wall, and posteriorly partly by viscera and partly by the parietal peritoneum of the posterior abdominal wall and pelvis. **Sac of the peritoneum, lesser [bursa omentalis (NA)].** The portion of the peritoneal cavity behind the liver, lesser omentum and stomach, above the transverse mesocolon and extending into the greater omentum. It communicates with the greater sac through a narrow opening below the liver. **Sac of the peritoneum, lesser, opening into the [foramen epiploicum (NA)].** The communication between the greater and lesser sacs, bounded anteriorly by the free border of the lesser omentum, superiorly by the caudate process of the liver and posteriorly by the peritoneum of the posterior abdominal wall covering the inferior vena cava. **Salt sac.** A bag of common salt formerly introduced into an open wound to facilitate drainage by encouraging the free passage by fluid osmosis. **Tubotympanic sac.** The recess of the embryonic pharynx which develops into the pharyngotympanic tube and tympanic cavity. **Umbilical sac.** Yolk sac (see below). **Vitelline sac.** Yolk sac (see foll.). **Yolk sac.** The entoderm-lined sac which is attached to the midgut of the embryo. It is one of the major fetal membranes. [Gk *sakkos* sack.]

See also: HILTON, LOWER.

saccades (sak·**ahdz**). Fast conjugate shifts of gaze as when altering fixation. Sometimes known as *voluntary eye movements.* [Fr. jerks.]

saccate (**sak**·ate). 1. Saccular; pouched. 2. Enclosed in a sac; encysted. [Gk *sakkos* sack.]

saccharamide (sak·ar·**am**·ide). An amide formed from saccharic acid by substitution in either or both of its terminal groups, e.g. $COOH(CHOH)_4CONH_2$.

saccharascope (sak·ar·ah·skope). A fermentation saccharimeter. [Gk *sakcharon* sugar, *skopein* to watch.]

saccharase (sak·ar·aze). Invertase, sucrase. An enzyme in plants, fungi and the intestinal secretion of animals, which brings about the hydrolysis of sucrose (saccharose) into equal parts of glucose and fructose (invert sugar). [Gk *sakcharon* sugar.]

saccharate (sak·ar·ate). 1. Any salt or ester of saccharic acid. 2. A compound formed by cane sugar with varying proportions of lime or strontia, e.g. calcium saccharate, $C_{12}H_{22}O_{11}CaO{\cdot}2H_2O$.

saccharated (sak·ar·a·ted). 1. Containing or mixed with sugar; sweetened. 2. Sugary. [Gk *sakcharon* sugar.]

saccharephidrosis (sak·ar·ef·e·dro'·sis). Excretion of sugar in the sweat. [Gk *sakcharon* sugar, ephidrosis.]

saccharic (sak·ar·ik). 1. Relating or belonging to sugar. 2. Derived from sugary substances. [Gk *sakcharon* sugar.]

saccharide (sak·ar·ide). 1. Any compound formed by the union of a sugar and a base. 2. General term applied to sugars, embracing the simple sugars or monosaccharides, the compound saccharides produced by the linkage of the latter, and the polysaccharides resulting from the condensation of monosaccharide units. **Saccharide ether.** A compound formed by the linkage with oxygen of 2 or more sugar units (compound saccharide), or a sugar and a non-sugar (glycoside). [see prec.]

sacchariferous (sak·ar·if·er·us). Yielding or containing sugar. [Gk *sakcharon* sugar, L *ferre* to carry.]

saccharification (sak·ar·if·ik·a'·shun). The process of converting starch into sugar. [Gk *sakcharon* sugar, L *facere* to make.]

saccharimeter (sak·ar·im·et·er). Any apparatus for the measurement of the concentration of sugars in solution. The term is commonly used to designate a polarimeter in which the scale is calibrated directly in units of sugar concentration instead of degrees of rotation; it is also applied to certain hydrometers devised to measure the concentration of sugar in solution by means of specific gravity, and to other apparatus used especially for determination of sugar. [Gk *sakcharon* sugar, meter.]

See also: CARWARDINE, EINHORN.

saccharimetry (sak·ar·im·et·re). The determination of the sugar content of a solution by the use of a saccharimeter.

saccharin (sak·ar·in). The chief of the synthetic sweetening agents, used by diabetics and to save sugar. It is a white crystalline powder, about 500 times as sweet as sugar, weight for weight, and harmless in small amounts even with repeated use (BP 1973). It has no food value. **Saccharin Sodium BP 1973, Soluble saccharin.** The sodium salt of saccharin, more soluble in water than the latter, and the form in which the sweetening agent is most commonly employed. [Gk *sakcharon* sugar.]

saccharine (sak·ar·een). 1. Sugary; relating to or containing sugar. Having a sweet taste. 2. Saccharin. [see prec.]

saccharins (sak·ar·inz). A series of lactones formed by the saccharinic acids; usually highly crystalline solids.

saccharinum (sak·ar·i·num). Saccharin.

Saccharobacillus (sak·ar·o·bas·il'·us). 1. A species of which *Lactobacillus pastorianus* is the only member now recognized [obsolete term.]. 2. *Clostridium butyricum* [obsolete term.]. [Gk *sakcharon* sugar, bacillus.]

saccharobiose (sak·ar·o·bi'·oze). Sucrose. [Gk *sakcharon* sugar, biose.]

saccharocoria (sak·ar·o·ko'·re·ah). Extreme dislike of sugar. [Gk *sakcharon* sugar, *koros* satiety.]

saccharogalactorrhoea (sak·ar·o·gal·ak·to·re'·ah). A condition in which excess of sugar is secreted in the milk. [Gk *sakcharon* sugar, *gala* milk, *rhoia* flow.]

saccharoids (sak·ar·oidz). A general term for polysaccharides which, though remotely resembling sugars, are not sweet, form colloidal solutions or are insoluble, and do not give sugar reactions. [Gk *sakcharon* sugar, *eidos* form.]

saccharolytic (sak·ar·o·lit'·ik). 1. Describing those enzymes which activate the hydrolysis of sugars into simpler units. 2. Applied to bacteria which break down carbohydrates in their metabolism. [Gk *sakcharon* sugar, *lysis* a loosing.]

saccharometabolic (sak·ar·o·met·ab·ol'·ik). Relating or belonging to saccharometabolism.

saccharometabolism (sak·ar·o·met·ab'·ol·izm). Sugar metabolism. [Gk *sakcharon* sugar, metabolism.]

saccharometer (sak·ar·om·et·er). Saccharimeter.

Saccharomyces Meyen 1837 (sak·ar·o·mi'·seez). A genus of yeasts which reproduce by budding and by formation of ascospores (sexual reproduction), but do not develop a mycelium. It includes species of importance in the baking and brewing industries. **Saccharomyces albicans** Reess 1877. *Candida albicans.* **Saccharomyces apiculatus** Reess. A common saprophyte belonging to a group of apiculate yeasts of the genus *Hansenia* Zikes 1911. **Saccharomyces blanchardi.** *Cryptococcus neoformans.* **Saccharomyces capillitii.** Oudemans and Pekelharing 1885. A species isolated from seborrhoea, and a synonym of *Pityrosporum ovale.* **Saccharomyces cerevisiae** Meyen 1870. The type species of the genus. The name has been applied indiscriminately to several species of industrial yeasts used in brewing and baking. **Saccharomyces ellipsoideus.** *Saccharomyces cerevisiae* (see above). **Saccharomyces exiguus** (Reess) Hansen 1888. A species isolated from pressed yeast. **Saccharomyces glutinis.** A common saprophytic pink yeast belonging to the genus *Rhodotorula.* **Saccharomyces granulomatogenes** Sanfelice 1898. A variety producing granulomatous tumours in pigs. **Saccharomyces guttulatus** Winter. A species cited by Rabenhorst 1881 and isolated from the digestive tracts of rabbits and from the faeces of guinea-pigs. **Saccharomyces hansenii** Zopf 1889. A species isolated from cotton pollen. **Saccharomyces hominis.** *Cryptococcus neoformans.* **Saccharomyces lithogenes.** *Cryptococcus neoformans.* **Saccharomyces mycoderma.** *Candida vini.* **Saccharomyces neoformans.** *Cryptococcus neoformans.* **Saccharomyces pastorianus** Hansen. A species isolated from the air near breweries; it gives a bitter taste and bad odour to beer. **Saccharomyces ruber.** *Rhodotorula rubra.* **Saccharomyces tumefaciens albus.** *Candida albicans.* [Gk *sakcharon* sugar, *mykes* fungus.]

See also: BUSSE.

saccharomycete (sak·ar·o·mi'·seet). A name often applied to any yeast or, in a restricted sense, to spore-forming yeast which does not form mycelium (the Saccharomycetaceae). [see prec.]

saccharomycetic (sak·ar·o·mi·se'·tik). Relating to or caused by fungi of the genus *Saccharomyces.*

saccharomycetolysis (sak·ar·o·mi·se·tol'·is·is). The destruction of saccharomycetic fungi. [saccharomyces, Gk *lysis* a loosing.]

saccharomycosis (sak·ar·o·mi·ko'·sis). Any morbid state due to the presence of a species of *Saccharomyces.* A rare cause of oral mycosis. [*Saccharomyces,* Gk *-osis* condition.]

saccharopinaemia (sak·ar·o·pin·e'·me·ah). Increased saccharopine in blood, cerebrospinal fluid and urine; found in short, mentally-retarded women. [saccharopine, Gk *haima* blood.]

saccharorrhoea (sak·ar·o·re'·ah). Glycosuria. **Saccharorrhoea cutanea.** Saccharephidrosis. **Saccharorrhoea lactea.** Saccharogalactorrhoea. **Saccharorrhoea pulmonalis.** The expectoration of sputum which has a sweetish taste. **Saccharorrhoea urinosa.** Diabetes mellitus. [Gk *sakcharon* sugar, *rhoia* flow.]

saccharosan (sak·ar·o·san). An anhydrosugar. [Gk *sakcharon* sugar.]

saccharosate (sak·ar·o·zate). Saccharate.

saccharose (sak·ar·oze). Sucrose. [Gk *sakcharon* sugar.]

saccharosuria (sak·ar·o·zewr'·e·ah). Sucrosuria. [Gk *sakcharon* sugar, urine.]

saccharum (sak·ar·um). Sucrose. **Saccharum album.** Sucrose. **Saccharum lactis.** Lactose. **Saccharum officinarum.** The sugar cane. **Saccharum purificatum.** Sucrose. **Saccharum ustum.** Burnt sugar, caramel; a dark mass prepared by heating sugar until it melts, then maintaining the temperature until carbonization has taken place. This is diluted with an equal volume of water to yield a solution of burnt sugar, used as a colouring in medicines and confectionery. [Gk *sakcharon* sugar.]

sacchorrhoea (sak·o·re·ah). Glycosuria. [Gk *sakcharon* sugar, *rhoia* flow.]

sacciform (sax·e·form). Sac-shaped. [Gk *sakkos* sack, form.]

Saccobranchus fossilis (sak·o·**brang**·kus fos·i·lis). A poisonous fish of India and Sri Lanka. [Gk *sakkos* sack, *branchion* gill, L *fossilis* dug up.]

saccular (sak·ew·lar). Sac-shaped. [L *sacculus* small sack.]

saccular nerve [nervus saccularis (NA)]. A terminal branch of the inferior branch of the vestibular nerve; it extends to the macula of the saccule.

sacculated (sak·ew·la·ted). Provided with saccules; having sac-like dilatations.

sacculation (sak·ew·**la**·shun). 1. The formation of a sac or pouch. 2. The state of being sacculated. 3. A sacculus or sac-like structure. **Anterior sacculation of the uterus.** A condition especially liable to occur with incarcerated retroversion of the pregnant uterus when the expansion of the uterus is almost entirely confined to the anterior wall. **Sacculations of the colon [haustra coli (NA)].** Sacculations produced on the medial sides of the ascending and descending parts of the colon and on the under surface of the transverse colon by contraction of the short longitudinal bands of fibres present. **Sacculation of the larynx.** Saccule of the larynx. [see foll.]

saccule [sacculus (NA)] (sak·ewl). The smaller of the 2 sacs within the vestibule of the ear, bulbous in form and connected below to the endolymphatic duct of the membranous labyrinth and the ductus reuniens. **Air saccule [sacculus alveolaris (NA)].** Air sac. *See* SAC. **Saccule of the larynx [sacculus laryngis (NA)].** The extension of the sinus of the larynx upwards outside the vestibular folds and internal to the lamina of the thyroid labyrinth. [L *sacculus* small sack.]

sacculocochlear (sak·ew·lo·**kok**'·le·ar). Relating to the vestibular saccule and the cochlea.

saccus (sak·us). A sac; a pouch. **Saccus reuniens.** The sinus venosus. **Saccus vitellinus.** The vitello-intestinal duct. *See* DUCT. [L sack.]

See also: VAN HORNE.

Sachs, Bernard (b. 1858). New York neurologist.

Sach's disease, Tay-Sachs disease. Amaurotic family idiocy, cerebromacular degeneration; a familial disease of infancy in which there is a progressive degeneration of nerve cells throughout the whole nervous system and in the retina. It is characterized clinically by progressive muscular weakness and paralysis, mental deterioration and blindness, usually leading to death in coma or convulsions towards the end of the second year. A characteristic cherry-red spot can be seen at the macula lutea on ophthalmoscopic examination. The degenerating nerve cells are filled with a lipoid similar to that in the Niemann-Pick form of phosphatide lipoidosis, but there is no enlargement of the liver and spleen.

Sachs, Hans (b. 1877). Heidelberg serologist.

Sach's antigen. Cholesterinized antigen, the acetone-insoluble fraction of an alcoholic extract of fresh normal beef heart to which an alcoholic solution of cholesterol is added to give 0.3-0.4 per cent of cholesterol. It is used as the antigen in the Wassermann reaction.

Sachs-Georgi test. A flocculation test for the serodiagnosis of syphilis.

Sackett, Guy E. 20th century Kansas biochemist.

Sackett's method. For cholesterol in blood. Serum or plasma (0.5 ml) is warmed with alcohol-ether and set aside for half an hour. The solution is then made to volume, mixed, filtered and an aliquot of filtrate evaporated to dryness. To the residue are added in succession 5 ml of chloroform, 2 ml of acetic anhydride and 0.1 ml of concentrated sulphuric acid. After standing for 10 min in the dark the colour is compared with cholesterol standards prepared similarly.

Sacks, Benjamin (b. 1896). New York physician.

Libman-Sacks disease or syndrome. Progressive anaemia in young people with slight persistent fever and purpuric and erythematous rash.

Libman-Sacks endocarditis. Non-bacterial verrucose endocarditis associated with systemic lupus erythematosus.

Osler-Libman-Sacks syndrome. Libman-Sacks endocarditis (see above).

sacra media (sa·krah **me**·de·ah). The median sacral artery. [sacrum, L *medius* middle.]

sacral (sa·kral). 1. Relating or belonging to the sacrum. 2. Occurring or situated near the sacrum. **Sacral plexus.** *See* PLEXUS. **Sacral sparing.** Retention of normal sensation in sacral dermatomes in spinal cord compression otherwise causing loss of sensation below the level of the lesion.

sacral arteries. Lateral sacral arteries [arteriae sacrales laterales (NA)]. Branches of the posterior division of the internal iliac artery, running along the lateral border of the sacrum, supplying the muscles and nerves in front of the sacrum, the structures within the sacral canal [rami spinales (NA)] and the muscles and skin in the gluteal region. **Median sacral artery [arteria sacralis mediana (NA)].** A small median branch of the abdominal aorta at its bifurcation, running down the front of the sacrum and coccyx; it may give off small lumbar branches. It corresponds to the caudal artery of many other vertebrates.

sacral nerves [nervi sacrales (NA)]. Segmental nerves, 5 in number, from the sacral portion of the spinal cord. The anterior primary rami [rami ventrales (NA)] of the upper 4 emerge through the anterior sacral foramina and the fifth between the sacral foramen and coccyx; the posterior primary rami [rami dorsales (NA)] through the posterior sacral foramina, except the last, which emerges between the sacral foramen and coccyx. Medial branches of the posterior primary rami [rami mediales (NA)] end in the multifidus muscle; the lateral branches [rami laterales (NA)] go to the dorsum of the sacrum. There are also gluteal branches to the buttocks [nervi clunium medii (NA)]. **Fourth sacral nerve, perineal branch of the.** A branch which pierces the coccygeus muscle, or passes between this and the levator ani muscle, to supply the sphincter ani externus muscle.

sacral veins. Lateral sacral veins [venae sacrales laterales (NA)]. Tributaries of the internal iliac vein. They follow the arteries of the same name. **Median sacral vein [vena sacralis mediana (NA)].** A tributary of one common iliac vein, or the commencement of the inferior vena cava.

sacralgia (sa·**kral**·je·ah). Pain affecting the sacrum. [sacrum, Gk *algos* pain.]

sacralization (sa·kral·i·**za**'·shun). Anomalous overgrowth of the transverse processes of the 5th lumbar vertebra and their apparent fusion with the sacrum.

sacrarthrogenic (sa·krar·thro·**jen**'·ik). Having origin in a lesion or injury of the sacrococcygeal or sacro-iliac joint. [sacrum, Gk *arthron* joint, *genein* to produce.]

sacrectomy (sa·**krek**·to·me). Excision of a part of the sacrum for the removal of a malignant rectum, as in the Kraske operation. [sacrum, Gk *ektome* excision.]

sacrococainization (sa·kro·ko·ka·ni·**za**'·shun). A coined word implying the anaesthetizing of the sacral region by the injection of cocaine or similar solution into the sacral canal.

sacrococcygeal (sa·kro·kok·**sij**'·e·al). Relating or belonging to the sacrum and the coccyx.

sacrococcygeus anticus (sa·kro·kok·**sij**'·e·us an·ti·kus). The sacrococcygeus ventralis muscle. [sacrococcyx, L *anticus* anterior.]

sacrococcygeus dorsalis muscle [musculus sacrococcygeus dorsalis (NA)] (sa·kro·kok·**sij**'·e·us dor·**sa**·lis musl). A vestigial muscle corresponding to the sacrococcygeus ventralis muscle, running from the posterior surface of the sacrum to the coccyx.

sacrococcygeus posticus (sa·kro·kok·**sij**'·e·us pos·ti·kus). The sacrococcygeus dorsalis muscle.

sacrococcygeus ventralis muscle [musculus sacrococcygeus ventralis (NA)] (sa·kro·kok·**sij**'·e·us ven·**tra**·lis musl). A vestigial muscle extending from the anterior surface of the sacrum to the coccyx.

sacrococcyx (sa·kro·**kox**·ix). The sacrum and the coccyx considered as one structure.

sacrocoxalgia (sa·kro·kox·**al**'·je·ah). Pain affecting the sacro-iliac joint. [sacrum, coccyx, Gk *algos* pain.]

sacrocoxitis (sa·kro·kox·i′·tis). Inflammation affecting the sacro-iliac joint. [sacrum, coccyx, Gk *-itis* inflammation.]

sacrodynia (sa·kro·**din**·e·ah). Pain in the region of the sacrum. [sacrum, Gk *odyne* pain.]

sacro-iliac (sa·kro·**il**·e·ak). Having reference to the sacrum and the ilium; more particularly describing the joints formed between the ilium and sacrum on either side.

sacro-iliitis (sa·kro·il·e·i·tis). Inflammation of the sacro-iliac joint. [sacrum, ilium, Gk *-itis* inflammation.]

sacrolisthesis (sa·kro·lis·**the**′·sis). A deformity in which the sacrum lies in front of the 5th lumbar vertebra. [sacrum, Gk *olisthanein* to slip.]

sacrolumbalis (sa·kro·lum·**ba**′·lis). The iliocostalis muscle. [sacrum, L *lumbus* loin.]

sacrolumbar (sa·kro·**lum**·bar). Relating or belonging to the sacrum and the lumbar region.

sacroperineal (sa·kro·per·in·e′·al). Relating or belonging to the sacrum and the perineum.

sacrosciatic (sa·kro·si·**at**′·ik). Belonging or referring to the sacrum and the ischium.

sacrospinal (sa·kro·**spi**·nal). Belonging to the sacrum and the vertebral column. [sacrum, spine.]

sacrospinalis muscle [musculus erector spinae (NA)] (sa·-kro·spi·**na**′·lis musl). A complex muscle which arises from the spines of the sacral and lumbar vertebrae, from the transverse tubercles of the sacrum and part of the iliac crest; it runs cranially lateral to the vertebral spines and is divided into 3 columns, iliocostocervicalis, longissimus and spinalis. It is in general an extensor of the vertebral column.

sacrotomy (sa·**krot**·o·me). Resection of the lower part of the sacrum. [sacrum, Gk *temnein* to cut.]

sacro-uterine (sa·kro·**ew**·ter·ine). Belonging to the sacrum and the uterus.

sacrovertebral (sa·kro·**ver**·te·bral). Relating to the sacrum and vertebrae.

sacrum [os sacrum (NA)] (sa·krum). The composite bone formed by the bony fusion of the sacral vertebrae, forming the back of the pelvis. It possesses a convex and very uneven dorsal surface [facies dorsalis (NA)] lying below the small of the back, and a concave and fairly smooth ventral surface [facies pelvina] which forms the back wall of the pelvis. **Apex of the sacrum [apex ossis sacri (NA)].** The lower surface of the 5th sacral vertebra. **Assimilation sacrum.** A sacrum with either lumbarization of the 1st sacral vertebra or sacralization of the 5th lumbar vertebra. **Base of the sacrum [basis ossis sacri (NA)].** The cephalic surface of the sacrum and hence of the 1st sacral vertebra. **Mass of the sacrum, lateral [pars lateralis (NA)].** The portion outside the anterior sacral foramen, formed of fused costal elements. **Surface of the sacrum, auricular [facies auricularis (NA)].** The joint surface on the lateral side of the first 3 sacral vertebrae for the ilium. **Tilted sacrum.** Sacro-iliac subluxation or dislocation resulting in tilting of the sacrum relative to the rest of the pelvis. [L sacred, because formerly believed imperishable.]

sactosalpinx (sak·to·**sal**·pingx). Gross distension of a uterine tube. **Sactosalpinx haemorrhagica.** Haematosalpinx. [Gk *saktos* stuffed, *salpigx* tube.]

saddle (sadl). 1. Any structure shaped like a saddle. 2. In dentistry, the narrow base of partial denture which extends across the roof of the mouth and covers only part of the palate. [AS *sadol.*]

sadism (sa·dizm). Sexual emotion associated with the wish to inflict and use violence. **Anal sadism.** The aggressive, instinctual quality associated with the anal region. **Oral sadism.** The aggressive instinctual quality associated with the oral region. [Donatien Alphonse François de *Sade* (Marquis de Sade), (b. 1740).

sadist (sa·dist). One who practises sadism.

sadistic (sad·is·tik). Relating or belonging to or characterized by sadism.

sadomasochism (sad·o·**mas**·o·kizm). Sexual emotion associated with both sadism and masochism.

sadomasochistic (sad·o·mas·o·**kis**′·tik). Pertaining to both sadism and masochism.

Saegesser, Max. 20th century Berne surgeon.

Saegesser's sign. Tenderness over the left phrenic nerve in rupture of the spleen.

Saemisch, Edwin Theodor (b. 1833). Bonn ophthalmologist.

Saemisch's operation or section, Graefe-Saemisch operation. For severe hypopyon ulcer. A paracentesis is performed by an incision with a Graefe knife through the centre of the ulcer, with extension into normal corneal tissue on each side and also through the whole length of the cornea. Still occasionally used.

Saemisch's ulcer. Ulcus serpens; hypopyon ulcer.

Saenger, Alfred (b. 1860). Hamburg neurologist.

Saenger's pupil reaction or sign. In neurosyphilis, other than tabes dorsalis, the reaction of the pupil to light which appears to be lost may return temporarily if the patient is kept in the dark for some time.

Saenger, Max (b. 1853). Prague gynaecologist.

Saenger's macula. Macula gonorrhoeica.

safflower (saf·flow·er). Carthamus, bastard saffron, American saffron; the flowers of *Carthamus tinctorius* Linn. (family Compositae), a plant indigenous to India. It is used as a domestic remedy for infant disorders such as measles, and as a colouring agent. [It. *safflore.*]

saffron (saf·ron). The dried stigmas and tops of *Crocus sativus* (family Iridaceae), used as a colouring agent in foodstuffs. **American saffron, Bastard saffron.** Safflower. **Bitter saffron.** Picrocrocin. **Meadow saffron.** The dried corm of *Colchicum autumnale* (family Liliaceae), containing the alkaloid colchicine. [Ar. *safra* yellow.]

safranine (saf·ran·een). Generic name for a group of dyestuffs derived from phenyldiaminophenazonium base, $NH_2C_6H_3NC_6H_5(N)C_6H_3NH_2$. They are fast dyes used for tanning cotton, and certain members are of value for staining animal tissue and as the reagent in testing for sugar in the urine. **Brilliant safranine.** $(CH_3)(NH_2)C_6H_2N_2(C_6H_5)C_6H_2(CH_3)(NH_2)Cl$. A safranine dye derived from aniline and toluidine; it is used to dye cotton and silk. [see prec.]

safranophil, safranophile (saf·ran·o·fil, saf·ran·o·file). Having affinity for safranine. [safranine, Gk *philein* to love.]

safrol, safrole (saf·rol, saf·role). 1-Allyl-3,4-methylenedioxybenzene, $CH_2O_2C_6H_3CH_2CH{=}CH_2$. A colourless oil occurring to the extent of 80 per cent in sassafras oil, but obtained mainly from essential oil of camphor. It is used in rubefacient mixtures and to destroy head parasites.

safu (sah·foo). Yaws with florid skin lesions, encountered in the Turks Islands.

safura (sah·**fewr**·ah). Ancylostomiasis.

sage (saje). Garden sage, red sage; the dried leaves of *Salvia officinalis* Linn. (family Labiatae). **Indian sage.** Thoroughwort, boneset; the dried herb *Eupatorium perfoliatum* Linn. (family Compositae). **Wood sage.** Garlic sage; the dried herb *Teucrium scordonia* (family Labiatae). [L *salvia.*]

sagittal [sagittalis (NA)] (saj·it·al). 1. Arrow-shaped. 2. In an anteroposterior direction, generally in the median plane (that of the sagittal suture of the skull). [L *sagitta* arrow.]

Sagnac, Georges (b. 1869). Paris physicist.

Sagnac rays. Electrons (β-rays) emitted by a metallic surface when γ-rays fall upon it.

sago (sa·go). The prepared pith starch of *Metroxylon rumphii* (family Palmaceae) which occurs in various forms and sizes in commerce. Commercial sago is also often made from potato starch. [Malay *sagu.*]

Sahli, Hermann (b. 1856). Berne physician.

Sahli's borax methylene blue. A mixture of methylene blue and borax in aqueous solution, used as a blood stain.

Sahli's method. A method for the estimation of haemoglobin by conversion to acid haematin with M/10 HCl and matching against either non-fading coloured glass or standard acid haematin solution.

Sahli's reagent. For free hydrochloric acid in gastric juice. Equal parts of a 48 per cent aqueous solution of potassium iodide and an 8 per cent aqueous solution of potassium iodate.

Sahli's whistle. A whistling or sizzling sound caused by gas and liquid being forced through a stenosis in the intestines. It may be heard some distance from the patient or through the stethoscope.

Sahli–Hellige haemoglobinometer. An instrument in which blood is treated with dilute acid, and the brown colour of the acid haematin diluted until it matches a brown glass wedge standard, as a means of estimating the haemoglobin content.

saimiri (sa·e·**me**·re). Seven-day fever of Japan. [Jap.]

St. Agatha's disease. Inflammation of the breasts.

St. Aignan's disease. Favus.

St. Anthony's disease. 1. Chorea; also called *St. Vitus' disease*. 2. Epidemic gangrene due to ergotism; often accompanied by severe mental changes and usually called *St. Anthony's fire*. The term has also been applied to erysipelas.

St. Appolonia's disease. Pain associated with a tooth; toothache.

St. Avertin's disease. Epilepsy; also called *St. Valentine's disease.*

St. Avidus' disease. Deafness.

St. Blasius' disease. Quinsy.

St. Dymphna's disease. Insanity.

St. Erasmus' disease. Colic.

St. Fiacre's disease. Haemorrhoids.

St. Francis' disease. Erysipelas.

St. Gervasius' disease. Rheumatism, juvenile or adult.

St. Gete's disease. Carcinoma.

St. Giles' disease. Leprosy.

St. Hubert's disease. Rabies.

St. John's wort. The perennial herb, *Hypericum perforatum*, formerly used as an astringent and diuretic.

St. Kilda's cold. Strangers' cold. *See* COLD.

St. Main's disease. Scabies.

St. Mathurin's disease. Idiocy.

St. Modestus' disease. Chorea; also called *St. Vitus' disease.*

St. Roch's disease. Plague.

St. Valentine's disease. Epilepsy; also called *St. Avertin's disease.*

St. Vitus' disease. Chorea.

St. Zachary's disease. Mutism.

sajina (saj·e·nah). An East Indian plant, *Moringa pterygosperma* (family Moringaceae). The seeds yield a fixed oil, ben oil, and the bark contains 2 alkaloids with an action similar to that of ephedrine.

saké, sakee (**sak**·e). An alcoholic liquor prepared in Japan from steamed rice (koji) fermented with the organism *Aspergillus oryzae.* [Jap.]

sal (sal). Salt; applied to a salt or any substance resembling a salt. **Sal acetosella.** Potassium binoxalate or quadroxalate which have similar properties to oxalic acid. **Sal aeratus.** 1. Potassium bicarbonate. 2. Sodium bicarbonate. **Sal alembroth.** A mercury salt obtained by crystallization from a solution of equal parts of ammonium and mercuric chlorides. **Sal amarum.** Magnesium sulphate. **Sal ammoniac.** Ammonium chloride salt. **Sal communis.** Common salt; sodium chloride. **Sal diureticum.** Potassium acetate. **Sal de duobus.** Potassium sulphate. **Sal enixum.** Potassium bisulphate. **Sal fossile.** Sodium chloride. **Sal glauberi.** Glauber salt; sodium sulphate. **Sal kissingense factitum.** Artificial Kissingen salt. **Sal marinum.** Sodium chloride. **Sal mirabile.** Sodium sulphate. **Sal peraltum.** Sodium phosphate. **Sal polychrestum.** Potassium sulphate. **Sal prunella.** A mixture of potassium nitrate and sulphur. **Sal rupium.** Rock salt; crude sodium chloride. **Sal seignette.** Potassium and sodium tartrate. **Sal sodae.** Sodium carbonate. **Sal vegetabile.** Potassium tartrate. **Sal vichyanum factitum.** Artificial Vichy salt. **Sal volatile, Sal volatilis.** Ammonium carbonate or a solution of ammonia and ammonium carbonate. [L.]

Salah. Egyptian physician.

Salah needle. For sternal puncture. A sternal puncture needle with an adjustable guard.

salamander (sal·am·**an**·der). A lizard-like animal of the family Salamandridae; used in certain laboratory experiments. [Gk *salamandra.*]

salamanderin (sal·am·**an**·der·in). A basic substance with toxic properties obtained from the skin of some salamanders.

Salazosulphadimidine (sal·a·zo·sul·fah·**dim**′·id·een). BP Commission approved name for 4′-(4,6-dimethylpyrimidin-2-ylsulphamoyl)-4-hydroxyazobenzene-3-carboxylic acid.

Salbutamol BP 1973 (sal·bew·tam·ol). 1-(4-Hydroxy-3-hydroxymethylphenyl)-2-(*tert*-butylaminoethanol), a sympathomimetic agent with predominantly beta-adrenergic activity. **Salbutamol Sulphate BP 1973.** The hemisulphate of salbutamol; used mainly as a bronchodilator, its action is similar to that of isoprenaline sulphate but more prolonged.

salep (sa·lep). The dried tubers of various species of orchid, including *Orchis mascula, O. maculata* and *O. latifolia*, used as a demulcent or as a food like sago. [Arabic *thaleb.*]

saleratus (sal·er·a·tus). 1. Potassium bicarbonate, $KHCO_3$. 2. Sodium bicarbonate, $NaHCO_3$. 3. A baking powder containing sodium bicarbonate, common salt and cream of tartar. [L *sal aeratus* aerated salt.]

salia effervescentia (sa·le·ah ef·er·ves·**en**′·she·ah). Effervescent salts; usually sodium sulphate or magnesium sulphate to which sodium bicarbonate and citric acid (or tartaric acid) have been added. The mixture effervesces upon the addition of water, and the taste of the aperient is thereby partially disguised. [L.]

Salicin BPC 1954 (sal·is·in). $C_6H_{11}O_5OC_6H_4CH_2OH$, an antipyretic and analgesic glycoside obtained from the bark of various species of willow (*Salix*) and poplar (*Populus*). It consists of colourless, odourless, bitter crystals or white powder, fairly soluble in cold water or alcohol, and is hydrolysed by acids or enzymes into glucose and salicyl alcohol (saligenin).

salicyl (sal·is·il). Name given to the radical OHC_6H_4CO- derived from salicylic acid. [Gk *salix* willow, *hyle* matter.]

salicylaemia (sal·is·il·e′·me·ah). Salicylates in the blood. [salicylate, Gk *haima* blood.]

salicylage (sal·is·il·aje). The use of salicylic acid in the preservation of foodstuffs or beverages.

salicylal (sal·is·il·al). Salicylic aldehyde. *See* ALDEHYDE. **Salicylal paraphenetidine.** Salicylide phenetidine.

Salicylamide (sal·is·il·**am**·ide). BP Commission approved name for *o*-hydroxybenzamide, the amide of salicylic acid, used for the same purposes as the acid itself.

salicylanilide (sal·is·il·**an**′·il·ide). $C_6H_4(OH)(CONHC_6H_5)$, a substance prepared from salicylic acid and acetanilide; used as an antipyretic.

salicylate (sal·is·il·ate). Any salt or ester of salicylic acid. Some salicylates, especially that of sodium, have an anti-pyretic and antirheumatic action internally. Others (e.g. methyl salicylate) are applied externally. In other cases the salicylate is merely used as a convenient acid radical and has no specific effects (e.g. bismuth salicylate and physostigmine salicylate). [Gk *salix* willow, *hyle* matter.]

salicylide (sal·is·il·ide). 1. Salicylic aldehyde. *See* ALDEHYDE. 2. Any anhydride of salicylic acid, especially tetrasalicylide, $(C_6H_4COO)_4$, a colourless compound formed by condensation. **Salicylide phenetidine.** Salicylal paraphenetidine, $C_2H_5OC_6H_4N{=}CHC_6H_4(OH)$, an antipyretic.

salicylism (sal·is·il·izm). Chronic poisoning due to an overdose or excessive use of salicylic acid or of its salts.

salicylize (sal·is·il·ize). 1. To add salicylic acid to a mixture. 2. To employ salicylic acid in the treatment of patients.

salicylol (sal·is·il·ol). Saligenin.

salifebrin (sal·e·**feb**·rin). $C_6H_4(OH)(CONHC_6H_5)$, an analogue of acetanilide; used as an antipyretic and antalgesic.

saliferous (sal·if·er·us). Containing or yielding salt. [L *sal* salt, *ferre* to bear.]

salifiable (sal·e·fi·abl). Having the ability to produce a salt by combination with an acid. [see foll.]

salify (sal·e·fi). 1. To change into a salt by the action of an acid or base. 2. To treat with a salt. [L *sal* salt, *facere* to make.]

saligenin (sal·ij·en·in). Salicyl alcohol, $C_6H_4(OH)(CH_2OH)$. An alcohol obtained by hydrolysis, of the glycoside, salicin. It is sometimes used in rheumatism.

saligenol (sal·ij·en·ol). Saligenin. [Obsolete term.]

salimeter (sal·im·et·er). Salinimeter. A type of hydrometer used to measure the specific gravity of salt solutions. [L *sal* salt, meter.]

salinaphthol (sal·e·naf·thol). β-Naphthyl salicylate, $C_6H_4(OH)COOC_{10}H_7$. A white powder with antiseptic properties; it has no medical use nowadays.

Salinazid (sal·in·a·zid). BP Commission approved name for *N*-isonic-otinoyl-*N'*-salicylidenehydrazine; used in the treatment of tuberculosis.

saline (sa·line). 1. Salty; pertaining to or having the characteristics of common salt. 2. Containing a salt of an alkali metal or earth, as in the case of natural waters. 3. A solution prepared for injection usually intravenous, of specified strength, usually 0.9 per cent, of sodium chloride or other salts. **Formol saline.** A common histological preservative and fixative containing 1 part of 40 per cent formaldehyde and 9 parts of normal saline. **Hypertonic saline.** A solution of sodium chloride or other salts of a strength higher than 0.9 per cent; a strength over 1.2 per cent is seldom used for intravenous injection. **Hypotonic saline.** A solution of sodium chloride or other salts of a strength less than 0.9 per cent; a strength less than 0.6 per cent is seldom used for intravenous injection. **Normal saline.** A 0.9 per cent sterile solution of sodium chloride in water, isotonic with blood and used for injection purposes. **Physiological saline.** Normal saline (see above). [L *sal* salt.]

salinimeter (sal·in·im·et·er). A special form of hydrometer so graduated that the strength of brine or seawater can be read-off directly. [saline, meter.]

salinometer (sal·in·om·et·er). 1. A salinimeter. 2. A conductivity cell used to determine the salt content of a solution by measurement of its resistance. [L *sal* salt, meter.]

saliphen, saliphenin (sal·e·fen, sal·if·en·in). Salicylide phenetidine.

Salisbury, James Henry (b. 1823). New York physician.

Salisbury treatment. A dietetic treatment, mainly of lean meat and hot water, used in the treatment of gout, obesity, psoriasis and certain other diseases.

saliva (sal·i·vah). The mixed secretions of the salivary glands (parotid, submaxillary and sublingual), and of the mucous membrane of the mouth, which may be regarded as the first of the digestive juices of the body to be brought into contact with food. It contains the amylase, ptyalin, which has some hydrolytic action upon the starch of foods, and it also serves to moisten food and to act as solvent and lubricant. In addition to ptyalin, saliva contains mucin, urea, inorganic ions, e.g. sodium, potassium, calcium, chlorides, phosphates and usually a trace of thiocyanate. *Groups* can be effected in those who secrete the blood group substances ABO, 75 per cent of all people secrete the water soluble group substances identical with their blood groups, and also H substance into saliva, semen, sweat, etc. **Chorda saliva.** Saliva secreted by the submaxillary glands as a result of stimulation of the chorda tympani nerves; the concentration of the saliva thus produced depends on the strength of the stimulation. **Ganglionic saliva.** Saliva secreted as a result of stimulation of the ganglionic cells which may be hilar (parasympathetic) or cervical (sympathetic). **Lingual saliva.** Saliva from the secretory glands of the tongue. **Parotid saliva.** Saliva secreted by the parotid glands; it is more watery than submaxillary or sublingual saliva but has a higher digestive power. **Resting saliva.** The normal saliva in the mouth when food is not being taken. **Sublingual saliva.** The secretion of the sublingual glands; it is more mucilaginous than either parotid or submaxillary saliva. **Submaxillary saliva.** Saliva secreted by the submaxillary glands. **Sympathetic saliva.** Saliva produced by stimulation of the sympathetic nerve supply of the submaxillary glands, such saliva being more mucilaginous than that produced without stimulation. **Viscid saliva.** Sticky saliva of high mucin content. [L spittle.]

salivant (sal·iv·ant). 1. Stimulating the flow of saliva; sialogenous. 2. An agent which increases the secretion of saliva; sialogogue.

salivary (sal·iv·ar·e). 1. Relating or belonging to saliva; sialic. 2. Producing saliva.

salivate (sal·iv·ate). To have a copious flow of saliva.

salivation (sal·iv·a·shun). 1. The process of salivating. 2. Secretion of saliva in excessive quantities, a condition that may be accompanied by soreness of mouth and gums.

salivator (sal·iv·a·tor). Sialogogue. [L *saliva* spittle.]

salivatory (sal·iv·a·tor·e). Giving rise to salivation; stimulating the production of saliva; sialogenous.

salivolithiasis (sal·iv·o·lith·i′·as·is). The condition characterized by formation of a salivary calculus. [saliva, Gk *lithos* stone.]

Salix (sa·lix). A genus of trees, the willows, belonging to the family Salicaceae. **Salix alba.** The European or white willow. **Salix nigra.** Black willow, pussy willow; like all species of *Salix* it contains salicin. [Gk.]

Salk, Jonas Edward (b. 1914). American virologist.

Salk vaccine. The first poliomyelitis vaccine. It contains poliovirus of types 1, 2 and 3 inactivated by formaldehyde and is given by intramuscular injection. It is adequate to protect the recipient against poliomyelitis but does not prevent spread of wild virus in the community; therefore, it is largely superseded by the oral Sabin vaccine, though preferred for routine vaccination in some countries.

Salkowski, Ernst Leopold (b. 1844). Berlin biochemist.

Salkowski's reagent. A solution used in testing urine for albumoses. It contains phosphotungstic acid.

Salkowski's test. 1. For cholesterol: mix a chloroform solution of substance with an equal volume of concentrated sulphuric acid. The chloroform shows shades of red to purple, and the acid exhibits a green fluorescence. 2. For creatinine; when excess acetic acid is added to the yellow solution obtained in Weyl's test and the solution is heated, a green colour changing to blue is given. 3. For carbon monoxide: add to blood, diluted with 20 volumes of water, a solution of sodium hydroxide (sp. gr. 1.34). In the presence of CO the sample turns cloudy and red.

Salmefamol (sal·mef·am·ol). BP Commission approved name for 1-(4-hydroxy-3-hydroxymethylphenyl)-2-(4-methoxy-α-methylphenethylamino)ethanol; a bronchodilator.

salmine (sal·meen). A protamine occurring in salmon sperm.

Salmonella (sal·mon·el·ah). A genus of the family Enterobacteriaceae; Gram-negative, non-sporing rods, usually motile, with peritrichate flagella. All species are active biochemically, and with one or two exceptions produce acid and gas from a number of carbohydrates; lactose is not fermented. The usual habitat is the gut of man and animals. They are pathogenic for man, animals and birds, causing typhoid fever, paratyphoid fever and food poisoning. Many somatic and flagellar antigens are shared by different species, and the majority of the species show diphasic variation of flagellar antigens, so that a final identification of an unknown organism can be made only by knowing its full antigenic formula. There are over 200 species, each identified by its antigenic structure. The Salmonellae are divisible into 2 main groups according to their primary hosts: 1. *Salmonella typhi, S. paratyphi A, B and C,* primary pathogens in man, which cause a clinical picture of a systemic infection with continued fever for 1-4 weeks and, usually, persistent diarrhoea. 2. All other Salmonellae, which are primary pathogens in a wide range of animals (mammals, birds, reptiles and amphibians) with a global distribution. Man may be secondarily infected, usually from heavily contaminated food, and the clinical picture is that of acute diarrhoea and vomiting of short duration and known as a form of bacterial food poisoning. The name of the city or area where an outbreak of Salmonella food poisoning has occurred, due to a newly identified serotype, is often attached to particular species, e.g. *Salmonella aberdeen, S. dublin, S. eastbourne, S. minnesota, S. montevideo, S. panama, S. poona, S. potsdam.* **Salmonella bovis mortificans.** A strain hitherto rare in the UK but it caused an extensive outbreak of food poisoning in Lancashire in 1953. **Salmonella brancaster.** A strain that caused an outbreak in a children's ward in a hospital in the London area in 1951. **Salmonella cholerae-suis.** The type species. **Salmonella dublin.** A natural pathogen of cattle which causes infection in man. **Salmonella enteritidis.** A species which causes food poisoning in man. **Salmonella infantis.** Probably identified with *S. virchow* (see below). **Salmonella london.** A food-poisoning strain isolated from various sources including spray-dried eggs. **Salmonella minnesota.** A strain that was responsible for an outbreak in Northamptonshire in 1951. **Salmonella paratyphi A, B and C.** The cause of paratyphoid fever. **Salmonella sendai.** A species isolated from cases of a typhoid-like fever in Japan, and again in Georgia. **Salmonella stanleyi.** A food-poisoning bacillus. **Salmonella typhi.** The cause of typhoid fever. **Salmonella typhimurium.** A natural pathogen of rodents which causes food poisoning in man. **Salmonella virchow.** A species isolated from a case of acute gastro-enteritis in Germany [Daniel Elmer *Salmon* (b. 1850), American pathologist.]

salmonellal (sal·mon·el·al). Caused by or pertaining to Salmonellae.

salmonellosis (sal·mon·el·**o**′·sis). Infection by Salmonellae. [*Salmonella*, Gk *-osis* condition.]

Salol BPC 1954 (**sa**·lol). Phenyl salicylate, $C_6H_4(OH)COOC_6H_5$. An internal antiseptic, once popular but now believed to be of little value. It was usually administered in cachets.

salolism (**sa**·lol·izm). Poisoning caused by excessive dosage of salol, the symptoms of phenol poisoning being more strongly predominant than those of salicylism.

Salomon, Hugo (b. 1872). German physician in Buenos Aires.

Salomon's test. *See* TEST FOR CANCER.

salop (**sa**·lop). Salep.

salophenin (sal·o·**fe**·nin). Acetylparamidosalol, $C_6H_4OHCOOC_6H_4NHCOCH_3$. A salicyl derivative of phenacetin, used in the treatment of sciatica, neuralgia, etc. but now obsolescent.

saloquinine salicylate (sal·o·**kwin**·een sal·**is**·il·ate). Rheumatin.

salpingectomy (sal·pin·**jek**·to·me). Excision of a uterine tube. [Gk *salpigx* tube, *ektome* a cutting out.]

salpingemphraxis (**sal**·pin·jem·**frax**′·is). 1. Obstruction of the uterine tube. 2. Obstruction of the pharyngotympanic tube. [Gk *salpigx* tube, emphraxis.]

salpingian, salpingic (sal·**pin**·je·an, sal·**pin**·jik). 1. Pertaining to a uterine tube. 2. Relating or belonging to a pharyngotympanic tube. [Gk *salpigx* tube.]

salpingion (sal·**pin**·je·on). In craniology, the apical point of the petrous part of the temporal bone on its inferior surface. [Gk *salpigx* tube.]

salpingitic (sal·pin·**jit**·ik). Relating or belonging to, or suffering from salpingitis.

salpingitis (sal·pin·**ji**·tis). Inflammation of the uterine (fallopian) tubes; sometimes applied also to inflammation of the pharyngotympanic (eustachian) tubes. **Acute salpingitis.** Acute inflammation of the uterine tubes. **Chronic salpingitis.** Chronic inflammation of the uterine tubes. **Follicular salpingitis.** Inflammation of the tube, leading to adhesions of the plicae and the formation of blind pockets within the tube. **Gonorrhoeal salpingitis.** Salpingitis caused by gonococci. **Salpingitis isthmica nodosa.** A condition in which there are nodular masses felt in the uterine tubes. The cause is uncertain. **Salpingitis profluens.** Salpingitis with a sudden discharge of fluid from secretions present in the uterine tubes. **Tuberculous salpingitis.** Infection of the uterine tubes with tuberculosis. This may be an endosalpingitis with the infection in the wall of the tube, or a perisalpingitis with subperitoneal tubercles only. [Gk *salpigx* tube, *-itis* inflammation.]

salpingocatheterism (**sal**·ping·go·**kath**′·et·er·izm). The procedure in which a catheter is passed into a pharyngotympanic (eustachian) tube. [Gk *salpigx* tube, catheter.]

salpingocele (sal·**ping**·go·seel). Hernia of a uterine tube. [Gk *salpigx* tube, *kele* hernia.]

salpingocyesis (sal·**ping**·go·si·e′·sis). Fallopian pregnancy. *See* PREGNANCY. [Gk *salpigx* tube, *kyesis* pregnancy.]

salpingogram (sal·**ping**·go·gram). The radiograph made during salpingography. [Gk *salpigx* tube, *gramma* record.]

salpingography (sal·ping·**gog**·raf·e). The radiographic visualization of the uterus and uterine tubes after the injection of an opaque oil or fluid through the neck of the uterus. [Gk *salpigx* tube, *graphein* to record.]

salpingolysis (sal·ping·**gol**·is·is). Breaking-down of adhesions in a uterine tube. [Gk *salpigx* tube, *lysis* a loosing.]

salpingomalleus (sal·**ping**·go·**mal**′·e·us). An obsolete name for the tensor tympani muscle. [Gk *salpigx* tube, malleus.]

salpingo-oöphorectomy (sal·**ping**·go·o·of·or·**ek**′·to·me). Excision of one of the uterine tubes and an ovary. [Gk *salpigx* tube, *oophoron* ovary, *ektome* a cutting out.]

salpingo-oöphoritis (sal·**ping**·go·o·of·or·**i**′·tis). Inflammation of a uterine tube and the associated ovary. [Gk *salpigx* tube, *oophoron* ovary, *-itis* inflammation.]

salpingo-oöphorocele (sal·**ping**·go·o·**of**′·or·o·seel). A hernia the contents of which are a uterine tube and its associated ovary. [Gk *salpigx* tube, *oophoron* ovary, *kele* hernia.]

salpingo-oöthecectomy (sal·**ping**·go·o·o·the·**sek**′·to·me). Salpingo-oöphorectomy. [Gk *salpigx* tube, *oon* egg, *theke* case, *ektome* a cutting out.]

salpingo-oöthecitis (sal·**ping**·go·o·o·the·**si**′·tis). Salpingo-oöphoritis. [Gk *salpigx* tube, *oon* egg, *theke* case, *-itis* inflammation.]

salpingo-oöthecocele (sal·**ping**·go·o·o·**the**′·ko·seel). Salpingo-oöphorocele. [Gk *salpigx* tube, *oon* egg, *theke* case, *kele* hernia.]

salpingo-ovariectomy, salpingo-ovariotomy (sal·**ping**·o·o·va·re·**ek**′·to·me sal·**ping**·go·o·va·re·**ot**′·o·me). Salpingo-oöphorectomy. [Gk *salpigx* tube, ovary, Gk *ektome* a cutting out.]

salpingo-ovaritis (sal·**ping**·go·o·var·**i**′·tis). Salpingo-oöphoritis. [Gk *salpigx* tube, ovary, Gk *-itis* inflammation.]

salpingopalatal, salpingopalatine (sal·**ping**·go·**pal**′·at·al, sal·**ping**·go·**pal**′·at·ine). Relating or belonging to a pharyngotympanic tube and the palate. [Gk *salpigx* tube, palate.]

salpingoperitonitis (sal·**ping**·go·per·e·ton·**i**′·tis). An inflammatory condition of that portion of peritoneum which is in association with a uterine tube. [Gk *salpigx* tube, peritonitis.]

salpingopexy (sal·**ping**·go·pex·e). Surgical fixation of the uterine tube. [Gk *salpigx* tube, *pexis* a fixation.]

salpingopharyngeal (sal·**ping**·o·far·**in**′·je·al). Relating or belonging to the pharyngotympanic tube and the pharynx. [Gk *salpigx* tube, pharynx.]

salpingopharyngeus muscle [musculus salpingopharyngeus (NA)] (sal·**ping**·go·far·**in**′·je·us musl). A muscle arising from the cartilage of the pharyngotympanic tube at its inner end and passing down in the wall of the pharynx to blend with the palatopharyngeus muscle. [Gk *salpigx* tube, pharynx.]

salpingoplasty (sal·**ping**·go·plas·te). Plastic surgery performed on a uterine tube. [Gk *salpigx* tube, *plassein* to form.]

salpingorrhaphy (sal·ping·**gor**·af·e). Operative repair by suture of the uterine tube. [Gk *salpigx* tube, *rhaphe* suture.]

salpingoscope (sal·**ping**·go·skope). An instrument used in the inspection of the pharyngotympanic tube and the nasal part of the pharynx. [Gk *salpigx* tube, *skopein* to watch.]

salpingoscopy (sal·ping·**gos**·ko·pe). Examination with a salpingoscope.

salpingostaphyline (sal·**ping**·go·**staf**′·il·ine). Relating or belonging to the pharyngotympanic tube and the uvula. [Gk *salpigx*, tube, *staphyle* uvula.]

salpingostaphylinus (sal·**ping**·go·staf·il·**i**′·nus). The tensor or levator palati muscles [Obsolete term.]. [see prec.]

salpingostenochoria (sal·**ping**·go·sten·o·**kor**′·e·ah). Stenosis of the pharyngotympanic tube. [Gk *salpigx* tube, stenochoria.]

salpingostomatoplasty (sal·ping·go·sto′·mat·o·plas·te). An operation in which a new abdominal ostium is made in the uterine tube. [Gk *salpigx* tube, *stoma* mouth, *plassein* to mould.]
salpingostomy (sal·ping·gos·to·me). An operation in which an opening is made into the uterine tube. [Gk *salpigx* tube, *stoma* mouth.]
salpingotomy (sal·ping·got·o·me). Incision of a uterine tube. [Gk *salpigx* tube, *temnein* to cut.]
salpingo-ureterostomy (sal·ping·go·ewr·e·ter·os′·to·me). The establishment of a passage between a uterine tube and a ureter. [Gk *salpigx* tube, ureter, Gk *stoma* mouth.]
salpingysterocyesis (sal·pin·jis·ter·o·si·e′·sis). Pregnancy at the uterine end of the uterine tube, within the uterus. [Gk *salpigx* tube, *hystera* womb, *kyesis* pregnancy.]
salpinx (sal·pingx). A tube; commonly the uterine (fallopian) tube, but also used for the pharyngotympanic (eustachian) tube. [Gk *salpigx.]*
salt (sawlt). 1. Common salt, sodium chloride. 2. A compound formed by a base with an acid, most commonly a metallic base with an inorganic acid; such salts are usually crystalline, soluble in water and good electrolytes, generally resembling common salt in appearance. 3. A mixture of several chemical salts, either natural or artificial, used in medicine. **Acid salt.** Any salt in which one or more of the acid hydrogen atoms remain unreplaced by basic atoms or radicals, e.g. $NaHSO_4$. **Alkaline salt.** A salt which shows an alkaline reaction with indicators. **Amphoteric salt.** A salt with both acid and base properties. **Bakers' salt.** Ammonium carbonate, sometimes used in baking. **Salts of barilla.** Impure sodium carbonate. **Basic salt.** A salt that contains oxygen or hydroxyl groups, and will combine with further acid to yield a neutral salt (see below); bismuth oxychloride, BiOCl, is an example. **Bay salt.** Sodium chloride from evaporated sea water, or sea salt. **Bile salt.** The sodium salts of glycocholic and taurocholic acids, occurring in bile. **Salt of bones.** Ammonium carbonate from the distillation of bones. **Buffer salt.** A salt of a weak acid with a strong base, or a weak base with a strong acid, which ionizes in solution in such a way that dilution or the addition of small quantities of acid or alkali do not affect the pH value of the solution. **Carlsbad salt.** A mixture of sodium sulphate, potassium sulphate, sodium chloride and sodium bicarbonate, obtained from the springs at Carlsbad or prepared artificially. It has diuretic and laxative properties, and is used in rheumatic diseases and as a tonic water. **Common salt.** Sodium chloride. **Complex salt.** A salt formed from 2 other salts but which gives a new ion in solution, e.g. potassium ferrocyanide which yields the ion $Fe(CN)_6^{4-}$. **Diuretic salt.** Potassium acetate. **Double salt.** Any salt formed from 2 other salts, but which still behaves as 2 salts in solution, though it may crystallize in a characteristic manner, e.g. alum, $K_2SO_4Al_2(SO_4)_3{\cdot}24H_2O$. **Effervescent salt.** A mixture of salts in an effervescent base of sodium bicarbonate with citric and tartaric acids. **Epsom salts.** Magnesium sulphate. **Halide salt, Haloid salt.** Any binary salt composed of a base and halogen element; a chloride, iodide, bromide or fluoride. **Kissingen salts.** The salts of the natural mineral springs at Kissingen in Germany. Artificial salts are made to resemble the natural salts in composition. **Salt of lemon.** Potassium quadroxalate. **Microcosmic salt.** Sodium ammonium phosphate. **Neutral salt, Normal salt.** A salt containing neither replaceable hydrogen atoms nor hydroxyl groups, e.g. Na_3SO_4. **Pancreatic salt.** A mixture of sodium chloride and pepsin, used as a digestant. **Peptic salt.** A mixture of sodium chloride and pepsin, used as a digestant. **Pink salt.** Tin ammonium chloride. **Potassium cyanide double salt.** Potassium sodium cyanide. **Rochelle salt.** Sodium potassium tartrate. **Rock salt.** Native sodium chloride with its impurities, as found in salt mines. **Sea salt.** Sodium chloride with other salts obtained when sea water is evaporated. **Secondary salt.** Neutral salt (see above). **Smelling salts.** Aromatized ammonium carbonate, with or without addition of ammonia, used as a stimulant and restorative, especially in the treatment of fainting. **Salt of soda.** Sodium carbonate. **Salt of sorrel.** Potassium quadroxalate. **Table salt.** Sodium chloride, with or without the addition of other salts or substances such as magnesium oxide, to make it free-running. *Iodized table salt* has had a small amount of iodide added to it and is valuable in districts where there is danger of endemic goitre due to low iodine content of the local drinking water. **Salt of tartar.** Potassium carbonate. **Tasteless purging salt.** Sodium phosphate. **Vichy salts.** The natural salts contained in Vichy water. Artifical salts are made to resemble the natural salts in composition. **Salt of vitriol.** Zinc sulphate. [AS *sealt.*]

See also: EVERITT, GLAUBER, MOHR, PLIMMER, PRESTON, REINECKE, SCHLIPPE.

salt sensitive (sawlt sen·sit·iv). Describing the spontaneous agglutination of certain bacteria when suspended in isotonic saline. [AS *sealt,* sensitive.]
saltation (sal·ta·shun). 1. Leaping movements, such as occur in saltatory spasm. 2. A genetic mutation; it is used when the difference between parent and offspring is relatively large. [L *saltare* to dance.]
saltative (sal·tat·iv). Of mutation or of evolution, proceeding by relatively large discrete steps. [see prec.]
saltatorial, saltatoric, saltatory (sal·tat·or·e·al, sal·tat·or·ik, sal·tat·or·e). Relating or belonging to saltation.
Salter, Robert B. 20th century Toronto orthopaedic surgeon.

Salter's osteotomy of the pelvis. Used in treatment of congenital dislocation of the hip. An osteotomy through the pelvis above the hip joint allowing the acetabulum to be redirected downwards, outwards and forwards and thus improving the cover of the head of the femur.

Salter, Sir Samuel James Augustus (b. 1825). London dental surgeon.

line of Salter. One of the incremental lines seen in cementum.

salting out (sawl·ting out). A procedure for the separating of protein fractions by precipitation, by the addition of salts (e.g. ammonium sulphate) of different degrees of concentration. The process is reversible, the precipitated protein redissolving if the salt is removed, e.g. by dialysis. [salt, As *ut.*]
saltpetre (sawlt·pe·ter). Nitre, potassium nitrate, KNO_3, used in pickling, medicine and the manufacture of gunpowder. **Air saltpetre.** Norge saltpetre (see below). **Chile saltpetre.** Sodium nitrate, $NaNO_3$, which occurs in vast deposits in Chile. **Norge saltpetre.** A fertilizer composed of calcium nitrate and nitrite produced in Norway by the arc process for the fixation of atmospheric nitrogen. **Wall saltpetre.** Calcium nitrate, $Ca(NO_3)_2$. [L *sal petrae* salt of the rock.]
saltrheum (sawlt·room). A colloquialism, particularly in the USA, meaning any of a variety of cutaneous eruptions, especially those of eczema. [salt, Gk *rheuma* stream.]
salts (sawltz). A saline cathartic. [AS *sealt.*]
salve (salv). An ointment. **Scarlet salve.** An ointment containing 5 per cent of scarlet red, which promotes epithelial growth, in a simple ointment base. [AS *sealf.*]
Salvia (sal·ve·ah). A genus of plants belonging to the family Labiatae, including sage, *Salvia officinalis* Linn. **Salvia reflexa.** Mint weed; a plant sometimes responsible for the poisoning of farm stock. [L sage.]
salvosal (sal·vo·sal). $C_6H_5OOCC_6H_4OPO(OH)_2$, a compound whose salts are used as diuretics. **Salvosal lithia.** A salt used in the treatment of gout. **Salvosal potash.** A salt with diuretic properties.
salysal (sal·is·al). Salicyl salicylate, $OHC_6H_4COOC_6H_4COOH$. A compound used for the same purposes as the other salicylates, but stated to have the advantage of not causing gastric disturbance as it is unaffected by gastric juice and is hydrolysed only in the duodenum.
Salzer, Fritz Adolf (b. 1858). Dutch surgeon.

Salzer's operation. An operation for large femoral hernias.

Salzman, Maximilian (b. 1862). Austrian ophthalmologist.

Salzman's nodular corneal dystrophy. Superficial corneal degeneration (non-familial) occurring in eyes previously affected by phlyctenular keratitis. Usually in females.

samandaridine (sam·an·dar·id·een). $C_{20}H_{31}ON$, a slightly toxic alkaloid obtained from the skin of salamanders.

samandarine (sam·an·der·een). $C_{19}H_{31}O_2N$, a toxic alkaloid obtained from the skin of salamanders.

samarium (sam·a·re·um). A rare-earth element of atomic weight 150.4, atomic number 62, and chemical symbol Sm. It is a very hard metal, with a high melting point, which occurs in the cerite earths and monazite sands. [Col. *Samarski,* Russian mining official.]

Sambucus (sam·bew·kus). 1. A genus of trees and shrubs, including the elder. 2. Sambuci flores, elder flowers, the dried corollas and stamens from the flowers of *Sambucus nigra* together with a proportion of buds, pedicels and ovaries. It contains about 3 per cent of volatile oil. *Aqua sambuci,* the distilled water, is a fragrant astringent used in eye and skin lotions. [L elder tree.]

sample (sahm·pl). A group of individuals drawn from a population. **Cluster sample.** A method of sampling that uses groups (or clusters) rather than individuals as the sampling unit. **Enriched sample.** A stratified sample in which the sampling fraction is disproportionately high in one or more strata. **Random sample.** A method of sampling in which each individual (or unit) in a population has an equal chance of being selected and in which the selection of one individual does not affect the chances of selection of other individuals in the population. **Stratified sample.** A method of sampling in which the population is divided into strata of known size according to some specified characteristic (e.g. sex, age, social class); random samples are then drawn from each stratum. [L *exemplum.*]

sampler (sahm·pler). **Slit sampler.** *See* SLIT-SAMPLER. [see prec.]

Sampson, John Albertson (b. 1873). Albany, New York, gynaecologist.

Sampson's cyst. A chocolate cyst of the ovary.

Sampson's endometrial implants. Small portions of the endometrium which by way of the uterine tubes reach the ovaries, the pelvic peritoneum or the uterus, and become implanted in them.

Sampson's cellular spill. In endometriosis: a theory of explanation of pelvic endometriosis where it is postulated that the endometrium cast off at menstruation passes through the uterine tubes by antiperistalsis and spills into the peritoneal cavity.

samshu (sam·shoo). A Chinese spirit prepared by the distillation of rice, or from sorghum. [*Samshui,* a port of southern China.]

Samways, Daniel West (b. 1857). English physician.

Samways' tourniquet. A rubber tourniquet kept taut by twisting one end around an anchor-like device attached to the other end.

Sanarelli, Guiseppe (b. 1864). Rome serologist.

Sanarelli virus. The virus of infectious myxomatosis; an infection of rabbits not known to be transmissible to man.

Sanarelli–Schwartzmann reaction. Schwartzmann reaction.

sanative (san·at·iv). Tending to heal; having a curative influence. [see foll.]

sanatorium (san·at·or·e·um). 1. An establishment for the treatment of persons suffering from chronic diseases, mental as well as physical, and as a place of recuperation for convalescent persons. In particular, the term is now used for those institutions where open-air treatment for tuberculous subjects is provided. 2. A locality in a tropical country selected as a health resort on account of its high altitude. 3. In institutions and large establishments, e.g. boarding schools, the room or rooms set aside for the treatment of the sick. [L *sanare* to restore to health.]

sanatory (san·at·or·e). Curative; sanative.

sand (sand). **Intestinal sand.** Small brown granules passed from the bowel and often associated with mucus casts. They consist of calcium soaps and calcium phosphate. [AS.]

sandal wood (san·dal wud). White sanders; the dried wood of the yellow sandal wood tree, *Santalum album* (family Santalaceae), a small tree indigenous to India. It yields a volatile oil, which gives it its strong fragrant odour, containing santalol, a stimulant and disinfectant of the urogenital system. **Red sandal wood.** Red sanders wood, pterocarpus, the heartwood of *Pterocarpus santalinus* Linn. which yields a red dye, santalin (santalic acid). [Sanskrit *candana* shining, AS *wudu.*]

sandarac (san·dar·ak). The resin obtained from *Tetraclinis articulata* (Vahl) Masters (family Cupressaceae), a small tree of North-west Africa. It contains a resin associated with traces of a volatile oil and a bitter principle; the chief constituent of the resin is pimaric acid. It is used for making varnishes. [Gk *sandarake* realgar.]

sandaracin (san·dar·as·in). An oleoresin from sandarac used in pill varnishes.

Sander, Wilhelm (b.1838). German psychiatrist.

Sander's disease. Paranoia.

Sanders, Murray (b. 1910). New York bacteriologist.

Sanders' disease. An infectious virus disease, starting with severe follicular conjunctivitis and followed by the formation of punctate corneal lesions; epidemic keratoconjunctivitis.

Sanders, R. D. 20th century American anaesthetist.

Sanders injector. An apparatus for the entrainment of air by a high-pressure jet of oxygen, used to ventilate the patient during bronchoscopy under general anaesthesia, in the presence of apnoea.

sanders (san·derz). Sandal wood.

sandfly (sand·fli). *Culicoides, Pericoma, Phlebotomus.*

sandix (san·dix). A form of red lead, Pb_3O_4, which occurs as a red powder and is used in paint as a pigment. [Gk vermilion.]

sandrock test. The application of friction to the skin normally results in dilatation of skin capillaries and a flush. This may be delayed or absent in the presence of disease of the skin vessels.

Sandström, Ivan Victor (b. 1852). Upsala anatomist.

Sandström's bodies or glands. The parathyroid glands. *See* GLAND.

Sandwith, Fleming Mant (b. 1853). British physician.

Sandwith's bald tongue. The deep-red, beefsteak tongue of advanced pellagra. The original use of the term has also been attributed to other tropical workers.

sangaree (sang·gar·ee). A cold drink containing wine, diluted with lemon water or spices, or both, and used in tropical countries. [Sp. *sangria.*]

sanguicolous (sang·gwik·o·lus). Applied to certain parasites that inhabit the blood of living organisms. [L *sanguis* blood, *colere* to dwell in.]

sanguifacient (sang·gwe·fa·shent). Taking part in or belonging to the formation of blood. [L *sanguis* blood, *facere* to produce.]

sanguiferous (sang·gwif·er·us). In physiology, containing or conveying blood; circulatory. [L *sanguis* blood, *ferre* to carry.]

sanguification (sang·gwif·ik·a'·shun). Haemopoiesis. [L *sanguis* blood, *facere* to produce.]

sanguinaria (sang·gwin·a·re·ah). Bloodroot; the dried rhizome, deprived of its roots, of *Sanguinaria canadensis* Linn. (family Papaveraceae), a small woodland plant found in eastern USA and Canada. Its chief constituent is the alkaloid, sanguinarine. [L *sanguis* blood.]

sanguinarine (sang·gwin·ar·een). $C_{20}H_{13}O_4N$, the principal alkaloid of bloodroot, *Sanguinaria canadensis* Linn. The name is also applied to a crude resinoid extractive of the root.

sanguine (sang·gwin). 1. Full-blooded; plethoric. 2. Full of vitality and confidence. 3. Blood-red. [L *sanguis* blood.]

sanguineous (sang·gwin·e·us). 1. Relating to or containing blood; bloody. 2. Belonging to the blood. 3. Full-blooded. [see prec.]

sanguinolent (sang·gwin·o·lent). Tinged with blood; of a blood-red tinge; bloody. [L *sanguinolentus* full of blood.]

sanguinopoietic (sang·gwin·o·poi·et'·ik). Haemopoietic. [L *sanguis,* Gk *poiein* to make.]

sanguirenal (sang·gwe·re·nal). Relating or belonging to the blood and the kidneys. [L *sanguis* blood, *ren* kidney.]

sanguivorous (sang·gwiv·or·us). Feeding on blood; applied to insects. [L *sanguis* blood, *vorare* to devour.]

sanies (sa·ne·eez). A thin fetid seropurulent discharge from a wound or ulcer. [L.]

saniopurulent (sa·ne·o·pewr′·ew·lent). Both sanious and purulent.

sanioserous (sa·ne·o·seer′·us). Of a discharge, both sanious and serous in character.

sanious (sa·ne·us). Relating to or having the character or appearance of sanies.

sanitarian (san·it·a·re·an). An authority on the science of sanitation and public health; a hygienist. [L *sanitas* health.]

sanitarium (san·it·a·re·um). Sanatorium.

sanitary (san·it·ar·e). 1. Relating or belonging to health and hygiene. 2. Conducive to the restoration or maintenance of health. [see foll.]

sanitation (san·it·a·shun). 1. The science of the maintenance of healthful and hygienic conditions of the environment. 3. The employment of sanitary measures. [L *sanitas* health.]

sanity (san·it·e). The state of being of sound mind. [see prec.]

sanoderma (san·o·der·mah). A bandage impregnated with bismuth subnitrate.

Sansevieria (san·sev·i·eer′·e·ah). A genus of East Indian liliaceous plants. **Sansevieria zeylanicum.** Bowstring hemp, murva, ghannasaphan; the juice of the roots and leaves is used as an expectorant and in snake bite, especially that of the Ghannas snake. [*Sanseviero* (b. 1710), Prince of Naples.]

Sansom, Arthur Ernest (b. 1838). London physician.

Sansom's sign. Dullness to percussion to the right and left of the sternum in the 2nd and 3rd intercostal spaces in pericardial effusion.

Sanson, Louis Joseph (b. 1790). Paris physician and surgeon.

Purkinje–Sanson images. The 3 images formed by the anterior surfaces of the cornea and the anterior and posterior surfaces of the lens, respectively, when a light source is held in front of the eye. They are of historical interest, as the alteration in the size and position of the latter 2 on accommodation proved that this was due to alteration in curvature of the lens.

santal (san·tal). Sandal wood.

santalal (san·tal·al). $C_{14}H_{23}CHO$, an aldehyde which is a constituent of oil of sandal wood.

santalin (san·tal·in). Santalic acid, santalenic acid, $C_{15}H_{25}O_5$. A red colouring matter obtained from red sandal wood, *Pterocarpus santalinus.*

santalol (san·tal·ol). $C_{15}H_{23}OH$, a mixture of 2 alcoholic sesquiterpene isomers found as the chief constituent of oil of sandal wood.

santalum (san·tal·um). Sandal wood. **Santalum rubrum.** The heartwood of *Pterocarpus santalinus* (family Leguminoseae) which contains a red colouring principle, santalin, used for colouring compound tincture of lavender. [Sanskrit *candana* shining.]

santalwood (san·tal·wud). Sandal wood.

santalyl (san·tal·il). The monovalent group, $C_{15}H_{23}$–, derived from santalol. **Santalyl salicylate.** The salicylic ester of santalol formerly used in gonorrhoea.

sante manoeuvre. A treatment procedure in collapse of the lung in which the patient is rolled from side to side until he coughs violently and causes re-expansion of the lung.

santheose (san·the·oze). An alternative and uncommon name for theobromine.

santobrite (san·to·brite). Sodium pentachlorophenate.

santonica (san·ton·ik·ah). Wormseed; the dried, unexpanded heads of *Artemisia cina* Berg. (family Compositae), a small shrub native to Turkestan. It contains from 2 to 3.5 per cent of santonin, and has been used as a vermifuge for roundworms. [Gk *santonikon* wormwood.]

Santonin BP 1963 (san·ton·in). $C_{15}H_{18}O_3$, a crystalline lactone of bicyclic sesquiterpene structure, obtained from the unexpanded flower heads of certain species of *Artemisia,* and a constituent of wormseed. It is insoluble in water, but soluble in alcohol, and is anthelminthic, being effective against roundworms but not against tapeworms. [see prec.]

santoninoxime (san·ton·in·ox′·ime). $C_{15}H_{18}O_2$=NOH, the oxime of santonin, used for the same purpose as the latter.

santonism (san·ton·izm). Poisoning caused by excessive dosage of santonin.

Santorini, Giovanni Domenico (b. 1681). Venice physician and anatomist.

Santorini's canal, duct of Santorini. The accessory pancreatic duct.

Santorini's capitulum. Santorini's tubercle (see below).

Santorini's cartilage. The corniculate cartilage of the larynx.

Santorini's carunculae. The caruncula major, that is the duodenal papilla, an elevation of mucous membrane surrounding the opening of the common bile duct and main pancreatic duct into the duodenum, and the caruncula minor, a similar elevation around the orifice of the accessory pancreatic duct.

Santorini's clefts, fissures or incisures. Clefts in the fibrocartilage of the tragus and external auditory meatus.

concha Santorini. The highest nasal concha; a small supernumerary concha in the spheno-ethmoidal recess of the nose, above the superior nasal concha.

corpus Santorini. Santorini's cartilage (see above).

Santorini's plexus. 1. The prostatic (venous) plexus. 2. The *retiform plexus of Santorini* is a term sometimes applied to the mandibular division and motor root of the trigeminal nerve where they are loosely fascicular in structure above the foramen ovale.

Santorini's tubercle. The elevation within the larynx caused by the corniculate cartilage.

Santorini's veins. The parietal emissary veins.

sap (sap). The fluid part of a cell; the fluid which circulates in the conducting tissues of a plant. **Cell sap.** The undifferentiated fluid portion of the cytoplasm of a cell. **Nuclear sap.** The fluid part of a cell nucleus surrounding the chromosomes and nucleolus. [AS *saep.*]

saphena (saf·e·nah). Referring to either the long or the short saphenous veins. [Gk *saphenes* manifest.]

saphenectomy (saf·e·nek·to·me). Resection of a part of one of the saphenous veins in the treatment of varicose veins. [saphenous vein, Gk *ektome* a cutting out.]

saphenous (saf·e·nus). Applied to certain structures in the leg, e.g. nerve vein. [Gk *saphenes* manifest.]

saphenous nerve [nervus saphenus (NA)]. A large sensory branch of the femoral nerve, given off in the subsartorial canal and descending medial to the knee to run close to the saphenous vein and supply the skin on the medial side of the leg and foot.

Infrapatellar branch [ramus infrapatellaris (NA)]. A branch of the saphenous nerve at the knee supplying the skin in front of the patella. It takes part in the formation of the infrapatellar plexus of nerves.

saphenous veins. Superficial veins of the foot and leg. **Accessory saphenous vein [vena saphena accessoria (NA)].** A frequent branch of the short saphenous vein which runs from the popliteal fossa to join the long saphenous vein in the thigh. **Long saphenous vein [vena saphena magna].** The main superficial vein of the lower limb, commencing at the dorsum of the foot and passing over the ankle to the back of the calf and knee and thence to the front of the thigh; a tributary of the femoral vein. This, and its tributaries, are frequently subject to thrombosis and varicosities. It possesses many valves, which are often incompetent, particularly in the elderly. **Short saphenous vein [vena saphena parva (NA)].** The main superficial vein draining the lateral side of the foot and the back of the leg. It begins at the lateral side of the dorsal venous arch of the foot and terminates by going deep to enter the popliteal vein.

sapid (sap·id). 1. Having or giving flavour; palatable. 2. Able to affect the organs of taste. [L *sapidus* savoury.]

sapidity (sap·id·it·e). The intrinsic factor in any substance that gives it its taste. [see prec.]

sapiphore (sap·e·for). Any chemical group considered to bestow sweetness on the molecule containing it. [L *sapor* taste, Gk *phorein* to bear.]

sapo (sa·po). Soap. **Sapo animalis.** Curd soap. *See* SOAP. **Sapo durus.** Hard soap. *See* SOAP. **Sapo kalinus.** Potash soap. *See*

SOAP. **Sapo mollis.** Soft soap. *See* SOAP. **Sapo mollis viridis, Sapo viridis.** Green soft soap. *See* SOAP, SOFT. [L.]

sapogenin (sap·oj·en·in). Any aglycone produced when a saponin is hydrolysed. It may be steriod or triterpenoid in structure, depending upon the original saponin. [L *sapo* soap, Gk *genein* to produce.]

Sapolini, Guiseppe (b. 1812). Italian anatomist.

Sapolini's nerve. The sensory root of the facial nerve.

saponaceous (sap·on·a·shus). Resembling or having the character or quality of soap. [L *sapo* soap.]

saponaria (sap·on·a·re·ah). Soaproot; the leaves and roots of *Saponaria officinalis* (family Caryophyllaceae). Its chief constituent is saponin. [see prec.]

saponatus (sap·on·a·tus). Mixed with soap. [L *sapo* soap.]

saponification (sap·on·if·ik·a'·shun). 1. The making of a soap; the action of an alkali on a fat to produce salts of the fatty acids present and free glycerol. 2. In general, the hydrolysis of an ester into an alcohol and acid, which latter forms a salt with the alkali producing the reaction. [L *sapo* soap, *facere* to make.]

saponiform (sap·on·e·form). Having the appearance and consistency of soap. [L *sapo* soap, form.]

saponify (sap·on·e·fi). 1. To make into a soap. 2. To bring about the chemical process of soap formation. [L *sapo* soap, *facere* to make.]

saponin, saponinum (sap·on·in, sap·on·i·num). A group of plant glycosides, so called because they lower the surface tension of aqueous solutions, like soap, and froth copiously when shaken. They are powerfully toxic and cause haemolysis of red blood corpuscles. On hydrolysis they yield 1 or more sugars and a sugar-free aglycone, or sapogenin. **Steroid saponin.** A saponin which yields a sapogenin related to cholesterol, i.e. of steroid structure. **Triterpenoid saponin.** A saponin which yields on hydrolysis a sapogenin which is a triterpene derivative; hederagenin is an example. [L *sapo* soap.]

saponule, saponulus (sap·on·ewl, sap·on·ew·lus). A pseudo-soap from an essential oil with an alkali. [see prec.]

saporific (sap·or·if·ik). 1. Capable of giving rise to the sensation of taste. 2. Applied to any substance that gives flavour or taste to another. [L *sapor* taste, *facere* to make.]

saporosity (sap·or·os·it·e). Sapidity. [L *sapor* taste.]

sapotalene (sap·o·tal·een). Trimethylnaphthalene, $C_{13}H_{14}$. A hydrocarbon derived from triterpenes, and also by the dehydrogenation of sapogenins of the triterpenoid type.

sapotoxin (sap·o·tox·in). $C_{17}H_{26}O_{10}$, a toxic saponin present in quillaia bark.

Sappey, Marie Philibert Constant (b. 1810). Paris anatomist.

Sappey's fibres. Smooth muscle fibres in the orbital check ligaments.

Sappey's plexus. A lymphatic plexus beneath the areola of the mammary gland.

accessory portal system of Sappey. A compensatory anastomosis between the veins in the liver or its capsule and general systemic veins such as the phrenic and intercostals. These are seen where the liver and diaphragm are uncovered by peritoneum, in the falciform ligament and in any peritoneal adhesions which may be present.

Sappey's veins. Veins in the falciform ligament which connect the portal and systemic venous systems.

sapphism (saf·izm). Homosexuality in the female. [Gk poetess *Sappho.*]

sapraemia (sap·re·me·ah). The form of toxaemia resulting from the absorption of bacterial toxins and the products of tissue destruction, without invasion of the blood stream by the organisms themselves which remain and multiply at the local site of invasion. [Gk *sapros* rotten, *haima* blood.]

sapraemic (sap·re·mik). Pertaining to, having the character of, or suffering from sapraemia.

saprodontia (sap·ro·don·she·ah). Dental caries. [Gk *sapros* rotten, *odous* tooth.]

saprogen (sap·ro·jen). Any micro-organism having putrefactive powers. [see foll.]

saprogenic, saprogenous (sap·ro·jen·ik, sap·roj·en·us). 1. Capable of producing, or resulting from putrefaction. 2. Relating or belonging to the instigation of a process of decay. 3. Originating in putrefying material. [Gk *sapros* rotten, *genein* to produce.]

saprophagous (sap·rof·ag·us). In zoology, feeding on decaying matter. [Gk *sapros* rotten, *phagein* to eat.]

saprophilous (sap·rof·il·us). Denoting certain micro-organisms which subsist on putrefying and dead matter. [Gk *sapros* rotten, *philein* to love.]

saprophyte (sap·ro·fite). Any vegetable organism that subsists on dead or putrefying organic matter and not on living tissue. Cf. AUTOPHYTE. [Gk *sapros* rotten, *phyton* plant.]

saprophytic (sap·ro·fit·ik). Relating, belonging to, or characteristic of a saprophyte.

Saprospira (sap·ro·spi·rah). A genus of the family Spirochaetaceae, characterized by a spiral protoplasm without evident axial filament. They are free-living in marine ooze, and are found in the intestinal canal of oysters. [Gk *sapros* rotten, *speira* coil.]

saprozoic (sap·ro·zo·ik). Living in dead or decaying organic matter, said of certain protozoa. [Gk *sapros* rotten, *zoon* animal.]

saprozoite (sap·ro·zo·ite). A non-parasitic protozoon, that is one that does not need a living host in order to maintain existence. [see prec.]

saraka (sar·ak·ah). Granules of bassora gum, a gum of uncertain origin, and frangula bark.

sarapus (sar·ap·us). A flat-footed person. [Gk *sarapous* splay-footed.]

Sarason's bath. A form of oxygen bath; an ozet bath.

Sarbó, Arthur von (b. 1867). Budapest neurologist.

Sarbó's sign. Analgesia in the distribution of the peroneal nerve, occasionally seen in tabes dorsalis, and often in sciatica due to a prolapsed intervertebral disc.

sarcidium (sar·sid·e·um). A fleshy outgrowth. [Gk *sarx* flesh.]

sarcin (sar·sin). A bacterial cell aggregation consisting of a packet of 8 cells in the form of a cube produced by the division of a bacterium in 3 planes. It typifies the genus Sarcina. [L *sarcina* bundle.]

Sarcina (sar·sin·ah). A genus of bacteria belonging to the family Micrococcaceae, characterized by division in 3 planes during multiplication, producing regular packets. They are usually Gram-positive, and their growth on agar is abundant, often with production of a yellow or orange pigment. 9 species have been fully described and investigated and a large number of other named species appear in the literature, mostly inadequately described, many of which are probably synonyms. **Sarcina aurantiaca.** A species which forms a yellow to orange-red growth on agar, is non-pathogenic and is found in air and water; it has also been isolated from beer. **Sarcina citrea.** A motile, non-pathogenic species which forms a citron-yellow to orange growth; it is found in the air. **Sarcina flava.** A species which produces a yellow pigment, is non-pathogenic and is found in air, water, soil and in beer and cheese. **Sarcina littoralis.** A species which produces a coral-red growth on starch media, is non-pathogenic and occurs in sea water. **Sarcina lutea.** A species which produces a yellow pigment, is non-pathogenic and is found in air, soil, water, on potatoes and on skin surfaces. **Sarcina maxima.** A species in which the cocci measure from 4 to 5 μm in diameter. It is non-pathogenic and is isolated from fermenting malt mash; it is also found in wheat bran and occasionally in soils. **Sarcina methanica.** A strict anaerobe, non-pathogenic and found in the sediment from methane fermentation, in mud and fermenting sewage sludge. **Sarcina ureae.** A species which forms a yellow growth, converts urea into ammonium carbonate and is non-pathogenic. It is isolated from urine. **Sarcina ventriculi.** The type species; it is non-pathogenic and is found in garden soil, dust, sand and in the human stomach. [L *bundle.]*

sarcine (sar·sine). A cube of 8 or 64 bacterial cells produced by the growth and multiplication of sarcinae in three planes. [see prec.]

sarcinic (sar·sin·ik). 1. Relating to the genus *Sarcina.* 2. Due to the presence of sarcinae.

sarcinuria (sar·sin·ewr·e·ah). The presence of sarcin in the urine.

sarcitis (sar·si·tis). Myositis. [Gk *sarx* flesh, *-itis* inflammation.]

sarco-adenoma (sar·ko·ad·en·o'·mah). Adenosarcoma; a tumour of mixed adenomatous and sarcomatous tissue.

sarcobiont (sar·ko·bi·ont). A micro-organism that lives on flesh. [Gk *sarx* flesh, *bios* life, *on* being.]

sarcoblast (sar·ko·blast). The primitive cellular element from which a muscle cell is derived. [Gk *sarx* flesh, *blastos* germ.]

sarcocarcinoma (sar·ko·kar·sin·o'·mah). 1. A mixed tumour composed of elements of carcinoma and sarcoma. 2. A tumour transitional between carcinoma and sarcoma.

sarcocele (sar·ko·seel). Any swelling or tumour of the testicles, whether of infective or neoplastic origin. **Syphilitic sarcocele.** A gummatous swelling of the testis. [Gk *sarx* flesh, *kele* tumour.]

Sarcocephalus (sar·ko·kef·al·us). A genus of the family Rubiaceae, including *Sarcocephalus esculentus,* the bark of which contains an alkaloid. [Gk *sarx* flesh, *kephale* head.]

sarcocyst (sar·ko·sist). Miescher's tube, Rainey's corpuscle; an elongated tubular body produced by species of *Sarcocystis.* They occur in the muscle fibres of many mammals.

sarcocystin (sar·ko·sis·tin). A toxic substance produced in the bodies of certain species of *Sarcocystis.*

Sarcocystis (sar·ko·sis·tis). A genus of Sarcosporidia; a group of muscle-inhabiting, spore-forming protozoa, found mainly in the muscle fibres of pigs, mice, sheep, cattle, horses and, rarely, in man. **Sarcocystis blanchardi.** A species found in cattle. **Sarcocystis lindemanni.** A species found as a parasite in man. **Sarcocystis muris.** A species found in mice. **Sarcocystis tenella.** A parasite of sheep, cattle and buffaloes. [Gk *sarx* flesh, *kystis* bladder.]

Sarcodina (sar·ko·di·nah). Rhizopoda, Amoeba; a class of Protozoa which move by protoplasmic protrusions called pseudopodia, and multiply by binary fission in the vegetative stage and by encystation. [Gk *sarkodes* fleshlike.]

sarco-enchondroma (sar·ko·en·kon·dro'·mah). A sarcoma with incorporation of cartilaginous elements; growth is usually rapid. [sarcoma, enchondroma.]

sarcogenic, sarcogenous (sar·ko·jen·ik, sar·koj·en·us). Flesh-forming. [Gk *sarx* flesh, *genein* to produce.]

sarcohydrocele (sar·ko·hi·dro·seel). A fleshy tumour of the testicle combined with a hydrocele. [Gk *sarx* flesh, hydrocele.]

sarcoid (sar·koid). A cutaneous lesion occurring as a manifestation of sarcoidosis. The term is also used as a synonym for sarcoidosis itself. **Multiple benign sarcoid.** Boeck's sarcoid. [Gk *sarx* flesh, *eidos* form.]

See also: BOECK (C. P. M.), DARIER, ROUSSY, SCHAUMANN, SPIEGLER.

sarcoidosis (sar·koid·o·sis). A generalized granulomatous disease, involving the reticulo-endothelial system, whose lesions predominate in the lymphatic system, the lymphatic glands, tonsils, bone marrow, spleen, lungs and liver; the skin may or may not be affected. The cause is disputed. Under this term may be included multiple benign sarcoid or miliary lupoïd of Boeck, the angiolupoid of Brocq and Pautrier, and lupus pernio. Schaumann's sarcoid is the same as sarcoidosis. Sarcoidosis may also affect the pituitary gland, causing hypopituitarism, and in some cases the thyroid and adrenals, as well as causing the "multiglandular syndrome". **Annular sarcoidosis.** Sarcoidal skin lesions with central clearing, leaving ring forms. **Beryllium sarcoidosis.** A serious pneumonitis, histologically identical with sarcoidosis, produced by exposure to beryllium dust. **Erythematous sarcoidosis.** A diffuse, maculopapular type of cutaneous sarcoidosis. **Erythrodermatous sarcoidosis.** A rare form of sarcoidosis, first described by Schaumann, in which there is erythroderma and widespread lymphadenopathy. **Nodular sarcoidosis.** Sarcoidosis nodules in the skin or, as in the Darier-Roussy type, under the skin. **Papular sarcoidosis.** A small nodular cutaneous sarcoidosis. **Scar sarcoidosis.** Sarcoidosis developing in a scar. [sarcoid, Gk *-osis* condition.]

sarcolactate (sar·ko·lak·tate). Any salt of sarcolactic acid.

sarcolemma (sar·ko·lem·ah). The plasma membrane of a smooth, striated or cardiac muscle fibre. [Gk *sarx* flesh, *lemma* sheath.]

sarcolemmic, sarcolemmous (sar·ko·lem·ik, sar·ko·lem·us). Relating or belonging to or having the character of sarcolemma.

sarcoleukaemia (sar·ko·lew·ke'·me·ah). Leucosarcoma, lymphosarcoma-cell leukaemia; a form of lymphosarcoma having a leukaemoid type of blood picture. [sarcoma, leukaemia.]

sarcology (sar·kol·o·je). 1. The anatomy of the soft tissues of the body. 2. Myology. [Gk *sarx* flesh, *logos* science.]

sarcolysis (sar·kol·is·is). Any breaking-up or maceration of fleshy tissue. [Gk *sarx* flesh, *lysis* a loosing.]

sarcolytic (sar·ko·lit·ik). 1. Relating or belonging to sarcolysis. 2. Able to disintegrate flesh. [see prec.]

sarcoma (sar·ko·mah) (pl. *sarcomata*). A malignant tumour of connective tissue or its derivatives. **Adipose sarcoma.** A sarcoma arising within adipose tissue. **Alveolar sarcoma.** Endothelioma. **Angiolithic sarcoma.** Psammoma. **Angioplastic sarcoma.** A sarcoma in which there is a striking tendency to form blood vessels; a testicular teratoma or syncytioma. **Botyroid sarcoma.** A sarcoma of the neck of the uterus which resembles clusters of grapes. **Sarcoma carcinomatodes.** A mixed tumour in which both sarcoma and carcinoma are found. **Chicken sarcoma.** Rous sarcoma, a fowl sarcoma caused by a filtrable virus. **Chloromatous sarcoma.** A green-pigmented lymphoma, usually malignant. **Cylindromatous sarcoma.** Perithelioma. **Deciduocellular sarcoma, Sarcoma deciduocellulare.** Chorionepithelioma. **Encephaloid sarcoma.** A soft, rapidly-growing sarcoma. **Sarcoma epithelioides.** An endothelioma of lymph glands resembling sarcoma and carcinoma in its cellular pattern. **Sarcoma epulis.** Osteoclastoma of the jaw. **Fusocellular sarcoma.** A sarcoma made up of elongated spindle-shaped cells. **Giant-cell sarcoma.** Osteoclastoma. **Glandular sarcoma.** Hodgkin's disease. **Granulation sarcoma.** A sarcoma composed of round cells. **Leucocytic sarcoma.** Leukaemia. **Sarcoma lipomatodes, Lipomatous sarcoma.** A sarcoma arising within adipose tissue; adipose sarcoma. **Sarcoma lymphadenoides.** Hodgkin's disease. **Lymphatic sarcoma.** Lymphangio-endothelioma. **Lymphoblastic sarcoma.** Lymphoblastic lymphoma; a highly malignant tumour composed of primitive lymphocytes or lymphoblasts, arising most often in lymph glands. **Mammary sarcoma.** Sarcomatous transformation of the connective tissue of the breast. **Mastoid sarcoma.** A sarcoma of the breast. **Medullary sarcoma.** Encephaloid sarcoma (see above). **Melanotic sarcoma.** A sarcoma in which the cells contain melanin. **Mixed-cell sarcoma.** A sarcoma composed of round, spindle and giant cells. **Sarcoma molle.** Lymphosarcoma. **Sarcoma molluscum.** Neurofibromatosis; von Recklinghausen's disease. **Multiple haemorrhagic sarcoma, Multiple idiopathic haemorrhagic sarcoma.** Kaposi's disease. **Myelogenic sarcoma, Myeloid sarcoma.** Osteoclastoma. **Sarcoma myxomatodes.** Myxosarcoma. **Net-cell sarcoma.** Malignant tumours of reticulo-endothelial cells, especially found in the lymph glands. **Neurogenic sarcoma.** A malignant tumour of nerve trunks. **Osteoblastic sarcoma.** A bone sarcoma composed of embryonic bone cells. **Osteogenic sarcoma.** A sarcoma which forms much new bone as it grows. **Osteoid sarcoma.** A variety of osteogenic sarcoma. **Osteolytic sarcoma.** A sarcoma which destroys bone as it grows. **Parosteal sarcoma.** An osteogenic sarcoma arising from the surface of a long bone and characterized by extensive and well-formed new bone developing over the outer cortex of the involved bone. It is usually well demarcated and is thought to have a better prognosis than other osteogenic sarcomata. **Periosteal sarcoma.** Sarcoma arising from the periosteum. **Periosteal spindle-cell sarcoma.** A sarcoma composed mainly of spindle-celled connective-tissue cells arising from periosteum. **Sarcoma phyllodes.** Adenofibroma of the breast. **Polymorphous sarcoma.** Mixed-cell sarcoma (see above). **Reticulo-endothelial sarcoma.** Reticulo-endothelioma; a tumour composed of reticulo-endothelial cells in the spleen, lymph nodes or skin. **Reticulum-cell sarcoma, Retothelial sarcoma.** The most primitive (in cell type) of lymphosarcoma. **Retroperitoneal sarcoma.** A rather slow-growing, mixed-cell sarcoma arising from the retroperitoneal tissues. **Round-cell sarcoma.** Granulation sarcoma (see above). **Sclerosing osteogenic sarcoma.** A sarcoma that forms much fibrous tissue and bone. **Sarcoma scroti.** Sarcocele. **Serocystic sarcoma.** Serous cystic disease of the ovary. **Spindle-cell sarcoma.** Fusocellular sarcoma (see above). **Telangiectatic sarcoma.** Angiosarcoma; a sarcoma in which the blood vessels are particularly large and prominent. **Thymic sarcoma.** A malignant tumour of the thymus gland that imitates sarcoma or carcinoma, or sometimes both together. [Gk *sarx* flesh, *-oma* tumour.]

See also: ABERNETHY, EWING, HODGKIN, JENSEN (C. O.), KAPOSI, MUELLER (J.), ROUS, WALKER.

sarcomagenic (sar·ko·mah·**jen**'·ik). Causing the development of sarcoma. [sarcoma, Gk *genein* to produce.]

sarcomatoid (sar·**ko**·mat·oid). Having the appearance of a sarcoma. [sarcoma, Gk *eidos* form.]

sarcomatosis (sar·ko·mat·**o**'·sis). The condition in which a number of sarcomata develop here and there on the body. **Sarcomatosis cutis.** A condition characterized by the formation of sarcomata on the skin. **General sarcomatosis.** The formation of multiple sarcomata in different parts of the body. [sarcoma, Gk *-osis* condition.]

sarcomatous (sar·**ko**·mat·us). 1. Relating or belonging to sarcoma. 2. Resembling sarcoma in character.

sarcomelanin (sar·ko·**mel**·an·in). The black pigmentary elements to be found in melanosarcoma. [sarcoma, *melas* black.]

sarcomere (**sar**·ko·meer). The repeating structural unit of a striated muscle fibre, the segment lying between two Z lines. [Gk *sarx* flesh, *meros* part.]

sarcomphalocele (sar·kom·**fal**·o·seel). A hard fleshy tumour of the umbilicus, or involving it. [Gk *sarx* flesh, omphalocele.]

sarcomyces (sar·ko·**mi**·seez). Any fleshy neoplasm with fungoid characteristics. [Gk *sarx* flesh, *mykes* fungus.]

Sarcophaga (sar·**kof**·ag·ah). A genus of flies of the family Sarcophagidae; flesh flies. All species are viviparous and most larviposit on decaying organic matter. The larvae of many species have occurred in intestinal and cutaneous myiasis throughout the world. They may also act as mechanical transmitters of infection. *S. carnaria* is the commonest flesh fly of Europe. Some of the more important species are *S. barbata, S. bullata, S. dux, S. fuscicauda, S. haemorrhoidalis, S. placida* and *S. ruficornis.* [Gk *sarx* flesh, *phagein* to eat.]

sarcophagid (sar·ko·**faj**·id). Flesh eating; applied to certain flies. [see foll.]

Sarcophagidae (sar·ko·**faj**·id·e). A family of flesh-feeding diptera, the larvae of some of which, e.g. *Wohlfahrtia magnifica,* may cause myiasis in man. [Gk *sarx* flesh, *phagein* to eat, *eidos* form.]

sarcoplasm (**sar**·ko·plazm). The cytoplasmic matrix of a smooth, striated or cardiac muscle cell in which the contractile elements are embedded.

sarcoplasmic (sar·ko·**plaz**·mik). 1. Relating or belonging to sarcoplasm. 2. Containing or composed of sarcoplasm.

sarcoplast (**sar**·ko·plast). An embryonic muscle cell or myoblast [Obsolete term.]. [Gk *sarx* flesh, *plassein* to form.]

sarcoplastic (sar·ko·**plas**·tik). Capable of forming muscle tissue. [see prec.]

sarcopoietic (sar·ko·poi·**et**'·ik). Sarcoplastic. [Gk *sarx* flesh, *poiein* to produce.]

sarcopsylla (sar·ko·**sil**·ah). *Tunga.* [Gk *sarx* flesh, *psylla* flea.]

Sarcoptes (sar·**kop**·teez). A genus of Acarina; scabies mites, itch mites, mange mites. The numerous forms are morphologically very alike, but usually host-specific and described as races of *Sarcoptes scabiei* var. *hominis,* the human itch mite. It is parasitic in all stages, the females burrowing in the epidermis, laying eggs within the burrow and causing scabies. Distribution is normally by close contact between hosts. [Gk *sarx* flesh, *koptein* to cut.]

Sarcoptidae (sar·**kop**·tid·e). A family of the acarine superfamily Sarcoptoidea; itch mites, mange mites. The genera *Notoëdres* and *Sarcoptes* are of medical interest. [Gk *sarx* flesh, *koptein* to cut, *eidos* form.]

sarcoptidosis (sar·kop·tid·**o**'·sis). Infestation with mites of the family Sarcoptidae. **Chorioptic sarcoptidosis.** Chorioptosis. **Psoroptic sarcoptidosis.** Psoroptosis. [*Sarcoptes,* Gk *-osis* condition.]

sarcoptoid (sar·**kop**·toid). One of the Sarcoptoidea.

Sarcoptoidea (sar·kop·**toid**·e·ah). A super-family of the order Acarina. The members are all minute parasites. The family Sarcoptidae is of medical interest. [Gk *sarx* flesh, *koptein* to cut, *eidos* form.]

sarcosinaemia (sar·ko·sin·e'·me·ah). Autosomal recessive inborn error of sarcosine metabolism with various clinical changes. [sarcosine, Gk *haima* blood.]

sarcosine (**sar**·ko·seen). Methylamino-acetic acid. *See* ACID.

sarcosis (sar·**ko**·sis). 1. A state generally marked by the presence of numerous fleshy growths in various parts of the body. 2. The excessive formation of flesh. 3. Sarcomata spread throughout an entire organ. [Gk *sarx* flesh, *-osis* condition.]

Sarcosporidia (sar·ko·spor·**id**'·e·ah). An order of Protozoa belonging to the class Sporozoa and reproducing by sporulation. All species are parasitic within the muscle tissues. [Gk *sarx* flesh, *spora* seed.]

sarcosporidiasis, sarcosporidiosis (sar·ko·spor·id·**i**'·as·is, sar·ko·spor·id·e·o'·sis). A condition, rarely found in human beings, marked by infection of striped muscle with Sarcosporidia. [Sarcosporidia, Gk *-osis* condition.]

sarcosporidium (sar·ko·spor·**id**'·e·um). Any protozoon of the order Sarcosporidia.

sarcostosis (sar·kos·**to**·sis). A degenerative process characterized by occurrence of bone elements in muscular tissue. [Gk *sarx* flesh, *osteon* bone.]

sarcostroma (sar·ko·**stro**·mah). A false membrane, thick and fleshy. [Gk *sarx* flesh, *stroma* mattress.]

sarcostyle (**sar**·ko·stile). One of a large number of fine longitudinal fibrils which compose a striped muscle fibre. [Gk *sarx* flesh, *stylos* pillar.]

sarcotherapeutics, sarcotherapy (sar·ko·ther·ap·**ew**'·tix, sar·ko·**ther**·ap·e). The use of meat or other extracts from animal tissues in the treatment of disease in man. [Gk *sarx* flesh, *therapeia* treatment.]

sarcotic (sar·**kot**·ik). 1. Relating or belonging to sarcosis. 2. Aiding or stimulating the growth of flesh. [Gk *sarx* flesh.]

sarcotome (**sar**·ko·tome). A spring devised for the crushing of tissue. [Gk *sarx* flesh, *temnein* to cut.]

sarcotripsy (**sar**·ko·trip·se). Histotripsy; the crushing of tissue by the use of a histotribe or an écraseur. [Gk *sarx* flesh, *tribein* to grind.]

sarcous (**sar**·kus). Relating or belonging to muscular tissue or flesh; fleshy. [Gk *sarx* flesh.]

sardonic (sar·**don**·ik). Descriptive of the strained grinning expression, risus sardonicus, caused by spasm of the facial muscles, typical of tetanus. [Gk *sardanios* prob. from *sardane,* a Sardinian plant said to screw up the facial muscles while it is being eaten.]

sarmentocymarin (sar·men·to·**si**'·mar·in). A cardioactive glycoside obtained from the African vine, *Strophanthus sarmentosus.* It yields sarmentogenin when hydrolysed. [L *sarmentosus* twiggy, cymarin.]

sarmentogenin (sar·men·**toj**·en·in). $C_{23}H_{34}O_5$, a sterol aglycone derived from the cardio-active glycoside sarmentocymarin. It has a hydroxyl group at the 11-position and has been used therefore as a starting point in the synthesis of cortisone.

Sarothamnus (sar·o·**tham**·nus). A genus of European leguminous plants, including broom, *Cytisus scoparius.* [Gk *saron* broom, *thamnos* shrub.]

Sarracenia (sar·ah·**se**·ne·ah). A genus of polypetalous flowers belonging to the family Sarraceniaceae, including the pitcher plant or saddle plant (*Sarracenia purpurea*), the root and leaves of which are used medicinally as a stomachic, diuretic and laxative. [Michel *Sarrazin* (b. 1659), Canadian physician.]

sarsa (sar·sah). The dried roots and rhizome of species of *Smilax* (family Liliaceae), climbing plants which grow in Central America. Its chief constituent is a crystalline glycoside, sarsasaponin. [Sp. *zarza* bramble.]

sarsaparilla (sar·sap·ar·il'·ah). Sarsa. [Sp. *zarzaparilla.*]

sarsasaponin (sar·sah·sap·on·in). $C_{44}H_{76}O_{20}·7H_2O$, a crystalline glycoside found in sarsaparilla root; it has emetic properties.

sartorius muscle [musculus sartorius (NA)] (sar·tor·e·us·musl). A long, strap-like muscle arising from the anterior superior spine of the ilium and passing obliquely across the front of the thigh to its insertion into the upper part of the medial surface of the tibia. [L *sartor* tailor.]

sassafras (sas·af·ras). The dried bark, deprived of most of the cork, of the root of *Sassafras variifolium* (Salisb.) O. Kuntze (family Lauraceae), a tree growing in the eastern states of North America. Its chief constituents are a volatile oil containing safrol, together with tannin and starch, which is used to destroy pediculi. [Sp. *sasafrás.*]

sassafrol (sas·af·rol). Safrole [sassafras, oil.]

sassolin (sas·o·lin). Boric acid. *See* ACID.

sassy bark (sas·e bark). Casca bark; the bark of *Erythrophloeum guineense* G. Don. (family Leguminoseae), used at one time in Africa as an arrow-poison. It contains the alkaloid, erythrophloeine.

satellite (sat·el·ite). 1. Applied to a vein which closely accompanies an artery for some distance. 2. In cytogenetics, a chromosomal agent (often relatively small) separated by a secondary constriction from the main body of the chromosome. **Bacterial satellite.** An organism which grows favourably in close proximity to a colony of another, often because of the liberation by the latter of chemical factors which stimulate the growth of the former, e.g. *Haemophilus influenzae* in the neighbourhood of staphylococci. **Satellite virus.** *See* VIRUS. [L *satelles* attendant.]

satellitism (sat·el·i·tizm). 1. A term used in bacteriology to indicate the enhancing effect on the growth of *Haemophilus influenzae* of another micro-organism, e.g. staphylococcus growing on the culture medium; the effect is due to the production by the latter of the V factor, a respiratory co-enzyme (*see* HAEMOPHILUS). 2. Symbiosis. [L *satelles* attendant.]

satellitosis (sat·el·i·to'·sis). The presence of free nuclei in the neighbourhood of the ganglion cells of the brain cortex. [L *satelles* attendant, *-osis* condition.]

Sato, Akira (b. 1871). Japanese physician.

Sato and Sekiya stain. A peroxidase stain containing copper sulphate and benzidine.

Satterthwaite, Thomas Edward (b. 1843). New York physician.

Satterthwaite's method. A method of artificial respiration involving alternate pressure and relaxation over the abdomen.

Sattler, Hubert (b. 1844). German ophthalmologist.

Sattler's couche. A layer of the choroid coat of the eye which is composed of elastic fibres, and which separates the vascular and choriocapillary layers.

Sattler's glands. The ciliary glands. *See* GLAND.

Sattler's layer. Part of the vascular layer of the choroid, made up of small blood vessels.

Sattler's veil. A diffuse corneal haze that may develop in a person wearing a contact lens.

saturated (sat·ewr·a·ted). 1. Referring to a chemical compound, one in which all valency bonds are fully utilized and which is unable therefore to form addition compounds. 2. Of solutions, that one which contains the maximum amount of solute that the given quantity of solvent will dissolve at the given temperature. 3. Applied to a vapour in contact with its liquid at a certain temperature. [L *saturare* to fill.]

saturation (sat·ewr·a·shun). 1. The state of being saturated. 2. The degree to which a liquid or gas is saturated. 3. In radiotherapy, a large dose of radiation followed by smaller doses to maintain the effect. **Haemoglobin oxygen saturation.** A measure of the degree to which oxygen is bound to haemoglobin expressed as a percentage of the maximum possible. In normal arterial blood it is not less than 94 per cent, and in normal venous blood 70–90 per cent. **Oxygen saturation.** The oxygen content divided by the oxygen capacity, multiplied by 100.

satureia (sat·ewr·e·ah). Garden savory; the dried herb *Satureia hortensis* (family Labiatae), used as a culinary herb and medicinally as an aromatic and carminative. [L.]

saturnine (sat·er·nine). Pertaining to or caused by lead. [*Saturn,* identified by alchemists with lead.]

saturnism (sat·er·nizm). Lead poisoning of chronic type; plumbism. [see prec.]

saturnotherapy (sat·er·no·ther'·ap·e). The treatment of disease by lead. [*Saturn,* identified by alchemists with lead, Gk *therapeia* treatment.]

Satvioni's cryptoscope. An early form of fluoroscope.

satyriasis, satyromania (sat·ir·i·as·is, sat·ir·o·ma'·ne·ah). Abnormally excessive sexual impulse in men. [Gk *satyros* satyr, mania.]

saucerization (saw·ser·i·za'·shun). The laying open of a cavity so as to produce a shallow, shelving depression, or the occurrence of such a depression as a result of trauma. [O Fr. *saussier.*]

saucerize (saw·ser·ize). An operation in which a cavity, e.g. of a bone, is laid widely open so that the adjacent muscle can fall in and obliterate any space. [see prec.]

Sauer, Louis Wendlin (b. 1885). Evanston, Illinois, paediatrician.

Sauer's vaccine. A whooping-cough vaccine prepared from freshly isolated strains of *Haemophilus pertussis,* introduced by Sauer, and found to be of distinct value in reducing incidence and severity of the disease.

Sauerbruch, Ernst Ferdinand (b. 1875). Berlin surgeon.

Sauerbruch's cabinet. A pressure-controlled cabinet for chest operations; of historical interest. It enabled the surgeon to open the thoracic cavity without the lung collapsing. This is achieved today by the positive pressure applied through an intratracheal tube by the anaesthetist.

Sauerbruch's prosthesis. An artificial limb in which movement is obtained by muscle and skin flaps.

Sauerbruch sternum splitter. A curved instrument with a sharp blade in its concavity and a percussion anvil on its convexity, the former being applied to the upper end of the sternum, and the latter struck with a mallet until the sternum splits downwards to afford access to the mediastinum.

Sauerbruch thoracoplasty. An extensive thoracoplasty involving the removal of the posterior parts of ribs 1-10, without apicolysis; it is done in 2 stages starting with the lower ribs. It was used in the treatment of pulmonary tuberculosis, but is now obsolete.

sauerkraut (sow·er·krowt). A preparation of cabbage made by cutting it into fine pieces and allowing it to ferment in a brine composed of its own juice and salt. [G.]

Saunders, Edward Watt (b. 1854). St. Louis physician.

Saunder's disease. An acute gastric disturbance suffered by infants as a result of dietetic starch intolerance. Vomiting causes early severe dehydration.

Saunders, John Cunningham (b. 1773). London ophthalmologist.

Saunders' needle. A type of cataract needle, or knife needle, with longer cutting edges than usual; used for discission of the cataractous lens or secondary cataract.

saunders (sawn·derz). Sandal wood.

sauriasis (saw·ri·as·is). Ichthyosis. [Gk *sauros* lizard.]

sauriderma (saw·re·der·mah). Saurodermia.

saurodermia (saw·ro·der·me·ah). Crocodile skin; severe ichthyosis. [Gk *sauros* lizard, *derma* skin.]

sauroid (saw·roid). Like a reptile. [Gk *sauros* lizard, *eidos* form.]

sausage (sos·ij). **Sigmoid sausage.** An elongated, sausage-shaped mass felt in the left iliac region and due to thickening of the walls of the sigmoid flexure. [L *salsus* salted.]

sausarism (saw·sar·izm). A paralysed and dry condition of the tongue. [Gk *sausarismos.*]

Saussure, Horace Benedict de (b. 1740). Geneva physicist and philosopher.

Saussure's hygrometer. Hair hygrometer: one which depends upon the lengthening of a hair in a humid atmosphere.

saussurea (saw·sewr·e·ah). An Indian drug consisting of the roots of *Saussurea lappa* (family Compositae) and probably also of *Saussurea hypoleuca.* It is used in India as an aromatic stimulant and as a tonic and aphrodisiac. [H. B. de *Saussure.*]

Sauvineau, Charles (b. 1862). French ophthalmologist.

Sauvineau's syndrome. Paralysis of the internal rectus muscle of one eye and spasm of the external rectus muscle of the other.

Savage, Henry (b. 1810). London gynaecologist and anatomist.

Savage's perineal body. The perineal body. *See* BODY.

Savill, Thomas Dixon (b. 1856). London physician.

Savill's disease. Dermatitis exfoliativa epidemica.

savin (sav·in). Sabina.

Saviotti's canals. Fine clefts between the acinar cells of the pancreas, seen best in stained preparations.

saw (saw). A cutting tool with a serrated edge. **Amputating saw.** A large saw used for amputations. **Chain saw.** A saw set upon a chain and used with 2 handles pulled upon alternately. **Crown saw.** A type of trephine, now obsolete. **Key-hole saw.** A saw with a long, narrow blade, used when access is restricted. **Nasal saw.** An instrument for sawing through nasal bones in plastic operations. **Separating saw.** A saw used for separating teeth. [AS *sagu.*]

See also: ADAMS (W.), ALBEE, BUTCHER, FARABEUF, GIGLI, HEY (W.), STRYKER.

Sawil syndrome. Generalized exfoliative dermatitis of unknown cause.

Saxer, Fritz (b. 1864). German pathologist.

Saxer's cells. Primitive mesamoeboid wandering cells found in the embryonic mesenchyme: their derivation and fate are uncertain but Saxer defended the view that they are derived from mesenchymal cells and develop into leucocytes.

saxifragant (sax·if·rag·ant). 1. Having the power to dissolve or crush calculi; lithotritic. 2. An agent capable of dissolving calculi. [L *saxum* stone, *frangere* to break.]

saxifrage (sax·e·fraje). Any of the numerous plants of the genus *Saxifraga* (family Umbelliferae). The root and herb of burnet saxifrage, *Pimpinella saxifrago,* are used as a carminative and stomachic. [L *saxifraga* spleenwort.]

Saxtorph, Mathias Hieronymus (b. 1772). Danish obstetrician.

Saxtorph's manoeuvre. A valuable contribution to obstetrics which was the forerunner of the axis-traction obstetric forceps. Downward pressure is exerted over the lock of the forceps at the same time as ordinary traction is applied.

Sayre, Lewis Albert (b. 1820). New York surgeon.

Sayre's apparatus. A gallows for suspending a patient during the application of a plaster-of-Paris jacket.

Sayre's jacket. A plaster-of-Paris spinal support used in the treatment of spinal disease.

Sayre's operation. Application of a plaster-of-Paris jacket for Pott's disease.

Sayre's splint. A metal splint used to immobilize the hip in hip-joint disease.

scab (skab). 1. The crust formed by the drying of the pus of an ulcer or of a superficial sore. 2. To form a scab or crust. **Transkeian scab.** Veldt sore. [ME.]

scabicide (ska·be·side). An agent which has the power to destroy *Sarcoptes scabiei* and is employed in the treatment of scabies. [scabies, L *caedere* to kill.]

scabies (ska·beez). Sarcoptic infestation of human skin, particularly a contagious skin disease caused by invasion of the epidermis with *Sarcoptes scabiei* var. *hominis,* characterized by burrows, follicular papules and various lesions due to scratching. It may occur in epidemic form, especially in war-time. Many mammals suffer from scabious infestations; the mites causing these diseases are named after their normal vertebrate hosts. If these mites obtain an impermanent lodging in human skin, various atypical forms of scabies are noted, as for example in cavalry-man's itch caused by *Sarcoptes scabiei* var. *equi.* **Bovine scabies.** Scabies of or contracted from cattle. **Cat scabies.** An eruption on human skin, usually of localized distribution, caused by *Notoëdres* or *Chevletiella parasitivorax* and contracted from cats. **Scabies crustosa.** Norwegian scabies (see foll.). **Norwegian scabies.** Severe scabies associated with crusting and scaling; the affected skin is densely infested. Itching may not be a prominent feature, and possibly the causal mite is not identical with *Sarcoptes scabiei* var. *hominis.* **Ovine scabies.** Scabies of sheep. **Scabies pustulosa.** Scabies with pustular lesions due to secondary infection. [L *scabere* to scratch.]

See also: BOECK (C. W.)

scabieticide (ska·be·et·is·ide). Scabicide.

scabiophobia (ska·be·o·fo′·be·ah). 1. A dread of scabies. 2. The delusion on the part of a person that he is suffering from scabies. [scabies, phobia.]

scabiosa (ska·be·o·sah). The herb of *Scabiosa succisa,* an infusion of which is used as a diaphoretic, demulcent and febrifuge. [L *scabiosus* rough.]

scabious (ska·be·us). 1. Relating to or affected with scabies. 2. Scabby; bearing scales. [see prec.]

scabrities unguium syphilitica (ska·brish·e·eez ung·gwe·um sif·il·it·ik·ah). Syphilis of the nail plate. [L roughness of the nails, syphilis.]

scaevolism (ske·vol·izm). Self-mutilation by burning. [*Scaevola* legendary Roman hero.]

scala (ska·lah). A staircase; applied to the spiral canals which are situated above (*scala vestibuli*) and below (*scala tympani*) the spiral lamina and the duct of the cochlea. Both are filled with perilymph. The scala vestibuli [NA] begins in the vestibule and is continuous through the helicotrema at the apex of the cochlea with the scala tympani [NA]. The latter ends at the fenestra cochleae which is closed by the secondary tympanic membrane. The duct of the cochlea may be known as the *scala media,* since it lies between the two. [L.]

See also: LOEWENBERG.

scald (skawld). 1. The lesion caused by contact with a hot liquid or vapour. 2. Scald head. *See* HEAD. **Acid scald.** An eruption in the napkin area caused by an acid stool due to high protein diet other than milk. [L *calidus* hot.]

scale (skale). 1. Any instrument for measurement, e.g. a slip of wood or other material, with lines engraved at regular intervals and numbered on its surface, for measuring or laying off distances. In plural, a pair of scales; a balance. [L *scala* ladder.] 2. Squama; an aggregation of superficial epidermal cells which at first is loosely attached to the surface of the skin, but which may become detached. 3. To remove with instruments salivary and subgingival calculus from the teeth. [O Fr. *escale.*] **Absolute gas scale.** A scale of temperature based on the expansion of a perfect gas, and identical with the absolute thermodynamic scale. **Absolute thermodynamic scale.** A scale of temperature which is independent of the physical properties of the material used and is based on defining the triple point of water as the fundamental fixed point, and assigning to it the temperature 273.16 kelvin exactly. The unit 'kelvin' is equal to the unit 'degree Celsius'. **Androgyny scale.** A scale used by anthropologists to measure the skeletal sex characteristics of men and women. The two measurements are the bi-iliac and the bi-acromial in centimetres, and a formula used is $3 \times$ bi-acromial $-$ bi-iliac $= x$. In males x is usually above 82, in females 82 or below. **Celsius scale.** The scale of a Celsius thermometer on which 0°C corresponds to the freezing point of water and 100°C to the boiling point of water, under normal atmospheric pressure. **Centigrade scale.** Celsius scale. **Dunfermline scale.** A method of classification of children according to their state of nutrition by clinical assessment. The grades described are superior, fair, requiring supervision, requiring medical attention; no scientific data are required. The scale was developed in the city of Dunfermline in Scotland. [L *scala* ladder.]

See also: BEAUMÉ, BENOIST, BINET, CELSIUS, CHARRIÈRE, CLARK (T.), FAHRENHEIT, GAFFKY, HALDANE, RÉAUMUR, SIMON (T.), SØRENSEN, TALLQVIST, THOMSON (W., LORD KELVIN).

scalene (ska·leen). 1. Relating to one of the scalenus muscles. 2. A triangle having three sides of unequal length. [Gk *skalenos* uneven.]

scalenectomy (ska·le·**nek**·to·me). Resection of any of the scalenus muscles. [scalenus, Gk *ektome* a cutting out.]

scaleniotomy, scalenotomy (ska·le·ne·**ot**·o·me, ska·le·**not**·o·me). Surgical division of one or more of the scalenus muscles adjacent to their insertions; it forms part of the operation of Semb's thoracoplasty, and is used in treatment of cervical rib syndrome. [scalenus, Gk *temnein* to cut.]

scalenus anterior muscle [musculus scalenus anterior (NA)] (ska·**le**·nus an·**teer**·e·or musl). A muscle arising from the anterior tubercles of the transverse processes of the 3rd to the 6th cervical vertebrae, and inserted into a tubercle near the anterior end of the 1st rib and on its posterior border.

scalenus medius muscle [musculus scalenus medius (NA)] (ska·**le**·nus **me**·de·us musl). A muscle arising from the anterior tubercles of the transverse processes of the 3rd to the 7th cervical vertebrae and from the transverse process of the axis. It is inserted into the upper surface of the 1st rib between its tubercle and the groove for the subclavian artery.

scalenus minimus muscle [musculus scalenus minimus (NA)] (ska·**le**·nus **min**·im·us musl). An occasional muscle running from the transverse process of the 7th cervical vertebra to the inner border of the 1st rib. It lies on the superior surface of the suprapleural membrane.

scalenus posterior muscle [musculus scalenus posterior (NA)] (ska·**le**·nus pos·**teer**·e·or musl). A small muscle arising from the posterior tubercles of the transverse processes of the 4th to the 6th cervical vertebrae, and inserted into the outer aspect of the 2nd rib.

scaler (**ska**·ler). 1. An instrument which records the number of electrical pulses produced by a radiation detector in a given time or, alternatively, the time required for a specified number of such pulses to be registered. 2. An instrument used in dentistry for the operation of scaling; it is made in many shapes and sizes. [O Fr. *escale.*]

scall (skawl). An eruption, particularly of the head, characterized by the formation of scabs or scurf. [Obsolete term.] **Dry scall.** A dry scab. **Honeycomb scall.** Probably this denoted impetigo. **Milk scall.** Milk-crust; the yellow seborrhoeic adherent crusts often seen on the scalp of infant. **Moist scall.** A moist scab covering an oozing area. [Old Norse *skalli* bare head.]

scalp (skalp). The layers covering the calvarium considered as one structure. **Washboard scalp.** A wrinkled condition of the skin of the scalp noted in acromegaly. [ME.]

scalpel (**skal**·pel). A small pointed knife with a convex edge. [L *scalprum* knife.]

scalprum (**skal**·prum). A raspatory, or periosteum elevator. [L knife.]

scaly (**ska**·le). 1. Resembling scales; squamous. 2. Composed of or covered with scales. 3. Scurfy.

scammoniae resina (skam·o·ne·e rez·i·nah). Ipomoea resin. *See* RESIN.

scammonin (**skam**·on·in). $C_{34}H_{56}O_{16}$, the ether-soluble (glycosidic) fraction of scammony and ipomoea resins. It is physiologically inactive.

scammony (**skam**·o·ne). The dried root of *Scammoniae radix* derived from the plant *Convolvulus scammonia* Linn. (family Convolvulaceae). The gum resin obtained by incising the living root and collecting the milky exudation is of chief importance; it consists of scammonin principally, and is used as a hydragogue and cathartic. **Scammony resin.** Ipomoea resin. *See* RESIN. **Scammony root.** Ipomoea. [Gk *skammonia.*]

scan (skan). 1. As a *noun* a diagrammatic representation of the distribution of ionizing radiation emanating from the whole body or from part of the body. 2. As a *verb,* the carrying out of the procedure by means of which the distribution of ionizing radiation emanating from the whole body or from a part of the body is determined. In both usages the term is employed whether or not a mechanical scanning process is used. Thus, the result of using a static imaging device is referred to as a *scan* and the process of using such a device is referred to as *scanning.* **Colour scan.** A scan where a series of colours is used to represent different radiation intensities detected by a scanner. **Contour scan.** A scan where lines are used to connect points where the radiation intensities detected by a scanner are equal. A contour map of radiation detected. **Derived scan.** A scan constructed after computation of the data derived from an imaging device. [L *scandere* to climb.]

scandium (**skan**·de·um). A rare-earth element of atomic weight 44.9559, atomic number 21 and chemical symbol Sc. It is a trivalent metal which resembles aluminium in chemical properties. [*Scandinavia,* birthplace of discoverer.]

scanner (**skan**·er). An instrument incorporating a radiation detector capable of movement in a regular manner relative to the body or part of the body, for determining the distribution of the radiation. It is usual for the body to remain stationary and for the detector to move, but the reverse has been utilized. It is also usual for the relative movement to be confined to straight parallel lines within a predetermined rectangular area (a rectilinear scanner), but other geometrical arrangements have been employed. A scanner normally incorporates arrangements for producing a representation of the radiation distribution, i.e. for producing a scan. This is one of a number of forms of imaging device used in nuclear medicine. [L *scandere* to climb.]

scanning (**skan**·ing). 1. Applied to a mode of utterance (scanning speech) in which there are distinct and generally rhythmic pauses between the syllables of words or between words. 2. The playing of an electron beam in successive bands over a surface, as in the cathode-ray tube. **Rectilinear scanning.** Scanning in which the transducer moves over the body or organ in parallel straight lines, usually back and forth. [L *scandere* to climb.]

scanogram (**skan**·o·gram). The graphic record produced by scanography. [scanning, Gk *gramma* record.]

scanography (skan·**og**·raf·e). The production of radiographs with a narrow beam of x-rays; this diminishes distortion of the image. [scanning, Gk *graphein* to record.]

Scanzoni, Friedrich Wilhelm (b. 1821). Prague/Würzburg gynaecologist.

Scanzoni's manoeuvre. The delivery of an occipitoposterior position with orthodox forceps occipito-anterior, using a double application of the blades.

scaphocephalic, scaphocephalous (skaf·o·kef·**al**′·ik, skaf·o·**kef**·al·us). Relating or belonging to scaphocephaly.

scaphocephalus (skaf·o·**kef**·al·us). Anyone with a scaphocephalic skull.

scaphocephaly (skaf·o·**kef**·al·e). The deformed condition of the skull produced by premature fusion at the sagittal suture, in which it is long and narrow and bears a ridge so that it has the appearance of an upturned boat with a keel. [Gk *skaphe* skiff, *kephale* head.]

scaphohydrocephalus (**skaf**·o·hi·dro·**kef**′·al·us). Hydrocephalus in which the skull is scaphocephalic in type. [Gk *skaphe* skiff, hydrocephalus.]

scaphohydrocephaly (**skaf**·o·hi·dro·**kef**′·al·e). The condition of scaphohydrocephalus.

scaphoid (**skaf**·oid, **ska**·foid). Boat-shaped. The term is applied to the bone on the radial side of the proximal row of carpal bones. The navicular bone of the tarsus was also known as the scaphoid, but this use of the name is now obsolete. [Gk *skaphe* skiff, *eidos* form.]

scaphoid bone [os scaphoideum (NA)]. The largest bone in the proximal row of carpal bones, on the lateral side.

scaphoiditis (skaf·oid·i·tis). Koehler's disease. [scaphoid, Gk *-itis* inflammation.]

See also: KOEHLER.

scapula [NA] (**skap**·ew·lah). A flattened triangular bone lying on the posteriolateral aspect of the chest wall. Its surfaces are dorsal [facies dorsalis (NA)] and ventral (costal) [facies costalis (NA)], the former carrying a triangular backwardly-projecting plate or spine and the latter being applied to the chest wall. Its angles are superior [angulus superior (NA)], inferior [angulus inferior (NA)] and lateral [angulus lateralis (NA)], the last named bearing the glenoid cavity for the head of the humerus, and the borders are upper [margo superior (NA)], medial [margo medialis (NA)] and lateral [margo lateralis (NA)]. The bone is attached to the trunk by the clavicle and several muscles. **Alar scapula, Scapula alata.** Winged scapula (see below). **Neck of the scapula [collum scapulae (NA)].** The constriction immediately behind the glenoid cavity. **Scaphoid scapula.** Hollowing over the scapula caused by muscular wasting. **Winged scapula.** An undue prominence or sticking out of the scapula. It is due to the projection of the posterior angles of the ribs because of their greater obliquity in long, flattened chests. It is also caused by paralysis of the serratus anterior muscle. [L *scapulae* shoulder-blades.]

See also: GRAVES.

scapulacromial (skap·ewl·ak·**ro**′·me·al). Belonging to the scapula and acromion process.

scapulalgia (skap·ewl·**al**·je·ah). Pain in the muscles and tissues adjacent to the scapula. [scapula, Gk *algos* pain.]

scapular (**skap**·ew·lar). Relating or belonging to the scapula; referring to the shoulder.

scapular arteries. Circumflex scapular artery [arteria circumflexa scapulae]. *See* SUBSCAPULAR ARTERY. **Descending scapular artery [arteria scapularis descendens].** *See* CERVICAL ARTERY, SUPERFICIAL.

scapular vein. Dorsal scapular vein [vena scapularis dorsalis (NA)]. A small vein which ascends along the medial border of the scapula and opens into the subclavian or external jugular veins.

scapulectomy (skap·ew·**lek**·to·me). Excision or resection of the scapula. [scapula, Gk *ektome* a cutting out.]

scapuloclavicular (skap·ew·lo·klav·**ik**′·ew·lar). Relating or belonging to the scapula and the clavicle.

scapulocoracoid (skap·ew·lo·**kor**′·ak·oid). Belonging to the scapula and the coracoid process.

scapulodynia (skap·ew·lo·**din**′·e·ah). Pain in the shoulder, especially in the scapular area. [scapula, Gk *odyne* pain.]

scapulohumeral (skap·ew·lo·**hew**′·mer·al). Relating or belonging to the scapula and the humerus.

scapulopexy (**skap**·ew·lo·pex·e). The operation of fixing the scapula to the ribs, usually by fascial slings. [scapula, Gk *pexis* a fixation.]

scapulothoracic (skap·ew·lo·thor·**as**′·ik). Relating or belonging to the scapula and the thorax.

scapulovertebral (skap·ew·lo·**ver**′·te·bral). Relating or belonging to the scapula and the vertebral column.

scar (skahr). Cicatrix; connective-tissue replacement of mesodermal or ectodermal tissue which has been destroyed by injury or disease. **Atrophic scar.** A scar having its surface depressed below the level of the surrounding skin. **Hypertrophic scar.** A thickened scar, its surface raised above the level of the adjacent skin; it does not extend beyond the boundaries of the original injury. **Keloidal scar.** Keloid. **Tissue-paper scar.** Thin scar-tissue, resembling tissue paper, usually at the site of healing of an ulcer, particularly a syphilitic ulcer. [Gk *eschara* scab.]

See also: REICHERT (K. B.).

scarabiasis (skar·ab·**i**·as·is). Infestation with beetles; dung beetles are passed in the motions and may within a few minutes emerge and crawl away. It has been associated with anorexia and emaciation in children. [L *scarabeus* beetle.]

scarification (skar·if·ik·**a**′·shun). The operation of making a number of small punctures or incisions in the superficial layer of the skin. [L *scarificare* to scratch.]

scarificator (**skar**·if·ik·a′·tor). An instrument used in scarifying skin, comprising a series of small concealed lancet-points which may be brought into action by pressure on a trigger.

scarifier (**skar**·if·i·er). Scarificator.

See also: HARRISON (L. W.).

scarify (**skar**·e·fi). To make a series of small punctures or incisions superficially in the skin. [L *scarificare* to scratch.]

scarlatina (skar·lat·e·nah). Scarlet fever. An acute infectious disease caused by strains of haemolytic streptococci, and characterized by fever, inflammation of the fauces and a punctate erythematous (scarlet) rash. Desquamation of the skin usually follows the disappearance of the eruption, and complications include otitis media, adenitis, arthritis and nephritis. The majority of cases are in children. The present mortality is low, although the disease was formerly very virulent. The organism produces a toxin which, when diluted, gives a positive Dick test in persons susceptible to scarlet fever. Toxin injected in appropriate doses immunizes Dick-positive persons; antitoxic serum, prepared against this toxin, and chemotherapy are often useful in treatment. **Scarlatina anginosa.** A form with extensive ulceration and necrosis of the fauces, and possible septic involvement of neighbouring parts. **Scarlatina cynanchica.** Scarlatina with severe inflammation and swelling of the throat, resembling quinsy. **Scarlatina haemorrhagica.** A very rare form with haemorrhages into the skin and from the mucous membranes; it is invariably fatal. **Scarlatina latens.** Scarlatina without obvious rash, but with other characteristic manifestations, including desquamation and possibly nephritis at the typical period of the disease. **Scarlatina maligna.** A highly-fatal form with severe constitutional symptoms and dusky, ill-defined rash: the fulminant toxic variety. **Scarlatina papulosa.** Scarlatina with small papular elevations, particularly on the legs. **Scarlatina pruriginosa.** A very rare form with papular rash and considerable irritation, suggestive of prurigo. **Puerperal scarlatina.** Infection of the generative tract with a toxigenic haemolytic streptococcus, before or during the puerperium. In other respects it is usually a scarlatina simplex. **Scarlatina pustulosa.** A variety with skin sepsis, due to extraneous bacterial infection. **Scarlatina rheumatica.** Arthritis and other rheumatic manifestations in association with scarlet fever. Also a synonym for *dengue.* **Scarlatina septica.** Scarlatina anginosa (see above). **Scarlatina simplex.** A term usually restricted to the so-called *simple* or benign variety, but also used for the mild, moderate and severe ordinary (uncomplicated) forms of scarlet fever. **Scarlatina sine angina.** Scarlatina with little faucial congestion, in which the haemolytic streptococci are present in some site other than the throat (wounds, burns, uterus, etc.). **Scarlatina sine eruptione, Scarlatina sine exanthemata.** A mild form with little or no rash. It may be due to partial immunity of the person infected. **Surgical scarlatina.** An erythematous eruption associated with an operation wound; one variety of scarlatina traumatica. **Scarlatina traumatica.** A variety following burns and wounds of the skin and mucous membranes which have become infected with the causal streptococcus. **Scarlatina typhosa.** A form with prolonged, remittent pyrexia and exhaustion, suggestive of typhoid fever. [It. *scarlattina.*]

scarlatinal (skar·**lat**·in·al). Relating or belonging to scarlatina.

scarlatinella (skar·lat·in·**el**′·ah). A non-typical, non-febrile and attenuated scarlet fever, the so-called *fourth disease.* [dim. of scarlatina.]

scarlatiniform, scarlatinoid (skar·lat·**in**·e·form, skar·**lat**·in·oid). Having resemblance to scarlatina, term applied to a rash. **Metadiptheritic scarlatinoid.** 1. Eruption that may occur during recovery from diphtheria, attended by scarlatinal symptoms. 2. Scarlatinella. [scarlatina, form, Gk *eidos* form.]

scarlet (**skar**·let). A bright red. **Scarlet G.** Sudan III. **Non-staining scarlet.** *o*-Amino-azotoluene, a compound soluble only in oils and fats. **Oil scarlet.** Sudan III. **Water-soluble scarlet.** Biebrich scarlet. [O Fr. *escarlate.*]

Scarpa, Antonio (b. 1747). Italian surgeon and anatomist.

Scarpa's fascia. *See* FASCIA OF THE ABDOMINAL WALL, SUPERFICIAL.

Scarpa's fluid. The fluid occupying the membranous labyrinth in the inner ear. More commonly known as *endolymph.*

Scarpa's foramen. Median incisive foramen; a foramen present sometimes in the midline of the incisive fossa of the hard palate.

Scarpa's ganglion. The vestibular ganglion; a ganglion in the vestibular division of the cochlear nerve.

Scarpa's hiatus. The helicotrema of the cochlea.

Scarpa's membrane. The secondary tympanic membrane. *See* MEMBRANE.

Scarpa's nerve. The long sphenopalatine nerve.

Scarpa's operation. Ligation of the femoral artery in the femoral triangle.

Scarpa's sheath. The cremasteric fascia. *See* CREMASTER MUSCLE AND FASCIA.

Scarpa's shoe. A right-angled metal splint used in the treatment of club-foot.

Scarpa's staphyloma. Thinning and bulging of the sclera, usually at the outer side of the optic disc, occurring in a highly myopic eye.

Scarpa's triangle. The femoral triangle. *See* TRIANGLE.

scatole (**ska**·tole). Skatole.

scatological (skat·o·**loj**·ik·al). Relating to the study of the faeces. [see foll.]

scatology (skat·**ol**·o·je). The study of the faeces; coprology. [Gk *skatos* of dung, *logos* science.]

scatoma (skat·o·mah). An accumulation of hardened faeces which presents the appearance of a tumour in the rectum or colon; stercoroma. [Gk *skatos* of dung, *-oma* tumour.]

scatophagous (skat·**of**·ag·us). 1. Having the habit of eating faeces, occurring in certain types of insanity. 2. In zoology, feeding on dung, as do certain beetles. [see foll.]

scatophagy (skat·**of**·ah·je). 1. In certain forms of insanity, the practice of eating faeces. 2. In zoology, the natural habit of feeding on excrement or dung. [Gk *skatos* of dung, *phagein* to eat.]

scatoscopy (skat·**os**·ko·pe). Examination of the bowel excreta for diagnostic purposes. [Gk *skatos* of dung, *skopein* to watch.]

scatoxyl (**ska**·tox·il). Skatoxyl.

scatter, scattering (**skat**·er, **skat**·er·ing). The diffusion and deviation of x-rays produced when they strike an object or of charged particles in an electric field. **Back scatter.** Reversal of the direction of motion of photons or particles by a scatterer. **Coherent scatter.** Scatter of photons or particles without change in energy. **Forward scatter.** Scatter of photons or particles at an angle equal to or less than 90 degrees to their original direction of motion. **Incoherent scatter.** Scattering of photons or particles with a change of energy. **Multiple scatter, Multiple scattering.** A term usually associated with the scattering of a charged particle, e.g. an electron, by a large number of encounters with the electric fields of other particles, such as nuclei. The resultant angles of scattering obey the gaussian distribution law. **Unmodified scatter.** Coherent scatter (see above). [ME.]

See also: COMPTON, COULOMB, RUTHERFORD.

Sceleth, Charles E. (b. 1873). Chicago physician.

Sceleth treatment. A treatment of drug addiction by saline cathartics and a mixture containing scopolamine, pilocarpine and ethyl morphine.

scelotyrbe (sel·o·**ter**·be). Clumsiness or weakness in walking, seen in a variety of paralytic conditions of the lower limbs [Obsolete term.]. **Scelotyrbe agitans, Scelotyrbe festinans.** Paralysis agitans; Parkinson's disease. **Scelotyrbe fibrilis.** Difficulty in walking, associated with involuntary twitching of the muscles; motor neurone disease. **Scelotyrbe pituitosa, Scelotyrbe spastica.** Spastic paraplegia. **Scelotyrbe tarantismus.** Chorea. [Gk *skellis* leg, *tyrbe* disorder.]

scent (sent). An effluvium emanating from living or inanimate matter and stimulating the olfactory sense. [L *sentire* to perceive.]

Schacher, Polycarp Gottlieb (b. 1674). Leipzig physician and anatomist.

Schacher's ganglion. The ciliary ganglion. *See* GANGLION.

Schachowa, Seraphina (fl. 1876). Russian histologist.

Schachowa's spiral tube. A portion of the nephron.

Schachowa's irregular tubule. The spiral segment of the renal tubule.

Schaeffer, Max (b. 1852). German neurologist.

Schaeffer's reflex. In spastic paralysis, pinching the middle third of the tendo calcaneus of the affected limb or limbs may produce flexion of the foot and toes.

Schaellibaum, Huldreich. 20th century Strasbourg microscopist.

Schaellibaum's solution. A solution of celloidin in clove oil used for attaching histological sections to slides.

Schafer, Sir Edward Albert Sharpey (b. 1850). Edinburgh physiologist and histologist.

dumb-bell of Schafer. Any one of the bodies shaped like a dumb-bell which are present in voluntary-muscle tissue and are visible only under a microscope.

Schafer's method. After decalcification, in nitric acid, sections of skeletal tissues are stained with safranine, followed by mercuric chloride. Cartilage appears orange, marrow and connective tissue appear red.

Schales, Otto (b. 1910). American biochemist.

Schales and Schales method. For chlorides in blood. Serum is diluted with water and titrated with standard mercuric-nitrate solution using diphenylcarbazide as indicator. At the end point the colour change is from pale-yellow to violet.

Schamberg, Jay Frank (b. 1870). Philadelphia dermatologist.

Schamberg's dermatitis or dermatosis. Grain itch; a dermatitis caused by a mite that lives in straw.

Schamberg's disease. 1. Progressive pigmentary disorder, with flat brown lesions having puncta resembling cayenne pepper around their borders. 2. Schamberg's dermatitis (see above).

Schanz, Alfred (b. 1868). Dresden orthopaedic surgeon.

Schanz's disease. Traumatic tendinitis of the Achilles tendon.

Schanz's osteotomy. A subtrochanteric osteotomy of the upper end of the femur with displacement and angulation. Years ago this was used in the treatment of ununited fracture of the neck of the femur and other hip disorders.

Schanz's syndrome. Vertebral insufficiency in juvenile scoliosis.

Schapiro, Heinrich (b. 1852). Russian physician.

Schapiro's sign. A sign of weakness of the heart muscle.

Schardinger, Franz. 20th century Vienna biochemist.

Schardinger's enzyme. An enzyme (dehydrogenase) occurring in milk which catalyses the oxidation of aldehydes. Thus, if an aldehyde is added to milk containing methylene blue the dye is rapidly decolorized; heated milk gives no reaction. It is identical with xanthine oxidase, an enzyme present in the liver, which catalyses the oxidation of the purines, xanthine and hypoxanthine, to uric acid.

Schardinger reaction. The decolorization of methylene blue by milk containing formaldehyde. The reaction is catalysed by Schardinger's enzyme present in milk.

scharlach R (**shar**·lak ar). Sudan IV, a red dye used as a fat stain in histology.

Schatz, Christian Friedrich (b. 1841). Rostock gynaecologist.

Schatz manoeuvre. An external method of converting a brow presentation into a vertex, by flexion of the head.

Schaumann, Jörgen Nilsen (b. 1879). Stockholm dermatologist.

Schaumann's sarcoid or syndrome, Besnier-Boeck-Schaumann disease or syndrome. Sarcoidosis.

Schauta, Friedrich (b. 1849). Vienna gynaecologist.

Schauta's operation. A radical and extended vaginal hysterectomy for carcinoma of the neck of the uterus.

Schede, Max (b. 1844). Bonn surgeon.

Schede's operation or resection. An operation designed to obliterate a chronic empyema cavity. It involves resection of several ribs and of the underlying thickened parietal pleura, so that the soft tissues are allowed to fall in, obliterating the cavity.

Scheele, Carl Wilhelm (b. 1742). Swedish chemist.

Scheele's acid. A dilute solution of hydrocyanic acid (4 per cent).

Scheele's green. Swedish green, cupric arsenite, $Cu_3(AsO_3)_2$

$\cdot 2H_2O$, a green pigment precipitated by copper salts from solutions of arsenites. It is also employed as an insecticide.

Scheibler's reagent. A solution used in testing for alkaloids. It contains phosphotungstic acid.

Scheie, Harold Glendon (b. 1909). American ophthalmologist.

Scheie's operation. A fistulizing operation for glaucoma by scleral cautery and peripheral iridectomy.

Scheie's syndrome. A genetic disease in which excess chondoitin sulphate is found in the urine, characterized by stiff joints, claw-hand and ocular changes.

Scheiner, Christoph (b. 1575). Jesuit mathematician and physicist.

Scheiner's experiment. To demonstrate the ability of the eye to focus. The eye looks at a needle through 2 pinholes in a card, whose distance apart is less than the diameter of the pupil. When focused, 1 needle only is seen; when unfocused, 2 needles are seen.

schema (ske·mah). 1. Shape, plan, scheme, outline or arrangement. 2. A schedule or table describing the contents and arrangement of a scientific or medical work of classification. **Body schema.** The neurophysiological disposition subserving the recognition of the posture of the body and changes in its posture. [Gk shape.]

schematic (ske·mat·ik). 1. Relating to a scheme. 2. Prepared or made according to a particular type of formula. 3. Representing in the main but without absolute precision, as an anatomical model or diagram. [see prec.]

schematogram (ske·mat·o·gram). An outline drawing of the body or parts of the body, in which details can be filled after examination of a patient. [Gk *schema* shape, *gramma* record.]

scheme (skeem). A plan. **Decay scheme.** Disintegration scheme (see foll.). **Disintegration scheme.** The detailed analysis of a radioactive disintegration in terms of the transitions between the various states of energy of parent and residual nucleus and their relative frequencies. **Level scheme.** A detailed plan of the possible states (or levels) of a system, usually a nucleus, atom or molecule, giving the energies and spins of the various states and the transition probabilities between states. [Gk *schema* shape.]

schemograph (ske·mo·graf). A graphical method of showing the outline of the visual field obtained by a perimeter. [Gk *schema* shape, *graphein* to record.]

Schenck, Benjamin Robinson (b. 1873). Detroit gynaecologist.

Schenck's disease. Sporotrichosis.

Schepelmann's sign. In dry pleurisy the pain is increased on bending sideways towards the sound side, whereas with intercostal neuralgia it is increased by bending towards the affected side.

Scherer, Johann Joseph von (b. 1814). Würzburg biochemist.

Scherer's test. For inositol in urine. Acidify the urine with concentrated nitric acid, evaporate almost to dryness and add a few drops of ammonia solution and of calcium chloride solution. Evaporate to dryness. A red colour indicates inositol.

scheroma (ske·ro·mah). A condition in which the eye is deprived of lacrimal fluid, e.g. in old trachoma, vitamin-A deficiency, etc. [Gk *scheros* dry, *-oma* tumour.]

Scheuermann, Holger Werfel (b. 1877). Copenhagen orthopaedic surgeon.

Scheuermann's disease or kyphosis. Osteochondritis of the epiphyses of the vertebral bodies.

Schick, Bela (b. 1877). Vienna and New York paediatrician.

Schick Control BP 1968. A preparation used in carrying out the Schick test. *See* SCHICK TEST TOXIN (below).

Schick reaction or test. A skin test for immunity to diphtheria, made by injecting intradermally a suitable dilution of diphtheria toxin, usually into the forearm. A similar amount of heated toxin is often injected as a control at the same time. Readings are usually made after 3–4 days. A local reaction to the toxin is regarded as positive (= susceptible).

Schick Test Toxin BP 1968. A fluid preparation containing the toxin produced by *Corynebacterium diphtheriae.* The concentration is adjusted so that 0.2 ml contains the test dose. It is injected intradermally to determine susceptibility to diphtheria. The result of the test is read by comparing the local reaction with that of a similar dose of the preparation which has been inactivated by heat; this preparation is called *Schick Control* (see above).

Schick's sign. An expiratory stridor heard over the front and back of a child suffering from any enlargement of the para-aortic and paratracheal lymph glands. It was at one time thought to be pathognomonic of tuberculous adenitis.

Schiefferdecker, Paul (b. 1849). Bonn anatomist.

Schiefferdecker's disc. An argentophilic substance found around the axis-cylinder at the node of Ranvier.

Schiefferdecker's symbiosis theory. There is interaction between the tissues of the body and the metabolic products of one tissue stimulate other tissues.

Schiff, A. 20th century Vienna physician.

Nirenstein and Schiff method. A modified form of Mett's method of testing for peptic activity in gastric juice.

Schiff, Hugo (b. 1834). German biochemist.

periodic acid-Schiff reaction. A histochemical reaction in which sections are treated with periodic acid to oxidize 1,2-glycol groups to dialdehydes which are then identified by treatment with Schiff's reagent; the method is used to study mucosubstances and is useful for staining basement membranes.

Schiff's biliary cycle. The passage into the bile of absorbed biliary constituents, notably of bile salts, demonstrated by Schiff about 1870.

Schiff's reagent. For aldehydes. Triturate 0.2 g of rosaniline hydrochloride (basic fuchsine or basic magenta) in a mortar with 10 ml of water, pour off the liquid and saturate with sulphur dioxide. Allow to stand for 24 h and dilute with water to 200 ml.

Schilder, Paul Ferdinand (b. 1886). Vienna and New York neurologist.

Schilder's disease or encephalitis, Flatau-Schilder disease. Encephalitis periaxalis diffusa; a cerebral demyelinating disease of infancy, beginning in the occipital lobes and giving rise to progressive blindness, deafness, dementia and paralysis. Also called *progressive subcortical encephalopathy.*

Schiller, Walter (b. 1887). American pathologist.

Schiller's test. For carcinoma of the neck of the uterus. The cervix is painted with Gram's solution and if it is normal it should stain a homogeneous brown. Unstained areas should make the observer suspicious of carcinoma. This is not a reliable test.

Schilling, Robert. 20th century American haematologist.

Schilling test. A test for vitamin B_{12} absorption using radioactive vitamin B_{12}.

Schilling, Victor (b. 1883). Berlin physician.

Schilling's classification, blood count, formula, haemogram, index or method. An elaboration of a simple differential leucocyte count affording a means for interpreting the significance of changes in the distribution and numbers of all leucocytes, but more especially of the numbers and form of maturation of presegmented granulocytes. It is based on the separation of the polymorphonuclear leucocytes into 4 groups, (*a*) myelocytes, (*b*) juvenile forms, (*c*) staff or stab cells or band forms and (*d*) segmented forms in which the nuclei have 2 or more lobes.

Schilling's leukaemia. A type of monocytic leukaemia involving the reticulo-endothelial system.

Schimmelbusch, Curt (b. 1860). Berlin surgeon.

Schimmelbusch's disease. Cystic disease of the breast.

Schimmelbusch's mask. An anaesthetic mask consisting of a metal frame over which gauze or lint is stretched.

Schindler, Rudolf (b. 1888). American surgeon.

Wolf-Schindler gastroscope. A flexible, side-vision type of gastroscope.

schindylesis (skin·dil·e·sis). A fibrous joint in which a ridge of bone is received into a groove on another bone, e.g. the articulation in which the rostrum of the sphenoid bone fits between the alae of the vomer. [Gk a splintering.]

Schinus (ski·nus). A genus of trees (family Anacardiaceae). The Peruvian peppertree, *Schinus molle*, yields a kind of mastic, American mastic, which is mildly purgative and aromatic. [Gk *schinos* mastic tree.]

Schiøtz, Hjalmar (1850). Oslo ophthalmologist.

Schiøtz tonometer. The first tonometer devised for measuring the intra-ocular tension in mmHg. A plunger with a concave footpiece rests vertically on the cornea. Various weights are placed on the plunger and the amount of indentation of the cornea is measured on a scale for each different weight. These readings are then converted into mmHg from a special graph produced by Schiøtz after calibrating his readings against known intra-ocular pressure.

Schiotz X tonometer. A slight modification of the original Schiotz tonometer in that the footplate is convex rather than concave and there is 1 fixed weight. It is more influenced by ocular rigidity.

Schirmer, Otto Wilhelm August (b. 1864). Greifswald ophthalmologist.

Schirmer's test. A method of estimating the amount of lacrimal secretion: a piece of filter paper 5 mm wide and 35 mm long with the last 5 mm hooked over and placed in the lower fornix of the conjunctiva for 5 min. The amount of wetted paper is then measured. Under 10 mm is suggestive of keratoconjunctivitis sicca.

schistasis (skis·tas·is). 1. The action of splitting. 2. A congenital cleft or fissured state of a part or limb. [Gk *schistos* cleft.]

schistocephalus (skis·to·**kef**·al·us). A monster with a cleft skull. [Gk *schistos* cleft, *kephale* head.]

schistocoelia (skis·to·**se**·le·ah). A congenital fissure of the wall of the abdomen. [Gk *schistos* cleft, *koilia* cavity.]

schistocormia (skis·to·**kor**·me·ah). A congenital condition marked by cleavage of the trunk. [Gk *schistos* cleft, *kormos* trunk.]

schistocormus (skis·to·**kor**·mus). A monster the trunk of which is either totally or partially cleft; the legs and feet may be absent or incompletely developed. [see prec.]

schistocystis (skis·to·**sist**·is). A vesical fissure. [Gk *schistos* cleft, *kystis* bag.]

schistocyte (skis·to·site). A fragmented or segmented red blood cell; it may be seen in prepared blood smears on slides. **Parasitiferous schistocyte.** A red-blood-cell fragment containing a parasite. [Gk *schistos* cleft, *kytos* cell.]

schistocytosis (**skis**·to·si·**to**′·sis). A condition marked by the presence of numbers of schistocytes in the blood. [schistocyte, Gk *-osis* condition.]

schistoglossia (skis·to·**glos**·e·ah). Congenital cleft of the tongue. [Gk *schistos* cleft, *glossa* tongue.]

schistomelia (skis·to·**me**·le·ah). Cleft limb or limbs, a congenital state. [Gk *schistos* cleft, *melos* limb.]

schistomelus (skis·**tom**·el·us). A monster with a cleft limb or limbs. [see prec.]

schistometer (skis·**tom**·et·er). An instrument for measuring the interval between the vocal cords. [Gk *schistos* cleft, meter.]

schistoprosopia (**skis**·to·pro·**so**′·pe·ah). A cleft of the face, the result of incomplete development. [Gk *schistos* cleft, *prosopon* face.]

schistoprosopus (skis·to·**pro**·so·pus). A monster with a cleft face. [see prec.]

schistorrhachis (skis·**tor**·ak·is). Spina bifida. [Gk *schistos* cleft, *rhachis* backbone.]

schistosis (skis·**to**·sis). The silicosis which occurs in workers in certain slate quarries. [schist (a type of rock), Gk *-osis* condition.]

Schistosoma (skis·to·**so**·mah). A genus of blood flukes. At least 3 species cause schistosomiasis (bilharziasis) in man, and the cercariae of these and other species may cause a dermatitis, swamp itch. The adults of the species which affect humans live in the veins of the lower abdomen: they are dioecious but the adults remain together in pairs, the cylindrical female in the gynaecophoric canal of the crescentic male. Eggs are shed in the small vessels of the intestine or bladder and pass into the lumen. Miracidia larvae bore into the snail hosts and form sporocysts in the digestive glands. These produce cercariae with bifid tails, without any intermediate redia stage. Cercariae bore actively through intact skin or through mucosa after entry *per os.* **Schistosoma bovis.** A species found in sheep and rarely, probably accidentally, in man; the intermediary host is *Bulinus truncatus.* **Schistosoma haematobium.** A species which occurs over much of Africa, including the Malagasy Republic, Egypt and the Sudan, and sporadically in the Mediterranean and Near East. The eggs, which have a terminal spine, are laid in valves of the bladder and pass out in urine. Secondary hosts are fresh-water snails of the genera *Bulinus, Physopsis* and, in Portugal, *Planorbis.* **Schistosoma incognitum.** A species known from pigs in India; its eggs have been found in human faeces. **Schistosoma intercalatum.** A species that is indistinguishable from *S. haematobium* except in its eggs, and occurs in man in Zaire. **Schistosoma japonicum.** A species which occurs in China, Japan and the Philippines. The eggs are small and unspined; they are laid in venules of the large intestine and pass in faeces. Secondary hosts are fresh-water and amphibious snails of the genera *Katayama, Oncomelania* and *Schistosomophora.* **Schistosoma mansoni.** A species which occurs over much of Africa and tropical America. The eggs, which have a lateral spine, are laid in venules of the large intestine and pass in faeces. Secondary hosts are fresh-water snails of the genus *Biomphalaria* in the Old World and *Australorbis glabratus* in the New World. **Schistosoma margrebowiei.** A species which occurs in cattle and game and perhaps in man in Rhodesia. **Schistosoma mattheei.** Probably the same as *S. bovis;* found in man in association with *S. haematobium;* intermediary host is *Physopsis africana.* **Schistosoma spindale.** A species which occurs in farm animals in India and has occurred in man, rarely. [Gk *schistos* cleft, *soma* body.]

Schistosomatidae (skis·to·so·**mat**′·id·e). A family of the trematode super-family Schistosomatoidea; blood flukes. The genus *Schistosoma* is of medical importance. [Gk *schistos* cleft, *soma* body, *eidos* form.]

Schistosomatoidea (**skis**·to·so·mat·**oid**′·e·ah). A super-family of Trematoda of the sub-order Strigeata. [see prec.]

schistosome (**skis**·to·some). A worm of the genus *Schistosoma.*

schistosomia (skis·to·**so**·me·ah). A congenital fissure of the abdominal wall. [Gk *schistos* cleft, *soma* body.]

schistosomiasis (**skis**·to·so·**mi**′·as·is). Bilharziasis; a group of diseases caused by trematode parasitic flukes of the family Schistosomatidae. They live in the veins of various internal organs and lay eggs of characteristic shapes which reach the exterior mainly by the urine or faeces. An essential stage in their life histories is passed in snails. **Asiatic schistosomiasis.** The variety caused by *Schistosoma japonicum.* **Cerebral schistosomiasis.** In any schistosomal infection, but particularly in *Schistosoma japonicum* infection, cerebral symptoms may occur as a result of ova lodging in the cerebral vessels. **Hepatic schistosomiasis.** Asiatic schistosomiasis (see above). **Intestinal schistosomiasis.** Manson's schistosomiasis, the variety caused by *Schistosoma mansoni;* symptoms of dysentery are found. **Schistosomiasis japonica.** Asiatic schistosomiasis (see above). **Oriental schistosomiasis.** Asiatic schistosomiasis (see above). **Rectal schistosomiasis.** Schistosomiasis involving the rectum; this normally occurs in *Schistosoma mansoni* infection but also in *S. japonicum* and *S. haematobium* infections. The ova can be found in rectal biopsies. **Urinary schistosomiasis.** The variety caused by *Schistosoma haematobium,* characterized by painful micturition with bleeding. **Vesical schistosomiasis.** Schistosomiasis affecting the bladder; *Schistosoma haematobium* infection. **Visceral schistosomiasis.** Intestinal schistosomiasis (see above).

See also: MANSON.

schistosomicide (skis·to·**so**·mis·ide). A specific drug used in the treatment of schistosomiasis. [schistosome, L *caedere* to kill.]

Schistosomidae (skis·to·**so**·mid·e). Schistosomatidae.

Schistosomophora (skis·to·so·**mof**′·or·ah). A genus of fresh-water pulmonate Gastropoda. Several species are intermediate hosts to the fluke *Schistosoma japonicum* in the Philippines. Most species are now classified in the genus *Oncomelania*. **Schistosomophora slateri.** *Oncomelania nosophora slateri.* [Gk *schistos* cleft, *soma* body, *phorein* to bear.]

schistosomus (skis·to·**so**·mus). A monster the body of which is cleft. [Gk *schistos* cleft, *soma* body.]

schistosternia (skis·to·**ster**·ne·ah). A congenital condition in which the sternum is fissured. [Gk *schistos* cleft, sternum.]

schistothorax (skis·to·**thor**·ax). A congenital cleft of the chest wall. [Gk *schistos* cleft, thorax.]

schistotrachelus (skis·to·**trak**·el·us). A monster the neck of which is fissured. [Gk *schistos* cleft, *trachelos* neck.]

schizaxon (skiz·**ax**·on). An axon which divides into 2 equal or almost equal branches. [Gk *schizein* to split, axon.]

schizo- (**ski**·zo, **skiz**·o). A combining term meaning a split or division. [Gk *schizein* to split.]

Schizoblastosporion (**ski**·zo·blas·to·**spor**′·e·on). A monospecific genus of asporogenous yeasts which reproduce by budding combined with fission. [Gk *schizein* to split, *blastos* germ, *sporos* seed.]

schizoblepharia (**ski**·zo·blef·**a**′·re·ah). A cleft of the eyelid. [Gk *schizein* to split, *blepharon* eyelid.]

schizocephalia (**ski**·zo·kef·**a**′·le·ah). The condition of a schizocephalus.

schizocephalus (**ski**·zo·**kef**·al·us). A monster the skull of which is fissured longitudinally. [Gk *schizein* to split, *kephale* head.]

schizocyte (**ski**·zo·site). Schistocyte. [Gk *schizein* to split, *kytos* cell.]

schizocytosis (**ski**·zo·si·**to**′·sis). Schistocytosis. [schizocyte, Gk *-osis* condition.]

schizogenesis (ski·zo·**jen**·es·is). In biology, reproduction by means of fission of cells; non-sexual reproduction. [Gk *schizein* to split, *genein* to produce.]

schizogenous (ski·**zoj**·en·us). Reproducing by schizogenesis.

schizognathism (ski·zo·**nath**·izm). A condition in which there is a cleft of either of the jaws. [Gk *schizein* to split, *gnathos* jaw.]

schizogonic (ski·zo·**gon**·ik). Relating or belonging to schizogony.

schizogony (ski·**zog**·on·e). Reproduction by fission, particularly that of the Sporozoa. [Gk *schizein* to split, *genein* to produce.]

schizogyria (ski·zo·**ji**·re·ah). A defective condition of the cerebral gyri in which continuity is broken owing to the presence of cuneiform fissures. [Gk *schizein* to split, gyrus.]

schizoid (**ski**·zoid). 1. Having qualities resembling those found in greater degree in schizophrenics, or qualities which may be found by catamnesis in schizophrenics before the onset of illness, or found in the relatives of schizophrenics, i.e. coldness, eccentricity, reserve, etc. 2. A person of schizoid personality. [schizophrenia, Gk *eidos* form.]

schizoidia, schizoidism (ski·**zoid**·e·ah, **ski**·zoid·izm). Schizophrenia. [see prec.]

schizoma sirenoides (ski·**zo**·mah si·ren·**oid**·eez). A fetal monster, superficially resembling a mermaid, in which 1 leg has failed to develop. There are associated abnormalities in the abdominal wall of the side where the limb is absent. [Gk *schizein* to split, *-oma* growth, *seiren* siren, *eidos* form.]

schizomycete (ski·zo·**mi**·seet). A micro-organism belonging to the class Schizomycetes.

Schizomycetes (**ski**·zo·mi·**se**′·teez). A class of micro-organisms embracing the bacteria or fission fungi. The class includes 5 orders, Actinomycetales, Chlamydobacteriales, Eubacteriales, Myxobacteriales and Spirochaetales. [Gk *schizein* to split, *mykes* fungus.]

schizomycetic (**ski**·zo·mi·**se**′·tik). Relating or belonging to schizomycetes, or caused by micro-organisms of the class Schizomycetes.

schizomycosis (**ski**·zo·mi·**ko**′·sis). Any disease caused by micro-organisms of the class Schizomycetes. [schizomycete, Gk *-osis* condition.]

schizont (**ski**·zont). The asexual dividing form of certain protozoa. It gives rise to young forms by division without conjugation, e.g. in the asexual cycle of malaria. [Gk *schizein* to split, *on* being.]

schizonticide (ski·**zon**·te·side). A certain class of antimalarial drug which is capable of destroying the malarial parasite at the schizont stage of its life cycle. Quinine and mepacrine are examples. [schizont, L *caedere* to kill.]

schizonychia (ski·zon·**ik**·e·ah). Splitting of the nails. [Gk *schizein* to split, *onyx* nail.]

schizophasia (ski·zo·**fa**·ze·ah). The unintelligible confused speech characteristically present in cases of schizophrenia. [Gk *schizein* to split, *phasis* speech.]

Schizophora (ski·**zof**·or·ah). A classificatory division of the insectan order Diptera. The families Calliphoridae, Gastrophilidae, Glossinidae, Hippoboscidae, Muscidae, Oestridae and Oscinidae are of medical interest. [Gk *schizein* to split, *pherein* to bear.]

schizophrenia (ski·zo·**fre**·ne·ah). A mental disorder characterized by a special type of disintegration of the personality: thought processes are directed by apparently random personal associations rather than logically to a goal, there is incongruity between the content of thought and the corresponding emotion, and an impaired relation to reality. Delusions, hallucinations and catatonia may be predominant features. [Gk *schizein* to split, *phren* mind.]

schizophreniac (ski·zo·**fre**·ne·ak). One affected with schizophrenia.

schizophrenic (ski·zo·**fren**·ik). 1. Relating or belonging to schizophrenia. 2. One affected with schizophrenia.

schizophrenogenic (**ski**·zo·fre·no·**jen**′·ik). Describing processes or conditions conducive to the appearance of schizophrenia or schizophrenic-like syndromes. [Gk *schizein* to split, *phren* mind, *genein* to produce.]

schizoprosopia (**ski**·zo·pro·**so**′·pe·ah). Congenital cleft of the face such as cleft palate or hare-lip. [Gk *schizein* to split, *prosopon* face.]

Schizosaccharomyces hominis (**ski**·zo·sak·ar·o·**mi**′·seez **hom**·in·is). An organism which has been shown by Dorrepaal to be a bacillus and not a yeast as at first supposed. [Gk *schizein* to split, saccharomyces, L *hominis* of man.]

schizosaccharomycosis pompholiciformis hominis (**ski**·zo·sak·ar·o·mi·**ko**′·sis pom·**fol**·is·if·**or**′·mis **hom**·in·is). An infection of the skin of the hands or feet associated with a dyshidrotic type of eruption, so named because it was reported to be caused by *Schizosaccharomyces hominis.* [Gk *schizein* to split, saccharomyces, Gk *-osis* condition, *pompholyx* bubble, L *forma* form, *hominis* of man.]

schizosis (ski·**zo**·sis). Excessive and morbid dislike of the society of others; a condition in which the individual tends to be morbidly self-centred. [Gk *schizein* to split, *-osis* condition.]

schizothorax (ski·zo·**thor**·ax). Congenital cleft of the chest wall. [Gk *schizein* to split, thorax.]

schizothymia (ski·zo·**thi**·me·ah). Schizophrenia. [Gk *schizein* to split, *thymos* soul.]

schizothymic (ski·zo·**thi**·mik). Schizophrenic. [see prec.]

schizotonia (ski·zo·**to**·ne·ah). Uneven tone in groups of muscles (hypertonia, hypotonia). [Gk *schizein* to split, *tonos* tension.]

schizotrichia (ski·zo·**trik**·e·ah). A disease of the hair in which the individual hairs are split at the tip. [Gk *schizein* to split, *thrix* hair.]

schizotropic (ski·zo·**trop**·ik). Attracted to schizonts. [schizont, Gk *trepein* to turn.]

schizotrypaniasis, schizotrypanosis (**ski**·zo·tri·pan·i′·as·is, **ski**·zo·tri·pan·**o**′·sis). Chagas' disease; American trypanosomiasis. [Gk *schizein* to split, trypanosome, Gk *-osis* condition.]

Schizotrypanum cruzi (**ski**·zo·**tri**·pan·um **kroo**·zi). *Trypanosoma cruzi;* a flagellated protozoon causing Chagas' disease in man in South and Central America. It is transmitted by the faeces of reduviid bugs.

schizozoite (ski·zo·**zo**·ite). The product of reproduction by fission of a schizont in the Sporozoa. [Gk *schizein* to split, *zoon* animal.]

schlammfieber (**shlam**·fe·ber). Mud fever; a form of spirochaetal jaundice which was described as occurring in young people who worked in the flooded areas around Breslau in 1891. [G slime fever.]

Schlange, Hans (b. 1856). Hanover surgeon.

Schlange's sign. Dilatation above, and absence of peristalsis below, the seat of obstruction in the intestine.

Schlatter, Carl (b. 1864). Zürich surgeon.

Schlatter's disease, Osgood-Schlatter disease. Osteochondritis of the epiphysis of the tibial tuberosity.

Schlemm, Friedrich (b. 1795). Berlin anatomist.

canal of Schlemm. The sinus venosus sclerae.

Schlesinger, Hermann (b. 1866). Vienna physician.

Schlesinger's sign. In tetany. Strong passive flexion at the hip joint will produce extreme extension of the knee and inversion of the foot; also called *leg phenomenon, leg sign.*

Schlesinger's type of syringomyelia. Syringomyelia of the dorsolumbar region of the spinal cord.

Schlesinger, Wilhelm (b. 1869). Vienna physician.

Schlesinger's test. For urobilin. To about 10 ml of urine add a few drops of solution of iodine (Lugol's) and an equal volume of saturated alcoholic zinc acetate. Mix and filter. The presence of urobilin is indicated by a greenish fluorescence in the filtrate. A more sensitive modification is: to 5 ml of urine in a small separator add a few crystals of ammonium persulphate, shake, add 5 ml of saturated alcoholic zinc acetate and mix. Add 10 ml of chloroform and shake gently for 10 s, allow to separate and run off the chloroform. Clarify the chloroform with a few drops of absolute alcohol and examine in filtered ultraviolet light. A golden-yellow fluorescence which is destroyed by addition of a crystal of trichloro-acetic acid indicates excess of urobilin.

Schlippe, K. F. (b. 1799). German chemist.

Schlippe's salt. Golden sulphide, $Na_3SbS_4{\cdot}9H_2O$, a yellow crystalline compound obtained by melting antimony trisulphide with sulphur, charcoal and sodium sulphate. It is used as a colouring for rubber.

Schloesser, Carl (b. 1857). Munich ophthalmologist.

Schloesser's injection, method or treatment. Injection of alcohol into the branches of the trigeminal nerve at their foramina, in the treatment of trigeminal neuralgia.

Schlossman, Abraham (b. 1918). American ophthalmologist.

Posner-Schlossman syndrome. Glaucomatocyclitic crises; recurrent unilateral non-congestive glaucoma characterized by an open angle and keratic precipitates.

Schmidt, Alexander (b. 1831). German physiologist.

Schmidt's fibrinoplastin. Serum globulin.

Schmidt's theory. Of blood coagulation. Coagulation of blood is the end-result of a series of factors reacting in sequence and culminating in the conversion of fibrinogen into fibrin under the influence of thrombin acting as a ferment.

Schmidt, Eduard Oskar (b. 1823). German anatomist.

Schmidt and Manz theory. To explain swelling of the optic disc in raised intracranial pressure. Accumulation of fluid in the intervaginal space causes a stasis of lymph in the trunk of the optic nerve, especially in the region of the lamina cribrosa sclerae; this causes compression of the central vessels, particularly the vein. This outflow of blood being obstructed, the disc becomes increasingly swollen.

Schmidt, Henry D. (b. 1823). New Orleans pathologist.

Schmidt's clefts or incisures, Schmidt-Lantermann clefts or incisures. Numerous irregular oblique notches or interruptions in the myelin sheath of a nerve fibre between the nodes of Ranvier.

Schmidt's node. The portion of a nerve fibre between successive nodes of Ranvier.

Schmidt-Lantermann segment. That portion of the myelin sheath of a nerve fibre that lies between successive incisures or clefts of Schmidt-Lantermann.

Schmidt, Johann Friedrich Moritz (b. 1838). Frankfurt laryngologist.

Schmidt's syndrome. The vago-accessory syndrome, due to a lesion of the nucleus ambiguus and the nucleus of the 11th cranial nerve; there is ipselateral paralysis of palatal, pharyngeal, and intrinsic laryngeal muscles and of sternocleidomastoid and trapezius muscles.

Schmidt-Rimpler, Hermann (b. 1838). German physician.

Schmidt-Rimpler's optometer. One of the earliest forms of optometer. Using the principle of indirect ophthalmoscopy, an image of a trellis-work marked on the source of light is focused sharply on the retina. From the distance of the condensing lens from the cornea can be measured the far point of the eye.

Schmiedel, Kasimir Christoph (b. 1716). German anatomist and botanist.

Schmiedel's anastomosis. Intercommunications between the tributaries of the inferior vena cava and those of the portal system.

Schmiedel's ganglion. A collection of ganglion cells in the carotid nerve of the cervical sympathetic system: it is situated in the cavernous sinus of the dura mater.

Schmincke, Alexander (b. 1877). Munich pathologist.

Schmincke tumour. A lympho-epithelioma of the lymphatic tissue in Waldeyer's ring around the nasopharynx.

Schmitz, Karl Eitel Friedrich (b. 1889). Greifswald physician.

Schmitz bacillus. *Shigella schmitzi.*

Schmorl, Christian Georg (b. 1861). Dresden pathologist.

Schmorl's body or node. *See* SCHMORL'S DISEASE (below).

Schmorl's disease. 1. Prolapse of the nucleus pulposus into the body of the vertebra. The protrusion is sometimes known as *Schmorl's body* or *node*, and the indentation in the border of the vertebra is referred to by radiologists as *Schmorl's nodule*. 2. Necrobacillosis of rabbits.

Schmorl's furrow. A groove about 2 cm below the apex of the lung, caused by a shortening of the 1st rib and consequent narrowing of the upper thoracic opening and pressure on the lung. It is not uncommon at birth, but normally disappears with the development of the chest at adolescence. Persistence has been regarded as predisposing to pulmonary tuberculosis.

Schmorl's groove. A groove produced by the bulging of intercostal spaces owing to underlying emphysema of the lung.

Schmorl's nodule. *See* SCHMORL'S DISEASE (above).

Schnabel, Isidor (b. 1842). Vienna ophthalmologist.

Schnabel's cavernous atrophy, excavation of the optic disc or caverns. Cupping of the optic disc not associated with glaucoma, but, according to Schnabel, with high myopia. A similar condition is sometimes seen as a result of sclerosis of the vessels supplying the optic nerve.

Schnabel's theory. The theory that myopia was due to a diminished rigidity of the coats of the eye due to a congenital defect.

Schnee bath. A bath designed to give a diathermy current treatment.

Schneeberg tumour. Cancer of the lung in cobalt miners.

Schneider, Edward Christian (b. 1874). Connecticut physiologist.

Schneider's indicator. An index of circulatory efficiency based on circulation data.

Schneider, Konrad Victor (b. 1614). Wittenberg anatomist.

Schneider's membrane, Schneiderian membrane. The mucous membrane lining the nasal cavities.

Schoemaker, Jan (b. 1871). The Hague surgeon.

Schoemaker's clamp. A fine crushing clamp with V-shaped blades for controlling the colon in aseptic excision.

Schoemaker's gastrectomy. A Billroth I type of gastrectomy in which the lesser curvature is reconstituted by the application of a special curved double crushing clamp to the upper part of the opening in the gastric remnant.

Schoemaker's line. A line connecting the greater trochanter of the femur to the anterior superior spine of the ilium. When the bones are in normal position a projection of this line runs above the umbilicus; when the trochanter is raised the projection runs below the umbilicus.

Schoemaker's operation. 1. Aseptic colectomy for carcinoma with the use of special fine crushing clamps. 2. Schoemaker's gastrectomy (see above).

Schoenheimer, Rudolf (b. 1898). American biochemist.

Schoenheimer and Sperry method. For cholesterol in blood. Serum is extracted with boiling acetone-alcohol (equal parts), cooled, made to volume and filtered. The free cholesterol in an aliquot of the filtrate is precipitated with digitonin, the precipitate purified and the cholesterol determined by the Liebermann-Burchard reaction. Another aliquot is saponified with potassium hydroxide and the total cholesterol precipitated with digitonin, purified and determined as before. The difference between total and free cholesterol gives cholesterol esters.

Schoenlein, Johannes Lucas (b. 1793). Berlin physician.

Schoenlein's disease or purpura. A purpura usually seen in young adults, associated with painful swollen joints; also called *purpura rheumatica.*

Henoch-Schoenlein disease, purpura or syndrome, Schoenlein-Henoch disease, purpura or syndrome. Allergic purpura. The term is used to include all the features of Schoenlein's and Henoch's purpuras.

Scholz, Willibald (b. 1889). German neurologist.

Scholz's disease. The juvenile form of diffuse cerebral sclerosis; a familial demyelinating encephalopathy related to Schilder's disease, Krabbe's disease and Pelizaeus-Merzbacher disease.

Schöngastia (shern·gas·te·ah). A genus of mites, 2 species of which cause mite dermatitis (scrub itch), namely, *Schöngastia blestowei* and *S. pusilla.*

Schott, Theodor (b. 1852). Nauheim physician.

Schott's treatment. Therapy of heart disorders by means of warm saline baths and regulated exercises. This is no longer a treatment for cardiovascular disease, but is a useful means of rehabilitating the patient who is convalescing from cardiac disease.

Schottmueller, Hugo (b. 1867). Hamburg physician.

Schottmueller's disease. Paratyphoid B fever [Obsolete term.].

Schottmueller's streptothrix. *Streptothrix muris,* now named *Actinomyces muris.*

Schramm's phenomenon. The funnel-neck deformity of the bladder due to dilatation of the proximal urethra with relaxation of the internal sphincter, so that the whole posterior urethra assumes a conical shape with the base of the cone directed towards the bladder. The condition is found in the neurogenic bladder of tabes, and is associated with certain other lesions on the spinal cord. It was originally described by Burns of Baltimore, and *funnel-neck deformity of the bladder neck* is the descriptive term of choice.

Schreger, Bernhard Gottlob (b. 1766). German anatomist.

Schreger's band, line or stria. One of the microscopic markings in dentine formed by the superimposition of the primary curvatures of the dentinal tubules.

Schreiber, Julius (b. 1848). Königsberg physician.

Schreiber's manoeuvre. The inner side of the upper part of the thigh is rubbed whilst the patellar reflex is tested.

Schridde, Hermann Robert August (b. 1875). Dortmund pathologist.

Schridde's disease. Congenital general dropsy.

Schridde's granules. Granules which stain with acid fuchsine dyes, and which have been described in certain lymphocytes and plasma cells.

Schridde's cancer hair. Dark coarse hairs found occasionally in the beard or on the temples of patients with cancer or cachexia.

Schroder's vaccine. An obsolete vaccine prepared from killed tubercle bacilli.

Schroeder, Karl Ludwig Ernst (b. 1838). Berlin gynaecologist.

Schroeder's ring. Bandl's ring.

Schroeder van der Kolk, Jacob Ludwig Conrad (b. 1797). Utrecht physician.

Schroeder's fibres. The fibres composing the reticular formation of the medulla oblongata.

Schroeder's law. Sensory fibres of a mixed nerve supply the parts which are moved by muscle activated by motor fibres of the same nerve.

Schroetter, Leopold (b. 1837). Vienna physician.

Schroetter's catheter. A firm rubber catheter for dilating a laryngeal stricture.

Schroth, Johann (b. 1800). German nature-curer.

Schroth's treatment. Of obesity. Reducing water to a minimum.

Schuchardt, Karl August (b. 1856). Stettin surgeon.

Schuchardt's operation. An extended paravaginal incision for facilitating access in vaginal surgery.

Schueffner, Wilhelm (b. 1867). German physician and parasitologist in Amsterdam.

Schueffner's culture medium. Fresh guinea-pig serum in buffered peptone: it is a medium used for *Leptospira.*

Schueffner's dots or stippling. Fine even stippling of the erythrocyte, characteristic of *Plasmodium vivax* and *P. ovale* infections.

Schueffner's granules. Schueffner's dots (see above); a term not commonly used.

Schuele, Heinrich (b. 1840). German psychiatrist.

Schuele's sign. Frowning, which is said to be characteristic of melancholia.

Schueller, Artur (b. 1874). Vienna neurologist.

Schueller's disease or syndrome, Christian-Schueller disease, Schueller-Christian disease, Hand-Schueller-Christian disease or syndrome. Hand's disease; xanthomatosis: a non-familial disturbance of lipoid (cholesterol) metabolism seen in young children, characterized by slight anaemia, defects in membranous bone, mainly skull, exophthalmos, diabetes insipidus, often with dwarfism, and a yellowish-brown colour (xanthomatosis) of the skin. Sometimes the liver, spleen and glands are enlarged to a moderate degree.

Schueller's phenomenon. A hemiplegic patient turns to the affected side on walking if the hemiplegia is organic, to the unaffected side if it is functional.

Schueller's projection. A radiographic position for examining the mastoid bone.

Schueller, Karl Heinrich Anton Ludwig Max (b. 1843). Berlin surgeon.

Schueller's ducts or glands. The para-urethral ducts of the female urethra. They transmit the secretion of small glands near the urethral orifice, believed to be homologues of the male prostatic glands.

Schueller's method. A method of artificial respiration in which the chest is raised rhythmically by the fingers hooked under the lower ribs.

Schueller's operation. For entropion [obsolete].

Schuetz, Johann Wilhelm (b. 1839). German bacteriologist.

Schuetz-Loeffler bacillus. *Pfeifferella mallei.*

Schultes (Scultetus), Johann (b. 1595). Ulm surgeon.

Scultetus' position. A position in which the body is in an inclined plane with head downwards.

Schultess, Ernst (fl. 1897). Jena physician.

Schultess' test. For proteose in urine. Acidify the urine with acetic acid and filter off any precipitate of mucoprotein. If coagulable protein is present, boil the filtrate and filter again. Add 5 ml of the filtrate to 150 ml of absolute alcohol and allow to stand overnight. Decant off the alcohol and dissolve the precipitate in a little hot water, filter and apply the biuret test. A positive reaction indicates proteose.

Schultz, Werner (b. 1878). Berlin physician.

Schultz angina, disease or syndrome, Werner Schultz disease. Agranulocytosis.

Schultz triad. Leucopenia, gangrenous stomatitis and jaundice; agranulocytic angina.

Schultz-Charlton phenomenon, reaction or test. A rash-extinction reaction or test, produced by injecting convalescent scarlet-fever serum or commercial streptococcus antitoxin intracutaneously into any area of bright red rash believed to be that of scarlet fever. Blanching at the site of injection indicates that the rash is that of scarlet fever.

Schultz-Dale reaction or test. Smooth muscle taken from an animal that has been made anaphylactic shows a powerful contraction in the presence of minute amounts of the same antigen: the smooth muscle is capable of being desensitized. Schultz used intestinal muscle, and Dale uterine muscle from virgin guinea-pigs.

Schultze, Bernhard Sigismund (b. 1827). Jena gynaecologist.

Schultze fold. A fold of the amnion where the umbilical cord attaches to the placenta and marking the site of the atrophic yolk sac.

Schultze powder. A mixture of calomel, talcum powder and zinc oxide, applied as a powder to the skin of newly-born infants.

Schultze, Ernst (b. 1860). Swiss physiologist.

Hardy-Schultze rule. In the coagulation of a lyophobic sol, instability is increased by the addition of electrolyte, the effect being proportionally greater with doubly- and triply-charged ions than with those bearing a single charge. The rule does not hold with lyophilic sols.

Schultze, Friedrich (b. 1848). Bonn neurologist.

Schultze sign. Chvostek's sign [Obsolete term.].

Schultze type. The simple form of acroparaesthesia tending to acrocyanosis.

Schultze, Maximilian Johann Sigismund (b. 1825). Bonn anatomist.

bundle of Schultze, Schultze tract. The comma tract or fasciculus interfascicularis; descending branches from the fibres of the cuneate and gracile fasciculi.

Schultze cells. Cells of the olfactory region of the nasal mucous membrane.

fasciculus of Schultze. The dorsal longitudinal fasciculus; a longitudinal bundle of fine, mostly non-medullated fibres in the central grey matter of the mid-brain, extending into the floor of the 4th ventricle and possibly to lower levels of the nervous system; they are said to arise in the hypothalamus.

Schultze membrane. The olfactory mucosa.

Schultze, Walter Hans Gustav (b. 1880). Göttingen pathologist.

Schultze's indophenol oxidase test. The original indophenol test, performed on formalin-fixed material, and of value in haematological studies of the bone marrow, because the granules of the myeloid series of cells give a positive reaction.

Schultze's phantom. A model of the female pelvis used to demonstrate and practise the manipulations employed in obstetrics.

Schulz, Hugo (b. 1853). German pharmacologist.

Arndt-Schulz law. A weak stimulus increases physiological activity, but a strong one abolishes or diminishes it.

Schumm, Otto (b. 1874). Hamburg biochemist.

Schumm's test. For methaemalbuminaemia. 10 parts of serum or plasma are covered with ether and 1 part of concentrated ammonium sulphide solution added. Spectroscopic examination will show absorption bands at 558 and 527 nm.

Schutz, H. (fl. 1902). German neurologist.

bundle of Schutz. The dorsal longitudinal fasciculus, mainly efferent from the hypothalamus to visceral nuclei of the brain stem.

Schwabach, Dagobert (b. 1846). Berlin otologist.

Schwabach's test. A test for comparison of normal hearing by bone conduction with that of a deaf patient. A vibrating tuning fork is placed on the vertex of a normal-hearing person's head. When no longer heard, it is transferred to the patient's vertex. If still heard by the patient, hearing by bone conduction is said to be prolonged. This occurs in impedance types of deafness, such as otosclerosis. If the sound is not heard, the test is repeated, the patient being tested first. If the examiner can hear the fork vibrating after the patient ceases to perceive it, hearing by bone conduction is recorded as being reduced. This occurs in cases of nerve deafness.

Schwalbe, Gustav Albert (b. 1844). Königsberg and Strasbourg anatomist.

Schwalbe's convolutions. The inferior lateral occipital gyrus. *See* GYRUS.

Schwalbe's corpuscles. The taste buds. *See* BUD.

Schwalbe's fissure. The choroidal fissure. *See* FISSURE.

Schwalbe's foramen. The pharyngeal bursa. *See* BURSA.

Schwalbe's line. The peripheral edge of Descemet's membrane from which the trabecular meshwork arises.

Schwalbe's nucleus. The medial vestibular nucleus. *See* NUCLEUS.

Schwalbe's sheath. The membrane covering an elastic fibre.

Schwalbe's space. A lymphatic space described on the outer surface of the dural sheath of the optic nerve.

Schwann, Friedrich Theodor (b. 1810). Louvain and Berlin anatomist.

Schwann's cell. A neurilemmal cell from the sheath of a peripheral nerve fibre.

Schwann's membrane, sheath of Schwann. The neurilemmal sheath of a nerve fibre, formed of nucleated cells. The inner endoneurium of the nerve fibres.

Schwann's nucleus. The nucleus of a neurilemmal cell.

white substance of Schwann. Myelin.

schwannoglioma, schwannoma (shwon·o·gli·o′·mah, shwon·o·-mah). An innocent tumour of a nerve derived from the neurilemma or sheath of Schwann. [F. T. *Schwann*, glioma.]

schwannosis (shwon·o·sis). Hypertrophy of the neurilemma or sheath of Schwann. [F. T. *Schwann*, Gk *-osis* condition.]

Schwartz, Samuel. Minneapolis physician.

Watson-Schwartz test. For porphyrinuria. A test similar to that of Waldenström.

Schwartze, Hermann (b. 1837). Halle otologist.

Schwartze's operation. The original operation for draining of the mastoid antrum and air cells.

Schwartzmann, Gregory (b. 1896). New York bacteriologist.

Schwartzmann phenomenon. Local haemorrhagic allergy to *Salmonella typhi* culture filtrate.

Schwartzmann reaction or test. A biological reaction to antigenic bacterial exotoxins. A bacterial filtrate is injected by any route; 24 h later the active substance is injected intravenously. Local haemorrhagic necrosis is produced at the site of the original injection.

Schweigger-Seidel, Franz (b. 1834). German histologist.

Schweigger-Seidel sheath. A sheath of elongated reticular cells surrounding the terminal branches of the splenic artery in the splenic pulp.

Schweitzer, Matthias Eduard (b. 1818). Zürich chemist.

Schweitzer's reagent. A solution formed by dissolving cupric hydroxide in ammonia. It contains the cuprammonium ion, and being a solvent for cellulose is used in the manufacture of rayon. It is also used in the waterproofing of cotton.

Schweninger, Ernst (b. 1850). Munich physician.

Schweninger's method. The treatment of obesity by the restriction of dietary fluid.

sciage (se·ahzh). In massage, a to-and-fro movement of medial border of the hand resembling that made in using a saw. [Fr. sawing.]

scialyscope (si·al·e·skope). An arrangement of mirrors and lenses to throw an image of an operation from the operating theatre into a darkened room. [Gk *skialos* shadowy, *skopein* to view.]

sciapody (si·ap·o·de). Macropodia. [Gk *skaios* clumsy, *pous* foot.]
sciatic (si·at·ik). Relating or belonging to the ischium or to the sciatic nerve. [Gk *ischiadikos* of the hip joint.]
sciatic nerve [nervus ischiadicus]. The largest nerve in the body; a branch of the sacral plexus (root value L4, 5 S1, 2, 3) consisting of 2 parts, the medial and lateral popliteal nerves, which may remain separate throughout. It supplies directly, or through its branches, the hamstring muscles, the muscles arising at or below the knee joint, the muscles of the foot and all the skin below the knee, except for a small area above and posteriorly and a large area on the medial side of the leg and foot.
sciatica (si·at·ik·ah). Pain in the course of the sciatic nerve, with tender points on pressure due to a neuritis of the nerve. [Gk *ischiadikos* of the hip joint.]
science (si·ens). A body of accepted fact; any system of knowledge covering a special field of investigation. **Christian Science.** A religious system of healing mind and body founded by Mary Baker Eddy (b. 1821). [L *scientia* knowledge.]
scieropia (si·er·o·pe·ah). Defect of vision in which objects are seen as if in a shadow. [Gk *skieros* shady, *ops* eye.]
scilla (sil·ah). Squill. The bulb of *Urginea maritima* Linn. Baker (family Liliaceae), divested of its dry membranous outer scales, cut into slices and dried. It contains the crystalline glycoside scillarin A, and an amorphous mixture of glycosides (scillarin B). [Gk *skilla.*]
scillaridin A (sil·ar·id·in a). $C_{24}H_{30}O_3$, an aglycone obtained by the hydrolysis of scillarin A. It is related to the aglycones from the digitalis glycosides.
scillarin (sil·ar·in). A mixture of the glycosides scillarin A and scillarin B. **Scillarin A, Scillarin B.** Glycosides occurring in squill and responsible for its cardiotoxic action. *Scillarin A*, $C_{36}H_{52}O_{13}$, is a crystalline compound which hydrolyses to scillaridin A, glucose and rhamnose: *scillarin B* is amorphous. Both are related to the digitalis glycosides.
scillism (sil·izm). Poisoning produced by squill. [scilla.]
scillitic (sil·it·ik). Of or relating to squill. [scilla.]
scillitoxin (sil·e·tox·in). A substance extracted from squill (scilla) which has some digitalis-like activity; it is not a pure glycoside. [scilla, Gk *toxikon* poison.]
scillocephaly (sil·o·kef·al·e). A small, conical-shaped head. [L *scilla* squill, Gk *kephale* head.]
scillonin (sil·on·in). An extract from squill (scilla) containing some of the active glycosides.
scintigram (sin·te·gram). A recording of the radioactivity emanating from an object or an organism, irrespective of the mode of introduction of the radionuclide or of the nature of the recording. [scintillation, Gk *gramma* record.]
scintigraphy (sin·tig·raf·e). The recording of an image of an organ by introduction of radioactive material which is detected by a scintillator detector. [L *scintillatio* a sparkling, Gk *graphein* to record.]
scintillascope (sin·til·ah·skope). A device for viewing the scintillations produced by α-particles on a fluorescent screen. [scintillation, Gk *skopein* to view.]
scintillation (sin·til·a·shun). The light flash produced when a quantum of ionizing radiation is absorbed in a crystal or in certain organic liquids or certain plastics. [L *scintillatio* a sparkling.]
scintillator (sin·til·a·tor). **Liquid scintillator.** An organic liquid which has the property of emitting light flashes when ionizing radiation is absorbed within it. Used as a liquid scintillation counter and, occasionally, in radiation detectors where the sensitive volume is required to be large. **Plastic scintillator.** A plastic with ingredients which confer upon it the property of emitting light flashes when ionizing radiation is absorbed within it. It is used in some forms of scintillation counter. [L *scintillatio* a sparkling.]
scintillography (sin·til·og·raf·e). Scintigraphy.
scintiscan (sin·te·skan). Strictly a scan composed of a series of dots, spots or dashes, the number of such per unit area representing the radiation intensity detected over the corresponding area of the body. The term is sometimes used more loosely as being synonymous with *scan.* [L *scintilla* spark, *scandere* to climb.]
scintiscanning (sin·te·skan·ing). The technique of recording the radioactivity emanating from a radio-isotope with an object, or part or organ of the body, by means of a scanning device. [scintillation, L *scandere* to climb.]
scirrhencanthis, scirrhencanthus (sir·en·kan·this, sir·en·kan·thus). A scirrhous tumour of the lacrimal gland. [scirrhus, Gk *en,* canthus.]
scirrhoblepharoncus (sir·o·blef·ar·ong'·kus). A scirrhus of the eyelid. [scirrhus, Gk *blepharon* eyelid, *ogkos* mass.]
scirrhocele (sir·o·seel). Hard cancerous growth of the testis. [scirrhus, Gk *kele* hernia.]
scirrhoid (sir·oid). Resembling a scirrhous tumour. [scirrhus, Gk *eidos* form.]
scirrhoma (sir·o·mah). Scirrhus. **Scirrhoma caminianorum.** Soot (chimney-sweeps') cancer. *See* CANCER. [scirrhus, Gk *-oma* tumour.]
scirrhophthalmia (sir·of·thal·me·ah). A scirrhous tumour of the eye. [scirrhus, Gk *ophthalmos* eye.]
scirrhosarca (sir·o·sar·kah). Sclerema neonatorum. [Gk *skirrhos* hard, *sarx* flesh.]
scirrhous (sir·us). Relating to or of the nature of a scirrhus; indurated.
scirrhus (sir·us). Hard and fibrous, usually applied to a hard, fibrous, slow-growing carcinoma. [Gk *skirrhos* hard.]
scissile (sis·ile). Suitable for cutting or dividing. [see foll.]
scission (sizh·un). Cutting; splitting; division. 1. In biology, the mitotic division of cells. 2. In chemistry, the fracture of a ring-structure or the splitting-off of part of a molecule as in the breaking-down of a carbon chain. [L *scindere* to split.]
scissiparity (sis·e·par·it·e). Reproduction by means of fission. [L *scindere* to split, *parere* to give birth.]
scissor (siz·er). **Scissor gait, Scissor leg.** A condition of adduction at both hips, which may be present after disease of the hip joints, resulting in crossing of the legs when walking. [see foll.]
scissors (siz·erz). A cutting instrument with apposed blades and handles on a central fulcrum. **Artery scissors.** Fine scissors with small blades used in vascular surgery. **Canalicular scissors.** Fine scissors with one blade probe-pointed for opening the lacrimal canaliculi. **Cannula scissors.** Probe-pointed scissors for laying open a canal. **Craniotomy scissors.** Strong scissors, double-curved on the flat, for opening the fetal head. **Iris scissors.** Fine scissors for iridectomy. **Jewish scissors.** A cutting instrument used in ritual circumcision. **Plaster scissors.** Strong scissors for removing plaster casts. [L *scindere* to cut.]
See also: LISTON, MAYO (C. H.), SMELLIE, WECKER.
scissura, scissure (sis·ewr·ah, sis·ewr). A cleft or fissure; a split. **Scissura pilorum.** Splitting at the tips of the individual hairs. [L a splitting.]
Sciurus argentinus (si·ewr·us ar·jen·ti·nus). The Argentine squirrel; a host of *Trypanosoma cruzi.* [L *sciurus* squirrel.]
Sclavo, Achille (b. 1861). Rome bacteriologist.
Sclavo's serum. Anti-anthrax serum, first prepared by Sclavo in sheep and later in the ass. It is useful in the treatment of human anthrax.
sclera [NA] (skleer·ah). The outer, opaque fibrous coat of the eyeball. It maintains the shape of the organ and provides attachment to the extrinsic ocular muscles. **Blue sclera.** An inherited trait in which the sclerotics show a bluish colour. [Gk *skleros* hard.]
scleradenitis (skleer·ad·en·i'·tis). Inflammatory hardening of a gland. [Gk *skleros* hard, *aden* gland, *-itis* inflammation.]
scleral (skleer·al). Relating or belonging to the sclera.
sclerangia (skleer·an·je·ah). 1. Sensation of hardness on palpation of a vein or artery. 2. Angiosclerosis. [Gk *skleros* hard, *aggeion* small vessel.]
scleratheroma (skleer·ath·er·o'·mah). Nodular arteriosclerosis; the outer coat is hyperplastic and there is adipose degeneration of the middle coat. [Gk *skleros* hard, *athere* meal, *-oma* tumour.]

scleratitis (skleer·at·i·tis). Scleritis.

scleratogenous (skleer·at·**oj**·en·us). 1. Producing or secreting sclerotic tissue. 2. Giving rise to sclerosis. [Gk *skleros* hard, *genein* to produce.]

sclerectasia, sclerectasis (skleer·ek·**ta**·ze·ah, skleer·**ek**·tas·is). A bulging or protrusion of the sclera. [sclera, Gk *ektasis* a stretching.]

sclerecto-iridectomy (skleer·**ek**·to·ir·id·**ek'**·to·me). An operation for the relief of glaucoma in which, in addition to iridectomy, a portion of sclera is also removed. It is associated with the name of Lagrange. [sclerectomy, iridectomy.]

sclerecto-iridodialysis (skleer·**ek**·to·ir·id·o·di·**al'**·is·is). Combined sclerectomy and iridodialysis, one of the operations performed for glaucoma.

sclerectome (**skleer**·ek·tome). An instrument used in sclerectomy.

sclerectomy (skleer·**ek**·to·me). An operation on the eye in which a piece of sclera is excised, either at the limbus as a drainage operation for glaucoma (e.g. Lagrange's operation with scissors, or Holth's with a punch) or where a circumferential strip is excised and the sclera sutured for retinal detachment. **Punch sclerectomy.** Holth's operation. [sclera, Gk *ektome* excision.]

See also: HOLTH, LAGRANGE.

sclerema, scleremia, scleremus (skleer·e·mah, skleer·e·me·ah, skleer·e·mus). Putty-like thickening of the skin and subcutaneous tissues. **Sclerema adiposum.** Sclerema neonatorum (see below). **Sclerema cutis.** Sclerema of the skin. **Sclerema neonatorum.** A malady of debilitated babies in which the skin of the lower extremities becomes smooth, shrunken, whitish, leathery and cold; the condition extends upward and the joints become immobile. The malady is a metabolic disease, associated with diminution of the olein content of the fat. The melting point of this abnormal fat is high and solidification of the fatty tissues occurs: death therefore ensues. A milder, non-fatal, variety of this disease, which occurs later in infancy, has been recognized. **Sclerema oedematosum.** Oedema neonatorum. [Gk *skleros* hard.]

sclerencephalia, sclerencephaly (**skleer**·en·kef·**a'**·le·ah, skleer·en·**kef**·al·e). A sclerotic condition with resultant shrinkage of the brain substance. [Gk *skleros* hard, *egkephalos* brain.]

sclerenchyma (skleer·en·**ki**·mah). In botany, the fibrous, woody substance in plants, e.g. that which composes the outer covering of a nut. [Gk *skleros* hard, enchyma.]

sclerenchymatous (skleer·en·**ki**·mat·us). Having the characteristics of sclerenchyma.

scleriasis (skleer·i·as·is). 1. Scleroderma. 2. An indurated condition of the eyelid. [Gk *skleros* hard.]

scleriritomy (skleer·i·**rit**·o·me). Incision of the iris and sclera; an operation for relief of anterior staphyloma. [sclera, iris, Gk *temnein* to cut.]

scleritic (skleer·it·ik). Sclerous.

scleritis (skleer·i·tis). Inflammation of the sclera, often of doubtful aetiology since it is frequently an allergic reaction to some infection such as tuberculosis, syphilis, focal disease (teeth, tonsils, etc.) and rheumatoid arthritis. It is also seen in gout. **Annular scleritis.** Scleritis in which the affection is limited to the area surrounding the margin of the cornea and forms a complete ring. **Anterior scleritis.** Scleritis affecting any portion or portions of the anterior half of the sclera. **Brawny scleritis.** A virulent form of diffuse annular scleritis, usually bilateral and associated with gelatinous swelling of the episcleral tissue. **Scleritis necroticans.** Scleromalacia perforans. **Posterior scleritis.** Scleritis in which the affection is limited to the posterior half of the globe and usually involves Tenon's capsule; it is associated with oedema of the eyelids and marked swelling of the bulbar conjunctiva (chemosis). [sclera, Gk *-itis* inflammation.]

sclero-adipose (skleer·o·**ad**·ip·oze). Applied to tissue composed of both fibrous and fatty elements. [Gk *skleros* hard, L *adeps* soft fat.]

sclero-atrophic (**skleer**·o·at·**rof'**·ik). Showing both sclerosis and atrophy.

scleroblastema (**skleer**·o·blas·**te'**·mah). The skeletogenous mesenchyme. [Gk *skleros* hard, *blastema* shoot.]

sclerocataract (skleer·o·**kat**·ar·akt). Hard cataract. *See* CATARACT. [Gk *skleros* hard, cataract.]

sclerochoroiditis (**skleer**·o·kor·oid·**i'**·tis). Inflammation of the sclera accompanied by choroiditis. **Sclerochoroiditis anterior.** That in which the anterior portion of the choroid is affected. **Sclerochoroiditis posterior.** That in which the posterior portion of the choroid is affected.

scleroconjunctival (**skleer**·o·kon·jungk·**ti'**·val). Belonging to the sclera and the conjunctiva.

scleroconjunctivitis (**skleer**·o·kon·jungk·tiv·**i'**·tis). Inflammation affecting the sclera and the conjunctiva. [sclera, conjunctiva, Gk *-itis* inflammation.]

sclerocornea (skleer·o·**korn**·e·ah). The sclera and cornea when considered together as forming 1 single coat of the eye; the sclerocorneal coat.

sclerocorneal (skleer·o·**kor**·ne·al). Relating or belonging to the sclera and the cornea.

sclerocyclotomy (**skler**·o·si·**klot'**·o·me). Division of the ciliary muscle through an incision in the sclera, an operation devised by Hancock. [sclera, Gk *kyklos* circle, *temnein* to cut.]

sclerodactylia (**skleer**·o·dak·**til'**·e·ah). Scleroderma involving the fingers or toes or both. **Sclerodactylia annularis ainhumoides.** A type of sclerodactylia which on occasion leads to destruction of the distal phalanges, as in ainhum. [Gk *skleros* hard, *daktylos* finger or toe.]

sclerodactyly (skleer·o·**dak**·til·e). Sclerodactylia.

scleroderma (skleer·o·**der**·mah). Progressive systemic sclerosis, one of the collagen group of disorders characterized by diffuse sclerosis of skin, alimentary tract, lungs and heart, and involvement of renal and other blood vessels. *Localized scleroderma* may occur in oval plaques (morphoea) or in guttate, linear and nodular forms. **Scleroderma circumscriptum.** Scleroderma affecting only a limited area or areas. **Diffuse scleroderma.** Systemic sclerosis. *See* SCLEROSIS. **Generalized scleroderma.** Widespread morphoea. **Scleroderma guttata.** White-spot disease; a variety of scleroderma characterized by multiple small white plaques which undergo atrophy. **Guttate scleroderma.** Lichen sclerosus et atrophicus. **Localized scleroderma.** Morphoea. **Scleroderma neonatorum.** 1. True scleroderma of the newborn child. 2. Fat necrosis of infants [obsolete usage]. **Systemic scleroderma.** Systemic sclerosis. *See* SCLEROSIS. [Gk *skleros* hard, *derma* skin.]

sclerodermatitis (**skleer**·o·der·mat·**i'**·tis). Inflammation and induration of the skin. [Gk *skleros* hard, dermatitis.]

sclerodermatous (skleer·o·**der**·mat·us). Having an indurated external covering. [see foll.]

sclerodesmia (skleer·o·**dez**·me·ah). Induration of ligaments. [Gk *skleros* hard, *desmos* band.]

scleroedema (skleer·e·**de**·mah). Myxoedema. **Scleroedema adultorum.** Buschke's scleroedema; rapidly spreading, non-pitting oedema, which commences on the head or cervical area, thence involving wide areas and terminating after 8-12 months, leaving no sequelae. The malady usually follows general infections or toxaemias, and also may be a complication of pyodermia. [Gk *skleros* hard, oedema.]

See also: BUSCHKE.

sclerogenous (skleer·**oj**·en·us). Giving rise to sclerosis. [Gk *skleros* hard, *genein* to produce.]

sclerogeny (skleer·**oj**·en·e). The process of formation of hard tissue. [see prec.]

sclerogummatous (skleer·o·**gum**·at·us). Applied to tissue which is composed of fibrous and gummatous elements. [Gk *skleros* hard, gumma.]

scleroid (**skleer**·oid). Hard or bony in texture; sclerous. [Gk *skleros* hard, *eidos* form.]

sclero-iritis (**skleer**·o·i·**ri'**·tis). Inflammation of the sclera and the iris. [sclera, iris, Gk *-itis* inflammation.]

sclerokeratitis (**skleer**·o·ker·at·**i'**·tis). Inflammation affecting the sclera and the cornea simultaneously. [sclera, Gk *keras* horn, *-itis* inflammation.]

sclerokerato-iritis (skleer·o·ker·at·o·i·ri′·tis). Inflammation in which the sclera, the cornea and the iris are all involved. [sclera, Gk *keras* horn, iritis.]

sclerokeratosis (skleer·o·ker·at·o′·sis). Sclerokeratitis. [sclera, Gk *keras* horn, *-osis* condition.]

scleroma (skleer·o·mah). An area of indurated tissue, particularly in the mucous membrane of the nose or larynx. **Scleroma adultorum.** Scleroderma adultorum. **Scleroma respiratorium, Respiratory scleroma.** Rhinoscleroma. [Gk *skleros* hard, *-oma* tumour.]

scleromalacia perforans (skleer·o·mal·a′·she·ah per·for·ans). A degenerative condition of the sclera, in which holes appear without signs of inflammation. It is found in the aged and may follow the breakdown of a nodule which forms rarely on the sclera in patients with rheumatoid arthritis. Also known as *scleritis necroticans.* [sclera, Gk *malakia* softening, L *perforare* to bore through.]

scleromeninx (skleer·o·men·ingx). The dura mater. [Gk *skleros* hard, *menigx* membrane.]

scleromere (skleer·o·meer). A mass of skeletogenous tissue in the embryo. [Gk *skleros* hard, *meros* part.]

sclerometer (skleer·om·et·er). Any instrument used to determine the relative hardness or density of substances. [Gk *skleros* hard, *metron* measure.]

scleromyxoedema (skleer·o·mix·e·de′·mah). A variety of lichen myxoedematosus in which diffuse thickening of the skin underlies the papules. [Gk *skleros* hard, *myxa* mucus, *oidema* swelling.]

scleronychia (skleer·on·ik·e·ah). A condition in which the nails become hard, thick and dry. [Gk *skleros* hard, *onyx* nail.]

scleronyxis (skleer·on·ix·is). Puncture of the sclera, e.g. to allow the escape of subretinal fluid in retinal detachment. [sclera, Gk *nyxis* puncture.]

sclero-oöphoritis, sclero-oöthecitis (skleer·o·o·of·or·i′·tis, skleer·o·o·the·si′·tis). Inflammation and induration of the ovary. [Gk *skleros* hard, *oophoron* ovary, *oon* egg, *theke* sheath, *-itis* inflammation.]

sclero-optic (skleer·o·op·tik). Relating or belonging to the sclera and the optic nerve.

sclerophthalmia (skleer·of·thal·me·ah). A developmental defect in which only the central portion of the cornea remains clear, owing to imperfect differentiation of its periphery from the sclera. [sclera, ophthalmia.]

scleroplasty (skleer·o·plas·te). Plastic repair of the sclera. [sclera, Gk *plassein* to mould.]

scleropoikiloderma (skleer·o·poi·kil·o·der′·mah). Poikiloderma associated with sclerodactylia.

scleroprotein (skleer·o·pro·te·in). Albuminoid; a class of proteins characterized by stability towards, and insolubility in, most chemical reagents. They occur in the skeletal system, and in connective and epidermal tissues. Typifying this class are the collagens of bone and cartilage, the elastins present in the elastic fibres of connective tissue and the keratins which occur in hair, nails, claws, horns and feathers. [Gk *skleros* hard, protein.]

sclerosal (skleer·o·sal). Sclerous.

sclerosant (skleer·o·zant). Producing sclerosis. [Gk *scleros* hard.]

sclerosarcoma (skleer·o·sar·ko′·mah). A hard, fleshy tumour of the gums; a type of epulis. [Gk *skleros* hard, sarcoma.]

sclerose (skleer·oze). To become hardened in a process of sclerosis; hence *sclerosed, sclerosing.* [Gk *skleros* hard.]

sclerosis (skleer·o·sis). Hardening of a tissue due to inflammation; more especially applied to increase of connective tissues in the nervous system. **Amyotrophic lateral sclerosis.** Wasting of the muscles due to degeneration in the anterior horn cells with sclerosis of the lateral columns; progressive muscular atrophy. **Anterolateral sclerosis.** Sclerosis of the anterior and lateral columns of the spinal cord. **Arterial sclerosis, Arteriocapillary sclerosis.** Thickening of the arteries; now called *atherosclerosis.* **Atrophic lobar sclerosis.** Atrophy and gliosis of a portion of each cerebral hemisphere, the pathological basis of one form of congenital cerebral diplegia. **Bone sclerosis.** Thickening and conversion of bone into an ivory-like mass. **Bulbar sclerosis.** Sclerosis of the medulla oblongata. **Central areolar choroidal sclerosis.** That in which the macular region and its surrounding area is chiefly affected; central senile areolar choroidal atrophy. **Cerebrospinal sclerosis.** Disseminated sclerosis (see below). **Choroidal sclerosis.** A vascular degenerative change in the vessels of the choroidal coat of the eye, giving rise to a secondary degeneration of the retina. The choroidal vessels are easily seen owing to the degenerate retina, and are sheathed with white lines. **Sclerosis circumscripta pericardii.** Progressive chronic pericarditis. **Combined sclerosis.** Sclerosis of the lateral and posterior columns of the spinal cord. **Sclerosis corii, Sclerosis dermatis.** Scleroderma. **Cutaneous sclerosis.** Scleroderma. **Diffuse sclerosis.** Sclerosis extending through a large part of the brain or spinal cord. **Diffuse choroidal sclerosis.** One in which the greater portion of the choroid and retina is affected. **Diffuse hyperplastic sclerosis.** A comprehensive term for arterial changes seen in hypertension; medial hypertrophy of medium arteries and intimal hyperplasia of arterioles. **Disseminated sclerosis.** A disease of unknown cause affecting adults in which patches of loss of myelin occur sporadically throughout the central nervous system, eventually followed by loss of axons and glial scarring. Symptoms often remit in the early stages and include optic neuritis, diplopia, paraesthesiae, weakness and ataxia. In severe cases there is terminal spastic paraplegia; multiple sclerosis. **Familial centrolobar sclerosis.** Hepatolenticular degeneration; Wilson's disease; pseudosclerosis (Westphal). **Generalized arteriolar sclerosis.** Widespread intimal hyperplasia of arterioles, seen in hypertension. **Hereditary cerebellar sclerosis.** Hereditary ataxia due to cerebellar degeneration. **Hereditary spinal sclerosis.** Friedreich's ataxia. **Intestinal sclerosis.** Involvement of the small intestine in scleroderma, causing malabsorption. **Lateral sclerosis.** Sclerosis of the lateral columns of the spinal cord as a primary disorder or secondary to a myelitis. **Lens sclerosis.** Nuclear sclerosis (see below). **Lichen sclerosis.** Lichen sclerosus et atrophicus; an atrophic condition of the skin, characterized by polygonal, flat-topped, ivory-coloured papules on the surface of which are comedo-like plugs or puncta. **Lobar sclerosis.** A sclerotic condition of the brain limited to a lobe. **Sclerosis of the middle ear.** Otosclerosis. **Multiple sclerosis, Multiple cerebrospinal sclerosis.** Disseminated, focal, or insular sclerosis; the occurrence of patches of sclerosis in the brain and spinal cord. Evidence, mostly serological, has been obtained from time to time suggesting that measles virus may play a part in causing this condition. However, conclusive proof has not been found and recently a transmissible agent, which may be a virus, has been discovered in the brains of MS patients. It is not yet known what role, if any, it plays in causation. **Nodular sclerosis.** Atherosclerosis. **Nuclear sclerosis.** A form of senile cataract in which there is a diffuse increase of density of the nucleus. Progress is slow and is marked by an increasing myopia; finally the sclerosis spreads to the cortex. Also known as *nuclear cataract, hard cataract* or *lens sclerosis.* **Sclerosis ossium.** Bone sclerosis (see above). **Peripapillary choroidal sclerosis.** One in which the choroid and retina around the optic disc are affected. **Posterior sclerosis, Posterior spinal sclerosis.** Sclerosis of the posterior columns of the spinal cord seen in various conditions. **Posterolateral sclerosis.** Sclerosis seen in subacute combined degeneration of the spinal cord. **Primary lateral sclerosis.** Lateral sclerosis (see above). **Progressive muscular sclerosis.** Pseudohypertrophic muscular dystrophy. *See* DYSTROPHY. **Progressive systemic sclerosis.** Scleroderma. **Renal sclerosis.** Chronic interstitial nephritis. *See* NEPHRITIS. **Renal arteriolar sclerosis.** Fibrosis of the arterioles of the kidney, seen in granular kidney. **Systemic sclerosis.** Raynaud's phenomenon followed by widespread scleroderma and a similar pathological condition affecting the heart, lungs, gastrointestinal tract, kidneys and muscles. There is also a widespread vasculitis and the course is slowly progressive. **Sclerosis telae cellularis et adiposae.** Scleroderma. **Tuberose sclerosis, Tuberous sclerosis.** A rare, inherited disease characterized in its fully developed form by mental defect, epilepsy, and adenoma sebaceum of the face. Sclerotic patches occur in the brain and benign tumours may be found in other organs (e.g. heart). **Unicellular sclerosis.** The growth of fibrous tissue between and isolating individual cells. **Vascular sclerosis.** Arterial degeneration. **Ventrolateral sclerosis.** Sclerosis of the ventral and lateral columns of the spinal cord. [Gk *sklerosis* a hardening.]

See also: ALZHEIMER, ERB, MARIE, MOENCKEBERG.

scleroskeletal (skleer·o·**skel**·et·al). Relating or belonging to the scleroskeleton.

scleroskeleton (skleer·o·**skel**·et·on). Those portions of the endoskeleton which are produced by ossification of fibrous structures such as tendons, ligaments and fasciae. [Gk *skleros* hard, skeleton.]

sclerostenosis (**skleer**·o·sten·**o'**·sis). 1. Hardening associated with stenosis and contraction of tissues. 2. Scleroderma. **Sclerostenosis cutanea.** Scleroderma. [Gk *skleros* hard, stenosis.]

sclerosteous (skleer·**os**·te·us). Describing ossification arising from a deposit of bony substance in a tendon. [Gk *skleros* hard, *osteon* bone.]

sclerostomy (skleer·**os**·to·me). An operation in which a portion of the sclera is removed, leaving a hole. [sclera, Gk *stoma* opening.]

sclerotenonitis (**skler**·o·ten·on·**i'**·tis). Posterior scleritis. *See* SCLERITIS. [Gk *skleros* hard, *tenon* tendon, *-itis* inflammation.]

sclerothrix (**skleer**·o·thrix). Excessive hardness, dryness and brittleness of the hair. [Gk *skleros* hard, *thrix* hair.]

sclerotic (skleer·**ot**·ik). 1. Hard, indurated or hardening; describing the seat of sclerosis. 2. The sclera of the eye or pertaining to the sclera. [Gk *skleros* hard.]

sclerotica (skleer·**ot**·ik·ah). Sclera.

scleroticectomy (skleer·**ot**·e·**sek'**·to·me). Surgical removal of a part of the sclera. [sclera, Gk *ektome* a cutting out.]

scleroticochoroiditis (skleer·**ot**·e·ko·kor·oid·**i'**·tis). Sclerochoroiditis.

scleroticonyxis (skleer·**ot**·e·ik·o·**nix'**·is). Operative puncture of the sclera. [sclera, Gk *nyssein* to pierce.]

scleroticopuncture (skleer·**ot**·ik·o·**punkt'**·tcher). Scleronyxis. [sclera, puncture.]

scleroticotomy (skleer·**ot**·ik·**ot'**·o·me). Sclerotomy.

sclerotidectomy (skleer·**ot**·id·**ek'**·to·me). Operative puncture of the sclera. [sclera, Gk *ektome* a cutting out.]

sclerotitis (skleer·ot·**i**·tis). Scleritis.

sclerotium (skleer·o·**she**·um). A firm, often rounded, mass of hyphae with or without spores, in or on it, of fungi of the class Pyrenomycetes. The only example of medical importance is ergot, the sclerotium of *Claviceps purpurea*. [Gk *skleros* hard.]

sclerotome (**skleer**·o·tome). 1. That part of a somite which becomes mesenchymal and migrates to surround the notochord; from it the axial skeleton is derived. 2. A special knife used in ophthalmic surgery for incising the sclera, the blade being guarded to obviate cutting too deep. [Gk *skleros* hard, *temnein* to cut.]

See also: LUNDSGAARD.

sclerotomy (skleer·**ot**·o·me). Incision of the sclera, performed for a variety of purposes (e.g. removal of an intra-ocular foreign body). **Anterior sclerotomy.** The operation in which the incision is anterior to the ciliary body and which was used at one time for relief of ocular tension in glaucoma. An anterior scleral incision is employed in various operations for glaucoma, e.g. iridencleisis. **Posterior sclerotomy.** That in which the incision is posterior to the ciliary body. It is used, for example, in the operation of cyclodialysis and in stab incision for temporary reduction of tension in acute glaucoma. [sclera, Gk *temnein* to cut.]

sclerotonyxis (**skleer**·o·to·**nix'**·is). A term for the couching or reclination of the lens, in which a broad needle is passed through the sclera behind the ciliary body between the iris and lens, and, by manipulating the handle, is made to depress the lens into the vitreous. [sclera, *nyxis* a pricking.]

sclerotrichia (skleer·o·**trik**·e·ah). Sclerothrix.

sclerous (**skleer**·us). Of a hard texture; indurated. [Gk *skleros* hard.]

sclero-uveitis (**skleer**·o·ew·ve·**i'**·tis). Inflammation of the sclera, associated with a severe iridocyclitis and sometimes choroiditis. [Gk *skleros* hard, uveitis.]

scobinate (**sko**·bin·ate). Having an uneven, irregular surface. [L *scobina* rasp.]

scoleciform (sko·**les**·e·form). Having resemblance to a scolex. [scolex, form.]

scolecoid (**sko**·lek·oid). Scoleciform. [scolex, Gk *eidos* form.]

scolecology (sko·le·**kol**·o·je). Helminthology. [Gk *skolex* worm, *logos* science.]

scolex (**sko**·lex). The head or attachment organ of the adult tapeworm. It is usually provided with hooks and suckers and used for attachment to the intestinal wall. [Gk worm.]

scoliokyphosis (**sko**·le·o·ki·**fo'**·sis). Associated scoliosis and kyphosis.

scoliolordosis (**sko**·le·o·lor·**do'**·sis). Scoliosis associated with lordosis.

scolioma (sko·le·**o**·mah). Scoliosis. [Gk *skolios* crooked, *-oma* tumour].

scoliorachitic (**sko**·le·o·rak·**it'**·ik). 1. Pertaining to a scoliotic and rachitic condition. 2. Suffering from scoliosis caused by rickets.

scoliosis (sko·le·**o**·sis). Lateral curvature of the spine. **Cicatricial scoliosis.** Scoliosis due to the contracture of scar tissue. **Congenital scoliosis.** Scoliosis due to congenital anomalies of the vertebrae. **Coxitic scoliosis.** Scoliosis due to hip-joint disease. **Empyematic scoliosis, Empyemic scoliosis.** Scoliosis secondary to empyema. **Fixed scoliosis.** Lateral curvature of the spine which cannot be corrected by suspension or manipulation. **Functional scoliosis.** Lateral curvature of the spine due to any pathological change in the spine or surrounding tissues; curvature occurring in a normal spine. **Habit scoliosis.** Lateral curvature as a result of persistent bad posture. **Idiopathic scoliosis.** Scoliosis for which there is no known cause. **Inflammatory scoliosis.** Scoliosis due to muscle spasm associated with acute inflammation. **Ischiatic scoliosis.** Lateral curve away or towards the affected leg in sciatica. **Mobile scoliosis.** Curvature which can be corrected by suspension or simple manipulation. **Myopathic scoliosis.** Curvature due to myopathy. **Neuropathic scoliosis.** Paralytic scoliosis (see below). **Ocular scoliosis, Ophthalmic scoliosis.** Lateral curvature of the spine secondary to defects of vision. **Osteopathic scoliosis.** Congenital scoliosis (see above). **Paralytic scoliosis.** Scoliosis due to nerve paralysis, e.g. poliomyelitis. **Rachitic scoliosis.** Curvature secondary to the bone deformities of rickets. **Rheumatic scoliosis.** Inflammatory scoliosis (see above). **Sciatic scoliosis.** Ischiatic scoliosis (see above). **Static scoliosis.** Curvature due to difference in the length of the legs. **Structural scoliosis.** Lateral curvature of the spine due to structural changes in the vertebrae. **Thoracogenic scoliosis.** Empyematic scoliosis (see above). [Gk *skoliosis* curvature.]

scoliosometer (**sko**·le·o·**som'**·et·er). An apparatus used in scoliosometry.

scoliosometry (**sko**·le·o·**som'**·et·re). The measurement of curvatures, in particular the degree of spinal curvature in scoliosis. [Gk *skolios* crooked, *metron* measure.]

scoliotic (sko·le·**ot**·ik). 1. Relating or belonging to, or characterized by scoliosis. 2. Suffering from scoliosis.

scoliotone (**sko**·le·o·tone). An instrument for correcting the curvature in scoliosis. [Gk *skoliosis* curvature, *tonos* stretching.]

Scolopendra (sko·lo·**pen**·drah). A genus of poisonous centipedes. [Gk *skolopendra*.]

scombrine (**skom**·breen). A protamine occurring in mackerel sperm. [see foll.]

scombrone (**skom**·brone). A histone occurring in the sperm of mackerel. [Gk *skombros* mackerel.]

scoop (skoop). An instrument shaped like a spoon and used to remove material from cavities. **Evisceration scoop.** A scoop similar to Mules' scoop. **Gall-bladder scoop.** A small shallow spoon mounted on a long, and often malleable, handle; used to remove stones from the bile passages and gall bladder. **Lens scoop.** An instrument shaped at the end like a shallow spoon, or with a wire loop of the same shape, used for delivering the lens during cataract extraction should there be vitreous loss or dislocation of the lens. The wire loop is also called a *vectis;* the solid spoon a *cataract spoon.* [ME *scope.*]

See also: DAVIEL, LANG, MULES.

scoparin (sko·**par**·in). $C_{22}H_{22}O_{11}$, a yellow crystalline substance with diuretic properties, present in the tops of broom, *Cytisus scoparius.*

scoparium (sko·**pa**·re·um). Broom tops; the fresh or dried tops of *Cytisus scoparius* (family Leguminoseae). It is a mild diuretic, due to the presence of the alkaloid sparteine, and is usually administered in the form of an infusion or decoction. [L *scopa* broom.]

scopine (**sko**·peen). $C_3H_5(OH)(CH)_2NHCH_3(CH)_2{=}O$, an intermediate base produced by the gentle hydrolysis of hyoscine (scopolamine). It is readily transformed into scopoline.

scopograph (**sko**·po·graf). A combined x-ray fluorescent screen and radiographic unit. [Gk *skopein* to view, *graphein* to record.]

scopolamine (sko·**pol**·am·een). Hyoscine. **Scopolamine hydrobromide.** Hyoscine Hydrobromide BP 1958.

scopolamini (sko·pol·**am**′·in·i). Scopolamine (hyoscine). **Scopolamini Hydrobromidum.** *European Pharmacopoeia* name for Hyoscine Hydrobromide BP 1973.

scopoleine (sko·**pol**·e·een). $C_{17}H_{21}NO_4$, an alkaloid obtained from *Scopolia japonica* and *S. carniolica.* It is a powerful mydriatic.

scopolia (sko·**po**·le·ah). The dried rhizome of *Scopolia carniolica* (family Solanaceae), used as an adulterant of and substitute for belladonna root. It contains hyoscyamine and hyoscine (scopolamine) totalling about 0.6–0.7 per cent. [Giovanni Antonio *Scopoli* (b. 1723), Pavia physician.]

scopoline (**sko**·pol·een). $C_8H_{13}O_2N$, a narcotic compound obtained by the hydrolysis of hyoscine (scopolamine).

scopometer (sko·**pom**·et·er). An instrument for estimating the density of a suspension by comparing its opalescence with a known standard. [Gk *skopein* to view, meter.]

scopometry (sko·**pom**·et·re). The quantitative estimation of precipitates, suspensions or turbidities, by the use of a scopometer.

scopomorphinism (sko·po·**mor**·fin·izm). Scopolamine–morphine addiction.

scopophilia (sko·po·**fil**·e·ah). The achievement of sexual pleasure from looking usually at nude persons or genital organs. **Passive scopophilia.** The desire to be looked at by others, a form of exhibitionism. [Gk *skopein* to view, *philein* to love.]

scopophobia (sko·po·**fo**·be·ah). Pathological fear of being looked at. [Gk *skopein* to view, phobia.]

Scopulariopsis (skop·ew·lar·e·**op**′·sis). A penicillin-like fungus. All species possess the ability to break down arsenious oxide and liberate arsene gas. *Scopulariopsis brevicaulis* is a known invader of nail tissue which has been previously damaged. Species have been isolated from gummatous lesions, but as they are common soil contaminants they must be carefully investigated before being designated as aetiological agents of disease; in most cases they are secondary invaders. [L *scopula* broom, Gk *opsis* appearance.]

scopulariopsosis (**skop**·ew·lar·e·op·**so**′·sis). A disease characterized by the presence of granulomata and due to the fungus *Scopulariopsis.* [*Scopulariopsis,* Gk *-osis* condition.]

scoracratia (skor·a·**kra**·she·ah). Incontinence of faeces. [Gk *skor* dung, *akrasia* incontinence.]

scorbutic (skor·**bew**·tik). 1. Relating or belonging to scurvy. 2. Affected with scurvy. [Fr. *scorbut* scurvy.]

scorbutigenic (skor·**bew**·te·**jen**′·ik). Giving rise to scurvy. [Fr. *scorbut* scurvy, Gk *genein* to produce.]

scorbutus (skor·**bew**·tus). Scurvy. [Fr. *scorbut* scurvy.]

scordinema (skor·din·**e**·mah). The stretching and yawning associated with languor and a sensation of heaviness in the head which occurs as one of the premonitory symptoms of an infectious disease. [Gk *skordinaomein* to feel tired.]

scorings (**skor**·ingz). Transverse lines in the metaphyses of growing bones, seen in x-rays and produced by areas of increased density representing periods of arrested growth. [AS *scoru.*]

Scorpio (**skor**·pe·o). A genus of scorpions. **Scorpio maurus.** A poisonous scorpion found in North Africa. [see foll.]

scorpion (**skor**·pe·on). A member of the arachnid order Scorpiones. Scorpions are characterized by the large chelate pedipalps and narrow metasomal region of the tail which terminates in a sting. The poison of all species is toxic and that of a few dangerous. [Gk *skorpios.*]

Scorpiones (skor·pe·o·neez). An order of the arthropod class Arachnida; scorpions. [see prec.]

Scorpoena scropha (skor·**pe**·nah **skro**·fah). A species of tropical sting-ray that may cause severe pain, oedema, collapse and even death. [Gk *skorpaina.*]

scotodinia (sko·to·**din**·e·ah). Dizziness associated with headache and visual impairment with appearance of black specks in front of the eyes; vertigo. [Gk *skotos* darkness, *dinos* whirl.]

scotogram, scotograph (**sko**·to·gram, **sko**·to·graf). 1. Any drawing or recording made in the dark. 2. A skiagraph; a photograph produced by x-rays. 3. Any effect recorded on a photographic plate in the dark by radiations of any kind. [Gk *skotos* darkness, *gramma* record, *graphein* to write.]

scotoma (sko·**to**·mah). An area in which the vision is depressed or abolished, situated within the visual field, so that it is surrounded by a normal or less depressed area. **Absolute scotoma.** One in which the vision is completely abolished. **Annular scotoma.** Ring scotoma (see below). **Arcuate scotoma.** One that is caused by a nerve fibre bundle defect on the temporal side of the optic disc. It arches round the fixation point from the top or bottom of the blind spot to end on the horizontal meridian on the nasal side, e.g. Bjerrum's scotoma. **Scotoma auris.** A trough of deafness; the term implies similarity to a loss in the visual field. **Central scotoma.** One situated in the centre of the visual field, taking in the fixation point. **Centrocaecal scotoma.** One that embraces both the fixation point and the blind spot, being oval in shape with the long axis horizontal. **Colour scotoma.** A form of relative scotoma, in which colour perception is lost, but that to white remains. **Cuneate scotoma.** One that is caused by an affection of a nerve fibre bundle on the nasal side of the optic disc, and is therefore wedge- or fan-shaped, extending outwards from the temporal side of the blind spot. **Eclipse scotoma.** That caused by observation of the sun; central and very small, and can be either relative or absolute. **Facultative scotoma.** One that is developed in alternating squints as a suppression of the central vision of the non-fixing eye, this being temporary and disappearing when this eye's turn comes for fixation. **Hemianopic scotoma.** One that covers half the central field, either nasal, temporal or altitudinal, above or below. **Junction scotoma.** A unilateral hemianopic or quadrantic central scotoma, due to a lesion where the optic nerve joins the chiasma. **Negative scotoma.** One that is invisible to, and not appreciated by, the patient. **Paracaecal scotoma.** One that is situated adjacent to the blind spot. **Paracentral scotoma.** One situated adjacent to the fixation point. **Pericaecal scotoma.** One occurring close to and surrounding the blind spot. **Pericentral scotoma.** One occurring close to and surrounding the fixation point. **Peripheral scotoma.** One that is situated in the periphery of the field, but does not break through to the outside. **Physiological scotoma.** Blind spot. *See* SPOT. **Positive scotoma.** One that is appreciated by the patient as a grey or misty area, and not just a gap. **Quadrantic scotoma.** One which occupies one of the four quadrants or sectors of the central field and is bounded by a vertical and a horizontal radius. **Relative scotoma.** One in which there is only partial and not complete loss of vision. **Ring scotoma.** One that encircles the fixation point, taking in the blind spot, as it is caused by a nerve fibre bundle defect, e.g. 2 arcuate scotomas. **Scintillating scotoma.** One that is positive and luminous, and often becomes hemianopic. Typically it appears in the visual aura of migraine. **Suppression scotoma.** One that is caused by the central suppression of the image of a squinting eye; if alternating, temporary (see FACULTATIVE SCOTOMA above); if a constant squint, permanent. **Wandering scotoma.** One that changes its position. **Zonular scotoma.** One that encircles the fixation point but does not follow the course of the nerve fibres, as in arcuate scotoma, and therefore need not include the blind spot. [Gk *skotos* darkness, *-oma* tumour.]

See also: BJERRUM, SEIDEL.

scotomagraph (sko·**to**·mah·graf). An instrument by means of which the shape and size of a scotoma may be recorded automatically. [scotoma, Gk *graphein* to record.]

scotomameter (sko·to·**mam**·et·er). An instrument used to determine the size of a scotoma. [scotoma, meter.]

scotomatous (sko·**to**·mat·us). Relating or belonging to, or affected with scotomata.

scotometer (sko·**tom**·et·er). An instrument, usually in the form of a screen and tangents, for finding and plotting scotomata. [scotoma, Gk *metron* measure.]

scotometry (sko·**tom**·et·re). The process of measuring isolated scotomata in the field of vision. [see prec.]

scotomization (**sko**·to·mi·**za**′·shun). The development of mental blind spots usually regarding attributes, facts or experiences which are unwanted or the subject of guilt or anxiety. [Gk *skotos* darkness.]

scotophilia (sko·to·**fil**·e·ah). Predilection for night; love of the hours of darkness. [Gk *skotos* darkness, *philein* to love.]

scotophobia (sko·to·**fo**·be·ah). Excessive dread of the darkness and silence of night, or of being in the dark. [Gk *skotos* darkness, phobia.]

scotopia (sko·**to**·pe·ah). The power of the eye to adjust itself for seeing in the dark; dark adaptation. [Gk *skotos* darkness, *opsis* sight.]

scotopic (sko·**to**·pik). Relating or belonging to scotopia.

scotoscopy (sko·**tos**·ko·pe). Retinoscopy. [Gk *skotos* darkness, *skopein* to watch.]

Scott, John (b. 1799). London surgeon.

Scott's dressing or ointment. Compound mercury ointment. *See* OINTMENT.

scourge (skerj). 1. Any severe disease which reaches epidemic proportions. 2. To use a light whip or knotted cord on the skin as a method of counter-irritation. [ME *escorge.*]

scraper (skra·per). An instrument used for producing a cutaneous abrasion. **Tongue scraper.** An instrument by which epithelial debris and other matter may be scraped from the tongue. [AS *scrapian.*]

scrapie (skra·pe). A progressive fatal neurological disease of sheep, starting with an intense pruritus and followed by tremors and inco-ordination. It is due to a transmissible agent which may be an atypical virus. Little is known of the agent. Its resistance to heat and formalin are much greater than that of other viruses.

scrattage (skrat·**ahzh**). Brossage; removal of trachoma granules from the conjunctiva by scratching them out with a pointed instrument. [Fr.]

screen (skreen). 1. A flat surface, which may or may not be a portable hard sheet or fabric, on which still or cinematograph pictures are projected. 2. A movable piece of furniture made of wood or other material used for interposition or as a protection or shield against draughts, heat or other rays, or simply observation, or a fixed partition for one or more of the same purposes. 3. To fluoroscope; to investigate radiologically with a fluorescent screen. 4. To subject to a process of preliminary selection by the observation of certain characteristics, e.g. in the examination of a population for certain diseases, picking out persons with certain clinical or serological characters: or in the selection of certain drugs by their antiparasitic action in infections in laboratory animals, as a preliminary to using them on man. **Campimeter screen.** Bjerrum's screen. **Fluorescent screen.** A flat surface on which is formed the shadow of an object or person examined by fluoroscopy. It consists of finely divided crystals of suitable material, such as zinc sulphide, spread evenly on cardboard and protected by lead glass. The screen lights up in a darkened room when x-rays pass through it. **Hand tangent screens.** Small, flat, portable screens on the same principle as the Bjerrum screen but held at a distance of 33 cm; useful only for rough estimations. **Intensifying screen.** A thin sheet of cardboard, celluloid or plastic, placed in contact with an x-ray film in a cassette, commonly used in pairs, one on either side of the film. The sheet is coated with a layer of finely divided crystals such as calcium tungstate, which converts x-ray energy into visible light; this intensifies the effect of radiation on the photographic emulsion. **Tangent screen.** A flat screen for investigating the central part of the visual field. The measurements will be on the tangent scale, and only accurate within 30 degrees from the fixation point. [ME *scren.*]

See also: BJERRUM, HESS (W. R.).

screening (**skreen**·ing). The carrying out of a test or tests in order to detect abnormalities. [ME *scren.*]

screws (skrooz). Caisson disease. *See* DISEASE. [O Fr. *escroe.*]

screw-worm (**skroo**·werm). Larva of any fly that occurs in wounds, particularly of *Cochliomyia hominivorax*, the New World screw-worm, and *Chrysomyia bezziana* and *Wohlfartia magnifica*, Old World screw-worms. [O Fr. *escroe*, AS *wyrm.*]

scribomania (skrib·o·**ma**·ne·ah). 1. Graphomania; a morbid desire or irresistible urge to be always writing. 2. Graphorrhoea; in psychiatric medicine, the insane condition of which the occasional writing down of long lists of unassociated and meaningless words is a characteristic. [L *scribere* to write, mania.]

scrobiculate (skro·**bik**·ew·late). Marked by numerous small, shallow depressions; pitted. [see foll.]

scrobiculus (skro·**bik**·ew·lus). A small cavity, depression or hollow. **Scrobiculus cordis.** The epigastric region. **Scrobiculus variolae.** A depressed scar left after the smallpox pustule has fallen or has been pulled off. [L little ditch.]

scrofula (**skrof**·ew·lah). An old name for a syndrome which is not recognized as such today. The most prominent feature of this syndrome was tuberculous cervical adenitis with or without ulceration; when the word is used today, it usually suggests this condition. Also called *King's evil.* [L *scrofa* brood sow; the name is probably derived from the resemblance to the folds in the neck of a fat sow or to its mammae.]

scrofulid, scrofulide (**skrof**·ew·lid, **skrof**·ew·lide). Scrofuloderma.

scrofulism (**skrof**·ew·lizm). The state in which there is predisposition to scrofula [Obsolete term.]

scrofuloderm (**skrof**·ew·lo·derm). Scrofuloderma.

scrofuloderma, scrofulodermia (**skrof**·ew·lo·**der**′·mah, **skrof**·ew·lo·**der**′·me·ah). Tuberculous infection of the skin secondary to tuberculous infection of an underlying lymphatic gland or bone. **Scrofuloderma gummosa.** A tuberculous gumma which develops in the skin or subcutaneous tissue, but which does not arise from infected lymphatic gland or bone. **Verrucous scrofuloderma.** A variety of scrofuloderma in which warty vegetations are noted. [scrofula, Gk *derma* skin.]

scrofulonychia (**skrof**·ew·lo·**nik**′·e·ah). Destruction or deformity of the nail, because of tuberculous infection arising in adjacent or underlying tissue. [scrofula, Gk *onyx* nail.]

scrofulophyma (**skrof**·ew·lo·**fi**′·mah). Tuberculosis varrucosa cutis. [scrofula, Gk *phyma* growth.]

scrofulosis (skrof·ew·**lo**·sis). A predisposition to scrofula [Obsolete term.] [scrofula, Gk *-osis* condition.]

scrofulotuberculosis (**skrof**·ew·lo·tew·ber·kew·**lo**′·sis). 1. Tuberculous scrofulodermia. 2. Attenuated tuberculosis. *See* TUBERCULOSIS. [scrofula, tuberculosis.]

scrofulotuberculous (**skrof**·ew·lo·tew·**ber**·kew·lus). Marked by the presence of scrofulous tubercles.

scrofulous (**skrof**·ew·lus). 1. Relating or belonging to, or having the character of scrofula. 2. Marked by the presence of, or suffering from scrofula.

scrotal (**skro**·tal). Relating or belonging to the scrotum.

scrotectomy (skro·**tek**·to·me). The operation of removing a portion of the scrotum. [scrotum, Gk *ektome* a cutting out.]

scrotitis (skro·**ti**·tis). An inflammatory condition of the scrotum. [scrotum, Gk *-itis* inflammation.]

scrotocele (**skro**·to·seel). Scrotal hernia. *See* HERNIA. [scrotum, Gk *kele* hernia.]

scrotopexy (**skro**·to·pex·e). A plastic operation combined with excision of part of the scrotum. [scrotum, Gk *pexis* a fixation.]

scrotoplasty (**skro**·to·plas·te). Plastic surgery as applied to the scrotum. [scrotum, Gk *plassein* to mould.]

scrotum [NA] (**skro**·tum). A pouch of skin and subcutaneous tissue, divided into two by a median septum, containing the testes, epididymides and the lower parts of the spermatic cords; it is situated below the root of the penis. **Lymph scrotum.** A scrotum in which the skin lymphatics are distended as a result of blockage of the efferent lymphatic channels; there is usually elephantoid overgrowth of the scrotum and continuous or frequent discharge from ruptured lymphatic vessels. **Watering-can scrotum.** An infected scrotum in which, as a result of a stricture and rupture of the urethra, there are numerous small sinuses on the under-surface and in the perineum which discharge urine. [L.]

scrumpox (**skrum**·pox). Impetigo contagiosa. [O Fr. *eskermir* hence skirmish, hence scrimmage, hence scrum (Rugby football term), AS *poc.*]

scruple (scroopl). In the Apothecaries system of weights, a unit equal to 20 grains (1.295 g). It is denoted by the symbol ℈. [L *scrupulus* small stone.]

scrupulosity (skroo·pew·**los**·it·e). Excessive conscientiousness in small affairs as noted in some insane types; abnormal fear of doing wrong or of overstepping the requirements of propriety; excessive punctiliousness. [L *scrupulosus* precise.]

scultetus. *See* SCHULTES.

scurf (skerf). Dandruff. [AS.]

scurvy (**sker**·ve). Avitaminosis C. A deficiency disease due to lack of vitamin C (ascorbic acid) in the diet. It is a general nutritional disorder shown by anaemia, sponginess and ulceration of the gums, and haemorrhages into the skin and subcutaneous tissues. Haemorrhages may also occur into joints, muscles and beneath the periosteum of bones. Hyperkeratosis of the hair follicles is an early sign. **Alpine scurvy, Scurvy of the Alps.** The local name applied to pellagra. **Button scurvy.** A skin disease with button-like nodules which was once common in Ireland; it has been suggested that the disease was yaws. **Infantile scurvy.** A condition due to a deficiency of vitamin C in infants, usually showing itself between the sixth and twelfth months. It is most often due to feeding on condensed milk. Occasionally it occurs with breast-fed infants when the mother's diet has been deficient in the vitamin. The most striking symptom is extreme tenderness of the legs due to subperiosteal haemorrhages. Haemorrhage into the orbit may occur and cause proptosis. Changes in the gums and cutaneous haemorrhages are uncommon. **Land scurvy.** Thrombocytopenic purpura. *See* PURPURA. **Sea scurvy.** Scurvy occurring in past times in seamen on long voyages, owing to the absence of fresh foods. **Subclinical scurvy.** A condition due to a diet with insufficient vitamin C. It can be detected by a quantitative examination of the excretion of the vitamin in the urine. It may be suspected in patients with slow healing of wounds, peptic ulcer, purpura or uterine haemorrhage. [scurf.]

See also: CRANDON.

scute (skewt). A cutaneous plate or scale, forming part of the dermal armour of various reptiles, fish and insects. **Tympanic scute.** The tegmen tympani of the temporal bone. [L *scutum* shield.]

scutellaria (skew·tel·a·re·ah). Scullcap, madweed; the dried tops of *Scutellaria galericulata* Linn. (family Labiatae). It contains a glycoside, scutellarin, and was formerly used for neuralgia and nervous disorders. [L *scutella* tray.]

scutellarin (skew·**tel**·ar·in). A glycoside, $C_{10}H_8O_3$, occurring in the leaves of *Scutellaria galericulata* Linn.

scutellum (skew·**tel**·um). Any flat or plate-like structure. [dim. of L *scutum* shield.]

scutiform (**skew**·te·form). Shaped like a shield. [L *scutum* shield, form.]

scutular (**skew**·tew·lar). Pertaining to, or marked by the presence of scutula.

scutulate (**skew**·tew·late). Shield-shaped. [see foll.]

scutulum (**skew**·tew·lum) (pl. *scutula*). The sulphur-yellow or straw-coloured adherent masses, formed chiefly of fungus, seen on the skin in favus. It is characteristic that these scutula have a central depression. [dim. of L *scutum* shield.]

scybalous (**sib**·al·us). Relating to or consisting of scybala.

scybalum (**sib**·al·um) (pl. *scybala*). An inspissated hard mass of faeces in the intestine, generally consisting of a small spherical unit like a marble; a number of these are generally to be found together. [Gk *skybalon* dung.]

scyphiform, scyphoid (si·fe·form, si·foid). Cup-shaped. [Gk *skyphos* cup, *eidos* form.]

scythropasmus (si·thro·**paz**·mus). A facial expression of extreme dullness and fatigue which, occurring in severe illnesses, is regarded as a grave symptom. [Gk *skythropazein* to look sullen.]

scytitis (si·**ti**·tis). Dermatitis. [Gk *skytos* skin, *-itis* inflammation.]

scytodephic, scytodepsic (si·to·**de**·fik, si·to·**dep**·sik). Pertaining to tannin or the process of tanning. [Gk *skytos* skin, *depsin* to soften.]

seal (seel). **Water seal.** The volume of water constantly maintained in the trap of a house drain, the purpose being to prevent foul gases reaching the house from the sewer. [O Fr. *seel.*]

searcher (**ser**·cher). A sound used in searching for stone in the bladder; called also *stone searcher.* [ME *serchen.*]

Seashore, Carl Emil (b. 1866). American psychologist.

Seashore test. A test of various aspects of musical talent.

seasickness (**se**·sik·nes). The type of motion sickness that may affect persons travelling by sea. It is marked by disordered gastric and intestinal function which may give rise to great distress and prostration, and may be due to excessive stimulation of the labyrinth, to which the victim is not accustomed, resulting from the irregular and repetitive motion of the ship. Apprehension and other psychological factors play a part. [AS *sae, seoc.*]

seatworm (**seet**·werm). The threadworm *Enterobius vermicularis.* [AS *sittan, wyrm.*]

seawrack (**se**·reck). Fucus. [AS *sae, wraec.*]

sebaceofollicular (se·**ba**·se·o·fol·**ik**′·ew·lar). Pertaining to sebaceous glands and hair follicles.

sebaceous (se·**ba**·shus). 1. Relating or belonging to sebum. 2. Secreting a fatty, greasy or oily substance. **Sebaceous gland.** *See* GLAND. [sebum.]

sebadilla (seb·ad·**il**·ah). Cevadilla.

sebastomania (se·**bas**·to·**ma**′·ne·ah). Religious mania bordering on insanity. [Gk *sebas* reverence, mania.]

sebiagogic (se·be·ag·**oj**′·ik). Stimulating the production of sebaceous or other similar matter. [sebum, Gk *agogos* leading.]

sebiferous (se·**bif**·er·us). Secreting fatty or sebaceous material. [sebum, L *ferre* to bear.]

Sebileau, Pierre (b. 1860). Paris anatomist and otolaryngologist.

Sebileau's bands or suspensory ligaments. 2 occasional fibromuscular bands inserted into the suprapleural membrane, one from the anterior tubercle of the 7th cervical vertebra, the other from the neck of the 1st rib.

Sebileau's hollow. A depression in the floor of the mouth between the tongue and the sublingual glands.

sebiparous (se·**bip**·ar·us). Sebiferous. [sebum, L *parere* to produce.]

sebocystoma (se·bo·sist·**o**′·mah). Sebaceous cyst. *See* CYST. [sebum, cystoma.]

sebocystomatosis (se·bo·sist·o·mat·**o**′·sis). A familial malady in which sebaceous cysts, varying in diameter from a few millimetres to 1 or more centimetres, develop on the upper anterior part of the trunk, the back, upper limbs, thighs and scrotum, but may occur in other areas also. The cysts may contain caseous material or a clear oily fluid. Usually, neither acne vulgaris nor seborrhoea is present. [sebocystoma, Gk *-osis* condition.]

sebolite, sebolith (**seb**·o·lite, **seb**·o·lith). Any stone-like aggregation occurring in a sebaceous gland; a sebaceous calculus. [sebum, Gk *lithos* stone.]

seborrhagia (seb·or·a·je·ah). Seborrhoea. [sebum, Gk *rhegnynein* to gush forth.]

seborrhoea (seb·or·e·ah). Hypersecretion of sebum which is said by some authorities also to be associated with excessive oily secretion from the sweat glands. **Seborrhoea capitis.** Seborrhoeic baldness. **Seborrhoea congestiva.** An archaic name for lupus erythematodes. **Seborrhoea corporis.** Duhring's name for circinate, or crescentic, yellowish-red, elevated, slightly scaly patches of seborrhoeic dermatitis on the trunk, particularly on the sternal and interscapular regions. **Eczematoid seborrhoea.** A seborrhoeic eruption having some resemblance to eczema. **Seborrhoea faciei.** A greasy state of the skin of the face caused by an exaggerated flow of sebum. **Seborrhoea nasi.** Cutis unctuosa nasi. **Seborrhoea oleosa.** Oiliness of the scalp accompanied by loss of hair. **Post-encephalitic seborrhoea.** A seborrhoea, chiefly on the face, that may develop from 6 to 18 months after an attack of encephalitis lethargica. **Seborrhoea sicca.** Hebra's name for pityriasis capitis. [sebum, Gk *rhoia* flow.]

seborrhoeal, seborrhoeic (seb·or·e·al, seb·or·e·ik). Pertaining to, affected with, or having the characteristics of seborrhoea.

seborrhoeid, seborrhoeide (seb·or·e·id, seb·or·e·ide). An anglicized version of the French term *séborrhéide,* meaning certain morbid conditions which occur on a seborrhoeic skin. MacLeod included under this term (*a*) seborrhoea capitis (seborrhoeic baldness); (*b*) seborrhoeic dermatitis, seborrhoea corporis or flannel rash, eczema seborrhoeicum; (*c*) acne vulgaris; (*d*) papular seborrhoids of the face, i.e. the perifollicular papules which occur in association with rosacea; and (*e*) seborrhoeic wart.

seborrhoid (**seb**·or·oid). A simple seborrhoeic lesion. [seborrhoea, Gk *eidos* form.]

sebotrophic (se·bo·**tro**·fic). Pertaining to a compound that causes or produces an excess of seborrhoea.

Sebrasez' breath-holding test. For anaesthetic risk: resting on a couch the patient takes a deep breath, closes his nose and mouth and holds his breath as long as he can. 25 s and over constitutes a normal; less than 15 s indicates severe impairment of function.

sebum (**se**·bum). The fatty secretion of the sebaceous glands; it is protective and water-repellent, and usually found in association with hairs. **Sebum cutaneum.** The fatty secretion from the sebaceous glands of the skin. **Sebum palpebrale.** The secretion of the sebaceous glands of the eyelids. **Sebum praeputiale.** Smegma, the secretion beneath the prepuce. [L *sevum* suet.]

Secale (se·**kale**). A genus of grasses (family Gramineae). **Secale cereale.** Rye. **Secale cornutum.** The international name for ergot. [L rye.]

secalin, secaline (**sek**·al·in, **sek**·al·een). An inert alkaloidal substance obtained from ergot, probably identical with crystalline ergotinine (Tanret). [L *secale* rye.]

Secbutobarbitone BP 1973 (**sek**·bew·to·**bar'**·be·tone). 5-*s*-Butyl-5-ethylbarbituric acid. A hypnotic comparable with butobarbitone; in smaller doses it is used as a sedative.

secernent (se·**sern**·ent). 1. Separating; secreting. 2. An organ which secretes or promotes secretion. [L *secernere* to separate.]

secerning, secernment (se·**sern**·ing, se·**sern**·ment). The act or process of secreting. [see prec.]

seclusion (see·**kloo**·zhun). **Seclusion of the pupil.** A sequel of iritis, in which adhesions between the posterior surface of the iris and anterior capsule of the lens extend all round the pupil margin. [L *secludere* to shut off.]

Secobarbitalum Natricum (**sek**·o·bar·bit·**a'**·lum **nat**·rik·um). *European Pharmacopoeia* name for Quinalbarbitone Sodium BP 1973.

secohm (**sek**·ome). An obsolete name for the *henry*, the unit of electrical inductance. [second (time unit), ohm.]

secohmmeter (sek·**ome**·me·ter). An instrument invented by Ayrton and Perry to measure the self-inductance of a coil of wire, given by the product of the time in seconds and the resistance in ohms. [secohm, meter.]

second intention (**sek**·und in·**ten**·shun). Referring to the healing of a wound, by granulations. [L *secundus* second, *intendere* to stretch.]

secondary (**sek**·un·dar·e). 1. Taking second place. 2. Of the nature of a metastasis. 3. A metastasis; more often used in the plural (*secondaries*). **Secondary structure.** *See* STRUCTURE. [L *secundus* second.]

secretagogue (se·**kre**·tag·og). 1. Causing secretion or exciting a more vigorous secretion. 2. A substance, e.g. a hormone, which stimulates a gland to secrete. [secretion, Gk *agogos* eliciting.]

Secrétan, Henri François (b. 1856). Lausanne physician.

Secrétan's disease. Severe traumatic oedema.

secrete (se·**kreet**). 1. To separate or form a particular substance from the blood, living organism or gland. 2. To pour out as a secretion. [L *secernere* to separate.]

secretin (se·**kre**·tin). 1. A hormone secreted by the upper small intestine in response to free fatty acids in the duodenum which causes the secretion of a dilute pancreatic juice rich in bicarbonate. It was discovered by Bayliss and Starling in 1902 and was the first hormone to be described. 2. BP Commission approved name for a hormone obtained from duodenal mucosa; it is used as a diagnostic aid. [L *secernere* to separate.]

secretion (se·**kre**·shun). 1. The function of glandular organs by which their epithelial cells manufacture certain chemical substances, especially enzymes, that are useful in further chemical processes. 2. The substance secreted. **Antilytic secretion, Antiparalytic secretion.** The secretion of saliva from the salivary glands on one side after the chorda tympani has been cut on the opposite side. **Blood-group secretion.** The ABO and Lewis blood group substances, according to the genetic constitution, may be secreted throughout the body in a water-soluble form. **External secretion.** Secretion in which the chemical products pass through ducts opening out on an epithelial surface. **Internal secretion.** Secretion in which the chemical products (hormones) pass from the gland directly into the blood stream. **Lab secretion.** The secretion of Lab enzyme by the stomach. **Menstrual secretion.** The discharge of menstrual fluid from the uterus. **Paralytic secretion.** Secretion which continues after the nerves of the gland have been cut. **Prostatic secretion.** A thin, slightly alkaline, opalescent fluid which dilutes the semen and activates the spermatozoa. **Sebaceous secretion.** The secretion of sebum by the sebaceous glands of the skin. [L *secernere* to separate.]

secretodermatosis (se·**kre**·to·der·mat·**o'**·sis). A cutaneous disease marked by a secretory disorder; a general term for functional disorder of the secretory apparatus of the skin. [secretion, dermatosis.]

secreto-inhibitory (se·**kre**·to·in·**hib'**·it·or·e). Inhibiting secretion.

secretomotor, secretomotory (se·**kre**·to·**mo'**·tor, se·**kre**·to·**mo'**·tor·e). Relating or belonging to nerves which influence or stimulate secretion. [secretion, motor.]

secretor (se·**kre**·tor). A person who secretes ABO blood group substances into mucous secretions, e.g. saliva, gastric juice. Over 80 per cent of humans are secretors, a genetically determined status related to the Lewis blood group system. [L *secernere* to separate.]

secretory (se·**kre**·tor·e). 1. Secreting. 2. Relating to or influencing secretion or the secretions.

sectile (**sek**·tile). 1. Of a character that can be cut or divided. 2. Bearing evidence of recent division or section. [L *sectilis* that can be cut.]

sectio (**sek**·she·o). Section. **Sectio abdominis.** Abdominal section. *See* SECTION. **Sectio alta.** Suprapubic cystotomy for stone (Douglas 1718). **Sectio cadaveris.** A post-mortem examination; an autopsy. **Sectio franconiana.** Suprapubic cytotomy for stone described by Franco (1556). **Sectio lateralis.** The earliest type of perineal lithotomy described originally by Celsus (53 B.C. to A.D. 7) and practised for the following 1400 years. **Sectio mariana, Sectio mediana.** Perineal lithotomy (Mariano 1531). [L.]

section (**sek**·shun). 1. The act of cutting. 2. A cut surface. 3. A thin slice of tissue prepared for microscopic examination (*histological section*). **Abdominal section.** The surgical opening of the abdominal cavity; laparotomy. **Caesarean section.** Delivery of the fetus by an incision into the uterus, usually through the abdominal wall. **Cataract section.** The incision made into the eye through which the lens is extracted. Classically this is through the upper half of the limbus, and is made with a Graefe knife. **Celloidin section.** A histological section from a tissue which has been impregnated with nitrocellulose. **Classical caesarean section.** Delivery of the fetus through an incision into the body of the uterus. **Coronal section.** A section cut in the plane of the coronal suture or parallel to it. **Section cutter.** A microtome; an instrument for cutting sections of tissues. **Extraperitoneal caesarean section.** Delivery of the child through the lower uterine segment, without opening the peritoneum. **Frontal section.** Coronal section (see above). **Frozen section.** A histological section from a tissue frozen with solid carbon dioxide. **Histological section.** *See* MAIN DEF. 3. (above). **Lower-segment caesarean section.** Delivery of the fetus by a retroperitoneal incision into the lower uterine segment. This incision may be transverse or longitudinal. **Paraffin section.** A histological section from a tissue embedded in paraffin wax. **Parasagittal section.** A section cut parallel to the sagittal suture. **Perineal section.** A surgical dissection of the perineum usually for exposure and incision of the male urethra. **Porro-caesarean section.** Caesarean section (see above) followed by subtotal hysterectomy. The uterine stump is fixed into the lower end of the abdominal wound. **Post-mortem caesarean section.** Delivery of the fetus by incision into the uterus after the death of the mother. **Root section.** Division of the sensory root of the 5th cranial nerve, for the relief of pain: also of the posterior roots of spinal nerves to relieve intractable pain or to interrupt the reflex arc in spastic paralysis. **Sagittal section.** A section cut in the sagittal plane. **Serial section.** In histology, one of a number of consecutive sections of tissue. **Section smoother.** A spatula for flattening tissue sections. **Trigeminal root section.** The cutting of the preganglionic root of the 5th cranial nerve for the relief of tic douloureux. **Vaginal section.** Delivery of the fetus *per vaginum* by incision of the lower uterine segment. [L *sectio.*]

See also: GRAEFE, PITRES, RANEY, SAEMISCH.

sectorial (sek·**tor**·e·al). Modified for cutting purposes. [L *sector* a cutter.]

secundae viae (se·**kun**·de **vi**·e). The lacteals, blood vessels, the second channels by which the products of foodstuffs pass into the body. [L second ways.]

secundigravida (se·**kun**·de·**grav**'·id·ah). A woman who is pregnant for the second time. [L *secundus* second, *gravidus* pregnant.]

secundines (**sek**·un·deenz). The placenta, umbilical cord and membranes expelled from the uterus after birth of the child. [L *secundus* second.]

secundipara (se·kun·**dip**·ar·ah). A woman who has had 2 children, in two different pregnancies. [L *secundus* second, *parere* to produce.]

secundiparity (se·**kun**·de·**par**'·it·e). The condition of being a secundipara.

secundiparous (se·kun·**dip**·ar·us). Describing a woman who is in labour with her second child or who has had 2 children. [L *secundus* second, *parere* to produce.]

sedans (se·**danz**) (pl. *sedantia*). Sedative; also any medicine with sedative properties. [L calming.]

sedation (se·**da**·shun). 1. The act of soothing or of allaying irritability. 2. The amelioration of pain or the production of calmness by means of a sedative. 3. The state of being tranquillized or of being in a condition of reduced pain. [L *sedatio* a calming.]

sedative (**sed**·at·iv). A substance the administration of which results in diminished activity of an organ or tissue, or of the whole animal or man. Whereas previously this term has been widely used with reference to almost every tissue or organ of the body, in recent years its use has been largely restricted to the nervous system. [L *sedare* to calm.]

sedentary (**sed**·en·tar·e). 1. Sitting; pertaining to the sitting posture. 2. Inclined to physical inaction. 3. Describing an occupation in which the worker does not move about but sits for the most part. [L *sedentarius* sitting.]

sediment (**sed**·im·ent). A spontaneous deposit of insoluble matter which settles at the bottom of a liquid; dregs. **Urinary sediment.** The solid matter which settles at the bottom of a sample of urine when this has been allowed to stand for some hours. [see foll.]

sedimentation (**sed**·im·en·**ta**'·shun). The deposition or settling to the bottom of solid particles in a fluid, which can be accelerated by centrifugation. **Blood sedimentation, Erythrocyte sedimentation.** The deposition or sedimentation of red blood cells when whole blood, made incoagulable, is allowed to stand. When this is permitted under standard conditions, the speed of sedimentation is termed the *erythrocyte sedimentation rate.* [L *sedimentum* a settling.]

sedimentator (**sed**·im·en·**ta**'·tor). A centrifuge by means of which the solid particles in urine are precipitated and formed into a composite mass. [see prec.]

sedimentin (sed·im·**en**·tin). A generic name for fibrinogen, serum globulin and similar substances in the plasma that together accelerate clumping and sedimentation of the red blood cells.

sedimentometer (**sed**·im·en·**tom**'·et·er). An apparatus used to measure the sedimentation rate of blood cells (erythrocyte sedimentation rate).

Seebeck, Thomas Johann (b. 1770). German physicist.

Seebeck effect. The electromotive force produced on account of a difference of temperature between 2 junctions of dissimilar materials in the same circuit.

seed (seed). 1. The structure resulting from the fertilization of the ovule of a plant of the Spermaphyta, from which the new plant grows. It includes the embryo and cotyledon or cotyledons enclosed in a seed-coat or testa. 2. Semen. 3. In bacteriology, to inoculate a culture medium with bacteria. 4. Secondary tumours growing close to a primary tumour as if seeded from the latter. 5. Radon seed. *See* RADON. **Celery seed.** Apium. **Flea seed.** Psyllium. **Millet seed.** An edible seed, about 2 mm in diameter: once a standard of measurement in pathology. **Pharbitis seeds.** Kaladana. **Plantago seed.** Psyllium. **Stavesacre seeds.** Staphisagria. [AS *saed.*]

seeker (se·ker). Vein seeker, an appliance with an infusion needle and teat bulb for finding veins. [AS *secan.*]

Seeligmueller, Otto Ludovicus Gustavus Adolphus (b. 1837). German neurologist.

Seeligmueller's neuralgia. Bilateral auriculotemporal neuralgia, characteristic of syphilis.

Seeligmueller's sign. Mydriasis on the affected side in tic douloureux.

seepage (**seep**·ij). 1. The slow percolation or oozing of fluid through a porous substance. 2. The amount of fluid so collected. 3. Rectal infusion of continuous type. [AS *sipian* to soak.]

Seessel, Albert (b. 1851). New York physician.

Seessel's pocket or pouch. A small ectodermal diverticulum from the developing foregut, close to the buccopharyngeal membrane. It persists in some marsupials, as part of the hypophysis, but disappears in man.

Séglas, Jules Ernest (b. 1856). French psychiatrist.

Séglas type. Paranoid type.

segment (**seg**·ment). 1. Any portion cut off. 2. A component or part of a structure, especially of a structure showing serial repetition. **Body segment.** A somite. **Bronchopulmonary segments [segmenta bronchopulmonalia (NA)].** Sub-divisions of the lobe of a lung, each constituting an isolated unit of lung tissue with its own branch of a bronchus, pulmonary artery and vein. They are the smallest sub-divisions of lung about which there is uniformity of arrangement. Each segment bears the same name as the branch of the bronchus which aerates it (*see* BRONCHUS). The pulmonary segments are named as follows: anterior segment of the superior lobes [segmentum anterius (NA)]; apical segment of the superior lobe of the right lung [segmentum apicale (NA)]; apical segment of the inferior lobes [segmentum apicale (superius) NA]; apicoposterior segment of the superior lobe of the left lung [segmentum apicoposterius

(NA)]; anterior basal segment of the inferior lobes [segmentum basale anterius (NA)]; lateral basal segment of the inferior lobes [segmentum basale laterale (NA)]; medial basal segment of the inferior lobes [segmentum basale mediale (cardiacum) NA]; posterior basal segment of the inferior lobes [segmentum basale posterius (NA)]; lateral segment of the middle lobe of the right lung [segmentum laterale (NA)]; inferior lingular segment of the superior lobe of the left lung [segmentum lingulare inferius (NA)]; superior lingular segment of the superior lobe of the left lung [segmentum lingulare superius (NA)]; medial segment of the middle lobe of the right lung [segmentum mediale (NA)]; posterior segment of the superior lobe of the right lung [segmentum posterius (NA)]; subapical segment of the inferior lobe [segmentum subapicale (subsuperius) NA]. **Ceratobranchial segment.** That portion of the 2nd pharyngeal arch of the embryo from which the lesser horn of the hyoid bone is derived. **Daughter segment.** One of the 2 products of cell division. **Epibranchial segment.** One of the segments of the skeleton of the pharyngeal arch, especially that of the 2nd arch which develops into the stylohyoid ligament. **Erythrocytic segment.** A fragment of an erythrocyte. **Hypobranchial segment.** The lower segment of the skeleton of a pharyngeal arch, especially that of the 2nd arch which develops into part of the body of the hyoid bone. **Interannular segment.** The internodal portion of a nerve fibre. **Intermediate segment of a cilium.** The middle piece of a cilium or hair-like process of a cell. **Liver segments.** The liver may be divided into lobes and segments according to the distribution of the intrahepatic bile ducts and the branches of the portal vein and hepatic artery. These do not correspond exactly to the anatomical lobes. On this basis, the latter is formed of a right lobe [lobus hepatis dexter (NA)] with anterior and posterior segments [segmenta anterius et posterius (NA)] and a left lobe [lobus hepatis sinister (NA)] with lateral and medial segments [segmenta laterale et mediale (NA)], the latter segment having a quadrate portion [pars quadrata (NA)]. **Lower uterine segment.** The thinned-out lower portion of the uterus which forms in labour, probably from the isthmus of the cervix, and may become of paper-like thickness in cases of obstructed labour. It is not active in normal labour; segment of Bandl, uterine segment. **Medullary segment.** Schmidt-Lantermann segment; that portion of the myelin sheath of a nerve fibre which lies between successive incisures of Schmidt-Lantermann. **Mesoblastic segment, Mesodermal segment.** A somite. **Muscle segment.** A myotome. **Neural segment.** A neuromere. **Pharyngobranchial segment.** One of the segments of the skeleton of a pharyngeal arch, especially that portion of the 2nd arch which develops into the styloid process. **Primitive segment.** A somite. **Protovertebral segment.** 1. A somite. 2. The sclerotome. **Renal segment [segmentum renalis (NA)].** One of the 5 segments into which the kidney may be divided, each of which is supplied by a segmental branch of the renal artery. The arteries of individual segments do not anastomose appreciably with each other but there is a free anastomosis between the veins. The segments are named as follows: apical [segmentum superius (NA)], upper (anterior) [segmentum anterius superius (NA)], lower (anterior) [segmentum anterius inferius (NA)], lower [segmentum inferius (NA)] and posterior [segmentum posterius (NA)]. **R(S)-T segment.** The interval between the end of the QRS complex of the electrocardiogram and the T wave, representing the period between the end of ventricular depolarization and the beginning of repolarization. Sometimes the interval is very short (i.e. when the rate is rapid) so that it constitutes merely a junction (RS-T junction). **Skin segment.** A segment the dermis of which is derived from a dermatome. **Spinal segment.** A portion of the spinal cord giving rise to 1 segmental nerve. **S-T segment.** R(S)-T segment (see above). **Uterine segment.** Lower uterine segment (see above). [L *segmentum* that which is cut off.]

See also: BANDL, LANTERMANN, RANVIER, SCHMIDT (H. D.).

segmental (seg·men·tal). Describing or pertaining to a structure which is repeated in similar form in successive segments of an organism, or which is undergoing segmentation.

segmentation (seg·men·ta·shun). 1. The process of becoming divided into segments of similar form. 2. Division into more or less similar parts, such as takes place in the developing parasite of malaria within the erythrocyte. 3. The process of sub-division of the fertilized ovum into a number of cells. **Centrolecithal segmentation.** The process of cell division and multiplication in an ovum such as that of an insect, where the yolk is centrally placed. **Complete segmentation.** That form of segmentation of an ovum where the cytoplasm is completely sub-divided at the first cell division. **Discoidal segmentation.** That form of segmentation of an ovum where only a small cap of cytoplasm above the yolk is sub-divided. **Duplicative segmentation.** A method of binary fission, the second division being in a plane at right angles to the first; exemplified by the gonococcus. **Germ segmentation.** The segmentation of the ovum. *See* MAIN DEF. 3 (above). **Haustral segmentation.** The condition of the colon in which the lumen is indented by projecting folds of mucous membrane due to the activity of the muscularis mucosae. **Holoblastic segmentation.** Complete segmentation (see above). **Incomplete segmentation, Meroblastic segmentation.** Discoidal segmentation (see above). **Metameric segmentation.** Segmentation of the body associated with the somites. **Partial segmentation.** Discoidal segmentation (see above). **Protovertebral segmentation.** Segmentation of the paraxial mesoderm into somites. **Regular segmentation.** Segmentation of the ovum where the daughter cells are equal in size. **Rhythmic segmentation.** Annular constrictions of the small intestine which occur rhythmically and divide the lumen into small distended segments. Each segment is then divided through its middle by the succeeding constriction. The segmenting movements have a rate of about 8 per minute, and help to bring the chyme into thorough mixture with the intestinal juices. **Total segmentation.** Complete segmentation (see above). **Unequal segmentation.** Segmentation of the ovum where the daughter cells are unequal in size. **Yolk segmentation.** Segmentation of the vitellus. [L *segmentum* that which is cut off.]

segmenter (seg·men·ter). A schizont. [see prec.]

Segmentina (seg·men·tin·ah). A genus of small, flattened, pulmonate Gastropoda. Several species are intermediate hosts to the fluke *Fasciolopsis buski* in the Far East. [L *segmentum* that which is cut off.]

segments (seg·ments). The series of units of which the spinal cord may be considered to be composed; one pair of nerves is connected to each. [see prec.]

segregation (seg·re·ga·shun). The separation in meiotic cell division of homologous chromosome pairs and their contained allelomorphic gene pairs. In consequence of this separation, the 2 component genes of an allelomorphic pair cannot be present in the same gamete. **Preferential segregation.** Non-random segregation of a particular chromosome or chromosome segment into cells giving rise to functional gametes. [L *segregare* to separate.]

segregator (seg·re·ga·tor). An instrument incorporating a double catheter which was inserted into the bladder and alleged to divide that cavity into 2 parts so that urine could be collected separately from each ureter. The instrument is now obsolete and has been superseded by retrograde catheterization of the ureters through the cystoscope. [see prec.]

Séguin, Edouard (b. 1812). French neurologist.

Séguin's sign or signal symptom. Muscular contraction as a premonitory sign of an epileptic seizure.

Seidel, Erich (b. 1882). German ophthalmologist.

Seidel's scotoma or sign. An enlargement of the blind spot above or below in an arcuate fashion, but becoming narrower as it goes away from the blind spot. The beginning of an arcuate scotoma, and a supposedly early sign of glaucoma.

Seidelin, Harald. 20th century Danish pathologist working in the West Indies.

Seidelin's bodies. *Paraplasma flavigenum.*

Seiler, Carl (b. 1849). Philadelphia laryngologist.

Seiler's cartilage. A small cartilage attached to the vocal process of the arytenoid cartilage.

seisaesthesia (si·ses·**the**·ze·ah). The sense perception of concussion. [Gk *seisis* concusssion, aesthesia.]

seismaesthesia (si·smes·**the**·ze·ah). The perception of vibratory impulses in liquid or aerial media by means of touch. [Gk *seismos* a shaking, aesthesia.]

seismotherapy (si·smo·**ther**·ap·e). The use of vibratory appliances in the treatment of disease. [Gk *seismos* a shaking, therapy.]

Seitz, Ernest (b. 1885). Bonn bacteriologist.

Seitz filter. A bacterial filter of fibrous material for use with either positive or negative pressure.

Seitz sign. Bronchial inspiratory sound beginning harshly and fading away, as a sign of a cavity in the lung.

seizure (**se**·zhewer). 1. A sudden attack of disease. 2. The sudden appearance of certain signs of disease, e.g. convulsions. **Audiogenic seizure.** One precipitated by a loud noise. **Cerebral seizure.** A focal epileptic seizure. **Epileptic seizure.** The clinical episode which results from an excessive neuronal discharge. **Erratic epileptic seizure.** A type of seizure peculiar to the newborn characterized by erratic electro-encephalographic discharges with perhaps associated clinical convulsions. **Evolved epileptic seizure.** An attack of epilepsy precipitated by some specific stimulus. **Fortuitous epileptic seizure.** Spontaneous epileptic seizure. **Gustatory epileptic seizure.** A partial epileptic attack consisting in hallucinations of taste, or in altered perception of taste. **Hallucinatory epileptic seizure.** A partial epileptic episode consisting in hallucinations involving one or more modalities of sensation. **Minor epileptic seizure.** Epileptic attacks of short duration or low intensity [Obsolete term.] **Non-convulsive epileptic seizure.** A seizure manifested clinically by a symptom other than convulsions. **Olfactory hallucinatory epileptic seizure.** A variety of epilepsy characterized by hallucinations of smell, usually unpleasant in character, commonly constituting the aura. **Self-induced epileptic seizure.** An attack deliberately brought about by the patient—usually a child—who provokes the seizure by some manoeuvre which he has discovered. **Spontaneous epileptic seizure.** A seizure occurring independent of any obvious provoking factor. **Sporadic epileptic seizure.** An attack occurring in a non-epileptic subject, caused by such factors as a convulsant drug, endogenous intoxication, sudden barbiturate withdrawal, or fever in infancy. **Subclinical epileptic seizure.** An attack where the manifestations are so slight as to pass unnoticed without the aid of appropriate electro-encephalographic techniques. **Unilateral epileptic seizure.** An attack in which the motor signs involved are predominantly on one side of the body. **Versine epileptic seizure.** A partial attack which produces conjugate deviation of the eyes, head and sometimes of the trunk, either towards the side opposite to that of the discharging lesion, less often towards the same side. **Larval seizure.** A masked or incomplete seizure. **Myoclonic seizure.** An isolated epileptic seizure of unusually brief duration. **Psychic seizure.** A seizure the manifestations of which are mental. [O Fr. *seisir.*]

sejunction (se·**jungk**·shun). The interruption of the continuity of association processes. [L *sejungere* to separate.]

Sekiya, S. 20th century Japanese physician.

Sato and Sekiya stain. A peroxidase stain containing copper sulphate and benzidine.

sel (sel). A salt. **Sel ammoniac.** Ammonium chloride, NH_4Cl, a compound frequently prescribed as an expectorant. **Sel d'Epsom.** Epsom salts. **Sel de Glauber.** Glauber salt, sodium sulphate, $Na_2SO_4 \cdot 10H_2O$, a colourless crystalline solid, readily soluble in water and administered orally as a saline purgative. **Sel de Saturne.** Lead acetate. **Sel de Sedlitz.** Magnesium sulphate, Epsom salts, $MgSO_4 \cdot 7H_2O$, a colourless crystalline solid, soluble in water to produce a solution that has a saline taste. It is administered orally as a saline purgative. [Fr.]

selaphobia (se·lah·**fo**'·be·ah). A morbid fear of lightning or of any flashing light. [Gk *selas* light, *phobein* to fear.]

selection (se·**lek**·shun). The process of selecting, e.g. for survival. **Artificial selection.** Natural selection (see below) in which the criterion of the fittest is controlled by man. **Selection of microbial mutants or recombinants.** By culturing in, or on, media which either lack an essential nutrient (e.g. an amino acid) or contain an antibacterial substance (e.g. an antibiotic) so that parental growth is suppressed and only the mutant or recombinant cells can grow. Such selection is the basis of fine structure genetic analysis since recombinants arising from genetic crosses at very low frequency (e.g. 1 per 10^6–10^8 parental cells) can be identified and counted. **Natural selection.** That which results in the survival and reproduction only of those most fitted to survive in the struggle for existence. Darwin postulated that, of the great reproductive potential of any organism, there would be a tendency for those better fitted to survive longer and reproduce more than those less fitted: since all organisms vary, those variations with greater survival value, provided that they were inheritable, would increase in the population at the expense of those with less survival value. This is the principal mechanism by which he believed evolution to have come about. **Sexual selection.** That in which individuals of one sex, usually the female, select for mates those of the other sex having certain characters while rejecting those with other characters. Such selection will be unimportant in evolution, except in cases of monogamy with unequal sex ratio or strict polyandry. [L *seligere* to choose from among.]

selector (se·**lek**·tor). An automatic electrical switching device serving to select a particular contact or contacts. [see prec.]

selenate (**sel**·en·ate). Any salt of selenic acid, H_2SeO_4.

selene unguium (sel·e·ne **ung**·gew·um). The lunula of a nail. [Gk *selene* moon, L *unguis* nail.]

selenic (sel·**e**·nik). Any compound of selenium in which the latter is hexavalent.

selenide (**sel**·en·ide). Any binary compound formed by the element selenium, with an electropositive element. It is analogous to a sulphide.

seleniferous (sel·en·**if**·er·us). 1. Containing selenium. 2. Yielding selenium. [selenium, L *ferre* to bear.]

selenite (**sel**·en·ite). 1. Any salt of selenious acid, H_2SeO_3. 2. A colourless transparent mineral form of calcium sulphate, $CaSO_4 \cdot 2H_2O$, used in optical instruments.

selenitic (sel·en·**it**·ik). 1. Pertaining to or containing selenium. 2. Subject to the influence of the moon. [see foll.]

selenium (sel·**e**·ne·um). An element of atomic weight 78.96, atomic number 34, and chemical symbol Se. It is a non-metal closely related to sulphur in chemical properties and existing in several allotropic forms; the grey crystalline, metallic, form varies in electrical resistance when exposed to light and is accordingly used in photo-electric cells. It occurs in many minerals as selenides, and some soils are so rich in selenium that grain and other plants grown upon it may contain relatively large amounts. Poisoning has been observed in animals feeding on such plants, giving a diverse picture of stunted growth, deformity of hooves and damage to the liver and nervous system (alkali disease); poisoning in man from this source has, however, not been proved. The element is used in industry in the manufacture of rubber, glass, electronic and photo-electric devices, and is a potential industrial hazard. [Gk *selene* moon.]

selenosis (sel·en·**o**·sis). Selenium poisoning. [selenium, Gk *-osis* condition.]

self-differentiation (**self**·dif·er·en·she·**a**'·shun). The theory that the differentiation or growth of cellular organisms is conditioned by their own internal forces and not by external influences, i.e. of the environment. [AS *self*, differentiation.]

self-digestion (self·di·**jes**·chun). 1. Autolysis; the self-destruction of the cells of an organism by its own serum, a condition encountered in certain pathological conditions and occurring after death. 2. Autodigestion; a condition found in disease of the stomach; the stomach walls are digested by the gastric juice. [AS *self*, digestion.]

self-encasement (self·en·**kase**·ment). The condition in which a portion of the small intestine is enclosed in a mesenteric pouch. [AS *self*, L *in*, *capsa* box.]

self-fertilization (self·fer·til·i·za'·shun). The fertilization of an ovule by the pollen of the same flower. [AS *self*, fertilization.]
self-hypnosis (self·hip·no·sis). The self-induction of hypnosis by mental concentration on one particular object or thought; or, in a susceptible subject who has often been hypnotized, by concentration on the fact of hypnosis; hence *self-hypnotism.* [AS *self*, hypnosis.]
self-inductance (self·in·duk·tans). An attribute of an electric circuit due to its self-induction, being the ratio of the electromotive force induced to the frequency of the current inducing it. The unit is the *henry.*
self-induction (self·in·duk·shun). An electrical phenomenon in which a variation in a current passing through a loop of a coil induces an opposing current in the neighbouring loops. [AS *self*, inductance.]
self-infection (self·in·fek·shun). Auto-infection, endogenous infection; a condition in which the infection arises from some focus within the patient's own body. [AS *self*, infection.]
self-limited (self·lim·it·ed). Pertaining to a disease which is restricted in duration by reason of its own peculiar characteristics not because of external influences. [AS *self*, L *limes* boundary.]
self-psychology (self·si·kol·o·je). A branch of psychology based on introspection. [AS *self*, psychology.]
self-suggestion (self·suj·es·chun). Autosuggestion. [AS *self*, L *suggerere* to supply.]
self-suspension (self·sus·pen·shun). Suspension of the body by the head alone or by the head and axillae in order to stretch or straighten the vertebral column. [AS *self*, suspension.]
Selivanoff, Feodor Feodorowitsch (b. 1859). Russian chemist.
Selivanoff's reaction or test. For laevulose (fructose) in urine. To 5 ml of 0.05 per cent resorcinol in dilute hydrochloric acid (1 part concentrated acid + 2 parts water) add 0.5 ml of urine and heat just to boiling. A red colour indicates laevulose.
sella turcica [NA] (sel·ah ter·sik·ah). A deep depression in the shape of a Turkish saddle in the upper surface of the body of the sphenoid bone, behind the tuberculum sellae, in the deepest part of which is lodged the hypophysis cerebri. [L Turkish seat.]
sellar (sel·ar). Relating or belonging to the sella turcica.
Sellards, Andrew Watson (b. 1884). Boston physician.
Sellard's test. Alkali tolerance test. *See* TEST.
Sellick, Brian Arthur. 20th century London anaesthetist.
Sellick manoeuvre. Backward pressure on the cricoid cartilage during tracheal intubation in the unconscious patient, to prevent passive regurgitation of stomach contents.
Selye, Hans (b. 1907). Canadian biochemist.
Selye hypothesis or syndrome. The hypothesis, which is not by any means universally accepted, that there is a response of the living organism to stress by a basic reaction that is the same irrespective of the agent causing the stress. It occurs in 3 stages: the alarm reaction, the stage of resistance and the stage of exhaustion. The alarm reaction has 2 phases: the shock phase, during which there are the low blood pressure, haemoconcentration, increased permeability, depressed temperature and other well-known features of clinical shock; and the countershock phase in which these are reversed. A stage of resistance follows when all the non-specific defence measures are brought into action. If the stress persists, or has been very heavy, the stage of exhaustion sets in and proceeds to decline and death; on the other hand the effect may be slight and shown by little more than a transient hyperglycaemia, tachycardia and leucocytosis. This basic pattern is complicated by other features which are specific to the particular stressor agents (*see* STRESS). The defence mechanism is initiated and co-ordinated by the hypothalamus which stimulates the nervous system and the anterior pituitary, in the latter increasing the output of adrenocorticotropic hormones (ACTH) at the expense of the other pituitary hormones. The cortex of the suprarenal gland responds in turn by the production of excessive amounts of glucocorticoid (including cortisone) and mineral corticoid hormones. It is considered that these are stimulated by separate pituitary hormones and are mutually antagonistic, but if adequate in amount and well balanced, health is maintained. Many disturbing factors may, however, distort the basic pattern; thus the hypothalamus may not respond, or an excess of mineral corticoids may be produced. A "disease of adaptation" then results: Addison's, Cushing's, and Simmonds' diseases are typically such, but the syndrome is concerned in many other diseases which may seem unrelated, e.g. rheumatic disorders, rheumatoid arthritis, gout, allergic states, nephrosclerosis, hypertension, ulcerative colitis and peptic ulcer, in which stress seems to play a part.
semanteme (se·man·teem). The smallest irreducible element or unit of meaning. **Pseudo-semanteme.** Utterances which wear the garment of true lexicon terms, cognate to the patient's original system, but not necessarily used appropriately. **Displaced semanteme.** Pseudo-semanteme. [Gk *semantikos* significant.]
semantics (se·man·tix). 1. The branch of linguistics concerned with the problems of meaning. 2. The science of signs (Syn: sermology or serniotics). 3. Signs and their relations to *designata* or the world experience, real or imagined. 4. The study of grammar or lexicon. **General semantics.** The scientific study of the difficulties of life as experienced by the individual, with special reference to the use of language as a means in adjustment; a method of treating aphasia and some psychological maladjustments. [Gk *semantikos* significant.]
semantophores (sem·an·to·forz). The informational macromolecules; usually applied to the nucleic acids (DNA and RNA) and proteins. [Gk *semantikos* significant, *pherein* to bear.]
semasiology (se·ma·se·ol'·o·je). That branch of semantics concerned with the historical study of changes in the meaning of words. [Gk *sema* sign, *logos* science.]
Semb, Carl Boye (b. 1895). Norwegian surgeon.
Semb's operation. 1. Gastrostomy by inversion of a cone of stomach wall into the lumen. 2. Extrafascial or extrapleural apicolysis for the collapse of a tuberculous cavity of the upper lobe; the apex of the pleura is depressed by blood-stained exudate after resection of one of the upper ribs and extrapleural stripping of the lung.
Semb's space. An artificial space left after the operation of apicolysis.
semeiography (sem·i·og·raf·e). A categorical statement of the symptoms and signs of any disease. [Gk *semeion* sign, *graphein* to record.]
semeiology (sem·i·ol·o·je). Symptomatology. [Gk *semeion* sign, *logos* science.]
semeiosis (sem·i·o·sis). The study of the signs and symptoms of disease. [Gk *semeion* sign.]
semeiotic (sem·i·ot·ik). 1. Relating or belonging to the symptoms or signs of disease. 2. Pathognomonic. [Gk *semeion* sign.]
semeiotics (sem·i·ot·ix). Symptomatology. [see prec.]
semen (se·men) (pl. *semina*). 1. A seed. 2. [Sperma (NA)]. The fecundating fluid of the male; it contains the spermatozoa together with secretions of the prostate and seminal vesicles. **Semen reflux.** A condition in which the semen is ejaculated into the bladder. It may be due to a congenital defect or be the result of a prostatectomy, a posterior urethral stricture or a lumbar sympathectomy. [L seed.]
semenuria (se·men·ewr·e·ah). A condition marked by the presence of semen in the urine.
semi-. Latin prefix meaning *half.*
semicanal (sem·e·kan·al'). A canal with an opening at one side. [L *semi-*, *canalis* water-pipe.]
semicanalis (sem·e·kan·a'·lis). Literally, a half-canal; a sulcus or groove. [see prec.]
semicartilaginous (sem·e·kar·til·aj'·in·us). Composed partly of cartilaginous tissue. [L *semi-*, cartilage.]
semicoma (sem·e·ko·mah). A state of coma which is not profound; the patient can be aroused. [L *semi*, coma.]
semicomatose (sem·e·ko·mat·oze). Marked by a condition of semicoma.

semiconductor (**sem**·e·kon·**duk**′·tor). A near insulator showing limited electrical conductivity which can be greatly varied by energy absorption. [L *semi-*, *conducere* to conduct.]
semiconscious (sem·e·**kon**·shus). A state of incomplete consciousness. [L *semi-*, consciousness.]
semiconservative (**sem**·e·kon·**serv**′·at·iv). In genetics, a term used to describe the mode of DNA replication postulated by Watson and Crick. This involves separation of the chains of the double helix, synthesis of the 2 chains complementary to the old ones, and the association of 1 old and 1 new complementary chain to form "daughter" double helices. [L *semi-*, *conservare* to keep together.]
semicretin (sem·e·**kre**·tin). Anyone affected with semicretinism.
semicretinism (**sem**·e·**kre**·tin·izm). A minor degree of cretinism in which the individual has sufficient intelligence to recognize the needs of the body and has some slight comprehension of the meaning and use of words. [L *semi-*, cretin.]
semicrista (sem·e·**kris**·tah). A small or imperfect crest or ridge. **Semicrista incisiva.** The nasal crest. *See* CREST. [L *semi-*, *crista* ridge.]
semidecussation (**sem**·e·de·kus·**a**′·shun). Partial decussation as of a tract of white matter, e.g. the pyramidal tracts in the medulla oblongata or the optic nerves at the chiasma. [L *semi-*, decussation.]
semiflexion (sem·e·**flek**·shun). Applied to a limb, a state in which the limb is in a position midway between full flexion and full extension. [L *semi-*, flexion.]
semilunar (sem·e·**loo**·nar). Shaped like a half moon; crescentic. [L *semi-*, *luna* moon.]
semilunare (**sem**·e·loo·**na**′·re). The lunate bone. [see prec.]
semiluxation (**sem**·e·lux·**a**′·shun). Subluxation; partial dislocation. [L *semi-*, luxation.]
semimembranosus muscle [musculus semimembranosus (NA)] (**sem**·e·mem·bran·**o**′·sus musl). One of the hamstring muscles which arises from the ischial tuberosity and is inserted into the groove on the back of the medial condyle of the tibia. [L *semi-*, *membrana* membrane.]
semimembranous (sem·e·**mem**·bran·us). Composed partly of membrane or fascia; e.g. applied to a muscle. [see prec.]
seminal (**sem**·in·al). 1. Relating or belonging to semen. 2. Consisting of, or contained in seed. [L *semen* seed.]
seminarcosis (**sem**·e·nar·**ko**′·sis). A half-conscious state, e.g. morphine-scopolamine anaesthesia. [L *semi-*, narcosis.]
semination (sem·in·a·shun). The deposition of semen in the vagina or uterus during coitus or by artificial means. [L *seminare* to sow.]
seminiferous (sem·in·**if**·er·us). 1. Conveying or producing semen, a term applied to the tubules of the testis. 2. In botany, seed-bearing. **Seminiferous tubules.** *See* TUBULE. **Seminiferous tubule dysgenesis.** Kleinfelter's syndrome. [L *semen* seed, *ferre* to bear.]
seminoma (sem·in·o·mah). A relatively undifferentiated form of teratoma of the testis. **Ovarian seminoma.** A teratoma of the ovary in which tissue with the structure of testis is found side by side with ovarian elements. [semen, Gk *-oma* tumour.]
seminormal (sem·e·**nor**·mal). Describing a volumetric solution which is half the normal or standard strength. [L *semi-*, normal.]
seminose (**sem**·in·oze). D-mannose. [L *semen* seed, glucose.]
semiography (sem·e·og·rag·e). Semeiography.
semiology (sem·i·**ol**·o·je). Symptomatology. [Gk *semeion* sign, *logos* science.]
semiotic (sem·i·**ot**·ik). Semantics. [Gk *semeion* sign.]
semipenniform (sem·e·**pen**·e·form). Shaped like a feather on one side, e.g. applied to a muscle in which the fibres are obliquely joined to one side of the tendon. [L *semi-*, *penna* feather, form.]
semipermeable (sem·e·**per**·me·abl). Partially permeable, term applied specifically to membranes that allow, in the process of osmosis, the passage of some molecules but prevent that of others. [L *semi-*, *permeare* to pass through.]
semiplegia (sem·e·**ple**·je·ah). Hemiplegia; paralysis of one side of the body. [L *semi-*, Gk *plege* stroke.]
semipronation (**sem**·e·pro·**na**′·shun). 1. The adoption of or the placing in a semiprone position. 2. The state of being in a semiprone position, as applied to the body generally; Sims' position.
semiprone (sem·e·**prone**). Applied to a position that is halfway between the mid-position and the prone position; threequarters prone. [L *semi-*, *pronus* leaning forward.]
semiptosis (sem·e·**to**·sis). Incomplete ptosis. [L *semi-*, ptosis.]
semirecumbent (**sem**·e·re·**kum**′·bent). Reclining or leaning back but not entirely recumbent. [L *semi-*, recumbent.]
semisideratio, semisideration (**sem**·e·sid·er·**a**′·she·o, **sem**·e·sid·er·**a**′·shun). Hemiplegia. [L *semi-*, *sideratio* stroke.]
semispeculum (sem·e·**spek**·ew·lum). A blunt gorget shaped like a half-speculum; used in perineal lithotomy, when the bladder neck was dilated and not cut. [L *semi-*, speculum.]
semispinalis muscle [musculus semispinalis (NA)] (**sem**·e·spi·**na**′·lis musl). Any of the muscles on the posterior aspect of the cervical and thoracic parts of the vertebral column, deep to the sub-divisions of the sacrospinalis muscle.
semispinalis capitis muscle [musculus semispinalis capitis (NA)] (**sem**·e·spi·**na**′·lis **kap**·it·is musl). A muscle arising from the transverse processes of the upper thoracic vertebrae and the articular processes of the lower cervical vertebrae; it is inserted into the occipital bone between the superior and inferior nuchal lines.
semispinalis cervicis muscle [musculus semispinalis cervicis (NA)] (**sem**·e·spi·**na**′·lis **ser**·vis·is musl). A muscle arising from the transverse processes of the upper thoracic vertebrae and inserted into the spines of the cervical vertebrae.
semispinalis thoracis muscle [musculus semispinalis thoracis (NA)] (**sem**·e·spi·**na**′·lis **thor**·as·is musl). A muscle arising by tendons from the transverse processes of the lower thoracic vertebrae and inserted into the spines of the upper thoracic and lower cervical vertebrae. [L *semi-*, *spinalis* of the spine.]
semisulcus (sem·e·**sul**·kus). A groove or channel on the edge of a bone or other structure which, when united with another groove on the opposing adjoining structure, forms a complete sulcus. [L *semi-*, sulcus.]
semisupination (**sem**·e·sew·pin·**a**′·shun). 1. The assumption of or the placing in a semisupine position. 2. A semisupine position.
semisupine (sem·e·**sew**·pine). Applied to a position that is halfway between the mid-position and the supine position; three-quarters supine. [L *semi-*, supine.]
semitendinosus muscle [musculus semitendinosus (NA)] (**sem**·e·ten·din·**o**′·sus musl). One of the hamstring muscles which arises from the ischial tuberosity and is inserted into the upper part of the medial surface of the tibia. [L *semi-*, *tendere* to stretch.]
semitendinous (sem·e·**ten**·din·us). Composed partly of tendon. [see prec.]
semivalent (sem·e·**va**·lent). Describing the single-electron link in certain compounds, unstable as compared with the normal link provided by electron pairs. [L *semi-*, valency.]
Semon, Sir Felix (b. 1849). London laryngologist.
Semon's law, Gerhardt-Semon law, Semon-Rosenbach law. In a progressive destructive lesion of the motor nerve supplying the intrinsic laryngeal muscles, the abductor mechanism is affected before the mechanism of adduction.
Semon, Richard Wolfgang (b. 1859). German naturalist.
Hering-Semon hypothesis, Semon-Hering theory. The mnemic theory. *See* THEORY.
sempervirine (sem·per·vi·reen). $C_{19}H_{16}N_2$, an alkaloid occurring in the rhizome and roots of *Gelsemium sempervirens* Linn. (family Loganiaceae).
Semple, Sir David (b. 1856). British army surgeon and bacteriologist.
Semple's method or treatment. A method of preparing anti-rabic vaccine that was used for many years in India; the spinal cord of an infected (fixed virus) rabbit is phenolized (1 per cent), pulverized and strained, and the filtrate used for injection.

Semple vaccine. A vaccine used for post-exposure immunization against rabies. It is a suspension of spinal cord from a rabbit or sheep infected with fixed virus, and inactivated with phenol. It is given as a course of 14 daily intramuscular injections during the incubation period and provides some degree of protection.

Sendroy, Julius, Jnr. (b. 1900). American biochemist.

Sendroy's method. For chlorides in blood. Serum or plasma is heated with phosphotungstic acid to precipitate proteins, and the mixture shaken with excess of solid silver iodate. After filtering, the iodate in the filtrate is determined by adding potassium iodide and titrating the liberated iodine with thiosulphate.

Senear, Francis Eugene (b. 1889). Chicago dermatologist.

Senear-Usher disease or syndrome, Usher-Senear disease. Pemphigus erythematodes; a relatively benign type of chronic pemphigus in which, besides bullae, lesions resembling lupus erythematodes or crusted seborrhoeic dermatitis may be noted.

Senecio (se·ne·she·o). A genus of plants of the family Compositae. When it forms one of the herbs in an infusion called "bush tea" it is held to be one of the causative factors in veno-occlusive disease. *Senecio* poisoning has caused hepatic damage in undernourished children in South Africa. **Senecio aureus.** Liferoot; used as an emmenagogue. **Senecio cineraria.** *Cineraria maritima;* a species used in the treatment of cataract. **Senecio jacoboea.** Ragwort; used as an emmenagogue. [L *senex* old man.]

senecionine (se·ne·se·o′·neen). $C_{18}H_{25}O_5N$, one of the constituent alkaloids of various species of *Senecio.*

senectitude (se·nek·te·tewd). Old age. [L *senex* old man.]

Senega BPC 1968 (sen·e·gah). Senegae radix, senega root; the dried root of *Polygala senega* Linn. (family Polygalaceae). It contains the saponins, senegin and polygalic acid, which resemble those of quillaia bark; there is also present a fixed oil and a trace of methyl salicylate. It is an expectorant, used in the treatment of bronchitis, usually as an infusion. [*Seneca* an Amer. Ind. tribe.]

senegin (sen·ej·in). A mixture of saponins of uncertain constitution present in senega root.

Senekjie (Senica), Harry. 20th century American parasitologist.

Senekjie's culture medium. A modification of NNN medium for the cultivation of *Leishmania.*

senescence (sen·es·ens). The bodily and mental state associated with advancing age. **Precocious senescence.** Progeria. [L *senescere* to become old.]

senescent (sen·es·ent). Growing old; ageing. [see prec.]

Senica. *See* SENEKJIE.

senile (se·nile). 1. Relating or belonging to old age. 2. Characteristic of old age. 3. Resulting from infirmity of old age. [L *senilis* aged.]

senilis (se·nil·is). 1. Belonging to old age. 2. Old. [L.]

senilism (se·nil·izm). Premature old age; progeria. [see foll.]

senility (se·nil·it·e). The general state resulting from the mental and physical weakness and enfeeblement which are the accompaniment of old age. [L *senilis* aged.]

senium (se·ne·um). Old age; senility. **Senium praecox.** Premature senility. [L weakness of old age.]

Senn, Emanuel John (b. 1869). Chicago surgeon.

Senn's operation, Kader-Senn operation. Gastrostomy by the inversion of the stomach wall around the gastrostomy tube in the form of an invertible ink-well.

Senn, Nicholas (b. 1844). Chicago surgeon.

Senn's bone plate. A plate of bone used during the 19th century in bowel anastomosis.

senna (sen·ah). The dried leaflets (Senna Leaf BP 1963) or the dried ripe fruits (Senna Fruit BP 1973, "senna pods") of *Cassia acutifolia* Delile or of *C. angustifolia* Vahl of the family Leguminosae. Both leaves and pods are effective purgatives, acting by irritation of the large intestine. **Alexandrian senna.** The leaves or pods of *Cassia acutifolia* Delile. **Sennae fructus acutifoliae, Sennae fructus angustifoliae.** *European Pharmacopoeia* names for Senna Fruit BP 1973. **Indian senna, Tinnevella senna.** The leaves or pods of *Cassia angustifolia.* [Ar. *sana.*]

senopia (se·no·pe·ah). Presbyopia. [L *senex* old man, *opsis* sight.]

Senoran's gastric aspirator or bottle. An aspirator by which negative pressure is produced in a bottle attached to a stomach tube.

sensation (sen·sa·shun). The effect in consciousness of stimulation of an afferent nerve. **Articular sensation.** Sensation of position and movement of the joints. **Cincture sensation.** Girdle sensation (see below). **Concomitant sensation.** A secondary sensation which develops as a by-product of a primary sensation. **Cutaneous sensation.** A sensation arising in the skin. **Delayed sensation.** A sensation localized in the skin in which there is an interval between the application of the stimulus and the registration of the sensation by the central nervous system. **Dermal sensation.** Cutaneous sensation (see above). **Eccentric sensation.** A sensation which gives an inaccurate impression of the location of the sensory stimulus. **Epileptic sensation.** A purely subjective experience, auditory, gustatory, olfactory, sensorial or visual, which represents a partial epileptic seizure, often taking its place. **External sensation.** Objective sensation (see below). **General sensation.** A sensation that cannot be localized but is felt throughout the body. **Girdle sensation.** A sensation of constriction around the body. **Gnostic sensation.** One of the more highly-developed forms of sensation, including light touch, tactile discrimination, stereognosis, position sense and the appreciation of vibration; a sensation mediated via the posterior column of the spinal cord. **Internal sensation.** Subjective sensation (see below). **Joint sensation.** Articular sensation (see above). **Kinaesthetic sensation.** Sensation associated with motion. **Negative sensation.** The effect of a subliminal stimulus. **Objective sensation.** The mental appreciation, as derived from the senses, of an external object. **Palmaesthetic sensation.** The appreciation of vibration applied to the skin. **Primary sensation.** Sensation that results directly from the reception of a stimulus. **Proprioceptive sensation.** The sensation of the position of limbs and joints that results from the automatic co-ordination of various stimuli from the periphery which individually seldom reach consciousness. **Psychovisual sensation.** A sensation of visual type arising in consciousness without retinal stimulation; a vision. **Radiating sensation.** An unpleasant sensation which spreads from a diseased part to an unaffected one. **Referred sensation, Reflex sensation.** A sensation not felt at the point of application of the stimulus, but elsewhere. **Secondary sensation.** 1. A radiating sensation (see above). 2. One form of sensation which accompanies another form; synaesthesia. **Special sensation.** A sensation which has its origin in one of the special senses. **Subjective sensation.** A sensation which does not result from, or depend upon, external stimuli. **Tactile sensation.** The sensation of touch. **Transferred sensation.** Referred sensation (see above). **Vascular sensation.** A sensation produced by changes in local vascular dilatation or contraction. [L *sentire* to feel.]

sense (sens). Any one of the faculties by which the body translates exogenous or endogenous stimuli into sensations which can be appreciated in consciousness. The main senses concerned with exogenous stimuli are vision, hearing, taste, smell and feeling; the first 4 of these are often referred to as the *special senses.* Pre-eminent among the many endogenous senses are those of hunger, thirst and sexual desire. **Acid sense.** A term applied to the reflex secretion of hydrochloric acid by the stomach in response to digestive needs. **Body sense.** The body image; the mental impression an individual obtains of the architecture and position of his own body, as a result of the summation and correlation of multiple sensory stimuli from the periphery. **Chemical sense.** The perception by the body of chemical agents, either in its environment or in direct contact with it; the term applies particularly to smell and taste. **Colour sense.** The sense through which colours are appreciated and distinguished. **Concomitant sense.** Concomitant sensation. *See* SENSATION. **Cutaneous sense, Dermal sense.** The appreciation of sensations resulting from stimuli applied to the skin. **Equilibrium sense.** The sense through which the equilibrium of the body is appreciated and maintained; static sense. **Form sense.** The faculty of recognizing the form of objects. **Genesic sense.** The procreative or sexual instinct. **Internal sense.** Any sense by which endogenous stimuli are translated into consciousness. **Kinaesthetic sense.** The faculty through which muscular position and movement are appreciated. **Labyrinthine sense.** The sense of equilibrium as mediated via the labyrinth. **Light sense.** The sense whereby graded intensities of light may be appreciated. **Muscle sense, Muscular sense.** Kinaesthetic sense (see above). **Pain sense.** The sense which mediates the perception of pain. **Sense of pitch.** Tone sense (see below). **Posture sense.** The ability to recognize the posture of the body and of its component parts, without the aid of vision; a combination of the kinaesthetic, proprioceptive and labyrinthine senses. **Pressure sense.** The faculty whereby pressure or weight applied to the body can be appreciated. **Proprioceptive sense.** The sense whereby a variety of sensory afferent impulses from the skin, muscles and joints, which fail to enter consciousness, are correlated in order to give conscious appreciation of position. **Reproductive sense.** Genesic sense (see above). **Respiratory sense.** The largely unconscious sense of the need to breathe. **Seventh sense.** The appreciation of sensations from the viscera [Obsolete term]. **Sixth sense.** A term originally employed to include all the components of proprioception, and all sensations concerned in the appreciation of position. In this context it is obsolete, but it is sometimes used in popular literature to imply supernatural powers of extrasensory perception. **Space sense.** The faculty whereby the position of objects in space can be appreciated. **Special sense.** Any one of the senses of vision, hearing, taste and smell. **Static sense.** Equilibrium sense (see above). **Stereognostic sense.** The appreciation of form without the aid of vision; applied particularly to the identification of objects placed in the hand. **Temperature sense.** The sense whereby variations in temperature can be appreciated; mediated via specialized skin receptors. **Time sense.** The appreciation of time; applied particularly to the ability to time auditory (e.g. musical) stimuli. **Tone sense.** The ability to distinguish between musical tones; the sense of pitch. **Visceral sense.** The sense whereby sensations arising in the viscera are appreciated; the sensory stimuli concerned travel by autonomic nerves. [L *sentire* to feel.]

sensibamine (sen·**sib**·am·een). A molecular compound of the two alkaloids, ergotamine and ergotaminine; it occurs in ergot.

sensibilisatrice (sen·sib·**il**·is·ah·**trees'**). The term used by Bordet and his school for *amboceptor.* [Fr.]

sensibility (sen·sib·**il**·it·e). The ability to receive, feel and appreciate sensations and impressions, whether physical or psychological. **Bone sensibility.** The ability to appreciate vibration, when a vibrating tuning fork is applied firmly to the skin overlying a bony prominence; also called *pallaesthesia.* **Common sensibility.** The appreciation of conscious existence and of the normal activity of body organs. **Cortical sensibility.** The ability of the cerebral cortex to receive, correlate and integrate sensory impressions. **Deep sensibility.** The awareness of sensations, such as those of pressure, tension and pain, which are appreciated by and transmitted from, structures deep to the skin. **Electromuscular sensibility.** Sensibility of a muscle to electrical stimulations. **Epicritic sensibility.** The ability to appreciate fine highly integrated sensations such as tactile discrimination [Obsolete term]. **Gnostic sensibility.** Those forms of somatic sensation mediated by the cerebral cortex. **Mesoblastic sensibility.** Deep sensibility (see above). **Organic sensibility.** The ability to receive and integrate sensory stimuli which do not enter conciousness [Obsolete term.] **Pallaesthetic sensibility, Palmaesthetic sensibility.** The ability to appreciate vibrations; *pallaesthetic sensibility* is usually used when the vibration is appreciated via bone, *palmaesthetic sensibility* when it is felt in the skin or soft tissues. **Proprioceptive sensibility.** Proprioceptive sensation; it is unsatisfactory to use sensibility in this context as proprioceptive sensations rarely reach consciousness. **Protopathic sensibility.** The ability to appreciate the more crude forms of sensation such as pain and temperature [Obsolete term]. **Range of sensibility.** *See* RANGE. **Recurrent sensibility.** The form of sensibility which arises in the anterior roots of spinal nerves but appears to depend upon the integrity of the posterior roots; the existence of this form of sensibility is in doubt and the term is little used. **Sensibility of the soma, Somataesthetic sensibility.** Consciousness of bodily position and movement. **Splanchnaesthetic sensibility.** Awareness of the viscera and of their activity, as mediated via the splanchnic nerves. **Vibratory sensibility.** The faculty of appreciating sensations of vibration; pallaesthetic and palmaesthetic sensibility. [L *sensibilis* perceptible by the senses.]

sensibilization (**sen**·sib·il·i·**za'**·shun). The process of rendering a cell or substance more sensitive; sensitization. [see prec.]

sensibilizer (**sen**·**sib**·**il**·i·zer). Amboceptor. [see foll.]

sensible (**sen**·sibl). 1. Capable of being perceived. 2. Able to receive impression through the senses. 3. Tending to be easily affected mentally or physically; sensitive. 4. Mentally perceptible. [L *sensibilis* perceptible by the senses.]

sensiferous (sen·**sif**·er·us). Arousing or conducting a sensation. [sensation, L *ferre* to carry.]

sensigenous (sen·**sij**·en·us). Causing the start of sensory impulses; causing sensation. [sensation, Gk *genein* to produce.]

sensimeter (sen·**sim**·et·er). An instrument for estimating the sensitiveness of the skin to a tactile stimulus. [sensitive, meter.]

sensitive (**sen**·sit·iv). 1. In a general sense, able to feel a sensation; responsive to or transmitting a stimulus. In a particular sense, capable of responding to a specified kind or degree of stimulus. 2. In chemistry, exhibiting a characteristic reaction in minute amounts or extreme dilution, e.g. a delicate test. 3. Responsive to minute changes in physical forces, e.g. a galvanometer. 4. In psychical research, a term applied to a medium; one able to manifest psychical phenomena; susceptible to extra-sensory stimuli. 5. Over-reactive to a psychological stimulus. 6. Of micro-organisms, readily inhibited by low concentrations of antibacterial substances. [L *sentire* to feel.]

sensitivity (sen·sit·**iv**·it·e). 1. The quality of being sensitive. 2. The extent to which a method gives results that are free from false negatives; the fewer the false negatives, the greater is the sensitivity (*see also* SPECIFICITY). **Antibiotic sensitivity.** The concentration of an antibiotic which will just suppress the growth of a standard inoculum of an organism. Of micro-organisms, the sensitivity with respect to a given drug is expressed numerically as the lowest concentration of drug which suppresses its growth in standard conditions.

sensitization (**sen**·sit·i·**za'**·shun). 1. A condition in which the response to second and later stimuli is greater than that to the original stimulus. 2. The process of rendering cells sensitive to lysis by complement, by pretreating them with the specific antibody. 3. The immune process by which individuals become hypersensitive to such substances as pollen, dandruff, etc. **Active sensitization.** Sensitization resulting when a dose of a particular antigen is injected into a susceptible person. **Auto-erythrocyte sensitization.** Allergic sensitivity to red blood cells in the tissues resulting in the painful-bruising syndrome. **Cross sensitization.** Sensitization to a primary allergen spreading to one or more secondary allergens which are of such closely similar chemical constitution to the primary allergen that the sensitized cells are unable to distinguish between them. This must be differentiated from *false cross sensitization* which occurs when the same chemical substance is present in different products. **Passive sensitization.** The sensitization which can be induced temporarily in a normal person by injecting serum from a sensitized person or animal. **Protein sensitization.** The state of hypersusceptibility or allergy which follows the introduction of a foreign protein into the body parenterally. After a period of 10 days the introduction of another dose of the same protein will produce certain symptoms of varying severity. The condition is the basis of serum sickness, some cases of asthma, hay fever, urticaria and other allergic diseases. **Rh sensitization.** The production of sensitization to the Rh factor as may arise after giving Rh-positive blood to an Rh-negative person, or from the presence of an Rh-positive fetus in an Rh-negative woman. **Skin sensitization.** The establishment of hypersensitivity of the skin to a chemical agent due to exposure to it, so that even minute amounts may provoke severe reactions. [L *sentire* to feel.]

sensitize (**sen**·sit·ize). To make sensitive.

sensitizer (**sen**·sit·i·zer). 1. In dermatology, a secondary irritant that makes a susceptible subject sensitive to the same, and in some cases to other, irritants. 2. Amboceptor. 3. In radiotherapy, an agent which potentiates the radiation effect. [L *sentire* to feel.]

sensitizin (**sen**·sit·i·zin). Anaphylactogen. [see prec.]

sensitometer (sen·sit·**om**·et·er). An arrangement for testing the sensitivity of a photographic emulsion. [sensitivity, meter.]

sensomobile (sen·so·**mo**·bile). Having power to respond to any afferent stimulus by moving. [sensation, mobile.]

sensomobility (**sen**·so·mo·**bil**′·it·e). The power which is intrinsic to animals, including human beings, to respond to sensory stimuli by movement. [see prec.]

sensomotor (sen·so·**mo**·tor). Sensory and motor; generally referring to nerves.

sensoparalysis (**sen**·so·par·**al**′·is·is). Paralysis affecting the sensory nerves.

sensorial (sen·**sor**·e·al). Relating or belonging to a sensorium.

sensoriglandular (**sen**·sor·e·**glan**′·dew·lar). Relating or belonging to glandular secretion or excretion occurring as reaction to a stimulus applied to the sensory nerves.

sensorimetabolism (**sen**·sor·e·met·**ab**′·ol·izm). The metabolic activity set up in response to sensory nerve stimulation.

sensorimotor (**sen**·sor·e·**mo**′·tor). Sensory and motor.

sensorimuscular (**sen**·sor·e·**mus**′kew·lar). Relating to or indicating reflex action in a muscle, produced as a result of sensory stimulus.

sensorium (sen·**sor**·e·sum). 1. Any sensory nerve centre. 2. The sensory nerve apparatus of the body as a whole, the centre or seat of sensation. **Sensorium commune.** A portion of the cerebral cortex which receives and controls the stimuli conveyed to the nerve centres. [L *sentire* to feel.]

sensorivascular, sensorivasomotor (**sen**·sor·e·**vas**′·kew·lar, **sen**·-sor·e·va·zo·**mo**′·tor). Indicating that changes in the blood vessels (contraction or dilatation) take place as the result of stimulation of the sensory nerves. [L *sentire* to feel, *vasculum* small vessel, *vas* vessel, motor.]

sensorivolitional (**sen**·sor·e·vo·**lish**′·un·al). Relating or belonging to sensation and volition.

sensory (**sen**·sor·e). 1. Belonging to sensation. 2. Instrumental in promoting sensation. 3. Relating to a sensorium.

sensualism (**sen**·sew·al·izm). The state of being dominated by, or of having poor control of, bodily passions or appetites. [L *sensualis* sensual.]

sentence (**sen**·tens). A number of words arranged grammatically and syntactically so as to constitute a grammatically complete sense-unit. A sequence of words or symbols which expresses a proposition, or which can be used to convey an assertion. A minimum complete utterance. [F.]

sentient (**sen**·she·ent). 1. Having the power to sense and to perceive. 2. Sensitive; possessing feeling. [L *sentire* to feel.]

sentiment (**sen**·tim·ent). An emotional feeling towards a person or object. [see prec.]

sepal (**sep**·al). One of the modified leaves forming the outer whorl, or calyx, of a flower. [L *separ* separate, petal.]

sepaloid (**sep**·al·oid). Having resemblance to a sepal. [sepal, Gk *eidos* form.]

separation (sep·ar·a·shun). In dentistry, the spacing of adjacent teeth. [see foll.]

separator (**sep**·ar·a·tor). An instrument used to force adjoining teeth apart. [L *separare* to lay aside.]

See also: HARRIS (M. LA S.), LUYS (G.).

Sepia (**se**·pe·ah). A genus of cephalopod Mollusca, cuttle-fish. *Sepia officinalis* is the commonest species in the North Atlantic; medicinal sepia is a product of the ink gland of this species. [Gk squid.]

sepium (**se**·pe·um). The internal shell (bone) of the cuttlefish *Sepia officinalis.* It is used in tooth powders as an abrasive.

sepsin, sepsine (**sep**·sin, **sep**·seen). A ptomaine formed in putrefying animal matter and decomposing yeast. [see foll.]

sepsis (**sep**·sis). 1. A term originally used to denote a putrefactive process in the body but now usually referring to infection with pyogenic micro-organisms. 2. A genus of Diptera. The larvae, which are normally saprophagous, have caused accidental intestinal myiasis. **Sepsis agranulocytica.** Agranulocytosis with necrotic ulceration in the mouth and alimentary canal. **Focal sepsis.** A local focus of infection giving rise to a toxaemia which manifests itself in general symptoms such as anaemia, fibrositis, arthritis, fever, etc. Common sites are the tonsils, teeth, nasal sinuses, gall bladder and the urinary tracts. **Gas sepsis.** Gas gangrene. *See* GANGRENE. **Sepsis intestinalis.** Food poisoning. **Sepsis lenta.** Infection with *Streptococcus viridans* resulting in subacute endocarditis. **Oral sepsis.** Excessive bacterial activity in the mouth, associated with such conditions as gingivitis, pyorrhoea alveolaris, dental abscesses, etc. **Puerperal sepsis.** Infection of the uterus after childbirth with organisms of which haemolytic streptococci are the most important. [Gk putrefaction.]

sepsometer (sep·**som**·et·er). An apparatus for measuring the number of micro-organisms in the air. [Gk *sepsis* putrefaction, meter.]

septa (**sep**·tah). *See* SEPTUM.

septaemia (sep·te·me·ah). Septicaemia.

septal (**sep**·tal). Relating or belonging to a septum.

septanose (**sep**·tan·oze). Heptose. [L *septem* seven.]

septate (**sep**·tate). Provided with a septum or partition; divided by partitions into compartments.

septation (sep·ta·shun). 1. Division into compartments by a septum; the state of being septate. 2. A septum.

septatome (**sep**·tat·ome). Septotome.

septavalent (sep·tah·va·lent). Septivalent. [L *septem* seven, *valens* powerful.]

septectomy (sep·tek·to·me). Resection of the nasal septum. **Atrial septectomy.** The surgical creation of an atrial septal defect, performed for the palliation of transposition of the great vessels; the Blalock-Hanlon operation. [septum, Gk *ektome* a cutting out.]

septic (**sep**·tik). 1. Pertaining to putrefaction. 2. Caused by or in a state of sepsis.

septicaemia (sep·te·**se**·me·ah). The severe type of infection in which the blood stream is invaded by large numbers of the causal bacteria which multiply in it and spread. It should be distinguished from bacteraemia in which organisms appear in the blood without the severe rapid generalization of infection characteristic of septicaemia. **Bronchopulmonary septicaemia.** Septicaemia following the aspiration of infected material into the lungs. **Cryptogenic septicaemia.** Septicaemia in which the original focus of infection is not discovered. **Melitensis septicaemia.** Undulant fever. *See* FEVER. **Metastasizing septicaemia.** Septicopyaemia. **Phlebitic septicaemia.** Pyaemia. **Plague septicaemia.** The septicaemic form of bubonic plague. **Puerperal septicaemia.** Septicaemia arising in the puerperium from septic infection of the uterus. **Typhoid septicaemia.** Septicaemia in typhoid fever. [Gk *septikos* putrid, *haima* blood.]

See also: BRUCE (D.).

septicaemic (sep·te·**se**·mik). Relating or belonging to, characterized by, or suffering from septicaemia.

septicine (**sep**·te·seen). A ptomaine obtained from putrid flesh. [Gk *septikos* putrid.]

septicophlebitis (**sep**·tik·o·fleb·**i**′·tis). Septic phlebitis, the result of a septicaemic condition.

septicopyaemia (**sep**·tik·o·pi·**e**′·me·ah). Septicaemia in which multiple abscesses have formed. **Cryptogenic septicopyaemia.** A form in which the original focus of infection is not obvious, or is so slight as to have been disregarded. **Metastatic septicopyaemia.** A condition in which abscesses form in the lungs, caused by embolism from septic thrombi. **Primary septicopyaemia.** One in which septicaemic symptoms have predominated from the beginning, the primary focus being trifling or hidden. **Secondary septicopyaemia.** Septicaemia secondary to a pre-existing septic lesion. **Spontaneous septicopyaemia.** Cryptogenic or primary septicopyaemia (see above). [septicaemia, pyaemia.]

septicopyaemic (sep·tik·o·pi·e'·mik). Relating or belonging to septicopyaemia.

septiferous (sep·**tif**·er·us). Spreading sepsis. [sepsis, L *ferre* to carry.]

septigravida (sep·te·**grav**·id·ah). A woman in her seventh pregnancy. [L *septem* seven, *gravida* pregnant.]

septile (**sep**·tile). Relating or belonging to a septum; septal.

septipara (sep·**tip**·ar·ah). A woman who has given birth to 7 children. [L *septem* seven, *parere* to produce.]

septivalent (sep·te·**va**·lent). Possessing a valency of 7. [L *septem* seven, valency.]

septomarginal (sep·to·**mar**·jin·al). Relating or belonging to the margin of a septum. **Septomarginal tract.** *See* TRACT.

septometer (sep·**tom**·et·er). 1. An instrument for measuring the width of the nasal septum. 2. A sepsometer.

septonasal (sep·to·**na**·zal). Relating or belonging to the nasal septum.

septostomy (sep·**tos**·to·me). The surgical procedure of creating a hole in a septum. **Atrial (balloon) septostomy.** The procedure of creating a hole in the atrial septum for the palliation of transposition of the great vessels; the Rashkind procedure. [L *saeptum* fence, Gk *stoma* mouth.]

septotome (**sep**·to·tome). A particular instrument with which the nasal septum may be incised or a part of it removed. [septum, Gk *temnein* to cut.]

septotomy (sep·**tot**·o·me). Incision of the nasal septum or of any other septum. [see prec.]

septulum [NA] (**sep**·tew·lum). A small septum.

septum [NA] (**sep**·tum) (pl. *septa*). A thin partition within or between anatomical structures or organs. **Alveolar septum.** The thin bone which separates the socket (alveolus) of one tooth from another. **Aortopulmonary septum.** The septum which develops in the truncus arteriosus of the embryo and divides it into the ascending aorta and the pulmonary trunk. **Atrial septum [septum interatriale (NA)].** The partition between the right and left atria of the heart. **Atrial septum, membranous part.** The lower and anterior portion of the atrial septum, formed from the septum primum. **Atrioventricular septum [septum atrioventriculare (NA)].** The part of the ventricular septum (see below) which separates the aortic vestibule from the right atrium. **Bulbar septum.** The septum which divides the bulbus cordis of the embryo into 2 parts which become the infundibulum of the right ventricle and the aortic vestibule of the left ventricle respectively. **Cloacal septum.** Urorectal septum (see below). **Septum of the corpora cavernosi of the clitoris [septum corporum cavernosorum (NA)].** The incomplete septum of the fibrous tissue between the 2 corpora cavernosa. **Crural septum.** Femoral septum (see below). **Enamel septum.** A septum in the pulp of the enamel organ of the developing tooth, dividing it into medial and lateral parts. **Femoral septum [septum femorale (NA)].** Connective tissue which closes the femoral ring. **Septum of the frontal sinuses [septum sinuum frontalium (NA)].** A bony septum separating the 2 frontal sinuses. It is often deflected to one side of the midline. **Gingival septum.** Gum septum (see below). **Septum of the glans [septum glandis (NA)].** A septum in the glans penis from the tunica albuginea to the urethra. **Gum septum.** The part of the gum between 2 adjacent teeth. **Hanging septum.** Undue thickening of the medial crura of the greater alar cartilages of the nose, giving a dependent appearance to the quadrilateral cartilage of the septum lying between them. **Septum inferius (of His).** The embryonic ventricular septum. **Interalveolar septum [septum interalveolare (NA)].** The bony plate between 2 adjacent tooth sockets. **Interauricular septum.** Atrial septum (see above). **Septum intermedium (of His).** The septum formed in the embryonic heart by the fusion of the endocardial cushions in the atrioventricular orifice. **Intermuscular septum.** Connective tissue which separates adjacent muscles or groups of muscles. **Interradicular septum [septum inter-radiculare (NA)].** That part of the alveolar bone of either the mandible or the maxilla which lies between the roots of teeth. **Intersegmental septum.** The mesenchymal partition between adjacent somites. **Interventricular septum.** Ventricular septum (see below). **Septum of the leg, anterior intermuscular [septum intermusculare anterius (cruris) NA].** The fascial septum between the extensor and peroneus groups of muscles in the calf. **Septum of the leg, posterior intermuscular [septum intermusculare posterius (cruris) NA].** The fascial septum between the peroneal and flexor groups of muscles in the calf. **Septa of the lens.** Partitions of amorphous material which separate the ends of the lens fibres and cause the appearance of sutural lines on the anterior and posterior surfaces of the lens. **Lingual septum.** Septum of the tongue (see below). **Septum lucidum [septum pellucidum (NA)].** A median partition, consisting of 2 lamellae, which separates the right from the left lateral ventricle; it is bounded by the anterior part of the corpus callosum and by the fornix. It gives tributaries [venae septi pellucidi] to the internal cerebral vein. **Mediastinal septum.** The mediastinum; the complex of tissues and organs between the vertebral column and the sternum which separates the 2 pleural cavities. **Septum of the nose [septum nasi (NA)].** The median partition in the nasal cavity made up of the vomer, the perpendicular plate of the ethmoid bone (together forming the osseous nasal septum [septum nasi osseum (NA)]) and the cartilage of the septum. **Septum of the nose, bony part [pars ossea (NA)].** The posterior part of the nasal septum, made up of the perpendicular plate of the ethmoid bone, the vomer and the nasal crests of the maxilla and the palatine bone. **Septum of the nose, cartilaginous part [pars cartilaginea (NA)].** Septal cartilage. *See* CARTILAGE. **Septum of the nose, membranous part [pars membranacea (NA)].** The lower anterior part of the nasal septum into which the septal processes of the lower nasal cartilages project. **Septum of the nose, movable part [pars mobilis septi nasi (NA)].** The anterior and inferior part of the nasal septum between the nostrils; it is formed by skin and septal processes of the lower nasal cartilages. **Orbital septum [septum orbitale (NA)].** A thin sheet of connective tissue attached to the periosteum at the supra-orbital margin and blending with the aponeurosis of the levator palpebrae superioris muscle in the upper eyelid and with the tarsal plate in the lower. **Pectiniform septum.** The septum of the penis (see following) or of the corpora cavernosa of the clitoris (see above). **Septum of the penis [septum penis (NA)].** The fibrous partition between the corpora cavernosa, deficient distally. **Pharyngeal septum.** The buccopharyngeal membrane of the embryo. **Posterior intermediate septum.** The septum, present only in the cervical part of the spinal cord [septum cervicale intermedium (NA)], which separates the fasciculus gracilis from the fasciculus cuneatus. **Posterior median septum.** The median partition in the spinal cord which separates the posterior columns. **Septum primum.** The first atrial septum to appear in the embryonic heart. **Rectovaginal septum [septum rectovaginale (NA)].** Loose areolar tissue between the vagina and the ampulla of the rectum. **Rectovesical septum [septum rectovesicale (NA)].** A layer of fascia between the ampulla of the rectum and the base of the bladder and prostate; it is formed from the lower part of the urorectal septum (see below). **Septum of the scrotum [septum scroti (NA)].** A median fibromuscular partition which divides the scrotal pouch into 2 cavities for the testes. **Septum secundum.** The second atrial septum to appear in the embryonic heart; it is formed on the right side of the septum primum and overlaps the ostium secundum. **Septum of the sphenoidal sinuses [septum sinuum sphenoidalium (NA).** The bony partition, usually asymmetrical and often incomplete, which separates the 2 parts of the sphenoidal sinus. **Spiral septum.** Aortopulmonary septum (see above). **Septum spurium.** A fold, formed by the fusion of the cranial ends of the venous valves in the embryo, which projects into the atrial cavity. **Subarachnoid septum.** A thin, incomplete fibrous partition in the medial plane of the subarachnoid space, posterior to the spinal cord. **Septa of the testis [septula testis (NA)].** Any of the septa which pass from the mediastinum testis to divide the organ into lobes. **Septum of the thigh, lateral intermuscular [septum intermusculare femoris laterale (NA)], Septum of the thigh, medial intermuscular [septum intermusculare femoris mediale (NA)].** Extensions from the fascia lata to the linea aspera; they separate the vasti muscles from the adductors of the thigh medially and the flexors and gluteus muscles laterally. **Septum of the tongue [septum linguae (NA)].** A medial fibrous partition which separates the 2 halves of the tongue and gives attachment to some of the intrinsic muscles. **Septum transversum.** Mesoderm found in the embryo, caudal to the pericardium; it forms the central tendon of the diaphragm and the connective tissue of the liver. **Septum of the upper arm, lateral intermuscular [septum intermusculare brachii laterale (NA)], Septum of the upper arm, medial intermuscular [septum intermusculare brachii mediale (NA)].** Fascial septa at each side of the arm between the flexor and extensor groups of muscles. **Urorectal septum.** A peritoneal pouch which grows caudally to divide the embryonic cloaca into the urogenital sinus anteriorly and the rectum behind. Its upper part persists as the rectovesical or recto-uterine pouch; its lower part is obliterated and represented in the adult by fascia only. **Ventricular septum [septum interventriculare (NA)].** The septum between the right and left ventricles of the heart. **Ventricular septum, membranous part [pars membranacea (NA)].** A small, oval area, composed of fibrous tissue covered with endothelium, in the upper part of the ventricular septum. **Ventricular septum, muscular part [pars muscularis (NA)].** The main muscular part of the ventricular septum, as opposed to the small membranous part. [L *saeptum* fence.]

See also: BIGELOW, CLOQUET (J. G.), DOUGLAS (J.), HIS (W. SNR.).

septuplet (sep·tew·plet). Any one of 7 born at one labour. [L *septuplum* group of seven.]

sequela (se·kwe·lah) (pl. *sequelae*). A disease or morbid condition resulting from or dependent upon another disease; generally used in the plural to indicate collectively the main complications arising from a certain disease. [L *sequi* to follow.]

sequenator (se·kwen·a·tor). An apparatus for the automated determination of the amino-acid sequence of a polypeptide chain. [L *sequi* to follow.]

sequence (se·kwens). The order of arrangement. **Amino-acid sequence.** The arrangement of amino-acid residues in a polypeptide chain between the amino and carboxyl ends. **Ancestral sequence.** A theoretical reconstructed sequence of a polypeptide or a polynucleotide thought to be the precursor, or ancestor, of other sequences. **Base sequence.** Nucleotide sequence (see below). **Nucleotide sequence.** The order of arrangement of nucleotide units in a polynucleotide chain from the 5′- to the 3′-end. [L *sequi* to follow.]

sequencer (se·kwen·ser). Sequenator. [L *sequi* to follow.]

sequential (se·kwen·shal). 1. Occurring in sequence. 2. Referring to sequelae. [see prec.]

sequester (se·kwes·ter). Sequestrum.

sequestral (se·kwes·tral). Relating or belonging to a sequestrum.

sequestration (se·kwes·tra·shun). 1. The development of a sequestrum. 2. A method of controlling or lessening haemorrhage in operations on the trunk or head by the tying of bands around the arms or thighs and so cutting off some portion of the blood from the general circulation. 3. In a case of infectious disease, isolation. **Pulmonary sequestration.** A non-functioning piece of lung provided with systemic circulation; possibly ectopic, e.g. below the diaphragm. [L *sequestrare* to lay aside.]

sequestrectomy (se·kwes·trek·to·me). Removal of necrosed bone by surgical means. [sequestrum, Gk *ektome* a cutting out.]

sequestrotomy (se·kwes·trot·o·me). To cut into a sequestrum and usually to remove the necrotic tissue. [sequestrum, Gk *temnein* to cut.]

sequestrum (se·kwes·trum). A portion of dead bone which has become detached from the healthy bone tissue, as occurs in necrosis. **Dental sequestrum.** A sequestrum arising from the jaws. **Primary sequestrum.** A sequestrum which is completely detached. **Secondary sequestrum.** One that is not entirely detached and can be retained. **Tertiary sequestrum.** A sequestrum which on account of slight damage is not displaced. [L deposit.]

Seractide (ser·ak·tide). BP Commission approved name for Ala^{26}-Gly^{27}-Ser^{31}-α^{1-39}-corticotrophin; a corticotrophic peptide.

seralbumin (seer·al·bew·min). Serum albumin.

serangitis (seer·an·ji·tis). Inflammation of the corpus cavernosum of the penis or corpus cavernosum of the clitoris. [Gk *seragx* hollow rock, *-itis* inflammation.]

seretin (ser·et·in). Carbon tetrachloride.

Sergent, Emile (b. 1869). Paris physician.

Sergent's line. Adrenal line; a white line which appears if the skin, e.g. of the abdomen, is lightly stroked with the fingernail. It appears after a short latent period, and after a minute or two gradually fades.

Bernard-Sergent syndrome. A term not in general use that has been employed to describe the abdominal symptoms of Addison's disease.

Sergentomyia (ser·jen·to·mi′·e·ah). A sub-genus of *Phlebotomus*. (= *Newsteadia*).

serialography (seer·e·al·og′·raf·e). Serial radiography. *See* RADIOGRAPHY. [series, radiograph.]

sericeps (ser·e·seps). An apparatus made of silk, used to apply traction to the fetal head. [L *sericum* silk, *caput* head.]

sericite (ser·is·ite). A silica compound that causes silicosis.

sericum (ser·ik·um). Silk; the prepared fibre obtained from the cocoons of the silkworm (*Bombyx* and *Antheroea* species). Silk thread is used as a surgical suture; waterproofed silk fabric, oiled silk, is a protective surgical dressing. [L.]

series (seer·eez). 1. Objects, numbers or quantities, arranged in such a way that some relationship is displayed. 2. In electricity, the connection of resistances or cells successively so that the total resistance or electromotive force is the sum of those possessed by the components. **Acetylene series.** A series of unsaturated hydrocarbons of which acetylene is the first member. They have the general formula C_nH_{2n-2}, and are characterized by a triple bond. **Actinide series.** The second rare-earth series of chemical elements beginning with actinium. **Actino-uranium series.** The natural radioactive series commencing with actino-uranium, U^{235}, which includes the eponymous member actinium Ac^{227}, and ends with stable lead Pb^{207}. The atomic mass numbers of members of this series are of the form $(4n + 3)$. **Aliphatic series.** In chemistry, any series of compounds with an open chain of carbon atoms. **Aromatic series.** Any series of organic compounds containing the benzene ring. **Closed-chain series.** Any series of organic compounds the members of which have molecules consisting of carbon atoms linked in a closed chain. **Contact series.** The arrangement of metals in a series such that contact between any particular metal and one below it in the series produces a positive potential difference. **Electrochemical series, Electromotive series.** A series of chemical elements arranged in the order of the potentials set up between the element and a solution of its ions. Beginning with the electropositive caesium and ending with the electronegative fluorine, the series gives the electromotive force obtainable from a cell composed of any 2 elements and their ions. The series also indicates which elements will displace others further down in the series from a solution of its ions. **Fatty series.** Any aliphatic series (see above), especially the series of hydrocarbons homologous with methane. **Homologous series.** In chemistry, a series of organic compounds which proceed from one member to the next by some constant grouping, usually CH_2. **Lyotropic series.** The arrangement of ions in a series indicating the diminishing magnitude of their effect when introduced into colloidal systems, e.g. in the salting-out of proteins. **Natural radioactive series.** A series of elements which are radioactive and are formed by a chain of disintegrations from a long-lived parent body. The occurrence "naturally" implies that the half-life of the parent is long on a geological scale, e.g. uranium, 4.4×10^9 years. **Neptunium series.** The radioactive series commencing with neptunium, Np^{237}, and ending with stable bismuth, Bi^{209}. The atomic mass numbers of this series are of the form $(4n + 1)$. **Open-chain series.** Any series of organic compounds the members of which have molecules of carbon atoms arranged in an open chain. **Radioactive series.** A radioactive atom on disintegration does not necessarily attain at once stability within its nucleus; one or more disintegrations may be necessary. The chain of elements from the starting point to the final stable product form a radioactive series. **Thorium series.** The natural radioactive series commencing with thorium, Th^{232}, and ending with stable lead, Pb^{208}. The atomic mass numbers of the members of this series are of the form $(4n + 1)$. [L a succession.]

seriflux (seer·e·flux). 1. Profuse watery or serous discharge. 2. A disease marked by a watery or serous discharge. [serum, flux.]

serine (ser·een). $CH_2(OH)CH(NH_2)COOH$, an amino acid occurring in protein hydrolysates.

serioscopy (seer·e·os·ko·pe). The x-ray visualization of a body in a series of parallel planes by means of multiple exposures taken in different directions. They are laid one on top of the other and moved until the projections of the various planes of the body coincide consecutively. [series, Gk *skopein* to view.]

seriscission (ser·e·sizh·un). A method of division of certain soft tissues by application of a silk ligature. [L *sericum* silk, *scindere* to cut.]

sero-anaphylaxis (seer·o·an·ah·fil·ax'·is). Anaphylaxis set up after the injection of blood serum.

seroche (ser·o·ke). Anoxia. [Sp.]

serochrome (seer·o·krome). The pigment of normal serum. [serum, Gk *chroma* colour.]

serocolitis (seer·o·kol·i'·tis). An inflammatory condition of the peritoneal covering (serous coat) of the colon. [serous coat, colitis.]

seroculture (seer·o·kul·tcher). A growth of bacteria on blood serum. [serum, culture.]

serocystic (seer·o·sist·ik). Comprised of serous cysts.

serodiagnosis (seer·o·di·ag·no'·sis). The use of serological reactions, e.g. precipitation, agglutination or complement fixation, in the diagnosis of disease.

sero-enteritis (seer·o·en·ter·i'·tis). Inflammation of the serous coat of the small intestine. [serum, enteritis.]

sero-enzyme (seer·o·en·zime). An enzyme present in the blood serum.

serofibrinous (seer·o·fi·brin·us). Consisting of serum and fibrin, generally used in referring to an exudate.

serofibrous (seer·o·fi·brus). Referring to serous and fibrous tissues.

seroglycoid (seer·o·gli·koid). A non-crystallizable mucoid which has been isolated from serum. [serum, Gk *glykys* sweet, *eidos* form.]

serohaemorrhagic (seer·o·hem·or·ah'·jik). Marked by the presence of serum and blood. [serum, haemorrhage.]

serohepatitis (seer·o·hep·at·i'·tis). Inflammation of the peritoneal investment of the liver. [serum, hepatitis.]

sero-immunity (seer·o·im·ewn'·it·e). Immunity conferred by administration of antiserum; passive immunity.

serolactescent (seer·o·lak·tes'·ent). Having the characters of both serum and milk. [serum, L *lac* milk.]

serolipase (seer·o·lip·aze). Lipase derived from blood serum.

serologist (seer·ol·o·jist). One who specializes in the science of serology.

serology (seer·ol·o·je). A branch of medical science which is concerned with the study of blood sera, identifying group-specific substances, protein and enzyme pattern. The application of serological methods in the study of other groupable tissues and fluids by antigen/antibody test, and of transfusion and injection antibody reactions by similar techniques. [serum, Gk *logos* science.]

serolysin (seer·ol·is·in). A lysin to be found in the blood serum.

seromembranous (seer·o·mem·bran·us). 1. Relating to or consisting of serous membrane. 2. Serous and membranous.

seromucoid (seer·o·mew·koid). A glycoprotein occurring to the extent of 0.1 per cent in blood plasma. It is precipitated by acetic acid. [serum, mucoid.]

seromucous (seer·o·mew·kus). Consisting of or containing both serum and mucus.

seromuscular (seer·o·mus·kew·lar). Referring or belonging to the serous and muscular coats of the intestine.

seronegative (seer·o·neg·at·iv). Giving a negative reaction to serological tests.

seroperitoneum (seer·o·per·it·o·ne'·um). 1. A membrane covering the lower visceral organs. 2. Ascites. [serum, peritoneum.]

serophysiology (seer·o·fiz·e·ol'·o·je). The study of serum in so far as it affects or is affected by the bodily activities. [serum, physiology.]

serophyte (seer·o·fite). A bacterium which thrives in the normal body fluids. [serum, Gk *phyton* plant.]

seroplastic (seer·o·plas·tik). Serofibrinous. [serum, plastic.]

seropneumothorax (seer·o·new·mo·thor'·ax). The condition in which serous fluid and air or gas has collected in the cavity of the pleura. [serum, pneumothorax.]

seropositive (seer·o·poz·it·iv). Giving a positive reaction to serological tests.

seroprophylaxis (seer·o·pro·fil·ax'·is). The injection of convalescent or immune serum as a prophylactic measure.

seropurulent (seer·o·pewr·ew·lent). Relating to or composed of serum and pus.

seropus (seer·o·pus). An exudate containing serum and pus.

seroreaction (seer·o·re·ak'·shun). A reaction in which serum is involved.

serorelapse (seer·o·re·laps'). A return to a positive serum reaction, after a period when it was negative or reduced in titre as a result of treatment.

seroresistance (seer·o·re·zis'·tans). The failure of a serum reaction to become negative or to be reduced in titre after treatment. [serum, resistance.]

serosa (seer·o·sah). A serous membrane; mainly applied to peritoneal covering.

serosanguineous (seer·o·sang·gwin'·e·us). Relating to or containing serum and blood. [serum, L *sanguis* blood.]

seroscopy (seer·os·ko·pe). Inspection of serum with the agglutinoscope for diagnostic purposes. [serum, Gk *skopein* to watch.]

serose (seer·oze). An albumose derived from serum albumin.

seroserous (seer·o·seer·us). Relating to 2 serous surfaces in apposition, as with sutures.

serositis (seer·o·si·tis). Inflammation affecting a serous membrane or coat. **Multiple serositis.** Polyorrhomenitis. [serous membrane, Gk *-itis* inflammation.]

serosity (seer·os·it·e). 1. The state or quality of being serous. 2. The serous quality of a fluid.

serosynovial (seer·o·si·no'·ve·al). Both serous and synovial.

serosynovitis (seer·o·si·no·vi'·tis). Synovitis associated with a serous effusion.

serotherapeutical (seer·o·ther·ap·ew'·tik·al). Relating or belonging to serum therapy.

serotherapist (seer·o·ther·ap·ist). One who practises serotherapy.

serotherapy (seer·o·ther·ap·e). The treatment of disease by injecting blood serum from immune individuals and immunized animals. [serum, Gk *therapeia* treatment.]

serothorax (seer·o·thor·ax). Hydrothorax. [serum, thorax.]

serotina (ser·o·ti·nah). The decidua basalis. [L late.]

serotonin (seer·o·to·nin). 5-Hydroxytryptamine (or 5 HT), found in high concentration in blood platelets and in the enterochromaffin cells of the gastro-intestinal tract. It is found in carcinoid tumours and in the central nervous system, especially in the hypothalamus. A breakdown product, 5-hydroxyindolacetic acid, is excreted in the urine. [serum, Gk *tonos* tone.]

serotoxin (seer·o·**tox**·in). 1. The substance postulated to explain the toxicity of homologous serum after treatment with substances such as kaolin and barium sulphate. 2. A synonym for *anaphylatoxin,* a hypothetical substance believed by some to be responsible for the symptoms of anaphylactic shock. [serum, toxin.]

serotype (**seer**·o·tipe). Serological type. *See* TYPE.

serous (**seer**·us). 1. Relating or belonging to serum. 2. Like serum, thin or watery. 3. Secreting or containing serum.

serovaccination (seer·o·vak·sin·**a**′·shun). A combination of serum therapy to produce immediate *passive* immunity, and of vaccination with a bacterial vaccine (or other prophylactic) to give more lasting *active* protection; combined active and passive immunization.

serozyme (**seer**·o·zime). The prothrombin in the blood plasma as described by Bordet; it is derived from the inactive form, proserozyme, in the presence of calcium, and then reacts with cytozyme to form thrombin. [serum, enzyme.]

serpens (**ser**·pens). Creeping; serpentine. [L.]

Serpentaria BPC 1949 (ser·pen·**ta**·re·ah). The dried rhizome and roots of *Aristolochia reticulata* Nutt. and of *A. serpentaria* Linn. (family Aristolochiaceae). It contains a volatile oil, tannin, and a bitter principle; it is used as a bitter tonic. [L *serpens* snake, from its use formerly in snakebite.]

serpentary (**ser**·pen·tar·e). Serpentaria.

serpentine (**ser**·pen·tine). Tortuous; sinuous; creeping. [L *serpere* to creep.]

serpiginous (ser·**pij**·en·us). Creeping from one part or surface to another. [see foll.]

serpigo (ser·**pi**·go). 1. Ringworm. 2. Herpes. 3. Any creeping eruption. [L *serpere* to creep.]

serpolet (**ser**·po·let). Wild thyme, *Thymus serpyllum,* and the camphoraceous oil produced therefrom. [L *serpyllum* thyme.]

Serpulia lacrimans (ser·**pew**·le·ah **lak**·rim·anz). A fungus which causes dry-rot of timber in buildings; the spores are reported to have caused severe bronchitis, by inhalation, and chronic gastro-intestinal disease by contaminating drinking water and food. [L *serpula* small serpent, *lacrimare* to weep.]

serrate, serrated (**ser**·ate, ser·**a**·ted). 1. Having notches or teeth on the edge as a saw has. 2. In botany, with marginal teeth pointing towards the apex. **Serrate suture.** *See* SUTURE. [L *serra* saw.]

Serratia (ser·**a**·she·ah). A genus of biochemically active organisms of the family Enterobacteriaceae; recognized in the USA but not generally in the UK where most species are placed in the genus *Chromobacterium.* They are small, Gram-negative, motile, aerobic rods which produce characteristic red pigments and are saprophytic on decaying plant and animal materials. **Serratia marcescens.** *Chromobacterium prodigiosum;* a species found on polenta and bread and producing a red pigment. **Serratia piscatoria.** A species which causes abscesses containing red pus on the hands of fishermen and sardine canners, when associated with an aerobe. By itself the organism is not pathogenic. [L *serra* saw.]

serration (ser·**a**·shun). 1. The condition of being serrated or toothed like a saw. 2. A formation like the toothed edge of a saw. 3. One of the tooth-like units in a serrate or toothed structure. [see prec.]

serratus (ser·**a**·tus). Serrated, like a saw; hence applied to muscles which arise or are inserted by a number of saw-toothed processes.

serratus anterior muscle [musculus serratus anterior (NA)]. A muscle with a serrated anterior border formed of digitations attached to the outer aspects of the upper 8 ribs and attached posteriorly along the vertebral border of the scapula.

serratus anterior muscle, nerve to the [nervus thoracicus longus (NA)]. A long nerve deriving its fibres from the 5th, 6th and 7th cranial nerves (roots of the brachial plexus) and supplying the serratus anterior muscle; the long respiratory nerve of Bell.

serratus posterior inferior muscle [musculus serratus posterior inferior (NA)]. A muscle arising from the lower 2 thoracic and upper lumbar vertebrae and inserted by digitations into the outer surfaces of the lower 4 ribs.

serratus posterior superior muscle [musculus serratus posterior superior (NA)]. A muscle which arises from the ligamentum nuchae and the 7th cervical and upper thoracic vertebral spines; it is inserted by digitations into the outer surfaces of the 2nd to the 5th ribs. [L *serra* saw.]

serrefine (sar·**feen**). A small spring-type of artery forceps. [Fr.]

serrenoeud (sar·**nerd**). An instrument for tightening knots, particularly those applied to bleeding vessels in a deep cavity and inaccessible to the fingers. [Fr.]

Serres, Antoine Etienne Renaud Augustin (b. 1786). Paris anatomist and philosopher.

Serres' glands. Aggregations of epithelial cells in the gingival mucosa of infants.

serrulate, serrulated (**ser**·ew·late, **ser**·ew·la·ted). Finely serrated or notched. [L *serrula* little saw.]

Sertoli, Enrico (b. 1842). Milan physiologist.

Sertoli's cell. One of the supporting cells of the seminiferous tubules, lying between clumps of germinal cells and having a number of spermatids partially buried in its cytoplasm.

column of Sertoli. The sustentacular or Sertoli cells in the wall of a seminiferous tubule.

Sertoli-cell tumour. A rare tumour in man; it causes feminism.

Sertoli–Leydig tumour. An ovarian tumour which usually causes masculinization and has varied histological structure.

serum (**seer**·um). 1. The yellowish fluid that remains after whole blood or plasma has been allowed to clot. It is free from cells and it will not clot again. 2. Immune serum (see below). 3. Loosely (and wrongly) used for all forms of injectable substances, especially vaccines. **ACS serum.** Anticytotoxic serum (see below). **Serum albumin.** The major protein of serum, normally present in a concentration of from 4 to 5 g per 100 ml. It has a molecular weight of 68 000 and is a typical albumin. **Antibotulinus serum.** Botulinum antitoxin. *See* ANTITOXIN. **Anticobra serum.** Antivenene prepared by the injection of cobra venom. **Anticomplementary serum.** A serum which interferes with complement-fixation tests by inactivating complement in a non-specific fashion. **Anticytotoxic serum.** A serum obtained from horses, after inoculation with extracts of human spleen or bone marrow, which is said to stimulate the reticulo-endothelial system when injected into man. It has a depressive effect on the system in large doses. **Antidiphtheritic serum.** Diphtheria antitoxin. *See* ANTITOXIN. **Antiglobulin serum.** An antibody prepared by injecting human globulin into rabbits or other animals used in the Coombs' test for detecting the presence of globulins on red cells. **Antilymphocytic serum.** Serum produced by injecting lymphocytes from one species into animals of another species. The lymphocyte-antibody is then used to create immunosuppression in the donor species to homografts. **Antimeningococcus serum.** A serum obtained from animals effective against strains of *Neisseria meningitidis.* It has largely been replaced by sulphonamides. **Antiplatelet serum.** Blood serum prepared, usually, by the injection of guinea-pig platelets into rabbits to produce platelet antibodies in the rabbit serum, which then has antiplatelet properties causing agglutination or lysis of platelets in the blood. **Antireticular cytotoxic serum.** Anticytotoxic serum (see above). **Anti-Rh serum.** Rh antiserum; a blood serum containing one or more of the specific Rh antibodies. **Antisnakebite serum.** A serum made by injecting the poison of venomous snakes into horses in increasing doses. The serum will protect against the bite of snakes of the genus from which it is made, e.g. that of North America against Crotalus, rattlesnakes, that of India against cobras and Russell's vipers. *See also* ANTIVENENE. **Antitetanus serum.** Horse-blood serum containing antibody to tetanus toxin. **Antivenomous serum.** Antivenene. **Artificial serum.** An aqueous solution of some of the salts found in normal blood, with acacia gum added to increase the viscosity. This solution is no longer in use. **Blister serum.** The serum of a blister; this has been used as a form of protein therapy. **Blood serum.** *See* MAIN DEF. 1 (above). **Convalescence serum, Convalescent serum, Convalescents' serum.** The serum from the blood of one or more patients convalescent from an acute infectious disease. It is used mainly as a prophylactic measure, by injection. **Cytotropic serum.** A serum which induces damage or death of cells because of an antibody-like component in it. **Despeciated serum.** A serum prepared from animal (ox or horse) blood that has been treated to remove its species specific protein so that it can be injected into human beings without producing anaphylaxis. **Dried Human Serum BP 1973.** A dried preparation of Liquid Human Serum BP 1958. **Serum equinum.** Horse-blood serum (see below). **Foreign serum.** Serum of a different species. **Serum globulin.** A collective term indicating the globulins of serum which are normally present to the extent of from 2 to 3 g per 100 ml. The globulins are separable into three main fractions termed α-, β- and γ-globulin, by electrophoresis, ultracentrifugation, or by fractional precipitation with salt solutions, e.g. at certain concentrations of sodium sulphate. **Haemolytic serum.** A serum containing haemolysins or haemolytic substances that destroy red cells, liberating haemoglobin; haemolytic sera are frequently present in haemolytic anaemias, but may be produced by the injection of foreign proteins, haemolysinogens or agglutinogens. **Heterologous serum.** Serum from the blood of an animal of another species; or an antiserum prepared by injecting a different, though allied, antigen from that against which it is being tested or used therapeutically. **Homologous serum.** Serum from the blood of an animal of the same species; or an antiserum prepared by injecting the identical antigen to that against which it is being tested or used therapeutically. **Horse serum.** Horse-blood serum (see following). **Horse-blood serum.** Either normal serum of the horse or an immunizing serum prepared from the blood of the horse. **Human measles immune serum.** The serum of blood from a healthy person who has had measles. Given to a child during the incubation period, it will modify the attack. **Human scarlet fever immune serum.** The serum of blood from a healthy person who has had scarlet fever. Given to a child during the incubation period, it will modify the attack. **Hyperimmune serum.** Immune serum (see following) in which some special measure has been adopted in making the antibody content particularly high. **Immune serum.** Any serum used in the treatment of a bacterial or virus disease, usually prepared in animals by extensive immunization with the causal organism or its products, e.g. anti-anthrax serum, antitetanus serum, etc., but also obtained from a human being or an animal that became naturally infected and has recovered from a particular infection, e.g. measles. **Serum lactis.** Whey. **Leucocytolytic serum.** Serum prepared from animal blood after intravenous injections of leucocytes, said to have the property of lysing leucocytes. **Leucocytotoxic serum.** Serum having leucocyte-destroying power. **Liquid Human Serum BP 1958.** The serum from human blood which has been allowed to clot in the absence of an anticoagulant. **Mercurialized serum.** Normal horse-blood serum to which mercuric chloride has been added. **Polyvalent serum.** A serum prepared as an antiserum to several types of the same bacterial species (e.g. pneumococci) in the hope that one of the antibodies produced will be specific for the organism causing the disease. **Pooled serum.** The mixed serum from several persons. **Prophylactic serum.** A serum containing specific antibody given to a subject to prevent the development of a particular disease. **Specific serum.** A serum containing antibodies to one type of organism only, sometimes to one antigen only. [L whey.]

See also: BARGEN, BEEBE, BEHRING, BULL, CADHAM, CALMETTE, CHANTEMESSE, COOPER (G.), DEGKWITZ, DICK, DOCHEZ, DOPTER, DUNBAR, FELIX, FELTON, FERRY, FLEXNER, FOSHAY, HAFFKINE, JOCHMANN, KITASATO, KOCH (R.), LECLAINCHE, LEYDEN, MARAGLIANO, MARMOREK, MENZER, MOSER, PANE, PETTIT, PRITCHETT, ROEMER, ROSENOW, ROUX (P. P. E.), SCLAVO, SOBERNHEIM, TAVEL, VALÉE, YERSIN.

serum-fast (seer·um·fahst). Describing bacterial organisms which cannot be destroyed by the action of serums. [serum, AS *faest.*]

serum-identical (seer·um·i·den'·tik·al). Having an identical action in regard to a particular immune serum.

serumal (seer·um·al). Relating or belonging to, or derived from serum.

sesame (ses·am·e). The seeds of *Sesamum indicum* Linn. (family Pedaliaceae). They contain about 50 per cent of an oil (sesame oil) related to olive oil, which is used in place of the latter in such preparations as liniments and ointments. [Gk *sesamon.*]

sesamoid (ses·am·oid). Having resemblance in shape or size to a sesame seed; nodular. [sesame, Gk *eidos* form.]

sesamoid bones [ossa sesamoidea (NA)]. Rounded nodules of bones embedded in certain tendons (e.g. of the hand or foot) and often related to and entering into the formation of joints.

sesamum (ses·am·um). Sesame. [L.]

Sesarma (se·sar·mah). A genus of fresh-water crabs of which some species act as intermediary hosts of *Paragonimus westermani.*

sesquibasic (ses·kwe·**ba**·sik). Describing any acid which has 3 hydrogen atoms replaceable by 2 atoms of a base. [L *sesqui-* one and a half, base.]

sesquibo (ses·kwe·bo). Term used in von Pirquet's index of nutritive intakes expressing a value 1½ times the nominal normal requirement based on the nutritive value of human milk. [L *sesqui-* one and a half, *bovinus* of an ox.]

sesquihora (ses·kwe·**hor**·ah). An hour and a half. [L.]

sesquioxide (ses·kwe·**ox**·ide). Any oxide in which 3 atoms of oxygen are combined with 2 atoms of another element, e.g. Fe_2O_3. [L *sesqui-* one and a half, oxide.]

sesquisalt (ses·kwe·sawlt). Any salt in which 3 radical groups from an acid are combined with 2 basic groups or atoms, e.g. $Al_2(SO_4)_3$. [L *sesqui-* one and a half, salt.]

sesquisulphate (ses·kwe·**sul**·fate). Any sulphate in which 3 SO_4 groups are combined with 2 basic groups or atoms, e.g. $Mn_2(SO_4)_3$. [L *sesqui-* one and a half, sulphate.]

sesquisulphide (ses·kwe·**sul**·fide). Any sulphide in which 3 atoms of sulphur are combined with 2 atoms of another element, e.g. Fe_2S_3. [L *sesqui-* one and a half, sulphide.]

sesquiterpene (ses·kwe·**ter**·peen). Any aromatic hydrocarbon of formula $C_{15}H_{24}$, so-called from its being composed of 1½ terpene molecules. [L *sesqui-* one and a half, terpene.]

sessile (ses·ile). 1. Attached directly by the base, denoting a tumour without peduncle or stalk. 2. In zoology, attached so that it is not possible to move about. [L *sessilis* sitting.]

set (set). 1. To reduce a fracture and apply appropriate dressings or splints. 2. To fix or be fixed securely in position. 3. To render hard or solid, or to become hard or solid. 4. In psychology, an attitude that makes a certain specified response likely. [AS *settan.*]

seta (se·tah). 1. A bristle. 2. A slender, rigid structure like a bristle. [L bristle.]

setaceous (se·ta·shus). 1. Bristly; provided with bristles or bristle-like appendages. 2. Having the character, or consisting of bristles. [see prec.]

Setchenov, Ivan Michailovich (b. 1829). Russian neurologist.

Setchenov's centre or nucleus. A number of centres in the spinal cord and medulla oblongata concerned with reflex inhibition of muscular and visceral activity.

setiferous, setigerous (se·tif·er·us, se·**tij**·er·us). Producing or having bristles. [L *seta* bristle, *ferre* to bear, *gerere* to have.]

seton (se·ton). 1. A thin strand of linen or silk drawn through a cutaneous wound in order to lay down the foundations of a drain. 2. The fistulous tract resulting from this procedure. [Fr.]

sevadilla (sev·ad·**il**·ah). Cevadilla.

Sever, James Warren (b. 1878). Boston surgeon.

Sever's disease. Osteochondritis of the epiphysis of the calcaneum.

seviparous (se·vip·ar·us). Sebiferous. [L *sebum* fat, *parere* to produce.]

sevum (se·vum). Suet; the prepared omental fat of the sheep, consisting of the glycerides of stearic, palmitic and oleic acids. It is a firm, white substance, melting at from 45 to 50°C, and is employed as a constituent of ointment bases for use in the tropics. **Sevum benzoinatum.** Benzoinated suet; suet digested with 3 per cent of benzoin as a preservative. **Sevum phosphoratum.** Phosphorated suet; suet containing 10 per cent of phosphorus. [L *sebum* fat.]

sewage (sew·ij). The excrementitious and other waste matter, liquid or solid, passing through a sewer. **Activated sewage.** That which is mixed with activated sludge. **Domestic sewage.** Sewage which is drained from domestic and public buildings, factories and so on. **Septic sewage.** That which is being subjected to an anaerobic putrefactive process.

sewer (sew·er). An artificial conduit which removes waste surface water, excreta and waste household matter. **Sewer swab.** *See* SWAB. [O Fr. *sewiere.*]

sewerage (sew·er·ij). The system of pipes by which all excrementitious and waste matter from a house or town is removed. [see prec.]

sex (sex). The totality of the structural and functional characteristics which distinguish the male from the female organism. **Chromosomal sex.** The sex of an individual as determined by the presence or absence of a Y chromosome. **Gonadal sex.** The sex of an individual as determined by the presence of a testis or an ovary. **Heterogametic sex.** That sex which produces 2 types of gamete (male- and female-determining gametes). This is often due to the presence of dissimilar sex chromosomes (X and Y or Z and W) in the cells of heterogametic individuals. The male is heterogametic in most animals but the female is heterogametic in all birds, Lepidoptera and a few others. **Homogametic sex.** That sex which only produces 1 type of gamete with regard to the sex-determining factors. **Somatic sex.** The sex of an individual as determined by the mode of development of the internal or external genitalia. **Sex intergrade.** *See* INTERGRADE. [L *sexus* male or female sex.]

sex-duction (sex·duk·shun). The process whereby bacterial genes are transferred from one cell to another by means of sex factors into which they are incorporated, i.e. F-prime factors. [sex, L *ducere* to lead.]

sex-limited (sex·lim·it·ed). **Sex-limited character.** A character which is expressed in one sex only, even though the potentiality for its expression, its controlling gene, may be present in both. [sex, L *limes* boundary.]

sex-linkage (sex·lingk·ij). The association of a gene or its expression with the sex of an individual, because the gene is carried on a sex chromosome. The heterogametic sex will receive only one X chromosome, and that from its homogametic parent. If the homogametic parent is heterozygous for any characters whose genes are carried on the sex chromosomes, one-half of the heterogametic offspring will show the recessive characters. It is for this reason that rare allelomorphs, such as haemophilia, are shown in men much more frequently than in women: in women they will be masked by dominant allelomorphs. [sex, Old Norse *link.*]

sex-linked (sex·lingkt). **Sex-linked character.** A character which is controlled by genes situated on the sex chromosomes. [see prec.]

sexidigital, sexidigitate (sex·e·dij·it·al, sex·e·dij·it·ate). With 6 digits on one foot or hand. [L *sex* six, digit.]

sexivalent (sex·e·va·lent). Hexavalent; possessing a valency of 6. [L *sex* six, valency.]

sexology (sex·ol·o·je). The branch of science that is concerned with sex and sex relations. [sex, Gk *logos* science.]

sextigravida (sex·te·grav·id·ah). A woman who is pregnant for the sixth time. [L *sextus* sixth, *gravida* pregnant.]

sextipara (sex·tip·ar·ah). A woman who has given birth to 6 children at the same number of labours. [L *sextus* sixth, *parere* to give birth.]

sextuplet (sex·tew·plet). One of 6 offspring born at one labour. [L *sextus* sixth.]

sexual (sex·ew·al). 1. Pertaining to sex. 2. Denoting eggs in which development takes place only after they have been fertilized.

sexuality (sex·ew·al·it·e). The quality of being sexual or having sex. **Pregenital sexuality.** An early stage in the development of sexuality when its object is the mouth, rectum or skin, not yet the genitals (psycho-analytic theory).

sexvalent (sex·va·lent). Hexavalent. [L *sex* six, valent.]

Sézary's reticulosis. A rare and fatal reticulosis showing an unusual type of giant cell *(Sézary cell)* in the blood, and also lesions of the skin. The cells are like very large monocytes with a narrow margin of monocyte-like cytoplasm and a densely staining nucleus.

SH antigen (es·aitch an·te·jen). Hepatitis B antigen.

shadow (shad·o). Relative darkness caused by the interception of an opaque body between the image and the source of light. A phantom; an attenuated remnant. **Blood shadow.** A colourless or very faintly staining red cell, a phantom or a ghost cell, commonly seen in severe hypochromic anaemia. **Butterfly shadow.** A characteristic brain scan appearance associated with a malignant glioma in both hemispheres joined through the corpus callosum. **Heart shadow.** The radiological opacity caused by the heart and great vessels seen radiographically or during fluoroscopy. **Retinoscopy shadow.** The light and shadow seen in the pupil during retinoscopy, the movement and axis of which is important in assessing the refractive error. **Sound shadow.** An interference with the normal progress of a sound wave as a result of some barrier between the source of the sound and the receiving ear. [AS *sceadu.*]

See also: GUMPRECHT, PONFICK.

shadow-casting (shad·o·kahst·ing). A technique used to improve the picture in electron microscopy. The specimen on the grid is sprayed from an oblique angle with a heavy metal. This leads to metal piling up on one side of any particles on the grid. When the specimen is photographed this gives the appearance of shadows cast by the particles. [shadow, Old Norse *casta.*]

Shadwell self-retaining gag. An adjustable, self-retaining mouth gag with a tongue-piece; it is suitable for use with endotracheal anaesthesia.

Shaffer, Philip Anderson (b. 1881). American biochemist.

Shaffer and Marriott method. For acetone bodies in urine. Urine is treated with basic lead acetate and the filtrate distilled. Acetone is determined in the filtrate iodimetrically; β-hydroxybutyric acid in the residue from distillation is oxidized with dichromate to acetone which is distilled off and estimated as before.

shaft (shahft). An elongated cylindrical structure, such as the part of a long bone between the epiphyses. [ME.]

shakes (sha·ks). Popular name for the rigor or shivering stage of intermittent fevers, or any condition in which there are tremors. **Hatters' shakes.** A fine tremor, notably in the hands, in those suffering from chronic mercurial poisoning. Mercuric nitrate was used, in the past, in the felting of hats, and workers absorbing mercury developed mercurialism, often with hatters' shakes. **Spelters' shakes.** Metal-fume fever. *See* FEVER. [AS *scacan.*]

shaking (sha·king). A form of massage which results in vibration of the tissue. [see prec.]

shamanism, shamanismus (sham·an·izm, sham·an·iz·mus). A religion of races of Northern Asia, involving a belief in good and evil spirits and the power of priests to propitiate them by magic; the excitement induced by the practices of such a religion. [Persian *shaman* idolater.]

Shambaugh, George Elmer, Jnr. (b. 1903). Chicago otolaryngologist.

Shambaugh's operation. A form of fenestration operation for the treatment of chronic deafness resulting from otosclerosis.

Sharman, Albert. 20th century Glasgow gynaecologist.

Sharman's curette. A small curette used to obtain endometrial biopsies in outpatient clinics.

Sharp, Ian Kerr. 20th century British orthopaedic surgeon.

Sharp's angle. A measurement of acetabular dysplasia. The angle is subtended between a horizontal line joining the inferior margin of the "tear drip" and a line drawn from the inferior margin of the tear drip to the upper and outer margin of the acetabulum.

Sharpey, William (b. 1802). London anatomist and physiologist. **Sharpey's fibre.** A connective-tissue fibre that passes from the exterior into the cortex of a bone.

shashitsu (shah·shit·zoo). Mite-borne typhus; tsutsugamushi disease. [Japanese.]

shearing (sheer·ing). A traumatic brain-surface stretching of the tethering membranes resulting in surface contusions and haemorrhages on the brain and also in deeper tortional haemorrhages; the common cause for traumatic subdural bleeding in the elderly and usually set on the opposite side to that injured by the contrecoup mechanism. [AS *scear* to cut.]

sheath [vagina (NA)] (sheeth). The covering of an organ or collection of organs or structures, usually composed of connective tissue which is part of the general fascial investments of the body, frequently tubular in character, as around nerves and blood vessels. **Adventitial sheath.** A sheath of connective tissue which is external to the structure covered, and not an essential part of it. **Axillary sheath.** The connective tissue covering the axillary artery and brachial plexus, derived from the prevertebral fascia of the neck. **Carotid sheath [vagina carotica (NA)].** The connective tissue which surrounds and binds together the common and internal carotid arteries, the internal jugular vein and the vagus nerve. **Chordal sheath.** A strong membrane surrounding the notochord. **Contraceptive sheath.** *See* CONDOM. **Crural sheath.** Femoral sheath (see below). **Dentinal sheath.** Neumann's sheath; a differentiated layer of dentine immediately adjacent to the canal of the dentinal tubules. **Endoneurial sheath.** Endoneurium; the delicate connective-tissue covering of individual nerve fibres outside the sheath of Schwann. **Epithelial sheath.** A downgrowth from the enamel organ around the root of a developing tooth which determines the form of the root. **Fascial sheath of the eyeball [vagina bulbi (NA)].** A sheath covering the posterior five-sixths of the eyeball, adherent anteriorly to the conjunctiva. **Femoral sheath.** The connective tissue derived from the transversalis and iliac fasciae which passes under the inguinal ligament enclosing the femoral artery and vein; the most medial part of the sheath contains only loose areolar tissue and forms the femoral canal. **Fibrous sheaths of a tendon [vaginae fibrosae tendinis (NA)].** Strong sheets of connective tissue, which bind a tendon to bone near the flexor surface of a joint, thus controlling the direction of its action. **Fibrous flexor sheaths of the tendons of the fingers [vaginae fibrosae digitorum manus (NA)].** Fibrous arches across the flexor tendons in the digits of the hand. They are attached to the sides of the phalanges and articular capsules, and are lined by synovial sheaths. They are thin at the joints and consist of annular [pars anularis vaginae fibrosae (NA)] and cruciate [pars cruciformis vaginae fibrosae (NA)] fibres. They prevent bow-stringing in flexion. **Fibrous flexor sheaths of the tendons of the toes [vaginae fibrosae digitorum pedis (NA)].** Tunnels of fibrous tissue on the plantar aspect of the toes whose edges are attached to the margins of the proximal and middle phalanges. The fibres in the region of the phalangeal shaft are transverse [pars anularis vaginae fibrosae (NA)]; those over the joints are obliquely disposed in a cruciform manner [pars cruciformis vaginae fibrosae (NA)]. **Intertubercular synovial sheath [vagina synovialis intertubercularis (NA)].** The tubular prolongation of the synovial membrane of the shoulder joint along the tendon of the long head of the biceps brachii muscle. **Medullary sheath, Myelin sheath.** The laminated sheath of a nerve fibre produced by the elongated spiralled mesaxon. It is interrupted at regular intervals at the nodes of Ranvier. **Neurilemmal sheath.** Neurilemma, sheath of Schwann; the sheath of a nerve fibre, formed of nucleated cells (cells of Schwann), one between each node of Ranvier. **Notochordal sheath.** Chordal sheath (see above). **Sheaths of the optic nerve, internal and external [vagina interna nervi optici, vagina externa nervi optici (NA)].** The extension of the meninges (dura, arachnoid and pia mater) around the optic nerve to the back of the eyeball. **Perivascular sheath.** Any sheath of connective tissue surrounding blood vessels; the adventitial sheath of blood vessels. **Primitive sheath.** Neurilemmal sheath (see above). **Sheath of the prostate [fascia prostatae (NA)].** Fascia of the pelvis condensed to form a sheath around the prostate outside its capsule. **Sheath of the rectus abdominis muscle [vagina musculi recti abdominis (NA)].** A fibrous-tissue sheath derived from the aponeuroses of the lateral muscles of the abdominal wall and enveloping each rectus muscle. The outer layer [lamina anterior (NA)] is complete but the inner layer [lamina posterior (NA)] is absent in the lower quarter of the muscle. It thus has a lower free border, the arcuate line, below which all the aponeurotic layers enter the anterior lamina. **Root sheath of a hair.** The downgrowth of surface epithelium forming a covering of that part of the shaft of a hair which lies below the surface and the bulb from which it grows. **Synovial sheath.** A thin, double-layered sheath generally found around tendons where they lie in contact with bone, or in osteofibrous tunnels; the opposed surfaces of the 2 layers of the sheath are covered with flattened cells similar to those of the synovial membrane of a joint and the intervening space contains a fluid of mucous character to facilitate the gliding of the tendons. **Synovial sheath of the extensor carpi ulnaris tendon [vagina tendinis musculi extensoris carpi ulnaris (NA)].** The synovial sheath of the tendon which begins just proximal to the extensor retinaculum and ends at its insertion. **Synovial sheath of the extensor digiti minimi tendon [vagina tendinis musculi extensoris digiti minimi (NA)].** The synovial sheath of the extensor digiti minimi muscle extending from the lower end of the forearm to the dorsum of the hand and partially covered by the extensor retinaculum. **Synovial sheath of the extensor digitorum and extensor indicis tendons [vagina tendinum musculorum extensoris digitorum et extensoris indicis (NA)].** The common synovial sheath for the extensor digitorum and extensor indicis muscles over the lower end of the radius and carpus, and partially covered by the extensor retinaculum. **Synovial sheath of the extensor digitorum longus tendons [vagina tendinum musculi extensoris digitorum pedis longi (NA)].** A sheath around these tendons under, and extending some distance on each side of, the inferior extensor retinaculum. **Synovial sheath of the extensor hallucis longus tendon [vagina tendinis musculi extensoris hallucis longi (NA)].** A long sheath around this tendon extending from the lower leg to the level of the base of the 1st metatarsal bone. **Synovial sheath of the extensor pollicis longus tendon [vagina tendinis musculi extensoris pollicis longi (NA)].** The sheath for this tendon on the back of the lower end of the radius and carpus and deep to the extensor retinaculum. **Synovial sheath of the flexor carpi radialis tendon [vagina synovialis tendinis musculi flexoris carpi radialis (NA)].** The sheath around this tendon as it passes under the flexor retinaculum. **Synovial sheath of the flexor digitorum longus tendons [vagina tendinum musculi flexoris digitorum pedis longi (NA)].** A synovial sheath for this tendon under the flexor retinaculum and behind the medial malleolus. **Synovial sheath of the flexor hallucis longus tendon [vagina synovialis tendinis musculi flexoris hallucis longi (NA)].** A synovial sheath for this tendon extending from the lower end of the tibia into the sole of the foot, partially under the flexor retinaculum. **Synovial sheath of the flexor pollicis longus tendon [vagina tendinis musculi flexoris pollicis longi (NA)].** A long sheath around this tendon and extending from the lower forearm, under the flexor retinaculum, to the insertion of the tendon in the thumb. **Synovial sheath of the flexor tendons, common [vagina synovialis communis musculorum flexorum (NA)].** A large common synovial sac for the long flexors of the digits, extending from the lower end of the forearm under the flexor retinaculum to the palm. It is usually continuous with the synovial sheath of the 5th digit. **Synovial sheaths of the flexor tendons of the fingers [vaginae synoviales digitorum manus (NA)].** Sheaths extending to the points of insertion of the tendons. They consist of a layer lining the sheath and one covering the tendon. **Synovial sheaths of the flexor tendons of the toes [vaginae synoviales digitorum pedis (NA)].** Sheaths extending from the heads of the metatarsals to the insertion of the tendons and consisting of a layer lining the fibrous sheath and one covering the tendon. The layers are connected by discrete strands of connective tissue covered with synovium (the vincula tendinum) which convey blood vessels to the tendon. **Synovial sheath of the peroneal tendons, common [vagina synovialis musculorum peroneorum (fibularium) communis (NA)].** The sheath around the peroneal tendons extending some distance above the lateral malleolus and carried below on to the tendon of the peroneus longus muscle to the lateral side of the cuboid bone. **Synovial sheath of the peroneus longus tendon, plantar [vagina tendinis musculi peronei (fibularis) longi plantaris (NA)].** A synovial sheath surrounding this tendon as it crosses the sole of the foot. **Synovial sheath of a tendon [vagina synovialis tendinis (NA)].** The tubular sac around a tendon, consisting of an inner layer over the tendon and an outer layer continuous with the former at the ends, and containing a mucoid material to facilitate movement of the tendon. **Synovial sheath of the tendons of the abductor pollicis longus and the extensor pollicis brevis muscles [vagina tendinum musculorum abductoris longi et extensoris brevis pollicis (NA)].** The common synovial sheath for these muscles between the extensor retinaculum and the groove on the lateral side of the lower end of the radius. **Synovial sheaths of the tendons of the foot, digital [vaginae synoviales tendinum digitorum pedis (NA)].** The common synovial sheaths for the tendons of the long and short flexors in each digit. **Synovial sheaths of the tendons of the hand, digital [vaginae synoviales tendinum digitorum (NA)].** The synovial sheaths which surround the long flexor tendons in the digits. **Synovial sheath of the tendons of the radial extensors of the wrist [vagina tendinum musculorum extensorum carpi radialium (NA)].** The common synovial sheath for the extensor carpi radialis brevis and longus muscles, deep to the extensor retinaculum. **Synovial sheath of the tibialis anterior tendon [vagina tendinis musculi tibialis anterioris (NA)].** The synovial sheath around this tendon extending from above the superior extensor retinaculum to the gap between the limbs of the inferior retinaculum. **Synovial sheath of the tibialis posterior tendon [vagina synovialis tendinis musculi tibialis posterioris (NA)].** A synovial sheath around this tendon under and extending a short distance on either side of the flexor retinaculum. [AS *scaeth.*]

See also: HENLE, HERTWIG (W. A. O.), KEY (E. A. H.), MAUTHNER, NEUMANN (E. F. C.), RETZIUS (M. G.), RUFFINI, SCARPA, SCHWALBE, SCHWANN, SCHWEIGGER-SEIDEL.

Sheehan, Harold Leeming (b. 1900). British pathologist.

Sheehan's syndrome. Hypopituitarism following ischaemic necrosis of the anterior pituitary at delivery; the lesion is due to a general circulatory collapse usually as a result of post-partum haemorrhage.

sheet (sheet). A large oblong piece of linen or cotton material, generally used as part of the bed covering in such a way as to protect the blankets. **Draw sheet.** A folded sheet which is longer than the width of the bed and usually made of absorbent cotton twill. It is placed across the bed, under the patient, and when soiled is easily replaced, or by a slight adjustment a cool patch may be provided. [AS *scete.*]

Sheldon, Joseph Harold. 20th century British geriatrician.

Sheldon's body types. Endomorphy, mesomorphy, ectomorphy.

Sheldon, Philip W. 20th century Oxford neurologist.

Sheldon's cannula. A cannula intended for use over a guide wire, in selective carotid arteriography.

Sheldon's needle. A terminal side-hole needle used exclusively for direct puncture of the vertebral artery in angiography.

shelf (shelf). Any shelf-like structure resembling a platform. **Rectal shelf.** The ridge of hard tissue felt *per rectum* and caused by metastases (usually transcoelomic and commonly from a stomach cancer) in the peritoneum at the bottom of the recto-vesical pouch or of the pouch of Douglas (recto-uterine). [AS *scylfe.*]

See also: BLUMER.

shell (shel). 1. In ophthalmology, a specially shaped shallow glass cup for placing in the conjunctival sac of the socket following enucleation and prior to the insertion of a permanent prosthesis. 2. In radiotherapy, a moulded device for radiation beam location. **K, L, M shells.** Electrons surrounding the nucleus of an atom are classified into shells, K, L, M, etc. [AS *scell.*]

Shellac BPC 1963 (shel·ac). Brown resinous transparent scales prepared from a secretion of the insect *Tachardia lacca* Kerr (family Coccidae). It is used in the preparation of varnishes and polishes and for the enteric coating of pills and tablets. [AS *scell,* lac.]

Shenton, Edward Warren Hine (b. 1872). London radiologist.

Shenton's arch or line. A line used for testing radiographically the relationship of the head and neck of the femur with the acetabulum. It follows the inferior border of the pubic ramus and continued outwards forms a regular curve down the medial border of the femoral neck.

Shepherd, Francis J. (b. 1851). Canadian surgeon.

Shepherd's fracture. Fracture of the external tubercle of the astragalus, sometimes confused with the os trigonum.

sherbet (sher·bet). Originally applied to a cooling drink in the East (Turkey, Persia, etc.) containing fruit juice, it is often used for Western imitations such as an effervescent drink made from *sherbet powder,* a mixture of sodium bicarbonate, tartaric acid, sugar and fruit flavouring. [Ar. *shariba* to drink.]

Sherman, Henry Clapp (b. 1875). New York chemist.

Bourquin-Sherman unit. A unit of measurement of riboflavine [Obsolete term.].

Sherman and Chase assay test. A test in which the aneurine hydrochloride content of a preparation was measured by noting its effect on the growth of rats kept on a diet deficient in aneurine. Now that crystalline preparations are available, the test is little used.

Sherman, William O'Neill. 20th century Pittsburgh orthopaedic surgeon.

Sherman plate. Vanadium bone plate.

Sherman screws. Vanadium steel tap screws.

Sherren, James (b. 1872). British surgeon.

Sherren's method, Ochsner-Sherren method or treatment. A method of non-operative management of established peritonitis due to acute appendicitis, which involves resting the intestine completely: used also nowadays in the treatment of the appendix mass.

Sherren's triangle. A triangle of skin marked by lines joining the right pubic tubercle, the umbilicus and the highest point of the iliac crest. Hyperaesthesia is often noted here, in acute appendicitis.

Sherrington, Sir Charles Scott (b. 1857). Oxford physiologist.

Sherrington's law. 1. Each posterior spinal nerve supplies a particular skin area, although there may be some overlap by fibres from adjacent segments. 2. The eyes are maintained in the primary position, by a state of slight contraction or tonus of all the extra-ocular muscles. When any movement takes place, some muscles relax and others contract.

Sherrington phenomenon, Vulpian-Heidenhain-Sherrington phenomenon. Following motor denervation by section of the ventral roots of the sciatic nerve, and after allowing time for degeneration, stimulation of the sciatic nerve causes a slow contraction of the muscles. This is thought to be due to diffusion of acetylcholine from the endings of undegenerated vasodilator nerve fibres running in the sciatic-nerve trunk.

Liddel and Sherrington reflex. Stretch reflex. *See* REFLEX.

Shevsky, Marian C. San Francisco biochemist.

Addis and Shevsky test. For kidney function. The patient abstains from fluid for 24 h; the urine is collected during the second 12 h of this period and the specific gravity determined. Normal function is shown by a specific gravity of more than 1.026.

Shibley, Gerald Spencer (b. 1890). American physician.

Shibley's sign. Aegophony in certain lung conditions.

shield (sheeld). 1. A protecting sheath or tube. 2. The metal tube enclosing the soft-iron core of the primary coil of a faradic machine, by the displacement of which the faradic current can be regulated. **Amputation shield.** A large, flat, metal shield which is used to retract the soft tissues at the time of division of the bone. **Arcing shield.** An arcing ring used to improve the voltage distribution across the units of a string of insulators. **Cartella shield.** A shallow cup made usually of stiff cardboard, sometimes aluminium, with small perforations, used to strap over the eye following operations. A similar shield to this can be fashioned from old x-ray film. **Circumcision shield.** A piece of metal with a slot into which the base of the foreskin is inserted to protect the glans penis during circumcision. **Cytherean shield.** A condom. **Earth shield.** A metal sheath immediately under and in contact with the lead sheath of a cable. **Embryonic shield.** The thin disc of cells which represents the early embryo of reptiles, birds and mammals, before the appearance of the embryonic mesoderm. **End shield.** A cover which partially or wholly encloses the end of a machine; it is fitted at the end of the frame and may carry a bearing. **Eye shield.** Usually a patch made of stiff material which is kept in position over the eye by tape or elastic. **Grading shield.** Arcing shield (see above). **Lead eye shield.** A form of contact lens, made of lead and lined with plastic, used for screening the eye when x-ray therapy of neighbouring structures is carried out. **Nipple shield.** A cover to protect the nipple of a lactating mother. **Phallic shield.** Circumcision shield (see above). **Skull shield.** A curved plate (often of perforated aluminium or of plastic) worn to cover a bony cranial defect, especially in the immediate postoperative period. **Test shield.** A metal sheath placed under and insulated from the lead sheath of a cable. [AS *scild.*]

See also: BULLER.

Shiels, Ethel M. 20th century American biochemist.

Reinhold and Shiels method. For blood cholesterol. A similar method to that of Myers and Wardell, anhydrous sodium sulphate being used instead of plaster of Paris for drying the serum prior to extraction.

Shiers, Leslie Gordon Percival. 20th century London orthopaedic surgeon.

Shiers' prosthesis. A hinged device used in arthroplasty of the knee.

shift (shift). 1. Alteration of position. 2. In cytogenetics, chromosome structural change resulting in the displacement of a chromosome segment to a different position within the same chromosome. **Axis shift.** Axis deviation. *See* DEVIATION. **Chloride shift, Chloride-bicarbonate shift.** The migration of chloride ions upon the entry of carbon dioxide into the blood stream. The carbon dioxide diffuses into the red corpuscles and the concentration of bicarbonate ions in the cells is increased above that of the plasma. A redistribution of ions then takes place, bicarbonate ions migrating from cells to plasma and chloride ions from plasma to cells. Oxygenation of blood in the lungs with its accompanying release of carbon dioxide causes a reversal of this process. **Degenerative blood shift to the left.** Term introduced by Schilling to indicate a failure of maturation of the myeloid leucocytes as a result of the depression of the bone-marrow function; there is an increase in numbers of immature myeloid leucocytes in the blood, and their nuclei are narrow, deeply staining and have little or no structural detail. **Shift to the left.** In Arneth's classification of myeloid leucocytes, an increase in the young polymorphonuclear or myeloid leucocytes having single and bilobate nuclei. **Regenerative shift.** Term used by Schilling to refer to a rapid, intense outpouring of mainly young, immature myeloid leucocytes. **Shift to the right.** In Arneth's classification of myeloid leucocytes, an increase in the older forms having from 3 to 5 lobed nuclei. [AS *sciftan* to divide.] *See also:* PURKINJE.

Shiga, Kiyoshi (b. 1870). Japanese bacteriologist.

Shiga's bacillus, Shiga-Kruse bacillus. *Shigella shigae.*

Shiga's dysentery. A severe bacillary dysentery caused by infection with *Shigella shigae* (not usually applied to the other *Shigella* infections).

Shigella (shig·el·ah). A genus of the family Enterobacteriaceae, the members of which cause bacillary dysentery in man and certain animals. They are Gram-negative, non-motile rods. Biochemically they are non-lactose fermenters and produce acid and, usually, no gas from various other carbohydrates; some species (e.g. *Shigella shigae*) produce powerful exotoxins. The genus is divided into 4 groups (A, B, C and D), partly on fermentation reactions but mainly on antigenic characters, viz: A—*S. dysenteriae* which includes *S. shigae, S. schmitzii* and 8 other non-mannitol fermenting serotypes; B—*S. flexneri* contains 6 serotypes; C—*S. boydii* contains 15 serotypes; D—*S. sonnei* contains only 1 serotype, but strains within this group may be further subdivided by colicine typing. *S. sonnei* is responsible for over 90 per cent of the notified cases of bacillary dysentery in the UK—the infection may be very mild and symptomless carriers are common; this species has become the most common *Shigella* in many countries with temperate climates. **Shigella alkalescens.** A species which is the possible cause of a mild type of enteritis, but its pathogenicity is not established. **Shigella ambigua.** *Shigella schmitzi* (see below). **Shigella boydi.** A species that causes dysentery in man; there are several types with a common group antigen which they share with some Flexner strains. **Shigella ceylonensis, Shigella dispar.** A late lactose-fermenting, indole-producing species which causes dysentery in man. **Shigella dysenteriae.** *Shigella shigae* (see below); *S. dysenteriae* is the form used in the USA. **Shigella flexneri.** A species that causes dysentery in man; many different serological types are recognized. **Shigella madampensis.** *Shigella ceylonensis* (see above). **Shigella newcastle.** A dysentery species closely related to *S. flexneri.* **Shigella paradysenteriae.** *Shigella flexneri* (see above); *S. paradysenteriae* is the form used in the USA. **Shigella parashigae.** A group of organisms that are biochemically associated with *S. shigae* but show antigenic differences. **Shigella schmitzi.** A species that causes a severe form of dysentery in man. **Shigella shigae.** A species that causes a severe form of dysentery in man, especially in Asia. **Shigella sonnei.** A late lactose-fermenting species that causes dysentery in man; the commonest cause of bacillary dysentery in the UK. [Kiyoshi *Shiga.*]

shigellosis (shig·el·o·sis). An infection with organisms of the genus *Shigella.* [*Shigella,* Gk *-osis* condition.]

shima-mushi, shimu-mushi (she·mah·**moo**·she, she·moo·**moo**·she). Mite-borne typhus; tsutsugamushi disease; Japanese river fever. [Japanese.]

shin (shin). The front of the leg below the knee; the tibia or the subcutaneous surface of the tibia. **Sabre shin.** Anterior bowing of the tibia due to syphilis or yaws. [AS *scinu.*]

shingles (**shing**·glz). Herpes zoster. [L *cingulum* girdle.]

ship (ship). *See* FABRICIUS AB AQUAPENDENTE.

Shipley, Walter Cleveland (b. 1903). Connecticut psychiatrist.

Shipley test, Shipley-Hartford test. A test of intellectual impairment, based on the comparison of scores on a vocabulary sub-test and a completion sub-test. [Hartford University.]

Shipway, Sir Francis Edward (b. 1875). British anaesthetist.

Shipway's apparatus. An anaesthesia apparatus in which a stream of air or of oxygen picks up ether and/or chloroform vapour, is warmed and delivered to the patient. Described in 1916.

shiver (**shiv**·er). 1. An involuntary contraction of the muscles of the skin. This may be physiological and occur in healthy persons whose skin is chilled, e.g. by swimming in cold water. Pathologically it occurs at the onset of fever when the heat balance is disturbed: although the body temperature is raised the cutaneous blood vessels are constricted so that the warm blood is excluded; the skin is pale, cold and may be cyanosed. The patient has the sensation of cold and this causes reflex contractions of muscles to produce heat to raise the temperature. Severe shivering is termed a *rigor.* The latter is characteristic of many febrile diseases when the temperature rapidly rises, such as pneumonia, cerebrospinal meningitis, malaria, pyelitis, pyaemia, etc. 2. To suffer such an involuntary contraction of the muscles of the skin. [ME *chiveren.*]

shock (shok). 1. The general bodily disturbance following a severe injury. A clinical syndrome characterized by a subnormal temperature, a fall of blood pressure, a feeble, rapid pulse, pallor, a cold moist skin, often vomiting, restlessness and anxiety. The causal agencies are numerous: trauma, haemorrhage, severe burns, coronary thrombosis, perforation of an abdominal viscus, dehydration, electrical currents of high voltage, etc. 2. An emotional or moral upset occasioned by some disturbing or unexpected experience. **Aerial shock.** Shock caused by the blast of bursting high-explosive shells. **Allergic shock.** The symptoms produced by the injection of a foreign protein to which the cells of the body are sensitized. **Anaesthesia shock.** Shock resulting from overdosage of an anaesthetic. **Anaphylactic shock.** Allergic shock (see above). **Anaphylactoid shock.** Symptoms resembling anaphylaxis produced by disturbance in the physical equilibrium of the colloids in the body, and attributed to the passage into the blood stream of unchanged colloids. **Apoplectic shock.** The depressed state of cerebral function which follows cerebral haemorrhage; the resulting hemiplegia is usually flaccid at first, but as shock wears off it may become spastic. **Bomb shock.** A state of emotional disturbance described in children after they have been repeatedly subjected to bombing. **Break shock.** The shock stimulus which occurs when an electric current is broken. **Burn shock.** A condition of shock which follows extensive burns; it may be manifest immediately after the burning or only after the passage of several hours. **Cardiac shock, Cardiogenic shock.** Acute peripheral circulatory failure following rapid and severe cardiac insufficiency and characterized by hypotension, tachycardia, peripheral vasoconstriction, sweating, restlessness, air hunger and sometimes loss of consciousness. The commonest cause is a sudden large coronary thrombosis in which there are thought to be 2 factors operating: acute left ventricular failure leading to sudden precipitous fall in cardiac output and peripheral failure resulting from widespread capillary dilatation, cutaneous arteriolar constriction being a compensatory mechanism. The peripheral component is possibly initiated by the stimulus of severe cardiac ischaemic pain. Other causes of cardiac shock are massive pulmonary embolism, acute fulminating carditis and arrhythmias such as paroxysmal ventricular tachycardia. **Colloid shock, Colloidoclastic shock.** Anaphylactoid shock (see above). **Cyclo shock.** A term not current in the UK; cyclopropane shock (see following). **Cyclopropane shock.** Shock resulting from improper administration of cyclopropane in anaesthesia. **Deferred shock, Delayed shock.** Shock which appears some time after the trauma, during which period there were no symptoms. **Diastolic shock.** When the heart, under the influence of a high venous filling pressure, suddenly meets the rigid pericardial sac in constrictive pericarditis, an early diastolic shock sound is produced. **Discharging shock.** The shock that occurs when a condenser is discharged. **Electric shock.** The effect of the passage of an electric current through the body. **Electrotherapeutic shock.** Treatment by the production of an electrically-induced epileptic convulsion. **Epigastric shock.** Shock following a severe blow on the epigastrium. **Erethismic shock.** Shock accompanied by excitement and restlessness. **Haematogenic shock.** Shock due to a fall in the volume of the circulating blood. **Haemoclastic shock, Haemolytic shock.** A form of protein shock in which leucopenia instead of leucocytosis may occur in certain patients suffering from liver disease after a test protein meal, used at one time as a test of liver function. **Haemorrhagic shock.** A shock which appears to be due mainly to blood loss, e.g. at operation or following injury. **Histamine shock.** Allergic shock resulting from the injection of histamine. **Hypoglycaemic shock.** Symptoms produced by hypoglycaemia, either spontaneous or following an overdose of insulin. **Hypovolaemic shock.** A state of circulatory depression due to a reduced circulating blood volume. **Induction shock.** A high-voltage low-amperage electrical shock from an induction coil. **Injection shock.** Fainting caused by the emotional disturbance of a subcutaneous injection. **Insulin shock.** Hypoglycaemic shock (see above). **Irreversible shock.** Shock which does not yield to the infusion of large volumes of blood [Obsolete term.]. **Liver shock.** Symptoms of collapse which sometimes follow the sudden relief of an obstruction of the common bile duct. **Mental shock.** Psychic shock (see below). **Metabolodispersion shock.** Shock due to an alteration in dispersion of the body colloids. **Neurogenic shock.** Shock of nervous origin. **Obstetric shock.** Shock occurring after childbirth. It is usually secondary to internal or external haemorrhage, operative intervention, precipitate delivery or excessive interference during the third stage. Occasionally there is no apparent cause. **Oligaemic shock.** Shock due to rapid loss of large quantities of blood. **Paralytic shock.** 1. The sudden onset of paralysis. 2. The depressed state of central nervous activity following upon a sudden severe lesion producing paralysis. **Peptone shock.** Symptoms following the intravenous injection of a solution of peptone. **Phenolic shock.** Haemoclastic shock (see above) produced by the injection of phenol. **Pink shock.** A form of protein shock accompanied by a blotchy erythematous rash. **Pleural shock.** A condition of hypotension, often associated with syncope, which may follow needling of the pleural space; it is occasionally fatal. Air embolism may be responsible in some cases. **Post-operative shock.** Surgical shock (see below) following operation. **Primary shock.** Shock immediately following trauma or other cause. **Protein shock.** A rigor and rise of temperature following intravenous injection of a protein. It is used as a therapeutic measure. **Psychic shock.** A shock to the mind. **Railway shock.** Shock following a railway accident: the subject is not necessarily physically hurt. **Secondary shock.** One which follows primary shock or comes on after a latent period. **Sense shock.** A nightmare occurring usually in the first stage of sleep. **Shell shock.** A psychoneurosis formerly attributed to the physical concussion from a shell burst, now attributed to the emotional stress of warfare. **Spinal shock.** The state of severe depression of spinal activity which may follow an injury to the spinal cord; below the level of the lesion all muscles are flaccid and tendon reflexes are absent. **Static shock.** The shock caused by contact with static electricity. **Surgical shock.** A condition in which there is a profound disturbance of bodily activities, following operation or injury. Reduction in the effective blood volume is a prominent feature, with failure of the peripheral circulation. Thirst, restlessness, sweating and cold blue extremities are usually evident. **Testicular shock.** A state of hypotension and often of syncope induced by a blow on the testicle or by its accidental needling, e.g. during tapping of a hydrocele. **Torpid shock.** Shock in which the patient is collapsed and immobile. **Traumatic shock.** Surgical shock following an injury, e.g. fractures of long bones. **Vasogenic shock.** Better known as *peripheral circulatory failure:* acute peripheral circulatory failure due to loss of capillary tone associated with a reduced circulating blood volume. There is splanchnic and cutaneous arteriolar constriction in order to direct the available circulating blood to the vital organs, and reduction of the cardiac output. Clinically, the condition is characterized by tachycardia, hypotension, pallor, weakness, sweating, restlessness, cold extremities and air hunger. It is produced by a variety of conditions: severe injuries, sudden massive haemorrhage or loss of fluid as a result of extensive burns or by copious vomiting or diarrhoea, as a sequel to perforation of a viscus, and conditions which are associated with sudden severe pain, such as acute pericarditis or coronary thrombosis; also in diabetic coma and in acute adrenal cortical insufficiency. **Wound shock.** Surgical shock resulting from a wound, especially in battle. [Fr. *choc.*]

shockproof (shok·proof). 1. Guarded against shock. 2. An apparatus designed to protect the user from the possibility of electric shock by surrounding all high-potential conductors with an earthed metallic screen. [shock, O Fr. *prueve.*]

shoe (shoo). *See* SCARPA. [AS *scoh.*]

Shohl, Alfred Theodore (b. 1889). American paediatrician.

Shohl and King method. For pH of gastric contents. To 2 ml

of filtered gastric contents are added 2 drops of 0.2 per cent thymol blue in 95 per cent alcohol. The colour is compared with that given by similar amounts of indicator and buffer solutions of pH 1.4, 1.6, 1.8, 2.0, 2.4 and 3.0 respectively in similar tubes.
Shohl and Pedley method. For calcium in urine. Urine is oxidized with sulphuric acid and ammonium persulphate, calcium is precipitated as oxalate, the calcium oxalate is filtered, washed and titrated with standard permanganate solution.

shook jong (shook jong). Koro. [Chinese.]

Shope, Richard Edwin (b. 1901). American virologist.
Shope papilloma. A benign virus-caused tumour of rabbits which frequently undergoes malignant change. The virus is a papovavirus of the papilloma genus.

short-sightedness (short·si·ted·nes). Myopia. [AS *sceort*, sight.]

short-windedness (short·**wind**·ed·ness). Dyspnoea. [AS *sceort*, wind.]

shoulder (**sho**·lder). 1. The region of the junction of the arm and the trunk. Its prominence is formed by the acromioclavicular arch and the upper end of the humerus clothed in the deltoid muscle. 2. In radiobiology, the first, non-exponential, part of a cell survival curve. **Shoulder blade.** The scapula. **Drop shoulder.** A condition in which one shoulder is lower than the other. **Frozen shoulder.** A condition of varied aetiology in which all movements of the shoulder are severely limited and very painful. It is a self-limiting condition, the shoulder returning to normal in about 2 years. **Shoulder girdle.** *See* GIRDLE. **Shoulder joint.** *See* JOINT. **Knocked-down shoulder.** Acromioclavicular dislocation. **Loose shoulder.** A manifestation of muscular weakness in the shoulder girdle, seen commonly in cases of progressive muscular dystrophy, rarely in progressive muscular atrophy of proximal type. On placing the hands in the patient's axillae and attempting to lift, because of muscular weakness the shoulders and arms ride upwards and the patient "slips through the hands". **Noisy shoulder.** A condition in which there is loud creaking on abduction of the shoulder due to irregularity of the costal surface of the scapula. [AS *sculder.*]

show (sho). 1. The discharge of blood from the vagina which occurs shortly before the onset of labour. 2. The first appearance of blood at the first menstrual period. [AS *sceawian.*]

shower (**show**·er). **Erythroblastic shower.** A marked or severe increase in numbers of erythroblasts (nucleated red cells) in the circulating blood in certain haemolytic anaemias, especially erythroblastic anaemia, Di Guglielmo's anaemia, erythroleukaemia and, rarely, in pernicious anaemia. [AS *scur.*]

Shrapnell, Henry Jones (d. 1834). English surgeon.
Shrapnell's membrane. The flaccid part of the tympanic membrane.

shudder (**shud**·er). Involuntary tremor or sudden shiver due to repugnance, cold or fear. [ME *shoderen.*]

shunt (shunt). 1. To divert. 2. A diversion; particularly a diversion of blood due to congenital defects, pathological processes or surgical procedures. 3. In electricity, a diversion, particularly a conductor connected in parallel with a section of an electrical circuit and carrying a portion of the main current. 4. A resistance put across the terminals of an instrument to reduce its sensitivity and increase its range. **Arteriovenous shunt.** The entry of arterial blood directly into the venous system via an abnormal channel. It may be *intracardiac* (ventricular or atrial septal defect) or *extracardiac* (patent ductus arteriosus or aortic septal defect); both cause increased pulmonary blood flow, and there is no cyanosis. **Bidirectional shunt.** The occurrence of arteriovenous and veno-arterial shunting of blood in the same patient, as occurs inevitably when there is complete mixing of all the venous return to the heart, or as may happen when shunting across a defect may be in one direction during one part of the cardiac cycle and in the opposite direction during another part of the cycle. **Blood shunt.** Any condition in which there is a passing of blood between arterial and venous systems, or between the portal and systemic systems, without its going through the capillaries. **Corpus cavernosum saphenous shunt.** Anastomosis of the saphenous vein to the corpus cavernosum for the relief of priapism. **Dialysis shunt.** An artificial connection between a peripheral artery and vein either in the arm or the leg, used for haemodialysis. **Left-to-right shunt.** Arteriovenous shunt (see above). **Peritoneocaval shunt.** A method of treating resistant ascites due to cirrhosis of the liver. Ascitic fluid is drained via a unidirectional low-pressure valve into the inferior vena cava by means of an indwelling catheter system. **Portacaval shunt, Portal-venous shunt, Post-caval shunt.** An anastomosis of the portal and the systemic circulations done to relieve certain types of portal hypertension. The 2 methods commonly used are (*a*) a direct anastomosis of the portal vein to the vena cava and (*b*) an anastomosis of the splenic vein to the renal vein. The term is sometimes used to cover the various anastomoses naturally formed between the 2 circulations in portal hypertension. **Reversed shunt.** A right-to-left shunt that was initially a left-to-right shunt, occurring as a result of increased pulmonary vascular resistance. **Right-to-left shunt.** Veno-arterial shunt (see below). **Veno-arterial shunt.** Unoxygenated venous blood passing directly into the arterial system without going through the lungs, with the production of central cyanosis. It occurs in the tetralogy of Fallot, Eisenmenger's syndrome, pulmonary arterial hypertension with ventricular septal defect and in arteriovenous aneurysm of the lung. [ME *shunten.*]

shunting (**shun**·ting). The method of diverting an electric current to an alternative path. [see prec.]

shuttle-bone (**shutl**·bone). The scaphoid bone. [AS *scytel*, bone.]

Sia, R. H. P. 20th century Chinese physician.
Sia's test. A serum test for kala-azar; 1 part of serum is added to 3 parts of distilled water; a flocculent precipitate indicates kala-azar.

siagonantritis (si·ag·on·an·**tri**′·tis). Inflammation of the maxillary sinus. [Gk *siagon* jaw, antritis.]

sialadenitis (si·al·ad·en·**i**′·tis). Sialo-adenitis.

sialadenoncus (si·al·ad·en·**ong**′·kus). A tumour of a salivary gland. [Gk *sialon* saliva, *aden* gland, *ogkos* tumour.]

sialaporia (si·al·ap·**or**′·e·ah). A condition in which too little saliva is secreted. [Gk *sialon* saliva, *aporia* poverty.]

sialectasis (si·al·**ek**·tas·is). Dilatation of the ducts of a salivary gland; usually demonstrated by sialography. **Globular sialectasis.** A more advanced stage of punctate sialectasis in which the diffuse radio-opaque areas have become larger. Sometimes also termed *saccular sialectasis.* **Punctate sialectasis.** A sialographic picture in the parotid gland characterized by the radio-opaque medium showing up as multiple, diffuse, punctate spots; due partly to dilatation of intralobular ducts and partly to extravasation of the radio-opaque medium through the weakened duct walls. [Gk *sialon* saliva, *ektasis* dilatation.]

sialemesia, sialemesis (si·al·em·**e**′·ze·ah, si·al·**em**·es·is). The vomiting of saliva in cases of hysteria. [Gk *sialon* saliva, emesis.]

sialic, sialine (si·**al**·ik, si·al·ine). Salivary. [Gk *sialon* saliva.]

sialidase (si·al·id·aze). The enzyme which catalyses the degradation of sialic acid.

sialism, sialismus (si·al·izm, si·al·**iz**·mus). Salivation. [Gk *sialon* saliva.]

sialitis (si·al·**i**·tis). 1. Sialo-adenitis. 2. Sialodochitis. [Gk *sialon* saliva, *-itis* inflammation.]

sialo-adenectomy (si·al·o·ad·en·**ek**′·to·me). Removal of one of the salivary glands. [Gk *sialon* saliva, *aden* gland, *ektome* a cutting out.]

sialo-adenitis (si·al·o·ad·en·**i**′·tis). Inflammation affecting a salivary gland. [Gk *sialon* saliva, adenitis.]

sialo-adenotomy (si·al·o·ad·en·**ot**′·o·me). The act of incising and draining one of the salivary glands. [Gk *sialon* saliva, *aden* gland, *temnein* to cut.]

sialo-aerophagy (si·al·o·a·er·**of**′·aj·e). The habit of swallowing frequently, causing saliva and air to be taken into the stomach. [Gk *sialon* saliva, *aer* air, *phagein* to eat.]

sialo-angiectasis (si·al·o·an·je·**ek**′·tas·is). Sialectasis. [Gk *sialon* saliva, *aggeion* vessel, *ektasis* dilatation.]

sialo-angiitis, sialo-angitis (si·al·o·an·je·i′·tis, si·al·o·an·ji′·tis). Inflammation of the ducts of the salivary glands. [Gk *sialon* saliva, *aggeion* vessel, *-itis* inflammation.]

sialocele (si·al·o·seel). A cyst or tumour of a salivary gland. [Gk *sialon* saliva, *kele* hernia.]

sialodochitis (si·al·o·do·ki′·tis). Inflammation of the ducts of the salivary glands from infection or the presence of a foreign body. There is usually associated inflammation of the glands themselves. [Gk *sialon* saliva, *doche* receptacle, *-itis* inflammation.]

sialodochium (si·al·o·do′·ke·um). A duct of a salivary gland. [Gk *sialon* saliva, *docheion* holder.]

sialodochogram (si·al·o·do′·ko·gram). Contrast outlining of the salivary ducts and branches, usually of the parotid or submaxillary glands. [Gk *sialon* saliva, *doche* receptacle, *gramma* record.]

sialodochoplasty (si·al·o·do′·ko·plas·te). Plastic surgery of the salivary duct. [Gk *sialon* saliva, *docheion* holder, *plassein* to mould.]

sialoductitis (si·al·o·duk·ti′·tis). Inflammation of the parotid duct. [Gk *sialon* saliva, duct, Gk *-itis* inflammation.]

sialogenous (si·al·oj·en·us). 1. Producing flow of saliva. 2. Sialogogue. [Gk *sialon* saliva, *genein* to produce.]

sialogogue (si·al·o·gog). An agent that increases the flow of saliva. [Gk *sialon* saliva, *agogos* leading.]

sialogram (si·al·o·gram). The radiograph visualizing the ducts and sometimes the acini of a salivary gland by the injection of an oily or watery radio-opaque medium; performed chiefly on the parotid but also on the submandibular gland. [Gk *sialon* saliva, *gramma* record.]

sialograph (si·al·o·graf). Sialogram. [Gk *sialon* saliva, *graphein* to record.]

sialography (si·al·og·raf·e). Visualization of the salivary glands by x-ray or radio-isotope means; e.g. *sialodochogram*, contrast outlining of the ducts and branches, and salivary *scintigram*, examination with radioactive isotopes. [see prec.]

sialoid (si·al·oid). Relating to or resembling saliva. [Gk *sialon* saliva, *eidos* form.]

sialolith (si·al·o·lith). A salivary calculus. [Gk *sialon* saliva, *lithos* stone.]

sialolithiasis (si·al·o·lith·i′·as·is). A condition characterized by the production or presence of salivary calculi. [see prec.]

sialolithotomy (si·al·o·lith·ot′·o·me). The surgical operation of incising a salivary gland or duct for the purpose of removing a calculus. [Gk *sialon* saliva, *lithos* stone, *temnein* to cut.]

sialoma (si·al·o·mah). A tumour of a salivary gland or duct. [Gk *sialon* saliva, *-oma* tumour.]

sialon (si·al·on). Saliva. [Gk.]

sialoncus (si·al·ong·kus). A sublingual tumour caused by obstruction of the duct of a salivary gland by catarrh or by a calculus. [Gk *sialon* saliva, *ogkos* a swelling.]

sialophagia (si·al·o·fa′·je·ah). The swallowing of an abnormal amount of saliva. [Gk *sialon* saliva, *phagein* to eat.]

sialorrhoea (si·al·o·re′·ah). An excessive flow of saliva. This is usually produced reflexly by irritative conditions of the mouth or oesophagus. It is common in parkinsonism and may be caused by drugs such as pilocarpine, iodides and mercury. [Gk *sialon* saliva, *rhoia* flow.]

sialoschesis (si·al·os·kes·is). Total stoppage of salivary secretion by a gland. [Gk *sialon* saliva, *schesis* a checking.]

sialosemeiology (si·al·o·sem·i·ol′·o·je). Salivary diagnosis; application of biochemical tests to the saliva or to other oropharyngeal secretions in order to assist in making a diagnosis. [Gk *sialon* saliva, semeiology.]

sialosis (si·al·o·sis). Profuse salivation. [Gk *sialon* saliva.]

sialostenosis (si·al·o·sten·o′·sis). Stenosis of the duct of a salivary gland. [Gk *sialon* saliva, stenosis.]

sialosyrinx (si·al·o·sir′·ingx). 1. A salivary fistula. 2. A tube for draining the salivary ducts. 3. A syringe for washing out the salivary ducts. [Gk *sialon* saliva, *syrigx* a tube.]

sialotic (si·al·ot·ik). Relating or belonging to, or characterized by a flow of saliva. [Gk *sialon* saliva.]

sialozemia (si·al·o·ze′·me·ah). The state of salivation in which there is excess and often dribbling with considerable loss. [Gk *sialon* saliva, *zemia* loss.]

sib (sib). Kindred; closely related by blood. [AS *sibb*.]

sibbens (sib·enz). A skin disease that occurred in Scotland during the 17th and 18th centuries, and which medical historians recognize to have been endemic non-venereal syphilis. [Gaelic *subhag* raspberry.]

sibilant (sib·il·ant). 1. Applied to a râle, the sound of which is shrill or whistling. 2. Applied to letters of the alphabet representing a hissing sound, e.g. *s*, *z*. [see foll.]

sibilation (sib·il·a·shun). 1. Utterance in which *s* is the predominant sound. 2. A hissing sound in utterance. [L *sibilare* to hiss.]

sibilismus (sib·il·iz·mus). 1. A hissing sound. 2. A sibilant râle. **Sibilismus aurium.** Tinnitus aurium. [see prec.]

sibilus (sib·il·us). A sibilant râle. [L a hissing.]

sibling (sib·ling). Offspring of the same parents. [AS *sibb*.]

Sibson, Francis (b. 1814). London physician.

Sibson's fascia. The suprapleural membrane, attached to the inner border of the 1st rib and to the transverse process of the 7th cervical vertebra and reinforcing the cupula of the pleura.

Sibson's furrow or groove. The groove between the lower border of the pectoralis major muscle and the chest wall.

Sibson's muscle. A common anomalous band of muscle fibres, arising from the lower cervical transverse processes, which is inserted into the suprapleural membrane and the 1st rib behind the subclavian artery.

Sibson's vestibule. The portion of the aortic orifice of the left ventricle proximal to the semilunar valves.

Sicard, Jean Athanase (b. 1872). Paris physician.

Sicard's sign. Bell sound. *See* SOUND.

Sicard syndrome, Collet–Sicard syndrome. Paralysis of palatal, intrinsic laryngeal, pharyngeal, tongue, sternomastoid and trapezius muscles on one side, due to a lesion of the 9th, 10th, 11th and 12th cranial nerves.

Sicard treatment. Bilateral anterolateral chordotomy (spinothalamic tractotomy) between the 1st and 2nd or 2nd and 3rd dorsal segments of the spinal cord, used for the relief of gastric crises of tabes dorsalis.

siccant, siccative (sik·ant, sik·at·iv). 1. Causing to become dry. 2. Having drying properties. 3. An agent which promotes drying. [L *siccare* to dry.]

sicchasia (sik·a·ze·ah). 1. Nausea. 2. The nausea which occurs during the early part of pregnancy. 3. A morbid aversion to food. [Gk *sikchainein* to loathe.]

siccolabile (sik·o·la·bile). Denoting a substance which is altered or destroyed by the process of drying. [L *siccus* dry, labile.]

siccostabile, siccostable (sik·o·sta·bile, sik·o·sta·bl). Referring to a substance which is neither altered nor destroyed in the process of drying. [L *siccus* dry, stabile.]

sicklaemia (sik·le·me·ah). The heterozygous form of sickle-cell anaemia; it is usually symptomless. [AS *sicol*, Gk *haima* blood.]

sickle-form (sikl·form). Sickle-shaped or crescentic. [AS *sicol*, form.]

sickling (sik·ling). The production of sickle-shaped red blood cells in the circulating or drawn blood, observed as a familial trait or in the chronic haemolytic disease peculiar to negroid subjects; sickle-cell anaemia. [AS *sicol*.]

sickness (sik·nes). 1. Disease; ill-health. 2. Vomiting. **Aerial sickness, Aeroplane sickness.** Air sickness (see below). **African sickness.** Trypanosomiasis. **Air sickness.** A form of motion sickness provoked by flying. **Altitude sickness.** Anoxia due to lowered oxygen pressure at heights. **Athletes' sickness.** Nausea and headache after severe exercise, caused by hypoglycaemia. **Aviation sickness, Aviators' sickness.** Anoxia of altitude. **Balloon sickness.** Altitude sickness (see above). **Black sickness.** Kalar-azar. **Borna sickness.** Borna disease. *See* DISEASE. **Car sickness.** Nausea and vomiting caused by the movements of a motorcar. **Ceylon sickness.** Beriberi. **Compressed-air sickness, Decompression sickness.** A syndrome caused by relatively rapid reduction of the ambient pressure which allows gases, chiefly nitrogen, dissolved in blood and tissues to come out of solution. Intravascular bubbles cause aeroembolism. Tissue gas collections cause aeroarthrosis and surgical emphysema. The pathogenesis of the bends, creeps, chokes, neurological symptoms and circulatory collapse (*see* NEUROCIRCULATORY COLLAPSE) is obscure. Arterial hypoxia is probably not a factor. Decompression sickness caused by reducing supra-atmospheric pressure is called *Caisson disease.* **Falling sickness.** Epilepsy. **Flying sickness.** Air sickness (see above). **Green sickness.** A chronic hypochromic anaemia seen in young girls (from 16 to 25 years of age) and termed chlorosis; a condition rarely seen now. **Indian sickness.** Gangrenous proctitis. **Jumping sickness.** Saltatory spasm. *See* SPASM. **Laughing sickness.** The severe emotional lability of pseudobulbar palsy. **Milk sickness.** An acute disease characterized by weakness, anorexia, vomiting, constipation and sometimes death. It is caused by the ingestion of milk, butter and the flesh of cattle suffering from a condition called *trembles.* **Miners' sickness.** Ancylostomiasis. **Monthly sickness.** The menses. **Morning sickness.** The typical nausea of early pregnancy. **Motion sickness.** A syndrome consisting of a tendency to yawning, increased salivation, gastro-intestinal discomfort, nausea, retching and vomiting, pallor, headache and vertigo, and mental depression; it may lead to severe dehydration, prostration and collapse. All forms of travel where there is irregular motion, and irregular motion especially in a vertical plane, other than that associated with travel, may induce it. *See also* SEASICKNESS. **Mountain sickness.** A syndrome seen when the ambient pressure is reduced on ascending a mountain to heights above 3000 m (10 000 ft). The *acute* symptoms include breathlessness, nausea, headache, weakness, impaired mental functions and unsteadiness. After several days, acclimatization begins due to changes in pulmonary ventilation, cardiac output and arterial oxygen capacity. Mountain dwellers become completely acclimatized but occasionally develop headache, hoarseness, anorexia, weakness and limb aches (*chronic* mountain sickness), the cause of which is obscure; it is not due to decompensation of the acclimatization mechanisms (*decompensated* mountain sickness). **Painted sickness.** Pinta. **Protein sickness.** Symptoms produced by the injection of foreign proteins. **Radiation sickness.** 1. X-ray sickness (see below). 2. The nausea and vomiting which is one of the early symptoms of the *acute radiation syndrome.* **Railway sickness.** Motion sickness (see above). **Sea sickness.** *See* SEASICKNESS. **Serum sickness.** A form of allergic or anaphylactic reaction which results from antigen/antibody reaction, often in prophylaxis, and which may be delayed. *See* ANAPHYLAXIS. **Sleeping sickness.** 1. Trypanosomiasis. 2. Encephalitis lethargica; more often called *sleepy sickness,* to distinguish it from 1. **Sleepy sickness.** A popular synonym for encephalitis lethargica. **Slum sickness.** General ill-health, mental and/or physical, associated with living in slum areas in big cities. **Spotted sickness.** 1. Pinta. 2. Cerebrospinal meningitis. *See* MENINGITIS. **Sweating sickness.** 1. An acute infectious disease reported in England in the 16th century. Cases were described by Foster and by Troy in France in World War I. It was characterized by fever, sweating and the formation of crops of papules succeeded by pustules. 2. Miliaria (miliary fever or prickly heat). **Talking sickness.** Talkative episodes with excitability and restlessness in cases of encephalitis lethargica. **Tin sickness.** Tin poisoning, the result of a prolonged diet of tinned foods. **Travel sickness.** Motion sickness (see above). **Trolley sickness.** Nausea from riding in electric trolley cars; motion sickness (see above). **Vomiting sickness.** Poisoning caused by eating unripe ackee fruit (*Blighia sapida*); once common in Jamaica. **X-ray sickness.** A general toxic reaction to the application of x-rays, leading to lassitude, nausea and vomiting. [AS *seoc.*]

side (side). 1. One of the 2 lateral surfaces of the body, midway between the anterior and posterior aspects. 2. One half of the body at either side of the median plane. [AS.]

side-effect (side·ef·**ekt**). A result of drug or other form of therapy in addition to the desired therapeutic effect. The term usually, but not necessarily, connotes an undesirable effect.

siderant (**sid**·er·ant). Of sudden occurrence; fulminant. [see foll.]

sideration (sid·er·**a**·shun). 1. An old name for erysipelas of the face. 2. Lightning stroke. *See* STROKE. 3. Sudden paralysis; sudden destruction of a part of the body. [L *sideri* to be struck down by disease through the baleful influence of a star (*sidus*).]

siderism, siderismus (**sid**·er·izm, sid·er·**iz**·mus.) Metallotherapy. [Gk *sideros* iron.]

siderocyte (**sid**·er·o·site). A red blood cell containing anything from 1 to 20 or more granules that are shown by staining with certain dyes; these non-haemoglobin iron granules may be extruded from the cell suggesting that it is an ageing red blood cell. Excessive numbers of siderocytes are noted most commonly in lead poisoning or industrial-solvent poisoning, haemolytic, pernicious or sickle-cell anaemias, and following splenectomy. [Gk *sideros* iron, *kytos* cell.]

siderofibrosis (**sid**·er·o·fi·**bro'**·sis). Splenic fibrosis characterized by the presence of deposits of iron. [Gk *sideros* iron, fibrosis.]

siderogenous (sid·er·**oj**·en·us). Forming or yielding iron. [Gk *sideros* iron, *genein* to produce.]

sideropenia (**sid**·er·o·**pe'**·ne·ah). A condition marked by deficiency in the amount of iron present in the blood. [Gk *sideros* iron, *penes* poor.]

siderophil (**sid**·er·o·fil). Siderophilous.

siderophilin (sid·er·**of**·il·in). A pseudoglobulin molecule that can carry iron. Ferrous iron is oxidized to ferric and, in the presence of CO_2, a complex of one CO_2 molecule for each ferric atom is attached to the protein molecule. [Gk *sideros* iron, *philein* to love.]

siderophilous (sid·er·**of**·il·us). 1. Capable of absorbing iron. 2. Referring to a cell or tissue which contains iron. [see prec.]

siderophone (**sid**·er·o·fone). A telephone-like magnetic instrument for the detection of intra-ocular foreign bodies containing iron. [Gk *sideros* iron, *phone* sound.]

siderophore (**sid**·er·o·for). A macrophage containing haemosiderin. [Gk *sideros* iron, *pherein* to bear.]

sideroscope (**sid**·er·o·skope). An instrument devised by Asmus and Hirschberg for the localization of magnetic foreign bodies in the eye by the deviation of a properly protected magnetic needle. [Gk *sideros* iron, *skopein* to view.]

siderosilicosis (**sid**·er·o·sil·ik·**o'**·sis). A form of pneumoconiosis due to inhalation of dust containing both iron and silica particles. [Gk *sideros* iron, silicosis.]

siderosis (sid·er·**o**·sis). Deposits of fine particles of iron in the lymphoid aggregations of the lungs, occurring in iron miners, arc welders and in other metal workers, who inhale the metallic dust. The particles do not, as a rule, lead to any reaction or change in the tissues; diffuse nodular shadows are seen in the lungs on x-ray examination, because the aggregations become relatively radio-opaque by reason of their metallic content. The term is also sometimes used for excessive amounts of iron in the blood or deposits of iron in other tissues of the body. **Bantu siderosis.** A type of iron overload of the hepatic cells and, later, the littoral cells often resulting in liver fibrosis, commonly found in Bantu inhabitants in South Africa. It is probably due to excessive iron intake from iron cooking pots; protein malnutrition and excessive alcohol intake may be predisposing factors. **Siderosis bulbi.** The deposition of iron in the tissues of the eye, following a retained intra-ocular foreign body, which is acted on by the tissue fluids. The condition usually goes on to blindness. **Siderosis conjunctivae.** A rust-coloured discoloration of the conjunctivae following a retained metallic foreign body. **Haematogenous siderosis.** The deposition of haemosiderin in various parts of the body as in haemochromatosis and some anaemias. **Hepatic siderosis.** Haemochromatosis; bronzed diabetes. **Urinary siderosis.** Haemosiderinuria; haemolytic anaemia with recurrent haemoglobinuria. [Gk *sideros* iron.]

siderotic (sid·er·**ot**·ik). Relating or belonging to, marked by, or suffering from siderosis.

siderous (**sid**·er·us). Composed of or containing iron. [Gk *sideros* iron.]

Siegert, Ferdinand (b. 1865). German paediatrician.

Siegert's sign. The deformity of the little finger found in mongolian idiocy; it is short and curves inwards.

Siegle, Emil (b. 1833). Stuttgart otologist.

Siegle's otoscope or speculum. An otoscope or speculum which is usually fitted with a magnifying lens. The pressure inside the speculum, and consequently the pressure on the tympanic membrane, can be varied by means of an air-bulb attachment to the instrument.

Siegriste's spots. Pigmented spots arranged along the course of a sclerosed choroidal vessel, seen in the fundus in albuminuric choroiditis.

Siemens, Hermann Werner (b. 1891). German dermatologist.

Siemens' syndrome. Ichthyosis congenita.

Christ-Siemens syndrome. Anhidrotic ectodermal dysplasia.

Siemerling, Ernst (b. 1857). German neurologist and psychiatrist.

Siemerling's nucleus. The ventromedial of the oculomotor group of nuclei, lying beneath the aqueduct of the mid-brain.

sierra salvia (se·er·ah **sal**·ve·ah). The mountain sage; the flowers of *Artemisia frigida*. [Sp. *sierra* mountain, salvia.]

Sieur, Célestin (b. 1860). French surgeon.

Sieur's sign. Bell sound. *See* SOUND.

sieve (siv). A reticulated screen enabling coarse particles to be separated from fine ones. A series of sieves of different mesh is used in grading powders; the sieves are numbered in accordance with the meshes per linear centimetre and the degree of fineness is given by this number. [AS *sife.*]

Sievert, R. M. 20th century Swedish physicist.

Sievert unit. An absolute unit of intensity of radiation equal to 8.4 r/h.

sigh (si). A prolonged, deep and audible complete respiration. [ME *sighen.*]

sighing (**si**·ing). 1. The utterance of a sigh. 2. Marked by sighs; applied to respiration in which air is inspired slowly and deeply, and audibly expelled. [see prec.]

sight (site). 1. The ability to see; the power of seeing; the faculty of vision. 2. An object seen. **Day sight.** Night blindness. *See* BLINDNESS. **Far sight, Long sight.** Hypermetropia. **Near sight.** Myopia. **Night sight.** Hemeralopia. **Old sight.** Presbyopia. **Second sight.** The improvement in near sight that occurs in age and may be caused by incipient cataract. **Short sight.** Myopia. **Weak sight.** Asthenopia. [AS *gesiht.*]

sigillation (sij·il·a·shun). The mark left on the skin by a healed cicatrix and generally characterized by a white fibrous contracted scar. [L *sigillum* small seal.]

sigillative (sij·il·a·tiv). Said of superficial wounds, progressing towards the stage of cicatrization. [see prec.]

sigma (**sig**·mah). The Greek letter σ; used as a symbol for Stefan's constant. It has been used as the symbol for a thousandth of a second, and in statistics for the standard deviation. The σ symbol is sometimes used for surface tension, electrical conductivity, radiation law constants, atomic cross-section and Poisson's ratio. The capital, Σ, is used in mathematics to denote summation of a series.

sigmatism (**sig**·mat·izm). 1. Imperfect pronunciation of the letter *s.* 2. Excessive use of the *s* sound. [see prec.]

Sigmodon (**sig**·mo·don). A genus of South American rodents. **Sigmodon hispidus.** The cotton rat; a laboratory animal. [sigma, Gk *-odous* tooth.]

sigmoid (**sig**·moid). S-shaped; shaped like the Greek letter sigma, Σ. [sigma, Gk *eidos* form.]

sigmoidectomy (sig·moid·**ek**·to·me). Surgical removal of the pelvic colon. [sigmoid, Gk *ektome* excision.]

sigmoiditis (sig·moid·**i**·tis). Inflammation of the pelvic colon. [sigmoid, Gk *-itis* inflammation.]

sigmoidopexy (sig·**moid**·o·pex·e). Fixation of the pelvic colon to the abdominal wall to correct its undue mobility, or to elevate a prolapsed rectum. [sigmoid, Gk *pexis* a fixation.]

sigmoidoproctostomy (sig·**moid**·o·prok·**tos**′·to·me). The operation of making an artificial anus in the region of the rectosigmoid junction. [sigmoid, Gk *proktos* anus, *stoma* mouth.]

sigmoidoscope (sig·**moid**·o·skope). A speculum used in inspection of the pelvic colon. [sigmoid, Gk *skopein* to watch.]

sigmoidoscopy (sig·moid·**os**·ko·pe). Inspection of the pelvic colon with the sigmoidoscope.

sigmoidosigmoidostomy (sig·**moid**·o·sig·moid·**os**′·to·me). The establishment of an anastomosis between 2 segments of the pelvic colon. [see foll.]

sigmoidostomy (sig·moid·**os**·to·me). The creation of an artificial anus in the third part of the pelvic colon. [sigmoid, Gk *stoma* mouth.]

sigmoidotomy (sig·moid·**ot**·o·me). Incision of the pelvic colon. [sigmoid, Gk *temnein* to cut.]

sigmoscope (**sig**·mo·skope). Sigmoidoscope.

Sigmund, Karl Ludwig (b. 1810). Austrian physician.

Sigmund's gland. The supratrochlear lymph gland. *See* GLAND.

sign (sine). Objective evidence of disease or deformity. **Accessory sign.** A sign which is not pathognomonic. **Achilles-tendon sign.** Absence of the ankle jerk in sciatica. **Anterior tibial sign.** When the thigh is forcibly flexed on the abdomen in a case of spastic paraplegia, contraction of the tibialis anterior muscle occurs. **Anticus sign.** Piotrowski's sign. **Assident sign.** Accessory sign (see above). **Bandage sign.** Similar to the Hess capillary resistance test, using a firm bandage round the arm above the elbow; in certain haemorrhagic conditions, especially purpura, a crop of fine petechiae will appear below the constrictive bandage. **Cardinal signs.** The chief or classical signs, or those signs peculiar to the disease itself and not just incidental. **Chair sign.** Pain shooting upwards from the anus on sitting down; it may be present in enterocolitis. **Chin-retraction sign.** Tracheal tug. *See* TUG. **Cobra-head sign.** A halo of radiolucent bladder wall on excretion urography, seen in ureterocele. **Cogwheel sign.** Cogwheel phenomenon. *See* PHENOMENON. **Commemorative sign.** A sign due to a previous disease. **Complementary opposition sign.** Grasset, Gaussel and Hoover sign. **Contralateral sign.** In a case of meningitis, passive flexion of one knee joint evokes a similar movement on the opposite side. **Dissociation sign.** Loss of the ability to appreciate painful and thermal stimuli, with retention of touch appreciation, tactile discrimination and position sense, seen particularly in syringomyelia but also in lesions of the spinothalamic tract and in centrally situated cord lesions of whatever type. **DTP sign.** Tinel's sign (DTP = distal tingling (on) pressure). **Duct sign.** Reddening from acute congestion at the orifice of Stensen's parotid duct in mumps. **Echo sign.** 1. The involuntary repetition of words the patient hears. 2. An echoing sound heard on percussion over a hydatid cyst. **External malleolar sign.** Chaddock's sign. **Extinction sign.** 1. Obliteration of the rash of scarlet fever by light pressure. 2. Schultz-Charlton phenomenon. **Fabere sign.** A clinical procedure devised by Patrick for the diagnosis of arthritis of the hip. The word is formed from the initial letters of the movements required to elicit this sign, namely, flexion, abduction, external rotation and extension. **Facial sign.** Chvostek's sign. **Fan sign.** The fanning of the 2nd to 5th toes which forms part of the extensor-plantar response (Babinski's reflex). **Femoral sign.** Psoas test. *See* TEST. **Flush-tank sign.** The sequence of intermittent hydronephrosis and the voiding of large quantities of urine associated with the disappearance of the hydronephrotic distension of the kidney in the loin. **Fontanelle sign.** Bulging of the anterior fontanelle in infants, caused by raised intracranial pressure. **Forearm sign.** Leri's sign. **Formication sign.** Tinel's sign. **Hyperkinesis sign.** Claude's hyperkinesis sign. **Interossei sign.** Finger phenomenon. *See* PHENOMENON. **Jugular sign.** Queckenstedt's sign. **Kink sign.** Tenderness on a line joining the umbilicus to the centre of Poupart's ligament, occurring with an ileal kink. **Leg sign.** 1. Neri's sign, 1st def. 2. Schlesinger's sign. **Ligature sign.** The development of purpuric spots below a ligature tied round the arm. **Mechanical grip sign.** If the examiner's finger be grasped by a patient, the

sign

grip relaxes when the wrist is flexed. **Meniscus sign.** A translucent zone separating a barium-filled crater from the main barium contents of the stomach, seen radiologically; it is due to the hard edge of the ulcer, and is commoner in malignant than in simple chronic ulcers. Known in the USA as *Carman's sign* and in the UK as *Kirklin's sign.* **Moulage sign.** A radiographic sign in which the mucosal pattern of the small intestines, coated with a barium-water solution, is altered from a normal feathery appearance to "clumping" of barium in sausage-shaped masses. It is due to excess mucus stimulated by the presence of fatty acids or lactic acid in the bowel, and is said to be constant in idiopathic steatorrhoea, rare in symptomatic sprue, and absent in pancreatic steatorrhoea. **Neck sign.** Brudzinski's sign, 1st def. **Negro sign.** 1. The apparent exaggeration of the upward movement of the eyeball noted in facial paralysis. 2. Cogwheel rigidity. *See* RIGIDITY. **Objective sign.** A sign that is appreciable to the examiner's senses. **Obturator sign.** Obturator test; internal rotation of the hip with resultant tightening of the obturator internus muscle may cause discomfort in acute pelvic appendicitis. **Orange-peel sign.** When the skin over a lipoma is pinched up by compressing the tumour between the thumb and fingers the skin becomes dimpled. **Orbicularis sign.** A hemiplegic subject may be unable to close the eye on the paralysed side without closing the other. **Palmoplantar sign.** Palmoplantar phenomenon. *See* PHENOMENON. **Physical sign.** An objective sign produced spontaneously by a patient or induced by some method such as percussion or palpation. **Plumb-line sign.** Sternal displacement in pleural effusion, as shown by a plumb line. **Pneumatic sign.** Hennebert's sign. **Signs of pregnancy.** The objective physical changes occurring in the pregnant woman by which pregnancy may be diagnosed. The positive signs are ballottement of fetal parts, auscultation of fetal-heart sounds and detection of fetal movements. Presumptive signs include breast changes and uterine enlargement. **Pronation sign.** Babinski's sign, 6th def. **Psoas sign.** Psoas test. *See* TEST. **Pyramid sign.** Any sign indicating pyramidal-tract disease. **Pyramidal sign.** Barré's pyramidal sign. **Radialis sign.** Struempell's sign, 2nd def. **Release sign.** When the hand is pressed gently over a tender area in the abdomen, there is a sharp pain as the hand is raised; mentioned as a sign of acute appendicitis, but it occurs in all forms of acute peritonitis. **Reservoir sign.** A clinical sign elicited in suppurative otitis media, which consists of the rapid return of discharge through a perforation in the tympanic membrane after thorough cleansing. It implies that pus is draining a fairly large abscess cavity which may either be a mastoid abscess or an extradural abscess. **Spine sign.** Resistance to passive flexion of the spine; seen in meningitis and poliomyelitis. **Stairs sign.** Difficulty in descending stairs; a characteristic feature of tabes dorsalis. **Sternomastoid sign.** Reflex spasm of the sternocleidomastoid muscle as a result of the presence of inflamed tuberculous glands along the muscle on the same side, or by a cold abscess with collar-stud connection with the underlying gland, or by an acute inflammatory condition of the lung or pleural membrane in the upper part of the chest as part of a "guarding" action, in which other thoracic muscles are involved. **String sign.** 1. The shadow of a narrow streak of barium caught in a string of mucus in the colon, sometimes seen during the later stages of a barium meal. Originally described by Crane as a sign of mucous colitis, it is now regarded as not specific for this condition. 2. Kantor's sign, the shadow of a narrow streak of barium seen in regional ileitis. **Subjective sign.** A symptom appreciable only by the patient. **Thermic sign.** Kashida's sign. **Tibialis sign.** Struempell's sign, 1st def. **Toe sign.** The extensor-plantar response; the Babinski reflex. **Tongue sign.** Dimpling of the tongue on tapping, occurring occasionally in tetany. **Trepidation sign.** Patellar clonus. *See* CLONUS. **Ulnar sign.** Anaesthesia in the distribution of the ulnar nerve as found in bed-ridden psychiatric patients, due presumably to pressure on the nerve in the ulnar groove. **Vallecular sign.** A radiological sign seen during a barium swallow: traces of barium persist in the piriform fossae and valleculae after the bolus has passed down the oesophagus. The sign is said to indicate a neuromuscular disorder of organic origin. **Vein sign.** A bluish cord in the midaxillary line caused by the junction of the dilated superficial epigastric and thoracic veins in the enlargement of the bronchial glands. **Vital signs.** The cardinal signs (see above). [L *signum.*]

See also: ABADIE, ABRAHAMS, AHLFELD, ANDRAL, ARNOUX, ARROYO, ASCHNER, AUENBRUGGER, AUFRECHT, BABINSKI, BACELLI, BAILLARGER, BALLET, BAMBERGER (H.), BÁRÁNY, BARRÉ, BARUCH, BASTIAN, BATTLE, BAUMÈS (J. B. T.), BECHTEREW, BECKER, BEEVOR, BÉHIER, BELL (C.), BENZADON, BERGER (E.), BETHEA, BEZOLD (F.), BIERMER, BIERNACKI, BINDA, BIOT, BIRD (S. D.), BJERRUM, BLUMBERG, BLUMER, BOAS, BONNET, BORDIER, BORSIERI DE KANILFELD, BOSTON, BOUVERET, BOYCE, BRAGARD, BRANHAM, BRAUN (H.), BRAXTON HICKS, BRICKNER, BRISSAUD, BROADBENT (W.), BROADBENT (W. H.), BRODIE (B. C.), BROWNE (J. C.), BRUDZINSKI, BRUNATI, BRUNS, BRYANT, BURGER, BURGHART, BURTON, BYCHOWSKI, CANTELLI, CARDARELLI, CARMAN, CARNETT, CASTELLANI, CASTELLINO, CATTANEO, ČEJKA, CESTAN, CHADDOCK, CHARCOT, CHASE, CHAUSSIER, CHEYNE (J.), CHOLEWA, CHVOSTEK (FRANTISEK), CLAUDE, CLAYBROOK, CLOQUET (J. G.), CODMAN, COMBY, COPE (V. Z.), CORRIGAN, COURTOIS, COURVOISIER, CROWE (S. J.), CRUVEILHIER, CULLEN (T. S.), CUMBO, CURSCHMANN (HEINRICH), CZIKY, DALRYMPLE, DAMOISEAU, DANCE, DAVIDSOHN, DAVIS, DÉJÈRINE, DE LA CAMP, DELBET (P.), DELMEGE, DEMARQUAY, DEMIANOFF, D'ESPINE, DEW, DORENDORF, DUCHENNE, DUCKWORTH, DUPUYTREN, DUROZIEZ, EBSTEIN, ELLIOT (G. T.), ELLIS (C.), ENROTH, EPSTEIN (A.), ERB, ERBEN, ESCHERICH, EWART, EWING, FAGET, FAJERSZTAJN, FEDERICI, FILIPOVITCH, FISHER (T.), FLINT, FODÉRÉ, FOIX, FORCHHEIMER, FOURNIER, FRAENKEL (A.), FRAENKEL, FRANK (J.), FRÉDÉRICQ, FRENKEL (HENRI), FRIEDREICH, FUERBRINGER, GARLAND, GAUSS, GAUSSEL, GERHARDT (C. C. A. J.), GIFFORD, GILBERT, GOLDSTEIN (H. I.), GOLONBOV, GOODELL, GOWERS, GRAEFE, GRANCHER, GRANGER, GRASSET, GREENE, GREGORY, GRIESINGER, GRISOLLE, GROCCO, GROSSMAN, GUBLER, GUÉNEAU DE MUSSY, GUENZBERG, GUILLAND, GUNN, GUTTMANN, GUYE, GUYON, HAENEL, HALL (J. N.), HALSTED, HAMMAN, HARDY, HASSIN, HATCHCOCK, HAUDEK, HEFKE, HEGAR, HEIM, HENNEBERT, HERNIG-LOMMEL, HERTWIG (K. W. T. R.), HERYNG, HIRSCHBERG (L. K.), HOCHSINGER, HOFFMANN (J.), HOLMES (G. M.), HOMANS, HOOVER, HORSLEY, HOWSHIP, HUCHARD, HUMAN, ITARD, JACCOUD, JACKSON (C.), JACKSON (J.), JAFFÉ (K.), JELLINEK, JENDRÄSSIK (ERNST), JOFFROY, KANAVEL, KANTER, KANTOR, KARPLUS, KASHIDA, KEHR, KEHRER (F. A.), KELLY (H. A.), KÉRANDEL, KERNIG, KIRKLIN, KLEIST, KLIPPEL, KOCHER, KOPLIK, KREYSIG, KUSSMAUL, LABORDE, LAËNNEC, LASÈGUE, LAUBRY, LEEDE, LE GENDRE, LEICHTENSTERN, LENNHOFF, LEOTTA, LERI, LESER, LESIEUR, LEUDET, LHERMITTE, LIAN, LICHTHEIM, LIEBERMEISTER, LINDER, LITTEN, LOEWI, LOMBARDI, LOW, LOWY, LUCAS, LUST, MCBURNEY, MCCARTHY (D. J.), MACEWEN, MCMURRAY, MADELUNG, MAGENDIE, MAGNUS, MANN (J. D.), MANNKOPF, MARAÑON, MARFAN, MARIE, MARINESCO, MARION, MASINI, MATHIEU, MENDEL (K.), MENNELL, MEUNIER, MILIAN, MINOR, MOEBIUS, MONTEVERDE, MORQUIO, MOSCHCOWITZ (E.), MOSLER, MUELLER (F.), MURAT, MURET, MURPHY (J. B.), MUSSET, NAUNYN, NERI, NIKOLSKY, NOTHNAGEL, O'CONNELL, OLIVER, ONANOFF, OPPENHEIM (H.), OPPOLZER, OSIANDER, OSLER, PARKINSON (JAMES), PARROT, PASTIA, PAYR, PFUHL, PILCZ (A.), PINS, PIOTROWSKI, PISKACEK, PITRES, PLUMMER, POOL, PORTER, POTAIN, POTTENGER, PREVEL, PREVOST, PRIVEY, QUANT, QUECKENSTEDT, QUÉNU, QUINCKE, QUINQUAUD, RADOVICI, RAIMIST, RAMOND (L.), RASCH, RAYNAUD, REICHMANN, REMAK (E. J.), REMLINGER, REVILLIOD, RICHARDSON, RIESMAN, RITTER (J. W.), ROCKLEY, ROGER, ROLLET (A.), ROMBERG, ROSENBACH (O.), ROSENHEIM (T.), ROSER, ROSSOLIMO, ROTCH, ROUTIER, ROVIGHI, ROVSING, RUGGERI, RUMPEL, RUMPF, SAEGESSER, SAENGER (A.), SANSOM, SARBÓ, SCHEPELMANN, SCHICK, SCHLANGE, SCHLESINGER (H.), SCHUELE, SCHULTZE (F.), SEELIGMUELLER, SÉGUIN, SEIDEL, SEITZ, SHIBLEY, SICARD, SIEGERT, SIEUR, SIGNORELLI, SIMON, SIMON (C. E.), SISTO, SKEER, SKODA, SMITH (E.), SNELLEN, SNOW, SOMAGYI, SOUQUES, SPALDING, SQUIRE, STELLWAG VON CARION, STERLE, STERNBERG (K.), STEWART (J. P.), STIERLIN, STILLER, STOKES (WILLIAM), STRAUS, STRAUSS, STRUEMPELL, SUKER, SZABO, TAR, THEIMICH, THIES, THOMAS (A.), THOMAS (H. O.), THOMAYER,

THOMSON (F. H.), TINEL, TOMMASI, TRÉLAT, TRENDELENBURG, TRESILIAN, TROEMNER, TROISIER, TROUSSEAU, TURNER (G. G.), TURNER (V. C.), TURYN, UHTHOFF, UNSCHULD, VANZETTI, VEDDER, VERCO, VERMEL, VIGOUROUX, VILLARET, VOHSEN, VOLTOLINI, WAHL, WALDENSTRÖM (J. H.), WARTENBERG, WEGNER, WEIL (M. P.), WEILL, WEISS (N.), WERNICKE (K.), WESTPHAL (C. F. O.), WIDOWITZ, WILLIAMS (C. J. B.), WILLIAMSON, WINTERBOTTOM, WINTRICH, WREDEN, WYNTER, ZAUFAL.

signature (sig·nah·tewr). That part of a prescription relating to dosage, and the manner and frequency of administration. [L *signare* to mark.]

signe (seen). Sign. **Signe du lacet.** Hess' test. [Fr.]

See also: LEGUEU.

significance (sig·nif·ik·ans). Importance. A difference is statistically significant if it is unlikely to have arisen by chance. [L *significare* to signify.]

Signorelli, Angelo (b. 1876). Italian physician.

Signorelli's sign. In meningitis, exquisite pain may be produced by pressure over the retromandibular point, beneath the lobe of the ear and in between the mandible and mastoid process of the temporal bone.

Signorini's tourniquet. Two padded metal cylinders carried on a hinge and approximated by screws.

sikimi (se·ke·me). Japanese star anise, bastard star anise; the fruits of *Ilicium religiosum* (family Magnoliaceae), used as an adulterant or substitute for star anise. They are toxic and contain no oil of anise; they have a balsamic smell attributed to safrol.

silane (sil·ane). General name for a series of organic silicon compounds analogous to the hydrocarbons, in which silicon replaces a carbon atom, e.g. SiH_4, $Si(CH_3)_4$, $(CH_3)_3SiC_6H_5$.

silent (si·lent). In clinical medicine, describing a disease which is symptomless. [L *silens.*]

silex (si·lex). 1. A highly refractory silica glass. 2. A form of silica used in paint manufacture. [L flint.]

silica (sil·ik·ah). Silicon dioxide, SiO_2. The anhydride of silicic acid which occurs widely in nature as quartz, flint, sand, rock crystal and in silicate rocks. It is a hard, white or colourless compound with a high melting point, used to make glass and refractory bricks. **Silica gel.** A coagulated form of hydrated silica which is employed as an absorbent and dehydrating agent. [see prec.]

silicate (sil·ik·ate). Any salt of silicic acid, H_2SiO_3. Most rocks and minerals are composed of the silicates of metallic bases.

silicatosis (sil·ik·at·o'·sis). Silicosis.

siliceous (sil·ish·us). Characterized by, or containing silica.

silicic (sil·is·ik). Pertaining to or containing silicon or silica.

silicide (sil·is·ide). Any binary compound of the element silicon with some other element, e.g. magnesium silicide, Mg_2Si.

silicious (sil·ish·us). Siliceous.

silicium (sil·ish·um). Silicon.

silico-anthracosis (sil·ik·o·an·thrah·ko'·sis). Silicosis. [silicosis, anthracosis.]

silicofluoride (sil·ik·o·floo'·or·ide). Any salt of hydrofluosilicic acid, H_2SiF_6, formed by the combination of silicon fluoride and the fluoride of a metal.

silicol (sil·ik·ol). General name given to organic hydroxy compounds of silicon. They readily polymerize with the elimination of water to form silicones.

silicon (sil·ik·on). An element of atomic weight 28.086, atomic number 14 and chemical symbol Si. It is a non-metal, related to carbon, and occurring in 2 allotropic forms, *amorphous silicon,* a light-brown powder, and *crystalline silicon,* orange, grey or black octahedral crystals. It is the most widely distributed element in nature, apart from oxygen, constituting a large proportion of clay and rocks; it also occurs in plant structural tissue, skeletal tissue of certain marine organisms and as a microconstituent in animal connective tissue. It does not occur free, but as silica and silicates. It is employed in the manufacture of alloys. **Silicon carbide.** Carborundum. **Silicon dioxide.** Silica. **Silicon fluoride.** SiF_4, a colourless fuming gas occasionally implicated in poisoning in the superphosphate industry. [L *silex* flint.]

silicone (sil·ik·one). General name applied to polymeric organic compounds of silicon with the general formula $(R_2SiO)_n$, where R represents an alkyl group. They are oils, greases, or plastics and are used on account of their non-reactivity and stability over wide ranges of temperature.

silicosiderosis (sil·ik·o·sid·er·o'·sis). A type of pneumoconiosis resulting from the inhalation of dust charged with particles of silicates and of iron. [silicate, Gk *sideros* iron.]

silicosis (sil·ik·o·sis). A type of pneumoconiosis caused by inhalation of particles of silica, quartz, gannister or slate. **Conglomerate silicosis.** A form of silicosis in which the fibrous nodules are increased in number and size, and coalesce. The affected lymph glands are often smaller than usual, owing to contraction of the infiltrated fibrous tissue. **Infective silicosis.** Tuberculosilicosis. [silica, Gk *-osis* condition.]

silicotic (sil·ik·ot·ik). Pertaining to or suffering from silicosis.

silicotuberculosis (sil·ik·o·tew·ber·kew·lo'·sis). Tuberculosilicosis.

siliculose (sil·ik·ew·loze). Siliquose.

silique (sil·eek). The slender pod of a cruciferous plant, e.g. the pod of the mustard. [Fr. from L *siliqua* pod.]

siliquose, siliquous (sil·ik·woze, sil·ik·wus). Bearing or resembling siliques. *See also* DESQUAMATION.

silk (silk). The prepared fibre from the cocoons of the silkworm *Bombyx mori* and other species of *Bombyx,* and of *Antheroea.* It is used as a haemostatic. **Artificial silk.** Rayon, an artificial textile fibre prepared principally from viscose or cellulose acetate and used as a substitute for silk in the manufacture of oiled silk. **Oiled Silk BPC 1954.** Silk treated with a suitable drying oil; it is used to prevent evaporation from moist dressings. [AS *seolc.*]

silkworm-gut (silk·werm·gut). A non-absorbent suture for surface wounds and incisions, obtained by drawing into a single strand a silkworm killed when about to spin its cocoon. [AS *seolc, wyrm, guttas.*]

sillonneur (se·yon·er). A scalpel with 3 blades, used in ophthalmic surgery. [Fr.]

Silphium (sil·fe·um). A genus of composite-flowered herbs. **Silphium laciniatum.** Rosin-weed, compass plant, polar plant; the dried herb and root is used as an antispasmodic and expectorant. **Silphium perfoliatum.** Indian cup plant, ragged cup; the root, which is a cylindrical crooked rhizome, is chiefly used as an extract. [Gk *silphion.*]

Siluridae (sil·ewr·id·e). A family of African fish that eat *Schistosoma*-carrying snails; they are known as *catfish.* [L *silurus* a river fish, Gk *eidos* form.]

silver (sil·ver). An element of atomic weight 107.868, atomic number 47 and chemical symbol Ag (*argentum*). It is a soft white metal, malleable and ductile, and a good conductor of electricity, occurring in the native state and also in various ores. It has been found in certain fungi and marine organisms, and is a constituent of sea water; it occurs in minute quantity in human tissue. The metal is used in alloys and jewellery, and its compounds are of importance in photography and medicine. The silver ion coagulates protein, and thus many of its compounds are applied locally as astringents, caustics and antiseptics; they are not used internally. Absorption of silver may occur from raw surfaces and mucous membranes, and be deposited in connective tissue: a bluish-grey line near the gum margins and a similar discoloration of the skin may result, the condition being called *argyria.* Once developed, this is generally permanent. **Silver arsenobenzol.** Silver arsphenamine (see following). **Silver arsphenamine.** The sodium salt of silver-3,3'-diamino-4,4'-dihydroxyarsenobenzene; a dark-brown powder, soluble in water, and formerly given by intravenous injection in the treatment of syphilis. **Silver chloride.** AgCl, a white insoluble compound which fuses to a horny mass known to the alchemists as *lunar cornea.* **Colloidal silver.** A term including preparations of silver such as the silver-protein compounds, which probably do not form true solutions but rather suspensions of very small particles. They ionize only slightly and thus are only weakly antiseptic, and little if at all astringent. **Silver Nitrate BP 1973.** $AgNO_3$, a colourless crystalline substance, astringent and caustic, and thus also antiseptic. It is used to destroy warts. Solutions are used as astringents in eczematous and ulcerated skin conditions, and as an antiseptic to the eye; they stain the skin. **Silver Nitrate, Mitigated BPC 1959.** A caustic stick used to destroy warts and other skin growths; the silver forms a proteinate with the tissues which become brown and eventually black. **Silver Nitrate, Toughened BP 1973.** Lunar caustic, a substance prepared by the fusion of silver nitrate (95 per cent) and potassium nitrate (5 per cent). It is usually prepared in the form of rods, greyish in colour, and used as a local caustic application, as in the removal of warts. **Silver nucleinate.** Mild silver protein (see below). **Silver picrate.** A yellow crystalline substance used for its astringent and germicidal actions, chiefly in vaginal trichomonas infection. If long-continued, it may cause argyria. **Silver Protein BP 1958.** Strong protein silver, a brown powder, a compound of silver and gelatin, which contains from 7.5 to 8.5 per cent of silver. In solution it has mild antiseptic properties; in this respect it is weaker than silver nitrate, but it is not caustic. It is used in solutions up to 10 per cent as a local application, mainly in nasal and conjunctival infections. **Silver Protein, Mild BPC 1968.** A compound of silver with a protein such as albumin or casein, containing from 19 to 23 per cent of silver. It may be a brown power, or a dark granular or scaly substance, with actions similar to silver protein, but weaker, and it is almost completely non-irritant. It is used for the same purposes, but in stronger solutions. **Silver trinitrophenate.** Silver picrate (see above). **Silver vitellin.** Mild silver protein (see above). [AS *seolfor.*]

Silverman, Irving (b. 1904). Brooklyn, New York, surgeon.

Vim–Silverman needle. An instrument by means of which a minute cylinder of liver tissue is obtained for histological examination during life.

silvestrene (sil·ves·treen). $C_{10}H_{16}$, a terpene hydrocarbon found in the turpentine of *Pinus silvestris.*

Simaba (sim·ah·bah). A genus of simarubaceous trees and shrubs. **Simaba cedron.** A species the dried seeds of which (cedron seeds), consisting of the separated cotyledons, are used as an antispasmodic and antipyretic. [simaruba.]

Simaruba (sim·ar·oo·bah). 1. A genus of tropical American trees belonging to the family Simarubaceae. 2. The dried root bark of *Simaruba amara* Aubl., used as a bitter stomachic. [Galabi (Guiana) *Simarauba.*]

Simerlin's type. The Leyden–Moebius type of muscular dystrophy.

simian (sim·e·an). Of the character of apes and monkeys. [L *simia* ape.]

Simmonds, Morris (b. 1855). German physician.

Simmonds' disease. A disease due to the partial or complete destruction of the anterior lobe of the pituitary gland, most commonly by thrombosis after post-partum haemorrhage. It is characterized by a combination of the signs of hypothyroidism, hypogonadism and hypo-adrenalism. Sometimes known as Sheehan's syndrome.

Simmons, James Stevens (b. 1890). American bacteriologist.

Simmons' citrate agar. A medium containing ammonium phosphate 1 g, dipotassium hydrogen phosphate 1 g, magnesium sulphate 0.2 g, sodium citrate 20 g, sodium chloride 5 g, agar 20 g, and water to 1 litre, with 5 ml of a 0.4 per cent aqueous solution of bromthymol blue as an indicator.

Simon, Charles Edmund (b. 1866). Baltimore physician.

Simon's septic factor. The production of polymorphonuclear leucocytosis and eosinophilic leucopenia in severe pyogenic infections.

Simon's sign. In the early stage of meningitis, the respiratory movements of the diaphragm and the thoracic cage may be irregular and out of step.

Simon, George. 20th century London radiologist.

Simon's focus. A primary haematogenous tuberculous focus at the apex of the lung in children, comparable to Assmann's focus.

Simon, Gustav (b. 1824). Heidelberg surgeon.

Simon's position. The dorsosacral position: the patient lies on his back with the legs flexed at the knees and the thighs flexed on to the abdomen with the legs abducted.

Simon's retractor. Two separate blades made especially to retract the anterior and posterior walls of the vagina.

Simon, Oskar (b. 1845). German anatomist.

Simon's lines. Surface manifestations of underlying orientation of dermal fibrous tissues. The cleavage lines. *See also:* LANGER'S LINE.

Simon, Theodore (b. 1873). French physiologist.

Binet–Simon scale or test. A test of intelligence devised by Binet to detect those children in the schools of Paris who were unable to benefit from the usual education. The underlying hypothesis was that it is possible to classify differences in intelligence by comparing individual scores in a series of tests with the scores obtained by average children of different ages, thus obtaining a mental age which could be compared with the chronological age. Initially the test comprised a wide variety of 30 sub-tests. It has been extensively revised, adapted and translated.

Simon's sign. Polyuria caused by a metastasis in the pituitary from a primary carcinoma of the breast.

Simons, Arthur (b. 1877). Berlin physician.

Simons' disease. Progressive lipodystrophy. *See* LIPODYSTROPHY.

Barraquer–Simons' disease. Partial lipo-atrophy.

Simonsiella (si·mon·se·el′·ah). A genus of algae. They have been found in the mouth.

simple (simpl). 1. Not compound; consisting of only 1 element or substance; single. 2. Straightforward, running a normal course; not complex. 3. An old term for a herb having medicinal value, commonly used in the plural *simples.* [L *simplex* unmixed, not complicated.]

Simpson, Sir James Young (b. 1811). Scottish obstetrician and pioneer in the use of anaesthesia in obstetrics.

Simpson's forceps. Obstetric forceps with a pelvic and cephalic curve.

Simpson's operation. A modification of Gilliam's operation, where the round ligaments are drawn through the internal abdominal rings.

Simpson, William Kelly (b. 1855). New York laryngologist.

Simpson's splint. A splint of cotton wool for packing into the nasal fossa.

Simpson, William Speirs (d. 1917). British civil engineer.

Simpson light. Ultraviolet light produced by an electric arc of which the electrodes are made of iron tungstate and manganese.

Sims, James Marion (b. 1813). New York gynaecologist.

Sims' depressor. A metal loop used to depress the anterior wall of the vagina during examination.

Sims' operation. The method of closure of vesicovaginal fistulae with silver wire.

Sims' position. A position in which the patient lies on the left side with the right knee and thigh drawn well up above the left. The left arm is put behind the back and allowed to hang over the edge of the couch. The chest and abdomen are permitted to fall forwards, thus creating a negative pressure in the abdomen and allowing the vagina to fill with air.

Sims' speculum. Duck-billed speculum; a U-shaped speculum having 2 spatulate blades of different sizes at each side of the U. It was devised by Sims for use in the repair of vesicovaginal fistula.

simulation (sim·ew·la·shun). 1. Assumption by a symptom or disease of the appearance of another symptom or disease. 2. Malingering. [L *simulare* to imitate.]

simulator (sim·ew·la·tor). A device for simulating the treatment beam and used for planning radiotherapy. [L *simulare* to imitate.]

Simuliidae (sim·ew·li·id·e). A family of the dipteran suborder Nematocera; black flies. The genus *Simulium* is of medical interest. [L *simulare* to imitate, Gk *eidos* form.]

Simulium (sim·ew·le·um). A genus of the dipteran family Simuliidae; black flies. The numerous species are all small, usually black, flies, with 11 segmented antennae. The larvae are aquatic, living only in fast-flowing waters. The females of all species feed on mammalian or avian blood, and several species bite man readily. The bites are very painful and, when numerous, may have severe toxic effects, but are very rarely fatal in man; however, livestock are sometimes killed in large numbers. Some species are known carriers of disease and others are under suspicion as such. Some species migrate up to 80 km (50 miles) from their breeding sites. **Simulium avidum.** *Simulium metallicum* (see below). **Simulium callidum.** A vector of *Onchocerca volvulus* in central America. **Simulium columbaczense.** The notorious columbacz fly of the Danube which kills animals in thousands and bites man. **Simulium damnosum.** An important man-biter in tropical Africa, and a vector of *Onchocerca volvulus* in Sierra Leone. **Simulium erythrocephalum.** A troublesome man-biter in central England. **Simulium indicum.** The potu fly; a troublesome man-biter in northern India. **Simulium metallicum.** A vector of *Onchocerca volvulus* in central America. **Simulium mooseri.** *Simulium callidum* (see above). **Simulium morsitans.** A troublesome man-biter in the New Forest, Hampshire. **Simulium naevei.** A vector of *Onchocerca volvulus* in central Africa. **Simulium ochraceum.** A vector of *Onchocerca volvulus* in central America. **Simulium reptans.** A troublesome man-biter in Wales and the Lake District in England. **Simulium tuberosum.** A troublesome man-biter in Scotland. [L *simulare* to imitate.]

sinal (si·nal). Sinusal.

sinalbin (sin·al·bin). A glucoside occurring in white mustard seeds. It yields acrinyl isothiocyanate and glucose on hydrolysis. [Gk *sinapi* mustard, L *albus* white.]

sinapeleum (sin·ap·el·e·um). Mustard oil. *See* OIL. [Gk *sinapi* mustard, *elaion* oil.]

sinapine (sin·ap·een). The alkaloid $C_{16}H_{25}O_6N$, obtained from black mustard seeds, *Brassica nigra.* [see foll.]

sinapis (sin·a·pis). Mustard. **Sinapis Alba BPC 1949.** White mustard; the dried seeds of *Brassica alba* Linn. (family Cruciferae) which contain a fixed oil and a crystalline glycoside, sinalbin, together with the enzyme, myrosin, which hydrolyses the glycoside into acrinyl isothiocyanate and glucose. **Sinapis Nigra BPC 1949.** Black mustard; the dried seeds of *Brassica nigra* which contain a fixed oil, a glycoside, sinigrin, and the enzyme, myrosin, which hydrolyses the glycoside into allyl isothiocyanate and glucose. [Gk *sinapi* mustard.]

sinapiscopy (sin·ap·is·ko·pe). The testing of abnormalities of the sensory field by the application of mustard to various areas of the skin. [sinapis, Gk *skopein* to watch.]

sinapize (sin·ap·ize). 1. To mix with mustard. 2. To apply mustard as a treatment. [sinapis.]

sincipital (sin·sip·it·al). Concerning the sinciput.

sinciput [NA] (sin·sip·ut). 1. The entire upper half of the skull. 2. The forehead. 3. The anterior and superior part of the head. 4. The bregma. [L half a head.]

Sinclair, Maurice (b. 1878). London orthopaedic surgeon.

Sinclair's glue. A special glue for applying extension in fractures, prepared from glue or gelatin, water and glycerin together with a small percentage of thymol as a preservative.

Sinding-Larsen, Christian Magnus Falsen (b. 1874). Norwegian surgeon.

Sinding-Larsen disease. Osteochondritis of the lower pole of the patella.

sinew (sin·ew). A tendon. **Weeping sinew.** An encysted ganglion which occurs chiefly on the back of the hand and contains synovia. [ME *sinewe.*]

Singer needle. An automatic needle for mechanical suturing.

singultation (sing·gul·ta·shun). The hiccuping reaction, which takes place just after the diaphragmatic spasm has passed. [see foll.]

singultient (sing·gul·she·ent). 1. Hiccuping. 2. Sighing; sobbing. [L *singultare* to hiccup.]

singultous (sing·gul·tus). Pertaining to or affected with hiccup. [see foll.]

singultus (sing·gul·tus). A hiccup. **Singultus gastricus nervosus.** Hiccup caused by gastric neurosis. [L hiccough.]

sinigrin (sin·ig·rin). A glucoside occurring in black mustard seeds. It yields allyl isothiocyanate and glucose on hydrolysis. [Gk *sinapi* mustard, L *niger* black.]

sinister, sinistra (sin·is·ter, sin·is·trah). On the left hand; left. [L.]

sinistral (sin·is·tral). 1. Relating or belonging to the left side. 2. Inclining to the left. 3. When there is a choice, preferring to use the left, e.g. eye, hand; left-handed. [see foll.]

sinistration (sin·is·tra·shun). 1. The state of inclining or turning to the left. 2. Left-handedness. [see prec.]

sinistraural (sin·is·traw·ral). Denoting an individual whose hearing is better in the left ear than in the right. [sinister, L *auris* ear.]

sinistrin (sin·is·trin). A carbohydrate present in squill and said to be identical with inulin. [L *sinister* left, because laevorotatory.]

sinistrocardia (sin·is·tro·kar′·de·ah). Displacement of the heart to the left. [sinister, Gk *kardia* heart.]

sinistrocardial (sin·is·tro·kar′·de·al). Relating or belonging to sinistrocardia.

sinistrocerebral (sin·is·tro·ser′·e·bral). Belonging to or found in the left cerebral hemisphere. [sinister, L *cerebrum* brain.]

sinistrocular (sin·is·trok·ew·lar). Relating to an individual whose left eye is stronger than the right or who uses his left eye in preference to the right when there is a choice, e.g. in microscopical work. [sinister, L *oculus* eye.]

sinistrogyration (sin·is·tro·ji·ra′·shun). The process of turning to the left, e.g. the eye. [sinister, L *gyrus* circuit.]

sinistrogyric (sin·is·tro·ji′·rik). Sinistrorse. [see prec.]

sinistrohepatal (sin·is·tro·hep′·at·al). Having the liver displaced to the left. [sinister, Gk *hepar* liver.]

sinistromanual (sin·is·tro·man′·ew·al). Left-handed. [sinister, L *manus* hand.]

sinistropedal (sin·is·trop·ed·al). Left-footed; using the left foot in preference to the right. [sinister, L *pes* foot.]

sinistrophoria (sin·is·tro·for′·e·ah). Tendency of the visual lines to turn to the left. [sinister, Gk *pherein* to bear.]

sinistrorsal, sinistrorse (sin·is·tror·sal, sin·is·trors). 1. Twisted or turned to the left. 2. In botany, winding spirally from right to left. [L *sinistrorsus* on the left hand.]

sinistrosplenic (sin·is·tro·splen′·ik). Having the spleen displaced to the left side. [sinister, spleen.]

sinistrotorsion (sin·is·tro·tor′·shun). A turning or twisting to the left. [sinister, L *torquere* to twist.]

sinistrous (sin·is·trus). 1. Sinistral. 2. Awkward; left-handed. [sinister.]

sinistrum (sin·is·trum). Sinister.

Sinkler, Wharton (b. 1845). Philadelphia neurologist.

Sinkler's phenomenon. In a paraplegic patient, sharply flexing the big toe may be followed by flexion of the hip and knee.

sino-atrial (si·no·a·tre·al). Between the sinus venosus and the atrium, or auricle, of the embryonic heart; it is applied to the nodal tissue in the wall of the right atrium which is situated between that part of the atrium which is developed from the sinus venosus and the part which corresponds to the embryonic atrium or auricle.

sino-auricular (si·no·aw·rik′·ew·lar). Sino-atrial. [sinus, auricle.]

sinobronchitis (si·no·brong·ki′·tis). Bronchitis associated with sinusitis.

sinogram (si·no·gram). The radiography made during sinography. [sinus, Gk *gramma* record.]

sinography (si·nog·raf·e). Radiographic visualization of a sinus track after the injection of a radio-opaque contrast medium into the skin opening. [sinus, Gk *graphein* to record.]

sinomenine (sin·o·men·een). An alkaloid, $C_{19}H_{23}O_4N$, from the Japanese plant *Sinomenium acutum.* It is a convulsive poison, used in small doses in Japan in the treatment of rheumatism.

Sinomenium (sin·o·me·ne·um). A genus of plants of the family Menispermaceae. The species *Sinomenium acutum* of Japan yields several alkaloids including sinomenine and tuduranine. [LL *Sinensis* Chinese, Gk *mene* moon.]

sinter (sin·ter). The silicious or calcareous encrustations formed by deposits of mineral springs. [G dross of iron.]

sintoc (sin·tok). The bark of *Cinnamomum sintoc* (family Lauraceae), which resembles cinnamon bark. [East Ind. *sintoq.*]

Sintonius (sin·to·ne·us). A sub-genus of *Phlebotomus.*

sinuate (sin·ew·ate). 1. Sinuous; tortuous. 2. In botany, having a wavy and deeply indented margin. [L *sinus* curve.]

sinu-atrial (si·new·a·tre·al). Belonging to one of the cardiac atria and the associated sinus venosus. **Sinu-atrial node.** *See* NODE.

sinu-auricular (si·new·aw·rik'·ew·lar). Sinu-atrial. [sinus, auricle.]

sinuitis (si·new·i·tis). Sinusitis.

sinuose (sin·ew·oze). Sinuous.

sinuosity (sin·ew·os·it·e). The quality or state of being sinuous.

sinuotomy (si·new·ot·o·me). Sinusotomy. [sinus, Gk *temnein* to cut.]

sinuous (sin·ew·us). Winding or bending in or out; tortuous. [L *sinus* curve.]

sinus (si·nus). 1. An infected tract communicating with the skin or with the lumen of a hollow viscus. Healing is usually prevented by the presence of a buried foreign body, often a non-absorbable suture or dead bone, constant reinfection of the wound, e.g. in a sinus near the rectum, or by the presence of a resistant infection, e.g. tuberculosis, actinomycosis. 2. An air sinus; a mucus-lined cavity in one of the bones of the face or skull which communicates with the nose (frontal, sphenoid, ethmoid, maxillary). These develop only late in childhood. When, as often happens, they become infected (sinusitis) either acutely or chronically, they may cause considerable invalidism. 3. Any wide, venous, blood space: applied especially to those of the dura, e.g. lateral, cavernous, sigmoid, superior and inferior sagittal. They are subject to thrombosis when infected (e.g. lateral sinus following mastoiditis or cavernous sinus in infections of the nose). Other named venous sinuses include coronary sinus, sinus venosus. 4. [NA] A pouch or recess: used frequently in anatomical description, e.g. sinus of the larynx, transverse and oblique sinuses of the heart (or pericardium), sinus tarsi. **Air sinus.** *See* MAIN DEF. 2 (above). **Anal sinuses [sinus anales (NA)].** The pocket-like recesses behind the anal valves. **Sinuses of the aorta [sinus aortae].** Three dilatations, 1 anterior and 2 posterior, in the root of the aorta, opposite the valve cusps and from 2 of which the coronary arteries arise. **Barbers' hair sinus.** An interdigital sinus due to hairs becoming embedded while haircutting. **Basilar sinuses, network of [plexus basilaris (NA)].** A network of veins on the base of the skull, between the inferior petrosal sinuses. **Branchial sinus.** During the complicated embryonic development of the neck, a recess lined with ectoderm from one of the branchial pouches (usually the 2nd) may be imprisoned deep to the skin. Following suppuration, incision or inadequate attempts at removal, this may acquire an opening on the skin. **Carotid sinus [sinus caroticus [NA)].** A dilatation of the upper end of the common carotid artery, usually involving the beginning of the internal carotid, and innervated by the glossopharyngeal nerve. It acts as a pressoreceptor, reflexly maintaining the intracranial blood pressure. **Cavernous sinus.** *See* SINUS OF THE DURA MATER, CAVERNOUS (below). **Cervical sinus.** Precervical sinus (see below). **Coccygeal sinus.** A sinus in the midline of the natal cleft (often multiple) over the coccyx, which is often complicated by infection in early adult life. It may be congenital or acquired, and may contain hair. Cf. PILONIDAL SINUS (below). **Coronary sinus [sinus coronarius (NA)].** A vein lying in the posterior atrioventricular groove, receiving most of the venous blood from the heart and opening into the right atrium by an orifice guarded by a valve, the valve of the coronary sinus. **Dental sinus.** A periapical abscess with a sinus opening up within the mouth or on the surface of the skin. **Dorsal sinus.** A congenital sinus resulting from failure of separation of the neural tube from the surface. **Sinus of the dura mater, cavernous [sinus cavernosus (NA)].** A bilateral large and important dural venous sinus lying at the side of the body of the sphenoid bone in the middle cranial fossa. It contains the internal carotid artery and abducent nerves in its lumen and several nerves in its lateral wall. It drains some cerebral veins and the superior ophthalmic veins, through which it communicates with the veins of the face and with the transverse sinus and internal jugular vein through the petrosal sinuses. **Sinuses of the dura mater, confluence of [confluens sinuum (NA)].** The site of meeting of the superior sagittal, transverse, straight and occipital dural venous sinuses. **Sinus of the dura mater, inferior petrosal [sinus petrosus inferior (NA)].** A venous sinus running in the groove between the petrous part of the temporal bone and the basilar part of the occipital bone, and connecting the cavernous sinus to the commencement of the jugular vein. **Sinus of the dura mater, inferior sagittal [sinus sagittalis inferior (NA)].** A venous sinus in the inferior margin of the falx cerebri; a tributary of the straight sinus. **Sinuses of the dura mater, intercavernous [sinus intercavernosi (NA)].** Usually 2 venous sinuses joining the cavernous sinuses in front and behind the pituitary gland. **Sinus of the dura mater, occipital [sinus occipitalis (NA)].** A venous sinus in the attached margin of the falx cerebelli, ending in the confluence of sinuses. **Sinus of the dura mater, sigmoid [sinus sigmoideus (NA)].** A continuation of the transverse sinuses along the posterior surface of the petrous part of the temporal bone to the jugular foramen where they join the jugular veins. **Sinus of the dura mater, straight [sinus rectus (NA)].** A venous sinus lying at the junction of the falx cerebri and the tentorium cerebelli, receiving the great cerebral vein, inferior sagittal sinus and veins from the cerebellum. It drains into the transverse sinuses (usually the left). **Sinus of the dura mater, superior petrosal [sinus petrosus superior (NA)].** A venous sinus along the posterior border of the petrous part of the temporal bone, in the attached margin of the tentorium cerebelli; it joins the cavernous to the transverse sinus. **Sinus of the dura mater, superior sagittal [sinus sagittalis superior (NA)].** A large venous sinus running along the attached border of the falx cerebri from the crista galli to the internal occipital protuberance where it joins the right or left or both transverse sinuses (usually the right). **Sinuses of the dura mater, transverse [sinus transversi (NA)].** Bilateral, usually asymmetrical, large venous sinuses lying along the attached margin of the tentorium cerebelli. They receive the superior sagittal and straight sinuses, and drain via the sigmoid sinuses to the internal jugular veins. **Sinuses of the dura mater, venous [sinus durae matris (NA)].** Venous channels lying between the 2 layers of the dura mater and draining the brain. **Sinus of the epididymis [sinus epididymidis (NA)].** A slit-like recess between the testis and body of the epididymis laterally, and lined with tunica vaginalis. **Ethmoidal sinuses [sinus ethmoidales (NA)].** A number of air cells within the ethmoid bone, grouped usually into anterior and middle [cellulae anteriores et mediae (NA)] groups (draining into the middle meatus) and posterior [cellulae posteriores (NA)] groups (draining into the superior meatus (NA)]. **Frontal sinus [sinus frontalis (NA)].** One of a pair of multi- or unilocular air cells separating the inner and outer tables at the junction of the frontal and orbital portions of the frontal bone and separated from its fellow by a thin septum. **Hair sinus.** A sinus formed when hair penetrates the skin and acts as a foreign body. **Intercavernous sinus.** *See* SINUSES OF THE DURA MATER, INTERCAVERNOUS (above). **Sinus of the kidney [sinus renalis (NA)].** The cavity within the kidney, occupied by the pelvis of the ureter, the calyces and the main renal vessels. **Lactiferous sinuses [sinus lactiferi (NA)].** Dilatations on the lactiferous ducts at the base of the nipple. **Sinus of the larynx [ventriculus laryngis (NA)].** A recess between the vestibular and vocal folds, extending upward outside the vestibular folds and internal to the lamina of the thyroid cartilage as the saccule of the larynx. It contains mucous glands which lubricate the vocal folds. **Lateral sinus.** Sinus of the dura mater, transverse (see above). **Longitudinal sinus.** Sinus of the dura mater, inferior, sagittal and posterior sagittal (see above). **Marginal sinus.** Placental sinus (see below). **Maxillary sinus [sinus maxillaris (NA)].** Antrum of Highmore, a large cavity containing air in the body of the maxilla and communicating with the nose in the middle meatus. The largest of the paranasal sinuses. **Oblique sinus.** *See* SINUS OF THE PERICARDIUM, OBLIQUE (below). **Occipital sinus.** *See* SINUS OF THE DURA MATER, OCCIPITAL (above). **Oral sinus.** The early embryonic mouth or stomatodaeum. **Paranasal sinuses [sinus paranasales (NA)].** Cavities within the skull bones, opening into the nasal cavity and lined by mucous membrane continuous with the nasal mucous membrane. **Sinus of the pericardium, oblique [sinus obliquus pericardii (NA)].** A pericardial-lined recess bounded by the inferior vena cava and right pulmonary veins on one side and the left pulmonary veins on the other, and lying between the posterior wall of the left atrium and the posterior wall of the pericardial sac. **Sinus of the pericardium, transverse [sinus transversus pericardii (NA)].** A pericardium-lined channel passing between the arterial trunks leaving the heart and the venous trunks entering it. **Sinus pericranii.** The air spaces in the bones of the base of the skull, each sinus being named after its containing bone, e.g. frontal, maxillary, ethmoid, sphenoid, mastoid. **Petrosal sinuses.** *See* SINUS OF THE DURA MATER, INFERIOR PETROSAL, AND SUPERIOR PETROSAL (above). **Pilonidal sinus.** A sinus containing hair, found in the natal cleft, the axilla, in the interdigital cleft of barbers and elsewhere; the hair is usually not growing but has become lodged in the sinus from without. Cf. COCCYGEAL SINUS (above). **Placental sinus.** A supposed venous sinus encircling the human placenta; it is not constantly present. **Portal sinus.** A vascular channel in the fetal liver into which open the portal vein and the umbilical vein, and from which leads the ductus venosus. **Posterior sinus [sinus posterior (NA)].** A depression in the posterior wall of the tympanic cavity above the pyramid. **Postoperative sinus.** A persisting sinus in an operation wound. It is most often due to infection round a non-absorbable suture, or to some specific infection like tuberculosis. **Sinus praecervicalis, Precervical sinus.** A deep ectoderm-lined pouch at the side of the neck of the early embryo, produced by the sinking in of the lower pharyngeal arches and their overgrowth by the 1st and 2nd arches and the epipericardial ridge. **Prostatic sinus [sinus prostaticus (NA).** The recess, on either side of the seminal colliculus, into which the prostatic ducts open. **Sinus of the pulmonary trunk [sinus trunci pulmonalis (NA)].** One of the dilatations in the pulmonary trunk, opposite to a cusp of the pulmonary valve. **Sacrococcygeal sinus.** *See* COCCYGEAL SINUS (above). It may on occasion be derived from the archenteric canal. **Sagittal sinus.** *See* SINUS OF THE DURA MATER, INFERIOR SAGITTAL, AND SUPERIOR SAGITTAL (above). **Sigmoid sinus.** *See* SINUS OF THE DURA MATER, SIGMOID (above). **Sphenoidal sinus [sinus sphenoidalis (NA)].** A paired, asymmetrical sinus in the body of the sphenoid bone. It drains into the spheno-ethmoidal recess. **Sphenoparietal sinus [sinus sphenoparietalis (NA)].** A small venous sinus along the lesser wing of the sphenoid bone; a tributary of the cavernous sinus. **Splenic sinus [sinus lienis (NA)].** One of the venous sinusoids in the splenic reticulum. **Straight sinus.** *See* SINUS OF THE DURA MATER, STRAIGHT (above). **Sinus tarsi [NA].** A tunnel lying between the inferior aspect of the neck of the talus and the dorsum of the calcaneum. **Terminal sinus.** The venous channel encircling the area vasculosa of the blastoderm or yolk sac. **Thyroglossal sinus.** A persistent thyrocervical duct, draining externally in the midline of the neck, usually as the result of rupture or surgical drainage or inadequate surgical removal of a thyroglossal cyst. **Tonsillar sinus.** The space between the palatoglossal and palatopharyngeal folds, occupied by the tonsils. **Transverse sinus.** 1. *See* SINUSES OF THE DURA MATER, TRANSVERSE (above). 2. *See* SINUS OF THE PERICARDIUM, TRANSVERSE (above). **Traumatic sinus.** A sinus which persists at the site of injury, e.g. due to a retained piece of clothing at the bottom of a puncture wound. **Sinus tympani [NA].** A depression in the tympanic cavity between the fenestra vestibuli and the fenestra cochleae. **Sinus unguis [NA].** The space between the projecting free border of the nail and the skin at the extremity of a digit. **Urogenital sinus [sinus urogenitalis (NA)].** 1. In embryology, the portion of the ventral division of the cloaca below the entrance of the genital ducts. It gives rise in the male to the urethra below the prostatic utricle and the bulbo-urethral glands, and in the female to the greater vestibular glands. 2. The common excretory channel for urinary and genital products in lower vertebrates. **Uterine sinus.** The venous spaces in the pregnant uterus. **Uteroplacental sinus.** The blood space formed in pregnancy between the placenta and the uterine wall. **Sinus of the venae cavae [sinus venarum cavarum (NA)].** That part of the right atrium which lies posterior and to the left of the crista terminalis. It receives the superior and inferior caval veins and is developed from the embryonic sinus venosus. **Sinus venarum.** The smooth part of the wall of the right atrium of the heart. **Sinus venosus.** The posterior chamber of the embryonic heart into which the cardinal, vitelline and umbilical veins drain. Its right half is absorbed into the right atrium; its left half becomes the coronary sinus. **Sinus venosus sclerae [NA].** An endothelially-lined circular canal in the sclera, close to the sclerocorneal junction, separated from the anterior chamber of the eye by trabecular tissue and draining into the anterior ciliary vein laterally. **Venous sinus [sinus venosus (NA)].** A dilated area containing venous blood. **Sinus ventriculi.** A space between mucosal folds in the pyloric antrum, seen radiographically. **Vertebral sinuses, longitudinal.** Paired longitudinal channels in front of and behind the spinal cord, forming part of the internal vertebral plexuses. [L *sinus* curve, hollow.]

See also: ARLT, BOCHDALEK, BRESCHET, CUVIER, FORSSELL, GUÉRIN (A. F. M.), HUGUIER, LAUTH (E. A.), LITTRÉ, LUSCHKA, MAIER, MORGAGNI, PALFYN, PETIT (F. P.), RIDLEY, TOURTUAL, VALSALVA.

sinusal (si·nus·al). Relating or belonging to a sinus.

sinusitis (si·nus·i·tis). Inflammation affecting the mural epithelium of a sinus, particularly of the paranasal sinuses. **Sinusitis abscendens.** Sinusitis associated with necrosis of the bone beneath the affected mucous membrane. **Chronic catarrhal sinusitis.** Mucocele. **Frontal sinusitis.** Inflammation affecting the paranasal frontal sinus or sinuses. **Serous sinusitis.** Mucocele. [sinus, Gk *-itis* inflammation.]

sinusoid (si·nus·oid). 1. Having resemblance to a sinus. 2. A small terminal blood vessel to be found in certain organs, e.g. spleen, pancreas. It is wider than a capillary and has an irregular lumen, with little or no connective tissue covering, the endothelium being in close contact with the cells of the organ. **Myocardial sinusoid.** A small terminal blood vessel which lies between the fibres of the myocardium. [sinus, Gk *eidos* form.]

sinusoidal (si·nus·oid·al). 1. Relating or belonging to a sinusoid. 2. Referring to a particular form of electric current. **Sinusoidal current.** *See* CURRENT.

sinusotomy (si·nus·ot·o·me). The operation of incising a sinus. [sinus, Gk *temnein* to cut.]

sinuventricular (si·new·ven·trik'·ew·lar). Relating to the sinus venosus of the atrium and the ventricle of the heart.

siphon (si·fon). A doubly-bent tube for the withdrawal of fluid by gravity through the upper end or neck of its container. **Carotid siphon.** Term used in angiography referring to the sigmoid shape of part of the intracavernous portion of the internal carotid artery. [Gk tube.]

See also: DUGUET.

siphonage (si·fon·ij). Gastric lavage or wound drainage by means of siphon action.

Siphonaptera (si·fon·ap·ter·ah). An order of insects, the fleas, characterized by the absence of wings, lateral flattening and hind legs modified for jumping. The larvae are apodal. Members of the genera *Ctenocephalides, Oropsylla, Pulex, Tunga* and *Xenopsylla* are of medical importance. [Gk *siphon* tube, *apteros* without wings.]

siphonoma (si·fon·o·mah). Cylindroma. [Gk *siphon* tube, *-oma* tumour.]

Siphonospora polymorpha (si·fon·**os**·por·ah pol·e·**mor**·fah). A name given by Brehmer to a micro-organism that he regarded as the cause of cancer. [Gk *siphon* tube, *spora* seed, *polymorphes* many-shaped.]

Siphunculata (si·**fun**·kew·**la'**·tah). An order of insects; the sucking lice. They are dorsoventrally flattened, wingless and with piercing and sucking mouth parts. All are parasites of mammals. The genera *Pediculus* and *Phthirus* are of medical importance. [L *siphunculus* little tube.]

Siphunculina (si·**fun**·kew·**li'**·nah). A genus of small flies. **Siphunculina funicola.** An important eye fly in the tropical Far East. [see prec.]

Sippy, Bertram Welton (b. 1866). Chicago physician.

Sippy's diet, method or treatment. A dietetic method of treatment of gastric ulcer which aims at neutralizing the free acid of the gastric juice, thereby allowing the ulcer to heal. It starts as a pure milk diet, and at intervals biscuits, cereals, eggs and puréed vegetables are added until the 28th day, when an ordinary diet is substituted.

Sippy powder. An alkaline powder used in the treatment of gastric ulcer. It consists of sodium bicarbonate mixed with an equal weight of calcium carbonate or magnesium carbonate. It is usually used in conjunction with olive oil, belladonna and Sippy's diet.

siqua (si·kwah). The unit introduced by von Pirquet to determine the area of the absorptive mucous surface of the intestine. It is the square of the sitting height calculated in centimetres. [L *sidentis altitudinis quadratio* square of sitting height.]

siren (si·ren). Sirenomelus.

sirenomelus (si·ren·**om**·el·us). A monster the legs of which are fused, the structure tapering to a blunt point without feet. [Gk *seiren* mermaid, *melos* limb.]

siriasis (si·**ri**·as·is). Heat stroke. *See* STROKE. [Gk *sieros* scorching (of summer heat).]

sisel (siz·el). Suslik. [Russian.]

sismotherapy (sis·mo·**ther**·ap·e). Seismotherapy.

Sisto, Genaro (d. 1923). South American paediatrician.

Sisto's sign. Continuous crying of infants suffering from congenital syphilis, presumably due to intracranial involvement. (Not generally accepted in the UK.)

Sistrunk, Walter Ellis (b. 1880). Rochester, Minnesota, surgeon.

Sistrunk's operation. Excision of a thyroglossal fistula with removal of the central part of the hyoid bone and a core from the tongue.

Sistrurus (sis·**troo**·rus). A genus of rattlesnakes of eastern North America. [Gk *seistron* rattle, *oura* tail.]

Sisymbrium (sis·**im**·bre·um). A genus of cruciferous plants. **Sisymbrium alliaria.** Hedge garlic; the herb and seeds contain a volatile oil with an alliaceous odour. **Sisymbrium officinale.** Hedge mustard; the dried herb is used for coughs. [Gk *sys* pig, *ombrios* wet, since the plant grows where pigs wallow.]

site (site). Position; situation. **Allosteric site.** A region of an allosteric protein which is specific for the binding of an effector molecule. **Placental site.** The placental area. *See* AREA. **Regulator sites.** *See* REGULATOR. [L *situs*.]

sitieirgia (si·te·**ire**·je·ah). An insane or hysterical refusal to take food. [Gk *sitos* food, *eirgein* to abstain from.]

sitiology (si·te·**ol**·o·je). Sitology.

sitiomania (si·te·o·**ma'**·ne·ah). Sitomania.

sitiophobia (si·te·o·**fo'**·be·ah). Sitophobia.

sitology (si·**tol**·o·je). Dietetics. [Gk *sitos* food, *logos* science.]

sitomania (si·to·**ma**·ne·ah). 1. Abnormal hunger or insane desire for food. 2. Attacks of bulimia which occur at intervals. [Gk *sitos* food, mania.]

sitophobia (si·to·**fo**·be·ah). 1. Aversion to food. 2. An insane or morbid fear of taking food. 3. Obstinate refusal to take food. [Gk *sitos* food, phobia.]

sitostane (**si**·to·stane). The hydrocarbon $C_{29}H_{52}$, which contains the characteristic steroid skeleton (cyclopentenophenanthrene-ring system) and can be regarded as the parent of the sitosterols. [Gk *sitos* food.]

sitosterol (si·to·**steer**·ol). $C_{29}H_{49}OH$, a sterol found in wheat embryo; it is a mixture of 3 isomers. [Gk *sitos* food, sterol.]

sitotaxis (si·to·**tax**·is). Sitotropism. [Gk *sitos* food, *taxis* a turning.]

sitotherapy (si·to·**ther**·ap·e). Dietotherapy; the application of the principles of dietetics in treatment. [Gk *sitos* food, therapy.]

sitotoxin (si·to·**tox**·in). Any basic food poison, particularly that developed in a grain or vegetable food by bacteria fungi. [Gk *sitos* food, toxin.]

sitotoxism (si·to·**tox**·izm). Food poisoning. *See* POISONING. [see prec.]

sitotropism (si·to·**trop**·izm). The tendency of living cells to be attracted or repelled by certain types of food. [Gk *sitos* food, *trope* a turning.]

situs (si·tus). A position or site. **Indeterminate situs.** An uncommon developmental abnormality in which it is not possible to determine whether the subject has situs solitus or situs inversus; the condition is associated with asplenia or polysplenia and severe malformation of the heart. **Situs inversus viscerum.** Lateral transposition of the abdominal and thoracic viscera. **Situs perversus.** Malposition of any viscus. **Situs solitus.** The normal position of any viscus. **Situs transversus.** Situs inversus viscerum (see above). [L place.]

sivvens (**siv**·ens). Sibbens.

Siwe, Sture August (b. 1897). Lund physician.

Letterer-Siwe disease. Systemic aleukaemic reticulo-endotheliosis or non-lipoid reticulo-endotheliosis in young children; it is characterized by a fatal progressive anaemia with haemorrhagic manifestations, splenomegaly, hepatomegalia, lymphadenopathy and a generalized hyperplasia of the reticulo-endothelial cells, resembling leukaemia clinically, but it is related in many ways to Hand-Schueller-Christian disease and to eosinophilic granuloma.

Sjögren, Henrik Samuel Conrad (b. 1899). Stockholm ophthalmologist.

Sjögren's disease. A syndrome characterized by deficient secretion of the lacrimal, salivary and other glands, giving rise to keratoconjunctivitis sicca, dry tongue and hoarse voice. It is frequently associated with rheumatoid arthritis and is chiefly confined to postmenopausal women. Now regarded as of the same nature as Mikulicz's disease.

skatole (**skat**·ole). 3-Methylindole, a crystalline foul-smelling substance present in faeces. It is formed in the intestine by the bacterial decomposition of tryptophan. [Gk *skatos* of dung.]

skatological (skat·o·**loj**·ik·al). Scatological.

skatology (skat·**ol**·o·je). Scatology.

skatophagia, skatophagy (skat·o·**fa**·je·ah, skat·**of**·ah·je). Scatophagia, scatophagy.

skatoxyl (skat·**ox**·il). 1. A radical which occurs in derivatives of skatole. 2. A compound which appears in urine pathologically. [Gk *skatos* of dung, oxygen.]

Skeer's sign. In tuberculous meningitis a narrow circular ring may be seen in both irises, close to the pupil.

skein (skane). A continuous tangled thread; a spireme. **Test skeins.** Skeins of coloured Berlin wool used in the colour-vision test originated by Holmgren. *See* TEST, WOOL. [O Fr. *escaigne*.]

skelalgia (skel·**al**·je·ah). Sensation of pain in the leg. [Gk *skelos* leg, *algos* pain.]

skelasthenia (skel·as·**the**·ne·ah). Lack of power in the muscles of the lower extremity, with consequent weakness of the legs. [Gk *skelos* leg, asthenia.]

skelatony (skel·**at**·on·e). Lowered tone of the vessels supplying the leg resulting in loss of normal heat, power and general comfort. [Gk *skelos* leg, atony.]

skeletal (**skel**·et·al). Relating or belonging to the skeleton. **Skeletal maturity.** Seen best in the appearance of the facial features, is under the control of hormones such as thyroid hormone, growth hormone and androgens.

skeletin (skel·e·tin). General term for gelatinous substances secreted by insects, e.g. chitin, which harden on exposure to form a skeletal frame.

skeletization (skel·et·i·za′·shun). 1. Extreme emaciation; the condition of being "reduced to a skeleton". 2. The process of removing the soft tissues from the skeleton, leaving the bones and remnants of ligaments.

skeletogenous (skel·et·oj·en·us). Producing skeletal tissue, structures or framework. [see foll.]

skeletogeny (skel·et·oj·en·e). The process of formation of the skeleton. [skeleton, Gk *genein* to produce.]

skeletology (skel·et·ol·o·je). The branch of anatomy and of mechanics which is concerned with the skeleton; osteology. [skeleton, Gk *logos* science.]

skeleton (skel·et·on). The framework around and within which the soft parts of the body are situated. This is the *endoskeleton,* consisting mainly of bones, but partly of cartilage, e.g. laryngeal cartilage, the cartilages of ribs, etc. The *exoskeleton,* hard tissues formed on the outer surface of the body, is well developed in some animals, e.g. invertebrates such as Crustacea, but is represented in man only by the nails and the enamel on the teeth. The fibrous framework of an organ may be referred to as its skeleton, e.g. the cardiac skeleton, consisting of the membranous part of the ventricular septum, the fibrous triangles and fibrous rings around the atrioventricular, pulmonary and aortic orifices. **Appendicular skeleton.** The skeleton of the appendages or limbs, including that of the pelvic and shoulder girdles. **Axial skeleton.** The skeleton of the trunk, including that of the head, but excluding the limb girdles. **Skeleton of the free lower limb [skeleton membri inferioris liberi (NA)].** The femur; tibia and fibula; the tarsus of 7 bones; 5 metatarsals; 14 phalanges, 2 in the big toe and 3 in each of the others. **Skeleton of the free upper limb [skeleton membri superioris liberi (NA)].** The humerus; radius and ulna; the carpus, containing 8 small bones arranged in 2 rows; 5 metacarpals; 14 phalanges, 3 in each finger and 2 in the thumb. **Visceral skeleton.** The bony framework enclosing the viscera; the sternum, ribs, vertebrae and pelvis. [Gk *skeletos* dried up.]

Skene, Alexander Johnston Chalmers (b. 1838). New York gynaecologist.

Skene's catheter. A glass, self-retaining catheter for the female bladder.

Skene's ducts, glands or tubules. The para-urethral ducts of the female urethra. Small ducts opening near the external urethral meatus, connected to vestigial glands believed to repesent the prostatic glands of the male.

skeneitis (skeen·i·tis). Inflammation of the para-urethral (Skene's) glands. [A. J. C. *Skene,* Gk *-itis* inflammation.]

skeneoscope (skeen·o·skope). An endoscope used in the examination of the para-urethral (Skene's) glands. [A. J. C. *Skene,* Gk *skopein* to view.]

skenitis (skeen·i·tis). Skeneitis.

skenoscope (skeen·o·skope). Skeneoscope.

skeocytosis (ske·o·si·to′·sis). The abnormal presence of immature or young forms of leucocytes (usually of the granular series) commonly noted as a deviation or shift to the left in the Arneth count. [Gk *skaios* left, *kytos* cell, *-osis* condition.]

skeptophylaxis (skep·to·fil·ax′·is). The desensitization of allergic individuals by the preliminary administration of small repeated doses of the allergen [Obsolete term.]. [Gk *skeptikos* doubtful, *phylax* guard.]

skevas-zerfus disease. Sponge-gatherers' disease, sponge-divers' disease; a disease of sponge-divers due to the poisonous secretion of a species of *Actinia* present in sea-water. The secretion on the skin causes an itching, a swelling, then a papule and finally a deep black ulcer, accompanied by shivering, pain and pyrexia.

Skey, Frederic Carpenter (b. 1798). London surgeon.

Skey's amputation. A variant of the mediotarsal amputation in which the 2nd metatarsal bone is divided at the level of the base of the 1st.

skiagram (ski·ah·gram). X-ray radiograph. [Gk *skia* shadow, *gramma* record.]

skiagraph (ski·ah·graf). X-ray radiograph. [Gk *skia* shadow, *graphein* to record.]

skiagraphy (ski·ag·raf·e). Radiography. [see prec.]

skialytic (ski·al·it·ik). Destroying or removing shadows. [Gk *skia* shadow, *lysis* a loosing.]

skiametry (ski·am·et·re). Retinoscopy. **Dynamic skiametry.** An objective method of measuring the accommodation by retinoscopy of the eyes in a state of active accommodation and convergence; this is achieved by the patient fixing a point on the retinoscope. More usually called *dynamic retinoscopy* in the UK. [Gk *skia* shadow, *metron* measure.]

skiaporescopy (ski·ap·or·es′·ko·pe). Retinoscopy, skiascopy; the procedure adopted in the objective determination of errors of refraction. [Gk *skia* shadow, *poros* opening, *skopein* to view.]

skiascope (ski·as·kope). 1. Retinoscope. 2. Retinoscopy rack. *See* RACK. [Gk *skia* shadow, *skopein* to view.]

skiascope-optometer (ski·ah·skope·op·tom′·et·er). An optometer used to determine errors of refraction by retinoscopy. [skiascope, optometer.]

skiascopy (ski·as·ko·pe). 1. Retinoscopy. 2. Fluoroscopy. [Gk *skia* shadow, *skopein* to view.]

skiatherapy (ski·ah·ther·ap·e). The treatment of disease by application of x-rays. [Gk *skia* shadow, therapy.]

skimmetin (skim·et·in). $C_9H_6O_3$, the aglycone obtained from skimmin by hydrolysis. It is a coumarin derivative.

Skimmia (skim·e·ah). A genus of shrubs of the family Rutaceae, endogenous to Japan. **Skimmia japonica.** A dwarf holly-like Japanese shrub containing the alkaloid skimmianine. [Jap. *skimmi.*]

skimmianine (skim·e·an·een). The alkaloid, $C_{14}H_{13}O_4N$, found in the leaves of *Skimmia japonica.*

skimmin (skim·in). $C_{15}H_{16}O_8$, the glucoside of skimmetin found in the bark of *Skimmia japonica.*

skin [cutis (NA)] (skin). The outer covering of the body, consisting of 2 layers, an inner, the dermis or corium, and an outer, the epidermis. **Anserine skin.** Goose flesh. *See* FLESH. **Citrine skin** (of Milian). Yellow, thickened, wrinkled skin due to prolonged exposure to the sun. **Crocodile skin.** A severe form of ichthyosis in which the skin consists of thick plaques like the skin of a crocodile. **Deciduous skin.** Exfoliated or shed skin. **Elastic skin.** Cutis hyperelastica. **Farmers' skin.** Pigmentation and keratosis of prominently exposed parts, e.g. the malar region, which may result in the development of rodent ulcers or epitheliomata; it is caused by continuous exposure to the elements, especially the ultraviolet rays of the sun. **Fish skin.** Ichthyosis. **Glossy skin.** Smooth, shiny skin caused by a trophic lesion. **Goose skin.** Goose flesh. *See* FLESH. **India-rubber skin.** Cutis hyperelastica. **Kava skin.** Swelling of the legs with coarse roughened skin, due to chronic intoxication with the drink produced from the Polynesian root, kava. **Lax skin.** Cutis laxa. **Leopard skin.** Extensive areas of depigmentation of the skin in onchocerciasis. **Lizard skin.** Thickened, lustreless, furrowed skin in onchocerciasis. **Marbled skin.** Cutis marmorata. **Paper skin, Parchment skin.** Thin, atrophic skin, sometimes wrinkled. **Piebald skin.** Unevenly depigmented skin, as in leucodermia and pinta. **Pig skin.** Dimpled skin as a result of lymphatic oedema. **Pink coloration of skin.** Due to post-mortem change upon exposure to cold and in CO and HCN poisoning. **Sailors' skin.** Farmers' skin (see above). **Scarf skin.** The epidermis. **Shagreen skin.** The appearance of connective tissue naevi, often seen with tuberous sclerosis (epiloia). **Toad skin.** Phrynoderma. **True skin.** Dermis. **Yolk skin.** The vitelline membrane which encloses the yolk. [AS *scinn.*]

Skinner's line. Shenton's line.

Sklowsky, E. L. 20th century German physician.

Sklowsky's symptom or test. A method suggested for the differential diagnosis of the vesicles of varicella and smallpox: light pressure by the index finger applied to the skin near, and then over, the lesion, ruptures the unilocular varicella vesicle but not the multilocular smallpox vesicle.

Skoda, Josef (b. 1805). Vienna physician.

Skoda's veiled puff. A faint inspiratory murmur which becomes suddenly loud and bronchial on deep inspiration. It is probably due to the sudden removal of an obstruction in a bronchial tube communicating with a cavity.

Skoda's sign. A high-pitched tympanitic percussion note heard above a pleural effusion; skodaic resonance.

skoliosis (sko·le·o·sis). Scoliosis. [Gk *skolios* curved.]

skoliosometer (**sko·le·o·som'·et·er**). Scoliosometer. [Gk *skolios* curved, *metron* measure.]

skopometer (sko·**pom**·et·er). Scopometer.

skotogram, skotograph (**sko**·to·gram, **sko**·to·graf). Scotogram, scotograph.

skull [cranium (NA)] (skul). The skeleton of the head, consisting of the calvaria overlying the brain, the facial skeleton (bony face) and the mandible [ossa cranii (NA)]. It is differentiated into an upper and a lower surface. **Base of the skull.** The floor of the calvaria. **Fenestrated skull.** Osteoporosis of the skull. **Geographical skull.** Map-like skull (see below). **Hot-cross bun skull.** The bossed head, with thickening of the frontal and parietal eminences, found in advanced rickets. **Map-like skull.** The radiographic appearance of the cranial bones in Hand-Schueller-Christian disease, due to irregularly shaped deposits of lipoid in both tables, causing map-like translucent areas. Also seen in Paget's disease (osteitis deformans). **Open-roofed skull.** A congenitally fissured skull. **Steeple skull.** Oxycephaly. **Stenobregmatic skull.** A skull in which the temporal region is abnormally narrow. **Surface of the skull, lower [basis cranii externa (NA)].** The irregular external surface of the base of the skull, including the hard palate in front and a broad flat plate of bone behind which bears the articular fossa for the mandible laterally and the foramen magnum centrally. **Surface of the skull, upper [basis cranii interna** (NA)]. The internal surface of the base of the skull, divided into anterior, middle and posterior cranial fossae. It bears many foramina for the passage of the cranial nerves and their branches and blood vessels, grooves for the meningeal vessels and shallow impressions for the cerebral gyri. **Tower skull.** Oxycephaly. [AS *skulle* bowl.]

See also: WEST (C.).

skull-cap (**skul**·cap). Calvaria. [skull, AS *caeppe*.]

slack (slak). A loose part. **Slack of the optic nerve.** The course of this nerve from the back of the eye to the optic foramen is somewhat sinuous, so as to prevent its being stretched during eye movements. The amount of slack is about 5.5 mm. [AS *sleac*.]

slake (slake). 1. To allay, cool or quench. 2. To mix with water so that disintegration occurs and a true chemical combination takes place. [AS *slacian*.]

slant (slahnt). The sloping surface of agar in a test-tube. [ME *slenten* to slope.]

slaver (**slav**·er). 1. To allow saliva to dribble from the mouth. 2. Saliva which flows involuntarily from the mouth. [Icelandic *slafur*.]

Slavianski's membrane. The basement membrane of a vesicular ovarian follicle.

sleep (sleep). The physiological process by which bodily functions are periodically rested. During sleep, consciousness and volition are partially or completely suspended and bodily activity generally is greatly reduced. **Crescendo sleep.** Sleep during which increasingly frequent muscular movements occur. **Electric sleep.** A state of anaesthesia instituted by passing a suitable electric current across the cerebral hemispheres. **Hypnotic sleep.** Sleep resulting from hypnosis. **Mesmeric sleep.** A state of anaesthesia induced by hypnosis. **Paroxysmal sleep.** Narcolepsy. **Prolonged sleep.** Prolonged narcosis. *See* NARCOSIS. **Twilight sleep.** A state of deep amnesia, analgesia and mental depression recommended by Gauss in 1906 for the relief of the pains of labour, produced by injections of morphine and hyoscine. [AS *slaep*.]

slide (slide). 1. A slip of glass on which objects are placed for microscopical examination. 2. A transparent rectangle on which is reproduced an illustration or other visual information for projection on to a viewing screen. **Histology slide.** A thin glass plate on which tissue sections are mounted prior to microscopical examination. **Microscope slide.** A thin glass plate on which objects are mounted for microscopical examination. [AS *slidan*.]

slime mould (**slime mo**·ld). Myxomycetes, forming the largest group of Mycetozoa. They are terrestrial organisms usually found in moist habitats on decaying wood, manure, decaying fungi, etc. [AS *slim*, mould.]

sling (sling). A bandage or other piece of cloth or material used for suspending a part. [ME.]

See also: GLISSON.

Slipules (**slip**·ewlz). A proprietary name for gelatin capsules for containing drugs that tend to cause vomiting if they dissolve in the stomach, e.g. emetine and bismuth iodide.

slit (slit). A narrow opening. **Filtration slit.** Slit pore. *See* PORE. **Gill slit.** One of a series of communications between the pharyngeal cavity and the exterior, separating successive pharyngeal arches, found in fishes and larval amphibians. **Slit of the microspectroscope.** A small, narrow opening, with parallel sides, limiting the light passing into the spectroscope used in conjunction with a microscope to examine the spectra of microscopical objects. [AS *slitan*.]

slit-sampler (**slit**·sahm·pler). A device for determining the bacterial population of samples of air. Air is sucked through a slit at a known rate, and is then made to impinge upon a segment of a rotating Petri dish. From the number of colonies of micro-organisms developing on the Petri dish after incubation, the bacterial content of the air sample can be calculated. [AS *slitan*, L *exemplum*.]

sloe (slo). The fruit of the blackthorn, *Prunus spinosa*. **Sloe gin.** A liqueur made by steeping sloes in gin. [AS *sla*.]

slope (slope). A tube of solid culture medium set in a sloping position; this allows the fluid to accumulate at the bottom and leave the surface of the medium dry, e.g. blood-agar slope, agar slope. **Potato slope.** A sterilized slice of potato used as a solid culture medium. [etym. dub.]

slough (sluf). 1. In general, any necrotic mass separated from the tissues, or the mass of dead tissue that is extruded from the surface of an ulcer. 2. To separate, as dead matter from living tissue. **Wash-leather slough.** A description given to the slough at the base of an ulcer, e.g. syphilitic, which consists of yellowish-green dead tissue. [ME *sluh* a husk.]

sloughing (**sluf**·ing). 1. The formation or separation of a slough. 2. Spermatogenesis developing in a disorderly fashion, so that the seminiferous tubules become choked with spermatozoa precursors and there is no lumen along which mature spermatozoa could pass if indeed they were formed.

Sluder, Greenfield (b. 1865). St. Louis laryngologist.

Sluder's guillotine. A guillotine for the tonsillectomy operation.

Sluder's method. 1. An operation for the evisceration of the ethmoidal labyrinth, for which Sluder designed special knives; an intranasal method for ablation of the ethmoidal labyrinth. 2. Injection of the sphenopalatine ganglion through the greater palatine foramen.

Sluder's operation. Enucleation of the tonsil.

Sluder's syndrome. A lower-half headache or unilateral facial pain, mainly in the orbital region and at the root of the nose. Also called *sphenopalatine ganglion neuralgia*.

sludge (sluj). The sediment obtained by treatment of sewage. **Activated sludge.** That which is produced by aeration of sewage and causes growth of oxidizing bacteria. **Dewatered sludge.** Sludge from which the water has been eliminated by a pressing or drying process. [etym. dub.]

sludging (**sluj**·ing). The settling of solid particles from suspension, forming a thick sludge at the bottom of a fluid. **Sludging of blood.** The settling or agglutination of blood corpuscles in and blocking the blood vessels, so that blood flow is impaired; it may occur in certain diseases or after injury and is believed to be an important factor in shock.

smallpox (**smawl**·pox). Variola; a generalized virus infection with a vesicular rash. Two main varieties, variola major and variola minor (alastrim), are described. They are clinically very similar but mortality in the major variety can be up to 30 per cent, while that in the minor is less than 1 per cent. This variable severity is a property of the infecting strain and strains of intermediate virulence also occur. The incubation period is 12 days, followed by a predromal influenza-like illness, which may be severe, and lasts 2-3 days. The rash appears 2 days later with deep-seated vesicles and showing a mainly centrifugal distribution. The rash progresses through the stages of macule, papule, vesicle, pustule and crust, with lesions in 1 area being at the same stage. Residual scarring is common. Death is mostly in the early stages and, in fulminating cases, may occur without the development of the rash. Treatment of cases is supportive (mostly correction of dehydration) while contacts should be vaccinated or given methisazone orally. The disease was the subject of a 10-year eradication campaign by the World Health Organisation started in 1966. By 1976 the only remaining endemic area in the world was Ethiopia where only a few foci remained, and it is likely to be the first major infectious disease to be eradicated as a deliberate act. **Abortive smallpox.** A term suggested for "illness among smallpox contacts", the modified disease occurring in persons previously vaccinated. Sometimes there is primary fever only and no rash *(variola sine variolis).* **African smallpox.** Variola major. **American smallpox.** Variola minor. **Black smallpox.** Haemorrhagic smallpox (see below). **Bovine smallpox.** Cowpox [obsolete term]. **Classical smallpox.** Variola major. **Confluent smallpox.** A severe form with confluent lesions, particularly on the face. **Haemorrhagic smallpox.** A form of smallpox with haemorrhages into the skin and mucosae. It indicates a severe infection and a bad prognosis. **Modified smallpox.** Mild clinical smallpox due to a partial immunity from vaccination. It can resemble mild chickenpox and is difficult to distinguish clinically. Such patients can shed fully infectious smallpox virus. (AS *smael, pocc*).

smartweed (**smart**·weed). Water pepper, pepperwort; the dried herb of *Polygonum hydropiper* (family Polygonaceae). [AS *smeortan, weod.*]

smegma (**smeg**·mah). 1. A sebaceous substance with a peculiar odour and secreted by small preputial glands on the corona glandis and neck of the penis. 2. The sebum. **Smegma of the clitoris.** The sebaceous substance secreted by the glands around the clitoris and labia minora. **Smegma embryonum.** The vernix caseosa. [Gk soap.]

smegmatic (smeg·**mat**·ik). Relating or belonging to, or characterized by smegma.

smegmolith (**smeg**·mo·lith). A preputial concretion. *See* CONCRETION. [smegma, Gk *lithos* stone.]

Smellie, William (b. 1697). London obstetrician.

Smellie's scissors. Strong scissors with cutting edges in the outer sides of the blades; used in craniotomy.

Mauriceau-Smellie-Veit manoeuvre, Smellie-Mauriceau-Veit manoeuvre or method. To deliver the after-coming head. The child is placed astride one arm and the middle and forefingers are placed over the upper jaw on each side of the nose. This maintains the head in an attitude of flexion. The ring and little finger of the other hand are applied over the child's right shoulder and the thumb is placed over the left shoulder. Traction is now exerted in a downward and backward direction until the head is brought into the pelvis. Gentle pressure suprapubically facilitates this manoeuvre. The child's body is now carried up towards the mother's abdomen and the head delivered slowly over the perineum.

Smilax (**smi**·lax). A genus of climbing smilaceous plants (family Liliaceae). The dried roots of *Smilax aristolochiaefolia* and other species are known as sarsaparilla. **Smilax pseudochina.** The rhizome of *Smilax china,* a plant endogenous to China and Japan and known as China-root; used like sarsaparilla. [Gk bindweed.]

smile (smile). **Levator smile, Nasal smile.** An expression peculiar to some patients with myasthenia gravis in which the normal movements observed at the angles of the mouth are absent. [ME.]

Smillie, Ian Scott. 20th century Scottish orthopaedic surgeon.

Smillie's knives. Special knives with an end cutting blade designed for the operation of meniscectomy.

Smith, Albert J. (fl. 1889). Dublin obstetrician.

Smith pessary. A vulcanite vaginal pessary used for maintaining the uterus in anteversion.

Smith, Erwin Frink (b. 1854). American bacteriologist.

Smith-Noguchi culture medium. A medium composed of fresh rabbit kidney tissue in sterile ascitic fluid under Vaseline in narrow tubes; it is prepared aseptically without heat.

Smith, Eustace (b. 1835). London physician.

Smith's disease. Mucous colitis. *See* COLITIS.

Eustace Smith's murmur or sign. A humming noise heard by auscultation over the manubrium sterni, produced by blood moving in the thoracic veins when the head is thrown backwards, in patients with bronchial obstruction.

Smith, Ferris (b. 1884). Grand Rapids, Michigan, otolaryngologist.

Ferris Smith operation. An external operation on the anterior group of air sinuses.

Smith, Sir Grafton Elliot (b. 1871). British anatomist and anthropologist.

Elliot Smith area paraterminalis. The paraterminal body. *See* BODY.

fasciculus of Elliot Smith. Fasciculus precommissuralis; fibres of various origins which pass through the septum in front of the anterior commissure and the lamina terminalis.

Smith, Henry (b. 1862). British surgeon in India.

Smith's clamp. A clamp with ivory-backed blades, for use in the cauterization of haemorrhoids.

Smith's operation. 1. The clamp and cautery treatment of haemorrhoids. 2. Extraction of a cataract with the capsule intact, by pressure on the cornea, below with an instrument like a squint hook, and above, at the posterior edge of the incision, with a special form of spatula. No capsule forceps are used; obsolete.

Smith-Indian method. Of cataract extraction. Smith's operation, 2nd def.

Smith, Nathan (b. 1762). American surgeon.

Smith's amputation. Semicircular-flap amputation.

Smith, Priestley (b. 1845). Birmingham ophthalmologist.

Priestley Smith tape. In strabismus. Two tapes are attached to a ring which is placed over an ophthalmoscope and the end of 1 tape, which is 1 m in length, is held by the patient to his nose; the second tape is marked in degrees and held horizontally at right angles to the first. The examiner then shines the light from the ophthalmoscope towards the patient's eyes and with the normal eye the patient watches his finger as it moves along the horizontal tape. The examiner watches the corneal reflex in the squinting eye, and when this becomes central or slightly nasal to the centre he reads off the angle of squint on the tape at the position of his finger.

Smith, Robert William (b. 1807). Irish surgeon.

Smith's fracture. A fracture of the lower end of the radius, with forward displacement of the lower fragment.

Smith, Sir Thomas (b. 1833). London surgeon.

Tom Smith's disease. Loss of the head of the femur from acute inflammation of the epiphysis in infancy.

Smith-Petersen, Marius Nygaard (b. 1886). Boston orthopaedic surgeon.

Smith-Petersen mould arthroplasty. An arthroplasty of the hip using a vitallium cup to reform the articular surfaces; cup arthroplasty.

Smith-Petersen nail or pin. A special metal 3-flanged nail used for fixing fractures of the neck of the femur.

Petersen's operation. Nailing of the neck of the femur after fracture.

Smithwick, Reginald Hammerick (b. 1899). American surgeon.

Smithwick's operation. Thoracicolumbar sympathectomy for hypertension.

smog (smog). A dark, dense form of fog which is heavily laden with smoke particles; of colloquial origin. [smoke, fog.]

smudging (**smuj**·ing). Faulty speech characterized by non-utterance of consonants which are difficult to pronounce. [ME *smogen.*]

snail (snale). Any gastropod mollusc with a spiral shell, but especially land and fresh-water forms. Many fresh-water and amphibious forms are secondary hosts of parasitic flukes. Laboratory-class snails are the garden snail and the Roman snail. [AS *snagel.*]

snake (snake). A serpent; a limbless reptile covered with characteristic scales from which the species can be recognized. Many are poisonous to man. **Coral snake.** A poisonous snake of the genera *Elaps* or *Callophis.* **Cottonmouth snake.** A poisonous snake of the sub-family Lachesinae, *Agkistrodon piscivorus,* found in America and Asia. **Sea snake.** Any snake of the family Hydrophinae; they are mostly poisonous. **Tiger snake.** A poisonous snake of the sub-family Elapinae, *Notechis scutatus,* found in Australia. For other snakes, see under their names. [AS *snacan* to creep.]

snake root (**snake** root). Name given to certain plants believed, with little reason, to be effective against snake bite. **Black snake root.** Cimicifuga. **Button snake root.** *Liastris spicata* (family Compositae), a plant indigenous to southern Ontario, the root of which has a warm, bitter taste and diuretic properties. **Canada snake root.** Asarum; the dried rhizome and roots of *Asarum canadense* (family Aristolochiaceae), containing a bitter acrid resin and a volatile oil. **Senega snake root.** Polygala; the dried root of *Polygala senega* (family Polygalaceae), containing saponins. **Texas snake root.** Serpentaria. **Virginian snake root.** Serpentaria. **White snake root.** The dried leaves and flowering tops of *Eupatorium rugosum* (family Compositae). [snake, AS *rot.*]

snakeweed (**snake**·weed). Pill-bearing spurge, cat's hair; the dried plant of *Euphorbia pilulifera* (family Euphorbiaceae), containing several glycosidic resins. [snake, AS *weod.*]

snakewort (**snake**·wert). Bistort, adder's weed; the dried rhizome of *Polygonum bistorta* (family Polygonaceae), a perennial herbaceous plant containing about 20 per cent of tannin. [snake, AS *wyrt.*]

snap (snap). A sharp clicking or cracking sound. **Opening snap.** In cases of mitral stenosis, a sharp clicking sound, as a rule to be heard in the fourth left intercostal space immediately after the beginning of the second heart sound. [ME *snappen.*]

snare (snare). A wire loop used in removing tumours and polypi. The loop is passed around the projection and drawn tight so that the mass is either removed by the roots or cut off at its base. **Cold snare.** An unheated snare. **Galvanocaustic snare.** Hot snare (see following). **Hot snare.** A wire snare which is raised to red or white heat by galvanic current and used for the burning-off of growths. [AS *sneare.*]

See also: FRANKFELDT, JARVIS.

sneeze (sneez). 1. To make a spasmodic, explosive and audible expiration of air through the nose and mouth. 2. An involuntary, explosive audible expiration through the mouth and nose; a reflex caused by irritation of the nasal mucosa. **Pregnancy sneeze.** Sudden attacks of sneezing occurring during pregnancy, caused by congestion of the nasal mucous membrane and resulting from circulatory disorder. [ME *snesen.*]

Snell, Esmond Emerson (b. 1914). Wisconsin biochemist.

Snell-Strong method. For riboflavine. A microbiological method in which the growth stimulation of *Lactobacillus casei* is measured by titration of the acid produced by the organism in a basal medium to which an extract of the sample has been added.

Snell, Simeon (b. 1851). Sheffield ophthalmologist.

Snell's law. In the case of a ray of light which passes from one medium to another, the sine of the angle of incidence bears a ratio to the sine of the angle of refraction that is a constant for the 2 given media.

Snell cell. A one-fluid voltaic cell with an anode of zinc and a cathode of platinized silver immersed in a dilute solution of sulphuric acid. It furnishes an emf of 0.75 V. Also known as *Smee cell.*

Snellen, Hermann (b. 1834). Utrecht ophthalmologist.

Snellen's chart or test-type. The usually accepted test for distant visual acuity, consisting of black capital letters on a white board, properly illuminated. The letters are of varied size and labelled in terms of the distance, e.g. the largest letter 60 (metres) and the smallest 4 (metres). The patient usually stands at 6 m and the visual acuity is recorded as a fraction, the nominator being the distance of the patient from the letters and the denominator the size of the smallest letters accurately read, e.g. 6/6.

Snellen's operation. 1. For senile and paralytic ectropion; also called *Snellen's ectropion suture*: a double-armed suture is inserted through the everted conjunctiva at the edge of the tarsus nearest to the lid margin. The suture is then passed through the eyelid, brought out, and tied over the skin 2 cm below the eyelid margin. 2. For entropion; also called *Snellen's entropion suture*: a double-armed suture is passed through the conjunctiva in the fornix, out through the skin of the lower lid, and then back beneath the skin of the eyelid to emerge just anterior to the lash margin where it is tied. 3. For entropion with deformed tarsal plate; a modification of Streatfield's operation: excision of a wedge-shaped strip of tarsus in its whole length about 5 mm above the eyelid margin, the apex of the wedge being deep, but the conjunctiva is not incised. When sutured the lash margin and lower tarsus segment are turned outward.

Snellen's reflex. Congestion of the ear resulting from stimulation of the cut end of the great auricular nerve.

Snellen's sign. Ocular bruit sometimes heard in exophthalmic goitre.

Snelling's reaction. For emetine: an orange-red colour changing to violet, resulting when a solution containing emetine is dropped on to a mixture of potassium chlorate and hydrochloric acid.

snore (snore). 1. To breathe during sleep or in coma, with a hoarse, rough sound caused by vibration of the uvula and the soft palate. 2. The hoarse, rough sound so produced. [AS *snora.*]

Snow's sign. A prominence of the upper part of the sternum, due to secondary carcinoma of the thymus from a primary in the breast.

snow (sno). **Carbon-dioxide snow.** Solid carbon dioxide, at a temperature of about −62°C (−80°F). By its intense cooling effect when applied locally it destroys tissues, and is therefore used in the treatment of warts and cutaneous vascular naevi. [AS *snaw.*]

snuff (snuf). Any powder which is inhaled through the nostrils and which is usually irritating to the nasal membrane. **Niopo snuff.** A narcotic snuff produced from the seeds of a Venezuelan plant, *Piptadenia peregrina.* Not used in orthodox medicine. [abbr. of D *snuiftabak* snuffing-tobacco.]

snuffbox (**snuf**·box). **Anatomical snuffbox.** The hollow on the radial side of the wrist formed between the tendons of the extensor pollicis brevis and extensor pollicis longus muscles when the thumb is extended. [snuff, L *buxum* boxwood.]

snuffles (**snuf**·lz). Obstruction of the nose accompanied by discharge of catarrh from the nasal mucosa, encountered chiefly in infants and usually those with congenital syphilis. [AS *snofl* mucus.]

soap (sope). A detergent substance prepared by boiling natural oils or fats with caustic alkali; used for cleaning the skin and also pharmaceutically in the preparation of liniments. **Animal soap.** Curd soap (see below). **Castile soap.** A hard soap prepared from olive oil and sodium hydroxide. **Curd Soap BPC 1963.** Sapo animalis, principally sodium stearate, prepared by the saponification of purified solid animal fats with sodium hydroxide. It is a yellowish or greyish-white solid, easily pulverizable when dry but can be moulded when heated. It is only slightly soluble in cold water but completely so in hot water and in alcohol. Used as a pill excipient. **G.11 soap.** An antiseptic soap containing G.11 (hexachlorophane), used for the cleansing of surgeon's hands. **Green soap.** Soft soap (see below). **Hard Soap BPC 1963.** Sapo durus, a soap prepared by the saponification of any vegetable oil with sodium hydroxide and usually consisting mainly of sodium oleate. It is a yellowish or greyish solid, easily powdered when dry but can be moulded when heated; soluble in cold water or in alcohol. It was formerly used as a laxative by oral administration in conjunction with purgatives such as rhubarb and aloes. It is employed in pharmacy as a pill excipient and also in the preparation of various soap plasters. **Soap Liniment BP 1958.** A liniment prepared by dissolving soft soap, camphor and rosemary oil in a mixture of alcohol (90 per cent) and distilled water. **Linseed-oil soap.** Potash soap (see below). **Soap plaster.** A plaster prepared from hard soap, lead plaster and colophony; often used as a protection for corns and bunions. **Potash soap.** Sapo kalinus, a soft soap prepared by heating linseed oil with aqueous potassium hydroxide. **Soft Soap BP 1973.** Sapo mollis, a soap prepared by the saponification of suitable vegetable oils with sodium or potassium hydroxide and concentration of the resultant solution so as to retain the glycerol. It may be anything from yellowish-white to brown in colour depending on the oil used in preparation, and if chlorophyll is added the product is known as *green soft soap.* It is readily soluble in cold water or in alcohol, and is used for cleaning the skin and scalp, and as a constituent of soap liniment for direct application in the treatment of sprains and bruises. **Soap spirit.** A solution of soft soap in alcohol (90 per cent) and containing 65 per cent w/v of soft soap. **Superfatted soap.** A soap containing more than the usual amount of fatty acids over and above that required for the neutralization of the alkali used in its preparation. **Zinc soap.** A soap obtained by the reaction between a soluble zinc salt, usually zinc sulphate, and sodium stearate; it consists mainly of zinc stearate but may also contain varying proportions of the oleate and palmitate. It is a white powder, used in the treatment of certain skin infections. [L *sapo.*]

soap bark (sope bark). Quillaia.

soaproot (sope·root). 1. Soapwort. 2. Yucca. [soap, AS *rot.*]

soapwort (sope·wert). Soaproot, bouncing bet, fuller's herb; the dried leaves and root of *Saponaria officinalis* (family Caryophyllaceae), which contains saponins. [soap, AS *wyrt.*]

sob (sob). 1. To draw breath in convulsive gasps, caused by diaphragmatic contraction and spasmodic closure of the glottis. 2. The sound so produced. [ME *sobben.*]

Sobernheim's serum. An anti-anthrax serum prepared in sheep or cattle.

Sobernheim's test. A test for the potency of smallpox vaccine lymph. A papilliform infiltration of the line of incision should appear 3 days after inoculation of the skin of a rabbit with a 1:1000 dilution of lymph.

sobrerole (sob·rer·ole). $C_{10}H_{16}(OH)_2$, a crystalline dihydric alcohol formed from pinene by exposure to the air and moisture in sunlight.

socia parotidis (so·she·ah par·ot·id·is). The accessory parotid gland. [L companion of the parotid.]

Social Security Act 1975. This Act consolidates the provisions of the Social Security Act 1973, which established a basic scheme of contributions and benefits, and the National Insurance (Industrial Injuries) Acts 1965 to 1974. The Act provides for a comprehensive and compulsory scheme of insurance against industrial injuries and industrial diseases, disablement, incapacity and death. The scheme covers all employed earners affected by any of the above misfortunes arising out of and in the course of employment. The benefits, payable in respect of the injury benefit period during which a person is incapable of work, may be enhanced during hospital treatment, or in respect of special hardship cases. Certain specific benefits in respect of prescribed diseases attributable to the employment and which ought to have been treated are also allowable. Regulations under the Act may provide for requiring claimants for injury benefit or disablement benefit to submit themselves to medical examination or treatment. The funds required for paying such benefits out of the National Insurance Fund are provided by means of four classes of contributions payable by earners, employers and others.

socialization (so·shal·i·za′·shun). The process by which the individual is adapted to his social environment, and becomes a recognized, co-operating, and efficient member of it. [L *socius* companion.]

Socin, August (b. 1837). Swiss surgeon.

Socin's operation. Enucleation of a thyroid adenoma.

sociology (so·she·ol·o·je). The science which is concerned with the development, constitution and laws of human society. [L *socius* companion, Gk *logos* science.]

sociomedical (so·she·o·med′·ik·al). Concerned with the relation of medicine and the other social services.

sock (sok). 1. A shortened stocking covering only the foot and ankle. 2. A loose inner sole for a boot or shoe. **Stump sock.** A conical woollen sock that is pulled over the end of an amputation stump to act as a buffer and to reduce the friction between the stump and the artificial limb. [AS *socc.*]

socket (sok·et). In dentistry, a cavity in the alveolar bone of the jaw [alveolus dentalis (NA)] which accommodates the root of a tooth. **Dry socket.** A tooth socket which, after a tooth extraction, is devoid of blood clot, either due to lack of formation of a clot or to its disintegration when formed owing to infection. It is accompanied by severe pain and a foul odour, and is a localized osteomyelitis. [O Fr. *soket.*]

socordia (so·kord·e·ah). Hallucination. [L folly.]

soda (so·dah). A loose term for alkaline sodium salts. Used without qualification, it usually means sodium carbonate. **Baking soda.** Sodium bicarbonate. **Caustic soda.** Sodium hydroxide. **Chlorinated soda.** An aqueous solution of sodium hypochlorite, NaOCl, prepared by the electrolysis of sodium chloride solution or by the action of sodium carbonate on chlorinated lime. A non-staining and non-irritant antiseptic solution. **Tartrated soda.** Soda potassium tartrate. **Washing soda.** Sodium carbonate. **Soda water.** Water charged with carbon dioxide under pressure; it may contain a small proportion of sodium bicarbonate. [etym. dub.]

soda-carmine (so·dah·kar·mine). A stain used for injection in bulk. [soda, carmine.]

sodaemia (so·de·me·ah). The presence of excess sodium in the blood. [sodium, Gk *haima* blood.]

sodic (so·dik). Relating to sodium or having sodium in its composition.

sodium (so·de·um). An element of atomic weight 22.9898, atomic number 11 and chemical symbol Na (*natrium*). It is a soft, white metal of the alkali series, related to potassium and extremely reactive, oxidizing rapidly in air and acting violently with water to generate hydrogen. It occurs as sodium chloride in sea water (1 per cent) and as the nitrate in the vast Chilean deposits. It is a microconstituent of practically all plant and animal tissue, and is considered essential to life. Physiologically, the sodium ion takes part in the ionic balance of the body, maintains tissue excitability, and because of the solubility of its salts plays an important rôle in the transport of metabolites. **Sodium acetanilide sulphonate.** An antipyretic used as a substitute for antipyrin. **Sodium acetarsol.** The sodium salt of acetarsol, used for similar purposes. **Sodium Acetate BP 1973.** CH_3COONa, a compound used as a diuretic and to increase the alkalinity of the urine. **Sodium Acetrizoate.** BP Commission approved name for sodium 3-acetylamido-2,4,6-tri-iodobenzoate, $C_6HI_3(COONa)(NHCOCH_3)$, an x-ray contrast medium used for the same purposes as diodone, but said to cause fewer and less severe side effects. **Sodium acetylarsanilate.** $C_6H_4NHCOCH_3AsO_3HNa$, a compound which has been used similarly to sodium aminoarsonate (see below). **Sodium acetylsalicylate.** $NaOOCC_6H_4OOCCH_3$, a soluble compound used similarly to aspirin. **Sodium acid borate.** A compound used in keratitis and conjunctivitis. **Sodium Acid Citrate BP 1973.** A compound with uses similar to those of the preceding salt, but it makes an acid solution with dextrose, and thus allows heating with less caramelization. **Sodium Acid Phosphate BP 1973.** Sodium dihydrogen phosphate, $NaH_2PO_4{\cdot}2H_2O$, a compound used for making the urine acid during the administration of hexamine. It is also employed as a diuretic. **Sodium acid sulphosalicylate.** Sodium sulphosalicylate (see below). **Sodium albuminate.** A sodium derivative of albumin in which the protein forms the anion. **Sodium Alginate BPC 1968.** The sodium salt of alginic acid extracted from species of seaweed. It is used as an emulsifying agent. **Sodium aminoarsonate, Sodium aminophenylarsenate.** $NH_2C_6H_4As(OH)ONa$, an arsenical derivative used in the treatment of syphilis and protozoal infections. **Sodium Aminosalicylate BP 1973, Sodium *p*-aminosalicylate.** $C_6H_3(NH_2)(OH)COONa{\cdot}2H_2O$, the sodium salt of *p*-amino salicylic acid (PAS). It is used in the treatment of tuberculosis, especially pulmonary; the best results are obtained when it is administered simultaneously with streptomycin. **Sodium amytal.** Sodium iso-amylethyl barbiturate, a short-acting barbiturate, used as a sedative, hypnotic and as a basal narcotic pre-operatively. **Sodium anhydromethylenecitrate.** An anti-lithaemic drug which liberates formaldehyde in the blood. **Anhydrous sodium arsenate.** Na_2HAsO_4, a compound used as a spirochaeticide and trypanocide. **Anhydrous Sodium Carbonate BPC 1959.** Na_2CO_3, sodium carbonate heated to dryness; it is used in pills and tablets. **Anhydrous Sodium Phosphate BPC 1959.** Sodium phosphate (see below) without water of crystallization. **Anhydrous Sodium Sulphate BPC 1959.** NA_2SO_4; its uses are similar to those of the crystalline salt, but it can be used in effervescent powders better in this form. **Sodium aniline arsenate.** Sodium aminoarsonate (see above). **Sodium aniline sulphonate.** Sodium sulphanilate (see below). **Sodium anisate.** An antiseptic and antipyretic. **Sodium Anoxynaphthonate BP 1963.** Sodium 4′-anilino-8-hydroxy-1,1′-azonaphthalene-3,6,5′-trisulphonate; a diagnostic aid. A dye of low toxicity used in measuring cardiac output and to define the position of cardiac shunts. **Sodium antimonyl tartrate.** Antimony sodium tartrate, $C_4H_6O_6SbONa$, a trivalent organic antimony compound used like antimony potassium tartrate (tartar emetic). *See* ANTIMONY. **Sodium antimonyl thioglycollate.** An organic antimony compound used in the treatment of granuloma inguinale. **Sodium Antimonylgluconate BP 1968.** A trivalent preparation of antimony that has been used in schistosomiasis and in cutaneous leishmaniasis (oriental sore) where the trivalent are more effective than the pentavalent preparations. **Sodium Apolate.** BP Commission approved name for poly(sodium ethylenesulphonate); an anticoagulant. **Sodium arsanilate.** Sodium aminoarsonate (see above). **Sodium arsenate.** Anhydrous sodium arsenate (see above). **Sodium arsenotartrate.** An arsenic salt used in skin diseases in place of potassium arsenite. **Sodium aurate.** $NaAuO_2$, a gold salt used as an antiseptic. **Sodium aurochloride.** $NaAuCl_4$, a gold salt used in syphilis. **Sodium Aurothiomalate BP 1973.** A soluble salt, mainly $COOHAuSCHCH_2COOH$, used in arthritis for which purpose it is replacing sodium aurothiosulphate. **Sodium aurothiosulphate.** Gold sodium thiosulphate, $Na_3Au(S_2O_3)_2{\cdot}2H_2O$, a compound used intravenously in the treatment of lupus erythematodes, and of value in syphilis and trypanosomiasis; also for gold therapy in the treatment of rheumatoid arthritis but great caution is necessary. **Sodium Benzoate BP 1973.** C_6H_5COONa, a soluble salt of benzoic acid used sometimes as an expectorant and as an antipyretic. It is chiefly employed as a urinary antiseptic. **Sodium benzosulphimide.** Saccharin. **Sodium benzoylglycine.** Sodium hippurate (see below). **Sodium betanaphthol.** Sodium naphtholate (see below). **Sodium biborate.** Sodium borate (see below). **Sodium Bicarbonate BP 1973.** $NaHCO_3$, a compound which reduces acidity in the stomach sometimes followed by an increased secretion of hydrochloric acid due to the stimulatory action of the carbon dioxide evolved. It is used extensively in lozenges and tablets for dyspepsia and flatulence, and also in effervescent preparations, mixed with citric and tartaric acids. **Sodium bi-iodosalicylate.** Sodium di-iodosalicylate (see below). **Sodium biphosphate.** Sodium acid phosphate (see above). **Sodium bismuth citropyroborate.** A compound used in dyspepsia and gastritis. **Sodium bismuthate.** $NaBiO_3$, a compound used in chemical analysis as a reagent for manganese. **Sodium bismuthyltartrate.** Bismuth sodium tartrate. **Sodium bisulphate.** $NaHSO_4{\cdot}H_2O$, a compound used for removing typhoid bacilli from drinking water and also internally as an antiferment. **Sodium bisulphite.** $NaHSO_3$, an anti-oxidant employed to stabilize pharmaceutical solutions. Medicinally, it has been used as an antiseptic in gastric fermentation and in parasitic skin diseases. **Sodium biurate.** A substance believed to be the deposit upon the joint tissues in gouty arthritis. **Sodium borate.** Borax. **Sodium borobenzoate.** A mixture of sodium borate and sodium benzoate used as an antiseptic and antilithic. **Sodium borosalicylate.** A soluble antiseptic and preservative. **Sodium borosulphate.** A compound used both internally and externally as an antiseptic. **Sodium Bromide BP 1973.** NaBr, a compound which, like potassium bromide, depresses the central nervous system in order of dosage from above down. It is used in nervous diseases, particularly in epilepsy, to diminish the excitability of the cerebral cortex, and also as a sedative in nervous anxiety and overwork. Prolonged overdosage may lead to symptoms of brominism, the drug being cumulative. **Sodium cacodylate.** $(CH_3)_2AsO_2Na{\cdot}3H_2O$, an organic arsenical that acts like an inorganic arsenic compound; no longer used therapeutically on account of its toxicity. **Sodium caffeine sulphate, Sodium caffeine sulphonate.** A compound used as a diuretic in cardiac oedema. **Sodium Calciumedetate BP 1973.** The chelate compound of calcium with the disodium salt of ethylenediamine *N,N,N′,N′*-tetra-acetic acid. **Sodium cantharidate.** A preparation of sodium hydroxide and cantharides that has been tried subcutaneously in tuberculosis. **Sodium carbolate.** Sodium phenate (see below). **Sodium Carbonate BP 1958.** $Na_2CO_3{\cdot}10H_2O$, crystalline sodium carbonate, a compound used chiefly externally, the non-irritant bicarbonate being preferred internally. Used in skin diseases as a lotion and occasionally as a mouth-wash. **Sodium carbonate monohydrate.** $Na_2CO_3{\cdot}H_2O$, sodium carbonate with 1 molecule of water of crystallization; used as a water softener. **Sodium Carboxymethylcellulose BPC 1968.** $[C_6H_{10-a}O_5(CH_2CO_2Na)_a]_m$, prepared from chloroacetic acid, cellulose and sodium hydroxide. It is used for suspending insoluble powders in aqueous preparations, including mixtures. Some grades of the substance are also used as bulk purgatives. **Sodium chlorate.** $NaClO_3$, a compound with medicinal properties similar to potassium chlorate. It may be used in stomatitis and in laryngitis as a gargle, or in pastilles or lozenges. **Sodium Chloride BP 1973.** Common salt, NaCl, a compound widely distributed in nature and essential in the diet. A 0.9 per cent solution is used for perfusions and irrigations (*physiological saline*). Excess loss of sodium chloride from the body due to excessive sweating causes heat cramps which are relieved by drinking weak salt solution. Hypertonic solutions are used as fomentations; large quantities of saline by mouth, particularly hypertonic, irritate the gastro-intestinal tract causing nausea and vomiting. **Sodium chloroborate.** A compound used as an antiseptic. **Sodium choleate.** Dried, purified ox gall used as a laxative in chronic constipation. **Sodium cinnamate.** $C_6H_5CH{=}CHCOONa$, the sodium salt of cinnamic acid; it has been used as a remedy for phthisis but is not a curative agent in tuberculosis. **Sodium Citrate BP 1973.** $COONaCH_2C(OH)(COONa)CH_2COONa{\cdot}2H_2O$, a compound that is oxidized in the tissues to alkali carbonate which is excreted; this renders the urine alkaline. It also has diuretic, diaphoretic, expectorant and sudorific actions. Added to shed blood it prevents clotting; it is also added to milk in infant feeding to prevent curdling by rennin in the stomach. **Sodium citrobenzoate.** A compound used in the treatment of asthma and bronchitis and as a diuretic and antilithic. **Sodium citrosphosphate.** A mixture of sodium phosphate, sodium nitrate and citric acid, used in liver complaints. **Sodium citrotartrate.** Granules containing sodium bicarbonate, citric acid and tartaric acid. **Sodium copaivate.** A yellow, water-soluble powder used as an antiseptic and diuretic. **Sodium cresylate.** An alkaline salt of cresol used as an antiseptic. **Sodium Cromoglycate BP 1973.** The disodium salt of 1,3-di(2-

carboxy-4-oxochromen-5-yloxy)propan-2-ol; used by inhalation in the treatment of asthma. **Sodium cyanide.** NaCN, an extremely poisonous compound acting like hydrocyanic acid; rarely used in medicine. **Sodium Cyclamate BP 1968.** Sodium cyclohexylsulphamate; a sweetening agent that is 30 times as sweet as sugar and leaves no bitter after-taste. It is useful for diabetics, but should be avoided where there is renal damage and in subjects on a low-salt diet. **Sodium desoxycholate.** The sodium salt of desoxycholic acid occurring in the bile salts. **Sodium Diatrizoate BP 1973.** Sodium 3,5-diacetamido-2,4,6-tri-iodobenzoate; an intravenous contrast medium used in urography. **Sodium dibromercurate.** A soluble mercurial compound occasionally injected hypodermically in syphilis. **Sodium Dibunate.** BP Commission approved name for sodium 2,6-di-*tert*-butylnaphthalenesulphonate; a cough suppressant. **Sodium dihydrogen phosphate.** Sodium acid phosphate (see above). **Sodium di-iodofluorescein.** A compound related to erythrosin. The particular compound containing the radioactive isotope of iodine is used in the localization of brain tumours. Injected intravenously, the solution tends to concentrate in brain-tumour cells. The site of the lesion is determined by measuring the radiation emitted at different points on the surface of the head. The method is unsuited to posterior-cranial-fossa tumours. **Sodium di-iodoparaphenol sulphonate.** Sodium sozoiodolate (see below). **Sodium di-iodosalicylate.** An analgesic and antiseptic used externally on parasitic sores. **Sodium dimethylarsonate.** Sodium cacodylate (see above). **Sodium dioxide.** Na_2O_2, a compound used as a bleaching agent and disinfectant. **Sodium diphenylhydantoinate.** An anticonvulsant with a variable or hypnotic action, used in the treatment of epileptic patients who are not benefited by phenobarbitone or bromides. **Sodium diphosphate.** Sodium acid phosphate (see above). **Sodium Diprotrizoate.** BP Commission approved name for sodium 3,5-dipropionamido-2,4,6-tri-iodobenzoate; a radio-opaque substance. **Sodium-2,6-ditertiarybutylnaphthalene monosulphonate.** A compound used in the form of a linctus for the treatment of all types of cough. **Sodium dithionate.** Sodium thiosulphate (see below). **Sodium dithiosalicylate.** A compound, the α salt of which is used externally as an antiseptic chiefly in veterinary practice. The β salt is used in the treatment of rheumatism. **Sodium Edetate BP 1963.** Disodium dihydrogen ethylenediamine-*N,N,N′,N′*-tetra-acetate dihydrate; it is used in the treatment of hypercalcaemia and in ophthalmology. **Effervescent sodium phosphate.** A mixture which contains 50 per cent sodium phosphate with sodium bicarbonate and tartaric acid; a pleasant way of giving sodium phosphate. **Effervescent sodium sulphate.** An effervescent preparation of sodium sulphate containing sodium bicarbonate, tartaric and citric acids; a pleasant way of administering sodium sulphate. **Sodium ethoxide.** Caustic alcohol, C_2H_5ONa, a very rapid and powerful caustic, used in alcoholic solution. **Sodium ethoxyphenyl succinamide.** Sodium phenosuccinate (see below). **Sodium ethyl sulphate.** $C_2H_5OSO_2ONa{\cdot}H_2O$, a crystalline substance used as a cathartic. **Sodium ethylate.** Sodium ethoxide (see above). **Exsiccated sodium arsenate.** Anhydrous sodium arsenate (see above). **Exsiccated sodium carbonate.** Anhydrous sodium carbonate (see above). **Exsiccated sodium phosphate.** Anhydrous sodium phosphate (see above). **Exsiccated sodium sulphate.** Anhydrous sodium sulphate (see above). **Sodium fluorescein.** A brownish-yellow dye which fluoresces strongly in solution. Solutions have been used in the diagnosis of corneal ulcers. **Sodium Fluoride BP 1973.** NaF, a compound which has been given internally in the form of a very dilute solution for the treatment of phthisis and toxic goitre. It destroys bacteria and vermin such as beetles and cockroaches. As a calcium precipitant it prevents blood clotting and is very toxic to tissues. **Sodium fluoroacetate.** Compound 1080, a substance used as a rodent poison. In action it interferes with the citric-acid cycle. **Sodium fluosilicate.** Sodium silicofluoride (see below). **Sodium formate.** $HCOONa{\cdot}H_2O$, a compound which has a marked diuretic action. It has also been used in lumbago and rheumatism. **Sodium Fusidate BP 1973.** The sodium salt of fusidic acid, an antimicrobial substance produced by the growth of *Fusidium coccineum*; an antibiotic active against Gram-positive organisms, including penicillin-resistant strains of *Staphylococcus aureus*. **Sodium Glucaldrate.** BP Commission approved name for sodium gluconatodihydroxyaluminate; it is used in the treatment of gastric hyperacidity. **Sodium Glucaspaldrate.** BP Commission approved name for octasodium tetrakis(gluconato)bis(salicylato)-μ-diacetatodialuminate(III) dihydrate; an analgesic. **Sodium glycerinoborate, Sodium glyceroborate.** A compound used for its antiseptic properties and for soothing and cleansing mucous membranes. **Sodium glycerophosphate, Sodium glycerylphosphate.** A compound claimed to be of value to aid metabolism, especially for providing phosphorus, and as a nerve tonic; its value is doubtful. **Sodium glycholate, Sodium glycocholate.** A bile salt used as a cholagogue for liver congestion, gall-stones and in constipation. **Gold sodium thiosulphate.** Sodium aurothiosulphate (see above). **Sodium guaiacol carbonate.** Sodium methylsalicylate, a compound used in the treatment of rheumatism. **Sodium gynocardate.** A compound used in leprosy. **Sodium hexametaphosphate.** Sodium polymetaphosphate (see above). **Sodium hippurate.** Sodium benzoylglycine, a compound which occurs in the urine of herbivorous animals, sometimes in man. It is used to increase the excretion of uric acid in gout and rheumatism. **Sodium hydnocarpate.** The sodium salts of part of the fatty acids of hydnocarpus oil, used for leprosy. It is given by hypodermic, intramuscular or intravenous injection. **Sodium hydrate, Sodium Hydroxide BP 1973.** NaOH, a powerful caustic which has been used externally to destroy naevi and warts. While a weak solution may be used as an antacid and diuretic, sodium bicarbonate is preferred. **Sodium hypobromite.** NaOBr, a compound used like sodium hypochlorite (see following) as an oxidizing agent. **Sodium hypochlorite.** NaOCl, a powerful disinfectant and deodorant with strong bleaching properties. Used for disinfection and for irrigation of infected wounds (Dakin's solution) and as a gargle or spray. **Sodium Hypophosphite BPC 1963.** NaH_2PO_2, a compound which, like the other hypophosphites, has no therapeutic value. **Sodium hyposulphite.** Sodium thiosulphate (see below). **Sodium ichthyol, Sodium ichthyolsulphonate, Sodium ichthyosulphonate.** A substance prepared by neutralizing ichthyolsulphonic acid with sodium hydroxide; it is used as a mild antiseptic in cutaneous disorders. **Sodium indigosulphate, Sodium indigotindisulphonate.** Indigo carmine; a compound used as a test for renal efficiency. **Sodium iodate.** $NaIO_3$, a compound used as a dusting-powder with boric acid, or in saturated solution as a dressing for ulcers. It is also employed like potassium chlorate in inflammatory conditions of mucous membranes. **Sodium Iodide BP 1973.** NaI, a compound with properties very similar to those of potassium iodide but less irritating to the stomach. **Sodium iodobismuthite.** Bismuth sodium iodide, Na_2BiI_5, a compound used as an antisyphilitic; claimed to penetrate the cerebrospinal canal. **Sodium iodohippurate.** Sodium ortho-iodohippurate (see below). **Sodium Ipodate.** BP Commission approved name for sodium 3-(3-dimethylaminomethylenamino-2,4,6-tri-iodophenyl)propionate; a radio-opaque substance. **Sodium Ironedetate.** BP Commission approved name for the iron chelate of the monosodium salt of ethylenediamine-*N,N,N′,N′*-tetra-acetic acid. **Sodium isoamylethyl barbiturate.** Sodium amytal (see above). **Sodium kussinate.** A compound used to expel tapeworms. **Sodium lactate.** $C_3H_5O_3Na$, a compound mainly used as an alkalinizing solution for parenteral use in the treatment of acidosis. It may also make the urine alkaline. **Sodium Lauryl Sulphate BP 1973.** A mixture of the sodium salts of sulphated normal aliphatic alcohols, mainly $C_{12}H_{25}OSO_2ONa$. It is an anionic detergent, stable in the presence of appreciable quantities of acids, alkalis and heavy metals. It also inhibits the growth of Gram-positive bacteria. **Sodium loser.** A patient who as the result of deficiency of cortisol or aldosterone has a loss of salt from the body. **Sodium lygosinate.** The sodium salt of dioxydibenzol acetone, used in gonorrhoea. **Sodium and magnesium borocitrate.** A white, antiseptic powder used in lithiasis. **Sodium mandelate.** $C_6H_5CHOHCOONa$, a salt used for the treatment of infections of the urinary tract, particularly those due to *Bacterium coli* and other bacillary organisms, also *Streptococcus faecalis*. **Sodium mercurophenyl disulphonate.** A compound used as an antiseptic and antisyphilitic. **Sodium Metabisulphite BP 1973.** $Na_2S_2O_5$, a compound which, in water, yields sodium bisulphite (see above). It is used as an anti-oxidant, e.g. in solutions of adrenaline. **Sodium meta-oxycyanocinnamate.** A substance used in dyspepsia and gastro-intestinal atony as an antiseptic stimulant. **Sodium metavanadate.** $NaVO_3$, an alterative and a substitute for arsenic. **Sodium methoxysalicylate.** Sodium guaiacol carbonate (see above). **Sodium Methyl Hydroxybenzoate BP 1973.** The sodium derivative of methyl 4-hydroxybenzoate; a preservative. **Sodium methylarsenite.** $Na_2(CH_3)AsO_3$, an arsenical compound used like sodium cacodylate. **Sodium methylsalicylate.** Sodium guaiacol carbonate (see above). **Sodium methylsulphate.** A compound used as a cathartic. **Sodium Metrizoate.** BP Commission approved name for sodium-3-acetamido-2,4,6-tri-iodo-5-*N*-methylacetamidobenzoate. **Sodium monosulphate.** Anhydrous sodium sulphate, Na_2SO_4, used as a purgative. **Sodium morrhuate.** A mixture of the sodium salts of the fatty acids of cod-liver oil. Most frequently used as a sclerosing agent in the treatment of varicose veins, haemorrhoids and hydrocele; it has also been employed in the treatment of lupus and leprosy. **Sodium naphthol, Sodium naphtholate, Sodium β-naphtholate.** A compound used externally as an antiseptic and internally as an antiseptic and antipyretic. **Neutral sodium borate.** An antiseptic for wounds and eye diseases. **Neutral sodium citrate.** A compound used as a purgative in genito-urinary diseases. **Sodium nitrate.** $NaNO_3$. Chile saltpetre, a compound rarely used in medicine. **Sodium Nitrite BPC 1968.** $NaNO_2$, a compound which slowly liberates the nitrite ion and is used in angina pectoris and asthma to lessen arterial tension and as a general vasodilator. **Sodium nitroferricyanide, Sodium nitroprusside.** A poisonous chemical reagent used to detect acetone bodies and aldehydes; it is also used to reduce blood pressure during hypotensive anaesthesia, because of its direct effect on the vessel walls. **Sodium nucleas, Sodium nucleinate.** A compound used in puerperal infections and in pneumonia. **Sodium Octoate BPC 1954.** $C_8H_{15}O_2Na$, a compound used as a fungicide. **Sodium oleate.** The sodium salt of oleic acid; a hard soap used internally in laxative pills, also in plasters to protect corns and bunions. **Sodium orthodinitrocresylate.** A compound used as an insecticide and in the treatment of scabies. **Sodium ortho-iodohippurate.** Sodium iodohippurate; a compound used in excretion urography. **Sodium orthophosphate.** Sodium phosphate (see below). **Sodium orthovanadate.** Sodium vanadate (see below). **Sodium ossalinate.** The sodium compound of the acid of ox marrow, used as a substitute for cod-liver oil. **Sodium oxide.** Sodium peroxide (see below). **Sodium oxyalphanaphtholate, Sodium α-oxynaphtholate.** An antiseptic and antipyretic. **Sodium oxybate.** Sodium gamma-hydroxybutyrate, an intravenous anaesthetic. **Sodium paracresotate.** The sodium salt of oxytoluic acid; it is used in acute rheumatism. **Sodium parafluorbenzoate.** A compound used in tuberculosis. **Sodium paranitrobenzoate.** An antistreptococcal compound. **Sodium pentachlorophenate.** $NaOC_6Cl_5$, a highly efficient molluscicide. **Sodium pentanucleotide.** A preparation of sodium pentose nucleotides obtained by the hydrolysis of nucleic acid with sodium hydroxide. **Sodium Perborate BPC 1968.** $NaBO_2,H_2O_2{\cdot}3H_2O$, an antiseptic and deodorant, used as a dusting-powder, and to prepare antiseptic solutions where it liberates oxygen. **Sodium percarbonate.** $Na_2CO_3{\cdot}1\frac{1}{2}H_2O_2$, an oxygen-antiseptic used in mouth-washes and in wound cleansing. Sodium perborate is usually preferred. **Sodium peroxide.** Sodium oxide, Na_2O_2, a yellow-white powder dissolving in water with the production of heat and liberating oxygen; it is used as a bleaching agent. **Sodium persulphate.** $Na_2S_2O_8$, a compound which has strong oxidizing and bleaching actions; it is used occasionally as an antiseptic gargle and as moist dressing for small wounds and ulcers. **Sodium phenate.** C_6H_5ONa, prepared by mixing phenol and sodium hydroxide; it is used as a gargle and disinfectant in solution. **Sodium phenolphthaleinate.** The sodium salt of phenolphthalein. **Sodium phenolsulphonate.** A substance which resembles phenol in its actions but is much less toxic. **Sodium phenosuccinate.** An antipyretic and antineuralgic. **Sodium Phosphate BP 1973.** Disodium hydrogen phosphate, $Na_2HPO_4{\cdot}12H_2O$, a comparatively tasteless, mild, saline cathartic. **Sodium Picosulphate.** BP Commission approved name for disodium 4,4′-(2-pyridyl)methylenedi(phenyl sulphate); a laxative. **Sodium polyborate.** Sodium borate (see above). **Sodium Polymetaphosphate BPC 1968.** A compound prepared from sodium acid phosphate by heating; it is used as a dusting powder. **Sodium polystyrene sulphonate.** A sodium-saturated ion-exchange resin for removing excess potassium ions. It is issued as a fine powder for use in hyperkaliaemia, and in chronic uraemia associated with high serum potassium. **Sodium potassium bismuthyl tartrate.** A basic water-soluble bismuth compound used in the treatment of syphilis, either in solution or in oil suspension. **Sodium Potassium Tartrate BPC 1968.** Rochelle salt, $COONa(CHOH)_2COOK{\cdot}4H_2O$, a saline cathartic producing a watery evacuation without irritation. Small doses are diuretic and make the urine less alkaline. Used in gout and rheumatism as a mild purgative. It is the active constituent in Seidlitz powders; also used in the preparation of Fehling's solution. **Sodium Propionate BPC 1954.** CH_3CH_2COONa, a compound used as a fungicide. **Sodium Propyl Hydroxybenzoate BP 1973.** The sodium derivative of propyl 4-hydroxybenzoate; a preservative. **Sodium pyroborate.** Sodium borate (see above). **Sodium pyrophosphate.** $Na_2P_4O_7{\cdot}10H_2O$, a compound which has a laxative action stronger than sodium phosphate but is rarely used. **Sodium pyrosulphite.** Sodium metabisulphite (see above). **Sodium quadriurate.** A urate found in urine during gout. **Sodium γ-resorcylate.** The sodium salt of 2,6-dihydroxy benzoic acid; $C_6H_3(OH)_2COONa$. It is claimed to be more effective than the salicylates in the treatment of rheumatic fever. **Sodium rhodonate.** Sodium thiocyanate (see below). **Sodium ricinoleate.** A mixture of the sodium salts of the fatty acids from castor oil. It reduces surface tension in solution, and is employed as an emulsifying agent. Solutions are used in infections of the mouth, and as sclerosing agents in the treatment of varicose veins. **Sodium rosanilinsulphonate.** Acid fuchsine, magenta, a dye used in the form of carbolfuchsine as a reagent in microscopy, also as a colouring agent, and in ointment form for impetigo. **Sodium rosolate.** A dyestuff used as an indicator. **Sodium saccharate, Sodium saccharinate.** Soluble saccharin, a sweetening agent and intestinal antiseptic. **Sodium Salicylate BP 1973.** $C_6H_4(OH)COONa$, a valuable antipyretic and antirheumatic drug; it also has a mild gastric antiseptic and mild cholagogue action. It has been employed as a sclerosing agent for varicose veins. **Sodium santoninate.** A combination of sodium carbonate or sodium hydroxide with santonin. Its use as a vermifuge should be avoided because of its liability to absorption. **Sodium silicate.** Water-glass, a substance used chiefly in industry and as an egg preservative. Medicinally it has been used as an antiseptic. **Sodium silicofluoride.** Na_2SiF_4, a toxic compound used as an insect exterminator and rat poison. **Sodium sozoiodolate.** An antiseptic used in phthisis. **Sodium stearate, Sodium stearinate.** A mixture of varying proportions of sodium stearate and sodium palmitate, used for pharmaceutical purposes as a substitute for wax in ointments, as a basis for vanishing creams and in glycerin suppositories. **Sodium Stibogluconate BP 1973.** A pentavalent antimony derivative of gluconic acid that is effective in the treatment of kala-azar. In solution it is stable and can therefore be supplied in ampules ready for injection. It can be given intravenously or intramuscularly. **Sodium succinate.** A compound which, injected hypodermically, increases the leucocytes in the blood. It is also used for alkalinizing the urine. **Sodium sulphanilate.** Sodium aniline sulphonate; a compound said to alleviate coryza. **Sodium sulphapyridine.** The sodium salt of sulphapyridine with properties similar to sulphanilamide but less readily absorbed and more readily giving rise to crystals in the urine. Sulphathiazole and sulphadiazine are now more widely used. **Sodium Sulphate BP 1973.** Glauber salt, $Na_2SO_4{\cdot}10H_2O$, a saline hydragogue cathartic, rapid in action, very little absorbed, that will abstract water from the tissues of the intestinal wall; used in habitual constipation due to deficient peristalsis. Mixed with sodium bicarbonate (Carlsbad salt) it is used in constipation associated with gout and hepatic disorders. **Sodium Sulphite BPC 1968.** $Na_2SO_3 \cdot 7H_2O$, a compound used as an antioxidant and reducing agent, also as an antiseptic and antizymotic. It has been used internally for fermentative dyspepsia and also as a mouth-wash in stomatitis; externally it is employed as a lotion in parasitic skin diseases. It liberates sulphur dioxide when mixed with acid and may be used as a food preservative. **Sodium sulphobenzoate.** A compound used as a urinary antiseptic. **Sodium sulphocarbolate.** Sodium phenolsulphonate. **Sodium sulphocyanate.** Sodium thiocyanate (see below). **Sodium sulphoichthyolate.** A dark-brown tarry substance used like ichthammol. **Sodium sulphoricinate.** A compound used as a detergent in soapless shampoos and as a wetting agent. It is an emulsifying agent and will dissolve iodine, resorcinol and naphthalene; it has been used in place of glycerin. **Sodium sulphosalicylate.** A compound used as an antiseptic and antipyretic. **Sodium sulphovinate.** Sodium ethyl sulphate (see above). **Sodium sulphurosobenzoate.** A relatively non-toxic antiseptic. **Sodium tartrate.** $NaOOC(CHOH)_2COONa \cdot 2H_2O$, a saline purgative like potassium tartrate. **Sodium taurocholate.** A bile salt used as a cholagogue and as an aid to pancreatic digestion in biliary deficiency. It is used externally with eucalyptus oil to destroy pediculi. **Sodium Tauroglycocholate BPC 1954.** Bile salts; prepared from ox or pig bile by extracting with alcohol, decolorizing with charcoal and precipitating the salt by the addition of excess of ether. It is given in capsules in cases of biliary deficiency. **Sodium tellurate.** A compound which is poisonous in large doses; small doses have a marked anhidrotic action. **Sodium tetraborate.** Sodium borate (see above). **Sodium tetrabromphenolphthalein, Sodium tetrabromphthalein.** A compound which has been used in cholecystography. **Sodium tetradecyl sulphate.** Sodium 7-ethyl-2-methyl-4-hendecanol sulphate, a white waxy water-soluble odourless anionic surface-active agent. It also has a sclerosing effect and is used in the treatment of varicose veins. **Sodium tetraiodophenolphthalein.** A compound administered internally as a contrast medium in x-ray of the gall bladder. **Sodium thiocarbonate.** Na_2CS_3, a compound analogous to sodium carbonate; it is a heavy brownish oil. **Sodium thiocyanate.** NaCNS, a compound used in essential hypertension. **Sodium thio-ethamyl.** Iso-amylethylthiobarbiturate. **Sodium thiolinate.** A soluble preparation of thiolin and soda used like ichthammol in skin diseases. **Sodium thiophenate.** A white powder used in ointment form for prurigo. **Sodium thiophene sulphonate.** A white scaly powder used as an antiseptic for prurigo and skin disease. **Sodium thiosulphate BPC 1968.** $Na_2S_2O_3 \cdot 5H_2O$, a compound chiefly used intravenously as an antidote in cases of overdosage with arsphenamine compounds, or salts of bismuth and gold. Used as a fixer in photographic processes, and industrially as an antichlor for removing chlorine. **Sodium thorium tartrate.** Thorium sodium tartrate. **Sodium trichlorocarbolate, Sodium trichlorophenol.** An antiseptic soluble in hot water, and more active but more irritant than phenol. **Sodium trioxybismuthobenzoate.** A soluble bismuth compound used as an antisyphilitic. **Sodium triphenylrosaniline.** Alkali blue, a dye used as an indicator in volumetric analysis. **Sodium tungstate.** A complex salt used as a laboratory reagent. **Sodium Tyropanoate.** BP Commission approved name for sodium 2-(3-butyramido-2,4,6-tri-iodobenzyl) butyrate; a contrast medium. **Sodium valerianate, Sodium valerate.** A compound used as a nerve sedative in hysteria and other neurotic conditions. **Sodium vanadate.** Na_3VO_4, a compound which has been used in anaemia, diabetes, tuberculosis and neurasthenia, with doubtful benefit. **Vinbarbital sodium.** Sodium 5-ethyl-(1-methyl-1-butenyl) barbiturate. A sedative and hypnotic. **Sodium xanthogenate.** An antiseptic. [soda.]

sodoku (so·do·koo). Rat-bite fever. *See* FEVER. [Jap. *so* rat, *doku* poison.]

sodomist, sodomite (sod·om·ist, sod·om·ite). An individual who practises sodomy.

sodomy (sod·om·e). Anal intercourse between men. [*Sodom*, a town of ancient Palestine, see Gen. xix. 4.]

Soemmering, Samuel Thomas von (b. 1755). Frankfurt physician.

Soemmering's foramen. The fovea centralis of the retina.

Soemmering's ganglion or grey substance. The substantia nigra of the mid-brain.

Soemmering's ligament. Fibres connecting the lacrimal gland with the orbital periosteum.

Soemmering's muscle. The levator glandulae thyroideae muscle.

Soemmering's nerve. The perineal branch of the posterior cutaneous nerve of the thigh.

Soemmering's ring or crystalline swelling. An annular swelling of the peripheral portion of the lens capsule following extracapsular cataract extraction. This is caused by the adherence of the anterior and posterior capsules in this region and the proliferation of the capsule cells inside.

Soerensen, Johann (b. 1862). Berlin surgeon.

Soerensen's operation. An operation for the radical excision of the larynx in malignant disease.

Glueck-Soerensen method or operation. Removal of the larynx performed from above downwards. The hypopharynx is entered and inspected during the early stages of the operation.

softening (sof·en·ing). A degenerative process whereby an organ or tissue loses its firmness, becomes soft, breaks down and is finally destroyed. **Acute gastric softening.** A post-mortem change in the stomach wall, due to acid digestion and leading to softening. **Anaemic softening.** Infarction or softening of a part of the central nervous system due to cessation or diminution of its blood supply. **Softening of the bones.** Any pathological condition in which the mineral content of the bones is diminished. **Softening of the brain.** 1. Actual softening of cerebral substance; encephalomalacia. 2. The term is sometimes applied colloquially to dementia paralytica in which there is generalized degeneration of the cerebral cortex. **Colliquative softening.** A form of necrosis in which the tissue is softened and converted into a semi-liquid mass. **Green softening.** The softening which occurs in purulent encephalitis, the green colour being due to the presence of pus. **Grey softening.** A form of softening of nervous tissue in which myelin is almost completely absorbed and the remaining tissue is grey in colour: seen in demyelinating diseases. **Haemorrhagic softening.** Degenerative changes accompanied by haemorrhage. **Softening of the heart.** Softening as the result of an infarct in the heart wall caused by obstruction of a coronary artery. **Inflammatory softening.** Softening as a result of any inflammatory process. **Mucoid softening.** Mucoid or myxomatous degeneration. **Oesophageal softening.** Ulceration of the oesophageal mucous membrane; post-mortem digestion with softening is common. **Pyriform softening.** Yellow softening (see below). **Red softening.** An infarct or area of softening into which haemorrhage has occurred; or an area of softening which is congested. **Softening of the spinal cord.** Softening of cord substance; myelomalacia. It may be due to infarction, inflammation or degeneration. **Softening of the stomach.** Destruction of the wall by degenerative or ulcerative changes; post-mortem digestion of the stomach. **Softening of a thrombus.** The digestion and break-down of a thrombus which may become partially or wholly absorbed. **White softening.** The terminal stage of the process of softening; degeneration of myelin ends in the deposition of white lipoid substance in the affected area. **Yellow softening.** A stage of degeneration in an area of softening preceding the end state (white softening, see above); the degenerating myelin is yellow in colour. [AS *softe*.]

soil (soil). 1. The top layer of earth in which plants and micro-organisms grow. It has been formed geologically by the weathering of rocks and minerals and consists mainly of inorganic silicates and decomposed organic matter (humus). Its chemical properties are the subject of much research for agricultural reasons. 2. Figuratively, the organism infected; used in contrast to the "seed", the infecting micro-organism. [L *solum* ground.]

soja (so·yah). Soya.

sokosho (so·**ko**·sho). Rat-bite fever. *See* FEVER. [Jap. *so* rat, *ko* bite, *sho* disease.]

sol (sol). Suspensoid. Any colloidal system in which the disperse phase is a solid suspended in a continuous liquid phase. Such colloids are of biological importance, comprising as they do the tissue proteins. **Metallic sol.** A sol formed by certain metals, principally gold, silver and copper, which is catalytic and is used as such in industry and in medicine. [contraction of *solution.*]

solandrine (so·**lan**·dreen). An alkaloid of uncertain composition obtained from the plant *Solandra laevis.* It resembles hyoscine in properties. [Charles *Solander* of Sweden.]

solaneine (so·lan·e·een). A mixture of the alkaloids solanine and solanidine, found in *Solanum dulcamara* (family Solanaceae), the bittersweet, woody nightshade or dulcamara.

solangustidine (so·lan·**gus**·tid·een). $C_{27}H_{43}O_2N$, an amorphous alkaloid occurring in *Solanum angustifolium.*

solangustine (so·lan·**gus**·teen). $C_{33}H_{53}O_7N$, a crystalline glycoside found in *Solanum angustifolium* (family Solanaceae). It hydrolyses into glucose and the alkaloid solangustidine.

solanidine (so·**lan**·id·een). $C_{27}H_{43}ON$, an alkaloid from the potato plant, *Solanum tuberosum* (family Solanaceae) and other species of *Solanum.* It is steroid in structure.

solanine (**so**·lan·een). $C_{42}H_{75}NO_{12}$, an alkaloidal glycoside present in the woody nightshade, *Solanum nigrum,* the potato, *S. tuberosum,* and other solanaceous plants. It hydrolyses into the alkaloid, solanidine, and a mixture of the monosaccharides, glucose, galactose and rhamnose. It is haemolytically toxic.

solanism (**so**·lan·izm). The condition of being poisoned by ingestion of solanine.

solanoid (**so**·lan·oid). Denoting a certain type of carcinoma which in texture resembles a raw potato. [solanum, Gk *eidos* form.]

solanoma (so·lan·**o**·mah). A carcinoma which resembles a potato in texture. [L *solanum* potato, Gk *-oma* tumour.]

Solanum (so·**la**·num). A genus of plants of the family Solanaceae, including the potato and the nightshades. **Solanum carolinense.** The horse-nettle, apple of Sodom, sandbrier or poisonous potato. **Solanum crispum.** A plant the leaves and shoots of which are a constituent of natri. **Solanum dulcamara.** Bittersweet, woody nightshade, dulcamara; a climbing plant with purplish cymose flowers with yellow anthers; all portions are poisonous, containing solanine and solanidine. **Solanum gayanum.** A constituent of the Chilean drug, natri. **Solanum insidiosum.** A Brazilian species. **Solanum mammosum.** Macaw bush; a plant indigenous to the West Indies. **Solanum nigrum.** Black nightshade, poison berry; an annual herb with small white flowers and globular fruits which has been used as an adulterant of belladonna leaf; it contains the alkaloidal glycoside, solanine. **Solanum oleaceae.** A herb of tropical America. **Solanum paniculatum.** A Brazilian species. **Solanum tomatillo.** A plant the leaves and shoots of which are constituents of the Chilean drug, natri. **Solanum tuberosum.** The potato; a perennial herb with swollen tubers which are used for food. The plant itself may contain solanine. [L nightshade.]

Solapsone BP 1968 (sol·**ap**·sone). $[C_6H_5CH(SO_3Na)CH_2CH(SO_3Na)NHC_6H_4]_2SO_2$, a water-soluble derivative of diaminodiphenyl sulphone used in the treatment of leprosy. It has also been used in tuberculosis, but it is inferior to combined treatment with PAS and streptomycin. Solapsone is a bacteriostatic of the sulphonamide type in so far as it is competitively inhibited by *p*-aminobenzoic acid. It is given by mouth or parenterally.

solar (**so**·lar). 1. Relating or referring to the sun, to sunlight or to the heat of the sun. 2. Produced by the action of the sun. [L *sol* sun.]

solarium (so·**la**·re·um). 1. A room or gallery enclosed in glass in which sun baths can be taken. 2. A room in which treatment by artificial light is given. [L balcony exposed to the sun.]

solarization (so·lar·i·za′·shun). 1. Exposure to sunlight. 2. Treatment by means of exposure to sunlight or electric light and the results of such treatment. 3. The loss of permeability to ultraviolet (short) rays of the sun that occurs with certain makes of glass after prolonged exposure to sunlight. [L *sol* sun.]

solarize (**so**·lar·ize). To expose to the rays of the sun. [see prec.]

solation (sol·a·shun). The formation of a sol by the liquefaction of a gel.

sole (sole). 1. [Planta (fibularis) (NA)]. The sole or plantar surface of the foot with its lateral [margo lateralis (NA)] and medial [margo medialis (tibialis) (NA)] borders. 2. [Planta pedis (NA)]. The region of the sole of the foot. 3. The sarcoplasm, containing several nuclei, of a motor end-plate on a striated muscle fibre. [L *solea.*]

sole-plate (**sole**·plate). A motor end-plate of striated muscle.

soleal (**so**·le·al). Relating to the soleus muscle. **Soleal line.** *See* LINE.

Solenoglypha (so·len·**og**·lif·ah). A name not now used taxonomically for those snakes which carry hollow poison fangs on the maxillae. [Gk *solen* tube, *glyphein* to carve.]

solenoid (**so**·len·oid). A hollow tube wound with a coil of wire: when an electric current is passed through the coil a magnetic field is created axially along the tube capable of drawing in a loose plunger or attracting an armature. It is used to operate switchgear. [Gk *solen* tube, *eidos* form.]

Solera's reaction or test. For thiocyanates in saliva: test papers are prepared by saturating filter paper with 0.5 per cent starch solution containing 1 per cent iodic acid, drying in the air and cutting into strips. The test paper is moistened with saliva and the appearance of a blue colour due to liberation of iodine from the iodate and formation of starch iodide indicates thiocyanate.

soleus muscle [musculus soleus] (**so**·le·us musl). A muscle of the calf arising from the posterior aspects of the tibia and fibula and inserted, in common with the gastrocnemius muscle, into the tuberosity of the calcaneum. [L *solea* sole of foot.]

solferino (sol·fer·e·no). Fuchsine. [*Solferino,* Italy.]

solid (**sol**·id). 1. A phase, neither gaseous nor liquid, in which the molecules are in close proximity and considerably reduced in motion. 2. Dense; free from holes or hollowness. 3. An object with 3 dimensions and occupying a definite volume. [L *solidus.*]

Solidago (sol·id·**a**·go). A genus of composite-flowered plants, the golden rods. **Solidago virgaurea.** Aaron's rod, the species chiefly used in medicine, the leaves being aromatic and carminative. [LL.]

Solifugae (sol·**if**·ew·ge). Solpugidae. [L *sol* sun, *fugare* to flee.]

solipsism (**so**·lip·sizm). In metaphysics, the belief or theory, (*a*) that the self can know only its own states and modifications, and (*b*) that there is only subjective reality. [L *solus* only, *ipse* self.]

solitary (**sol**·it·ar·e). 1. Single; alone. 2. Not associated with other organisms in a group. [L *solitarius* standing alone.]

Solovieff's phenomenon. Spasmodic contractions of the diaphragm in tetany.

Solpugidae (sol·**pew**·jid·e). An order of Arachnida, the sun spiders. The species are principally desert forms and are characterized by the relatively enormous chelicerae. Their bites are not poisonous but very painful. Solifugae. [L *solpuga* venomous spider.]

solubility (sol·ew·**bil**·it·e). The ability of a solute to dissolve in a specified solvent: defined as the number of grams of the former required to saturate 100 g of the latter at a given temperature. **Solubility curve.** The expression graphically of the variation with temperature of the solubility of a given substance in a specified solvent. [see foll.]

soluble (**sol**·ewbl). Able to dissolve. [L *solubilis.*]

solum [NA] (**so**·lum). The lowest part of a structure; the sole. [L.]

solute (**sol**·ewt). The substance which dissolves in a solvent to form a solution. [L *solutus* dissolved.]

solution (sol·**ew**·shun). 1. The dispersion of a substance (the solute) throughout a liquid (the solvent) to form a homogeneous mixture, from which the solute may be recovered by purely physical processes such as crystallization or distillation, though ionization may have occurred whilst it was in solution. 2. The homogeneous molecular mixture formed by one or more substances, whether solid, liquid or gaseous, with another substance, usually a liquid, but also sometimes a solid (e.g. the solution of one metal in another to form an alloy). 3. Specifically, in pharmacy, a liquor, or in chemistry, a reagent used in a particular test, e.g. Fehling's solution. 4. Resolution, e.g. the solving of a problem, or the termination of an inflammation; separation, e.g. of the continuity of solid tissue such as bone. **Acid solution.** A solution containing an excess of hydrogen ions, i.e. of pH value lower than 7. **Adrenaline Solution BP 1973.** A solution of adrenaline and chlorbutol in sodium chloride and metabisulphite with hydrochloric acid. **Alcoholic solution.** A solution of any substance in alcohol; in pharmacy, a spirit or tincture. **Alibour solution.** Eau d'Alibour; an antiseptic solution of the sulphates of zinc and copper in camphor water. **Alkaline solution.** A solution containing an excess of hydroxyl ions, i.e. of pH value higher than 7. **Solution of Amaranth BPC 1959.** A solution of amaranth in chloroform water used as a colouring agent. **Ammonia Solution, Dilute BP 1958.** A solution of 10 per cent w/w of ammonia in distilled water, used as a restorative. **Ammonia Solution, Strong BP 1958.** A solution of 32.5 per cent ammonia in distilled water. **Ammoniacal silver solution.** A solution of silver nitrate and excess ammonia used in testing for reducing substances, e.g. tartrates, which cause silver to be deposited. **Ammonium thiocyanate solution.** A reagent used by analysts for detecting iron and determining silver, mercury, halogens, etc. **Anaesthetic solution.** A solution of a drug to be used as an anaesthetic. Various solutions are applied to the surface or injected subcutaneously for local anaesthesia, injected into or round the nerve trunk for regional anaesthesia, into the subarachnoid space for spinal anaesthesia, into the rectum for basal narcosis, or into a vein for general anaesthesia. **Aqueous solution.** A solution of any substance in water; in pharmacy, a liquor or aqua. **Arsenical Solution BPC 1959.** A neutral solution of arsenic trioxide in potassium hydroxide with dilute hydrochloric acid to neutralize; used in stomatitis and Vincent's angina. Fowler's solution. **Basic lead-acetate solution.** Lead subacetate solution (see below). There are 2 solutions of basic lead acetate in the *British Pharmacopoeia;* one is 80 times the strength of the other. They are used in lotions for the treatment of bruises. **Buffer solution.** A solution of a weak acid and its salt or of a weak base and its salt, which maintains its pH value against dilution or the addition of small quantities of acid or alkali. **Calcium Hydroxide Solution BP 1968.** A solution formed by shaking calcium hydroxide with distilled water. It is used as an antacid. **Colloidal solution.** A solution in which particles of colloid dimensions (disperse phase) are homogeneously distributed through a solvent (continuous phase); such a solution has characteristic properties differing from those of a true solution (see below), e.g. brownian movement, and displays electrophoresis, interface phenomena and sedimentation. **Solution of contiguity.** Separation of parts originally in contact. **Solution of continuity.** Separation into 2 or more fragments of a tissue originally 1. **Contrast solution.** A soluble contrast medium opaque to x-rays, introduced into the body for radiographic visualization of certain organs. **Cresol and Soap Solution BP 1968.** A solution of cresol and linseed oil in potassium hydroxide solution, used as a disinfectant. **Decimolar solution.** A solution which contains one-tenth of the gram-molecular weight (mol) of a reagent per litre. **Disclosing solution.** A solution containing iodine, which when applied to the surface of a tooth stains any debris or bacterial plaques, which are thereby rendered visible. **Eutectic solution.** A particular solution in which the proportions of solute and solvent are such that the solution has the lowest freezing point or melting point of all other solutions composed of the same substances. **Formaldehyde Solution BP 1973.** A solution of formaldehyde in water with ethyl alcohol, used as a disinfectant. **Gram-molecular solution.** A solution which contains the gram-molecular weight of a reagent per litre. **Gum solution.** An injection of sodium chloride and acacia, formerly used in shock therapy [obsolete]. **Heavy solution.** Hyperbaric solution (see below). **Hydrogen Peroxide Solution BP 1973.** An antiseptic and deodorant solution of hydrogen peroxide in water 5-7 per cent w/v. **Hyperbaric solution.** Heavy solution; a solution containing anaesthetics for spinal anaesthesia, of higher specific gravity than the cerebrospinal fluid, so that it will fall to the lowest parts of the canal. **Hyperosmotic solution, Hypertonic solution.** Any solution having a higher osmotic pressure than that of blood serum. **Hypobaric solution.** Light solution; a solution of lower specific gravity than the cerebrospinal fluid so that it will tend to rise. **Hypotonic solution.** Any solution having a lower osmotic pressure than that of blood serum. **Iodine Solution, Aqueous BP 1973.** A solution of 5 per cent w/v iodine in potassium iodide and water. **Iodine Solution, Strong BP 1958.** A solution of 10 per cent w/v iodine in an alcoholic solution of potassium iodide. **Iodine Solution, Weak BP 1973.** A solution of 2.5 per cent iodine in alcoholic potassium iodide solution. **Isobaric solution.** A solution of the same specific gravity as the cerebrospinal fluid. **Isohydric solution.** A solution of equal hydrogen-ion concentration. **Isotonic solution.** A solution having the same osmotic pressure as blood serum. **Javelle solution.** A solution of sodium hypochlorite. **Lead Subacetate Solution, Dilute BP 1973.** A diluted solution of strong solution of lead subacetate (see following) used for the same purposes. **Lead Subacetate Solution, Strong BP 1963.** Goulard's extract; a clear solution prepared by dissolving lead monoxide in a solution of lead acetate. It is used externally in lotions and as a soothing astringent for application to bruises and sprains. **Light solution.** Hypobaric solution (see above). **Meralluride sodium solution.** An equimolecular mixture of theophylline and a complex organic mercurial, $HgOHCH_2CH(OCH_3)CH_2NHCONHCOCH_2CH_2COOH$; a diuretic similar to mersalyl. The theophylline reduces the local irritant action of the mercurial. **Molal solution.** A solution which contains 1 mol of reagent per 1000 g of solvent. **Molar solution.** A solution which contains 1 mol of reagent per litre of solution. **Molecular disperse solution.** A colloidal solution in which the particles of the disperse phase are of the order of molecular dimensions and can be sedimented only by ultracentrifugal methods. **Molybdate solution.** A solution of ammonium molybdate in diluted nitric acid, used for the detection and determination of phosphate and the detection of arsenic. **Morphine Hydrochloride Solution BP 1968.** A solution of morphine hydrochloride in dilute hydrochloric acid and alcohol, with distilled water. It contains 0.76 per cent w/v of anhydrous morphine. **Neutral solution.** A solution in which the concentration of hydrogen ions exactly equals that of hydroxyl ions; a solution with a pH value of 7. **Normal solution.** A solution which contains the gram-equivalent weight of a reagent per litre; denoted by N/1 or N. **Normal oxidizing solution.** A solution of an oxidizing agent 1 l of which will completely oxidize a litre of solution which contains 1 gram-ion of the element whose valency is increased, e.g. Fe^{2+}. **Normal reducing solution.** A solution of a reducing agent 1 l of which will completely reduce a litre of a solution which contains 1 gram-ion of the element whose valency is reduced, e.g. Fe^{3+}. **Normal saline solution, Normal salt solution.** Physiological saline solution; a sterile 0.9 per cent w/v solution of sodium chloride in distilled water. It is isotonic with the body fluids and is used as a solvent for drugs injected parenterally; also injected intravenously to increase blood volume and pressure in severe haemorrhage and surgical shock or to prevent dehydration in acute diarrhoea. **Nuclear solution.** The solution of nuclear material following the death of a cell. **Physiological saline solution, Physiological salt solution.** Normal saline solution (see above). **Potassium Hydroxide Solution BP 1973.** A solution of potassium hydroxide in distilled water containing 5 per cent w/v of alkali; it is used occasionally as an antacid. **Saline solution, Salt solution.** A solution of sodium chloride; normal saline solution is 0.9 per cent w/v. **Saturated solution.** A solution which contains the maximum amount of solute that a given quantity of solvent will dissolve at a given temperature. **Sclerosing solution.** A solution for injection with a view to obliterating a varicose vein or a hernial sac. **Solid solution.** A mixture of 2 or more solids homogeneously combined, as in an alloy. **Standard solution.** Any solution used in analysis or assay which contains a specified amount of reagent per volume or weight of solution, e.g. molal, molar and normal solutions. **Supersaturated solution.** A solution which contains more than the maximum amount of solute that a given quantity of solvent would normally dissolve at a given temperature. **Surgical Chlorinated Soda Solution BP 1958.** A solution of chlorinated lime, sodium carbonate and boric acid, yielding about 0.5 per cent w/v of chlorine. It is used as a surgical antiseptic; Dakin's solution. **True solution.** A solution as generally understood by the term, in which the particles of solute are of molecular size and comparable with those of the solvent with which they form a homogeneous mixture. Such a solution can not be separated into its constituents by mechanical means, e.g. filtration or centrifugalization, as distinct from a suspension or colloidal solution (see above). **Volumetric solution.** Any solution containing the whole or a stated fraction of the gram-equivalent weight of a reagent per litre. It is used in volumetric analysis. **Water-glass solution.** A solution of sodium silicate, used mainly for preserving eggs. [L *solutus* dissolved.]

See also: ALSEVER, BANNERMAN, BARKER (A. E. J.), BENEDICT (S. R.), CALLISON, CRAMER (W.), CURSCHMANN (HANS), CUTLER (N. L.), CZAPEK-DOX, CZOCOR, DAKIN, DARROW, DISCOMBE, DOBELL, DONOVAN (M.), DUNHAM (E. K.), FEHLING, FLEMMING, FOL, FONIO, FOWLER (T.), GÉNÉVRIER, GOLGI, GOWERS, GRAM, HAMDI, HARRINGTON, HARTMANN (A. F.), HAYEM, HUBL, KAISERLING, LEMPERT (H.), LOCKE, LOEFFLER (F. A. J.), LUGOL, MANDL, MANSON, MAYER (F. F.), MONSEL, ORTH, PACINI, PASTEUR, PATRICK, PEARSON (G.), PERÉNYI, PIAZZA, PITFIELD, RABLE, RANDOLPH, RINGER, RUGE, SCHAELLIBAUM, STARTIN, SUBY, SWIETEN, TAKAYAMA, TOISON, TYRODE, VAN GIESON, VLEMINCKX, VOLHARD (J.), WIJ, ZENKER (K.).

solution-tablets (sol·ew·shun·**tab'**·lets). Tablets containing a drug or drugs, and which are dissolved in water for external or local use. [solution, tablets.]

solvable (**sol**·vabl). Soluble. [see foll.]

solvate (**sol**·vate). A union of the molecules of a solvent with the molecules or ions of a solute to form a complex, postulated to explain phenomena peculiar to certain solutions. [L *solvere* to dissolve.]

solvation (sol·**va**·shun). The formation of a complex, or solvate, by the association of the molecules of a solvent with the ions or molecules of a solute in solution.

solvellae (sol·**vel**·e). Solution-tablets.

solvend (**sol**·vend). Term applied to a solute. [Obsolete term.] [see foll.]

solvent (**sol**·vent). The medium, usually a liquid, which dissolves a solute to form a solution. [L *solvere* to dissolve.]

solvin (**sol**·vin). Sodium sulphoricinate, a solvent with antiseptic properties, which haemolyses red blood corpuscles.

solvolysis (sol·**vol**·is·is). 1. General term for reactions in the nature of double-decompositions which take place in solutions, e.g. hydrolysis. 2. The influence of the ionization of the solvent itself upon the dissociation of the solute dissolved in it. [L *solvere* to dissolve, *lysis* a loosing.]

soma (**so**·mah). 1. The body as distinct from the mind. 2. All the body tissue except the germ cells. 3. All the axial body, i.e. excluding the arms and legs. [Gk body.]

somaesthesia (so·mes·**the**·ze·ah). Somataesthesia.

somaesthetic (so·mes·**thet**·ik). Somataesthetic.

somaesthetopsychic (so·mes·the·to·**si'**·kik). An epithet applied to the association areas of the somatic sensory cortex. [Brodman's areas 5 and 7.) [Gk *soma* body, aesthesia, *psyche* soul.]

Somagyi's reflex or sign. Dilatation of the pupils during deep inspiration, and contraction on full expiration; thought to be due to vagal instability.

somal (**so**·mal). Relating or belonging to the body. [Gk *soma* body.]

somantin (**so**·man·tin). A peptide component of growth hormone which is also diabetogenic.

somaplasm (**so**·mah·plazm). Somatoplasm. [Gk *soma* body, *plasma* something formed.]

somasthenia (so·mas·**the**·ne·ah). Somatasthenia.

somataesthesia (**so**·mat·es·**the'**·ze·ah). The state of consciousness of the body. [Gk *soma* body, aesthesia.]

somataesthetic (**so**·mat·es·**thet'**·ik). Relating or belonging to somataesthesia.

somatalgia (so·mat·**al**·je·ah). Any sensation of pain. [Gk *soma* body, *algos* pain.]

somatasthenia (**so**·mat·as·**the'**·ne·ah). A condition of chronic physical weakness, associated with insomnia and lack of appetite and as a rule with low blood pressure, in which the individual is unable to live a life of normal activity without suffering fatigue. [Gk *soma* body, asthenia.]

somatic (so·**mat**·ik). 1. Of or pertaining to the body *(soma)* as opposed to the mind *(psyche)*. 2. Of or pertaining to the body as opposed to the germ cells. 3. Of or pertaining to the framework of the body as opposed to the viscera. [Gk *soma* body.]

somaticosplanchnic (so·**mat**·ik·o·**splangk'**·nik). Somaticovisceral. [Gk *soma* body, *splagchna* viscera.]

somaticovisceral (so·**mat**·ik·o·**vis'**·er·al). Relating or belonging to the body and the viscera. [Gk *soma* body, viscera.]

somatist (**so**·mat·ist). One who regards mental disorders as having an organic cause. [Gk *soma* body.]

somatization (**so**·mat·i·**za'**·shun). The process by which a mental event is expressed in a disturbance of bodily function. [see prec.]

somatoceptor (so·mat·o·**sep'**·tor). A sensory organ responding to stimuli from the body itself as opposed to the outside world. [Gk *soma* body, receptor.]

somatodidymus (so·mat·o·**did'**·im·us). A twin monster the bodies of which are fused. [Gk *soma* body, *didymos* twin.]

somatogenesis (so·mat·o·**jen'**·es·is). The development of bodily structure from hereditary sources with active environmental influences at work; origination in or formation out of somatic cells. [Gk *soma* body, *genein* to produce.]

somatogenetic, somatogenic (so·mat·o·jen·**et'**·ik, **so**·mat·o·**jen'**·ik). 1. Relating or belonging to somatogenesis. 2. Having origin in the body cells. [see prec.]

somatogeny (so·mat·**oj**·en·e). Somatogenesis.

somatological (**so**·mat·o·**loj'**·ik·al). Relating or belonging to somatology.

somatology (so·mat·**ol**·o·je). The science of the body, including anatomy and physiology. [Gk *soma* body, *logos* science.]

somatomammotrophin (so·mat·o·**mam**·o·**tro**·fin). Human chorionic-HCS. A placental extract that has properties of growth hormone and prolactin.

somatome (**so**·mat·ome). 1. A somite. 2. Any cutting instrument used in embryotomy; embryotome. [Gk *soma* body, *temnein* to cut.]

somatomedin (**so**·mat·o·**med**·in). Intermediary in somatotrophic action. Identical with the sulphation factor. A peptide with a molecular weight of 4000.

somatomegaly (so·mat·o·**meg'**·al·e). Gigantism. [Gk *soma* body, *megas* large.]

somatometry (so·mat·**om**·et·re). Measurement of the size of the body. [Gk *soma* body, *metron* measure.]

somatomic (so·mat·**om**·ik). Relating or belonging to a somatome.

somatopagus (so·mat·**op**·ag·us). A monster with a double trunk. [Gk *soma* body, *pegos* fixed.]

somatopathic (so·mat·o·**path'**·ik). Caused by organic or bodily lesions, as opposed to neuropathic or psychopathic. [Gk *soma* body, *pathos* disease.]

somatopathy (so·mat·**op**·ath·e). A disorder of organic origin. [see prec.]

somatophrenia (**so**·mat·o·**fre'**·ne·ah). A neurosis in which the patient exaggerates the severity of a bodily disorder or imagines that he is suffering from one. [Gk *soma* body, *phren* mind.]

somatoplasm (**so**·mat·o·plasm). The protoplasm of the general body cells as opposed to that of the germ cells. [Gk *soma* body, protoplasm.]

somatopleural (so·mat·o·**ploor'**·al). Relating or belonging to the somatopleure.

somatopleure (**so**·mat·o·ploor). The ventral part of the body wall of the early embryo and the fetal membranes continuous with it, composed of an outer layer of ectoderm and an inner layer of somatic mesoderm. Sometimes the term refers to the mesodermal component only. [Gk *soma* body, *pleura* side.]

somatopsychic (so·mat·o·si'·kik). Relating or belonging to the mind as well as the body. [Gk *soma* body, *psyche* soul.]

somatopsychosis (so·mat·o·si·**ko'**·sis). Any mental disorder symptomatic of bodily (non-neurological) disease (Southard). [Gk *soma* body, *psyche* soul, *-osis* condition.]

somatoschisis (so·mat·**os**·kis·is). Splitting of the vertebral bodies. [Gk *soma* body, *schisis* a cleaving.]

somatoscopy (so·mat·**os**·ko·pe). Visual examination of the body. [Gk *soma* body, *skopein* to watch.]

somatosplanchnopleuric (so·mat·o·splangk·no·**ploor'**·ik). Relating or belonging to both the somatopleure and the splanchnopleure.

somatotomy (so·mat·**ot**·o·me). 1. Anatomy of the body. 2. Dissection. [Gk *soma* body, *temnein* to cut.]

somatotonia (so·mat·o·**to'**·ne·ah). A variety of temperament described by Sheldon as being characterized by bodily assertiveness and by desire for muscular activity. [Gk *soma* body, *tonos* tension.]

somatotridymus (so·mat·o·**tri'**·dim·us). A triple-bodied monster. [Gk *soma* body, *tridymos* triplet.]

somatotrophin (so·mat·o·**trof'**·in). The growth hormone secreted by the eosinophil cells of the anterior lobe of the pituitary gland. [Gk *soma* body, *trophe* nourishment.]

somatotrophic (so·mat·o·**trof'**·ik). 1. Exerting an influence on the body or body cells. 2. Pertaining to or possessing the qualities of a somatotrophin. [Gk *soma* body, *trophe* nourishment.]

somatotype (so·**mat**·o·tipe). Classification of bodily constitution. [Gk *soma* body, type.]

somatotyping (so·mat·o·**ti'**·ping). Studying and classifying the different physical types of man. [see prec.]

somatotypy (so·**mat**·o·ti·pe). The ascertainment of the class of body build, with categorization according to type.

somite (**so**·mite). One of the paired blocks of mesoderm present in each segment of the early embryo, lying on either side of the notochord and neural tube. Each somite gives rise to a dermatome from which the dermis of a skin segment is derived, a myotome which produces a striated muscle segment and a sclerotome which forms one-half of a vertebra and its associated rib. A distinction is sometimes made between the somites of lowly vertebrates, which give rise to all the mesoderm of one-half of the embryonic segments, and those of higher vertebrates, which only give rise to the axial mesoderm. [Gk *soma* body.]

somitic (so·**mit**·ik). Relating or having resemblance to a somite.

somnal (**som**·nal). Ethylchloralurethane, $CCl_3CH(OC_2H_5)NHCO OC_2H_5$. A hypnotic related chemically to chloral hydrate, and similar in action.

somnambulance (som·**nam**·bew·lans). Somnambulism.

somnambulation (som·**nam**·bew·**la'**·shun). The act of walking in the sleep. [L *somnus* sleep, *ambulare* to walk.]

somnambulator (som·**nam**·bew·la·tor). Somnambulist.

somnambulism (som·**nam**·bew·lizm). A sleep disorder in which an individual walks and performs other acts while asleep; a condition of hypnotic sleep in which some of the individual's senses are awake but he cannot later recall any acts he has performed. [L *somnus* sleep, *ambulare* to walk.]

somnambulist (som·**nam**·bew·list). One who walks in his sleep. [see prec.]

somnambulistic (som·**nam**·bew·**lis'**·tik). Pertaining or subject to somnambulism.

somnial (**som**·ne·al). Relating or belonging to dreams or to sleep. [see foll.]

somniation (som·ne·**a**·shun). Sleep accompanied by dreams. [L *somniare* to dream.]

somniculous (som·**nik**·ew·lus). 1. Inducing sleep. 2. Drowsy. [L *somniculosus* sleepy.]

somnifacient (som·ne·**fa**·shent). 1. Soporific; hypnotic. 2. An agent that causes or induces sleep. [L *somnus* sleep, *facere* to produce.]

somniferine (som·**nif**·er·een). A narcotic alkaloid from *Withania somnifera* (family Solanaceae). [see foll.]

somniferous (som·**nif**·er·us). Soporific; hypnotic. [L *somnus* sleep, *ferre* to produce.]

somnific (som·**nif**·ik). Somnifacient.

somnifugous (som·**nif**·ew·gus). Driving away sleep. [L *somnus* sleep, *fugare* to put to flight.]

somniloquence, somniloquism (som·**nil**·o·kwens, som·**nil**·o·kwizm). 1. Habitual talking during sleep. 2. Talking by a person in a state of hypnosis. [see foll.]

somniloquist (som·**nil**·o·kwist). An individual who habitually talks in his sleep. [L *somnus* sleep, *loqui* to speak.]

somniloquous (som·**nil**·o·kwus). Tending to talk while asleep. [see prec.]

somniloquy (som·**nil**·o·kwe). Somniloquence.

somnipathist (som·**nip**·ath·ist). 1. One who suffers from somnipathy. 2. An individual susceptible to hypnotism or one in whom a hypnotic state has been induced. [see foll.]

somnipathy (som·**nip**·ath·e). 1. Any sleep disorder. 2. The state of being hypnotized. [L *somnus* sleep, *pathos* disease.]

somnol (**som**·nol). A synthetic product of chloralurethane with a polyatomic alcohol; it is used as a hypnotic and sedative. [L *somnus* sleep.]

somnolence, somnolency (**som**·no·lens, **som**·no·lens·e). 1. Sleepiness. 2. Abnormal drowsiness or inclination to sleep. [L *somnolentia* sleepiness.]

somnolent (**som**·no·lent). 1. Sleepy; drowsy; inclined to sleep. 2. Inducing drowsiness. 3. Semicomatose. [see prec.]

somnolescent (som·no·**les**·ent). 1. Inclined to be drowsy or sleepy. 2. An agent which induces sleep. [see foll.]

somnolism (**som**·no·lizm). The hypnotic trance. [L *somnus* sleep.]

somnopathist (som·**nop**·ath·ist). 1. A sufferer from somnopathy. 2. Anyone in whom a state of hypnosis has been induced. [see foll.]

somnopathy (som·**nop**·ath·e). Any sleep disorder. [L *somnus* sleep, Gk *pathos* disease.]

somnovigil (som·no·**vij**·il). Coma vigil. [L *somnus* sleep, vigil.]

Somogyi, Michael (b. 1883). St. Louis biochemist.

Somogyi unit. Of serum amylase. 1 mg of reducing sugar (as glucose) produced by 100 ml of serum from starch at 40° C in 30 min represents 1 unit of amylase activity.

somopsychosis (so·mo·si·**ko'**·sis). A term not in common use denoting any psychosis with predominantly bodily symptoms. [Gk *soma* body, psychosis.]

sonde coudé (sond koo·**da**). A catheter angled or elbowed near its tip. [Fr.]

sone (sone). A subjective estimate of loudness or loudness function. One sone can be defined as the loudness of 1000 Hz (c/s) tone 40 decibels above normal threshold. A sound which appears to a listener to be twice as loud as this sound is said to have a loudness of 2 sones. [L *sonus* sound.]

sonitus (**son**·it·us). Tinnitus aurium. [L noise.]

Sonne, Carl Olaf (b. 1882). Copenhagen bacteriologist.

Sonne's bacillus. *Shigella sonnei.*

Sonne dysentery. A form of dysentery, usually mild, found especially in childhood epidemics in many temperate countries and due to *Shigella sonnei.* It is especially prevalent in the autumn and winter, and in adults may be severe and accompanied by high pyrexia. The stools have been compared to tomato juice. This form of dysentery is not so amenable to sulphonamide treatment as others of the group, but sulphonamides, such as phthalylsulphathiazole are effective when combined with streptomycin.

Sonnenschein, Franz Leopold (b. 1819). German pharmacist.

Sonnenschein's reagent. A solution of phosphomolybdic acid used in testing for alkaloids.

sonocardiometry (son·o·kar·de·om′·et·re). The technique of using ultrasound echo detection to measure the size of the cardiac cavities. *See* ECHOCARDIOGRAPHY. [L *sonus* sound, Gk *kardia* heart, *metron* measure.]

sonography (son·og·raf·e). Visible speech. [L *sonus* sound, Gk *graphein* to record.]

sonometer (so·nom·et·er). 1. One of the many instruments used in testing auditory acuity. 2. An instrument used for measuring the frequency of sound vibrations and establishing the pitch of muscial notes. [L *sonus* sound, meter.]

sonorous (so·nor·us). 1. Resonant. 2. Loud in sound. [L *sonor* noise.]

sonvelography (son·vel·og·raf·e). The technique of recording the heart sounds and murmurs in the form of a diagram representing the envelope enclosing the normal type of phonocardiograms. [L *sonus* sound, Fr. *enveloppe*, Gk *graphein* to record.]

sophisticate (so·fis·tik·ate). To adulterate; to render impure by the intentional addition of foreign material. [Gk *sophistikos* deceitful.]

sophistication (so·fis·tik·a′·shun). Adulteration. [see prec.]

sophomania (sof·o·ma·ne·ah). A type of megalomania in which the patient thinks he is far wiser than in reality he is. [Gk *sophia* wisdom, mania.]

Sophora (so·for·ah). The coral bean; a genus of Texan trees (family Leguminoseae), with poisonous berries containing sophorine. [Arabic *sofara.*]

sophorine (so·for·een). Cytisine, $C_{11}H_{14}ON_2$. An alkaloid found in the seeds of various species of *Sophora* as well as other genera, e.g. *Baptisia* and *Cytisus.* It is highly poisonous, having an action like nicotine.

sopor (so·por). Sleep that is deep or profound, or that is abnormally deep as in stupor. [L deep sleep.]

soporifacient (so·por·e·fa′·shent). 1. Inducing sleep. 2. Any drug which induces sleep. [L *sopor* deep sleep, *facere* to make.]

soporiferous (so·por·if·er·us). Soporific. [L *sopor* deep sleep, *ferre* to bear.]

soporific (so·por·if·ik). 1. Tending to cause or causing deep sleep. 2. Hypnotic. 3. An agent that produces sleep. [L *sopor* deep sleep, *facere* to make.]

soporose, soporous (so·por·oze, so·por·us). 1. Relating to or found in association with deep sleep or stupor. 2. Comatose. [L *sopor* deep sleep.]

sorbefacient (sor·be·fa·shent). 1. Causing or subserving absorption. 2. An agent which either causes absorption or renders it easier. [L *sorbere* to suck in, *facere* to make.]

sorbic (sor·bik). Concerned with the mountain ash, *Sorbus aucuparia* (family Rosaceae), e.g. sorbic acid. [L *sorbus* mountain ash.]

Sorbide Nitrate (sor·bide ni·trate). BP Commission approved name for 1,4-3,6-dianhydrosorbitol dinitrate; it is used in the treatment of angina pectoris.

sorbin, sorbinose (sor·bin, sor·bin·oze). Sorbose.

sorbitans (sor·bit·anz). A general name for esters of sorbitol used as surface active emulsifying agents. BP Commission approved names are Sorbitan Monolaurate, Sorbitan Mono-oleate, Sorbitan Monopalmitate, Sorbitan Monostearate, Sorbitan Sesquioleate, Sorbitan Trioleate and Sorbitan Tristearate.

sorbite (sor·bite). Sorbitol.

Sorbitol BP 1973 (sor·bit·ol). A hexahydric alcohol isomeric with mannitol. It is a sweetening agent and may be used by diabetics in place of sucrose. It is also used in dialysis fluid instead of dextrose.

sorbose (sor·boze). $CH_2OH(CHOH)_3COCH_2OH$, a ketohexose derived from the sorbitol in the berries of the mountain ash by the action of the sorbose bacterium. It is a sweet-tasting sugar, non-fermentable by yeast and of importance in the synthesis of ascorbic acid.

Sorby's cell. A receptacle made from barometer tubing, used for the spectroscopic examination of blood.

sordes (sor·deez). Dark brown or nearly black crusts which accumulate on the teeth, lips and gums in patients with low fevers, and having origin in general oral debris, epithelium, food and bacteria. **Sordes aurium.** Ear wax. **Sordes gastricae.** Undigested mucus and food in the stomach. [L filth.]

sore (sore). A popular word applied to any lesion of the skin or mucous membrane. When associated with the name of a place it forms a loose medical term applied to a characteristic cutaneous lesion common in that place. Such a name was usually a cloak for ignorance of the true aetiology of the lesion at the time when it was originally described. In many such places more than one type of cutaneous lesion is now prevalent, and the names have lost their value, but in others the names have been adopted to indicate specific sores of known aetiology, e.g. Delhi sore, Sart sore. *See also:* ULCER. **Ashkabad sore, Baghdad sore.** Cutaneous leishmaniasis. **Bed sore.** Decubital ulcer. *See* ULCER. **Canker sores.** Aphthae. **Chrome sore.** Chrome ulcer; ulceration and destruction of the nasal septum and deep ulcers on the hands, seen in chrome workers. It is due to the caustic action of chromic acid and the chromates of potassium and sodium. **Cochin China sore.** Ulcus tropicum. **Cold sore.** Lesions of herpes simplex, especially those occurring on or near the lips during menstruation; originally used to denote herpetic lesions on this site during the course of a cold or during any disease associated with fever. **Decubitus sore.** Decubitus ulcer. *See ulcer.* **Delhi sore.** Cutaneous leishmaniasis. **Desert sore.** An infective ulcer occurring in the desert; a variant of ecthyma. It is sometimes caused by diphtheria bacilli. **Gallipoli sore.** Desert sore. **Hard sore.** An ulcer with indurated margin and base; usually restricted to a syphilitic chancre. **Jungle sore.** An indolent, erythematous lesion, of multiple aetiology, originating in miliaria, insect bites, abrasions, etc., and complicated by superinfection by pyogenic and other bacteria; it occurs in hot, humid countries. **Kandahar sore, Lahore sore.** Cutaneous leishmaniasis. **Madagascar sore, Naga sore.** Ulcus tropicum. **Natal sore.** Desert sore. **Oriental sore.** Cutaneous leishmaniasis. **Pendeh sore, Pendinski sore, Pendinsky sore.** Cutaneous leishmaniasis. (Pendinski or Pendinsky is the adjectival form of Pendeh). **Pressure sore.** An ulcer or any skin lesion caused by pressure from the bed or from any appliance, e.g. a plaster-of-Paris or other splint. **Sart sore.** Cutaneous leishmaniasis. **Soft sore.** A non-indurated ulcer; usually restricted to a chancroid ulcer. **Umballa sore.** Cutaneous leishmaniasis. **Veldt sore.** Desert sore. **Venereal sore.** An ulcer of venereal origin; syphilis or chancroid. **Water sore.** Ground itch; the skin manifestation at the point of entry of the larva in hookworm infection. [AS *sar.*]

sore throat (sore throte). Any form of inflammation of the larynx or pharynx, including also tonsillitis. **Clergyman's sore throat.** A sore throat producing dysphonia, resulting from abuse or overuse of the voice in professional voice users, including clergymen. **Cyclists' sore throat.** Sore throat said to result from the inhalation of road dust in cyclists. **Diphtheria sore throat.** Sore throat resulting from infection with *Corynebacterium diphtheriae.* **Epidemic streptococcal sore throat.** A sore throat, epidemic in character, resulting from an infection by a streptococcus. The organism has been known to be spread by means of infected milk. **Hospital sore throat.** Inflammation of the pharynx and fauces affecting people who work in hospitals, particularly nurses and medical students in the early part of hospital training. **Putrid sore throat.** A gangrenous ulceration of the pharynx. **Septic sore throat.** A severe form of throat infection, usually of streptococcal origin. **Spotted sore throat.** Follicular tonsillitis. *See* TONSILLITIS. **Streptococcus sore throat.** A sore throat resulting from streptococcal infection. **Surgical sore throat.** Hospital sore throat (see above). **Ulcerated sore throat.** Painful ulcers of the throat, from any cause. [AS *sar*, throat.]

See also: FOTHERGILL (J.).

Sørensen, Søren Peter Lauritz (b. 1868). Copenhagen chemist.

Sørensen's method. 1. A method of determining amino acids by formol titration. 2. The determination of pH by addition of indicators to unknown solutions and comparing the colours with those given by standard buffer solutions with the same indicators.

Sørensen's scale. A scale to measure alkalinity and acidity; a scale of hydrogen-ion concentration in which the values are expressed in pH.

Henriques and Sørensen method. For amino-acid nitrogen in urine. The urine is treated with barium chloride and barium hydroxide to remove carbonates and phosphates, and any large amount of ammonia distilled off *in vacuo.* The filtrate is neutralized to phenolphthalein, neutral formaldehyde solution is added and the acidity produced is titrated with standard alkali.

Soret, Celestin (d. 1931). French radiologist.

Soret effect. The difference in concentration of a solution produced by maintaining a higher temperature in the upper part of the solution.

sorghum (sor·gum). Sugar-producing grasses of the family Gramineae, e.g. *Andropogon sorghum,* from which sorghum syrup is obtained; the meal is used as both human food and cattle feed. **Sorghum saccharatum.** Chinese sugar cane; a source of sugar. [It. *sorgo.*]

Sorgius, Wilhelm. 19th century German anatomist.

glands of Sorgius. Part of the anterior group of axillary lymph glands occasionally found on the anterior surface of the pectoralis major muscle near its lower border. They drain the breast tissue.

soroche (so·ro·cha). A term used in the Andes for a form of mountain sickness. [Sp antimony, as the disease was attributed to that metal.]

sororiation (sor·o·re·a'·shun). Development of the mammary glands at puberty. [L *sororiare* to swell together.]

sorption (sorp·shun). Adsorption. The concentration of the molecules of a solute upon a surface or interface within the solution. [L *sorbere* to suck in.]

sorrel (sor·el). A plant of the genus *Rumex, R. acetosa* (family Polygonaceae). **Salt of sorrel.** Salts of lemon, used to remove stains, e.g. rust, ink. [O Fr. *sur* sour.]

sorroche (so·ro·cha). Soroche.

soterocyte (so·ter·o·site). A platelet. [Gk *soter* saviour, *kytos* cell.]

Sottas, Jules (b. 1866). Paris neurologist.

Déjérine-Sottas atrophy, disease or neuropathy, Sottas-Déjérine atrophy, disease or neuropathy. Progressive hypertrophic intersitial neuritis of infants.

souffle (soo·fl). A soft, blowing sound or murmur heard on auscultation. **Cardiac souffle.** A cardiac murmur. **Electric souffle.** A breezy sensation derived from the slight discharge of electricity from a static electric machine in action. **Fetal souffle, Funic souffle.** A blowing noise heard in the region of the umbilical cord during pregnancy. **Splenic souffle.** A murmur sometimes heard over the spleen. **Umbilical souffle.** Fetal souffle (see above). **Uterine souffle.** The hissing noise made by the blood passing through the uterine vessels during pregnancy. [Fr a puff.]

soul (sole). 1. The essential substance or activating part of individual existence, usually shown in psychical behaviour; it is separable from the body and is supposed to have a separate existence from it. 2. A term metaphorically applied to man's psychical and emotional nature and to the psychical and spiritual side of things, e.g. the soul of the universe or the spirit and patriotism of a country; also, to a leader or inspirer of a religion or enterprise. 3. Spirit, courage, noble or moral behaviour. 4. A person or human being. 5. A spirit or disembodied being. [AS *sawel.*]

See also: STAHL (G. E.).

soulal (soo·lal). A severe scabietic infestation in Arabs.

Souligoux, Antoine Léone Charles (b. 1865). French surgeon.

Souligoux-Morestin method. A method of lavage of the peritoneal cavity in acute peritonitis.

sound (sownd). 1. A stimulus which excites the function of hearing; it is produced by vibrations transmitted through the air or other medium. 2. The noise of some bodily function, normal or abnormal, detectable either directly by the ear or with the aid of an instrument, e.g. heart, fetal heart, bowel, cracked-pot. 3. An instrument used in exploring cavities (e.g. passing a bladder sound to detect stone), or in the detection and dilatation of strictures (e.g. urethral sound), or in demonstrating the patency of channels (e.g. bile duct and ampulla of Vater). 4. To use a sound, e.g. for detecting stone in the bladder. **Amphoric sound.** The sound produced when one breathes or speaks into the opening of a wide-mouthed bottle. **Anasarcous sound.** A sound heard on auscultation over oedematous skin. **Aortic second sound.** The component of the second heart sound (see below) which is produced by closure of the aortic valve; it is audible all over the precordium. **Atrial sound.** The fourth heart sound; a sound associated with atrial systole and therefore occurring shortly before the first heart sound. It is probably produced by vibrations in the ventricular wall set up by the thrust of blood into the chamber by atrial contraction. Although often detectable by the phonocardiogram, it cannot normally be heard by auscultation; an audible sound is always abnormal and indicative of ventricular disease. **Auscultatory sound.** A sound heard on auscultation. **Bandbox sound.** The resonant percussion note heard over an emphysematous lung. **Bell sound.** The sound heard with a stethoscope over a pneumothorax cavity when a coin placed on the chest some distance away is struck by another coin. **Bladder sound.** A curved metal instrument passed along the urethra to aid the detection of bladder stone. *See also* URETHRAL SOUND (below). **Bottle sound.** Amphoric sound (see above). **Breath sound.** The respiratory sound in auscultation. **Bronchial sounds.** The sounds heard on auscultation over a bronchus, or over consolidated lung when the bronchial breath sounds are transmitted without loss. **Cardiac sound.** Heart sound (see below). **Coin sound.** Bell sound (see above). **Cracked-pot sound.** The sound sometimes heard on percussion over a cavity with an opening to a bronchus. **Cranial cracked-pot sound.** The change in note on percussion of the skull which is supposed to occur when distension has caused widening of the sutures. **Curved sound.** A curved bougie of varying type for calibrating and dilating the urethra. **Diastolic-shock sound.** An early diastolic sound that can be heard and occasionally felt over the right ventricle when the heart, under the influence of high venous filling pressure, suddenly meets the resistance of a rigid pericardial sac, as in constrictive pericarditis. The term *diastolic shock* may also be used to denote the palpable second heart sound sometimes felt in the pulmonary artery in pulmonary hypertension. **Dive bomber sound.** The crescendo sound elicited in the loudspeaker of the electromyograph when the recording needle is moved in a myotonic muscle. **Ejection sound.** Ejection click. *See* CLICK. **Falling-drop sound.** A sound sometimes heard on auscultation over a hydropneumothorax and due to a drop of liquid falling into the accumulated liquid at the base of the pleural cavity. **Fetal-heart sounds.** The beats of the fetal heart as heard on auscultation. **Friction sound.** The sound heard over an area of dry pleurisy or pericarditis. **Funicular bellows sound.** Funic souffle. *See* SOUFFLE. **Gallop sound.** A sound occurring in diastole and, added to the first and second sounds, producing a gallop rhythm. **Heart sounds.** The sounds produced by the action of the heart. There are 4 in each cardiac cycle, of which only the first and second are usually audible in health. *First:* the sound at the beginning of the ventricular systole, caused mainly by closure of the atrioventricular valves and partly by contraction of the ventricular muscle and the turbulence of the blood in the ventricles; it has a low-pitched prolonged quality. *Second:* the sound which follows the first and occurs at the onset of ventricular diastole. It is produced by closure of the aortic and pulmonary valves, closure of the former occurring slightly before the latter so that the second sound is duplicated. *Third:* a sound occurring during early ventricular diastole in the phase of rapid ventricular filling, and due to the vibration of the ventricular walls. It is commonly heard at the apex of the heart in healthy children, and less frequently in adults unless the heart is disordered. *Fourth:* atrial sound (see above). **Hippocratic sound.**

The succussion splash which is heard over a hydropneumothorax on shaking the patient. **Lacrimal sound.** Lacrimal probe. *See* PROBE. **Metallic sound.** A metallic or consonating quality of a râle which is produced in a cavity. **Metallic heart sounds.** An accentuated metallic quality to the heart sounds which may occur when the normally aerated lung lying between the heart and the chest wall is absent or diseased, i.e. in pneumothorax or cavitation. When the pressure in the systemic circulation is increased (systemic hypertension) the aortic valve closes with increased speed and force, so that the first (aortic) element of the second heart sound may have a loud ringing quality. The same phenomenon may be applied to the second (pulmonary) element of the second heart sound in the presence of pulmonary arterial hypertension. **Metamorphosing breath sound.** A breath sound which alters its quality during its course. **Mid-diastolic sound.** A sound heard in the middle period of ventricular diastole: in heart failure the third and fourth heart sounds may be audible, but in the presence of a tachycardia the shortening of the ventricular diastole causes the 2 sounds to merge into each other. If the atrioventricular conduction time is considerably lengthened the fourth (atrial) sound is usually audible and falls in the mid- instead of the pre-systole; this constitutes another type of mid-diastolic sound. **Muscle sound.** The sound heard over contracting muscle. **Oesophageal sound.** An instrument seldom used nowadays consisting of a length of whalebone carrying a metal olive; used in the management of oesophageal stricture. **Osseous sound.** The sound heard on percussion over bone, e.g. the ribs in percussion of the chest; it is a short, slightly resonant note which modifies the sound produced by percussion over an intercostal space. **Peacock sound.** A change in the quality of the voice due to disease of the larynx or air passages. **Percussion sound.** The sound produced by percussion. **Physiological sounds.** Subjective sounds in the ear, only appreciated in normal people when the external auditory meatus is blocked. These sounds arise from vessels in the neighbourhood of the ear with the movement of the jaw and grinding of the teeth. **Pistol-shot sound.** A sharp, loud sound heard over the femoral or other arteries with each pulse beat in case of free aortic incompetence or large patent ductus arteriosus. The sound corresponds to the apex of the ascending limb of the arterial pulse, and is due to the increased volume of blood from the left ventricle being ejected rapidly into the arteries and striking the arterial wall forcibly. **Pulmonary sound.** A sound produced in the lungs. **Pulmonary second sound.** The component of the second heart sound (see above) which is produced by closure of the pulmonary valve; normally it is audible only in the so-called pulmonary area, the upper left sternal edge, but when accentuated it may be more widely heard. It occurs a little later than the aortic second sound and normally this is more so in inspiration. **Respiratory sound.** Breath sound (see above). **Shaking sound.** The succussion splash; hippocratic sound (see above). **Sizzling sound.** The sound produced by small bubbles in the stomach. **Straight sound.** A straight bougie of varying size for calibrating the urethra. **Subjective sound.** The sound produced by the blood flowing through vessels near the ears. **Succussion sound.** Hippocratic sound (see above). **Tic-tac sounds.** The cadence produced when both the first and second heart sounds in each cycle are equally spaced as a result of shortening of diastole due to tachycardia, and of equal muffled intensity. It occurs in severe circulatory failure, particularly when the blood volume is reduced. Also known as *fetal rhythm* or *embryocardia* from its resemblance to the normal fetal-heart sounds. **To-and-fro sound.** A sound produced during both systole and diastole as pericardial friction. **Tracheal sounds.** The breath sounds produced in the trachea. **Tubular sound.** High-pitched bronchial breathing. **Urethral sound.** A slender steel instrument bent distally to correspond to the curve of the posterior urethra; sometimes the tip is conical and the proximal end may be weighted to provide balance. Such instruments have been used from the earliest times for the examination and calibration of the urethra, the dilatation of strictures, or for "the sounding of the bladder for stone", before cystoscopes and x-rays were available. **Uterine sound.** A graduated instrument for measuring the length of the uterine cavity. **Water-wheel sound.** *Bruit de moulin*; a splashing sound synchronous with the heart beat heard in cases of pneumohydropericardium. **Water-whistle sound.** The whistling sound produced by air passing in and out of a bronchial fistula. **White sound.** A composite sound composed of pure tones, harmonics and discordants, of equal intensity throughout the range of hearing, used as a background noise in tests of speech intelligibility. It is named from the analogy of the spectrum of white light. [L *sonus.*]

See also: BÉNIQUÉ, BRIGHT, KOROTKOFF.

Souques, Achille Alexandre (b. 1860). French neurologist.

Souques' phenomenon. Finger phenomenon. *See* PHENOMENON.

Souques' sign. 1. Souques' phenomenon; finger phenomenon. 2. In disease of the corpus striatum (e.g. parkinsonism), if a patient in a chair is pushed backwards there is loss of the normal extension of the legs that occurs to prevent overbalancing; a sign due to loss of associated movements.

source (sors). **Gamma-ray source.** A radioactive substance emitting γ-rays, usually in a container convenient for use in radiology. **Ion source.** A source of gaseous ions of the desired element, as in a mass spectrometer or cyclotron. **Radiation source.** The source of the radiation of interest. In nuclear medicine, often used to designate a quantity of radioactive material used as a source of ionizing radiation. [O Fr. *sourse.*]

Sourdille, G. 20th century French ophthalmologist.

Sourdille's operation. For ptosis. Division of the levator palpebrae superioris muscle some distance behind its insertion and attaching the distal end to the occipitofrontalis muscle just above the eyebrow with two X sutures. [Obsolete.]

sourwood (sow·er·wud). Elk tree, sorrel tree; a small tree of South America, *Oxydendrum arboreum* (family Ericaceae), the leaves of which are used for their diuretic properties. [O Fr. *sur,* AS *wudu.*]

Sousa, Manuel Bento de (b. 1835). Lisbon surgeon and anatomist.

Sousa's nerve. The palatal taste fibres within the greater superficial petrosal nerve.

southernwood (suth·ern·wud). Old man's tree, boy's love, slovern wood; a species of the genus *Artemisia, A. abrotanum* (family Compositae). It is used as a stimulant, emmenagogue. antiseptic and detergent. [AS *suth, wudu.*]

Southey, Reginald (b. 1835). London physician.

Southey's capillary drainage cannula or tube. A thin rubber tube threaded along a special cannula into the subcutaneous tissues, usually of the legs, to relieve severe cardiac oedema.

Souttar, Sir Henry Sessions (b. 1875). London surgeon.

Souttar's cautery. A steam-heated cautery.

Souttar's tube. A tube consisting of a spiral cylinder of wire introduced into the lumen of the oesophagus at the site of a carcinoma as a palliative measure to relieve dysphagia.

Soxhlet, Franz Ritter von (b. 1848). Munich biochemist.

Soxhlet apparatus. An apparatus which allows continuous extraction of a solid material with a fixed volume of solvent. It is employed in biochemical analysis for extracting fats and plant principles.

soya (soi·ah). Soy beans; the seeds of several varieties of *Glycine,* including *G. max* (Linn.) Merr., *G. soja* and *Soja hispida* of the family Leguminoseae, grown in America and the Far East and sometimes known as *Chinese beans.* The chief constituents are protein (albuminoids) and a fixed oil (soya oil). There is very little starch, and it is therefore a valuable food for diabetics; in the East it is an important article of diet. From it is prepared soybean milk and soybean cheese; it is also used as a cattle food before or after the extraction of the oil. Its protein constituents are used in the plastics industry, and it contains an enzyme, urease, which converts urea into ammonium carbonate and is therefore employed in the assay of blood urea. [Hind. fennel.]

space [spatium (NA)] (spase). An area or region; a cavity. **Accommodation space.** The loose tissue round the acini of the breast which accommodates the cellular proliferation of the menstrual cycle and pregnancy. **Antecubital space.** Cubital fossa. *See* FOSSA. **Cartilage space.** One of the cell-containing cavities of cartilaginous tissue. **Cathode dark space.** A dark space in a discharge tube when the discharge is passing, between the cathode glow and the negative glow; Brookes' dark space. **Cell space.** Unstained cell-containing cavities in preparations of loose connective tissue. **Circumlental spaces.** Zonular spaces (see below). **Dead space.** 1. That volume of the tidal air (usually one-third) which, at the end of inspiration, goes no farther than the bronchial tubes; at expiration it is the first air to be expelled. Its resting (and anatomical) value is about 140 ml, and this air does not exchange gases with the blood. 2. Any unobliterated space in the body, e.g. following excision of a tumour. It is liable to become filled by blood, and to delay healing. **Distal pulp space.** A multilocular fascial compartment on the palmar aspect of the terminal phalanx. **Effective dead space.** The volume of inspired air which does not mingle with the alveolar air at inspiration, as determined by analysis of expired and alveolar airs and by the volume of the inspiration. It is larger than the anatomical dead space, especially in deep breathing. **Epidural space.** Extradural space (see below). **Episcleral space [spatium episclerale (NA)].** A tissue space between the sclera and the fascial sheath of the eyeball. **Extracellular space.** The volume of fluid calculated from markers which freely diffuse throughout the extracellular fluid but do not penetrate the inside of the cell. **Extradural space [cavum epidurale (NA)].** The potential space between the spinal dura mater and the walls of the vertebral canal, occupied by fat and the extensive internal spinal plexus of veins. **Gaussian space.** The narrow space surrounding the principal axis of a system of lenses. **H space.** A radiographically translucent area, 25-50 mm (1-2 in) wide, between the posterior border of the heart shadow and the spine, in the right anterior oblique position. Also known as *Holzknecht's space.* **Haversian space.** A widened haversian canal resulting from bone resorption. **Hypothenar space.** The fascial compartment of the palm which contains the palmaris brevis muscle. **Intercellular space.** The region between adjacent cells. **Intercostal space [spatium intercostale (NA)].** The interval between adjacent ribs and cartilages. **Interdental space.** The space between the necks of adjacent teeth. **Interfascicular space.** The space between bundles of nerve or connective-tissue fibres. **Interglobular spaces [spatia interglobularia (NA)].** Small, irregular spaces in the dentine of the tooth, supposed to be due to imperfection in calcification. **Intermesoblastic space.** The coelom. **Interosseous space.** The region between 2 adjacent bones. **Interosseous spaces of the metacarpus or of the metatarsus [spatium interosseum metacarpi, spatium interosseum metatarsi (NA)].** The interval between 2 adjacent metacarpal or metatarsal bones. **Interseptal space.** Part of the cavity of the embryonic right atrium of the heart lying between the septum primum and the septum spurium. **Intervaginal spaces [spatia intervaginalia].** The extension of the subarachnoid spaces around the optic nerve. **Intervillous space.** The space filled with maternal blood surrounding the villi of the human placenta. **Spaces of the iridocorneal angle [spatia anguli iridocornealis (NA)].** Spaces in the trabecular tissue, forming the inner wall of the sinus venosus sclerae and intervening between the latter and the anterior chamber of the eye. **Joint space.** A radiological term for that space between the 2 bony articular surfaces of a joint. **Marrow space, Medullary space.** A marrow-containing cavity in cancellous bone. **Mid-palmar space, Middle palmar space.** The medial of the 2 potential spaces in the palm of the hand, deep to the flexor tendons of the digits and superficial to the metacarpals and interossei. It is bounded medially by the palmaris muscles and laterally by a fasical septum attached to the third metacarpal; distally it communicates with the fascial covering of the 2nd, 3rd and 4th lumbrical muscles, and proximally with Parona's space. **Palmar space.** The mid-palmar and thenar spaces, *q.v.* **Pelvocrural space.** The interval between the inguinal ligament and the hip bone through which structures pass from the false pelvis to the thigh. **Perichoroidal space [spatium perichoroideale (NA)].** Any of the endothelially lined spaces in the suprachoroid lamina. **Perilymphatic space [spatium perilymphaticum (NA)].** The space between the membranous and bony labyrinth. **Perineal space, deep [spatium perinei profundum (NA)].** The potential space between the superior and inferior fasciae of the urogenital diaphragm, containing the membranous part of the urethra, the deep transversus perinei muscle and the sphincter urethrae muscle. **Perineal space, superficial [spatium perinei superficiale (NA)].** The potential space between the membranous fascia in the perineum and the perineal membrane. **Perineuronal space.** The fluid-filled space around a nerve-cell body in the central nervous system, supposed to be continuous, through the perivascular spaces of Virchow-Robin, with the subarachnoid space. It is thought to act as a nutritive and excretory channel for the nerve cell. **Perivascular spaces.** Virchow-Robin spaces. **Perivitelline space.** The space between the egg proper and the egg membrane, which appears after fertilization. **Physiological dead space.** That fraction of the tidal volume which is not available for gaseous exchange and is therefore wasted; it includes the anatomical dead space (see above). **Placental blood space.** Intervillous space (see above). **Pleuroperitoneal space.** That portion of the embryonic coelom between the pericardial and peritoneal cavities into which the lung initially expands, and which forms the basis of the pleural cavity. **Popliteal space.** Popliteal fossa. *See* FOSSA. **Prevertebral space.** H space (see above). **Prezonular space.** The part of the eye bounded by the iris in front and the anterior zonular fibres behind. **Pulp space.** The part of the finger consisting of fat and connective tissue which lies on the palm side of the fingers, especially the tip. It is a common site of infection (whitlow or felon). **Retrocardiac space.** H space (see above). **Retrolental space.** That immediately behind the crystalline lens of the eye, previously considered empty but now known to contain the anterior expansion of the primary vitreous. **Retroperitoneal space [spatium retroperitoneale (NA)].** The potential space in the loose fascia outside the parietal peritoneum. **Retropharyngeal space.** A cellular interval separating the pharynx from the prevertebral layer of the cervical fascia. **Retropubic space [spatium retropubicum (NA)].** A potential space, occupied by a pad of fat, the retropubic pad, between the urinary bladder and the symphysis and body of the pubis and below the level of the reflection of the peritoneum from the anterior abdominal wall to the bladder; the cave of Retzius. **Retrozonular space.** That part of the eye bounded by the zonular fibres in front, the vitreous behind and the ciliary body laterally. Also called *canal of Petit.* **Space medicine.** *See* MEDICINE. **Space probe.** *See* PROBE. **Subarachnoid space [cavum subarachnoideale (NA)].** The space between the arachnoid and pia mater containing cerebrospinal fluid showing dilatations or subarachnoid cisterns, in various places in the cranium and extending caudally to the level of the 2nd sacral vertebra. It is crossed by delicate trabeculae joining the arachnoid and pia mater. **Subdural space.** The potential space between the inner layer of the cranial dura mater (or the spinal dura mater) and the arachnoid mater. **Subhepatic spaces.** Two potential peritoneal spaces below the liver. The *right* subhepatic space corresponds to Morison's pouch and the *left* to the lesser sac of the peritoneum. **Subphrenic spaces.** The peritoneal recesses which lie between the upper surface of the liver and the lower surface of the diaphragm. They lie one on either side of the falciform ligament. **Suprasternal space.** A space between the layers of the deep cervical fascia where they are attached to the anterior and posterior borders of the manubrium sterni. **Thenar space.** The lateral of the 2 potential spaces in the palm of the hand, deep to the flexor tendons of the digits and superficial to the metacarpals and interossei. It is bounded laterally by the thenar muscles and medially by a fascial septum attached to the third metacarpal; distally it communicates with the fascial covering of the first (and occasionally the second) lumbrical muscle. **Venous spaces of the corpora cavernosa [cavernae corporum cavernosorum (NA)].** The intertrabecular venous spaces of the corpora cavernosa of the penis or the clitoris. **Venous spaces of the corpus spongiosum [cavernae corporis spongiosi (NA)].** The intertrabecular venous spaces in the corpus spongiosum. **Yolk space.** Perivitelline space (see above). **Zonular spaces of the ciliary zonule [spatia zonularia (NA)].** Irregular spaces in the ciliary zonule linked to form a canal behind the suspensory ligament of the lens, encircling the lens equator. [L *spatium*.]

See also: BLESSIG, BOGROS (A. J.), BROCA, BURNS (A.), CHASSAIGNAC, CLOQUET (J. G.), COLLES, COTUGNO (COTUNNIUS), CROOKES, CZERMAK (J. N.), DESSE, DOUGLAS (J.), FARADAY, FONTANA (F.), HENKE, HIS (W., SNR.), HOLZKNECHT, KANAVEL, KIERNAN, KRETSCHMANN, LARREY, MAGENDIE, MALACARNE, MOHRENHEIM, NUEL, PARONA, POISEUILLE, PROUST (P. T.), PRUSSAK, RETZIUS (A. A.), ROBIN (C. P.), SCHWALBE, SEMB, TARIN, TENON, TRAUBE (L.), TRAUTMANN, TROELTSCH, VIRCHOW, WESTBERG, ZANG.

space-retainer (spase·re·ta·ner). An apparatus for maintaining the space left by deciduous teeth which have been prematurely lost, into which the permanent teeth can erupt. [space, L *retinere* to keep.]

Spaeth, Edmund Benjamin (b. 1890). Philadelphia ophthalmologist.

Spaeth's operation. For epicanthus. Two adjoining crescentic-shaped vertical incisions are made just medial to the epicanthal folds; these form an X shape. Two lateral incisions from the lateral tips of the two X's are made towards the upper and lower lid. The two triangular flaps are then swung laterally towards the upper and lower lid respectively and sutured in to the position of the 2 lateral incisions whose edges have been undermined and retracted to receive them.

spagirism (spaj·ir·izm). Spagyrism.

spagyric (spaj·ir·ik). Relating or belonging to spagyrism.

spagyrism (spaj·ir·izm). The paracelsian or alchemistic school or theory of medicine. [Fr. *spagirie* alchemy.]

spagyrist (spaj·ir·ist). An alchemist or paracelsian; an iatrochemist. [see prec.]

Spahlinger, Henry (b. 1882). Geneva bacteriologist.

Spahlinger treatment. The treatment of tuberculosis by a special method of vaccine and serum therapy.

Spalding, Alfred Baker (b. 1874). San Francisco gynaecologist.

Spalding's sign. The overlapping of the fetal skull bones seen on x-ray examination when there is fetal death *in utero*.

Spallanzani, Lazaro (b. 1729). Italian physiologist.

Spallanzani's law. Young cells have more power to regenerate than older ones.

spanaemia (span·e·me·ah). Anaemia. [Gk *spanos* scarce, *haima* blood.]

Spangler's treatment. The use of injections of rattlesnake venom in cases of epilepsy. [Obsolete.]

spanopnoea (span·op·ne·ah). Slow and deep respiration associated with dyspnoea. [Gk *spanos* scarce, *pnoia* breath.]

sparadrap (spar·ad·rap). A plaster. [It. *sparadrappo*.]

sparer (spa·rer). A foodstuff which, by replacing another foodstuff, reduces the need for it. [AS *spaer*.]

sparganosis (spar·gan·o·sis). Infestation with a species of the pseudogenus, Sparganum. [*Sparganum*, Gk *-osis* condition.]

Sparganum (spar·gan·um). A pseudogeneric name given to plerocercoids of species of tapeworms belonging to the genus *Diphyllobothrium*. It is used particularly when the adult is unknown, but also as a general term for larvae of this form. The procercoids of all species develop in copepods of the genus *Cyclops*. The specific identity of the named forms is not yet clear. **Sparganum baxter.** A plerocercoid from the Far East, rarely recorded in man. **Sparganum erinacei.** A plerocercoid from Europe which develops best in Amphibia and has been recorded in human muscle. **Sparganum mansoni.** A plerocercoid from India and the Far East generally; it develops best in frogs, and infestations around the eye are common in man following the placing of freshly killed frogs on sore eyes. **Sparganum mansonoides.** A plerocercoid from America which develops best in mice and has been recorded from human muscle. **Sparganum proliferum.** A species recorded from Florida and Japan which multiplies in superficial human muscle, forming thousands of small attached individuals in an elongate irregular mass. It is believed to result from the effects of abnormal environments. [Gk *sparganon* swaddling clothes.]

spargosis (spar·go·sis). 1. Abnormal swelling of a part. 2. A condition in which the skin is swollen or thickened. 3. Distension of the mammary glands with milk. 4. Elephantiasis. [Gk *spargaein* to swell.]

Sparmannia africana (spar·man·e·ah af·rik·ah·nah). A mucilaginous plant grown in Africa.

sparteine (spar·te·een). $C_{15}H_{26}N_2$, an alkaloid obtained from the broom, *Cytisus scoparius*. It was introduced as a substitute for digitalis in cardiac diseases, but its effect is very different; it lessens both the irritability and conductivity of the cardiac muscle and the frequency and amplitude of its contractions are diminished. Only excessively large doses show diuretic properties. It is used chiefly in medicine for the treatment of irregularities of the heart, such as tachycardia and functional palpitation, but is only of limited usefulness. **Sparteine hydrochloride.** The hydrochloride of sparteine which is soluble in water and alcohol. **Sparteine sulphate.** The commonest form in which sparteine is used; it is soluble in water. **Sparteine tri-iodide.** A compound of sparteine and iodine used like the sulphate. [L *spartium* broom.]

spartism (spar·tizm). Poisoning caused by ingestion of sparteine.

spartium (spar·she·um). Scoparium. [L broom.]

spasm (spazm). A sudden, powerful, involuntary contraction of muscle. **Spasm of accommodation.** Undue contraction of the ciliary muscle, sometimes causing a state of artificial myopia, caused by an attempt to overcome a weak accommodation, as in early presbyopia or reading too close. It also follows the administration of strong miotic drugs. **Athetoid spasms.** The spasmodic movements of athetosis. **Blacksmiths' spasm.** Hephestic spasm (see below). **Bronchial spasm.** Asthma; contraction of the bronchoconstrictor muscles. **Cadaveric spasm.** The instant contraction of voluntary muscle at the moment of death, especially under emotional tension, e.g. resulting in a victim gripping the knife used to kill in a vice-like grasp. Wrongly used to describe post-mortem rigidity or rigor mortis. **Canine spasm.** Risus sardonicus; spasm of the facial muscles in tetanus. **Carpopedal spasm.** Muscular spasms of the hands and feet in tetany. **Cerebral spasm.** Muscular spasm of cerebral origin. **Ciliary spasm.** Spasm of accommodation (see above). **Clonic spasm.** Alternating involuntary contractions and relaxations of muscles. **Spasm of convergence.** An excess of convergence which it is difficult to relax; it can be due to an irritative cerebral lesion or hysteria, or associated with an accommodative spasm. **Convulsive tic spasm.** Habit spasm (see below). **Cyclic oculomotor spasm.** A rare condition in which one eye shows first almost total ophthalmoplegia, with ptosis, followed by contraction of the pupil, slight convergence, upper lid retraction and spasm of accommodation. These 2 phases continue alternating in a rhythmic fashion. **Cynic spasm.** Canine spasm (see above). **Dancing spasm.** Saltatory spasm (see below). **Drivers' spasm.** A fatigue spasm (see below) of drivers; first described as cramps in the arms of drivers of horse-drawn carriages when they took the reins. **Facial spasm.** Involuntary spasmodic movements in the muscles innervated by the facial nerve; it may be generalized throughout the facial musculature on one side, but often begins in the orbicularis oculi, and is called *facial hemispasm*. In many cases it is due to an irritative lesion of the facial nerve. **Fatigue spasm.** Incapacitating cramp-like spasm of the muscles involved most frequently in the individual's occupation; e.g. writers' cramp, tailors' cramp, etc.; now known not to be due to fatigue but to be a manifestation of occupational neurosis. **Fixed spasm.** A permanent rigidity of a muscle. **Flexor spasm.** Involuntary flexion of the lower limbs in paraplegia. **Functional spasm.** Fatigue spasm (see above). **Glottic spasm.** Spasm of the constrictor mechanism of the larynx resulting in laryngeal obstruction and stridor. **Habit spasm.** Spasmodic movements, particularly of the muscles of the face or shoulder girdles, which are originally voluntary but later become so habitual as to be almost involuntary, though they may sometimes be stopped temporarily by an effort of the will. They occur particularly in tense, anxious individuals, and are also called *tics.* **Hammer spasm.** Fatigue spasm (see above) in the operative arm of workers who wield hammers. **Handicraft spasm.** Any fatigue spasm (see above). **Hemifacial spasm.** A disorder of the facial nerve giving rise to involuntary spasmodic contractions of the muscles of facial expression. **Hephestic spasm.** Spasmodic muscular movements in hemiplegic limbs; post-hemiplegic chorea alleged to be common in blacksmiths. **Histrionic spasm.** Habit spasm of the facial muscles giving rise to exaggerated facial expressions. **Idiopathic muscular spasm.** Spontaneous cramps. **Infantile spasm.** A form of epilepsy comprising brief attacks of flexion of the trunk and major fits in infancy, accompanied by progressive mental and motor defect; *syn.* hypsarrhythmia. There is a characteristic appearance in the EEG. **Inspiratory spasm.** Bronchial spasm occurring during inspiration. **Intention spasm.** A muscular spasm brought on by a voluntary movement. **Laryngeal spasm.** Reflex reduction in size of the rima glottidis, causing stridor and respiratory obstruction. **Laryngeal congenital spasm.** A spasmodic narrowing of the laryngeal airway in infancy, resulting in inspiratory stridor. It is not associated with developmental errors in the larynx, and tends to disappear at the age of 2 years. **Lingual spasm.** A rare condition in which anarthria is due to bilateral spasm of muscles innervated by the hypoglossal nerve; also called *aphthargia.* **Lock spasm.** Writers' cramp in which the finger locks around the pen; fatigue spasm (see above). **Malleatory spasm.** Sharp muscular twitching of the hands, like taps of a hammer. **Masticatory spasm.** Spasm of the jaw muscles. **Milkers' spasm.** An occupational neurosis occurring sometimes in milkers. **Mimic spasm.** Facial tic or habit spasm (see above). **Mobile spasm.** Slow, irregular spasmodic movements of hemiplegic limbs. **Movement spasm.** Fatigue spasm (see above). **Myopathic spasm.** Myotonia. **Nictitating spasm.** Blinking of the eyelids; spasmodic contractions of the orbicularis oculi muscle. **Nodding spasm.** Clonic contractions of the anterior neck muscles, particularly the sternocleidomastoids, giving head-nodding. In its most severe form, the frequent bowing movements have led to the term *salaam spasm* being used. **Occupational spasm.** Fatigue spasm (see above). **Oculogyric spasms.** Conjugate tonic spasmodic deviation of the eyes, usually upwards, found in postencephalitics. Usually called *oculogyric crises.* **Pantomimic spasm.** Tic; habit spasm (see above). **Penman's spasm.** Writers' cramp; a form of fatigue spasm (see above). **Peripheral vascular spasm.** Spasm of the muscles controlling the peripheral blood vessels. **Phonatory spasm.** A sudden closure of the glottis when the individual attempts to phonate. It may be hysterical, but is sometimes seen in professional voice users, due to faulty voice production. **Progressive torsion spasm.** Dystonia musculorum deformans; a syndrome characterized by torsion of the limbs and trunk with involuntary, spasmodic muscular movements. It is due to disease of the basal ganglia and is usually called *torsion spasm* or *torsion dystonia.* **Respiratory spasm.** Spasm of the diaphragm; hiccup. **Retrocollic spasm.** Spasmodic contraction of the posterior neck muscles, giving head retraction. **Rotatory spasm.** Rotatory movements of the head due to intermittent contraction of the splenius capitis muscle. **Salaam spasm.** Spasmodic bowing movements; nodding spasm (see above). **Saltatory spasm.** Spasmodic contractions of the leg muscles giving a peculiar leaping, jumping action; also called *palmus, choromania, jumping disease, jumping sickness, dancing spasm,* etc. It is sometimes a manifestation of hysteria, sometimes of psychosis. **Sewing spasm.** Fatigue spasm (see above) of tailors, cobblers and seamstresses, and of others whose work involves sewing. **Smiths' spasm.** Hephestic spasm or blacksmiths' spasm (see above). **Sobbing spasm.** A syncopal attack in infancy occurring after protracting sobbing leading to panting bradypnoea culminating in transient asphyxia. **Spinal accessory spasm.** Clonic contraction of muscles innervated by the spinal accessory nerve, particularly the sternocleidomastoid muscle; spasmodic torticollis. **Static reflex spasm.** Saltatory spasm (see above). **Stutter spasm.** Speech difficulty allied to stutter due to spasm of the lingual and palatal muscles. **Synclonic spasm.** Clonic spasms affecting more than one muscle. **Telegraphists' spasm.** Fatigue spasm (see above) of telegraphists, involving particularly the muscles of the "tapping" finger. **Tetanic spasm.** 1. A spasm in which muscular contraction persists unchanged for some time; also called *tonic spasm.* 2. A muscular spasm in a case of tetanus. **Tonic spasm.** A sustained contraction (of muscle) as opposed to a clonic or intermittent contraction. **Torsion spasm.** Involuntary movements causing twisting of the limbs and spine, occurring in a number of disorders. **Toxic spasm.** Spasms or convulsions caused by poisoning. **Winking spasm.** Nictitating spasm (see above). **Writers' spasm.** Writers' cramp; a form of fatigue spasm (see above). [Gk *spasmos.*]

See also: BELL (C.), FRIEDREICH, ROMBERG.

spasmodic (spaz·**mod**·ik). 1. Relating or referring to spasm. 2. Affected with spasm. 3. Characterized by a spasm or spasms. [Gk *spasmodes.*]

spasmodism (**spaz**·mod·izm). Spasmodic conditions of the muscles, due to medullary centres being stimulated or subjected to excitation. [see prec.]

spasmodyspnoea (**spaz**·mo·**disp**′·ne·ah). Dyspnoea caused by spasm; generally of the diaphragm or intercostal muscles.

spasmolygmus (spaz·mo·**lig**·mus). Spasmodic hiccup. [spasm, Gk *lygx* hiccup.]

spasmolysant (spaz·mo·**li**·sant). 1. Relieving spasms. 2. A drug which relieves or relaxes spasm. [see foll.]

spasmolysis (spaz·**mol**·is·is). Arrest of a convulsive attack or of a spasm. [spasm, Gk *lysis* a loosing.]

spasmolytic (spaz·mo·**lit**·ik). Arresting spasm. [see prec.]

spasmomyxorrhoea (**spaz**·mo·mix·o·**re**′·ah). Myxorrhoea intestinalis; a mucoid discharge from the bowel occurring in neurotic persons suffering undue mental strain. [spasm, myxorrhoea.]

spasmophemia (spaz·mo·**fe**·me·ah). A fitful type of dysphemia in which no utterance of any kind can be made, there apparently being a nervous obstruction which the sufferer is for a time unable to overcome. [spasm, Gk *pheme* speech.]

spasmophile (**spaz**·mo·file). Spasmophilic.

spasmophilia (spaz·mo·**fil**·e·ah). The spasmophilic diathesis; a morbid state in which there is abnormal response of the motor nerves to electrical or mechanical excitation, shown by a tendency to tetany, convulsions and spasm. [spasm, Gk *philein* to love.]

spasmophilic (spaz·mo·**fil**·ik). Having a tendency to, or characterized by spasmodic seizures. [see prec.]

spasmotin (**spaz**·mo·tin). $C_{20}H_{21}O_9$, a poisonous acid principle from ergot.

spasmotoxin (spaz·mo·**tox**·in). The toxin tetanospasmin produced by *Clostridium tetani.* [spasm, toxin.]

spasmous (**spaz**·mus). Having the characteristics of spasm.

spasmus (**spaz**·mus). Spasm. **Spasmus bronchialis.** Asthma. **Spasmus caninus.** Risus sardonicus; the spasm of facial muscles in tetanus. **Spasmus glottidis.** Glottic spasm. *See* SPASM. **Spasmus intestinorum.** Intestinal colic. *See* COLIC. **Spasmus muscularis.** A muscular spasm. **Spasmus nictitans.** A clonic spasm of the orbicularis oculi muscle, causing prolonged and excessive blinking associated with irritative conditions of the eye, the facial nerve or the trigeminal nerve. **Spasmus nutans.** Nodding spasm. *See* SPASM. **Spasmus oculi.** Nystagmus [obsolete term]. **Spasmus ventriculi.** A gastric spasm. [Gk *spasmos.*]

spastic (**spas**·tik). 1. Relating or belonging to spasm, particularly tonic spasm; spasmodic. 2. Produced by spasm; convulsive; tetanic. 3. One affected with spasticity, often applied to children with cerebral palsy. [Gk *spastikos* drawing in.]

spasticity (spas·**tis**·it·e). 1. The quality of being spastic. 2. Strongly marked hypertonicity of muscles, characterized by rigidity and increased reflexes. **Clasp-knife spasticity.** Rigid tonic contraction of muscle in response to attempted stretch; when sufficient force is applied, sudden complete relaxation occurs. **Spasticity of conjugate gaze.** Conjugate lateral deviation of the eyes on forced closure of the lids, caused by a cerebral lesion on the contralateral side. [see prec.]

spatial (**spa**·shal). Relating or belonging to space or to any space. [L *spatium* space.]

spatula (**spat**·ew·lah). A flat, blunt knife, of metal or plastic, used for mixing or transferring powders or ointments. [dim. of L *spatha* paddle.]

See also: ROUX (P. P. E.).

spatular (**spat**·ew·lar). Spatulate.

spatulate, spatulated (**spat**·ew·late, **spat**·ew·la·ted). 1. Shaped like a spatula. 2. Spoon-shaped.

spatule (**spat**·ewl). A spatulate structure, organ or part.

Spatz, Hugo (b. 1888). Giessen neurologist.

Hallervorden-Spatz disease or syndrome. A progressive disease of childhood, characterized by progressive rigidity, athetotic movements and mental and emotional dulling, and pathologically by degeneration of the globus pallidus and reticular part of the substantia nigra.

spay (spa). To excise the ovaries; to castrate a female animal. [O Fr. *espeier*.]

spearmint (**speer**·mint). Mint, garden mint; the dried leaf and flowering tops of *Mentha viridis* Linn. (family Labiatae). It yields a volatile oil containing L-limonene and L-carvone. [ME *spere*, Gk *mintha*.]

specialism (**spesh**·al·izm). In medicine, concentration on 1 special branch of medical science. [see foll.]

specialist (**spesh**·al·ist). In medicine, one who concentrates on 1 special branch of medical science. [L *specialis* individual.]

specialization (**spesh**·al·i·za′·shun). In medicine, the act of concentrating on 1 special branch of medical science. [see prec.]

species (**spe**·sheez). 1. A taxonomic class category below the genus and composed of individuals; a group of actually or potentially interbreeding natural populations which are reproductively isolated from other such groups. 2. A popular name applied to certain herb preparations, e.g. *aromatic species*, a mixture of garden thyme, wild thyme, peppermint, lavender, cubebs and cloves. **Di-ovulatory species.** Species that discharge 2 eggs at 1 ovulation. **Monovulatory species.** Species that discharge 1 egg at 1 ovulation. **Morphological species.** A community, or number of related communities, the distinctive morphological characters of whose individuals are sufficiently definite to entitle them to a specific name. **Polyovulatory species.** Species that discharge many eggs at 1 ovulation. [L form.]

specific (spes·**if**·ik). 1. Of or pertaining to any particular thing; reacting with any particular class of compound, e.g. a specific enzyme. 2. Of or pertaining to any class category composed of individuals; pertaining to a taxonomic species. 3. A remedy that cures a particular ailment, because, for example, it acts on a particular causal organism or supplies a particular deficiency. [L *species* form, *facere* to make.]

specificity (spes·if·**is**·it·e). 1. The quality of being specific. 2. Of antigens, the affinity for the corresponding antibody; these may be group specific, type specific or species specific. 3. Specific phase; used of *Salmonellae* which are subject to diphasic variation of their flagellar antigens. 4. The extent to which a method gives results that are free from false positives; the fewer the false positives, the greater is the specificity (*see also* SENSITIVITY).

specillum (spe·**sil**·um). A probe or sound. [L *specere* to look.]

specimen (**spes**·im·en). A part of anything taken as a sample for the purpose of diagnosis, identification, study or demonstration. [L sample.]

spectacles (**spek**·taklz). Framed or rimless glasses fitted with side pieces (temples). **Bifocal spectacles.** Spectacles in which each lens has 2 parts of different focal lengths. The commonest type is that in which the upper part is a correction for distant vision and the lower contains a presbyopic addition for reading and close work. **Bloomed spectacles.** Spectacles of which the lenses are coated with a thin film that diminishes surface reflection, thus allowing more light to pass through them. **Compound spectacles.** Spectacles fitted with additional lenses. These may be tinted for protection from glare and are then plane, or they may have dioptric power, e.g. convex to convert distance into reading glasses, or concave to convert reading into distance glasses. **Decentred spectacles.** Those in which the optical centres of the lenses do not coincide with the geometrical centres and so produce a prismatic effect. **Divided spectacles.** Term usually applied to Franklin's split bifocals. **Galilean spectacles.** Telescopic spectacles (see below). **Mica spectacles.** Goggles fitted with sheets of mica to protect the eyes from foreign bodies. It is usual now to employ transparent plastic material which can, if necessary, be moulded into the shape of the lenses required for correction of errors of refraction. **Orthoscopic spectacles.** Spectacles used for fine, close work: each lens is combined with a prism, base in, of corresponding dioptric strength to which may be added any correction needed for ametropia. **Pantoscopic spectacles.** Reading spectacles with ᴗ-shaped lenses which enable the user to look over the top of them. **Periscopic spectacles.** Spectacles containing lenses so designed as to enable the wearer to see distinctly when ranging his eyes up and down or from side to side. **Prismatic spectacles.** Spectacles the lenses of which contain prisms for the purpose of overcoming the strain and diplopia caused by defective movements of the eyes. **Protective spectacles.** A variety of forms of spectacles designed to protect the eye from trauma. A simple example is the use of lenses made of plastic material in place of glass, so that breakage is avoided. **Pulpit spectacles.** Pantoscopic spectacles (see above). **Stenopeic spectacles.** Spectacles the lenses of which are replaced by opaque discs pierced by 1 or more small holes; slits are sometimes used. They are of use in cases of corneal opacities and for focusing simultaneously objects at different distances, e.g. in sighting a rifle. **Telescopic spectacles.** Those designed on the principle of the galilean telescope, that is with a convex lens as objective and a concave as eyepiece, separated by the difference in their focal length. This gives magnification and is particularly useful in high myopia and in cases with retinal degeneration; galilean spectacles. **Tinted spectacles.** Spectacles the lenses of which are tinted variously according to the purposes for which they are required, e.g. to keep out ultraviolet light, to reduce the amount of visible light or to keep out heat rays. Some tinted spectacles depend to a large extent on reflection for their efficiency, e.g. those incorporating a thin film of platinum or gold, and are cooler to wear than the ordinary dark glasses. **Wire-framed spectacles.** Protective spectacles made of fine-mesh wire gauze. [L *spectaculum* a show.]

See also: FRANKLIN, MASSELON.

Spectinomycin (**spek**·tin·o·**mi**′·sin). BP Commission approved name for an antibiotic produced by *Streptomyces spectabilis*.

spectral (**spek**·tral). 1. Relating or belonging to the spectrum or to a spectrum. 2. Made by the spectrum. 3. Carried out by means of the spectrum.

spectrochrome (**spek**·tro·krome). A form of treatment which consists of exposing a patient to various colours of the spectrum. [spectrum, Gk *chroma* colour.]

spectrocolorimeter (**spek**·tro·kol·or·**im**′·et·er). A form of spectroscope used for detecting perception of 1 colour. [spectrum, colour, meter.]

spectrograph (**spek**·tro·graf). 1. An optical arrangement designed to record spectra upon a photographic plate. 2. Any such photograph of a spectrum. **Mass spectrograph.** An apparatus by means of which a beam of mixed ions of different weights or charges may be deflected by electrical and magnetic fields into a band like an optical spectrum. It is used to identify and determine the mass of individual atoms and to separate isotopes. **Sound spectrograph.** Sonograph. **Quartz spectrograph.** One in which the prisms and lenses are of quartz for use with ultraviolet light. **X-ray spectrograph.** One used in crystal analysis with x-rays. [spectrum, Gk *graphein* to record.]

See also: LITTROW.

spectrometer (spek·**trom**·et·er). A graduated spectroscope by means of which the angle that light is refracted can be measured and the wavelength of any part of a spectrum deduced therefrom. It may also be used to determine refractive indices. **Constant deviation spectrometer.** One incorporating a right-angled prism so that the spectrum is produced at a fixed angle to the light source. **Infrared spectrometer.** An instrument which produces a spectrum in the infrared region on which intensity and wavelength measurements may be made. It is generally used for the investigation of infrared absorption spectra. **Isotopic mass spectrometer.** A physical instrument in which a beam of ions of fixed isotopic weight may be collected and measured in intensity. The instrument may be used for the exact comparison of isotopic weights, the comparison of the relative percentages of the isotopes of an element, or for the measurement of very small quantities of a stable isotope. **Neutron spectrometer.** An apparatus for the production and measurement of Bragg reflections from a crystal of a neutron beam. **X-ray spectrometer.** An apparatus for the production and measurement of Bragg reflections from a crystal of an x-ray beam. [spectrum, meter.]

spectrometry (spek·**trom**·et·re). 1. The determination of refractive indices by means of the spectrometer. 2. The estimation of the wavelengths of light rays with a spectrometer, and the recognition of the spectra characteristic of certain elements and compounds.

spectromicroscope (spek·tro·**mi**·kro·skope). 1. A spectroscope used in conjunction with a microscope to examine absorption bands of tissues. 2. A microscope eyepiece fitted to a spectroscope in order to examine the spectral lines more closely. [spectrum, microscope.]

spectrophobia (spek·tro·**fo**·be·ah). 1. Morbid fear of seeing oneself in a mirror. 2. Fear of spectres or ghosts. [spectrum, phobia.]

spectrophone (**spek**·tro·fone). An instrument adapted for use in spectrometry, whereby the visible spectrum is converted into a succession of sounds. [spectrum, Gk *phone* sound.]

spectrophotometer (**spek**·tro·fo·**tom**'·et·er). An instrument used to compare the intensities of 2 differently coloured light sources by resolving their light into spectra and measuring the relative intensities of those spectra, wavelength by wavelength. **Infrared absorption spectrophotometer.** An instrument for the measurement of the variation of the intensity with wavelength of the absorption spectrum produced by a substance in the infrared region. [spectrum, Gk *phos* light, meter.]

spectrophotometry (**spek**·tro·fo·**tom**'·et·re). The ultraviolet, infrared and fluorescent methods of chemical analysis used in the detection and measurement of toxic substances in body tissues and fluids. Absorption curves for most substances enable accurate quantitative and qualitative data to be obtained. [spectrum, Gk *phos* light, meter.]

spectropolarimeter (**spek**·tro·po·lar·**im**'·et·er). A combination of a spectroscope and a polarimeter for determining the optical rotation of light of different wavelengths.

spectropyrheliometer (**spek**·tro·pire·he·le·**om**'·et·er). An apparatus for measuring the energy corresponding to different parts of the sun's spectrum. [spectrum, Gk *pyr* fire, *helios* sun, meter.]

spectroscope (**spek**·tro·skope). An instrument for producing and examining the spectra of luminous bodies in order to determine the composition of the latter. **Direct-vision spectroscope.** A convenient form of spectroscope having an arrangement of crown and flint glass prisms to give dispersion without deviation of the mean ray. It is used for the qualitative examination of luminous bodies. **Reversion spectroscope.** A spectroscope which gives 2 spectra of the same solution under examination arranged so that 1 spectrum is in the reverse direction to the other. [spectrum, Gk *skopein* to view.]

See also: HARTRIDGE.

spectroscopic (spek·tro·**skop**·ik). Relating or belonging to the spectroscope or spectroscopy.

spectroscopy (spek·**tros**·ko·pe). The use of the spectroscope in chemical analysis or physics.

spectrotherapy (spek·tro·**ther**·ap·e). The use of various rays of the spectrum for therapeutic purposes.

spectrum (**spek**·trum). 1. The band of colours formed when white light is passed through a glass prism. 2. A range of wavelengths of electromagnetic radiation extending from the shortest gamma rays to the longest waves used in wireless telegraphy. The *visible spectrum* includes radiation of wavelengths between about 400 to 800 nm (4000 to 8000 Å) (from violet to red); the *invisible spectrum* extends below 400 nm (4000 Å) (ultraviolet, grenz rays, x-rays and gamma rays) and above 800 nm (8000 Å) (infrared rays and radio waves). **Absorption spectrum.** A plan of the amount of absorption of light in terms of wavelength, specific for each chemical substance. **Acoustic spectrum.** The range of sounds that are audible, i.e. from 16 to 24 000 Hz (c/s). **Active spectrum.** A plan of the effectiveness of various wavelengths producing a given biological effect. **Bacterial spectrum.** 1. Referring to an antibiotic or chemotherapeutic agent, the range of bacteria usually susceptible to its action. 2. A range of bacterial species found in a given situation, e.g. in urinary infections. **Band spectrum.** A spectrum consisting of a number of bright bands of light, one edge of a band being sharp, the other edge being less well defined; it gives a fluted appearance and is often referred to as *fluted spectrum.* **Chemical spectrum.** The part of the spectrum which includes the ultraviolet or actinic rays. **Chromatic spectrum.** That part which includes the visible rays. **Continuous spectrum.** A spectrum containing all wavelengths between the limits of the spectrum. **Diffraction spectrum.** A spectrum formed when light is passed through a diffraction grating. **Dispersion spectrum.** That produced by refraction of light by a glass prism and in which the deviation is *not* proportional to the wavelength. **Electromagnetic spectrum.** The complete range of wavelengths of electromagnetic radiation. **Emission spectrum.** The spectrum of radiation emitted from a source, e.g. spectrum of sunlight (*see* SOLAR SPECTRUM, below). **Energy spectrum.** All the wavelengths representing radiant energy, from the long radio waves, infrared or heat waves, visible light waves, ultraviolet waves, down to the very short x-rays and cosmic rays. **Fluted spectrum.** Band spectrum (see above). **Fortification spectrum.** The zig-zag of bright, coloured light seen in the visual aura of migraine; it may be part of, or the beginning of the scintillating scotoma. **Gaseous spectrum.** The spectrum of light given out by glowing gases in a discharge tube and consisting of a number of bright lines in different parts of the spectrum. **Grating spectrum.** Diffraction spectrum (see above). **Line spectrum.** A spectrum consisting of sharp, bright lines given by elements heated to incandescence if solid, or submitted to an electric discharge if gaseous. **Normal spectrum.** Diffraction or grating spectrum, the characteristic of which is that the deviation of each colour from the direction of the incident light is proportional to its wavelength. **Prismatic spectrum.** Dispersion spectrum (see above). **Pure spectrum.** A spectrum in which there is no mixing of colours. **Series spectrum.** A spectrum in which the arrangement of the lines is regular. **Solar spectrum.** The spectrum of sunlight which is a continuous spectrum crossed by a number of dark lines (the Fraunhofer lines) all of which occupy the exact positions of the emission spectrum lines of certain elements. **Thermal spectrum.** That part of the spectrum where the red and infrared rays lie. **Toxin spectrum.** A diagram used by Ehrlich to demonstrate the neutralizing power of antitoxins against toxins and various modified toxins. **Visible spectrum.** All those wavelengths 800–400 nm (8000–4000 Å) of radiant energy that are visible as light to the human eye. **X-ray spectrum.** The spectrum of a heterogeneous beam of x-rays produced by diffraction at a crystal lattice. [L image.]

See also: SWAN, VAUBAN.

speculum (**spek**·ew·lum). Any instrument used in the inspection of a normally closed tube or passage. They vary in type according to their intended use. Many are named after the person who invented them. **Anal speculum.** A speculum for the examination of the anal canal. **Aural speculum.** An instrument inserted into the external auditory meatus to facilitate its examination and to allow inspection of the tympanic membrane. **Duck-billed speculum.** A U-shaped speculum having 2 spatulate blades of different sizes at each side of the U; devised by Sims for use in the repair of vesicovaginal fistula. **Eye speculum.** An instrument designed for automatic retraction of the eyelids during ophthalmic surgery. **Lacrimal-sac speculum.** A spring speculum with teeth designed to keep apart the skin and orbicularis oculi muscle in lacrimal-sac surgery. **Nasal speculum.** An instrument inserted within the anterior nares to facilitate inspection of the nasal cavity. **Rectal speculum.** A hollow, cylindrical, metal instrument, usually with a handle, and an obturator, used to inspect the cavity of the rectum. **Urethral speculum.** A narrow, hollow cylinder with an obturator used in the examination of the female urethra. **Vaginal speculum.** An instrument of which there is a wide variety of types, used in the inspection of the vaginal cavity and cervix, e.g. bivalved, consisting of 2 opening blades which are articulated at one end. [L mirror.]

See also: ARRUGA, AUVARD, CUSCO, FERGUSSON, HELMHOLTZ, HELMONT, KELLY (H. A.), LANG, LAWFORD, SIEGLE, SIMS, TERSON, VAUBAN.

Spee, Ferdinand Graf von (b. 1855). Kiel embryologist.

Spee's curve. A curved line passing through the tips of the buccal cusps of the premolar and molar teeth.

speech (speech). The expression and reception of ideas and feelings by way of verbal symbols. **Ataxic speech.** The dysarthria of cerebellar ataxia. **Bulbar speech.** Thick, slurring dysarthria due to paralysis of articulatory muscles from a bulbar or suprabulbar lesion. **Clipped speech.** Speech in which each word is clipped. **Echo speech.** 1. A tendency to repeat words pronounced or recently heard. 2. Repetitive speech produced by stimuli during a hypnotic state. **Explosive speech.** Sudden loud utterances met with in mental cases. **Incoherent speech.** Disconnected utterances while semiconscious or delirious. **Inner speech.** The silent process of thought. **Interjectional speech.** Emotional expression by expletives or inarticulate cries: found in motor aphasia. **Jumbled speech.** Incoherent speech (see above). **Mirror speech.** Speech in which the order of syllables may be reversed. **Oesophageal speech.** A type of speech which may be used following laryngectomy; the sound produced by the regurgitation of air swallowed into the oesophagus is modified into speech by movements of the tongue, lips, cheeks and palate. **Plateau speech.** Speech characterized by high, even, monotonous tone. **Speech reading.** Lip reading by a deaf person. **Scamping speech.** Clipped speech (see above). **Scanning speech.** Slow deliberate speech in which syllables are separated. **Slurred speech.** Speech in which the words are not completed and tend to run into each other, met with in general paralysis (dementia paralytica). **Staccato speech.** Jerky speech with syllables separated, met with in multiple sclerosis. **Syllabic speech.** Scanning speech (see above). [AS *spaec.*]

speedwell (speed·wel). Bird's eye, cat's eye; the dried leaves and flowering tops of *Veronica officinalis* (family Scrophulariaceae). It is used as an expectorant and diuretic. [AS *spedan, wel.*]

speliotomy (spe·le·ot·o·me). The external drainage made for a large tuberculous cavity in the lung. The operation is done in 2 stages, the first to secure adhesion of the pleural layers by applying an iodine pack to the outer layer, and the second by incision into and cleaning of the wall of the cavity and subsequent daily packing. Healing occurs only slowly, but symptoms are much relieved. [Gk *spelaion* cave, *temnein* to cut.]

spelter (spel·ter). The name given to commercial zinc containing 1–3 per cent of lead, 0.1 per cent of iron and traces of arsenic and cadmium. [etym. dub.]

Spemann, Hans (b. 1869). German embryologist.

Spemann's induction. The process whereby tissue and cellular differentiation is initiated as a result of influences emanating from neighbouring cells of a different type, or as the result of artificial stimulation.

Spence, James (b.1812). Edinburgh surgeon.

Spence's axillary tail. The axillary tail of the breast.

Spencer, Roscoe Ray (b. 1888). American physician.

Spencer–Parker vaccine. A vaccine of Rocky Mountain spotted fever made from ground-up ticks.

Spencer, Walter George (b. 1860). London surgeon.

Spencer's area. An area of the cerebral cortex which, on stimulation, influences respiratory movements. It lies in the frontal lobe, anterior to the point where the olfactory tract joins the sphenoid part of the temporal lobe of the cerebrum.

Spencer Wells. *See* WELLS, SIR THOMAS SPENCER.

Spengler, Carl (b. 1861). Swiss physician.

Spengler's fragments. Small globular bodies found in the sputum of patients with pulmonary tuberculosis.

Spens, Thomas (b. 1764). Edinburgh physician.

Spens' syndrome. Syncope or transient dulling of consciousness due to ventricular asystole. Originally described by Morgagni in 1700, it is usually called the *Stokes-Adams syndrome.* Typically transient ventricular arrest occurs when partial heart block becomes complete, the sensitivity of the atrioventricular node being impaired. The severity of the attack varies directly with the duration of ventricular asystole. Attacks may also occur when it is paroxysmal, in which event cardiac conduction is normal between attacks. A seizure may be succeeded by an episode of ventricular tachycardia or fibrillation. A similar type of syncope can result from any condition in which the cardiac output suddenly falls to a low level, as in paroxysmal ventricular arrhythmias.

Sperino's operation. For cataract: by repeated paracentesis [obsolete].

sperm (sperm). 1. The semen. 2. A spermatozoon. **Sperm agglutination.** In which the sperms in the ejaculate are found to be (auto-) agglutinated. [Gk *sperma* seed.]

Spermaceti BPC 1968 (sper·mah·se·te). Cetaceum; a translucent crystalline wax, consisting cheifly of cetyl palmitate, $C_{15}H_{31}COOC_{16}H_{33}$. It is obtained from the head of the sperm and bottle-nosed whales, and was used in the preparation of cold creams and ointments. [Gk *sperma* seed, *ketos* sea-monster.]

spermase (sper·maze). An enzyme present in barley seeds. [Gk *sperma* seed.]

spermaster (sper·mas·ter). The aster which forms in the neighbourhood of the sperm nucleus within the fertilized egg.

spermatacrasia (sper·mat·ak·ra'·ze·ah). A defect in the number and activity of the spermatozoa in the semen. [Gk *sperma* seed, *akrasia* without mixture.]

spermatemphraxis (sper·mat·em·frax'·is). Obstruction to the passage of semen. [Gk *sperma* seed, *emphraxis* a blocking up.]

spermatheca (sper·mah·the·kah). An organ of the female reproductive system of many animals in which mature sperm is stored after copulation. [Gk *sperma* seed, *theke* sheath.]

spermatic (sper·mat·ik). Relating or belonging to sperm; seminal.

spermaticidal (sper·mat·e·si'·dal). Spermatocidal.

spermatid (sper·mat·id). The penultimate stage in the development of the spermatozoon; it is derived from the division of a secondary spermatocyte in the wall of a seminiferous tubule. It is at first a spherical cell, and undergoes a lengthy process of rearrangement of external form and internal structure, termed *spermatogenesis,* during its maturation.

spermatine (sper·mat·een). An organic base, the phosphate of which has been isolated from semen and stated to have the formula $(C_2H_5N)_2HPO_4$. It has been reported in brain, in the bone marrow and in the blood in leukaemia.

spermatitis (sper·mat·i·tis). Inflammation of the spermatic cord. [spermatic cord, Gk *-itis* inflammation.]

spermatoblast (sper·mat·o·blast). A Sertoli cell with developing spermatids in its cytoplasm. [Obsolete term.] [spermatid, Gk *blastos* germ.]

spermatocele (sper·mat·o·seel). Cystic dilatation of the ducts of the upper part of the epididymis or in the rete testis; the cyst is well defined. The fluid aspirated is cloudy and contains spermatozoa, so that rupture of the cyst into the tunica vaginalis produces a hydrocele containing spermatozoa. [spermatozoa, Gk *kele* tumour.]

spermatocelectomy (sper·mat·o·se·**lek'**·to·me). Surgical removal of a spermatocele. [spermatocele, Gk *ektome* a cutting out.]

spermatocidal (sper·mat·o·**si'**·dal). Having the capacity to destroy spermatozoa. [sperm, L *caedere* to kill.]

spermatocide (sper·mat·o·side). An agent which is destructive to spermatozoa. [see prec.]

spermatocyst (sper·mat·o·sist). 1. A seminal vesicle. 2. A spermatocele. [sperm, Gk *kystis* bag.]

spermatocystectomy (sper·mat·o·sist·**ek'**·to·me). Surgical removal of the seminal vesicles. [spermatocyst, Gk *ektome* a cutting out.]

spermatocystic (sper·mat·o·**sist'**·ik). Relating or belonging to a spermatocyst.

spermatocystitis (sper·mat·o·sist·**i'**·tis). Inflammation of the seminal vesicles; seminal vesiculitis [spermatocyst, Gk *-itis* inflammation.]

spermatocystotomy (sper·mat·o·sist·**ot'**·o·me). The act of incising a seminal vesicle in order to promote drainage. [spermatocyst, Gk *temnein* to cut.]

spermatocytal (sper·mat·o·**si'**·tal). Relating or belonging to a spermatocyte.

spermatocyte (sper·mat·o·site). An early stage in the development of a spermatozoon; a spherical cell in the wall of a seminiferous tubule, usually exhibiting some stage of meiosis, i.e. reduction division. **Primary spermatocyte.** A large cell in the outer part of the wall of a seminiferous tubule, formed by the mitotic division and subsequent enlargement of a spermatogonium; it contains the full diploid number of chromosomes (e.g. 46 in man). **Secondary spermatocyte.** A cell derived from the meiotic division of a primary spermatocyte; it contains the haploid number of chromosomes (e.g. 23 in man). [Gk *sperma* seed, *kytos* cell.]

spermatocytogenesis (sper·mat·o·si·to·**jen'**·es·is). The first stage in the formation of spermatozoa from spermatogonia, in which first primary spermatocytes, then secondary spermatocytes and finally spermatids, are formed as the result of a complex series of mitotic and reduction (meiotic) divisions. [spermatocyte, Gk *genein* to produce.]

spermatogenesis (sper·mat·o·**jen'**·es·is). The formation and development of spermatozoa. [sperm, Gk *genein* to produce.]

spermatogenic, spermatogenous (sper·mat·o·**jen'**·ik, sper·mat·**oj**·en·us). 1. Relating or belonging to spermatogenesis. 2. Forming spermatozoa. [see prec.]

spermatogonium (sper·mat·o·**go'**·ne·um). The primordial male germ cell in the outer zone of the wall of a seminiferous tubule. Through repeated mitotic divisions, generations of primary spermatocytes are produced from them in the course of normal spermatogenesis. [Gk *sperma* seed, *gone* generation.]

spermatoid (sper·mat·oid). 1. Bearing a similarity to a sperm. 2. The flagellated male form of malaria parasites; the microgamete. [Gk *sperma* seed, *eidos* form.]

spermatolysis (sper·mat·**ol**·is·is). Destruction of spermatozoa, with fluid disintegration. [sperm, Gk *lysis* a loosing.]

spermatolytic (sper·mat·o·**lit'**·ik). Destructive to spermatozoa. [see prec.]

spermatorrhoea (sper·mat·o·**re'**·ah). Copious emission of semen taking place frequently without orgasm. **Spermatorrhoea dormientum.** A nocturnal discharge of semen. **False spermatorrhoea.** Spermatorrhoea in which spermatozoa are absent from the semen. **True spermatorrhoea.** Spermatorrhoea occurring with spermatozoa present in the semen. [sperm, Gk *rhoia* flow.]

spermatotoxin (sper·mat·o·**tox'**·in). A cytotoxin which causes destruction of spermatozoa; in particular, an antibody formed in animals which have been injected with spermatozoa.

spermatozoa (sper·mat·o·**zo'**·ah). *See* SPERMATOZOON.

spermatozoal, spermatozoan (sper·mat·o·**zo'**·al, sper·mat·o·**zo'**·an). Relating or belonging to a spermatozoon or spermatozoa.

spermatozoid (sper·mat·o·**zo'**·id). 1. Having resemblance to a spermatozoon. 2. In botany, the type of male sexual cell that occurs in algae and mosses. [spermatozoon, Gk *eidos* form.]

spermatozoon (sper·mat·o·**zo'**·on) (pl. *spermatozoa*). The mature male germ cell, consisting of a disc-shaped head, a short middle-piece and an elongated motile tail (end-piece). In man, the head is approximately 5 μm in diameter, the tail about 60 μm long. [Gk *sperma* seed, *zoon* animal.]

spermicidal (sper·mis·i·dal). Able to destroy spermatozoa. [see foll.]

spermicide (sper·mis·ide). Spermatocide; any agent that has a destructive effect on spermatozoa. [sperm, L *caedere* to kill.]

spermiduct (sper·me·dukt). The vas deferens and ejaculatory duct. [sperm, duct.]

spermine (sper·meen). $NH_2(CH_2)_3NH(CH_2)_4NH(CH_2)_3NH_2$, a base occurring in sperm and in various animal tissues, notably in the human prostate. **Spermine phosphate.** A phosphate of spermine and calcium.

spermiogram (sper·me·oh·gram). Examination of the sperms in a specimen of semen. [Gk *sperma* seed, Gk *gramma* record.]

spermolith (sper·mo·lith). A calculus in a spermatic duct or seminal vesicle. [sperm, Gk *lithos* stone.]

spermolysin (sper·**mol**·is·in). Spermatotoxin. [sperm, Gk *lysis* a loosing.]

spermolysis (sper·**mol**·is·is). Spermatolysis.

spermolytic (sper·mo·**lit**·ik). Spermatolytic.

Spermophilus (sper·**mof**·il·us). A genus of small burrowing rodents of eastern Asia. Several species are important reservoirs of field plague. [Gk *sperma* seed, *philein* to love.]

Sperry, Warren Myron (b. 1900). American biochemist.

Schoenheimer and Sperry method. For cholesterol in blood. Serum is extracted with boiling acetone-alcohol (equal parts), cooled, made to volume and filtered. The free cholesterol in an aliquot of the filtrate is precipitated with digitonin, the precipitate purified and the cholesterol determined by the Liebermann–Burchard reaction. Another aliquot is saponified with potassium hydroxide and the total cholesterol precipitated with digitonin, purified and determined as before. The difference between total and free cholesterol gives cholesterol esters.

spes phthisica (spes thi·zik·ah). The optimism and confidence in recovery that is characteristic of most sufferers from pulmonary tuberculosis, and particularly of those on whom the disease has a fatal hold. [L *spes* hope, Gk *phthisis* a wasting.]

sphacelate (sfas·el·ate). 1. Gangrenous. 2. To become gangrenous; to undergo mortification; to slough. [Gk *sphakelos* gangrene.]

sphacelation (sfas·el·a·shun). The process of becoming gangrenous; mortification; necrosis. The formation of a sphacelus or slough. [see prec.]

sphacelism (sfas·el·izm). 1. A gangrenous condition; necrosis. 2. Encephalitis. [Gk *sphakelos* gangrene.]

sphaceloderma (sfas·el·o·**der'**·mah). Gangrene of the skin. [Gk *sphakelos* gangrene, *derma* skin.]

sphaceloid (sfas·el·oid). Resembling gangrene or a sphacelus. [Gk *sphakelos* gangrene, *eidos* form.]

sphacelotoxin (sfas·el·o·**tox'**·in). A poisonous, yellow resin obtained from ergot. [Gk *sphakelos* gangrene, *toxikon* poison.]

sphacelous (sfas·el·us). Of gangrenous nature; necrotic; sloughing. [see foll.]

sphacelus (sfas·el·us). A mass of necrotic or gangrenous tissue; a slough. [Gk *sphakelos* gangrene.]

Sphaeranthus (sfer·an·thus). A genus of plants belonging to the family Compositae. **Sphaeranthus indicus.** A herbaceous plant indigenous to Africa, Asia and Australia, used as an aphrodisiac. [Gk *sphaira* sphere, *anthos* flower.]

Sphaerococcus (sfer·o·**kok**·us). An obsolete genus now included in the genus *Streptococcus.* [Gk *sphaira* sphere, coccus.]

Sphaerotilus (sfer·**ot**·il·us). A genus of the family Chlamydobacteriaceae. They are saprophytic water bacteria. **Sphaerotilus bovis.** An old name for *Actinomyces bovis.* [Gk *sphaira* sphere, *tilos* flock-like.]

sphage (sfage). The anterior part of the neck. [Gk *sphage* throat.]

sphagiasmus (sfa·je·**az'**·mus). Contraction of neck muscles in a major epileptic convulsion. [see prec.]

sphagitis (sfa·**ji**·tis). 1. Any inflammatory condition of the throat. 2. Inflammation affecting one or other of the jugular veins. [Gk *sphage* throat, *-itis* inflammation.]

sphagnum (**sfag**·num). A group of mosses belonging to the family Sphagnaceae, found in bogs where they decay to form peat; bog moss, peat moss. Dried sphagnum moss was formerly used as an absorbent dressing. [Gk *sphagnos* moss.]

sphenencephalus (sfe·nen·**kef**·al·us). Sphenocephalus.

sphenic (**sfe**·nik). Like a wedge in shape; sphenoid. [Gk *sphen* wedge.]

sphenion (**sfe**·ne·on). Pterion. [Gk *sphen* wedge.]

sphenobasilar (sfe·no·**ba**·sil·ar). Relating to the sphenoid bone and the basilar part of the occipital bone.

sphenocephalus (sfe·no·**kef**·al·us). A monster, the head of which is shaped like a wedge. [Gk *sphen* wedge, *kephale* head.]

sphenocephaly (sfe·no·**kef**·al·e). The type of teratism in which the head is wedge-shaped. [see prec.]

spheno-ethmoidal (sfe·no·eth·**moid**′·al). Relating or belonging to the sphenoid and the ethmoid bones. **Spheno-ethmoidal recess.** *See* RECESS.

sphenofrontal (sfe·no·**frun**·tal). Relating to the sphenoid and the frontal bones.

sphenoid bone [os sphenoidale (NA)] (**sfe**·noid bone). A complicated unpaired bone forming the central part of the base of the skull. It separates the frontal and ethmoidal bones and maxillae in front from the temporal and occipital bones behind, and articulates with most of the other cranial bones. It consists of a central body, 2 greater and 2 lesser wings, and 2 vertical pterygoid processes, extending down from the junctions of body and greater wings, each made up of a medial and lateral plate fused anteriorly. [Gk *sphen* wedge, *eidos* form.]

body [corpus (NA)]. The central portion lying between the basilar part of the occipital bone and the ethmoid bone; it contains the sphenoidal sinuses.

frontal border [margo frontalis (NA)]. The border which articulates with the frontal bone.

parietal border [margo parietalis (NA)]. The border which articulates with the parietal bone.

squamous border [margo squamosus (NA)]. The border which articulates with the squamous part of the temporal bone.

zygomatic border [margo zygomaticus (NA)]. The border which articulates with the zygomatic bone.

cerebral surface. *See* WINGS OF THE SPHENOID BONE.

infratemporal surface. *See* WINGS OF THE SPHENOID BONE.

orbital surface. *See* WINGS OF THE SPHENOID BONE.

sphenomaxillary surface. *See* WINGS OF THE SPHENOID BONE.

temporal surface. *See* WINGS OF THE SPHENOID BONE.

sphenoidal (sfe·**noid**·al). Relating or belonging to the sphenoid bone. **Sphenoidal sinus.** *See* SINUS.

sphenoiditis (sfe·noid·**i**·tis). Inflammation affecting the sphenoidal sinus, often with necrosis of part of the bone. [sphenoidal sinus, Gk *-itis* inflammation.]

sphenoidostomy (sfe·noid·**os**·to·me). The operation of making an opening into the sphenoidal sinus. [sphenoidal sinus, Gk *stoma* opening.]

sphenoidotomy (sfe·noid·**ot**·o·me). The operation of incising the sphenoidal sinus. [sphenoidal sinus, Gk *temnein* to cut.]

sphenomalar (sfe·no·**ma**·lar). Belonging to the sphenoid and malar (zygomatic) bones.

sphenomandibular (sfe·no·man·**dib**′·ew·lar). Belonging to the sphenoid bone and the mandible.

sphenomaxillary (sfe·no·max·**il**′·ar·e). Belonging to the sphenoid bone and the maxilla.

sphenometer (sfe·**nom**·et·er). An instrument for measuring the size of a wedge of bone to be removed in the operation of cuneiform osteotomy. [Gk *sphen* wedge, meter.]

spheno-occipital (sfe·no·ok·**sip**′·it·al). Belonging to the sphenoid and occipital bones.

spheno-orbital (sfe·no·**or**·bit·al). Belonging to the sphenoid bone and the orbit.

sphenopalatine (sfe·no·**pal**·at·ine). Belonging to the sphenoid bone and the palate. **Sphenopalatine ganglion.** *See* GANGLION.

sphenopalatine artery [arteria sphenopalatina]. *See* MAXILLARY ARTERY.

sphenopalatine nerves. Branches of the sphenopalatine ganglion. **Long sphenopalatine nerve [nervus nasopalatinus (NA)].** A branch from the sphenopalatine ganglion which runs along the septum of the nose and enters the mouth through the incisive canal; Scarpa's nerve. It supplies the mucous membrane of these parts. **Short sphenopalatine nerves [rami nasales posteriores superiores laterales, rami nasales posteriores superiores mediales (NA)].** Branches to the upper and posterior part of the nose and to the ethmoidal sinuses from the sphenopalatine ganglion.

sphenopalatine veins. Veins draining the nose into the pterygoid plexus.

sphenoparietal (sfe·no·par·**i**′·et·al). Relating or belonging to the sphenoid and parietal bones.

sphenopetrosal (sfe·no·pet·**ro**′·sal). Belonging to the sphenoid bone and the petrous part of the temporal bone.

sphenopterygoid (sfe·no·**ter**·e·goid). Belonging to the body of the sphenoid bone and the pterygoid process.

sphenosalpingostaphylinus (sfe·no·sal·ping·go·staf·il·**i**′·nus). The tensor palati muscle [Obsolete term.]. [sphenoid bone, Gk *salpigx* tube, *staphyle* uvula.]

sphenosis (sfe·**no**·sis). A condition in which the fetus is wedged in the pelvis. [Gk *sphen* wedge, *-osis* condition.]

sphenosquamosal (sfe·no·skwa·**mo**′·sal). Belonging to the sphenoid bone and the squamous part of the temporal bone.

sphenotemporal (sfe·no·**tem**·por·al). Belonging to the sphenoid and temporal bones.

sphenotic (sfe·**no**·tik). The lingula of the sphenoid bone, which lies lateral to the internal carotid artery. [sphenoid bone, Gk *ous* ear.]

sphenotresia (sfe·no·**tre**·ze·ah). Perforation of the base of the fetal skull during craniotomy. [Gk *sphen* wedge, *tresis* a boring.]

sphenotribe (**sfe**·no·tribe). In obstetrics, an instrument designed for crushing the base of the fetal skull. [Gk *sphen* wedge, *tribein* to grind.]

sphenotripsy (**sfe**·no·trip·se). The act of crushing the base of the fetal skull with the sphenotribe.

sphenoturbinal (sfe·no·**ter**·bin·al). The sphenoidal conchae; 2 thin plates of bone anterior to the body of the sphenoid in the posterosuperior part of the nasal cavity. They are perforated by the openings of the sphenoidal sinus. [sphenoid bone, turbinate.]

sphenovomerine (sfe·no·**vo**·mer·ine). Relating or belonging to the sphenoid bone and the vomer.

sphenozygomatic (sfe·no·zi·go·**mat**′·ik). Relating to the sphenoid and zygomatic bones.

spheraesthesia (sfer·es·**the**·ze·ah). A perverted sensation as of contact with a spherical body such as a ball. [Gk *sphaira* ball, aesthesia.]

sphere (sfeer). 1. A ball or globe-shaped object. 2. The solid generated by a circle revolving on a diameter as axis. 3. A range of influence. **Attraction sphere.** The centrosome or cell centre; an area of specialized cytoplasm near the nucleus and containing the centriole. **Embryonic sphere, Segmentation sphere.** The spherical segmented ovum or morula, or one of the more or less spherical cells composing it. [Gk *sphaira* ball.]

See also: MORGAGNI.

spherical (**sfer**·ik·al). 1. Relating or belonging to a sphere. 2. Resembling a sphere in shape; globular.

spherocylinder (sfeer·o·**sil**·in·der). A lens having 1 spherical surface and 1 cylindrical surface.

spherocyte (**sfeer**·o·site). An erythrocyte which is abnormally thick and tends to be biconvex instead of biconcave. [sphere, Gk *kytos* cell.]

spherocytic (sfeer·o·**sit**·ik). 1. Relating or belonging to a spherocyte. 2. Denoting a morbid condition of which the presence of spherocytes in the blood is a feature.

spherocytosis (sfeer·o·si·to′·sis). A condition in which there are abnormally thick, almost spherical, red blood cells or spherocytes in the blood. This is seen most commonly in haemolytic spherocytic anaemia and acholuric jaundice. [spherocyte, Gk *-osis* condition.]

spheroid, spheroidal (sfeer·oid, sfeer·oid·al). Resembling a sphere, but with 1 axis elongated. [Gk *sphaira* ball, *eidos* form.]

spheroiding (sfeer·oid·ing). In dentistry, the formation of globules of amalgam causing defective margins in a filling in a tooth. It is due to incorrect preparation of the filling material. [see prec.]

spheroma (sfeer·o·mah). A spherical tumour. [sphere, Gk *-oma* tumour.]

spherometer (sfeer·om·et·er). An instrument used to determine the degree of convexity of surfaces. [sphere, Gk *metron* measure.]

spherophakia (sfeer·o·fak·e·ah). Spherical lens. [Gk *sphaira* ball, *phakos* lens.]

Spherophorus (sfer·of·or·us). A genus of Gram-positive, non-motile, non-sporing rods. Synonymous with the genus *Fusiformis*. **Spherophorus necrophorus.** *Fusiformis necrophorus*. [sphere, Gk *pherein* to carry.]

spheroplast (sfeer·o·plast). A cell surrounded solely by its limiting membrane. Applied to yeast cells where the outer coat has been removed by digestion with cellulose or other lytic enzymes. [Gk *sphaira* ball, *plassein* to form.]

spherule (sfer·ewl). A small spherical body. **Paranuclear spherule.** The area of cytoplasm adjacent to the nucleus and occupied by the Golgi apparatus and associated bodies, especially in developing spermatozoa. [dim. of Gk *sphaira* ball.]

sphincter (sfingk·ter). Any annular muscle closing an orifice. **Sphincter of the bile duct [musculus sphincter ductus choledochi (NA)].** A sphincter of smooth muscle which surrounds the lower end of the bile duct where it joins the pancreatic duct. **Sphincter of the ampulla of the bile duct [musculus sphincter ampullae hepatopancreaticae (NA)].** A sphincter of smooth muscle surrounding the common opening of the bile and pancreatic ducts; the sphincter of Oddi. **Cardiac sphincter.** The ring of muscle that surrounds the oesophagus at its entrance into the cardiac end of the stomach. **Precapillary sphincter.** The small collection of smooth muscle fibres which surround the origin of a capillary from a metarteriole. **Sphincter of the pupil [musculus sphincter pupillae (NA)].** The circular muscle fibres in the iris. **Pyloric sphincter [musculus sphincter pylori (NA)].** The thickening of the circular muscle layer of the stomach at the pyloric orifice. [Gk *sphigkter* one who binds.]

See also: GIORDANO, GLISSON, HENLE, HYRTL, NÉLATON, O'BEIRNE, OCHSNER, ODDI, VILLEMIN (F.).

sphincter ani externus muscle [musculus sphincter ani externus (NA)] (sfingk·ter a·ni ex·ter·nus musl). A flat sheet of muscle encircling the anal orifice, subdivided into 3 parts, subcutaneous [pars subcutanea (NA)], superficial [pars superficialis] and deep [pars profunda (NA)].

sphincter ani internus muscle [musculus sphincter ani internus (NA)] (sfingk·ter a·ni in·ter·nus musl). A sphincter formed of the thickened inner circular coat of the bowel.

sphincter urethrae muscle [musculus sphincter urethrae] (sfingk·ter ewr·eth·re musl). A flat muscle surrounding the membranous portion of the urethra in the male and the terminal part of the urethra in the female. Its outermost fibres are attached to the ischiopubic rami; the innermost fibres are circular.

sphincteral (sfingk·ter·al). Relating or belonging to, or having the characters of a sphincter.

sphincteralgia (sfingk·ter·al·je·ah). Pain affecting the sphincter ani muscles. [sphincter, Gk *algos* pain.]

sphincterectomy (sfingk·ter·ek·to·me). 1. Excision of a sphincter. 2. In ophthalmology, the releasing of the iris sphincter when it is adherent to the back of the cornea by dividing the anterior synechiae. [sphincter, Gk *ektome* excision.]

sphincteric (sfingk·ter·ik). Sphincteral.

sphincterismus (sfingk·ter·iz·mus). Spasmodic contraction of muscles of the sphincter ani, as a rule due to the presence of an anal ulcer or fissure.

sphincteritis (sfingk·ter·i·tis). Inflammation affecting a sphincter, especially the sphincter of Oddi. [sphincter, Gk *-itis* inflammation.]

sphincterolysis (sfingk·ter·ol·is·is). The separation of adhesions between the anterior surface of the iris and the back of the cornea. [sphincter, Gk *lysis* a loosing.]

sphincteroplasty (sfingk·ter·o·plas·te). Plastic surgery of any sphincter muscle. [sphincter, Gk *plassein* to form.]

sphincterotomy (sfingk·ter·ot·o·me). Division of a sphincter by surgical methods. [sphincter, Gk *temnein* to cut.]

sphingogalactoside (sfing·go·gal·ak′·to·side). A cerebroside present in relatively large quantities in the spleen, marrow and other organs in Gaucher's disease, of which disease it is a diagnostic feature. [Gk *sphiggein* to bind, galactoside.]

sphingomyelin (sfing·go·mi·el·in). A type of phospholipide occurring chiefly in the brain, distinguished from lecithin and cephalin by its insolubility in ether. The sphingomyelin molecule is formed by combination of one molecule each of sphingosine, choline, phosphoric acid and a fatty acid. [Gk *sphiggein* to bind, *myelos* marrow.]

sphingosine (sfing·go·seen). $CH_3(CH_2)_{12}CH{=}CHCH(OH)CH(NH_2)CH_2OH$, an amino alcohol which occurs as a molecular constituent of sphingomyelin and the cerebrosides, and from which it is released by hydrolysis.

sphingosinol (sfing·go·sin·ol). Sphingosine.

sphoerogyna (sfe·ro·ji·nah). Pediculoides.

sphygmic (sfig·mik). The second (ejection) phase of ventricular contraction of the heart, between the opening and closing of the pulmonary and aortic valves, during which time blood is expelled into the pulmonary artery and aorta. [Gk *sphygmos* pulse.]

sphygmobologram (sfig·mo·bo·lo·gram). The record or tracing made by the sphygmobolometer. [Gk *sphygmos* pulse, *bolos* mass, *gramma* a record.]

sphygmobolometer (sfig·mo·bo·lom′·et·er). An instrument used to determine and register the strength of the pulse wave; the systolic force may thus be also ascertained. [Gk *sphygmos* pulse, *bolos* mass, *metron* measure.]

sphygmobolometry (sfig·mo·bo·lom′·et·re). Determination of the force of the pulse wave by means of the sphygmobolometer.

sphygmocardiogram (sfig·mo·kar·de·o·gram). The tracing made by a sphygmocardiograph. [Gk *sphygmos* pulse, *kardia* heart, *gramma* record.]

sphygmocardiograph (sfig·mo·kar·de·o·graf). An apparatus which records simultaneously the heart beat and the pulse waves. [Gk *sphygmos* pulse, *kardia* heart, *graphein* to record.]

sphygmodic (sfig·mod·ik). Resembling the pulse; pulsating. [Gk *sphygmos* pulse.]

sphygmodynamometer (sfig·mo·di·nam·om′·et·er). An instrument used to measure the force of the pulse. [Gk *sphygmos* pulse, dynamometer.]

sphygmogram (sfig·mo·gram). A record of the arterial pulse waves obtained by a sphygmograph. The normal arterial pulse record consists of a sharp upstroke, the anacrotic wave, and a gradually declining downstroke, the catacrotic wave. The former represents the advancing head and the latter the retreating tail of the pulse wave. On the catacrotic limb is a well-marked incisura, followed by a sharp positive wave, the dicrotic notch and catacrotic wave, respectively; the dicrotic notch and wave are due to the elastic recoil of the artery following closure of the aortic valve. [Gk *sphygmos* pulse, *gramma* record.]

sphygmograph (sfig·mo·graf). An instrument for recording the form of the arterial pulse. One type consists of a light lever which lies upon a palpable artery (e.g. radial) and records the pulsation upon a moving paper surface. The record produced is known as the *sphygmogram*. [Gk *sphygmos* pulse, *graphein* to record.]

sphygmographic (sfig·mo·graf·ik). Relating or belonging to a sphygmograph.

sphygmography (sfig·mog·raf·e). 1. The recording of the arterial pulse by means of a sphygmograph. 2. A description of the pulse. **Jugular pulse sphygmography.** The recording of the pressure changes in the jugular vein.

sphygmoid (sfig·moid). Having resemblance to the pulse. [Gk *sphygmos* pulse, *eidos* form.]

sphygmology (sfig·mol·o·je). The science and study of the pulse. [Gk *sphygmos* pulse, *logos* science.]

sphygmomanometer (sfig·mo·man·om′·et·er). An instrument for measuring the arterial blood pressure. By means of an inflatable cuff which encircles the limb, air pressure within the cuff is balanced against the pressure in the artery (usually the brachial artery); the pressure is estimated by means of a mercury or aneroid manometer. Various types of instrument bear the names of their originators. [Gk *sphygmos* pulse, manometer.]

sphygmomanometry (sfig·mo·man·om′·et·re). Measurement of the blood pressure by the use of a sphygmomanometer.

sphygmometer (sfig·mom·et·er). Sphygmograph. [Gk *sphygmos* pulse, *metron* measure.]

sphygmometrograph (sfig·mo·met·ro·graf). An instrument by which the maximum and minimum pressure of the arterial pulse may be ascertained. [Gk *sphygmos* pulse, *metron* measure, *graphein* to record.]

sphygmometroscope (sfig·mo·met·ro·skope). Sphygmomanometer. [Gk *sphygmos* pulse, *metron* measure, *skopein* to view.]

sphygmo-oscillometer (sfig·mo·os·il·om′·et·er). A type of oscillometer used in the measurement of the oscillations of the blood stream, in which the disappearance and return of the pulse are marked by a vibrating needle. [Gk *sphygmos* pulse, oscillometer.]

sphygmopalpation (sfig·mo·pal·pa′·shun). The act of "taking" the pulse. [Gk *sphygmos* pulse, palpation.]

sphygmophone (sfig·mo·fone). An apparatus by the use of which the sound of each individual pulse beat may be heard. [Gk *sphygmos* pulse, *phone* sound.]

sphygmoplethysmograph (sfig·mo·pleth·iz′·mo·graf). An instrument which produces a graphic record of the arterial pulse curve and measures the blood flow in a limb. [Gk *sphygmos* pulse, *plethysmos* increase, *graphein* to record.]

sphygmoscope (sfig·mo·skope). An instrument for recording the form of the arterial pulse wave. [Gk *sphygmos* pulse, *skopein* to view.]

See also: BISHOP.

sphygmoscopy (sfig·mos·ko·pe). 1. The use of the sphygmoscope. 2. Examination of the pulse. [see prec.]

sphygmosignal (sfig·mo·sig·nal). A form of sphygmograph. [Gk *sphygmos* pulse, signal.]

sphygmosystole (sfig·mo·sis·to·le). That section of the sphygmogram which refers to the cardiac systole. [Gk *sphygmos* pulse, systole.]

sphygmotonogram (sfig·mo·to·no·gram). The record produced by the sphygmotonograph.

sphygmotonograph (sfig·mo·to·no·graf). A device for simultaneously recording and timing the arterial blood pressure, the jugular or carotid pulse and the brachial pulse. [Gk *sphygmos* pulse, *tonos* tension, *graphein* to record.]

sphygmotonometer (sfig·mo·to·nom′·et·er). An instrument by which the degree of elasticity of the arterial wall may be estimated. [Gk *sphygmos* pulse, tonometer.]

sphygmous (sfig·mus). 1. Relating or belonging to the pulse. 2. Having the character of a pulse. [Gk *sphygmos* pulse.]

sphygmoviscosimetry (sfig·mo·vis·kos·im′·et·re). The procedure of measuring the pressure and viscosity of the blood. [Gk *sphygmos* pulse, viscosity, Gk *metron* measure.]

sphygmus (sfig·mus). 1. The pulse. 2. A pulsation. [Gk *sphygmos* pulse.]

sphyra (sfi·rah). The malleus. [Gk *sphyra* hammer.]

sphyrectomy (sfi·rek·to·me). The operation of excising the malleus. [Gk *sphyra* hammer, *ektome* a cutting out.]

sphyrion (sfi·re·on). An anthropometric point; the lowest point on the medial malleolus. [Gk *sphyra* hammer.]

sphyrotomy (sfi·rot·o·me). Resection of any part of the malleus. [Gk *sphyra* hammer, *temnein* to cut.]

spica (spi·kah). A figure-of-eight bandage; applied to a joint it bears a resemblance to an ear of wheat. [L ear of wheat.]

spice bush (spise bush). A tall shrub of North America, *Lindera benzoin;* it has an aromatic bark that is used as a diaphoretic. [L *species* kind, ME *busk.*]

spicular (spik·ew·lar). 1. Relating or belonging to a spicule. 2. Having the character of a spicule; dart-like. 3. Bearing spicules.

spicule, spiculum (spik·ewl, spik·ew·lum). 1. A minute sharp-pointed body, like a needle. 2. In zoology, a spike-like organ. 3. In botany, any small secondary spike as in grasses. **Bony spicule.** A spiked bone or portion of bone. [L *spiculum* sharp point.]

spider (spi·der). 1. An arthropod of the natural order Aranea having a head-chest (cephalothorax) and abdomen, the former bearing 6 pairs of appendages, i.e. a pair of poison claws, a pair of palpi and 4 pairs of walking legs. The eyes are usually 8 in number. 2. A qualification applied to structures that bear some resemblance to spider's legs, e.g. spider naevus. **Black-widow spider.** *Latrodectus mactans,* causes generalized (spastic contractions) and localized (necrosis) conditions in man. **Funnelweb spider.** *Atrax robustus,* a poisonous spider found in Australia. **Karakurt spider.** A poisonous spider found in Turkestan, *Latrodectus tredecimguttatus.* **Knoppie spider.** The popular name of poisonous South African spiders, e.g. *Latrodectus geometricus.* **Pruning spider.** *Glyptocranium gasteracanthoides.* **Shoe-button spider.** Black-widow spider (see above). **Vascular spider.** Naevus araneus. [ME *spithre.*]

spider burst (spi·der berst). A skin area on the leg in which the capillaries are visible in lines radiating from a central point; the capillary congestion is based on a dilated, but non-varicose, condition of the veins in the neighbourhood. [spider, AS *berstan.*]

spider lick (spi·der lik). A linear eruption on the skin, generally on the face or neck, with vesication and pustulation. It occurs in India, and is believed to be due to an irritant poison secreted by an insect. [spider, AS *liccian.*]

Spieghel [Spigelius], Adriaan van (b. 1578). Flemish anatomist.

Spigelian hernia. Hernia through the linea semilunaris at the lateral border of the sheath of the rectus abdominis muscle.

Spigelius' line. The linea semilunaris; a groove on the abdominal wall marking the lateral border of the rectus abdominis muscle.

Spigelius' lobe or lobus. The caudate lobe of the liver.

Spiegler, Eduard (b. 1860). Vienna dermatologist.

Spiegler's tumour. Multiple benign epitheliomata of the scalp.

Spiegler-Fendt sarcoid. A variety of lymphosarcoma occurring in 2 forms, localized and disseminate.

Spielmeyer, Walther (b. 1879). Munich neurologist.

Spielmeyer-Stock disease, Stock-Spielmeyer disease. The retinal atrophy observed in Spielmeyer-Vogt disease.

Spielmeyer-Vogt disease, Vogt-Spielmeyer disease. The juvenile form of cerebromacular degeneration.

Spigelia (spi·je·le·ah). Pink root, wormweed, wormroot; a genus of loganaceous plants. The dried rhizomes of *Spigelia marilandica* and *S. anthelmia* are used in the treatment of worms. [Adriaan van *Spieghel.*]

Spigelius. *See* SPIEGHEL.

spike (spike). The main peak in the oscillographic record of the action potential wave; the secondary peak is referred to as the *after-potential.* **Spike and wave, Spike and slow wave.** Stereotyped electroencephalographic discharges consisting of a fast and slow component, occurring at 3Hz (c/s) in petit mal epilepsy. **Focal spike.** A fast component in the electroencephalographic record originating in a localized area. [L *spica.*]

spikenard (spike·nard). The plant, *Nardostachys jatamansi,* and other valerianaceous plants; oils and ointments made from them were used in the Orient as perfumes and medicines. **American spikenard.** The plant, *Aralia racemosa,* used as a diaphoretic.

False spikenard. An East Indian grass, *Andropogon nardus.* [L *spica* spike, *nardus* aromatic balsam.]

Spilanthes (spi·**lan**·theez). A genus of composite-flowered plants. **Spilanthes oleracea.** A plant of tropical America which is chewed and produces a copious flow of saliva. It is valuable in tooth-ache. The flowers contain spilanthole. [Gk *spilos* spot, *anthos* flower.]

spilanthole (spi·**lan**·thole). $C_{14}H_{25}NO$, a pungent compound obtained from *Spilanthes oleracea.* It has strong local anaesthetic properties and is employed in tooth-ache.

spill (spil). A naevus. [Gk *spilos* spot.]
See also: SAMPSON.

Spiller, William Gibson (b. 1863). Philadelphia neurologist.
Frazier-Spiller operation. Intracranial trigeminal nerve section in the treatment of neuralgia.

spill-over (spil·o·ver). Secondary adjacent abscesses in a case of pulmonary abscess. [AS *spillan, ofer.*]

spiloma (spi·**lo**·mah). A naevus. [Gk *spilos* spot, *-oma* tumour.]

spiloplania (spi·lo·**pla**·ne·ah). A condition of temporary erythema of the skin characterized by the appearance and disappearance here and there of areas of hyperaemia or discoloured spots or patches. [Gk *spilos* spot, *plane* a wandering about.]

spiloplaxia (spi·lo·**plax**·e·ah). Leprous spots on the skin. [Gk *spilos* spot, *plax* plate.]

spilus (**spi**·lus). Spiloma.

spina (NA) (**spi**·nah). 1. The spine; the vertebral column. 2. A process or projection resembling a spine. **Spina bifida.** A defect in development of the vertebral column in which there is a central deficiency of the vertebral lamina; the condition often affects several vertebrae, and is most common in the lumbar region. Variable protrusion of the meninges and of other contents of the spinal canal occurs through the gap, giving rise to a meningocele or a meningomyelocele. *See also:* RACHISCHISIS. **Spina bifida occulta.** A spina bifida in which there is no protrusion of the meninges or the cord, and there is no external evidence of its existence. **Spina nodosa.** Osteo-arthritis of the spine. **Spina ventosa.** Tuberculosis of bone in which the bone is expanded and the cortex thinned. It usually occurs in the phalanges. [L backbone.]

spinal (**spi**·nal). 1. Relating or belonging to the vertebral column. 2. Relating to a spine or to any spinous process. [L *spina* backbone.]

spinal arteries. Anterior spinal artery [arteria spinalis anterior (NA)]. A small branch of the first part of the vertebral artery. It unites with its fellow anterior to the medulla and runs as a single median artery as far as the filum terminale. **Posterior spinal artery [arteria spinalis posterior (NA)].** A branch of the posterior inferior cerebellar artery or of the main vertebral artery at the side of the medulla. It divides into 2 longitudinal vessels running respectively anterior and posterior to the posterior spinal roots. It is reinforced by many segmental branches, especially from the lumbar and posterior intercostal arteries.

spinal nerves [nervi spinales (NA)]. Segmental nerves, 31 in number and mixed in character, formed by the union of anterior (motor) and posterior (sensory) roots which arise from the spinal cord. They are grouped according to the region of the spinal cord from which they arise into 8 cervical, 12 thoracic, 5 lumbar, 5 sacral and 1 coccygeal nerves. They emerge from the vertebral canal through the intervertebral foramina. The 1st cervical nerve is an exception, as it may not possess a posterior root and emerges between the atlas and the skull.

grey communicating branches. Connections between the ganglion sympathetic chain with the trunks of the spinal nerves. They consist of postganglionic non-medullated fibres having their cells of origin mainly in the ganglion. The fibres are distributed to the blood vessels, sweat glands and the arrectores pilorum muscles.

meningeal branch [ramus meningeus (NA)]. A small branch to the meninges from the trunk of a spinal nerve.

white communicating branches. Connections between the spinal nerve trunks, or the commencement of the anterior primary rami, and the sympathetic ganglion in the thoracic region and the pelvic splanchnic nerves (parasympathetic) in the sacral region. They consist of the axons of motor cells lying in the lateral column in these regions (preganglion medullated fibres), and of sensory fibres with their cells of origin in the posterior root ganglion.

anterior primary ramus [ramus ventralis (NA)]. One of the primary divisions of a spinal nerve after it has emerged from the vertebral canal, consisting of motor and sensory fibres. Collectively these rami are responsible for the nerve supply of the ventral and lateral skin and musculature of the trunk and entirely for the supply of the skin and muscle of the limbs.

posterior primary ramus [ramus dorsalis (NA)]. The posterior of the 2 primary divisions of the spinal nerve, supplying the skin and musculature on the back of the trunk. They mainly divide into *medial* and *lateral branches,* the former supplying the muscle of the sacrospinalis mass and the latter supplying divisions of this muscle and the skin. Their distribution differs, however, in detail in the different regions.

anterior root [radix ventralis (NA)]. Axons of large motor cells lying in the anterior horn of the spinal cord. These emerge in several bundles or rootlets and unite to form a compact bundle, the anterior root, in each segment, which joins the posterior root to form the corresponding spinal nerve.

posterior root [radix dorsalis (NA)]. The sensory root of the spinal nerve, the axons of which arise in the cells of the spinal ganglion and pass laterally as a compact bundle, or posterior root, to join the anterior root and form the corresponding spinal nerve.

spinal veins [venae spinales (NA)]. A venous plexus in the pia mater of the spinal cord, draining blood from the cord into the internal and intervertebral veins.

spinalgia (spi·**nal**·je·ah). Pain in the neighbourhood of the vertebral column. [L *spina* backbone, Gk *algos* pain.]
See also: PETRUSCHKY.

spinalis muscle [musculus spinalis (NA)] (spi·**na**·lis musl). The most medial part of the sacrospinalis muscle. It consists of 3 portions: capitis, cervicis and thoracis.

spinalis capitis muscle [musculus spinalis capitis (NA)] (spi·**na**·lis **kap**·it·is musl). A few muscular fasciculi blended with the semispinalis capitis.

spinalis cervicis muscle [musculus spinalis cervicis (NA)] (spi·**na**·lis **ser**·vis·is musl). An inconstant muscle arising from the lower part of the ligamentum nuchae, the 7th cervical and 1st and 2nd thoracic spines, and inserted into the spine of the axis.

spinalis thoracis muscle [musculus spinalis thoracis (NA)] (spi·**na**·lis **thor**·as·is musl). A muscle arising from the spines of the upper lumbar and lower thoracic vertebrae, and inserted into the spines of the upper thoracic vertebrae.

spinate (**spi**·nate). 1. Thorn-shaped. 2. Bearing spines or thorns. [L *spina* thorn.]

spinawl (**spin**·awl). A sharp-edged awl for puncturing skin before the insertion of a lumbar-puncture needle. [spine, AS *ael.*]

spindle (spindl). An elongated structure which has tapered extremities and a thick central portion. **Achromatic spindle.** A fusiform body composed of viscous cytoplasm or nuclear sap and having a fibrillar appearance in fixed preparations, found in dividing cells. The chromosomes become attached to it in metaphase. **Central spindle.** The centre portion of an achromatic spindle (see above) between the asters. **Cleavage spindle.** Achromatic spindle (see above). **Enamel spindle.** The continuation of a dentinal tubule across the amelodentinal junction into the substance of the enamel beneath a cusp or the incisive edge of a tooth. **Karyokinetic spindle.** Achromatic spindle (see above). **Mitotic spindle.** Achromatic spindle (see above). **Muscle spindle.** A specialized sensory organ in voluntary muscle composed of a bundle of fine, striated, intrafusal muscle fibres, innervated by gamma fibres; their nuclei are collected together near the centre of each fibre to form a nuclear bag. The latter is surrounded by sensory, annulospiral nerve-endings, and the intrafusal fibres by sensory flower-spray endings. The whole is enclosed in a fibrous sheath and forms a proprioceptive receptor. **Neuromuscular spindle.** Muscle spindle (see prec.). **Neurotendinal spindle.** The tendon spindle (corpuscle) of Golgi, analogous to the muscle spindle; it consists of an encapsulated group of small tendon fibres richly innervated with sensory nerve-endings, and responsive to stretch. **Nuclear spindle.** Achromatic spindle (see above). **Segmentation spindle.** The achromatic spindle of the fertilized ovum at the time of the first cell division. **Tendon spindle.** A specialized sensory nerve-ending in tendon, activated by tension. **Tigroid spindle.** Supposed fusiform elements composing the Nissl substance of nerve cells. [AS *spinel.*]

See also: AXENFELD, BUETSCHLI, HIS (W. JNR.), KRUKENBERG (F. E.), KUEHNE (W.), NISSL.

spine [spina (NA)] (spine). 1. A sharp-pointed bony projection. 2. The vertebral column. **Bamboo spine.** A descriptive term for the radiographic appearance in spondylitis ankylopoietica. **Cleft spine, Cloven spine.** Spina bifida. **Spine of the helix [spina helicis (NA)].** A small pointed projection on the anterior border of the auricular cartilage at the point where the helix turns upwards. **Hysterical spine.** A variety of psychoneurosis, with symptoms of pain and deformity referred to the spinal column. **Iliac spine, anterior inferior [spina iliaca anterior inferior (NA)].** A projection on the anterior border of the ilium just below the anterior superior iliac spine, giving attachment to the rectus femoris and to the iliofemoral ligament. **Iliac spine, anterior superior [spina iliaca anterior superior (NA)].** The projection at the anterior end of the iliac crest. It gives attachment to the inguinal ligament. **Iliac spine, posterior inferior [spina iliaca posterior inferior (NA)].** The point at which the posterior border of the ilium makes a sharp bend forwards into the greater sciatic notch. **Iliac spine, posterior superior [spina iliaca posterior superior (NA)].** The projection at the posterior end of the iliac crest, marked in the living by a dimple in the lower back region. **Irritable spine.** Pain in the back or tenderness over the vertebrae, associated with fatigue on exertion; a neurotic manifestation. **Ischial spine [spina ischiadica (NA)].** A pointed projection on the posterior margin of the ischium which gives attachment to the sacrospinous ligament. **Kissing spines.** Contact between the tips of any 2 lumbar vertebrae or between the 5th lumbar and 1st sacral. This causes lower back pain that is localized in the midline and is increased on extension of the spine. **Nasal spine [spina nasalis (NA)].** A median ridge projecting downwards from the nasal part of the frontal bone. **Nasal spine, anterior [spina nasalis anterior (NA)].** The pointed median prominence of the maxillary bones on the lower margin of the bony external nares. **Nasal spine, posterior [spina nasalis posterior (NA)].** A projection at the medial end of the posterior border of the horizontal plate of the palatine bone. **Palatine spine [spina palatinae (NA)].** A sharp process at the anterior end of the nasal crest, which with the fellow of the opposite side forms the anterior nasal spine. **Poker spine.** A complete rigidity of the spinal column, generally the result of ankylosing spondylitis or of rheumatoid arthritis. **Railway spine.** A form of hysterical spine (see above) following involvement in a railway accident. **Rigid spine.** Poker spine (see above). **Spine of the scapula [spina scapulae (NA)].** The triangular shelf of bone projecting from the dorsal surface of the scapula continuous with the acromion process laterally. **Spine of the sphenoid bone [spina ossis sphenoidalis (NA)].** A spine on the inferior surface of the greater wing of the sphenoid bone at the lateral end of its posterior border, to which the sphenomandibular ligament is attached. **Suprameatal spine [spina supra meatum (NA)].** A small projection of bone in the suprameatal triangle, giving attachment to part of the external ear cartilage. **Thoracic spine.** That particular portion of the spinal column which lies within and forms part of the chest. **Trochlear spine [spina trochlearis (NA)].** Trochlear fossa. *See* FOSSA. **Tympanic spine, greater [spina tympanica major (NA)].** The upper anterior part of the tympanic ring. **Tympanic spine, lesser [spina tympanica minor (NA)].** The upper posterior part of the tympanic ring. **Typhoid spine.** A painful condition in the lumbar and sacral regions of the spine occurring after typhoid fever, possibly even a mild attack. Nervous and hysterical symptoms are often present. Recovery is complete in from 1 to 12 months. **Spine of a vertebra [processus spinosus (NA)].** The backwardly directed bony process from the junction of the laminae. [L *spina.*]

See also: CIVININI, ERICHSEN, HENLE, SPIX.

spinibulbar (spi·ne·**bul**·bar). Spinobulbar.

spinicerebellar (**spi**·ne·ser·e·**bel**′·ar). Spinocerebellar.

spinicerebrate (spi·ne·**ser**·e·brate). Having a brain and a spinal cord. [spinal cord, cerebrum.]

spinifugal (spi·**nif**·ew·gal). Conducting impulses away from the spinal cord, as the efferent fibres of the spinal nerves. [spinal cord, L *fugere* to run away from.]

spiniperipheral (**spi**·ne·per·**if**′·er·al). Spinoperipheral.

spinipetal (spi·**nip**·et·al). Conducting impulses towards the spinal cord, as the afferent fibres of the spinal nerves. [spinal cord, L *petere* to reach towards.]

spinitis (spi·**ni**·tis). Myelitis. [spinal cord, Gk *-itis* inflammation.]

spinning top (**spin**·ing top). An obsolete method of checking the calibration of an x-ray time-switch. Photographic film is placed on the disc of a top and spun in the x-ray beam during a short exposure. The number of spots on the film gives the exposure, measuring the frequency of alternation of the supply. [AS *spinnan*, top.]

spinobulbar (spi·no·**bul**·bar). Relating or belonging to the spinal cord and the medulla oblongata. [spinal cord, bulb.]

spinocellular (spi·no·**sel**·ew·lar). Pertaining to, composed of, or having resemblance to prickle cells. [L *spina* thorn, cell.]

spinocerebellar (**spi**·no·ser·e·**bel**′·ar). Relating or belonging to the spinal cord and the cerebellum. **Spinocerebellar tract.** *See* TRACT.

spinocortical (spi·no·**kor**·tik·al). Relating or belonging to the spinal cord and the cerebral cortex.

spinocostalis (**spi**·no·kos·**ta**′·lis). The serratus posterior inferior and the serratus posterior superior muscles considered as 1 muscle. [spinal cord, L *costa* rib.]

spinogalvanization (**spi**·no·gal·van·i·**za**′·shun). The application of the galvanic (constant) current to the spine for therapeutic purposes.

spinoglenoid (spi·no·**gle**·noid). Belonging to the spine of the scapula and the glenoid cavity. **Spinoglenoid notch.** *See* NOTCH.

spinomuscular (spi·no·**mus**·kew·lar). Belonging to the spinal cord and the muscles.

spinoneural (spi·no·**newr**·al). Belonging to the spinal cord and the peripheral nerves. [spinal cord, Gk *neuron* nerve.]

spinoperipheral (**spi**·no·per·**if**′·er·al). Relating to the spinal cord and the surface of the body. [spinal cord, periphery.]

spinose (**spi**·noze). Spinous.

spinotectal (spi·no·**tek**·tal). Tectospinal. **Spinotectal tract.** *See* TRACT. [spinal cord, L *tectum* roof.]

spinothalamic (**spi**·no·thal·**am**′·ik). Pertaining to the spinal cord and the thalamus. **Spinothalamic tract.** *See* TRACT.

spinotransversarius (**spi**·no·trans·ver·**sa**′·re·us). The splenius capitis and the obliquus capitis superior muscles considered as 1 muscle. [spinal cord, L *transversus* across.]

spinous (**spi**·nus). 1. Like a spine or thorn in shape. 2. Belonging to the vertebral column or to a spiny process. 3. Having spines.

spinthariscope (spin·**thar**·is·kope). A device for viewing the scintillations produced by α-particles on a fluorescent screen. Of historical interest only. [Gk *spinther* spark, *skopein* to view.]

spintherism (**spin**·ther·izm). A sensation of light, as of flashes or sparks, associated with disease of the retina. [Gk *spinther* spark.]

spintheropia (spin·ther·**o**·pe·ah). The condition in which spintherism is present. [Gk *spinther* spark, *ops* eye.]

spinulosin (spin·ew·**lo**·sin). 3,6-Dihydroxy-4-methoxy-2,5-toluquinone, $CH_3C_6O_2OCH_3(OH)_2$. A pigmented compound formed by the growth of the mould, *Penicillium spinulosum*, in glucose. It has antibiotic properties.

Spiperone (**spi**·per·one). BP Commission approved name for 8-[3-(4-fluorobenzoyl)propyl]-1-phenyl-1,3,8-triazaspiro[4,5]decan-4-one; a tranquillizer.

spiradenitis (spi·rad·en·i′·tis). Hidradenitis suppurativa. [Gk *speira* coil, adenitis.]

spiradenoma (spi·rad·en·o′·mah). Adenoma of the sweat glands. [Gk *speira* coil, adenoma.]

spiral (spi·ral). 1. Winding; screw-like. 2. A screw-like curve. [Gk *speira* coil.]

See also: CURSCHMANN (HEINRICH), GOLGI, PERRONCITO.

Spiramycin (spi·rah·mi·sin). BP Commission approved name for an antibiotic obtained from *Streptomyces ambofaciens.* It is active against Gram-positive cocci and does not tend to act on the normal Gram-negative organisms of the intestinal canal, and it is therefore unlikely to provoke intestinal infections with *Candida.* It is administered orally.

Spiranthes (spi·ran·theez). A genus of orchidaceous plants. **Spiranthes autumnalis.** A British orchid, said to have aphrodisiac properties. **Spiranthes diuretica.** A plant of Chile, believed to be diuretic. [Gk *speira* coil, *anthos* flower.]

spirem (spi·rem). Spireme.

spireme (spi·reem). The tangled mass of chromosomes visible in the prophase of mitosis, or meiosis, thought at one time to constitute a single continuous thread. It is now known that the chromosomes remain discrete throughout cell division. [Gk *speirema* coil.]

Spirilene (spi·ril·een). BP Commission approved name for 8 - [4 - (4 -fluorophenyl)pent - 3 - enyl] - 1 - phenyl - 1,3,8 - triazaspiro [4,5]decan-4-one; a tranquillizer.

spirilla (spi·ril·ah). *See* SPIRILLUM.

spirillaemia (spi·ril·e·me·ah). A condition characterized by the existence of spirilla in the blood. **Spirillaemia minus.** Rat-bite fever. *See* FEVER. [spirillum, Gk *haima* blood.]

spirillicidal (spi·ril·e·si′·dal). Having a destructive effect on spirilla. [see foll.]

spirillicide (spi·ril·e·side). An agent which is capable of destroying spirilla. [spirillum, L *caedere* to kill.]

spirillicidin (spi·ril·e·si′·din). A spirillicidal substance formed in the blood of patients who have undergone immunization against spirilla.

spirillolysis (spi·ril·ol·is·is). The destruction of spirilla by disintegration or dissolution. [spirillum, Gk *lysis* a loosing.]

spirillosis (spi·ril·o·sis). Any morbid state which is due to the existence of spirilla in the blood or tissues. [spirillum, Gk *-osis* condition.]

spirillotropic (spi·ril·o·tro′·pik). 1. Relating or belonging to spirillotropism. 2. Having the property of attracting spirilla. [see foll.]

spirillotropism (spi·ril·o·trop′·izm). Having an affinity for spirilla. [spirillum, Gk *trope* a turning.]

Spirillum (spi·ril·um) (pl. *spirilla*). A bacterial genus in the family Spirillacea (order Pseudomonadales), non-flexuous spiral filaments (to be distinguished from spirochaetes) mostly saprophytic. **Spirillum buccale.** *Borrelia buccalis.* **Spirillum cholerae.** *Vibrio cholerae.* **Spirillum duttoni.** *Borrelia duttoni.* **Spirillum metchnikovi.** *Vibrio metchnikovi.* **Spirillum minus.** A species found naturally in rats and other rodents; it is the cause of one form of rat-bite fever in man, a relapsing febrile illness with a local inflammatory lesion and enlargement of regional glands. **Spirillum pseudocholera.** A non-pathogenic vibrio. **Spirillum undula.** The type species, found in stagnant water. [Gk *speira* coil.]

spirit (spir·it). 1. Any solution of a volatile oil or other volatile substance (e.g. camphor) in alcohol (*simple spirit*). 2. Any liquid prepared by distillation, of varying composition (*complex spirit*). **Aromatic Spirit of Ammonia BPC 1959.** A solution containing 3 per cent of ammonium carbonate in approximately 70 per cent alcohol, flavoured with oils of lemon and nutmeg. It is administered, mixed with water, as a stimulant and carminative. **Spirit of Camphor BPC 1959.** A 1 in 10 solution of camphor in alcohol (90 per cent) for internal administration. **Chloroform Spirit BP 1968.** A 1 in 20 solution of chloroform in alcohol (90 per cent), used as a flavouring for mixtures and emulsions. **Cologne spirit.** Spiritus coloniensis. **Compound spirit of bay.** Spiritus myrciae compositus. **Compound spirit of ether.** Spiritus aetheris compositus. **Compound spirit of juniper.** A solution containing oil of juniper 8, oil of caraway 1, oil of fennel 1, alcohol (99 per cent) 1400 and water to 2000. **Compound Spirit of Orange BPC 1959.** An alcoholic solution of oils of orange, lemon, coriander and anise. **Compound spirit of pimento.** Spiritus myrciae compositus. **Spirit of Ether BP 1953.** A solution of anaesthetic ether 1 in 3 in alcohol (90 per cent), for internal administration. **Industrial Methylated Spirit BP 1968.** Ethyl alcohol (95 per cent) rendered non-potable by the addition of 1/19 of its volume of wood naphtha (impure methyl alcohol). **Industrial Methylated Spirit (Acetone-Free) BPC 1968.** Similar to the above but acetone, which is incompatible with iodine and otherwise objectionable, is absent from the denaturant. **Spirit of juniper.** Spiritus juniperi. **Methylated spirit.** An industrial and domestic mixture of methyl (5 per cent) and ethyl (95 per cent) alcohols tinted, by law, with magenta in some countries, and commonly used by degenerate or impoverished alcohol addicts owing to its low cost. A dangerously toxic alcoholic drink causing optic nerve damage in particular. In its metabolism, formic acid and formaldehyde may be identified. **Nitrous Ether Spirit BPC 1959.** A solution containing 1.5-2.5 per cent of ethyl nitrite together with a little acetylaldehyde in approximately 85 per cent alcohol. It is diaphoretic, diuretic and stimulant. **Peppermint Spirit BP 1958.** Essence of peppermint; a solution of peppermint oil 1 in 10 in alcohol (90 per cent), used as a flavouring agent and as a carminative. **Petroleum spirit.** Light petroleum. *See* PETROLEUM. **Potato spirit.** Crude amyl alcohol. **Proof spirit.** Ethyl alcohol (57.1 per cent v/v). **Pyroligneous spirit.** Crude methyl alcohol. **Rectified Spirit BP 1973.** Ethyl alcohol 95 per cent v/v in water. **Spirit of sal volatile.** Aromatic spirit of ammonia (see above). **Spirit of salt.** Hydrochloric acid. *See* ACID. **Spirit of Soap BPC 1959.** A solution of soft soap in alcohol (90 per cent) and containing 65 per cent w/v of soft soap. **Sweet spirit of nitre.** Nitrous ether spirit (see above). **Spirit of wine.** Ethyl alcohol. **Wood spirit.** Crude methyl alcohol. [L *spiritus* breath.]

See also: MINDERERS.

spirituous (spir·it·ew·us). 1. Containing a considerable quantity of alcohol. 2. Having the character of spirit; alcoholic. [see prec.]

spiritus (spir·it·us). Spirit. Before 1953 all spirits were officially classified as *Spiritus.* **Spiritus Aetheris Compositus BPC 1949.** A preparation containing ether in approximately 65 per cent alcohol, for internal administration. **Spiritus Anisi BPC 1949.** Spirit of anise, 1 in 10 solution of oil of anise in alcohol (90 per cent), used as a flavouring agent and carminative. **Spiritus Coloniensis BPC 1949.** A solution of orange-flower water and oils of bergamot, lemon, neroli, rosemary and thyme in alcohol (90 per cent). It is a refreshing external application similar to eau de Cologne. **Spiritus frumenti.** Whisky. **Spiritus Juniperi BPC 1949.** A solution of oil of juniper, 1 in 10 in alcohol (90 per cent), for internal use. **Spiritus Myrciae Compositus BPC 1949.** A solution of oils of bay, orange and pimento, with dry extract of quassia and saponin in alcohol (55-58 per cent), used externally as a wash for the hair and as an astringent after shaving. **Spiritus tenuior.** Proof spirit. *See* SPIRIT. **Spiritus vini gallici.** Brandy. [L.]

Spirochaeta (spi·ro·ke·tah). 1. A genus of the family Spirochaetaceae. They are flexible spiral micro-organisms, saprophytic and found in water. 2. More generally, though this use is now obsolete, any member of the order Spirochaetales. **Spirochaeta bronchialis, Spirochaeta carteri.** *Borrelia carteri.* **Spirochaeta duttoni.** *Borrelia duttoni.* **Spirochaeta hebdomadis.** *Leptospira hebdomadis.* **Spirochaeta icterohaemorrhagiae.** *Leptospira icterohaemorrhagiae.* **Spirochaeta obermeiri.** *Borrelia recurrentis.* **Spirochaeta pallida.** *Treponema pallidum.* **Spirochaeta persica.** *Borrelia persica.* **Spirochaeta recurrentis.** *Borrelia recurrentis.* **Spirochaeta refringens.** *Borrelia refringens.* **Spirochaeta sogdiana.** *Borrelia sogdianum.* **Spirochaeta vincenti.** *Borrelia vincenti.* [Gk *speira* coil, *chaite* hair.]

Spirochaetaceae (spi·ro·ke·ta′·se·e). A family of the order Spirochaetales. It contains the genera *Spirochaeta* and *Saprospira.* These organisms are found in fresh or salt water and in the intestinal tract of molluscs. They are not known to be pathogenic to man.

spirochaetaemia (spi·ro·ke·te′·me·ah). The presence of spirochaetes in the blood. [spirochaete, Gk *haima* blood.]

spirochaetal (spi·ro·ke·tal). 1. Relating or belonging to spirochaetes. 2. Indicative of injection with spirochaetes.

Spirochaetales (spi·ro·ke·ta′·leez). An order of the class Schizomycetes, whose members are distinguished by the presence of a slender flexuous cell body with at least 1 complete turn. Some species are pathogenic, some saprophytic. It includes the families Spirochaetaceae and Treponemataceae. [Gk *speira* coil, *chaite* hair.]

spirochaete (spi·ro·keet). A term applied colloquially to members of the bacterial order Spirochaetales, which differs from other bacterial orders in the possession of long filaments applied to their bodies; to these structures the spirochaetes owe their shape, elasticity and movement. There are no flagella. There are many commensal species of spirochaetes. The 3 genera with species pathogenic to man are *Treponema, Borrelia* and *Leptospira*; they constitute the family Treponemataceae (the small spirochaetes). [Gk *speira* coil, *chaite* hair.]

spirochaeticidal (spi·ro·ke·te·si′·dal). 1. Relating or belonging to a spirochaeticide. 2. Capable of destroying spirochaetes. [see foll.]

spirochaeticide (spi·ro·ke·te·side). Any agent which is destructive to spirochaetes. [spirochaete, L *caedere* to kill.]

spirochaetogenous (spi·ro·ke·toj′·en·us). Brought about by spirochaetes. [spirochaete, Gk *genein* to produce.]

spirochaetolysin (spi·ro·ke·tol′·is·in). An agent which effects lysis of spirochaetes. [see foll.]

spirochaetolysis (spi·ro·ke·tol′·is·is). The destruction of spirochaetes by chemotherapy, by specific antibodies or by other lysins. [spirochaete, Gk *lysis* a loosing.]

spirochaetolytic (spi·ro·ke·tol·it′·ik). Capable of destroying spirochaetes. [spirochaete, Gk *lysis* a loosing.]

spirochaetosis (spi·ro·ke·to′·sis). Any disease caused by spirochaetes. **Spirochaetosis arthritica.** Any affection of the joints, occurring during the course of one of the diseases caused by infection with a spirochaete, e.g. syphilis. **Bronchopulmonary spirochaetosis.** Infection of the bronchial tract with spirochaetes. **Icterogenic spirochaetosis.** Leptospirosis. **Spirochaetosis icterohaemorrhagica.** Leptospirosis icterohaemorrhagica. **Spirochaetosis riverensis.** A form of meningitis found in Brazil and believed to be due to a chronic spirochaetal infection. [spirochaete, Gk *-osis* condition.]

spirochaetotic (spi·ro·ke·tot′·ik). 1. Relating or belonging to spirochaetosis. 2. Marked by spirochaetosis.

spirochaeturia (spi·ro·ke·tewr′·e·ah). The presence of spirochaetes in the urine.

spirogram (spi·ro·gram). The curve or tracing made by the spirograph. [L *spirare* to breathe, Gk *gramma* record.]

spirograph (spi·ro·graf). An apparatus by which graphic records of depth and rapidity of the respirations are made. [L *spirare* to breathe, Gk *graphein* to record.]

spirography (spi·rog·raf·e). The registration of breathing movements and of lung capacity by means of the spirograph.

spiroid (spi·roid). Having resemblance to a spiral or a screw. [spiral, Gk *eidos* form.]

spiro-index (spi·ro·in·dex). The index obtained by dividing the vital capacity measured in cubic centimetres of a person by his height in centimetres. [L *spirare* to breath, index.]

spiroma (spi·ro·mah). Spiradenoma. [Gk *speira* coil, *-oma* tumour.]

spirometer (spi·rom·et·er). An apparatus used to determine the sum of the tidal, complemental and supplemental air (vital capacity) of the lungs. **Tidal spirometer.** An apparatus for measuring a patient's respiratory tidal volume. [L *spirare* to breathe, meter.]

Spirometra (spi·ro·me·trah). **Spirometra houghtoni.** A pike-like fish, the barracuta, which is poisonous when eaten in certain seasons. **Spirometra mansoni, S. mansonoides.** Tapeworms whose larvae (spargana) cause the tissue infection sparganosis. [Gk *speira* coil, *metron* measure.]

spirometric (spi·ro·met·rik). Relating or belonging to spirometry or to the spirometer.

spirometry (spi·rom·et·re). Measurement of the vital capacity of the lungs by means of the spirometer. **Bronchoscopic spirometry.** Measurement with a special instrument of the air capacity and function of each lung separately.

Spironema (spi·ro·ne·mah). An obsolete generic name for the spirochaetes that are now placed in the genera *Borrelia* and *Treponema.* [Gk *speira* coil, *nema* thread.]

Spironolactone BP 1973 (spi·ron·o·lak′·tone). β-(7α-Acetylthio-17β-hydroxy-3-oxoandrost-4-en-17α-yl)propionic acid lactone; used in the treatment of resistant oedema.

spirophore (spi·ro·fore). A particular type of cabinet used in the induction of artificial respiration. The patient is placed inside, only his head remaining outside. Inhalation and exhalation are induced by alternately increasing and decreasing the pressure of the air within the cabinet. [L *spirare* to breathe, Gk *pherein* to carry.]

spiroscope (spi·ro·skope). A type of spirometer used for the observation of the effectiveness of breathing exercises; the patient is able to see the quantity of water which is displaced in a certain time and so measure his breathing capacity. [L *spirare* to breathe, Gk *skopein* to view.]

spiroscopy (spi·ros·ko·pe). The use of the spiroscope.

Spirosoma (spi·ro·so·mah). An obsolete genus now included in the genus *Spirillum.* [Gk *speira* coil, *soma* body.]

Spirurata (spir·ew·ra·tah). Filariata; a sub-order or order or sub-class Spirurida. The super-families or sub-orders Filarioidea and Spiruroidea are of medical interest. [Gk *speira* coil, *oura* tail.]

Spiruridae (spir·ew·rid·e). A family of the nematode super-family Spiruroidea. The genus *Gongylonema* is of medical interest. [Gk *speira* coil, *oura* tail, *eidos* form.]

Spiruroidea (spir·ew·roi·de·ah). A super-family or sub-order of the nematode sub-order or order Spirurata. [see prec.]

spissated (spis·a·ted). Inspissated; made thicker, drier or less fluid by means of evaporation. [L *spissare* to make thick.]

spissitude (spis·it·ewd). A degree of dryness or inspissation in which a substance is almost solid because of evaporation of liquid constituents. [L *spissitudo* density.]

spit (spit). 1. Saliva. 2. Sputum. 3. To expectorate. [AS *spittan.*]

Spitzer, Alexander (b. 1868). Austrian anatomist.

Spitzer's theory. The hypothesis that the development of the lungs brings about the septation of the heart.

Spitzka, Edward Anthony (b. 1876). New York neurologist.

Spitzka's nucleus. Oculomotor nucleus. *See* NUCLEUS.

Spitzka, Edward Charles (b. 1852). New York neurologist.

Spitzka's bundle. 1. Fibres in the medial longitudinal bundle connecting the oculomotor and abducens nerve nuclei. 2. The most medial fibres of the medial lemniscus, marked in the cetacea, containing sensory fibres which appear to pass direct to the internal capsule.

Spitzka's tract, column of Spitzka–Lissauer. The posterolateral tract of the spinal cord. It lies at the apex of the posterior horn of the spinal grey matter.

Spivack, Julius Leo (b. 1889). Chicago surgeon.

Spivack's operation. 1. A form of gastrostomy in which a subcutaneous tube is made from the anterior stomach wall. 2. A similar form of cystostomy.

Spivack's rule. When the terminal part of the ileum is attached to the brim of the pelvis the appendix is retrocaecal or retrocolic in position.

Spix, Johann Baptist (b. 1781). Munich anatomist.

Spix's ossicle or spine. The lingula; a bony process at the posterior orifice of the mandibular canal, to which is attached the sphenomandibular ligament.

splanchnaesthesia (splangk·nes·**the**·ze·ah). Visceral sensation. [Gk *splagchna* viscera, aesthesia.]

splanchnaesthetic (splangk·nes·**thet**·ik). Relating or belonging to splanchnaesthesia.

splanchnectopia (splangk·nek·**to**·pe·ah). Displacement of a viscus. [Gk *splagchna* viscera, *ektopos* out of the way.]

splanchnemphraxis (splangk·nem·**frax**·is). Obstruction of any of the viscera, and in particular, of the intestine; intestinal obstruction. [Gk *splagchna* viscera, emphraxis.]

splanchneursyma (splangk·newr·**iz**·mah). Intestinal distention. [Gk *splagchna* viscera, aneurysm.]

splanchnic (**splangk**·nik). 1. Relating or belonging to the viscera; visceral. 2. An agent used for the treatment of intestinal disorders. [Gk *splagchna* viscera.]

splanchnic nerves. Nerves going to the cardiac and aorticorenal ganglia composed mainly of preganglionic fibres. **Greater splanchnic nerve [nervus splanchnicus major (NA)].** A nerve formed by branches from the 5th to the 9th thoracic ganglia and going to the ganglion. It is composed mainly of preganglionic fibres. **Lesser splanchnic nerve [nervus splanchnicus minor (NA)].** A nerve formed by branches from the 9th and 10th thoracic ganglia and going to the aorticorenal ganglion. It is composed mainly of preganglionic fibres. **Lowest splanchnic nerve [nervus splanchnicus imus (NA)].** A branch from the 12th thoracic ganglion to the renal plexus. **Lumbar splanchnic nerves [nervi splanchnici lumbales (NA)].** Branches from the lumbar part of the sympathetic trunk to the hypogastric plexus. **Pelvic splanchnic nerves [nervi splanchnici pelvini (nervi erigentes) (NA)].** Visceral branches of the 2nd, 3rd and 4th sacral nerves to the rectum, urinary bladder, uterus and penis or clitoris. **Sacral splanchnic nerves [nervi splanchnici sacrales (NA)].** Branches from the sacral part of the sympathetic trunks to the pelvic plexuses. They are distributed through these to the pelvic viscera.

splanchnicectomy (splangk·nis·**ek**·to·me). Resection of part of the splanchnic nerves. [splanchnic nerve, Gk *ektome* a cutting out.]

splanchnicotomy (splangk·nik·**ot**·o·me). The procedure of dividing one of the splanchnic nerves. [splanchnic nerve, Gk *temnein* to cut.]

splanchnoblast (**splangk**·no·blast). In the embryo, the rudiment of any viscus. [Gk *splagchna* viscera, *blastos* germ.]

splanchnocele (**splangk**·no·seel). Herniation of any of the abdominal viscera. [Gk *splagchna* viscera, *kele* hernia.]

splanchnocoele (**splangk**·no·seel). That part of the embryonic coelom which surrounds the alimentary canal and gives rise to the pericardial, pleural and peritoneal cavities. [Gk *splagchna* viscera, *koilos* hollow.]

splanchnocranium (splangk·no·**kra**·ne·um). Splanchnoskeleton. [Gk *splagchna* viscera, cranium.]

splanchnoderm (**splangk**·no·derm). Splanchnopleure. [Gk *splagchna* viscera, *derma* skin.]

splanchnodiastasis (**splangk**·no·di·**as'**·tas·is). Displacement or separation of any of the viscera. [Gk *splagchna* viscera, *diastasis* a standing apart.]

splanchnodynia (splangk·no·**din**·e·ah). Pain in any of the abdominal organs. [Gk *splagchna* viscera, *odyne* pain.]

splanchnography (splangk·**nog**·raf·e). A description of or a treatise on the viscera. [Gk *splagchna* viscera, *graphein* to record.]

splanchnolith (**splangk**·no·lith). Any calculus or concretion formed or present in the intestine. The nucleus may be a hard foreign body such as the stone of a fruit. [Gk *splagchna* viscera, *lithos* stone.]

splanchnolithiasis (**splangk**·no·lith·**i'**·as·is). A stone in the intestinal canal. [see prec.]

splanchnology (splangk·**nol**·o·je). That section of medical science which is concerned with the viscera. [Gk *splagchna* viscera, *logos* science.]

splanchnomegaly (splangk·no·**meg**·al·e). Abnormal increase in the size of any viscus. [Gk *splagchna* viscera, *megas* great.]

splanchnomicria (splangk·no·**mi**·kre·ah). Exceptional smallness of any viscus. [Gk *splagchna* viscera, *mikros* small.]

splanchnopathy (splangk·**nop**·ath·e). Any diseased condition of the viscera. [Gk *splagchna* viscera, *pathos* disease.]

splanchnopleural (splangk·no·**ploor**·al). Relating or belonging to the splanchnopleure.

splanchnopleure (**splangk**·no·ploor). The wall of the primitive gut and yolk sac of the embryo, composed of entoderm and mesoderm. The term is sometimes applied to the mesoderm only, where it lies in contact with entoderm. In the very early embryo the splanchnopleure is the first tissue to show blood-vessel and blood-cell formation. **Extra-embryonic splanchnopleure.** That part of the wall of the yolk sac which is well supplied with blood vessels. [Gk *splagchna* viscera, *pleura* side.]

splanchnoptosis (splangk·nop·**to**·sis). A condition in which the viscera are displaced downward. [Gk *splagchna* viscera, *ptosis* a falling.]

splanchnosclerosis (**splangk**·no·skler·**o'**·sis). Hardening of any viscus. [Gk *splagchna* viscera, *skleros* hard.]

splanchnoscopy (splangk·**nos**·ko·pe). Examination of any of the viscera by means of an endoscope. [Gk *splagchna* viscera, *skopein* to watch.]

splanchnoskeleton (splangk·no·**skel**·e·ton). The visceral arch skeleton of the head, namely the skeleton of the mandibular, hyoid and the 3rd, 4th, 5th and possibly 6th visceral arches; it is represented in the adult by the auditory ossicles (malleus, incus and stapes), and hyoid bone and its cornua, the laryngeal cartilages, and probably the cartilage of the trachea. It is sometimes referred to as the splanchnocranium in contrast to the neurocranium. [Gk *splagchna* viscera, skeleton.]

splanchnosomatic (**splangk**·no·so·**mat'**·ik). Relating or belonging to the viscera and to the body. [Gk *splagchna* viscera, *soma* body.]

splanchnostaxis (splangk·no·**stax**·is). Leaking of blood from small splanchnic veins or arteries. [Gk *splagchna* viscera, *staxis* a trickling.]

splanchnotomy (splangk·**not**·o·me). The anatomy or dissection of the internal organs. [Gk *splagchna* viscera, *temnein* to cut.]

splanchnotribe (**splangk**·no·tribe). A crushing instrument used to occlude the intestine temporarily, before resection of the organ is performed. [Gk *splagchna* viscera, *tribein* to grind.]

splash (splash). The sound produced by the free movement of fluid in an air-containing space. **Gastric splash.** The sound heard over a dilated stomach containing fluid when the hand is suddenly dipped over it. **Hippocratic succussion splash.** The sound heard with a stethoscope over a hydropneumothorax when the patient is shaken. [onomat.]

spleen [lien (NA)] (spleen). The largest endocrine (ductless) gland. Soft, highly vascular and dark-purple in colour, it lies between the fundus of the stomach and the diaphragm, mainly behind the midaxillary plane with its long axis along the 10th rib. The lienorenal ligament contains its blood supply and connects it to the posterior abdominal wall. The gastrosplenic ligament connects it to the greater curvature of the stomach. It has a peritoneal [tunica serosa (NA)] and fibro-elastic [tunica fibrosa (NA)] coat; from the latter numerous trabeculae arise which penetrate and form the main support of the splenic pulp. **Accessory spleen [lien accessorius (NA)].** Small nodules of splenic tissue occurring near the spleen, usually in the gastrosplenic ligament and the greater omentum. **Ague-cake spleen.** A dark-coloured, fibrotic spleen caused by repeated attacks of malaria. **Amyloid spleen.** A spleen in which the cut surface shows translucent, homogenous, oily areas. Other forms of amyloid spleen are *diffuse waxy spleen, lardaceous spleen, sago spleen* and *waxy spleen.* **Bacon spleen.** Amyloid spleen (see above). **Border of the spleen, lower [margo inferior (NA)].** The inferior of the 2 borders separating the visceral from the diaphragmatic surfaces. **Border of the spleen, upper [margo superior (NA)].** A border which usually contains 1 or 2 notches palpable in enlargement. It separates the diaphragmatic surface from the gastric impression. **Cyanotic spleen.** The spleen of chronic venous congestion. **Diffuse waxy spleen.** Amyloid spleen (see above). **End of the spleen, lateral [extremitas anterior (NA)].** The pole at which the upper and lower borders meet anterolaterally. **End of the spleen, medial [extremitas posterior (NA)].** The pole at which the upper and lower borders meet posteromedially. **Enlarged spleen.** Splenomegaly; a spleen which can be palpated below the ribs. **Flecked spleen.** A spleen mottled with small necrotic areas which are the result of ischaemia from arteriosclerosis. **Floating spleen.** A movable spleen which is usually part of a general visceroptosis. **Hard-baked spleen.** Hodgkin's disease of the spleen producing firm, white infiltrations of granulomatous tissue. **Hilum of the spleen [hilus lienis (NA)].** The fissure at the lower border of the gastric impression by which the blood vessels enter and leave the organ. **Iced spleen.** Chronic perisplenitis; thickening of the splenic capsule due to the laying down of hyaline connective tissue in the course of arteriosclerosis or chronic infection of the spleen. **Indian spleen.** Chronic enlargement of the spleen in malaria. **Lardaceous spleen.** Amyloid spleen (see above). **Movable spleen.** Floating spleen (see above). **Porphyry spleen.** Lymphadenoma of the spleen showing large areas of necrosis. **Sago spleen.** Amyloid spleen (see above). **Speckled spleen.** Flecked spleen (see above). **Surface of the spleen, diaphragmatic [facies diaphragmatica (NA)].** The rounded external surface. **Surface of the spleen, visceral [facies visceralis (NA)].** The hollowed internal surface containing the hilum, by which the blood vessels leave and enter the organ. It is divided into areas in contact with the stomach [facies gastrica (NA)], left kidney [facies renalis (NA)], left colic flexure [facies colica (NA)] and tail of the pancreas. **Wandering spleen.** Floating spleen (see above). **Waxy spleen.** Amyloid spleen (see above). [Gk *splen*.]

See also: FEITIS, GANDY-GAMNA.

splenadenoma (**splen**·ad·en·**o'**·mah). Hyperplasia of the splenic tissue and consequent enlargement of the spleen. [spleen, Gk *aden* gland, *-oma* tumour.]

splenalgia (splen·**al**·je·ah). Pain in the spleen. [spleen, Gk *algos* pain.]

splenatrophia, splenatrophy (splen·at·**tro**·fe·ah, splen·**at**·ro·fe). Splenic atrophy.

splenauxe (splen·**aux**·e). Enlargement of the spleen. [spleen, Gk *auxe* increase.]

splenectasis (splen·**ek**·tas·is). Abnormal splenic enlargement. [spleen, Gk *ektasis* a stretching.]

splenectomize (splen·**ek**·to·mize). To excise the spleen. [spleen, Gk *ektome* a cutting out.]

splenectomy (splen·**ek**·to·me). The operation of excising the spleen. **Subcapsular splenectomy.** Incision of the splenic capsule, removal of the splenic pulp within and packing of the cavity with gauze (Szendy). [see prec.]

splenectopia, splenectopy (splen·ek·**to**·pe·ah, splen·**ek**·to·pe). 1. A condition in which the spleen is more than normally mobile; floating spleen. 2. Displacement of the spleen; malposition of the spleen. [spleen, ectopia.]

splenelcosis (splen·el·**ko**·sis). Abscess of the spleen. [spleen, *helkosos* ulceration.]

splenemphraxis (splen·em·**frax**·is). Congestion of the spleen. [spleen, emphraxis.]

spleneolus (splen·e·o·lus). An accessory spleen. [dim. of L *splen* spleen.]

splenial (**sple**·ne·al). Relating or belonging to the splenium of the corpus callosum or to one of the splenius muscles.

splenic (**splen**·ik). Relating or belonging to the spleen.

splenic artery [arteria lienalis (NA)]. A division of the coeliac artery which courses in a tortuous fashion to the hilum of the spleen [rami lienales (NA)]. As it passes along the upper border of the pancreas it gives small pancreatic branches [rami pancreatici (NA)], a larger dorsal pancreatic artery [arteria pancreatica dorsalis (NA)] which passes behind the pancreas, a great pancreatic artery [arteria pancreatica magna (NA)] and an artery of the tail [arteria cauda pancreatis (NA)]. The inferior pancreatic artery [arteria pancreatica inferior (NA)] connects the dorsal and great pancreatic arteries. The splenic artery also supplies the stomach and greater omentum [rami epiploici (NA)] by means of the short gastric arteries [arteriae gastricae breves (NA)] and the left gastro-epiploic artery [arteria gastro-epiploica sinistra (NA)].

splenic vein [vena lienalis (NA)]. One of the main tributaries of the portal vein, draining the spleen, the veins from the greater curvature of the stomach (short gastric and left gastro-epiploic), the pancreatic veins and the inferior mesenteric vein.

splenicogastric (**splen**·ik·o·**gas'**·trik). Relating or belonging to both the spleen and the stomach. [Gk *splenikos* of the spleen, *gaster* stomach.]

splenicopancreatic (**splen**·ik·o·pan·kre·**at'**·ik). Relating or belonging to both the spleen and the pancreas. [Gk *splenikos* of the spleen, pancreas.]

splenicterus (splen·**ik**·ter·us). Splenitis associated with jaundice. [splenitis, Gk *ikteros* jaundice.]

spleniculus (splen·**ik**·ew·lus). An accessory spleen. [dim. of L *splen* spleen.]

splenification (**splen**·if·ik·**a'**·shun). Splenization. [spleen, L *facere* to make.]

spleniform (**splen**·e·form). Having resemblance to the spleen. [spleen, form.]

splenin (**sple**·nin). A splenic extract that in small doses reduces bleeding time but in large doses increases it. **Splenin A.** Probably a derivative of ascorbic acid. It is found in the normal blood. **Splenin B.** A fatty acid ester with a complex alcohol; it may occur in the serum in haemolytic states, thyrotoxicosis and in rheumatoid arthritis. It never occurs in healthy persons. Splenins A and B are opposed to one another pharmacologically.

spleniserrate (sple·ne·**ser**·ate). Relating or belonging to the splenius and the serratus muscles.

splenitis (sple·**ni**·tis). Inflammation affecting the spleen. [spleen, Gk *-itis* inflammation.]

splenium (**sple**·ne·um). 1. [Splenium corporis callosis (NA)]. The thickest part of the corpus callosum. 2. A compress or bandage. [Gk *splenion* bandage.]

splenius (**sple**·ne·us). 1. A bandage. 2. Applied in anatomy to 2 muscles which are wrapped round the neck somewhat like a bandage. [see prec.]

splenius capitis muscle [musculus splenius capitis (NA)] (**sple**·ne·us **kap**·it·is musl). A muscle which arises from the ligamentum nuchae and upper thoracic vertebral spines and is inserted into the mastoid process, just below the lateral third of the superior nuchal line under cover of the sternocleidomastoid muscle.

splenius cervicis muscle [musculus splenius cervicis (NA)] (**sple**·ne·us **ser**·vis·is musl). A muscle which arises from the spines of the 3rd to 6th thoracic vertebrae and is inserted into the posterior tubercles of the transverse processes of the upper cervical vertebrae.

splenization (splen·i·za·shun). Applied to the appearance of a congested and oedematous lung which resembles that of a soft and vascular spleen. **Hypostatic splenization.** The passively congested and partially consolidated condition of hypostatic pneumonia.

splenoblast (**sple**·no·blast). A cell from which a splenocyte develops. [spleen, Gk *blastos* germ.]

splenocele (**sple**·no·seel). 1. Hernial protrusion of the spleen. 2. A splenic tumour. [spleen, Gk *kele* hernia.]

splenocleisis (sple·no·**kli**·sis). Rawing the surface of the spleen, or transplanting the spleen to the abdominal wall, to encourage the development of venous anastomosis between portal and systemic venous tributaries and so relieve portal hypertension, as in the Talma-Morison operation. [spleen, Gk *kleisis* closure.]

splenocolic (sple·no·**kol**·ik). Relating or belonging to the spleen and the colon.

splenocyte (**sple**·no·site). A large mononuclear phagocyte found by Pappenheim in the spleen. [spleen, Gk *kytos* cell.]

splenodynia (sple·no·**din**·e·ah). Pain in the spleen. [spleen, Gk *odyne* pain.]

splenogenic, splenogenous (sple·no·**jen**·ik, sple·**noj**·en·us). Produced by or having origin in the spleen. [spleen, Gk *genein* to produce.]

splenogram (**sple**·no·gram). 1. The radiograph made during splenography. 2. A differential cell count of material obtained by splenic puncture. [spleen, Gk *gramma* record.]

splenogranulomatosis siderotica (**sple**·no·gran·ew·lo·mat·**o**'·sis sid·er·**ot**·ik·ah). Gamna's disease, a condition associated with enlargement of the spleen, thickening of the splenic capsule and periarterial haemorrhages which become fibrosed and infiltrated with deposits of iron-containing pigments, forming brown areas in the splenic pulp (the so-called Gandy-Gamna nodules). [spleen, granulomatosis, Gk *sideros* iron.]

splenography (sple·**nog**·raf·e). Radiography of the spleen.

splenohepatomegalia, splenohepatomegaly (**sple**·no·hep·at·o·meg·**a**'·le·ah, **sple**·no·hep·at·o·**meg**'·al·e). Concurrent increase in the size of the spleen and the liver. [spleen, Gk *hepar* liver, *megas* great.]

splenoid (**sple**·noid). Having resemblance to the spleen. [spleen, Gk *eidos* form.]

splenokeratosis (**sple**·no·ker·at·**o**'·sis). Fibrous induration of the spleen. [spleen, keratosis.]

splenolaparotomy (**sple**·no·lap·ar·**ot**'·o·me). Incision of the spleen through an abdominal opening, e.g. in order to drain a splenic abscess or cyst. [spleen, laparotomy.]

splenology (sple·**nol**·o·je). The branch of medical science that is concerned with the spleen. [spleen, Gk *logos* science.]

splenolymph (**sple**·no·limf). Splenic and lymphatic.

splenolymphatic (**sple**·no·limf·**at**'·ik). Relating to the spleen and the lymph glands.

splenolymphoma (**sple**·no·limf·**o**'·mah). Splenadenoma. [spleen, lymph, Gk *-oma* tumour.]

splenolysis (sple·**nol**·is·is). Lysis of the spleen tissue. [spleen, Gk *lysis* a loosing.]

splenoma (sple·**no**·mah). A splenic tumour. [spleen, Gk *-oma* tumour.]

splenomalacia (**sple**·no·mal·**a**'·she·ah). Softening of the spleen. [spleen, malacia.]

splenomedullary (**sple**·no·med·**ul**'·ar·e). Relating or belonging to the spleen and the bone marrow. [spleen, L *medulla* marrow.]

splenomegalia (**sple**·no·meg·**a**'·le·ah). Splenomegaly.

splenomegaly (sple·no·**meg**·al·e). Enlargement of the spleen. This may occur in association with many diseases of different types: (*a*) acute and chronic inflammatory conditions such as glandular fever, subacute bacterial endocarditis, lupus, typhoid, septicaemia, malaria, syphilis, Hodgkin's disease, Boeck's sarcoid, kala-azar and helminthic infections; (*b*) congestive conditions, Banti's disease, thrombosis of splenic or portal veins, cirrhosis of the liver; (*c*) the haemolytic anaemias, chronic anaemias such as pernicious anaemia, thalassaemia, chronic hypochromic anaemia, purpura, polycythaemia vera; (*d*) leukaemias; (*e*) primary splenic neutropenia; (*f*) disturbances of lipoid metabolism (Niemann-Pick, Gaucher and Hand-Schueller-Christian diseases, amyloidosis); (*g*) various benign and malignant tumours and cysts. **Bilharzial splenomegaly.** Splenomegaly resulting from infection with *Schistosoma* (*Bilharzia*). *See* SCHISTOSOMA. **Chronic congestive splenomegaly.** Splenic anaemia, Banti's disease; a condition of splenomegaly with hepatomegaly, slight anaemia and often associated with oesophageal varices and haemorrhoids. Portal hypertension is one aetiological factor. **Chronic malarial splenomegaly.** Splenomegaly resulting from frequent attacks of malaria, for which inadequate or no treatment has been given. **Egyptian splenomegaly.** Schistosomiasis, splenomegaly with a diffuse hyperplastic periportal cirrhosis of the liver, perisplenic-vein fibrosis and splenic-vein thrombosis, due to infestation with *Schistosoma mansoni* or *S. japonicum*. **Haemolytic splenomegaly.** Chronic haemolytic anaemia; acholuric jaundice. **Hypercholesterolaemic splenomegaly.** A splenomegaly associated with an increased amount of cholesterol in the blood (hypercholesterolaemia). **Infantile splenomegaly.** Infantile pseudoleukaemia. **Infectious splenomegaly.** Splenomegaly associated with a severe infection. **Myelophthisic splenomegaly.** Splenomegaly with fibrotic changes and diminution in the amount of myeloid tissue. **Siderotic splenomegaly.** Splenogranulomatosis siderotica. **Spodogenous splenomegaly.** Enlargement of the spleen caused by the presence of excessive quantities of red blood cells. **Thrombophlebitic splenomegaly.** Splenomegaly due to thrombophlebitis of the splenic vein. **Tropical febrile splenomegaly.** Kala-azar. [spleen, Gk *megas* large.]

See also: GAUCHER, NIEMANN.

splenomyelogenous (**sple**·no·mi·el·**oj**'·en·us). Splenomedullary. [spleen, Gk *myelos* marrow, *genein* to produce.]

splenomyelomalacia (**sple**·no·mi·el·o·mal·**a**'·she·ah). Morbid softening of the spleen and the bone marrow. [spleen, Gk *myelos* marrow, malacia.]

splenoncus (sple·**nong**·kus). A splenic swelling or tumour. [spleen, Gk *ogkos* a swelling.]

splenonephric (sple·no·**nef**·rik). Relating to the spleen and the kidney. [spleen, Gk *nephros* kidney.]

splenonephroptosis (**sple**·no·nef·rop·**to**'·sis). Ptosis of both the spleen and the kidney. [spleen, Gk *nephros* kidney, ptosis.]

splenopancreatic (**sple**·no·pan·kre·**at**'·ik). Relating or belonging to the spleen and the pancreas.

splenoparectasia, splenoparectasis (**sple**·no·par·ek·**ta**'·ze·ah, **sple**·no·par·**ek**'·tas·is). Gross enlargement of the spleen. [spleen, Gk *parektasis* stretching.]

splenopathia, splenopathy (sple·no·**path**·e·ah, sple·**nop**·ath·e). Any diseased state of the spleen. **Splenopathia leucocythaemia.** Myeloid leukaemia. *See* LEUKAEMIA. [spleen, Gk *pathos* disease.]

splenopexia, splenopexis (sple·no·**pex**·e·ah, sple·no·**pex**·is). Splenopexy.

splenopexy (**sple**·no·pex·e). The operation of fixing a misplaced or floating spleen to the wall of the abdomen by sutures. [spleen, Gk *pexis* fixation.]

splenophrenic (sple·no·**fren**·ik). In anatomy, relating or belonging to the spleen and the diaphragm. [spleen, Gk *phren* diaphragm.]

splenoportography (**sple**·no·port·**og**'·raf·e). Demonstration of the splenic and portal veins by the injection of a radio-opaque medium into the spleen. [spleen, portal vein, Gk *graphein* to record.]

splenoptosis (sple·nop·**to**·sis). Prolapse of the spleen. [spleen, Gk *ptosis* a falling.]

splenorenal (sple·no·**re**·nal). Relating to the spleen and kidney. [spleen, L *ren* kidney.]

splenorrhagia (sple·no·**ra**·je·ah). Haemorrhage from the spleen. [spleen, Gk *rhegnynein* to gush forth.]

splenorrhaphy (sple·**nor**·af·e). 1. The procedure of suturing a ruptured spleen or a wound of the spleen. 2. Splenopexia. [spleen, Gk *rhaphe* suture.]

splenosis (sple·**no**·sis). Multiple splenic implants in the peritoneum. [spleen, Gk *-osis* condition.]

splenotomy (sple·**not**·o·me). 1. Operative incision into the spleen. 2. Anatomy or dissection of the spleen. [spleen, Gk *temnein* to cut.]

splenotoxin (sple·no·**tox**·in). A toxin that has a particular affinity for the spleen, or a problematic toxin produced in the spleen in certain circumstances.

splenulus, splenunculus (**splen**·ew·lus, splen·**ung**·kew·lus). An accessory or rudimentary spleen. [dim. of L *splen* spleen.]

splint (splint). A rigid appliance used for the immobilization of a part or for the correction of deformity. **Acrylic splint.** A splint made of acrylic material used especially in dentistry and facial surgery. **Aeroplane splint.** A splint for holding the arm in abduction at the shoulder. **Ambulatory splint.** A splint in which a patient can walk. **Anchor splint.** A splint for fracture of the mandible. The teeth are fixed by wire loops to a bar. **Angular splint.** A metal splint designed to hold a particular part at any desired angle. **Balkan splint.** Balkan beam. *See* BEAM. **Banjo traction splint.** A splint for the provision of extension to the fingers and consisting of a wire bent to the shape of a banjo. **Bavarian splint.** A splint formed of alternate layers of plaster and flannel. **Caliper splint.** A metal splint designed to support the leg and allow walking, e.g. Thomas' caliper. **Cap splint.** A cast-metal splint which fits accurately over the crowns of the teeth in a fractured jaw and is cemented into position to produce immobilization of the fragments. **Cock-up splint.** A splint for fractures of the hand or wrist; arranged so that the wrist is in slight dorsiflexion; the optimum position. **Halo splint.** A device for the immobilization of the cervical spine using a metallic ring screwed into the outer table of the skull. **Infusion splint.** A splint applied to an infant's leg (or arm) to facilitate the giving of an infusion. **Open-cap splint.** A cap splint which does not cover the occlusal surfaces of the teeth to which it is attached. **Plaster splint.** A splint made of plaster of Paris. **Plastic splint.** Any splint made of moulded plastic material. **Pneumatic splint.** An inflatable splint used in the temporary immobilization of long bone fractures. **Poroplastic splint.** A splint which can be softened and moulded on the limb. **Silicone-foam splint.** A splint formed by the catalysis of basic silicone liquids and capable of being moulded to fit accurately the part to be splinted. **Tobruk splint.** A method of immobilization of the leg by a combination of plaster and a Thomas' splints. **Toronto splints.** Arm and leg splints made for attachment to a Bradford frame and used in poliomyelitis. [Middle D *splinte.*]

See also: ANDERSON (R.), ANGLE, BROWNE (D.), CRAMER (F.), DEPUY, GIBSON, GILMER, GOOCH (B.), GUNNING (T. B.), HODGEN, JONES (R.), KANAVEL, KINGSLEY, LISTON, MCINTYRE, MIDDELDORPF, PHELPS, SAYRE, SIMPSON (W. K.), STADER, THOMAS (H. O.), ZIMMER.

splinter (**splin**·ter). A sharp-pointed fragment of wood, glass, bone, metal or other hard substance. **Bone splinter.** Any sharp piece of bone which has been detached in a fracture. [see prec.]

splinter-bone (**splin**·ter·bone). A popular name for the fibula. [splinter, bone.]

splinting (**splin**·ting). The application of splints.

splitting (**split**·ing). In chemistry, the breaking-up of the molecule of a more complex compound into 2 or more simpler compounds, e.g. by hydrolysis. **Splitting of the atom.** The bombardment of the nucleus of an atom with protons, neutrons, deuterons or high-energy α-particles, resulting in its disruption. **Fee splitting.** Dichotomy, 3rd def. **Splitting of the heart sound.** A duplication of the first or second heart sounds. Splitting of the first heart sound may result from unequal closure of the mitral and tricuspid valves, as in bundle-branch block; splitting of the second is due to asynchronous closure of the pulmonary and aortic valves. Increase in the normal physiological split occurs in conditions with a low pulmonary-artery pressure, e.g. pulmonary stenosis, or with delayed contraction of the right ventricle, e.g. right bundle-branch block. [Middle D *splitten.*]

spodography (spo·**dog**·raf·e). Micro-incineration of sections of tissue for the localization of ash in such tissue. [Gk *spodos* wood ash, *graphein* to record.]

Spoendli, Heinrich (b. 1824). Zürich obstetrician.

Spoendli's foramen. A small foramen between the ethmoid and sphenoid cartilages of the developing skull.

spogel seeds (**spo**·gl seedz). Ispaghula.

spoke bone (**spoke** bone). The radius [obsolete term]. [AS *spaca*, bone.]

spoke-shave (**spoke**·shave). A knife designed on the pattern of the carpenter's spoke-shave, formerly used for the radical removal of the turbinal bones. [AS *spaca, scafan.]*

spondylalgia (spon·dil·**al**·je·ah). Pain affecting a vertebra or located in some part of the vertebral column. [Gk *sphondylos* vertebra, *algos* pain.]

spondylarthritis (**spon**·dil·ar·**thri**'·tis). A condition occurring most commonly in children by narrowing of intervertebral disc spaces and some destruction of adjacent vertebrae, followed by slow healing over a period of months. **Spondylarthritis ankylopoietica.** Spondylarthritis marked by a gradual ankylosis of the articular surfaces of the spine, associated with atrophy of the vertebral bodies. **Spondylarthritis synovialis.** Inflammation affecting the synovial membranes of the articular process of the vertebrae. [Gk *sphondylos* vertebra, arthritis.]

spondylarthrocace (**spon**·dil·ar·**throk**'·as·e). Carious disease of a vertebra or of several neighbouring vertebrae. [Gk *sphondylos* vertebra, arthrocace.]

spondyle (**spon**·dile). A vertebra. [Gk *sphondylos* vertebra.]

spondylexarthrosis (**spon**·dil·ex·ar·**thro**'·sis). Dislocation of a vertebra. [Gk *sphondylos* vertebra, *ex*, arthrosis.]

spondylitic (spon·dil·**it**·ik). 1. One who is affected with spondylitis. 2. Pertaining to or having the character of spondylitis.

spondylitis (spon·dil·**i**·tis). Inflammation of the spine. **Spondylitis ankylopoietica, Ankylosing spondylitis.** Poker spine; a condition in which the ligaments of the spine ossify and the lateral joints become ankylosed. The sacro-iliac joints are also affected. **Spondylitis deformans.** Arthritis of the spine, resulting in severe fixed kyphosis. **Hypertrophic spondylitis.** Spondylitis with hypertrophy and lipping at the joints. **Spondylitis muscularis.** Deformity due to muscular weakness. **Spondylitis ossificans ligamentosa.** Spondylitis ankylopoietica (see above). **Post-traumatic spondylitis.** Arthritis of the spine following injury. **Rheumatoid spondylitis.** Ankylosing spondylitis (see above). **Spondylitis rhizomelica.** Spondylitis ankylopoietica (see above). **Spondylitis tuberculosa.** Tuberculous infection of the spine; Pott's disease. **Spondylitis typhosa.** Infection of the spine by the typhus bacillus. [Gk *sphondylos* vertebra, *-itis* inflammation.]

See also: KUEMMELL, MARIE, STRUEMPELL.

spondylo-arthrosis (**spon**·dil·o·ar·**thro**'·sis). Osteo-arthritis of the spine. [Gk *sphondylos* vertebra, arthrosis.]

spondylocace (spon·dil·**ok**·as·e). Destruction of the body of a vertebra, usually in Pott's disease. [Gk *sphondylos* vertebra, *kake* badness.]

spondylodesis (**spon**·dil·o·**de**'·sis). The operation of fusion of the spine, usually by a bone graft. [Gk *sphondylos* vertebra, *desis* a binding.]

spondylodidymia (**spon**·dil·o·did·**im**'·e·ah). In teratism, the condition in which the vertebral columns of twin monsters are fused. [Gk *sphondylos* vertebra, *didymos* twin.]

spondylodymus (spon·dil·**od**·im·us). The twin monsters in spondylodidymia. [see prec.]

spondylodynia (**spon**·dil·o·**din**'·e·ah). Pain in a vertebra. [Gk *sphondylos* vertebra, *odyne* pain.]

spondylolisthesis (**spon**·dil·o·lis·**the**'·sis). Forward displacement of one vertebra upon the vertebra below, usually occurring between the 5th lumbar vertebra and the sacrum, and due either to injury or to a congenital defect of the pedicles of the vertebra. [Gk *sphondylos* vertebra, *olisthanein* to slip.]

spondylolisthetic (**spon**·dil·o·lis·**thet**'·ik). Pertaining to or characterized by spondylolisthesis.

spondylolysis (spon·dil·**ol**·is·is). 1. The breaking-down of a vertebra. The condition is characterized by a laminar cleft separating the upper and lower articular processes. 2. Loosening of the normally stable attachment existing between one vertebra and the next. [Gk *sphondylos* vertebra, *lysis* a loosing.]

spondylomalacia (**spon**·dil·o·mal·**a**'·she·ah). Softening of the vertebra. **Spondylomalacia traumatica.** Kuemmell's disease. [Gk *sphondylos* vertebra, malacia.]

spondylometer (spon·dil·**om**·et·er). A device for measuring the range of spinal movement. [Gk *sphondylos* vertebra, meter.]

spondylomyelitis (**spon**·dil·o·mi·el·**i**'·tis). Spondylitis. [Gk *sphondylos* vertebra, myelitis.]

spondylopathy (spon·dil·**op**·ath·e). Any diseased or deformed state of the vertebrae. **Traumatic spondylopathy.** Post-traumatic spondylitis. *See* SPONDYLITIS. [Gk *sphondylos* vertebra, *pathos* disease.]

spondyloptosis (**spon**·dil·op·**to**'·sis). Spondylolisthesis. [Gk *sphondylos* vertebra, *ptosis* a falling.]

spondylopyosis (**spon**·dil·o·pi·**o**'·sis). Inflammation of suppurative type of one or more of the vertebrae, particularly the bodies. [Gk *sphondylos* vertebra, pyosis.]

spondyloschisis (spon·dil·**os**·kis·is). Congenital cleft of a vertebral arch or arches. [Gk *sphondylos* vertebra, *schisis* a cleaving.]

spondylosis (spon·dil·**o**·sis). A term now largely reserved for non-inflammatory and degenerative disease of the spine, for example osteo-arthrosis. [Gk *sphondylos* vertebra, *-osis* condition.]

spondylosyndesis (**spon**·dil·o·**sin**'·de·sis). Arthrodesis of the spine. [Gk *sphondylos* vertebra, syndesis.]

spondylotherapy (**spon**·dil·o·**ther**'·ap·e). Treatment of diseased conditions of the vertebral column. [Gk *sphondylos* vertebra, therapy.]

spondylotomy (spon·dil·**ot**·o·me). 1. Incision for the purpose of laying bare the spinal cord. 2. Division of the vertebral column of the fetus in order to make delivery easier. [Gk *sphondylos* vertebra, *temnein* to cut.]

spondylous (**spon**·dil·us). Relating or belonging to a vertebra; vertebral. [Gk *sphondylos* vertebra.]

sponge (spunj). The elastic fibrous skeleton of certain non-mobile marine animals of the order Porifera; its basis is a protein substance, spongin, with lime and silica. Used for washing and absorbing purposes, it has been largely replaced by synthetic plastic products. **Fibrin sponge.** Dry fibrin in the form of pledgets or wads for application to oozing surfaces at operation, reducing bleeding partly by mild pressure, partly by the encouragement of clotting; left in the wound, the sponge is slowly absorbed. **Gauze sponge.** A piece of folded gauze used during a surgical operation, especially to swab bleeding surfaces so that the bleeding points can be picked up. **Gelatin Sponge, Absorbable BP 1973.** Gelatin used in a similar manner to the fibrin sponge (see above). [Gk *spoggia.*]

spongeitis (spon·je·i·tis). Inflammation affecting the corpus spongiosum penis. [corpus spongiosum, Gk *-itis* inflammation.]

spongia (**spun**·je·ah). Sponges; invertebrate marine animals of the order Porifera, the dried skeleton of which forms the sponges of commerce. **Spongia officinalis.** The official name for a sponge. [L.]

spongiform (**spun**·je·form). Having resemblance to a sponge. [sponge, form.]

spongiitis (spon·je·i·tis). Spongeitis.

spongin (**spun**·jin). A scleroprotein occurring in sponge.

spongioblast (**spon**·je·o·blast). An embryonic neuroglial cell which will give rise to astroblasts and finally to astrocytes. **Spongioblast of the retina.** Cells of the embryonic retina which will give rise to the neuroglial elements of the retina, e.g. Mueller's fibres. [Gk *spoggia* sponge, *blastos* germ.]

spongioblastoma (**spon**·je·o·blas·**to**'·mah). A variety of malignant glioma derived from spongioblasts which are embryonic derivatives of the epithelium of the neural canal. **Spongioblastoma multiforme.** A pleomorphic spongioblastoma. **Spongioblastoma unipolare.** A rare variety of spongioblastoma in the optic nerves or pons, composed of unipolar spongioblasts. [spongioblast, Gk *-oma* tumour.]

spongiocyte (**spon**·je·o·site). 1. A neuroglial cell. 2. A vacuolated cell which occurs in the cortex of the suprarenal gland.

spongiocytoma (**spon**·je·o·si·**to**'·mah). A tumour or neoplasm containing neuroglial cells. [spongiocyte, Gk *-oma* tumour.]

spongioid (**spun**·je·oid). Spongiform. [sponge, Gk *eidos* form.]

spongioplasm (**spon**·je·o·plazm). The reticular component of the cell cytoplasm in fixed histological preparations, now known to be an artefact resulting from the precipitation of part of the protein complex of the protoplasm. [Gk *spoggia* sponge, *plasma* plasm.]

spongiosa (spon·je·o·sah). Cancellous or spongy bone (spongy substance), as found in the ends of long bones, in the bodies of vertebrae, etc. [Gk *spoggia* sponge.]

spongiose (**spun**·je·oze). Full of small holes, like a sponge; spongy. [see prec.]

spongiosis (spon·je·o·sis). Oedema in the epidermis with separation of the prickle cells, and stretching and ultimate rupture of their prickles; a characteristic histological finding in eczema. [Gk *spoggia* sponge, *-osis* condition.]

spongiositis (**spon**·je·o·**si**'·tis). Spongeitis. [corpus spongiosum, Gk *-itis* inflammation.]

spongious (**spun**·je·us). Spongiose.

spool (spool). 1. A reel on which suture material is wound. 2. A tubular structure used in intestinal anastomosis. [Middle D *spoele.*]

See also: CARASSINI.

spoon (spoon). 1. A small oval bowl with a handle, used for transferring and measuring liquids or powders. 2. Any instrument shaped like a spoon. **Cataract spoon.** A shallow, spoon-shaped instrument used in cataract extraction when vitreous loss or dislocation of the lens occurs. It is passed behind the lens and lifts it out assisted by counter-pressure on the cornea. **Chalazion spoon.** A small, spoon-shaped instrument with sharp edges, used for curetting out chalazions. **Excavator spoon.** Spoon excavator; a spoon-shaped dental excavator. **Sharp spoon, Surgical spoon.** A surgical instrument with a heavily built spoon-shaped end, used for scraping away granulations and scooping away dead tissue, especially from cavities. [AS *spon* chip.]

See also: DAVIEL, VOLKMANN (R.).

sporadic (spor·**ad**·ik). Scattered; separate; occurring singly; not epidemic. [Gk *sporaden* scattered about.]

sporadoneure (spor·**ad**·o·newr). An isolated nerve cell not associated with the central nervous system or the peripheral ganglia. [Gk *sporaden* scattered about, *neuron* nerve.]

sporangia (spo·**ran**·je·ah). *See* SPORANGIUM.

sporangial (spo·**ran**·je·al). Belonging to, or having the character of a sporangium.

sporangiophore (spo·**ran**·je·o·for). The fertile hypha or stalk which bears a sporangium or sporangia. [sporangium, Gk *pherein* to bear.]

sporangiospore (spo·**ran**·je·o·spore). A spore produced within a sporangium.

sporangium (spo·**ran**·je·um) (pl. *sporangia*). A closed receptacle, often of globose shape, in which asexual spores of a fungus are formed by successive nuclear divisions and septation of the protoplasm; a spore case. **Resting sporangium.** One which requires a rest period before liberating its spores. These sporangia have thick walls and are found in some plant parasites which have to tide over an unfavourable period between seasons. [spore, Gk *aggeion* vessel.]

spore (spor). A relatively resistant dormant body (a seed) produced by micro-organisms and by certain higher plants, as a means of multiplication or of survival. They may be formed in numbers or singly, and as a result of conjugation of cells (sexual) or asexually. **Arthrogenous spore.** An arthrospore. **Asexual spore.** One produced vegetatively without the fusion of nuclei. **Bacterial spore.** The highly resistant spore produced by bacteria. **Spore case.** The structure in which endospores are developed. **Compound spore.** A spore made up of 2 or more cells, as in some Uredinales and the macroconidium of the dermatophytes. **Daughter spore.** Secondary spore (see below). **Mother spore.** In the Ascomycetes the ascus is sometimes referred to as the *spore mother cell.* **Naked spore.** One without a definite cell wall; an amoeboid spore, as in the Myxomycetes. **Primary spore.** A spore borne on a sporophore which is part of the fungal plant. **Resting spore.** A spore which is dormant for a period before germinating. **Spore sac.** A thin-walled sac which is extruded when a certain type of sporangium ruptures and into which the spores pass before being liberated; a situation found in some lower fungi. **Secondary spore.** A spore borne exogenously by another spore without the intermediate production of a fungal plant. **Sexual spore.** A spore produced usually after the fusion of 2 haploid nuclei from either 2 dissimilar or 2 similar cells. **Swarm spore.** A flagellated spore. **Washed spores.** Spores suspended in liquid and then retrieved by centrifugalization or sedimentation in order to remove extraneous matter. [Gk *sporos* seed.]

See also: ROSS (R.).

sporenrest (**spo**·ren·rest). Sporal residuum. [G.]

sporicidal (spo·re·si·dal). Capable of destroying spores. [see foll.]

sporicide (spo·re·side). A substance or agent which kills spores. [spore, L *caedere* to kill.]

sporidiosis (spo·rid·e·o'·sis). Infection by sporidia. [sporidium, Gk *-osis* condition.]

sporidium (spo·rid·e·um) (pl. *sporidia*). The spore stage of a protozoon. **Sporidium vaccinale.** *Cytoryctes vacciniae.* [dim. of Gk *sporos* seed.]

sporiferous (spo·rif·er·us). Bearing or producing spores. [spore, L *ferre* to bear.]

sporification (spo·rif·ik·a'·shun). The process of forming spores. [spore, L *facere* to make.]

sporiparous (spo·rip·ar·us). 1. Reproducing by sporulation. 2. Sporiferous. [spore, L *parere* to produce.]

sporo-agglutination (spo·ro·ag·loo·tin·a'·shun). Agglutination of a spore suspension with a serum containing antibodies; used in a special sense for the non-specific serum agglutination of spores of *Sporotrichum* as a test for fungus infections.

sporoblast (spo·ro·blast). A stage in the life-cycle of Sporozoa of the genus *Plasmodium.* It is one of the bodies derived from the oöcyte within the oöcyst, and gives rise to the sporozoites. [spore, Gk *blastos* germ.]

sporocyst (spo·ro·sist). 1. A stage in the life-cycle of many Protozoa, especially Sporozoa. It is a cyst-like form in which the spores develop and are later liberated. 2. A stage in the life-cycle of Trematoda, between the miracidium and the redia; it occurs within the secondary host. [spore, Gk *kystis* bladder.]

sporogenesis (spo·ro·jen·es·is). 1. Reproduction by means of spores. 2. The development or formation of spores. [spore, Gk *genein* to produce.]

sporogenic (spo·ro·jen·ik). Relating or belonging to sporogenesis.

sporogenous (spo·roj·en·us). Reproducing by means of spores. [spore, Gk *genein* to produce.]

sporogeny, sporogony (spo·roj·en·e, spo·rog·o·ne). Sporogenesis.

sporomycosis (spo·ro·mi·ko'·sis). A morbid condition due to invasion of the lungs by the spores of a fungus. [spore, Gk *mykes* fungus, *-osis* condition.]

sporont (spo·ront). A sexually mature protozoal parasite. [spore, Gk *on* being.]

sporonticide (spo·ron·tis·ide). A drug which, while not necessarily being gametocytocidal, will prevent the process of sporogony developing to the complete maturation of the oöcyst of the malaria parasite. [sporont, L *caedere* to kill.]

sporophore (spo·ro·fore). The spore-bearing portion of an organism. [spore, Gk *pherein* to bear.]

sporophyte (spo·ro·fite). The generation which bears asexual spores in those plants in which there is alternation of generations. [spore, Gk *phyton* plant.]

sporoplasm (spo·ro·plazm). Reproduction cell protoplasm [spore, Gk *plasma* something formed.]

sporotheka (spo·ro·the·kah). The membrane surrounding developing sporozoites in the anopheles mosquito. [spore, Gk *theke* sheath.]

Sporothrix schenckii (spo·ro·thrix shen·ke·i). The causative organism of sporotrichosis (Hektoen and Perkins, 1900), formerly called *Sporotrichum schenckii.* In tissues the fungus is present as scanty yeasts or cigar-shaped bodies. In culture at room temperature the fungus grows as a moist, wrinkled, membranous colony of septate hyphae. On enriched media at 37°C, the yeast form is grown. [Gk *sporos* seed, *thrix* hair.]

sporotrichosis (spo·ro·trik·o'·sis). A chronic mycotic infection caused by *Sporothrix schenckii* (although formerly believed to be caused by the species *Sporotrichum*) which usually commences in a wound and is characterized by the formation of indolent nodules, abscesses and ulcers; these often develop along the course of the lymphatic channels which drain the primary site of infection. [Gk *sporos* seed, *thrix* hair, *-osis* condition.]

Sporotrichum (spo·ro·trik·um). This species was formerly thought to be the causative agent of sporotrichosis, now known to be due to *Sporothrix schenckii.* Species of the genus *Sporotrichum* are cosmopolitan and destroy organic materials in nature. [Gk *sporos* seed, *thrix* hair.]

Sporozoa (spo·ro·zo·ah). A class of the phylum Protozoa, characterized by the absence of organs of locomotion in the adults, an alternation of sexual and asexual generations and a parasitic mode of life. The genera *Isospora, Plasmodium* and *Toxoplasma* are of medical importance. [spore, Gk *zoon* animal.]

sporozoan (spo·ro·zo·an). Relating to a member of the class Sporozoa.

sporozoite (spo·ro·zo·ite). In the Sporozoa the product of schizogony of the zygote. In *Plasmodium* species the elongate zygote in the mosquito stomach wall, by repeated divisions of the cytoplasm, forms the oöcyst containing many thousand sporozoites, which are the infective forms. [spore, Gk *zoon* animal.]

sporozooid (spo·ro·zo·oid). One of the falciform bodies produced by every spore of the true coccidia; any oöspore. [spore, Gk *zoon* animal, *eidos* form.]

sporozoon (spo·ro·zo·on). Any protozoon of the class Sporozoa. **Sporozoon furunculosum.** The name given by Firth in 1891 to bodies found in oriental sore that are now known as *Leishmania tropica.* [obsolete term.]

sporozoosis (spo·ro·zo·o'·sis). An infection due to the presence of sporozoa. [sporozoa, Gk *-osis* disease.]

sport (sport). Mutation. [ME *desport.]*

sporular (spor·ew·lar). Resembling, relating to, or having the character of a spore or sporule.

sporulation (spor·ew·la·shun). The formation of spores; a process of reproduction exercised by certain protozoa in which the original cell divides into a number of daughter forms. **Arthrogenous sporulation.** Fungal spores produced by simple fragmentation of the mycelium. **Endogenous sporulation.** Spore formation within the definitive host. **Exogenous sporulation.** Spore formation outside the definitive host. [sporule.]

sporule (spor·ewl). 1. A small spore. 2. A very small particle within a spore. 3. In mycology, a spore that is contained within a perithecium. [dim. of Gk *sporos* seed.]

sporuliferous (spor·ew·lif·er·us). Bearing sporules. [sporule, L *ferre* to bear.]

spot (spot). A small part of the surface of anything, distinguished by colour or texture; a mark or stain. **Black spots.** Dark areas occurring on cold-storage meat, caused by the growth of species of *Cladosporium.* **Blind spot.** The physiological scotoma present in the visual field to the temporal side of the fixation point, due to absence of the perceptive retinal elements where the optic nerve enters the eye. Also called *punctum caecum* and *Mariotte's blind spot.* **Blue spot.** Macula caeruleae. **Café-au-lait spots.** Spots of patchy cutaneous pigmentation in generalized neurofibromatosis (von Recklinghausen's disease). **Cayenne pepper spots.** Reddish-brown macules due to haemosiderin arising from extravasation from superficial capillaries, e.g. in Schamberg's disease. **Cherry-red spot at the macula.** 1. The appearance of the macula as a bright red spot surrounded by a milky-white oedematous retina in the early stages following a sudden occlusion of the central retinal artery. 2. A small red or brown spot surrounded by a white slightly raised area of the retina, resembling the above picture, seen in Tay–Sachs disease or the infantile form of amaurotic familial idiocy. **Cold spot.** A small area of skin specially sensitive to cold. **Deaf spot.** Deaf field. *See* FIELD. **Embryonic spot.** The early blastoderm of large-yolked eggs as it appears to the naked eye. **Eye spot.** The position on the surface of the embryo overlying the optic cup. **Focal spot.** The cross-sectional area of the cathode beam in an x-ray tube, where it strikes the target face. **Germinal spot.** Embryonic spot (see above). **Herald spot.** Herald patch. *See* PATCH. **High spot.** In radiotherapy, a tissue point so related to one or more radiation sources as to receive a dose substantially above the general level in the treated volume. **Hot spot.** A small area of skin specially sensitive to heat. **Hypnogenetic spot.** An area on the surface of the body which, when stimulated, induces sleep. **Interpalpebral spot.** The yellowish triangular spot commonly seen in the conjunctiva near the limbus in the horizontal meridian. More commonly called *pinguecula.* **Lenticular spot.** Rose spot (see below). **Liver spots.** Pityriasis (tinea) versicolor. **Milk spot.** A white opaque area seen on the visceral pericardium at post-mortem examination, situated over the right ventricle usually in persons who have passed middle age. The aetiology is still unknown. **Mongolian spot.** A blue, brown or dark spot noted on the lower sacral region in mongolian children. The lesions may be single or multiple, or a small oval or round area may be involved. The spot or spots are present at birth, and usually disappear in the third or fourth years of life. The pigment cells of mongolian spots may be demonstrated in Europeans between the fifth and ninth months of intra-uterine life, which may explain why the lesions are noted in infants of the white races suffering from mongolism. **Mother's spot.** A naevus. **Pain spot.** A small area of skin especially sensitive to pain stimuli. **Pelvic spots.** Small round or oval opacities seen radiographically internal to the shadow of the pelvic brim. Usually due to phleboliths, they sometimes represent concretions in an appendix or colonic diverticula. They may simulate ureteral calculi. **Plague spots.** 1. Reddish spots on the skin of patients suffering from plague. They are caused by flea bites. 2. Disease-ridden areas. **Rose spots.** Roseola typhosa; the rose-coloured rash in typhoid fever. Spots appear on the abdomen and thighs, usually from the seventh to tenth day of illness. **Ruby spot.** A bright red petechial spot seen on the skin of old people. Its significance is not understood. **Sacral spot.** Mongolian spot (see above). **Temperature spot.** A hot or cold spot (see above). **Tendinous spot.** Macula albida. **Trigger spot.** A focal point of increased sensitivity in the soft tissues from which pain radiates or may be referred. **Typhoid spot.** Rose spot (see above). **Warm spot.** Hot spot (see above). **White spots.** Raised white or greyish areas found on the ventricular surface of the anterior segment of the mitral valve. **Wine spot.** A small port-wine stain; naevus flammeus. **Yellow spot.** Macula lutea. [ME.]

See also: BIER, BITOT, CARLETON, CHRISTOPHERS, DALEN, DE MORGAN, ELSCHNIG, FILATOV, FLINDT, FUCHS (E.), GAULE, JANEWAY (E. G.), KOPLIK, MARIOTTE, ROTH (M.), SIEGRISTE, STEPHENS, TARDIEU, TAY, TROUSSEAU.

sprain (sprane). Injury by sudden traction to the muscles, ligaments or articular capsule of a limb, not sufficiently severe to produce rupture of these structures. The condition is most common in the immediate neighbourhood of joints. **Riders' sprain.** Sprain of the adductor muscles of the thigh, following riding horseback. [etym. dub.]

spray (spra). A suspension of minute drops of liquid in air or other gas, used for the medication of the throat and nasal passages. **Ether spray.** The spraying of ether on the body surface to produce local anaesthesia by the cooling effect of its rapid evaporation. **Vichy spray.** Fine streams of water, at a temperature of 39°C (102°F), directed on to the recumbent body from a series of rose jets. [ME.]

spread (spred). 1. The act of spreading out an inoculum on a bacteriological plate. 2. Of an epidemic, the spreading of a disease, either directly or indirectly, from one individual to another. **Metaphase spread.** The chromosomes of a cell in metaphase spread out by cytological procedures designed to help the morphological analysis of chromosomes (that is, hypotonic treatment, air drying, squashing). [see foll.]

spreader (spred·er). 1. An instrument used for distributing inoculated bacteria on the surface of a solid medium so as to obtain separate colonies. A curved, smooth glass rod is commonly used. 2. A culture which spreads over the surface of a solid medium, e.g. *Proteus;* even small inocula may spread over a large area. **Bladder-neck spreader.** A surgical instrument used in retropubic prostatectomy for maintaining exposure of the bladder neck and prostatic cavity. [AS *spraedan.*]

spreading (spred·ing). 1. The smearing or laying out of anything over a surface. 2. Extending, as for example the edge of a bacterial colony which advances across the surface of the medium away from the point of inoculation. [see prec.]

Sprengel, Otto Gerhard Karl (b. 1852). German surgeon.

Sprengel's deformation or deformity. Congenital upward displacement of the scapula.

springhaas (spring·has). *Pedetes caffer,* the giant jerboa; a reservoir of plague in South Africa. [Afrikaans.]

sprue (sproo). 1. A non-febrile tropical disease of uncertain origin. It is characterized by steatorrhoea, macrocytic anaemia, multiple vitamin deficiencies and also deficient absorption of iron and calcium. The jejunal and ileal mucosa shows villous atrophy of varying degree. Wasting is a marked feature. 2. In dentistry, a hole through which molten metal is poured or forced in making a casting for an artificial restoration for the mouth. [D *sprouw.*]

spud (spud). 1. An instrument used to separate the mucous membrane in flaps of tissue in surgical procedures which involve the excision of bone. 2. A short, flat, bevelled blade used in removal of a foreign body. [etym. dub.]

spur (sper). 1. A projecting portion of bone. 2. In dentistry a piece of metal projecting from a dental plate or appliance. **Calcanean spur.** A small outgrowth of bone arising from the under-surface of the calcaneum, sometimes associated with a painful heel. **Occipital spur.** An abnormal process of bone projecting from the occipital bone. **Olecranon spur.** An abnormal piece of bone projecting from the olecranon process of the ulna. **Scleral spur.** A spur for the origin of the radial fibres of the ciliary muscle and the insertion of the trabecular meshwork. **Spur of the septum.** A projection on the septum of the nose, usually near its base. It sometimes gives rise to nasal obstruction. [AS *spura.*]

See also: MORAND.

spurge (sperj). Common name for species of *Euphorbia.* **Spurge flax, Spurge laurel.** The dried bark of *Daphne mezereum, D. gnidium* or *D. laureola* (family Thymeleaceae). The bark contains a bitter glycosidal principle associated with wax, an acrid resin and colouring matter. [O Fr. *espurge.*]

Spurway, John (fl. 1917). British physician.

Spurway syndrome. Fragilitas ossium.

sputa (spew·tah). *See* SPUTUM.

sputtering (sput·er·ing). A technique for the deposition of thin layers of metal or other conductor on a surface. The substance in question is exposed in a low-pressure electrical glow discharge to the bombardment of positive ions, leading to a slow mechanical disintegration and deposition as a coherent film on nearby surfaces. [onomat.]

sputum (spew·tum) (pl. *sputa*). The material expelled from the respiratory passages by coughing or clearing the throat. It is of mixed origin being derived from the nose, pharynx, trachea, bronchi and lung alveoli, with saliva from the mouth and any extraneous matter such as blood or pus which may have entered the respiratory tract from neighbouring tissues. It may therefore contain such varied material as watery or mucoid secretions, desquamated epithelial cells, blood, pus, caseous matter, elastic fibres and disintegrated tissues from destruction of the lung, bacteria, fungi and other microparasites. **Sputum aeroginosum, Aeruginous sputum.** Green sputum, the colour of verdigris. **Albuminoid sputum.** A thin, watery, frothy sputum, often blood-stained, containing albumin from the blood serum exuded in oedema of the lungs. **Black-pigmented sputum.** Sputum which may occur in coal miners. **Sputum coctum.** The mucopurulent sputum of the later stages of bronchitis. **Sputum crudum.** Clear, tenacious sputum produced in early laryngitis. **Sputum cruentum.** Blood-stained sputum. **Egg-yolk sputum.** Bright yellow sputum seen with jaundice. **Globular sputum.** Sputum consisting of spherical lumps which flatten and become nummular. **Green sputum.** That which may be seen in chronic jaundice, when a liver abscess has ruptured into the lung, and in cases of chloroma. **Icteric sputum.** Sputum stained with bile. **Mucopurulent sputum.** A mixture of mucus and pus. **Mucous sputum.** Sputum consisting of mucopurulent lumps which sink to the bottom of the sputum cup and flatten out into coin-like masses;

in pulmonary tuberculosis it is suggestive of lung cavities. **Pearly sputum.** A sputum seen in some cases of asthma in which small pearly globules or sago-like grains appear in the sputum. These can be unrolled into the convoluted threads called *Curschmann's spirals.* **Prune-juice sputum.** A watery, dark-brown sputum from altered blood in pneumonic plague and some other conditions. **Purulent sputum.** Sputum that consists mainly of pus. **Red-currant-jelly sputum.** The self-explanatory name given to the characteristic sputum in new growths of the lung. **Rusty sputum.** Sputum in which altered blood pigment is diffused through the sputum; it occurs in pneumonia. **Sputum tuberculosum.** A sputum in which ragged mucopurulent lumps surrounded by mucus are found. Caseous material, blood and tubercle bacilli may also be present. **Yellow sputum.** A sputum which may be seen with jaundice or the rupture of a liver abscess into the lung. [L spittle.]

sputum-negative (spew·tum·**neg**·at·iv). Applied to cases of actual or suspected pulmonary tuberculosis in which the sputum on test is found to be free from tubercle bacilli. [sputum, negative.]

sputum-positive (spew·tum·**poz**·it·iv). Applied to cases of pulmonary tuberculosis in which the sputum on test is found to contain tubercle bacilli. [sputum, positive.]

squama (**skwa**·mah) (pl. *squamae*). A flattened scale (e.g. fish); hence the thin expanded part of a bone, particularly in the wall of the cranial cavity. **Frontal squama [squama frontalis (NA)].** The part of the frontal bone that forms the anterior part of the calvaria. [L scale.]

squamate (**skwa**·mate). Scaly; squamous. [see prec.]

squamatization (**skwa**·mat·i·**za'**·shun). Keratinization. [L *squama* scale.]

squamofrontal (skwa·mo·**frun**·tal). Relating or belonging to the orbital plate. [L *squama* scale, frontal.]

squamoid (**skwa**·moid). Having resemblance to a squama. [L *squama* scale, Gk *eidos* form.]

squamomandibular (**skwa**·mo·man·**dib'**·ew·lar). Relating to the squamous part of the temporal or occipital bones and the mandible.

squamomastoid (skwa·mo·**mas**·toid). Relating or belonging to the squamous and mastoid parts of the temporal bone.

squamo-occipital (**skwa**·mo·ok·**sip'**·it·al). Relating or belonging to the squamous part of the occipital bone.

squamoparietal (**skwa**·mo·par·**i'**·et·al). Pertaining to the squamous part of the temporal bone and to the parietal bone.

squamopetrosal (**skwa**·mo·pet·**ro'**·sal). Relating or belonging to the squamous and petrous parts of the temporal bone.

squamosa (skwa·**mo**·sah). The squamous part of the occipital or temporal bones, and of the latter in particular. [L *squama* scale.]

squamosal (skwa·**mo**·sal). Squamous; relating or belonging to the squamous part of the temporal bone.

squamosphenoid (skwa·mo·**sfe**·noid). Relating to the squamous part of the temporal bone and to the sphenoid bone.

squamotemporal (skwa·mo·**tem**·por·al). Relating or belonging to the squamous part of the temporal bone.

squamotympanic (**skwa**·mo·tim·**pan'**·ik). Pertaining to the squamous part of the temporal bone and to the tympanic ring or plate. **Squamotympanic fissure.** *See* FISSURE.

squamous (**skwa**·mus). 1. Resembling a scale; platelike. 2. Scaly; covered with scales. [L *squama* scale.]

squamozygomatic (**skwa**·mo·zi·go·**mat'**·ik). Relating or belonging to the squamous part, and the zygomatic process of, the temporal bone.

squarra (**skwar**·ah). A rugose, tineal crust. [Gk *eschara* scab.]

squarrose, squarrous (**skwar**·oze, **skwar**·us). 1. Scurfy; covered with dandruff. 2. In botany and zoology, bearing rough scaly processes. [see prec.]

squash-bite (skwosh·bite). Mushbite. [O Fr. *esquasser,* bite.]

squatting (**skwot**·ing). In cardiology, the typical posture adopted by many children with cyanotic congenital heart disease, especially *Fallot's tetralogy,* to obtain relief from the distress produced by exercise. [O Fr. *esquatir* to press down.]

squaw vine (**skwaw** vine). Squaw berry, twin berry, winter clover; the dried herb *Mitchella repens* found in North America (family Rubiaceae). No active principles have been discovered in it and its therapeutic value is doubtful. [Amer. Ind. *squa,* L *vinea.]*

squeeze (skweez). Term sometimes used for caisson disease. **Tussive squeeze.** The act of coughing which compresses the lungs so that mucus and other fluids are forced into the bronchi. [AS *cwesan.*]

Squill BPC 1968 (skwil). The sliced and dried scale-leaves from the bulb of *Urginea maritima* (Linn.) Baker (family Liliaceae). It contains a crystalline glycoside, scillarin A, and an amorphous mixture of glycosides named scillarin B. **Red squill.** A variety of *Urginea maritima* containing a red anthocyanin colouring matter. [L *squilla.*]

squillitic (skwil·**it**·ik). Prepared from squills.

squint (skwint). A condition in which one eye deviates from the point of fixation. **Accommodative squint.** Squint due to excessive accommodation in hypermetropes. It usually reacts well to treatment (adequate glasses and orthoptic training). **Alternating squint.** Squint which may appear in either eye. **Comitant squint, Concomitant squint.** One in which the angle of squint remains relatively unaltered on conjugate movement of the eyes. **Convergent squint.** One in which the deviating eye looks inwards towards the nose. **Divergent squint.** One in which the deviating eye looks outwards. This often occurs in a blind eye or in one with defective vision. **Intermittent squint.** One in which the squint is not always present; a condition seen sometimes in early stages of squint. **Latent squint.** A condition similar to heterophoria, the eye deviating when covered but becoming straight again when the cover is removed. **Manifest squint.** Tropia. **Occasional squint.** Intermittent squint (see above). **Paralytic squint.** One in which the deviation is non-comitant, i.e. it varies as the direction of gaze is shifted, being greatest when the affected eye attempts to look in the direction of action of the paralysed muscle. **Periodic squint.** Intermittent squint (see above). **Psychological squint.** That due primarily to an emotional disturbance, e.g. jealousy, fear, imitation. **Uni-ocular squint.** One in which the squint remains confined to a particular eye; this will usually take up fixation on covering the sound eye, but returns to its deviated position when the cover is removed. **Upward-and-downward squint.** Usually classified as *vertical squint.* **Vertical squint.** The deviation is in a vertical direction. Many of the cases are non-comitant, the commonest cause being overaction of one or both inferior oblique muscles which causes the eye to shoot up on adduction. **Voluntary squint.** A squint produced voluntarily, a faculty not uncommon. It is done by converging excessively and then making a conjugate lateral movement of the eyes. [ME.]

Squire's sign. Spontaneous alternate contraction and dilation of the pupil, indicative of basilar meningitis.

squirrel (**skwir**·el). A medium-sized rodent of the family Sciuridae; most species are arboreal, but the ground squirrel is one that burrows and does not climb. African, east Asian and North American species may be important reservoirs of field plague. [Gk *skiouros.*]

squirting cucumber (**skwert**·ing **kew**·kum·ber). A perennial vine, *Ecballium elaterium* (family Cucurbitaceae), indigenous to Mediterranean regions. The fruit is like a small cucumber covered with hairs and prickles; when ripe it throws out its juice and seeds with considerable force through an opening at the base. The juice deposits a substance, elaterium, which contains a purgative principle, elaterin. [*squirt* onomat., L *cucumis.*]

Ssabanejew, J. F. 19th century Russian surgeon.

Ssabanejew-Frank operation. Gastrotomy performed by withdrawing a cone of stomach through the chest wall and inserting a tube in it.

stab (stab). 1. A stab wound. 2. To puncture with a sharp narrow-bladed instrument. 3. In bacteriology, the line produced by thrusting a needle into the culture. **Stab culture.** *See* CULTURE. **Stab form.** A neutrophil leucocyte having an unsegmented rod-shaped nucleus. [etym. dub.]

stabile (sta·bile). Stable; constant; fixed. In electrotherapy, applied to electrodes that remain in position. **Heat stabile.** Thermostabile, resistant to heat at certain temperatures. [see foll.]

stability (stab·il·it·e). 1. The power to remain unchanged, displayed by an object, situation or event. 2. Chemically, the ability of a compound to resist decomposition either spontaneous or in the face of conditions tending to bring it about. [L *stabilis* firm.]

stabilizer (sta·bil·i·zer). 1. In a chemical action, any substance employed to maintain an equilibrium or moderate the velocity. 2. Any compound which improves the stability of another compound. 3. A distilling apparatus used for sharp fractionating. 4. An apparatus for automatically maintaining a variable at a desired constant value, e.g. a voltage or current stabilizer. **Froth stabilizer.** Any substance which renders a froth more permanent. [see prec.]

stable (sta·bl). Firmly fixed; not moving; stabile. [L *stabilis* firm.]

staccato (stak·**ah**·to). Denoting a form of speech in which the words and syllables are uttered sharply and jerkily with a brief pause between them. [It. disconnected.]

stachydrine (stak·e·dreen). $C_7H_{13}NO_2$, an alkaloid found in the roots of *Stachys tuberifera* and in many other plants including the chrysanthemum. It is a betaine of the amino acid, proline.

Stacke, Ludwig (b. 1859). Erfurt otologist.

Stacke's operation. One of the early radical operations for the complete drainage of the middle-ear cleft.

stactometer (stak·**tom**·et·er). A glass pipette having a small bore used for measuring fluid in drops. [Gk *staktos* oozing out in drops, *metron* measure.]

Stader, Otto. American veterinary surgeon.

Stader splint. A splint used in the external fixation of fractures. Two pins are driven into the fragments and connected by a bar; the fragments can be drawn into apposition by adjusting a screw on the bar.

Staderini, Rutilio (b. 1869). Florence neurologist.

Staderini's nucleus. The nucleus intercalatus; a small nucleus lying between the hypoglossal and dorsal vagal nuclei.

stadium (sta·de·um). The stage reached in the progress of a disease. **Stadium acmes.** The height of a disease. **Stadium amphiboles.** The stage after a disease has reached its height but before it declines. **Stadium augmenti.** The period of increasing symptoms. **Stadium caloris.** The hot stage of a febrile illness, especially malaria. **Stadium contagii.** The period during which a fever is contagious. **Stadium convalescentiae.** The period of gradual recovery. **Stadium decrementi.** The stage of decreasing symptoms. **Stadium decrustationis.** The stage in an eruptive fever when the eruption is drying and becoming crusted. **Stadium defervescentia.** The defervescent stage, the stage of declining fever. **Stadium desquamationis.** The period of desquamation in the exanthemata. **Stadium eruptionis.** The eruptive stage, the stage during which the rash appears. **Stadium exsiccationis.** Stadium decrustationis (see above). **Stadium floritionis.** The period when the eruption is fully developed. **Stadium fluorescentiae.** The eruptive stage of an exanthematic fever. **Stadium frigoris.** The cold shivering stage of a febrile disease. **Stadium incrementi.** Stadium augmenti (see above). **Stadium incubationis, Stadium invasionis.** The incubation period. **Stadium maniacale.** The period of great excitement and restlessness when delirium is at its height. **Stadium prodromum.** The prodromal stage. **Stadium sudoris.** The sweating stage of a fever. **Stadium suppurationis.** The pustular stage of smallpox. **Stadium ultimum.** The last stage of a febrile disease. [Gk *stadion* race-course.]

Staehelin, Rudolf (b. 1875). Basle clinician.

Staehelin's test. Of myocardial reserve. The increase in heart rate on exercise is greater in subjects with cardiac insufficiency than in normal persons.

Staehli, Jean. 20th century Zürich ophthalmologist.

Staehli's line. Hudson's line.

staff (staf). A grooved sound passed *per urethram* either through or to the face of a urethral stricture, and used as a guide in perineal operations, e.g. external urethrotomy. **Lithotomy staff.** A grooved instrument for passage along the urethra, used in exposing the bladder by the perineal route. [AS *staef.*]

See also: AESCULAPIUS, WHEELHOUSE.

stage (sta·j). 1. The platform of a microscope, on which the object to be examined is mounted. 2. A distinct period or phase in the course or progress of a disease. **Algid stage.** The stage of rigor or chilliness at the commencement of a fever. **Amphibolic stage.** The period between the climax of a disease and its decline. **Asphyxial stage.** The early phase of an attack of cholera, with painful muscular cramps and cyanosis of the face and extremities. **Cold stage.** The initial stage of a typical attack of malaria, with rigors and a feeling of intense cold. **Defervescent stage.** The stage of fever in which the temperature falls to normal, either rapidly by *crisis* or more gradually by *lysis.* **Eruptive stage.** The stage during which a rash is present. **Expulsive stage.** Second stage of labour. *See* STAGES OF LABOUR (below). **Stage of fervescence.** A stage of fever where the temperature is rising. **Hot stage.** The second stage of a typical attack of malaria, with intense flushing of the skin, severe thirst and a high temperature. **Incubative stage.** A confusing term used in 2 senses: prodromal stage (see below) and incubation period. **Stage of invasion.** The incubation period. **Stages of labour.** *First stage:* the time from the commencement of regular contractions of the uterus until full dilatation of the cervix. *Second stage:* from complete dilatation of the cervix to expulsion of the child. *Third stage:* from the birth of the child to delivery of the placenta. *Fourth stage:* following delivery of the placenta, when post-partum haemorrhage may occur. **Stage of latency.** The incubation period. **Mechanical stage.** In microscopy, a device by which the slide can be moved in 2 directions slowly and accurately on the stage of the microscope; it may be built in or attachable. **Microscope stage.** The stage or platform that forms part of a compound microscope and on which the slide or the object to be examined is placed. **Placental stage.** Third stage of labour. *See* STAGES OF LABOUR (above). **Precystic stage.** A stage of the life of an amoeba immediately before it becomes rounded and secretes a cyst wall. **Pre-eruptive stage.** The stage after infection and before the development of the rash. **Premenstrual stage.** The secretory phase of the endometrium. It is more usual to speak of this as a *premenstrual phase.* **Prodromal stage.** The premonitory period during which some manifestations of an impending disease are observed, but not the specific and characteristic symptoms. **Progestation stage.** Premenstrual stage (see above). **Proliferative stage.** The building up of the uterine mucosa which follows menstruation and precedes ovulation. It is more usual to speak of this as a *proliferative phase.* **Pyretogenic stage, Pyrogenic stage.** The stage of onset of fever. **Resting stage.** The phase in the cell cycle which lies between successive cell divisions, when the chromosomes are not visible. **Ring stage.** The stage in which the young trophozoite of the malarial plasmodium appears like a signet ring. **Sauroid stage.** A stage of maturation of the nucleated red cells at which the normoblasts or sauroid cells (resembling the nucleated normal red cells of the reptile) are present [obsolete term]. **Senile leucocyte stage.** The stage of complete maturation with maximal lobulations of the nucleus of the polymorphonuclear leucocyte. **Stepladder stage.** An early stage of typhoid and possibly other fevers, when the temperature curve shows step-like gradations. **Sweating stage.** The sweating stage of a fever, but especially the third and final stage of a typical attack of malaria, with profuse perspiration and a critical fall in the temperature of the body. **Vegetative stage.** Resting stage (see above). **Zoogloea stage.** A stage in the life cycle of certain micro-organisms in which a mass of cells embedded in a jelly-like matrix is formed. [O Fr. *estage.*]

See also: RANKE (K.E.).

staging (sta·jing). **Clinical staging.** Staging in which only clinical factors are taken into account. **Clinico-histological staging.** A more accurate form than clinical staging, but only possible after examination of the operation specimen in which both clinical and histological factors are taken into account. **TNM staging.** A method of clinical staging originally devised for carcinoma of the breast in which numerical values are given for the character of the primary tumour (*T*), the lymph nodes (*N*), and according to the presence or absence of demonstrable metastases (*M*). **Staging of tumours.** A subdivision of malignant tumours according to the degree of their development and spread, with the object of being able to compare like with like in assessing the results of treatment.

stagnation (stag·na·shun). 1. The slowing down or stoppage of the current of a circulating fluid, leading to an accumulation. 2. In dentistry, the accumulation of debris around the teeth, due to lack of oral hygiene or to lack of function of the teeth. [L *stagnare* to become standing water.]

Stahl, Friedrich Karl (b. 1811). Würzburg psychiatrist.

Stahl ears. Two specific deformities of the ears described by Stahl; variations in the relative size of the landmarks, including the helix and antihelix.

Stahl, Georg Ernst (b. 1660). German physiologist.

Stahl's soul or theory. Animism; the theory of control of the body by the perceptive soul, as demonstrated by activity and movement.

Stahr, Hermann (b. 1869). Danzig pathologist.

Stahr's gland. A lymph gland sometimes found beside the facial artery as the latter crosses the mandible.

stain (stane). 1. A discoloration. 2. To impart colour to cells or tissues, and thus facilitate their microscopic examination. 3. In histology and bacteriology, any dyestuff or other chemical substance used to colour tissues, tissue components, bacteria, etc., so as to render them more easily visible, identifiable and in some cases to indicate also their chemical nature. Stains may be used singly or in combination on living or fixed material, with or without special mordanting procedures and differentiations. *Simple stains,* such as methylene blue, may be used to study the morphology of cells. *Differential stains,* such as Gram's stain, are of value in the identification of organisms; they depend upon the principle that if certain dyes are mordanted on to bacteria and an attempt is then made to decolorize the cells, organisms of certain genera will hold the dye whilst those of other genera will be decolorized and can be counterstained with a counterstaining dye. *Acid stains* have a special affinity for the more basic tissue elements, *basic stains* for the more acidic. *Selective stains* are relatively specific in their affinities. *Nuclear* and *protoplasmic stains* have a special affinity for these respective cellular components. A *primary stain,* relatively specific in its action, is often combined with a *counterstain* to colour the background in an unspecific manner. *Metachromatic stains* colour certain tissue components a markedly different colour from that of the staining solution employed. *Negative stains* such as nigrosin or Indian ink stain background so that the bacterial cells show up white. **Claret stain, Port-wine stain.** Port-wine mark; a capillary vascular naevus having the colour of port wine spilled on a table-cloth. The name is loosely applied to capillary naevi which, in fact, may vary in hue from faint pink to livid purple or plum. [see foll.]

stains and staining methods (sta·nz, sta·ning meth·odz). **Absolute-alcohol stain.** Any dye used for staining which is dissolved in absolute alcohol. **Acid stain.** A dye salt whose acid radical combines with the basic groups of tissue components, staining them selectively. **Acid fuchsine.** *See* FUCHSINE. **Alcohol stain.** Any stain employed in alcoholic, as opposed to aqueous, solution. **Alcoholic borax-carmine solution.** A mixture of carmine, borax and alcohol, used in the bulk staining of embryos. **Alum carmine.** A mixture of potassium or ammonium alum and carmine, used in the bulk staining of embryos. **Alum-haematoxylin.** A stain for amoebae and other protozoa in faeces. **Aniline fuchsine.** A solution of acid fuchsine in aniline water, used to stain mitochondria. **Aqueous borax-carmine solution.** An aqueous solution of borax and carmine, used as a nuclear stain in tissue sections. **Basic stain.** A dye salt in which the basic radical combines with the acidic radicals of the tissue components stained by it. **Benzopurpurine.** An acid dye, used to stain cytoplasm dark red as a counterstain to haematoxylin. It has also been used to stain spirochaetes. **Bismarck brown.** *See* BISMARCK BROWN. **Blue mass.** A mixture of Berlin blue and gelatin, used for the injection of blood vessels, lymphatics and other hollow structures. **Borax-carmine solution.** Alcoholic and aqueous borax-carmine solutions (see above). **Carbol gentian violet.** A solution of gentian violet and phenol in alcohol, used for the staining of bacteria in tissue sections. **Carbolfuchsine.** *See* CARBOLFUCHSINE. **Carmine bleu de Lyon.** The combination of carmine as a nuclear stain and bleu de Lyon (spirit blue) as a counterstain. Used for the bulk staining of protozoa, small animals and embryos. **Chloride and copper acetate.** A useful fixative for fresh objects in aqueous media: objects so fixed will stain well with methyl green. Of value in cytological research. **Contrast stain.** A stain of a different colour, used after the primary stain to demonstrate structures left unstained by the latter. **Corrosive sublimate.** Mercuric chloride; a component of many fixing solutions where it is desired to preserve cellular granules, especially in glandular tissues. It also acts as a mordant for many common stains employed in histology. **Differential stain.** *See* STAIN, 2nd def. (above). **Double stain.** Two dyes of contrasting colour used either mixed together or successively. Commonly an acid and a basic stain are combined. **Eau de labarraque.** Hypochlorite of soda; a solution which dissolves chitin, or in dilute solution renders chitin transparent and permeable to staining fluids. **Eosin.** One of a group of pink or red dyes used as general counterstains. Eosin has special affinity for erythrocytes, muscle fibres and the granules of many types of cell. **Fuchsine.** *See* FUCHSINE. **Gelatin carmine.** An injection mass for blood vessels, containing carmine and gelatin. **Gentian violet.** *See* VIOLET, GENTIAN. **Gold-chloride stain.** The use of gold chloride for the staining of nerve-endings and connective-tissue fibres. **Green stain.** An extrinsic green stain found mainly at the necks of the upper anterior teeth. **Haemalum.** *See* HAEMALUM. **Haematoxylin.** *See* HAEMATOXYLIN. **Haematoxylin-eosin method.** The most widely used of all tissue stains. There are numerous modifications. Essentially, sections are first stained with one of the alum-haematoxylin solutions, differentiated with acidulated alcohol, and counterstained with one of the eosins. Nuclei are stained blue, cytoplasm pink. **Haematoxylin-safranine method.** Chrome-fixed sections are first stained with haemotoxylin, and then counterstained with safranine and differentiated in absolute alcohol. A general tissue stain, but particularly valuable for cartilage and mucopolysaccharides. **Indian-ink method.** For spirochaetes. Mix a loopful of the material to be examined with a loopful of Indian ink, spread on a thin film on a slide, dry and examine with 2 mm objective. The spirochaetes stand out white against a black background. **Iron haematoxylin.** 1. Heidenhain's. Tissues are mordanted in iron alum, stained in aqueous haematoxylin and differentiated in iron alum; a general tissue stain. 2. Weigert's. A mixture of alcoholic haematoxylin and ferric chloride; a nuclear stain. **Japanese method.** A method for fixing paraffin sections to glass slides in which a thin layer of glycerin-albumin is first applied to the slide and coagulated by heat before the sections are floated on with water. **Metachromatic stain, Metachromatic staining.** Certain basic dyes, such as toluidine blue, have the property of staining highly polymerized substances such as mucopolysaccharides red, while the other constituents are stained the normal blue colour. A metachromatic stain is one capable of exhibiting this property under suitable conditions. A cell constituent is said to exhibit metachromatic staining or metachromasia, if it stains a different colour from that of the stain employed. The property of metachromasia is made use of in the histochemical detection of mucopolysaccharides. **Methyl green.** *See* GREEN, METHYL. **Methyl-violet solution.** 0.5 per cent aqueous solution of the dye, used in Jensen's modification of Gram's method of staining. **Negative stain.** A staining technique used in light microscopy (see *Indian-ink stain* (above) and *Nigrosin stain* (below)) and electron microscopy whereby the background is stained and organelles, bacteria, viruses, etc. are contrasted as unstained areas. In electron microscopy, solutions of heavy metal salts are used, most commonly potassium phototungstate. *Negative* *contrast* is a synonym. **Neutral stain.** A stain produced by a chemical combination of an acid and a basic stain, and employed in alcoholic solution. Eosin-methylene-blue combinations are frequently so employed. **Nigrosin method.** For cellular morphology. Used to pick out possible diphtheria bacilli from Loeffler slopes. A loopful of the culture is mixed with a loopful of nigrosin and a thin smear made. The organisms are white against a black background. **Nuclear stain.** A stain whose predominant affinity is for the chromatin of the nucleus. Nuclear stains are usually basic dyes, such as haematoxylin or methylene blue. **Orcein.** *See* ORCEIN. **Osmic acid stain.** *See* ACID, OSMIC. **Paracarmine.** *See* PARACARMINE. **Peroxidase stain.** For demonstrating the peroxidase-containing granules which are found in leucocytes of marrow origin but not in those derived from lymphatic tissue. **Picric acid.** Trinitrophenol; a yellow dye much used as a component of fixing solutions, and in staining combinations such as that of Van Gieson. Muscle is stained bright yellow. **Picrofuchsine.** Van Gieson's solution: a solution of acid fuchsine in saturated aqueous picric acid, used as a connective-tissue stain after iron haematoxylin. **Picronigrosin.** *See* PICRONIGROSIN. **Plasmatic stain, Plasmic stain.** A dyestuff which has a special affinity for the cell cytoplasm, such as eosin. **Polychrome methylene blue.** *See* BLUE. **Pre-agonal staining.** Vital staining (see below). **Protoplasmic stain.** A dyestuff with an affinity for cells as opposed to intercellular matrices. **Safranine.** *See* SAFRANINE. **Selective stain.** One having a special affinity for one or more tissue components, leaving others unstained. **Sudan stains.** *See* SUDAN. **Supravital stains.** Substances such as brilliant cresyl blue, janus green B and neutral red, used for staining cells in the living state before they have been killed by fixation, desiccation or lapse of time. Used especially for blood cells. **Tetrachrome stain.** Romanovsky stain. **Thionin.** *See* THIONIN. **Vital stains.** Stains used to colour living tissues by injection of the organism. [O Fr. *desteindre* to dye.]

See also: ALBERT (H.), ALZHEIMER, ANDERSON (J.), BENDA (C.), BEST, BETHE (A.), BIELSCHOWSKY, BIONDI, BIRCH-HIRSCHFIELD (F. V.), BOEHMER, BULLARD, CASTAÑEDA, CZOCOR, DELAFIELD, DONALDSON, DORNER, EHRLICH, ERLICKI, FARRANT, FEULGEN, FLEMMING, FOL, FONTANA (A.), FREUD, FRIEDLAENDER, GIEMSA, GOLGI, GOODPASTURE, GRAHAM (G. S.), GRAM, GRENACHER, GRUENWALD, HAUG, HEIDENHAIN, HELD, HELLER (A. L. G.), HERMANN, HERXHEIMER, HISS, HOFBAUER, HORTEGA, HOYER, JENNER (L. L.), JENSEN (O.), KAISERLING, KALLIUS, KLOTZ, KRONECKER, KUTSCHER, LEISHMAN, LEVADITI, LOEFFLER (F. A. J.), LOEWIT, LORRAIN SMITH, MCCORD, MAGYARY-KOSSA, MALASSEZ, MALL, MALLORY, MANN (G.), MARCHI, MARX, MAY (R.), MAYER (P.), MOELLER (A.), MUELLER (H. F.), MUIR (R.), NEELSEN, NEISSER (M.), NICOLLE, NISSL, NOCHT, PAL, PAPPENHEIM, PIORKOWSKI, RABLE, RAMON Y CAJAL, RANVIER, RIBBERT, RIPART, ROBINOW, ROMANOVSKY, ROUX (P. P. E.), RUZICKA, SAHLI, SATO, SEKIYA, STIEDA (L.), STROEBE, TAENZER, UNNA, VAN GIESON, VERHOEFF, WALDEYER-HARTZ, WEIGERT, WHEAL, WOOD (F. C.), WRIGHT (J. H.), YAMAGIWA, ZIEHL.

staircase (sta·er·kase). Treppe; increase in force of muscular contraction in response to the first few of a series of constant stimuli. The phenomenon is due to the beneficial accumulation of products of contraction, until finally a steady state is reached. [AS *staeger*, O Fr. *casse*.]

stalactite (stal·ak·tite). 1. An icicle-like formation hanging from the roof of a cave. 2. Applied to any similar formation, e.g. a bacterial colony hanging from the surface film of a fluid culture. [Gk *stalaktos* dripped.]

stalagmometer (stal·ag·mom·et·er). An apparatus employed to produce and measure drops of a liquid with a view to calculating therefrom the surface tension of the latter. [Gk *stalagmos* drop, meter.]

stalagmometry (stal·ag·mom·et·re). The measurement of the relative surface tension of liquids by a comparison of the weight of drops formed at the same orifice. [see prec.]

stalk (stawk). A cylindrical tissue bridge. **Abdominal stalk, Body stalk.** The bridge of extra-embryonic mesoderm connecting the posterior end of the embryo to the chorion and acting as the forerunner of the umbilical cord. **Stalk of the epiglottis [petiolus epiglottidis [NA]).** The inferior narrowed extremity of the epiglottis attached to the interior surface of the angle formed by the 2 laminae of the thyroid cartilage just below the thyroid notch. **Optic stalk.** The forerunner of the optic nerve of the embryo. **Pituitary stalk.** Consists of the pathway of nerve fibres that runs from the supra-optic and paraventricular nuclei in the hypothalamus to the posterior lobe of the pituitary. **Yolk stalk.** The connection between the yolk sac and the mid-gut of the embryo. [ME *stalke*.]

Stallard, Hyla Bristow (b. 1901). London ophthalmologist.

Stallard's operation. 1. For epiphora; when the lower canaliculus is damaged: the lacrimal sac having been dissected free, the upper part is brought into the inner canthus through the conjunctiva. The tip of the sac is excised and the edges sutured to the cut edges of conjunctiva. 2. Conjunctivodacryocystostomy.

Stallard's corneoscleral suture. A form of mattress suture placed through the cornea and sclera at the 12 o'clock position, which allows the section in cataract extraction to be made after it has been inserted.

stamen (sta·men). The male organ of flowering plants, consisting of the anther (pollen sac) and filament (stalk). [L thread.]

Stamm, Martin (b. 1847). Fremont, Ohio, surgeon.

Stamm gastrostomy or operation. The insertion of a rubber tube in the stomach, the wall of the organ being angled round the tube like an invertible ink-well.

stammer (stam·er). 1. A disorder of speech in which there is either hesitation before pronunciation of a word or syllable or repetition of the word, or in which certain consonants, such as *l, r, s*, are transposed or mispronounced. 2. To use such a form of speech. [AS *stamerian*.]

stammering (stam·er·ing). **Urinary stammering.** Spasm of the urethral muscles due to psychic causes and rendering urination difficult. [see prec.]

stanch (stahnsh). Staunch; to check or stop the flowing of blood or other fluid from any wound. [ME *stanchen*.]

standard (stan·dard). That which is established as a measure or model, to which others of similar nature should conform. **Standard candle.** *See* CANDLE. **Standard cell.** *See* CELL. **Standard deviation.** *See* DEVIATION. **Standard error.** *See* ERROR. **League of Nations standard.** A standard laid down by a committee of the Health Organization of the League of Nations. This work is now undertaken by the World Health Organization. **Standard million.** A population numbering 1 000 000 which is divided, proportionally, into similar age groups to those present in the population of a certain country, e.g. England and Wales, in some specified year. It is employed in the preparation of Life Tables and in the calculation of standardized death rates. **Standard temperature and pressure.** A pressure of 101 325 Pa (760 mmHg) and temperature 0°C. [O Fr. *estandart*.]

See also: AUB, BENEDICT (F. G.), DU BOIS (E. F.), PIGNET, TALBOT (F. B.).

standardization (stan·dard·i·za'·shun). 1. The preparation of anything to a predetermined standard. 2. The establishment of standards, or standard methods, for future reference, e.g. the evaluation of drugs and preparations by their physiological effect upon living creatures.

standardize (stan·dard·ize). 1. To test or assay by reference to pre-established standards. 2. To lay down standards for the future.

standstill (stand·stil). A cessation or suspension of active function. **Atrial standstill.** Complete cessation of atrial activity, a subsidiary pacemaker, usually junctional (junctional rhythm), taking over and maintaining ventricular activity but without retrograde stimulation of the atria. **Cardiac standstill.** Cardiac arrest; complete cessation of cardiac activity, due to ventricular asystole either as a result of vagal inhibition or ventricular fibrillation. **Expiratory standstill.** The cessation of breathing at the end of expiration. **Inspiratory standstill.** The cessation of breathing at the end of inspiration. **Respiratory standstill.** The cessation of respiratory movements. **Ventricular standstill.** Complete cessation of the action of the ventricles of the heart. [AS *standan, stille.*]

Stange's test. Henderson's test.

Stanley, Edward (b. 1793). London anatomist and surgeon.

Stanley's cervical ligaments. The retinaculae of the femoral neck; groups of fibres reflected along the neck from the capsule of the hip joint.

Stannard, William. 20th century London laboratory technician.

Bunyan-Stannard envelope. A bag of plastic material or waterproof silk for application to a burned extremity. The mouth of the bag, which contains saline fluid, is sealed around the proximal part of the extremity above the burned area, and the part lying within the bag is bathed in the fluid.

Bunyan-Stannard treatment. For burns. The area is enclosed in a Bunyan-Stannard air-tight envelope of oiled silk. Through openings in the covering, irrigation with 5 per cent hypochlorite solution is carried out.

stannate (stan·ate). Any salt derived from stannic acid, H_2SnO_3.

stannic (stan·ik). 1. Having the characteristics of tin or containing it. 2. Chemically, any compound of tin in which the latter is tetravalent. **Stannic chloride.** Occurs as a hydrate, $SnCl_4{\cdot}5H_2O$; also known as *tin oxymuriate* and *butter of tin.* It is used as a mordant in silk dyeing. **Stannic oxide.** Tin dioxide. [L *stannum* tin.]

stanniferous (stan·if·er·us). Yielding or containing tin. [L *stannum* tin, *ferre* to bear.]

stannite (stan·ite). 1. Any salt derived from the hypothetical stannous acid, H_2SnO_2. 2. Tin pyrites, bell-metal ore, SnS_2Cu_2S FeS, a native mineral found in tin-bearing veins. [L *stannum* tin.]

Stannius, Hermann Friedrich (b. 1808). Rostock physiologist.

ligature of Stannius. A ligature tied round the frog's heart so as to interrupt the conduction of impulses from the auricles to the ventricles, so that each of them continues to beat at its own intrinsic and independent rate.

stannous (stan·ous). 1. Having the characteristics of tin or containing it. 2. Chemically, any compound of tin in which the latter is divalent. **Stannous oxide.** Tin oxide. [L *stannum* tin.]

Stanolone (stan·o·lone). BP Commission approved name for 17β-hydroxy-5α-androstan-3-one; an anabolic agent.

Stanozolol (stan·o·zo·lol). BP Commission approved name for 17β-hydroxy-17α-methyl-5α-androstano [3,2-*c*] pyrazole; an anabolic agent.

Stanton, Sir Thomas Ambrose (b. 1875). Kuala Lumpur and London physician.

Stanton's disease. Melioidosis.

stapedectomy (sta·pe·dek·to·me). Excision of the stapes. [stapes, Gk *ektome* a cutting out.]

stapedial (sta·pe·de·al). Relating or belonging to the stapes or the stapedius muscle.

stapediolysis (sta·pe·de·ol'·is·is). Surgical mobilization of a pathologically fixed stapes. [stapedius muscle, Gk *lysein* to loosen.]

stapediotenotomy (sta·pe·de·o·ten·ot'·o·me). Division of the tendon of the stapedius muscle. [stapedius muscle, Gk *tenon* tendon, *temnein* to cut.]

stapediovestibular (sta·pe·de·o·ves·tib'·ew·lar). Relating or belonging to the stapes and the vestibule.

stapedius muscle [musculus stapedius (NA)] (sta·pe·de·us musl). A small muscle which arises from the walls of a cavity in the pyramid on the posterior wall of the tympanic cavity; its tendon passes anteriorly to an insertion into the neck of the stapes. It acts reflexly with the tensor tympani in damping excessive vibration, thereby protecting the internal ear.

stapedius muscle, nerve to the [nervus stapedius (NA)] A branch of the facial nerve, given off in the posterior wall of the middle ear.

stapes [NA] (sta·peez). One of the chain of 3 movable ossicles in the tympanic cavity which has a resemblance to a stirrup. Its head [caput stapedis (NA)] articulates with the lentiform nodule of the incus and the base [basis stapedis (NA)], which resembles the footplate of the stirrup, is fitted to the margin of the fenestra vestibuli. [L *stapes* stirrup.]

staphisagria (staf·is·ag·re·ah). The ripe seeds of *Delphinium staphisagria* Linn., louse-wort or stavesacre (family Ranunculaceae). They contain several alkaloids and are very toxic; their only use is for killing lice in the hair. [Gk *staphis* raisin, *agrios* wild.]

staphylagra, staphylagrum (staf·il·ag·rah, staf·il·ag·rum). A forceps for grasping the uvula. [Gk *staphyle* uvula, *agra* a catching.]

staphyle (staf·il·e). The uvula. [Gk.]

staphylectomy (staf·il·ek·to·me). Surgical removal of the uvula. [Gk *staphyle* uvula, *ektome* a cutting out.]

staphyleus (staf·il·e·us). Staphyline.

staphylin (staf·il·in). A lytic substance produced by certain strains of staphylococci.

staphyline (staf·il·ine). 1. Having resemblance to a bunch of grapes. 2. Relating or belonging to the uvula; uvular. [Gk *staphyle* bunch of grapes, uvula.]

staphylinopharyngeus (staf·il·i·no·far·in'·je·us). The palatopharyngeus muscle. [Gk *staphyle* uvula, pharynx.]

staphylion (staf·il·e·on). 1. In craniometry, the point on the posterior border of the hard palate at the median line. 2. The uvula. 3. A nipple or teat. [Gk *staphyle* uvula, bunch of grapes.]

staphylitis (staf·il·i·tis). Uvulitis. [Gk *staphyle* uvula, *-itis* inflammation.]

staphylo-angina (staf·il·o·an·ji'·nah). A mild form of inflammation of the throat characterized by a pseudomembranous deposit which is caused by infection with staphylococci. [staphylococcus, angina.]

staphylocide (staf·il·o·side). Staphylococcicide.

staphylocoagulase (staf·il·o·ko·ag'·ew·laze). A substance produced by pathogenic strains of staphylococci, which has the property of coagulating human or rabbit plasma. [staphylococcus, coagulase.]

staphylococcaemia (staf·il·o·kox·e'·me·ah). The presence of staphylococci in the blood. [staphylococcus, Gk *haima* blood.]

staphylococcal, staphylococcic (staf·il·o·kok'·al, staf·il·o·kox'·ik). Relating to or caused by staphylococci.

staphylococcicide (staf·il·o·kox'·is·ide). Any agent capable of destroying staphylococci. [staphylococcus, L *caedere* to kill.]

staphylococcus (staf·il·o·kok'·us). A bacterial genus in the family Micrococcaceae. They are Gram-positive cocci growing in grape-like clusters. Many species produce pigment. The pathogenic species *Staphylococcus aureus* (or *pyogenes*) is distinguished by its production of coagulase and various toxins; it usually forms a golden pigment *(S. aureus)* but white or cream-coloured variants occur. It is the common causal organism of boils, carbuncles, abscesses and of some deep-seated septic infections, e.g. osteomyelitis. The common saprophytic staphylococcus, *S. epidermidis,* a skin commensal, usually forms white *(albus)* colonies, but lemon *(citreus),* yellow *(flavus)* and red-coloured *(roseus)* variants occur. [Gk *staphyle* bunch of grapes, coccus.]

staphyloderma (staf·il·o·der'·mah). A staphylococcal lesion of the skin. **Bullous staphyloderma.** A bullous eruption caused by staphylococci. [staphylococcus, Gk *derma* skin.]

staphylodermatitis (staf·il·o·der·mat·i'·tis). Inflammation affecting the skin and due to infection with staphylococci. [staphylococcus, dermatitis.]

staphylodialysis (staf·il·o·di·al'·is·is). Relaxed and elongated condition of the uvula. [Gk *staphyle* uvula, dialysis.]

staphylohaematoma (staf·il·o·he·mat·o'·mah). An effusion of blood into the uvula. [Gk *staphyle* uvula, haematoma.]

staphylohaemia (staf·il·o·he'·me·ah). The presence of staphylococci in the blood. [staphylococcus, Gk *haima* blood.]

staphylolysin (staf·il·**ol**·is·in). A haemolytic substance produced by staphylococci. [staphylococci, lysin.]

staphyloma (staf·il·**o**·mah). Protrusion of the contents of the eye through an area where the sclera or cornea is thin or deficient. Scleral protrusions are lined by uveal pigment, look black and have a fanciful resemblance to a grape, whence the name. **Staphyloma aequatoriale, Staphyloma aequatoris.** One or more protrusions in the equatorial region of the eyeball. **Annular staphyloma.** Applied to the area of atrophy in high myopia when it surrounds the disc and is not limited only to the temporal side. **Anterior staphyloma.** Staphyloma in which the protrusion is in the region of the corneal margin. **Ciliary staphyloma.** Staphyloma in the region of the ciliary body, the ciliary vessels emerging in front of the protrusion. **Staphyloma corneae, Corneal staphyloma.** That due to thinning or rupture of the cornea and frequently lined by iris tissue. **Staphyloma corneae racemosum.** Bulging of the cornea with the iris prolapsed through small holes in it. **Equatorial staphyloma.** Staphyloma aequatoriale (see above). **Intercalary staphyloma.** Staphyloma in which the protrusion is limited to the narrow zone corresponding with the angle of the anterior chamber, the ciliary vessels emerging behind it. **Posterior staphyloma.** Protrusion of the sclera at the posterior pole of the eye, occurring in high myopia. **Staphyloma posticum.** 1. Ammon's: protrusion of the sclera below the posterior pole of the eye, in association with a coloboma of the choroid. 2. Scarpa's: thinning and bulging of the sclera, usually at the outer side of the optic disc, occurring in a highly myopic eye. **Projecting staphyloma.** A tautological term applied to staphyloma of the cornea. **Retinal staphyloma.** A localized protrusion forward of the retina. **Scleral staphyloma.** Staphyloma not involving the cornea. **Uveal staphyloma.** Hernia of part of the uveal tract through the ruptured eyeball. [Gk *staphyle* bunch of grapes, *-oma* tumour.]

See also: AMMON, SCARPA.

staphylomatous (staf·il·**o**·mat·us). Pertaining to or characterized by staphyloma, or having resemblance to staphyloma.

staphyloncus (staf·il·**ong**·kus). An enlargement or tumour of the uvula. [Gk *staphyle* uvula, *ogkos* swelling.]

staphylo-oedema (**staf**·il·o·e·**de**'·mah). An oedematous condition of the uvula. [Gk *staphyle* uvula, oedema.]

staphylophage (**staf**·il·o·faje). A bacteriophage which parasitizes staphylococci. Different staphylophages are type specific, though 2 or more phages may infect the same bacterial type. Use of this is made in phage-typing strains of staphylococci. [staphylococcus, Gk *phagein* to eat.]

staphylopharyngorrhaphy (**staf**·il·o·far·in·**gor**'·af·e). A term used to cover a number of different types of operation on the uvula and soft palate, including a form of repair in cases of cleft palate, and also the modification of this technique which has been used for the lengthening of a short soft palate. [Gk *staphyle* uvula, pharynx, Gk *rhaphe* suture.]

staphyloplasty (**staf**·il·o·plas·te). Reparative surgery of the uvula or soft palate. [Gk *staphyle* uvula, *plassein* to mould.]

staphyloptosia, staphyloptosis (**staf**·il·op·**to**'·ze·ah, **staf**·il·op·**to**'·sis). A relaxed and elongated condition of the uvula. [Gk *staphyle* uvula, *ptosis* fall.]

staphylorrhaphy (staf·il·**or**·af·e). Suture of a cleft palate. [Gk *staphyle* uvula, *rhaphe* suture.]

staphyloschisis (staf·il·**os**·kis·is). A cleft state of the uvula or of the uvula and soft palate. [Gk *staphyle* uvula, *schisis* division.]

staphylostreptococcia (**staf**·il·o·strep·to·**kok**'·e·ah). A combined staphylococcal and streptococcal infection.

staphylostreptoderma (**staf**·il·o·strep·to·**der**'·mah). Any eczematous skin eruption which lacks the characteristics of impetigo or ecthyma, and is due to a mixed staphylococcal and streptococcal infection. [staphylococcus, streptococcus, Gk *derma* skin.]

staphylotome (**staf**·il·o·tome). A surgical instrument used in staphylotomy.

staphylotomy (staf·il·**ot**·o·me). 1. Incision of the uvula. 2. Amputation of the uvula. 3. Excision of a staphyloma. [Gk *staphyle* uvula, *temnein* to cut.]

staphylotoxin (**staf**·il·o·**tox**'·in). A toxin produced in staphylococcal cultures.

staphylotropic (**staf**·il·o·**trop**'·ik). Having attraction for staphylococcal bacteria. [staphylococcus, Gk *trope* turn.]

staphylygroma (**staf**·il·e·**gro**'·mah). Staphylo-oedema. [Gk *staphyle* uvula, *hygros* moist, *-oma* tumour.]

staphysina (staf·is·**i**·nah). A substance yielded by the seeds of *Delphinium staphisagria* Linn.

star (star). Any radiate figure similar in appearance to the conventional representation of a star. **Blazing star.** Helonias. **Daughter star.** One of the asters of a dividing cell. **Star figure at the macula.** Small spots of white exudate radiating from the macula in the form of a star, sometimes incomplete and shaped like a fan, found usually in severe retinopathies due to nephritis, malignant hypertension or toxaemia of pregnancy. **Mother star.** An undivided aster. **Polar star.** One of the asters of a dividing cell which has reached its definitive position near one extremity of the cell. [AS *steorra*.]

See also: VERHEYEN, WINSLOW.

star anise (star **an**·is). Illicium; the ripe fruit of *Illicium verum* Hook. f. (family Magnoliaceae), a small tree indigenous to China. From it is distilled a volatile oil, anise oil, which contains from 80 to 90 per cent of anethole. [star, anise.]

starch (starch). 1. $(C_6H_{10}O_5)_n$, a carbohydrate occurring widely in plant tissues as the main form of carbohydrate reserve. It is present in the form of granules of varying size and shape which, together with certain other physical features, are characteristic of the plant, and starches from different sources may thus be identified microscopically. Primary cleavage of the starch molecule yields 2 fractions termed *amylase* and *amylopectin*, the former being water-soluble and non-viscous whilst the latter is insoluble in cold water but gelatinizes and forms a paste with hot water. Further hydrolysis of starch leads to the successive production of dextrins, maltose and, finally, glucose. The structure of starch is generally regarded as consisting of a long chain of glucose residues in pyranose form bonded by α-glucoside linkages. 2. Amylum, a starch obtained from the grains of wheat, maize or rice, or from potatoes. It is a fine white powder or friable masses, insoluble in cold water and in organic solvents, but forming a translucent viscous solution on boiling with water. It is used as a constituent of dusting powders (BP 1973) and of the protective applications, starch glycerin. Mucilage of starch is the basis of some enemata. **Animal starch.** Glycogen. **Corn starch.** Starch obtained from maize. **Starch gel.** A medium for the electrophoretic techniques used in the identification of the protein blood groups of human serum called *haptoglobins*. **Iodized starch.** Starch containing 5 per cent of iodine; it is a suggested treatment for poisoning by hydrogen sulphide. **Maize starch.** Corn starch (see above). **Soluble starch.** Starch treated with hydrochloric acid which renders it readily soluble in hot water. **Sterilizable Maize Starch BP 1973.** Maize starch treated by chemical and physical means so that it does not gelatinize on exposure to moisture or steam sterilization. It is used as a lubricant for surgeons' gloves and as a vehicle for medicated dusting powders. [AS *stearc* strong.]

stare (sta·er). **Postbasic stare.** A characteristic sign in postbasic meningitis of infants, in which the eyeballs are turned downwards and the upper lids are retracted. [AS *starian*.]

Stargardt, Karl Bruno (b. 1875). German ophthalmologist.

Stargardt's disease. A familial form of retinal degeneration involving the macula, occurring at puberty and unassociated with mental symptoms. It was first described by Rayner Batten.

Starling, Ernest Henry (b. 1866). English physiologist.

Starling's law. The force of contraction of the heart is dependent on the length of the muscle just before contraction. It results from variable amount of overlap of the actin and myosin filaments.

starter (**star**·ter). The initial inoculum of a pure culture of a micro-organism used for fermentation or similar industrial processes. [ME *sterte*.]

Startin, James (b. 1851). British dermatologist.

Startin's solution. Magnesium sulphate, ferrous sulphate, ginger syrup, with dilute sulphuric acid and water.

starvation (star·va·shun). The condition induced by continuous lack of sufficient food. **Salt starvation.** Deprivation of salts leading to serious symptoms. Simple deficiency causes renal failure with nitrogenous retention in the blood and development of alkalaemia. Muscular cramps, a feeling of great fatigue, dyspnoea and mental apathy follow. [ME *sterven* to die.]

Stas, Jean Servais (b. 1813). Belgian chemist.

Stas-Otto method. A method used in toxicological analysis for the isolation of non-volatile organic poisons from viscera and other biological material. The material is thoroughly minced, acidified with tartaric acid and extracted several times with alcohol. The alcohol is removed from the extract and the residue dissolved in dilute acid. The acid solution is extracted with a non-miscible solvent, usually chloroform, which removes acidic and neutral substances, and is then made alkaline and re-extracted to remove basic substances. The latter include the alkaloids with the exception of morphine. Morphine is finally removed by adding an equal volume of alcohol to the alkaline aqueous solution and extracting with chloroform.

stasibasiphobia (sta·se·ba·se·**fo'**·be·ah). Insensate belief on the part of anyone that he can neither stand nor walk, and abnormal dread of attempting to do either. [Gk *stasis* standing, *basis* stepping, phobia.]

stasidynic (sta·sid·in·ik). Active in an acid or an alkaline medium. [Gk *stasis* standing, *dynamis* power.]

stasimetry (sta·**sim**·et·re). The determination of the consistency of soft bodies. [Gk *stasis* standing, *metron* measure.]

stasiphobia (sta·se·**fo**·be·ah). A delusion on the part of anyone that he cannot stand upright, and morbid fear of attempting to do so. [Gk *stasis* standing, phobia.]

stasis (sta·sis). The slowing down or stoppage of the flowing of any fluid. **Diffusion stasis.** Circulatory stasis with diffusion of lymph. **Foot stasis.** Trench foot. *See* FOOT. **Ileal stasis.** Delay in the passage of the contents of the ileum. **Intestinal stasis.** Delay in the passage of faeces through the bowel. **Papillary stasis.** A little-used term for *papilloedema.* **Pressure stasis.** Obstruction to circulation by pressure. [Gk standing.]

state (state). A condition. **Anelectrotonic state.** The state of diminished excitability and conductivity occurring at or near the anode when a constant current is passed through a nerve. **Anxiety state, Anxious state.** A mental reaction characterized essentially by the dominant presence of an anxious state of mind; the latter term indicates a less specific mental reaction, possibly a temporary phase. **Carrier state.** The state in which the subject is acting as host to some potentially pathogenic micro-organism or worm, is capable of passing on the infection, but is not suffering from the disease at the time. **Catarrhal state.** Catarrhal infection of a mucous membrane. **Catelectrotonic state.** The state of increased excitability occurring at or near the cathode when a constant current is passed through a nerve. **Central excitatory state.** A state of supernormal excitability of nerve cells which follows the application of a subthreshold stimulus. **Central inhibitory state.** A state which is antagonistic to the central excitatory state, and may be due either to the application of an inhibitory volley to the central neurones concerned or to the withdrawal of the normal subliminal bombardment which maintains the excitatory state. **Colloidal state.** The condition in which a substance is dispersed in a solvent in particles of ultramicroscopic size. **Compulsive state.** A mental disorder characterized by the repetition of an action or actions, with a mental compulsion to act in this way. There is a recognition that the action is unreasonable, but a feeling of tension arises if the compulsion is resisted. **Constitutional psychopathic state.** A condition characterized by disorder of conduct of an antisocial type. **Correlated state.** Dynamic equilibrium. *See* EQUILIBRIUM. **Depressive state.** Any mental state in which depression is dominant. **Dream state.** A state of impaired consciousness in which the environment is perceived as if in a dream; if persistent it is often hysterical. **Dreamy state.** An expression often used in lay terminology to describe the condition of a person who is deep in thought and oblivious to his surroundings. **Epileptic state.** Status epilepticus. **Fatigue state.** Neurasthenia. **Ground state.** The state of lowest energy of a system. **Hypnogogic state.** The state of consciousness midway between sleep and wakefulness, noted during the onset of sleep; the identical state which occurs during the process of awakening is called a *hypnopompic state.* **Hypnoidal state, Hypnodic state.** A rudimentary splitting of consciousness in hysteria. **Hypnoleptic state.** A state characterized by narcolepsy. **Hypnopompic state.** The state of partial consciousness which occurs on arousal from sleep, before the individual is fully awake. **Isomeric states.** States of a nucleus having different energies and observable half-lives. **Local excitatory state.** A state of supernormal excitability following the application of a subthreshold stimulus. **Marble state.** Status marmoratus. **Metastable states.** In a nucleus, isomeric states with energies above that of the ground state. **Obsessive ruminative state.** A mental state characterized by the recurrent emergence in consciousness of a thought or idea, against the will of the subject, and with his recognition of its apparent meaninglessness. **Postepileptic state.** The stuporous state which commonly follows an epileptic fit. **Pre-blackwater state.** A recognizable clinical state, preceding an attack of blackwater fever, in which there is a sallow complexion, an icteric tinge of the conjunctivae, a large congested liver, furred tongue and enlarged spleen, in a subject who has had several attacks of malignant tertian malaria during the preceding year or so. **Refractory state.** A state of inexcitability following excitation of either a muscle or nerve. **Resting state.** A state in which there is no activity, e.g. the cystic stage of amoebae. **Seborrhoeic state.** A state in which there is excessive discharge of sebum from the sebaceous glands, especially those on the face; the subject develops a greasy complexion. **Steady state.** Dynamic equilibrium. *See* EQUILIBRIUM. **Subscurvy state.** A state in which there is insufficient intake of vitamin C, but in which the symptoms are latent. If such a person is wounded or operated upon, the deficiency may become apparent by the slow healing of the wounds. **Twilight state.** An impaired state of consciousness in which a patient may perform detailed purposive acts and may have no memory of them afterwards; this may occur as a complication of the hypnopompic state (see above) physiologically, but is also seen in disease. **Typhoid state.** The syndrome associated with a severe toxaemia, sometimes seen in typhus, typhoid and other continued fevers: muscular weakness, stupor, muttering delirium, rapid feeble pulse, dry fissured tongue, sordes of lips, incontinence of urine and faeces. The prostration may advance to death or may gradually mend. **Ultragaseous state.** A term used formerly to describe the luminous radiation which appears during electrical discharges in gases at very low pressures. **Varicose state.** A number of varices regarded as a group. [L *status* condition.]

See also: BARBER.

static (**stat**·ik). Stationary; at rest, as opposed to dynamic. [Gk *statikos* causing to stand.]

Statice (**stat**·is·e). A genus of plumbagineous plants. **Statice limonium.** Sea lavender, marsh rosemary, inkroot; a maritime plant found in salt marshes. The root contains 12 per cent of tannic acid and is a powerful astringent. [Gk *statike.*]

statics (**stat**·ix). The study of matter in equilibrium under forces which produce no motion. [Gk *statikos* causing to stand.]

station (**sta**·shun). Position when standing; stance. **Station of the fetus.** A term indicating the degree of descent of the fetus in the pelvic cavity. [L *stare* to stand.]

See also: ROMBERG.

statistics (stat·**is**·tix). 1. The systematic collection of numerical facts and data for use as examples, or for making general deductions on any subject. 2. The science of compiling, classifying and tabulating such data, and expressing the results in a mathematical or graphical form. **Medical statistics.** That branch of statistics concerned with mathematical facts and data relating to health, preventive medicine and disease. **Vital statistics.** That branch of statistics which chiefly deals with births, deaths, human populations and the incidence of disease. The main uses of vital statistics are the ascertainment of conditions appertaining to the health and welfare of communities over a period of years, to determine the probable causes of such conditions and, consequently, to assist in the study of the prevention of mortality and disease. [L *status* condition.]

statocyst (**stat**·o·sist). The utricle or saccule of the membranous labyrinth. [Obsolete term.] [Gk *statos* standing, *kystis* bladder.]

statokinetic (**stat**·o·kin·**et**'·ik). Relating to the balance and posture of the body in movement. [Gk *statos* standing, *kinesis* movement.]

statolith (**stat**·o·lith). Otolith; minute crystals of calcium carbonate adhering to the hair cells of the maculae of the utricle and saccule in the inner ear; it subserves the function of orientation to gravity and comparable forces. [Gk *statos* standing, *lithos* stone.]

statometer (stat·**om**·et·er). An instrument for measuring proptosis. [Gk *statos* standing, meter.]

statosphere (**stat**·o·sfeer). Centrosome. [Gk *statos* standing, *sphaira* sphere.]

statural (**stat**·ewr·al). Relating or belonging to stature.

stature (**stat**·ewr). 1. The natural height of anyone standing upright. 2. A person's standing or importance in society. [L *statura* height of a man.]

status (**sta**·tus). State or condition. **Status anginosus.** A condition in which ischaemic cardiac pain is induced by the slightest stimulus, e.g. emotion, cold, digestion or bodily environment, and may be constantly present. It occurs in acute coronary thrombosis and cardiac infarction, in acute coronary artery insufficiency, in prolonged paroxysmal tachycardia and in aortic valvular disease. Although it may be induced by any condition which reduces the coronary artery flow, there is invariably serious underlying heart disease, and the prognosis is generally poor. **Status arthriticus.** The nervous and other manifestations which are believed to precede an attack of acute gout in certain persons. **Status asthmaticus.** A severe and continuous attack of asthma in which there is marked dyspnoea and finally exhaustion and collapse. **Status calcifames.** Calcium deficiency. **Status catarrhalis.** The catarrhal state; catarrhal infection of a mucous membrane. **Status choleraicus.** The stage of collapse in cholera, with cold clammy skin, feeble pulse and suppression of urine. **Status choreicus.** A severe and prolonged attack of chorea. **Status convulsivus.** Status epilepticus (see below). **Status cribralis, Status cribrosus.** A sieve-like condition of the brain (mainly microscopic) due to widespread dilation of the perivascular spaces; the appearances may result mainly from post-mortem change. **Status criticus.** Repeated and severe tabetic crises. **Status dysmyelinisatus.** 1. A pathological condition of the basal ganglia in children, in which iron pigment accumulates in the globus pallidus and substantia nigra. It gives rise to mental defect and progressive rigidity of the extremities, and is known as *Hallevorden-Spatz disease.* 2. Demyelination involving the hypothalamic nuclei, the dentate nucleus, the ventral nucleus of the thalamus and the globus pallidus. **Status dysraphicus.** Delayed closure of the sutures of the skull. **Status epilepticus.** Repeated and prolonged epileptic seizures without recovery of consciousness between attacks. **Status hemicranicus.** Very frequent and severe attacks of migraine. **Status lacunaris, Status lacunosis.** The pathological condition of the brain resulting from multiple small cortical infarcts. **Status lymphaticus.** The condition of hyperplasia of lymphatic tissue, at one time thought to be a common cause of sudden death in infants. **Status marmoratus.** The marble state or *état marbré* of the corpus striatum which has a "marbled" appearance on section; histologically, ganglion cells may be replaced by strands of myelin. Clinically, it may give rise to a variety of syndromes characterized by rigidity of limbs and involuntary movements. Changes of this type have been discovered in cases with the clinical picture of Little's disease, Vogt's disease and torsion spasm. **Status nervosus.** Typhoid state. *See* STATE. **Status parathyreoprivus.** Hypoparathyroidism. [Obsolete term.] **Petit mal status.** A form of epilepsy characterized by prolonged disturbance of consciousness accompanied by electroencephalographic discharges of the type seen in petit mal. **Status praesens.** The present condition. **Status raptus.** A state of ecstasy. **Status spongiosus.** Multiple vacuoles in the cerebral cortex; a state resembling status lacunaris (see above) and usually due to multiple infarcts. **Status thymicolymphaticus.** Status lymphaticus (see above). **Status thymicus.** Persistent enlargement of the thymus gland, generally with lymphatic hyperplasia. **Status typhosis.** Typhoid state. *See* STATE. **Status verminosus.** A verminous condition; lousiness. **Status vertiginosus.** Repeated attacks of vertigo, often of labyrinthine origin; or a single prolonged episode of vertigo. [L.]

statuvolence (stat·**ew**·vol·ens). A self-induced state of hypnotism. [L *status* condition, *volens* willing.]

statuvolent, statuvolic (stat·**ew**·vol·ent, stat·ew·**vol**·ik). Characterized by statuvolence, or having the ability to enter such a state.

Staub, Hans (b. 1890). Basle pharmacologist.

Staub-Traugott effect. The observation that if a normal person has been given a dose of glucose by mouth, a similar dose an hour later is not followed by a corresponding rise in the blood sugar level.

staunch (stawnsh). To check or stop the flowing of blood or other fluid from a wound. [ME *stanchen.*]

stavesacre (**sta**·vza·ker). Staphisagria. [corruption of *staphisagria.*]

staxis (**stax**·is). 1. Slow haemorrhage occurring in drops. 2. Drop-by-drop flow of liquid. [Gk a dropping.]

steal (steel). The diversion of blood flow from its normal territory of distribution through collateral vesicles to supply another territory which is ischaemic because of obstruction of its normal artery of supply. **Subclavian steal.** The steal phenomenon occurring in the presence of subclavian arterial obstruction with diversion of blood flow from the brain stem down the vertebral artery; the clinical manifestations are episodes of brain-stem ischaemia occurring when the arm is exercised. [AS *stelan* take away.]

steapsin (ste·**ap**·sin). Lipase. [Gk *stear* fat, *pepsis* digestion.]

stearate (**ste**·ar·ate). Any salt or ester of stearic acid.

steariform (ste·**ar**·e·form). Resembling hard fat or stearin. [Gk *stear* fat, form.]

stearin (**ste**·ar·in). Tristearin, $C_3H_5(OOCC_{17}H_{35})_3$. A solid compound occurring in tallow and other natural fats, and produced by the hydrogenation of liquid fats and oils. [see foll.]

stearine (**ste**·ar·een). Name given to a mixture of fatty acids, predominantly stearic acid, obtained by the hydrolysis with superheated steam of various fats. It is a white, hard, semi-crystalline mass, insoluble in water, soluble in alcohol, ether, chloroform and in other fats. It is used alone, or partly neutralized, in the preparation of vanishing creams and ointment bases. [Gk *stear* fat.]

stearodermia (ste·ar·o·**der**'·me·ah). A disordered state of the skin in which the sebaceous glands are involved. [Gk *stear* fat, *derma* skin.]

stearol (**ste**·ar·ol). Stearyl alcohol, $C_{17}H_{35}CH_2OH$. The alcohol corresponding to stearic acid.

stearoptene (ste·ar·**op**·teen). That constituent of an essential oil which is solid or crystalline, such as camphor. [Gk *stear* fat, *ptenos* volatile.]

stearoyl (**ste**·ar·o·il). The monovalent acyl radical $C_{17}H_{35}CO$-, derived from stearic acid. [Gk *stear* fat, *hyle* matter.]

stearrhoea (ste·ar·e·ah). Steatorrhoea.

stearyl (**ste**·ar·il). The monovalent radical $CH_3(CH_2)_{17}$, derived from stearyl alcohol.

steatadenoma (ste·at·ad·en·**o**'·mah). Sebaceous adenoma. *See* ADENOMA. [Gk *stear* fat, adenoma.]

steatitis (ste·at·i·tis). Inflammation of fatty tissue. [Gk *stear* fat, *-itis* inflammation.]

steatocele (ste·**at**·o·seel). A fatty tumour in the scrotum. [Gk *stear* fat, *kele* hernia.]

steatocryptosis (**ste**·at·o·krip·**to**'·sis). 1. Irregularity of function of the sebaceous glands. 2. Stearodermia. [Gk *stear* fat, *kryptos* hidden, *-osis* condition.]

steatocystoma multiplex (**ste**·at·o·sist·**o**'·mah **mul**·tip·lex). Steatomatosis. [Gk *stear* fat, cystoma, L manifold.]

steatogenous (ste·at·**oj**·en·us). 1. Causing steatosis. 2. Giving rise to disease of the sebaceous glands. 3. Producing fat. [Gk *stear* fat, *genein* to produce.]

steatoid (**ste**·at·oid). Resembling fat. [Gk *stear* fat, *eidos* form.]

steatolysis (ste·at·**ol**·is·is). The hydrolysis of fat. [Gk *stear* fat, *lysis* a loosing.]

steatolytic (**ste**·at·o·**lit**'·ik). Relating or belonging to steatolysis.

steatoma (ste·at·**o**·mah). 1. Lipoma. 2. A sebaceous cyst. [Gk *stear* fat, *-oma* tumour.]

See also: MUELLER.

steatomatosis (**ste**·at·o·mat·**o**'·sis). A morbid condition characterized by the presence of multiple sebaceous cysts. [steatoma, Gk *-osis* condition.]

steatopyga, steatopygia (**ste**·at·o·**pi**'·gah, **ste**·at·o·**pij**'·e·ah). An excessive accretion of fat on the buttocks affecting *inter alia* the women of certain African races; sometimes referred to as *Hottentot bottom.* [Gk *stear* fat, *pyge* buttocks.]

steatopygous (ste·at·**op**·ig·us). Having an excessive accumulation of fat on the buttocks. [see prec.]

steatorrhoea (**ste**·at·or·**e**'·ah). 1. A condition in which an excess of split fat appears in the stools, as in coeliac disease. 2. Seborrhoea; over-secretion of sebum. **Steatorrhoea flavescens.** Seborrhoea in which the sebum develops a yellow coloration. **Idiopathic steatorrhoea.** Coeliac disease in adults; steatorrhoea which is not recognized until adolescence or adult life, although usually beginning in childhood. **Steatorrhoea nigricans.** Chromhidrosis of the melanhidrotic type. **Steatorrhoea simplex.** Seborrhoea. [Gk *stear* fat, *rhoia* flow.]

steatosis (ste·at·**o**·sis). 1. Fatty degeneration. 2. Excess of fat to an abnormal degree in any place. **Steatosis cardiaca.** Cardiomyolipoşis; fatty degeneration of the musculature of the heart. **Cholesterin steatosis.** Deposition of cholesterol as amorphous esters or crystals within reticulo-endothelial cells throughout the body, or as a localized mass. [Gk *stear* fat, *-osis* condition.]

stechiology (stek·e·**ol**·o·je). Stoichiology.

stechiometry (stek·e·**om**·et·re). Stoichiometry.

steel (steel). Name applied to varieties of iron containing different proportions of carbon (from 0.5 to 1.5 per cent) in the form of iron carbide, Fe_3C (cementite). It is manufactured by removing part of the carbon from cast iron (pig iron), and certain other metals (e.g. manganese, chromium, nickel) may be added to confer desired qualities, which are further dependent on the heat treatment the steel has received. [AS *style.*]

Steell, Graham (b. 1851). Manchester physician.

Steell's murmur, Graham Steell murmur. A soft, high-pitched early diastolic murmur heard in the 2nd intercostal space to the left of the sternum and arising from the pulmonary valve. It indicates valvular regurgitation in patients with severe mitral stenosis which has led to right ventricular and pulmonary hypertension.

Stefan, Josef (b. 1835). Austrian physicist.

Stefan's constant. σ, the ratio of the energy radiated per unit area per second by a black body to the fourth power of the absolute temperature of the body.

stegnosis (steg·**no**·sis). 1. Stenosis. 2. The arrest of any excretion or secretion. 3. Constipation. [Gk stoppage.]

stegnotic (steg·**not**·ik). 1. Pertaining to stegnosis. 2. Astringent. 3. An astringent agent that checks secretion or excretion. [see prec.]

Stegomyia (steg·o·**mi**·e·ah). A sub-genus of the mosquito genus, Aëdes. *Aëdes (Stegomyia) aegypti* is the vector of yellow fever, and widely distributed in the tropics and subtropics. *A. (S.) albopictus* and *A. (S.) scutellaris* are house mosquitoes in south-east Asia and vectors of dengue. **Stegomyia calopus.** *Aëdes aegypti.* **Stegomyia fasciata.** *Aëdes aegypti.* [Gk *stegos* roof, *myia* fly.]

Stehle, Raymond Louis (b. 1888). Canadian pharmacologist.

Stehle's method. Urea in urine is determined by measurement of the nitrogen evolved upon treatment with hypobromite.

Stein, Irving F. (b. 1887). American gynaecologist.

Stein-Leventhal syndrome. A syndrome affecting women and characterized by obesity, hirsutism, infertility, oligomenorrhoea or amenorrhoea, and infrequent ovulation. Typically, but not always, both ovaries are slightly enlarged with a pale smooth surface and contain multiple subcapsular cysts derived from unruptured follicles. Hormone biosynthesis by the ovaries is disturbed.

Stein, Stanislav Aleksandr Fyodorovich von (b. 1855). Russian otologist.

Stein's test. In labyrinthine disorders. The patient falls over when requested to stand on one leg with the eyes closed.

Stein's antigen. An antigen used in the serological diagnosis of relapsing fever.

Steinach, Eugen (b. 1861). Vienna surgeon.

Steinach method or operation. Ligation of the vas deferens to produce atrophy of the spermatogenic apparatus of the testis and consequently, it was thought, proliferation of the interstitial tissue and increased production of testosterone.

Steinbrocker, Otto (b. 1898). New York rheumatologist.

Steinbrocker criteria. Criteria for functional classification of patients suffering from rheumatoid arthritis.

Steindler, Arthur (b. 1878). Iowa City orthopaedic surgeon.

Steindler's operation. For pes cavus. Correction of pes cavus by separation of the short sole muscles from their origin from the calcaneum.

Steinert, Hans. 20th century Leipzig physician.

Steinert disease. Dystrophia myotonica.

Steinmann, Fritz (b. 1872). Berne surgeon.

Steinmann's extension. Traction applied to a limb by weight attached to a nail or pin transfixing a bone, usually the os calcis or the tibia.

Steinmann's nail or pin. A pin to which a weight can be attached by way of a stirrup for extension on a bone.

Stellaria (stel·a·re·ah). A genus of caryophyllaceous plants; the chickweeds. **Stellaria media.** Chickweed; the dried herb is occasionally used as a demulcent. [L *stella* star.]

stellate (**stel**·ate). 1. Shaped like the traditional representation of a star; radiating or branching from a centre. 2. Arranged as stars are in a group. **Stellate ganglion.** *See* GANGLION. [L *stella* star.]

stellate veins [venulae stellatae (NA)]. A convergence on the surface of the kidney of subcapsular vessels; they form an interlobar vein.

stellectomy (stel·**ek**·to·me). The operation of excising the stellate ganglion. [stellate ganglion, Gk *ektome* a cutting out.]

stellite (**stel**·ite). A hard, non-corroding alloy, containing usually cobalt (50 per cent), chromium (30 per cent), carbon (2½ per cent) and tungsten (17½ per cent). It is employed in the manufacture of surgical instruments and high-speed tools.

stellulae winslowii (**stel**·ew·le win·**slo**·e·i). Stars of Winslow; venous capillary whorls found in the choriocapillaries of the choroidal coat of the eye. [dim. of L *stella* star.]

Stellwag von Carion, Carl (b. 1823). Vienna ophthalmologist.

Stellwag's operation. For symblepharon. Removal of the adherent conjunctiva and grafting of the bare area with conjunctiva from the other eye or with mucosa from the mouth or vagina.

Stellwag's sign. Infrequency of blinking in thyrotoxic exophthalmos.

gelatinous trachoma of Stellwag. A late stage of mixed trachoma when the conjunctiva becomes gelatinous.

stem (stem). 1. The supporting stalk of a leaf or a plant. 2. To check or arrest bleeding, e.g. by finger pressure. **Stem cells.** The cells in the genital ridge which give rise to the primordial ova present at birth. [AS *stemm.*]

stenagma (sten·**ag**·mah). A sigh. [Gk groan.]

stenagmus (sten·**ag**·mus). The act of sighing. [Gk *stenagmos* a groaning.]

Stenger, P.

Stenger's test. For simulated unilateral deafness. The patient's eyes are covered. Two tuning-forks of the same pitch and vibrating at the same intensity are placed at a short distance from each ear. A patient genuinely suffering from unilateral deafness will state that he can hear some sound. A malingerer, not knowing that both ears are under test, frequently denies that he can hear anything.

Wells–Stenger test. A hearing test for distinguishing real from simulated unilateral deafness: preliminary tests are carried out to indicate the relative distances at which a vibrating tuning-fork can be appreciated in each ear. A tuning-fork inserted into a length of tube connected to the supposedly deaf ear is then vibrated, and the distance at which the original tuning-fork can now be appreciated from the good ear is then recorded. If this is perceived at the same distance as before, the opposite ear is probably truly deaf. If it has to be approximated more closely to the good ear, a diagnosis of malingering can be supported.

stenion (**sten**·e·on). In craniometry, a point in the temporal fossa marking the termination of the shortest transverse diameter in that area. [Gk *stenos* narrow.]

steno. *See* STENSEN (NIELS).

stenobregmate, stenobregmatic (sten·o·**breg**·mate, **sten**·o·breg·**mat'**·ik). Of a skull, being narrowed in the upper and anterior part. [Gk *stenos* narrow, bregma.]

stenocephalia (**sten**·o·kef·**a'**·le·ah). Stenocephaly.

stenocephalous (sten·o·**kef**·al·us). Having a markedly narrow head. [see foll.]

stenocephaly (sten·o·**kef**·al·e). Abnormal narrowness of the head; craniosynostosis. [Gk *stenos* narrow, *kephale* head.]

stenochoria (sten·o·**kor**·e·ah). Stenosis; contraction. **Stenochoria saccilacrimalis.** Contraction of the lacrimal sac; usually applied to stenosis of the nasolacrimal duct. [Gk *stenos* narrow, *choros* space.]

stenocoriasis (**sten**·o·kor·i'·as·is). A contracted condition of the pupil. [Gk *stenos* narrow, *kore* pupil.]

stenocrotaphia, stenocrotaphy (**sten**·o·kro·**taf'**·e·ah, sten·o·**krot'**·af·e). The condition in which the skull in the temporal region is abnormally narrow, as in the case of a stenobregmatic skull. [Gk *stenos* narrow, *krotaphos* side of forehead.]

stenodont (**sten**·o·dont). A person who has abnormally narrow teeth. [Gk *stenos* narrow, *odous* tooth.]

stenomycteria (**sten**·o·mik·**teer'**·e·ah). Stenosis of the nostrils. [Gk *stenos* narrow, *mykter* nostril.]

stenopaeic, stenopaic (sten·o·**pe**·ik, sten·o·**pa**·ik). Stenopeic.

stenopeic (sten·o·**pe**·ik). Denoting optical devices which have a narrow opening or slit, as those used in measurement of astigmatism or as a certain type of snow-goggles. [Gk *stenos* narrow, *ope* opening.]

stenosal (sten·**o**·sal). 1. Relating or belonging to stenosis. 2. Due to stenosis.

stenosed (sten·**o**·zd). Narrowed; constricted; affected with stenosis. [see foll.]

stenosis (sten·**o**·sis). The constriction or narrowing of an orifice or the lumen of a hollow or tubular organ. **Aortic stenosis.** Any form of narrowing of the left ventricular outflow. The different forms are *aortic valvar (valvular) stenosis, aortic subvalvar stenosis, aortic supravalvar stenosis,* which are all fixed anatomical lesions, and *functional aortic stenosis.* **Aortic subvalvar (subvalvular) stenosis.** Narrowing of the left ventricular outflow below the aortic valve. This may be a developmental abnormality with a fibrous ring or diaphragm immediately below the valve cusps, or a functional obstruction secondary to muscle hypertrophy (*functional aortic stenosis,* see below). Fixed subvalvar aortic stenosis is usually associated with some aortic incompetence. **Aortic supravalvar (supravalvular) stenosis.** A rare condition in which there is a constriction of the aorta immediately above the aortic valve. It occurs familially and sporadically. Usually it is found as part of a syndrome which is characterized by atypical facies with redundancy of the upper lip, mental retardation, arterial stenoses elsewhere and sometimes idiopathic hypercalcaemia in infancy. **Aortic valvar (valvular) stenosis.** Narrowing of the aortic valve occurring as a developmental abnormality, as a result of rheumatic carditis or because of calcific degenerative changes in a congenitally abnormal, but not obstructive, valve (e.g. a bicuspid valve). Some incompetence is commonly associated with the 2 latter varieties. **Aqueduct stenosis.** Gross narrowing to almost complete obliteration of the aqueduct of the mid-brain, leading to hydrocephalus of the lateral and third ventricles. **Cardiac stenosis.** Obstruction to the flow of blood through any of the heart chambers which is not due to valvular narrowing. It may occur when there is a pedunculated or sessile organized thrombosis in the left atrium in cases of mitral stenosis (pseudomyxoma, ball thrombus) or more rarely, in the case of intracardiac neoplasms, such as myxomata or invasion of the heart by secondary spread from mediastinal neoplasms. **Cicatricial stenosis.** Obstruction caused by the contraction of scar tissue. **Fixed aortic stenosis.** Narrowing of the left ventricular outflow tract by a fixed anatomical lesion. **Functional aortic stenosis.** Hypertrophic (obstructive) cardiomyopathy is almost always the cause but, rarely, severe left ventricular hypertrophy, secondary to hypertension or fixed aortic stenosis, can cause systolic obstruction between the apex of the ventricle and the outflow tract. **Granulation stenosis.** Obstruction by the formation of granulation tissue. **Idiopathic hypertrophic subaortic stenosis.** Hypertrophic cardiomyopathy. *See* CARDIOMYOPATHY. **Infundibular stenosis.** Pulmonary infundibular stenosis (see below). **Mitral stenosis.** Narrowing of the orifice of the mitral valve, which in almost every case is the result of rheumatic endocarditis, the very rare exceptions being of congenital origin. The valve leaflets are fused together, and the papillary muscles and chordae tendineae thickened and shortened. Often calcification is present, and there may be some degree of mitral incompetence. **Postdiphtheritic stenosis.** Constriction or narrowing of the larynx or trachea following diphtheria. **Post-tracheotomy stenosis.** Stenosis after tracheotomy. **Pulmonary stenosis.** Any form of narrowing of the right ventricular outflow. The different forms are *pulmonary valvar (valvular) stenosis, pulmonary infundibular stenosis* and, rarely, *supravalvar (supravalvular) stenosis.* Very rarely the outflow tract may be compressed by mediastinal expanding lesions. **Pulmonary arterial branch stenosis.** Narrowing of 1 or more branches of the pulmonary artery. Most commonly this occurs with Fallot's tetralogy but also with aortic supravalvar stenosis and as an isolated abnormality. It is probably a congenital developmental abnormality. **Pulmonary infundibular stenosis.** Narrowing of the infundibulum of the right ventricle. This occurs most commonly as a part of Fallot's tetralogy but is also found in other more complex cardiac abnormalities and, uncommonly, it occurs as an isolated abnormality. Usually it is a congenital developmental abnormality but it has been shown to develop after birth in the presence of a ventricular septal defect. As a rule the stenosis is fixed but often there is a significant muscular (functional) element. **Pulmonary supravalvar (supravalvular) stenosis.** Narrowing of the pulmonary artery. In a form comparable to aortic supravalvar stenosis with the narrowing immediately above the valve, it is a very rare condition, but more distal stenoses at the bifurcation of the pulmonary artery or of 1 or more of its branches *(pulmonary arterial branch stenosis)* are more common. **Pulmonary valvar (valvular) stenosis.** Narrowing of the pulmonary valve which almost always occurs as a developmental abnormality. Rare cases of rheumatic pulmonary stenosis have been described. Most commonly it occurs with a ventricular septal defect, as part of *Fallot's tetralogy;* less commonly the ventricular septum is intact but in these cases an atrial septal defect or a patent foramen ovale is often present. **Pyloric stenosis.** Narrowing of the pyloric opening; it may be *congenital* (hypertrophic) due to thickened muscle in infants under 6 weeks old or *cicatricial,* usually due to ulcer or cancer. **Subaortic stenosis.** Aortic subvalvar stenosis (see above). **Tricuspid stenosis.** Narrowing of the orifice of the tricuspid valve as the result of rheumatic endocarditis, or very rarely, congenital maldevelopment. The valve leaflets are fused and some regurgitation is usually present. [Gk *stenos* narrow, *-osis* condition.]

See also: DITTRICH.

stenostegnosis (sten·o·steg·no′·sis). Stenostenosis.

stenostenosis (sten·o·sten·o′·sis). Stenosis of the parotid (Stensen's) duct. [Niels *Stensen,* stenosis.]

stenostomatous (sten·o·**sto**·mat·us). Having an abnormally narrow mouth. [see foll.]

stenostomia, stenostomy (sten·o·**sto**·me·ah, sten·**os**·to·me). Abnormal narrowness of the mouth. [Gk *stenos* narrow, *stoma* mouth.]

stenothorax (sten·o·**thor**·ax). A short, narrow thorax or chest. [Gk *stenos* narrow, thorax.]

stenotic (sten·**ot**·ik). Relating or belonging to stenosis; narrowed, strictured. [Gk *stenos* narrow.]

Stensen, Niels (Nicolaus Steno) (b. 1638). Danish physician and theologian.

Stensen's (Steno) canal or foramen. The lateral incisive foramen. *See* FORAMEN.

Stensen's duct. The parotid duct. *See* DUCT.

Stensen's experiment. The demonstration that when the abdominal aorta is compressed the blood supply to the lower part of the spinal cord is greatly reduced, so that the nerves arising in that part no longer conduct and localized paralyses result.

Stensen's plexus. A venous network on the surface of the parotid duct.

Stent's composition. A proprietary form of composition used in dentistry and in skin grafting.

stentorophonous (sten·tor·**of**·on·us). Loud-voiced. [*Stentor,* a loud-voiced herald in Homer's *Iliad,* Gk *phone* voice.]

step (step). **Nasal step.** Rönne's nasal step. [AS *staepe.*]

See also: RÖNNE.

stephanial, stephanic (stef·**an**·e·al, stef·**an**·ik). Relating or belonging to the stephanion.

stephanion (stef·**an**·e·on). In craniometry, the point of intersection of the temporal line and the coronal suture. [Gk *stephanos* crown.]

Stephens, John William Watson (b. 1865). Liverpool physician.

Stephens' dots or spots. Dots in erythrocytes found only in association with heavy infections of the subtertian malaria parasite *(Plasmodium falciparum).* With Romanovsky stains they take on a reddish tinge in the protoplasm of the corpuscle.

Kanthack and Stephens serum agar. *See* AGAR, SERUM.

steppage (**step**·ij). Steppage gait. *See* GAIT. [AS *staepe.*]

stercobilin (ster·ko·**bi**·lin). $C_{33}H_{46}O_6N_4$, a dark brown pigment formed in faeces upon exposure to air as a result of the oxidation of stercobilinogen.

stercobilinogen (ster·ko·bi·**lin**′·o·jen). A reduction product of bilirubin in the intestinal canal. [L *stercus* dung, bilinogen.]

stercolith (**ster**·ko·lith). A faecal concretion. [L *stercus* dung, Gk *lithos* stone.]

stercoporphyrin (ster·ko·**por**·fir·in). $C_{36}H_{38}N_4O_8$, a porphyrin pigment which is a by-product in normal haemopoiesis. It is excreted largely by the liver in bile and thence in normal faeces and urine. Increased excretion occurs in porphyria and porphyrinuria, and has been reported in various other disorders. [L *stercus* dung, porphyrin.]

stercoraceous (ster·kor·**a**·shus). Faecal; containing faeces. [see foll.]

stercoral, stercorary (**ster**·kor·al, **ster**·kor·ar·e). Faecal. [L *stercus* dung.]

stercorin, stercorol (**ster**·kor·in, **ster**·kor·ol). $C_{27}H_{47}OH$, a sterol occurring in faeces. It is fully saturated and is apparently formed by hydrogenation of cholesterol in the intestine, probably by the action of bacteria. [see prec.]

stercorolith (**ster**·**kol**·o·lith). A hard mass of faeces in the bowel. [L *stercus* dung, Gk *lithos* stone.]

stercoroma (ster·kor·o·mah). An accumulation of hardened faeces which on inspection and palpation gives the impression that there is a tumour in the rectum. [L *stercus* dung, Gk *-oma* tumour.]

stercorous (**ster**·kor·us). Faecal. [L *stercus* dung.]

Sterculia (ster·kew·le·ah). A genus of trees and shrubs, chiefly tropical, of the family Sterculiaceae. Sterculia (BPC 1968) is the gum obtained from *Sterculia urens* and possibly other species, and is used as a substitute for tragacanth. [L *Sterculius,* the Roman god of manuring.]

stereo-agnosis (steer·e·o·ag·no′·sis). Inability to recognize objects by the feel of them or by touching them. Lack of the stereognostic sense. [Gk *stereos* solid, *a, gnosis* knowledge.]

stereo-anaesthesia (steer·e·o·an·es·the′·ze·ah). The condition in which ability to recognize the shape of objects by touch has been lost. [Gk *stereos* solid, anaesthesia.]

stereo-arthrolysis (steer·e·o·ar·throl′·is·is). The surgical procedure of making a new joint capable of movement in a case of bony ankylosis. [Gk *stereos* solid, arthrolysis.]

stereo-auscultation (steer·e·o·aw·skul·ta′·shun). A method of auscultation in which 2 phonendoscopes are used at different positions; 1 tube of each instrument is inserted into an ear whilst the other tube is closed with the fingers. [Gk *stereos* solid, auscultation.]

stereocampimeter (steer·e·o·kam·pim′·et·er). An instrument like a stereoscope designed by Lloyd for plotting out uni-ocular scotomata; the eye not being examined maintains fixation. [Gk *stereos* solid, L *campus* field, meter.]

stereochemical (steer·e·o·kem′·ik·al). Relating to stereochemistry.

stereochemistry (steer·e·o·kem′·is·tre). The study of the structure of chemical compounds from a three-dimensional point of view; the spatial disposition of the atoms in a molecule. [Gk *stereos* solid, chemistry.]

stereocilium (steer·e·o·sil′·e·um). One of a group of non-motile processes which project from the free end of certain epithelial cells, e.g. those of the epididymis. [Gk *stereos* solid, L *cilium* eyelash.]

stereocognosy (steer·e·o·kog′·no·se). Stereognosis.

stereo-encephalotome (steer·e·o·en·kef′·al·o·tome). An instrument used for placing cerebral lesions by stereotaxic surgery. [Gk *stereos* solid, encephalon, Gk *temnein* to cut.]

stereo-encephalotomy (steer·e·o·en·kef·al·ot′·o·me). The production of lesions in the brain by stereotaxic surgery. [Gk *stereos* solid, encephalon, Gk *temnein* to cut.]

stereofluoroscopy (steer·e·o·floo·or·os′·ko·pe). Stereoscopic fluoroscopy. [Gk *stereos* solid, fluoroscopy.]

stereognosis (steer·e·og·no′·sis). Ability to recognize the shape and character of an object by means of touch. [Gk *stereos* solid, *gnosis* knowledge.]

stereognostic (steer·e·og·nos′·tik). Relating to stereognosis.

stereogram, stereograph (steer·e·o·gram, steer·e·o·graf). A stereoscopic radiograph.

stereo-isomer (steer·e·o·i′·so·mer). A particular form of isomer arising out of stereochemical considerations, in which 2 compounds may possess the same groups of atoms linked in the same way but arranged differently in space so that one can in no way be superimposed upon the other. Such a stereo-isomer is often characterized by optical activity and the possession of 1 or more asymmetric atoms. [Gk *stereos* solid, isomer.]

stereo-isomeric (steer·e·o·i·so·mer′·ik). Relating or belonging to stereo-isomerism.

stereo-isomerism (steer·e·o·i·som′·er·izm). Chemical isomerism due to the dissimilarity in spatial arrangement of the same groups of atoms in the molecule. This phenomenon produces stereo-isomers which may be mirror-images of one another, or otherwise incapable of being superimposed, and may have the property of optical activity associated with an asymmetric atom. [Gk *stereos* solid, isomerism.]

stereometer (steer·e·**om**·et·er). An apparatus for measuring the volumes of small solids; it is also used in the determination of the specific gravities of powders, or of substances that would dissolve if the water method were used. [see foll.]

stereometry (steer·e·**om**·et·re). The measuring of the volume of a solid body, or of the cavity within a solid body. [Gk *stereos* solid, meter.]

stereo-ophthalmoscope (steer·e·o·of·**thal**′·mo·skope). A special ophthalmoscope with 2 eyepieces, by which the fundus is examined stereoscopically.

stereo-orthopter (steer·e·o·or·**thop**′·ter). A form of reflecting stereoscope used in orthoptic training.

stereophantoscope (steer·e·o·**fan**′·to·skope). A stereoscope in which the pictures are replaced by rotating discs. [Gk *stereos* solid, *phanein* to appear, *skopein* to view.]

stereophorometer (steer·e·o·for·**om**′·et·er). A modified stereoscope fitted with prisms and used for measurement of the angle of squint. [Gk *stereos* solid, *pherein* to bear, meter.]

stereophotomicrograph (steer·e·o·fo·to·**mi**′·kro·graf). A stereoscopic photomicrograph.

stereopsis (steer·e·**op**·sis). The condition of having stereoscopic vision. [Gk *stereos* solid, *opsis* vision.]

stereoradiography (steer·e·o·ra·de·**og**′·raf·e). The taking of a stereoscopic x-ray photograph. [Gk *stereos* solid, radiography.]

stereoroentgenometry (steer·e·o·runt·yen·**om**′·et·re). The measurement of a solid radio-opaque body, obtained from its stereoscopic radiographs. [Gk *stereos* solid, roentgenometry.]

stereoscope (steer·e·o·skope). An instrument used in stereoscopy.

stereoscopic (steer·e·o·**skop**′·ik). Giving the impression of depth and solidity: applied to the effect produced by combining 2 two-dimensional pictures in an optical device and presenting them to the eyes as a three-dimensional view. [see foll.]

stereoscopy (steer·e·**os**·ko·pe). A radiographic technique by which a pair of radiographs may be viewed with stereoscopic vision. Two separate exposures are made with different positions of the tube focus 6.5 cm (2.5 in) apart. The films are placed in a stereoscope and viewed at 43–50 cm (17–20 in) distance. For viewing at greater distances, the tube shaft must be correspondingly increased. [Gk *stereos* solid, *skopein* to view.]

stereoskiagraphy (steer·e·o·ski·**ag**′·raf·e). Stereoradiography. [Gk *stereos* solid, skiagraphy.]

stereostroboscope (steer·e·o·**stro**′·bo·skope). An apparatus used in physiology for investigating the perception of points moving in 3 dimensions. [Gk *stereos* solid, *strobos* a whirling, *skopein* to view.]

stereotaxis (steer·e·o·**tax**′·is). 1. A method of locating structures in the brain during life. 2. Stereotropism. [Gk *stereos* solid, *taxis* arrangement.]

stereotropic (steer·e·o·**trop**′·ik). Pertaining to or characterized by stereotropism.

stereotropism (steer·e·o·**trop**′·izm). In biology, the tendency shown by small organisms to move or grow in a particular direction under stimulus of mechanical contact with a larger object. **Negative stereotropism.** The tendency to grow or move away from the stimulating object. **Positive stereotropism.** The tendency to grow or move towards the stimulating object. [Gk *stereos* solid, *trope* a turning.]

stereotypy (steer·e·o·**ti**′·pe). Unvarying repetition, as of speech or movement, or unvarying persistence, as of attitude. **Verbal stereotypy.** Monophasia. [Gk *stereos* solid, *typos* impression.]

stereovectorcardiography (steer·e·o·**vek**·tor·kar·de·**og**′·raf·e). Three-dimensional vectorcardiography. [Gk *stereos* solid, vectorcardiography.]

Sterges' carditis. Combined endocarditis and pericarditis.

steric, sterical (steer·ik, steer·ik·al). Due to the positioning of atoms in three-dimensional space. **Steric effect.** Any chemical phenomenon ascribable to the disposition of atoms in space. **Steric hindrance.** The slowing or prevention of the normal reactions expected of a certain chemical group due to the spatial disposition of other groups around it in the molecule. [Gk *stereos* solid.]

sterid (steer·id). Steroid.

sterigma (ster·ig·mah). A specialized spore-bearing cell, usually flask-shaped, from the narrow tubular neck of which spores arise in chains by a process of successive apical growth and abstriction cutting off the terminal segment. [Gk support.]

sterigmatocystis, sterigmocystis (ster·**ig**·mat·o·**sist**′·is, ster·**ig**·mo·**sist**′·is). Those species of the Aspergillaceae which produce both primary and secondary sterigmata, formerly set apart in this genus but now usually included in the genus *Aspergillus*. [sterigma, Gk *kystis* bag.]

sterilamp (ster·e·lamp). A low-power electric bulb emitting rays capable of sterilizing solutions. [Obsolete term.] [sterile, lamp.]

sterile (ster·ile). 1. Infertile; incapable of producing offspring. 2. Free from all living micro-organisms. [see foll.]

sterility (ster·il·it·e). The condition of being infertile by reason of failure to conceive or reproduce the species. **Facultative sterility.** Sterility produced voluntarily. **Idiopathic sterility.** Sterility of unknown causation. **One-child sterility.** Sterility occurring in a woman who has previously borne 1 child. **Relative sterility.** Sterility in which there is no absolute bar to the occurrence of pregnancy but where 1 or several factors operate to depress fertility below the threshold of conception. **Revocable sterility.** Sterility caused by a contraceptive measure which can be discontinued. [L *sterilis* barren.]

sterilization (ster·il·i·**za**′·shun). 1. The production of sterility. 2. The complete removal of living micro-organisms from materials. This can be achieved by physical or chemical methods, e.g. by any physical agent, such as heat (dry or moist), ultraviolet light, x-rays, supersonic waves, or by mechanical methods such as filtration through materials which hold back micro-organisms, shaking with glass beads, grinding, etc. or by antiseptic solutions. **Electronic sterilization.** Sterilization by high-velocity electrons. **Eugenic sterilization.** Sterilization undertaken for eugenic reasons. **Fractional sterilization, Intermittent sterilization.** The intermittent exposure of materials to moist heat, under conditions which allow any spores of micro-organisms present to germinate between treatments. First described by Tyndall in 1877. [see foll.]

sterilize (ster·il·ize). 1. To render sterile or aseptic. 2. To castrate. 3. To render powerless to reproduce. [L *sterilis* barren.]

sterilizer (ster·il·i·zer). An apparatus used in sterilization. **Steam sterilizer.** An apparatus that renders objects aseptic by exposing them to the action of live steam raised to atmospheric pressure.

Sterle's sign. Increased pulsation in the cardiac region in intrathoracic tumours.

Stern, Heinrich (b. 1862). New York physician.

Stern's position. A position in which a body is supine with the head lowered over the end of a table.

sternal (ster·nal). Relating or belonging to the sternum.

sternalgia (ster·**nal**·je·ah). 1. Pain affecting the sternum. 2. Angina pectoris. [sternum, Gk *algos* pain.]

sternalis muscle [musculus sternalis (NA)] (ster·**na**·lis musl). A superficial muscle only occasionally present on the front of the chest; it arises below from the sheath of the rectus abdominis muscle and ends above in fascia, or by blending with the sternal head of the sternocleidomastoid muscle. It may be a vestige of the panniculus carnosus. [Gk *sternon* chest.]

Sternberg, Karl (b. 1872). Vienna pathologist.

Sternberg's giant cell, Sternberg-Reed cell. The giant cell of Hodgkin's disease.

Sternberg's disease. 1. Leucosarcoma. 2. Tuberculous pseudoleukaemia.

Sternberg's sign. Tenderness of the shoulder muscles on palpation in cases of pleurisy.

Paltauf-Sternberg disease. Lymphadenoma.

Sternberg, William H. (b. 1913). New Orleans pathologist.

Albright-McCune-Sternberg syndrome. A name not in general use. *See* ALBRIGHT'S SYNDROME.

sternebra (ster·ne·bra) (pl. *sternebrae*). Any one of the several parts of the sternum before fusion takes place. [sternum, vertebra.]

sternochondroscapularis muscle (ster·no·**kon**·dro·skap·ew·**la'**·ris musl). A muscle, occasionally present, which arises from the sternum and the 1st costal cartilage and runs to the scapula. It is probably part of the infrahyoid muscular sheet from which the infrahyoid muscles are developed. [Gk *sternon* chest, *chondros* cartilage, scapula.]

sternoclavicular (ster·no·klav·**ik'**·ew·lar). Belonging to the sternum and the clavicle.

sternoclavicularis muscle (ster·no·klav·ik·ew·**la'**·ris musl). A slip of muscle occasionally present. It arises from the upper border of the manubrium sterni and passes laterally behind the sternocleidomastoid muscle to be inserted in the upper surface of the clavicle. It is part of the infrahyoid muscular sheet from which the sternohyoid, sternothyroid and omohyoid muscles are developed.

sternocleidal (ster·no·**kli**·dal). Sternoclavicular. [sternum, Gk *kleis* key.]

sternocleidomastoid muscle [musculus sternocleidomastoideus (NA)] (ster·no·**kli**·do·**mas'**·toid musl). A muscle of the neck attached to the mastoid process and superior nuchal line, and below by 2 heads to the manubrium sterni and to the medial end of the clavicle. [sternum, Gk *kleis* key, mastoid.]

sternocleidomastoid vein [vena sternocleidomastoidea (NA)] (ster·no·**kli**·do·**mas'**·toid vane). A tributary from the muscle to the superior thyroid vein. It accompanies the sternomastoid branch of the occipital artery.

sternocoracoid (ster·no·**kor**·ak·oid). Relating or belonging to the sternum and the coracoid process.

sternocostal (ster·no·**kos**·tal). Relating or belonging to the sternum and the ribs. [sternum, L *costa* rib.]

sternocostalis muscle (ster·no·kos·**ta'**·lis musl). The anterior part of the transversus thoracis muscle running from the sternum to the 2nd to 6th costal cartilages. It lies between the internal mammary artery and the pleura.

sternodymia (ster·no·**dim**·e·ah). In teratism, the condition in which the 2 bodies of a twin monster are fused at the anterior chest wall or the sternum. [sternum, Gk *didymos* twin.]

sternodymus (ster·**nod**·im·us). A twin monster the 2 bodies of which are united at the sternum. [see prec.]

sternodynia (ster·no·**din**·e·ah). Pain in the sternum. [sternum, Gk *odyne* pain.]

sternofascialis muscle (ster·no·fash·e·**a'**·lis musl). A muscle occasionally present, arising from the manubrium sterni behind the sternocleidomastoid muscle and ending in the fascia of the omohyoid muscle; it belongs to the infrahyoid group of muscles. [sternum, fascia.]

sternoglossal (ster·no·**glos**·al). Relating or belonging to the sternum and the tongue. [sternum, Gk *glossa* tongue.]

sternogoniometer (ster·no·go·ne·**om'**·et·er). An instrument used to ascertain the degree of the sternal angle. [sternum, Gk *gonia* angle, *metron* measure.]

sternohyoid (ster·no·**hi**·oid). Relating or belonging to the sternum and the hyoid bone.

sternohyoid muscle [musculus sternohyoideus (NA)]. A strap-like muscle attached above to the body of the hyoid bone and below to the posterior surface of the manubrium sterni, the sternoclavicular joint and the adjacent clavicle.

sternoid (ster·noid). Having resemblance to the sternum. [sternum, Gk *eidos* form.]

sternomastoid (ster·no·**mas**·toid). Belonging to the sternum and the mastoid process. **Sternomastoid muscle.** Sternocleidomastoid muscle.

sterno-omphalodymia (ster·no·om·fal·o·**dim'**·e·ah). In teratism, the type of twin monster in which there is fusion at the sternal and umbilical regions. [sternum, Gk *omphalos* navel, *didymos* twin.]

sternopagia (ster·no·**pa**·je·ah). Sternodymia. [sternum, Gk *pagos* fixed.]

sternopagus (ster·**nop**·ag·us). Sternodymus. [see prec.]

sternopericardiac, sternopericardial (ster·no·per·e·**kar'**·de·ak, ster·no·per·e·**kar'**·de·al). Relating or belonging to the sternum and the pericardium.

sternoscapular (ster·no·**skap**·ew·lar). Relating or belonging to the sternum and the scapula.

sternothyroid (ster·no·**thi**·roid). Relating or belonging to the sternum and the thyroid gland or thyroid cartilage.

sternothyroid muscle [musculus sternothyroideus (NA)]. A short muscle from the manubrium sterni to the thyroid cartilage.

sternotomy (ster·**not**·o·me). The surgical procedure of making an incision into or through the sternum. [sternum, Gk *temnein* to cut.]

sternotracheal (ster·no·trak·e'·al). Relating or belonging to the sternum and the trachea.

sternotrypesis (ster·no·tri·**pe'**·sis). The operation of perforating or trephining the sternum. [sternum, Gk *trypaein* to pierce through.]

sternoxiphoid (ster·no·**zif**·oid). Pertaining to the sternum and the xiphoid process.

sternum [NA] (ster·num). Breast bone; a long flat bone forming the anterior wall of the thorax in the middle line, articulating with the clavicles above and with the other 7 pairs of costal cartilages marginally. It consists of 3 parts, the manubrium, the body and the xiphoid process, and is composed of anterior and posterior dense bony plates enclosing a medullary cavity which contains red bone marrow. [Gk *sternon* chest.]

angle [angulus sterni (NA)]. The angle between the manubrium and the body of the sternum; the angle of Louis.

body [corpus sterni]. The middle and largest piece of the sternum.

sternum splitter (ster·num **split**·er). *See* SAUERBRUCH. [sternum, Middle D *splitten.*]

sternutatio convulsiva (ster·new·**ta**·she·o kon·vul·**si**·vah). Sneezing which occurs in paroxysms. [L convulsive sneezing.]

sternutation (ster·new·**ta**·shun). Sneezing. [see foll.]

sternutator (ster·new·**ta**·tor). A substance which causes sneezing. [L *sternutare* to sneeze.]

sternutatory (ster·new·**ta**·tor·e). 1. Causing sneezing. 2. A substance that causes sneezing. **Sternutatory absence.** A complex absence characterized by sneezing. [see prec.]

sternzellen (shtern·tzel·en). Star-shaped cells, especially the Kupffer cells of the hepatic sinusoids. [G star cell.]

sterochemistry (steer·o·**kem**·is·tre). Stereochemistry.

steroid (steer·oid). A group of organic compounds related to cholesterol and containing a cyclopentenophenanthrene ring system. Derivatives of the latter include the important sex hormones, cardiac glycosides, bile acids, cortical hormones, saponins, toad poisons and the D vitamins. [sterol, Gk *eidos* form.]

steroidogenesis (steer·oid·o·**jen'**·es·is). The process of steroid synthesis from acetyl CoA. [Gk *stereos* solid, *genesis* origin.]

sterol (steer·ol). Any alcohol of the cholane series, characterized by the cyclopentenophenanthrene skeleton. They may be saturated or unsaturated, and comprise the *zoosterols* of animal origin (e.g. cholesterol) and the *phytosterols* and *zymosterols* of plants. They are waxy, insoluble substances entirely distinct from the lipide alcohols, and of considerable biological importance. [Gk *stereos* solid, alcohol.]

sterolytic (steer·o·**lit**·ik). Capable of dissolving a sterol. [sterol, Gk *lysis* a loosing.]

sterone (steer·one). General name given to steroids which contain 1 or more keto-groups, =CO, e.g. androsterone, testosterone.

stertor (ster·tor). Snoring or noisy breathing associated with mucoid obstruction of the air passages during deep sleep or in coma. **Hen-cluck stertor.** A breathing sound which resembles the clucking of a hen and occurs in cases of postpharyngeal abscess. [L *stertere* to snore.]

stertorous (ster·tor·us). 1. Pertaining to stertor. 2. Characterized by deep snoring or stertor, as in apoplexy.

stetharteritis (steth·ar·ter·**i'**·tis). Inflammation affecting the arteries of the thorax. [Gk *stethos* chest, arteritis.]

stethendoscope (steth·en·do·skope). A fluoroscopic apparatus for examination of the chest by x-ray. [Gk *stethos* chest, *endon* within, *skopein* to view.]

stethophone (**steth**·o·fone). 1. Stethoscope. 2. An instrument by which several persons can listen to stethoscopic sounds at the same time. [Gk *stethos* chest, *phone* sound.]

stethophonometer (**steth**·o·fo·**nom**′·et·er). An instrument by which the intensity of stethoscopic sounds can be measured. It contains an adjustable slit which can be gradually reduced until the sound becomes inaudible. [Gk *stethos* chest, *phone* sound, meter.]

stethopolyscope (steth·o·**pol**·e·skope). Stethophone, 2nd def. [Gk *stethos* chest, *polys* many, *skopein* to view.]

stethoscope (**steth**·o·skope). An instrument invented by Laennec for conducting sounds from the chest wall to the ear. It is used in *mediate auscultation* as distinct from *immediate (direct) auscultation* when the ear is applied directly to the chest wall. **Binaural stethoscope.** One which has 2 earpieces, each connected by a flexible rubber tube to the chestpiece. **Differential stethoscope.** A binaural stethoscope designed so that sounds produced at 2 different parts of the chest can be compared. **Monaural stethoscope, Straight stethoscope.** A stethoscope consisting of a hollow stem of wood or vulcanite with a small funnel-shaped chestpiece at one end and a larger flat piece at the other which is applied to the ear. **Oesophageal stethoscope.** A special rubber tube which is inserted into the oesophagus and through which the rate, force and rhythm of the cardiac action can be heard and harmlessly monitored. [Gk *stethos* chest, *skopein* to view.]

See also: CAMMANN.

stethoscopic (steth·o·**skop**·ik). 1. Relating or belonging to the stethoscope. 2. Effected or obtained by means of a stethoscope. 3. Relating or belonging to examination of the chest. [see prec.]

stethoscopy (steth·**os**·ko·pe). Examination by means of the stethoscope.

Stevens, Albert Mason (b. 1884). New York paediatrician.

Stevens–Johnson disease or syndrome. Erythema multiforme with a purulent conjunctivitis, complicated often with corneal ulceration and perforation, associated with fever and vesicles in the mouth (stomatitis), nose, genito-urinary orifices and anal canal.

Stevens, George Thomas (b. 1832). New York ophthalmologist.

Stevens' operation. 1. For squint: a method of muscle resection; a triangular piece of the muscle is excised with its base parallel and near to the insertion and the apex posteriorly. The muscle is then sutured vertically. The shortening is central only; obsolete. 2. A method of tenotomy: a buttonhole is made in the centre of the tendon of the muscle and the rest of the tendon divided above and below to the amount required.

Stewart, George Neil (b. 1860). Canadian physiologist.

Stewart's test. Calorimeter test; a method of determining the blood flow through a limb by measuring the transfer of heat from the limb to water in which it is immersed, using a calorimeter.

Stewart, Sir James Purves (b. 1869). London neurologist.

Stewart–Holmes sign. Rebound phenomenon; spring-like phenomenon. *See* PHENOMENON.

Stewart–Morel syndrome. Morgagni's syndrome.

sthenia (**sthe**·ne·ah). A condition of strength, vigour or forcefulness; the abnormal activity which characterizes some fevers. [Gk *sthenos* power.]

sthenic (**sthen**·ik). 1. Relating or belonging to sthenia. 2. Characterized by sthenia.

Stibamine Glucoside (stib·am·een **gloo**·ko·side). BP Commission approved name for a glucoside of sodium *p*-aminophenylstibonate. It was at one time used in the treatment of kala-azar, but it proved rather toxic in susceptible persons and has largely been replaced by other antimony compounds. [L *stibium* antimony, glucoside.]

stibiacne (stib·e·**ak**·ne). A follicular rash caused by antimony. [L *stibium* antimony, acne.]

stibial (**stib**·e·al). Antimonial. [see foll.]

stibialism (**stib**·e·al·izm). Poisoning by antimony. [L *stibium* antimony.]

stibiated (**stib**·e·a·ted). Containing or impregnated with antimony. [see prec.]

stibiation (stib·e·**a**·shun). Treatment with antimonials in high doses. [L *stibium* antimony.]

stibium (**stib**·e·um). Antimony. [L.]

Stibocaptate (stib·o·**kap**·tate). BP Commission approved name for antimony(III) sodium *meso*-2,3-dimercaptosuccinate; it is used in the treatment of schistosomiasis.

stibonium (stib·**o**·ne·um). The radical (SbH_4) in which antimony is quinquivalent; it forms a series of compounds analogous to ammonium, (NH_4). [see prec.]

Stibophen BP 1968 (**stib**·o·fen). Sodium antimony bispyrocatechol-3,5-sodium disulphonate, $C_{12}H_4O_{13}S_4SbNa_5 \cdot 7H_2O$. A colourless, crystalline powder soluble in water, used by intramuscular injection in the treatment of schistosomiasis.

stichochrome (**stik**·o·krome). A nerve cell with the chromidial substance arranged in layers or striae. [Gk *stichos* a row, *chroma* colour.]

Sticker, Georg (b. 1860). German physician.

Sticker's disease. Infectious erythema. *See* ERYTHEMA.

Sticta (**stik**·tah). A genus of lichens. **Sticta pulmonaria.** Lungwort; a lichen used as an astringent. [Gk *stiktos* pointed.]

Stieda, Alfred (b. 1869). Königsberg surgeon.

Pellegrini–Stieda disease. Ossification in the upper part of the medial collateral ligament of the knee as a result of injury.

Stieda, Ludwig (b. 1837). German anatomist and histologist.

Stieda's method. A method for simultaneous demonstration of nuclei and iron salts, employing lithium carmine and the Prussian-blue reaction.

Stieda's process. The posterior tubercle of the talus.

Stieglitz, Edward J. (b. 1899). Chicago physician.

Stieglitz test. A pharmacological test for assessing the presence or absence of cerebral atherosclerosis; the patient's blood pressure is recorded before and after the inhalation of amyl nitrite. In the normal individual the diastolic blood pressure falls, but in patients with cerebral atherosclerosis it remains unchanged. (This test is unreliable and so has become obsolete.)

Stierlin, Eduard (b. 1878). Zürich and Munich surgeon.

Stierlin's image or sign. A radiological sign of caecal tuberculosis. When the ileocaecal region is outlined by a barium meal, a gap is present between the terminal ileum and ascending colon. The gap may be due to spasm, organic stricture, or to a combination of both. The sign is now recognized as not exclusive to tuberculosis.

Stifel's figure. A black disc with a central white dot, used for the investigation of the physiological blind spot.

stiffness (**stif**·nes). Rigidity. **Morning stiffness.** A period of muscular stiffness which occurs on waking in patients with rheumatoid arthritis and other inflammatory polyarthritides. [OE *stif.*]

stigma (**stig**·mah) (pl. *stigmas, stigmata*). 1. A small spot, mark or scar on the skin. 2. A space seen microscopically between the endothelial cells of a capillary when the specimen is stained with silver nitrate. 3. The part of the pistil of a flower which receives pollen. 4. A matter for moral reproach. 5. Any spot, mark or small hole. 6. A sign, diagnostically, especially a physical defect accompanying mental deficiency. **Bakers' stigma.** A corn on the hand common among bakers from kneading bread. **Costal stigma.** A floating 10th rib. **Stigmata croci.** Saffron. **Stigma of degeneracy.** One of several physical abnormalities (e.g. attached ear lobes) once thought to be associated with mental degeneracy. **Follicular stigma, Stigma of a graafian follicle.** The spot on the surface of an ovary indicating the site of future rupture of a graafian follicle. **Hereditary stigma.** An inherited stigma. **Hysterical stigma.** Neurasthenic stigma (see below). **Malpighian**

stigmata. Apparent intervals in the walls of capillaries between the endothelial cells; the intervals are closed by intercellular substance. **Stigmata maydis.** Corn-silk; the fresh styles and stigmas of *Zea mays;* slender purplish-brown or greenish-yellow filaments containing maizenic acid, a fixed oil, resin and chlorophyll. They have been used in acute and chronic cystitis and urethritis and are believed to have diuretic properties, though their value is doubtful. **Neurasthenic stigma.** A skin rash of psychogenic origin or an artefact. **Stigmata nigra.** Black spots on the skin caused by a close-up discharge of a fire-arm; they are caused by small particles of gunpowder on the skin. **Stigma ovarii.** Follicular stigma (see above). **Professional stigmata.** Changes in the skin which do not impair its functional ability. Oppenheimer is quoted by Prosser White as classifying these as (*a*) stains or colouring; (*b*) stratifications; (*c*) excoriations; (*d*) nail changes; (*e*) pigmentation; (*f*) callosities; (*g*) telangiectases; (*h*) bursae; (*i*) cicatrices; (*j*) tattooing. **Psychic stigma.** A mental stigma. **Somatic stigma.** A physical sign of a nervous disease. **Syphilitic stigmata.** Certain visible signs of inherited syphilis, including saddleback nose, rhagades, sabre-shaped tibiae, Hutchinson's teeth and bosses on the frontal bones. **Stigmata ventriculi.** Stigmata of Benecki; small petechial haemorrhages and erosions in the mucous membrane of the stomach. [Gk tattoo-mark.]

See also: BENECKI.

stigmal (stig·mal). Stigmatic.

stigmasterol (stig·mas·ter·ol). $C_{29}H_{47}OH$, a phytosterol present in Calabar bean, *Physostigma venenosum* Balf., soya bean and cocoa butter.

stigmata (stig·mah·tah). *See* STIGMA.

stigmatic (stig·mat·ik). 1. Pertaining to or characterized by a stigma. 2. Emmetropic.

stigmatism (stig·mat·izm). 1. A condition which is caused or characterized by the presence of stigmata. 2. Emmetropia.

stigmatization (stig·mat·i·za'·shun). 1. Formation of cutaneous impressions or stigmata. 2. Production of red lines or bleeding points on the skin due to hypnotic suggestion or to hysteria.

stigmatometer (stig·mat·om·et·er). An instrument for measuring astigmatism, in which a point source of light is reflected into the eye by a cover-glass. The observer looks through this at the fundus reflex in the patient's pupil and, on moving his head, obtains the same effects as in retinoscopy with the plane mirror. The word might also apply to some forms of electric ophthalmoscope which can be used for measuring astigmatism. [Gk *stigma* spot, *metron* measure.]

stigmatose (stig·mat·oze). Stigmatic.

stilbamidine isethionate (stil·bam·id·een i·se·thi·on·ate). 4,4'-Diamidinostilbene di-(β-hydroxy-ethane-sulphonate), $(NH_2C(=NH)C_6H_4)_2(CH)_2(C_2H_6SO_4)_2$. A drug used for the treatment of visceral leishmaniasis which, though very effective, causes a troublesome neuropathy in a large percentage of patients treated and is therefore contra-indicated except in patients very resistant to other forms of treatment. *Stilbamidine* is a BP Commission approved name.

Stilbazium Iodide (stil·ba·ze·um i·o·dide). BP Commission approved name for 1-ethyl-2,6-di-[4-(pyrrolidin-1-yl)styryl] pyridinium iodide; an anthelmintic.

stilbene (stil·been). $C_6H_5CH{=}CHC_6H_5$, an unsaturated hydrocarbon which forms the nucleus of the molecule of stilboestrol.

Stilboestrol BP 1973 (stil·be·strol). 4,4'-Dihydroxystilbene, $OHC_6H_4CH{=}CHC_6H_4OH$. An artificial oestrogen which does not possess the steroid structure of the natural oestrogens. The name is also used as a shortened form of diethylstilboestrol, 4,4'-dihydroxy-α,β-diethylstilbene, a synthetic substance with oestrogenic properties, active when given by mouth.

Stiles, Sir Harold Jalland (b. 1863). Edinburgh surgeon.

Stiles' intraperitoneal transplantation of ureters. Direct transperitoneal ureterocolic anastomosis, the divided ureter being secured within the colon through a simple stab incision.

stilette (stil·et). 1. Wire inserted into the lumen of a catheter in order to stiffen it during its passage or to remove an obstruction. 2. A fine probe. 3. Wire of small calibre used to keep the canal of a hypodermic needle free from corrosion when not in use. [Fr.]

Still, Sir George Frederic (b. 1868). London paediatrician.

Still's disease, Chauffard-Still syndrome, Still-Chauffard syndrome. Rheumatoid arthritis occurring in children.

stillbirth (stil·berth). The lifeless state of birth. Failure to breathe or show any other sign of a separate existence upon expulsion from the body of the mother. Term commonly used only for gestations of 28 weeks or more (prior to this, referred to as products of abortion). Certified by either midwife or doctor in attendance or examining the body after birth, or by a coroner or the pathologist examining the body. [AS *stille,* ME birth.]

stillborn (stil·born). Dead at birth; any child issuing from the mother after the 28th week of pregnancy which does not at any time after being expelled breathe or show any other signs of life. [AS *stille,* born.]

Stiller, Berthold (b. 1837). Budapest physician.

Stiller's disease. General asthenia.

Stiller's sign or theory. Undue mobility of the 10th rib in enteroptosis.

stillicidium (stil·is·id·e·um). The dribbling or flowing of a liquid drop-by-drop. **Stillicidium lacrimarum.** Epiphora. **Stillicidium narium.** Coryza. **Stillicidium urinae.** The passing of urine drop-by-drop as in cases of vesical spasm. [L a dropping moisture.]

Stilling, Benedict (b. 1810). Cassel anatomist.

Stilling's bundle. The fasciculus solitarius.

Stilling's canal. The hyaloid canal. *See* CANAL.

Stilling's cell, Stilling-Clarke cell. Large rounded or fusiform cells in the thoracic nucleus of the spinal cord.

Stilling's column, Stilling-Clarke column. The thoracic nucleus of the spinal cord.

Stilling's fibres. The fibres forming the reticular formation of the medulla oblongata.

Stilling's fleece. A network of white fibres around the dentate nucleus.

Stilling's nucleus. 1. The red nucleus. *See* NUCLEUS. 2. The sacral portion of the gelatinous matter of the spinal cord. 3. That part of the hypoglossal-nerve nucleus underlying the fourth ventricle.

Stilling's raphe. The intermingled bundle of nerve fibres seen on the anterior surface of the medulla oblongata, formed by the decussation of the pyramids.

Stillingia (stil·in·je·ah). A genus of euphorbiaceous trees, shrubs and herbs. **Stillingia sylvatica.** Queen's delight, queen's root, yaw-root; the root has been used as a laxative and diuretic. [Benjamin *Stillingfleet* (b. 1702), English botanist.]

Stimson, Lewis A. 20th century New York orthopaedic surgeon.

Stimson's manoeuvre. A method of reduction of dislocation of the hip. The manipulation is carried out with the patient lying face downwards on a table with the affected limb flexed over the end of the table.

stimulant (stim·ew·lant). 1. Producing stimulation. 2. Any drug or agent which causes stimulation. **Alcoholic stimulant.** Any drink containing ethyl alcohol, such as brandy, wine, whisky, rum and fermented malt preparations. **Bronchial stimulant.** Any drug which increases bronchial secretion; any expectorant, including ammonium acetate, ammonium carbonate, ammonium chloride, antimony potassium tartrate, apomorphine, benzoin, codeine, ipecacuanha, squill, senega and potassium iodide. **Cardiac stimulant.** Any drug which increases the action of the heart, e.g. digitalis, strophanthus, adrenaline and the sympathomimetics, and belladonna. **Cerebral stimulant.** Any drug which stimulates the higher centres of the brain, e.g. amphetamine, caffeine, picrotoxin, leptazol, nikethamide, atropine, cocaine and alcohol. **Cutaneous stimulant.** Any diaphoretic agent which stimulates the skin and induces sweating, including alcohol, ammonia, antimony potassium tartrate, ipecacuanha, opium, pilocarpine, sodium salicylate and spirit of nitrous ether. **Diffusible stimulant.** A stimulant which acts promptly and strongly, e.g. ammonia. **Gastric stimulant.** Any agent promoting the flow of gastric juice, including stomachics or carminatives (e.g. ether, alcohol), bitters (e.g. gentian, quinine, strychnine), volatile oils (e.g. caraway, fennel, dill and peppermint) and dilute acids (e.g. hydrochloric, phosphoric, hydrocyanic). Histamine is a gastric stimulant. **General stimulant.** A stimulant which acts on the whole body, e.g. cold water. **Genital stimulant.** An agent increasing sexual desire; an aphrodisiac, including alcohol, cannabis, cantharides, strychnine and yohimbine. **Hepatic stimulant.** A drug which increases the secretion of bile; a cholagogue, including oleic acid, olive oil, ox bile, bile salts and magnesium sulphate. **Intestinal stimulant.** Any drug which increases intestinal movement, including cathartics, cholagogues (e.g. oleic acid, ox bile, mercurous chloride, magnesium sulphate, podophyllum resin, soap, sodium taurocholate and olive oil), laxatives (e.g. cassia, euonymus, figs, sulphur, tamarind), bulk-producing stimulants (e.g. agar, ispaghula, linseed, psyllium, tragacanth), saline aperients (e.g. magnesium salts, potassium acid tartrate, sodium acid tartrate, sodium phosphate, sodium sulphate), stimulants acting on the colon (e.g. aloe, aloin, cascara, rhubarb, senna) or on the small intestine (e.g. castor oil, phenolphthalein), drastic purgatives (e.g. aloe, aloin, colocynth, mercury, ipomoea, jalap, magnesium sulphate, croton oil, castor oil, podophyllum and scammony), or those given by injection (e.g. ergot, pituitary extract, physostigmine). **Local stimulant.** A drug which affects only the part to which it is applied, e.g. mustard, camphor, turpentine, chloral hydrate, cantharides, methyl salicylate. **Nervous stimulant.** An agent which acts mainly on the nerve centres; cerebral or spinal stimulants, e.g. strychnine, picrotoxin, leptazol, nikethamide, camphor, caffeine, theophylline, cocaine. **Paradoxical stimulant.** A warm object applied to one of the cold spots of the body, producing a sensation of cold. **Renal stimulant.** Any agent increasing renal secretion, including saline salts (e.g. ammonium chloride, potassium acetate, potassium tartrate, sodium benzoate), kidney irritants (e.g. buchu, copaiba, juniper, turpentine, mercurial salts), cardiac stimulants (e.g. digitalis, strophanthus, squill), and purine derivatives (e.g. caffeine, theobromine and theophylline). **Respiratory stimulant.** A drug increasing respiratory movements, e.g. carbon dioxide, nikethamide, leptazol, hexazole, picrotoxin, lobeline, amphetamine and methylamphetamine. Stimulation of the sensory nerves may also be a respiratory stimulant. **Spinal stimulant.** A drug acting upon or through the spinal cord (e.g. strychnine, caffeine). **Stomachic stimulant.** Gastric stimulant (see above). **Topical stimulant.** Local stimulant (see above). **Uterine stimulant.** A drug increasing uterine movement, e.g. quinine, ergot, posterior pituitary extract, hydrastis. **Vascular stimulant.** A drug acting on the vasomotor centre, e.g. ammonia, ergot, strychnine, opium, belladonna, picrotoxin, leptazol, nikethamide, amphetamine. **Vasomotor stimulant.** Vascular stimulant (see preceding). [L *stimulare* to incite.]

stimulate (stim·ew·late). 1. To apply a stimulus to a structure. 2. To arouse to more vigorous functional activity, either the system in general or a particular system or organ; in the restoration of animation, to arouse by administration of alcohol or other drink or drug. [see prec.]

stimulation (stim·ew·la·shun). 1. The state of being stimulated. 2. The act of stimulation. **Paradoxical stimulation.** The subjective sensation of cold in response to a warm stimulus. **Punctual stimulation.** Stimulation of a single receptor or sensory point.

stimulator (stim·ew·la·tor). Anything that stimulates. **Electric stimulator.** An instrument used for the production of electrical pulses of potential for physiological stimulation. The pulses may be varied in duration, amplitude, polarity and repetition frequency. **Long-acting thyroid stimulator (LATS).** An IgG globulin which maintains hyperthyroidism. [L *stimulare* to incite.]

stimulin (stim·ew·lin). A factor in the blood serum said (by Metchnikoff) to stimulate or accelerate phagocytic action.

stimulus (stim·ew·lus) (pl. *stimuli*). 1. Any act or agent which produces an effect upon nervous tissue, leading either to the recording of a sensation or to a motor response. 2. Any change in environment that produces a response in a living organism. **Adequate stimulus.** A stimulus sufficient to produce a response; a liminal or supraliminal stimulus (see below). **Chemical stimulus.** A stimulus due to, or produced by, a chemical substance as, for example, the stimulation of postganglionic neurones, parasympathetic effector organs and motor endplates, by acetylcholine, and of most sympathetic effector organs by noradrenaline. **Conditioned stimulus.** A stimulus to which the reflex response has been conditioned by previous experience. **Electric stimulus.** A stimulus applied by an electric current. **Heterologous stimulus.** A stimulus which does not require a specific end-organ but which can excite any form of nervous tissue. **Heterotopic stimulus.** In cardiology, an impulse initiating cardiac contraction and arising from a focus in the heart other than the sinu-atrial or atrioventricular nodes. **Homologous stimulus.** A stimulus which requires a specific end-organ for its reception and transmission; e.g. light can only be perceived by the retina. **Liminal stimulus.** A stimulus just sufficient to produce a response. **Normotopic stimulus.** The natural stimulus to cardiac contraction, arising in the sinu-atrial node. **Noxious stimulus.** A harmful stimulus. **Subliminal stimulus.** Less than a threshold stimulus: it will produce no response. **Supraliminal stimulus.** Above a threshold stimulus. **Threshold stimulus.** Liminal stimulus (see above). [L goad.]

sting (sting). 1. Any sharp organ of insects or plants that, puncturing the skin, gives rise to burning, pricking pain because of the poison carried by the sting. 2. To give rise to acute pain or a burning smart. [AS *stingan.*]

sting-ray (sting·ra). Any individual of the family Trygonidae, particularly *Trygon pastinaca.* A sharp spine on the tail can inflict painful wounds. [sting, L *raia* ray-fish.]

Stintzing, Roderich (b. 1854). Jena physician.

Stintzing's table. A table giving average values of the normal electrical excitability of nerves and muscles.

stippling (stip·ling). A dotted appearance in cells on staining. **Malarial stippling.** Red dots in blood cells stained by eosin-haematoxylin stains, occurring in malaria. [D *stippen* to prick.]

See also: MAURER, SCHUEFFNER, ZIEMANN.

Stirimazole (sti·**rim**·az·ole). BP Commission approved name for 2-(4-carboxystyryl)-5-nitro-1-vinylimidazole; it is used in the treatment of amoebiasis, trichomoniasis and trypanosomiasis.

stirpicultural (ster·pe·**kul**·tcher·al). Relating or belonging to stirpiculture.

stirpiculture (ster·pe·kul·tcher). The continuous raising of the quality of a race or stock by application of the principles of scientific selection in breeding. [L *stirps* stock, culture.]

stirps (sterps). 1. The aggregation of hereditary organic units in the impregnated ovum (Galton). 2. Family; race; stock. [L *stirps* stock.]

stirrup (stir·up). A U-shaped steel rod used with a pin or wire for skeletal traction in the treatment of certain fractures. **Swivel stirrup.** A metal stirrup for attachment to a bone transfixion pin for the purpose of weight extension. The stirrup is provided with swivels to prevent movement of the pin. [AS *stirap.*]

stirrup bone (stir·up bone). The stapes. [AS *stirap,* bone.]

stitch (stich). 1. Suture. 2. A momentary, sudden sharp pain, often at the costal margin on one side, sometimes occurring after running or eating. 3. To join together with a needle threaded with catgut, silk or wire. **Glovers' stitch.** A continuous stitch. *See* SUTURE. **Stitch in the side.** A pain in the side that occurs after severe or relatively severe unaccustomed exercise, especially running. It is probably due to spasm of some of the muscle fibres of the diaphragm as a result of hyperventilation. [ME *stiche.*]

See also: GOODSALL, MARCY, MOYNIHAN.

Stivalius (sti·va·le·us). A genus of fleas, of which several are vectors of plague.

Stock, Wolfgang (b. 1874). Jena ophthalmologist.

Spielmeyer-Stock disease, Stock-Spielmeyer disease. The retinal atrophy observed in Spielmeyer-Vogt disease.

stocking (stok·ing). A close-fitting knitted or woven garment for the leg and foot. **Elastic stocking.** A rubberized stocking designed for therapeutic support of the leg, sometimes used in the treatment of varicosities. [AS *stocc.*]

Stoddard, James Leavitt (b. 1889). Boston pathologist.

Stoddard and Drury method. For total fatty acids in blood. Whole blood, plasma or serum is extracted with hot alcohol-ether. The filtered extract is boiled with alkali to saponify the free and combined fatty acids; the fatty acids are then separated, washed, dissolved in alcohol and titrated with standard alkali using phenol blue as indicator.

Stoerk, Karl (b. 1832). Vienna laryngologist

Stoerk's blennorrhoea. Blennorrhoea and ensuing morbid enlargement of the nasal, pharyngeal and laryngeal mucous membrane, with associated profuse and chronic discharge of pus.

Stoffel, Adolf (b. 1880). Mannheim orthopaedic surgeon.

Stoffel operation. Resection of a portion of a motor nerve to reduce the spasticity of muscle in spastic paralysis.

Stohr, Philipp (b. 1849). Würzburg and Zürich anatomist and histologist.

Stohr's cellules. Metachromatic cells in the pyloric gastric mucosa.

stoichiology (stoi·ke·**ol**·o·je). The study of cell physiology. [Gk *stoicheion* element, *logos* science.]

stoichiometry (stoi·ke·**om**·et·re). Chemical calculation; the study of the combining proportions of elements by weight and volume. [Gk *stoicheion* element, meter.]

stoke (stoke). A unit of viscosity equal to $10^{-4}\,m^2\,s^{-1}$. [Sir George G. *Stokes*.]

stoker's treatment. Continuous inhalation of oxygen in the treatment of bronchiectasis.

Stokes, Sir George Gabriel (b. 1819). Cambridge physicist.

Stokes' law. The velocity attained by a small sphere sinking under gravity through a viscous medium is given by the formula

$$\frac{2gr^2(d_1-d_2)}{9\eta}$$

where r is the radius of the sphere, d_1 its density, d_2 the density of the medium, g the acceleration due to gravity and η the coefficient of viscosity of the medium.

Stokes, William (b. 1804). Dublin physician.

Stokes' disease. Graves' disease [obsolete term].

Stokes' law. Paralysis may affect a muscle underlying an inflamed mucous or serous membrane.

Adams-Stokes attack, disease or syndrome, Morgagni-Adams-Stokes disease or syndrome, Stokes-Adams syndrome. Disturbance of consciousness due to inadequate central blood flow, accompanying extreme slowing of the heart or ventricular standstill; in severe cases complete loss of consciousness and even epileptiform convulsions may result. As soon as ventricular beating is resumed consciousness is rapidly regained, followed by a widespread flush (reactive hyperaemia). It occurs not infrequently when partial atrioventricular heart block is becoming complete, and less frequently in cases of established complete heart block. Ventricular asystole may sometimes follow an episode of ventricular paroxysmal tachycardia with a similar clinical syndrome, but this is not strictly the Morgagni-Adams-Stokes syndrome. Originally described by Morgagni in 1700, it is usually called the *Stokes-Adams syndrome.*

Cheyne-Stokes nystagmus. Nystagmus the eye movements of which resemble Cheyne-Stokes respiration in rhythm.

Cheyne-Stokes phenomenon, respiration or sign. Rhythmical waxing and waning of respiration, consisting of alternating periods of hyperpnoea (increased depth and rate of respiration) and apnoea (cessation of respiration). Respiration steadily increases in depth, then wanes, until finally it ceases entirely. After a few moments the cycle is repeated. During apnoea the pupils contract and consciousness is often lost: during hyperpnoea the pupils dilate and consciousness is regained. Cheyne-Stokes respiration is due to an altered sensitivity of the respiratory centre, connected with reduced cerebral blood flow. It occurs in cerebral tumour, raised intracranial pressure, cerebral vascular accidents; in congestive cardiac failure (usually of the left ventricle); after narcotics such as morphine derivatives and barbiturates; and in uraemia. Occasionally it occurs in normal persons during sleep.

Cheyne-Stokes psychosis. A confusional state associated with Cheyne-Stokes respiration.

Stokes, Sir William (b. 1839). Dublin surgeon.

collar of Stokes. In obstruction of the superior vena cava, dilatation of the veins in the area between the neck and the diaphragm, with thickening of the soft tissues of the thorax and neck due to the presence of fluid.

Stokes' operation. Amputation at the hip.

Gritti-Stokes amputation. Supracondylar amputation of the femur, the patella being retained, denuded of its articular cartilage, and applied to the end of the stump.

Stokes, William Royal (b. 1870). Baltimore pathologist.

Stokes' reagent. For the reduction of haemoglobin and its derivatives. Dissolve 2 g of ferrous sulphate and 3 g of tartaric acid in 100 ml of water. For use, add ammonium hydroxide to a portion of this solution until the precipitate first formed redissolves to form ammonium ferrotartrate.

Stokvis, Barend Joseph (b. 1834). Dutch physician.

Stokvis' disease. Enterogenous cyanosis. *See* CYANOSIS.

Stoll, Norman Rudolph (b. 1892). Princeton parasitologist.

Stoll's count or method. A method for estimating the number of ova in a faecal specimen by adding to a weighted portion of faeces decinormal caustic soda up to a specified level.

stolonization (sto·lon·i·za'·shun). The process of transforming in certain organisms one organ into another through external influences such as contact, light or gravity. [L *stolo* a shoot.]

Stoltz, Joseph Alexis (b. 1803). Strasbourg gynaecologist.

Stoltz operation. An operation for cystocele, done by denuding a patch on the anterior vaginal wall and running a purse-string suture around the edge.

stoma (sto·mah) (pl. *stomata*). 1. A mouth-like opening, or pore, or communication between cavities. 2. An opening which leads into the gastro-intestinal tract from the outside or from one part of the intestine into another, e.g. gastrojejunal stoma, abdominal or perineal stoma. 3. One of the hypothetical openings from the peritoneal cavity into the diaphragmatic lymphatics. [Gk mouth.] *See also:* FUCHS (E.).

stomacace (sto·**mak**·as·e). Stomatocace.

stomach [ventriculus (gaster) (NA)] (**stum**·ak). The enlarged part of the alimentary tract immediately succeeding the oesophagus, varying in position and form with the position of the subject and state of distension, but usually occupying the epigastric, left hypochondriac and umbilical regions of the abdomen. The walls are designated anterior [paries anterior (NA)] and posterior [paries posterior (NA)]. **Aviators' stomach.** A gastric neurosis in airmen attributed to anoxia and emotional strain. There is gastric discomfort with nervous irritability and insomnia. **Bilocular stomach.** Hour-glass stomach; a stomach divided into 2 compartments by a constriction. **Body of the stomach [corpus ventriculi (NA)].** That part of the organ between the fundus and the pyloric antrum; the main central part of the stomach. **Cascade stomach.** A physiological loculation in the upper part of the stomach, seen sometimes in radiological examination in the erect position. The posterior wall forms a shelf on which barium spills; when the shelf is full barium cascades anteriorly or anterolaterally into the pyloric portion. **Coat of the stomach, mucous [tunica mucosa (NA)].** The innermost coat of the stomach consisting of a simple tall columnar epithelium from which branched tubular glands project into the thick subjacent connective-tissue layer, limited on its deep aspect by a layer of smooth muscle. It is thick and loosely attached to the underlying tissue, thus enabling it to be thrown into folds in the empty organ. **Coat of the stomach, muscular [tunica muscularis (NA)].** The middle circular [stratum circulare (NA)], outer longitudinal [stratum longitudinale (NA)] and inner oblique [fibrae obliquae (NA)] layers of smooth muscle fibres. **Coat of the stomach, serous [tunica serosa (NA)].** The visceral peritoneum covering the anterior and posterior walls of the stomach. **Coat of the stomach, submucous [tela mucosa (NA)].** A layer of connective tissue containing large blood and lymph vessels and venous plexuses. It connects the mucous and muscular coats. **Desiccated stomach.** A preparation from the vacuum-dried defatted stomach of the pig, *Sus scrofa* Linn. (family Suidae). It is used in the treatment of pernicious anaemia as an alternative to liver, but as there is no means of assaying it, it is usually only employed when liver does not bring about a response. **Drain-tap stomach.** A stomach with a sharp bend of the lesser curvature and a high pylorus. **Dumping stomach.** Following partial gastric resection for peptic ulcer (especially Billroth II or its modification) food may leave the small remaining stomach very rapidly and distend the jejunum; this happening seems often to cause disabling symptoms. **Fish-hook stomach.** J stomach; an elongated stomach shaped like a J. **Fundus of the stomach [fundus ventriculi (NA)].** The cul-de-sac of the stomach, which lies above the level of the cardiac orifice. **Hour-glass stomach.** Bilocular stomach (see above). **J stomach.** Fish-hook stomach (see above). **Leather-bottle stomach.** A diffuse sclerosis of the stomach, with much thickening of its walls and a shrunken lumen; of malignant origin. **Miniature stomach.** Pavlov's stomach. **Portion of the stomach, cardiac [pars cardiaca (NA)].** That part of the organ to the left of a vertical line passing through the angular notch on the lesser curvature. It consists of the body and fundus. **Portion of the stomach, pyloric [pars pylorica (NA)].** That part of the organ to the right of a vertical line through the angular notch. **Steer-horn stomach.** A transversely disposed stomach. **Thoracic stomach.** A condition in which the stomach is situated above the diaphragm. **Trifid stomach.** A stomach with 2 constrictions, forming 3 compartments. **Wallet stomach.** A dilated stomach, like a bag. **Waterfall stomach.** Cascade stomach (see above); a term not used in the UK. **Water-trap stomach.** Drain-tap stomach (see above). [Gk *stomakhos* gullet.]

See also: HOLZNECHT, PAVLOV.

stomachalgia (stum·ak·**al**·je·ah). Any pain in the stomach. [stomach, Gk *algos* pain.]

stomachic (**stum**·ak·ik). 1. Relating or belonging to the stomach; gastric. 2. Promoting digestion by stimulating gastric action. 3. A medicine that acts as a tonic on the stomach, improving appetite and assisting the digestive process; a cordial.

stomadeum (sto·mah·**de**·um). Stomatodaeum.

stomal (**sto**·mal). Stomatal.

stomata (**sto**·mah·tah). *See* STOMA.

stomatal (**sto**·mat·al). Relating to 1 or more stomata.

stomatalgia (sto·mat·**al**·je·ah). Pain in the mouth. [Gk *stoma* mouth, *algos* pain.]

stomatic (sto·**mat**·ik). Belonging to the mouth. [Gk *stoma* mouth.]

stomatitis (sto·mat·**i**·tis). Inflammation of the mucous membrane of the mouth. **Allergic stomatitis.** An allergic reaction within the mouth to denture materials, dentifrices, chewing gum or other substances. **Angular stomatitis.** Inflammation and ulceration of the lips and cracks at the corners of the mouth due to a deficiency of riboflavine. **Aphthous stomatitis.** Small, slightly raised vesicles occurring on the mucous membrane of the cheeks and lips and rupturing to form greyish painful ulcers with a red margin. Frequently caused by the virus of herpes simplex. **Blackberry stomatitis.** Bleeding granulomatous lesions in the mouth in South American blastomycosis (paracoccidioidomycosis). **Catarrhal stomatitis.** Simple inflammation causing a red, swollen, mucous membrane with excess of mucus. It may be present in poorly nourished children during dentition, in specific fevers or as a result of excessive smoking or consumption of alcohol. **Epidemic stomatitis.** Foot and mouth disease; this may rarely occur in man, causing blebs and ulcers. **Epizootic stomatitis.** Foot and mouth disease in animals. **Erythematous stomatitis.** Redness due to simple inflammation. **Stomatitis exanthematica.** Catarrhal stomatitis (see above) occurring in the exanthemata. **Follicular stomatitis.** Inflammation of the mucous follicles producing painful ulcers. **Gangrenous stomatitis.** Noma, cancrum oris; sloughing ulceration of the cheeks and gums which spreads rapidly and forms brawny thickening of the subcutaneous tissues that may become gangrenous and perforate the cheek. It is now a very rare disease, but may occur in children living under insanitary conditions, especially during convalescence from measles or scarlet fever. **Herpetic stomatitis.** A term applied to aphthous stomatitis (see above) but should now be applied to the form caused by the virus of herpes simplex (herpes labialis) of which it may be the primary lesion. The latter is accompanied by fever and may then become latent, being thereafter carried by persons for years and only manifested occasionally by recurrent herpes labialis. **Stomatitis hyphomycetica.** Mycotic stomatitis (see below). **Infectious pustular stomatitis.** Foot and mouth disease caused by a virus which attacks cattle, pigs, sheep, goats, etc. **Stomatitis intertropica.** The stomatitis of sprue, in which the tongue is clean, red and sore, with atrophy of the mucous membrane and papillae, and superficial ulceration. **Irritant stomatitis.** Stomatitis caused by a primary irritant. **Stomatitis medicamentosa.** Stomatitis caused by a drug taken internally. **Mercurial stomatitis.** A form occurring in chronic mercurial poisoning: the gums become red and swollen and ulcerate, especially around carious teeth; there is considerable fetor and salivation. **Mycotic stomatitis, Parasitic stomatitis.** Thrush; caused by the fungus *Candida albicans*, it occurs in debilitated bottle-fed young infants and is manifested by small white patches on the mucous membrane of the cheeks, lips, gums, tongue and palate which are rather firmly adherent and tend to spread into larger areas; it also occurs after the administration of antibiotics. **Scorbutic stomatitis.** Swelling and bleeding of the gums with loosening of the teeth, occurring in scurvy. **Stomatitis simplex.** Simple catarrhal stomatitis (see above). **Syphilitic stomatitis.** Erythema and mucous patches in the mouth, occurring in the secondary stage of syphilis. **Stomatitis traumatica.** Inflammatory lesions produced by irritant substances. **Tropical stomatitis.** Stomatitis of sprue. **Ulcerative stomatitis of sheep.** An affection of sheep caused by *Actinomyces necrophorus*. **Ulceromembranous stomatitis.** Vincent's stomatitis; a severe spreading stomatitis which may occur in epidemic form. It is caused by infection with Vincent's organisms. **Vulcanite stomatitis.** An erythematous and vesicular inflammation caused by vulcanite dental plates. [Gk *stoma* mouth, *-itis* inflammation.]

See also: VINCENT.

stomatocace (sto·mat·**ok**·as·e). Ulcerative stomatitis. [Gk *stoma* mouth, *kake* badness.]

stomatocatharsis (**sto**·mat·o·kath·**ar**'·sis). 1. Ptyalism. 2. Cleansing or disinfection of the cavity of the mouth. [Gk *stoma* mouth, catharsis.]

stomatodaeal, stomatodeal (**sto**·mat·o·**de**'·al). Pertaining to the stomatodaeum.

stomatodaeum, stomatodeum (**sto**·mat·o·**de**'·um). The surface depression lined with ectoderm which forms the primitive mouth cavity of the early embryo. [Gk *stoma* mouth, *odaios* pertaining to a way.]

stomatodynia (**sto**·mat·o·**din**'·e·ah). Pain in the mouth. [Gk *stoma* mouth, *odyne* pain.]

stomatodysodia (**sto**·mat·o·dis·**o**'·de·ah). An offensive odour having origin in the mouth. [Gk *stoma* mouth, *dysodes* ill-smelling.]

stomatogastric (**sto**·mat·o·**gas**'·trik). Relating or belonging to the stomach and the mouth. [Gk *stoma* mouth, *gaster* stomach.]

stomatolalia (**sto**·mat·o·**la**'·le·ah). A condition in which the individual speaks through the mouth with the nares closed or obstructed as in adenoids. [Gk *stoma* mouth, *lalein* to talk.]

stomatological (**sto**·mat·o·**loj**'·ik·al). Pertaining to stomatology.

stomatologist (sto·mat·**ol**·o·jist). A specialist in diseases of the oral region. [see foll.]

stomatology (sto·mat·**ol**·o·je). The branch of medical science concerned with the mouth and its diseases. [Gk *stoma* mouth, *logos* science.]

stomatomalacia (**sto**·mat·o·mal·**a'**·she·ah). Morbid softening of any of the oral structures. [Gk *stoma* mouth, malacia.]

stomatomenia (**sto**·mat·o·**me'**·ne·ah). Bleeding in the mouth in association with menstrual disorders. [Gk *stoma* mouth, *men* month.]

stomatomia (sto·mat·**o**·me·ah). Incision of the mouth of an organ. [Gk *stoma* mouth, *temnein* to cut.]

stomatomy (sto·**mat**·o·me). Stomatotomy. [see prec.]

stomatomycosis (**sto**·mat·o·mi·**ko'**·sis). Any morbid condition of the mouth which is caused by a microscopical fungus, e.g. thrush. [Gk *stoma* mouth, mycosis.]

stomatonecrosis, stomatonoma (sto·mat·o·nek·**ro'**·sis, **sto**·mat·o·**no'**·mah). Gangrenous stomatitis. *See* STOMATITIS. [Gk *stoma* mouth, necrosis, Gk *noma* spreading.]

stomatopathy (sto·mat·**op**·ath·e). Any diseased condition of the mouth. [Gk *stoma* mouth, *pathos* disease.]

stomatophylaxis (**sto**·mat·o·fil·**ax'**·is). Oral prophylaxis. [Gk *stoma* mouth, *phylaxis* a guarding.]

stomatoplastic (**sto**·mat·o·**plas'**·tik). Relating or belonging to stomatoplasty.

stomatoplasty (**sto**·mat·o·plas·te). 1. Plastic surgery of the mouth. 2. Reparative surgery of the os uteri. [Gk *stoma* mouth, *plassein* to mould.]

stomatopoiesis (**sto**·mat·o·poi·**e'**·sis). Stomatoplasty. [Gk *stoma* mouth, *poiein* to make.]

stomatorrhagia (**sto**·mat·o·**ra'**·je·ah). Bleeding from the mouth or any part of the oral cavity. **Stomatorrhagia gingivarum.** Bleeding from the gums. [Gk *stoma* mouth, *rhegnynein* to gush forth.]

stomatoscope (sto·**mat**·o·skope). An illuminating instrument for inspection of the oral cavity. [Gk *stoma* mouth, *skopein* to view.]

stomatosis (sto·mat·**o**·sis). Any disease or disorder of the mouth. [Gk *stoma* mouth, *-osis* condition.]

stomatosyrinx (**sto**·mat·o·**sir'**·ingx). The pharyngotympanic tube. *See* TUBE. [Gk *stoma* mouth, *syrigx* pipe.]

stomatotomy (sto·mat·**ot**·o·me). In obstetrics, surgical incision of the neck of the uterus.

stomenorrhagia (**sto**·men·o·**ra'**·je·ah). Stomatorrhagia.

stomocephalus (sto·mo·**kef**·al·us). A monster the head and jaws of which are undeveloped, the skin falling in folds round the snout-like mouth. [Gk *stoma* mouth, *kephale* head.]

stomodaeum, stomodeum (sto·mo·**de**·um). Stomatodaeum.

stomoschisis (sto·**mos**·kis·is). Hare-lip. [Gk *stoma* mouth, *schisis* a cleaving.]

Stomoxys (sto·**mox**·is). A genus of muscid flies closely resembling house flies but with piercing mouth parts. Many species bite man painfully. **Stomoxys calcitrans.** The stable fly or biting house fly. It is world wide and breeds in straw or similar litter. It may possibly act as a mechanical transmitter of the *Leishmania* of oriental sore, bacteria of anthrax and tetanus, and some trypanosomes. [Gk *stoma* mouth, *oxys* sharp.]

stone (stone). A concretion; in particular, a calculus. **Bezoar stone.** *See* BEZOAR. **Stone in the bladder.** Urolithiasis; a concretion in the bladder cavity. **Blue stone.** Crystalline copper sulphate; it has astringent and antiseptic properties and is used locally for this purpose. **Chalk stone.** A gouty concretion composed of sodium urate and calcium salts. **Stone child.** Lithopaedion. **Dental stone.** Pulp stone (see below). **Ear stone.** Otolith. **Gall stone.** *See* GALL-STONE. **Lung stone.** Minute concretions in the smaller bronchi that form around foreign bodies or altered lung secretions. **Metabolic stone.** Cholesterol stone in the gall bladder. **Pulp stone.** A mass of calcified material found within the substance of the tooth pulp. **Skin stone.** A calcified nodule within the subcutaneous tissue. **Stag-horn stone.** A branched calculus within the pelvis of the ureter and calyces. **Tear stone.** Dacryolith; a concretion usually found in the lacrimal canaliculus and more rarely in the lacrimal sac, sometimes multiple. **Vein stone.** Phlebolith; a calcified thrombus in a vein. **Womb stone.** A uterine calculus. [AS *stan.*]

Stookey, Byron Polk (b. 1887). New York neurosurgeon.

Stookey reflex. If the leg is held semiflexed at the knee joint, further flexion results from tapping the tendons of the hamstrings; this reflex has little clinical value but is analogous to the other deep reflexes.

stool (stool). The faecal matter discharged from the bowels. **Acholic stool.** A stool containing no bile pigment, as in complete obstruction of the common bile duct. **Bilious stool.** Bright yellow or green stool due to excess of bilirubin or biliverdin. **Fatty stool.** A stool containing an abnormal amount of fat. **Lead-pencil stool.** A narrow, pencil-like stool from stricture of the rectum. **Lienteric stool.** One that contains much undigested food. **Pea-soup stool.** The characteristic thin, copious evacuation often observed in typhoid fever. **Pipe-stem stool.** Lead-pencil stool (see above). **Ribbon stool.** A long, flattened, firm stool seen in obstruction in the rectum. **Rice-water stool.** A watery stool with fine white flocculi in suspension. It is chiefly found in cholera. **Schafkoth stool, Sheep-dung stool.** A stool consisting of small, hard, rounded balls, as in spastic constipation. **Silver stool.** The passing of a pale watery stool which, when shaken or swirled round the inside of the receptacle, gives the appearance of silver or aluminium paint. This condition is usually associated with an excess of fatty-acid crystals. It occurs in several conditions in which there is a disturbance of fat metabolism. A similar appearance is also claimed for stools in cancer of the ampulla of Vater, in which case it is thought to be a combination of the pale stool of obstructive jaundice with the black stool of melaena. **Spinach stool.** An abnormal stool of infants. It resembles in colour and consistency the appearance of spinach purée, and is caused by infection, or by drugs such as mercury powders. **Tarry stools.** Stools that are black, like tar, due to changed blood, e.g. as in a bleeding peptic ulcer, or to the taking of bismuth, barium, iron and certain other medicaments. [AS *stol* seat.]

Stopes, Marie Carmichael (b. 1880). London palaeobotanist and pioneer in birth control.

Stopes' cap. An occlusive diaphragm for contraceptive purposes.

stopping-power (**stop**·ing·pow·er). A measure of the rate at which a moving particle loses energy in a medium, i.e. energy lost per unit path length. **Atomic stopping-power.** The comparison of stopping-power on the basis of equal numbers of atoms along the path traversed. **Linear stopping-power.** The comparison of energy loss rates (stopping-power) made on the basis of equal path lengths traversed. **Mass stopping-power.** The comparison of stopping-power on the basis of equal masses traversed. **Relative stopping-power.** The ratio of stopping power for a given substance, to that for a standard substance, usually air. [AS *stoppian,* ME *poer.]*

storax (**sto**·rax). **Prepared Storax BP 1958.** The purified balsam obtained from the trunk of the hamamelidaceous tree *Liquidambar orientalis* Mill. The secretion is induced by wounding the tree, and is purified by solution in alcohol followed by filtration and evaporation. It contains a resin, storesinol, and an oily liquid consisting of a mixture of cinnamic acid, cinnamic esters and vanillin. It is an ingredient of Friars' balsam, and is also used as a parasiticide in ointments. [Gk *styrax.*]

storesin (sto·rez·in). Storesinol.

storesinol (sto·**rez**·in·ol). An amorphous resin which occurs in storax, free and also combined with cinnamic acid.

Storm van Leeuwen, Willem (b. 1882). Leyden pharmacologist.

Storm van Leeuwen chamber. A room constructed to prevent the entrance of dust or air-borne allergens, used in the treatment of asthma.

strabilismus (strab·il·**iz**·mus). Strabismus; squint.

strabism (**strab**·izm). Strabismus; squint.

strabismal, strabismic (strab·**iz**·mal, strab·**iz**·mik). Relating or belonging to, having the character of, or affected with strabismus.

strabismometer (strab·iz·**mom**·et·er). An instrument for measuring the angle of squint. [Gk *strabismos* squinting, meter.]

strabismometry (strab·iz·**mom**·et·re). The process of measuring the degree of strabismus by means of the strabismometer.

strabismus (strab·**iz**·mus). Squint. [Gk *strabismos.*]

strabometer (strab·**om**·et·er). Strabismometer.

strabometry (strab·**om**·et·re). Strabismometry.

strabotome (**strab**·o·tome). A scalpel used especially in ocular tenotomy. [see foll.]

strabotomy (strab·**ot**·o·me). The surgical division of 1 or more of the muscles of the eyeball or their tendons for the correction of strabismus. [strabismus, Gk *temnein* to cut.]

Strachan, William Henry Williams (b. 1857). British physician.

Strachan's disease. A form of polyneuritis observed in Jamaica and described by Strachan; now thought to have been pellagra.

straggling (**strag**·ling). The small variations which occur in the range of charged identical particles of the same initial energy. They arise from the statistical nature of the mechanism of energy loss of a particle in passing through matter. [ME *straken* to roam.]

strain (strane). 1. A subdivision of a species, usually defined in terms of a particular characteristic. 2. To overtax a faculty or part of the body; the result of such an overtaxing. 3. To separate a solid from a liquid in which it is suspended, by passing the latter through a fine mesh of material. **Brunhilde strain.** The prototype strain of type I poliomyelitis virus. (The name is taken from that of a chimpanzee from which the strain was recovered.) **Cardiac strain.** A cardiac disorder that is the direct result of physical strain in a person whose heart was previously normal; an outmoded concept. **Heterologous strain.** A strain with a different antigenic constitution from the type strain. **Homologous strain.** A strain with an identical or very similar antigenic constitution to that of the type strain. **Lansing strain.** The prototype strain of type II poliomyelitis virus. (This strain was isolated from a fatal case of poliomyelitis at Lansing, Michigan.) **Left ventricular strain.** A term sometimes used to indicate the ST and T wave changes that may occur in the electrocardiogram with left ventricular hypertrophy from any cause. There is downward-sloping ST depression which merges smoothly into an inverted T wave in leads I, aVL and the left chest leads. **Leon strain.** The prototype strain of type III poliomyelitis virus. (The name is that of a patient who died of poliomyelitis and from whom the strain was isolated.) **Right ventricular strain.** A term sometimes used to indicate the ST and T wave changes that may occur in the electrocardiogram with right ventricular hypertrophy from any cause. There is downward-sloping ST depression which merges smoothly into an inverted T wave in the right chest leads. **Rough strain.** A strain of bacteria in which the majority of the organisms are in the rough phase. **Sacro-iliac strain.** Strain of the posterior sacro-iliac ligaments causing backache. **Smooth strain.** A strain of bacteria in which the majority of the organisms are in the smooth phase. **Vi strain.** A strain of *Salmonella typhi* or other members of the Enterobacteriaceae carrying a Vi antigen. [ME *streinen.*]

Stramonii Folium. *European Pharmacopoeia* name for Stramonium BP 1973.

Stramonium BP 1973 (stra·**mo**·ne·um). Stramonium leaves, thornapple leaves; the dried leaves and flowering tops of *Datura stramonium* Linn. and *Datura tatula* Linn. (family Solanaceae). It contains the alkaloid, hyoscyamine. [Gk *strychnos* nightshade, *manikos* mad.]

strand (strand). **Lateral enamel strand.** A band of epithelial tissue which forms an additional attachment between the enamel organ and the tooth band. [O Fr. *estran* rope.]

See also: BILLROTH.

Strandberg, James. Swedish dermatologist.

Groenblad-Strandberg syndrome. The association of angioid streaks with pseudoxanthoma elasticum (yellow patches seen on the skin of the neck and flexures).

strangle (**strang**·gl). To compress or constrict the trachea as with a rope or the hands so that respiration is impossible. [L *strangulare* to choke.]

strangling (**strang**·gling). Strangulation.

strangulated (**strang**·gew·la·ted). Of the contents of a hernial sac, having been constricted at the neck, with arrest of the circulation. In general, having had the blood supply interrupted. [L *strangulare* to choke.]

strangulation (strang·gew·**la**·shun). 1. The condition of being strangulated, as e.g. a hernia. 2. Extreme compression or constriction of the trachea or of any part, causing a suspension of respiration or congestion in the part, from which death may result. 3. A state of excessive constriction. **Manual strangulation.** Strangulation by the hand, necessarily either accidental or homicidal, owing to the impossibility of maintaining a self-strangling hold to the moment of death. [see prec.]

stranguria, strangury (strang·**gewr**·e·ah, **strang**·gewr·e). A painful excretion of urine, slowly and drop-by-drop, due to spasmodic contraction of the urethra and bladder. [Gk *stranx* drop, *ouron* urine.]

strap (strap). 1. A strip or band of leather, adhesive plaster or any material used for securing apparatus, in surgical extension of a limb or immobilization of a part of the body. 2. The act of binding or strapping. [AS *stropp.*]

See also: WYMAN.

strapping (**strap**·ing). 1. Application of overlapping strips of adhesive plaster, covering a part and compressing it for the protection of a lesion. 2. The material used in such procedure. [see prec.]

Strasburger, Eduard Adolf (b. 1844). German histologist.

Strasburger's cell plate. A row of granules formed across the equator of a dividing cell just before separation of the daughter cells.

Strassmann, Paul Ferdinand (b. 1866). German gynaecologist.

Strassmann's phenomenon. Pressure on the fundus uteri when the placenta is undelivered and the cord ligated results in distension of the umbilical vein if the placenta is still attached to the uterine wall.

strata (**stra**·tah). *See* STRATUM.

stratification (strat·if·ik·**a**'·shun). Arrangement in layers of strata. [stratum, L *facere* to make.]

stratified (**strat**·e·fide). Formed, laid down or arranged in layers of strata, e.g. in stratified epithelium. [see prec.]

stratiform (**strat**·e·form). 1. Arranged in the form of strata. 2. Composed of layers or strata.

stratigram (**strat**·e·gram). The x-ray radiograph of a selected layer of the body made by stratigraphy.

stratigraphy (strat·**ig**·raf·e). Tomography or body-section radiography. [stratum, Gk *graphein* to record.]

Stratiomyidae (stra·she·o·**mi**'·e·de). A family of brachyceran Diptera, mostly shining metallic flies of medium size. The genus *Hermetia* is of medical interest. [Gk *stratios* warlike, *myia* fly.]

stratum [NA] (**stra**·tum) (pl. *strata*). A layer. **Stratum basale.** The deepest layer of the uterine decidua, containing the narrow terminal portions of the uterine glands. **Stratum compactum.** The innermost layer of the uterine decidua, containing the necks of the uterine glands. **Stratum corneum of the skin.** The outer layer of the epidermis consisting of dead, scaly cells. **Strata of the cortex.** The layers of nerve cells in the cerebral cortex, varying in thickness from one functional region to another. **Stratum germinativum of the skin.** The deepest layer of the epidermis consisting of living polyhedral cells. **Stratum granulosum [NA].** The layer of cells surrounding the ovum and lining the ovarian follicle. **Stratum granulosum of the skin.** The thin layer of polyhedral cells in the epidermis, containing keratohyalin granules, which lies between the stratum germinativum internally and the stratum lucidum externally. **Stratum lucidum of the skin.** The thin, clear layer of dead and dying cells just outside the stratum granulosum of the skin. **Stratum mucosum of the skin.** Stratum germinativum of the skin (see above). **Stratum opticum.** The outermost layer of the retina. **Stratum papillare of the skin.** Corpus papillare. **Stratum spinosum of the skin.** The stratum germinativum of the skin (see above), so termed because of the spines which project from the surface of the cells and connect with neighbouring cells. **Stratum spongiosum.** The middle layer of the uterine decidua, containing dilated portions of the uterine glands. **Stratum spongiosum urethrae of the female urethra.** The vascular erectile tissue deep to the mucous membrane. **Stratum zonale** [NA]. A thin sheet of nerve fibres covering the superior surface of the thalamus. [L.]

See also: ARLT, BECCARI, OEHL.

Straus, Isidore (b. 1845). Strasbourg and Paris pathologist.

Straus' phenomenon or sign. In facial paralysis of central origin equal sweating occurs on the 2 sides of the face after an injection of pilocarpine; if the paralysis is caused by a lesion distal to the facial ganglion, sweating on the affected side is greatly impaired.

Straus' test. A laboratory reaction for the diagnosis of glanders. If a male guinea-pig is inoculated intraperitoneally with pathological material from a case of glanders or with a recently isolated culture of *Pfeifferella mallei*, swelling of the testis is noted. The test is not altogether reliable since swelling may also occur after the injection of *Brucella abortus* and certain other organisms.

Strauss, Hermann (b. 1868). Berlin physician.

Strauss' sign. A projecting shelf in the pouch of Douglas due to a tumour metastasis.

Strauss' test. For lactic acid: to 5 ml of strained gastric contents in a separatory funnel add 20 ml of ether, shake thoroughly and allow to separate. Run off the lower layer completely and discard. To the ether add 20 ml of water and 2 drops of 10 per cent ferric chloride solution, mix gently. If 0.1 per cent of lactic acid or more is present the aqueous layer is coloured an intense greenish yellow.

streak (streek). A line, narrow band, furrow or stripe. **Angioid streaks.** Breaks in Bruch's membrane, seen ophthalmoscopically as brown or red branching streaks around the disc. Sometimes found in association with pseudoxanthoma elasticum, senile elastosis, sickle-cell anaemia or Paget's disease. **Germinal streak.** Primitive streak (see below). **Medullary streak.** The embryonic medullary plate or groove. **Meningitic streak.** Tache cérébrale. **Primitive streak.** A midline thickening of the posterior part of the embryonic disc along which mesodermal cells migrate from the surface to form the middle germ layer. It is formed in various ways; in lower vertebrates, by fusion of the lateral lips of the blastopore; in higher vertebrates, by local proliferation and accumulation of migrating cells. **Reflex streak.** The bright light reflex seen along the fundal vessels when they are examined with an ophthalmoscope. This becomes wider and more pronounced in arteriosclerosis of the vessels. [AS *strica.*]

See also: WEISS (L.).

stream (streem). The steady flow or current of any fluid. **Axial stream.** In a blood vessel, the main concentration of erythrocytes suspended in the middle of the blood stream, with the plasma on either side. **Hair streams [flumina pilorum].** Tracts along which the hairs are regularly arranged in various parts of the body, all hairs in any one tract or stream sloping in the same direction. [AS.]

Streatfield, John Fremlyn (b. 1828). British ophthalmologist.

Streatfield's operation. 1. For entropion: a modification of Snellen's operation; a wedge-shaped strip of tarsus, from 2 to 3 mm wide, with apex deep, is excised along the whole length of the lid, just above the lid margin. The strip of overlying skin and muscle is also excised. It is left unsutured to granulate. 2. For absent or occluded lacrimal punctum: the fellow punctum is dilated and the canaliculus slit up to the sac. A bent wire is then passed up the occluded canaliculus, and by cutting down on the tip of the wire this canaliculus can also be slit. 3. For division of posterior synechia: a small hook is passed into the anterior chamber through a suitable incision and synechiae detached. Obsolete.

streblomicrodactyly (**streb**·lo·mi·kro·**dak**′·til·e). Streptomicrodactyly. [Gk *streblos* crooked, microdactylous.]

strephosymbolia (**stref**·o·sim·**bo**′·le·ah). 1. A condition in which objects seen appear to be reversed as if they are reflected in a mirror. 2. A condition in which the individual has difficulty in learning to read although he has no apparent mental abnormality; alexia. 3. A reversal in the direction of reading. [Gk *strephein* to alter, symbol.]

strepitus (**strep**·it·us). A sound heard on auscultation. **Strepitus aurium.** Tinnitus. **Strepitus coriaceus.** *Bruit de cuir neuf.* **Strepitus uterinus.** Uterine souffle. *See* SOUFFLE. [L loud noise.]

strepsinema (strep·sin·**e**·mah). The chromosomes at that stage of meiosis in which they become closely wrapped together in pairs (pachytene). [Obsolete term.] [Gk *strepsis* twist, *nema* thread.]

strepsitene (**strep**·sit·een). The pachytene stage of meiotic division. [Obsolete term.] [Gk *strepsis* twist, *tainia* ribbon.]

streptamine (**strep**·tam·een). Diamino-tetrahydroxycyclohexane, $NH_2C_6H_6(OH)_4NH_2$. A breakdown product of streptomycin.

strepticaemia (strep·te·**se**·me·ah). Streptococcaemia. [streptococcus, Gk *haima* blood.]

streptidine (**strep**·tid·een). $C_8H_{18}N_6O_4$, a guanidine derivative of cyclohexane produced by the breakdown of streptomycin.

strepto-angina (strep·to·**an**·jin·ah). A false membrane found in the throat as a result of streptococcal infection. [streptococcus, angina.]

streptobacillus (strep·to·bas·**il**′·us). A classificatory term in bacteriology, now obsolete except in so far as it is applied to *Streptobacillus moniliformis.* **Streptobacillus moniliformis.** An organism belonging to the family Bacteroidaceae; it is a Gram-negative pleomorphic bacillus growing in chains and is found in the throat of rats, causing one form of *rat-bite fever* in man, either by a bite or after ingestion of contaminated food (Haverhill fever). [Gk *streptos* curved, bacillus.]

streptobacterin (strep·to·**bak**·ter·in). A general term for any vaccine prepared from streptococci. [streptococcus, bacterin.]

streptococcaemia (strep·to·kok·**se**′·me·ah). The presence of streptococci in the blood. [streptococcus, Gk *haima* blood.]

streptococcal (strep·to·**kok**·al). 1. Relating or belonging to any streptococcus. 2. Caused by infection due to any species of streptococcus.

Streptococceae (strep·to·**kox**·e·e). Collective name for the tribe of organisms including the genera *Leuconostoc, Streptococcus* and *Staphylococcus.* [Gk *streptos* curved, *kokkos* berry.]

streptococcic (strep·to·**kok**·sik). Streptococcal.

streptococcicide (strep·to·**kox**·e·side). Any agent that destroys streptococci. [streptococcus, L *caedere* to kill.]

streptococcicosis (**strep**·to·kox·e·**ko**′·sis). Any infection due to the presence of streptococci. [streptococcus, Gk *-osis* condition.]

streptococcolysin (**strep**·to·kok·**ol**′·is·in). Streptolysin.

Streptococcus (strep·to·**kok**·us). A bacterial genus in the family Lactobacillaceae; they are Gram-positive, spherical or oval cocci, occurring in chains of varying length; most are facultative aerobes but a few species are anaerobic. A useful primary division of the aerobic streptococci is based on the ability to produce a soluble haemolysin; some non-haemolytic species produce partial clearing around individual colonies grown on a blood-agar medium (α-haemolytic). The truly haemolytic strains are divisible into groups on antigenic analysis of the somatic (C) polysaccharide of the cell wall; these groups (named after Rebecca *Lancefield*) are numbered alphabetically from A to R; Lancefield group A streptococci *(Streptococcus pyogenes)* is responsible for over 90 per cent of streptococcal infections in man, the remainder are mostly associated with groups B, C, D and G. Some groups are causally related to infections in cattle, horses, dogs, etc. Group A streptococci may be further subdivided into serotypes (Griffith) on the basis of their surface protein antigens (M, T, R) and this subdivision is useful epidemiologically in tracing sources and modes of spread of infection. The most common streptococcal infections are sore throat and scarlet fever, otitis media, skin infections (impetigo, erysipelas), puerperal fever, wound infections and other suppurative conditions. Acute rheumatic fever may occur as a non-septic sequela of streptococcal sore throat or streptococcal impetigo. Non-haemolytic streptococci, e.g. *S. viridans,* are causally related to subacute bacterial endocarditis. *S. faecalis,* present in the gut, may be associated with urinary tract infections. **Streptococcus faecalis** (Enterococcus). A group D streptococcus arranged in pairs or chains, possessing the ability to grow in the presence of bile salts and resisting heating to 60°C for 30 min. It is found in the human intestine, and is usually resistant to penicillin. **Streptococcus haemolyticus.** *Streptococcus pyogenes.* **Streptococcus mitis.** A strain of streptococcus found in the human mouth. **Streptococcus pneumoniae.** Pneumococcus; ovoid cocci arranged in pairs or short chains, non-motile and sensitive to heat and soluble in bile. The pneumococci are divided into over 70 antigenic types on the basis of their species-specific capsular carbohydrate antigens. It causes pneumonia and certain other infections in man; it is usually sensitive to penicillin. **Streptococcus pyogenes.** This label is usually applied to those strains which fall into Lancefield's group A, and are β-haemolytic. This includes many of the important pathogenic strains for man; they are usually sensitive to penicillin. **Streptococcus viridans.** A coccus similar in morphology and growth requirement to *Streptococcus pyogenes.* It produces a zone of α-haemolysis in blood agar. It commonly causes subacute bacterial endocarditis in man, as well as other minor infections. [Gk *streptos* curved, *kokkos* berry.]

streptocolysin (strep·to·**kol**·is·in). Streptococcolysin.

streptoderma (strep·to·**der**·mah). A skin lesion due to streptococci. [streptococcus, Gk *derma* skin.]

streptodermatitis (**strep**·to·der·mat·**i**'·tis). Dermatitis due to the presence of streptococci.

Streptodornase (strep·to·**dor**·naze). BP Commission approved name for an enzyme obtained from cultures of various strains of *Streptococcus haemolyticus* and capable of catalysing the depolymerization of polymerized deoxyribonucleoproteins.

Streptoduocin (strep·to·**dew**·o·sin). BP Commission approved name for a mixture of streptomycin sulphate and dihydrostreptomycin sulphate. It is used in the treatment of tuberculosis and non-tuberculous infections which do not respond to penicillin.

Streptokinase (strep·to·**kin**·aze). BP Commission approved name for an enzyme obtained from cultures of various strains of *Streptococcus haemolyticus* and capable of changing plasminogen into plasmin. [streptococcus, Gk *kinein* to move.]

streptolysin (strep·**tol**·is·in). Two haemolytic toxins are produced by *Streptococcus pyogenes: Streptolysin O* which is antigenic and oxygen labile, and *Streptolysin S* which is antigenic only when present in the whole organism (see TEST: *Antistreptolysin O test*). [Gk *streptos* curved, *kokkos* berry, *lysein* to loosen.]

Streptomicini Sulfas (strep·to·**mi**·sin·i **sul**·fas). *European Pharmacopoeia* name for Streptomycin Sulphate BP 1973.

streptomicrodactylia (**strep**·to·mi·kro·dak·**til**'·e·ah). Permanent immobility of 1 or more flexed joints, affecting the little fingers only. [Gk *streptos* curved, microdactylia.]

Streptomyces (strep·to·**mi**·seez). A genus of the family Streptomycetaceae, several species of which were the original sources of certain antibiotics. The species *Streptomyces madurae, S. pelletieri, S. somaliensis* are causative agents of actinomycotic mycetoma in man. **Streptomyces albus.** The source of actinomycetin. **Streptomyces ambofaciens.** The antibiotic, spiramycin, is obtained from growth of this species. **Streptomyces antibioticus.** The source of actinomycin; *Actinomyces (Streptothrix) antibioticus.* **Streptomyces argillaceus.** A source of the antibiotic, mithramycin. **Streptomyces aureofaciens.** A species which is the source of aureomycin. **Streptomyces caeruleorubidus.** A species from which the antibiotic, daunorubicin, is obtained. **Streptomyces canus.** The species from which amphomycin is obtained. **Streptomyces capreolus.** The species from which capreomycin is obtained. **Streptomyces chrysomallus.** A source of antinomycin. **Streptomyces decaris.** The species from which framycetin is obtained. **Streptomyces fradiae.** The species from which the antibiotic, neomycin, is obtained. **Streptomyces griseus.** A species from which streptomycin was obtained. **Streptomyces hachijoensis.** The source of the antibiotic, hachimycin. **Streptomyces halstedi.** A soil actinomycete from which carbomycin is obtained. **Streptomyces hygroscopicus** var. **azalomyceticus.** The species from which azalomycin is obtained. **Streptomyces kanamyceticus.** The species from which kanamycin is obtained. **Streptomyces lincolnensis.** The species from which the antibiotic, lincomycin, is obtained. **Streptomyces mediterranei.** The species from which rifamycin is obtained. **Streptomyces mitakaensis.** The source of the antibiotic, mikamycin. **Streptomyces natalensis.** The source of the antibiotic, natamycin. **Streptomyces niveus.** A source of the antibiotic, novobiocin. **Streptomyces nodosus.** The source of the antibiotic, amphotericin. **Streptomyces orientalis.** The source of vancomycin. **Streptomyces peuceticus** var. **caesius.** The species from which doxorubicin is produced. **Streptomyces pristina spiralis.** The source of the antibiotic, pristinamycin. **Streptomyces rimosus.** The source of oxytetracycline. **Streptomyces rufochromogenus.** The source of the antibiotic, rufocromomycin. **Streptomyces spectabilis.** The species from which spectinomycin is obtained. **Streptomyces tanashiensis.** A source of the antibiotic, mithramycin. **Streptomyces tenebrarius.** The species from which the antibiotic tobramycin is obtained. **Streptomyces venezuelae.** The mould from which chloramphenicol was prepared. **Streptomyces verticillus.** The species from which bleomycin is produced. **Streptomyces virginiae.** The source of the antibiotic, virginiamycin. [Gk *streptos* curved, *mykes* fungus.]

Streptomycetaceae (**strep**·to·mi·set·**a**'·se·e). A family of the Actinomycetes of which *Streptomyces* is a genus. [Gk *streptos* curved, *mykes* fungus.]

streptomycin (strep·to·**mi**·sin). A group of antibiotics produced by cultures of *Streptomyces griseus.* Streptomycin, $C_{21}H_{37}N_7O_{12}$, is effective in the treatment of a large number of infections, but primarily in tuberculosis. Its 2 main disadvantages are its tendency to produce streptomycin-resistant strains of organisms, and the toxic effects occurring from its administration over prolonged periods. For these reasons streptomycin is usually restricted to the combating of penicillin-resistant organisms apart from its use in pulmonary and miliary tuberculosis and tuberculous meningitis, where its employment has revolutionized the prognosis of these diseases. **Streptomycin Sulphate BP 1973.** The most suitable salt of streptomycin. When streptomycin is prescribed, streptomycin sulphate is dispensed.

streptomycosis (**strep**·to·mi·**ko**'·sis). An infection caused by micro-organisms of the genus *Streptomyces.* [*Streptomyces,* Gk *-osis* condition.]

Streptonicozid (strep·to·**nik**·o·zid). BP Commission approved name for a chemical compound of streptomycin and isonicotinic acid hydrazide, used in tuberculosis therapy.

Streptopus amplexifolius (**strep**·to·pus **am**·plex·e·**fo**'·le·us). A plant of the family Liliaceae. The seeds are used to prepare an astringent gargle; the root is used in salads. [Gk *streptos* curved, *pous* foot, L *amplexus* embrace, *folium* leaf.]

streptosepticaemia (**strep**·to·sep·te·**se**'·me·ah). Septicaemia which is due to streptococci.

streptothrichal (strep·to·**thrik**·al). Pertaining to or due to the presence of a streptothrix.

streptothricin (strep·to·**thri**·sin). An antibiotic substance derived from culture filtrates of *Actinomyces lavendulae.* It is soluble in water and dilute mineral acids but not in ether or chloroform. It is inactivated by concentrated mineral acids but unaffected by blood, peptone or vitamin B and will withstand boiling for 15 min. It is bacteriocidal as well as bacteriostatic. It is active against both Gram-positive and Gram-negative bacteria. [*Streptothrix.*]

Streptothrix (**strep**·to·thrix). A genus of bacteria, the pathogenic species of which have been transferred to other genera, *Actinomyces* or *Fusiformis.* **Streptothrix moniliformis, Streptothrix muris ratti.** *Actinomyces muris.* [Gk *streptos* curved, *thrix* hair.]

See also: SCHOTTMUELLER.

streptothrycin (strep·to·**thri**·sin). Streptothricin.

stress (stres). 1. Any potentially damaging strain, force or agent, which stimulates a physiological defence reaction and is capable under certain circumstances of producing pathological lesions. Adaptations to the various kinds of stress to which man is exposed is a condition of his survival, and in the course of evolution defence mechanisms have become part of his physiology. It is considered (Selye) that a living organism responds to stress by the same basic reaction, irrespective of the nature of the agent causing the stress. This basic reaction is complicated by other features which are specific to the particular stress or agents; these may be climatic, traumatic, allergic, surgical, obstetric, infective, toxic, etc. *See* GENERAL ADAPTATION SYNDROME and SELYE'S HYPOTHESIS. 2. In dentistry, the pressure exerted by the teeth of one jaw on those of the other during biting and mastication. [O Fr. *estrecier.*]

stretch (strech). 1. To lengthen or make broader by extending or drawing out. 2. To strain, tense or over-extend. 3. To distend forcibly. 4. The farthest distance to which a limb may be extended from the body or one limb separated from the other corresponding limb. [AS *streccan.*]

stretcher (stretch·er). An appliance, often of canvas, stretched on an oblong wooden or metal frame with a handle at each corner, used to carry sick or disabled persons. [see prec.]

stria [NA] (stri·ah). A line, thin band, streak or stripe. **Stria atrophica.** One of the whitish, wrinkled scars on the skin of the abdomen and elsewhere, caused by gross stretching of the skin and rupture of the elastic fibres, as in pregnancy or obesity. Before delivery they are pinkish in colour but this fades during the post-partum period. **Auditory striae [striae medullares ventriculi quarti (NA)].** Conspicuous bundles crossing each half of the floor of the 4th ventricle at its widest part. **Brown striae.** Retzius' parallel striae. **Striae ciliares.** Narrow striae running on the surface of the ciliary body from the ora serrata to between the ciliary processes. **Stria cutis distensae, Striae of distension.** Stria atrophica (see above). **Stria gravidarum.** Stria atrophica (see above). **Stria habenularis of the thalamus [stria medullaris thalami (NA)].** A band of white fibres running along the junction of the medial and superior surfaces of the thalamus; its fibres end in both habenular nuclei. **Longitudinal stria, lateral [stria longitudinalis lateralis (NA)].** Anteroposteriorly running white fibres in the floor of the callosal sulcus, forming part of the rhinencephalon. **Longitudinal stria, medial [stria longitudinalis medialis (NA)].** Anteroposteriorly running white fibres on the surface of the corpus callosum, forming part of the rhinencephalon. **Stria mallearis [NA].** The line of attachment of the manubrium of the malleus to the tympanic membrane. **Stria medullaris [NA].** A thin band of white matter subdividing a mass of grey matter in the central nervous system. **Meningitic stria.** Tache cérébrale. **Olfactory stria [stria olfactoria (NA)].** Any one of the medial, intermediate or lateral roots of the olfactory tract. **Retinal stria.** 1. Angioid streaks. 2. White concentric lines sometimes seen in the fundus in retinal detachment and situated where the retina has become reattached; a sort of high-water mark. **Stria semicircularis [stria terminalis (NA)].** A bundle of white fibres running from the amygdaloid nucleus along the roof of the inferior horn and then in a groove between the caudate nucleus and the thalamus, partly to the anterior commissure and partly to the hypothalamus. **Stria vascularis [NA].** A network of blood vessels beneath the periosteum above the crista basilaris of the cochlea. [L furrow.]

See also: AMICI, BAILLARGER, FRANCKE, FROMMANN, GENNARI, GIACOMINI, HEIDENHAIN, LANCISI, LANGHANS, LIESEGANG, NITABUCH, PRUSSAK, RETZIUS (M. G.), ROHR, SCHREGER, WICKHAM.

striatal (stri·a·tal). Relating or belonging to the corpus striatum.

striate (stri·ate). 1. Marked in parallel with striae; striped. 2. Bearing structural lines, as a fibre. 3. Associated with any striated structure.

striate vein [vena striata (NA)]. A tributary of the basal vein, draining the part of the corpus striatum adjacent to the anterior perforated substance.

striation (stri·a·shun). 1. The presence of stripes. 2. One or more streaks or scratches. 3. A structure characterized by numerous striae. *See* BAILLARGER. **Tabby-cat striation, Tigroid striation.** Streaking or mottling on muscles which have undergone adipose degeneration, particularly the heart muscle. [stria.]

See also: BAILLARGER.

striatum (stri·a·tum). Term applied to those elements of the corpus striatum that have a common origin and structure, the caudate nucleus and putamen.

stricture (strik·tewr, strik·tcher). The narrowing of a duct or passage. It varies in length and in degree, and may be due to a variety of causes, e.g. congenital, inflammatory, neoplastic. **Anal stricture.** Stricture of the anal orifice or of the anal canal, due most often to congenital causes or following an operation for haemorrhoids or fissure. **Annular stricture.** A stricture affecting the entire circumference of a passage, e.g. colon. **Bridle stricture.** A stricture in which a band of tissue crosses the lumen narrowing it; seen almost only in the urethra. **Cicatricial stricture.** A narrowing by scar tissue, e.g. after a corrosive burn of the oesophagus or injury to the urethra. **Common-bile-duct stricture.** A stricture due most often to injury to the duct during the course of a cholecystectomy: a most intractable condition. **Congestive stricture.** A localized ureteral spasm, ureteritis or constriction of the ureter, described by Hunner in 1911. The histological changes associated with the condition are minimal, but may lead to alterations in the sensitivity of the ureter which may give rise to pain. **Contractile stricture.** One which can be dilated instrumentally but which promptly relapses. **False stricture, Functional stricture.** Spasmodic stricture (see below). **Hourglass stricture.** That due to a double stricture, 2 dilated spaces resulting, connected by a narrow segment. **Hysterical stricture.** A hysterical manifestation when there is dysphagia without any apparent oesophageal obstructions; globus hystericus. **Impassable stricture, Impermeable stricture.** A stricture which resists every effort to negotiate it with even the finest of probes. **Irregular stricture.** An uneven stricture which is usually difficult to negotiate. **Irritable stricture.** A stricture where spasm and discomfort follow attempts at instrumentation. **Linear stricture.** A stricture where only one aspect of the channel is affected, and that over some length. **Oesophagus stricture.** That commonly due to the swallowing of corrosive substances; it may also follow operation. **Organic stricture.** A stricture where structural, and usually irreversible, changes have occurred in the wall. **Passable stricture.** A stricture which can be negotiated by an instrument. **Permanent stricture.** Organic stricture (see above). **Permeable stricture.** Passable stricture (see above). **Rectal stricture.** A stricture of the rectum, such as may follow lymphogranuloma, radiation, operation or cancer. **Ring stricture.** Annular stricture (see above). **Spasmodic stricture, Spastic stricture.** A stricture where there is no organic change but only muscle spasm. **String stricture.** A term commonly applied to the narrowing of a short segment of the colon, found in some cases of cancer of the colon. **Temporary stricture.** Spasmodic stricture (see above). **Tortuous stricture.** A stricture which leads to a tortuous channel. **Ureteral stricture.** A stricture of the ureter most often due to tuberculosis, less often to stone or to injury at operation (e.g. hysterectomy). **Urethral stricture.** A form of stricture common only in the male; it often follows gonorrhoea, instrumentation or injury. **Valvular stricture.** One where there is usually only a fibrous fold, which allows fluid to pass in 1 direction only. [L *strictura* compression.]

See also: HUNNER.

strident (stri·dent). Harsh and grating in sound; stridulous. [L *stridere* to make a harsh sound.]

stridor (stri·dor). The loud, harsh, vibrating sound produced by partial obstruction of the larynx or trachea. **Congenital stridor, Congenital laryngeal stridor.** An inspiratory stridor in a newborn infant, caused by a congenital defect of the upper aperture of the larynx combined with flaccidity so that the parts are sucked together during inspiration. It tends to disappear after 12 months or so. **Stridor decutium, Stridor dentium.** The noise produced by grinding the teeth. **Inspiratory stridor.** Stridor occurring on inspiration only. **Laryngeal stridor.** Stridor caused by laryngeal spasm, usually associated with simple catarrhal laryngitis, in young children. **Stridor serraticus.** The sound produced by breathing through a tracheotomy tube resembling that of filing a saw. **Thymic stridor.** Stridor produced by pressure of an enlarged thymus gland upon the trachea. [L.]

stridulous (**strid**·ew·lus). 1. Relating to or affected with stridor. 2. Having a creaking or hissing sound. [L *stridulus* creaking.]

Strigeata (strij·e·a·tah). A sub-order of the trematode order Prostomata. The super-families Schistosomatoidea and Strigeoidea are of medical interest. [L *strigatus* striped.]

Strigeidae (strij·e·i·de). A family of Trematoda of the sub-order Strigeoidea. The genus *Prohemistomum* is of medical interest. [see foll.]

Strigeoidea (strij·e·**oid**·e·ah). A super-family of the trematode sub-order Strigeata, or a sub-order of the order Prostomata. The family Strigeidae in the super-family, and the families Schistosomatidae and Strigeidae in the sub-order, are of medical interest. [Strigeata, Gk *eidos* form.]

stringent (**strin**·jent). 1. Drawing tight; binding. 2. Restrictive, rigid. [L *stringere* to bind tight.]

striocellular (stri·o·**sel**·ew·lar). 1. Relating or belonging to striped muscle fibres and cells. 2. Made up of striated tissue. [stria, cell.]

striocerebellar (**stri**·o·ser·e·**bel**'·ar). Relating or belonging to the corpus striatum and the cerebellum.

striomuscular (stri·o·**mus**·kew·lar). Consisting of striated muscle.

striospinoneural (**stri**·o·spi·no·**newr**'·al). Applied to a system of nerve fibres which passes through the corpus striatum and the spinal cord. [corpus striatum, spinal cord, Gk *neuron* nerve.]

strip (strip). **Bimetallic strip.** A strip of 2 metals with different coefficients of expansion, used for temperature compensation in vaporizers for volatile anaesthetics. [LG *strippe* strap.]

stripe (stripe). A streak; a stria. **Colliers' stripes.** Blue-grey linear stripes in the skin caused by inground coal dust. [Middle D.]

See also: BAILLARGER, D'AZYR, GENNARI, HENSEN, MEES.

stripper (**strip**·er). *See* MASSON. [see foll.]

stripping (**strip**·ing). Uncovering; unsheathing; the expressing of the contents from a flexible tube or canal such as the urethra, by passing the finger along it. **Stripping of the pleura.** In thoracic surgery the removal of part of the pleura. The term is also used for the removal of the lining membrane of the thorax of an animal, by meat vendors, to obliterate any evidence of pulmonary tuberculosis or inflammation of the pleura. [AS *strypan* to rob.]

strobic (**stro**·bik). Associated with spinning like a top. [Gk *strobos* whirling.]

strobila (stro·**bi**·lah). The adult form of tapeworms, consisting of scolex, neck, proliferating region and proglottides. The first proglottides behind the region of proliferation are small, those behind becoming progressively larger. The number varies from 3 to 4 up to many hundreds; each is a protandrous hermaphrodite, and the ultimate ones are filled with the enlarged uterus containing embryos. Each proglottis contains discrete reproductive and muscular systems, but there is a continuity of nervous and excretory systems. [Gk *strobile* twist.]

strobilation (stro·bil·**a**·shun). Segmentation of the type found in the body of a tapeworm. [Gk *strobile* twist.]

strobilization (**stro**·bil·i·**za**'·shun). The formation of a strobila in a tapeworm by budding off new proglottides at the region of proliferation.

strobiloid (**stro**·bil·oid). Having the appearance of a twisted chain, e.g. tapeworm segments. [Gk *strobile* twist, *eidos* form.]

stroboscope (**stro**·bo·skope). Any instrument for studying or observing the successive phases of any body which is in a state of periodic vibration, by means of interrupted light falling on the object. In this way it appears to slow down the rate of vibration. [Gk *strobos* whirling, *skopein* to view.]

stroboscopic (stro·bo·**skop**·ik). Relating or belonging to the stroboscope.

strobostereoscope (stro·bo·**steer**·e·o·skope). Stereostroboscope.

Stroebe's aniline blue method. A method for the staining of nerve fibres in sections employing aniline blue, differentiation in potassium hydroxide and counterstaining with safranine.

Stroganov, Vasilii Vasilyevich (b. 1857). Russian obstetrician.

Stroganov's treatment. A method of treating eclampsia with morphine and magnesium sulphate.

stroke (stroke). A sudden seizure; the commonly used lay term for apoplexy. **Apoplectic stroke.** An attack of apoplexy. **Back stroke.** The recoil of the ventricles of the heart at the time of ejection of blood. **Cold stroke.** Drowsiness, a fall of body temperature and coma, due to exposure to cold. At low temperatures the dissociation of oxyhaemoglobin is greatly impaired and there is consequent oxygen starvation of the tissues, especially of the brain. **Heat stroke.** A breakdown of the temperature-regulating mechanism due to climatic conditions of exposure to heat and humidity, and being distinguished from heat exhaustion due to prolonged sweating and chloride depletion in those working in buildings, ships' holds, mines, etc. **Light stroke.** Narcosis or death following the exposure to light of sensitized animals. **Lightning stroke.** Shock, muscular spasms and coma, caused by severe damage to the nervous system by lightning. **Paralytic stroke.** A sudden attack of paralysis due to disease or injury of the brain or spinal cord. [AS *strac.*]

stroma (NA) (**stro**·mah). The connective-tissue basis or framework of an organ. **Stroma of the erythrocytes.** The non-pigmented, protein framework of the erythrocyte that forms the disintegrated residue after removal of the haemoglobin. **Stroma of the iris [stroma iridis** (NA)**].** The connective-tissue basis of the iris. **Stroma of the ovary [stroma ovarii** (NA)**].** The framework in which the ovarian follicles are embedded, richly vascular and composed of spindle-shaped cells and a small amount of connective tissue. **Stroma of the thyroid gland [stroma glandulae thyroideae** (NA)**].** *See* THYROID GLAND. **Stroma of the vitreous body [stroma vitreum**(NA)**].** The framework of the vitreous, believed to be prolonged inwards from the hyaloid membrane. [Gk covering.]

See also: HIS (W. SNR.), ROLLET (A.).

stromal, stromatic (**stro**·mal, stro·**mat**·ik). Of the nature of or belonging to stroma.

stromatin (**stro**·mat·in). The protein of which stroma is formed.

stromatogenous (stro·mat·**oj**·en·us). Originating from connective tissue. [Gk *stroma* covering, *genein* to produce.]

stromatolysis (stro·mat·**ol**·is·is). Destruction by solution of the stroma of a cell, such as a red cell during haemolysis. [stroma, Gk *lysein* to loosen.]

Stromeyer, Georg Friedrich Ludwig (b. 1804). German surgeon.

Stromeyer's cephalhaematocele. Cephalhaematoma communicating with the intracranial venous sinuses and so distending on straining.

Stromeyer's operation. For strabotomy; obsolete.

Stromeyer-Little operation. Evacuation of a chronic liver abscess which is located by a cannula and incised by a knife introduced alongside the cannula.

stromuhr (**shtro**·moor). The instrument devised by Ludwig for measuring the velocity of the blood flow; rheometer. [G stream clock.]

Strong, Frank Morgan (b. 1908). Wisconsin biochemist.

Snell-Strong method. For riboflavine. A microbiological method in which the growth stimulation of *Lactobacillus casei* is measured by titration of the acid produced by the organism in a basal medium to which extract of the sample has been added.

Strong, Richard Pearson (b. 1872). Harvard physician and parasitologist.

Strong's cholera vaccine. A vaccine made from nucleoproteins of *Vibrio cholerae.*

Strongylata (stron·jil·a·tah). A sub-order of the nematode order Rhabditata. The super-families Metastrongyloidea, Strongyloidea and Trichostrongyloidea are of medical interest. It is sometimes treated as an order. [Gk *stroggylos* round.]

strongyliasis (stron·jil·i·as·is). A morbid condition due to infestation with a species of *Strongylus.*

Strongylidae (stron·jil·id·e). A family of the nematode super-family or sub-order Strongyloidea. The genera *Oesophagostomum* and *Ternidens* are of medical interest. [Gk *stroggylos* round, *eidos* form.]

strongyliform (stron·jil·e·form). Of larval hookworms, having resemblance to *Strongylus;* characteristic of third instar larvae. [Gk *stroggylos* round, form.]

Strongyloidea (stron·jil·oid·e·ah). A super-family or sub-order of the nematode sub-order or order Strongylata. The families Ancylostomidae, Strongylidae and Syngamidae are of medical interest. [see foll.]

Strongyloides (stron·jil·oid·eez). A genus of nematode worms. **Strongyloides fullerborne.** A species that rarely infects man. **Strongyloides stercoralis.** A small, very common intestinal parasite of man in tropical and subtropical regions. The adults occur anywhere in the intestinal canal, burrowing in the mucosa and, when numerous, causing severe damage. Eggs, passed in the faeces, hatch into rhabditiform larvae which may develop in either of 2 ways: in direct (homogenic) development they moult into a filariform larva which is retained in the rhabditiform cast until opportunity occurs to penetrate the skin; in indirect (heterogenic) development the rhabditiform larvae produce free-living males and females. These latter lay eggs which hatch to rhabditiform larvae which produce the infective filariform stage. These larvae migrate to the lungs, where they may cause haemorrhage, and thence to the intestine. Occasionally rhabditiform larvae moult to become invasive filariform larvae within the colon or on the perianal skin, penetrate the skin and wander through it to give a linear urticarial rash called *larva currens.* [Gk *stroggylos* round, *eidos* form.]

strongyloidiasis, strongyloidosis (stron·jil·oid·i′·as·is, stron·jil·oid·o′·sis). Infection with *Strongyloides stercoralis.* [*Strongyloides,* Gk *-osis* condition.]

strongyloplasm (stron·jil·o·plazm). An obsolete synonym for a virus. [Gk *stroggylos* round, *plasma* anything formed.]

strongylosis (stron·jil·o·sis). Strongyliasis.

Strongylus (stron·jil·us). A genus of hookworms. The species are parasitic in horses and their relatives, not in man. The name has been used in the past for numerous species which do not belong to it. [Gk *stroggylos* round.]

strontia, strontian (stron·she·ah, stron·she·an). Strontium oxide, SrO, one of the alkaline earths.

strontium (stron·she·um, stron·te·um). An element of atomic weight 87.62, atomic number 38 and chemical symbol Sr. It is a metal of the alkaline earths, similar to calcium in chemical properties, and occurring in the minerals strontianite ($SrCO_3$) and celestine ($SrSO_4$). It is present in sea-water and hence occurs in the ash of marine plants; it has also been found in minute quantities in the human tissues. The salts have been used in medicine, but their use is now obsolete; they are of importance in the manufacture of pyrotechnics and in the refining of sugar. **Strontium bromide.** $SrBr_2$, a colourless deliquescent crystalline substance with a bitter taste; it has the general actions of the bromides. **Strontium iodide.** SrI_2, a colourless deliquescent crystalline substance which has the general actions of the iodides. **Strontium oxide.** SrO, one of the alkaline earths. [*Strontian,* Scotland, the place where the mineral carbonate was first found.]

strophanthidin (stro·fan·thid·in). A steroid aglycone occurring in *Strophanthus* species and in lily-of-the-valley.

strophanthin (stro·fan·thin). Usually refers to *strophanthin-K,* a mixture of glycosides from the seeds of *Strophanthus kombé* of varying composition and requiring biological assay; it may also refer to *strophanthin-G,* ouabain, a pure crystalline glycoside from *S. gratus* or *strophanthin-H,* a glycoside from *S. hispidus.* The pharmacological actions are identical with those of digitalis but more rapid and more transient: when rapid digitalization is demanded, either of the strophanthins may be injected intravenously and are to be preferred to digitalis, especially as there is less danger of a cumulative effect.

strophanthobiose (stro·fan·tho·bi′·oze). $C_{12}H_{22}O_{11}$, a disaccharide occurring in strophanthus glycosides.

Strophanthus (stro·fan·thus). A genus of plants of Africa and Asia (family Apocyanaceae). **Brown strophanthus.** The seeds of *Strophanthus hispidus* D.C. which contain strophanthin-H. **Strophanthus gratus.** A species found in East Africa, the seeds of which are a source of ouabain. **Green strophanthus.** The dried ripe seed of *Strophanthus kombé* Oliver freed from the awns. It contains strophanthin-K, a mixture of cardiac glycosides. **Strophanthus sarmentosus.** A species found in East Africa, the seeds of which yield sarmentogenin. [Gk *strophe* twist, *anthos* flower.]

strophocephalus (stro·fo·kef·al·us). A monster in which there is distortion or displacement of portions of the face and head. [Gk *strophe* twist, *kephale* head.]

strophocephaly (stro·fo·kef·al·e). The condition of a strophocephalus.

strophulus (strof·ew·lus). A name seldom used now. It had various meanings, including milium, prickly heat, papular urticaria. **Strophulus albidus.** Grutum. **Strophulus infantum.** Heat rash; red gum; a sweat rash resembling miliaria, occurring in infants and children in temperate climates. **Strophulus pruriginosus** (Hardy). Hebra's prurigo. [dim. of Gk *strophos* colic, with which these symptoms were associated.]

Stroud, Bert Brenette (fl. 1896). American physiologist.

Stroud's pecten or pectinated area. The area of anal mucosa between the anal valves and the mucocutaneous junction in the anal canal.

structure (struk·tewr, struk·tcher). 1. The arrangement of the component parts and constituent tissues of an organism. 2. The way in which a part is constructed. 3. Any formation, tissue or organ composed of related parts. **Alveolar structure.** One that has small, shallow depressions or alveoli, as in the gastric mucosa. **Primary structure.** The first level of organization of protein or nucleic acid molecules; the amino-acid sequence of a polypeptide and the nucleotide sequence of a polynucleotide. **Quaternary structure.** The fourth level of organization of those proteins which exist, in the native state, as aggregates of more than one polypeptide chain that are not linked to each other by disulphide bonds or by any other type of covalent linkage. **Secondary structure.** The second level of organization of a protein or nucleic acid molecule. In proteins it is determined by the components of the peptide bonds forming hydrogen bonds which may be *intermolecular* and give rise to a pleated sheet structure, or *intramolecular* and give rise to a helical structure. In nucleic acids it results from hydrogen bonds between complementary base pairs and may also be inter- or intra-molecular. **Tertiary structure.** The third level of organization of proteins; it results from the properties of the amino-acid side chains and the formation of globular or fibrous shapes. [L *structura* arrangement.]

Struempell, Ernst Adolf Gustav Gottfried von (b. 1853). Leipzig neurologist.

Struempell's disease, Struempell-Leichtenstern disease. Acute encephalitis of infancy; acute polioencephalitis.

Struempell phenomenon or reflex. Struempell's sign, 1st def.

Struempell's sign. 1. In a leg showing spastic paralysis, when the thigh is flexed, dorsiflexion and eversion of the foot occur; also called the *tibialis sign.* 2. In hemiplegia the fist cannot be closed on the affected side without marked extension of the wrist; also called the *radialis sign.* 3. In hemiplegia passive flexion of the forearm causes pronation of the arm; also called the *pronation sign.*

Struempell's type. Familial spastic paraplegia.

Fleischer–Struempell ring. Kayser–Fleischer ring.

Marie–Struempell arthritis, disease or spondylitis, Struempell–Marie disease. Ankylosing spondylitis, spondylitis ankylopoietica; sometimes known as *rheumatoid spondylitis.*

Marie–Struempell polio-encephalitis. Acute infantile hemiplegia.

Struempell–Westphal pseudosclerosis, Westphal–Struempell

disease. Pseudosclerosis spastica; hysteria with symptoms of disseminated sclerosis.

struggle (strugl). Violent movements of the body and limbs. They may be produced voluntarily, as in an attempt to overcome resistance, or involuntarily, as in convulsive fits. **Death struggle.** Convulsive movements immediately preceding death, as in cases of asphyxia, strychnine poisoning, etc. [ME *strogelen.*]

struma (**stroom**·ah). An obsolescent term which has been used with 2 different meanings. 1. The equivalent of goitre. 2. The equivalent of scrofula; tuberculous swellings of the lymph glands which caseate, break down and discharge, so forming fistulous channels. **Struma aberranta.** Goitre of an accessory thyroid gland. **Adrenal struma.** Adenoma of the suprarenal gland. **Struma aneurysmatica.** A very vascular goitre with dilated pulsating arteries. **Struma basedowificata.** Toxic goitre; exophthalmic goitre. **Struma calculosa.** A calcified goitre. **Struma colloides.** Colloid goitre. **Struma colloides cystica.** Colloid goitre showing many cysts. **Struma congenita.** Congenital goitre. **Struma cystica ossea.** A goitre showing bone formation. **Struma endothoracica.** A substernal goitre. **Struma fibrosa.** A goitre with fibrous hyperplasia. **Struma follicularis.** Parenchymatous goitre. **Struma gelatinosa.** Colloid goitre. **Struma lingualis.** Persisting thyroid glandular tissue in the caecal foramen of the tongue. **Struma lymphomatosa.** Hashimoto's goitre; a goitre with considerable lymphatic tissue, going on to fibrosis and atrophy. **Struma maligna.** Carcinoma of the thyroid. **Struma mollis.** Parenchymatous goitre. **Struma nodosa.** A nodular adenoma of the thyroid. **Struma ovarii.** A very rare teratoma in which the predominant tissue is thyroid and which secretes thyroid hormones. **Struma postbranchialis.** A thyroid cancer whose component cells suggest their origin from remnants of the lateral thyroid anlage or postbranchial body. **Retrosternal struma, Substernal struma.** An enlarged thyroid behind the upper part of the sternum. **Thymus struma.** An enlarged persistent thymus gland. **Struma vasculosa.** A very vascular goitre. [L a scrofulous tumour.]

See also: HASHIMOTO, RIEDEL.

strumectomy (stroom·**ek**·to·me). 1. Excision of a goitre or of all or a part of a goitrous tumour. 2. Excision of a scrofulous gland. **Median strumectomy.** Excision of the enlarged median portion of a thyroid gland or of a hypertrophied isthmus. [struma, Gk *ektome* a cutting out.]

strumiform (**stroom**·e·form). Having resemblance to scrofula or goitre. [struma, form.]

strumiprival, strumiprivic, strumiprivous (stroom·e·**pri**·val, stroom·e·**pri**·vik, stroom·e·**pri**·vus). Term applied to the constitutional state or to symptoms resulting from surgical removal of a goitre. [struma, L *privare* to deprive of.]

strumitis (stroom·**i**·tis). Inflammation of a goitrous thyroid gland. [struma, Gk *-itis* inflammation.]

strumoderma (stroom·o·**der**·mah). Scrofuloderma. [struma, Gk *derma* skin.]

strumose (**stroom**·oze). 1. Having an enlargement on one side. 2. Protruding like a sebaceous cyst. [struma.]

strumositas (stroom·**os**·it·as). 1. The strumous diathesis. 2. The goitrous diathesis. [struma.]

strumous (**stroom**·us). 1. Scrofulous. 2. Relating or belonging to, or suffering from goitre. [struma.]

Struthers, Sir John (b. 1823). Aberdeen anatomist.

Struthers' ligament. A fibrous band sometimes seen passing from the lowest attachment of the coracobrachialis muscle to the medial epicondyle of the humerus. It occasionally contains muscle fibres. It may be considered to represent the vestige of coracobrachialis muscle of primates.

Strutt, John William (Lord Rayleigh). *See* RAYLEIGH.

struxine (**strux**·een). $C_{21}H_{30}O_4N_2$, a decomposition product of strychnine or brucine, obtainable from spoilt nux vomica seeds.

strychnia (**strik**·ne·ah). Strychnine.

strychnicine (**strik**·nis·een). A white crystalline alkaloid obtained from the leaves of *Strychnos nux-vomica* Linn. (family Loganiaceae). It is slightly poisonous.

Strychnine BPC 1959 (**strik**·neen). $C_{21}H_{22}O_2N_2$, an alkaloid obtained from nux vomica, the seeds of various species of *Strychnos.* It occurs as colourless crystals or as a white crystalline powder, with an extremely bitter taste. It has a powerful stimulant effect on the central nervous system, particularly on the spinal cord, and, to a less degree, on the medulla. Toxic amounts of strychnine cause convulsions, and death may occur from subsequent medullary depression. In therapeutics, strychnine preparations are used internally as bitters, to stimulate the appetite (generally as the tincture of nux vomica) or for their supposed "tonic" action, for which there is no rational basis. Strychnine salts are sometimes used parenterally in the treatment of barbiturate poisoning, though they have been largely superseded by picrotoxin for this purpose. **Strychnine Hydrochloride BP 1958.** $C_{21}H_{22}O_2N_2HCl$, a colourless crystalline substance with a very bitter taste. Its actions and uses are those of strychnine. **Iron, quinine and strychnine citrate.** A green or yellow deliquescent scaly preparation, containing approximately 1 per cent of strychnine, and used as a haematinic and bitter. **Iron and strychnine citrate.** A green, scaly preparation containing about 1 per cent of strychnine, employed as a haematinic and bitter. **Strychnine Sulphate BPC 1959.** $C_{21}H_{22}O_2N_2H_2SO_4$, a colourless or white crystalline substance with a very bitter taste. Its actions and uses are those of strychnine. [Gk *strychnos* nightshade.]

strychninism (**strik**·nin·izm). The condition of ill health that results from overuse of strychnine.

strychninization (**strik**·nin·i·za'·shun). Induction of the state of strychninism.

strychninum (strik·**ni**·num). Strychnine. [L.]

strychnism (**strik**·nizm). Strychninism.

Strychnos (**strik**·nos). A genus of loganaceous tropical trees with very poisonous seeds. Species yield nux vomica seeds *(Strychnos nux-vomica),* St. Ignatius beans *(S. ignatii)* and curare. [Gk nightshade.]

Stryker saw. A mechanical saw with a blade which rocks quickly from side to side and has none of the hazards of a circular saw.

stub-thumb (**stub**·thum). A thumb with a short thick terminal phalanx. [AS *stybb,* thumb.]

stump (stump). The end of the limb after amputation. **Conical stump.** A cone-shaped stump caused by excessive retraction of the divided muscles, often due to infection. **Stump of the eyeball.** That part of the eyeball remaining following amputation of the anterior segment, or of a staphylomatous cornea, e.g. Critchett's operation. **Painful stump, Tender stump.** An amputation stump which is painful or tender due to disease or neuroma. **Stump of a tooth.** A colloquial term for the root of a tooth. [ME *stumpe.*]

stump-foot (**stump**·fut). Talipes. [stump, AS *fot.*]

stupe (stewp). A hot medical fomentation to which is added a few drops of an irritant such as turpentine. Used as a counter-irritant for the relief of pain. [L *stupa* tow.]

stupefacient, stupefactive (stew·pe·**fa**·shent, stew·pe·**fak**·tiv). Narcotic; soporific; causing stupor. [stupor, L *facere* to make.]

stupemania (stew·pe·**ma**·ne·ah). Insanity associated with symptoms of stupor. [stupor, mania.]

stupor (**stew**·por). A state characterized either by a lowering of consciousness or by mutism, or both, usually accompanied by a profound diminution of spontaneous movement. **Anergic stupor.** A stupor with diminution of spontaneous movement. **Benign stupor.** Any stupor with a good outlook for recovery [obsolete term]. **Delusion stupor.** Stupor accompanied by delusions [obsolete term]. **Epileptic stupor.** The stuporose state which commonly follows an epileptic fit; also called *postepileptic stupor* or *state.* **Episodal stupor.** The name given to a condition that may occur in persons subjected to portacaval anastomosis. **Lethargic stupor.** Any stupor accompanied by lethargy [obsolete term]. **Stupor melancholicus.** Stupor due to a depressive state. **Postconvulsive stupor, Postepileptic stupor.** Epileptic stupor (see above). **Stupor vigilans.** Catalepsy. [L numbness.]

stuporous (**stew**·por·us). 1. Relating or belonging to stupor. 2. Characterized by stupor. 3. In a condition of stupor.

stupp (stup). Mercurial soot; a deposit formed in the condensers in the distillation of mercury ores. It contains up to 80 per cent of finely divided metallic mercury along with mercurial compounds, other mineral residues and sooty products.

Sturge, William Allen (b. 1850). British physician.

Sturge–Weber syndrome. The association of a port wine naevus in the skin of the face with a vascular abnormality in the meninges of the same side.

sturine (**stew**·reen). A protamine occurring in the sperm of the sturgeon. [L *sturio* sturgeon.]

Sturm, Johann Christoph (b. 1635). Altdorf mathematician.

Sturm's conoid. The imaginary three-dimensional figure enclosing rays of light after their passage through an astigmatic lens system. Successive sections show an ellipse, a circle or a straight line. The distance between the 2 linear images of a point source of light formed by the astigmatic system of lenses is called *Sturm's interval.* The first of these lines is parallel with the meridian of the lesser curvature, the second at right angles to it.

stuttering (**stut**·er·ing). Hesitant, jerky, intermittent speech, due to an inability to enunciate and join together syllables; also called *stammering.* **Labiochoreic stuttering.** Choreiform movements of the lips during speech, giving rise to stuttering. **Urinary stuttering.** The hesitancy or involuntary interruption in the urinary stream which becomes apparent unless the effort is sustained. Associated with the condition may be atony of the vesical musculature or a urethral obstruction. [ME *stutten.*]

sty, stye (sti). A small abscess in the eyelid due to infection of one of the glands of Zeis which opens into the lash follicle. [etym. dub.]

style (stile). Stylet.

stylet, stylette (**sti**·let, sti·**let**). 1. Wire inserted into the lumen of a catheter in order to stiffen it during its passage or to remove an obstruction. 2. A fine probe. 3. Wire of small calibre used to keep the canal of a hypodermic needle free from corrosion when not in use. **Lacrimal stylet.** A particular type of probe for the relief of stricture of the nasolacrimal duct. [It. *stiletto* dagger.]

styliform (**sti**·le·form). Shaped like a bodkin or a peg. [Gk *stylos* pillar, form.]

stylion (**sti**·le·on). An anthropometric point; the tip of the styloid process of the radius.

styliscus (sti·**lis**·kus). A thin, cylindrical tent for plugging a wound. [Gk *stylos* pillar.]

stylo-auricularis (sti·lo·aw·rik·ew·**la**′·ris). A muscular slip occasionally present; it arises from the cartilage of the external auditory meatus and passes to the styloid process of the temporal bone. [styloid process, L *auricularis* pertaining to the ear.]

styloglossal (sti·lo·**glos**·al). Pertaining to the styloid process of the temporal bone and to the tongue. [styloid process, Gk *glossa* tongue.]

styloglossus muscle [musculus styloglossus (NA)] (sti·lo·**glos**·us musl). A slender muscle arising near the tip of the styloid process of the temporal bone and passing downwards and forwards into the side of the tongue. [see prec.]

stylohyal (sti·lo·**hi**·al). Relating or belonging to the styloid process of the temporal bone and to the hyoid bone.

stylohyoid (sti·lo·**hi**·oid). 1. Relating or belonging to the styloid process of the temporal bone and to the hyoid bone. 2. Relating or belonging to the stylohyoid muscle.

stylohyoid muscle [musculus stylohyoideus (NA)]. A slender muscle which arises from the posterior surface of the styloid process of the temporal bone and is inserted into the hyoid at the junction of the greater horn with the body.

styloid (**sti**·loid). 1. Having the appearance of a stylet or pen; long and tapered. 2. Peg-shaped. **Styloid process.** *See* PROCESS. [Gk *stylos* pillar, *eidos* form.]

styloiditis (sti·loid·**i**·tis). Inflammation affecting the tissues surrounding the styloid process; in particular inflammation of the stylohyoid branch of the facial nerve as a result of constant friction between the nerve and the styloid process. [styloid process, Gk *-itis* inflammation.]

stylolaryngeus muscle (**sti**·lo·lar·**in**′·je·us musl). That part of the stylopharyngeus muscle which is attached to the thyroid cartilage. [styloid process, larynx.]

stylomandibular (**sti**·lo·man·**dib**′·ew·lar). Relating to the styloid process of the temporal bone and to the mandible.

stylomastoid (sti·lo·**mas**·toid). Belonging to the styloid and mastoid processes of the temporal bone.

stylomastoid artery [arteria stylomastoidea (NA)]. *See* ARTICULAR ARTERY, POSTERIOR.

stylomastoid vein [vena stylomastoidea (NA)]. A vein draining into the posterior auricular vein.

stylomaxillary (sti·lo·max·**il**′·ar·e). Belonging to the styloid process of the temporal bone and to the maxilla.

stylomyloid (sti·lo·**mi**·loid). Belonging to the styloid process of the temporal bone and to the area around the molar teeth. [Gk *stylos* pillar, *myle* mill, *eidos* form.]

stylopharyngeus muscle [musculus stylopharyngeus (NA)] (**sti**·lo·far·**in**′·je·us musl). A slender muscle arising from the medial side of the base of the styloid process of the temporal bone and passing into the pharyngeal wall between the superior and middle constrictor muscles of the pharynx.

Stylosanthes (sti·lo·**san**·theez). A genus of leguminous herbs, chiefly found in South America. **Stylosanthes elatior.** Pencil flower; a species of North America, an extract of which is used as a uterine sedative. [Gk *stylos* pillar, *anthos* flower.]

stylostaphyline (sti·lo·**staf**·il·ine). Relating or belonging to the styloid process of the temporal bone and to the uvula. [Gk *stylos* pillar, *staphyle* uvula.]

stylosteophyte (sti·**los**·te·o·fite). A peg-shaped outgrowth of bone. [Gk *stylos* pillar, osteophyte.]

stylus (**sti**·lus). 1. A stylet. 2. A medicated preparation shaped like a pencil, e.g. a stick of silver nitrate or other caustic substance. 3. In zoology, a style. [Gk *stylos* pillar.]

styma (**sti**·mah). Priapism. [Gk stiffness.]

stymatosis (sti·mat·o·sis). Priapism of extreme degree accompanied by haemorrhage into the urethral canal. [styma, Gk *-osis* condition.]

stypage (**sti**·page). The production of local anaesthesia by applying a stype (or pledget of wool) soaked in an appropriate anaesthetic solution.

stype (stipe). A tampon or pledget. [Gk *stype* tow.]

stypsis (**stip**·sis). 1. Astringency. 2. The application of an astringent in treatment. 3. Styptic action. [Gk *stypsis* a steeping in an astringent.]

styptic (**stip**·tik). 1. Astringent; having the power to arrest bleeding either by mechanical or chemical means. 2. A substance with astringent and haemostatic properties. [Gk *styptikos* astringent.]

stypticity (stip·**tis**·it·e). The quality of being astringent. [see prec.]

styracin (**sti**·ras·in). Cinnamyl cinnamate, $C_6H_5CH{=}CHCOO$ $CH_2CH{=}CHC_6H_5$. A constituent of the balsam, styrax, obtained from the bark of *Liquidambar orientalis.*

styracitol (sti·**ras**·it·ol). An alcohol obtained from a species of *Styrax.*

Styramate (**sti**·ram·ate). BP Commission approved name for 2-hydroxy-2-phenylethyl carbamate; a muscle relaxant.

Styrax (**sti**·rax). A genus of styraceous trees, chiefly important for the gum resins they contain, e.g. *Styrax benzoin* yields gum benzoin. **Styrax praeparatus.** Prepared storax. *See* STORAX. [Gk storax.]

styrene (**sti**·reen). Vinyl benzene, phenylethylene, cinnamene, $C_6H_5CH{=}CH_2$. An unsaturated liquid hydrocarbon obtained from storax or prepared industrially by the catalysed interaction of benzene and ethylene. It polymerizes readily and the polymers are of value as plastics.

styrol (**sti**·rol). Phenylethylene, cinnamene, $C_6H_5CH{=}CH_2$. A colourless aromatic liquid found in storax.

styrolene (**sti**·rol·een). Styrol.

styrone (sti·rone). Cinnamyl alcohol, phenylallyl alcohol, $C_6H_5CH{=}CHCH_2OH$. A compound prepared by the saponification of cinnamyl cinnamate (styracin) with potassium hydroxide. It is used as a microscopical reagent and as an antiseptic.

sub-. Prefix, from the Latin preposition *sub*, meaning *under, less than normal.*

subabdominal (sub·ab·**dom**·in·al). Occurring below or near the abdomen. [L *sub*, abdomen.]

subabdominoperitoneal (sub·ab·**dom**·in·o·per·it·o·**ne'**·al). Below or deep to the abdominal peritoneum. [L *sub*, abdomen, peritoneum.]

subacetabular (**sub**·as·et·**ab'**·ew·lar). Situated below the acetabulum. [L *sub*, acetabulum.]

subacetal (sub·**as**·et·al). The solution of lead subacetate and alum which yields aluminium acetate.

subacetate (sub·**as**·et·ate). Of the several acetates formed by a metal, that one which contains the least proportion of acetic radical; a basic acetate, such as $Pb(C_2H_3O_2)_2{\cdot}2Pb(OH)_2$. [Obsolete term.] [L *sub*, acetate.]

subacid (**sub**·as·id). 1. Describing anything that has acidic properties below normal. 2. Acidulous. [L *sub*, acid.]

subacidity (sub·as·**id**·it·e). 1. Less than normal acidity. 2. Slight acidity. [see prec.]

subacrocentric (**sub**·ak·ro·**sen'**·trik). Of a chromosome or chromatid, with the centromere within one of the terminal quarters of the chromosome but with rather elongated arms. [L *sub*, Gk *akros* extreme, *kentron* centre.]

subacromial (sub·ak·**ro**·me·al). Below the acromion. **Subacromial bursa.** *See* BURSA. [L *sub*, acromion.]

subacute (sub·ak·**ewt**). Applied to a disease that runs a moderately rapid and severe course for which the word acute would not be appropriate, but not necessarily a chronic course. [L *sub*, acute.]

subalimentation (**sub**·al·im·en·**ta'**·shun). The condition resulting from an inadequate diet.

subanal (sub·a·nal). Occurring below the anus. [L *sub*, anus.]

subanconeal (sub·an·**ko**·ne·al). Beneath the anconeus muscle. [see foll.]

subanconeus (sub·an·**ko**·ne·us). A few fibres from the deep surface of the triceps brachii muscle which are inserted into the articular capsule of the elbow joint. [L *sub*, Gk *agkon* elbow.]

subapical (sub·a·pik·al). Below the apex, e.g. of the lung. [L *sub*, *apex* summit.]

subaponeurotic (**sub**·a·po·newr·**ot'**·ik). Beneath an aponeurosis. [L *sub*, aponeurosis.]

subarachnoid (sub·ar·**ak**·noid). Situated deep to the arachnoid mater of the brain. **Subarachnoid space.** *See* SPACE. [L *sub*, arachnoid.]

subarachnoiditis (**sub**·ar·ak·noi·**di'**·tis). Inflammation in the space underlying the arachnoid membranes. [L *sub*, arachnoid, Gk *-itis* inflammation.]

subarcuate (sub·**ar**·kew·ate). 1. Slightly arched or bowed. 2. Below the arcuate ligament. [L *sub*, arcuate.]

subareolar (sub·ar·e·o·lar). Beneath the areola of the mammary gland. [L *sub*, areola.]

subastragalar, subastragaloid (sub·as·**trag**·al·ar, sub·as·**trag**·al·-oid). Beneath the talus (astragalus). [L *sub*, astragalus.]

subastringent (sub·as·**trin**·jent). Astringent in a moderate or slight degree. [L *sub*, astringent.]

subatom (**sub**·at·om). Any particle less than atomic in size and weight. [L *sub*, atom.]

subatomic (sub·at·**om**·ik). Applied to the particles and phenomena of the region within the atom. [see prec.]

subaudition (sub·aw·**dish**·un). The act of mentally supplying what is not expressed. [L *sub*, *audire* to hear.]

subaural (sub·**aw**·ral). Beneath the ear. [L *sub*, *auris* ear.]

subauricular (sub·aw·**rik**·ew·lar). Below an auricle, particularly that of the ear. [L *sub*, auricle.]

subaxial (sub·**ax**·e·al). Below the axis. [L *sub*, axis.]

subaxillary (sub·ax·**il**·ar·e). Below the axilla. [L *sub*, axilla.]

Subbarow, Yellapragada (b. 1896). Boston biochemist.

Fiske and Subbarow method. 1. For phosphate in urine: 0.5 ml urine is diluted to 5 ml with water, 0.7 ml of 60 per cent perchloric acid, 0.7 ml of 5 per cent aqueous ammonium molybdate and 0.5 ml of aminonaphtholsulphonic acid reagent (0.2 g 1,2,4-aminonaphtholsuphonic acid; 12 g sodium metabisulphite; 2.4 g crystalline sodium sulphite; water to 100 ml) are added. The solution is diluted to 10 ml and the colour compared with standards after 10 min. 2. For inorganic phosphate in blood: 2 ml blood, serum or plasma are added to 8 ml 10 per cent trichloro-acetic acid. The mixture is shaken, filtered and 5 ml of filtrate treated as for urine.

sub-basal (sub·**ba**·sal). Below the base. [L *sub*, base.]

sub-brachial, sub-brachiate (sub·**bra**·ke·al, sub·**bra**·ke·ate). 1. Beneath the inferior or superior brachium of the mid-brain. 2. Subpectoral. [L *sub*, brachium.]

sub-brachycephalic (sub·**brak**·e·kef·**al'**·ik). Slightly brachycephalic; noting a skull with a cephalic index of from 78 to 79. [L *sub*, Gk *brachys* short, *kephale* head.]

subcalcareous (sub·kal·**ka**·re·us). Below normal calcium content. [L *sub*, *calx* lime.]

subcalcarine (sub·**kal**·kar·een). Beneath the calcarine sulcus. [L *sub*, calcarine sulcus.]

subcallosal (sub·kal·**o**·sal). Below the corpus callosum. [L *sub*, corpus callosum.]

subcalorism (sub·**kal**·or·izm). A pathological condition due to the circulation being affected by exposure to extreme cold over a considerable length of time. [L *sub*, *calor* animal heat.]

subcapital (sub·**kap**·it·al). 1. Occurring below the head. 2. Below the head of the femur. [L *sub*, *caput* head.]

subcapsular (sub·**kap**·sew·lar). Underneath a capsule. [L *sub*, capsule.]

subcapsuloperiosteal (sub·**kap**·sew·lo·per·e·**os'**·te·al). Beneath the capsule and periosteum of a joint. [L *sub*, capsule, periosteum.]

subcarbonate (sub·**kar**·bon·ate). Of the several carbonates formed by a metal, that one which contains the least proportion of carbonic radical; a basic carbonate, such as lead carbonate, $2PbCO_3Pb(OH)_2$. [Obsolete term.] [L *sub*, carbonate.]

subcartilaginous (**sub**·kar·til·**aj'**·in·us). 1. Partially cartilaginous. 2. Beneath a cartilage. [L *sub*, cartilage.]

subcentral (sub·**sen**·tral). 1. Near any centre. 2. Located anterior to the central sulcus of the cerebrum. [L *sub*, centre.]

subception (sub·**sep**·shun). Subliminal perception. *See* PERCEPTION.

subcerebellar (**sub**·ser·e·**bel'**·ar). Beneath the cerebellum. [L *sub*, cerebellum.]

subcerebral (sub·**ser**·e·bral). Beneath the cerebrum. [L *sub*, cerebrum.]

subchloride (sub·**klor**·ide). Of the several chlorides of a metal, that one which contains the least proportion of chlorine, such as mercury subchloride, HgCl. [L *sub*, chloride.]

subchondral (sub·**kon**·dral). Beneath a cartilage. [L *sub*, Gk *chondros* cartilage.]

subchordal (sub·**kord**·al). 1. Ventral to the notochord. 2. Below the vocal folds. [L *sub*, chord.]

subchorioidal (**sub**·kor·e·**oid'**·al). Subchoroidal.

subchorionic (**sub**·ko·re·**on'**·ik). Beneath the chorion. [L *sub*, chorion.]

subchoroidal (sub·kor·**oid**·al). Lying beneath the choroid. [L *sub*, choroid.]

subchromatid (sub·kro·**mat**·id). A subunit into which a chromatid may be longitudinally divided. [L *sub*, chromatid.]

subchronic (sub·**kron**·ik). More chronic than acute but not truly chronic. [L *sub*, chronic.]

subclavian (sub·**kla**·ve·an). Beneath the clavicle. **Subclavian plexus.** *See* PLEXUS. **Subclavian trunk.** *See* TRUNK. [L *sub*, clavicle.]

subclavian artery [arteria subclavia (NA)]. The main artery supplying the upper limb, arising on the right side from the innominate artery and on the left from the arch of the aorta; it becomes the axillary artery at the outer border of the 1st rib. Its 3 parts lie respectively medial to, behind and lateral to the scalenus anterior muscle.

subclavian vein [vena subclavia (NA)]. The main vein draining the upper limb, a continuation of the axillary vein and a tributary of the innominate vein. It receives the external and sometimes the anterior jugular veins in the neck.

subclavicular (sub·klav·**ik**·ew·lar). Subclavian.

subclavius muscle [musculus subclavius (NA)] (sub·**kla**·ve·us musl). A muscle with a tendinous origin from the anterior end of the 1st rib and the adjacent costal cartilage, and an insertion into a groove on the under-surface of the middle third of the clavicle. [L *sub*, clavicle.]

subclavius muscle, nerve to the [nervus subclavius(NA)]. A branch of the upper trunk of the brachial plexus, carrying fibres from the 5th and 6th cervical segments of the spinal cord to the subclavius muscle. It often connects also with the phrenic nerve. [see prec.]

subclinical (sub·**klin**·ik·al). 1. Of a disease, one in which, while the characteristic pathological changes are present and may be developing, (*a*) there are no clinical symptoms at all, or (*b*) there are no clinical symptoms giving any indication of the nature of the disease; especially applied to the early stages of a disease in which at a later date symptoms may develop. 2. Of an infection, one that produces no material pathological changes but is present and possibly multiplies in the body, or one that produces minor pathological changes that are not reflected in the clinical picture. [L *sub*, clinical.]

subconjunctival (**sub**·kon·jungk·**ti**′·val). Lying beneath the conjunctiva. [L *sub*, conjunctiva.]

subconscious (sub·**kon**·shus). 1. The part of the mind containing mental processes not present in consciousness at any given moment, yet available to introspection. More exact terms are *foreconscious* or *preconscious.* 2. The term is used less exactly for *unconscious.* [L *sub*, conscious.]

subconsciousness (sub·**kon**·shus·nes). The condition of incomplete consciousness. [see prec.]

subcontinuous (sub·kon·**tin**·ew·us). Almost but not quite continuous. [L *sub*, continuous.]

subcoracoid (sub·**kor**·ak·oid). Beneath the coracoid process. [L *sub*, coracoid.]

subcortex (sub·**kor**·tex). The white matter of the brain which lies immediately beneath the cortex. [L *sub*, cortex.]

subcortical (sub·**kor**·tik·al). Lying underneath the cerebral cortex. [see prec.]

subcostal (sub·**kos**·tal). Beneath a rib. [L *sub*, *costa* rib.]

subcostal arteries [arteriae subcostales (NA)]. The last pair of arteries from the thoracic aorta, in series with the posterior intercostal arteries and branching similarly [ramus dorsalis, ramus spinalis (NA)].

subcostal muscles [musculi subcostales (NA)]. Part of the transversus thoracis muscle. They vary greatly in number and size, and pass from one rib to another near their angles.

subcostal nerve [nervus subcostalis (NA)]. The last thoracic nerve, running below the 12th rib. It supplies the abdominal muscles and the skin of the lower abdomen and front of the buttock.

subcostal vein [vena subcostalis (NA)]. A tributary of the ascending lumbar vein or vena azygos; it runs below the last rib and drains the abdominal wall.

subcostalgia (sub·kos·**tal**·je·ah). Pain over the course of the subcostal nerve or beneath the ribs. [L *sub*, *costa* rib, Gk *algos* pain.]

subcranial (sub·**kra**·ne·al). Beneath the cranium. [L *sub*, cranium.]

subcrepitant (sub·**krep**·it·ant). Pertaining to a râle which is faintly crepitant. [see foll.]

subcrepitation (**sub**·krep·it·**a**′·shun). 1. A sound or râle which is faintly crepitant in character. 2. A condition in which subcrepitant râles are present. [L *sub*, crepitation.]

subcruraeus, subcruralis (sub·kroo·**re**·us, sub·kroo·**ra**·lis). The articularis genu muscle; a few fibres which arise from the lower part of the anterior surface of the femur and are inserted into the synovial membrane of the knee joint above the patella. [L *sub*, *crus* thigh.]

subculture (sub·**kul**·tcher). A secondary culture of an organism, derived by inoculation from the primary culture. [L *sub*, culture.]

subcutaneous (sub·kew·**ta**·ne·us). 1. Beneath the skin. 2. Hypodermic; for introduction under the skin. [L *sub*, *cutis* skin.]

subcutaneus colli (sub·kew·**ta**·ne·us **kol**·i). The platysma. [L under the skin of the neck.]

subcuticular (sub·kew·**tik**·ew·lar). Subepidermal. [see foll.]

subcutis (sub·**kew**·tis). 1. The true skin, the corium. 2. The layer of vascular connective tissue beneath the skin. [L *sub*, *cutis* skin.]

subdelirium (sub·de·**lir**·e·um). Slight or intermittent delirium. [L *sub*, delirium.]

subdermal, subdermic (sub·**der**·mal, sub·**der**·mik). Subcutaneous. [L *sub*, Gk *derma* skin.]

subdiaphragmatic (**sub**·di·ah·frag·**mat**′·ik). Underneath the diaphragm. [L *sub*, diaphragm.]

subdolichocephalic (sub·**dol**·ik·o·kef·**al**′·ik). Denoting a skull with a cephalic index of more than 75 but less than 78. [L *sub*, dolichocephalic.]

subdorsal (sub·**dor**·sal). Situated inferior to the dorsal region. [L *sub*, *dorsum* back.]

subduction (sub·**duk**·shun). Infraduction. [L *sub*, *ducere* to lead.]

subdural (sub·**dewr**·al). Beneath the dura mater. **Subdural space.** *See* SPACE. [L *sub*, dura mater.]

subectodermal (**sub**·ek·to·**der**′·mal). Beneath the ectoderm. [L *sub*, ectoderm.]

subendocardial (**sub**·en·do·**kar**′·de·al). Beneath the endocardium. [L *sub*, endocardium.]

subendothelial (**sub**·en·do·**the**′·le·al). Beneath an endothelial structure or the endothelium. [L *sub*, endothelium.]

subendymal (sub·**en**·dim·al). Beneath the ependyma. [L *sub*, ependyma.]

subepicardial (**sub**·ep·e·**kar**′·de·al). Beneath the epicardium. [L *sub*, Gk *epi*, *kardia* heart.]

subepidermal, subepidermic (**sub**·ep·e·**der**′·mal, **sub**·ep·e·**der**′·mik). Beneath the epidermis. [L *sub*, epidermis.]

subepiglottic (**sub**·ep·e·**glot**′·ik). Beneath the epiglottis. [L *sub*, epiglottis.]

subepithelial (**sub**·ep·e·**the**′·le·al). Immediately beneath the epithelium. [L *sub*, epithelium.]

suberin (**sew**·ber·in). A modified form of cellulose observed in cork. [L *suber* cork.]

suberosis (sew·ber·**o**·sis). Hypersensitivity reaction of pulmonary and bronchial tissues in workers handling cork; it is possibly due to thermophilic actinomycetes. [L *suber* cork, Gk *osis* condition.]

subexcite (sub·ex·**ite**). To induce a state of mild stimulation or irritation. [L *sub*, excite.]

subextensibility (**sub**·ex·ten·sib·**il**′·it·e). Decreased power of extension. [L *sub*, extend.]

subfalcial (sub·**fal**·se·al). Lying beneath the falx cerebri. [L *sub*, falx cerebri.]

sub-family (sub·**fam**·il·e). A sub-division of the family in the classification of plants and animals. [L *sub*, family.]

subfascial (sub·**fash**·e·al). Beneath a fascia. [L *sub*, fascia.]

subfebrile (sub·**feb**·rile). Any condition in which the temperature is raised only slightly above the normal, generally 37.5-38.5°C (99-101°F). [L *sub*, *febris* fever.]

subfecundity (sub·fek·**un**·dit·e). Reduced production of young, short of complete sterility, on the part of the female. [L *sub*, *fecunditas* fertility.]

subfertility (sub·fer·**til**·it·e). Reduced power of producing young, short of complete sterility, on the part of the male or female. [L *sub*, *fertilis* fertile.]

subfoliar (sub·**fo**·le·ar). Relating or belonging to a subfolium.

subfolium (sub·**fo**·le·um). One of the secondary, leaf-like divisions of the cerebellar folia. [L *sub*, folium.]

subfornical (sub·**for**·nik·al). Beneath the fornix cerebri. [L *sub*, fornix.]

subfrontal (sub·**frun**·tal). Beneath a frontal gyrus or lobe. [L *sub*, *frons* forehead.]

subgaleal (sub·**ga**·le·al). Beneath the epicranial aponeurosis. [L *sub*, galea.]

subgallate (sub·**gal**·ate). A basic gallate, such as bismuth subgallate, $Bi(OH)_2C_7H_5O_5$. [L *sub*, gallate.]

subgemmal (sub·**jem**·al). Beneath a taste bud or any gemma or bud. [L *sub*, *gemma* bud.]

sub-genus (sub·**je**·nus). A division of the genus, containing some of the species of the genus which have a combination of characters not possessed by the rest. In biological nomenclature, sub-generic names are printed between the generic and the trivial, in parentheses with an upper case initial. [L *sub*, genus.]

subgingival (sub·**jin**·jiv·al). Lying beneath the surface of the gums. [L *sub*, *gingiva* gum.]

subglenoid (sub·**gle**·noid). Lying below the glenoid cavity or fossa. [L *sub*, glenoid.]

subglossal (sub·**glos**·al). Pertaining to the structures or parts beneath the tongue. [L *sub*, Gk *glossa* tongue.]

subglossitis (sub·glos·**i**·tis). Inflammation of the undersurface of the tongue or of the tissues lying beneath it. [L *sub*, Gk *glossa* tongue, *-itis* inflammation.]

subglottic (sub·**glot**·ik). Beneath the glottis. [L *sub*, glottis.]

subgranular (sub·**gran**·ew·lar). Denoting a substance or tissue the granular content of which is small. [L *sub*, granule.]

subgrondation, subgrundation (sub·gron·**da**·shun, sub·grun·**da**·shun). The sinking of one fragment of a fractured cranial bone beneath the other. [L *suggrunda* the eaves of a house.]

subgyrus (sub·**ji**·rus). A gyrus that is partially screened by, or lies beneath another or others. [L *sub*, gyrus.]

subhepatic (sub·hep·**at**·ik). Beneath the liver. [L *sub*, Gk *hepar* liver.]

subhumeral (sub·**hew**·mer·al). Below the humerus. [L *sub*, humerus.]

subhyaloid (sub·**hi**·al·oid). Beneath the hyaloid membrane. [L *sub*, hyaloid.]

subhyoid, subhyoidean (sub·**hi**·oid, sub·hi·**oid**·e·an). Below the hyoid bone. [L *sub*, hyoid.]

subicteric (sub·ik·**ter**·ik). Hyperbilirubinaemia without actual jaundice or with barely perceptible jaundice. [L *sub*, Gk *ikteros* jaundice.]

subicular (sew·**bik**·ew·lar). Relating or belonging to the subiculum.

subiculum (sew·**bik**·ew·lum). An obsolete term (in full, subiculum cornu ammonis) originally synonymous with the hippocampal gyrus. Its precise delimitation in modern works varies. **Subiculum promontorii** [NA]. A ridge of bone forming the posterior boundary of the fenestra vestibuli. [L *subex* layer.]

subiliac (sub·**il**·e·ak). Below the ilium. [see foll.]

subilium (sub·**il**·e·um). The lowest part of the iliac bone. [L *sub*, ilium.]

subincision (sub·in·**sizh**·un). A custom among savage tribes, particularly Australian aborigines, of making an incision into the penile urethra. It does not prevent normal intercourse, and fertility is unaffected. [L *sub*, incision.]

subinfection (sub·in·**fek**·shun). A mild infection with only slight clinical manifestations; a mild chronic infection with occasional exacerbations. [L *sub*, infection.]

subinflammation (sub·in·flam·**a**′·shun). A slight degree of inflammation. [L *sub*, inflammation.]

subinflammatory (sub·in·**flam**·at·or·e). Pertaining to or characterized by mild inflammation. [see prec.]

subintegumental, subintegumentary (sub·in·teg·ew·**men**′·tal, sub·in·teg·ew·**men**′·tar·e). Pertaining to the tissues beneath the common integument. [L *sub*, integument.]

subintimal (sub·**in**·tim·al). Beneath the tunica intima. [L *sub*, tunica intima.]

subintrant (sub·**in**·trant). Anticipating; overlapping; as in temperature charts of subtertian or malignant tertian malaria where successive paroxysms tend to overlap. [L *subintrare* to enter stealthily.]

subinvolution (sub·in·vol·**ew**′·shun). Incomplete involution of an organ or part, such as the uterus after labour; partial involution. [L *sub*, involution.]

subiodide (sub·**i**·o·dide). Of the several iodides formed by a metal, that one which contains the least proportion of iodine. [L *sub*, iodide.]

subject (**sub**·jekt). 1. A human being or animal under treatment or upon whom experiments are being carried out for the purposes of research. 2. A cadaver for dissection. 3. To be liable to attacks of a particular disease. [L *subjicere* to expose.]

subjective (sub·**jek**·tiv). Of symptoms or sensations, evident to the person affected but not to anyone else. [see prec.]

subjectoscope (sub·**jek**·to·skope). An instrument employed in the investigation of subjective sensations in the eye. [subjective, Gk *skopein* to view.]

subjee (**sub**·je). Name given to the capsules and larger leaves of *Cannabis indica*. [Hind. *sabzi* greenness.]

subjugal (sub·**joo**·gal). Below the zygomatic arch. [L *sub*, *jugum* yoke.]

sublation (sub·**la**·shun). The detachment, displacement, elevation or removal of a part. [L *sublatus* taken away.]

sublethal (sub·**le**·thal). Of drugs, poisons or radiation, a dose which is not quite sufficient to cause death. [L *sub*, *letum* death.]

subleukaemia (sub·lew·**ke**·me·ah). Subleukaemic leukaemia, aleukaemic leukaemia; leukaemic conditions in which the leucocyte count is normal or subnormal with only a few immature white cells in the peripheral blood. The clinical manifestations are those seen in the corresponding leukaemias with increased leucocyte counts. [L *sub*, leukaemia.]

sublimate (**sub**·lim·ate). Any solid prepared by sublimation. **Corrosive sublimate.** Mercuric chloride. **Formol sublimate.** A histological fixative containing formaldehyde and mercuric chloride.

sublimation (sub·lim·**a**·shun). 1. In chemistry, the passing of a solid on heating at ordinary pressure directly into vapour and, on cooling of the latter, back into the solid state without any intermediate liquid phase. 2. In psycho-analysis, the directing by instinct of itself towards an aim other than and remote from that of sexual gratification. [L *sublimare* to elevate.]

sublime (sub·**lime**). To convert a solid directly into vapour by heating it, and to re-condense it on a cold surface without any liquid phase. [see prec.]

subliminal (sub·**lim**·in·al). Below the threshold of sensation or perception. [L *sub*, *limen* threshold.]

sublimis (sub·**li**·mis). 1. Near or on the surface; elevated. 2. At the top. 3. The flexor digitorum sublimis muscle. [L high.]

sublingual (sub·**ling**·gwal). 1. Beneath the tongue. 2. Relating to the structures under the tongue. [L *sub*, *lingua* tongue.]

sublingual vein [vena sublingualis]. A vein that drains the sublingual gland into the vena comitans of the hypoglossal nerve.

sublinguitis (sub·ling·**gwi**·tis). Inflammation affecting the sublingual salivary gland. [L *sub*, *lingua* tongue, Gk *-itis* inflammation.]

sublobe (**sub**·lobe). Any one of the divisions of a lobule. [L *sub*, lobe.]

sublobular (sub·**lob**·ew·lar). Lying beneath a lobule. [L *sub*, lobule.]

sublumbar (sub·**lum**·bar). Below the lumbar region. [L *sub*, lumbar.]

subluxation (sub·lux·**a**·shun). Incomplete dislocation; a general hypermobility of a joint with actual displacement of the parts. [L *sub*, luxation.]

sublymphaemia (sub·limf·**e**·me·ah). Hypolymphaemia. [L *sub*, lymphaemia.]

submalleolar (sub·mal·**e**·o·lar). Below a malleolus. [L *sub*, malleolus.]

submammary (sub·**mam**·ar·e). Beneath a mammary gland. [L *sub*, mammary.]

submandibular (sub·man·**dib**·ew·lar). Below the mandible. **Submandibular fossa.** *See* FOSSA. **Submandibular lymph gland.** *See* GLAND. [L *sub*, mandible.]

submania (sub·**ma**·ne·ah). A minor degree of manic excitement. [L *sub*, mania.]

submarginal (sub·**mar**·jin·al). 1. Near the margin or border of a part. 2. Situated next to a marginal structure. [L *sub*, margin.]

submaxilla (sub·max·**il**·ah). The mandible. [L *sub*, maxilla.]

submaxillaritis (**sub**·max·il·ar·**i**'·tis). Inflammation affecting the submandibular gland; mumps. [L *sub*, maxilla, Gk *-itis* inflammation.]

submaxillary (sub·max·il·ar·e). 1. Mandibular. 2. Situated beneath the mandible or the lower jaw. [L *sub*, maxilla.]

submaxillitis (**sub**·max·il·**i**'·tis). Submaxillaritis.

submedial, submedian (sub·**me**·de·al, sub·**me**·de·an). Lying near or under the middle; not exactly in the middle but very close to it. [L *sub*, medial.]

submembranous (sub·**mem**·bran·us). Consisting partly or almost entirely of membranous tissue. [L *sub*, membrane.]

submeningeal (sub·men·**in**·je·al). Beneath the meninges of the brain and spinal cord. [L *sub*, meninges.]

submental (sub·**men**·tal). Under the chin. [L *sub*, *mentum* chin.]

submental artery [arteria submentalis (NA)]. The largest cervical branch of the facial artery running along the lower margin of the mandible to reach the chin and lower lip.

submental vein [vena submentalis (NA)]. A vessel draining the region of the chin into the anterior facial vein.

submentale (sub·men·**ta**·le). The deepest point on the bony profile between the infradentale and the pogonion. [L *sub*, *mentum* chin.]

submerge (sub·**merj**). To plunge under water or place under the surface of a liquid. [L *submergere* to plunge under.]

submersion (sub·**mer**·shun). 1. The act of plunging anything under the surface of water or other liquid. 2. The state of being submerged. [see prec.]

submesaticephalic (**sub**·mes·at·e·kef·**al**'·ik). Of a skull, having a cephalic index of from 75 to 76. [L *sub*, mesaticephalic.]

submetacentric (**sub**·met·ah·**sen**'·trik). Of a chromosome or chromatid, with the centromere within the 2 inner (proximal) quarters, but away from the middle. [L *sub*, Gk *meta*, *kentron* centre.]

submetallic (sub·met·**al**·ik). Exhibiting only limited metallic properties. [L *sub*, metal.]

submicron (sub·**mi**·kron). Any particle so small that it is beyond the limit of the ordinary microscope, but visible under the ultramicroscope: between 0.2 μm and 5 nm in diameter. [L *sub*, micron.]

submicroscopic, submicroscopical (**sub**·mi·kro·**skop**'·ik, **sub**·mi·kro·**skop**'·ik·al). Referring to any particle which can be differentiated by the ultramicroscope. [L *sub*, microscope.]

submorphous (sub·**mor**·fus). Partly amorphous and partly crystalline; said of some calculi. [L *sub*, Gk *morphe* shape.]

submucosa (sub·mew·**ko**·sah). A layer of areolar tissue beneath a mucous membrane. [L *sub*, mucous.]

submucosal (sub·mew·**ko**·sal). 1. Relating or belonging to the submucosa. 2. Submucous.

submucous (sub·**mew**·kus). Occurring beneath the mucosa or a mucous membrane. [L *sub*, mucous.]

subnarcotic (sub·nar·**kot**·ik). Having a mildly narcotic effect. [L *sub*, narcotic.]

subnasal (sub·**na**·zal). Occurring or in a position under the nose. [L *sub*, *nasus* nose.]

subnasale (sub·na·**za**·le). In craniometry, the apex of the angle formed by the lower border of the nasal septum and the philtrum. [L *sub*, nasal septum.]

subnitrate (sub·**ni**·trate). Of the several nitrates formed by a metal, that one which contains the least proportion of the nitric radical; a basic nitrate such as $Bi(OH)_2(NO_3)$. [Obsolete term.] [L *sub*, nitrate.]

subnormal (sub·**nor**·mal). 1. Less than the normal. 2. Term now used to define diminished responsibility under the Homicide Act 1957. [L *sub*, normal.]

subnormality (sub·nor·**mal**·it·e). The state of being subnormal. **Mental subnormality.** A state of arrested or incomplete development of mind such that the patient is, and will continue to be, incapable of living an independent life or of guarding himself against serious exploitation and which requires medical treatment or other special care or training.

subnotochordal (**sub**·no·to·**kord**'·al). Ventral to the notochord. [L *sub*, notochord.]

subnucleus (sub·**new**·kle·us). A secondary nucleus formed by the separation of a number of nerve cells from a larger nucleus. [L *sub*, nucleus.]

subnutrition (sub·new·**trish**·un). A mild degree of malnutrition. [L *sub*, nutrition.]

suboccipital (sub·ok·**sip**·it·al). Below the occipital bone or the occiput. **Suboccipital plexus.** *See* PLEXUS. [L *sub*, occiput.]

suboccipital nerve [nervus suboccipitalis]. *See* CERVICAL NERVES.

suboesophageal (**sub**·e·sof·ah·**je**'·al). Occurring or lying beneath the oesophagus. [L *sub*, oesophagus.]

suboperculum (sub·o·**per**·kew·lum). The orbital operculum. [L *sub*, operculum.]

suboptic (sub·**op**·tik). Infra-orbital. [L *sub*, optic.]

suboptimal (sub·**op**·tim·al). Relating or belonging to the suboptimum.

suboptimum (sub·**op**·tim·um). Not quite optimal; below the optimum; applied to a temperature which is lower than that most favourable to the development of an organism. [L *sub*, *optimus* best.]

suborbital (sub·**or**·bit·al). Infra-orbital. [L *sub*, orbit.]

subordination (**sub**·or·din·**a**'·shun). The condition in which one organ is controlled by or is dependent on another organ. [L *sub*, *ordo* rank.]

suboxidation (**sub**·ox·id·**a**'·shun). Deficient oxidation. [L *sub*, oxidation.]

suboxide (sub·**ox**·ide). Of the several oxides formed by a metal, that one which contains the least proportion of oxygen. [L *sub*, oxide.]

subpapular (sub·**pap**·ew·lar). Indicating an eruption of which the lesions are only slightly elevated and slightly papular, or of which the papules are sparse and scattered. [L *sub*, papule.]

subparalytic (**sub**·par·al·**it**'·ik). Applied to a paralysis which is not complete. [L *sub*, paralysis.]

subparietal (sub·par·**i**·et·al). Situated beneath or below any parietal structure. [L *sub*, parietal.]

subpatellar (sub·pat·**el**·ar). Under the patella. [L *sub*, patella.]

subpectoral (sub·**pek**·tor·al). Beneath either the pectoralis major or pectoralis minor muscles. [L *sub*, *pectus* chest.]

subpenduncular (sub·ped·**ung**·kew·lar). Beneath one of the cerebral or cerebellar peduncles. [L *sub*, peduncle.]

subpericardial (**sub**·per·e·**kar**'·de·al). Beneath the pericardium. [L *sub*, pericardium.]

subpericranial (**sub**·per·e·**kra**'·ne·al). Beneath the pericranium. [L *sub*, pericranium.]

subperiosteal (**sub**·per·e·**os**'·te·al). In a position deep to the periosteum. [L *sub*, periosteum.]

subperiosteocapsular (**sub**·per·e·os·te·o·**kap**'·sew·lar). Subcapsuloperiosteal. [L *sub*, periosteum, capsule.]

subperitoneal (**sub**·per·it·on·**e**'·al). Lying beneath the peritoneum. [L *sub*, peritoneum.]

subperitoneopelvic (**sub**·per·it·o·ne·o·**pel**'·vik). Under the peritoneum of the pelvis. [L *sub*, peritoneum, pelvis.]

subpharyngeal (sub·far·**in**·je·al). Below the pharynx. [L *sub*, pharynx.]

subphrenic (sub·**fren**·ik). Below the diaphragm. [L *sub*, Gk *phren* diaphragm.]

subpial (sub·**pe**·al). Lying beneath the pia mater. [L *sub*, pia mater.]

subplacenta (sub·plas·**en**·tah). The decidua parietalis. [L *sub*, placenta.]

subplacental (sub·plas·**en**·tal). 1. Beneath the placenta. 2. Relating to the decidua parietalis. [see prec.]

subplantigrade (sub·**plan**·te·grade). Denoting a gait in which the sole of the foot is placed on the ground, the heel being slightly raised. [L *sub*, *planta* sole of the foot, *gradi* to step.]

subpleural (sub·**ploor**·al). Between the pleura and the thoracic parietes. [L *sub*, pleura.]

subplexal (sub·**plex**·al). Beneath any plexus. [L *sub*, plexus.]

subpontile, subpontine (sub·**pon**·tile, sub·**pon**·tine). Below the pons. [L *sub*, pons.]

subpreputial (sub·pre·**pew**·shal). Beneath the prepuce. [L *sub*, prepuce.]

subprostatic (sub·pros·**tat**·ik). Beneath the prostate gland. [L *sub*, prostate.]

subpubic (sub·**pew**·bik). Below the pubic symphysis or pubic arch. [L *sub*, pubis.]

subpulmonary (sub·**pul**·mon·ar·e). Below a lung or the lungs, towards the abdominal cavity. [L *sub*, *pulmo* lung.]

subpulpal (sub·**pul**·pal). Beneath the pulp of the teeth. [L *sub*, pulp.]

subpyramidal (sub·pir·**am**·id·al). 1. Occurring below a pyramid. 2. Almost pyramidal in shape. [L *sub*, pyramid.]

subrectal (sub·**rek**·tal). Below the rectum. [L *sub*, rectum.]

subreniform (sub·**ren**·e·form). Having a certain resemblance in shape to the kidney, but not truly kidney-shaped. [L *sub*, *ren* kidney, form.]

subresin (sub·**rez**·in). That part of a resin which is soluble in boiling alcohol but precipitates again on cooling. [L *sub*, resin.]

subretinal (sub·**ret**·in·al). Beneath the retina. [L *sub*, retina.]

subrostral (sub·**ros**·tral). Beneath the rostrum of the corpus callosum. [L *sub*, rostrum.]

subsacral (sub·**sa**·kral). Under the sacrum. [L *sub*, sacrum.]

subsalt (**sub**·sawlt). Any basic salt. [Obsolete term.] [L *sub*, salt.]

subsartorial (sub·sar·**tor**·e·al). Under the sartorius muscle. [L *sub*, sartorius.]

subsaturation (**sub**·sat·ewr·**a**'·shun). Applied to the state of any solution which is below saturation. [L *sub*, saturation.]

subscaphocephaly (**sub**·skaf·o·**kef**'·al·e). The condition of being slightly scaphocephalic. [L *sub*, scaphocephaly.]

subscapular (sub·**skap**·ew·lar). 1. Pertaining to the deep surface of the scapula. 2. Belonging to or supplying the subscapularis muscle. [L *sub*, scapula.]

subscapular artery [arteria subscapularis (NA)]. The largest branch of the axillary artery, from the third part. It runs along the lower margin of the subscapularis muscle to the angle of the scapula, giving off a large circumflex scapula branch [arteria circumflexa scapulae (NA)] to the infraspinous fossa.

subscapular nerves [nervi subscapulares (NA)]. Two branches, the upper and lower, from the posterior cord of the brachial plexus to the subscapularis and teres major muscles.

subscapularis muscle [musculus subscapularis] (**sub**·skap·ew·**la**'·ris musl). A muscle arising from most of the surface of the subscapular fossa and inserted into the lesser tuberosity of the humerus.

subscleral (sub·**skleer**·al). Beneath the sclera. [L *sub*, sclera.]

subsclerotic (sub·skleer·**ot**·ik). 1. Subscleral. 2. Sclerotic or sclerosed to mild degree. [L *sub*, sclerotic.]

subscription (sub·**skrip**·shun). That part of a prescription which gives the list of contents and the form the medicament is to take when compounded. It also includes directions for administration. [L *sub*, *scribere* to write.]

subseptal (sub·**sep**·tal). Beneath a septum. [L *sub*, septum.]

subserosa (sub·seer·**o**·sah). The tissue just underneath a serous membrane. [L *sub*, serous.]

subserous (sub·**seer**·us). Under a serous coat or a serous gland. [see prec.]

subserrate (sub·**ser**·ate). Having a moderately serrated edge or margin. [L *sub*, serrate.]

subsibilant (sub·**sib**·il·ant). Designating a râle the sound of which is between blowing and whistling in character. [L *sub*, *sibilans* hissing.]

subsoil (**sub**·soil). The stratum or bed of more compact material which lies beneath the surface earth or soil. [L *sub*, soil.]

sub-species (sub·**spe**·sheez). A taxonomic grouping below the species. Used of morphologically-distinct populations with some degree of isolation, usually geographical, but nevertheless capable of interbreeding with other members of the same species. Sub-specific names are printed in italic after the species name, giving trinomials. [L *sub*, species.]

subspinale (sub·spi·**na**·le). The deepest point on the bony profile between the nasal spine and crest of the maxilla. [L *sub*, spine.]

subspinous (sub·**spi**·nus). Beneath a spine, particularly the spine of the scapula. [see prec.]

substage (**sub**·staje). That part of a microscope which is below the stage and carries the illuminating unit (diaphragm, condenser, mirror, etc.). [L *sub*, stage.]

substance (**sub**·stans). 1. Matter; particularly solid matter. 2. [Substantia (NA)] Tissue. **Ad substance.** That substance effecting the passage of a nervous impulse across a synapse. **Agglutinable substance.** The substance in cells, such as erythrocytes and bacteria, that reacts with its specific agglutinin leading to agglutination of the cells concerned. **Agglutinating substance.** Agglutinin. **Alpha substance.** The reticular substance in erythrocytes. **Anterior pituitary-like substance.** A substance having a gonadotrophic activity similar to that of pituitary gonadotrophin; serum gonadotrophin, chorionic gonadotrophin. **Bactericidal substance.** A substance lethal to bacteria. **Basic substance.** An alkaline material; a cell constituent having an affinity for basic dyes. **Beta substance.** Heinz bodies. **C substance.** C substance of streptococci; the carbohydrate which is used as an antigen in the Lancefield group. All members of a given Lancefield group produce the same C substance. **Cell substance.** Protoplasm. **Cement substance.** Hyaline material which binds cells or fibres together, especially the cement between the endothelial cells of blood vessels. **Chromophilic substance.** Any cell constituent having a marked affinity for dyes. **Compact substance [substantia compacta (NA)].** The dense exterior portion of a bone. **Contact substance.** Any substance employed as a contact catalyst, e.g. platinized asbestos. **Contractile substance.** The contractile proteins of muscle fibres. **Cortical substance [substantia corticalis (NA)].** The outer portion of an organ, especially of the kidney, the brain or of a bone. **Ground substance.** The mucoid material in which connective-tissue cells and fibres are embedded, composed of hyaluronic acid, chondroitin sulphate and other mucopolysaccharides together with salts and water. **Group-specific substances.** Substances specific to a particular group, but usually the haemagglutinogens, e.g. the blood group-specific substances A and B, and other agglutinogens which are found in red cells, serum tissue cells and secretions such as saliva, gastric mucin, fluid from certain types of ovarian cysts, peptone and pepsin. **H substance.** The name given by Lewis to the substance released locally by an irritant stimulus applied to the skin, and which causes local redness and weal formation very similar to the effects of histamine. **Haemolytic substance.** The haemolysin or substance (cytase) in a haemolytic serum that lyses or destroys erythrocytes when added to it. **Interfilar substance.** Interfibrillar substance of Flemming. **Interprismatic substance.** The calcified tissue which lies between adjacent enamel prisms and unites them to form a solid mass. **Interspongioplastic substance.** Interfibrillar substance of Flemming. **Interstitial substance.** The ground substance of connective tissue; the cell matrix. **Isotelic substance.** A substance which has a physiological action because it contains a certain molecular group or arrangement of groups. **Ketogenic substance.** Any substance producing ketone bodies; applied to a high-fat diet. **Living substance.** Any essential part of a living cell. **Medullary substance.** The marrow or soft internal material of a bone, lymph gland or other organ with a well-defined firm outer cortex and a softer interior. **Metachromatic substance.** Fine lipoid granules seen in erythrocytes under certain conditions, such as after supravital staining. **Metaplastic substance.** Non-essential inclusions with a living cell. **Molecular substance.** The non-cellular components of grey matter. **Non-threshold substance.** Any substance in the blood which is excreted in the urine and has no renal threshold level. **Onychogenic substance.** The fibrous keratinous material composing the matrix of the developing nail. **Parietal substance.** The material composing the wall or cortex of an organ or cell. **Perforated substance, anterior [substantia perforata anterior (NA)].** An area on the under-surface of the brain between the optic tract and the uncus, bound anteriorly by the roots of the olfactory tract and laterally by the limen insulae. It lies below the corpus striatum, and is perforated by central branches of the anterior and middle cerebral arteries. **Perforated substance, posterior [substantia perforata posterior (NA)].** A layer of grey matter in the posterior part of the interpeduncular fossa perforated by branches of the posterior cerebral arteries. **Prelipoid substance.** Partially-broken-down myelin found during the early stages of degeneration of a tract or nerve. **Receptive substance.** A substance supposed to exist in motor end-plates, effecting the passage of the nervous impulse from nerve to muscle. **Reticular substance.** The reticulated or basket-like threads or network seen in some supravitally stained erythrocytes, as in reticulocytes. **Sarcous substance.** The cytoplasm of a muscle fibre. **Sensibilizing substance, Sensitizing substance.** Amboceptor. **Specific capsular substance, Specific soluble substance.** A polysaccharide produced by micro-organisms, e.g. pneumococci, and found in their capsules. It is upon this material that their antigenic specificity depends. **Spongy substance [substantia spongiosa (NA)].** The spongy bone underlying the compact substance. **Threshold substance.** A substance in the circulating blood that is only excreted in the urine when its blood level exceeds its specific renal threshold value. **Thromboplastic substance.** A substance that accelerates blood coagulation. **Tigroid substance.** Nissl substance. **Zymoplastic substance.** Thromboplastic substance (see above). [L *substantia* essence.]

See also: FLEMMING, NISSL, REICHSTEIN, ROLANDO, ROLLET (A.), ROVIDA, SCHWANN, SOEMMERING.

substantia [NA] (sub·stan·she·ah). Substance. **Substantia ferruginea [NA].** A collection of nerve cells in the lateral part of the floor of the 4th ventricle at the level of the middle of the pons. **Substantia gelatinosa.** The poorly-staining translucent grey matter which caps the dorsal extremity of the dorsal horn of grey matter of the spinal cord; Rolando's fasciculus or substance. **Substantia gelatinosa centralis.** The diffuse grey matter which surrounds the central canal of the spinal cord. **Substantia hyalina.** A chronic degenerative condition of collagen or elastic fibres in scar tissue, especially of small blood vessels during arteriosclerosis. **Substantia intermedia centralis [NA].** The band of grey matter in the spinal medulla which is situated immediately around the central canal; it is gelatinous in appearance and is the central part of the transverse grey commissure. **Substantia intermedia lateralis [NA].** The lateral and main portion of the transverse grey commissure of the spinal medulla. **Substantia lentis [NA].** The substance of the lens, apart from its epithelium and capsule. It consists of a firm central nucleus and a cortex. **Substantia metachromaticogranularis.** Heinz bodies. **Substantia nigra [NA].** A dark-brown band of grey matter lying between the tegmentum and basis pedunculi in the mid-brain. **Substantia opaca.** Substantia hyalina (see above). **Substantia propria [substantia propia corneae (NA)].** Superimposed lamellae of transparent fibrous tissue with their cells, the corneal corpuscles, forming the bulk of the thickness of the cornea. **Substantia propria sclerae [NA].** The white fibrous tissue of the sclera. [L essence.]

substernal (sub·ster·nal). Located below or deep to the sternum. [L *sub*, sternum.]

substernomastoid (sub·ster·no·mas′·toid). Under the sternocleidomastoid muscle. [L *sub*, sternomastoid.]

substitute (sub·stit·ewt). A replacement. **Blood substitute.** An artificial or natural fluid or mixture of fluids used as a replacement for blood in transfusion; they include plasma, serum, solutions of glucose, gelatin, gum, saline, isinglass, pectin, polymerized polysaccharides (dextran) and polyvinylpyrrolidine. [see foll.]

substitution (sub·stit·ew·shun). 1. The replacement of anything by another thing similar to it, or serving a similar function. 2. In chemistry, the replacement of certain atoms or radicals in a molecule by other atoms or radicals, sometimes closely related. 3. In pharmacy, the replacement of one drug by another in dispensing; it is only fraudulent when performed without regard to the wishes of the prescriber, and deliberately for gain. 4. In psycho-analysis, the formation of a substitute for the original aim of an instinct. [L *substituere* to put in place of.]

substitutive (sub·stit·ew·tiv). Substituting; capable of bringing about a change or substitution.

substrate (sub·strate). The term used in enzyme chemistry to denote the compound which is acted upon by an enzyme. **Renin substrate.** A serum globulin fraction which is acted upon by renin to produce hypertension. [L *sub*, *stratum* layer.]

substriate (sub·stri·ate). Partially striate; having striae that are imperfectly formed. [L *sub*, striate.]

subsulcus (sub·sul·kus). A sulcus that is hidden by overlapping. [L *sub*, sulcus.]

subsulphate (sub·sul·fate). Of the several sulphates of a metal, that one which contains the least proportion of sulphate radical, such as basic mercuric sulphate, $HgSO_4 \cdot 2HgO$. [L *sub*, sulphate.]

subsultory (sub·sul·tor·e). Convulsive; jerking; twitching. [L *sub*, *saltire* to leap.]

subsultus (sub·sul·tus). A convulsive or twitching movement. **Subsultus clonus, Subsultus tendinum.** A twitching of the muscles and tendons, particularly of the wrist, occurring in typhoid and asthenic fevers. [see prec.]

subsylvian (sub·sil·ve·an). Beneath the lateral sulcus of the cerebrum. [L *sub*, sylvian.]

subsynovial (sub·si·no·ve·al). Located beneath a synovial membrane or fold. [L *sub*, synovial.]

subtaenial (sub·te·ne·al). Occurring beneath any of the taenia of the brain, or of the large intestine. [L *sub*, taenia.]

subtalar (sub·ta·lar). Below the talus. [L *sub*, talus.]

subtarsal (sub·tar·sal). Located below the tarsus. [L *sub*, tarsus.]

subtegumental (sub·teg·ew·men′·tal). Subcutaneous; beneath the skin. [L *sub*, *tegumentum* cover.]

subtelocentric (sub·tel·o·sen′·trik). An improper term sometimes used to indicate acrocentric chromosomes. [L *sub*, Gk *telos* end, *kentron* centre.]

subtemporal (sub·tem·por·al). Located beneath the temple or temporal bone, or in the lower portion of the temporal lobe. [L *sub*, temple.]

subtentorial (sub·ten·tor·e·al). Situated beneath a tentorium. [L *sub*, tentorium.]

subterminal (sub·ter·min·al). Occurring near the end of a body. [L *sub*, *terminus* end.]

subtertian (sub·ter·shan). An intermittent malarial fever that deviates from the course of an ordinary tertian, applied specifically to malignant tertian malaria. [L *sub*, *tertius* third.]

subtetanic (sub·tet·an·ik). Having a slight tetanic quality; applied to convulsions which are remittently tonic and yet not clonic. [L *sub*, tetanus.]

subthalamic (sub·thal·am·ik). Located beneath the thalamus. **Subthalamic nucleus.** *See* NUCLEUS. [see foll.]

subthalamus (sub·thal·am·us). The region of the diencephalon between the thalamus above and the hypothalamus below; it includes the zona incerta, the fields of Forel, the subthalamic nucleus and the cranial ends of the red nucleus and substantia nigra. It contains many fibre systems connected mainly with the corpus striatum, thalamus and hypothalamus. [L *sub*, thalamus.]

subtilin (sub·ti·lin). An antibiotic, biosynthesized by a strain of *Bacillus subtilis*, which has been used in medicine, e.g. against Gram-positive bacteria, Gram-negative cocci and *Entamoeba* *histolytica;* in these rôles it has been surpassed by other antibiotics, but it has maintained its place in agriculture as a seed disinfectant.

subtotal (sub·**to**·tal). Not complete. [L *sub, totus* whole.]

subtrapezial (sub·trap·e·**ze**·al). Beneath the trapezius muscle. [L *sub,* trapezius.]

subtrochanteric (**sub**·tro·kan·**ter'**·ik). Below a trochanter. [L *sub* trochanter.]

subtrochlear (sub·**trok**·le·ar). Below the trochlea. [L *sub,* trochlea.]

subtropical (sub·**trop**·ik·al). Relating to a geographical region which borders on the tropical zone, or to the climate associated with it. [L *sub,* tropical.]

subtympanic (sub·tim·**pan**·ik). 1. Beneath the tympanic cavity. 2. Having a slightly resonant quality. [L *sub,* Gk *tympanon* drum.]

subtypical (sub·**tip**·ik·al). Not completely typical. [L *sub,* typical.]

subumbilical (sub·um·**bil**·ik·al). Below the umbilicus. [L *sub,* umbilicus.]

subungual, subunguial (sub·**ung**·gwal, sub·**ung**·gwe·al). Beneath a nail. [L *sub, unguis* nail.]

suburethral (sub·ewr·**e**·thral). Beneath the urethra. [L *sub,* urethra.]

subvaginal (sub·**vaj**·in·al). Below any sheath, particularly the vagina. [L *sub, vagina* sheath.]

subvalval (sub·**val**·val). Underneath a valve. [L *sub,* valve.]

subvertebral (sub·**ver**·te·bral). 1. Below a vertebra. 2. Towards the anterior or ventral aspect of the vertebral column. [L *sub,* vertebra.]

subvirile (sub·**vir**·ile). Lacking in virility. [L *sub,* virile.]

subvitaminosis (sub·vi·tam·in·**o'**·sis). Hypovitaminosis; a state brought on by deficiency of vitamin. **Subvitaminosis B_1.** Beriberi. [L *sub,* vitamin, Gk *-osis* condition.]

subvitrinal (sub·**vit**·rin·al). Beneath the vitreous body. [L *sub,* vitreous.]

subvolution (sub·vol·**ew**·shun). Turning under; applied to operations on the conjunctiva, e.g. McReynold's, where the pterygium, after being freed from the cornea, is tucked under the lower lip of the conjunctival wound. [L *sub, volvere* to turn.]

Suby, Howard I. 20th century Massachusetts urologist.

Suby's solution G. A solution of citric acid, magnesium oxide and sodium carbonate, used as a phosphatic solvent in bladder lavage.

subzonal (sub·**zo**·nal). Below any zone. [L *sub,* zone.]

subzygomatic (**sub**·zi·go·**mat'**·ik). Located below the zygomatic bone. [L *sub,* zygomatic.]

succagogue (**suk**·ag·og). Stimulating glandular secretion, or a substance capable of stimulating glandular secretion. [L *succus* juice, Gk *agogos* a leading.]

succedaneous (sux·e·**da**·ne·us). Pertaining to a succedaneum; serving as a substitute.

succedaneum (sux·e·**da**·ne·um). 1. A substitute. 2. Any drug which has the same therapeutic properties as another, and may be used instead of the latter. **Caput succedaneum.** An area of passive oedema forming on the presenting part of the fetus during labour. It is due to pressure on veins and lymphatics. [L *succedere* to replace.]

succenturiate (sux·en·**tewr**·e·ate). Employed as a substitute; accessory. [L *succenturiare* to receive a replacement.]

succiferous (sux·**if**·er·us). Yielding or bearing sap. [L *succus* juice, *ferre* to bear.]

succinamide (sux·**in**·am·ide). $NH_2COCH_2CH_2CONH_2$, a derivative of succinic acid with ammonia; used in organic synthesis.

succinate (**sux**·in·ate). $(CH_2COOH)_2$, an intermediate of the citric-acid cycle. **Succinate dehydrogenase.** The flavoprotein-linked dehydrogenase which catalyses the formate of fumarate from succinate. **Succinate thiokinase.** The enzyme which catalyses the formation of succinate and GTP from succinyl CoA and GDP during citric-acid cycle turnover.

succinic dehydrogenase (sux·**in**·ik de·**hi**·droj·en·aze). An enzyme occurring in most animal and plant tissues which catalyses the oxidation of succinic acid, yielding fumaric acid.

succinimide (sux·**in**·im·ide). $(CH_2CO)_2NH$, a derivative of succinic acid which is readily reduced to pyrrole. It is used in the manufacture of certain drugs, and its chloralimide is employed in the sterilization of drinking water.

succinonitrile (**sux**·in·o·**ni'**·trile). Ethylene dicyanide, $CNCH_2CH_2CN$. A compound derived from ethylene bromide and hydrolysed to succinic acid, in the artificial synthesis of the latter.

succinous (**sux**·in·us). Of the nature of or relating to amber. [L *succinum* amber.]

succinum (**sux**·in·um). Amber. [L.]

succinyl CoA (**sux**·in·il). An intermediate in the citric-acid cycle. Also a precursor of *S*-amino-laevulinic acid and the porphyrins.

succinylcholine (**sux**·in·il·**ko'**·leen). Suxamethonium.

succinyldicholine (**sux**·in·il·di·**ko'**·leen). A derivative of choline which is hydrolysed by true cholinesterase at high substrate concentrations and by pseudocholinesterase at both low and high concentrations, to form first succinylmonocholine and then succinic acid and choline.

succinylmonocholine (**sux**·in·il·mon·o·**ko'**·leen). A derivative of choline which is hydrolysed by true cholinesterase at low substrate concentrations. In rabbits in high doses it has a relaxant effect which can be controlled by intravenous pseudo-cholinesterase.

Succinylsulfathiazolum (suk·sin·il·**sul**·fah·thi·az·**o'**·lum). *European Pharmacopoeia* name for Succinylsulphathiazole BP 1973.

Succinylsulphathiazole BP 1973 (**sux**·in·il·sul·fah·**thi'**·az·ole). 2-(*p*-Succinylaminobenzene sulphonamide), $HOOC(CH_2)_2CONHC_6H_4SO_2NHC_3H_2NS$. A derivative of sulphanilamide in which both the amino- and amido- groups are substituted. It is absorbed with difficulty, about 95 per cent remaining in the alimentary canal, and for this reason is used mainly to treat bacterial infections of the gut. It causes a marked reduction in *Bacterium coli* and related organisms, and is employed in bacillary dysentery and to prepare patients for extensive surgery of the gastro-intestinal tract where there would be increased risk of peritonitis.

succorrhoea (suk·or·e·ah). An increase in the flow of a digestive juice. **Pancreatic succorrhoea.** An abnormal increase of pancreatic juice where there is undue stimulation of the nerves supplying the pancreas. [L *succus* juice, *rhoia* flow.]

succory (**suk**·or·e). Chicory; the root of *Cichorium intybus* Linn. (family Compositae), of Europe and Asia. It resembles dandelion root. Dried, roasted and ground, it is used to adulterate coffee and as a substitute for the latter. [corruption of *chicory.*]

succus [NA] (**suk**·us). Juice. **Succus allii.** The juice of *Allium sativum* preserved by the addition of alcohol; it has been used in the treatment of lupus. **Succus prostaticus.** Prostatic fluid. [L.]

succussion (suk·**ush**·un). A method of ascertaining the presence of free fluid and gas in any of the body cavities by shaking the patient; the splashing is heard. **Hippocratic succussion.** A splashing sound in the pleural cavity, heard in cases of hydro-, pyo- or sero-pneumothorax; also the sound of fluid in a dilated stomach. [L *succutere* to shake up.]

suckle (sukl). 1. To nurse at the breast. 2. To suck from the breast. [L *sugere* to suck.]

suckling (**suk**·ling). An unweaned child. [see prec.]

Sucquet, J. P. (fl. 1840–1870). Paris anatomist.

Sucquet's anastomoses or canals, Sucquet-Hoyer anastomoses or canals. Communications between preterminal branches (glomic branches) of cutaneous arterioles and venules found in the digits.

Sucralox (**sew**·kral·ox). BP Commission approved name for a polymerized complex of sucrose and aluminium hydroxide.

sucramine (**sew**·kram·een). The ammonium salt of saccharin, used as a sweetening agent. It is said to be 700 times as sweet as sugar. [see foll.]

sucrase (**sew**·kraze). Saccharase, invertase. An enzyme in plants, fungi and the intestinal secretion of animals. It brings about the hydrolysis of sucrose into equal parts of glucose and fructose (invert sugar). [Fr. *sucre* sugar.]

sucrate (sew·krate). A saccharosate; any compound formed by cane sugar (sucrose) with a base.
sucrene (sew·kreen). Sucrol.
sucroclastic (sew·kro·klas·tik). Describing any enzyme or organism that breaks down sugars into simpler compounds. [sucrose, Gk *klastis* a breaking.]
sucrol (sew·krol). $C_2H_5OC_6H_4NHCONH_2$, a compound used as a sweetening agent. It is moderately soluble in water, and is about 200 times as sweet as sugar. [Fr. *sucre* sugar.]
sucrosaemia (sew·kro·se·me·ah). A morbid condition marked by the presence of sucrose in the blood. [sucrose, Gk *haima* blood.]
Sucrose BP 1973 (sew·kroze). Saccharose, saccharobiose, cane sugar, beet sugar, $C_{12}H_{22}O_{11}$. A disaccharide (fructofuranose α-glucoside) found in sugar cane, sugar beet, sugar maple and other plants. It is a colourless crystalline substance, very soluble in water, giving a solution that is non-reducing and dextrorotatory. Hydrolysed by dilute acids and invertase to a laevorotatory mixture of glucose and fructose (invert sugar). It is used in confectionery and preserves, and as a food and sweetening agent. [Fr. *sucre* sugar.]
Sucrosum (sew·kro·sum). *European Pharmacopoeia* name for Sucrose BP 1973.
sucrosuria (sew·kro·sewr·e·ah). The presence of sucrose in the urine. [sucrose, Gk *ouron* urine.]
suction (suk·shun). 1. The process of sucking; aspiration. 2. The combined forces of adhesion and cohesion which retain an artificial denture in position in the mouth. **Post-tussive suction.** A sucking noise heard immediately after a cough when the stethoscope is placed over a cavity whose walls are not too rigid. It is due to the re-entry of air into the cavity which has been partially compressed. [L *sugere* to suck.]
See also: BIER, WANGENSTEEN.
Suctoria (suk·tor·e·ah). An order of insects; Aphaniptera, Siphonaptera; fleas. [Obsolete term.] [see prec.]
suctorial (suk·tor·e·al). 1. Relating to suction or sucking. 2. Serving or adapted to produce suction.
sucuuba (soo·koo·oo·bah). *Plumeria phagedenica* (family Apocyanaceae), a medicinal plant found in South America.
sudamen (sew·da·men) (pl. *sudamina*). A minute non-inflammatory white vesicle formed in the ducts of sweat glands or under the epidermis after fevers and copious sweating. **Sudamina crystallina.** Miliaria alba. [L *sudare* to sweat.]
sudaminal (sew·dam·in·al). Characterized by or relating to sudamina.
Sudan (soo·dan). A series of fat stains used in histology, especially *Sudan I, II, III* and *IV* and *Sudan black.* They are azo, diazo or polyazo dyes, insoluble in water, slightly soluble in alcohol and dissolving freely in liquid fatty substances; they are therefore usually employed in alcoholic solution on frozen sections of tissue. **Sudan III.** Oil scarlet, benzeneazobenzeneazo-β-naphthol; it is also sometimes used as a substitute, in the treatment of wounds, for scarlet red (Sudan IV) and has a similar action. **Sudan IV.** Scarlet red, Biebrich scarlet medicinal, $CH_3C_6H_4N{=}NC_6H_3(CH_3)N{=}NC_{10}H_6OH$. It is also used in the form of an ointment to hasten epithelial growth.
sudanophil, sudanophile (soo·dan·o·fil, soo·dan·o·file). Capable of taking up Sudan stains (Sudan III); usually associated with leucocytes or other tissue cells that have undergone fatty degeneration. [Sudan, Gk *philein* to love.]
sudanophilia (soo·dan·o·fil'·e·ah). A condition in which the white blood cells contain certain fatty or lipoid structures or particles that can be stained with Sudan red dyes. [see prec.]
sudanophilic (soo·dan·o·fil'·ik). Sudanophil.
sudation (sew·da·shun). 1. Sweating. 2. Hyperhidrosis. [see foll.]
sudatoria (sew·dat·or·e·ah). 1. Hyperhidrosis; ephidrosis. 2. Miliaria. [L *sudare* to sweat.]
sudatorium (sew·dat·or·e·um). 1. A sweat bath or hot-air bath, which produces copious sweating. 2. A room in which hot-air baths are given; a Turkish bath. [see prec.]
Sudeck, Paul Hermann Martin (b. 1866). Hamburg surgeon.
Sudeck's atrophy or disease, Sudeck-Leriche syndrome. Acute atrophy of bone at the site of an injury showing radiographically as an area of osteoporosis and probably caused by reflex local vasospasm; it occurs most commonly in the small bones of the hand or foot.
point of Sudeck. The site of division of the inferior mesenteric artery in distal colon resection so that the blood supply is preserved; a point on the inferior mesenteric artery directly below the first inferior left colic branch.
sudokeratosis (sew·do·ker·at·o'·sis). Sudorikeratosis.
sudolorrhoea (sew·do·lor·e'·ah). Seborrhoea. [L *sudor* sweat, *oleum* oil, Gk *rhoia* flow.]
sudomotor (sew·do·mo·tor). Of nerves, stimulating the secretion of sweat. [L *sudor* sweat, *movere* to move.]
sudor [NA] (sew·dor). Sweat; perspiration. **Sudor anglicus.** Miliaria rubra; miliary fever. **Sudor cruentis.** Haemathidrosis. **Sudor nocturnus.** Night sweat. **Sudor sanguineus, Sudor sanguinosus.** Haemathidrosis. **Sudor urinosus.** Urhidrosis. [L.]
sudoral (sew·dor·al). Pertaining to or caused by sweat. [L *sudor* sweat.]
sudoresis (sew·dor·e·sis). Hyperhidrosis; copious sweating; diaphoresis. [see prec.]
sudoriferous (sew·dor·if·er·us). Excreting or yielding sweat. [L *sudor* sweat, *ferre* to bear.]
sudorific (sew·dor·if·ik). Diaphoretic; giving rise to perspiration. [L *sudor* sweat, *facere* to make.]
sudorikeratosis (sew·dor·e·ker·at·o'·sis). Keratosis of the ducts of the sweat glands. [L *sudor* sweat, keratosis.]
sudoriparous (sew·dor·ip·ar·us). Sudoriferous. [L *sudor* sweat, *parere* to produce.]
sudorrhoea (sew·dor·e·ah). Hyperhidrosis; undue sweating. [L *sudor* sweat, Gk *rhoia* flow.]
Sudoxicam (sew·dox·e·kam). BP Commission approved name for 4-hydroxy-2-methyl-*N*-thiazol-2-yl-2*H*-1,2-benzothiazine-3-carboxamide 1,1-dioxide; an anti-inflammatory agent.
suet (sew·et). Prepared suet, sevum; a fat obtained from the fresh omentum of the sheep. It is used in the preparation of a few ointments. **Benzoinated suet.** Suet melted with 3 per cent of benzoin. [O Fr. *seu.*]
suffocate (suf·o·kate). To stop respiration and cause asphyxia. [see foll.]
suffocation (suf·o·ka·shun). Interference with respiration which causes a deprivation of air. It usually refers to obstruction to the entrance of air into the mouth, nose, larynx or trachea by mechanical impediments, and so includes smothering, overlying, foreign bodies in the air passages, the result of natural disease, accident or intention, and the effect of irrespirable gases. [L *suffocare* to choke.]
suffumigation (suf·few·mig·a'·shun). 1. The act of fumigating with smoke or vapour. 2. Any preparation used in fumigation. [L *sub, fumigare* to smoke.]
suffusion (suf·ew·zhun). 1. The spreading of a body fluid into the adjoining tissues. 2. An extravasation of blood. 3. The treatment by pouring water or any other fluid over the affected part. [L *sub, fundere* to pour out.]
sugar (shug·er). 1. The ordinary name for sucrose. 2. The common general name for carbohydrates that have a sweet taste, are soluble in water and are mostly crystallizable with more or less ease; they may be of animal origin, plant origin or formed artificially by organic synthesis. They are divided into *simple sugars* (monosaccharides) and *compound sugars*, which are composed of 2 or more monosaccharides. All simple sugars contain either aldehyde or ketone groups and thus reduce alkaline solutions of cupric salts; compound sugars are non-reducing or reducing, according to whether these groups are or are not involved in the linkage of the monosaccharide units. The presence of an asymmetric carbon atom confers optical activity on all sugars. In the animal, sugars are the source of energy (heat, muscular activity); in the plant they go to build tissue (cellulose). **Acid of sugar.** Oxalic acid; so-called because of its preparation by the oxidation of cane sugar. **Acorn sugar.** Quercitol, a cyclic sugar found in acorns. **Actual sugar.** The true

sugars of the blood. **Anhydrous sugar.** Anhydrosugar. **Barley sugar.** An amorphous form of cane sugar obtained by melting it. **Beechwood sugar.** Wood sugar (see below). **Beet sugar.** Sucrose obtained from sugar beet, *Beta vulgaris* var. *rapa*. **Blood sugar.** The sugars of the blood; mainly glucose, with small quantities of fructose, galactose and sometimes pentoses. **Brain sugar.** Galactose, the sugar of the cerebrosides. **Brown sugar.** Cane sugar not fully refined. **Burnt Sugar BPC 1968.** Caramel, a dark mass prepared by heating sugar; used as a colouring. **Cane sugar.** Sucrose obtained from the juice of the sugar cane, *Saccharum officinarum*. **Cellulose sugar.** Cellobiose, a disaccharide obtained from cellulose by hydrolysis. **Collagen sugar.** Gelatin sugar (see below). **Corn sugar.** A mixture of glucose, maltose and dextrin, obtained by the hydrolysis of starch. **Date sugar.** The sugar obtained from the date, *Phoenix dactylifera*. **Diabetic sugar.** Glucose observed in the urine in diabetes mellitus; sometimes applied wrongly to the saccharin used by diabetics as a sweetening agent. **Fruit sugar.** Fructose, so called from its occurrence in fruits. **Gelatin sugar.** The simple amino acid, glycine, obtained by the hydrolysis of collagens and gelatin; it is sweet tasting, but not a true sugar. **Grape sugar.** Glucose; so-called from its occurrence in grape juice. **Gum sugar.** Arabinose; so-called from its occurrence in gum arabic and other gums. **Heart sugar.** Muscle sugar (see below). **Honey sugar.** Glucose; so-called from its occurrence in honey. **Invert sugar.** The mixture of glucose and fructose produced by the hydrolysis of sucrose; so-called because of the inversion of optical rotation from the dextrorotation of sucrose to the laevorotation of the mixture. **Sugar of lead.** Lead acetate. **Liver sugar.** Glycogen, found stored in the liver and muscles; it is a polysaccharide and not a true sugar. **Malt sugar.** Maltose, the disaccharide occurring in germinated barley (malt). **Manna sugar.** Mannose. **Maple sugar.** Sucrose obtained from maple syrup. **Meat sugar.** Muscle sugar (see below). **Milk sugar.** Lactose, a disaccharide occurring in the milk of all mammals. **Muscle sugar.** Inositol, a sweet-tasting hexahydroxy alcohol occurring in muscle; it is not a true sugar. **Pectin sugar.** Arabinose. **Reducing sugar.** Name applied to any sugar which reduces alkaline solutions of cupric salts, e.g. Fehling's solution: all simple sugars and certain compound sugars. **Refined sugar.** Sucrose, whether cane or beet sugar, that has been fully refined. **Simple sugar.** Any monosaccharide. **Starch sugar.** Dextrin, an intermediate in the hydrolysis of starch and not a true sugar. **Sulphur sugar.** A synthetic sugar in which sulphur has replaced the oxygen of the aldehyde group, e.g. thioglucose. **Virtual sugar.** Reducing substances of blood released on hydrolysis and estimable as sugar. **Wood sugar.** Xylose, the pentose occurring in wood as the polymeric xylans. [Gk *sakcharon*.]

See also: HISS, LEO.

sugarin (shug·ar·in). Methyl saccharin, a sweetening agent said to be 500 times as sweet as sugar.

suggestibility (suj·es·tib·il'·it·e). A state of mind in which the individual is abnormally receptive to the ideas and suggestions of others. **Negative suggestibility.** Negativism.

suggestible (suj·es·tibl). Open to be influenced by suggestion.

suggestion (suj·es·chun). 1. The insinuation into the mind of a person of certain ideas or sensations originating externally and producing such a condition that he is influenced thereby in his actions, or experiences such sensations as are suggested to him. 2. The idea or sensation suggested. **Hypnotic suggestion.** A suggestion implanted in the mind of an individual under hypnosis. **Posthypnotic suggestion.** One made to an individual under hypnosis, causing him to carry out the particular act suggested after he has emerged from the hypnotic state. **Self suggestion.** Autosuggestion. **Traumatic suggestion.** A condition arising after accidental injury in which all subsequent injuries, however slight, produce exaggerated hysterical symptoms. [L *suggerere* to suggest.]

suggillation (suj·il·a·shun). 1. A bruise or ecchymosis. 2. A livedo. [L *suggilare* to render black and blue.]

suicide (sew·is·ide). 1. The act of killing oneself. Now no longer a crime since the passing of the Suicide Act 1961. 2. An individual who had voluntarily and deliberately taken his own life. [L *sui* of himself, *caedere* to kill.]

suint (swint). The crude potash soap obtained from the washings of wool and from which wool fat is prepared. [Fr. wool fat.]

suit (sewt). **Anti-G suit, G suit.** A garment which prevents pooling of blood in the lower half of the body when increased G force makes the blood heavier. **Pressure suit.** A garment designed to maintain pressure upon the lungs and the body so that the respiration and circulation of the blood may continue in low ambient pressures. **Space suit.** A pressure suit designed for extravehicular activities.

Suker's sign. Inability to hold fixation on extreme lateral movements of the eyes, as seen in thyrotoxic exophthalmos.

sulcal (sul·kal). Of the nature of or pertaining to a sulcus.

sulciform (sul·se·form). Similar to a sulcus in form.

sulculus (sul·kew·lus) (pl. *sulculi*). A small sulcus. [L.]

sulcus [NA] (sul·kus). A furrow, especially of the cerebral hemispheres. **Ampullary sulcus [sulcus ampullaris].** *See* AMPULLA, MEMBRANOUS. **Anterolateral sulcus [sulcus lateralis anterior** (NA)**].** The groove between the olive and the pyramid, from which the hypoglossal rootlets emerge. **Sulcus of the antihelix, transverse [sulcus anthelicis transversus** (NA)**].** A furrow on the cranial surface of the cartilage, corresponding to the inferior crus of the antihelix. **Arterial sulci [sulci arteriosi** (NA)**].** Markings on the interior surface of the skull produced by the middle meningeal artery. **Sulcus of the auricle, posterior [sulcus auriculae posterior** (NA)**].** A sulcus separating the lower end of the antihelix from the antitragus. **Basilar sulcus.** Sulcus of the pons, basilar (see below). **Bulboventricular sulcus.** The groove between the bulbus and ventricle of the embryonic heart. **Calcarine sulcus [sulcus calcarinus** (NA)**].** A deep, horizontal fissure on the medial surface of the cerebral hemisphere, continuous with the postcalcarine sulcus and lying in front of the parieto-occipital sulcus. **Callosal sulcus [sulcus corporis callosi** (NA)**].** A fissure on the medial surface of the cerebral hemisphere, separating the corpus callosum from the gyrus cinguli. **Carpal sulcus [sulcus carpi** (NA)**].** The concavity on the front of the carpus. **Central sulcus.** Sulcus of the cerebrum, central (see below). **Cerebral sulci [sulci cerebri** (NA)**].** Enfoldings of the surface of the cerebral cortex. **Sulcus of the cerebral peduncle, lateral.** A groove on the lateral surface of the cerebral peduncle separating it into a tegmental and a basal portion. **Sulcus of the cerebral peduncle, medial [sulcus medialis cruris cerebri** (NA)**].** A longitudinal furrow on the medial surface of the cerebral peduncle from which the fibres of the oculomotor nerve emerge. **Sulcus of the cerebrum, central [sulcus centralis** (NA)**].** A deep fissure on the superolateral surface of the cerebrum extending downwards and forwards from just behind the middle of the superior border to near the lateral sulcus. It separates the frontal from the parietal lobe. **Sulcus of the cerebrum, lateral [sulcus lateralis** (NA)**].** A deep fissure on the superolateral surface separating the temporal lobe below from the frontal and parietal lobes above. It contains the insula and the middle cerebral artery. **Sulcus cinguli [NA].** A sulcus situated anteriorly on the medial surface of the cerebral hemisphere curving around the corpus callosum; it separates the gyrus cinguli from the medial frontal gyrus. **Circular sulcus.** Sulcus of the insula, circular (see below). **Collateral sulcus [sulcus collateralis** (NA)**].** A sulcus on the tentorial surface and bounding the lingual gyrus inferolaterally. It runs parallel to the calcarine and postcalcarine sulci. **Sulcus of the crus of the helix [sulcus cruris helicis** (NA)**].** A furrow on the cranial surface of the cartilage, corresponding to the crus. **Sulcus of the frontal lobe, inferior frontal [sulcus frontalis inferior** (NA)**].** The lower of 2 parallel sulci on the surface of the frontal lobe. **Sulcus of the frontal lobe, precentral [sulcus precentralis** (NA)**].** A sulcus in front of and parallel to the central sulcus of the cerebrum, usually in 2 parts. **Sulcus of the frontal lobe, superior frontal [sulcus frontalis superior** (NA)**].** The superior of 2 horizontal sulci lying between the superior and middle frontal gyri. **Gingivolabial sulcus.** The pouch formed at the junction of the mucosa on the labial aspect of the join with that of the cheek. **Hemispherical sulcus.** The groove separating the rudiment of a cerebral hemisphere from the diencephalon in the early embryo. **Hippocampal sulcus [sulcus hippocampi (NA)].** A sulcus on the medial side of the hippocampal gyrus. It produces a bulge in the floor of the inferior horn of the lateral ventricle called the *hippocampus.* **Hypothalamic sulcus.** Sulcus of the third ventricle, hypothalamic (see below). **Infrapalpebral sulcus [sulcus infrapalpebralis (NA)].** The depression below the lower eyelid. **Sulcus of the insula, central [sulcus centrale insulae (NA)].** A deep sulcus which runs upwards and backwards across the insula, dividing it into a larger anterior and a smaller posterior part. **Sulcus of the insula, circular [sulcus circularis insulae (NA)].** A depression surrounding the insula in the floor of the lateral sulcus; Reil's sulcus. **Interatrial sulcus.** The groove on the surface of the embryonic heart at the junction of the right and left atria as these begin to be differentiated from the common atrial chamber. **Intraparietal sulcus.** Sulcus of the parietal lobe, intraparietal (see below). **Labiodental sulcus.** The furrow which appears on the upper surface of the mandibular arch of an embryo, defining the boundary between lip and jaw. **Lateral sulcus.** 1. Sulcus of the cerebrum, lateral (see above). 2. Sulcus of the cerebral peduncle, lateral (see above). 3. Sulcus of the occipital lobe, lateral (see below). **Sulcus limitans** [NA]. A longitudinal furrow which develops in the early embryo on the inner surface of each lateral wall of the spinal medulla and brain stem and divides this into 2 functionally distinct areas termed the alar and basal laminae. **Sulcus limitans of the fourth ventricle [sulcus limitans (NA)].** A laterally placed groove in the floor of the 4th ventricle extending from the cerebral aqueduct through the superior and inferior foveae to the central canal of the closed part of the medulla oblongata. In the embryo it separates the alar and basal laminae. **Lunate sulcus.** Sulcus of occipital lobe, lunate (see below). **Medial sulcus.** Sulcus of the cerebral peduncle, medial (see above). **Median sulcus.** A sulcus in the midline. **Sulcus medianus of the fourth ventricle [sulcus medianus (NA)].** The midline groove that extends the whole length of the floor of the 4th ventricle from the aqueduct to the central canal in the closed part of the medulla oblongata. **Nasofrontal sulcus.** The furrow between the forehead and the nose on the face of an early embryo before the bridge of the nose has appeared. **Sulcus of the occipital lobe, lateral.** A variable fissure on the lateral surface of the occipital lobe, forming the superior and inferior occipital gyri. **Sulcus of the occipital lobe, lunate [sulcus lunatus (NA)].** A curved sulcus on the lateral surface which forms the anterior limit of the visual cortex. **Sulcus of the occipital lobe, transverse [sulcus occipitalis transversus (NA)].** A sulcus from the occipital branch of the intraparietal sulcus of the parietal lobe continuing over the occipital lobe. **Occipitotemporal sulcus [sulcus occipitotemporalis (NA)].** A sulcus on the tentorial surface, lateral and parallel to the collateral and rhinal sulci. It separates the medial and lateral occipitotemporal gyri. **Olfactory sulcus [sulcus olfactorius (NA)].** A sulcus on the inferior surface of the frontal lobe parallel to the inferomedial border and in which the olfactory lobe and tract lie. **Sulci of the orbital surface of the cerebral hemisphere, orbital [sulci orbitales (NA)].** A composite furrow of great variety, separating the orbital gyri. **Palatinovaginal sulcus [sulcus palatinovaginalis (NA)].** A groove on the lower surface of the vaginal process of the pterygoid process of the sphenoid bone which, with a similar groove on the sphenoidal process of the palatine bone, forms the palatinovaginal canal. **Sulcus of the parietal lobe, intraparietal [sulcus intraparietalis (NA)].** An irregular horizontal sulcus dividing the posterior part of the parietal lobe into a superior and inferior parietal lobule. **Sulcus of the parietal lobe, postcentral [sulcus postcentralis (NA)].** A sulcus parallel to and behind the central sulcus of the cerebrum. **Parieto-occipital sulcus [sulcus parieto-occipitalis (NA)].** A deep sulcus on the medial surface of the cerebral hemisphere running downwards and forwards from the superomedial border to meet the junction of the calcarine and postcalcarine sulci. **Parolfactory sulcus, anterior.** A shallow groove on the medial surface of the cerebral hemisphere bounding the parolfactory area anteriorly. **Parolfactory sulcus, posterior.** A shallow groove on the medial surface of the cerebral hemisphere between the parolfactory area and paraterminal gyrus. **Sulcus of the pons, basilar [sulcus basilaris (NA)].** A median groove on the anterior surface of the pons, lodging the basilar artery. **Postcalcarine sulcus.** The posterior part of a deep horizontal fissure which runs from the occipital pole to the parieto-occipital sulcus on the medial surface of the cerebral hemisphere. **Postcentral sulcus.** Sulcus of the parietal lobe, postcentral (see above). **Posterolateral sulcus [sulcus lateralis posterior (NA)].** The longitudinal groove that passes posterior to the olive, from the bottom of which the glossopharyngeal, vagus and accessory nerves emerge. **Pre-auricular sulcus.** A groove in front of the auricular surface of the ilium present in some female bones. **Precentral sulcus.** Sulcus of the frontal lobe, precentral (see above). **Prelunate sulcus.** Sulcus of the occipital lobe, lateral (see above). **Prenodular sulcus.** The sulcus between the posterior lobe and the rest of the cerebellum. Its middle portion lies between the nodule and uvula of the vermis. **Sulcus of the pterygoid hamulus [sulcus hamuli pterygoidei (NA)].** A groove on the hamulus in which the tendon of the tensor palati muscle lies. **Pterygopalatine sulcus [sulcus palatinus major (NA)].** That part of the pterygoid process that forms the posterior wall of the pterygopalatine fossa. **Pulmonary sulcus [sulcus pulmonalis (NA)].** The broad groove lying on either side of the vertebral column in the thorax, resulting from the backward and lateral direction of the ribs from their heads to their angles. **Rhinal sulcus [sulcus rhinalis (NA)].** A sulcus on the tentorial surface in line with, and sometimes continuous with, the collateral sulcus. It lies between the temporal pole and the uncus. **Sulcus sclerae** [NA]. A circular furrow between the sclerocorneal junction and the iris. **Sulcus of the spinal cord, posterior intermediate [sulcus intermedius posterior (NA)].** A longitudinal furrow present on the surface of the cervical and upper thoracic region of the spinal medulla and marking the junction of the fasciculi gracilis and cuneatus. **Sulcus of the spinal cord, posterior lateral [sulcus lateralis posterior (NA)].** A longitudinal furrow on the surface of the spinal medulla along which the bundles of the posterior nerve roots enter. **Sulcus of the spinal cord, posterior median [sulcus medianus posterior (NA)].** A shallow midline groove on the back of the spinal cord, from which the posterior median septum projects deeply into the white matter of the cord. **Spiral sulci.** Grooves lying immediately above the crista basilaris (external groove [sulcus spiralis externus (NA)]) or the tympanic lip (internal groove [sulcus spiralis internus (NA)]). **Suprasplenial sulcus [sulcus subparietalis (NA)].** A shallow groove surrounding the parasplenial area. **Suprasylvian sulcus.** A sulcus present in many mammals above the lateral sulcus; it does not occur in man. **Sulcus of the temporal lobe, inferior temporal [sulcus temporalis inferior (NA)].** The lower of 2 sulci parallel to the lateral sulcus; it is often subdivided and irregular. **Sulcus of the temporal lobe, superior temporal [sulcus temporalis superior (NA)].** A sulcus parallel to and below the lateral sulcus; it separates the superior and middle temporal gyri. **Sulci of the temporal lobe, transverse temporal [sulci temporales transversi (NA)].** Transverse fissures on the floor of the posterior ramus of the lateral sulcus. **Sulcus terminalis** [NA]. A V-shaped sulcus, open forwards, at the junction of the anterior two-thirds and posterior one-third of the tongue; at the apex of the V is a small pit. The sulcus marks the junction of developmentally distinct parts of the organ. **Sulcus terminalis of the right atrium [sulcus terminalis (NA)].** A groove on the lateral surface of the right atrium, running between the right sides of the entrances of the venae cavae. It marks the division between the embryonic atrium and sinus venosus. **Sulcus of the third ventricle, hypothalamic [sulcus hypothalamicus (NA)].** A shallow groove on the side wall of the 3rd ventricle separating the thalamus from the hypothalamus, thought by some to be the rostral continuation of the sulcus limitans. **Sulcus of the tongue, median [sulcus medianus linguae (NA)].**

The furrow on the dorsum of the tongue in the midsagittal plane. **Venous sulci [sulci venosi (NA)].** Markings on the interior surface of the skull produced by venous channels. **Vermicular sulci.** The grooves on each side of the vermis of the cerebellum. **Vomerovaginal sulcus [sulcus vomerovaginalis (NA)].** A groove on the upper surface of the vaginal process of the pterygoid process of the sphenoid bone which, with a similar groove on the ala of the vomer, forms the vomerovaginal canal. [L.]

See also: EBERSTALLER, ECKER, HARRISON (E.), JACOBSON (L. L.), MONRO II, PANSCH, REIL, ROLANDO, SYLVIUS, TURNER (W.), WALDEYER-HARTZ.

Sulfacytine (sul·fah·si·teen). BP Commission approved name for 1-ethyl-*N*-sulfanilylcytosine; an antibacterial agent.

Sulfadimidinum (sul·fah·**dim**·id·in·um). *European Pharmacopoeia* name for Sulphadimidine BP 1973.

Sulfadoxine (sulf·ah·**dox**·een). BP Commission approved name for 4-(4-aminobenzenesulphonamido)-5,6-dimethoxy-pyrimidine; it is used in sulphonamide therapy.

Sulfametopyrazine (**sul**·fah·met·o·**pi**′·raz·een). BP Commission approved name for 2-(4-aminobenzenesulphonamido)-3-methoxypyrazine; it is used in sulphonamide therapy.

sulfhaemoglobin (**sulf**·he·mo·**glo**′·bin). *See* SULPHAEMOGLOBIN.

Sulglycotide (sul·**gli**·ko·tide). BP Commission approved name for the sulphuric polyester of a glycopeptide isolated from pig duodenum; it is used in the treatment of peptic ulcer.

Sulkowitch, Hirsh Wolf (b. 1906). Boston physician.

Sulkowitch reagent. For calcium. Dissolve 2.5 g of oxalic acid, 2.5 g of ammonium oxalate and 5 ml of glacial acetic acid in water, and dilute to 150 ml.

Sulkowitch's test. For calcium in urine. Mix equal volumes of urine and Sulkowitch reagent. No precipitate indicates hypocalcaemia, a fine white cloud indicates a normal serum calcium, while if the liquid looks like milk hypercalcaemia is probable.

sullage (**sul**·ij). Sewage. [O Fr. *soillage.*]

Sullivan, Michael Savier (b. 1875). Georgetown biochemist.

Sullivan's test. For cysteine. To 5 ml of test solution add 1 ml of 1 per cent sodium cyanide in 0.8 M sodium hydroxide. Add 1 ml of a freshly prepared aqueous solution of 1,2-naphthoquinone-4-sodium sulphonate and then, after 5 min, 5 ml of 0.5 M sodium sulphite in 0.5 M sodium hydroxide. Allow to stand for 20 min. Add 1 ml of freshly prepared 0.1 M sodium hydrosulphite ($Na_2S_2O_4$) in 0.5 M sodium hydroxide. Mix and add 5 ml of 2.5 M sodium hydroxide. An orange to red colour indicates cysteine. For cystine, allow to stand for 10 min after addition of cyanide to ensure reduction to cysteine.

sulpha drugs (**sul**·fah drugz). Sulphanilamide and its derivatives, used extensively in the chemotherapy of bacterial infections. They are effective against Gram-positive cocci (e.g. haemolytic streptococci and pneumococci), and to a lesser degree against staphylococci; their greatest value is against Gram-negative meningococci and gonococci. They are not effective against Gram-negative bacilli, viruses or the spirochaetes of syphilis.

Sulphacetamide BPC 1959 (sul·fah·**set**·am·ide). *p*-Aminobenzenesulphonacetamide, $NH_2C_6H_4SO_2NHOCCH_3$. A sulphonamide compound which is very soluble, especially the sodium salt (Sulphacetamide Sodium BP 1973) which readily penetrates the cornea and conjunctiva and also the skin. Its chief value is for local application, especially for surface lesions of the cornea or conjunctiva. The sterile powder is also applied to wounds or burns. Internally it is relatively non-toxic, but its therapeutic activity is less than that of sulphathiazole and sulphadiazine, which are to be preferred. It has been used in *Bacterium coli* infections of the urinary tract and in meningitis since it penetrates the cerebrospinal fluid.

sulphacid (sulf·**as**·id). Sulpho-acid.

sulphadiazine (sul·fah·**di**·az·een). 2-(*p*-Aminobenzenesulphonamido)-pyrimidine. A sulphonamide compound which is slowly but completely absorbed and slowly excreted. It is more active *in vivo* than sulphathiazole, and is one of the least toxic sulphonamides. Only sparingly soluble in the urine and tending to crystallize, it may cause haematuria and anuria and is therefore not advisable for use routinely. It readily penetrates the cerebrospinal fluid and into the eye, and is valuable in conjunction with sulphathiazole and sulphamerazine in the treatment of meningitis (BP 1973). It is especially employed for local application when slow absorption is required. **Sulphadiazine Sodium BP 1968, Soluble sulphadiazine.** The sodium salt of sulphadiazine.

Sulphadimethoxine BP 1973 (**sul**·fah·di·meth·**ox**′·een). 6-*p*-Aminobenzenesulphonamido-2,4-dimethoxypyrimidine; used in sulphonamide therapy.

sulphadimethylpyrimidine (**sul**·fah·di·**meth**·il·pir·**im**′·id·een). Sulphadimidine.

sulphadimidine (sul·fah·**dim**·id·een). 2-(*p*-Aminobenzenesulphonamido)-4,6-dimethylpyrimidine. A dimethyl derivative of sulphadiazine which has the advantage of a high solubility; absorption is fairly rapid and urinary excretion slow. It combines a high therapeutic activity with a low toxicity and absence of side effects: the sulphonamide of choice for routine use, particularly in pneumococcal infections. Since it does not readily diffuse into the cerebrospinal fluid, it is unsuitable for meningitis; though its high solubility in the urine, together with the high concentration, make it valuable for urinary infections (BP 1973). **Sulphadimidine Sodium BP 1973, Soluble sulphadimidine.** The water-soluble sodium derivative of sulphadimidine, given by injection as a 33 per cent solution when oral administration of sulphadimidine gives an insufficiently high blood level.

sulphaemoglobin (**sulf**·he·mo·**glo**′·bin). A greenish pigmentary derivative of haemoglobin produced by its reaction with soluble inorganic sulphides or by the absorption of hydrogen sulphide or of sulphides from the alimentary tract. It is the cause of the greenish discoloration seen particularly in the abdomen of cadavers; it is produced under the influence of many substances such as nitrates, chlorates and nitrites, or coal-tar derivatives such as phenacetin, acetanilide, sulphonamides, etc., causing enterogenous cyanosis or sulphaemoglobinaemia. [sulphide, haemoglobin.]

sulphaemoglobinaemia (**sulf**·he·mo·glo·bin·e′·me·ah). The presence of sulphaemoglobin in the blood. It is caused by the absorption of hydrogen sulphide in the intestine, and is often present after treatment with drugs of the sulphonamide group. It is either endogenous, that is, caused by absorption of hydrogen sulphide from the intestinal tract after sensitization by some drug, e.g. acetanilide, phenacetin, antipyrin, potassium chlorate and nitrites have been incriminated, or exogenous due to direct absorption of the sulpha molecule from administered sulphonamides. [sulphaemoglobin, Gk *haima* blood.]

Sulphaethidole (sul·fah·**eth**·id·ole). BP Commission approved name for 5-*p*-aminobenzenesulphonamido-2-ethyl-1,3,4-thiadiazole; used in the treatment of infections of the respiratory tract.

Sulphafurazole BP 1973 (sul·fah·**fewr**·az·ole). 5(4-Aminobenzenesulphonamido)-3,4-dimethylisoxazole; NU445. A highly soluble sulphonamide used in infections of the urinary tract.

Sulphaguanidine BP 1958 (sul·fah·**gwan**·id·een). *p*-Aminobenzenesulphonylguanidine, one of the least potent of the sulphonamides. Absorption is rapid but very incomplete; about half of it remains in the intestine, and the high concentration in the bowel makes it of value in bacillary dysentery and for reducing the bacterial count prior to operation.

sulphaldehyde (sulf·**al**·de·hide). Thio-acetaldehyde, CH_3CHS. A colourless liquid with a characteristic and powerful odour. It is a hypnotic, its actions being similar to, but rather stronger than, paraldehyde.

sulphamerazine (sul·fah·**mer**·az·een). 2-(*p*-Aminobenzenesulphonamido)-4-methylpyrimidine, the methyl derivative of sulphadiazine, being more rapidly absorbed than the latter and about as active though quicker and more sustained (BP 1958); it is also slightly more toxic and renal complications are common. It penetrates the cerebrospinal fluid readily and is of value in meningitis. Best used as one of the sulphonamides in a mixture so as to lower the risk of renal impairment, it is valuable for maintaining a high and prolonged blood concentration, rendering dosage less frequent. **Sulphamerazine Sodium BPC 1959.** The sodium derivative of sulphamerazine.

sulphamethazine (sul·fah·**meth**·az·een). Sulphadimidine.

Sulphamethizole BP 1973 (sul·fah·**meth**·iz·ole). 2-*p*-Aminobenzenesulphonamido-5-methyl-1,3,4-thiadizole, a sulpha drug used for infections of the urinary tract, including *Bacterium coli* infections.

Sulphamethoxazole BP 1973 (**sul**·fah·meth·**ox**′·az·ole). 3-(4-Aminobenzenesulphonamido)-5-methylisoxazole; a sulphonamide preparation.

Sulphamethoxydiazine BP 1973 (**sul**·fah·meth·ox·e·**di**′·az·een). 2-(4-Aminobenzenesulphonamido)-5-methoxypyrimidine; an antibacterial agent.

Sulphamethoxypyridazine BP 1973 (**sul**·fah·meth·**ox**·e·pi·**rid**′·az·een). 3-*p*-Aminobenzenesulphonamido-6-methoxypyridazine; used in sulphonamide therapy.

sulphamethylthiazole (**sul**·fah·meth·il·**thi**′·az·ole). 2(*p*-Aminobenzenesulphonamido)-4-methylthiazole, $NH_2C_6H_4SO_2NHC_3HNSCH_3$. A sulphonamide compound which is as active as sulphathiazole but which has fallen into disrepute because of its tendency to cause peripheral neuritis.

sulphamezathine (sul·fah·**mez**·ah·theen). Sulphadimidine.

sulphamide (**sulf**·am·ide). 1. Sulphuric acid diamide, $SO_2(NH_2)_2$, a compound formed by ammonia with sulphuryl chloride. 2. Any organic compound derived from sulphuric acid diamide by replacement of the hydrogen atoms with alkyl groups.

sulphamido- (sulf·**am**·id·o). A prefix denoting a compound which contains the group, $-SO_2NH_2$.

sulphamine (**sulf**·am·een). Sulphonamide.

Sulphamoprine (sulf·**am**·o·preen). BP Commission approved name for 2-(4-aminobenzenesulphonamido)-4,6-dimethoxypyrimidine; it is used in sulphonamide therapy.

Sulphamoxole (sul·fam·**ox**·ole). BP Commission approved name for 2-(4-aminobenzenesulphonamido)-4,5-dimethyloxazole; it is used in sulphonamide therapy.

sulphanaemia (sul·fan·e·**me**·ah). An anaemic state brought on by treatment with drugs of the sulphonamide group. [sulphonamide, Gk *haima* blood.]

sulphanilamide (sul·fan·**il**·am·ide). *p*-Aminobenzenesulphonamide, $NH_2C_6H_4SO_2NH_2$. The first of the simple sulphonamides to be used in medicine and the first systemic bactericide (BPC 1968). It is a compound of low potency but high solubility, rapidly and completely absorbed from the intestine and readily penetrating the tissues including the cerebrospinal fluid. Its therapeutic properties are typical of all the sulphonamides, but its use is now almost confined to the combating of streptococci, other drugs of the same group being employed for specific infections. Mixed with sulphathiazole or penicillin it is sometimes applied to wounds and burns. **Dodecanoyl sulphanilamide.** A lipide derivative of sulphanilamide. **Sulphanilamide quinine.** A compound of sulphanilamide and quinine which is more soluble than sulphanilamide itself.

sulphanilate (sul·**fan**·il·ate). Any salt or ester of sulphanilic acid. [sulphur, aniline.]

sulphanilylguanidine (sul·**fan**·il·il·**gwan**′·id·een). Sulphaguanidine.

sulphanuria (sul·fan·**ewr**·e·ah). Anuria caused by treatment with drugs of the sulphonamide group.

Sulphaphenazole (sul·fah·**fen**·az·ole). BP Commission approved name for 5-*p*-aminobenzenesulphonamido-1-phenylpyrazole; used in sulphonamide therapy.

Sulphaproxyline (sul·fah·**prox**·il·een). BP Commission approved name for *N*′-(4-isopropoxybenzoyl)-*p*-aminobenzenesulphonamide.

Sulphapyridine BP 1973 (sul·fah·**pir**·id·een). 2-(*p*-Aminobenzenesulphonamido)-pyridine, a sulphonamide compound with a low solubility, and slow and erratic in absorption. It has a moderate potency and a low renal clearance; its toxic effects are marked and it tends to crystallize in the urine. Not now used to any great extent routinely, it is still valuable for the treatment of dermatitis herpetiformis.

sulpharsenobenzene (**sulf**·ar·sen·o·**ben**′·zeen). Sulpharsphenamine.

Sulpharsphenamine BP 1953 (sulf·ars·**fen**·am·een). 3,3′-Diamino - 4,4′ - dihydroxyarsenobenzene - *N*- *N*′ - dimethylene bisulphite, $NaSO_3CH_2NHC_6H_3(OH)As{=}AsC_6H_3(OH)NHCH_2SO_3Na$. A compound used like neoarsphenamine in the treatment of syphilis. It is less toxic and less irritant and may be given by intramuscular injection, an advantage in children, and adults with poor veins.

sulphas (**sul**·fas). Sulphate. [L.]

Sulphasalazine (sul·fah·**sal**·az·een). BP Commission approved name for 4-hydroxy-4′-(pyrid-2-ylsulphamoyl)azobenzene-3-carboxylic acid; used in the treatment of ulcerative colitis.

sulphasolucin (sul·fah·**sol**·ew·sin). $NH_2C_6H_4SO_2NHCH(SO_3Na)CH_2CH(SO_3Na)C_6H_5$, one of the lesser-known sulpha drugs; more effective ones are available.

Sulphasomidine BP 1963 (sul·fah·**so**·mid·een). 4-(4-Aminobenzenesulphonamido) - 2,6 - methylpyrimidine, $NH_2C_6H_4SO_2NHC{=}NC(CH_3){=}NC(CH_3){=}CH$. A compound which acts as a typical sulphonamide drug, being effective in meningococcal, pneumococcal and gonococcal infections, and in rheumatic fever. It does not damage the kidney and is useful in kidney infections; it is of low toxicity and it is tolerated in single doses up to 10 g daily. It is administered by mouth.

Sulphasomizole (sul·fah·**so**·miz·ole). BP Commission approved name for 5-*p*-aminobenzenesulphonamido-3-methylisothiazole.

sulphasuxidine (sul·fah·**sux**·id·een). Succinylsulphathiazole, 2-(*p*-succinyl-aminobenzenesulphonamide)-thiazole. $HOOC(CH_2)_2CONHC_6H_4SO_2NHC_3H_2NSH_2O$. A compound which is itself inactive but slowly liberates sulphathiazole which exerts a bacteriostatic action. It acts chiefly against coliform organisms in the bowel, also against many strains of dysentery; typhoid and paratyphoid are resistant. It is used extensively to exterminate *Bacillus coli* prior to operation on the bowel.

sulphataemia (sul·fa·te·**me**·ah). A condition marked by the retention of sulphates in the blood. [sulphate, Gk *haima* blood.]

sulphatase (**sul**·fa·taze). 1. An enzyme of the esterase class occurring in animal and plant tissues, which catalyses the hydrolysis of phenolic esters of sulphuric acid, yielding sulphuric acid and the phenol. 2. An enzyme distinct from 1. (above) occurring in certain micro-organisms, which catalyses the hydrolysis of conjugate sulphates.

sulphate (**sul**·fate). Any salt or ester of sulphuric acid. **Acid sulphate.** A bisulphate, one which retains a hydrogen atom of the original sulphuric acid, e.g. $MHSO_4$. **Basic sulphate.** A subsulphate, one in which the sulphuric acid radical is combined with a base and a hydroxyl group. **Conjugate sulphate.** Any sulphate of phenolic origin excreted in the urine. **Dimethyl sulphate.** *See* DIMETHYL. **Ethereal sulphate.** Conjugate sulphate (see above). **Sulphate of lime.** Calcium sulphate. **Mineral sulphate.** Any inorganic sulphate, especially those of sodium and potassium, appearing in the urine. **Neutral sulphate.** A sulphate in which the base has completely replaced the hydrogen of the original acid. **Sulphate of potash.** Potassium sulphate. **Preformed sulphate.** Mineral sulphate (see above).

sulphation factor (**sul**·fah·shon **fak**·tor). A peptide produced by the liver and kidney, incorporating sulphate into growing cartilage cells. May stimulate the hypothalamus to produce growth-hormone-releasing factor. Sulphation factor is present in large amounts in the plasma of acromegalics and absent from the plasma of hyposomatotrophic dwarfs. It is sometimes referred to as somatomedin.

sulphathiazole (sul·fah·**thi**·az·ole). 2-(*p*-Aminobenzenesulphonamido)-thiazole, the most active of the sulphonamides. Absorption is rapid so that it is quick acting, but it is rapidly excreted making blood concentrations difficult to control and generally low, as are the concentrations in the tissues. It is excreted in the urine in the acetylated form which is very insoluble with risk of haematuria and oliguria. Drug fever and rashes are particularly liable to occur; applied to the skin there is a risk of sensitization dermatitis. The difficulty of controlling blood levels, together with the incidence of side effects, have led to its disuse, sulphadiazine being preferred systemically. It is used, however, in combination with sulphanilamide and penicillin for application to wounds (BPC 1968). **Sulphathiazole Sodium BP 1953, Soluble sulphathiazole.** The water-soluble sodium derivative of sulphathiazole, used where injections of aqueous solutions are required. **Succinyl sulphathiazole.** Sulphasuxidine.

Sulphathiourea (sul·fa·thi·o·ewr·e′·ah). BP Commission approved name for *p*-aminobenzenesulphonylthiourea; used in the treatment of infected wounds.

sulphatide (sul·fat·ide). Sulpholipide.

Sulphatolamide (sul·fah·tol·am·ide). BP Commission approved name for *p*-aminobenzenesulphonylthiourea salt of *p*-sulphamoylbenzylamine; used in the treatment of leucorrhoea.

Sulphaurea (sul·fah·ewr·e′·ah). BP Commission approved name for *p*-aminobenzenesulphonylurea; a bactericide.

sulphestol (sul·fes·tol). A detergent and wetting agent consisting of a mixture of sodium secondary alkyl sulphates. It is especially used for laboratory apparatus and surgical instruments.

sulph-hydrate (sulf·hi·drate). 1. Incorrectly, a sulphide. 2. A hydrosulphide or mercaptan; any organic compound containing the -SH group, analogous to a hydroxide.

sulph-hydryl (sulf·hi·dril). The monovalent thiol group, -SH, so-called by analogy with hydroxyl.

sulphide (sul·fide). Any compound of sulphur with an element or base; usually a binary compound of a metal with sulphur having a characteristic colour of value in qualitative analysis. **Alkyl sulphide.** Thio-ether.

sulphindigotate (sulf·in·dig·o·tate). Any salt or ester of sulphindigotic (indigodisulphonic) acid.

sulphine (sul·feen). Name given to any sulphur compound.

sulphinide (sul·fin·ide). Saccharin.

sulphino- (sul·fin·o). Prefix denoting a compound containing the group $-SO_2H$.

Sulphinpyrazone BP 1973 (sul·fin·pi·raz·one). 1,2-Diphenyl-4-(2-phenylsulphinylethyl)pyrazolidine-3,5-dione; used in the treatment of chronic gout.

sulphinyl (sul·fin·il). The divalent group, -OS-.

sulphite (sul·fite). Any salt or ester of sulphurous acid, H_2SO_3.

sulphmethaemoglobin (sulf·met·he·mo·glo′·bin). Sulphaemoglobin. [sulphide, methaemoglobin.]

sulpho group (sul·fo groop). The monovalent acidic radical, $-SO_2OH$, which enters into organic compounds to form sulphonic acids.

sulpho-azotized (sul·fo·az·ot·i·zd). Describing any organic compound which contains both sulpho- and azo- groups.

sulphobromophthalein sodium (sul·fo·bro·mo·thal′·e·in so·de·um). The disodium salt of tetrabromophenolphthalein disulphonic acid, $OCOC_6Br_4C{=}[C_6H_3(OH)SO_3Na]_2$. It is a dye used for testing liver function.

sulphocarbanilide (sul·fo·kar·ban′·il·ide). Thiocarbanilide, diphenylthio-urea, $C_6H_5NHCSNHC_6H_5$. A compound derived from aniline with carbon disulphide. It is used as an accelerator in the manufacture of rubber.

sulphocarbolate (sul·fo·kar·bol·ate). Any salt or ester of sulphocarbolic (paraphenolsulphonic) acid; a phenolsulphonate. **Zinc sulphocarbolate.** $(HOC_6H_4SO_2O)_2Zn{\cdot}8H_2O$. A solution employed as an astringent and antiseptic.

sulphocarbonate (sul·fo·kar·bon·ate). Thiocarbonate. Any salt formed by the union of sulphides and carbon disulphide. They are used in the treatment of vines for *Phylloxera*.

sulphocarbonated (sul·fo·kar·bon·a·ted). Treated with carbon disulphide to form a sulphocarbonate.

sulphocarbonism (sul·fo·kar·bon·izm). Carbon disulphide poisoning.

sulphoconjugation (sul·fo·kon·joo·ga′·shun). The union of indoxyl or other phenolic compounds with sulphate to form conjugated compounds, such as indican, which are excreted in the urine. [sulphate, conjugate.]

sulphocyanate (sul·fo·si·an·ate). A former name for a thiocyanate.

sulphogel (sul·fo·jel). A gel in which the dispersed liquid phase consists of sulphuric acid.

sulphoguaiacol (sul·fo·gwi·ah·kol). Potassium guaiacolsulphonate.

sulphohydrate (sul·fo·hi·drate). Sulph-hydrate.

sulpholipide (sul·fo·lip·ide). A class of lipides in which fatty acids are combined with sulphuric acid and a nitrogenous base.

sulpholysis (sul·fol·is·is). A reaction analogous to hydrolysis, in which sulphuric acid takes part. [sulphur, Gk *lysis* a loosing.]

Sulphomyxin Sodium BP 1973 (sul·fo·mix·in so·de·um). A mixture of sulphomethylated polymyxin B and sodium bisulphite; an antibiotic with actions and uses similar to those of polymyxin B sulphate.

Sulphonal BPC 1949 (sul·fo·nal). Sulphonemethane, diethylsulphonedimethylmethane, $(CH_3)_2C(SO_2C_2H_5)_2$. A hypnotic possessing no analgesic properties. It has been superseded by more effective, safer, drugs.

sulphonalism (sul·fo·nal·izm). 1. A toxic state caused by the excessive use of sulphonal. 2. Addiction to sulphonal.

sulphonamidaemia (sul·fon·am·i·de′·me·ah). Sulphonamide in the blood. [sulphonamide, Gk *haima* blood.]

sulphonamide (sul·fon·am·ide). Denoting the group $-SO_2NH_2$; the name has come to be applied to a number of organic derivatives containing this group, including the bactericides known as *sulpha drugs*, prontosil, etc. **Sulphonamide P.** Sulphanilamide.

***p*-sulphonamidobenzylamine** (par·ah sul·fon·am·id·o·ben·zil·am′·een). Maphenide.

sulphonamidocholia (sul·fon·am·id·o·ko′·le·ah). Sulphonamide in the bile. [sulphonamide, Gk *chole* bile.]

sulphonamidotherapy (sul·fon·am·id·o·ther′·ap·e). Sulphonamide therapy.

sulphonamiduria (sul·fon·am·id·ewr′·e·ah). The presence of sulphonamide compounds in the urine.

sulphonate (sul·fon·ate). Any salt or ester of a sulphonic acid.

sulphonation (sul·fon·a·shun). The preparation of organic sulphonic acids by the substitution of sulpho groups, SO_3H, for the hydrogen atoms of hydrocarbons. It is usually achieved by the use of fuming sulphuric acid, and is a process of importance in the synthesis of drugs and dyestuffs.

sulphone (sul·fone). One of a family of organic compounds formed by oxidation of the corresponding sulphides, in which the divalent group, $=SO_2$, is united to 2 alkyl radicals, e.g. methyl ethyl sulphone, $(CH_3)SO_2(C_2H_5)$.

sulphonemethane (sul·fone·me′·thane). Sulphonal.

sulphonephenolphthalein (sul·fone·fe·nol·thal′·e·in). Phenol sulphonephthalein; phenol red.

sulphonethylmethane (sul·fon·eth·il·me′·thane). Methylsulphonal, $(C_2H_5)(CH_3)C(SO_2C_2H_5)_2$, a hypnotic drug related to sulphonal. This and other drugs of this group are now largely replaced by barbiturates.

sulphonic (sul·fon·ik). Denoting an organic compound in which the sulpho group, SO_3H, has replaced a hydrogen atom.

sulphonyl (sul·fon·il). Sulphuryl. The divalent group, $=SO_2$.

sulphonylurea (sul·fon·il·u·rea). An orally active group of antidiabetic compounds.

sulphoparaldehyde (sul·fo·par·al′·de·hide). Trithio-acetaldehyde, $(CH_3CHS)_3$. A hypnotic drug.

sulphophenate (sul·fo·fe·nate). 1. Phenolsulphonate. 2. The name is also sometimes applied to a phenylsulphate, e.g. phenyl potassium sulphate, $C_6H_5OSO_2OK$.

sulphophenol (sul·fo·fe·nol). Paraphenolsulphonic acid. *See* ACID.

sulphophenylate (sul·fo·fe·nil·ate). Sulphophenate.

sulphoprotein (sul·fo·pro·te·in). Any albumin containing a high percentage of sulphur. [sulphur, protein.]

sulphopyretotherapy (sul·fo·pi·re·to·ther′·ap·e). The production of fever by the intramuscular injection of sulphur solutions. [sulphur, Gk *pyretos* fever, therapy.]

sulphosalt (sul·fo·sawlt). 1. A salt of any acid derived from sulphur. 2. Any salt or ester of a sulphonic acid.
sulphosol (sul·fo·sol). A sol in which the continuous liquid phase consists of sulphuric acid.
sulphosote (sul·fo·sote). Potassium creosote sulphonate. A preparation which has been used in tuberculosis.
sulphoxide (sulf·ox·ide). Any organic compound consisting of two alkyl radicals and united to the divalent sulphinyl group, -SO-, e.g. diethyl sulphoxide, $(C_2H_5)_2SO$; formed by gentle oxidation of the corresponding sulphide.
sulphugator (sul·few·ga·tor). Cloth impregnated with sulphur and used for fumigation purposes.
sulphur (sul·fer). An element of atomic weight 32.06, atomic number 16 and chemical symbol S. It is a non-metal which exists in several allotropic forms, the crystalline yellow α- and *β-sulphur*, the *amorphous* or *plastic sulphur* (γ- or *μ-sulphur*) and *colloidal sulphur* (see below). The element occurs free in Italy, Sicily and the USA; also in the form of sulphides in many important metallic ores, e.g. galena, iron pyrites. It is a constituent of plant protein, of animal scleroprotein (skin, hair, etc.), of muscle, of skin pigments, of sulpholipides and of mucoitin and chondroitin sulphates, as well as various plant products such as mustard and garlic oils. The allotropic forms differ slightly in solubility, but in general sulphur is insoluble in water or alcohol, soluble in carbon disulphide and partly soluble in benzene, ether, chloroform, light petroleum or turpentine oil. It is used for the manufacture of sulphuric acid, dyes, drugs, parasiticides and fumigants, as well as in the vulcanizing of rubber. Medicinally, it is used internally as a mild intestinal antiseptic and stimulant; externally it acts as an antiseptic and parasiticide, sublimed sulphur being employed in the form of an ointment, precipitated sulphur in lotions and dusting powders. The fumes of burning sulphur are used for fumigation. **Colloidal sulphur.** Sulphur prepared in colloidal form by precipitation in the presence of a protective colloid; it is used externally, orally or by intramuscular or intravenous injection. **Sulphur dioxide.** SO_2, a gas prepared by the combustion of sulphur or by the reaction of copper and sulphuric acid. It is supplied compressed in cylinders or in siphons and is used as a preservative for foodstuffs and certain medicinal products. A solution (1-2 per cent SO_2) is applied externally as a lotion and as a throat spray. **Flowers of sulphur.** Sublimed sulphur (see below). **Hepar sulphur.** Liver of sulphur (see below). **Sulphur iodide.** A compound of sulphur and iodine used in the treatment of parasitic skin diseases. **Lac sulphur.** A mixture of sulphur and calcium sulphate obtained on precipitation of a solution of calcium polysulphides and calcium thiosulphate by the addition of sulphuric acid. **Liver of sulphur.** A mixture of the sulphide, polysulphides, sulphite and thiosulphate of potassium, obtained by fusing potassium carbonate with sulphur. It is a hard, brittle solid, greenish-yellow outside, with a liver-brown fracture. It is soluble in water, and the aqueous solution is used locally as a parasiticide and in the treatment of acne and eczema; it is also employed in sulphur baths in the treatment of rheumatism. **Sulphur lotum.** Sublimed sulphur (see below) digested with water and ammonia solution for 24 h, then well washed and dried at moderate temperature; it is used internally as a mild antiseptic and stimulant. **Milk of sulphur.** Precipitated sulphur (see below). **Sulphur monochloride.** S_2Cl_2, a fuming red liquid with a pungent smell; it dissolves sulphur. **Neutral sulphur.** A term embracing those sulphur compounds other than sulphates which occur in the urine, e.g. cystine, mercaptans and derivatives of taurine. **Sulphur nigrum.** Impure sulphur obtained as the residue after the preparation of sublimed sulphur; it is a dark grey or black powder, used in veterinary medicine. **Precipitated Sulphur BP 1973.** An impalpable pale-yellow powder prepared by the precipitation of sulphur from solution. **Roll sulphur.** Brimstone, a brittle yellow solid, being sulphur melted and cast into cylinders. **Sublimed Sulphur BP 1958.** Flowers of sulphur, a yellow gritty powder formed by the condensation of sulphur vapour. **Sulphur trioxide.** SO_3, a white crystalline solid which forms sulphuric acid with water. **Washed sulphur.** Sulphur lotum (see above). [L.]
sulphuraria (sul·fer·a·re·ah). A sulphurous sediment obtained from springs in Italy, containing sulphur, sulphides of calcium, silica, etc. It is used in skin diseases.
sulphurated (sul·fewr·a·ted). Sulphuretted.
sulphuration (sul·fewr·a·shun). The process of combining anything with sulphur; treating or dressing with sulphur.
sulphuret (sul·fewr·et). An old name for a sulphide.
sulphuretted (sul·fewr·et·ed). Treated with sulphur or having sulphur in its composition.
sulphuric (sul·fewr·ik). Applied to any compound of sulphur in which the latter is hexavalent; any derivative of sulphur trioxide, SO_3. **Sulphuric anhydride.** Sulphur trioxide. **Sulphuric ester.** Any organic ester formed by sulphuric acid.
sulphuricity (sul·fewr·is·it·e). Sulphur content; the amount of sulphur present in a compound.
sulphurine (sul·fewr·een). A preparation of sulphur with the higher sulphides of sodium and potassium.
sulphurize (sul·fewr·ize). To introduce sulphur chemically into combination.
sulphurous (sul·fewr·us). 1. Having the characteristics of, or containing sulphur. 2. Applied to any compound of tetravalent sulphur; any compound derived from sulphur dioxide, SO_2. **Sulphurous ester.** Any organic ester formed by sulphurous acid.
sulphuryl (sul·fewr·il). The divalent group, $=SO_2$.
sulphydryl (sul·fi·dril). Sulph-hydryl.
Sulpiride (sul·pir·ide). BP Commission approved name for *N*-(1-ethylpyrrolidin-2-ylmethyl)-2-methoxy-5-sulphamoylbenzamide; an antidepressant and anxiolytic agent.
sultan (sul·tan). Benzopurpurine, a diazo dye derived from toluidine, used as a stain in microscopy and as a pH indicator (3.1–4.4).
Sulthiame BP 1973 (sul·thi·ame). 4-(Tetrahydro-2*H*-1,2-thiazin-2-yl)benzenesulphonamide *S,S*-dioxide, an anticonvulsant used in suppressing focal epilepsy, myoclonic seizures and hyperkinetic behaviour; it is not the drug of choice in the common forms of epilepsy—grand mal and petit mal.
Sulzberger, Marion B. (b. 1895). New York dermatologist.
Sulzberger-Garbe disease. A chronic, extensive, exudative, discoid and lichenoid eruption, mostly occurring in males.
sumac (sew·mak). Sumach.
sumach (sew·mak). Name given to a number of species of *Rhus* (family Anacardiaceae) and other plants. **Chinese sumach.** The dried bark of *Ailanthus glandulosa*, Tree of Heaven. **Poison sumach.** Swamp sumach (see below). **Smooth sumach.** The bark and berries of *Rhus glabra*. **Swamp sumach.** Poison elder; the shrub *Rhus vernix (R. venenata)*; it has poisonous properties. **Sweet sumach.** The root bark of *Rhus aromatica*. **Venetian sumach.** *Rhus cotinus*, a species which yields fustic. [Arabic *summaq*.]
sumbul (sum·bul). Musk root; the rhizome and roots of *Ferula sumbul* Hook. (family Umbelliferae) and other species of Ferula, possessing a characteristic musk-like odour. It contains resinous matter and a volatile oil. [Arabic *sumbul*.]
summation (sum·a·shun). The aggregation of a number of parts. **Central summation.** The condition in which repeated subliminal stimuli finally so increase the reactivity of nerve cells by an accumulation of small metabolic changes that the same stimulus becomes liminal and effective. **Multifibre summation, Quantal summation.** When a strong, as compared with a weak, stimulus is applied to a motor nerve, there is an increased contraction of the muscle due to an increase in the number of motor units contracting. **Summation of stimuli.** Neural or muscular reactions which result from several subliminal stimuli. [L *summa* total.]
Summerson, W. H.
Summerson-Barker method. For lactic acid in blood. A protein-free blood filtrate is treated with copper-sulphate solution and powdered calcium hydroxide to remove interfering substances. An aliquot of filtrate is heated with concentrated sulphuric acid to convert lactic acid to acetaldehyde

and the latter is determined colorimetrically with *p*-hydroxydiphenyl.

Sumner, James Batcheller (b. 1887). American biochemist.

Sumner's method. For sugar in urine. The urine is heated with Sumner's reagent (see below), and the colour produced by reduction is compared with that given by standard solutions of glucose.

Sumner's reagent. For glucose in urine. To 10 g of crystallized phenol add 22 ml of 10 per cent sodium hydroxide solution, dissolve in a little water and dilute to 100 ml. To 6.9 g of sodium bisulphide add 69 ml of the alkaline phenol solution and then 300 ml of 4.5 per cent sodium hydroxide solution, 255 g of Rochelle salt and 880 ml of 1 per cent dinitrosalicylic acid.

sunburn (**sun**·bern). A dermatitis associated with redness and often blistering of the skin, caused by exposure to the rays of the sun. [AS *sunne, baernan.*]

sunstroke (**sun**·stroke). Term confined to exposure to environmental conditions of heat and humidity causing the heat-regulating mechanism to break down. *Heat exhaustion* refers to breakdown due to prolonged sweating as in buildings, ships' holds, mines, etc. [AS *sunne, strac.*]

suntan (**sun**·tan). Pigmentation of the skin resulting from stimulation of the melanocytes by ultraviolet irradiation. [AS *sunne*, O Fr. *tanner.*]

super-. Prefix, from the Latin preposition *super*, meaning *over, above.*

superabduction (sew·per·ab·**duk'**·shun). Abnormal abduction of a limb. [L *super*, abduction.]

superacid (sew·per·**as**·id). Of higher acidity than normal. [L *super*, acid.]

superacidity (sew·per·as·**id'**·it·e). Hyperacidity; acidity beyond the normal. In particular, the increased acidity of the gastric juice; hyperchlorhydria. [see prec.]

superacromial (sew·per·ak·ro'·me·al). Supra-acromial.

superalbal (sew·per·**al**·bal). Pertaining to the region of the white brain tissue; situated in the white matter. [L *super*, substantia alba.]

superalbuminosis (sew·per·al·bew·min·**o'**·sis). A condition characterized by the production of an excess of albumin. [L *super*, albumin, Gk *-osis* condition.]

superalimentation (sew·per·al·im·en·**ta'**·shun). Overfeeding as a therapeutic measure; gavage; the treatment of neurasthenia, tuberculosis and certain wasting diseases by forced feeding in excess of appetite or normal nutritional requirements. [L *super, alimentum* nourishment.]

superalkalinity (sew·per·al·kal·**in'**·it·e). Alkalinity above the normal. [L *super*, alkaline.]

supercallosal (sew·per·kal·**o'**·sal). Pertaining to the region above the corpus callosum. [L *super*, corpus callosum.]

supercarbia (sew·per·**kar**·be·ah). A condition occurring when the blood carbon dioxide tension reaches 53 kPa (400 mmHg), which may be associated with a zone of acute tolerance in animals. [L *super, carbo* coal.]

supercarbonate (sew·per·**kar**·bon·ate). Bicarbonate. [L *super*, carbonate.]

supercentral (sew·per·**sen**·tral). 1. Situated above a central part. 2. Pertaining to the region above the central sulcus of the cerebrum. [L *super*, centre.]

supercerebellar (sew·per·ser·e·**bel'**·ar). Supracerebellar; located in or pertaining to the upper part of the cerebellum. [L *super*, cerebellum.]

supercerebral (sew·per·**ser**·e·bral). Supracerebral; located in or pertaining to the upper part of the cerebrum. [L *super*, cerebrum.]

superciliary (sew·per·**sil**·e·ar·e). Referring to the region of the eyebrow. **Superciliary arch.** *See* ARCH. [L *super, cilium* eyelash.]

superconception (sew·per·kon·**sep'**·shun). Superfetation. [L *super*, conception.]

supercooled (sew·per·**koold**). The state of a liquid which is at a temperature below its normal freezing point. The condition is unstable and the liquid will solidify at once if a small particle of solid is added. [L *super*, AS *col.*]

superdicrotic (sew·per·di·**krot'**·ik). Hyperdicrotic; having a marked double beat. [L *super*, Gk *dikrotos* double beat.]

superdistension (sew·per·dis·**ten'**·shun). Distension much beyond the normal. [L *super*, distension.]

superduction (sew·per·**duk**·shun). The elevation of the visual axis of an eye. [L *super, ducere* to draw.]

superdural (sew·per·**dewr**·al). Supradural; pertaining to the upper part of the dura mater. [L *super*, dura mater.]

super-ego (sew·per·e·go). A division of the mind developed from the representation of parents as figures of authority, concerned with the management of the instincts and acting as a conscience from the unconscious mind (psycho-analysis). [L *super, ego* I.]

superexcitation (sew·per·ek·si·**ta'**·shun). 1. Undue stimulation; excessive excitation. 2. A condition of over-excitement. [L *super, excitare* to arouse.]

superextended (sew·per·ex·**ten'**·ded). Hyperextended; extended beyond the normal confines. [see foll.]

superextension (sew·per·ex·**ten'**·shun). The extension of any part beyond its accustomed confines. Applied particularly to the forcible extension employed in orthopaedics. [L *super, extendere* to stretch out.]

super-family (sew·per·**fam**·il·e). In the classification of plants and animals, a division between the order and the family. [L *super*, family.]

superfatted (sew·per·**fat**·ed). Containing an excess of fat. Of a soap, one that has more fat than the alkali will take up. [L *super*, fat.]

superfecundation (sew·per·fek·un·**da'**·shun). The successive fertilization by separate acts of coitus of 2 or more ova produced during the same menstrual cycle. [L *super, fecundare* to fertilize.]

superfecundity (sew·per·fek·**un'**·dit·e). Fertility much above the ordinary. [see prec.]

superfemale (sew·per·fe·male). *See* METAFEMALE and XXX FEMALE.

superfetation (sew·per·fe·**ta'**·shun). The conception of a second fetus by a woman already pregnant, owing to the fertilization of an ovum produced at a later ovulation. [L *super*, fetus.]

superfibrination (sew·per·fi·brin·**a'**·shun). The appearance of an excess of fibrin in the blood. [L *super*, fibrin.]

superficial (sew·per·**fish**·al). 1. [Superficialis (NA)] Confined to the surface; not penetrating deeply. 2. Of an examination, one that is cursory. [L *superficialis.*]

superficialis (sew·per·fish·e·**a'**·lis). Superficial; applied to nerves, blood vessels and other structures immediately deep to the skin. **Superficialis colli.** The anterior cutaneous nerve of the neck arising from the 2nd and 3rd cervical nerves. **Superficialis volae.** A branch of the radial artery which forms part of the anterior carpal arch. [L.]

superfissure (sew·per·**fish**·ewr). Any fissure or sulcus between 2 overlapping cerebral gyri. [L *super*, fissure.]

superflexion (sew·per·**flek**·shun). The bending of a limb beyond the normal extent. [L *super, flectere* to bend.]

superfrontal (sew·per·**frun**·tal). Above and at the front; as when describing the upper region of the frontal lobe of the cerebrum. [L *super, frons* forehead.]

superfunction (sew·per·**fungk**·shun). The overactivity of any organ or gland. [L *super*, function.]

supergenual (sew·per·**jen**·ew·al). Located above the knee. [L *super, genu* knee.]

supergyre (**sew**·per·jire). Any cerebral gyrus that overlaps another. [L *super*, gyre.]

superinfection (sew·per·in·**fek'**·shun). Reinfection by the introduction of organisms of the same species as those already causing the infection. [L *super*, infection.]

superinvolution (sew·per·in·vol·**ew'**·shun). The contraction of a uterus after parturition to a size less than normal. [L *super*, involution.]

superior (sew·**peer**·e·or). 1. [NA] Situated above in relation to another structure when the body is in the anatomical position;

directed upward. 2. Better in quality or value. 3. More useful. [L higher.]

superlactation (sew·per·lak·**ta**′·shun). 1. The secretion of an excessively abnormal amount of milk. 2. The prolongation of lactation beyond the usual term. [L *super*, lactation.]

superlethal (sew·per·**le**·thal). Describing a dose of a drug that is greater than that required to cause death. [L *super*, *letalis* fatal.]

superligamen (sew·per·**lig**·am·en). A surgical bandage applied over a dressing. [L *super*, *ligare* to bind.]

supermale (**sew**·per·male). In *Drosophila*, a male with a ratio of X chromosomes to autosome sets lower than ½; for example, a triploid with only one X chromosome. [L *super*, *mas* male.]

supermedial (sew·per·**me**·de·al). Superomedial.

supermicroscope (sew·per·**mi**·kro·skope). Electron microscope. [Obsolete term.] *See* MICROSCOPE. [L *super*, microscope.]

supermoron (sew·per·**mor**·on). A dull-witted person who is nevertheless higher mentally than a moron. [L *super*, *moros* dull.]

supermotility (sew·per·mo·**til**′·it·e). Hypermotility. [L *super*, motile.]

supernatant (sew·per·**na**·tant). 1. Floating; borne upon the surface of a liquid. 2. The clear liquid left above when a precipitate settles. [L *super*, *natare* to swim.]

supernate (**sew**·per·nate). Supernatant fluid. [see prec.]

supernutrition (sew·per·new·**trish**′·un). Over-nourishment. [L *super*, nutrition.]

superoccipital (sew·per·ok·**sip**′·it·al). Supra-occipital. [L *super*, occiput.]

superofrontal (sew·per·o·**frun**′·tal). Superfrontal.

superol (**sew**·per·ol). A form of 8-hydroxyquinoline used as a bactericide and deodorant.

superolateral (sew·per·o·**lat**′·er·al). Located at the side and above. [L *super*, *latus* side.]

superomedial (sew·per·o·**me**′·de·al). Located above the middle line. [L *super*, *medius* middle.]

superovulation (sew·per·ov·ew·**la**′·shun). Increased frequency of ovulation. [L *super*, ovulation.]

superoxide (sew·per·**ox**·ide). Any oxide containing more oxygen than that required by normal valencies; a peroxide. [L *super*, oxygen.]

superoxidize (sew·per·**ox**·id·ize). To oxidize above the normal; to convert into a superoxide. [see prec.]

superoxygenation (sew·per·ox·e·jen·**a**′·shun). 1. The process of inducing any substance (e.g. blood) to take up more oxygen than normal. 2. The resulting condition. [L *super*, oxygen.]

superpalite (sew·per·**pal**·ite). Surpalite, diphosgene, trichloromethylchloroformate, $ClCOOCCl_3$. A choking gas with severe irritant effect upon the lungs; used in chemical warfare. Also known as *perstoff.*

superparasite (sew·per·**par**·ah·site). A parasite that preys upon another parasite. [L *super*, parasite.]

superparasitic (sew·per·par·ah·**sit**′·ik). Characterized by superparasitism.

superparasitism (sew·per·**par**·ah·sit·izm). The preying of one parasite upon another. [L *super*, parasite.]

superphosphate (sew·per·**fos**·fate). An acid phosphate. **Superphosphate of lime.** An agricultural fertilizer consisting of a mixture of the acid phosphate of calcium, $CaH_4(PO_4)_2H_2O$, with calcium sulphate. [L *super*, phosphate.]

superpigmentation (sew·per·pig·men·**ta**′·shun). The presence of an excess of pigmentation. [L *super*, pigment.]

supersalt (**sew**·per·sawlt). An acid salt. [L *super*, salt.]

supersaturate (sew·per·**sat**·ewr·ate). To produce a supersaturated solution.

supersaturated (sew·per·**sat**·ewr·a·ted). Containing solute above the saturation point. [L *super*, saturation.]

superscription (sew·per·**skrip**·shun). The sign ℞ at the head of a prescription. It is a traditional symbol for the word *recipe.* [L *super*, *scribere* to write.]

supersecretion (sew·per·se·**kre**′·shun). The production of an abnormally large amount of secretion. Overactivity of a secretory gland. [L *super*, secrete.]

supersensitive (sew·per·**sen**·sit·iv). Extremely sensitive. [see foll.]

supersensitization (sew·per·sen·sit·i·**za**′·shun). The production of a high degree of reactivity to a foreign protein by a previous injection of it. [L *super*, *sentire* to feel.]

supersoft (**sew**·per·soft). Describing x-rays of long wavelength and hence of low penetrating power, e.g. grenz rays. [L *super*, soft.]

supersonic (sew·per·**son**·ik). Applied to speed greater than the speed of sound through any particular medium. [L *super*, *sonus* sound.]

supersphenoid (sew·per·**sfe**·noid). The region located above the sphenoid bone. [L *super*, sphenoid.]

supersulcus (sew·per·**sul**·kus). Superfissure. [L *super*, sulcus.]

supertemporal (sew·per·**tem**·por·al). Supratemporal. [L *super*, temporal.]

supervenosity (sew·per·ve·**nos**′·it·e). The state in which the blood is abnormally venous owing to imperfect oxidation. [L *super*, *vena* vein.]

superversion (sew·per·**ver**·zhun). The turning of any part upwards, particularly the eyes. [L *super*, *vertere* to turn.]

supervirulent (sew·per·**vir**·ew·lent). Of extreme virulence. [L *super*, virulent.]

supervitaminosis (sew·per·vi·tam·in·**o**′·sis). A condition due to the administration of an excess of vitamins. [L *super*, vitamin, Gk *-osis* condition.]

supinate (**sew**·pin·ate). 1. To rotate the forearm and hand, so that the palm faces anteriorly. 2. Similarly, to rotate the leg outward. [see foll.]

supination (sew·pin·**a**·shun). 1. The rotation of the forearm and hand so that the palm faces anteriorly. 2. Lying on the back so that the face is upward. [L *supinus* lying on the back.]

supinator muscle [musculus supinator (NA)] (sew·pin·a·tor musl). A muscle of the forearm which arises from the ulna immediately distal to the radial notch, from the lateral epicondyle of the humerus and from the radial collateral ligament of the elbow joint; it is inserted into the lateral and anterior aspect of the proximal third of the radius. [see prec.]

supine (sew·**pine**). In a position of supination, referring to a limb or the body.

suppedaneous (sup·ed·**a**·ne·us). Relating to the sole of the foot. [L *sub*, *pes* foot.]

suppedanium (sup·ed·**a**·ne·um). A local application made to the sole of the foot. [see prec.]

supplemental (sup·le·**men**·tal). Additional; in the nature of a supplement. [L *supplere* to complete.]

support (sup·**ort**). *See* JONES (R.). [L *supportare* to bring up to.]

suppositorium (sup·oz·it·**or**·e·um). Suppository.

suppository (sup·**oz**·it·or·e). A small cone-shaped medicament having cocoa butter or gelatin as its basis and usually intended for the treatment of local conditions in the rectum. The basis is of such consistency that it is solid and can be handled at ordinary room temperature, but melts at the temperature of the body. [L *sub*, *ponere* to place.]

suppression (sup·**resh**·un). 1. The prevention or inhibition of a natural function, especially that of a secretory or excretory organ, e.g. suppression of urine. 2. The voluntary removal from consciousness of undesired mental material. 3. In genetics, the reversion of a mutant phenotype by a second mutation at a site different from that of the original mutation, i.e. the mutant phenotype is suppressed but the original mutation remains and can be recovered as a mutant recombinant in crosses between wild-type and revertant. 4. The mental inhibition of visual sensations from one eye in favour of those from the other, when both eyes are open. [L *supprimere* to press down.]

suppressor (sup·**res**·or). Anything which produces suppression. **Genetic suppressor.** The name given to a gene, or its product, which is responsible for suppression of a mutant phenotype.

Surge suppressor. Any electrical device which protects an equipment from damage by surges of current above normal.

suppurant (sup·ewr·ant). 1. In a state of suppuration. 2. A suppurantium.

suppurantium (sup·ewr·an·she·um) (pl. *suppurantia*). Any substance that promotes suppuration. [see foll.]

suppuration (sup·ewr·a·shun). The production or exudation of pus. **Alveolodental suppuration.** Pyorrhoea alveolaris. [L *suppurare* to form pus.]

suppurative (sup·ewr·a·tiv). Pus-forming; having a tendency towards suppuration.

supra-. A prefix, from the Latin preposition *supra,* meaning *above.*

supra-acromial (sew·prah·ak·ro′·me·al). Upon or superior to the acromion. [L *supra,* acromion.]

supra-acromiohumeralis (sew·prah·ak·ro·me·o·hew·mer·a′·lis). The deltoid muscle. [L *supra,* acromiohumeral.]

supra-anal (sew·prah·a·nal). Above the anus. [L *supra,* anus.]

supra-auricular (sew·prah·aw·rik′·ew·lar). Above the pinna of the ear, or over the auricle of the heart. [L *supra,* auricle.]

supra-axillary (sew·prah·ax·il′·ar·e). Above the axilla. [L *supra,* axilla.]

suprabuccal (sew·prah·buk·al). In the upper part of the buccal region. [L *supra, bucca* cheek.]

supracephalic (sew·prah·kef·al′·ik). Situated on top of the head. [L *supra,* Gk *kephale* head.]

supracerebellar (sew·prah·ser·e·bel′·ar). Located in or pertaining to the upper part of the cerebellum. [L *supra,* cerebellum.]

supracerebral (sew·prah·ser·e·bral). Located in or pertaining to the upper part of the cerebrum. [L *supra,* cerebrum.]

suprachoroid (sew·prah·kor·oid). Located on the outer part of the choroid of the eye. **Suprachoroid lamina.** *See* LAMINA. [see foll.]

suprachoroidea (sew·prah·kor·oid′·e·ah). Suprachoroid lamina. *See* LAMINA. [L *supra,* choroid.]

supraciliary (sew·prah·sil·e·ar·e). Superciliary. [L *supra, cilium* eyelash.]

supraclavicular (sew·prah·klav·ik′·ew·lar). Located above the clavicle. **Supraclavicular fossa.** *See* FOSSA. [L *supra,* clavicle.]

supraclavicular nerves [nervi supraclaviculares]. Branches, generally 3 in number, the medial [nervi supraclaviculares mediales (NA)], intermediate [nervi supraclaviculares intermedii (NA)] and lateral [nervi supraclaviculares laterales posteriores (NA)] supraclavicular nerves, arising by a common trunk from the 3rd and 4th cervical nerves, through the cervical plexus, and descending over the clavicle to supply the skin over the upper part of the chest and the upper part of the deltoid muscle.

supraclavicularis (sew·prah·klav·ik·ew·la′·ris). The sternoclavicularis muscle. [L *supra,* clavicle.]

supracondylar, supracondyloid (sew·prah·kon·di′·lar, sew·prah·kon·di′·loid). Above a condyle. [L *supra,* condyle.]

supracostal (sew·prah·kos·tal). Above or superficial to the ribs. [L *supra, costa* rib.]

supracotyloid (sew·prah·kot·il·oid). Above the cotyloid cavity or acetabulum. [L *supra,* cotyloid.]

supracranial (sew·prah·kra·ne·al). On the upper surface of the skull. [L *supra,* cranium.]

supracristal (sew·prah·kris·tal). Above the crista of the right heart. [L *supra,* crista.]

supradiaphragmatic (sew·prah·di·ah·frag·mat′·ik). Above or upon the upper surface of the diaphragm. [L *supra,* diaphragm.]

supraduction (sew·prah·duk·shun). The turning upwards of any part of the eye; rotation of the eyeball upwards. [L *supra, ducere* to lead.]

supradural (sew·prah·dewr·al). Pertaining to the upper part of the dura mater. [L *supra,* dura mater.]

supra-epicondylar (sew·prah·ep·e·kon′·dil·ar). Above an epicondyle. [L *supra,* epicondyle.]

supra-epitrochlear (sew·prah·ep·e·trok′·le·ar). Above the medial epicondyle of the humerus. [L *supra,* epitrochlea.]

supraglenoid (sew·prah·gle·noid). Above the glenoid cavity. [L *supra,* glenoid.]

supraglottic (sew·prah·glot·ik). Above the glottis. [L *supra,* glottis.]

suprahepatic (sew·prah·hep·at′·ik). Above the liver. [L *supra,* Gk *hepar* liver.]

suprahyoid (sew·prah·hi·oid). Above the hyoid bone. [L *supra,* hyoid.]

suprahyoid artery [ramus suprahyoideus (NA)]. *See* LINGUAL ARTERY.

suprahyoid muscles [musculi suprahyoidei (NA)]. Muscles lying above the hyoid bone and attached to it; the digastric, stylohyoid, mylohyoid and geniohyoid muscles, but not the tongue muscles.

supra-iliac (sew·prah·il·e·ak). At the upper end of the ilium. [L *supra,* ilium.]

supra-inguinal (sew·prah·ing·gwin·al). Above the groin. [L *supra, inguen* groin.]

supra-intestinal (sew·prah·in·tes′·tin·al). Above the intestine. [L *supra,* intestine.]

supralabial (sew·prah·la·be·al). In the region above the upper lip. [L *supra, labium* lip.]

supraliminal (sew·prah·lim·in·al). Above the threshold of perception. [L *supra, limen* threshold.]

supralumbar (sew·prah·lum·bar). Above the lumbar region, or in the upper part of the region. [L *supra,* lumbar.]

supramalleolar (sew·prah·mal·e′·o·lar). Above a malleolus. [L *supra,* malleolus.]

supramammary (sew·prah·mam·ar·e). Above a mammary gland. [L *supra, mamma* breast.]

supramandibular (sew·prah·man·dib′·ew·lar). Situated high in the mandibular region; above the mandible. [L *supra,* mandible.]

supramarginal (sew·prah·mar·jin·al). Above any edge or margin. [L *supra,* margin.]

supramastoid (sew·prah·mas·toid). Above the mastoid process of the temporal bone. [L *supra,* mastoid.]

supramaxilla (sew·prah·max·il′·ah). The upper jaw; the maxilla. [L *supra,* maxilla.]

supramaxillary (sew·prah·max·il′·ar·e). 1. Relating to the upper jaw or maxilla. 2. Above the maxilla. [see prec.]

supramaximal (sew·prah·max·im·al). Over the maximum. [L *supra,* maximum.]

suprameatal (sew·prah·me·a′·tal). Above any meatus. [L *supra,* meatus.]

supramental (sew·prah·men·tal). Above the region of the chin. [L *supra, mentum* chin.]

supranasal (sew·prah·na·zal). Above the nose. [L *supra, nasus* nose.]

supraneural (sew·prah·newr·al). Above a nerve or neural axis. [L *supra,* Gk *neuron* nerve.]

supranuclear (sew·prah·new·kle·ar). In general, referring to nerve fibres situated above a nucleus; more especially used in relation to the pyramidal tracts. [L *supra,* nucleus.]

supra-occipital (sew·prah·ok·sip′·it·al). Located in the region above the occiput. [L *supra,* occiput.]

supra-occlusion (sew·prah·ok·loo′·zhun). The state of a tooth which projects beyond the normal occlusal plane, usually due to over-eruption resulting from absence of an opposing tooth. [L *supra, occludere* to close up.]

supra-ocular (sew·prah·ok·ew·lar). Above the eyeball. [L *supra* above, *oculus* eyeball.]

supra-optic nuclei (sew·prah·op·tik nu·cli·i). A collection of nuclei lying in the hypothalamus which send nerve fibres down the pituitary stalk together with the fibres from the paraventricular tracts conveying the so-called posterior pituitary hormones to the posterior lobe. Is probably responsible for the synthesis of vasopressin.

supra-optimal, supra-optimum (sew·prah·op·tim·al, sew·prah·op·tim·um). Above the optimum. [L *supra,* optimum.]

supra-orbital (sew·prah·or·bit·al). 1. Above the orbit. 2. Relating to the supra-orbital nerve. **Supra-orbital foramen.** *See* FORAMEN.

Supra-orbital margin. *See* MARGIN. **Supra-orbital notch.** *See* NOTCH. **Supra-orbital ridge.** Superciliary arch. *See* ARCH. [L *supra*, orbit.]

supra-orbital artery [arteria supra-orbitalis (NA)]. A large branch of the ophthalmic artery. It is the main supply to the forehead and front of the scalp.

supra-orbital nerve [nervus supra-orbitalis (NA)]. The larger and more lateral of the branches of the frontal nerve. It crosses the supra-orbital margin to the forehead. It has 2 branches, the lateral and larger on the forehead [ramus lateralis (NA)], and the medial and smaller [ramus medialis (NA)].

supra-orbital vein [vena supra-orbitalis (NA)]. A tributary of the anterior facial vein, from the forehead and scalp.

suprapatellar (sew·prah·pat·**el'**·ar). Above the patella. [L *supra*, patella.]

suprapelvic (sew·prah·**pel**·vik). Above the pelvic plane. [L *supra*, pelvis.]

suprapineal (sew·prah·**pin**·e·al). Above the pineal body. [L *supra*, pineal.]

suprapontine (sew·prah·**pon**·tine). Above or in the upper part of the pons. [L *supra*, pons.]

suprapubic (sew·prah·**pew**·bik). Above the pubic arch. [L *supra*, pubis.]

suprarenal (sew·prah·**re**·nal). Now more often referred to as "adrenal". 1. Above a kidney. 2. Relating to the suprarenal capsule or gland. **Suprarenal body, Suprarenal capsule, Suprarenal gland.** *See* GLAND. [L *supra*, *ren* kidney.]

suprarenal arteries. The arteries that supply the suprarenal gland. **Inferior suprarenal artery [arteria suprarenalis inferior (NA)].** *See* RENAL ARTERY. **Middle suprarenal arteries [arteria suprarenalis media (NA)].** Small paired arteries from the side of the abdominal aorta lying in front of the crura of the diaphragm. **Superior suprarenal artery [arteria suprarenalis superior (NA)].** A branch of the phrenic artery to the suprarenal gland.

suprarenal vein. A tributary of the inferior vena cava on the right [vena suprarenalis dextra (NA)] and the renal vein on the left [vena suprarenalis sinistra (NA)].

suprarenalaemia (sew·prah·re·nal·**e'**·me·ah). An increase in the amount of adrenaline secreted into the blood. [suprarenal, Gk *haima* blood.]

suprarenalectomy (sew·prah·re·nal·**ek'**·to·me). Surgical excision of a suprarenal gland. [suprarenal, Gk *temnein* to cut.]

suprarenalism (sew·prah·**re**·nal·izm). A condition caused by hyperactivity of the suprarenal glands.

suprarenalopathy (sew·prah·re·nal·**op'**·ath·e). Any disease of the suprarenal glands or morbid condition resulting from their dysfunction. [suprarenal, Gk *pathos* disease.]

suprascapular (sew·prah·**skap**·ew·lar). Situated above or in the upper part of the scapula. **Suprascapular ligament.** *See* LIGAMENT. **Suprascapular notch.** *See* NOTCH. [L *supra*, scapula.]

suprascapular artery [arteria suprascapularis (NA)]. A branch of the thyrocervical trunk running behind the clavicle, across the brachial plexus to the back of the scapula, taking part in the scapular anastomosis. Its acromial branch [ramus acromialis (NA)] pierces the trapezius and anastomoses over the acromion with the acromiothoracic artery.

suprascapular nerve [nervus suprascapularis (NA)]. The nerve of supply to the supraspinatus and infraspinatus muscles, and to the acromioclavicular and shoulder joints. It carries fibres from the 5th and 6th cervical segments of the cord through the upper trunk of the brachial plexus.

suprascapular vein [vena suprascapularis (NA)]. A tributary of the external jugular vein.

suprascleral (sew·prah·**skleer**·al). On the outer surface of the sclera. [L *supra*, sclera.]

suprasellar (sew·prah·**sel**·ar). Above the sella turcica. [L *supra*, sella turcica.]

supraseptal (sew·prah·**sep**·tal). Above a septum. [L *supra*, septum.]

suprasonic (sew·prah·**son**·ik). Ultrasonic. [L *supra*, *sonus* sound.]

suprasonics (sew·prah·**son**·ix). Ultrasonics. [see prec.]

supraspinal (sew·prah·**spi**·nal). Above the spinal column or any spine. [L *supra*, spine.]

supraspinatus muscle [musculus supraspinatus (NA)]. (sew·prah·spi·**na'**·tus musl). A muscle arising in the supraspinous fossa of the scapula and passing above the shoulder joint to an insertion on the greater tuberosity of the humerus.

supraspinous (sew·prah·**spi**·nus). Above the spinous process of a vertebra or of the scapular. **Supraspinous fossa.** *See* FOSSA. [L *supra*, spine.]

suprasplenial (sew·prah·**sple**·ne·al). Above the spleen. **Suprasplenial sulcus.** *See* SULCUS. [L *supra*, spleen.]

suprastapedial (sew·preh·sta·**pe'**·de·al). Above the stapes. [L *supra*, stapes.]

suprasternal (sew·prah·**ster**·nal). Above the sternum. **Suprasternal notch.** *See* NOTCH. [L *supra*, sternum.]

suprasternal bones [ossa suprasternalia (NA)]. Ossicles which occur occasionally in the ligaments of the sternoclavicular joint.

suprasternale (sew·prah·ster·**na'**·le). An anthropometric point; the middle of the suprasternal notch.

suprasterol (sew·prah·**steer**·ol). A class of substance produced by over-irradiation of vitamin D. Suprasterols I and II are known and are devoid of antirachitic activity, if not actually toxic. [L *supra*, sterol.]

suprasylvian (sew·prah·**sil**·ve·an). Above the lateral sulcus of the cerebrum. **Suprasylvian sulcus.** *See* SULCUS. [L *supra*, sylvian.]

supratemporal (sew·prah·**tem**·por·al). In the upper part of the temporal region or above it. [L *supra*, temporal.]

suprathoracic (sew·prah·thor·**as'**·ik). Above or in the upper part of the thorax. [L *supra*, thorax.]

supratonsillar (sew·prah·**ton**·sil·ar). Above a tonsil. [L *supra*, tonsil.]

supratrochlear (sew·prah·**trok**·le·ar). Above a trochlea, especially above the trochlea of the humerus. [L *supra*, trochlea.]

supratrochlear arteries. 1. [Arteria collateralis ulnaris inferior.] A branch from the brachial artery arising 5 cm (2 in) above the elbow, giving branches that descend in front of and behind the medial epicondyle to take part in the anastomosis around the elbow. 2. [Arteria supratrochlearis.] *See* OPHTHALMIC ARTERY.

supratrochlear nerve [nervus supratrochlearis]. The medial and smaller terminal branch of the frontal nerve. It goes above the pulley of the superior oblique muscle to the upper eyelid and the forehead.

supratrochlear veins [venae supratrochleares]. Tributaries of the anterior facial vein, from the forehead and temple.

supraturbinal (sew·prah·**ter**·bin·al). The superior nasal concha (superior turbinate bone). [L *supra*, turbinate.]

supratympanic (sew·prah·tim·**pan'**·ik). Above the tympanic cavity. [L *supra*, tympanum.]

supra-umbilical (sew·prah·um·**bil'**·ik·al). Above the umbilicus. [L *supra*, umbilicus.]

supravaginal (sew·prah·**vaj**·in·al). Above or outside any sheath; particularly applied to the area above the vagina. [L *supra*, *vagina* sheath.]

supravalvar (sew·prah·**val**·var). Above, and therefore distal to, the aortic or pulmonary valve; the term is usually applied to rare forms of stenosis affecting the vessels at these sites. [L *supra*, *valva* leaf of a door.]

supraverge (sew·prah·**verj**). Vertical divergence, particularly the divergence of the visual axes of the eyes. [L *supra*, *vergere* to incline.]

supravergence (sew·prah·**ver**·jens). Disjunctive reciprocal motion of the eyes in the vertical meridian while fusion is still maintained. The eye which moves upwards is performing supravergence. **Left supravergence.** Supravergence with the left eye. **Right supravergence.** Supravergence with the right eye. [see prec.]

supravital (sew·prah·**vi**·tal). Applied to the staining or other investigation of living cells or tissues removed from the organism. [L *supra, vita* life.]

supraxiphoid (sew·prah·**zif**·oid). Above the xiphoid process of the sternum. [L *supra*, xiphoid.]

sural (**sewr**·al). Relating to the calf of the leg. [L *sura* calf of the leg.]

sural artery. *See* POPLITEAL ARTERY.

sural nerve [nervus suralis (NA)]. A branch of the medial popliteal nerve to the skin of the lateral and posterior sides of the lower part of the leg. It is joined by the sural communicating branch [nervus cutaneus surae mediales (NA)] from the lateral popliteal nerve; the nerve resulting from this union is known in NA terminology as the sural nerve [nervus suralis (NA)].

lateral calcanean branches [rami calcanei laterales (NA)]. Branches of the sural nerve supplying the lateral aspect of the heel.

medial calcanean branches [rami calcanei mediales (NA)]. Branches to the medial aspect of the heel.

suralimentation (ser·al·e·men·**ta**′·shun). Superalimentation.

Suramin BP 1968 (**sewr**·am·in). Suramin sodium. A complex urea compound used by intravenous injection to treat trypanosomiasis and onchocerciasis. It is most effective if given early in the course of the infection, but it does not penetrate to the central nervous system and tryparsamide is more effective in the later stages; frequently both drugs are used in combination. Suramin combines with serum proteins and may remain in the body for weeks, consequently occasional doses are effective in preventing sleeping sickness. It is a potent nephrotoxin.

surdimutism (ser·dim·**ewt**·izm). Deaf-mutism. [L *surdus* deaf, *mutus* dumb.]

surditas (**ser**·dit·as). Deafness. **Surditas verbalis.** Word deafness, a form of aphasia. [L.]

surdity (**ser**·dit·e). Deafness. [see prec.]

surdomute (**ser**·do·mewt). 1. A deaf-mute. 2. Deaf and dumb. [L *surdus* deaf, *mutus* dumb.]

surdomutitas (ser·do·**mew**·tit·as). Deaf-mutism. [see prec.]

surexcitation (**ser**·ek·si·**ta**′·shun). Superexcitation.

surface (**ser**·fis). 1. A two-dimensional outermost part of a solid body or the uppermost part of a fluid substance when it is in contact with a gas. 2. Facies [NA]. **Articular surface.** A joint surface. **Extensor surface.** The surface of a limb under which lie the extensor muscles. **Flexor surface.** The surface of a limb under which lie the flexor muscles. **Glenoid surface.** A glenoid cavity. **Isocount surface.** A surface in space in the region of a radioactive source on all points of which the count rate obtained with a radiation detector is the same. **Isodose surface.** A surface on which all points receive equal doses. **Respiratory surface.** The surface within the alveoli through which there is exchange between the inspired air and the blood of oxygen and other gases. **Tentorial surface.** The surface of the cerebrum that lies on the tentorium cerebelli. [L *superficies* surface.]

surfactant (ser·**fak**·tant). An agent which reduces the surface tension, a wetting agent, e.g. detergents, emulsifiers, etc. **Pulmonary surfactant.** A phospholipid with a hydrophilic "head" and 2 hydrophilic "tails", which forms a liquid surface lining to the alveoli. When an alveolus becomes smaller during expiration, the surface tension is reduced by the presence of the surfactant, so that it does not collapse. There is a deficiency in hyaline membrane disease. [L *superficies* surface.]

surfusion (ser·**few**·zhun). The cooling of a liquid to a temperature below its normal freezing point without solidification. [L *super, fundere* to pour.]

surgeon (**ser**·jun). A medical practitioner who treats disease, injury or deformity of the body by operative means. One qualified to practise surgery. **House surgeon.** A surgeon resident in a hospital who acts under the orders of the attending surgeon. [Gk *cheirourgos.*]

surgery (**ser**·jer·e). 1. That part of the art of medicine which deals with the treatment of disease and injuries, mainly by manipulative and operative methods. 2. A practitioner's consulting room (the American "office"). **Abdominal surgery.** The branch of surgery which deals with operations on the abdominal contents, mainly the viscera (usually taken to exclude those of the urinary tract). **Antiseptic surgery.** Operative procedure where existence of bacterial contamination is admitted, but where steps are taken to destroy bacteria by the use of appropriate antiseptics. **Aseptic surgery.** The ideal surgical method where bacterial contamination is studiously avoided at every stage of the operative procedure. **Aural surgery.** The art of surgery as applied to the organ of hearing. **Battle surgery.** Emergency surgery in a battle area. **Brain surgery.** Cerebral surgery (see below). **Cancer surgery.** The surgery of malignant tumours. **Cardiac surgery.** Surgery of the heart and great vessels mostly concerned with congenital and acquired anatomical lesions of the heart but also applied to vascular disease involving the aorta and coronary arteries. **Cerebral surgery.** Surgery applied to the treatment and investigation of intracranial disease or injury. **Clinical surgery.** That aspect of surgery (especially in relation to teaching by lecture and at the bedside) which has to do with the treatment of patients. **Closed-heart surgery.** Cardiac surgery performed without more than transient interruption of the cardiac action. **Conservative surgery.** Any method of surgery which encourages the preservation and reconstruction of structures wherever possible. **Conservative dental surgery.** Operative dental surgery (see below). **Cosmetic surgery.** That branch of plastic surgery which deals mainly with attempts to improve the appearance, especially of face, hands and breast. **Definitive surgery.** Planned or elective surgery, as distinct from emergency surgery. **Dental surgery.** That branch of the practice of surgery which deals with the treatment of the teeth and the surrounding oral tissues. **Elective (cold) surgery.** Definitive surgery (see above). **Emergency surgery.** Surgery which has by necessity to be undertaken immediately. **General surgery.** A term embracing every type of surgical work encountered in a community and including orthopaedic, urological and other similar special branches of surgical practice. **Heroic surgery.** Hazardous surgery undertaken by an intrepid surgeon, in the expectation that only by so doing can he promise any prospect of cure. **Major surgery.** The type of work which involves formidable operations and which can properly be conducted only where adequate hospital facilities are available. **Manipulative surgery.** Surgical treatment mainly by non-operative manipulation. **Military surgery.** The surgical care of soldiers on active service, including the care of battle casualties. **Minor surgery.** The type of surgery which can reasonably be undertaken even when no hospital facilities are available. **Open-heart surgery.** Cardiac surgery which involves arresting the heart and opening the heart or great vessels, thereby leading to interruption of the natural circulation to the body which is usually replaced by the use of a pump oxygenator. **Operative surgery.** That branch of surgery which involves the display or removal of structures by incising the skin. **Operative dental surgery.** The science and practice of restoring teeth which have been damaged. **Ophthalmic surgery.** The art of surgery as applied to the organ of sight. **Oral surgery.** That part of surgery which concerns operations upon the jaws and associated soft tissues. **Orthopaedic surgery.** A term originally applied to surgery concerned in the correction of deformities in children, it is now used in a much wider sense to include every aspect of the surgery of the musculoskeletal system (at least of the trunk and extremities) whether due to congenital deformity, injury or disease. **Palliative surgery.** Surgery which aims only at relief of pain or disability, and not a cure, especially in relation to inoperable cancer. **Pelvic surgery.** Surgery of the pelvic organs. **Plastic surgery.** That branch of surgery which deals with the reconstruction, or with the correction, of deformities of soft tissues. **Radical surgery.** A term applied almost only to extensive surgical operations designed to circumvent cancerous growth. **Reconstructive surgery.** Surgery which aims at the rebuilding of severely damaged or of lost tissues, often by multistage operations, e.g. in reconstructing the nose or a thumb. **Rectal surgery.** The surgery of the rectum, as well as the anus, anal canal and usually also the distal colon. **Reparative surgery.** Reconstructive surgery (see above). **Veterinary surgery.** The surgery of animals other than humans. [see prec.]

surgical (ser·jik·al). 1. Relating to surgery or surgeons. 2. Employed in, or performed by, surgery. **Surgical neck.** *See* HUMERUS.

Surinam bark (sew·ri·nam bark). The bark of *Andira retusa* (family Leguminosae). [*Surinam*, Dutch Guiana, bark.]

surinamine (sew·rin·am·een). Methyltyrosine, β-*p*-hydroxyphenyl-α-methylaminopropionic acid, $HOC_6H_4CH_2CH(NHCH_3)COOH$. An organic base occurring naturally in plants.

Surmay's operation. Jejunostomy.

surpalite (ser·pal·ite). Superpalite.

surra (soor·ah). Trypanosomiasis of horses and camels, caused by *Trypanosoma evansi*, which is transmitted by Tabanidae. [Marathi, wheezing.]

surrogate (ser·o·gate). A person or thing acting for and representing another. The term is used more specifically in psychoanalysis for a person or thing representing someone or something in the unconscious mind. [L *surrogare* to elect as substitute.]

sursumduction (ser·sum·**duk**·shun). Vertical upward movement of one eye, the fellow remaining stationary. [L *sursum* up, *ducere* to lead.]

sursumvergence (ser·sum·**ver**·jens). Supravergence. [L *sursum* up, *vergere* to turn.]

sursumversion (ser·sum·**ver**·zhun). Parallel motion of the eyes upwards. [L *sursum* up, *vertere* to turn.]

surumpe (soo·**room**·pe). Retinal hypersensitiveness occurring at high altitudes. [Sp.]

survey (ser·va). A detailed examination or investigation. **Cross-sectional survey.** A study of the characteristics of a population at one particular point of time. **Malarial survey.** An investigation into all the factors concerned in the causation of malaria in a population, including the incidence of malaria in the various age groups, the physiography of the terrain and the incidence of actual and potential malaria-carrying mosquitoes. **Prospective (longitudinal) survey.** A study of the characteristics of a population over a period of time, the study being set up at the beginning of this period. **Radiation survey.** An investigation of those factors associated with an installation or process which could give rise to a radiation hazard. **Retrospective survey.** A study of the characteristics of a population in which the previous experience of the population is examined. [O Fr. *surveeir*.]

survivorship (ser·vi·ver·ship). In forensic medicine, the survival of 1 or more persons after the death of the other or others. [Fr. *survivre*.]

"Susa" fixative (soo·zah **fix**·at·iv). A histological fixative composed of mercuric chloride, acetic and trichloro-acetic acids, and formalin. It gives rapid fixation and only slight shrinkage of connective tissue.

susceptibility (sus·**ep**·tib·**il**'·it·e). The opposite of immunity; the condition of being susceptible or lacking the power to resist a particular disease or infection; sensitivity. **Acquired susceptibility.** That acquired after birth; not congenital. **Anaphylaxis susceptibility.** Sensitization to a particular foreign substance. **Familial susceptibility.** That which occurs in some families. **Individual susceptibility.** Susceptibility occurring in only 1 individual out of many. **Inherited susceptibility.** That conveyed to the child through the germ cells of the parents; congenital. **Racial susceptibility.** That which occurs in individuals belonging to a certain race or group. **Specific susceptibility.** Susceptibility to a certain particular disease. [see foll.]

susceptible (sus·**ep**·tibl). 1. Having a predisposition to react to an influence; sensitive. 2. Liable to infection. [L *suscipere* to undertake.]

suscitability (sus·it·ab·**il**'·it·e). Excitability; the capacity for being aroused or stimulated. [L *suscitare* to lift up.]

suslik (suz·lik). A small ground squirrel of the genus *Citellus*, particularly *Citellus pygmaeus* of south-east Russia. They are important plague reservoirs. [Russian.]

susotoxin (sus·o·**tox**·in). The toxin from the hog cholera bacillus, once believed to be the cause of swine fever. [L *sus* hog, toxin.]

suspensiometer (sus·pen·she·**om**'·et·er). An instrument for standardizing bacterial suspensions in terms of turbidity; it is now called a *nephelometer*. [suspension, meter.]

suspension (sus·**pen**·shun). 1. Temporary cessation of a function. 2. The treatment of spinal disorders by traction, with the body weight as counter-traction. 3. A system consisting of a solid dispersed in a liquid medium in which the size of the solid particles is greater than 100 nm, i.e. larger than in colloidal systems. **Cephalic suspension.** Suspension by the head to straighten a spinal deformity, usually before application of plaster. **Insulin Zinc Suspension BP 1973, Insulin Zinc Suspension (Amorphous) BP 1973, Insulin Zinc Suspension (Crystalline) BP 1973.** Sterile, buffered suspensions of the specific antidiabetic principle of the mammalian pancreas with zinc chloride. **Suspension stability.** The stability of the suspension of the blood corpuscles in blood plasma; this varies considerably in pregnancy and various physiological and pathological conditions. **Tendon suspension.** Tenodesis. **Suspension of the uterus.** An operation to replace the uterus in a normal position by shortening its ligamentous attachments in various ways. [L *suspendere* to hang.]

suspensoid (sus·**pen**·soid). Applied to substances which in colloidal solution are readily precipitated by small amounts of electrolytes. Typical suspensoid sols are those formed by certain metals and metallic salts. [suspension, Gk *eidos* form.]

suspensorium (sus·pen·**so**·re·um). An old name for a support. **Suspensorium hepatis.** The coronary and triangular ligaments of the liver. **Suspensorium testis.** The cremaster muscle. [see foll.]

suspensory (sus·**pen**·sor·e). 1. Pertaining to a suspension. 2. Supporting a part; applied to a muscle, bone, ligament or surgical appliance such as a bandage or sling, which supports a dependent part. [L *suspendere* to hang.]

suspiration (sus·pi·**ra**·shun). A sigh. [L *suspirare* to sigh.]

suspirious (sus·**pi**·re·us). Breathing that is heavy, like sighing. [see prec.]

sustentacular (sus·ten·**tak**·ew·lar). 1. Pertaining to a sustentaculum. 2. Serving to support. [L *sustentare* to support.]

sustentaculum (sus·ten·**tak**·ew·lum) (pl. *sustentacula*). Any structure which supports another. **Sustentaculum lienis.** The phrenicocolic ligament supporting the left flexure of the colon. **Sustentaculum tali [NA].** A projection from the medial surface of the calcaneum which serves to support the talus. [see prec.]

sustoxin (sus·**tox**·in). Susotoxin.

susurration (sus·er·**a**·shun). A murmur. [L *susurrus* murmur.]

sutho (**sew**·tho). A local Korean name for leprosy.

sutika (**sew**·tik·ah). A disease of pregnancy and the puerperium, occurring in India, and characterized by persistent diarrhoea and macrocytic anaemia.

Sutton, Henry Gawen (b. 1837). London physician.

Gull and Sutton disease, Sutton and Gull disease. Arteriosclerosis.

Sutton, Richard Lightburn (b. 1878). Kansas City dermatologist.

Sutton's disease or naevus. Leucoderma acquisitum centrifugum.

Sutton's ulcer. Mucosal aphthosis with ulceration.

sutura (sew·tewr·ah). Suture. **Sutura harmonia.** Simple apposition of 2 or more bones. **Sutura limbosa.** Contact of bevelled bone surfaces. **Sutura serrata.** Accurate apposition of 2 serrated bone edges. **Sutura squamosa.** A suture where 1 bone overlaps another. [L.]

sutural (sew·tewr·al). Of the nature of, or relating to a suture.

sutural bones [ossa suturarum (NA)]. Small accessory bones that sometimes develop in the sutures between the bones of the cranial vault; wormian bones.

suturation (sew·tewr·a·shun). The act of applying sutures; stitching.

suture (**sew**·tewr). 1. A surgical stitch, or group or row of such stitches. 2. To insert a surgical stitch; to sew. 3. The material used for stitching. Also used as an adjective, as in *suture material*. 4. [Sutura (NA)]. The interlocking lines of fusion of the separate bones which unite to form the cranium. **Absorbable suture.** Suture material which is gradually and completely removed by tissue phagocytes. **Apposition suture.** A suture which maintains the margins of an incision closely together. **Approximation sutures.** Sutures which are often provisional and which draw the edges of an incision towards each other, usually as a preliminary to their more exact fixation. **Arterial suture.** A fine suture, commonly of silk or of catgut, used in arterial anastomosis. **Atraumatic suture.** A suture which is fused into the head of the needle so that only a single thickness is pulled through each needle puncture. **Baseball suture.** A form of continuous suture (see below). **Blanket suture.** A form of continuous suture (see below). **Bridle suture.** Superior rectus suture (see below). **Bulb suture.** Direct suture of neuromata (bulbs) in divided nerve without previous trimming, to conserve nerve length. **Buried suture.** Any suture inserted to bring together neither skin nor the mucous lining of any viscus, but the soft tissues in-between. **Button sutures.** Sutures tied over a button to prevent their cutting into the skin, e.g. in reconstruction of the urethra in hypospadias. **Buttonhole suture.** A continuous suture used in intestinal anastomosis to prevent slipping and puckering. **Catgut suture.** A suture made of catgut which is an absorbable material; used in situations where, mainly because of inaccessibility, it is not planned to remove the suture subsequently. **Chain-stitch suture.** A continuous suture like a sewing-machine stitch. **Circular suture.** A continuous suture which runs all the way round the circumference as, for example, in small intestine or in arterial anastomosis. **Coaptation suture.** A suture which brings the skin edges closely together; apposition suture. **Cobblers' suture.** A suture with a needle on each end which are passed in the opposite direction. **Conchiform suture.** The junction within the hard palate of the paired maxillary and palatine bones. **Continuous (running) suture.** A single suture which runs backwards and forwards without interruption, joining 2 tissues together. Cf. INTERRUPTED SUTURE (below). **Corneoscleral suture.** A suture commonly used in cataract extraction to obtain quick and firm union of the section. Various methods of insertion are employed, some before the section is made and some after. **Coronal suture [sutura coronalis** (NA)**].** The suture between the posterior border of the frontal bone and the anterior borders of the parietal bones. **Cruciform suture.** A suture between the palatine processes of the maxillae and the horizontal plates of the palatine bones, the intermaxillary and interpalatine parts lying in the sagittal plane and the palatomaxillary parts in the coronal. **Delayed suture.** The practice of leaving a wound open and then suturing it later when the risk of infection has diminished, especially applicable to battle wounds. Cf. PRIMARY SUTURE (below). **Delayed primary suture.** Wound closure undertaken a few days after wounding, when the risk of serious infection has passed. **Denticulate suture.** A suture present in a series of tooth-like processes, wider at their free margin than at their bases. **Dermal suture.** A special fine suture material. **Ethmoidomaxillary suture [sutura ethmoideomaxillaris** (NA)**].** A suture between the lower border of the orbital plate of the ethmoid bone and the medial edge of the orbital surface of the maxilla. **Everting suture.** A suture which turns the edge of a wound outwards, usually to facilitate more accurate apposition. Cf. INFOLDING SUTURE (below). **Fascial suture.** A strip of fascia taken from the same patient and used as suture material. **Figure-of-eight suture.** A suture which takes a bite of the deepest layer on each side of a wound and then crosses over to pass through the superficial layers on the opposite side before being tied. **Flat suture [sutura plana** (NA)**].** A suture where there is simple apposition of the adjoining surfaces. **Frontal suture [sutura frontalis (metopica)** (NA)**].** The suture separating the two halves of the frontal bone in infancy and occasionally persisting in the adult; the metopic suture. **Fronto-ethmoid suture [sutura fronto-ethmoidalis** (NA)**].** The suture joining the crista galli and alae of the cribriform plate of the ethmoid bone to the nasal spine and the anterior border of the ethmoidal notch of the frontal bone. **Frontolacrimal suture [sutura frontolacrimalis** (NA)**].** The suture between the anterior part of the medial border of the orbital plate of the frontal bone and the upper border of the lacrimal bone. **Frontomaxillary suture [sutura frontomaxillaris** (NA)**].** The suture between the nasal part of the frontal bone and the frontal process of the maxilla. **Frontonasal suture [sutura frontonasalis** (NA)**].** The suture between the nasal notch of the frontal bone and the upper border of the nasal bones. **Frontozygomatic suture [sutura frontozygomatica** (NA)**].** The suture between the zygomatic process of the frontal bone and the frontal process of the zygomatic bone. **Granny-knot suture.** A suture tied with the clumsy, weak, granny knot, and not the more compact and more secure reef knot. **Guy sutures.** Sutures inserted in a wound to divide it into small subsections and to support it while further sutures are inserted primarily to control bleeding, e.g. in the margin of the divided scalp. **Hare-lip suture.** An operation to close a congenital defect in the upper lip. **Horizontal mattress suture.** *See* MATTRESS SUTURE (below). **Incisive suture [sutura incisiva** (NA)**].** The suture, present at birth and later disappearing, which separates the incisive bone from the maxilla. **Infolding suture.** A suture so placed as to turn the edges of a wound inwards, e.g. in intestinal anastomosis. Cf. EVERTING SUTURE (above). **Infra-orbital suture [sutura infra-orbitalis** (NA)**].** A suture between the infra-orbital foramen and the orbit, present for a short time after the groove has been converted into a canal. **Intermaxillary suture [sutura intermaxillaris** (NA)**].** The intermaxillary part of the cruciform suture (see above). **Internasal suture [sutura internasalis** (NA)**].** A suture between the medial borders of the nasal bones. **Interpalatine suture.** The interpalatine part of the cruciform suture (see above). **Interrupted suture.** A single suture tied separately. Cf. CONTINUOUS (RUNNING) SUTURE (above). **Intradermic suture.** A suture inserted into the deepest part of the true skin (dermis); occasionally used in plastic surgery on the face. **Invaginating suture.** Infolding suture (see above). **Lacrimoconchal suture [sutura lacrimoconchalis** (NA)**].** A suture between the inferior border of the lacrimal bone and the lacrimal process of the inferior nasal concha. **Lacrimomaxillary suture [sutura lacrimomaxillaris** (NA)**].** A suture between the anterior border of the lacrimal bone and the frontal process of the maxilla. **Lambdoid suture [sutura lambdoidea** (NA)**].** A suture between the posterior borders of the parietal bones and the anterior border of the squamous part of the occipital bone. **Lens sutures.** The lines seen in the centre of the crystalline lens of the eye. They take the form of 2 letters Y, the anterior being erect, the posterior being inverted. Also called *Y sutures.* **Lid sutures.** Those inserted into the upper and lower eyelids, which when traction is applied to them act as lid retractors. **Limbous suture.** A serrated suture where one bone overlaps another. **Living suture.** A fascial suture, occasionally also of skin. **Loop-on mucosa suture.** Connell suture. **Mattress suture.** A suture so inserted that there is a loop on each side; this loop may be parallel with the edge of the incision *(horizontal mattress)* or at right angles to it *(vertical mattress).* This latter is an excellent everting suture. **Mendosal suture.** An accessory suture of the occipital bone. **Metopic suture.** Frontal suture (see below). **Nasomaxillary suture [sutura nasomaxillaris** (NA)**].** A suture between the lateral border of the nasal bone and the frontal process of the maxilla. **Nerve suture.** Very fine material, often of silk, used to bring together with meticulous care the supporting sheath of a divided nerve. **Non-absorbable suture.** A suture which resists all attempts made by the tissues to digest and remove it, e.g. silk, thread, nylon, steel. Those in the skin are removed; those buried in the tissues and in the viscera are left *in situ.* **Occipitomastoid suture [sutura occipitomastoidea** (NA)**].** A suture between the squamous part of the occipital bone and the mastoid part of the temporal bone. **Palatine suture, median [sutura palatina mediana** (NA)**].** The suture between the medial borders of the horizontal plates of the palatine bones. **Palatine suture, transverse [sutura palatina transversa** (NA)**].** The suture between the anterior borders of the horizontal plates of the palatine bones and the palatine processes of the maxillae. **Palato-ethmoidal suture [sutura palato-ethmoidalis** (NA)**].** A suture between the ethmoidal crest on the nasal surface of the perpendicular plate of the palatine bone and the middle nasal concha of the ethmoid bone. **Palatomaxillary**

suture [sutura palatomaxillaris (NA)]. The palatomaxillary part of the cruciform suture (see above). **Parietomastoid suture [sutura parietomastoidea (NA)].** A suture between the posterior part of the lower border of the parietal bone and the upper border of the mastoid part of the temporal bone. **Peg-and-socket suture [gomphosis (NA)].** The suture between a conical process and a corresponding socket. **Petrobasilar suture.** A suture between the petrous part of the temporal bone and the basilar part of the occipital bone; a thin plate of cartilage separates the bones. **Petro-occipital suture.** A suture between the petrous part of the temporal bone and the condylar part of the occipital bone. **Petrosquamous suture.** A suture between the lateral part of the anterior border of the petrous part of the temporal bone and its squamous part. **Plane suture.** Flat suture (see above). **Plicating suture.** A continuous suture that is pulled tight so that there is puckering and folding of the wound. **Primary suture.** Suturing completed at the time of the first operation, e.g. in the repair of war wounds. Cf. DELAYED SUTURE (above). **Primary delayed suture.** Delayed primary suture (see above). **Pulley suture.** A suture combining a relaxation suture with a coaptation suture. The needle passes through the tissues well away from one side of the wound, then out a similar distance from the opposite wound edge; then through the tissues close to the first edge and out close to the opposite margin. Finally the ends are tied. **Purse-string suture.** A continuous suture inserted so as to form a circle round a small wound in a viscus, e.g. appendix stump. On being drawn tight it closes the opening. **Relaxation suture, Relief suture.** A suture which takes a wide bite and which is adjusted to take the strain off a sutured operation wound during healing, e.g. in the abdomen. **Sagittal suture [sutura sagittalis (NA)].** The suture between the upper borders of the parietal bones. **Secondary suture.** The repair of a wound which has been allowed to remain open until it is covered with healthy granulations, e.g. following a partial wound disruption. Cf. PRIMARY SUTURE (above). **Serrate suture [sutura serrata (NA)].** A suture with saw-like edges. **Shotted suture.** A suture consisting of a single strand each end of which is anchored by a lead shot. **Silkworm-gut suture.** A non-absorbable, monofilamentous suture made from the intestine of the silkworm and often used to unite skin. **Sutures of the skull [suturae cranii (NA)].** Immovable joints between the bones of the skull; these become obliterated with advancing years. **Spheno-ethmoidal suture [sutura spheno-ethmoidalis (NA)].** The suture between the anterior border of the body of the sphenoid bone and the posterior border of the cribriform plate of the ethmoid bone. **Sphenofrontal suture [sutura sphenofrontalis (NA)].** A suture between the anterior border of the lesser wing of the sphenoid bone and the posterior border of the orbital plate of the frontal bone. **Sphenomaxillary suture [sutura sphenomaxillaris (NA)].** An occasional suture between the pterygoid process of the sphenoid bone and the posterior surface of the maxilla. **Spheno-orbital suture.** A suture between the body of the sphenoid bone and the orbital process of the palatine bone. **Sphenoparietal suture [sutura sphenoparietalis (NA)].** A suture between the body of the sphenoid bone and the orbital process of the palatine bone. **Sphenoparietal suture [sutura sphenoparietalis (NA)].** A suture between the upper border of the greater wing of the sphenoid bone and the anterior part of the lower border of the parietal bone. **Sphenosquamous suture [sutura sphenosquamosa (NA)].** A suture between the posterior border of the greater wing of the sphenoid bone and the squamous part of the temporal bone. **Sphenozygomatic suture [sutura sphenozygomatica (NA)].** A suture between the anterior border of the greater wing of the sphenoid bone and the zygomatic bone. **Squamomastoid suture [sutura squamomastoidea (NA)].** A suture present during development between the petromastoid and squamous elements of the temporal bone. It fuses about the first postnatal year, but remnants may persist into adult life. **Squamous suture [sutura squamosa (NA)].** 1. A suture between flat overlapping bones. 2. A suture between the upper border of the squamous part of the temporal bone and the lower border of the parietal bone in its middle part. **Subcuticular suture.** A continuous suture carefully placed so as to bring together the tissues immediately under the skin; it may be of non-absorbable material which can be removed later by pulling on one end, leaving a wound without any suture mark. **Superior rectus suture.** A suture placed through the belly of the superior rectus muscle of the orbit, so that when traction is applied the eye is held steady looking downwards; a valuable adjunct to intra-ocular surgery, especially cataract extraction. **Temporozygomatic suture [sutura temporozygomatica (NA)].** A suture between the zygomatic process of the temporal bone and the temporal process of the zygomatic bone. **Tension suture.** Relaxation suture (see above). **Through-and-through sutures.** Sutures inserted through the entire thickness of the abdominal wall. **Track corneoscleral suture.** A suture inserted through the cornea and sclera in cataract extraction, then withdrawn to allow the section to be made, and then reinstated through the old track with a minimum of pressure on the eye. **Transfixion suture.** A suture which is first carried on a needle to transfix the structure round which it is then drawn tight, e.g. neck of hernial sac. **Tympanomastoid suture.** A suture between the tympanic plate and the mastoid part of the temporal bone lateral to the tympanomastoid fissure. **Uninterrupted suture.** Continuous (running) suture (see above). **Vertical mattress suture.** *See* MATTRESS SUTURE (above). **Vomero-ethmoidal suture.** The suture between the upper half of the anterior border of the vomer and the posterior border of the perpendicular plate of the ethmoid bone. **Wedge-and-groove suture.** A suture where a ridge of one bone fits into a groove on another. **Y suture of the lens.** Lens suture (see above). **Zygomaticomaxillary suture [sutura zygomaticomaxillaris (NA)].** A suture between the maxillary border of the zygomatic bone and the zygomatic process of the maxilla. **Zygomaticotemporal suture.** Temporozygomatic suture (see above). [L *sutura*.]

See also: ARLT, AXENFELD, BUNNELL (S.), CONNELL (F. G.), CUSHING (HAYWARD W.), CZERNY (V.), GAILLARD, HALSTED, KALT, LEMBERT, LESPINASSE, MCLEAN (J. M.), PAGENSTECHER, SNELLEN, STALLARD.

suxamethonium (sux·a·meth·o′·ne·um). Succinylcholine. A bis-choline ester of succinic acid used by anaesthetists in the form of the iodide, bromide or chloride. **Suxamethonii Chloridum.** *European Pharmacopoeia* name for Suxamethonium Chloride BP 1973. **Suxamethonium Bromide BP 1973.** Succinylcholine bromide bis-2-dimethylaminoethyl succinate bismethobromide. A short-acting muscle relaxant used to produce relaxation during operations or manipulations. **Suxamethonium Chloride BP 1973.** Succinylcholine chloride, bis-2-dimethylaminoethyl succinate bismethochloride. A muscle relaxant of ultra-short action. **Suxamethonium iodide.** Bis-2-dimethylaminoethyl succinate bismethiodide. This is a synthetic quaternary ammonium compound which has a neuromuscular blocking action similar to C10 (decamethonium) but of short duration. It causes depolarization of the muscle end-plate and differs in being broken down by cholinesterase in the body; there is also a stimulation of the muscle before paralysis which may later cause stiffness, but which may be avoided by slow administration. Though chemically related to acetycholine it is free from the muscarinic actions of the latter and thus does not cause bradycardia. High doses do, however, show the nicotinic effect on blood pressure. It is particularly valuable for profound but brief muscular relaxation; its main indications therefore are in intubation, convulsive shock therapy and manipulations. For long operations it can be given by repeated injections or by constant infusion. A narcotic should always precede its administration, and artificial respiration is usually necessary during the paralysis. There is no antidote, the brevity of its action rendering this unnecessary. Since the drug is broken down by cholinesterase, the use of neostigmine is contra-indicated; in a few individuals with an abnormally low serum cholinesterase or a genetically determined abnormal type of serum cholinesterase the duration of action may be prolonged.

Suxethonium Bromide (sux·eth·o·ne·um **bro**·mide). BP Commission approved name for bis-2-dimethylaminoethyl succinate bisethobromide, a short-acting muscle relaxant chemically similar to the suxamethonium chloride of the BP 1973. It is said to be especially useful in short surgical procedures requiring relaxation.

Suzanne, Jean Georges (b. 1859). Bordeaux physician.

Suzanne's gland. A mucous gland in the oral mucous membrane near the midline underneath the tongue.

Svedberg, Theodor (b. 1884). Swedish chemist. Nobel Prize winner. Inventor of the ultracentrifuge for the determination of sedimentation rates of proteins.

Svedberg unit. The unit of sedimentation rate; a sedimentation coefficient of 1×10^{-13} s.

swab (swob). An absorbent pad, sometimes on the end of a stick, by means of which materials may be applied to or removed from parts of the body, e.g. from the throat. **NIH** (National Institutes of Health, USA) **swab.** A cellophane square attached to a glass rod, used for collecting material for direct examination from *Enterobius* ova. **Radio-opaque swab.** A surgical swab that has woven into it a thread opaque to x-rays. **Sewer swab.** A large swab of absorbent cotton wool or similar material immersed in a sewage system for 1-4 days and then examined bacteriologically for the presence of intestinal pathogens. [D *zwabber,* a ship's drudge.]

See also: GRAHAM, WEST (J. M.).

swab stick (**swob** stik). A piece of wood, bamboo or wire, to the end of which is attached a cotton-wool pledget. [swab, AS *sticca.*]

swage (swaje). In dentistry, to shape metal on a die; to exert pressure on the margins of a gold filling in order to make a watertight junction with the tooth structure. Also applied to the counter-die used in the process. [O Fr. *souage.*]

swager (**swa**·jer). An apparatus having a die and a counter-die, used in dentistry for shaping the base of a crown or artificial denture. [see prec.]

swallow's nest (**swol**·oze **nest**). A depression either side of the lower surface of the cerebellum for the cerebellar tonsils. [AS *swalewe, nest.*]

swallowing (**swol**·o·ing). Deglutition; the passing of food down the oesophagus into the stomach. **Air swallowing.** Aerophagy; the commonest cause of gastric flatulence. It may be hysterical, but is common in functional and organic dyspepsias. **Tongue swallowing.** A popular misnomer based on the misinterpretation of the falling back of the mandible and the flaccidity of the tongue which produce respiratory obstruction during profound unconsciousness. [AS *swelgan.*]

Swammerdam, Jan (b. 1637). Leyden and Amsterdam anatomist.

Swammerdam's corpora heterogenia or glands. The suprarenal glands in amphibia.

Swan, Harold James Charles (b. 1922). Los Angeles physician.

Swan-Ganz catheter. A soft catheter with a balloon near its tip which can be passed from a vein through the right heart chambers to the pulmonary artery without the aid of fluoroscopy; the blood flow carries the balloon along and so guides the catheter to its intended position. Once in the pulmonary artery, inflation of the balloon may serve to block the artery proximal to the catheter tip, permitting a record to be obtained of the left atrial pressure transmitted back through the pulmonary vascular bed.

swan spectrum. A banded emission spectrum.

swarming (**swarm**·ing). Applied to bacteria which spread across the surface of a solid culture medium. [AS *swearm.*]

Swartzia madagascariensis (**swawt**·ze·ah **mad**·ah·gas·kar·e·**en**'·sis). An African plant the fruits of which have molluscicidal properties.

swayback (**swa**·bak). A congenital demyelinizing disease of lambs. [LG *swajen,* back.]

swearing (**swa**·er·ing). **Compulsive swearing.** The compulsive repetition of obscene words; a part of the Gilles de la Tourette's disease. [AS *swerian.*]

sweat (swet). 1. [Sudor (NA)] The watery secretion of the sweat glands which contains sodium chloride and urea in solution. 2. To secrete sweat; to perspire. **Bloody sweat.** Haemathidrosis; sweat containing blood. It is exceedingly rare but undoubted cases have been described. **Blue sweat.** That which may be caused by the presence of *Pseudomonas pyocyanea.* **Colliquative sweat.** A profuse cold perspiration. **Coloured sweat.** Chromhidrosis; it has also been produced by hysterical girls and malingerers from the use of dyes and can be due to aniline dyes soaked out of clothing by excessive sweating. **English sweat.** The sweating sickness which appeared in epidemic form in England at the end of the 15th century. **Fetid sweat.** Bromhidrosis; it may occur from the feet, axillae, groins and pubes. It is produced by excessive sweating, maceration of epithelium and bacterial decomposition. **Green sweat.** That which may be seen from copper compounds in workers with this metal. **Night sweats.** Sweating occurring as a result of nocturnal fever, as in phthisis. **Phosphorescent sweat.** That which is probably due to phosphorescent bacteria but has been described after eating certain fish. **Red sweat.** That which may be due to the presence of *Chromobacterium prodigiosum.* **Urinary sweat.** Crystalline frosty deposits of urea which may occur on the skin in chronic renal disease. **Yellow sweat.** That occurring in jaundice. [AS *swaetan.*]

sweating (**swet**·ing). The excretion of sweat. **Gustatory sweating.** 1. Sweating on eating or in response to other stimuli. 2. Auriculotemporal syndrome. *See* SYNDROME. [AS *swaetan.*]

sweetbread (**sweet**·bred). The thymus (neck or throat sweetbread), the pancreas (stomach or abdominal sweetbread) or the testes of an animal; prized as a food delicacy. [AS *swete, bread.*]

swelling (**swel**·ing). An enlargement, elevation or protuberance, usually associated with a disease process. **Albuminous swelling.** Albuminous degeneration, albuminoid degeneration; an early degenerative change in the cellular protoplasm of parenchymatous tissues, epithelium, endothelium and leucocytes, mainly associated with the toxaemia of an infection. The cells become enlarged, with irregular outline, coarsely granular protoplasm and indistinct nuclei. When the cause is removed, there is a reversion to normal appearances. **Arytenoid swelling.** One of the paired swellings appearing on the floor of the embryonic pharynx from which the posterior wall of the larynx is derived. **Bulbar swelling.** One of the paired ridges appearing on the inner endocardial wall of the embryonic bulbus cordis which will later fuse and form a complete septum separating the pulmonary trunk from the ascending aorta. **Calabar swelling.** An allergic transient swelling of various sizes usually on the forearms, legs or face, caused by *Loa loa,* the eye worm of West Africa. **Cloudy swelling.** Albuminous swelling (see above). **Fugitive swelling.** A swelling that only lasts for a short time and usually reappears. **Genital swelling.** Labial swelling (see below). **Giant swelling.** Angioneurotic oedema. *See* OEDEMA. **Glassy swelling.** Hyaline or amyloid degeneration. *See* DEGENERATION. **Hunger swelling.** Nutritional oedema. *See* OEDEMA. **Kamerun swelling.** Calabar swelling (see above). **Labial swelling, Labioscrotal swelling.** The outer pair of folds which flank the urogenital portion of the cloacal membrane of the embryo, representing the future labia majora or scrotum. **Lateral lingual swelling.** One of the paired swellings arising from the mandibular arches on either side of the midline in the floor of the embryonic pharynx from which the anterior two-thirds of the tongue is formed. **Sexual swelling.** Labial swelling (see above). **Tympanic swelling.** Swelling of the ear-drum from any cause. **White swelling.** Tumour albus, the swelling of the soft tissues produced by tuberculous arthritis [obsolete term]. [AS *swellan.*]

See also: SOEMMERING.

Swenson, Orvar (b. 1909). Boston, Massachusetts, surgeon.

Swenson's operation. Rectosigmoidectomy for megacolon.

Swieten, Gerhard van L. B. (b. 1700). Vienna physician.

van Swieten's solution. A solution of mercuric chloride 0.1 per cent w/v.

Swift, Homer Fordyce (b. 1881). New York physician.

Swift-Ellis treatment. Autoserosalvarsan treatment.

Swift, Joly. *See* JOLY, JOHN SWIFT.

switch (swich). **Selector switch.** A switch by means of which connection can be made to any one of a number of alternative electric currents. [LG *zwuksen.*]

sycoma (si·**ko**·mah). A condyloma or wart; fig-like growths on soft tissues. [Gk *sykon* fig, *-oma* tumour.]

sycosiform (si·**ko**·se·form). Having a similarity to sycosis.

sycosis (si·**ko**·sis). A chronic pustular perifolliculitis, usually affecting the beard and moustache areas, commonly attributed to staphylococcal infection, characterized by the formation of follicular papulopustules, inflammatory nodules and indurated swellings, with some tendency to scarring and destruction of the hair follicles. The chronicity of many infections has been attributed not only to the infection but also to hypersensitivity of the skin to the infecting bacteria. **Bacillogenic sycosis.** Tommasoli (1889) described a case of sycosis in which a bacillus was proved to be the causal agent; the name has been applied to cases of similar aetiology. **Sycosis barbae.** Sycocis of the beard area. **Coccogenic sycosis.** Sycosis caused by infection with cocci. **Sycosis contagiosa.** Tinea barbae. **Sycosis framboesiformis.** Hebra's term for dermatitis papillaris capillitii. **Hyphomycotic sycosis.** Tinea barbae. **Keloid sycosis.** Dermatitis papillaris capillitii. **Lupoid sycosis.** Milton's name for a rare type of sycosis which usually affects only limited parts of the beard or moustache areas, characterized by the destruction of the hair follicles and the formation of smooth atrophic skin; ulerythema sycosiforme. **Sycosis mentagra.** Tinea barbae. **Mycotic sycosis.** Tinea barbae. **Non-parasitic sycosis.** Coccogenic sycosis (see above). **Sycosis nuchae.** Dermatitis papillaris capillitii. **Sycosis nuchae necrotisans.** Ehrmann's name for dermatitis papillaris capillitii. **Sycosis palpebrae marginalis.** One affecting the eyelash follicles at the eyelid margin; also called *sycotic blepharitis.* **Parasitic sycosis, Sycosis parasitica.** Tinea barbae. **Schizomycetic sycosis.** Folliculitis attributed to invasion of the pilosebaceous follicles by schistosome cercariae. Many authorities deny that these cercariae enter the follicles. **Seborrhoeic sycosis.** Seborrhoeic dermatitis associated with follicular pustulation. **Sycosis sous-narinaire.** One affecting the hair follicles of the upper lip, secondary to a sycotic blepharitis, the infection spreading via the nasolacrimal duct to the nose. **Sycosis staphylogenes.** Sycosis caused by staphylococci. **Sycosis tarsi.** Blepharitis. **Sycosis vulgaris.** Sycosis, usually of the beard or moustache areas. [Gk *sykon* fig, *-osis* condition.]

Sydenham, Thomas (b. 1624). English physician.

Sydenham's chorea. Acute chorea, ordinary chorea, a disease chiefly affecting children and characterized by irregular involuntary movements of the limbs and face, commonest between the ages of 5 and 15 years and occurring in females more frequently than in males. It is often associated with signs of acute endocarditis and with symptoms or history of rheumatism. Some emotional instability may be exhibited, even actual mania.

Sydenham gag. A type of incisor gag.

syllabic utterance (sil·**ab**·ik **ut**·er·ans). Scanning speech; slow staccato speech. [Gk *syllabe* syllable, AS *ut* out.]

syllabize (**sil**·ab·ize). To split words into syllables when speaking.

syllable stumbling (**sil**·abl **stum**·bling). Dysphasia, in which the enunciation of certain syllables causes difficulty resulting in stuttering; a symptom of dementia paralytica. [Gk *syllabe.*]

syllepsiology (sil·ep·se·**ol**'·o·je). That branch of physiology concerned with conception and pregnancy. [Gk *syllepsis* conception, *logos* science.]

syllepsis (sil·**ep**·sis). Conception or fertilization of the ovum. [Gk.]

sylvatic (sil·**vat**·ik). Sylvan, relating to woods and forests. **Sylvatic plague.** *See* PLAGUE. [L *sylva* woodland.]

sylvestrine (sil·**ves**·treen). A terpene occurring in Swedish and Russian oil of turpentine.

sylviduct (**sil**·ve·dukt). Sylvius' aqueduct.

Sylvius (de le Boë), Franciscus (b. 1614). Dutch anatomist.

Sylvius' angle. The angle between the posterior ramus of the lateral cerebral sulcus, and a line perpendicular to the upper margin of the cerebral hemisphere.

Sylvius' aqueduct. The aqueduct of the mid-brain.

Sylvius' artery, Sylvian artery. The middle cerebral artery.

Sylvius' fissure or sulcus, Sylvian sulcus. The lateral sulcus of the cerebral hemisphere.

muscle of Sylvius. The flexor digitorum accessorius muscle.

Sylvius' ventricle. The cavity of the septum lucidum.

symballophone (sim·**bal**·o·fone). A special form of stethoscope with 2 chestpieces; it enables one to compare and localize sounds. [Gk *syn, ballein* to throw, *phone* sound.]

symbion, symbiont (**sim**·bi·on, **sim**·bi·ont). Any organism existing in symbiosis with another. [Gk *syn, bios* life.]

symbiosis (sim·bi·**o**·sis). The intimate association of 2 organisms of different species; in the usual, more restricted sense, to their mutual advantage, an advantage which may be so important that one could not live without the other; commensalism, mutualism. In the widest sense it also includes parasitism. **Antagonistic symbiosis, Antipathetic symbiosis.** Parasitism. **Conjunctive symbiosis.** Symbiosis with some bodily union. **Constructive symbiosis.** A symbiosis that assists the metabolism of one of the symbions. **Disjunctive symbiosis.** Symbiosis without bodily union. [Gk *syn, bios* life.]

symbiote (**sim**·bi·ote). A symbion.

symbiotic (sim·bi·**ot**·ik). 1. Characterized by symbiosis; concerned with symbiosis. 2. Existing in symbiosis.

symblepharon (sim·**blef**·ar·on). Adhesion of the eyelid to the eyeball which may be congential, or the result of disease or injury. The adhesion may affect only the anterior part of one lid, the posterior part, or involve the whole or both. [Gk *syn, blepharon* eyelid.]

symblepharopterygium (sim·**blef**·ar·o·ter·**ij**'·e·um). Pterygium occurring in association with symblepharon. Also applied to cases of symblepharon in which the adhesion between the eyelid and the eyeball resembles a pterygium.

symblepharosis (sim·**blef**·ar·**o**'·sis). A condition marked by adhesion of the eyelids to the eyeball or to one another. [Gk *syn, blepharon* eyelid, *-osis*, condition.]

symbol (**sim**·bol). 1. Any letter, character or sign, recognized as standing for any concept or attribute. 2. In chemistry, a capital letter (e.g. S, sulphur) or abbreviation (e.g. Na, *natrium* sodium) used to represent an atom of an element; or a similar abbreviation representing a group of atoms (e.g. Me, methyl, CH_3). The symbol is often used in the literature as a shorthand for the element concerned. 3. In psycho-analysis, something which represents and stands for something else in the unconscious mind. **Isotopic symbols.** Numbers placed conventionally in relation to the chemical symbol of the element. At the upper left of the symbol is the mass number of the atom; at the lower left is the nuclear charge of the atom; at the lower right is the number of atoms in a molecule. The upper right position is reserved for symbols indicating the ionic state. Thus, the commonest isotope of hydrogen is ${}^{1}_{1}H$, and if this is part of a molecule of water it is ${}^{1}_{1}H_2O$. **Phallic symbol.** Something which represents, in disguise, the male organ of generation. [Gk *symbolon* sign.]

symbolia (sim·**bo**·le·ah). The capacity to perceive and understand the shape and nature of external objects by touch. [see prec.]

symbolism (**sim**·bol·izm). 1. The representation of something by a sign standing for it. 2. The mechanism by which complexes repressed into the unconscious mind evade the censorship and are expressed symbolically in the conscious mind (psycho-analysis). 3. The study of the influence of language on thought. [Gk *symbolon* sign.]

symbolization (**sim**·bol·i·**za**'·shun). The act of representation by a symbol.

symbrachydactylia (sim·**brak**·e·dak·**til**'·e·ah). Webbing of the fingers or toes with shortening of the digits. [Gk *syn, brachys* short, *daktylos* finger or toe.]

Syme, James (b. 1799). Edinburgh surgeon.

Syme's amputation. Amputation at the ankle joint; the malleoli are sawn off and the stump is covered by a skin flap from the heel.

Syme's operation. 1. Syme's amputation. 2. Median translingual pharyngotomy. 3. A method of external urethrotomy for passable stricture of the urethra, using a special staff.

Symington, Johnson (b. 1851). Scottish surgeon in Belfast.

Symington's anococcygeal body. The anococcygeal body; a mass of muscular and fibrous tissue, behind the anal canal, in front of the coccyx.

symmelia (sim·e·le·ah). A condition in which the legs and feet are fused. [Gk *syn, melos* limb.]

symmelic (sim·el·ik). Having the form of a symmelus.

symmelus (sim·el·us). A fetal monstrosity in which there is defective development of the pelvis and partial or complete fusion of the feet and legs. [Gk *syn, melos* limb.]

Symmers, Douglas (b. 1879). New York pathologist.

Brill–Symmers disease. Giant follicular reticulosis. *See* RETICULOSIS.

Brown–Symmers disease. Serous encephalitis, a rapidly fatal encephalitis of children below the age of 7 years.

symmetric, symmetrical (sim·et·rik, sim·et·rik·al). Having symmetry.

symmetromania (sim·et·ro·ma'·ne·ah). A manic compulsion to make symmetrical movements, such as moving both arms when the movement of only one is called for.

symmetry (sim·et·re). 1. The equality of parts on each side of an imaginary dividing line or point. 2. Anatomically, the correspondence of opposite parts of the body. 3. Chemically, the arrangement of atoms within a molecule so that similar groups are disposed equally about a central atom or ring. 4. In crystals, the regularity displayed by the positions of similar faces or edges. 5. The hypothesis that constitutional disease may attack either side of the body equally. **Bilateral symmetry.** Symmetry of the two halves of an organism. [Gk *syn, metron* measure.]

symparalysis (sim·par·al·is·is). Conjugate paralysis; the loss of synkinetic movements, especially those of the eyes. [Gk *syn*, paralysis.]

sympathectomy (sim·path·ek·to·me). The operation for the removal of the dorsal and lumbar sympathetic trunk or parts thereof. **Cervical sympathectomy.** Removal of the cervical and/or stellate ganglia. **Chemical sympathectomy, Medical sympathectomy.** Administration of drugs which completely or partially block conduction via the sympathetic ganglia. **Periarterial sympathectomy.** The operation for stripping the sympathetic plexus from around main arteries. **Postganglionic sympathectomy, Preganglionic sympathectomy.** Sympathectomy where the excision is done either distal or proximal to sympathetic ganglia. [sympathetic, Gk *ektome* excision.]

sympatheoneuritis (sim·path·e·o·newr·i'·tis). Sympathiconeuritis.

sympathesis (sim·path·e·sis). Those sympathies and synergies which act together to the detriment of the body. [Gk *sympathein* to feel with.]

sympathetectomy (sim·path·et·ek'·to·me). Sympathectomy.

sympathetic (sim·path·et·ik). 1. Relating to or displaying sympathy. 2. Relating to the autonomic nervous system. **Sympathetic ganglia, Sympathetic nerve.** *See* SYSTEM, SYMPATHETIC. **Sympathetic plexus.** *See* PLEXUS. **Sympathetic system.** *See* SYSTEM. [Gk *sympathein* to feel with.]

sympatheticalgia (sim·path·et·ik·al'·je·ah). Pain arising from the cervical ganglia of the sympathetic nervous system. [sympathetic, Gk *algos* pain.]

sympatheticectomy (sim·path·et·is·ek'·to·me). Sympathectomy.

sympatheticism (sim·path·et·is·ism). Sympathism.

sympatheticoma (sim·path·et·ik·o'·mah). Sympathoma.

sympatheticomimetic (sim·path·et·ik·o·mim·et'·ik). Producing an effect similar to that obtained by stimulation of the sympathetic nervous system. [sympathetic, Gk *mimesis* imitation.]

sympatheticoparalytic (sim·path·et·ik·o·par·al·it'·ik). Arising out of paralysis of the sympathetic nervous system.

sympatheticotonia (sim·path·et·ik·o·to'·ne·ah). Sympathicotonia.

sympatheticotonic (sim·path·et·ik·o·ton'·ik). Sympathicotonic.

sympatheticotonus (sim·path·et·ik·o·to'·nus). Sympathicotonia.

sympathetoblast (sim·path·et·o·blast). An embryonic cell which can develop into a sympathetic neurone. [sympathetic, Gk *blastos* germ.]

sympathicectomy (sim·path·is·ek'·to·me). Sympathectomy.

sympathicoblast (sim·path·ik·o·blast). Sympathetoblast.

sympathicoblastoma (sim·path·ik·o·blas·to'·mah). An innocent or malignant tumour derived from sympathetic ganglia, terminal sympathetic filaments, and the chromaffin tissue of the suprarenal gland [sympathetic, blastoma.]

sympathicodiaphtheresis (sim·path·ik·o·di·af·the·re'·sis). Doppler's operation. [sympathetic, Gk *diaphtheirein* to destroy.]

sympathicogonioma (sim·path·ik·o·go·ne·o'·mah). A more differentiated variety of sympathicoblastoma. [sympathetic, gonioma.]

sympathicolytic (sim·path·ik·o·lit'·ik). 1. Inimical to sympathetic nerve fibres. 2. Exerting an inhibitory effect on nerve impulses in the sympathetic system. [sympathetic, Gk *lysein* to loosen.]

sympathicomimetic (sim·path·ik·o·mim·et'·ik). Sympathomimetic.

sympathiconeuritis (sim·path·ik·o·newr·i'·tis). Inflammation of any of the nerves of the sympathetic system. [sympathetic, Gk *neuron* nerve, *-itis* inflammation.]

sympathicopathy (sim·path·ik·op'·ath·e). Any morbid condition resulting from disturbance of the sympathetic nervous system. [sympathetic, Gk *pathos* disease.]

sympathicotonia (sim·path·ik·o·to'·ne·ah). A state produced by stimulation of the autonomic (sympathetic) system. [sympathetic, Gk *tonos* tension.]

sympathicotonic (sim·path·ik·o·ton'·ik). Characterized by sympathicotonia.

sympathicotonus (sim·path·ik·o·to'·nus). Sympathicotonia.

sympathicotripsy (sim·path·ik·o·trip'·se). Operative crushing of a sympathetic ganglion. [sympathetic, Gk *tribein* to crush.]

sympathicotrope (sim·path·ik·o·trope). Anything which is sympathicotropic.

sympathicotropic (sim·path·ik·o·trop'·ik). Possessing a particular affinity for the sympathetic nervous system. [sympathetic, Gk *trepein* to turn.]

sympathin (sim·path·in). A name formerly given to noradrenaline.

sympathism (sim·path·izm). Suggestibility; susceptibility to hypnotic suggestion. [Gk *sympatheia* sympathy.]

sympathoblast (sim·path·o·blast). Sympathetoblast.

sympathoblastoma (sim·path·o·blas·to'·mah). Sympathicoblastoma.

sympathochromaffin (sim·path·o·kro·maf'·in). Referring to certain postganglionic neurones of the sympathetic nervous system which give a chromaffin reaction.

sympathoglioblastoma (sim·path·o·gli·o·blas·to'·mah). A mixed variety of sympathicoblastoma, in which fibrils and neuroglial cells are numerous. [sympathetic, neuroglia, blastoma.]

sympathogonia (sim·path·o·go'·ne·ah). Embryonic cells which are transformed into the nerves of the sympathetic system. [sympathetic, Gk *gonos* seed.]

sympathogonioma (sim·path·o·gon·e·o'·mah). A malignant tumour formed of sympathogonia. **Sympathogonioma purum.** A sympathogonioma composed wholly of sympathetic cells. **Sympathogonioma tenuifibrillare.** A tumour composed of sympathetic cells and fibres. [sympathogonia, Gk *-oma* tumour.]

sympatholytic (sim·path·o·lit'·ik). Sympathicolytic.

sympathoma (sim·path·o·mah). A tumour in which the tissue is similar to that comprising the sympathetic nervous system. [sympathetic, Gk *-oma* tumour.]

sympathomimetic (sim·path·o·mim·et'·ik). Adrenergic; producing an effect similar to that obtained by stimulation of the sympathetic nervous system. [sympathetic, Gk *mimesis* imitation.]

sympathy (**sim**·path·e). 1. The pathological change produced in an organ, part or structure, by the occurrence of disease in another and perhaps distant part. 2. The relationship between mind and body which results in the one being influenced by the other. 3. The influence exercised by one person over another, as seen in hypnotism. 4. Mental contagion; the spread of hysterical symptoms from one person to another. [Gk *sympathein* to feel with.]

sympectothiene, sympectothion (sim·pek·to·**thi**·een, sim·pek·to·**thi**·on). Former names for thioneine. [Gk *syn, pexis* a fixation, *theion* sulphur.]

symperitoneal (**sim**·per·it·o·**ne**′·al). Pertaining to the operation in which portions of the peritoneum are joined together, as in the Talma–Morison operation. [Gk *syn, peritoneum.*]

sympexia, sympexion, sympexis (sim·**pex**·e·ah, sim·**pex**·e·on, sim·**pex**·is). 1. The disposition of erythrocytes under the influence of surface tension. 2. The formation of concretions in certain glands such as the prostate, seminal vesicles, lymphatics and thyroid. [Gk *syn, pexis* fixation.]

symphalangia, symphalangism (sim·fal·**an**·je·ah, sim·fal·**an**·jizm). 1. Ankylosis of the joints of neighbouring phalanges. 2. Syndactylism, a condition in which 2 or more fingers or toes are fused. [Gk *syn, phalagx* finger.]

symphorol (**sim**·for·ol). Salts of caffeine sulphonic acid used as diuretics. **Symphorol lithium, Symphorol L.** Lithium caffeine sulphonate $C_8H_9N_4O_2SO_2OLi$, a diuretic used in gout and rheumatism. **Symphorol N (sodium).** A compound analogous to the lithium derivative and also used as a diuretic. **Symphorol strontium.** Strontium caffeine sulphonate, a diuretic.

symphyocephalus (**sim**·fe·o·**kef**′·al·us). Syncephalus. [Gk *symphyes* growing together, *kephale* head.]

symphyogenetic (**sim**·fe·o·jen·**et**′·ik). Relating to the associated influence of heredity and environment upon the form and function of an organism. [Gk *symphyes* growing together, *genein* to produce.]

symphyseal (sim·**fiz**·e·al). Relating to a symphysis. **Symphyseal surface.** *See* PUBIS.

symphyseorrhapy (**sim**·fiz·e·**or**′·af·e). Symphysiorrhaphy.

symphyseotome (sim·**fiz**·e·o·tome). An instrument employed in symphyseotomy.

symphyseotomy (**sim**·fiz·e·**ot**′·o·me). The enlargement of the pelvic diameter by dividing the fibrocartilage of the pubic symphysis. [symphysis, Gk *temnein* to cut.]

symphysial (sim·**fiz**·e·al). Symphyseal.

symphysic (sim·**fiz**·ik). Relating to a symphysis, or the pathological fusion of neighbouring parts.

symphysiectomy (**sim**·fiz·e·**ek**′·to·me). Removal of a portion of the pubic symphysis to avoid difficulty at a future delivery. [symphysis, Gk *ektome* excision.]

symphysiolysis (**sim**·fiz·e·**ol**′·is·is). The parting or slipping of a symphysis, particularly the pubic symphysis. [symphysis, Gk *lysis* a loosing.]

symphysion (sim·**fiz**·e·on). A craniometric point on the lower jaw; the middle of the anterior border of the alveolar process. [Gk *symphysis* a growing together.]

symphysiorrhaphy (**sim**·fiz·e·**or**′·af·e). The suturing of the parts of a separated symphysis. [symphysis, Gk *raphe* suture.]

symphysiotome (sim·**fiz**·e·o·tome). Symphysectome.

symphysiotomy (**sim**·fiz·e·**ot**′·o·me). Symphyseotomy.

symphysis (**sim**·fis·is). A secondary cartilaginous joint in which the opposed surfaces of the bones are covered by thin layers of hyaline cartilage between which they are connected by fibrocartilage. Symphyseal joints are found between the bodies of the vertebrae, between the two pubic bones and between the manubrium and the body of the sternum. **Cardiac symphysis.** Adhesion of the pericardia to one another and to the mediastinum. **Symphysis mandibulae, Symphysis menti.** The junction between the two halves of the body of the mandible, forming the prominence of the chin; it is at the beginning fibrous, but is ossified during the first year after birth. **Pubic symphysis [symphysis pubica (NA)].** The symphysis between the pubic bones. [Gk a growing together.]

symphysodactylia (**sim**·fiz·o·dak·**til**′·e·ah). Syndactylism. [symphysis, *daktylos* finger or toe.]

symphysopsia (sim·fiz·**op**·se·ah). A congenital malformation in which the conceptus has only one eye. [symphysis, Gk *ops* eye.]

symphysoskelia (**sim**·fiz·o·**ske**′·le·ah). A condition in which there is partial or complete fusion of the lower limbs. [symphysis, Gk *skelos* leg.]

Symphytum (**sim**·fit·um). A genus of boraginaceous plants, including *Symphytum officinale* Linn., comfrey; used in homoeopathy. [Gk *syn, phyton* plant.]

symplasm (**sim**·plazm). A living, nucleated tissue without apparent cellular structure. [Gk *syn, plasma* something formed.]

symplasmatic (sim·plaz·**mat**·ik). Characterized by the fusion of the protoplasmic components. [see prec.]

symplast (**sim**·plast). Symplasm.

symplex (**sim**·plex). Any chemical compound, usually of high molecular weight, that has residual valencies which enable it to form loose combinations, as in the case of haemoglobin. [Gk *syn, plakein* to twine.]

Symplocarpus foetidus (sim·plo·**kar**·pus **fe**·tid·us). Skunkweed, meadow cabbage; the plant *Dracontium foetidum* (family Araceae). The dried root is known as *skunk cabbage:* used in homoeopathy. [Gk *symplokos* twined, *karpos* fruit, L stinking.]

Symplocos (**sim**·plo·kos). A genus of plants of the family Styraceae. **Symplocos alstonia.** A species of South America; its leaves are used as maté. **Symplocos platyphylla.** Sweetleaf, a species of South America. **Symplocos racemosa.** An East Indian tree the root of which is mildly astringent. **Symplocos tinctoria.** A species indigenous to South Carolina, containing a yellow dye. [Gk *symplokos* twined.]

sympodia (sim·**po**·de·ah). The fusion of both feet into one. [Gk *syn, pous* foot.]

symptom (**simp**·tom). The consciousness of a disturbance in a bodily function; the subjective feeling that there is something wrong in the working of the body and of which the patient complains, e.g. shortness of breath, pain, fatigue, palpitation, etc. The symptom may or may not be accompanied by observable signs. **Abstinence symptom.** Withdrawal symptom (see below). **Accessory symptom, Accidental symptom, Assident symptom.** One which is not essential or pathognomonic. **Cardinal symptoms.** Cardinal signs. *See* SIGN. **Characteristic symptom.** An effect which is peculiar to the administration of a drug in homoeopathic practice. **Concomitant symptom.** One which accompanies the main symptoms, but is not an essential one. **Consecutive symptom.** A symptom which follows, and may be the result of another. **Constitutional symptom.** One which affects the whole body and is not merely local. **Deficiency symptom.** One due to a deficiency of an essential substance in the food, such as a vitamin or mineral salt, or of a chemical substance manufactured in the body, such as a hormone. **Delayed symptom.** One whose manifestation is delayed for an appreciable time after the cause, such as delayed shock. **Direct symptom.** One that can be attributed to a definite cause. **Dissociation symptom.** Loss of the ability to appreciate painful and thermal stimuli, with retention of touch appreciation, tactile discrimination and position sense. It is seen particularly in syringomyelia, but also in lesions of the spinothalamic tract and in centrally situated cord lesions of whatever type. **Drug symptom.** Any effect exhibited by a patient on whom a drug is being "proved" in homoeopathic practice. **Endothelial symptom.** Rumpel-Leede phenomenon. **Equivocal symptom.** A doubtful symptom or one which can be attributed to more than one cause. **General symptom.** Constitutional symptom (see above). **Guiding symptom.** A symptom which is characteristic of a certain disorder and guides towards diagnosis. **Indirect symptom.** One that cannot be attributed directly to a definite cause. **Induced symptom.** One that is produced by an action of the observer, e.g. pain on pressure. **Keynote symptom.** An effect which is peculiar to the administration of a drug in homoeopathic practice. **Labyrinthine symptom.** Anything untoward related to the labyrinth or internal ear. **Local symptom.** One which is localized to a part and not general. **Localizing symptom.** One which assists in localizing the lesion. **Negatively pathognomonic symptom.** A symptom which is constantly absent in a certain condition, and if present would be against the diagnosis of this particular condition. **Neighbourhood symptom.** A symptom which is referred to a part but is caused by a lesion in a neighbouring part. **Nostril symptom.** A movement of the ala of the nose, recognized in some forms of nasal obstruction and in the oxygen want of laryngeal obstruction or chest infection. **Objective symptom.** A symptom accompanied by signs from which the existence of the symptom can be deduced. **Oesophagosalivary symptom.** Excessive salivation in cancer of the oesophagus. **Passive symptom.** Static symptom (see below). **Pathogenic symptom.** Drug symptom (see above). **Precursory symptom, Premonitory symptom.** An early symptom giving warning of further developments. **Presenting symptom.** The symptom of which the patient complains, and which causes him to seek medical advice. **Pressure symptom.** Any manifestation of pressure upon the brain or spinal cord. This term may include pain, convulsions, hyperaesthesia, hypo-aesthesia, hypo-algesia, flaccid or spastic paralysis, and many other symptoms or signs. **Rational symptom.** Subjective symptom (see below). **Reflex symptom.** One which is caused reflexly in a part remote from the lesion. **Signal symptom.** A premonitory symptom, especially one such as an aura which gives warning of an approaching epileptic attack. **Static symptom.** A quiet stationary symptom. **Subjective symptom.** One appreciated by the patient only; all symptoms are, strictly speaking, subjective. **Sympathetic symptom.** One referred to a part, when the actual lesion is in a different part. **Symptom turpitudinis.** Nymphomania. **Withdrawal symptom.** Features, often severe, of withdrawal from addiction habits; marked by a sensation of cold, feeling of unease, yawning, rhinorrhoea, laboured respirations, goose flesh, tremors, tachycardia, cramps in the legs, perspiration and diarrhoea. [Gk *symptoma* that which happens.]

See also: ANTON, BÉHIER, BERNHARDT (M.), BUERGER, CHARCOT, COLLIVER, EPSTEIN (ALOIS), GOWERS, GUÉNEAU DE MUSSY, HARDY, JONAS (S.), KUSSMAUL, MAGNAN, MARIE, MURAT, NOTHNAGEL, OEHLER, REMAK (E. J.), SÉGUIN, SKLOWSKY, TRUNECEK, WARTENBERG.

symptom complex (simp·tom **kom**·plex). A syndrome; the symptoms of a particular disease taken as a whole. [symptom, complex.]

See also: AVELLIS, BERNHARDT (M.), DANA, ESCHERICH, FRIEDMANN (M.), PUTNAM, ROTH (V. K.).

symptomatic (simp·to·**mat**·ik). 1. Having the characteristics of a symptom. 2. Indicating a specific disease. 3. Directed towards a symptom as in symptomatic treatment.

symptomatology (simp·to·mat·**ol**′·o·je). 1. The science of symptoms, being the study of the symptoms of disease. 2. The symptoms of any particular disease regarded as a whole. [symptom, Gk *logos* science.]

symptomatolytic (simp·to·mat·o·**lit**′·ik). Eliminating symptoms. [symptom, Gk *lysein* to loosen.]

symptosis (simp·**to**·sis). A progressive emaciation of the body as a whole or in part; atrophy, marasmus. [Gk *syn, ptosis* a falling.]

sympus (**sim**·pus). A fetal monster with fused lower limbs. **Sympus apus.** A sirenomelus, having only toes. **Sympus dipus.** A sympus with 2 more or less distinct feet. **Sympus monopus.** A sympus with only 1 foot. [Gk *syn, pous* foot.]

syn-. Prefix, from the Greek preposition *syn,* meaning *together.*

synactosis (sin·ak·**to**·sis). Defective development due to the fusion of parts. [Gk *synaktos* fused, *-osis* condition.]

synadelphus (sin·ad·**el**·fus). A fetal monster with 1 head and trunk but possessing 4 arms and 4 legs. [Gk *syn, adelphos* brother.]

synaesthesia (sin·es·**the**·ze·ah). 1. A condition in which a certain stimulus produces not only the normal sensation, but also a secondary one of dissimilar character. Thus, the perception of a sound may excite a sensation of colour. Sometimes the secondary response replaces the normal one completely. 2. A sensation experienced in one part, due to the application of a stimulus to another part. **Synaesthesia algica.** Painful synaesthesia, sensory disturbance caused by neuritis. [Gk *syn, aisthesis* sensation.]

synaesthesialgia (sin·es·the·ze·**al**′·je·ah). 1. A condition in which pain is experienced on the affected side with stimulation, although there is no sensation felt on the healthy side, or if any, a pleasurable one. 2. Synaesthesia resulting from neuritis. [Gk *syn, aisthesis* sensation, *algos* pain.]

synalgia (sin·**al**·je·ah). Referred pain; the experience of pain in a point remote from the lesion causing the pain. [Gk *syn, algos* pain.]

synalgic (sin·**al**·jik). Having the characteristics of synalgia.

synanastomosis (sin·an·as·to·**mo**′·sis). Anastomosis of several veins or arteries. [Gk *syn,* anastomosis.]

synanche (**sin**·an·ke). Cynanche; a sore throat that obstructs breathing. [Gk *syn, anchein* to choke.]

synanthem, synanthema (sin·**an**·them, sin·an·**the**·mah). An eruption of papules on the skin, consisting of several kinds together. [Gk *syn, anthein* to bloom.]

synanthrin (sin·**an**·thrin). Inulin.

synanthrose (sin·**an**·throze). Laevulin, $(C_6H_{10}O_5)_n$. A carbohydrate isomeric with inulin, occurring in the rhizomes of *Helianthus tuberosus.*

synaphymenitis (sin·**ap**·hi·men·**i**′·tis). Conjunctivitis. [Gk *synaptein* to join, *hymen* membrane, *-itis* inflammation.]

synapse (**sin**·aps). The microscopic area of proximity between 2 neurones; i.e. between axon and dendrite or axon and cell body. [Gk *synaptein* to join.]

synapsis (sin·**ap**·sis). 1. Synapse. 2. At meiosis, the pairing of homologous chromosomes. [Gk *synaptein* to join.]

synaptase (sin·**ap**·taze). Emulsin.

synaptene (sin·**ap**·teen). That stage of meiosis in which the homologous chromosomes come together in pairs. [Gk *synaptein* to join.]

synaptic (sin·**ap**·tik). Pertaining to, or of the nature of a synapse.

synaptolemma (sin·**ap**·to·**lem**′·ah). The membrane separating the interior of an axon from the interior of a nerve cell body or dendrite at a synapse. [Gk *synaptein* to join, *lemma* sheath.]

synapton (sin·**ap**·ton). Synaptinemal complex. *See* COMPLEX.

synarthrodia (sin·ar·**thro**·de·ah). Synarthrosis.

synarthrodial (sin·ar·**thro**·de·al). Having the characteristics of synarthrosis.

synarthrophysis (sin·ar·thro·**fi**′·sis). 1. Progressive ankylosis of the joints. 2. The process of ankylosis. [Gk *syn, arthrodia* joint, *physis* growth.]

synarthrosis (sin·ar·**thro**·sis). A fixed joint; a joining of 2 bones immovably without intervening tissue. [Gk *syn, arthrosis* joining.]

synathresis, synathroisis (sin·ath·**re**·sis, sin·ath·**roi**·sis). Congestion or localized hyperaemia. [Gk *syn* together, *athroisis* collection.]

syncaine (**sin**·kane). Procaine hydrochloride, a synthetic local anaesthetic resembling cocaine in action.

syncanthus (sin·**kan**·thus). The formation of pathological adhesions between the eyeball and the surrounding orbital structures. [Gk *syn,* canthus.]

syncephalus (sin·**kef**·al·us). A fetal twin monster having a fused head and 2 bodies. **Syncephalus assymetros.** Iniops. [Gk *syn, kephale* head.]

syncephaly (sin·**kef**·al·e). In teratism, the state in which the 2 heads are fused into one. [see prec.]

syncheilia (sin·**ki**·le·ah). Atresia of the mouth. [Gk *syn, cheilos* lip.]

syncheiria (sin·**ki**·re·ah). A sensory disorder in which a stimulus applied to one side of the body is felt on both sides. [Gk *syn, cheir* hand.]

synchesis (**sin**·ke·sis). Synchysis.

syncholia (sin·**ko**·le·ah). The secretion of a substance in the bile not normally found there and derived from some external source. [Gk *syn, chole* bile.]

synchondroseotomy (sin·kon·dro·se·**ot**′·o·me). Synchondrotomy.

synchondrosis (sin·kon·**dro**·sis). A cartilaginous joint formed when 2 bones are connected by cartilage; such joints may be primary or secondary. In a primary joint the bones are connected by hyaline cartilage and this type of connection is usually temporary, as between the epiphyses and diaphyses of long bones, or between the bodies of the sphenoid and occipital bones. A secondary cartilaginous joint is more complex and is called a *symphysis;* it is permanent throughout life. **Intra-occipital synchondrosis, anterior [synchondrosis intra-occipitalis anterior** (NA)]. The primary cartilaginous joints between the basilar and lateral (condylar) parts of the occipital bone. **Intra-occipital synchondrosis, posterior [synchondrosis intra-occipitalis posterior** (NA)]. The primary cartilaginous joint between the squamous and the lateral (condylar) parts of the occipital bone. **Sternal synchondrosis.** Manubriosternal joint. *See* JOINT. [Gk *syn, chondros* cartilage.]

synchondrotomy (sin·kon·**drot**·o·me). A surgical operation dividing a synchondrosis. [Gk *syn, chondros* cartilage, *temnein* to cut.]

synchronia (sin·**kro**·ne·ah). 1. Synchronism. 2. The development or functioning of tissues or organs either simultaneously or at the normal time. [see foll.]

synchronism (sin·kron·izm). Occurring at the same time. [Gk *synchronos* simultaneous.]

synchronous (**sin**·kron·us). Occurring simultaneously. [see prec.]

synchysis (**sin**·kis·is). Liquefaction of the vitreous body. **Synchysis scintillans.** The presence of glittering crystals in liquefied vitreous, often consisting of cholesterol, and due to long-standing degenerative changes. [Gk mixing together.]

syncleisis (sin·**kli**·sis). Occlusion. [Gk *syn, kleisis* a closing.]

synclinal (sin·**kli**·nal). Inclined in the same direction towards a common point. [Gk *syn, klinein* to lean.]

synclisis (**sin**·klis·is). Synclitism.

synclitic (sin·**klit**·ik). Characterized by synclitism.

synclitism (**sin**·klit·izm). 1. Parallelism; equal inclination. 2. The situation in which the planes of the fetal head and the pelvis are parallel. [Gk *syn, klinein* to lean.]

synclonus (**sin**·klo·nus). 1. Muscular tremor; the clonic contraction of several muscles simultaneously. 2. Any disease of which muscular tremor is a symptom, e.g. chorea. **Synclonus ballismus.** Paralysis agitans. **Synclonus beriberica.** Beriberi. [Gk *syn, klonos* tumult.]

syncoelom (sin·se·lom). The cavities surrounding the viscera regarded as a unit, comprising the peritoneum, pleurae, pericardial cavity and the tunica vaginalis testis. [Gk *syn,* coelom.]

syncopal (**sin**·ko·pal). Relating to or resembling syncope,

syncope (**sin**·ko·pe). Transient loss of consciousness due to inadequate cerebral blood flow. **Syncope anginosa.** Syncope occurring with anginal (cardiac ischaemic) pain. Any of the conditions given below under cardiac syncope may produce cardiac pain owing to reduced coronary-artery flow. **Cardiac syncope.** Syncope due to a sudden fall in cardiac output such as occurs in cardiac standstill, ventricular asystole, ventricular tachycardia or fibrillation, massive pulmonary embolus or cardiac infarction, ball-valve thrombus of the left auricle, aortic stenosis and acute haemopericardium causing cardiac compression. It may occur on effort in patients who cannot increase their cardiac output sufficiently to meet the demands of exercise, e.g. in severe mitral stenosis. **Carotid syncope.** Carotid sinus syndrome. **Cerebral syncope.** Syncope due to local changes in the cerebral vascular system which reduce the cerebral blood flow, or to anoxia. The former may occur when there is a lack of carbon dioxide resulting from prolonged hyperpnoea; the latter when there is insufficient oxygen in the blood reaching the brain, as with impairment of oxygenation in the lungs, or right to left intracardiac shunt in cyanotic congenital heart disease. **Cough syncope.** Fainting occurring in relation to a bout of coughing which raises intrathoracic pressure sufficiently to impede venous return (as in the *Valsalva manoeuvre*) so leading to cerebral anoxia. **Laryngeal syncope.** Cough syncope (see above). **Local syncope.** Acute ischaemia leading to loss of sensation in a limb or part of a limb. **Micturition syncope.** Syncope occurring in middle-aged men after micturating in the upright posture after rising from a warm bed. **Tussive syncope.** Laryngeal syncope (see above). **Vasomotor syncope, Vasovagal syncope.** Syncope due to a sudden fall in blood pressure as a result of failure of the peripheral resistance. The commonest cause is the psychogenic "faint"; other causes include haemorrhage, extreme pain, perforated hollow viscus, agents which lower central venous pressure rapidly or cause peripheral vasodilatation, prolonged standing erect (orthostatic hypotension) and sensitive carotid sinus. The symptoms and signs depend upon stimulation of the vagus producing vasodilatation and slowing of the heart. [Gk fainting.]

syncopic (sin·**kop**·ik). The blue pigment produced by *Pseudomonas syncyanea.*

syncytial (sin·**sit**·e·al). Of the nature of a syncytium.

syncytiolysin (**sin**·sit·e·**ol**′·is·in). A cytolysin produced by injections of an emulsion of placental tissue. [syncytium, Gk *lysein* to loosen.]

syncytioma (**sin**·sit·e·**o**′·mah). A tumour composed of syncytial tissue, usually uterine and highly malignant. **Syncytioma malignum.** Chorionic carcinoma. [syncytium, Gk *-oma* tumour.]

syncytiotrophoblast (sin·**sit**·e·o·**tro**′·fo·blast). The outer syncytial layer of the chorionic epithelium. [syncytium, trophoblast.]

syncytium (sin·**sit**·e·um). 1. A tissue composed of a mass of nucleated protoplasm without cell boundaries, e.g. the outer layer of the trophoblast of a placenta. 2. A mass of cells united by protoplasmic bridges. [Gk *syn, kytos* cell.]

syncytoid (**sin**·sit·oid). Of the nature of a syncytium. [syncytium, Gk *eidos* form.]

syndactyl, syndactyle (sin·**dak**·til, sin·**dak**·tile). Syndactylous; having fingers or toes partially or completely fused. [Gk *syn, daktylos* finger or toe.]

syndactylia, syndactylism (sin·dak·**til**·e·ah, sin·**dak**·til·izm). A condition in which 2 or more fingers or toes are fused. [see prec.]

syndactylous (sin·**dak**·til·us). Syndactyl.

syndactylus (sin·**dak**·til·us). A person with webbed fingers or toes. [Gk *syn, daktylos* finger or toe.]

syndactyly (sin·**dak**·til·e). Syndactylia.

syndectomy (sin·**dek**·to·me). An operation usually performed for the relief of trachomatous pannus, in which a ring of conjunctiva surrounding the cornea is excised. [Gk *syn, dein* to bind, *ektome* excision.]

syndelphus (sin·**del**·fus). Synadelphus.

syndesis (**sin**·de·sis). 1. Arthrodesis. 2. Synapse. [Gk *syn, dein* to bind.]

syndesmectomy (sin·des·**mek**·to·me). The operation of excising the whole part of a ligament. [Gk *syndesmos* ligament, *ektome* excision.]

syndesmectopia (**sin**·des·mek·**to**′·pe·ah). The state in which a ligament is out of place. [Gk *syndesmos* ligament, *ektopos* displaced.]

syndesmitis (sin·des·**mi**·tis). Inflammation of a ligament. [Gk *syndesmos* ligament, *-itis* inflammation.]

syndesmochorial (sin·des·mo·**kor**′·e·al). Describing a type of placenta in which the fetal villi are separated from the maternal blood vessels by a layer of maternal connective tissue, as in the sheep and the goat. [Gk *syndesmos* bond, chorion.]

syndesmodiastasis (**sin**·des·mo·di·**as**′·tas·is). Rupture of a ligament. [Gk *syndesmos* ligament, *diastasis* separation.]

syndesmology (sin·des·**mol**·o·je). The anatomical study of ligaments. [Gk *syndesmos* ligament, *logos* science.]

syndesmoma (sin·des·**mo**·mah). A tumour formed from connective tissue. [Gk *syndesmos* ligament, *-oma* tumour.]

syndesmo-odontoid (sin·**des**·mo·o·**don**′·toid). The articulation between the transverse ligament of the atlas and the odontoid process of the axis. [Gk *syndesmos* bond, odontoid.]

syndesmopexy (sin·**des**·mo·pex·e). Operative fixation of a joint by reconstruction of ligaments. [Gk *syndesmos* ligament, *pexis* a fixation.]

syndesmophyte (sin·**des**·mo·fite). A bony bridge occurring between adjacent vertebrae in ankylosing spondylitis or ankylosing vertebral hyperostosis. [Gk *syndesmos* ligament, *phyton* plant.]

syndesmoplasty (sin·des·mo·**plas**·te). Plastic repair of a ligament. [Gk *syndesmos* ligament, *plassein* to form.]

syndesmorrhaphy (sin·des·**mor**·af·e). Suture of a ligament. [Gk *syndesmos* ligament, raphe.]

syndesmosis [NA] (sin·des·**mo**·sis). A fibrous joint in which the opposing surfaces are held together by a ligament of connective tissue, such as occurs in the inferior tibiofibular joint. **Tibiofibular syndesmosis.** The tibiofibular joint. See JOINT. **Tympanostapedial syndesmosis [syndesmosis tympanostapedia (NA)].** The ring of ligamentous fibres which connects the margin of the fenestra vestibuli with the base of the stapes. [Gk *syndesmos* ligament.]

syndesmotomy (sin·des·**mot**·o·me). The operation of dividing a ligament. [Gk *syndesmos* ligament, *temnein* to cut.]

syndesmus (sin·**des**·mus). A ligament. [Gk *syndesmos.*]

syndrome (**sin**·drome, **sin**·dro·me). A distinct group of symptoms or signs which, associated together, form a characteristic clinical picture or entity. **Abdominal syndrome.** A term not now used in clinical medicine: abdominal signs or symptoms are of daily occurrence, but there is no particular combination of these which can be called a syndrome. **Absent abdominal muscle syndrome.** A rare condition particularly affecting males in which absence of muscle in the lower abdomen wall is associated with genito-urinary abnormalities. **Accelerated conduction syndrome.** An alternative name for the electrocardiographic anomaly of short P-R interval and wide QRS complex known as the *Wolff-Parkinson-White syndrome* or *pre-excitation syndrome.* The anomaly is considered to be due to conduction of impulses, not subject to delay in the atrioventricular node, through accessory pathways in the atrioventricular rings. **Acute radiation syndrome.** The collection of symptoms and signs of disease which follows within several hours to a few days the absorption by the whole body, or by a substantial part of the trunk, of a large single dose of ionizing radiation. In man the LD_{50} is probably about 500 rem to the whole body. **Adaptation syndrome.** General adaptation syndrome (see below). **Addisonian syndrome.** The syndrome of Addison's disease. **Adiposogenital syndrome.** The syndrome of obesity and genital underdevelopment. When this is due to a tumour pressing on the anterior pituitary gland, it is known as *Fröhlich's syndrome.* **Adrenocortical syndrome.** A syndrome due to overactivity of the adrenal cortex. It occurs in 2 forms, the adrenogenital syndrome (see below) and Cushing's syndrome. **Adrenogenital syndrome.** Masculinization in women, due to adrenal cortical overactivity. **Adrenosympathetic syndrome.** Paroxysmal hypertension; episodic hypertension, glycosuria, tachycardia, pallor, sweating and occasional other symptoms due to phaeochromocytoma of the adrenal medulla. **Afferent-loop syndrome.** Stasis in the afferent loop of a partial gastrectomy due to kinking of the loop at the junction with the stomach, clinically characterized by a bitter taste in the mouth and regurgitation of yellow, green or brown bile, unmixed with any food, within an hour of taking a meal. **Amnesic syndrome, Amnestic syndrome.** The clinical state in which there is failure to retain and/or recall recent events. **Amyostatic syndrome.** A rare usage for hepatolenticular degeneration; Wilson's disease. **Anginal syndrome, Anginose syndrome.** Angina pectoris. **Anorectal syndrome.** A syndrome (pruritus, perianal soreness and rectal burning and diarrhoea) that not infrequently follows tetracycline administration. It is apparently due to the overgrowth of fungi replacing the bacteria that have been eliminated by the tetracycline and it responds to yoghourt or vitamin-B complex. **Anterior cerebral artery syndrome.** The clinical features of occlusion of the anterior cerebral artery, varying according to its site. The commonest is contralateral hemiplegia with predominant involvement of the leg. **Anterior cornual syndrome.** Atrophy of muscles due to lesions of the anterior horn (anterior cornua) of the spinal cord. Poliomyelitis and motor neurone disease are prominent causes of this syndrome. **Anterior tibial syndrome.** Ischaemic necrosis of the muscles in the anterior tibial compartment of the leg associated with a lesion of the anterior tibial nerve. It occurs mainly in fit young men after severe unaccustomed exercise, but also as a result of arterial embolism. Pain, swelling and redness of the front of the leg with inability to dorsiflex the foot and toes, and sensory loss of the dorsum of the foot are the prominent symptoms. **Anterolateral syndrome.** A syndrome caused by combined lesions of the anterior horn and lateral columns of the spinal cord; the amyotrophic anterolateral-sclerosis form of motor neurone disease is the most common cause of this picture. **Antibody deficiency syndrome.** Immunological deficiency either genetically determined or secondary to other disease; it is characterized by low immunoglobulin levels and inability to produce antibody normally on antigenic challenge. **Anxiety syndrome.** Palpitation, rapid pulse, shallow breathing, sweating, trembling, dry mouth, feeling of panic, etc., accompanying the anxiety state. **Aortic arch syndromes.** Syndromes of vascular insufficiency resulting from chronic occlusion of branches of the aortic arch. Causes include atherosclerosis, collagen disease, syphilis, Takayasu's disease. **Apical syndrome.** The clinical picture associated with lesions of the upper cervical vertebrae; there may be pain in the neck and stiffness, interference with diaphragmatic movement and long tract signs. **Apoplectic syndrome.** Sudden loss of consciousness followed by signs of a massive focal cerebral lesion, usually due to a cerebrovascular accident. **Arterial pulmonary syndrome.** The condition of pulmonary hypertension; an increase in pressure in the pulmonary artery. **Asphyctic syndrome.** A combination of slow pulse, rapid breathing, cyanosis and anxiety. **Asplenia syndrome.** A complex developmental abnormality with absence of the spleen, indeterminate visceral situs and complex cardiac abnormalities, often with dextrocardia and apparent isolated laevocardia. **Auriculotemporal syndrome.** Sweating on eating, sometimes accompanied by redness, on the side of the cheek in the area of distribution of the auriculotemporal nerve. A sequel of operations on, and rarely diseases of, the parotid gland. **Basal-cell naevus syndrome.** Naevi, usually multiple, with basal-cell carcinoma histology. There are usually cysts of the jaws, bifid ribs and numerous other abnormalities. **Syndrome of basilar impression.** Young's syndrome. **Battered baby syndrome.** A condition due to maltreatment and characterized by multiple fractures in ribs and in the metaphyseal areas of long bones. **Blind-loop syndrome.** Steatorrhoea, abdominal pain and megaloblastic anaemia due to stasis in the lumen of the gut, occurring in cases of diverticula of the small intestine, gastrojejunocolic fistula or Crohn's disease. **Blue rubber-bleb naevus syndrome.** Rubbery, blue, subcutaneous, cavernous, haemangiomatous naevi, with submucous haemangiomata in the gastro-intestinal tract or haemangiomata in other organs. **Blue-sclera syndrome.** Osteogenesis imperfecta. **Bradycardia-tachycardia syndrome.** Sick-sinus syndrome (see below). **Branchial-arch syndrome.** Developmental defects of the first branchial arch, including mandibulofacial dysostosis, mandibular dysostosis, mandibulo-oculofacial dyscephaly and oculo-auriculovertebral dysplasia. **Bulbar syndrome.** Lesions in the lower part of the bulb giving rise to a homolateral hypoglossal palsy and a contralateral hemiplegia; lesions situated more superiorly give paralysis of palatal and laryngeal muscles and sometimes contralateral hemianaesthesia; also referred to as *Déjérine's syndrome.* **Capsular thrombosis syndrome.** Thrombosis of the branches of the middle cerebral artery which supply the anterior limb of the internal capsule, resulting in hemiplegia on the contralateral side of the body. **Capsulothalamic syndrome.** A syndrome resulting from damage to the internal capsule and the thalamus, usually due to cerebral haemorrhage. There is contralateral hemiplegia and hemianaesthesia (often the cruder sensations such as pain and temperature are particularly impaired) and marked emotional hyperactivity with involuntary laughing and crying. **Carcinoid syndrome.** A clinical syndrome associated with metastases from a particular type of intestinal syndrome

tumour termed carcinoid or argentaffinoma. The features include chronic facial cyanosis, flushing episodes of the face and body of several minutes' duration, palpitations and hyperperistalsis; valvular heart disease, particularly of the pulmonary valve, has been described. The syndrome appears to be associated with the production of serotonin (5-hydroxy-tryptamine) by the tumour cells. **Cardiac-asthma syndrome.** Paroxysmal dyspnoea at rest, usually at night, waking the patient from sleep, and resulting from failure of the left ventricle. It is usually precipitated by the patient sliding down into the recumbent posture, and commences with pulmonary congestion, often with bronchial spasm, and may progress to acute pulmonary oedema. **Cardiac-limb syndrome.** Autosomal dominant defects in the upper limbs and cardiac septa. **Carotid-sinus syndrome.** Undue sensitivity of the carotid sinus, stimulation of which causes vagal overaction, resulting in syncope. Attacks may occur spontaneously in rare instances, due to pressure on the sinus by a tight collar or sudden movement of the neck. Seizures may be of 4 types; syncope due to cardiac standstill, due to precipitous fall of blood pressure and bradycardia, due to acute hypotension without bradycardia, or due to a cerebral factor unassociated with bradycardia or alteration in blood pressure and probably akin to epilepsy. **Carpal-tunnel syndrome.** A syndrome caused by compression of the median nerve in the carpal tunnel; the main symptom is acroparaesthesia, usually nocturnal. **Cat-cry syndrome.** Cri-du-chat syndrome (see below). **Cat-eye syndrome.** Hypertelorism and coloboma with antimongoloid palpebral slant, perhaps due to small extra achrocentric chromosome. **Cauda equina syndrome.** Interference with the action of the bladder and anal sphincters due to abnormality of the cauda equina as from infection, neoplasm or injury. **Cavernous-sinus syndrome.** Proptosis, oedema of the conjunctiva and eyelid, together with paralysis of the oculomotor (3rd, 5th, 6th) cranial nerves, due to thrombosis of the cavernous sinus. **Centroposterior syndrome.** Dissociated anaesthesia with vasomotor and trophic changes, due to a lesion of the posterior commissure of grey matter of the spinal cord, near to the central canal; the most common disease causing this syndrome is syringomyelia. **Cerebellar syndrome.** A syndrome indicating disease of the cerebellar hemispheres or their central connections, characterized by ataxia, dysmetria, dyssynergia, hypotonia, dysarthria, inco-ordination and nystagmus. Also called *Nonne's syndrome.* **Cerebellopontine angle syndrome.** Lesions of the eighth, fifth and seventh cranial nerves with ipsilateral cerebellar ataxia, most commonly due to an acoustic neurofibroma. **Syndrome of the cerebral peduncle.** Weber's syndrome. **Cerebrohepatorenal syndrome.** Flat facies, large liver, weakness and death in early infancy. **Cerebroretinal syndromes.** A group of diseases, usually hereditary, presenting with degenerations in the retina and cerebrum, e.g. Tay-Sachs disease. **Cervical-rib syndrome, Cervicobrachial syndrome.** A syndrome produced by compression of the lower cord of the brachial plexus by a cervical rib. There is pain down the medial aspect of the arm and forearm, with wasting of small hand muscles and hypo-aesthesia on the medial aspect of the palm. It is suggested that an identical syndrome may result when the cord is compressed by the tendons of the scalenus anterior or scalenus medius muscles (*scalenus syndrome*), or even by compression between the clavicle and 1st rib (*costoclavicular syndrome*). **Chiasma syndrome, Chiasmal syndrome, Chiasmatic syndrome.** A syndrome due to a lesion of the optic chiasma; there is variable visual impairment depending upon the extent of the lesion, and visual-field defects are also variable, though they are never congruous in the two eyes; central scotomata are common. **Chorea syndrome.** A syndrome due to atrophy or degeneration of the neostriatum (mainly the globus pallidus); spontaneous choreiform movements occur and tend to be stereotyped and repetitive. This is one form of senile chorea and is one of Hunt's striatal syndromes. **Coeliac syndrome.** Coeliac disease. *See* DISEASE. **Compression syndrome.** Shock, haematuria and oliguria, caused by long-continued compression of a limb such as occurred in bombed buildings. **Concussion syndrome.** Acute traumatic encephalopathy; irritability is a feature, coma or semicoma may occur, and on recovery of the senses there is often retrograde amnesia. **Congenital ectodermal-defect syndrome. Congenital alopecia.** *See* ALOPECIA. **Conn's syndrome.** *See* ALDOSTERONISM. **Cor-pulmonale syndrome.** Pulmonary heart disease; cardiac involvement secondary to lung disease, consisting of pulmonary hypertension, right ventricular hypertrophy or failure, systemic cardiac oedema, cyanosis and often polycythaemia, due to chronic lung disease. **Syndrome of the corpus striatum.** Vogt's syndrome. **Costoclavicular syndrome.** Pain in the arm, wasting and weakness of hand muscles, distal sensory loss and sometimes ischaemia, due to compression or stretching of the neurovascular bundle at the thoracic outlet. **Cough syndrome.** Vertigo, dimming of consciousness or syncope, following a paroxysm of coughing. Originally described by Charcot, who believed the condition to be a form of epilepsy, the syncope is now known to be due to cerebral anoxia; prolonged coughing raises the intrapleural pressure above that in the venae cavae, so that filling to the right auricle is impeded. This results in a sudden fall in cardiac output and in cerebral blood flow. **Craniometaphyseal syndrome.** Pyle's syndrome. **Cri-du-chat syndrome.** A syndrome of mental retardation and mild congenital malformations (moon-like face with hypertelorism, epicantic folds, low-set malformed ears, micrognathia, sometimes associated with congenital heart disease and/or skeletal abnormalities) characterized, in the neonatal period, by a high-pitched mewing cry. It is usually due to deficiency of part of the short arm of chromosome No.5. Deficiency of the short arm of chromosome No.4 produces a syndrome which seems to overlap to a large extent with the cri-du-chat syndrome but is somewhat more severe and may partly resemble the Patau syndrome; the mewing cry is usually absent. Better discrimination between these syndromes will be forthcoming due to improved techniques of chromosome analysis and more complete ascertainment. **Syndrome of crocodile tears.** Lacrimation on gustatory stimulation: it occurs particularly after a severe facial paralysis of lower motor-neuron type and may be due to crossed reinnervation, fibres of the chorda tympani reaching the lacrimal gland. **CRST syndrome.** Calcinosis, Raynaud's phenomenon, sclerodactylia and telangiectasis as occurring in systemic sclerosis. **Crush syndrome.** Compression syndrome (see above). **Cutaneo-intestinal syndrome.** A bullous and crusted skin condition with oropharyngeal ulceration and intestinal ulcers which may perforate. **Syndrome of the decussation of the pyramids.** Spastic weakness of the ipsilateral arm and contralateral leg, hemiplegia cruciata, due to a lower medullary lesion. **Defibrination syndrome.** A haemolytic state due to extensive destruction or utilization of fibrinogen *in vivo.* **Deletion syndromes** (the best known are ANTIMONGOLISM and the *Cri-du-chat syndrome*): *4p-syndrome* is the cri-du-chat syndrome (see above); *18p-syndrome* is characterized by short stature, webbing of the neck and often mental retardation and other somatic anomalies suggestive of the Bonnevie-Ulrich syndrome, which is associated with deletions of the short arm of chromosome No. 18; *18q-syndrome* is characterized by mental retardation, microcephaly, abnormal facies with midline dystrophy and associated with deletions of the long arm of chromosome No.18; *13q-syndrome* is characterized by mental deficiency and head deformity (microcephaly, trigonocephaly, micrognathia, microphthalmos, large malformed ears, etc.) often accompanied by retinoblastoma and associated with deletions of the long arm of chomosome No.13. **Diencephalic syndrome.** A syndrome defined by A. Russell, with increased appetite followed by anorexia, failure to grow and euphoria. It is usually due to a neoplasm affecting the diencephalon. **Syndrome of double athetosis.** Vogt's syndrome. **Dumping syndrome.** Rapid passage of gastric contents into the jejunum causing fainting, sweating and diarrhoea after eating or drinking; it may follow gastrectomy, vagotomy or gastro-enterostomy. Symptoms late after eating may be due to low blood-sugar levels. **Dystocia dystrophia syndrome.** A name given by DeLee to indicate a case associated with masculine pelvis and signs of pituitary hypofunction, aged primiparity, postmaturity, non-engagement of the head at the start of labour, occipitoposterior position, premature rupture of the membranes, weak pains, a tendency to eclampsia and a history of family dystocia. **Effort syndrome.** Neurocirculatory asthenia; Da Costa's syndrome; soldier's heart; disordered action of the heart; a condition in which the main symptoms are fatigue, shortness of breath, pain under the heart and palpitation; usually part of an anxiety neurosis. **Egg-white syndrome.** Egg-white injury. *See* INJURY. **EMG syndrome.** Exomphalos, macroglossia and gigantism. **Encephalotrigeminal vascular syndrome.** Angiomata of the brain and face; Sturge's syndrome; Sturge-Weber syndrome. **Endocrine candidosis syndrome.** Candidosis of skin, nails and mouth with diabetes mellitus, hypoparathyroidism, Addison's disease, pancreatitis or hypothyroidism. **Epidemic vomiting syndrome.** Winter vomiting disease occurring amongst schoolchildren in small epidemics, of viral origin and of 1-2 days' duration. **Epiphyseal syndrome.** One due to a lesion of the pineal body; there is premature development of the body, especially of the genitalia and long bones, and signs of internal hydrocephalus. Also called *Pellizzi's syndrome.* **Extrapyramidal syndrome.** Any syndrome attributed to disease of the extrapyramidal system, particularly Parkinson's disease. **Facet syndrome.** A form of osteo-arthritis in which the articular facets of the spinal vertebrae are mainly affected. **Fibro-fatty syndrome.** Panniculitis. **Frontal-lobe-tumour syndrome.** Headache and progressive dementia, with the late development of signs of increased intracranial pressure. **Gastro-cardiac syndrome.** Disturbance of cardiac function said to be connected with derangement of gastric function or displacement of the stomach. Hiatus hernia of the oesophagus is frequently associated with substernal pain suggesting cardiac ischaemia, but related to position rather than effort. Attacks of severe pain with peripheral circulatory failure and minor electrocardiographic changes may occur, simulating cardiac infarction. It is not known whether hiatus hernia or oesophagitis do in fact have any direct effect on the coronary circulation or cardiac function. **General adaptation syndrome.** The sum of all non-specific systematic reactions of the body which ensue upon long-continued exposure to stress. Selye divides it into 3 stages, the alarm reaction (shock and counter-shock), the stage of resistance and the stage of exhaustion. **Syndrome of the globus pallidus.** Juvenile paralysis agitans. *See* PARALYSIS. **Grey (or gray) syndrome.** Cardiovascular collapse in the newborn due to chloramphenicol. (The term is derived from the ash colour of the children affected.) **Grey spinal syndrome.** Any syndrome resulting from a lesion of the grey matter of the spinal cord; if the anterior horns are involved, there will be muscular atrophy, if the posterior horns, loss of reflexes, and if the lateral horns, vasomotor disturbances, while lesions near the central canal will give dissociated anaesthesia. **Haemogenic syndrome.** Thrombocytopenic purpura. *See* PURPURA. **Haemoglobinopathic syndromes.** Syndromes arising from defects in haemoglobin synthesis. **Haemohistioblastic syndrome.** Reticulo-endotheliosis. **Haemolytic-uraemia syndrome.** An acute disease of children with haemolytic anaemia, distorted red corpuscles, low platelet limit and high blood urea, and casts, red corpuscles and protein in the urine. **Haemopleuropneumonic syndrome.** Haemoptysis, dyspnoea, rapid pulse and fever associated with dullness at the base of the chest and tubular breath sounds over the mid-zones, suggesting pneumonia and haemothorax, caused by punctured wounds of the chest. **Hemiparaplegic syndrome.** Brown-Séquard's syndrome. **Hepatorenal syndrome.** Symptoms of combined hepatic and renal failure. **Syndrome of high-titre cold haemagglutination.** A syndrome in which the Raynaud phenomenon, to the extent of gangrene of the finger tips, and intravascular haemolysis, to the extent of a severe haemolytic anaemia and haemoglobinuria, occur on exposure to cold. **Humoral syndrome.** Deficiency of blood chloride and tissue dehydration due to intestinal obstruction. **Hunterian glossitis syndrome.** Pernicious anaemia. *See* ANAEMIA. **Hydrallazine syndrome.** A clinical syndrome caused by hydrallazine, closely resembling lupus erythematosus with many LE cells in the blood. **Hyperabduction syndrome.** A syndrome which includes pain down the arm, numbness, redness and swelling of the hand, and sometimes weakness and paralysis, caused by hyperabduction of the shoulder during an anaesthetic or during sleep. **Hyperadduction syndrome.** Symptoms due to compression of the main vessels and nerves due to prolonged hyperabduction of the arm. **Hyperkinetic syndrome.** Effort syndrome (see above). **Hypermotility syndromes.** A group of disorders such as the Ehlers-Danlos syndrome and Marfan's syndrome in which there is hypermotility of the joints due to excess elastic tissue. Joint pain and swelling may ensue. **Hypoplastic left-heart syndrome.** A group of developmental abnormalities of the heart which have in common imperfect development of the structures of the left side of the heart; the individual elements include mitral atresia, aortic stenosis or atresia, aortic hypoplasia, coarctation of the aorta and hypoplasia of the left ventricle, often with endocardial fibro-elastosis. **Hypoplastic right-heart syndrome.** A group of developmental abnormalities of the heart which have in common imperfect development of the structures of the right side of the heart; the individual elements include tricuspid atresia, pulmonary stenosis or atresia, pulmonary arterial stenosis or hypoplasia and hypoplasia of the right ventricle. **Hypothalamic syndrome.** Any syndrome in which signs and symptoms are present as a result of damage to the hypothalamus. There is usually a combination of neurological, autonomic and endocrine abnormalities. **Incarceration syndrome.** The sequence of pain and swelling of the kidney which may accompany a severe degree of nephroptosis and may be relieved when the patient assumes the recumbent posture and the kidney slips back to its normal position. **Inspissated bile syndrome.** Persistent obstructive jaundice following haemolytic jaundice. **Internal carotid artery syndrome.** Ipsilateral blindness and crossed hemiplegia due to thrombosis of the internal carotid artery. **Irritable-bowel syndrome.** A disorder of intestinal mobility associated with emotional stress; alternating diarrhoea and constipation with pain and often mucus in the stools. It may follow infection but with no organic disease present. It is sometimes called *spastic colon* or *mucous colitis.* **Jaw-winking syndrome.** Unilateral ptosis at rest followed by a rapid exaggerated elevation of the lid when the mandible is depressed or deviated to the opposite side. The condition is occasionally familial and the cause is unknown. **Jejunal syndrome.** Dumping syndrome (see above). **Jugular-foramen syndrome.** The syndrome produced by damage to the 9th, 10th and 11th cranial nerves as they leave the skull via the jugular foramen. There is unilateral flaccid paralysis of palatal, pharyngeal and intrinsic laryngeal muscles and of the sterno-cleidomastoid and trapezius muscles; nasal speech, hoarseness of the voice and dysphagia result. In addition there is loss of taste sensibility on the posterior third of the tongue on the affected side. Also called *Vernet's syndrome.* **Karroo syndrome.** Pyrexia, lymphadenitis and gastro-enteritis occurring amongst white inhabitants of the Karroo in South Africa. **Katayama syndrome.** The acute febrile condition arising during the invasive phase of *Schistosoma japonicum,* accompanied by diverse allergic manifestations. **Kissing-spine syndrome.** *See* SPINE. **Knuckle pad syndrome.** Hale-White's syndrome; fibrous pads over the knuckles of the fingers mimicking arthritis. **Laevulosuric syndrome.** Laevulosuria with mental symptoms such as insomnia, melancholia and impotence. **Lateral cord and associated anterior cornual syndrome.** Anterolateral syndrome (see above). **Lateral medullary syndrome.** Ipsilateral palatal, pharyngeal and laryngeal palsies, analgesia of the face, Horner's syndrome and cerebellar ataxia, with crossed analgesia of the limbs; usually due to medullary infarction. Wallenberg's syndrome. **Liver-death syndrome, Liver-kidney syndrome.** Hepatorenal syndrome (see above). **Syndrome of locking.** An acute pain associated with fixation of a joint, usually in a partially flexed position. This may occur in joints with intra-articular cartilages, e.g. the knee, or in joints without these; in the latter case the phenomenon is less easy to explain. **Loculation syndrome.** Froin's syndrome. **Low-horizon syndrome.** Break-off phenomenon. *See* PHENOMENON. **Lower-nephron syndrome.** Acute renal failure with oliguria, occurring in a variety of conditions, e.g. limb-crushing injuries,

syndrome

concealed accidental haemorrhages, mismatched blood transfusions. Pathological changes are found in the loop of Henle and the distal convoluted renal tubules. **Lumbago-sciatica syndrome.** Low backache followed by sciatic pain, commonly due to intervertebral-disc prolapse. **Malabsorption syndrome.** A group of symptoms and signs resulting from steatorrhoea and malabsorption of vitamins, proteins, carbohydrates, minerals and water. Manifestations include malnutrition, anaemia, hyperpigmentation, follicular hyperkeratoses, purpura, ecchymoses, haematuria, dermatitis, glossitis, peripheral neuritis, oedema, ichthyosis and defective hair and nails. **Mediastinal syndrome.** Dyspnoea, stridor and paroxysmal cough, with signs of pressure on arteries, veins and nerves. **Meningitic syndrome.** 1. A syndrome in which symptoms of meningeal irritation are the most prominent. 2. A manifestation of subarachnoid haemorrhage in which consciousness is not lost, but headache, stiffness of the neck, Kernig's sign and other signs and symptoms of meningeal irritation, are present. **Menopausal syndrome.** A combination of subjective phenomena occurring in some women about the time of the menopause. The symptoms include irritability, depression, insomnia and paroxysmal flushing and sweating. **Metameric syndrome.** A syndrome suggesting a lesion of a single segment of the spinal cord; also called *segmental syndrome.* **Middle-lobe syndrome.** Subacute inflammation of the middle lobe of the right lung, generally due to compression of the bronchus by hilar lymph nodes. **Middle radicular syndrome.** Paralysis of the triceps brachiia and wrist extensors, due to a lesion of the middle root of the brachial plexus. **Milk-alkali syndrome.** A syndrome following milk diet with excessive amounts of absorbable alkali, such as sodium bicarbonate, causing a non-renal uraemia (alkalosis). **Multifidus-triangle syndrome.** A lower back pain localized in the multifidus triangle. It is characterized by acute episodes, with recurrence after periods of quiescence. There are points of much tenderness, usually just below the posterior superior iliac spine. The cause is probably an injury to the muscle and its fascia, and the treatment is by local injections. **Nail-patella syndrome.** An inherited anomaly with defective nails, rudimentary patellae and bony iliac spines. **Nephrotic syndrome.** Increasing oedema, albuminuria, often raised blood pressure and increase of the $alpha_2$ $beta_2$ serum globulin fraction. **Neuro-anaemic syndrome.** Pernicious anaemia with posterolateral sclerosis. **Neurocutaneous syndrome.** Strawberry naevi associated with vascular malformations of the central nervous system (and sometimes in the bones). **Nonsense syndrome.** A condition resembling the Ganser syndrome but without any disturbance of consciousness. **Syndrome of the nucleus ambiguus and spinal fillet.** Avellis' syndrome. **Oculodentodigital syndrome.** Microphthalmos, narrow nose, bent fifth digits on hands, enamel hypoplasia and perhaps glaucoma. **Orbital apex syndrome.** Involvement of the optic nerve and nerves passing through the superior orbital fissure. **Orofacial digital syndrome.** Hypoplastic alae nasi, hypertrophic frenulae of lip and tongue, multilobed tongue, cleft palate, dental defects, deformed hands and, sometimes, polycystic disease of the liver and kidneys. **Otolith syndrome.** The otolithic catastrophe; an affection of the internal ear, accompanied by sudden momentary alterations in muscle tone. The patient falls suddenly to the ground without loss of consciousness, vertigo or malaise, and almost immediately feels normal again. In involvement of the utricle, collapse occurs in the anteroposterior plane. When the saccule is affected, the collapse is to one side or the other. In combined conditions in which both saccular and utricular function is disturbed, attacks may occur in either the sagittal or the coronal plane. Hearing by bone conduction is reduced in the ear involved. **Otopalatodigital syndrome.** Taybi's syndrome of nerve deafness, cleft soft palate, small mouth and broad ends of digits. **Painful bruising syndrome.** Auto-erythrocyte sensitization presenting as painful bruises, mostly on the thighs. Intradermal injections of red cells reproduce the lesions. **Palaeostriatal syndrome.** The manifestations of any disease of the palaeostriatal system as distinct from those due to disease of the neostriatum; the commonest is paralysis agitans. **Pallidal syndrome.** The clinical manifestations of disease of the globus pallidus; prominent among these are rigidity of muscles and tremor, e.g. paralysis agitans. **Pallidomesencephalic syndrome.** The clinical manifestations of any disease of the globus pallidus and mid-brain (particularly the substantia nigra). **Paralysis-agitans syndrome.** The name given to a palaeostriatal syndrome described by Hunt, now believed to be indistinguishable from paralysis agitans. **Paratrigeminal syndrome.** Horner's syndrome, with affection of the trigeminal nerve on the same side. **Parkinsonian syndrome.** Mask-like facies, excessive salivation, loss of emotional and associated movements, static tremor inhibited by movement and a festinating gait, due to a lesion of the globus pallidus and often the substantia nigra (the palaeostriatum). If due to degeneration it is called *paralysis agitans,* if to chronic encephalitis lethargica, *post-encephalitic parkinsonism.* **Penta-X syndrome.** Mental deficiency, short stature, patent ductus arteriosus and small hands, with five X and no Y chromosomes. **Pericolic-membrane syndrome.** Symptoms simulating those of appendicitis, caused by the pressure of pericolic membrane. **Perinatal distress syndrome.** Pulmonary hyaline-membrane disease. *See* DISEASE. **Periodic syndrome.** A caretaker name for a recurrent syndrome of childhood in which bilious and migrainous attacks occur, and which has in the past been referred to by unsatisfactory names such as *cyclic vomiting, abdominal migraine* and *acidosis.* When the aetiology is more fully understood, a more satisfactory name may be found. **Phrenogastric syndrome.** Accumulation of gas in the fundus of the stomach, with elevation of the left dome of the diaphragm, sometimes seen in patients with coronary-artery disease, at the onset of cardiac infarction, due either to air swallowing in an attempt to relieve pain, or to dilatation of the stomach occurring reflexly as a result of the pain. **Pickwickian syndrome.** Extreme obesity, with cardiorespiratory distress and polycythaemia. **Pineal syndrome.** Epiphyseal syndrome (see above). **Pluriglandular syndrome, Polyglandular syndrome.** One due to combined endocrine deficiencies. **Polysplenia syndrome.** A complex developmental abnormality with multiple splenunculi, instead of a single properly-formed spleen, indeterminate visceral situs and complex cardiac abnormalities, often with dextrocardia or apparent isolated laevocardia. **Pontine syndrome.** There are numerous pontine syndromes, including the Babinski-Nageotte, Cestan-Chenais, Millard-Gubler, Foville syndromes and others, but this term is usually applied to the Raymond-Cestan syndrome. **Popliteal web syndrome.** Popliteal web, pits in the lower lip and cleft palate. **Porphyrin syndrome.** A disease of the prophyrin metabolism, congenital or acquired, in which porphyrins of abnormal kinds and in abnormal amounts are produced and excreted. It may be associated with red urine, light sensitivity of the skin and gastrointestinal and nervous disturbances. **Postcardiotomy syndrome** (PCS). A rare complication of heart surgery. Symptoms are fever, pleuropericarditis, raised erythrocyte sedimentation rate and spontaneous resolution; rarely arthralgia and relapse. Corticosteroids are used for prophylaxis and treatment. **Postconcussion syndrome.** A syndrome often following closed head injury and including irritability, memory defect, headaches, giddiness and poor concentration. **Posterior-cord syndrome.** The clinical manifestations of a lesion in the posterior columns of the spinal cord; there is sensory ataxia and impairment of appreciation of position, vibration and tactile discrimination. **Posterolateral syndrome.** Any syndrome due to lesions of the posterior and lateral columns of the spinal cord; the term applies particularly to subacute combined degeneration of the cord; *see* LICHTHEIM'S SYNDROME. **Postgastrectomy syndromes.** A small percentage of patients have unpleasant postprandial symptoms following gastrectomy. Immediately after food there may be the *dumping syndrome* (see above). Later, symptoms of hypoglycaemia with flushing, sweating and prostration. **Post-tachycardia syndrome.** The persistence of T-wave inversion in the electrocardiogram for a period after a paroxysm of tachycardia, which may lead to the incorrect diagnosis of myocardial ischaemia or infarction. **Post-thrombotic syndrome.** The changes in a leg after deep venous thrombosis. They include oedema, eczema, contact allergic reactions, woody induration, ulceration and hyperpigmentation. Periphlebitis, thrombophlebitis and recurrent cellulitis may occur and solid oedema may finally result. **Post-traumatic syndrome.** Postconcussion syndrome (see above). **Pre-excitation syndrome.** Physiological bundle-branch block with short P-R interval; a condition in which the duration of the QRS complex of the electrocardiogram is greater than 0.1 s (bundle-branch block), in association with a short P-R interval. It is thought to be due to early excitation of one or other ventricle, the impulse from the sinu-atrial node having short circuited through anomalous conducting tissue (bundle of Kent). The condition is often congenital, and is associated with a liability to paroxysmal tachycardia. The heart is generally normal, but cases may occur in association with congenital heart disease. The syndrome may also complicate acquired heart disease. **Premenstrual syndrome.** A syndrome characterized by irritability, emotional disturbance, nervous tension, headache, tender swelling of the breasts and a variety of other symptoms. A number of factors have been suggested in its aetiology, but water retention is probably an important feature. **Premotor syndrome.** The syndrome resulting from a lesion of the frontal premotor cortex; there is a spastic hemiplegia, with sometimes contralateral forced grasping, conjugate deviation of the head and eyes, and variable vasomotor disturbance. **Pronator syndrome.** Compression of the median nerve between the 2 heads of the pronator teres muscle. **Prune-belly syndrome.** Congenital deficiency of the abdominal muscle accompanied by serious urogenital malformation. **Punch-drunk syndrome.** Friedmann's complex. **Pyloric-channel syndrome.** Inflammation of the prepyloric region and pylorus resulting in muscle hypertrophy and narrowing of the pyloric canal, giving rise to pyloric obstruction and, if an ulcer occurs, to stenosis. Clinical signs are those of recurrent peptic ulcer and pyloric obstruction. **Radial aplasia-thrombocytopenia syndrome.** Autosomal recessive congenital absence of radial bones with megakaryocytopenia and thrombocytopenia, with or without cardiac anomaly. **Radicular syndrome.** Any syndrome due to a lesion of a nerve root or roots. Commonly there is pain, motor weakness and sensory loss in the distribution of the affected root or roots. An example is the brachial neuralgia produced by lateral prolapse of a cervical intervertebral disc. **Release syndrome.** Compression syndrome (see above). **Retraction syndrome.** A congenital condition in which the external rectus muscle of the orbit is replaced by a fibrous band. On adduction of the eye the eyeball retracts and the palpebral fissure becomes narrower. Also called *Duane's syndrome.* **Retroparotid-space syndrome.** Villaret's syndrome. **Rolandic-vein syndrome.** Hemiplegia due to cortical infarction as a result of thrombosis of the veins of the area of Rolando. **Sanfilippo syndrome.** Mucopolysaccharidosis type III. **Scalded-child syndrome.** Dermatitis exfoliativa in the infant, due to staphylococcal infection; Ritter's disease. **Scalenus syndrome, Scalenus-anticus syndrome.** Pain down the medial border of the arm with sometimes sensory loss over the hypothenar eminence and wasting of small hand muscles, due to compression of the lower cord of the brachial plexus by the scalenus anterior muscle. The manifestations due to compression by a cervical rib are similar. Also called *Naffziger's syndrome.* **Scimitar syndrome.** In cardiology, a radiological appearance on the chest x-ray in isolated anomalous drainage of a lower pulmonary vein where the distended vein running up the right atrium has an appearance likened to a scimitar. **Seabright bantam syndrome.** *See* PSEUDOHYPOPARATHYROIDISM. **Segmental syndrome, Segmentary syndrome.** Metameric syndrome (see above). **Shoulder-hand syndrome.** A painful stiff shoulder, associated with trophic changes in the arm and hand, occurring in elderly persons as a result of subdeltoid bursitis, or following painful conditions of the chest and/or upper extremity, or after immobilization of the arm. It is said to occur more frequently after coronary thrombosis than in association with other conditions, but often no precipitating cause is found. The movements of the shoulder joints are grossly restricted, and calcification may occur in the supraspinatus muscle or in the subdeltoid bursa. **Sicca syndrome.** Dryness of the mouth due to deficient formation of saliva often associated with deficient tear formation (*syn:* Sjögren's syndrome). **Sick-sinus syndrome.** A name which has been applied to a condition characterized by progressive disturbance of function of the sinu-atrial node, resulting in episodes of sinus bradycardia, supraventricular tachycardia and atrial fibrillation, often leading eventually to sinus arrest. It is sometimes associated with degeneration of the conducting system leading to heart block. **Sphenoidal-fissure syndrome.** Pain and later anaesthesia in the area supplied by the ophthalmic branch of the 5th cranial nerve, associated with ocular muscle palsies and later proptosis. It is caused by pressure on the 3rd, 4th, 6th and the 1st branch of the 5th cranial nerves as they pass through the fissure. **Sphenopalatine syndrome.** Unilateral oedema of the face with unilateral lacrimation, rhinitis and recurrent redness and swelling of the affected side. **Splenic-flexure syndrome.** A benign syndrome that has to be considered in the differential diagnosis of coronary disease. The symptoms are a feeling of pressure and fullness in the precordium, shortness of breath and palpitation. It is caused by gas in, and spasm of, the splenic flexure. The attack is predisposed by emotional disturbances and constipation, and relieved by the passing of wind or faeces or by a change of position. **Stasis syndrome.** The changes in the legs caused by chronic venous insufficiency; they include oedema, aching discomfort, pigmentation due to extravasation of blood, thickening of the skin, scaling and itching, vesicular eczema and, when arteriolar insufficiency co-exists, there is also patchy white atrophy with telangiectasia. Varicose veins may or may not be present. **Stiff-man syndrome.** A syndrome that starts during the fifth decade of life with increasing muscular stiffness and rigidity, and painful muscular spasms. It is a progressive disease that does not respond to antispasmodics and it is thought to be due to specific metabolic defect. It may, however, possibly be associated with dystonia musculorum deformans, which is caused by degenerative changes in the basal ganglia. **Striatal syndrome.** Hunt's striatal syndrome. **Striocortical syndrome.** Intellectual impairment, stiffness of muscles during voluntary activity and marked emotional lability, particularly with regard to facial movements; it is due to concurrent degeneration of the frontal cortex and of the corpus striatum, and often due to atherosclerosis. **Subclavian steal syndrome.** Disturbance of blood flow sometimes resulting from obstruction of the subclavian artery proximal to the origin of the vertebral artery whereby the direction of flow in the latter is reversed, particularly when the ipsilateral arm is exercised, causing episodic brain-stem dysfunction. **Superior oblique tendon sheath syndrome.** A congenitally short tendon sheath at the trochlea, resulting in limited elevation in abduction. **Supine hypotensive syndrome of late pregnancy.** A state of hypotension and cardiovascular depression due to the bulk of the pregnant uterus pressing on the inferior vena cava and preventing adequate venous return to the heart when the patient lies on her back. **Suprarenogenic syndrome.** That resulting from disturbance of the normal functioning of the suprarenal glands; it is characterized by hairiness, adiposity and pigmentation. **Supraspinatus syndrome.** Pain during the middle degrees of abduction of the arm, due to tenderness of the tendon of the supraspinatus muscle. **Surdocardiac syndrome.** The combination of deafness with cardiac disease; the latter is usually manifested by a prolonged QT time and attacks of syncope due to recurrent episodes of ventricular fibrillation. **Tarsal tunnel syndrome.** Compression of the posterior tibial nerve behind the medial malleolus, causing pain and paraesthesiae in the sole of the foot. **Tegmental syndrome, Tegmental syndrome of the midbrain.** Benedikt's syndrome. **Temporomandibular joint pain dysfunction syndrome.** Pain and tenderness in the temporomandibular joints and muscles of mastication due to disturbance in normal reflex jaw function often associated with trismus. Causes include anxiety habits such as bruxism, painful teeth and malocclusion. **Testicular feminizing syndrome.** An individual with male chromosomes but with feminized body; the breasts swell at puberty but the uterus is absent. Testes may be found in the inguinal region and, if left, may develop germinomata. There is thought to be a "target organ" failure to testosterone. **Thalamic syndrome.** A syndrome, usually of vascular origin, in which damage occurs to the ventral and posterolateral nuclei of the thalamus and thalamocortical pathways. There is raising of the threshold to all forms of sensation on the opposite side of the body, but all stimuli, however minimal, excite an exaggerated unpleasant burning response called *hyperpathia.* There may be associated hemiplegia and hemianopia, and sometimes ataxia, choreo-athetosis and emotional lability. Also called the *syndrome of Déjérine-Roussy.* **Uveoparotid syndrome.** A condition in which enlargement of the parotid gland is associated with uveitis and facial paralysis. There is sometimes slight intermittent fever. **Vago-accessory syndrome.** Schmidt's syndrome. **Syndrome of vago-accessory hypoglossal paralysis.** Jackson's syndrome. **Vasovagal syndrome.** Recurrent vasovagal attacks. **Winking-jaw syndrome.** A brisk movement of the mandible to the contralateral side when the cornea is touched. **XXXXY syndrome.** The clinical features shown by XXXXY males. *See* MALE. **Yellow nail syndrome.** Slowly-growing yellow nails, curved on their long axes, with defective cuticle and oncholysis, associated with lymphoedema due to atresia or varicosity of lymphatics. **YY or double Y syndrome.** In man, males with two Y chomosomes have a variable phenotype and some are essentially normal. The extra Y, however, has a positive effect on height and a negative effect on mental and psychological development leading fairly often to social maladjustment and criminal behaviour. The karyotypes associated with this syndrome are essentially the 47,XYY and 48,XXYY. [Gk *syn, dromos* course.]

See also: ABERCROMBIE, ACHARD, ADAMS (R.), ADIE, ALBRIGHT, ALZHEIMER, ANDERSEN, ANGELUCCI, APERT, ARNOLD (F.), ARNOLD (J.), AVELLIS, AYERZA, BABINSKI, BANNICK, BANTI, BARD, BARDET, BARRÉ, BAUMGARTEN (W.), BEAU, BEHÇET, BENEDIKT, BERNARD (C.), BERNARD (L.), BERNHARDT (M.), BERNHEIM, BERTOLOTTI, BESNIER, BIANCHI (L.), BIEDL, BLUM, BOECK (C. P. M.), BONNIER, BOUILLAUD, BOUVERET, BRAILSFORD, BRIQUET, BRISSAUD, BRISTOWE, BROWN-SÉQUARD, BRUGSCH, BRUNS, BUDD, CAPGRAS, CAPLAN, CATHELINEAU, CESTAN, CHARCOT, CHAUFFARD, CHENAIS, CHIARI, CHRISTIAN, CLARK (C.), CLERAMBAULT, CLÉRAT, CLOUGH, COLLET, CONN, COSTEN, COTARD, COURVOISIER, CROSFILL, CRUVEILHIER, CUSHING (HARVEY W.), CYRIAX, DA COSTA, DANA, DANLOS, DEBRÉ, DÉJÉRINE, DÉJÉRINE-KLUMPKE, DE TONI, DIGHTON, DRESBACH, DUANE, DUCHENNE, DUPLAY, DUPRÉ, EBSTEIN, EDDOWES, EHLERS, EISENLOHR, EISENMENGER, EPSTEIN (A. A.), ERB, ESCHERICH, FABER, FANCONI, FELTY, FITZ (R. H.), FORSSMAN, FOVILLE, FRANK (J.), FREY (L.), FRIDERICHSEN, FRIEDMANN (M.), FRÖHLICH, FROIN, FUCHS (E.), GAILLARD, GAISBOECK, GANSER, GÉLINEAU, GERLIER, GERSTMANN, GOLDFLAM, GOUGEROT, GOWERS, GRADENIGO, GROENBLAD, GUBLER, GUILLAIN, GUNN, HADFIELD, HALLEVORDEN, HAND, HARE (E. S.), HASSIN, HAYEM, HENCH, HENOCH, HERTWIG (K. W. T. R.), HEYD, HINES, HOLMES (G. M.), HOMÉN, HOPPE, HORNER (J. F.), HORTON, HOUSSAY, HUNT (J. R.), HURLER, HUTCHISON, JACKSON (J. H.), JACQUET, JAKSCH, JOHNSON (F. C.), KANDINKSY, KARTAGENER, KELLY (A. B.), KENNEDY, KENT (A. F. S.), KIMMELSTIEL, KLEINE-LEVIN, KLINEFELTER, KLIPPEL, KOENIG (FRITZ), KORSAKOFF, LANDRY, LAUNOIS, LAURENCE, LERICHE, LERMOYEZ, LESCHKE, LÉVI, LÉVY, LHERMITTE, LIBMAN, LICHTHEIM, LINDAU, LOBSTEIN, LOEFFLER (W.), LORAIN, LUTEMBACHER, LUYS (J. B.), MCCUNE, MACKENZIE (S.), MAFFUCCI, MAGENDIE, MARAÑON, MARCHIAFAVA, MARFAN, MARIE, MEIGE, MEIGS (J. V.), MENIÈRE, MICHELI, MIKULICZ-RADECKI, MILIAN, MILKMAN, MILLARD, MILROY, MINKOWSKI, MOEBIUS, MOON (R. C.), MOORE (M. T.), MOREL, MORGAGNI, MORQUIO, MORVAN, MOSSE, MUNCHAUSEN, MURCHISON, NAFFZIGER, NAGEOTTE, NIEMANN, NONNE, NOTHNAGEL, OGILVIE, OSLER, PAESSLER, PANCOAST (H. K.), PARINAUD, PARKES, PARKINSON (JAMES), PARKINSON (JOHN), PATERSON (D. R.), PEL, PELLIZZI, PEPPER, PIC, PICK (F.), PLUMMER, POTAIN, PROFICHET, PUTNAM, RAYMOND, RAYNAUD, REICHMANN, REITER, RICHTER (I. M.), ROGER (G. H.), ROMBERG, ROQUE, ROSENBACH (O.), ROSENBERG, ROTH (V. K.), ROUSSY, RUST, SACKS, SAUVINEAU, SAWIL, SCHAUMANN, SCHMIDT (J. F. M.), SCHOENLEIN, SCHUELLER (A.), SCHULTZ, SELYE, SENEAR, SERGENT, SICARD, SIEMENS, SLUDER, SPATZ, SPENS, SPURWAY, STERNBERG (W. H.), STEVENS (A. M.), STEWART (J. P.), STILL, STOKES (WILLIAM), STRANDBERG, STURGE, SUDECK, TAPIA, TERRIER, THAON, THIBIERGE, THIERS, TOMMASELLI, TROISIER, TROTTER, TURNER (H. H.), USHER, VAN DER HOEVE, VAQUEZ, VERNET, VILLARET, VINSON, VOGT (C.), VOGT (O.), WALLENBERG, WATERHOUSE (R.), WEBER (F. P.), WEBER (H. D.), WEINGARTNER, WERNER (C. W. O.), WERNICKE (K.), WHITE (P. D.), WIDAL, WILKS, WILSON (C.), WILSON (S. A. KINNIER), WOLFF (L.), WRIGHT (I. S.), YOUNG.

syndromic (sin·**dro**·mik). Having the characteristics of, or pertaining to syndrome.

synechia (sin·e·ke·ah). Adhesion; in ophthalmology, an adhesion formed between the iris and the posterior surface of the cornea, or the anterior capsule of the lens, following attacks of iritis. **Annular synechia.** One binding the whole edge of the pupil to the anterior lens capsule and so shutting off the posterior chamber from the anterior. Also called *seclusion of the pupil.* **Anterior synechia.** One in front of the iris to the posterior surface of the cornea. **Anterior peripheral synechia.** One forming in front of the iris at the periphery of the anterior chamber and so blocking the drainage angle. **Synechiae pericardii.** Pericardial adhesions which anchor the heart to the surrounding mediastinal structures and chest wall. They may result in constrictive pericarditis in which the heart is compressed by the adhesions. **Posterior synechia.** One between the iris and the anterior lens capsule. **Ring synechia.** Annular synechia (see above). **Total synechiae.** Those when the whole of the posterior surface of the iris is bound down to the anterior lens capsule. **Synechia vulvae.** Congenital fusion of the labia minora. [Gk a continuity.]

synechiotomy (sin·e·ke·**ot**'·o·me). The operation of dividing a synechia. [synechia, Gk *temnein* to cut.]

synechotome (sin·**ek**·o·tome). An instrument used in synechiotomy.

synechotomy (sin·e·**kot**·o·me). Synechiotomy.

synechtenterotomy (**sin**·ek·ten·ter·**ot**'·o·me). A dividing of intestinal adhesions. [Gk *synechein* to hold together, *enteron* intestine, *temnein* to cut.]

synencephalia (sin·en·kef·**a**'·le·ah). A condition of having 2 bodies but a fused head; as in syncephalus. [Gk *syn, egkephalos* brain.]

synencephalocele (sin·en·**kef**·al·o·seel). An encephalocele characterized by adhesions to the neighbouring parts. [Gk *syn, egkephalos* brain, *kele* tumour.]

synencephalus (sin·en·**kef**·al·us). A monster displaying synencephalia.

syneresis (sin·**er**·es·is). A phenomenon observed in the clotting of milk or blood. It is due to the contraction of a gel upon itself, which squeezes out some of the dispersed liquid phase. **Syneresis of the vitreous.** Condensation of the collagenous framework into strands and membranes, leaving pockets of fluid vitreous. [Gk *syn, hairein* to draw.]

synergenesis (sin·er·**jen**·es·is). Syngenesis.

synergetic (sin·er·**jet**·ik). Synergic.

synergia (sin·**er**·je·ah). Synergy.

synergic (sin·**er**·jik). Acting or working together, as when several muscles co-operate in the performance of a movement. [Gk *syn, ergein* to work.]

synergism (**sin**·er·jizm). Synergy.

synergist (**sin**·er·gist). 1. A medicament which supplements the action of another, often to such an extent that the combined action is greater than the sum of the effects of the 2 drugs independently administered. 2. An organ the action of which is co-ordinated with that of another organ. 3. A muscle acting synergically. **Pituitary synergist.** A substance said to be present in pituitary extracts which enhances the action of chorionic gonadotrophin. [Gk *syn, ergein* to work.]

synergistic (sin·er·**jis**·tik). 1. Pertaining to synergy. 2. Synergetic.

synergy (**sin**·er·je). 1. Co-ordination in the action of muscles, organs or drugs. 2. The faculty of the nervous system to combine muscular functions in such a way that specialized actions requiring particular movements can be carried out. [Gk *syn*, *ergein* to work.]

Syngamidae (sin·**gam**·id·e). A family of the nematode superfamily or sub-order Strongyloidea; gapeworms. The genus *Syngamus* is of medical interest. [Gk *syn*, *gamos* marriage, *eidos* form.]

syngamous (**sin**·gam·us). Concerned with the idea that the future sex of an organism is determined at the moment of fertilization of the ovum. [Gk *syn*, *gamos* marriage.]

Syngamus (**sin**·gam·us). A genus of strongyloid nematode worms. The species occur in the upper respiratory tracts always in permanently attached pairs. **Syngamus kingi.** A species that has been recorded once from man in the West Indies. **Syngamus laryngeus.** A species whose normal hosts are cattle, and which has occurred occasionally in man. [see prec.]

syngamy (**sin**·gam·e). Sexual reproduction; the union of gametes. [Gk *syn*, *gamos* marriage.]

syngenesioplasty (sin·jen·e·se·o·plas·te). The transplantation of tissue from one person to another, when the latter are blood relations. [Gk *syn*, *genesis* origin, *plassein* to form.]

syngenesious (sin·jen·e·se·us). Derived from the same species. [see foll.]

syngenesis (sin·**jen**·es·is). 1. Sexual reproduction. 2. The theory that every gamete contains in itself the seeds of all subsequent generations. [Gk *syn*, *genesis* origin.]

syngenetic (sin·jen·**et**·ik). Relating to syngenesis.

syngenic (sin·**jen**·ik). Congenital.

syngonic (sin·**gon**·ik). Syngamous. [Gk *syn*, *gone* seed.]

synizesis (sin·iz·e·sis). A falling in; an occlusion, aggregation or agglutination. **Synizesis pupillae.** Closure of the pupil [obsolete term]. [Gk a falling in.]

synkaryon (sin·**kar**·e·on). A cell nucleus produced by fusion of 2 gametes or, in general, by the fusion of 2 nuclei. [Gk *syn*, *karyon* nut.]

synkinesis (sin·kin·e·sis). An involuntary movement occurring in one part of the body at the same time as a deliberate movement is made in another part. **Imitative synkinesis.** An involuntary movement occurring on the healthy side of the body when movement on the paralysed side is attempted. **Mouth-and-hand synkinesis.** Children on opening the mouth wide make associated movements with their hands, opening them and spreading the fingers. **Spasmodic synkinesis.** A movement occurring on the affected side of the body when a deliberate movement is made on the normal side. [Gk *syn*, *kinesis* movement.]

synkinetic (sin·kin·et·ik). Characterized by synkinesis.

synocha, synochus (sin·o·kah, **sin**·o·kus). Any continued fever. [Gk *synochos* lasting.]

synoecology (sin·e·**kol**·o·je). The study of environmental factors in relation to groups of organisms associated together considered as a whole. [Gk *syn*, oecology.]

synonym (**sin**·o·nim). One of 2 names for 1 species or other taxonomic grouping. [Gk *synonymos* of similar name.]

synophridia (sin·of·**rid**·e·ah). Synophrys.

synophrys (sin·**of**·ris). A meeting of the eyebrows across the middle line. [Gk *syn*, *ophrys* eyebrow.]

synophthalmia (sin·of·**thal**·me·ah). Congenital cyclopia; the complete or partial blending of both eyes into one. [Gk *syn*, *ophthalmos* eye.]

synophthalmus (sin·of·**thal**·mus). Cyclops; a fetal monster with both eyes blended into one. [see prec.]

synopsy (sin·**op**·se). The production of sensations of colour when the individual hears certain tones; a form of synaesthesia. [Gk *syn*, *opsis* vision.]

synoptophore (sin·**op**·to·for). A modified form of stereoscope used in squint training. [Gk *syn*, *opsis* vision, *pherein* to bear.]

synorchidism (sin·or·kid·izm). Synorchism.

synorchism (sin·**or**·kism). Complete or partial fusion of the testes. [Gk *syn*, *orchis* testis.]

synoscheos (sin·**os**·ke·os). The abnormal joining of the penis and scrotum. A congenital malformation observed in hermaphroditism. [Gk *syn*, *osche* scrotum.]

synosteology (**sin**·os·te·**ol**′·o·je). Arthrology; the study of joints and articulations. [Gk *syn*, *osteon* bone, *logos* science.]

synosteophyte (sin·**os**·te·o·fite). Congenital bony ankylosis. [Gk *syn*, *osteon* bone, *phyton* growth.]

synosteosis (**sin**·os·te·**o**′·sis). Synostosis.

synosteotomy (**sin**·os·te·**ot**′·o·me). Arthrotomy; the surgical dissection of joints and articulations. [Gk *syn*, *osteon* bone, *temnein* to cut.]

synostosis (sin·os·**to**·sis). 1. Bony ankylosis; the joining of bones by the ossification of the connecting tissues. 2. The joining of contiguous and separate bones by osseous tissue. **Synostosis congenita.** Synosteophyte. **Cranial synostosis.** Union by bone formation across sutures of cranial bones. **Radio-ulnar synostosis.** Union of the upper ends of the radius and ulna. **Transphalangeal synostosis.** Union of phalanges by ossification of interphalangeal joints. **Tribasilar synostosis.** Union of the 3 basal bones of the skull in infancy, with, owing to the shortening of the base of the skull, resultant idiocy. [Gk *syn*, *osteon* bone.]

synostotic (sin·os·**tot**·ik). Characterized by synostosis.

synotia (sin·o·she·ah). Union of the ears in agnathous monsters. [Gk *syn*, *ous* ear.]

synotus (sin·**o**·tus). An agnathous monster in which the lower jaw is missing and the ears are fused beneath the skull. [see prec.]

synovectomy (si·no·**vek**·to·me). The cutting away of part or all of a synovial membrane. [synovia, Gk *ektome* excision.]

synovia [NA] (si·**no**·ve·ah). The glairy fluid secreted by synovial membranes. The fluid contains small quantities of albumin, mucin, extractives and salts. [a word invented by Paracelsus, perhaps from Gk *syn*, L *ovum* egg (referring to egg-white).]

synovial (si·**no**·ve·al). 1. Secreting synovia. 2. Relating to or consisting of synovia. **Synovial bursa.** *See* BURSA. **Synovial fluid.** Synovia. **Synovial joint.** *See* JOINT. **Synovial membrane.** *See* MEMBRANE. **Synovial sheath.** *See* SHEATH.

synovialis (si·**no**·ve·**a**′·lis). A synovial membrane.

synovialoma (si·**no**·ve·al·**o**′·mah). Synovioma.

synovin (si·**no**·vin). A mucinous substance found in synovia.

synovioblast (si·**no**·ve·o·blast). The predominant connective-tissue cell of synovial membrane, closely related to, if not identical with, the fibroblast of ordinary connective tissue. [synovia, Gk *blastos* germ.]

synovioma (si·**no**·ve·**o**′·mah). A tumour derived from a synovial membrane. **Malignant synovioma.** A malignant tumour arising within the synovial membrane of joints or occasionally of tendons. [synovia, Gk *-oma* tumour.]

synoviparous (si·no·**vip**·ar·us). Secreting synovia. [synovia, L *parere* to produce.]

synovitis (si·no·**vi**·tis). Inflammation of the synovial membrane of a joint. The condition is usually associated with an effusion of fluid within the synovial cavity. **Acute suppurative synovitis.** Acute inflammation of a synovial membrane with production of pus; it is due to an infection. **Bursal synovitis.** Inflammation of a bursa; bursitis. **Chronic purulent synovitis.** An inflammatory condition of a synovial membrane of low virulence, but with pus formation; it is commonly due to infection with the tubercle bacillus. **Chronic serous synovitis.** Long-standing effusion into a synovial cavity, usually of the knee. **Dendritic synovitis.** Synovitis in which villous outgrowths develop from the walls of the cavity. **Dry synovitis.** Synovitis without effusion. **Exanthematous synovitis.** Inflammation of a synovial membrane secondary to an eruptive fever. **Fibrinous synovitis.** Synovitis in which multiple fibrinous bodies develop in the cavity. **Fungous synovitis.** An archaic synonym for tuberculous synovitis or arthritis. **Gonorrhoeal synovitis.** Acute or chronic inflammation of synovial cavities mostly in association with joints; it is due to infection with the gonococcus. **Synovitis hyperplastica.** Synovitis that is usually tuberculous. **Lipomatous synovitis.** Synovitis associated with an excessive deposit of subsynovial fat. **Pigmented villonodular synovitis.** A disease in which there is tumour-like proliferation of the synovium, sometimes haemorrhagic, giving rise to pain and swelling of 1 or more joints and leading to destruction of cartilage and bone erosion. **Purulent synovitis.** Synovitis with pus within the synovial cavity. **Scarlatinal synovitis.** Synovitis complicating scarlet fever. **Serous synovitis.** Synovitis with serous fluid in the sac. **Synovitis sicca.** Dry synovitis (see above). **Simple synovitis.** Traumatic synovitis with clear synovial effusion. **Syphilitic synovitis.** Synovitis due to syphilis. **Tendinous synovitis.** Inflammation of a tendon sheath; tenosynovitis. **Traumatic synovitis.** Synovitis resulting from injury or over-use. **Tuberculous synovitis.** Synovitis due to infection by the tubercle bacillus. **Urethral synovitis.** Gonorrhoeal rheumatism. **Vaginal synovitis.** Tenosynovitis. [synovia, Gk *-itis* inflammation.]

synovium (si·**no**·ve·um). A synovial membrane.

synphalangism (sin·**fal**·an·jizm). A condition in which the joints of certain fingers or toes are fused. [Gk *syn, phalagx* finger or toe.]

syntactics (sin·**tak**·tiks). The branch of semantics which concerns signs and the relations between signs. [Gk *syn, taxis* arrangement.]

syntasis (**sin**·tas·is). Stretching. [Gk *syn, teinein* to stretch.]

syntaxis (sin·**tax**·is). 1. Articulation; the ordering of words in speech. 2. The reduction of a dislocation or hernia. 3. A suture. [Gk *syn, taxis* arrangement.]

syntectic (sin·**tek**·tik). Pertaining to syntexis.

syntenosis (sin·ten·**o**·sis). A hinge joint, such as a phalangeal articulation, which is protected by tendons. [Gk *syn, tenon* tendon.]

syntexis (sin·**tex**·is). Wasting; emaciation; cachexia. [Gk melting together.]

synthermal (sin·**ther**·mal). Isothermal; possessing the same temperature. [Gk *syn, therme* heat.]

synthescope (**sin**·thes·kope). An apparatus for observing the phenomena taking place at the interface between 2 liquids. [Gk *synthesis* a placing together, *skopein* to watch.]

synthesis (**sin**·thes·is). 1. In chemistry, the building up in the laboratory of a more complex compound from simpler compounds or from its elements; the term is also applied to similar building up of compounds in plant or animal tissues. 2. The building up of a unit from separate items; more specifically in psycho-analysis, the building up of the structure of the personality, especially with material from the subconscious. **Co-ordinated enzyme synthesis.** The rates of synthesis of 2 or more enzymes are observed to vary together on induction or repression because they are subject to a common system of genetic regulation, e.g. they belong to the same operon. **DNA repair synthesis.** DNA synthesis which takes place as a result of DNA repair. **Morphological synthesis.** The differentiation of cells, tissues and organs, in development or regeneration. [Gk a placing together.]

See also: FOURIER.

synthesize (**sin**·thes·ize). To form by synthesis.

synthetase (**sin**·thet·aze). An enzyme that catalyses the synthesis of a substance. **Fatty acid synthetase.** The enzyme complex which converts acetyl CoA and malonyl CoA into fatty acid CoA, utilizing NADPH. **Glutamine synthetase.** The enzyme responsible for glutamine synthesis from glutamate and ammonia. ATP is simultaneously converted to ADP and phosphate. **Glycogen synthetase.** The enzyme responsible for glycogen synthesis from UDP glucose. It exists in 2 forms, one active, the other physiologically inactive. The interconversion is affected by glucose, insulin and glycogen. [synthesis, *-ase* enzyme.]

synthetic (sin·**thet**·ik). 1. Formed by or relating to synthesis. 2. Produced artificially.

synthetize (**sin**·thet·ize). Synthesize.

synthorax (sin·**thor**·ax). A twin monster fused at the sternum. [Gk *syn*, thorax.]

syntone (**sin**·tone). The condition of harmonious adjustment to the environment. [see foll.]

syntonic (sin·**ton**·ik). Reacting to the environment with spontaneity, directness and immediacy, and with warm emotional tone. The syntonic personality is frequently used to include all forms of the cycloid personality, but especially denotes the more balanced types. [Gk *syn, tonos* tone.]

syntonin (**sin**·to·nin). Acid albumin; a substance formed by the action of dilute acids on albumin.

syntopic (sin·**top**·ik). Applied to any anatomical description locating an organ with reference to its surrounding organs. [see foll.]

syntopy (**sin**·to·pe). The situation of an organ relative to the surrounding organs. [Gk *syn, topos* place.]

syntoxoid (sin·**tox**·oid). Toxoid having the same affinity for antitoxin as the toxin from which it was derived. [Gk *syn*, toxoid.]

syntripsis (sin·**trip**·sis). A comminuted fracture; the comminution of a bone. [Gk *syn, tribein* to rub.]

syntrophism (**sin**·tro·fizm). The ability of 2 strains of bacteria to grow in mixed culture in a medium which will not allow growth of either alone. This is due to the excretion by each organism of growth factors required by the other. [Gk *syn, trophe* nourishment.]

syntrophoblast (sin·tro·fo·blast). Syncytiotrophoblast.

syntrophus (**sin**·tro·fus). An inherited or congenital disease. [Gk *syntrophos* reared together.]

syntropic (sin·**trop**·ik). 1. Characterized by syntropy; inclined or orientated in 1 direction, as in the case of the ribs. 2. Denoting a well-balanced personality. [see foll.]

syntropy (**sin**·tro·pe). The tendency towards a common point, as when physical features incline the same way, or when diseases augment one another. [Gk *syn, trepein* to turn.]

synulosis (sin·ew·**lo**·sis). The formation of a cicatrix. [Gk *syn, oule* scar, *-osis* condition.]

synulotic (sin·ew·**lot**·ik). 1. Favourable to cicatrization. 2. Applied to anything which promotes cicatrization. [see prec.]

Synura (sin·**ewr**·ah). A genus of flagellate Protozoa. The species are notorious for giving an unpleasant taste of ripe cucumbers to drinking water.

syphilelcos, syphilelcus (sif·il·**el**·kos, sif·il·**el**·kus). A syphilitic chancre. [syphilis, Gk *helkos* ulcer.]

syphilid, syphilide (**sif**·il·id, **sif**·il·ide). Bullous; an eruption occurring during the secondary or tertiary stage of syphilis or as a manifestation of inherited syphilis. **Acneiform syphilid.** Acuminate or rounded pustules, resembling the lesions of both acne vulgaris and variola; the eruption is widespread and usually is seen in the early secondary stage. **Acuminate papular syphilid.** An eruption of large or small, pointed follicular papules; less common than the flat papular eruption. **Annular syphilid.** Ring-like lesions formed by clusters of papules, which usually form on the face or neck in association with a typical secondary eruption in other areas. **Bullous syphilid.** An eruption formerly called *syphilitic pemphigus;* the lesions, which are relatively few in number, are discrete blebs each surrounded by a red areola. The contents of the blisters rapidly become pustular; healing occurs after desiccation. **Syphilide cornée.** Circumscribed horny accumulations on the palms. **Conymbose syphilid.** An eruption consisting of relatively large papules, each surrounded by a cluster of small papules. **Echthymatous syphilid.** An eruption of large flat pustules, from the contents of which yellow-brown crusts form; these cover shallow ulcers. **Erythematous syphilid.** A rose-coloured macular eruption. **Flat papular syphilid.** An accurate descriptive term for one of the commoner secondary eruptions. **Follicular syphilid.** Papular lesions arising in association with the follicles. **Framboesiform syphilid.** An eruption which usually occurs on the face, scalp or neck, formed by aggregations of hypertrophic papules, resembling a raspberry. **Gummatous syphilid.** Lesions of tertiary syphilis formed by gummata. **Impetiginous syphilid.** An eruption formerly called impetigo syphilitica; a variety of pustulocrustaceous eruption. **Lenticular syphilid.** An eruption of small flat papules. **Lichenoid syphilid.** One characterized by flat-topped papules resembling lichen. **Macular syphilid.** One characterized by flat stains without papulation, usually red or coppery in hue. **Maculoroseo-**

lar syphilid. One characterized by a rosy discoloration, often resembling pityriasis rosea. **Miliary syphilid.** An eruption of small follicular papules, often closely aggregated in groups. **Nodular syphilid.** Few or numerous superficial gummata which tend to be aggregated in small irregular groups, or to be arranged in annular or serpiginous patterns, or to coalesce and form plaques. **Nummular syphilid.** A syphilitic eruption in which the lesions tend to be grouped in small discs. **Palmar syphilid.** A syphilitic eruption on the palms, usually of the macular, maculopapular or papulosquamous variety. **Papular syphilid.** A secondary syphilitic eruption characterized by the formation of papules. **Papulopustular syphilid.** One characterized by the presence of papules and pustules. **Papulosquamous syphilid.** An eruption of papules, each of which is covered with yellowish-white scales. **Pemphigoid syphilid.** Bullous syphilid (see above). **Plantar syphilid.** A syphilitic eruption on the soles, similar to palmar syphilid. **Psoriasiform syphilid.** A papulosquamous syphilid having some resemblance to psoriasis. **Pustular syphilid.** A pustular syphilitic eruption, the lesions of which may be small or large, flat or pustulocrustaceous. **Pustulocrustaceous syphilid.** An eruption in which the lesions become pustular; crusts are formed under which ulceration usually occurs. **Roseolar syphilid.** A widespread, symmetric eruption of pinkish-red macules; one of the commonest early syphilids. **Rupial syphilid.** A pustulorcrustaceous eruption associated with superficial ulceration. **Secondary syphilid.** Any eruption due to syphilis seen during the secondary stage. **Serpiginous syphilid.** An eruption, usually of limited extent, in which the lesions (which are superficial gummata) form a sinuous pattern. **Squamous syphilid.** A dry, scaly eruption. **Tertiary syphilid.** An eruption formed by gummata. **Tubercular syphilid.** Occasionally used to refer to forms of papular syphilid; it usually connotes a gummatous eruption, tubercular meaning nodular. **Tuberoserpiginous syphilid.** A condition due to syphilis, characterized by nodules and tumours of serpiginous shapes within the skin. **Varicelliform syphilid.** A vesicular eruption resembling chickenpox, occurring as a symptom of secondary syphilis. Although described by Jonathan Hutchinson, Radcliffe Crocker, Duhring and others, its existence has often been doubted. **Varioliform syphilid.** A generalized pustular syphilid resembling smallpox. **Vegetating syphilid.** Hypertrophic papular lesions, occurring particularly on the mucocutaneous junctions on the genitalia on the perianal area and elsewhere; condylomata lata. Stelwagon described the formation of vegetations arising from gummatous ulcers and included this condition, now very rare, as a form of vegetating syphilid. **Vitiligoid syphilid.** Round, oval or irregular areas of depigmentation of the skin, occurring as a symptom of secondary syphilis. The neck is the site of election, and the condition is seen most frequently in women. There may be some increase in pigmentation of the adjacent skin. Localized areas of pigmentation may develop to mark the sites where papules have been present. Generalized pigmentation due to syphilis has been described. [Fr. *syphilide.*]

syphilidophthalmia (sif·il·id·of·**thal'**·me·ah). Ophthalmia caused by syphilitic infection.

syphilimetry (sif·il·**im**·et·re). A term employed only in relation to the quantitative serological test for syphilis devised by Vernes [obsolete term]. [syphilis, meter.]

syphilis (**sif**·il·is). Lues venerea. A contagious venereal disease affecting primarily the skin or mucous membrane of the genitalia, later involving any organ or tissue and following a prolonged course, with intermissions and recrudescences, over many years. Syphilis is not known to affect any animal in the natural state, but the higher apes and the rabbit are susceptible to experimental inoculation. The specific agent is a slender spiral organism, the *treponema pallidum* (*Spirochaeta pallida*), which is present in large numbers in the lesions of the early stages of the disease. It is stained with difficulty and is most accurately detected by dark-ground microscopy. The spirochaete of syphilis is indistinguishable on microscopy from that of yaws or of pinta. The disease is divided in its natural history into 2 phases, *Early syphilis* and *Late syphilis.* The early phase lasts for 2 years, the patient remaining contagious. In the late phase the patient is not contagious, but cure with serological reversal is not attained as non-virulent, but antigenic, treponema persist in the lymph nodes. **Acquired syphilis.** Syphilitic infection occurring at any time after birth. **Acute meningeal syphilis.** Cerebrospinal involvement in the secondary stage. **Congenital syphilis.** Generalized syphilitic disease in the infant due to infection *in utero.* It is characterized by wasting, coryza (snuffles), rashes and osteitis in the first few months of life, and in later childhood by interstitial keratitis, deafness and notches in the cutting edge of the permanent incisor teeth (Hutchinson's triad). Signs of syphilis may be absent in infancy yet appear in late childhood or adolescence (*syphilis hereditaria tarda*). **Constitutional syphilis.** Generalized distribution of the infection throughout the body. **Syphilis d'emblée.** Constitutional syphilis developing without the formation of a primary sore. **Extragenital syphilis.** Syphilis commencing from a primary lesion situated on any part of the body other than the genital organs. Chancres may appear on the lip, cheek, finger, tonsil or tongue, and, rarely, on other parts of the skin. **Syphilis innocentum, Syphilis insontium.** Syphilis acquired by accidental transmission and not by coitus. **Marital syphilis.** Syphilis acquired from a spouse. **Meningovascular syphilis.** Acute meningeal syphilis (see above). **Non-venereal syphilis.** Endemic syphilis occurring in primitive communities. [The name is derived from H. Fracastoims' medieval poem "Syphilis sive Morbus Gallicus", 1530, which sums up the knowledge of the time concerning the disease. The shepherd hero of the poem is named "Syphilus". Etymology doubtful, possibly Gk *syn, philein* to love.]

syphilitic (sif·il·**it**·ik). Of the nature of, characterized by, or affected with syphilis.

syphilization (**sif**·il·i·**za'**·shun). 1. Attempted immunization against syphilis by inoculation with *Treponema pallidum.* 2. The gradual development of a relative immunity to syphilis that develops in a community as a result of generations of experience of the disease.

syphiloderm, syphiloderma (**sif**·il·o·derm, sif·il·o·**der**·mah). A syphilid; any syphilitic infection of the skin. [*syphilis,* Gk *derma* skin.]

syphilodermatous (**sif**·il·o·**der'**·mat·us). Characterized by syphilitic skin lesions. [see prec.]

syphilogenesis (**sif**·il·o·**jen'**·es·is). The origin and development of syphilis. [syphilis, Gk *genein* to produce.]

syphilogenous (sif·il·**oj**·en·us). Causing syphilis. [see prec.]

syphiloid (**sif**·il·oid). Resembling syphilis. [syphilis, Gk *eidos* form.]

syphiloma (sif·il·**o**·mah). Any tumour of a syphilitic nature; a gumma. [syphilis, Gk *-oma* tumour.]

syphilomania (**sif**·il·o·**ma'**·ne·ah). A morbid dread of contracting syphilis. [syphilis, mania.]

syphilomatous (sif·il·**o**·mat·us). Of the nature of a syphiloma; gummatous.

syphilonychia (**sif**·il·on·**ik'**·e·ah). Syphilis affecting 1 or more nails; it may occur at any stage of the disease. **Syphilonychia exulcerans.** Syphilitic infection with ulceration affecting a nail or nails; usually the signs are of an ulcerative perionyxis. **Syphilonychia sicca.** Abnormality of the nails, without ulceration, due to syphilis. [syphilis, Gk *onyx* nail.]

syphilopathy (sif·il·**op**·ath·e). Any syphilitic manifestation. [syphilis, Gk *pathos* disease.]

syphilophobe (**sif**·il·o·fobe). An individual affected with syphilophobia.

syphilophobia (**sif**·il·o·**fo'**·be·ah). A morbid dread of becoming infected with syphilis, or a condition in which the individual believes, incorrectly, that he is infected with syphilis. [syphilis, Gk *phobos* fear.]

syphilophobic (**sif**·il·o·**fo'**·bik). Affected with syphilophobia.

syphilopsychosis (**sif**·il·o·**si'**·ko·sis). Any mental disease arising from syphilitic infection. [syphilis, psychosis.]

syphilosis (sif·il·o·sis). Any generalized syphilitic disease. [syphilis, Gk *-osis* condition.]
syphilotherapy (sif·il·o·ther'·ap·e). Treatment of syphilis. [syphilis, Gk *therapeia* treatment.]
syphilotropic (sif·il·o·trop·ik). Having a predisposition to the effects of the syphilitic virus; applied to certain tissues. [syphilis, *trepein* to turn.]
syphonoma (si·fon·o·mah). Cylindroma.
syrigmophonia (sir·ig·mo·fo'·ne·ah). 1. A sibilant râle. 2. A whistling sound which accompanies the *s*-sound in speech. 3. A whistling voice. [Gk *syrigmos* whistle, *phone* sound.]
syrigmus (sir·ig·mus). Tinnitus; a subjective ringing sound in the ears. [Gk *syrigmos* whistle.]
syringadenoma (sir·ing·ad·en·o'·mah). A tumour of the ducts of the sweat glands. **Syringadenoma papilliferum.** A single warty plaque, usually on the scalp, with areas of crusting and occasionally tiny cysts; histologically, a naevoid adenoma of the ducts of sweat glands. [Gk *syrigx* tube, *aden* gland, *-oma* tumour.]
syringadenosus (sir·ing·ad·en·o'·sus). Syringadenous.
syringadenous (sir·ing·ad·en·us). Peculiar to the sweat glands. [Gk *syrigx* tube, *aden* gland.]
syringe (sir·inj). An instrument designed to direct fluid, usually under some pressure, into a cavity or into the tissues. Commonly a cylinder fitted with a piston plunger. **Aural syringe.** A large capacity syringe, usually of metal, used mainly in washing wax from the external auditory meatus. **Chip syringe.** A syringe with a rubber bulb, used to project a stream of air into a cavity in a tooth which is being prepared for a filling in order to remove debris. **Continuous-flow syringe.** A syringe designed for tissue infiltration; by pulling back the piston the barrel of the syringe is refilled from an adjacent reservoir of solution. An example of this type of syringe is that devised by Dunn. **Dental syringe.** One of the many forms of syringe used in the practice of dental surgery. **Ear syringe.** Aural syringe (see above). **Enema syringe.** A syringe designed for giving enemata, e.g. Higginson's syringe. However there is a tendency now to give enemata with a funnel and rubber tube and to depend on gravity rather than manual force for introducing the fluid. **Hypodermic syringe.** A syringe, commonly of glass or of glass and metal, which delivers immediately under the skin an injection of fluid through a fine hollow needle. **Lacrimal syringe.** A small syringe, with a special cannula fitted, for washing through the lacrimal canaliculi, sac and nasolacrimal duct. **Micrometer syringe.** A hypodermic syringe fitted with a micrometer screw, and utilized in the measurement and delivery of minimal quantities of fluid for injection, e.g. into a living cell in micromanipulation. **Pyorrhoea syringe.** A syringe with a fine nozzle used for irrigating pyorrhoea pockets. **"Record" syringe.** A graduated metal and glass syringe of various sizes. The name was originally a proprietary one, but the term has come to be used for any metal and glass syringe. **Rectal syringe.** Enema syringe (see above). **Tooth syringe.** A form of dental syringe. **Tuberculin syringe.** A narrow, small-capacity, carefully calibrated syringe, used to deliver small doses of tuberculin. **Two-way (three-way) syringe.** A syringe with an adjustable tap which allows of the deviation of fluid in 2 or 3 directions; used in aspiration of pleural effusion and in direct donor/patient transfusion. **Urethral syringe.** A conical glass syringe with a rubber bulb, used in anaesthetizing the urethra; Canny Ryall syringe. **Vaginal syringe.** A glass syringe used in vaginal irrigations. **Wound syringe.** A glass syringe with a conical nozzle and a rubber or cotton plunger. [Gk *syrigx* tube.]

See also: ANEL, CANNY RYALL, DUNN, HIGGINSON, LABAT, LUER, MARTIN, ROUX (P. P. E.), WAITE.
syringeal (sir·in·je·al). 1. Pertaining to the pharyngotympanic tube. 2. Of the nature of a fistula. [Gk *syrigx* tube.]
syringectomy (sir·in·jek·to·me). The operation of excising the walls of a fistula. [Gk *syrigx* tube, *temnein* to cut.]
syringenin (sir·in·jen·in). Dimethoxyconiferyl alcohol, $OHC_6H_2(OCH_3)_2CH{=}CHCH_2OH$. The aglycone present in syringin.
syringin (sir·in·jin). $C_{17}H_{24}O_9$, a glucoside of the lilac, *Syringa vulgaris,* said to be of value as an antiperiodic in malaria. It hydrolyses to glucose and syringenin.
syringious (sir·in·je·us). Fistulous. [Gk *syrigx* tube.]
syringitis (sir·in·ji·tis). Inflammation of the pharyngotympanic tube. [Gk *syrigx* tube, *-itis* inflammation.]
syringobulbia (sir·ing·go·bul'·be·ah). Cavitation within the medulla oblongata analogous to, and often accompanying, syringomyelia, and causing progressive lower cranial nerve palsies. [Gk *syrigx* tube, bulb.]
syringocele, syringocoele (sir·ing·go·seel). 1. The normal central canal of the spinal cord. 2. A meningomyelocele in which there is a cavity in the ectopic spinal cord. [Gk *syrigx* tube, *koilia* hollow.]
syringocystadenoma (sir·ing·go·sist·ad·en·o'·mah). A condition first described by Biesiadecki and Kaposi in 1872 as lymphangioma tuberosum multiplex; chronic, painless, soft, white or pink, slightly elevated, small, dome-shaped lesions, usually seen in adult women in the axillae or on the shoulders or chest. These benign, cystic, epithelial tumours are derived from the ducts of sweat glands. [Gk *syrigx* tube, cystadenoma.]
syringocystoma (sir·ing·go·sist·o'·mah). A cystic tumour of the sweat glands; one originating in the hair follicles. [Gk *syrigx* tube, *kystis* cyst, *-oma* tumour.]
syringo-encephalia (sir·ing·go·en·kef·a'·le·ah). Abnormal cavitation in the substance of the brain. [Gk *syrigx* tube, *egkephalos* brain.]
syringo-encephalomyelia (sir·ing·go·en·kef·al·o·mi·e'·le·ah). A condition characterized by the formation of cavities in the brain substance and in the spinal cord. [Gk *syrigx* tube, *egkephalos* brain, *myelos* marrow.]
syringoid (sir·ing·goid). Of the nature of a tube; fistulous. [Gk *syrigx* tube, *eidos* form.]
syringoma (sir·ing·go·mah). Adenoma of the sweat glands. [Gk *syrigx* tube, *-oma* tumour.]
syringomeningocele (sir·ing·go·men·ing'·go·seel). A meningocele which connects with the central canal of the spinal cord. [Gk *syrigx* tube, *menigx* membrane, *kele* tumour.]
syringomyelia (sir·ing·go·mi·e'·le·ah). The presence in the spinal cord, particularly the cervical region, of elongated central fluid-containing cavities surrounded by gliosis and probably resulting from congenital partial obstruction of the flow of cerebrospinal fluid. Symptoms commonly present in early adult life include muscular wasting in the upper limbs, spastic weakness of the legs and extensive loss of pain and thermal sensibility. The disease is usually progressive but may sometimes be treated successfully by surgery. [Gk *syrigx* tube, *myelos* marrow.]

See also: SCHLESINGER (H.).
syringomyelitis (sir·ing·go·mi·el·i'·tis). An inflammatory condition of the spinal cord marked by the development of cavities in its substance. [Gk *syrigx* tube, *myelos* marrow, *-itis* inflammation.]
syringomyelocele (sir·ing·go·mi'·el·o·seel). A form of spina bifida including protrusion of membranes and spinal cord. [Gk *syrigx* tube, *myelos* marrow, *kele* hernia.]
syringomyelus (sir·ing·go·mi'·el·us). A condition of dilatation of the central canal of the spinal cord marked by the transformation of the grey matter into connective tissue and the formation of a cavity. [Gk *syrigx* tube, *myelos* marrow.]
syringopontia (sir·ing·go·pon'·she·ah). A cavity formed in the pons in similar fashion to that formed in syringomyelia. [Gk *syrigx* tube, pons.]
Syringospora (sir·ing·go·spor'·ah). The generic name proposed by Quinquand (1868) for the thrush fungus group now known as *Candida.* [Gk *syrigx* tube, *sporos* seed.]
syringosystrophy (sir·ing·go·sis'·tro·fe). Tubotorsion; the torsion of a tube, such as the uterine tube. [Gk *syrigx* tube, *systrophe* a twisting.]
syringotome (sir·ing·go·tome). An instrument used in incising a fistula. [Gk *syrigx* tube, *temnein* to cut.]

syringotomy (sir·ing·got·o·me). Operative treatment incising a fistula, especially an anal fistula. [see prec.]

syrinx (sir·ingx). 1. The pharyngotympanic (eustachian) tube. 2. A fistula. [Gk *syrigx* tube.]

Syrosingopine (si·ro·sin·go·peen). BP Commission approved name for methyl 18-(4-ethoxycarbonyloxy-3,5-dimethoxybenzoyl) reserpate; it is used in the treatment of hypertension.

Syrphidae (ser·fid·e). A family of the dipteran sub-order Cyclorrhapha; hover flies. The genus *Eristalis* is of medical interest. [Gk *syrphos* a fly, *eidos* form.]

Syrphus (ser·fus). A genus of Diptera; hover flies. The larvae, normally free-living and carnivorous, have been recorded in accidental intestinal myiasis. [Gk *syrphos* a fly.]

syrup (sir·up). A liquid medicament for oral administration, containing a large percentage of sugar either for the purpose of flavouring or as a preservative, or both. **Syrup of Ferrous Phosphate with Quinine and Strychnine BPC 1959.** A syrup composed of the phosphates of ferrous iron, quinine and strychnine, with glycerin; Easton's syrup. It was at one time a most popular tonic, but is now replaced by tablets of ferrous sulphate. **Compound Syrup of Figs BPC 1959.** A syrup containing extracts of rhubarb, senna, cascara and fig; a laxative. **Ginger Syrup BP 1963.** Strong tincture of ginger (5 per cent) in simple syrup; a carminative. **Syrup of Liquid Glucose BPC 1959.** A syrup composed of liquid glucose (1 part) and simple syrup (2 parts); used in massing pills. **Compound Syrup of Hypophosphites BPC 1959.** A tonic syrup containing the hypophosphites of calcium, manganese, potassium, quinine, strychnine and iron, flavoured with a little chloroform water. **Lemon Syrup BP 1958.** An alcoholic extract of fresh lemon peel mixed with citric acid and syrup; used in cough mixtures and as a flavouring. **Orange Syrup BP 1963.** Tincture of orange (1 part) diluted with simple syrup to 8 parts; a flavouring. **Simple Syrup BP 1958.** Sugar (2 parts by weight) dissolved by gentle heat in water (1 part by weight) and used as a basis for many medicated syrups. **Syrup of Squills BPC 1959.** Vinegar of squill mixed with simple syrup; used in cough mixtures. **Syrup of Tolu BP 1968.** A syrup containing tolu balsam; the fragrant volatile oil in this balsam makes it an agreeable constituent of "cough mixtures". **Syrup of Virginian Prune, Syrup of Wild Cherry BPC 1959.** An aqueous extract of wild cherry bark mixed with glycerin, sugar and water; used to alleviate coughs. [Arabic *sharab.*]

See also: DUSART, EASTON, GIBERT, PARRISH.

syrupus (sir·up·us). Syrup. Before 1953 syrups were listed officially as *Syrupi.* **Syrupus Allii BPC 1949.** A syrup containing about 18 per cent of the expressed juice of *Allium sativum* Linn.; it has an expectorant action and can be used in bronchitis and whooping-cough. Claims for its use in tuberculosis have not been substantiated. **Syrupus Calcii Lactophosphatis BPC 1949.** Calcium lactate and phosphoric acid in a syrup flavoured with orange-flower water; a tonic. **Syrupus Cocillanae Compositus BPC 1949.** A syrup containing cocillana, euphorbia, senaga, squill, tartar emetic, codeine phosphate, menthol and glycerin; for coughs in adults. **Syrupus Papaveris BPC 1949.** A syrup containing liquid extract of poppy; a sedative incorporated in cough mixtures. [L.]

sys specific (sis spes·if·ik). An Indian "cure" for dysentery and diarrhoea, consisting of powders of calcium carbonate and sometimes containing opium.

syspasia (sis·pa·ze·ah). Inability to speak owing to muscle spasm. [Gk *syspasis* a contracting.]

syssarcosis (sis·sar·ko·sis). Muscular articulation; the union of bones by muscular tissue as in the connection between the patella and the femur. [Gk *syn, sarx* flesh, *-osis* condition.]

syssomus (sis·so·mus). A twin monster in which the bodies are completely or partially joined, but the 2 heads are separate. [Gk *syn, soma* body.]

systaltic (sis·tal·tik). Contracting and dilating alternately; pulsating. [Gk *systaltikos* contracting.]

systasis (sis·tas·is). Consistency; density. [Gk bringing together.]

systatic (sis·tat·ik). Characterized by the simultaneous affection of several sensory faculties. [see prec.]

system (sis·tem). 1. A set of connected things, a combination of parts. 2. The body as a whole. 3. A method of arrangement or classification. 4. A group of organs united in a common function; as the digestive system. 5. A term employed for a particular cult or method of instruction in medicine, often associated with the name of its propounder, e.g. the paracelsian system, enunciated by Paracelsus. **ABO system.** *See* BLOOD GROUP (under GROUP). **Accessory portal system.** A compensatory anastomosis between the veins in the liver or its capsule and general systemic veins such as the phrenic and intercostals. These are seen where the liver and diaphragm are uncovered by peritoneum, in the falciform ligament and in any peritoneal adhesions which may be present. **Aesthesiodic system.** The sensory pathways of the spinal cord. **Alimentary system.** Digestive system (see below). **Arch-loop-whorl system.** The primary classification of fingerprints, based upon the arrangement of the lines of the skin pattern into 4 types, arch-, loop-, whorl- or composite form. **Autonomic nervous system [systema nervosum autonomicum (NA)].** That part of the central and peripheral nervous system which regulates the activity of structures not normally under voluntary control, e.g. smooth muscle wherever found and gastric glands. It is divided into 2 complementary parts, sympathetic and parasympathetic, having opposite action. **Blood vascular system.** The whole of the closed system of vessels, including arteries, arterioles, capillaries, venules and veins, in which the blood is circulated by the heart which also forms part of the system. **Borstal system.** A system of detention of young criminals based upon the idea of removing them from bad environment and allowing the exertion of wholesome influences and discipline. **Buffer system.** A mixture of buffers designed to produce a determined buffer action. **Bulbospiral system.** The muscle bundles of the heart which are associated with the primitive infundibulum and the root of the aorta. **Cardiovascular system.** The heart and blood vessels with their nerve supply. **Case system.** The method of clinical instruction which is based upon the thorough study, analysis and logical deduction of a diagnosis of reported cases. **Centimetre-gram-second system.** A system of physical units in which the unit of length is the centimetre, the unit of weight the gram, and the unit of time the second. **Central nervous system [systema nervosum centrale (NA)].** The brain and spinal cord; the main system by means of which sensations are co-ordinated and responses organized. **Cerebellorubral system.** The efferent system of the dentate nucleus, which relays in the opposite red nucleus. **Cerebellorubrospinal system.** The pathway by which impulses from the cerebellum reach the spinal cord via the red nucleus. **CGS system.** Centimetre-gram-second system (see above). **Chromaffin system.** The system of cells which give a chromaffin reaction due to their contents of adrenaline and its derivatives, including the medulla of a suprarenal gland and the paraganglia of the autonomic nervous system. **Circulatory system.** Cardiovascular system (see above). **Closed ecological system.** A system which provides living conditions in a closed space by re-using all waste products. A *closed respiratory gas system* is a closed space in which carbon dioxide is washed from the expired air and oxygen is added to a pressure adequate to support life. **Colloidal system.** The disperse and continuous phases of a colloidal solution considered together; such a system may be a combination of any 2 of the 3 states of matter, e.g. liquid/gas, as in mists, solid/gas, as in smokes, solid/liquid, as in sols, or liquid/liquid, as in emulsions. **Corticopontocerebellar system, Corticostrionigral system.** Extrapyramidal system (see below). **Craniosacral autonomic nervous system.** The parasympathetic division of the autonomic nervous system, so called because its outflow occurs in the 3rd, 7th, 9th, 10th and 11th cranial nerves and the 2nd, 3rd and 4th sacral nerves. **Dentinal system.** The tubes radiating in the dentine from the surface of the tooth pulp. **Dermal system, Dermoid system.** The skin and appendages. **Digestive system [apparatus digestorius (systema digestorium) (NA)].** A collective term for the organs concerned with the process of conversion of food into material suitable for absorption, with the absorption of these and other materials ingested by mouth, and with the elimination of those constituents which are unabsorbed or excreted intact. **Dioptric system.** A system of lenses or other refracting surfaces and media, for the purpose of refracting light and having a certain dioptric power, e.g. the eye. **Disperse system, Dispersion system.** Colloidal system (see above). **Endocrine system.** The system comprising the glands of internal secretion. **Endothelial system.** Reticulo-endothelial system (see below). **Exteroceptive nervous system.** That part of the nervous system concerned in the perception of external stimuli. **Exterofective nervous system.** The nervous mechanisms concerned in adaptation to the external environment. **Extrapyramidal system.** A widespread motor system including all motor pathways from the brain that do not run in the pyramidal tracts; applied especially to the outflow from the basal ganglia. **Fogging system.** A procedure in subjective testing for errors of refraction. In hypermetropes fogging of the test types is brought about by placing an excessively convex lens in front of the eye, in myopes by placing a too weak concave lens in front of the eye, so as to prevent unconscious accommodation. **Genital system.** Reproductive system (see below). **Haemolytopoietic system.** The mechanism or system supposed to control the formation and destruction (haemolysis) of the cellular elements in the circulating blood and haemopoietic system. **Haemopoietic system.** The system (which includes the blood, bone marrow, spleen and, to less extent, possibly other organs) concerned with the formation and functioning of blood and its cellular constituents. **Haversian system.** An osteon; a cylindrical unit of compact bone structure built around a central vascular canal and composed of concentric bony lamellae. **Hepatic portal system.** Portal system (see below). **Heterogeneous system.** Any system the components of which may be separated by mechanical means, e.g. a colloidal solution. **Homogeneous system.** Any system the components of which cannot be separated by mechanical means, e.g. a true solution. **Hypophyseal portal system.** A series of vessels which pass from the hypothalamus to the anterior lobe of the pituitary and convey releasing factors to it. **Integumentary system.** Dermal system (see above). **Intermediary system.** A fragmentary haversian system between 2 or more complete haversian systems. **Interofective nervous system.** The autonomic nervous system, concerned in adaptation to the internal environment. **Involuntary nervous system.** Autonomic nervous system (see above). **Kinesodic system.** The motor tracts of the spinal cord. **Kinetic system.** The motor system concerned in reflex, associated and involuntary movements of skeletal muscle. **Labyrinthine system.** The internal ear, consisting of the membranous labyrinth, a hollow, tortuous structure containing fluid known as endolymph, lying within the bony labyrinth containing perilymph. Its most important components are the cochlea and the vestibular apparatus comprising the 3 semicircular canals, the saccule and the utricle. **Life-support system.** A complex which provides the food, water, air and waste-disposal facilities necessary to support life in space. **Limbic system.** A functionally related set of neural structures in the region of the mid-brain activated during motivated behaviour and emotional arousal. **Locomotor system.** Those structures in the body concerned with locomotion; the muscles, bones, joints, vascular and nerve supply of the lower limb. **Lymphatic system [systema lymphaticum (NA)].** A closed vascular system forming an alternative route for the absorption of tissue fluid and its return to the blood. It is composed of lymph vessels and glands and lymphoid tissue in the alimentary canal. The vessels are widely distributed throughout all tissues except the central nervous system and avascular structures. Their presence is doubtful in bone and striped muscle. **Macrophage system.** Reticulo-endothelial system (see below). **Manchester system.** Paterson and Parker system. **Metric system.** The system of weights and measures based upon the metre; the cgs system is derived from it. **Muscular system.** The muscles of the body; usually applied only to the striped muscles. **Neokinetic system.** The corticospinal system regulating voluntary movement. **Nervous system [systema nervosum (NA)].** The nervous tissues of the body; includes the peripheral nerves, spinal cord, ganglia and nerve centres. **Non-rebreathing system.** A system of breathing tubes used in anaesthesia in which all the exhalations of the patient are vented into the air and none of the expired gases is re-inhaled. **Osseous system.** The bones of the body. **Oxidation-reduction system.** Any system in which 1 or more components can undergo reversible oxidation and reduction. The enzyme systems present in living cells provide important examples of oxidation-reduction systems. **Palaeokinetic system.** The phylogenetically old motor systems arising from subcortical structures. **Pallidal system.** The effective neurones of the corpus striatum, located in the globus pallidus. **Palm-and-sole system of identification.** An extension of the Galton system to include the palmar and plantar prints. **Parasympathetic nervous system [pars parasympathica (NA)].** A division of the autonomic nervous system consisting of a cranial part, whose fibres run in the 3rd, 7th, 9th, 10th and possibly 11th cranial nerves, and a spinal part, whose fibres emerge with the anterior primary rami of the 2nd to the 4th sacral nerves which they leave to form the pelvic splanchnic nerves, which enter each pelvic plexus. The emerging fibres of both parts synapse with their postganglionic neurones in, or near, the viscera they supply. **Pedal system.** The caudate nucleus with the anterior and posterior caudate fibres. **Peripheral nervous system [systema nervosum periphericum (NA)].** All the nervous tissue lying outside the central nervous system. **Periscopic lens system.** A series of lenses placed in a tube to transmit the wide field of view obtained at one end of the tube to the other end. **Pin-index system.** An arrangement of pins and slots designed to prevent a patient from receiving a wrong gas from an anaesthetic apparatus when gas cylinders are attached. **Pipeline system.** An arrangement whereby gases used in intensive care and in anaesthesia are supplied to the patient from central stores via gas pipes. **Plenum system.** The forcing of a regulated volume of fresh air into a room, thus expelling the vitiated air. By means of filters, radiators and wet screens the air is cleansed, warmed and moistened, that is "conditioned", as required. In some installations the entering air is warmed and no radiators are provided. **Portal system.** A vessel (or vessels) which breaks up into capillaries at either end, such as the portal vein or the hypophyseal portal system. **Projection system.** Fibre tracts linking the cerebral cortex with the thalamus and lower nervous structures. **Pyramidal system.** The corticospinal system arising in the motor cortex and subserving voluntary movement. **Redox system.** An abbreviation of oxidation-reduction system (see above). **Reproductive system.** The organs and structures associated with reproduction and with the necessarily preceding procreative act, in men and women; the testes, the external genitalia, the seminal vessels and the prostate in men, and the vulva, vagina, uterine tubes and ovaries in women. **Respiratory system [apparatus respiratorius (systema respiratorium) (NA)].** The lungs and air passages, including the nasal cavities, pharynx, larynx, trachea and main bronchi. **Reticulo-endothelial system.** The collection of specialized endothelial and reticular cells found throughout the body which phagocytose particulate matter and injected colloidal dyes such as trypan blue. Such cells are concentrated in the spleen, bone marrow, liver and lymph glands. **Rubrospinal system.** The efferent pathway from the red nucleus to the spinal cord. **SI system.** The internationally agreed system of units based on the metre, kilogram, second, ampere, kelvin, mole and candela. **Sinospiral system.** The muscle bundles of the heart which are connected with the primitive sinus venosus. **Somatic nervous system.** The entire nervous system apart from the autonomic nervous system. **Static system.** The motor system concerned in postural muscle contraction. **Supra-opticohypophyseal system.** The efferent pathway from the supra-optic nucleus of the hypothalamus to the neurohypophysis, which regulates the secretion of antidiuretic hormone. **Sympathetic nervous system [pars sympathica (NA)].** A larger subdivision of the autonomic nervous system, consisting of collections of ganglia, nerve cords and plexuses, and supplying the viscera, glands, heart, blood vessels, and unstriped muscle in general. It consists of medullated nerve fibres, white communicating branches [rami communicantes], which run to the ganglia, where they synapse with cells, which in turn give rise to non-medullated fibres, grey communicating branches [rami communicantes (NA)], to supply the structures mentioned with motor fibres; it also contains less well-understood sensory fibres. *See also* GANGLION TRUNK. **Sympathetic nervous system, cephalic and cervical parts [pars cephalica et cervicalis systematis autonomici (NA)].** The part of the autonomic nervous system distributed to the head and neck. It includes the upper thoracic preganglionic fibres of the sympathetic nervous system that are so distributed after relaying in 1 of the 3 cervical ganglia, and those fibres of the cranial parasympathetic nervous system incorporated in the oculomotor, facial and glossopharyngeal nerves. **Sympathetic nervous system, lumbar part [pars abdominalis systematis autonomici (NA)].** Part of the sympathetic trunk in the abdomen, in front of the psoas muscle and behind the peritoneum. **Sympathetic nervous system, oesophageal branches.** Contributions from the greater splanchnic nerves to the oesophageal plexus. **Sympathetic nervous system, pelvic part [pars pelvina systematis autonomici (NA)].** Two converging trunks, each generally containing 4 ganglia, lying on the pelvic surface of the sacrum and coccyx. They may unite inferiorly. Grey communicating branches are given to all sacral and the coccygeal nerves, and branches from the second and third ganglia to the ipsilateral pelvis plexus. **Sympathetic nervous system, thoracic part [pars thoracica systematis autonomici (NA)].** Part of the sympathetic trunk, with the corresponding ganglia which lie on the thorax, on the heads of the ribs and covered by pleura. Differentiated parts are the renal branch [ramus renalis (NA)] and the pulmonary branches of the thoracic ganglia. **Systemic system.** Systemic circulation. *See* CIRCULATION. **Transition system.** An intermediate colloidal system. **Triaxial reference system.** *See* BAYLEY'S TRIAXIAL REFERENCE SYSTEM. **Urinary system.** The organs and viscera whose function is the concentration, filtration and excretion of urine; the kidneys, ureters, bladder and urethra. **Urogenital system [apparatus urogenitalis (systema urogenitale) (NA)].** The excretory system (the organs for the secretion and passage of urine) together with the organs of reproduction. **Vagal autonomic system.** Autonomic nervous system (see above). **Vascular system.** The blood vessels of the body. **Vasomotor system.** The nerve centres, the ganglia and the nerves that control the blood vessels of the body. **Vegetative system.** Autonomic nervous system (see above). **Vestibular system.** Labyrinthrine system (see above). [Gk *systema.*]

See also: BAYLEY, BERTILLON, CONOLLY, GALTON, GRANCHER, HAVERS, HUGUENIN, LING, MCCARTHY (J. F.), MEYER (A.), PARKER (H. M.), PATERSON (J. R. K.), PINEL, RADEMACHER, SAPPEY, WARING.

systematic (sis·tem·**at**·ik). Pertaining to a system or formed in accordance with a system.

systematization (sis·tem·at·i·**za**'·shun). The process of reduction to an organized whole. [system.]

systematize (**sis**·tem·at·ize). To classify in accordance with a system.

systematology (sis·tem·at·**ol**'·o·je). The science of classification. [system, Gk *logos* science.]

systemic (sis·**tem**·ik). 1. Systematic. 2. Relating to the body as a whole, rather than to its individual parts. 3. In cardiology, the circulation supplied by the aorta and its branches, as opposed to the pulmonary circulation.

systemoid (**sis**·tem·oid). 1. Like a system. 2. Describing a tumour that is composed of several kinds of tissue, like a system. [system, Gk *eidos* form.]

systogene (**sis**·to·jeen). Tyramine.

systole (**sis**·to·le). The period during which the heart contracts. **Systole alternans.** Alternate weak and powerful ventricular contractions with regular rhythm. Less blood is injected into the aorta during the weak contractions, and this gives rise to alternating weak and strong pulse waves (alternating pulse). It occurs in association with failure of the left ventricle and other serious cardiac lesions, and usually indicates a poor prognosis. **Anticipated systole.** Premature systole (see below). **Arterial systole.** The period from the commencement of the upstroke of the pulse to the dicrotic notch. **Atrial systole.** The contraction of the atria of the heart which precedes ventricular systole. Its duration is about 0.1 s when the heart rate is 70 per min. **Electrical systole.** The period during which there is electrical activity relating to the stimulation and recovery of the myocardium. The term is applicable to either the atria or the ventricles but is difficult to define in relation to the artria because of the small amplitude of the atrial repolarization potentials; in the ventricle, electrical systole is usually equated with the time from the commencement of the QRS complex to end of the T wave (the QT time), strictly the ill-defined U wave also represents the final part of the repolarization process. **Premature systole.** Systole occurring prematurely as a result of a discharge of an ectopic focus in the atria, atrioventricular node or ventricle (ectopic heart beat). **Ventricular systole.** The contraction of the ventricles of the heart which succeeds atrial systole. Its commencement is signalled by the first heart sound; at a heart rate of 70 per min its duration is about 0.3 s. [Gk contraction.]

systolic (sis·**tol**·ik). Relating to or resulting from a systole.

systremma (sis·**trem**·ah). Muscular cramp in the calf of the leg, producing a hard knot of muscles. [Gk twist.]

syzygial (siz·**ij**·e·al). Relating to a syzygy.

syzygiology (siz·ij·e·**ol**'·o·je). The study of the interrelationship of the parts of an entity rather than the study of the individual parts or functions themselves. [Gk *syzygia* yoke, *logos* science.]

syzygium (siz·**ij**·e·um). 1. Syzygy. 2. A genus of myrtaceous trees including *Syzygium jambolana,* jambul, the bark of which was erroneously believed to be of value in diabetes. The bark and seeds have been used in India as an astringent in diarrhoea. [see foll.]

syzygy (**siz**·ij·e). (pl. *syzygies*). 1. The fusion of parts or organs, each however maintaining its individuality. 2. A micro-organism believed to be produced by conjugation of larval parasites. 3. A zygote. [Gk *syzygia* yoke.]

Szabo, Diorys (fl. 1878). Budapest physician.

Szabo's sign. Sensory loss on the lateral surface of the foot in sciatica.

Szondi test. A personality test in which from each of 6 sets of the pictures of patients (one in each set representing a homosexual, a sadistic murderer, an epileptic, a hysteric, a catatonic, a paranoic, a depressive and a maniac) the subject must select the 2 most liked and most disliked pictures, and must tell stories about the 4 most liked and disliked of the entire series.

Szymanowski, Julius von (b. 1829). Russian surgeon.

Szymanowski operation, Kuhnt-Szymanowski operation. An operation for transverse shortening of the lower eyelid in cases of ectropion: the lateral half of the lid is split between the tarsal and cutaneous layers, a triangle or tarsus from the medial part and a similar triangle of skin from the lateral part are removed, and the wounds are sutured. The lid is shortened by an amount equal to the base of these triangles.

T

tabacism (tab·as·izm). Tabacosis.

tabacosis (tab·ak·o·sis). Tobacco poisoning caused by over-indulgence in the use of tobacco, or by inhaling tobacco dust. **Tabacosis pulmonum.** Pneumoconiosis arising as an occupational disease among workers in tobacco factories. [tobacco, Gk *-osis* condition.]

tabacum (tab·ak·um). Tobacco.

tabagism (tab·aj·izm). Nicotinism; a form of tabacosis resulting from an over-indulgence in tobacco.

tabanid (tab·an·id). A member of the dipterous family Tabanidae.

Tabanidae (tab·an·id·e). A family of Diptera; clegs, horseflies. They are large flies with flat bodies, and the females of many are vicious biters of man. The genera *Chrysops, Haematopota, Pangonia,* and *Tabanus* are of medical interest. [see foll.]

Tabanus (tab·a·nus). A genus of flies of the family Tabanidae; clegs, horseflies. It is world wide and the females of many of the species bite man painfully. They are not known to be secondary hosts of any human parasites, but may act as passive carriers when interrupted feeding causes them to move from host to host rapidly. [L gadfly.]

tabardillo (tab·ar·de·yo). Typhus fever occurring in the elevated regions of Mexico. [Sp. typhus.]

tabasheer (tab·ash·eer). A substance obtained from certain kinds of bamboo; it is used in India for coughs. [Hind.]

tabaxir (tab·ax·eer). Tabasheer.

tabefaction (ta·be·fak·shun). Wasting; emaciation; atrophy. [tabes, L *facere* to make.]

tabella (tab·el·ah). A tablet. The official name before the *British Pharmacopoeia* of 1953. [L.]

tabes (ta·beez). 1. A wasting condition, either of the whole body or of part of it. 2. The term is most commonly used as an abbreviated form of tabes dorsalis (see below). **Abortive tabes.** Tabes that has been arrested in an early stage. **Burnt-out tabes.** Rudimentary tabes (see below). **Cerebral tabes.** Dementia paralytica. **Cervical tabes.** Tabes dorsalis in which the pathological process is most active in the cervical part of the spinal cord and hence the upper extremities are most affected. **Diabetic tabes.** Diabetic peripheral neuropathy with pain, absent reflexes, and sometimes Charcot joints in the lower limbs, associated with absence of the pupillary reaction to light; due to a neuropathic process in the ciliary ganglia and usually called *diabetic pseudotabes.* **Tabes diuretica.** Diabetic neuritis. *See* NEURITIS. **Tabes dolorosa.** Tabes dorsalis in which pain is severe and persistent. **Tabes dorsalis.** A degenerative condition at the root entry zone of posterior roots of the spinal cord and hence of the posterior columns, as a result of neurosyphilis. The patients complain of shooting pains in the limbs and of difficulty in walking, particularly in the dark, and there are often severe paroxysmal attacks of pain and disturbance of function in many organs called *crises.* On examination there is sensory ataxia; bilateral ptosis and Argyll Robertson pupils are found, with loss of deep-pain sensibility, particularly in the tendo calcaneus, loss of deep reflexes, and often Charcot's joints. Also called *locomotor ataxia.* **Tabes ergotica.** A condition due to ergotism, resembling tabes dorsalis. **Hereditary tabes.** 1. Friedreich's ataxia. 2. Tabes dorsalis due to congenital neurosyphilis. **Tabes infantum.** Tabes dorsalis in children with congenital syphilis. **Tabes inferior.** Tabes dorsalis in which the pathological changes are predominant in the lumbar part of the spinal cord and hence the lower limbs are affected most. **Interstitial tabes.** Tabes dorsalis in which there is neuroglial proliferation in the posterior columns and the pathological changes result in part from syphilitic endarteritis of the arterial branches supplying the posterior columns. **Marantic tabes.** Severe cachexia in tabes dorsalis. **Tabes mesenterica.** Tuberculous lymphadenitis of the lymph glands of the mesentery: the *acute* type is usually a sequel to acute infection of the upper respiratory tract; the *chronic* is associated with chronic or recurrent infections of the glands draining the whole of the alimentary canal. **Monosymptomatic tabes.** Tabes dorsalis which presents with only one symptom. **Nerve tabes.** Tabes dorsalis in which the predominant pathological changes are in the posterior columns of the spinal cord as distinct from the root entry zones. **Peripheral tabes.** Pseudotabes due to a peripheral neuropathy, as in diabetes. **Rudimentary tabes.** Abortive tabes; tabes dorsalis in which only a few manifestations of the disease have appeared and it has then stopped progressing. This state of affairs is sometimes referred to as *burnt-out tabes.* **Spasmodic tabes.** Tabes dorsalis in which severe crises occur. **Tabes spinalis.** Tabes dorsalis (see above). **Tabes superior.** Cervical tabes (see above). **Vessel tabes.** A syndrome resembling tabes dorsalis, resulting from syphilitic endarteritis of the arteries supplying the posterior columns of the cord. [L wasting.]

See also: FRIEDREICH.

tabescence (ta·bes·ens). Progressive wasting away; withering; marasmus. [see foll.]

tabescent (ta·bes·ent). Becoming progressively emaciated. [L *tabescere* to waste away.]

tabetic (ta·bet·ik). 1. Relating to or characterized by tabes. 2. Affected with tabes, particularly tabes dorsalis.

tabetiform (ta·bet·e·form). Similar in symptoms to tabes. [tabes, form.]

tabic, tabid (ta·bik, ta·bid). Tabetic.

tabification (ta·bif·ik·a'·shun). The progressive wasting of the body. [tabes, L *facere* to make.]

tablature (tab·lah·tewr). The peculiar formation of the cranial bones consisting as they do of outer and inner tables with an intervening spongy diploë. [see foll.]

table (ta·bl). 1. A flat-topped article of furniture. 2. Any structure that is flat, e.g. in anatomy, table of bone. 3. A setting-out of data in columns, for easy reference. **Operating table.** A long table, usually of metal, on which the patient is positioned for operation. It is usually so constructed that a wide variety of positions can be maintained, so as to give the best access for differing operating procedures. **Periodic table.** An arrangement of the chemical elements in order of their atomic weights, originally made by Mendeléeff in 1869, whereby he was able to demonstrate the occurrence of related elements at regular intervals, and to predict the properties of then unknown elements. The modern arrangement is in order of atomic numbers, and the table is of considerable importance in the theories of atomic structure and valency. **Table of the skull, inner [lamina interna (NA)].** The inner of the two layers of compact bone that enclose the diploë of the skull. **Table of the skull, outer [lamina externa (NA)].** The outer of the two layers of compact bone that enclose the diploë of the skull. **Spin table.** A device designed to investigate the effects of angular motion. **Tilt table.** A platform capable of seesaw motion used to study the response of the circulatory system to gravitational force. **Tilting table.** A variety of prosthesis on which the patient really sits when the site of amputation has been at or about the level of the hip joint. **Water table.** The level at which rock is saturated with water (ground water) which flows over an underlying impervious stratum. [L *tabula* board.]

See also: BERKOW, STINTZING.

tablespoon (**ta**·bl·spoon). A rough measure: a medicinal tablespoon holds 15 ml (0.5 fl. oz). Most domestic tablespoons are too large and should not be used for measuring liquid medicaments. [table, AS *spon.*]

tablet (**tab**·let). A solid disc containing one or more medicaments and prepared by compressing a granulated powder in the die of a suitable machine. The powdered medicament is usually mixed with a disintegrating agent such as starch which swells and causes the tablet to break up when in contact with the gastric fluid. Talc or stearic acid is incorporated to prevent the compressed tablet from sticking to the punches of the machine, and a granulating agent such as syrup, or emulsion of cocoa butter, is necessary to yield a fine flowing material that will not block the machine. Tablets have almost entirely replaced pills as a convenient means of administering medicaments orally (BP 1958). Before 1953 tablets were listed officially as *Tabellae.* The BP 1973 lists tablets of the following: Acetazolamide, Acetomenaphthone, Allopurinol, Alprenolol, Aluminium Hydroxide, Aluminium Phosphate, Aminophylline, Amitriptyline, Amodiaquine, Amphetamine Sulphate, Amylobarbitone, Amylobarbitone Sodium, Antazoline, Ascorbic Acid, Aspirin, Aspirin Phenacetin and Codeine, Atropine Sulphate, Azathioprine, Barbitone Sodium, Bendrofluazide, Benzhexol, Benztropine, Benzylpenicillin, Betamethasone, Betamethasone Sodium Phosphate, Bethanidine, Bisacodyl, Busulphan, Butobarbitone, Calcium Lactate, Caramiphen (68), Carbamazepine, Carbenoxolone, Carbimazole, Carbromal (68), Cascara, Cephalexin, Chlorambucil, Chlorcyclizine, Chloroquine Phosphate, Chloroquine Sulphate, Chlorothiazide, Chlorotrianisene, Chlorpheniramine, Chlorproguanil, Chlorpromazine, Chlorpropamide, Chlorthalidone, Choline Theophyllinate, Clomiphene, Codeine Phosphate, Colchicine, Colistin, Compound Sodium Bicarbonate, Cortisone, Co-trimoxazole, Cyclizine, Cyclobarbitone, Cyclopenthiazide, Cyclophosphamide, Cycloserine, Cyproheptadine, Dapsone, Desipramine, Dexamethasone, Dexamphetamine, Dextromethorphan, Dextromoramide, Diazepam, Dichloralphenazone, Dichlorophen, Dichlorphenamide, Dicyclomine, Dienoestrol, Diethylcarbamazine, Digitoxin, Digoxin, Dihydrocodeine, Di-iodohydroxyquinoline, Diloxanide Furoate, Dimenhydrinate, Dimethisterone, Dydrogesterone, Emetine and Bismuth Iodide, Ephedrine Hydrochloride, Ergometrine, Ergotamine, Erythromycin, Erythromycin Stearate, Ethambutol, Ethinyloestradiol, Ethionamide, Ethisterone, Ethacrynic Acid, Ethopropazine, Ethotoin, Fenfluramine, Ferrous Fumarate, Ferrous Gluconate, Ferrous Succinate, Ferrous Sulphate, Fludrocortisone, Fluoxymesterone, Fluphenazine, Folic Acid, Frusemide, Glutethimide, Glyceryl Trinitrate, Griseofulvin, Guanethidine, Haloperidol, Hydrochlorothiazide, Hydroflumethiazide, Hydroxychloroquine, Hyoscine, Imipramine, Iopanoic Acid, Isocarboxazid, Isoniazid, Isoprenaline, Levodopa, Levorphanol, Liothyronine, Lithium Carbonate, Lucanthone (68), Mecamylamine (68), Meclozine, Melphalan, Mepacrine, Meprobamate, Mepyramine, Mercaptopurine, Metformin, Methadone, Methandienone, Methoin, Methoserpidine, Methotrexate, Methylamphetamine, Methyldopa, Methylergometrine, Methylprednisolone, Methyltestosterone, Methylthiouracil, Methyprylone, Metronidazole, Morphine Sulphate, Nealbarbitone (68), Neomycin, Neostigmine, Nialamide, Niclosamide, Nicotinic Acid, Nicoumalone, Nitrazepam, Nitrofurantoin, Norethandrolone, Norethisterone, Nortriptyline, Novobiocin, Nystatin, Orciprenaline, Orphenadrine Hydrochloride, Oxyphenbutazone, Oxyphencyclimine, Oxytetracycline, Oxytocin, Paracetamol, Pempidine (68), Penicillamine, Pentaerythritol, Pentobarbitone, Perphenazine, Pethidine, Phenazocine, Phenelzine, Phenethicillin, Phenformin, Phenindamine, Phenindione, Phenmetrazine, Phenobarbitone, Phenobarbitone Sodium, Phenolphthalein, Phenoxymethylpenicillin, Phenylbutazone, Phenytoin, Phthalylsulphathiazole, Phytomenadione, Piperazine Adipate, Piperazine Phosphate, Poldine, Potassium Chloride, Practolol, Prednisolone, Prednisone, Prepared Digitalis, Primaquine, Primidone, Probenecid, Procainamide, Prochlorperazine, Procyclidine, Proguanil, Promazine, Promethazine Hydrochloride, Promethazine Theoclate, Propantheline, Propicillin, Propranolol, Propylthiouracil, Protriptyline, Pyrazinamide, Pyridostigmine, Pyrimethamine, Quinalbarbitone, Quinidine Sulphate, Quinine Bisulphate, Quinine Sulphate, Reserpine, Salbutamol, Senna, Slow Lithium Carbonate, Slow Orphenadrine Citrate, Sodium Aminosalicylate, Sodium Calciumedetate, Sodium Chloride, Sodium Citrate, Solapsone (68), Soluble Aspirin, Soluble Aspirin Phenacetin and Codeine, Spironolactone, Stilboestrol, Strong Calciferol, Succinylsulphathiazole, Sulphadiazine, Sulphadimethoxine, Sulphadimidine, Sulphafurazole, Sulphamethizole, Sulphamethoxydiazine, Sulphamethoxypyridazine, Sulphapyridine, Sulphinpyrazone, Sulthiame, Tetracycline, Thiambutosine, Thiamine Hydrochloride, Thioridazine, Thyroid, Thyroxine, Tolazoline, Tolbutamide, Tranylcypromine, Triclofos, Tricyclamol (68), Trifluoperazine, Trimipramine, Triprolidine, Viprynium, Warfarin. **Solution-tablets.** *See* SOLUTION-TABLETS. **Tablet triturate.** A solution-tablet, used for convenience in making injections; it consists of a medicament made into a tablet with lactose, which is to be dissolved in sterilized water immediately prior to injection. [Fr. *tablette.*]

tablier (tab·le·a). Pudendal apron; enlarged nymphae. [Fr. apron.]

taboo (tab·**oo**). 1. Something which is both sacred and forbidden. 2. A prohibition imposed by religion or social custom upon any particular thing. [Polynesian *tabu.*]

taboparalysis (**ta**·bo·par·**al**'·is·is). Taboparesis. [tabes, paralysis.]

taboparesis (**ta**·bo·par·**e**'·sis). The association of the symptoms of general paralysis of the insane (general paresis) with those of tabes dorsalis.

tabophobia (ta·bo·**fo**·be·ah). A morbid dread of being affected with tabes. [tabes, Gk *phobos* fear.]

tabula (**tab**·ew·lah). Table. [L board.]

tabular (**tab**·ew·lar). 1. Pertaining to a list. 2. Having the characteristics of a table; laminar. 3. Like a table in shape. [see prec.]

tacahout (tak·ah·**hoot**). A gall obtained from tamarisk trees; it contains gallic acid. [Arabic.]

tache (tash). A spot or mark. **Tache anastomotique.** Little's area. **Taches blanches.** White spots associated with the infiltration of leucocytes and bacteria, observed on the liver in certain infectious diseases. **Taches bleuâtres.** Bluish spots said to occur on the skin of certain typhoid fever patients, and usually caused by lice. **Tache cérébrale.** In certain diseases of the brain and meninges, such as meningitis, skin capillaries may be unduly irritable and a line of congestion, sometimes with petechial haemorrhage, may develop on scratching the skin; also called the *meningeal streak.* **Tache laiteuse.** Small localized white areas of adhesion in the serous membranes, especially the pericardium, or small collections of reticulo-endothelial cells in the peritoneum and pleura. **Tache méningéale.** Tache cérébrale (see above). **Tache motrice.** A motor end-plate in unstripped muscle. **Tache noir.** A local lesion occurring at the point of infection in certain rickettsial fevers, e.g. fièvre boutonneuse and tsutsugamushi disease. It consists of a small ulcer covered by a necrotic scab. **Tache spinale.** The formation of bullae, like burn blisters, on the skin, in disease of the spinal cord. **Tache vierge.** A small circular area of clearing produced on a plate culture by bacteriophage. [Fr.]

tacheometer (tak·e·**om**·et·er). An apparatus for determining the speed of the blood in the vessels. [Gk *tachos* speed, meter.]

tachetic (tak·**et**·ik). Characterized by bluish or purple blotches. [Fr. *tache* spot.]

tachistoscope (tak·**is**·to·skope). An instrument used to register the speed of visual perception, by displaying visual stimuli briefly and then increasing the exposure until identification is attained. [Gk *tachistos* very swift, *skopein* to view.]

tachogram (**tak**·o·gram). A tracing made by a tacheometer. [Gk *tachos* speed, *gramma* record.]

tachography (tak·**og**·raf·e). The recording of the speed of the flow of the blood in the vessels. [Gk *tachos* speed, *graphein* to write.]

tachometer (tak·**om**·et·er). TACHEOMETER.

tachyarrhythmia (**tak**·e·a·**rith'**·me·ah). A rapid abnormal cardiac rhythm. [Gk *tachys* swift, *a*, *rhythmos* rhythm.]

tachyauxesis (**tak**·e·awx·e'·sis). Heterauxesis. [Gk *tachys* swift, *auxesis* increase.]

tachycardia (tak·e·**kar**·de·ah). Rapid action of the heart; there are wide limits of normality for adults, from 40 to 100 beats per minute. It may occur as a result of widespread influences which act upon the heart, e.g. exercise, fever, emotion, hypotension, or increased metabolic rate (reflex tachycardia); it may also result from primary disorders of the heart such as cardiac failure, and paroxysmal disorders of rhythm. It only becomes abnormal when it is outside the normal range for the individual under the circumstances in which it occurs. **Atrial tachycardia, Auricular tachycardia.** Regular tachycardia due to rapid discharge of impulses from an ectopic focus in the atrium. The atrial rate is from 140 to 240 per minute and the ventricles usually respond to each atrial contraction. Attacks commence and terminate suddenly and may be stopped by vagal stimulation, e.g. pressure upon the carotid sinus; they do not usually endanger life and cardiac disease is often absent. The condition is closely akin to atrial flutter, with electrocardiographic and clinical differences. **Atrioventricular tachycardia, Auriculoventricular paroxysmal tachycardia, Auriculoventricular paroxysmal nodal tachycardia.** Paroxysmal tachycardia due to the rapid discharge of impulses from an ectopic focus in or near the atrioventricular node. There is usually retrograde conduction to the auricles, with P waves falling on the QRS complex; occasionally the P wave may precede the QRS complex, with short P–R intervals if the focus is high in the node. The attacks begin and terminate suddenly and the heart is usually normal. **Circus movement tachycardia.** Tachycardia maintained by the continuing passage of a stimulating wavefront round a pathway which results in its re-entry to the beginning of the pathway with each circuit. **Coronary-sinus tachycardia.** A form of high nodal tachycardia with inverted P waves in the electrocardiogram due to a focus near the coronary sinus. **Idioventricular tachycardia.** Paroxysmal tachycardia from a pacemaker in or below the atrioventricular node, or in one or the other ventricle. **Junctional tachycardia.** A rapid cardiac rhythm resulting from the regular discharge of impulses from a focus in tissue in the region of the atrioventricular node. This term is sometimes used in preference to (atrioventricular) nodal tachycardia, as commonly precise location of the focus to the atrioventricular node is not possible. **Nodal tachycardia.** Paroxysmal tachycardia due to a rapid succession of discharges from an ectopic focus in the region of the atrioventricular node. Clinically it usually has the same characteristics and complications as atrial tachycardia, but there are electrocardiographic differences. **Paroxysmal tachycardia.** Any tachycardia due to a rapid succession of impulses arising from an ectopic focus, e.g. atrial, nodal, ventricular. **Paroxysmal tachycardia in Wolff–Parkinson–White syndrome.** Supraventricular tachycardia occurring in patients with this syndrome. Attacks tend to be repetitive and difficult to terminate, although the prognosis is good. Paroxysms may occur in which the QRS complex of the electrocardiogram is widened or of normal duration. **Re-entry tachycardia.** Tachycardia in which the mechanism is the continued re-entry of the stimulating wavefront into the pathway exciting the heart, thus maintaining a 'circus' movement. **Reflex tachycardia.** Increase in heart rate due to stimulation of the sinu-atrial pacemaker as a result of reflex changes acting through the autonomic nervous system, e.g. increase in pressure in great veins (Bainbridge reflex), fall in systemic blood pressure (Marey's law), or stimulation of the sympathetic nervous system. Reflex tachycardia may be initiated by exercise, fever, emotion, etc. **Repetitive paroxysmal tachycardia.** An uncommon rhythm disturbance in which short runs of ectopic beats occur frequently after a few normally conducted beats. **Sinus tachycardia.** Increase in heart rate due to stimulation of the sinu-atrial pacemaker. **Tachycardia strumosa exophthalmica, Thyrotoxic tachycardia.** Sinus tachycardia arising in patients with thyrotoxicosis, due to stimulation of the sinu-atrial node by increased sympathetic activity. The heart may be affected, particularly in the elderly, and paroxysmal tachycardia, or more usually atrial fibrillation, occurs (thyrotoxic heart disease). **Supraventricular tachycardia.** Any rapid cardiac rhythm resulting from impulses originating above the ventricles. **Ventricular tachycardia.** Paroxysmal tachycardia due to a rapid succession of impulses from an ectopic focus in the ventricle. Unlike atrial tachycardia, the ventricular rate is often slightly irregular, and the attacks do not respond to vagal stimulation and occur in the presence of severe cardiac damage, i.e. coronary thrombosis. There are also notable electrocardiographic differences, and the prognosis is grave. [Gk *tachys* swift, *kardia* heart.]

See also: HIS (W. JNR.).

tachycardiac (tak·e·**kar**·de·ak). Relating to or affected with tachycardia.

tachygraph (**tak**·e·graf). A form of tacheometer for recording the speed of the blood. [Gk *tachys* swift, *graphein* to write.]

tachygraphy (tak·**ig**·raf·e). Tachography.

tachylalia (tak·e·**la**·le·ah). Very rapid speaking. [Gk *tachys* swift, *lalein* to speak.]

tachylogia (tak·e·**lo**·je·ah). Tachyphrasia. [Gk *tachys* swift, *logos* word.]

tachymeter (tak·**im**·et·er). 1. Any device employed to measure the speed of a body in motion. 2. Tacheometer. [Gk *tachys* swift, meter.]

tachyphagia (tak·e·**fa**·je·ah). Quickness in eating; bolting food. [Gk *tachys* swift, *phagein* to eat.]

tachyphasia (tak·e·**fa**·ze·ah). Tachyphrasia. [Gk *tachys* swift, *phasis* speech.]

tachyphemia (tak·e·**fe**·me·ah). Tachyphrasia. [Gk *tachys* swift, *pheme* speech.]

tachyphrasia (tak·e·**fra**·ze·ah). Volubility, or quickness of speech. [Gk *tachys* swift, *phrasis* speaking.]

tachyphrenia (tak·e·**fre**·ne·ah). Excessive activity of the mind. [Gk *tachys* swift, *phren* mind.]

tachyphylaxis (**tak**·e·fil·**ax'**·is). 1. Rapid desensitization against the effects of toxic doses of an extract or serum by the previous injection of subtoxic doses of the same extract or serum. 2. A condition produced by a drug in which repeated doses produce progressively smaller effects or in which progressively larger doses are required to produce the initial effect. [Gk *tachys* swift, phylaxis.]

tachypnoea (tak·ip·**ne**·ah). Unduly rapid breathing. **Nervous tachypnoea.** A hysterical symptom in which the breathing is quick and shallow. [Gk *tachys* swift, *pnoia* breath.]

tachypragia (tak·e·**pra**·je·ah). Quickness of action. [Gk *tachys* swift, *pragos* deed.]

tachypsychia (tak·e·**si**·ke·ah). A state in which thought processes are accelerated. [Gk *tachys* swift, *psyche* mind.]

tachyrhythmia (tak·e·**rith**·me·ah). Tachycardia. [Gk *tachys* swift, *rhythmos* rhythm.]

tachysterol (tak·e·**steer**·ol). $C_{28}H_{44}O$, an isomer of ergosterol from which it is formed by irradiation with ultraviolet light.

tachysystole (tak·e·**sis**·to·le). Tachycardia; rapid systole. **Auricular tachysystole.** Auricular flutter. *See* FLUTTER. [Gk *tachys* swift, *systole* contraction.]

tachytrophism (tak·e·**trof**·izm). Rapidity of metabolic assimilation. [Gk *tachys* swift, *trophe* nutrition.]

Tacrine (**tak**·reen). BP Commission approved name for 9-amino-1,2,3,4-tetrahydroacridine, a stimulant of the respiratory centre, an analeptic and anticholinesterase which will antagonize the actions of non-depolarizing myoneural blocking agents and will potentiate those of suxamethonium.

tactile (**tak**·tile). 1. Concerned with touch or the sense of touch. 2. Capable of being felt. [L *tactus* touch.]

tactilogical (tak·til·**oj**·ik·al). Concerned with touch. [L *tactus* touch, Gk *logos* science.]

taction (**tak**·shun). 1. The sense of touch. 2. Touching. [L *tactus* touch.]

tactometer (tak·**tom**·et·er). An apparatus for estimating the keenness of touch. [L *tactus* touch, meter.]

tactor (**tak**·tor). Any tactile organ. [L *tactus* touch.]

tactual (**tak**·tew·al). Tactile.

tactus eruditus, tactus expertus (**tak**·tus er·ew·**di**·tus, **tak**·tus ex·**per**·tus). The acute sense of touch developed by experience. [L skilled touch, experienced touch.]

taedium vitae (te·de·um **vi**·te). Tiredness of life; suicidal inclination. [L.]

Taenia (te·ne·ah). A genus of tapeworms. It contains the two true human tapeworms as well as many others, normal to domestic animals, which occasionally infest man. In early literature many other tapeworms were lumped in *Taenia*, and the name is sometimes used almost as a synonym of tapeworm. **Taenia africana.** A species resembling *T. saginata* which has been recorded rarely in East Africa. **Taenia bremneri.** A form described from man in West Africa; it is perhaps a form of *T. saginata*. **Taenia coenurus.** *Multiceps multiceps.* **Taenia confusa.** A form of doubtful specific identity recorded from man in Africa and America. It is perhaps a form of *T. saginata* but its life cycle is unknown. **Taenia hydatigena.** A species normally infesting dogs, which has perhaps occurred in man. **Taenia lata.** *Diphyllobothrium latum.* **Taenia multiceps.** *Multiceps multiceps.* **Taenia saginata.** The beef tapeworm. Man is the normal host of the adult and very rarely of the cysticercus; secondary hosts are cattle and some wild ungulates. It is of more frequent occurrence than the following species and often abundant in cattle-rearing communities where meat is traditionally seared and not sufficiently heated throughout. The adult is about 7 m long. The ripe proglottides have about 20 main branches to the uterus and are shed singly; they move actively and deposit eggs as they move. The cysticerci, so-called Cysticercus bovis, are chiefly found in the muscles of the heart and mouth. **Taenia solium.** The pork tapeworm. Man is the only host of the adult and frequently harbours the cysticercus also. Secondary hosts, other than man, are principally pigs, but many other mammals can serve. It is an uncommon species in civilized areas, though cysticercus infections are often more common. The adult bears a rostellar ring of alternating large and small hooks; it reaches about 3 m. The mature proglottides closely resemble those of the preceding species, but have only about 10 main branches to the uterus. These are shed singly, or in chains, and are inactive. The cysticerci, the so-called Cysticercus cellulosae, cause the characteristic appearance of measly pork. In man they may occur not only in muscles but in the brain, the subcutaneous tissues, and the eyes. **Taenia taeniaeformis.** A common species in cats, which has been recorded from man very rarely. [Gk *tainia* band.]

taenia [tenia (NA)] (te·ne·ah). Any structure band-like in form. **Tenia choroidea [NA].** The slight thickening along the upper surface of the thalamus marking the attachment there of the ependyma covering the choroid plexus of the lateral ventricle. The term is also used to include the taeniae of the 3rd and 4th ventricles. **Teniae coli [NA].** Band-like thickenings, three in number, of the longitudinal muscle layer of the colon and caecum. They are respectively the mesocolic band [tenia mesocolica (NA)], the omental band [tenia omentalis (NA)], and the free band [tenia libera (NA)]. **Taenia of the fimbria.** The recurved part of the fimbria to the lateral edge of which the epithelium covering the choroid plexus of the inferior horn of the lateral ventricle is attached. **Taenia of the fornix [tenia fornicis (NA)].** The medial edge of the fimbria of the hippocampus (taenia of the fimbria, see above). The term is also applied to the stria habenularis of the thalamus, which consists of fibres from the columns of the fornix coursing along the surface of the thalamus. **Taenia of the fourth ventricle [tenia ventriculi quarti (NA)].** The thickened ridge at the attachment of the tela chorioidea to the lower lateral border of the 4th ventricle. **Taenia of the hippocampus.** Fimbria of the hippocampus. **Taenia libera [tenia libera (NA)], Taenia mesocolica [tenia mesocolica (NA)], Taenia omentalis [tenia omentalis (NA)].** *See* TENIAE COLI (above). **Taenia of the pons.** A frequently occurring thin white band winding around the cerebral peduncle just rostral to the pons and entering the cerebellum; they are detached pontine fibres. **Taenia telae [tenia telae (NA)].** A general term including any taeniae in the central nervous system. **Taenia of the thalamus [tenia thalami (NA)], Taenia of the third ventricle.** The thickened ridges at the lateral attachment of the roof of the 3rd ventricle to the thalamus. [see prec.]

taeniacide (te·ne·ah·side). Any remedy that kills tapeworms. [taenia, L *caedere* to kill.]

taeniafuge (te·ne·ah·fewj). Anything that will expel tapeworms. [taenia, L *fugare* to put to flight.]

taenial (te·ne·al). Pertaining to tapeworms. [taenia.]

Taeniarhynchus (te·ne·ah·**ring**'·kus). A generic name occasionally used for those species of *Taenia* in which the scolex is unarmed, e.g. *T. saginata*. [Gk *tainia* band, *rhynchos* snout.]

taeniasis (te·ni·as·is). 1. Infestation by tapeworms. 2. The symptoms caused by tapeworm infestation. **Intestinal taeniasis.** Taeniasis due to adult tapeworms in the intestine, e.g. of *Taenia saginata*. **Somatic taeniasis.** Taeniasis due to larval worms in the tissues, e.g. the cysticercus of *T. solium*. [taenia.]

taeniatus (te·ne·a·tus). Taenial; relating to taeniae.

taenicide (te·ne·side). A vermicide that is active against tapeworms. [taenia, L *caedere* to kill.]

taeniform (te·ne·form). Taenioid. [taenia, form.]

taenifugal (te·ne·**few**·gal). Possessing the ability to expel tapeworms. [taenia, L *fugare* to put to flight.]

Taeniidae (te·ne·id·e). A family of the cestode order Cyclophyllidea. The genera *Echinococcus, Multiceps*, and *Taenia* are of medical interest.

taenioid (te·ne·oid). 1. Like a ribbon. 2. Having a resemblance to a tapeworm. [taenia, Gk *eidos* form.]

taeniola (te·ne·o·lah). A thin structure like a band or ribbon. **Taeniola cinerea.** One of the narrow white bands of nerve matter located in the floor of the 4th ventricle. **Taeniola corporis callosi.** A slender extension of the corpus callosum down the anterior commissure towards the paraterminal gyrus. [L dim. of Gk *tainia* band.]

taeniophobia (te·ne·o·**fo**·be·ah). Obsessional fear of being infested with tapeworms. [taenia, Gk *phobein* to fear.]

Taeniorhynchus (te·ne·o·**ring**'·kus). A genus of mosquitoes of world-wide, mostly tropical, distribution. Alone among noxious mosquitoes, the larvae and pupae obtain air by tapping underwater plants, particularly *Pistia stratiotes*. **Taeniorhynchus africanus.** A secondary host of *Wuchereria bancrofti* in Nigeria, and a potential vector of yellow fever. **Taeniorhynchus annulatus.** A secondary host of *W. bancrofti* from Malaysia to the Philippines. **Taeniorhynchus annuliferus.** An important secondary host of *W. malayi* in India and Sri Lanka. **Taeniorhynchus fuscopennatus.** A secondary host of *Dipetalonema perstans*, which transmits Rift Valley fever in tropical Africa. **Taeniorhynchus indianus.** Probably a secondary host to *W. malayi* in Malaysia, Java, Indo-China, and Thailand. **Taeniorhynchus juxta mansonius.** A potential vector of *W. malayi*. **Taeniorhynchus longipalpis.** An important secondary host of *W. malayi* in Malaysia and Indo-China. **Taeniorhynchus pseudotitillans.** A secondary host of *W. bancrofti* in the Guianas and Brazil. **Taeniorhynchus uniformis.** A secondary host for *Acanthocheilonema perstans, W. bancrofti*, and *W. malayi*, and a mechanical transmitter of *Trypanosoma gambiense* in West Africa. [Gk *tainia* band, *rhynchos* snout.]

taeniotoxin (te·ne·o·**tox**'·in). A toxin derived from tapeworms. [taenia, toxin.]

Taenzer, Paul Rudolf (b. 1858). Bremen dermatologist.

Taenzer's disease. Ulerythema ophryogenes.

Taenzer's stain, Unna–Taenzer stain. For elastic fibres: sections are stained in an alcoholic solution of orcein, and counterstained with haematoxylin or methylene blue. Elastic fibres are stained a reddish-brown.

tag (tag). A small pendant piece of tissue attached to the main structure along one margin or by a pedicle. [etym. dub.]

tagatose (tag·at·oze). $CH_2OH(CHOH)_3COCH_2OH$, a ketohexose isomeric with fructose. It is synthesized from galactose.

Tagetes (taj·e·teez). A genus of composite-flowered plants. *Tagetes patula* and *T. erecta*, are French and African marigold respectively, indigenous to Mexico. [*Tages* Etruscan god.]

tagged (tag·d). Labelled; made identifiable. A compound is rendered physically distinguishable from the normal compound by the presence of the tagged element. This may be a radioactive or non-radioactive isotope of the normal element, and whilst the tagged compound is chemically indistinguishable from the normal compound its presence can be detected and its amount quantitatively estimated. [etym. dub.]

Tagliacozzi, Gasparo (b. 1546). Bologna surgeon.

tagliacotian operation. A plastic operation on the nose.

tail (tale). 1. The caudal extremity. [Cauda (NA).] 2. Applied to anything tail-like in form. **Axillary tail of the breast.** That portion of the upper and outer quadrant of the breast which may lie in the axilla. **Tail of the caudate nucleus.** *See* NUCLEUS. **Tail of the epididymis.** *See* EPIDIDYMIS. **Faun tail.** A tuft of hair occurring over the lumbosacral region as a developmental abnormality. **Tail of the helix [cauda helicis (NA)].** A sharp downwardly projecting process at the posterior end of the helix, separated from the rest of the auricular cartilage by the fissura antitragohelicina. **Tail of an incision.** End of an incision; sometimes applied to its lower end. **Tail of the pancreas.** *See* PANCREAS. [AS *taegel.*]

See also: SPENCE.

tail-gut (tale·gut). A transient diverticulum of the entodermal cloaca, passing into the tail in early embryos. [tail, gut.]

Taillefer, Horace Auguste (b. 1802). French physician.

Taillefer's valve. A fold of mucous membrane sometimes present halfway down the nasolacrimal duct.

taint (ta·nt). A blemish; applied to an infection, particularly a syphilitic one. [Fr. *teindre* to tinge.]

taipan (ta·pan). *Pseudechis scutellatus*, a large poisonous snake of Australasia.

Tait, Robert Lawson (b. 1845). English surgeon and gynaecologist.

Tait's knot. Staffordshire knot; a method of securing a pedicle. A double-threaded needle is passed through the stump, leaving a loop of thread which is passed round the stump. One end of the thread is passed through the loop, and the other round the pedicle, and they are tied in a reef knot.

Tait's law. In every case of disease in the pelvis or abdomen in which life is in danger, unless the cause is known to be malignant, an exploratory laparotomy should be performed.

Tait's operation. A method of repairing a lacerated perineum with two flaps brought from either side. [obsolete.]

taka-koji (tah·kah·ko·je). A diastatic enzyme produced by the organism *Aspergillus oryzae.* It plays a part in the fermentation of steamed rice, koji, in the manufacture of saké, the Japanese drink. [Jap.]

taka-moashi (tah·kah·mo·ash·e). Taka-koji. [Jap.]

taka panna (tah·kah pan·ah). Pistia stratiotes. [Jap.]

Takata, Maki (b. 1892). Japanese pathologist.

Takata's reagent. A mixture of mercuric chloride solution (0.5 per cent) with an equal part of basic fuchsine solution (0.02 per cent). It is used in the diagnosis of liver disease.

Takata-Ara test. For liver function: place 1 ml of normal saline in each of eight small tubes. To the first add 1 ml of serum, mix and transfer 1 ml of the diluted serum to tube 2. Continue the serial dilution discarding 1 ml from tube 8. To each tube add with mixing 0.25 ml of 10 per cent sodium carbonate followed by 0.15 ml of 0.5 per cent mercuric chloride. Allow the tubes to stand for 24 hours. A positive reaction is shown by a thick flocculent precipitate in at least three tubes, one of which should be the 1:32 dilution or higher. Any fine granular precipitate is disregarded. Positive results are usually obtained in advanced liver disease, especially in cirrhosis.

Takayama, Masao (b. 1871). Japanese physician.

Takayama's reagent, or solution. For the recognition of blood stains: it consists of 10 per cent sodium hydroxide solution, 3 ml; pyridine, 3 ml; saturated aqueous glucose, 3 ml; water 7 ml. When a drop of solution is applied to suspected material, if it is a blood stain haemochromogen, crystals will form.

Takayasu, U. (b. 1871). Japanese physician.

Takayasu's disease. An inflammatory occlusive disease of the aorta, especially of the arch and the vessels arising from it, of unknown aetiology, producing absence of peripheral pulses and ischaemic lesions, especially in the head, including the eyes (the last being the feature described by Takayasu); pulseless disease.

take (take). The semi-popular term for a satisfactory response, e.g. of a vaccination, to show the characteristic vesicle formation, or of a graft, to become organized. [AS *tacan.*]

talalgia (ta·lal·je·ah). Pain experienced in the heel. [talus, Gk *algos* pain.]

Talampicillin (tal·am·pe·sil'·in). BP Commission approved name for phthalidyl 6-[D(−)-α-aminophenylacetamido]penicillanate; an antibiotic.

talantropia (tal·an·tro·pe·ah). Nystagmus. [Gk *talanton* balance, *trepein* to turn.]

talar (ta·lar). Pertaining to the talus.

Talauma elegans (tal·aw·mah el·eg·anz). A Javanese plant of the family Magnoliaceae. It is used medicinally in Java. [Javanese *talauma*, L *elegans* elegant.]

Talbot, Fritz Bradley (b. 1878). Boston paediatrician.

Benedict-Talbot standards. Tables of the calorie or joules output per hour of children based on their weight in kilograms.

talc, talcum (talk, tal·kum). Purified Talc BP 1973, French chalk; a native magnesium silicate, $3MgO{\cdot}4SiO_2{\cdot}H_2O$ purified by treatment with a mineral acid followed by washing with water. It is a fine white powder used usually in admixture with starch, zinc oxide, and boracic acid, as a dusting-powder. It is also employed as an adsorbent in clarifying liquids. [Arabic *talq.*]

talectomy (ta·lek·to·me). Surgical excision of the talus. [talus, Gk *ektemnein* to cut out.]

taliped (tal·ip·ed). Club-footed; a person suffering from talipes.

talipedic (tal·ip·ed·ik). Club-footed; having the deformity of talipes.

talipes (tal·ip·eez). Club-foot; a deformity of the foot: the foot is of abnormal shape and is habitually held in an abnormal position. **Talipes adductus.** Pes adductus. **Talipes arcuatus.** An abnormally high arched foot. **Talipes calcaneovalgus.** A combined deformity of talipes calcaneus and talipes valgus (see below). **Talipes calcaneovarus.** A combination of talipes calcaneus and talipes varus. **Talipes calcaneus.** Talipes in which the heel is depressed and the forefoot elevated so that the patient walks on the heel; it is commonly the result of paralysis of the calf muscles. **Talipes cavus.** An abnormally high arched foot. **Talipes equinovalgus.** A combination of talipes equinus and talipes valgus. **Talipes equinovarus.** A combination of talipes equinus and talipes varus; the common congenital variety of talipes. **Talipes equinus.** A deformity in which the foot is fixed in plantar flexion (extension) so that the subject can only walk on the toes of the affected foot. **Talipes planus.** Flat foot. **Spasmodic talipes planus.** Flat foot associated with spasm of the peroneus muscles. **Talipes valgus.** Foot deformity in which the patient walks on the inner border of the foot. **Talipes varus.** A deformity of the foot, in which the patient walks on the outer border, the forefoot being displaced and rotated inwards. [L.]

talipomanus (tal·ip·o·man'·us). Club-handed; a deformity of the hand corresponding to club-foot. [talipes, L *manus* hand.]

Tallerman, Lewis A. British inventor.

Tallerman's apparatus. An apparatus for the application of hot air to an extremity.

tallow (**tal**·o). The internal fat of certain ruminant animals, used in the manufacture of candles and soap. **Bayberry tallow, Virola tallow.** A vegetable fat from the wax myrtle *Myrica cerifera*; it is not a tallow. [ME *talgh*.]

Tallqvist, Theodor Waldemar (b. 1871). Finnish physician.

Tallqvist's scale. A very inaccurate method of direct colour comparison for the determination of the blood haemoglobin value; a drop of fresh blood is collected on a piece of absorbent paper and the colour is compared with a series, or scale, of colours devised by Tallqvist representing haemoglobin values from 10 to 100 per cent.

Talma, Sape (b. 1847). Utrecht physician.

Talma's disease. Tonic muscular spasm which has developed as a result of injury or secondarily to some other disease.

Talma-Morison operation. A combination of splenectomy, rawing of the surfaces of the viscera, and implantation of the omentum in the abdominal wall, to encourage collateral venous anastomosis in portal obstruction.

talocalcanean (ta·lo·kal·**ka**'·ne·an). Involving both the talus and the calcaneum. **Talocalcanean joint.** *See* JOINT.

talocalcaneonavicular (ta·lo·kal·**ka**·ne·o·nav·**ik**'·ew·lar). Involving the talus, calcaneum, and the navicular bone. **Talocalcaneonavicular joint.** *See* JOINT.

talocrural (tal·o·**kroo**·ral). Involving both the talus and the bones of the leg. [L *talus* ankle, *crus* leg.]

talofibular (ta·lo·**fib**·ew·lar). Involving both the talus and the fibula.

talon (**tal**·on). In the tritubercular theory of evolution of the modern mammalian tooth, the backward extension of the trigone from which the postero-internal cusp of an upper molar tooth is formed. [L bird claw.]

talonavicular (ta·lo·nav·**ik**'·ew·lar). Concerned with the articulation of the talus and the navicular bone. **Talonavicular joint.** *See* JOINT.

talonid (**tal**·on·id). In the tritubercular theory of evolution of the modern mammalian tooth, the backward extension of the trigonid from which the distal cusps of a lower molar tooth are formed. [talon.]

taloscaphoid (ta·lo·**skaf**·oid). Talonavicular. [L *talus* ankle, scaphoid.]

talose (**tal**·oze). $CH_2OH(CHOH)_4CHO$, an aldohexose isomeric with glucose; it is a liquid sugar.

talotibial (ta·lo·**tib**·e·al). Relating to the talus and the tibia.

Taloximine (tal·**ox**·im·een). BP Commission approved name for 4 - (2 - dimethylaminoethoxy) - 1,2 - dihydro - 1 - hydroxyiminophthalazine; a respiratory stimulant.

Talpa (**tal**·pah). 1. The genus including the common European mole, *Talpa europea*. 2. A sebaceous cyst or wen. [L mole.]

talpiform (**tal**·pe·form). Resembling a wen. [talpa, form.]

talus [NA] (**ta**·lus). The ankle bone; the bone connecting the bones of the foot with those of the leg, forming the ankle joint.

Body [corpus tali (NA)]. The posterior part of the bone, transmitting the body weight from the tibia to the calcaneum and lying between the malleoli.

Head [caput tali (NA)]. The distal part of the talus, joined to the body by the neck, and articulating with the navicular bone, the sustentaculum tali, and the plantar calcaneonavicular ligament.

Neck [collum tali (NA)]. That portion of the bone joining the head to the body and articulating with the sustentaculum tali.

Anterior surface. That to which the neck is attached.

Lateral surface. The outer surface, mostly occupied by a large, triangular, articular facet for the lateral malleolus.

Lower surface. The surface which rests on the calcaneum; it bears a large oval facet for articulation with the posterior articular facet on the upper surface of the calcaneum.

Medial surface. The inner surface; it bears a comma-shaped facet for the medial malleolus above, elsewhere it is roughened and pitted.

Posterior surface. The narrow surface behind, bearing a groove for the tendon of the flexor hallucis longus muscle. On either side of the groove are tubercles, the medial and posterior tubercles. The posterior tubercle may be connected to the remainder of the bone by cartilage only and is then called the os trigonum.

Upper surface [facies superior (NA)]. That portion of the body bearing the articular surface which forms part of the ankle joint.

Tamarind BPC 1959 (**tam**·ar·ind). The fruit of *Tamarindus indica* freed from the outer pericarp and preserved by being mixed with sugar. It forms a dark, brownish, sugary mass, and contains tartaric acid, cream of tartar, glucose, and fructose, and the sucrose in which it is preserved. It is a mild laxative and an ingredient of confection of senna. [Arabic *tamr Hindi* Indian date.]

tamarindus (tam·ar·**in**·dus). Tamarind.

tambour (**tam**·boor). A cylindrical drum covered with an elastic membrane and connected by an air-tube to a stylus which records alterations in the pressure within the drum. It is used in physiology. [Fr. drum.]

tamisage (**tam**·is·aje). Examination of stools for infection.

Tamoxifen (tam·**ox**·e·fen). BP Commission approved name for 1 - *p* - β - dimethylaminoethoxyphenyl - *trans* - 1,2 - diphenylbut - 1 - ene; it is used in the treatment of mammary carcinoma.

tampan (**tam**·pan). An African name for the tick *Ornithodorus moubata*.

tampol (**tam**·pol). A tampon impregnated with a medicinal substance.

tampon (**tam**·pon). A plug, e.g. of cotton wool, used to occlude an orifice in the control of bleeding, or to mop up secretions. **Kite-tail tampon.** A tampon which consists of several small balls of gauze or wool strung together on a string. **Vaginal tampon.** A tampon usually made from wool or cellulose with a cord attached for its removal, used to apply medication to the vaginal wall and cervix, and also to absorb the menstrual discharge. [Fr. plug.]

See also: CORNER (E. M.).

tamponade (**tam**·pon·ade). The inserting of a tampon. **Cardiac tamponade.** Heart tamponade (see below). **Chronic tamponade.** Constrictive pericarditis. *See* PERICARDITIS. **Heart tamponade.** The compressive effect upon the heart of blood or fluid that has accumulated in the pericardium. [Fr. *tamponnade*.]

See also: ROSE (E.).

tamponage, tamponing, tamponment (**tam**·pon·ij, **tam**·pon·ing, **tam**·pon·ment). Tamponade.

Tamus (**ta**·mus). A genus of plants of the family Dioscoreaceae.

Tamus communis. Black bryony root; a species the root of which is used in the fresh state as a rubefacient and diuretic. The pulp is applied to bruises. [L *tamnus* wild vine.]

tan (tan). 1. To acquire a brown pigmentation of the skin as the result of exposure to the sun or to ultraviolet light. 2. The pigmentation so acquired. [OFr. *tanner*.]

tanacetin (tan·as·e·tin). $C_{11}H_{16}O_4$, a bitter principle from *Tanacetum vulgare*, tansy.

tanacetum (tan·as·e·tum). Tansy. [LL.]

tanaka (tan·**ak**·ah). A Japanese plant, *Digenia simplex*, used medicinally.

tanalum (tan·**al**·um). Aluminium tannotartrate. A compound used in nose and throat diseases.

tandem (**tan**·dem). A linear arrangement of radium sources used for intracavitary radiotherapy.

tanghin (**tang**·gin). The seed, or an extract from the seeds, of the Madagascan tree *Cerbera tanghin* (family Apocynaceae). It contains a cardiac poison with properties like strophanthin. [Malagasy *tanging*.]

tangle (**tang**·gl). 1. A confused interlacing of fibres, such as those of nerve cells. 2. *Laminaria*; a genus of the brown algae (Phaeophyceae). [ME.]

tango-foot (**tang**·go·fut). Tenosynovitis from excessive dancing. [tango, the South American dance, foot.]

tangoreceptor (**tang**·go·re·**sep**'·tor). Any sensory organ that responds only to touch. [L *tangere* to touch, receptor.]

tank (tangk). A receptacle constructed to hold and store water or other liquid; a cistern. **Activated sludge tank.** A tank receiving screened or filtered sewage, and provided with pipes at the bottom through which large volumes of air are forced. In this way the mixed sewage is agitated with a mixture of 15 per cent or more of its volume of biologically-active liquid sewage in the presence of an ample supply of oxygen from the air for an adequate time to coagulate most of the colloidal substances present. This is followed by a sedimentation which precipitates the sludge flocculi, the activated sludge being previously produced by aeration of successive portions of sewage. The process may be continuous, but is more usually intermittent. **Anaerobic tank.** Septic tank (see below). **Biological tank.** A septic tank (see below) modified to allow more prolonged action of anaerobic organisms on the sewage. **Digestion tank.** A deep septic tank (see below) in which the sludge is removed and acted on by anaerobic organisms without rendering the more liquid portion of the sewage putrescent as in the ordinary septic tank. **Dortmund tank.** A deep tank into which the sewage flows downwards and at a slow rate, thus allowing time for the sludge to settle. **Hydrolytic tank.** Septic tank (see following). **Septic tank.** A tank receiving sewage in a disposal system. The suspended or floating particles of the sewage settle as sludge, and part of this disappears through the action of anaerobic organisms. The scum or film on the top is acted on by aerobic organisms in the presence of atmospheric oxygen. After a sufficient time, the liquid sewage flows into a contact bed for further purification. **Settling tank.** A tank into which liquid sewage passes at a slow rate of flow, thus allowing a proportion of solid particles to settle as sludge. The rest of the sewage passes on to a septic tank. [Port. *tanque.*]

See also: EMSHER, HUBBARD, IMHOFF.

tannal (tan·al). Aluminium tannate. **Insoluble tannal.** A basic aluminium tannate, $Al_2(OH)_4(C_{14}H_9O_9)_2{\cdot}10H_2O$, used as an astringent for chronic catarrh. **Soluble tannal.** A soluble aluminium tannate containing the tartrate radical; it is an astringent.

tannase (tan·aze). An enzyme capable of hydrolysing tannins.

tannate (tan·ate). Any salt or ester of tannic acid.

Tanner, Norman Cecil (b. 1906). London surgeon.

Tanner's operation. An operation for bleeding oesophageal varices; the lower end of the oesophagus and the upper 5 cm of the stomach are freed, dividing all vessels entering the parts, and the stomach divided 2 cm below the cardio-oesophageal orifice and resutured. The object of the operation is to sever the portal azygos venous connections.

tannic (tan·ik). Pertaining to tannin. [Celtic *tann* oak.]

tannin (tan·in). A general term used to describe two different types of naturally-occurring compounds: the *pyrogallol tannins* which are glycosides of glucose with *m*-digallic acid and occur in oak galls, etc.; and the *pyrocatechol tannins* which are sugar-free derivatives of catechol and occur in catechu, eucalyptus, kino, rhatany, etc. Tannin for medicinal purposes is that obtained from oak galls by extracting them with water-saturated ether, and is known as *tannic acid.* **Catechol tannin.** Phlobatannin. **Diacetyl tannin.** Acetannin, $C_{14}H_8O_7(COOCH_3)_2$, a greyish insoluble powder used in diarrhoea. **Pathological tannin.** A tannin produced by pathological conditions, e.g. that of oak galls. **Physiological tannin.** Tannin which occurs normally, e.g. that in oak bark. **Tannin proteinate.** A brown insoluble compound of tannin and albumin used as an intestinal disinfectant.

Tanret, Charles (b. 1847). French physician.

Tanret's reagent. For protein: a reagent made by the addition of 1.35 g of mercuric chloride dissolved in 25 ml of water to 3.32 g of potassium iodide dissolved in 25 ml of water, made up to 60 ml with water and added to 20 ml of glacial acetic acid.

Tanret's test. For protein in urine: a white precipitate is given by protein with Tanret's reagent; obsolete.

Tanret–Mayer test. A modification of Tanret's test adapted for testing for quinine in urine, in order to check whether a patient is actually taking quinine that has been prescribed. A solution of 1.45 g of mercuric chloride in 80 ml of undistilled water is added to a solution of 5 g of potassium iodide in 20 ml of distilled water, the mixture being agitated during the process. The urine is first boiled and filtered, and to 5 ml of the filtrate a few drops of reagent are added; an immediate precipitate forms if the alkaloid, quinine, is present in the urine.

Tansini, Iginio (b. 1855). Pavia surgeon.

Tansini's operation. Removal of the malignant breast with involved overlying skin, and repair by skin flap from the back.

Tansley, J. O. (fl. 1894). American surgeon.

Tansley's operation, Hunt–Tansley operation. For ptosis: a central vertical strap of skin, attached only below, is fashioned in the upper lid, by excising an area of skin to the nasal and temporal side of this strap. This is passed subcutaneously up to the eyebrow and stitched to the occipitofrontalis muscle.

tansy (tan·ze). The plant *Tanacetum vulgare* (family Compositae). The dried herb is used as an anthelmintic and tonic. [Gk *athanasia* immortality.]

tantalum (tan·tal·um). An element of atomic weight 180.95, atomic number 73, and chemical symbol Ta. It occurs in the mineral tantalite from which it gets its name, and other rare minerals. A grey ductile metal of high melting point, and non-corrosive, it was formerly used for the filaments of electric lamps. Its alloys are valuable for cutting tools, laboratory ware and surgical instruments; the metal itself is utilized in surgery. [Gk *Tantalos,* legendary hero tortured by thirst; refers to element's non-absorption.]

tantrum (tan·trum). An exhibition of uncontrolled temper afforded by children and mental patients. [etym. dub.]

taon (tah·on). Beriberi in infants in South-east Asia. [Philippine name.]

tap (tap). 1. To strike lightly with the finger or a hammer as in percussion or when evoking reflexes. 2. To draw off fluid by means of a hollow needle, trocar, or cannula. 3. A local East Indian name for a jungle fever, possibly mite typhus. **Bloody tap.** A lumbar puncture in which a pink-tinged or bloody fluid is obtained. **Front tap.** A light blow delivered to the anterior muscles of the leg which produces contraction of the calf muscles in cases of spinal irritability. **Heel tap.** A reflex movement of the toes elicited by tapping the heel; it is seen in disseminated sclerosis and certain other diseases of the cerebrospinal tract. [ME *tappen.*]

tape (tape). *See* SMITH (PRIESTLEY). [AS *taeppe.*]

tapeinocephalic (tap·i·no·kef·al′·ik). Having the features of tapeinocephaly.

tapeinocephaly (tap·i·no·kef′·al·e). A flattened head in which the vertical index of the skull is less than 72. [Gk *tapeinos* low, *kephale* skull.]

tapetal (tap·e·tal). Relating to the tapetum.

tapetum (tap·e·tum). A carpet; hence a layer that can be thought to have something of the texture of a carpet. **Tapetum of the corpus callosum.** The layer formed by the fibres of the corpus callosum which run laterally over the lateral ventricle and interesect with the fibres of the corona radiata. **Tapetum of the eye, Tapetum lucidum.** A layer of tissue in the chorioidea of the eye, between its vascular and capillary layers. It may be cellular (*tapetum cellulare*) in carnivora, or fibrous (*tapetum fibrosum*) in ruminants, and may contain crystals. It reflects the light strongly and is responsible for the green reflex, e.g. in cats. There is no tapetum in the human eye. **Tapetum nigrum.** Pigmented layer of the retina. *See* LAYER. [L *tapeta.*]

tapeworm (tape·werm). The adult of any member of the class Cestoidea of the phylum Platyhelminthes. They are characterized, except for some primitive forms living in fish, by the presence of an anterior scolex, often furnished with suckers and hooks, followed by a neck and region of proliferation from which are budded a series of proglottides which form the tape. The number of proglottides in mature worms varies according to the species from three to four to several thousand. The total length of the tape ranges from a few mm up to 50 m. Each proglottis contains a discrete set of reproductive organs; all tapeworms are hermaphrodite and most protandrous. All tapeworms live in the intestines of vertebrates and their life histories include one or two secondary hosts. In most, the eggs are shed in the faeces within a ripe proglottis and develop to form an onchosphere. If the egg is eaten by a secondary host, it hatches and the onchosphere passes through the intestinal wall into the blood stream and settles in muscles. Here it forms the cysticercus or other larval form, which on ingestion by the primary host evaginates the scolex, sheds the bladder, and develops to the adult. **Beef tapeworm.** *Taenia saginata*, perhaps the commonest human tapeworm; man is the primary host, cattle secondary. **Broad tapeworm.** *Diphyllobothrium latum*; its primary hosts are fish-eating mammals including man. Secondary hosts are copepoda and then fish. **Dog tapeworm.** *Dipylidium caninum*; its primary host is the dog but it is not uncommon in children. Secondary hosts are dog fleas and lice. **Dwarf tapeworm.** *Hymenolepis nana*; its primary hosts are commensal rats and mice, and man; secondary hosts are usually absent, infection being caused by direct ingestion of eggs. **Fish tapeworm.** Broad tapeworm (see above). **Hydatid tapeworm.** *Echinococcus granulosus*; its primary host is the dog. Secondary hosts are sheep, cattle and man in some agricultural regions. The cysticercus is very large with numerous scolices, the hydatid cyst. **Mouse tapeworm.** *Hymenolepis diminuta*, which occasionally infects man. Infection is usually from mouse droppings in food. **Pork tapeworm.** *Taenia solium*; its primary host is man and secondary the pig. **Rat tapeworm.** *Hymenolepis diminuta*, a species occurring rarely in man, or *H. nana*, dwarf tapeworm (see above). [AS *taeppe, wyrm.*]

taphephobia, taphiphobia (taf·e·fo·be·ah). Taphophobia.

taphophobia (taf·o·**fo**·be·ah). An obsessional dread of premature burial. [Gk *taphos* grave, *phobein* to fear.]

Tapia, Antonio Garcia (b. 1875). Madrid neurologist.

Tapia's operation. An operation for the radical excision of the larynx in malignant disease.

Tapia's syndrome. Paralysis of the vocal cord associated with a paralysis of the tongue, both occurring on one side.

tapinocephaly (**tap**·in·o·**kef**'·al·e). Tapeinocephaly.

tapiroid (**ta**·pir·oid). Like the snout of a tapir; applied to an abnormally long cervix uteri. [Brazilian *tapira*, Gk *eidos* form.]

tapotage (tah·po·**tahzh**). A sign sometimes produced in pulmonary tuberculosis; a loose cough elicited by percussion of the supraclavicular region. [Fr. patting.]

tapôtement (tah·pote·**mahn**). The use of percussion in massage. [Fr.]

Tar, Aloys (b. 1886). Budapest physician.

Tar's sign. In health the lower margin of the lungs in a person lying down during moderate expiration is as low as when standing with deep inspiration; with infiltrating disease of the lungs this is not the case.

tar (tahr). 1. General name applied to the dark viscid organic mixtures obtained by the distillation of coals, shales, or vegetable matter. 2. (BP 1973) Stockholm tar (see below). **Birch tar.** The tar obtained by the distillation of the wood of the birch, *Betula alba*; it separates into a tar and an oil which is used in ointments for eczema. **Coal tar.** The tar obtained by the destructive distillation of coal at about 1000°C. It is the source of many aromatic hydrocarbons, phenols, etc., and of pitch. It has itself antiseptic properties and is used for skin affections (BPC 1968). **Gas tar.** Coal tar, particularly that obtained in the manufacture of coal gas. **Juniper tar.** Cade Oil BP 1958, the dark oily liquid obtained by the destructive distillation of the wood of *Juniperus oxycedrus* L. It is an antiseptic stimulant, usually employed in the form of ointments to relieve skin conditions, especially psoriasis and dry eczema. **Oil of tar.** A brownish mobile liquid obtained by the redistillation of certain wood tars and containing all ingredients except the pitch; it is used for veterinary purposes. **Prepared Coal Tar BP 1973.** A product of heating coal tar for one hour at 50°C. It is used in skin diseases. **Spirit of tar.** The lower boiling fraction of oil of tar, which is colourless or light yellow. **Stockholm tar.** A bituminous liquid obtained by the destructive distillation of the Scotch fir, *Pinus sylvestris* and allied species. It is used to relieve coughs, and for skin diseases, and its aqueous extract has an acid reaction as against coal tar which is alkaline. **Syrup of tar.** A filtered mixture of wood tar, alcohol, sugar, and water, containing much of the volatile part of tar but none of the pitch; it is used in coughs. **Wood tar.** Stockholm tar (see above); the tar which must be supplied when the word is unqualified. [AS *teoru.*]

tarabagan (tar·ab·a·gan). Siberian marmot, *Arctomys bobac*; a large rodent that is susceptible to a chronic form of *Pasteurella pestis* infection and constitutes the reservoir of plague infection in northern Asia. [Siberian.]

Taraktogenos (tar·ak·**toj**·en·os). A genus of tropical trees. **Taraktogenos kurzii.** The species from the seeds of which chaulmoogra oil is obtained. [Gk *taraktos* disturbed, *genein* to produce.]

tarantism, tarantismus (**tar**·an·tizm, tar·an·**tiz**·mus). A type of choromania ascribed to tarantula bite.

tarantula (tar·**an**·tew·lah). 1. A popular name for any large, free-living spider, particularly *Lycosa tarantula* of southern Europe, whose bite causes superficial lysis. 2. A genus of whip scorpions which are harmless. **Black tarantula.** *Sericopelma communis* of Panama. **European tarantula.** *Lycosa tarantula* (see above). [L *Tarentum* town in Italy.]

tarassis (**tar**·as·is). Hysteria in male subjects. [Gk *taraxis* disturbance.]

taraxaci radix (tar·**ax**·ah·se **rad**·ix). Taraxacum BPC 1949.

taraxacin (tar·**ax**·as·in). A crystalline bitter substance obtained from the root of the dandelion, *Taraxacum officinale* Weber (family Compositae).

Taraxacum (tar·**ax**·ak·um). 1. A genus of plants of the family Compositae. 2. Taraxacum BPC 1949, taraxacum root, dandelion root; the fresh or dried root and rhizome of *Taraxacum officinale* Weber. It yields a milky juice (latex) containing taraxacin, a bitter principle. It is used as a tonic and bitter, also as a mild laxative. [Pers. *tarashqun* dandelion.]

tarbadillo (tar·bah·**deel**·yo). Tabardillo. [Sp. *tabardillo* typhus.]

tarbagan (**tar**·bag·an). Tarabagan.

Tardieu, Auguste Ambroise (b. 1818). Paris hygienist and medicolegal expert.

Tardieu's spots or petechiae. Minute spots of bleeding from venules and capillaries engorged and distended by venous stasis or obstruction and thus rendered penetrable to whole blood, described as characteristic of asphyxia; commonly seen in the scalp, face, eyelids or conjunctivae following strangling, but not confined to cases of violence.

Tardieu's test. The presence of air bubbles in the gastric mucosa after the establishment of breathing, as evidence of a separate existence of the fetus. This is historical, and the presence of air in the stomach by itself is not regarded as significant from a medicolegal point of view.

tardive (**tar**·div). Tardy; delayed. Denoting a disease in which a period elapses before recognizable symptoms appear. [L *tardus* late.]

tare (**ta**·er). A counterpoise weight equal to that of a container, which is placed in the opposite pan of the balance when weighings involving the container are made. [see foll.]

tared (**ta**·erd). Weighed and allowed for; in chemistry, describing a vessel or container whose predetermined weight is deducted from any subsequent weighings in which it takes part. [Obsolete term.] [Ar. *taraha* to reject.]

target (**tar**·get). In radiobiology, a concept of the critical locus for radiation interaction. [OFr. *targuete.*]

Tarin, Pierre (b. 1725). Paris anatomist.

Band of Tarin. That part of the stria semicircularis which lies in the medial part of the roof of the inferior horn of the lateral ventricle.

Tarin's fasciculus. The molecular stratum of the dentate gyrus of the cerebrum.

Tarin's foramen. The opening through which the greater superficial petrosal nerve leaves the temporal bone.

Tarin's fossa. Interpeduncular fossa. *See* FOSSA.

Tarin's recess. That part of the interpeduncular fossa underlying the posterior perforated substance.

Tarin's space. The posterior perforated substance of the cerebrum.

Tarin's valves. Thickenings of the inferior medullary velum, in continuity with parts of the vermis of the cerebellum.

Tarin's velum. The inferior medullary velum. *See* VELUM.

Tarnier, Etienne Stéphane (b. 1828). Paris obstetrician.

Tarnier's forceps. A variety of obstetrical forceps.

taro (**tah**·ro). The root of *Colocasia antiquorum*; a food substance eaten extensively by some poor populations in the eastern tropics. It has been blamed as a cause of leprosy on very inadequate grounds. [Tahitian.]

Tarozzi and Radaeli white mycetoma. *See* MYCETOMA, WHITE.

Tarpeia (tar·**pe**·e·ah). A suggested generic name for viruses of the influenza group, but not generally accepted.

tarsadenitis (tar·sad·en·**i**′·tis). An affection of the tarsi of the eyelids and the tarsal glands. [tarsus, adenitis.]

tarsal (**tar**·sal). Relating to the tarsi of the eyelids, or of the foot.

tarsal arteries [arteriae tarseae laterales (NA)]. Branches of the dorsalis pedis artery to the dorsum of the foot and the extensor digitorum brevis muscle. The medial arteries [arteriae tarsae mediales (NA)] go to the medial border.

tarsal bones [ossa tarsi (NA)]. A group of seven small irregular bones forming the posterior part of the skeleton of the foot.

tarsal muscles. Bundles of muscle fibres, superior [musculus tarsalis superior (NA)] and inferior [musculus tarsalis inferior (NA)], close to the margin of each eyelid, derived from the orbicularis oculi muscle.

tarsale (tar·**sa**·le). Any of the bones of the tarsus.

tarsalgia (tar·**sal**·je·ah). Pain experienced in the tarsus of the foot, usually associated with flattening of the arch. [tarsus, Gk *algos* pain.]

tarsalia (tar·**sa**·le·ah). The bones of the tarsus regarded as a whole.

tarsalis (tar·**sa**·lis). Either of the tarsal muscles.

tarsectomy (tar·**sek**·to·me). 1. An operation for the excision of a bone from the tarsus of the foot. 2. An operation for the removal of a portion of the tarsal cartilage of the eyelid. [tarsus, Gk *ektome* excision.]

tarsectopia (tar·sek·**to**·pe·ah). Dislocation of one or more of the bones of the tarsus. [tarsus, Gk *ektopos* out of place.]

tarsitis (tar·**si**·tis). Inflammation of the margin of the eyelids; marginal blepharitis. [tarsus, Gk *-itis* inflammation.]

tarsocheiloplasty (tar·so·**ki**·lo·plas·te). Marginal blepharoplasty; plastic surgery of the edge of the eyelids. [tarsus, Gk *cheilos* lip, *plassein* to mould.]

tarsoclasis (tar·so·**kla**·sis). Remedial breaking of the tarsus of the foot to cure club-foot. [tarsus, Gk *klassein* to break.]

tarsomalacia (**tar**·so·mal·**a**′·she·ah). Softening of the tarsi of the eyelids. [tarsus, Gk *malakia* softening.]

tarsomegaly (tar·so·**meg**·al·e). Morbid engagement of the calcaneum. [tarsus, Gk *megas* great.]

tarsometatarsal (tar·so·met·ah·**tar**′·sal). Involving both the tarsus and the metatarsus. **Tarsometarsal joint.** *See* JOINT.

Tarsonematoidea (**tar**·so·nem·at·**oid**′·e·ah). A super-family of the arachnid order Acarina. The family Tarsonemidae is of medical interest. [Gk *tarsos* sole of foot, *nema* thread, *eidos* form.]

Tarsonemidae (tar·so·**nem**·id·e). A family of the acarine super-family Tarsonematoidea. The genera *Pediculoides* and *Tarsonemus* are of medical interest. [see prec.]

Tarsonemus (tar·so·**ne**·mus). A genus of mites of which some species have been found in sputum: the significance of their presence is not known. [Gk *tarsos* sole of foot, *nema* thread.]

tarso-orbital (tar·so·**or**·bit·al). Relating to the tarsi of the eyelids and the walls of the orbit.

tarsophalangeal (**tar**·so·fal·**an**′·je·al). Involving the tarsus of the foot and the phalanges.

tarsophyma (tar·so·**fi**·mah). Any growth on the tarsi of the eyelids. [tarsus, Gk *phyma* growth.]

tarsoplasia, tarsoplasty (tar·so·**pla**·ze·ah, **tar**·so·plas·te). Blepharoplasty; plastic surgery of the tarsi of the eyelids. [tarsus, Gk *plassein* to mould.]

tarsoptosia, tarsoptosis (tar·sop·**to**·se·ah, tar·sop·**to**·sis). Flat foot; dropping of the tarsus. [tarsus, Gk *ptosis* a falling.]

tarsorrhaphy (tar·**sor**·af·e). An operation for producing union of the upper and lower eyelids. The commonest indication for its performance is anaesthesia of the cornea. **Lateral tarsorrhaphy.** An operation in which the lateral parts only of the upper and lower lids are united. [tarsus, Gk *rhaphe* suture.]

tarsotarsal (tar·so·**tar**·sal). Denoting the articulations between the two rows of tarsal bones.

tarsotibial (tar·so·**tib**·e·al). Involving the tarsus and the tibia.

tarsotomy (tar·**sot**·o·me). 1. An operation performed upon the tarsus of the foot. 2. Operative incision of the tarsi of the eyelids. **Cuneiform tarsotomy.** Removal of a wedge-shaped piece from one of the tarsal bones. [tarsus, Gk *temnein* to cut.]

tarsus [NA] (**tar**·sus). 1. The seven bones of the foot which intervene between the tibia and fibula and the metatarsals. They consist of the talus and calcaneum proximally, the former articulating with the tibia and fibula, the latter forming the prominence of the heel; distal to the calcaneum on the lateral side is the cuboid bone, and to the talus medially, the navicular bone, in front of which are the three cuneiform bones. The cuboid articulates with the 4th and 5th metatarsals, the three cuneiforms with the 1st, 2nd, and 3rd metatarsals respectively. [Gk *tarsos* sole of the foot.] 2. A plate of condensed fibrous tissue in the upper and lower eyelids in which the tarsal glands are embedded. [Gk *tarsos* edge of eyelid.]

tartar (**tar**·tar). 1. The sediment of crude acid potassium tartrate occurring in wine casks. 2. A mass of calcium and magnesium salts deposited around the teeth and upon artificial dentures; calculus. **Cream of tartar.** Potassium acid tartrate. [Fr. *tartre.*]

tartarated (**tar**·tar·a·ted). Treated with, or containing tartaric acid.

tartarize (**tar**·tar·ize). To mix with tartaric acid.

tartarus (**tar**·tar·us). Tartar. **Tartarus boraxatus.** Sodium borotartrate; an antiseptic and diuretic obtained by the evaporation of a mixture of borax (2 parts), potassium acid tartrate (5 parts), and water (15 parts). **Tartarus depuratus.** Potassium acid tartrate. **Tartarus natronatus.** Sodium potassium tartrate.

tartrate (**tar**·trate). Any salt or ester of tartaric acid. **Acid tartrate.** Bitartrate; any tartrate in which one COOH group of the original tartaric acid remains. **Normal tartrate.** One in which the acid hydrogens of tartaric acid have both been replaced by a base.

tartrated (tar·**tra**·ted). Tartarated.

Tartrazine BPC 1954 (**tar**·traz·een). $NaSO_3C_6H_4N{=}N{-}C_3HON_2(NaOOC)C_6H_4SO_3Na$, a disulphonate derived from pyrazolone; a yellow azo-dyestuff used to colour foods.

tartrobismuthate (tar·tro·**biz**·muth·ate). Bismuthotartrate.

tartronate (**tar**·tron·ate). $CHOH(COOH)_2$, hydroxymalonate; an inhibitor of malate transport across the mitochondrial membrane.

tasikinesia (ta·se·kin·**e**′·se·ah). An obsessional impulse to walk about; inability to sit still. [Gk *tasis* straining, *kinesis* motion.]

taste (**ta**·st). The sensation produced in the mouth by certain chemical substances. The sense organs responsible for taste (*taste buds*) are situated on the posterior part of the tongue and in the walls of the pharynx; the nerve of taste is the 9th cranial, though the 5th and 7th may contribute. **Taste buds.** *See* BUD. **Colour taste.** Pseudogeuaesthesia. **Taste deficiency.** A hereditary or acquired inability to taste. Lesions of the 5th and 7th cranial nerves may cause a taste defect of the anterior two-thirds of the tongue, and lesions of the 9th may affect the posterior third. **Taste end, Taste ending.** A taste bud with its accompanying nerve fibres. **Franklinic taste.** A sour taste resulting from electrical stimulation of the tongue. [OFr. *taster.*]

Tatera (**tah**·te·rah). A genus of gerbils, several species of which are reservoirs of sylvatic plague. *Tatera brantsi* and *T. schinzi* in

South Africa, *T. indica* in India and Iran, and *T. nigrita* in Zaire are the most important.

tattooing (tat·oo·ing). Indelible markings in the skin, arranged in decorative patterns; they are produced by puncturing the skin and inserting a suitable pigment. Descriptive also of the powder markings around a firearm entry wound delivered at close range. **Tattooing of the cornea.** Coloration of the cornea to conceal a leucoma. **Electrolytic tattooing.** The treatment of naevus or angioma by the use of an electrode consisting of several needles. [Tahitian *tatu.*]

Tauber, Henry (b. 1897). American biochemist.

Tauber's test. For pentose in urine: to 0.1 ml of urine add 0.5 ml of 0.5 per cent benzidine in glacial acetic acid. Heat to boiling, cool rapidly under the tap and add 1 ml of water. A pink to red colour indicates pentose.

tauranga (taw·rang·gah). A disorder occurring in New Zealand among cattle and sheep which causes progressive anaemia.

taurine (taw·reen). 2-Amino ethylsulphonic acid, $NH_2CH_2CH_2SO_3H$. A derivative of the amino acid, cysteine, present in bile in combination with cholic acid as taurocholic acid.

taurocholaemia (taw·ro·ko·le′·me·ah). A condition characterized by the appearance of taurocholic acid in the blood. [taurocholic acid, Gk *haima* blood.]

taurocholaneresis (taw·ro·ko·lan·er′·es·is). Increase of taurocholic acid in the bile. [taurocholic acid, Gk *a-*, *eresis* removal.]

taurocholanopoiesis (taw·ro·ko·lan·o·poi·e′·sis). The production by the liver of taurocholic acid. [taurocholic acid, Gk *ano* upwards, *poiesis* production.]

taurocholate (taw·ro·ko·late). Any salt or ester of taurocholic acid.

Taurolin (taw·ro·lin). BP Commission approved name for 4,4′ - methylenedi(tetrahydro - 1,2,4 - thiadiazine - 1 - dioxide); an antibacterial agent.

Taurultam (tor·ul·tam). BP Commission approved name for tetrahydro-1,2,4-thiadiazine 1,1-dioxide; its action is antibacterial and antifungal.

Taussig, Helen Brook (b. 1898). Baltimore physician.

Taussig-Bing syndrome. A developmental abnormality of the heart, falling within the group of transposition of the great vessels in which the aorta arises from the right ventricles and the pulmonary artery overrides the ventricular system, a septal defect being present.

Blalock-Taussig operation. The operation devised by Blalock to achieve, as suggested by Taussig, an increase in the blood-flow to the lungs in patients with cyanotic heart disease; a systemic artery, usually the subclavian but sometimes the innominate, is divided and the proximal end anastomosed to the side or the distal end of the pulmonary artery on the same side.

tautomeral, tautomeric (taw·tom·er·al, taw·to·mer·ik). In chemistry, of the nature of or characterized by tautomerism.

tautomerism (taw·tom·er·izm). A form of dynamic isomerism in which two isomers may exist in equilibrium, one passing into the other reversibly according as the equilibrium is disturbed by any outside factor. Such isomerism involves changes in linkage; a classical example is aceto acetic ester, of which the keto form, $CH_3COCH_2COOC_2H_5$, is in equilibrium with the enol form, $CH_3C(OH){=}CHCOOC_2H_5$. [Gk *tautos* same, *meros* part.]

tautorotation (taw·to·ro·ta′·shun). Mutarotation. [Gk *tautos* same, rotation.]

Tavel, Ernst (b. 1858). Berne surgeon.

Tavel's serum. An antityphoid serum.

Tawara, Sunao (b. 1873). Japanese pathologist.

Node of Tawara, His-Tawara node. Atrioventricular node. *See* NODE.

taxis (tax·is). The manual reduction of a hernia or dislocation. **Bipolar taxis.** The correction of a retroverted uterus by drawing the cervix down the vagina, at the same time pushing the fundus upwards by means of a finger in the rectum. **Negative taxis, Positive taxis.** The movement of cells respectively away from or towards other cells. [Gk arrangement.]

Taxodium distichum (tax·o·de·um dis·tik·um). The North American black cypress, the resin of which has been used in rheumatism treatment. [Gk *taxos* yew, *eidos* form, *dis* twice, *stichos* row.]

taxology (tax·ol·o·je). Taxonomy. [Gk *taxis* arrangement, *logos* science.]

taxonomic (tax·on·om·ik). Pertaining to taxonomy.

taxonomy (tax·on·o·me). In biology, the classification of plants and animals. [Gk *taxis* arrangement, *nomos* law.]

Taxus (tax·us). A genus of coniferous trees (family Taxaceae). **Taxus baccata.** The common yew. [Gk *taxos* yew.]

Tay, Warren (b. 1843). London ophthalmologist.

Tay's central guttate choroiditis, disease, or spots. The development of yellowish-white raised spots, usually in the macular region around the disc, but sometimes peripherally and often unassociated with visual loss. Caused by wart-like excrescences of Bruch's membrane, a degenerative condition usually senile but occasionally seen in young people.

Tay-Sachs disease. Amaurotic family idiocy, cerebromacular degeneration; a familial disease of infancy in which there is a progressive degeneration of nerve cells throughout the whole nervous system and in the retina. It is characterized clinically by progressive muscular weakness and paralysis, mental deterioration, and blindness, usually leading to death in coma or convulsions towards the end of the second year. A characteristic cherry-red spot can be seen at the macula lutea on ophthalmoscopic examination. The degenerating nerve cells are filled with a lipoid similar to that in the Niemann-Pick form of phosphatide lipoidosis, but there is no enlargement of the liver and spleen.

Taylor, Charles Bell (b. 1829). British ophthalmologist.

Bell Taylor's knife. A modified keratome or lance-shaped knife for iridectomy. It is angled, has slightly curved edges, and the upper side has a bevelled to a central ridge. In common use.

Bell Taylor's operation. For cataract: a method of cataract extraction in which a peripheral incision was made in the iris through which the lens was delivered. Of historical interest.

Taylor, Charles Fayette (b. 1827). New York surgeon.

Taylor's brace. A steel support for the spine, used in Pott's disease.

Taylor, Hermon (b. 1905). London surgeon.

Hermon Taylor gastroscope. A rigid type of gastroscope.

Schranz-Taylor gastroscope. An instrument which can be actively flexed by turning a wheel on the proximal end. It transmits more light and gives a larger image than the Wolf-Schindler gastroscope.

Taylor, Robert William (b. 1842). New York dermatologist.

Taylor's disease. 1. Dermatitis chronica atrophicans. 2. Idiopathic atrophy of the skin.

tea (tee). The prepared young leaves and leaf-buds of *Thea sinensis* Linn. (*Camellia thea* Linn.) of the family Theaceae, cultivated in India, Sri Lanka, China, and Japan. Its main constituents are caffeine and tannin; there is also a little essential oil and traces of theobromine and theophylline. **Beef tea.** An infusion of beef; obsolete, as it is now considered to be of little or no nutritional value. **Hottentot tea.** Buchu. **Maté tea.** The leaves of *Ilex paraguayensis* (family Aquifoliaceae); they contain caffeine and chlorogenic acid. **Paraguay tea.** Maté tea (see prec.). [Chinese *ch'a.*]

teaberry (te·ber·e). Gaultheria, wintergreen; the leaves of *Gaultheria procumbens* (family Ericaceae), containing the essential oil, oil of wintergreen, which is obtained by maceration and steam distillation.

Teacher, John Hammond (b. 1869). Glasgow pathologist.

Bryce-Teacher ovum. One of the classical early human embryos.

Teague, Oscar (b. 1878). New York bacteriologist.

Teague and Clurman agar. Brilliant-green eosin agar. *See* AGAR.

Holt-Harris and Teague agar. Eosin methylene blue agar. *See* AGAR.

teak (teek). The timber tree *Tectona grandis.* The wood yields a medicinal oil and a tar. [Malayalam *tekka.*]

Teal's test. For simulated unilateral deafness: bone conduction on the allegedly deaf side is tested with a vibrating tuning fork over the mastoid process of the temporal bone. Usually the candidate states that this is heard. He is then told that the test will be repeated. This time, however, the non-vibrating fork is held close to the meatus. If now, he still states that he can hear vibrations, he is presumed to be malingering.

Teale, Thomas Pridgin (b. 1801). London surgeon.

Teale's amputation. Amputation by two rectangular flaps of skin and muscle, one long and one short.

Teale's hernia. Prevascular femoral hernia; femoral hernia entering the thigh in front of the femoral sheath.

Teale's operation. For symblepharon: two vertical pedicle flaps of conjunctiva are cut with the bases below, one on the inner and one on the outer side. They are then swung down to cover the bare area produced by the excision of the scarred conjunctiva.

Teare, Robert Donald (b. 1911). London forensic pathologist.

Teare's cardiomegaly. An asymmetrical left ventricular muscle thickening pronounced under the aortic valve, commonly causing stenosis of the outflow of the left ventricle. A familiar disorder emerging as a clinical entity in adult life.

tears (teerz). 1. The watery fluid secreted by the lacrimal glands, which moistens the conjunctiva. 2. Small round drops of natural gum or resin. **Crocodile tears.** The copious secretion of tears on eating due to misdirection of regenerating nerve fibres in recovery from Bell's palsy. [AS.]

tease (teez). To disintegrate the fibres of biological tissue by pulling apart with needles, preparatory to microscopical examination. [AS *taesan* to pluck.]

teaspoon (tee·spoon). A domestic measure for liquids; considered roughly equal to 5 ml (1 fluid drachm). [tea, AS *spon.*]

teat (teet). A nipple. [OFr. *tete.*]

teatulation (teet·ew·**la**·shun). The development of a protuberance resembling a nipple [see prec.]

technetium (tek·**ne**·she·um). The element of atomic number 43, atomic weight 98.91 and chemical symbol Tc. It was obtained (1937) by the bombardment of molybdenum by neutrons in a cyclotron. It has a half-life of one million years, and was originally named masurium. No stable isotope is known so that the prefix radio- is not used. The isotope of technetium of medical interest is ^{99}Tc, which is very widely used especially in the form pertechnetate (TcO_4). [Gk *technetos* artificial.]

technical (tek·nik·al). Concerned with the technique of an operation or procedure, or resulting from it.

technician (tek·**nish**·un). One skilled in technical work. [see foll.]

technique (tek·**neek**). The detailed steps in completing any procedure, e.g. in a surgical operation. **DCF technique.** *See* LANE, C. A. **Epidural technique.** A technique of local analgesia in which the solution is injected into the epidural or extradural space. **Invasive technique** (of investigation). A method which involves breaching the patient's skin in order to achieve the desired result, and which therefore may involve discomfort and risk. **Non-invasive technique** (of investigation). A method which does not involve breaching the patient's skin, and which therefore does not involve discomfort or risk. **Paris technique.** In cervical carcinoma. Regaud and Lacassagne technique. **Stockholm technique.** In cervical carcinoma. Heyman's technique. **Time-diffusion technique.** A form of spinal anaesthesia in which the upward level of the anaesthesia is controlled by sitting the patient upright for a measured number of seconds after the intrathecal injection of a hypobaric solution of an anaesthetic drug; Etherington-Wilson technique. **T-piece anaesthetic technique.** Endotracheal inhalation anaesthesia in which the expired gases escape freely via the open vertical limb of the T-piece tube, as devised by Dr. Ayre. [Gk *technikos* skilful.]

See also: ADAMSON, COLT, ETHERINGTON-WILSON, HARTEL, HEYMAN, KIENBOECK, KRISTELLER, LACASSAGNE, LANE (C. A.), PATRICK, PEER, REGAUD, TRUETA, WANGENSTEEN, WOODHALL.

technocausis (tek·no·**kaw**·sis). Actual cautery by heat. [Gk *techne* art, *kausis* a burning.]

technologist (tek·**nol**·o·jist). One versed in technology.

technology (tek·**nol**·o·je). The study of the manufacturing processes whereby natural resources are converted to the use of man. [Gk *techne* art, *logos* science.]

technometer (tek·**nom**·et·er). An instrument which measures and registers the amount of an x-ray exposure.

Teclothiazide (tek·lo·**thi**·az·ide). BP Commission approved name for 6 - chloro - 3,4 - dihydro - 3 - trichloromethyl - 1,2,4 - benzothiadiazine - 7 - sulphonamide 1,1 - dioxide; a diuretic.

tecnoctonia (tek·nok·**to**·ne·ah). Child-murder; infanticide. [Gk *teknon* child, *ktonos* murder.]

tecnocyte (**tek**·no·site). Teknocyte.

tectiform (**tek**·te·form). Shaped like a roof. [L *tectum* roof, form.]

tectocephalic (**tek**·to·kef·**al**'·ik). Scaphocephalic; having a lengthy skull with a ridge along the top. [L *tectum* roof, Gk *kephale* skull.]

tectology (tek·**tol**·o·je). Structural morphology; the study of the structure of plants and animals. [Gk *tekton* builder, *logos* science.]

tectonic (tek·**ton**·ik). Concerned with plastic surgery, or the replacement of tissues by grafting. [Gk *tekton* builder.]

tectorial (tek·**tor**·e·al). Roof-like, or pertaining to a roof or cover. [see foll.]

tectorium (tek·**tor**·e·um). A roof; applied to any structure that serves as a roof. [L.]

tectospinal (tek·to·**spi**·nal). Connected with the tectum (quadrigeminal bodies) of the mid-brain and the spinal cord. **Tectospinal tract.** *See* TRACT.

tectum (**tek**·tum). A roof or cover. **Tectum of the mid-brain [tectum mesencephali (NA)].** The quadrigeminal bodies which develop in the roof plate of the mid-brain. [L.]

teeth (teeth). *See* TOOTH.

teething (**tee**·thing). The process of cutting the teeth of the deciduous dentition.

tegmen [NA] (**teg**·men). A covering. **Tegmen tympani [NA].** A thin plate of bone which forms the roof of the tympanic cavity and antrum and covers also the bony part of the pharyngotympanic tube. [L.]

tegment (**teg**·ment). The tegmentum.

tegmental (teg·**men**·tal). Of the nature of a tegmen, or relating to a tegmentum.

tegmentum [NA] (teg·**men**·tum). A covering; a term applied to the part of the mid-brain between the cerebral peduncles ventrally and the tectum (quadrigeminal bodies) dorsally. It contains the red nucleus, oculomotor nucleus, etc., and extends cranially into the diencephalon below the thalamus as the *subthalamic tegmentum* and caudally above the transverse fibres of the pons, forming the floor of the 4th ventricle, as the *tegmentum of the pons.* **Tegmentum of the hind-brain [tegmentum rhombencephali].** The dorsal portion of the pons and the medulla oblongata; the term excludes the basilar portion of the pons with its longitudinal and tranverse fibres and nuclei pontis. **Tegmentum of the pons.** *See* MAIN DEF. (above). **Subthalamic tegmentum.** *See* MAIN DEF. (above). [L.]

tegumen (**teg**·ew·men). Tegmen.

tegument (**teg**·ew·ment). The common integument; the skin. [L *tegumentum* cover.]

tegumental, tegumentary (teg·ew·**men**·tal, teg·ew·**men**·tar·e). Having the character of or pertaining to an integument; cutaneous. [see prec.]

Teichmann-Stawiarski, Ludwig (b. 1823). Cracow histologist.

Teichmann's crystals. Haemin crystals; yellow to chocolate-brown rhombic microcrystals of haematin chloride, formed by the action of hot glacial acetic acid on dried blood in the presence of sodium chloride, and separating out on cooling. The reaction is used to detect blood stains.

Teichmann's networks. The lymphatic plexuses of the stomach wall.

Teichmann's test. For blood. *See* HAEMIN TEST (under TEST).

teichopsia (ti·**kop**·se·ah). Fortification spectra; zig-zag appearances before the eyes, in migraine. [Gk *teichos* wall, *opsis* vision.]

teknocyte (**tek**·no·site). A young or early neutrophil leucocyte. [Gk *teknon* child, *kytos* cell.]

tela [NA] (**te**·lah). A web; in anatomy, a web-like membrane or layer. **Tela choroidea [NA].** A layer of pia mater which, together with blood vessels, is invaginated into one of the ventricles of the brain as a choroid plexus; hence the tela choroidea of the 3rd [tela choroidea ventriculi terti (NA)] and 4th [tela choroidea ventriculi quarti (NA)] ventricles. Its ventricular surface is covered with modified ependymal cells which secrete cerebrospinal fluid. [L.]

telaesthesia (tel·es·**the**·ze·ah). Perception of objects at a distance without normal sensory contact. [Gk *tele* far off, *aisthesis* sensation.]

telaesthetoscope (tel·es·**thet**·o·skope). An electrically amplified stethoscope for the audible demonstration of symptomatic sounds. [Gk *tele* far off, *aisthesis* sensation, *skopein* to observe.]

telalgia (tel·**al**·je·ah). Referred pain; pain experienced at a different point from that in which the lesion is situated. [Gk *tele* far off, *algos* pain.]

telangiectasia (tel·**an**·je·ek·**ta'**·ze·ah). A condition of dilated capillary blood vessels, often multiple in character and forming angiomata. **Arborizing telangiectasia.** Generalized essential telangiectasia (see below). **Branching linear telangiectasia.** A leash of venules often seen on the thighs. **Essential telangiectasia.** Telangiectasia arising from mechanical abnormalities causing stasis in, and therefore dilatation of, the capillary vessels. **Telangiectasia faciei.** Acne rosacea. **Familial telangiectasia, Hereditary haemorrhagic telangiectasia.** Rendu-Osler-Weber disease, a hereditary disease characterized by recurrent bleeding from multiple telangiectases (dilated capillaries), usually in mucous membranes or skin, with normal platelet count, coagulation and bleeding times, clot retraction, etc., but there is often a secondary anaemia. **Generalized essential telangiectasia.** A widespread telangiectasia of undetermined cause. **Telangiectasia lymphatica.** A condition of dilatation of lymphatic vessels causing lymphangiomata. It may be congenital, or arise from various chronic mechanical or other obstructive causes. **Telangiectasia macularis eruptiva perstans.** An urticarial type of skin lesion accompanied by a persisting red macular appearance. **Postradiation telangiectasia.** A permanent discoloration of the skin due to the formation of multiple telangiectases which may follow heavy doses of radiotherapy. **Radiogenic telangiectasia.** The telangiectatic component of chronic radiodermatitis. **Spider telangiectasia.** Naevus araneus. **Telangiectasia verrucosa.** A telangiectatic condition of the skin, which may be associated with wart-like growths and thickening of the epidermis. It is seen most commonly on the legs and feet of children. [Gk *telos* end, *aggeion* vessel, *ektasis* dilatation.]

telangiectatic (tel·**an**·je·ek·**tat'**·ik). Concerned with telangiectasia, or having its characteristics.

telangiectodes (tel·**an**·je·ek·**to'**·deez). Term applied to tumours displaying telangiectasia. [telangiectasia, Gk *eidos* form.]

telangiectoma (tel·**an**·je·ek·**to'**·mah). 1. A birthmark or naevus. 2. A telangioma. [telangiectasia, Gk *-oma* tumour.]

telangiitis (tel·**an**·je·**i'**·tis). Inflammation of the capillaries. [Gk *telos* end, *aggeion* vessel, *-itis* inflammation.]

telangioma (tel·**an**·je·**o'**·mah). An angioma of the capillaries. [Gk *telos* end, *aggeion* vessel, *-oma* tumour.]

telangion (tel·**an**·je·on). A capillary; a terminal arteriole. [Gk *telos* end, *aggeion* vessel.]

telangiosis (tel·**an**·je·**o'**·sis). Any diseased state of the capillaries. [Gk *telos* end, *aggeion* vessel, *-osis* condition.]

telar (**te**·lar). Relating to or having the characteristics of a tela or web.

telarche (tel·**ar**·ke). Enlargement of the breasts at puberty. Cf. MENARCHE. [Gk *telos* end, *archaios* from the beginning.]

telebinocular (tel·e·bin·**ok'**·ew·lar). An instrument containing prisms, used for exercises to cure squint. [Gk *tele* far off, binocular.]

telecardiogram (tel·e·**kar**·de·o·gram). A form of electrocardiogram which produces a record at a distance from the patient. [Gk *tele* far off, cardiogram.]

telecardiography (**tel**·e·kar·de·**og'**·raf·e). A method of studying the actions of the heart by means of the telecardiogram.

telecardiophone (tel·e·**kar**·de·o·fone). A form of cardiophone which broadcasts heart sounds to listeners at a distance from the patient. [Gk *tele* far off, cardiophone.]

teleceptive (tel·e·**sep**·tiv). Relating to a telereceptor.

teleceptor (**tel**·e·sep·tor). Telereceptor.

telecinesia, telecinesis (**tel**·e·sin·**e'**·ze·ah, **tel**·e·sin·**e'**·sis). Telekinesia.

teledactyl (tel·e·**dak**·til). An apparatus to enable crippled people to pick up objects from the floor. [Gk *tele* far off, *daktylos* finger.]

teledendrite, teledendron (tel·e·**den**·drite, tel·e·**den**·dron). Telodendron.

telediastolic (**tel**·e·di·as·**tol'**·ik). Referring to the final stage of the cardiac diastole. [Gk *telos* end, diastole.]

telegony (tel·**eg**·o·ne). The appearance in offspring of subsequent matings with a different male of characters derived from the male of a previous mating. A discarded doctrine which has a long back history; the famous Penycuik experiments between zebra and horses were designed to prove or disprove it and were thought to have proved it, but it is not accepted today. [Gk *tele* far off, *gone* seed.]

telekinesia, telekinesis (**tel**·e·kin·**e'**·ze·ah, tel·e·**kin**·e·sis). The movement of a physical object through space without physical contact with the object or physical influence upon it. The power is claimed by certain spiritualistic mediums. [Gk *tele* far off, *kinesis* movement.]

telelectrocardiogram (tel·el·ek·tro·**kar'**·de·o·gram). Telecardiogram. [Gk *tele* far off, electrocardiogram.]

telelectrocardiography (tel·el·**ek**·tro·kar·de·**og'**·raf·e). Telecardiography. [Gk *tele* far off, electrocardiography.]

Telemann, W. (fl. 1908). German parasitologist.

Telemann method. A method for detecting schistosoma ova when they are scanty. A portion of stool is shaken with a mixture of concentrated hydrochloric acid, water, and ether (two parts), strained, and the filtrate centrifuged. The deposit is mixed with water so that the miracidia hatch out and these are easily detected by means of a hand lens and indirect lighting.

telemeter (tel·**em**·et·er). To measure from afar with the help of an intermediary agent, usually radio. [Gk *tele* far off, *metron* measure.]

telemnemonike (tel·e·ne·**mon'**·ik·e). The process of becoming conscious of the contents of another person's memory. [Gk *tele* far off, *mnemonikos* concerned with memory.]

telencephalic (tel·en·kef·**al'**·ik). Relating to the telencephalon.

telencephalization (**tel**·en·kef·al·i·**za'**·shun). The evolutionary process whereby the forebrain assumes an increasing measure of control over nervous functions formerly mediated by lower nerve centres. [Gk *tele* far off, *egkephalos* brain.]

telencephalon [NA] (tel·en·**kef**·al·on). The cerebral hemispheres; that part of the brain which develops as paired outgrowths from the anterior end of the forebrain and includes the cerebral cortex, olfactory lobes, and corpora striata. [Gk *telos* end, *egkephalos* brain.]

teleneurite (tel·e·**newr**·ite). The branching end of an axon. [see foll.]

teleneuron (tel·e·**newr**·one). Any nerve-ending. [Gk *telos* end, *neuron* nerve.]

teleodendron (**tel**·e·o·**den'**·dron). Telodendron.

teleological (**tel**·e·o·**loj'**·ik·al). Pertaining to teleology.

teleology (tel·e·**ol**·o·je). The doctrine of ends or final causes; the theory that everything is directed towards some final purpose. [Gk *telos* end, *logos* science.]

teleomitosis (tel·e·o·mi·to′·sis). The completion of mitosis. [Gk *telos* end, mitosis.]

tele-organic (tel·e·or·gan′·ik). Devoted to the purpose of organic existence. [Gk *telos* end, *organon* organ.]

teleoroentgenography (tel·e·o·runt·yen·og′·raf·e). Teleradiography. [Gk *tele* far off, roentgenography.]

teleotherapeutics (tel·e·o·ther·ap·ew′·tix). Suggestion therapy. See THERAPY. [Gk *tele* far off, therapeutics.]

telepathine (tel·e·path·een). Banisterine, yageine, $C_{13}H_{12}ON_2$. An alkaloid obtained from the South American plant yagé, *Banisteria caapi*. It would seem to be identical with harmine.

telepathy (tel·ep·ath·e). The transference of thought from one mind to another without ordinary physical communication. [Gk *tele* far off, *pathos* feeling.]

teleradiograph (tel·e·ra·de·o·graf). A radiograph made by the teleradiographic technique.

teleradiography (tel·e·ra·de·og′·raf·e). Radiography with the x-ray tube approximately 1.8–2.1 m (6–7 ft) away from the radiograph, in order to secure parallel x-rays and the absence of distortion. [Gk *tele* far off, radiography.]

teleradiotherapy (tel·e·ra·de·o·ther′·ap·e). Treatment with radiation, employing a long target or source-skin distance. [Gk *tele* far off, radiotherapy.]

teleradium (tel·e·ra·de·um). Radium at a distance. [Gk *tele* far off, radium.]

telereceptor (tel·e·re·sep′·tor). Any sensory nerve-ending, such as those of the nose, ears, and eyes, which receives stimuli from objects at a distance. [Gk *tele* far off, receptor.]

telergic (tel·er·jik). Producing an effect at a distance. [Gk *tele* far off, *ergein* to work.]

telergy (tel·er·je). 1. Action at a distance; movements of a subject under the influence of another mind some distance away. 2. Automatism. [see prec.]

teleroentgenotherapy (tel·e·runt·yen·o·ther′·ap·e). Teleradiotherapy. [Gk *tele* far off, roentgenotherapy.]

telescope (tel·es·kope). An optical device for obtaining magnified images of distant objects. **Galilean telescope.** A refracting telescope composed of two convex lenses, first used for astronomical purposes by Galileo Galilei (1564–1642). **Reflecting telescope.** A telescope in which a concave mirror is used to produce a magnified real image of the distant object, which is viewed with a refracting eyepiece. **Refracting telescope.** A combination of a convex lens as objective and an eyepiece with which the magnified real image is viewed. [Gk *tele* far off, *skopein* to view.]

telestereoradiography (tel·e·ster·e·o·ra·de·og′·raf·e). Stereoradiography with the x-ray tube 1.8–2.1 m (6–7 ft) away from the plate. [Gk *tele* far off, stereoradiography.]

telestereoroentgenography (tel·e·steer·e·o·runt·yen·og′·raf·e). Telestereoradiography. [Gk *tele* far off, stereoroentgenography.]

telesystolic (tel·e·sis·tol′·ik). Referring to the final stage of the cardiac systole. [Gk *telos* end, systole.]

teletactile (tel·e·tak·tile). The appreciation of sound by means of touch. [Gk *tele* far off, L *tactus* touch.]

teletactor (tel·e·tak·tor). An aid for the deaf in which vibrations are received through the sense of touch. [see prec.]

teletherapy (tel·e·ther·ap·e). 1. Teleradiotherapy. 2. The treatment of mental disease from a distance. [Gk *tele* far off, therapy.]

telicherry bark (tel·e·cher·e bark). Conessi bark; the bark of *Holarrhena antidysenterica* Wall. (family Apocyanaceae). It is a spongy rust-coloured substance, used in dysentery and diarrhoea and contains the alkaloid, conessine, among others.

tellurate (tel·ewr·ate). Any salt of telluric acid, H_2TeO_4.

telluric (tel·ewr·ik). 1. Associated with the soil. 2. Associated with tellurium. [L *tellus* earth.]

tellurism (tel·ewr·izm). The idea that a pathogenic influence is to be attributed to the soil. [L *tellus* earth.]

tellurite (tel·ewr·ite). 1. Any salt of tellurous acid, H_2TeO_3. 2. A mineral form of tellurium dioxide, TeO_2.

tellurium (tel·ewr·e·um). An element of atomic weight 127.60, atomic number 52, and chemical symbol Te. It is a silver-white non-metal closely allied to sulphur in chemical properties though a good conductor of electricity. It also occurs in a number of allotropic forms. The soluble salts of tellurium are poisonous, causing inflammation of the bowels and kidneys, whilst potassium tellurate has a marked antihidrotic action. The metal and its compounds find their chief use in industry. [L *tellus* earth.]

Tellyesniczky, Kalmar (b. 1868). Budapest histologist.

Tellyesniczky's mixture. A fixing solution consisting of potassium dichromate and acetic acid.

telocentric (tel·o·sen·trik). Of a chromosome or chromatid, with the centromere at one end. [Gk *telos* end, *kentron* centre.]

telocinesia, telocinesis (tel·o·sin·e′·ze·ah, tel·o·sin·e′·sis). Telophase. [Gk *telos* end, karyokinesis.]

telodendrion (tel·o·den·dre·on). Telodendron.

telodendron (tel·o·den·dron). The terminal branching of a dendrite. [Gk *telos* end, dendrite.]

telogen (tel·o·jen). The resting phase in the cycle of hair growth which lasts for about 3 months. At any one time, between 4 and 24 per cent of scalp hairs are in the telogen phase. [Gk *telos* end, *genein* to produce.]

teloglia (tee·log·le·ah). Cells which cover the outer surface of motor end-plates. [Gk *telos* end, *glia* glue.]

telokinesis (tel·o·kin·e′·sis). Telophase. [Gk *telos* end, karyokinesis.]

telolecithal (tel·o·les·ith·al). Describing an egg in which there is a large mass of yolk with a small germinal disc at one end. [Gk *telos* end, *lekithos* yolk.]

telolemma (tel·o·lem·ah). The membrane covering a motor end-plate, consisting of the sarcolemma of the muscle fibre fused with the endoneurium of the nerve fibre. [Gk *telos* end, *lemma* sheath.]

telolysosome (tel·o·li′·so·some). A membrane-bound body containing the end-products of the digestive processes which take place in heterolysosomes or autolysosomes. [Gk *telos* end, *lysis* a loosing, *soma* body.]

telomere (tel·o·meer). A hypothetical structure specific for the ends of eukaryotic chromosomes. Its absence would prevent normal chromosome behaviour. [Gk *telos* end, *meros* part.]

telophase (tel·o·faze). The last stage in mitotic and meiotic karyokinesis when the daughter chromosomes, which have completed their migration, lose their identity and are surrounded by a newly-formed nuclear membrane. [Gk *telos* end, *phasis* appearance.]

telophragma (tel·o·frag·mah). Krause's membrane, or intermediate disc, which separates adjacent sarcomeres in a muscle fibre. [Gk *telos* end, *phragma* enclosure.]

teloreceptor (tel·o·re·sep′·tor). Telereceptor.

Telosporidia (tel·o·spor·id′·e·ah). A sub-class of Sporozoa including the orders Coccidia, Gregarinida, and Haemosporidia: spore formation ends the life of the individual. [Gk *telos* end, spore.]

Temazepam (tem·az·e·pam). BP Commission approved name for 7 - chloro - 3 - hydroxy - 1 - methyl - 5 - phenyl - 1*H* - 1,4 - benzodiazepin - 2′(3*H*) - one; a tranquillizer.

Temin, Howard. 20th century molecular biologist.

Temin's enzyme. Reverse transcriptase; RNA-dependent-DNA polymerase.

temperament (tem·per·am·ent). That aspect of personality which denotes a person's emotional disposition. The Greeks (Hippocrates, Aristotle) believed that the body was composed of four humours, blood, phlegm, yellow bile, and black bile. This humoral doctrine in some guise held sway until the middle of the 19th century when it was replaced by the cell theory of Virchow. In mediaeval times the humours were correlated with the temperaments of which four were described, *sanguine, phlegmatic, melancholic*, and *choleric*, according to which of the humours predominated in a particular constitution; others such as the *nervous* and *lymphatic* were added later. These terms are now only of historic interest although attempts are still made to correlate them with various bodily characteristics. [L *temperamentum* mixture in proper proportions.]

temperature (tem·per·at·cher, tem·per·at·ewr). A measure of the hotness of a body. **Absolute temperature.** A scale of temperature based on the properties of a hypothetical perfect gas. Measured in degrees Kelvin (K). On this scale the melting point of ice is 273.16 K, the boiling point of water 373.16 K. **Basal temperature.** Body temperature, under basal conditions, at rest, taken on waking. Used to determine whether ovulation is taking place. **Biphasic temperature.** An indication that ovulation is taking place. The temperature is relatively low before and relatively high after ovulation. **Body temperature.** The internal temperature of the body. This depends upon the balance between heat production and heat loss. **Critical temperature.** That temperature above which a gas cannot be liquefied. **DNA melting temperature.** The temperature at the midpoint of the melting curve for a particular deoxyribonucleic acid. **Temperature equivalents.** Conversion formulae:

$$^{\circ}\text{C}=\frac{(^{\circ}\text{F}-32)}{9}\times 5,\ ^{\circ}\text{F}=\frac{9}{5}\,^{\circ}\text{C}+32.$$

Maximum temperature. In bacteriology, the highest temperature, in some specified circumstances. **Mean temperature.** The arithmetic mean of a number of temperature observations. **Minimum temperature.** In bacteriology, the lowest temperature, in some specified circumstances. **Normal temperature.** For ordinary clinical purposes, the temperature of a normal person at rest as recorded by a clinical thermometer placed in the axilla, mouth, or rectum with due precautions. The mean normal temperature in the mouth is usually given as 37°C (98.6°F), but as the temperature is constantly varying with such factors as rest, exercise, sleep, eating and drinking, metabolic processes, the evaporation of sweat, the temperature of the air, and so on, it is more accurate to speak of the normal range of temperature. The mouth temperature ranges from about 36.6-37.2°C (97.8-99°F); rectal temperatures are about 0.3-0.4°C (0.5-0.75°F) higher. Axillary temperatures are the lowest and are generally inaccurate. **Optimum temperature.** In bacteriology, the most favourable temperature, for some specified purpose. **Room temperature.** The air temperature at a point in a room. **Subnormal temperature.** A temperature with a range below normal. **Zero temperature.** The point on a thermometer scale from which measurements are made. On the Celsius thermometers, zero measures the melting point of ice. On the Fahrenheit thermometer, zero is 212° below the boiling point of water and 32° above the melting point of ice. [L *temperatura.*]

template (tem·plate). 1. A mould or cast. In immunology, referring to the template hypothesis started by Ehrlich that antibodies are formed as the mirror images of the antigen structure by condensation of the protein on the surface of the antigen so that a close fit results. 2. A macromolecule on which is assembled another macromolecule (e.g. messenger RNA in the synthesis of polypeptides, RNA or DNA in the synthesis of RNA or DNA, respectively). [L *templum* rafter.]

temple [temporum (NA)] (tem·pl). The flat region on either side of the head above the zygomatic arch. [L *tempus.*]

tempolabile (tem·po·la·bile). Unstable with respect to time; usually applied to a serum. [L *tempus* time, *labilis* unstable.]

temporal (tem·por·al). 1. Located in the region of the temple or pertaining to the temporal bone. [L *tempus* temple.] 2. Related to time. [L *tempus* time.]

temporal arteries. Deep temporal arteries [arteriae temporales profundae (NA)]. Branches, anterior and posterior, of the maxillary artery to the temporal muscle. **Middle temporal artery [arteria temporalis media (NA)].** *See* TEMPORAL ARTERY, SUPERFICIAL (following). **Superficial temporal artery [arteria temporalis superficialis (NA)].** The terminal branch of the external carotid artery, supplying mainly the temple and scalp. It also sends twigs to the auricle [rami auriculares anteriores (NA)], the parotid gland [rami parotidei (NA)], the masseter muscle, and the temporomandibular joint and, having divided into a small anterior [ramus frontalis (NA)] and a larger posterior [ramus parietalis (NA)] branch, anastomoses freely on the scalp with other arteries. Other named branches of the superficial temporal artery are the transverse facial artery [arteria transversa faciei (NA)], which passes forward above the parotid duct to supply the masseter muscle and overlying skin, the zygomatic branch [arteria zygomatico-orbitalis (NA)], which runs to the lateral angle of the orbit, and the middle temporal artery [arteria temporalis media (NA).].

temporal bone [os temporale (NA)]. One of a pair of bones lying in the side wall of the vault and base of the skull and housing the middle and internal ear. It is divided into squamous, petrous, tympanic, and mastoid portions and the styloid process, and articulates with the sphenoid, parietal, occipital, and zygomatic bones.

Mastoid part. That part which lies behind the external auditory meatus and below the supramastoid crest, and bears the mastoid process.

Petrous part [pars petrosa (NA)]. The part that projects into the base of the skull between the greater sphenoid wing and the basi-occiput, and contains the middle and internal ears.

Apex [apex partis petrosae (NA)]. The point at which the three surfaces and borders of the petrous part meet. It abuts on the basisphenoid.

Anterior border. The border separating the anterior and inferior surfaces, which articulates with the greater wing of the sphenoid bone.

Occipital border [margo occipitalis (NA)]. That border which articulates with the occipital bones.

Posterior border [margo posterior partis petrosae (NA)]. The border separating the posterior and inferior surfaces. It articulates with the lateral border of the basi-occipital bone.

Superior border [margo superior partis petrosae (NA)]. The border separating the anterior from the posterior surface, and the middle from the posterior cranial fossa.

Anterior surface [facies anterior partis petrosae (NA)]. The surface between the superior and anterior borders, which forms part of the middle cranial fossa.

Inferior surface [facies inferior partis petrosae (NA)]. The irregular undersurface forming part of the inferior surface of the skull.

Posterior surface [facies posterior partis petrosae (NA)]. The surface between the superior and posterior borders. It contains the orifice of the internal auditory meatus, and forms part of the posterior cranial fossa.

Squamous part [pars squamosa (NA)]. That part which contributes to the side-wall of the vault below the parietal bone and bears the zygomatic process. Its inner surface, the cerebral surface [facies cerebralis (NA)], forms the side-wall of the middle cranial fossa, its outer or temporal surface [facies temporalis (NA)] gives origin to the temporal muscle, whilst in front and below the zygomatic process there is a small area, the infratemporal surface, which contributes to the infratemporal fossa. Its inferior surface [facies articularis (NA)] forms part of the articular fossa. Its named borders are the parietal [margo parietalis] and the sphenoidal [margo sphenoidalis (NA)].

Tympanic part [pars tympanica]. A quadrilateral plate forming the anterior, inferior, and part of the posterior walls of the bony external auditory meatus.

temporal muscle [musculus temporalis (NA)]. A muscle which closes the jaw; it arises from the side of the cranium (temporal fossa) and is inserted into the coronoid process of the mandible.

temporal nerves, deep [nervi temporales profundi (NA)]. Branches, usually two in number, from the mandibular nerve to the temporal muscle.

temporal veins. Deep temporal veins [venae temporales profundae (NA)]. Veins which empty into the pterygoid plexus. **Middle temporal vein [vena temporalis media (NA)].** A vein which joins the superficial temporal vein to form the posterior facial vein. **Superficial temporal veins [venae temporales super-**

ficiales (NA)]. The main drainage of the temple and middle part of the scalp; tributaries of the posterior facial vein.

temporo-auricular (**tem**·por·o·aw·**rik'**·ew·lar). Referring to the associated temporal and auricular regions.

temporofacial (**tem**·por·o·**fa'**·she·al). Concerned with the temples and the face.

temporofrontal (**tem**·por·o·**frun'**·tal). Concerned with the temporal and frontal regions. **Temporofrontal tract.** *See* TRACT.

temporohyoid (**tem**·por·o·**hi'**·oid). Connecting the temporal and hyoid bones.

temporomalar (**tem**·por·o·**ma'**·lar). Temporozygomatic. [temporal, malar.]

temporomandibular (**tem**·por·o·man·**dib'**·ew·lar). Connecting the temporal bone and the mandible; pertaining to the articulation of the lower jaw.

temporomastoid (**tem**·por·o·**mas'**·toid). Concerned with the temporal and mastoid regions.

temporomaxillary (**tem**·por·o·max·**il'**·ar·e). Concerned with the temporal bone and the maxilla.

temporo-occipital (**tem**·por·o·ok·**sip'**·it·al). Concerned with the temporal and occipital regions or bones.

temporoparietal (**tem**·por·o·par·**i'**·et·al). Concerned with the temporal and parietal regions or bones.

temporoparietal muscle [musculus temporoparietalis (NA)]. An occasional muscle occurring in the lateral part of the epicranial aponeurosis.

temporopontine (**tem**·por·o·**pon'**·tine). Located between the temporal lobes of the cerebrum and the pons.

temporosphenoid (**tem**·por·o·**sfe'**·noid). Concerned with the temporal and sphenoid bones.

temporozygomatic (**tem**·por·o·zi·go·**mat'**·ik). Concerned with the temporal and zygomatic regions or bones.

tempostabile (tem·po·**sta**·bile). Describing a chemical compound that remains stable with the passage of time. [L *tempus* time, *stabilis* stable.]

tempus (**tem**·pus). 1. Temple. 2. Time. [L.]

temulence (**tem**·ew·lens). Alcoholic intoxication. [L *temulentia.*]

tenacious (ten·a·shus). Glutinous; adhesive; remaining firmly attached. [see foll.]

tenacity (ten·**as**·it·e). The ability to remain attached or coherent; persistence. **Cellular tenacity.** The tendency of cells to continue in the same form of activity. [L *tenax* holding fast.]

tenaculum (ten·**ak**·ew·lum). 1. A surgical fine-pointed hook employed to pick up and hold tissue divided in the course of an operation. 2. A fibrous band, which maintains structures in position. **Tenaculum tendinum.** Vinculum tendinum. [L holder.]

tenalgia (ten·**al**·je·ah). Tenodynia. [Gk *tenon* tendon, *algos* pain.]

tenderness (**ten**·der·nes). Soreness; abnormal and painful sensitivity to the touch. **Rebound tenderness.** Pain when pressure is released. [OFr. *tendre.*]

tendinitis (ten·din·i·tis). Inflammation affecting a tendon and its muscular attachments; tenonitis, tenontitis. **Tendinitis ossificans traumatica.** A condition resulting from trauma, in which ossified areas appear in tendons. **Tendinitis stenosans, Stenosing tendinitis.** Tendinitis affecting the flexor tendons of the fingers with narrowing of the tendon sheaths. [L *tendo* tendon, Gk *-itis* inflammation.]

tendinoplasty (**ten**·din·o·plas·te). Tenoplasty.

tendinosuture (**ten**·din·o·**sew'**·tewr). The suturing of a tendon. [L *tendo* tendon, suture.]

tendinous (**ten**·din·us). Pertaining to or having the nature of a tendon. [L *tendo* tendon.]

tendo [NA] (**ten**·do). **Tendo calcaneus [tendo calcaneus (Achillis) NA].** The Achilles tendon; the common tendon of the gastrocnemius and soleus muscles and attached to the back of the calcaneum; the largest tendon in the body. [L.]

tendolysis (ten·**dol**·is·is). Loosening a tendon from its adhesions. [L *tendo* tendon, Gk *lysis* a loosing.]

tendomucin, tendomucoid (ten·do·**mew**·sin, tend·do·**mew**·koid). A mucinous substance found in tendons. [L *tendo* tendon, mucin, mucoid.]

tendon [tendo (NA)] (**ten**·don). A discrete band of connective tissue mainly composed of parallel bundles of collagenous fibres by which muscles are attached, or two muscle bellies joined. Tendons, or leaders, occur where space is restricted, muscles change direction or play over bone, or bony attachment is restricted. *For named tendons other than those mentioned below, see relevant muscles.* **Achilles tendon.** Tendo calcaneus. **Central tendon of the diaphragm [centrum tendineum (NA)].** A centrally situated trefoil-shaped aponeurotic sheath with its base directed posteriorly. **Conjoint tendon of the transversus abdominis muscle [falx inguinalis (tendo conjunctivus) NA].** The lower tendinous fibres of the internal oblique and transversalis muscles, which form a common tendon of insertion into the crest and pectineal line of the pubis. It lies deep to the superficial inguinal ring. **Crico-oesophageal tendon [tendo crico-esophageus (NA)].** The attachment of the muscle fibres of the oesophagus at the back of the cricoid cartilage. **Kangaroo tendon.** Strips of the tendon of the kangaroo's tail used when great strength is required in a suture; for example, for the suture of bone. **Pulled tendon.** Strain of a tendon; usually of the tendon of the semitendinosus muscle. **Riders' tendon.** Rupture of the adductor tendons of the thigh. [L *tendo.*]

See also: ACHILLES, GERLACH, TODARO, ZINN.

tendophony (ten·**dof**·on·e). Tenophony.

tendoplasty (**ten**·do·plas·te). Tenoplasty.

tendosynovitis (**ten**·do·si·no·**vi'**·tis). Tenosynovitis.

tendotome (**ten**·do·tome). Tenotome.

tendotomy (ten·**dot**·o·me). Tenotomy.

tendovaginal (ten·do·**vaj**·in·al). Concerning a tendon and its sheath. [L *tendo* tendon, *vagina* sheath.]

tendovaginitis (**ten**·do·vaj·in·**i'**·tis). 1. Inflammation of a tendon and its sheath. 2. Tenosynovitis. **Tendovaginitis crepitans.** Tenosynovitis. **Tendovaginitis granulosa.** Tuberculosis of a tendon sheath with the formation of granular tissue. [L *tendo* tendon, *vagina* sheath, Gk *-itis* inflammation.]

Tenebrio (te·**neb**·re·o). A genus of beetles. **Tenebrio molitor.** A species whose larva, the common meal worm, is a secondary host of the tapeworm *Hymenolepis diminuta.* [L lover of darkness.]

tenectomy (ten·**ek**·to·me). The operation of excising a part of a tendon or its sheath. [Gk *tenon* tendon, *ektome* excision.]

tenesmic (ten·**ez**·mik). Characterized by tenesmus.

tenesmus (ten·**ez**·mus). Straining; a painful endeavour to defaecate or urinate, or pain associated with defaecation or urination. **Rectal tenesmus.** Spasm of the sphincter ani muscles rendering defaecation painful and difficult. **Vesical tenesmus.** Painful difficulty in urinating. [Gk *teinesmos.*]

tenodesis (ten·**od**·e·sis). Fixation of a tendon; the suture of the end of a tendon to a new point. [Gk *tenon* tendon, *desis* fixation.]

tenodynia (ten·o·**din**·e·ah). Pain experienced in a tendon. [Gk *tenon* tendon, *odyne* pain.]

tenofibril (ten·o·**fi**·bril). A fine thread observed in the cytoplasm of epithelial cells. [Gk *tenon* tendon, fibril.]

tenolysis (ten·**ol**·is·is). The freeing of a tendon from adhesions. [Gk *tenon* tendon, *lysis* a loosing.]

tenomyoplasty (ten·o·**mi**·o·plas·te). A plastic operation for the lengthening or shortening of muscle together with its tendon, or involving the surgical displacement of a muscle with its tendon attached. [Gk *tenon* tendon, *mys* muscle, *plassein* to mould.]

tenomyotomy (**ten**·o·mi·**ot'**·o·me). An operation involving the excision of part of a tendon and the muscle. [Gk *tenon* tendon, *mys* muscle, *temnein* to cut.]

Tenon, Jacques René (b. 1724). Paris surgeon.

Tenon's capsule, fascia, or membrane. The fascial sheath of the eyeball.

Tenon's space. The episcleral space, a tissue space between the sclera and the fascial sheath of the eyeball.

tenonitis (ten·on·i·tis). 1. Tendinitis. 2. Inflammation of the fascial sheath of the eyeball (Tenon's capsule). [Gk *tenon* tendon, *-itis* inflammation.]

tenonostosis (ten·on·os·to′·sis). Tenostosis.

tenontagra (ten·on·tag·rah). Gout affecting the tendons. [Gk *tenon* tendon, *agra* seizure.]

tenontitis (ten·on·ti·tis). Tendinitis. **Tenontitis prolifera calcarea.** Tendinitis producing degeneration of the tendon with calcification. [Gk *tenon* tendon, *-itis* inflammation.]

tenontodynia (ten·on·to·din′·e·ah). Tenodynia.

tenontolemmitis (ten·on·to·lem·i′·tis). Tenosynovitis. [Gk *tenon* tendon, *lemma* sheath, *-itis* inflammation.]

tenontomyoplasty (ten·on·to·mi′·o·plas·te). Tenomyoplasty.

tenontomyotomy (ten·on·to·mi·ot′·o·me). Tenomyotomy.

tenontophyma (ten·on·to·fi′·mah). Tenophyte. [Gk *tenon* tendon, *phyma* growth.]

tenontothecitis (ten·on·to·the·si′·tis). Tenosynovitis. **Tenontothecitis prolifera calcarea.** Tenosynovitis with necrosis and the formation of calcareous matter. [Gk *tenon* tendon, *theke* sheath, *-itis* inflammation.]

tenontotomy (ten·on·tot·o·me). Tenotomy.

tenophony (ten·of·o·ne). A heart murmur attributed to the chordae tendineae. [Gk *tenon* tendon, *phone* sound.]

tenophyte (ten·o·fite). A bony or cartilaginous growth in a tendon of a bony or cartilaginous nature. [Gk *tenon* tendon, *phyton* growth.]

tenoplastic (ten·o·plas·tik). Concerned with tenoplasty.

tenoplasty (ten·o·plas·te). Plastic surgery performed on a tendon. [Gk *tenon* tendon, *plassein* to mould.]

tenoreceptor (ten·o·re·sep′·tor). The proprioceptive nerve-ending of a tendon, which is sensitive to changes in tension. [Gk *tenon* tendon, receptor.]

tenorrhaphy (ten·or·af·e). An operation for the suturing of the divided ends of a tendon. [Gk *tenon* tendon, *rhaphe* suture.]

tenositis (ten·o·si·tis). Tendinitis.

tenostosis (ten·os·to·sis). Ossification occurring in a tendon. [Gk *tenon* tendon, *osteon* bone.]

tenosuspension (ten·o·sus·pen′·shun). An operation for stabilizing a joint, using a tendon as an artificial ligament. [Gk *tenon* tendon, suspension.]

tenosuture (ten·o·sew·tewr). Tenorrhaphy. [Gk *tenon* tendon, suture.]

tenosynitis (ten·o·si·ni′·tis). Tenosynovitis.

tenosynovectomy (ten·o·si·no·vek′·to·me). The operation of excising a part of a tendon sheath. [Gk *tenon* tendon, synovia, Gk *ektome* excision.]

tenosynovitis (ten·o·si·no·vi′·tis). Inflammation of a tendon sheath. **Tenosynovitis acuta purulenta.** Acute suppurative inflammation of a tendon sheath. **Adhesive tenosynovitis.** Chronic inflammation of a tendon sheath, resulting in adhesions between the tendon and the sheath. **Tenosynovitis crepitans.** Tenosynovitis accompanied by a creaking sensation on movement of the tendon. **Gonorrhoeal tenosynovitis.** Tenosynovitis due to gonococcal infection. **Tenosynovitis granulosa.** Tenosynovitis due to infection by the tubercle bacillus. **Tenosynovitis stenosans.** 1. Painful thickening of the sheaths of the abductor pollicis longus and extensor pollicis brevis muscles at the wrist (de Quervain's disease). 2. Contraction of the fibrous flexor tendon sheath of a finger or thumb resulting in the phenomenon of trigger finger or trigger thumb. **Tuberculous tenosynovitis.** Tenosynovitis granulosa (see above). [Gk *tenon* tendon, synovia, Gk *-itis* inflammation.]

tenotic (ten·ot·ik). Concerned with a tendon. [Gk *tenon* tendon.]

tenotome (ten·o·tome). An instrument used in tenotomy. [Gk *tenon* tendon, *temnein* to cut.]

tenotomy (ten·ot·o·me). The cutting of a tendon; in ophthalmology the cutting of the tendon of one of the extra-ocular muscles in the treatment of manifest or latent squint. **Central tenotomy.** That in which the central part of the tendon only is cut. **Controlled tenotomy.** One in which the cut tendon is controlled by a suture, which can be adjusted if necessary following the operation. **Fenestrated tenotomy.** That in which a central and marginal cut is made, but still leaving part of the tendon intact. **Guarded tenotomy.** Controlled tenotomy (see above). **Marginal tenotomy.** That in which the marginal part only of the tendon is cut. **Open tenotomy.** Division of a tendon after full exposure through an adequate incision. **Partial tenotomy.** That in which only a part of the tendon is cut. **Subconjunctival tenotomy.** One performed under the conjunctiva without full exposure of the tendon. **Subcutaneous tenotomy.** Division of a tendon through a puncture wound. **Two-stage tenotomy.** A partial tenotomy in which the central part is cut first and the marginal parts at a later operation. [Gk *tenon* tendon, *temnein* to cut.]

tenovaginitis (ten·o·vaj·in·i′·tis). Tenosynovitis. [Gk *tenon* tendon, L *vagina* sheath, Gk *-itis* inflammation.]

tensio-active (ten·she·o·ak′·tiv). Affecting surface tension, either increasing or decreasing it. (Obsolete term.) [tension, active.]

tensiometer (ten·she·om·et·er). A device for estimating the surface tension of a liquid by the amount of force necessary to pull away a metal ring resting on its surface. [tension, meter.]

tension (ten·shun). 1. A force in a material tending to produce extension. 2. The state of being stretched, or the amount to which anything is stretched. **Arterial tension.** The tension exerted on the arterial wall of the column of blood within the artery. **Electric tension.** Electric potential. *See* POTENTIAL. **Gaseous tension.** The pressure of a gas, or the partial pressure of a gaseous component of a mixture of gases. **Interfacial tension.** The tension between two substances, numerically equal to the work done in producing unit area of contact surface. This may be positive or, in the case of a liquid which wets a solid surface, negative. For a liquid and gas it becomes the surface tension. **Intravenous tension.** The tension within the veins. **Muscular tension.** The amount of tension appearing when a muscle is passively stretched. **Ocular tension.** The tension of the eyeball as estimated with the fingers or tonometer by the impressibility of the walls of the globe. This is effected mainly by the intra-ocular pressure, but also by other factors such as scleral rigidity and eyeball size which have to be allowed for in the calibration of tonometers in mm of mercury. **Premenstrual tension.** The physical and mental disturbances experienced before menstruation. **Surface tension.** The effect due to molecular attraction in a fluid, which gives rise to an apparent tension in the free surface of the fluid. It accounts for the phenomenon of capillary rise of a liquid, and is expressed in newtons per metre (dynes/cm or ergs/cm^2). **Tissue tension.** The condition of equilibrium found in a tissue. [L *tendere* to stretch.]

tensiophone (ten·she·o·fone). A form of sphygmomanometer for measuring blood pressure by combined auscultation and palpation. [tension, Gk *phone* sound.]

tensive (ten·siv). Having the feeling of being stretched. [see foll.]

tensor (ten·sor). A muscle which stretches any structure or makes it tense. [L *tendere* to stretch.]

tensor fasciae latae muscle [musculus tensor fasciae latae (NA)] (ten·sor fash·e·e la·te). A muscle which arises from the anterior part of the external lip of the iliac crest and a narrow strip of the external surface of the ilium below this; it is inserted between the two layers of the iliotibial tract of the fascia lata.

tensor palati muscle [musculus tensor veli palatini (NA)] (ten·sor pal·at·i). The tensor of the soft palate, arising from the scaphoid fossa on the sphenoid bone and the pharyngotympanic tube.

tensor palati muscle, nerve to the [nervus tensoris veli palatini (NA)]. A branch from the otic ganglion.

tensor tympani muscle [musculus tensor tympani] (ten·sor tim·pan·i). A muscle arising from the walls of the small canal above the bony pharyngotympanic tube. Its tendon turns laterally around the processus cochleariformis to insert into the upper end of the handle of the malleus.

tensor tympani muscle, nerve to the [nervus tensoris tympani (NA)]. A branch of the otic ganglion.

tent (tent). 1. A cylindrical or conical plug, usually of absorbent material, used to dilate or keep open an orifice, wound, or sinus: it is sometimes used to dilate the neck of the uterus and induce labour. 2. A canvas or plastic cover placed over a bed or cot, either to provide an environment containing a higher concentration of oxygen than the atmosphere, or for the administration of inhaled medicaments which may be gaseous or particulate. **Laminaria tent.** A plug made of *Laminaria*, a seaweed. **Oxygen tent.** A tent-like canopy which surrounds the head and neck of a patient and which contains a high tension of oxygen. It is sometimes used in oxygen therapy, especially in small children. **Sponge tent.** A plug made of compressed sponge. **Steam tent.** A cover into which steam from a kettle is led. **Tupelo tent.** A plug made from the root of the water-tupelo tree. [ME *tente.*]

tentacle (ten·takl). An elongated thin flexible appendage in the invertebrates and lower vertebrates, used in locomotion, in grasping, or for feeling. [L *tentare* to feel.]

tentigo (ten·**ti**·go). Pathologically increased sexual desire. [L *tendere* to stretch.]

tentorial (ten·**to**·re·al). Relating to the tentorium cerebelli.

tentorium (ten·**to**·re·um). A tent; hence applied in anatomy to any tent-like structure. **Tentorium cerebelli [NA].** A double fold of dura mater between the undersurface of the occipital lobes of the cerebrum and the cerebellum; it forms an incomplete roof over the posterior cranial fossa. **Tentorium of the hypophysis.** The diaphragma sellae; a fold of dura mater covering the hypophyseal fossa and pierced by the stalk of the hypophysis. [L.]

tentorium, nerve to the [ramus tentorii (NA)]. A branch from the ophthalmic nerve to the dura mater.

tenuate (ten·ew·ate). To thin out; to reduce in thickness or density. [see foll.]

tenuis (ten·ew·is). Thin; fine; delicate. **Tenuis mater.** The pia mater. [L.]

tenuity (ten·**ew**·it·e). Slenderness; thinness. [see prec.]

tephromalacia (tef·ro·mal·**a**′·she·ah). A condition in which the grey matter of the brain or spinal cord becomes soft. [Gk *tephros* ash-grey, *malakia* softness.]

tephromyelitis (tef·ro·mi·el·**i**′·tis). Inflammation of the grey matter of the spinal cord; poliomyelitis. [Gk *tephros* ash-grey, *myelos* marrow, *-itis* inflammation.]

Tephrosia vogelii (tef·**ro**·ze·ah vo·**gel**·e·i). An African plant, the fruits of which have molluscicidal properties. [Gk *tephros* ash-grey.]

tephrosis (tef·**ro**·sis). Cremation. [Gk.]

tepid (**tep**·id). Lukewarm. [L *tepidus.*]

tepidarium (tep·id·a·re·um). A warm bath, or a room in which a warm bath is taken. [see prec.]

tepor (te·por). Moderate heat. [L.]

teramorphous (ter·ah·**mor**·fus). Monster-like. [Gk *teras* monster, *morphe* shape.]

teras (ter·as) (pl. terata). A mis-shapen fetus; a monster. [Gk.]

teratic (ter·**at**·ik). Concerning a monster; having the form of a monster, or severe congenital deformity. [see foll.]

teratism (**ter**·at·izm). The occurrence of a congenital developmental abnormality resulting in the formation of a monster. **Allantoido-angiopagous teratism.** A fetal monster with another rudimentary fetus attached to it by the umbilical vessels. **Atresic teratism.** Deformity resulting in an imperforate condition of one or more natural body openings. **Ceasmic teratism.** A developmental abnormality in which the embryonic fissures persist after birth. **Ectogenic teratism.** Teratism in which certain body parts are absent or defective. **Ectopic teratism.** The form in which organs or parts of organs are abnormally sited. **Hypergenetic teratism.** The form in which there is excessive size of certain organs. **Symphysic teratism.** The abnormal fusion of organs or adjacent parts. [Gk *teras* monster.]

teratoblastoma (ter·at·o·blas·**to**′·mah). A highly malignant, almost undifferentiated teratoma. [teratoma, blastoma.]

teratocarcinoma (**ter**·at·o·kar·sin·**o**′·mah). A carcinoma which has developed from one of the epithelial elements of a teratoma. [Gk *teras* monster, *karkinos* crab, *-oma* tumour.]

teratogenesis (ter·at·o·**jen**′·es·is). Teratogeny: the development and birth of a monster. [Gk *teras* monster, *genein* to produce.]

teratogenetic, teratogenic (ter·at·o·jen·**et**′·ik, **ter**·at·o·**jen**′·ik). Characterized by teratogenesis.

teratogenous (ter·at·**oj**·en·us). Composed of fetal elements; monstrously formed. [Gk *teras* monster, *genein* to produce.]

teratogeny (ter·at·**oj**·en·e). Teratogenesis. [see prec.]

teratoid (**ter**·at·oid). Like a monster. [Gk *teras* monster, *eidos* form.]

teratological (ter·at·o·**loj**′·ik·al). Relating to teratology.

teratology (ter·at·**ol**·o·je). The scientific study of the development and form of monsters and their classification. [Gk *teras* monster, *logos* science.]

teratoma (ter·at·**o**·mah). A group of tumours, some innocent, others malignant, composed of recognizable tissues (e.g. fat) and complex organs (e.g. teeth) derived from more than one germinal layer of the embryo. Special examples include dermoids and epidermoids. **Adult teratoma.** A teratoma in which there is considerable differentiation of the component tissues. **Autochthonous teratoma.** A true dermoid. **Congenital teratoma.** An epidermoid arising from congenital misplacement of epithelium. **Ovarian teratoma.** A highly malignant tumour arising usually in childhood and secreting chorionic gonadotrophin, oestrogen and progesterone. Similar to chorionepithelioma. **Polypoid teratoma.** A dermoid cyst showing many papillae in its wall. **Tridermal teratoma.** A teratoma in which derivatives of all three germinal layers of the embryo are represented. [Gk *teras* monster, *-oma* tumour.]

teratomatous (ter·at·**o**·mat·us). Characterized by or relating to a teratoma.

teratophobia (ter·at·o·**fo**′·be·ah). 1. Dread of monsters; unreasoning aversion to deformity in others. 2. Obsessional fear on the part of a pregnant woman that she may give birth to a deformed child. [Gk *teras* monster, *phobein* to fear.]

teratosis (ter·at·**o**·sis). Teratism.

teratospermia (ter·at·o·**sper**′·me·ah). Abnormality of the spermatozoa. [Gk *teras* monster, sperm.]

terbium (**ter**·be·um). A rare-earth element of atomic weight 158.93, atomic number 65, and chemical symbol Tb, found in gadolinite. [*Yterby* in Sweden.]

Terbutaline (ter·**bew**·tal·een). BP Commission approved name for 1-(3,5-dihydroxyphenyl)-2-(*t*-butylamino)ethanol; a bronchodilator.

terebene (**ter**·eb·een). A mixture of dipentene and other hydrocarbons obtained by steam distillation of the substance produced by the action of sulphuric acid on turpentine oil. It is a stimulant expectorant used in bronchitis, taken internally or inhaled; it is also used in dyspepsia and as a deodorant (BPC 1959). It has weak antiseptic properties. **Terebene glycerin, Terebene glycerol.** A mixture of 4 parts of terebene, 7 parts of glycerin, and 1 part of water used on purulent wounds by external application. [Gk *terebinthinos* turpentine.]

terebentene, terebenthene (ter·e·**ben**·teen, ter·e·**ben**·theen). L-Pinene, $C_{10}H_{16}$. The optically-active terpene occurring in French oil of turpentine.

terebinth (**ter**·e·binth). 1. The Mediterranean tree, *Pistacia terebinthus*, from which a turpentine is extracted. 2. Turpentine. **Terebinth canadensis.** Canada turpentine, Canada balsam; an oleoresin obtained from the stem of the balsam fir *Abies balsamea* and used to cement glass. **Terebinth oil.** Turpentine oil. [Gk *terebinthinos* turpentine.]

terebinthinate (ter·e·**bin**·thin·ate). Having turpentine as a constituent. [see prec.]

terebinthine (ter·e·**bin**·theen). 1. Of the nature of turpentine. 2. Gum thus, American thus, common frankincense; the oleoresin obtained from various species of *Pinus*, from which turpentine oil is distilled. [Gk *terebinthinos* turpentine.]

terebinthinism (ter·e·**bin**·thin·izm). Poisoning by turpentine. [see prec.]

terebrachesis (teer·e·brak·**e**′·sis). The surgical shortening of the round ligaments of the uterus. [teres, Gk *brachys* short.]

terebrant, terebrating (**ter**·e·brant, **ter**·e·bra·ting). Characterized by piercing pain. [see foll.]

terebration (ter·e·**bra**·shun). 1. Boring; trephination. 2. A piercing pain. [L *terebrare* to bore.]

teres (teer·eez). 1. Round and elongated. 2. A muscle or ligament that is cylindrical in shape. [L.]

teres major muscle [musculus teres major (NA)] (teer·eez ma·jor). A muscle which arises on the dorsal surface of the scapula and is inserted into the humerus. It adducts the arm and rotates it inwards.

teres minor muscle [musculus teres minor (NA)] (teer·eez mi·nor). A muscle arising from the dorsal surface of the scapula and inserted into the greater tuberosity of the humerus. It adducts the arm and rotates it outwards.

tergal (ter·gal). Relating to the back; dorsal. [L *tergum* back.]

tergolateral (ter·go·lat·er·al). Indicating the back and side. [L *tergum* back, *latus* side.]

tergum (ter·gum). The back. [L.]

term (term). 1. A defined compass or period; particularly understood to mean the normal gestation period. 2. In the plural, old name for menses. [Gk *terma* limit.]

Terman, Lewis Madison (b. 1877). American psychologist.

Terman test. *See* STANFORD TEST (under TEST).

Terman-Merrill test. A later revision of the Stanford test.

terminal (ter·min·al). 1. An end, or relating to an end. 2. A device for making an electrical connection. **Terminal redundancy.** Referring to the genetic material of certain bacteriophages which contains more than a complete genome, the two ends of the linear chromosome comprising short duplicated regions. [L *terminalis* of a boundary.]

Terminalia (ter·min·a·le·ah). 1. A genus of trees common in India, of the family Combretaceae. 2. Myrobalan; the dried immature fruits of *Terminalia chebula.* It contains tannin and is used as an astringent. [see prec.]

termination (ter·min·a·shun). 1. The distal end of a structure. 2. The conclusion of anything. **Chain termination.** *See* CHAIN and MUTATION. [L *terminus* end.]

ternary (ter·nar·e). 1. Three in number, or third successively. 2. In chemistry, applied to a compound composed of three elements only, or one in which three identical radicals have been substituted. [L *terni* three each.]

Terni, Camillo (b. 1864). Naples pathologist.

Bandi and Terni vaccine. A prophylactic vaccine against plague, made from the peritoneal exudate of rats and rabbits inoculated with *Pasteurella pestis.*

Ternidens (ter·nid·enz). A genus of nematode worms. **Ternidens diminutus.** A species which forms nodules in the intestinal wall. It is a not uncommon form in man in East Africa. [L *terni* three each, *dens* tooth.]

ternitrate (ter·ni·trate). Trinitrate. Any nitrate that contains three nitric groups, e.g. $Al(NO_3)_3$. (Obsolete term.) [L *ter* thrice, nitrate.]

teropterin (ter·op·ter·in). Pteroyl-γ-glutamyl-γ-glutamyl glutamic acid, $C_{28}H_{33}N_9O_{10}$. A synthetic analogue of folic acid, used for the treatment of malignant disease in man. It produces responses in pernicious anaemia and sprue similar to those produced by folic acid.

terpene (ter·peen). Any member of a family of isomeric unsaturated hydrocarbons, all with formula $C_{10}H_{16}$, which occur in essential oils and resins. They may be *acyclic* (open-chain), e.g. myrcene from oil of bay, *monocyclic,* e.g. limonene from oil of citron, *dicyclic,* e.g. pinene from turpentine oil, or *tricyclic* such as tricyclene derived from sandal-wood oil. They are mostly liquids with a fragrant odour. **Terpene hydrate.** Terpin hydrate. **Terpene hydriodide.** Iodoterpene, $C_{10}H_{16}·HI$; it is used as an antiseptic. **Terpene hydrochloride.** Pinene hydrochloride, artificial camphor, $C_{10}H_{16}·HCl$, from turpentine; it is used as an antiseptic in tuberculosis and skin diseases. [turpentine.]

terpenism (ter·pen·izm). Poisoning by a terpene or its derivatives.

terpilene dihydrochloride (ter·pil·een di·hi·dro·klor·ide). $C_{10}H_{16}·2HCl$, a camphor-like substance derived from eucalyptus oil.

terpin (ter·pin). *p*-Mentha-1,8-diol, $C_{10}H_{18}(OH)_2$. A diterpene alcohol obtained from turpentine oil. It occurs in two stereoisomeric forms, the *cis-* and *trans-*; the *cis*-compound is a solid which readily absorbs water to form terpin hydrate, and its anhydride is cineole. **Terpin Hydrate BPC 1968.** $C_{10}H_{18}(OH)_2·H_2O$, a colourless crystalline compound, slightly soluble in water, more so in alcohol (90 per cent), and used as an expectorant in the form of an elixir or as pills.

Terpineol BP 1958 (ter·pin·e·ol). $C_{10}H_{17}OH$, a mixture of isomeric alcohols obtained from terpin. The α-form occurs naturally, and has the odour of lilac; it is an aromatic solvent antiseptic and is also employed in the manufacture of perfumes.

terpinol (ter·pin·ol). A mixture of terpenes with variable proportions of terpineol and cineole, prepared by the distillation of terpin hydrate and dilute sulphuric acid. It has a hyacinth-like odour and is used in perfumery.

terra (ter·ah). **Terra alba.** 1. Kaolin. 2. Barium sulphate. **Terra fullonica.** Fuller's earth; a clay closely related to kaolin and used largely for its absorbent properties in decolorizing and purifying fats and oils. It is also used as an absorbent dusting-powder. **Terra japonica.** Catechu. **Terra ponderosa.** Barium sulphate. **Terra silicea purificata.** The official US name for diatomite (kieselguhr). [L.]

terracing (ter·as·ing). In surgery, the sewing of a wound in a thickness of tissue by means of sutures in rows or superimposed upon one another in layers. [L *terra* earth.]

terrein (ter·e·in). $C_8H_{10}O_2$, one of the metabolic products of the mould *Aspergillus terreus.*

Terrier, Louis-Félix (b. 1837). Paris surgeon.

Terrier's promontory, or valve. The uppermost of the oblique ridges of mucous membrane lining the neck of the gall bladder.

Courvoisier-Terrier syndrome. Obstructive jaundice, distension of the gall bladder, and clay-coloured faeces, indicating obstruction of the common bile duct, e.g. by a tumour of the ampulla of Vater.

Terry, Theodore Lasater (b. 1899). American ophthalmologist.

Terry's syndrome. Retrolental fibroplasia. *See* FIBROPLASIA.

Terson, Albert (b. 1867). Paris ophthalmologist.

Terson's capsule forceps. Fine curved forceps for removing part of the anterior lens capsule in cataract extraction.

Terson's glands. Small acinar glands opening into the conjunctival fornices.

Terson's operation. For ectropion: excision of the hypertrophied conjunctiva combined with a triangle of skin lateral to the outer canthus, the base vertical and the apex outwards.

Terson's speculum. A retractor for performing double eversion of the upper eyelid.

tertian (ter·shan). The term applied to paroxysms of fever occurring every 48 h; such periodicity is characteristic of benign tertian malaria due to *Plasmodium vivax* and *P. ovale.* **Double tertian.** Daily paroxysms (quotidian fever) caused by the alternation of two generations of these parasites. **Malignant tertian.** A malarial fever caused by *Plasmodium falciparum* in which the 48 h periodicity is usually maintained, but in which the intermissions may not be complete; also called *subtertian.* [L *tertianus* third.]

tertiary (ter·she·er·e). The third in any series. **Tertiary structure.** *See* STRUCTURE. [L *tertius* third.]

tertigravida (ter·she·grav·id·ah). A woman in her third pregnancy. [L *tertius* third, *gravida* pregnant.]

tertipara (ter·she·par·ah). A woman who has had three children. [L *tertius* third, *parere* to bear.]

tervalent (ter·va·lent). Trivalent.

Tesla, Nikola (b. 1856). New York electrical engineer.

Tesla's current. A high-frequency current of high voltage, but of a lower voltage than Oudin's current.

tesla (tes·la). The unit of magnetic flux density. [Nikola *Tesla.*]

teslaization (tes·la·i·za·shun). Electric treatment by Tesla's currents. [Nikola *Tesla.*]

tessellated (tes·el·a·ted). Composed of small squares. **Tessellated epithelium.** Simple squamous epithelial cells fitting at their edges like a mosaic. [L *tessella* a small square stone.]

test (test). 1. A term that has a number of different applications in medicine which do not differ fundamentally from its non-medical applications. A means of trial to determine the presence of, the identity of, the quality of, the constitution of, or the amount of, a substance, state, or function. *See also* REACTION *and* TESTS. 2. In protozoology, a case, shell, or covering. **Absorption test.** An immunological test for differentiating closely-related species of bacteria, used in classifying the *Salmonellae.* **Acetic-acid test.** For protein in urine: half fill a test-tube with urine, heat the upper part to boiling and acidify with dilute acetic acid; a turbidity or precipitate in the upper part of the tube indicates protein. This method is useful for detection of a trace of protein, which appears as a haze contrasting with the clear lower layer of urine. **Acetylmethylcarbinol test.** A biological test to distinguish *Bacterium coli* from *B. aerogenes.* **Acidosis test.** *See* ALKALI TOLERANCE TEST (below). **Acrolein test.** For detection of glycerol, oils, and fats: heat a little of the substance with powdered potassium bisulphate in a dry tube; acrolein is formed by dehydration and is recognized by its extremely irritating odour. **Adrenaline test.** Injection of dilute solutions (e.g. 1:100 000) of adrenaline into the skin to test the contractile excitability of metarterioles and capillary sphincters. **After-image test.** For demonstrating the presence or survival of normal retinal correspondence in cases of squint. The patient fixes a bright linear light, first with the straight eye when the light is horizontal, then with the squinting eye when the light is vertical. If normal retinal correspondence is present the after-image of both eyes will form a cross. **Agglutination test.** A serological test widely applied in bacteriology and haematology, in which clumping of bacteria, red blood corpuscles, or other particles, is produced by a corresponding antiserum containing specific antibodies (agglutinins or haemagglutinins). The test is used, for example, to identify an unknown organism, by finding that it is clumped by a known agglutinating serum, and, conversely, to identify unknown agglutinins in the serum of a patient or animal by finding that known bacteria are clumped by this serum. The agglutination reaction is most commonly practised in typhoid and paratyphoid fevers, in *Brucella* affections, and in the determination of blood groups. *See also:* COOMBS' TEST, PAUL-BUNNELL TEST. **Aldehyde test.** A serum test for kala-azar. One drop of commercial formalin is added to 1 ml of serum: in a well-established case of kala-azar (of at least 4 months' duration) the mixture turns into a solid opaque gel; in the earlier stages of the disease varying degrees of cloudiness and opalescence develop. **Alkali tolerance test.** For acidosis: 5 g of sodium bicarbonate in 100 ml water is given every half hour until the urine is alkaline to litmus, the total amount given being calculated to g/kg body weight. Normally up to 0.5 g/kg is sufficient to render the urine alkaline. **Allergy test.** Any form of skin, patch, nasal, or conjunctival test used to detect allergy or minimize the danger of allergic shock. This includes serum sensitivity tests, e.g. the preliminary subcutaneous injection of diluted serum (trial dose) before the main therapeutic dose, pollen tests in hay fever, and tuberculin tests. **Alpha test.** An intelligence test introduced for the purpose of classifying American recruits in World War I, comprising a variety of verbal and performance tests. It has now fallen out of use. **Amyl nitrite test.** A pharmacological test for spinal block: the pressure of the cerebrospinal fluid in the lumbar theca is measured manometrically before and after the inhalation of amyl nitrite. The absence of an increase in pressure after administration of the drug is taken to indicate a block in the spinal subarachnoid space. **Anaesthetic test.** A test used to assess a patient's physiological state and his fitness to undergo the administration of an anaesthetic. *See also:* BARACH'S INDEX, CRAMPTON'S TEST, HENDERSON'S TEST, MOOTS' FORMULA, SABRASÉZ' TEST. **Antimony test.** A serum test for kala-azar of moderate specificity, depending upon changes in the serum proteins. Serum diluted ten times is placed in a narrow-bore test tube (1.5 mm) and a 4 per cent solution of urea stibamine in distilled water added; an immediate heavy flocculent precipitate indicates a strongly positive reaction. False positives may be given in other conditions, e.g. malaria, when the spleen is grossly enlarged. Also known as *Chopra's test.* **Antimony trichloride test.** *See* CARR-PRICE TEST. **Antinuclear factor test.** A test for detecting antibodies to nuclear material, usually performed using an immunofluorescence technique. **Antistreptolysin test.** For measuring the titre of antibodies to streptolysin O of *Streptococcus pyogenes*; if the titre is above an arbitrary level (say 1:200), the finding is suggestive of recent streptococcal infection and, more particularly, of rheumatic fever. Other serological tests of a similar nature measure antibodies to streptococcal DNA-ase, hyaluronidase, etc. **Anvil test.** A test for disease of a bone or joint, when if the affected limb is jarred by a blow distal to the suspected area, pain is experienced in the diseased joint. Thus, in early disease of the hip a blow on the heel with the leg extended produces pain in the hip. **Aptitude test.** A test designed to estimate an individual's potential ability for the performance of a certain type of activity of a specialized kind and within a restricted range. **Arm-lung time test.** A test to determine the pulmonary circulation time. It is done by means of an injection into the cubital vein of substances such as ether or acetone which are detectable in the breath after arrival at the lungs. Normal time, about 6 s. The time is reduced in exercise, hyperthyroidism, and anaemia, and is increased in cardiac disorders, myxoedema, and polycythaemia. **Arm-tongue time test.** A test to determine the circulation time from arm to tongue, i.e. vein-heart-capillary time. It is done by means of injection into the cubital vein of a substance such as dehydrocholic acid (2 per cent solution) which causes a bitter taste on arrival at the tongue. A 20 per cent saccharin solution can also be used. Normal time, about 11-14 s. The time is reduced in exercise, hyperthyroidism, and anaemia, and increased in cardiac disorders, myxoedema, and polycythaemia. **Association test.** Any test in which the subject is required to respond to a series of test words by replying as quickly as possible with the first word or words that come to his mind. A delayed or unusual response is thought to follow a stimulus word which touches an emotional complex. **Atropine test.** A test in which the subject is given 2 mg atropine sulphate by subcutaneous injection and the heart rate counted at intervals of 1 min for 30 min after administration. If the cardiac vagus is intact, the heart rate should rise appreciably and by at least 15 beats per minute above the pre-injection rate. Originally devised as a test for typhoid fever, the test now has little application except in the investigation of bradycardia, heart blocks, certain cardiac arrhythmias, and disorders of the autonomic nervous system. **Bacteriolytic test.** *See* PFEIFFER'S PHENOMENON. **Balance test.** A metabolic test in which excretion of a constituent of the diet is compared with intake. If the former is less than the latter there is a positive balance, and if greater, a negative balance. **Bar reading test.** A test for binocular vision first described by Javal: a bar or bars are intervened between the eyes and the book, so that words are occluded for one eye, but seen by the other. If the patient can read easily without moving the head, then good binocular vision is present. **Basophil degranulation test** (Shelley). An *in vitro* test designed to demonstrate allergy to penicillin. **Basophilic aggregation test.** A staining method used to facilitate estimation of the proportion of stippled erythrocytes in the detection and control of lead poisoning. The red cells in one half of an evenly spread film are haemolysed before staining the film with brilliant cresyl blue. The basophilic material is more easily stained in the haemolysed area, and the proportion of cells which originally contained this material is computed on the basis of the number of red cells in the non-haemolysed part occupying the same area. **Belt test.** *See* GLÉNARD'S TEST. **Benzidine test.** For occult blood: a thin suspension of faeces in water is boiled to inactivate enzymes, and after cooling 1 ml is added to about 3 ml of benzidine reagent; a blue colour develops at once if blood is present. The benzidine reagent consists of 2 ml of freshly prepared 3 per cent benzidine in cold glacial acetic acid mixed with 1 ml of 10 volumes hydrogen peroxide. Now obsolete. **Benzidine and nitroprusside peroxidase test.** 1. A test for detecting peroxidases that occur in granular white blood corpuscles, and therefore of great value in differentiating early granular (myeloid) cells from non-granular (lymphoid) cells. The test depends on the formation of a coloured substance from the benzidine under the influence of hydrogen peroxide. The stain consists of sodium nitroprusside (0.05 g) in distilled water (2 ml), added to 95 per cent alcohol (100 ml) containing benzidine (0.05 g), basic fuchsine (0.05 g), and hydrogen peroxide (0.5 ml); this is put on the blood film, and in one minute an equal volume of freshly prepared 0.2 per cent hydrogen peroxide added, the peroxidase-containing granules staining deep blue. 2. A test to demonstrate haemoglobin and its derivatives in tissues. Of several methods, Pickworth's technique is to place the tissue section for 5-10 min in a solution of benzidine (0.2 g), a small crystal of sodium nitroprusside, and glacial acetic acid (four drops) in 15 ml methyl alcohol; it is washed with ozonic ether in which it is left for 10 min, and then counterstained with 1 per cent aqueous neutral red for 3 min. Haemoglobin and most of its derivatives stain dark blue, but the cell nuclei are red. **Beta test.** An intelligence test devised for the purpose of classifying those American recruits in World War I who were illiterate or who did not speak English. It includes image, cube analysis, symbol-digit combination, picture completion, and geometric sub-tests. **Bicarbonate tolerance test.** *See* ALKALI TOLERANCE TEST (above). **Bile solubility test.** A biochemical test for the differentiation between pneumococci and streptococci: add 5 ml broth culture to each of two tubes; add 0.5 ml ox bile to one tube and 0.5 ml saline to the other (control) tube. Pneumococci usually lyse, and the culture loses its opacity; cultures of streptococci remain turbid. **Biuret test.** A violet colour is formed when any substance containing two carbamoyl groups (—$CONH_2$) joined either together or to the same carbon or nitrogen atom is treated with sodium or potassium hydroxide and copper sulphate. The reaction is given by proteins, polypeptides, oxamide, and biuret directly, and by urea after heating to 180°C. Its chief biochemical application is the detection and determination of proteins in body fluids. **Bracelet test.** The occurrence of pain on moderate lateral compression of the lower ends of the radius and ulna. It used to be employed as a diagnostic confirmatory test in cases of rheumatoid arthritis. **Breath-holding test.** *See* MYOCARDIAL-RESERVE TESTS, 1st def. (below). **Bromine test.** 1. For melanin in urine: to 50 ml of urine add 50 ml of bromine water. A yellow precipitate which darkens gradually and eventually becomes black indicates melanin present (Zeller's test). 2. For tryptophan: to 5 ml of a solution containing tryptophan add bromine water drop by drop. A pink colour is formed which disappears when excess bromine is present. 3. For uracil; add excess of bromine to an aqueous solution and remove excess by boiling. Add barium hydroxide; a purple colour indicates uracil or cytosine. **Bromsulphthalein test.** For liver function; 2 mg of dye per kg body weight of the patient is injected intravenously. After 30 min, 10 ml of blood are taken from the other arm and the serum separated. The dye is estimated in the serum by adding 2 ml of 0.1 M sodium hydroxide to 2 ml of serum and measuring the bright red colour in an absorptiometer with a green light filter against a blank prepared by mixing 2 ml of serum with 2 ml of 0.1 M hydrochloric acid. 2 ml of a standard solution containing 4 mg of bromsulphthalein per 100 ml are treated with 2 ml of 0.1 M sodium hydroxide and the colour measured against a blank consisting of 2 ml standard +2 ml 0.1 M hydrochloric acid and the reading is taken as 100 per cent. The amount of dye remaining in the serum after 30 min is normally not more than 5 per cent; in liver dysfunction 10 per cent or more, the dye is retained. The test is sufficiently sensitive for use in the examination of non-icteric patients. **Brucellergin test.** A test for sensitivity analogous to the brucellin test (see foll.). Brucellergin, a *Brucella* nucleoprotein extract, is used for intradermal injection. **Brucellin test.** An allergic skin test used for the control of the treatment of undulant fever. Brucellin, the filtrate of a 20-day-old broth culture of different types of *Brucella*, is injected intradermally, subsequent doses for treatment being regulated in accordance with the extent of the reaction. **Caffeine test.** *See* COFFEE TEST (below). **Calorimeter test.** Stewart's test. **Capillary fragility test, capillary resistance test.** *See* HESS' TEST. **Carbohydrate tolerance test.** *See* GALACTOSE TOLERANCE TEST, GLUCOSE TOLERANCE TEST, LAEVULOSE TOLERANCE TEST (below). **Carbon monoxide haemoglobin test.** For carbon monoxide in blood: a dilution of the suspected blood in dilute ammonia is compared with a similar dilution of normal blood in the Hartridge reversion spectroscope. The presence of carbon monoxide is shown by a shift of the absorption bands towards the violet. **Cardiac output test.** *See* CIRCULATORY-EFFICIENCY TESTS, GENERAL, 1st def. (below). **Cardiovascular efficiency tests.** *See* CIRCULATORY EFFICIENCY TESTS, MYOCARDIAL-RESERVE TESTS (below). **Cephalin-cholesterol flocculation test.** *See* HANGER'S TEST. **Chair test.** *See* BÁRÁNY'S CHAIR TEST. **Chicago test.** A test of supposed primary mental abilities, number facility, verbal meaning, spatial perception, word fluency, reasoning, and note memory. **Chromic acid test.** For alcohol: the solution under test is warmed with dilute sulphuric acid and a few drops of very dilute solution of potassium dichromate added. The colour is changed from orange to green, and an odour of acetaldehyde is produced. **Circulation-time test.** *See* CIRCULATORY-EFFICIENCY TESTS, GENERAL, 2nd def. (below). **Circulatory-efficiency tests, general.** 1. Cardiac output test: the amount of blood ejected by the heart per minute (minute volume) may be measured in several ways, the most usual being based on the application of the Fick principle that the amount of blood passing through the pulmonary capillaries in unit time is a measure of the output of the right ventricle. The pulmonary blood flow can therefore be determined from the amount of oxygen absorbed in unit time, and the difference in oxygen concentration in the blood before and after leaving the lungs (arteriovenous oxygen difference). The cardiac output is given by:

$$\frac{\text{Oxygen consumption (ml/min)}}{\text{Arterial oxygen} - \text{Mixed venous blood oxygen (ml/l)}}$$

Other methods of measuring cardiac output include the inhalation of foreign gases such as nitric oxide or acetylene, and the intravenous injection of dyes such as Evans' blue. The output is usually reduced in congestive cardiac failure, myxoedema, and peripheral circulatory failure. It is raised during exercise and fever, in thyrotoxicosis, severe anaemia, arteriovenous fistula, Paget's disease, beriberi, and certain forms of pulmonary heart diease. 2. Circulation-time test: the shortest time taken by a substance injected into a vein to reach a distal point in the circulation in sufficient concentration to produce a measurable effect, either subjective or objective, e.g. taste on the tongue (sodium dehydrocholate), fluorescence in the lips (fluorescein), or Geiger-counter responses to radioactive sodium. The circulation time of the arterial side of the pulmonary circuit may be determined by the intravenous injection of volatile substances which cause a cough or odour on arrival in the lungs, e.g. ether or paraldehyde. Injection in each case is into the median cubital vein. The arm-to-tongue time, measuring the total circulation time (systemic and pulmonary) is prolonged in congestive left ventricular failure, while the arm-to-lung time, measuring the speed of circulation between the cubital vein and the arterial side of the lung capillaries, remains normal if there is no associated right ventricular failure. In purely right-sided congestive failure the arm-to-tongue and arm-to-lung times are prolonged, but the lung-to-tongue time may be normal. In combined right and left ventricular failure greatly prolonged arm-to-tongue and arm-to-lung times occur. The test is therefore of limited value in the diagnosis of dyspnoea. The circulation times have also been used to investigate intracardiac shunts in congenital heart disease: shortening of the arm-to-tongue time suggests a right-to-left shunt. The arm-to-tongue time is shortened in diseases associated with high cardiac output, such as hyperthyroidism, severe anaemia, certain types of heart failure due to pulmonary disease, arteriovenous fistula, beriberi, and Paget's disease. *See also* BING'S TEST. **Circulatory-efficiency tests, local peripheral.** 1. Reactive hyperaemia test: *see* LEWIS AND PICKERING TEST. 2. Reflex vasodilatation test: *see* GIBBON AND LANDIS TEST. 3. Sweating tests: tests to determine the integrity of sweat glands and their control by the autonomic nervous system. Sweating is induced by the application of body heat, and the area to be tested is dusted with starch powder after being painted with a mixture containing iodine. The presence of sweat causes the iodine to act upon the starch, producing a blue colour. Sweating can also be detected by the change in electrical resistance of the skin. 4. Calorimeter test: *see* STEWART'S TEST. 5. Skin temperature tests: determination of the amount of blood flowing through an extremity by measuring the temperature of the skin with a skin thermometer employing copper-constantin thermocouples. A decrease in skin blood flow due to vasospastic or organic vascular disease is shown by a reduction in skin temperature in the affected limb as compared with its normal fellow. 6. Plethysmography test: measurement of the amount of blood flow in a limb by detecting the increase in size of the limb which occurs when the venous return is temporarily occluded. The limb is inserted in the plethysmograph and sealed off. The outside of the plethysmograph is connected to a recording device which measures changes in volume within the instrument. When venous occlusion is applied, the limb swells because of the arterial blood entering it, and the increase in volume represents the blood flow at that time. 7. Oscillometry test: *see* PACHON TEST. 8. Fluorescein test: a test to determine the speed of circulation to the lower extremities in cases of suspected peripheral vascular disease. Sodium fluorescein is injected into a vein in the antecubital area and the time taken for fluorescence to appear at various points on the limbs is measured by a stopwatch, the fluorescence being detected by an ultraviolet lamp in a darkened room. The injection of small amounts of histamine into the skin at selected points facilitates detection of the end-point. 9. Histamine flare test; the injection of histamine into the skin. This normally causes a small local "flare" and a weal, but these reactions are diminished in patients in whom the blood supply to the skin is impaired. A drop of a solution of 1:1000 histamine acid phosphate is placed on the skin in selected areas, the skin is pricked through each drop, and the reaction is noted. *See also* ALLEN'S TEST, BRODIE-TRENDELENBURG TEST, BUERGER'S TEST, MATAS' TEST, MOSCHCOWITZ TEST, SANDROCK TEST, TRENDELENBURG TEST. **Cis-trans test.** A genetic complementation test in which two mutations, usually involving the same phenotype, are introduced into the same diploid cell or organism in two difference configurations. In the *cis* (on this side of) configuration which acts as control for the test, the mutations are on the same chromosome, the other chromosome containing both wild-type alleles, so that the organism should display the wild phenotype. In the *trans* (on the other side of) configuration, the two mutations are on opposite chromosomes; if the mutations are in different genes, the organism will possess one complete set of good genes and will be of wild phenotype, but if the mutations are in the same gene the organism will display the mutant phenotype. **Clearance test.** *See* UREA-CLEARANCE TEST (below). **Coagulase test.** A test for the presence of a specific plasma-coagulating enzyme in staphylococci. Most pathogenic staphylococci are coagulase-positive, and coagulase-negative strains are usually avirulent. **Coccidioidin test.** The intracutaneous test of specific dermal sensitivity to an allergenic extract of the fungus *Coccidioides immitis*, the cause of coccidioidomycosis. The test has a particular value in epidemiological surveys to determine the incidence and infection rate of the disease and the extent of its endemic distribution. It is also used as a diagnostic test in the primary stage of the disease. **Cock's-comb test.** For ergot preparations: a test which depends on the darkening in colour of a cock's comb caused by ergotoxine and allied alkaloids. The effect of the sample is compared with that obtained by definite quantities of ergotoxine. **Coffee test.** A provocative test for doubtful glaucoma. Ocular tension is taken before and after taking 45 g of coffee in 150 ml of water. Caffeine can also be given either by the intravenous or by the intramuscular route. Rise of tension of from 15 to 25 mg in 20–40 min is suggestive of glaucoma. Also called the *caffeine test.* **Coin test.** A test for pneumothorax, made by placing a silver coin flat on the chest and tapping it at right angles with another coin. On auscultation a metallic ringing sound is heard if pneumothorax is present. It is unreliable if the pneumothorax is shallow or loculated. **Cold agglutination test.** An immunological test for the presence of autohaemagglutinating antibodies that exert their effect in the cold. A high titre of such antibodies is found in some diseases, particularly in primary atypical pneumonia. **Cold pressor test.** *See* HINES AND BROWN TEST. **Colloidal gold test.** 1. *See* LANGE'S COLLOIDAL GOLD TEST. 2. Serum colloidal gold test, for liver function: to 0.05 ml of serum in a small clean tube add 0.5 ml of barbitone buffer solution (pH 7.8) and 2.5 ml of colloidal gold solution. Allow to stand overnight. A positive reaction, which is shown by precipitation of the gold, occurs in cirrhosis and infective hepatitis. **Colostrum test.** For pregnancy: squeezing the base of the nipple and breast with the finger and thumb causes a minute amount of colostrum to appear in the pregnant subject. **Compatibility tests.** In transfusion, *in vitro* investigation of the recipient's serum for the presence of antibodies which react with potential donor's red cells. **Complement-fixation test.** A test based on the fact that many antibodies when they combine with their specific antigen are able to fix complement so that it cannot be detected in another test system. It is a widely applicable test in serology. **Complementation test.** A test to determine whether two mutations involve the same or different genes, i.e. whether they are functionally allelic, by introducing them into the same cell or organism on opposite chromosomal homologues and observing whether the mutant or wild phenotype is expressed; equivalent to the *cis-trans* test, but the *cis* control is usually omitted in practice. **Concentration test.** *See* URINE CONCENTRATION TEST (below). **Confrontation test.** A rough method of testing the visual fields without specialized apparatus. The patient sitting opposite the examiner closes the left eye and fixes the left eye of the examiner, who also shuts his right eye. The examiner then moves a white-headed hat pin, held midway between him and the patient, in from the periphery from all directions. The patient states when he first sees the white pinhead, and the examiner compares this with his own field of vision. The left field is then examined similarly. **Congo-red test.** *See* BENNHOLD'S TEST. **Conjunctival test.** A serological test for allergic sensitivity: the antigenic extract is dropped into the conjunctival sac, and where sensitivity exists it produces reddening, with considerable itching and discomfort. **Contact test.** *See* PATCH TEST (below). **Contradictory response tests.** For feigned partial deafness: the better ear is occluded with a finger, and the ear under test subjected to tuning fork, whispered voice, watch tick, audiometric and other tests. The tests are repeated *ad infinitum* and the responses carefully recorded. A malingerer will produce varying and contradictory answers on different occasions. **Copper-pyridine test.** For the detection of barbituric acid derivatives: a solution of copper sulphate (3 per cent) in aqueous pyridine yields a precipitate, usually pink to violet in colour, when added to a 1 per cent solution of the drug in 10 per cent aqueous pyridine (Zwikker test). **Cover test.** A method of detecting manifest or latent squint: one eye is covered and the other fixes an object. On uncovering, the movement necessary for this eye to take up fixation shows a latent squint or heterophoria, while if no movement takes place until the opposite eye is covered this shows a manifest squint. **Creatine-tolerance test.** The diagnosis of myxoedema and hyperthyroidism by the urinary excretion of creatine following a standard dose. **Creatinine-clearance test.** For kidney function: a measure of the filtration rate of creatinine when the quantity of blood cleared of creatinine per minute is referred to as the *creatinine clearance.* The urine volume in ml per minute is divided by the number of mg of creatinine in 100 ml of blood. **Cyanine dye test.** For vitamin B_6: a colorimetric assay depending upon the blue dye formed by interaction between pyridoxine and 2,6-dichloroquinone chloroimide. **Dark-adaption test.** For vitamin-A deficiency: the ability to see in the dark depends upon the speed of the reformation of visual purple which is impaired in vitamin-A deficiency. A special photometer is used, and the technique must be carefully controlled. **Dark-room test.** A provocative test for glaucoma of the narrow angle type: the intra-ocular tension is taken with a Schiøtz tonometer before and after one hour in a dark room. A rise of 1.2 kPa (9 mmHg) or more, or a second reading of over 4.1 kPa (31 mmHg) strongly suggest glaucoma of this type. **Dehydrocholate test.** *See* CIRCULATION-TIME TEST (CIRCULATORY-EFFICIENCY TESTS, GENERAL). **Denver development screening test.** A simple method of assessing whether or not a child under the age of 7 years is within the normal range of mental development. **Dexamethasone suppression test.** After one or more 24-hour collections of urine in which the 17-hydroxycorticosteroids (17-OHCS) are estimated, 0.5 mg of dexamethasone is given 6-hourly for 2 days. The 17-OHCS is suppressed to below 50 per cent in normal cases and is also greatly impaired in cases of Cushing's syndrome due to bilateral adrenal hyperplasia. The high dose consists in giving 2 mg 6-hourly for 2 days. This completely suppresses 17-OHCS in Cushing's syndrome due to hyperplasia. In cases due to adrenal cortical tumours the tumour is autonymous and neither the low nor the high dose suppresses 17-OHCS output. **Dextrose tolerance test.** *See* GLUCOSE TOLERANCE TEST (below). **Diacetic acid test.** *See* GERHARDT'S TEST. **Diacetyl test.** For citrulline in proteins: to 2 ml protein solution add three drops of 3 per cent diacetyl monoxime followed by 3 ml of concentrated hydrochloric acid. Boil for half a minute, cool, add one or two drops of 1 per cent potassium persulphate. If citrulline is present a carmine colour develops which deepens on heating. Other monosubstituted ureas give the same colour, and urea itself gives a yellow colour when tested by this method. **Dilution test.** For kidney function: a test that depends upon the observation that if a normal individual drinks 1200 ml of water within half an hour, he or she will eliminate about the same volume during the next 4 h, most of it being excreted within 2 h. When water elimination is impaired, very much smaller volumes, e.g. 200 ml or less, are excreted. This test is of little value unless combined with the urine-concentration test, to eliminate extrarenal causes such as cardiac failure or oedema. **Dimethylamino-azobenzene test.** *See* TOEPFER'S TEST. **Dinitrobenzene test.** For neutral 17-ketosteroids in urine: a 24-h specimen of urine is collected with a little hydrochloric acid as preservative. 100 ml are boiled with 15 ml of concentrated hydrochloric acid under a reflux condenser for 10 min and cooled in running water. The liquid is extracted three times with 50 ml of anaesthetic ether and the combined ether extracts washed twice with 50 ml of 10 per cent sodium hydroxide solution and then twice with 50 ml of water. The ether extract is evaporated to dryness and the residue dried for about an hour *in vacuo.* The residue is dissolved in 4 ml of pure absolute ethyl alcohol. 0.2 ml of the alcoholic solution is mixed with 0.2 ml of 2 per cent alcoholic *m*-dinitrobenzene and 0.2 ml of 2.5 N alcoholic potash. The colour developed after one hour at 25°C in the dark is read after addition of 10 ml of alcohol in an absorptiometer using a green and then a violet screen. A reagent blank (0.2 ml alcohol) and a standard (0.1 mg androsterone in 0.2 ml alcohol) are prepared concurrently, as also is a urine blank (0.2 ml test solution; 0.2 ml alcohol; 0.2 ml alcoholic potash). The test and standard are corrected for reagent blank; the former also for urine blank and then by formula (green − 0.6 violet) ÷ 0.73 for non-specific colour. The final values of test and standard are used for calculation of mg of ketosteroid excreted in 24 h. Normal ranges: men, 10–24 mg; women, 5–15 mg. **Diplopia test.** A test for double vision: a light is looked at by the patient wearing a red glass in front of one eye and a green glass in front of the other. The position of the red and green images can then be charted in all positions of gaze. **Direct-matching test.** The direct cross-matching technique of testing donor's and recipient's bloods against each other. This provides a complete safeguard against incompatibility; the donor's cells are tested against the recipient's serum, and the recipient's cells against the donor's serum. **Duochrome test.** A test for checking the spherical lens correction of the eye in refraction: two rows of black letters printed on red and green glass, suitably illuminated from behind, are used. Owing to chromatic aberration the red rays come to a focus behind the green. Therefore in hypermetropia the green letters will be clearer, and in myopia the red. When the refraction of the eye is accurately neutralized both rows of letters should appear equally plain but slightly blurred. Accurate to 0.25 dioptre sphere. **Dye exclusion test.** A test with vital stains for viability of cells *in vitro.* Living cells exclude dyes such as trypan blue, whereas dead cells take them up and are stained. **"E" test.** A test for visual acuity for young children and illiterates. The test is similar to Snellen's, but the letters are replaced by "E's" in different positions, reversed, upside down, etc. The child is given a cardboard "E" and asked to turn it to the same position as the one indicated on the test-type. **Ear specula test.** For simulated deafness: words spoken at varying distances are repeated by the patient who is blindfolded, after the insertion of an aural speculum on each side. The tests are repeated with the substitution of similar speculae filled with wax. **Edestin test.** For peptic activity in the diagnosis of gastric cancer: gastric juice is neutralized and then rendered slightly alkaline with sodium carbonate. Edestin is added and the mixture incubated at 37°C for 4 h. The undigested edestin is precipitated by neutralization with acetic acid and is estimated by the degree of turbidity. **Effort-tolerance test.** *See* MYOCARDIAL-RESERVE TESTS, 2nd def. (below). **Erythrocyte fragility test.** Osmotic fragility test; saline fragility test; for fragility of red blood corpuscles: a quantitative measure of the amount of haemolysis which occurs when red corpuscles are placed in serial concentrations of saline ranging from 0.3 to 0.75 per cent. Normal corpuscles begin to show haemolysis between 0.4 and 0.45 per cent, whereas the spherocytes of congenital haemolytic icterus and other haemolytic anaemias are ruptured by higher concentrations. **Erythrocyte-sedimentation test.** A measure of the amount of settling of corpuscles which takes place in a given time when a column of fresh citrated (or oxalated) blood is allowed to stand in a strictly vertical position, the extent and velocity of which varies greatly under various physiological and pathological conditions (sedimentation rate). **Ethyl acetate test.** For ethyl alcohol: add an equal volume of concentrated sulphuric acid and a little glacial acetic acid. Heat in boiling water for a few minutes, cool and pour into a beaker of water. The characteristic fragrant odour of ethyl acetate indicates ethyl alcohol. **Ethyl butyrate test.** For pancreatic lipase: neutral pancreatic extract or juice is added to a substrate of water, litmus powder, and ethyl butyrate, and incubated at 40°C. The action of lipase liberates butyric acid which turns the litmus red. **Exercise test.** 1. In cardiology, observation of the effect of exercise on the electrocardiogram, recorded either during or immediately after the exercise; it is usually performed to investigate the possibility of myocardial ischaemia produced by exercise. *Graded exercise test* is a study of the effects of measured, increasingly strenuous exercise, using a treadmill or bicycle ergometer, on the electrocardiogram or other aspects of cardiac function. *Maximal exercise test* is a graded exercise test continued to the limit of the patient's ability, to determine the patient's exercise tolerance and to observe the cardiovascular effects of maximal exercise. 2. A rise of rectal temperature after exercise which persists after more than half an hour's complete rest, may be indicative of an active form of tuberculosis in the lung. **Extinction test.** *See* SCHULTZ-CHARLTON TEST. **Fermentation test.** For fermentable sugars: yeast which has been thoroughly washed with water is mixed with the solution so as to form a well dispersed suspension. The mixture is transferred to a U-tube having one closed limb so that the air in the latter is completely displaced by the liquid, and the U-tube is incubated at 37°C. If fermentable sugar is present gas will collect in the closed limb within 4 h, and fermentation will usually be complete within 24 h. The test is applied to urine which has first been boiled to kill organisms and cooled. A positive fermentation test with urine indicates that the sugar present is either glucose or fructose, and these can then be distinguished by Selivanoff's test. **Ferric chloride test.** 1. For acetoacetic acid in urine: *see* GERHARDT'S TEST. 2. For homogentisic acid in urine: to 5 ml of urine add 1 per cent ferric chloride solution drop by drop. A transient green or blue colour is produced in alkaptonuria. 3. For melanogen in urine: to 5 ml of test

urine add about 1 ml of 10 per cent ferric chloride in 10 per cent HCl. If melanogen is present the colour of the urine becomes dark-brown to black. 4. For salicylates in urine: a violet colour, obtained as in Gerhardt's test with urine which has been thoroughly boiled to remove any acetoacetic acid, indicates salicylates. 5. For thiocyanate in saliva: to a little saliva add a few drops of dilute ferric chloride solution and make just acid with dilute HCl. A red colour which is discharged by addition of a drop of mercuric chloride solution indicates that thiocyanate is present. 6. For lactic acid: *see* KELLING'S TEST. **Figlu test.** A test for folic-acid deficiency based on the excretion of formiminoglutamic acid (Figlu) in urine. The test is usually carried out after histidine loading, the patient being given histidine orally and the urine collected over the period 3–8 h after administration. Figlu is separated by electrophoresis or chromatography, converted to glutamic acid with ammonia, and this is then detected with ninhydrin. **Finger-to-finger test.** A clinical test of co-ordination and position or joint sense in the upper limbs: the patient is asked to approximate the tips of both index fingers in space; an intention tremor occurring almost at the completion of the act indicates inco-ordination due to disease of the cerebellum or of cerebellar connections. If carried out with the eyes shut the test can be used to assess whether position and joint sense is intact in the hands; if this sense is impaired, the fingers cannot be approximated. **Finger-nose test.** A clinical test of co-ordination in the upper limbs: the patient is asked to bring the tip of the index finger quickly to touch the nose, first with the eyes open, then with them shut. Inco-ordination due to cerebellar disease may produce intention tremor or inaccurate judgment of distance, giving past pointing. **Fingerprint sweat test.** A test for fibrocystic disease of the pancreas by estimation of the sweat electrolytes: an agar medium containing silver nitrate and potassium chromate is used to receive the imprint. **Fistula test.** To determine the presence of a communication between the middle ear and labyrinth: when positive, compression of the air in the external auditory meatus either by presenting the tragus over the meatal orifice or by means of a pneumatic speculum produces a sensation of vertigo, and ocular nystagmus may be visible. In cases of suppurative otitis media, it indicates erosion of the labyrinthine capsule and is only elicited when the labyrinth is still active. It is a valuable sign in post-fenestrated otosclerotics and indicates the continued patency of the novovalis. In these cases it can be induced by gentle probing in the region of the fenestra. **Flaginac test.** Flaginac reaction. *See* REACTION. **Flicker test.** The ability to differentiate separate flashes of light depending upon the integrity of the retinal vessels. The threshold for flicker-fusion has been used as an index of retinal arterial disease, and indirectly of systemic hypertension. **Flicker-fusion test.** At a certain critical rate regular intermittent flashes of light instead of being separately perceived are fused into a continuous brightness. This rate is altered in conditions of fatigue or anoxaemia. **Flicking test.** Flicking of the forearm with the finger during venous occlusion of the arm with a sphygmomanometer cuff produces petechiae in subjects with various forms of purpura. **Flocculation test.** Any serological test in which the combination of antigen and antibody produces floccules, e.g. the test for diphtheria toxin. **Fluctuation test** (Luria and Delbrück, 1943). A statistical test to determine the clonal nature (e.g. mutation) of variation in micro-organisms by observing whether the fluctuation between the number of variants arising in multiple individual fluid cultures, started from small inocula, exceeds that found between different samples of the same culture. **Fluorescein test.** *See* CIRCULATORY-EFFICIENCY TESTS, LOCAL PERIPHERAL, 8th def. (above). **Foam test.** For bile pigments: shake the suspected urine in a stoppered tube vigorously and compare the colour of the foam with that produced similarly in a normal urine. When bile pigments are present the foam has a distinct yellow tint. **Formol-gel test.** 1. A serum test for syphilis, introduced by Gaté and Papacosta (1920): found to be of little value. 2. (Especially in French literature), aldehyde test, for kala-azar. **Fragility test.** *See* ERYTHROCYTE-FRAGILITY TEST (above). **Friend test.** For binocular vision: the word, FRIEND, with alternate letters illuminated in green and red is looked at by the patient, who wears red and green glasses, at a distance of 6 m in a dark room. If binocular vision is present the patient sees the whole word; if not, either FIN or RED. **Frog test.** A test used to indicate pregnancy, in which a frog is used. **FTA 200 test.** A fluorescent antibody test for the detection of specific antibodies to *Treponema pallidum* in a patient's serum. **Galactose tolerance test.** For liver function: the principle of this test is that galactose cannot be utilized by the body directly but must first be converted to glycogen in the liver. In patients with moderately severe liver damage the rate of removal of galactose from the blood is very much slower than in normal individuals and there is also much greater excretion of galactose in the urine. 40 g of galactose are given orally in water: urine is collected for 5 h after ingestion and the galactose determined; if more than 3 g are excreted in this period there is some impairment of liver function. Blood is taken before ingestion and at half-hourly periods during the 2 h following ingestion; the galactose is determined. The blood galactose falls to less than 10 mg per 100 ml in 2 h in normal individuals, but remains above this concentration in patients with liver damage. **Gall-bladder function test.** *See* GRAHAM TEST. **Galvanic test.** For differentiating labyrinthine from vestibular nerve lesions: one electrode is applied to the mastoid process of the temporal bone, the other to the hand. A current increasing from 2 to 16 mA is passed until nystagmus is elicited. With the anode applied to the mastoid, the nystagmus is to the opposite ear; the cathode results in nystagmus to the same side. A positive reaction indicates stimulation of the whole vestibular pathway; a negative reaction indicates a lesion of the vestibular neural pathways. **Globulin test.** *See* NONNE-APELT REACTION, PANDY'S TEST. **Glucose tolerance test.** The patient after fasting for at least 12 h is given 50 g of glucose in water orally: blood is taken before ingestion at half-hourly intervals and afterwards for 2 h. Urine is collected before ingestion and at hourly intervals afterwards. The test is usually prolonged to 4 or 6 h when hypoglycaemia is suspected. A normal blood sugar curve shows a fasting level between 3 and 6 mmol/l (60 and 100 mg per 100 ml) which rises to a peak of less than 10 mmol/l (180 mg per 100 ml) in 0.5–1 h and returns to fasting level in 2 h; no glycosuria should occur in the test. In diabetes mellitus the fasting level is usually above the normal range; after ingestion the level rises to a peak of above 10 mmol/l (180 mg per 100 ml) and then falls slowly, so that after two hours it is still well above the fasting level. There is also glycosuria. In addition to diabetes mellitus, decreased sugar tolerance may also be observed in hepatic dysfunction, thyrotoxicosis, Cushing's syndrome, and after prolonged treatment with cortisone. When glycosuria occurs with a normal blood sugar curve it denotes a lowered renal threshold for glucose. Flat blood sugar curves are not necessarily abnormal but are obtained with marked hypoglycaemia in such conditions as Addison's and Simmonds' diseases. **Glyoxylic acid test.** *See* ADAMKIEWICZ TEST, HOPKINS-COLE TEST. **Gonococcal complement-fixation test.** A widely used test for the presence of complement-fixing antibodies to the gonococcus in patients' sera. **Group test.** Any test which is administered to a group of subjects collectively, rather than to each subject individually. **Guaiac test, Guaiacum test.** For occult blood: dissolve 2 g of powdered guaiac in 10 ml of 95 per cent ethyl alcohol. Make a smear of the faeces upon filter paper and add one or two drops of guaiac solution followed by one or two drops of hydrogen peroxide solution. A dark green to blue colour developing within 30 s is regarded as positive. **Haemagglutination test.** An agglutination test using red blood cells which can be agglutinated by antibody either to the cells themselves or to antigens passively attached to their surfaces (as in tanned red cell agglutination). Alternatively, some chemicals and many viruses can agglutinate red cells directly and this effect can be prevented by specific antibody in a *haemagglutination inhibition test.* **Haemin test.** For blood: to a drop of aqueous extract of the stain upon a slide add a particle of sodium chloride and evaporate to dryness. Add a drop of glacial acetic acid, heat gently until bubbles appear and examine under the microscope.

If positive, haemin crystals will be seen as yellowish-brown rhombic plates (Teichmann's test). **Haemophilus influenzae antibody test.** A test for the typing of *Haemophilus influenzae*, which depends on swelling of the capsules of the organisms on exposure to the appropriate type serum, a reaction comparable to the Neufeld phenomenon or test in typing pneumococci (Alexander test). **Haemosiderin test.** A test for the presence of iron-containing breakdown products of haemoglobin, such as are found in the liver, spleen, bone marrow, etc., in cases of rapid blood destruction. On treatment with potassium ferrocyanide and hydrochloric acid the Prussian-blue reaction is given. **Hammer test.** A complement-fixation test for tuberculosis in which the antigen employed is a mixture of Koch's old tuberculin with an extract of tuberculous granulation tissue. **Heel-knee test.** A clinical test for co-ordinated movements of the lower extremities: the patient is asked to place one heel on the opposite knee and then move the heel down the front of the shin to touch the tip of the great toe. A normal person can do this readily but in an ataxic patient the movement is performed clumsily and jerkily and the heel continually slips off the leg. **Heel-tap test.** A clinical test for pyramidal-tract disease: extension of the great toe on tapping the heel; as with Crafts' test, a positive response simply indicates that an extensor-plantar response is obtainable by stimulation over a wide field. **Heparin tolerance test.** *See* DE TAKATS' TEST. **Hepatic function test.** *See* BROMSULPHTHALEIN TEST, COLLOIDAL GOLD TEST, 2nd def. (above), THYMOL TURBIDITY TEST (below), and HANGER'S TEST. **Heterophil antibody test.** *See* PAUL-BUNNELL TEST. **Hippuric acid test.** For liver function: 6 g of sodium benzoate in 30 ml of water followed by a further 100 ml of water are given orally. Urine is collected over the next 4 h, acidified with acetic acid and concentrated if necessary to 120 ml. The urine is then saturated with salt, acidified with 50 per cent sulphuric acid to congo red and left to stand overnight. The precipitated hippuric acid is filtered by suction, washed with cold saturated salt solution, dissolved in distilled water and titrated with 0.4 N sodium hydroxide to phenolphthalein; 1 ml NaOH≡0.061 g of hippuric acid as benzoic acid. A correction of 0.1 g is added to the total for loss of hippuric acid by non-precipitation. Normally 2.5 g or more are excreted; less than this amount suggests liver damage (Quick's test). **Histamine test.** 1. For achylia gastrica: the contents of the resting stomach are first aspirated and the stomach washed out with tepid water until clear and empty. 0.5 mg of histamine is then injected subcutaneously and the stomach contents are continuously aspirated, the volume and acidity of each 10-min sample are estimated. Care must be taken that the saliva is not swallowed. The test may be dangerous in cases of low blood pressure, and if the initial pressure is below 15 kPa (110 mmHg) the dose of histamine must be reduced. If no acid is produced there is proof of achylia. 2. A pharmacological test for lesions of the sympathetic nervous system: an area of skin is cleaned, a drop of a 1 in 1000 solution of histamine phosphate is dropped upon it and is introduced into the skin by multiple needle punctures. In the normal individual the triple response consists of firstly, a local reddish spot caused by capillary dilatation owing to the local effect of histamine; secondly, a weal due to transudation of serum, and thirdly, widespread flushing of the skin around the lesion, due to reflex dilatation of arterioles. In disease of the sympathetic nervous system the third element of the response is absent. **Hormone test.** *See* ASCHEIM-ZONDEK TEST. **Hydrostatic test.** For the expansion of the lungs: if the lungs of a dead child float when they are put in water, then the infant was not stillborn. **Hyperpnoea test.** A clinical test for epilepsy: the alkalosis produced by hyperventilation for 2-3 min may produce an epileptic seizure in a susceptible subject. The test is particularly effective in evoking petit mal seizures. **Hypo-oxaemia test.** *See* MYOCARDIAL-RESERVE TESTS, 3rd def. (below). **Icterus index test.** A measure of the amount of bilirubin in blood plasma by comparing the colour with that of a 1 in 10 000 solution of potassium dichromate, which is regarded as 1. Normal blood has a range of 4-7. **Indigo carmine test.** For kidney impermeability: a test for kidney function following the intravenous injection of indigo carmine. The dye should appear in the urine in health within a few minutes. The injection of indigo carmine may also be used during a cystoscopic examination to enable the observer to visualize the ureteric orifice (chromocystoscopy). **Indophenol test.** A histochemical test for the presence of oxidizing enzymes in cells, particularly cytochrome oxidase. In the presence of such an enzyme, dimethylparaphenylenediamine reacts with α-naphthol to give a bluish colour. The mixture of dimethylparaphenylenediamine and α-naphthol is known as the *Nadi reagent*. **Ink-blot test.** Any projection test in which the stimulus material is a bisymmetrical ink blot. **Insulin-glucose tolerance test.** 0.1 unit of insulin per kg body weight is injected intravenously into the fasting patient. Blood is taken before injection and 30 min after, or before if hypoglycaemic symptoms develop. 0.8 g glucose per kg body weight is given orally at this point and blood is taken at 1, 1½, 2 and 3 h after the insulin injection. In normal subjects the blood sugar level falls to about 45 per cent of the fasting level in the 30-min specimen. It then rises to a peak of about 150 per cent usually at 1½ h and returns in 3 h to slightly below the fasting level. In Addison's and Simmonds' diseases there is an exaggerated response to insulin and a subnormal response to glucose after insulin. In Cushing's syndrome and acromegaly there is a subnormal response to insulin, and after glucose an exaggerated rise in the blood sugar with delayed falling. **Insulin tolerance test.** 0.1 unit of insulin per kg body weight is given intravenously. Blood is taken before injection and at 60, 90, and 120 min. In patients suspected of having panhypopituitarism, Addison's disease, or hyperinsulinism, one-half or one-third of the calculated dose of insulin should first be tried as a precaution against inducing coma. A normal response is a fall in the blood sugar level to about 50 per cent of the fasting level in from 20-30 min and then a return to the fasting level in from 90-120 min after injection. Two types of abnormality occur: (*a*) insulin resistant, the fall in sugar level does not reach 50 per cent of the fasting level or does not do so for 45 min or more; (*b*) hypoglycaemic unresponsiveness, where the subsequent rise is absent or delayed. The latter response occurs in hyperinsulinism, and Addison's disease (possibly with insulin resistance in addition) and in panhypopituitarism with increased response to insulin. **Intelligence test.** Any test which is designed to measure the general intelligence, or special aspects of the intelligence of the subject. *See* PSYCHOLOGICAL TEST (below). **Intracutaneous test.** *See* MANTOUX TEST, MENDEL'S TEST. **Intradermal test.** *See* MCCLURE-ALDRICH TEST. **Inulin clearance test.** Inulin is excreted through the glomerular filter without reabsorption in the tubules; its rate of excretion therefore can be used as a direct measure of glomerular filtration. 10 g of inulin in 100 ml of sterile saline solution are given intravenously at the rate of 10 ml per min. Urine is collected at 1 and 2 h after injection and blood is taken before and at 1½ and 2½ h after injection. Inulin is determined in all the specimens and the clearance rate calculated as ml of blood per min per square metre of body surface. The normal figure is about 70. **In vitro immobilization test.** A test for syphilis in which the serum of the patient, plus complement, is added to a suspension of *Treponema pallidum*. **Iodine test.** 1. For polysaccharides: a dilute solution of iodine added to the test solution produces a deep-blue colour with starch, and red with glycogen or dextrin. The colour disappears upon heating or making alkaline, and reappears upon cooling or reacidifying. 2. For bilirubin in urine: 1 per cent tincture of iodine is layered upon the urine. If bilirubin is present a green ring develops at the junction of the liquids. **Iodoform test.** For alcohol and acetone: these substances are separated by distillation before testing. To 2 ml of distillate add five drops of 10 per cent sodium hydroxide solution and then Lugol's solution of iodine drop by drop until a faint yellow persists. If acetone is present a precipitate of iodoform forms in the cold and may be recognized by the characteristic odour, and by its crystalline form when examined under the microscope. Ethyl alcohol gives iodoform under similar conditions when the final mixture is warmed. **Irrigation test.** For turbidity of urine: a test employed to determine whether a urethral discharge arises from the anterior or posterior urethra. After irrigation of the anterior urethra, the patient voids urine which, if turbid, indicates that the exudate has arisen from the posterior urethra above (Jadassohn test). **Laevulose tolerance test.** For liver function: 50 g of laevulose are given orally. Blood is taken before ingestion and at half-hourly intervals afterwards for 2 h, and the sugar determined. Normally the blood sugar shows little rise after laevulose and the curve is generally considered to be abnormal if the rise is greater than 30 mg per cent. The test is not very sensitive, and is of most use in cases with toxic liver damage. **Latex test.** A laboratory test for the presence of rheumatoid factor in serum or other fluids. A positive result is produced by agglutination of latex particles which have been previously coated with human gamma globulin. **LE cell test.** A laboratory test for the diagnosis of systemic lupus erythematosus. In a positive test, nuclear material from damaged white blood cells is seen to have been phagocytosed by other cells, usually polymorphs, in a peripheral blood smear. **Leg-raising test.** Lasègue's test. **Leishmania test.** A test for oriental sore by the injection of 0.1 ml of a suspension of killed *Leishmania* flagellates intradermally. **Leprolin test.** Lepromin test (see foll.). **Lepromin test.** A specific test for the actual or potential capacity of the body to put up a successful defence against leprosy. It consists of the observation of the skin reaction to the intracutaneous injection of sterilized extract of leprosy bacilli (*Mycobacteria leprae*). It is analogous to the Mantoux test in tuberculosis. Also called *Mitsuda test, Mitsuda-Rost test, leprolin test.* **Litmus-milk test.** For pancreatic lipase: milk to which litmus has been added is incubated at 40°C with the pancreatic preparation. The litmus turns red as fatty acids are liberated from the milk fat by the action of lipase. **Loss of resistance test.** The loss of resistance to the injection of air or fluid when the point of a lumbar puncture needle passes from the tough ligamentum flavum into the extradural space. Used in the location of the extradural space. **Loud-voice test.** For simulated unilateral deafness: the patient is blindfolded and his better ear occluded. Words and numbers are repeated at louder and louder intensities. If he still denies hearing anything when the sounds are loud enough to be detected by his good ear, this presupposes that he is malingering. **Magnet test.** To find out whether an intra-ocular foreign body is magnetic: a Mellinger or similar type of powerful electromagnet is placed almost touching the eye and the patient asked if he feels any pain when the current is switched on. **Malachite green (leuco-malachite green) test.** A test similar to the benzidine test, indicating the presence of blood by the development of a bright green colour. **Mallein test.** A method of diagnosis of latent or chronic glanders in horses, using mallein, which is a preparation from *Pfeifferella mallei* analogous to tuberculin. Subcutaneous injection into a glandered horse produces a local swelling after 24 h and a general reaction with elevation of temperature. In the conjunctival mallein test, mallein rubbed into the eyelids produces an inflammatory response. In the intradermal palpebral test, the reagent is injected into the cutaneous surface of the eyelid. Swelling associated with conjunctivitis constitutes a positive reaction. **Mecholyl test.** The subcutaneous injection of 25 mg of mecholyl induces a rise in blood pressure in patients with phaeochromocytoma and a fall in normal persons. **Melitin test.** *See* BRUCELLIN TEST (above). **Methyl red test.** For coliform organisms: a chemical test used in differentiating organisms of the coliform group, by detecting the acidity produced by cultures growing in glucose phosphate medium. A red colour (MR+) indicates a strongly acid reaction and is given by *Escherichia coli* (*Bacterium coli*); a yellow colour (MR−) is given by *Aerobacter aerogenes* (*B. aerogenes*) which gives a less strongly acid reaction. **Methylamine test.** For lactose: 1 ml of 0.2 per cent solution of methylamine hydrochloride and 0.2 ml of 10 per cent sodium hydroxide solution are added to 5 ml urine and heated to 56°C for half an hour. A red coloration denotes more than 0.5 per cent of lactose. **Methylene blue test.** For bacterial quality of milk: 1 ml of standard methylene blue solution (prepared from standard tablets) is added to 10 ml of milk in a test-tube, mixed by slow inversion, and incubated at from 37-38°C. The tube together with controls is inspected every half-hour until decolorization is complete, being inverted once at each inspection. Milks of good bacterial quality will not decolorize the methylene blue in less than 4½ h in summer, or 5½ h in winter. **Microprecipitation test.** Any precipitation test in which minimal quantities of serum are used. **40-Millimetre test.** The nose is closed with a clamp and the subject expires through a mouthpiece, sustaining a column of mercury at a height of 40 mm as long as possible. The pulse rate is taken every 5 s. In a physically fit person the pulse rate is unaltered for a minute or more. **Minnesota multiphasic personality inventory test.** A test in which the subject is required to answer "true", "false", or "cannot say", to each of 550 statements, depending on the applicability of each statement to himself. From the answers the subject can be rated for depression, hypomania, hypochondriasis, hysteria, psychopathic personality, paranoia, psychasthenia, schizophrenia, and masculinity-feminity. The validity, reliability, and honesty of the answers can also be assessed. **Minnesota pre-school scale test.** An intelligence test with a variety of items, designed for use with children between the ages of 18 months and 6 years. **Mirror test.** A laryngeal mirror is placed at an angle of 45° to the larynx and the patient made to cough; the mirror is then washed with about 2 ml sterile saline which is injected into a guinea-pig. If the animal develops tuberculosis within 6 weeks the test is positive. If obvious specks of sputum can be seen on the mirror, a direct microscopical examination may be made by mixing these on the mirror with one drop of saline and preparing a slide from the fluid. **Monochord test.** A test of hearing, particularly for establishing the upper tone limit. The Monochord is used, but this is now really a museum piece as modern methods of audiometry have rendered this instrument more or less obsolete. **Mouse-protection test.** A test for yellow-fever immunity, in which the subject's serum mixed with an emulsion of the brain of a mouse that has previously been infected with a neurotropic strain of virus is injected into other (conditioned) mice; if antibodies are present in the serum the mice will survive. **Mucic acid test.** For lactose in urine: add 10 ml of concentrated nitric acid to 50 ml of urine and concentrate on the water bath to about 10 ml, cool, add 10 ml of water and allow to stand overnight. A white, sandy precipitate of mucic acid separates if lactose or galactose is present. Galactose is distinguished from lactose by Tollens' test. **Murexide test.** For uric acid and other purines: moisten a little of the solid with concentrated nitric acid and dry on a water bath. The residue is coloured bright orange. Addition of a drop of dilute ammonia gives a purple-red, or of potassium hydroxide solution a purple-violet colour. It is a very useful test for the detection of uric acid in calculi. **Myocardial-reserve tests.** These tests all depend upon the response of pulse rate, blood pressure, respiratory rate, oxygen consumption, or electrocardiogram to procedures which place a strain on the heart and circulation. 1. Breath-holding test: a test to measure the time during which the subject can hold his breath. Normal persons can hold their breath for 30 s or longer; those with cardiac insufficiency can rarely do so for more than 20 s. 2. Effort-tolerance test; to detect ischaemic heart disease: the patient performs a variable number of ascents of two steps, each 25 cm in height, the number of climbs being previously calculated from tables based on height, age, sex, and weight. An electrocardiogram is taken immediately before, immediately after, and at subsequent short intervals up to 5 min. The test is terminated if anginal pain or distress of any kind occurs. If ischaemic heart disease is present, the electrocardiogram shows distinctive changes consisting of S-T segment depression and flattening or inversion of the T waves, due to myocardial ischaemia. 3. Hypo-oxaemia test; anoxaemia is induced by the inhalation of a mixture of 10 per cent oxygen and 90 per cent nitrogen for 20 min (unless cardiac pain appears sooner), electrocardiograms being recorded before and after. The specific changes of myocardial ischaemia indicate ischaemic heart disease. The test is less accurate and more dangerous than the effort-tolerance test. *See also* CRAMPTON'S TEST, MASTER'S

TOLERANCE TEST, MENDELSOHN'S TEST, MESSINGER'S TEST, NYLIN'S TEST, STAEHELIN'S TEST, WOOD'S EFFORT-TOLERANCE TEST. **Naphthoquinone test.** For indole; to 10 ml of test solution add two drops of 2 per cent β-naphthoquinone sodium monosulphonate and 2 ml of 10 per cent sodium hydroxide. Allow to stand for 15 min, add 2 ml of chloroform and mix gently. The chloroform is coloured reddish pink if indole was present in the test solution (Herter's test). **Nasal allergy test.** By insufflating or inhaling pollen or other dusts into the nose. A positive reaction is shown by intense sneezing and a watery secretion. **Neutralization test.** A test of the ability of antibody to neutralize a toxic or infective agent, applied particularly to toxins and viruses. The test can be used to quantitate antibody and to identify toxins or viruses. It is a very sensitive test. **Nicotine test.** A test for diabetes insipidus which depends on the fact that patients with this disease do not show any diminution of urinary flow after the ingestion of amounts of nicotine which would produce antidiuresis in normal subjects. **Ninhydrin test.** For proteins and protein derivatives: *see* TRIKETOHYDRINDENE HYDRATE TEST (below). **Nitric acid test.** *See* HELLER'S TEST. **Nitric acid-magnesium sulphate test.** *See* ROBERTS' TEST. **Nitrite test.** For urorosein; to 10 ml of urine add 2 ml of concentrated hydrochloric acid and a little dilute solution of potassium nitrite. A rose-red colour indicates urorosein. **Nitroprusside test.** 1. For acetone bodies: *see* LEGAL'S TEST, ROTHERA'S TEST. 2. For creatinine. *See* WEYL'S TEST. **Nitroso test.** For indole and skatole: acidify the test solution with nitric acid and add a few drops of potassium nitrite solution. A red colour indicates indole, a white turbidity skatole. **Non-verbal test.** Any mental test in which the substance and responses, and occasionally the directions, do not involve the use of language. **Nystagmus test.** For testing vestibular function: the patient is placed in a rotating chair with his head inclined forwards at an angle of 30°. His eyes are closed and he is rotated to the right 10 times in 20 s. On stopping, the eyes are opened and a horizontal nystagmus lasting from 14-36 s occurs in a normal case. The test is repeated in the opposite direction. **Obturator test.** With the patient in the dorsal position, flexion of the right thigh with internal rotation of the hip joint, by tightening of the obturator internus muscle, may cause pain in the hypogastrium if the appendix is inflamed. Also known as *Cope's test.* **Occlusion test.** For muscle imbalance of the eyes: in cases of heterophoria, occlusion of one eye will decide whether the symptoms complained of are due to the heterophoria or to some other cause, such as refractive error. **Oidiomycin test.** A test of dermal sensitivity by intracutaneous injection of oidiomycin, an allergenic extract of the thrush fungus, *Candida albicans.* The test has little value in diagnosis and is seldom used. **Opsonocytophagic test.** A test dependent on the capacity of leucocytes to engulf bacteria, e.g. strains of *Brucella.* An opsonocytophagic power of from 0-40 per cent of cell suggests infection, whereas a power of from 60-100 per cent indicates immunity from past infection. It is regarded as of little value by British workers. A similar test has been employed in tularaemia and other infections. **Orcinol test.** *See* BIAL'S TEST. **Organoleptic test.** Any test of the function of the senses. **Orthotolidine test.** A test for blood pigment, resulting in green or blue colour similar to the benzidine test. **Osazone test.** For sugar. 1. Mix 0.1 g of the sugar, 0.2 g of phenylhydrazine hydrochloride, 0.3 g of sodium acetate, and 2 ml of water in a test-tube. Place in boiling water for 10 min, and allow to cool slowly. The osazones of glucose and laevulose crystallize from the hot solution, those of lactose and maltose appear on cooling. The crystals are identified by microscopic examination, glucose and laevulose give bundles in wheat-sheaf form, lactose forms long thin needles arranged like burrs, and maltose gives stellate clusters of long thin plates. 2. Mix 4 ml of urine with 1 ml of acetate buffer pH 5 and add 50 mg phenylhydrazine hydrochloride. Heat in boiling water for about an hour and then allow to cool slowly. If an osazone forms, identify microscopically. The test is made upon urine which reduces Benedict's solution, to provide confirmatory evidence of glucose. A negative Selivanoff test and positive fermentation test will then definitely identify glucose. *See also:* COLE'S TEST. **Oscillometry test.** Pachon test. **Osmotic fragility test.** Erythrocyte-fragility test (see above). **Oxalic acid paper test.** For indole in cultures: the use of filter-paper strips soaked in oxalic acid and placed in culture tubes above the medium to indicate the production of indole. The presence of indole causes the oxalic acid paper to turn pink. **Pain-reproduction test.** The injection of fluid during retrograde pyelography in the conscious patient until pain is caused, to discover if it is similar to that occurring in nephralgia. **Para-aminohippuric acid clearance test.** This test is usually combined with the thiosulphate clearance test. PAH clearance provides a measure of the effective renal plasma flow (ERPF), and thiosulphate clearance of the glomerular filtration rate (GFR). ERPF divided by GFR gives the filtration factor (FF). The patient has no breakfast but drinks sufficient water to provide a urine flow greater than 2 ml per minute. 10 g of thiosulphate are injected intravenously slowly (10-15 min) to avoid nausea, and 1 g of PAH is given subcutaneously. Blood and urine are collected before the injections, to provide blanks. After 30 min the bladder is emptied and blood taken, and the first clearance period commences. At the end of about 30 min (timed exactly) the bladder is emptied and washed with water by catheterization; blood is taken. A second clearance period is then run similarly. All the blood and urine samples are analysed for PAH and thiosulphate, the volume of urine plus washings is measured for each period, and clearances are expressed as ml plasma cleared per minute (ERPF), and ml plasma filtered per minute (GFR). Values observed in normal individuals (surface area 1.73 m^2) show some variation between the sexes, average figures for ERPF being 697 (male) and 594 (female); for GFR, 131 (male), 117 (female). The FF is about the same in both sexes and varies between 0.17 and 0.23. The ERPF and GFR are low in nearly all kidney diseases; the FF is high in hypertension and low in acute nephritis. **Paradimethylaminobenzaldehyde test.** *See* EHRLICH'S TEST. **Paraffin glove test.** A test for detecting firearm powder particle residues in the skin or clothing. **Passive transfer test.** *See* PRAUSNITZ-KUESTNER TEST. **Pasteurization test.** *See* PHOSPHATASE TEST (below). **Patch test.** A test of epidermal sensitivity devised by Jadassohn, in which suspected allergens are applied to the skin under small patches of e.g. lint and plaster. Often small pieces of lint, gauze, or blotting paper are soaked in dilutions of the allergen and applied to the skin under a suitable cover. Controls must always be used. **Patency test.** With a tourniquet round the upper thigh, the patient walks briskly. If the deep veins are not patent, pain occurs in less than 10 min. **Paternity test.** A test based upon the genetic interpretation of blood groups, used medicolegally to exclude the possibility of a man being the father of a particular child. A blood group is the product of a pair of genes, one received from the mother and the other from the father. Specific sera are available that cause agglutination of red blood corpuscles of persons possessing the corresponding gene. If, after every contribution of genes that can have been received from the mother has been considered the child has one or more genes that the alleged father does not possess and, therefore, cannot have given, paternity is excluded. Tests on the child and alleged father may be sufficient; a group-AB person cannot have a group-O child, or a group-O person a group-AB child; a group-M person cannot have a group-N child, or *vice versa,* and a group CDe/CDe-person cannot have a cde/cde child, etc. **Pattern perception test.** A test of adult intelligence devised by Penrose, consisting of a series of problems in which in each case the inappropriate member of the series must be crossed out. **Peppermint test.** The vapour of peppermint spirit is injected into the pneumothorax space from a large syringe in which a drop of the spirit has been placed. An almost immediate smell of peppermint indicates a perforation of the lung. **Perchlorate discharge test.** Before iodide trapped by the thyroid cells can be built up to form the thyroid hormone it has to be converted to organic iodine. This process is known as organification. If defective, the patient is to some extent hypothyroid. Potassium perchlorate prevents the trapping of iodide and all the iodide which has not been converted to organic iodine diffuses out of the gland. The ^{132}I uptake is determined. (^{132}I is used generally because the patient is usually a child, the dysorganification being a congenital defect.) A dose of potassium perchlorate is then given to stop trapping. A subsequent repeat ^{132}I uptake test shows a fall of more than 10 per cent in 60 or 90 min. **Percutaneous test.** A test such as the Moro test or Vollmer's patch test, in which the ointment or jelly is applied to the surface of the skin. *See also:* WOLF'S TEST. **Performance test.** Any non-verbal mental test. **Peroxidase test.** *See* BENZIDINE TEST, NITROPRUSSIDE PEROXIDASE TEST (above). **Personality test.** Any test designed to give an estimated rating of assessment of personality. **Phenolphthalein test.** *See* KASTLE-MEYER TEST. **Phenolsulphonephthalein test.** Of kidney function: 6 mg of phenolsulphonephthalein contained in 1 ml of solution is given by intramuscular injection in the lumbar region. Urine is collected in hourly specimens and the dye estimated by adding sodium hydroxide drop by drop to produce the maximum red colour and matching against standards. Normally 60-85 per cent of drug is excreted in 2 h, 40-60 per cent in the first hour, and 20-25 per cent in the second. **Phenylhydrazine test.** 1. For sugars. *See* OSAZONE TEST (above). 2. For formaldehyde. *See* BUCHANAN AND SCHRYVER TEST. **Phloroglucin test.** *See* TOLLENS' TEST. **Phosphatase test.** 1. A test for the pasteurization of raw milk. The enzyme phosphatase undergoes a 96 per cent reduction in heat at 63°C (145°F) applied for 30 min. Phosphatase being more resistant than the tubercle bacillus and other pathogenic organisms which may occur in milk, its absence indicates adequate heat treatment of the milk. It is thus used as an official test for the efficacy of pasteurization. Phosphatase activity is estimated by the hydrolysis of disodium phenylphosphate and colorimetry of the free phenol by Folin-Ciocalteau reagent (aqueous solution of sodium tungstate, sodium molybdate, phosphoric acid, and hydrochloric acid). Also known as Kay-Graham test. 2. A test for the presence of seminal fluid which depends on the high level of acid phosphatase in prostatic secretion and is measured in King-Armstrong units, reaching 400-8000 units per ml. Other body fluids have values around 20 units per ml. **Photo-patch test.** A closed patch test with a substance suspected of being a light sensitizer, followed by irradiation of the test area with ultraviolet light. **Phytopharmacological tests.** Tests carried out on the effects of drugs on the growth of plants. **Plasmacrit test.** A rapid test for screening large population groups for syphilis. **Plasma-proteins test.** The estimation of the plasma-protein fractions. **Plethysmography test.** *See* CIRCULATORY-EFFICIENCY TESTS, LOCAL PERIPHERAL, 7th def. (above). **Pointing test.** *See* BÁRÁNY'S POINTING TEST. **Polyuria test.** *See* ALBARRAN'S TEST. **Porphobilinogen test.** *See* WALDENSTRÖM'S TEST. **Postcycloplegic test.** Postmydriatic test (see foll.). **Postmydriatic test.** A test which is necessary when the refraction of the eyes has been carried out under a mydriatic. The usual subjective tests are repeated after a suitable interval to allow for the ciliary muscle and pupil to return to their physiological state. **Potassium tolerance test.** An obsolete test for Addison's disease which depended on the fact that patients with this disease show an abnormally steep rise in plasma potassium after administration of potassium. **Precipitin test.** Precipitin reaction. *See* REACTION. **Prism cover test.** A method of measuring the angle of squint, manifest or latent: the patient fixes an object, and increasing prisms are held before the squinting eye until no movement takes place when this eye takes up fixation of the object by the covering of the straight eye. **Progressive matrices test.** A test of adult intelligence devised by Penrose and Raven, consisting of a series of problems in which in each case the subject is required to select that one of a series of figures which will complete a pattern or system of relations. **Projection intelligence test.** *See* MASSELON TEST. **Prostatic-bead test.** A test for gonorrhoea: after the urethra has been washed out with saline the prostate is massaged *per rectum* and any secretion examined. **Protein-tyrosine test.** Devised by Proske and Watson: a simple colorimetric test based on the fact that proteins possess chromogenic properties which can be measured quantitatively against the colour produced by pure tyrosine in the presence of a phenol reagent. The chromogenic value is constant for a given protein, and the intensity of colour produced is an indication of the amount of protein present. The test is non-specific, but its high sensitivity in malaria has led to its adoption as an aid to diagnosis of this disease. **Prothrombin test, Prothrombin consumption test.** A method of measuring the amount of thromboplastin in the plasma that reacts with the prothrombin, determined by estimating the amount of prothrombin present in the serum during and after coagulation of the blood. *See also* QUICK'S TEST. **Prussian-blue test.** For cyanide: to 5 ml of solution or distillate add 3 ml of sodium hydroxide (25 per cent), a few drops of ferrous sulphate solution and a few drops of ferric chloride solution. Warm, cool, and add concentrated hydrochloric acid drop by drop until the precipitate dissolves. A blue colour or precipitate indicates cyanide. **Psoas test.** When an acute appendix lies on the psoas major muscle, pain may be elicited by passive hyperextension of the hip. **Psychological test.** Any test providing an estimate of one or more aspects of a subject's psychological make-up or mental performance. *See* ALPHA TEST, APTITUDE TEST, ASSOCIATION TEST, BETA TEST, CHICAGO TEST, GROUP TEST, INK-BLOT TEST, INTELLIGENCE TEST, MINNESOTA MULTIPHASIC PERSONALITY INVENTORY TEST, MINNESOTA PRE-SCHOOL SCALE TEST, NON-VERBAL TEST, PATTERN PERCEPTION TEST, PERFORMANCE TEST, PERSONALITY TEST, PROGRESSIVE MATRICES TEST (above), PSYCHOMETRIC TEST, PSYCHOMOTOR TEST, RECKONING TEST, SOCIOMETRIC TEST, STANFORD TEST, STANFORD-BINET TEST, STANFORD SCIENTIFIC APTITUDE TEST, THEMATIC APPERCEPTION TEST, THREE-PAPER TEST, VINELAND SOCIAL MATURITY SCALE TEST, VOCABULARY TEST (below), *and* BABCOCK TEST, BENDER VISUAL-MOTOR GESTALT TEST, BERNREUTER TEST, BINET TEST, BINET-SIMON TEST, CATTELL CULTURE-FREE TEST, CORNELL INDEX TEST, DEARBORN TEST, GELB-GOLDSTEIN TEST, GESELL'S DEVELOPMENTAL SCHEDULE TEST, GOLDSTEIN-GELB-WEIGL-SCHEERER TEST, GOLDSTEIN-SCHEERER TEST, HANFMANN-KASANIN TEST, HARROWER-ERICKSON TEST, HERRING TEST, HERRING-BINET TEST, HUNT-MINNESOTA TEST, KENT TESTS, KOHS' TEST, KUDER PREFERENCE RECORD TEST, KUHLMANN TEST, KUHLMANN-ANDERSON TEST, MARIE'S TEST, MASSELON TEST, MERRILL-PALMAR TEST, MURRAY'S TEST, MURRAY-HARVARD TEST, PINTNER-PATERSON TEST, PORTEOUS MAZE TEST, RORSCHACH TEST, ROSENZWEIG PICTURE-FRUSTRATION TEST, SEASHORE TEST, SHIPLEY TEST, SHIPLEY-HARTFORD TEST, SZONDI TEST, TERMAN TEST, TERMAN-MERRILL TEST, VIGOTSKY TEST, WECHSLER-BELLEVUE TEST, WEIGL TEST, YERKES' TEST, YERKES-BRIDGES TEST. **Psychometric test.** Any test giving a measure of any mental performance of the subject. The term is usually restricted to tests of intelligence. **Psychomotor test.** Any test involving the co-ordination of mental and voluntary motor activity. **Purified protein test.** For tuberculosis: a modified Mantoux test in which a purified protein derivative is used; this has the advantage of a more constant potency. **Quinine test.** *See* THALLEOQUIN TEST (below). **Rash-extinction test.** Schultz-Charlton test. **Reactive hyperaemia test.** Lewis and Pickering test. **Reckoning test.** Any test involving the use of calculation as its basis. **Reflex vasodilatation test.** Gibbon and Landis test. **Resazurin test.** A dye reduction test which, like the methylene blue test, is used to determine the hygienic quality of milk. **Resorcinol-hydrochloric acid test.** *See* SELIVANOFF'S TEST. **Ring test.** 1. A plate test for antibiotic activity; the solution is placed in a hole in an agar plate previously seeded with a suspension of a sensitive test organism. After overnight incubation, the size of the surrounding clear zone of growth inhibition is an indication of the strength of the antibiotic solution. 2. Any chemical qualitative test in which the test solution and reagent are layered without mixing, so that a characteristic colour or turbidity is formed at the junction of the two liquids. **Rose-bengal test.** For liver function: 5-10 ml of 2 per cent solution of dye are injected, and blood taken after 2 and 8 min. The plasmas are treated with acetone and sodium hydroxide and centrifuged, and the colour of the filtrates measured. The colour of the second (8-min) specimen should be at least 50 per cent less than that of the 2-min specimen; if higher than 50 per cent, hepatic dysfunction is indicated. **Salicylaldehyde test.** *See* BEHRE'S TEST. **Saline fragility test.** Erythrocyte-fragility test (see above). **Saliva test.** A test carried out on the saliva of a pregnant woman which was claimed to determine the sex of the child before delivery. Experience has not so far fully supported the claim. **Scarification test.** *See* von PIRQUET'S TEST. **Scratch test.** One form of test for skin sensitivity to protein extracts, horse serum, etc. After cleansing the site, breaks in the skin are made very lightly with a Hagedorn needle, and the test protein applied. A typical positive reaction is an urticarial weal, with surrounding erythema. **Sedimentation test.** 1. A test in which there is deposition of particles, e.g. an agglutination test or an erythrocyte-sedimentation test. 2. A test for dirt in fresh milk: a standard glass sedimentation vessel is employed, and a carefully standardized procedure is followed for the separation by sedimentation and centrifugation, washing, and measurement sedimentation and centrifugalization, washing, and measurement of the dirt. Clean milk generally contains less than 1 part per 100 000 by volume of moist dirt. **Seidlitz powder test.** 1. A method used radiologically for demonstrating diaphragmatic hernia. The stomach is distended by CO_2 which rises into and outlines the herniated portion of stomach. (This test is not now used.) 2. A radiological method of determining the distensibility of the oesophagus and stomach in cases of suspected cancer, by the use of the above principle. **Self-balancing test.** A test used in the examination of candidates for the air services. The candidate, in boots or shoes, stands with feet close together, heels and toes touching, and arms to the sides. He then flexes one knee to a right angle without moving the hip, and, having obtained his balance, shuts his eyes tightly and endeavours to remain steady in this position for 15 s. The knees must not touch. In the event of failure at the first attempt, two further tests are allowed. The result of the test is recorded for each leg separately as: S., steady (no appreciable movement of the body away from the vertical axis); F.S., fairly steady (a slight oscillation away from this axis); U., unsteady (the lateral sway considerable, but corrected); O., failure (the raised foot touches the ground, the candidate touches some object in his surroundings, the supporting foot is moved from its original position, or the eyes are opened). Unsteadiness in the balancing tests indicates defective higher nervous control. Except in the case of old injury to the lower limbs, marked unsteadiness or failure in the self-balancing test is regarded as unfavourable, even in the absence of other signs of instability. **Serological test.** Any test with serum. **Serum test.** An immunological test for blood, meat, or sperms: the suspected material is treated with physiological saline to dissolve some of the protein, and added to specific rabbit antiserum prepared against the substance in question. The mixture will become cloudy if the suspected specimen is of the same species as the antigen used to prepare the antiserum. *See also* PRECIPITIN REACTION (*under* REACTION), and BORDET'S TEST. **Serum-neutralization test.** Mouse-protection test (see above). **Shadow test.** Retinoscopy. **Sheep red-cell agglutination test.** *See* ROSE WAALER TEST. **Skin test.** *See* ALVES' SKIN TEST, MCCLURE ALDRICH TEST, RODRIGUEZ' TEST, SANDROCK TEST, SCHICK TEST. **Skin temperature test.** *See* CIRCULATORY-EFFICIENCY TESTS, LOCAL PERIPHERAL, 5th def. (above). **Smear test.** The identification of cancer cells, by means of cytological characteristics and reaction to certain stains, in body secretions, especially vaginal. **Sociometric test.** Any test designed to elucidate by questionnaire the social structure of a group. **Sodium tetraiodophenolphthalein test.** *See* GRAHAM TEST. **Spectroscopic test.** 1. Any test in which the spectroscope is used to identify absorption bands. 2. A most reliable test for carbon monoxide in blood. A drop of normal blood is diluted until the solution is yellow. A drop of blood suspected to contain CO is similarly diluted: if CO is present this will remain pink. Each sample is examined spectroscopically; both will show bands between D and E, but on adding a drop of ammonium sulphide to each test-tube, the normal blood will show the normal blood spectrum of oxyhaemoglobin whereas the sample containing the CO will show only one band of reduced haemoglobin. **Sphenopalatine test.** A clinical test in which one sphenopalatine ganglion is anaesthetized in order to determine whether that one or the other is responsible for transmitting impulses giving rise to the symptoms noted. **Spot test.** Any test in which a drop of the substance to be identified is put on a piece of paper, blotting paper, or glass. **Squatting test.** The patient with beriberi is unable to rise from the squatting position without using his hands. **Stanford test, Stanford-Binet test.** A revision of the Binet-Simon intelligence test, made under the direction of Terman at Stanford University. **Stanford scientific aptitude test.** A test designed to predict success in scientific studies. **Station test.** A clinical test for disturbances of postural tone and sensibility in the lower limbs: the patient is asked to stand erect with the heels and toes together; inability to do so or undue swaying and unsteadiness indicates disturbed postural tone (in cerebellar ataxia) or impaired postural sensibility (in sensory ataxia). Unsteadiness may only be severe when the eyes are closed; this modification is known as *Romberg's sign* or *test.* **Sulphosalicylic acid test.** For protein in urine, etc.: to 1 volume of urine add 3 volumes of 3 per cent sulphosalicylic acid solution. A turbidity or precipitate indicates protein. **Sulphur test.** For cystine and protein containing cystine: to the solution add a drop of lead acetate solution and sufficient sodium hydroxide solution to redissolve the precipitate. A brown or black colour on boiling indicates cystine. **Sweat test.** In fibrocystic disease (mucoviscidosis), there is excessive sodium chloride in the sweat. The limits of normal vary with age but generally the result is positive if there is over 50 mol/l (average normal 27 mol/l). *See also* FINGERPRINT SWEAT TEST (above). **Sweating test.** A procedure for testing the conductivity of the autonomic (sudomotor) fibres of a nerve. The whole area is dusted with quinizarin powder; the areas where sweating occurs show a deep mauve coloration. **Tannic acid test.** *See* OTT'S TEST. **Tannin test.** For carboxyhaemoglobin; dilute blood with 4 volumes of distilled water and divide into two parts; to each add 1 ml of 10 per cent potassium ferrocyanide. Shake one vigorously for a period of about 10 min to oxygenate. Add 5 drops of yellow ammonium sulphide and 10 ml of 10 per cent tannin solution to each. A dirty olive-green precipitate forms in the shaken portion, whilst if carboxyhaemoglobin was present in the blood a bright red precipitate forms in the unshaken portion. **Tape test.** Moro's reaction: an ointment made of equal parts of Koch's old tuberculin and anhydrous lanolin is rubbed into the skin between the shoulder blades after thorough cleansing with alcohol-ether and a control patch is treated with lanolin alone. If positive after 48 h, the Moro's ointment area becomes reddened and papular and sometimes indurated. It is used mainly in young children. **Tellurite test.** *See* MANZULLO'S TEST. **Thalleoquin test.** For quinine and quinidine: dissolve a little of the substance in water or in decinormal acid, add 2 drops of bromine water and then 1 ml of dilute ammonia solution. An emerald green colour is given by quinine and quinidine. **Thematic apperception test.** A projection test in which the subject is presented with a series of ambiguous pictures one by one, is told that the test is one of imagination, and is required to tell a story based on each picture. The story is thought to reveal the content of the subject's personality, in particular those aspects that he will not or cannot discuss. **Thermoprecipitin test.** A serological test for specific animal species: the minced organ or part is heated with 5 volumes of water, filtered, and the filtrate layered with specific antiserum. A precipitate forming in a few minutes indicates that the organ belongs to the same species as that to which the antiserum was prepared. It is very useful in forensic medicine. **Thiochrome test.** For aneurine: to a solution of the substance in 2M sodium hydroxide add 10 ml of 5 per cent potassium ferrocyanide and 5 ml of *n*-butyl alcohol, shake for 2 min and allow to separate. An intense blue fluorescence (thiochrome) in the alcohol layer, which disappears upon acidification and reappears upon making alkaline, indicates aneurine. **Thiosulphate clearance test.** *See* PARA-AMINOHIPPURIC ACID CLEARANCE TEST (above). **Three-glass test.** In urethritis and chronic prostatitis: the early morning specimen of urine is passed into three coniform glasses. The urine in the first glass contains pus when there is anterior urethritis. Specimens 2 and 3 will remain clear. In posterior urethritis the urine in all three specimens contains pus. If the urine in the third glass is that which completed the act of voiding and contains shreds, there is prostatitis. **Three-paper test.** *See* MARIE'S TEST. **Thymol test.** For carbohydrates: to 0.5 ml of solution add 3 drops of 3 per cent alcoholic thymol solution, 5 ml of concentrated hydrochloric acid and 2 g of solid sodium chloride. Boil gently over a microburner. A carmine colour indicates carbohydrates. **Thymol turbidity test.** For liver function: to 0.05 ml of serum add 3 ml of thymol buffer reagent and allow to stand for 30 min. Measure the turbidity by the protein standards for urine in arbitrary units (1 unit ≡ 10 mg protein). The normal range is 0-4 units. Abnormally high values are usually obtained in hepatitis and cirrhosis but not in obstructive jaundice. *Thymol buffer*: add 500 ml of water to 1.03 g of sodium barbitone, 1.38 g of barbitone, and about 3 g of thymol. Heat just to boiling, shake well, and cool thoroughly. Seed with a few crystals of thymol and stand overnight at 20-25°C. Shake and filter. **Thyroid clearance test.** A test of thyroid function in which the uptake of radioactive iodine by the thyroid in a specified time is calculated from the concentrations in the plasma and in the region of the thyroid by means of counting apparatus. In its simplest form the clearance of iodide by the thyroid is obtained by comparing the count given at the neck with that at the thigh. **Free thyroxine index test.** Calculated from product of PBI (protein-bound iodine) in μg per cent and resin uptake ratio. Normal = 3.41-5.89. **Toad test.** *See* HOGBEN TEST. **Toluidine test.** For blood. *See* RUTTAN AND HARDISTY TEST. **Tongue test.** A sharp blow on the tongue will sometimes produce fibrillary contraction in patients with tetany due to hypocalcaemia. **Tourniquet test.** *See* HESS' TEST. **Toxoplasmin test.** A skin test using *Toxoplasma* antigen. **Trapeze test.** Suspension of the patient from a bar will abolish postural spinal deformity but will have no effect upon a structural deformity. **Treponema pallidum immobilization test.** A serological test for syphilis dependent upon immobilization of *Treponema pallidum*, in a suspension prepared from rabbit syphiloma, when incubated with a syphilitic serum in the presence of complement. Immobilization occurs in serum from cases of secondary, late, and congenital syphilis, but not consistently in serum from cases of primary syphilis. The reaction appears to be independent of the Wassermann reaction, and is found positive in cases of undoubted late syphilis in which the Wassermann reaction is persistently negative. **Trichophytin test.** An intracutaneous test of dermal sensitivity to trichophytin, an allergenic extract of one or more species of *Trichophyton*. The test is used to detect and measure the state of allergic sensitivity rather than for the diagnosis of ringworm infection. **Tri-iodothyronine (T_3) resin uptake test.** ^{131}I-labelled, diluted human serum albumin added to resin is counted and compared with the original serum after the addition of T_3 and the difference is expressed as the resin uptake. Normal range = 0.82-1.28. A test of thyroid function which is convenient because it does not require the presence of the patient (only a specimen of his blood). **Triketohydrindene hydrate test.** For proteins and protein derivatives: to 5 ml of the approximately neutral solution add 0.5 ml of a 0.1 per cent solution of ninhydrin, boil for a minute or two and cool. A blue colour is given by proteins, proteoses, peptones, polypeptides and amino acids (ninhydrin test). **Trypsin test.** The faeces or fluid are suspended or mixed with 1 per cent crystalline sodium carbonate and a drop is placed upon the emulsion side of a small strip of photographic film together with a drop of the sodium carbonate solution as control. The film is placed upon a piece of moist filter paper in a Petri dish, covered, and incubated for 30 min at 37°C. The dish is then placed in a refrigerator until thoroughly cooled. The film is then removed and washed in a gentle stream of water. If the material examined contained trypsin the test spot shows a circular hole where gelatin has been digested to soluble products which have dissolved in the water. If trypsin is absent the test spot is similar to the control which usually shows slight swelling but no solution in water. This test may be used to detect intestinal contents in abdominal exudates, and is also a test of pancreatic secretion in faeces. **Tuberculin test.** Any test in which an allergic reaction is produced by percutaneous, intracutaneous, or subcutaneous use of tuberculin, e.g. Moro's reagent, Mantoux or von Pirquet tests, etc. **Tuberculin patch test.** *See* VOLLMER'S PATCH TEST. **Tuberculin titre test.** *See* ELLERMANN AND ERLANDSEN TEST. **Turmeric test.** For boric acid or borates in foodstuffs: the foodstuff is ashed after addition of a little alkali and the ash dissolved in hydrochloric acid. A strip of turmeric paper is soaked in this solution and dried. A red colour turning green when the paper is moistened with alkali solution indicates the presence of boric acid or borates. **Two-glass test.** For urethritis. *See* THOMPSON'S TEST. **Urea clearance test.** For kidney function: the patient is kept at rest after a moderate breakfast. The bladder is emptied and the urine discarded. A glass of water is given and urine is collected during the next hour. Blood is then taken, another glass of water given, and urine again collected during the next hour. The volumes of urine specimens are accurately measured, and the urea in both blood and urine determined. The urea clearance is calculated from the formula $(UV/B) \times 1.33$, where U is the urine urea in mg per 100 ml, V the volume of urine passed in ml per minute, and B the blood urea in mg per 100 ml. If V is less than 2 the formula is $(U\sqrt{[V]}/B) \times 1.85$. Normal renal function is shown by a clearance of 70 or more, whilst figures below this indicate renal failure in proportion to the diminution in urea clearance. **Urea concentration test.** For kidney function: the patient receives no fluids for 8-12 h before the test, and then drinks 15 g of urea in 100 ml of water. Urine passed during the next 3 h is collected in hourly specimens and the urea determined in each. If the highest concentration of urea is greater than 2.5 per cent, renal function is regarded as satisfactory. A maximum concentration below 2 per cent indicates inadequate renal function. **Urease test.** For urea: incubation at 55°C of the neutral solution with an extract of soya or jack-bean meal causes liberation of ammonia if urea is present. The ammonia may be detected and determined by various methods, e.g. with Nessler's reagent. **Urine concentration test.** For kidney function: this test is carried out similarly to the urea concentration test (see above), except that no urea is given. The specific gravity of the hourly specimens is determined, and in at least one of them should exceed 1020 if renal efficiency is normal. **VDRL test.** A microflocculation serological test for syphilis, using cardiolipin, designed by the Venereal Disease Research Laboratory, US Marine Hospital, Staten Island, New York. **Vineland social maturity scale test.** A rating scale of maturity in the fields of self-help, self-direction, locomotion, occupation, communication, and socialization. **Virulence test.** A test for the poisonous or invasive properties of organisms, made by injecting pure cultures into susceptible laboratory animals. For example, true virulent diphtheria bacilli cause the death of guinea-pigs on subcutaneous injection, or produce characteristic necrotic lesions on intracutaneous injection. Control animals receiving a protective dose of antitoxin are unharmed by the cultures. **Vocabulary test.** Any test in which the score depends on the number of test words of which the subject knows the meaning, thus giving an estimate of intelligence. **Watch-tick test.** For hearing: a rough estimate of hearing ability may be obtained by noting the distance at which a watch can be heard from the meatus. Bone conduction can be tested by placing it on the skull, mastoid processes, or teeth. **Water test.** A provocative test for doubtful cases of glaucoma. The ocular tension is taken before and after drinking a litre of water. The test is suggestive of glaucoma if the rise of tension is more than 1.2 kPa (9 mmHg) within one hour. **Water-gurgle test.** When water is swallowed, a gurgling sound is heard with a stethoscope placed posteriorly to the left of the dorsal spine above the 6th dorsal vertebra and to the right below that level. If oesophageal obstruction is present the sound is not heard below the level of obstruction. **Water-vasopressin test.** A pharmacological test for epilepsy: it is known that in about 50 per cent of epileptic individuals fluid intoxication will produce a seizure. In the test the patient is made to drink a large volume of water and injections of vasopressin are given to inhibit diuresis. If a seizure is produced this gives valuable confirmation of the diagnosis of epilepsy, but a negative result is of no clinical value. **Whisper test (vox afona).** Test of hearing: the patient is turned with one ear facing the examiner. The opposite meatus is occluded in a vibrate manner by the forefinger of an assistant. The patient's eyes are shielded to exclude lip reading. The examiner stands at a measured distance, and, employing a forced whisper, asks the patient to repeat a series of selected words and numbers. He approaches nearer and nearer until the words are repeated correctly. Words are selected to include low- and high-pitched comments. A useful test for estimating the degree of deafness, and for differentiating low- and high-tone deafness. Both ears can be tested at once, the patient standing with his back to the examiner. **Wool test.** For colour blindness: 3 skeins of Berlin wool, green, red, and rose, have to be matched to a number of other variously coloured skeins. Devised by Holmgren. **Xanthoproteic test.** Xanthoproteic reaction: to 5 ml of protein solution add about 1 ml of nitric acid. A precipitate forms which dissolves upon heating to give a yellow colour. Cool and make alkaline with ammonia or caustic soda. The yellow colour deepens to orange. This test is given by amino acids such as tyrosine and tryptophan which contain phenyl groups. **Xenopus pregnancy test.** *See* HOGBEN TEST. **Zinc sulphate test.** A test that depends on the addition of buffered zinc sulphate to serum to give a turbidity, which Kunkel (1947) claims is more specifically related to gamma globulin than other flocculation and turbidity tests. The normal range is 2-8 units, and deviations, in general, follow those observed with the more widely used thymol turbidity test, except that it is more sensitive in the detection of residual hepatitis. [L *testum* crucible.]

tests:

Test for acetoacetic acid in urine. *See* GERHARDT'S TEST.

Test for acetone. *See* IODOFORM TEST (above), *and* DENIGÈS' TEST.

Test for acetone and acetoacetic acid in urine. *See* ROTHERA'S TEST.

Test for acetone bodies in urine. *See* BEHRE'S TEST, LEGAL'S TEST, LIEBEN'S TEST.

Test for achylia gastrica. *See* HISTAMINE TEST (above).

Test for acidosis. *See* ALKALI TOLERANCE TEST (above).

Test for acids in urine. *See* FERRIC CHLORIDE TEST (above).

Test for Addison's disease. *See* POTASSIUM TOLERANCE TEST (above), *and* CUTLER, POWER, AND WILDER TEST, ROBINSON-POWER-KEPLER TEST.

Test for adrenaline. *See* VULPIAN'S TEST.

Test for albumin. *See* ACETIC ACID TEST, SULPHOSALICYLIC ACID TEST (above), *and* HELLER'S TEST, OSGOOD-HASKINS TEST, ROBERTS' TEST.

Test for alcohol. *See* CHROMIC ACID TEST, ETHYL ACETATE TEST, IODOFORM TEST (above).

Test for alcoholic intoxication. 1. Clinical tests for inebriety. 2. Laboratory tests of breath, blood or urine for their alcoholic content; by breathalyser, chemical (Widmark) analysis, or gas chromatography.

Test for alkaloids. *See* FROHN'S TEST, MAYER'S TEST, VITALI'S TEST.

Test for amylase in urine. *See* FABRICUS-MOLLER URINE TEST.

Test for amyloidosis and nephrosis. *See* BENNHOLD'S TEST.

Test for aneurine. *See* THIOCHROME TEST (above), *and* SHERMAN AND CHASE ASSAY TEST.

Test for aneurysm. *See* KOROTKOFF'S TEST, TUFFIER'S TEST.

Test for angle of squint. *See* PRISM COVER TEST (above), *and* HIRSCHBERG'S TEST.

Test for antimony. *See* MARSH TEST, REINSCH'S TEST.

Test for aplastic anaemia. *See* BENDA'S TEST.

Test for appendicitis. *See* OBTURATOR TEST, PSOAS TEST (above), *and* COPE'S TEST.

Test for arsenic. *See* GUTZEIT TEST, MARSH TEST, MARSH-BERZELIUS TEST, REINSCH'S TEST.

Test for ascites. *See* BLAXLAND'S TEST.

Test for ataxia. *See* STATION TEST (above), *and* FOURNIER TEST, ROMBERG'S TEST.

Test of auditory fatigue. *See* GRADENIGO'S TEST.

Test of aural sensitivity. *See* GRUBER'S TEST.

Test for barbituric acid (barbiturates). *See* COPPER-PYRIDINE TEST (above), *and* ZWIKKER TEST.

Test for beriberi. *See* SQUATTING TEST (above), *and* AALSMEER'S TEST.

Test for bile acids (bile salts). *See* MYLIUS' TEST, PETTENKOFER'S TEST, UDRÁNSZKY'S TEST.

Test for bile pigments. *See* FOAM TEST (above), *and* GMELIN'S TEST, HAMMARSTEN'S TEST, HUPPERT'S TEST, ROSENBACH-GMELIN TEST.

Test for bilirubin. *See* IODINE TEST (above), *and* van den BERGH'S TEST, FOUCHET'S TEST.

Test for binocular vision. *See* BAR READING TEST, FRIEND TEST (above), *and* WORTH'S FOUR-DOT TEST.

Test for blood. *See* BENZIDINE TEST, GUAIAC TEST, HAEMIN TEST, TOLUIDINE TEST (above), *and* BORDET'S TEST, KASTLE-MEYER TEST, MALACHITE GREEN TEST, NIPPE'S TEST, ORTHO-TOLIDINE TEST, RUTTAN AND HARDISTY TEST, TEICHMANN'S TEST.

Test for boric acid (and borates) in foodstuffs. *See* TURMERIC TEST (above).

Test for butter fat. *See* VALENTA TEST.

Test for calcium in urine. *See* SULKOWITCH'S TEST.

Test for cancer. The following are advanced as tests for cancer but their value has not so far received scientific confirmation; Aron's, Bendien's, Botelho's, von Dungern's, Friedman-Hamburger, Fuchs', Gruskin, Kahn's, Neubaure and Fischer, Roffo's, Salomon's, Thomas-Binetti. *See also* EDESTIN TEST, SMEAR TEST (above).

Test for carbohydrates. *See* THYMOL TEST (above), *and* MOLISCH'S TEST.

Tests for carbon monoxide. 1. Spectroscopic test. *See* SPECTROSCOPIC TEST, 2nd def. (above). *See also:* CARBON MONOXIDE HAEMOGLOBIN TEST. 2. Chemical tests. *See* BOETTGER'S TEST, DEJUST'S TEST, HOPPE-SEYLER'S TEST, KATAYAMA'S TEST, KUNKEL'S TEST, RUBNER'S TEST, SALKOWSKI'S TEST, ZALESKI'S TEST.

Test for carboxyhaemoglobin. *See* TANNIN TEST.

Test for carcinoma of the cervix. *See* SCHILLER'S TEST.

Test for cerebellar lesion. *See* BÁRÁNY'S POINTING TEST.

Test for cerebral atherosclerosis. *See* STIEGLITZ TEST.

Test for chancroid infection. *See* ITO-REENSTIERNA TEST.

Test for cholesterol. *See* LIEBERMANN-BURCHARD TEST, SALKOWSKI'S TEST.

Test for citrulline in proteins. *See* DIACETYL TEST (above).

Test for colour vision. *See* WOOL TEST (above), *and* EDRIDGE-GREEN TEST, ISHIHARA'S TEST.

Test for creatinine. *See* SALKOWSKI'S TEST, WEYL'S TEST.

Test for cyanide. *See* PRUSSIAN BLUE TEST.

Test for cyclophoria. *See* MADDOX DOUBLE-PRISM TEST.

Test for cysteine. *See* SULLIVAN'S TEST.

Test for cystine and protein containing cystine. *See* SULPHUR TEST (above).

Test for cystosine. *See* TEST FOR URACIL (above).

Test for deafness. *See* LOUD-VOICE TEST, WATCH-TICK TEST, WHISPER TEST (above), *and* DOERFLER-STEWART TEST, GAULT'S COCHLEOPALPEBRAL REFLEX, KABATSCHNIK'S TEST, POLITZER'S TEST, RINNE'S TEST, SCHWABACH'S TEST, WEBER-LIEL TEST.

Test for death. *See* BALFOUR'S TEST, ICARD'S TEST, MAGNUS' SIGN, WINSLOW'S TEST.

Test for deoxyribonucleic acid. *See* FEULGEN'S TEST.

Tests of dermal sensitivity. *See* COCCIDIOIDIN TEST, OIDIOMYCIN TEST, TRICHOPHYTIN TEST (above).

Test for diabetes insipidus. *See* NICOTINE TEST.

Test for diastase in urine. *See* WOHLGEMUTH'S TEST.

Test for diphtheria. *See* TELLURITE TEST (above), *and* MANZULLO'S TEST, REH'S TEST, SCHICK TEST.
Test for diphtheria antitoxin. *See* RAMON'S FLOCCULATION TEST.
Test for diplopia. *See* DIPLOPIA TEST (above), *and* LANCASTER PROJECTION TEST.
Test for dirt in fresh milk. *See* SEDIMENTATION TEST (above).
Test for disease of the cerebellum. *See* FINGER-TO-FINGER TEST, FINGER-NOSE TEST (above).
Test for disease of the pyramidal tract. *See* HEEL-TAP TEST (above), *and* CRAFTS' TEST.
Test for dislocation of the shoulder. *See* CALLAWAY'S TEST, DUGAS' TEST, HAMILTON'S TEST.
Test for enteroptosis. *See* GLÉNARD'S TEST.
Test for epilepsy. *See* HYPERPNOEA TEST, WATER-VASOPRESSIN TEST (above).
Test for ergot alkaloids. *See* COCK'S-COMB TEST (above).
Test for ethyl alcohol. *See* ETHYL ACETATE TEST (above).
Test for fat in milk. *See* ADAMS' METHOD.
Test for fibrocystic disease of the pancreas. *See* FINGERPRINT SWEAT TEST, SWEAT TEST (above).
Test for formaldehyde. *See* BUCHANAN AND SCHRYVER TEST, JORISSEN'S TEST, LEACH'S TEST.
Test for fragility of skin capillaries. *See* DALLDORF'S TEST.
Test for free hydrochloric acid in gastric contents. *See* GUENZBERG TEST, TOEPFER'S TEST.
Test for fructose (laevulose) in urine. *See* BORCHARDT'S TEST, SELIVANOFF'S TEST.
Test for functional anaesthesia. *See* JANET'S TEST.
Test for glanders. *See* MALLEIN TEST (above), *and* STRAUS TEST.
Test for glandular fever. *See* PAUL-BUNNELL TEST.
Test for glaucoma. *See* COFFEE TEST, DARK-ROOM TEST, WATER TEST (above).
Test for globulin. *See* NOGUCHI'S TEST, PANDY'S TEST.
Test for glucose (dextrose). *See* FERMENTATION TEST, OSAZONE TEST (above).
Test for glucose in urine. *See* BRAUN'S TEST, JOHNSON'S TEST.
Test for glucuronic acid (glucuronates). *See* TOLLENS' TEST.
Test for glycerol, oils, and fats. *See* ACROLEIN TEST (above), *and* MAUMENÉ'S TEST.
Test for gonorrhoea. *See* PROSTATIC-BEAD TEST (above).
Test for haemoglobin. *See* BENZIDINE AND NITROPRUSSIDE PEROXIDASE TEST (above).
Test for haemophilia and jaundice. *See* QUICK'S TEST.
Test for haemorrhagic diathesis. *See* KOCH'S TEST.
Test for haemosiderin in urine. *See* ROUS' TEST.
Test for hernia. *See* KELLY'S TEST.
Test for hot spots. *See* GOLDSCHEIDER'S TEST.
Test for hydatid disease. *See* CASONI TEST.
Test for Indian hemp. *See* GAYER TEST.
Test for indican. *See* JAFFÉ'S TEST, JOLLES' TEST, OBERMAYER'S TEST.
Test for indole. *See* NAPHTHOQUINONE TEST, NITROSO TEST, OXALIC ACID PAPER TEST (above), *and* EHRLICH'S TEST, HERTER'S TEST.
Test for indole in cultures. *See* OXALIC ACID PAPER TEST (above).
Test for inositol. *See* SCHERER'S TEST.
Test for intracranial tumour. *See* AYALA'S TEST.
Test for intrinisic factor. *See* CASTLE'S TEST.
Test for iron in the tissues. *See* BRUGSCH'S TEST, TIZZONI'S TEST.
Test for jaundice. *See* QUICK'S TEST.
Test for kala-azar. *See* ALDEHYDE TEST, ANTIMONY TEST (above), *and* BRAHMACHARI'S TEST, SIA'S TEST; tests dependent on changes in the proportion of serum proteins.
Test for ketosteroids in urine. *See* DINITROBENZENE TEST (above).
Test for kidney disease. *See* MURPHY'S TEST.
Test for kidney function. *See* CREATININE-CLEARANCE TEST, DILUTION TEST, INDIGO-CARMINE TEST, PARA-AMINOHIPPURIC ACID CLEARANCE TEST, PHENOLSULPHONEPHTHALEIN TEST, UREA CLEARANCE TEST, UREA CONCENTRATION TEST, URINE CONCENTRATION TEST (above), *and* ACHARD-CASTAIGNE TEST, ADDIS AND SHEVSKY TEST, ALBARRAN'S TEST, MOELLER, MCINTOSH AND VAN SLYKE TEST, MOSENTHAL'S TEST, ROWNTREE AND GERAGHTY TEST, VOELCKER AND JOSEPH TEST.
Test for labyrinthine disease. *See* BABINSKI-WEIL TEST, EITELBERG'S TEST, HITZIG'S GALVANIC TEST, MITTERMAIER'S TEST, STEIN'S TEST.
Test of lacrimal secretion. *See* SCHIRMER'S TEST.
Test for lactic acid. *See* KELLING'S TEST, STRAUSS' TEST, UFFELMANN'S REAGENT.
Test for lactose in urine. *See* METHYLAMINE TEST, MUCIC ACID TEST (above), *and* COLE'S TEST, RUBNER'S TEST.
Test for laevulose. *See* BORCHARDT'S TEST, SELIVANOFF'S TEST.
Test for latent squint. *See* COVER TEST (above).
Test for lead. *See* BLYTH'S TEST.
Test for lead poisoning. *See* BASOPHILIC AGGREGATION TEST (above).
Test for leishmaniasis. *See* TEST FOR KALA-AZAR, LEISHMANIA TEST (above), *and* MONTENEGRO'S TEST.
Test for leprosy. *See* LEPROMIN TEST (above), *and* RODRIGUEZ' TEST.
Test for lesions of the optic cortex. *See* WILBRAND'S PRISM TEST.
Test for life. *See* TEST FOR DEATH (above).
Test for liver function. *See* BROMSULPHTHALEIN TEST, CEPHALIN-CHOLESTEROL TEST, COLLOIDAL GOLD TEST, GALACTOSE TOLERANCE TEST, HIPPURIC ACID TEST, LAEVULOSE TOLERANCE TEST, ROSE BENGAL TEST, THYMOL TURBIDITY TEST (above), *and* HANGER'S TEST, QUICK'S TEST, TAKATA-ARA TEST.
Test for lymphogranuloma. *See* FREI TEST.
Test for malaria. *See* PROTEIN-TYROSIN TEST (above), *and* HENRY'S MELANOFLOCCULATION TEST, URRIOLA'S TEST.
Test for maltose. *See* OSAZONE TEST.
Test for melanin in urine. *See* THORMAEHLEN'S TEST, ZELLER'S TEST.
Test of memory. *See* MARIE'S TEST.
Test for mercury. *See* REINSCH'S TEST.
Test for metatarsalgia. *See* MORTON'S TEST.
Test for methaemalbuminaemia. *See* SCHUMM'S TEST.
Test for middle-ear disease. *See* EITELBERG'S TEST, GARDINER-BROWN TEST.
Test for monosaccharide. *See* BARFOED'S TEST.
Test for muscle balance of the eyes. *See* MADDOX HAND-FRAME TEST, MADDOX ROD TEST, MADDOX WING TEST.
Test for muscle imbalance of the eyes. *See* OCCLUSION TEST (above).
Test for myocardial ischaemia. *See* MYOCARDIAL-RESERVE TESTS (above).
Test for nitrites. *See* ILOSVAY'S REAGENT.
Test for nucleoprotein in urine. *See* OTT'S TEST.
Test for oesophageal obstruction. *See* WATER-GURGLE TEST (above).
Test for oils and fats (temperature reaction). *See* MAUMENÉ'S TEST.
Test for olfactory acuity. *See* PROETZ TEST.
Test of olfactory function. *See* ELSBERG'S TEST.
Test for opium alkaloids. *See* MARQUIS' TEST.
Test for organic nitrogen. *See* LASSAIGNE'S TEST.
Test for osteo-arthritis. *See* JANSEN'S TEST.
Test for pancreatic function. *See* GLUCOSE TOLERANCE TEST (above), *and* WOHLGEMUTH'S METHOD.
Test for pancreatic lipase. *See* ETHYL BUTYRATE TEST, LITMUS-MILK TEST (above).
Test for pasteurization of milk. *See* PHOSPHATASE TEST (above).
Test for patency of deep veins. *See* PATENCY TEST (above).
Test for patent ductus arteriosus. *See* PLESCH'S TEST.
Test for pentose in urine. *See* BIAL'S TEST, TAUBER'S TEST.
Test for peptic activity in the diagnosis of gastric cancer. *See* EDESTIN TEST (above).

Test for phaeochromocytoma. *See* MECHOLYL TEST (above).
Test for phenols in urine. *See* MILLON'S TEST.
Test for pneumococci. *See* NEUFELD TEST.
Test for polysaccharides. *See* IODINE TEST (above).
Test for porphyrinuria. *See* WALDENSTRÖM'S TEST, WATSON-SCHWARTZ TEST.
Test for pregnancy. *See* ASCHHEIM ZONDEK TEST.
Test for the presence of pus. *See* WATERHOUSE TEST.
Test for protein in urine. *See* ACETIC ACID TEST, SULPHOSALICYLIC ACID TEST (above), *and* HELLER'S TEST, OSGOOD-HASKINS TEST, ROBERTS TEST, TANRET'S TEST.
Test for proteins containing tyrosine. *See* MILLON'S TEST.
Test for proteose in urine. *See* SCHULTESS' TEST.
Test for purpura. *See* FLICKING TEST (above), *and* GROCCO'S TEST, HESS' TEST, PECK'S TEST.
Test for quinine and quinidine. *See* THALLEOQUIN TEST (above).
Test for quinine in urine. *See* TANRET-MAYER TEST.
Test for reducing sugar in urine. *See* FEHLING'S TEST.
Test for renal function. *See* TEST FOR KIDNEY FUNCTION (above).
Test for renal inadequacy. *See* ALBARRAN'S TEST.
Test for respiratory efficiency. *See* FLACK TEST.
Test for rheumatic fever. *See* WELTMANN'S SERUM TEST.
Test for rheumatoid arthritis. *See* LATEX TEST (above), *and* ROSE WAALER TEST.
Test for salicylic acid (salicylates). *See* FERRIC CHLORIDE TEST (above).
Test for sarcoidosis. *See* KVEIM.
Test for scalenus anticus syndrome. *See* NAFFZIGER'S TEST.
Test for scarlet-fever immunity. *See* DICK TEST.
Test for schistosomiasis. *See* ALVES' SKIN TEST, FAIRLEY'S FIXATION TEST.
Test for sciatica. *See* BECHTEREW'S TEST, LASÈGUE'S TEST.
Test for seminal fluid. *See* FLORENCE TEST, PHOSPHATASE TEST.
Test for separate existence of the fetus. *See* TARDIEU'S TEST.
Test for serum phosphatase. *See* BODANSKY METHOD, GUTMAN AND GUTMAN METHOD, KING AND ARMSTRONG METHOD.
Test for simulated deafness. *See* CONTRADICTORY RESPONSE TESTS, EAR SPECULA TEST, LOUD-VOICE TEST (above), *and* BLOCKSTENGER TEST, BURCKHARDT-MERIAN TEST, CALLAHAN'S TEST, CHIMANI-MOOS TEST, COGGINS TEST, ERHARD'S TEST, GAULT'S COCHLEOPALPEBRAL REFLEX, LOMBARD'S TEST, LUCAE-TEUBER TEST, STENGER'S TEST, TEAL'S TEST, WELLS-STENGER TEST.
Test for skatole. *See* NITROSO TEST (above), *and* EHRLICH'S TEST.
Test for spinal block. *See* AMYL NITRITE TEST (above), *and* AYER'S TEST, QUECKENSTEDT TEST, TOBEY-AYER TEST.
Test for stapes fixation. *See* GELLÉ'S TEST.
Test for stereoscopic vision. *See* HERING'S DROP TEST.
Test for sugar. *See* OSAZONE TEST (above).
Tests for sugars in urine. *See* FERMENTATION TEST, METHYLAMINE TEST, MUCIC ACID TEST, OSAZONE TEST (above), *and* BARFOED'S TEST, BENEDICT'S METHOD, BIAL'S TEST, BORCHARDT'S TEST, FEHLING'S TEST, RUBNER'S TEST, SELIVANOFF'S TEST, TAUBER'S TEST, TOLLENS' TEST.
Test for sympathetic nervous lesions. *See* HISTAMINE TEST (above), *and* BROWN'S FEVER TEST.
Test for syphilis. *See* FORMOL-GEL TEST, IN VITRO IMMOBILIZATION TEST, TREPONEMAL IMMOBILIZATION TEST, VDRL TEST (above), *and* CANTANI TEST, CASILLI'S TEST, DOWNIE'S TEST, KAHN TEST, SACHS-GEORGI TEST, WASSERMANN TEST, PLASMACRIT TEST.
Test for systemic lupus erythematosus. *See* ANTINUCLEAR FACTOR TEST *and* LE CELL TEST (above).
Test for tennis elbow. *See* MILLS' TEST.
Test for thiamine. *See* THIOCHROME TEST (above), *and* SHERMAN AND CHASE ASSAY TEST.
Test for thiocyanates in saliva. *See* FERRIC CHLORIDE TEST (above), *and* SOLERA'S TEST.
Test for thrombosis. *See* DE TAKATS' TEST, TOBEY-AYER TEST.
Test for tinea versicolor. *See* ALLEN'S TEST.
Test of topognostic sensibility. *See* FOERSTER'S CUTANEOUS NUMERAL TEST.
Test for trichiniasis. *See* BACHMAN TEST.
Test for tryptophan and proteins containing tryptophan. *See* BROMINE TEST (above), *and* ADAMKIEWICZ'S TEST, HOPKINS-COLE TEST.
Test for tubal patency. *See* RUBIN'S TEST.
Test for tuberculosis. *See* COIN TEST, EXERCISE TEST, HAMMER TEST, MIRROR TEST, PEPPERMINT TEST, PURIFIED PROTEIN TEST, SCARIFICATION TEST, TAPE TEST, TUBERCULIN TEST, TUBERCULIN PATCH TEST, TUBERCULIN TITRE TEST (above), *and* ARLOING-COURMONT TEST, BLUMENAU'S TEST, DARÁNYI TEST, ELLERMANN AND ERLANDSEN TEST, ESCHERICH'S TEST, GAIRDNER'S COIN TEST, GRUSKIN'S TEST, HAMBURGER'S TEST, HEAF TEST, LAUTIER'S TEST, LESIEUR-PRIVEY TEST, LIGNIÈRES' TEST, MANTOUX TEST, MENDEL'S TEST, MÉRIEUX-BAILLON TEST, TRIBOULET'S TEST, VALSALVA'S TEST, VOLLMER'S PATCH TEST.
Test for tularaemia. *See* FOSHAY'S TEST.
Test for tumour. *See* PAGET'S TEST.
Test for typhoid fever. *See* DREYER'S TEST, WIDAL'S TEST.
Test for tyrosine. *See* HOFMANN'S TEST, MILLON'S TEST, MOERNER'S TEST, PIRIA'S TEST.
Test for uracil. *See* BROMINE TEST (above).
Test for urea. *See* BIURET TEST, UREASE TEST (above).
Test for urea (salivary). *See* HENCH-ALDRICH TEST.
Test for urethritis. *See* THREE-GLASS TEST, TWO-GLASS TEST (above), *and* THOMPSON'S TEST.
Test for uric acid and other purines. *See* MUREXIDE TEST (above).
Test for urobilin. *See* SCHLESINGER'S TEST.
Test for urobilinogen. *See* EHRLICH'S TEST.
Test for urochromogen. *See* WEISS' TEST.
Test for urorosein. *See* NITRITE TEST (above).
Test for varicose veins. *See* LINTON'S TEST.
Test for vestibular function. *See* NYSTAGMUS TEST (above).
Test for visual acuity. *See* "E" TEST, POSTMYDRIATIC TEST (above), *and* LANDOLT'S RING TEST, WORTH'S IVORY-BALL TEST.
Test for vitamin A. *See* CARR-PRICE TEST, ROSENHEIM-DRUMMOND TEST.
Test for vitamin-A deficiency. *See* DARK-ADAPTATION TEST (above), *and* FRIEDERICHSEN'S TEST.
Test for vitamin B_1. *See* PREBLUDA AND MCCOLLUM TEST.
Test for vitamin-B_1 deficiency. *See* SQUATTING TEST (above), *and* JONGCK TEST.
Test for vitamin B_6. *See* CYANINE DYE TEST (above).
Test for vitamin-C deficiency. *See* ROTTER'S TEST.
Test for white phosphorus. *See* MITSCHERLICH'S TEST.
Test for whooping-cough vaccine. *See* KENDRICK MOUSE INTRACEREBRAL TEST.
Test for xanthine. *See* WEIDEL'S TEST.

test-breakfast (test·brek·fast). Test-meal. [test, AS *brecan, faestan.*]

test-card (test·kard). **Stigmatometric test-card.** A card with designs on it for the subjective estimation of astigmatism. [test, Gk *chartes* papyrus.]

test-dinner (test·din·er). Test-meal. [test, Fr. *dîner.*]
See also: LEUBE, RIEGEL.

test-meal (test·meel). A standard meal given to test the secretory function of the stomach. The gastric contents are withdrawn at intervals afterwards for inspection and analysis. The meal varies in type, but is commonly either gruel or 7 per cent alcohol. **Motor test-meal.** A meal containing an opaque substance, the progress of which through the alimentary canal can be followed by x-rays. [test, AS *mael.*]
See also: BOAS, EWALD.

test-object (test·ob·jekt). 1. An object having a fine structure which is used as a test of the optical resolution of a microscope. 2. Flat, circular discs coloured white, red, green, and blue, and varying in diameter from 1 to 70 mm and mounted on slender holders. They are used in estimating the size and state of the visual fields in conjunction with a perimeter or screen. [test, object.]

test-plate (test·plate). *See* ABBÉ, E. K.

test-spoon (test·spoon). A small spatula-like spoon used for handling substances in chemistry, e.g. in weighing or analysis. [test, AS *spon.*]

test-tube (test·tewb). A small cylindrical vessel with rounded bottom, made of thin glass, used to hold substances and solutions, especially in qualitative chemical analysis. [test, tube.]

test-types (test·ti·pz). White cards with black letters, pictures, or other devices printed on them in varying sizes as a test for visual acuity both for near and distance. [test, type.]

See also: JAEGER (E. R. J.), SNELLEN.

testa (tes·tah). A shell. **Testa ovi.** Crushed egg-shell. **Testa praeparata.** Powdered oyster-shell used as an antacid. [L.]

testaceous (tes·**ta**·shus). 1. Possessing a shell. 2. Shell-like, or concerned with a shell. [L *testa* shell.]

testalgia (tes·**tal**·je·ah). Testicular pain. [testis, Gk *algos* pain.]

testectomy (tes·**tek**·to·me). Surgical removal of a testis; orchidectomy; male castration. [testis, Gk *ektome* excision.]

testicle (tes·tikl). The male gonad where, in adult life, spermatozoa develop; the testis. **Atrophic testicle.** A small and usually functionless testis not uncommonly a sequel to injury to its blood supply at operation, e.g. varicocele or undescended testicle. **Ectopic testicle.** A testis which is not situated either in its adult position in the scrotum or along the line of normal descent from the abdomen; it may lie in the perineum, groin, thigh, or above the pubis. **Imperfectly descended testicle.** Undescended testicle (see below). **Inverted testicle.** A testis which is not fixed in the normal position in the scrotum and so is liable to torsion, e.g. in superior inversion the long axis of the testis disposed horizontally. **Pigeon's egg testicle.** A painless enlargement of the testis, occasionally found in infancy in congenital syphilis. **Retained testicle.** A testicle which has failed to complete its descent into the scrotum and is retained inside the abdominal parietes; cryptorchism. **Scrofulous testicle.** A tuberculous testicle, almost always involved secondary to epididymitis. **Supernumerary testicle.** A rare happening where there is a third testicle, usually elsewhere than in the scrotum. **Syphilitic testicle.** Involvement of the testis either in early life in congenital syphilis (see pigeon's egg testicle, above) or as a tertiary manifestation in acquired disease. **Undescended testicle.** Cryptorchidism. A testis which during the process of descent has never reached the scrotum but has been arrested in the inguinal canal or abdomen. To be distinguished from a retractile testis which has retracted from the scrotum to the inguinal canal or abdomen as the result of a strong cremaster reflex. An ectopic testis has descended, but not into the scrotum. It has usually been diverted into the superficial inguinal pouch, lying between the skin and the underlying inguinal canal. [L *testiculus.*]

testicular (tes·**tik**·ew·lar). Concerned with or derived from the testes. [L *testiculus* testicle.]

testicular artery [arteria testicularis (NA)]. A long, slender, ventrolateral branch from the aorta, passing obliquely downwards and laterally across the psoas major muscle and ureter (which it supplies) [rami ureterici (NA)] to the deep inguinal ring, where it joins the other constituents of the spermatic cord. It ends in the back and sides of the testis.

testicular feminization (tes·**tik**·ew·lar fem·in·i·za′·shun). A condition in which a genetic male with normal XY chromosomes appears to be a phenotypic female because his body is unable to respond to normal amounts of androgen produced by his testes.

testicular (ovarian) veins [venae testiculares et venae ovaricae (NA)]. Tributaries of the inferior vena cava on the right [dextra (NA)], and of the renal vein on the left [sinistra (NA)]. They commence below in plexuses, the radicals of which gradually unite to form single veins.

testiculoma (tes·tik·ew·**lo**′·mah). A tumour formed of testicular tissue. **Testiculoma ovarii.** Arrhenoblastoma. [testicle, Gk *-oma* tumour.]

testis [NA] (tes·tis). The male gonad suspended in the scrotum by the spermatic cord. It is covered by a dense fascial coat, the tunica albuginea [NA], from the posterior thickened portion of which, the mediastinum testis, septa pass into the organ dividing it into lobes containing seminiferous tubules. The epididymis is attached to its posterior border. It has an upper [extremitas superior (NA)] and lower [extremitas inferior (NA)] pole. The lateral surface [facies lateralis (NA)] is the outer convex surface, and the medial surface [facies medialis (NA)] the inner convex. The convex front border [margo anterior (NA)] faces forwards and slightly downwards, whilst the straight back border [margo posterior (NA)] faces backwards and slightly upwards. **Lobe of the testis [lobulus testis (NA)].** One of the subdivisions of the testis produced by the passage into its interior of the septula from the mediastinum. It contains 2 to 4 seminiferous tubules. **Testis redux.** A testis which is drawn up to the upper pole of the scrotum, e.g. on exposure to cold. **Retractile testis.** A testis that is retracted into the inguinal canal by a strong cremaster reflex and therefore is often incorrectly diagnosed as an undescended testis. [L.]

testitis (tes·ti·tis). Orchitis. [testis, Gk *-itis* inflammation.]

testitoxicosis (tes·te·tox·ik·o′·sis). A condition known to arise as the result of ligaturing the vasa deferentia. [testis, Gk *toxikon* poison.]

testoid (tes·toid). Resembling a testis; applied in particular to the rudimentary testicle sometimes observed in the female. [testis, Gk *eidos* form.]

testopathy (tes·**top**·ath·e). Any morbid condition of the testes. [testis, Gk *pathos* disease.]

testosterone (tes·to·**steer**·one, tes·**tos**·ter·one). $C_{19}H_{28}O_2$, the hormone secretion of the testicles. By far the most potent natural androgenic hormone. It is a steroid, the systematic name of which is Δ^4-androstene-3-one-17(α)-ol (BP 1973). **Ethinyl testosterone.** Ethisterone BP 1973, pregneninolone, an orally active steroid having the actions of progesterone. **Testosterone Implants BP 1973.** Sterile cylinders prepared by fusion or heavy compression of testosterone. **Methyl testosterone.** An orally active derivative of testosterone having similar properties to the latter. **Testosterone Phenylpropionate BP 1973.** The ester of testosterone with phenylpropionic (hydrocinnamic) acid. **Testosterone Propionate BP 1973.** Δ^4-androsten-17(α)-propionate-3-one, an ester of testosterone having a prolonged action when injected parenterally.

Testosteroni Propionas (tes·**tos**·ter·**o**′·ni **pro**·pe·on·as). *European Pharmacopoeia* name for Testosterone Propionate BP 1973.

tetania (tet·a·ne·ah). Tetany. **Tetania epidemica.** Epidemic tetany. *See* TETANY. **Tetania gravidum.** Tetany associated with pregnancy. **Tetania parathyreopriva.** Parathyroid tetany. *See* TETANY. **Tetania rheumatica.** Epidemic tetany. *See* TETANY. **Tetania strumipriva.** An old name applied to a parathyroid tetany when it was thought to be caused by removal of the thyroid. [Gk *tetanos* convulsive tension.]

tetanic (tet·**an**·ik). 1. Having the characteristics of, or relating to tetanus. 2. Any poison which produces symptoms like tetanus.

tetaniform (tet·**an**·e·form). Tetanoid. [tetanus, form.]

tetanigenous (tet·an·**ij**·en·us). Causing tetanus or giving rise to tetanus-like spasms. [tetanus, Gk *genein* to produce.]

tetanilla (tet·an·**il**·ah). 1. Tetany. 2. Myoclonus. [dim. of tetanus.]

tetanine (tet·an·een). Tetanotoxine.

tetanism (tet·an·izm). A hypertonicity in the muscles of young infants, having long duration and certain of the features of tetanus, but not due to the tetanus bacillus.

tetanization (tet·an·i·za′·shun). The bringing on of tetanic spasms.

tetanize (tet·an·ize). To produce a tetanic spasm in a muscle.

tetanode (tet·an·ode). The quiet period between tonic spasms in tetanus.

tetanoid (tet·an·oid). Having a similarity to tetanus. [tetanus, Gk *eidos* form.]

tetanolysin (tet·an·**ol**·is·in). A thermolabile haemolytic toxin produced by *Clostridium tetani*; it probably plays little part in the natural disease. [tetanus, lysin.]

tetanometer (tet·an·**om**·et·er). A device for the measurement of muscular spasm of tetanus.

tetanomotor (**tet**·an·o·**mo'**·tor). An instrument for producing tetanic spasms of muscle. [tetanus, L *movere* to move.]

tetanophil, tetanophilic (**tet**·an·o·fil, tet·an·o·**fil**·ik). Possessing an attraction for tetanus toxin. [tetanus, Gk *philein* to love.]

tetanophobia (**tet**·an·o·**fo'**·be·ah). The dread of becoming infected with tetanus. [tetanus, Gk *phobein* to fear.]

tetanospasmin (tet·an·o·**spaz'**·min). An extremely powerful neurotoxin produced by *Clostridium tetani*, which causes the characteristic violent convulsions of tetanus. [tetanus, spasm.]

tetanotoxine (**tet**·an·o·**tox'**·een). The crude bacterial filtrate of a culture of *Clostridium tetani*, containing at least two toxins, tetanospasmin and tetanolysin. [tetanus, toxin.]

tetanus (**tet**·an·us). 1. An infective disease due to the toxins of the *Clostridium tetani*, the organisms entering through an abrasion or wound of the skin. Symptoms are produced by the extremely powerful soluble toxin elaborated by the bacilli, the earliest being trismus or tonic spasm of the masseter muscles; other muscles become involved until the spasms are general. 2. A sustained tonic spasm of muscle. **Acoustic tetanus.** Tetanus produced in a muscle-nerve preparation by rapidly repeated induction shocks, so-named because the rate of stimulation is measured against standard tuning forks. **Acute tetanus.** The acute infective disease due to *Clostridium tetani*. **Tetanus anticus.** Tetanus in which the body is arched forwards during a spasm. **Artificial tetanus.** Convulsions produced by a drug such as strychnine which causes tonic spasms, or experimentally by electrical stimulation of motor nerves. **Cephalic tetanus.** A form of tetanus due to wounds of the head; the symptoms are confined to the head. **Cerebral tetanus.** That form of tetanus which may arise from wounds of the head in particular and which results in stiffness of the muscles of the jaw and paralysis of the facial muscles on the same side as the wound. **Chronic tetanus.** A form of tetanus of delayed onset, slow progress, and more favourable prognosis than usual. **Cryptogenic tetanus.** A form of tetanus in which the site of entrance cannot be found. **Descending tetanus.** Tetanus in which the muscular spasms gradually spread downwards, that is, after starting in the face and neck, they later involve the muscles of the chest and upper limbs. **Tetanus dolorificus.** Tetanus with very painful spasms. **Tetanus dorsalis.** Tetanus in which the body is arched backwards during a spasm. **Drug tetanus.** Artificial tetanus (see above). **Extensor tetanus.** Tetanus in which the extensor muscles are principally affected. **Flexor tetanus.** Tetanus in which the flexor muscles are especially affected. **Head tetanus, Hydrophobic tetanus.** Tetanus following a wound of the head, especially of the eyebrow region. It is characterized by trismus, facial paralysis on one side, and marked dysphagia. The symptoms superficially resemble those of rabies. **Idiopathic tetanus.** Tetanus without obvious cause. **Imitative tetanus.** Hysterical pseudotetanus. **Tetanus infantum.** Tetanus neonatorum (see below). **Inoculation tetanus.** Experimental tetanus produced by inoculation with a culture of the causal organism. **Kopf tetanus.** Head tetanus (see above). **Tetanus lateralis.** Tetanus in which the body is arched sideways. **Localized tetanus.** Localization of the muscular spasms to the neighbourhood of the wound without general spasms. **Tetanus neonatorum.** Infection of the newborn baby by the tetanus organism, usually through the umbilical cord or stump. Symptoms usually appear at the end of the first week and consist of dysphagia, spasms of the muscles of the face and neck, leading to generalized convulsions and later rigidity. Death results from spasm of the respiratory muscles. Since the introduction of modern aseptic wound treatment the disease has practically died out in civilized countries. **Tetanus paradoxus.** Cephalic tetanus in which trismus is combined with paralysis of the facial or some other cranial nerve. **Paralytic tetanus.** Head tetanus (see above). **Partial tetanus.** An undesirable term for tetany. **Tetanus posticus.** Tetanus in which the body is arched backwards during spasms. **Postoperative tetanus.** Tetanus following an operation. **Postserum tetanus.** Tetanus following an injection of horse serum. **Puerperal tetanus.** The tetanic state occurring during the puerperium, common in native communities. **Splanchnic tetanus.** Tetanus in which the muscles concerned with deglutition and respiration are severely affected. **Surgical tetanus.** Postoperative tetanus (see above). **Toxic tetanus.** The effects of an overdose of a drug causing tonic spasms, such as with an overdose of strychnine. **Traumatic tetanus.** Tetanus following a wound. **Uterine tetanus.** Puerperal tetanus (see above). [Gk *tetanos* convulsive tension.]

See also: JANIN, KLEMM, RITTER (J. W.), ROSE (E.), WUNDT.

tetany (**tet**·an·e). A disease caused by a decrease of calcium in the blood serum and marked clinically by a hyperexcitability of the neuromuscular system. The reduction of calcium may be due to a deficiency of parathyroid secretion from atrophic disease of the glands, their operative removal, or damage after thyroidectomy. In other cases there is deficient absorption or utilization of calcium as in rickets, steatorrhoea, osteomalacia, or alkalosis. **Epidemic tetany.** A form of 2 or 3 weeks' duration, occurring occasionally in Europe. **Gastric tetany.** A form of tetany occurring in cows and which is often fatal. It is said to be due to feeding on lush pastures. **Hyperventilation tetany.** Tetany caused by the alkalaemia due to excessive pulmonary ventilation. **Lactation tetany.** A form due to the increased demands for calcium during lactation which brings to light a latent tetany due to other causes, such as deficient absorption of calcium. **Latent tetany.** A tetany which is only made apparent by mechanical or electrical stimulation. **Parathyroid tetany.** That due to a deficiency of parathyroid secretion. **Rheumatic tetany.** Epidemic tetany (see above). **Thyroprival tetany.** That which follows thyroidectomy. [see prec.]

tetartanopia, tetartanopsia (**tet**·ar·tan·**o'**·pe·ah, **tet**·ar·tan·**op'**·se·ah). Homonymous loss of a quadrant of the field of vision. [Gk *tetartos* fourth, anopia.]

tetra-amylose (tet·rah·**am**·il·oze). Tetramylose, $(C_{12}H_{20}O_{10})_2$. A compound isolated from starch paste, consisting of two bisamylose units. [Gk *tetra* four, amylose.]

tetrabasic (tet·rah·**ba**·sik). 1. Applied to an acid that has four atoms of hydrogen replaceable by a metal or radical. 2. Of an alcohol, one containing 4 hydroxyl groups. [Gk *tetra* four, base.]

Tetrabenazine (tet·rah·**ben**·az·een). BP Commission approved name for 3 - isobutyl - 1,2,3,4,6,7 - hexahydro - 9,10 - dimethoxybenzo[α]quinolizin - 2 - one; it is used in the treatment of neuroses.

tetrablastic (tet·rah·**blas**·tik). Describing an embryo possessing four germ layers. [Gk *tetra* four, *blastos* germ.]

tetrabrachius (tet·rah·**bra**·ke·us). A fetal monster with four arms. [Gk *tetra* four, *brachion* arm.]

tetrabromofluorescein (tet·rah·**bro**·mo·floo·or·**es'**·e·in). $C_{20}H_8Br_4O_5$, the parent substance of the various forms of eosin used as dyes for silk and wool, in the manufacture of red inks, and as stains in pathological work.

tetrabromophenolphthalein (tet·rah·**bro**·mo·fe·nol·**thal'**·e·in). $CO{=}C_6H_4O{=}C(C_6H_2Br_2OH)_2$, an indicator used in alkalimetry.

tetrabromophenolsulphonephthalein (**tet**·rah·bro·mo·**fe**·nol·sul·fone·**thal'**·e·in). Bromphenol blue. *See* BLUE.

tetracaine hydrochloride (**tet**·rah·kane hi·dro·**klor**·ide). Amethocaine Hydrochloride BP 1958.

Tetracainii Chloridum. *European Pharmacopoeia* name for Amethocaine Hydrochloride BP 1973.

tetracetate (tet·**ras**·et·ate). Any acetate which contains four acetic radicals. [Gk *tetra* four, acetate.]

tetracheirus (tet·rah·**ki**·rus). A fetal monster with four hands. [Gk *tetra* four, *cheir* hand.]

Tetrachilomastix (**tet**·rah·ki·lo·**mas'**·tix). A genus of flagellate Protozoa. **Tetrachilomastix bengalensis.** *Chilomastix mesnili.* **Tetrachilomastix intestinalis.** A coprozoic organism occasionally observed in human faeces. It is possible that there has been confusion with some species of *Trichomonas*. [Gk *tetra* four, *cheilos* lip, *mastix* whip.]

tetrachlorethane (**tet**·rah·klor·**eth'**·ane). 1,1,2,2-Tetrachloroethane. A dense liquid used for dissolving oils, sulphur, phosphorus, and cellulose acetate. It is also of value as an insecticide.

tetrachlorethylene (tet·rah·klor·**eth**′·il·een). 1,1,2,2-Tetrachloroethene.

tetrachloride (tet·rah·**klor**·ide). Any chloride which contains four atoms of chlorine. [Gk *tetra* four, chloride.]

tetrachlormethane (tet·rah·klor·**me**′·thane). Carbon tetrachloride, CCl_4, a colourless liquid used as a solvent, fire extinguisher, and also as an anaesthetic and anthelmintic.

Tetrachloroethylene BP 1973 (tet·rah·klor·o·**eth**′·il·een). 1,1,2,2-Tetrachloroethene, $Cl_2C{=}CCl_2$. A colourless mobile liquid, insoluble in water and miscible with most organic solvents. It is administered orally in the form of capsules, or an emulsion, as an all-round anthelmintic in the treatment of worm infections in man but especially in hookworm infections, and against roundworm and hookworm in animals.

tetrachromic (tet·rah·**kro**·mik). Having the ability to recognize only 4 of the 6 spectral colours of Edridge-Green's classification of colour blindness. [Gk *tetra* four, *chroma* colour.]

tetracid (tet·**ras**·id). Referring to a base, one which has four available hydroxyl groups, or is capable of neutralizing two molecules of a dibasic acid. [Gk *tetra* four, acid.]

tetracoccus (tet·rah·**kok**·us). Any coccus which divides by binary fission in two different planes, thus forming a tetrad of four cells. [Gk *tetra* four, *kokkos* berry.]

Tetracosactrin (tet·rah·ko·**sak**′·trin). BP Commission approved name for β^{1-24}-corticotrophin; a synthetic corticotrophin. **Tetracosactrin Acetate BP 1973.** A synthetic polypeptide identical with the first 24 of the 39 amino acids of corticotrophin. Given intravenously, 1 mg of tetracosactrin is equal in activity to about 100 units of corticotrophin. Depot injections, intramuscularly, produce corticotrophin effects for 1-2 days.

tetracrotic (tet·rah·**krot**·ik). Referring to a pulse tracing, one that has two secondary waves in addition to the dicrotic on the downstroke, making four in all. [Gk *tetra* four, *krotos* beat.]

Tetracycline (tet·rah·**si**·kleen). BP Commission approved name for the basic skeleton of aureomycin and oxytetracycline. Tetracyline is itself an antibiotic, and solutions are more stable than those of either of the others. **Tetracycline Hydrochloride BP 1973.** The official form of tetracyline. **Tetracycline Phosphate Complex.** BP Commission approved name for a relatively soluble complex of sodium metaphosphate and tetracycline; it has the same action and uses as tetracycline.

tetrad (**tet**·rad). 1. Any element with a valency of four, e.g. carbon. 2. A group of four; the group of four cells as produced by *Micrococcus tetragenus.* 3. The four cells resulting from meiotic division of a gametocyte. 4. The four chromatids of a bivalent at meiosis. [Gk *tetras* quadrant.]

See also: FALLOT.

tetradactyl (tet·rah·**dak**·til). Tetradactylous.

tetradactylous (tet·rah·**dak**·til·us). Possessing only four digits in each hand or foot. [Gk *tetra* four, *daktylos* digit.]

tetraethylammonium (tet·rah·eth·il·am·**o**′·ne·um). The organic group, $N(C_2H_5)_4$, analogous with ammonium NH_4. **Tetraethylammonium Bromide BPC 1954.** $(C_2H_5)_4NBr$, a smooth-muscle relaxant owing to its ability to block the transmission of nerve impulses at the autonomic ganglia. It is usually injected as a 10 per cent solution. **Tetraethylammonium chloride.** $(C_2H_5)_4NCl$, a compound which possesses similar properties as tetraethylammonium bromide. **Tetraethylammonium hydroxide.** $N(C_2H_5)_4OH$, a ganglionic blocking agent preventing the transmission of the nerve impulse across sympathetic and parasympathetic ganglia. It obliterates vasoconstrictor tone, causing on injection an increase in skin temperature, a transient decrease in both systolic and diastolic blood pressure, postural hypotension, and increase in heart rate and cardiac output, dilatation of the pupil, and decrease in tone of the bladder. It has been used in Raynaud's disease, causalgia, hypertension, and to assess the possible vaue of sympathectomy.

tetraethylpyrophosphate (tet·rah·**eth**·il·pi·ro·**fos**′·fate). $(C_2H_5O)_2(P_2O_3)(OC_2H_5)_2$, a compound which is administered orally for the treatment of myasthenia gravis owing to its inhibiting action on cholinesterase. It is also used as a systemic insecticide in horticulture.

tetraethylthiuram disulphide (tet·rah·eth·il·thi·**ewr**′·am di·**sul**·fide). $(C_2H_5)_2NCSSSSCN(C_2H_5)_2$, a compound used in the treatment of chronic alcoholism. It is itself non-toxic, but when alcohol is subsequently administered extremely unpleasant symptoms develop. These include flushing, tachycardia, vomiting, hypotension, syncope, and coma, and are thought to be due to the production of acetaldehyde in the blood. Deaths have been reported and the drug must be used with extreme caution; its use is contra-indicated when renal, cardiac, and respiratory diseases are present, or when alcohol has recently been administered.

tetragenic (tet·rah·**jen**·ik). Derived from *Micrococcus tetragenus.* [see foll.]

tetragenous (tet·**raj**·en·us). Divided in groups of four, as do certain bacteria. [Gk *tetra* four, *genein* to produce.]

tetragon, tetragonum (**tet**·rag·on, tet·rag·**o**·num). A quadrilateral; a figure with four sides. **Tetragonum lumbale.** The lumbar quadrangle, the irregular four-sided space between the serratus posterior inferior muscle above, the internal oblique muscle below, medially the sacrospinalis muscle, and laterally the external oblique muscle. [Gk *tetra* four, *gonia* angle.]

tetragonus (tet·rag·o·nus). 1. Quadrangular. 2. The platysma muscle. [see prec.]

tetrahydric (tet·rah·**hi**·drik). Referring to an alcohol that contains four OH groups. [Gk *tetra* four, hydroxyl.]

tetrahydrocortisol (tet·ra·hi·dro·cor·tis·ole). Cortisol to which four atoms of hydrogen have been added in the process of degradation of Ring A during the biosynthesis of cortisol.

tetrahydrofurfuryl (tet·rah·hi·dro·**fer**′·fewr·il). An organic group derived from furfuryl.

tetrahydronaphthalene (tet·rah·hi·dro·**naf**′·thal·een). Tetralin.

tetrahydronaphthyl imidazoline hydrochloride (tet·rah·hi·dro·**naf**′·thil im·id·**az**·o·leen hi·dro·**klor**·ide). 2-(1,2,3,4-tetrahydro-1-naphthyl) imidazoline hydrochloride. A vasoconstrictor and decongestant useful for relieving inflammation and obstruction of sinuses and nasal mucosa in common cold, rhinitis, and hay fever.

tetrahydroparaquinanisol (tet·rah·**hi**·dro·par·ah·kwin·**an**′·is·ol). Thalline, *p*-methoxytetrahydroquinoline, $C_9H_{10}NOCH_3$. A compound obtained from coal tar, with antiseptic and antipyretic properties.

Tetrahydrozoline (tet·rah·hi·**droz**′·o·leen). BP Commission approved name for 2-(1,2,3,4-tetrahydro-1-naphthyl)-imidazoline; used in the treatment of nasal congestion.

tetraiodophenolphthalein (tet·rah·i·o·do·fe·nol·**thal**′·e·in). A compound, the disodium salt of which, iodophthalein, $C_{20}H_8O_4I_4Na_2{\cdot}3H_2O$, is used as a contrast medium in the radiography of the biliary tract, being excreted by the liver into the gall bladder, which it renders opaque to x-rays. It has now been largely superseded by pheniodol, which is less toxic. **Tetraiodophenolphthalein sodium.** Iodophthalein, $C_{20}H_8O_4I_4Na{\cdot}3H_2O$. A diagnostic medium which renders the gall bladder opaque to x-rays. It is administered orally or by intravenous injection.

tetraiodopyrrole (tet·rah·i·o·do·**pir**′·ole). C_4I_4NH, a greyish-brown crystalline powder used as a surgical dusting-powder in place of iodoform. It is free from odour.

tetraiodothyronine (tet·rah·i·o·do·**thi**′·ro·neen). Thyroxine.

tetralin (tet·ral·in). Tetrahydronaphthalene, $C_{10}H_{12}$. A liquid formed by the hydrogenation under pressure of naphthalene. It is an important solvent for fats, waxes, and resins.

tetralogy (tet·**ral**·o·je). A series of four related writings. [Gk *tetra* four, *logos* word.]

See also: FALLOT.

tetramastia (tet·rah·**mas**·te·ah). The possession of four breasts. [Gk *tetra* four, *mastos* breast.]

tetramastigote (tet·rah·**mas**·tig·ote). Furnished with four flagella, as in the case of certain micro-organisms. [Gk *tetra* four, *mastix* whip.]

tetramazia (tet·rah·**ma**·ze·ah). Tetramastia. [Gk *tetra* four, *mazos* breast.]

tetramelus (tet·**ram**·el·us). Four-legged. [Gk *tetra* four, *melos* limb.]

tetrameric (tet·rah·**mer**·ik). Tetramerous.

tetramerism (tet·**ram**·er·izm). Division into four parts. [see foll.]

tetramerous (tet·**ram**·er·us). Divided into four parts, or having parts arranged in fours. [Gk *tetra* four, *meros* part.]

tetramethyl (tet·rah·**meth**·il). Denoting any compound that has four methyl groups in its structure. [Gk *tetra* four, methyl.]

tetramethylammonium hydroxide (tet·rah·**meth**·il·am·**o**′·ne·um hi·**drox**·ide). $N(CH_3)_4OH$, a compound which acts on sympathetic and parasympathetic nervous systems like nicotine, causing first stimulation and then paralysis. It produces first a peripheral muscarine-like inhibition of the heart, leading to a fall of blood pressure, followed by a nicotine-like stimulation of sympathetic ganglion cells producing a rise in blood pressure. Finally there is a nicotine-like paralysis of ganglion cells, causing a fall in blood pressure. Because of its complex actions the tetraethylammonium compound is preferred for blocking ganglia.

tetramethylbenzene (tet·rah·meth·il·**ben**′·zeen). $C_6H_2(CH_3)_4$, a compound which occurs in three isomeric forms; the 1,2,4,5 isomer is known as *durene*.

tetramethylenediamine (tet·rah·**meth**·il·een·**di**′·am·een). Putrescine.

tetramethylputrescine (tet·rah·meth·il·**pew**′·tres·een). $(CH_3)_2N(CH_2)_4N(CH_3)_2$, a crystalline base derived from putrescine, with toxic properties stimulating the action of muscarine.

tetramethylthionine chloride (tet·rah·meth·il·**thi**′·o·neen **klor**′·ide). Methylene blue. *See* BLUE.

tetramitiasis (tet·rah·mit·**i**′·as·is). Infestation of the intestine with the protozoan *Chilomastix* (*Tetramitus*) *mesnili*.

tetramitus (tet·rah·**mi**·tus). *Chilomastix*. [Gk *tetra* four, *mitos* thread.]

tetramylose (tet·**ram**·il·ose). Tetra-amylose.

tetranitrol (tet·rah·**ni**·trol). Erythrityl tetranitrate.

tetranophthalmos (tet·ran·of·**thal**′·mos). A fetal monster with a double face, four eyes, and two ears. [Gk *tetra* four, *ophthalmos* eye.]

tetranopia, tetranopsia (tet·ran·**o**·pe·ah, tet·ran·**op**·se·ah). Loss of a quadrant of field in one eye. [Gk *tetra* four, anopia.]

Tetranthera (tet·**ran**·the·rah). A genus of Indian trees. The bark of *Tetranthera laurifolia* is used as an astringent. [Gk *tetra* four, *antheros* flowery.]

Tetranychus (tet·**ran**·ik·us). A genus of mites. *Tetranychus molestissimus* of South America and *T. telarius* of Europe bite man, causing intense irritation. [Gk *tetra* four, *onyx* nail.]

tetra-ophthalmus (tet·rah·of·**thal**′·mus). Tetranophthalmos.

tetra-otus (tet·rah·**o**·tus). A fetal monster with four ears and four eyes, the two heads being almost separate. [Gk *tetra* four, *ous* ear.]

tetrapeptide (tet·rah·**pep**·tide). A simple compound formed by the union of four amino acids by peptide linkages. Such a compound is to be found among the products of protein hydrolysis. [Gk *tetra* four, peptide.]

tetraphenylmethane (tet·rah·fe·nil·**me**′·thane). $C(C_6H_5)_4$, a stable, colourless, crystalline hydrocarbon.

tetraplegia (tet·rah·**ple**·je·ah). Paralysis of both arms and both legs. [Gk *tetra* four, *plege* stroke.]

tetraploid (tet·rah·ploid). Of chromosome complements, cells or organisms having four sets of chromosomes (symbol 4*n*). [Gk *tetraploos* fourfold, *eidos* form.]

tetrapodesis (tet·rah·po·**de**′·sis). Progression on all fours, as in the case of very young children. [see foll.]

tetrapus (tet·rah·pus). 1. Four-footed. 2. A fetal monster possessing four feet. [Gk *tetra* four, *pous* foot.]

tetrascelus (tet·**ras**·el·us). A fetal monster possessing four legs. [Gk *tetra* four, *skelos* leg.]

tetraschistic (tet·rah·**skis**·tik). Tetragenous. [Gk *tetra* four, *schisis* fission.]

tetrasomic (tet·rah·**so**·mik). Of cells or individuals, fundamentally diploid but with four copies of a chromosome. [Gk *tetra* four, *soma* body.]

tetraster (tet·**ras**·ter). An abnormal mitotic figure in which two amphiasters, or achromatic figures, are present. [Gk *tetra* four, *aster* star.]

tetrastichiasis (tet·rah·stik·**i**′·as·is). An abnormal development of the eyelashes which are arranged in four rows. [Gk *tetra* four, *stichos* row.]

tetrathionate (tet·rah·**thi**·on·ate). Any salt of tetrathionic acid; they are usually formed by treating a thiosulphate with iodine.

Tetrathyridea (tet·rah·thi·**rid**′·e·ah). A pseudogenus, like Sparganum, in which are put the larvae of *Mesocestoides* spp. [Gk *tetra* four, *thyris* window.]

tetratomic (tet·rat·**om**·ik). 1. Describing a compound composed of four atoms. 2. Applied to an acid that has four replaceable hydrogen atoms, or an alcohol or base with four replaceable hydroxyl groups. (Obsolete term.) [Gk *tetra* four, atom.]

Tetratrichomonas buccalis (tet·rah·trik·**om**′·on·as buk·**a**·lis). The old name for *Trichomonas buccalis*. [Gk *tetra* four, *thrix* hair, *monas* unit, L *bucca* cheek.]

tetravaccine (tet·rah·**vak**·seen). Literally, a quadruple vaccine. An unsatisfactory term, formerly applied to Typhoid-paratyphoid A and B and Cholera vaccine. [Gk *tetra* four, vaccine.]

tetravalent (tet·rah·**va**·lent). Quadrivalent; having a valency of four. [Gk *tetra* four, valency.]

tetrelle (tet·**rel**). A device used in cases where an infant is too weak to suckle naturally. It comprises a nipple-shield provided with two tubes one of which the mother sucks, the milk passing along the other to the child. [Fr. *têter* to suck.]

tetrophthalmos, tetrophthalmus (tet·rof·**thal**·mos, tet·rof·**thal**·mus). Tetranophthalmos.

tetrose (**tet**·roze). Any simple sugar of genera formula $C_4H_8O_4$. Structurally, it may be either an aldotetrose, $CH_2OH(CHOH)_2CHO$, or a ketotetrose, $CH_2OHCHOHCOCH_2OH$. [Gk *tetra* four.]

tetrotus (tet·**ro**·tus). Tetra-otus.

tetroxide (tet·**rox**·ide). Any oxide which contains four atoms of oxygen. [Gk *tetra* four, oxide.]

tetryl (**tet**·ril). Tetranitromethylaniline, $(NO_2)_3C_6H_2N(CH_3)(NO_2)$. An explosive solid which causes yellow staining of the skin, dermatitis, nasal irritation and, rarely, epistaxis. Sometimes conjunctivitis and oedema of the eyelids may be produced, but constitutional symptoms are rare.

tetter (**tet**·er). An archaic noun indicating any of various vesicular skin diseases, e.g. herpes, eczema, ringworm, or a pimple, pustule, or blister. **Wet tetter.** Vesicular eczema. [AS *teter*.]

Teucrium (**tew**·kre·um). A genus of labiate plants. **Teucrium chamaedrys.** A species the dried herb of which has tonic, diaphoretic, and diuretic properties. **Teucrium scordium.** Water germander; a herb used as an antiseptic, diaphoretic, and stimulant. It has a bitter taste and an alliaceous odour. **Teucrium scorodonia.** Wood sage, garlic sage; a herb used as a diaphoretic, astringent, and tonic. [Gk *teukrion* germander.]

Teutleben, E. von (fl. 1877). Leipzig anatomist.

Teutleben's ligament. The pulmonary ligament of the pleura.

Texan snake root (**tex**·an snake root). Serpentaria.

textiform (**tex**·te·form). Web-like; reticulated. [L *textum* web, form.]

textoblastic (tex·to·**blas**·tik). Applied to cells which form regenerative tissues. [L *textum* web, Gk *blastos* germ.]

textoma (tex·**to**·mah). A neoplasm formed of fully differentiated cells. [L *textum* web, Gk *-oma* tumour.]

textural (**tex**·tewr·al). Concerning the texture of tissues.

texture (**tex**·tewr). 1. The disposition of tissue in an organ or part. 2. The nature of the organized tissue itself. [see foll.]

textus (**tex**·tus). Tissue. [L.]

thalamencephalic (thal·am·en·kef·**al**′·ik). Referring to the thalamencephalon.

thalamencephalon [NA] (thal·am·en·**kef**′·al·on). The thalamic brain or interbrain: the hindmost part of the forebrain, comprising the thalamus, hypothalamus, epithalamus, and metathalamus. [thalamus, Gk *egkephalos* brain.]

thalamic (thal·am·ik). Relating to the thalamus.

thalamocele, thalamocoele (thal·am·o·seel). A former name for the 3rd ventricle. (obsolete term.) [thalamus, Gk *koilia* hollow.]

thalamocortical (thal·am·o·kor'·tik·al). Concerning both the thalamus and the cerebral cortex.

thalamocrural (thal·am·o·kroo'·ral). Thalamopeduncular. [thalamus, crus.]

thalamolenticular (thal·am·o·len·tik'·ew·lar). Concerning both the thalamus and the lenticular nucleus.

thalamomamillary (thal·am·o·mam·il'·a·re). Concerning the thalamus and the mamillary bodies.

thalamopeduncular (thal·am·o·ped·ung'·kew·lar). Concerning the thalamus and one of the cerebral peduncles.

thalamostriate vein [vena thalamostriata (NA)] (thal·am·o·stri'·ate vane). A vein draining parts of the thalamus and caudate nucleus. [thalamus, stria.]

thalamotegmental (thal·am·o·teg·men'·tal). Referring to the thalamus and the tegmentum.

thalamotomy (thal·am·ot·o·me). The production of focal lesions within the thalamic nuclei by electrical, chemical or thermal means in the treatment of diseases of the basal ganglia and of otherwise intractable pain. [thalamus, Gk *temnein* to cut.]

thalamus [NA] (thal·am·us). A large mass of grey matter in the upper part of the lateral wall of the 3rd ventricle of the brain. It is subdivided by the internal medullary laminae [laminae medullares thalami (NA)] into many nuclei, nearly all of which give efferent connections to the cerebral cortex. It receives as its afferent connections ascending sensory tracts from the brain stem and spinal cord (spinothalamic tracts, medial lemniscus), and tracts from the cerebellum, hypothalamus, and corpus striatum. The medial and lateral geniculate bodies, receiving secondary auditory and optic fibres respectively and relaying them to the cerebral cortex, are differentiated parts of the thalamus. **Nucleus of the thalamus, anterior [nucleus anteriores thalami (NA)].** A nucleus which lies under the anterior tubercle. Its afferents form the mamillothalamic tract and its efferents run to the gyrus cinguli. **Nucleus of the thalamus, centromedial [nucleus medialis centralis (centromedianus) NA].** A small collection of nerve cells within the internal medullary lamina. **Nuclei of the thalamus, intralaminar [nuclei intralaminares (NA)].** Small collections of nerve cells within the internal medullary lamina. **Nucleus of the thalamus, lateral [nucleus lateralis thalami (NA)].** The largest part of the thalamus, consisting of ventral and lateral groups of nuclei. The former comprise an anterior nucleus [nucleus ventralis anterolateralis (NA)] which receives afferent fibres from the globus pallidus and sends efferents to the cerebral cortex, an intermediate nucleus [nucleus ventralis intermedius (NA)] which receives afferents from the cerebellum via the red nucleus and sends efferents to the cerebral cortex, a posteromedial (arcuate) nucleus [nucleus ventralis posteromedialis (NA)] which receives the trigeminal lemniscus, and a posterolateral nucleus [nucleus ventralis posterolateralis (NA)] which receives the lateral spinothalamic tract and the medial lemniscus. These posterior nuclei send efferents to the sensory area of the cerebral cortex. The lateral group of nuclei extend posteriorly to reach the pulvinar [nucleus posterior (pulvinar thalami) NA] and receive afferents from other parts of the thalamus. **Nucleus of the thalamus, medial [nucleus medialis thalami].** A dark area forming the upper part of the medial surface. Its efferents end in the frontal cortex, and its afferents arise in the hypothalamus. **Nucleus of the thalamus, reticular [nucleus reticularis thalami (NA)].** A thin sheet of cells on the lateral aspect of the thalamus. **Nucleus of the thalamus, ventral [nucleus ventralis thalami].** An ill-defined nucleus in the ventral part of the thalamus, receiving impulses from the lemnisci and the cerebellum and sending efferents to the postcentral gyrus and the motor cortex. It is divided into a posterior part [nucleus ventralis thalami posterior] which receives the somatic afferent pathways and intermediate [nucleus ventralis thalami intermedius] and anterior [nucleus ventralis thalami anterior] parts which receive the cerebellorubral and cerebellothalamic tracts. **Optic thalamus, Thalamus opticus.** Obsolete names for the thalamus. [Gk *thalamos* chamber.]

thalassaemia (thal·as·e·me·ah). Cooley's anaemia, erythroblastic anaemia, Mediterranean disease, familial microcytic anaemia, target-cell anaemia: a chronic, progressive anaemia of congenital, familial, and racial incidence, showing splenomegaly, bone changes, mongoloid facies and typical target cells or thin, poorly staining red cells (leptocytes) in the circulating blood. The condition appears commonly in peoples from countries in a broad tropical belt extending from the Mediterranean basin through the Middle East and Far East. Thalassaemia is not a single disease entity, but a group of disorders resulting from an inherited defective rate of production of one of the types of polypeptide chains involved in haemoglobin structure. In *alpha thalassaemia,* the alpha-type chains are under-produced with a concomitant excess of gamma- or beta-type chains leading to the production of the unstable haemoglobins Bart's (δ_4) or H(β_4). In *beta thalassaemia* there is an under-production of beta-type chains, the excess of alpha-type chains precipitating inside freshly-produced red blood cells in the bone marrow, and fetal haemoglobin persists beyond the neonatal period. Each of these main types of thalassaemia consists of several genetically distinct disorders which can be distinguished by the electrophoretic pattern of the haemoglobin and by the associated haematological findings. Treatment is still mainly symptomatic. **Thalassaemia major.** Cooley's anaemia; the severest form of thalassaemia usually seen in children when both parents are suffering from minor forms of the disease. It is usually fatal. **Thalassaemia minima.** A condition in which persons who are carriers of the trait have no clinical symptoms whatever but show recognizable haematological evidence. **Thalassaemia minor.** A mild form of thalassaemia in which there is mild clinical as well as haematological evidence of the disease usually recognized in adults and adolescents; the persons thus affected are carriers of the thalassaemia trait. [Gk *thalassa* sea, anaemia.]

thalassanaemia (thal·as·an·e'·me·ah). Thalassaemia.

thalassin (thal·as·in). A substance obtained from the sea anemone *Anemone scultetus.* It irritates the skin and mucous membranes. [Gk *thalassa* sea.]

thalassophobia (thal·as·o·fo'·be·ah). Morbid dread of the sea. [Gk *thalassa* sea, *phobein* to fear.]

thalassotherapy (thal·as·o·ther'·ap·e). Treatment of disease by sea air, sea bathing, or a sea voyage. [Gk *thalassa* sea, *therapeia* treatment.]

thalidomide (thal·id·o·mide). α-Phthalimidoglutarimide, a non-barbiturate sedative and hypnotic. This drug has been withdrawn from general use on account of serious side effects.

thalleoquin (thal·e·o·kwin). An intensely green compound produced when quinine or quinidine are treated in aqueous solution with bromine followed by ammonia. It is characteristic of these alkaloids. [Gk *thallos* young green shoot, quinine.]

thallic (thal·ik). Referring to compounds of thallium in which the latter is quadrivalent.

thalline (thal·een). Tetrahydroparaquinanisol, *para*-methoxy-tetrahydroquinoline, $C_9H_{10}NOCH_3$. An antiseptic and antipyretic derived from coal tar. The use of thalline and its salts has now been entirely abandoned.

thallium (thal·e·um). An element of atomic weight 204.37, atomic number 81, and chemical symbol Tl. It is a soft grey metal resembling lead in properties, and is used in the manufacture of optical glass. In its compounds it is an active poison nearly as toxic as arsenic and showing cumulative effects. **Thallium acetate.** CH_3COOTl, a compound which given internally or applied in the form of an ointment causes a rapid falling of the hair. It has been widely used for depilation of the skin in the treatment of ringworm, but because of numerous serious toxic effects its use has now been largely abandoned. **Thallium sulphate.** Tl_2SO_4, a compound with similar properties to the acetate. [Gk *thallos* young green shoot, from colour of spectral line.]

Thallophyta (thal·**of**·it·ah). The lowest division of the plant kingdom, in which the vegetative body is not differentiated into root, stem, or leaf, i.e. algae, fungi, bacteria. [Gk *thallos* young green shoot, *phyton* plant.]

thallophyte (**thal**·o·fite). One of the group of cryptogams, including algae, fungi, lichens, and bacteria. [see prec.]

thallospore (**thal**·o·spor). A spore formed directly from the thallus or vegetative element of a fungus, by septation (arthrospore) or by budding (blastospore).

thallotoxicosis (**thal**·o·tox·ik·**o**′·sis). Thallium poisoning; gastro-enteritis and peripheral neuritis caused by the absorption of thallium compounds. [thallium, Gk *toxikon* poison, *-osis* condition.]

thallus (**thal**·us). The vegetative part of a member of the lower plant kingdom (Thallophyta) which may be unicellular or multicellular but is never differentiated into root, stem, or leaf. [Gk *thallos* young green shoot.]

thalposis (thal·**po**·sis). Sensitivity to warmth. [Gk *thalpos* warmth.]

thalpotic (thal·**pot**·ik). Able to feel warmth. [see prec.]

Thamnidium (tham·**nid**·e·um). A genus of moulds in the order Mucorales in which two sizes of sporangia are borne (one large terminal sporangium and several small lateral ones, or sporangiola) on each sporophore. [Gk *thamnos* bush.]

Thamnomys surdaster surdaster (**tham**·no·mis sewr·**das**·ter sewr·**das**·ter). The Congo tree-rat from which *Plasmodium bergei* was first isolated. [Gk *thamnos* bush, *mys* rat.]

thanatobiological (**than**·at·o·bi·o·**loj**′·ik·al). Concerned with the phenomenon of life and death. [Gk *thanatos* death, *bios* life, *logos* science.]

thanatognomonic (**than**·at·o·no·**mon**′·ik). Denoting approaching death. [Gk *thanatos* death, *gnomon* sign.]

thanatoid (**than**·at·oid). 1. Death-like. 2. Lethal; mortal. [Gk *thanatos* death, *eidos* form.]

thanatology (than·at·**ol**·o·je). The scientific study of death. [Gk *thanatos* death, *logos* science.]

thanatomania (**than**·at·o·**ma**′·ne·ah). Suicidal or homicidal madness. [Gk *thanatos* death, *mania* frenzy.]

thanatometer (than·at·**om**·et·er). Any instrumental means of confirming death, such as the insertion of a thermometer into the body to confirm the fall in bodily temperature. [Gk *thanatos* death, meter.]

thanatophidia (**than**·at·o·**fid**′·e·ah). A collective term for the venomous snakes. [Gk *thanatos* death, *ophis* snake.]

thanatophidial (**than**·at·o·**fid**′·e·al). Relating to thanatophidia.

thanatophobia (**than**·at·o·**fo**′·be·ah). 1. An unjustified fear that death is imminent. 2. Exaggerated fear of death. [Gk *thanatos* death, *phobein* to fear.]

thanatos (**than**·at·os). The death instinct (Freud). [Gk death.]

thanatosis (than·at·**o**·sis). Necrosis; gangrene. [Gk *thanatos* death.]

Thane, Sir George Dancer (b. 1850). British anatomist.

Thane's method. A method for the surface marking of the central sulcus of the cerebrum.

Thaon, Louis Albert (b. 1846). Paris physician.

Guillain–Thaon syndrome. Cerebrospinal involvement in the secondary stage of syphilis.

Thapsia (**thap**·se·ah). A genus of umbelliferous plants. **Thapsia garganica.** A North African species, the root bark of which yields an intensely irritant resin which is used in plasters as a counter-irritant. [Gk deadly carrot.]

thaumatrope (**thaw**·mah·trope). An instrument used in physiology to demonstrate the persistence of visual impressions. Rotation of a board with figures on opposite sides gives the effect of the figures merging. [see foll.]

thaumatropy (thaw·**mat**·ro·pe). The changing of one form of tissue into another; the metamorphosis of an organ. [Gk *thauma* wonder, *trepein* to turn.]

thaumaturgic (thaw·mat·**er**·jik). Miraculous. [Gk *thauma* wonder, *ergein* to work.]

Thayer, Sidney Allen (b. 1902). American physician.

Thayer–Doisy unit. Mouse unit. *See* UNIT.

Thaysen, Thorwald Einar Hess (b. 1883). Copenhagen physician.

Thaysen's disease. Chronic circumscribed induration of the corpus cavernosum.

Gee–Thaysen disease. Coeliac disease or the infantile form of idiopathic steatorrhoea.

thea (**the**·ah). Tea.

Thebacon (the·**ba**·son). BP Commission approved name for acetyldihydrocodeinone, an analgesic and cough depressant of the morphine series.

thebaic (the·**ba**·ik). Having the characteristics of or derived from opium. [see foll.]

thebaica (the·**ba**·ik·ah). A name for opium, derived from Thebes where opium was prepared.

thebaine (the·**ba**·een). $C_{19}H_{21}O_3N$, a minor alkaloid of opium with a slight narcotic action. [see prec.]

thebaism (the·**ba**·izm). Addiction to opium; opiumism. [thebaica.]

Thebesius, Adam Christian (b. 1686). Leyden anatomist and pathologist.

Thebesius' foramina. Foramina venarium minimarum.

Thebesius' valve. The valve of the coronary sinus.

Thebesius' veins. The venae cordis minimae; very small veins in the myocardium opening directly into the atria or ventricles.

theca (**the**·kah). A sheath or envelope. **Theca cell tumour.** A rare ovarian tumour similar to granulosa cell tumour and secretes oestrogen. **Theca cerebri.** An obsolete name for the dura mater. **Theca folliculi [NA].** The capsule of an ovarian follicle, derived from the surrounding ovarian stroma; it consists of an inner vascular layer [tunica interna (NA)], and an outer layer [tunica externa (NA)] which is less vascular and contains some smooth muscle. **Theca interna.** The layer of cells adjacent to the membrana granulosa of the ovarian follicle. After ovulation it invades the follicle with luteal cells which stain yellow and become the corpus luteum (yellow body) and in addition to oestradiol secrete progesterone. **Theca vertebralis.** A name for the dura mater. [Gk *theke* sheath.]

thecal (**the**·kal). Relating to a theca. **Thecal abscess.** Tenosynovitis; whitlow.

thecate (**the**·kate). Provided with a sheath. [Gk *theke* sheath.]

thecitis (the·**si**·tis). Tenosynovitis. [Gk *theke* sheath, *-itis* inflammation.]

thecoma (the·**ko**·mah). An ovarian tumour which may easily be confused with fibroma, but its cut surface shows varying amounts of yellow streaking due to the lipoid content of its component thecal cells. [theca, Gk *-oma* tumour.]

thecostegnosis (**the**·ko·steg·**no**′·sis). The shrinking or narrowing of the sheath of a tendon. [Gk *theke* sheath, *stegnosis* a narrowing.]

Theden, Johann Christian Anton (b. 1714). German military surgeon.

Theden's vulnerary. A mixture of vinegar, alcohol, dilute sulphuric acid, honey, and water; at one time used in the treatment of wounds.

Theile, Friedrich Wilhelm (b. 1801). Weimar anatomist.

Theile's canal. The transverse sinus of the pericardium.

Theile's glands. Mucous glands in the neck of the gall bladder and the cystic duct.

Theile's muscle. Occasional muscular slips lying subcutaneously below the superficial transverse perineal muscles.

Theiler, Max (b. 1889). Boston immunologist and Nobel prize winner.

Theiler's disease. Encephalomyelitis of mice, caused by a virus and having in its anatomical distribution some resemblance to human poliomyelitis.

Theiler's virus. Mouse poliomyelitis virus.

Theileria (thi·**leer**·e·ah). A genus of protozoa, parasitic in many species of mammals but not in man. **Theileria parva.** The causal organism of East African fever in cattle, an extremely fatal disease carried by ticks. **Theileria tsutsugamushi.** *Rickettsia orientalis.* [Sir Arnold *Theiler*, 1867-1936, South African veterinary pathologist.]

theileriasis (thi·leer·i·as·is). East Coast fever, Rhodesian fever; a disease of cattle prevalent in East Africa and caused by *Theileria (Babesia) parva.*

Theimich's lip sign. Pouting of the lips on tapping the orbicularis oris muscle; it is exaggerated in upper motor neuron paralysis.

theine (**the**·een). Caffeine. [thea.]

theinism (**the**·in·izm). Theism.

Theis, Ruth C. New York biochemist.

Benedict and Theis method. For phenols in blood: proteins are precipitated by tungstic acid. 10 ml of filtrate are mixed with 1 ml of 1 per cent gum acacia solution, 1 ml of 50 per cent sodium acetate solution and 1 ml of diazotized *p*-nitroaniline reagent (1.5 g *p*-nitroaniline, 40 ml conc. HCl, water to 500 ml; to 25 ml add 0.75 ml of 10 per cent sodium nitrite solution). After 2–4 min, compare with standard (10 ml of phenol solution containing 0.0025 mg per ml).

theism (**the**·izm). A state of chronic dyspepsia and headache attributed to too much drinking of tea. [thea.]

thelalgia (the·**lal**·je·ah). Pain experienced in the nipple. [Gk *thele* nipple, *algos* pain.]

thelasis, thelasmus (the·**las**·is, the·**laz**·mus). Sucking; suckling. [Gk *thelazein* to suck.]

Thelazia (the·**la**·ze·ah). A genus of nematode worms. The adults inhabit the nasolacrimal ducts and conjunctival sacs of the mammalian eye, sometimes moving across the conjunctiva, causing scarring. **Thelazia californiensis.** A species which has been recorded rarely from man in western North America. **Thelazia callipoeda.** A species recorded rarely from man in China. [see prec.]

thelaziasis (the·laz·i·as·is). Infection of the eye with thelazia.

Thelaziidae (the·la·**zi**·id·e). A family of nematodes including the genus *Thelazia.* [Gk *thelazein* to suck, *eidos* form.]

thele (**the**·le). A nipple. [Gk.]

thelectomy (the·**lek**·to·me). Excision of the nipple. [Gk *thele* nipple, *ektome* a cutting out.]

theleplasty (**the**·le·plas·te). A plastic operation on the nipple. [Gk *thele* nipple, *plassein* to mould].

thelerethism (the·**ler**·eth·izm). An erection of the nipple brought about by the contraction of the muscular fibres on mechanical stimulation. [Gk *thele* nipple, *erethisma* a stirring.]

thelitis (the·**li**·tis). Inflammation of the nipple. [Gk *thele* nipple, *-itis* inflammation.]

thelium (**the**·le·um) (pl. *thelia*). 1. A nipple. 2. A papilla of any sort. 3. A layer of tissue cells. [Gk *thele.*]

Thelohania magna (the·lo·**ha**·ne·ah **mag**·nah). A microsporidium which is parasitic in the larva of the mosquito *Culex pipiens.*

theloncus (the·**long**·kus). A growth on the nipple. [Gk *thele* nipple, *ogkos* swelling.]

thelophlebostemma (**the**·lo·fleb·os·**tem**'·ah). The ring of veins around the base of the nipple; the circulus venosus. [Gk *thele* nipple, *phleps* vein, *stemma* wreath.]

thelorrhagia (the·lo·**ra**·je·ah). A flow of blood from the nipple. [Gk *thele* nipple, *rhegnynein* to gush forth.]

thelothism, thelotism (**the**·lo·thizm **the**·lo·tizm). Thelerethism.

thelyblast (**thel**·e·blast). The nucleus of the fertilized ovum. [Gk *thelys* female, *blastos* germ.]

thelyblastic (thel·e·**blas**·tik). Having the characteristics of a thelyblast.

thelygenic (thel·e·**jen**·ik). Giving birth to females only. [Gk *thelys* female, *genein* to produce.]

thelygonia (thel·e·**go**·ne·ah). The development of ova producing females only, such as occurs in parthenogenesis. [Gk *thelys* female, *gone* seed.]

thelymania (thel·e·**ma**·ne·ah). Satyriasis. [Gk *thelys* female, *mania* madness.]

thelyotoky (thel·e·**ot**·o·ke). Thelygonia. [Gk *thelys* female, *tokos* birth.]

thelyplasm (**thel**·e·plazm). That constituent of the germ cell which carries the female-determining factor. [Gk *thelys* female, *plasma* something formed.]

thelyplasty (**thel**·e·plas·te). Theleplasty.

thelytocia (thel·e·**to**·she·ah). Thelygonia. [Gk *thelys* female, *tokos* birth.]

thelytocous (thel·**it**·o·kus). Thelygenic. [see prec.]

thelytoky (thel·**it**·o·ke). Thelygonia. [Gk *thelys* female, *tokos* birth.]

thenal (**the**·nal). Concerned with the palm of the hand. [Gk *thenar* palm of the hand.]

Thenalidine (then·**al**·id·een). BP Commission approved name for 1-methyl-4-*N*-(2-thenyl)anilinopiperidine. It is used in the treatment of allergic conditions.

thenar (**the**·nar). 1. The ball of the thumb; the lateral or thumb side of the palm of the hand. 2. Thenal. **Thenar muscles.** The flexor and abductor pollicis brevis and the opponens pollicus. [Gk palm of the hand.]

Thenium Closylate (**the**·ne·um **klo**·sil·ate). BP Commission approved name for dimethyl - (2 - phenoxyethyl)-2-thenylammonium-4-chlorobenzenesulphonate; an anthelmintic.

Thenyldiamine (then·il·**di**·am·een). BP Commission approved name for *N'N'*-dimethyl-*N*-2-pyridyl-*N*-3-thenyl-ethylenediamine; an antihistamine.

thenylpyramine hydrochloride (then·il·**pir**·am·een hi·dro·**klor**·-ide). *N,N* - dimethyl - *N'*(2 - thenyl)-*N'*(2 - pyridyl)-ethylenediamine, $C_4H_3SCH_2N(C_5H_4N)CH_2CH_2N(CH_3)_2{\cdot}HCl$. An antihistaminic drug of moderate intensity.

Theobaldia (the·o·**bawl**·de·ah). A genus of mosquitoes which provides many species in temperate and arctic zones. [Frederic Vincent *Theobald* (b. 1868), British zoologist.]

Theobroma (the·o·**bro**·mah). A genus of sterculaceous plants. **Theobroma cacao.** A species the seeds of which are the source of cocoa; they contain theobromine and cocoa butter. **Prepared Theobroma BPC 1968.** Roasted theobroma seed deprived of most of its shell, pressed to remove a portion of its fat, and finely ground. It may be flavoured with vanillin or cinnamon, but must not have undergone any process of alkalinization. It is used as a basis for some tablets and lozenges and as a flavouring in barium meals. [Gk *theos* god, *broma* food.]

Theobromine BP 1968 (the·o·**bro**·meen). 3,7-Dimethylxanthine, $C_7H_8N_4O_2$. A purine derivative which occurs in cocoa bean. It is a white crystalline powder, soluble about 1 in 1000 of water. It has some stimulant action on heart muscle and dilates the coronary arteries, thus improving the blood supply to the organ; it also dilates blood vessels peripherally, and this action is partly responsible for its diuretic effect. Other effects of the drug which probably contribute to its diuretic action are an increase in the number of active glomeruli, and inhibition of the reabsorption of water, though it has the weakest diuretic effect of all three purine derivatives in the tubules. It causes very little stimulation of the central nervous system. **Theobromine and sodium acetate.** A mixture of sodium theobromine and sodium acetate; its advantage over the theobromine base is its solubility in water (1 in 2), its pharmacological actions being the same. **Theobromine and Sodium Salicylate BP 1953.** A mixture of sodium theobromine and sodium salicylate in molecular proportions. Its pharmacological effects are the same as those of theobromine, and it is the most commonly used of the salts because of its great solubility in water (1 in 1). [theobroma.]

Theodrenaline (the·o·**dren**·al·een). BP Commission approved name for 7-[2-(3,4,β-trihydroxyphenylethylamino)ethyl]theophylline; an analeptic.

theomania (the·o·**ma**·ne·ah). 1. Religious mania. 2. A form of insanity in which the patient has the impression that he is possessed by a divine spirit. [Gk *theos* god, *mania* madness.]

theomaniac (the·o·**ma**·ne·ak). A person affected with theomania.

theophobia (the·o·**fo**·be·ah). A morbid dread of divine punishment, or of the deity. [Gk *theos* god, *phobein* to fear.]

Theophylline BP 1973 (the·**of**·il·een). 1,3-Dimethylxanthine, $C_7H_8N_4O_2$. A purine derivative which occurs in tea-leaves. It has properties similar to those of theobromine and produces diuresis by the same mechanism but more powerfully. It causes more stimulation of the central nervous system than theobromine but less than caffeine, which is trimethylxanthine. **Theophylline Hydrate BP 1973.** The monohydrate of 1,3-dimethylxanthine; it has the same actions and uses as the base. [thea, Gk *phyllon* leaf.]

Theophyllinum (the·of·il·i′·num). *European Pharmacopoeia* name for Theophylline BP 1973. **Theophyllinum et Ethylenediaminum.** *European Pharmacopoeia* name for Aminophylline BP 1973. **Theophyllinum Monohydricum.** *European Pharmacopoeia* name for Theophylline Hydrate BP 1973.

theorem (the·or·em). Any proposition which can be demonstrated (proved) by argument from certain accepted axioms or premises. [Gk *theorema* speculation.]

See also: GIBBS.

theory (the·or·e). 1. An explanation or reasonable supposition upon which the abstract principles of an art or science, e.g. medicine, are based. 2. The abstract systematized mass of knowledge upon which a science is based, as distinct from the practical work to which it owes its existence and by means of which it is taught. 3. An explanation of the process underlying a group of phenomena, based usually upon the experimental verification of a priori hypothesis. **Action theory.** The theory that movement, though unconscious, is an essential factor in sensory perception. **Apposition theory.** The doctrine that bone cannot expand interstitially but only by surface deposition of new bone. **Atomic theory.** The theory that all matter is composed of elements which, combining, form the molecules of compounds. The atoms of any particular element are identical and remain unchanged in their chemical combinations, but they differ from the atoms of other elements in mass and internal structure. Within the atom there is a nucleus constituted of neutrons and protons, and this is surrounded by "shells" of electrons which, under normal conditions, render the atom neutral as a whole. **Avalanche theory.** The theory that nerve impulses are reinforced, and therefore increase in strength as they travel peripherally. **Brunonian theory.** The system of medicine devised by John Brown; this regarded all diseases as either sthenic, depending on an excess of stimulation, or asthenic, lacking in stimulation. The former were to be treated by sedative medicines, e.g. opium, and the latter by stimulants (wine or brandy). For a time this theory gained considerable support, especially in Germany and Italy. **Cell theory.** The doctrine that living matter is composed of discrete units, or cells, capable of independent activity. **Cell-chain theory.** The theory that nerve fibres are derived from a chain of cells rather than from the nerve cell. **Theory of central analysis.** Rutherford's theory. Also called telephone theory. **Chiasmatype theory.** The theory maintaining that chiasmata are either the cause or consequence of crossing-over. **Clonal selection theory.** A selective theory of antibody production, proposed by Burnet, whereby an antigen acts by affecting the population dynamics of antibody-producing cells, selecting those clones of cells already modified by somatic mutation to react to that antigen and causing them to multiply and produce specific antibody and cell-mediated immunity. **Theory of concrescence.** In dentistry, a theory used to explain the development of the mammalian tooth. **Corpuscular theory.** A theory formerly held that light is composed of corpuscles. It was discredited by the wave theory (see below) but the modern view tends to regard light as both corpuscular and wave-like in nature. **Darwinian theory.** The theory that evolution has occurred by survival of the fittest individuals in the struggle for existence by means of natural selection. Individuals which vary from the rest are continually occurring, and, if some of these are more fitted to survive, the variations that they show will become normal to the population. **Dimer theory.** A theory propounded by Bolk to explain the development of the mammalian tooth. **Dualistic theory of blood-cell formation.** A theory that all blood cells are derived from two differentiated mother cells or blast cells. **Duplicity theory.** The theory that there are two different mechanisms in the visual process: one, the rods with visual purple, which are responsible for scotopic vision taking place in light of reduced intensity; the other, the cones responsible for photopic vision taking place in light of greater intensity. **Electron theory.** The theory that the atom consists of a positively-charged nucleus composed of protons and neutrons round which, in orbits or shells, rotate electrons equal in number to the protons. It describes an electric current as a stream of electrons moving in a conductor, and affords an explanation of phenomena such as valency, ionization, and oxidation-reduction. **Electrosome theory.** The view that the mitochondria are cytoplasmic organs performing specialized chemical syntheses. **Emigration theory.** Cohnheim's theory. **Freudian theory.** *See* FREUD. **Germ theory.** The reasonable assumption that all contagious and infectious diseases are caused by living micro-organisms. **Germ-layer theory.** The view that each cell type in the adult organism can be traced back to only one of the three primary germ layers, viz. ectoderm, entoderm, and mesoderm, of the early embryo, and that the germ layers are homologous in any major group of animals. Thus, nerve cells are said to be always of ectodermal origin, bone cells of mesodermal origin, and liver cells of entodermal origin. **Gestalt theory.** The theory that perception and mental phenomena in general cannot be analysed into their component parts without loss, and that the proper object of study is the organized whole. **Ground-water theory.** Pettenkofer's theory. **Hahnemannian theory.** Like cures like, *similia similibus curantur.* **Humoral theory.** *See* HUMOURS. **Information theory.** The mathematical and theoretical principles of communication engineering. These principles may be applied to biological systems. **Instructive theories of immunity.** Theories of immunity which hold that the function of antigen in the immune response is to instruct or direct uncommitted cells to form a new antibody which reflects the nature of the antigen itself. **Ionic theory.** The theory that the molecules of all electrolytes in solution are dissociated to some degree into free, electrically-charged ions, the degree increasing with the dilution. It explains electrolysis as a migration of ions to the oppositely charged poles, acidity and alkalinity as an excess respectively of hydrogen and hydroxyl ions, and many other phenomena, including those of such biological importance as buffering, chloride shift, and the Donnan equilibrium. **Lateral-chain theory.** Ehrlich's side-chain theory. **Lymphatic permeation theory.** Concerns the mode of spread of cancer, particularly of the breast. A theory which postulated a centrifugal growth of cancer cells from the periphery of the primary tumour in solid continuous columns in the lymphatic vessels (Handley, W.S.). **Theory of medicine.** The knowledge of the principles, reasons, and theoretical considerations upon which the art and science of medicine are based. **Mendelian theory.** The theory that the characters of sexually-reproducing organisms are handed on to the offspring in fixed ratios and without blending. **Migration theory.** To explain the spread of sympathetic ophthalmia from one to the other eye: Deutschmann suggested that the causal organism travelled via the lymph channels along the intervaginal spaces of the optic nerves and chiasma. **Mnemic theory.** The theory that a long-lasting stimulus or irritant produces in the cells concerned a change that persists, even after removal of the stimulus or irritation, thus tending to the creation of habit. **Monophyletic theory of blood-cell formation.** The theory of blood-cell formation based on the view that a totipotential primitive blood cell, the haemocytoblast, is the first recognizably differentiated cell, and is the mother cell giving rise to all the cellular elements of the blood, red cells and white cells, as required. **Myogenic theory.** The theory that it is the inherent rhythmicity and tonicity of cardiac muscle which enables it to maintain contraction and tone. **Neo-unitary theory of haemopoiesis.** A modification of the monophyletic theory of blood-cell formation postulating that all cells arise from one primitive mother cell, that normally only the myeloblast acts as the myeloid mother cell, while the lymphocyte does not change to other types of cell, but this latter may happen under abnormal conditions. **Neural quantum theory.** The theory that the relationship between physical stimuli and sensory responses is of a discontinuous step-like nature. **Neurogenic theory.** The theory that contraction of the heart muscle is a result of nervous stimuli. **Neuron theory.** The doctrine that the nervous system is composed of discrete cellular units, the neurons. **Opponent-colours theory.** Hering's theory. **Over-production theory.** The hypothesis that regenerating tissues form in excess of the tissues they are replacing. **β-Oxidation theory.** In the metabolism of the fatty acids, oxidation always takes place at the carbon atom in the β-position with respect to the terminal carboxyl group, making the fatty acid chain less by two carbon atoms. **Paralytic theory.** The theory that hyperaemia is the essential factor in inflammation, and that it is due to a paralysis of the vasomotor nerves. **Place theory of hearing.** The theory that the basilar membrane consists of localized units each vibrating to a sound of a particular frequency. **Plasma relation theory.** The hypothesis that the ratio of nuclear and cytoplasmic volumes tends to be constant for a given cell type. **Point de repère theory.** The theory that hallucinations are determined by environmental stimuli. **Polyphyletic theory of blood-cell formation.** The theory of blood-cell formation that depends on the first recognition of precursor blast cells for all the different series of blood cells, each capable of producing only its own specific mature blood cell (e.g. erythroblast, myeloblast, lymphoblast, monoblast). Partial polyphyletism includes the dualistic (see above) and the trialistic (see below) theories. **Quantum theory.** The theory that energy is emitted or absorbed by atoms discontinuously in discrete quanta measured by the product hv, where h is Planck's constant and v the frequency of the radiation. It has been considerably modified by the more recent ideas of wave mechanics. **Recapitulation theory.** The theory that ontogenesis recapitulates phylogenesis. **Resonance theory.** A theory of hearing propounded by Helmholtz in which the cochlea contains fibres each having its own natural frequency, being set into resonant vibration by sound of that frequency. **Static theory.** A theory that postulates a positional function for the semicircular canals: varying head positions cause the endolymph to exert varying degrees of pressure upon the ampullae, thereby assisting in the control of equilibration (Goltz theory). **Telephone theory.** Rutherford's theory. **Template theory.** An instructive theory of antibody formation which proposes that the antigen enters the antibody-forming cell and there directly influences the characteristics of the antibody molecules produced. **Trialistic theory of haemopoiesis.** A theory of blood-cell formation that considers there are three classes of mother or blast cells giving rise to the lymphoid, myeloid, and erythroid types of blood cells. Schilling considers these are the myeloblast (also giving rise to the erythrocyte), lymphoblast, and monoblast. **Trichromatic theory.** *See* BLINDNESS, COLOUR, 1st def. **Tritubercular theory.** A theory which suggests that the modern mammalian tooth is derived from a tooth bearing three cusps. **Undulatory theory.** Wave theory (see below). **Unitarian theory.** Monophyletic theory of blood-cell formation (see above). **Unitarian theory of antibodies.** The theory that for a given antigen the different types of antigen-antibody reaction which may be observed are caused by a single antibody, the type of reaction (e.g. precipitation, agglutination, or lysis) depending on the physical state of the antigen. **Unitary theory.** 1. The hypothesis that disease is not made up of a number of separate morbid components, but is the manifestation of a single entity. 2. The postulation of one complement only in the serum of any particular animal. **Wave theory.** The theory that light and other electromagnetic radiations are propagated as waves. It has been considerably modified by the quantum theory (see above) and by the new theories of wave mechanics. **Zeistic theory.** The old theory that pellagra was caused by eating diseased maize. [Gk *theoria* speculation.]

See also: ABBÉ, ADAMI, ADLER, ALTMANN, ARRHENIUS, AVOGADRO, BOLK, BOWMAN, BROWN (J.), BUERGI, CANNON, COHNHEIM, DARWIN, DEUTSCHMANN, DE VRIES, EHRLICH, FRERICHS, FREUD, GIFFORD, GOLGI, GOLTZ, HAHNEMANN, HAMMARSTEN, HARTRIDGE, HELMHOLTZ, HERING (K. E. K.), HINSHELWOOD, KEPLER (J.), KNOOP, LADD-FRANKLIN, LAMARCK, LUDWIG (K. F. W.), MACDOUGAL, MCDOUGALL, MANZ, MENDEL (G. J.), METCHNIKOFF, MEYER (H. H.), MONAKOW, MORAWITZ, NERNST, OVERTON, PASTEUR, PEKELHARING, PETTENKOFER, RIBBERT, ROAF, ROEMER, RUTHERFORD, SCHIEFFERDECKER, SCHMIDT (A.), SCHMIDT (E. O.), SCHNABEL, SEMON (R. W.), SPITZER, STAHL (G. E.), STILLER, TRAUBE (L.), TSCHERNING, VILLEMIN (J. A.), VIRCHOW, WEISMANN, YOUNG (T.), ZUNTZ.

theotherapy (the·o·ther·ap·e). The healing of disease by prayer. [Gk *theos* god, *therapeia* treatment.]

therapeusis (ther·ap·ew·sis). Therapeutics.

therapeutic (ther·ap·ew·tik). Concerned with therapeutics; curative.

Therapeutic Substances Act, 1956. Part II of this Act imposes restrictions on the sale and supply, and on administration for treatment, of penicillin and such other therapeutic substances as may be prescribed from time to time, in regulations made jointly by the Health Minister of England and Wales, Scotland, and Northern Ireland, after consultation with the Medical Research Council. The additional substances to which these provisions may be applied are those which appear to be capable of causing danger to the health of the community if used without proper safeguards.

therapeutical (ther·ap·ew·tik·al). Therapeutic.

therapeutics (ther·ap·ew·tix). That branch of medicine which is concerned with the treatment of disease, palliative or curative; in common usage this refers mainly to the use of drugs, physiotherapy, etc. **Alimentary therapeutics.** Treatment by dietary means. **Cellular therapeutics.** Treatment of disease by the use of animal organs or their extracts; an expression more or less obsolete and not now applied to endocrinological methods. **Dental therapeutics.** Treatment of diseases of the teeth. **Dynamic therapeutics.** Treatment based on the use of individual drugs for a distributive purpose. **Empirical therapeutics.** Treatment which, though lacking a scientific basis, seems effective on the grounds of clinical experience. **Massive sterilizing therapeutics.** Therapia magna sterilisans. **Mediate therapeutics.** Treatment by giving drugs to a nursing mother so that the infant imbibes them in the milk; an inexact method of treatment for which there can be little use now, and one of historical interest only. **Mental therapeutics.** Treatment of which hypnotism is the best example, directed at influencing the patient's condition by way of the mind. **Rational therapeutics.** Treatment based on the scientific application of proved remedies to suitable cases. **Ray therapeutics.** Radiotherapy. **Specific therapeutics.** The use of specific drugs in disease (e.g. antimalarials; or arsenicals in syphilis). **Spinal therapeutics.** Treatment of diseased conditions of the vertebral column. **Stomatological therapeutics.** Treatment of diseases of the mouth. **Suggestive therapeutics.** The use of hypnotism in the treatment of disease. **Vibratory therapeutics.** The use of vibrations in massage and other forms of physiotherapy. [Gk *therapeutike* medical practice.]

therapeutist (ther·ap·ew·tist). One versed in any particular form of therapy.

therapia magna sterilisans (ther·ap·e·ah mag·nah ster·il·i·zanz). An expression devised by Ehrlich. It refers to a guiding principle he adopted of finding a chemical drug which would destroy all the parasites in the tissues if possible in a single dose. [Gk *therapeia* treatment, L *magnus* great, *sterilis* barren.]

therapic (ther·ap·ik). Therapeutic.

therapist (ther·ap·ist). Therapeutist.

therapy (ther·ap·e). Treatment. **Anti-gametocyte therapy.** The giving of a drug to destroy the plasmoidal gametocytes in the blood of a malarial subject, or to affect them in such a way that they will not develop fully in the mosquito. This is effected by very small doses of pamaquin and by certain other, but not all, antimalarial drugs. **Artificial-fever therapy.** Fever therapy (see below). **Autoserum therapy.** The injection of a patient's own serum in treatment. **Aversion therapy.** A form of treatment, particularly for chronic alcoholism, in which two stimuli are presented simultaneously, e.g. apomorphine and alcohol; one stimulus is unpleasant, the other is related to the symptom being treated. The stimuli are thereby associated, and subsequent presentation of the other stimulus leads to the experience of an unpleasant effect, and hence aversion to it. **Bacterial therapy.** Treatment with bacterial vaccines, viz. the bacteria (usually killed by heat or chemicals) of a disease, or their products. Opsonins, or substances in the blood which prepare microbes for phagocytosis, were supposed to be increased by this treatment. It is a variety of vaccine therapy (see below). **Beam therapy.** Radium-beam therapy (see below). **Behaviour therapy.** Behavioural treatment methods derived from experimental psychology and applying the principles of learning, especially those of classical and operant conditioning. **Blunderbuss therapy.** The polypharmacy of former days in which a number of drugs were given together. Warburg's tincture, or antiperiodic tincture is an example; it contains the alcohol-soluble constituents of 18 separate drugs. **Collapse therapy.** A form of therapy used in pulmonary tuberculosis, whereby the volume of the affected portion of the lung is reduced. This produces relaxation and aids in healing of the diseased tissue. Methods commonly used are pneumothorax, pneumoperitoneum, phreniclasia, extrapleural or extrafascial plombage with polythene spore or spheres, and thoracoplasty. **Contact therapy.** Low-voltage x-ray therapy in which the source of radiation is brought close to the part to be treated (short target-skin distance). **Converging-beam therapy.** A form of rotation therapy (see below) in which the axis of rotation is in the short axis of the body. The patient rotates in the horizontal position beneath an angled beam, or the angled beam describes a circular or spiral movement above the recumbent patient. **Convulsive shock therapy.** Treatment by the artificial production, by electrical or chemical means, of an epileptiform convulsion. **Deep x-ray therapy.** The range of x-ray therapy between superficial and supervoltage, usually taken to indicate the 0.2–1.0 MV range. **Deleading therapy.** Treatment employed to remove lead from the bones and so promote its excretion in patients who have suffered from manifestations of lead poisoning. Periods of low calcium intake together with acid-forming drugs alternate with periods of high calcium intake. **Diathermic therapy.** The therapeutic heating of deep tissues by diathermy. **Duplex therapy.** The therapeutic employment of the diathermic and galvanic currents in combination, both being applied to the body simultaneously through the same electrodes. **Electric-shock therapy.** Treatment by the production of an electrically-induced epileptiform convulsion. **Electrocoma therapy, Electroshock therapy.** Electric-shock therapy (see preceding). **Electron therapy.** Radiotherapy by means of electron beams. **Emanation therapy.** Treatment by gaseous disintegration products given off by radioactive substances. **Endocrine therapy.** Treatment by means of hormones. **Existential therapy.** A form of psychotherapy derived from existentialist philosophy. **Fever therapy.** Therapeutic fever; the treatment of disease by induced fever, in particular, the therapy of general paralysis of the insane by induced malaria or by direct heating of the body. **Fly-larvae therapy.** Maggot therapy (see below). **Glandular therapy.** Endocrine therapy (see above). **Grid therapy.** X-ray sieve therapy (see below). **Group therapy.** Group discussion methods of psychotherapy. **Heterovaccine therapy.** Vaccine therapy with some microbe which does not cause the specific disease. **High-voltage x-ray therapy.** Deep x-ray therapy (see above). **Hunger therapy.** Treatment by a reduced diet or fasting. **Hyperbaric oxygen therapy.** A method of treatment whereby the oxygen tension in the blood is raised, because of its administration in a circumambient pressure, greater than normal. **Hypoglycaemic therapy.** The therapy of disease by lowering the blood-sugar level, in particular the therapy of schizophrenia by the repeated production of comas from the injection of insulin. **Immunization therapy.** The use of vaccines or antisera to render a person immune against a specific infection. **Insulin-shock therapy.** Treatment by the induction of a series of comas by injection of insulin, with subsequent recovery from coma by the administration of glucose. **Intensive arsenical therapy.** The treatment of syphilis by continuous intravenous drip, or multiple short-period intravenous injections of arsphenamine. **Interstitial therapy.** Interstitial irradiation; treatment by the insertion of radioactive materials into the tissues, either naturally radioactive (e.g. radium needles, or radon seeds), or artificially radioactive (e.g. cobalt-60, tantalum-182, or gold-198). **Intracavitary therapy.** Intracavitary irradiation; treatment by the insertion of radioactive materials into body cavities, e.g. radium, radon, or other radioactive isotopes in solid or fluid form. **Intra-osseous therapy.** Transfusion or infusion of fluids into the medullary cavity of the sternum, tibia, or other bone. **Intravenous therapy.** Treatment by injection of a therapeutic substance into a vein. **Isotope therapy.** Therapy by the radiation from internally or externally applied radioactive isotopes which have been artificially produced, usually by neutron irradiation in an atomic pile. **Larval therapy.** Maggot therapy (see below). **Light therapy.** The application to the body for therapeutic purposes of radiations in the visible spectrum. **Maggot therapy.** A method, now seldom practised, of treating chronic osteomyelitis by introducing maggots to remove offensive slough and discharge. **Malarial therapy.** The therapy of general paralysis of the insane by induced malaria. **Mantle therapy.** Specially-shaped radiation field used in the treatment of lymph node areas above the diaphragm in lymphomatous disorders such as Hodgkin's disease. **Massive intravenous-drip therapy.** A method of treatment of early syphilis by a single massive dose of an antisyphilitic drug, chemotherapeutic or antibiotic, considerably diluted and given over a long period by intravenous drip. **Megavoltage therapy.** Supervoltage therapy (see below). **Microwave therapy.** A form of diathermy based on the absorption of electromagnetic waves by the body. **Moving-field therapy.** Rotation therapy (see below). **Non-specific therapy.** Paraspecific therapy (see below). **Nuclein therapy.** The injection of nuclein in order to increase leucocytosis in infectious diseases. **Occupational therapy.** The employment of patients on work or hobby, e.g. sketching, specially planned to stimulate and promote recovery. **Opsonic therapy.** Bacterial therapy (see above). **Oxygen therapy.** The use of oxygen in the treatment of anoxic conditions. **Paraspecific therapy.** Treatment by the injection of proteins, bacterial vaccines, or other substances that act by stimulating generally the body responses to infection. **Physical therapy.** The treatment of pathological conditions and the restoration of function by physical methods. **Protective therapy.** Treatment aimed at protecting an organ by reducing its activity as much as possible. **Protein therapy, Protein-shock therapy, Proteose therapy.** Non-specific therapy by the parenteral injection of proteins or their derivatives. **Psychic therapy.** The therapy of mental disorder by psychological methods. **Pyrexial therapy.** Fever therapy (see above). **Radium therapy.** The use of radium and its emanations in the treatment of disease. **Radium-beam therapy.** Telecurie therapy with radium as the source. **Reflex therapy.** Treatment that produces its effects by reflex action upon an organ, e.g. by counter-irritation. **Replacement therapy.** The use, in treatment, of natural body products or substances, or their synthetic analogues, to replace a deficiency. **Rotation therapy.** X-ray and telecurie therapy in which either the patient rotates in the beam of radiation or the beam rotates about the patient. **Salicyl therapy.** The treatment of rheumatism with compounds of salicylic acid. **Serum therapy.** The treatment of disease with the blood serum of immune animals or persons which contains antibodies. **Shock therapy.** Convulsive shock therapy (see above). **Short-wave therapy.** The therapeutic heating of the deep tissues by short-wave diathermy. **Simultaneous multifield therapy.** The use of multiple x-ray or telecurie-therapy beams at one and the same time in treatment. **Solar therapy.** The therapeutic use of the solar spectrum. **Spa therapy.** Treatment at a spa. The name of the specific spa is usually introduced. **Sparing therapy.** Protective therapy (see above). **Specific therapy.** Treatment by administration of a substance that has a direct selective action upon the specific cause of a disease, e.g. a specific antiserum or a specific drug, or that calls forth a specific antibody response, e.g. a specific vaccine, in contrast to paraspecific therapy and supporting or symptomatic treatment. **Substitution therapy.** Therapy by the provision of a substance, e.g. an endocrine extract, through the deficiency of which the disease is caused. **Suggestion therapy.** Treatment of disease by means of suggestion, with or without hypnosis. **Superficial x-ray therapy.** Low-voltage x-ray therapy below an arbitrary limit, usually taken at 200 kV. **Supervoltage therapy, Supervoltage x-ray therapy.** High-voltage x-ray therapy above an arbitrary limit, usually taken as 1 MV. **Telecurie therapy.** Treatment with a beam of radiation from a large source of some radioactive element (usually radium, but also 60 Co or 137 Cs) at some distance from the patient. **Teleradium therapy.** Radium-beam therapy (see above). **Vaccine therapy.** Treatment aimed at the production of active immunity against a disease by the injection of a vaccine, usually a suspension of the specific micro-organisms or their products; protective inoculation against a bacterial or virus disease. **X-ray therapy.** Treatment with x-rays. **X-ray sieve therapy.** Radiotherapy given through a perforated layer of protective material (usually lead rubber, lead sheet, or tungsten alloy) to produce an inhomogeneous field of irradiation. **Zomo therapy.** Treatment with meat juices and extracts. **Zone therapy.** The treatment by counter-irritation of a skin area situated in the same zone as a disordered organ. [Gk *therapeia* treatment.]

See also: CHAOUL, CURIE, GUELPA.

Theria (the·re·ah). A sub-class of the class Mammalia that contains Marsupialia and Eutheria. [Gk *ther* beast.]

theriaca (the·ri·ak·ah). Treacle. **Theriaca andromachi.** Venice treacle. [Gk *theriake* antidote.]

theriacal (the·ri·ak·al). Relating to theriaca: relating to antidotes.

Theridiidae (ther·ri·di·id·e). A family of spiders; it includes the poisonous black spider, *Latrodectus.* [Gk *theridion* small animal.]

theriodic (the·re·od·ik). Malignant. [Gk *therion* wild beast.]

therioma (the·re·o·mah). A malignant tumour or ulcer. [Gk *therion* wild beast, *-oma* tumour.]

theriomimicry (the·re·o·mim'·ik·re). The imitation of the behaviour of animals. [Gk *therion* wild beast, *mimesis* imitation.]

therm (therm). A unit of heat equal to 105.506 MJ, defined as being 100 000 Btu. [Gk *therme* heat.]

thermacogenesis (ther·mak·o·jen'·es·is). The action of a drug causing pyrexia. [Gk *therme* heat, L *con*, Gk *genein* to produce.]

thermae (ther·me). 1. Hot springs; warm baths. 2. Places where the therapeutic benefits of hot baths or mineral springs may be obtained. [Gk *thermai.*]

thermaerotherapy (therm·a·er·o·ther'·ap·e). The treatment of disease by the use of hot air. [Gk *therme* heat, *aer* air, *therapeia* treatment.]

thermaesthesia (therm·es·the·ze·ah). The capacity for feeling heat and cold, or the ability to recognize variations in temperature. [Gk *therme* heat, *aisthesis* sensation.]

thermaesthesiometer (therm·es·the·se·om'·et·er). An apparatus with which the sensitivity of the skin to heat may be determined. [Gk *therme* heat, *aisthesis* sensation, meter.]

thermal (ther·mal). Pertaining to warmth and heat; hot. [Gk *therme* heat.]

thermalgesia (therm·al·je·ze·ah). Thermo-algesia.

thermalgia (therm·al·je·ah). A feeling of intense and burning pain felt in nerve injuries. [Gk *therme* heat, *algos* pain.]

thermanaesthesia (therm·an·es·the'·ze·ah). Thermo-anaesthesia.

thermanalgesia (therm·an·al·je'·ze·ah). Thermo-analgesia.

thermatology (ther·mat·ol·o·je). The study of heat in its application to the treatment of disease. [Gk *therme* heat, *logos* science.]

thermhypaesthesia (therm·hi·pes·the'·ze·ah). Thermohypo-aesthesia.

thermic (ther·mik). Of the nature of heat. [Gk *therme* heat.]

thermion (therm·i·on). An ion or electron emitted by any hot body. [see foll.]

thermionics (therm·i·on·ix). The science which studies the electrons and ions emitted by hot bodies. [Gk *therme* heat, ion.]

thermistor (ther·mis·tor). A device whose electrical resistance decreases with an increase of temperature. It can be used to measure and control temperature. The thermistor has the advantage over an ordinary thermometer in that it can be extremely small and can be sterilized by heat. [*therm*ally sensitive res*istor.*]

thermo-aerophore (ther·mo·a·er·o·for). An apparatus for the local application of hot air. [Gk *therme* heat, *aer* air, *pherein* to bear.]

thermo-aesthesia (ther·mo·es·the'·ze·ah). Thermaesthesia.

thermo-aesthesiometer (ther·mo·es·the·ze·om'·et·er). Thermaesthesiometer.

thermo-algesia (ther·mo·al·je'·ze·ah). Extreme sensitivity to heat, or the sensation of pain produced by heat. [Gk *therme* heat, *algos* pain.]

thermo-anaesthesia (ther·mo·an·es·the'·ze·ah). Loss of sensibility to heat; the inability to recognize the difference between heat and cold or to feel variations in temperature. [Gk *therme* heat, anaesthesia.]

thermo-analgesia (ther·mo·an·al·je'·ze·ah). Thermo-anaesthesia. [Gk *therme* heat, analgesia.]

thermobiosis (ther·mo·bi·o'·sis). The capacity to maintain life at higher temperatures. [Gk *therme* heat, *bios* life.]

thermobiotic (ther·mo·bi·ot'·ik). Capable of maintaining existence at higher temperatures, as in the case of certain bacteria. [see prec.]

thermocauterectomy (ther·mo·kaw·ter·ek'·to·me). Excision by means of the thermocautery. [thermocautery, Gk *ektome* excision.]

thermocautery (ther·mo·kaw·ter·e). 1. Actual cautery; cauterization with a hot wire or heated metal instrument. 2. Paquelin's cautery; cauterization with a hollow platinum instrument heated by benzene vapour mixed with air. [Gk *therme* heat, cautery.]

thermochemistry (ther·mo·kem·is·tre). The study of heat changes during chemical reactions. [Gk *therme* heat, chemistry.]

thermochroic (ther·mo·kro·ik). Having the ability to absorb heat rays of a certain wavelength, transmitting or reflecting the remainder. [Gk *therme* heat, *chroa* colour.]

thermochroism, thermochrosis (ther·mo·kro·izm, ther·mo·kro·sis). The ability of some substances to absorb heat of certain wavelengths, reflecting or transmitting the remainder. [see prec.]

thermochrosy (ther·mo·kro·ze). The phenomenon of being thermochroic.

thermocoagulation (ther·mo·ko·ag·ew·la'·shun). The production of coagulation by the heating effect of a high-frequency current. [Gk *therme* heat, coagulation.]

thermocouple (ther·mo·kupl). An instrument for measuring temperatures, particularly very high or very low temperatures. It consists of two wires or rods of dissimilar metals forming a junction which is subjected to the temperature to be determined; the other junction is maintained at a fixed temperature, and the current set up in the circuit is a measure of the temperature difference. [Gk *therme* heat, couple.]

thermocurrent (ther·mo·kur·ent). A current generated by thermoelectric means. [Gk *therme* heat, current.]

thermode (ther·mode). An arrangement used for the transfer of heat to or from a localized region in order to increase or decrease its temperature. [Gk *therme* heat, *hodos* way.]

thermodiffusion (ther·mo·dif·ew'·zhun). The diffusion of a liquid or gas caused by the increased kinetic energy imparted to its molecules by a rise in temperature. [Gk *therme* heat, diffusion.]

thermodilution (ther·mo·di·lew'·shun). Thermal dilution. *See* DILUTION.

thermodin (ther·mo·din). Acetyl-*p*-ethoxyphenylurethane, C_2H_5O $C_6H_4N(COCH_3)COOC_2H_5$. A derivative of ethyl carbamate used as an antipyretic.

thermoduric (ther·mo·dewr·ik). Able to survive comparatively high temperatures. [Gk *therme* heat, L *durus* enduring.]

thermodynamics (ther·mo·di·nam'·ix). That branch of physics concerned with the laws relating to heat changes and the convertibility of heat into other forms of energy. [Gk *therme* heat, *dynamis* power.]

thermo-electric (ther·mo·el·ek'·trik). Concerned with thermoelectricity.

thermo-electricity (**ther**·mo·el·ek·**tris'**·it·e). Electricity produced by the effect of heat on a thermocouple. [Gk *therme* heat, electricity.]

thermo-excitory (**ther**·mo·ek·**si'**·tor·e). Having the ability to promote heat production in the body. [Gk *therme* heat, L *excitare* to arouse.]

thermogen (**ther**·mo·jen). 1. An appliance for raising the general temperature of a patient or the local temperature of a part. 2. An electrically-heated mattress for an operating table or bed.

thermogenesis (ther·mo·**jen**·es·is). Heat production; specifically the physiological process of heat production in the body. [Gk *therme* heat, *genein* to produce.]

thermogenetic (**ther**·mo·jen·**et'**·ik). Thermogenic.

thermogenic (ther·mo·**jen**·ik). 1. Heat producing. 2. Concerned with the production of heat. [see foll.]

thermogenics (ther·mo·**jen**·ix). 1. The study of heat production. 2. The treatment of disease by raising the temperature of the body. [Gk *therme* heat, *genein* to produce.]

thermogenous (ther·**moj**·en·us). Thermogenic.

thermogram (**ther**·mo·gram). The record produced by a thermograph. [Gk *therme* heat, *gramma* record.]

thermograph (**ther**·mo·graf). An apparatus in which an inked stylus connected with a thermometer furnishes a continuous record of temperature changes upon a rotating chart. [Gk *therme* heat, *graphein* to write.]

thermography (ther·**mog**·raf·e). The technique of measuring the amount of heat radiated from the surface of the body by means of a unit with detector cells which convert thermal energy into electronic signals, or by a heat-sensitive photographic plate. It is used in the diagnosis of tumours in the breast and for identifying any communication between veins and subcutaneous varicose veins. [Gk *therme* heat, *graphein* to record.]

thermohyperaesthesia (**ther**·mo·hi·per·es·**the'**·ze·ah). Extreme thermaesthesia. [Gk *therme* heat, *hyper*, *aisthesis* sensation.]

thermohyperalgesia (**ther**·mo·hi·per·al·**je'**·ze·ah). Extreme and painful sensitiveness to even moderate heat. [Gk *therme* heat, *hyper*, *algos* pain.]

thermohypo-aesthesia (**ther**·mo·hi·po·es·**the'**·ze·ah). Reduced sensitiveness to heat and cold, or to variations in temperature. [Gk *therme* heat, *hypo*, *aisthesis* sensation.]

thermo-inhibitory (**ther**·mo·in·**hib'**·it·or·e). Checking or preventing heat production in the body. [Gk *therme* heat, L *inhibere* to restrain.]

thermo-integrator (ther·mo·**in**·te·gra·tor). An instrument consisting of a heated cylinder furnished with recording thermocouples with which environmental warmth may be measured. [Gk *therme* heat, L *integrare* to make whole.]

thermolabile (ther·mo·**la**·bile). Easily decomposed, or otherwise altered, by heat. [Gk *therme* heat, L *labilis* slipping.]

thermolaryngoscope (**ther**·mo·lar·**ing'**·go·skope). A laryngoscope in which the mirror is electrically heated to prevent clouding. [Gk *therme* heat, laryngoscope.]

thermology (ther·**mol**·o·je). The study of heat and its phenomena. [Gk *therme* heat, *logos* science.]

thermoluminescence (**ther**·mo·lew·min·**es'**·ens). A property of certain materials which luminesce after exposure to radiation only after heating. [Gk *therme* heat, L *lumen* light.]

thermolysis (ther·**mol**·is·is). 1. In chemistry, dissociation brought about by heat. 2. The loss of heat from the body by evaporation, excretion, and radiation. [Gk *therme* heat, *lysis* a loosing.]

thermolytic (ther·mo·**lit**·ik). 1. Concerned with thermolysis. 2. Responsible for dissipating heat from the body. [see prec.]

thermomassage (**ther**·mo·mas·**ahzh'**). Massage accompanied by heat. [Gk *therme* heat, massage.]

thermometer (ther·**mom**·et·er). An instrument for the measurement of temperature. **Air thermometer.** A thermometer containing air as the thermometric substance, in which the scale of temperature is obtained by measurement of the variation with temperature of the pressure of a fixed mass of air at constant volume, or the variation of the volume at constant pressure. **Alcohol thermometer.** One in which the expansible indicator is alcohol; this is usually coloured. **Axilla thermometer.** A thermometer suitable for taking the temperature in the axilla; an ordinary clinical thermometer. **Celsius (Centigrade) thermometer.** A thermometer calibrated by the Celsius scale. **Clinical thermometer.** A bedside thermometer; one suitable for taking a patient's temperature. **Depth thermometer.** A thermometer adapted for the determination of the temperature of the internal organs of the body or of the muscles. Frequently, specially designed thermocouples are used. **Differential thermometer.** 1. A thermometer used to measure small temperature differences which may be set to any desired temperature range, e.g. Beckmann's thermometer. 2. One which measures the temperature difference between two points, e.g. paired thermocouples. **Fever thermometer.** Clinical thermometer (see above). **Half-minute thermometer.** A clinical thermometer that registers rapidly, reputedly in half a minute. **Kata thermometer.** *See* KATATHERMOMETER. **Maximum thermometer.** One that registers the maximum temperature reached since it was last set. **Mercurial thermometer.** One in which the expansible indicator is mercury. **Metallic thermometer.** One in which temperature is measured by the bending of a bimetallic strip. **Metastatic thermometer.** Differential thermometer, 1st def. (see above). **Minimum thermometer.** One that registers the minimum temperature reached since it was last set. **Pentane thermometer.** A thermometer filled with pentane; it is used in low-temperature work. **Resistance thermometer.** A thermometer calibrated according to a scale of temperature obtained by measurement of the variation of the electrical resistance of a metal, generally platinum. It may be used up to a temperature of 1100°C. **Self-registering thermometer.** One having some type of recording mechanism. **Spirit thermometer.** One containing coloured alcohol as thermometric substance. **Surface thermometer.** A thermometer adapted for the determination of the temperature of the surface of the body. Usually, specially designed thermocouples are used. **Wet and dry bulb thermometer.** An instrument for the determination of the relative humidity of the atmosphere. The temperature of a thermometer, the bulb of which is kept moist with water, is compared with that of a similar dry thermometer. Evaporation from the wet thermometer causes a depression of its reading, and the temperature difference between the two decreases with increasing humidity. [Gk *therme* heat, *metron* measure.]

See also: BECKMANN, CELSIUS, FAHRENHEIT, RÉAUMUR, THERMISTOR.

thermometric (ther·mo·**met**·rik). 1. Relating to thermometry or to a thermometer. 2. Anything determined by thermometry.

thermometry (ther·**mom**·et·re). The technique of measuring temperatures. [Gk *therme* heat, *metron* measure.]

thermoneurosis (**ther**·mo·newr·**o'**·sis). A hysterical symptom in which the temperature of the body is raised by vasomotor action. [Gk *therme* heat, neurosis.]

thermopalpation (**ther**·mo·pal·**pa'**·shun). Feeling the temperature of the body by applying the palm or back of the hand. [Gk *therme* heat, palpation.]

thermopenetration (**ther**·mo·pen·e·**tra'**·shun). The production of heat in the deeper tissues by the application of high-frequency (diathermy) current to the body. [Gk *therme* heat, penetration.]

thermophagy (ther·**mof**·aj·e). The habit of eating excessively hot food. [Gk *therme* heat, *phagein* to eat.]

thermophil, thermophilic (**ther**·mo·fil, ther·mo·**fil**·ik). Liking heat; describing those organisms which grow best at elevated temperatures (from 40° to 70°C). [Gk *therme* heat, *philein* to love.]

thermophobia (ther·mo·**fo**·be·ah). An unreasoning fear of heat; aversion to warmth. [Gk *therme* heat, *phobein* to fear.]

thermophore (**ther**·mo·for). An obsolete method of applying local heat, using a bag containing certain chemical substances which evolve heat when water is added. [Gk *therme* heat, *pherein* to bear.]

thermophylic (ther·mo·**fi**·lik). Heat resistant; applied to certain organisms that are unaffected by comparatively high temperatures. [Gk *therme* heat, *phylassein* to guard.]

thermopile (**ther**·mo·pile). An instrument for measuring radiant heat. It consists of a series of thermocouple junctions, usually rods of antimony and bismuth, alternate junctions being arranged closely on a flat surface and on a surface parallel to it, and the whole embedded in an insulating material. When one surface is exposed to radiant heat the difference in temperature between the two surfaces gives rise to a thermo-electric current which is measured by a galvanometer. [Gk *therme* heat, pile.]

thermoplegia (ther·mo·**ple**·je·ah). Heat stroke. *See* STROKE. [Gk *therme* heat, *plege* stroke.]

thermopolypnoea (**ther**·mo·pol·ip·**ne**'·ah). Increased rate of breathing caused by fever; panting brought on by exposure to heat. [Gk *therme* heat, *polys* many, *pnein* to breathe.]

thermopolypnoeic (**ther**·mo·pol·ip·**ne**'·ik). Characterized by rapid breathing due to fever or heat; exhibiting thermopolypnoea.

thermoprecipitation (**ther**·mo·pre·sip·it·**a**'·shun). Precipitation brought about by heating. [Gk *therme* heat, precipitation.]

thermoprecipitin (**ther**·mo·pre·**sip**'·it·in). A little-used term; it refers particularly to the extract used in the diagnosis of anthrax. [Gk *therme* heat, precipitin.]

thermoprecipitinogen (**ther**·mo·pre·sip·it·**in**'·o·jen). The extract prepared by Ascoli (1911) by heating anthrax-infected tissues with saline; it will react specifically with an anthrax antiserum. [Gk *therme* heat, precipitin, Gk *genein* to produce.]

thermoradiotherapy (**ther**·mo·ra·de·o·**ther**'·ap·e). Radiotherapy combined with heating of the tissues. [Gk *therme* heat, radiotherapy.]

thermoreceptor (**ther**·mo·re·**sep**'·tor). The nerve-endings that receive stimuli from hot or cold objects. [Gk *therme* heat, L *recipere* to receive.]

thermoregulation (**ther**·mo·reg·ew·**la**'·shun). The regulation of heat. [Gk *therme* heat, regulation.]

thermoregulator (ther·mo·**reg**·ew·la·tor). 1. Thermostat. 2. Anything which controls heat or heat production. [see prec.]

thermoresistant (**ther**·mo·re·**zis**'·tant). Able to resist heat: applied to bacteria, capable of surviving comparatively high temperatures. [Gk *therme* heat, resistance.]

thermoscope (**ther**·mo·skope). A differential thermometer; one which demonstrates a difference in temperature between bodies, though not actually measuring the amount. [Gk *therme* heat, *skopein* to view.]

thermostabile (ther·mo·**sta**·bile). 1. Stable at moderate temperatures. [Gk *therme* heat, L *stabilis* stable.]

thermostat (**ther**·mo·stat). Any device which automatically regulates heat, or maintains an apparatus at a given temperature. [Gk *therme* heat, *statos* standing.]

thermosteresis (**ther**·mo·ster·**e**'·sis). The removal or deprivation of heat or warmth. [Gk *therme* heat, *steresis* deprivation.]

thermostromuhr (ther·mo·**stro**·moor). An instrument (Rein's) for measuring the volume of blood flowing through a vessel. An exposed blood vessel is heated by two electrodes through which passes a high-frequency current. By means of a thermocouple the temperature of the blood is measured above and below the heated portion: from the difference the blood flow can be calculated. [Gk *therme* heat, G *Stromuhr* stream clock.]

thermosystaltic (**ther**·mo·sis·**tal**'·tik). Contracting when stimulated by heat, as in the case of a muscle; exhibiting thermosystaltism.

thermosystaltism (ther·mo·**sis**·tal·tizm). The phenomenon of contraction under the influence of heat, such as is displayed in muscles; contracture under thermal stimuli. [Gk *therme* heat, *systellein* to contract.]

thermotactic, thermotaxic (ther·mo·**tak**·tik, ther·mo·**tax**·ik). Concerned with thermotaxis.

thermotaxis (ther·mo·**tax**·is). 1. The mechanism of heat regulation in the body. 2. Thermotropism. [Gk *therme* heat, *taxis* arrangement.]

thermotherapy (ther·mo·**ther**·a·pe). The use of heat in the treatment of disease. [Gk *therme* heat, *therapeia* treatment.]

thermotics (ther·**mot**·ix). Thermology.

thermotolerant (ther·mo·**tol**·er·ant). Able to withstand elevated temperatures; describing thermophilic bacteria. [Gk *therme* heat, tolerance.]

thermotonometer (**ther**·mo·to·**nom**'·et·er). Any device for measuring the contracture of a muscle under heat stimuli. [Gk *therme* heat, *tonos* tension, *metron* measure.]

thermotoxin (ther·mo·**tox**·in). Any toxin produced in tissue which is exposed to excessive heat. [Gk *therme* heat, toxin.]

thermotracheotomy (**ther**·mo·trak·e·**ot**'·o·me). Tracheotomy in which actual cautery is employed. [Gk *therme* heat, tracheotomy.]

thermotropic (ther·mo·**trop**·ik). Describing living cells which are attracted towards heat. [see foll.]

thermotropism (ther·**mot**·ro·pizm). The movement of certain bacteria towards or away from heat. [Gk *therme* heat, *trepein* to turn.]

theroid (**the**·roid). Having the instincts or characteristics of a wild animal; bestial. [Gk *ther* beast, *eidos* form.]

theromorphia, theromorphism (ther·o·**mor**·fe·ah, ther·o·**mor**·fizm). The presence of malformation in a higher animal which closely resembles the normal counterpart in an animal of a lower order. [Gk *ther* beast, *morphe* shape.]

thesaurismosis (**the**·saw·riz·**mo**'·sis). A general term for a group of metabolic disorders in which there is an abnormal storage of some substance in the reticulo-endothelial cells, e.g. lipoidosis. [Gk *thesauros* treasure, *-osis* condition.]

thesaurosis (the·saw·**ro**·sis). The accumulation of any substance by the body, whether normal or foreign to it. [Gk *thesauros* treasure.]

theta (**the**·tah). The eighth letter of the Greek alphabet, θ. **Theta rhythm.** *See* RHYTHM.

Thevetia (thev·e·she·ah). A genus of apocynaceous plants; the dogbanes.

thevetin (**thev**·et·in). A cardiac glycoside resembling those of strophanthus and digitalis, and obtained from species of *Thevetia*. It hydrolyses to digitoxigenin, glucose, and thevetose.

thevetose (**thev**·et·oze). A sugar occurring in the glycosides of *Thevetia* species.

Thiabendazole (thi·ah·**ben**·daz·ole). BP Commission approved name for 2-(thiazol-4-yl)benzimidazole; an anthelmintic.

Thiacetazone (thi·**as**·et·az·one). BP Commission approved name for 4-acetamidobenzaldehyde thiosemicarbazone; a compound used with streptomycin in the treatment of tuberculosis to prevent the production of drug-resistant bacteria.

thiaemia (thi·e·me·ah). The presence of an abnormal amount of sulphur in the blood. [Gk *theion* sulphur, *haima* blood.]

Thialbarbitone (thi·al·**bar**·bit·one). BP Commission approved name for 5-allyl-5-(cyclohex-2-enyl)-2-thiobarbituric acid; an anaesthetic.

Thialbarbitone Sodium BPC 1959 (thi·al·**bar**·bit·one **so**·de·um). 5-Allyl-5-cyclohex-2′-enyl-2-thiobarbituric acid; an intravenous anaesthetic that is reported to cause less respiratory depression and is less likely to produce laryngeal spasm than most other barbiturates.

Thiambutosine BP 1973 (thi·am·**bew**·to·seen). *N-p*-butoxyphenyl-*N′-p*-dimethylaminophenylthiourea; used in the treatment of leprosy.

thiamin (**thi**·am·in). Thiamine.

thiamine (**thi**·am·een). An essential vitamin forming part of an enzyme system in the biochemistry of carbohydrate by catalysing the oxidation and decarboxylation of pyruvic acid. The richest natural sources are yeast, food grains and pulses; acute deficiency results in Wernicke's encephalopathy and cardiovascular beriberi, and chronic deficiency leads to sensorimotor polyneuritis. **Thiamine Hydrochloride BP 1973.** 3 - (4 - Amino - 2 - methyl - 5 - pyrimidinylmethyl) - 5 - (2 - hydroxyethyl) - 4 - methylthiazolium chloride hydrochloride, vitamin B_1; it is administered orally in tablets or by supplementation in food substances, or by injection. **Thiamine phosphate.** Co-carboxylase. **Thiamine pyrophosphate.** The pyrophosphate of thiamine which is required for the activity of a number of enzymes including pyruvate dehydrogenase, 2-oxoglutarate dehydrogenase, transketolase, glycogen phosphorylase and pyruvate decarboxylase and which was known as *co-carboxylase.*

Thiaminii Chloridum. *European Pharmacopoeia* name for Thiamine Hydrochloride BP 1973.

thiasine (**thi**·as·een). A sulphur-containing substance present in blood which interferes with the estimation of blood uric acid (Benedict). [Gk *theion* sulphur.]

Thiazesim (thi·**az**·e·sim). BP Commission approved name for 5 - (2 -dimethylaminoethyl) - 2,3 - dihydro - 2 - phenyl - 1,5 - benzothiazepin - 4 - one; an antidepressant.

thiazole (**thi**·az·ole). Any member of a large family of organic compounds based structurally upon a heterocyclic five-membered ring composed of three carbon atoms and one atom each of sulphur and nitrogen. [Gk *theion* sulphur, azote.]

Thibierge, Georges (b. 1856). French dermatologist.

Thibierge-Weissenbach syndrome. Calcinosis.

thickness (**thik**·nes). **Half-value thickness.** The thickness of a material required to reduce the intensity of an x-ray beam to half its original value. **Mean corpuscular average thickness.** The mean value for the average thickness of the red blood corpuscle (erythrocyte) (in μm) as measured by

$$\frac{\text{mean corpuscular volume}}{\pi(0.5\times\text{mean corpuscular diameter})^2\ \text{microns}}\ .$$

The average thickness for the normal corpuscle is 1.7-2.5 μm (mean 2.1 μm). **Tenth-value thickness.** That thickness of an absorber which reduces the intensity of radiation emerging from it to one-tenth of its initial value. [AS *thicce.*]

Thielmann, Karl Heinrich (b. 1802). St. Petersburg physician.

Thielmann's mixture. A diarrhoea mixture consisting of tincture of opium, tincture of valerian, ether, peppermint oil, fluid extract of ipecacuanha, and alcohol.

Thiers, Joseph (b. 1873). Paris physician.

Achard-Thiers syndrome. Diabetes and hypertrichosis in women; a form of adrenal cortical over-activity.

Thiersch, Karl (b. 1822). Leipzig surgeon.

Thiersch's grafts. Split-skin grafts, grafts of part of the thickness of the skin originally cut rather thin and by razor; the term is now commonly applied to the thicker split-skin graft, or Ollier-Thiersch graft.

Thiersch's method. Split-skin grafting.

Thiersch's operation. 1. Split-skin grafting. 2. Insertion of a subcutaneous silver encircling stitch around the anus, for rectal prolapse. 3. A method of repair of epispadias.

Ollier-Thiersch graft. Thick split-skin graft; free grafts of large sheets of skin, usually one-half to almost full thickness, and commonly employed to replace skin defects after burns.

Thies' sign. A paralytic sympathetic miosis associated with disease of the sigmoid flexure and rectum.

Thiethylperazine (thi·**eth**·il·**per**'·az·een). BP Commission approved name for 2-ethylthio-10-[3-(4-piperazin-1-yl)propyl]-phenothiazine; an antemetic.

thigh [femur] (thi). The part of the leg between the hip and the knee. Named surfaces are the anterior [facies anterior], the posterior [facies posterior], the lateral [facies lateralis], and the medial [facies medialis]. **Thigh bone.** The femur. [AS *theoh.*]

thigh, cutaneous nerves of the. Nerves supplying the skin of the thigh. **Intermediate cutaneous nerve of the thigh [ramus cutaneus anterioris (NA)].** A sensory branch of the femoral nerve to the skin on the front of the thigh. **Lateral cutaneous nerve of the thigh [nervus cutaneus femoris lateralis (NA)].** A sensory branch of the lumbar plexus (root value L2 and L3) which supplies the skin over the lateral side and adjacent part of the front of the thigh. **Medial cutaneous nerve of the thigh [ramus cutaneus cruris medialis (NA)].** A sensory branch of the femoral nerve to the skin on the medial side of the thigh. **Posterior cutaneous nerve of the thigh [nervus cutaneus femoris posterioris (NA)].** A sensory branch from the sacral plexus (root value S2 and S3) to the skin of the lower part of the buttock [nervi clunium inferiores (NA)], perineum [rami perineales (NA)], and the back of the thigh and leg.

thigmaesthesia (thig·mes·**the**·ze·ah). Sensitiveness to touch. [Gk *thigma* touch, *aisthesis* sensation.]

thigmocyte (**thig**·mo·site). Blood platelet. [Gk *thigma* touch, *kytos* cell.]

thigmotaxis (thig·mo·**tax**·is). The response of a motile cell to contact stimulation, whether of attraction or repulsion. [Gk *thigma* touch, *taxis* arrangement.]

thigmotropism (thig·mo·**trop**·izm). The cellular property of reaching to contact stimulation. [Gk *thigma* touch, *trepein* to turn.]

thimble (thimbl). **Obstetric thimble.** An obstetric device; a metal thimble with a sharp point at the end. It is used for rupturing the membranes. [AS *thymel.*]

thio-acetaldehyde (**thi**·o·as·et·**al**'·de·hide). $(CH_3CHS)_3$, a polymerized solid, analogous to acetic aldehyde.

thio acid (thi·o **as**·id). Any acid in which sulphur has replaced an oxygen atom. Inorganic acids one or other, or both, of the oxygen atoms of the carboxyl group may be replaced. They are distinguished accordingly, RCOSH (thiolic), RCSOH (thionic), and RCSSH (thion-thiolic or dithionic), where R is an organic group. [Gk *theion* sulphur, acid.]

thio alcohol (thi·o **al**·ko·hol). Any member of a family of organic compounds analogous to the alcohols in which the oxygen of the OH group is replaced by sulphur, e.g. ethyl mercaptan, C_2H_5SH. [Gk *theion* sulphur, alcohol.]

thio-arsenite (thi·o·**ar**·sen·ite). Any salt of thio-arsenious acid, H_3AsS_3. They are formed by the solution of arsenic trisulphide in a solution of an alkali sulphide.

Thiobacillus (**thi**·o·bas·**il**'·us). A genus of bacteria which can derive energy from the oxidation of sulphur to sulphuric acid. [Gk *theion* sulphur, bacillus.]

thiobacteria (thi·o·bak·**teer**'·e·ah). Members of the genus *Thiobacillus,* characterized by the presence of sulphur granules in their protoplasm. [Gk *theion* sulphur, bacteria.]

thiocarbamide (thi·o·kar·bam·ide). Thiourea.

thiocarbanilide (**thi**·o·kar·**ban**'·il·ide). Sulphocarbanilide, C_6H_5NH $CSNHC_6H_5$. A compound derived from aniline by reaction with carbon disulphide. It is used as an accelerator in the manufacture of rubber.

thiocarbonate (thi·o·**kar**·bon·ate). Any salt of thiocarbonic acid.

Thiocarlide (thi·o·**kar**·lide). BP Commission approved name for *N,N'*-di-(4-isopentyloxyphenyl)thiourea; it is used in the treatment of tuberculosis.

thiochrome (**thi**·o·krome). $C_{12}H_{14}ON_4S$, a yellow pigment found in yeast and produced by the oxidation of vitamin B_1. It fluoresces in ultraviolet light.

thiochromogen (thi·o·**kro**·mo·jen). Aureolin, primuline yellow; a dyestuff derived from *p*-toluidine; it is a sulphonated mixture of *p*-aminobenzo di- and tri- thiazoles. [Gk *theion* sulphur, *chroma* colour, *genein* to produce.]

thiocyanate (thi·o·si·an·ate). Any salt or ester of thiocyanic acid.

thiocyanogen (**thi**·o·si·**an**'·o·jen). The compound NCSSCN which is used in the assay of fats.

thiodiphenylamine (**thi**·o·di·fen·il·**am**'·een). Phenothiazine.

thiodotherapy (**thi**·o·do·**ther**'·ap·e). Treatment involving both sulphur and iodine. [Gk *theion* sulphur, iodine, therapy.]

thioesters (thi·o·es·terz). An important class of compounds in biochemistry formed between carboxylic acids and hydrosulphides, especially in coenzyme A. Important examples of coenzyme A thioesters include acetyl, succinyl and palmitoyl derivatives of coenzyme A. [Gk *theion* sulphur, ester.]

thio ether (thi·o e·ther). Alkyl sulphide; any organic sulphide analogous to an ether, in which sulphur has replaced the oxygen atom. [Gk *theion* sulphur, ether.]

thio-ethylamine (**thi**·o·eth·il·**am**'·een). $SHCH_2CH_2NH_9$, a decarboxylation product of cysteine.

thioflavine (thi·o·**fla**·veen). 1. One of the yellow thiazole dyestuffs. 2. $C_{17}H_{19}N_2SCl$, a methyl derivative of primuline used to dye tannined cotton and silk. [Gk *theion* sulphur, flavine.]

thiogenic (thi·o·**jen**·ik). Describing certain bacteria which have the power to convert H_2S into higher compounds of sulphur. [Gk *theion* sulphur, *genein* to produce.]

thioglucose (thi·o·**gloo**·kose). $CH_2OH(CHOH)_4CSH$, a synthetic sugar in which sulphur has replaced the oxygen of the aldehyde group. [Gk *theion* sulphur, glucose.]

Thioguanine (thi·o·**gwan**·een). BP Commission approved name for 2-aminopurine-6-thiol; an antineoplastic agent.

thiolin (**thi**·o·lin). A dark-green substance prepared from sulphur and linseed oil. It is employed in the treatment of skin diseases. **Thiolin sodium.** A compound prepared by treating thiolin with soda, and used in skin diseases. [Gk *theion* sulphur, linseed.]

Thiomersal BP 1973 (thi·**om**·er·sal). Sodium ethylmercurithiosalicylate, $C_2H_5HgSC_6H_4{=}COON$; a fungicide and a bactericide for non-sporing bacteria. It is used for sterilizing the skin and instruments before surgical operations and in fungicidal creams for application to the skin.

Thiomesterone (thi·o·**mes**·ter·one). BP Commission approved name for 1α,7α-bis(acetylthio)-17β-hydroxy-17α-methylandrost-4-en-3-one; an anabolic steroid.

thioneine (thi·on·e·een). Thiolhistidine betaine, $HSC_3H_2N_2CH_2CHCOON(CH_3)_3$. A cyclic base derived from histidine and observed in red blood corpuscles. It also occurs in ergot (ergothioneine).

thionic (thi·**on**·ik). Of or pertaining to sulphur. (Obsolete term.) [Gk *theion* sulphur.]

thionin, thionine (**thi**·on·in, **thi**·on·een). 3,6-Diaminophenthiazine, $NH_2C_6H_3{=}NS{=}C_6H_3NH_2$. A purplish stain used in microscopy because of its affinity for acidic constituents of cells and intercellular matrices, such as nucleoproteins and mucopolysaccharides. It is often used to stain the Nissl substance of nerve cells.

thionyl (**thi**·on·il). 1. Sulphinyl; the divalent group -OS-. 2. Denoting any compound incorporating the group OS, e.g. thionyl bromide, $SOBr_2$.

thiopectic (thi·o·**pek**·tik). Able to achieve the fixation of sulphur, as in the case of sulphur bacteria which convert H_2S and free sulphur into soil sulphates. [Gk *theion* sulphur, *pexis* fixation.]

thiopental sodium (thi·o·**pen**·tal **so**·de·um). Thiopentone sodium.

Thiopentalum Natricum (**thi**·o·pen·**ta'**·lum **nat**·rik·um). *European Pharmacopoeia* name for Thiopentone Sodium BP 1973.

thiopentobarbital (**thi**·o·pen·to·**bar'**·bit·al). Thiopentone sodium.

Thiopentone Sodium BP 1973 (thi·o·**pen**·tone **so**·de·um). Sodium ethyl-L-methylbutyl thiobarbiturate. A pale yellow powder dissolved and used as a general anaesthetic by intravenous injection, and as a basal narcotic by rectal injection.

thiopexic (thi·o·**pex**·ik). Thiopectic.

thiopexy (**thi**·o·pex·e). The conversion of sulphur, either free or in the form of H_2S, into tissue-building compounds or soil sulphates by bacteria such as *Beggiatoa alba*. [Gk *theion* sulphur, *pexis* fixation.]

thiophanium (thi·o·**fa**·ne·um). A group of organic derivatives one of which (trimetaphan) has been found recently to be a suitable agent for the production of hypotension during anaesthesia.

thiophene (**thi**·o·feen). C_4H_4S, a colourless oily liquid present in coal tar and commercial benzene. Several halogen derivatives have been used as antiseptics. **Thiophene di-iodide.** $C_4H_2I_2S$, a yellow crystalline powder, with antiseptic properties. **Thiophene sodium sulphonate.** $C_4H_3S{\cdot}NaSO_3$, a white crystalline powder, used in prurigo. **Thiophene tetrabromide.** C_4Br_4S, a yellow crystalline powder with antiseptic properties.

thiophil, thiophilic (**thi**·o·fil, thi·o·**fil**·ik). Having an affinity for sulphur; particularly applied to those bacteria which require sulphur or its compounds for existence. [Gk *theion* sulphur, *philein* to love.]

Thiopropazate (thi·o·**pro**·paz·ate). BP Commission approved name for 10 - {3 - [4 - (2 - acetoxyethyl)piperazin - 1 - yl]-propyl} - 2 - chlorophenothiazine. **Thiopropazine Hydrochloride BPC 1968.** The dihydrochloride of thiopropazate. Its action and uses resemble those of chlorpromazine but weight for weight it is more potent and it is less liable to produce toxic effects on bone marrow and liver.

Thioproperazine (**thi**·o·pro·**per'**·az·een). BP Commission approved name for 2 - dimethylsulphamoyl - 10 - [3 - (4 - methylpiperazin - 1 - yl) - propyl]phenothiazine.

Thioridazine (thi·or·**id**·az·een). BP Commission approved name for 10 - [2 - (1 - methyl - 2 - piperidyl)ethyl] - 2 - methylthiophenothiazine. **Thioridazine Hydrochloride BP 1973.** The hydrochloride of thioridazine, a tranquillizer used mainly for the treatment of schizophrenia and to control mania and agitation. Its action resembles that of chlorpromazine, but it has no anti-emetic or hypothermic effects.

thiosemicarbazone (**thi**·o·sem·e·**kar'**·baz·one). General name for a derivative of a ketone prepared by condensing it with thiosemicarbazide, and possessing the general formula $R'R''C{=}NNHCSNH_2$. Certain thiosemicarbazones are of use in the treatment of tuberculosis.

thiosinamine (thi·o·**sin**·am·een). Rhodallin, allylthiourea, $CH_2{=}CHCH_2NHCSNH_2$. A white compound, fairly soluble in water, and prepared from volatile oil of mustard. It has the property of absorbing scar tissue, and has been used to promote resolution of excessive fibrous tissue.

thiosulphate (thi·o·**sul**·fate). Any salt of thiosulphuric acid.

Thiotepa BP 1973 (thi·o·**te**·pah). Triaziridin-1-ylphosphine sulphide, a cytotoxic agent used in the treatment of neoplastic disease; it is administered intravenously.

Thiothixene (thi·o·**thix**·een). BP Commission approved name for *N,N*-dimethyl - 9 - [3 - (4 - methylpiperazine - 1 - yl)-propylidene]thioxanthen - 2 - sulphonamide; a psychotomimetic.

Thiothrix (**thi**·o·thrix). A genus of bacteria found in fresh and salt water and in mud. They are colourless, and are characterized by globules of sulphur in their cells. They grow by oxidizing H_2S chemosynthetically in the presence of O_2 and CO_2 to S and H_2SO_4, and play an important part in the sulphur cycle. [Gk *theion* sulphur, *thrix* hair.]

thiouracil (thi·o·**ewr**·as·il). 2-Mercapto-4-hydroxypyrimidine, a compound derived from thiourea, which inhibits the formation of thyroxine in the thyroid gland. It is effective in all types of hyperthyroidism, whether due to diffuse or nodular goitres, causing a slow remission of symptoms and gain in body weight; the symptoms, however, tend to return when treatment is discontinued. While it may be used in the preparation of the hyperthyroid patient for thyroidectomy, it may cause an enlarged vascular thyroid, and it is usual to replace the drug with iodine treatment for a fortnight before operating. Its toxic effects are chiefly due to the incidence of granulocytopenia and leucopenia during treatment, and skin rashes and urticaria are common. These effects are greatly reduced by the employment of the methyl, ethyl, or propyl derivatives which are also more active.

thiourea (**thi**·o·ewr·**e'**·ah). $(NH_2)_2C{=}S$, a colourless crystalline substance which has been used as an antithyroid drug in thyrotoxicosis. In this respect it has now been displaced by its derivatives, the thiouracils. [Gk *theion* sulphur, urea.]

thiourethane (thi·o·**ewr**·e·thane). 1. $C_2H_5SCONH_2$, the ethyl ester of thiocarbamic acid. 2. Any urethane in which sulphur has replaced an oxygen atom.

Thioxolone (thi·**ox**·o·lone). BP Commission approved name for 6-hydroxy-1,3-benzoxathiol-2-one; a keratolytic agent.

thiozine (**thi**·o·zeen). Thioneine.

thirst (therst). A strong desire for water or any other liquid. **Excessive thirst.** Polydipsia. **Morbid thirst.** Dipsosis. [AS *thurst.*]

Thiry, Ludwig (b. 1817). Austrian physiologist.

Thiry-Vella fistula. An isolated loop of bowel communicating with the intestinal canal on the one hand and with the exterior on the other.

thiuret (**thi**·ewr·et). $C_8H_7N_3S_2$, an antiseptic which liberates nascent sulphur.

thixolabile (thix·o·**la**·bile). Thixotropic. [Gk *thixis* touch, labile.]

thixotropic (thix·o·**trop**·ik). Displaying thixotropism.

thixotropism, thixotropy (thix·**ot**·rop·izm, thix·**ot**·rop·e). Change in viscosity of a colloid; a phenomenon displayed by gels which become liquid when shaken and revert to gel form again when allowed to stand. An increase in viscosity on standing is observed in the case of paint. When stirred or agitated, the viscosity is reduced again. [Gk *thixis* touch, *trepein* to turn.]

thlipsencephalus (thlip·sen·kef·al·us). A fetal monster in which the occipital bone and the upper cervical vertebrae are lacking, and the base of the brain protrudes. [Gk *thlipsis* pressure, *egkephalos* brain.]

Thoma, Richard (b. 1847). German histologist.

Thoma's ampulla. The terminal dilatation in the pulp of the splenic arterioles.

Thoma's fluid. A decalcifying agent consisting of 5 per cent nitric acid in alcohol.

Thoma's method. For the enumeration of leucocytes: blood, diluted 1 in 10, or 1 in 20, with a suitable fluid in a leucocyte-counting pipette, is well shaken and filled into a glass chamber of the Thoma-Zeiss counting cell (see below). The number of leucocytes lying upon 1 mm^2 ($\equiv$ 400 small squares) multiplied by 100 (or 200 according to dilution) is the number of leucocytes per mm^3 of undiluted blood. A modification of this method is now usually used.

Thoma-Zeiss counting cell. For counting blood corpuscles: this consists of a glass slide and a rigid cover-glass. The slide is ground in such a way that when the cover-glass is placed in position there is a 0.1 mm space between the cover-glass and the slide. The slide is etched with a series of lines at right angles to one another, so that the sides of the squares thus formed are exactly 0.05 mm long, the square area is $0.05 \times 0.05 = 2.5 \times 10^{-3}$ mm^2, and the cubic capacity $0.05 \times 0.05 \times 0.1 = 2.5 \times 10^{-4}$ mm^3. Diluted blood is run between the cover-glass and the slide and the number of red cells within a number of these squares is counted and recorded; the squares are arranged in groups of 16 to facilitate the calculations. The counting chamber can also be used for counting leucocytes.

Thomas, André (b. 1867). French neurologist.

André Thomas sign. 1. The rebound phenomenon, a manifestation of cerebellar hypotonia: if the patient raises his arm and then allows it to fall suddenly, a marked rebound will occur. 2. In a transverse lesion of the spinal cord, pinching the trapezius muscle gives goose flesh above the level of the lesion.

Thomas, Hugh Owen (b. 1834). Liverpool surgeon.

Thomas' caliper. A Thomas' splint modified for use on ambulatory patients.

Thomas' knee splint. A splint for immobilization of the knee, consisting of two lateral iron bars connected by a leather-covered ring which is passed over the leg to rest against the ischial tuberosity. The lateral irons project beyond the foot and are connected together.

Thomas' posterior or hip splint. A splint made of malleable iron, extending down the back of the trunk and leg from the nipple line to the foot for the purpose of immobilization of the hip.

Thomas' sign. With the patient supine, the sound leg is fully flexed at the hip: if the painful leg rises from the bed the sign is positive of hip-joint disease.

Thomas, Joseph (b. 1892). Paris physician.

Thomas-Binetti test. *See* TEST FOR CANCER.

Thomas, Theodore Gaillard (b. 1831). New York gynaecologist.

Thomas' pessary. A cradle-like pessary which holds back the uterus in anteflexion and in addition stretches the vaginal walls.

Thomayer, Josef (b. 1853). Prague surgeon.

Thomayer's sign. In chronic peritonitis with ascites, contraction of the mesentery draws the intestines over to the right side, and when the patient lies on his back the right side is resonant and the left side dull from the fluid.

Thompson, Gershom Joseph (b. 1901). Rochester, Minnesota, urologist.

Thompson's children's lithotrite. An instrument of F.10 Charrière scale which may be used for crushing stones in young children.

Thompson's operation. A method of lithotrity.

Thompson's cold punch. An instrument used in transurethral resection.

Gershom Thompson prostatic punch. A direct-vision cold punch in which a tubular knife removes portions of the prostate made to project through a fenestrum near the tip of the sheath of the endoscope. Bleeding points are controlled by electrocoagulation, and there is an irrigating system.

Thompson, Sir Henry (b. 1820). London surgeon.

Thompson's test. For urethritis: an early-morning specimen of urine is passed and collected in two coniform glasses. In anterior urethritis the urine contained in the first glass is turbid, while that in the second glass is clear. When the urethritis extends to the posterior urethra both specimens remain turbid (two-glass test).

Thompson, Theophilus (b. 1807). London physician.

Thompson's line. A red line on the margin of the gum in cases of pulmonary tuberculosis.

Thomsen, Asmus Julius Thomas (b. 1815). Danish physician.

Thomsen's disease. Myotonia congenita.

Thomson, Allen (b. 1809). Glasgow anatomist.

Thomson's fascia. The iliopectineal fascia. *See* FASCIA.

Thomson, Frederick Holland (b. 1867). London physician.

Thomson's sign. Transverse lines in the creases of the skin at the bend of the elbow which are observed in scarlet fever after the rash has faded elsewhere. They are of some diagnostic value in late cases. Also called *Pastia's lines.*

Thomson, Matthew Sydney (b. 1894). London dermatologist.

Thomson's disease, Rothmund-Thomson syndrome. Poikiloderma congenitale.

Thomson, Sir St. Clair (b. 1859). London laryngologist.

St. Clair Thomson's quinsy opener. Sharp-pointed bayonet-shaped forceps which open and drain a peritonsillar abscess in one procedure.

Thomson, William (b. 1833). American ophthalmologist.

Thomson's lantern. A special lantern designed to test colour vision. It has one aperture behind which can be rotated two superimposed discs each with seven apertures containing glasses of various colours and different-sized openings.

Thomson, William (Lord Kelvin) (b. 1824). Glasgow physicist.

Thomson (Kelvin) effect. 1. The liberation or absorption of heat when an electric current flows from a hotter to a colder portion of the same material. 2. The production of an electromotive force due to a difference of temperature between two portions of the same conductor.

Kelvin scale. A scale of absolute thermodynamic temperatures each degree of which is the same as a degree on the Celsius scale, with absolute zero (0K) − 273 °C.

Joule-Thomson effect. The change in temperature which occurs when a gas passes through a porous plug which separates two regions at different pressures.

Thomson-Walker, Sir John William (b. 1870). London urologist.

Thomson-Walker's operation. Suprapubic transvesical prostatectomy with the insertion of haemostatic sutures at the bladder neck.

Walker's modification of Maisonneuve's urethrotome. An internal urethrotome in which the triangular knife in its passage through the groove in the staff is firmly controlled within the groove, and the face of the stricture only is engaged and divided. The apex of the triangular knife is bevelled and non-cutting.

Thonzylamine (thon·zil·am·een). BP Commission approved name for *N*-4-methoxybenzyl-*N'N'*-dimethyl *N*-2-pyrimidylethylenediamine, a well tolerated antihistaminic similar to mepyramine maleate.

thoracalgia (thor·ak·al·je·ah). Pain in the thorax; pleurodynia. [thorax, Gk *algos* pain.]

thoracectomy (thor·as·**ek**·to·me). An operation involving the removal of part of a rib. [thorax, Gk *ektome* excision.]

thoracentesis (**thor**·ah·sen·**te**'·sis). Thoracocentesis.

thoracic (thor·as·ik). Referring to the chest; located in the thorax. **Thoracic aorta.** The particular part of the aorta that lies in the thorax. **Thoracic axis.** Acromiothoracic artery. **Thoracic index.** *See* INDEX.

thoracic arteries. Lateral thoracic artery [arteria thoracica lateralis (NA)]. A branch from the second part of the axillary artery, running along the lower margin of the pectoralis minor muscle to the side of the chest. In the female it gives off a large external mammary branch [rami mammarii laterales (NA)] to the breast. **Superior thoracic artery [arteria thoracica suprema (NA)].** A small branch from the first part of the axillary artery, ramifying on the chest wall above the pectoralis minor muscle.

thoracic nerves [nervi thoracici (NA)]. Segmental nerves, 12 in number, given off the thoracic part of the spinal cord. Each nerve emerges from the vertebral canal below the corresponding thoracic vertebra.

Anterior primary ramus [ramus ventralis (nervi intercostales) NA]. One of the two branches into which each thoracic nerve divides. They traverse the body wall below the corresponding rib and form 11 intercostal nerves and one subcostal nerve. Each anterior primary ramus terminates as an anterior cutaneous branch [ramus cutaneus anterior (pectoralis et abdominalis) NA], and gives off a lateral cutaneous branch [ramus cutaneus lateralis (pectoralis et abdominalis) NA] of which the second, crossing the axilla to reach the arm, is called the intercostobrachial nerve. The mammary gland and the skin over it are supplied by branches of the lateral cutaneous branch [rami mammarii laterales (NA)] and of the anterior cutaneous branch [rami mammarii mediales (NA)].

Posterior primary ramus [ramus dorsalis (NA)]. One of two branches into which each thoracic nerve divides as it emerges from the intervertebral foramen. They pass dorsally into the sacrospinalis muscle in which they divide into medial [ramus cutaneus medialis (NA)] and lateral [ramus cutaneus lateralis (NA)] branches. Both branches supply the muscle, but the overlying skin is supplied by medial branches in the upper thorax and lateral branches in the lower.

thoracic vein, lateral [vena thoracica lateralis (NA)]. The vein accompanying the artery of the same name and draining the lateral wall of the chest, mammary gland, and structures in the axilla, into the axillary vein.

thoracico-abdominal (thor·as·ik·o·ab·**dom**'·in·al). Concerning both the thorax and the abdomen.

thoracico-acromial (thor·**as**·ik·o·ak·**ro**'·me·al). Concerning the chest and the shoulder, the thorax and the acromion.

thoracico-acromialis (thor·**as**·ik·o·ak·ro·me·**a**'·lis). The acromiothoracic artery.

thoracicohumeral (thor·**as**·ik·o·**hew**'·mer·al). Relating to the thorax and the humerus.

thoracispinal (thor·**as**·e·**spi**'·nal). Relating to the thoracic portion of the vertebral column or of the spinal cord.

thoraco-abdominal (**thor**·ak·o·ab·**dom**'·in·al). Thoracico-abdominal.

thoraco-acephalus (**thor**·ak·o·a·**kef**'·al·us). Thoracopagus parasiticus in which there is an acephalic parasite.

thoracobronchotomy (**thor**·ak·o·brong·**kot**'·o·me). The operation of cutting into a bronchus through the wall of the thorax. [thorax, bronchus, Gk *temnein* to cut.]

thoracocautery (**thor**·ak·o·**kaw**'·ter·e). The cauterization of thoracic adhesions to complete the pulmonary collapse initiated by artificial pneumothorax.

thoracocentesis (**thor**·ak·o·sen·**te**'·sis). Puncture of the wall of the thorax with a view to removing fluid. [thorax, Gk *kentesis* puncture.]

thoracocoeloschisis (**thor**·ak·o·se·**los**'·kis·is). A congenital fissure involving both the chest and the abdomen. [Gk *thorax* chest, *koilia* hollow, *schisis* a splitting.]

thoracocyllosis (**thor**·ak·o·sil·**o**'·sis). Any deformity of the walls of the thorax. [thorax, Gk *kyllosis* a crippling.]

thoracocyrtosis (**thor**·ak·o·ser·**to**'·sis). A bulging of the chest wall, or exaggerated curvature of the thorax. [thorax, Gk *kyrtosis* curvature.]

thoracodelphus (**thor**·ak·o·**del**'·fus). A fetal monster possessing four legs, but only two arms and one head, the bodies being united above the umbilicus. [thorax, Gk *adelphos* brother.]

thoracodidymus (**thor**·ak·o·**did**'·im·us). A twin monster joined at the thorax. [thorax, Gk *didymos* twin.]

thoracodorsal artery [arteria thoracodorsalis (NA)] (**thor**·ak·o·**dor**'·sal **ar**·ter·e). One of the terminal branches of the subscapular artery. It continues in the line of the parent trunk to the inferior angle of the scapula and is accompanied in the distal part of its course by the nerve to the latissimus dorsi muscle.

thoracodynia (**thor**·ak·o·**din**'·e·ah). Pain in the thorax; pleurodynia. [thorax, Gk *odyne* pain.]

thoraco-epigastric veins [venae thoraco-epigastricae (NA)] (**thor**·ak·o·ep·e·**gas**'·trik **va**·nz). Veins connecting the lateral thoracic and femoral vein directly or indirectly through the superficial epigastric vein.

thoracogastrodidymus (**thor**·ak·o·gas·tro·**did**'·im·us). A twin monster joined at the chest and abdomen. [thorax, Gk *gaster* belly, *didymos* twin.]

thoracogastroschisis (**thor**·ak·o·gas·**tros**'·kis·is). Thoracocoeloschisis. [thorax, Gk *gaster* belly, *schisis* a splitting.]

thoracograph (thor·**ak**·o·graf). An instrument with which the contour of the thorax may be plotted, and its expansion and contraction during respiration recorded. [thorax, Gk *graphein* to write.]

thoracolaparotomy (**thor**·ak·o·lap·ar·**ot**'·o·me). A surgical approach to the peritoneal cavity by a wound through the chest wall and diaphragm, with or without an extension of the wound through the abdominal wall. [thorax, Gk *lapara* loin, *temnein* to cut.]

thoracolumbar (**thor**·ak·o·**lum**'·bar). Concerning the thoracic and lumbar regions or the corresponding portions of the vertebral column. Used particularly to denote the thoracic and upper lumbar ganglia and fibres of the sympathetic nervous system.

thoracolysis (thor·ak·**ol**·is·is). The operation of stripping pleural adhesions by excision of the ribs of the precordium. **Thoracolysis praecordia.** Cardiolysis. [thorax, Gk *lysis* a loosing.]

thoracomelus (thor·ak·**om**·el·us). A fetal monster with an arm or a leg attached to its chest. [thorax, Gk *melos* extremity.]

thoracometer (thor·ak·**om**·et·er). An instrument with which the expansion of the chest may be measured. [thorax, meter.]

thoracometry (thor·ak·**om**·et·re). The measurement of the expansion of the chest in respiration. [see prec.]

thoracomyodynia (**thor**·ak·o·mi·o·**din**'·e·ah). Pain experienced in the muscles of the thorax. [thorax, Gk *mys* muscle, *odyne* pain.]

thoracopagus (thor·ak·**op**·ag·us). A twin fetal monster united in the sternum. **Thoracopagus parasiticus.** Twins united in the thoracic region. **Thoracopagus tribrachius.** One in which two of the arms are fused. **Thoracopagus tripus.** One in which two of the legs are fused. [thorax, Gk *pagos* fixed.]

thoracoparacephalus (**thor**·ak·o·par·a·**kef**'·al·us). Thoracopagus twins one of which has a rudimentary head. [thorax, paracephalus.]

thoracoparasitus (**thor**·ak·o·par·as·**i**'·tus). Thoracopagus parasiticus.

thoracopathy (thor·ak·**op**·ath·e). Any morbid condition of the thorax or of the organs and tissues contained therein. [thorax, Gk *pathos* disease.]

thoracoplasty (thor·**ak**·o·plas·te). An operation devised to secure permanent collapse of the lung in cases of chronic pulmonary tuberculosis with adhesions and in some other pulmonary diseases. It consists of the partial or complete resection of a number of ribs; this causes the thoracic wall to fall in and obliterate the pleural cavity. According to the site selected, the operation may also be described as apical, anterior, lateral, posterior, anteroposterior, etc. **Costoversion thoracoplasty.** A modification of thoracoplasty in which several ribs are completely divided anteriorly, but posteriorly are left with a periosteal hinge during division. The ribs thus treated are twisted round and then fixed by pulling the lower one into a vertical position so as to form a firm, concave, bony cage which holds the underlying lung in a collapsed position. **Lateral thoracoplasty.** The removal of almost the whole length of varying numbers of ribs, without apicolysis, used principally to obliterate empyema spaces. [thorax, Gk *plassein* to mould.]

See also: HOLST, SAUERBRUCH.

thoracopneumograph (thor·ak·o·new'·mo·graf). An apparatus for demonstrating and recording the chest respiratory movements. [thorax, Gk *pneumon* lung, *graphein* to write.]

thoracopneumoplasty (thor·ak·o·new'·mo·plas·te). Thoracoplasty. [thorax, Gk *pneumon* lung, *plassein* to mould.]

thoracoschisis (thor·ak·**os**·kis·is). A congenital fissure of the thorax. [thorax, Gk *schisis* a splitting.]

thoracoscope (thor·**ak**·o·skope). 1. An instrument employed to view the interior of the pleural cavity. 2. A stethoscope. [thorax, Gk *skopein* to view.]

thoracoscopy (thor·ak·**os**·ko·pe). 1. General examination of the chest. 2. Examination of the interior of the pleural cavity by the thoracoscope. [see prec.]

thoracostenosis (thor·ak·o·sten·**o**'·sis). Extreme narrowing of the thorax. [thorax, Gk *stenosis* contraction.]

thoracostomy (thor·ak·**os**·to·me). 1. An opening made in the chest wall, e.g. for the draining of an empyema. 2. Excision of part of a rib or ribs over an enlarged heart. [thorax, Gk *stoma* opening.]

thoracotomy (thor·ak·**ot**·o·me). The operation of incising the wall of the thorax. [thorax, Gk *temnein* to cut.]

thoradelphus (thor·ad·**el**·fus). Thoracodelphus.

Thoraeus, Robert. Swedish physicist.

Thoraeus filter. A composite filter for hardening a beam of x-rays, often made of 0.44 mm tin, 0.25 mm copper, and 1.0 mm aluminium.

thorax [NA] (thor·ax). The part of the trunk between the neck and the abdomen; the chest. **Amazon thorax.** A chest with the absence of one or both breasts. There are usually other associated abnormalities. **Thorax asthenicus.** An elongated flat chest with increased obliquity of the ribs. **Barrel-shaped thorax.** The chest in emphysema, with increased anteroposterior diameter, elevated ribs, rounded back, increased costal angle, and prominent sternomanubrial junction. **Fusiform thorax.** A chest constricted in its lower portion by tight lacing. **Infrasternal angle of the thorax [angulus infrasternalis (NA)].** The angle formed on the front of the body between the right and left subcostal margins as they approach the sternum. **Inlet of the thorax [apertura thoracis superior (NA)].** The upper entrance into the thorax, bounded by the first thoracic vertebra behind, the upper border of the manubrium in front, and the first rib on either side. **Outlet of the thorax [apertura thoracis inferior (NA)].** The lower opening of the thorax, bounded by the last thoracic vertebra behind, the costal margins at the sides, and the xiphisternum in front. **Paradoxical thorax.** That seen in paralysis of one half of the diaphragm; the paralysed half rises during inspiration and falls with expiration, the reverse of the normal movements. **Thorax paralyticus.** Thorax asthenicus; flat chest. **Vapour thorax.** At ambient pressures below 6.25 kPa (47 mmHg), water vaporizes. Animals exposed to ambient pressures below 6.25 kPa (47 mmHg) develop water vapour bubbles in the pleural space. [Gk chest.]

See also: PEYROT.

Thorel, Christen (b. 1868). Nuremberg physician.

Thorel's bundle. A myocardial bundle connecting the sinuatrial and atrioventricular nodes, passing medial to the orifice of the inferior vena cava.

thoriagram (thor·e·ah·gram). A radiograph made after the introduction of a thorium compound as contrast medium. Thorium compounds are now seldom used for this purpose on account of their danger. The term is not a good one and is avoided by many radiologists. [thorium, radiogram.]

thorium (thor·e·um). A radioactive element of atomic weight 232.04, atomic number 90, and chemical symbol Th. It occurs as a silicate in thorite, as the oxide in thorianite, and in monazite sand. It was extensively used in the manufacture of gas mantles. The parent of a series of radioactive elements, it emits α, β, and γ rays while changing through the stages of mesothorium, radiothorium, and thorium X. **Thorium A, B, C, C′, C″, D.** Disintegration products of thorium in the series of radioactive elements produced from the latter. **Thorium dioxide.** ThO_2, a radioactive substance used in diagnostic radiography. It has been employed to outline the blood vessels and also the liver and spleen, but is rarely used now because of the potential danger of delayed irradiation effects. It is still of value for the outlining of cerebral abscesses where the thorium salt is largely expelled with the discharging pus and is not retained in the body. **Thorium sodium tartrate.** A compound occasionally used instead of barium sulphate, as a contrast medium in radiology of the colon. When an aqueous solution is injected as an enema, thorium is precipitated evenly on the colonic mucous membrane, showing fine detail of the mucosa. This technique has been superseded by the use of tannic acid added to the barium solution. **Thorium X.** A disintegration product of thorium identified as the radium isotope, Ra^{224}. [*Thor*, god of thunder.]

Thormaehlen, Johann (fl. 1910). German physician.

Thormaehlen's test. For melanin in urine: to 5 ml of urine add 3 or 4 drops of a dilute aqueous solution of sodium nitroprusside and 0.5 ml of 40 per cent sodium hydroxide solution and shake. Acidify with acetic acid (33 per cent). A deep-blue or green-blue colour indicates melanin.

Thorn, George Widmer (b. 1906). Baltimore physician.

Thorn's test. The administration of corticotrophin causes a rapid fall in the number of circulating eosinophil cells in normal people, but not in those suffering from adrenal deficiency.

Thorn, Wilhelm (b. 1857). Magdeburg gynaecologist.

Thorn's manoeuvre. A method of correcting a face presentation requiring two attendants, one attendant flexing the head with a vaginal hand pressing on the occiput and the other hand pressing on the chest wall of the fetus through the abdominal wall; the second attendant pulls the breech towards the child's chest.

thornapple leaves (thorn·apl le·vz). Stramonium. [AS *thorn*, *aeppel*, leaf.]

Thornwaldt (Tornwaldt), Gustav Ludwig (b. 1843). Danzig physician.

Thornwaldt's (Tornwaldt's) bursitis. Pharyngeal bursitis. *See* BURSITIS.

thoron (thor·on). Thorium emanation. *See* EMANATION.

thoroughwort (thor·o·wert). Indian sage. *See* SAGE. [AS *thurh*, *wyrt*.]

Thrassis (thras·is). A genus of fleas, some species of which are vectors of plague. [Gk *thrassein* to disturb.]

thread (thred). **Clap thread.** A slender filamentous structure, composed of epithelial cells, leucocytes, and mucus, occurring in the urine in chronic gonorrhoea. **Mycelial thread.** A hypha or filamentous thallus of a fungus. **Nuclear thread.** An elongated portion of the precipitated chromatin in a cell nucleus. [AS *thraed*.]

See also: GOLGI.

threadworm (thred·werm). *Enterobius vermicularis*; also applied to other slender nematode worms. [AS *thraed*, *wyrm*.]

thremmatology (threm·at·**ol**·o·je). The study of heredity and breeding, e.g. experimental cross-breeding of plants and animals. [Gk *thremma* nursling, *logos* science.]

threonine (thre·o·neen). 1-amino-2-hydroxy butanoic acid, $CH_3CH(OH)CH(NH_2)COOH$. An amino acid occurring in the hydrolysates of certain proteins, notably of blood fibrin. It is essential in diet for the maintenance of health.

threose (thre·oze). $CH_2OH(CHOH)_2CHO$, an aldotetrose isomeric with erythrose.

threpsology (threp·sol·o·je). The study of nutrition. [Gk *threpsis* nutrition, *logos* science.]

threptic (threp·tik). 1. Concerned with nutrition. 2. Describing the relationship between parents and their offspring. [Gk *threpsis* nutrition.]

Thresh, J. C. 19th-20th century public health expert.

Thresh disinfector. A steam-pressure sterilizer used for disinfecting clothes.

threshold (thresh·hold). 1. Literally, the sill of a doorway that prevents substances, e.g. grain, inside the room, from falling out until they have reached a certain depth (the height of the sill). 2. The point at which increasing stimuli are first detected, differentiated, or produce these specific effects. 3. The level of concentration of a substance (threshold substance) in a fluid reached before that substance is excreted, e.g. renal threshold (see below). **Absolute threshold.** The lowest value at which a given stimulus can be perceived. **Achromatic threshold.** The intensity at which the sensation of colour arises; below this intensity only a sensation of brightness exists. **Auditory threshold.** The least intensity at which a given sound can be perceived. **Threshold of consciousness.** The lowest limit of perception. **Convulsant threshold.** In convulsive shock therapy, the minimum amount (e.g. electric current or insulin) that will produce a convulsion. **Differential threshold.** The lowest limit of discrimination of two stimuli. **Double-point threshold.** The least distance apart at which two stimuli can be perceived as distinct. **Flicker-fusion threshold.** The maximum interval between flashes of light that allows them to appear as a continuous light. **Galvanic threshold.** The minimal galvanic current necessary to stimulate muscle through its nerve-ending. **Neuron threshold.** That strength of stimulus which, when applied to a neuron, is just sufficient to induce activity in the tissue it innervates. **Pain threshold.** The level in the sensorium where the minimal stimulus will produce pain. **Relational threshold.** The ratio of the strength of two stimuli when the difference between them is just perceptible. **Renal threshold.** The level of concentration of certain substances in the blood above which urinary excretion commences or becomes abnormally large. Of chief significance in this respect is glucose, the normal renal threshold for which is about 10 mmol/l (180 mg/100 ml). **Resolution threshold.** The minimum angular or spatial separation between two points which produces a visual sensation of two points. **Sensitivity threshold, Stimulus threshold.** Absolute threshold (see above). **Sugar threshold.** *See* RENAL THRESHOLD (above). **Threshold of visual sensation.** The least intensity of light that is visible. [AS *therscold.*]

thridacium (thri·da·she·um). Lactucarium; lettuce opium. [Gk *thridax* lettuce.]

thrill (thril). 1. A series of fine vibrations perceptible to the touch. They may also cause audible sound waves. 2. A palpable murmur; if sufficiently loud it will produce vibrations which can be felt through the skin. **Aneurysmal thrill.** A vibration which can be felt over an aneurysm, due to the movement of blood between the sac and the lumen. In the case of arterial aneurysms the thrill is in systole, but with arteriovenous aneurysms it is felt through systole and diastole. **Aortic thrill.** A vibration, usually in systole, felt in the 2nd intercostal space to the right of the sternum (aortic area). It is due to disease of the aortic valve (stenosis), or rarely to aortic aneurysm. Incompetence of the aortic valve produces a diastolic murmur that is seldom intense enough to produce a thrill. **Diastolic thrill.** A vibration in ventricular diastole, felt over the heart or great vessels in certain conditions. It may occur in mitral stenosis (felt at the apex of the heart), or with a patent ductus arteriosus (felt in the 2nd intercostal space to the left of the sternum), and, rarely, in pulmonary incompetence. **Fat thrill.** Slight vibrations transmitted through fatty tissue which may sometimes be felt on palpation of an obese abdomen. **Fluid thrill.** Vibrations transmitted across a collection of fluid in a cavity by sharply flicking the cavity wall with the finger. One of the signs of ascites. **Hydatid thrill.** A thrill sometimes felt over a large hydatid cyst of the liver or lung when, with three fingers placed flat over the overlying skin, the middle finger is percussed. It is caused by the shaking together of daughter cysts inside the hydatid cyst. **Presystolic thrill.** A thrill with crescendo in late diastole, felt at the apex of the heart in mitral stenosis with regular rhythm. When auricular fibrillation is present, the thrill becomes mid-diastolic. **Purring thrill.** A thrill which resembles that felt when the hand is placed over the body of a cat whilst it is purring. **Systolic thrill.** A thrill in systole, felt in the aortic area in aortic valvular stenosis, in the 2nd intercostal space to the left of the sternum in pulmonary stenosis, in the 3rd and 4th spaces to the left of the sternum in ventricular septal defect, and at the apex in mitral incompetence. [AS *thyrlian.*]

thrix annulata (thrix an·ew·la·tah). Trichonosus versicolor; ringed hair: hair that is banded in alternate patches of pigment and white. [Gk *thrix* hair, L ringed.]

throat (throte). 1. The front part of the neck. 2. The pharynx and the fauces. 3. Hence, a constricted passage. **Smokers' throat.** A chronic hyperaemia and oedematous condition of the pharyngeal and glossal mucous membrane, associated with excessive tobacco smoking. **Sore throat.** *See* SORE THROAT. **Trench throat.** Infection of the mucous membrane of the buccal cavity and tonsils by Vincent's organisms. [AS *throte.*]

Throckmorton, Tom Bentley (b. 1885). Philadelphia neurologist.

Throckmorton's reflex. An extensor-plantar response in pyramidal-tract disease, elicited by percussion on the dorsum of the foot in the metatarsophalangeal region; a variant of the Babinski reflex.

thrombase (throm·baze). Thrombin.

thrombasthenia (throm·bas·the·ne·ah). Thrombo-asthenia.

thrombectomy (throm·bek·to·me). The operation of removing a thrombus. [thrombus, Gk *ektome* excision.]

thrombin (throm·bin). An albumin-like protein having very powerful clotting activity when added to whole blood or to solutions of fibrinogen. It is formed during the clotting of blood from prothrombin under the influence of thromboplastin, calcium, and probably other factors in the blood. It is not present in the unclotted circulating blood. **Dried Human Thrombin BP 1973.** The enzyme obtained from human plasma by precipitation with suitable salts and organic solvents under controlled conditions of pH, ionic concentration, and temperature. It converts human fibrinogen into fibrin. **Topical thrombin.** A thrombin preparation applied locally as a haemostatic. [thrombus.]

thrombinogen (throm·bin·o·jen). Prothrombin. [thrombus, Gk *genein* to produce.]

thrombo-angiitis (throm·bo·an·je·i'·tis). Inflammation of the coats of blood vessels with associated thrombosis and destruction of the intima. **Thrombo-angiitis obliterans.** A disease characterized by inflammation of the coats of arteries and veins, associated with thrombosis, destruction of the intima, and occlusion of the lumen. The wall of the blood vessel shows leucocytic infiltration and formation of giant cells; periarteritis or phlebitis occurs, causing adhesions between the vessel and surrounding tissues. Recanalization of the affected vessel may take place. The disease affects mainly the distal vessels of the lower limbs, but may also occur in the upper extremities and involve larger vessels or, rarely, visceral vessels. Its distribution is segmental, i.e. normal segments alternate with diseased ones. The condition is encountered in adult males under the age of 45, and is known also as *Buerger's disease.* [thrombus, Gk *aggeion* vessel, *-itis* inflammation.]

thrombo-arteritis (throm·bo·ar·ter·i'·tis). Thrombosis in association with arteritis. **Thrombo-arteritis obliterans.** Virtually the same as thrombo-angiitis obliterans. **Thrombo-arteritis purulenta.** The breaking down of an arterial thrombus with the formation of pus and inflammation of the walls of the artery. [thrombus, arteritis.]

thrombo-asthenia (**throm**·bo·as·**the**′·ne·ah). 1. A form of hereditary haemorrhagic diathesis occurring in either sex having normal bleeding and clotting times, poor clot retraction, normal platelet count, and characterized by multiple haemorrhagic manifestations. 2. A functional deficiency of platelets. **Hereditary thrombo-asthenia, Hereditary haemorrhagic thrombo-asthenia.** Hereditary haemorrhagic diathesis. *See* DIATHESIS. [thrombus, asthenia.]

thromboblast (**throm**·bo·blast). A giant cell from which the blood platelets are derived. [thrombocyte, Gk *blastos* germ.]

thrombocinase (throm·bo·**sin**·aze). Thromboplastin.

thromboclasis (throm·bo·**kla**·sis). Thrombolysis. [thrombus, Gk *klasis* a breaking.]

thromboclastic (throm·bo·**klas**·tik). Thrombolytic. [see prec.]

thrombocyst, thrombocystis (**throm**·bo·sist, throm·bo·**sist**·is). The membrane found enveloping a thrombus. [thrombus, Gk *kystis* bladder.]

thrombocyte (**throm**·bo·site). Blood platelet. *See* PLATELET. [thrombus, Gk *kytos* cell.]

thrombocythaemia (**throm**·bo·si·**the**′·me·ah). Thrombocytosis. [thrombocyte, Gk *haima* blood.]

thrombocytocrit (throm·bo·**si**·to·krit). An apparatus for counting blood platelets. [thrombocyte, Gk *krinein* to separate.]

thrombocytolysis (**throm**·bo·si·**tol**′·is·is). The breaking-up of the blood platelets. [thrombocyte, Gk *lysis* a loosing.]

thrombocytopen (throm·bo·**si**·to·pen). A thrombocytopenic substance said to be present in the spleens of patients suffering from thrombocytopenic purpura and capable of causing a decrease in the numbers of platelets (thrombocytopenia) in the circulating blood when injected into the rabbit. A similar thrombocytopenic substance can be extracted from other organs and normal urine. [see foll.]

thrombocytopenia (**throm**·bo·si·to·**pe**′·ne·ah). Reduction in the number of platelets present in the blood. It is associated with haemorrhage into the skin and from the mucosa, and plays an important part in some types of purpura. **Essential thrombocytopenia.** Thrombocytopenic purpura. *See* PURPURA. **Malignant thrombocytopenia.** A form of aplastic anaemia in which the platelets are affected; leucopenia is nearly always present. [thrombocyte, Gk *penia* poverty.]

See also: FRANK (A. E.).

thrombocytopoiesis (**throm**·bo·si·to·poi·**e**′·sis). The formation of blood platelets. [thrombocyte, Gk *poiesis* a making.]

thrombocytopoietic (**throm**·bo·si·to·poi·**et**′·ik). Involved in the production of blood platelets. [see prec.]

thrombocytosin (**throm**·bo·si·**to**′·sin). A lipid substance said to be liberated from body fats by various factors and having the property of increasing the numbers and adhesiveness of platelets. [thrombocyte.]

thrombocytosis (**throm**·bo·si·**to**′·sis). An increase above the normal in the number of blood platelets present in the blood. [thrombocyte, Gk *-osis* condition.]

thrombocytozyme (throm·bo·**si**·to·zime). Platelet factor; a so-called *enzyme* produced when the blood platelets lyse in contact with a foreign surface, such as when bleeding occurs. [thrombocyte, enzyme.]

thrombo-embolism (throm·bo·**em**·bol·izm). Thrombosis producing embolism in the blood vessel.

thrombo-embolization (**throm**·bo·em·bol·i·**za**′·shun). Embolism of a blood vessel by means of a detached thrombus.

thrombo-endarterectomy (**throm**·bo·end·ar·ter·**ek**′·to·me). The surgical removal of a thrombus together with the inner layer of the media and the diseased intima of an artery. [thrombus, Gk *endon* within, artery, Gk *ektome* a cutting out.]

thrombo-endarteritis (**throm**·bo·end·ar·ter·**i**′·tis). Thrombo-arteritis. [thrombus, Gk *endo* within, arteritis.]

thrombo-endocarditis (**throm**·bo·en·do·kar·**di**′·tis). Inflammation of the endocardium, involving the formation of thrombi on the valves; thrombi will form on any acutely damaged valve, as in acute rheumatic carditis, or bacterial endocarditis.

thrombogen (**throm**·bo·jen). Ac globulin, labile factor, factor V; a constituent normal blood plasma that is essential for the formation of thrombin from prothrombin. It is unstable, being oxidized during storage, but is not affected by vitamin-K deficiency or anticoagulant therapy with dicoumarol and similar substances. It is regarded as a plasma conversion factor in the formation of thrombin. [thrombin, Gk *genein* to produce.]

thrombogenesis (throm·bo·**jen**·is·is). Clot formation; the production of a thrombus. [thrombus, Gk *genein* to produce.]

thrombogenic (throm·bo·**jen**·ik). 1. Pertaining to a thrombus or to thrombogen. 2. Causing thrombosis or clotting. [see prec.]

thromboid (**throm**·boid). Having the characteristics of a thrombus; clot-like. [thrombus, Gk *eidos* form.]

thrombokinesis (**throm**·bo·kin·**e**′·sis). The process of blood clotting. [thrombosis, Gk *kinein* to set in motion.]

thrombolymphangitis (**throm**·bo·lim·fan·**ji**′·tis). Lymphangitis associated with a lymph clot. [thrombus, lymphangitis.]

thrombolysis (throm·**bol**·is·is). The dissolution of a thrombus. [thrombus, Gk *lysis* a loosing.]

thrombolytic (throm·bo·**lit**·ik). 1. Concerned with thrombolysis. 2. Having the effect of breaking-up a thrombus. [see prec.]

thrombon (**throm**·bon). That part of the haemopoietic system concerned with the platelets and their precursors (megakaryocytes) and the mechanism of their production. [thrombus.]

thrombopathy (throm·**bop**·ath·e). A lack of clotting power in the blood, due to some cause other than thrombopenia. **Constitutional thrombopathy.** von Willebrand's thrombopathy; a rare form of hereditary haemorrhagic diathesis or pseudohaemophilia. **Granulopenic thrombopathy.** A disease resembling von Willebrand's constitutional thrombopathy, but showing structural abnormalities such as poorly granular cytoplasm in the platelets. [thrombus, Gk *pathos* disease.]

See also: FONIO, WILLEBRAND.

thrombopenia (throm·bo·**pe**·ne·ah). Thrombocytopenia.

thrombophilia (throm·bo·**fil**·e·ah). A tendency of the blood towards clotting. **Essential thrombophilia.** A condition of recurring thrombosis of the blood vessels, due to an unusual coagulability of unknown aetiology but apparently not related to infection, inflammatory conditions, or stasis. [thrombus, Gk *philein* to love.]

thrombophlebitis (**throm**·bo·fleb·**i**′·tis). Phlebitis following the formation of an intravascular clot, caused by an alteration of the blood. **Thrombophlebitis migrans.** Successive attacks of thrombophlebitis in various sites. **Portal vein thrombophlebitis.** A severe complication of appendicitis causing purulent inflammation in the portal vein; it is usually fatal. [thrombus, *phleps* vein, *-itis* inflammation.]

thromboplastic (throm·bo·**plas**·tik). Concerned with the coagulation of the blood. [thrombus, Gk *plassein* to mould.]

thromboplastid (throm·bo·**plas**·tid). A blood platelet. [see prec.]

thromboplastin (throm·bo·**plas**·tin). A substance which, in the presence of cations and with possible help from a lipid activator, converts prothrombin to thrombin, which then combines with fibrinogen to form a clot. It is probably not present in circulating blood, but is set free from disintegrating platelets when blood is shed. [thrombin, Gk *plassein* to mould.]

thromboplastinogen (**throm**·bo·plas·**tin**′·o·jen). A substance occurring in blood plasma and said to be the inactive precursor of thromboplastin which is produced under the influence of thromboplastinogenase. This substance may be the antihaemophilic globulin. [thromboplastin, Gk *genein* to produce.]

thromboplastinogenase (**throm**·bo·plas·tin·**oj**′·en·aze). An enzyme-like substance said by some to be liberated from platelets when blood is shed and capable of converting thromboplastinogen into thromboplastin at the beginning of the blood-clotting process.

thromboplastinopenia (**throm**·bo·plas·tin·o·**pe**′·ne·ah). Reduction in the amount of thromboplastin in the blood. [thromboplastin, Gk *penia* poverty.]

thrombopoiesis (**throm**·bo·poi·**e**′·sis). 1. The formation of thrombocytes. 2. The production of a thrombus. [thrombus, Gk *poiesis* a making.]

thrombopoietic (**throm**·bo·poi·**et'**·ik). 1. Concerned with the production of thrombocytes. 2. Clot-forming. [see prec.]

thrombose (**throm**·boze). 1. To clot. 2. To bring about the formation of a clot. [Gk *thrombos* lump.]

thrombosin (throm·**bo**·sin). Thrombin.

thrombosinusitis (**throm**·bo·si·nus·**i'**·tis). Thrombosis occurring in sinuses of the dura mater. [thrombosis, sinusitis.]

thrombosis (throm·**bo**·sis). Intravascular coagulation during life, producing a thrombus. Coagulation within a vessel after death, or outside a vessel during life, produces a *coagulum* or *clot.* The causes are not fully understood, but important factors include infection, stasis of the blood stream, and disorganization of the normal mechanisms in the blood which prevent clotting. **Agonal thrombosis.** Coagulation of blood within the vascular system just before or at the moment of death. It occurs in the right side of the heart and in the pulmonary artery; the thrombi are tough and stringy and do not adhere to the endothelium. **Atrophic thrombosis.** Thrombosis associated with wasting, dehydration, reduced blood flow, increased blood viscosity, or infection. The term is also applied to thrombosis occurring usually in the superior sagittal sinus in infants suffering from severe infections. **Ball-valve thrombosis.** Thrombosis in the left atrium in subjects with mitral stenosis, producing a pedunculated spherical thrombus which is motile within the atrium and blocks the orifice of the mitral valve for short periods like the action of a ball-valve. Attacks of syncope result, and showers of systemic emboli may be thrown off from the thrombus. **Calcarine thrombosis.** Thrombosis of the posterior cerebral artery with ischaemia of the calcarine cortex and consequent crossed homonymous hemianopia. **Cardiac thrombosis.** Intracardiac thrombosis (see below). **Cavernous-sinus thrombosis.** Thrombosis of the cavernous sinus, usually associated with infection spreading from the orbit or arising from the area of the face drained into the sinus. **Cerebellar thrombosis.** Thrombosis of a cerebellar artery, the clinical features depending on the artery involved. **Cerebral thrombosis.** Thrombosis of a cerebral artery, with ischaemia and loss of function of the area of brain supplied: the commonest type of cerebrovascular accident. **Compression thrombosis.** Thrombosis in a vessel, usually a vein, resulting from occlusion from without producing stasis of blood within. Some other factor, such as infection, or disease of the vein wall, is generally required for the thrombosis. **Coronary thrombosis.** Thrombosis occurring within a coronary artery, causing myocardial ischaemia, and usually, but not invariably, cardiac pain (angina pectoris) and myocardial infarction. The common cause is atherosclerotic disease of the coronary arteries, but occasionally syphilis, trauma, dissecting aneurysm of the aorta, or, very rarely, coronary artery embolism, may be aetiological factors. **Creeping thrombosis.** Slowly progressive thrombosis. **Dilatation thrombosis.** Thrombosis within a vein which is chronically dilated and incompetent, and in which there is stasis of blood flow, as in varicose veins. **Embolic thrombosis.** Thrombosis occurring at the site of impaction of an embolus in a vessel. **Foam thrombosis.** Thrombosis partly resulting from the admixture of air and blood; some additional factor, e.g. disease of the vessel wall, is required to induce thrombosis. **Infective thrombosis.** Thrombosis due to infection of the vessel wall, or to impaction of an infected embolus. **Intracardiac thrombosis.** Cardiac thrombosis; thrombosis at the heart valves or within the chambers of the heart; the latter is commonly seen in the left atrium in patients with mitral stenosis and atrial fibrillation, but it may also occur in the ventricle (especially the left after a large cardiac infarct). More rarely it is secondary to atrial fibrillation from any cause, protracted congestive heart failure, or in association with intracardiac tumours and endocardial fibrosis. It commonly occurs on the damaged valve cusps during bacterial endocarditis; infected thrombi may become detached and cause systemic arterial embolism. **Intraventricular thrombosis.** That resulting from large myocardial infarcts, especially transmural. **Jumping thrombosis.** Migrating thrombosis (see below). **Marantic thrombosis, Marasmic thrombosis.** Atrophic thrombosis (see above). **Migrating thrombosis.** Thrombosis which wanders from vein to vein; also known as *thrombophlebitis migrans,* which is due to disease of isolated portions of superficial and deep veins, and is common in thrombo-angiitis obliterans. **Placental thrombosis.** Thrombi in the placenta and veins of the uterus. **Plate thrombosis, Platelet thrombosis.** Thrombosis produced by an abnormal accumulation or agglutination of blood platelets, as in thrombocytosis after splenectomy. **Thrombosis of the portal vein.** Thrombosis in the extrahepatic course of the vein, due either to acquired disease or to congenital malformation. In the former case the cause is often unknown. The condition produces the clinical syndrome of portal hypertension. **Postoperative thrombosis.** Thrombosis involving chiefly the deep venous plexuses of the calf and the femoral vein which may occur following any operation but is most common after abdominal, particularly pelvic, operations, and fractures of or operations on the femur. **Puerperal thrombosis, Puerperal venous thrombosis.** Thrombosis of the veins of the legs or pelvis after childbirth. **Sinus thrombosis.** Thrombosis of an intracranial venous sinus (superior sagittal, transverse, or cavernous). **Traumatic thrombosis.** Thrombosis of a vessel, usually a vein, as a result of trauma or irritation. The latter may result from intravenous procedures, e.g. infusion of physiological fluids, especially glucose which is irritant to the vein wall. **Venous thrombosis.** Thrombosis of a vein. [Gk *thrombos* lump, *-osis* condition.]

See also: RIBBERT.

thrombostasis (throm·bo·**sta**·sis). Stoppage of the flow of blood, with associated thrombosis. [thrombus, Gk *stasis* a standing still.]

thrombotic (throm·**bot**·ik). Characterized or caused by thrombosis.

thrombus (**throm**·bus). A blood clot formed in and remaining in a blood vessel or the heart. **Agglutinative thrombus.** Hyaline thrombus (see below). **Agonal thrombus, Agony thrombus.** A clot in the heart cavities immediately before or at the time of death. **Annular thrombus.** A clot shaped like a ring. **Ante-mortem thrombus.** A white or red thrombus formed in the heart or vessel cavities during life. **Autochthonous thrombus.** Blood-plate thrombus (see below). **Ball thrombus.** A loose, rounded thrombus in a heart cavity. **Bile thrombus.** A plug of bile-stained detritus within a small bile duct. **Blood-plate thrombus.** An agglutinated mass of blood platelets forming a thrombus in a vein. **Calcified thrombus.** A phlebolith. **Coral thrombus.** An ante-mortem thrombus (see above) in which the platelet deposits are very prominent, giving a microscopic coralline effect. **Coronary thrombus.** An ante-mortem thrombus (see above) in a coronary artery. **Currant-jelly thrombus.** A soft, red, jelly-like post-mortem clot. **Ferment thrombus.** A clot formed by the action of fibrin ferment. **Fibrinous thrombus.** A clot composed chiefly of fibrin. **Fibrolaminar thrombus.** Ante-mortem thrombus (see above). **Globulin thrombus, Haematoblastic thrombus.** A deposit of globulin inside a blood vessel. **Haemostatic thrombus.** A thrombus that has formed at a site of stagnation in a vessel. **Hyaline thrombus.** Hyaline degeneration in a thrombus. **Infective thrombus.** Septic thrombus (see below). **Laminated thrombus.** A thrombus in which the constituents are arranged in layers. **Lateral thrombus.** A thrombus attached to the side of a vessel. **Marantic thrombus, Marasmic thrombus.** A thrombus formed during the course of a wasting disease. **Mechanical thrombus.** A thrombus resulting from mechanical obstruction to a blood vessel. **Mixed thrombus.** Laminated thrombus (see above). **Mural thrombus.** An ante-mortem thrombus (see above) attached to the endocardium as distinct from a valve. **Obstructing thrombus, Obstructive thrombus.** One that obstructs completely the vessel lumen. **Organized thrombus.** A thrombus that has been replaced by reparative scar tissue. **Pale thrombus.** White thrombus (see below). **Parasitic thrombus.** A blocking mass of malarial parasites and pigment in the brain capillaries. **Parietal thrombus.** Lateral thrombus (see above). **Phagocytic**

thrombus. A thrombus composed of mononuclear leucocytes. **Pigmentary thrombus.** A mass of free pigment in the brain capillaries. **Plate thrombus.** A thrombus composed of blood platelets. **Post-mortem thrombus.** A clot formed in the heart cavities or vessels after death. **Primary thrombus.** A thrombus located at its site of origin. **Progressive thrombus, Propagated thrombus.** A thrombus which has spread for some distance from its site of origin. **Red thrombus.** A thrombus composed largely of red blood corpuscles. **Septic thrombus.** A thrombus that is infected with bacteria and causes a severe inflammatory reaction in the vessel and the surrounding tissues. **Stratified thrombus.** Laminated thrombus (see above). **Traumatic thrombus.** One that results from an injury. **Valvular thrombus.** A thrombus attached to the wall of a vessel or a heart cavity so as to form a valve. **White thrombus.** A thrombus composed mainly of platelets and leucocytes. [Gk *thrombos* lump.]

throwback (thro·bak). An individual organism which has characteristics not normally present in other contemporary members of the same stock or species, but which are known, or assumed, to have been present in more or less remote ancestors. The term has no genetic connotation, and such forms are usually mutants or homozygotes for rare recessives. [AS *threow, baec.*]

thrush (thrush). Aphthous stomatitis; a disease common in emaciated children and in debilitated adults. It is due to infection with species of fungi of the genus *Candida*, and is characterized by the formation of pearly-white spots in the mouth with accompanying gastro-intestinal symptoms and fever. [etym. dub.]

thrypsis (thrip·sis). A comminuted fracture. [Gk a breaking in pieces.]

Thuja (thew·jah). 1. A genus of coniferous trees (family Pinaceae). 2. The fresh tops of the white cedar, *Thuja occidentalis* Linn.; arbor vitae. **Thuja articula.** A species which yields sandarac. **Thuja occidentalis.** White cedar; a species of North America. **Thuja oil.** Cedar-leaf oil; an oil obtained from *T. occidentalis.* The name is sometimes also applied to the empyreumatic oil from *Callitris quadrivalvis.* [Gk *thyia* fragrant cedar.]

thujin (thew·jin). A flavone glycoside found in *Thuja occidentalis.*

thujol (thew·jol). A volatile oil obtained from *Thuja occidentalis.* It has antipyretic properties.

thujone (thew·jone). $C_{10}H_{16}O$, a bridged terpene ketone obtained from the oils of thuja, tansy, wormwood, and sage. A colourless oil with a menthol odour which occurs in two optically-active forms.

thulium (thew·le·um). A rare-earth element of atomic weight 168.93, atomic number 69, and chemical symbol Tm. It occurs in samarskite and monazite sand. [*Thule*, old name for Shetland.]

thumb [pollex (digitus I) NA] (thum). The first digit on the radial side of the hand. It has only two phalanges. **Bifid thumb.** One characterized by bifurcation of the distal phalanx. **Broad thumbs.** Thumbs are broad in Leri's pleonostosis, Mohr's syndrome, Rubinstein-Taybi syndrome and Taybi's otopalatal-digital syndrome. **Thumb centre.** A cerebral centre responsible for thumb movements. **Tennis thumb.** Tendinitis with calcification in the flexor pollicis longus muscle, caused by friction and strain. **Trigger thumb.** The temporary fixation of the thumb in flexion, due to a narrowing of the fibrous flexor tendon sheath and a secondary thickening of the tendon, which on active or passive extension is overcome with a sudden jerk. [AS *thuma.*]

thumb-print (thum·print). An imprint made by the thumb. [thumb, ME *prent.*]

Thurfyl Nicotinate (ther·fil nik·o·tin·ate). BP Commission approved name for tetrahydrofurfuryl nicotinic acid ester. An ester of nicotinic acid said to be of some benefit in rheumatic conditions when applied locally, usually as a cream (5 per cent).

thus (thus). Gum thus, American thus, common frankincense (not to be confused with genuine frankincense): the concrete oleoresin obtained as an exudation from the trees of various species of *Pinus.* [L.]

thuya (thoo·yah). Thuja.

thuyone (thoo·yone). Thujone.

thylakentrin (thi·lak·en·trin). The follicle-stimulating hormone of the anterior pituitary gland. [Gk *thylax* bag, *kentron* goad.]

thymacetin (thi·mas·et·in). $C_6H_2(CH_3)(C_3H_7)(OC_2H_5)NH(C_2H_3O)$, a thymol analogue of phenacetin used as an antalgesic.

thyme (time). The dried leaves and flowering tops of *Thymus vulgaris* Linn. (family Labiatae). **Thyme camphor.** Thymol. **Oil of thyme.** Origanum oil, a colourless, yellow or red, volatile oil obtained from *T. vulgaris* Linn. and containing cymene, pinene, thymol, and carvacrol. **Wild thyme.** *T. serpyllum*, a species which yields oil of thyme. [Gk *thymon.*]

thymectomy (thi·mek·to·me). The surgical excision of the thymus. [thymus, Gk *ektome* excision.]

thymene (thi·meen). $C_{10}H_{16}$, a terpene occurring in oil of thyme.

thymergasia (thi·mer·ga·ze·ah). General term in the Meyer system for the group of affective-reaction types of psychoses, e.g. manic-depressive. [Gk *thymos* mind, *ergein* to work.]

thymergastic (thi·mer·gas·tik). Relating to thymergasia, or characterized by the affective-reaction type of psychosis (Meyer).

thymiasis (thi·mi·as·is). Thymiosis.

thymic (thi·mik). 1. Concerned with the thymus gland. 2. Derived from thyme.

thymic veins [venae thymicae (NA)]. Tributaries of the left innominate and/or inferior thyroid veins.

thymicolymphatic (thi·mik·o·lim·fat'·ik). Concerned with the relationship between the thymus and the lymph glands, as in status lymphaticus.

thymidine (thi·mid·een). $CH_3C_4H_2N_2O_2C_5H_9O_3$, a nucleoside formed by condensation of thymine with deoxyribose. There is some evidence that the conversion of thymine to thymidine biologically is catalysed by vitamin B_{12} and it has been suggested that failure to synthesize thymidine in this way constitutes the primary biochemical deficiency in pernicious anaemia. **Tritiated thymidine.** Thymidine labelled with the isotope tritium and used as a marker for the synthetic phase of cell mitoses.

thymine (thi·meen). Methyl uracil, 2,6-dioxy-5-methyl pyrimidine, $C_5H_6O_2N_2$. A base occurring in the nucleoside, thymidine, derived from the hydrolysis of nucleoproteins. [Gk *thymos* thymus.]

thymion (thi·me·on). A cutaneous wart. [Gk.]

thymiosis (thi·mi·o·sis). 1. Yaws. 2. Warts. [Gk *thymion* wart, *-osis* condition.]

thymitis (thi·mi·tis). Inflammation of the thymus. [thymus, Gk *-itis* inflammation.]

thymocrescin (thi·mo·kres·in). Describing a growth-promoting substance in thymus extracts; its actual existence is in doubt. [thymus, L *crescere* to grow.]

thymocyte (thi·mo·site). A thymus-gland cell. [thymus, Gk *kytos* cell.]

thymokesis (thi·mo·ke·sis). Persistence of the thymus into adult life, sometimes with enlargement.

thymokinetic (thi·mo·kin·et'·ik). Stimulating the thymus. [thymus, Gk *kinesis* movement.]

thymol (thi·mol). 1 - Methyl - 4 - isopropyl - 3 - hydroxy-benzene, $(CH_3)_2CHC_6H_3(CH_3)OH$. A colourless crystalline substance, which is obtained from oil of thyme (*Thymus vulgaris* Linn.), and from the oils of *Monarda punctata* Linn. and *Trachyspermum ammi* Linn. Sprague; it may also be prepared synthetically. It has a strong and characteristic aromatic taste and odour, with antiseptic properties, being more powerful than phenol in this respect, but may irritate raw surfaces (BP 1973). It is a constituent of various mildly antiseptic mouth-washes and gargles such as Compound Glycerin of Thymol BPC 1959 and Compound Solution-tablets of Thymol BPC 1959. It was formerly used extensively in the treatment of hookworm infestation, but has now been largely replaced by less toxic substances. It is liable to cause abdominal pain and vomiting, and sometimes stimulation followed by depression of the central nervous system. **Thymol iodide.** A brownish powder with a slight aromatic odour, almost insoluble in water, alcohol, and glycerin, and with practically no antiseptic activity. It is sometimes used as a dusting-powder for its protective and absorbent properties. It is a mixture of iodine derivatives of thymol.

thymolipoma (thi·mo·lip·o'·mah). A benign tumour in the anterior mediastinum, especially in children 10–15 years of age. [thymus, Gk *lipos* fat, *-oma* tumour.]

thymolphthalein (thi·mol·**thal**·e·in). A derivative of phthalic anhydride used as an indicator (pH 9.3–10.5).

thymolsulphonephthalein (thi·mol·sul·fone·**thal**'·e·in). Thymol blue. *See* BLUE.

thymolysin (thi·**mol**·is·in). An antibody that has a destructive effect on the cells of the thymus. [see foll.]

thymolysis (thi·**mol**·is·is). The breaking down of the tissue of the thymus. [thymus, Gk *lysis* a loosing.]

thymolytic (thi·mo·**lit**·ik). Destructive to the tissue of the thymus. [see prec.]

thymoma (thi·**mo**·mah). A tumour formed from thymic tissue. [thymus, Gk *-oma* tumour.]

thymometastasis (thi·mo·met·**as**'·tas·is). A metastasis from the thymus.

thymonoic (thi·mon·o·ik). Describing a type of affective mental disorder with marked systematization of thought. [Gk *thymos* mind, *nous* thought.]

thymopathy (thi·**mop**·ath·e). 1. Disease of the thymus. 2. Any mental disorder or neurosis. [thymus, Gk *thymos* mind, *pathos* disease.]

thymopexy (thi·mo·pex·e). Suture of an enlarged thymus to the edges of an incision. [thymus, Gk *pexis* a fixation.]

thymoprivic, thymoprivous (thi·mo·**pri**·vik, thi·mo·**pri**·vus). Conditioned by premature atrophy or excision of the thymus. [thymus, L *privus* deprived of.]

thymopsyche (thi·mo·**si**·ke). Affective mental processes. [Gk *thymos* mind, *psyche* soul.]

thymotoxic (thi·mo·**tox**·ik). Damaging to the tissue of the thymus. [thymus, Gk *toxikon* poison.]

thymotoxin (thi·mo·**tox**·in). Thymolysin. [see prec.]

Thymoxamine (thi·**mox**·am·een). BP Commission approved name for 4 - (2 - dimethylaminoethoxy) - 5 - isopropyl - 2 - methylphenyl acetate; a peripheral vasodilator.

thymus [NA] (**thi**·mus). A soft, pinkish, lobulated gland; large at birth, it increases in relative size up to late childhood and then gradually involutes. It consists of a right and left lobe [lobus (dexter et sinister) NA], in contact along their median borders, and stretching from just below the larynx to the 4th costal cartilages. It is composed of small lobules [lobuli thymi (NA)] separated by septa derived from the capsule. Each lobule has a framework of epithelial cells and is divided into a densely packed cortex containing large numbers of lymphocytes and a looser medulla which contains the concentric corpuscles and in which the epithelial cells are prominent. The latter are probably the source of a lymphopoietic factor. The thymus plays an important role in the development and maintenance of the lymphatic system. **Persistent thymus, Thymus persistens hyperplastica.** One that persists beyond the normal age; it may simply fail to atrophy, or it may actually hypertrophy. [Gk *thymos* a warty excrescence which looks like a bunch of thyme flowers.]

Thymus (**thi**·mus). A genus of plants of the family Labiatae. **Thymus serpyllum.** Wild thyme; it yields an oil similar to that of *T. vulgaris.* **Thymus vulgaris.** Sweet thyme; a herb used as a condiment, and the source of oil of thyme and thymol. [Gk *thymos.*]

thymusectomy (thi·mus·**ek**·to·me). Thymectomy.

thynnin (**thin**·in). A protamine occurring in the sperm of the tunny fish, *Thymnus thynnus.* [Gk *thynnos* tunny.]

thyratron (**thi**·rat·ron). A gas- or vapour-filled triode valve used for a variety of control operations, e.g. starting and stopping heavy currents. It can be used as a relay, or rectifier of alternating currents; its action is different from that of the high-vacuum triode valve. [Gk *thyreos* oblong shield, electron.]

thyro-active (thi·ro·**ak**·tiv). Stimulating the thyroid gland and increasing its internal secretion. [thyroid, active.]

thyro-adenitis (**thi**·ro·ad·en·**i**'·tis). Inflammation of the thyroid gland. [thyroid, Gk *aden* gland, *-itis* inflammation.]

thyro-arytenoid (**thi**·ro·ar·**it**'·en·oid). Pertaining to the thyroid and arytenoid cartilages.

thyro-arytenoid muscle [musculus thyro-arytenoideus (NA)]. A muscle running from the lower half of the angle of the thyroid cartilage to the anterolateral surface of the arytenoid cartilage, passing lateral to the vocal fold and the sinus and saccule of the larynx. The lower and deeper fibres, which are attached to the vocal process of the arytenoid cartilage, constitute the vocalis muscle. Many of these fibres are inserted directly into the vocal ligament instead of reaching the thyroid cartilage. The whole muscle shortens and relaxes the vocal folds and helps to approximate them by rotating the arytenoids medially. The vocalis portion makes tense the anterior parts of the folds, thus raising the pitch of the voice.

thyrocalcitonin (**thi**·ro·kal·sit·**o**'·nin). A peptide hormone produced by the C-cells present mainly in the thyroid in lower mammals and additionally perhaps in the parathyroid and thymus in man and in the ultimobranchial body in birds and reptiles. The hormone lowers plasma calcium and phosphate by actions on bone and kidney.

thyrocardiac (thi·ro·**kar**·de·ak). 1. Concerned with the heart and the thyroid gland. 2. A person with cardiac affection due to hyperthyroidism. [thyroid, Gk *kardia* heart.]

thyrocarditis (**thi**·ro·kar·**di**'·tis). Any cardiac disorder attributable to hyperthyroidism. [thyroid, Gk *kardia* heart, *-itis* inflammation.]

thyrocele (**thi**·ro·seel). Tumour or enlargement of the thyroid gland; goitre. [thyroid, Gk *kele* tumour.]

thyrochondrotomy (**thi**·ro·kon·**drot**'·o·me). The operation of dividing the thyroid cartilage. [thyroid, Gk *chondros* cartilage, *temnein* to cut.]

thyrocolloid (thi·ro·**kol**·oid). The colloid substance of the thyroid gland.

thyrocricotomy (**thi**·ro·kri·**kot**'·o·me). Tracheotomy by division of the cricovocal membrane. [thyroid, cricoid, Gk *temnein* to cut.]

thyro-epiglottic (**thi**·ro·ep·e·**glot**'·ik). Concerning both the thyroid cartilage and the epiglottis.

thyro-epiglottic muscle [musculus thyro-epiglotticus (NA)]. Fibres derived from the upper part of the thyro-arytenoid muscle, extending in the aryepiglottic fold as far as the margin of the epiglottis. It widens the inlet of the larynx.

thyrofissure (thi·ro·**fish**·ewr). The establishment of an opening through the thyroid cartilage. [thyroid, fissure.]

thyrogenic, thyrogenous (thi·ro·**jen**·ik, thi·**roj**·en·us). Derived from the thyroid gland or having the latter as origin. [thyroid, Gk *genein* to produce.]

thyroglobulin (thi·ro·**glob**·ew·lin). An iodized protein synthesized and stored in the thyroid gland, in which it constitutes the principal constituent of the colloid of the vesicles. It represents the storage form of the thyroid hormones, and upon hydrolysis yields the biologically active amino acids, thyroxine and triiodothyronine [thyroid, globulin.]

thyroglossal (thi·ro·**glos**·al). Connecting the thyroid gland and the tongue. [thyroid, Gk *glossa* tongue.]

thyrohyal (thi·ro·**hi**·al). The greater horn of the hyoid. [thyroid, hyoid.]

thyrohyoid (thi·ro·**hi**·oid). Concerned with the thyroid cartilage and the hyoid bone.

thyrohyoid muscle [musculus thyrohyoideus (NA)]. One of the infrahyoid muscles, attached to the greater horn of the hyoid bone and to the oblique line on the lamina of the thyroid cartilage.

thyroid (**thi**·roid). 1. Thyroid BP 1973; the thyroid glands of oxen, sheep, or pigs, after removal of connective tissue, drying, powdering, and defatting by means of light petroleum. The product is diluted with lactose to contain 0.09–0.11 per cent of iodine. 2. The thyroid gland. *See* GLAND. **Aberrant thyroid.** A thyroid gland in an abnormal position, or a mass of thyroid tissue detached from the main gland and situated in some other part of the body. **Accessory thyroid.** Accessory thyroid gland. *See* GLAND. **Thyroid acropachy.** *See* ACROPACHY. **Thyroid crisis.** Extreme tachycardia, fever, vomiting and diarrhoea. There may be generalized erythema and hypotension and the patient may be delirious and death may occur. Since adequate therapy for thyrotoxicosis has been available thyroid crisis (or "storm") rarely occurs. **Intrathoracic thyroid.** A thyroid gland that is situated much lower than its normal position in the neck and behind the sternum. **Lingual thyroid.** A mass of thyroid tissue found on the dorsum of the tongue at the foramen caecum due to failure of the embryonic thyroid outgrowth to descend. **Retrosternal thyroid, Substernal thyroid.** Intrathoracic thyroid (see above). [Gk *thyreos* oblong shield, *eidos* form.]

thyroid arteries. Arteries of supply of the thyroid gland that give branches to other structures. **Inferior thyroid artery [arteria thyroidea inferior (NA)].** A branch of the thyrocervical trunk supplying the lower and posterior parts of the thyroid gland, and sending twigs to the larynx [arteria laryngea inferior (NA)], pharynx [rami pharyngei (NA)], trachea [rami tracheales (NA)], oesophagus [rami oesophagei (NA)], and neck muscles. It also gives off the ascending cervical artery [arteria cervicalis ascendens (NA)] which passes up medial to the phrenic nerve to supply the deep neck muscles by muscular branches and the spinal cord and membranes by spinal branches [rami spinales]. There is also a deep branch. **Superior thyroid artery [arteria thyroidea superior (NA)].** A branch of the external carotid artery, entering the apex of the lateral lobe of the thyroid gland. It communicates with its partner across the isthmus, and also with branches of the inferior thyroid arteries, and supplies branches to the larynx [arteria laryngea superior (NA)] and sternocleidomastoid muscles [ramus sternocleidomastoideus (NA)] and a small infrahyoid branch [ramus infrahyoideus (NA)] along the lower margin of the hyoid bone. The cricothyroid branch [ramus cricothyroideus (NA)] crosses the cricothyroid ligament in its upper part. The glandular branches are the terminal thyroid branches and consist of an anterior branch [ramus anterior (NA)] to the upper pole and anterior surface, and a posterior branch [ramus posterior (NA)] running behind the gland and anastomosing with the inferior thyroid artery.

thyroid veins. Veins draining the thyroid gland. **Inferior thyroid vein [vena thyroidea inferior (NA)].** A tributary of the innominate vein; it crosses in front of the trachea. **Middle thyroid vein [vena thyroidea media (NA)].** One of the veins draining the thyroid gland; it is a tributary of the internal jugular vein and has no accompanying artery. **Superior thyroid vein [vena thyroidea superior (NA)].** A vein accompanying the artery of the same name from the thyroid gland. It is a tributary of the common facial or internal jugular veins.

thyroidea (thi·roid·e·ah). Thyroid. **Thyroidea accessoria, Thyroidea ima.** The accessory thyroid gland. *See* GLAND.

thyroidea ima artery [arteria thyroidea ima (NA)] (thi·roid·e·ah i·mah ar·ter·e). An inconstant artery, usually small, arising most commonly from the innominate artery and ending in the thyroid isthmus.

thyroidectomize (thi·roid·ek·to·mize). To subject to thyroidectomy.

thyroidectomy (thi·roid·ek·to·me). The operation of excising the thyroid gland. **Partial thyroidectomy.** Leaving about 8 mm of thyroid tissue behind; the usual operation for thyrotoxicosis. [thyroid, Gk *ektome* excision.]

thyroiditis (thi·roid·i·tis). Inflammation of the thyroid gland. The term has been loosely used for non-inflammatory conditions such as goitre. **Acute thyroiditis.** A condition which may occur with various infectious diseases. **Acute suppurative thyroiditis.** A form which may occur in pyaemia with the production of abscesses in the gland, or may be due to extension from a neighbouring suppurative lesion. **Parasitic thyroiditis.** Thyroiditis occurring in Chagas' disease (American trypanosomiasis). [thyroid, Gk *-itis* inflammation.]

See also: HASHIMOTO, RIEDEL.

thyroigenous (thi·roi·jen·us). Attributable to disease of the thyroid gland. [thyroid, Gk *genein* to produce.]

thyrolaryngeal (thi·ro·lar·in′·je·al). Pertaining to the thyroid gland and the larynx.

thyrolingual (thi·ro·ling·gwal). Thyroglossal. [thyroid, L *lingua* tongue.]

thyrolytic (thi·ro·lit·ik). Destructive to the tissue of the thyroid gland. [thyroid, Gk *lysis* a loosing.]

thyromegaly (thi·ro·meg·al·e). Enlargement of the thyroid gland. [thyroid, Gk *megas* large.]

thyroparathyroidectomy (thi·ro·par·ah·thi·roid·ek′·to·me). The surgical removal of the thyroid and parathyroid glands. [thyroid, parathyroid, Gk *ektome* excision.]

thyropathy (thi·rop·ath·e). Disease or dysfunction of the thyroid gland. [thyroid, Gk *pathos* disease.]

thyroprival (thi·ro·pri·val). Describing any effect or symptom resulting from the removal of the thyroid or the abolition of its function. [thyroid, L *privus* deprived.]

thyroptosis (thi·rop·to·sis). Downward displacement of the thyroid. [thyroid, Gk *ptosis* fall.]

thyrotherapy (thi·ro·ther·ap·e). The treatment of disease by administration of thyroid extract. [thyroid, therapy.]

thyrotome (thi·ro·tome). An instrument used in thyrotomy.

thyrotomy (thi·rot·o·me). 1. Surgical incision of the thyroid cartilage, as in laryngotomy. 2. Incision of the thyroid gland. [thyroid, Gk *temnein* to cut.]

thyrotoxaemia (thi·ro·tox·e′·me·ah). Thyrotoxicosis. [thyroid, toxaemia.]

thyrotoxia (thi·ro·tox·e·ah). Thyrotoxicosis.

thyrotoxic (thi·ro·tox·ik). 1. Relating to or derived from thyrotoxin. 2. Characterized by thyrotoxicosis.

thyrotoxicosis (thi·ro·tox·ik·o′·sis). Graves' disease. Any toxic condition attributable to hyperactivity of the thyroid gland. **Primary thyrotoxicosis.** Thyrotoxicosis in which the goitre and the thyrotoxicosis appear together. **Secondary thyrotoxicosis.** Thyrotoxicosis appearing in a patient who already has a goitre. [thyroid, Gk *toxikon* poison, *-osis* condition.]

thyrotoxin (thi·ro·tox·in). A cytotoxin developed by the thyroid gland. [thyroid, Gk *toxikon* poison.]

Thyrotrophin (thi·ro·trof·in). BP Commission approved name for the thyrotrophic hormone; used in thyroid therapy.

thyrotrophin, thyrotropin (thi·ro·trof·in, thi·ro·trop·in). Thyroid-stimulating hormone (TSH); the hormone secreted by the basophil cells of the anterior lobe of the pituitary gland, which stimulates the secretion of thyroid hormone by the thyroid gland. [thyroid, Gk *trophe* nutrition, *trepein* to turn.]

thyrotropism (thi·ro·tro·pizm). A constitution characteristic of thyroid influence. [thyroid, Gk *trepein* to turn.]

thyroxinaemia (thi·rox·in·e′·me·ah). The presence of excess thyroxine in the blood. [thyroxine, Gk *haima* blood.]

thyroxine (thi·rox·een). β - [3,5 - Di-iodo - 4 - (3′,5′ - di-iodo-4′-hydroxyphenoxy)phenyl]-α-aminopropionic acid, $OHC_6H_2I_2OC_6H_2I_2CH_2CH(NH_2)COOH$. A crystalline iodine compound, the active hormone of the thyroid gland, now prepared synthetically. It is chiefly used in the form of the sodium salt, thyroxine sodium, in the treatment of myxoedema and cretinism and in other conditions where it is desired to increase the basal metabolic rate. Thyroxine has the advantage of accurate standardization of activity. There is delay in metabolic response and repeated doses at short intervals may lead to accumulation. **Thyroxine Sodium BP 1973.** The sodium salt of thyroxine; a compound which is sparingly soluble in water but more so in sodium carbonate solution, and is used for that reason in place of thyroxine, which is very insoluble, both by mouth and hypodermically. A simplified synthesis has enormously reduced its cost, enabling it to be used to increase lactation in cattle as a practical proposition.

thyroxinic (thi·rox·in·ik). Relating to or derived from thyroxine.

thysanothrix (thi·san·o·thrix). *Trichostasis spinulosa.* [Gk *thysanos* tassel, *thrix* hair.]

Thysanura (thi·san·ewr·ah). An order of primitively wingless insects. *Lepisma saccharina*, the silver fish, and *Thermobia domesticus*, the fire brat, are members of it. [Gk *thysanos* tassel, *oura* tail.]

tibia [NA] (tib·e·ah). The long bone on the medial and pre-axial border of the leg, articulating with the fibula laterally, the femur above, and the talus below. **Articular surface of the tibia, fibular [facies articularis fibularis (NA)].** A facet in the postero-inferior aspect of the lateral condyle for articulation with the head of the fibula. **Articular surface of the tibia, inferior [facies articularis inferior (NA)].** The area at the lower end of the tibia, concave from before backwards, and convex from side to side, to articulate with the upper surface of the body of the talus. **Articular surfaces of the tibia, superior [facies articulares superiores (NA)].** The roughly oval articular surfaces on the condyles of the tibia bearing the medial and lateral menisci and articulating with the condyles of the femur. **Intercondylar area of the tibia [area intercondylaris anterior et area intercondylaris posterior (NA)].** An irregularly roughened and laterally compressed area between the articular surfaces on the upper end of the tibia, bearing anteriorly two small tubercles or spines and giving attachment to the horns of the semilunar cartilages and the cruciate ligaments. **Sabre tibia, Sabre-scabbard tibia, Sabre-shaped tibia.** Curved tibia due to syphilitic periostitis; it also occurs in yaws. **Shaft of the tibia [corpus tibiae (NA)].** The main part of the bone supporting the upper and lower ends. It is triangular in cross-section, with three borders, anterior, interosseous, and medial, separating three surfaces, posterior, medial, and lateral, a surface opposite each border. The anterior border [margo anterior (NA)] is a sharp crest, the shin, which gives attachment to the deep fascia of the leg; the interosseous border [margo interossea (NA)] is well defined and gives attachment to the interosseous membrane, while the medial border [margo medialis (NA)] is less well defined and gives attachment to the fascia which covers the deep muscles of the back of the leg and to the medial ligament of the knee above. The medial surface [facies medialis (NA)] is subcutaneous, the lateral surface [facies lateralis (NA)] gives origin to the tibialis anterior muscle, and the posterior surface [facies posterior (NA)] gives attachment to the popliteus muscle and the deep flexor muscles of the ankle and foot. **Tibia valga.** A bowed tibia with the convexity towards the midline. **Tibia vara.** Bowed tibia with the convexity to the outer side. [L shin-bone, flute.]

See also: LANNELONGUE.

tibia, nutrient artery to the [arteria nutritea tibiae]. A branch of the posterior tibial artery to the tibia.

tibial [tibialis (NA)]. (tib·e·al). Concerning the tibia.

tibial arteries. Terminal branches of the popliteal artery that with the peroneal artery supply blood to the leg and foot. **Anterior tibial artery [arteria tibialis anterior (NA)].** One of the terminal branches of the popliteal artery. It passes from the popliteal fossa to the front of the leg, where it descends to the foot. It has a recurrent branch [arteria recurrens tibialis anterior (NA)] to the patellar network. The posterior recurrent branch [arteria recurrens tibialis posterior (NA)] does not always exist. **Posterior tibial artery [arteria tibialis posterior (NA)].** One of the terminal branches of the popliteal artery which descends along the back of the leg to midway between the medial malleolus [rami malleolares mediales (NA)] and calcaneum [rami calcanei (NA)], where it divides into medial and lateral plantar arteries. The circumflex fibular branch [ramus circumflexus fibulae (NA)] winds round the neck of the fibula to anastomose with the lateral inferior genicular artery.

tibial nerves. Nerves that constitute the main nerve supply of the leg and foot. **Anterior tibial nerve [nervus peroneus (fibularis) profundus (NA)].** One of the terminal branches of the lateral popliteal nerve supplying the muscles of the extensor compartment of the leg [rami musculares (NA)], the extensor digitorum brevis muscle, and the skin bordering the first interdigital cleft in the foot [nervi digitales dorsales, hallucis lateralis et digiti secundi medialis (NA)]. **Posterior tibial nerve.** The continuation of the medial popliteal nerve from the lower border of the popliteus along the back of the leg to the interval between the heel and the lateral malleolus where it divides into medial and lateral plantar nerves. It supplies the deep muscles on the back of the leg, and the skin on the medial side of the heel. The medial calcaneal branches to the skin on the medial side of the heel pierce the flexor retinaculum.

tibial veins. Deep veins of the lower limb; they are tributaries of the popliteal vein. **Anterior tibial veins [venae tibiales anteriores (NA)].** The venae comitantes of the anterior tibial artery; tributaries of the popliteal vein. **Posterior tibial veins [venae tibiales posteriores (NA)].** The venae comitantes of the posterior tibial arteries; tributaries of the popliteal vein.

tibiale (tib·e·a·le). An anthropometric point; the upper border of the medial condyle of the tibia.

tibialgia (tib·e·al·je·ah). Pain in the shin. A specific syndrome associated with lymphocytosis and eosinophilia, and believed to be due to vitamin deficiency. [tibia, Gk *algos* pain.]

tibialis muscles (tib·e·a·lis muslz). **Tibialis anterior muscle [musculus tibialis anterior (NA)].** A muscle arising from the lateral surface of the tibia and the interosseous membrane and inserted into the base of the 1st metatarsal and 1st cuneiform bones. It is a dorsiflexor and invertor of the foot. **Tibialis posterior muscle [musculus tibialis posterior (NA)].** A muscle arising from both the tibia and the fibula and from the posterior surface of the interosseous membrane, and inserted into the navicular bone and several other bones of the tarsus. It is a plantar flexor and invertor of the foot.

tibiocalcanean (**tib**·e·o·kal·**ka'**·ne·an). Concerning both the tibia and calcaneum.

tibiofemoral (**tib**·e·o·**fem'**·or·al). Concerning the tibia and the femur.

tibiofibular (**tib**·e·o·**fib'**·ew·lar). Connecting the tibia and the fibula, as in the tibiofibular articulation.

tibionavicular (**tib**·e·o·nav·**ik'**·ew·lar). Concerning the tibia and the navicular bone of the tarsus.

tibioperoneal (**tib**·e·o·per·o·**ne'**·al). Tibiofibular. [tibia, Gk *perone* brooch, fibula.]

tibioscaphoid (**tib**·e·o·**skaf'**·oid). Tibionavicular. [tibia, scaphoid.]

tibiotarsal (**tib**·e·o·**tar'**·sal). Concerning the tibia and the tarsus, as in the ankle joint.

tic (tik). A co-ordinated repetitive movement, usually involving a number of muscles which follow their normal rôles of prime mover, antagonist, and synergist. Tics commonly involve the face and shoulders, occur in people of neurotic disposition, and usually develop early in life. Also called *habit spasm.* The term was once applied to any spasmodic muscular movement, particularly of the face, and because of this usage it was used in naming various syndromes. **Bowing tic.** Repetitive bowing movements; salaam spasm. **Cheek-biting tic.** A habitual sucking and chewing of a cheek, causing a thickened whitish, sometimes eroded, epithelium in the line of occlusion within the mouth. **Convulsive tic.** Hemifacial spasm. *See* SPASM. **Degenerative tic.** Any tic which may occur in a degenerative nervous disease. **Diaphragmatic tic.** Repetitive spasmodic diaphragmatic contractions. **Tic douloureux.** Paroxysmal trigeminal neuralgia; the pain is brief, strictly unilateral, limited to the distribution of the trigeminal nerve, and is provoked by chewing, speaking, touching the face, or a variety of other stimuli. **Facial tic.** Any tic involving the facial musculature. **Gesticulatory tic.** A tic in which dramatic gesticulatory movements occur. **Habit tic.** Habit spasm; according to modern usage this term is tautologous, as tic means habit spasm. **Impulsive tic.** Psychomotor tic (see below). **Laryngeal tic.** A tic of the laryngeal muscles, giving explosive expulsion of air. **Local tic.** A tic limited to a very small area of a muscle, say a part of the orbicularis oculi. **Mimic tic.** Mimic spasm; this name was given to facial tics because of the apparent element of mimicry. **Motor tic.** A tic whose manifestations are limited to the motor system and consist of spasmodic muscular contractions with no overt mental manifestations. According to modern usage all tics fall into this group, but the term was once used to exclude psychomotor tics (see below). **Tic non-douloureux.** Myoclonic epilepsy. *See* EPILEPSY. **Occupation tic.** Occupational neurosis; fatigue spasm. **Painless tic.** An obsolete term used to describe any habit spasm which is not painful. **Tic de pensée.** The habit of automatically putting one's thoughts into spoken words. **Progressive choreic tic.** A term sometimes applied to torsion spasm or dystonia musculorum deformans; it can also be applied to any progressive disease of the basal ganglia which gives rise to choreiform involuntary movements. **Psychomotor tic.** Spasmodic exaggerated muscular contractions, often giving rise to jumping, leaping, or dancing movements, and associated with mental abnormality. Some authorities believe that this group of diseases are hysterical; others that they are psychotic illnesses. Into this group fall the variety of similar conditions known as saltatory spasm, latah, choromania, palmus, mental torticollis, jumping disease, and Gilles de la Tourette's disease. **Respiratory tic.** Diaphragmatic tic (see above). **Rotatory tic.** Rotatory spasm. *See* SPASM. **Saltatory tic.** Saltatory spasm. *See* SPASM. **Simple tic.** Repeated twitching co-ordinated movements of the same nature in the same place (usually of the face and in children) in which the prognosis is good. **Tic de sommeil.** Involuntary twitching movements, particularly of the head, which may occur during sleep. **Spasmodic tic.** Any tic in which spasmodic contractions of muscle groups occur at variable intervals of time. [Fr.]

See also: GUINON.

Ticarcillin (ti·**kar**·sil·in). BP Commission approved name for 6 - [2 - carboxy - 2 - (3 - thienyl)acetamido] - penicillanic acid; an antibiotic.

tick (tic). A blood-sucking arachnid of the order Acarina and super-family Ixodoidea; the largest of the Acarina, many are important vectors of human disease. **Bandicoot tick.** *Haemaphysalis humerosa.* **Bont tick.** *Amblyomma hebraeum.* **Castor-bean tick.** *Ixodes ricinus.* **Dog tick.** *Haemaphysalis leachi.* **Ear tick.** *Otobius megnini.* **Lone-star tick.** *Amblyomma americanum.* **Miana tick.** *Argas mianensis.* **Paralysis tick.** Any tick the female of which produces tick paralysis. **Scrub tick.** *Ixodes holocyclus.* **Seed tick.** The six-legged larva of any tick. **Sheep tic.** *Ixodes ricinus.* **Tampan tick.** *Ornithodorus moubata.* [ME *tike.*]

tickle (tickl). 1. To stimulate the surface of the skin gently and in such a way as to produce results ranging from pleasurable reflexes such as laughter, to pain and convulsions. 2. The sensation of tickling. [ME *tikelle.*]

tictology (tik·**tol**·o·je). Obstetrics. [Gk *tiktein* to give birth, *logos* science.]

tide (tide). Lapse of time; rise and fall; ebb and flow. **Acid tide.** Temporary increase in acidity of the urine after fasting. **Alkaline tide.** Temporary decrease in acidity of the urine after a meal. **Fat tide.** The physiological increase of fat in the blood after a fatty meal. [AS *tid* time.]

Tidy, Sir Henry Letheby (b. 1877). London physician.

Tidy type of non-thrombotic phlebitis. A phlebitis with periphlebitis, quite unrelated to thrombophlebitis migrans, which is characterized by spindle-shaped swellings that develop along the course of veins, usually of the upper extremities, but are not accompanied by thrombosis. The swellings are associated with an inflammatory reaction only for a short time. They tend to migrate in a distal direction, but eventually clear up completely.

Tiedemann, Friedrich (b. 1781). Würzburg anatomist.

Tiedemann's gland. The greater vestibular gland.

Tiedemann's nerve. Nerve fibres said to arise from the ciliary ganglion and accompany the central artery of the retina.

Tiemann, George. New York instrument maker.

Tiemann's catheter. A hard, white-rubber catheter with a fixed curve at its tapering proximal end.

Tiemonium Iodide (ti·em·o·ne·um i·o·dide). BP Commission approved name for 4 - [3 - hydroxy - 3 - phenyl - 3 - (2 - thienyl)propyl] - 4 - methylmorpholinium iodide; an antispasmodic and anticholinergic.

Tietze, Alexander (b. 1864). German surgeon.

Tietze disease. Enlargement of the costochondral junctions, commonly affecting the second rib, of unkown aetiology.

tigering (ti·ger·ing). An appearance of the heart muscle produced by irregular streaks of pale, friable areas of fatty degeneration resembling the stripes of a tiger. It occurs particularly in severe and prolonged anaemia, but may result from any condition which causes anoxaemia. Also known as *tiger heart, tiger-lily heart, tabby-cat heart,* and *thrush-breast heart.* [Gk *tigris* tiger.]

tiglic aldehyde (tig·lik **al**·de·hide). 2 - methylbut - 2 - en - 1 - al $CH_3CH{=}C(CH_3)CHO$. An unsaturated aldehyde obtained by the distillation of guaiacum resin.

tiglium (tig·le·um). The croton oil plant, *Croton tiglium.* [etym. dub.]

Tigloidine (tig·**lo**·id·een). BP Commission approved name for tiglylpseudotropeine; it is used in the treatment of spasticity and muscle spasm.

tigretier (tig·ret·e·er). A form of choromania. [*Tigre,* district in Abyssinia.]

tigroid (ti·groid). Streaked; spotted. [Gk *tigris* tiger, *eidos* form.]

tigrolysis (ti·**grol**·is·is). The breaking up of tigroid spindles in a nerve cell. [tigroid, Gk *lysis* a loosing.]

tikitiki (te·ke·te·ke). A crude preparation of rice polishings used in the Far East in the prophylaxis or cure of beriberi. It is rich in vitamins of the B_2 complex. [Japanese.]

Tilbury Fox. *See* FOX, WILLIAM TILBURY.

Tiletamine (ti·**let**·am·een). BP Commission approved name for 2-ethylamino-2-(2-thienyl)cyclohexanone; an anticonvulsant and anaesthetic.

Tilia (**til**·e·ah). A genus of trees belonging to the family Liliaceae; the lindens. **Tilia europaea.** The linden, or lime tree, the flowers of which are used in the form of an infusion for their antispasmodic and diaphoretic properties. [L.]

tiliacin (til·e·a·sin). A glycoside of the linden tree, *Tilea europaea.*

Tilidate (ti·lid·ate). BP Commission approved name for ethyl 2 - dimethylamino - 1 - phenylcyclohex - 3 - ene - 1 - carboxylate; an analgesic.

Tillaux, Paul Jules (b. 1834). Paris surgeon.

Tillaux's disease. Chronic mastitis with formation of tumour-like nodules.

Tilletia (til·e·she·ah). A genus of fungi responsible for smut on cereals.

tiltometer (til·**tom**·et·er). A simple instrument showing the degree of tilt of the operating table; used for the gravimetric control of subarachnoid analgesia. [AS *tealt* unsteady, meter.]

timbo (**tim**·bo). Lonchocarpus.

timbre (timber, tahmbr). The characteristic quality of a voice, musical note, or instrument. **Timbre metallique.** Metallic second sound heard in dilatation of the aorta. [Fr.]

time (time). A measure of duration. **Apex time.** The interval of time between the two peaks of muscular contraction in a summated contraction. **Arm-to-lung time, Arm-to-tongue time.** *See* CIRCULATION TIME (below). **Association time.** The time between a verbal stimulus and the verbal response. **Bleeding time.** The time required for bleeding to cease spontaneously when a moderately deep cut is made into the skin or lobe of the ear under standardized conditions; normally it is 1-3 min. It is prolonged in certain diseases of the blood, and is primarily a measure of the capillary contractility but may be associated with a thrombocytopenia. **Calcium time.** A test formerly employed to determine whether there is a deficiency of blood calcium; it is obtained by comparing the clotting time of the whole blood with whole blood to which additional excess calcium has been added. **Cell generation time.** The time taken by the cell to go through the cell cycle. **Circulation time.** The time taken by a particle of blood to pass once round the entire circulation (*total circulation time*), or to pass once through the pulmonary circuit (*pulmonary circulation time*). The former is measured by the time taken for a substance (saccharin or dehydrocholic acid) to pass from the median cubital vein to the tongue, where its arrival is appreciated by a characteristic taste (*arm-to-tongue time*); the latter is measured by the use of a volatile substance (ether or paraldehyde) which is excreted in the lungs, and the time is measured from the moment of injection into the median cubital vein until the characteristic odour appears in the subject's breath (*arm-to-lung time*). A decrease in cardiac output entails an increase in circulation time, which is prolonged in congestive heart failure. **Clot-retraction time.** A measure of the time taken for the blood clot to contract firmly or retract from the wall of the test-tube or container, expressing serum; it is normally 30–60 min. A semi-quantitative method depends on the measurement of the volume of serum expressed. **Clotting time.** 1. Of whole blood: a measure of the coagulability of whole blood, determined by withdrawing blood quickly under very careful standardized conditions and determining the time taken for clotting to occur; normally it is from 4 to 15 min, according to the method employed, but may be markedly prolonged in patients with haemophilia, and in other haemorrhagic diseases due to deficiencies of calcium, fibrinogen, prothrombin, vitamin K. 2. Of recalcified plasma; a measure of the clotting time of blood plasma that has been recalcified by the addition of a slight excess of calcium chloride to remove or overcome the anticoagulant previously added; the normal time is from 90 s to 2 min. **Coagulation time.** Clotting time (see above). **Dead time.** The time following the absorption of a quantum of radiation by a radiation detector during which the instrument cannot detect a further quantum. It is of particular importance when a Geiger-Muller counter is used. **Ejection time.** In cardiology, the time during which blood is being ejected from the left ventricle in any one systole. **Generation time.** The mean time interval between successive generations; in micro-organisms, the duration of the cellular division cycle. **Inertia time.** In a muscle or sense organ, the time necessary to overcome inertia between the arrival of a stimulus and the response. **Insensitive time.** The time duration following actuation of a counter in which it is insensitive to further actuation. **Overall treatment time.** The total time, from beginning to end, of a single radiation treatment, or of a whole series of treatments if fractionated. **Paralysis time.** Dead time (see above). **Perception time.** The time needed for the process of perceiving and recognizing a stimulus. **Persistence time.** An obsolete term denoting the duration of ventricular systole, from its onset to the beginning of diastole. It consists of isometric contraction and maximal and reduced ejection phases. **Pre-ejection time.** In cardiology, the time between the commencement of the electrical activation of the ventricles to the onset of ejection of blood from the left ventricle; it represents the electromechanical delay before ejection starts. **Prothrombin time of plasma.** A measure of the prothrombin in the blood plasma determined by one-stage or two-stage methods. The general principle of the determination is to carry out the coagulation test in the presence of adequate or optimal amounts of all the factors necessary for blood coagulation, with only the prothrombin already present in the plasma to be tested; the plasma prothrombin time, normally 10–25 s, is inversely proportional to the prothrombin content of the blood tested. It is necessary to run parallel tests with normal blood before the prothrombin time can be converted into the actual prothrombin concentration. **Psychophysical time.** Stimulus-response time (see below). **Pulmonary circulation time.** *See* CIRCULATION TIME (above). **QT time.** The duration of the electrical activity related to ventricular systole, measured from the beginning of the Q wave to the end of the T wave in the electrocardiogram. The normal QT time is related to the heart beat. **QTc time.** The QT time as measured, adjusted to correct it to the value it would have been at a heart rate of 60 per minute. **Reaction time.** The time between the application of a stimulus and the beginning of a response. **Recognition time.** Perception time (see above). **Recovery time.** The time taken for an electronic circuit to rest after actuation to prepare for further actuation. **Resolution time.** The minimum (time) duration between two consecutive pulses which a scaler will accept as separate pulses. **Resolving time.** Dead time (see above). **Sedimentation time.** The time taken for the sedimentation of erythrocytes in a vertical column. **Stimulus-response time.** The time taken for a mental stimulus to produce a physical response. **Thermal death time.** Of bacteria: the time of exposure to a given temperature needed to sterilize a culture. **Total circulation time.** *See* CIRCULATION TIME (above). **Time of unconsciousness.** The time interval between the loss of oxygen supply and unconsciousness. **Time of useful consciousness.** The time interval between the loss of oxygen supply and clouding of consciousness to a point that makes efficient skilled response impossible. **Ventricular activation time.** The time taken for the electrical impulse to pass through the ventricular muscle mass of the heart. It is represented by the interval between the beginning of the down stroke of the R wave and the beginning of the Q wave in semidirect precordial leads. [AS *tima.*]

time-switch (time·switch). A mechanical or electrical instrument for carrying out a sequence of switching operations at fixed time intervals or for performing switching operations at a fixed time of day. It has a special use for initiating or terminating an x-ray exposure.

timer (ti·mer). A time-switch. The term may also include a mechanism which indicates duration of time without operating a switch. **Clockwork timer.** A timer or time-switch driven by a spring clock mechanism. **Electronic timer.** A timer in which the time element is an electrical circuit, usually the rise of potential on a condenser charged through a high resistance. It is used for radiographs, exposure being finished automatically when the potential reaches a fixed value. **Impulse timer.** Synchronous timer (see below). **Photo-electric timer.** A time-switch for the automatic correct exposure of a radiograph. X-rays passing through the film fall on a fluorescent screen the light output from which is electrically integrated. The exposure is terminated automatically when the film has received the correct x-ray dose. **Synchronous timer.** A timer or time-switch driven from a.c. mains by a synchronous motor the speed of which depends only upon the frequency of the supply. Switching operations are carried out by a rotating disc driven by the motor.

Timofeew, D. A. 19th century Kazan histologist.

Apparatus of Timofeew. The mass of axonal filaments within a lamellated corpuscle.

Timofeew's corpuscle. A form of laminated nerve-ending said to exist in the submucous coat of the posterior urethra.

Timolol (tim·o·lol). BP Commission approved name for (−) - *t* - butylamino - 3 - (4 - morpholino - 1,2,5 - thiadiazol - 3 - yloxy) - propan - 2 - ol; a beta adrenergic blocking agent.

tin (tin). An element of atomic weight 118.69, atomic number 50, and chemical symbol Sn (*stannum*). It is a soft white metal, malleable and slightly ductile, which resists corrosion in air and water, and is used for plating, the making of alloys and tinplate, and the silvering of mirrors. It has valencies of two and four. **Tin ammonium chloride.** Pink salt, $(NH_4)_3SnCl_6$, a mordant used in dyeing. **Butter of tin.** Stannic chloride, $SnCl_4$. **Tin chloride.** Stannous chloride, $SnCl_2$. **Tin dioxide.** Stannic oxide, SnO_2, a white powder used as a polishing medium. **Tin oxide.** A compound administered, usually in tablets, for the treatment of boils, carbuncles, and acne, but its efficacy is suspect. **Tin powder.** Finely divided tin, used similarly to tin oxide (above). **Precipitated tin.** A precipitate formed electrolytically; it is used as a taenicide. [AS.]

tincal (tin·kal). An impure form of borax containing lime, magnesia, and other substances. It is obtained by evaporation of the water of alkaline lakes in California and Tibet. [Persian *tinkal.*]

tinction (tingk·shun). 1. A stain. 2. Staining. [see foll.]

tinctorial (tingk·tor·e·al). Concerned with staining or colouring. [L *tingere* to tint.]

tinctura (tingk·tewr·ah). Tincture. All tinctures were listed officially as *Tinctura* before 1953. [L.]

tincture (tingk·tewr, tingk·tcher). An alcoholic extract of a vegetable or animal drug prepared usually by a percolation or maceration process. The strength is usually such that 10 parts by volume of tincture contains the active constituents of one part by weight of the dry drug. Simple alcoholic solutions of pure substances such as quinine or iodine are no longer known by this term. Tinctures listed as official in the BP 1973 include those of the following substances to which reference should be made: Belladonna, Camphorated Opium, Colchicum, Compound Cardamon, Compound Rhubarb, Hyoscyamus, Ipecacuanha, Nux Vomica, Opium, Stramonium, Strong Ginger, Weak Ginger. **Antiperiodic tincture.** Warburg's tincture; the most outstanding example remaining of the blunderbuss therapy or polypharmacy of former days. It contains the alcohol-soluble constituents of 18 separate drugs. **Ethereal tincture.** Any tincture in which spirit of ether is employed as menstruum instead of the usual alcohol-water mixture. [L *tinctura* a dyeing.]

See also: WARBURG (C.).

tinea (tin·e·ah). Ringworm; mycotic infection of the skin, hair, or nails. **Tinea alba.** A form of tinea versicolor said to occur in the tropics. **Tinea albigena.** A malady noted in Java by Nieuwenhuis (1908), attributed to infection of the skin with *Trichophyton albiciscans*, causing parasitic pseudo-achromia, i.e. vitiligo-like depigmentation. **Tinea amiantacea, Tinea asbestina, Asbestos-like tinea.** Pityriasis amiantacea. **Tinea axillaris.** Ringworm of the axillae, usually caused by *Epidermophyton floccosum*, *Trichophyton interdigitale*, or *T. rubrum*. **Tinea barbae.** Ringworm affecting the skin and hairs of the beard area and sometimes also the moustache area of the face, usually caused by an ectothrix variety of *Trichophyton*, e.g. *T. verrucosum*, or occasionally by an endothrix variety. **Tinea capitis.** Ringworm affecting the skin and hairs of the scalp. In children it is caused usually by *Microspora* (e.g. *Microsporan audouini, M. canis*). **Tinea ciliorum.** Tinea of the eyelashes and of the adjacent skin of the eyelids. **Tinea circinata.** Ringworm of the glabrous skin caused rarely by *M. canis* or *M. audouini*. **Tinea corporis.** Ringworm of the body. **Tinea cruris.** Ringworm of the groin and adjacent areas, so-named because it usually appears to commence on the leg at the level of the lowest-hanging testis. It is caused typically by the fungi that also cause tinea axillaris. **Tinea decalvans.** 1. Archaic name for alopecia areata. 2. Term used by Tilbury Fox for suppurative types of ringworm in which the hairs are shed so that a bald area results. **Tinea favosa.** Favus. **Tinea ficosa.** Archaic name for favus. **Tinea flava.** A tropical variety of tinea versicolor in which the lesions are yellowish in colour. **Tinea glabrosa.** Tinea corporis (see above). **Tinea imbricata.** Bowditch Island ringworm, Burmese ringworm, Chinese ringworm, Malabar itch, Tokelau ringworm; a tropical ringworm, endemic chiefly in the Malay Peninsula and South Sea Islands, but well known in some other hot countries. It is caused by *Trichophyton concentricum*, and is characterized by the formation of greyish-white imbricated scales arranged in concentric circles with the bases of the scales towards the periphery and the free margins towards the centre, or in wavy parallel lines like watered silk. In severe cases very large areas of skin may be involved, but the scalp often escapes. The nails may be affected. **Tinea inguinalis.** Tinea of the inguinal region; tinea cruris. **Tinea interdigitalis.** A variety of tinea pedis in which the infecting organism is *T. interdigitale*; not a generally accepted name. **Tinea kerion.** Kerion, a more or less bald, rounded, inflammatory, boggy, carbuncle-like, cutaneous tumour, discharging purulent fluid from the patulous follicles on its surface; caused usually by trichophytic infection. **Tinea lupinosa.** Archaic name for favus. **Tinea nigra.** A superficial infection of the skin by *Cladosporium werneckii*, a dematiaceous fungus. **Tinea nodosa.** Leptothrix. **Tinea pedis.** Ringworm of the feet. It is caused by the same organisms as tinea axillaris and tinea cruris. **Tinea profunda.** A rare type of ringworm in which indolent nodules and plaques form in the skin; ulceration may occur. It is usually due to *T. verrucosum*. **Tinea sycosis.** Tinea barbae (see above). **Tinea tarsi.** Ringworm of the eyelids. **Tinea tondens, Tinea tonsurans.** Tinea capitis (see above). **Tinea trichophytina.** In the older literature signifying *ringworm*, all types of the malady were thought to be due to one fungus, the *Trichophyton*. Later it was used as a synonym for trichophytosis. The term is now regarded as archaic. **Tinea unguium.** Ringworm of the nails caused by *Trichophyta*, especially *Trichophyton rubrum*, or by *Epidermophyton floccosum*; it is rarely caused by *Microsporum* spp. **Tinea vera.** Archaic name for favus. **Tinea versicolor.** Pityriasis versicolor; a cutaneous infection, due to *Malassezia furfur*, characterized by variously sized and shaped, furfuraceous, macular patches of yellow or fawn colour, usually occurring on the upper part of the trunk, and sometimes associated with pseudo-achromia. [L worm.]

Tinel, Jules (b. 1879). Paris neurosurgeon.

Tinel's sign. During nerve regeneration, percussion over or just below the point of original section gives rise to tingling sensations in the periphery; also called *formication sign* and *D.T.P. sign*.

tingibility (tin·jib·il·it·e). The ability to be stained. [L *tingere* to tint.]

tingible (tin·jibl). Able to be stained with a dye. [see prec.]

tingle (ting·gl). A slight pricking or stinging sensation felt in the skin. [ME *tink* to tinkle.]

tingling (ting·gling). A pricking sensation caused by cold or injury to a nerve. **Distal tingling.** Tinel's sign, tingling at the end of an extremity on percussing a partially divided or regenerating nerve. [see prec.]

Tinidazole (ti·ni·daz·ole). BP Commission approved name for ethyl 2 - (2 - methyl - 5 - nitroimidazol - 1 - yl) - ethyl sulphone; an antitrichomonal agent.

tinkle (ting·kl). Tinkling.

See also: BOUILLAUD.

tinkling (ting·kling). Musical, bell-like, metallic, adventitious sounds heard over large pulmonary cavities or pneumothorax. [ME *tink*.]

tinnitus (tin·i·tus). Subjective noise in the ear. **Clicking tinnitus.** A clicking sound in the ear which may be due to spasm of the tensor palati muscle or the tensor tympani muscle. **Non-vibratory tinnitus.** Tinnitus produced as a result of biochemical abnormalities affecting the internal ear, its neural pathways, or central connections. **Objective tinnitus.** Tinnitus which can be heard by an examiner as well as by the patient. **Telephone tinnitus.** A noise in the ear which follows long use of the telephone, particularly when the telephone is associated with loud voices. **Vibratory tinnitus.** Tinnitus due to muscle contractions or vascular pulsations transmitted to the internal ear. [L *tinnire* to tinkle.]

See also: LAUDET.

tint B (tint be). A colour change produced in a pastille under irradiation, said to indicate the dose which will cause epilation. The method is inaccurate, and the term is now obsolete. [L *tingere* to tint.]

tintometer (tin·tom·et·er). A colorimeter; a graded colour scale used for the estimation of colouring matter in a fluid. [tint, meter.]

See also: LOVIBOND.

tintometric (tin·to·met·rik). Concerned with tintometry.

tintometry (tin·tom·et·re). Colorimetric estimation of substances in blood and other fluids by use of a tintometer.

Tiprenolol (tip·ren·o·lol). BP Commission approved name for 3 - isopropylamino - 1 - [2 - (methylthio)phenoxy] - propan - 2 - ol; an adrenergic beta receptor blocking agent.

Tipula (ti·pew·lah). A genus of Diptera; crane flies. The larvae, normally burrowing and herbivorous, have been recorded in accidental intestinal myiasis. [L water spider.]

tiqui-tiqui (te·ke·te·ke). Tikitiki.

tisane (te·zahn). An infusion of a vegetable herb, usually about one-tenth the strength of the original. Tisanes are used largely by peasants in Europe. [Fr.]

Tisdall, Frederick Fitzgerald (b. 1893). Toronto paediatrician.

Kramer and Tisdall method. For calcium in serum: calcium is precipitated directly from diluted serum by addition of ammonium oxalate solution. After standing for half an hour, the precipitate is separated and washed with dilute ammonia by centrifugation, dissolved in hot dilute sulphuric acid, and titrated with M/100 potassium permanganate.

Tiselius, Arne (b. 1902). Uppsala biochemist.

Tiselius apparatus. An apparatus for the study of electrophoresis, i.e. for determining the rate of movement of charged particles or ions in an electric field.

tissue (**tis**·ew, **tish**·ew). A basic anatomical and physiological component of the living organism, consisting of a collection of cells and their intracellular matrices, one cell type predominating, e.g. muscular tissue, nervous tissue, adipose tissue, etc. **Accidental tissue.** A normal tissue found in an abnormal situation, or a tissue which is not normally found at all. **Adenoid tissue.** Lymphatic or lymphoid tissue, consisting of a collection of lymphocytes in a supporting framework of reticular cells and fibres. **Adipose tissue.** A tissue largely composed of fat cells. **Analogous tissue.** An accidental tissue (see above) similar to normal tissue in other parts of the body. **Animal tissue.** A tissue found in or derived from animal rather than plant sources. **Areolar tissue.** A loose type of connective tissue containing relatively sparse collagenous elastic and reticular fibres, fibroblasts, macrophages and other wandering cells, with supporting blood vessels, nerves and lymphatics, and an intercellular semifluid matrix containing mucopolysaccharides. **Basement tissue.** A membranous structure supporting an epithelium composed of plaited collagenous fibres and mucoproteins. **Blubbery tissue.** Tissue in which the tissue spaces are distended with lymph as in elephantiasis of an extremity. **Bony tissue.** A hard form of connective tissue consisting of a matrix of collagenous fibres, mucopolysaccharide cement and calcium phosphate, in which are buried characteristic spidery osteocytes which lie in cell spaces known as *lacunae* from which canaliculi, containing the cell processes, branch. **Brown-fat tissue.** A special form of adipose tissue (see above) in which the cells contain numerous small fatty droplets and a brown pigment. It is found in the interscapular region of rodents and hibernating animals. **Cancellous tissue.** Spongy bone, containing numerous marrow cavities, found especially towards the end of the long bones and in the interior of most flat bones. **Cartilaginous tissue.** A firm connective tissue in which the collagenous matrix is highly impregnated with mucopolysaccharide, and therefore having a special affinity for basic dyes which stain the matrix metachromatically. The cells are spherical, and usually occur in small groups of 2 to 8. **Cavernous tissue.** Erectile tissue (see below). **Cellular tissue.** One in which the cells predominate over the intercellular matrix. **Chondroid tissue.** A form of connective tissue having some of the properties of cartilage, but in which the cells predominate over the matrix. It is found in the embryonic stages of cartilage development, and in the lower vertebrates as a permanent feature of the skeleton. **Chordal tissue.** The tissue composing or derived from the notochord, as the nucleus pulposus of the intervertebral disc. The cells are large, vesicular, and the matrix gelatinous. **Chromaffin tissue.** A tissue which stains brown in the fresh state with chromium salts, due to the presence of adrenaline derivatives. It is found in the medulla of the suprarenal gland and the sympathetic paraganglia. **Cicatricial tissue.** Scar tissue (see below). **Compact tissue.** A dense form of bone composing most of the shaft of the long bones and the external layer of all bones. **Connective tissue [tela conjunctiva (NA)].** The derivatives of the embryonic mesenchyme, comprising the bones, cartilages, ligaments, tendons, fascias, and aponeuroses as well as the looser supporting tissues within and around the definitive organs. Collagenous and/or elastic fibres are universally present in the matrices of connective tissues and the basic cell type is the fibroblast, or its near relatives, the osteoblast, osteocyte, chondrocyte, and reticular cell. **Corneous tissue.** Any hard, transparent tissue. **Cribriform tissue.** Areolar tissue which has a lacy appearance when spread. **Tissue culture.** *See* CULTURE. **Dartoid tissue.** A tissue resembling the dartos layer of the scrotum which is chiefly composed of thin interlacing smooth-muscle fibres. **Dental tissue.** One of the tissues of a tooth or providing the attachment of the tooth to the jaw. **Elastic tissue [tela elastica (NA)].** A form of connective tissue containing many elastic fibres, giving the tissue elasticity and a yellowish colour. It is found characteristically in the ligamenta flava of the spinal column and in the walls of the larger blood vessels. **Embryonal connective tissue.** Mesenchyme; a loose cellular form of connective tissue, containing stellate cells and an abundant gelatinous matrix. **Endothelial tissue.** The lining epithelium of the blood vessels and lymphatics. **Episcleral tissue.** The loose connective tissue between the sclera and the conjunctiva. **Epithelial tissue.** Epithelium; the single or stratified layer of cells covering the body and lining its cavities, canals, ducts, and passages. **Erectile tissue.** A highly vascular tissue capable of engorgement with blood, or erection, such as is found in the external genitalia, the nipple, the nose, and elsewhere. **Extraperitoneal tissue [tela subserosa (NA)].** Fibro-areolar tissue between the parietal peritoneum and the abdominal wall. It varies greatly in amount at different sites, and in places contains much fat. **Fatty tissue.** Adipose tissue (see above). **Fibro-areolar tissue.** Areolar tissue (see above) in which fibres predominate. **Fibrocartilaginous tissue.** A firm connective tissue containing dense collagenous-fibre masses interspersed with islands of cartilage or chondroid tissue; or cartilage in which bands of fibrous tissue are visible in the matrix. It is found principally in the intervertebral discs. **Fibro-elastic tissue.** Elastic tissue (see above) in which the yellow fibres predominate. **Fibrohyaline tissue.** A pathological tissue in which the collagenous fibres are matted together and swollen by a mucoid substance. **Fibrous tissue, Fibrous connective tissue.** A dense form of connective tissue in which the matrix consists of closely packed strands of collagenous fibres. The term includes ligaments, tendons, and fascial membranes. **Gelatigenous tissue.** A tissue which yields gelatin on boiling, such as bone, cartilage, or any of the denser, more fibrous, connective tissues. **Gelatinous tissue.** A loose connective tissue whose matrix contains large amounts of mucoids, such as Wharton's jelly of the umbilical cord. **Glandular tissue.** A collection of epithelial secreting cells, either in small groups, or in large masses, composing the definitive glandular organs such as the liver, thyroid, etc. **Granulation tissue.** Tissue consisting of young sprouting blood vessels and cells of different types which appears in the early stages of wound healing; known to laymen as *proud flesh.* **Haemopoietic tissue.** Blood-cell-forming tissue, as in the medulla of long bones. **Heterologous tissue.** An accidental tissue (see above) not normally found anywhere in the organism. **Homologous tissue.** Tissue identical in structure and function with another in the same or another organism. **Hylic tissue.** An old term for a non-epithelial component of an embryo. **Indifferent tissue.** A tissue composed of undifferentiated cells such as those of the early embryo. **Inflammatory tissue.** In the presence of infection, profound changes occurring in the tissues, especially in the formation of new blood vessels and in the aggregation of different types of cells, mostly phagocytes. The exact type of cellular response depends on the nature of the infecting organisms. **Interstitial tissue.** 1. A specialized tissue found in the interstices of an organ, e.g. between the seminiferous tubules, or between the ovarian follicles. 2. The connective tissue within an organ surrounding and supporting the major functional elements. **Intertubular tissue.** The calcified tissue lying between the dentinal tubules in a tooth. **Junctional tissue.** The portions of the specialized conducting tissue of the heart which connect the auricles with the ventricles. It consists of the atrioventricular node and the atrioventricular bundle. **Keratinized tissue.** Epithelial tissue in which some of the cells have died and become converted into horny scales. **Laminated tissue.** A tissue in which the components are arranged in layers, such as the elastic tissue of the wall of a large blood vessel. **Lardaceous tissue.** A tissue that is occupied by amyloid. **Lepidic tissue.** An old term for an epithelial tissue of an embryo. **Lymphatic tissue.** A tissue containing more or less permanent accumulations of lymphocytes supported by a framework of reticular cells and fibres. **Lymphoid tissue.** A tissue consisting of masses of developing and mature lymphocytes supported on a framework of reticular cells and fibres. Examples are the tonsils, adenoids, and Peyer's patches of the intestine. **Mesenchymal tissue.** The embryonic mesenchyme, or a loose primitive connective tissue resembling it. **Metanephrogenic tissue.** The cells of the lower end of the intermediate mesoderm of the embryo which are differentiated into the uriniferous tubules of the metanephros, or permanent kidney. **Mucoid tissue, Mucous tissue.** A loose form of connective tissue in which the matrix appears gelatinous, due to the presence of mucopolysaccharides. It is characteristic of the early embryonic connective tissues. **Muscular tissue.** A tissue composed principally of plain, striated, voluntary, or cardiac muscle fibres. **Myeloid tissue.** The red marrow which forms both red and white blood cells. **Nephrogenic tissue.** The cells of the intermediate mesoderm of the embryo which give rise to the secretory tubules of the pronephros, mesonephros, and metanephros, in the course of development. **Nerve tissue, Nervous tissue.** Tissue from the central nervous system or the peripheral nerves, consisting of nerve cells and/or their processes, and supporting elements such as neuroglial cells and fibres, Schwann cells, and neurilemmal sheath, blood vessels, and connective tissue. **Nodal tissue.** Those portions of the specialized conducting tissue of the heart which constitute the sinu-atrial node, which acts as the cardiac pacemaker, and the atrioventricular node which initiates ventricular contraction. **Osseous tissue.** Bony tissue (see above). **Osteogenetic tissue.** A form of connective tissue which is capable of, or actually engaged in, bone formation. **Osteoid tissue.** Uncalcified bone, either as a transient stage in normal bone formation, or more permanently in rickets and some other bone diseases. **Parenchymatous tissue.** 1. The principal components of an organ, as opposed to the supporting elements such as blood vessels and connective tissue. 2. In botany, a soft cellular tissue in which cellulose walls are feebly developed. **Periodontal tissue.** The tissue immediately surrounding a tooth *in situ*; the periodontal membrane. **Primitive-pulp tissue.** 1. Hylic tissue (see above). 2. The vascular mesenchyme of the interior of a developing tooth. **Reticular tissue, Retiform tissue.** A form of connective tissue found in lymph glands, bone marrow, spleen, and elsewhere, consisting of a framework of fine reticular fibres and stellate phagocyte cells, in the meshes of which developing blood cells are found. **Rubber tissue.** Sheets of thin rubber used mainly for maintaining postoperative drainage. **Scar tissue.** When tissue has been destroyed either by injury or infection, a tough, white, inelastic, and avascular fibrous tissue which eventually fills the gap. If scar formation is excessive there may be considerable impairment of function, e.g. in the fingers. **Sclerous tissue.** The firm connective tissues such as bone, cartilage, or dense fibrous tissue. **Shock tissue.** The tissue which is most affected in anaphylactic reactions. This varies from one species of animal to another. **Simple tissue.** One with few component cell types. **Skeletal tissue.** 1. Bone or cartilage. 2. Any connective tissue. **Splenic tissue.** Splenic pulp; highly vascular tissue consisting of sinusoids lined by endothelial cells and controlled by muscular sphincters. **Subcutaneous tissue [tela subcutanea (NA)].** The loose, usually fatty, connective tissue lying just beneath the skin. **Subcutaneous fatty tissue [panniculus adiposus (NA)].** The superficial fascia; a loose connective tissue containing lobules of adipose tissue (see above), found just beneath the skin. **Sustentacular tissue.** The supporting framework of the retina, consisting mainly of Mueller's fibres, fine fibrils of which form fibre baskets, and also spider cells. **Symplastic tissue.** A mass of cytoplasm containing many nuclei without definite cell boundaries. **Vesicular supporting tissue.** Chondroid tissue (see above). **White fibrous tissue.** A connective tissue largely composed of white collagenous fibres. **Yellow elastic tissue.** A connective tissue largely composed of yellow elastic fibres. [OFr. *tissu.*]

See also: GAMGEE, HALLER, HUMAN TISSUE ACT 1961.

titanium (tit·a·ne·um). An element of atomic weight 47.90, atomic number 22, and chemical symbol Ti. It is a white metal found in certain ores, and as a micro-constituent of plants and higher animals. It is used for the making of alloys with iron, and with copper. **Titanium Dioxide BPC 1968.** Titanium oxide, TiO_2, a white powder used in paint and porcelain manufacture and to tint artificial teeth. It has an action on the skin similar to zinc oxide, and is employed in the treatment of dermatoses with exudation and to relieve pruritus. It is also used as an ingredient of face powders and other cosmetics, and to prevent sunburn, as it absorbs ultraviolet rays. **Titanium salicylate.** A compound used similarly to the sulphate. **Titanium sulphate.** $Ti_2(SO_4)_3$, a compound which has been used as a local remedy in the treatment of lupus, eczema, and conjunctivitis. **Titanium trichloride.** $TiCl_3$, a violet compound used as a reducing agent and as a reagent for the estimation of iron or nitro compounds. [Gk *Titan* giant.]

titillation (tit·il·a·shun). Tickling. [L *titillare* to tickle.]

titrate (ti·trate). To estimate by titration.

titration (ti·tra·shun). The estimation of the weight of a solute in solution by running into a measured volume of it a standard solution of a reagent from a graduated burette. The end-point, or complete equivalence of reactants, is shown either by a colour change in a suitable indicator or by the alteration in electrical state. [Fr. *titre* standard.]

titre (ti·ter). 1. The result of a titration, usually giving the amount of one substance required to equilibrate with a known amount of another substance. 2. The normality of a solution estimated by titration and usually expressed in grams or gram-molecules (moles) of solute per litre of solution. 3. A test for oils and waxes based on the solidifying point of the fatty acids obtained by saponification. 4. The extent to which an antibody containing biological substance can be diluted before losing its power of reacting specifically with the appropriate antigen; e.g. the agglutination titre of a serum. **Agglutination titre.** The highest dilution of a specified serum which will produce clumping or agglutination of a stated micro-organism. **Antistaphylococcal titre.** A serological test for staphylococcal infection. [Fr. standard.]

titrimetry (ti·trim·et·re). Analysis by the method of titration. [titre, meter.]

titubant (tit·ew·bant). A person who stumbles either in walking or in speech. [see foll.]

titubation (tit·ew·ba·shun). 1. Stumbling in walking, especially in cases of spinal lesion. 2. Restless movement observed in spinal and cerebellar diseases. **Lingual titubation.** Stammering. [L *titubare* to stagger.]

Tityus (tit·e·us). A genus of scorpions, many species of which are poisonous. **Tityus bahienis.** A tropical scorpion whose bite may be fatal in a child. **Tityus servulatus.** A poisonous scorpion. [L Illyrian river.]

tixol (tix·ol). An arsenical sheep-dip.

Tizzoni, Guido (b. 1853). Pisa physician.

Tizzoni's test. A chemical test for iron in the tissues: a section is treated with 2 per cent potassium ferrocyanide solution and, afterwards, with 0.5 per cent hydrochloric acid solution. A blue stain shows the presence of iron.

tjettek (chet·ek). A strychnine-containing arrow poison. [Javanese.]

toadhead (tode·hed). A fetal malformation of the head, approaching acephalia. [AS *tadige*, head.]

tobacco (to·bak·o). The dried and prepared leaves of the plant *Nicotiana tabacum* Linn. (family Solanaceae). The chief alkaloid present is nicotine. **Indian tobacco.** Lobelia BPC 1959. [Sp. *tabaco.*]

tobaccoism (to·bak·o·izm). Poisoning due to over-indulgence in tobacco; nicotinism.

Tobey, George Loring (b. 1881). Boston otolaryngologist.

Tobey-Ayer test. For thrombosis of the lateral cerebral sinus: pressure on one or both jugular veins normally causes a rise in pressure of the cerebrospinal fluid, and this rise can be measured by a manometer connected to a lumbar-puncture needle. In cases of lateral sinus thrombosis, no rise occurs on the affected side.

tobramycin (to·brah·mi·sin). O^6 - (3 - amino - 3 - deoxy - α - D - glycopyranosyl) - O^4 - (2,6 - diamino - 2,3,6 - trideoxy - α - D - ribohexopyranosyl) - 2 - deoxystreptamine; an antibiotic obtained from cultures of *Streptomyces tenebrarius* or the same substance obtained by any other means.

tochil (to·chil). Paragonimiasis; parasitic haemoptysis.

tocodynagraph (to·ko·**di**·nah·graf). An instrument devised to give a visual record of uterine contractions. [Gk *tokos* birth, *dynamis* power, *graphein* to record.]

tocodynamometer (to·ko·di·nam·**om**'·et·er). Tocometer. [Gk *tokos* birth, *dynamis* force, meter.]

toco-ergometry (to·ko·er·**gom**'·et·re). Measurement of the expulsive force of the uterus in labour. [Gk *tokos* birth, *ergein* to work, meter.]

tocograph (to·ko·graf). A tocometer which furnishes a continuous record of the force and frequency of uterine contractions in labour. [Gk *tokos* birth, *graphein* to write.]

tocography (to·**kog**·raf·e). The recording of the force and frequency of uterine contractions in labour. [see prec.]

tocokinin (to·ko·**ki**·nin). An oestrogenic substance prepared from yeast. [Gk *tokos* birth, *kinein* to move.]

tocology (to·**kol**·o·je). Obstetrics. [Gk *tokos* birth, *logos* science.]

tocomania (to·ko·**ma**·ne·ah). Disturbance of the mind after childbirth. [Gk *tokos* birth, *mania* madness.]

tocometer (to·**kom**·et·er). An instrument which affords a comparative indication of the force of uterine contractions in labour. [Gk *tokos* birth, meter.]

tocopherol (to·**kof**·er·ol). General chemical name for the alcohols associated as so-called antisterility factors in wheat-germ oil and designated vitamin E. They are fat-soluble oils, also occurring in lettuce and watercress, and in cotton-seed and hemp-seed oils. The most potent is α-tocopherol, $C_{29}H_{50}O_2$, also prepared synthetically, the acetate of which is used as the standard of vitamin-E activity. Others are β-tocopherol, $C_{28}H_{48}O_2$, and its isomer γ-tocopherol. [Gk *tokos* birth, *pherein* to bear, alcohol.]

tocopheryl (to·**kof**·er·il). The monovalent radical $C_{29}H_{49}O$, derived from tocopherol. **Tocopheryl Acetate BPC 1954.** $C_{31}H_{52}O_3$, the acetate of natural α-tocopherol obtainable from wheat-germ oil, or of synthetic (±)-α-tocopherol. It is one of the forms of vitamin E; as a deficiency of vitamin E seriously affects the normal pregnancy, tocopheryl acetate is used in the treatment of habitual abortion. The results are, however, conflicting.

tocophobia (to·ko·**fo**·be·ah). Unreasoning dread of childbirth. [Gk *tokos* birth, *phobein* to fear.]

tocus (to·kus). Childbirth. [Gk *tokos* birth.]

Tod, David (fl. 1832).

Tod's muscle. Auricularis posterior muscle.

Todaro, Francesco (b. 1839). Florence, Messina and Rome anatomist.

Todaro's tendon. A flat, fibrous band attached to the right margin of the trigone of the fibrous skeleton of the heart.

Todd, Frank C. (b. 1869). American ophthalmologist.

Todd's operation. For squint: a method of tendon lengthening by making three vertical cuts in the tendon stretched between two squint hooks.

Todd, John Lancelot (b. 1876). British bacteriologist.

Todd-Hewitt broth. A medium prepared from beef infused at a temperature not higher than 85°C, to which is added peptone 2 per cent, sodium chloride 0.2 per cent, sodium hydrogen phosphate 0.1 per cent, dextrose 0.1 per cent, and sodium bicarbonate 0.2 per cent.

Todd, Robert Bentley (b. 1809). London physician.

Todd's cirrhosis. Hypertrophic cirrhosis. *See* CIRRHOSIS.

Todd's paralysis. Transient postepileptic paralysis of a limb which is involved in jacksonian convulsions.

Todd's ascending process. The membranous layer of superficial fascia of the anterior abdominal wall.

Toddalia (tod·a·le·ah). A genus of rutaceous shrubs. The root of *Toddalia aculeata* has been used as an aromatic stomachic in East Indian medicine.

toddy (tod·e). 1. Whisky or gin with hot water and sugar added. 2. The sap, fermented or plain, of various species of palm trees. [Hind. *tādi.*]

todophthalein (to·do·**thal**·e·in). The disodium salt of tetra-iodophenolphthalein.

Todrazoline (to·**draz**·o·leen). BP Commission approved name for ethyl 3-phthalazin-1-ylcarbazate; an antihypertensive agent.

toe [digitus pedis (NA)] (to). A digit of the foot. The dorsal [facies dorsalis (NA)] and plantar [facies plantaris (NA)] surfaces are differentiated, as are the lateral [facies laterales (NA)] and medial [facies mediales (NA)] margins. **Big toe [hallux (digitus I) NA].** The first toe; the toe on the medial side of the foot. **Clawed toes.** Fixed flexion deformity of the interphalangeal joints of the toes. **First toe.** Big toe (see above). **Flexed toe.** Deformity of the toe in which both interphalangeal joints are fixed in flexion. **Great toe.** Big toe (see above). **Hammer toe.** A deformed toe in which the terminal interphalangeal joint is hyperextended, the proximal interphalangeal joint hyperflexed and the metatarsophalangeal joint hyperextended. The condition nearly always affects the second toe. **Hong Kong toe.** Fungous infection of the big toe by *Epidermophyton floccosum.* **Little toe [digitus minimus (digitus V) NA].** The small toe on the lateral side of the foot. **Mallet toe.** Hammer toe (see above). **Mango toe.** Hong Kong toe (see above); so-called because in India the condition is prevalent in the mango season. **Ostlers' toe.** A toe in which the nail becomes thick and curved. It is the result of trauma, e.g. a horse treading on it, and is also called *onychogryphosis.* **Pigeon toe.** Pes adductus. **Second, third and fourth toes [digiti II-IV (NA)].** The toes between the big toe and the little toe. **Webbed toes.** A condition in which the toes are connected together by webs of skin. [AS *tá.*]

See also: MORTON (T. G.).

Toepfer, Alfred Eduard (b. 1858). German physician.

Toepfer's reagent. For free hydrochloric acid in gastric juice: dissolve 0.5 g of dimethylamino-azobenzene in 100 ml of 95 per cent alcohol.

Toepfer's test. For free hydrochloric acid in gastric contents: a bright red colour upon addition to gastric contents of a few drops of 0.5 per cent alcoholic dimethyl yellow indicates free mineral acid.

Tofenacin (to·**fen**·as·in). BP Commission approved name for *N*-methyl-2-(2-methylbenzhydryloxy)-ethylamine; it is used in the treatment of Parkinson's syndrome.

togaviruses (to·gah·vi·rus·ez). Arboviruses (groups A and B).

Togna exercises. A system of self-applied massage and exercises carried out in the bath and reputed to improve circulatory efficiency; named after the originator.

toilet (toi·let). The cleansing of the parts after childbirth or of a wound after an operation, involving the removal of damaged tissue and foreign bodies and the washing of raw surfaces of the skin around them. [Fr. *toilette.*]

Toison, Jules (b. 1858). French histologist.

Toison's diluting fluid, mixture, or solution. A diluting solution containing sodium chloride 1 g, sodium sulphate 8 g, methyl violet 5B 0.025 g, neutral glycerin 30 ml, distilled water 180 ml, used as a diluent in the counting of red blood corpuscles.

toko-. For words beginning with *Toko-, see* TOCO-.

Tolamolol (tol·**am**·o·lol). BP Commission approved name for 4 - [2 - (2 - hydroxy - 3 - *o* - tolyloxypropylamino) - ethoxyl]-benzamide; an adrenergic beta receptor blocking agent.

Tolazamide (tol·**az**·am·ide). BP Commission approved name for 1,1 - hexamethylene - 4 - toluene - *p* - sulphonylsemicarbazide; an oral hypoglycaemic agent.

Tolazoline Hydrochloride BP 1973 (tol·**az**·o·leen hi·dro·**klor**·ide). 2-Benzyliminazoline hydrochloride; a vasodilator which stimulates the secretion of hydrochloric acid. It is used in bedsores and slow-healing ulcerations, and as a substitute for histamine.

Tolbutamide BP 1973 (tol·**bew**·tam·ide). *N*-Butyl-*N'*-toluene-*p*-sulphonylurea; it is used in the treatment of certain types of diabetes mellitus in adults.

Tolbutamidum (tol·bew·**tam**·id·um). *European Pharmacopoeia* name for Tolbutamide BP 1973.

Toldt, Karl (b. 1840). Prague and Vienna anatomist.

Toldt's fascia. A fascial plane behind the pancreas.

Toldt's membrane. The anterior layer of the renal fascia.

tolerance (**tol**·er·ans). 1. Lessened response to the action of a drug, so that a larger dose than usual must be given to produce its characteristic effect. 2. The degree of response to a drug or test substance, e.g. insulin or glucose, in comparison with the normal. **Acquired tolerance.** Tolerance which has developed as a result of the repeated use of a drug. **Cross tolerance.** Tolerance which has been acquired to one drug, and which is manifested also towards other drugs generally closely related chemically or in their pharmacological actions. **G tolerance.** The greatest inertial force that an individual or an animal can tolerate without significant loss of function. It is expressed as the number of G acting on the body times duration of action. **Glucose tolerance.** The ability of the body to maintain the blood sugar within normal limits after the ingestion or injection of glucose. **Immunological tolerance.** An immunological unresponsiveness or tolerance of the lymphoid tissues to an antigen ordinarily capable of inducing a humoral or cell-mediated response; it may follow contact with the antigen in fetal or neonatal life, or in adults after very large or very small doses of certain antigens (*acquired tolerance*). **Individual tolerance.** Unusually slight (or absent) response to a drug occurring in a particular person or animal. **Insulin tolerance.** The response of the blood sugar level to the intravenous injection of a standard dose of insulin, compared with the normal response. **Species tolerance.** Individual tolerance (see above) present as a characteristic of a particular species of animal. **Sugar tolerance.** The ability of the body to deal with ingested sugar; it is measured as the maximum amount of sugar that can be taken without its causing an undue increase of blood sugar or appearing in the urine. [L *tolerare* to endure.]

tolerant (**tol**·er·ant). Possessing tolerance.

toleration (tol·er·**a**·shun). Tolerance.

tolerific (tol·er·**if**·ik). Promoting tolerance. [tolerance, L *facere* to make.]

tolidine (**tol**·id·een). Dimethyldiaminodiphenyl, $(CH_3)_2C_6H_3C_6H_3(NH_2)_2$. A compound which occurs in four isomeric forms. The *ortho* form is used in the manufacture of dyes.

tolite (**tol**·ite). The explosive, trinitrotoluene.

Tollens, Bernhard Christian Gottfried (b. 1841). German chemist.

Tollens' test. 1. For glucuronic acid in urine: to 5 ml of urine add 1 ml of 1 per cent naphthoresorcinol in 95 per cent alcohol and 5 ml of concentrated hydrochloric acid. Boil for 1 min, stand 4 min, cool and extract with an equal volume of ether. A violet-red colour in the ether layer indicates glucuronic acid. 2. Phloroglucin–hydrochloric acid reaction: to the solution add an equal volume of hydrochloric acid (sp.gr. 1.09) and a little phloroglucinol. Heat in boiling water. A red colour indicates galactose, pentose, or glucuronic acid.

tollwut (tol·**voot**). Rabies. [G.]

Tolnaftate BP 1973 (tol·**naf**·tate). *O*-2-naphthyl *N*-methyl-*m*-tolylthiocarbamate; it is used in the treatment of fungal infections.

Tolpentamide (tol·**pen**·tam·ide). BP Commission approved name for *N* - cyclopentyl - *N'* - toluene - *p* - sulphonylurea; a hypoglycaemic agent.

Tolperisone (tol·**per**·iz·one). BP Commission approved name for 2 - methyl - 3 - piperidino - 1 - *p* - tolylpropan - 1 - one; a muscle relaxant.

Tolpiprazole (tol·**pip**·raz·ole). BP Commission approved name for 5-methyl - 3 - [2 - (4 - *m* - tolylpiperazin - 1 - yl) - ethyl]pyrazole; a tranquillizer.

Tolpronine (**tol**·pro·neen). BP Commission approved name for 1 - (1,2,3,6 - tetrahydropyridino) - 3 - *o* - tolyloxypropan - 2 - ol; an analgesic.

Tolpropamine (tol·**pro**·pam·een). BP Commission approved name for *N,N* - dimethyl - 3 - phenyl - 3 - *p* - tolylpropylamine; an antihistaminic agent.

toluene (**tol**·ew·een). Toluole, methylbenzene, $C_6H_5CH_3$. An aromatic volatile liquid, homologous with benzene and found with it in coal tar. It also occurs in Tolu balsam, whence the name. It is highly inflammable, and is used as a solvent; it is also employed in the manufacture of drugs, dyestuffs, and explosives.

toluenediamine (tol·ew·een·**di**'·am·een). Tolylenediamine.

toluene-sodium-sulphochloramide (tol·ew·een·**so**·de·um·sul·fo·**klor**'·am·ide). Chloramine-T.

toluenesulphodichloramide (tol·ew·een·sul·fo·di·**klor**'·am·ide). Dichloramine-T.

toluidine (tol·**ew**·id·een). Aminotoluene, $C_6H_4(CH_3)(NH_2)$. A derivative of toluene occurring in three isomers, the *ortho*, the *meta*, and the *para*. The first two are liquid; the last a solid. They are intermediates in the synthesis of certain drugs and dyestuffs.

Toluidine blue. A stain used in microscopy.

toluole (**tol**·ew·ole). Toluene.

tolusafranine (tol·ew·**saf**·ran·een). Brilliant safranine, $(CH_3)(NH_2)C_6H_2N_2(C_6H_5)C_6H_2(CH_3)(NH_2)Cl$. A safranine dye derived from aniline and toluidine; used to dye cotton and silk.

toluyl (**tol**·ew·il). The acyl group $CH_3C_6H_4CO$, derived from toluic acid.

toluylene (**tol**·ew·il·een). Cresylene; the group $CH_3C_6H_3$, derived from toluene. **Toluylene blue.** An indamine dyestuff used as an indicator in oxidation-reduction reactions. **Toluylene red.** An azine dyestuff.

Tolycaine (**tol**·e·kane). BP Commission approved name for methyl 2-diethylaminoacetamido -*m*-toluate; a local anaesthetic.

tolyl (**tol**·il). The group $CH_3C_6H_4$, derived from toluene; isomeric with the benzyl group. **Tolyl hydroxide.** Cresol, $CH_3C_6H_4OH$. **Tolyl salicylate.** $C_6H_4(OH)COOC_6H_4(CH_3)$, an antiseptic derived from cresol.

tolylantipyrine (tol·il·an·te·**pi**'·reen). A toluene analogue of phenazone (antipyrin), used as an analgesic. **Tolylantipyrine salicylate.** The salicylate of tolylantipyrine used in rheumatic conditions.

tolylenediamine (tol·il·een·**di**'·am·een). Toluenediamine, $CH_3C_6H_3(NH_2)_2$. A compound used in the manufacture of dyestuffs. It is reputed to have a cholagogue action.

tolypyrine (tol·e·**pi**·reen). Tolylantipyrine.

tolysal (**tol**·e·sal). Tolylantipyrine salicylate.

tomato (tom·**ah**·to). The edible fruit of the plant *Lycopers cum esculentum* (family Solanaceae). It is rich in vitamin C. [Mexican *tomatl*.]

tomentum (to·**men**·tum). The mass of minute blood vessels between the pia mater and the brain cortex. [L stuffing.]

Tomes, Sir Charles Sissmore (b. 1846). London dental surgeon.

Tomes' processes. Ameloblastic processes; short processes, hexagonal in shape, found at the basal ends of the ameloblasts.

Tomes, Sir John (b. 1815). London dental surgeon.

Tomes' fibre, or fibril. A process of an odontoblast whose ramifications occupy a dentinal tubule of a tooth.

granular layer of Tomes. A zone produced by a number of irregular spaces contained in the outermost layer of dentine of the root of a tooth.

Tommaselli, Salvatore (b. 1830). Italian physician.

Tommaselli's disease, or syndrome. Quinine poisoning causing haematuria and pyrexia.

Tommasi, L. Italian physician.

Tommasi's sign. Alopecia of the posterolateral aspects of the legs, indicative of gout in males.

tomogram (**to**·mo·gram). A radiograph produced by tomography. [Gk *tome* section, *gramma* record.]

tomograph (**to**·mo·graf). An x-ray apparatus which makes a radiograph of a layer of the body tissue at any required depth. [Gk *tome* section, *graphein* to record.]

tomography (to·**mog**·raf·e). Body-section radiography. **Hypocycloid tomography.** Body-section radiography in which the x-ray tube traverses a non-linear pathway. **Linear tomography.** Body-section radiography in which the x-ray tube traverses a linear pathway. **Ultrasonic tomography.** Scanning various parts of the body by ultrasound. *See* RADIOGRAPHY. [see prec.]

tomotocia (to·mo·to·she·ah). Caesarean birth. [Gk *tome* section, *tokos* birth.]

tonaphasia (ton·af·a·ze·ah). A form of aphasia in which the patient has lost the power of singing. [Gk *tonos* stretching, a-, *phasis* speech.]

tonco bean (tong·ko been). Tonka seed.

tone (tone). 1. The quality of a sound which primarily depends upon the frequency of vibrations, or pitch. 2. The state of bodily organs that are functioning normally in a person in good health. 3. A mental or moral attitude or atmosphere. **Feeling tone.** The mental state or feeling which accompanies a thought or action. **Finger tone.** The sound heard when a finger is placed on the diaphragm of a phonendoscope. **Heart tone.** The state of the heart muscle in which the fibres do not fully relax but maintain their position in partial contraction, **Jecoral tone.** The note produced by percussion over the liver. **Muscle tone.** The state of partial contraction in which the muscles maintain their posture without fully relaxing. It is due to low-frequency asynchronous impulses from the anterior horn cells which produce a partial tetanus. **Plastic tone.** The condition of muscles which enables them to maintain their position indefinitely, e.g. a limb may remain in the position in which it has been placed by an observer. **Stomach tone.** The postural activity of the muscles of the stomach which enables the organ to adapt itself to the volume of its contents. **Summational tones.** Theoretically, when two pure tones are sounded in unison, a tone whose frequency is the sum of the exciting tones should be produced. This summational tone is difficult for the human ear to perceive, possibly because it is of higher frequency than the other two tones, and also because of their masking effect. [Gk *tonos* stretching.]

tonga (tong·gah). 1. A mixture of medicinal barks from Fiji, taken for neuritis. 2. A local name for yaws in New Caledonia.

tongs (tongz). **Ice tongs.** In orthopaedic surgery, a steel caliper used for skeletal traction. The spikes of the caliper are driven into the bone and a weight is attached. [AS *tange.*]

tongue [lingua (NA)] (tung). A muscular organ, partly in the mouth, partly in the pharynx, for mastication, swallowing, tasting, and speaking. **Adherent tongue.** A tongue which is attached by adhesions or folds of mucous membrane to the floor and sides of the mouth. **Apex of the tongue.** Tip of the tongue (see below). **Baked tongue.** The dry tongue, with brown fur, in certain severe cases of typhoid fever. **Bald tongue.** A smooth tongue in which the filiform papillae have been destroyed from chronic glossitis, as in idiopathic hypochromic anaemia. **Bifid tongue.** A tongue divided by a longitudinal fissure. **Black tongue, Black hairy tongue.** A brown or black patch on the dorsum of the tongue, or discoloured elongated filiform papillae; usually due to heavy smoking or broad spectrum antibiotic therapy. **Body of the tongue [corpus linguae (NA)].** The main part of the tongue excluding the apex and root. **Bulky tongue.** An excessively large tongue, particularly in its anterior portion, which can cause irregularities of the anterior teeth. **Burning tongue.** Glossodynia. **Cardinal tongue.** A bright-red inflamed tongue; it is seen in pellagra. **Cerebriform tongue.** Scrotal tongue (see below). **Choreic tongue.** The tongue in chorea, which is abruptly protruded and withdrawn, thrust into one cheek or smacked against the palate. **Cleft tongue.** Bifid tongue (see above). **Coated tongue.** A furred tongue in which the surface is covered with a whitish or brown accumulation of desquamated epithelial cells, food debris, bacteria, mycelia, etc. **Cobblestone tongue.** Leucoplakia. **Crocodile tongue.** Scrotal tongue (see below). **Dorsum of the tongue [dorsum linguae (NA)].** The upper surface of the tongue. **Dotted tongue.** A tongue which is stippled with fur deposited on the papillae. **Double tongue.** Bifid tongue (see above). **Dry tongue.** The tongue in conditions of dehydration, **Earthy tongue.** A tongue coated with rough calcareous material. **Encrusted tongue.** A heavily coated tongue. **Fern-leaf tongue.** A tongue with a central furrow from which branch-off lateral furrows. **Frog tongue.** Ranula. **Furred tongue.** A tongue coated with fur. **Furrowed tongue.** Scrotal tongue (see below). **Geographical tongue.** A tongue bearing rounded red patches with grey margins. The patches are inconstant, change their shape in a short time and fuse with other patches, thus resembling the outlines of a map. **Glassy tongue, Glazed tongue.** The smooth shining tongue of chronic superficial glossitis. **Grooved tongue.** Scrotal tongue (see below). **Hairy tongue.** A tongue with a blackish patch on the dorsum on which the filiform papillae are much elongated and thickened like bristly hairs. **Lobulated tongue.** A congenital condition in which the tongue is divided into lobules by deep fissures. **Magenta tongue.** A tongue with a magenta coloration; it occurs in riboflavine deficiency. **Mappy tongue.** Geographical tongue (see above). **Parrot tongue.** A dry, shrunken, horn-like tongue which is protruded with difficulty; it is seen in low fevers. **Plastered tongue.** A thickly coated tongue. **Plicated tongue.** Scrotal tongue (see below). **Raspberry tongue.** *See* STRAWBERRY TONGUE (below). **Raw-beef tongue.** A bright-red tongue that occurs in certain conditions, e.g. macrocytic anaemia in remission, and diabetes. **Root of the tongue [radix linguae (NA)].** The attachment of the tongue to the hyoid bone, mandible, and floor of the mouth. **Scrotal tongue.** A tongue much furrowed and corrugated like the skin of the scrotum. **Slit tongue.** Bifid tongue (see above). **Smokers' tongue.** Leucoplakia. **Sprue tongue.** The characteristic tongue of sprue; it consists of aphthous vesicles, atrophy of the filiform papillae, and inflammation of the fungiform papillae. **Stamp-lickers' tongue.** Glossitis from the irritation of gum. **Stippled tongue.** A tongue in which the papillae are covered with fur. **Strawberry tongue.** A tongue with swollen, red, prominent papillae protruding throught the white fur, called by some the *white strawberry tongue*; seen typically in the stage of invasion of scarlet fever and in other diseases such as diphtheria and measles. About the fourth day of scarlet fever, the tongue is mainly clean, hyperaemic, and vivid red in colour; this is the characteristic *red strawberry* or *raspberry* tongue. **Sulcated tongue.** Scrotal tongue (see above). **Surface of the tongue, inferior [facies inferior (linguae) NA].** The under surface of the tongue bearing the frenulum and the fimbriated folds. **Surface of the tongue, superior.** Dorsum of the tongue (see above). **Tip of the tongue [apex linguae (NA)].** The anterior part of the tongue that rests against the incisor teeth. **Transition tongue.** The intermediate stage between the *strawberry* and *raspberry* tongues, when the features of both are seen in different areas of the tongue. **White tongue.** 1. A tongue coated with white fur. 2. A tongue coated with a film of thrush fungus (*Candida albicans*). **Wooden tongue.** A hard tongue affected with actinomycosis; it occurs in cattle. [AS *tunge.*]

See also: SANDWITH.

tongue, muscles of the [musculi linguae (NA)]. Those on which the shape and movements of the tongue depend. **Longitudinal muscles of the tongue, superior and inferior [musculi longitudinales, superior et inferior (NA)].** Two bands of longitudinally running intrinsic muscles of the tongue. When contracting they shorten the tongue, and raise (superior muscle) or depress (inferior muscle) the tip. **Transverse muscle of the tongue [musculus transversus linguae (NA)].** A transversely coursing intrinsic muscle of the tongue; when contracting, it narrows and lengthens the organ. **Vertical muscle of the tongue [musculus verticalis linguae (NA)].** A vertically coursing intrinsic muscle of the tongue, lying close to the tip; when contracting, it flattens and broadens the organ.

tongue-swallowing (tung·swol·ow·ing). The slipping back of the tongue into the pharynx in an unconscious person lying on his back; respiration is thus seriously impeded. [tongue, swallow.]

tongue-tie (tung·ti). A congenital shortening of the frenulum which prevents the tongue from being protruded. [tongue, AS *tigan.*]

tonic (ton·ik). 1. Possessing tone; in a state of partial and continuous contraction. 2. A drug, or pharmaceutical preparation of drugs, which sustains, strengthens, or improves the functions of the body, or of any of its organs or tissues; or more generally, which increases the patient's feeling of well-being. The use of most so-called *tonics* lacks pharmacological justification. **Bitter tonic.** A drug or preparation with a bitter taste, whose chief action and use is to stimulate the appetite. **Cardiac tonic.** A drug which increases the contractile power of the myocardium, e.g. digitalis. [Gk *tonikos* of stretching.]

tonicity (ton·is·it·e). 1. The normal state of muscular tension; the healthy elasticity of the tissues. 2. The osmotic tension of a fluid. [Gk *tonikos* of stretching.]

tonicoclonic (**ton**·ik·o·**klon**′·ik). Tonoclonic.

tonitrophobia (**ton**·it·ro·**fo**′·be·ah). An abnormal fear of thunder. [L *tonitrus* thunder, Gk *phobein* to fear.]

tonka, tonka seed (**tong**·kah, **tong**·kah seed). The seed of *Dipteryx odorata* (Aubl.) Willd., a large tree native to Brazil (Dutch tonka bean), and of *D. oppositifolia* (Aubl.) Willd., a tree indigenous to Brazil (English tonka bean), both of the family Leguminosae. The active constituent is coumarin, used as a flavouring agent. [Guiana *tonca.*]

tonnenem (ton·e·nem). A term used in von Pirquet's system to denote the nutritive value of 1 kg of human milk; it is equivalent to 1000 nems. [Fr. *tonne* ton, nem.]

tonoclonic (ton·o·**klon**·ik). Describing muscular spasms that are both tonic and clonic.

tonofibril (ton·o·**fi**·bril). Thin fibrils or striae observed in epithelial cells and thought to be supporting in function. [Gk *tonos* stretching, fibril.]

tonogram (**to**·no·gram). A record made by a recording tonometer, an apparatus for determining the partial pressure of gases in the blood. [Gk *tonos* stretching, *gramma* record.]

tonograph (**to**·no·graf). A tonometer that affords a continuous record of tensions. [Gk *tonos* stretching, *graphein* to write.]

tonometer (to·**nom**·et·er). 1. An instrument for measuring tension. There are many types, e.g. for measuring the partial pressure of gases in solution, of muscle, and of blood vessels. 2. In ophthalmology, an instrument for measuring the intra-ocular tension by the impressibility of the globe. **Applanation tonometer.** One which measures the force necessary to flatten a given area of cornea. It is more accurate than the impression tonometer. **Impression tonometer.** One which measures the amount of indentability of the cornea with certain weights, e.g. Schiøtz and McLean's. [Gk *tonos* stretching, *metron* measure.]

See also: GAERTNER (G.), MCLEAN, MUSKENS, RECKLINGHAUSEN, SCHIØTZ.

tonometry (to·**nom**·et·re). The measurement of tension. **Digital tonometry.** Estimation of intra-ocular pressure by pressing a finger on the eyeball. [see prec.]

tonoplast (to·no·plast). An intracellular vacuole surrounded by a semipermeable membrane and capable of osmotic swelling. [Gk *tonos* stretching, *plassein* to mould.]

tonoscillograph (to·**nos**·il·o·graf). An apparatus that affords a record of the arterial pressure with the corresponding pulse tracing. [Gk *tonos* stretching, L *oscillare* to swing, Gk *graphein* to write.]

tonquin bean (**tong**·kwin been). Tonka seed. [Tonka, AS *bean.*]

tonquinol (**tong**·kwin·ol). Trinitrobutyltoluene $C_6H(CH_3)(C_4H_9)(NO_2)_3$. An artificial musk used in perfumery.

tonsil (**ton**·sil). 1. A mass of lymphoid tissue, in particular the palatine tonsil. 2. Any anatomical structure similar to the palatine tonsil. **Buried tonsil.** A tonsil in which the greatest mass is buried in the palate, with little projection of the tonsil body beyond the faucial pillars. **Tonsil of the cerebellum [tonsilla cerebelli].** A rounded, circumscribed part of the inferior surface of each cerebellar hemisphere adjoining the uvula of the inferior vermis. **Lingual tonsil [tonsilla lingualis].** A collection of lymphoid tissue in the submucous layer of the posterior one-third, or pharyngeal, part of the tongue. **Nasopharyngeal tonsil [tonsilla pharyngea].** A mass of lymphoid tissue in the roof and posterior wall of the nasopharynx. It is often referred to, when enlarged, as *adenoids.* **Palatine tonsil [tonsilla palatina].** A mass of lymphoid tissue on the side wall of the oral part of the pharynx between the palatoglossal and palatopharyngeal arches. **Submerged tonsil.** Buried tonsil (see above). **Tube tonsil [tonsilla tubaria].** The lymphoid tissue surrounding the opening of the pharyngotympanic tube. [L *tonsilla.*]

See also: GERLACH, LUSCHKA.

tonsillar (**ton**·sil·ar). Relating to a tonsil.

tonsillar artery [ramus tonsillaris]. The main blood supply of the tonsil, entering the lower lateral part. It arises from the facial artery, and pierces the superior constrictor muscle.

tonsillectome (ton·sil·**ek**·tome). A surgical instrument employed in tonsillectomy.

tonsillectomy (ton·sil·**ek**·to·me). Surgical excision of a tonsil. **Suction tonsillectomy.** A method of removing the tonsils by suction; it is reputed to obviate undue haemorrhage, but it is not a generally accepted method. [tonsil, Gk *ektome* excision.]

tonsillith (**ton**·sil·ith). Tonsillolith.

tonsillitic (ton·sil·**it**·ik). Referring to tonsillitis.

tonsillitis (ton·sil·**i**·tis). Inflammation of the tonsil. **Acute catarrhal tonsillitis.** A mild form of tonsillitis associated with a catarrhal exudate over the tonsil. **Acute parenchymatous tonsillitis.** A severe form of tonsillitis similar to quinsy. **Caseous tonsillitis.** An inflammation of the tonsil associated with the discharge of caseous material from the crypts. **Diphtheritic tonsillitis.** Tonsillitis associated with the deposit of diphtheritic membrane on the tonsil. **Erythematous tonsillitis.** A mild acute tonsillitis. **Follicular tonsillitis.** Tonsillitis associated with purulent infection of the tonsillar crypts. **Herpetic tonsillitis.** A herpes which forms on, or in the region of, the tonsil. **Lacunar tonsillitis.** Tonsillitis associated with the formation of caseous material in the crypts. **Lingular tonsillitis.** Inflammation of the lymphoid tissue on the base of the tongue, on the lingual tonsil. **Mycotic tonsillitis.** Inflammation of the tonsil resulting from a fungus infection. **Phlegmonous tonsillitis.** A severe gangrenous inflammation of the tonsil associated with profound constitutional disturbances. **Pustular tonsillitis.** A condition resembling follicular tonsillitis (see above). **Streptococcus tonsillitis.** Tonsillitis resulting from infection by one of the streptococcal organisms. **Suppurative tonsillitis.** Acute parenchymatous tonsillitis (see above). [tonsil, Gk *-itis* inflammation.]

See also: VINCENT.

tonsillohemisporosis (**ton**·sil·o·hem·e·spo·**ro**′·sis). Mycosis of the tonsils due to infection by the fungus *Hemispora stellata.* [tonsil, hemisporosis.]

tonsillolith (**ton**·sil·o·lith). A stone or calculus in the crypt of a tonsil. [tonsil, Gk *lithos* stone.]

tonsillomoniliasis (**ton**·sil·o·mon·il·**i**′·as·is). Infection of the tonsils by species of the fungus *Candida (Monilia).* [tonsil, moniliasis.]

tonsillomycosis (**ton**·sil·o·mi·**ko**′·sis). Any infection of the tonsils caused by a fungus. [tonsil, mycosis.]

tonsillopathy (ton·sil·**op**·ath·e). Any morbid condition of the tonsils. [tonsil, Gk *pathos* disease.]

tonsilloscope (**ton**·sil·o·skope). Any device for examining the tonsils. [tonsil, Gk *skopein* to view.]

tonsilloscopy (ton·sil·**os**·ko·pe). Examination of the tonsils by means of a tonsilloscope.

tonsillotome (**ton**·sil·o·tome). A surgical instrument employed in tonsillectomy.

tonsillotomy (ton·sil·**ot**·o·me). 1. The surgical operation for the removal of a part of a tonsil. 2. Incision of a tonsil. [tonsil, Gk *temnein* to cut.]

tonsilsector (ton·sil·**sek**·tor). A form of tonsillotome, being a pair of round scissor blades within a guard ring. [tonsil, L *secare* to cut.]

tonsolith (**ton**·so·lith). Tonsillolith.

tonus (**to**·nus). A state of slight tension usually present in muscles even when they are not undergoing active contraction. In skeletal muscle the tonus is neurogenic, in involuntary muscle it is myogenic. **Acerebral tonus.** Usually called decerebrate rigidity; a state of tonic contraction in both flexor and extensor skeletal muscle after removal of the cerebrum. **Chemical tonus.** The state of slight chemical activity occurring in resting muscles. **Muscle tonus.** Muscle tone. *See* TONE. **Myogenic tonus.** The state of tonus such as is seen in involuntary muscle; it is intrinsic, i.e. independent of the nervous system. **Neurogenic tonus.** The state of tonus such as is seen in skeletal muscle; it is dependent on low-frequency nerve impulses. [Gk *tonos* tension.]

Tooke, Frederick T. Montreal ophthalmologist.

Tooke's corneal splitter. An instrument with a flat, rounded, sharp blade in common use in ophthalmic surgery for splitting the corneal lamella at the limbus in order to expose the part of the cornea for excision in the corneoscleral trephine or similar procedure. It can be straight or angled.

Tooth, Howard Henry (b. 1856). London neurologist.

Tooth's type, Charcot–Marie–Tooth atrophy, disease, or type, Marie–Tooth disease. Peroneal muscular atrophy; a familial disease of the spinal cord characterized by wasting and weakness of distal muscles in the lower and upper limbs; there is usually pes cavus, and appreciation of vibration and position may be impaired in the lower limbs.

tooth [dens (NA)] (tooth) (pl. *teeth*). One of the hard structures for cutting and mastication of food; in mammals they occur only in the jaws. They are composed of dentine, covered on the crown by enamel and on the root by cementum, which is attached to the alveolar bone by the periodontal membrane. **Anterior tooth.** Either an incisor or a canine tooth. **Auditory teeth [dentes acustici (NA)].** The auditory teeth of Huschke. *See* HUSCHKE. **Barred tooth.** A tooth with splayed roots, and therefore difficult to extract. **Biscuspid tooth.** Premolar tooth (see below). **Buccal tooth.** Either a molar or a premolar tooth. **Canine teeth [dentes canini (NA)].** The dog teeth, so-called because they are the most prominent teeth in dogs. There are four, two in the upper and two in the lower jaw. The upper canine teeth are the teeth immediately behind the premaxillary sutures; the lower canine teeth are the teeth which bite immediately in front of the upper canine teeth. **Cheek tooth.** Either a molar or a premolar tooth. **Conical tooth.** A tooth with a cone-shaped crown. **Crown of a tooth [corona dentis (NA)].** The portion of a tooth which is covered by enamel. **Cuspid teeth.** Canine teeth (see above). **Dead tooth.** Devitalized tooth (see below). **Deciduous tooth [dens deciduus (NA)].** A tooth of the first, or milk, dentition, which is completed by about 2 years of age and comprises two incisors, one canine and two milk molars in each half of each jaw. These teeth are replaced by teeth of the permanent dentition by about 12 years of age. **Devitalized tooth.** A tooth whose pulp has been removed; a dead tooth. **Dog teeth.** Canine teeth (see above). **Eye tooth.** A canine tooth in the upper jaw. **Functionless tooth.** A tooth that is unopposed as a result of extraction of the antagonist in the opposite jaw without replacement by an artificial substitute. **Geminated teeth.** Teeth which are joined together, as in true or physiological gemination, when fusion occurs between two tooth germs each of which forms a tooth, or in false or pathological gemination, when two completely formed teeth, usually the upper second and third molar teeth, are united by secondary or pathological cementum formed around their roots. **Hypoplastic tooth.** A tooth whose enamel is grooved or pitted, and whose dentine presents an abnormally large number of interglobular spaces as a result of disturbances of calcification. **Impacted tooth.** An abnormally placed tooth that from its position cannot erupt normally; commonly a lower, third molar tooth. **Incisor tooth [dens incisivus (NA)].** One of the front biting teeth, four in number in each jaw and characterized by a chisel-shaped crown and a single root lying anterior to the canine teeth in the arch. **Labial tooth.** Either an incisor or a canine tooth. **Malacotic tooth.** An imperfectly formed tooth which is very liable to decay. **Malposed tooth.** An abnormally placed tooth. **Mandibular tooth.** One of the teeth of the lower jaw. **Maxillary tooth.** One of the teeth of the upper jaw. **Milk tooth.** Deciduous tooth (see above). **Molar tooth [dens molaris (NA)].** One of the grinding teeth, with a broad tuberculated crown and cusps on its occlusal surface. There are four in the deciduous dentition and six in the permanent dentition in each jaw. Each usually has two or three roots. **Mottled tooth.** A tooth whose enamel shows irregular patches of white or brownish pigmentation usually associated with drinking water containing more than 0.9 parts per million of fluorides during tooth calcification. **Mulberry tooth.** Mulberry molar. *See* MOLAR. **Neck of a tooth [collum (cervix) dentis (NA)].** The part of the tooth between the crown and root, usually constricted and normally surrounded by the gum. **Notched tooth.** A normal newly erupted incisor tooth with two notches and three tubercles on its incisive edge; a permanent incisor tooth whose middle tubercle is absent, the incisive edge taking the shape of a crescentic notch in a patient with hereditary syphilis; a hutchinsonian incisor. **Peg-top tooth.** A conical tooth. **Permanent tooth [dens permanens (NA)].** A tooth of the second dentition, which is complete by 25 years of age and can persist for the remainder of life. They total 32 in all, comprising two incisors, one canine, two premolars and three molars in each half of each jaw. **Pink teeth.** A post-mortem staining of the teeth due to coloration by dissolved blood pigments, commonly seen in immersion and burial. **Plastic tooth.** An artificial tooth made of synthetic resins. **Porcelain tooth.** An artificial tooth made of porcelain. **Premolar tooth [dens premolaris (NA)].** One of the two teeth on each side of each jaw immediately behind the canine tooth in the permanent dentition, characterized by the possession of two cusps on the crown and generally a single or double root. It is preceded by a deciduous molar tooth. **Pulp of a tooth [pulpa dentis (NA)].** The highly vascular and sensitive loose connective tissue occupying the pulp cavity in the centre of the crown, neck, and root of a tooth. **Rake teeth.** Teeth with unduly wide spaces between them. **Root of a tooth [radix dentis (NA)].** The part of the tooth embedded in the jaw bone. **Successional teeth.** The permanent teeth which replace those of the deciduous or temporary dentition. **Superior tooth.** Maxillary tooth (see above). **Supernumerary tooth.** A tooth additional to the normal dentition which resembles the general shape of the adjacent teeth. **Supplemental tooth.** A tooth additional to the normal dentition which is dissimilar in shape to that of the adjacent teeth. **Surface of a tooth, axial.** A surface that lies parallel to its long axis. **Surface of a tooth, buccal.** Vestibular surface (see below). **Surface of a tooth, contact [facies contactus (NA)].** That surface which is in contact with the corresponding surface of the next tooth in the same jaw. With incisor and canine teeth, this gives rise to a medial and a lateral surface. With the premolars and molars, the surfaces are anterior and posterior. **Surface of a tooth, distal [facies distalis (NA)].** That surface which is in contact with the tooth behind it in the dental arch. **Surface of a tooth, facial.** The buccal or labial surface. **Surface of a tooth, labial.** The surface which comes in contact with the mucous membrane of the lips or cheek. **Surface of a tooth, lingual [facies lingualis (NA)].** The surface which faces the tongue. **Surface of a tooth, masticatory.** Occlusal surface (see below). **Surface of a tooth, mesial [facies mesialis (NA)].** The surface which is in contact with the tooth in front of it in the dental arch. **Surface of a tooth, morsal.** Occlusal surface (see foll.). **Surface of a tooth, occlusal [facies occlusalis (NA)].** The biting surface that comes in contact with the corresponding surfaces of the teeth in the opposite jaw when the mouth is closed. **Surfaces of a tooth, proximal.** The surfaces in contact; the mesial or distal surfaces. **Surface of a tooth, vestibular [facies vestibularis (facialis) NA].** That surface of a tooth which is in contact with the cheek. **Temporary tooth.** Deciduous tooth (see above). **Unerupted tooth.** A tooth that has not erupted. **Vital tooth.** A tooth in which a vital pulp is present. **Wisdom tooth.** The third permanent molar tooth in each jaw. It is often absent, and when present, may fail to erupt. [AS *toth.*]

See also: CORTI, HUSCHKE, HUTCHINSON, MOON (H.).

tooth-ache (tooth·ake). Pain in a tooth, generally due to caries producing pulpitis. [tooth, AS *aeca.*]

toothed (tooth·d). 1. Furnished with teeth; dentate. 2. Having indentations; serrated.

topaesthesia (to·pes·the·ze·ah). Topo-aesthesia.

topagnosis (top·ag·no·sis). Inability to identify the exact spot where a sensation is felt. [Gk *topos* place, *a-*, *gnosis* recognition.]

topalgia (to·**pal**·je·ah). Topo-algia.

topectomy (to·**pek**·to·me). Excision of limited areas of frontal cortex, usually in Brodmann's areas 9 and 10, in the treatment of mental disorders. [Gk *topos* place, *ektome* excision.]

tophaceous (to·**fa**·shus). 1. Exhibiting the characteristics of a tophus. 2. Gritty; sandy. [L *tophus* tufa.]

topholipoma (to·fo·lip·o'·mah). A lipoma in which tophi are present.

tophus (to·fus) (pl. *tophi*). A localized deposit of sodium biurate usually found in the region of joints in gouty patients. It generally occurs in cartilage or bone. **Auricular tophus.** A tophus of the pinna. [L tufa.]

topical (**top**·ik·al). Localized. [Gk *topos* place.]

Topinard, Paul (b. 1830). French anthropologist.

Topinard's angle. The angle of intersection at the anterior nasal spine between lines from the external auditory meatus and the glabella.

Topinard's line. A line from the glabella passing through the most anterior part of the symphysis menti.

topo-aesthesia (to·po·es·**the**'·ze·ah). The ability to identify a spot where touched, purely by tactile sense. [Gk *topos* place, *aisthesis* sensation.]

topo-algia (to·po·**al**·je·ah). A neurasthenic or hysterical state in which pain is experienced at a particular spot without any lesion or trauma to account for it. [Gk *topos* place, *algos* pain.]

topo-anaesthesia (to·po·an·es·**the**'·ze·ah). Inability to identify the exact spot where touched. [Gk *topos* place, anaesthesia.]

topodysaesthesia (to·po·dis·es·**the**'·ze·ah). Imperfect sensation or dysaesthesia experienced in one particular area. [Gk *topos* place, *dys* difficult, *aisthesis* sensation.]

topognosis (to·**pog**·no·sis). The ability to localize a sensation. [Gk *topos* place, *gnosis* recognition.]

topographic, topographical (to·po·**graf**·ik, to·po·**graf**·ik·al). Referring to special regions. [Gk *topos* place, *graphein* to write.]

topography (to·**pog**·raf·e). The anatomical description of any particular part of the body in terms of the region in which it lies and its surrounding structures. [see prec.]

topology (to·**pol**·o·je). 1. The study of topographical anatomy. 2. The orientation of the presenting part of a fetus to the pelvic canal. [Gk *topos* place, *logos* science.]

toponarcosis (to·po·nar·**ko**'·sis). Local anaesthesia. [Gk *topos* place, *narkosis* a numbing.]

toponeurosis (to·po·newr·**o**'·sis). Localized neurosis. [Gk *topos* place, neurosis.]

toponym (to·po·nim). A regional designation as distinguished from the name of a structure or organ. [Gk *topos* place, *onyma* name.]

toponymy (to·**pon**·im·e). Regional nomenclature in anatomy, as distinct from the nomenclature of organs and structures. [see prec.]

topoparaesthesia (to·po·par·es·**the**'·ze·ah). Sensation arising of its own accord in a particular part of the body. [Gk *topos* place, paraesthesia.]

topophobia (to·po·**fo**·be·ah). Unreasoning fear of certain places. [Gk *topos* place, *phobein* to fear.]

topophone (to·po·fone). An instrument used to trace the source of a sound. [Gk *topos* place, *phone* sound.]

topothermaesthesiometer (to·po·therm·es·**the**·ze·**om**'·et·er). An instrument for comparing the sensibility to heat of various parts of the body. [Gk *topos* place, *therme* heat, *aisthesis* sensation, meter.]

topovaccinotherapy (to·po·vak·sin·o·**ther**'·a·pe). Local immunity achieved by the use of vaccines. [Gk *topos* place, vaccinotherapy.]

torcula herophili (tor·kew·lah he·**rof**·il·i). The confluence of the sinuses at the internal occipital protuberance; the superior sagittal, straight, right and left transverse, and occipital sinuses all communicate at this point. [L the wine press of Herophilus.]

Torek, Franz J. A. (b. 1861). New York surgeon.

Torek operation. 1. Orchidopexy; an operation for undescended testicle in which, after mobilization of the cord, the testis is firmly secured under the skin of the thigh to prevent retraction of the cord during healing. 2. Excision of the thoracic part of the oesophagus by way of the pleural cavity.

Keetley-Torek operation. Torek operation, 1st def. (see above).

toric (**tor**·ik). Curved in the form of a torus.

Torkildsen, Arne. Oslo neurosurgeon.

Torkildsen's operation. Insertion of a tube to drain the cerebrospinal fluid from the lateral ventricle to the cerebellomedullary cisterna for hydrocephalus.

tormen (**tor**·men) (pl. *tormina*). An acute pain in the bowel; griping spasm. **Tormina alvi.** Colic. **Tormina celsi.** Dysentery. **Tormina intestinorum.** Griping pains in the abdomen; dysentery. **Post-partum tormina.** After-pains. **Tormina ventricula nervosa.** Increased peristalsis of the bowel. [L.]

tormentil (tor·**men**·til). The dried root and herb of *Potentilla tormentilla* (family Rosaceae). The rhizome contains a red colouring principle, and also considerable quantities of tannin, and is used as a tonic and astringent in diarrhoea. [L *tormentum* torment.]

torminal, torminous (**tor**·min·al, **tor**·min·us). Characterized by acute intestinal pain. [tormen.]

Tornwaldt. *See* THORNWALDT.

torose, torous (to·rose, to·rus). Bulging; knobby. [L *torosus* bulging.]

torpent (**tor**·pent). 1. Torpid. 2. Allaying irritation. [L *torpere* to be numb.]

torpescence (tor·**pes**·ens). The state of becoming torpid or numb. [L *torpescere* to grow numb.]

torpid (**tor**·pid). Lacking vigour; apathetic; sluggish; numb. [L *torpidus.*]

torpidity (tor·**pid**·it·e). Torpor.

torpify (**tor**·pe·fi). To make torpid or to render numb. [torpor, L *facere* to make.]

torpitude (**tor**·pe·tewd). Torpor.

torpor (**tor**·por). 1. Sluggishness; apathy; numbness. 2. Slowness or lack of response to the usual stimuli. **Torpor intestinorum.** Constipation. **Torpor retinae.** Lack of retinal response except to very bright lights. [L.]

torque (tork). A force producing rotation; in dentistry, the rotation of a tooth around its long axis. [L *torquere* to twist.]

torquing (**tor**·king). The mechanical rotation of a tooth which is twisted along its long axis, into its normal position. [see prec.]

torrefaction (tor·e·**fak**·shun). The roasting of drugs to dry them and render them friable. [see foll.]

torrefication (tor·e·fik·**a**'·shun). Roasting. [L *torrefacere* to dry by heating.]

torrefy (**tor**·e·fi). To parch; to dry by roasting. [see prec.]

torres-teixeira body. The inclusion body found in lesions of alastrim or variola minor.

torsiometer (tor·she·**om**·et·er). An instrument for measuring the amount of torsion of the eye around its anteroposterior axis.

torsion (**tor**·shun). 1. The act of twisting or rotating. 2. In ophthalmology, rotation of the eyeball around its fixation axis; *extorsion* when the upper end of the vertical meridian of the cornea rotates outwards, and *intorsion* when it rotates inwards. There is an element of torsion in all oblique movements of the eyes. **Torsion of an artery.** A method of arresting bleeding by catching the cut end of an artery with forceps and twisting it round. **Torsion of the brain.** Twisting and deep twisting damage to the brain, especially the brain stem, as a result of violent impact to the head causing torsional strain. A cause of post-traumatic bleeding into the brain when asymmetrical (twisting) bleeding occurs in one cerebral hemisphere. **Torsion of the gall bladder.** Twisting of a mobile gall bladder, usually found in older women. **Lateral torsion.** Twisting to one side, especially with reference to the eye in which the vertical meridian is diverted to one or the other side. **Negative torsion.** Rotation in an anti-clockwise direction. **Positive torsion.** Rotation in a clockwise direction. **Torsion of teeth.** In dentistry, the act of rotating a tooth around its long axis. **Torsion of the uterus.** Rotation of the uterus upon its axis, usually to the right. [L *torquere* to twist.]

torsionometer (tor·shun·**om**·et·er). An apparatus used to measure the amount of rotation of the vertebral column. [torsion, meter.]

torsive (**tor**·siv). Twisted spirally. [L *torquere* to twist.]

torsiversion (tor·se·**ver**·shun). In dentistry, the state of a tooth which is rotated along its long axis into an abnormal position. [L *torquere* to twist, *vertere* to turn.]

torso (**tor**·so). The trunk; the body considered without the head and limbs. [It.]

torsoclusion (tor·sok·**loo**·zhun). 1. A method of acupressure in which a needle is inserted originally parallel to the artery and twisted over its surface and brought round at right angles before being embedded in the tissues opposite. 2. Torso-occlusion. [L *torquere* to twist, *claudere* to close.]

torso-occlusion (**tor**·so·ok·**loo**'·zhun). The condition of a tooth which is abnormally rotated along its long axis from its normal position. [L *torquere* to twist, *occludere* to shut together.]

tort (tort). To rotate the eyeball around its visual axis. [L *tortus* twisted.]

torticollar (tor·te·**kol**·ar). Characterized by torticollis.

torticollis (tor·te·**kol**·is). Spasm of the neck muscles, drawing the head to one side and twisting the neck. **Congenital torticollis.** A torticollis due to the formation of a haematoma in a sternocleidomastoid muscle at birth; absorption and fibrosis later occur and the muscle fails to lengthen as other neck structures grow, so that the torticollis increases. **Dermatogenic torticollis.** Torticollis due to scarring and contracture of the skin of the neck. **Fixed torticollis.** Torticollis in which the shortening of the affected muscle or muscles is so great that the head is virtually fixed in one position. **Hysterical torticollis.** Hysterical contraction of neck muscles on one side giving rise to the position of torticollis; the contraction can be overcome by suggestion or by hypnosis. **Intermittent spasmodic torticollis.** Spasmodic torticollis (see below). **Labyrinthine torticollis.** Spasmodic torticollis resulting from disease of the semicircular canals. **Mental torticollis.** A tic or habit spasm of the neck muscles giving rise to twisting or tilting of the head. **Myogenic torticollis.** Transient torticollis due to muscular fibrositis or to cold; the common "stiff neck". **Neurogenic torticollis.** Torticollis which results from contraction of the sternocleidomastoid muscle due to irritation of or pressure upon the 11th cranial (accessory) nerve. **Ocular torticollis.** A tilting of the head on the neck, either in order to obtain binocular vision with fusion in cases of vertical ocular muscle paresis, usually congenital, or an attempt to straighten objects seen in marked oblique astigmatism, or when the axis of the correcting cylindrical lens is not accurate. **Reflex torticollis.** The torticollis which may result from reflex spasm of the sternocleidomastoid muscle due to suppuration or inflammation in the tissue of the neck and particularly in the lymph nodes which underly the muscle. **Rheumatoid torticollis.** Torticollis due to involvement of the cervical spine in rheumatoid arthritis. **Spasmodic torticollis.** Intermittent spasmodic torticollis, due to powerful involuntary contraction of the neck muscles, particularly the sternocleidomastoid; a fragmentary form of torsion spasm, it results from disease in the corpus striatum. **Spurious torticollis.** An abnormal twisted or tilted position of the head and neck resulting from disease in the cervical vertebrae. **Symptomatic torticollis.** Torticollis due to local disease in the neck; myogenic torticollis, reflex torticollis, rheumatoid torticollis, and spurious torticollis can be included under this heading. [L *tortus* twisted, *collum* neck.]

tortipelvis (tor·te·**pel**·vis). 1. Dystonia musculorum deformans: spasm in children, producing distortion of the spine and hips. 2. Deformed pelvis. [L *tortus* twisted, pelvis.]

tortua facies (**tor**·tew·ah **fa**·se·eez). Neuralgia of the trigeminal nerve. [L facial agony.]

tortuous (**tor**·tew·us). Having many twists or turns. [L *tortus* twisted.]

Torula (**tor**·ew·lah). A generic name often applied incorrectly to asporogenic yeast fungi of the genus *Cryptococcus* (Kützing) Vuillemin (syn. *Torulopsis* Berlese) which includes the pathogenic species *C. neoformans* (syn. *Torula histolytica*). This is *Torula* in the sense of Turpin (1838). By priority the name should be reserved for dematiaceous fungi (black yeasts) named *Torula* by Persoon (1796). **Torula capsulatus.** *C. neoformans.* **Torula cerevisiae.** *Saccharomyces cerevisiae.* **Torula histolytica.** Name proposed by Stoddard and Cutler (1916) for *C. neoformans* (Sanfelice) Vuillemin, the cause of *Cryptococcus* meningitis and other forms of cryptococcosis. **Torula jeanselmei.** Name proposed by Langeron (1928) for a fungus isolated from a case of mycetoma with black grains. The species has been transferred to the genus *Phialophora* as *P. jeanselmei* by Emmons. **Torula mansoni.** *Cladosporium werneckii.* [L *torulus* small swelling.]

See also: PASTEUR.

toruliform (**tor**·ew·le·form). Beaded or knotted in form; having the characteristics of fungi of the genus *Cryptococcus (Torulopsis).* [L *torulus* small swelling, form.]

Torulopsis (tor·ew·**lop**·sis). The generic name of a group of asporogenous yeasts closely related to *Candida* species. **Torulopsis glabrata.** A species implicated in rare cases as a secondary infection in patients with severe debilitating diseases or who are receiving steroids, antibiotics, or immunosuppressive therapy. **Torulopsis neoformans.** *Cryptococcus neoformans.* [L *torulus* small swelling, Gk *opsis* appearance.]

torulopsosis (**tor**·ew·lop·**so**'·sis). A rare fungal disease caused by *Torulopsis glabrata* in compromised patients. [L *torulus* small swelling, Gk *opsis* appearance, *-osis* condition.]

torulosis (tor·ew·**lo**·sis). Cryptococcosis, an infection caused by *Cryptococcus neoformans* in which tubercles and gelatinous cystic structures containing numerous torulae appear in the brain with accompanying leptomeningitis. The cerebrospinal system is primarily involved, but there is also sometimes infection of the skin, mucosa, liver, kidneys, and spleen. [L *torulus* small swelling, Gk *-osis* condition.]

torulus (**tor**·ew·lus). A small swelling or papilla. **Torulus tactilis.** A tactile elevation, a minute raised area on the skin that is especially sensitive to touch. [L small swelling.]

torus [NA] (**tor**·us). A linear elevation or prominence; a ridge. **Torus levatorius [NA].** The elevation caused by the levator palati muscle underlying the mucous membrane of the lateral wall of the nasopharynx. **Torus mandibularis.** An exostosis of the inner surface of the mandible. **Torus manus.** The carpus. **Palatine torus [torus palatinus (NA)].** A bony ridge along the hard palate at the site of the intermaxillary suture, frequently present in some races. **Torus uretericus.** A ridge along the upper border of the trigone of the urinary bladder, connecting the ureteric orifices. [L a swelling.]

Totaquine BP 1953 (**to**·tah·kween). A mixture of the total alkaloids of cinchona bark, obtained from *Cinchona succirubra* Pavon or *C. robusta* Howard, for example; this is standardized to contain at least 70 per cent of the four crystallizable alkaloids, quinine, cinchonine, cinchonidine, and quinidine, of which at least 15 per cent must be quinine, and not more than 20 per cent of amorphous alkaloids. The standard was originally laid down by the Health Organization of the League of Nations in order to provide a cheap but efficient antimalarial for the people of poorer countries. The hardy cinchona plants from which it could be prepared could be grown in many countries including many malarious countries; in this way these countries would become self-supporting. The advent of the synthetic antimalarials made this cheap, natural antimalarial largely redundant.

Toti, Addeo (b. 1861). Florence otolaryngologist.

Toti's operation. For epiphora: the formation of a new channel into the nose from the lacrimal sac. *See* MOSHER-TOTI OPERATION (below). The original Toti's operation differed in that the sac was all preserved and sutured to the nasal mucosa. **Mosher-Toti operation.** For epiphora: a method of dacryocystorrhinostomy; the bone between the lacrimal sac and nose is resected and the nasal mucosa underneath removed and also the middle turbinate. The medial wall of the sac is removed and the lateral wall pushed into the opening in the nose. No sutures are employed.

totipotence (to·**tip**·o·tens). The potentiality inherent in the germ cell to produce the many and varied cells of the complete individual. [see foll.]

totipotent, totipotential (to·**tip**·o·tent, **to**·te·po·**ten'**·shal). Describing a cell such as a fertilized ovum in which there is promise of the complete individual to come, with all his many different kinds of cells. [L *totus* all, *potentia* power.]

touch (tuch). 1. Tactile sense. 2. Palpation; various methods of examination by the tactile sense are described as *abdominal touch, double touch* (vaginal and abdominal, or vaginal and rectal), *rectal touch,* and *vaginal touch.* [Fr. *toucher.*]

touch-me-not (**tuch**·me·not). 1. Any of various types of ulcerating skin disease of the face, especially lupus exedens (lupus exulcerans). 2. (*a*) Any plant of the genus *Impatiens,* especially the European touch-me-not, (*b*) the squirting cucumber.

tour de maître (toor de **ma**·tr). A classical method of passing a metal catheter or sound through the urethra into the bladder in the male. The operator introduces the beak of the catheter or sound to the anterior urethra with its convexity upwards, while the shaft lies above and parallel to the inguinal ligament. Thereafter the handle is swung over to the umbilicus with the shaft still parallel to the abdominal wall. As the beak is felt to engage the membranous urethra the handle is carried upwards with a circular movement and the beak is made to enter the bladder by depressing the shaft between the patient's thighs. [Fr. a master's turn.]

Tourette. *See* GILLES DE LA TOURETTE.

Tournay, Auguste (b. 1878). French ophthalmologist.

Tournay's reaction. Inequality of the pupils sometimes found when the eyes are turned to the extreme right or left. The pupil of the abducted eye dilates, and that of the adducted eye is thought by some to contract.

tournesol (**toor**·ne·sol). Litmus. [Fr. *tourner* to turn, *soleil* sun.]

tourniquet (**toor**·ne·ka). An instrument for the circular compression of a limb with interruption of its blood supply. It is intended to stop the circulation in the limb and prevent haemorrhage from a wound, or during a surgical operation performed upon some part of the limb. **Field tourniquet.** A strap, fitted with a pad, which can be tightened by a screw after application. **Forceps tourniquet.** A clamp with one flat blade and one blade probe-pointed; the former lies externally, the latter is passed deep to the femoral artery which is controlled by closure of the two blades. It is employed in disarticulation of the hip. **Garrotte tourniquet.** A windlass type of tourniquet. **Pneumatic tourniquet.** An elongated rubber balloon bound round a limb and inflated to occlude the main artery. **Provisional tourniquet.** A tourniquet placed loosely around a limb, to be tightened if bleeding should occur. **Screw tourniquet.** A tourniquet rendered taut by a windlass device. **Spanish tourniquet, Torcular tourniquet.** A windlass tourniquet. **Windlass tourniquet.** Spanish windlass, a tourniquet made by tying a handkerchief or similar article round a limb and exerting pressure by inserting a small stick or pencil in the knot and twisting it. [Fr.]

See also: DUPUYTREN, ESMARCH, FINOCHIETTO, FOULI, LYNN THOMAS, SAMWAYS, SIGNORINI.

Touroff, Arthur Sigmund Wood. New York surgeon.

Touroff's operation. An operation for pulmonary abscess.

Tourtual, Kaspar Theobald (b. 1802). Munster anatomist.

Tourtual's canal. The greater palatine canal. *See* CANAL.

Tourtual's membrane. The aryepiglottic fold. *See* FOLD.

Tourtual's sinus. The intratonsillar cleft. *See* CLEFT.

tousey (**tow**·ze). An obsolete unit of x-ray power, being the radiance which produced on a photographic film a density equal to that produced by one candle power of electric light.

Touton, Karl (b. 1858). Breslau dermatologist.

Touton giant cells. Large multinucleated giant cells rich in lipoid material, found in xanthomata.

tow (to). Coarse broken flax or hemp used in surgical dressings. [ME.]

Towns, Charles Barnes (b. 1862). American insurance official.

Towns-Lambert treatment. For drug addiction: systematic purging, gradual withdrawal of the drug, and the prescribing of belladonna, hyoscyamus, and xanthoxylum.

Townsend, Joseph (b. 1739). English clergyman.

Townsend's mixture. Red mercuric oxide, potassium iodide, syrup of orange, tincture of cardamom, and water.

toxaemia (tox·e·me·ah). The condition of general poisoning caused by the entrance of soluble bacterial toxins into the blood. **Alimentary toxaemia.** The condition of ill-health caused by the absorption of bacterial toxins from the alimentary canal. **Eclamptic toxaemia.** Toxaemia of pregnancy accompanied by convulsions. **Eclamptogenic toxaemia.** Toxaemia of pregnancy causing convulsions. **Hydatid toxaemia.** General symptoms caused by the rupture of a hydatid cyst; they comprise urticaria, erythema, prutitus, diarrhoea, vomiting, asthma, etc., and are allergic in origin. **Menstrual toxaemia.** Untoward symptoms at the time of the menses attributed to a toxin in the shedding endometrium. **Pre-eclamptic toxaemia.** A syndrome characterized by hypertension, albuminuria, and generalized oedema, occurring only in pregnancy. Any two of these three signs are usually sufficient to establish the diagnosis. **Toxaemia of pregnancy.** A series of conditions affecting women in pregnancy, such as hypertensive disease, renal disease, pre-eclampsia and eclampsia, vomiting of pregnancy, and other unclassifiable toxaemias. [toxin, Gk *haima* blood.]

toxaemic (tox·e·mik). Relating or due to toxaemia.

toxalbumic (tox·al·**bew**·mik). Of the nature of a toxic albumin.

toxalbumin (tox·al·**bew**·min). Any albumin with toxic properties. Some, such as snake venom, are active only when injected. Others, such as ricin of the castor-oil seed and phallin of the toadstool *Amanita phalloides,* are absorbed from the alimentary canal.

toxalbumose (tox·al·**bew**·moze). A toxic albumose.

toxamine (**tox**·am·een). Term applied by Mellanby to hypothetical substances in foods which antagonize vitamin action. It was used in particular of the supposed antirachitic substance in cereals held to be responsible for their effect in intensifying vitamin-D deficiency. It has been shown, however, that this last effect is due to the presence of phosphate in the form of phytic acid which produces insoluble calcium salts and is itself relatively insoluble; there is thus poor absorption of calcium and phosphate ions in the intestine and the defective calcification of the bones is aggravated. [Gk *toxikon* poison, amine.]

toxanaemia (tox·an·e·me·ah). Anaemia caused by a haemolytic toxin.

Toxascaris (tox·**as**·kar·is). A genus of the roundworm (family Ascaridae). *Toxascaris leonina* found in cats and dogs, has been recorded rarely from man. [Gk *toxon* bow, *askaris* intestinal worm.]

toxic (**tox**·ik). 1. Poisonous. 2. Of the nature of or related to a toxin. 3. Produced by a toxin, e.g. symptoms. [Gk *toxikon* poison.]

toxicaemia (tox·is·e·me·ah). Toxaemia.

toxicant (**tox**·ik·ant). 1. Toxic; poisonous. 2. Any drug or agent, particularly alcohol, which causes intoxication.

toxicarol (tox·ik·**ar**·ol). One of the insecticidal ingredients of derris root.

toxication (tox·ik·**a**·shun). Poisoning. [Gk *toxikon* poison.]

toxicide (**tox**·is·ide). Having a destructive action on toxins; an antidote. [toxin, L *caedere* to kill.]

toxicity (tox·**is**·it·e). 1. The quality of being poisonous. 2. The amount and strength of toxin produced by a micro-organism. [Gk *toxikon* poison.]

toxicodendrol (**tox**·ik·o·**den'**·drol). A non-volatile poisonous oil obtained from toxicodendron.

toxicodendron (tox·ik·o·**den'**·dron). Poison oak, poison ivy; the leaves of *Rhus toxicodendron* (family Anacardiaceae), a North American species of sumach. Its toxic properties are attributed to the non-volatile oil, toxicodendrol. [Gk *toxikon* poison, *dendron* tree.]

toxicoderma (tox·ik·o·**der**′·mah). Toxicodermia.

toxicodermatitis (tox·ik·o·der·mat·**i**′·tis). Skin affection produced by the action of a poisonous substance. [Gk *toxikon* poison, dermatitis.]

toxicodermia (tox·ik·o·**der**′·me·ah). Any affection of the skin caused by a toxin. [Gk *toxikon* poison, *derma* skin.]

toxicodermitis (tox·ik·o·der·**mi**′·tis). Toxicodermatitis.

toxicogenic (tox·ik·o·**jen**′·ik). 1. Producing a toxin or poison. 2. Produced by a toxin or poison. [Gk *toxikon* poison, *genein* to produce.]

toxicohaemia (tox·ik·o·**he**′·me·ah). Toxaemia.

toxicoid (tox·ik·oid). Transiently poisonous; resembling a poison or toxin in action. [Gk *toxikon* poison, *eidos* form.]

toxicological (tox·ik·o·**loj**′·ik·al). Concerned with toxicology.

toxicologist (tox·ik·**ol**·o·jist). An expert on poisons and their antidotes. [see foll.]

toxicology (tox·ik·**ol**·o·je). The study of poisons, with special reference to their preparation, identification, physiological action, and antidotes. [Gk *toxikon* poison, *logos* science.]

toxicomania (tox·ik·o·**ma**′·ne·ah). 1. Toxicophobia. 2. An insane desire for poison. [Gk *toxikon* poison, *mania* madness.]

toxicomucin (tox·ik·o·**mew**′·sin). A toxic mucin formed in cultures of the tubercle bacillus.

toxicopathic (tox·ik·o·**path**′·ik). Describing any disease that is due to a toxic agent. [see foll.]

toxicopathy (tox·ik·**op**·ath·e). Any disease caused by the action of a toxic substance. [Gk *toxikon* poison, *pathos* disease.]

toxicopeptone (tox·ik·o·**pep**′·tone). Toxin, a breakdown product of peptone, especially that produced by *Vibrio cholerae* when growing in peptone water.

toxicophloea (tox·ik·o·**fle**′·ah). Acocanthera. [Gk *toxikon* poison, *phloios* bark.]

toxicophobia (tox·ik·o·**fo**′·be·ah). An unreasoning fear of being poisoned. [Gk *toxikon* poison, *phobein* to fear.]

toxicosis (tox·ik·**o**·sis). The pathological condition caused by the absorption of poisons. It usually refers to poisons of metabolic or bacterial origin. **Alimentary toxicosis.** Poisoning by products formed in the alimentary canal. **Endogenous toxicosis.** Poisoning by substances produced within the body. **Exogenous toxicosis.** Poisoning by substances introduced from without the body. **Haemorrhagic capillary toxicosis.** A haemorrhagic condition due to weakening of the capillaries by some toxic factor (Frank). **Retention toxicosis.** Poisoning by the retention of waste products normally excreted from the body. [Gk *toxikon* poison, *-osis* condition.]

toxidermatosis (tox·e·der·mat·**o**′·sis). Any cutaneous abnormality due to toxaemia. [Gk *toxikon* poison, dermatosis.]

toxidermia (tox·e·**der**·me·ah). Toxicodermia.

toxidermitis (tox·e·der·**mi**′·tis). Toxicodermatitis.

toxiferous (tox·**if**·er·us). Describing organisms which carry or produce toxins. [toxin, L *ferre* to bear.]

toxigenic (tox·i·**jen**·ik). Producing toxins. [toxin, Gk *genein* to produce.]

toxigenicity (tox·e·jen·**is**′·it·e). The measure of the virulence of a micro-organism through the toxin it produces. [see prec.]

toxigenous (tox·**ij**·en·us). Toxigenic.

toxignomic (tox·ig·**nom**·ik). Symptomatic of a toxin or poison. [Gk *toxikon* poison, *gnome* sign.]

toxi-infection (tox·e·in·**fek**′·shun). Toxinfection.

toxi-infectious (tox·e·in·**fek**′·shus). Toxinfectious.

toximucin (tox·e·**mew**·sin). Toxicomucin.

toxin (**tox**·in). 1. Any poisonous substance of biological origin. 2. An antigenic product of bacterial metabolism which is capable of causing symptoms when administered apart from the intact organism. It is usual to recognize *endotoxins*, which are only released on the dissolution of the bacterial bodies, and *exotoxins*, which diffuse freely out of living bacterial cells. **Alpha toxin.** 1. Of staphylococci: a haemolysin active against rabbit red blood cells, but not against human erythrocytes. 2. Of *Clostridium welchii*: an exotoxin produced by all strains of *C. welchii*. It appears to be a lecithinase, and shows haemolytic, lethal, and necrotizing activity. **Amanita toxin.** The poisonous principle of the fungus *Amanita phalloides*. **Botulinum toxin.** The exotoxin produced by *Clostridium botulinum*. **Dermonecrotic toxin.** A toxin that causes skin necrosis, e.g. certain staphylococci give rise to such a toxin. **Diphtheria toxin.** The filtrate of a broth culture toxic to men, guinea-pigs, rabbits, and many other animals (not rats or birds). A small quantity of freshly prepared standardized toxin on intradermal injection into man or guinea-pig gives a flare reaction (Schick test positive), unless there is circulating antitoxin in the blood stream (as in an immune person) when a negative reaction is obtained. **Dysentery toxin.** The exotoxin of *Shigella dysenteriae*. **Erythrogenic toxin.** Any toxin causing a red reaction in the skin at the site of injection. **Necrotizing toxin.** Dermonecrotic toxin (see above). **Plant toxin.** A poisonous substance derived from a plant, e.g. ricin. **Scarlatinal toxin.** The toxic substance produced in cultures of haemolytic streptococci isolated from cases of scarlet fever. It is used in the Dick test for demonstrating susceptibility to scarlet fever. **Tetanus toxin.** The exotoxin of *Clostridium tetani*. **Vegetable toxin.** Plant toxin (see above). [Gk *toxikon* poison.]

See also: COLEY, DICK, FERRY, TUNNICLIFF.

toxin–antitoxin (**tox**·in·an·te·**tox**′·in). A mixture of toxin and antitoxin. Diphtheria toxin–antitoxin mixture was formerly much used for active immunization in the USA. Its action was explained on the basis that toxin held in an unstable union with antitoxin was gradually liberated in the human body.

toxinaemia (tox·in·e·me·ah). Toxaemia.

toxinfection (tox·in·**fek**·shun). A disease with toxic symptoms the bacterial cause of which cannot be detected. [toxin, infection.]

toxinfectious (tox·in·**fek**·shus). Having the nature of a toxin-fection.

toxinic (tox·**in**·ik). Toxin in character, or attributable to a toxin.

toxinicide (tox·**in**·is·ide). Anything that will destroy toxins. [toxin, L *caedere* to kill.]

toxinosis (tox·in·**o**·sis). Toxicosis.

toxinotherapy (tox·in·o·**ther**′·ap·e). The treatment of disease by means of toxins. [toxin, therapy.]

toxintoxoid (tox·in·**tox**·oid). A mixture of toxin and toxoid.

toxipathy (tox·**ip**·ath·e). Toxicopathy.

toxipeptone (tox·e·**pep**·tone). Toxicopeptone.

toxiphobia (tox·e·**fo**·be·ah). Toxicophobia.

toxiphoric (tox·e·**for**·ik). Having the ability to link with a toxin. [toxin, Gk *pherein* to bear.]

toxiphrenia (tox·e·**fre**·ne·ah). A confusional state occurring in schizophrenia. [Gk *toxikon* poison, *phren* mind.]

toxisterol (tox·e·**steer**·ol). $C_{28}H_{44}O$, a sterol isomeric with ergosterol from which it is produced by ultraviolet irradiation to a stage beyond the formation of calciferol. It has no antirachitic properties but produces toxic calcification of soft tissues, and was probably the cause of the high toxicity of certain early preparations of irradiated ergosterol used therapeutically.

toxitherapy (tox·e·**ther**·ap·e). Toxinotherapy.

toxituberculid, toxituberculide (tox·e·tew·**ber**′·kew·lid, tox·e·tew·**ber**′·kew·lide). A lesion of the skin attributed to the toxin of tuberculosis.

Toxocara (tox·o·**ka**·rah). A genus of ascarid nematodes. *T. canis* and *T. mystax* (= *cati*), the common ascarids of dog and cat respectively, may infect man, especially children, and cause intestinal and respiratory symptoms (migration of larvae) with eosinophilia and enlargement of the spleen and liver (toxocariasis). [Gk *toxon* bow, *kara* head.]

toxocariasis (tox·o·ka·**ri**′·as·is). Infection in children by larvae of *Toxocara* from the dog or cat, causing granulomatous swellings with eosinophilia. [*Toxocara*, Gk *-osis* condition.]

toxogen (**tox**·o·jen). Anything that produces a toxin. [toxin, Gk *genein* to produce.]

toxogenin (tox·**oj**·en·in). The factor which, it is suggested, develops in serum after sensitization by an injection of antigen, and which, although itself inactive, causes anaphylaxis on further injection of the antigen. [see prec.]

toxoglobulin (tox·o·**glob**·ew·lin). A toxic globulin.

toxoid (**tox**·oid). The material resulting from the treatment of toxin in such a way that the toxic properties are inactivated whilst the antigenic potency remains intact. **Alum-precipitated toxoid.** APT, a suspension of the precipitate formed by the addition of alum to formol toxoid (diphtheria toxoid). The toxoid protein adheres to the insoluble alumina, and on injection this permits slow release of the antigen into the blood stream, producing a high level of antitoxic immunity. The process can be applied to several toxoids, but when abbreviated, APT refers exclusively to diphtheria. **Diphtheria toxoid.** Diphtheria culture filtrates to which have been added small amounts of formalin; the product is devoid of toxicity but is still an extremely effective prophylactic agent. **Formol toxoid.** FT. Diphtheria toxoid (see prec.). **Purified toxoid aluminium phosphate.** PTAP, a diphtheria-immunizing preparation made by adding to purified formol toxoid a suspension of hydrated aluminium phosphate in saline. **Staphylococcus Toxoid BP 1968.** A toxoid prepared from the toxic filtrates of staphylococcus. Its use has not been attended with the same success as diphtheria toxoid. **Tetanus toxoid.** Tetanus Vaccine BP 1973, the toxin of *Clostridium tetani*, rendered harmless by formalin and heat. It has been used to produce immunity in soldiers, agricultural workers, and others who may be exposed to the danger of tetanus, but is not administered to all volunteer infants and children as part of the triple vaccine (diphtheria, tetanus and pertussis); it is also injected into horses for the production of tetanus antitoxin or antitetanic serum. [toxin, Gk *eidos* form.]

toxoid-antitoxin (**tox**·oid·an·te·**tox**′·in). A saline-suspended precipitate of toxoid with the equivalent neutralizing dose of antitoxin.

toxo-infection (tox·o·in·**fek**′·shun). Toxinfection.

toxo-infectious (tox·o·in·**fek**′·shus). Toxinfectious.

toxolysin (tox·**ol**·is·in). Antitoxin. [toxin, Gk *lysis* a loosing.]

toxomucin (tox·o·**mew**·sin). Toxicomucin.

toxonosis (tox·o·**no**·sis). Toxicosis.

toxopeptone (tox·o·**pep**·tone). Toxicopeptone.

toxophile (**tox**·o·file). 1. Possessing an affinity for a toxin. 2. Readily affected by a toxin. [toxin, Gk *philein* to love.]

toxophilous (tox·**of**·il·us). Toxophile.

toxophore (**tox**·o·for). That part of the toxin molecule which is responsible for its poisonous action. This can be modified by various reagents, so that the toxic effect is greatly reduced whilst the capacity of the toxin molecule to stimulate antitoxin production is unimpaired; such modified toxins are called *toxoids*. [toxin, Gk *pherein* to bear.]

toxophorous (tox·**of**·or·us). Concerned with the action of the toxophore.

Toxoplasma (tox·o·**plaz**·mah). A genus of protozoa of the class Sporozoa which is found in endothelial cells of mammals and birds and which has been reported in man as a congenital infection of the nervous system, and as an acquired infection. The species found in man has been called *Toxoplasma hominis* and those found in animals by other names, e.g. *T. gondii*, according to the host; it seems probable that these are all one species. [Gk *toxikon* poison, *plasma* anything formed.]

toxoplasmatic, toxoplasmic (tox·o·plaz·**mat**′·ik, tox·o·**plaz**·mik). Referring to *Toxoplasma*.

toxoplasmosis (tox·o·plaz·**mo**′·sis). An infection caused by the protozoal parasite *Toxoplasma gondii (hominis)*. It occurs naturally in mice, guinea-pigs, rabbits, and several other small animals and birds; man becomes infected from the faeces of such animals. The most serious results of infection are found in young infants and stillborn, that have become infected *in utero*. They may show a variety of serious conditions including encephalomyelitis, hydrocephalus, or microcephaly, cerebral calcification, and choroidoretinitis. The mother of such an infant usually shows no symptoms, but antibodies are present in her blood. Subclinical and mild infections are relatively common, but an acute eruptive fever may occur. [*Toxoplasma*, Gk *-osis* condition.]

toxoprotein (tox·o·**pro**·te·in). 1. A toxic protein. 2. A mixture of a toxin and a protein.

toxosis (tox·**o**·sis). Any affection due to toxic causes. [Gk *toxikon* poison, *-osis* condition.]

Toynbee, Joseph (b. 1815). London otologist.

Toynbee's corpuscles. The corneal corpuscles.

Toynbee's experiment. Reduction of the pressure on the tympanic membrane by swallowing with both nose and mouth closed.

Toynbee's law. Intracranial spread of infection from otitis media reaches the transverse sinus and/or the cerebellum via the mastoid, and the temporal lobe via the tympanic plate.

Toynbee's ligament. The anterior ligament of the malleus.

Toynbee's muscle. The tensor tympani muscle.

T-piece. *See* AYRE.

trabecula [NA] (trab·**ek**·ew·lah). A wooden beam or rib; hence in anatomy, the bony lamellae of cancellous bone which are arranged somewhat like beams or struts. **Trabeculae carneae [NA].** The ridges or strands of muscle found on the inner aspect of the chambers of the heart. **Trabecula cerebri.** An obsolete term for the corpus callosum. **Trabeculae cordis.** Trabeculae carneae (see above). **Trabeculae cranii.** Two bars of cartilage that develop in the base of the chondrocranium anterior to the parachordal cartilage which forms around the anterior part of the notochord. **Trabeculae of the penis.** Fibromuscular strands [trabeculae corporum cavernosorum (NA)] which divide the corpora cavernosa into numerous small cavernous spaces that are lined by endothelium and filled with blood, and the fibrous septa separating the cavernous spaces of the corpus spongiosum [trabeculae corporis spongiosi (NA)]. **Trabecula of the spleen [trabecula lienis (NA)].** The fibro-elastic framework attached to the capsule and to the sheaths of blood vessels, in the meshes of which the splenic pulp lies. [L little beam.]

See also: RATHKE.

trabecular (trab·**ek**·ew·lar). 1. Referring to a trabecula. 2. Characterized by trabeculae. **Trabecular meshwork.** The sieve-like inner aspect of the canal of Schlemm, consisting of trabeculae arising from Schwalbe's line and being inserted into the scleral spur.

trabecularism (trab·**ek**·ew·lar·izm). The existence of trabeculae in the supporting tissue of a structure or organ.

trabeculate (trab·**ek**·ew·late). Consisting of trabeculae; trabecular.

trabeculation (trab·**ek**·ew·**la**′·shun). The development of trabeculae in a structure or organ.

trabeculectomy (trab·**ek**·ew·**lek**′·to·me). An operation for glaucoma, consisting of removal of part of the trabecular meshwork of the anterior chamber. [L *trabecula* little beam, Gk *ektome* a cutting out.]

trabeculotomy (trab·**ek**·ew·**lot**′·o·me). The operation of incising the trabecular meshwork for the relief of glaucoma. Goniotomy is one variant used extensively for the treatment of buphthalmos. *Trabeculotomy ab externo* has had some success in adult simple glaucoma. [L *trabecula* little beam, Gk *ektome* a cutting out.]

tracer (**tra**·ser). 1. A blunt instrument for the dissection of vessels and nerves. 2. Any radioactive isotope the progress of which, through the body, can be followed by means of a detector such as a Geiger counter. It is used to trace the course of the element the isotope of which has been employed. [Fr.]

traces (**tra**·sez). **Contact traces.** A medicolegal term that includes traces left by the suspected criminal, e.g. fingerprints, semen, and traces left on the suspected criminal, e.g. blood stains. [see prec.]

trachea [NA] (**tra**·ke·ah, trak·e·ah). The windpipe; a rigid tube, 10 cm long, extending from the cricoid cartilage to the upper border of the 5th thoracic vertebra (or lower during deep inspiration) where it divides into the two main bronchi. Its wall is strengthened by 15-20 cartilages, each resembling a horseshoe in form, the deficiency lying posteriorly. The membranous wall [paries membranaceus (NA)] is a fibro-elastic membrane in two layers, one on each surface of the cartilaginous rings. Between the rings the layers fuse; where the rings are deficient posteriorly the two layers enclose the muscles. **Coat of the trachea and**

bronchi, mucous [tunica mucosa (NA)]. The inner coat composed of two layers, a pseudostratified columnar ciliated epithelium containing numerous goblet cells mounted on a basement membrane, and a layer of connective tissue containing lymphoid tissue, blood vessels, and elastic fibres. **Coat of the trachea and bronchi, submucous [tela submucosa (NA)].** A thin layer of connective tissue between the lamina propria of the mucous layer and the muscular layer. **Scabbard trachea.** Flattening of the trachea by lateral compression due to tumours or other swellings. [Gk *tracheia* the rough artery.]

trachea-ectasy (tra·ke·ah·**ek**′·tas·e). Dilatation of the trachea. [trachea, Gk *ektasis* extension.]

tracheal (tra·ke·al). Referring to the trachea or having origin there.

tracheal veins [venae tracheales (NA)]. Tributaries of the inferior thyroid vein.

trachealgia (tra·ke·al·je·ah). 1. Pain experienced in the trachea. 2. Croup. [trachea, Gk *algos* pain.]

trachealis muscle [musculus trachealis (NA)] (tra·ke·a·lis). Smooth muscle fibres which run transversely on the posterior aspect of the trachea.

tracheitis (tra·ke·i·tis). Inflammation of the membrane lining the trachea; tracheal catarrh. [trachea, Gk *-itis* inflammation.]

trachelagra (trak·el·ag·rah). Gout or rheumatism in the muscles of the neck. [Gk *trachelos* neck, *agra* seizure.]

trachelectomopexy (trak·el·**ek**·to·mo·pex·e). Partial amputation and fixation of the neck of the uterus. [Gk *trachelos* neck, *ektome* excision, *pexis* a fixation.]

trachelectomy (trak·el·**ek**·to·me). Amputation of the neck of the uterus. [Gk *trachelos* neck, *ektome* excision.]

trachelhaematoma (**trak**·el·he·mat·**o**′·mah). Haematoma of the neck, particularly of the sternocleidomastoid muscle. [Gk *trachelos* neck, *haima* blood, *-oma* tumour.]

trachelism, trachelismus (**trak**·el·izm, trak·el·**iz**·mus). Spasmodic contraction of the neck muscles which bends the head backwards, as in epilepsy. [Gk *trachelismos.*]

trachelitis (trak·el·i·tis). Inflammation of the lining of the neck of the uterus. [Gk *trachelos* neck, *-itis* inflammation.]

trachelo-achromial (**trak**·el·o·ak·**ro**′·me·al). Concerning the neck and the scapula. [Gk *trachelos* neck, *akron* tip, *omos* shoulder.]

trachelobregmatic (**trak**·el·o·breg·**mat**′·ik). Concerning the neck and the bregma. [Gk *trachelos* neck, bregma.]

trachelocele (**trak**·el·o·seel). Tracheocele.

tracheloclavicular (**trak**·el·o·klav·**ik**′·ew·lar). Connecting the neck and the clavicle. [Gk *trachelos* neck, clavicle.]

trachelocyllosis (**trak**·el·o·sil·**o**′·sis). Torticollis. [Gk *trachelos* neck, *kyllosis* a bending.]

trachelocyrtosis (**trak**·el·o·ser·**to**′·sis). Trachelokyphosis. [Gk *trachelos* neck, *kyrtos* curved.]

trachelocystitis (**trak**·el·o·sist·**i**′·tis). Inflammation of the neck of the bladder. [Gk *trachelos* neck, cystitis.]

trachelodynia (**trak**·el·o·**din**′·e·ah). Pain experienced in the neck. [Gk *trachelos* neck, *odyne* pain.]

trachelokyphosis (**trak**·el·o·ki·**fo**′·sis). Anterior curvature of the cervical vertebrae. [Gk *trachelos* neck, *kyphosis* humpback.]

trachelologist (trak·el·**ol**·o·jist). A specialist on diseases and injuries of the neck. [see foll.]

trachelology (trak·el·**ol**·o·je). The study of diseases and injuries of the neck. [Gk *trachelos* neck, *logos* science.]

trachelomastoid (**trak**·el·o·**mas**′·toid). An obsolete name for the longissimus capitis muscle. [Gk *trachelos* neck, mastoid.]

trachelomyitis (**trak**·el·o·mi·**i**′·tis). Inflammation of the neck muscles. [Gk *trachelos* neck, *mys* muscle, *-itis* inflammation.]

trachelo-occipitalis (**trak**·el·o·ok·sip·it·**a**′·lis). An obsolete name for the semispinalis capitis muscle. [Gk *trachelos* neck, occiput.]

trachelopexia, trachelopexy (**trak**·el·o·**pex**′·e·ah, **trak**·el·o·pex·e). Surgical fixation of the neck of the uterus. [Gk *trachelos* neck, *pexis* a fixation.]

tracheloplasty (trak·el·o·plas·te). Surgical repair of the neck of the uterus. [Gk *trachelos* neck, *plassein* to mould.]

trachelorrhaphy (trak·el·**or**·af·e). An operation for repair of the neck of the uterus by suturing. [Gk *trachelos* neck, *rhaphe* suture.]

trachelorrhectes (**trak**·el·o·**rek**′·teez). An instrument used in embryotomy to crush the cervical vertebrae. [Gk *trachelos* neck, *rhectes* a breaker.]

tracheloschisis (trak·el·**os**·kis·is). Congenital opening in the neck as the result of a branchial cleft which has failed to close. [Gk *trachelos* neck, *schisis* fissure.]

trachelotomy (trak·el·**ot**·o·me). Surgical incision of the neck of the uterus. [Gk *trachelos* neck, *temnein* to cut.]

tracheo-aerocele (**trak**·e·o·**a**′·er·o·seel). A saccular protrusion of the trachea, containing air. [trachea, Gk *aer* air, *kele* hernia.]

tracheoblenorrhoea (**tra**·ke·o·blen·o·**re**′·ah). Copious discharge of mucus from the trachea. [trachea, Gk *blennos* mucus, *rhoia* flow.]

tracheobronchial (**tra**·ke·o·**brong**′·ke·al). Concerning the trachea and bronchi.

tracheobronchitis (**tra**·ke·o·brong·**ki**′·tis). Inflammation of the bronchi, spreading to the trachea. [trachea, bronchus, Gk *-itis* inflammation.]

tracheobronchogram (**tra**·ke·o·**brong**′·ko·gram). Radiographic visualization of the upper respiratory passages, either by means of tomography or following contrast injection. [trachea, bronchus, Gk *gramma* record.]

tracheobronchoscopy (**tra**·ke·o·brong·**kos**′·ko·pe). Internal examination of the trachea and bronchi. [trachea, bronchus, Gk *skopein* to view.]

tracheocele (**tra**·ke·o·seel). Extrusion of the tracheal lining through a weakness in the wall of the trachea. [trachea, Gk *kele* hernia.]

tracheofissure (**tra**·ke·o·**fish**′·ewr). The establishment of a fissure in the trachea.

tracheofistulization (**tra**·ke·o·fis·tew·li·**za**′·shun). Introduction of any medicinal agent directly into the trachea through an artificial fistula established in the wall.

tracheolaryngeal (**tra**·ke·o·lar·**in**′·je·al). Concerned with the trachea and the larynx.

tracheolaryngotomy (**tra**·ke·o·lar·in·**got**′·o·me). Surgical incision made into the larynx and the wall of the trachea. [trachea, larynx, Gk *temnein* to cut.]

tracheomalacia (**tra**·ke·o·mal·**a**′·she·ah). Softening of the cartilaginous rings of the trachea. [trachea, Gk *malakia* softness.]

tracheo-oesophageal (**tra**·ke·o·e·sof·ah·**je**′·al). Concerning the trachea and the oesophagus.

tracheopathia, tracheopathy (**tra**·ke·o·**path**′·e·ah, tra·ke·**op**·ath·e). Any morbid condition of the trachea. **Tracheopathia osteoplastica.** The development of bone and cartilage in the mucous lining of the trachea. [trachea, Gk *pathos* disease.]

tracheopharyngeal (**tra**·ke·o·far·**in**′·je·al). Concerning the trachea and the pharynx.

tracheophony (tra·ke·**of**·on·e). A hollow sound heard in auscultation over the trachea. [trachea, Gk *phone* sound.]

tracheoplasty (tra·ke·o·plas·te). Plastic surgery of the trachea. [trachea, Gk *plassein* to mould.]

tracheopyosis (**tra**·ke·o·pi·**o**′·sis). Tracheitis with suppuration. [trachea, Gk *pyon* pus, *-osis* condition.]

tracheorrhagia (**tra**·ke·o·**ra**′·je·ah). Haemorrhage from the lining of the trachea. [trachea, Gk *rhegnynein* to gush forth.]

tracheorrhaphy (tra·ke·**or**·af·e). Surgical suture of the trachea. [trachea, Gk *rhaphe* suture.]

tracheoschisis (tra·ke·**os**·kis·is). Any fissure occurring in the trachea. [trachea, Gk *schisis* fissure.]

tracheoscopic, tracheoscopical (**tra**·ke·o·**skop**′·ik, **tra**·ke·o·**skop**′·ik·al). Concerned with tracheoscopy.

tracheoscopy (tra·ke·**os**·ko·pe). The inspection of the interior of the trachea. **Percervical tracheoscopy.** Tracheoscopy by way of a tracheotomy wound. **Peroral tracheoscopy.** Tracheoscopy by way of the mouth and larynx. [trachea, Gk *skopein* to view.]

tracheostenosis (**tra**·ke·o·sten·**o**′·sis). Narrowing of the trachea. [trachea, Gk *stenosis* contraction.]

tracheostome (tra·ke·o·stome). The artificial opening made into the trachea by the operation of tracheostomy. [trachea, Gk *stoma* mouth.]

tracheostomy (tra·ke·os·to·me). An artificial opening made into the trachea through the neck. [trachea, Gk *stoma* mouth.]

tracheotome (tra·ke·o·tome). Surgical instrument employed in tracheotomy.

tracheotomy (tra·ke·ot·o·me). The surgical establishment of an opening from the exterior into the interior of the trachea. **High tracheotomy.** Tracheotomy above the level of the isthmus of the thyroid gland. **Inferior tracheotomy, Low tracheotomy.** Tracheotomy through a wound below the level of the isthmus of the thyroid gland. **Superior tracheotomy.** High tracheotomy (see above). [trachea, Gk *temnein* to cut.]

trachielcosis (tra·ke·el·ko'·sis). Formation of ulcers in the trachea. [trachea, Gk *helkos* ulcer.]

trachielcus (tra·ke·el·kus). An ulcer of the trachea. [see prec.]

Trachinus draco (tra·ki·nus dra·ko). A poisonous fish found in the Mediterranean. [LL *trachinus* horse-mackerel, L dragon.]

trachitis (tra·ki·tis). Tracheitis.

trachoma (trak·o·mah) (pl. *trachomata*). A chronic contagious disease affecting the conjunctiva and the cornea, running a prolonged course, and characterized by follicle formation and papillary hypertrophy in the conjunctiva, vascularization, and infiltration of the cornea known as *pannus*, and finally scarring of the lids and cornea, caused by the TRIC (trachoma-inclusion conjunctivitis) agent, now classified as *Bedsonia*. It is sensitive to tetracyclines. Also called *Egyptian ophthalmia* or *granular conjunctivitis*. For convenience it is divided into four stages: *stage* 1, the early stage of infiltration, indistinguishable from ordinary conjunctivitis; *stage* 2, the stage of active inflammation when clinical diagnosis can be made; *stage* 3, the healing stage when scarring takes place; and *stage* 4, when the condition is healed and no further inflammatory changes take place. **Acute trachoma.** When the disease starts with an acute onset: this may sometimes be due to secondary infection. **Follicular trachoma, Trachoma folliculare.** Trachoma in which the follicles in the conjunctiva are particularly marked, appearing granular, like sago grains. **Granular trachoma, Trachoma granulosum.** Synonyms for trachoma folliculare (see above), when trachoma was considered to be two diseases, this and trachoma papillare. **Trachoma mixtum.** A combination of the papillary and follicular types. Microscopically, all cases show both types. **Papillary trachoma, Trachoma papillare.** That in which there is papillary hypertrophy of the conjunctiva especially covering the upper tarsus, it becomes red and velvety. **Trachoma verum.** Trachoma folliculare (see above). [Gk roughness.]

See also: ARLT, STELLWAG VON CARION.

trachomatous (trak·o·mat·us). Exhibiting the characteristics of trachoma; affected with trachoma.

Trachybdella (tra·ke·del·ah). A genus of New World leeches. **Trachybdella bistriata.** A species recorded as feeding on man in Brazil. [Gk *trachys* rough, *bdella* leech.]

trachychromatic (tra·ke·kro·mat'·ik). Describing tissue that stains intensely; particularly applied to the chromatin of the cell nucleus. [Gk *trachys* rough, *chroma* colour.]

trachyphonia (tra·ke·fo·ne·ah). Hoarseness; roughnes of the voice. [Gk *trachys* rough, *phone* sound.]

track (trak). 1. The path of an ionizing particle, e.g. in a cloud chamber or photographic emulsion. 2. The path of a mechanical component, e.g. a groove in a gramophone record. **Fog track.** A visible track in a Wilson cloud chamber showing the path of an ionizing particle. It is caused by condensation of supersaturated vapour on the ions in the track. [OFr. *trac.*]

tract [tractus (NA)] (trakt). A part of some structure, usually that part along which something passes, e.g. air, secreta, or nervous impulses. **Afferent tract.** Ascending tract (see below). **Alimentary tract.** Alimentary canal. *See* CANAL. **Ascending tract.** One conveying impulses rostrally in the nervous system. **Association tract [tractus nervosus associationis (NA)].** One linking areas of the cortex of the same cerebral hemisphere. **Biliary tract.** The tract along which bile flows, from the bile canaliculi in the liver to the opening of the bile duct into the duodenum. **Bulbar tract.** A tract of the medulla oblongata. **Central tegmental tract.** Central tegmental fasciculus. *See* FASCICULUS. **Cerebellorubral tract [tractus cerebellorubralis (NA)].** A tract from the dentate nucleus to the red nucleus. **Cerebellothalamic tract [tractus cerebellothalamicus (NA)].** Fibres from the dentate nucleus to the medial nucleus of the thalamus. **Cerebropontine tracts [tractus corticopontinus (NA)].** Fibres arising in the cerebral cortex and ending in the nuclei pontis. They consist of frontopontine and temporopontine fibres. **Cerebrospinal tract, anterior [tractus corticospinalis (pyramidalis) anterior (NA)].** The fibres of the main motor pathway in the anterior white column that do not cross in the pyramidal decussation, **Cerebrospinal tract, lateral [tractus corticospinalis (pyramidalis) lateralis (NA)].** The main motor pathway (pyramidal tract) in the lateral white column which arises in the motor cortex (and in areas anterior to this), decussates at the level of the lower medulla, and terminates around the anterior horn cells in the cord. **Comma tract.** Fasciculus interfascicularis. **Commissural tract [tractus nervosus commissuralis (NA)].** Fibres connecting the opposite hemispheres of the brain. **Corticobulbar tract.** Those fibres of the pyramidal tract that pass to the cranial motor nuclei instead of the anterior horn cells of the spinal cord. **Corticohypothalamic tract [tractus corticohypothalamicus (NA)].** Descending fibres from the frontal lobe to the hypothalamus. **Corticonuclear tract [tractus corticonuclearis (NA)].** The fibres of the pyramidal tract (see below) which terminate around cells of the motor nuclei of the cranial nerves in the brain stem. **Dead tract.** Those dentinal tubules which are shut off from the tooth pulp by a hyaline layer of calcified tissue in dental caries. **Dentatorubral tract.** Cerebellorubral tract (see above). **Descending tract.** One conveying impulses caudally in the nervous system. **Digestive tract.** Alimentary canal. *See* CANAL. **Dorsolateral tract.** Posterolateral tract (see below). **Efferent tract.** Descending tract (see above). **Fibre tract.** A bundle of nerve fibres having a similar origin, termination, and function. **Frontopontine tract [tractus frontopontinus (NA)].** Descending fibres from cells in the frontal cortex; they terminate around cells of the nuclei pontis of the same side. **Gastro-intestinal tract.** The stomach and the intestines considered as a continuous canal. **Generative tract.** The female genital system. **Geniculocalcarine tract.** The optic radiation. *See* RADIATION. **Genito-urinary tract.** The urogenital system. *See* SYSTEM. **Gracile tract.** The fasciculus gracilis. **Hypothalamo-hypophyseal tract.** A tract of nerve fibres running mainly from the supra-optic and paraventricular nuclei of the hypothalamus to the posterior lobe of the hypophysis. It is responsible for the transport and release of the posterior lobe hormones. **Iliopubic tract.** The deep crural arch. *See* ARCH. **Iliotibial tract [tractus iliotibialis (NA)].** A thickened portion of the fascia lata, extending from the iliac crest to the lateral condyle of the tibia and receiving the whole insertion of the tensor fasciae latae and part of that of the gluteus maximus muscle. **Internodal tracts.** The hypothetical pathways of preferential conduction between the sinu-atrial node and the atrioventricular node in the heart. **Internuncial tract.** A tract connecting two, usually neighbouring, nuclei. **Intersegmental tracts [fasciculi proprii medullae spinalis (fasciculi intersegmentales) NA].** The fibrous tracts linking spinal segments, comprising the anterior, lateral, and posterior intersegmental tracts. **Intersegmental tract, anterior [fasciculus proprius (NA)].** Fibres of variable length in the anterior white column connecting spinal cells of different levels. Some continue cranially into the medial longitudinal bundle. **Intersegmental tract, lateral [fasciculus proprius (NA)].** Fibres of varying length in the lateral white column connecting spinal cells of different levels. **Intersegmental tract, posterior [fasciculus proprius (NA)].** Fibres of varying length in the posterior white column connecting cells of the spinal cord at different levels. **Intestinal tract.** Intestinal canal. *See* CANAL. **Mamillopeduncular tract.** The ascending tract in the brain stem, possibly coming partly from the nucleus of the tractus solitarius and ending in the mamillary body; the peduncle of the mamillary body. **Mamillotegmental tract [fasciculus mamillotegmentalis (NA)].** A bundle of fibres from the mamillary body to the tegmentum. **Mamillothalamic tract [fasciculus mamillothalamicus (NA)].** A compact bundle of fibres which passes from the mamillary body to the anterior nucleus of the thalamus. **Mesencephalic tract.** Tract of the trigeminal nerve, mesencephalic (see below). **Motor tract.** One conveying impulses regulating movement. **Occipitopontine tract [tractus occipitopontinus (NA)].** Descending fibres from cells in the occipital cortex; they terminate around cells of the nuclei pontis of the same side. **Olfactory tract [tractus olfactorius (NA)].** The fibres of the olfactory system which connect the olfactory bulb to the cerebral hemispheres. It divides posteriorly to form the roots, medial and lateral. **Olfactory tract, intermediate root of the.** Partly developed fibres to the anterior perforated substance. **Olfactory tract, lateral root of the.** Fibres which skirt the anterior perforated substance and run to the limen insulae where they turn on themselves and proceed to the uncus. **Olfactory tract, medial root of the.** Fibres which run medial to the anterior perforated substance on to the medial surface of the hemisphere; it appears to end in the parolfactory area. **Olivocerebellar tract [tractus olivocerebellaris (NA)].** Fibres passing medially from the olive, especially from the hilar region, to enter the inferior cerebellar peduncle of the other side. **Olivospinal tract.** A small tract passing from the olive to the anterior horn cells in the cervical region, usually said to lie in the lateral white column. It is part of the extrapyramidal motor system. **Optic tract [tractus opticus (NA)].** A flattened band of nerve fibres running backwards and laterally, around each cerebral peduncle, from the optic chiasma to the lateral geniculate body. **Optic tract, lateral root of the.** The true optic tract which ends in the lateral geniculate body and the superior colliculus. **Optic tract, medial root of the.** Non-visual fibres believed to connect the two medial geniculate bodies. **Parietopontine tract [tractus parietopontinus (NA)].** Descending fibres from cells in the parietal cortex; they terminate around the cells of the nuclei pontis of the same side. **Posterolateral tract [tractus dorsolateralis (NA)].** The non-myelinated or finely myelinated fibres in the lateral white column, carrying impulses concerned with painful and thermal sensibility, which run from the posterior nerve root along the apex of the posterior grey column before ending in the gelatinous substance. **Projection tract [tractus nervosus projectionis (NA)].** Fibres connecting the cerebral cortex with the lower parts of the brain and spinal cord. **Pyramidal tract [tractus pyramidalis (NA)].** Lateral cerebrospinal tract; the pathway by which the cortex controls contralateral voluntary movement: arising in the motor cortex, it runs through the brain stem to decussate in the medulla, finally occupying part of the lateral column of the spinal cord, a few fibres remaining uncrossed in the anterior column. Its superficial position produces a pyramidal elevation on the ventral surface of the medulla oblongata. **Respiratory tract.** Respiratory system. *See* SYSTEM. **Reticulospinal tract [tractus reticulospinalis (NA)].** A descending tract formed by axons of the cells in the reticular formation in the brain stem; its fibres terminate around the motor cells of the anterior grey column of the spinal medulla. **Rubrospinal tract [tractus rubrospinalis (NA)].** Fibres in the lateral white column arising in the red nucleus of one side, decussating in the tegmentum, and terminating around the contralateral anterior horn cells, especially in the cervical region. It is part of the extrapyramidal system. **Semilunar tract [fasciculus septomarginalis (NA)].** A comma-shaped tract in the posterior white column, probably intersegmental. **Seminal tract.** The seminal vesicle and its duct. **Sensory tract.** A tract conveying impulses originating in peripheral sense organs or plexuses. **Septomarginal tract.** A collective name for intersegmental fibres in the posterior white column, running close to the posterior median sulcus. **Speech tract.** One linking the cortex with the nuclei innervating the organs of speech. **Spinal tract.** Tract of the trigeminal nerve, spinal (see below). **Spinocerebellar tract, anterior [tractus spinocerebellaris anterior (NA)].** A tract in the lateral white column carrying axons of cells in the thoracic nucleus (or adjacent nuclei) to the cerebellum, entering by the superior cerebellar peduncle; both homolateral and contralateral connections exist. **Spinocerebellar tract, posterior [tractus spinocerebellaris posterior (NA)].** A tract in the lateral white column carrying axons of the cells of the thoracic nucleus to the cerebellum, which it enters by the inferior cerebellar peduncle; it is reputed to be entirely homolateral. **Spinotectal tract [tractus spinotectalis (NA)].** A tract in the lateral white column arising in the posterior grey column and ending in the opposite superior quadrigeminal body. It is a pathway for reflexes that produce movements of the head and eyes. **Spinothalamic tract, anterior [tractus spinothalamicus anterior (NA)].** One of the ascending fibre tracts in the anterior white column, mediating tactile sensations. **Spinothalamic tract, lateral [tractus spinothalamicus lateralis (NA)].** A tract in the lateral white column made up of fibres that have arisen in the vicinity of the posterior grey column (especially in the gelatinous substance) and have crossed to the opposite side of the spinal cord. It ends in the thalamus and mediates painful and thermal sensibility. **Supra-opticohypophyseal tract [tractus supra-opticohypophysialis (NA)].** Fibres from the supra-optic, tuberal, and paraventricular nuclei of the hypothalamus which pass to the posterior lobe of the hypophysis cerebri. **Tectocerebellar tract.** A tract arising in the tectum of the mid-brain and passing with the superior cerebellar peduncle to the cerebellum. **Tectospinal tract [tractus tectospinalis (NA)].** Fibres in the lateral white column arising in each superior quadrigeminal body and ending around the anterior horn cells, mainly of the opposite side. **Temporofrontal tract.** A tract of white fibres from the temporal lobe to the frontal lobe of the brain. **Temporopontine tract [tractus temporopontinus (NA)].** Descending fibres from cells in the temporal cortex; they terminate around the cells of the nuclei pontis of the same side. **Thalamo-olivary tract.** The tract that carries afferent fibres from the thalamus, interstitial nucleus, red nucleus, and tegmental nuclei to the olive. **Tracheobronchial tract.** That part of the respiratory tract that traverses the trachea and bronchi. **Transverse peduncular tract.** Fibres passing from the inferior brachium ventrally around the mid-brain in the groove rostral to the superior quadrigeminal body. **Tract of the trigeminal nerve, mesencephalic [tractus mesencephalicus nervi trigemini (NA)].** A column of cells lateral to the aqueduct of the mid-brain, for reception of proprioceptive fibres from the muscles of mastication. **Tract of the trigeminal nerve, spinal [tractus spinalis nervi trigemini (NA)].** A tract, accompanied by a corresponding nucleus [nucleus tractus spinalis nervi trigemini (NA)] lying on its medial side, which runs downwards from the mid-pons level (near the lateral margin of the floor of the 4th ventricle) to the level of the spinal cord, where its nucleus is continuous with the gelatinous matter. It conveys painful and thermal impulses from the trigeminal area. **Urinary tract.** The tract from the pelvis of the ureter to the urinary orifice considered as a continuous canal. **Urogenital tract.** Urogenital system. *See* SYSTEM. **Uveal tract.** The vascular and pigmented tissues forming the middle coat of the eye: the iris, ciliary body, and choroid. **Vestibulospinal tract [tractus vestibulospinalis].** The tract in the anterior white column derived from the large cells of the lateral vestibular nuclei and ending around the anterior horn cells, mainly of the same side. [L *tractus.*]

See also: ALLEN, BECHTEREW, BRUCE (A.), BURDACH, CIAGLINSKI, COLLIER, D'AZYR, DEITERS, FLECHSIG, FOVILLE, GOLL, GOMBAULT, GOWERS, HELWEG, HOCHE, LISSAUER, LOEWENTHAL, MAISSIAT, MEYNERT, MONAKOW, MUIR (J. C.), MUNZER, PHILIPPE, SCHULTZE (M. J. S.), SPITZKA (E. C.), WALDEYER-HARTZ.

tractellum (trak·tel·um). An anterior flagellum of a flagellate protozoan, or other motile body, which propels the body by traction. [dim. of L *tractus* tract.]

traction (trak·shun). The act of pulling. **Axis traction.** Traction made on the fetus in the direction of the birth canal. **Elastic traction.** Traction by an elastic appliance. **Gallows traction.** Traction on the legs of a child by suspending the child from an overhead frame, resembling a gallows. Traction is applied to the legs by means of strapping, the strapping then being attached to the overhead bar of the gallows. **Head traction.** Traction exerted on the head, e.g. in the treatment of injuries of the cervical vertebrae. **Intermaxillary traction, Intramaxillary traction.** Reciprocal anchorage in one jaw. **Skeletal traction.** Traction directly upon the bone by a weight attached to a pin or wire transfixing the bone, or by an ice-tong caliper attached to the bone. **Tongue traction.** A manoeuvre which consists of pulling the tongue forward to maintain a free upper air passage; it is used in anaesthesia, during epileptiform convulsions, and in any state of unconsciousness in which the airway is in danger of becoming obstructed by the tongue falling backwards. **Weight traction.** Traction applied to a limb by means of a suspended weight attached to the limb. **Windlass traction.** Traction applied to a limb by means of extension tapes of adhesive strapping attached to that limb. The tapes are then fixed to a Thomas' splint by means of a small wooden bar, thus producing a pull upon the limb. [L *trahere* to draw.]

See also: ANDERSON (R.), BOEHLER, PUGH, RUSSELL (R. H.).

tractor (**trak**·tor). A traction machine. [see prec.]

See also: PERKINS.

tractotomy (trak·**tot**·o·me). The operation for cutting nerve tracts in the spinal cord or mid-brain (*mesencephalic tractotomy*). It is used chiefly in the relief of severe intractable pain (e.g. *spinothalamic tractotomy*). *Pyramidal tractotomy* has been used for certain motor disorders with spastic and athetotic symptoms. When the cut is at the level of the cerebral peduncles the operation is known as *peduncular tractotomy.* [tract, Gk *temnein* to cut.]

tractus [NA] (**trak**·tus). Tract. **Tractus solitarius [NA].** A slender tract lying in the lateral part of the upper medulla near its dorsal surface. It is made up of gustatory fibres from the 7th, 9th, and 10th cranial nerves, which terminate in cells, lying alongside the tract, constituting its nucleus [nucleus tractus solitarii (NA)]. **Tractus spiralis foraminosus [NA].** A series of spirally arranged holes surrounding the central canal of the cochlear in the lower part of the vertical plate at the lateral end of the internal auditory meatus; these and the central canal transmit the fibres of the cochlear nerve. [L tract.]

tragacanth (**trag**·ak·anth). The dried gummy exudation obtained by incision from *Astragalus gummifer* and allied species. It occurs in flattened ribbon-like flakes which are white, translucent, and marked on the flat sides with concentric rings. The powdered drug forms a viscous mucilage with water even in concentrations as low as 1 per cent; used as a suspending agent in pharmacy, both for powders and for resinous tinctures (BP 1973). **False tragacanth.** A gum obtained from a species of *Prunus* and used as a substitute for tragacanth. **Indian tragacanth.** Sterculia. [Gk *tragos* goat, *akantha* thorn.]

tragal (**tra**·gal). Concerning the tragus.

tragi (**tra**·ji). Hairs of the external auditory meatus. [Gk *tragos* goat.]

tragicus muscle [musculus tragicus (NA)] (**tra**·gik·us musl). An intrinsic muscle of the auricle on the lateral surface; it is a quadrate muscle whose vertically running fibres cover the tragus.

tragomaschalia (tra·go·mas·**ka**'·le·ah). Unpleasant odour of perspiration from the armpits. [Gk *tragos* goat, *maschale* armpit.]

tragophonia, tragophony (tra·go·**fo**·ne·ah, tra·**gof**·o·ne). A bleating kind of voice symptomatic of hydrothorax and heard in auscultation. [Gk *tragos* goat, *phone* sound.]

tragopodia (tra·go·**po**·de·ah). Knock knee; genu valgum. [Gk *tragos* goat, *pous* foot.]

tragus [NA] (**tra**·gus). The small extension of the auricular cartilage in front of the orifice of the external auditory meatus. [Gk *tragos* goat.]

Trainor's operation. For ptosis: a modification of Motais' operation. A horizontal strip of the upper border of the tarsal plate is fashioned, being left attached at one end. This is passed under the superior rectus tendon and sutured back to the tarsal plate, so forming a sling.

trait (tra). 1. A special, relatively stable feature of body, mind, or character, inherited or developed. 2. An inherent tendency towards the development of such a special feature. **Sickle-cell trait.** The expression of the heterozygous inheritance of the gene determining sickle haemoglobin (HbS). The subject possesses both HbA and HbS in his red blood cells, though the latter is in a concentration too low to cause intravascular sickling at oxygen tensions obtaining in the tissues in health. **Thalassaemic trait.** A trait resulting from the heterozygous occurrence of the thalassaemia gene; thalassaemia results from its homozygous occurrence. [Fr.]

See also: COOLEY, JADELOT.

trajector (traj·**ek**·tor). An instrument for seeking a bullet in a wound. [L piercer.]

Tramazoline (tram·**az**·o·leen). BP Commission approved name for 2 - (5,6,7,8 - tetrahydro - 1 - naphthylamino) - 2 - imidazoline; a sympathomimetic agent.

Trambusti, Arnaldo (b. 1863). Italian pathologist.

Trambusti's reaction. Endodermoreaction; the response to a test in which tuberculin is introduced into the layers of the skin on a needle inserted tangentially. Reddening, 3 days later, is a positive result.

tramitis (tram·**i**·tis). The radiological appearance of a late form of tuberculosis, characterized by fibrosis, collapse, and calcification. [obsolete term.]

trance (trahns). 1. A state of altered consciousness, often with absence of voluntary movement, or with automatism. 2. A state of mental abstraction from environment. **Alcoholic trance.** Trance (in the sense of def. 1. above) due to alcoholic intoxication. **Trance coma.** A trance state in which the degree of impairment of consciousness approaches coma. **Death trance.** Trance simulating death. **Ecstatic trance.** Trance in which the mental content is one of ecstasy. **Hypnotic trance.** Trance induced by hypnosis. **Hysterical trance.** Trance due to hysteria. **Induced trance.** Trance induced by some external event. [L *transire* to pass over.]

tranquillizer (**tran**·kwil·i·zer). A drug which has a depressant action on the central nervous system and has the ability to relieve emotional distress and disturbed behaviour and symptoms without causing clouding of consciousness. [L *tranquillus* calm.]

trans-. Latin prefix meaning *through* or *across.*

transaminases (trans·**am**·in·azez). Aminotransferases; a group of enzymes which catalyse reaction between an amino acid and a 2-oxo acid to form a new amino acid and a new 2-oxo acid. Pyridoxal phosphate is required as coenzyme. Common examples include glutamate, aspartate, aminotransferase (glutamate + oxaloacetate ⇌ 2-oxoglutarate + aspartate) and glutamate alanine aminotransferase (glutamate + pyruvate ⇌ 2-oxoglutarate + alanine). The blood plasma activities of transaminase give an estimate of cell damage, e.g. in liver disease or myocardial infarction. **Glutamic-oxalacetic transaminase.** GO-T, an enzyme of the citric-acid cycle which catalyses the reaction aspartate ⇌ oxalacetate. It is abundant in heart muscle and in the liver, and is released into the blood in myocardial infarction and in liver disease. It is determined in the serum as an aid to the diagnosis of these conditions. **Glutamic-pyruvic transaminase.** GP-T, an enzyme which catalyses the reaction alanine ⇌ pyruvate. It is distributed in the body similarly to glutamic-oxalacetic transaminase but is more concentrated in the liver, and its determination in serum is of chief significance in liver disease.

transamination (**trans**·am·in·**a**'·shun). The transfer, through the agency of an enzyme (transaminase), of an amino group, NH_2, from one compound to another, e.g. from glutamic acid to a keto acid which is thereby converted to an amino acid. [L *trans*, amino.]

transanimation (**trans**·an·im·**a**'·shun). Artificial respiration applied to a stillborn child to induce it to breathe. [L *trans, anima* breath.]

transaudient (trans·**aw**·de·ent). Describing any substance that allows sound waves to pass through it. [L *trans, audire* to hear.]

transcalent (trans·**ka**·lent). Allowing the passage of radiant heat. [L *trans, calere* to be warm.]

transcervical (trans·ser·**vi**·kal, trans·**ser**·vik·al). Across the neck. Chiefly used in relation to the neck of the femur. [L *trans, cervix* neck.]

transcoelomic (trans·se·**lo**·mik). Across a body cavity. [L *trans,* Gk *koiloma* hollow.]

transcolumellar (**trans**·kol·um·**el**·ar). Across the columella nasi. [L *trans, columella* little column.]

transcondylar (trans·kon·**di**·lar). Through the condyles; a surgical term. [L *trans,* condyle.]

transcondyloid (trans·kon·**di**·loid). Transcondylar. [L *trans,* condyle, Gk *eidos* form.]

transcortical (trans·**kor**·tik·al). 1. Through the cortex of an organ. 2. Describing connections between different parts of the cerebral cortex. [L *trans,* cortex.]

transcortin (trans·**kor**·tin). An α-globulin plasma protein with a high affinity for cortisol and corticosterone. [L *trans,* corticosterone.]

transcriptase (tran·**skrip**·taze). The class of RNA polymerases which are dependent for their activity on the presence of DNA. They function in the transcription of DNA in living cells by converting a DNA base sequence into its complementary RNA base sequence. **Reverse transcriptase.** An RNA-dependent DNA polymerase; it is present in RNA tumour viruses and is thought to be involved in the transformation of normal cells to tumour cells. [L *transcriptum,* a reproduction.]

transcription (tran·**skrip**·shun). The process by which the nucleotide sequence of a strand of DNA is converted into a complementary nucleotide sequence of a strand of RNA; the synthesis of RNA using, as template, a strand of DNA. [L *transcriptum,* a reproduction.]

transcutaneous (trans·kew·**ta**·ne·us). Percutaneous. (L *trans, cutis* skin.]

transdeamination (**trans**·de·am·in·a′·shun). In the metabolism of proteins, the removal of an NH_2 group from an amino acid and its transference to another compound. [L *trans,* deamination.]

transdehydro-iso-androsterone (trans·de·**hi**·dro·is·o·an·dro·**steer**′·one). A steroid obtained from the urine of male animals, female animals with adrenal tumours, and pregnant animals. Its systematic name is Δ^5-androstene-3(β)-ol-17-one.

transducer (trans·**dew**·ser). In biophysics, a measuring device for converting one type of energy into another, e.g. pressure or mechanical energy into electrical energy, or electrical energy into sound. [L *trans, ducere* to lead.]

transduction (trans·**duk**·shun). Genetic transfer among bacteria, mediated by particles of temperate bacteriophage grown in the donor strain and subsequently used to infect a recipient strain. Of the phage particles liberated by the donor strain, only about one in 10^2–10^3 carry fragments of bacterial chromosome and are transducing. The length of the carried transducing fragments varies, but is of the order 0.1-0.01 of the bacterial chromosome. Transducing phages for a wide range of bacterial genera and species are now known. **Abortive transduction.** Occurs when the transferred donor fragment of DNA is neither replicated nor integrated into the recipient chromosome to form a stable recombinant (complete transductant), but expresses its genes and is inherited unilinearly among the recipient progeny for a limited number of generations. It occurs only in generalized transduction where the majority of transfers tend to be abortive. **Generalized transduction.** Any fragment of the chromosome may be transferred in a random manner; a property of the phage, e.g. phage P1 of *Escherichia coli,* phage P22 of *Salmonella.* The transducing particles probably contain no phage DNA, fragments of bacterial DNA of the right size being accidentally incorporated into the phage head by a process of phenotypic mixing. The transduced fragments replace their homologues in the recipient chromosome to yield haploid transductants. **Localized (or specialized) transduction.** Only a particular fragment of donor chromosome, located adjacent to the site of integration of the prophage in lysogeny, is transduced, e.g. transduction of the *E. coli* galactose region to phage *lambda.* Transducing particles arise only following the induction of lysogenic bacteria and usually contain a defective phage genome into which the fragment of bacterial chromosome is incorporated. When transferred to a recipient cell this structure becomes circular and, by recombinaton, can be alternately inserted into and released from the chromosome (*see* CAMPBELL MODEL); the recipient homologue is not lost so that the cell is diploid (heterogenote) for the transduced region (exogenote). [L *trans, ducere* to lead.]

transduodenal (**trans**·dew·o·**de**′·nal). Through the duodenum. [L *trans,* duodenum.]

transection (tran·**sek**·shun). Cross-section. [L *trans, secare* to cut.]

transfection (trans·**fek**·shun). Infection of competent bacterial cells by transformation with purified viral DNA. [L *trans, inficere* to stain.]

transfer (trans·fer). **Peptidyl transfer.** The process catalysed by the enzyme peptidyl transferase during protein synthesis in living cells. [L *transferre* to bring across.]

transference (**trans**·fer·ens). 1. The mental process occurring during the course of psycho-analytical treatment when the patient sees in the analyst the reincarnation of people from his past, and transfers to the analyst emotions that applied to those people. 2. The act of transferring. *See also:* NICOLADONI. **Negative transference, Positive transference.** *See* TRANSFERENCE NEUROSIS (*under* NEUROSIS). **Transference of sensation.** The faulty localization of a sensation to a place at which the stimulus was not applied. [L *transferre* to bring across.]

transferrin (trans·**fer**·in). A β-globulin found in the plasma which acts as a carrier for iron. [L *trans, ferrum* iron.]

transfix (trans·**fix**). To impale; to pierce completely with a sharp point. [L *trans, figere* to fix.]

transfixion (trans·**fik**·shun). 1. The act of transfixing. 2. In surgery, the method of amputation by passing the knife through the soft tissues from one side to the other as near to the bone as possible, and cutting the muscles from within outwards. [see prec.]

transforation (trans·for·**a**·shun). Perforation, particularly the piercing of the fetal skull in craniotomy. [L *trans, forare* to pierce.]

transforator (**trans**·for·a·tor). An instrument employed in transforation.

transformation (trans·for·**ma**·shun). 1. A change in form or function. 2. The change of one nuclide into another. **Asbestos transformation.** A silky appearance of hyaline cartilage produced by accentuation or new formation of the fibres. **Bacterial transformation.** The transfer of genetic characters from donor to recipient bacteria, mediated by donor DNA molecules. First described, but not understood, by F. Griffith (1928) in the case of transformation of capsular type specificity in *Pneumococcus.* Valuable in genetic analysis of bacterial species in which other mechanisms of genetic transfer are not available, e.g. *Haemophilus, Aerobacter,* some *Bacillus* spp; also valuable in assessing the effect of various treatments of DNA on its biological function, as judged by ability to transform. Uptake of DNA by recipient bacteria depends on attainment of a physiological state of *competence.* **G-F transformation, Globular-fibrous transformation.** The reversible change of actin from its globular to its polymerized fibrous, or filamentous, form. [see foll.]

transformer (trans·**form**·er). An apparatus without continuously moving parts which, by electromagnetic induction, changes alternating or intermittent electrical energy at one voltage into electrical energy of the same frequency at a different voltage. **Closed-core transformer.** A transformer having a closed unbroken core of laminated magnetic material, usually soft iron. **Filament transformer.** A step-down transformer (see below) to supply low-voltage current for heating the cathode filament of an x-ray tube. **Open-core transformer.** A transformer having a core of laminated magnetic material open at both ends, as in an induction coil. **Resonance transformer.** A high-voltage transformer designed so that the secondary winding resonates at the supply frequency applied to the primary. It is used for high-voltage x-ray machines and is smaller than the conventional transformer. **Step-down transformer.** One transforming electrical energy from a higher to a lower voltage. **Step-up transformer.** One transforming electrical energy from a lower to a higher voltage, with diminution of current. **Tripler transformer.** An electrical transformer for converting a three-phase alternating supply into a single-phase supply of three times the frequency. [L *transformare* to change in shape.]

transfuse (trans·**fewz**). To give a transfusion.

transfusion (trans·**few**·zhun). The introduction into the blood vessels of the circulatory system of sterile fluids such as blood, plasma, serum, blood substitutes and other solutions, but normally implying the administration of blood or its fractions by various continuous or intermittent techniques. Cf. INFUSION. **Arterial transfusion.** The transfusion of blood into an artery of the recipient. **Direct transfusion.** The transfer of whole blood directly from the vein of the donor to the vein of the recipient without exposure to the air or intermediate collection in a vessel, thus obviating defibrination or the use of anticoagulants. **Drip transfusion.** The administration of blood or packed red cells slowly over a long period so adjusted that a required number of drops per minute are given. **Exchange transfusion, Exsanguination transfusion.** Replacement transfusion (see below). **Immediate transfusion.** Direct transfusion (see above). **Indirect transfusion.** The transfusion of blood or its fractions into the recipient after its previous withdrawal from the donor and preparation by addition of anticoagulants, defibrinating, etc. **Leucocyte transfusion.** The transfusion of a large volume of separated white blood cells into a patient suffering from any disease characterized by very small numbers of, or no, white cells in the circulating blood. **Mediate transfusion.** Indirect transfusion (see above). **Peritoneal transfusion.** The infusion of blood serum, fractions, or other solutions, into the peritoneal cavity. **Plasma transfusion.** The transfusion of blood plasma. **Replacement transfusion.** The removal of most or all of the recipient's blood with the simultaneous transfusion of an equal volume of normal blood, a technique usually performed in young children suffering from acute leukaemia or erythroblastosis. **Serum transfusion.** The transfusion of blood serum. **Sternal transfusion.** Transfusion into the medullary cavity of the sternum. **Subcutaneous transfusion.** The slow infusion of fluids in large quantities into the subcutaneous tissues, usually with the object of combating dehydration. **Substitution transfusion.** Replacement transfusion (see above). **Total transfusion.** Replacement transfusion (see above). **Vaccinating transfusion.** The transfusion into a patient who is severely ill with an infectious disease, of blood or serum taken from a patient in the convalescent stage of the same disease, in order to produce a rapid immunity. **Venous transfusion.** The transfusion of blood or blood substitutes into the recipient's vein. [L *transfundere* to pour through.]

transgression (trans·**gresh**·un). The passage of a substance from one solvent to another through a medium in which it may be almost insoluble. [L *transgredi* to advance across.]

transients (trans·e·ents). Quantities, e.g. electrical signals or mechanical movements, which occur and are then not repeated. [L *transire* to go through.]

transiliac (trans·**il**·e·ak). Extending from one ilium to the other. [L *trans*, ilium.]

transilient (trans·**il**·e·ent). Passing across from one point to another, as with association fibres of the cerebral cortex which link convolutions that are not adjacent. [L *trans*, *salire* to leap.]

transillumination (**trans**·il·ew·min·**a**'·shun). The examination of a translucent part by placing a strong light behind it, when the presence of fluid, lesions, or cavities is made apparent. [L *trans*, *illuminare* to light up.]

transilluminator (trans·il·**ew**·min·a·tor). Ophthalmodiaphanoscope. [see prec.]

transinsular (trans·**in**·sew·lar). Across the insula of the brain. [L *trans*, insula.]

transischiac (trans·**is**·ke·ak). Passing across from one ischium to the other. [L *trans*, ischium.]

transisthmian (trans·**isth**·me·an). Crossing any isthmus, referring particularly to the isthmus of the gyrus cinguli. [L *trans*, isthmus.]

transistor (trans·**is**·tor). An electronic device made from semiconductor materials which performs the same functions as thermionic valves, but is smaller and consumes less power.

transition (trans·**ish**·un). **Isomeric transition.** IT, a transition between two isomeric states of a nucleus. [L *transire* to go through.]

transitional (trans·**ish**·un·al). Transient; passing from one state to another. **Transitional epithelium.** Epithelium in which cells of the lower layers are continually being transformed to replace those lost by the upper layers. **Transitional zone.** That part of the crystalline lens where the epithelial capsule cells change into lens fibres. [L *transire* to go through.]

transitionals (trans·**ish**·un·alz). An old name for large monocytes with indented nuclei, formerly supposed to undergo transition into granulocytes.

translation (trans·**la**·shun). In molecular biology, the process whereby the ribosomes, in association with transfer-RNA molecules, read and convert the sequence of nucleotide base triplets (codons) in messenger-RNA molecules into the sequence of amino acids in polypeptide chains. [L *translatio*, a handing over.]

translocase (trans·lo·**kaze**). The enzyme activity responsible for the movement of ribosomes during protein synthesis. [L *trans*, *locus* place.]

translocation (trans·lo·**ka**·shun). Chromosome aberration due to the transfer of a chromosome segment either to another chromosome or to a different position within the same chromosome. The latter, however, is more usually called *shift* or *intrachange*. The reciprocal exchange of chromosome material between two chromosomes is called *reciprocal translocation* or *interchange*. Translocations resulting in the intercalary incorporation of a chromosome segment into another are called *insertions*. **Robertsonian translocation** (or *centric fusion*). Translocation involving two acrocentric chromosomes and leading to their fusion at the centromere or nearby regions. **Tandem translocation.** A translocation resulting from a break near the centromere of a chromosome and the end of another, and leading to the fusion of an arm from the first to the terminal portion of the second. [L *trans*, *locus* place.]

translucency (trans·**lew**·sens·e). The quality of being translucent. **Root translucency.** The extending translucency of the root of a tooth which provides an indication of age. One of the Gustafson data.

See also: Regression LINE.

translucent (trans·**lew**·sent). Allowing light to pass to a limited extent, so that an illuminated field is seen but no distinct objects. Cf. TRANSPARENT. [L *trans*, *lucens* shining.]

translucid (trans·**lew**·sid). Translucent.

transmembrane (trans·**mem**·brane). Across a membrane, usually the membranous wall of a cell and applied to differences of electrical potential, concentrations of ions, metabolites, etc. [L *trans*, *membrana* membrane.]

transmethylation (**trans**·meth·il·**a**'·shun). The process of biological methylation carried on chiefly in the liver, in which methyl groups are transferred from methionine to other substances in the biosynthesis of such essential compounds as choline and creatine. [L *trans*, methylation.]

transmigration (trans·mi·**gra**·shun). 1. Diapedesis. 2. A movement from one position to another, as in the change of position from one side of the body to another. **External transmigration.** Migration of an ovum across the abdominal cavity into the uterine tube of the opposite side. **Internal transmigration.** Migration of the ovum from one uterine tube to the other by way of the uterus. [L *transmigrare* to migrate.]

transmissibility (trans·**mis**·ib·il′·it·e). The degree to which a disease may be transmitted from one person or place to another.

transmissible (trans·**mis**·ibl). Capable of being passed from one person or place to another, as in the case of a disease. [see foll.]

transmission (trans·**mish**·un). The passing or sending of anything from one person or place to another. **Arthropod transmission.** The transmission of a disease to a man or other animal from another by the agency of an insect or other arthropod. **Cyclical transmission.** Transmission after a cycle of development within the host. **Direct transmission.** The transmission of infection by insects immediately after acquisition without any intervening period during which it undergoes a cycle of development. **Duplex transmission.** The passage of impulses along a nerve in two directions. **Hereditary transmission.** The passing of heritable characters or of infection to offspring. **Hereditary arthropod transmission.** The transmission of acquired infection to the next generation, e.g. the *Rickettsia* of scrub typhus in mites. **Insect transmission.** Arthropod transmission (see above). **Placental transmission.** The transference of a substance or gas across the placental barrier. **Synaptic transmission.** Transmission across a synapse. [L *transmittere* to transmit.]

transmutation (trans·mew·**ta**·shun). 1. Mutation; the change brought about in a species by evolution. 2. The conversion of one element into another. This takes place in radioactivity and can be achieved artificially by bombardment with atomic projectiles. [L *transmutare* to change.]

transocular (trans·**ok**·ew·lar). Passing across the eye. [L *trans, oculus* eye.]

transonance (trans·**o**·nans). The passing of sound from one organ through another, e.g. when the heart is heard through the lungs and chest wall. [L *trans, sonare* to sound.]

transparent (trans·**pare**·ent). Allowing light to pass through, so that objects beyond may be clearly seen. Cf. TRANSLUCENT. [L *trans, parere* to appear.]

transperitoneal (trans·per·it·o·**ne**′·al). Across the peritoneum. [L *trans,* peritoneum.]

transphosphorylation (trans·fos·for·il·**a**′·shun). The direct transfer of phosphate groups between organic phosphates without the intermediate appearance of inorganic phosphates. [L *trans,* phosphorylation.]

transpiration (trans·pir·**a**·shun). Perspiration; the passage of water or a solution through a membrane or the skin, with subsequent evaporation. **Pulmonary transpiration.** The transfer of water from the blood to form vapour in the air of the pulmonary alveoli. [L *trans, spirare* to breathe.]

transplacental (trans·plas·**en**·tal). Conveyed through the placenta, as in the case of certain infections. [L *trans,* placenta.]

transplant (**trans**·plahnt). 1. To transfer a piece of tissue from one site to another, qualified as *autotransplant* (the donor being also the recipient), *homotransplant* (from one individual to another of the same species, e.g. mother to child), *heterotransplant* (from one species to another, e.g. monkey testis to human), *organ transplant* (transfer of a complete organ such as the kidney). 2. The tissue so transferred. *See also* GRAFT. **Digit transplant.** Staged transfer of a digit, usually from one part of the hand to another, e.g. in the formation of a new thumb. [L *transplantare.*]

See also: GALLIE, MCREYNOLDS.

transplantar (trans·**plan**·tar). Extending across the sole of the foot, as in the case of muscles and ligaments. [L *trans, planta* sole of foot.]

transplantation (trans·plan·**ta**·shun). The operation of transfer of tissue from one site to another. **Autologous transplantation.** Transfer of tissue to a new site in the same individual. **Autoplastic transplantation.** Autologous transplantation (see above). **Cardiac transplantation.** The operation of transference of the heart from a previously healthy individual immediately after death to replace the grossly diseased heart of another individual. **Transplantation of the cornea.** The replacement of a portion of the cornea of the eye, either the whole or partial thickness, with a graft of cornea taken from another eye, recently enucleated or one removed soon after death. Also called *corneal graft, keratoplasty.* **Heterologous transplantation.** Transfer of tissue from an animal to man or from one animal to another of a different species. **Heteroplastic transplantation.** Heterologous transplantation (see above). **Heterotopic transplantation.** Transplantation in which the graft is taken from a part of the body of the donor other than that on which it is transplanted in the recipient. **Homoeoplastic transplantation.** Homologous transplantation (see foll.). **Homologous transplantation.** Transfer of tissue from one human being to another or between one animal and another of the same species. **Homoplastic transplantation.** Homologous transplantation (see prec.). **Isologous transplantation.** Transfer of tissue to another genetically identical individual. In man, it is only possible between identical twins. **Organ transplantation.** The transfer of an entire organ to a new site, involving the re-establishment of its arterial, venous and other attachments. **Syngenesioplastic transplantation.** The transference of tissue to a recipient who is closely related to the donor. **Transplantation of teeth.** The act of implanting a tooth from one person into a tooth socket of another. **Tendon transplantation.** 1. An operation by which a tendon is altered in its point of insertion or in its direction of pull, especially in the correction of nerve palsies and following poliomyelitis. 2. In ophthalmology, an operation used in the surgery of paralysis of the external ocular muscles, the tendon or part of a tendon of an unaffected muscle being transplanted to the insertion of a paralysed one; O'Connor's operation, Hummelsheim's operation. **Tenoplastic transplantation.** Transplantation in which the donor and the recipient are of widely differing species. [L *transplantare* to transplant.]

See also: NESBIT, STILES.

transpleural (trans·**ploor**·al). Across the pleural cavity. [L *trans,* pleura.]

transport (**trans**·port). The movement or transference of biochemical substances. **Active transport.** Transport which requires the expenditure of energy. **Passive transport.** Transport which is non-energy dependent, e.g. diffusion down a gradient. [L *trans, portare* carry.]

transposition (trans·po·**zish**′·un). 1. In cardiology, a term which applies to conditions in which parts of the heart are interchanged in their positions or relationships as the result of abnormal embryonic development; it is most commonly used with reference to the roots of the aorta and pulmonary artery. 2. An operation which involves a change in the relative positions of two structures, especially in plastic surgery in the fashioning and swinging of skin flaps. **Transposition of the great arteries.** A developmental abnormality of the heart in which the roots of the aorta and pulmonary artery do not bear their normal relationship to each other; there are several varieties with no generally accepted terminology and there are almost always other associated structural abnormalities of the heart. **Transposition of the great vessels.** Transposition of the great arteries (see above). **Complete transposition of the great vessels.** A transposition of the aorta and pulmonary artery whereby their normal anterior-posterior relationships are reversed so that the aorta rises anteriorly from the right ventricle and the pulmonary artery posteriorly from the left ventricle. **Corrected transposition of the great vessels.** 1. *Physiological.* Anatomical transposition of the aorta and pulmonary artery which is physiologically corrected, so that the aorta receives the pulmonary venous return and the pulmonary artery the systemic venous return as the result of associated inversion of other parts of the heart, usually the ventricles. 2. *Anatomical.* A rare form of transposition in which the aorta arises to the left of the pulmonary artery but is still connected to the left ventricle, and the pulmonary artery still arises from the right ventricle. **D-Transposition of the great vessels.** Those forms of transposition in which, characteristically, the pulmonary root lies to the left of the aorta and the ventricles have developed from a *d*-loop type of primitive cardiac tube. **Inverted transposition of the great vessels.** Those forms of transposition of the great vessels in which the main abnormality of the relationship of the roots of the aorta and pulmonary artery to each other is that the aorta lies to the left of (lateral to) the pulmonary artery. L-Transposition of the great vessels. Those forms of transposition in which, characteristically, the pulmonary root lies to the right of the aorta, which has its root to the left; this is most commonly associated with ventricular inversion developing from an *l*-loop type of primitive cardiac tube, forming the commonest variety of physiologically corrected transposition of the great vessels. **Partial transposition of the great vessels.** A condition in which one of the arterial roots is normally placed but the other is displaced in relation to the ventricles. [L *transponere* to transpose.]

trans-sexualism (trans·**sex**·ewe·al·ism). Sexual aberration in which the person attempts to assume the physical characteristics of the opposite sex.

trans-sphenoidal (trans·sfe·**noid**·al). Across the sphenoid bone. [L *trans*, sphenoid bone.]

trans-substantiation (**trans**·sub·stan·she·a′·shun). The replacement of tissue of one kind by another. [L *trans*, *substantia* substance.]

transtemporal (trans·**tem**·por·al). Taking a course across the temporal lobe of the cerebrum. [L *trans*, temporal.]

transthalamic (trans·thal·**am**·ik). Traversing the thalamus. [L *trans*, thalamus.]

transthermia (trans·**ther**·me·ah). Diathermy. [L *trans*, Gk *therme* heat.]

transthoracic (trans·thor·**as**·ik). Across the thorax. [L *trans*, thorax.]

transtracheal (trans·trak·**e**·al). The route whereby a local analgesic solution can be injected into the lumen of the trachea by a needle inserted between the tracheal rings. [L *trans*, Gk *tracheia* the rough artery.]

transudate (**trans**·ew·date). Any fluid that has passed through a membrane or the skin with certain of its dissolved salts. [see foll.]

transudation (trans·ew·**da**·shun). The passage of a fluid through a membrane as a transudate. [L *trans*, *sudare* to sweat.]

transude (trans·**ewd**). To pass or be passed through a membrane as a transudate. [see prec.]

transuranium (trans·ewr·**a**·ne·um). Describing the elements with higher atomic numbers than that of uranium, 92. [L *trans*, uranium.]

transurethral (trans·ewr·**e**·thral). Passing through the urethra, or describing any operation performed via the urethra. [L *trans*, urethra.]

transvaginal (trans·**vaj**·in·al). Passing through the vagina, or pertaining to any operation performed through the vagina. [L *trans*, vagina.]

transverse [transversalis, transversus (NA)] (**trans**·vers). Crosswise; across the long axis of the body or an organ. **Transverse process of a vertebra.** *See* PROCESS. **Transverse sinus.** *See* SINUS. **Transverse sulcus of the temporal lobe.** *See* SULCUS. [L *transversus.*]

transversectomy (trans·ver·**sek**·to·me). The operation of removing a transverse process of a vertebra. [transverse, Gk *ektome* excision.]

transversion (trans·**ver**·shun). The condition of a tooth which is transposed with another in the jaw. [L *transvertere* to turn across.]

transversocostal (**trans**·ver·so·**kos**′·tal). Pertaining to the ribs and their transverse processes. [transverse, L *costa* rib.]

transversospinalis muscle [musculus transversospinalis (NA)] (trans·**ver**·so·spi·**na**′·lis musl). The layer of muscles deep to the sacrospinalis muscle of the back; it includes the semispinalis, multifidus, etc. [transverse, spinalis.]

transversostomy (trans·vers·**os**·to·me). Colostomy involving the transverse colon. [transverse, Gk *stoma* mouth.]

transversotomy (trans·vers·**ot**·o·me). Incision of the transverse process of a vertebra. [transverse, Gk *temnein* to cut.]

transverso-urethralis (trans·**ver**·so·ewr·**e**·**thra**′·lis). An obsolete name for the muscles of the deep pouch of the perineum; the deep transverse perinei muscle and the sphincter urethrae muscle.

transversus abdominis muscle [musculus transversus abdominis (NA)] (trans·**ver**·sus ab·**dom**·in·is musl). The deepest of the three flat muscles of the abdomen. Its fibres run transversely from the lateral part of the inguinal ligament, iliac crest, lumbar fascia, and inner surfaces of the lower ribs to an aponeurotic insertion into the linea alba, and to the pectineal line and crest of the pubis as part of the conjoint tendon.

transversus menti muscle [musculus transversus menti (NA)] (trans·**ver**·sus **men**·ti musl). Occasional slips which connect the depressor anguli oris of either side.

transversus nuchae muscle [musculus transversus nuchae (NA)] (trans·**ver**·sus **new**·ke musl). An occasional small muscle extending from the external occipital protuberance to the upper end of the sternocleidomastoid muscle.

transversus perinei muscles (trans·**ver**·sus per·**in**·e·i muslz). **Deep transversus perinei muscle [musculus transversus perinei profundus (NA)].** A muscle which runs from the ramus of the ischium transversely across the perineum to meet its fellow. It lies in the deep perineal pouch between the perineal membrane and the visceral pelvic fascia. **Superficial transversus perinei muscle [musculus transversus perinei superficialis (NA)].** A muscle arising from the front of the tuberosity of the ischium and inserted into the perineal body, where it meets its fellow. It lies superficial to the perineal membrane.

transversus thoracis muscle [musculus transversus thoracis (NA)] (trans·**ver**·sus **thor**·as·is musl). A lining for the thoracic cage composed of three sheets of muscle, the sternocostalis, the innermost intercostals, and the subcostals, connected by an aponeurosis. It corresponds to the transversus abdominis muscle.

transvesical (trans·**ves**·ik·al). Passing through the bladder. [L *trans*, *vesica* bladder.]

transvestite (trans·**vest**·ite). A person who dresses in clothes of the opposite sex. [L *trans*, *vestis* garment.]

transvestitism (trans·**vest**·it·izm). Sexual aberration taking the form of dressing in clothes of the opposite sex.

Trantas, Alexios (b. 1867). Greek ophthalmologist.

Trantas' dots. Chalky concretions found in the conjunctiva around the limbus in vernal conjunctivitis.

Tranylcypromine (tran·il·**si**·pro·meen). BP Commission approved name for (±)*trans*-2-phenylcyclopropylamine. **Tranylcypromine Sulphate BP 1973.** A mono-amine oxidase inhibitor used in the treatment of depressive states, including endogenous, reactive and psychoneurotic depression.

trap (trap). **Iodide trap.** The thyroid gland traps iodide circulating in the blood and converts it into thyroid hormone. The saliva, gastric juice and milk of lactating women also contain large quantities of iodine, but do not form thyroid hormones. **Radiation trap.** A safety device on sinks where radioactive containers are cleaned to prevent accidental escape of radioactive materials into the drains. Sometimes also used for a system of protective walls (radiation maze) giving indirect access to rooms containing sources of radiation. **Sanitary trap.** A U-shaped device interposed in the continuity of a waste or sanitary pipe to prevent the back-escape into a room of noxious gases. [AS *treppe.*]

Trapa (**tra**·pah). A genus of fresh-water flowering plants. *Trapa bicornis* and *T. natans* of the tropical Far East are known as *horn nuts.* The cercariae of *Fasciolopsis buski* encyst on the nuts, which are eaten raw by man.

trapezial (trap·e·ze·al). Referring to a trapezium.

trapeziform (trap·e·ze·form). Shaped like a trapezium. [Gk *trapezion* small table, form.]

trapeziometacarpal (trap·e·ze·o·met·ah·**kar**′·pal). Concerning the trapezium and metacarpus of the thumb.

trapezium (trap·e·ze·um). 1. A four-sided figure, none of the sides of which are parallel. 2. The carpal bone on the radial side of the distal row, articulating with the base of the metacarpal bone of the thumb [os trapezium (NA)]. 3. The trapezoid decussation in the lower part of the pontine region of the brain stem [Gk *trapezion* small table.]

trapezius muscle [musculus trapezius (NA)] (trap·e·ze·us musl). A large, flat muscle of the back arising from the superior nuchal line, external occipital protuberance, ligamentum nuchae, and the spines and supraspinous ligaments of the thoracic vertebra. It is inserted into the upper border of the spine of the scapula, the acromion, and the posterior border of the outer third of the clavicle. [Gk *trapezion* small table.]

trapezoid (trap·e·zoid). Trapeziform. [Gk *trapezion* small table, *eidos* form.]

trapezoid bone [os trapezoideum (NA)]. A small bone in the distal row of carpal bones, placed between the trapezium and the capitate bone.

Traube, Ludwig (b. 1818). Berlin physician.

Traube's corpuscle. Ghost corpuscle. *See* CORPUSCLE.

Traube's curve, Traube-Hering curve, or waves. Slow rhythmical waves on the blood-pressure record when the blood supplying the medulla is deficient in oxygen or contains an excess of carbon dioxide. The waves are due to periodic variations in the tone of the vasomotor centre.

Traube's membrane. A semipermeable membrane of cupric ferrocyanide made by allowing solutions of potassium ferrocyanide and copper sulphate to come into contact, usually in the walls of a porous vessel, the latter giving rigidity to the delicate membrane. It is used for measuring osmotic pressure.

Traube's murmur. Gallop rhythm. *See* RHYTHM.

Traube's phenomenon. In conditions associated with high arterial pulse pressure (aortic incompetence) a systolic murmur is heard over the femoral or other large artery when the vessel is compressed. If compression just distal to the stethoscope is increased to a critical level, a diastolic murmur is also heard.

Traube's plugs. Small, foul-smelling, yellowish masses seen in the deeper layers of the sputum in fetid bronchiectasis after standing in a sputum glass.

Traube's space. An area on the chest wall over which it is possible to percuss the resonance of the gastric air bubble. The area is bounded above by the lower border of the left lung; below by the left costal margin; to the right by the left lobe of the liver; and behind and to the left by the upper border of the spleen.

Traube's resonance theory. Resonance theory. *See* THEORY.

Traube, Moritz (b. 1826). German chemist.

Traube's rule. The adsorption of homologous organic compounds from a solution is proportional to the number of CH_2 groups present in the compounds, i.e. to their molecular weights.

Traugott, Karl (b. 1885). Frankfurt physician.

Staub-Traugott effect. The observation that if a normal person has been given a dose of glucose by mouth, a similar dose an hour later is not followed by a corresponding rise in the blood-sugar level.

traulism, traulismus (traw·lizm, traw·liz·mus). Lisping; an affection of the speech. [Gk *traulismos.*]

trauma (traw·mah). Injury. **Actual trauma.** In dentistry, a pathological alteration of the supporting tissues of a tooth due to abnormal occlusion. **Auditory trauma.** Damage to the ear (and hearing) caused by excessive noise, e.g. blast injury. **Birth trauma.** Damage to the fetus, especially the head, during birth. **Psychic trauma.** A disturbing psychological stress. [Gk.]

traumatic (traw·mat·ik). 1. Concerning a wound or injury. 2. Arising out of a wound or injury. [Gk *trauma* wound.]

traumatism (traw·mat·izm). 1. A trauma. 2. Any condition arising out of a wound or injury.

traumatogenic (traw·mat·o·jen'·ik). Originating in trauma. [Gk *trauma* wound, *genein* to produce.]

traumatopnoea (traw·mat·op·ne'·ah). 1. Partial asphyxia accompanied by collapse of the patient as the result of a wound opening into the pleura. 2. The respiration of air through a wound in the chest wall. [Gk *trauma* wound, *pnein* to breathe.]

traumatosis (traw·mat·o·sis). Traumatism. [trauma, Gk *-osis* condition.]

traumatotropism (traw·mat·o·trop'·izm). The attraction of micro-organisms to damaged tissue. [Gk *trauma* wound, *trepein* to turn.]

Trautmann, Moritz Ferdinand (b. 1832). Berlin aural surgeon.

Trautmann's triangle, or triangular space. A triangle in the temporal bone, the sides of which are formed above by the superior petrosal sinus, posteriorly by the anterior border of the lateral sinus, and anteriorly by a tangent drawn to the posterior semicircular canal. By removing the bone of this triangle, the area can be used as an approach to the cerebellum, the posterior semicircular canal, and the endolymphatic sac.

Travers, Benjamin (b. 1783). English surgeon.

Travers' operation. A method of cataract extraction; now obsolete.

tray (tra). A shallow vessel to contain instruments. **Annealing tray.** A mica or quartz tray on which gold foil may be placed when being heated for annealing. **Impression tray.** A device used for conveying impression material to the cavity of the mouth for the purpose of obtaining an impression of the teeth and surrounding tissues. [AS *treg.*]

Trazodone (traz·o·done). BP Commission approved name for 2 - [3 - (4 - *m* - chlorophenyl - 1 - piperazinyl)propyl] - 1,2,4 - triazolo[4,3 - a]pyridin - 3(2*H*) - one; a central nervous system stimulant.

Treacher-Collins. *See* COLLINS, EDWARD TREACHER.

treacle (tre·kl). The uncrystallizable residue from sugar refining; it is a thick, brown, sweet syrup. A mixture of treacle and hot milk (equal parts) has been used as an enema. **Venice treacle.** A mixture of over 60 drugs used in mediaeval days as an antidote to poisoning. [Gk *theriake* antidote.]

treatment (treet·ment). The course of action adopted to deal with illness, and the control of the patient. **Active treatment.** That in which active steps, e.g. by giving specific drugs or by surgical measures, are taken. Cf. EXPECTANT TREATMENT (below). **Albumose treatment.** An obsolete treatment of typhoid fever by the intravenous injection of a solution of albumose. **Antigen treatment.** An unusual term that includes all methods of immunization with toxoids, vaccines, and other substances which stimulate the production of antibodies. **Autoserosalvarsan treatment.** The intradural injection of a patient's own serum which has been taken after an intravenous injection of arsphenamine; used as treatment for dementia paralytica by Swift and Ellis and often termed the *Swift-Ellis treatment.* **Autoserous treatment.** Autoserum therapy. *See* THERAPY. **Bee-venom treatment.** The use of bee stings or subcutaneous injections of bee venom for the treatment of chronic rheumatism. **Bomb treatment.** A colloquial alternative term for telecurie therapy. **Bulgarian treatment.** The treatment of parkinsonism, particularly the postencephalitic variety, with Bulgarian belladonna. A decoction (5 per cent) of the belladonna is made with white wine and 5-15 ml of the mixture is given thrice daily. **Causal treatment.** Treatment which is aimed at removing the cause of a disease. **Choline treatment.** The intravenous injection of choline borate and the use of radioactive substances in the treatment of cancer. **Closed-plaster treatment.** The management of a wound after excision, or an osteomyelitis after drainage, in a closed-plaster case which is left intact for a prolonged period. The part is rested, and saprophytic organisms displace pathogenic bacteria. **Conservative treatment.** In medicine, treatment aimed at preserving the strength whilst the body builds up resistance against the disease; in surgery, treatment that preserves a large portion of the limb or tissue in the hope that it will be possible to restore function. Cf. RADICAL TREATMENT (below). **Cross-fire treatment.** The irradiation of tissues at a depth in the body with beams of radiation from several directions designed to raise the dose in the deep tissues and spare the overlying structures. **Curative treatment.** Treatment concerned with the cure of a disease, as opposed to preventive treatment. **Danish treatment.** Treatment of scabies by the use of an ointment containing polysulphides, known as *Marcussen's ointment.* **Dietetic treat-**

ment. Treatment by the regulation of the diet. **Drip treatment.** Treatment by infusion or transfusion of fluids into the body at a slow rate; the rate is measured in drops per minute. **Drug treatment.** The use of drugs in treatment. **Electric-light treatment.** The same as infrared baths, except that the source of heat is electric-light bulbs instead of infrared elements. **Electric-shock treatment.** Treatment by the administration of an electric shock, in particular the treatment of mental disorder in this way through electrodes placed on the temples, leading to an epileptiform convulsion. **Electrocoma treatment, Electroshock treatment.** Electric-shock treatment (see above). **Empiric treatment, Empirical treatment.** Treatment which is based on experience only without any rational or scientific basis. **Envelope treatment.** *See* BUNYAN-STANNARD TREATMENT. **Erlangen treatment.** Erlangen method. *See* METHOD. **Expectant treatment.** Treatment to relieve symptoms while awaiting the body's natural response to infection, or a firmer diagnosis. **Exposure treatment.** Treatment of wounds, particularly burns, by leaving them exposed to the air so that a dry coagulum may form. **Fever treatment.** The treatment of disease by induced fever; in particular, the treatment of general paralysis of the insane by induced malaria or by direct heating of the body. **Fractionated treatment.** In radiotherapy; a course of treatment in which the dose is given in fractions over a period of time. Cf. COUTARD'S METHOD. **High-frequency treatment.** Treatment by high-frequency currents. **Hot-air treatment.** Local treatment by hot dry air with the limb in a closed chamber. **Hygienic treatment.** Treatment of the environment of the patient so as to place him in the best possible position to overcome his disease, e.g. by the provision of fresh air, an equable temperature, wholesome food, a comfortable bed, and cleanliness. **Hypoglycaemic-shock treatment, Insulin treatment.** The treatment of disease by lowering of the blood-sugar level, in particular the treatment of schizophrenia by the repeated production of comas from the injection of insulin. **Intralesional treatment.** Treatment by injection of a corticosteroid into a lesion; it is carried out mostly in the skin, around tendons, and into joints. **Isoserum treatment.** Treatment by the use of serum taken from another individual with the same disease, or one who has had the same disease. **Light treatment.** Treatment by light; phototherapy. **Maintenance treatment.** The treatment of a chronic disease which is aimed at maintaining a patient's condition at the highest level possible. It usually follows a preliminary investigation and stabilization of the patient's condition so that the necessary treatment required to maintain this is ascertained, e.g. insulin treatment of diabetes, liver in pernicious anaemia, digitalis in auricular fibrillation, etc. **Malarial treatment.** Treatment by induction of malaria, in particular the treatment of general paralysis of the insane. **Medicinal treatment.** Treatment by drugs. **Multiple-field treatment.** Irradiation through multiple ports of entry. **Palliative treatment.** The relief of pain and distressing symptoms in cases of incurable disease. **Perennial treatment.** Treatment throughout the year. Cf. PRESEASONAL TREATMENT (below). **Planchna treatment.** The treatment of leprotic infiltration of the skin by repeated injections of antileprol or other esters of chaulmoogra. Now totally superseded by chemotherapy. **Plombière treatment.** Colonic lavage. **Preseasonal treatment.** Prophylactic treatment a short time before the expected time of onset of a seasonal disease, e.g. hay fever. **Preventive treatment, Prophylactic treatment.** Treatment aimed at the prevention of disease. This may be general, such as improvement of the social environment, improved hygienic conditions, and better housing and feeding, or specific, such as prophylactic injections for infections such as diphtheria or typhoid fever, vaccination for smallpox, or a drug, e.g. for malaria. **Protein shock treatment.** Intravenous injection of TAB vaccine, sterile milk or certain other protein substances producing a considerable pyretic reaction. Used in chronic infections, sinuses, and in lymphopathia venereum. **Protracted treatment.** In radiotherapy; a long course of treatment spread over many weeks, each fraction often given at a low dose-rate. Cf. COUTARD'S METHOD. **QAP treatment.** The army treatment of malaria in World War II by a combination of quinine, mepacrine, and pamaquin in order to prevent relapses of benign tertian malaria. **Quinine-calcium treatment.** The intramuscular injection of a solution of quinine-calcium laevulinate in the treatment of lobar pneumonia. **Radical treatment.** Treatment aimed at complete eradication of the disease, or diseased part, e.g. by chemotherapy, by surgery. **Rational treatment.** Treatment which is based upon a rational understanding of the disease and the action of the proposed remedy. **Root-canal treatment.** The treatment of the root canal of a tooth from which the pulp tissue has been removed. **Rotunda treatment.** A method of treating eclampsia used at the Rotunda Hospital, Dublin. **Salicyl treatment.** The treatment of rheumatism with compounds of salicylic acid. **Sewage treatment.** The process to which sewage is subjected to purify it and to render it non-infective and safe for disposal. The usual methods in use are: emptying into an estuary or the sea; addition of chemical substances to precipitate solid material, the liquid portion passing on to a water-course; the application of biological processes (aerobic and anaerobic bacteria) to promote the production of a pure effluent; and irrigation and filtration through land before passing into a river. **Shock treatment.** Treatment by a variety of methods involving a violent reaction, in particular electric-shock treatment and hypoglycaemic-shock treatment (see above). **Slush treatment.** Treatment of cutaneous lesions with applications of a slush made by adding acetone or ether to solid carbon dioxide. **Sodoku treatment.** The treatment of dementia paralytica by fever, produced by the inoculation of the patient with the organism of rat-bite fever (*Spirillum minus*). **Solar treatment.** Heliotherapy. **Specific treatment.** Treatment which acts directly upon the specific cause of a disease, e.g. a specific serum or vaccine, or a selective drug. **String-method treatment.** A method of negotiating a difficult oesophageal stricture by first passing a string weighted by a bead and then threading a bougie along the string: it has also been used to saw through a stricture. **Supporting treatment.** Treatment which keeps up the patient's strength whilst other remedies are being applied. **Surgical treatment.** Treatment which involves the use of surgical methods, commonly operative. **Symptomatic treatment.** Treatment of symptoms as they arise. **Teleradium treatment.** Radium-beam therapy. *See* THERAPY. **Terrain treatment.** Oertel's treatment. **Tonic treatment.** Treatment which is supposed to increase the function or tone of organs. **Triple-dye treatment.** A solution containing gentian violet, brilliant green, and acriflavine, used in the treatment of burns. **Underwater treatment.** Treatment of weak or paralysed muscles and rheumatic conditions in the deep pool. **Venous-heart treatment.** McPheeters' treatment. [Fr. *traitment.*]

See also: ALBERTINI, ALLEN (F. M.), APOSTOLI, ASCOLI, BABÈS, BACELLI, BALFOUR (G. W.), BARGEN, BAUNSCHEIDT, BEARD, BERGONIÉ, BIER, BIRD (G.), BLAIR-BELL, BLANCHARD, BLUEMEL, BOUCHARDAT, BREHMER, BUELAU, BUNYAN, CALOT, CARREL, CHERVIN, CLARK (A.), COFFEY (W. B.), COMBY, CORDIER, DANCEL, DÉBOVE, DUBOIS (P. C.), EBSTEIN, EHRLICH, ELLIOTT (C. R.), ELLIS (A. W. M.), FELSEN, FELT, FERMI (C.), FERRIER, FICHERA, FILATOV, FINSEN (N. R.), FISCHER (M. H.), FLECHSIG, FORLANINI, FOWLER (G. R.), FRAENKEL (A.), FRENKEL (H. S.), FRIEDMANN (F. F.), GENNERICH, GIRARD, GUELPA, GUINARD, HASSIN, HATA, HEISER, HÖGYES, HUCHARD, HUMBER, JAROTSKY, KARELL, KAUFMANN, KELLGREN, KENNY, KITTEL, KLAPP, KNOPF, KOGA, KORÁNYI (A.), KROMAYER, LAMBERT (A.), LANDERER, LARAT, LEES, LENHARTZ, LERICHE, LEUBE, LOMHOLT, MCPHEETERS, MATAS, MAYO (C. H.), MELTZER, METCHNIKOFF, MINOT, MITCHELL, MØLLGAARD, MORO, MUIRHEAD, MURPHY (J. B.), MURPHY (W. P.), NOORDEN, OCHSNER, OERTEL, OPPENHEIMER, ORR, PERCY, PETREN, PILCZ (J.), PLAYFAIR, POLITZER, POTTER (C. A.), PROETZ, QUINTIN, RETAN, ROEDER, ROGERS, ROLLIER, SALISBURY, SCELETH, SCHLOESSER, SCHOTT, SCHROTH, SEMPLE, SHERREN, SICARD, SIPPY, SPAHLINGER, SPANGLER, STANNARD, STOKER, STROGANOV, SWIFT, TOWNS, TRUETA, TUFFNELL, VALSALVA, VIDAL (J. B. E.), WAGNER von JAUREGG, WIDAL, WOODBRIDGE, WYETH, YEO, ZELLER, ZIEMSSEN, ZUNDBURGUET.

trehalase (tre·**ha**·laze). An enzyme which hydrolyses the disaccharide trehalose into two molecules of glucose. [Turkish *trehala* manna.]

trehalose (tre·**ha**·loze). $C_{12}H_{22}O_{11}$, a disaccharide occurring in yeast, fungi, and seaweeds. It is non-reducing and is not hydrolysed by the enzyme sucrase, but is hydrolysed by acids and by a specific enzyme, trehalase, one molecule yielding two molecules of glucose. [see prec.]

Treitz, Wenzel (b. 1819). Austrian physician.

Treitz arch. A vascular fold in the peritoneum between the third part of the duodenum and the left kidney. It contains the superior left colic artery and the inferior mesenteric vein.

Treitz fascia. A layer of fascia which lies behind the head of the pancreas and separates it from the aorta, the right crus of the diaphragm, the inferior vena cava, and the right renal vein.

Treitz fossa. The inferior duodenal fossa.

Treitz hernia. Hernia at the situation of the fossa of Treitz behind the inferior duodenal fold of the peritoneum.

Treitz ligament, or muscle. The superior retention band of the developing mid-gut, the so-called suspensory muscle (ligament) of the duodenum.

Trélat, Ulysse (b. 1828). Paris surgeon.

Trélat's sign. The presence of small yellow spots adjacent to tuberculous ulcers of the mouth.

Leser-Trélat sign. The (quite incorrect) belief that senile angiomata, seborrhoeic warts, and pigmented areas are evidence of carcinoma.

Trematoda (trem·at·o·dah). A class of the phylum Platyhelminthes. As adults they are external or internal parasites of, usually, vertebrates; when there are secondary hosts, they are fresh-water snails. Flukes of medical importance belong to the sub-class Digenea, which have two hosts and an asexual generation. [Gk *trematodes* pierced.]

trematode (**trem**·at·ode). A member of the platyhelminth class Trematoda; a fluke.

trematodiasis (**trem**·at·o·**di**'·as·is). Infection by a trematode. **Pulmonary trematodiasis.** Paragonimiasis of the lungs.

trematoid (**trem**·at·oid). Relating to a trematode. [trematode, Gk *eidos* form.]

tremble (**trem**·bl). To shake involuntarily, as with fear, excitement, or agitation. [L *tremere* to tremble.]

tremmeloid, tremmelose (**trem**·el·oid, **trem**·el·oze). Resembling jelly; gelatinous. [L *tremere* to tremble, Gk *eidos* form.]

tremogram (**trem**·o·gram). The recording obtained by the use of a tremograph. [tremor, Gk *gramma* record.]

tremograph (**trem**·o·graf). An apparatus designed to afford a continuous recording of tremors. [tremor, Gk *graphein* to write.]

tremolabile (trem·o·**la**·bile). Describing anything that is destroyed or rendered inactive by shaking. [L *tremor* shaking, *labilis* slipping.]

tremophobia (trem·o·**fo**·be·ah). An unreasoning fear of trembling. [L *tremor* shaking, Gk *phobein* to fear.]

tremor (**trem**·or). A rhythmic, involuntary, purposeless, oscillating movement resulting from the alternate contraction and relaxation of opposing groups of muscles. **Arsenic tremor.** A tremor of the hands occurring as a result of arsenic poisoning. **Tremor artuum.** The tremor of paralysis agitans. **Asynergic family tremor.** Essential tremor (see below). **Tremor capitis.** Any tremor affecting head and neck muscles. **Coarse tremor.** A tremor in which the oscillatory movements are slow or coarse. **Continuous tremor.** A persistent tremor, continuously present, e.g. paralysis agitans. **Convulsive tremor.** Paramyoclonus multiplex; a form of myoclonic epilepsy. **Tremor cordis.** An obsolete term signifying cardiac palpitation. **Epileptoid tremor.** Tremor due to intermittent clonic contractions of muscles, resembling the movements of myoclonic epilepsy. **Essential tremor.** A familial tremor that is exaggerated by stress and tends to increase with age; it is unassociated with any other nervous symptoms. **Familial heredity tremor.** A fine tremor which is increased by voluntary movement and by exertion and which involves particularly the hands, lips, and tongue. It usually develops in the first 25 years of life, involves several members of the family, and is not associated with other neurological abnormalities. **Fascicular tremor, Fasciculation tremor, Fibrillary tremor.** Muscular fasciculation due to involuntary contraction of individual muscle bundles or fasciculi. If occasional it may be physiological, but if profuse, giving widespread muscular twitching, it may be a manifestation of motor neurone disease. **Fine tremor.** A tremor which occurs after completion of a violent voluntary movement, or one which develops as a result of fatigue after long-continued muscle fixation. **Heredofamilial tremor.** A tremor of varying characteristics, unaccompanied by any other neurological symptoms, with a marked familial tendency; it has been noted in families in which paralysis agitans occurs. It has been suggested that it is an abortive form of olivopontocerebellar atrophy. **Hysterical tremor.** This may be of two types; one is a fine tremor resembling the shaking of severe fear, the other is a coarse irregular tremor, made worse by voluntary movement. Characteristically the tremor is irregular and variable, diminishing when the patient's attention is distracted, and increasing when the affected limb is the subject of discussion. **Intention tremor.** A tremor which arises or is intensified by voluntary movement; it may be most evident at the end of the movement, particularly during over-reaching. **Intermittent tremor.** A tremor which is intermittent, or one which only appears on attempted voluntary movement, e.g. intention tremor (see preceding). **Kinetic tremor.** A tremor which is accentuated by voluntary movement. **Lenticulostriate tremor.** Tremor due to disease of the basal ganglia. **Tremor linguae.** Tremor of the tongue; a feature of dementia paralytica and alcoholism. **Tremor mercurialis.** A fine tremor of the hands which is seen, together with erethism, in chronic mercury poisoning. **Metallic tremor.** A tremor resulting from poisoning with a metal, e.g. mercury. **Motofacient tremor.** Tremulous movements of individual muscles which participate in a particular voluntary activity. **Muscular tremor.** Minute regular contractions of muscle fasciculi; fascicular or fibrillary tremor (see above). **Tremor opiophagorum.** The characteristic tremor of opium addicts, accentuated by withdrawal of the drug. **Passive tremor.** A tremor which occurs only when the member involved is at rest. **Persistent tremor.** A continuous tremor; one which occurs whether the affected parts are moving or at rest. **Physiological tremor.** Tremor due to physiological causes, e.g. exhaustion, fear, cold, etc. **Tremor potatorum.** The shaking hands of the chronic alcoholic. **Purring tremor.** An obsolete term denoting a palpable murmur or thrill. **Tremor saturninus.** The tremor of the extremities seen in cases of chronic lead poisoning. **Static tremor.** A tremor which develops when an attempt is made to hold a limb in one particular position. **Striocerebellar tremor.** A tremor with components arising from disease of both the cerebellum and the corpus striatum; a combination of passive tremor and intention tremor. **Tremor tendinum.** Subsultus tendinum; involuntary twitching of the muscles of the hands and feet, seen in the typhoid state of low fevers. **Toxic tremor.** A tremor resulting from poisoning or intoxication by toxic substances. **Trombone tremors.** Coarse tremors of the tongue, lips, and facial muscles. **Vibratile tremor.** Fremitus; a palpable vibration, as of the thoracic cage during phonation. **Volitional tremor.** A trembling during voluntary effort; the tremulous movements may spread to involve the entire body. An exaggeration of an intention tremor, it may be seen in cerebellar disease and in multiple sclerosis. **Zinc-poisoning tremor.** Metal-fume fever. *See* FEVER. [L shaking.]

See also: HUNT (J. R.), MINOR, RENDU.

tremorgram (**trem**·or·gram). Tremogram.

tremulation (trem·ew·**la**·shun). A state of trembling. [L *tremulare* to tremble.]

tremulor (**trem**·ew·lor). An apparatus for giving vibratory treatment to the body. [see prec.]

Trenaunay, Paul (b. 1875). French physician.

Klippel-Trenaunay-Weber syndrome. Haemangiectatic hypertrophy.

trend (trend). The tendency to proceed in a certain direction; the likely prognosis. **Benign trend.** A favourable prognosis; the tendency of a disease to subside. **Malignant trend, Pernicious trend.** A fatal prognosis; the tendency of a disease towards a fatal termination. [AS *trendan.*]

Trendelenburg, Friedrich (b. 1844). Leipzig surgeon.

Trendelenburg cannula. A tube with an inflatable rubber collar to close the trachea after tracheotomy.

Trendelenburg limp. Unstable gait due to instability of the hip joint.

Trendelenburg's operation. Ligation of the saphenous vein in the treatment of varix.

Trendelenburg's position. A position with the table tilted head down, the patient being prevented from slipping off by shoulder, or preferably pelvic, supports, and by having the legs hanging over the end of the table. It is very commonly used in gynaecological operations.

Reversed Trendelenburg position. A position when the head is high and the body slopes downwards towards the feet. It is sometimes used to lessen bleeding in operations on the head and neck.

Trendelenburg's sign. In cases of instability of the hips from dislocation, fracture of the femoral neck, or paralysis of the gluteus medius muscle, if the patient stands on the affected leg then the pelvis drops towards the opposite leg.

Trendelenburg test, Brodie-Trendelenburg test. A test to determine the integrity of the saphenous and deep veins of the lower limb. The subject lies recumbent, and the leg is elevated to drain the venous blood. Pressure is applied over the upper part of the saphenous vein in order to occlude it, then the patient stands up, and the pressure is released suddenly. The procedure is repeated, but pressure is maintained for 35 s. The test is positive, and indicates incompetence of the valve of the deep saphenous vein, if the veins (or varices) fill rapidly when pressure is released as soon as the patient stands, fill slowly when the pressure is maintained, and are not distended fully at the end of 35 s. The test is negative if they fill slowly when the pressure is maintained, and do not fill more rapidly when it is immediately released.

Treosulfan (tre·o·sul·fan). BP Commission approved name for L-threitol 1,4-dimethanesulphonate; a cytostatic agent.

trepan (tre·pan). 1. To trephine. 2. An obsolete form of trephine. [Gk *trypan* to bore.]

trepanatio (tre·pan·a·she·o). Trepanation.

trepanation (tre·pan·a·shun). The operation of trepanning.

trepanning (tre·pan·ing). The removing of a bone disc from the skull for limited intracranial exploration; now largely archaic. [Gk *trypan* to bore.]

trephination (tref·in·a·shun). The surgical operation of removing a circular disc of bone or other tissue with a trephine.

trephine (tref·ine, tref·een). 1. Any instrument with a circular cutting edge that is rotated either with the fingers, hand, or mechanically, and cuts out a disc of tissue, especially the crown saw for removing a circular bone disc from the skull. 2. The using of such an instrument. **Conical trephine.** A trephine with cutting edges sloping inwards so that the bone disc removed is a conic section. **Corneal trephine.** One used for cutting a disc of cornea in keratoplasty. **Corneoscleral trephine.** One used for cutting out a disc of cornea and sclera at the limbus in Elliot's operation for glaucoma. It has a diameter of 1.5–2 mm. **Dacryocystorrhinostomy trephine.** A manual instrument with teeth about 8 mm in diameter, used for cutting the bony opening into the nose in order to suture the lacrimal sac to the nasal mucous membrane. **Mechanical trephine.** One rotated by electricity or clockwork. [Gk *trypan* to bore.]

See also: ELLIOT (R. H.), HIPPEL, HORSLEY.

trephinement (tref·ine·ment). Trephination.

trephocyte (tref·o·site). A nurse cell, e.g. a Sertoli cell of the seminiferous tubule in which spermatids are embedded and receive nourishment during their maturation. [Gk *trephein* to nourish, *kytos* cell.]

trepidatio (trep·id·a·she·o). Trepidation. **Trepidatio cordis.** Palpitation of the heart.

trepidation (trep·id·a·shun). 1. Trembling; tremor. 2. A state of alarm or anxiety. [L *trepidare* to tremble.]

Treponema (trep·o·ne·mah). A genus of organisms of the family Treponemataceae, order Spirochaetales, consisting of slender, spiral, motile organisms, 3–18 μm long. Their spirals may be closely or loosely wound, regular or irregular, and are weakly refractile under dark-ground illumination. They are strict anaerobes, and some are pathogenic for man and animals. **Treponema calligyrum.** A non-pathogenic species found in the pudenda and smegma. **Treponema carateum.** The cause of pinta, occurring in the cutaneous lesions. **Treponema cuniculi.** The cause of rabbit spirochaetosis, causing papular lesions in the genitals and perineum. **Treponema duttoni.** *Borrelia duttoni.* **Treponema genitalis.** A non-pathogenic species found in human genitalia. **Treponema gracilis.** A non-pathogenic species, very like *T. pallidum.* **Treponema macrodentium, Treponema microdentium.** A non-pathogenic species occurring in the human mouth and gums. **Treponema mucosum.** A species found in pus from pyorrhoea alveolaris. **Treponema pallidum.** The cause of syphilis in man, readily found in the acute primary lesion. **Treponema pertenue.** A species indistinguishable from *T. pallidum* and the cause of yaws or tropical framboesia. **Treponema recurrentis.** *Borrelia obermeieri.* **Treponema refringens.** *Borrelia refringens.* **Treponema vincenti.** *Borrelia vincenti.* [Gk *trepein* to turn, *nema* thread.]

Treponemataceae (trep·o·ne·mat·a'·se·e). A family of micro-organisms more closely related to the bacteria than to the protozoa which include many pathogens, of the genera *Spirochaeta, Treponema,* and *Leptospira.* [see prec.]

treponematosis (trep·o·ne·mat·o'·sis). A term applied to a group of diseases caused by spirochaetes of the genus *Treponema,* the latter being the generic name introduced by Schaudinn for the organism of syphilis, *T. pallidum,* and the allied species, *T. pertenue,* of yaws. Some authorities include also the relapsing fever group, *T. recurrentis, T. duttoni,* etc., but more recently they have been relegated to the genus *Borrelia.* **Tropical treponematosis.** Yaws, bejel, and pinta. [treponema, Gk *-osis* condition.]

treponemicidal (trep·o·ne·mis·i'·dal). 1. Capable of destroying treponema. 2. Antisyphilitic. [treponema, L *caedere* to kill.]

trepopnoea (trep·op·ne·ah). A condition in which the patient finds he is able to breathe more easily when lying in some particular way. [Gk *trepein* to turn, *pnein* to breathe.]

treppe (trep·ah). Staircase phenomenon described by Bowditch. The rise in tension in succeeding contractions observed on stimulating a muscle after a quiescent period. *See* PHENOMENON. [G staircase.]

Tresilian, Frederick James (b. 1862). London physician.

Tresilian's sign. Duct sign. *See* SIGN.

tresis (tre·sis). Perforation. **Tresis causis.** A burn. **Tresis punctura.** A puncture. **Tresis vulnus.** A wound. [Gk a boring.]

Tretamine (tret·am·een). BP Commission approved name for 2,4,6-tri(1-aziridinyl)-1,3,5-triazine, a general cytotoxic agent, useful in chronic leukaemias and Hodgkin's disease, but of no use in acute leukaemias.

Trethinium Tosylate (treth·in·e·um tos·il·ate). BP Commission approved name for 2-ethyl-1,2,3,4-tetrahydro-2-methylisoquinolinium toluene-*p*-sulphonate; a hypotensive agent.

Tretinoin (tret·in·o·in). BP Commission approved name for 3,7 - dimethyl - 9 - (2,6,6 - trimethyl-cyclohex - 1 - enyl)nona - 2,4,6,8 - all-*trans*-tetraenoic acid; a dermatic agent.

Treves, Sir Frederick (b. 1853). London surgeon.

Treves' folds. The ileocaecal and ileocolic folds. *See* FOLD.

Treves' hernia. Ileo-appendicular hernia; an internal hernia in a fossa between the ileum and the appendix.

Treves' operation. Evacuation of a psoas abscess.

Trevor, David (b. 1906). British orthopaedic surgeon.

Trevor's disease. Tarso-epiphyseal aclasis; a congenital error of epiphyseal development affecting one or other side of the knee and/or ankle.

tri-. A Greek (and Latin) prefix signifying *three*.

triacetate (tri·as·et·ate). Any acetate that contains three acetic groups, e.g. $(CH_3COO)_3Al$. [Gk *tri-*, acetic.]

triacetin (tri·as·et·in). $C_3H_5(OCOCH_3)_3$, an oily liquid widely used as a plasticizer.

Triacetyloleandomycin (tri·as·et·il·o·le·an·do·**mi**'·sin). BP Commission approved name for the triacetyl ester of the antibiotic oleandomycin. It is more rapidly absorbed from the gastro-intestinal tract.

triacid (tri·as·id). Applied to a base with three available hydroxyl groups; one capable of neutralizing three molecules of a monobasic acid. [Gk *tri-*, acid.]

triacontanol (tri·ak·**on**·tan·ol). $C_{30}H_{59}OH$, an unsaturated alcohol, obtained from species of lucerne. [Gk *triakonta* thirty.]

triad (tri·ad). 1. A group of three identical or closely related objects, signs, or symptoms. 2. Any element or radical with a valency of three. 3. Trivalent. **Triad of anaesthesia.** Narcosis, reflex suppression, and relaxation (*Gray*). [Gk *trias* the number three.]

See also: BECK (C. S.), BEZOLD (F.), CHARCOT, GRANCHER, HERZ, HUTCHINSON, JACOB, KARTAGENER, LUCIANI, OSLER, SCHULTZ.

trial (tri·al). Process or mode of testing the qualities of a thing. **Controlled clinical trial.** A method of assessing results of two different types of treatment by allotting patients in equal numbers to each group by random sampling.

trialism (tri·al·izm). Trialistic theory of haemopoiesis.

trialkylamine (tri·al·kil·**am**'·een). Alkylamine.

triallylamine (tri·al·il·**am**'·een). $(CH_2{=}CHCH_2)_3N$, a tertiary amine.

Triamcinolone (tri·am·**sin**·o·lone). BP Commission approved name for 9α-fluoro-16α-hydroxyprednisolone. **Triamcinolone Acetonide BP 1973.** 9α - Fluoro - 11β,21 - dihydroxy - 16α,17α - isopropylidenedioxypregna - 1,4 - diene - 3,20 - dione; it has the actions and uses of hydrocortisone applied topically as a cream, lotion, ointment, or dental paste. **Triamcinolone Hexacetonide.** BP Commission approved name for 21 - (3,3 - dimethylbutyryloxy)-9α - fluoro - 11 β - hydroxy - 16α,17α - isopropylidenedioxypregna - 1,4 - diene - 3,20 - dione.

triamine (tri·am·een). Any organic compound possessing three amino NH_2 groups. [Gk *tri-*, amino.]

Triamterine BP 1973 (tri·**am**·ter·een). 2,4,7-Triamino-6-phenylpteridine, a diuretic which antagonizes aldosterone and is somewhat weaker than the thiazides. It leads to potassium retention.

triamylose (tri·**am**·il·oze). $(C_6H_{10}O_5)_3$, a compound isolated from the amylopectin of starch.

triangle (tri·ang·gl). 1. A three-sided geometrical figure. 2. [Trigonum.] Any three-sided area bearing resemblance to a triangle. **Anal triangle.** The posterior part of the perineum behind the transversus perinei muscles. It contains the termination of the anal canal. Also known as the *anal region*, or *rectal triangle*. **Anterior triangle.** Triangle of the neck, anterior (see below). **Triangle of auscultation.** A triangular area bounded by the lower border of the trapezius muscle, the upper border of the latissimus dorsi muscle, and the vertebral border of the scapula. **Bladder triangle.** Trigone of the bladder. **Cardiohepatic triangle.** Cardiohepatic angle. *See* ANGLE. **Carotid triangle, inferior.** A triangle bounded by the midline of the neck, the superior belly of the omohyoid muscle above and the sternocleidomastoid muscle behind; nowadays it is generally known as the *muscular triangle*. In its floor lie the sternohyoid and sternothyroid muscles. **Carotid triangle, superior [trigonum caroticum (NA)].** A triangle bounded behind by the sternocleidomastoid muscle, in front and below by the superior belly of the omohyoid muscle, and above by the stylohyoid muscle and posterior belly of the digastric muscle. It contains the terminal part of the common, and commencement of the external and internal, carotid arteries. Now generally known as the *carotid triangle*. **Digastric triangle.** The triangle bounded by the mandible and by the diverging bellies of the digastric muscle. **Triangle of the elbow.** The triangular hollow at the bend of the elbow bounded by the supinator muscle laterally, the pronator teres medially, and a line joining the two humeral condyles above. Nowadays known as the *cubital fossa*, it contains the termination and division of the brachial artery and the median nerve. **Triangle of election.** Carotid triangle, superior (see above). **Extravesical triangle.** Pawlik's triangle or trigone. **Facial triangle.** The triangle included by the line from the basion, alveolar point, and nasion. **Femoral triangle [trigonum femorale (NA)].** An area bounded by the medial sides of the sartorius and the adductor longus muscles and the inguinal ligament, containing the femoral vessels and nerve and marked in the adult by a slight depression below the fold of the groin. **Hypoglossal triangle [trigonum nervi hypoglossi (NA)].** An elevation in the floor of the 4th ventricle beside the midline and posterior to the auditory striae; the nucleus of the hypoglossal nerve is subjacent. **Infraclavicular triangle.** The area bounded by the middle one-third of the clavicle above, the anterior border of the deltoid muscle behind, and the superior border of the pectoralis major muscle in front. It is marked by a slight depression in the living. **Inguinal triangle [trigonum inguinale (NA)].** The area of the anterior abdominal wall between the inferior epigastric artery laterally, the lateral margin of the rectus abdominis muscle medially, and the inguinal ligament below. It is often termed *Hesselbach's triangle*. **Lumbar triangle [trigonum lumbale (NA)].** A triangular interval occurring immediately above the iliac crest between the posterior free border of the external oblique muscle of the abdomen and the adjacent border of the latissimus dorsi muscle. **Lumbosacral triangle.** A triangular space bounded by the body of the 5th lumbar vertebra, the ala of the sacrum, and medial border of the psoas major muscle. **Lymphoid triangle.** Waldeyer's tonsillar ring. **Multifidus triangle.** The inverted right-angled triangle the base of which extends from the midline to the posterior superior spine of the ilium and whose apex is the lowest point of origin of the multifidus muscle. **Muscular triangle.** The area in the neck bounded by the sternocleidomastoid muscle, the anterior belly of the omohyoid muscle and the midline. **Triangle of necessity.** Carotid triangle, inferior (see above). **Triangle of the neck, anterior.** The triangle bounded by the median line of the neck in front, the lower border of the mandible, and a line continuing it back to the sternocleidomastoid muscle above and the anterior border of the sternocleidomastoid muscle behind. It can be subdivided into the muscular, carotid, and submental triangles. **Triangle of the neck, posterior.** The triangle bounded in front by the posterior border of the sternocleidomastoid muscle, behind by the anterior border of the trapezius muscle, and below by the middle one-third of the clavicle. The upper part of the brachial plexus lies in the floor of the triangle. **Nodal triangle.** A triangle of enlarged lymphatics on the inner aspect of the knee in glandular fever: discovered usually by digital pressure. **Occipital triangle.** The upper subdivision of the posterior triangle of the neck, bounded in front by the upper two-thirds of the border of the sternocleidomastoid muscle, behind by the anterior border of the trapezius muscle, and below by the posterior belly of the omohyoid muscle. **Omoclavicular triangle [trigonum omoclaviculare (fossa supraclavicularis major) NA].** The depression in the root of the neck above the body of the clavicle; the supraclavicular fossa. **Paravertebral triangle.** A paravertebral triangular area of dullness found posteriorly on the side opposite to a pleural effusion. The apex of the triangle is at the level where the dullness due to the effusion reaches the vertebral spine, and the base is at the level of the tenth vertebra, extending outwards for 2–5 cm. **Posterior triangle.** Triangle of the neck, posterior (see above). **Pubo-urethral triangle.** The triangle on each side on the front part of the perineum bounded by the ischiocavernosus, bulbospongiosus, and transversus perinei muscles; the route formerly used for lateral lithotomy. **Rectal triangle.** Anal triangle (see above). **Sternocostal triangle.** The interval between the sternal and costal fibres of the diaphragm, containing the superior epigastric vessels. **Subclavian triangle.**

Supraclavicular triangle (see below). **Submandibular triangle, Submaxillary triangle [trigonum submandibulare (NA)].** A subdivision of the anterior triangle of the neck, bounded by the posterior belly of the digastric below, the lower border of the mandible above, and the midline in front. Not strictly triangular, it contains the submandibular gland. **Submental triangle.** The triangle bounded by the hyoid bone, the anterior belly of the digastric muscle, and the midline of the neck. **Suboccipital triangle.** The area bounded above and medially by the rectus capitis posterior major muscle, above and laterally by the obliquus capitis superior muscle, and below and laterally by the obliquus capitis inferior muscle. In its floor is the posterior arch of the atlas and the vertebral artery; in its roof is the semispinalis capitis muscle. **Supraclavicular triangle.** The lower and anterior part of the posterior triangle of the neck, bounded by the posterior border of the sternocleidomastoid muscle in front, the posterior belly of the omohyoid muscle above, and the clavicle below. In its floor is the 1st rib, insertion of the scalenus medius muscle, and the first digitation of the serratus anterior muscle and the subclavian artery. **Suprameatal triangle.** The triangle on the squamous part of the temporal bone below the level of the suprameatal crest. It is bounded by the suprameatal crest above, the posterosuperior quadrant of the external auditory meatus below, and a tangent to the most posterior part of the external auditory meatus behind. It is an important guide to the tympanic antrum, which lies 3-20 mm deep to the surface of the bone here. **Tracheal triangle.** The inferior carotid triangle (see above). **Urogenital triangle.** The anterior part of the perineum, with a line joining the anterior parts of the ischial tuberosities as its base. **Vagal triangle [trigonum nervi vagi (NA)].** The triangular area between the diverging grooves of the inferior fovea; the dorsal vagal nucleus is subjacent. **Vaginal triangle.** Pawlik's triangle or trigone. **Vertebrocostal triangle.** A triangular gap sometimes occurring behind the crura of the diaphragm and the fibres of that muscle arising from the 12th rib. The triangular area is bounded below and behind by the 12th rib. This deficiency is congenital, and through it abdominal contents may herniate into the thorax. Also called the *lumbocostal trigone.* **Vesical triangle.** Trigone of the bladder. [L *triangulus* three-cornered.]

See also: ALSBERG, AMMON, ASSÉZAT, BÉCLARD, BONWILL, BRYANT, BUROW, CALOT, EINTHOVEN, ELAUT, FARABEUF, GARLAND, GERHARDT (C. C. A. J.), GOMBAULT, GROCCO, GRYNFELTT, HENKE, HESSELBACH, JACKSON (C.), KANAVEL, KOCH (W.), KORÁNYI (F.), LABBÉ (L.), LANGENBECK (B. R. K.), LESSER, LESSHAFT, LIEUTAUD, MacEWEN, MALGAIGNE, MARCILLE, MIDDELDORPF, PAWLIK, PETIT (J. L.), PIROGOFF, RAUCHFUSS, REIL, SCARPA, SHERREN, TAUTMANN, WEBER (W. E.), WERNICKE (K.).

triangularis (tri·ang·gew·**la'**·ris). Triangular. **Triangularis sterni.** The sternocostalis or transversus thoracis muscle, arising from the posterior surface of the lower part of the body of the sternum, the lower costal cartilages, and the xiphisternum. Its fibres pass upwards and laterally to be inserted into the costal cartilages from the 2nd to the 6th. [see prec.]

Triatoma (tri·**at**·o·mah). A genus of blood-sucking bugs of the family Reduviidae. The species are particularly numerous in the New World tropics, and are important as vectors of *Trypanosoma cruzi.* Several species are house bugs in the southern parts of North America. The following species are among the numerous potential vectors of *Trypanosoma cruzi: Triatoma barberi, T. brasiliensis, T. brasiliensis melanica, T. carrioni, T. chagasi, T. dimidiata, T. gerstaeckeri, T. heidemanni, T. indictiva, T. longipennis, T. longipes, T. maculata, T. maculipennis, T. nigromaculata, T. oswaldoi, T. patagonica, T. phyllosoma, T. picturata, T. platensis, T. protracta, T. protracta woodi, T. rosenbuschi, T. rubida, T. rubrovaria, T. sanguisuga, T. sanguisuga ambigua, T. spinolai, T. uhleri,* and *T. vitticeps.* **Triatoma infestans.** The principal vector of *Trypanosoma cruzi* in the Argentine, southern Brazil, Paraguay, and Uruguay. **Triatoma megista.** *Panstrongylus megistus,* the principal vector of *Trypanosoma cruzi* in Brazil. **Triatoma rubrofasciata.** An important house bug throughout the New World tropics, and an experimental vector of *Trypanosoma cruzi.* **Triatoma sordida.** A house bug of Brazil which is a vector of *Trypanosoma cruzi* of lesser importance than *Triatoma megista.* [Gk *tri, atomos* uncut.]

triatomic (tri·at·**om**·ik). 1. Describing a molecule in which there are three atoms. [Gk *tri-*, atom.]

Triatomidae (tri·at·**om**·id·e). A family of the insectan order Hemiptera, sometimes included in Reduviidae. The genera *Rhodnius* and *Triatoma,* including *Panstrongylus,* are of medical interest. [Gk *tri-, atomos* uncut, *eidos* form.]

Triaziquone (tri·**az**·e·kwone). BP Commission approved name for tri(aziridin-1-yl)-1,4-benzoquinone; an antineoplastic agent.

triazol 156 (tri·**az**·ol). Hexazole, 4-cyclohexyl-3-ethyl-1,2,4-triazole. A convulsant used in the treatment of mental disorders by convulsive shock therapy.

triazole (tri·**az**·ole). Name given to a number of isomeric five-membered heterocyclic compounds containing three nitrogen atoms in the ring. The most important is 1,2,4-triazole, $\overline{NHN{=}CNN{=}C}H$, a colourless compound occurring in three tautomeric forms and the parent of nitron, a reagent used in the estimation of nitrates with which it forms an insoluble precipitate.

tribade (**trib**·ade). A woman given to tribadism.

tribadism, tribady (**trib**·ad·izm, **trib**·ad·e). Sexual perversion in women, who obtain satisfaction by the friction of each others genitals. [Gk *tribein* to rub.]

tribasic (tri·**ba**·sik). Describing an acid which has three replaceable hydrogen atoms. [Gk *tri-*, base.]

Tribe (tribe). In biology, a subdivision of a Family. [L *tribus* a division of the people.]

Tribolium (tri·**bo**·le·um). A genus of Coleoptera; flour beetles. The adults are secondary hosts to the tapeworm *Hymenolepis diminuta. T. castaneum* and *T. confusum* are pests of flour and have been used as laboratory animals. [Gk *tribolos* three-pointed.]

tribology (trib·**ol**·o·je). The science that deals with the design, friction, wear and lubrication of interacting surfaces in relative motion (as in bearings or gears.). The study of joint lubrication. [Gk *tribo* to rub.]

Tribondeau, Louis Mathieu Frédéric Adrien (b. 1872). French naval physician.

Law of Bergonié and Tribondeau. A statement about radio-sensitivity of tissues in general, evolved from work on the testes. It is either stated as: "The biological action of Roentgen rays is greater the higher the reproductive activity of the cell, the longer the period of its mitosis, and the less the degree of differentiation of the cell in respect to its morphology and function" or as, "The biological effect of x-rays varies directly as the mitotic activity of the cell and inversely as the stage of embryonic development and degree of differentiation".

Triboulet, Henri (b. 1864). French physician.

Triboulet's reagent, and test. A lump of faeces, the size of a walnut, is well mixed with 20 ml distilled water and filtered; 3 ml of the filtrate is mixed with 12 ml distilled water and 20 ml of Triboulet's reagent (3.5 per cent solution of perchloride of mercury with 1 per cent acetic acid). A control mixture is made without the reagent. Both are shaken and compared after 5 h and 24 h. A positive reaction, indicated by a cloudy grey or brown deposit, suggests ulcerative tuberculosis of the intestines.

tribrachius (tri·**bra**·ke·us). A fetal monster with three arms. [Gk *tri-, brachion* arm.]

tribromethanol (tri·brom·**eth**·an·ol). Tribromoethanol. CBr_3CH_2OH, a white crystalline substance used in solution of amylene hydrate as a basal anaesthetic.

tribromide (tri·**bro**·mide). Any bromide that contains three bromine atoms, e.g. $FeBr_3$. [Gk *tri-*, bromide.]

tribromobenzene, tribromobenzol (tri·bro·mo·**ben'**·zeen, tri·bro·mo·**ben'**·zol). $C_6H_3Br_3$, a substituted derivative of benzene that exists in three isomeric forms.

tribromoethanol (tri·bro·mo·**eth**′·an·ol). Tribromethanol.
tribromomethane (**tri**·bro·mo·**me**′·thane). Bromoform, $CHBr_3$. A colourless liquid with a pleasant odour, used as an antispasmodic in whooping-cough.
tribromphenol (tri·brom·**fe**·nol). Bromol $C_6H_2(OH)Br_3$. A silky crystalline substance used as an intestinal disinfectant. **Tribromphenol bismuth.** $(C_6H_2OBr_3)BiOH{\cdot}Bi_2O_3$, the basic bismuth derivative of tribromphenol used for the same purpose.
tributyrin (tri·**bew**·ter·in). $C_3H_5(CO_2C_3H_7)_3$, one of the fats present in butter and other fatty foods.
tributyrinase (tri·**bew**·ter·in·aze). An enzyme of the lipase type occurring in saliva. It catalyses the liberation of butyric acid from tributyrin.
tricalcic (tri·**kal**·sik). Any compound that contains three calcium atoms, e.g. $Ca_3(PO_4)_2$. [Gk *tri-*, calcium.]
tricaprin (tri·**kap**·rin). The most important of the glyceryl caprates that occur in butter. [Gk *tri-*, caprin.]
tricaproin (tri·**kap**·ro·in). The most important of the glyceryl caproates that occur in butter. Cf. CAPROIN.
tricaprylin (tri·**kap**·ril·in). The most important of the glyceryl caprylates that occur in butter. Cf. CAPRYLIN.
tricellular (tri·**sel**·ew·lar). Having three cells. [Gk *tri-*, cell.]
tricentric (tri·**sen**·trik). Of a chromosome, with three centromeres. [Gk *tri-*, *kentron* centre.]
tricephalus (tri·**kef**·al·us). A three-headed monster. [Gk *tri-*, *kephale* head.]
triceps (**tri**·seps). Three-headed. [L.]
triceps brachii muscle [musculus triceps brachii (NA)] (**tri**·seps **bra**·ke·i musl). A muscle of the arm which arises by three heads, two, the lateral head [caput laterale (NA)] and the medial head [caput mediale (NA)] from the humerus, and one, the long head [caput longum (NA)], from the infraglenoid tubercle of the scapula. It is inserted into the olecranon process of the ulna.
triceps surae muscle [musculus triceps surae (NA)] (**tri**·seps **sewr**·e musl). The two heads of the gastrocnemius muscle and the soleus muscles of the calf, all being inserted into the tendo calcaneus (Achilles).
Tricercomonas (tri·ser·ko·**mo**′·nas). A questionable genus of flagellate Protozoa. **Tricercomonas intestinalis.** A rare intestinal parasite of man; *Enteromonas hominis.* [Gk *tri-*, *kerkos* tail, *monas* unit.]
trichalgia (trik·**al**·je·ah). Pain experienced when the hair is touched. [Gk *thrix* hair, *algos* pain.]
trichangiectasis (**trik**·an·je·**ek**′·tas·is). Dilatation of the capillaries. [Gk *thrix* hair, angiectasis.]
trichatrophia (trik·at·**ro**·fe·ah). Atrophy of the hair bulbs, rendering the hair brittle and causing it to split and fall out. [Gk *thrix* hair, atrophy.]
trichauxe, trichauxis (trik·**awx**·e, trik·**awx**·is). Abnormally increased growth of hair on any particular part. [Gk *thrix* hair, *auxe* increase.]
trichiasis (trik·**i**·as·is). 1. Ingrowing of the hair around an orifice, particularly eyelashes, which set up an irritation of the conjunctiva. 2. Minute hair-like filaments in the urine. **Trichiasis of the anus.** Irritation of the anal mucous membrane by hair growing inwards. [Gk *thrix* hair.]
Trichina (trik·**i**·nah). An earlier, but inadmissible, name for *Trichinella.*
Trichinella (trik·in·**el**·ah). A genus of nematode worms. **Trichinella spiralis.** The causal agent of trichiniasis, and an important human parasite: pigs, rats, cats, and dogs are also true hosts. The adult worms live in the intestinal mucosa, the females shedding hatched embryos in the tissues; after laying, the females emerge into the lumen and are passed out with faeces. The larvae are carried by the blood throughout the body, but further development takes place only in striped muscle. They remain alive in the muscle for many years but are gradually enclosed in a calcareous cyst secreted by the host; subsequent development depends upon their being ingested. Pigs are almost the sole source of human infestation, but rats may act as reservoirs from which pigs may be infested. [Gk *thrix* hair.]
trichinelliasis, trichinellosis (**trik**·in·el·**i**′·as·is, **trik**·in·el·**o**′·sis). Etymologically more correct but seldom used terms for trichiniasis.
trichiniasis (trik·in·**i**·as·is). A disease caused by larvae of the parasitic nematode *Trichinella spiralis* in the muscles, as the result of eating infected pork. The symptoms are nausea, diarrhoea, and fever, leading to painful swelling of the muscles, oedema, sweating, and insomnia.
trichiniferous (trik·in·**if**·er·us). Infested with or bearing *Trichinella.* [trichina, L *ferre* to bear.]
trichinization (**trik**·in·i·**za**′·shun). Invasion of the tissues by *Trichinella.*
trichinophobia (**trik**·in·o·**fo**′·be·ah). Morbid fear of *Trichinella* infection. [*Trichinella*, Gk *phobein* to fear.]
trichinosis (trik·in·**o**·sis). Trichiniasis.
trichinotic (trik·in·**ot**·ik). Trichinous.
trichinous (**trik**·in·us). Concerned with *Trichinella* or containing this parasite.
trichion (**trik**·e·on). The midpoint of the hairline at the upper limit of the forehead. [Gk *thrix* hair.]
trichismus (trik·**iz**·mus). 1. A hair-like fracture. 2. A capillary fissure. [Gk *thrix* hair.]
trichite (**trik**·ite). A rod-like body in the surface layer of a ciliate; it is of unknown function. [Gk *thrix* hair.]
trichitis (trik·**i**·tis). Inflammation of the hair bulbs. [Gk *thrix* hair, *-itis* inflammation.]
trichloraldehyde (tri·klor·**al**·de·hide). 1. Trichloracetic aldehyde; chloral. 2. Sometimes used loosely as a synonym for chloral hydrate.
trichlorbutyl alcohol (**tri**·klor·bew·til **al**·ko·hol). Chlorbutol, $(CH_3)_2C(OH)CCl_3$. A mild analgesic and sedative; it is used widely to prevent travel sickness.
trichlorbutylaldehyde (**tri**·klor·bew·til·**al**′·de·hide). Butylchloral hydrate $CH_3CHClCCl_2CH(OH)_2$. A rarely-used substitute for chloral hydrate, being weaker in its hypnotic action. It is sometimes given for facial analgesia.
trichlorethylene (tri·klor·**eth**·il·een). Trichloroethylene BP 1973.
trichloride (tri·**klor**·ide). Any chloride that contains three chlorine atoms, e.g. $AlCl_3$. [Gk *tri-*, chlorine.]
trichlormethane (tri·klor·**me**·thane). Chloroform.
trichlorobutylaldehyde (tri·**klor**·o·bew·til·**al**′·de·hide). Trichlorbutylaldehyde.
trichlorobutylidene glycol (**tri**·klor·o·bew·**til**′·id·een **gli**·kol). Butylchloral hydrate.
Trichloroethylene BP 1968 (**tri**·klor·o·**eth**′·il·een). CCl_2CHCl, a colourless transparent liquid with a characteristic odour not unlike that of chloroform, and burning, sweet taste. It decomposes when exposed to light and air. It produces depression of the central nervous system, and is used by inhalation as a general anaesthetic; it is less potent than ether, but is non-irritant, and non-inflammable when used with air. Induction is rapid, but it is difficult to obtain deep anaesthesia unless some other agent is used as well. It may cause cardiac arrhythmias, and must never be given in a closed circuit as toxic products are formed. It may be used by self-administration to produce light temporary anaesthesia or analgesia during labour pains. The drug is employed sometimes also by inhalation from a gauze swab as an analgesic in trigeminal neuralgia, angina pectoris, and migraine: habituation may occur. Its industrial use as a solvent may lead to poisoning, the chief feature of which is cranial-nerve damage, especially trigeminal disturbance and blindness.
Trichlorofluoromethane BPC 1968 (trik·**klor**·o·floo·or·o·**me**′·thane). CCl_3F. A refrigerant and aerosol propellant.
trichloromethane (**tri**·klor·o·**me**′·thane). Chloroform.
trichloromethylchloroformate (**tri**·klor·o·**meth**·il·klor·o·**for**′·mate). Diphosgene, $ClCOOCCl_3$. A choking gas with a severely irritant effect on the lungs; used in chemical warfare under the names *perstoff* and *superpalite.*

trichloronitromethane (tri·klor·o·ni·tro·me′·thane). CCl_3NO_2, a dense liquid with a suffocating lacrimatory vapour that also causes vomiting; used as a choking gas in chemical warfare.

trichloroquinone (tri·klor·o·kwin′·one). $C_6HO_2Cl_3$, a yellow compound formed from quinone by substitution.

trichlorotoluene (tri·klor·o·tol′·ew·een). Benzotrichloride.

trichlorotrivinylarsine (tri·klor·o·tri·vi·nil·ar′·seen). As(CHCl CH)$_3$, a toxic but non-irritating substance used in chemical warfare as a poison gas.

tricho-aesthesia (trik·o·es·the′·ze·ah). 1. Hair sensitivity; sensation experienced when the hair of a part is touched. 2. The feeling of a hair in the mouth or on the eyeball when there is no real cause for the impression. [Gk *thrix* hair, *aisthesis* sensation.]

tricho-aesthesiometer (trik·o·es·the·ze·om′·et·er). An electrical apparatus which can be used to measure the sensibility of single hairs. [Gk *thrix* hair, *aisthesis* sensation, meter.]

tricho-anaesthesia (trik·o·an·es·the′·ze·ah). Inability to feel anything when the hair of a part is touched. [Gk *thrix* hair, *a-*, *aisthesis* sensation.]

trichobacteria (trik·o·bak·teer′·e·ah). 1. Bacteria possessing flagella. 2. A general term for the group of filamentous bacteria. [Gk *thrix* ahir, bacteria.]

Trichobacterium (trik·o·bak·teer′·e·um). A sub-genus of the genus *Bacterium* in the classification of bacteria, proposed by Janke, 1930. [see prec.]

trichobezoar (trik·o·be·zo·ar). A concretion in the stomach or intestine composed mainly of hair; hair ball. [Gk *thrix* hair, bezoar.]

Trichobilharzia szidati (trik·o·bil·harts′·e·ah zi·da·te). A schistosome of ducks that occasionally causes a dermatitis in man. [Gk *thrix* hair, bilharzia.]

trichocardia (trik·o·kar·de·ah). Villous heart; shaggy pericardium; hair-like exudate on the heart due to pericarditis. [Gk *thrix* hair, *kardia* heart.]

Trichocephalus (trik·o·kef·al·us). A superseded name of a nematode genus. **Trichocephalus dispar.** *Trichuris trichiura.* **Trichocephalus hepaticus.** *Capillaria hepatica.* [Gk *thrix* hair, *kephalos* head.]

trichochromogenic (trik·o·kro·mo·jen′·ik). Capable of producing the colour in hair. [Gk *thrix* hair, *chroma* colour, *genein* to produce.]

trichoclasia, trichoclasis (trik·o·kla·ze·ah, trik·ok·las·is). Brittle hair. [Gk *thrix* hair, *klasis* a breaking.]

trichoclasmania (trik·o·klaz·ma′·ne·ah). A morbid desire to pull out the hair, usually of the head. [Gk *thrix* hair, *klasis* a breaking, *mania* madness.]

trichoclasty (trik·o·klas·te). Any nervous tic involving the hair, such as pulling at the eyebrows or stroking the beard. [Gk *thrix* hair, *klasis* a breaking.]

trichocryptosis (trik·o·krip·to′·sis). Any morbid condition of the hair follicles. [Gk *thrix* hair, *kryptos* concealed.]

trichodangeitis, trichodangiitis (trik·o·dan·je·i′·tis). Inflammation of the fine, hair-like capillaries. [Gk *trichodes* hair-like, *aggeion* vessel, *-itis* inflammation.]

trichodarteriitis (trik·o·dar·ter·e·i′·tis). Inflammation of the arterioles. [Gk *trichodes* hair-like, artery, Gk *-itis* inflammation.]

Trichodectes (trik·o·dek·teez). A genus of Mallophaga; biting lice. **Trichodectes canis.** A common dog louse, and a secondary host of *Dipylidium caninum.* [Gk *thrix* hair, *dektes* beggar.]

trichodophlebitis (trik·o·do·fle·bi′·tis). Inflammation of the venules. [Gk *trichodes* hair-like, phlebitis.]

trichodynia (trik·o·din·e·ah). Pain experienced when the hair is touched. [Gk *thrix* hair, *odyne* pain.]

tricho-epithelioma (trik·o·ep·e·the·le·o′·mah). 1. Small benign papular lesions in the skin about the eyes, arising from hair follicles and varying in size from 1 to 4 mm. They are the colour of the normal skin or a little paler, and are more frequently seen in adult females than in males. 2. Carcinoma (usually basal-cell) arising from the hair follicles. **Tricho-epithelioma papulosum multiplex.** Acanthoma adenoides cysticum (Unna), epithelioma adenoides cysticum (Brooke), multiple benign cystic epithelioma; a malady, often familial, in which few or many round, firm, translucent nodules appear on the face and occasionally on the scalp, neck, and chest. The lesions arise from the outer walls of the hair follicles, and, rarely, some of them become basal-cell epitheliomata. Certain authorities regard the tumours as epithelial naevi. [Gk *thrix* hair, epithelioma.]

trichofolliculoma (trik·o·fol·ik·ew·lo′·mah). A developmental tumour (hair follicle naevus) composed of multiple malformed hair roots arising from an enlarged follicular canal. There is a firm, pearly tumour, usually on the face, with a central pit containing keratin or hairs. [Gk *thrix* hair, L *folliculus* a small bag, Gk *-oma* tumour.]

trichogen (trik·o·jen). Anything that promotes hair growth. [Gk *thrix* hair, *genein* to produce.]

trichogenous (trik·oj·en·us). Stimulating hair growth. [see prec.]

trichoglossia (trik·o·glos·e·ah). Hairy tongue; a condition in which the papillae of the tongue are thickened, giving the latter a hairy appearance. [Gk *thrix* hair, *glossa* tongue.]

trichographism (trik·og·raf·izm). Contractions of the pilomotor muscles of the skin, i.e. so-called *goose flesh,* when the skin is stroked. [Gk *thrix* hair, *graphein* to draw.]

trichohyaline (trik·o·hi·al·een). The hyaline of the hair. [Gk *thrix* hair, hyaline.]

trichoid (trik·oid). Resembling a hair; having the characteristics of hair. [Gk *thrix* hair, *eidos* form.]

trichokryptomania (trik·o·krip·to·ma′·ne·ah). A neurotic habit of breaking the hair of the face or scalp by nipping it with the fingernails. [Gk *thrix* hair, *kryptos* secret, *mania* madness.]

tricholabion, tricholabis (trik·o·la·be·on, trik·ol·ab·is). Tweezers for the removal of hair. [Gk *thrix* hair, *labis* forceps.]

tricholith (trik·o·lith). A hard nodule on the hair observed in cases of piedra. [Gk *thrix* hair, *lithos* stone.]

trichologia (trik·o·lo·je·ah). 1. Insane plucking-out of the hair, also a symptom of delirium. 2. Carphologia; floccilation. [Gk *thrix* hair, *legein* to pull.]

trichology (trik·ol·o·je). 1. The study of the hair. 2. Trichologia. [Gk *thrix* hair, *logos* science.]

trichoma (trik·o·mah). 1. Entropion; introversion of the margin of the eyelid. 2. Plica polonica; matting of the hair. 3. Trichiasis; ingrowing hairs. [Gk hairy growth.]

trichomadesis (trik·o·ma·de′·sis). Alopecia. [Gk *thrix* hair, *madesis* a falling out.]

trichomania (trik·o·ma·ne·ah). Trichotillomania.

Trichomastix cuniculi (trik·o·mas·tix kew·nik·ew·li). A common intestinal flagellate of the rabbit that may be mistaken for *Trichomonas* parasites of man. [Gk *thrix* hair, *mastix* whip, L *cuniculus* rabbit.]

trichomatose (trik·o·mat·oze). Trichomatous.

trichomatosis (trik·o·mat·o′·sis). Matting of the hair attributable to fungus infection, as in plica polonica. [trichoma, Gk *-osis* condition.]

trichomatous (trik·o·mat·us). Affected with trichoma.

trichomegaly (trik·o·meg·al·e). Long and coarse eyebrows. [Gk *thrix* hair, *megas* large.]

trichomonacidal (trik·o·mo·nas·i′·dal). Capable of destroying *Trichomonas.* [*Trichomonas,* L *caedere* to kill.]

trichomonacide (tri·ko·mo·nas·ide). A drug that kills protozoa of the genus *Trichomonas,* especially *T. vaginalis.* [see prec.]

trichomonad (trik·o·mo·nad). A protozoon parasite of man which is a member of the genus *Trichomonas.* It causes diarrhoea, vaginitis, and urethritis in man and animals. [Gk *thrix* hair, *monas* unit.]

trichomonadicidal (trik·o·mo·nad·is·i′·dal). Capable of destroying trichomonads. [trichomonad, L *caedere* to kill.]

trichomonal (trik·o·mo·nal). Relating or due to the presence of *Trichomonas.*

Trichomonas (trik·o·mo·nas). A genus of flagellate Protozoa, class Flagellata (Mastigophora). It is characterized by having from three to five anterior flagella, an axostyle, a single posterior flagellum, and a distinct cytosome. Many of the numerous species are parasitic or coprozoic. Reproduction is by fission only, and cysts are not known. The species are difficult to differentiate; individuals vary much in form and in the number of flagella. **Trichomonas buccalis, Trichomonas elongata.** *T. tenax* (see below). **Trichomonas hominis.** A species which occurs commonly in the lower intestines of man and may cause diarrhoea. **Trichomonas pulmonalis.** A species recorded from human sputum, probably identical with *T. tenax* (see foll.). **Trichomonas tenax.** A species which occurs in the human mouth, particularly around tooth roots, and is one of the organisms found in cases of pyorrhoea. **Trichomonas vaginalis.** A species which occurs commonly in the human vagina and causes a copious leucorrhoea. It does not, however, invade the uterus. [Gk *thrix* hair, *monas* unit.]

trichomoniasis (trik·o·mo·**ni**'·as·is). The condition of being infected by *Trichomonas.* It is usually sexually transmitted, producing vaginitis in women and urethritis in both sexes. The organism, which is isolated by moist-slide and culture, is more easily identified in women than in men.

trichomonicide (trik·o·**mo**·nis·ide). A chemotherapeutic agent against parasites of the genus *Trichomonas.* [*Trichomonas*, L *caedere* to kill.]

trichomyces (trik·o·**mi**·seez). The parasitic fungus *Trichophyton* which causes ringworm.

trichomycosis (**trik**·o·mi·**ko**'·sis). Chromotrichomycosis, tinea nodosa, trichomycosis axillaris, trichomycosis axillaris flava, trichomycosis nodosa, trichomycosis nodularis, trichomycosis palmellina; infection of the axillary (less often of pubic) hair by *Corynebacterium tenuis* (Crissey, 1952), with or without associated chromogenic cocci. It is not a fungal infection (*see* PIEDRA). The infected hairs are not brittle; on examination they present soft sheaths or nodular excrescences, black, yellow or red in colour. In the black and red varieties *Micrococcus* species are present in association with the *Corynebacterium* and impart the pigmentation to the nodules. In the yellow variety only *Nocardia* is present. The disease occurs often in temperate regions, but is more widespread in the tropics where heat and moisture favour the growth of the organism. There are usually no symptoms except discoloration of the hair; this stains the clothing. The condition is not highly infectious. [Gk *thrix* hair, *mykes* fungus, *-osis* condition.]

trichon (**trik**·on). Trichophytin.

trichonocardiasis, trichonocardiosis (**trik**·o·no·kar·**di**'·as·is, **trik**·o·no·kar·de·**o**'·sis). Trichomycosis axillaris. [Gk *thrix* hair, *Nocardia*, Gk *-osis* condition.]

trichonodosis (**trik**·o·no·**do**'·sis). Trichorrhexis nodosa. [Gk *thrix* hair, L *nodosus* nodulated.]

trichonosis, trichonosus (trik·o·**no**·sis, trik·o·**no**·sus). Any diseased condition of the hair. **Trichonosis cana, Trichonosis discolor.** Canities, greying of the hair. **Trichonosis furfuracea.** Ringworm of the scalp. **Trichonosis versicolor.** Ringed hair, hair with alternate bands of white and pigment. [Gk *thrix* hair, *nosos* disease.]

trichopathic (trik·o·**path**·ik). Concerned with trichopathy.

trichopathophobia (**trik**·o·path·o·**fo**'·be·ah). Undue anxiety over the growth and care of the hair. [Gk *thrix* hair, *pathos* disease, *phobein* to fear.]

trichopathy (trik·**op**·ath·e). Any morbid condition of the hair. [Gk *thrix* hair, *pathos* disease.]

trichophagia, trichophagy (trik·o·**fa**·je·ah, trik·**of**·aj·e). The neurotic habit of biting the hair. [Gk *thrix* hair, *phagein* to eat.]

trichophobia (trik·o·**fo**·be·ah). Aversion to hair; morbid disgust evoked by the sight of loose hairs on the person. [Gk *thrix* hair, *phobein* to fear.]

Trichophyta (trik·o·**fi**·tah). *See* TRICHOPHYTON.

trichophytic (trik·o·**fi**·tik). 1. Of the nature of trichophytosis. 2. Concerning the fungus *Trichophyton.* 3. Trichogenous. 4. Trichogen. [see foll.]

trichophytid, trichophytide (trik·o·**fi**·tid, trik·o·**fi**·tide). An eruption of widespread or limited extent caused by haematogenous diffusion of *Trichophyton*, or of toxins derived from a focus of infection with a fungus of that genus. The eruption occurs only if the patient is allergic or hypersensitive to the fungus or its toxins. If the eruption is generalized, it may be associated with systemic disturbances such as fever, lymphadenopathy, and enlargement of the spleen. Careless authors have incorrectly used the term to denote "-id" reactions due to infections with fungi other than *Trichophyta.* [Gk *thrix* hair, *phyton* plant.]

trichophytin (trik·o·**fi**·tin). An extract of cultures of species of *Trichophyton*, used by intradermal injection as a test for specific dermal sensitivity in cases of ringworm infections.

trichophytobezoar (**trik**·o·**fi**·to·**be**'·zo·ar). A ball composed of vegetable matter and hair found in the stomach or intestine. [Gk *thrix* hair, *phyton* plant, bezoar.]

Trichophyton (trik·o·**fi**·ton) (pl. *Trichophyta*). A genus of fungi which attack hair, skin, and nails. In the hair they may produce large or small spores in chains, and the lesion may be endothrix, ectothrix, or ecto-endothrix. The genus includes both human and animal parasites. **Trichophyton acuminatum.** *T. sabouraudi* (see below). **Trichophyton albiciscans.** A species which causes a parasitic pseudo-achromia. **Trichophyton album.** *T. discoides* (see below). **Trichophyton asteroides.** *T. mentagrophytes* (see below). **Trichophyton cerebriforme.** *T. epilans* (see below). **Trichophyton concentricum.** A tropical ringworm which causes tinea imbricata. **Trichophyton crateriforme.** *T. tonsurans* (see below). **Trichophyton cruris.** *Epidermophyton floccosum.* **Trichophyton discoides.** A common cause of ringworm of cattle; it also affects man. **Trichophyton epilans.** An ecto-endothrix species probably animal in origin but it affects man. **Trichophyton equinum.** A large-spored species affecting horses and man. **Trichophyton erinacei.** A species isolated from hedgehogs and from lesions in man. **Trichophyton ferrugineum.** A small-spored infection found in eastern Asia and tropical Africa. **Trichophyton flavum.** *T. epilans* (see above). **Trichophyton gallinae.** A ringworm infection causing fowl favus or white comb and which rarely infects man. **Trichophyton glabrum.** Probably a non-pigmented variety of *T. violaceum* (see below) and usually regarded as a synonym. **Trichophyton gourvilii.** A cause of endothrix scalp ringworm in Africa. **Trichophyton gypseum.** *T. mentagrophytes* (see below). **Trichophyton interdigitale.** A species closely related to *T. mentagrophytes* (see below) and possibly a synonym. **Trichophyton megalosporon.** Any large-spored *Trichophyton.* **Trichophyton megnenii.** A large-spored ectothrix parasite of man, especially in the Mediterranean area of Portugal and Sardinia. **Trichophyton mentagrophytes.** Two varieties are recognized: *T. mentagrophytes* var. *granulare*, a small-spored ectothrix species parasitic on horses, dogs, rodents and other small mammals, and which can affect man; *T. mentagorophytes* var. *interdigitale*, the anthropophilic form commonly associated with tinea pedis. Passage of the human variety on laboratory animals results in conversion to the granular, animal form. **Trichophyton microsporon.** *Microsporum audouini.* **Trichophyton ochraceum.** *T. discoides* (see above). **Trichophyton persicolor.** A small ectothrix species very closely related to *T. mentagrophytes.* **Trichophyton purpureum.** *T. rubrum* (see below). **Trichophyton quinckeanum.** Mouse favus; infections have been reported in man. **Trichophyton rosaceum.** *Achorion gallinae*; it has been isolated from fowls. **Trichophyton rubrum.** A worldwide parasite of man causing chronic infections of hands, feet and nails often intractable to therapy. It affects all parts of the body but only rarely invades the hair. **Trichophyton sabouraudi.** A parasite of man which causes black-dot ringworm and also affects the skin and nails. **Trichophyton schoenleinii.** The cause of favus in man. **Trichophyton simii.** Common in the Indian subcontinent where it infects monkeys and fowls; it has been isolated with increasing frequency in man. **Trichophyton soudanense.** A cause of endothrix infection in man, occurring predominantly in Africa. **Trichophyton sulphureum.** A cause of endothrix infection in man, especially in North America and Europe; considered to be a yellow variant of *Trichophyton tonsurans.* **Trichophyton tonsurans.** The cause of endothrix infections in man; kerion may occur in some cases, usually non-inflammatory. It is a worldwide species. **Trichophyton verrucosum.** A common cause of ringworm in cattle, invading hairs in the large-spored ectothrix form. It also affects man where kerion formation is commonly associated with beard and scalp infections. **Trichophyton vinosum.** A large-spored parasite which produces a velvety colony and is probably a synonym of *T. rosaceum* (see above). **Trichophyton violaceum.** An important cause of scalp ringworm in Europe, the Near East and Africa, although isolations occur worldwide. It is an endothrix hair invader and may cause favus-like crusts; it also affects skin and nails. **Trichophyton yaoundei.** A species causing endothrix hair invasions in man; it occurs predominantly in West Africa. [Gk *thrix* hair, *phyton* plant.]

trichophytosis (**trik**·o·fi·**to**'·sis). Infection of the skin, hair, or snails with any fungus of the genus *Trichophyton.* **Trichophytosis barbae.** Trichophytic infection of the beard area; the moustache area is sometimes involved. **Trichophytosis capitis.** Trichophytic infection of the scalp. **Trichophytosis corporis.** Trichophytic infection of the skin of the body. **Trichophytosis cruris.** Trichophytic infection of the groin, e.g. tinea cruris. **Granulomatous trichophytosis.** A nodular granulomatous condition of the legs caused by trichophytic infection. **Trichophytosis unguium.** Trichophytic infection of the nails. [*Trichophyton*, Gk *-osis* condition.]

trichopoliosis (**trik**·o·pol·e·**o**'·sis). Canities, greying of the hair. [Gk *thrix* hair, *poliosis* greyness.]

trichoptilosis (**trik**·op·til·**o**'·sis). 1. Trichorrhexis nodosa. 2. A condition of the hair in which the shaft splits along its length into a feathery form. [Gk *thrix* hair, *ptilosis* plumage.]

trichorrhexis (trik·o·**rex**·is). Brittleness of the hairs, causing them to split and break off. **Trichorrhexis invaginata.** Bamboo hairs. *See* HAIR. **Trichorrhexis nodosa.** The formation of nodes in the hairs and the subsequent splitting of the shafts at these points. [Gk *thrix* hair, *rhexis* fracture.]

trichorrhexomania (**trik**·o·rex·o·**ma**'·ne·ah). A neurotic habit of breaking off the hair of the face or scalp by nipping it with the fingernails. [Gk *thrix* hair, *rhexis* breaking, *mania* madness.]

trichorrhoea (trik·o·**re**·ah). Rapid falling-out of the hair. [Gk *thrix* hair, *rhoia* flow.]

trichoschisis (trik·**os**·kis·is). Splitting of the hairs. [Gk *thrix* hair, *schisis* a splitting.]

trichoscopy (trik·**os**·ko·pe). The examination of the hair. [Gk *thrix* hair, *skopein* to view.]

trichosis (trik·**o**·sis). Any morbid condition or abnormal growth of the hair. **Trichosis athrix.** Alopecia. **Trichosis carunculae.** An anomalous growth of hair on the lacrimal caruncle. **Trichosis decolor.** A condition of the hair marked by discoloration. **Trichosis distrix.** Trichorrhexis nodosa. **Trichosis hirsuties.** Hirsuties. **Trichosis plica.** 1. Plica polonica. 2. Trichomatosis. **Trichosis poliosis.** Canities. **Trichosis sensitiva.** Hyperaesthesia of the scalp. **Trichosis setosa.** A condition characterized by thickening and coarsening of the hair. [Gk *thrix* hair, *-osis* condition.]

Trichosporon (trik·o·**spor**·on). A genus of yeast fungi having budding cells and true mycelium and arthrospores. **Trichosporon beigelii.** The aetiologic agent of white piedra in man. **Trichosporon cutaneum.** The common commensal of man, it has been reported from gummatous lesions in man. [Gk *thrix* hair, *sporos* seed.]

trichosporosis (**trik**·o·spor·**o**'·sis). Piedra. [Gk *thrix* hair, *spora* seed, *-osis* condition.]

trichostasis spinosa, trichostasis spinulosa (trik·**os**·tas·is spin·o·sah, spin·ew·**lo**·sah). Bundelhaar, lanugo comedones, pinselhaare, thysanothrix; blockage of the pilosebaceous follicles, particularly on the shoulders, back, sides of thorax, and upper abdomen, with comedo-like plugs containing large numbers (10–40) of lanugo hairs. The apices of the lesions are raised above the level of the skin. [Gk *thrix* hair, *stasis* standing, L *spinosus* prickly.]

trichostrongyliasis (**trik**·o·stron·jil·**i**'·as·is). Trichostrongylosis.

Trichostrongylidae (**trik**·o·stron·**jil**'·id·e). A family of the nematode super-family or sub-order Trichostrongyloidea. The genera *Haemonchus*, and *Trichostrongylus* are of medical interest. [Gk *thrix* hair, *stroggylos* round, *eidos* form.]

Trichostrongyloidea (**trik**·o·stron·jil·**oid**'·e·ah). A super-family or sub-order of the nematode sub-order or order Strongylata. The family Trichostrongylideae is of medical interest. [see prec.]

trichostrongylosis (**trik**·o·stron·jil·**o**'·sis). Infestation by the nematode *Trichostrongylus.* [*Trichostrongylus,* Gk *-osis* condition.]

Trichostrongylus (trik·o·**stron**·jil·us). A genus of nematode worms. The adults, which are very small, live in the intestines of mammals, burrowing in the mucosa. Many species occur in domestic animals and have occurred in man; *T. colubriformis* is one of the commonest species found in man. **Trichostrongylus orientalis.** A species from Japan and the Far East and known only in man. [Gk *thrix* hair, *stroggylos* round.]

trichotillomania (**trik**·o·til·o·**ma**'·ne·ah). 1. Insane plucking of the hair. 2. The nervous habit of pulling out the hairs of the face. [Gk *thrix* hair, *tillein* to pull, *mania* madness.]

trichotomous (tri·**kot**·o·mus). Divided into three. [Gk *tricha* threefold, *temnein* to cut.]

trichotrophy (trik·**ot**·ro·fe). The nourishment of the hair. [Gk *thrix* hair, *trophe* nourishment.]

trichroic (tri·**kro**·ik). Characterized by trichroism.

trichroism (tri·**kro**·izm). The phenomenon in which a crystalline substance displays a different colour when viewed along each of three axes. [Gk *tri-*, *chroa* colour.]

trichromat (tri·**kro**·mat). A person who perceives the three primary colours; red, blue, and green. **Anomalous trichromat.** A person who can appreciate the three primary colours, red, blue, and green, but in whom either the red or green is only partially appreciated: if red, he is called a *deuteranomalous trichromat,* or *red blind*; if green, a *protanomalous trichromat.* Very rarely the perception of blue is affected; such a person is called a *tritanomalous trichromat.* **Normal trichromat.** A person who can appreciate all three primary colours normally, and has normal colour vision. [Gk *tri-*, *chroma* colour.]

trichromatic (tri·kro·**mat**·ik). 1. Consisting of three colours. 2. Able to distinguish the three fundamental colours, red, blue, and green. [see prec.]

trichromatism (tri·**kro**·mat·izm). Trichroism.

trichromatopsia (**tri**·kro·mat·**op**'·se·ah). Normal colour vision; the ability to distinguish the three fundamental colours, red, blue, and green. [Gk *tri-*, *chroma* colour, *opsis* vision.]

trichromic (tri·**kro**·mik). Trichromatic. [Gk *tri-*, *chroma* colour.]

Trichurata (trik·ewr·a·tah). A sub-order of the nematode order Enoplata. The families Capillariidae, Trichinellidae, and Trichuridae are of medical interest. It is sometimes treated as an order. [Gk *thrix* hair, *oura* tail.]

trichuriasis (trik·ewr·i·as·is). Invasion of the large intestine by the nematode *Trichuris trichiura.*

Trichuridae (trik·**ewr**·id·e). A family of the nematode sub-order Trichurata. The genus *Trichuris* is of medical interest. [Gk *thrix* hair, *oura* tail, *eidos* form.]

Trichuris (**trik**·ewr·is). A genus of nematode worms; whip worms. **Trichuris trichiura.** The whip worm of man, a widely distributed form, which is commonest in warm countries where the rainfall is high. Adults, which have the anterior two-thirds of the body very narrow, live in the caecum and, to a lesser extent, the large intestine. Eggs, passed in faeces, develop slowly, and may remain viable for long periods; on ingestion they hatch in the small intestine. Light infestations are harmless, but heavy are often associated with severe diarrhoea. [Gk *thrix* hair, *oura* tail.]

tricipital (tri·**sip**·it·al). 1. Applied to anything that has three heads, such as a muscle. 2. Concerning the triceps muscles (triceps brachii or triceps surae). [Gk *tri-*, L *caput* head.]

Triclofos (tri·klo·fos). BP Commission approved name for 2,2,2-trichloroethyl dihydrogen phosphate. **Triclofos Sodium BP 1973.** The monosodium salt of Triclofos, a sedative and hypnotic of the chloral group.

tricornute (tri·**kor**·newt). Possessing three horns. [Gk *tri-*, *cornu* horn.]

tricresol (tri·**kre**·sol). A crude mixture of the three isomeric cresols, $CH_3C_6H_4OH$, used as an antiseptic. **Tricresol phosphate.** Tricresyl phosphate, $(CH_3C_6H_4)_3PO_4$; a compound used as a plasticizer in cellulose varnishes and lacquers. It is an industrial risk, as it produces degeneration of nervous tissue.

tricresyl phosphate (tri·**kre**·sil **fos**·fate). Tricresol phosphate.

tricrotic (tri·**krot**·ik). Characterized by tricrotism.

tricrotism (tri·**krot**·izm). In a pulse tracing, the presence of two secondary waves in the downstroke. [Gk *tri-*, *krotos* beat.]

tricuspid (tri·**kus**·pid). 1. Possessing three points or cusps. 2. Referring to the tricuspid valve. **Tricuspid area.** The region of the chest where the sounds of the tricuspid valve are best heard. **Tricuspid valve.** The right atrioventricular valve. *See* VALVE. [Gk *tri-*, L *cuspis* point.]

Tricyclamol Chloride BP 1968 (tri·**si**·klam·ol **klor**·ide). (±) - 1 - (3 - Cyclohexyl - 3 - hydroxy - 3 - phenylpropyl) - 1 - methylpyrrolidinium chloride, a cholinergic blocking agent with atropine-like action used in the treatment of duodenal and gastric ulcers, pylorospasm, and ulcerative colitis.

tridactyl (tri·**dak**·til). Possessing three fingers or toes. [Gk *tri-*, *daktylos* digit.]

trident, tridentate (**tri**·dent, tri·**den**·tate). Formed into three points. [Gk *tri-*, L *dens* tooth.]

tridermal, tridermic (tri·**der**·mal, tri·**der**·mik). Possessing or derived from all three germ layers, ectoderm, entoderm, and mesoderm. [Gk *tri-*, *derma* skin.]

tridermogenesis (**tri**·der·mo·**jen**'·es·is). The process of formation of the three primary embryonic germ layers. [Gk *tri-*, *derma* skin, *genein* to produce.]

tridermoma (tri·der·**mo**·mah). A teratoma in which derivatives of all three germ layers of the embryo are represented. [Gk *tri-*, *derma* skin, *-oma* tumour.]

Tridihexethyl Chloride (**tri**·di·hex·**eth**'·il **klor**·ide). BP Commission approved name for 1-cyclohexyl-3-diethylamino-1-phenylpropan-1-ol ethochloride; a cholinergic blocking agent.

tridymite (**tri**·dim·ite). A crystalline form of silica, SiO_2, which occurs naturally in fine-grained igneous rocks. [Gk *tridymos* threefold.]

trielcon (tri·**el**·kon). A trifid hook for removing bullets from wounds. [Gk *tri-*, *elkein* to draw.]

triencephalus (tri·en·**kef**·al·us). A fetal monster with a deformed head from which the nose, eyes, and ears are missing. [Gk *tri-*, *egkephalos* brain.]

Triethanolamine BPC 1968 (tri·eth·an·**ol**·am·een). $N(CH_2CH_2OH)_3$, an oily base miscible with water and forming crystalline salts with acids; those salts formed with the higher fatty acids behave like the soaps of alkali metals and are used as emulsifying agents in pharmacy.

triethanomelamine (tri·**eth**·an·o·**mel**'·am·een). Tretamine.

triethylene (tri·**eth**·il·een). **Triethylene glycol.** $HOCH_2(CH_2OCH_2)_2CH_2OH$, a solvent for nitrocellulose, resins, oils, etc., and a valuable antifreeze. **Triethylene melamine.** Tretamine.

triethylenephosphoramide (tri·**eth**·il·een·fos·**for**'·am·ide). A compound the thio derivative of which, triethylenethiophosphoramide, has been used in the treatment of leukaemic diseases.

triethylenethiophosphoramide (tri·**eth**·il·een·thi·o·fos·**for**'·am·ide). A nitrogen mustard preparation which is used in the treatment of chronic or subacute myeloid and lymphatic leukaemia, Hodgkin's disease, polycythaemia, and various reticuloses.

trifacial (tri·**fa**·she·al). An obsolete name for the trigeminal nerve. [Gk *tri-*, face.]

trifid (**tri**·fid). Split into three parts, or having three clefts. [Gk *tri-*, L *findere* to split.]

triflagellate (tri·**flaj**·el·ate). Possessing three whip-like flagella. [Gk *tri-*, L *flagellum* whip.]

Trifluoperazine (tri·floo·o·**per**'·az·een). BP Commission approved name for 10 - [3 - (4 - methylpiperazin - 1 - yl)propyl] - 2 - trifluoromethylphenothiazine. **Trifluoperazine Hydrochloride BP 1973.** The dihydrochloride of trifluoperazine; one of the chlorpromazine group of drugs but it has a stimulating rather than a sedative effect. It suppresses nausea and vomiting.

Trifluperidol (tri·floo·**per**·id·ol). BP Commission approved name for 1 - [3 - (4 - fluorobenzoyl)propyl] - 4 - (3 - trifluoromethylphenyl)piperidin - 4 - ol; a neuroleptic agent.

Trifolium (tri·**fo**·le·um). A genus of leguminous plants; the clovers. The flowers of *Trifolium arvense*, hare's-foot clover, and of *T. pratense*, red clover, have been used medicinally. [Gk *tri-*, L *folium* leaf.]

triformol (tri·**for**·mol). Paraformaldehyde.

trigastric (tri·**gas**·trik). Describing anything, such as a muscle, that has three bellies. [Gk *tri-*, *gaster* belly.]

trigeminal (tri·**jem**·in·al). 1. Triple; divided into three. 2. Referring to the trigeminal nerve. [Gk *tri-*, L *geminus* twin.]

trigeminal artery. An embryonic artery lying close to the trigeminal nerve which may persist into adult life to form an anastomosis between the intracranial portion of the internal carotid and basilar arteries.

trigeminal nerve [nervus trigeminus (NA)]. The 5th cranial nerve. It arises from the cells in the pons, mid-brain, and trigeminal ganglion. Emerging from the side of the pons as two roots, motor [radix motoria (NA)] and sensory [radix sensoria (NA)], it is distributed through its three main branches, ophthalmic, maxillary, and mandibular, to the skin of the face and scalp, conjunctiva, mucous membranes of the nose and mouth, and to the muscles of mastication.

Mesencephalic nucleus [nucleus tractus mesencephalici nervi trigemini (NA)]. A collection of nerve cells in the lateral part of the grey matter of the mid-brain whose fibres form the mesencephalic tract.

Motor nucleus [nucleus motorius nervi trigemini (NA)]. A nucleus in the upper part of the pons close to its dorsal surface near the lateral margin of the 4th ventricle; the source of impulses to the muscles of mastication.

Spinal nucleus [nucleus tractus spinalis nervi trigemini]. A nucleus lying on the medial side of the spinal tract of the trigeminal nerve.

Superior sensory nucleus [nucleus sensorius principalis nervi trigemini (NA)]. The principal nucleus of reception for tactile fibres arising in the trigeminal area. It lies in the pons, lateral to the motor nucleus.

trigeminus (tri·**jem**·in·us). The trigeminal nerve.

trigeminy (tri·**jem**·in·e). Occurring in threes. Usually used in cardiology to describe heart beats occurring in sets of three, most commonly consisting of a normally conducted ventricular beat followed by two ectopic beats, but also occurring in some forms of second degree heart block. [Gk *tri-*, L *geminus* twin.]

trigger material (**trig**·er mat·**eer**·e·al). Any substance which initiates a function. [D *trekker*, material.]

triglyceride (tri·**glis**·er·ide). A combination of glycerol with the acid radical of three different fatty acids, e.g. stearic, oleic, and palmitic. Most animal and vegetable fats are triglyceride esters.

trigocephalus (tri·go·**kef**·al·us). Trigonocephalus.

trigonal (**tri**·go·nal). 1. Triangular. 2. Referring to a trigone. [see foll.]

trigone [trigonum (NA)] (**tri**·gone). A triangle; hence a triangular space, eminence, or swelling. **Trigone of the bladder [trigonum vesicae (NA)].** A triangular area on the base of the bladder bounded behind by the interureteric ridge and, at the sides, by lines joining the ureteral orifices with the internal urethral orifice, which forms the apex of the area. **Cerebral trigone.** An old name for the fornix. **Collateral trigone [trigonum collaterale (NA)].** An eminence in the floor of the lateral ventricle between the posterior and inferior horns. **Deltopectoral trigone.** The narrow triangular depression between the deltoid and the clavicular head of the pectoralis major muscle. **Femoral trigone [trigonum femorale].** A triangular area on the front of the upper part of the thigh, bounded by the inguinal ligament, the adductor longus muscle, and the sartorius muscle. **Hypoglossal trigone.** Hypoglossal triangle. *See* TRIANGLE. **Interpeduncular trigone.**

The fossa on the base of the brain between the two cerebral peduncles. **Lumbar trigone.** Lumbar triangle. *See* TRIANGLE. **Lumbocostal trigone.** Vertebrocostal triangle. *See* TRIANGLE. **Olfactory trigone.** The small triangular eminence at the root of the olfactory peduncle and anterior to the anterior perforated space. **Trigone of the vagus.** Vagal triangle. *See* TRIANGLE. [Gk *trigonos* three-cornered.]

See also: HENKE, LIEUTAUD, MUELLER (H.), PAWLIK.

trigonectomy (tri·go·**nek**·to·me). Excision of part of the trigone to relieve obstruction of the neck of the bladder. [trigone, Gk *ektome* excision.]

Trigonella (trig·on·**el**·ah). A genus of plants of the Leguminosae. **Trigonella foenumgraecum.** Fenugreek; a species the seeds of which are used for making poultices in medical and veterinary practice. They contain the alkaloid, trigonelline. Other species, e.g. *T. elatior* and *T. monspeliaca*, have also been used medicinally. [Gk *trigonos* three-cornered.]

trigonelline (trig·on·**el**·een). *N*-Methyl-nicotinic-betaine, $C_7H_7NO_2$. A base present in the reeds of the fenugreek, *Trigonella foenumgraecum*.

trigonid (tri·**go**·nid). The triangle formed by the three primary cusps of a lower molar tooth. [Gk *trigonos* three-cornered.]

trigonitis (tri·go·**ni**·tis). Inflammation of the trigone of the urinary bladder. **Pseudomembranous trigonitis.** Inflammation of the trigone of the bladder in the female, as a result of which a greyish-pink false membrane is formed, consisting of semi-organized inflammatory debris. [trigonum, Gk *-itis* inflammation.]

trigonocephalic (tri·go·no·kef·**al**′·ik). Characterized or pertaining to trigonocephaly.

trigonocephalus (tri·go·no·**kef**′·al·us). A fetal monster with a triangular head due to the premature closing of the coronal suture and arrested development of the frontal bone. [Gk *trigonos* three-cornered, *kephale* head.]

trigonocephaly (tri·go·no·**kef**′·al·e). The state of trigonocephalus in which development of the frontal bone has been arrested.

trigonotome (tri·**go**·no·tome). An instrument employed in cutting the trigone of the bladder. [trigonum, Gk *temnein* to cut.]

trigonum [NA] (tri·**go**·num). Triangle; trigone. **Trigona fibrosa [NA].** Name applied to two triangular masses of dense fibrous tissue, right and left, between the aortic arterial ring and the right and left atrioventricular rings respectively. **Trigonum habenulae [NA].** The small triangular eminence above the thalamus and imediately lateral and anterior to the stalk of the pineal body. It marks the position of the habenular nucleus, or epithalamus. [Gk *trigonos* three-cornered.]

trihexyphenidyl (tri·hex·e·**fen**′·id·il). 1 - Cyclohexyl - 1 - phenyl - 3 - piperidine - 1 - propanol, $C_{21}H_{31}ON$; benzhexol hydrochloride. A compound used in the form of the hydrochloride; it blocks transmission of autonomic impulses and is the most satisfactory drug for the treatment of extrapyramidal parkinsonism, being least liable to cause side reactions, and suitable for use by old and debilitated patients. In addition to its peripheral effects it has a central stimulant action against the depression which is common in parkinsonism. It may also be used in the treatment of spasmodic torticollis, facial spasm, and other dyskinesias.

trihybrid (tri·**hi**·brid). A hybrid which displays variation from the parents in three respects. [Gk *tri-*, hybrid.]

trihydrate (tri·**hi**·drate). 1. A trihydroxide. 2. Any compound that has crystallized with three molecules of water. [Gk *tri-*, *hydor* water.]

trihydric (tri·**hi**·drik). Applied to an alcohol that contains three OH groups. [Gk *tri-*, hydroxyl.]

trihydrol (tri·**hi**·drol). The associated molecule, $(H_2O)_3$, which is present in cold water and ice. [Gk *tri-*, *hydor* water.]

trihydroxide (tri·hi·**drox**·ide). Any compound which contains three OH groups. [Gk *tri-*, hydroxyl.]

trihydroxyanthraquinone (tri·hi·**drox**·e·an·thrah·**kwin**′·one). Anthragallol.

tri-iniodymus (tri·in·e·**od**·im·us). A three-headed fetal monster with a single body, the heads being united at the back. [Gk *tri-*, *inion* nape, *didymos* twin.]

tri-iodide (tri·i·o·dide). Any iodide that contains three atoms of iodine, e.g. BiI_3. [Gk *tri-*, iodine.]

tri-iodomethane (tri·i·o·do·**me**′·thane). Iodoform, CHI_3. A yellow compound used as an antiseptic for wound dressing, also in the treatment of tuberculosis and as a taenicide.

tri-iodothyronine (tri·i·o·do·**thi**′·ro·neen). 3,5,3′-Tri-iodothyronine, one of the two thyroid hormones, the other being tetra-iodothyronine (thyroxine). It seems probable that tri-iodothyronine accounts for some 40 per cent of the total thyroid hormone activity and thyroxine for 60 per cent.

triketohydrindene hydrate (tri·**ke**·to·hi·**drin**′·deen **hi**·drate). Ninhydrin.

triketopurine (tri·ke·to·**pewr**′·een). Uric acid. The keto form of hydroxy-purine, $(CONH)_2C_2(NH)_2CO$, which occurs in urine.

trilaminar (tri·**lam**·in·ar). Composed of three layers. [Gk *tri-*, L *lamina* plate.]

trilateral (tri·**lat**·er·al). Possessing three sides. [Gk *tri-*, L *latus* side.]

trilaurin (tri·**law**·rin). Glyceryl trilaurate, $C_3H_5(OCOC_{11}H_{23})_3$. One of the chief constituents of coconut and palm-kernel oils.

trilinolein (tri·lin·o·le·in). Glyceryl triolein, $C_3H_5(OCOC_{17}H_{31})_3$. An unsaturated glyceride found in linseed and other drying oils, such as those of hemp and sunflower.

Trillium (**tril**·e·um). A genus of liliaceous plants. **Trillium erectum.** The wake-robin, bethroot; the dried rhizome is used as an expectorant and astringent. [etym. dub.]

trilobate, trilobed (tri·**lo**·bate, tri·**lo**·bd). Possessing three lobes. [Gk *tri-*, lobe.]

trilocular (tri·**lok**·ew·lar). Composed of three cells. [Gk *tri-*, L *loculus* cell.]

trilogy (**tril**·o·je). A series of three related writings. [Gk *tri-* three, *logos* word.]

See also: FALLOT.

trimanual (tri·**man**·ew·al). Performed with three hands, as in certain obstetrical manoeuvres. [Gk *tri-*, L *manus* hand.]

Trimastigamoeba gruberi (tri·**mas**·tig·am·e′·bah **groo**·ber·i). A common free-living amoeba often encountered in stale specimens of stools. It has both amoeboid and flagellate forms. [Gk *tri-*, *mastix* whip, amoeba.]

trimastigate, trimastigote (tri·**mas**·tig·ate, tri·**mas**·tig·ote). Furnished with three whip-like flagellae. [Gk *tri-*, *mastix* whip.]

trimensual (tri·**men**·sew·al). Occurring every 3 months. [Gk *tri-*, L *mensis* month.]

Trimeperidine (tri·mep·**er**·id·een). BP Commission approved name for 1,2,5-trimethyl-4-phenyl-4-propionyloxypiperidine; an analogue of pethidine, having similar morphine-like actions.

Trimeprazine (tri·**mep**·raz·een). BP Commission approved name for 10-(3-dimethylamino-2-methylpropyl)phenothiazine. **Trimeprazine Tartrate BPC 1968.** The tartrate of dimeprazine; it acts as an antihistamine and also has effects on the central nervous system resembling those of chlorpromazine. A valuable anti-pruritic, but drowsiness is troublesome and some serious toxic effects have occurred.

trimercuric (tri·mer·**kewr**·ik). Denoting a compound of divalent mercury that contains three molecules of the latter. (Obsolete term.) [Gk *tri-*, mercury.]

Trimeresurus (**trim**·er·e·**sewr**′·us). A genus of poisonous snakes that includes the habu or *T. flavoviridis*. [Gk *tri-*, *meros* part, *oura* tail.]

trimester (tri·**mes**·ter). A period of 3 months. [L *trimestris* of three months.]

Trimetaphan BP 1968 (tri·**met**·ah·fan). 4,6 - Dibenzyl - 5 - oxo - 1 - thia - 4,6 - diaza-tricyclo-[6.3.0.0^{3,7}]undecanium (+)-camphor-sulphonate; a ganglion-blocking agent with the actions, uses and side-effects of pempidine tartrate. Its action is brief and it is used in surgery to induce controlled hypotension.

Trimetazidine (tri·met·**az**·id·een). BP Commission approved name for 1-(2,3,4-trimethoxybenzyl)piperazine; a vasodilator.

trimethadione (tri·meth·ad·i′·one). Troxidone.

Trimethidinium Methosulphate (tri·meth·id·in′·e·um meth·o·sul·fate). BP Commission approved name for (+) - 3 - (3 - dimethylaminopropyl) - 1,8,8 - trimethyl - 3 - azabicyclo[3,2,1]-octane di(methyl methosulphate).

Trimethoprim BP 1973 (tri·meth·o·prim). 2,4-Diamino-5-(3,4,5-trimethoxybenzyl)pyrimidine; an antimicrobial agent.

trimethylene (tri·meth·il·een). Cyclopropane.

trimethylenediamine (tri·meth·il·een·di′·am·een). $CH_2(CH_2NH_2)_2$, a poisonous ptomaine formed in cultures of the *Vibrio cholerae*.

trimethylethylene (tri·meth·il·eth′·il·een). Iso-amylene.

trimethylglycine (tri·meth·il·gli′·seen). Betaine. **Trimethylglycine hydrochloride.** Betaine hydrochloride.

trimethylglycocoll (tri·meth·il·gli′·ko·kol). Betaine.

trimethylxanthine (tri·meth·il·zan′·theen). Caffeine.

Trimipramine (tri·mip·ram·een). BP Commission approved name for 5 - (3 - dimethylamino - 2 - methylpropyl) - 10,11 - dihydrodibenz[*b,f*]azepine. **Trimipramine Maleate BP 1973.** The hydrogen maleate, an antidepressant.

trimorphic (tri·mor·fik). Characterized by trimorphism.

trimorphism (tri·mor·fizm). Existence in three distinct forms. [Gk *tri-, morphe* form.]

Trimustine (tri·mus·teen). BP Commission approved name for tri-(2-chloroethyl)amine; used in chronic lymphatic and myeloid leukaemias, and Hodgkin's disease.

trineural (tri·newr·al). Concerning three nerves. [Gk *tri-, neuron* nerve.]

trinitrate (tri·ni·trate). Any nitrate that contains three nitrate groups, e.g. $Al(NO_3)_3$. [Gk *tri-*, nitric.]

trinitrine (tri·ni·treen). Trinitroglycerine, $C_3H_5(NO_3)_3$.

trinitrocellulose (tri·ni·tro·sel′·ew·loze). One of the group of cellulose nitrates of general formula $[C_6H_7O_5(NO_2)_3]_x$ formed by the treatment of wood pulp with a mixture of nitric and sulphuric acids. It is employed in the manufacture of guncotton and celluloid; dissolved in acetone it constitutes collodion.

trinitrocresol (tri·ni·tro·kre′·sol). $(CH_3)C_6H(OH)(NO_2)_3$, a compound formed by the nitration of cresol; it has antiseptic properties.

trinitroglycerine (tri·ni·tro·glis′·er·een). Glyceryl trinitrate, $C_3H_5(NO_3)_3$. An oily liquid manufactured by mixing glycerol with concentrated sulphuric and nitric acids. It is an explosive; absorbed in diatomite or wood pulp, it is known as *dynamite*.

trinitrol (tri·ni·trol). Erythrityl tetranitrate.

Trinitrophenol BPC 1959 (tri·ni·tro·fe′·nol). Picric acid, carbazotic acid, $C_6H_2(NO_2)_3OH$, yellow crystals, only slightly soluble in water, and used as an explosive (lyddite), a yellow dye, and a stain in microscopy; employed to precipitate albumin (Esbach's reagent) and to detect glucose in urine. Medicinally, it is no longer given by mouth owing to toxicity. It is a strong antiseptic and has been used in burn dressings, but there is the danger of absorption; this may result in anaemia, nephritis, and/or hepatitis. It should not be applied to large areas. It must be stored in quantities of less than 500 g in non-metal containers.

trinitrotoluene (tri·ni·tro·tol′·ew·een). $C_6H_2CH_3(NO_2)_3$, a pale-yellow crystalline solid obtained by the nitration of toluene and used as a high explosive. It is absorbed mainly through the skin, causing yellow staining and papular contact dermatitis, with intense irritation; methaemoglobinaemia ensues with livid cyanosis, often without symptoms. Aplastic anaemia is rare, but when it occurs is nearly always fatal; there may be toxic jaundice, either of sudden onset or preceded by drowsiness, gastritis, and dark urine, and the liver shows necrotic changes.

trinucleate (tri·new·kle·ate). Possessing three nuclei. [Gk *tri-*, nucleus.]

trinucleotide (tri·new·kle·o·tide). A combination of three nucleotide units found in nucleoprotein. [Gk *tri-*, nucleotide.]

triolein (tri·o·le·in). Olein, glycerol trioleate, $(C_{17}H_{33}COO)_3C_3H_5$. A liquid fat which occurs in many natural fats and oils. It is unsaturated and may be hardened catalytically with hydrogen into tristearin.

triophthalmos (tri·of·thal·mos). A double-faced fetal monster with three eyes. [Gk *tri-, ophthalmos* eye.]

triopodymus (tri·op·od·im·us). A fetal monster with three faces and a single head. [Gk *tri-, ops* face, *didymos* twin.]

triorchid, triorchis (tri·or·kid, tri·or·kis). An individual with three testicles. [Gk *tri-, orchis* testicle.]

triorthocresyl phosphate (tri·or·tho·kre′·sil fos·fate). A colourless liquid, $(CH_3C_6H_4)_3PO_4$, found in Jamaican ginger and causing paralysis.

triose (tri·oze). The simplest of the monosaccharide true sugars. It is produced by the oxidation of glycerol and is in two isomeric forms, the *aldotriose*, glycerose, $CH_2OHCHOHCHO$, and the *ketotriose*, dihydroxyacetone, $CH_2OHCOCH_2OH$. **Triose phosphate.** The general name given to the two compounds, glyceraldehyde phosphate and dihydroxyacetone phosphate, which play an important part in muscle glycogenolysis, sugar fermentation, and photosynthesis.

triotus (tri·o·tus). A double-faced fetal monster with three ears and usually four eyes. [Gk *tri-, ous* eye.]

trioxide (tri·ox·ide). Any oxide which contains three atoms of oxygen, e.g. Fe_2O_3. [Gk *tri-*, oxide.]

trioxymethylene (tri·ox·e·meth′·il·een). Paraformaldehyde.

trioxypurine (tri·ox·e·pewr′·een). Uric acid. *See* ACID.

tripalmitin (tri·pal·mit·in). Palmitin, $(C_{15}H_{31}COO)_3C_3H_5$. A solid fat found in palm oil and other natural oils; it is used in soap-making.

tripara (trip·ar·ah). A woman who has given birth to children three times. [Gk *tri-*, L *parere* to give birth.]

Triparanol (tri·par·an·ol). BP Commission approved name for 2 - (4 - chlorophenyl) - 1 - (4 - diethylaminoethoxyphenyl) - 1 - *p* - tolylethanol; a cholesterol inhibitor.

Tripelennamine (tri·pel·en·am·een). BP Commission approved name for *N*-benzyl-*N′N′*dimethyl-*N*-2-pyridylethylenediamine. An antihistaminic drug which has been successful in urticaria and agioneurotic oedema when other antihistaminic drugs have failed.

tripeptide (tri·pep·tide). A polypeptide derived by the condensation of any three amino acids by means of peptide linkages. [Gk *tri-*, peptide.]

triphalangia (tri·fal·an·je·ah). A deformity of the hand or foot in which there are three phalanges in the thumb or big toe. [Gk *tri-, phalagx* digit.]

triphasic (tri·fa·zik). Having three phases. [Gk *tri-, phasis* appearance.]

triphenylchlorethylene (tri·fe·nil·klor·eth′·il·een). $(C_6H_5)_2C=C(C_6H_5)Cl$, a synthetic oestrogen with the systematic name of 1,1,2-triphenyl-2-chlorostilbene.

triphenylethylene (tri·fe·nil·eth′·il·een). 1,1,2-triphenylstilbene, $(C_6H_5)_2C=CH(C_6H_5)$. A hydrocarbon, derivatives of which are oestrogenic without possessing the steroid structure of the natural oestrogens.

triphenylmethane (tri·fe·nil·me′·thane). $CH(C_6H_5)_3$, a colourless crystalline hydrocarbon which is the parent of a family of dyes.

triphenylstibinsulphide (tri·fe·nil·stib·in·sul′·fide). $(C_6H_5)_3SbS$, a compound which readily liberates sulphur, and is a strong reducing agent. It has been used in dermatology, e.g. in seborrhoea.

Tripier, Léon (b. 1842). French surgeon.

Tripier's amputation. A method resembling the mediotarsal amputation, but with removal of part of the tarsus.

Tripier operation. A double-pedicle skin flap of the "bucket-handle" type, taken from the upper eyelid and transposed to the lower lid for certain cases of skin loss.

triplegia (tri·ple·je·ah). Paralysis of one side of the body associated with paralysis of an arm or leg on the other side. [Gk *tri-, plege* stroke.]

triplet (trip·let). 1. One of three delivered at a birth. 2. A combination of three, such as lenses in a microscope. **Chain-termination triplet, Termination triplet.** Termination codon. *See* CODON. [Gk *triploos* triple.]

triploblastic (trip·lo·**blas**·tik). Pertaining to an embryo with three germ layers, namely, ectoderm, entoderm, and mesoderm. [Gk *triploos* triple, *blastos* germ.]

triplocoria (trip·lo·**kor**·e·ah). A variety of polycoria in which there are three pupils. [Gk *triploos* triple, *kore* pupil.]

triploid (**trip**·loid). Of chromosome complements, cells or individuals having three sets of chromosomes (symbol 3*n*). [Gk *triploos* triple, *eidos* form.]

triploidy (tri·**ploid**·e). The state characteristic of triploids. [Gk *triploos* triple, *eidos* form.]

triplopia (trip·**lo**·pe·ah). A visual defect in which the sufferer sees three images of the same object. [Gk *triploos* triple, *ops* eye.]

tripod (**tri**·pod). A vessel or other object which rests upon three feet or legs; three-legged. **Anatomical tripod.** The three points on which the foot rests: the heel, the three medial metatarsal heads, and the two lateral metatarsal heads. **Tripod of life, Vital tripod.** The brain, heart, and lungs, so regarded because they are essential for the maintenance of life. [Gk *tri-*, *pous* foot.]

See also: HALLER.

tripositive (tri·**poz**·it·iv). Having three positive charges, e.g. the ferric ion, Fe^{3+}. [Gk *tri-*, positive.]

Triprolidine (tri·**prol**·id·een). BP Commission approved name for *trans*-1-2′-pyridyl-3-pyrrolidino-1-*p*-tolylprop-1-ene, a highly potent, quick-acting antihistaminic, with an effect lasting about 12 hours. Useful in serum sickness, hay fever, vasomotor rhinitis, and other respiratory allergic disorders. It is usually administered in the form of the hydrochloride (BP 1973).

triprosopus (tri·**pros**·o·pus). A fetal monster with three faces fused into one. [Gk *tri-*, *prosopon* face.]

tripsis (**trip**·sis). 1. Trituration. 2. Massage. [Gk rubbing.]

triptocoria (trip·to·**kor**·e·ah). Triplocoria.

tripus (**tri**·pus). 1. Tripod. 2. A monster having three feet. **Tripus coeliacus, Tripus halleri.** The coeliac artery. [Gk *tri-*, *pous* foot.]

triquetral (tri·**kwe**·tral. Triangular; three-cornered. [L *triquetrus*.]

triquetral bone [os triquetrum (NA)]. The most medially placed bone in the proximal row of carpal bones; the cuneiform bone.

triquetrous (tri·**kwe**·trus). Triquetral; three-cornered. **Triquetrous bone.** 1. A wormian bone of a cranial suture. 2. The cuneiform bone of the hand. [L *triquetrus* triangular.]

triquetrum (tri·**kwe**·trum). A triquetrous bone.

triradial, triradiate (tri·**ra**·de·al, tri·**ra**·de·ate). Radiating three ways; having three rays. [Gk *tri-*, L *radius* ray.]

triradiation (tri·ra·de·**a**′·shun). Spread or extension in three directions. [see prec.]

triradius (tri·**ra**·de·us). The point of convergence of dermal ridges running in three different directions. [Gk *tri-*, L *radius* ray.]

trisaccharidase (tri·**sak**·ar·id·aze). An enzyme which activates the hydrolysis of trisaccharides, e.g. raffinase.]

trisaccharide (tri·**sak**·ar·ide). The general term for a carbohydrate formed by the union of any three monosaccharide units. They have the general formula $C_{18}H_{32}O_{16}$, and include raffinose and melezitose. [Gk *tri-*, saccharide.]

trismic (**triz**·mik). Having the characteristics of trismus.

trismus (**triz**·mus). Inability to open the mouth due to tonic contracture of the muscles of the jaw. **Trismus capistratus.** A fixing of the jaws by adhesions between the cheeks and gums. **Trismus cynicus.** The risus sardonicus of tetanus—"lockjaw". **Trismus nascentium, Trismus neonatorum.** Trismus in the new-born owing to tetanus infection of the navel. **Trismus uteri.** Trismus arising out of infection during the puerperium. [Gk *trismos* gnashing.]

trisnitrate (tris·**ni**·trate). Trinitrate. [Gk *tris* thrice, nitrate.]

trisomic (tri·**so**·mik). Of cells, tissues or individuals essentially diploid but with three copies of a chromosome. **Double trisomic.** Of trisomics, having three copies of two different chromosomes. **Interchange trisomic.** A pseudodiploid cell or individual with three doses of nearly all the material of a chromosome, but with the additional segment attached by translocation to another member of the complement. **Partial trisomic.** A cell or individual with only part of a chromosome present in triplicate. **Primary trisomic.** A trisomic whose additional chromosome is completely homologous to the other two, i.e. a normal member of the chromosome complement. **Secondary trisomic.** A trisomic whose additional chromosome is an isochromosome. In this case the cell or individual is virtually tetrasomic for one chromosome arm. **Tertiary trisomic.** A trisomic whose additional chromosome is the product of a reciprocal translocation. [Gk *tri-*, *soma* body.]

trisomy (**tri**·so·me). The state of trisomics. **Trisomy 21.** The trisomy responsible for Down's syndrome. **Trisomy C.** The trisomy of an autosome belonging to the C group (nos. 6-12). If the chromosome involved can be positively identified, a more specific notation should be used (e.g. trisomy 9). **Trisomy D_1, 13–15 or 13.** The trisomy responsible for Patau's syndrome; the chromosome responsible for this syndrome has been recently identified as chromosome no. 13. **Trisomy E_1, 17–18 or 18.** The trisomy responsible for Edward's syndrome; due to involvement of chromosome no. 18. [Gk *tri-*, *soma* body.]

tristearin (tri·**ste**·ar·in). Stearin, glycerol tristearate, $(C_{17}H_{35}COO)_3C_3H_5$. A solid fat found in lard, suet, and other natural fats; also manufactured by the catalytic hydrogenation of triolein. [Gk *tri-*, stearin.]

tristemania (tris·te·**ma**·ne·ah). Melancholia. [L *tristis* sad, Gk *mania* madness.]

tristichia, tristichiasis (tri·**stik**·e·ah, tri·stik·**i**·as·is). A rare anomaly in which there are three rows of eyelashes on each lid. [Gk *tri-*, *stichos* row.]

trisubstituted (tri·**sub**·stit·ew·ted). Describing a compound in the molecule of which three atoms or substituent groups have been replaced by others. [Gk *tri*, substitute.]

trisulcate (tri·**sul**·kate). Possessing three grooves or furrows. [Gk *tri-*, L *sulcus* groove.]

trisulphanilamide (**tri**·sul·fan·**il**′·am·ide). A loose term applied to a mixture of equal parts of the three sulphonamide drugs, sulphadiazine, sulphathiazole, and sulphamerazine.

trisulphide (tri·**sul**·fide). Any sulphide which contains three atoms of sulphur, e.g. Fe_2S_3. [Gk *tri-*, sulphide.]

tritanomalopia (**trit**·an·om·al·**o**′·pe·ah). Tritanomaly. [Gk *tritos* third, anomaly, Gk *opsis* sight.]

tritanomaly (trit·an·**om**·al·e). A form of partial colour blindness of the anomalous trichromatic type, in which the blue portion of the spectrum is only imperfectly perceived. [Gk *tritos* third, anomaly.]

tritanope (**trit**·an·ope). A dichromat who is unable to appreciate the blue portion of the spectrum; a blue-blind person, a very rare condition. [Gk *tritos* third, *ops* eye.]

tritanopia, tritanopsia (trit·an·**o**·pe·ah, trit·an·**op**·se·ah). A form of partial colour blindness of the dichromatic type in which the blue portion of the spectrum is not perceived; a rare form of colour blindness in which blue and yellow are confused. [Gk *tritos* third, anopia.]

triterpene (tri·**ter**·peen). Any member of a family of isomeric hydrocarbons of formula $C_{30}H_{48}$.

trithioacetaldehyde (tri·**thi**·o·as·et·**al**′·de·hide). Sulphoparaldehyde, $(CH_3CHS)_3$, a hypnotic drug.

tritiated (**trit**·e·a·ted). Used to describe a chemical compound which has been labelled with radioactive hydrogen, tritium.

triticeoglossus (trit·is·e·o·**glos**′·us). A small muscle occasionally present; it runs from the cartilago triticea into the side of the tongue. [triticeum, Gk *glossa* tongue.]

triticeous (tri·**tish**·us). Like a grain of wheat. **Triticeous nodule.** Triticeum. [see foll.]

triticeum (trit·**is**·e·um). The cartilago triticea, a cartilaginous nodule in the lateral thyrohyoid ligament. [L *triticum* wheat.]

triticin (**trit**·is·in). $(C_6H_{10}O_5)_x$, a polysaccharide resembling inulin and composed of fructose units. It occurs in the rhizome of couch grass, *Triticum repens.*

Triticum (**trit**·ik·um). 1. A genus of grasses of the family Gramineae, e.g. couch grass. 2. Agropyrum, the dried rhizome of *Agropyron* (Triticum) *repens* Linn. (Beauvois), used as a diuretic. [L wheat.]

tritium (trit·e·um). Hydrogen, the nuclei of the atoms of which consist of a proton and two neutrons: ^3H, a radioactive isotope of hydrogen. [Gk *tritos* third.]

tritol (tri·tol). The name given in Germany and Austria to a preparation of filix-mas extract and malt extract, often with castor oil. It is administered in the treatment of tapeworm.

triton (tri·ton). 1. Trinitrotoluene. 2. Tetramethyl ammonium hydroxide, $N(CH_3)_4OH$, a compound used in soap manufacture. 3. The nucleus of an atom of tritium; a particle consisting of a proton and two neutrons.

tritoxide (trit·ox·ide). Trioxide.

tritrichomonas (tri·trik·o·mo′·nas). An obsolete term used to indicate a trichomonas with three anterior flagella; the number of flagella is not a constant characteristic. [Gk *tri-*, *thrix* hair, *monas* unit.]

tritubercular (tri·tew·ber·kew·lar). Possessing three tubercles or cusps; tricuspid. [Gk *tri-*, tubercle.]

triturable (trit·ewr·abl). Lending itself to trituration.

triturate (trit·ewr·ate). 1. To reduce to a fine powder by grinding. 2. To make evenly distributed mixtures of powders with a pestle and mortar. [L *triturare* to thresh.]

trituration (trit·ewr·a·shun). 1. The reduction of a solid to a fine powder. 2. A finely ground powder, or, more usually, finely ground and evenly mixed powders. [see prec.]

triturium (trit·ewr·e·um). An apparatus for separating immiscible liquids by their different densities. [L *triturare* to thresh.]

trivalent (tri·va·lent). Having a valency of three; describing an element or radical which is capable of combining with or replacing three atoms of hydrogen or other monovalent element. Applied also to sera and vaccines. [see prec.]

trivalerin (tri·val·er·in). Phocenine.

trivalve, trivalvular (tri·valv, tri·val·vew·lar). Provided with three valves. [Gk *tri*, valve.]

trocar (tro·kar). A sharp instrument carrying a cannula around it for piercing body cavities and withdrawing fluid. **Piloting trocar.** A handled trocar for the insertion of a jointed Durham's tracheotomy tube. [Fr. *trois* three, *carres* sides.]

See also: DUCHENNE, DURHAM (A. E.), KIDD, MORSON.

trochanter (tro·kan·ter). Either of the two bony prominences at the upper end of the femur, so called perhaps from their movements in the action of running. **Greater trochanter [trochanter major (NA)].** A large projection from the lateral aspect of the proximal end of the shaft of the femur to which the gluteus medius and gluteus minimus muscles are attached. **Lesser trochanter [trochanter minor (NA)].** A projection on the posteromedial aspect of the shaft of the femur just below the neck, giving insertion to the psoas major muscle. **Third trochanter [trochanter tertius (NA)].** A term applied to the gluteal ridge on the femur when it is particularly prominent. It receives part of the insertion of the gluteus maximus muscle. [Gk runner.]

trochanteric (tro·kan·ter·ik). Concerned with a trochanter particularly with the greater trochanter.

trochanterion (trok·an·te·re·on). An anthropometric point; the upper border of the greater trochanter.

trochanteroplasty (tro·kan·ter·o·plas′·te). Removal and reimplantation of the greater trochanter as part of a reconstruction operation at the upper end of the femur. [trochanter, Gk *plassein* to mould.]

troche (tro·ke). A lozenge, having a drug incorporated in a sugar and gum basis causing it to set hard. It is most commonly used to treat local conditions of the mouth and throat, but may be used to administer drugs required to have an action in the alimentary canal, or even for drugs required to produce systemic effects. [Gk *trochos* pill.]

trochiscus (tro·kis·lus) (pl. *trochisci*). A troche; a lozenge. [Gk *trochiskos* lozenge.]

trochlea [NA] (trok·le·ah). A pulley; applied in anatomy to a surface convex in one direction and concave in a direction at right angles, and allowing movement around a transverse axis. It is also applied to structures round or through which another structure, such as a tendon, may pass, thus altering the direction of its pull. **Trochlea of the astragalus.** Trochlea of the talus (see below). **Trochlea of the femur.** The grooved surface on the front of the distal end of the femur for articulation with the patella. **Trochlea of the humerus [trochlea humeri (NA)].** The grooved surface at the distal end of the humerus which articulates with the trochlear notch of the ulna. **Muscular trochlea.** Muscular pulley. *See* PULLEY. **Trochlea of the orbit.** Trochlea of the superior oblique muscle of the orbit (see below). **Trochlea of a phalanx.** The pulley-shaped head of a proximal or middle phalanx. **Trochlea of the superior oblique muscle of the orbit [trochlea musculi obliquus superior (NA)].** A fibrocartilaginous ring attached to the medial side of the roof of the orbit; the tendon of the superior oblique muscle passes through the ring as it changes its direction. **Trochlea of the talus [trochlea tali (NA)].** The superior articular surface of the talus which articulates with the tibia. [L pulley.]

trochlear (trok·le·ar). 1. Pulley-shaped. 2. Relating to a trochlea. 3. Concerned with the trochlear nerve. **Trochlear fossa.** *See* FOSSA. **Trochlear notch.** *See* NOTCH. **Trochlear spine.** Trochlear fossa. *See* FOSSA. [see prec.]

trochlear nerve [nervus trochlearis (NA)]. The 4th cranial nerve. It arises from cells in the mid-brain, emerges from the superior medullary velum, passes to the orbit through the superior orbital fissure, and supplies the superior oblique muscle.

nucleus [nucleus nervi trochlearis (NA)]. A small group of cells situated ventrally in the central grey matter of the mid-brain near the midline at the level of the inferior quadrigeminal body.

trochleariform (trok·le·ar·e·form). Trochlear. [trochlea, form.]

trochlearis (trok·le·a·ris). The old name for the superior oblique muscle of the orbit. [L *trochlea* pulley.]

trochocardia (trok·o·kar·de·ah). Displacement of the heart brought about by its turning on its longest axis. [Gk *trochos* wheel, *kardia* heart.]

trochocephalia, trochocephalus, trochocephaly (trok·o·kef·a′·le·ah, trok·o·kef·al·us, trok·o·kef·al·e). A deformed skull attributed to synostosis of the frontal and parietal bones. [Gk *trochos* wheel, *kephale* head.]

trochoginglymus (trok·o·jing·gli·mus). A trochoid or pivot joint combined with a ginglymus or hinge joint, e.g. the elbow joint. [Gk *trochos* wheel, *gigglymos* hinge.]

trochoid (tro·koid). Permitting rotation; like a pulley or pivot. [Gk *trochos* wheel, *eidos* form.]

trochoides (tro·koi·deez). A pivot joint, e.g. the joint between the head of the radius and the humerus. [see prec.]

trochorizocardia (trok·or·izo·kar′·de·ah). Trochocardia with horizocardia.

Troeltsch, Anton Friedrich von (b. 1829). Wurzburg otologist.

Troeltsch's depressions, pockets, pouches, recesses, or spaces. The three recesses, anterior, posterior, and superior, of the tympanic membrane, formed by the folding of the mucous membrane on the internal surface of the tympanic membrane.

Troeltsch's folds. The anterior and posterior malleolar folds.

Troemner, Ernest L. O. (b. 1868). Hamburg neurologist.

Troemner's sign. Digital reflex, 2nd def. *See* REFLEX.

Troglotrematidae (trog·lo·trem·at′·id·e). A family of the trematode sub-order Distomata or Fascioloidea, lung flukes. The genus *Paragonimus* is of medical interest. [Gk *trogle* hole, *trema* perforation, *eidos* form.]

troilism (tro·il·izm). Sexual practice involving three people, two males and a female, or one male and two females.

Troisier, Charles Emile (b. 1844). Paris physician.

Troisier's ganglion, or sign. Enlargement of the lymph glands above the clavicle, on the left side with abdominal malignant growths and on the right with intrathoracic growths.

Troisier's node. Signal node. *See* NODE.

Troisier's syndrome. Bronze pigmentation with glycosuria; haemochromatosis.

Trolard, Paulin (b. 1842). Paris anatomist.

Trolard's net, or plexus. A collection of about five small veins which surround the hypoglossal nerve in the anterior condylar canal and communicate with the inferior petrosal sinus of the dura mater.

Trolard's vein. An anastomotic vein which runs from the superior saggital sinus of the dura mater to the base of the cranium where it terminates by joining either the superior petrosal sinus or the cavernous sinus.

Trolnitrate Phosphate (trol·**ni**·trate **fos**·fate). BP Commission approved name for triethanolamine *O,O′,O″*-trinitrate diorthophosphate; a vasodilator.

Trombicula (trom·**bik**·ew·lah). A genus of mites of the super-family Trombidioidea; harvest mites, red bugs. The larvae are parasitic and adults free-living, the former having been described in the genus *Leptus* when the adults were unknown. They are very important vectors of typhus Rickettsiae of the Felix-Weil group, i.e. tsutsugamushi disease and its allies. All species cause irritation and rash. The principal species are as follows: *T. akamushi*, the principal vector of tsutsugamushi disease in Japan and Taiwan (it has been described from other Far Eastern countries, perhaps in error); *T. alfreddugesi*, see *Eutrombicula; T. autumnalis*, the common harvest mite of Europe, causes mite dermatitis (scrub itch); *T. brumpti* and *T. buloloensis* cause mite dermatitis (scrub itch); *T. deliensis*, an important vector of rural typhus in India, Malaysia, and Sumatra, occurs in Australia; *T. fletcheri*, a species probably confused with *T. akamushi* in Malaysia and a vector of mite-borne typhus; *T. irritans, T. irritans uruguayensis* and *T. mansoni* causes mite dermatitis (harvest itch); *T. minor*, the itch mite of Australia, causes mite dermatitis (harvest itch) and is a vector of mite-borne typhus; *T. walchi*, a vector of rural typhus; and *T. wichmanni*, the gonone of Celebes, Borneo, and New Guinea, and a vector of rural typhus. [invented dim. from Gk *tromein* to tremble.]

trombiculiasis (trom·**bik**·ew·**li**′·as·is). Trombiculosis.

Trombiculidae (**trom**·bik·ew·**li**′·de). A family of trombidiiform mites. The genera *Eutrombicula* and *Trombicula* are of medical importance. [*Trombicula*, Gk *eidos* form.]

trombiculosis (trom·**bik**·ew·**lo**′·sis). Infestation with mites of the genus *Trombicula* [*Trombicula*, Gk *-osis* condition.]

trombidiiasis (**trom**·bid·e·**i**′·as·is). Trombidiosis.

Trombidiidae (trom·bid·i·id·e). A family of trombidiiform mites. Their larvae are parasitic on insects and of no medical importance. The Trombiculidae, which are medically important, were once included here. [*Trombidium*, Gk *eidos* form.]

trombidiiform (trom·bid·i·e·form). Of the nature of the Trombidiidae. [Trombidiidae, form.]

Trombidioidea (**trom**·bid·e·**oid**′·e·ah). A super-family of the arachnid order Acarina. The family Trombiculidae is of medical interest. [*Trombidium*, Gk *eidos* form.]

trombidiosis (**trom**·bid·e·**o**′·sis). Lesions of the skin caused by the harvest mite *Trombicula autumnalis*. [*Trombidium*, Gk *-osis* condition.]

Trombidium (trom·**bid**·e·um). A genus of mites. The medically important species are now placed in *Trombicula*. [invented dim. from Gk *tromein* to tremble.]

Trometamol (tro·**met**·am·ol). BP Commission approved name for 2-amino-2-hydroxymethylpropane-1,3-diol; it is used in the treatment of gastric hyperacidity.

tromomania (trom·o·**ma**·ne·ah). Delirium alcoholicum. [Gk *tromos* trembling, *mania* madness.]

tromophonia (trom·o·**fo**·ne·ah). Dysphonia in which the voice is tremulous. [Gk *tromos* trembling, *phone* voice.]

tropacocaine (**tro**·pah·ko·**kane**′). A local analgesic from coca leaves grown in Java. It is the ester of the base, pseudotropine, with benzoic acid. **Tropacocaine hydrochloride.** $C_8H_{14}ON$ $C_6H_5CO{\cdot}HCl$, the water-soluble salt of the alkaloid.

tropaeolin (tro·**pe**·o·lin). Any one of a series of orange dyestuffs derived from *p*-hydroxyazobenzene, and used as indicators in alkalimetry. Called after the garden nasturtium (*Tropaeolum*) because of their colours. **Tropaeolin D.** Methyl orange, helianthine, sodium dimethylaminobenzene *p*-sulphonate, $(CH_3)_2NC_6H_4N{=}NC_6H_4SO_3Na$; used as an indicator in volumetric analysis (pH 3.0–4.5). **Tropaeolin G.** Metanil yellow. **Tropaeolin O.** Resorcinol yellow, sodium dihydroxyazobenzene sulphonate, $(OH)_2C_6H_4N{=}NC_6H_4SO_3Na$; used as an indicator (pH 11.0–12.5). **Tropaeolin OO.** Orange IV, sodium diphenylaminoazobenzene sulphonate, $(C_6H_5)_2NC_6H_4N{=}NC_6H_4SO_3Na$; an indicator (pH 1.5–2.5), and also used in dyeing wool and silk. **Tropaeolin OOO.** Orange II, sodium β-naphthol azobenzene sulphonate, $OHC_{10}H_6N{=}NC_6H_4SO_3Na$; an indicator (pH 7.5–8.5). **Tropaeolin R.** Resorcinol yellow. *See* YELLOW. [Gk *tropaios* changing.]

tropate (**tro**·pate). Any salt or ester of tropic acid.

tropeine (**tro**·pe·een). Any ester formed by tropine with an organic acid. They include atropine, homatropine, and other mydriatic alkaloids.

tropeinism (tro·**pe**·in·izm). Poisoning by a tropeine or a tropeine derivative. The symptoms range from dysphagia and increased pulse rate to clonic spasms and eventually to loss of consciousness followed by cardiac and respiratory paralysis.

tropeolin (tro·**pe**·o·lin). Tropaeolin.

tropesis (tro·**pe**·sis). An inclination; a tendency. [Gk *trope* a turning.]

trophectoderm (tro·**fek**·to·derm). Trophoblast. [Gk *trophe* nutrition, *ektos* outer, *derma* skin.]

trophesy (**tro**·fes·e). Defective nutrition due to the loss of trophic nervous activity. [obsolete term.] [Gk *trophe* nutrition.]

trophic (**trof**·ik). Concerned with nutrition. [Gk *trophe* nutrition.]

trophism (**trof**·izm). 1. A trophic influence. 2. Nutrition. [Gk *trophe* nutrition.]

trophoblast (**tro**·fo·blast). The outer cellular and syncytial layer of mammalian blastocysts which makes contact with the uterine wall and through which nutritive materials and waste products are exchanged between the fetal and maternal circulations. In some species, such as man, it is responsible for erosion of the uterine wall during implantation of the ovum and during the growth of the chorionic villi and placenta. [Gk *trophe* nutrition, *blastos* germ.]

trophoblastic (tro·fo·**blas**·tik). Concerning the trophoblast.

trophoblastoma (**tro**·fo·blas·**to**′·mah). A malignant tumour derived from cells of the syncytium and chorion at the site of the placenta in the pregnant uterus. [Gk *trophe* nutrition, *blastos* germ, *-oma* tumour.]

trophochromatin (tro·fo·**kro**·mat·in). Trophochromidia.

trophochromidia (**tro**·fo·kro·**mid**′·e·ah). The non-germinal chromatin found outside the nucleus in certain protozoa and concerned with nutrition. [Gk *trophe* nutrition, chromidia.]

trophocyte (**tro**·fo·site). A Sertoli cell of the testis which supports and nourishes the developing spermatozoa. [Gk *trophe* nutrition, *kytos* cell.]

trophoderm (**tro**·fo·derm). Trophoblast. [Gk *trophe* nutrition, *derma* skin.]

trophodermatoneurosis (tro·fo·**der**·mat·o·newr·**o**′·sis). Fugitive skin rash seen in psychosomatic conditions. [Gk *trophe* nutrition, *derma* skin, neurosis.]

trophodynamics (**tro**·fo·di·**nam**′·ix). The equilibria and the chemical and physical forces involved in the processes of nutrition of the organism. [Gk *trophe* nutrition, *dynamis* force.]

trophoedema (tro·fe·**de**·mah). Chronic oedematous swelling of the legs and feet due to faulty or under-nutrition. [Gk *trophe* nutrition, oedema.]

trophology (tro·**fol**·o·je). The study of nutrition in the body. [Gk *trophe* nutrition, *logos* science.]

trophoneurosis (**tro**·fo·newr·**o**′·sis). Alteration in any tissue due to failure of nutrition from defective nerve influence. **Disseminated trophoneurosis.** Sclerodermia. **Facial trophoneurosis.** Facial hemiatrophy. *See* HEMIATROPHY. **Lingual trophoneurosis.** A type showing hemiatrophy of the tongue. **Muscular trophoneurosis.** Muscular wasting due to nerve defect. [Gk *trophe* nutrition, *neuron* nerve, *-osis* condition.]

See also: ROMBERG.

trophoneurotic (tro·fo·newr·**ot'**·ik). Marked by or relating to trophoneurosis.

trophonosis, trophonosus (tro·fo·**no**·sis, tro·fo·**no**·sus). Disease arising out of nutritional defect. [Gk *trophe* nutrition, *nosos* disease.]

trophonucleus (tro·fo·**new**·kle·us). Of the two nuclei of certain protozoa, the one which is concerned primarily with metabolic rather than reproductive functions. [Gk *trophe* nutrition, nucleus.]

trophopathia, trophopathy (tro·fo·**path**·e·ah, trofe·**op**·ath·e). Trophonosis. [Gk *trophe* nutrition, *pathos* disease.]

trophospongia (tro·fo·**spun**·je·ah). An old term for the decidua, or maternal placenta (Hubrecht). [Gk *trophe* nutrition, *spoggia* sponge.]

trophospongium (tro·fo·**spun**·je·um). A system of intracellular canals (Holmgren) found in certain cells, e.g. the parietal cells of the gastric mucosa. Their significance is unknown. [see prec.]

trophotaxis (tro·fo·**tax**·is). The movement of cells positively towards, or negatively away from, substances that are nutritive. [Gk *trophe* nutrition, *taxis* arrangement.]

trophotherapy (tro·fo·**ther**·ap·e). Treatment of disease by control of the diet. [Gk *trophe* nutrition, *therapeia* treatment.]

trophotropic (tro·fo·**trop**·ik). Pertaining to cell movements in response to nutritional stimuli, e.g. nutriment in solution. [Gk *trophe* nutrition, *trepein* to turn.]

trophotropism (tro·fo·**trop**·izm). A tropism in relation to nutritive materials. **Negative trophotropism.** Movement of cells away from nutrient materials. **Positive trophotropism.** Movement of cells towards nutrient materials. [see prec.]

trophozoite (tro·fo·**zo**·ite). A stage in the reproduction of protozoa. The parasite feeds and grows, giving rise to daughter individuals; in the case of the malaria parasites the merozoite enters the red blood corpuscle, the young parasite becomes a trophozoite which when fully developed becomes a schizont, or alternatively may initiate a sexual cycle and give rise to a sporont (gametocyte). [Gk *trophe* nutrition, *zoon* animal.]

tropia (**tro**·pe·ah). A manifest deviation of the fixation axis of one eye or other when both eyes are uncovered: *esotropia* when the deviation is inwards, *exotropia* when outwards, *hypermetropia* when upwards, and *hypotropia* when downwards. Also called *manifest squint, strabismus*, or *heterotropia.* [Gk *trope* turn.]

tropical (**trop**·ik·al). Characteristic of or relating to the tropical regions of the earth. [Gk *tropikos.*]

Tropicamide BP 1973 (tro·**pik**·am·ide). *N*-Ethyl-*N*-(4-piperidylmethyl)tropamide; a parasympatholytic agent. Its action resembles that of atropine, but its mydriatic and cycloplegic effects are more rapid in onset and less prolonged. It is used mainly in ophthalmology.

tropicopolitan (**trop**·ik·o·**pol'**·it·an). Occurring in tropical countries. [tropical, Gk *polites* citizen.]

Tropicorbis (trop·ik·**or**·bis). A genus of snails, which has now been merged into the genus *Biomphalaria.* **Tropicorbis centrimetalis.** An intermediary host of *Schistosoma mansoni.* **Tropicorbis havanensis.** Occurs in Louisiana, Texas, and the West Indies; a potential host of *Schistosoma mansoni.* [Gk *tropikos* tropical, L *orbis* world.]

tropics (**trop**·ix). Literally, that part of the world that lies between the Tropic of Cancer and the Tropic of Capricorn. Within this zone, the mid-day sun is at some time during the year directly overhead. While generally speaking this is the hottest part of the earth there are some anomalies, e.g. some of the Sahara desert and of the hottest parts of India do not fall within this zone. [Gk *tropikos* tropical.]

tropidine (**tro**·pid·een). $C_8H_{13}N$, an oily base obtained by the dehydration of tropine.

Tropigline (**tro**·pig·leen). BP Commission approved name for tiglyltropeine; it is used in the treatment of Parkinson's syndrome.

tropin (**tro**·pin). Any antibody occurring in serum which increases the rate of phagocytosis of bacteria. [Gk *trepein* to turn.]

tropine (**tro**·peen). $CH_3NC_6H_{10}CHOH$, a dicyclic alcoholic tertiary amine occurring in species of *Belladonna, Hyoscyamus, Stramonium,* and other genera of the family Solanaceae, usually in the form of esters, e.g. atropine, hyoscyamine, all of which have antispasmodic properties.

tropism (**tro**·pizm). Movement of living cells or organisms under the influence of an external agency, e.g. towards or away from light (positive or negative phototropism). [Gk *trepein* to turn.]

tropochrome (**tro**·po·krome). Pertaining to those serous cells of the salivary glands which do not stain for mucin after formol-bichromate fixation. [Gk *trepein* to turn, *chroma* colour.]

tropococaine (**tro**·po·ko·**kane'**). Tropacocaine.

tropometer (tro·**pom**·et·er). 1. An instrument for measuring the torsion of a bone. 2. An instrument for measuring the movements of the eye, by observations through a form of telescope. (Obsolete.) [Gk *trepein* to turn, *metron* measure.]

tropomyosin (tro·po·**mi**·o·sin). A muscle protein which lies in the groove of the α-helix actin and which is concerned with the formation of cross-bridges during muscle contraction. [Gk *trepein* to turn, *mys* muscle.]

troponin (**tro**·po·nin). A muscle protein which is attached to the actin–tropomyosin complex with a periodicity of 400 Å. It has probably three parts concerned with: (*a*) inhibition of cross-bridge formation, (*b*) Ca^{2+} binding, (*c*) tropomyosin binding. [Gk *trepein* to turn.]

Trotter, Wilfred Batten Lewis (b. 1872). London surgeon.

Trotter's laminectomy forceps. An angled bone-nibbling forceps.

Trotter's operation. A method of removal of cancer of the pharynx by way of an incision in the neck.

Trotter syndrome. Deafness, palatal paralysis, and facial neuralgia, usually due to a nasopharyngeal carcinoma.

trotyl (**tro**·til). Trinitrotoluene.

trough (trof). A groove or channel. **Gingival trough.** The groove or sulcus round the neck of a tooth, bounded externally by the epithelium of the gum. **Synaptic trough.** The recess in a muscle fibre which is occupied by the axon termination in a motor end-plate. [AS *trog.*]

Trousseau, Armand (b. 1801). Paris physician.

Trousseau's disease. Haemochromatosis.

Trousseau's phenomenon. A sign of latent tetany; spasm of the hand and wrist with adduction of the thumb, bunching of the fingers, and flexion of the wrist, produced by compression of the forearm in subjects having undue neuromuscular excitability as a result of deficiency of ionized calcium.

Trousseau's apophysiary points. Sensitive points in relation to the dorsal and lumbar vertebrae in cases of lumbago.

Trousseau's sign. 1. Trousseau's phenomenon (see above). 2. A streak of congestion produced by scratching the skin; the tache cérébrale. It occurs in a variety of cerebral diseases.

Trousseau's spot. Trousseau's sign, 2nd def.

Trousseau's twitching. Repeated tic-like facial twitching.

Lallemand–Trousseau body. A cylindrical body in coagulated seminal-vesicle secretion.

Troxerutin (trox·e·**roo**·tin). BP Commission approved name for 7,3′,4′-tri[*O*-(2-hydroxyethyl)]rutin; it is used in the treatment of venous disorders.

Troxidone BP 1973 (**trox**·e·done). 3,5,5-trimethyloxazolidine-2,4-dione, an anticonvulsant used in epilepsy, but only of value in the petit mal type. It is also an analgesic.

Troxonium Tosylate (trox·o·ne·um **tos**·il·ate). BP Commission approved name for triethyl-2-(3,4,5-trimethoxybenzoyloxy)-ethylammonium toluene-*p*-sulphonate; a hypotensive agent.

Troxypyrrolium Tosylate (**trox**·e·pir·**o'**·le·um **tos**·il·ate). BP Commission approved name for *N*-ethyl-*N*-2-(3,4,5-trimethoxy-benzoyloxy)-ethylpyrrolidinium toluene-*p*-sulphonate; a hypotensive agent.

Truemmerfeld line, or zone. The line of rarefaction lying immediately adjacent to the calcified matrix at the growing ends of the long bones, which occurs in scurvy. Fracture through this zone may lead to displacement of the epiphysis.

Trueta, Joseph (b. 1897). Spanish orthopaedic surgeon.

Trueta method, technique, or treatment. The treatment of wounds, especially of the extremities, by their adequate excision followed by complete encasement of the limb in plaster of Paris: popularized in the Spanish Civil War.

truncal (trung·kal). 1. Referring to the trunk of the body. 2. Concerned with the trunk of an artery or nerve.

truncate (trung·kate). 1. To amputate, or to take the limbs from the trunk. 2. Describing anything that has had its end cut off at right angles to its axis. [L *truncare* to cut off.]

truncus (trung·kus). Trunk. **Truncus arteriosus.** A continuation of the bulbus cordis of the embryonic heart which becomes divided by a spiral septum to form the aorta and the pulmonary trunk.

Trunecek, Karel (b. 1865). Paris physician.

Trunecek's symptom. Pulsation of the subclavian artery at the insertion of the sternocleidomastoid muscle in individuals with atherosclerosis and unfolding of the aorta.

trunk [truncus (NA)] (trungk). The main stem from which branches spring; in anatomy, used principally for large arteries and nerves from which many branches take origin. **Trunk of the atrioventricular bundle [truncus (fasciculi atrioventricularis) NA].** The undivided part of the atrioventricular bundle, extending from the atrioventricular node to the upper border of the muscular part of the interventricular septum. **Trunk of the brachial plexus, lower.** Part of the brachial plexus formed by the union of the 8th cervical and 1st thoracic root behind the subclavian artery. **Trunk of the brachial plexus, middle.** Part of the brachial plexus in the neck, formed by the 7th cervical root, and lying behind the scalenus anterior muscle. **Trunk of the brachial plexus, upper.** Part of the brachial plexus in the neck formed by the union of the 5th and 6th cervical roots. It lies behind the scalenus anterior muscle. **Bronchomediastinal trunks, right and left.** *See* MEDIASTINAL TRUNK (below). **Trunk of the corpus callosum [truncus corporis callosi (NA)].** That portion of the corpus callosum which lies between the genu anteriorly and the splenium posteriorly. **Costocervical trunk [truncus costocervicalis (NA)].** A large artery arising from the back of the subclavian (second part on the right side first part on the left) which arches over the cervical pleura to divide, above the neck of the 1st rib, into the superior intercosta artery and the deep cervical artery. **Intestinal trunk [truncus intestinalis (NA)].** A tributary of the cisterna chyli, receiving efferents from the coeliac, superior, and inferior mesenteric glands which drain the fore-, mid-, and hind-gut and their derivatives. **Jugular trunk [truncus jugularis (NA)].** The terminal lymph vessel draining its own half of the head and neck. The right drains into the right lymphatic duct, the left into the thoracic duct, but either may drain into any adjacent vein. **Linguofacial trunk [truncus linguofacialis (NA)].** The common trunk by which the lingual and facial arteries frequently arise from the external carotid artery. **Lumbar trunks, right and left [trunci lumbales (dexter et sinister) NA].** A pair of tributaries of the cisterna chyli draining the lower limbs and the trunk below the umbilicus, the genito-urinary organs, and the pelvic viscera. **Lumbosacral trunk [truncus lumbosacralis (NA)].** The nerve trunk formed by the union of a branch from the anterior primary ramus of the 4th lumbar nerve and the whole of that of the 5th lumbar nerve. It descends into the pelvis to join the sacral plexus. **Mediastinal trunk [truncus bronchomediastinalis (NA)].** The terminal lymph vessel draining the internal mammary, tracheobronchial, and innominate lymph glands. The right may enter the right lymphatic trunk and the left the thoracic duct, but commonly the trunk enters the venous system independently. **Pulmonary trunk [truncus pulmonalis].** The stem from which the right and left pulmonary arteries arise. **Subclavian trunk [truncus subclavius (NA)].** One of the pair of terminal lymph vessels draining the arms. The right drains into the right lymphatic duct, the left into the thoracic duct, but either may drain into any adjacent vein. **Sympathetic trunk [truncus sympathicus (NA)].** One of two more or less symmetrical chains of ganglia connected by sympathetic fibres [rami interganglionares (NA)] situated alongside the vertebral column from the skull to the coccyx. The ganglia are classified as cervical, thoracic, lumbar, and sacral, according to the region in which they lie. The two cords meet in front of the coccyx in a terminal ganglion, the ganglion impar. **Thyrocervical trunk [truncus thyrocervicalis (NA)].** A short, wide trunk from the first part of the subclavian artery. It divides into three terminal branches; the inferior thyroid, the suprascapular, and the transverse cervical arteries. **Vagal trunk, anterior [truncus vagalis anterior (NA)].** A branch from the oesophageal plexus which descends on the front of the oesophagus to the anterior surface of the stomach. **Vagal trunk, posterior [truncus vagalis posterior (NA)].** A branch of the oesophageal plexus which descends behind the oesophagus to the posterior surface of the stomach. [L *truncus*.]

trusion (troo·zhun). In dentistry, malposition of a tooth or of a group of teeth. **Bimaxillary trusion.** Malposition of teeth in both jaws. **Mandibular trusion.** Malposition of teeth in the lower jaw. **Maxillary trusion.** Malposition of teeth in the upper jaw. [L *trudere* to push.]

truss (trus). An external appliance designed to control a hernia. **Adder-headed truss.** A spring inguinal truss, the effective end of which is slightly expanded. **Bag truss.** A cloth bag, now rarely used, suspended from the neck or trunk to support a large, irreducible and inoperable scrotal hernia. **Ball-and-socket truss.** A truss consisting of a metal support coming round from the patient's back, and articulating at a ball-and-socket joint with a pad which lies flat over the hernial site. **Double truss.** A truss for the control of a bilateral (usually inguinal) hernia. **Horseshoe truss.** A double truss usually made of rubber, used for inguinal hernia in infants. **Nasal truss.** A splint for fractured nasal bones. **Opposite-sided truss.** A truss designed for the control of a femoral hernia: applied round the opposite side of the trunk and quite ineffective. **Rat-tailed truss.** An inguinal truss, the head of which is continued down as a perineal strap. **Single truss.** A truss for the control of a unilateral hernia. **Spring truss.** A truss which incorporates a long strip of metal designed to maintain pressure over the hernia from a far distant counter-point. **Suspensory truss.** A bag truss designed to relieve the pull of a large irreducible (usually scrotal) hernia. **Vulcanite truss.** A truss of vulcanite which can be worn while bathing. [OFr. *trusser*.]

truxillines (trux·il·eenz). Ecgonine derivatives found in crude extracts of cocaine. They are respectively α- and β-truxilline, and have the formula $C_{38}H_{46}O_8N_2$.

trypagar (trip·a·gar). A bacterial culture medium. It is prepared by the digestion of meat by trypsin at alkaline pH, filtration, and solidification of the clear filtrate by agar.

trypan-atoxyl (tri·pan·at·ox'·il). Trypanotoxyl.

trypanblau (tri·pan·blow). Trypan blue. *See* BLUE. [trypanosome, G *blau* blue.]

trypanid, trypanide (tri·pan·id, tri·pan·ide). A skin eruption occurring in trypanosomiasis.

trypanocidal (tri·pan·o·si'·dal). Able to destroy trypanosomes. [trypanosome, L *caedere* to kill.]

trypanocide (tri·pan·o·side). Anything that will destroy trypanosomes. [see prec.]

trypanolysis (tri·pan·ol·is·is). The dissolution and destruction of trypanosomes. [trypanosome, Gk *lysis* a loosing.]

trypanolytic (tri·pan·o·lit'·ik). Able to bring about the destruction of trypanosomes. [see prec.]

Trypanoplasma (tri·pan·o·plaz'·mah). A genus of protozoa, none of which are parasitic to man. [Gk *trypanon* borer, *plasma* formation.]

Trypanosoma (tri·pan·o·so'·mah). A genus of the class Flagellata (Mastigophora), phylum Protozoa, members of which are parasites of the blood or tissues of vertebrates. The typical structure is an elongated body containing a nucleus, kinetoplast, undulating membrane, and a single free flagellum. Species pathogenic for humans and for most animals undergo part of a complex life cycle in insects. Transmission is usually by insect bites but may occur by ingestion or by scratching. **Trypanosoma brucei.** The cause of nagana especially in cattle and horses in

Africa. **Trypanosoma congolense.** A species causing disease in domestic animals in Africa. **Trypanosoma cruzi.** The cause of American trypanosomiasis, transmitted by the rubbing of the infected faeces of a bug of the genus *Triatoma* into the bite wound, or by the contamination of mucous membranes. **Trypanosoma equinum.** The cause of "mal de caderas", a fatal disease of horses in South America. **Trypanosoma equiperdum.** The cause of dourine of horses, transmitted by coitus. **Trypanosoma evansi.** The cause of surra in horses and cattle in the Orient. **Trypanosoma gambiense.** The cause of African sleeping sickness; transmitted by the bite of *Glossina* flies. **Trypanosoma lewisi.** A species causing a non-fatal infection of rats. **Trypanosoma rangeli.** A trypanosome very similar to *T. cruzi,* found on American triatomes. **Trypanosoma rhodesiense.** A cause of African sleeping sickness; the infection tends to run a more acute course than that of the *T. gambiense* infection. **Trypanosoma vivax.** A cause of widespread disease of domestic and wild animals in Africa. [Gk *trypanon* borer, *soma* body.]

trypanosomacide (tri·pan·o·so′·mas·ide). Trypanocide. [trypanosome, L *caedere* to kill.]

trypanosomal, trypanosomatic (**tri**·pan·o·**so′**·mal, **tri**·pan·o·so·**mat′**·ik). Concerned with or attributable to trypanosomes.

trypanosomatosis (**tri**·pan·o·so·mat·**o′**·sis). Trypanosomiasis. [trypanosome, Gk *-osis* condition.]

trypanosomatotropic (tri·pan·o·so·mat·o·**trop′**·ik). Possessing a specific affinity for trypanosomes. [trypanosome, Gk *trepein* to turn.]

Trypanosome (tri·**pan**·o·some). A member of the genus *Trypanosoma.* [Gk *trypanon* borer, *soma* body.]

trypanosomiasis (**tri**·pan·o·so·**mi′**·as·is). The diseases caused by infection with protozoal parasites of the genus *Trypanosoma.* Several species infect cattle and other animals, but only three infect humans; *T. gambiense* and *T. rhodesiense* in tropical Africa and *T. cruzi* in tropical America. The trypanosomes are transmitted by tsetse flies in Africa and by winged bugs in America. The Gambian illness is the less severe in that its progress is slower. The early stage constitutes a febrile condition resulting from a generalized blood and tissue infection following a local proliferation at the site of the bite. The late stage is induced when the trypanosomes invade the brain and central nervous system, resulting in a somnolent condition leading to coma or other nervous manifestations. The Rhodesian illness presents a more rapid but somewhat similar invasion of the nervous system so that early diagnosis is essential if a cure is to be achieved. **African trypanosomiasis.** *See* MAIN DEF. (above). **American trypanosomiasis, Brazilian trypanosomiasis, South American trypanosomiasis.** Chagas' disease.

See also: CRUZ.

trypanosomic (tri·pan·o·**so′**·mik). Trypanosomal.

trypanosomicidal (**tri**·pan·o·so·mis·**i′**·dal). Able to destroy trypanosomes. [trypanosome, L *caedere* to kill.]

trypanosomicide (tri·pan·o·**so′**·mis·ide). Trypanocide.

trypanosomid, trypanosomide (tri·pan·o·**so′**·mid, **tri**·pan·o·**so′**·mide). A skin eruption characteristic of trypanosomiasis.

trypanosomonas (**tri**·pan·o·so·**mo′**·nas). Trypanosoma. [Gk *trypanon* borer, *soma* body, *monas* unit.]

trypanosomosis (**tri**·pan·o·so·**mo′**·sis). Trypanosomiasis. [trypanosome, Gk *-osis* condition.]

trypanotoxyl (tri·pan·o·**tox′**·il). A hypothetical substance postulated by Levaditi to account for the trypanocidal properties which arise when sodium aminoarsonate and liver emulsion are incubated together at 37 °C. The activating substance is probably a reducing agent allied to glutathione.

trypanozoon (tri·pan·o·**zo′**·on). Trypanosome. [Gk *trypanon* borer, *zoon* animal.]

trypanrot (**tri**·pan·rot). Trypan red. *See* RED. [trypanosome, G *rot* red.]

tryparosan (tri·**par**·o·san). A chloro- derivative of parafuchsine, of uncertain composition. It was formerly used in trypanosomiasis.

Tryparsamide BP 1968 (tri·**par**·sam·ide). The sodium salt of *N*-phenylglycineamide-4-arsonic acid, $AsO(OH)(ONa)C_6H_4NH CH_2CONH_2{\cdot}H_2O$. It is a trypanocidal and spirochaeticidal reagent capable of penetrating the central nervous system and hence of great value in the treatment of neurosyphilis; it is however of no value for primary and secondary syphilis. Though often administered orally, it is more effective and gives rise to fewer unpleasant reactions when given intravenously. It is one of the most effective drugs in the treatment of African sleeping sickness.

trypesis (tri·**pe**·sis). Trephination. [Gk boring.]

trypochete (**tri**·po·keet). Small round inclusion bodies described by Doehle and by others in polymorphonuclear leucocytes in the circulating blood in certain infectious diseases.

trypsin (**trip**·sin). A proteolytic enzyme occurring in the intestinal canal, which catalyses the hydrolysis of proteins to peptones and peptides. It has optimum activity in alkaline solution with a pH range 8–11. It is of the nature of protein and has been prepared in crystalline form. [etym. dub.]

trypsinized (**trip**·sin·i·zd). Having been subjected to digestion with trypsin; it may refer to the destruction of antitryptic factors, and also to the enzymatic alteration of the protein constituents of blood serum that may take place under the influence of the trypsin-like enzymes liberated from disintegrating white blood cells.

trypsinogen (trip·**sin**·o·jen). The inactive form of trypsin secreted in the pancreatic juice. It is activated to trypsin by the enzyme enterokinase present in the intestine. [trypsin, Gk *genein* to produce.]

tryptase (**trip**·taze). Any enzyme of the proteinase type, having optimum activity in alkaline solution.

tryptic (**trip**·tik). Concerned with or produced by trypsin.

tryptolysis (trip·**tol**·is·is). The hydrolysis of protein, especially by the enzyme, trypsin. [tryptone, Gk *lysis* a loosing.]

tryptolytic (trip·to·**lit**·ik). Describing a hydrolytic action on proteins, especially that of trypsin. [see prec.]

tryptonaemia (trip·to·**ne**·me·ah). A state marked by the presence of tryptones in the blood. [tryptone, Gk *haima* blood.]

tryptone (**trip**·tone). A peptone created by the action of trypsin on albuminates.

tryptophan, tryptophane (**trip**·to·fan, **trip**·to·fane). Amino-indole-propionic acid, an amino acid present in hydrolysates of most proteins, which is essential in diet for growth and maintenance of health. It is the dietary source of the putrefactive products, indole, skatole, and indican and the principal precursor of 5-hydroxyindoles which are excreted in the carcinoid syndrome. **Tryptophane 5-hydroxylase.** The enzyme which converts tryptophane to 5-hydroxytryptophane.

tryptophanuria (**trip**·to·fan·**ewr′**·e·ah). A condition in which tryptophan appears in the urine.

Tscherning, Marius Hans Erik (b. 1854). Copenhagen ophthalmologist.

Tscherning's theory of accommodation. A theory that on accommodation the ciliary muscle contracted and tightened the suspensory ligament, pulled the choroid forwards, and so with it the vitreous. This pressed on the lens from behind and made it bulge and become more globular in the centre anteriorly where it had no support; of historical interest.

tsetse (**tet**·se). A fly of the genus *Glossina.* The species are confined to central Africa and south-western Arabia. They are larviparous, and both sexes feed on vertebrae blood. They are secondary hosts of the trypanosomes of sleeping sickness and several diseases of animals. [Tswana name.]

Tsuga (**tsoo**·gah). A genus of coniferous trees (family Pinaceae). **Tsuga canadensis.** Hemlock spruce, a species which yields a resinous exudation, Canada pitch, containing resin and a trace of essential oil. [Jap. larch.]

Tuaminoheptane (tew·am·in·o·**hep′**·tane). BP Commission approved name for 1-methylhexylamine; a vasoconstrictor.

tuba (**tew**·bah). A tube. **Tuba acustica.** The pharyngotympanic tube. **Tuba root.** Derris. [L.]

tubage (tew·bij). The introduction of a tube into a cavity or any other part of the body tissues, usually for the purpose of draining the exudate. **Tubage of the glottis.** Intubation.

tubal (tew·bal). Referring to a tube, in particular to the uterine tube or the pharyngotympanic tube.

tubba, tubboe (tub·ah, tub·o). Crab yaws, attacking the soles of the feet and the palms.

tube (tewb). 1. A long, hollow appliance, especially used for conducting fluids; made in glass, rubber, metal, polythene, etc. 2. [Tuba (NA).] Any structure resembling such an appliance. **Air tube.** Any respiratory tube, e.g. a bronchus. **Alcotest tube.** A tube containing chromic acid and sulphuric acid through which persons suspected of drinking inflate a bag; the alcoholic breath sample changes the colour of the crystals from yellow to green to a distance along the tube which is commensurate with the alcohol level. **Alimentary tube.** Alimentary canal. *See* CANAL. **Blood-sedimentation tube.** Erythrocyte-sedimentation tube (see below). **Bronchial tube.** A bronchus, or one of its ramifications. **Capillary tube.** A fine, hair-like tube. **Cardiac tube.** The embryonic heart before the separation of the atria and ventricles. **Cathode-ray tube.** An evacuated tube carrying a terminal cathode and side anode. Under the influence of a potential gradient a stream of electrons is caused to impinge on the distant end of the tube, producing a spot of fluorescence. The position of the spot may be varied by the application of electromagnetic, magnetic, or electrostatic fields at right angles to the electron stream. High-frequency oscillations imposed on the fields by electronic circuits produce wave traces and transform the cathode-ray tube into an oscilloscope or oscillograph. **Cerebromedullary tube.** Neural tube (see below). **Digestive tube.** Alimentary canal. *See* CANAL. **Discharge tube.** Any evacuated vessel containing two electrodes between which electrical conduction may take place through the residual gas in the tube. It is specifically used for describing tubes which do not contain a thermionic electron source. **Double-lumen tube.** A breathing tube consisting of two tubes fused together, one ventilating the right bronchus, the other the left bronchus. **Drainage tube.** A tube usually introduced at operations to conduct blood, inflammatory material, or secretions to the surface; it is commonly made of rubber. **Dressed tube.** A rubber tube surrounded by gauze, such as may be used after haemorrhoidectomy. **Duodenal tube.** A flexible rubber tube which can be passed into the duodenum for withdrawal of its contents. **Empyema tube.** A curved rubber tube with a flange, designed for maintaining drainage of an empyema cavity. **Endobronchial tube.** A breathing tube placed in one or other of the main bronchi. **Endotracheal tube.** *See* Intratracheal tube (below). **Erythrocyte-sedimentation tube.** A graduated tube of narrow uniform bore used for estimating the rate of sedimentation of erythrocytes. **Eustachian tube.** Pharyngotympanic tube (see below). **Fallopian tube.** Uterine tube (see below). **Feeding tube.** A stomach tube for introducing food. **Fermentation tube.** A U-shaped tube closed at one end, used to study gas production by bacterial cultures. **Flatus tube.** A rubber tube passed *per rectum* to facilitate the passage of flatus after operation. **Fusion tubes.** An apparatus designed by Priestley Smith for investigating and training binocular vision and fusion. **Gas tube.** 1. An x-ray tube in which the electrons are obtained by cumulative ionization of the residual gas in the tube. (Obsolete in medical practice.) 2. Any electronic valve in which the residual gas in the valve has a specific function, e.g. thyratron trigger valve. **Gastric biopsy tube.** A tube for obtaining biopsies of gastric mucosa. There are several types, but the general principle of each is the same, namely that, when a tube is passed into the empty stomach and the opening at or near one end is applied on the mucosa, any suction applied at the other end will cause the mucosa to be drawn into the opening, so that by means of a built-in knife under distant control a piece is cut off. **Hot-cathode tube.** A discharge tube in which the thermo-electrons are emitted from a heated cathode. This can be of two types: (*a*) directly heated, as in an x-ray tube, where a heated filament emits electrons; (*b*) indirectly heated, where a cathode coated with a mixture of oxides of the alkaline earths is heated by an electrical heater not in electrical contact with it. Electron emission from such a cathode occurs at a much lower temperature than from (*a*). **Illuminated sucker tube.** A sucker tube (see below) with an electric lamp attached at the distal end. **Intratracheal tube.** An artificial airway inserted into the trachea from the nose or mouth to facilitate general anaesthesia. More correctly named *endotracheal tube.* **Intubation tube.** A tube introduced through the vocal cords directly into the trachea. Special intubation tubes, such as O'Dwyer's, are used in laryngeal obstruction or diphtheria. Tubes and catheters of various designs are used in endotracheal anaesthesia. **Meatus tube.** The tubular skeletal structure composed of bone and cartilage which surrounds and supports the pharyngotympanic and middle-ear cavities of the embryo. **Medullary tube.** Neural tube (see below). **Nasopharyngeal tube.** A rubber or plastic breathing tube inserted from the nose into the trachea. Used in anaesthesia and intensive therapy. **Nasotracheal tube.** A nasal catheter. **Neural tube.** The embryonic basis of the central nervous system in the form of a tube lined with ectodermal cells running the length of the embryo. **Oesophageal tube.** Souttar's tube. **Orotracheal tube.** A breathing tube which is passed from the mouth into the larynx and trachea. **Ovarian tube.** An ingrowth of germinal epithelium from the surface of the ovary in the form of a cord or tube, from which the primitive ovarian follicles are derived. **Oxford tube.** A tracheal tube moulded with a right-angle bend in order to prevent kinking as it passes from the mouth into the pharynx and trachea. (Described by Alsop in 1955.) **Pharyngotympanic tube [tuba auditiva (NA)].** A passage connecting the tympanic cavity with the nasopharynx, so equalizing pressures on either side of the tympanic membrane. Its general direction is downwards, forwards, and medially. It has a bony part [pars ossea tubae auditivae (NA)] in the petrous part of the temporal bone and a longer cartilaginous part [pars cartilaginea tubae auditivae (NA)] attached to the groove between the petrous part of the temporal and the greater wing of the sphenoid bone. The latter is shaped like a flattened cone; the superior and medial walls are of fibrocartilage and the lateral and inferior of fibrous tissue. The larger medial and lateral walls are separated during swallowing by attached palate muscles. The tympanic opening [ostrium tympanicum tubae auditivae (NA)] is on the anterior wall of the middle ear and the pharyngeal opening [ostium pharyngeum tubae auditivae (NA)] is on the lateral wall of the nasopharynx level with the hard palate. It is lined with ciliated columnar mucous membrane [tunica mucosa (NA)] with, in the cartilaginous part, numerous mucous glands [glandulae tubariae (NA)], and near the pharyngeal orifice [ostium pharyngeum tubae (NA)], some adenoid tissue. It is also known as the *eustachian tube.* **Pus tube.** A uterine tube distended with pus; pyosalpinx. **Radium tube.** A radium container in the form of a tube, usually for intracavitary application. **Roll tube.** A test-tube in which the solidifying culture medium coats the inside of the tube; this is made by rapid rotation of the tube, e.g. between the palms. **Sedimentation tube.** 1. A tube which usually narrows towards its lower end, used for collecting and/or estimating the amount of sediment suspended in a fluid, e.g. urine. 2. Erythrocyte-sedimentation tube (see above). **Shutter tube.** A device, generally made of lead, fixed to an x-ray tube to intercept the useful beam when required. **Stomach tube.** A flexible tube passed into the stomach for washing out or withdrawing its contents. **Sucker tube.** A metal tube of which the proximal end is connected with some apparatus for producing negative pressure and the distal end applied to a surgical operation field to clear blood, exudate, or applied solutions, in order to enable the operator to see bleeding points. **T-tube.** A hollow-drainage tube in the shape of a T; used especially in drainage of the common bile duct, so that the flow of the bile into the duodenum need not be interrupted. **Tampon tube.** A dressed rubber tube introduced into the rectum, especially after primary or secondary bleeding following haemorrhoidectomy. **Tracheal tube.** A breathing tube introduced from the mouth or the nose into the trachea. Also known as an *endo*tracheal or an *intra*tracheal tube. **Tracheotomy tube.** A curved hollow metal (or rubber) tube introduced into the trachea, usually to relieve respiratory obstruction, temporary or permanent. **U-tube.** A U-shaped tube, used in laboratory work. **Urogenital tube.** The ventral cloaca; the ventral division of the embryonic cloaca which forms the bladder and urethra. **Uterine tube [tuba uterina (NA)].** The oviduct, a muscular tube about 10 cm long, lying in the upper border of the broad ligament; the fallopian tube. Its lateral end [ostrium abdominale tubae uterinae (NA)] opens into the peritoneal cavity lateral to the ovary, its medial end traverses the uterine wall and opens into the superior angle of the uterine cavity [ostium uterinum tubae (NA)]. **Uterine tube, mucous coat of the [tunica mucosa (NA)].** A coat continuous with the mucosa of the uterus. It is composed of ciliated columnar epithelium thrown into longitudinal folds, especially developed in the ampulla. **Uterine tube, muscular coat of the [tunica muscularis (NA)].** The coat composed of involuntary muscle continuous with that of the uterus. It is arranged in a circular and an outer longitudinal layer. **Uterine tube, serous coat of the [tunica serosa (NA)].** A mesothelium continuous with the peritoneum of the broad ligament. **Uterine tube, submucous coat of the.** A layer of connective tissue between the mucous and muscular coats; the absence of a well-defined deep surface of the lamina propria renders the boundary between it and the submucosa ill-defined. **Uterine tube, subserous coat of the [tunica subserosa (NA)].** A layer of loose areolar tissue containing peritoneum. **Uterine tube, uterine part of the [pars uterina (NA)].** The portion of the tube lying in the uterine wall, about 1 cm long. **Vacuum tube.** An evacuated vessel containing two or more electrodes. **X-ray tube.** In medical practice, a highly evacuated tube containing a tungsten wire filament which may be electrically heated, and a metal target, usually tungsten, which is bombarded by the electrons produced from the filament. The electrons are accelerated on to the target by application of a high positive potential to the target, and most of the x-ray energy is produced by the deceleration of the electrons on striking the target. [L *tubus.*]

See also: ABBOTT (W. O.), AYRE, BELLOCQ, BILLROTH, BLAKEMORE, BLAKEMORE-SENGSTAKEN, BOCHDALEK, BOUCHUT, BUCHNER, CANTOR, CARREL, CHAOUL, CHAUSSIER, COOLIDGE, CRAIGIE, CROOKES, DAKIN, DEBOVE, DEPAUL, DOMINICI, DURHAM (A. E.), DURHAM (H. E.), ESBACH, EUSTACHIO, FALLOPIO, FOLIN, GEIGER, GEISSLER, HENLE, JUTTE, KIDD, KOBELT, LEITER, LENARD, LEVIN, LINZENMEIER, LORD, LYSTER, METT, MIESCHER, MILLER (T. G.), MUELLER (W.), O'DWYER, PAUL (F. T.), PFLUEGER, REHFUSS, ROTHBERG-EVANS, RUYSCH, RYLE, SCHACHOWA, SOUTHEY, SOUTTAR, VALENTIN, VEILLON, WANGENSTEEN, WESTERGREN, WINSBURY-WHITE, WINTROBE.

tube housing (tewb how·zing). An enclosure which covers the x-ray tube and sometimes also other portions of the x-ray equipment (transformer) and which limits the major portion of radiation emitted from the tube to the useful beam. **Diagnostic-type protective tube housing.** A tube housing in which the direct radiation is reduced to, at most, 0.1 R/h to 28 μR/s at a distance of 1 m from the tube target when the tube is operated at its maximum rated voltage and current. **Fully protective tube housing.** Tube housing in which the leakage radiation is reduced to, at most, 6.25 mR/h, corresponding to 300 mR/week for 48 h exposure time, at contact with the tube housing when the tube is continuously operated with closed window at its maximum rated voltage and current. **Highly protective tube housing.** Tube housing in which the leakage is reduced to, at most, 100 mR/h, corresponding to 300 mR/week for 3 h exposure time, at contact with the tube housing when the tube is continuously operated with closed window at its maximum rated voltage and current. **Therapeutic-type protective tube housing.** A tube housing through which the direct radiation is reduced to, at most, 1 R/h or 280 μR/s at a distance of 1 m from the tube target when the tube is operated at its maximum rated voltage and current. [tube, AS *hus*.]

tubectomy (tew·bek·to·me). Excision of a uterine tube. [tube, Gk *ektome* excision.]

tuber [NA] (tew·ber). A swelling. **Tuber cinereum [NA].** A part of the hypothalamus which forms an eminence behind the optic chiasma and in front of the mamillary bodies; it is connected by the infundibulum with the posterior lobe of the hypophysis cerebri. **Tuber impar.** A median swelling in the floor of the embryonic mouth between the two lingual swellings of the mandibular arches; it is later incorporated in the tongue. **Tuber ischii.** Ischial tuberosity. *See* TUBEROSITY. **Tuber omentale of the liver [tuber omentale (NA)].** A swelling on the visceral surface of the left lobe of the liver which projects into the concavity of the lesser curvature of the stomach. **Tuber omentale of the pancreas [tuber omentale (NA)].** A blunt process on the upper border of the body of the pancreas which projects forwards into contact with the posterior surface of the lesser omentum. [L.]

tubercle (tew·ber·kl). 1. A nodule. 2. [Tuberculum (NA).] A rounded elevation on a bone or other structure. 3. The specific lesion of tuberculosis. **Adductor tubercle [tuberculum adductorium (NA)].** A small projection on the upper part of the medial condyle of the femur which gives attachment to the lowermost (ischial) part of the adductor magnus muscle. It marks the site of epiphyseal cartilage in the young bone. **Anal tubercle.** Anal hillock; one of paired swellings which appear at the sides of the anal portion of the cloacal membrane, and, by their fusion, give rise to the wall of the lower part of the anal canal. **Anatomical tubercle.** A variety of tuberculosis verrucosa cutis usually seen in anatomists, pathologists, and butchers. Tubercle bacilli are inoculated into a wound; within 24 h a zone of erythema appears, and this is followed by the formation of a chronic warty tuberculous lesion. **Tubercle of the aryepiglottic fold, corniculate [tuberculum corniculatum (NA)].** The elevation produced by the corniculate cartilage. **Tubercle of the aryepiglottic fold, cuneiform [tuberculum cuneiforme (NA)].** The elevation produced by the cuneiform cartilage. **Tubercle of the atlas, anterior [tuberculum anterius (NA)].** A small, median bony projection on the front of the anterior arch of the atlas. **Tubercle of the atlas, posterior [tuberculum posterius (NA)].** A small, backwardly directed median projection from the posterior arch of the atlas. **Tubercle of the auricle [tuberculum auriculae (NA)].** A small swelling on the helix at the point where it turns downwards posteriorly. **Tubercle of the calcaneum, anterior.** A lip on the anterior end of the inferior surface near the medial border. **Tubercle of the calcaneum, lateral [processus lateralis tuberis calcanei (NA)].** A small tubercle on the posterior end of the inferior surface. **Tubercle of the calcaneum, medial [processus medialis tuberis calcanei (NA)].** A large tubercle on the posterior end of the inferior surface. **Carotid tubercle [tuberculum caroticum (vertebrae cervicalis VI (NA)].** The enlarged anterior tubercle of the 6th cervical vertebra against which the common carotid artery can be compressed. **Tubercle of a cervical vertebra, anterior [tuberculum anterius (vertebrarum cervicalium) NA].** The rough projection at the tip of the anterior root of the transverse process of a cervical vertebra for muscular attachments. **Tubercle of a cervical vertebra, posterior [tuberculum posterius (vertebrarum cervicalium) NA].** The rounded projection at the tip of the posterior root of the transverse process of a cervical vertebra for muscular attachment. **Cloacal tubercle.** Genital tubercle (see below). **Conglomerate tubercles.** Fused tubercles. **Conoid tubercle [tuberculum conoideum (NA)].** A well-defined prominence on the inferior surface of the clavicle, near to the acromial end, to which is attached the conoid part of the coracoclavicular ligament. **Corniculate tubercle.** Tubercle of the aryepiglottic fold, corniculate (see above). **Cuneate tubercle.** Tubercle of the medulla oblongata, cuneate (see below). **Cuneiform tubercle.** Tubercle of the aryepiglottic fold, cuneiform (see above). **Dissection tubercle.** Anatomical tubercle (see above). **Dorsal tubercle.** A bony projection on the posterior surface of the lower end of the radius; Lister's tubercle. **Epiglottic tubercle [tuberculum epiglotticum (NA)].** A projection from the lower part of the posterior surface of the epiglottis.

Epithelial tubercle. An epithelial tag on the glans penis or glans of the clitoris of the embryo at the distal end of the urethral groove. **Fibrous tubercle.** Fibrous tissue replacement of a tubercle. **Genial tubercle [spina mentalis (NA)].** A nodule on either side of the symphysis menti, on the inner surface of the mandible. **Genital tubercle, Genito-anal tubercle.** A swelling at the ventral end of the cloacal membrane of the embryo, which later becomes the penis or the clitoris. **Gracile tubercle [tuberculum nuclei gracilis (NA)].** A swelling on the dorsal surface of the medulla on each side of the lower extremity of the 4th ventricle, overlying the gracile nucleus. **Grey tubercle.** A greyish mass of tuberculous tissue. **Hepatic tubercle.** A swelling composed of entodermal cells, found ventrally at the junction of the embryonic fore- and mid-gut, from which the liver and biliary passage are later derived. **Tubercle of the iliac crest.** A prominence on the outer lip of the iliac crest about 5 cm behind the anterior superior iliac spine. **Infraglenoid tubercle [tuberculum infraglenoidale (NA)].** A roughened prominence at the upper end of the lateral border of the scapula, giving origin to the long head of the triceps brachii muscle. **Intercondylar tubercle, lateral [tuberculum intercondylare laterale (NA)].** The less prominent of the two bony eminences on the intercondylar area of the tibia. **Intercondylar tubercle, medial [tuberculum intercondylare mediale (NA)].** The more prominent of the two bony eminences on the intercondylar area of the tibia. **Intervenous tubercle [tuberculum intervenosum (NA)].** A projection from the posterior wall of the right atrium just below the superior vena caval orifice. It is believed to direct the blood from the superior vena cava towards the tricuspid orifice during fetal life. **Intravascular tubercle.** A tubercle of the inner layers of a blood vessel. **Jugular tubercle [tuberculum jugulare (NA)].** An elevation medial to the jugular foramen. **Labial tubercle [tuberculum (NA)].** The slight elevation on the upper lip at the base of the philtrum. **Lymphoid tubercle.** A tubercle composed mainly of lymphocytes. **Marginal tubercle [tuberculum marginale (NA)].** A rounded eminence on the posterior border of the zygomatic bone just below the frontozygomatic suture. **Tubercle of the medulla oblongata, cuneate [tuberculum nuclei cuneati (NA)].** A swelling on the dorsal surface of the medulla at the upper termination of each fasciculus cuneatus, overyling the cuneate nucleus. **Mental tubercle [tuberculum mentale (NA)].** A small tubercle on each side of the symphysis menti. **Tubercle of the 1st metatarsal bone [tuberositas ossis metatarsalis I (NA)].** A tubercle to which is attached the tendon of the peroneus longus muscle. **Tubercle of the 5th metatarsal bone [tuberositas ossis metatarsalis V (NA)].** The projection from the base of the 5th metatarsal, to which the peroneus brevis muscle is attached. **Miliary tubercle.** A tuberculous collection, about the size of a millet seed. **Obturator tubercle, anterior [tuberculum obturatorium anterius (NA)].** A small tubercle sometimes present on the anterior edge of the groove for the obturator vessels. The free edge of the obturator membrane attaches to it. **Obturator tubercle, posterior [tuberculum obturatorium posterius (NA)].** A small tubercle sometimes present in the posterior edge of the groove for the obturator vessels. The free edge of the obturator membrane attaches to it. **Olfactory tubercle.** A small elevation behind the olfactory pyramid; it is rarely seen in man. **Painful tubercle.** A tender mass in the subcutaneous tissues about the joints. **Tubercle of the palatine bone [processus pyramidalis (NA)].** The part of the palatine bone which projects downwards and backwards to articulate with the medial and lateral pterygoid plates. **Pathological tubercle.** Anatomical tubercle (see above). **Peroneal tubercle [trochlea peronealis (fibularis) NA].** A tubercle on the lateral surface of the calcaneum separating the tendons of the peroneus longus and brevis muscles. **Pharyngeal tubercle [tuberculum pharyngeum (NA)].** A small bone elevation on the inferior surface of the basilar part of the occipital bone. **Post-mortem tubercle.** Anatomical tubercle (see above). **Pubic tubercle [tuberculum pubicum (NA)].** A small projection at the lateral end of the pubic crest giving attachment to the inguinal ligament. It is palpable at the inner end of the fold of the groin. **Rabic tubercle.** A collection of cells around degenerated neurones in the medulla and spinal ganglia in cases of rabies. **Tubercle of a rib [tuberculum costae (NA)].** The prominence on the posterior surface of a rib at the junction of the neck and shaft, and articulating in true ribs with the transverse process of a thoracic vertebra at the articular facet [facies articularis tuberculi costae (NA)]. **Tubercle of the root of the zygoma.** The tubercle on the lateral end of the eminentia articularis for the temporomandibular ligament. **Sacral tubercle.** Sacral tuberosity. *See* TUBEROSITY. **Tubercle of the sacrum, articular [crista sacralis intermedia (NA)].** The bony projection marking the fused articular processes of adjacent sacral vertebrae. **Tubercle of the sacrum, spinous [crista sacralis mediana (NA)].** One of the low bony projections in the midline crest on the dorsal surface of the sacrum, representing the tips of the spines. **Tubercle of the sacrum, transverse [crista sacralis lateralis (NA)].** A bony projection marking the tip of a fused transverse process on the dorsum of the sacrum. **Scalene tubercle [tuberculum musculi scaleni anterioris (NA)].** A small projection or roughness on the inner border of the 1st rib for the scalenus anterior muscle. **Tubercle of the scaphoid [tuberculum ossis scaphoidei (NA)].** A rounded elevation on the lower part of the anterior surface of the scaphoid, giving attachment to the flexor retinaculum. **Tubercle of the serratus anterior muscle [tuberositas musculi serrati anterioris (NA)].** A rough tubercle on the outer surface of the second rib. **Spinous tubercle.** Tubercle of the sacrum, spinous (see above). **Supraglenoid tubercle [tuberculum supraglenoidale (NA)].** A rough area just above the glenoid cavity of the scapula, giving origin to the long head of the biceps brachii muscle. **Supratragal tubercle [tuberculum supratragicum (NA)].** A rounded prominence sometimes present on the upper part of the tragus. **Tubercle of the talus, lateral [processus lateralis tali (NA)].** The prominent apex of the triangular facet on the lateral surface. **Tubercle of the talus, medial [tuberculum mediale (NA)].** A rudimentary tubercle on the posterior surface, medial to the groove for the flexor hallucis longus muscle. **Tubercle of the talus, posterior [processus posterior tali (NA)].** A prominent tubercle on the posterior surface, medial to the groove for the flexor hallucis longus muscle; lateral to the groove for this muscle is the lateral tubercle [tuberculum laterale (NA)]. **Tubercle of the thalamus, anterior [tuberculum anterius thalami (NA)].** An elevation on the anterior end of the dorsum, produced by the anterior nucleus. **Thyroid tubercle, inferior [tuberculum thyroideum inferius (NA)].** A tubercle on the lower border of the lamina at the lower end of the oblique line. **Thyroid tubercle, superior [tuberculum thyreoideum superius (NA)].** A tubercle on the superior border of the lamina at the upper end of the oblique line. **Tubercle of the tibia [tuberositas tibiae (NA)].** The low bony eminence on the front of the upper end of the tibia, giving attachment to the patellar tendon. It bears the weight at the knee in kneeling. **Tubercles of a tooth [tubercula (coronae) dentis (NA)].** Small projections on the masticating surface of the molar and premolar teeth. **Yellow tubercle.** A yellow, fatty mass of tuberculous tissue. **Zygomatic tubercle.** Tubercle of the root of the zygoma (see above). [dim. of L *tuber* swelling.]

See also: BABES, CARABELLI, CHASSAIGNAC, DARWIN, FARRE (J. R.), GERDY, GHON, HIS (W. SNR.), LISFRANC, LISTER (J.), LOWER, MONTGOMERY, MORGAGNI, MUELLER (J.), PRINCETEAU, ROLANDO, SANTORINI, VATER, WHITNALL, WOOLNER, WRISBERG.

tubercular (tew·**ber**·kew·lar). Having the characteristics of or relating to tubercles or nodules. Cf. TUBERCULOUS.

tuberculase (tew·**ber**·kew·laze). An obsolete vaccine prepared from tubercle bacilli.

tuberculate, tuberculated (tew·**ber**·kew·late, tew·**ber**·kew·**la**′·ted). Possessing nodules or tubercles; nodular.

tuberculation (tew·**ber**·kew·**la**′·shun). 1. The appearance of nodules or tubercles in a part. 2. Affection with tubercles.

tuberculid, tuberculide (tew·**ber**·kew·lid, tew·**ber**·kew·lide). One of a group of cutaneous eruptions occurring in tuberculous patients in which, although the histology of the lesions is tuberculous, the tubercle bacillus is absent. **Acneiform tuber-**

culid. Acne scrofulosorum; an eruption of small red papules each surmounted by a pustule. Tiny ulcers form at the sites of each lesion, and eventually scarring ensues. **Indurative subcutaneous tuberculid.** Bazin's disease. **Lichenoid tuberculid.** 1. A generalized exanthematous lichenoid eruption. The lesions are most numerous on the extremities. 2. Lichen scrofulosorum. **Micronodular tuberculid, Micropapular tuberculid.** Varieties of rosacea-like tuberculid (see below). **Nodular tuberculid.** An indurated subcutaneous tuberculid. **Papulonecrotic tuberculid.** Toxituberculid (Hallopeau); paratuberculoses (Johnston): an eruption of small, round, purplish-red papules lying in the deeper parts of the skin. Usually a small pustule forms on each papule and eventually the site is marked by a scar. In general there are two varieties named *acnitis* and *folliclis.* **Tuberculid en plaque** (Sweitzer). An eruption of annular plaques occurring on the extremities. **Rosacea-like tuberculid, Rosaceous tuberculid** (Lewandowsky). A facial eruption, usually occurring in adults, resembling rosacea. The lesions are bluish or brown-red papules or papulopustules, associated with hyperaemia and telangiectasia. It is not of tuberculous origin but is a foreign-body type of granuloma occurring in rosacea.

tuberculigenous (tew·ber·kew·**lij'**·en·us). Causing or tending to cause tuberculosis. [tuberculosis, Gk *genein* to produce.]

tuberculin (tew·**ber**·kew·lin). A general term for some fraction or extract of the tubercle bacillus, formerly used in the treatment of tuberculous patients by Koch. Such preparations are now restricted for use in the Mantoux test and similar tests for tuberculin sensitivity. There are innumerable modifications of the method for preparing the tuberculin. **Old Tuberculin BP 1973.** The original preparation of tuberculin by Koch from the glycerin-broth culture of *Mycobacterium tuberculosis* after filtration and concentration of the liquid. **Perlsucht tuberculin original, Perlsucht tuberculin rest.** Two early forms of bovine tuberculin. **Tuberculin Purified Protein Derivative BP 1973, Tuberculin PPD.** A concentrate of a culture of tubercle bacilli on synthetic medium, purified by ultrafiltration and precipitation of the protein material with trichloro-acetic acid.

tuberculination (tew·**ber**·kew·lin·**a'**·shun). The use of tuberculin in skin testing or the therapy of tuberculosis.

tuberculine (tew·**ber**·kew·leen). A crude filtrate of the tubercle bacillus containing proteins and capable of eliciting the tuberculin reaction in tissues sensitized to tuberculosis.

tuberculinization (tew·**ber**·kew·lin·i·**za'**·shun). Tuberculination.

tuberculinotherapy (tew·**ber**·kew·lin·o·**ther'**·ap·e). The use of tuberculin in the treatment of tuberculosis. [tuberculin, Gk *therapeia* treatment.]

tuberculinum (tew·**ber**·kew·**li'**·num). Tuberculin. **Tuberculinum Crudum.** *European Pharmacopoeia* name for Old Tuberculin BP 1973. **Tuberculini Derivatum Proteinosum Purifactum.** *European Pharmacopoeia* name for Tuberculin Purified Protein Derivative BP 1973.

tuberculitis (tew·ber·kew·**li'**·tis). Inflammation of a tubercle and the surrounding tissues. [tubercle, Gk *-itis* inflammation.]

tuberculization (tew·**ber**·kew·li·**za'**·shun). 1. The formation of tubercles in tissues. 2. Applied to a race or population, the process over years of being subjected to infection with tuberculosis, and of developing a degree of immunity to this infection.

tuberculo-albumin (tew·**ber**·kew·lo·al·**bew'**·min). One of the proteins that can be extracted from the body of the tubercle bacillus. [tubercle, albumin.]

tuberculocele (tew·**ber**·kew·lo·seel). Tuberculosis of the testis. [tuberculosis, Gk *kele* tumour.]

tuberculocidal (tew·**ber**·kew·lo·**si'**·dal). Capable of destroying the causal organism of tuberculosis, *Mycobacterium tuberculosis.* [tubercle, L *caedere* to kill.]

tuberculocide (tew·**ber**·kew·lo·side). Any agent that will destroy tubercle bacilli. [see prec.]

tuberculoderm, tuberculoderma (tew·**ber**·kew·lo·derm, tew·**ber'**·kew·lo·**der'**·mah). Any tuberculous lesion of the skin. [tuberculosis, Gk *derma* skin.]

tuberculofibroid (tew·**ber**·kew·lo·**fi'**·broid). Applied to a tubercle that has fibrosed.

tuberculofibrosis (tew·**ber**·kew·lo·fi·**bro'**·sis). Fibroid tuberculosis. *See* TUBERCULOSIS.

tuberculoid (tew·**ber**·kew·loid). Resembling tuberculosis or a tubercle in form. [tubercle, Gk *eidos* form.]

tuberculoidin (tew·ber·kew·**loid'**·in). A modified form of tuberculin. (obsolete term.) [tuberculin, Gk *eidos* form.]

tuberculol (tew·**ber**·kew·lol). A modified form of tuberculin. (obsolete term.)

tuberculoma (tew·ber·kew·**lo'**·mah). A well-defined, tumour-like mass of tuberculous tissue. **Tuberculoma en plaque.** Plaques of tuberculous granulation tissue. [tuberculous, Gk *-oma* tumour.]

tuberculomania (tew·**ber**·kew·lo·**ma'**·ne·ah). A morbid and unfounded impression that one has tuberculosis. [tuberculosis, Gk *mania* madness.]

tuberculo-opsonic (tew·**ber**·kew·lo·op·**son'**·ik). Concerning the opsonin of the tubercle bacillus.

tuberculophobia (tew·**ber**·kew·lo·**fo'**·be·ah). Unreasoning fear of becoming infected with tuberculosis. [tuberculosis, Gk *phobein* to fear.]

tuberculoprotein (tew·**ber**·kew·lo·**pro'**·te·in). Any of the proteins occurring in the body of the tubercle bacillus. [tubercle, protein.]

tuberculosaccharide (tew·**ber**·kew·lo·**sak'**·ar·ide). A saccharide derived from *Mycobacterium tuberculosis.*

tuberculose (tew·**ber**·kew·lose). Tuberculate.

tuberculosilicosis (tew·**ber**·kew·lo·sil·ik·**o'**·sis). Silicosis with a superimposed tuberculous infection.

tuberculosis (tew·**ber**·kew·**lo'**·sis). The disease caused by infection with the *Mycobacterium tuberculosis.* The characteristic lesion is the tubercle, a microscopic collection of epitheloid cells, leucocytes, mainly lymphocytes, and a few giant cells. The tubercles may regress and heal, or increase in size and caseate at the centre. Healing is by fibrosis with or without calcification. The disease may run an acute course but is usually a chronic granulomatous disease; it may be localized or generalized and varies greatly in intensity and its manifestations, according to the organs involved and the degree of resistance shown by the tissues. Infection is almost invariably either by inhalation or ingestion of the organism, and once established may spread locally by direct invasion, or more widely by the blood stream or lymphatics. **Aerogenic tuberculosis.** Tuberculosis caused by inhalation of air-borne infective material. **Anthracotic tuberculosis.** Pulmonary tuberculosis supervening on anthracosis in the lungs of coal miners working in siliceous mines. The determining factor is the formation of a silica colloid which favours secondary infection by tubercle bacilli (Kettle and Gye). **Attenuated tuberculosis.** Infection with a weak strain of the bacillus, as in lupus. **Avian tuberculosis.** Tuberculosis in birds caused by *M. avium.* **Basal tuberculosis.** Applied to tuberculosis involving the basal portion of the lung. **Bovine tuberculosis.** Tuberculosis of cattle caused by *M. tuberculosis bovis,* most commonly causing pulmonary tuberculosis or glandular lesions including mastitis. **Bronchogenic tuberculosis.** Pulmonary tuberculosis in which infection originates in the smaller bronchi. **Bronchopneumonic tuberculosis.** An acute tuberculous inflammatory process starting in the smaller bronchioles which become blocked, so that the distal lobule is airless and filled with secretion which may become caseous. The process is multiple, and adjacent areas fuse to produce patches of consolidation. **Caseous pneumonic tuberculosis.** Large areas of consolidation involving a lobe or whole lung which becomes airless, yellowish-white in colour, and cheesy in consistency. **Cerebral tuberculosis.** Tuberculosis of the brain; it may be general, in miliary tuberculosis, or local, forming a tuberculoma. Rupture of a tuberculoma through the pia mater results in tuberculous meningitis. **Chicken tuberculosis.** Avian tuberculosis (see above). **Chronic ulcerative tuberculosis.** An area of tuberculosis with some consolidation, in which the bronchioles and alveoli lose their lining membrane by ulceration and which usually results in cavity formation. The ulceration may extend to the larger bronchi or the trachea and larynx. **Closed tuberculosis.** Tuberculosis in which tubercle bacilli do not occur, or for practical purposes are not demonstrable by ordinary bacteriological methods after repeated (three) examinations, in the sputum or stomach contents. **Tuberculosis colliquativa.** Scrofulodermia; cutaneous tuberculosis arising by direct extension from tuberculous disease in underlying structures, particularly lymph glands, joints, and bones. **Tuberculosis cutis.** Infection of the skin by *M. tuberculosis*: it is said that 40 per cent of the cases are due to the human variety of the organism and 60 per cent to the bovine type. **Disseminated tuberculosis.** Miliary tuberculosis (see below). **Endogenous tuberculosis.** Tuberculosis originating from a tuberculous infection in some other part of the body of the patient. **Endothelial tuberculosis.** Tuberculosis predominantly affecting lymphatic canals or glands or serous membranes such as pleural or peritoneal sacs. **Exogenous tuberculosis.** Tuberculosis originating from an infection acquired from outside the body, e.g. from another person. **Fibrocaseose tuberculosis.** A chronic condition in which the elastic tissue of the lung has been replaced by fibrous tissue and solid avascular areas of disease have become necrotic and cheesy in appearance. **Fibroid tuberculosis.** Tuberculosis of the lung with extensive fibrosis but little caseation, so that the infection is only very slowly progressive. **Fowl tuberculosis.** Avian tuberculosis (see above). **Tuberculosis fungosa cutis.** A localized form of fungating tuberculosis of the skin associated with tuberculosis of underlying bone or gland. **Glandular tuberculosis.** Tuberculosis of the lymphatic glands, often bovine in origin. **Haematogenous tuberculosis.** Tuberculosis in which the infection has been blood-borne. **Inactive tuberculosis.** An arbitrary term for the stage of tuberculosis in which there are no symptoms, the sputum is repeatedly negative for tubercle bacilli, and the x-ray taken at intervals shows no increased shadows or signs of progressive cavitation. **Tuberculosis indurativa, Tuberculosis indurativa subcutanea.** Bazin's disease, purplish nodules, frequently ulcerating, situated on the legs of young women suffering from tuberculosis. **Inhalation tuberculosis.** Infection through the air passages. **Ischiorectal tuberculosis.** An abscess in the ischiorectal fatty tissues, almost always secondary to tuberculosis of the lung, bowel, or prostate, chronic in type which may lead to internal or external fistula, or both. It may be the first presenting symptom of tuberculosis elsewhere. **Tuberculosis lichenoides.** Groups of minute punctiform papules of reddish-brown colour, many capped with horny tips; the condition occurs in young people suffering from tuberculosis. **Lobar pneumonic tuberculosis.** Consolidation affecting a whole lobe which is usually accompanied by toxaemia and may pass on to caseation or excavation of the whole or part of the lobe. It occurs mainly in children. **Tuberculosis luposa.** Lupus vulgaris. **Lymphoid tuberculosis.** Tuberculosis in which lymphocytes and their precursors are very numerous. **Tuberculosis miliaris cutis.** A rare form of tuberculosis resulting from haematogenous dissemination and lodging of tubercle bacilli in the skin, giving a papular or pustular rash. It is associated sometimes with tuberculous meningitis. **Miliary tuberculosis.** A form in which miliary tubercles are disseminated either as a general infection or localized to certain organs such as the lungs or the meninges. **Minimal tuberculosis.** A term now standardized to include tuberculous infiltration in which the radiological shadows occupy not more than the area of two intercostal spaces, without cavitation, the apex of the upper lobe being regarded as equal to one intercostal space. It may not be of recent origin, and may quickly become extensive. **Moderately advanced tuberculosis.** Tuberculosis in which, although there may be extensive disease and cavitation, there is enough functioning lung tissue to maintain easy respiration at rest and accompanied by a moderate degree of toxaemia. **Tuberculosis necrogenica.** Tuberculosis verrucosa cutis acquired from a human or animal corpse. **Open tuberculosis.** Any form of tuberculosis in which there is a discharge of tubercle bacilli from the body. **Tuberculosis orificialis.** Tuberculosis ulcerosa (see below). **Tuberculosis papulonecrotica.** Various eruptions occurring in tuberculous subjects in which the fundamental lesion is a small intradermal erythematous papule which in time is surmounted by a vesicopustule. If this is ruptured, a small necrotic pit is exposed. The lesions appear in crops, and when they disappear are replaced by scars. Acnitis or acne agminata, acne scrofulosorum or acneiform tuberculid, acne cachecticorum, and folliclis are all varieties of the condition. **Pelvic tuberculosis.** A term including tuberculous salpingitis, oöphoritis, endometritis, prostatitis, and localized peritonitis. **Primary tuberculosis.** The changes which occur as a result of the first infection with the tubercle bacillus. For the most part these are of little clinical significance since they generally occur and heal without detection, but a change from negative to positive tuberculin reaction occurs within 8 weeks from the time of infection. Very occasionally they fail to heal, and the focus spreads with production of malaise and may even be disseminated to produce acute miliary or meningeal tuberculosis or pleural effusion and extensive glandular involvement. An unhealed primary focus may also give rise to skeletal and renal lesions, but if well healed the primary focus appears to confer some degree of immunity to subsequent infection. **Pulmonary tuberculosis.** Phthisis; any form of tuberculosis involving the lungs, caused in man by either the human or bovine type of tubercle bacillus. **Re-infection tuberculosis.** Lesions resulting from infection by the tubercle bacillus after a primary infection and healing has occurred. It may be of exogenous origin, but residual bacilli may escape from a so-called healed lesion and produce endogenous infection elsewhere. **Renal tuberculosis.** Tuberculosis of the kidney and renal tract. **Spinal tuberculosis.** Tuberculosis of the spine and spinal cord. **Surgical tuberculosis.** Tuberculosis of the bones and joints and other parts amenable to treatment by surgery. **Tuberculosis ulcerosa.** Tuberculous ulceration of the mucocutaneous margins of an orifice such as the nose, mouth, or anus. **Uveoparotid tuberculosis.** Enlargement of the parotid glands with uveitis and facial paralysis. This syndrome is now considered to be a manifestation of sarcoidosis, but some cases appear to be due to true tuberculosis. **Tuberculosis verrucosa.** Infections of skin or mucous membranes by *Mycobacterium tuberculosis*, characterized by the formation of warty lesions. **Tuberculosis verrucosa cutis.** Lupus verrucosus; a variety of cutaneous tuberculosis, usually due to local inoculation from without of the tubercle bacillus, in which the lesions have a wart-like appearance. Anatomical tubercle is a variety of the malady. **Zoogleic tuberculosis.** Pseudotuberculosis; this includes a number of diseases in animals having a superficial resemblance to tuberculosis but caused by a variety of organisms, e.g. streptothrices, pasteurellae, diphtheroids, etc. [tubercle, Gk *-osis* condition.]

tuberculostatic (tew·**ber**·kew·lo·**stat**'·ik). Arresting the growth of the tubercle bacillus. [tubercle, Gk *statikos* causing to stand.]

tuberculotherapy (tew·**ber**·kew·lo·**ther**'·ap·e). A term used for the treatment of tuberculosis with the flesh of tuberculous animals. It is now considered to be an outmoded form of therapeutics.

tuberculotoxin (tew·**ber**·kew·lo·**tox**'·in). A toxin derived from *Mycobacterium tuberculosis.*

tuberculotropic (tew·**ber**·kew·lo·**trop**'·ik). Possessing a specific affinity for the tubercle bacillus. [tubercle, Gk *tropos* turning.]

tuberculous (tew·**ber**·kew·lus). Referring to tuberculosis, or to infection caused by *Mycobacterium tuberculosis.*

tuberculum [NA] (tew·**ber**·kew·lum). Tubercle. **Tuberculum arthriticum.** An archaic term denoting a gouty tophus. **Tuberculum dolorosum.** Painful tubercle. **Tuberculum impar.** A swelling of the floor of the embryonic pharynx, just behind the meeting-place of the ventral ends of the mandibular arches in the region of the developing tongue. It disappears as a distinct entity later, and its contribution to the development of the tongue is difficult to assess. **Tuberculum sebacea, Tuberculum sebaceum.** Milium. **Tuberculum sellae [NA].** A transversely disposed oval elevation separating the sella turcica from the optic groove.

tuberiferous (tew·ber·**if**·er·us). Producing or bearing tubers. [tuber, L *ferre* to bear.]

tuberin (tew·ber·in). A globulin occurring in potatoes in which it constitutes about 50 per cent of the total protein.

tuberose (tew·ber·oze). Tuberous.

tuberosis cutis pruriginosa (tew·ber·o·sis **kew**·tis **proo**·rij·in·o′·-sah). Prurigo nodularis. [tuber, Gk *-osis* condition, L *cutis* skin, *prurigo* itch.]

tuberositas (tew·ber·**os**·it·as). Tuberosity.

tuberosity [tuber (NA)] (tew·ber·**os**·it·e). A rounded swelling, generally on a bone. **Bicipital tuberosity.** Tuberosity of the radius (see below). **Tuberosity of the calcaneum.** The swollen posterior extremity of the calcaneum which forms the projection of the heel. **Coracoid tuberosity.** The conoid tubercle of the clavicle. **Costal tuberosity.** The rough projection on the under surface of the inner end of the clavicle to which the costo-clavicular ligament is attached. **Tuberosity of the cuboid bone [tuberositas ossis cuboidei (NA)].** A smooth projection on the lateral and plantar aspect of the cuboid bone over which passes the tendon of the peroneus longus muscle. **Deltoid tuberosity [tuberositas deltoidea (NA)].** A rough, slightly raised area on the lateral aspect of the shaft of the humerus to which the deltoid muscle is attached. **Tuberosity of a distal phalanx of a finger [tuberositas phalangis distalis (NA)].** The horseshoe-shaped expanded portion of a distal phalanx supporting the pulp of the finger and the finger nail. **Tuberosity of the distal phalanx of a toe [tuberositas phalangis distalis (NA)].** A roughened eminence on the plantar aspect of the distal end of the distal phalanx. **Gluteal tuberosity [tuberositas glutea (NA)].** A broad, rough area on the posterior aspect of the upper end of the shaft of the femur which can be followed distally into the lateral lip of the linea aspera; the third trochanter. **Tuberosity of the humerus.** 1. Greater [tuberculum majus (NA)]: the projection from the lateral and posterior surface of the upper end of the shaft of the humerus to which the supraspinatus, infraspinatus, and teres minor muscles are attached. 2. Lesser [tuberculum minus (NA)]: the projection on the humerus at its upper end to which the subscapularis muscle is attached. **Iliac tuberosity [tuberositas iliaca (NA)].** The rough everted swelling on the lateral lip of the iliac crest a short distance posterior to the anterior superior spine. **Infraglenoid tuberosity.** The infraglenoid tubercle, giving origin to the long head of the triceps. **Ischial tuberosity [tuber ischiadicum (NA)].** The enlarged rough lower part of the ischium on which the body rests in the sitting position. **Malar tuberosity.** A blunt projection on the lateral aspect of the zygomatic bone. **Masseteric tuberosity [tuberositas masseterica (NA)].** An occasional tuberosity in the area of insertion of the masseter muscle. **Maxillary tuberosity [tuber maxillae (NA)].** The swollen posterior part of the maxilla. **Tuberosity of the 1st metatarsal bone.** Tubercle of the 1st metatarsal bone. **Tuberosity of the 5th metatarsal bone.** Tubercle of the 5th metatarsal bone. **Tuberosity of the navicular bone [tuberositas ossis navicularis (NA)].** The projection on the navicular bone of the tarsus to which the tibialis posterior muscle is attached. **Tuberosity of the palatine bone.** Tubercle of the palatine bone. **Pterygoid tuberosity [tuberositas pterygoidea (NA)].** An occasional tuberosity in the area of insertion of the medial pterygoid muscle. **Tuberosity of the radius [tuberositas radii (NA)].** A broad prominence on the shaft of the radius immediately below the neck, to which the tendon of the biceps brachii muscle is attached. **Sacral tuberosity [tuberositas sacralis (NA)].** The area above and behind the auricular surface of the sacrum to which the interosseous sacro-iliac ligament is attached. **Tuberosity of the sacrum.** The roughened posterior aspect of the lateral mass of the sacrum, lateral to the posterior sacral foramina. **Supraglenoid tuberosity.** Supraglenoid tubercle. *See* TUBERCLE. **Tuberosity of the tibia.** Tubercle of the tibia. **Tuberosity of the ulna [tuberositas ulnae (NA)].** A swelling on the coronoid process to which part of the brachialis muscle is attached. **Unguicular tuberosity.** The roughened head of a distal phalanx which underlies the nail bed. [L *tuber* swelling.]

tuberous (tew·ber·us). Of the nature of a tuber; having tuberosities.

tubiferous (tew·**bif**·er·us). Tuberiferous.

tubo-abdominal (**tew**·bo·ab·**dom**′·in·al). Concerning the uterine tube and the abdomen.

tubocurarine (**tew**·bo·kew·**rah**′·reen). An alkaloid which is responsible for the activity of tube curare, and consists of a mixture of D- and L- forms, i.e. it is racemic. **D-Tubocurarine.** An alkaloid that has been used surgically to induce muscular relaxation of the non-depolarizing type without deep anaesthesia, also in convulsive shock therapy, and in the treatment of tetanus and certain spastic disorders. **Tubocurarine Chloride BP 1973.** $C_{38}H_{44}O_6N_2Cl_2 \cdot 5H_2O$, the chloride of the alkaloid, D-tubocurarine, obtained from extracts of the stems of species of *Chondrodendron* (family Menispermaceae). It paralyses skeletal muscle, and is used chiefly for securing muscle relaxation in surgical operations. Since ether has a curare-like action, smaller doses of tubocurarine chloride are used with this than with other general anaesthetics.

Tubocurarinii Chloridum. *European Pharmacopoeia* name for Tubocurarine Chloride BP 1973.

tubogastrostomy (**tew**·bo·gas·**tros**′·to·me). Gastrostomy established by fashioning a tube of stomach wall and bringing it through the abdomen.

tuboligamentous (tew·bo·lig·am·**en**′·tus). Concerning the uterine tube and the broad ligament of the uterus.

tubo-ovarial, tubo-ovarian (**tew**·bo·o·**va**′·re·al, **tew**·bo·o·**va**′·re·-an). Relating to the ovary and the uterine tube.

tubo-ovariotomy (tew·bo·o·va·re·**ot**′·o·me). Surgical excision of a uterine tube and the ovary. [tube, ovary, Gk *temnein* to cut.]

tubo-ovaritis (**tew**·bo·o·var·**i**′·tis). Salpingo-oöphoritis. [tube, ovary, Gk *-itis* inflammation.]

tuboperitoneal (**tew**·bo·per·it·o·**ne**′·al). Concerning the uterine tube and the peritoneum.

tuborrhoea (tew·bo·**re**·ah). Discharge from the pharyngotympanic tube. [tube, Gk *rhoia* flowing.]

tubotorsion (tew·bo·**tor**·shun). The twisting of any tube, particularly of the uterine tube. [tube, L *torquere* to twist.]

tubotympanal (tew·bo·**tim**·pan·al). Concerning the pharyngotympanic tube and the tympanic cavity.

tubo-uterine (**tew**·bo·**ew**·ter·ine). Relating to the uterus and a uterine tube.

tubovaginal (tew·bo·**vaj**·in·al). Relating to the uterine tube and the vagina.

tubular (**tew**·bew·lar). Having the form of a tube, or relating to a tubule.

tubule [tubulus (NA)] (**tew**·bewl). A small tube. **Dentinal tubule.** One of the many tubules, each containing a dentinal fibril and fluid, radiating in dentine from the surface of the pulp to its margins. **Epigenital tubule.** One of the tubules of the mesonephros lying adjacent to the gonad which, in the male, becomes an aberrant tubule of the epididymis, and in the female, one of the tubules of the epoöphoron. **Tubules of the epoöphoron [ductuli transversi (NA)].** The persistent mesonephric tubules. **Mesonephric tubule.** A tubule of the mesonephros, or secondary kidney. **Paragenital mesonephric tubule.** A tubule of the mesonephros adjacent to the testes or ovary which becomes an efferent ductule of the testes or a tubule of the paroöphoron. **Renal tubule [tubulus renalis (NA)].** The part of the nephron which leads from the glomerulus to the collecting ducts. It is divided into the convoluted and straight parts of the proximal tubule, the descending and ascending limbs of the loop of Henle, and the distal convoluted tubule. The last-named tubule leads into the collecting ducts and ducts of Bellini. **Segmental tubule.** One of the segmental tubules of the pronephros or mesonephros draining into the pronephric or mesonephric duct. **Seminiferous tubules, convoluted [tubuli seminiferi contorti (NA)].** The contents of the lobes of the testis each of which contains from two to four of these long thread-like tubes loosely packed in areolar tissue. **Seminiferous tubules, straight [tubuli seminiferi recti (NA)].** A number of short tubes formed by the union of several seminiferous tubules and draining into the rete testis. **T tubule.** One of a system of minute transverse tubules which are found at the level of the Z lines of striated muscle. **Uriniferous tubule.** A collecting tubule of the kidney which conveys the urine from the renal tubules to Bellini's duct. **Vertical tubule.** One of the tubules of the epoöphoron, running vertically into the duct of epoöphoron. [L *tubulus*.]

See also: ALBARRAN, BELLINI, FERREIN, HENLE, KOBELT, MIESCHER, SCHACHOWA, SKENE.

tubulin (**tew**·bew·lin). A substance isolated from kidney tissue. It is known to have some effect on lowering of blood pressure. [tubule.]

tubulization (**tew**·bew·li·**za'**·shun). The apposition of the divided ends of an injured nerve in a sleeve of absorbable material which guides growing nerve fibres from the proximal to the distal cut end. [L *tubulus* small tube.]

tubulocyst (**tew**·bew·lo·sist). The cystic dilatation of a functionless duct or canal. [tubule, cyst.]

tubulodermoid (**tew**·bew·lo·**der'**·moid). A dermoid cyst arising from fetal tubular structures or ducts.

tubuloracemose (**tew**·bew·lo·**ras'**·em·ose). Having both tubular and racemose character.

tubulorrhexis (**tew**·bew·lo·**rex'**·is). Focal tubular ruptures occurring in association with tubular necrosis of the kidney. [tubule, Gk *rhexis* a breaking.]

tubulosaccular (**tew**·bew·lo·**sak'**·ew·lar). Having both tubular and saccular character.

tubulose, tubulous (**tew**·bew·loze, **tew**·bew·lus). Composed of tubules.

tubus (**tew**·bus). A tube or canal. **Tubus medullaris.** The vertebral canal. *See* CANAL [L.]

tuduranine (tew·**dur**·an·een). $C_{18}H_{19}O_3N$, an alkaloid obtained from species of *Sinomenium.*

Tuerck, Ludwig (b. 1810). Vienna neurologist.

Tuerck's bundle, column, or fasciculus. Parieto- and possibly temporo-pontine fibres in the lateral part of the cerebral peduncle.

Tuerck's degeneration. Secondary degeneration in fibre tracts of the spinal cord.

Tuerk, Wilhelm (b. 1871). Vienna physician.

Tuerk irritation cell. A cell resembling very closely the plasma cell and said to occur in the blood when the bone marrow is irritated, but its presence does not appear to have any diagnostic significance.

Tuffier, Marin Théodore (b. 1857). Paris surgeon.

Tuffier's operation. 1. The repair of an artery by insertion of a metal tube. 2. Apicolysis.

Tuffier's test. In the presence of an aneurysm of a major limb artery, venous filling distal to the aneurysm following compression of the main proximal artery and vein will only occur if the collateral circulation is intact.

Tuffnell, Thomas Joliffe (b. 1819). Dublin surgeon.

Tuffnell's treatment. Treatment of aortic aneurysm by rest and low-calorie diet.

tuft (tuft). A tassel-like structure. **Enamel tufts.** Extensions into the enamel of a tooth, from the amelodentinal junction, of poorly calcified rods with much cement substance between them. **Hair tuft.** A circumscribed aggregation of hairs. **Malpighian tuft, Renal tuft.** A glomerulus of the kidney. [Fr. *touffe.*]

See also: FISCHER (E.).

tufting (**tuf**·ting). Osteophytic outgrowths that occur at the distal ends of the terminal phalanges in acromegaly. [see prec.]

tug (tug). To pull. **Tracheal tug.** 1. In thoracic aneurysm, pulsation of the aorta transmitted through the trachea, when the cricoid cartilage is grasped between the finger and thumb, and steady and gentle upward pressure exercised on it. The patient should be in the erect position, his mouth closed and chin elevated. 2. A downward jerking of the larynx and lower jaw by the action of the accessory muscles of respiration, observed in deep general anaesthesia. [ME *toggen.*]

tugging (**tug**·ing). Violent pulling. **Tracheal tugging.** A symptom of aortic aneurysm, the trachea being tugged downwards with each heart beat. [see prec.]

tularaemia (too·lar·e·me·ah). An acute infectious plague-like disease caused by *Brucella tularensis,* first reported as an epizootic of squirrels in Tulare, California, in 1911. Human cases have occurred widely in the Northern hemisphere, mainly among persons handling wild rabbits, but several animal species besides rabbits are implicated. Ticks and other blood-sucking insects may transmit the infection. Laboratory workers may contract the disease. The incubation period is usually 3 days, but varies within wide limits: in the commonest type, in man, the primary lesion develops into an ulcer, with enlargement of the regional lymphatic glands and influenza-like general symptoms. Mortality is 5-8 per cent. Antibiotics are useful in treatment. Also known as *rabbit fever, deer-fly fever, tick fever,* and *Francis disease.* [*Brucella tularensis,* Gk *haima* blood.]

tulase (**tew**·laze). A form of tuberculin introduced by Behring for combating tuberculosis.

tulle gras (tewl **grah**). A coarse-meshed gauze soaked with soft paraffin containing 1 per cent Peru balsam. It is a dressing used for the emergency treatment of burns and in some abdominal operations. [Fr. fatty tulle.]

Tullio, Pietro. 20th century Sardinian physician.

The Tullio phenomenon. Vestibular disturbances resulting from auditory stimuli seen sometimes after fenestration operations. Tullio first described this phenomenon in 1916 during some experiments carried out on the semicircular canals of the pigeon.

Tully, William (b. 1785). American physician and botanist.

Tully's powder. Compound powder of morphine.

tulose (**tew**·loze). Tulase.

Tulp (Tulpius), Nicolaes (b. 1593). Amsterdam physician; the central figure in Rembrandt's *Lesson in Anatomy.*

Tulp's valve. The ileocolic valve. *See* VALVE.

tumefacient (tew·me·**fa**·shent). Causing swelling. [see foll.]

tumefaction (tew·me·**fak**·shun). 1. A swelling or oedema. 2. A state of being swollen. [L *tumere* to swell, *facere* to make.]

tumefy (**tew**·me·fi). To swell up, or to bring about swelling. [see prec.]

tumenol (**tew**·men·ol). An artificial substitute for ichthammol. It is no longer used.

tumentia (tew·**men**·she·ah). Swelling. **Vasomotor tumentia.** Oedematous swellings on the legs and arms due to disturbance of the vasomotor system. [L *tumere* to swell.]

tumescence (tew·**mes**·ens). Tumefaction. [L *tumescere* to begin to swell.]

tumescent (tew·**mes**·ent). Becoming swollen. [see prec.]

tumid (**tew**·mid). Swollen; distended; puffy. [see foll.]

tumidity (tew·**mid**·it·e). The condition of being swollen. [L *tumidus* swollen.]

tumoraffin (tew·mor·**af**·in). Applied to anything that has selective affinity for tumour cells. [tumour, L *affinis* related.]

tumorcidin (tew·mor·**si**·din). The serum of an animal treated by injections of gonad extract. Claims have been made for its use in malignant disease, without substantiation. [tumour, L *caedere* to kill.]

tumorigenesis (tew·mor·e·**jen'**·es·is). The origin and development of tumours. [tumour, Gk *genein* to produce.]

tumorigenic (tew·mor·e·**jen'**·ik). Producing tumours. [see prec.]

tumorous (**tew**·mor·us). Swollen; having the characteristics of a tumour.

tumour (tu·mer). A swelling. **Acoustic-nerve tumour.** Neurofibroma occurring on the course of the 8th cranial nerve in the cerebellopontine angle in the posterior cranial fossa. **Acute splenic tumour.** Swelling of the spleen in acute infections. **Adenoid tumour.** Adenoma. **Adenomatoid tumour.** A benign tumour found in the epididymis and, more rarely, in the arteries. It is composed of clefts and tubular spaces lined by flattened cells; these are associated with a fibrous stroma in which are groups of cells of epithelial type. **Adipose tumour.** Lipoma. **Tumour albus.** White swelling; tuberculosis of a joint. **Amyloid tumour.** A localized collection of amyloid. **Anaplastic polygonal-cell tumour.** Anaplastic carcinoma. *See* CARCINOMA.

Aniline tumour. Cancer of the bladder in aniline workers. **Argentaffin tumour.** A slowly growing, and occasionally metastasizing tumour composed of cells that stain deeply with silver salts, found most frequently in the appendix and stomach. Symptoms suggestive of endocrine disorder have been associated with this tumour. **Basal cell tumour.** A tumour, e.g. carcinoma, papilloma or naevus, arising from basal cells of the epidermis. **Benign tumour.** Simple, non-malignant, innocent tumour; a tumour, one important feature of which is its inability to infiltrate locally and to spread discontinuously to a distance (to metastasize). Cf. MALIGNANT TUMOUR (below). **Blood tumour.** Haematoma. **Carcinoid tumour.** A tumour which, though locally invasive, only rarely behaves in a malignant fashion. It is found in the gastro-intestinal tract and occasionally in the bronchus. **Cartilaginous tumour.** Chondroma. **Cavernous tumour.** Cavernous haemangioma. *See* HAEMANGIOMA. **Cellular tumour.** One rich in cells. **Chromaffin tumour.** Paraganglioma. **Chromophil tumour.** An adenoma of the pituitary gland, composed either of eosinophil or basophil cells. **Colloid tumour.** Either a colloid carcinoma or a myxoma. **Connective-tissue tumour.** Such tumours as fibroma, lipoma, chondroma, sarcoma. **Craniopharyngeal-duct tumour.** Craniopharyngioma. **Cystic tumour.** A hollow tumour. **Dentinoid tumour.** An odontome composed mainly of dentine; a dentinoma. **Dermoid tumour.** Dermoid cyst. *See* CYST. **Desmoid tumour.** A type of locally recurring fibrous-tissue tumour, commonly seen in the muscles of the abdomen in women. *See also* PAGET'S RECURRENT FIBROID. **Desmoid tumour of the mediastinum.** Mediastinal fibroma. **Dumb-bell tumour.** 1. A rare tumour, commonly a neurofibroma, consisting of two parts, one lying inside the vertebral canal, and the other outside (usually in the mediastinum). 2. A rare variety of pleomorphic adenoma (mixed tumour) of the parotid gland growing both outwards to present behind the mandible and inwards to cause a bulge of the soft palate, and constricted in its middle by the styloid and stylomandibular ligament. **Eiloid tumour.** A cutaneous tumour resembling a coil of intestine: turban tumour. **Encysted tumour.** An encapsulated tumour. **Epithelial tumour.** One composed of epithelium, such as papilloma, adenoma, or carcinoma. **Erectile tumour.** One composed of erectile tissue. **Faecal tumour.** A tumour due to a mass of inspissated faeces. **False tumour.** A tumour which, on further investigation, proves to be due to a normal structure, e.g. pancreas. **Fatty tumour.** A lipoma, or fat hernia. **Fibrocellular tumour.** Fibroma. **Fibroplastic tumour.** Fibrosarcoma. **Fibrous tumour.** Fibroma. **Fluid tumour.** A fluid-containing tumour. **Follicular tumour.** An archaic name for sebaceous cyst. **Fungating tumour.** 1. A tumour which has erupted through the overlying skin and presents externally. 2. Any tumour which presents as an exuberant surface growth. **Gelatinous tumour.** Myxoma. **Giant-cell tumour.** Osteoclastoma, or benign synovioma of a tendon sheath. **Glomus jugulare tumour.** A rare vascular tumour arising in a chemoreceptor organ, the glomus jugulare, in the roof of the jugular foramen. **Glomus tumour.** (Syn. glomangioma.) A tumour involving the arteriovenous anastomoses of the skin, often painful. It consists of many small vascular channels surrounded by *glomus* cells which are often intimately involved in the vascular walls. Glomus cells occasionally develop into smooth muscle cells. The ratio of glomus cells to vessels is very variable and in some tumours their presence can be easily missed. **Granulation tumour.** Granuloma. **Granulosa-cell tumour.** A tumour arising from the granulosa cells of the ovarian follicles. Its stroma is often composed of thecal cells; oestrin is secreted. **Gummatous tumour, Gummy tumour.** Gumma. **Heterologous tumour, Heterotypic tumour.** One composed of tissue different from that in which it has arisen. **Histoid tumour.** One composed of a single tissue. **Homoeotypical tumour.** Homologous tumour (see foll.). **Homologous tumour.** A tumour that resembles the surrounding tissues in its structure. **Hour-glass tumour.** Dumb-bell tumour (see above). **Hypernephroid tumour.** Hypernephroma. **Hypophyseal-duct tumour.** Craniopharyngioma. **Infiltrating tumour.** One that spreads some distance from its site of origin into the surrounding region. **Innocent tumour.** A slow-growing localized tumour that shows no tendency to spread. **Islet tumour.** A tumour of the islets of Langerhans. **Ivory-like tumour.** Osteoma eburneum. **Tumour lienis.** Splenic enlargement. **Limbal tumour.** A tumour of the corneal limbus. **Malignant tumour.** A tumour, one important feature of which is its invasion and destruction of neighbouring tissue. Cf. BENIGN TUMOUR (above). **March tumour.** A neuroma of a digital nerve of the foot. **Margaroid tumour.** Cholesteatoma. **Mast-cell tumour.** A tumour composed of mast cells. The granules of the cells stain metachromatically with toluidine blue. **Metastatic tumour.** A tumour originating from a metastasis from some other tumour in the body. **Migrated tumour, Migratory tumour.** A metastasis or secondary growth. **Mixed mesodermal tumour.** A tumour of the female genital tract, most common in the uterus of elderly patients. The tumour forms a large mass, often with a relatively narrow pedicle attached to the uterine wall. It consists of a mass of mesenchymal tissues with islands of striped muscle, cartilage and atypical epithelial proliferations. Secondary deposits may be composed either of the sarcomatous or of the carcinomatous elements, or may show both types of tissue. **Mixed tumour.** One composed of more than one type of neoplastic tissue. **Mother-of-pearl tumour.** Cholesteatoma. **Mucous tumour.** Myxoma. **Muscular tumour.** Myoma. **Nerve tumour.** Neuroma. **Neuro-ectodermal tumour.** Retinal anlage tumour, melanotic ameloblastoma; a tumour of the maxilla in infancy, usually presenting as a pigmented mass in the mouth. **Neuromyarterial glomus tumour.** A painful tiny tumour arising from the glomus bodies in the fingers or toes. **Oat-celled tumour of bronchi.** A variety of carcinoma of the lung, in which many of the cancer cells present a blunted and a pointed end resembling in shape an oat-seed. **Organoid tumour.** Teratoma. **Papillary tumour.** Papilloma. **Pearl tumour, Pearly tumour.** Cholesteatoma, epidermoid. **Phantom tumour.** Distension of the abdomen with gas, producing a swelling which may be mistaken for an organic tumour. **Potato tumour.** A hard, carotid-body tumour. **Pulmonary-sulcus tumour.** Pancoast's tumour. **Ranine tumour.** A cystic swelling beneath the tongue caused by the blocking of a duct of a salivary gland. **Recurrent tumour.** A tumour that recurs after extirpation. **Retinal anlage tumour.** Neuro-ectodermal tumour (see above). **Sacrococcygeal tumour.** A dermoid or teratoma of the sacrococcygeal region, arising from remnants of the archenteric canal. **Sand tumour.** Psammoma. **Schneeburg tumour.** Cancer of the lung in cobalt miners. **Sebaceous tumour.** Sebaceous cyst. *See* CYST. **Secondary tumour.** A tumour arising as a metastasis of a primary tumour. **Sheath tumour.** Meningioma. **Splenic tumour.** An enlarged spleen. **Stercoral tumour.** Faecal tumour (see above). **Superior-sulcus tumour.** Pancoast's tumour. **Teratoid tumour.** Teratoma. **Tomato tumour.** The physical lesion of the tumour stage of mycosis fungoides. **Transition tumour.** One that recurs after removal, and then behaves as a malignant growth. **Tridermic tumour.** A dermoid cyst derived from the three embryonic layers. **True tumour.** Any tumour arising by proliferation of cells. **Tuberous tumour.** One that resembles a tuber. **Turban tumour.** Cylindroma, endothelioma capitis; a raised, solid tumour, more frequently seen on the scalp than elsewhere, red or skin-colour in hue, having a distinctive histological appearance and varying in diameter from a few millimetres to several centimetres. Numerous tumours may occur in a single individual and cover the scalp like a turban. **Varicose tumour.** A tumour consisting of a mass of veins. **Vascular tumour.** 1. An aneurysm. 2. An angioma. 3. Any tumour which has a rich blood supply. **Villous tumour.** Papilloma. **Warty cicatricial tumour.** A warty tumour arising, often in parallel masses, on the surface of a scar. **White tumour.** Chronic tuberculous arthritis. [L *tumor.*]

See also: ABRIKOSOV, BRENNER, BRODIE (B. C.), BROOKE, BROWN-PEARCE, COCK, EWING, GRAWITZ, HUERTHLE, KROMPECHER, KRUKENBERG (F. E.), NÉLATON, PANCOAST (H. K.), POTT, RATHKE, RECKLINGHAUSEN, SCHMINCKE, SCHNEEBERG, SERTOLI, SPIEGLER, WILMS.

tumultus (tew·**mul**·tus). Over-activity; agitated movement; upheaval. **Tumultus cordis.** Irregular heart action. **Tumultus sermonis.** Stuttering in reading due to pathological lesion. [L.]

Tunga (**tung**·gah). A genus of fleas. **Tunga penetrans.** The chigoe or jigger flea, which is South American in origin and introduced into tropical Africa. Males and virgin females behave like other flea species. Impregnated females burrow in the skin, particularly of the feet, until only the posterior abdominal segments are visible; the anterior abdomen swells to a sphere of about 7 mm diameter. They give rise to serious inflammation, and secondary infections may occur.

tungiasis (tung·gi·**as**·is). Infestation with the sand-flea, *Tunga penetrans.* The feet are the parts most commonly infected.

Tungidae (**tung**·gi·de). The chiggers, a family of the Siphonaptera (fleas). [*Tunga*, Gk *eidos* form.]

tungstate (**tung**·state). Any salt of tungstic acid.

tungsten (**tung**·sten). An element of atomic weight 183.85, atomic number 74, and chemical symbol W (*wolfram*). It is an extremely hard metal with a high melting point, which occurs in wolframite and tungstite. It is used for electric lamp filaments and in alloys for high-speed tools. [Swedish, heavy stone.]

tunic (**tew**·nik). A coat or membrane. *See* TUNICA. [L *tunica* tunic.]

See also: BICHAT, BRUECKE, RUYSCH.

tunica [NA] (**tew**·nik·ah). A coat or covering; in anatomy, applied to any layer of tissue covering an organ or lining a space. **Tunica adnata.** The part of the conjunctiva which covers the eyeball directly. **Tunica adventitia [tunica externa (NA)].** The external coat of an artery or vein, consisting mainly of white connective-tissue fibres. **Tunica albuginea [NA].** A covering of white (collagenous) fibrous tissue. 1. Of the eye; the sclerotic coat and the cornea. 2. Of the ovary; the fibrous coat beneath the surface epithelium. 3. Of the penis; the fibrous coat of the corpora cavernosa [tunica albuginea corporum cavernosorum (NA)] and that of the corpus spongiosum [tunica albuginea corporis spongiosi (NA)]. 4. Of the spleen; the fibrous capsule of the spleen. 5. Of the testis; that immediately beneath the tunica vaginalis testis (see below). **Tunica elastica.** Tunica media (see below). **Tunica fibrosa.** Tunica albuginea (see above). **Tunica interna.** 1. Of blood vessels; the tunica intima (see below). 2. Of the eye; the retina and the epithelium of the ciliary body and iris. **Tunica intima [NA].** The inner coat of an artery or vein, consisting of endothelium and varying amounts of connective and elastic tissue. **Tunica media [NA].** The middle coat of an artery or vein, containing varying amounts of smooth muscle and elastic tissue. **Tunica propria [NA].** The particular covering of a part as distinct from a general investment. **Tunica propria of the corium [tunica propria (NA)].** The deeper, dense, connective-tissue layer of the skin; also called the *dermis* or *cutis.* **Tunica uvea.** Tunica vasculosa of the eye (see below). **Tunica vaginalis testis [NA].** The distal portion of the processus vaginalis of the peritoneum, forming a sac surrounding the front and sides of the testis composed of a visceral layer [lamina visceralis (NA)] on the organ and a parietal layer [lamina parietalis (NA)] lining the internal spermatic fascia. **Tunica vasculosa.** Any vascular covering. 1. Of the eye; the uveal coat, consisting of the choroid, the ciliary body, and the iris. 2. Of the lens; a covering of vascular mesenchyme which invests the developing lens in the embryo. 3. Of the testis; loose vascular connective tissue beneath the tunica albuginea of the testis. [L tunic.]

See also: BRUECKE, HALLER, RUYSCH.

tunicary (**tew**·nik·ar·e). Covered with a tunic, or of the nature of a tunic.

tuning fork (**tew**·ning fork). A steel fork with two equal prongs the length of which is so adjusted that the fork emits a note of definite pitch when set into vibration. Used to test deafness and bone conduction. [tone, L *furca.*]

tunnel (**tun**·el). A canal. **Carpal tunnel [canalis carpi (NA)], Flexor tunnel.** The osteofibrous tunnel bounded by the carpus and the flexor retinaculum through which flexor tendons and the median nerve enter the hand. [OFr. *tonnel.*]

See also: CORTI.

Tunnicliff, Ruth (b. 1876). Chicago bacteriologist.

Tunnicliff's test. The intradermal injection of a broth filtrate (toxin) of a Gram-positive diplococcus (*Tunnicliff coccus*), associated with measles, or an antigen prepared from this coccus. The skin reactions obtained failed to distinguish measles-immune from susceptible persons. Largely obsolete. **Tunnicliff's toxin.** A product from an anaerobic diplococcus assumed by Tunnicliff to be the cause of measles. It was once used in diagnostic testing and prophylaxis, but is now obsolete.

Tuohy, E. B. American anaesthesiologist.

Tuohy needle. A lumbar puncture needle designed in 1945 for continuous spinal analgesia but now generally used for continuous extradural block. Through it, a catheter can be introduced so that serial injections can be given.

turacin (tew·**ras**·in). A copper-porphyrin compound which occurs as a red pigment in the feathers of a South African bird, the Touraco. It is the only known instance of a copper-porphyrin compound occurring in an animal species.

turanose (tew·ran·oze). $C_{12}H_{22}O_{11}$, a disaccharide, α-glucose β-fructoside, which occurs naturally in the trisaccharide, melitriose.

Turbatrix aceti (ter·**ba**·trix **as**·et·i). A nematode worm, the vinegar worm, that has been reported in the vaginal exudate and urine of women. [L disturber of vinegar.]

turbid (**ter**·bid). 1. Clouded; obscured by solids in suspension. 2. Confused mentally. [L *turbidus* confused.]

turbidimeter (ter·bid·**im**·et·er). An instrument with which the turbidity of a fluid may be estimated. [turbidity, meter.]

turbidimetric (ter·bid·im·**et**'·trik). Concerned with turbidimetry, or with a turbidimeter.

turbidimetry (ter·bid·**im**·et·re). The estimation of the amount of solids suspended in a liquid by comparing the light that a given thickness of the liquid will transmit with that transmitted by the same thickness of a standard liquid containing a known quantity of suspended solids. [turbidity, meter.]

turbidity (ter·**bid**·it·e). The state of being turbid.

turbinal (**ter**·bin·al). 1. Turbinate. 2. Any of the nasal conchae.

turbinate, turbinated (**ter**·bin·ate, **ter**·bin·a·ted). Scroll-like, or shaped like an inverted cone. **Turbinate bone.** One of the three thin bony plates within the nasal fossa; the conchae. [L *turbinatus* like a top.]

turbinectomy (ter·bin·**ek**·to·me). Surgical excision of a turbinate bone. [turbinate, Gk *ektome* excision.]

turbinotome (ter·**bin**·o·tome). An instrument employed in turbinectomy and turbinotomy.

turbinotomy (ter·bin·**ot**·o·me). Surgical incision of a turbinate bone. [turbinate, Gk *temnein* to cut.]

turbulence (**ter**·bew·lens). Irregular, tumultuous movement of a gas or liquid. It is produced by high velocities of flow or by irregularities in the channels containing the flowing material. Turbulence in blood flow is the origin of cardiac murmurs. [L *turbulentia.*]

turgescence (ter·**jes**·ens). The swelling-up of a part. [L *turgescere* to begin to swell.]

turgescent (ter·**jes**·ent). Becoming swollen. [see prec.]

turgid (**ter**·jid). Swollen; inflated; congested. [L *turgidus.*]

turgometer (ter·**gom**·et·er). A device for measuring the amount of swelling of a part. [L *turgere* to swell, meter.]

turgor (**ter**·gor). The state of being swollen or extended to fullness, normal or otherwise. **Turgor vitalis.** The normal distension of blood vessels. [L *turgere* to swell.]

turiopin (tew·re·**o**·pin). An alcoholic extract of the Austrian pine, *Pinus nigricans* (family Pinaceae) used in the treatment of bronchitis.

turmeric (**ter**·mer·ik). Curcuma; the dried rhizome of *Curcuma longa* Linn. (family Zingiberaceae). It contains the colouring matter, curcumin. [etym. dub.]

turmerol (ter·mer·ol). An oily substance obtained from turmeric.

Turnbull's blue. The deep blue compound formed when a solution of a ferrous salt is added to a solution of potassium ferricyanide.

Turner, George Grey (b. 1877). Newcastle upon Tyne and London surgeon.

Grey Turner's sign, Turner's sign. Two or three days after the onset of acute pancreatitis, bruising may be observed in the loin on one or both sides.

Turner, Henry Hubert (b. 1892). Oklahoma physician.

Turner's syndrome. Gonadal dysgenesis associated with webbing of the neck, short stature, and sometimes with coarctation of the aorta, cubitus valgus, scoliosis, and absence of upper lateral incisors. This condition is most frequently due to the presence of only one X chromosome (46,X). Other karyotypes found in this condition are: 45,X/46,XX; 45,X/46,XX/47,XXX; 45,X/46,Xr(X); 45,X/46,Xi(Xq); 45,X/46,Xi(Xp); 45,X/46,XXp-; 45,X/46,XXq-; 45,X/46,XY.

Turner's syndrome in the male. A syndrome presented by males with prepubertal or post-pubertal gonadal or genital anomalies associated with the somatic abnormalities of Turner's syndrome. Males with this syndrome have, usually, a normal chromosome complement.

Pseudo-Turner syndrome. A condition with signs of Turner's syndrome but with normal chromosome count, in males and females.

Ullrich-Turner syndrome. *See* BONNEVIE-TURNER SYNDROME.

Turner, Philip (b. 1873). London surgeon.

Turner-Ombredanne orchidopexy. An operation performed for mal-descent of the testis. In this operation, after mobilization of the cord, the imperfectly descended testis is secured in the contralateral compartment of the scrotum between the septum and the inner side of the normal testis.

Turner, Vernon C. Milwaukee orthopaedic surgeon.

Hefke-Turner sign. Shenton's line.

Turner, Sir William (b. 1832). Edinburgh anatomist.

Turner's sulcus. The intraparietal sulcus of the parietal lobe which joins the postcentral sulcus horizontally.

turnera (ter·ner·ah). Damiana. [W. *Turner,* 1520-1568, English physician and botanist.]

turning (ter·ning). Version in obstetrics. [AS *tyrnan.*]

turnsol (tern·sol). Tournesol; litmus. [Fr *tournesol* sunflower.]

turpentine (ter·pen·tine). An oleoresin obtained from the bark of various species of *Pinus.* It is the essential oil (turpentine oil) distilled from this oleoresin that is used in medicine. Turpentine oil irritates the skin and causes hyperaemia of the part to which it is applied; consequently it finds its most frequent use in medicine as an ingredient of liniments. It has been taken internally as a carminative and expectorant, but its action in the latter case is dependent upon its excretion in the lungs, and since a great deal is excreted by the kidneys, it is more efficient to inhale the vapour when it is added to hot water. The use of turpentine oil as an anthelminthic is obsolete and dangerous. **Bordeaux turpentine.** A variety of turpentine obtained from France. **Canada turpentine.** Canada balsam; used as a mounting medium in microscopy. **Common turpentine.** Turpentine unrefined for medicinal use. **Larch turpentine, Venice turpentine.** The turpentine obtained from the bark of the larch. [Gk *terebinthinos.*]

turrecephaly, turricephaly (ter·e·kef·al·e). A skull with a high peaked crown; oxycephaly. [L *turris* tower, Gk *kephale* head.]

turunda, turundula (tur·un·dah, tur·un·dew·lah). 1. A surgeon's tent. 2. A suppository. [L.]

Turyn, Felix (b. 1899). Warsaw physician.

Turyn's sign. Passive dorsiflexion of the great toe in a case of sciatica gives pain in the gluteal region.

tussal (tus·al). Relating to a cough; tussive. [L *tussis* cough.]

tussedo (tus·e·do). Tussis.

tussicula (tus·ik·ew·lah). Slight coughing. [L.]

tussicular (tus·ik·ew·lar). Relating to a cough; tussive. [L *tussicula* a slight cough.]

tussiculation (tus·ik·ew·la'·shun). A short hacking cough. [see prec.]

Tussilago (tus·il·a·go). A genus of plants of the family Compositae. **Tussilago farfara.** Coltsfoot; the dried leaves are tonic and demulcent on account of their mucilage. [L.]

tussis (tus·is). Cough. **Tussis convulsiva.** Pertussis. [L.]

tussive (tus·iv). Concerned with a cough or caused by coughing. [L *tussis* cough.]

tutamen (tew·ta·men) (pl. *tutamina*). Any structure that has a protective function. **Tutamina cerebri.** The skull, cerebral membranes, scalp, and hair, all of which protect the brain. **Tutamina oculi.** Eyelids, eyebrows, and eyelashes, which protect the eyes. [L protection.]

Tuthill, Elizabeth.

Butler and Tuthill method. For sodium in blood: organic matter of serum is destroyed by wet oxidation and the sodium precipitated with zinc uranyl acetate. The precipitate is washed with alcohol and ether, dried in a desiccator, and weighed as $(UO_2)_3ZnNa(CH_3COO)_9{\cdot}6H_2O$.

tutin (too·tin). $C_{17}H_{20}O_7$, a glycoside found in the New Zealand toot-plant which closely resembles *Coriaria ruscifolia.* It is highly poisonous.

Tuttle, James Percival (b. 1857). New York surgeon.

Tuttle's proctoscope. A proctoscope bearing a small electric bulb at its extremity and a balloon device for inflating the interior of the rectum.

tweens (tweenz). Non-ionic emulsifying agents consisting of polyoxyethylene esters or ethers of sorbitol. They are yellow to brown liquids of varying viscosity, stable to pH changes and to high concentrations of electrolytes. The tweens are given different numbers according to their composition, viscosity, etc. **Tween 80.** Polyoxyethylene sorbitan mono-oleate; one of the series of tweens. [trade name.]

twin (twin). 1. One of a pair of individuals developing or which have developed together *in utero,* in animals which usually produce only one offspring at a time. In animals which normally produce two or more at a time the correct term is *litter-mate.* 2. Characterized by or appertaining to such an individual. **Allantoido-angiopagous twin.** Unequal separate twins, of which one is normal and the other an acardiac monster attached to the fetal membranes. **Binovular twins.** Twins developing from separate eggs. **Conjoined twins.** United twins, as in Siamese twins. **Dichorial twins.** Twins developing in separate chorionic sacs. **Dizygotic twins.** Binovular twins (see above). **Enzygotic twins.** Identical twins (see below). **Fraternal twins.** Binovular twins (see above). **Identical twins.** Twins developing from the same egg. **Monochorionic twins.** Twins developing within a single chorionic sac. **Monozygotic twins.** Identical twins (see above). **Omphalo-angiopagous twins.** Allantoido-angiopagous twins (see above). **Polyembryonic twin.** Enzygotic twin (see above). **Unequal twins.** Twins in which only one is fully developed. **Uniovular twins.** Identical twins (see above). **Unlike twins.** Unequal twins (see above). [AS *twinn* double.]

Twining, Edward. 20th century Manchester radiologist.

Twining's apparatus. A simple attachment enabling tomography to be carried out on any x-ray couch of the usual pattern. Twining did not originate the principle of tomography, but his simplified apparatus brought the method into more general use.

Twining's line. A measurement made on a lateral pneumoencephalogram by joining the tuberculum sellae to the internal occipital protuberance, devised to indicate abnormal displacement of the mid-brain and hind-brain structures.

twinning (twin·ing). 1. The production of twins. 2. The formation of similar structures by equal subdivision of the parent structure.

twitch (twich). The contraction of a small muscular unit. [AS *twiccian.*]

twitching (twich·ing). A succession of contractions of small portions of a muscle. **Fascicular twitching.** Twitching involving large groups of muscle fibres. **Fibrillar twitching.** Twitching. [see prec.]

See also: TROUSSEAU.

Twort, Frederick William (b. 1877). London bacteriologist.

Twort-d'Herelle phenomenon. The lysis of a bacterial culture by bacteriophage; it is transmissible and specific.

Tybamate (ti·bam·ate). BP Commission approved name for 2-methyl-2-propyltrimethylene butylcarbamate carbamate; a tranquillizer.

Tyformin (ti·for·min). BP Commission approved name for 4-guanidinobutyramide; an oral hypoglycaemic agent.

tyloma (ti·lo·mah). Callus; a localized area of hyperkeratosis due to intermittent pressure and friction. [Gk *tylos* knot, *-oma* tumour.]

Tylophora asthmatica (ti·lof·or·ah as·mat·ik·ah). A plant of south Asia (family Asclepiadaceae). The dried leaves (tylophorae folia) contain the alkaloids, tylophorine and tylophorinine. [Gk *tylos* knot, *pherein* to bear, asthma.]

tylophorine (ti·lof·or·een). $C_{24}H_{27}O_4N$, an alkaloid that occurs in the plant *Tylophora asthmatica*.

tylophorinine (ti·lof·or·in·een). $C_{23}H_{27}O_4N$, an alkaloid that occurs in the plant *Tylophora asthmatica*.

tylosis (ti·lo·sis). 1. A callosity. 2. Tylosis palmarum et plantarum, keratosis palmaris et plantaris, symmetrical keratoderma of the extremities, congenital keratoma of the palms and soles; symmetrical thickening of the horny layer of the epidermis of the palms and soles. Most authorities reserve the term for a congenital hyperkeratosis of the palms and soles, but others state that the malady may be acquired. 3. Drooping and thickening of the eyelid margin in long-standing ulcerative blepharitis. Also called *hypertrophic blepharitis.* **Tylosis linguae.** Leucoplakia of the tongue. [Gk a rendering callous.]

tylositas articuli (ti·lo·sit·as ar·tik·ew·li). Knuckle pads. [Gk *tylos* knot, L *articulatio* joint.]

tylosteresis (ti·lo·ster·e'·sis). The excision of a callosity. [Gk *tylos* knot, *sterein* to deprive.]

tylotic (ti·lot·ik). Callous or affected with callosity. [Gk *tylos* knot.]

Tyloxapol (ti·lox·ap·ol). BP Commission approved name for oxyethylated *t*-octylphenol formaldehyde polymer; a surface-active agent.

Tymazoline (ti·maz·o·leen). BP Commission approved name for 2-thymyloxymethyl-2-imidazoline; a vasoconstrictor.

tympanal (tim·pan·al). Tympanic.

tympanectomy (tim·pan·ek·to·me). Surgical removal of the tympanic membrane. [tympanic membrane, Gk *ektome* excision.]

tympania (tim·pan·e·ah). Tympanites.

tympanic (tim·pan·ik). 1. Concerned with the tympanic cavity and membrane. 2. Resonant. **Tympanic angle.** *See* ANGLE. **Tympanic antrum.** Mastoid antrum. *See* ANTRUM. **Tympanic bone.** The bony ring at the inner end of the external auditory meatus to which the drum is attached. **Tympanic canal.** The scala tympani. **Tympanic cavity.** *See* CAVITY. **Tympanic ganglion.** *See* GANGLION. **Tympanic lip.** *See* LIP. **Tympanic membrane.** *See* MEMBRANE. **Tympanic plate.** *See* PLATE. **Tympanic plexus.** *See* PLEXUS. **Tympanic ring.** *See* RING.

tympanic arteries. Anterior tympanic artery [arteria tympanica anterior (NA)]. *See* MAXILLARY ARTERY. **Inferior tympanic artery [arteria tympanica inferior (NA)].** *See* PHARYNGEAL ARTERY, ASCENDING. **Posterior tympanic artery [arteria tympanica posterior (NA)].** *See* AURICULAR ARTERY, POSTERIOR. **Superior tympanic artery [arteria tympanica superior (NA)].** *See* MENINGEAL ARTERY, MIDDLE.

tympanic nerve [nervus tympanicus (NA)]. A branch from the glossopharyngeal nerve to the tympanic plexus; it supplies sensory fibres to the mucous membrane of the middle ear and sends twigs to the greater and lesser superficial petrosal nerves.

tympanic veins [venae tympanicae (NA)]. Veins draining into the posterior facial vein.

tympanicity (tim·pan·is·it·e). The possession of tympanic or drum-like features.

tympaniform (tim·pan·e·form). Resembling a drum. [Gk *tympanon* drum, form.]

tympanism (tim·pan·izm). Tympanites.

tympanites (tim·pan·i·teez). Swelling of the abdomen due to gas in the intestine or the cavity of the peritoneum. **Uterine tympanites.** Gas in the uterine cavity of the peritoneum. [Gk *tympanon* drum.]

tympanitic (tim·pan·it·ik). 1. Of the nature of tympanites. 2. Tympanic or resonant.

tympanitis (tim·pan·i·tis). Otitis media; inflammation of the middle ear. [Gk *tympanon* drum, *-itis* inflammation.]

tympanohyal (tim·pan·o·hi'·al). 1. Concerning the typanic cavity and the hyoid arch. 2. The proximal part of the styloid process of the temporal bone which ossifies from a separate centre.

tympanolabyrinthopexy (tim·pan·o·lab'·e·rin·tho·pex·e). An operation for the fistulization of the labyrinth; an attempt to combat obstructive deafness, such as otosclerosis, and the forerunner of the modern fenestration operation. [Gk *tympanon* drum, labyrinth, Gk *pexis* a fixation.]

tympanomalleal (tim·pan·o·mal'·e·al). Concerning the tympanic bone and the malleus.

tympanomandibular (tim·pan·o·man·dib'·ew·lar). Referring to the tympanic cavity and the mandible.

tympanomastoid (tim·pan·o·mas'·toid). Concerning both the tympanic cavity and the mastoid air cells.

tympanomastoiditis (tim·pan·o·mas·toid·i'·tis). Otitis media extending to the mastoid air cells. [tympanic cavity, mastoid, Gk *-itis* inflammation.]

tympanophonia, tympanophony (tim·pan·o·fo'·ne·ah, tim·pan·of·o·ne). 1. Tinnitus aurium; subjective noises in the ears. 2. Autophony; amplified voice, breath, and arterial sounds, heard in otitis media. [Gk *tympanon* drum, *phone* voice.]

tympanoplastic (tim·pan·o·plas'·tik). Relating to the operation of tympanoplasty.

tympanoplasty (tim·pan·o·plas'·te). Surgical operation on the tympanic cavity and mastoid, including reconstruction of the conductive mechanism of hearing. [Gk *tympanum* drum, *plassein* to mould.]

tympanosclerosis (tim·pan·o·skler·o'·sis). Thickening of the tympanic membrane. [tympanum, sclerosis.]

tympanosis (tim·pan·o·sis). Tympanites. [Gk *tympanon* drum, *-itis* inflammation.]

tympanosquamosal (tim·pan·o·skwa·mo'·sal). Referring to the tympanic and squamous parts of the temporal bone.

tympanostapedial (tim·pan·o·sta·pe'·de·al). Relating to the tympanic cavity and the stapes.

tympanosympathectomy (tim·pan·o·sim·path·ek'·to·me). Surgical ablation of the tympanic plexus situated on the surface of the promontory for intractable tinnitus, in the belief that this condition may be due to ganglionitis affecting the plexus. [tympanic plexus, sympathetic, Gk *ektome* excision.]

tympanotemporal (tim·pan·o·tem'·por·al). Concerning the tympanic cavity and the temporal bone.

tympanotomy (tim·pan·ot·o·me). Surgical exploration of the middle ear. [tympanic membrane, Gk *temnein* to cut.]

tympanous (tim·pan·us). Tympanitic; distended with gas.

tympanum (tim·pan·um). The old name, still commonly used, for the tympanic cavity (middle ear) and the tympanic membrane (ear-drum) combined. [Gk *tympanon* drum.]

tympany (tim·pan·e). A low-pitched, resonant, drum-like note obtained on percussion over a large air-containing space such as a pneumothorax or distended abdomen. *See* RESONANCE. [see prec.]

Tymphonotomus microptera (tim·fon·ot·o·mus mi·krop·ter·ah). A snail that lives in brackish fresh water and is an intermediary host of *Heterophyes heterophyes.*

Tyndall, John (b. 1820). London physicist.

Tyndall effect, or phenomenon. The making visible of a beam of light passing through a transparent medium by the scattering of light from the beam, by suspended particles in the medium. Light (*Tyndall light*) scattered at right angles to the beam is plane-polarized.

tyndallization (tin·dal·i·za'·shun). Intermittent or fractional sterilization, with repetition of heating at intervals so that spore-forming bacteria are attacked in an adult phase. [John *Tyndall.*]

tynorman (tin·or·man). An antithyroid substance in the blood (Blum).

type (tipe). A class or group of persons, diseases, or substances, that can be recognized by a characteristic combination of features that the members have in common. It is a word with a wide use; the following are only examples. **Allotropic type.** 1. A variable type. 2. A type of individual who is not self-centred, but is preoccupied with other people and their affairs. **Amyostatic-kinetic type.** A form of encephalitis lethargica in which there is increasing apathy, muscular rigidity, and slowing of movement, with sometimes tremor of the limbs. **Apoplectic type.** Habitus apoplecticus. **Asthenic type.** A type of person with a long, narrow, flat chest and poor muscular development. **Athletic type.** A type of person with a broad and deep chest, flat abdomen, and good muscular development. **Aztec type.** A type of microcephalic idiocy, named after a pair of American sibs who toured Europe and America in exhibitions. **Bird's-head type.** A type of microcephalic idiocy in which the head resembles that of a bird. **Blood type.** The blood group of an individual. **Buffalo type.** The form of obesity seen in Cushing's syndrome; excessive fat deposits develop, particularly on the head, neck, and trunk. **Cycloid type.** A personality type in touch with and affected by the environment, tending to alternate in mood between depression and elation. **Dysplastic type.** A habitus unlike any of the other recognized ones, e.g. sthenic type. **Kalmuk type.** Mongol. **Koinotropic type.** A personality type where the subject's interests are identified with those of the common people. **Leg type.** Peroneal muscular atrophy; the Charcot–Marie–Tooth type. **Leptosome type.** Asthenic type (see above). **Organic-reaction type.** The type of mental break-down occasioned by organic disease of the brain, characterized by intellectual impairment and disorder of behaviour. **Overactive type.** The type of personality characterized by excess of physical and mental activity. **Phthinoid type, Phthisic type.** Flat and narrow-chested type: habitus phthisicus. **Pneumococcal type.** Antigenic subdivisions of the species *Streptococcus pneumonia*, the type-specific antigen of which is found in the capsule. **Pyknic type.** A rounded body with thick chest, short stout neck, broad head, and a tendency to obesity. **Scapulohumeral type.** Erb's juvenile type of progressive muscular dystrophy. **Schizoid type.** A personality type concerned less with the environment than with his inner mental life, tending to have minor degrees of traits shown in full by patients with schizophrenia. **Sendai type.** *See* SALMONELLA. **Serological types.** Individual types of micro-organisms which are identifiable by type-specific sera. **Sthenic type.** The muscular, strong type of person. **Sympathicotonic type.** A type of bodily constitution characterized by overactivity of the sympathetic nervous system. **Syntonic type.** A personality type in harmony with and responding adequately to the environment. **Vagotonic type.** The type in which parasympathetic activity predominates over sympathetic activity. The pulse is slow, blood pressure is low, sugar tolerance is high; there is localized sweating, and a tendency to allergic phenomena. **Vesanic type.** A term applied diffusely to any type of psychosis. **Visual type.** The type of person who thinks predominantly in visual images. **Wild type.** Phenotype which is characteristic of the wild populations of any organism; used of laboratory stocks. [Gk *typos* mark.]

See also: ARAN, BOYD, CHARCOT, DÉJÈRINE, DOWNEY, DUCHENNE, EICHHORST, ERB, FALRET, FAZIO-LONDE, GRIFFITH (F.), JAEGER (E. R. von J.), KRETSCHMER, LANDOUZY, LÉVI, LEYDEN, LORAIN, MANN (L.), MARIE, MOEBIUS, NOTHNAGEL, PENDE, PEPPER, RAYMOND, REMAK (E. J.), SCHLESINGER (H.), SCHULTZE (F.), SÉGLAS, SIMERLIN, SNELLEN, STRUEMPELL, WERDNIG, ZIMMERLIN.

typembryo (tip·em·bre·o). An embryo at the stage of development when specific, generic, familial, or class characteristics are identifiable. [type, embryo.]

typhaceae (ti·fa·se·e). An obsolete name for *Salmonella.* [typhoid fever.]

typhlatonia, typhlatony (tif·lat·o·ne·ah, tif·lat·o·ne). A persistent contraction of the muscles of the caecum. [typhlon, Gk *a-*, *tonos* tone.]

typhlectasia (tif·lek·ta·ze·ah). Typhlectasis.

typhlectasis (tif·lek·tas·is). Dilatation of the caecum. [typhlon, Gk *ektasis* dilatation.]

typhlectomy (tif·lek·to·me). Surgical excision of the caecum. [typhlon, Gk *ektome* excision.]

typhlenteritis (tif·len·ter·i'·tis). Typhlitis. [typhlon, Gk *enteron* intestine, *-itis* inflammation.]

typhlitis (tif·li·tis). Inflammation of the caecum. Before the recognition of appendicitis as a distinct entity, abscess in the right iliac region was thought to be due to typhlitis. [typhlon, Gk *-itis* inflammation.]

typhlocele (tif·lo·seel). A hernia involving the caecum. [typhlon, Gk *kele* hernia.]

typhlocolitis (tif·lo·kol·i'·tis). Inflammation of the lining of the caecum. [typhlon, colitis.]

typhlodicliditis (tif·lo·dik·lid·i'·tis). Inflammation of the ileocolic valve. [typhlon, Gk *diklis* valve, *-itis* inflammation.]

typhlo-enteritis (tif·lo·en·ter·i'·tis). Typhilitis. [typhlon, enteritis.]

typhloid (tif·loid). Having impaired vision. [Gk *typhlos* blind, *eidos* form.]

typhlolexia (tif·lo·lex·e·ah). Visual aphasia, word blindness; loss of the power to understand the written or printed word. [Gk *typhlos* blind, *lexis* speech.]

typhlolithiasis (tif·lo·lith·i'·as·is). The occurrence of calculi or faecal concretions in the caecum. [typhlon, Gk *lithos* stone.]

typhlology (tif·lol·o·je). Investigation of blindness in all its aspects. [Gk *typhlos* blind, *logos* science.]

typhlomegaly (tif·lo·meg·al·e). Hypertrophy of the caecum. [typhlon, Gk *megas* large.]

typhlomyxorrhoea (tif·lo·mix·o·re'·ah). The passage of mucus from the bowels, thought to be derived from the caecum. [typhlon, Gk *myxa* mucus, *rhein* to flow.]

typhlon (tif·lon). The caecum. [Gk *typhlos* blind.]

typhlopexia, typhlopexy (tif·lo·pex·e·ah, tif·lo·pex·e). Fixation at a normal level of an unduly mobile or unnaturally low caecum. [typhlon, Gk *pexis* a fixation.]

typhloptosis (tif·lop·to·sis). A condition in which the caecum is displaced downwards. [typhlon, Gk *ptosis* a falling.]

typhlorrhaphy (til·lor·af·e). Surgical suture of the caecum. [typhlon, Gk *rhaphe* suture.]

typhlosis (tif·lo·sis). Blindness. [Gk *typhlos* blind.]

typhlospasm (tif·lo·spazm). Spasm of the caecum. [typhlon, spasm.]

typhlostenosis (tif·lo·sten·o'·sis). Narrowing of the caecum. [typhlon, Gk *stenosis* a narrowing.]

typhlostomy (tif·los·to·me). The surgical operation for making an artificial fistula in the caecum. [typhlon, Gk *stoma* mouth.]

typhlotomy (tif·lot·o·me). The operation of cutting into the caecum. [typhlon, Gk *temnein* to cut.]

typhlo-ureterostomy (tif·lo·ewr·e·ter·os'·to·me). The operation of implanting the ureter into the caecum. It is now known that, in addition to the danger of ascending infection to the kidney, serious chemical imbalance may follow the introduction of urine to the proximal colon. [typhlon, ureter, Gk *stoma* mouth.]

typhobacillosis (ti·fo·bas·il·o'·sis). An obsolete vague term for the general symptoms of typhoid infection. **Typhobacillosis tuberculosa.** An obsolete, indefinite term for tuberculous infection with typhoid-like symptoms. [typhoid, bacillus, Gk *-osis* condition.]

typhogenic (ti·fo·jen·ik). Causing or producing typhus or typhoid fever. [typhus, typhoid, Gk *genein* to produce.]

typhoid (ti·foid). *See* FEVER, TYPHOID. **Cholera typhoid.** Typhoid-like symptoms occurring in the defervescent stage of cholera, possibly allergic. Usually they are severe. **Pellagra typhoid.**

Typhoid-like symptoms occurring in acute pellagra and usually fatal; also called *pellagra typhus.* [typhus, Gk *eidos* form.]

typhoidal (ti·**foid**·al). Exhibiting features similar to typhoid fever.

typholumbricosis (ti·fo·lum·brik·**o'**·sis). A feverish condition simulating typhoid fever, caused by infection with *Ascaris lumbricoides.* [typhoid, lumbricosis.]

typhomalaria (ti·fo·mal·**a'**·re·ah). A form of subtertian malaria (*Plasmodium falciparum*) with high remittent fever which, together with the symptoms this fever sometimes evokes, may resemble and/or be mistaken for typhoid fever and treated accordingly. By others the term is reserved for the complication of typhoid fever by coincident malaria.

typhomalarial (ti·fo·mal·**a'**·re·al). Pertaining to typhomalaria.

typhomania (ti·fo·**ma**·ne·ah). Delirium and coma characteristic of typhoid, typhus, and other fevers. [Gk *typhos* stupor, *mania* madness.]

typhopaludism (ti·fo·**pal**·ew·dizm). Typhomalaria. [typhoid, paludism.]

typhopneumonia (ti·fo·new·**mo'**·ne·ah). 1. Pneumonia associated with typhoid fever. 2. Pneumonia with stupor and exhaustion.

typhotoxin (ti·fo·**tox**·in). A poisonous ptomaine, $C_7H_{17}NO_2$, released into the medium in old cultures of the typhoid bacillus by autolysis of bacterial cells. It causes diarrhoea, muscular paralysis, and dilatation of the pupil in animals. The typhoid bacillus does not produce an exotoxin in the ordinary sense of that term. [typhoid, toxin.]

typhus (ti·fus). In the restricted sense this word refers to the classical epidemic or louse-borne disease. It is, however, now usual to refer to the typhus group of fevers which includes all the fevers caused by rickettsiae, except possibly Q fever and rickettsial pox, and any one of these may be referred to loosely as *typhus* without the specific qualifying adjective, tick-borne, flea-borne, etc. On the European continent typhoid fever is often referred to as *typhus* or *typhus abdominalis.* **Abdominalis typhus, Typhus abdominalis.** Typhoid fever. **Amarillic typhus.** An old term for yellow fever. **Benign typhus.** 1. Any mild form of typhus. 2. Sometimes applied to Brill's disease. **Collapsing typhus.** A typhoid-like fever; the im-pyeng of Korea. **Endemic typhus.** Flea-borne or murine typhus (see below). **Epidemic typhus, Exanthematic typhus.** A febrile disease caused by *Rickettsia prowazeki* and transmitted to man by the agency of the louse, *Pediculus humanus.* The onset is sudden with fever rising to 39.5°C (103°F) or so within 48 h and continuing for 10–14 days. A macular morbiliform rash appears about the fifth day on the trunk, limbs, and sometimes the face, and may become haemorrhagic. The disease runs a severe often fatal course, but is usually amenable to treatment by chloramphenicol. **Flea-borne typhus.** An endemic form of typhus transmitted by fleas from rodents; also called *murine typhus.* **Fleck typhus.** Epidemic typhus (see above). **Typhus icteroides.** Yellow fever. **K Typhus.** Mite-borne typhus, or tsutsugamushi disease. **Typhus levissimus.** 1. A mild form of typhus. 2. Brill's disease. **Louse-borne typhus.** Epidemic typhus (see above). **Mexican typhus.** Tabardillo, or epidemic typhus in Mexico. **Mite-borne typhus.** A relatively severe form of typhus transmitted by larval mites, e.g. *Trombicula akamushi* and *deliensis.* **Mouse typhus.** An epizootic disease of mice caused by *Salmonella typhimurium.* **Murine typhus.** Flea-borne typhus (see above). **Pellagra typhus.** Pellagra typhoid. *See* TYPHOID. **Queensland tick typhus.** Typhus caused by *Rickettsia australis* and acquired from small marsupials. **Rat typhus.** Flea-borne typhus (see above). **Typhus recurrens.** A recurrent form of exanthematic typhus. **Rocky Mountain tick typhus.** Rocky Mountain spotted fever. *See* FEVER. **Rural typhus.** Mite-borne typhus (see above). **São Paulo typhus.** Tick-borne typhus of Brazil; it may be an analogue of Rocky Mountain spotted fever. It is transmitted by the tick *Amblyomma cajennense.* **Scrub typhus.** Mite-borne typhus, or tsutsugamushi disease. **Ship typhus.** Flea-borne typhus (see above). **Shop typhus.** Flea-borne typhus in Malaya. **Typhus siderans.** An acute form of epidemic typhus. **Tick-borne typhus.** A typhus fever transmitted by ticks, as for example Rocky Mountain spotted fever. **Toulon typhus.** Flea-borne typhus that occurred on battleships in Toulon (1936). **Urban typhus, W typhus.** Flea-borne typhus, in Malaysia. [Gk *typhos* stupor.]

See also: GUBLER, ROBIN (E. C. R.).

typing (ti·ping). **Blood typing.** Blood grouping. [type.]

typoscope (ti·po·skope). A rectangle of dull black material with an opening 8 mm high and 15 cm long. When placed on a book, it may aid those with defective vision to read, and is especially useful in cases of cataract. [type, Gk *skopein* to view.]

typus (ti·pus). Type. **Typus degenerativus amstelodamensis.** Dwarfism, mental defect, eyebrows which tend to meet in the middle, upturned nose and thin, downturning upper lip. Described by Cornelia de Lange of Amsterdam, but not restricted to that city. **Typus inversus.** Applied to a temperature chart, one in which the morning recording is higher than the evening, as sometimes occurs in grave tuberculosis. [L.]

tyramine (ti·ram·een). Hydroxyphenylethylamine, $NH_2CH_2CH_2C_6H_4OH$. A sympathomimetic amine which releases the actively circulating catecholamines but has little effect on the storage of catecholamines which are degraded mainly by monoamine oxidase. Tyramine test for phaeochromocytoma, *see* TEST. [Gk *tyros* cheese, amine.]

tyrannism (**tir**·an·izm). Morbid and psychopathic cruelty; sadism. [Gk *tyrannos* tyrant.]

tyrein (ti·re·in). Coagulated casein. [Gk *tyros* cheese.]

tyriasis (ti·**ri**·as·is). 1. Elephantiasis. 2. Alopecia. [Gk *tyros* cheese.]

tyrocidin, tyrocidine (ti·ro·**si**·din, ti·ro·**si**·deen). An antibiotic which occurs with gramicidin in the tyrothricin obtained from species of *Bacillus.*

Tyrode, Maurice Vejux (b. 1878). Cambridge pharmacologist.

Tyrode's solution. An aqueous solution of the following percentage composition; sodium chloride 0.8, potassium chloride 0.02, calcium chloride 0.02, sodium bicarbonate 0.1, disodium hydrogen phosphate 0.005, glucose 0.1, magnesium chloride 0.01, water to 100. This solution is useful for experiments on mammalian gut.

Ringer–Tyrode solution. An aqueous solution of sodium chloride, potassium chloride, calcium chloride, magnesium chloride, dextrose, sodium acid phosphate, and sodium bicarbonate, used for physiological experiments.

tyrogenous (ti·**roj**·en·us). Derived from cheese. [Gk *tyros* cheese, *genein* to produce.]

Tyroglyphidae (ti·ro·**glif**·id·e). A family of the acarine super-family Tyroglyphoidea. The genera *Glyciphagus, Tyroglyphus,* and *Tyrophagus* are of medical interest. [Gk *tyros* cheese, *glyphein* to carve.]

Tyroglyphoidea (ti·ro·glif·**oi'**·de·ah). A super-family of the arachnid order Acarina. The family Tyroglyphidae is of medical interest. [Gk *tyros* cheese, *glyphein* to carve, *eidos* form.]

Tyroglyphus (ti·ro·**glif**·us). A genus of acarids. **Tyroglyphus farinae.** The flour mite, a cause of grocers' itch. It may also cause inflammation and diarrhoea if ingested in large quantity. It has been found in the sputum in man. **Tyroglyphus longior.** A mite of dry-stored products. The usual form may be a causative agent of grocers' itch. The form *castellanii* is the causative agent of copra itch. **Tyroglyphus siro.** The cheese mite, which also occurs in other foodstuffs. It may cause severe irritation of the alimentary canal if eaten in large quantities, and is also the causal agent of cutaneous vanillism. [Gk *tyros* cheese, *glyphein* to carve.]

tyroid (ti·roid). Resembling cheese; of the nature of cheese. [Gk *tyros* cheese, *eidos* form.]

tyroma (ti·**ro**·mah). A tumour or growth containing cheese-like matter. [Gk *tyros* cheese, *-oma* tumour.]

tyromatosis (ti·ro·mat·**o'**·sis). Caseation; the formation of cheese-like masses in the tissues. [Gk *tyros* cheese, *-oma* tumour, *-osis* condition.]

Tyrophagus (ti·**rof**·ag·us). A genus of mites of the family

Tyroglyphidae. Some species of *Tyroglyphus* are sometimes placed here. [Gk *tyros* cheese, *phagein* to eat.]

tyrosal (ti·ro·sal). Phenazone salicylate, $C_{11}H_{12}ON_2C_6H_4(OH)COOH$. A compound formerly used as an anodyne and antipyretic.

tyrosinase (ti·ro·sin·aze). Monophenol oxidase; an enzyme present in various animal and plant tissues which converts tyrosine into a red indole compound and thence to melanin, or monohydroxyphenols generally into catechols and thence to quinones.

tyrosine (ti·ro·seen). *p*-Hydroxyphenylalanine, $OHC_6H_4CH_2CH(NH_2)COOH$. An amino acid occurring in protein hydrolysates, which is essential in the diet for the maintenance of health. It is required by the body for the production of the hormones thyroxine and adrenaline, and is also the source of the pigment melanin. It occurs as a crystalline deposit in urine in certain conditions, chiefly in acute yellow atrophy of the liver, whilst the rare condition alkaptonuria results from an inborn disorder of tyrosine metabolism. [Gk *tyros* cheese.]

tyrosinosis (ti·ro·sin·o′·sis). Breakdown in the tyrosine metabolism with the appearance of dihydroxyphenylalanine in the urine. At least three faults in tyrosine metabolism have been described, one in infants causing vomiting, bleeding and death due to hepatic or hepatorenal failure. [tyrosine, Gk *-osis* condition.]

tyrosinuria (ti·ro·sin·ewr′·e·ah). The presence of tyrosine in the urine.

Tyrothricin (ti·ro·thri·sin). BP Commission approved name for a complex antibiotic substance produced by a species of *Bacillus,* first described by Dubos 1939. It consists of a mixture of gramicidin and tyrocidin. This antibiotic has a wide spectrum of activity, but is very toxic and is therefore only used for topical application. [see foll.]

Tyrothrix (ti·ro·thrix). A generic name of a group of bacteria now placed in several genera, *Bacillus, Lactobacillus,* and *Clostridium.* [Gk *tyros* cheese, *thrix* hair.]

tyrotoxicon (ti·ro·tox·ik·on). Name given by Vaughan to a crystallizable ptomaine isolated from putrefying cheese in the Michigan epidemic of cheese poisoning of 1883–4. The substance occurs in putrid milk and egg products and has the chemical and pharmacological reactions of diazobenzene. [Gk *tyros* cheese, *toxikon* poison.]

tyrotoxicosis (ti·ro·tox·ik·o′·sis). Tyrotoxism. [Gk *tyros* cheese, *toxikon* poison, *-osis* condition.]

tyrotoxism (ti·ro·tox·izm). Poisoning caused by cheese or by the decomposition products of milk. [Gk *tyros* cheese, *toxikon* poison.]

Tyrrell, Frederick (b. 1793). London surgeon and anatomist.

Tyrrell's fascia. Denonvilliers' fascia; the rectovesical fascia.

Tyrrell's hook. A blunt-ended instrument used for hooking up the iris, strands of capsule, or lens matter in intra-ocular operations.

Tyson, Edward (b. 1650). London physician and anatomist.

Tyson's glands. Rudimentary sebaceous glands of the corona glandis and the inner layer of the prepuce. Their secretion forms one of the constituents of smegma.

tysonitis (ti·son·i·tis). Inflammation of the preputial (Tyson's) glands. [Tyson's glands, Gk *-itis* inflammation.]

Tzanck, Arnault (b. 1886). Paris dermatologist.

Tzanck cells. Large multinucleate giant cells seen in scrapings from the floor of vesicles in viral infections, predominantly in those caused by herpes simplex and chicken-pox viruses.

Tzanck test. When the floor of a pemphigus bulla is scraped and the debris stained, the epithelial cells are found to be atypical; their cytoplasm is rounded and sharply defined, they stain deeply at the periphery and the nucleus is pyknotic.

U

uber (ew·ber). A mammary gland. **Uberis apex.** The nipple. [see foll.]

uberous (ew·ber·us). Prolific; fruitful; fertile. [L *uber* udder.]

uberty (ew·ber·te). Fertility. [see prec.]

Udránszky, Laszlo (b. 1862). Budapest physiologist.

Udránszky's test. For bile acids: to 5 ml of solution add a few drops of 0.1 per cent aqueous furfural solution, and shake to produce a thick foam. Add a drop or two of concentrated sulphuric acid to the foam. A pink coloration indicates bile acids.

Uffelmann, Julius August Christian (b. 1837). Rostock physician.

Uffelmann's reagent. For lactic acid: to 50 ml of 2 per cent phenol add 10 per cent ferric chloride solution drop by drop until a purple colour is produced. This reagent is extremely unstable.

Uhl, Henry Stephen Magraw (b. 1921). Rhode Island physician.

Uhl's anomaly. Uhl's syndrome (see below).

Uhl's syndrome. A rare condition characterized by congenital hypoplasia of the wall of the right ventricle, with almost total absence of the ventricular muscle, presenting as right heart failure in infancy.

Uhthoff, Wilhelm (b. 1853). Breslau ophthalmologist.

Uhthoff's sign. Nystagmus as a manifestation of disseminated sclerosis.

Uhthoff's symptom. Reduction in visual acuity following exercise, hot baths or hot drinks. Seen in patients who have optic neuropathy due to multiple (disseminated) sclerosis.

ukambin (oo·kam·bin). An alkaloid similar to digitalis and strophanthus, used by Africans as an arrow poison. In small doses intravenously it acts as a cardiac stimulant.

ula (ew·lah). The gums; the gingiva. [Gk *oulon* gum.]

ulaemorrhagia (ewl·e·mor·a'·je·ah). Haemorrhage of the gums. [Gk *oulon* gum, haemorrhage.]

ulaganactesis (ew·lag·an·ak·te'·sis). Irritation of the gums. [Gk *oulon* gum, *aganaktesis* irritation.]

ulcer (ul·ser). A localized necrotic lesion of the skin or a mucous surface, in which the superficial epithelium is destroyed and deeper tissues are exposed in an open sore. *See also* SORE. **Aden ulcer.** Not a clinical entity, probably either ulcus tropicum or veldt sore. **Adherent ulcer.** A cutaneous ulcer, the base of which is adherent to underlying tissue. **Amoebic ulcer.** An ulcer, usually in the large intestine, caused by or maintained by the parasitic protozoon, *Entamoeba histolytica.* Such an ulcer is always heavily infected with bacteria also; therapy is best directed against both protozoa and bacteria. Primary amoebic ulcers are usually in the caecum, but the infection spreads to other parts of the large bowel, especially the iliopelvic colon and the flexures, points where there is likely to be stasis. Amoebic ulcers also occur in the skin, usually around the anus or a colostomy ostium. **Anal ulcer.** Anal fissure. *See* FISSURE. **Anastomotic ulcer.** A peptic ulcer which occurs at the site of an anastomosis between the stomach and the small intestine, commonly after gastro-enterostomy. **Annam ulcer.** Ulcus tropicum. **Aphthous ulcers.** Small pinhead vesicles upon the tongue, inner surface of lips and cheeks, or on the palate, which break down into shallow painful ulcers. They occur in young children as the first manifestation of infection with the virus of herpes simplex; in later life the subjects are liable to recurrent herpes. **Arrosion ulcer.** An ulcer of the deeper respiratory passages, usually tuberculous in origin. **Arterial ulcer.** An ulcer of the skin caused by obstruction of an artery. **Arteriosclerotic ulcer.** An ulcer (usually on the leg) due to a defective blood supply following arteriosclerosis. **Atheromatous ulcer.** 1. An ulcer resulting from the destruction of the endothelial coat over an atheromatous patch in a large artery. 2. A corneal ulcer forming in an old, dense, degenerate scar, and usually progressing rapidly. **Atonic ulcer.** An indolent, slow-healing ulcer with unhealthy granulations. **Bahia ulcer, Bauru ulcer.** Mucocutaneous leishmaniasis. *See* LEISHMANIASIS. **Bilharzia ulcer.** An ulcer in the bowel or bladder mucous membrane resulting from infection with the worms *Schistosoma mansoni* or *japonicum.* **Buruli ulcer.** A sclerotic ulcerative lesion of the skin and subcutaneous tissue due to *Mycobacterium ulcerans,* apparently acquired from sedges and reeds growing along river margins. Though first recognized in Victoria (Australia) it is named after Buruli county in Uganda. It has now been reported from tropical Africa, Mexico, Malaya and New Guinea. The disease responds to antituberculous therapy, and BCG vaccination gives some protection. **Caecal ulcer.** An ulcer in the caecum which may be a solitary lesion usually of obscure aetiology, or multiple, as a sequel to colonic obstruction (stercoral ulcer). **Callous ulcer.** An ulcer with a hard, indurated, avascular base and thick inelastic margins, e.g. in a chronic oedematous leg. **Catarrhal ulcer.** 1. A superficial ulcer of a mucous membrane, secondary to catarrhal infection. 2. A superficial corneal ulcer situated near the limbus, usually associated with an acute catarrhal conjunctivitis. **Central indolent ulcer.** A bilateral, central, corneal ulcer occurring in very ill children. There is little local reaction and the ulcers, although not deep, are obstinate in healing. **Chancroid ulcer.** A soft, painful, venereal ulcer occurring in the genital area due to infection with Ducrey's bacillus (*Haemophilus ducreyi*). **Chiclero ulcer.** Cutaneous and mucocutaneous leishmaniasis. *See* LEISHMANIASIS. **Chrome ulcer.** Chrome sore; ulceration and destruction of the nasal septum and deep ulcers on the hands, seen in chrome workers. It is due to the caustic action of chromic acid and the chromates of potassium and sodium. **Chronic ulcer.** Any ulcer that runs a chronic course. **Cochin-China ulcer.** Ulcus tropicum. **Contact ulcer.** Ulcer produced by the rubbing together of two adjacent surfaces, or by the transfer of an infective agent between such surfaces. **Corroding ulcer.** Ulceration associated with gangrene. **Corrosive ulcer.** Gangrenous stomatitis. *See* STOMATITIS. **Crateriform ulcer.** Specifically, an epithelioma of the face, somewhat conical in shape and having an ulcer at its apex, the whole resembling a tiny volcano. The term also is used of any ulcer having an appearance in its flanks and its bowl-shaped cavity that resembles the popular conception of a vol. ano. **Creeping ulcer.** Serpiginous ulcer (see below). **Curling ulcer.** An acute or subacute ulcer in the duodenum developing soon after shock from burns or scalds. Less frequently gastric or multiple. **Decubital ulcer, decubitus ulcer.** A breakdown of skin and subcutaneous tissues, usually infected and later sloughing, in parts of the body under prolonged pressure; commonly over shoulder blades, spine, base of back or heels. A trophic ulceration. **Dendritic ulcer.** A superficial, fissure-like, corneal ulcer shaped like a dendrite due to its peculiar branching method of spreading; caused by the herpes virus. Also known as *herpes simplex cornealis, dendritic keratitis.* **Dental ulcer.** An ulcer produced in the mouth by some form of trauma, such as an ill-fitting denture or a jagged tooth. **Diphtheritic ulcer.** 1. An ulcer due to infection with virulent, toxigenic diphtheria bacilli, possibly following detachment of diphtheritic membrane. 2. One form of skin ulcer, apparently a cutaneous diphtheria. 3. A loose term for any ulcer with a fibrinous exudate. **Duodenal ulcer.** A peptic ulcer situated in the duodenum near the pylorus. **Eczematous ulcers.** Phlyctenular ulcers (see below). **Elusive ulcer.** Hunner's ulcer. **Erythrocyanotic ulcer.** Ulceration of perniotic skin. **Exuberant ulcer.** An ulcer having abundant tissue growing from its base. **Factitial ulcer.** Self-inflicted ulcer; an ulcer which is caused by the patient himself, commonly by burning or by the application of caustics. **Fascicular ulcer.** A small, superficial, corneal ulcer that extends slowly towards the centre, having a sheaf of superficial vessels connecting it to the limbus. **Fissured ulcer.** An ulcer which is neither circular nor oval in shape, but linear. **Follicular ulcer.** 1. A small ulcer on the skin formed in the neighbourhood of a pilosebaceous follicle. 2. A small ulcer on mucous membrane commencing in a lymphatic follicle. **Gaboon ulcer.** Ulcus tropicum. **Gastric ulcer.** An ulcer of the gastric mucous membrane which may proceed to destruction of the deeper layers of the stomach wall. **Gastrojejunal ulcer.** Anastomotic ulcer (see above). **Girdle ulcer.** An ulcer which spreads circularly in the intestine. **Gouty ulcer.** An ulcer over or near a gouty joint, due to tissue damage resulting from underlying tophi. **Granulocytopenic ulcer.** An ulcer that develops on mucous membranes, especially of the mouth, in the course of granulocytopenic conditions. **Gravitational ulcer.** Varicose ulcer (see below). **Gummatous ulcer.** The ulceration of syphilitic gummatous tissue through skin or mucous membrane. **Gwalior ulcer.** Ulcus tropicum. **Haemorrhagic ulcer.** An ulcer the base or walls of which bleed easily. **Hard ulcer.** Any ulcer exhibiting induration; often restricted to syphilitic chancre. **Hypertensive ischaemic ulcer of the leg.** Ulceration of the lower third of the leg, due to arteriosclerosis and hypertension. **Hypopyon ulcer.** An acute suppurative form of corneal ulcer with a yellowish-white, sloughing advancing edge, associated with pus in the anterior chamber of the eye. It is commonly caused by the pneumococcus. It is also known as *serpiginous ulcer, ulcus serpens, pneumococcal ulcer.* **Indolent ulcer.** Correctly used the term *indolent* means painless. Any painless ulcer therefore can be called *indolent.* Commonly the term is applied to any chronic or slothful ulcer which is reluctant to heal. **Jeddah ulcer.** Cutaneous leishmaniasis. *See* LEISHMANIASIS. **Jejunal ulcer.** Anastomotic ulcer (see above). **Kissing ulcer.** An ulcer that forms on opposed surfaces constantly or intermittently in contact, especially applied to peptic ulcers situated opposite each other on the anterior and posterior walls of the first part of the duodenum. **Kurunegala ulcer.** Pyosis tropica. **Lahore ulcer.** Cutaneous leishmaniasis. *See* LEISHMANIASIS. **Leprous ulcer.** A skin or mucosal ulcer, resulting from infection with *Mycobacterium leprae* locally, or a trophic ulcer resulting from a leprous nerve lesion. **Lupoid ulcer.** An ulcer of the skin resembling the ulceration formerly seen in some types of lupus vulgaris. **Lymphatic ulcer.** An ulcer having a lymph-like exudate. **Malabar ulcer.** Ulcus tropicum. **Marginal ulcer.** A superficial type of corneal ulcer, often crescentic in shape, occurring near the limbus; sometimes secondary, as in catarrhal conjunctivitis, sometimes primary, of doubtful aetiology. **Mercurial ulcer.** An ulcer formed by the corrosive action of a mercurial salt or as a result of chronic mercurial poisoning. **Mozambique ulcer.** Ulcus tropicum. **Mycobacterial ulcer.** A term applied to ulceration caused by Mycobacteria other than *Mycobacterium tuberculosis* and *M. leprae.* **Mycotic ulcer.** 1. One caused by fungus infection. 2. A chronic superficial corneal ulcer with a yellowish edge and associated with a hypopyon; caused by a fungus. **Neurogenic ulcer.** In neurological diseases, particularly those like syringomyelia which cause cutaneous analgesia, painless ulceration of the skin may occur and may give rise to extensive destruction of surrounding tissues. **Neurotic ulcer of the buccal mucosae.** Periadenitis mucosa necrotica recurrens; a chronic, intractable malady which usually begins in childhood, characterized by the appearance on the buccal and laryngeal mucosae of painful small areas of necrosis and moderately extensive ulcers. The cause is unknown, and the malady persists for many years with remissions and exacerbations. **Neurotrophic ulcer.** Neurogenic ulcer (see above). **Oyster-shell ulcer.** An ulcer overlying an area of subcutaneous or muscular calcinosis. The base has a grey, hard, irregular surface. **Pendeh ulcer, Pendinsky ulcer.** Cutaneous leishmaniasis. *See* LEISHMANIASIS. **Peptic ulcer.** An ulcer in the causation of which the stomach secretions are believed to play some part. It is found mainly in the stomach or duodenum, and less often at other sites. **Perforating ulcer.** 1. An intractable, deep, painless ulcer, usually on the sole and often extending down to the bone, when the skin is insensitive, e.g. in diabetic neutritis, tabes dorsalis, sciatic-nerve palsy. 2. An ulcer that penetrates the whole thickness of the wall of a hollow viscus. **Persian ulcer.** Cutaneous leishmaniasis. *See* LEISHMANIASIS. **Phagedenic ulcer.** Ulcer tropicum. **Phlegmonous ulcer.** An ulcer associated with a submucous, spreading, suppurative inflammation. **Phlyctenular ulcers.** Small superficial corneal ulcers seen in phlyctenular keratoconjunctivitis and allergic in nature. **Pneumococcal ulcer.** Hypopyon ulcer (see above). **Post-operative serpiginous ulcer** (Cullen). Pyoderma gangraenosum. **Post-thrombic ulcer.** Varicose ulcer (see below). **Pressure ulcers.** Trophic blebs of the skin developing as a result of pressure necrosis of tissues, commonly at the base of the back or over the bony prominences and leading to gangrene in the deeper parts, owing to infection. **Putrid ulcer.** An offensive ulcer. **Ring ulcers.** 1. Marginal corneal ulcers that become confluent and form a complete ring, seen in phlyctenular keratoconjunctivitis, a serious condition sometimes complicated by sloughing of the whole cornea. 2. Girdle ulcer (see above). **Rodent ulcer.** A basal-celled carcinoma, arising from the basal cells of the skin or their derivatives, which grows slowly and destroys tissues as it grows. It commonly occurs on the face. **Rodent ulcer of the cornea.** Mooren's ulcer. **Roentgen ulcer.** Radionecrosis; ulceration caused by exposure to ionizing irradiation. **Rosacea ulcer.** Superficial corneal ulceration occurring in rosacea keratitis. Greyish-white subepithelial infiltrates appear first, finally breaking-down into ulcers; associated with vascularization. **Scorbutic ulcer.** Ulceration of the skin or mucous surfaces due to deficiency of vitamin C. **Scrofulous ulcer.** Phlyctenular ulcer (see above). **Sea-anemone ulcer.** A deep intestinal ulcer with raised frayed necrotic margins, as in amoebiasis. **Self-inflicted ulcer.** Factitial ulcer (see above). **Serpiginous ulcer.** An ulcer with an irregular crescentic margin, seen typically in tertiary syphilis; an ulcer which heals in one area, only to extend to another. **Sickle-cell anaemia ulcers.** Single or multiple, punched-out ulcers of the legs, seen particularly in negroes, characteristic of sickle-cell anaemia. **Snail-track ulcers.** Secondary syphilitic ulcers of the mucous membranes of the mouth, fauces, anus, and vulva, that spread rapidly, leaving a track that is coated with shiny mucus. **Stasis ulcer.** An ulcer of the lower limbs due to venous stasis, e.g. a varicose ulcer. **Stercoral ulcer.** Ulceration of the mucous membrane found above the level of an unrelieved intestinal obstruction, especially in the colon. It may perforate and precipitate peritonitis. **Stoma ulcer, stomal ulcer.** Anastomotic ulcer (see above). **Streptococcal ulcer.** A chronic ulcer following streptococcal infection of an abrasion or insect bite. **Symptomatic ulcer.** Ulceration which indicates the presence of a general disease such as syphilis, tuberculosis, or scurvy. **Syphilitic ulcer.** An ulcer due to syphilis, encountered in a variety of forms in congenital as well as in all three stages of the acquired disease. **Syrian ulcer.** A cutaneous ulcer described in Syria and associated with various bacteria, notably *Corynebacterium diphtheriae.* **Tanner's ulcer.** Chrome ulcer (see above), occurring in tanners using chromium salts. **Taschkent ulcer, Tashkend ulcer.** Cutaneous leishmaniasis. *See* LEISHMANIASIS. **Trachomatous ulcers.** Chronic superficial corneal ulcers associated with pannus in trachoma. **Traumatic ulcer.** Ulceration due to injury. **Trophic ulcer.** An intractable ulcer found in areas of skin when the sensory innervation is defective, e.g. in syringomyelia. **Trophoneurotic ulcer.** Neurogenic ulcer (see above). **Tropical ulcer.** Ulcus tropicum. **Tuberculous corneal ulcer.** A chronic corneal ulceration of varying types caused by infection with *Mycobacterium tuberculosis,* and associated with much vascularization; rare. **Vagabonds' ulcer.** A neglected ulcer, commonly on the leg, and typically in the aged. **Varicose ulcer.** The common ulcer in the lower third of the leg or near the ankle, especially in parous women, often associated with eczema, varicose veins, and oedema; commonly a sequel to venous thrombosis. **Venereal ulcer.** Chancre or chancroid. **Warty ulcer.** Marjolin's ulcer. **Weak ulcer.** An ulcer which is lined with pale sodden granulations, and which shows no sign of healing. **Zambesi ulcer.** Ulcus tropicum. [L *ilcus.*]

See also: BAZIN, BOUVERET, CURLING, FENWICK (E. H.), HUNNER, JACOB, LIPSCHUETZ, MARJOLIN, MOOREN, PARROT, PLAUT, SAEMISCH.

ulcerate (ul·ser·ate). To form an ulcer.

ulceration (ul·ser·a·shun). The process of formation of an ulcer. **Phagedenic ulceration.** Chronic indurated skin ulceration that spreads and shows little tendency to spontaneous healing; large areas of skin may be destroyed. **Rheumatoid ulceration.** Ulceration of the pyoderma gangraenosum type sometimes occurring with rheumatoid arthritis. **Ulceration of the stomach.** A localized destructive lesion of the gastric mucous membrane caused by the digestion of a devitalized area by the acid gastric juice.

See also: BOUVERET, DUGUET.

ulcerative (ul·ser·a·tiv). 1. Referring to ulcers. 2. In a state of ulceration.

ulcerogranuloma (ul·ser·o·gran·ew·lo′·mah). Ulcerating granuloma of the pudenda; granuloma inguinale.

ulceromembranous (ul·ser·o·mem′·bran·us). Exhibiting both ulcers and a false membrane.

ulceronodular (ul·ser·o·nod′·ew·lar). Ulceration characterized by nodules.

ulcerous (ul·ser·us). 1. Having the characteristics of an ulcer. 2. In a state of ulceration.

ulcus (ul·kus). An ulcer. **Ulcus cancrosum.** An ulcerating cancer. **Ulcus cruris.** Ulcer of the leg. **Ulcus durum.** Hard ulcer. *See* ULCER. **Ulcus exedens.** Ulcus rodens (see below). **Ulcus grave.** Ulcus tropicum (see below). **Ulcus hypostaticum.** A bedsore. **Ulcus induratum.** Hard ulcer. *See* ULCER. **Ulcus molle, ulcus molle cutis.** Chancroid ulcer. *See* ULCER. **Ulcus penetrans.** A perforating ulcer. **Ulcus rodens.** Rodent ulcer. *See* ULCER. **Ulcus rodens corneae.** Mooren's ulcer. **Ulcus scorbuticum.** Ulcers caused by scurvy. **Ulcus septicus.** Hypopyon ulcer. *See* ULCER. **Ulcus serpens.** An ulcer having a serpiginous outline. **Ulcus terebrans.** A rodent ulcer which invades the periosteum, the bones of the face, or even the meninges. **Ulcus tropicum.** An indolent ulcer that occurs usually on the lower limbs in the humid tropics. The causal organism is a fusiform bacillus, *Fusiformis fusiformis*, but a spirochaete, *Borrelia vincenti*, is frequently found in association with it. The infection is superimposed on a scratch, insect bite, or other abrasion. A punched-out ulcer covered by a slough develops and extends to about 30 mm (1¼ in) in diameter, when it usually stops extending, but it may grow bigger and coalesce with adjacent ulcers to form a large area of ulceration that may even extend around the whole circumference of the leg. It usually responds to treatment with penicillin. **Ulcus tuberculosum.** A tuberculous ulcer. **Ulcus tuberculosum cutis.** Tuberculous ulcer of the skin; it normally occurs near natural orifices and in subjects with pulmonary tuberculosis. **Ulcus venereum molle.** Chancroid ulcer. *See* ULCER. **Ulcus ventriculi.** Gastric ulcer. *See* ULCER. **Ulcus ventriculi perforans.** A perforating gastric ulcer. **Ulcus ventriculi rotundum.** A round ulcer of the stomach. **Ulcus vulvae acutum.** Lipschuetz's acute ulcer of the vulva. [L.]

ule (ew·le). A scar or cicatrix. [Gk *oule* scar.]

ulectomy (ew·lek·to·me). 1. The cutting out of scar tissue, as in secondary iridectomy. [Gk *oule* scar, *ektome* excision.] 2. The surgical removal of gum tissue; gingivectomy. [Gk *oulon* gum, *ektome* excision.]

ulegyria (ew·le·ji·re·ah). Scarring of the cerebral gyri. [Gk *oule* scar, gyre.]

ulerythema (ewl·er·ith·e′·mah). A descriptive name for any eruption characterized by scarring associated with erythema. **Ulerythema acneiforme.** Atrophoderma vermiculatum, atrophoderma reticulatum symmetricum faciei, folliculitis ulerythematosa reticulata, honeycomb acne; a malady of unknown cause, characterized by erythema of both cheeks, and associated with follicular comedo-like lesions: eventually typical honeycomb pattern scarring of the areas is noted. **Ulerythema centrifugum** (Unna). Lupus erythematodes. **Ulerythema ophryogenes.** Erythema of the eyebrows associated with the formation of follicular papules. The hairs are thin and may break off. Follicular and interfollicular atrophy may occur causing a cicatricial alopecia. The malady may be akin to keratosis pilaris, and may develop on the scalp or upper arms. **Ulerythema sycosiforme** (Unna). Lupoid sycosis (Milton), the severe, usually localized type of coccogenic sycosis in which the hair follicles are destroyed and permanent alopecia ensues. [Gk *oule* scar, erythema.]

uletic (ew·let·ik). 1. Characterized by scars; cicatricial. [Gk *oule* scar.] 2. Concerning the gums; gingival. [Gk *oulon* gum.]

uletomy (ew·let·o·me). Surgical incision made into scar tissue. [Gk *oule* scar, *temnein* to cut.]

uliginous (ew·lij·in·us). Slimy; damp. [L *uliginosus* moist.]

Ullrich, Otto (b. 1894). German physician.

Ullrich's syndrome. *See* BONNEVIE-ULLRICH SYNDROME.

Ullrich-Turner syndrome. *See* BONNEVIE-ULLRICH SYNDROME.

Bonnevie-Ullrich syndrome in the male. A syndrome presented by males with normal genital and gonadal development but with the somatic anomalies of Turner's syndrome.

ulmin (ul·min). 1. $C_{40}H_{16}O_{14}$, a gum found in slippery elm, *Ulmus fulva*. 2. A compound in peat and coal resulting from organic decomposition. [see foll.]

Ulmus (ul·mus). A genus of trees (family Ulmaceae); the elms. **Ulmus fulva.** A species the dried inner bark of which contains a mucilage and is known as slippery elm. [L, elm.]

ulna [NA] (ul·na). The long and medial bone of the forearm. The upper end bears the olecranon and coronoid processes and articulates with the humerus and radius; the lower end possesses a head which articulates with the radius. [L, elbow.]

Head [caput ulnae (NA)]. The rounded part of the lower end of the ulna, bearing an articular surface distally for the articular disc in the wrist joint, and a semilunar articular surface on its anterior and lateral sides, the articular circumference [circumferentia articularis (NA)], for the ulnar notch of the radius.

Shaft [corpus ulnae]. The main part of the bone carrying the upper and lower ends. It is triangular in cross-section with a prominent interosseous border [margo interossea (NA)] for the interosseous membrane adjacent to the radius, and blunt anterior [margo anterior (NA)] and posterior [margo posterior (NA)] borders. The last named is subcutaneous and can be felt easily in the living from the olecranon above to the styloid process below. The anterior [facies anterior (NA)] and medial [facies medialis (NA)] surfaces, bounded by the interosseous and the anterior and posterior borders, respectively, give attachment to the flexor digitorum profundus and pronator quadratus muscles. The remaining surface [facies posterior (NA)] is for attachment of the deep extensor muscles of the forearm.

ulnar [ulnaris (NA)] (ul·nar). Referring to the ulna, or to the arteries and nerves associated with it. **Ulnar notch.** *See* NOTCH. **Ulnar phenomenon.** Analgesia of the ulnar nerve observed in certain psychoses.

ulnar artery [arteria ulnaris (NA)]. The larger of the two terminal branches of the brachial artery. It passes downwards and medially between the superficial and deep flexors of the forearm, enters the hand by passing superficial to the flexor retinaculum, and terminates as the superficial palmar arch. In the forearm, it gives off the ulnar recurrent artery [arteria recurrens ulnaris (NA)] (dividing into the anterior ulnar recurrent artery [ramus anterior (NA)] and the posterior ulnar recurrent artery [ramus posterior (NA)], and taking part in the anastomosis around the elbow) and then the large common interosseus artery [arteria interossea communis (NA)], which supplies an interosseous recurrent artery [arteria interossea recurrens (NA)], and then divides into the anterior [arteria interossea anterior (NA)] and posterior interosseous [arteria interossea posterior (NA)] arteries to supply the deep tissues of the front and back of the forearm. The ulnar artery supplies multiple palmar, carpal, and digital branches, and a deep branch [ramus palmaris profundus (NA)] that completes the deep palmar arch.

Anterior carpal branch [ramus carpeus palmaris (NA)]. *See* CARPAL ARCH, ANTERIOR (under ARCH).

Posterior carpal branch [ramus carpeus dorsalis (NA)]. *See* CARPAL ARCH, POSTERIOR (under ARCH).

ulnar collateral artery [arteria collateralis ulnaris superior (NA)] (ul·nar kol·at·er·al ar·ter·e). A small branch of the brachial artery that accompanies the ulnar nerve and takes part in the anastomosis around the elbow.

ulnar nerve [nervus ulnaris (NA)]. One of the principal nerves of the upper limb, arising from the medial cord of the brachial plexus and receiving fibres from the 8th cervical and 1st thoracic roots. It supplies the flexor carpi ulnaris and part of the flexor digitorum muscles in the forearm, and the muscles of the hypothenar eminence, the interosseous and adductor pollicis muscles and the medial two lumbrical muscles.

Deep terminal branch [ramus profundus (NA)]. One of the terminal branches of the ulnar nerve which passes deeply amongst the palmaris muscles (which it supplies) and then across the palm of the hand to supply the medial two lumbricals, the interosseous and adductor pollicis muscles.

Dorsal branch [ramus dorsalis nervi ulnaris (NA)]. A branch of the ulnar nerve, given off in the lower forearm and passing dorsally to supply the dorsum of the medial one and a half fingers or more [nervi digitales dorsales] and the corresponding part of the dorsum of the hand.

Muscular branches [rami musculares (NA)]. Branches to the flexor carpi ulnaris and flexor digitorum profundus muscles and the muscles of the hypothenar eminence.

Palmar branch [ramus palmaris nervi ulnaris (NA)]. The part of the nerve between the dorsal branch and the terminal branches.

Palmar cutaneous branch [ramus cutaneus palmaris (NA)]. A branch of the ulnar nerve given off in the forearm and passing down to supply the skin on the medial side of the palm.

Superficial terminal branch [ramus superficialis (NA)]. One of the terminal branches of the ulnar nerve, mainly cutaneous to the medial one and a half digits.

ulnar recurrent artery [arteria recurrens ulnaris (NA)] (ul·nar re·kur·ent ar·ter·e). *See* ULNAR ARTERY.

ulnar veins [venae ulnares (NA)]. Vessels accompanying the ulnar artery; they join with the radial veins to form the brachial veins.

ulnare (ul·na·re). The bone on the ulnar side of the proximal row of carpal bones.

ulnocarpal (ul·no·kar·pal). Concerning the ulna and the carpus, or denoting the ulnar part of the wrist.

ulnoradial (ul·no·ra·de·al). Relating to the ulna and the radius or to the ligaments and articulations thereof.

ulodermatitis (ew·lo·der·mat·i'·tis). Dermatitis with the formation of scar tissue. [Gk *oule* scar, dermatitis.]

uloid (ew·loid). 1. Having scar-like features, but not caused by a preceding superficial lesion. 2. A lesion resembling a scar in the deeper part of the skin, due to degeneration and characteristic of syphilis and lupus. [Gk *oule* scar, *eidos* form.]

ulosis (ew·lo·sis). The formation of a scar. [Gk *oule* scar, *-osis* condition.]

ulotic (ew·lot·ik). 1. Referring to a scar. 2. Concerning or causing scar formation. [Gk *oule* scar.]

ulotomy (ew·lot·o·me). 1. The incision of scarring tissue to prevent deformity. [Gk *oule* scar, *temnein* to cut.] 2. Incision of the gums. [Gk *oulon* gum, *temnein* to cut.]

ulotriches (ew·lot·rik·eez). One of Haeckel's two main types of mankind, indicating races with woolly hair. Cf. LEIOTRICHES. [see foll.]

ulotrichous (ew·lot·rik·us). Characterized by woolly hair, as in the negro. Cf. LEIOTRICHOUS. [Gk *oulos* crisp, *thrix* hair.]

ultex (ul·tex). A form of multifocal spectacle lens, made by grinding two or more different curves on one of its surfaces.

ultracentrifuge (ul·trah·sen·trif·ewj). Any high-speed centrifuge that gives a centrifugal force 100 000 times gravity, or greater. [L *ultra* beyond, centrifuge.]

ultrafiltration (ul·trah·fil·tra'·shun). Filtration through collodion membranes of known pore diameter by which viruses or other colloid particles with a mean diameter larger than a given value may be held back. [L *ultra* beyond, filter.]

ultraligation (ul·trah·lig·a'·shun). The ligation of an artery distal to the origin of one of its branches. [L *ultra* beyond, ligation.]

ultramicrochemistry (ul·trah·mi·kro·kem'·is·tre). Chemical experiments, e.g. analysis, atomic-weight determinations, employing minute quantities of compounds. [L *ultra* beyond, microchemistry.]

ultramicron (ul·trah·mi·kron). The least particle that can be seen under an ultramicroscope; a colloid particle 5 nm (5×10^{-9} m) in diameter. [L *ultra* beyond, micron.]

ultramicroscope (ul·trah·mi·kro·skope). An arrangement whereby a strong beam of light is focused on to a liquid being examined under an ordinary microscope. The beam is at right angles to the optical axis of the microscope. By this method particles beyond the range of the ordinary microscope can be seen as illuminated specks. [L *ultra* beyond, microscope.]

ultramicroscopic, ultramicroscopical (ul·trah·mi·kro·skop'·ik, ul·trah·mi·kro·skop'·ik·al). 1. Concerned with the ultramicroscope or ultramicroscopy. 2. Applied to anything that is beyond the range of the ordinary microscope but within that of the ultramicroscope.

ultramicroscopy (ul·trah·mi·kros'·ko·pe). The technique and use of the ultramicroscope.

ultrared (ul·trah·red). Infrared. [Obsolete term.] [L *ultra* beyond, AS *read.*]

ultrashortwave (ul·trah·short·wave). A form of diathermy using ultra-high-frequency currents. [L *ultra* beyond, AS *sceort, wafian.*]

ultrasome (ul·trah·some). Anything too small to be seen in the microscope. [L *ultra* beyond, Gk *soma* body.]

ultrasonic (ul·trah·son·ik). Ultrasound. **Ultrasonic diathermy.** *See* DIATHERMY. **Ultrasonic tomography.** *See* TOMOGRAPHY. [see foll.]

ultrasonics (ul·trah·son·ix). Ultrasound; the science of sound waves of so high a frequency that they cannot be appreciated by the human ear. *High-intensity ultrasonics.* Used to produce cavitation, heating, drilling, etc., often producing irreversible changes in tissues. *Low-intensity ultrasonics.* Used to investigate the physical properties of tissues without causing permanent damage. [L *ultra* beyond, *sonus* sound.]

ultrasonocardiography (ul·trah·son·o·kar·de·og'·raf·e). Echocardiography. [L *ultra* beyond, *sonus* sound, Gk *kardia* heart, *graphein* to record.]

ultrasonogram (ul·trah·son·o·gram). The recording obtained with ultrasonic cameras. [ultrasonic, Gk *gramma* record.]

ultrasonography (ul·trah·son·og'·raf·e). A display of ultrasonic echoes particularly used in the examination of soft tissues. The recording is one-dimensional in the A-scan, and two-dimensional in the B-scan. Three-dimensional images can be obtained by the complex technique of ultrasonic holography. [L *ultra* beyond, *sonus* sound, Gk *graphein* to record.]

ultrasound (ul·trah·sownd). Ultrasonics or ultrasonic waves. Used *diagnostically* in such techniques as echo-encephalography, biometry and measurement of the fetus. Used *therapeutically*, for example, in the removal of scar tissue as in Dupuytren's contracture, the resolution of haematoma, and the destruction of the vestibular apparatus in Ménière's disease. [L *ultra* beyond, sound.]

ultrasonotherapy (ul·trah·son·o·ther'·ap·e). Use of ultrasound or ultrasonic waves in treatment. [ultrasonics, therapy.]

ultratoxon (ul·trah·tox·on). A toxin with a low degree of combining power. [L *ultra* beyond, toxin.]

ultraviolet (ul·trah·vi·o·let). Rays found immediately beyond the violet end of the visible spectrum, with wavelengths extending to the x-rays, i.e. from 390 to 20 nm (3900–200 Å). They have powerful photochemical and photoerythemal effects; biotic rays. They are necessary or helpful to normal growth, promoting the vitamin D calcium metabolism. **Far ultraviolet.** Ultraviolet rays with wavelengths extending from 290 to 20 nm (2900–200 Å); abiotic rays. **Near ultraviolet.** Ultraviolet rays with wavelengths extending from 390 to 290 nm (3900–2900 Å;) the biotic rays. [L *ultra* beyond, OFr. *violette.*]

ululation (ul·ew·**la**·shun). Hysterical wailing in certain psychotic conditions. [L *ululare* to howl.]

Umbelliferae (**um**·bel·**if**·er·ae). A family of plants to which the parsley, carrot and parsnip belong; they bear white or yellow flowers in umbels. [L *umbella* sunshade, *ferre* to bear.]

umbelliferone (um·bel·**if**·er·one). 4-Hydroxycinnamic acid lactone, $OHC_6H_3CHCHCOO$. A derivative of α-pyrone which occurs in the bark of the spurge laurel and which is obtained from the resinous matter of species of *Ferula* (family Umbelliferae). Its formation and characteristic blue fluorescence with ammonia is used to distinguish asafoetida and galbanum from the similar oleo gum resin, ammoniacum. [L *umbella* sunshade, *ferre* to bear.]

Umbellularia (**um**·bel·ew·**la'**·re·ah). A genus of trees of the family Laurineae. **Umbellularia californica.** Californian laurel, California sassafras, spice tree; an evergreen shade tree of California, the leaves of which yield on distillation a brownish volatile oil containing pinene, cineole, eugenol, and umbellulone. [dim. of L *umbella* sunshade.]

umbellulone (um·**bel**·ew·lone). A ketone which occurs in the volatile oil derived from the Californian laurel, *Umbellularia californica.*

umbilectomy (um·bil·**ek**·to·me). Surgical removal of the umbilicus. [umbilicus, Gk *ektome* excision.]

umbilical (um·**bil**·ik·al, um·bil·i·kal). Concerning the umbilicus. **Umbilical ligaments.** *See* LIGAMENT.

umbilical artery [arteria umbilicalis (NA)]. A continuation of the internal iliac artery of the fetus, passing along the deep surface of the anterior abdominal wall to the umbilicus where it enters the umbilical cord and carries deoxygenated blood to the placenta. It is converted to a fibrous cord, the lateral umbilical ligament, after birth.

umbilical vein [vena umbilicalis sinistra (NA)]. The single vein draining the placenta, corresponding to the left member of a pair present in the first third of fetal life. It empties via the ductus venosus into the inferior vena cava.

umbilicate, umbilicated (um·**bil**·ik·ate, **um**·bil·ik·**a'**·ted). Resembling the umbilicus in shape; dimpled; possessing a pit, like the umbilicus.

umbilication (**um**·bil·ik·**a'**·shun). 1. Being or becoming umbilicate. 2. Any depression resembling the umbilicus in form.

umbilicus [NA] (um·**bil**·ik·us, um·bil·i·kus). The navel; the cicatricial depression in the surface of the abdomen where, in the fetus, the umbilical cord was attached. **Decidual umbilicus.** A small scar appearing on the ovum after becoming embedded in the decidua and thought to be the site of the decidua capsularis. **Posterior umbilicus.** Pilonidal sinus, a sinus in the coccyx marked by a hairy tuft. [L, navel.]

umbo (**um**·bo) (pl. *umbones*). Any convex projection on a surface. **Umbo of the tympanic membrane [umbo membranae tympani (NA)].** The projection on the inner surface of the ear-drum where the handle of the malleus is attached. [L, boss.]

umbonate (**um**·bo·nate). Resembling an umbo; possessing a knob or convex elevation.

umbonation (um·bo·**na**·shun). The development of rounded eminences like umbones.

Uncaria (un·**ka**·re·ah). A genus of rubiaceous tropical plants. **Uncaria gambier.** The species which yields pale catechu (gambir), a dried aqueous extract prepared from the leaves and twigs. [L *uncus* hook.]

unchuca (un·**chuk**·ah). The local name in Argentina for *Triatoma infestans,* a vector of *Trypanosoma cruzi.*

unciform (**un**·se·form). Hook-like. **Unciform bone.** The hook-shaped bone in the carpus; the hamate bone. [L *uncus* hook, form.]

unciforme (un·se·**for**·me). The hamate bone of the wrist which has a hook-like process. [see prec.]

uncinal (**un**·sin·al). Uncinate.

uncinariasis, uncinariosis (**un**·sin·ar·**i'**·as·is, **un**·sin·a·re·**o'**·sis). Obsolete terms for ancylostomiasis or hookworm disease. [LL *uncinus* hook, Gk *-osis* condition.]

uncinate (**un**·sin·ate). Hooked. [LL *uncinus,* hook.]

uncipressure (**un**·se·presh·er). Pressure with a blunt hook on a blood vessel to stop bleeding. [L *uncus* hook, pressure.]

unconscious (un·**kon**·shus). 1. In a state of unconsciousness. 2. Pertaining to "the unconscious". 3. In psycho-analysis, that part of the mind inaccessible to deliberately directed thought and containing repressed wishes. [see foll.]

unconsciousness (un·**kon**·shus·nes). The state in which the higher functions of the cerebrum are in abeyance, and there is a lack of appreciation of sensory impulses reaching the cerebrum. This may be physiological, as in sleep, or pathological, as in conditions interfering with the blood supply (temporarily as in fainting, or persistent as with compression). It may also be due to toxic causes. Severe unconsciousness, in which the patient cannot be roused, is termed *coma.* [AS *un-* not, L *conscius* aware.]

unction (**ungk**·shun). 1. An ointment. 2. The process of anointing. [L *ungere* to anoint.]

unctuous (**ungk**·tew·us). Oily. [see prec.]

uncus [NA] (**ung**·kus). The hook-like anterior end of the hippocampal gyrus on the medial side of the temporal lobe of the cerebrum. [L, hook.]

undecane (**un**·dek·ane). $C_{11}H_{24}$, a saturated hydrocarbon, eleventh in the homologous series of paraffins. It is a colourless liquid which occurs in petroleum. [L *undecim* eleven.]

under-compensation (**un**·der·kom·pen·**sa'**·shun). In cardiology, the state of affairs when the heart functions without evidence of failure despite the presence of heart disease, usually valvular. [AS *under,* L *compensare* to weigh together.]

undercut (**un**·der·kut). A condition produced by overhanging tissue. In dentistry, the condition of a cavity prepared in a tooth so as to provide retention for a filling. [AS *under,* ME *cut.*]

underexposure (**un**·der·ex·**po'**·zewr). A radiographic term used to describe a radiograph that has been made with too small a quantity of x-rays, usually in the milliampere-seconds range. [AS *under,* L *exponere* to lay out.]

underhung, underjawed (**un**·der·hung, **un**·der·jawd). Describing a lower jaw which projects beyond the maxilla. Inferior protrusion. [AS *under, hangian.*]

under-nutrition (**un**·der·new·**trish'**·un). Inadequate nutrition from any cause. [AS *under,* nutrition.]

under-penetration (**un**·der·pen·e·**tra'**·shun). A radiographic term denoting the use of too small a kilovoltage, so that the radiograph lacks contrast. [AS *under,* L *penetrare* to penetrate.]

under-productivity (**un**·der·prod·uk·**tiv'**·it·e). Diminution and retardation of mental activity. [AS *under,* productivity.]

undertaker (**un**·der·ta·ker). A person who attends to the preparation of the dead for burial and the funeral arrangements. [AS *under, tacan.*]

undertoe (**un**·der·to). Displacement of the big toe under the outer toes. [AS *under,* toe.]

under-ventilation (**un**·der·ven·til·**a'**·shun). A state in which tidal exchange in the lungs is inadequate to keep the blood gases within normal limits. [AS *under,* L *ventilare* to wave.]

Underwood, Michael (b. 1737). London physician.

Underwood's disease. Sclerema neonatorum.

undifferentiation (**un**·dif·er·en·she·**a'**·shun). The return of cells to a lower and more primitive form, as in malignancy. [AS *un-* not, differentiate.]

undine (**un**·deen). A small glass vessel used in irrigation of the eye. [see foll.]

undinism (un·din·izm). Sexual excitation aroused by running water, urine, or the act of urination. [L *unda* wave.]

undulant (un·dew·lant). Wave-like; rising and falling as with waves; fluctuating. [see prec.]

undulation (un·dew·la·shun). A wave, vibration, oscillation, or fluctuation. **Jugular undulation.** The venous pulse. **Respiratory undulation.** The rhythmic cycle of changes in blood pressure that accompanies respiration. [L *unda* wave.]

unfit to plead (un·fit to pleed). Said of a person whose state of mind at the time of the trial was such that he (or she) was unable to understand the nature of the charge or the proceedings, to instruct counsel or to challenge a juror. This is decided by a duly sworn jury after having medical evidence.

ungual (ung·gwal). 1. Concerning the finger nails. 2. Resembling a finger nail in form. [L *unguis* nail.]

unguent (ung·gwent). An ointment. [L *ungere* to anoint.]

unguentum (ung·gwen·tum) (pl. *unguenta*). Ointment. Prior to the *British Pharmacopoeia* of 1953, all official ointments were classed as unguenta. **Unguentum acidi benzoici compositum.** Compound ointment of benzoic acid. *See* OINTMENT. **Unguentum acidi borici.** Ointment of boric acid. **Unguentum Acidi Borici Flavum BPC 1949.** Yellow ointment of boric acid; boric acid in yellow soft paraffin. **Unguentum acidi carbolici.** Unguentum phenolis (see below). **Unguentum acidi salicyli.** Salicylic acid ointment. *See* OINTMENT. **Unguentum acidi salicyli et sylphuris.** Ointment of salicylic acid and sulphur. **Unguentum Acidi Tannici BPC 1949.** Ointment of tannic acid, an ointment consisting of tannic acid, glycerin, and simple ointment; it is used as an external application in the treatment of haemorrhoids, anal prolapse, and for some forms of ulcer. **Unguentum Adipis Lanae Hydrosi BPC 1949.** Ointment of hydrous wool fat, lanolin ointment, an ointment consisting of a mixture of hydrous wool fat and soft paraffin; it is used as a skin emollient, and as a hydrous ointment base. **Unguentum alcoholium lanae.** Wool alcohols ointment. *See* OINTMENT. **Unguentum Aquae Rosae BPC 1949.** Ointment of rosewater, cold cream; a water-in-oil emulsion of rosewater, white beeswax, borax, almond oil, and oil of rose; it is used as an emollient for chapped and irritated skin, also as a base for more active ingredients. **Unguentum argenti nitratis compositum.** An ointment consisting of silver nitrate and Peru balsam in yellow soft paraffin; it has been used in the treatment of eczema. **Unguentum Belladonnae BPC 1949.** An ointment composed of liquid extract of belladonna in a basis of wool fat and benzoinated lard; it has a mild anodyne action and is applied externally to allay pain, though of doubtful value. **Unguentum benzocanae compositum.** Compound ointment of benzocaine. *See* OINTMENT. **Unguentum betulae compositum.** Compound ointment of methyl salicylate. *See* OINTMENT. **Unguentum calaminae.** Ointment of calamine. *See* OINTMENT. **Unguentum calaminae compositum.** Compound ointment of calamine. *See* OINTMENT. **Unguentum Camphorae Durum BPC 1949.** Hard ointment of camphor, camphor ice, camphor in a mixture of hard and soft paraffins, used as a rubefacient and mild counter-irritant. **Unguentum capsici.** Ointment of capsicum. **Unguentum Capsici Compositum BPC 1949.** Compound ointment of capsicum, chilli paste, an ointment of oleoresin of capsicum with menthol, chloral hydrate, and camphor, in soft paraffin; it is used as a counter-irritant in the treatment of rheumatism, lumbago, and neuralgia. **Unguentum Cetacei BPC 1949.** Ointment of spermaceti, spermaceti in white beeswax and liquid paraffin, used as a basis for ointments. **Unguentum Chrysarobini BPC 1949.** Ointment of chrysarobin, chrysarobin in a simple ointment base; it is used in the treatment of psoriasis, ringworm, and other skin diseases, but it may irritate the skin and, if large quantities are absorbed, may lead to renal irritation. **Unguentum Cinchocainae Compositum BPC 1949.** Compound ointment of cinchocaine, an ointment consisting of cinchocaine with aluminium acetate solution and hamamelis in a basis of soft paraffin and wool fat; it is used for its local anaesthetic and astringent properties. **Unguentum colophonii.** Ointment of colophony. **Unguentum dithranolis.** Dithranol ointment. *See* OINTMENT. **Unguentum dithranolis forte.** Strong dithranol ointment. *See* OINTMENT. **Unguentum emulsificans.** Emulsifying ointment. *See* OINTMENT. **Unguentum Eucalypti BPC 1949.** Ointment of eucalyptus, an ointment consisting of oil of eucalyptus in hard and soft paraffins; it has been used in the treatment of first-degree burns. **Unguentum gallae.** Ointment of gall. **Unguentum gallae et opio.** Ointment of gall and opium. **Unguentum Glycerini Plumbi Subacetatis BPC 1949.** Ointment of glycerin of lead subacetate, an ointment consisting of glycerin of lead subacetate in a paraffin ointment base; it is used as an emollient and astringent in the treatment of eczema, pruritus, and haemorrhoids. **Unguentum hamamelidis.** Hamamelis ointment. *See* OINTMENT. **Unguentum hydrargyri ammoniati.** Ammoniated mercury ointment. *See* OINTMENT. **Unguentum hydrargyri ammoniati et picis carbonis.** Ointment of ammoniated mercury and coal tar. **Unguentum hydrargyri compositum.** Compound ointment of mercury. *See* OINTMENT. **Unguentum hydrargyri dilutum.** Dilute ointment of mercury. *See* OINTMENT. **Unguentum hydrargyri nitratis dilutum.** Dilute ointment of mercuric nitrate. *See* OINTMENT. **Unguentum hydrargyri nitratis forte.** Strong ointment of mercuric nitrate. *See* OINTMENT. **Unguentum hydrargyri oleati.** Ointment of oleated mercury. **Unguentum hydrargyri oxidi flavi.** Pagenstecher's ointment, golden ointment, yellow mercuric oxide ointment, an ointment composed of yellow mercuric oxide in yellow soft paraffin, chiefly used for conjunctivitis and blepharitis, especially styes. It has mild antiseptic properties. **Unguentum Hydrargyri Oxidi Rubri BPC 1949.** Red mercuric oxide ointment, an ointment consisting of red mercuric oxide in a paraffin ointment base; it is used in seborrhoea, alopecia, and as a parasiticide. It is too irritant to be employed ophthalmically. **Unguentum Hydrargyri, Plumbi et Zinci BPC 1949.** Ointment of mercury, lead, and zinc, an ointment composed of strong ointment of mercuric nitrate, ointment of lead subacetate, and zinc ointment. **Unguentum Hydrargyri Subchloridi BP 1948.** Calomel ointment, a mixture of mercurous chloride in simple ointment; it has a disinfectant and antisyphilitic action, and has been used locally as a prophylactic against syphilis, though it is not entirely reliable. It has also been used in various ulcerated conditions, more especially venereal ulcer. **Unguentum hydrocortisoni.** Hydrocortisone ointment. *See* OINTMENT. **Unguentum hydrocortisoni acetatis.** Hydrocortisone acetate ointment. *See* OINTMENT. **Unguentum ichthammolis.** Ointment of ichthammol. **Unguentum Iodi BPC 1949.** Ointment of iodine, an ointment prepared by dissolving iodine in water with potassium iodide and incorporating in a simple ointment base; it may be used as a counter-irritant in the treatment of fibrositis, chilblains, and swollen or inflamed glands. **Unguentum iodi denigrescens.** Non-staining ointment of iodine. *See* OINTMENT. **Unguentum iodi denigrescens cum methylis salicylate.** Non-staining ointment of iodine with methyl salicylate. *See* OINTMENT. **Unguentum Kaolini BPC 1949.** Ointment of kaolin, an ointment composed of kaolin in a hard paraffin base; it allays irritation when applied to abraded skin. **Unguentum lanolini.** Unguentum Adipis Lanae Hydrosi (see above). **Unguentum metallorum.** Unguentum Hydrargyri, Plumbi et Zinci (see above). **Unguentum methylis salicylatis.** Ointment of methyl salicylate. **Unguentum methylis salicylatis compositum.** Compound ointment of methyl salicylate. *See* OINTMENT. **Unguentum methylis salicylatis compositum forte.** Compound ointment of methyl salicylate. *See* OINTMENT. **Unguentum methylis salicylatis forte.** Ointment of methyl salicylate. **Unguentum Olei Cadini BPC 1949.** Ointment of oil of cade, an ointment consisting of oil of cade in a beeswax and soft paraffin base; it is used in the treatment of psoriasis, eczema, and seborrhoeic conditions of the scalp. **Unguentum oleoresinae capsici compositum.** Unguentum Capsici Compositum (see above). **Unguentum paraffini.** Paraffin ointment. *See* OINTMENT. **Unguentum penicillini.** Ointment of penicillin. *See* OINTMENT. **Unguentum Phenolis BP 1948.** An ointment of phenol in lard and paraffin base; it has been largely used as an antipruritic in various skin diseases, and for its local analgesic action. Phenol has little antiseptic or caustic action when dissolved in an oily base. **Unguentum physostigminae.** Physostigmine ointment. *See* OINTMENT. **Unguentum picis carbonis compositum.** Ointment of ammoniated mercury and coal tar. **Unguentum picis liquidae.** Ointment of tar. **Unguentum Plumbi Subacetis BPC 1949.** Ointment of lead subacetate, an ointment prepared from strong solution of lead subacetate in a wool fat, hard paraffin and white soft paraffin base; it is used for its astringent and protective action on the skin. **Unguentum potassi polysulphidi.** Danish ointment, Marcussen's ointment, Lomholt's ointment, potassium polysulphide ointment, an ointment composed of polysulphides of potassium, zinc hydroxide, and benzaldehyde in a wool fat and paraffin base; it has been used in the treatment of scabies. **Unguentum resinae.** Ointment of colophony. **Unguentum resorcini.** Unguentum Resorcinolis (see below). **Unguentum resorcini et bismuthi compositum.** Unguentum Resorcinolis et bismuth Compositum (see below). **Unguentum resorcini compositum.** Compound ointment of resorcinol. *See* OINTMENT. **Unguentum Resorcinolis BPC 1949.** Ointment of resorcinol, an ointment composed of resorcinol and glycerin in a wool fat and white soft paraffin base; it is used in the treatment of psoriasis, eczema, seborrhoea, and other skin affections. **Unguentum resorcinolis et acidi salicylici.** Castellani's ointment, an ointment composed of resorcinol and salicylic acid in a lanolin and soft paraffin base; it is used for the treatment of dhobie itch and other fungal diseases of the skin. **Unguentum Resorcinolis et Bismuthi Compositum BPC 1949.** Compound ointment of resorcinol and bismuth, an ointment containing resorcinol, zinc oxide, bismuth oxychloride, cade oil, and starch as important constituents; it is used in the treatment of fungal diseases of the skin. **Unguentum resorcinolis compositum.** Compound ointment of resorcinol. *See* OINTMENT. **Unguentum rubri scarlatini, unguentum rubrum.** Ointment of scarlet red. **Unguentum Rusci Compositum BPC 1949.** Compound ointment of birch tar, an ointment composed of birch-tar oil with resorcinol, zinc oxide, and starch, in a hydrous ointment and wool fat base. It is used in the treatment of eczema and psoriasis. **Unguentum salol cum menthol.** An ointment of salol and menthol in an olive and wool fat base; it is used in fissures of the skin, e.g. chapped hands. **Unguentum sedativum.** Compound ointment of calamine. *See* OINTMENT. **Unguentum simplex.** Simple ointment. *See* OINTMENT. **Unguentum sodii perboratis.** Sodium perborate ointment. *See* OINTMENT. **Unguentum sulphuris.** Sulphur ointment. *See* OINTMENT. **Unguentum thymolis.** Thymol ointment. *See* OINTMENT. **Unguentum undecylenati.** Zinc undecenoate ointment. *See* OINTMENT. **Unguentum zinci.** Zinc ointment. *See* OINTMENT. **Unguentum zinci et olei ricini.** Zinc and castor oil ointment. *See* OINTMENT. **Unguentum Zinci Oxidi cum Benzoino BPC 1949.** Ointment of zinc oxide with benzoin, an ointment prepared from compound tincture of benzoin in ointment of zinc oxide; it is used to stimulate the healing of small fissures and ulcers, and of cracked nipples. [L.]

unguiculate (ung·**gwik**·ew·late). Possessing nails, or in the case of animals, denoting those with claws. [see foll.]

unguiculus (ung·**gwik**·ew·lus). A diminutive nail or claw. [L, a small nail.]

unguinal (**ung**·gwin·al). Concerning the nails; ungual. [L *unguis* nail.]

unguis (**ung**·gwis). 1. The inelastic, translucent, horny plate formed of flat cornified epidermal cells, classified as an epidermal appendage and commonly known as a nail. *See* NAIL. 2. An old name for what is now termed *hypopyon*, or pus in the anterior chamber of the eye, so-called because the outline was shaped like the crescent of white at the base of the finger nail; onyx. **Unguis incarnatus.** An ingrowing nail. [L.]

ungula (**ung**·gew·lah). In obstetrics, an instrument used to extract a dead fetus from the uterus. [L, claw, hoof.]

Ungulata (ung·gew·**la**·tah). A zoological class that includes all hooved animals. [see prec.]

uni-articular (ew·ne·ar·**tik**'·ew·lar). Relating to one joint; monarticular. [see foll.]

uni-articulate (ew·ne·ar·**tik**'·ew·late). Possessing only a single joint. [L *unus* one, articulation.]

uni-aural (ew·ne·**aw**·ral). Concerned with only one ear. [L *unus* one, *auris* ear.]

uni-axial (ew·ne·**ax**·e·al). 1. Possessing only one axis, as of hinge joints. 2. Growing out or progressing in only one direction. [L *unus* one, axis.]

unibasal (ew·ne·**ba**·sal). Possessing a single base. [L *unus* one, base.]

unicamerate (ew·ne·**kam**·er·ate). Characterized by one cavity only. [L *unus* one, *camera* chamber.]

unicellular (ew·ne·**sel**·ew·lar). Composed of a single cell. [L *unus* one, cell.]

unicentral (ew·ne·**sen**·tral). Possessing one centre, as in growth or ossification. [L *unus* one, centre.]

uniceps (**ew**·ne·seps). Anything that has a single head or origin, as in the case of certain muscles. [L *unus* one, *caput* head.]

unicorn (**ew**·ne·korn). Unicornous.

unicornous (ew·ne·**kor**·nus). Possessing only one horn or cornu. *See* HORN. [L *unus* one, *cornu* horn.]

unicuspid, unicuspidate (ew·ne·**kus**·pid, ew·ne·**kus**·pid·ate). Possessing only one point or cusp; a tooth which has a single cusp, such as an incisor or canine. [L *unus* one, *cuspis* point.]

unifamilial (**ew**·ne·fam·**il**'·e·al). Occurring in one family only. [L *unus* one, *familia* family.]

unifilar (ew·ne·**fi**·lar). 1. Possessing only one thread or filament. 2. Attached by a single thread or filament. [L *unus* one, *filum* thread.]

uniflagellate (ew·ne·**flaj**·el·ate). Furnished with only a single flagellum. [L *unus* one, flagellum.]

unifocal (ew·ne·**fo**·kal). Capable of being brought to a single focus; having only one focus. [L *unus* one, focus.]

unigeminal (ew·ne·**jem**·in·al). Concerning only one of twins. [L *unus* one, *geminus* twin.]

unigerminal (ew·ne·**jer**·min·al). Relating to a single ovum or germ. [L *unus* one, germ.]

uniglandular (ew·ne·**glan**·dew·lar). Concerned with or composed of a single gland. [L *unus* one, gland.]

unigravida (ew·ne·**grav**·id·ah). Describing a woman in her first pregnancy. [L *unus* one, *gravida* pregnant.]

unilaminar, unilaminate (ew·ne·**lam**·in·ar, ew·ne·**lam**·in·ate). Composed of only one layer. [L *unus* one, *lamina* layer.]

unilateral (ew·ne·**lat**·er·al). One-sided; involving one side only. [L *unus* one, *latus* side.]

unilobar, unilobed (ew·ne·**lo**·bar, ew·ne·**lo**·bd). Composed of one lobe only. [L *unus* one, lobe.]

unilocular (ew·ne·**lok**·ew·lar). Characterized by a single loculus or cavity. [L *unus* one, *loculus* compartment.]

uninuclear, uninucleated (ew·ne·**new**·kle·ar, ew·ne·**new**·kle·a·-ted). Possessing a single nucleus. [L *unus* one, nucleus.]

uni-ocular (ew·ne·**ok**·ew·lar). Concerning or possessing a single eye. [L *unus* one, *oculus* eye.]

union (**ew**·ne·on). 1. The joining of anything. 2. The joining together of tissues; healing. **Bony union.** 1. A fracture healed by the laying-down of new bone. 2. The union of two bones at a joint, following disease, injury, or operation. **Delayed union.** Healing of a fracture which appears to be unduly slow. **False union.** Healing of a fracture by scar tissue only. **Faulty union.** A condition where tissues have joined together but not in their correct positions. **Immediate union, primary union.** Healing which occurs promptly and without complicating infection; healing by first intention. **Mal-union.** Faulty union (see above). **Non-union.** A fracture in which the opposing fracture surfaces have become sclerosed and remain ununited. **Syngamic nuclear union.** The fusion of the nuclei of spermatozoon and ovum during fertilization. [L *unus* one.]

uni-oval, uni-ovular (ew·ne·**o**·val, ew·ne·**ov**·ew·lar). Concerning a single ovum; developing from a single ovum as with certain twins. [L *unus* one, ovum.]

unipara (ew·**nip**·ar·ah). A woman who has given birth once only. [L *unus* one, *parere* to bear.]

uniparous (ew·**nip**·ar·us). 1. Referring to a unipara. 2. Normally producing one offspring at a birth. [see prec.]

unipolar (ew·ne·**po**·lar). 1. Possessing a single pole, as in the case of certain nerve cells. 2. Located at one pole or tip. [L *unus* one, pole.]

unipotent, unipotential (ew·**nip**·o·tent, ew·ne·po·**ten**'·shal). Describing a cell whose fate has been completely determined so that it is capable of only one line of development. [L *unus* one, *potens* able.]

uniseptate (ew·ne·**sep**·tate). Provided with a single septum. [L *unus* one, septum.]

unisexual (ew·ne·**sex**·ew·al). 1. Concerning one sex only. 2. Having one sex, or the reproductive organs of only one sex. [L *unus* one, sex.]

unit (**ew**·nit). 1. Anything which may be regarded as single and complete in itself, and into which larger and more complex structures may be broken down, e.g. hexose unit, amino-acid unit, unit of society. 2. Any standard by means of which a thing may be measured. **Alexinic unit.** Minimum haemolytic dose of complement. *See* DOSE. **Amboceptor unit.** Minimum haemolytic dose of amboceptor. *See* DOSE. **Antigen unit.** The smallest quantity of antigen that will fix one minimum haemolytic dose of complement. **Antitoxic unit, antitoxic serum unit,** au. A unit or "yard-stick" for expressing the potency of an antitoxin. First introduced by Ehrlich (1897) for diphtheria antitoxin, this unit is now defined as a certain weight of a dried diphtheria antitoxin, preserved as an international standard at the direction of the League of Nations Health Commission. This serum was compared with Ehrlich's standard serum to maintain continuity of unitage; Ehrlich's original unit was defined as the smallest amount of diphtheria antitoxin that would neutralize 100 times the guinea-pig minimal lethal dose of toxin (one particular toxic filtrate). The unit of tetanus antitoxin was originally defined as that amount of antitoxin which would protect a guinea-pig against 1000 fatal doses of toxin. A considerable number of *units* have now been set up for antisera and microbic products. These units have been arbitrarily chosen as measured amounts of standard preparations, for which the World Health Organization is responsible. **Atomic mass unit.** One-twelfth of the mass of a neutral atom of carbon-12. Symbol amu. **Atomic weight unit.** One-twelfth of the mean mass of the neutral atoms of naturally occurring carbon. Symbol awu. **Avena unit.** The unit of plant growth hormone in use before pure crystalline auxins were available. **British thermal unit** (B.Th.U) an obsolete unit of heat being the amount of heat required to raise the temperature of one pound of water 1° F. It is equal to about 1055 joules. **Cardiac care unit.** A hospital unit designed for the expert care of severe cardiac disease, e.g. infarction. **Cat unit.** A unit of biological standardization, defined as the potency of a digitalis preparation which is just lethal enough to kill a cat intravenously, divided by the animal's weight in kilograms, i.e. dose per kilogram. It is now obsolete. **Centimetre-gram-second unit (cgs unit).** Any unit of the centimetre-gram-second system of physical units. **Cobalt 60 beam therapy unit.** An apparatus for irradiating a patient at a distance (usually several cm) with a beam of radiation from a large source of radioactive cobalt (^{60}Co). **Coincidence unit.** In radiation technique, a device which counts coincident pulses produced by the simultaneous occurrence of two atomic particles at a particular point. **Columbia unit.** A unit for the measurement of bacitracin. **Complement unit.** Minimum haemolytic dose of complement. *See* DOSE. **Cornell unit of riboflavine.** A unit equal to 1 μg of the vitamin. **Dental unit.** 1. A complicated apparatus embodying the instruments and machinery necessary for carrying out the practice of operative dental surgery. 2. A single tooth. **Digitalis unit.** The specific activity contained in such an amount of the standard preparation of digitalis as the Medical Research Council may from time to time indicate as the quantity exactly equivalent to the unit accepted for international use. **Unit of electrical capacitance.** The farad; the capacitance of a capacitor the potential of which is raised one volt by a charge of one coulomb. **Unit of electrical current.** The ampere; that constant current which, if maintained in two parallel conductors of infinite length, of negligible circular cross-section, and placed one metre apart in vacuum, would produce between these conductors a force equal to 2×10^{-7} newton per metre length. **Unit of electrical quantity.** The coulomb; the amount of electricity passed by a current of one ampere in one second. **Unit of electricity.** Any of the units employed in electrical measurements. The practical ones are the ampere (current), the coulomb (quantity), the volt (electromotive force), the ohm (resistance), the farad (capacity), the henry (inductance), and watt (power). **Electromagnetic unit (emu).** Any fundamental electrical unit of the cgs system. **Unit of electromotive force.** The volt; the potential difference between two points of a conducting wire carrying a constant current of one ampere, when the power dissipated between these points is equal to one watt. **Electrostatic unit (esu).** Any fundamental electrical unit based upon the unit electrostatic charge of the cgs system. **Unit of energy or work.** The joule; the work done when the point of application of a force of one newton moves a distance of one metre in the direction of the force. **Energy unit.** The original name suggested for the *roentgen-equivalent physical* or *rep.* **Unit of force.** The newton; the force which gives to a mass of one kilogram an acceleration of one metre per second, per second. **Frog unit.** In animal experiments, the smallest amount of digitalis that, given to a frog weighing 30 g, will bring about its death in 30 min. **Gram-roentgen unit of dose.** A unit of total energy absorption for ionizing radiation. The energy absorbed per gram of substance composed of light elements is approximately independent of the precise atomic composition, and in particular the energy absorption in tissue is approximately the same as in air. Since the roentgen is a unit of energy absorption per unit mass of air and corresponds to 83.8×10^{-7} joule/gram (83.8 erg/gram), the total energy absorbed may l expressed as the product of dose in roentgens times irradiated mass, in gram-roentgen units. One gram-roentgen thus equals 83.8×10^{-7} joules (83.8 ergs). **Haemolytic unit.** Minimum haemolytic dose of amboceptor. *See* DOSE. **Haemorrhagin unit.** That quantity of viper venom which will produce haemorrhages in the vascular network of a 3-day chick embryo. **Unit of heat.** The same as the unit of energy or work (see above). In the cgs system, the calorie; the amount of heat which will raise the temperature of one gram of water 1°C, and is equal to approximately 4.2 joules. **Immunizing unit,** iu. Antitoxic unit (see above). **Intensive care unit.** A department of a modern hospital specializing in the care of acutely ill patients, mainly those with respiratory, cardiac, renal or nervous abnormalities, and those suffering from multiple injuries or trauma, where sophisticated methods of management and monitoring are employed. **International unit of antitoxin,** iu. Antitoxic unit (see above). **International unit of gonadotropic activity.** 1. Chorionic gonadotrophin; the specific activity contained in 0.1 mg of a standard preparation. 2. Serum gonadotrophin; the specific activity contained in 0.25 mg of a standard preparation. Both standard preparations are stored at the National Institute for Medical Research, London. **International unit of heat.** The quantity of heat necessary to raise the temperature of one gram of water from 14.5°C to 15.5°C; the gram-calorie, now being replaced by the joule. **International insulin unit.** The specific activity contained in 0.0455 mg of pure, dried, crystalline insulin hydrochloride. Variation in the amount of standard preparation may be indicated from time to time by the Medical Research Council, London. **International unit of male hormone.** The specific activity contained in 0.1 mg of pure androsterone. **International unit of penicillin.** The activity of 0.6 μg of a sample of dried crystalline benzylpenicillin. Pure sodium benzylpenicillin contains 1675 units per mg. **International unit of progestational activity.** The specific activity contained in 1 mg of pure crystalline progesterone. **International tuberculin unit.** 0.00002 mg of purified protein derivative. **International unit of vitamin A.** The specific activity contained in an amount of standard preparation equivalent to 0.3 μg of all-*trans* vitamin-A alcohol. **International unit of vitamin B$_1$.** The specific antineuritic activity contained in 3.125 μg of pure synthetic crystalline aneurine hydrochloride. **International unit of vitamin C.** The antiscorbutic activity contained in 0.05 mg of pure ascorbic acid. **International unit of vitamin D.** The specific antirachitic activity contained in 0.025 μg of a standard preparation. **J unit of dose.** A proposed radiological unit of dose. One J unit has been received at any point in a medium when the ionization in an infinitesimal cavity containing the point is 1.58×10^{12} ion pairs per gram of air enclosed in the cavity. **Unit of light.** The lumen; the luminous flux emitted in unit solid angle by a uniform point source having a luminous intensity of one candela. **Lung unit.** All of the histological structures distal to a respiratory bronchiole. **Mass unit.** 1. Since the masses of nuclei are all approximately integral multiples of the mass of the proton, it is convenient to work in terms of such a unit. For reasons of practical convenience, the actual mass unit was originally defined as one-sixteenth of the mass of the oxygen atom, but is now defined in terms of carbon. (See Atomic mass unit). 2. A term used in radiotherapy to denote a teletherapy unit or bomb using large quantities of radium or radiocobalt. **Metre-kilogram-second unit.** Any unit of the metre-kilogram-second system of physical units. **Monosaccharide unit.** The group $C_6H_{11}O_5$ which enters into the composition of higher saccharides. **Motor unit.** The unit of the voluntary motor system, formed by a motor neurone and the muscle fibres which it innervates. **Mouse unit.** Mouse units and rat units as measurements of oestrogen activity are obsolete, as pure oestrogens are now available. **Nerve unit.** The neurone; a single nerve cell with its cell body and processes. **Unit of oestrogenic activity.** 1 mg of oestrone contains 10 000 units of oestrogenic activity (oestrone standard); 1 mg of oestradiol monobenzoate contains 10 000 units of oestrogenic activity (benzoate standard). These units are defined by the Permanent Commission on Biological Standards of the World Health Organization. **Oxford unit.** The first unit for penicillin activity defined in 1940 by the Oxford workers as "that amount of penicillin contained in one millilitre of a certain phosphate buffer solution containing ether". This solution, which was the first standard, was replaced in 1941 by a solid standard, and again in the following year by a stable standard. Today the standard for penicillin is the International Penicillin Standard, a defined weight of which contains 1 unit which is approximately equivalent to the original Oxford unit. **Probe unit.** A pre-amplifier or quenching unit, used with a Geiger counter. **Quantum unit.** Planck's constant; the constant *h* in the product $h\nu$ which measures the quantum of energy associated with a radiation of frequency ν. It equals 6.6256×10^{-34} joule-seconds. **Quenching unit.** Probe unit (see above). **R unit.** The roentgen; that quantity of x- or γ-radiation such that the associated corpuscular emission per 0.001293 g of air produces, in air, ions carrying 1 electrostatic unit of quantity of electricity of either sign: (0.001293 g is the mass of 1 ml of dry air at NTP). Also **R unit,** Behnken's unit; an obsolete unit of radiation equal to 1.06 roentgen. **Unit of radioactivity.** The curie; the quantity of any radioactive substance in which there are 3.7×10^{10} disintegrations per second. **Rat unit.** *See* MOUSE UNIT (above). **Unit of resistance.** The ohm; the resistance of a conductor in which an electromotive force of one volt produces a current of one ampere. **Sealing unit.** Water seal. *See* SEAL. **SI unit.** *Système International d'Unités.* A coherent system of units based on the metre, kilogram, second, ampere, kelvin, candela and mole. **Skin test unit.** The amount of scarlet-fever toxin which, on intradermal injection, gives positive (Dick) reactions in persons susceptible to the disease, and negative reactions in those who are immune. The minimum area of reddening of a positive Dick test should be 1 cm in diameter. **Specific smell unit.** Or olfact; a measure in grams per litre of the smallest concentration of a substance (minimum perceptible odour) which can be appreciated by a person with normal olfaction. **Spermatocyte unit.** The minimal quantity of tuberculin which on injection into the testicle of a guinea-pig will prevent spermatogenesis. **Thermal unit.** *See* BRITISH THERMAL UNIT (above). **Toronto unit.** A unit of anticoagulant activity equivalent to 10^{-5}g of barium heparin. **Toxic unit, toxin unit.** A little-used and erroneous term for the minimal lethal dose of toxin. The potency of toxic filtrates is correctly expressed in terms of combining power with antitoxin, and not in toxin units. **USP unit.** A *United States Pharmacopeia* measure of the potency of a liver extract for the treatment of pernicious anaemia. It is determined by the biological trial of its curvature effects on relapsing uncomplicated cases of pernicious anemia, and is assessed as the minimal amount of the liver extract necessary to produce, when given daily, adequate clinical and haemopoietic responses in such cases. **Vitamin A unit.** *See* INTERNATIONAL UNIT OF VITAMIN A (above). **Vitamin B_1 unit.** *See* INTERNATIONAL UNIT OF VITAMIN B_1 (above). **Vitamin C unit.** *See* INTERNATIONAL UNIT OF VITAMIN C (above). **Vitamin D unit.** *See* INTERNATIONAL UNIT OF VITAMIN D (above). **Unit of work.** *See* UNIT OF ENERGY (above). In the cgs system, the erg; the work done by a force of one dyne acting over one centimetre, and equal to 10^{-7} joules. In the UK the foot-pound was used, being the work done by a force of one poundal acting over one foot, and is equal to approximately 4.2×10^{-2} joules. [L *unus* one.]

See also: ÅNGSTRÖM, ARMSTRONG (A. R.), BEHNKEN, BODANSKY, BOURQUIN, CARR, DOISY, FELTON, FLOREY, HAMPSON, HANSON, HOLZKNECHT, KING (E. J.), LOVIBOND, MCCARTHY (J. F.), MACHE, NOON, PRICE (E. A.), SHERMAN (H. C.), SIEVERT, SOMOGYI, THAYER, VOEGTLIN.

unitary (ew·nit·ar·e). Referring to a single unit.

uniterminal (ew·ne·**ter**·min·al). Having only one terminal or pole. [L *unus* one, terminal.]

unitubercular (ew·ne·tew·**ber**′·kew·lar). Having a single tubercle or cusp. [L *unus* one, tubercle.]

univalent (ew·ne·**va**·lent). 1. Possessing a valency of one. 2. In cytogenetics, a body formed at the first meiotic division by an unpaired chromosome. Univalents may be formed by chromosomes lacking a pairing partner, by premature dissociation of paired configurations (*desynapsis*) or by failure of homologous pairing (*asynapsis*). [L *unus* one, valent.]

univitelline (ew·ne·vi·**tel**′·ine). Concerned with or developing from a single ovum. [L *unus* one, *vitellus* yoke.]

unmedullated (un·**med**·ew·la·ted). Having no medullary sheath, as in the case of some nerve fibres. [AS *un-* not, medulla.]

Unna, Paul Gerson (b. 1850). Hamburg dermatologist.

Unna's paste boot. Alternate layers of cotton bandage and Unna's paste applied to a leg to give support to a sufferer from varicose ulcers.

Unna's pityriasis maculata. Pityriasis alba.

Unna's plasma cell. Any connective-tissue cell with basophilic cytoplasm resembling a plasma cell.

Unna's disease. Eczema seborrhoeicum.

Unna's layer. The deepest layer of the epidermis.

Unna's method. 1. For connective-tissue fibrils: sections are stained with polychrome methylene blue, followed by an alcoholic solution of orcein. Cells and muscle fibres are stained blue, collagenous elastic fibres and most cell granules red. 2. For elastic fibres: sections are stained in an alcoholic solution of orcein containing hydrochloric acid. Elastic fibres are stained a deep brown colour. 3. For hyalin and colloid: sections are stained in acid fuchsine, followed by picric acid. Hyalin and connective-tissue fibres are red, colloid yellow. 4. For keratohyalin: sections are stained in haemalum, and differentiated with potassium permanganate. Keratohyalin granules are stained dark blue.

Unna's naevus. Naevus flammeus nuchae; a capillary naevus on the nape of the neck or lower part of the occiput.

Unna's paste. Zinc oxide (15 per cent) in a glycogelatin base. It is melted prior to use and applied with a brush; other ingredients, such as ichthammol, are often added.

Unna's differential stain. For plasma and mast cells: sections are stained in polychrome methylene blue and differentiated in glycerin ether. Most cell granules are stained red, plasma cells blue.

Unna's isolated stains. For mast cells: polychrome methylene blue containing alum, used to stain mast cell granules red.

Unna–Pappenheim stain. A stain containing methyl green and pyronine, used especially for demonstrating plasma cells.

Unna–Taenzer stain. For elastic fibres: sections are stained in an alcoholic solution of orcein, and counterstained with haematoxylin or methylene blue. Elastic fibres are stained a reddish-brown, nuclei blue.

unofficial (un·o·**fish**·al). Referring in medicine to a drug or preparation which does not occur in the *Pharmacopoeia.* There is no definite ruling about the application of the word, but in Great Britain it is usually understood to refer to drugs which do not occur in the *British Pharmacopoeia* or the *British Pharmaceutical Codex.* Cf. OFFICIAL. [AS *un-* not, official.]

unorganized (un·**or**·gan·i·zd). 1. Having no logical structure. 2. Lacking organs. [AS *un-* not, organ.]

unorientation (un·**or**·e·en·**ta**′·shun). Disorientation; the inability to remember surroundings or find one's way, due to mental confusion. [AS *un-* not, orientation.]

unphysiological (un·**fiz**·e·o·**loj**′·ik·al). Contrary to physiological principles. [AS *un-* not, physiology.]

unrest (un·**rest**). Lack of regularity; instability. **Peristaltic unrest.** Spasmodic movements of the stomach or intestine. [AS *un-* not, rest.]

unsatisfied (un·**sat**·is·fide). In the chemical terms of valency, referring to the potential of a compound, or part of a compound (e.g. an atom) to combine with other compounds or atoms with a similar potential. [AS *un-* not, satisfy.]

unsaturated (un·**sat**·ewr·a·ted). 1. Applied to a solution that is able to dissolve further quantities of the substance it has already in solution, without requiring to be raised in temperature. 2. In organic chemistry, any compound which contains double or triple valency bonds which, by opening and uniting with more atoms, render the compound saturated. [AS *un-* not, saturate.]

Unschuld, Paul (b. 1835). German physician.

Unschuld's sign. Cramp in the calves of the legs in diabetes.

unsharpness (un·**sharp**·nes). Blurring of the edges of the various shadows in a radiograph or on a fluorescent screen. It is produced by many technical factors, the more important of which are a broad-tube focus, mobility of the object, short focus–film distance and long object–film distance. [AS *un-* not, *scearp.*]

unstriated (un·**stri**·a·ted). Possessing no striations. [AS *un-* not, striated.]

unstriped (un·**stri**·pd). Having no stripes or striations, as in the case of involuntary muscles. [AS *un-* not, stripe.]

Unverricht, Heinrich (b. 1853). Magdeburg physician.

Unverricht's disease, or myoclonus. A rare, fatal, hereditary form of diffuse neuronal disease, beginning in late childhood with major epilepsy and widespread myoclonus, and ending in dementia with tetraplegia and pseudobulbar palsy.

upas (**ew**·pas). A poisonous Javanese tree, *Antiaris toxicaria* (family Urticaceae). It yields a resin (bohun upas). **Upas antiar.** A gum-resinous exudation from *Antiaris toxicaria.* [Malay, poison.]

upsiloid (**up**·si·loid). U- or V-shaped. [Gk *ypsilon* letter *u, eidos* form.]

uptake (**up**·take). A term used to indicate the absorption by a tissue of some substance, food material, mineral, etc. [AS *up-*, *tacan.*]

urachal (ewr·a·kal). Referring to the urachus.

urachovesical (ewr·a·ko·**ves**′·ik·al). Concerning the urachus and the urinary bladder. [urachus, L *vesica* bladder.]

urachus [NA] (**ewr**·a·kus). A fibrous cord stretching from the apex of the bladder to the umbilicus, representing the obliterated allantoic duct. It is sometimes called the *median umbilical ligament* or *median false ligament of the bladder.* **Patent urachus.** Persistence of the allantoic duct as a patent tube between the apex of the bladder and the umbilicus. [Gk *ourachos* the urinary canal.]

uracil (**ewr**·as·il). 2,6-Dioxypyrimidine, a pyrimidine base which gives rise to the uridine nucleotides and their derivatives.

uracrasia, uracratia (ewr·a·**kra**·ze·ah, ewr·a·**kra**·she·ah). Inability to hold the urine; enuresis. [Gk *ouron* urine, *akrasia* incontinence.]

uradal (**ewr**·ad·al). Carbromal.

uraemia (ewr·**e**·me·ah). The condition which results from severe renal failure, and is associated with the retention of normal and abnormal metabolic products in the blood and disturbance of the acid-base ratio of the latter. **Azotaemic uraemia.** Uraemia associated with the retention of urea and other nitrogenous substances in the blood. **Convulsive uraemia.** The cerebral type of uraemia with convulsions. **Eclamptic uraemia.** Convulsive uraemia (see above). **Extrarenal uraemia.** Uraemia in which the primary cause of renal failure lies outside the kidney. This may occur in alkalosis from excessive ingestion of alkalis or repeated vomiting. **Ischaemic uraemia.** Uraemia due to ischaemia of the kidney, causing autolysis and consequent damage to the renal tubules as in the crush syndrome and concealed uterine haemorrhage. **Prerenal uraemia.** Extrarenal uraemia (see above). **Renal uraemia.** The terminal stage of severe renal disease. [Gk *ouron* urine, *haima* blood.]

uraemic (ewr·**e**·mik). Concerned with uraemia.

uraemigenic (ewr·**e**·me·**jen**′·ik). Arising out of or causing uraemia. [uraemia, Gk *genein* to produce.]

uragogue (**ewr**·ag·og). Promoting the secretion of urine. [Gk *ouron* urine, *agogos* leading.]

urali (oo·**rah**·le). Curare.

uramil (**ewr**·am·il). $CO(NHCO)_2CHNH_2$, a compound prepared from violuric acid. It is converted by ammonia into murexide, or oxidized to alloxan.

uramine (**ewr**·am·een). Guanidine, $HN{=}C(NH_2)_2$. A toxic compound occurring in vetch seeds, and produed by the oxidation of the guanine of nucleoprotein.

Uramustine (ewr·ah·**mus**·teen). BP Commission approved name for 5-di-(2-chloroethyl)-aminouracil; an antineoplastic agent.

uran-gallein (ewr·an·**gal**·e·in). A staining combination for elastic tissue, containing gallein and a uranium salt.

uranianism (ewr·a·ne·an·izm). Uranism.

uranin (**ewr**·a·nin). An old term for sodium fluorescein, a brownish-yellow dye which fluoresces strongly in solution. Solutions have been used in the diagnosis of corneal ulcers.

uraninite (ewr·**an**·in·ite). Pitchblende. A mineral containing uranium oxides, lead, thorium, and rare-earth metals.

uraniscochasma (ewr·an·is·ko·**kaz**′·mah). Cleft palate. *See* PALATE. [Gk *ouraniskos* palate, *chasma* cleft.]

uraniscolalia (ewr·**an**·is·ko·**la**′·le·ah). Indistinctness of speech caused by a cleft palate. [Gk *ouraniskos* palate, *lalia* speech.]

uraniscoпitis (ewr·**an**·is·ko·**ni**′·tis). Inflammation of the palate. [Gk *ouraniskos* palate, *-itis* inflammation.]

uraniscoplasty (ewr·**an**·is·ko·plas·te). The remedial operation for cleft palate. [Gk *ouraniskos* palate, *plassein* to mould.]

uraniscorrhaphy (ewr·**an**·is·**kor**′·af·e). Surgical suture of a cleft palate; staphylorrhaphy. [Gk *ouraniskos* palate, *rhaphe* suture.]

uraniscus (ewr·an·is·kus). The palate. [Gk *ouraniskos* palate.]

uranism (**ewr**·an·izm). Homosexuality. [Gk *ouranios,* heavenly, an epithet of Aphrodite, patroness of homosexuals.]

uranist (**ewr**·an·ist). A homosexual. [see prec.]

uranium (ewr·a·ne·um). A radioactive element of atomic weight 238.029, atomic number 92, and chemical symbol U. It is a hard white metal occurring in pitchblende and carnotite as the oxide and vanadate, respectively. It exists in three isotopes; one of them, ^{235}U, undergoes nuclear fission when bombarded by thermal neutrons, with the release of enormous energy. The element disintegrates radioactively with a half life of 4.4×10^9 years, emitting an α-particle to form *uranium* X_1, and is the parent of the uranium series of radioactive elements. Its salts have no medical uses; they are corrosive, and after absorption are very toxic, causing renal and hepatic damage. **Uranium nitrate.** $UO_2(NO_3)_2{\cdot}6H_2O$, a yellow crystalline compound, soluble in water, with astringent properties. **Uranium oxide.** U_3O_8, the form in which uranium occurs naturally in pitchblende. **Uranium X.** A disintegration product of uranium that emits beta and gamma rays. **Uranium X_1.** A decay product of uranium; it has a half life of 24.5 days, emitting a β-particle. **Uranium X_2.** A decay product of uranium X_1; it has a half-life of 1.14 min, emitting a β-particle. **Uranium Z.** A decay product of uranium X_1; it has a half life of 6.7 h, emitting a β-particle. [Called after the planet *Uranus.*]

uranocoloboma (ewr·an·o·kol·o·**bo'**·mah). Uranoschisma. [Gk *ouranos* palate, *koloboma* a mutilated part.]

uranomania (ewr·an·o·**ma'**·ne·ah). Religious mania. [Obsolete term.] [Gk *ouranos* heaven, *mania* madness.]

uranoplastic (ewr·an·o·**plas'**·tik). Concerned with uranoplasty.

uranoplasty (ewr·an·o·plas·te). Plastic surgery of the roof of the mouth; the operation for cleft palate. [Gk *ouranos* palate, *plassein* to mould.]

uranoplegia (ewr·an·o·**ple'**·je·ah). Paralysis affecting the soft palate. [Gk *ouranos* palate, *plege* stroke.]

uranorrhaphy (ewr·an·**or**·af·e). The suture of the palate for cleft palate. [Gk *ouranos* palate, *rhaphe* suture.]

uranoschisis (ewr·an·**os**·kis·is). Cleft palate. *See* PALATE. [see foll.]

uranoschism (ewr·an·os·kizm). A fissure in the palate; cleft palate. [Gk *ouranos* palate, *schisis* fissure.]

uranoschisma (ewr·an·o·**skiz'**·mah). Congenital cleft of the palate. [see prec.]

uranostaphyloplasty (ewr·an·o·**staf'**·il·o·plas·te). Surgical repair of cleft palate. [Gk *ouranos* palate, *staphyle* uvula, *plassein* to mould.]

uranostaphylorrhaphy (ewr·an·o·staf·il·**or'**·af·e). Surgical repair of cleft palate. [Gk *ouranos* palate, *staphyle* uvula, *rhaphe* suture.]

uranostaphyloschisis (ewr·an·o·staf·il·**os'**·kis·is). Fissure extending from the hard to the soft palate. [Gk *ouranos* palate, *staphyle* uvula, *schisis* fissure.]

uranosteoplasty (ewr·an·**os**·te·o·plas·te). Uranoplasty. [Gk *ouranos* palate, *osteon* bone, *plassein* to mould.]

uranyl (ewr·a·nil). The term applied to salts of uranium in which the group UO_2 takes the place of the metallic radical. These salts are greenish-yellow in colour, and are freely soluble in water giving fluorescent solutions. They form complex salts with a number of other metallic salts. **Uranyl acetate.** $UO_2(CO_2CH_3)_2·2H_2O$, a yellow crystalline salt prepared by dissolving uranium trioxide in acetic acid. It is used as a reagent in the determination of sodium in serum and other biological materials. **Uranyl nitrate.** $UO_2(NO_3)_2·6H_2O$, a yellow crystalline salt prepared by dissolving uranium trioxide in nitric acid. It has been used in the treatment of diabetes and cancer but with no evident benefit.

urapostema (ewr·ap·**os**·te·mah). An abscess which contains urine. [Gk *ouron* urine, *apostema* abscess.]

urari (oo·**rah**·re). Curare.

urataemia (ewr·at·e·me·ah). A condition marked by the accumulation of urates in the blood. [urate, Gk *haima* blood.]

urate (ewr·ate). Any salt of uric acid. Urates occur commonly in urinary deposits and calculi, chiefly as the ammonium and sodium salts.

uratic (ewr·**at**·ik). Relating to urates and in particular to gout.

uratohistechia (ewr·a·to·his·**te'**·ke·ah). Urea, uric acid, or urates in excess in the tissues. [urate, Gk *histos* tissue, *echein* to hold.]

uratolysis (ewr·at·**ol**·is·is). The dissolving or breaking-up of urates in the treatment of gout. [urate, Gk *lysis* a loosing.]

uratolytic (ewr·at·o·**lit'**·ik). Referring to anything that is able to dissolve or break up urates and remove them from the system. [see prec.]

uratoma (ewr·at·**o**·mah). A concretion of urates appearing round the joints; a tophus. [urate, Gk *-oma* tumour.]

uratosis (ewr·at·**o**·sis). Any morbid state due to formation of uric crystals in the tissues. [urate, Gk *-osis* condition.]

uraturia (ewr·at·**ewr**·e·ah). The appearance of an abnormal amount of urates in the urine.

urazole (ewr·a·zole). $(CONH)_2NH$, a crystalline derivative of urea.

Urbach, Erich (b. 1893). Philadelphia dermatologist.

Urbach's extracellular cholesterolosis. A rare, maculopapular and nodular skin condition with extracellular infiltrations of cholesterol.

Urbach-Oppenheim disease. Xanthoma diabeticorum.

Urbach-Wiethe disease. Lipoid proteinosis. *See* PROTEINOSIS.

Urban's operation. Removal of a malignant breast, together with the axillary glands, the upper costal cartilages, and the underlying pleura.

urea (ewr·e·ah). Carbamide, $CO(NH_2)_2$. A colourless crystalline, solid, soluble in water and alcohol, insoluble in ether (BP 1958). It occurs in the blood and tissue fluids of all vertebrates, and of some invertebrates, and is the chief nitrogenous constituent of mammalian urine. It is the end-product of protein metabolism and is formed exclusively in the liver. The manner of its formation is uncertain, but the ornithine cycle theory has found some measure of acceptance. In this process arginine is converted by the action of the enzyme arginase to ornithine and urea; ornithine condenses with ammonia and carbon dioxide to form citrulline which then takes up a second molecule of ammonia to form arginine. The concentration of urea in human blood, normally 3.3–6.7 mmol per litre (20–40 mg per 100 ml), becomes abnormally high in renal disease, and in heart failure. The average daily excretion of urea in the urine is 25–35 g, but determinations of urea concentration in urine are only of major clinical significance if made under the prescribed conditions of kidney-function tests such as the urea-clearance and urea-concentration tests. **Diethyl malonyl urea.** Barbitone. **Malonyl urea.** Barbituric acid. *See* ACID. **Mesoxalyl urea.** Alloxan, $CO(NHCO)_2CO$; a crystalline substance, soluble in water and alcohol, produced by oxidation of uric acid and nitric acid. Injection into animals causes alloxan diabetes by reason of its destructive action upon the pancreatic-islet tissue. **Urea nitrogen.** The amount of nitrogen in the form of urea, as distinct from nitrogen combined in protein. **Urea peroxide.** A compound of urea and hydrogen peroxide which splits into its components on hydrolysis. [Gk *ouron* urine.]

ureabromine (ewr·e·ah·**bro'**·meen). A combination of calcium bromide and urea, used like the bromides.

ureagenesis (ewr·e·ah·**jen'**·is·is). The processes by which urea becomes the final product of the metabolism of amino acids in the body of mammals. Ureagenesis is confined almost entirely to the liver, its essential purpose being detoxication of the ammonia formed from amino-acid metabolism. [urea, Gk *genein* to produce.]

ureagenic (ewr·e·ah·**jen'**·ik). Having the property of producing urea. [see prec.]

ureal (ewr·**e**·al). Concerned with urea or composed of it.

ureameter (ewr·e·**am**·et·er). An apparatus for estimating the urea-content of urine by measuring the volume of nitrogen liberated from a sample. [urea, meter.]

ureametry (ewr·e·**am**·et·re). The estimation of the urea-content of urine by means of a ureameter.

ureapoiesis (ewr·e·ah·poi·**e'**·sis). The formation of urea. [urea, Gk *poiein* to form.]

urease (ewr·e·aze). An enzyme of the aminase class which catalyses the conversion of urea into ammonium carbonate; its principal sources are the jack bean and soya bean. It is a water-soluble substance of the nature of protein and has been prepared in crystalline form. It is destroyed by pepsin. It is largely used in the determination of urea in blood, urine, and other biological materials, as its action upon urea is quite specific.

urecchysis (ewr·**ek**·is·is). Extravasation of urine into the areolae of the tissue. [urine, Gk *ekchysis* a pouring out.]

Urechites suberecta (ewr·**ek**·it·eez sub·er·**ek**·tah). Savannah flower, yellow-flowered nightshade; a woody plant of the family Apocyanaceae, indigenous to Colombia and grown in the West Indies. The leaves contain a toxic alkaloid, and a less poisonous glycoside. The plant is a powerful cardiac poison of the digitalis type. [Gk *yrichos* wicker basket, L *sub* almost, *erectus* erect.]

Uredinales (ew·red·in·**a'**·leez). An order of parasitic fungi; the rusts. They form coloured rust-like spots on the leaves and stems of plants. [L *uredo* blight.]

uredo (ewr·e·do) (pl. *uredines*). 1. An itching or burning sensation in the skin. 2. Urticaria. [L, blight.]

ureide (**ewr**·e·ide). Any organic compound derived from urea by the replacement of one or more of its hydrogen atoms by acyl groups. **Cyclic ureide.** A ring compound formed by the union of both carboxyl groups of a dibasic acid with urea, e.g. barbituric acid, CONHCONHCOCH$_2$; of considerable importance medically.

urelcosis (ewr·el·**ko**·sis). Ulceration of the urinary passages. [Gk *ouron* urine, *elkosis* ulceration.]

ureometer (ewr·e·**om**·et·er). Ureameter.

ureosecretory (**ewr**·e·o·se·**kre'**·tor·e). Concerned with the secretion of urea.

ureotelic (**ewr**·e·o·**tel'**·ik). Uricotelic.

uresiaesthesis (**ewr**·e·se·es·**the'**·sis). A feeling of wanting to urinate; the normal urge to pass urine. [Gk *ouresis* urination, *aisthesis* sensation.]

uresis (ewr·e·sis). Urination. [Gk *ouresis.*]

uretal (ewr·e·tal). Referring to the ureter.

ureter [NA] (ewr·e·ter). The duct conveying urine from the kidney to the bladder. **Aberrant ureter.** One that discharges urine into some other viscus than the bladder. **Coat of the ureter, adventitious [tunica adventitia (NA)].** The connective-tissue sheath surrounding the muscular coats. **Coat of the ureter, mucous [tunica mucosa (NA)].** Fibro-elastic tissue covered with transitional epithelium; it is thrown into folds when the ureter is empty. **Coat of the ureter, muscular [tunica muscularis (NA)].** In the upper part, consisting of outer circular and inner longitudinal coats; in the lower part there is an outer longitudinal layer, a middle circular and an inner (mainly) longitudinal layer. **Golf-hole ureter.** The retracted and widely gaping ureteric orifice which is characteristic of tuberculous ureteritis. This descriptive term was used by Edwin Hurry Fenwick. **Part of the ureter, abdominal [pars abdominalis (NA)].** The portion extending from the pelvis of the ureter to the brim of the true pelvis. **Part of the ureter, pelvic [pars pelvina (NA)].** The part lying within the true pelvis. **Postcaval ureter, retrocaval ureter.** A congenital anomaly in which the right ureter passes behind the inferior vena cava and may become constricted at that point. The ureter is displaced medially. **Truant ureter.** A congenital anomaly in which the ureter has an abnormal insertion to the lower urinary tract or outside it, e.g. posterior urethra, seminal vesicle, or the vagina. [Gk *oureter.]*

ureteral (ewr·e·ter·al). Concerning the ureter, or any operation relating thereto.

ureteralgia (ewr·e·ter·**al'**·je·ah). Pain experienced in the ureter. [ureter, Gk *algos* pain.]

uretercystoscope (ewr·e·ter·**sist'**·o·skope). A cystoscope which incorporates a separate channel in its wall through which a ureteric catheter may be introduced to either ureter. Most modern cystoscopes have a separate catheterizing telescope so that the structure of the sheath of the cystoscope is uncomplicated by additional channels in its wall.

ureterectasia, ureterectasis (ewr·e·ter·ek·**ta'**·ze·ah, ewr·e·ter·**ek'**·tas·is). Distention or dilatation of the ureter. [ureter, Gk *ektasis* dilatation.]

ureterectomy (ewr·e·ter·**ek'**·to·me). The surgical excision of the whole or part of a ureter. [ureter, Gk *ektome* excision.]

ureteric (ewr·e·**ter**·ik). Ureteral.

ureteritis (ewr·e·ter·**i'**·tis). Inflammation of a ureter. [ureter, Gk *-itis* inflammation.]

ureterocele (ewr·e·ter·o·seel). 1. A hernia involving a ureter. 2. A dilatation of the lower part of a ureter. [ureter, Gk *kele* hernia.]

ureterocervical (ewr·e·ter·o·**ser'**·vik·al). Involving both a ureter and the neck (cervix) of the uterus, as in the case of a fistula.

ureterocolostomy (ewr·e·ter·o·ko·**los'**·to·me). The surgical establishment of an opening for a ureter into the colon. [ureter, colon, Gk *stoma* mouth.]

ureterocystanastomosis (ewr·e·ter·o·sist·an·as·to·**mo'**·sis). The surgical establishment of a new and alternative opening for a ureter into the bladder. [ureter, Gk *kystis* bladder, anastomosis.]

ureterocystic (ewr·e·ter·o·**sist'**·ik). Pertaining to the bladder and the ureter. [ureter, Gk *kystis* bladder.]

ureterocystoneostomy (ewr·e·ter·o·sist·o·ne·**os'**·to·me). Ureteroneocystostomy. [ureter, Gk *kystis* bladder, *neos* new, *stoma* mouth.]

ureterocystoscope (ewr·e·ter·o·**sist'**·o·skope). Uretercystoscope.

ureterocystostomy (ewr·e·ter·o·sist·**os'**·to·me). The surgical establishment of an alternative opening for a ureter into the bladder. [ureter, Gk *kystis* bladder, *stoma* mouth.]

ureterodialysis (ewr·e·ter·o·di·**al'**·is·is). The rupture of a ureter. [ureter, Gk *dialysis* a breaking.]

uretero-enteric (ewr·e·ter·o·en·**ter'**·ik). Involving both a ureter and the intestine. [ureter, Gk *enteron* intestine.]

uretero-entero-anastomosis (ewr·e·ter·o·**en**·ter·o·an·as·to·**mo'**·sis). Uretero-enterostomy. [ureter, Gk *enteron* intestine, *anastomosis* opening.]

uretero-enterostomy (ewr·e·ter·o·en·ter·**os'**·to·me). The formation surgically of an opening for a ureter into the intestine. [ureter, Gk *enteron* intestine, *stoma* mouth.]

ureterogram (ewr·e·ter·o·gram). A radiograph taken during ureterography. [ureter, Gk *gramma* a record.]

ureterography (ewr·e·ter·**og'**·raf·e). Radiography of the lumen of the ureter by the injection of a contrast medium. [ureter, Gk *graphein* to record.]

ureterohydronephrosis (ewr·e·ter·o·hi·dro·nef·**ro'**·sis). Pathological distension of the ureter and kidney pelvis due to obstruction. [ureter, Gk *hydor* water, *nephros* kidney, *-osis* condition.]

uretero-ileostomy (ewr·e·ter·o·i·le·**os'**·to·me). Implantation of the ureters into an isolated loop of ileum which is brought out as an isolated urinary conduit onto the abdominal wall. [ureter, ileum, Gk *stoma* mouth.]

uretero-intestinal (ewr·e·ter·o·in·**tes'**·tin·al). Concerning both a ureter and the neighbouring intestine, as in the case of a fistula.

ureterolith (ewr·e·ter·o·lith). A calculus appearing in the ureter. [ureter, Gk *lithos* stone.]

ureterolithiasis (ewr·e·ter·o·lith·**i'**·as·is). The formation or occurrence of a calculus in a ureter. [see prec.]

ureterolithotomy (ewr·e·ter·o·lith·**ot'**·o·me). Surgical incision of a ureter for the removal of a calculus. [ureter, Gk *lithos* stone, *temnein* to cut.]

ureterolysis (ewr·e·ter·**ol'**·is·is). 1. Rupture or paralysis of a ureter. 2. Surgical division of ureteral adhesions. [ureter, Gk *lysis* a loosing.]

ureteroneocystostomy (ewr·e·ter·o·ne·o·sist·**os'**·to·me). The surgical establishment of a new opening for a ureter into the bladder. [ureter, Gk *neos* new, *kystis* bladder, *stoma* mouth.]

ureteroneopyelostomy (ewr·e·ter·o·ne·o·pi·el·**os'**·to·me), Surgical removal of a diseased part of a ureter and the connection of what remains with the pelvis of the ureter. [ureter, Gk *neos* new, *pyelos* pelvis, *stoma* mouth.]

ureteronephrectomy (ewr·e·ter·o·nef·**rek'**·to·me). Surgical removal of a kidney together with its ureter. [ureter, Gk *nephros* kidney, *ektome* excision.]

ureteropathy (ewr·e·ter·**op'**·ath·e). Any diseased state of a ureter. [ureter, Gk *pathos* disease.]

ureteropelvioneostomy (ewr·e·ter·o·pel·ve·o·ne·**os'**·to·me). Ureteroneopyelostomy. [ureter, pelvis, Gk *neos* new, *stoma* mouth.]

ureteroplasty (ewr·e·ter·o·plas·te). Plastic surgery performed upon a ureter, particularly to relieve stricture. [ureter, Gk *plassein* to mould.]

ureteroproctostomy (ewr·e·ter·o·prok·**tos'**·to·me). Surgical establishment of an opening for a ureter into the rectum. [ureter, Gk *proktos* anus, *stoma* mouth.]

ureteropyelitis (ewr·e·ter·o·pi·el·**i'**·tis). Inflammation of a ureter, extending from a pyelitic kidney. [ureter, Gk *pyelos* pelvis, *-itis* inflammation.]

ureteropyelography (ewr·e·ter·o·pi·el·**og**′·raf·e). Pyelography covering both a ureter and its pelvis.

ureteropyeloneostomy (ewr·e·ter·o·pi·el·o·ne·**os**′·to·me). Ureteroneopyelostomy.

ureteropyelonephritis (ewr·e·ter·o·pi·el·o·nef·**ri**′·tis). Inflammation extending from the pelvis of the kidney to the ureter. [ureter, Gk *pyelos* pelvis, *nephros* kidney, *-itis* inflammation.]

ureteropyelonephrostomy (ewr·e·ter·o·pi·el·o·nef·**ros**′·to·me). Ureteroneopyelostomy. [ureter, Gk pyelos pelvis, *nephros* kidney, *stoma* mouth.]

ureteropyeloplasty (ewr·e·ter·o·**pi**′·el·o·plas·te). Plastic surgery performed on a ureter and the pelvis of the kidney. [ureter, Gk *pyelos* pelvis, *plassein* to mould.]

ureteropyelostomy (ewr·e·ter·o·pi·el·**os**′·to·me). Ureteroneopyelostomy.

ureteropyosis (ewr·e·ter·o·pi·**o**′·sis). Inflammation of a ureter with the formation of pus. [ureter, Gk *pyon* pus.]

ureterorectoneostomy (ewr·e·ter·o·rek·to·ne·**os**′·to·me). Ureterorectostomy. [ureter, rectum, Gk *neos* new, *stoma* mouth.]

ureterorectostomy (ewr·e·ter·o·rek·**tos**′·to·me). The surgical establishment of an outlet for a ureter into the rectum. [ureter, rectum, Gk *stoma* mouth.]

ureterorrhagia (ewr·e·ter·o·**ra**′·je·ah). Haemorrhage from a ureter. [ureter, Gk *rhegnynein* to gush forth.]

ureterorrhaphy (ewr·e·ter·**or**′·af·e). Surgical suture of a ureter in the case of fistula or injury. [ureter, Gk *rhaphe* suture.]

ureterosalpingostomy (ewr·e·ter·o·sal·ping·**gos**′·to·me). The establishment surgically of communication between a ureter and an oviduct. [ureter, Gk *salpigx* tube, *stoma* mouth.]

ureterosigmoidostomy (ewr·e·ter·o·sig·moid·**os**′·to·me). The surgical establishment of an opening for a ureter in the sigmoid flexure. [ureter, sigmoid, Gk *stoma* mouth.]

ureterostegnosis (ewr·e·ter·o·steg·**no**′·sis). Ureterostenosis. [ureter, Gk *stegnosis* contraction.]

ureterostenoma (ewr·e·ter·o·sten·**o**′·mah). The narrowed part of a ureter in a case of stricture. [ureter, Gk *stenoma* narrow part.]

ureterostenosis (ewr·e·ter·o·sten·**o**′·sis). A narrowing of a ureter; stricture. [ureter, Gk *stenosis* construction.]

ureterostoma (ewr·e·ter·**os**′·to·mah). 1. The opening of the ureter into the urinary bladder. 2. A fistula of the ureter. [ureter, Gk *stoma* mouth.]

ureterostomatic (ewr·e·ter·os·to·**mat**′·ik). Pertaining to a ureteral orifice or fistula. [see prec.]

ureterostomosis (ewr·e·ter·os·to·**mo**′·sis). Ureterostomy.

ureterostomy (ewr·e·ter·**os**′·to·me). The establishment of a permanent opening from a ureter to the surface or into another viscus. **Cutaneous ureterostomy.** The establishment of a ureteral fistula by bringing the ureter to the surface of the skin through an incision made in the iliac region. [ureter, Gk *stoma* mouth.]

ureterotomy (ewr·e·ter·**ot**′·o·me). Surgical incision made into a ureter. [ureter, Gk *temnein* to cut.]

ureterotrigonosigmoidostomy (ewr·e·ter·o·tri·go·no·sig·moid·**os**′·to·me). Implantation into the sigmoid flexure of the colon of the trigone of the bladder and the ureters entering it. This is one of the earliest types of uretero-intestinal anastomosis and it has been superseded by the implanting of the ureters individually to the bowel. [ureter, trigone, sigmoid, Gk *stoma* mouth.]

uretero-ureteral (ewr·e·ter·o·ewr·**e**′·ter·al). Concerning two parts of a ureter, or corresponding parts of the two ureters, and any artificial connection between them.

uretero-ureterostomy (ewr·e·ter·o·ewr·e·ter·**os**′·to·me). The establishment surgically of a connection between two parts of the same ureter or between one ureter and the other. [ureter, Gk *stoma* mouth.]

uretero-uterine (ewr·e·ter·o·**ew**′·ter·ine). Describing any connection, such as a fistula, between a ureter and the uterus.

ureterovaginal (ewr·e·ter·o·**vaj**′·in·al). Concerning a ureter and the vagina.

ureterovesical (ewr·e·ter·o·**ves**′·ik·al). Concerning a ureter and the urinary bladder. [ureter, L *vesica* bladder.]

ureterovesicostomy (ewr·e·ter·o·ves·ik·**os**′·to·me). The establishment of a new opening for a ureter into a bladder. [ureter, L *vesica* bladder, Gk *stoma* mouth.]

urethane (ewr·e·thane). 1. General name given to esters of carbamic acid. 2. Urethane BP 1963; ethyl carbamate, $NH_2COOC_2H_5$, a colourless compound, soluble in water, alcohol, or ether; it is a safe hypnotic, especially suitable for administration to children and the aged. It has also been used successfully in the treatment of certain types of leukaemia. A solution of quinine hydrochloride and urethane is given by injection in the treatment of varicose veins.

urethra [NA] (ewr·e·thrah). The canal through which the urine passes on its way from the bladder to the exterior. **Coat of the urethra, mucous [tunica mucosa (NA)].** The lining of the urethra; its epithelium is transitional in the prostatic portion, then columnar, and finally in the last 2.5 cm, stratified squamous. **Coat of the urethra, muscular [tunica muscularis (NA)].** The thin muscular layers, outer circular and inner longitudinal in the wall of the prostatic and membranous parts of the urethra. **Coat of the urethra, submucous.** The layer of vascular erectile tissue. **Female urethra [urethra feminina (NA)].** A short channel, 2.5-4 cm (1-1½ in) in length, which leads from the bladder to the external urethral orifice, the latter lying within the vulva immediately in front of the vaginal orifice. **Male urethra [urethra masculina (NA)].** The channel which leads from the bladder to the external urethral orifice in the male. It is approximately 20 cm (8 in) in length, and is divided into three parts: the first, or prostatic part [pars prostatica] (2.5 cm) traverses the prostate and ends at the level of the superior fascia of the urogenital diaphragm; the second or membranous part [pars membranacea (NA)] (1.3 cm) lies within the urogenital diaphragm and ends by piercing its inferior fascia (perineal membrane) to become continuous with the third, or penile part (15 cm) which traverses the bulb and corpus spongiosum urethrae [pars spongiosa (NA)] to open at the external orifice on the glans penis. **Primary urethra.** That portion of the embryonic urethra which lies above the openings of the muellerian and wolffian ducts. It forms the whole of the definitive female urethra, but only the proximal half of the prostatic urethra in the male. [Gk *ourethra.*]

urethral (ewr·e·thral). Concerning the urethra.

urethral artery [arteria urethralis (NA)]. A branch of the internal pudendal artery. It arises deep to the perineal membrane, which it pierces to reach the corpus spongiosum penis in which it passes forward to the glans penis.

urethralgia (ewr·e·**thral**·je·ah). Pain experienced in the urethra. [urethra, Gk *algos* pain.]

urethrascope (ewr·e·thrah·skope). Urethroscope.

urethratresia (ewr·e·thrah·**tre**′·ze·ah). Lack of free passage through the urethra due either to congenital imperforation or to occlusion. [urethra, Gk *a*, *tresis* a boring.]

urethrectomy (ewr·e·**threk**·to·me). Surgical operation for removing the urethra as a whole or in part. [urethra, Gk *ektome* excision.]

urethremphraxis (ewr·e·threm·**frax**′·is). Any stoppage in the urethra. [urethra, Gk *emphraxis* stoppage.]

urethrism, urethrismus (ewr·e·thrizm, ew·re·**thriz**·mus). Urethral spasm associated with urethritis or urethrotrigonitis.

urethritis (ewr·e·**thri**′·tis). Inflammation of the urethra, associated with a purulent discharge from the external meatus. **Anterior urethritis.** An inflammation affecting the urethra distally to the triangular ligament or urogenital diaphragm. **Chemical urethritis.** Urethritis due to chemical irritants. **Gonorrhoeal urethritis.** Urethritis due to infection by the gonococcus. **Gouty urethritis.** A non-specific urethritis associated with gout. **Urethritis granulosa.** A chronic urethritis in which patchy areas of granulation tissue may present from inflamed and blocked lacunae. **Non-specific urethritis.** A urethritis which is non-gonococcal and not due to the tubercle bacillus or other specific micro-organisms, but may be due to a virus infection. The infection may be acute or chronic and may be transmitted during coitus. It may be recurrent and is often found in individuals of a neurasthenic type. **Posterior urethritis.** Inflammation of the posterior part of the urethra, including the prostatic urethra and the membranous urethra between the two layers of the triangular ligament. **Prophylactic urethritis.** A mild urethritis which may be induced by chemical irritation by solutions used during urethral irrigation. **Simple urethritis.** A urethritis not due to the gonococcus but to the urethral infection from an indwelling catheter or to a pyogenic organism introduced in some other way. **Specific urethritis.** Urethritis due to a specific micro-organism; it is usually restricted to gonorrhoea. [urethra, Gk *-itis* inflammation.]

urethro-atresia (ewr·e·thro·at·**re**′·ze·ah). Urethratresia.

urethroblenorrhoea (ewr·e·thro·blen·o·**re**′·ah). A discharge from the urethra, usually purulent. [urethra, Gk *blennos* mucus, *rhoia* flow.]

urethrobulbar (ewr·e·thro·**bul**′·bar). Concerning the urethra and the bulb of the penis.

urethrocele (ewr·e·thro·seel). 1. A true prolapse of the urethral mucosa in the female through the external urinary meatus. 2. A small diverticulum or pouch in the floor of the female urethra following infection, or more commonly due to the trauma of the urethra caused by the fetal head during prolonged labour. The weakened portion of the urethra dilates under the pressure associated with micturition. [urethra, Gk *kele* hernia.]

urethrocystitis (ewr·e·thro·sist·**i**′·tis). Cystitis extending to inflammation of the urethra.

urethrocystogram (ewr·e·thro·**sist**′·o·gram). An x-ray picture of the urethra and the urinary bladder after opacification of these structures with a contrast medium. [urethra, Gk kystis bladder, *gramma* a record.]

urethrocystography (ewr·e·thro·sist·**og**′·raf·e). Radiographic visualization of the urinary bladder and urethra after injection of a radio-opaque contrast medium, either retrograde or anterograde. [urethra, Gk *kystis bladder, graphein* to record.]

urethrocystopexy (ewr·e·thro·sist·o·**pex**′·e). The operation of slinging up the junction of the urethra and bladder for the treatment of stress incontinence in women. [urethra, Gk *kystis* bag, *pexis* fixation.]

urethrodynia (ewr·e·thro·**din**′·e·ah). Pain experienced in the urethra. [urethra, Gk *odyne* pain.]

urethrogram (ewr·e·thro·gram). An x-ray picture of the urethra. [urethra, Gk *gramma* a record.]

urethrograph (ewr·e·thro·graf). An instrument for recording in graphic form the size or contractility of the urethra. [urethra, Gk *graphein* to record.]

urethrography (ewr·e·**throg**·raf·e). Radiography of the urethra after filling its lumen with an opaque medium. [see prec.]

urethrometer (ewr·e·**throm**·et·er). An instrument for measuring the calibre of the lumen of the urethra. [urethra, Gk *metron* measure.]

urethropenile (ewr·e·thro·**pe**′·nile). Concerning the urethra and the penis.

urethroperineal (ewr·e·thro·per·in·**e**′·al). Concerned with the urethra and the perineum.

urethroperineoscrotal (ewr·e·thro·per·in·e·o·**skro**′·tal). Referring to the urethra, perineum, and scrotum.

urethropexy (ewr·e·thro·pex·e). A surgical procedure for buttressing or lifting and suspending the female urethra forward and upwards. [urethra, Gk *pexis* a fixation.]

urethrophraxis (ewr·e·thro·**frax**′·is). Obstruction occurring in the urethra. [urethra, Gk *phrassein* to obstruct.]

urethrophyma (ewr·e·thro·**fi**′·mah). Any tumour or swelling round the urethra. [urethra, Gk *phyma* tumour.]

urethroplasty (ewr·e·thro·plas·te). Plastic surgery performed on the urethra to remedy wounds or malformation. [urethra, Gk *plassein* to mould.]

urethroprostatic (ewr·e·thro·pros·**tat**′·ik). Concerning the urethra and the prostate gland.

urethrorectal (ewr·e·thro·**rek**′·tal). Involving both the urethra and the rectum.

urethrorrhagia (ewr·e·thro·**ra**′·je·ah). Haemorrhage from the urethra. [urethra, Gk *rhegnynein* to gush forth.]

urethrorrhaphy (ewr·e·**thror**·af·e). Suture of the urethra in the case of a wound, or fistula. [urethra, Gk *rhaphe* suture.]

urethrorrhoea (ewr·**e**·thro·**re**′·ah). The passage of any morbid discharge from the urethra. [urethra, Gk *rhein* to flow.]

urethroscope (ewr·e·thro·skope). An instrument with which the urethra may be inspected internally. [urethra, Gk *skopein* to view.]

See also: HARRISON (L. W.), JOLY.

urethroscopic (ewr·e·thro·**skop**′·ik). Concerning the urethroscope, or connected with urethroscopy.

urethroscopy (ewr·e·**thros**·ko·pe). Inspection of the lining of the urethra, making use of a urethroscope.

urethrospasm (ewr·e·thro·spazm). Chronic spasm of the muscles around the urethra; spasmodic stricture of the urethra.

urethrostaxis (ewr·e·thro·**stax**′·is). The exudation of blood from the mucous lining of the urethra; slow bleeding from the urethra. [urethra, Gk *staxis* a trickling.]

urethrostenosis (ewr·e·thro·sten·**o**′·sis). Urethral stricture. [urethra, Gk *stenosis* a narrowing.]

urethrostomy (ewr·e·**thros**·to·me). Surgical section of the urethra, usually just distal to its membranous portion, in order to establish a permanent urethral opening in the perineum which will be continent owing to the preservation of the external sphincter. [urethra, Gk *stoma* mouth.]

urethrotome (ewr·e·thro·tome). An instrument used for performing internal urethrotomy. **Dilating urethrotome.** A combined urethrotome and dilator, of doubtful practicability.

See also: MAISONNEUVE, THOMPSON-WALKER.

urethrotomy (ewr·e·**throt**·o·me). The operation of making an incision in the urethra. **External urethrotomy.** Exposure of the urethra through an incision in the perineum; thereafter a staff is passed as a guide and the urethra opened. The stricture may be incised or excised. The operation may be performed to facilitate the passage of a resectoscope to the bladder in order to avoid trauma to the anterior urethra; it is also used for the surgical removal of a calculus impacted in the urethra. **Internal urethrotomy.** An operation carried out solely for urethral stricture, by means of a urethrotome. [urethra, Gk *temnein* to cut.]

urethrotrigonitis (ewr·e·thro·tri·go·**ni**′·tis). Inflammation of the urethra and the trigone of the urinary bladder. [urethra, trigone, Gk *-itis* inflammation.]

urethro-ureteral (ewr·e·thro·ewr·**e**′·ter·al). Concerning the urethra and the ureter.

urethrovaginal (ewr·e·thro·**vaj**′·in·al). Referring to the urethra and the vagina.

urethrovesical (ewr·e·thro·**ves**′·ik·al). Concerning the urethra and the urinary bladder. [urethra, L *vesica* bladder.]

Urginea (er·**jin**·e·ah). A genus of liliaceous plants. **Urginea indica.** Indian squill, a species the dried bulbs of which constitute squill. [*Ben Urgin* name of Algerian tribe.]

urhidrosis (ewr·hid·**ro**′·sis). The excretion of urea in the sweat. Urea is normally present in trifling amounts, but it is much increased in uraemia when it may be deposited in crystalline form on the skin. [Gk *ouron* urine, *hidros* sweat.]

uric (ewr·ik). Concerning the urine.

uricacidaemia (ewr·ik·as·id·**e**′·me·ah). The occurrence of an abnormal amount of uric acid in the blood. [uric acid, Gk *haima* blood.]

uricaciduria (ewr·ik·as·id·**ewr**′·e·ah). The state marked by an abnormal increase in the amount of uric acid appearing in the urine.

uricaemia (ewr·is·e·me·ah). Uricacidaemia.

uricase (ewr·ik·aze). Uricolytic enzyme; an enzyme present in the liver of most mammals and the kidney of some, which oxidizes uric acid to allantoin and carbon dioxide.

uricocholia (ewr·ik·o·**ko**′·le·ah). The excretion of uric acid in the bile. [uric acid, Gk *chole* bile.]

uricolysis (ewr·ik·**ol**·is·is). The process of destruction of uric acid by oxidation or hydrolysis. [see foll.]

uricolytic (ewr·ik·o·**lit**·ik). Having the property of destroying uric acid. [uric acid, Gk *lysein* to loosen.]

uricosuria (ewr·ik·o·**sewr'**·e·ah). Urinary excretion of uric acid. [uric acid, Gk *ouron* urine.]

uricotelic (ewr·ik·o·**tel'**·ik). Characterized by the excretion of uric acid as the chief end-product of nitrogen metabolism. [see foll.]

uricotelism (ewr·ik·**ot**·el·izm, **ewr**·ik·o·**te'**·lizm). The excretion of uric acid as the chief end-product of nitrogen metabolism. [uric acid, Gk *telos* end.]

uridine (**ewr**·id·een). Uridine nucleotides; uracil in combination with ribose and phosphoric acid residues giving uridine mono-, di- and triphosphates. The uridine nucleotides are important in metabolism, especially through the formation of uridine diphosphate derivatives of sugars such as glucose which are involved as precursors in the biosynthesis of polysaccharides, glycoproteins, glycosaminoglycans, and in the interconversion of galactose and glucose.

uridrosis (ewr·id·**ro**·sis). Urhidrosis.

urinaemia (ewr·in·e·me·ah). The accumulation in the blood of substances, such as urea, that are normally excreted in the urine. [urine, Gk *haima* blood.]

urinal (**ewr**·in·al). Any vessel or place used for urination.

urinalysis (ewr·in·**al**·is·is). The analysis of urine, chemically or bacteriologically.

urinary (**ewr**·in·ar·e). Concerned with urine.

urinary bladder [vesica urinaria (NA)]. The sac situated in the anterior part of the pelvis which receives the ureters posteriorly, and from which the urethra arises. Its wall is composed largely of smooth muscle, and it is lined by transitional epithelium.

Apex [apex vesicae (NA)]. The apex of the bladder to which the urachus is attached.

Base [fundus vesicae (NA)]. The posterior surface of the bladder separated from the rectum by the rectovesical pouch, and to which the seminal vesicles and the terminal parts of the ureters and vasa deferentia are applied.

Body [corpus vesicae (NA)]. The whole of the organ.

Mucous coat [tunica mucosa (NA)]. The vascular mucous membrane, lined with transitional epithelium. When the bladder is empty it is thrown into folds (rugae) except over the trigone.

Muscular coat [tunica muscularis (NA)]. Three indefinite coats of smooth muscle fibres, circular between longitudinal; the detrusor urinae.

Serous coat [tunica serosa (NA)]. The peritoneal covering applied to the superior surface, the upper parts of the inferolateral surfaces and, in the male, the upper part of the base.

Submucous coat [tela submucosal (NA)]. The loose areolar tissue between the mucous and muscular coats.

Neck [cervix vesicae (NA)]. The part of the bladder related to the upper surface of the prostate gland.

Inferolateral surfaces, right and left. The surfaces of the bladder in contact with the pubis in front and the levator ani muscle posteriorly.

Superior surface. The peritoneal covered surface that is directed upwards. Its enlargement is the main contribution to increased capacity of the organ. Coils of small intestine or sigmoid colon lie above it in the male and the body of the uterus in the female.

urinate (**ewr**·in·ate). To pass urine freely from the bladder; to micturate.

urination (ewr·in·**a**·shun). The act of passing urine; micturition. **Precipitant urination.** A sudden and overwhelming urge to pass urine. **Stuttering urination.** Jerky flow in urination due to spasmodic contractions of the bladder.

urinative (**ewr**·in·a·tiv). Any agent which promotes the flow of urine; a diuretic.

urine (**ewr**·in). The fluid secretion of the kidneys which is excreted by way of the bladder, in which it is stored, and the urethra. It is normally a clear, light-yellow to amber liquid having an acid reaction and a specific gravity of 1.010 to 1.025. The volume excreted daily is influenced by the fluid intake, but averages 900–1,500 ml by adults and 400–600 ml by children. The solids present in urine are derived almost wholly from the blood, being end-products of the metabolic processes of the body or salts surplus to its requirements, and for this reason the examination of urine is of considerable clinical significance. The amount of solids excreted in urine is usually 50–70 g per day, the bulk of which is made up of organic nitrogenous compounds, chiefly urea, creatine, and uric acid, and inorganic salts, chiefly chlorides, phosphates, and sulphates of sodium and potassium with smaller amounts of those of calcium and magnesium. Other constituents, such as certain steroids and vitamins and their metabolities, are present in comparatively small amounts but have achieved important clinical significance. In some pathological conditions abnormal constituents may appear in the urine, e.g. glucose and acetone in diabetes, protein in nephritis, bile pigments in jaundice, whilst in other conditions a normal component may be decreased or increased. **Black urine.** Urine containing melanine. **Chylous urine.** An opaque, milky urine containing chyle from the lymphatic system. **Diabetic urine.** Urine containing excessive amounts of glucose. **Febrile urine.** Deep-orange, strong-smelling urine which characterizes most pyrexic conditions. **Milky urine.** Chylous urine (see above). **Residual urine.** The urine remaining in the bladder after micturition. [Gk *ouron.*]

uriniferous (ewr·in·**if**·er·us). Having as its function the conveyance of urine. [urine, L *ferre* to bear.]

urinific (ewr·in·**if**·ik). Concerned with the secretion of urine; uriniparous. [urine, L *facere* to make.]

uriniparous (ewr·in·**ip**·ar·us). Effecting the secretion of urine. [urine, L *parere* to produce.]

urinocryoscopy (ewr·in·o·kri·**os'**·ko·pe). The determination of the freezing point of urine as an indication of the amount of solids in solution. [urine, Gk *kryos* cold, *skopein* to view.]

urinod (**ewr**·in·od). A substance, believed to be 3-cyclohexene-1-one, to which the characteristic odour of urine has been attributed. [urine, odour.]

urinogenital (ewr·in·o·**jen'**·it·al). Concerning the urinary and genital organs.

urinogenous (ewr·in·**oj**·en·us). 1. Devoted to the secretion or excretion of urine. 2. Originating in the urinary system. [urine, Gk *genein* to produce.]

urinolepsia (ewr·in·o·**lep'**·se·ah). Micturition syncope. *See* SYNCOPE.

urinology (ewr·in·**ol**·o·je). The study of urine and the urinary system. [urine, Gk *logos* science.]

urinoma (ewr·in·**o**·mah). A cyst which contains urine. [urine, Gk *-oma* tumour.]

urinometer (ewr·in·**om**·et·er). A form of hydrometer calibrated to measure the specific gravity of urine.

urinometry (ewr·in·**om**·et·re). The measurement of the specific gravity of urine by means of a urinometer.

urinosanguineous (ewr·in·o·sang·**gwin'**·e·us). Consisting of both urine and blood. [urine, L *sanguis* blood.]

urinoscopy (ewr·in·**os**·ko·pe). The examination of the urine diagnostically. [urine, Gk *skopein* to view.]

urinose (**ewr**·in·oze). 1. Possessing characteristics associated with urine, such as smell or colour. 2. Consisting of or containing urine.

urinous (**ewr**·in·us). Urinose.

urisolvent (ewr·e·**sol**·vent). Able to dissolve uric acid.

Urist, Marshall. 20th century American orthopaedic surgeon.

Urist cup. A metallic cup fixed with intramedullary prongs, used to resurface the acetabulum in arthroplasty of the hip.

uro-acidimeter (ewr·o·as·id·**im'**·et·er). Any device for estimating the acidity of a sample of urine. [Gk *ouron* urine, acid, meter.]

uro-ammoniac (ewr·o·am·**o'**·ne·ak). Containing both uric acid and ammonia, as in the case of certain calculi.

urobilin (ewr·o·**bi**·lin). $C_{33}H_{46}O_6N_4$, a brown pigment formed from urobilinogen by oxidation upon exposure to air. It is identical with stercobilin.

urobilinaemia (ewr·o·bi·lin·**e**'·me·ah). The appearance of urobilin in the blood. [urobilin, Gk *haima* blood.]

urobilinicterus (ewr·o·bi·lin·**ik**'·ter·us). A jaundiced state of the skin, associated with urobilinaemia. [urobilin, icterus.]

urobilinogen (ewr·o·bi·**lin**'·o·jen). $C_{33}H_{48}O_6N_4$, a colourless derivative of bilirubin from which it is produced by bacterial reduction in the intestine and excreted in traces in the urine. It is identical with the stercobilinogen present in faeces. In liver diseases it may appear in the urine in excessive amounts. [urobilin, Gk *genein* to produce.]

urobilinogenaemia (ewr·o·bi·**lin**·o·jen·**e**'·me·ah). The appearance of urobilinogen in the blood. [urobilinogen, Gk *haima* blood.]

urobilinogenuria (ewr·o·bi·**lin**·o·jen·**ewr**'·e·ah). A condition marked by the presence of an abnormal amount of urobilinogen in the urine.

urobilinoid (ewr·o·**bi**·lin·oid). Having a similarity to urobilin. [urobilin, Gk *eidos* form.]

urobilinuria (ewr·o·bi·lin·**ewr**'·e·ah). A condition marked by the occurrence of an abnormal amount of urobilin in the urine, e.g. in cirrhosis of the liver.

urocele (ewr·o·seel). The escape of urine into the scrotum, causing distension of the sac. [Gk *ouron* urine, *kele* hernia.]

urocheras (ewr·**ok**·er·as). Gravel or sediment in the urine. [Gk *ouron* urine, *cheras* gravel.]

urochesia (ewr·o·**ke**·ze·ah). The passage of urine through the rectum. [Gk *ouron* urine, *chezein* to defaecate.]

urochrome (ewr·o·krome). $C_{43}H_{51}O_{26}N$, the yellow pigment to which urine owes its colour. It is a derivative of urobilin formed with a polypeptide. [Gk *ouron* urine, *chroma* colour.]

urochromogen (ewr·o·**kro**·mo·jen). A substance of unknown constitution, absent from normal urine but reported to be present in urine in various pathological states, notably pulmonary tuberculosis in which condition it has been claimed to have diagnostic and prognostic significance. Its presence is shown by the appearance of a yellow colour upon oxidation with potassium permanganate (Weiss test). The connection of urochromogen with normal urinary pigments is obscure, but it is thought to arise from a defect in oxidation. [Gk *ouron* urine, *chroma* colour, *genein* to produce.]

urocinetic (ewr·o·sin·**et**'·ik). Urokinetic.

uroclepsia (ewr·o·**klep**·se·ah). Involuntary urination, without being aware of the fact. [Gk *ouron* urine, *kleptein* to steal.]

urocrisia (ewr·o·**kris**·e·ah). Diagnosis resulting from observation and testing of the urine. [Gk *ouron* urine, *krinein* to separate.]

urocrisis (ewr·o·**kri**·sis). 1. A stage in the progress of a disease when copious urination begins. 2. Severe pain in the urinary bladder, characteristic of tabes dorsalis; vesical crisis. [Gk *ouron* urine, crisis.]

urocyanosis (ewr·o·si·an·**o**'·sis). The condition in which the urine is blue, due to the presence of indican. [Gk *ouron* urine, *kyanos* blue.]

urocyst, urocystis (ewr·o·sist, ewr·o·**sist**·is). The urinary bladder. [Gk *ouron* urine, *kystis* bladder.]

urocystitis (ewr·o·sist·**i**'·tis). Inflammation of the bladder. [Gk *ouron* urine, *kystis* bladder, *-itis* inflammation.]

urodialysis (ewr·o·di·**al**'·is·is). The complete or partial arrest of urinary secretion. [Gk *ouron* urine, *dialysis* a cessation.]

urodynia (ewr·o·**din**·e·ah). Pain experienced when urinating. [Gk *ouron* urine, *odyne* pain.]

uroedema (ewr·e·**de**·mah). Swelling and puffiness of the tissues caused by extravasation of urine. [Gk *ouron* urine, oedema.]

uroerythrin (ewr·o·**er**·ith·rin). A reddish pigment, one of the normal pigments of urine, responsible for the staining of amorphous urate deposits to give the characteristic "brick-dust" appearance. It is normally present in urine in small amount but may be increased in various pathological conditions, giving the urine a deep orange-red colour. [Gk *ouron* urine, *erythros* red.]

uroflavin (ewr·o·**fla**·vin). A fluorescent lyochrome excreted in the urine in persons taking riboflavin and at one time considered to be a degradation product of riboflavin, but later this was contradicted. [Gk *ouron* urine, L *flavus* yellow.]

uroflowmeter (ewr·o·**flo**·me·ter). An instrument for measuring the rate of urinary flow during micturition. [Gk *ouron* urine, AS *flowan* flow, Gk *metron* measure.]

urogastrone (ewr·o·**gas**·trone). A hormone found in the urine and secreted in the duodenum. It inhibits gastric secretion. [Gk *ouron* urine, *gaster* belly.]

urogenital (ewr·o·**jen**·it·al). Referring to the urinary and genital organs.

urogenous (ewr·**oj**·en·us). 1. Concerned with the secretion and excretion of urine. 2. Derived from urine. [Gk *ouron* urine, *genein* to produce.]

Uroglena (ewr·o·**gle**·nah). A genus of protozoa; they are flagellate and free-swimming.

uroglycosis (ewr·o·gli·**ko**'·sis). Excretion of sugar in the urine. [Gk *ouron* urine, *glykys* sweet.]

urogram (ewr·o·gram). An x-ray radiograph of the urinary tract obtained in urography. [Gk *ouron* urine, *gramma* a record.]

urography (ewr·**og**·raf·e). The radiographic examination of the urinary tract. **Ascending urography.** Instrumental urography (see below). **Contrast urography.** The use of contrast media for demonstrating radiographically the lumina of the urinary tract. **Cytoscopic urography.** Instrumental urography (see below). **Descending urography, excretion urography, excretory urography.** Contrast urography in which the opaque medium is introduced by either the intravenous (usual), intramuscular, subcutaneous, oral, or intramedullary route. It is excreted in the urine. **Instrumental urography.** Retrograde urography (see below). **Intravenous urography.** Excretory urography (see above). **Retrograde urography.** Contrast urography in which the medium is introduced directly into the lumen of the lower urinary tract, either urethra or bladder. [Gk *ouron* urine, *graphein* to record.]

urohaematonephrosis (ewr·o·he·mat·o·nef·**ro**'·sis). Over-distension of the pelvis of the ureter with blood and urine, usually as the result of the presence of a stone or tumour in the upper urinary tract. [Gk *ouron* urine, *haima* blood, *nephros* kidney, *-osis* condition.]

Urokinase (ewr·o·**kin**·aze). BP Commission approved name for a plasminogen activator isolated from human urine.

urokinetic (ewr·o·kin·**et**'·ik). Denoting any condition that can be attributed to reflex from the urinary system, e.g. when dyspepsia results from disease of the bladder. [Gk *ouron* urine, *kinesis* movement.]

urokymography (ewr·o·ki·**mog**'·raf·e). X-ray kymography used in the study of movement in the organs of urinary excretion, the urine being opacified by suitable contrast media. [Gk *ouron* urine, kymography.]

urolagnia (ewr·o·**lag**·ne·ah). Sexual perversion centred on urine, urination, or the sight of another person urinating. [Gk *ouron* urine, *lagneia* lust.]

urolite (ewr·o·lite). Urolith.

urolith (ewr·o·lith). A urinary stone or calculus. [Gk *ouron* urine, *lithos* stone.]

urolithiasis (ewr·o·lith·**i**'·as·is). The production of urinary calculi, and the morbid state due to the presence of calculi in the urinary system. [see prec.]

urolithic (ewr·o·**lith**·ik). Referring to urinary calculi or to urolithiasis.

urologic, urological (ewr·o·**loj**·ik, ewr·o·**loj**·ik·al). Concerned with urology.

urologist (ewr·**ol**·o·jist). A specialist in urology.

urology (ewr·**ol**·o·je). The study of the urinary system. [Gk *ouron* urine, *logos* science.]

urolytic (ewr·o·**lit**·ik). Applied to any agent or process that will effect the breaking-up and solution of urinary calculi. [Gk *ouron* urine, *lysis* a loosing.]

uromelus (ewr·**om**·el·us). A fetal monster with legs fused into one and having a single foot. [Gk *oura* tail, *melos* limb.]

urometer (ewr·**om**·et·er). Urinometer.

uromphalus (ewr·**om**·fal·us). A fetal deformity in which the urachus protrudes from the umbilicus. [urachus, Gk *omphalos* navel.]

uron (ewr·on). Proton. [Obsolete term.]

uroncus (ewr·**ong**·kus). A urinary cyst, a swelling caused by extravasation of urine into the tissues. [Gk *ouron* urine, *ogkos* tumour.]

Uronema nigricans (ewr·o·**ne**·mah **ni**·grik·anz). A free-living coprozoic ciliate. [Gk *ouron* urine, *nema* thread, L *niger* black.]

uronephrosis (ewr·o·nef·**ro**'·sis). Hydronephrosis. [Gk *ouron* urine, *nephros* kidney.]

uronology (ewr·on·**ol**·o·je). Urology.

uropathy (ewr·**op**·ath·e). A general term for any pathological change in the urinary tract. **Obstructive uropathy.** A sequence of pathological changes in the urinary tract proximal to an obstruction. [Gk *ouron* urine, *pathos* disease.]

uropenia (ewr·o·**pe**·ne·ah). Reduction in the amount of urine secreted. [Gk *ouron* urine, *penia* poverty.]

urophan (ewr·o·fan). Any substance that after ingestion appears in the urine in an unchanged condition. [Gk *ouron* urine, *phanein* to appear.]

urophanic (ewr·o·**fan**·ik). Pertaining to urophan.

urophosphometer (ewr·o·fos·**fom**'·et·er). An appliance for estimating phosphorus in the urine. [Gk *ouron* urine, phosphorus, meter.]

uropittin (ewr·o·**pit**·in). $C_9H_{10}O_3N_2$, a compound derived from the decomposition of urochrome. [Gk *ouron* urine, *pitta* pitch.]

uroplania (ewr·o·**pla**·ne·ah). The presence of urine in organs and tissues that are outside the urogenital tract. [Gk *ouron* urine, *planos* a wandering.]

uropoiesis (ewr·o·poi·**e**'·sis). The formation of urine in the metabolism. [Gk *ouron* urine, *poiein* to make.]

uroporphyrin (ewr·o·**por**·fir·in). $C_{40}H_{38}O_{16}N_4$, a porphyrin occurring in the urine in congenital porphyrinuria. it may also occur, as a result of treatment with certain hypnotics, in the urine of patients who are especially sensitive to these drugs.

uropsammus (ewr·o·**sam**·us). Sand-like sediment in the urine. [Gk *ouron* urine, *psammos* sand.]

uropterin (ewr·**op**·ter·in). A xanthopterin-like substance found in the urine.

uropyonephrosis (ewr·o·pi·o·nef·**ro**'·sis). The pathological accumulation of pus and urine in the pelvis of the ureter. [Gk *ouron* urine, *pyon* pus, *nephros* kidney.]

uropyoureter (ewr·o·pi·o·ewr·**e**'·ter). Pus and urine which accumulates in an infected ureter. [Gk *ouron* urine, *pyon* pus, ureter.]

urorhythmography (ewr·o·rith·**mog**'·raf·e). A graphic recording of the efflux of urine from the ureteric orifices. [Gk *ouron* urine, rhythm, Gk *graphein* to record.]

urorosein (ewr·o·**ro**·ze·in). A rose-red pigment occurring in certain pathological urines in the form of a chromogen which has been identified with indole-acetic acid. The colour is produced upon addition of hydrochloric acid and a solution of nitrite to the fresh urine, but may be produced by addition of hydrochloric acid alone in stale urines owing to the presence of preformed nitrite. Positive reactions have been reported in typhoid fever, pulmonary tuberculosis, nephritis, and pellagra. [Gk *ouron* urine, L *roseus* rosy.]

urorrhagia (ewr·o·**ra**·je·ah). The passing of abnormally large quantities of urine, such as is observed in cases of diabetes insipidus. [Gk *ouron* urine, *rhegnynein* to gush forth.]

urorrhoea (ewr·o·**re**·ah). 1. Involuntary urination; bedwetting; enuresis. 2. The passing of large amounts of urine; polyuria. [Gk *ouron* urine, *rhein* to flow.]

uroscheocele (ewr·**os**·ke·o·seel). Extravasation of urine into the scrotum. [Gk *ouron* urine, *oscheon* scrotum, *kele* tumour.]

uroschesis (ewr·**os**·kes·is). 1. Involuntary retention of the urine. 2. Cessation of urinary secretion. [Gk *ouron* urine, *schesis* a holding.]

uroscopic (ewr·o·**skop**·ik). Concerned with the diagnostic examination of the urine. [Gk *ouron* urine, *skopein* to view.]

uroscopy (ewr·**os**·ko·pe). The examination of the urine diagnostically. [see prec.]

urosemeology (ewr·o·sem·e·**ol**'·o·je). Urology. [Gk *ouron* urine, *semeion* sign, *logos* science.]

urosepsis (ewr·o·**sep**·sis). A general toxic state arising in the urinary tract. [Gk *ouron* urine, *sepsis* putrefaction.]

uroseptic (ewr·o·**sep**·tik). Referring to urosepsis.

urostealith (ewr·o·**ste**·al·ith). A urinary calculus rich in fatty material. [Gk *ouron* urine, *stear* fat, *lithos* stone.]

urosteatoma (ewr·o·ste·at·**o**'·mah). Urostealith. [Gk *ouron* urine, *stear* fat, *-oma* tumour.]

urothelium (ewr·o·**the**·le·um). The transitional-cell epithelium of the urinary tract. [Gk *ouron* urine, *thele* nipple.]

urotherapy (ewr·o·**ther**·ap·e). Auto-urotherapy.

urotoxicity (ewr·o·tox·**is**'·it·e). The toxic nature of the urine. [Gk *ouron* urine, *toxikon* poison.]

uro-ureter (ewr·o·ewr·**e**'·ter). The retention of urine in a ureter, with swelling of the latter. [Gk *ouron* urine, ureter.]

uroxanic (ewr·ox·**an**·ik). Pertaining to alloxantin (uroxin).

uroxin (ewr·**ox**·in). Alloxantin. [Gk *ouron* urine, *oxys* sour.]

Urriola's test. Aro Luis Urriola, acting President of the Republic of Panama, was convinced that he had found in serum and urine special pigments diagnostic of malaria. These consisted of coal-black pigment in fine grains of the urine; in the sediment are found fine grains of yellow pigment. By addition of 7 per cent solution of chlorate of potash to blood he claimed that crescents developed. There is no evidence that these observations have any foundations in fact.

ursin (er·sin). Arbutin.

Urtica (er·tik·ah). A genus of plants of the family Urticaceae, including the nettles. **Urtica dioica.** The stinging nettle, an important source of chlorophyll. [L, a nettle.]

urticant (er·tik·ant). Any agent that produces stinging or itching of the skin. [see prec.]

urticaria (er·tik·a·re·ah). Hives; nettle rash: an acute or chronic affection of the skin characterized by the formation of evanescent whitish, pink, or red elevations or weals, attended by itching, stinging, or burning. **Allergic urticaria.** Urticaria due to hypersensitivity to some ingested, injected, or contact, allergen. **Urticaria bullosa.** 1. A form of urticaria in which the weals become capped with blebs. This anomaly is seen most frequently on the extremities. 2. Papular urticaria in which the lesions are capped or replaced by bullae. **Cholinergic urticaria.** Urticaria caused by exercise, heat, or emotion, the symptoms of which are believed to be due to release of choline by the cholinergic nerves in the skin. **Cold urticaria.** Urticaria caused by external cold. **Urticaria evanida.** Urticaria characterized by rapid evolution of the lesions. **Urticaria factitia, factitious urticaria.** Wealing of the skin caused by a minimal degree of trauma. **Urticaria geographica.** A form of urticaria that spreads peripherally. **Giant urticaria, urticaria gigans.** 1. Urticaria characterized by the formation of large weals. 2. Angioneurotic oedema. *See* OEDEMA. **Urticaria gyrata.** Urticaria geographica (see above). **Urticaria haemorrhagica.** An eruption in which haemorrhage occurs in the weals. It usually occurs as a complication of severe systemic disease, e.g. nephritis or septicaemia. Occasionally weals occur as a complication of purpura in which the bleeding occurs first and the weal formation is superimposed (purpura urticans). **Urticaria medicamentosa.** Urticaria due to ingestion of certain drugs, e.g. antipyrin or quinine. **Menstrual urticaria.** Urticaria which recurs at each menstrual period. **Urticaria oedematosa.** Angioneurotic oedema. *See* OEDEMA. **Papular urticaria, Urticaria papulosa.** Prurigo simplex acutus; strophulus: a malady of the skin of infants and young children characterized by the formation of reddish macules on which papules arise. In some cases a short weal disguises the papule; in others the papules are capped by a vesicle. The condition is usually caused by insect bites. **Urticaria perstans.** Urticaria in which the lesions instead of being evanescent persist for several days or weeks. **Urticaria perstans pigmentosa.** Urticaria pigmentosa (see below). **Urticaria petechialis.** Urticaria haemorrhagica (see above). **Urticaria photogenica.** Urticaria caused by exposure to light. **Urticaria pigmentosa.** A persistent, cutaneous affection which usually begins in early infancy, affecting males more frequently than females, in which macules, papules, or nodules develop; these become urticarial when rubbed. Histologically the lesions are characterized by the large number of mast cells in the corium. Cases have been recorded in which similar eruptions have developed in adult life, but it is doubtful whether these are manifestations of the same disease. **Serum urticaria.** An urticarial rash caused by the injection of serum; an anaphylactoid phenomenon, **Urticaria solaris.** Urticaria developing after exposure to sunlight. **Urticaria vesiculosa.** A form of papular urticaria in which the lesions are replaced by vesicles. [L *urtica* nettle.]

See also: MILTON.

urticarial (er·tik·a·re·al). Characterized by urticaria, or referring to the latter.

urticariogenic (er·tik·a·re·o·**jen'**·ik). Likely to cause an urticarial response. [urticaria, Gk *genein* to produce.]

urticarious (er·tik·a·re·us). Urticarial.

urticate (**er**·tik·ate). 1. To treat by urtication. 2. To be marked by weals or blisters as in urticaria. [L *urticare* to sting.]

urtication (er·tik·a·shun). 1. Counter-irritation set up by means of stinging nettles. 2. The stinging or burning itch of urticaria. 3. The eruption of urticaria. [see prec.]

Uschinsky, Nicolaus (b. 1863). Leningrad bacteriologist.

Uschinsky's protein-free broth. A protein-free synthetic culture medium containing asparagine, ammonium lactate, sodium chloride, magnesium sulphate, calcium chloride. potassium phosphate, and glycerin.

Usher, Barney David (b. 1899). Quebec dermatologist.

Senear-Usher disease, or syndrome, Usher-Senear disease. Pemphigus erythematodes; a relatively benign type of chronic pemphigus, in which besides bullae, lesions resembling lupus erythematosus or crusted seborrhoeic dermatitis may be noted.

Uskow, N. 19th century German anatomist.

Uskow's pillars. The upper degenerated portions of the mesonephros on each side of the back of the coelomic cavity of the embryo which contribute towards the closing of the pleuroperitoneal canals and are eventually incorporated in the back of the diaphragm.

ustilaginism (us·til·**aj**·in·izm). A disorder caused by eating maize contaminated by a smut fungus, *Ustilago maydis.* Species of *Ustilago* can cause hypersensitivity reactions in bronchopulmonary tissues in sensitive individuals. [L *ustulare* to scorch.]

Ustilago (us·til·a·go). A genus of fungi of the order Basidiomycetes, parasitic on plants; smuts. **Ustilago maydis, Ustilago zeae.** Corn smut, produced on Indian corn grains (maize). It has an oxytocic action on the uterus, like ergot, but has little therapeutic value. [L *ustulare* to scorch.]

ustion (**ust**·shun). Burning; actual cautery. [L *urere* to burn.]

usure (ew·zhewr). Localized atrophy of a part caused by pressure of a tumour. [L *uti* to wear out.]

uta (**oo**·tah). Mucocutaneous leishmaniasis; *uta* is the name given to the form of mucocutaneous leishmaniasis that occurs in the foot-hills in tropical and sub-tropical South and Central America. Nasopharyngeal ulceration is relatively rare and usually occurs by direct extension from a skin ulcer rather than metastatically. Cf. ESPUNDIA. The names *uta* and *espundia* are often used synonymously, but in South America the distinction is more frequently observed. **Uta hembra.** Ulcerative mucocutaneous leishmaniasis. **Uta macho.** Tuberculoid mucocutaneous leishmaniasis. This and the preceding name are accepted locally, but are little known elsewhere. [Sp.]

uteralgia (ew·ter·**al**·je·ah). Pain experienced in the uterus. [uterus, Gk *algos* pain.]

uterectomy (ew·ter·**ek**·to·me). Surgical excision of the uterus. [uterus, Gk *ektome* excision.]

uterine (**ew**·ter·ine). Concerning or referring to the uterus.

uterine artery [arteria uterina (NA)]. A branch of the anterior division of the internal iliac artery which runs through the base of the broad ligament to supply the uterus, vagina, and uterine tube [ramus tubarius (NA)]; it anastomoses with the ovarian artery [ramus ovaricus (NA)].

uterine motility (**ew**·ter·ine mo·**til**·it·e). The degree of tonic contraction of the uterine muscle.

uterine veins [venae uterinae (NA)]. Veins which commence in the uterine plexus. They are tributaries of the internal iliac veins.

uterismus (ew·ter·**iz**·mus). A painful spasm of the uterus.

uteritis (ew·ter·**i**·tis). Inflammation of the uterus. [uterus, Gk *-itis* inflammation.]

utero-abdominal (**ew**·ter·o·ab·**dom'**·in·al). Concerning the uterus and the abdomen.

uterocele (**ew**·ter·o·seel). A hernia of or involving the uterus. [uterus, Gk *kele* hernia.]

uterocervical (**ew**·ter·o·**ser'**·vik·al). Concerning the uterus and the neck (cervix) of the uterus.

uterocolic (**ew**·ter·o·**kol'**·ik). Pertaining to the uterus and the adjacent colon.

uterocystostomy (**ew**·ter·o·sist·**os'**·to·me). The surgical establishment of a communication between the neck of the uterus and the urinary bladder. [uterus, Gk *kystis* bladder, *stoma* mouth.]

uterodynia (**ew**·ter·o·**din'**·e·ah). Pain experienced in the uterus. [uterus, Gk *odyne* pain.]

uterofixation (**ew**·ter·o·fix·**a'**·shun). The surgical fixation of a misplaced uterus by attachment to the anterior wall of the abdomen or to the vaginal peritoneum.

uterogestation (**ew**·ter·o·jes·**ta'**·shun). A normal pregnancy; one in which the fetus develops within the uterus, as distinguished from an extra-uterine pregnancy. [uterus, Gk *gestare* to bear.]

uterography (ew·ter·**og**·raf·e). Radiography of the uterus. [uterus, Gk *graphein* to record.]

utero-intestinal (**ew**·ter·o·in·**tes'**·tin·al). Concerning the uterus and the intestine.

uterolith (**ew**·ter·o·lith). 1. A calculus occurring in the uterus. 2. A calcified uterine myoma. [uterus, Gk *lithos* stone.]

uteromania (**ew**·ter·o·**ma'**·ne·ah). Excessive sexual urge in women. [uterus, Gk *mania* madness.]

uterometer (ew·ter·**om**·et·er). An instrument for measuring the depth of the cavity of the uterus.

uterometry (ew·ter·**om**·et·re). Measurement of the size of the uterus.

utero-ovarian (ew·ter·o·o·**va'**·re·an). Concerning both the uterus and the ovary.

uteroparietal (**ew**·ter·o·par·**i'**·et·al). Involving the uterus and the wall of the abdomen, as in abdominal hysteropexy. [uterus, Gk *paries* wall.]

uteropelvic (**ew**·ter·o·**pel'**·vik). Connecting the uterus and the pelvis.

uteropexia, uteropexy (**ew**·ter·o·**pex'**·e·ah, **ew**·ter·o·pex·e). Uterofixation. [uterus, Gk *pexis* fixation.]

uteroplacental (**ew**·ter·o·plas·**en'**·tal). Concerning the uterus and the placenta.

uteroplasty (**ew**·ter·o·plas·te). Plastic surgery of the uterus. [uterus, Gk *plassein* to mould.]

uterorectal (**ew**·ter·o·**rek'**·tal). Involving the uterus and the rectum.

uterosacral (**ew**·ter·o·**sa'**·kral). Connecting the uterus and the sacrum, as with the uterosacral ligaments.

uterosalpingography (ew·ter·o·sal·ping·**gog'**·raf·e). X-ray examination of the uterus and uterine tubes. [uterus, Gk *salpigx* tube, *graphein* to record.]

uteroscope (**ew**·ter·o·skope). An instrument used to visualize the uterine cavity. [uterus, Gk *skopein* to view.]

uterothermometry (**ew**·ter·o·ther·**mom'**·et·re). The measurement of the temperature within the uterus. [uterus, Gk *therme* heat, *metron* measure.]

uterotome (ew·ter·o·tome). An instrument used in uterotomy.

uterotomy (ew·ter·**ot**·o·me). Incision of the uterus, as in caesarean section. [uterus, Gk *temnein* to cut.]

uterotonic (ew·ter·o·**ton**'·ik). 1. Applied to any agent that restores tone to the uterine muscles. 2. Maintaining the tone of the uterus.

uterotractor (ew·ter·o·**trak**'·tor). A special type of forceps with multiple teeth on each blade, used to apply traction to the neck of the uterus during hysterectomy.

uterotubal (ew·ter·o·**tew**'·bl). Concerning the uterus and the uterine tubes.

uterotubography (ew·ter·o·tewb·**og**'·raf·e). Uterosalpingography. [uterus, tube, Gk *graphein* to record.]

uterovaginal (ew·ter·o·**vag**'·in·al). Involving both the uterus and the vagina.

uteroventral (ew·ter·o·**ven**'·tral). Referring to the uterus and the abdomen. [uterus, L *venter* belly.]

uterovesical (ew·ter·o·**ves**'·ik·al). Involving the uterus and the urinary bladder. [uterus, L *vesica* bladder.]

uterus [NA] (ew·ter·us). A hollow, thick-walled, muscular organ in which the impregnated ovum is developed into the child. In the nonpregnant women it is about 75 mm in length, pyriform in shape, and flattened in the coronal plane. It is divided into a broad body [corpus uteri (NA)] above, flexed ventrally by a few degrees on the narrower cervix below which projects into the vagina. The uterine tubes enter the body at the upper end of each lateral border [margo uteri (dexter et sinister (NA)]. **Uterus acollis.** A uterus without a cervix. **Uterus arcuatus.** A uterus with a depression in the centre of the fundus, giving it an arched appearance. **Uterus bicornis.** A uterus which is divided into two halves which are separate at the upper ends and united to some extent at the lower end. **Uterus bicornis unicollis.** A uterus bicornis with a single cervix. **Bifid uterus.** A uterus which is divided into two parts by a septum. **Uterus biforis.** A uterus in which the external os of the cervix is divided by a septum. **Uterus bilocularis, uterus bipartitus.** Bifid uterus (see above). **Uterus bipartitus unicollis.** A bifid uterus with a single cervix. **Coat of the uterus, mucous [tunica mucosa (endometrium) NA].** The endometrium; it is surfaced with columnar epithelium, ciliated before puberty, lying on a thick cellular connective-tissue layer in which lie the numerous tubular uterine glands [glandulae uterinae (NA)] lined with columnar ciliated epithelium and opening on to its surface. In the upper cervix the mucosa is thinner and the glands fewer. In the lower cervix the surface is covered with tall, columnar, mucus-secreting cells which are continued into the numerous branching cervical glands [glandulae cervicales (uteri) NA]. At the external os this becomes stratified squamous epithelium. **Coat of the uterus, muscular [tunica muscularis (NA)].** A thick coat formed of interlacing unstriped muscle fibres indistinctly separable into three layers. The middle is the thickest, and the outer mainly longitudinal. **Coat of the uterus, serous [tunica serosa (perimetrium) NA].** The peritoneal coat which invests the fundus and body and the posterior surface of the supravaginal cervix. Traced laterally it is continuous with the broad ligament on either side. **Cochleate uterus.** An under-developed uterus showing acute anteflexion. **Uterus cordiformis.** A uterus bicornis showing only a very slight depression at the fundus. **Uterus didelphys, uterus duplex.** A double uterus, but having only one tube to each uterus. **Fetal uterus.** A small uterus with the cervix relatively bigger than the body. **Fundus of the uterus [fundus uteri (NA)].** The portion of the body situated above the plane of the entering uterine tubes. **Gravid uterus.** A pregnant uterus. **Uterus incudiformis.** A uterus in which the normal convexity of the uterine fundus is absent and there is a straight line joining the two uterine tubes. **Infantile uterus.** A uterus which retains the characteristics of late ante-natal life. **Irritable uterus.** Usually applied to a uterus exhibiting the hypertonic type of uterine inertia. **Neck of the uterus [cervix uteri (NA)].** The lower, more cylindrical segment of the uterus, the vaginal [portio vaginalis (cervicis) NA] or lower portion of which projects at an angle into the upper part of the anterior vaginal wall. The supravaginal part [portio supravaginalis (cervicis) NA] lies between this part and the body. The thicker anterior lip [labium anterius (NA)] and the thinner posterior lip [labium posterius (NA)] are formed by the neck of the uterus at the external os uteri. **Uterus parvicollis.** One in which the body of the uterus is normal, but the cervix is atrophied or absent. **Pubescent uterus.** A uterus which retains the pubescent shape present before menstruation in adult life, the cervix and the body of the uterus being of equal length. **Sacculated uterus.** A condition especially liable to occur with an incarcerated retroversion of the pregnant uterus when the expansion of the uterus is almost entirely confined to the anterior wall; known also as *anterior sacculation of the uterus.* **Uterus septus.** Bifid uterus (see above). **Uterus subseptus.** A developmental abnormality of the uterus, where a septum is found arising in the midline of the fundus and extending for a short distance into the cavity. **Surface of the uterus, intestinal [facies intestinalis (NA)].** The posterior peritoneal covered surface of the uterus, in contact usually with coils of the small intestine. **Surface of the uterus, vesical [facies vesicalis (NA)].** The peritoneal covered anterior surface of the body, in contact with the superior surface of the bladder. **Unicorn uterus, uterus unicornis.** A malformation of the uterus in which only one half of the two fused paramesonephric ducts is fully developed, the other half being very small or absent. [L womb.]

See also: COUVELAIRE.

utricle [utriculus (NA)] (ew·trikl). A membranous sac occupying the elliptical recess of the bony labyrinth, into which the semicircular canals open. **Prostatic utricle [utriculus prostaticus (NA)].** A blind sac extending backwards into the substance of the prostate from its orifice on the crest of the prostatic urethra. It is alleged to represent the remains of the fused ends of the paramesonephric ducts in the male, and the openings of the ejaculatory ducts lie on either side of it. [L *utriculus* small bag.]

utricular (ew·**trik**·ew·lar). Referring to or shaped like a utricle.

utricular nerve [nervus utricularis (NA)]. A branch of the vestibular nerve which supplies the utricle.

utriculitis (ew·trik·ew·**li**'·tis). Inflammation of the utricle of the ear, or of the prostatic utricle. [utricle, Gk *-itis* inflammation.]

utriculo-ampullar (ew·**trik**·ew·lo·am·**pul**'·ar). Concerning the utricle of the ear and the ampullae.

utriculo-ampullar nerve [nervus utriculoampullaris (NA)]. The superior branch of the vestibular nerve. It is given off in the internal auditory meatus and ends in the macula of the utricle and the ampullary crests of the superior and lateral semicircular canals.

utriculoplasty (ew·**trik**·ew·lo·plas·te). A plastic operation by which the size of the uterine body and cavity are reduced by excision of a wedge of the uterine wall at the fundus of the uterus. [L *utriculus* small bag, Gk *plassein* to mould.]

utriculosaccular (ew·**trik**·ew·lo·**sak**'·ew·lar). Concerning the utricle of the ear and the saccule.

utriform (ew·tre·form). Resembling a small bag in shape. [L *utriculus* small bag.]

uva (ew·vah). The raisin; the dried fruit of the grape vine, *Vitis vinifera* (family Vitaceae). **Uvae passae.** Dried grapes, or raisins; they contain glucose, sucrose, and tartaric acid. **Uvae passae minores.** Commercial currants, a variety of small raisins. [L, grape.]

uvaeformis (ew·ve·**for**·mis). The middle layer of the choroid coat of the eye, comprising the lamina vasculosa and the lamina choriocapillaris. [L *uva* grape, form.]

uvea (ew·ve·ah). The vascular middle coat of the eye which is divided, from behind forwards, into the choroid, the ciliary body, and the iris. [L *uva* grape.]

uveal (ew·ve·al). Referring to the uvea.

uveitic (ew·ve·**it**·ik). Characterized by uveitis.

uveitis (ew·ve·i·tis). Inflammation of part or whole of the uveal tract, which comprises the iris, ciliary body, and choroid. **Anterior uveitis.** Iritis, or iridocyclitis. **Heterochromic uveitis.** A chronic form of uni-ocular iridocyclitis producing discoloration of the affected iris. **Posterior uveitis.** Inflammation of the choroid coat of the eye and the ciliary body, shown clinically by vitreous opacities, keratic precipitates, and perhaps a patch of choroiditis. **Sympathetic uveitis.** A severe form of bilateral uveitis of unknown aetiology, often terminating in blindness and almost invariably due to a perforating wound frequently associated with prolapse of the uveal tract in the so-called "exciting eye". **Toxoplasmic uveitis.** A uveitis caused by *Toxoplasma gondii*; the condition responds to pyrimethamine. [uvea, Gk *-itis* inflammation.]

See also: FOERSTER (R.).

uveoparotid (ew·ve·o·par·ot′·id). Involving the uvea and the parotid glands.

uveoparotitis (ew·ve·o·par·o·ti′·tis). Heerfordt's disease. [uvea, parotid, Gk *-itis* inflammation.]

uveoplasty (ew·ve·o·plas·te). Plastic surgery of the uvea. [uvea, Gk *plassein* to mould.]

uveoscleritis (ew·ve·o·skleer·i′·tis). Inflammation of the sclera due to extension from uveitis.

uviform (ew·ve·form). Resembling a grape or bunch of grapes. [L *uva* grape, form.]

uviometer (ew·ve·om·et·er). An instrument for measuring ultraviolet radiations. [Obsolete term.] [ultraviolet, meter.]

uvioresistant (ew·ve·o·re·zis′·tant). Resistant to the effects of ultraviolet radiation. [Obsolete term.] [ultraviolet, resistant.]

uviosensitive (ew·ve·o·sen′·sit·iv). Sensitive to the effects of ultraviolet radiations. [Obsolete term.] [ultraviolet, sensitive.]

uvula [NA] (ew·vew·lah). Uvula palatinae; specifically, the tongue-like process which projects from the middle of the posterior edge of the soft palate. **Bifid uvula.** A condition in which the uvula is split into two halves owing to failure of union of the posterior ends of the palatine folds. **Uvula of the bladder [uvula vesicae (NA)].** A projection into the interior of the bladder immediately posterior to the internal urethral orifice, produced by the underlying middle lobe of the prostate; it is usually confined to the elderly. **Uvula of the cerebellum.** Uvula of the vermis (see below). **Uvula palatinae.** *See* MAIN DEF. (above). **Uvula of the vermis [uvula vermis (NA)].** That portion of the inferior vermis which lies between the nodule in front and the pyramid behind. [dim. of L *uva* grape.]

uvular (ew·vew·lar). Referring to or concerning the uvula.

uvularis (ew·vew·la·ris). The musculus uvulae.

uvulatome (ew·vew·lat·ome). Uvulotome.

uvulatomy (ew·vew·lat·o·me). Uvulotomy.

uvulectomy (ew·vew·lek·to·me). Surgical removal of the uvula. [uvula, Gk *ektome* excision.]

uvulitis (ew·vew·li·tis). Inflammation of the uvula. [uvula, Gk *-itis* inflammation.]

uvuloptosis (ew·vew·lop·to·sis). A relaxed state of the uvula, which hangs long and pendulous. [uvula, Gk *ptosis* a falling.]

uvulotome (ew·vew·lo·tome). An instrument used in excision of the uvula. [see foll.]

uvulotomy (ew·vew·lot·o·me). Surgical incision of the uvula, or removal of part of it. [uvula, Gk *temnein* to cut.]

V

vaccigenous (vak·sij·en·us). Vaccine producing, or concerned with the production of vaccine. [vaccine, Gk *genein* to produce.]

vaccinal (vak·sin·al). Referring to vaccines or to vaccination, and also, but less correctly, to vaccinia.

vaccinate (vak·sin·ate). 1. To inoculate against smallpox with vaccine lymph (vaccinia virus). 2. To inject any viral or bacterial vaccine in order to stimulate immunity to an infection.

vaccination (vak·sin·a·shun). The process or act of immunizing for preventive purposes, less commonly for the treatment of disease. The term is applied particularly to the use of vaccinia virus against smallpox. The virus is propagated on the epidermis of sheep or calves (animal or vaccine lymph) or in the tissue of the chick embryo. The lymph contains glycerol to reduce bacterial contamination and permit storage unfrozen at −20°C. More commonly, freeze-dried vaccine is prepared; it keeps better in the tropics and can be stored in an ordinary refrigerator. Vaccination against smallpox is usually by multiple pressure or linear scratch through a drop of lymph placed on the skin. The primary reaction on first vaccination is a single vesicle which proceeds through pustulation to crusting, and heals usually with scarring. The response on revaccination is very variable. A significant flare around the site 5 days later is usually taken as indicating a satisfactory revaccination, but results are best interpreted with experience. The complications of vaccination include severe local lesions which rarely spread progressively, generalized vaccinia, encephalomyelitis or, in eczematous persons, eczema vaccinatum. An adequate immunity lasting 3-5 years follows successful vaccination. **Jennerian vaccination.** Successful vaccination against smallpox introduced in the 18th century by Edward Jenner, who used matter from cowpox lesions to protect against smallpox. [L *vaccinus* of a cow.]

vaccine (vak·seen). Originally applied only to the matter or vesicle fluid of cowpox (vaccinia), first used as an immunizing agent against smallpox by Edward Jenner. Pasteur, in honour of Jenner, suggested its use as a generic term for any preparation employed to produce active immunity. Vaccines may be bacterial or viral. **Bacterial vaccines.** May consist of the organisms themselves alive but attentuated (as in BCG vaccine) or killed (as in typhoid vaccine), or they may contain a bacterial toxin inactivated with formaldehyde (as in tetanus vaccine). **Viral vaccines.** May contain live attenuated virus (as in Sabin-type poliomyelitis vaccine), killed virus (as in some influenza vaccines), viral antigens (as in some other influenza vaccines) or an antigenically related live virus that is relatively harmless (as in smallpox vaccine). **Acne vaccine.** Vaccine once much used in the treatment of acne vulgaris, prepared from acne bacilli and white and yellow staphylococci; obtained either from autogenous or stock cultures. **Adenovirus vaccine.** Vaccine prepared from adenovirus (types 4 and 7) used in the prevention of infection by these organisms of the upper respiratory tract. **Adsorbed Diphtheria Vaccine BP 1973.** Prepared from diphtheria formol toxoid containing not less than 1500 flocculation equivalents (1500 L_f) per mg of protein nitrogen and a mineral carrier which may be aluminium hydroxide or aluminium phosphate. It is used for the prophylaxis of diphtheria when primary immunization is required. For the reinforcement of primary immunization, diphtheria vaccine or adsorbed diphtheria vaccine is used. **Adsorbed Diphtheria and Tetanus Vaccine BP 1973.** Prepared from diphtheria and tetanus formol toxoid and a mineral carrier (see Adsorbed Diphtheria Vaccine BP 1973), it is used for the prophylaxis of diphtheria and tetanus. **Adsorbed Diphtheria, Tetanus and Pertussis Vaccine BP 1973.** Adsorbed Diphtheria and Tetanus Vaccine (see above) to which has been added a suspension of killed *Bordetella pertussis*; it is used for the prophylaxis of diphtheria, tetanus and pertussis. **Adsorbed Tetanus Vaccine BP 1973.** Prepared from tetanus formol toxoid and a mineral carrier (aluminium hydroxide or aluminium phosphate), it is used for the prophylaxis of tetanus. **Anthrax vaccine.** Attenuated cultures of *Bacillus anthracis* produced by growing the organisms at 42°C, used for actively immunizing sheep, horses, and cattle. **Antirabic vaccine.** Rabies vaccine (see below). **Antityphoid vaccine.** A sterile suspension of the bacillus *Salmonella typhi*, killed by heat or by a bactericide. It is used as a prophylactic against typhoid fever for members of the armed forces, the staffs of fever hospitals, and persons in countries in which typhoid fever is endemic. It is one constituent of typhoid-paratyphoid A and B vaccine. **Aqueous vaccine.** A vaccine in which the antigenic material is suspended in water or salt solution. **Autogenous vaccine.** A vaccine prepared from cultures of organisms already infecting the patient. **Bacillus-Calmette-Guérin Vaccine BP 1973, BCG vaccine.** A vaccine of living bovine tubercle bacilli obtained from a strain originally isolated in 1906 by Calmette and Guérin, and attenuated by repeated subculture under standard conditions on a glycerin-bile-potato medium. The strain was proved to remain avirulent, and was first used for vaccination of infants in 1922. It is now given by intradermal injection to increase resistance to tuberculosis in those found to be tuberculin-negative. Successful vaccination results in a positive tuberculin skin reaction from four to six weeks later. **Bacillus Calmette-Guérin Vaccine, Percutaneous, BP 1973.** Suspension of living cells of an authentic strain of the bacillus of Calmette-Guérin but with a higher viable bacterial count than bacillus Calmette-Guérin vaccine. It is used as a prophylactic against tuberculosis by percutaneous administration, and must not be given by the intradermal route. **Cholera Vaccine BP 1973.** The standard cholera vaccine now employed, containing 8 000 million *Vibrio cholerae* per ml. **Cowpox vaccine.** Vaccine lymph containing cowpox virus, or more usually vaccinia virus, prepared in the calf or sheep, the eruption being scraped off, ground up and treated with 50 per cent glycerol to form a suspension. Cultivated virus (vaccinia virus grown in tissue cultures or infertile eggs) is replacing vaccine lymph. **Defatted tubercle vaccine.** Vaccine, now obsolete, prepared after treating tubercle bacilli with formaldehyde and defatting with acetone. **Diphtheria Vaccine BP 1973.** Diphtheria prophylactic; diphtheria toxin detoxicated with formaldehyde solution and thus converted into toxoid. It is used in various forms (e.g. Formol Toxoid, FT; Alum Precipitated Toxoid, APT; Purified Toxoid Aluminium Phosphate, PTAP; and Toxoid-Antitoxin Floccules, TAF) to produce active immunity to diphtheria. The term was formerly applied to a sterile suspension of killed diphtheria bacilli. **Diphtheria and Tetanus Vaccine BP 1973.** Mixture of diphtheria vaccine formol toxoid and tetanus vaccine in simple solution, or of the constituent toxoids with aluminium hydroxide or aluminium phosphate. Used to immunize simultaneously against diphtheria and tetanus. **Diphtheria, Tetanus, Pertussis and Poliomyelitis Vaccine BP 1973.** Mixture of diphtheria vaccine formol toxoid, tetanus vaccine in simple solution, pertussis vaccine and poliomyelitis vaccine (inactivated). Used by injection for the prophylaxis of diphtheria, tetanus, pertussis and poliomyelitis. **Diphtheria, Tetanus and Poliomyelitis Vaccine BP 1973.** Mixture of diphtheria vaccine formol toxoid, tetanus vaccine in simple solution and poliomyelitis vaccine (inactivated). Used by injection for the prophylaxis of diphtheria, tetanus and poliomyelitis only when the reinforcement of primary immunization is required. **Eltor Vaccine BP 1973.** Sterile suspension of suitable strains of the cholera vibrio (*Vibrio cholerae* biotype *eltor*). Used by injection for the prophylaxis of cholera. **Dmelcos vaccine.** A vaccine prepared from *Haemophilus ducreyi.* **Heterologous vaccine.** A vaccine made from a micro-organism other than the one against which the vaccine is used. **Homologous vaccine.** A vaccine from an organism recovered from some other person. **Humanized vaccine.** Smallpox vaccine obtained from vaccinia vesicles in man. **Hydrophobia vaccine.** Rabies vaccine (see below). **Influenza vaccines.** Prepared against influenza A and influenza B, separately and in combination. Vaccines containing live attenuated strains have been prepared but are still experimental. Most vaccines contain virus grown in fertile eggs and inactivated with formalin. Others contain separated haemagglutinin antigen, and both types are given by intramuscular injection. Live attenuated vaccines for intranasal instillation have been prepared and have been used in the USSR. Current influenza A vaccines, however efficacious, suffer from the disadvantage of being prepared against the particular strain of the virus and may be of no use against new antigenic strains which appear and supplant the old. **Jennerian vaccine.** *See* COWPOX VACCINE (above) and JENNERIAN VACCINATION (under VACCINATION. **Lipodysentery vaccine.** A vaccine of heat-killed dysentery bacilli suspended in almond oil, used for the prevention of the disease. **Mixed vaccine.** A vaccine prepared from cultures of several species of micro-organisms. **Multi-partial vaccine, Multivalent vaccine.** Polyvalent vaccine (see below). **Mumps vaccine.** Live attenuated vaccine which has been tried with some success in America but is not generally available in the UK. **Paratyphoid vaccine.** A sterile suspension of the bacilli *Salmonella paratyphi A, B,* and sometimes *C,* killed by heat or by a bactericide. It is used as a prophylactic against the para-typhoid fevers for members of the armed forces and others likely to be exposed to infection. It is a constituent of typhoid-paratyphoid vaccines. **Pertussis Vaccine BP 1973.** Bordet-Gengou bacillus vaccine, a sterile suspension of killed *Haemophilus pertussis* bacilli; it should contain not less than 10 000 million killed bacilli per ml. **Plague Vaccine BP 1973.** A standard plague vaccine made from cultures of *Pasteurella pestis.* It contains 3 000 million killed bacilli per ml. **Poliomyelitis Vaccine (Inactivated) BP 1973.** Aqueous suspension of strains of poliomyelitis viruses, types I, II, and III, used to produce active immunity to poliomyelitis. **Poliomyelitis vaccines.** Two vaccines are available. The earlier to be developed was of Salk and contains poliovirus inactivated with formaldehyde; it induces good humoral antibody but does little to limit the spread of wild virus in the community. The later is Sabin's vaccine and contains live attenuated virus grown in monkey renal cell cultures and generally contains all 3 serotypes of the virus; a full course of 3 doses given orally usually induces good immunity to all 3 serotypes and also limits virus spread in the community. **Polyvalent vaccine.** A vaccine prepared from several antigenic types within a species. **Pure vaccine.** Univalent vaccine (see below). **Rabies Vaccine BP 1968.** Used in man for post-exposure immunization, of 2 types: simple vaccine contains fixed virus grown in rabbit brain and inactivated with phenol; duck embryo vaccine is grown in the yolk sac of fertile eggs. **Rubella vaccine.** Live virus attenuated by passage in cell culture. Given by intramuscular injection it induces a satisfactory immunity without significant excretion of the virus. British practice is to immunize only females, preferably before puberty or under contraceptive cover in the child-bearing period, leaving the unimmunized males to act as a reservoir for infection to give periodic boosts to immunity. **Sensitized vaccine.** A vaccine prepared by suspending organisms in homologous immune serum. **Smallpox Vaccine BP 1973.** A lymph preparation from animals inoculated with vaccinia virus cutaneously. It should contain not more than 1 000 micro-organisms per ml. **Smallpox Vaccine, Dried, BP 1973.** Freeze-dried smallpox vaccine used as a prophylactic against smallpox by scarification or pressure inoculation. **TAB vaccine.** Typhoid-paratyhpoid A and B vaccine (see below). **TABC vaccine.** Typhoid-paratyphoid A, B, and C vaccine (see below). **TABT vaccine.** Typhoid, Paratyphoid A and B, and Tetanus Vaccine BP 1973 (see below). **TABTD vaccine.** Combined TAB vaccine, tetanus toxoid, and diphtheria toxoid or other diphtheria prophylactic. **Tetanus Vaccine BP 1973.** Tetanus toxoid; tetanus toxin detoxicated with formaldehyde solution and thus converted into toxoid. It is used in simple solution or in alum-precipitated form to produce active immunity to tetanus. **Tetanus and Pertussis Vaccine BP 1973.** Mixture of tetanus vaccine in simple solution and pertussis vaccine. Used by injection for the prophylaxis of tetanus and pertussis. **Turtle vaccine.** A tuberculosis vaccine made from acid-fast bacilli recovered from the lungs of the turtle. It was used in much the same way as BCG vaccine, but was discredited and is now of historical interest only. **Typhoid vaccine.** Antityphoid vaccine (see above). **Typhoid Vaccine BP 1973.** Sterile suspension of *Salmonella typhi, S. paratyphi A, S. paratyphi B* and *S. paratyphi C.* Used by injection for the prophylaxis of enteric fevers. **Typhoid-Paratyphoid A and B Vaccine BP 1973.** A sterile suspension of the bacteria *Salmonella typhi, S. paratyphi A* and *S. paratyphi B* killed by heat or by a bactericide. **Typhoid-Paratyphoid A and B Vaccine, Intracutaneous, BP 1973.** Suspension of killed *Salmonella typhi* and *S. paratyphi A and B* that are smooth and have the full complement of O and H antigens, *S. typhi* containing also the Vi antigen. It is used for the prophylaxis of enteric fevers and administered by intracutaneous injection. **Typhoid-Paratyphoid A and B, and Cholera Vaccine BPC 1973.** A mixture of a sterile suspension of *Salmonella typhi, S. paratyphi A,* and *S. paratyphi B,* and *Vibrio cholerae.* It is used to produce active immunity to typhoid and paratyphoid fevers, and tetanus. **Typhoid-Paratyphoid A and B, and Tetanus Vaccine BP 1973.** A mixture of a sterile suspension of typhoid, paratyphoid A and paratyphoid B bacilli with tetanus vaccine in simple solution. It is used to produce active immunity to the enteric group of fevers and tetanus. **Typhoid and Tetanus Vaccine BP 1973.** Mixture of a suspension of killed *Salmonella typhi* and tetanus formol toxoid. **Typhus Vaccine BP 1973.** A sterile suspension of killed typhus rickettsiae. **Univalent vaccine.** A vaccine prepared from a culture of one antigenic type within a species. **Vole vaccine.** A vaccine made from *Mycobacterium muris,* the causal organism of natural tuberculosis in the vole. This vaccine has been used prophylactically against tuberculosis in the same way that BCG vaccine is used. **Yellow Fever Vaccine BP 1973.** A serum-free suspension in water of chick embryo tissue which has been infected with the 17D strain of the yellow fever virus. It gives a long lasting immunity. [L *vaccinus* of a cow.]

See also: ALIVISATOS, ARAGÃO, BANDI, BLANC, CALMETTE, CARONIA, CASTAÑEDA, CASTELLANI, CHANTEMESSE, CLAYPOLE, COX (H. R.), CROWE (H. W.), DANYSZ, DESSY, DURAND, GALEOTTI, GAY (F. P.), HAFFKINE, JENNER, KELSER, KLIMMER, LAIGRET, LUSTIG, MARTINOTTI, OTTEN, PARKER (R. R.), PASTEUR, RUCK, SABIN, SALK, SAUER, SCHRODER, SEMPLE, SPENCER (R. R.), TERNI, WEIGL (R.), WRIGHT (A. E.), ZINSSER.

vaccinella (vak·sin·el·ah). Mild vaccinia [obsolete term.]

vaccinia (vak·sin·e·ah). A virus disease of cows affecting the udders and teats. *Poxvirus officinale* (vaccinia virus) is probably a mutant of cowpox virus. Vaccinia in man is an acute infection with vaccinia virus caused by its deliberate or accidental inoculation. **Accidental vaccinia.** Vaccinia that may occur on the vaccinated individual, particularly with atopic dermatitis, or on a contact. **Vaccinia gangrenosa.** Local gangrene of the skin and subcutaneous tissues when the local reaction to vaccination has been of exceptional severity. **Generalized vaccinia.** The commoner form (eczema vaccinatum) occurs in individuals with skin disease, particularly atopic dermatitis. In the rarer form the eruption is due to a delayed antibody response to vaccinia. There is no previous skin abnormality and the eruption starts at about 10 days after vaccination. **Prenatal vaccinia.** Vaccinia resulting from vaccination performed during pregnancy; the fetus becomes infected and is stillborn with generalized vaccinia. **Progressive vaccinia.** Condition resulting from the individual's failure to form specific antibodies to the virus. There is no inflammatory response, the primary lesion fails to heal and viraemia leads to metastatic lesions on skin and mucous membranes, with gangrene. It is always fatal unless treated with hyperimmune vaccinial gamma globulin. [L *vaccinus* of a cow.]

vaccinial (vak·**sin**·e·al). 1. Pertaining to vaccinia. 2. Vaccinal.

vaccinid, vaccinide (**vak**·sin·id, **vak**·sin·ide). The cutaneous eruption which appears at a point of vaccination, sometimes consisting of several vesicles.

vaccinifer (vak·**sin**·e·fer). The animal, usually calf or sheep, from which vaccine lymph is taken. [vaccine, L *ferre* to bear.]

vacciniform (vak·**sin**·e·form). Having the character of vaccinia. [vaccine, form.]

vacciniola (**vak**·sin·e·**o**'·lah). A type of secondary vesicle occurring somehwere on the body, and possibly due to accidental inoculation from a successful vaccination on the same individual. It may resemble the eruption of smallpox. [dim. of *vaccinia.*]

vaccinium (vak·**sin**·e·um). A genus of plants of the family Ericaceae, including the whortleberry, cranberry, and bilberry, all of which are edible. The leaves of several species have been used in medicine. **Vaccinium crassifolium.** The creeping blueberry. **Vaccinium myrtillus.** The bilberry, whortleberry, or huckleberry. [L, whortleberry.]

vaccinization (**vak**·sin·i·**za**'·shun). The repetition of smallpox vaccination until reaction is absent and immunity complete [obsolete term].

vaccinogen (vak·**sin**·o·jen). The animal or other source from which a vaccine is obtained. [vaccine, Gk *genein* to produce.]

vaccinogenous (vak·sin·**oj**·en·us). Vaccigenous.

vaccinoid (**vak**·sin·oid). Resembling vaccinia; vacciniform. [vaccinia, Gk *eidos* form.]

vaccinophobia (**vak**·sin·o·**fo**'·be·ah). An unreasoning and morbid dread of being vaccinated. [vaccine, Gk *phobein* to fear.]

vaccinostyle (vak·**sin**·o·stile). A small metal lancet employed for vaccination. [vaccine, L *stylus* point.]

vaccinotherapeutics, vaccinotherapy (vak·sin·o·ther·ap·**ew**'·tix, **vak**·sin·o·**ther**'·ap·e). The use of vaccines for therapeutic purposes.

vaccinum (**vak**·sin·um). Vaccine. **Vaccinum Influenzae Inactivatum.** *European Pharmacopoeia* name for Influenza Vaccine BP 1973. **Vaccinum Morbillorum.** *European Pharmacopoeia* name for Measles Vaccine (Live Attenuated) BP 1973. **Vaccinum Pertussis.** *European Pharmacopoeia* name for Pertussis Vaccine BP 1973. **Vaccinum Poliomyelitidis Inactivatum.** *European Pharmacopoeia* name for Poliomyelitis Vaccine (Inactivated) BP 1973. **Vaccinum Poliomyelitidis Perorale.** *European Pharmacopoeia* name for Poliomyelitis Vaccine (Oral) BP 1973. **Vaccinum Tuberculesis.** *European Pharmacopoeia* name for BCG Vaccine BP 1973. **Vaccinum Typhoidi.** *European Pharmacopoeia* name for Typhoid Vaccine BP 1973. **Vaccinum Variolae Cryodesiccatum Dermicum.** *European Pharmacopoeia* name for Smallpox Vaccine (Dried) BP 1973. **Vaccinum Variolae Fluidum Dermicum.** *European Pharmacopoeia* name for Smallpox Vaccine BP 1973.

vacuolar (**vak**·ew·o·lar). Having the nature of or relating to a vacuole.

vacuolate, vacuolated (**vak**·ew·o·late, **vak**·ew·o·**la**'·ted). Containing vacuoles.

vacuolation (**vak**·ew·o·**la**'·shun). 1. A condition marked by the presence of vacuoles. 2. The process of development of vacuoles in tissue or cells.

vacuole (**vak**·ew·ole). A fluid-filled cavity within the cytoplasm of a cell. **Autophagic vacuole.** Autophagosome. **Contractile vacuole.** A vacuole in the cytoplasm of amoeba and other protozoa, which swells and collapses rhythmically in connection with its function as an excretory organ and regulator of the water and salt content of the organism. **Diffusion vacuole.** A cell vacuole coloured by a dyestuff diffusing in from the surrounding medium. **Food vacuole.** A drop of fluid within the cytoplasm of certain protozoa within which food particles are enclosed and digested. **Water vacuole.** A droplet of water ingested into the cytoplasm of a cell from the surrounding medium. [L *vacuus* empty.]

See also: BARRIER.

vacuolization (**vak**·ew·o·li·**za**'·shun). Vacuolation.

vacuome (**vak**·ew·ome). An intracellular organelle consisting either of a system of vacuoles, or a system of canals. Originally described by light microscopists, it is now seen to be equivalent to the various membrane-bound organelles which can be recognized by electron microscopy. [L *vacuus* empty, Gk *-oma* tumour.]

vacuum (**vak**·ew·um). Theoretically, a space devoid of atoms or molecules. It is unattainable in practice, and the term is therefore applied to any space in which the air or gas has been reduced to a very low pressure. **High vaccum.** A space containing gas at very low pressure. It is produced by rotary vacuum pumps supplemented by condensation of the remaining gas with liquid air or hydrogen. **Torricellian vacuum.** The space above the column of mercury in a barometer tube; it contains only mercury vapour at its low vapour pressure. (Named after Evangelista *Torricelli,* 15th century Italian physicist.) **Uteroplacental vacuum.** The vacuum created between the detached placenta and the uterine wall in traction. [L *vacuus* empty.]

vagal (**va**·gal). Referring to or concerning the vagus nerve.

vagectomy (va·**jek**·to·me). Excision of part of the vagus nerve in the treatment of peptic ulcer. [vagus, Gk *ektome* excision.]

vagina [NA] (vaj·**i**·nah). 1. Any structure resembling a sheath. 2. Specifically, a passage directed downwards and forwards from the external os uteri to open at the vulva (vaginal orifice) immediately posterior to the external urethral orifice. Its anterior wall [paries anterior (NA)] is related to the bladder and the uterus; its posterior wall [paries posterior (NA)] to the lower part of the rectum and the anal canal. It accommodates the penis during sexual intercourse. **Coat of the vagina, mucous [tunica mucosa (NA)].** Stratified squamous epithelium forming the vaginal mucosa which is thrown into an anterior and a posterior median longitudinal fold or column from which numerous transverse ridges arise. **Coat of the vagina, muscular [tunica muscularis (NA)].** A coat formed of an inner circular layer and an outer, thicker longitudinal layer continuous with the superficial uterine musculature. **Vaginae fixura.** Colpopexy. **Vagina pili.** The sheath surrounding the root of a hair. **Septate vagina.** One that is divided into two chambers by a septum. **Vagina synovialis trochleae.** The sheath surrounding the tendon of the superior oblique muscle of the orbit. [L.]

vaginal (vaj·i·nal, vaj·in·al). 1. Having the characteristics of a sheath. 2. Referring to the vagina. 3. Referring to the tunica vaginalis testis. **Vaginal smear.** Smear taken from the vagina, mainly to determine the extent of influence of oestrogen, progestogen and androgen. [L *vagina* sheath.]

vaginal artery [arteria vaginalis (NA)]. A branch of the anterior division of the internal iliac artery; it supplies the vagina and adjacent parts of the bladder and rectum.

vaginal nerves [nervi vaginales (NA)]. Branches from the pelvic plexus to the wall of the vagina and the erectile tissue of the vestibule.

vaginal vein. A vein which drains the vaginal plexus into the internal iliac vein.

vaginalectomy (**vaj**·in·al·**ek**'·to·me). Surgical removal of the tunica vaginalis testis as a whole or in part. [tunica vaginalis, Gk *ektome* excision.]

vaginalitis (**vaj**·in·al·**i**'·tis). Inflammation of the tunica vaginalis testis. [tunica vaginalis, Gk *-itis* inflammation.]

vaginapexy (vaj·i·nah·pex·e). 1. Suture of the vagina to the abdominal wall. 2. Vaginal hysteropexy; fixation of the vagina by surgical attachment of its membranous covering to the uterus. 3. Fixation of the tunica vaginalis testis after transplantation of the testis in varicocele. [vagina, Gk *pexis* fixation.]

vaginate (vaj·in·ate). Describing any structure that is invested in a sheath. [L *vagina* sheath.]

vaginectomy (vaj·in·**ek**·to·me). 1. The surgical removal of the vagina. 2. Excision of the whole or part of the tunica vaginalis testis; vaginalectomy. [vagina, Gk *ektome* excision.]

vaginiferous (vaj·in·**if**·er·us). Producing or bearing a sheath. [L *vagina* sheath, *ferre* to bear.]

vaginiperineotomy (vaj·in·e·per·in·e·**ot**'·o·me). Vaginoperineotomy.

vaginismus (vaj·in·**iz**·mus). Painful spasm of the muscles surrounding the vagina. **Deep vaginismus.** That caused by spasm of the levator ani muscle. **Mental vaginismus.** Vaginismus arising from extreme aversion to sexual intercourse. **Perineal vaginismus.** Spasm of the perineal muscles. **Posterior vaginismus.** Deep vaginismus (see above). **Superficial vaginismus.** Spasm of the muscles surrounding the vaginal entrance.

vaginitis (vaj·in·i·tis). Inflammation of the vagina or of a sheath. **Vaginitis adhaesiva.** Inflammation of the vagina resulting in the formation of adhesions between its walls. **Atrophic vaginitis.** Postmenopausal degenerative changes in the vaginal mucous membrane. **Candidal vaginitis.** Pruritic vaginitis with leucorrhoea and vulvitis, caused by *Candida albicans.* **Diphtheritic vaginitis.** The type in which a false membrane is formed. **Emphysematous vaginitis.** Vaginitis in which gas bubbles form in the connective tissue of the vagina. **Granular vaginitis.** The form which has a granular appearance due to inflammatory enlargement of the papillae. **Papulous vaginitis.** Vaginitis with the formation of papules. **Senile vaginitis.** An atrophic condition of the vagina resulting from inadequate oestrogen secretion. It usually only occurs in women after menopause. **Vaginitis testis.** Inflammation of the tunica vaginalis testis. **Trichomonas vaginitis.** The variety caused by the parasitic flagellate protozoa *Trichomonas vaginalis.* [vagina, Gk *-itis* inflammation.]

vagino-abdominal (vaj·in·o·ab·**dom**'·in·al). Referring to the vagina and the abdomen.

vaginocele (vaj·in·o·seel). A hernia or tumour obtruding into the vagina. [vagina, Gk *kele* tumour.]

vaginodynia (vaj·in·o·**din**'·e·ah). Pain experienced in the vagina. [vagina, Gk *odyne* pain.]

vaginofixation (vaj·in·o·fix·**a**'·shun). The operative fixation of the vagina. The usual method employed is to suture the retroflexed uterine fundus to the vagina.

vaginogenic (vaj·in·o·**jen**'·ik). Developing from the vagina, or having its origin there. [vagina, Gk *genein* to produce.]

vaginogram (vaj·in·o·gram). Radiographic visualization of the vagina after the injection of a radio-opaque contrast medium. [vagina, Gk *gramma* record.]

vaginolabial (vaj·in·o·**la**'·be·al). Concerning the vagina and the labia.

vaginometer (vaj·in·**om**·et·er). An instrument with which the length and diameter of the vagina may be measured.

vaginomycosis (vaj·in·o·mi·**ko**'·sis). A condition of mycotic or fungous infection of the vagina.

vaginopathy (vaj·in·**op**·ath·e). Denoting any disease of the vagina. [vagina, Gk *pathos* disease.]

vaginoperineal (vaj·in·o·per·in·**e**'·al). Concerning the vagina and the perineum.

vaginoperineorrhaphy (vaj·in·o·per·in·e·**or**'·af·e). The suture of a torn vagina and perineum. [vagina, perineum, Gk *rhaphe* suture.]

vaginoperineotomy (vaj·in·o·per·in·e·**ot**'·o·me). Surgical incision of the vagina and perineum to enlarge the vaginal orifice. [vagina, perineum, Gk *temnein* to cut.]

vaginoperitoneal (vaj·in·o·per·it·o·**ne**'·al). Concerning the vagina and its investing peritoneum.

vaginopexy (vaj·in·o·pex·e). Fixation of the vagina. [vagina, Gk *pexis* a fixation.]

vaginoplasty (vaj·in·o·plas·te). Plastic surgery performed on the vagina. [vagina, Gk *plassein* to mould.]

vaginoscope (vaj·in·o·skope). A speculum designed for the examination of the vagina. [vagina, Gk *skopein* to view.]

vaginoscopy (vaj·in·**os**·ko·pe). Examination of the vagina with a vaginal speculum. [see prec.]

vaginotome (vaj·in·o·tome). An instrument used in vaginotomy for incising the vagina.

vaginotomy (vaj·in·**ot**·o·me). Surgical incision of the vagina. [vagina, Gk *temnein* to cut.]

vaginovesical (vaj·in·o·**ves**'·ik·al). Concerning both the vagina and the urinary bladder. [vagina, L *vesica* bladder.]

vaginovulvar (vaj·in·o·**vul**'·var). Referring to the vulva and the orifice of the vagina.

vagitis (va·gi·tis). Inflammation of the vagus nerve. [vagus nerve, Gk *-itis* inflammation.]

vagitus (vaj·i·tus). The cry of an infant. **Vagitus uterinus.** The crying of a child in the uterus before birth. **Vagitus vaginalis.** The crying of a child while the head is still in the vagina during labour. [L.]

vago-accessorius (va·go·ak·ses·**or**'·e·us). The vagus and the spinal accessory nerves, considered as a single unit.

vagoglossopharyngeal (va·go·glos·o·far·**in**'·je·al). Referring to the vagus and glossopharyngeal nerves.

vagogram (va·go·gram). A record of the electrical variations in the vagus nerve. [vagus nerve, Gk *gramma* record.]

vagomimetic (va·go·mim·**et**'·ik). Having an effect similar to that due to stimulation of the vagus nerve. [vagus nerve, Gk *mimesis* an imitation.]

vagosplanchnic (va·go·**splangk**·nik). Vagosympathetic. [vagus nerve, splanchnic.]

vagosympathetic (va·go·sim·path·**et**'·ik). Relating to the vagus and the cervical part of the sympathetic system.

vagotomized (va·**got**·o·mi·zd). Denoting an animal in which the vagus nerve has been divided for experimental purposes. [vagus nerve, Gk *temnein* to cut.]

vagotomy (va·**got**·o·me). Division of the vagus nerves in the lower thorax or upper abdomen in order to diminish the secretory and motor activity of the stomach. It is usually performed in the treatment of duodenal or gastric ulcer. It may be *truncal* (whole nerve) or *selective* (only branches to the stomach and duodenum divided). **Selective vagotomy.** Trans-abdominal vagotomy limited to branches of nerve supplying the stomach in the endeavour to avoid the complication of post-operative diarrhoea. [vagus nerve, Gk *temnein* to cut.]

vagotonia (va·go·**to**·ne·ah). Hyperexcitability of the parasympathetic nervous system, as opposed to sympatheticotonia. [vagus nerve, Gk *tonos* tension.]

vagotonic (va·go·**ton**·ik). Relating to vagotonia, or exhibiting its characteristics.

vagotonin (va·go·**to**·nin). A substance, probably not a true hormone, derived from the pancreas; it stimulates the vagus nerve, lowers the blood pressure, and causes a drop in the blood sugar. [vagus nerve, gk *tonos* tension.]

vagotony (va·**got**·o·ne). Vagotonia.

vagotrope (**va**·go·trope). Vagotropic.

vagotropic (va·go·**trop**·ik). Possessing a specific affinity for the vagus nerve. [see foll.]

vagotropism (va·**got**·ro·pizm). The specific action or affinity displayed by a drug or agent towards the vagus nerve. [vagus nerve, Gk *trepein* to turn.]

vagovagal (va·go·**va**·gal). Reflex activity mediated entirely through the vagus nerve.

vagus nerve [nervus vagus (NA)] (va·gus **nerv**). The 10th and longest of the cranial nerves. It is a mixed motor and sensory nerve, arising from the medulla oblongata, supplying motor fibres to the muscles of the pharynx, and larynx [nervus laryngeus inferior (NA)], motor and sensory fibres to the trachea [rami tracheales (NA)], bronchi [rami bronchiales (NA)], heart, oesophagus [rami oesophagei (NA)], stomach and small intestine, and sensory fibres [ramus meningeus (NA)] to the taste buds of the epiglottis and vallecula, and a sensory twig to the back of the auricle and the posterior wall of the external auditory meatus. **Auricular branch [ramus auricularis (NA)].** A branch from the superior ganglion of the vagus nerve to the skin at the back of the auricle and in the posterior wall of the external auditory meatus. **Cardiac branches, cervical [rami cardiaci cervicales inferiores et superiores (NA)].** Branches arising in the neck from the vagus nerve and distributed to the heart via the deep cardiac plexus; they belong to the craniosacral division of the autonomic nervous system. When stimulated they produce slowing, or with stronger stimuli stoppage, of the heart. **Coeliac branches [rami celiaci (NA)].** Branches from the posterior gastric plexus to the coeliac ganglion. **Gastric branches.** Branches from the vagus nerve to the stomach, those to the anterior surface [rami gastrici anteriores (NA)] of the organ arising from the left nerve, and those to the posterior surface [rami gastrici posteriores (NA)] from the right nerve. **Hepatic branches [rami hepatici (NA)].** Filaments from the anterior gastric plexus passing in the lesser omentum to the hepatic (autonomic) plexus. **Pharyngeal branches [rami pharyngei (NA)].** The chief motor supply to the muscles of the pharynx, arising from the inferior ganglion of the vagus nerve and passing into the pharyngeal plexus between the superior and middle constrictor muscles. **Renal branches [rami renales (NA)].** Branches to the renal (autonomic) plexus. **Splenic branches.** Branches to the splenic (autonomic) plexus. **Thoracic cardiac branches [rami cardiaci thoracici (NA)].** Cardiac branches of the vagus or recurrent laryngeal nerves which arise within the thorax. **Nuclei [nuclei nervi vagi (NA)].** The nuclei of the vagus nerve; they include the dorsal nucleus, nucleus ambiguus, and the nucleus of the tractus solitarius. **Dorsal nucleus [nucleus dorsalis nervi vagi (NA)].** A group of cells lying lateral to the nucleus of the hypoglossal nerve. It gives rise to vagal fibres innervating unstriped muscle and probably receives splanchnic afferent impulses.

vagusstof (va·gus·shtof′). Acetylcholine. [vagus nerve, G *Stoff* substance.]

valence (va·lens). Valency.

valency (va·len·se). Combining power. 1. In chemistry it is defined as the number of atoms of hydrogen that any one atom of an element will combine with or replace; the term is extended to the combining power of radicals or groups which act as units in chemical combinations. Valencies may have all values from 0 to 8, and many elements have more than one value. 2. The number of antigens with which an antibody will unite. **Valency bond.** The hypothetical link between atoms due to their valencies. **Co-ordinate valency.** A form of valency achieved by the sharing of a pair of electrons both from the same atom. Such a linkage gives rise to a number of complex compounds. **Electronic valency.** The interpretation of valency in terms of electrons, the types of linkage being: (*a*) electrovalent, involving the transfer of electrons from one atom to another; (*b*) covalent, necessitating the sharing of a pair of electrons, one from each atom; and (*c*) co-ordinate, or the sharing of a pair of electrons both from the same atom. [L *valere* to be worth.]

valent (va·lent). Having valency.

valenta test. For purity of butter fat: equal volumes (3 ml) of butter fat and glacial acetic acid are warmed until the mixture is clear, and then allowed to cool until the first appearance of turbidity, when the temperature is noted. Pure butter gives a figure of about 34°C, but this figure is raised by the presence of other oils and fats except coconut oil, which will lower it if present.

Valentin, Gabriel Gustav (b. 1810). Berne physiologist.

Valentin's ganglion. A ganglion occasionally found on a branch of the posterior superior dental nerve.

Valentin's nerve. One of the short sphenopalatine nerves.

Valentin's tube. One of the ingrowing columns of cells arising from the germinal epithelium of the fetal ovary, which contain primordial ova.

Valentine, Ferdinand C. (1851–1909). New York surgeon.

Valentine's position. A modified position with the patient supine and hips slightly flexed in order to facilitate urethral instrumentation.

valeral, valeraldehyde (val·er·al, val·er·al·de·hide). Valeric aldehyde. *See* ALDEHYDE. [valerian.]

valerate (val·er·ate). Any salt or ester of valeric acid.

valerene (val·er·een). Amylene, C_5H_{10}. A liquid olefine hydrocarbon, occurring in several isomeric forms.

Valerian BPC 1963 (val·eer·e·an). The dried rhizome and roots of *Valeriana officinalis* Linn. (family Valerianaceae). It contains about 1 per cent of volatile oil, the main constituent of which is bornyl isovalerianate; the latter is slowly decomposed by an enzyme present yielding isovaleric acid with a characteristic odour. It is used in hysteria as a sedative and in neurotic states. **Greek valerian.** The plant *Polemonium caeruleum* (family Polemoniaceae); Jacob's ladder. **Japanese valerian.** Kesso; the rhizome of *Valeriana angustifolia* which is smaller and more aromatic than *Valeriana officinalis* and yields a different volatile oil. [L *valeriana*.]

valeriana (val·eer·e·ah′·nah). 1. A genus of plants of the family Valerianaceae. 2. Valerian. [L.]

valerianate (val·eer·e·an·ate). Any salt or ester of valeric acid.

valeric (val·eer·ik). Describing a preparation of valerian.

valeridin (val·er·id·in). $C_2H_5OC_6H_4NHCOC_4H_9$, the valeryl derivative of phenetidin, analogous to phenacetin. It is used as an analgesic.

valerolactone (val·er·o·lak′·tone). A cyclic compound which occurs in several isomeric forms, the most common being the α-isomer, $CH_3CH_2CH_2CHCOO$, derived from wood vinegar.

valerone (val·er·one). Di-isobutyl ketone, $(CH_3)_2CHCH_2COCH_2CH(CH_3)_2$. A liquid derived from isovaleric acid.

valerydine (val·er·id·een). Valeridin.

valeryl (val·er·il). The organic acyl radical, $CH_3CH_2CH_2CH_2CO—$, derived from *n*-valeric acid.

valerylene (val·er·il·een). Methylethyl acetylene, $CH_3C{\equiv}CCH_2CH_3$. One of the acetylene hydrocarbons; a liquid.

valetudinarian (val·e·tew·din·a′·re·an). A weak or infirm person; an invalid. [L *valetudo* ill health.]

valetudinarianism (val·e·tew·din·a′·re·an·izm). A condition of poor health or infirmity. [L *valetudo* ill health.]

valgoid (val·goid). Having a resemblance to the valgus. [valgus, Gk *eidos* form.]

valgus (val·gus). 1. Talipes valgus. 2. In general, displaced outwards from the central line of the body. **Acute spasmodic valgus.** Painful flat foot associated with spasm of the peroneal tendons. [L, bowlegged.]

valinaemia (val·in·e·me·ah). Retarded mental and physical growth found in 1 child with raised levels of valine in plasma and urine. [valine, Gk *haima* blood.]

valine (val·een). α-Amino-isovaleric acid, $(CH_3)_2CHCH(NH_2)COOH$. An amino acid occurring in hydrolysates of proteins, which is essential in diet for the maintenance of health.

valinomycin (va·lin·o·mi′·sin). An antibiotic which renders mitochondria permeable to potassium ion.

vallate (val·ate). Surrounded by a raised rim; enclosed as if by a wall; cupped. [L *vallum* a rampart.]

vallecula [NA] (val·ek·ew·lah). A small depression below the general surface level of a part. **Vallecula of the cerebellum [vallecula cerebelli (NA)].** A deep depression which separates the two hemispheres on the inferior aspect of the cerebellum. **Vallecula of the cerebrum.** The depression on the lateral side of the optic chiasma, the floor of which is formed by the anterior perforated substance. **Vallecula epiglottica [NA].** A depression behind the root of the tongue, between the median and lateral glossoepiglottic folds. **Vallecula unguis.** The groove occupied by the root and lateral edges of the nail. [dim. of L *valles* valley.]

vallecular (val·ek·ew·lar). Concerning a vallecula.

Vallée, Henri (b. 1874). Paris veterinarian.

Vallée's serum, Leclainche-Vallée serum. A serum used for anthrax.

Valleix, François Louis Isidore (b. 1807). Paris physician.

Valleix's aphthae. Small ulcerated patches found on the hard palate and gingival margins in cases of marasmus, and caused by local infection of damaged mucosa as a result of sucking infected articles.

Valleix's points, Beard–Valleix points. In cases of neuralgia in the distribution of a particular nerve, exquisitely tender points along the course of the nerve. These are also known as *puncta dolorosa.*

Valli, Eusebio (b. 1755). Italian physiologist.

Ritter–Valli law. When section separates a portion of nerve from its parent nerve cell, irritability is first increased and later lost; both changes travel centrifugally.

vallum (val·um). The eyebrow. [L, rampart.]

valonia (val·o·ne·ah). The acorn cups of *Quercus aegilops* (family Cupuliferae); they have astringent properties due to the large percentage of tannin they contain. [Gk *balanos* acorn.]

Valsalva, Antonio Maria (b. 1666). Bologna surgeon and anatomist.

Valsalva's experiment, or manoeuvre. The demonstration that, if the pharyngotympanic (eustachian) tubes are patent, a forcible expiratory effort with both nose and mouth closed produces an increased pressure on the tympanic membrane. At the same time an increase of intrathoracic pressure occurs, so that the return of blood to the heart may be momentarily reduced and the veins in the neck become engorged. Valsalva's observation has been adapted for many purposes: 1. As a therapeutic procedure by the otolaryngologist; 2. In x-ray diagnostic work by the blowing out of the hypopharynx and occasionally of the larynx; 3. In testing the patency of the pharyngotympanic (eustachian) tubes, the mobility of the tympanic membrane can be observed by direct examination, and air entry heard on auscultation; 4. For determining the inflatability of the collapsed lung after artificial pneumothorax treatment.

Valsalva's eustachian tube inflation. *See* VALSALVA'S EXPERIMENT OR MANOEUVRE 3. (above).

Valsalva's ligaments. The extrinsic ligaments of the auricle.

Valsalva's sinuses. The sinuses of the aorta.

Valsalva's test. *See* VALSALVA'S EXPERIMENT OR MANOEUVRE 4. (above).

Valsalva's treatment. Treatment of aneurysms by rest, low-calorie diet and venesection. These measures were designed to minimize the work of the heart and the strain on the aneurysm wall, in order to prevent rupture: more specific measures are now available and venesection has no place in treatment.

Valsuani, Emilio (fl. 1870). Italian physician.

Valsuani's disease. Macrocytic anaemia of pregnancy; a severe anaemia resembling pernicious anaemia, occurring in lactating women.

value (val·ew). The relative number, quantity, or measure. **Absolute value.** An expression of the actual number present, as opposed to a ratio or percentage. Cf. RELATIVE VALUE (below). **Acetyl value.** Acetyl number; the measure of the oxyacids and alcohols contained in a fat or oil. It is expressed as the number of milligrams of potassium hydroxide necessary to neutralize the acetic acid produced by one gramme of the fat or oil previously acetylated and then saponified. **Acid value.** Acid number; the measure of the free fatty acids of a fat or oil. It is expressed as the number of milligrams of potassium hydroxide necessary to neutralize one gramme of the fat or oil. **Buffer value.** The buffer action of a solution measured in terms of the standard acid or alkali necessary to effect a change in the pH value of the solution. **Calorific value, Energy value, Fuel value.** The amount of heat liberated when foodstuffs are burned in the body. In arriving at the value for a particular food the protein, fat, and carbohydrate contents are separately determined and the calorific value calculated from the data that protein and carbohydrate yield 17.2 kJ (4.1 large calories) per gramme, and fat 40 kJ (9.3 large calories) per gramme. **Globular value.** The amount of haemoglobin in a red blood corpuscle, expressed as a percentage of the normal value. **Iodine value.** The weight of iodine absorbed by 100 parts of an oil or fat under specified conditions. Wij's solution is universally used as the reagent in this determination. It is essentially a measure of the constituent unsaturated fatty acids. **Liminal value.** That amount of a substance, or that degree of stimulation, that will just produce a response. **pH value.** The acidity or alkalinity of a solution expressed in a scale ranging from 0 for maximum acidity to 14 for the opposite extreme of alkalinity, true neutrality being midway, 7. It is defined as the negative value of the power to which the numerical base 10 must be raised to equal the concentration of hydrogen ions in grammes per litre. **Relative value.** The expression of a value in relation to some other value, e.g. as a ratio or percentage. Cf. ABSOLUTE VALUE (above). **Saponification value.** Saponification number; the number of milligrams of potassium hydroxide necessary to neutralize the free acids and completely saponify one gramme of a fat or oil. **Thiocyanogen value.** A test similar to the iodine value, applied to oils and fats by use of a special thiocyanogen reagent. This value is expressed in terms of iodine absorbed, and the difference between the iodine and thiocyanogen values divided by the factor 0.905 gives the percentage of linoleic acid. **Threshold value.** Liminal value (see above). [L *valere* to be worth.]

See also: POLENSKÉ, REICHERT (J. S.).

valval (val·val). Valvar.

valvar (val·ver). Pertaining to a valve. [L *valva* leaf.]

valvate (val·vate). Having the form of a valve, or acting as a valve; furnished with a valve or valves.

valve (valv). 1. Any device which regulates the flow of a liquid or gas through a pipe, particularly one which limits the flow to a single direction. 2. [Valva (NA)]. In anatomy, any structure that performs the above function and certain fold-like structures that simulate valves but do not necessarily have a valvular structure. The term has been extended to electrical devices which produce unidirectional current, e.g. thermionic valve. **Anal valves [valvulae anales (NA)].** Semilunar folds of mucous membrane joining the lower ends of the anal columns. **Aortic valve [valva aortae (NA)].** A valve composed of three semilunar cusps, one anterior and two posterior [valvula semilunaris sinistra, dextra, et posterior (NA)], situated at the beginning of the artery. In the centre of each free border is a nodule [nodulus valvulae semilunarium (NA)], on either side of which the thin semilunar border is called the lunule. **Atrioventricular (mitral) valve, left [valva atrioventricularis sinistra (valva mitralis) NA].** The valve guarding the left atrioventricular orifice, composed of a large anterior cusp [cuspis anterior (NA)] placed between the mitral and aortic orifices, and a smaller posterior cusp [cuspis posterior (NA)]. **Atrioventricular (tricuspid) valve, right [valva atrioventricularis dextra (valva tricuspidalis) NA].** The valve guarding the right atrioventricular orifice, composed of three cusps, a posterior, a medial (septal), and an anterior [cuspis posterior, septalis, anterior (NA)], the latter placed between the atrioventricular orifice and the infundibulum. **Bicuspid valve.** A developmental abnormality in which a semilunar valve, which normally has 3 cusps, has only 2 cusps; it is a common abnormality of the aortic valve, undetectable in early life, but may become the site of bacterial endocarditis or, later, undergo calcific degeneration. **Cold cathode valve.** An electronic valve which does not contain a thermionic electron source. **Congenital urethral valve.** A modification of the mucous membrane folds at the urinary meatus that may cause obstruction and retention. **Valve of the coronary sinus [valvula sinus coronarii (NA)].** A thin semicircular fold of endocardium guarding the lower part of the orifice of the sinus. **Demand valve.** A valve in a breathing circuit which only admits gases when the patient breathes in. **Diode valve.** A thermionic valve containing only a cathode and anode. **Eustachian valve.** Valve of the inferior vena cava (see below). **Expiratory valve.** A valve in a breathing circuit which opens during expiration but remains closed during inspiration. **Fallopian valve.** Ileocolic valve (see below). **False valves.** Pseudovalves. **Valves of the foramen ovale [valvula foraminis ovalis (falx septi) NA].** The portion of the septum primum which overlaps the foramen ovale on its left side and acts as a valve during fetal life. **Valve of the fossa terminalis [valvula fossae navicularis (NA].** The fold of mucous membrane which demarcates the lacuna magna; it lies in the superior wall of the fossa terminalis. **Gas valve.** An electronic valve containing a gas at low pressure, the gas entering into the function of the valve by providing ions for passage of current between the electrodes, e.g. thyratron. **Hot cathode valve.** A thermionic valve with a heated cathode electron source. **Ileocolic valve [valvula ileocaecalis (NA)].** The valve guarding the ileocolic orifice, and consisting of two folds of mucous membrane, the upper and lower frenula, which join to form ridges on either side of the opening. **Valve of the inferior vena cava [valvula venae cavae inferioris (NA)].** A semilunar fold of endocardium attached to the anterior border of the vena-caval opening. It is large in fetal life, and directs blood from the inferior vena cava into the left atrium through the foramen ovale. **Inspiratory valve.** A valve used in anaesthesia which closes during expiration and opens during the patient's inspirations. **Lymphatic valve [valvula lymphatica (NA)].** A valve-like fold of the intima of a lymph vessel which controls the direction of the lymph flow. Such folds are numerous in the large lymph vessels. **Mitral valve.** Left atrioventricular (mitral) valve (see above). **Non-return valve.** A valve in a breathing circuit which prevents the expired gases from reaching the reservoir bag. **One-way valve.** A valve in a breathing circuit which ensures that the gases flow in 1 direction only. **Pressure-reducing valve.** A valve designed to reduce the pressure of a gas issuing from a storage cylinder from a high to a lower pressure; it is used on anaesthetic apparatus and on oxygen and nitrous oxide cylinders. **Pulmonary valve [valva trunci pulmonalis (NA)].** A valve composed of three semilunar cusps, two anterior and one posterior [valvula semilunaris anterior, sinistra, et dextra (NA)], situated at the beginning of the artery. In the centre of each free border is a nodule [nodulus valvulae semilunaris (NA)], on either side of which the thin semilunar region is called the lunule. **Semilunar valves.** The pulmonary and aortic valves, so called from their half-moon shape. **Spiral valve [plica spiralis (NA)].** An enfolding of the mucous membrane of the neck of the gall bladder and the cystic duct, forming an irregular spiral. **Switch valve.** A valve used in a circuit to switch current on or off through a load. **Thermionic valve.** A vacuum tube designed to rectify and amplify oscillating currents. It consists of a glass or metal tube, evacuated and containing as cathode a heated filament which produces a stream of electrons. These pass towards the anode (plate) through a grid or system of grids which regulate the electrons eventually reaching the anode. **Tricuspid valve.** Right atrioventricular (tricuspid) valve (see above). **Triode valve.** A thermionic valve containing a grid in addition to the cathode and anode. **Venous valves [valvulae venosae (NA)].** Membranous semilunar folds of the intima which project into the lumen of a vein. They point in the direction of the blood stream and enclose pockets between themselves and the main wall of the vessel. They occur singly or in pairs (rarely in triplicate) and when competent prevent the back-flow of blood. [L *valva* leaf of a door.]

See also: AMUSSAT, BALL, BAUHIN, BÉRAUD, BIANCHI (G. B.), BOCHDALEK, CRUVEILHIER, EUSTACHIO, FALLOPIO, FOLTZ, GERLACH, GUBARER, GUÉRIN (A. F. M.), HASNER, HEISTER, HOLOKENIUS, HOUSTON, HUSCHKE, KERCKRING, KOHLRAUSCH (O. L. B.), KRAUSE (W. J. F.), MERCIER, MORGAGNI, O'BEIRNE, ROSENMUELLER, TAILLEFER, TARIN, TERRIER, THEBESIUS, TULP, VAROLIO, VIEUSSENS, WILLIS.

valved (val·vd). Valvate; furnished with valves.

valveless (valv·les). Possessing no valves, as in the case of certain veins like the portal.

valviform (val·ve·form). Resembling a valve in shape or function. [valve, form.]

valvotomy (val·**vot**·o·me). Valvulotomy.

valvula (val·vew·lah). A small valve or valve-like structure. **Valvulae conniventes.** The circular folds of mucous membrane of the small intestine. [dim. of L *valva* leaf of a door.]

valvular (val·vew·lar). 1. Concerning a valve, or originating in one. 2. Behaving like a valve.

valvulation (val·vew·**la**·shun). Having the form or function of a valve. [see foll.]

valvule [valvula (NA)] (val·vewl). A small valve. [dim. of L *valva* leaf of a door.]

See also: BRAUNE, FOLTZ, GUÉRIN (A. F. M.), KERCKRING.

valvulitis (val·vew·**li**·tis). Inflammation of a valve or valves, particularly of one of the valves of the heart. **Rheumatic valvulitis.** Rheumatic infection of the valves of the heart. [valvule, Gk *-itis* inflammation.]

valvuloplasty (val·vew·lo·plas·te). A plastic operation on a valve. **Cardiac valvuloplasty.** A surgical operation on a heart valve, e.g. on the mitral valve in stenosis. [valvule, Gk *plassein* to mould.]

valvulotome (val·vew·lo·tome). An instrument employed in valvulotomy.

valvulotomy (val·vew·**lot**·o·me). The operation of splitting, usually with the finger, or cutting with instruments a valve, especially the mitral valve of the heart in mitral stenosis. [valvule, Gk *temnein* to cut.]

valzin (val·zin). Dulcine.

vampire (**vam**·pire). One of two species of bat which feed exclusively on mammalian blood, including that of man. *Desmodus rufus*, the common vampire occurs throughout tropical and subtropical America; *Diphylla ecaudata* occurs in Brazil. They may transmit rabies. [Magyar *vampir.*]

Van Buren, William Holme (b. 1819). New York surgeon.

Van Buren's disease. Induration of the corpora cavernosa.

Van Buren's operation. Cauterization of the prolapsed rectum.

Van Creveld, Simon (b. 1894). Dutch paediatrician.

Ellis-Van Creveld syndrome. Chondro-ectodermal dysplasia; a syndrome of bilateral manual polydactylism, chondrodysplasia of the long bones resulting in acromelic dwarfism, hidrotic ectodermal dysplasia affecting the nails and hair, and congenital malformation of the heart.

Van de Graaff, Robert Jemison (b. 1901). American physicist.

Van de Graaff machine. An electrostatic generator for the production of a high potential. Electric charge is sprayed on to a continuously moving belt of insulating material and transferred by the belt to an insulated sphere, which reaches a high potential.

Van den Bergh. *See* BERGH.

Van der Hoeve's syndrome. Conductive deafness due to otosclerotic-like foci in the temporal bone associated with blue sclera and osteogenesis imperfecta.

Van Gieson, Ira Thompson (b. 1866). New York neuropathologist.

Van Gieson's method. For connective tissue: sections are stained in iron haematoxylin followed by Van Gieson's solution. Nuclei are stained bluish-black, muscle fibres yellow, connective-tissue fibres red.

Van Gieson's solution, or contrast stain. A solution of acid fuchsine in saturated aqueous picric acid, used as a connective-tissue stain.

Van Gieson's stain. For nervous tissue: a method very similar to the method for connective tissue (above); perivascular connective tissue is stained, but neuroglial tissue is not.

Van Hook, Weller (b. 1862). Chicago surgeon.

Van Hook's operation. Uretero-ureterostomy, largely on the experimental basis, 1893. He originated modern methods of ureteral repair.

Van Horne (Heurnius). *See* HORNE.

Van Milligan, Edwin (b. 1851). British ophthalmologist.

Van Milligan's operation. For trichiasis: the eyelid is split in its whole length along the grey line posterior to the eyelashes for a depth of 3 mm. A free graft of buccal mucosa is then cut and placed in the raw area.

Van Neck's disease. Osteochondrosis of the epiphysis of the pubic symphisis.

Van Slyke, Donald Dexter (b. 1883). New York biochemist.

Van Slyke apparatus. A form of manometer adapted to gas analysis. The gases are liberated or absorbed in a special chamber under reduced pressure, and the alterations in pressure are read from the height of the mercury column in the graduated manometric tube. The volume of gas can be calculated from the pressure readings.

Van Slyke's method. 1. For alkali reserve: plasma is saturated with carbon dioxide by treatment with alveolar air and 1 ml is transferred to a special apparatus where it is shaken with acid under reduced pressure. The liberated carbon dioxide is measured, the volume is corrected to s.t.p. and the result expressed as ml CO_2 per 100 ml plasma. 2. For amino-acid nitrogen: the solution containing amino acids is treated with nitrous oxide in a special apparatus in which the nitrogen evolved can be purified and measured. 3. For the specific gravity of plasma and serum: plasma or serum is added drop by drop to a series of copper-sulphate solutions of known specific gravity. Surface combination of copper and protein causes the drops to retain their form and the gravity of the drops relative to the solutions is shown by a rise or fall. Where no rise or fall occurs, the gravity of the plasma or serum is the same as that of the solution. The protein content in g per 100 ml is calculated from the formula: Protein = 365 (SG—1.007). 4. For chlorides in blood and tissues: the chloride is precipitated, and organic matter oxidized, by heating with silver nitrate and nitric acid. The excess silver nitrate is titrated with thiocyanate.

Van Slyke and Cullen method. For urea in blood: blood is treated with urease and the mixture is made alkaline with potassium carbonate and aerated. The ammonia is absorbed in standard acid and the excess of acid titrated with standard alkali.

Van Slyke and Fitz method. For alkali reserve: urine is collected for 24 h, the volume is measured and the ammonia and titratable acidity determined as ml 0.1 M per litre of urine. The sum of the latter figures multiplied by the 24-h volume in litres gives the rate of excretion per 24 h, *D*. The plasma carbon dioxide capacity $= 80-5\sqrt{D/W}$ where *W* is the body weight of the patient.

Van Slyke, MacFadyean, and Hamilton ninhydrin method. For α-amino-acid nitrogen in urine: the urine is treated with urease to destroy urea, and is then heated with ninhydrin in a closed vessel at 100°C. The carbon dioxide evolved is then determined by transferring to the Van Slyke apparatus. The amino-acid nitrogen is calculated upon the basis that 1 mol of carbon dioxide is given by 1 mol of α-amino-acid nitrogen.

Møller, McIntosh, and Van Slyke test. Urea clearance test. *See* TEST.

Van Slyke and Neill method. For the manometric analysis of gases in blood and other solutions: the sample solution is introduced into a specially designed apparatus and the gas or gases to be determined are liberated by treating with a suitable reagent under reduced pressure. The gas volume is then adjusted to a set value and the pressure read from a manometer. The gas is removed by ejection or absorption and the pressure again read at the same gas volume. The difference between the two readings gives the partial pressure of the gas at the given volume, from which the gas volume at s.t.p. can be calculated.

Van Slyke and Palmer method. For organic acids in urine: carbonates and phosphates are precipitated by adding slaked lime, the filtrate is neutralized to phenolphthalein, and is then titrated with standard acid using tropaeolin OO as indicator.

vanadate (van·ad·ate). General term for a salt of vanadic acids.

vanadiotherapy (van·a·de·o·**ther**′·ap·e). Treatment by vanadium preparations in syphilis; now obsolete.

vanadium (van·a·de·um). An element of atomic weight 50.94, atomic number 23, and chemical symbol V. It is a hard white metal resembling tantalum and found in certain rare ores. It is present in the blood of some marine animals (holothurians and ascidians). Its principal use is in steel alloys. It has no medical uses, but cases of industrial poisoning have been reported. These cases show bronchitis, and damage to the kidneys and colon. [Old Norse *Vanadis*, a goddess.]

vanadiumism (van·a·de·um·izm). Chronic vanadium poisoning occurring among those handling the metal or its compounds.

Vancomycin (van·ko·**mi**·sin). BP Commission approved name for an antibiotic produced by *Streptomyces orientalis*. **Vancomycin Hydrochloride BP 1973.** Antibiotic produced by the growth of *Streptomyces orientalis*, or by any other means. It is effective against Gram-positive cocci and used mainly in the treatment of systemic infections due to staphylococci which are resistant to other antibiotics.

Vanghetti, Guiliano (b. 1861). Italian orthopaedic surgeon.

Vanghetti's prosthesis. An artificial limb in which movement is obtained by muscle and skin flaps.

vanilla (van·il·ah). The cured, full-grown, but unripe fruits of *Vanilla planifolia* Andr. (family Orchidaceae). They contain an aromatic constituent, vanillin, and are used in confectionery and perfume manufacture. **False vanilla.** The plant *Liatris odoratissima* (family Compositae). [Sp. *vainilla* a small pod.]

Vanillin BP 1958 (van·**il**·in). 4-Hydroxy-3-methoxy-benzaldehyde, $CH_3OC_6H_3(OH)CHO$. The odorous principle of vanilla; a white, crystalline substance, only slightly soluble in water but readily in most organic solvents, used as a flavouring agent in confectionery. It may be prepared synthetically from eugenol or guaiacol.

vanillism (van·il·izm). A disease sometimes seen in workers with vanilla plants. The persons affected feel unwell, and have catarrh of the nose, running from the eyes, and dermatitis. It is due to a tyroglyphid mite. **Nervous vanillism.** A toxic manifestation arising in vanilla workers.

Van't Hoff. *See* HOFF.

Vanzetti, Tito (b. 1809). Padua surgeon.

Vanzetti's sign. In sciatica, even though there is marked scoliosis the pelvis is always horizontal; in other conditions giving scoliosis, the pelvis is usually tilted.

vapocauterization (va·po·kaw·ter·i·**za**′·shun). Cauterization carried out with steam or heated vapour.

vaporimeter (va·por·**im**·et·er). A device for estimating the volatility of oils by vaporizing them in a current of air. [vapour, meter.]

vaporization (va·por·i·**za**′·shun). The changing of a liquid or solid into vapour.

vaporize (va·por·ize). 1. To pass from the liquid into the gaseous phase, as when a liquid evaporates. 2. To cause a liquid to be converted to vapour. [vapour.]

vaporizer (va·por·i·zer). 1. An atomizer, for producing a fine vaporous spray. 2. A still, for vaporizing and recondensing volatile liquids. **Oxford vaporizer.** An apparatus giving a controlled percentage of ether vapour for inhalation anaesthesia. It was devised by the Nuffield Department of Anaesthesia at Oxford and was of great value in wartime emergencies (1939–1945). **Oxford miniature vaporizer.** A small non-thermocompensated vaporizer for use with volatile anaesthetics. (Described by Parkhouse in 1966.)

vapotherapy (va·po·**ther**·ap·e). The therapeutic use of vapours, steam, or sprays.

vapour (va·per). A gaseous phase of matter formed when a liquid is raised in temperature or placed in conditions that permit the free escape of molecules from its surface. [L *vapor* steam.]

vapours (va·perz). An archaic name for depression, hypochondria, or hysteria. [L *vapor* steam.]

Vaquez, Louis Henri (b. 1860). Paris physician.

Vaquez' disease. Polycythaemia vera.

Babinski-Vaquez syndrome. Babinski's syndrome; the association of luetic aortic incompetence, and possibly aortic aneurysm, with neurosyphilis.

Osler-Vaquez disease, Vaquez-Osler disease. Polycythaemia vera.

varec (var·ek). The local name in Normandy for the ash of seaweeds gathered and burnt for potash and iodine; kelp.

variability (va·re·ab·**il**′·it·e). 1. The ability to diverge from a given standard. 2. The amount by which anything diverges from a normal. 3. The evolutionary adaptation in structure or function of any living organism to circumstances. [L *variare* to diversify.]

variable (va·re·abl). Any attribute that is not constant, but liable to change with circumstances. Variables may be qualitative (being allocated to a particular class) or quantitative (being a number). It is often related to another variable, which relationship can be expressed usually in mathematical or graphic form. [see prec.]

variance (va·re·ans). In a statistical sample, the errors in the correct value tend to be distributed in a recognized method, known as the *normal law of frequency of error* or the *normal distribution.* The liability to error in the sample is termed the *variance*; it is expressed by calculating the mean value of the squares of these errors, and diminishes in increasing samples in inverse proportion to the number in the sample. [see foll.]

variant (va·re·ant). In bacteriology, a strain that varies in some usually minor way from the strain from which it originated. **Chromosome variant.** An alternative form of a chromosome, presumably arisen from mutational events of unknown nature, which produces either a small or no deviation from the "wild" phenotype. [L *variare* to diversify.]

variate (va·re·ate). A variable.

variation (va·re·a·shun). Differences, particularly between the individuals of a species, or between individual populations of a species. **Bacterial variation.** The appearance within a clone, of individuals with different phenotypic characters from the normal. Variants may arise either by mutation or by adaptation. **Continuous variation.** That in which the steps between one form and the next are very small. **Double variation.** The biphasic change in electrical potential produced in a muscle by a single induction shock. **Genotypic variation.** That which is caused by inherited differences in genic material. **Host-controlled variation.** Alteration of immigrant viral or plasmid DNA molecules by specific host enzymes, often by methylation or glucosylation, so that they are no longer recognized as foreign and broken down by endonucleases. Such variations are not inheritable and may be lost following replication when the progeny phages or plasmids are transferred to a new host. **Impressed variation.** A variation occurring only in the presence of a specific environmental factor. **Inborn variation.** Genotypic variation (see above). **Meristic variation.** That of number as opposed to kind. **Negative variation.** The negative phase of the change in potential produced in a muscle by a single induction shock. **Phase variation.** In bacteria, the switching of a character between one and the other of 2 alternate states; not due to mutation but to a poorly understood genetic regulatory mechanism, e.g. diphasic flagellar variation in some *Salmonella* serotypes. **Phenotypic variation.** That which is caused by differences in the environment during the life of the individuals. **Random variation.** An unbiased form of error whose mean, in repeated measurements, tends towards zero. Also known as *random error.* **Saltatory variation.** That in which the steps between one form and the next are relatively large. [L *variare* to diversify.]

varicated (var·ik·a·ted). Affected with varices.

varication (var·ik·a·shun). 1. The occurrence or formation of varices. 2. A number of varices regarded as a group; the varicose state.

varicectomy (var·is·ek·to·me). Surgical excision of a varicose vein. [varix, Gk *ektome* excision.]

varicella (var·is·el·ah). Chickenpox, crystal pox, glass pox. *See* CHICKENPOX. **Varicella bullosa.** A very rare type resembling pemphigus. Large bullae or vesicles develop, and are associated with severe itching and general symptoms. **Varicella gangraenosa, Varicella gangrenosa.** Dermatitis gangraenosa infantum; an unusual form of varicella with gangrenous lesions. Fulminating and subacute subvarieties are described; the former may be fatal within a few hours, and is due to secondary infection with a haemolytic streptococcus. **Varicella haemorrhagica.** Varicella in which there is bleeding not only into the vesicles but into the skin and mucous membranes; a severe, often fatal form. **Varicella inoculata.** Abortive chickenpox produced, with difficulty and not without danger, by artificial inoculation with virus from a vesicle. It is an unreliable method of specific prophylaxis. **Pustular varicella, Varicella pustulosa.** An unusual form of chickenpox in which few or many of the lesions become pustular from infection with associated staphylococci or streptococci. When scarlatina and chickenpox are concurrent, pustulation may be severe and lead to death from septic bronchopneumonia. **Vaccination varicelle.** Unsuccessful attempts to pass on chickenpox by artificial inoculation from a vesicle; varicella inoculata (see above); varicellation. **Varioloid varicella.** Alastrim or variola minor. [dim. of L *varius* spotted.]

varicellation (var·is·el·a'·shun). Inoculation with chickenpox (varicella) virus as a prophylactic measure.

varicelliform (var·is·el·e·form). Resembling the vesicles of varicella in shape and appearance. [varicella, form.]

varicellization (var·is·el·i·za'·shun). Varicellation.

varicelloid (var·is·el·oid). Resembling chickenpox (varicella). [varicella, Gk *eidos* form.]

varices (va·ris·eez). *See* VARIX.

variciform (var·is·e·form). Of the nature of a varix; varicose. [varix, form.]

varicoblepharon (var·ik·o·blef'·ar·on). A varicose condition of the eyelid. [varix, Gk *blepharon* eyelid.]

varicocele (var·ik·o·seel). Varicosity of the testicular veins producing swelling of the scrotum. **Varicocele of the nipple.** Condition in which dilatation of the ducts under the nipple and areola give, on palpation, a sensation comparable to that of a varicocele. **Ovarian varicocele, Pelvic varicocele, Tubo-ovarian varicocele, Utero-ovarian varicocele.** Varicosity of the pampiniform plexus in the female. [varix, Gk *kele* tumour.]

varicocelectomy (var·ik·o·se·lek'·to·me). Surgical treatment of variocele by removal of the affected veins. [varicocele, Gk *ektome* excision.]

varicography (var·ik·og·raf·e). X-ray visualization of varicose veins. [varix, Gk *graphein* to record.]

varicoid (var·ik·oid). Like a varix; variciform. [varix, Gk *eidos* form.]

varicômphalos (var·ik·om·fal·os). A varicose condition around the navel. [varix, Gk *omphalos* navel.]

varicophlebitis (var·ik·o·fleb·i'·tis). Inflammation of veins that are already varicose. [varix, phlebitis.]

varicose (var·ik·oze). 1. Swollen and knotted; having the nature of a varix. 2. Characterized by varicose veins, or arising out of them.

varicosis (var·ik·o·sis). Varicosity of the veins of any part. [varix, Gk *-osis* condition.]

varicosity (var·ik·os·it·e). 1. A morbid state marked by varices. 2. A varix or varicose vein. [see prec.]

varicotomy (var·ik·ot·o·me). Surgical treatment of a varix or varicose vein by incision. [varix, Gk *temnein* to cut.]

varicula (var·ik·ew·lah). A conjunctival varix. [dim. of L *varix* dilated vein.]

variety (var·i·et·e). A taxonomic term for individuals within a population of a species, which differ from the normal form or colour pattern of that population; a term without exact meaning.]L *varius* diverse.]

variform (va·re·form). Existing in several different forms. [L *varius* diverse, form.]

variola (var·i·o·lah). Smallpox. **Black variola.** Haemorrhagic smallpox. *See* SMALLPOX. **Bovine variola.** Cowpox [obsolete term]. **Canadian variola.** Mild smallpox (alastrim) due to a strain of virus harboured in Canada [obsolete term]. **Coherent variola.** Variola in which the pocks remain separate but are very closely set. **Confluent variola.** Confluent smallpox. *See* SMALLPOX. **Variola crystallina.** Varicella. **Discrete variola.** Discrete smallpox. *See* SMALLPOX. **Equine variola.** Horse pox, also known as *grease* or *sore heels* in horses. It may occur as a stomatitis with a pustular eruption in the mouth, and is due to a virus of the pox group, distinct from cowpox virus. **Haemorrhagic variola.** Haemorrhagic smallpox. *See* SMALLPOX. **Variola haemorrhagica pustulosa.** Variola in which the haemorrhages accompanying the vesicles infiltrate their bases and appear within the pustules, as well as between them. **Variola inserta.**

Inoculation smallpox. *See* SMALLPOX. **Variola major.** The major, more severe form of smallpox. **Malignant variola.** Malignant smallpox. *See* SMALLPOX. **Variola miliaris.** Smallpox in which the skin lesions are small (literally, like millet seeds). **Variola minor.** Alastrim or less severe form of smallpox. **Variola mitigata.** An unusual synonym for mild smallpox or alastrim. **Mouse variola.** Mouse pox; infectious ectromelia. **Ovine variola.** Sheep pox, which is due to a virus peculiar to sheep. It is characterized by papulo-vesicular eruption and marked general symptoms, and is endemic in south-eastern Europe and elsewhere. **Variola pemphigosa.** A variety of smallpox with large blebs. **Semiconfluent variola.** Coherent variola (see above). **Variola siliquosa.** Smallpox in which the pustules become empty from absorption of their contents. **Variola sine eruptione.** Smallpox modified by vaccination so that no rash occurs but the patient may excrete infectious virus from the nose, mouth and, rarely, the eyes (*see* SMALLPOX). **Variola sine variolis.** An abortive form of smallpox in which the typical rash does not appear. **Variola vera.** Ordinary smallpox, to be differentiated from the severe haemorrhagic variety and also from varioloid, or smallpox modified by vaccination. **Variola verrucosa.** A form in which the smallpox eruption does not develop beyond the stage of papules. [dim. of L *varius* spotted.]

variolar (var·i·o·lar). Referring to smallpox (variola). [see prec.]

variolate (va·re·o·late). 1. Pustulated like smallpox. 2. To inoculate with the virus of smallpox. [see foll.]

variolation (va·re·o·la′·shun). Inoculation with the virus of smallpox (variola). [variola.]

variolic (var·i·ol·ik). Referring to smallpox; variolar. [see prec.]

varioliform (va·re·o·le·form). Resembling smallpox (variola). [variola, form.]

variolin, variolinum (var·i·o·lin, var·i·o·li′·num). A homoeopathic preparation from smallpox virus. [variola.]

variolization (va·re·o·li·za′·shun). Variolation.

varioloid (va·re·o·loid). 1. Having a resemblance to smallpox (variola). 2. A true form of smallpox, but of a mild nature, in persons who have a certain immunity naturally or acquired from a previous infection or by vaccination. [variola, Gk *eidos* form.]

variolous (var·i·o·lus). Characterized by smallpox (variola) or relating to it. [variola.]

variolovaccine (var·i·o·lo·vak′·seen). A vaccine prepared by inoculating a heifer with virus smallpox.

variolovaccinia (var·i·o·lo·vak·sin′·e·ah). Vaccinia developed by a cow as the result of inoculation with the virus of human variola.

varix (va·rix) (pl. *varices*). An enlarged, dilated, and tortuous venous channel; such a vein is described as *varicose*. **Anastomotic varix.** A system of communicating varicose channels. **Aneurysmal varix, Aneurysmoid varix.** A varix in which dilatation is of aneurysmal proportions. **Arterial varix.** Any condition in which blood passes from artery to vein without traversing the intervening capillaries. It may be acquired as the result of trauma, or be congenital. It is also known as *arteriovenous fistula, arteriovenous aneurysm, cirsoid aneurysm* (*cirsoid varix*), *varicose aneurysm*, and *cavernous angioma*. *Cirsoid aneurysm* and *cavernous angioma* are usually reserved for the congenital lesions. **Chyle varix.** A varix of chyle-conveying lymphatic vessels in the neighbourhood of the pelvis of the ureter. Such a varix occurs in filariasis, and leads to several complications, such as chyluria, and chyliform ascites. **Cirsoid varix.** *See* ARTERIAL VARIX (above). **Varix lymphaticus.** Lymphatic varices occurring in the axilla as well as the groin, associated with lymph stasis and infection with *Wuchereria bancrofti*; another form of lymph varix is a congenital abnormality. **Oesophageal varix.** A dilatation of the portal-systemic venous anastomoses between tributaries of the left gastric vein and the veins of the thorax, found in portal hypertension. **Papillary varix.** A localized naevus, e.g. de Morgan's spots. **Turbinal varix.** Dilated vessels on the turbinal bones, less common here than on the nasal septum. **Varicose varix.** *See* ARTERIAL VARIX (above). [L.]

varnish (var·nish). A solution containing gums and resins in a volatile solvent which evaporates to leave a hard flexible film. *Surgical varnishes* form a protective antiseptic coating on the skin; *pill varnishes* mask the unpleasant taste of certain ingredients and minimize deterioration on storage. Varnishes are also used in the preservation of permanent mounts in microscopy. **Benzoin varnish.** A solution of benzoin, colophony, and Tolu balsam in ether. **Sandarac varnish.** A solution of sandarac in alcohol, used in dentistry as a separating medium when casting plaster models. [Fr. *vernisser.*]

See also: WHITEHEAD (W.).

varolian (va·ro·le·an). Concerning or described by Costanzo Variolo.

Varolio (Varolius), Costanzo (b. 1543). Italian surgeon and anatomist.

Bridge, or pons of Varolius. The pons.

Varolius' valve. The ileocolic valve.

varus (va·rus). 1. A deformity in which the legs are bent outwards; genu varus. 2. Inversion of the foot so that the weight is brought on to the outer part of the sole; talipes varus. [L, bent outwards.] 3. Inflammation of the sebaceous glands of the face. [L, pimple.]

vas [NA] (vas) (pl. *vasa*). A vessel. **Vas aberrans.** A vessel taking an aberrant or abnormal course. **Vas aberrans of the epididymis.** A diverticulum from the lower end of the duct of the epididymis. **Vas afferens [NA].** A small arterial twig to a glomerulus of the kidney. **Vasa afferentia.** 1. Vessels carrying blood to a part, e.g. the vasa afferentia of the glomeruli of the kidney. 2. The vessels conveying lymph to a lymph gland. **Vasa brevia.** Short gastric arteries; branches of the splenic artery which supply the upper end of the greater curvature of the stomach. **Vasa centralia retinae.** The central artery and vein of the retina. **Vas deferens [ductus deferens (NA)].** A long (46 cm) muscular tube, the continuation of the duct of the epididymis, which traverses the inguinal canal and side wall of the pelvis, ending by joining the duct of the corresponding seminal vesicle to form the ejaculatory duct. It conveys the semen from the testis to the prostatic urethra. **Vas deferens, adventitious coat of the [tunica adventitia (NA)].** A sheath of connective tissue external to the muscular coats. **Vas deferens, mucous coat of the [tunica mucosa (NA)].** A coat covered with columnar epithelium, ciliated in parts, and arranged in longitudinal folds, except in the ampulla which has a honeycomb appearance. **Vas deferens, muscular coat of the [tunica muscularis (NA)].** A thick coat divided into an inner and an outer longitudinal coat, and separated by a thicker intermediate circular coat. **Vas efferens [NA].** The vessel leaving a glomerulus of the kidney to enter the capillary plexus around the tubules. **Vasa efferentia.** 1. The blood vessels draining a part, or the lymph vessels draining a lymph gland. 2. The ductules which connect the rete testis with the duct of the epididymis. **Vasa intestinae tenuis.** The blood vessels of the small intestine. **Vasa praevia.** The terminal branches of the placental ends of the umbilical vessels. **Vas prominens [NA].** A blood vessel underlying the spiral prominence of the outer wall of the cochlear duct. **Vasa propria.** Vessels associated with the early amnion. **Vasa recta.** The branches of the efferent arterioles of the juxtamedullary glomeruli which supply the renal medulla (*descending vasa recta*), the long ascending vessels which drain the medulla into the arciform or interlobular veins (*ascending vasa recta*). **Vas spirale [NA].** A large vessel found on the under-surface of the basilar membrane of the organ of Corti. **Vasa vasorum [NA].** Minute blood vessels supplying the outer and middle coats of the larger arteries and veins. **Vasa vorticosa.** The venae vorticosae which drain the choroid coat of the eye. [L.]

See also: FERREIN, HALLER, JUNGBLUTH.

vas deferens, artery of the [arteria ductus deferentis (NA)]. A branch of the superior or inferior vesical arteries.

vasa (va·zah). *See* VAS.

vasal (va·sal). Concerning a vas or vessel.

vasalgia (vas·al·je·ah). Pain in a vessel of any kind. [L *vas* vessel, Gk *algos* pain.]

vascular (**vas**·kew·lar). 1. Concerned with a vessel or vessels. 2. Containing or provided with vessels. [L *vasculum* small vessel.]

vascularity (vas·kew·**lar**·it·e). The state of being vascular or provided with vessels.

vascularization (**vas**·kew·lar·i·za′·shun). The development of vessels in a part, particularly of new blood capillaries. [L *vasculum* small vessel.]

vascularize (**vas**·kew·lar·ize). To render vascular by the development of vessels.

vasculature (**vas**·kew·lat·ewr). The system of distribution of blood vessels to an organ or part. [L *vasculum* small vessel.]

vasculitis (vas·kew·**li**·tis). Inflammation of a blood vessel. **Allergic vasculitis.** Form of vasculitis affecting the skin and other organs. In the skin there may be one or more of erythema, urticaria, purpura, ecchymoses, papules, vesicohaemorrhagic papules, haemorrhagic blisters, nodules, necroses and ulceration. There is often fever, malaise, arthralgia and gastro-intestinal or renal symptoms. Involvement of the heart or the kidneys has a serious effect on the prognosis. **Cutaneous vasculitis.** Vasculitis affecting the skin without involvement of other organs. **Nodular vasculitis.** Cutaneous vasculitis presenting with nodules, mostly on the legs. [L *vasculum* small vessel, Gk *-itis* inflammation.]

vasculogenesis (**vas**·kew·lo·**jen**′·es·is). The development of vessels in a part. [L *vasculum* small vessel, Gk *genein* to produce.]

vasculolymphatic (**vas**·kew·lo·lim·**fat**′·ik). Concerning the blood or lymph vessels. [L *vasculum* small vessel, lymph.]

vasculomotor (**vas**·kew·lo·**mo**′·tor). Controlling the dilatation or constriction of vessels. [L *vasculum* small vessel, *movere* to move.]

vasectomy (vas·**ek**·to·me). Division of the vas deferens. Bilateral vasectomy results in sterility. [L *vas* vessel, Gk *ektome* a cutting out.]

vasicine (va·se·seen). Peganine.

vasifaction (vas·e·**fak**·shun). The formation of new blood vessels. [L *vas* vessel, *facere* to make.]

vasifactive (vas·e·**fak**·tiv). The ability to form new blood vessels, and tissues rich in them. [L *vas* vessel, *facere* to make.]

vasiform (**vas**·e·form). Tubular in form, or shaped like a vessel. [L *vas* vessel, form.]

vasitis (vas·**i**·tis). Inflammation affecting the vas deferens. [vas deferens, Gk *-itis* inflammation.]

vaso- (va·zo, va·so, **vas**·o, **vaz**·o). A combining form used in terms relating to the vascular system.

vasoconstriction (va·zo·kon·**strik**′·shun). The narrowing of the lumen of a blood vessel. [L *vas* vessel, constriction.]

vasoconstrictive (va·zo·kon·**strik**′·tiv). Bringing about vasoconstriction.

vasoconstrictor (va·zo·kon·**strik**′·tor). 1. Inducing vasoconstriction. 2. Any nerve or agent that brings about vasoconstriction.

vasocorona (va·zo·kor·**o**′·nah). Arteries running radially through the spinal cord. [L *vas* vessel, *corona* crown.]

vasodentine (va·zo·**den**·teen). Vascular dentine. [L *vas* vessel, dentine.]

vasodepression (va·zo·de·**presh**′·un). The depression of vasomotor action.

vasodepressor (va·zo·de·**pres**′·or). 1. Exerting a depressor effect on the vasomotor centres. 2. Any agent exerting such an effect.

vasodilatation (va·zo·di·lat·**a**′·shun). Dilatation of a blood vessel. **Reflex vasodilatation.** Dilatation of a blood vessel due to inhibition of its constrictor or stimulation of its dilator nerves, the nerve activity having been induced by psychic or physical stimulation of the afferent, or sensory, side of the reflex arc. [L *vas* vessel, *dilatare* to spread out.]

vasodilatin (va·zo·di·**la**′·tin). Histamine [obsolete term]. [see prec.]

vasodilation (va·zo·di·**la**′·shun). Vasodilatation.

vasodilative (va·zo·di·**la**′·tiv). Causing vasodilatation.

vasodilator (va·zo·di·**la**′·tor). 1. Bringing about dilatation of the blood vessels. 2. Any nerve or agent which induces dilatation of the blood vessels. [L *vas* vessel, *dilatare* to spread out.]

vaso-epididymostomy (**va**·zo·ep·e·did·im·**os**′·to·me). Surgical establishment of a communication between the vas deferens and the epididymis. [vas deferens, epididymis, Gk *stoma* mouth.]

vasofactive, vasoformative (va·zo·**fak**·tiv, va·zo·**for**·mat·iv). Vasifactive.

vasoganglion (va·zo·**gang**·gle·on). Any mass of blood vessels forming themselves into a rete or glomus. [L *vas* vessel, ganglion.]

vasography (va·**zog**·raf·e). Radiographic or radio-isotopic visualization of the blood vessels or lymphatics. A term not in general use. [L *vas* vessel, Gk *graphein* to record.]

vasohypertonic (va·zo·hi·per·**ton**′·ik). Causing increased tonicity in the plain muscle of blood vessels. [L *vas* vessel, Gk *hyper*, *tonos* tone.]

vasohypotonic (va·zo·hi·po·**ton**′·ik). Decreasing the tonicity of the plain muscles of the blood vessels. [L *vas* vessel, Gk *hypo*, *tonos* tone.]

vaso-inhibitor (va·zo·in·**hib**′·it·or). Any drug or agent which reduces or arrests the action of the vasomotor nerves. [L *vas* vessel, inhibit.]

vaso-inhibitory (va·zo·in·**hib**′·it·or·e). Reducing or arresting the action of the vasomotor nerves. [see prec.]

vasoligation, vasoligature (va·zo·lig·**a**′·shun, va·zo·**lig**·at·ewr). Ligature of the vas deferens.

vasoliment (va·**so**·lim·ent). A liniment prepared from liquid paraffin, oleic acid, ammoniated alcohol, and alcohol (90 per cent).

vasoliniment (va·so·**lin**·im·ent). Vasoliment.

vasomotion (va·zo·**mo**·shun). Alteration in the internal diameter of a blood vessel brought about by modification of the tonus of the plain muscle of the walls through the action of constrictor or dilator nerves. [L *vas* vessel, *movere* to move.]

vasomotor, vasomotorial, vasomotory (va·zo·**mo**·tor, **va**·zo·mo·**tor**′·e·al, va·zo·**mo**·tor·e). 1. Involved in the mechanism of vasomotion. 2. Any drug or agent which affects vasomotions. 3. A nerve of the sympathetic or parasympathetic system, or an antidromic fibre, which causes dilatation or constriction of a blood vessel.

vasoneuropathy (va·zo·newr·**op**′·ath·e). Disorder caused by disease of the vasomotor nerves. **Peripheral vasoneuropathy after chilling.** The peripheral changes occurring in the limbs after exposure to cold and damp, e.g. in immersion foot and trench foot. [L *vas* vessel, Gk *neuron* nerve, *pathos* disease.]

vasoneurosis (va·zo·newr·**o**′·sis). Any disorder of the vasomotor system. [L *vas* vessel, Gk *neuron* nerve.]

vaso-orchidostomy (va·zo·or·kid·**os**′·to·me). Surgical establishment of a communication between the vas deferens and the body of the testis. [L *vas* vessel, Gk *orchis* testicle, *stoma* mouth.]

vasoparalysis (va·zo·par·**al**′·is·is). Vasomotor paralysis. *See* PARALYSIS. [L *vas* vessel, paralysis.]

vasoparesis (va·zo·par·**e**′·sis). Paresis of the vasomotor nerves. [L *vas* vessel, paresis.]

vasopressin (va·zo·**pres**·in). A hormone produced by the posterior pituitary which is identical with antidiuretic hormone. Its main effect is to increase the permeability of the collecting ducts of the kidney, leading to increased reabsorption of water. In large amounts it produces a rise in the blood pressure when injected intravenously, but it is unlikely that it is secreted in sufficient amounts for this to happen normally. [L *vas* vessel, *premere* to press.]

vasopressor (va·zo·pres·or). An agent which raises the blood pressure when given intravenously. [L *vas* vessel, *premere* to press.]

vasopuncture (va·zo·**pungk**·tcher). Puncture of the vas deferens.

vasoreflex (va·zo·**re**·flex). Reflex action affecting a blood vessel. [L *vas* vessel, reflex.]

vasorelaxation (va·zo·re·lax·**a**′·shun). Reduction in the automatic tonus of the plain muscle of a blood vessel; fall in vascular pressure. [L *vas* vessel, relaxation.]

vasoresection (va·zo·re·**sek**′·shun). The removal of a part of the vas deferens. [vas deferens, resection.]

vasorrhaphy (va·zor·af·e). Suture of the vas deferens, particularly the rejoining of a divided or resected vas. [vas deferens, Gk *rhaphe* suture.]

vasosection (va·zo·sek·shun). Severance of the vas deferens. [vas deferens, section.]

vasosensory (va·zo·sen·sor·e). Concerned with sensation in the blood vessels; describing certain afferent nerve fibres. [L *vas* vessel, sensory.]

vasospasm (va·zo·spazm). Spasmodic constriction of the small arteries causing cramp and claudication. [L *vas* vessel, spasm.]

vasospastic (va·zo·spas·tik). Characterized by or causing vasospasm. [L *vas* vessel, Gk *spastikos* a stretching.]

vasostimulant (va·zo·stim·ew·lant). 1. Promoting vasomotor activity. 2. Any drug or agent which stimulates the vasomotor system. [L *vas* vessel, stimulant.]

vasostomy (va·zos·to·me). The establishment surgically of an opening in the vas deferens. [vas deferens, Gk *stoma* mouth.]

vasothrombin (va·zo·throm·bin). A factor reputed to be produced by the endothelial cells and resembling leucothrombin in that it combines with so-called hepatothrombin to form thrombin. [L *vas* vessel, thrombin.]

vasotomy (va·zot·o·me). Surgical incision of the vas deferens. [vas deferens, Gk *temnein* to cut.]

vasotonia (va·zo·to·ne·ah). The tonus of a blood vessel. [L *vas* vessel, tonus.]

vasotonic (va·zo·ton·ik). 1. Concerning the normal and automatic tonus of the blood vessels. 2. Vasostimulant. [see prec.]

vasotribe (va·zo·tribe). Surgical forceps employed to stop haemorrhage from an artery by crushing it into the surrounding tissue. [L *vas* vessel, Gk *tribein* to crush.]

vasotripsy (va·zo·trip·se). The use of the vasotribe to prevent haemorrhage from an artery.

vasotrophic (va·zo·trof·ik). 1. Concerned with the nutrition of blood and lymph vessels. 2. Affecting the nutrition of a part by controlling the blood supply of that part. [L *vas* vessel, Gk *trophe* nourishment.]

vasotropic (va·zo·trop·ik). With an attraction for blood vessels; with selective action on blood vessels. [L *vas* vessel, Gk *trepein* to turn.]

vasovagal (va·zo·va·gal). Vascular and vagal. **Vasovagal attacks.** Non-epileptic seizures, or convulsive syncope, due to cerebral ischaemia secondary to a systemic hypotension. [Obsolete term.] [L *vas* vessel, vagus.]

vasovasostomy (va·zo·va·zos′·to·me). Anastomosis between two divided ends of the vas deferens. [vas deferens, Gk *stoma* mouth.]

vasovesiculectomy (va·zo·ves·ik·ew·lek′·to·me). Removal of the vas deferens together with the seminal vesicle on the same side. [vas deferens, vesicle, Gk *ektome* excision.]

vasovesiculitis (va·zo·ves·ik·ew·li′·tis). Inflammation involving both the vas deferens and the seminal vesicles. [vas deferens, vesicle, Gk *-itis* inflammation.]

vastus (vas·tus). Very large; vast. [L.]

vastus muscles (vas·tus muslz). **Vastus intermedius muscle [musculus vastus intermedius (NA)], Vastus lateralis muscle [musculus vastus lateralis (NA)], Vastus medialis muscle [musculus vastus medialis (NA)].** Three muscles which, together with the rectus femoris muscle, comprise the quadriceps femoris muscle of the thigh. [L, very large.]

Vater, Abraham (b. 1864). Wittenburg anatomist and botanist.

Vater's ampulla, or diverticulum. An ampulla at the end of the common bile duct in the greater duodenal papilla.

Vater's corpuscles, Vater-Pacini corpuscles. Lamellated corpuscles. *See* CORPUSCLE.

Vater's tubercle. The greater duodenal papilla. *See* PAPILLA.

vateria indica (vat·er·e·ah in·dik·ah). Indian copal tree, white dammar; an East Indian tree (family Dipterocarpeae) which yields Indian copal, an amber resin. [Abraham *Vater*, L *Indicus* of India.]

Vauban, Sebastien le Prestre, Marquis de, (b. 1633). French military engineer.

Vauban's fortification pictures, Vauban's fortification spectra. Teichopsia.

vault (vawlt). An arched cavity, e.g. the hard palate of the oral cavity. **Vault of the pharynx.** Pharyngeal fornix. *See* FORNIX. [O Fr. *vaute.*]

Veau, Victor (b. 1871). Paris surgeon.

Veau's operation. A repair for congenital cleft palate using palatal flaps which are retroposed on the V-Y operation principle. They depend for their blood supply on the posterior palatine arteries, and tension is avoided by fracture of the pterygoid hamulus. The mucosa of the floor of the nose is dissected up, and the repair is completed by a two-layer suture of oral and nasal mucosa.

vectis (vek·tis). A curved instrument, similar to the blade of the obstetric forceps, for applying traction to the fetal head to assist its delivery at caesarean section or vaginally. A similarly-shaped instrument is used in delivering a lens from the eye. [L bar.]

vector (vek·tor). 1. In physics, a quantity having both magnitude and direction. 2. In biology, an animal which carries other organisms from one place to another, particularly one which carries a parasite from one host to another, inter- or intraspecifically. **Biological vector.** One in which a parasitic organism can live normally; a host. **Cardiac vector.** The sum of all the electrical forces acting on the heart at any given instant in magnitude and direction. The electrical events of the cardiac cycle are made up of an infinite number of instantaneous vectors from which a mean three-dimensional vector can be obtained; there is one for the atrial cycle (P-wave vector), for the ventricular depolarization (QRS-wave vector), and for ventricular repolarization (T-wave factor). **Mechanical vector, Passive vector.** A vector in which no development of the parasite takes place, but which merely conveys the parasite, e.g. on its legs or proboscis, to a potential host. [L, carrier.]

vectorcardiogram (vek·tor·kar·de·o·gram). A tracing of the mean direction and magnitude of all the instantaneous vectors occurring in the frontal plane during the cardiac cycle, recorded as a loop beginning and ending at the centre of the heart. It is obtained by the simultaneous recording of the three standard limb leads, employing a cathode-ray oscilloscope. The form of the loop is derived from measurements of the areas enclosed by the simultaneous P, QRS, and T deflexions. **Spatial vectorcardiogram.** A vectorcardiogram which records the vector simultaneously in all three dimensions. [vector, Gk *kardia* heart, *gramma* a record.]

vectorcardiography (vek·tor·kar·de·og′·raf·e). A method of recording the magnitude and direction of the electrical forces acting on the heart (P-, QRS-, and T-wave vectors) in the form of a continuous loop for each vector (vector-cardiogram, monocardiogram). **Spatial vectorcardiography, Three-dimensional vectorcardiography.** A method of recording the movement of the cardiac vectors in three planes, frontal, horizontal, and sagittal. [vector, Gk *kardia* heart, *graphein* to record.]

vectorial (vek·tor·e·al). Referring to a vector.

Vedder, Edward Bright (b. 1878). American physician.

Vedder's starch agar. Starch agar. *See* AGAR.

Vedder's sign. In beriberi: pain on pressure over the calf muscles, anaesthesia of the anterior aspect of the legs, loss of knee jerk, and difficulty in rising from the squatting position.

vegan (vej·an). An extreme vegetarian who eats no animal food of any kind, not even milk or other dairy products.

vegetable (vej·e·tabl). 1. Having the characteristics of a plant, or derived from plant life. 2. Any plant used as a food. **Vegetable albumin.** Phyto-albumin. **Vegetable base.** An alkaloid. **Vegetable gelatin.** Agar. **Vegetable sulphur.** Lycopodium. [L *vegetare* to animate.]

vegetal (vej·e·tal). Concerned with plants; plant-like; vegetable. **Vegetal function.** Any biological activity that is common to plants and animals alike, as distinct from mental functions which are possessed by animals alone. [see prec.]

vegetarian (vej·e·ta·re·an). A person whose diet is restricted to fruit and vegetables, or to foods of purely vegetable origin.

vegetarianism (vej·e·ta·re·an·izm). The cult of living on a diet composed of fruit and vegetables; in certain cases the diet is extended to include milk and eggs, but flesh is rigidly excluded.

vegetation (vej·e·ta·shun). Any growth that is plant-like, e.g. neoplasm, papilloma. **Adenoid vegetation.** Hypertrophy of the adenoid mass of the post-nasal space; the so-called pharyngeal, or Luschka's tonsil. **Bacterial vegetation.** An irregular excrescence on a cardiac valve, or septum, or in great vessels, composed of fibrin, blood platelets, red and white blood cells, and bacteria. The most common sites are the mitral and aortic valves, a defective interventricular septum, and patent ductus arteriosus. When occurring on a valve there is usually an underlying abnormality, congenital or acquired. **Dendritic vegetation.** Shaggy, villous masses seen in certain cancers or fibrinous deposits on serous membranes. **Verrucous vegetation.** A small nodular warty excrescence on a heart valve, such as occurs in rheumatic heart disease or a similar growth elsewhere, e.g. on the skin surface. [L *vegetare* to animate.]

vegetative (vej·e·ta·tiv). 1. Involved in the processes of growth and nutrition, or relating to these functions. 2. Growing or living like a vegetable, without will or consciousness; functioning involuntarily. **Vegetative disturbance.** Disorder of growth and nutrition. [see prec.]

vegulin (vej·ew·lin). An extract from cabbage reputed to cause reduction of the blood sugar in rabbits when injected or given by mouth. These observations have not yet been substantiated.

vehicle (ve·ikl). 1. Any substance used in pharmacy to convey or give bulk to a medicine, without itself necessarily possessing therapeutic properties; an excipient. 2. Anything which conveys an impulse. [L *vehiculum* conveyance.]

veil (vale). A veil-like appendage or screen. **Acquired veil.** A loss of ring or timbre in the singing voice, due to vocal strain or infection of the singing organs. **Hottentot veil.** The elongated labia minora seen in Hottentot women. **Uterine veil.** Any device covering the neck of the uterus to prevent conception. [L *velum.*]

See also: JACKSON (J. N.), SATTLER.

Veillon, Adrien (b. 1864). Paris bacteriologist.

Veillon tube. A tube of inoculated agar, closed at one end with a cork, used for the isolation of anaerobic organisms.

Veillonella (va·yon·el·ah). A genus of the family Neisseriaceae; Gram-negative anaerobic cocci, whose normal habitat is the mouth of man and animals. They include the species *Veillonella gazogenes* and *V. parvula.* [Adrien *Veillon.*]

vein [vena (NA)] (vane). A vessel conducting blood from the capillary bed to the heart. (For specific veins, see under qualifying adjective or the organ concerned.) **Allantoic veins.** Paired veins draining the allantois of the early embryo; they become the umbilical veins once the allantochorial circulation is established. **Cardinal veins, anterior.** A pair of large veins in the embryo which drain the head region. Each joins with a posterior cardinal vein to form a common cardinal vein or duct of Cuvier. **Cardinal veins, common.** Paired veins of the embryo opening into the sinus venosus. In man, the right one becomes the terminal portion of the superior vena cava, the left one the oblique vein of the left atrium. **Cardinal veins, posterior.** paired embryonic veins draining the region of the embryo behind the heart. They empty into the common cardinal veins and are closely associated with the mesonephros. Part of the right vein is incorporated in the terminal part of the vena azygos. **Communicating vein.** A vein which perforates the deep fascia to connect the deep and superficial venous systems. **Cutaneous vein [vena cutanea (NA)].** Any vein lying in the skin. **Emissary vein.** A vein passing through a foramen in the skull and linking a sinus within the skull to a vein outside it. **Omphalomesenteric veins.** Paired embryonic veins which pass through the liver to end in the sinus venosus of the heart. They are formed from earlier vitelline veins after they have established connection with the mesenteric veins. **Para-ureteric veins.** Lateral sympathetic veins (see below). **Primary head vein.** The forward continuation of the anterior cardinal vein which drains the brain. It runs medial to the trigeminal ganglion but lateral to the acousticofacial ganglion. Part of it, persists as the cavernous sinus and superior petrosal sinus of the adult. **Subcardinal veins.** Paired embryonic veins which lie ventromedial to the mesonephros and replace part of the posterior cardinal veins. Part of the right vein forms the portion of the inferior vena cava between the kidney and the liver. **Supracardinal veins.** Lateral sympathetic veins (see foll.). **Sympathetic veins, lateral.** Paired embryonic veins which lie lateral to the sympathetic chains on the posterior wall of the thorax and abdomen. Part of the right vein becomes the subrenal part of the inferior vena cava. **Sympathetic veins, medial.** Paired embryonic veins lying medial to the sympathetic chains of the posterior thoracic and abdominal walls. They persist in part as the venae azygos and hemiazygos of the adult. **Umbilical veins.** Paired veins of the umbilical cord of the early embryo, or the persisting left vein of the later embryo, which drains oxygenated blood from the placenta into the liver circulation. In the adult it is represented by the fibrous round ligament. **Varicose veins.** Permanently dilated or tortuous veins superficially situated and therefore with little support from other tissues; usually of the lower limbs. **Vitelline veins.** Paired veins of the early embryo which drain the yolk sac, through the liver, into the sinus venosus of the heart. Parts of the vitelline veins are incorporated in the portal vein and terminal inferior vena cava as well as the liver sinusoids of the adult. **Vorticose veins.** The whorl of veins on the outer layer of the choroid of the eye. [L *vena.*]

See also: BRESCHET, BUROW, GALEN, KOHLRAUSCH (O. L. B.), KONSTANTINOWICH, KRUKENBERG (A.), LABBÉ (C.), LATARGET, MARSHALL (J.), MAYO (W. J.), RETZIUS (A. A.), ROSENTHAL (F. C.), RUYSCH, SANTORINI, SAPPEY, THEBESIUS, TROLARD, VIEUSSENS, ZUCKERKANDL.

veinography (va·nog·raf·e). X-ray examination of the veins. [vein, Gk *graphein* to record.]

Veit, Gustav (b. 1824). Bonn gynaecologist.

Mauriceau-Smellie-Veit manoeuvre, Smellie-Mauriceau-Veit manoeuvre, or method. To deliver the aftercoming head: the child is placed astride one arm and the middle and forefingers are placed over the upper jaw on each side of the nose. This maintains the head in an attitude of flexion. The ring and little finger of the other hand are applied over the child's right shoulder and the thumb is placed over the left shoulder. Traction is now exerted in a downward and backward direction until the head is brought into the pelvis. Gentle pressure suprapubically facilitates this manoeuvre. The child's body is now carried up towards the mother's abdomen and the head delivered slowly over the perineum.

vela (ve·lah). *See* VELUM.

velamen (ve·la·men). A membranous covering of any kind; a velum or tegument. **Velamen nativum.** The skin. **Velamen vulvae.** The pudendal apron. *See* APRON. [L, veil.]

velamentous (ve·lam·en·tus). Hanging down or spread over; draped like a veil. [see foll.]

velamentum (ve·lam·en·tum). Any membranous covering; a velum or velamen. **Velamentum abdominale.** The peritoneum. **Velamentum cerebrale.** Any of the membranes covering the brain or spinal cord; a meninx. **Velamentum corporis commune.** The skin. **Velamentum infantis.** Any of the fetal membranes. **Velamentum linguae.** Any of the lateral or medial folds of mucous membrane between the tongue and the epiglottis. [L, veil.]

velar (ve·lar). Referring to a velum, particularly that of the palate.

veliform (ve·le·form). Velamentous. [velum, form.]

Vella, Luigi (b. 1825). Bologna physiologist.

Thiry-Vella fistula. An isolated loop of bowel communicating with the intestinal tract on the one hand and with the exterior on the other.

vellicate (vel·ik·ate). To jerk or twitch; to contract spasmodically. [L *vellicare* to twitch.]

vellication (vel·ik·a·shun). Jerky twitching of the fibrillary muscles. [see prec.]

vellus (vel·us). Soft unmedullated hair up to 2 cm long and usually unpigmentated. [L fleece.]

velonoskiascopy (ve·lo·no·ski·**as**′·ko·pe). A subjective test for errors of refraction, developed from Scheiner's experiment by Trantas and Lindner. A wire cross with narrow arms (0.75 mm) is placed close to an eye viewing a white cross on a black background similarly orientated. If the eye is emmetropic, no shadow is seen; if it is not, the arms of the wire cross produce a shadow on those of the white one. [L *velum* veil, Gk *skia* shadow, *skopein* to view.]

velosynthesis (ve·lo·**sin**·thes·is). Repair of a cleft soft palate. [L *velum* veil, Gk *synthesis* a putting together.]

Velpeau, Alfred Armand Louis Marie (b. 1795). Paris surgeon.

Velpeau's hernia. Femoral hernia in front of the femoral vessels.

Velpeau's diarrhoea mixture. Tincture of opium, camphor, and tincture of gambir.

velum [NA] (**ve**·lum) (pl. *vela*). Veil. **Velum interpositum.** The tela chorioidea of the 3rd ventricle. **Medullary velum, inferior, right and left [velum medullare inferius (NA)].** A thin, white lamina forming part of the roof of the 4th ventricle. **Medullary velum, superior [velum medullare superius (NA)].** A thin, white lamina constituting part of the roof of the 4th ventricle. **Velum palatinum [NA].** The part of the fauces that comprises the uvula, the palatoglossal arch, and the palatopharyngeal arch. **Velum transversum.** In the embryonic brain, the fold in the tela chorioidea between the diencephalon and the telencephalon. [L.]

See also: TARIN.

vena [NA] (**ve**·nah) (pl. *venae*). Vein. **Venae advehentes.** Branches of the vitelline veins taking blood into the liver sinusoids. **Vena azygos [NA].** A tributary of the superior vena cava; it begins in the abdomen and courses along the back of the thorax on the right side before entering the superior vena cava. The main venous drainage of the chest wall and thoracic part of the oesophagus, it communicates freely by its tributaries with the veins within the spinal canal. **Vena azygos, phrenic branches of the [venae phrenicae superiores (NA)].** Small veins accompanying the arteries to the diaphragm, and ending in the inferior vena cava, the vena azygos, and the renal or suprarenal veins. **Vena cava, inferior [vena cava inferior (NA)].** The main vein of the lower half of the body, formed in the lower abdomen by the union of the common iliac veins and terminating immediately above the diaphragm in the right atrium. **Vena cava, superior [vena cava superior (NA)].** The main venous drainage of the head, neck, and upper limbs. It is formed in the chest by the union of the two innominate veins and opens into the right atrium of the heart. **Vena comitans of the hypoglossal nerve [vena comitans nervi hypoglossi (NA)].** The main vein of the tongue, accompanying the nerve and drainage into the common facial vein, venae comitantes of the lingual artery, or internal jugular vein. **Venae comitantes [NA].** Two or more venous channels accompanying an artery and connected to each other by numerous cross communications. **Venae comitantes of the lingual artery.** Tributaries of the internal jugular vein. **Venae cordis minimae [NA].** Small veins in the substance of the heart which open directly into the cavities over which they lie. **Vena hemiazygos, inferior [vena hemiazygos (NA)].** A tributary of the vena azygos, draining the lower intercostal spaces of the left side and some oesophageal veins. **Vena hemiazygos, superior [vena hemiazygos accessoria (NA)].** A tributary of the vena azygos, draining the middle intercostal spaces of the left side and some bronchial veins. **Venae revehentes.** Branches of the vitelline veins which drain blood from the liver sinusoids into the inferior vena cava. They later become the hepatic veins. **Venae vorticosae [venae vorticosae (venae choroidea oculi) NA].** Veins of the choroid of the eye; their tributaries are arranged in groups which converge on four or five veins which pierce the sclera and enter the ophthalmic veins. [L.]

Venable, Charles Scott (b. 1877). San Antonio orthopaedic surgeon.

Venable plate. Vitallium bone plate.

vena-caval (ve·nah·**ka**·val). Pertaining to the vena cava.

venation (ve·**na**·shun). The system of distribution of veins within a part. [L *vena* vein.]

venectasia (ve·nek·**ta**·ze·ah). A varicosed state of a vein. [L *vena* vein, Gk *ektasis* dilatation.]

venectomy (ve·**nek**·to·me). The surgical excision of a vein. [L *vena* vein, Gk *ektome* excision.]

venenation (ven·en·**a**·shun). Poisoning, or the condition resulting from poisoning. [L *venenum* poison.]

venene (**ven**·een). A mixture of the venoms of poisonous snakes, formerly used empirically in various diseases, and now used to produce antivenene. [see prec.]

veneniferous (ven·en·**if**·er·us). Bearing poison; toxiferous. [L *venenum* poison, *ferre* to bear.]

venenific (ven·en·**if**·ik). Poison-forming; toxicogenic. [L *venenum* poison, *facere* to make.]

venenosalivary (ven·en·o·sal·i′·var·e). Having a poisonous saliva. [L *venenum*, saliva.]

venenose (**ven**·en·oze). Venenous.

venenosity (ven·en·**os**·it·e). Toxicity. [see foll.]

venenous (**ven**·en·us). Poisonous; toxic. [L *venenosus* full of poison.]

venepuncture (ve·ne·**pungk**·tcher). Puncture of a vein. [L *vena* vein, *pungere* to prick.]

venereal (ven·**eer**·e·al). Transmitted by sexual intercourse. [L *Venus* goddess of love.]

Venereal Disease Act 1917. This Act prohibits the treatment of venereal diseases by any person other than a qualified medical practitioner, and the advertisements of any offer to treat such diseases or to give advice thereon.

venereologist (ven·**eer**·e·**ol**′·o·jist). One who specializes in the treatment of veneral diseases. [see foll.]

venereology (ven·**eer**·e·**ol**′·o·je). The branch of medicine devoted to the study and treatment of venereal disease. [venereal, Gk *logos* science.]

venereophobia (ven·**eer**·e·o·**fo**′·be·ah). 1. A morbid fear of venereal disease, or the unreasoning and unfounded impression that venereal disease has been contracted. 2. Morbid dread of sexual intercourse. [venereal, Gk *phobein* to fear.]

venerology (ven·er·**ol**·o·je). Venereology.

venesection (ve·ne·**sek**·shun). Surgical blood-letting by the opening of a vein. [L *vena* vein, section.]

venesuture (ve·ne·**sew**·tewr). Suture of a vein. [L *vena* vein, suture.]

venin, venine (**ven**·in, **ven**·een). Venene.

venipuncture (ve·ne·**pungk**·tcher). Venepuncture.

venisuture (ve·ne·**sew**·tewr). Venesuture.

venitis (ven·**i**·tis). Inflammation of the veins. [L *vena* vein, Gk *-itis* inflammation.]

veno-auricular (ve·no·aw·**rik**′·ew·lar). Pertaining to the vena cava and the auricle.

venoclysis (ve·**nok**·lis·is). The introduction of nutritive fluid or a solution of a drug directly into a vein. [L *vena* vein, Gk *klysis* injection.]

venofibrosis (ve·no·fi·**bro**′·sis). A fibrosed state of a vein. [L *vena* vein, fibrosis.]

venogram (**ve**·no·gram). 1. The radiograph made during venography. 2. A recording of the pressure variation in one of the veins nearest the heart; a venous pulse tracing or phlebogram. [L *vena* vein, Gk *gramma* record.]

venography (ve·**nog**·raf·e). 1. Radiographic visualization of veins after injection of a radio-opaque contrast medium into the lumen. 2. Investigation of the venous pulse. **Splenic venography.** A method of demonstrating radiologically the splenic vein and part of the portal circulation, e.g. by the injection of a contrast medium. [L *vena* vein, Gk *graphein* to record.]

venom (**ven**·om). A poisonous fluid secreted by any animal. **Venom Antiserum BPC 1959.** An antitoxin obtained from animals immunized against the particular venom. **Bee venom.** That produced by the poison glands and injected by the sting of hive and wild bees. It contains neurotoxic and haemoly[illegible] proteins. **Moccasin venom.** Venomin. **Snake venom.** That produced by the poison glands of the mouth and injected by the fangs of poisonous snakes. It varies greatly in constitution, but usually contains powerful proteolytic enzymes, neurotoxins, and phosphatases. **Spider venom.** That produced by the cheliceral glands and injected by the bite of many spiders. **Toad venom.** That produced by the skin glands of many species of toad. It contains digitalis-like heart glycosides. **Viper venom.** The venom of Russell's viper, used as a haemostatic, and useful in dental surgery and in nose and throat surgery. The solution is applied on a pledget of cotton wool. [L *venenum* poison.]

venomin (ven·o·min). Moccasin venom; an extract of the venom obtained from two species of moccasin snakes occurring in the southern USA, the water moccasin and the cotton-mouth. It is claimed to have an analgesic effect, and is administered intradermally in the treatment of arthritis, lumbago, neuralgia, sciatica, and similar disorders.

venomosalivary (ven·o·mo·sal·i′·var·e). Referring to any creature that secretes a poisonous saliva. [L *venenum* poison, saliva.]

venomotor (ve·no·mo·tor). Describing any factor that brings about an alteration in the internal diameter of a vein; relating to the sympathetic vasoconstrictor fibres to veins. [L *vena* vein movere to move.]

venomous (ven·om·us). 1. Poisonous. 2. Applied to creatures that have venom-secreting glands. [L *venenum* poison.]

venoperitoneostomy (ve·no·per·it·o·ne·os′·to·me). A now-abandoned operation for ascites in which a pouch of peritoneum in the region of the femoral canal was anastomosed to the upper end of the long saphenous vein. [L *vena* vein, peritoneum, Gk *stoma* mouth.]

venopressor (ve·no·pres·or). Concerned with the pressure in the veins, particularly with pressure variations in the great veins nearest the heart. [L *vena* vein, pressure.]

venosclerosis (ve·no·skler·o′·sis). Hardening of the walls of veins. [L *vena* vein, Gk *sklerosis* a hardening.]

venose (ve·noze). Furnished with veins. [L *venosus.*]

venosinal (ve·no·si·nal). Concerning the openings of the venae cavae, the right atrium, and the coronary sinus.

venosity (ve·nos·it·e). 1. Applied to blood in a part of the body, the degree to which it shows venous characteristics. 2. The accumulation of blood in the venous system with the fall in cardiac output, as in circulatory shock.

venospasm (ve·no·spazm). A contraction of the veins that may follow the transfusion of cold blood or other substance. [L *vena* vein, Gk *spasmos* spasm.]

venostasis (ve·no·sta·sis). The compression of an extremity to decrease the return flow of blood in the veins. [L *vena* vein, Gk *stasis* a standing.]

venostat (ve·no·stat). An appliance for effecting venostasis.

venothrombotic (ve·no·throm·bot′·ik). A substance that will produce venous thrombosis.

venotomy (ve·not·o·me). Surgical section of a vein. [L *vena* vein, Gk *temnein* to cut.]

venous (ve·nus). Concerned with a vein or veins, or characterized by veins. [L *venosus* veiny.]

venovenostomy (ve·no·ve·nos′·to·me). Anastomosis between two veins. [L *vena* vein, Gk *stoma* mouth.]

vent (vent). An outlet to the exterior, e.g. the anus. [O Fr. *fente* cleft.]

venter (ven·ter) (pl. *ventres*). Belly. **Venter propendens.** A pendulous abdomen such as that seen in late pregnancy. [L.]

ventilate (ven·til·ate). 1. To maintain atmospheric conditions which are healthful and comfortable, usually by renewal of the air in a room at regular intervals. 2. A term sometimes applied to the process of oxygenating the blood in the lungs. [L *ventilate* to wave.]

ventilation (ven·til·a·shun). 1. The science of maintaining atmospheric conditions which are healthful and comfortable to the human body. 2. The cleansing or purification of the air of a room. 3. The maintenance of tidal exchange in the lungs. **Assisted ventilation.** Intermittent positive pressure ventilation synchronous with the patient's inadequate inspirations. **Controlled ventilation.** Intermittent positive pressure ventilation in the apnoeic patient. **Downward ventilation.** A system of ventilation in which the outlets for air are placed lower than the inlets for fresh air. **Exhausting ventilation, Exhaustion ventilation.** A system of ventilation in which the foul air is extracted by one or more fans and then conveyed, at a suitable velocity, to some central point in the building or factory. It is essential for the removal of fumes or dust in various manufacturing processes. **Expired-air ventilation.** Inflation of the lungs of an apnoeic patient by the attendant's expired air; the "kiss of life". **Intermittent positive pressure ventilation** (IPPV). Rhythmic inflation of the lungs during apnoea, allowing expiration to occur by the natural processes. **Mechanical ventilation.** Ventilation of the apnoeic or hypoventilating patient by a machine able to produce intermittent positive pressure ventilation. It is used in anaesthesia and intensive therapy. **Natural ventilation.** The admittance and exit of atmospheric air to a room or building through simple inlets and outlets. It is dependent on diffusion, winds (perflation or aspiration), and the movement of masses of air of unequal temperature. **Plenum ventilation.** In the plenum system, a regulated volume of fresh air is forced into a room, thus expelling the vitiated air. By means of filters, radiators, and wet screens, the air is cleansed, warmed, and moistened, that is, "conditioned", as required. In some installations the entering air is warmed and no radiators are provided. **Upward ventilation.** A system of ventilation in which the incoming air enters a room at a lower level than the outlets. **Vacuum ventilation.** A system of ventilation in which a vacuum is employed for the forcible extraction of vitiated air. [see prec.]

ventilators (ven·til·a·torz). Mechanical respirators which can deliver high concentrations of oxygen to patients with impaired respiration or apnoea, or following heart surgery. **Barnet ventilator.** Electrical time-cycled ventilating machine devised by technicians at the Barnet group of hospitals. It is more practical to transport and is easier to operate than the oxygen tent. **Bird ventilator.** An apparatus used in anaesthesia and to assist respiration. **East-Radcliffe ventilator.** A popular apparatus for artificial ventilation of the lungs. **Patient-triggered ventilator.** An artificial ventilating machine so devised that it will inflate the lungs of a patient in response to a feeble inspiratory effort. **Pressure-cycled (or preset) ventilator.** An artificial ventilating machine set to deliver gases to the patient at a preset pressure; it can compensate for small leaks in the circuit. **Time-cycled ventilator.** An artificial ventilating machine set to produce inspiration and expiration at regular intervals and independently of other factors. **Triggered ventilator.** An artificial ventilating machine in which a feeble inspiratory effort of the patient will initiate intermittent positive pressure breathing. **Volume-cycled ventilator.** An artificial ventilating machine in which the volume of inflating gases is preset.

ventouse (vawn·tooz). A cupping glass. [Fr.]

ventral [ventralis (NA)] (ven·tral). 1. Referring to the belly; abdominal. 2. Towards the front; anterior. [L *venter* belly.]

ventres (ven·treez). *See* VENTER.

ventricle (ven·trikl). A small cavity, chamber, or compartment. **Ventricles of the brain.** The ependymal-lined dilatations of the central canal of the brain of which there are four, two lateral, a third, and a fourth. **Common ventricle.** Single ventricle (see below). **Ventricle of the cord [ventriculus terminalis (NA)].** A dilatation of the central canal of the spinal cord at the lower end of the conus medullaris. **Double-inlet left ventricle.** A rare developmental abnormality in which both mitral and tricuspid orifices open into the left ventricle. **Double-inlet right ventricle.** A rare developmental abnormality in which both mitral and tricuspid orifices open into the right ventricle. **Double-outlet left ventricle.** A rare developmental abnormality in which both aorta and pulmonary artery arise from the left ventricle. **Double-outlet right ventricle.** An uncommon developmental abnormality in which both aorta and pulmonary artery arise from the right ventricle. **Fifth ventricle.** Cavity of the septum lucidum; a cavity contained between the two laminae of the septum lucidum. In brains lacking a rostrum of the corpus callosum it communicates directly with the median interhemispheral space. **Fourth ventricle [ventriculus quartus (NA)].** An ependymal-lined cavity within the hind-brain, communicating below with the central canal of the spinal cord and above with the aqueduct of the mid-brain. Its diamond-shaped floor [fossa rhomboidea (NA)] is formed by the dorsal surfaces of the medulla and pons, and its roof [tegmen ventriculi quarti (NA)] from above downwards by the superior medullary velum, cerebellum, inferior medullary velum, and tela chorioidea. The vestibular area on the floor of the 4th ventricle overlies the vestibular nuclei. It communicates through the lateral and medial apertures with the subarachnoid space. **Ventricles of the heart [ventriculi cordis (NA)].** The two major pumping chambers of the heart, the *left ventricle* and *right ventricle* (see below). **Ventricle of the larynx.** Sinus of the larynx. **Lateral ventricle [ventriculus lateralis (NA)].** An ependymal-lined cavity within each cerebral hemisphere which communicates with the third ventricle through the interventricular foramen. It is divided into a central part [pars centralis (NA)], or body, and three horns; anterior [cornu anterius (NA)], posterior [cornu posterius (NA)], and inferior [cornu inferius (NA)], which extend respectively into the frontal, occipital, and temporal lobes. The bulb of the posterior horn is a swelling on the medial wall formed by the forceps major. **Left ventricle [ventriculus sinister (NA)].** The thick-walled muscular chamber which forms the left border and apex of the heart. Normally it receives oxygenated blood from the left atrium through the mitral orifice and ejects it into the aorta. **Pineal ventricle.** The pineal recess of the third ventricle. **Right ventricle [ventriculus dexter (NA)].** The muscular chamber which lies to the right and in front of the left ventricle, forming most of the front of the heart. Normally it receives venous blood from the right atrium through the tricuspid orifice and ejects it into the pulmonary artery. **Single ventricle.** A developmental abnormality of the heart in which there is anatomically or functionally a single ventricular chamber. **Sixth ventricle.** A space between the corpus callosum and the body of the fornix cerebri. **Terminal ventricle.** Ventricle of the cord (see above). **Third ventricle [ventriculus tertius (NA)].** A median ependymal-lined cavity bounded on either side by the corresponding thalamus and hypothalamus and communicating anteriorly with the lateral ventricles, and posteriorly with the aqueduct of the mid-brain. It is limited anteriorly by the lamina terminalis and optic chiasma; posteriorly, it narrows to join the aqueduct, while its floor is formed by the tuber cinereum, mamillary body, the posterior perforated substance, and the tegmentum of the cerebral peduncle. The roof is ependymal and is overlain by the tela chorioidea. [L *ventriculum*.]

See also: ARANZIO, DUNCAN (J. M.), GALEN, KRAUSE (W. J. F.), MORGAGNI, SYLVIUS, VERGA, VIEUSSENS, WENZEL (J.).

ventricornu (ven·tre·**kor**·new). The anterior horn of grey matter of the spinal cord. [L *venter* belly, *cornu* horn.]

ventricular (ven·**trik**·ew·lar). Appertaining to a ventricle. **Ventricular muscle.** The thyro-epiglottic muscle.

ventricularis (ven·trik·ew·**la**'·ris). A minute bundle of muscle fibres extending between the lateral edge of the arytenoid cartilage and the corresponding part of the epiglottic cartilage. [ventricle.]

ventriculitis (ven·trik·ew·**li**'·tis). Inflammation of the ventricles of the brain. [ventricle, Gk *-itis* inflammation.]

ventriculocisternostomy (ven·**trik**·ew·lo·sis·ter·**nos**'·to·me). Ventriculostomy. [ventricle, cisterna, Gk *stoma* mouth.]

ventriculocordectomy (ven·**trik**·ew·lo·kord·**ek**'·to·me). An operation for the relief of laryngeal stenosis, following double abductor paralysis. The operation is carried out by means of punch forceps, removing the entire ventricular floor but leaving the vocal processes *in situ.* [ventricle, cord, Gk *ektome* excision.]

ventriculogram (ven·**trik**·ew·lo·gram). 1. In cardiology, a radiograph of one of the ventricles of the heart obtained by injection of a contrast medium into its cavity. 2. A radiograph of the ventricles of the brain taken during the examination of ventriculography. [ventricle, Gk *gramma* a record.]

ventriculography (ven·trik·ew·**log**'·raf·e). 1. In cardiology, the technique of visualizing the ventricles of the heart by the injection of a radio-opaque contrast medium through a catheter introduced into the ventricle through the vascular system. 2. A radiographic method of demonstrating the ventricles of the brain by direct injection of contrast medium (usually air) through a trephine opening. [ventricle, Gk *graphein* to record.]

ventriculomastoidostomy (ven·**trik**·ew·lo·mas·toid·**os**'·to·me). The surgical procedure of establishing a communication, usually by means of a polyethylene tube, between the inferior horn of the lateral ventricle and the tympanic antrum. It is used in the treatment of hydrocephalus.

ventriculometry (ven·**trik**·ew·**lom**'·et·re). Measurement of pressure in or capacity of, the ventricles of the brain.

ventriculonector (ven·**trik**·ew·lo·**nek**'·tor). Referring to the atrioventricular bundle. [ventricle, L *nector* joiner.]

ventriculopuncture (ven·**trik**·ew·lo·**pungk**'·tcher). The passage of a brain needle into the ventricles of the brain, a diagnostic procedure for examining the pressure and/or contents of the ventricular fluid. [ventricle, puncture.]

ventriculoscope (ven·**trik**·ew·lo·skope). An instrument for viewing the inside of the ventricles of the brain directly. **Coagulating ventriculoscope.** A partially insulated ventriculoscope whose tip can also be used for applying coagulating current. [ventricle, Gk *skopein* to view.]

ventriculoscopy (ven·**trik**·ew·**los**'·ko·pe). The operation of using the ventriculoscope.

ventriculostium (ven·**trik**·ew·**los**'·te·um). An opening made at the operation of ventriculostomy. [ventricle, L *ostium* mouth.]

ventriculostomy (ven·trik·ew·**los**'·to·me). The neurosurgical procedure for making an opening in the ventricles of the brain to allow drainage of cerebrospinal fluid, usually by fitting a tube from the ventricles to the subarachnoid cisternae: hence, lateral or 3rd ventricular ventriculostomy, etc., according to the ventricle drained. [ventricle, Gk *stoma* mouth.]

ventriculosubarachnoid (ven·**trik**·ew·lo·sub·ar·**ak**'·noid). Concerning the ventricles of the brain and the subarachnoid spaces.

ventriculotomy (ven·trik·ew·**lot**'·o·me). A cutting into a ventricle, e.g. of the heart as part of an intracardiac surgical procedure, or of the brain during the surgical treatment of hydrocephalus. [ventricle, Gk *temnein* to cut.]

ventriculus (ven·**trik**·ew·lus). 1. Ventricle. 2. The stomach. **Ventriculus cerebri.** Ventricle of the brain. **Ventriculus Desiccatus BPC 1949.** Desiccated stomach, dried pig stomach used in the treatment of pernicious anaemia. **Ventriculus medius.** Third ventricle. *See* VENTRICLE. **Ventriculus tricornis cerebri.** Lateral ventricle. *See* VENTRICLE. [L.]

ventricumbent (ven·tre·**kum**·bent). Lying prone on the belly. [L *venter* belly, *cumbere* to lie.]

ventriduction (ven·tre·**duk**·shun). The drawing of a part towards the belly, as in flexing the thigh. [L *venter* belly, *ducere* to lead.]

ventrifixation (ven·tre·fix·**a**'·shun). Ventrofixation.

ventriflexion (ven·tre·**flek**·shun). The bending of a part towards the belly. [L *venter* belly, *flectere* to bend.]

ventrimesal (ven·tre·**me**·zal). Ventromedian. [L *venter* belly, Gk *mesos* in the middle.]

ventrimeson (ven·tre·**mes**·on). The ventral middle line. [see prec.]

ventrocystorrhaphy (ven·tro·sist·**or**'·af·e). The fixation by a suture of the anterior wall of the bladder to the abdominal parietes, sometimes employed to prevent retraction of the bladder following permanent suprapubic cystotomy. [L *venter* abdomen, Gk *kystis* bladder, *rhaphe* suture.]

ventrodorsal (ven·tro·**dor**·sal). Referring to the anterior and posterior surfaces, or extending between them. [L *venter* belly, *dorsum* back.]

ventrofixation (ven·tro·fix·**a**'·shun). An operation, usually for retroversion, in which the body of the uterus is fixed by stitches to the fascia of the abdominal wall. [L *venter* belly, fixation.]

ventrohysteropexy (ven·tro·**his**·ter·o·pex·e). Suture of a displaced uterus to the wall of the abdomen. [L *venter* belly, Gk *hystera* uterus, *pexis* a fixation.]

ventro-inguinal (ven·tro·**ing**·gwin·al). Concerning the abdomen and the groin. [L *venter* belly, *inguen* groin.]

ventrolateral (ven·tro·**lat**·er·al). At the side and towards the front; ventral and lateral. [L *venter* belly, *latus* side.]

ventromedian (ven·tro·**me**·de·an). At the front and towards the centre; ventral and median. **Ventromedian nucleus.** Which plays a part in stimulation and suppression of appetite. [L *venter* belly, *medius* middle.]

ventroptosis (ven·trop·**to**·sis). Downward displacement of the stomach. [L *venter* belly, Gk *ptosis* a falling.]

ventroscopy (ven·**tros**·ko·pe). Visualization of the contents of the abdomen by an optical instrument introduced into the peritoneal cavity. [L *venter* belly, Gk *skopein* to view.]

ventrosuspension (ven·tro·sus·**pen**′·shun). The surgical fixing of the uterus forward by using some sort of peritoneal attachment or shortening of the round ligaments; this is to achieve anteversion. [L *venter* belly, *suspendere* to hang.]

ventrotomy (ven·**trot**·o·me). Surgical incision of the abdominal wall; laparotomy. [L *venter* belly, Gk *temnein* to cut.]

ventrovesicofixation (ven·tro·**ves**·ik·o·fix·**a**′·shun). The surgical fixation of the uterus to the bladder and anterior abdominal wall. [L *venter* belly, *vesica* bladder, fixation.]

venturimeter (ven·tewr·**im**·et·er). An instrument for measuring the velocity of fluid flow through pipes by observing differences of pressure on each side of a constriction placed in the flow. [Giovanni Battista *Venturi*, (b. 1746) Italian physicist.]

venula [NA] (**ven**·ew·lah) (pl. *venulae*). A small vein or venule. **Venulae rectae [NA].** Venules transmitting blood back to the interlobular veins after passage around the descending limbs of Henle's loops. [L.]

venular (**ven**·ew·lar). Referring to or concerning venulae.

venule [venula (NA)] (**ven**·ewl). A very small vein, especially one merging into a capillary. [L *venula* small vein.]

verabroine (veer·**ab**·ro·een). Verine.

Verapamil (ver·**ap**·am·il). BP Commission approved name for 5 - [*N* - (3,4 - dimethoxyphenethyl)methylamino] - 2 - (3,4 - dimethoxyphenyl) - 2 - isopropylvaleronitrile; a coronary dilator.

veratria (ver·**at**·re·ah). Veratrine.

veratridine (ver·**at**·rid·een). $C_{36}H_{51}O_{11}N$, an amorphous alkaloid present in sabadilla.

veratrine (ver·**at**·reen). A mixture of alkaloids from cevadilla (sabadilla), including cevadine (*crystallized veratine*), $C_{32}H_{49}O_9N$, cevine (sabadinine), $C_{27}H_{43}O_8N$, veratridine (*amorphous veratrine*), $C_{37}H_{53}O_{11}N$, cevadilline (sabadilline), $C_{34}H_{53}O_8N$, and sabadine, $C_{29}H_{53}O_8N$. The name has also been applied to veratridine itself, and to indefinite mixtures of cevadine and veratridine. The mixture occurs as a white or greyish powder which is exceedingly irritating, especially to the mucous membranes, and which must be handled with care. It has an intense local irritant action and some anaesthetic action; applied to the skin it causes warmth and hence is used as a counter-irritant in neuralgia and arthritis. Internally it is exceedingly poisonous, causing violent irritation of the gastro-intestinal tract, with intense burning in the mouth and throat, violent vomiting, and purging. It is a powerful muscle poison causing an extraordinary prolongation of the contraction of voluntary muscles. On the heart it prodces a marked bradycardia. It is seldom given internally; externally its chief use is as a parasiticide and counter-irritant. [L *veratrum* hellebore.]

veratrinize, veratrize (ver·**at**·rin·ize, **ver**·at·rize). To give veratrine.

veratroidine (ver·at·**roi**·deen). $C_{26}H_{43}O_2N$, a physiologically inert alkaloidal constituent of green hellebore, *Veratrum viride*.

veratrum (ver·a·trum). A genus of poisonous liliaceous plants. **Veratrum album.** White hellebore; it has similar constituents to green hellebore, *Veratrum viride* (see below). **American veratrum.** **V. viride** (see below). **Veratrum sabadilla.** A species from which at one time it was believed sabadilla was obtained. **Veratrum viride.** Green hellebore, the dried rhizome contains several alkaloids, including protoveratrine and jervine. [L, hellebore.]

Verazide (**ver**·az·ide). BP Commission approved name for *N*-isonicotinoyl - 2 - veratrylidenehydrazine; it is an anti-infective drug used like isoniazid.

Verbascum (ver·**bas**·kum). A genus of plants of the foxglove family (Scrophulariaceae). **Verbascum thapsus.** Great mullein, mullein dock, Aaron's rod; the dried leaves and flowers contain several saponins and have been used medicinally as a demulcent. [L, mullein.]

Verbena (ver·**be**·nah). A genus of herbs and shrubs belonging to the family Verbenaceae. **Verbena hastata, Verbena officinalis.** Vervain, wild hyssop; the dried herb is used and contains a glycoside, verbenalin. [L, sacred bough.]

verbenalin (ver·**be**·nal·in). A glycoside that occurs in the wild hyssop, *Verbena officinalis.*

verbigeration (ver·bij·er·**a**′·shun). Obsessional reiteration of words which have no meaning or significance. [L *verbigerare* to chatter.]

verbomania (ver·bo·**ma**·ne·ah). Ceaseless chattering; psychotic loquacity. [L *verbum* word, Gk *mania* madness.]

Verco, Sir Joseph Cooke (b. 1851). English physician in Australia.

Verco's sign. Striae or punctae of haemorrhage under the nails in erythema nodosum.

verdigris (**ver**·de·gris, **ver**·de·grees). 1. Any green deposit of cupric salts on a copper surface due to weathering, etc. 2. Copper oxyacetate; blue scales or needles of indefinite composition, approximating to $Cu(CH_3COO)_2Cu(OH)_25H_2O$. It has similar medicinal properties to copper sulphate. [O Fr. *vert de Grece* green of Greece.]

verdoflavin (ver·do·**fla**·vin). A flavin of grass, similar to riboflavine. [L *viridis* green, flavin.]

verdoglobin (ver·do·**glo**·bin). *See* HEINZ BODIES.

verdoperoxidase (ver·do·per·**ox**′·id·aze). A green-coloured enzyme occurring in leucocytes and taking part in certain biological oxidations. It is responsbile for the colour of purulent sputum in bronchial diseases. [L *viridis* green, peroxidase.]

Verga, Andrea (b. 1811). Milan neurologist.

Verga's lacrimal groove. A groove in the lateral wall of the inferior meatus of the nose which is occasionally present below the opening of the nasolacrimal duct. It runs downwards, or downwards and backwards and prolongs the lower orifice of the duct.

Verga's ventricle. The sixth ventricle; a space between the corpus callosum and the body of the fornix cerebri.

vergence, vergency (**ver**·jens, **ver**·jen·se). Disjunctive reciprocal motion of the eyes. [L *vergere* to bend.]

verger (**ver**·jer). *See* MADDOX.

vergetures (**ver**·jet·ewrz). Striae atrophicae. [L *virga* stripe.]

Verheyen, Philippe (b. 1648). Louvain anatomist.

Stars of Verheyen. The stellate veins of the kidney.

Verhoeff, Frederick Hermann (b. 1874). Boston ophthalmologist.

Verhoeff's operation. For squint: advancement combined with resection of the muscle, using Prince's forceps and a double-armed mattress suture to attach the muscle to the sclera.

Verhoeff's stain. For elastic fibres: a mixture of haematoxylin, alcohol, ferric chloride, and Lugol's solution. Elastic fibres are stained blue-black.

verine (**ver**·een). $C_{27}H_{43}O_8N$, a base obtained on the alkaline hydrolysis of veratridine.

verjuice (**ver**·joos). The juice of green or unripe dates, etc. [Fr. *vert* green, *jus* juice.]

Vermel's sign. Visible pulsation of the superficial temporal artery on the affected side in unilateral (migrainous) headache.

vermetoid (**ver**·me·toid). Resembling worms; vermiform. [L *vermis* worm, Gk *eidos* form.]

vermian (**ver**·me·an). 1. Concerning a worm or worms. 2. Referring to the vermis of the cerebellum. [L *vermis* worm.]

vermicidal (ver·me·si·dal). Capable of killing worms, particularly those which invade the intestine. [see foll.]

vermicide (ver·me·side). Any drug or agent which kills the parasitic worms that invade the intestine; an anthelminthic. [L *vermis* worm, *caedere* to kill.]

vermicular (ver·mik·ew·lar). Resembling a worm or worms in appearance and character; vermiform. [see foll.]

vermiculate (ver·mik·ew·late). Like a worm. [L *vermiculus* small worm.]

vermiculation (ver·mik·ew·la′·shun). Crawling or rippling movement suggestive of a worm; applied to intestinal peristaltic movements. [see prec.]

vermicule (ver·mik·ewl). 1. A very small worm, or a sinuous structure resembling a small worm. 2. An oökinete. [L *vermiculus* a small worm.]

vermiculose, vermiculous (ver·mik·ew·loze, ver·mik·ew·lus). 1. Vermiform. 2. Wormy; having worms, or infested with larvae. [see prec.]

vermiculus (ver·mik·ew·lus). A very small worm. [L.]

vermiform (ver·me·form). Resembling a worm in appearance. [L *vermis* worm, form.]

vermifugal (ver·mif·ew·gal). Able to expel worms from the intestine. [L *vermis* worm, *fugare* to put to flight.]

vermifuge (ver·me·fewj). 1. Any substance which causes the expulsion of parasitic worms. 2. Causing the expulsion of parasitic worms. [L *vermis* worm, *fugare* to put to flight.]

vermilingual (ver·me·ling·gwal). Having a long wormlike tongue. [L *vermis* worm, *lingua* tongue.]

vermilion (ver·mil·e·on). Cinnabar, mercuric sulphide, HgS. A red mineral used as a source of mercury and as a pigment. [L *vermilium.*]

vermilionectomy (ver·mil·e·on·ek′·to·me). Excision of part of the vermilion (red) border of the lip as part of a plastic procedure on the mouth orifice. [vermilion, Gk *ektome* a cutting out.]

vermin (ver·min). Parasitic insects and worms, and depredating rodents. [L *vermis* worm.]

verminal (ver·min·al). Concerned with worms or vermin.

vermination (ver·min·a·shun). 1. Infestation of the body by worms or vermin. 2. The multiplication of vermin.

verminosis (ver·min·in·o·sis). A morbid state set up by infestation with worms or vermin, [vermin, Gk *-osis* condition.]

verminotic (ver·min·ot·ik). Relating to or attributable to worms or vermin infestation.

verminous (ver·min·us). Referring to worms or vermin; infested with vermin.

vermiphobia (ver·me·fo·be·ah). 1. A morbid dread of becoming infested with worms or vermin. 2. An unreasoning and unfounded conviction that one has intestinal worms. [L *vermis* worm, Gk *phobein* to fear.]

vermis (ver·mis). A wormlike structure; usually refers to the vermis of the cerebellum. **Vermis of the cerebellum [vermis (NA)].** The median portion connecting the two lateral hemispheres of the cerebellum. It is subdivided into a *superior* and an *inferior vermis.* [L, worm.]

vermouth, vermuth (ver·muth). A beverage prepared in France and Italy by adding a vinous infusion of wormwood and other aromatics to a white wine. It contains about 16 per cent of ethyl alcohol, and is usually taken as an apertif. Vermouth finds little or no use in British medicine. [G *Wermuth* wormwood.]

Vernet, Maurice (b. 1887). French neurologist.

Vernet's syndrome. Jugular foramen syndrome. *See* SYNDROME.

Verneuil, Aristide Auguste Stanislas (b. 1823). Paris surgeon.

Verneuil's neuroma. A plexiform or cirsoid neuroma.

vernier (ver·ne·a). A scale auxiliary to the main scale on an instrument, which enables an accurate interpolation between the smallest divisions on the main scale to be made. [Pierre *Vernier,* (b. 1580) French physicist.]

vernine (ver·neen). A nucleoside appearing in the products of the hydrolysis of yeast-nucleic acid, and also occurring in leguminous seedlings such as vetch, *Vicia sativa.*

vernix caseosa (ver·nix ka·se·o·sah). The fatty covering of the skin of the fetus during the final three months of pregnancy; it results from desquamation of the epidermis, and contains sebaceous secretion. [L, cheese-like varnish.]

vernonia (ver·no·ne·ah). A genus of plants of the family Compositae. **Vernonia anthelmintica.** A species of East India, the seeds of which are used as an anthelminthic. [William *Vernon,* 17th century British botanist.]

veronica (ver·on·ik·ah). A genus of plants of the family Scrophulariaceae; the speedwells. **Veronica officinalis.** Speedwell; the dried herb is used as an astringent. [traditional name of the woman cured of an issue of blood, Mark v. 25.]

verruca (ver·oo·kah). Wart. *See also:* WART. **Verruca acuminata.** Venereal wart. **Verruca carnea.** A fleshy wart. **Verruca digitata.** Digitate wart. **Verruca filiformis.** Filiform wart. **Verruca necrogenica.** Anatomical wart. **Verruca peruana, Verruca peruviana.** Veruga peruana. **Verruca plana, Verruca plana juvenilis.** Plane wart. **Verruca plantaris.** Plantar wart. **Verruca seborrhoeica.** Seborrhoeic wart. **Verruca senilis.** Senile wart. **Verruca simplex.** Verruca vulgaris (see below). **Verruca tuberculosa.** Anatomical wart. **Verruca vulgaris.** A small, circumscribed, epidermal tumour, having a filiform surface and caused by infection with a papillomavirus: common on exposed surfaces. A similar or identical virus causes plantar and venereal warts and may also be involved in laryngeal warts.

verruciform (ver·oo·se·form). Resembling a wart in appearance. [L *verruca* wart, form.]

verrucoid (ver·oo·koid). Wart-like. [L *verruca* wart, Gk *eidos* form.]

verrucose (ver·oo·koze). Having warts or wart-like growths; warty. [L *verruca* wart.]

verrucosis (ver·oo·kos·sis). The state of being affected with warts. **Lymphostatic verrucosis.** A papillomatous condition of the soles of the feet occurring in Nigeria and Uganda. [L *verruca* wart, Gk *-osis* condition.]

verrucous (ver·oo·kus). Verrucose.

verruga peruana, verruga peruviana (ver·oo·gah per·oo·ah·nah, per·oo·ve·ah·nah). The nodular eruptive stage of Oroya fever (Carrion's disease). Cherry pink bleeding nodules appear on the face and limbs. [Sp, Peruvian wart.]

verrugas (ver·oo·gas). Verruga peruana. [Sp, warts.]

versene (ver·seen). Ethylenediaminetetra acetic acid. *See* ACID.

versicolour, versicoloured (ver·se·kul·er, ver·se·kul·erd). 1. Variegated; having many colours. 2. Exhibiting different colours according to the light. [L *versicolor* changing colour.]

version (ver·shun). An alteration of the lie of the fetus in the uterus by the act of turning so that the presentation is changed. **Abdominal version.** External version (see below). **Bimanual version.** Combined version (see below). **Bipolar version.** A combined movement effected by one hand on the abdomen and two fingers of the other hand in the uterus, so that both poles of the fetus are manipulated. **Cephalic version.** Turning of the fetus so as to make the head present. **Combined version.** Version combining internal and external manipulations. **External version.** That which is performed by manipulation through the abdominal wall. **Forced version.** A type of accouchement forcé. **Internal version.** Turning the fetus by the hand introduced into the uterine cavity. **Lateral version.** The state of being deflected to one or other side. **Mixed version.** Combined version (see above). **Ocular version.** Conjugate movement of the eyes. **Podalic version.** That which causes a breech presentation. **Spontaneous version.** A version which occurs naturally in the absence of fetal manipulations. [L *vertere* to turn.]

See also: BRAXTON HICKS, POTTER (I. W.).

vertebra (ver·te·brah). A bony unit of the segmented spinal column, typically composed of an anterior part, the body [corpus vertebrae (NA)], and a posterior vertebral arch made up of paired pedicles and laminae. Transverse processes spring from the junction of the pedicle and lamina, articular processes project above and below the posterior ends of the pedicles, and a spine projects backwards from the junction of the paired laminae. The vertebrae are grouped according to their situation into seven cervical [vertebrae cervicales (NA)], twelve thoracic [vertebrae thoracicae (NA)], five lumbar [vertebrae lumbales (NA)], five sacral [vertebrae sacrales (NA)], and four coccygeal vertebrae [vertebrae coccygeae (NA)]. **Anticlinal vertebra.** The vertebra in which the spine points directly dorsally, marking the junction between the upper vertebrae where the spines point caudally and the lower vertebrae where the spines point cranially; usually the 11th thoracic in man. **Block vertebra.** Where 2 or more vertebral bodies are congenitally fused, there being no intervening intervertebral disc. **Butterfly vertebra.** A radiological sign where the 2 lateral halves of a vertebral body do not fuse (congenital). **Cranial vertebra.** One of the vertebrae sometimes postulated as incorporated within the skull bones, especially the basi-occiput and basi-sphenoid. **Dorsal vertebra.** A thoracic vertebra. **Vertebra plana.** The radiographic term applied to a vertebral body crushed to a thin plate, as seen in severe cases of Calvé-Perthes disease, eosinophilic granuloma of bone, and Hand-Schueller-Christian disease. **Primitive vertebra.** One of a series of condensed mesenchymal masses surrounding the notochord, formed by the fusion of right and left sclerotomes from the somites of a particular body segment. **Vertebra prominens [NA].** The 7th cervical vertebra, the spine of which is the first bony prominence to be felt at the lower end of the nuchal furrow. [L, joint.]

vertebral (ver·te·bral). 1. Concerning a vertebra, or relating to vertebrae. 2. Possessing vertebrae. **Vertebral ribs.** The floating ribs. *See* RIBS.

vertebral artery [arteria vertebralis (NA)]. A large branch from the first part of the subclavian artery, passing through the foramina in the upper six cervical transverse processes, entering the skull through the foramen magnum and joining its fellow at the lower border of the pons to form the basilar artery. It gives off spinal [rami spinales (NA)] and meningeal [ramus meningeus (NA)] branches, and a large branch to the under-surface of the cerebellum and the side of the medulla, the posterior inferior cerebellar artery.

vertebral nerve. The vertebral branch of the inferior cervical ganglion.

vertebral vein [vena vertebralis (NA)]. The venous drainage of the plexus around the vertebral artery. It is a tributary of the innominate vein. **Accessory vertebral vein [vena vertebralis accessoria (NA)].** A branch of the plexus around the vertebral artery which passes through the foramen transversarium of the seventh cervical vertebra before joining the innominate vein. **Anterior vertebral vein [vein vertebralis anterior (NA)].** A small vein accompanying the ascending cervical artery and ending in the vertebral vein.

vertebrata (ver·te·**bra**·tah). A division or sub-phylum of the phylum Chordata, which contains all those forms in which a cartilaginous or bony vertebral column is developed. It includes all fish, amphibia, reptiles, birds, and mammals. The less usual term *Craniata* is more correct.

vertebrate (ver·te·brate). 1. Possessing a vertebral column. 2. Any animal of the phylum Vertebrata.

vertebrated (ver·te·**bra**·ted). 1. Vertebrate. 2. Describing a flexible instrument composed of small jointed segments, such as a vertebrated catheter.

vertebrectomy (ver·te·**brek**·to·me). The surgical removal of part of a vertebra. [vertebra, Gk *ektome* excision.]

vertebro-arterial (ver·te·bro·ar·**teer**′·e·al). Pertaining to a vertebra and an artery, or to the vertebral artery.

vertebrobasilar (ver·te·bro·**ba**′·sil·ar). Pertaining to the vertebrae and the base of the skull, or to the vertebral and basilar arteries. **Vertebrobasilar insufficiency.** *See* INSUFFICIENCY.

vertebrochondral (ver·te·bro·**kon**′·dral). Concerning a vertebra and a costal cartilage. [vertebra, Gk *chondros* cartilage.]

vertebrocostal (ver·te·bro·**kos**′·tal). Concerning a vertebra and a rib, or a vertebra and a costal cartilage. [vertebra, L *costa* rib.]

vertebrodidymia (ver·te·bro·did·**im**′·e·ah). A fetal monster consisting of twins united by their spinal columns. [vertebra, Gk *didymos* twin.]

vertebrofemoral (ver·te·bro·**fem**′·or·al). Concerning the spinal column and the femur. [vertebra, femur.]

vertebro-iliac (ver·te·bro·**il**′·e·ak). Connecting the spinal column and the ilium, as with the iliolumbar ligament. [vertebra, ilium.]

vertebromammary (ver·te·bro·**mam**′·ar·e). Referring to the region of the thorax between the vertebral column and the mammae.

vertebrosacral (ver·te·bro·**sa**′·kral). Concerning the lumbar vertebrae and the sacrum.

vertebrosternal (ver·te·bro·**ster**′·nal). Connecting the vertebrae and the sternum, as with the true ribs.

vertex [NA]. (ver·tex) (pl. *vertices*). The highest point or summit, e.g. the vertex of the skull. **Vertex coccygeus.** Vortex coccygeus. **Vertex cordis.** The apex of the heart, formed by the left ventricle. **Vertex of the cornea [vertex corneae (NA)].** The most prominent point on the curvature of the cornea. **Vertex of the lens.** The point at which the axis of the lens meets the surface. [L, summit.]

vertical [verticalis (NA)]. (ver·tik·al). 1. Straight up and down; perpendicular. 2. Referring to the vertex. [see prec.]

vertices (ver·tis·eez). *See* VERTEX.

verticil (ver·tis·il). A whorl; a circle of leaves, tentacles, hairs, processes, etc., radiating from an axis on the same horizontal plane. [L *verticillus* the whirl of a spindle.]

verticillate (ver·tis·**il**·ate). Characterized by verticilis; whorled.

Verticillium (ver·tis·**il**·e·um). A genus of moulds. **Verticillium cinnabarinum.** *Acrostalagmus cinnabarinus.* **Verticillium graphii.** *Glenospora graphii.* A mould which has been observed in the internal auditory meatus. [L *verticillus* the whirl of a spindle.]

verticomental (ver·tik·o·**men**′·tal). Referring to the crown of the head and the chin, as with the craniometric measurement. [L *vertex* summit, *mentum* chin.]

vertiginous (ver·**tij**·in·us). Relating to or simulating vertigo.

vertigo (ver·tig·o). Giddiness, swimming in the head, a sense of instability, often with a sensation of rotation. It is associated with middle-ear disease, eye disorders, and cerebellar disease. **Vertigo ab aure laeso.** Auditory vertigo (see below). **Angiopathic vertigo.** That due to vascular causes. **Arteriosclerotic vertigo.** Cardiovascular vertigo (see below). **Auditory vertigo, Aural vertigo.** Vertigo due to ear disease. This always includes a sensation of rotation and, when severe, is prostrating and accompanied by vomiting. **Benign postural vertigo.** Severe but brief vertigo induced by change of posture, particularly lying down, thought to be due to disease of the utricle sometimes resulting from head injury. **Cardiac vertigo.** Vertigo with organic heart disease. **Cardiovascular vertigo.** That due to arteriosclerosis, or heart disease. **Cerebral vertigo.** That due to organic brain disease. **Endemic paralytic vertigo, Epidemic vertigo.** Gerlier's disease. **Epidemic vertigo.** An acute disease, possibly due to viral infection, causing severe aural vertigo without loss of hearing; vestibular neuronitis. **Epileptic vertigo.** The aura of the epileptic fit. **Essential vertigo.** Vertigo with no discoverable organic basis. **Gastric vertigo.** Vertigo with stomach disorders. **Height vertigo.** The sensation of falling on looking down from a height. **Horizontal vertigo.** That experienced on lying down, probably associated with labyrinthine disorder. **Hysterical vertigo.** That associated with hysterical symptoms. **Labyrinthine vertigo.** That associated with labyrinthine disorder; auditory vertigo. **Laryngeal vertigo.** Paroxysmal attacks of coughing followed by a brief period of unconsciousness; cough syncope. **Lateral vertigo.** Vertigo noted on passing a succession of similar objects, probably due to an eye disorder. **Mechanical vertigo.** That due to a repetition of change of position, as in seasickness. **Nocturnal vertigo.** A sensation of falling when on the point of sleep. **Objective vertigo.** The sensation of objects revolving round the patient. **Ocular vertigo.** That due to lack of eye muscle balance. **Organic vertigo.** Vertigo with cerebellar lesions or due to lack of sense of position, as in tabes dorsalis or gross peripheral neuritis. **Paralysing vertigo.** Gerlier's disease. **Riders' vertigo.** A form noted in riders in motor-cars; lateral vertigo (see above). **Rotatory vertigo.** Vertigo in which the body seems to be rotating, as opposed to objective vertigo in which objects around appear to be moving. **Smokers' vertigo.** That which is the result of excessive smoking. **Subjective vertigo.** Rotatory vertigo (see above). **Systematic vertigo.** Rotatory vertigo (see above). **Tenebric vertigo, Vertigo tenebricosa.** Vertigo in darkness, as in locomotor ataxia. **Toxaemic vertigo, Toxic vertigo.** Vertigo as a result of consuming some toxic agent, e.g. alcohol. **Vertical vertigo.** That caused by looking up or down. **Vestibular vertigo.** That due to a lesion in the labyrinth or vestibule. [L.]

See also: CHARCOT.

verumontanum (ver·ew·mon·ta'·num). The urethral crest, a median elevation in the posterior wall of the prostatic urethra on which the ejaculatory ducts and the prostatic utricle open. [L *veru* spit, *montanus* mountainous.]

vervain (ver·vain). A species of verbena, extract of which is used as an expectorant. [O Gr. *verveine.*]

vesalianum (ves·a·le·a·num). A separation of the tuberosity at the base of the 5th metatarsal bone to form a distinct bony element. It also refers to the bone occasionally formed by ossification within the tendon of the peroneus longus muscle as it passes over the lateral border of the cuvoid bone. [Andreas *Vesalius.*]

Vesalius, Andreas (b. 1514). Brussels anatomist.

Bone of Vesalius. An accessory ossicle in the foot produced by separation of the tuberosity of the 5th metatarsal bone.

Foramen of Vesalius. An inconstant foramen in the greater wing of the sphenoid bone transmitting a vein.

Glands of Vesalius. The bronchopulmonary lymph glands.

vesanic (ve·san·ik). Mentally disordered. [L *vesania* madness.]

vesica (ves·i·kah). A bladder. **Vesica prostatica.** Prostatic utricle. [L.]

vesical (ves·ik·al). Referring to the urinary bladder, or to the gall bladder. [L *vesica* bladder.]

vesical arteries. Branches of the anterior division of the internal iliac artery. **Inferior vesical artery [arteria vesicalis inferior (NA)].** A branch of the anterior division of the internal iliac artery to the bladder, prostate, seminal vesicle, and ureter. **Superior vesical arteries [arteriae vesicales superiores (NA)].** Branches of the anterior division of the internal iliac artery to the bladder, vas deferens, and ureter. They arise from the parent vessel in common with the lateral umbilical ligament. **Ureteric branches of the vesical arteries [rami ureterici (NA)].** Branches from the superior and inferior vesical arteries.

vesical veins, inferior [venae vesicales (NA)]. Veins draining the vesical (venous) plexus into the internal iliac veins.

vesicant (ves·ik·ant). 1. Blistering or producing blisters. 2. Any agent that causes blisters. [L *vesica* blister.]

vesication (ves·ik·a·shun). 1. The production of blisters. 2. A blister or blistered surface. [L *vesica* blister.]

vesicatory (ves·ik·a·tor·e). Blistering or producing blisters.

vesicle (ves·ikl). 1. A small bladder. 2. A small, rounded blister formed by accumulation of fluid in the epidermis, associated with disintegration of the cells in the affected area. Usually a vesicle is filled with serous fluid. 3. [Vesicula (NA).] Any structure that has the appearance of 1. or 2. (above). **Acoustic vesicle.** Auditory vesicle (see below). **Allantoic vesicle.** A sac-like fetal membrane connected with the bladder and subserving respiratory and excretory functions; the allantois. **Amniocardiac vesicle.** That portion of the embryonic coelom enveloping the cardiac tubes which develops into the pericardial cavity. **Amnioembryonic vesicle.** The early amnion. **Amnionic vesicle.** The amnion. **Anhidrotic vesicle.** A vesicle formed in the skin during exertion, in cases of tropical anhidrosis; the lesions (they are always multiple) are formed by accumulations of sweat which cannot reach the surface of the skin because of the blockage of the sweat pores. **Archoplasmic vesicle.** A vesicle derived from the centrosome of a spermatid whose contents appear to be contributed to the tail of the spermatozoon. **Auditory vesicle.** An ectoderm-lined vesicle at the side of the embryonic hind-brain, which is derived from the invagination of the auditory placode. It develops into the lining and special sensory epithelia of the internal ear. **Blastodermic vesicle.** The blastocyst; a hollow ball of cells formed by the segmenting ovum of mammals. **Brain vesicle.** One of the subdivisions of the early embryonic brain, produced by alternate dilatations and constrictions of the anterior part of the neural tube. **Cephalic vesicle, Cerebral vesicle.** One of the two lateral outgrowths at the front end of the embryonic neural tube which become the cerebral hemispheres. **Cervical vesicle.** A transient, ectoderm-lined vesicle in the embryonic neck region, formed by the sinking in and closing over of the cervical-sinus ectoderm. If persistent it may give rise to a branchial fistula. **Chorionic vesicle.** The outer villus-covered layer of the early embryo enclosing the amnion, umbilical cord, yolk sac, and embryo proper. **Compound vesicle.** A multilocular vesicle. **Encephalic vesicle.** Cephalic vesicle (see above). **Germinal vesicle.** The nucleus of an ovum [obsolete term]. **Graafian vesicle.** Graafian follicle; a vesicle in the ovary which contains and discharges the ovum. It is lined with epithelial cells, and outside this is a stromal capsule. **Lens vesicle.** A small sac-like structure lined with ectodermal cells, which becomes the lens of the eye. **Lung vesicle.** Pulmonary alveoli. **Medullary coccygeal vesicle.** The dilated terminal portion of the embryonic spinal cord. **Ocular vesicle.** Optic vesicle (see below). **Olfactory vesicle.** A hollow outgrowth from the front end of the cerebral hemisphere of the embryo, which develops into the olfactory bulb and tract. **Ophthalmic vesicle.** Optic vesicle (see following). **Optic vesicle [vesicula ophthalmica (NA)].** A hollow outgrowth from the lateral aspect of the forebrain of the early embryo, from which the retina and the optic nerve are derived. **Otic vesicle.** Auditory vesicle (see above). **Pituitary vesicle.** Rathke's pouch; an ectoderm-lined diverticulum from the primitive mouth, from which the anterior lobe of the pituitary is derived. **Primary brain vesicle.** One of the three vesicles into which the early embryonic brain is at first subdivided, viz. forebrain, mid-brain, and hind-brain vesicles. **Seminal vesicle [vesicula seminalis (NA)].** One of a pair of hollow, sacculated diverticula placed between the base of the bladder and the ampulla of the rectum. Their lower ends join at an acute angle with the ampulla of the vas deferens. **Seminal vesicle, adventitious coat of the [tunica adventitia (NA)].** A sheath of connective tissue external to the muscular coats. **Seminal vesicle, mucous coat of the [tunica mucosa (NA)].** A coat covered with columnar epithelium thrown into folds and depressions resembling a honeycomb. **Seminal vesicle, muscular coat of the [tunica muscularis (NA)].** A thin coat indistinctly divided into inner and outer longitudinal layers separated by a middle circular layer. **Sense vesicle.** A rudimentary sense organ in the embryo. **Sex vesicle.** A body formed in the nucleus of mammalian primary spermatocytes by the association of the condensed X and Y chromosome during the pachytene and diplotene stages of meiosis. **Synaptic vesicle.** A small vesicle, 20–50 nm in diameter, large numbers of which are found in terminal boutons. They are believed to contain the chemical mediator for the synapse. **Umbilical vesicle.** The yolk sac, or that part of it which lies outside the embryo and is connected to the mid-gut by the vitello-intestinal duct. [L *vesicula* small bladder.]

See also: BAER (K. E.), MALPIGHI, NABOTH, PURKINJE.

vesico-abdominal (ves·ik·o·ab·dom'·in·al). Concerning the urinary bladder and the abdominal wall. [L *vesica* bladder, abdomen.]

vesicocavernous (ves·ik·o·kav'·er·nus). Vesiculocavernous.

vesicocele (ves·ik·o·seel). A hernia involving the bladder. [L *vesica* bladder, Gk *kele* hernia.]

vesicocervical (ves·ik·o·ser'·vik·al). Concerning the urinary bladder and the neck of the uterus. [L *vesica* bladder, *cervix* neck.]

vesicoclysis (ves·ik·ok·lis·is). Flushing of the urinary bladder by an injection. [L *vesica* bladder, Gk *klysis* a washing out.]

vesicofixation (ves·ik·o·fix·a'·shun). 1. The surgical suture of the uterus to the wall of the urinary bladder. 2. Suture of the urinary bladder or of the gall bladder to the abdominal wall. [L *vesica* bladder, fixation.]

vesicoprostatic (ves·ik·o·pros·**tat'**·ik). Concerning the urinary bladder and the prostate gland. [L *vesica* bladder, prostate.]

vesicopubic (ves·ik·o·**pew'**·bik). Referring to the urinary bladder and the pubis, as with the band of muscles from the lower part of the bladder passing on each side to the pubis. [L *vesica* bladder, pubis.]

vesicopustule (ves·ik·o·**pus'**·tewl). A vesicle that is becoming pustulous.

vesicorectal (ves·ik·o·**rek'**·tal). Concerning the urinary bladder and the rectum. [L *vesica* bladder, rectum.]

vesicorenal (ves·ik·o·**re'**·nal). Involving the urinary bladder and the kidney. [L *vesica* bladder, *ren* kidney.]

vesicosigmoid (ves·ik·o·**sig'**·moid). Concerning the urinary bladder and the sigmoid flexure. [L *vesica* bladder, sigmoid.]

vesicosigmoidostomy (ves·ik·o·sig·moid·**os'**·to·me). The surgical establishment of a communicating passage between the urinary bladder and the sigmoid flexure. [L *vesica* bladder, sigmoid, Gk *stoma* mouth.]

vesicospinal (ves·ik·o·**spi'**·nal). Connecting the spinal cord with the urinary bladder, as in the case of the nerves controlling urination. [L *vesica* bladder, spine.]

vesicotomy (ves·ik·**ot**·o·me). Surgical incision of the urinary bladder or of the gall bladder; cystotomy. [L *vesica* bladder, Gk *temnein* to cut.]

vesicotubular (ves·ik·o·**tew'**·bew·lar). Having both vesicular and tubular qualities, as with a respiratory sound.

vesico-umbilical (ves·ik·o·um·**bil'**·ik·al). Referring to the urinary bladder and the umbilicus. [L *vesica* bladder, umbilicus.]

vesico-urachal (ves·ik·o·**ewr'**·a·kal). Concerning the urinary bladder and the remains of the urachus, as with the median umbilical ligament. [L *vesica* bladder, urachus.]

vesico-ureteral (ves·ik·o·ewr·**e'**·ter·al). Referring to the urinary bladder and the ureters. [L *vesica* bladder, ureter.]

vesico-urethral (ves·ik·o·ewr·**e'**·thral). Referring to the urinary bladder and the urethra. [L *vesica* bladder, urethra.]

vesico-uterine (ves·ik·o·**ew'**·ter·ine). Referring to the urinary bladder and the uterus. [L *vesica* bladder, uterus.]

vesico-uterovaginal (ves·ik·o·ew·ter·o·**vaj'**·in·al). Referring to the urinary bladder, the uterus, and the vagina. [L *vesica* bladder, uterus, vagina.]

vesicovaginal (ves·ik·o·**vaj'**·in·al). Referring to both the urinary bladder and the vagina, as in the case of a fistula. [L *vesica* bladder, vagina.]

vesicovaginorectal (ves·ik·o·vaj·in·o·**rek'**·tal). Involving the urinary bladder, the vagina, and the rectum, as with a fistula. [L *vesica* bladder, vagina, rectum.]

vesicula [NA] (ves·**ik**·ew·lah). Vesicle. **Vesicula germinativa.** Germinal vesicle. *See* VESICLE. **Vesicula graafiana.** Graafian follicle. **Vesicle ophthalmica, Vesicula optica.** Optic vesicle. *See* VESICLE. **Vesicula proligera.** Daughter cysts budded off from a cysticercus cyst. **Vesicula serosa.** The chorion, or false amnion of the developing ovum. [L.]

vesicular (ves·**ik**·ew·lar). Referring to a vesicle, or made up of vesicles; originating in or attributed to a vesicle.

vesiculate, vesiculated (ves·**ik**·ew·late, ves·**ik**·ew·**la'**·ted). Made up of vesicles.

vesiculation (ves·ik·ew·**la'**·shun). 1. The process of forming vesicles. 2. The state of being vesicular.

vesiculectomy (ves·ik·ew·**lek'**·to·me). The surgical excision of a vesicle, particularly that of a seminal vesicle as a whole or in part. [L *vesicula* small bladder, Gk *ektome* excision.]

vesiculiform (ves·**ik**·ew·le·form). Resembling a vesicle in shape. [vesicle, form.]

vesiculitis (ves·ik·ew·**li'**·tis). Inflammation of a vesicle. **Seminal vesiculitis.** Inflammation of a seminal vesicle. [vesicle, Gk *-itis* inflammation.]

vesiculobronchial (ves·**ik**·ew·lo·**brong'**·ke·al). Having both vesicular and bronchial qualities, as with a respiratory sound.

vesiculocavernous (ves·**ik**·ew·lo·**kav'**·er·nus). Having both vesicular and cavernous qualities, as with a respiratory sound indicating a cavity in otherwise healthy lung tissue.

vesiculogram (ves·ik·ew·lo·gram). A radiograph taken during vesiculography. [vesicle, Gk *gramma* a record.]

vesiculography (ves·ik·ew·**log'**·raf·e). Radiography of the lumen of the seminal vesicle, vas deferens, and ejaculatory duct by the injection of a contrast medium. [vesicle, Gk *graphein* to record.]

vesiculopapular (ves·ik·ew·lo·**pap'**·ew·lar). Describing a skin eruption that exhibits both vesicles and papules.

vesiculopustular (ves·ik·ew·lo·**pus'**·tew·lar). Describing a skin eruption consisting of both vesicles and pustules.

vesiculose (ves·**ik**·ew·lose). Vesicular.

vesiculotomy (ves·ik·ew·**lot'**·o·me). Surgical incision into a vesicle. **Seminal vesiculotomy.** Surgical incision into a seminal vesicle. [vesicle, Gk *temnein* to cut.]

vesiculotympanic (ves·**ik**·ew·lo·tim·**pan'**·ik). Having both vesicular and tympanic qualities, as with a sound in percussion.

vespa (ves·pah). A genus of social Hymenoptera, strictly including only the hornets but used for social wasps. **Vespa crabro.** European hornet. [L, wasp.]

vespajus (ves·pa·jus). A folliculitis of the scalp. [L *vespa* wasp, *jus* juice.]

vesperal (ves·per·al). Referring to the evening; occurring only in the evening. [L *vespera* evening.]

vespula (ves·pew·lah). A genus of social Hymenoptera which includes the common black and yellow banded wasps. [L, little wasp.]

vessel (vesl). 1. A container for fluids. 2. [Vas (NA)]. A vessel carrying a body fluid. **Afferent vessels of a lymph gland [vasa afferentia (NA)].** Vessels conveying lymph to a lymph gland. Perforating the capsule, they empty into the peripheral lymph sinus. **Anastomotic vessel [vas anastomoticum (NA)].** A branch of an artery which is directly continuous with a branch of the same or another artery. **Arterioluminal vessels.** Small branches of the coronary arteries which run through the myocardium between muscle bundles, and communicate directly with the left ventricular cavity. **Arteriosinusoidal vessels.** Small branches of the coronary arteries which communicate with the left ventricular cavity by means of sinusoids which lie between the muscle bundles and muscle fibres. **Bile vessel.** A vessel that carries bile in the biliary canaliculi and ducts. **Blood vessel.** A vessel that carries blood; an artery, arteriole, capillary, venule, or vein. **Capillary vessel [vas capillare (NA)].** A fine network of thin-walled vessels connecting arterioles and venules and forming the site of maximum metabolic exchange between blood and tissue fluid. **Chyliferous vessel.** A vessel that conveys chyle from the intestinal lacteals to the thoracic duct. **Collateral vessel [vas collaterale (NA)].** A branch running parallel to the artery from which it arose. **Efferent vessels of a lymph gland [vasa efferentia (NA)].** Vessels draining a lymph gland, which they leave by the hilum. **Haemorrhoidal vessel.** 1. An artery or vein of the rectum and anal canal, e.g. the superior rectal artery and vein, and the rectal (venous) plexus. 2. A varicosed vein of the last-named. **Lacteal vessel.** A lymph vessel that collects the chyle from the intestinal villi. **Lymph vessels [vasa lymphatica (NA)].** Fine transparent valved channels, forming a network in most tissues; their irregular calibre gives them a beaded appearance. The collecting vessels form two groups, one superficial to the deep fascia, and tending to run with superficial veins [vasa lymphatica superficialia (NA)], the other below the deep fascia mainly grouped around arteries [vasa lymphatica profunda (NA)], those from the small intestine are called *lacteals.* They ultimately form two channels, the thoracic duct and the right lymphatic duct, which drain into the venous system at the root of the neck. **Lymphatic vessel.** Lymph vessel (see above). **Nutrient vessel.** A vessel that penetrates into and nourishes bone. [L *vascellum* small vase.]

See also: LEXER.

vestibular (ves·**tib**·ew·lar). Concerning a vestibule.

vestibular nerve [pars vestibularis (nervi octavi) NA]. One of the main divisions of the auditory nerve, concerned with equilibrium, and arising in the vestibular ganglion. It splits into superior [pars superior (NA)] and inferior [pars inferior (NA)] branches. The peripheral fibres carry impulses from the maculae of the utricle and saccule, and ampullae of the semicircular canals; the central fibres lie around a group of nuclei in the floor of the 4th ventricle of the medulla.

vestibular veins [venae vestibulares (NA)]. Tributaries of the internal auditory vein.

vestibulate (ves·**tib**·ew·late). Provided with a vestibule; resembling a vestibule; vestibular.

vestibule [vestibulum (NA)] (ves·tib·ewl). 1. A minor subdivision of, or extension from, a cavity. 2. A space leading to the entrance of a canal. **Aortic vestibule.** The upper and anterior part of the cavity of the left ventricle leading to the aortic orifice; its walls consist mainly of fibrous tissue. **Vestibule of the bursa omentalis [vestibulum bursae omentalis (NA)].** That portion of the cavity of the bursa omentalis lying just within the epiploic foramen and continuous beyond the right gastropancreatic fold with the main portion of the cavity. **Vestibule of the ear.** The central portion of the osseous labyrinth which lodges the utricle and saccule. **Vestibule of the larynx [vestibulum laryngis (NA)].** The uppermost part of the cavity of the larynx lying above the false vocal cords. **Vestibule of the mouth [vestibulum oris (NA)].** That portion of the oral cavity lying between the lips and cheeks on the one hand and the teeth and gums on the other. **Vestibule of the nose [vestibulum nasi (NA)].** A subdivision of the nasal cavity lying just within the nostril and limited above by the limen nasi. **Vestibule of the perineum.** Vestibule of the vagina (see foll.). **Vestibule of the vagina [vestibulum vaginae (NA)].** The space enclosed between the labia minora. **Vestibule of the vulva.** Vestibule of the vagina (see prec.). [L *vestibulum* forecourt.]

See also: SIBSON.

vestibule, artery of the. *See* PENIS, ARTERY OF THE BULB OF THE.

vestibule, vein of the. *See* PENIS, VEIN OF THE BULB OF THE.

vestibulotomy (ves·tib·ewl·**ot'**·o·me). Surgical incision into the vestibule of the ear. [vestibule, Gk *temnein* to cut.]

vestibulo-urethral (ves·**tib**·ew·lo·ewr·**e'**·thral). Concerning the vestibule of the vagina and the urethral orifice.

vestibulum (ves·**tib**·ew·lum). Vestibule. [L.]

vestige [vestigium (NA)] (**ves**·tij). A relic or remnant of some structure more fully developed in embryonic life, or in an ancestral form. **Caudal medullary vestige.** A remnant of the medullary coccygeal vesicle found in the subcutaneous tissues of the tip of the coccyx. It is derived from the epithelium of the dilated termination of the embryonic spinal cord. **Coccygeal vestige.** Caudal medullary vestige (see prec.). **Vestige of the vaginal process [vestigium processus vaginalis (NA)].** A fibrous process within the spermatic cord between the peritoneum and the tunica vaginalis of the scrotum, a remnant of the vaginal process of the embryo. [L *vestigium*.]

vestigial (ves·**tij**·e·al). Having the characteristics of a vestige; rudimentary.

vestigium (ves·**tij**·e·um). Vestige.

vesuvin (ve·**sew**·vin). Bismarck brown, a dye sometimes used as a histological counterstain. [*Vesuvius*, volcano in Italy.]

veta (**va**·tah). Altitude sickness common in rail travellers in the Andes. [Sp.]

vetch (vech). A leguminous plant of the genus *Vicia*, particularly the common tare, *Vicia sativa*. [L *vicia*.]

veterinary drug. A medicinal product which is manufactured, sold, supplied, imported or exported for the purpose of being administered to animals, but not for the purpose of being administered to human beings.

viability (vi·ab·**il**·it·e). The ability to go on living. [see foll.]

viable (**vi**·abl). 1. The state when the fetus has reached a sufficient degree of maturity that independent survival outside the uterus is possible. Theoretically about the 28th week of pregnancy. 2. Term used in surgery to denote that an organ or tissue that has been damaged by injury or disease is capable of surviving and therefore need not be excised, e.g. a strangulated loop of intestine. [Fr. from L *vita* life.]

viadril (**vi**·ad·ril). The water-soluble sodium salt of the hemisuccinate ester of the steroid, 21-hydroxypregnanedione. It is an anaesthetic agent free from any hormonal action, and is reputed to give more efficient and more complete anaesthesia than thiopentone.

vial (**vi**·al). A small bottle; a phial. [Gk *phiale* drinking cup.]

vibesate (**vi**·bes·ate). A polyvinyl plastic used as a spray to form a film to cover wounds.

vibex, vibix (**vi**·bex, **vi**·bix). Narrow linear mark; a linear subcutaneous effusion of blood. [L, weal.]

vibration (vi·**bra**·shun). An oscillatory to-and-fro movement. [L *vibrare* to vibrate.]

vibrative (**vi**·brat·iv). Capable of vibration, or characterized by it; describing a sound produced by air setting parts of the respiratory tract into vibration.

vibratode (**vi**·brat·ode). The applicator of a vibratory appliance (vibrator).

vibrator (vi·**bra**·tor). An instrument designed to produce vibrations for use in massage.

vibratory (**vi**·brat·or·e). In a state of vibration, or causing vibration.

vibrio (**vib**·re·o). Muller 1773. A genus of the family Pseudomonadaceae; short, curved cells, motile by a polar flagellum, and Gram-positive. Most species are water saprophytes, and a few are pathogenic. The type species is *Vibrio cholerae*. **Vibrio agarliquefaciens.** A soil vibrio. **Vibrio cholerae** (synonym *V. comma* Schroeten 1886). The cholera vibrio, the cause of cholera first isolated by Koch in 1884. The El Tor vibrio which was isolated from cases of dysentery in 1905 by Gotschlich is probably a variant of this with which it shares H and O antigens; it is differentiated by the production of soluble haemolysins for sheep and goat red cells. There are three recognized strains, Inaba the type strain, and two variants, Ogawa and Hikojema. **Vibrio cuneatus.** A soil vibrio. **El Tor vibrio.** *See* VIBRIO CHOLERAE (above). **Vibrio fetus** (M'Fadyean and Stockman, Smith and Taylor 1919). A cause of infectious abortion in sheep and cows. Human infections have been described. **Vibrio granii.** A salt-water vibrio. **Vibrio liquefaciens.** A water vibrio. **Vibrio metchnikovi** (Gamaléia 1888). The cause of a cholera-like disease of chickens. **Vibrio neocistes.** A soil vibrio. **Paracholera vibrio.** A word loosely applied to certain water saprophytes that are causally unassociated with cholera, or of very dubious pathogenicity, e.g. *V. berolinensis*, *V. danubicus*, *V. helocogenes*, *V. ivanoff*, *V. phosphorescens*, and *V. proteus*. **Vibrio strictus.** A large water vibrio. [L *vibrare* to vibrate.]

See also: KOCH (R.).

vibrion septique (**vib**·re·on **sep**·teek). *Clostridium septicum*, [obsolete term]. [Fr., septic vibrio.]

vibrissae (**vib**·ris·e). Stiff, coarse hairs at the muzzle of many animals and in the nostrils of man. [L *vibrare* to shake.]

vibrocardiogram (vi·bro·**kar**·de·o·gram). An instrument which records the vibration of the heart sounds. [vibration, cardiogram.]

vibrolode (**vi**·bro·lode). Vibratode.

vibromassage (**vi**·bro·mas·**ahj'**). Massage given with a mechanical vibrator, or by rapid oscillatory movements of the fingertips.

vibromasseur (**vi**·bro·mas·**er'**). An instrument used in the vibratory massage of the ear.

vibrometer (vi·**brom**·et·er). An instrument for the treatment of deafness resulting from adhesions of the middle ear. It is a form of massage treatment. [L *vibrare* to vibrate, meter.]

vibrophone (**vi**·bro·fone). A form of vibrometer. [L *vibrare* to vibrate, Gk *phone* voice.]

vibrotactile (vi·bro·**tak**·tile). Teletactile. [L *vibrare* to vibrate, *tactus* touch.]

vibrotherapeutics (**vi**·bro·ther·ap·**ew'**·tix). The therapeutic use of vibratory appliances.

viburnin (vi·**ber**·nin). A bitter principle present in the bark of the black haw, *Viburnum prunifolium* Linn. [see foll.]

viburnum (vi·**ber**·num). A genus of plants of the family Caprifoliaceae. **Viburnum opulus.** High bush cranberry bark, true camp bark; the dried bark contains a volatile oil reputed to have a depressant action on the uterus. **Viburnum prunifolium.** Black haw; the dried bark of the root or stem contains salicin and a volatile oil. [L, the wayfaring tree.]

vicarious (vi·**ka**·re·us). 1. Acting as a substitute. 2. Occurring in circumstances where not normally expected. [L *vicarius* substituted.]

vicia (**vis**·e·ah). A genus of plants of the family Leguminosae, including the broad bean. **Vicia faba, Vicia fava.** An Italian lentil to which has been attributed favism, a form of haemolytic anaemia. **Vicia sativa.** The common tare, a vetch that grows as a contaminant of *Lathyrus sativus.* It contains a toxic substance, divicine, which acts as an alkaloid and is thought to be responsible for the condition known as lathyrism. [L, vetch.]

vicianin (vis·e·**an**·in). A glucoside occurring in the vetch or common tare, *Vicia sativa.*

vicianose (**vis**·e·an·oze). $C_{10}H_{20}O_{10}$, a disaccharide formed from glucose and arabinose which occurs in vicianin.

vicilin (vis·**il**·in). A globulin occurring in the seeds of leguminous plants. [L *vicia* vetch.]

vicinal (**vi**·sin·al). In chemistry, denoting an isomer in which the substituent radicals occupy neighbouring positions, e.g. 1, 2, 3, on the benzene ring. [L *vicinus* neighbour.]

Vicq D'Azyr. *See* D'AZYR.

Vidal, Auguste Theodore (b. 1803). Paris surgeon.

Vidal's operation. Subcutaneous ligation of the veins for varicocele.

Vidal, Jean Baptiste Emile (b. 1825). Paris dermatologist.

Vidal treatment. 1. Treatment by scarification with a many-bladed knife of an area of lupus vulgaris. 2. Treatment of the non-ulcerative type of lupus vulgaris by oil of cashew nut applied with friction every three to four days.

Vidarabine (vi·**dar**·ab·een). BP Commission approved name for 9β-D-arabinofuranosyladenine; an antiviral agent.

Vidian (**vid**·e·an). Referring to any anatomical structure named by or after Vidius. *See* GUIDI, GUIDO (VIDIUS).

Vierordt, Karl von (b. 1818). Tübingen physiologist.

Vierordt's haemotachometer. An apparatus designed for the measurement of the rate of blood flow in blood vessels.

Vieth's ratio. The ratio of the percentage of lactose: protein: ash in normal cows' milk, approximating closely to 13:9:2. It is of use in distinguishing between genuine abnormalities and adulteration with water.

Vieussens, Raymond de (b. 1641). French physician and anatomist.

Vieussens' annulus. Annulus ovalis.

Vieussens' ansa. Ansa subclavia.

Centrum ovale of Vieussens. The central white matter of the cerebrum as seen when a horizontal section is cut at the level of the dorsal border of the corpus callosum.

Vieussens' foramina. The openings of the small cardiac veins into the right atrium.

Vieussens' valve. 1. The superior medullary velum. 2. The valve at the junction of the great cardiac vein and the coronary sinus.

Vieussens' veins. The small veins of the heart; most of them drain the anterior and posterior surfaces of the right ventricle and open directly into the right atrium.

Vieussens' ventricle. The cavity of the septum lucidum.

vigil (**vij**·il). Insomnia. **Coma vigil.** Semiconscious delirium, often with the eyes open and staring. [L, waking.]

vigilambulism (vij·il·**am**·bew·lizm). Automatism in the waking state, with impairment of consciousness. [L *vigil* waking, *ambulare* to walk about.]

vigintinormal (vij·**in**·te·**nor**'·mal). One-twentieth normal strength. [L *viginti* twenty, normal.]

Vignal, Guillaume (b. 1852). Paris histologist.

Vignal's cell. An embryonic cell associated with the formation of the myelin sheath around nerve axons.

Vigo, Giovanni da (b. 1460). Italian surgeon.

Vigo's powder. Red mercuric oxide.

Vigotsky, L. S. 20th century Russian psychologist.

Vigotsky test. The original test from which the Hanfmann-Kasanin test was derived.

vigour (**vig**·er). Body energy. **Hybrid vigour.** Increase in size, rate of growth, fertility, or viability, appearing in the offspring of a cross between two species or stocks of the same species. [L *vigor.*]

Vigouroux, Auguste 19th century Paris neurologist.

Vigouroux' sign, Charcot-Vigouroux sign. Diminished electric resistance of the skin, said to be present in thyrotoxicosis.

Villaret, Maurice (b. 1877). Paris physician.

Villaret's sign. In a lesion of the sciatic nerve, percussion on the tendo calcaneus gives flexion of the great toe.

Villaret's syndrome. Ipsilateral paralysis of the 9th, 10th, 11th, and 12th cranial nerves, and of the cervical sympathetic nervous system, due to a lesion in the retropharyngeal or retroparotid space. On the affected side there is paralysis of palatal, pharyngeal, and laryngeal muscles, and of the sternocleidomastoid and trapezius muscles, with Horner's syndrome and loss of taste sensation on the posterior third of the tongue.

Villemin, Fernand (fl. 1913). French anatomist.

Villemin's sphincter. A sphincter reputed to be present at the lower end of the duodenum.

Villemin, Jean Antoine (b. 1827). Paris physician.

Villemin's theory. The doctrine of the infectiousness of tuberculosis, which originated from Villemin's successful transmission of the disease to animals by direct inoculation of infectious material (1868).

villi (**vil**·i). *See* VILLUS.

villiferous (vil·**if**·er·us). Bearing villi. [villus, L *ferre* to bear.]

villiform (**vil**·e·form). Resembling villi. [villus, form.]

villikinin (vil·**ik**·in·in). A substance obtained by acid extraction of intestinal mucous membrane. It stimulates the movements of the intestinal villi. [villus, Gk *kinein* to move.]

villoma (vil·**o**·mah). A villous tumour, e.g. of the bladder or rectum. [villus, Gk *-oma* tumour.]

villose (**vil**·oze). Provided with villi.

villositis (vil·o·**si**·tis). Inflammation of the placental villi. [villus, Gk *-itis* inflammation.]

villosity (vil·**os**·it·e). 1. A villus. 2. The state of being villous.

villous (**vil**·us). Of a surface, covered with villi.

villus [NA] (**vil**·us) (pl. *villi*). A small finger-like process projecting from a surface, usually that of a mucous membrane. **Amniotic villi.** Irregular tags of epithelium on the surface of the amnion. **Anchoring villus.** A placental villus which passes across the placenta from chorion to decidua. **Arachnoid villus.** A protrusion of the cerebral arachnoid into the dural wall of a venous sinus or its lateral lacuna. As age proceeds some become hypertrophied to form arachnoid granulations (*pacchionian bodies*). **Chorionic villi.** Minute finger-like processes on the surface of the chorion which project into the intervillous space; when fully developed (*secondary villus*) each consists of a mesodermal core, a central blood vessel, and a covering of trophoblast. The majority lie free within the intervillous space but some (*anchoring villi*) bridge it to become attached to the basal layer of trophoblast. **Diffuse villus.** One of the villi found evenly spaced over the surface of the early chorion in man, or as a permanent feature of the chorion of the pig, horse, and some other animals. **Intestinal villi [villi intestinales (NA)].** Minute processes covering the mucous membrane of the small intestine. Each consists of a covering layer of columnar epithelium, a network of blood vessels, and a central lymphatic or lacteal. **Labial villus.** One of the small villous projections of the inner margins of the lips of fetuses and suckling infants. **Pleural villus.** A process projecting from the surface of the pleura in the costomediastinal recess. **Primary villus.** A finger-shaped process of cellular and syncytial trophoblast, without mesoderm or blood vessels, which is the forerunner of a definitive chorionic villus. **Secondary villus.** *See* CHORIONIC VILLI (above). **Synovial villus [villus synovialis**

(NA)]. A tuft-like projection of the synovial membrane into the joint cavity. [L, shaggy hair.]

villusectomy (vil·us·**ek**·to·me). Removal of a synovial villus. [villus, Gk *ektome* excision.]

Viloxazine (vil·**ox**·az·een). BP Commission approved name for 2-(2-ethoxyphenoxymethyl)tetrahydro-1,4-oxazine; it is used in the treatment of certain mental diseases.

Vim-Silverman needle. An instrument by means of which a minute cylinder of liver tissue is obtained for histological examination during life.

Vimtrup, B. 20th century Scandinavian physiologist.

Vimtrup's cell. A flattened cell with numerous processes wrapped around the capillaries of frogs and other amphibia which are thought to contract and constrict the vessels when stimulated by the sympathetic nervous system.

vinbarbital (vin·**bar**·bit·al). Vinbarbitone.

Vinbarbitone (vin·**bar**·bit·one). BP Commission approved name for 5-ethyl-5-(1-methyl-1-butenyl)-barbituric acid, $C_{11}H_{16}N_2O_3$. A compound used as a sedative and mild hypnotic for pre-operative and pre-anaesthetic sedation, and in obstetric practice in which it is a valuable amnestic. It can be given orally, rectally, or intravenously. The toxic effects are those usually caused by barbiturates. It is the sodium derivative that is usually employed.

Vinblastine (vin·**blas**·teen). BP Commission approved name for an alkaloid extracted from *Vinca rosea*. **Vinblastine Sulphate BP 1973.** Sulphate of vinblastine; a cytotoxic agent used in the treatment of neoplastic disease.

vincennite (vin·**sen**·ite). A mixture of toxic substances, including hydrocyanic acid and arsenic trichloride; used as a poison gas in chemical warfare.

Vincent, Jean Hyacinthe (b. 1862). Paris physician and bacteriologist.

Vincent's angina. Infection of the tonsil associated with ulceration and the formation of membrane. It often occurs in epidemic forms in schools, camps, and public institutions. The causal organisms are the fusiform bacillus, *Fusiformis fusiformis*, and the spirochaete, *Borrelia vincenti*; they also affect the gums and the mouth generally. Trench mouth has the same aetiology.

Vincent's disease. Infection of the mouth and/or throat with Vincent's organisms.

Vincent's mixture. 1. Stearin, paraffin, and petroleum, used to lubricate tubes, as in the collection of blood samples. 2. A powder consisting of sodium hypochlorite and boric acid, used as a wound dressing.

Vincent's organisms. *Borrelia vincenti* and *Fusiformis fusiformis.*

Vincent's powder. Vincent's mixture, 2nd def. (see above).

Vincent's stomatitis. Infection of the mouth with Vincent's organisms.

Vincent's tonsillitis. Infection of the tonsils with Vincent's organisms.

Vincetoxicum (vin·se·**tox**·ik·um). A genus of plants of the order Asclepiadaceae. **Vincetoxicum officinale.** White swallow-wort; the dried root is used as an emetic. [L *vincere* to conquer, Gk *toxikon* poison.]

Vincristine (vin·**kris**·teen). BP Commission approved name for an alkaloid obtained from *Vinca rosea*; an antineoplastic agent, also used in acute cases of leukaemia.

vinculum (vin·kew·lum) (pl. *vincula*). A connecting band, or fold. **Vinculum linguae.** The frenulum of the tongue. **Vincula lingualia cerebelli.** Lateral extensions of the cerebellum. **Vinculum praeputii.** The frenulum of the prepuce. **Vincula tendinum [NA].** Bands of fibrous tissue enclosed in folds of the mucous synovial sheaths of the flexor tendons of the fingers [manus (NA)] and toes [pedis (NA)]. They are of two types: vincula longa [NA] and vincula brevia [NA], and besides connecting the tendons to the ventral aspects of the phalanges they also convey small blood vessels to them. **Vinculum umbilicale.** Umbilical cord. *See* CORD. [L, bond.]

Vineberg, Arthur M. 20th century Montreal cardiac surgeon.

Vineberg's operation. The implantation of an internal mammary artery into the myocardium.

vinegar (**vin**·e·gar). 1. Acetum; an aqueous solution containing from 4 to 6 per cent of acetic acid, prepared by the oxidation of fermented alcoholic liquors under the action of bacteria. 2. Any preparation made by dissolving a medicament in vinegar (as above) or in acetic acid. **Apple vinegar.** Cider vinegar (see below). **Aromatic vinegar.** Glacial acetic acid containing oils of bergamot, cinnamon, clove, lavender, orange, and thyme. **Vinegar of cantharides.** Cantharides extracted with acetic acid (50 per cent). **Vinegar of cantharidin.** A solution of cantharidin (1 in 2000) and glacial acetic acid, in aqueous acetic acid (33 per cent), used in the preparation of hair lotions. **Cider vinegar.** Apple vinegar; vinegar made from the juice of apples: in the USA "vinegar" without qualification means cider vinegar. **Vinegar of honey.** Oxymel. **Vinegar of ipecacuanha.** A solution of liquid extract of ipecacuanha and alcohol, in aqueous acetic acid, used as an expectorant. **Vinegar of Squill BPC 1959.** Squill macerated with aqueous acetic acid (33 per cent). It is used as an expectorant, either alone or as a constituent of syrup of squills. **Toilet vinegar.** An aqueous solution containing acetic acid, with ethyl alcohol, tinctures of tolu and benzoin, and oils of bergamot, cassia, clove, lavender, and lemon. **White-wine vinegar.** A vinegar prepared from white wine and containing 6 per cent of acetic acid. [Fr. *vin aigre* sour wine.]

vinous (**vi**·nus). 1. Appertaining to wine. 2. Containing wine, or of the nature of wine. [L *vinum* wine.]

Vinson, Porter Paisley (b. 1890). Rochester, Minnesota, physician.

Plummer-Vinson anaemia, or syndrome, Vinson-Plummer syndrome. Chronic hypochromic microcytic anaemia with dysphagia, glossitis, and achylia gastrica, due to iron deficiency.

vinum (**vi**·num). Wine; the fermented juice of the grape, or of some other fruits, used medicinally as a vehicle for the administration of medicaments such as tonics, purgatives, sedatives, and expectorants. Such use is declining. [L.]

vinyl (**vi**·nil). The monovalent unsaturated chemical grouping, CH_2=CH-. Compounds containing this grouping form polymers of importance in the plastics industry. **Vinyl chloride.** CH_2=CHCl, a gas prepared from acetylene which polymerizes to form vinylite, a plastic used in x-ray films. **Vinyl Ether BP 1973.** $(CH_2=CH)_2O$, a volatile anaesthetic about four times as active as diethyl ether and more rapid in its action. Approximately 4 per cent of alcohol and a stabilizer are usually added to the pure substance when it is used medicinally. **Vinyl sulphide.** $(CH_2=CH)_2S$, a constituent of volatile oil of garlic. **Vinyl thio-oxazolidine.** $CH_2=CHC_3H_6NS$, a goitrogenic compound found in yellow turnip and other vegetables. [L *vinum* wine, Gk *hyle* substance.]

Vinylbitone (vi·nil·bit·one). BP Commission approved name for 5-(1-methylbutyl)-5-vinylbarbituric acid; a hypnotic and sedative.

Viola (vi·o·lah). A genus of herbaceous plants; the violets and pansies.

violaquercitrin (vi·o·lah·**kwer**'·sit·rin). A glycoside present in *Viola odorata* root.

violation (vi·o·la·shun). Illegal carnal knowledge, with or without force. [L *violare* to outrage.]

violet (vi·o·let). 1. A flower of the genus *Viola*. 2. The colour of the shortest end of the visible spectrum; light of wave-lengths between 39 and 45 nm. 3. A number of synthetic dyestuffs, e.g. methyl violet, crystal violet, etc., used to stain biological material violet. **Amethyst violet.** Heliotrope B. **Cresyl violet, Cresylecht violet.** A violet dye used in staining the central nervous system. **Crystal Violet BP 1968.** Methylrosaniline chloride, medicinal gentian violet, hexamethylpararosaniline hydrochloride, $[(CH_3)_2NC_6H_4]_2C=C_6H_4=N(CH_3)_2Cl$; a greenish-bronze crystalline powder, fairly soluble in water, very soluble in alcohol and chloroform. It is a powerful antiseptic, specifically active against Gram-positive organisms. It acts against the causative organism of Vincent's angina, and against many strains of *Candida, Torula, Epidermophyton,* and *Trichophyton*; it is relatively ineffective against streptococci. Externally it is used in the form of a paint or jelly, sometimes in conjunction with brilliant green, as an antiseptic dressing for the treatment of infected wounds, in the treatment of burns, chronic ulcers, and mycotic skin infections. Internally, it is a valuable anthelminthic, especially against *Strongyloides.* It is also used in oxyuriasis and liver-fluke infestation. It should be given in enteric-coated tablets. It has been given intravenously in staphylococcal septicaemia and chronic cystitis. **Gentian violet.** Principally hexamethylene pararosaniline chloride, used as a primary stain and as a bacteriostatic for Gram-positive organisms. **Hexamethyl violet.** Crystal violet (see above). **Medicinal gentian violet.** Crystal violet (see above). **Methyl violet.** A mixture of methylpararosanilines, principally the tetra-, penta-, and hexamethyl derivatives, used in a modification of Gram's staining technique. **Methylene violet.** Crystal violet (see above). **Visual violet.** Visual purple. *See* PURPLE. [L *viola.*]

Viomycin (vi·o·**mi**·sin). BP Commission approved name for an antibiotic produced by strains of *Streptomyces griseus.* **Viomycin Sulphate BP 1973.** Sulphate of the base; it is an antibiotic effective against streptomycin-resistant strains of *Mycobacterium tuberculosis.*

viosterol (vi·o·**steer**·ol). A general name for irradiated ergosterol which contains one of the vitamins of the D group. The name followed by, say, 50D, infers that the sample is 50 times as active as regards vitamin D as a standard, biologically assayed cod-liver oil. This term is less often used now that pure crystalline calciferol is obtainable.

viper (**vi**·per). Any member of the sub-family Viperinae of the family Viperidae; a poisonous snake of the Old World, particularly of the genus *Vipera.* **European viper,** *Vipera berus.* The only British species. **Horned viper.** *Cerastes cornutus* of North Africa. **Pit viper.** A member of the sub-family Crotalinae of the family Viperidae, which includes copperheads, moccasins, and rattlesnakes. They have a sensory uveal pit between the eyes and nostrils. [L *vipere.*]

See also: RUSSELL (P.).

vipera (**vi**·per·ah). A genus of Old World viperine snakes, all species of which are poisonous. **Vipera berus.** The European viper, or adder. **Viper russelli.** A large, very poisonous snake of India, Burma, and Thailand. [L.]

viperidae (vi·**per**·id·e). A family of snakes that includes many poisonous species. [viper, Gk *eidos* form.]

viperinae (vi·**per**·in·e). A sub-family of poisonous snakes that includes the adder, the Russell's viper, and the phoorsa.

viperine (**vi**·per·een). 1. Referring to a viper. 2. Serpentaria, Virginian snake root, used as a diaphoretic. 3. An extract of viper venom.

Viprynium Embonate BP 1973 (vi·**pri**·ne·um **em**·bo·nate). 6 - Dimethylamino - 2 - [2 - (2=5 - dimethyl - 1 - phenyl - 3 - pyrrolyl)vinyl] - 1 - methylquinolinium embonate; an anthelminthic.

viraemia (vi·**re**·me·ah). A virus in the blood. [virus, Gk *haima* blood.]

viraginity (vir·aj·**in**·it·e). The possession by a woman of physical qualities which are characteristically male. [L *virago* an amazon.]

viral (**vi**·ral). Of or pertaining to viruses.

virales (vi·**ra**·leez). The order of viruses.

Virchow, Rudolf Ludwig Karl (b. 1821). Berlin pathologist.

Virchow's angle. The angle at the nasion between lines joining the latter and the basion and the subnasal point, respectively.

Virchow's cell. Lepra cell; a mononuclear phagocyte full of leprosy bacilli.

Virchow's crystals. Yellow or orange needle-shaped or rhombic crystals observed in faeces that indicate recent haemorrhage into the bowel.

Virchow's degeneration. Amyloid degeneration. *See* DEGENERATION.

Virchow's disease. Leontiasis ossea.

Virchow's gland, or node. Signal node. *See* NODE.

Virchow's law. All cells are derived from normal, pre-existing cells: "*omnis cellulae e cellula*".

Virchow's line. A line from the nasion to the lambda.

Virchow's space, Virchow-Robin space. The perivascular space that surrounds blood vessels as they enter the brain substance and communicates with the subarachnoid space.

Virchow's theory. The theory that it is the cell that is involved in disease. This theory replaced the humoral doctrine in the middle of the 19th century.

vires (**vir**·eez). *See* VIS.

virgin (**ver**·jin). 1. A female (or male) without experience of sexual intercourse. 2. Untouched; unused; uncontaminated. **Virgin generation.** Parthenogenesis. **Virgin's milk.** Tincture of benzoin and rose water used for toilet purposes. [L *virgo* a maid.]

virginal (**ver**·jin·al). 1. Of the nature of a virgin; pure. 2. Relating to virginity. **Virginal membrane.** The hymen.

virginia creeper (ver·**jin**·e·ah **kre**·per). *Vitis hederacea,* a plant of the family Vitaceae. The bark and twigs are astringent. [*Virginia,* State in the USA.]

Virginiamycin (ver·**jin**·e·ah·**mi**′·sin). BP Commission approved name for an antibiotic produced by *Streptomyces virginiae.*

virginity (ver·**jin**·it·e). The state of being a virgin.

virginium (ver·**jin**·e·um). Name given to a radioactive element now called Francium. [*Virginia,* State in the USA.]

virgo intacta (**ver**·go in·**tak**·tah). A pure virgin. It does not necessarily mean an unruptured hymen, although this is the most commonly accepted meaning of the words. [L, untouched maid.]

viricidal (vir·is·**i**·dal). Virucidal. [virus, L *caedere* to kill.]

viridobufagin (**vir**·id·o·**boo**′·faj·in). A secretion of the skin glands of the toad *Bufo viridis.* It has a toxic action on the heart.

virile (**vir**·ile). Having male qualities; pertaining to the male sex; able to procreate. **Virile member.** The penis. [L *virilis* masculine.]

virilising (**vir**·il·ize·ing). Something which increases the tendency to masculinization.

virilism (**vir**·il·izm). A condition in women in which male characteristics are present. It differs from hirsutism in that in addition to excessive hair growth there is one or more signs of masculinity such as clitoral hypertrophy, deepening of the voice, temporal hair recession and male bodily habitus. [L *virilis* masculine.]

virility (vir·**il**·it·e). 1. The prime of manhood. 2. Potency in the male. [see prec.]

virion (**vir**·e·on). A complete, mature, infectious virus particle.

virologist (vi·**rol**·o·jist). A specialist in virology.

virology (vi·**rol**·o·je). The study of viruses and the diseases they produce. [virus, Gk *logos* science.]

viropexis (vi·ro·**pex**·is). The process by which a virus enters a cell. It may be an aggressive action by the virus or ingestion by the cell, or both, and varies with different viruses and different host cells. [virus, Gk *pexis* a fixation.]

virose, virous (**vi**·roze, **vi**·rus). Of a poisonous nature; virulent. [L *virus* poison.]

virucidal (vi·rus·**i**·dal). Able to inactivate viruses. [virus, L *caedere* to kill.]

virucidin (vi·rus·**i**·din). A substance lethal to viruses. [see prec.]

virulence (**vir**·ew·lens). The capacity of any organism to produce disease in any stated host; a host/parasite relationship. **Mucin virulence.** The enhancement of virulence produced by simultaneously injecting mucin with the organism. It is due to the prevention of phagocytosis by coating the bacteria with mucin. [L *virulentus* full of poison.]

virulent (**vir**·ew·lent). Very toxic or poisonous. [see prec.]

virulicidal (vir·ew·**lis**·id·al). Virucidal.

virus (**vi**·rus). One of a large group of micro-organisms, between 20 nm and 250 nm in diameter, whose structure can only be seen in detail with the electron microscope. They are obligate intracellular parasites containing predominantly only one kind of nucleic acid (DNA or RNA) which is surrounded by at least one layer of protein. Recent research on bacterial, animal and plant viruses has shown that infection is a genetic phenomenon due to virus

release of the viral genetic material, which may be DNA or RNA, into the cell. This genetic material then uses the synthetic machinery of the cell to replicate its nucleic acid and to make new viral capsid components which are later assembled into new, mature virus particles. A. Lwoff (1959) redefined viruses by the three criteria of: infectivity, dependence for their reproduction on the biochemical machinery of the host, and the possession of only one type of nucleic acid. Viruses are widely disseminated in nature, being found as parasites on most animal species and many plants, including bacteria and mycoplasmas. They are the cause of several infectious diseases in man but their intimate association with cells during replication has made it difficult to find drugs which will inactivate the virus without also damaging the host. (In addition to the viruses defined below, *see* ADENOVIRUS, ARBOVIRUS, ARENAVIRUS, CORONAVIRUS, CYTOMEGALOVIRUS, ECHOVIRUS, ENTEROVIRUS, HERPESVIRUS, MYXOVIRUS, PAPILLOMAVIRUS, PAPOVAVIRUS, PARAMYXOVIRUS, PICORNAVIRUS, POLIOVIRUS, POLYOMAVIRUS, POXVIRUS, REOVIRUS, RHABDOVIRUS, RHINOVIRUS. **Adenoidopharyngoconjunctival virus.** *See* ADENOVIRUS. **Adeno satellite virus.** Adenovirus-associated virus (see below). **Adenovirus-associated virus** (AAV). A small, 20 nm, virus found in association with some serotypes of adenovirus. It contains DNA but insufficient to replicate the virus completely and requires the presence of the adenovirus to supply a missing function. It is not known to cause disease in man. Also known as *adeno satellite virus.* **Alastrim virus.** Smallpox virus (see below). **Attenuated virus.** A virus whose virulence for a particular species has been lowered either by physical or chemical action or by repeated passage through cells of another species. This process may select naturally occurring mutants of low virulence and may be encouraged by chemical mutagens. **Avian leucosis viruses.** A group of RNA-containing tumour viruses which may cause epidemics of a leukaemia-like disease in chickens, though often they cause no overt disease. Useful as a model for research into cancer mechanisms, the viruses may be transmitted vertically through the egg and horizontally to other susceptible birds. **B virus.** A virus causing ascending myelitis in man; it causes a generalized exanthematic infection in the monkey, but is not apparently neurotropic in this animal. **Brunhilde strain of poliomyelitis virus.** The prototype of type I poliomyelitis virus. The name is taken from that of a chimpanzee from which the strain was recovered. **Bunyamwera virus.** A member of the Bunyamwera supergroup of arboviruses. *See* ARBOVIRUS. **Castañeda-positive virus.** A name given to psittacosis and allied viruses which are stained by Castañeda's method. **Coxsackie virus.** One of the RNA-containing enteroviruses which affect man. Coxsackie viruses comprise 30 serotypes divided into two groups, A (24 serotypes) and B (6 serotypes), on the basis of biological characteristics. They, like other enteroviruses, primarily invade the cells of the gut but may cause a generalized febrile illness. This can lead to aseptic meningitis with or without paralysis (groups A and B), herpangina (group A), hand, foot and mouth disease (group A), pleurodynia (group B), or myocarditis (group B). The members of the group are distinguished serologically by neutralization or complement-fixation tests. Coxsackie is a village in New York State where the first outbreak was identified. **Cubic virus.** A virus whose protein shell surrounding the nucleic acid has axes of symmetry similar to those of a cube. Such viruses usually appear more or less spherical. **Cytopathic virus.** A virus which damages beyond recovery the cells it infects. **Dehumanized virus.** A strain of vaccinia virus obtained by inoculation of a calf with material from a human case. **Dermotropic virus.** A virus which tends to produce lesions in the skin. **EB virus** (Epstein and Barr). Belonging to the *Herpesvirus* group; possibly a cause of infectious mononucleosis. **Egg virus.** Vaccinia virus propagated on the developing chick embryo. **Enveloped virus.** A virus whose outer surface is a membrane usually derived from host cell membrane modified to include viral antigens. **Equine encephalomyelitis virus.** An insect-borne virus, of which there are at least two varieties, that causes encephalomyelitis in horses; its relation to the virus of human encephalomyelitis is not fully understood. **Filtrable virus.** *See* MAIN DEF. 2 (above). **Virus fixé, Fixed virus.** The virus of rabies (the original *street virus*) exalted in virulence by passage through successive rabbits until it kills in from five to six days; its killing period for rabbits has become "fixed". This virus is used in preparing rabies vaccine. **Genital inclusion virus.** A virus found in the male and female genital canals and also in the conjunctival sacs of the newborn. **Haemagglutinating virus.** A virus which has surface antigens capable of attaching to red blood cells and thereby agglutinating them. The haemagglutinin is virus specific but is not always part of the virion. **Helical virus.** A virus whose protein shell surrounding the nucleic acid has a spiral form like a screw thread with a single axis of helical symmetry down its centre. **Hepatitis virus.** The viruses of infectious and serum hepatitis are usually regarded as distinct (types A and B respectively), though insufficient is known about the viruses to be certain what distinctions there are and whether they are significant. *See also* Australia ANTIGEN and Dane PARTICLES. **Hepatotropic virus.** The virus, or one of the viruses responsible for infective hepatitis (or catarrhal jaundice). **Humanized virus.** Humanized vaccine. *See* VACCINE. **Icosahedral virus.** A virus whose shape is based on an icosahedron (a 20-sided regular solid). They are cubic viruses. **Inactivated virus.** A virus which has been treated by physical or chemical methods and is no longer capable of replication unaided. **Inclusion virus.** The virus which is postulated as the cause of inclusion cervicitis, arthritis, and conjunctivitis. **Influenza virus.** The causative virus of influenza. It is an RNA-containing virus, very pleomorphic in appearance, about 90 nm in size, and divided antigenically, on the basis of the internal nucleoprotein antigen, into three groups A, B and C. *Influenza A,* the virus of epidemic influenza, due to its ability to undergo periodic antigenic alteration. The virus has two surface antigens, a haemagglutinin and a neuraminidase, both of which undergo independent variation. Influenza virus is unique among viruses in that new antigenic variants replace the old completely, making existing vaccines obsolete. Influenza A types possess a similar internal nucleoprotein antigen, which does not elicit any protective antibody in the host; they have been isolated from numerous species of birds, horses and bovines, as well as man. Generally, there is a barrier to spread from one species to another but haemagglutinin and neuraminidase antigens indistinguishable from some human strains have been found in animal strains. Influenza A types, sufficiently different from previous strains to cause pandemics, may acquire names of their own, e.g. *Spanish influenza* in 1918 and *Asian influenza* in 1957. *Influenza B,* morphologically identical with influenza A but antigenically distinct. It possesses haemagglutinin and neuraminidase surface antigens which show a gradual alteration (antigenic drift). Major alterations as seen with influenza A do not occur and influenza B does not, therefore, cause pandemics. *Influenza C* differs slightly, but significantly, in morphology from influenza A and B. It has been associated with influenza-like illnesses but does not readily cause clinical influenza. Consequently, its designation as an influenza virus may have to be reconsidered. **JH virus.** A virus associated with the common cold and used in successful vaccination experiments; the virus was isolated at Johns Hopkins University. **Lansing strain of poliomyelitis virus.** The prototype strain of type II poliomyelitis virus. This strain was isolated from a fatal case of poliomyelitis at Lansing, Michigan. **Latent virus.** A virus which has become integrated into host cells so that it is no longer detectable, but which can be reactivated under suitable circumstances. **Leon strain of poliomyelitis virus.** The prototype strain of type III poliomyelitis virus. The name is that of a patient who died of poliomyelitis and from whom the strain was isolated. **Marburg virus.** The causative virus of Marburg disease, a severe febrile illness with a case mortality of over 20 per cent. It appeared in 1967 as a laboratory outbreak in Marburg, Frankfurt and Belgrade among workers who had handled tissues from African green monkeys. It is an RNA virus, rod-shaped in appearance which causes a maculopapular rash with haemorrhages. **Measles virus.** The causative agent of measles. It is an enveloped RNA-containing virus, morphologically resembling the para-influenza viruses though unrelated serologically. It has a haemagglutinin probably using a different mechanism to other similar viruses. Different isolates are antigenically uniform. It is not particularly easy to cultivate in the laboratory, but passage-attenuated strains are used in live vaccines. **Meningo-encephalomyelitis virus.** A virus isolated in Uganda; it causes paralysis in man and monkeys. **Milker's nodule virus.** The virus of cowpox. **Mouse leukaemia viruses.** A group of RNA-containing viruses which cause leukaemia in mice. Fresh isolates will usually only induce leukaemia in newborn mice but repeated passage, especially in inbred strains, increases the virulence so that they induce leukaemia more quickly and also in older mice. Apart from some similarities in physical properties, the group, which includes Gross, Graffi, Moloney, Rauscher and Friend viruses, also shows serological cross-reactivity but no group specific antigen has been described. **Mumps virus.** An enveloped RNA-containing virus, indistinguishable in morphology from para-influenza, Newcastle disease or measles viruses. It possesses haemagglutinin and neuraminidase antigens as well as an internal nucleoprotein (S) antigen. Antibodies to the S antigen develop more quickly than to the V or surface antigens and decline more quickly. Their presence in serum is indicative, therefore, of recent infection. **Neurotropic virus.** A virus with a predilection for multiplication in the central nervous system. **Newcastle disease virus.** The causative agent of one form of fowl pest. It is a paramyxovirus, different strains of which vary widely in their pathogenicity for their natural host, the chicken. The virus may occasionally be transmitted to man, in whom it causes conjunctivitis. Lymphadenitis and some generalized symptoms may also occur, but recovery without sequelae is usual and quick. **Oncogenic virus.** A tumour virus (see below). **Orphan virus.** A virus that has been isolated and is identifiable but has not been, or was not originally, associated with any particular pathological condition. **Pantropic virus.** One that attacks tissues of all three embryonic layers. **Para-influenza virus.** An enveloped RNA-containing virus associated with upper respiratory tract infections in man and morphologically identical with other paramyxoviruses. It is pleomorphic in appearance and there are four stable serological types: *type 1* - haemadsorption virus type 2, newborn pneumonitis virus, haemagglutinating virus of Japan, Sendai; *type 2* - croup-associated virus; *type 3* - haemadsorption virus type 1, bovine shipping fever virus; and *type 4* - Simian virus type 5 found as an apparent commensal in monkey tissues, is closely related to para-influenza type 2 and may be identical with it. Para-influenza viruses have surface haemagglutinin and neuraminidase antigens, and most can fuse cells in culture even when inactivated with formalin. **Parrot virus.** The virus of psittacosis. **Plaque-forming virus.** A virus that forms discrete, countable foci of cell necrosis in cell cultures. Such foci can be used to titrate the virus. **Poliomyelitis virus.** One of the smallest recognized pathogenic viruses, from 25 to 32 nm; there are at least three types, or groups, of this virus, each consisting of many strains, namely, type I (the prototype of which is the Brunhilde strain), type II (the prototype of which is the Lansing strain), and type III (the prototype of which is the Leon strain). **Rabies virus.** The causative agent of rabies. It is an RNA-containing virus of the rhabdovirus group, probably bullet-shaped (though more pleomorphic than other members of the group), about 150 nm long and 100 nm wide. Only one antigenic type has been described; marked differences in virulence are found between wild (street) strains and strains passed in the laboratory (fixed strains). Phenolized vaccines have been made from infected rabbit or sheep brain (Semple), and inactivated vaccines from virus grown in duck embryos and after passage in eggs. No vaccine is entirely satisfactory for use in man at present but work on attenuated strains shows promise. **Respiratory syncytial virus.** An RNA-containing pleomorphic enveloped virus about 100 nm in size though larger forms are found. In adults it causes a mild upper respiratory tract infection but in children, especially infants, it can cause a severe, and sometimes fatal, lower tract infection with bronchiolitis, bronchitis, or bronchopneumonia. An adequate vaccine is being sought but inactivated virus has not proved suitable. In cell culture the virus typically causes multinucleate giant syncytia. It is not related antigenically to other viruses, in particular not to the paramyxovirus group which it resembles superficially in morphology. **Rubella virus.** A pleomorphic enveloped RNA-containing virus about 75 nm in size. The cause of rubella, it has marked teratogenic properties in pregnancy, particularly in the first three months. Only one antigenic type is known and live attenuated vaccines with minimum post vaccination excretion of the virus are available. Vaccination is usually offered to pre-puberty girls or post-partum to adult women, but with women of child-bearing age vaccination should normally only be given under adequate contraceptive cover. **Salivary gland virus.** Cytomegalovirus. **Satellite virus.** A partially defective virus unable to replicate itself, requiring a helper. **Semliki forest virus.** A virus found in African mosquitoes during yellow-fever investigations. It is pathogenic to many animals and man, and other animals living in the area possess antibodies against this virus in their blood. **Sendai virus.** A virus recovered from patients during an outbreak of pneumonitis among newborn infants, 12 out of 17 of whom died. Antibodies have been identified in the blood of convalescents from both mild and severe respiratory disease in the UK and the USA. **Simian virus type 40** (SV40). A papovavirus of the papilloma genus. Frequent commensal in Old World monkeys and hence of cell cultures derived from their tissues, including kidneys. It has been found as a contaminant of vaccines grown in monkey kidney cells but has not been shown to be pathogenic for man, though it can induce tumours in suckling hamsters, rhesus monkeys, grivets and baboons under laboratory conditions. In man, the virus induces antibody but no tumours. Synonyms: *Simian vacuolating virus* or *agent*. **Sindbis virus.** A group of A arbovirus which may cause a benign influenza-like illness. The natural hosts are probably birds and mosquitoes with occasional spread to man. **Slow virus.** A member of a heterogeneous group of viruses which cause slowly developing chronic degenerative diseases, with a long incubation period (up to several years) and usually fatal. The members of the group are not known to have any features in common and some, e.g. scrapie agent, have properties markedly different from those of most viruses. The viruses are transmissible but difficult to isolate or assay. **Smallpox virus.** The virus of smallpox (variola major), closely related to the viruses of alastrim (variola minor) and cowpox. By successive passage through susceptible animals any of these viruses may mutate into the laboratory variant *vaccinia virus*; this does not occur naturally. Various vaccinia strains are in use for the preparation of smallpox vaccine, and are maintained by passage in the epidermis of the calf, sheep, or rabbit. The virus has been propagated also on the chorioallantoic membranes of developing chick embryos, and in tissue culture; it can also be dried in the frozen state, and should be stored as a stable product. **Street virus.** Rabies virus taken from a dog suffering from rabies naturally acquired. **Tumour virus.** A virus which is capable of inducing tumour formation either directly (inoculation of the virus into an experimental animal causes tumours) or indirectly (the virus transforms normal cells in culture into abnormal ones capable of initiating tumours when inoculated into a suitable experimental host). In the indirect case, the virus may become integrated into the transformed cells and may not be readily detected. Tumour viruses may be either DNA- or RNA-containing and have only an oncogenic potential in common. Most RNA-containing tumour viruses have been shown to contain a little DNA as well as the enzyme reverse transcriptase whose function may be to integrate the virus genome into that of the host cell as an essential part of transformation. The only tumours in man unequivocally caused by viruses are benign (warts, molluscum contagiosum). EB virus is associated with Burkitt's lymphoma but probably not as sole cause. **Ultra-microscopic virus.** *See* MAIN DEF. 2 (above). **Vaccine virus, Vaccinia virus.** The virus used for vaccination against smallpox. It is related antigenically to the viruses of cowpox and variola (smallpox). It is distinct from both although it has some properties in common with each. Its origin is obscure but it is probably a cowpox-variola hybrid and it is a typical DNA-containing poxvirus. Many strains are maintained for vaccine production in different countries. All are probably identical antigenically but differ in some properties such as the presence or absence of haemorrhage in the pocks formed on the chorio-allantoic membrane of the egg and in neurovirulence for mice. **Varicella virus.** The causative virus of chickenpox (varicella). It is a herpesvirus which may have minor antigenic relationships with herpes B of monkeys and also with herpes simplex virus. It is relatively difficult to cultivate; it will grow slowly in cells of human origin and from some monkey tissues. **Variola virus.** The causative virus of smallpox (variola). Strains of different virulence (variola major, variola minor) are found and are indistinguishable antigenically. They differ only in the maximum ceiling temperature at which they will grow on the chorio-allantoic membrane of the fertile egg. A temperature of 38°C inhibits variola minor but variola major will produce pocks at 38.5°C, though not at 40°C. The virus is related closely to those of vaccinia and cowpox but has a more restricted host range, which may be due to its lower temperature ceiling. It is probably one of the genetic parents of vaccinia virus. **Venezuelan virus.** Equine encephalomyelitis virus (see above). **Vesicular stomatitis virus.** A naturally occurring virus disease of domestic hoofed animals which closely resembles foot and mouth disease, although it is more mild. It is caused by a rhabdovirus and a wide variety of species can be infected experimentally. Accidental laboratory infection of man has occurred, the infection causing an influenza-like illness. **Viscerotropic virus.** One that attacks the viscera, but not the nervous system, and causes active disease. **Wart virus.** A papillomavirus about 50 nm in diameter. It can cause infectious warts on the skin, soles of the feet, genital area (acuminata) and probably the larynx. It is present in large numbers in the superficial layers of common warts but is more difficult to demonstrate in genital and laryngeal warts. It has not been grown artificially except by transplantation into volunteers and probably only one serotype exists. **West Nile virus.** An encephalitis virus isolated from a patient in Uganda. **Yellow fever virus.** A group B arbovirus transmitted by *Aëdes* mosquitoes. It can be grown readily in mice, cell culture and fertile eggs. In the chick embryo, attenuation of virulence occurs and the 17D vaccine strain is derived from mouse and egg passage. [L, poison.]

See also: BITTNER, DURAND (P.), EPSTEIN (M. A.), FRIEND, GRAFFI, GROSS (L.), MOLONEY (J. B.), RAUSCHER (F. J.), ROUS, SANARELLI, THEILER.

virusaemia (vi·rus·e·me·ah). Viraemia.

vis (vis) (pl. *vires*). Energy, power. **Vis conservatrix.** The innate strength of an organism enabling it to withstand disease or injury. **Vis formativa.** Reparative energy, healing power, creating new tissue to replace that destroyed. **Vis a fronte.** A force in front, pulling or impeding. **Vis inertia.** The inertia that keeps a body at rest. **Vis in situ.** Power inherent in the body. **Vis medicatrix naturae.** The natural ability of the organism to prevail over disease without external assistance. **Vis a tergo.** A force behind, pushing or retarding. **Vis vitae, Vis vitalis.** The life force. [L, force.]

See also: HELD.

visammin (vis·am·in). Khellin.

viscera (vis·er·ah). *See* VISCUS.

visceral (vis·er·al). Concerned with a viscus; of the nature of a viscus; splanchnic.

visceralgia (vis·er·al·je·ah). Pain experienced in a viscus. [viscus, Gk *algos* pain.]

visceralism (vis·er·al·izm). The theory that disease is visceral in origin.

viscerimotor (vis·er·e·mo'·tor). Visceromotor.

viscerogenic (vis·er·o·jen'·ik). Having origin in the viscera, as in certain reflexes. [viscus, Gk *genein* to produce.]

viscerography (vis·er·og·raf·e). Radiography of the viscera. A term not used in the UK.

viscero-inhibitory (vis·er·o·in·hib'·it·or·e). Inhibiting the movement or function of an organ. [viscus, inhibition.]

visceromotor (vis·er·o·mo'·tor). 1. Activating or controlling the functional movements of a viscus, as with the nerves involved in peristalsis. 2. Describing any movement in a part due to reflex stimulation from a viscus. [viscus, L *movere* to move.]

visceroparietal (vis·er·o·par·i'·et·al). Referring to any relationship between a viscus and the wall of the abdomen, as when an organ is sutured to the abdominal wall to remedy displacement. [viscus, L *paries* wall.]

visceropericardial (vis·er·o·per·e·kar'·de·al). Concerning the visceral portion of the serous pericardium.

visceroperitoneal (vis·er·o·per·it·o·ne'·al). Referring to the portion of the peritoneum that is reflected over the viscera.

visceropleural (vis·er·o·ploor'·al). Relating to that part of the pleura that invests the surface of the lung. [viscus, pleura.]

visceroptosis (vis·er·op·to·sis). A falling or displacement of the abdominal viscera, usually due to loss of tone by the pelvic and abdominal muscles. **Virginal visceroptosis.** The type of visceroptosis that occurs in the very thin person of the asthenic habitus and which is usually constitutional. [viscus, Gk *ptosis* a falling.]

viscerosensory (vis·er·o·sen'·sor·e). Concerning sensation in the viscera, or pain in a part attributable to disease in the underlying viscera.

visceroskeletal (vis·er·o·skel'·et·al). Pertaining to the visceral skeleton.

viscerosomatic (vis·er·o·so·mat'·ik). Concerning viscera and the body. [viscus, Gk *soma* body.]

viscerotome (vis·er·o·tome). 1. An instrument used at autopsies for cutting out a specimen from the liver or other internal organs for microscopic examination. 2. That part of an abdominal organ which has an afferent nerve supply from a single posterior root. [viscus, Gk *temnein* to cut.]

viscerotomy (vis·er·ot·o·me). The removal of a piece of liver *post mortem* by means of a viscerotome for examination for yellow fever. **Viscerotomy service.** A public health organization under whose auspices pieces of liver are taken from cadavers by means of a viscerotome, and examined histologically for evidence of yellow fever. In some South American countries this organization is supported by the Government and the examination is made compulsory in the case of death after a febrile illness. [see prec.]

viscerotonia (vis·er·o·to'·ne·ah). A variety of temperament described by Sheldon as being characterized by relaxation, conviviality, and gluttony for food, for company, and for affection, or social support. [viscus, Gk *tonos* tone.]

viscerotropic (vis·er·o·trop'·ik). Displaying attraction towards the viscera, as in the case of certain viruses. [viscus, Gk *trepein* to turn.]

viscid (vis·id). Sticky; semiliquid; having a glutinous consistency. [see foll.]

viscidity (vis·id·it·e). The quality of being viscid, glutinous, or gummy. [L *viscidus* sticky.]

viscidosis (vis·id·o·sis). Fibrocystic disease of the pancreas. [L *viscidus* sticky, Gk *-osis* condition.]

viscin (vis·in). A glutinous substance found in the berries of the mistletoe, *Viscum album*. [L *viscus* mistletoe.]

viscogel (vis·ko·jel). A gel which yields a viscid sol.

viscolizer (vis·ko·li·zer). Homogenizer. [L *viscosus* sticky.]

viscometer (vis·kom·et·er). An instrument for determining viscosity; used particularly with reference to the viscosity of the blood. [viscosity, meter.]

viscometry (vis·kom·et·re). Viscosimetry: the measurement and study of viscosity; used particularly with reference to viscosity of the blood. [see prec.]

viscose (vis·koze). A gelatinous substance obtained by the solution of cellulose in carbon disulphide and sodium hydroxide. It contains cellulose xanthate, and hardens in air to form a horny mass used as substitute for celluloid. If purified and pressed through dies, it forms artificial silk. [L *viscosus* sticky.]

viscosimeter (vis·ko·**sim**·et·er). Viscometer.

viscosimetry (vis·ko·**sim**·et·re). Viscometry.

viscosity (vis·**kos**·it·e). The property of a fluid whereby it resists the relative motion of its parts; the quality of being viscid or sticky. The term is also applied to the coefficient of viscosity, the ratio of the shearing force per unit area between two parallel layers of a liquid in motion, to the velocity gradient between the layers. This is usually symbolized by η. *Kinematic viscosity* is the ratio η/ρ where ρ is the density of the liquid. [L *viscosus* sticky.]

viscous (**vis**·kus). Sticky; glutinous; viscid; having marked viscosity. [see prec.]

viscum (**vis**·kum). A genus of plants of the family Loranthaceae. **Viscum album.** The European species of mistletoe; a parasitic shrub, particularly on the apple and other rosaceous fruit trees. It contains a glutinous substance, viscin, gum, and tannin. **Viscum flavescens.** The American species. [L *viscus* mistletoe.]

viscus [NA] (**vis**·kus) (pl. *viscera*). A term applied to the internal organs of the body which are closely related to, or contained within, one of the great serous cavities, pleural, pericardial, or peritoneal, and which are innervated by autonomic nerves. Some other organs, similarly innervated but not related to a serous cavity (e.g. the salivary glands), may also be referred to as viscera. [L.]

vision (**vizh**·un). In ophthalmology, the ability to see, and sometimes, loosely, the acuity of vision, commonly designated by *V*. Outside ophthalmology it is also used as a synonym for dreams, phantoms, prophetic insight, and apparitions. **Achromatic vision.** Vision without perception of colour, the world appearing as it does in a monochromatic photograph. It occurs in complete colour blindness, and in scotopic vision. **After vision.** Awareness of an after-image. **Anomalous trichromatic vision.** *See* TRICHROMATIC VISION (below). **Binocular vision.** That in which the retinal images from the two eyes are seen simultaneously either fused as one, double, or with part of one image suppressed. The following grades of binocular vision are recognized: *simultaneous macular perception, fusion, stereopsis.* **Central vision.** The ability to see with the central (macular) portion of the retina. **Chromatic vision.** Chromatopsia. **Daylight vision.** The type of vision experienced with a light-adapted (photopic) eye. **Defective vision.** Vision which fails to reach the accepted standard of normal in respect of perception of form or colour. **Dichromatic vision.** A form of colour blindness in which only two of the three primary colours are appreciated. **Direct vision.** Central vision (see above). **Double vision.** Diplopia. **Entoptic vision.** Visual perception of objects within the eyeball or produced by non-visual stimulation of the retina. **Facial vision.** Stimulation of the skin of the face by heat, enabling the subject to determine the location of its source. **Foveal vision.** The result of stimulation of the foveal (central) portion of the retina. **Half vision.** Hemianopia. **Halo vision.** The presence of an apparent coloured ring resembling a rainbow round a small source of light. It occurs in punctate cataract, some cases of glaucoma, and occasionally in conjunctivitis. **Haploscopic vision.** Perception of depth; stereoscopic vision. **Indirect vision.** Sensation aroused by stimulation of the extramacular portion of the retina. **Iridescent vision.** Halo vision (see above). **Monocular vision.** Seeing with one eye; preferably called *uni-ocular vision.* **Multiple vision.** Polyopia. **Night vision.** Vision in light of low intensity, using rods and visual purple. **Visual nul.** The presence in the visual field of a blind area of which the subject is not conscious. **Vision obscure.** The awareness of scotomata in the visual field. **Oscillating vision.** A state in which an object used in perimetry appears and disappears several times in the same meridian; usually a manifestation of hysteria, but it can occur in retinal exhaustion. **Panoramic vision.** A condition in which only a small fraction of the visual fields overlap. It occurs in the lower animals and is associated with an almost complete decussation of visual nerve fibres at the chiasma. **Peripheral vision.** That in which the image falls on the periphery of the retina, stimulating mostly rods and giving good appreciation of movement, but poor detail and no colour. **Photerythrous vision.** The type of dichromatic vision in which green is not appreciated; deuteranopia. **Photopic vision.** That which takes place in strong illumination, e.g. daylight. There is good appreciation of detail. It is chromatic and is carried out by the cones. **Pseudoscopic vision.** An illusion produced by reversing the pictures in a stereoscope so that far objects appear near, near ones far, and convex ones concave, or *vice versa.* **Qualitative vision.** Vision sufficient to permit the distinction of the qualities of objects (shape, size, colour, etc.). **Quantitative vision.** The power of distinguishing light from darkness. **Rainbow vision.** Halo vision (see above). **Rod vision.** The contribution of the rods to visual perception; also applied to states in which the cones are little, if at all, stimulated, e.g. in scotopic vision. **Scoterythrous vision.** The type of dichromatic vision in which red is not appreciated; protanopia. **Scotopic vision.** Vision in the dark-adapted eye. This is achromatic, from 50 to 100 000 times more sensitive than in the light-adapted eye, and occurs mainly in the peripheral rod-bearing retina. **Shaft vision.** Narrowing of the field of vision. **Solid vision, Stereoscopic vision.** Accurate depth perception in the presence of binocular single vision, due to the slight disparity in the two retinal images of the same object; also called *stereopsis.* **Trichromatic vision.** That in which all three primary colours, red, green, and blue, are appreciated normally; if there is only a partial appreciation of red or green it is known as *anomalous trichromatic vision.* **Tubular vision.** A term sometimes regarded as synonymous with *shaft vision* (see above) and *tunnel vision* (see below), but should be limited to a condition seen in hysteria. In this the area of field is the same whatever distance the eye is from the perimeter or screen, whereas in the normal person the area of field is proportional to the square of the distance at which it is taken, provided the target is not too small. **Tunnel vision.** That in which the visual fields show extreme general constriction to about 10 degrees from the fixation point. It is common in advanced chronic glaucoma and retinitis pigmentosa. Although the central visual acuity may remain good it is very incapacitating. It is sometimes used as a synonym for *tubular vision* which has a more specialized meaning. **Twilight vision.** Scotopic vision (see above). **Uni-ocular vision.** Monocular vision (see above). **Word vision.** The ability to see words. [L *visio* a seeing.]

See also: PICK (A.).

visna (**vis**·nah). A disease of Icelandic sheep of the Karakul breed, due to a *slow virus.* It is extinct as a wild disease following a slaughter policy, and is maintained only in virus laboratories. The incubation period ranges from months to years and is followed by a chronic progressive paralysis, ultimately leading to total paralysis and death. The virus contains ribonucleic acid, can be grown in sheep choroid plexus cells in culture, and is the best characterized slow virus to date. The virion is spherical and about 85 nm in diameter.

Visnadine (vis·nad·een). BP Commission approved name for 10 - acetoxy - 9,10 - dihydro - 8,8 - dimethyl - 9 - α - methylbutyryloxy - 2*H*,8*H* - benzo[1,2 - *b*=3,4 - *b*′] - dipyran - 2 - one; a coronary vasodilator.

visual (**vizh**·ew·al). Concerned with sight. The adjective is also employed in other senses, e.g. with regard to memory, when visual impressions are remembered better than auditory. **Visual acuity.** A measure of the resolving power of the eye, usually with regard to its power of distinguishing letters. Normal acuity of vision is taken as being the ability to distinguish block letters adequately lighted which subtend an angle of 5′ at the eye, the width of each stroke of the letter being 1′. In Europe the test is usually carried out at a distance of 6 m and the result expressed as a fraction, of which the numerator is the distance at which the test was performed, the denominator, the distance at which the letters seen should be read by a normal eye; 6/6 therefore is normal vision, 6/12, that the eye at 6 m reads letters which should be discernible at 12 metres. In America the distance is expressed in feet, and we have 20/20, 20/40 etc. **Visual efficiency.** A wider term than visual acuity, but applicable also to other functions of the eye such as colour vision, stereoscopic vision, power of dark adaptation, and size of fields of vision. **Visual reflex epilepsy.** A variety of epilepsy wherein attacks are precipitated by visual stimuli. Syn: light-sensitive epilepsy; photogenic epilepsy; photosensitive epilepsy. [L *visus* vision.]

visualization (**vizh**·ew·al·i·**za'**·shun). The process of formation of a visual mental image. **Double contrast visualization.** Mucosal-relief radiography. *See* RADIOGRAPHY.

visuo-auditory (**vizh**·ew·o·**aw'**·dit·or·e). Concerning seeing and hearing, as with the association fibres linking the visual and auditory areas of the brain. [L *visus* vision, *audire* to hear.]

visuognosis (**vizh**·ew·og·**no'**·sis). Knowing through visual characteristics. [L *visus* vision, Gk *gnosis* a knowing.]

visuometer (vizh·ew·**om**·et·er). An instrument devised by Smee in 1847 to measure the distance between the optical and geometrical centres of lenses. [L *visus* vision, meter.]

visuopsychic (**vizh**·ew·o·**si'**·kik). Pertaining to the visual association areas of the occipital cortex (Brodmann's areas 18 and 19). [L *visus* vision, Gk *psyche* mind.]

visuosensory (**vizh**·ew·o·**sen'**·so·re). Relating to the reception of visual impressions. [L *visus* vision, sensory.]

vitaglass (vi·tah·glahs). A special glass capable of transmitting ultraviolet rays which are absorbed by ordinary glass. It contains a high percentage of quartz. [L *vita* life, glass.]

vitagonist (vi·**tag**·on·ist). A vitamin antagonist.

Vitali, Dioscoride (b. 1832). Bologna pharmacologist.

Vitali's reaction, or test. For certain alkaloids: evaporate a small amount of alkaloid with a few drops of nitric acid to dryness in a porcelain dish. To the residue add a drop or two of alcoholic potassium hydroxide (10 per cent). A violet colour changing to red is given by atropine, hyoscine, and hyoscyamine, but not by homatropine. Strychnine and yohimbine also give violet colours.

vitalism (vi·tal·izm). A theory that ascribes the phenomenon of life to a specific vital force that is independent of physical or chemical causes. [L *vita* life.]

vitalist (vi·tal·ist). An exponent of the theory of vitalism.

vitalistic (vi·tal·**is**·tik). Concerned with the theory of vitalism.

vitality (vi·**tal**·it·e). 1. The capacity for living; being alive. 2. The vital principle of the theory of vitalism. [L *vita* life.]

vitallium (vi·**tal**·e·um). An alloy of cobalt, chromium, and molybdenum used in surgery, especially for making movable joints in ossified conditions such as rheumatoid arthritis. [L *vita* life, alloy.]

vitamer (vi·tam·er). A term which has been applied to natural or synthetic compounds which are structurally related to particular vitamins and possess some degree of specific biological activity. [L *vita* life, Gk *meros* part.]

vitameter (vi·**tam**·et·er). An instrument which has been especially adapted to the determination of a vitamin. [vitamin, meter.]

vitamin (vi·tam·in). Any constituent of diet other than protein, fat, carbohydrate, and inorganic salts, which is necessary for maintenance of normal growth and activity and which the body must obtain from external sources. An inadequate dietary supply of a vitamin leads to a typical deficiency disease. **Anti-dermatitis vitamin.** Vitamin B_6. **Anti-haemorrhagic vitamin.** Vitamin K. **Anti-infection vitamin.** Vitamin A. **Anti-neuritic vitamin.** Vitamin B_1. **Anti-pellagra vitamin.** Nicotinic acid: *see* VITAMIN B. **Anti-rachitic vitamin.** Vitamin D. **Anti-scorbutic vitamin.** Vitamin C. **Anti-sterility vitamin.** Vitamin E. **Anti-xerophthalmic vitamin.** Vitamin A. **Fertility vitamin.** Vitamin E. **Pellagra-preventing vitamin, P-P vitamin.** Nicotinic acid: *see* VITAMIN B. **Permeability vitamin.** Vitamin P. [L *vita* life, amine.]

vitamin A. $(CH_3)_3C_6H_6CH{=}CHC(CH_3){=}CHCHCHC(CH_3){=}CHCH_2OH$, a fat-soluble unsaturated alcohol, two molecules of which are formed by hydrolysis of one molecule of β-carotene. Carotenes are converted to vitamin A in the liver, and the carotene of vegetable foods therefore forms a valuable source of the vitamin. Vitamin A is present in butter fat and in yolk of egg, but the most prolific source is fish-liver oil, particularly that of the halibut. The characteristic effects of vitamin-A deficiency are xeroma and night blindness, keratinization of the epithelial tissues, and susceptibility to infection. Excessive amounts of the vitamin are toxic. **Vitamin A_1.** Vitamin A (see above). **Vitamin A_2.** Type of vitamin A occurring in the tissues of fresh-water fish and not present in salt-water fish or mammals. It has specific vitamin-A activity, and is distinguished by differences in its ultraviolet-absorption spectrum. **Vitamin A ester concentrate.** "An ester or a mixture of esters of vitamin A alcohol, or a solution of the ester or mixture of esters in arachis oil or other suitable vegetable oil; esters of natural or synthetic origin or mixtures of such esters may be used" (BP 1968). Its action and uses are those of vitamin A.

vitamin B. Originally thought to be a mixture of watersoluble substances and is now referred to as the *vitamin-B complex.* Factors so far identified are: 1. Thiamine (*see* VITAMIN B_1); 2. Riboflavine (*see* VITAMIN B_2); 3. Pyridoxine (*see* VITAMIN B_6); 4. Folic acid (*see* VITAMIN B_c); 5. Biotin (*see* VITAMIN H); 6. *p*-Aminobenzoic acid (*see* VITAMIN B_x); 7. Vitamin B_{12}; 8. Nicotinic acid, pyridine β-carboxylic acid C_5H_4NCOOH: a substance essential in human nutrition, deficiency of which gives rise to pellagra; normal adult daily requirement is from 10 to 20 mg. (*See* ACID, NICOTINIC); 9. Pantothenic acid, $HOCH_2C(CH_3)_2CHOHCONHCH_2COOH$. A substance, deficiency of which produces in animals dermatitis, keratitis, adrenal atrophy, and haemorrhage, growth arrest, and depigmentation of hair. (*see* ACID, PANTOTHENIC); 10. Inositol, hexahydroxycyclohexane, $C_6H_6(OH)_6$. 11. Choline, ethanol-trimethylammonium hydroxide, $HON(CH_3)_3C_2H_4OH$. This substance is chiefly effective in the mobilization of fat in the body. Deficiency leads to fatty liver ultimately developing into hepatic cirrhosis, and also to renal haemorrhages (*see* CHOLINE). **Vitamin B_1.** Thiamine Hydrochloride BP 1968; thiamine hydrochloride; a water-soluble compound built up from a combination of pyrimidine and thiazole nuclei and having the structural formula $CH{=}NC(CH_3){=}NC(NH_2){=}CCH_2N(Cl){=}CHSC(CH_2CH_2OH){=}C(CH_3)$. Its chief sources are yeast and the germ and bran of cereals from which concentrates are made, whilst meat and animal products, fruit and vegetables all provide moderate amounts. Deficiency of vitamin B_1 gives rise to beriberi, minimal daily requirement being from 1 to 2 mg. Excessive doses have toxic effects. **Vitamin B_2.** Riboflavine BP 1968, lactoflavine, vitamin G, 6,7-dimethyl-9(D-1'-ribityl)-isoalloxazine, $C_{17}H_{20}O_6H_4$. A yellow crystalline powder, soluble in normal saline, slightly soluble in alcohol, but insoluble in ether. Its physiological function lies in its importance in flavoprotein enzyme systems, and it is required by all young animals for growth. It occurs chiefly in yeast, eggs, milk, and malt. Deficiency is characterized by any or all of the following symptoms: cheilosis, glossitis, stomatitis, seborrhoeic dermatitis, photophobia, and corneal vascularization. Minimal daily requirement is from 1.8 to 3 mg. **Vitamin B_6.** Pyridoxine Hydrochloride BPC 1959, 2-methyl-3-hydroxy-4,5-di(hydroxymethyl)-pyridine hydrochloride, $(CH_2OH)_2C_5HN(OH)(CH_3)HCl$. A white, crystalline powder, soluble in water, occurring in yeast, liver, cereals, legumes, and milk. Its absence from the diet produces dermatitis in rats, but there is little evidence with regard to its effect in human nutrition. **Vitamin B_8.** Adenylic acid: the term vitamin B_8 has been used in this connection, but it has not been satisfactorily proved that adenylic acid is actually a vitamin. **Vitamin B_{12}.** Cyanocobalamin BP 1968. Several fractions of vitamin B_{12} have been separated and claims made for their heterogeneity, e.g. vitamin $B_{12}a$, hydroxocobalamin, probably the anhydro- form of vitamin $B_{12}b$; vitamin $B_{12}b$, aquocobalamin, probably identical with vitamin $B_{12}a$; vitamin $B_{12}c$, nitritocobalamin; vitamin $B_{12}d$, almost certainly identical with vitamin $B_{12}b$. **Vitamin B_c.** Folic Acid BP 1968, pteroylglutamic acid, $C_{15}H_{15}O_8N_5$, a bright-yellow crystalline solid, slightly soluble in water, occurring in liver, in the green leaves of plants, and in yeast. It is present in the form of various conjugates which possess differing chemical and physical properties as well as different physiological potency, and has therefore been described under a number of names. Deficiency in animals gives rise to anaemia, leucopenia, and agranulocytosis. It is used in the treatment of pernicious anaemia, sprue, nutritional anaemia, and macrocytic anaemias of infancy and pregnancy. **Vitamin B_c conjugate.** Folic acid conjugate; folic acid occurs naturally in animal and plant materials chiefly in the form of conjugates from which free folic acid is liberated by the action of specific enzymes. The conjugates are microbiologically inactive. **Vitamin B_x.** *p*-Aminobenzoic acid, $NH_2C_6H_4COOH$, a compound essential to the growth of certain micro-organisms including *Streptococcus pyogenes* and *Brucella abortus.* There is no evidence of any human dietary requirement of this substance.

vitamin C. Ascorbic Acid BP 1968, cevitamic acid, COC(OH)= C(OH)CHCHOHCH$_2$OH (ring closed through O); the enol form of 3-keto-*l*-gulofuranolactone. A colourless, crystalline substance, soluble in water, occurring chiefly in fruits and vegetables. It is specific in the treatment of scurvy, and is given as a prophylactic in all conditions where metabolism is accelerated or where diet is restricted. The minimum daily requirement is 30 mg.

vitamin D. A term applied to substances having antirachitic properties which are produced by ultraviolet irradiation of certain sterols. The most important compounds are those obtained by irradiation of ergosterol and 7-dehydrocholesterol. The chief natural sources of vitamin D are the fish-liver oils, animal fats such as butter, and eggs. **Vitamin D_1.** The name given to the particular form of vitamin D first isolated. It was a mixture of calciferol and lumisterol. **Vitamin D_2.** Calciferol BP 1968, viosterol, irradiated ergosterol, $C_{28}H_{43}OH$. The colourless, odourless, tasteless, crystalline, antirachitic substance obtained by ultraviolet irradiation of ergosterol. Insoluble in water, but soluble in oils and most organic solvents; it is specific in the treatment of rickets, spasmophilia, and osteomalacia. Excessive dosage leads to toxic symptoms. **Vitamin D_3.** $C_{27}H_{44}O$, an antirachitic substance, prepared by the ultraviolet irradiation of 7-dehydrocholesterol, which has greater biological activity than calciferol. It has been isolated from tunny-liver oil.

vitamin E. The oil-soluble substance, occurring in the germ oil of cereals and in green leaves, which has been termed the antisterility factor. It is essential to normal reproductivity in rats in both male and female, but the value of vitamin-E therapy in humans is indefinite. The chief active principle of vitamin-E preparations is α-tocopherol; β- and γ-tocopherols are also present, but possess less biological activity.

vitamin G. Riboflavine. [Obsolete term.]

vitamin H. Biotin, co-enzyme R, 2-keto-3,4-imidazolido-2-tetrahydrothiophene-*n*-valeric acid, $C_{10}H_{16}N_2O_3S$. A crystalline substance occurring in liver and yeast. It is essential for the growth of yeast and is the anti-egg-white factor which prevents dermatitis in rats fed upon raw egg-white. There is no definite information with regard to human requirements of this substance.

vitamin K. A factor necessary for the biosynthesis of prothrombin and for maintaining the level of plasma prothrombin. Two natural substances having the specific activity have been isolated, vitamin K_1 from lucerne and horse-chestnut leaves, and vitamin K_2 from rotted fishmeal. Both are derivatives of 1,4-naphthoquinone, vitamin K_1 being the 2-methyl-3-phytyl derivative and vitamin K_2 the 2-methyl-3-farnesyl derivative. A synthetic substance menaphthone, 2-methyl-1,4-naphthoquinone, is prepared commercially for use in the treatment of the haemorrhage of obstructive jaundice, neonatal haemorrhage, and to combat hypoprothrombinaemia produced by drug therapy. Other substituted 1,4-naphthoquinones show vitamin-K activity.

vitamin L. Two factors, L_1 and L_2, have been reported to be essential to lactation in rats, but are so far unidentified.

vitamin M. An anti-anaemia factor in monkeys, identified as folic acid.

vitamin P. A factor regulating the permeability of the blood capillaries. Its exact nature is in dispute, the present choice being between hesperidin and rutin. Both substances have been used in the treatment of increased capillary fragility, but rutin has the more favourable reports.

vitaminogenic (vi·tam·in·o·**jen**′·ik). 1. Producing vitamins. 2. Attributable to vitamins. [vitamin, Gk *genein* to produce.]

vitaminoid (vi·tam·in·oid). Having the characteristics of a vitamin; vitamin-like. [vitamin, Gk *eidos* form.]

vitanition (vi·tan·**ish**·un). Malnutrition due to a deficiency of vitamins: an unsatisfactory word. [vitamin, Gk *an-* without.]

vitellarium (vi·tel·a·re·um). An accessory sexual gland which secretes food reserves for eggs, particularly a diffuse gland in tapeworms. [L *vitellus* yolk.]

vitellary (vi·**tel**·ar·e). Pertaining to the vitellus; vitelline.

vitellin (vi·**tel**·in). The major protein of egg yolk. It is a phosphoprotein containing 15.2 per cent of nitrogen and 2.29 per cent of phosphorus pentoxide. [see foll.]

vitelline (vi·**tel**·ine). Referring to the yolk of an egg. [L *vitellus* yolk.]

vitellogenesis (vi·tel·o·**jen**′·es·is). Yolk production. [L *vitellus* yolk, Gk *genein* to produce.]

vitellomesenteric (vi·tel·o·mes·en·**ter**′·ik). Relating to the yolk sac and the mesentery. [L *vitellus* yolk, mesentery.]

vitellus (vi·**tel**·us). The yolky part of an egg, consisting chiefly of fatty substances, including phospholipide and cholesterol esters, and various conjugated proteins, pigments, salts and water. The vitellus serves as a reserve store of nutriment for the developing embryo. [L.]

vitex (vi·tex). A genus of shrubs of the family Verbenaceae. Several species are stated to act as febrifuges. **Vitex agnuscastus** Linn. A Mediterranean species used as a poultice. [L, the chaste-tree.]

vitiligines (vit·il·**ij**·in·eez). The glistening white lines seen in the abdominal wall as a result of abdominal distension. Usually caused by pregnancy. [vitiligo.]

vitiliginous (vit·il·**ij**·in·us). Having the features of vitiligo, or affected with it.

vitiligo (vit·il·**i**·go). Idiopathic leucoderma; an acquired failure of pigmentation in which sharply demarcated areas of skin become depigmented, giving a piebald appearance. **Vitiligo acquisita syphilitica.** Syphilitic vitiligo (see below). **Vitiligo capitis.** 1. Vitiligo of the scalp with depigmentation of the hairs on the leucodermatous areas. 2. Alopecia areata. **Vitiligo iridis.** Small white patches seen in the iris due to depigmentation. They often follow tuberculous and herpetic iritis, and occasionally smallpox. **Perinaevic vitiligo.** Vitiligo surrounding a naevus. **Syphilitic vitiligo.** Leucoderma, especially of the neck, occurring during the secondary stage of syphilis. [L, a cutaneous eruption.]

See also: CELSUS.

vitiligoid (vit·**il**·ig·oid). Resembling vitiligo in appearance. [vitiligo, Gk *eidos* form.]

vitiligoidea (vit·il·ig·**oid**′·e·ah). An archaic word used by Addison and Gull to denote xanthoma. **Vitiligoidea planum.** Xanthelasma palpebrarum. **Vitiligoidea tuberosum.** Xanthoma tuberosum multiplex. [vitiligo, Gk *eidos* form.]

vitis (vi·tis). A genus of plants which includes the common grape vine. [L.]

vitium (**vish**·e·um). A defect or vice. **Vitium caducum.** Epilepsy. **Vitium conformationis.** A malformation. **Vitium cordis.** Organic deformity of the heart. **Vitium primae formationis.** Deformity arising before birth. [L, vice.]

vitochemical (vi·to·**kem**·ik·al). Biochemical; of the nature of the chemistry of living matter. Organic. [L *vita* life, chemistry.]

vitodynamic (vi·to·di·**nam**′·ik). Relating to active vital processes. [L *vita* life, *dynamis* force.]

vitreocapsulitis (vit·re·o·kap·sew·**li**′·tis). A condition supposed to be caused by inflammation of the posterior capsule of the lens where it lies in contact with the vitreous [obsolete term]. [vitreous, capsule, Gk *-itis* inflammation.]

vitreous (**vit**·re·us). 1. Resembling glass; hyaline. 2. The vitreous body. **Anterior vitreous.** The embryonic substance lying between the lens vesicle and the surface epithelium, later giving rise to the ectodermal basis of the cornea. **Artificial vitreous.** The glass ball inserted into the sclera following evisceration. *See* MULES' OPERATION. **Fluid vitreous.** That which is of fluid consistency instead of jelly-like. It is caused by degeneration and is most commonly seen in high myopia, senility, and inflammatory conditions of the eye. Also called *synchysis.* **Primary vitreous.** That which originally lies between the neural ectoderm and the surface ectoderm. This becomes vascularized by the hyaloid artery and is finally pushed forwards to the centre of the eye behind the lens by the formation behind it of the secondary vitreous. **Secondary vitreous.** That formed behind the anterior vitreous (see above) by the inner layer of the optic cup; it fills the remainder of the vitreous cavity. **Tertiary vitreous.** That formed after the secondary vitreous (see prec.), and anterior to it in the ciliary region. It later forms the fibres of the zonule. [L *vitreus* glassy.]

vitrescence (vit·res·ens). The state of becoming like glass. [L *vitrum* glass.]

vitreum (vit·re·um). The vitreous body of the eyeball; a mass of jelly-like consistency lying between the retina and the crystalline lens. [L *vitreus* glassy.]

vitriol (vit·re·ol). 1. Sulphates of certain metals [obsolete term]. 2. Sulphuric acid. **Blue vitriol.** Blue stone, copper sulphate, $CuSO_4.5H_2O$. **Green vitriol.** Copperas, ferrous sulphate, $FeSO_4.7H_2O$. **White vitriol.** Zinc sulphate, $ZnSO_4$. [L *vitrum* glass.]

vitriolated (vit·re·ol·a′·ted). 1. Mixed with a sulphate or sulphuric acid. 2. Converted into a sulphate or sulphuric acid. [vitriol.]

vitriolation (vit·re·ol·a′·shun). 1. The transformation of a substance into a glass-like form. [L *vitrum* glass.] 2. The conversion of a substance into a sulphate or sulphuric acid; admixture with the latter. [vitriol.]

vitritis (vit·ri·tis). Glaucoma [obsolete term]. [L *vitrum* glass, Gk *-itis* inflammation.]

vitrodentine (vit·ro·den·teen). A coarse type of dentine containing very few tubules. [L *vitrum* glass, dentine.]

vitropression (vit·ro·presh·un). Blanching of the skin by pressure with a strip of glass, in order to reveal any abnormal discoloration not due to hyperaemia. [L *vitrum* glass, pressure.]

vitrosin (vit·ro·sin). A collagen-like component of the vitreous humour of the eye. [L *vitreus* glassy.]

vitular, vitulary, vituline (vit·ew·lar, vit·ew·lar·e, vit·ew·line). Concerning a calf or calving. [L *vitellus* calf.]

vividialysis (viv·e·di·al′·is·is). Dialysis through a living membrane. [L *vivus* alive, dialysis.]

vividiffusion (viv·e·dif·ew′·zhun). The removal of diffusable substances from the blood of living animals by passing it through collodion tubes in continuity with the blood vessels. The tubes are immersed in a saline solution so constituted that only waste substances dialyse out of the blood. [L *vivus* alive, diffusion.]

viviparity (viv·ip·ar·it·e). The ability to produce living young without preliminary hatching. [see foll.]

viviparous (viv·ip·ar·us). Able to produce young that require no hatching and which move about from birth. [L *vivus* alive, *parere* to bring forth.]

vivipation (viv·ip·a·shun). Generation that proceeds fully in the womb and produces young which display life from birth. [see prec.]

vivisect (viv·e·sekt). To perform an operation on a living animal. [L *vivus* alive, *secare* to cut.]

vivisection (viv·e·sek·shun). The use of living animals for experimental purposes; essentially the performance of experimental surgical operations upon living animals. [see prec.]

vivisectionist, vivisector (viv·e·sek·shun·ist, viv·e·sek·tor). A person who performs vivisection, or an advocate of vivisection for its experimental value.

Vladimiroff, Vladimir Dmitriyevich (b. 1837). Moscow surgeon.

Vladimiroff-Mikulicz amputation, or operation. An osteoplastic resection of the heel; the talus and the calcaneum are removed and to the lower end of the tibia is apposed the anterior row of tarsal bones.

Vleminckx, Jean François (b. 1800). Brussels military surgeon.

Vleminckx's solution. A solution of sulphuretted lime, prepared by boiling sulphur with slaked lime and water. It is used in scabies and as a fungicide in horticulture.

vocal (vo·kal). 1. Pertaining to the voice or the organs of speech. 2. Uttered by or performed with the voice. **Vocal muscle.** The thyro-arytenoid muscle. [L *vocalis* of the voice.]

vocalis muscle [musculus vocalis (NA)] (vo·ka·lis musl). The lower and deeper fibres of the thyro-arytenoid muscle which are attached to the vocal processes of the arytenoid cartilage.

vodka (vod·kah). The Russian national beverage, prepared by the distillation of fermented liquors obtained from maize, potatoes, rye, or barley. It is neither matured, flavoured, nor coloured, and contains about 46 per cent v/v ethyl alcohol. Vodka is not used in medicine. [Russian.]

Voegtlin, Carl (b. 1879). Washington pharmacologist.

Voegtlin unit. That quantity of a substance which must be used to produce a contraction of the isolated guinea-pig uterus of the same size as would 0.5 mg of standard posterior pituitary powder.

Voelcker, Fritz (b. 1872). Heidelberg surgeon.

Voelcker and Joseph test. Indigocarmine test. *See* TEST.

Voges, Otto (b. 1867). Berlin physician.

Voges-Proskauer reaction. A reaction involving the production of acetylmethylcarbinol by the typhoid group of organisms, and not by the coliform group. A culture of the organism in glucose broth is made alkaline with potassium hydroxide; a red colour slowly develops when positive.

Vogt, Alfred (b. 1879). Zürich ophthalmologist.

Posterior saucer-shaped cataract of Vogt. Posterior corneal opacities which appear saucer-shaped on slit-lamp examination. It is a common type of senile corneal cataract.

Arcuate line of Vogt. A small, white, crescentic line seen at the posterior pole of the lens of the eye and thought to represent the reflection of Cloque's canal.

Vogt's operation. 1. For detached retina: galvanic current using the cathode as a penetrating needle, i.e. electrolysis. 2. For glaucoma: diathermy over the region of the ciliary body. Also called *cyclodiathermy.*

Vogt, Cécile (b. 1875). German neurologist.

Vogt-Koyanagi syndrome. Uveitis, alopecia, detachment of the retinae, deafness, and vitiligo of the hands and feet.

Spielmeyer-Vogt disease, Vogt-Spielmeyer disease. The juvenile form of cerebromacular degeneration.

Vogt, Karl (b. 1817). German naturalist and physiologist.

Vogt's angle. The angle at the nasion between lines joining the latter and the prosthion and basion, respectively.

Vogt, Oskar (b. 1870). Berlin neurologist.

Vogt's disease, or syndrome. Emotional lability, bilateral athetosis and rhythmical movements of the limbs with no paralysis, sensory loss, or mental impairment, due to degeneration of the corpus striatum. Also called the *syndrome of double athetosis.*

Vogt, Paul Friedrich Emmanuel (b. 1847). Greifswald surgeon.

Vogt's point, Vogt-Hueter point. A point at the intersection of a horizontal line two finger-breadths above the zygoma with a vertical line a thumb-breadth behind the external angular process of the frontal bone. It is one site for trephining to arrest middle meningeal haemorrhage.

voice (vois). The sounds produced by the vocal cords and given quality and timbre by resonance. **Amphoric voice, Cavernous voice.** Exaggerated bronchophony heard over a large cavity. **Double voice.** A vocal freak; an extensive vocal range covering as much as four octaves and the timbre of the voice changing throughout the register. **Eunuchoid voice.** Failure of the development of the adult male voice at puberty, due to some disturbance of the sex glands. **Nasal voice.** A speech defect usually an imperfect nasal resonance, but it may be functional. If the resonance is too great, the condition is known as *hyperrhinolalia* or *rhinolalia aperta,* and occurs in such conditions as cleft palate. Too little resonance, as may occur in obstructions due to polypi or adenoid hypertrophy, is accompanied by the voice defect of *hyporhinolalia* or *rhinolalia clausa.* **Ventricular-**

fold voice. Abnormal voice produced by the ventricular folds (false vocal cords) or as a substitute for the note normally produced by the true vocal cords. **Whispered voice.** Articulated voice sounds in which the glottis plays no part. It is used in vocal resonance for pectoriloquy. [L *vox*.]

Voigt, Christian August (b. 1809). Vienna anatomist.

Voigt's lines. Lines marking the boundary of peripheral nerves.

Voillemier, Léon Clémont 20th century French urologist.

Voillemier's point. A point on the linea alba from 6 to 7 cm below a line joining the anterior superior iliac spines, designating the site for suprapubic puncture of the bladder in fat or oedematous individuals.

Voisenet-Rhode reaction. The reaction of aromatic aldehydes with tryptophan.

Voit, Karl von (b. 1831). Munich physiologist.

Voit's nucleus. A nucleus accessory to the dentate nucleus of the cerebellum.

Voit, Max (b. 1876). Göttingen anatomist.

Voit's nerve. A branch of the vestibular division of the auditory nerve supplying the macula of the saccule.

vola (vo·lah). The palm; the sole. **Vola manus.** The palm of the hand. **Vola pedis.** The sole of the foot. [L.]

volar (vo·lar). Concerning the palm of the hand or the sole of the foot; palmar, plantar. **Volar surface.** The flexor surface of the forearm or the wrist. [see prec.]

volardorsal (vo·lar·dor·sal). Referring to volar and dorsal surfaces.

volatile (vol·at·ile). Having a ready tendency to evaporate; having a high vapour pressure. [L *volatilis* flying.]

volatility (vol·at·il·it·e). The capacity of a liquid to volatilize. **Volatility product.** The product of the concentrations of vapours when in equilibrium with their liquids.

volatilization (vol·at·il·i·za′·shun). The passing of a liquid into vapour form. [L *volatilis* flying.]

volatilize (vol·at·il·ize). 1. To cause a liquid to vaporize. 2. To become a vapour. [see prec.]

volatilizer (vol·at·il·i·zer). An apparatus designed to achieve the volatilization of liquids.

vole (vole). Small rodents of the genera *Clethrionomys* and *Microtus*. Species of *Microtus* have been found infected with sylvatic plague in north-western America. The European short-tailed field vole is *Microtus agrestis*. [Scand. *voll* field.]

Volhard, Franz (b. 1872). **German physician.**

Volhard's test. Urine-concentration test. *See* TEST.

Volhard and Arnold method. For chlorides in urine: the urine is acidified with nitric acid, excess of standard silver nitrate solution is added, and the solution is filtered. The excess silver nitrate in the filtrate is determined by titration with thiocyanate, using ferric alum solution as indicator.

Fahr–Volhard disease, Volhard–Fahr disease. Malignant hypertension. *See* HYPERTENSION.

Volhard and Harvey method. For chlorides in urine: the same as Volhard and Arnold method (above) except that filtration of the precipitated chloride is omitted.

Volhard, J. (b. 1834). German chemist.

Volhard's solution. A decinormal solution of potassium or ammonium thiocyanate, used for the determination of silver nitrate, mercury, and halides.

volition (vo·lish·un). The exercise of the will in choosing to perform or abstain from any action. [L *velle* to wish.]

volitional (vo·lish·un·al). Referring to volition; performed by volition.

Volkmann, Alfred Wilhelm (b. 1800). Halle physiologist.

Volkmann's canals. Canals in bone which transmit blood vessels from the surface to the more deeply situated and smaller haversian canals.

Volkmann, Richard von (b. 1830). German surgeon.

Volkmann's cheilitis. The suppurative form of glandular cheilitis.

Volkmann's contracture. Fixed deformity due to fibrosis of muscle following injury to its blood supply, usually affecting the hand.

Volkmann's operation. An incision of the tunica vaginalis testis for hydrocele.

Volkmann's paralysis. Ischaemic paralysis. *See* PARALYSIS.

Volkmann's spoon. A spoon with a sharp edge, used to scrape away granulations.

volley (vol·e). The simultaneous discharge of nerve impulses arising from a group of central neurones and passing along a number of different axons to a single organ. **Antidromic volley.** Any volley of impulses travelling along a nerve in a direction opposite to the usual one, e.g. centrifugal impulses in a sensory nerve. It may be naturally or experimentally induced. [Fr. *volée*.]

Vollmer, Hermann (b. 1896). New York paediatrician.

Vollmer's patch test. A test consisting of a strip with three small squares of thin lint, of which the two outer squares have been treated with (*a*) human- and (*b*) bovine-type tuberculin. The centre patch is a control with uninoculated broth medium. The strip, which has adhesive edges, is then applied to the cleansed skin between the shoulder blades. A reddened papular reaction under either of the tuberculinized squares occurs in 48 hours if the patient has had a tuberculous lesion. Used mainly in small children. The patches are supplied as a proprietary preparation.

volsella (vol·sel·ah). Vulsella; a forceps whose blades are tipped with sharp right-angled points directed inwards. [L, pincers.]

volt (volt). The unit of potential difference or electromotive force; defined as the potential difference between two points of a conducting wire carrying a constant current of 1 ampere, when the power dissipated between these points is equal to 1 watt. Symbol V. **Electron volt.** A unit of energy equal to the kinetic energy acquired by an electron in passing through a potential difference of 1 volt in vacuum; 1 $eV = 1.60219 \times 10^{-19} J$ (1.60×10^{-12}erg). Symbol eV. [Count Alessandro *Volta*.]

Volta, Count Alessandro (b. 1745). Italian physicist and physiologist.

Volta effect. When two dissimilar metals are placed in contact with one another in air, one acquires a positive potential with respect to the other.

voltage (volt·ij). Electrical potential expressed in volts. **Constant voltage.** In radiological practice, a term applied to a unidirectional voltage which has small periodic variations. The periodic component is called the *ripple voltage*. **Effective voltage.** For an alternating potential, equal to the root mean square value; for a sine wave this equals $1/\sqrt{2}$ of the peak value. **Inverse voltage.** The voltage applied to an electrical component from an alternating supply during the half-cycle in which conduction through the component is a minimum. **Peak voltage.** The maximum voltage of a direct pulsating supply, or of an alternating supply usually taken in the half-cycle in which conduction occurs. **Pulsating voltage.** A unidirectional potential which undergoes periodic variations in magnitude at a frequency related to that of the mains supply. **Ripple voltage.** *See* CONSTANT VOLTAGE (above). **Unidirectional voltage.** A constant or pulsating voltage which does not change in polarity.

voltagram (volt·ah·gram). A voltaic battery designed to give an approximately constant voltage. [voltaic, Gk *gramma* a record.]

voltaic (volt·a·ik). A term used formerly to distinguish the phenomena of the current electricity produced by a primary battery from those of static electricity. [Count Alessandro *Volta*.]

voltaism (volt·a·izm). Galvanism. Chemical electricity; the phenomena peculiar to the electricity generated by the voltaic cell.

voltameter (vol·tam·et·er). Coulometer. A U-tube fitted with electrodes and used for the electrolysis of water; also extended to include cells in which electrolytic deposition of metals takes place. So-called because the amount of gas liberated, or metal deposited, can serve to measure the current that has passed. [voltaic, meter.]

voltammeter (vol·tam·et·er). An electrical measuring instrument which gives readings of both the voltage and amperage of a current.

voltampere (volt·**am**·pare). The product of a volt and an ampere.

voltmeter (**volt**·me·ter). An electrical measuring instrument which gives direct readings of electromotive force in volts. It is a form of moving-coil galvanometer with a high-resistance incorporated, and is used in parallel with the circuit. **Electrostatic voltmeter.** An instrument for the measurement of potential which works by the electrostatic forces existing between electric charges; steady reading may be obtained on the instrument without taking current from the source of potential. **Sphere gap voltmeter.** An instrument for determination of the peak voltage of a high-potential supply, as used for an x-ray tube. The distance between polished metal spheres at which a spark will pass determines the peak voltage under known atmospheric conditions.

Voltolini, Friedrich Eduard Rudolph (b. 1819). Breslau otorhinolaryngologist.

Voltolini's disease. Otitis media purulenta chronica.

Voltolini's sign, Voltolini–Heryng sign. Heryng's sign.

volume (vol·ewm). The space occupied by anything; cubic capacity. **Atomic volume.** The atomic weight of a liquid or solid element divided by its density (specific gravity); the volume in cubic centimetres of the atomic weight in grams. **Blood volume.** The volume of whole blood in the body, comprising the volume of the red and white cells (*cell volume*) and the plasma volume. The blood volume weighs approximately 9 per cent, the cell volume 4 per cent, and the plasma volume 5 per cent of the total body weight. The whole blood volume of an average adult is in the region of 6 litres, and comprises the blood in rapid circulation (*circulating blood volume*) and that which is in reserve in blood depots, in extensive capillary networks in the skin, and in the spleen and liver. **Cell volume.** *See* BLOOD VOLUME (preceding). **Circulating blood volume, Circulation volume.** The volume of blood which is in rapid circulation in the vascular compartment at any one time. **Dead-space volume.** 1. *Anatomical*: extending from the nostrils or mouth down to, but not including, the alveoli. 2. *Physiological*: a space occupied by air not available for respiratory exchange; it cannot be measured directly but can be estimated from the Bohr equation: physiological dead space equals

$$V_T \; \frac{P_aCO_2 - P_ECO_2}{P_aCO_2}$$

where V_T equals the tidal volume, P_aCO_2 equals tension of CO_2 in arterial blood, and P_ECO_2 equals the tension of CO_2 in expired air. **Gram-molecular volume.** The volume of one gram-molecule of a gas, which is the same for all gases at 0°C and 760 mm; 22.415 litres. **Mean corpuscular volume.** MCV, the mean volume of a single erythrocyte (in cubic microns) and obtained from

$$\frac{\text{Vol. of packed erythrocytes (ml per litre blood).}}{\text{No. of erythrocytes (millions per cu.mm).}}$$

The normal range is 78 to 94 c.μm (mean 86 c.μm). **Minute volume.** 1. The volume of air inspired per minute. 2. The volume of blood expelled from the left ventricle in one minute; also known as the *cardiac output*. **Molecular volume.** The volume of the gram-molecular weight of a substance. The molecular volumes of all gases are equal at a given pressure and temperature. **Packed-cell volume.** PCV, in a measured quantity of blood to which an anticoagulant has been added, the volume of red cells after being "packed" by means of a centrifuge revolving at 2000 revolutions per minute. It is usually expressed as a percentage; the normal is from 45 to 48 per cent. Also called the *haematocrit reading*. **Plasma volume.** The volume of the plasma in the body (about 5 per cent of the total body weight). *See also* BLOOD VOLUME (above). **Residual volume.** The volume of air remaining in the lungs at the end of a maximal expiration. **Specific volume.** The volume in ml of a gramme of a substance. **Stroke volume.** The volume of blood expelled from the left ventricle with each beat of the heart; it is estimated by dividing the minute volume by the heart rate. **Tidal volume.** In respiration, the volume of the tidal air. [L *volumen* roll of papyrus.]

volumebolometer (**vol**·ewm·bo·**lom**'·et·er). Volume-sphygmobolometer.

volumenometer (**vol**·ew·men·**om**'·et·er). Volumometer.

volumesphygmobolometer (**vol**·ewm·sfig·mo·bo·**lom**'·et·er). An apparatus designed by Sahli for measuring the volume of the pulse. [volume, Gk *sphygmos* pulse, *bolos* mass, meter.]

volumetric (vol·ew·**met**·rik). 1. Pertaining to the measurement of liquid or gaseous volumes. 2. Achieved by the measurement of liquid volumes, as in volumetric analysis.

volumometer (vol·ew·**mom**·et·er). 1. A specific-gravity bottle; a pyknometer. 2. A device for measuring the volume occupied by any solid body. 3. Any apparatus for measuring the growth of a plant or animal. 4. A device for measuring the tidal exchange of the lungs. [volume, meter.]

voluntary (**vol**·un·tar·e). Under the power of the will. [L *voluntarius* voluntary.]

voluntomotory (**vol**·un·to·**mo**'·tor·e). Concerned with volitional movement. [L *voluntas* will, *movere* to move.]

volute (**vol**·ewt). 1. A scroll or scroll-shaped formation. 2. Furled like a scroll; convoluted. [L *voluta* scroll.]

volutin (vol·**ew**·tin). Granules of uncertain composition found in some bacteria.

volvulus (**vol**·vew·lus). Obstruction of a hollow abdominal viscus by torsion; usually a part of the intestine but occasionally the stomach. In the intestine the torsion is around its mesenteric axis, but in the stomach around its longitudinal axis. It is commonest in loops of small intestine, the mesentery of which has been contracted by adhesions. It also occurs in sigmoid colon and the ileocaecal region. **Volvulus of the stomach.** Rotation of the stomach, usually congenital, found mainly in adults often with defects of the diaphragm. [L *volvere* to turn.]

vomer [NA] (**vo**·mer). The thin bony inferior part of the septum of the nose extending from the sphenoid bone to the palatine bone. **Cartilaginous vomer.** The cartilage of the septum of the nose. [L, ploughshare.]

vomerine (**vo**·mer·ine). Pertaining to the vomer.

vomerobasilar (**vo**·mer·o·**ba**'·sil·ar). Referring to the vomer and the sphenoid bone in the base of the skull.

vomeronasal (**vo**·mer·o·**na**'·zal). Referring to the vomer and the nasal bone.

vomica (**vom**·ik·ah). A cavity, especially a cavity in the lung. [L, abscess.]

vomicine (**vom**·is·een). $C_{22}H_{24}O_4N_2$, an alkaloid present in nux vomica (*Strychnos nux-vomica*). It is not used in medicine in its isolated form.

vomit (**vom**·it). 1. To expel forcibly the contents of the stomach through the mouth. 2. The material so vomited. **Barcoo vomit.** A disorder in which vomiting, nausea, and bulimia occur. It has been described among persons in South Australia. **Bilious vomit.** Vomit stained yellow or green from the presence of biliverdin. **Black vomit.** The vomited material containing blood which has been altered by the action of the gastric juice. It was regarded as a fatal sign in yellow fever. **Bloody vomit.** Vomit containing blood. **Coffee-ground vomit.** Darkened fluid vomit containing fine particles of clotted acid-darkened blood from the stomach; common to bleeding ulcers or growth, to corrosive acid poison damage, and after aspirin and arsenic have been swallowed. [L *vomere* to vomit.]

vomiting (**vom**·it·ing). The forcible expulsion of the contents of the stomach through the mouth. **Bilious vomiting.** Vomiting of green-yellow matter; it is due to a regurgitation through the pylorus of the contents of the duodenum. **Cerebral vomiting.** Spontaneous vomiting occurring without nausea in cases of increased intracranial pressure. **Cyclical vomiting.** Periodic attacks of vomiting, beginning in childhood, usually with headache and sometimes with ketosis; it is often inherited and associated with migraine. **Dry vomiting.** Nausea with attempts at vomiting, without result. **Faecal vomiting.** The vomiting caused by intestinal obstruction, when the excessive secretions of the upper part of the intestine contaminated with *Bacterium coli* overflow into the stomach. **Hyperacid vomiting.** Vomiting with hyperchlorhydria. **Hysterical vomiting.** Vomiting in hysteria, without organic disease of the stomach. **Incoercible vomiting.** Uncontrollable vomiting. **Nervous vomiting.** Vomiting due to a gastric neurosis. **Periodic vomiting.** Cyclic vomiting (see above). **Pernicious vomiting.** Severe vomiting in pregnancy, which endangers life. **Postanaesthetic vomiting.** An occasional but unfortunate sequel of anaesthesia and operations. **Vomiting of pregnancy.** Vomiting occurring in the early months of pregnancy. **Projectile vomiting.** The stomach contents are forcibly projected from the stomach. It occurs with congenital pyloric stenosis. **Recurrent vomiting.** Cyclic vomiting (see above). **Stercoraceous vomiting.** Faecal vomiting in intestinal obstruction. [see prec.]

vomitive (**vom**·it·iv). Emetic. [L *vomere* to vomit.]

vomitory (**vom**·it·or·e). 1. An emetic. 2. A vessel for matter vomited. [see prec.]

vomitus (**vom**·it·us). Vomiting; also used for the material vomited. **Vomitus cruentus.** Blood-stained vomit. **Vomitus marinus.** Seasickness. **Vomitus matutinus.** Morning vomiting seen in chronic gastritis, especially of alcoholic origin. **Vomitus niger.** Black vomit. *See* VOMIT. [L.]

Von Gies joint. A chronic syphilitic chondro-osteoarthritis. It is a very rare condition.

Von Pirquet. *See* PIRQUET.

Von Rosen, Sophus Swedish orthopaedic surgeon.

Von Rosen splint. A splint used to treat congenital dislocation of the hip in the newborn.

Von Stockert's phenomenon. Rapid induction of sleep by visual stimuli; a sequel of encephalitis lethargica.

vonulo (**von**·ew·lo). A West African disease of the bronchi, which is associated with severe substernal and subscapular pain.

Voorhees, James Ditmars (b. 1869). New York obstetrician.

Voorhees' bag. A rubber bag inflatable with water, used for dilating the neck of the uterus.

Voronoff, Serge (b. 1866). Russian physician in Paris.

Voronoff's operation. Transplantation into man of the testes of an anthropoid ape.

vortex [NA] (**vor**·tex) (pl. *vortices*). A rapid movement of particulate matter around a central axis; a whorl; especially applied to the spiral arrangement of the muscle fibres of the heart wall. **Vortex coccygeus.** Coccygeal whorl. *See* WHORL. **Vortex cordis [NA].** The spiral arrangement of the superficial fibres of the myocardium at the apex of the heart. **Vortex lentis.** The spiral patterns on the surface of the lens of the eye. **Vortex pilorum.** Hair whorl. *See* WHORL. [L, whirl.]

vorticella (vor·tis·**el**·ah). A free-living ciliate. [dim. of L *vortex* whirl.]

vortices (**vor**·tis·eez). *See* VORTEX.

vorticose (**vor**·tik·oze). Having whorl-like formation. [L *vortex* whirl.]

Vossius, Adolf (b. 1855). Giessen ophthalmologist.

Vossius' cataract, or ring. A ring of minute dark dots on the anterior capsule just outside the pupil margin, usually following contusion. The dots are pigment or blood derivatives.

voussure (**voo**·sewr). Undue prominence or bulge of the precordium due to hypertrophy of the right ventricle in infancy as a result of congenital heart disease. [Fr., arch.]

vox (vox). The voice. **Vox abscissa.** Loss of the voice. **Vox capitis.** The upper voice register. **Vox cholerica.** A peculiar voice associated with cholera. **Vox rauca.** A hoarse voice. [L.]

voyeur (**vwoi**·er). One who practises voyeurism.

voyeurism (**vwoi**·er·izm). The practice of obtaining sexual gratification from looking at others' sexual actions or organs. [Fr. *voyeur* an onlooker.]

vrolik, prenatal fracture of. Multiple fractures that occur *in utero* in osteogenesis imperfecta.

vuerometer (vew·er·**om**·et·er). An instrument to measure the interpupillary distance. [Fr. *vue* sight, meter.]

vulcanite (**vul**·kan·ite). A hard substance prepared from indiarubber by treatment with sulphur. [L *Vulcan* god of fire.]

vulnerability (**vul**·ner·ab·**il**'·it·e). Weakness; the state of being open to infection or trauma. [L *vulnus* wound.]

vulnerant (**vul**·ner·ant). Wounding; capable of injuring. [see prec.]

vulnerary (**vul**·ner·ar·e). 1. Pertaining to or healing wounds. 2. An agent which heals wounds. [see foll.]

See also: THEDEN.

vulnerate (**vul**·ner·ate). To wound or to injure. [L *vulnus* wound.]

vulpes fulva (**vul**·peez **ful**·vah). The silver fox, a host of *Dracunculus medinenis* in North America where man is never infected. [L, tawny fox.]

Vulpian, Edmé Félix Alfred (b. 1826). Paris physiologist.

Vulpian's atrophy. A form of progressive spinal muscular atrophy which affects the scapula and the humerus.

Vulpian's law. When a part of the brain is destroyed its functions are transferred to other areas.

Vulpian's reaction. or test. For adrenaline: a green colour is produced with ferric chloride solution.

Vulpian–Heidenhain–Sherrington phenomenon. Following motor denervation by section of the ventral roots of the sciatic nerve, and after allowing time for degeneration, stimulation of the sciatic nerve causes a slow contraction of the muscles. This is thought to be due to diffusion of acetylcholine from the endings of undegenerated vasodilator nerve fibres running in the sciatic-nerve trunk.

vulsella, vulsellum (vul·**sel**·ah, vul·**sel**·um). A forceps whose blades are tipped with sharp right-angled points directed inwards. [L *volsella* pincers.]

vulva (**vul**·vah). The pudendum; the female external genitalia, comprising the mons pubis, labia majora and minora, the clitoris, the vestibule of the vagina, the bulb of the vestibule, and the greater vestibular glands. [L, a wrapper.]

vulval (**vul**·val). Vulvar.

vulvar (**vul**·var). Concerning the vulva.

vulvectomy (vul·**vek**·to·me). Surgical excision of the vulva. [vulva, Gk *ektome* excision.]

vulvismus (vul·**viz**·mus). Spasm of the vulva; vaginismus.

vulvitis (vul·**vi**·tis). Any inflammatory condition of the vulva; inflammation of the vulva. **Vulvitis blenorrhagica.** Vulvitis with mucopurulent discharge usually due to gonorrhoea. **Diabetic vulvitis.** That form caused by diabetes mellitus. **Diphtheric vulvitis, Diphtheritic vulvitis.** Vulvitis with a grey false membrane which can be caused by the organism of diphtheria. **Eczematiform vulvitis.** That type with vesicular pustules. **Erythematous vulvitis.** An inflammatory condition of the vulva in female infants. **Follicular vulvitis.** Inflammation of the vulval skin follicles. **Leucoplakic vulvitis.** A specific type of inflammatory change produced in the vulval skin by leucoplakia. The cause is unknown. It appears in two stages: the first is a whitening and thickening of the skin with the development of fissures and bleeding; later atrophy occurs and parchment-like areas appear. It is a precancerous disease. **Pseudo-leucoplakic vulvitis.** Vulvitis in which the skin is white and opaque without the presence of true leucoplakic changes. **Ulcerative vulvitis.** Vulvitis marked by the formation of ulcers. [vulva, Gk *-itis* inflammation.]

vulvocrural (vul·vo·**krewr**·al). Concerning the vulva and the crura of the clitoris.

vulvopathy (vul·**vop**·ath·e). Any morbid state of the vulva. [vulva, Gk *pathos* disease.]

vulvo-uterine (vul·vo·**ew**·ter·ine). Concerning both the vulva and the uterus.

vulvovaginal (vul·vo·**vaj**·in·al). Pertaining to the vulva and the opening of the vagina.

vulvovaginitis (vul·vo·vaj·in·**i**′·tis). 1. Inflammation of the vulva extending to the vagina. 2. An inflamed state of Bartholin's glands. **Mycotic vulvovaginitis.** This is usually due to *Candida albicans*; it is occasionally caused by other *Candida* species and only rarely by other genera of yeasts. [vulva, vagina, Gk *-itis* inflammation.]

W

Waage, Peter (b. 1833). Norwegian chemist.

Guldberg and Waage law. Law of mass action.

wabain (wah·ba·in). Ouabain, $C_{29}H_{44}O_{12}·8H_2O$. A crystalline cardiac glycoside obtained from the seeds of *Strophanthus gratus* and other sources. It is administered by intravenous injection, but digitalis is safer. Also known as *Strophanthin G.*

Wachendorf, Evert Jacob (b. 1703). Utrecht botanist and anatomist.

Wachendorf's membrane. 1. Pupillary membrane. *See* MEMBRANE. 2. Plasma membrane. *See* MEMBRANE.

wadding (wod·ing). A form of lightly carded raw wool or cotton supplied in rolled sheets for surgical dressings; cotton wool. [ME.]

wads (wodz). Discs comprising an integral part of the content of a live round for bullet- or shot-firing weapons, notably the latter, separating the propellant charge from the missile, or covering the latter; a forensic term. [etym. dub.]

Waechter, Hermann Julius Gustav (b. 1878). Freiburg physician.

Bracht–Waechter body. Focal collections of round cells and polymorphonuclear leucocytes found in the myocardium in subacute bacterial endocarditis; they probably represent miliary abscesses but do not suppurate.

Waelsch urethritis. A non-specific urethritis possibly due to a virus or a pleuropneumonia-like organism.

wafer (wa·fer). A cachet made of rice paper between the two halves of which medicament is enclosed. [O Fr. *vaufre.*]

Wagner, Ernst Leberecht (b. 1829). Leipzig pathologist.

Wagner's disease. Colloid milium. See MILIUM.

Wagner, Johann Phillipp (b. 1799). German physicist.

Wagner's hammer. An interrupting device designed for the rapid opening and closing of an electric circuit.

Wagner, Rudolf (b. 1805). Gottingen physiologist.

Wagner's corpuscle. Meissner's corpuscle; an encapsulated sensory nerve-ending found in the dermal papillae of the skin of the palm, fingers, sole of foot and toes. It is thought to be a receptor for the sensation of touch.

Wagner, Wilhelm (b. 1848). Konigshütte surgeon.

Wagner's operation. Osteoplastic craniotomy. *See* CRANIOTOMY.

Wagner-Jauregg, Julius (b. 1857). Vienna neurologist.

Wagner–Jauregg treatment. The treatment of dementia paralytica by inoculation of the subject with malaria.

wagnerism (vahg·ner·izm). The production of fever for purposes of treatment, by inoculation of malaria parasites by hypodermic syringe. [Julius *Wagner-Jauregg.*]

wagogo (wag·o·go). An African arrow poison obtained from the juice of a tree of the *Euphorbia* genus. It is not used medicinally.

Wagstaffe, William (b. 1834). British surgeon.

Wagstaffe's fracture. Vertical fracture of the anterior margin of the fibular malleolus.

Wahl, Eduard von (b. 1833). Dorpat surgeon.

von Wahl's sign. Local distension on the proximal side of an intestinal obstruction.

wahoo bark (wah·hoo bark). Euonymus. [Amer. Ind. name.]

waist (wa·st). That part of the trunk between the lowermost ribs and the iliac crests. **Wasp waist.** Thoracostenosis. [AS *weaxt.*]

Waite, W. H. 19th–20th century British dental surgeon.

Waite's pattern dental syringe. A type of syringe used to inject local anaesthetic solution.

wakamba (wa·kam·bah). An arrow poison used in Zanzibar. It causes vasomotor stimulation with a marked rise of blood pressure.

wakefulness (wake·ful·ness). An alert state of the mind in which sleep is impossible; insomnia. [AS *wacian.*]

waking epilepsy (wake·in ep·il·ep·se). Epilepsy in which attacks take place soon after waking from sleep, whether nocturnal or diurnal. Syn: *morning epilepsy*; mosphoric epilepsy.

Walcher, Gustav Adolf (b. 1856). Stuttgart gynaecologist.

Walcher's position. A position in which the patient has the hips on the edge of the table and the legs are allowed to hang down.

Walden, Paul (b. 1863). German chemist.

Walden inversion. In chemistry, the changing of a compound into another of opposite optical rotation with a rearrangement of the atoms within the molecule about a central atom.

Waldenström, Jan Gösta (b. 1906). Upsala biochemist.

Waldenström's purpura hyperglobulinaemia. A haemorrhagic disease in which the patient suffers from recurrent crops of purpuric spots that leave brown stains, especially after a period of undue exertion; the blood proteins show a flat peak in the γ-globulin region. The disease is self-limiting. Chromosome abnormalities are often found in the bone marrow of individuals with this condition and a large metacentric or submetacentric marker chromosome has been found in several cases.

Waldenström's test. For porphyrinuria. Mix equal parts of urine and 2 per cent *p*-dimethylaminobenzaldehyde in dilute hydrochloric acid (1+2). A red colour indicates urobilinogen or porphobilinogen. Shake with amyl acetate and centrifuge. A red colour remaining in the aqueous layer, the latter showing an absorption band at 562 nm, indicates porphyrinuria.

Waldenström, Johann Henning (b. 1877). Stockholm surgeon.

Waldenström's sign. A radiological sign observed in osteochondritis of the hip, a widening of the joint space between the head of the femur and the floor of the acetabulum, attributed by Waldenström to an effusion in the joint, but later shown to be due to thickening of the ligament of the head of the femur.

Legg–Calvé–Waldenström disease. Coxa plana; osteochondritis of the upper femoral epiphysis.

Waldeyer-Hartz, Heinrich Wilhelm Gottfried von (b. 1836). Berlin anatomist.

Waldeyer's plasma cells. Spheroidal cells found in areolar tissue.

Waldeyer's fluid. A decalcifying agent in histology. *See* WALDEYER'S METHOD FOR BONE (below).

Waldeyer's fossae. The inferior and superior duodenal fossae.

Waldeyer's glands. Sweat glands of the eyelids; they are most numerous in the attached margin of the lower lid.

Waldeyer's layer. The germinal epithelium.

Waldeyer's line. Farre–Waldeyer line (see below).

Waldeyer's method for bone. A mixture of hydrochloric acid and palladium chloride, used to fix and decalcify bone.

Waldeyer's organ. The paradidymis.

Waldeyer's tonsillar ring. The oropharyngeal ring of lymphoid tissue.

Waldeyer's sulcus. The grooved extremity of the osseous spiral lamina.

Waldeyer's tract. The dorsolateral fasciculus of the spinal cord.

Farre-Waldeyer line. The boundary between the germinal epithelium of the ovary and the peritoneum of the ovarian mesentery.

walk (wawk). *See* GAIT. [AS *wealcan* to rove.]

Walker, Arthur Earl. 20th century American neurologist.

Dandy-Walker syndrome. Obstruction of the foramina in the roof of the fourth ventricle by a congenital septum, causing hydrocephalus.

Walker, J. T. Ainslie (b. 1868). English chemist.

Rideal-Walker coefficient. A number intended to represent the ratio of bactericidal effectiveness of a substance compared to phenol as a standard.

Rideal-Walker method. A method of assessing efficiency of disinfectants, in relation to phenol as a standard.

Walker sarcoma. A transplantable sarcoma or carcinoma of rats, used in cancer research.

wall [paries] (wawl). The internal surface of a cavity; a boundary. **Axial wall.** The wall of a cavity prepared in a tooth which is parallel to the long axis of the tooth. **Cavity wall.** The dentine wall which surrounds a cavity in a tooth. **Cell wall.** 1. The living plasma membrane bounding the cell cytoplasm externally. 2. The non-living, hardened secretion of the cell, lying outside the plasma membranes, e.g. the cellulose wall of a plant cell. **Germinal wall.** A ridge surrounding the blastoderm, or germinal area on the surface of the yolk, representing the advancing margin of cellular expansion and yolk dissolution. **Nail wall.** *See* NAIL. **Parietal wall.** Denoting the outer somatopleuric lining of the coelom of the embryo, or of any of the serous cavities derived from it. **Periotic wall.** The periotic capsule. *See* CAPSULE. **Splanchnic wall.** Denoting the inner splanchnopleuric lining of the coelom of the embryo, or of any of the serous cavities derived from it. **Subpulpal wall.** The floor of the pulp chamber of a tooth. **Visceral wall.** Splanchnic wall (see above). [L *vallum* rampart.]

wall-eye (wawl·i). An eye which is deformed by having a conspicuous white opacity of the cornea, an iris which is whitish, parti-coloured or different in colour from that of the fellow eye, or by a divergent squint. [Old Norse *vagleygr.*]

Wallace, Alfred Russell (b. 1823). British zoologist.

Wallace's line. An imaginary line in the Indonesian seas running between Borneo and Celebes and Bali and Lombok. The fauna to the east of the line is Australasian and to the west Oriental; for example there are marsupials in Lombok but not in Bali.

Wallace, George Bradley (b. 1874). New York pharmacologist.

Wallace and Diamond method, for urobililogen in urine. Urine is diluted step by step until the red colour obtained with Ehrlich's reagent is just discernible, the result being expressed as the limiting dilution.

Walldius, Börje. 20th century Swedish orthopaedic surgeon.

Walldius knee prosthesis. A metallic hinge device used in arthroplasty of the knee.

Wallenberg, Adolf (b. 1862). Danzig neurologist.

Wallenberg's bundle. A bundle which arises in the olfactory centres and runs through the lateral part of the hypothalamus.

Wallenberg's syndrome. The syndrome of thrombosis of the posterior inferior cerebellar artery; infarction of the lateral aspect of the medulla occurs and gives ipsilateral paralysis of palatal and pharyngeal muscles with dysphagia and dysphonia, ipsilateral facial anaesthesia and Horner's syndrome, ipsilateral dyssynergia and hypotonia, and contralateral loss of pain and temperature sensibility in the limbs and trunk.

Waller, Augustus Volney (b. 1816). London physician.

wallerian degeneration. Adipose degeneration in nerve fibres following their transection or rupture.

Waller's law. A nerve fibre divided from its cell of origin loses its normal structure and function.

Wallgren, Arvid Johann (b. 1889). Gothenburg paediatrician.

Wallgren's meningitis. Benign lymphocytic meningitis. *See* MENINGITIS.

Wallhauser, Andrew (b. 1892). Pittsburg physician.

Wallhauser and Whitehead method. A method of treatment of Hodgkin's disease by a soluble extract of an autogenous gland.

walnut (wawl·nut). The seed of *Juglans regia* (family Juglandaceae). The distilled spirit has antispasmodic properties. [AS *wealh* foreign, nut.]

Walsham's forceps. A forceps designed to manipulate the nasal bones. One blade is introduced into the nasal cavity and the other along the lateral side of the nose; control of the bone is thus obtained.

Walter, Johann Gottlieb (Theophilus) (b. 1734). Frankfurt and Berlin anatomist.

Walter's nerve. The lowest splanchnic nerve; sometimes known as the *nerf rénal postérieur.*

Walthard, Max (b. 1867). Swiss gynaecologist.

Walthard's inclusions. Embryological nests of cells resembling squamous epithelium and sometimes converted into tiny cysts that may be found in the superficial part of the ovaries, the tubes and uterine ligaments, especially in the newborn and young child and sometimes in adults. These nests are thought to be the origin of the Brenner tumour. Also known as *Walthard's islets* and *Walthard's cell rests.*

Walther, Augustin Friedrich (b. 1688). Leipzig anatomist.

Walther's canal or ducts. The multiple ducts of the sublingual salivary gland: these ducts are usually attributed to Rivinus, but it was Walther who in 1724 established by demonstration that the ducts were multiple.

Walther's ganglion. Ganglion impar.

Walther's plexus. A nervous plexus within the cavernous sinus of the dura mater.

Walton's law. Law of reciprocal proportions.

wandering (won·der·ing). Movement from one place to another. **Wandering of a tooth.** The pathological movement of a tooth whose bony support has been lost owing to disease. [AS *wandrian.*]

Wangensteen, Owen Harding (b. 1898). Minneapolis surgeon.

Wangensteen apparatus and tube. A suction apparatus connected with a slender tube for continuous aspiration of the stomach and duodenum.

Wangensteen drainage, suction or technique. Continuous suction applied to the distended gastro-intestinal tract above an obstruction, by way of a tube passed through the nose or mouth, oesophagus and stomach, combined with controlled fluid replacement.

Wangensteen's operation. Excision of the malignant breast, together with axillary and internal mammary glands, with resection of rib cartilages.

Wanscher, Oscar (b. 1846). Danish physician.

Wanscher's mask. A mask used in anaesthesia; it is now obsolete.

waras (war·as). The hairs and glands of the fruits of *Flemingia congesta,* used as a substitute for the taenicide, kamala. [African name.]

warble (wor·bl). A fly of the genus *Hypoderma*; botfly. The larvae are skin parasites of ruminants. Several species have occurred casually in man. [Scand. *varbulde* boil.]

warbles (wor·blz). *Hypoderma.* [see prec.]

Warburg, Carl (b. 1804). Austrian physician.

Warburg's tincture. Antiperiodic tincture; the most outstanding example remaining of the blunderbuss therapy or polypharmacy of former days. It contains the alcohol-soluble constituents of 18 separate drugs.

Warburg, Otto Heinrich (b. 1883). Berlin biochemist.

Warburg's apparatus. A manometric apparatus designed to measure respiration of minced or thinly-sliced tissues.

Warburg's respiratory enzyme. Cytochrome oxidase, an iron-containing factor which, in the processes of tissue respiration, oxidizes reduced cytochrome to cytochrome thus restoring to the latter its capacity as hydrogen carrier.

Warburg's yellow enzyme or ferment. A complex flavoprotein in which riboflavine is linked by a phosphoric-acid molecule to a specific protein. Isolated from yeast by Warburg and Christian in 1932, it acts as a hydrogen carrier in tissue respiration.

Warburg's factor. A term originally applied to an organic iron catalyser which made available the free oxygen essential to cell respiration. It is similar to or identical with the cytochromes.

Warburg's manometer. Warburg's apparatus (see above).

Ward, Sir Terence George. 20th century British oral surgeon.

Ward's osteotomy. Of the mandibular condylar neck, designed to reposition the condylar head in temporomandibular joint disorders.

Wardell, Emma Louise (b. 1886). Baltimore biochemist.

Myers and Wardell method, for cholesterol in blood. The blood is dried on plaster of Paris, extracted with chloroform in a Soxhlet apparatus, and the cholesterol determined in the extract by the Liebermann–Burchard reaction.

Wardill, William Edward Mandall (b. 1894). British surgeon.

Wardill's operation. An operation for the repair of cleft palate.

Wardrop, James (b. 1782). English surgeon.

Wardrop's disease. Onychia maligna.

Wardrop's operation. 1. Distal ligation of an artery for the relief of aneurysm. 2. For entropion [obsolete].

Warfarin (war·far·in). BP Commission approved name for 3-(2-acetyl-1-phenylethyl)-4-hydroxycoumarin; it is used as an anticoagulant. **Warfarin Sodium BP 1973.** The sodium derivative of 4-hydroxy-3-(3-oxo-1-phenylbutyl)coumarin; an anticoagulant that has been found useful in several conditions, including coronary thrombosis.

Waring, George Edward (b. 1833). American hygienist.

Waring's method or system. One of the methods for the land treatment of sewage on the broad irrigation principle by subsoil drainage.

warm-blooded (worm·**blud**·ed). Homothermic; able, by internal mechanisms, to maintain body temperature relatively constant; usually, in temperate climates, above that of the surrounding atmosphere. It is characteristic of mammals and birds. [AS *wearm,* blood.]

Warren, Jonathan Mason (b. 1811). American surgeon.

Warren's operation. An operation for the repair of cleft palate.

wart (wort). Verruca. 1. A circumscribed, cutaneous excrescence having a papilliferous surface. 2. A small, circumscribed, epidermal tumour, caused by localized hypertrophy of the prickle-cell layer, resulting from an infection with a virus; it may be soft or hard, rounded, flat, acuminate or filiform. **Acuminate wart.** Venereal wart (see below). **Anatomical wart.** Verruca necrogenica, verruca tuberculosa; a variety of tuberculosis verrucosa cutis caused by local inoculation of the tubercle bacillus. **Asbestos wart.** A warty reaction to a particle of asbestos in the skin. **Common wart.** Verruca vulgaris; a lesion usually seen on the back of a finger or hand caused by a localized hypertrophy of the prickle-cell layer of the epidermis and associated with some thickening of the horny layer. It is due to infection with a virus and is contagious. It is a small. circumscribed, epidermal excrescence, which may have a grey or black surface from dirt; this surface is rough from the presence of small horny points. **Digitate wart.** Verruca digitata; a variety of wart which usually occurs on the face, scalp or neck, consisting of several short finger-like projections, each having a horny cap, closely grouped on a narrow base. The lesions may be sessile or have a short peduncle. **Fig wart.** Venereal wart (see below). **Filiform wart.** Verruca filiformis; a discrete, threadlike, epidermal outgrowth, usually noted on the neck or eyelids. The lesions, which are usually multiple and may be grouped, are often 6 mm in length or larger. **Flat wart.** Plane wart (see below). **Gonorrhoeal wart.** Venereal wart (see below). **Juvenile wart.** Plane wart (see below). **Moist wart.** Venereal wart (see below). **Mosaic wart.** A dry, progressive, radio-resistant, wart-like patch, irregular in outline and variable in size, occurring on the sole. **Necrogenic wart.** Anatomical wart (see above). **Palmar wart.** A lesion similar to the plantar wart, affecting the palm. **Para-ungual wart.** A wart at the nail fold, at the side of the nail or near the free border of the nail. **Peruvian wart.** Verruga peruana; warty lesions on the skin and mucosae occurring as a symptom of Carrion's disease (bartonellosis). **Pitch wart.** A warty excrescence developing on skin that has been exposed to pitch. The lesions are either malignant from the beginning or else become malignant. **Plane wart.** Verruca plana juvenilis, a small, rectangular or polygonal, flat-topped, yellow or brownish, excrescence on the skin; usually multiple, the lesions tending to coalesce. They are caused by a virus and are usually seen on the backs of the hands and fingers in children, but may occur in older persons. The face may be affected. **Plantar wart.** Papilloma of the sole, verruca plantaris; a small, tender, round or oval, flattened, yellowish-white, deeply embedded lesion occurring in the skin of the sole or of the plantar aspect of a toe, caused by a virus. **Pointed wart.** Venereal wart (see below). **Post-mortem wart.** Anatomical wart (see above). **Prosectors' wart.** Anatomical wart (see above). **Seborrhoeic wart.** Keratosis seborrhoeica, seborrhoeic naevus (Unna), verruca seborrhoeica; a small, benign, raised, round or oval, yellowish or brown tumour, probably a naevus, occurring on the skin of the trunk in elderly people. The lesions are usually multiple, each covered by a greasy, adherent scale. **Senile wart.** Verruca senilis, keratosis senilis; a flat, dry, circumscribed area of keratosis which develops on an exposed area of skin, particularly on the backs of the hands of white-skinned persons who have been much exposed to tropical sunlight. The lesion is covered by a brown or black, adherent scale. It is seldom seen in young people. Usually the lesions are multiple and may become malignant. **Soft wart.** A fibro-epithelial polyp. **Soot wart.** A papilliferous lesion on skin that has been much exposed to soot. It is usually multiple and the lesions are very similar to pitch warts (see above). **Telangiectatic wart.** Angiokeratoma. **Tuberculous wart.** Tuberculosis verrucosa cutis. **Venereal wart.** Condyloma acuminatum, verruca acuminata; usually seen as an exuberant, pink or red, soft, moist, cauliflower-like mass developing near the mucocutaneous junctures in moist areas such as the vulva or prepuce. It is caused by a virus and is very contagious, so that several lesions in various stages of development are usually noted. The virus is probably the same as that which causes common warts. An analogous lesion may occur on the tongue (or on the buccal mucosa) and has been named condyloma acuminatum linguae. There is also an extreme variety of venereal wart noted by Castellani among Tamil women. **Vitreous warts.** Warts which may develop as localized thickenings on the back of the cornea in Descemet's membrane, in the capsule of the lens, or in Bruch's membrane on the inner surface of the choroid where they give rise to Drüsen bodies visible ophthalmoscopically as yellow spots. [AS *wearte.*]

See also: HASSALL, HENLE.

Wartenberg, Robert (b. 1887). San Francisco neurologist.

Wartenberg's disease. Cheiralgia paraesthetica.

Wartenberg's phenomenon. If light pressure is exerted with the ball of the thumb on the upper eyelid, on closure of the eyes a fine vibration will be felt. The reaction is equal on the two sides in normal individuals but is diminished on the affected side in facial palsy.

Wartenberg's sign. 1. In ulnar palsy there is abduction of the little finger. 2. In pyramidal and more particularly extrapyramidal disease (e.g. parkinsonism) which is unilateral, the affected arm does not swing when the patient walks. 3. Active flexion against resistance of the terminal phalanges of the fingers of a hand affected by pyramidal-tract disease gives adduction, flexion and opposition of the thumb; similar to Hoffmann's sign.

Wartenberg's symptom. In certain cases of cerebral tumour, the development of irritability of the nostrils and of the tip of the nose.

Warthin, Aldred Scott (b. 1866). Indiana pathologist.

Warthin-Finkeldey giant cell. A multinucleated giant cell identified in the lymphatic tissue of tonsils, appendix and elsewhere, and formerly believed to be pathognomonic of early measles. The claim is unconfirmed; giant cells are not seen in autopsies of fatal cases.

Warthin's tumour. Adenolymphoma.

wash (wosh). An aqueous lotion, often containing solid matter in suspension. **Black wash.** A lotion of mercurous chloride in lime water, formerly used for syphilis. **Eye wash.** Collyrium. **Red wash.** A lotion of zinc sulphate in compound tincture of lavender. **Yellow wash.** A suspension of mercuric oxide obtained by precipitating a solution of mercuric chloride with calcium hydroxide. [AS *wascan.*]

Washbourn's blood agar. Solid nutrient agar over which fresh sterile blood has been spread.

Waskia (was·ke·ah). The name given to a genus of flagellate protozoa; the name *Embadomonas* Mackinnon 1911, however, has priority. *Embadomonas intestinalis* Wenyon and O'Connor 1917 is the commonest species.

wasp (wosp). Any member of the hymenopteran super-family Vespoidea. More generally, a yellow and black banded, social insect with poisonous sting in workers and queens. Most wasps of the Old World belong to the genus *Vespula,* but in tropical countries many others are represented. [L *vespa.*]

Wassén, Erik (b. 1901). Copenhagen physician.

Wassén test. A test for the virus of lymphopathia venereum;a fatal encephalitis is produced in mice injected with the material containing the virus.

wassercelle (vas·er·sel). Clear cell. *See* CELL. [G. water-clear, cell.]

Wassermann, August Paul von (b. 1866). Berlin bacteriologist.

Wassermann's ascitic-fluid agar. *See* AGAR.

Wassermann reaction, or test. A complement-fixation test for syphilis using as antigen an alcoholic extract of beef heart together with an alcohol solution of cholesterol.

provocative Wassermann reaction. A Wassermann test carried out after an arsphenamine injection which will sometimes provoke a positive reaction in a person with syphilis who previously gave a false negative reaction.

Harrison-Wassermann test. A modification of the Wassermann test.

Wassermann-fast (vas·er·man·fahst'). The persistence of a positive Wassermann reaction despite antisyphilitic treatment.

Wassilieff, Nikolai Porfirievich (b. 1861). Russian physician.

Wassilieff's disease. Leptospirosis.

Wassmund, Martin. 20th century Berlin oral surgeon.

Wassmund's maxillary osteotomy. To enable the correction of premaxillary protrusion.

waste (wa·st). 1. To lose weight; to become thin or emaciated. 2. Anything for which there is no further use; rubbish; detritus; excrement. [L *vastare* to destroy.]

water (waw·ter). The oxide of hydrogen, H_2O, existing also as probably aggregates, $(H_2O)_2$, (H_2O_3), etc. It solidifies under normal pressure at 0°C, becoming ice, and is converted into steam at 100°C. It forms up to 80 per cent of animal and vegetable tissues, and more than 90 per cent of the natural secretions. Its functions biologically are to give rigidity to the tissues, transport nutritional materials in solution; take part in metabolic processes (e.g. synthesis, enzyme action), promote ionization and the phenomena thereof, and regulate heat by evaporation. Tap water is permissible for the compounding of medicaments for oral use, except where calcium and magnesium salts (hardness) would result in incompatibility; for parenteral administration only distilled water can be used. **Aerated water.** Water containing dissolved carbon dioxide under pressure. **Alibour water.** Eau d'Alibour, copper sulphate 1 per cent, zinc sulphate 3.5 per cent, in camphor water; it is used as an astringent in eye affections, e.g. conjunctivitis. **Anise Water, Concentrated, BPC 1959.** A solution of 2 per cent v/v anise oil in a mixture of alcohol and water; diluted 1 to 40 with distilled water, it is used as a flavouring agent. **Apollinaris water.** A German effervescent water. **Aromatic waters.** Solutions of essential oils or other substances in water, used principally for flavouring. The BP 1958 includes Camphor Water, Chloroform Water, Concentrated Cinnamon Water, Concentrated Dill Water and Concentrated Peppermint Water. The BPC 1959 includes Concentrated Anise Water, Concentrated Caraway Water, Concentrated Chloroform Water, Double-strength Chloroform Water and Concentrated Spearmint Water. **Barley water.** A decoction of barley, containing starch and used in diarrhoea of infants and invalids. **Bound water.** A term used to differentiate the water in cellular organisms bound by adsorption to proteins and tissues from that which is in the free state. **Water on the brain.** Hydrocephalus. **Camphor Water BP 1958.** A 1 in 1000 solution of camphor in distilled water containing 2 per cent of alcohol. **Capillary water.** The water that ascends by capillary attraction into the soil above the water table of the ground water. **Caraway water.** A saturated solution of caraway oil in water, obtained by distilling the fruit with water. It is used as a carminative. **Caraway Water, Concentrated, BPC 1959.** A solution of 2 per cent caraway oil in dilute alcohol; it is used as a carminative and flavouring agent. **Carbonated water, Carbonic water.** Aerated water (see above). **Carlsbad water.** A mineral water from the Bohemian Forest. Like most natural mineral waters its use is now obsolescent. **Chalybeate water.** A mineral water containing iron salts. **Cherry-laurel water.** Aqua Lauro-cerasi BPC 1949. **Water on the chest.** Hydrothorax; pleural effusion: a lay term. **Chloroform Water BP 1958.** A 0.25 per cent v/v solution of chloroform in water; used as a flavouring and preservative. **Chloroform Water, Concentrated, BPC 1959.** A 1 in 10 solution of chloroform in water and alcohol. **Chloroform Water, Double Strength, BPC 1959.** A 1 in 200 solution of chloroform in water. **Cinnamon Water, Concentrated, BP 1958.** A solution of 2 per cent v/v of cinnamon oil in dilute alcohol. Diluted 1 to 40 with distilled water it is used as a carminative and flavouring agent. **Water of combustion.** Water formed by the combustion of foodstuffs within the body. **Contrexeville water.** An alkaline French mineral water. **Water of crystallization.** The water loosely bound in the crystal lattice of salts. It can usually be removed by drying the salt at 100°C. **Dalibour water.** Alibour water (see above). **Dill Water, Concentrated, BP 1958.** A solution of 2 per cent v/v dill oil in a mixture of alcohol and water; 1 part diluted with 39 parts of distilled water is used as a carminative in flavouring gripe mixtures for babies. **Distilled water.** Potable water freed from its non-volatile impurities and most of its volatile by distillation in a suitably baffled still. **Elder-flower water.** A solution of essential oil obtained by the steam distillation of elder flowers; it is used as a basis for eye lotions and cosmetic preparations. **Fennel water.** Aqua foeniculi concentrata. **Free water.** *See* BOUND WATER (above). **Ground water.** The water which flows under the soil above an impervious stratum. *See* WATER TABLE (under TABLE). **Hamamelis Water BPC 1968.** Distilled extract of witch hazel; the distillate obtained by distilling a macerate of the young dormant twigs. It is widely used as a cooling application and as a constituent of eye lotions. **Hard water.** Water containing dissolved calcium and magnesium salts. Tap water varies in hardness according to its source. **Heavy water.** Deuterium oxide, ^2H_2O. Often used to denote water containing a proportion of deuterium oxide larger than occurs naturally. **Hunyadi János water.** A Hungarian mineral water. **Water of hydration.** 1. Water of crystallization (see above). 2. The bound water of the tissues associated hydrophilically with proteins, soaps and ions. **Water for Injections BP 1973.** Sterilized distilled water, used for parenteral injection. **Javelle water.** A chlorinated soda solution used as an antiseptic. **Joint water.** Synovia. **Water on the knee.** Synovitis of the knee with effusion into the joint. **Lead water.** A dilute solution of lead subacetate. **Lime water.** A saturated aqueous solution of calcium hydroxide. **Metabolic water.** Water of combustion (see above). **Mineral water.** A natural water obtained from a mineral spring. Such waters contain small amounts of metallic salts in solution, varying with the source, and were formerly consumed for a number of diseases. They are now rapidly falling out of use. **Orange-flower water.** Aqua Aurantii Floris Concentrata BPC 1949. **Peppermint Water, Concentrated, BP 1973.** A solution of 2 per cent v/v peppermint oil in dilute alcohol. Diluted 1 to 40 with distilled water, it is used as a carminative and flavouring agent. **Peptone water.** 1 per cent solution of peptone in 0.5 per cent saline, used in the indole test for *Bacterium coli.* **Potable water.** Any water sufficiently free from mineral, bacterial and fungal impurity to be passed by a local authority as fit for human consumption. **Potash water.** A mineral water containing potassium. **Purified Water BP 1973.** Distilled water (see above). **Pyrogen-free water.** Water that is not only distilled and sterile, but is entirely free from the dead bodies of bacteria or from other particulate or dissolved matter that when injected into man might give rise to a sharp febrile reaction. **Radioactive water.** Tritiated water (see below). **Saline water.** A water containing any salt in solution. **Seltzer water.** A Prussian effervescent mineral water. **Serum water.** Serum-water culture medium. *See* CULTURE MEDIUM. **Serum-dextrose water.** Serum-dextrose culture medium. *See* CULTURE MEDIUM. **Soda water.** An aerated water; it contains no sodium salts. **Soft water.** A water containing no salts of calcium or magnesium. Sodium or potassium salts may be present, but they do not render the water "hard", i.e. do not precipitate with soap solutions. **Subsoil water.** Water that is trapped by shallow wells; the water that lies above the first impervious layer. **Tritiated water,** ^3H_2O. Radioactive water. Often used to denote water containing only a small proportion of its molecules incorporating radioactive hydrogen (^3H). **Vichy water.** A natural water from Vichy, France. [AS *waeter.*]

See also: DURHAM (H. E.), FOULARD, HISS, PASTEUR.

water-bite (waw·ter·bite). Immersion foot; trench foot. *See* FOOT. [water, AS *bitan.*]

water-borne (waw·ter·born). Conveyed by water, describing certain diseases transferred by contaminated water. [water, AS *beran.*]

water-glass (waw·ter·glahs). A solution of sodium or potassium silicate used for many domestic purposes (e.g. preserving eggs), but also used to add stiffening to surgical bandages. [water, AS *glaes.*]

waterbrash (waw·ter·brash). Eructation of dilute acid from the stomach, causing a burning sensation at the back of the throat; heartburn.

Waterhouse, Benjamin (b. 1754). American physician.

Waterhouse test. If the pain in a local inflammatory swelling is increased by applying a constricting bandage, pus is present.

Waterhouse, Rupert (b. 1873). Bath physician.

Waterhouse-Friderichsen syndrome. A feature of meningococcal septicaemia in which the adrenal glands become disintegrated by haemorrhage and an acute adrenal insufficiency develops with alarming rapidity.

waterlogging (waw·ter·log·ing). The saturation with water to such an extent that deterioration is caused. [water, ME *logge.*]

Waters, Charles Alexander (b. 1885). American radiologist.

Waters' position. Prone position of the head for x-rays of the frontal region [obsolete].

Waters' projection. The occipitomental position for x-ray examination of the skull, to view the maxillary antra and facial skeleton.

Waters, Edward Gilman (b. 1898). Jersey City obstetrician.

Waters' operation. A type of extraperitoneal caesarean section where the bladder is retracted downwards.

Waters, Ralph Milton (b. 1883). Wisconsin anaesthetist.

Waters' to-and-fro closed circuit. A system of anaesthetic breathing tubes consisting of a reservoir bag and a canister containing soda lime through which rebreathed gases are passed for carbon-dioxide absorption in closed anaesthesia.

waters (waw·terz). The amniotic fluid which escapes during the second stage of labour. [AS *waeter.*]

watersheds (waw·ter·shedz). **Abdominal watersheds.** In the supine position, cavities formed in the abdomen by the lumbar fossae and pelvis accentuated by the projecting brim of the pelvis and the forward prominence of the lumbar vertebrae. Free effusions into the peritoneal cavity tend to gravitate into these positions. [water, AS *sceadan.*]

Waterston, David James (b. 1910). London paediatric surgeon.

Waterston anastomosis. An anastomosis created between the posterior aspect of the ascending aorta and the adjacent anterior aspect of the right pulmonary artery, used for the palliation of cyanotic congenital heart disease with reduced pulmonary blood flow.

Watkins, John Armstrong (b. 1888). Asheville, North Carolina, physician.

Bass-Watkins test. A slide agglutination method for the diagnosis of typhoid fever; now obsolescent.

Watkins, Thomas James (b. 1863). Chicago gynaecologist.

Watkins' operation. Interposition operation: an operation for the treatment of cystocele and uterine prolapse. The positions of uterus and bladder are transposed. [Obsolete].

Watson, Benjamin Philip (b. 1880). American obstetrician.

Watson's method. A method of induction of labour by the use of castor oil and quinine by mouth and extract of pituitary by injection. [Obsolete].

Watson, Cecil James (b. 1901). Minneapolis physician.

Watson-Schwartz test, for porphyrinuria. A test similar to that of Waldenström.

Watson, James Dewey (b. 1928). American biologist and geneticist. Nobel Prize winner 1962.

Watson-Crick DNA double helix. The model of DNA structure in which the molecule is represented as consisting of 2 right-handed helical polynucleotide chains coiled around the same axis to form a double helix, the purine and pyrimidine bases of each strand being on the inside of the double helix and paired accordingly to the base-pairing rule such that adenine can only pair with thymine, and cytosine only with guanine.

Watson-Crick pair. The complementary nucleoside bases: adenine and guanine, cytosine and thymine or uracil.

Watson-Crick pairing. The formation of hydrogen bonds between complementary nucleoside base pairs.

Watson, Thomas Alistair. 20th century New Zealand radiotherapist in Canada.

Lambert-Watson operation. A method of treating malignant disease of the larynx by the application of x-rays direct to the growth, after the removal of the thyroid ala on the affected side.

Watson, William Spencer (b. 1836). English ophthalmologist.

Watson's operation, for trichiasis at inner or outer parts of the eyelid. Two narrow flaps are formed along the eyelid, one at the margin, taking in the lashes and based at the lid centre, the other directly above and with the base at the canthus. The flaps are dissected free and interchanged, so moving the lash margin up.

Watson-Farrar, John. 20th century British orthopaedic surgeon.

McKee-Farrar arthroplasty. A prosthesis for total hip replacement consisting of a false acetabulum and a false femoral head, both fixed in position with acrylic cement.

Watson-Jones, Sir Reginald (b. 1902). London orthopaedic surgeon.

Watson-Jones' two-stage arthrodesis. Fusion of the hip by removal of the articular cartilages, followed by fixation of the joint by means of a long 3-flanged nail introduced at a second operation.

watt (wot). The unit of power defined as that which in one second gives rise to energy of 1 joule (10^7 ergs per second). Symbol W. One horse-power equals 746 watts. **Watt hour.** The energy expended or generated in 1 hour when the power is 1 watt; equals 3600 joules. [J. *Watt,* 18th–19th century British engineer.]

wattage (wot·ij). The number of watts produced by a generator or consumed by an electrical appliance.

wattmeter (wot·me·ter). An electrical measuring instrument for the direct reading in watts of the power generated or consumed in an electrical circuit.

Waugh, George Ernest (b. 1875). British surgeon.

Waugh gag. A molar gag specially designed so as not to slip or turn when in position.

wave (wave). 1. A periodic disturbance of the particles of a medium by which energy is propagated progressively through the medium. 2. Referring to the graphic recording obtained by an instrument such as an electro-encephalograph. **A wave.** Alpha wave (see below). **"a" wave.** *See* WAVES OF THE PHLEBOGRAM (below). **Alpha (α) waves.** Those waves in the electro-encephalograph which have a frequency of from 8 to 13 Hz (c/s). Also called *alpha rhythm* or *Berger rhythm. See also* ELECTRO-ENCEPHALOGRAPH. **Anacrotic wave, Anadicrotic wave.** A secondary fluctuation on the upstroke or anacrotic limb of the arterial pulse tracing (sphygmogram) found in subjects with aortic valvular stenosis. In this disease the anacrotic limb is a gradual slope of low amplitude. **Arrow-head T wave.** Cove-plane T wave; coronary T wave (see below). **Arterial wave.** An artefact occurring in the jugular phlebogram due to the vibration produced by the carotid pulse. **Beta (β) waves.** Those waves in the electro-encephalograph that have a frequency of from 15 to 60 Hz (c/s), and a lower voltage than the alpha waves. Also called *beta rhythm. See also* ELECTRO-ENCEPHALOGRAPH. **"c" wave.** *See* WAVES OF THE PHLEBOGRAM (below). **Cannon waves.** Large waves in the venous pulse produced by atrial contraction in the face of a closed tricuspid valve, as may occur during ventricular ectopic beats or with heart block. **Carrier wave.** Radio frequency. *See* FREQUENCY. **Catacrotic wave, Catadicrotic wave.** The positive wave which follows the negative wave on the descending (catacrotic) limb of the normal arterial pulse tracing. **Contraction wave.** The progressing wave of the contraction of a muscle fibre. It arises at the point where the stimulus enters the muscle. **Coronary T wave.** Extreme inversion of the T wave of the electrocardiogram recorded from leads which face ischaemic myocardium, indicating disturbance of repolarization due to coronary insufficiency or coronary thrombosis. **Cove-plane T wave.** Sharp inversion of the T wave of the electrocardiogram in leads facing ischaemic myocardium. The R(S)-T segment, when elevated, as in coronary thrombosis, is straight instead of concave, and the T wave becomes convex or cove-shaped when it regains the iso-electric line. **Deep Q wave.** Pathological Q wave; a large deep Q wave of the electrocardiogram, found in leads which face a myocardial infarct. A Q wave with an amplitude of more than 25 per cent of the total QRS complex and measuring more than 0.04 s is suspicious of infarction. **Delta (δ) wave.** In cardiology, the abnormal wave at the commencement of the QRS complex of the electrocardiogram in patients with the Wolff-Parkinson-White syndrome. *See also* ELECTRO-ENCEPHALOGRAM. **Dicrotic wave.** Catacrotic wave (see above). **Electrocardiographic waves.** The deflections of the electrocardiogram, consisting of the P wave, representing activation of the atria, the QRS complex, representing depolarization of the ventricles, and the T and U waves, representing repolarization of the ventricles. **Electromagnetic wave.** One in which the disturbance is an electrostatic and electromagnetic field mutually perpendicular and in a plane perpendicular to the direction of progression of the wave. **Excitation wave.** The wave-like progression of contraction from one muscle fibre to another. **F wave.** Fibrillary wave (see below). **ff waves.** The small, rapid, irregular deflections of the electrocardiogram which replace the P waves of normal atrial contraction when atrial fibrillation is present. **Fibrillary wave.** A continuous succession of small undulations seen in the jugular phlebogram and electrocardiogram, due to atrial fibrillation. **Frequency wave.** Radio frequency. *See* FREQUENCY. **"h" wave.** *See* WAVES OF THE PHLEBOGRAM (below). **Hertzian waves.** Radio wave (see below). **Kappa (κ) wave.** *See* ELECTRO-ENCEPHALOGRAPH. **Lamba (λ) wave.** *See* ELECTRO-ENCEPHALOGRAPH. **Light waves.** So-called waves travelling from the source of light in all directions, varying in length according to their colour between 723 and 397 nm which stimulate the retinal perceptive elements and are therefore visible. **Longitudinal wave.** One in which the direction of disturbance of the particles is parallel to the direction of propagation of the wave, e.g. sound. **Micro waves.** Those electromagnetic waves of wavelengths between 1 mm and 30 cm; they thus bridge the gap between radio waves and heat waves (infrared radiation). **Mitral P wave.** The abnormally broadened, notched or biphasic P wave in the electrocardiogram seen with left atrial enlargement and which is most commonly the consequence of mitral valve disease. **Outflow remainder wave, Overflow wave.** The initial portion of the descending limb of the sphygmogram between the apex of the pulse wave and the catacrotic wave. **P wave.** The deflection of the electrocardiogram produced by atrial depolarization. **Papillary wave.** The ascending wave of the pulse tracing. **Pardee wave.** Elevation of the S-T segment, which is straight, and inversion of the T wave in leads facing a myocardial infarct; the T wave is convex, resembling an arrow head. **Percussion wave.** Papillary wave (see above). **Peridicrotic wave.** Outflow remainder wave (see above). **Peristaltic wave.** A wave of alternate contraction and relaxation of a tube, such as the intestine, which impels the contents forward. **Waves of the phlebogram.** *"a" Wave:* the first wave, representing the rise of pressure in the great veins, due to contraction of the atria. *"c" Wave:* the wave immediately following the "a" wave, denoting the beginning of ventricular systole and closure of the tricuspid valve. *"v" Wave:* the third wave, representing the increase in pressure produced by the flow of blood into the atria and great veins while the tricuspid valve is closed; it reaches its maximum just before the valve opens, after which the pressure falls rapidly forming the descending limb of the wave. Also known as *"h" wave.* **Phrenic wave.** Diaphragm phenomenon. *See* PHENOMENON. **Postdicrotic wave.** A small wave which follows the catadicrotic wave (see above). **Predicrotic wave.** A small wave preceding the catadicrotic wave on the dicrotic limb of the sphygmogram. **Pulmonary P wave.** The abnormally tall, pointed P wave in the electrocardiogram seen with right atrial enlargement associated with right ventricular hypertrophy, most commonly secondary to pulmonary hypertension or pulmonary valve stenosis. **Pulse wave.** The pressure change which is produced by the passage of blood from the left ventricle into the full aorta and is propagated as a wave through the column of blood and the walls of the arteries to the periphery. The form of the pulse wave consists of an abrupt upstroke, the anacrotic limb, which represents the head of the advancing pulse wave, followed by a more gently sloping downstroke, the catacrotic limb. The descending limb shows a depression, the dicrotic notch, followed by a positive wave, the catacrotic wave; the slope of the anacrotic limb depends upon the duration of ventricular ejection, the stroke volume, the level of the diastolic blood pressure and the elasticity of the arterial walls. If the ejection is slow, as in aortic valvular stenosis, the upstroke is gradual and may show a secondary wave (anacrotic wave); when the output is large, the ejection rapid or the diastolic pressure low, as in aortic incompetence, the anacrotic limb is steep and of high amplitude. The dicrotic notch is produced in the following way; the elastic rebound of the aortic wall following closure of the aortic valve propels the column of blood centrally as well as peripherally, and the central swing produces a negative fluctuation in the peripheral pulse which causes the notch. The rebound of the blood column from the closed taut aortic-valve cusps causes a positive pressure change and produces the catacrotic wave; this is exaggerated when the diastolic pressure is low, the arterial system underfilled or if there is vasodilatation. The dicrotic limb is abrupt when the diastolic pressure is low and is gradual if the pulse pressure is low, as in aortic stenosis. **Q wave.** The initial negative deflection of the electrocardiogram due to ventricular depolarization, representing invasion of the ventricular septum from left to right. **QRS wave.** QRS complex. *See* COMPLEX. **QRST wave.** QRST complex. *See* COMPLEX. **QS wave.** A monophasic negative deflection recorded from leads which face the tail of the ventricular depolarization wave or a ventricular cavity. QS deflections may be recorded from leads facing the right ventricle in left bundle branch block and occasionally in left ventricular hypertrophy; those recorded from leads facing the left ventricle or septal region indicate coronary thrombosis. **R wave.** The principal positive wave of ventricular depolarization representing invasion of the ventricular muscle mass. The beginning of the downstroke of the R wave is sometimes called the *intrinsicoid deflection,* and the interval between this and the beginning of the Q wave in semidirect precordial leads, the *ventricular activation time,* and has been used to represent the time taken for the electrical impulse to pass through the ventricular muscle mass. The height of the R wave in a semidirect precordial lead is roughly proportional to the thickness of the ventricular muscle facing the electrode. **Radio wave.** Electromagnetic wave with radio frequency. **Random wave.** Alpha wave (see above). **Recoil wave.** Catacrotic wave (see above). **Respiratory wave.** A rhythmic variation in the arterial blood pressure with respiration; it rises during inspiration and falls during expiration. **S wave.** The negative deflection of the ventricular complex of the electrocardiogram representing the passing of the electrical impulse away from the electrode. **Short wave.** Describing a band of wavelengths of electromagnetic waves used in radio; approximately from 60 m to 10 m. Also used loosely to describe high-frequency diathermy. **Sonic wave.** A sound wave (see following). **Sound wave.** A travelling wave system passing through a medium by longitudinal displacement of the particles of the medium, which when received by the ear is heard as a sound. **Stimulus wave.** The wave of excitation which passes along a muscle as the result of applied stimulus. **Supersonic wave.** 1. A wave of sound vibration higher than audible frequency, arbitrarily above 20 Hz [obsolete term]. 2. In aviation, a shock wave generated by a body moving with a velocity greater than sound. **T wave.** The deflection of the electrocardiogram which is produced by the electrical forces caused by the retreat of the excitation wave through the ventricular muscle during the latter part of systole (ventricular repolarization). **Ta wave.** The deflection of the electrocardiogram produced by the terminal phase of auricular systole (atrial repolarization). It is usually hidden in the QRS waves of the ventricular complex. **Theta (θ) wave.** *See* ELECTRO-ENCEPHALOGRAPH. **Transverse wave.** A wave in which the particle disturbance is perpendicular to the direction of propagation of the wave. **U wave.** A small rounded positive wave immediately following the T wave of the electrocardiogram. **Ultrashort wave.** An arbitrary term used in radio to describe electromagnetic waves of wavelengths less than 3 m. **Ultrasonic wave.** A sound wave of frequency higher than 20 kHz. **"v" waves.** *See* WAVES OF THE PHLEBOGRAM (above). **Ventricular waves.** The waves of the venous pulse tracing which indirectly represent ventricular events. **X-descent wave.** The negative wave (depression) during atrial diastole that succeeds the positive wave of auricular systole seen in the jugular venous pulse; also known as *auricular depression.* **Y-descent wave.** The negative wave which follows the "v" wave in the venous pulse as the ventricles relax and blood begins to flow into them from the atria. [AS *wafian.*]

See also: BERGER (H.), ERB, HERING (K. E. K.), HERTZ, MAYER, TRAUBE (L.).

wave-form (wave·form). 1. The mode of variation of a periodic function, e.g. the electric potential of the a.c. mains if plotted as a function of time gives a sinusoidal wave-form. 2. The shape of a wave, such as a water wave. [wave, form.]

wavelength (wave·length). An attribute of any wave motion, being the measurement from any point on a wave to a corresponding point on the next wave, e.g. crest to crest. It is defined as the velocity of the wave divided by its frequency, and is denoted by the symbol λ. **Critical absorption wavelength.** That wavelength at which a sudden change in the x-ray absorption coefficient of a material occurs, a small decrease in wavelength causing a large increase in absorption coefficient. **Effective wavelength.** The single wavelength which most nearly represents the quality of a heterogeneous beam of radiation. **Minimum wavelength.** Of the many wavelengths comprising a spectrum, that one which is the shortest. [wave, AS *lengthu.*]

See also: BROGLIE.

wavemeter (wave·me·ter). An instrument used for the determination of the wavelength of electromagnetic radiation. [wave, meter.]

wax (wax). An ester or mixture of esters, of a higher fatty acid with a higher aliphatic alcohol; free acids and alcohols are usually present. **Bayberry wax.** A green wax from the bark of *Myrica cerifera.* **Bone wax.** Aseptic surgical wax; a mixture of wax, oil and carbolic acid applied to the cut surface of bone to stop bleeding. **Carnauba wax.** Wax from a Brazilian palm, used as a substitute for beeswax and in the manufacture of candles, shoe polish, etc. **Cetomacrogol Emulsifying Wax BP 1973.** A non-ionic emulsifying wax prepared by melting together 2 parts of cetomacrogol 1000 and 8 parts cetostearyl alcohol. **Ear wax [cerumen (B.N.A.)].** A product of the modified sweat glands of the external auditory meatus. **Emulsifying Wax BP 1973.** Cetostearyl alcohol and sodium laural sulphate or similar sodium salts of sulphated higher primary aliphatic alcohols, prepared in an emulsifying ointment and aqueous cream and used as a water-miscible cream basis. **Grave wax.** Adipocere. **Mineral wax.** Ceresine. **Vegetable wax.** A waxy substance occurring as a bloom on certain fruits; used instead of beeswax. **White wax.** White Beeswax BP 1973; cera alba; bleached beeswax. **Yellow wax.** Yellow Beeswax BPC 1959; cera flava. [AS *weax.*]

See also: HORSLEY.

wax myrtle bark (wax mertl bark). Bayberry bark, myrica. [wax, Gk *myrtos,* bark.]

waxy (wax·e). Of the nature of wax; wax-like.

weal (weel). A hard raised patch on the skin produced by an acute irritation such as the sting of a nettle or the bite of an insect. The intradermal effusion that causes the swelling is under pressure and makes the patch bloodless and decolorized. It is also observed in urticaria. [AS *walu.*]

wean (ween). To break an infant of the habit of suckling and to accustom the child to ordinary food. [AS *wenian* to accustom.]

web (web). Any membranous structure; an open-weave tissue; a tela. **Web of the brain.** The supporting network for the nervous tissue of the brain and spinal cord; neuroglia. **Choroid web.** The tela chorioidea forming the roof of the third ventricle. **Web of the fingers.** The folds of skin joining the proximal segments of the fingers on the palmar aspect. **Oesophageal web.** A rare abnormality in which a fold of tissue partially obstructs the lumen of the oesophagus at the level of the bifurcation of the trachea. **Web of the toes.** The folds of skin joining the proximal segments of the toes on the plantar aspect. [AS *wefan* to weave.]

web-eye (web·i). Pterygium; a triangular thickening of the conjunctiva of the eye extending from the canthus to the pupil. [web, eye.]

web-fingered (web·fing·gerd). Having the fingers joined for most of their length by a fold of skin. [web, finger.]

web-foot (web·fut). A condition in which the toes are joined by a fold of skin. [web, foot.]

web-toed (web·tode). Affected with the condition of web-foot. [web, toe.]

webbed (web·d). Describing any part of the body that is united to an adjacent part by a web-like fold of tissue.

Weber, Adolph (b. 1829). German ophthalmologist.

Weber's operation. 1. For cataract extraction [obsolete]. 2. For lacrimal stricture: an obsolete modification of Bowman's operation.

Weber, Ernst Heinrich (b. 1795). Leipzig anatomist and physiologist.

Weber's sensory circles. A hypothetical arrangement of nerve-endings in the skin designed to account for the phenomenon of 2-point tactile discrimination.

Weber's glands. Mucous glands of the lateral borders of the tongue.

Weber's law. The increase in stimulus necessary to produce the smallest perceptible increase in sensation bears a constant ratio to the strength of the stimulus already acting.

Weber's paradox. When a muscle is stretched to more than a certain extent it can no longer contract in response to stimulation.

Weber-Fechner law. Psychophysical law. *See* LAW.

Weber, Frederick Parkes (b. 1863). London physician.

Weber's disease, Weber-Dimitri disease, Sturge-Weber disease or syndrome, Sturge-Kalischer-Weber disease. Naevoid amentia; congenital cerebral hemiatrophy due to diffuse capillary angiomatous change and subcortical calcification, producing fits, mental impairment and hemiplegia. It is associated with a port-wine naevus of the face (usually on the side of the cerebral lesion) and often unilateral buphthalmia.

Christian-Weber disease. Nodular, pyrexial, non-suppurative panniculitis.

Klippel-Trenaunay-Weber syndrome. Haemangiectatic hypertrophy.

Rendu-Osler-Weber disease. Hereditary haemorrhagic telangiectasia. *See* TELANGIECTASIA.

Weber, Sir Hermann David (b. 1823). London physician.

Weber's paralysis or syndrome, Weber-Gubler syndrome. A lesion of the cerebral peduncle involving the 3rd cranial nerve and the corticospinal pathway and giving rise to an ipsilateral paralysis of the 3rd cranial nerve with a contralateral spastic hemiplegia; also called the *syndrome of the cerebral peduncle* and *superior alternating hemiplegia.*

Weber, Moritz Ignatz (b. 1795). Bonn anatomist.

Weber's artery. The anterior tympanic branch of the maxillary artery.

Weber's corpuscle or organ. The prostatic utricle.

Weber, Wilhelm Eduard (b. 1804). Gottingen physicist.

Weber's point. A point 1 cm below the promontory of the sacrum believed by Weber to correspond to the centre of gravity of the body.

Weber's triangle. A triangular area bound by a line drawn through the 1st and 5th metatarsal heads and having as its apex the midpoint of the plantar aspect of the heel.

weber (va·ber, web·er). The unit of magnetic flux defined as the magnetic flux which, linking a circuit of one turn, would produce in it an electromotive force of 1 volt if it were reduced to zero at a uniform rate in 1 second. [Wilhelm Eduard *Weber.*]

Weber-Liel, Friedrich Eugen (b. 1832). Berlin and Jena otologist.

Weber's test. In unilateral deafness: a vibrating tuning-fork placed on the vertex of the skull is normally heard in the midline. In unilateral conductive types of deafness, the vibrations are heard more intensely on the diseased side; in perceptive deafness, in the sound ear.

Webster, John Clarence (b. 1863). Canadian gynaecologist in Chicago.

Baldy-Webster operation. A seldom-used operation for correction of retrodisplacement of the uterus. The round ligaments are passed through the perforated broad ligaments and fixed to the posterior surface of the uterus.

Wechsberg, Friedrich (b. 1873). Vienna physician.

Neisser-Wechsberg phenomenon. Deviation of complement; when more specific amboceptor is added to a mixture of antigen and complement than can be absorbed by the antigen the excess amboceptor may combine with the complement. This prevents the complement from acting on the antigen-amboceptor complex.

Wechsler, David (b. 1896). New York psychologist.

Wechsler-Bellevue test. A test of adult intelligence comprising 11 sub-tests: Comprehension, Information, Digit Span, Arithmetic, Similarities, Vocabulary, Picture Arrangement, Picture Completion, Block Design, Object Assembly and Digit Symbol. The scores on each of the sub-tests tend to deviate from the mean in a characteristic scatter pattern in various psychiatric and intellectual disorders.

Wecker, Louis de (b. 1832). Paris ophthalmologist.

de Wecker's operation. 1. For squint: (*a*) advancement of the muscle combined with shortening by tucking; the muscle is not cut; (*b*) advancement of a muscle by advancing Tenon's capsule and not cutting the tendon. 2. For after-cataract: de Wecker's iris scissors are introduced through a keratome incision and the capsule divided. 3. For glaucoma: (*a*) broad iridectomy by cutting only the pillars of the iris and tearing the root; (*b*) anterior sclerotomy; 2 incisions are made simultaneously through the sclera 1 mm outside the limbus, by the puncture and counter-puncture of a Graefe knife, the section not being completed [obsolete]; (*c*) combined anterior sclerotomy with iridodialysis; iris forceps are introduced through a small keratome incision and the iris pulled downwards towards the centre of the pupil [obsolete]. 4. For epicanthus: removal of a fold of skin over the bridge of the nose by transfixing with sutures, then cutting off the fold and finally tying sutures. 5. For division of anterior synechia: with scissors introduced through a keratome incision. 6. For staphyloma of the cornea: excision of the staphyloma, extraction of the lens through the wound, suture of the corneal gap and finally suturing of the mobilized conjunctiva over the cornea. 7. For trichiasis: the eyelid margin is split as far up as the upper border of the tarsus; the eyelash margin is then stitched in this new position.

de Wecker's scissors. A delicate scissors, spring operated, for operations on the eyeball.

Wedensky, Nicolai Igorevich (b. 1844). Russian neurologist.

Wedensky facilitation. A facilitation similar to that seen across a nerve block, but in this case involving summation of endplate potentials by means of successive stimuli, until an intensity is attained that can break through a curare block and cause muscular contraction.

Wedensky inhibition or phenomenon. The phenomenon of total or partial block to conduction that occurs in a nerve when repetitive stimuli are so spaced that each falls in the refractory period of its predecessor.

wedge (wej). **Wedge filter.** *See* FILTER.

Weeks, John Elmer (b. 1853). New York ophthalmologist.

Koch-Weeks bacillus. *Haemophilus influenzae.*

Koch-Weeks conjunctivitis. An acute epidemic mucopurulent bilateral form of conjunctivitis, very contagious and therefore commonly seen in institutions. It is caused by the Koch-Weeks bacillus. Also known as *acute epidemic mucopurulent conjunctivitis* or *pink eye.*

weep (weep). 1. To shed tears; to lacrimate. 2. To exude fluid slowly. [see foll.]

weeping (weep·ing). 1. Lacrimation. 2. The exudation of a fluid from a surface. [AS *wepan* to cry.]

Wegner, Friedrich Rudolf Georg (b. 1843). Berlin pathologist.

Wegner's sign. Deformity of the epiphyseal line in infants suffering from untreated congenital syphilis; not usually recognized in the UK.

Wehnelt, Arthur (b. 1871). Berlin physicist.

Wehnelt's interrupter. An electrolytic device for very rapid and regular interruption of large electric currents. It is usually employed to interrupt the primary current of an induction coil when used with heavy currents.

Weichardt, Wolfgang. 19th century German pathologist.

Weichardt's antikenotoxin. A hypothetical antitoxin said to be produced in response to the presence of an equally hypothetical toxin which is supposed to develop in active tissues and cause their fatigue.

Weichselbaum, Anton (b. 1845). Vienna pathologist.

Weichselbaum's diplococcus. *Neisseria meningitidis.*

Fraenkel-Weichselbaum pneumococcus. *Streptococcus pneumoniae.*

Weidel, Hugo (b. 1849). Austrian chemist.

Weidel's reaction or test, for xanthine. Treat a little of the substance with bromine water and evaporate to dryness on the water bath. Moisten the yellow residue with caustic potash solution and heat. A red colour becoming purple-red upon heating, becoming yellow upon addition of a little water and leaving a red residue upon evaporation, indicates xanthine.

Weigert, Karl (b. 1843). Frankfurt histologist.

Weigert's differentiating fluid. A mixture of borax and potassium ferricyanide, used to differentiate haematoxylin staining in the myelin-sheath techniques.

Weigert's alcohol haematoxylin. *See* HAEMATOXYLIN.

Weigert's iron haematoxylin. *See* HAEMATOXYLIN.

Weigert's law. Reparative processes call forth new tissue in excess of that which has been lost.

Weigert's method. Gram–Weigert method (see below).

Weigert's method for neuroglia. A long and complicated method employing mordanting with a copper acetate and chrome-alum mixture after formalin fixation, reduction with potassium permanganate, followed by formic acid, and staining with alcoholic methyl violet and an iodine in potassium-iodide solution.

Weigert's quick method for mordanting myelin sheaths. Tissues are fixed in formalin and mordanted in a mixture of chrome alum and potassium dichromate.

Weigert's mixture. A clearing agent containing either phenol or aniline in xylene.

Weigert's picrocarmine. A mixture of carmine, ammonia and picric and acetic acids, used as a nuclear stain.

Weigert's stain. A modified form of Gram staining, using gentian violet and Lugol's solution for the demonstration in sections of fibrin and Gram-positive bacteria.

Weigert's elastic-tissue stain. A mixture of acid fuchsine, resorcinol, ferric chloride, alcohol and hydrochloric acid. Elastic fibres are stained blue-black.

Weigert's myelin-sheath stain. Tissues are fixed in Mueller's fluid, mordanted in a mixture of copper acetate, acetic acid and chrome alum, stained in a lithium carbonate-haematoxylin solution and differentiated in borax-ferricyanide.

Gram–Weigert method, for bacteria in celloidin sections. Sections are first stained with lithium carmine to demonstrate cell nuclei, then with aniline gentian violet, and differentiated with iodine to show bacteria. For *Trichophyton* in hair: the technique is as outlined, but the differentiation is effected very slowly by iodized aniline oil. The fungus is stained dark blue.

Pal's modification of Weigert's myelin-sheath stain, Weigert-Pal method. After fixation in formalin, followed by mordanting in a mixture of potassium dichromate and chrome alum, sections are stained in Weigert's haematoxylin, blued with lithium carbonate and differentiated with potassium permanganate followed by oxalic acid. Myelin sheaths are stained blue-black against a clear background.

weight (wate). 1. The force exerted on a body by gravitation; the pull on a body towards the earth's centre due to the earth's gravitation, lessened by the opposing centrifugal force. Cf. MASS. 2. An accurately standardized piece of metal or other substance used for weighing objects in a balance. 3. In statistics, an addition to any term or terms to take into account an extraneous factor. **Apothecaries' weight.** The weight in a system of weighing in which a pound (lb) equals 5760 grains (0.373 kg); formerly the official system used by apothecaries. **Atomic weight.** For a given specimen of an element, the mean weight of its atoms expressed in either atomic mass units (physical scale) or atomic weight units (chemical scale). **Avoirdupois weight.** The weight in a system of weighing in which a pound (lb) equals 7000 grains (0.453 kg). **Combining weight.** Equivalent weight (see following). Chemical reactions take place between elements or compounds in proportions that are simple multiples of their combining weights (equivalents). **Equivalent weight.** The weight of an element in any chosen unit (usually grams) which will displace a unit weight of hydrogen from a compound containing the latter, e.g. an acid, or combine with or replace a unit weight of hydrogen. The equivalent weight of a compound either itself contains unit weight of hydrogen or will react completely with another compound containing unit weight of hydrogen. **Gram-molecular weight.** The numerical molecular weight of a substance expressed in grams. **Imperial weight.** Avoirdupois weight (see above). **Isotopic weight.** The weight of an atom of an isotope compared with the weight of the standard atom of carbon (12). **Molecular weight.** The weight of a molecule of a substance, being the sum of the weights of the atoms composing it as compared with a standard atom of carbon (12). **Troy weight.** The weight in a system of weighing used by jewellers, in which pounds, ounces and grains are the same as in the Apothecaries' system, but the pennyweight (dwt) = 24 grains (1.555 g) is used in the place of the drachm = 60 grains (3.887 g). [AS *gewiht.*]

Weigl, Egon. 20th century German psychologist.

Weigl test. A psychological test in which 12 coloured blocks must be sorted according to colour and to shape.

Weigl, R. 20th century Polish virologist.

Weigl's method. The preparation of typhus vaccine by infecting lice with rickettsiae rectally.

Weigl vaccine. A typhus vaccine made from infected lice.

Weil, Adolf (b. 1848). Wiesbaden physician.

Weil's disease. Leptospirosis icterohaemorrhagica.

Weil, Edmund (b. 1880). Austrian physician and bacteriologist.

Weil's meat-potato agar. A nutrient agar containing potato extract.

Weil-Felix test. An agglutination test, originally for typhus fever but now extended to some other rickettsial infections, in which the patient's serum is reacted with suspensions of proteus strains (OX19, OXa, OXk) containing a heterophile antigen.

Weil, L. A. 19th century German dentist.

basal layer of Weil. That part of the tooth pulp which lies immediately beneath the odontoblast cells.

Weil, Mathieu Pierre (b. 1884). Paris physician.

Klippel-Weil sign. In disease of the pyramidal tract with flexion contracture of the fingers, passive extension of the fingers produces flexion and adduction of the thumb.

Weill, Edmond (b. 1858). Lyons paediatrician.

Weill's sign. Diminished movement of the subclavicular region of the chest in acute lobar pneumonia; not used in the UK.

Weinbach, Ancel Pavès (b. 1911). Baltimore biochemist.

Weinbach method, for sodium in blood. Sodium in a protein-free serum filtrate is precipitated with zinc uranyl acetate in alcoholic solution. The precipitate is washed, dissolved in water and titrated with standard sodium hydroxide using phenophthalein as indicator.

Weingartner, R. J. 20th century German physician in India.

Weingartner's disease or syndrome. Tropical eosinophilia; Weingartner was not, however, the first to describe this disease.

Weir, Robert Fulton (b. 1838). New York surgeon.

Weir's operation. Appendicostomy.

Weir Mitchell. *See* MITCHELL, SILAS WEIR.

Weisbach, Augustin (b. 1837). Austrian anatomist.

Weisbach's angle. Angle between a line passing from the basion to the prosthion and one from the nasion to the prosthion.

Weismann, August Friedrich Leopold (b. 1834). Frankfort biologist.

Weismann's bundle. The intrafusal fibres of a muscle spindle.

Weismann's fibre. One of the small muscle fibres of a muscle spindle.

Weismann's theory. The germ plasma is independent of the soma, and thus acquired characters are not inherited.

weismannism (vise·man·izm). The doctrine that acquired characteristics are not inherited. [A. F. L. *Weismann.*]

Weiss, Leopold (b. 1849). Heidelberg ophthalmologist.

Weiss reflex, reflex streak of Weiss. A light reflex crescentic in shape seen on the nasal side of the optic disc in early and sometimes advanced myopia, during ophthalmoscopy.

Weiss, Moriz (b. 1877). Vienna physician.

Weiss' test, for urochromogen. Dilute urine with 2 volumes of distilled water and add 3 drops of 1 per cent potassium-permanganate solution. A yellow colour indicates urochromogen.

Weiss, Nathan (b. 1851). Vienna physician.

Weiss' sign, Chvostek-Weiss sign. In tetany, e.g. after total parathyroidectomy, tapping the 7th cranial nerve or facial muscles results in twitching of these muscles. Also called *Chvostek's sign.*

Weiss, Soma (b. 1899). American physician.

Mallory-Weiss syndrome. Massive haematemisis due to acute rupture of the mucosa at the gastro-oesophageal junction after straining and vomiting. Hiatus hernia may be associated.

Weissenberg, K. (fl. 1922). German radiologist.

Weissenberg camera. An x-ray camera developed from the single-crystal camera; moving-film camera.

Weitbrecht, Josias (b. 1702). St. Petersburg anatomist.

Weitbrecht's cartilage. The meniscus of the acromioclavicular joint.

Weitbrecht's cord or ligament. The oblique cord connecting the radius and ulna.

Weitbrecht's fibres or retinacula. Fibrous strands anchoring the synovial membrane to the neck of the femur.

Weitbrecht's foramen. An opening in the articular capsule of the shoulder joint.

Welch, Francis Henry (b. 1839). British Army surgeon.

Welch's aortitis. Syphilitic aortitis. *See* AORTITIS.

Welch, William Henry (b. 1850). Baltimore pathologist.

Welch's bacillus. *Clostridium welchii.*

Welcker, Hermann (b. 1822). German physiologist.

Welcker's sphenoidal angle. The angle between the two basicranial axes.

Welcker's method. A method of determining total blood volume by complete exsanguination and subsequent washing out of the vascular system.

Welker's biuret reagent, for proteins. To 40 per cent sodium-hydroxide solution add 1 per cent copper-sulphate solution drop by drop with stirring until the solution is a deep blue colour. It gives a purple reaction with the higher proteins.

Wells, Charles Alexander (b. 1898). Liverpool surgeon.

Wells' tidal irrigator and cystometer. A tidal irrigator and cystometer which may be used at the bedside; the bladder automatically fills and empties through a siphon bottle, and the irrigating fluid may contain an antibiotic or phosphate solvent. The intravesical tension may be measured on a meter-stick placed alongside a vertical glass tube which is connected to the siphon bottle and so acts as a cystometer.

Wells, Sir Thomas Spencer (b. 1818). London surgeon and gynaecologist.

Spencer Wells cannula. An ovarian-cyst cannula with side-tube and a handle pierced to carry the trocar.

Wells' facies. Facies ovarica; the drawn and pinched face seen in women with an ovarian tumour.

Spencer Wells forceps. Scissor-shaped surgical forceps, used for gripping tissues or needles, with a locking device so that they continue to grip when they are no longer held.

Wells-Stenger test. A hearing test for distinguishing real from simulated unilateral deafness: preliminary tests are carried out to indicate the relative distances at which a vibrating tuning-fork can be appreciated in each ear. A tuning-fork inserted into a length of tube connected to the supposedly deaf ear is then vibrated, and the distance at which the original tuning-fork can now be appreciated from the good ear is again recorded. If this is perceived at the same distance as before, the opposite ear is probably truly deaf. If it has to be approximated more closely to the good ear, a diagnosis of malingering can be supported.

Welsh, David Arthur (b. 1875). Edinburgh and Sydney pathologist.

Welsh's cells. Cells of the parathyroid gland.

Weltmann, Oskar (b. 1885). Vienna physician.

Weltmann's serum test. Coagulation of blood serum by solutions of calcium chloride. It was formerly used as a prognostic test in rheumatic fever.

weltmerism (welt·mer·izm). A system of suggestion which aims at producing complete harmony between the body and mind. [Cyrus Ernst *Weltmer* (b. 1880), self-styled "mental scientist" of Nevada, Mo.]

wen (wen). A benign tumour, usually on the scalp, which contains sebaceous matter. **Explosive wen.** An inflamed wen that subsequently becomes malignant. [AS *wenn.*]

Wenckebach, Karel Frederik (b. 1864). Dutch physician in Vienna.

Wenckebach's bundle. A bundle of cardiac muscle fibres passing from the superior vena cava into the wall of the right atrium.

Wenckebach phenomenon. The term applied to a form of block in the cardiac conduction system in which conduction becomes longer with each successive beat until conduction is completely blocked, after which conduction is restored to its initial velocity and the whole cycle is repeated. It is most commonly seen, and most easily recognized, when it affects the main His bundle so that the P-R interval lengthens with each beat until a beat is dropped; this is a form of second-degree heart block. There is evidence that the phenomenon can occur in other parts of the conducting system, such as one of the bundle branches.

Wenzel, Joseph (b. 1768). Mainz anatomist and physiologist.

Wenzel's ventricle. The cavity of the septum lucidum.

Wenzel, Michael Jean Baptiste de (d. 1790). French ophthalmologist.

Wenzel's operation, for cataract. A flap section is made below, the knife cutting through the iris and also opening the anterior lens capsule. Historical.

Wepfer, Johann Jacobus (b. 1620). German physician.

Wepfer's disease. Cerebral haemorrhage due to rupture of an atherosclerotic artery.

Wepfer's glands. Brunner's glands.

Werdnig, Guido (b. 1862). Graz neurologist.

Werdnig-Hoffman disease. Familial progressive spinal muscular atrophy of infancy.

Werlhof, Paul Gottlieb (b. 1699). Hanover physician.

Werlhof's disease. Idiopathic thrombocytopenic purpura. *See* PURPURA.

Werneking, Friedrich Christian Gregor (b. 1798). Swiss anatomist.

Werneking's commissure. A decussation of efferent cerebellar fibres constituting the superior cerebellar peduncles.

Werner, C. W. O. 20th century German physician.

Werner's syndrome. A hereditary disorder characterized by cataracts, osteoporosis, sexual immaturity, early arteriosclerosis, shortness in height and premature greying of the hair.

Werner, Heinrich (b. 1874). German physician in South Africa.

His-Werner disease, Werner-His disease. Trench fever. *See* FEVER.

Wernicke, Karl (b. 1848). Breslau neurologist.

Wernicke's aphasia. That caused by lesions of the posterior branch of the sylvian artery and, according to the extent of the lesion, described as *sensory aphasia, Wernicke's aphasia* or *total aphasia.*

Wernicke's area, centre, field or zone. The sensory speech centre situated in the posterior third of the superior temporal gyrus and adjacent angular gyrus in the dominant hemisphere; it is concerned with the recognition, recall and interpretation of words and other auditory symbols, and with their translation into language.

Wernicke's disease. Wernicke's encephalopathy (see below).

Wernicke's encephalopathy. Encephalopathy associated with a deficiency of thiamine (vitamin B_1). It is found in chronic alcoholism, hyperemesis gravidarum or in carcinoma of the stomach. There are petechial haemorrhages in the region of the third or fourth ventricles.

Wernicke's fibres. Gratiolet's radiation; the optic radiation.

Wernicke's fissure. An occasional fissure which separates the occipital lobe of the cerebrum from the parietal and temporal lobes.

Wernicke's hemianopic pupil reaction, reflex or sign. In hemianopia due to a lesion of the optic tract a light thrown on the side of the retina involved in the hemianopia gives no contraction of the pupil, while on stimulation of the unaffected half of the retina the pupils contract.

Wernicke's syndrome. A disease picture characterized aetiologically by a deficiency of the vitamin-B complex (in particular aneurine), pathologically by multiple cerebral petechial haemorrhages, in particular in the region of the mamillary bodies, neurologically by disturbances of ocular movements of pupillary responses and of tendon reflexes, and mentally by a Korsakoff syndrome.

Wernicke's triangle. A triangular area in the posterior part of the posterior limb of the internal capsule lying between the fibres of the posterior thalamic radiation and the optic radiation.

lateral zone of Wernicke. The region of the brain lying lateral to the lateral geniculate body and containing fibres from the optic tract and the optic radiation.

Wernicke-Mann type. Partial hemiplegia; paraesthesia.

Wernicke, Robert Johann (b. 1873). Buenos Aires pathologist.

Posada-Wernicke disease. Coccidioidomycosis.

Wertheim, Ernst (b. 1864). Vienna gynaecologist.

Wertheim's hysterectomy or operation. Radical abdominal hysterectomy; removal of the uterus and its appendages, with as much cellular tissue of the pelvis and as many regional glands as possible, together with an ample vaginal cuff.

Wertheimer, Ernst (b. 1893). Halle cytologist.

Wertheimer's serum agar. *See* SERUM AGAR.

West, Charles (b. 1816). British physician.

West's skull, West-Engstler skull. A form of craniotabes giving a honeycomb appearance of the cranium which is sometimes associated with spina bifida or encephalocele.

West, John Montgomery (b. 1876). American otolaryngologist.

West's operation. Dacryocystorrhinostomy by the nasal route.

West's swab. A postnasal swab enclosed in a curved glass tube.

West, Randolph (b. 1890). New York physician.

Dakin and West liver fraction. An extract of liver containing the haemopoietic factor and used in the treatment of pernicious anaemia.

West's syndrome. Infantile myoclonic encephalopathy with hypsarrhythmia.

Westberg, Friedrich (b. 1868). Breslau physician.

Westberg's disease. Morphoea guttata.

Westberg's space. A space enclosed by the reflection of the parietal pericardium on to the ascending aorta; the aortic recess.

Westergren, Alf (b. 1891). Swedish physician.

Westergren method. A method for estimating the rate of erythrocyte sedimentation in whole blood to which an anticoagulant has been added. Readings are taken after 1 h and 2 h, in millilitres, the distance of the red cell column from the top of the fluid (the 0 mark) being read off.

Westergren tube. A narrow-bore (2.5 mm) tube, similar to a 1 ml pipette, used for estimating the rate of sedimentation of erythrocytes. It is calibrated downwards from zero to 200, the zero mark being 200 mm from the lower end of the tube.

Weston, Edward (b. 1850). American engineer.

Weston cell. Cadmium cell. *See* CELL.

Westphal, Alexander Karl Otto (b. 1863). German neurologist.

Westphal's contraction. Fixation contraction; reflex contraction of a muscle on maximum passive shortening, said to occur in paralysis agitans.

Westphal's pupillary reflex, Pilcz-Westphal phenomena or reaction, Westphal-Pilcz phenomenon, reaction or pupillary reflex. Contraction of the pupil of the eye on attempted closure of the lids while they are being held open; unilateral. Also called *von Graefe's lid reaction.*

Westphal, Carl Friedrich Otto (b. 1833). Berlin neurologist.

Westphal's neurosis or pseudosclerosis, Struempell-Westphal pseudosclerosis, Westphal-Struempell disease. A hysterical condition with symptoms of disseminated sclerosis but without the lesions.

Westphal's nucleus, Edinger-Westphal nucleus. A nucleus ventrolateral to the upper end of the aqueduct of the midbrain giving origin to oculomotor nerve fibres to the sphincter of the pupil and ciliary muscles.

Westphal's phenomenon or sign, Erb-Westphal sign, Westphal-Erb sign. Loss of the patellar reflex; as first described, this applies particularly to cases of tabes dorsalis.

wet (wet). Damp, moist. [AS *waet.*]

wetting agent (wet·ing a·jent). A surface-active compound which, by virtue of certain hydrophilic groups, e.g. OH, COOH, SO_3H, acts as a detergent and promotes the wetting of a surface by water. [wet, agent.]

Wever, Ernest Glen (b. 1902). Princeton psychologist.

Wever-Bray phenomenon. When sounds fall upon the ear, the auditory nerve shows changes of potential directly and closely related to the incident sound.

Weyl's test. For creatinine: a solution of sodium nitroprusside is added and then a few drops of sodium hydroxide. A ruby-red colour is obtained, which changes to yellow.

Wharton, Thomas (b. 1614). English physician and anatomist.

Wharton's duct. Submandibular duct. *See* DUCT.

Wharton's gelatin or jelly. The primitive connective tissue of the umbilical cord, containing large quantities of the mucopolysaccharide, hyaluronic acid.

whartonitis (wor·ton·i·tis). Inflammation of the duct of the submandibular salivary gland (Wharton's duct). [Thomas *Wharton.*]

wheal (hweel). Weal.

wheal and clown method. A special stain for the club bodies of *Actinomyces.* The clubs are stained red by carbol fuchsine, and the mycelium greenish-blue, by haematoxylin and picric acid.

wheat (hweet). The ripe fruit of *Triticum aestivum* (family Graminae). It is an important food on account of its protein and carbohydrate content. **Wheat germ.** The embryo of the wheat seed. It is valuable as a source of vitamin E which is often administered in the form of wheat germ oil. [AS *hwaete.*]

wheatmeal (hweet·meel). Wheat flour almost entirely (85 per cent) free from chaff. **National wheatmeal.** The standard flour directed by the British Government to be used for bread-making during World War II. Its composition varied from time to time; it contained calcium carbonate, and standards were laid down for fibre and vitamin-B_1 content. [wheat, meal.]

Wheatsone, Sir Charles (b. 1802). British physicist.

Wheatstone bridge. An instrument consisting of a graduated resistance wire and a known resistance, used to measure electrical resistance.

Wheeler, John Martin (b. 1879). New York ophthalmologist.

Wheeler's knife. *See* WHEELER'S OPERATION 7 (below).

Wheeler's operation. 1. Tarsorrhaphy of the canthal angle: the lash margin is removed from each eyelid and tongue fashioned from the tarsal plate of one lid is sutured into the intermarginal groove of the other. It can be combined with a narrowing of the palpebral fissure by resuturing the external palpebral ligament further out. 2. For repair of eyelid colobomata: an external canthotomy is performed and at the same time the orbicularis fibres going to the lid are cut subcutaneously in this position with scissors. The coloboma edges are cleaned, and split and sutured in the deep and superficial layers, the lines of suture being offset. A small Ammon triangle of skin is excised at the outer canthus. 3. Tarsectomy: excision of the tarsal plate; the levator palpebrae superioris muscle is then sutured to the lower tarsal rim that is left, and to the skin of the lid. 4. For cicatricial ectropion; for one or both lids: all scar tissue is resected, lid margins brought back to normal position and tarsorrhaphy performed. The bare area is covered with an epidermal or Thiersch graft. 5. For entropion: (*a*) A strip of orbicularis muscle is dissected free in the whole length of the lid. This is left attached at the ends but divided in the centre, and the two ends overlapped and sutured together and to the tarsal plate. (*b*) A strip of orbicularis muscle is dissected free and left attached medially, but cut laterally. This end is then pulled laterally and upwards and sutured to the periosteum of the zygomatic bone. 6. For ptosis: a strip of orbicularis muscle is dissected free in the upper lid at its medial and lateral ends, being left attached in the centre. These two free ends are passed through above the tarsal plate each side of the levator and sutured to each side of the superior rectus muscle. 7. For discission: *Wheeler's knife*, shaped like a small Graefe knife, is passed into the anterior chamber at the limbus, cutting edge downwards, and with 1 sweep it passes through the capsule into the vitreous; the movement is reversed and the knife withdrawn. 8. For glaucoma: a cyclodialysis combined with a broad iridectomy in the same quadrant.

Wheelhouse, Claudius Galen (b. 1826). Leeds surgeon.

Wheelhouse's operation. A method of perineal section for impermeable stricture of the urethra by incising the urethra immediately distal to the stricture against the shoulder of the Wheelhouse staff. Thereafter the stricture is incised under vision.

Wheelhouse's perineal staff. An instrument used in the operation of external urethrotomy for impermeable stricture of the urethra.

wheeze (hweez). 1. To breathe with an audible whistling. 2. The sound produced during difficult breathing, by the air in the glottis. **Asthmatoid wheeze.** Jackson's sign, a symptom of obstruction in the trachea or in a bronchus, the sound heard resembling that characteristic of asthma. [Old Norse *hvaesa* to hiss.]

wheezing (hweez·ing). Laboured and noisy breathing such as that observed in asthma. [see prec.]

whelk (hwelk). 1. Acne. 2. A pimple or pustule. [AS *hwylca*.]

whey (hwa). The liquid separated from milk after coagulation with rennet or by the lactic acid on souring. The greater part of the protein and fat has been removed, and the chief constituents are lactalbumin and lactose. It may be used in the preparation of humanized milk and of special diets. **Alum whey.** The liquid separated from milk after coagulation by boiling with alum. **Wine whey.** A preparation of milk coagulated with white wine, with the curd removed and sugar added to sweeten. It may be used as an invalid diet. [AS *hwaeg*.]

whip (hwip). *See* HARRISON (L. W.). [ME *whippen*.]

whiplash (hwip·lash). A violent forward and backward movement of the head upon the neck, occurring in sudden acceleration or deceleration involving passengers in motor and other vehicles upon impact. [AS *hwaeg*, O Fr. *lasche*.]

Whipple, Allen Oldfather (b. 1881). New York surgeon.

Whipple's incision. A curved incision, convex upwards, between the xiphoid process and umbilicus, with division of both rectus muscles.

Whipple's operation. Excision of the head of the pancreas together with the duodenum.

Whipple's triad. The triad of clinical features in the Zollinger-Ellison syndrome.

Whipple, George Hoyt (b. 1878). Baltimore pathologist.

Whipple's disease. A lipoid disorder in which the lymph spaces of the intestines and mesentery are enlarged and filled with lipides. There is steatorrhoea with associated abdominal symptoms, loss of weight, discoloration of the skin suggesting Addison's disease, and joint symptoms. There is usually achlorhydria, a flat glucose tolerance curve, hypocalcaemia and hypokalaemia, and the barium meal shows a deficiency pattern.

whipworm (hwip·werm). *Trichuris trichiura.* [ME *whippen*, worm.]

whiskey (hwis·ke). Whisky.

whisky (hwis·ke). A spirit prepared by distillation of a fermented mash made from grain, followed by maturation for at least 4 years in sherry casks. Barley is used for the preparation of Scotch whisky, wheat, rye or maize for other whiskies. Whisky contains about 40 per cent v/v of ethyl alcohol and is used medicinally for the oral administration of the latter. [Gael. *uisgebeatha* water of life.]

whisper (hwis·per). 1. The soft sibilant speech produced by tongue and lips alone, without the setting of the vocal cords into vibration. 2. The auscultatory sound heard when the patient whispers. [AS *hwisprian*.]

whistle (hwisl). 1. A tubular wind instrument that makes a shrill note. Whistles are used for testing the upper tones of hearing: some of the sounds produced are beyond the range of human appreciation. 2. To produce a shrill sound either by contracting the lips, by the aid of a tubular wind instrument, or by some other means. **Water whistle.** Sahli's whistle; an abdominal sound caused by flatus in the intestine. [AS *hwistle*.]

See also: SAHLI.

White, James Clarke (b. 1833). Boston dermatologist.

White's disease. Keratosis follicularis.

White, James William (b. 1850). Philadelphia surgeon.

White's operation. Castration for hypertrophy of the prostate.

White, Paul Dudley (b. 1886). Boston cardiologist.

Wolff-Parkinson-White syndrome. This consists of physiological bundle-branch block with short P-R interval, probably as a result of an abnormal short conducting pathway between auricles and ventricles. This results in premature excitation of one ventricle (usually the right) and gives rise to functional block of the left bundle. It occurs as a congenital anomaly in an otherwise normal heart and is associated with a liability to repeated paroxysms of tachycardia. A similar electrocardiographic appearance may sometimes be seen as a result of nodal rhythm resulting from acquired cardiac lesions.

white (hwite). **Egg white.** The viscous colourless fluid, consisting essentially of water and proteins, which surrounds the yolk. The proteins are ovalbumin, ovoglobulin and ovomucoid. [AS *hwit*.]

white-cap (hwite·kap). Witkop. [white, AS *caeppe*.]

Whitehead, John M. (b. 1899). Indiana physician.

Wallhauser and Whitehead method. A method of treatment of Hodgkin's disease by a soluble extract of an autogenous gland.

Whitehead, Walter (b. 1840). Manchester surgeon.

mucous disease of Whitehead. Mucous colitis.

Whitehead's operation. 1. Circular resection of haemorrhoids. 2. Removal of one half of the tongue for carcinoma.

Whitehead's varnish. An antiseptic surgical varnish containing iodoform, benzoin, storax and Tolu balsam in ether.

Whitehorn, John Clare (b. 1894). American biochemist.

Whitehorn's method, for chlorides in blood. To 10 ml Folin-Wu filtrate add 5 ml of standard silver nitrate (1 ml = 1 mg NaCl) and 5 ml of concentrated nitric acid. Mix and titrate with standard thiocyanate (1.7 g KCNS per litre), using ferric alum as indicator.

whites (hwi·tz). Leucorrhoea. [AS *hwit*.]

Whitfield, Arthur (b. 1868). English dermatologist.

Whitfield's ointment. Compound ointment of benzoic acid.

whitlow (hwit·low). Infection of the finger pulp. **Herpetic whitlow.** A group of blisters near a finger nail, usually in nurses, caused by *Herpesvirus hominis.* **Melanotic whitlow.** A malignant melanoma of the nail bed. **Thecal whitlow.** Infection of a digital flexor synovial sheath. [etym. dub.]

Whitman, Royal (b. 1857). New York orthopaedic surgeon.

Whitman's frame. A frame for the nursing of tuberculosis of the spine; it is similar to Bradford's frame.

Whitman's operation. 1. An arthroplasty of the hip. 2. A method of immobilization of an intracapsular fracture of the neck of the femur by plaster of Paris. 3. Astragalectomy for the treatment of a paralytic calcaneus deformity.

Whitman's plaster. A plaster spica used in the treatment of intracapsular fracture of the femoral neck.

Whitmore, Alfred (b. 1876). British Army pathologist in Burma.

Whitmore's bacillus. *Pfeifferella whitmori.*

Whitnall, Samuel Ernest (b. 1876). British and Canadian anatomist.

Whitnall's tubercle. A tubercle of varying size and form on the orbital aspect of the frontal process of the zygomatic bone giving attachment to the lateral palpebral ligament.

whoop (hoop). The crowing inspiration at the end of the paroxysm in whooping-cough. [O Fr. *houper.*]

whooping-cough (**hoop·ing·kof**). Pertussis, a specific infectious disease caused by *Haemophilus pertussis* or the Bordet-Gengou bacillus. It is characterized by respiratory catarrh and paroxysms of coughing which may be accompanied by long-drawn inspirations (whoops) and vomiting. Endemic in countries with temperate climates (also occasional epidemics), it is pre-eminently a disease of infants and children under 5 years of age. The incubation period to the onset of catarrhal stage is from 7 to 14 days; the paroxysmal stage commences from 7 to 14 days later, the severity and duration of the latter stage being very variable. The paroxysms are most severe and often most numerous at night. Complications and sequelae include bronchopneumonia, emphysema, pulmonary collapse, digestive troubles, convulsions and cardiac dilatation. One attack usually protects; second and even third attacks may occur in adults, but tend to be atypical and mild. There is little or no immunity transferred to the newborn. General measures of treatment include fresh air, good nursing and chemotherapy. Vaccines offer protection, and are given preferably in infancy. [O Fr. *houper,* cough.]

whorl (hworl). One of the patterns formed by the dermal ridges on the finger tips. This is characterized by the presence of 2 triradii. **Bone whorl.** Enostosis. **Coccygeal whorl [vortex coccygeus (BNA)].** The hair whorl at the tip of the coccyx. **Hair whorls [vortices pilorum].** Areas where the hairs are arranged spirally, or have their free ends directed inwards, towards a centre. They are seen at the navel and at the tip of the coccyx. [ME *hwarwyl.*]

Whytt, Robert (b. 1714). Scottish physician.

Whytt's disease. 1. Internal hydrocephalus. 2. Tuberculous meningitis in infancy and childhood.

Whytt's reflex. Loss of pupillary constriction in response to light; described by Whytt in destruction of the superior quadrigeminal bodies.

Wiart, Pierre (b. 1870). Paris anatomist.

Wiart's duodenal notch. An impression on the anterior surface of the pancreas formed by the duodenum.

Wickerkiewicz's operation. 1. For epicanthus: an arrow-shaped area of skin pointing to the nose is removed from the nasal side of the fold. The edges are undermined and sutured. 2. For colobomata of the upper eyelid: the conjunctiva and tarsal plate are first sutured and then a triangular skin flap, base down, is dissected from the lower lid and sutured into the gap in the upper lid.

Wickersheimer, J. (b. 1832). Berlin anatomist.

Wickersheimer's fluid or medium. A fluid, used at one time for anatomical preservation, containing arsenic trioxide, potassium salts and sodium chloride in an alcohol, glycerin and water solution.

Wickham, Louis Frédéric (b. 1861). Paris dermatologist.

Wickham's striae. Whitish striae on the surface of the flat-topped papules of lichen planus, noted by Wickham and ascribed by Darier to localized thickenings of the granular layer of the epidermis. The striae may be arranged like the spokes of a wheel, or like a river with tributaries; or the papules may be cross-hatched by striae; occasionally a single stria is seen.

Widal, Georges Fernand Isidore (b. 1862). Paris physician.

Widal's reaction or test, Gruber-Widal reaction, Grünbaum-Widal reaction or test. An agglutination test for typhoid fever in which a selected living culture of the typhoid bacillus was agglutinated in test-tubes or on glass slides by dilutions of the patient's serum or other immune serum. The reaction has now been adapted for the diagnosis of typhoid and paratyphoid cases and carriers. The Vi, H and O antigens of the enteric group organisms are all considered.

Widal's syndrome. Acholuric jaundice. *See* JAUNDICE.

Widal's treatment. Treatment of cardiovascular disease (congestive heart failure, hypertension) by restricting the intake of sodium chloride (salt) in food and drink. Salt is retained in the body in congestive heart failure and favours the formation of oedema, while a very small intake of salt is said to lower systemic blood pressure. (Salt restriction forms the basis of the management of congestive cardiac failure at the present time.)

Widal-Abrami disease. Acquired haemolytic jaundice.

Hayem-Widal anaemia or syndrome. A haemolytic anaemia.

Widowitz's sign. Cantelli's sign.

Wieiver-Saver operation. For epiphora: dacryocystorrhinostomy through the nose.

Wiener, Alexander Solomon (b. 1907). Brooklyn, New York, serologist and expert in blood grouping.

Wiener notation. *See* CDE NOTATION.

Wiesel, Josef (b. 1876). Vienna physician.

Wiesel's paraganglion. Chromaffin tissue found in the cardiac plexus of the sympathetic nervous system.

Wiesner, R. (b. 1875). Vienna anatomist.

Wiesner's paraganglion. Wiesel's paraganglion.

Wiethe, Camillo. 20th century Austrian otolaryngologist.

Urbach-Wiethe disease. Lipoid proteinosis. *See* PROTEINOSIS.

Wigand, Justus Heinrich (b. 1769). Hamburg gynaecologist.

Wigand's manoeuvre. A method of flexing the fetal head in breech delivery.

Wij's solution and test. A solution of iodine monochloride in glacial acetic acid, used for determining the iodine value or number (degree of unsaturation) of fixed oils and fats.

Wilbrand's prism test. For differentiating between lesions of the visual cortex and optic tract: a patient with hemianopia is asked to fix a small point on a uniform ground and its image is then thrown on to the blind side by placing 14 degree prisms in front of each eye; when this is done an abrupt movement of the eyes may bring the image on to the seeing side again. Wilbrand felt that this was a reflex response seen only in intracerebral lesions, particularly those of the cortex, and not in disease of the tract. It is now believed that the movement is voluntary and not reflex; the test is of historical interest, but of no clinical value.

Wildbolz, Hans (b. 1873). Swiss physician.

Wildbolz reaction. A local reaction following the intradermal injection of the patient's own urine; regarded as indicative of tuberculosis [obsolete].

Wilde, Sir William Robert Wills (b. 1815). Dublin surgeon.

Wilde's cone of light. The reflection of a source of light on the tense portion of the tympanic membrane.

Wilde's cords. Fibres of the corpus callosum passing horizontally and connecting the cerebral hemispheres.

Wilde's operation. An incision 12 mm behind the attachment of the auricle down to the periosteum, used in subperiosteal abscess or mastoid disease.

Wilder, Russell Morse (b. 1885). Rochester, Minnesota, physician.

Cutler, Power and Wilder test. A chemical test for Addison's disease which depended upon the induction of an exacerbation of the disease by the withholding of salt. It is now obsolete because of its danger.

Wilder, William (b. 1860). American ophthalmologist.

Wilder's sign. Jerky, horizontal movements of the eyes in endocrine exophthalmos.

Wilder's law. The more nearly an organ is working at maximal capacity the less easily can it be stimulated to do further work, though it may be depressed or inhibited without difficulty.

Wildermuth, Hermann (b. 1852). Stuttgart psychiatrist.

Wildermuth's ear. A deformity of the ear with variations in landmarks and contours.

Wilkie, Sir David Percival Dalbreck (b. 1882). Edinburgh surgeon.

Wilkie's classification of appendicitis. A system which distinguishes obstructive from mural appendicitis.

Wilkie's manoeuvre. In splenectomy, mobilization of the spleen by division of the left (posterior) layer of the lienorenal ligament.

Wilkinson, John Frederick (b. 1897). Manchester haematologist.

Wilkinson's anaemia. Achrestic anaemia. *See* ANAEMIA.

Wilkinson's haemopoietin. A heat-labile enzyme-like substance (anti-pernicious-anaemia factor), probably a mucoprotein present in normal human and pig gastric secretions that reacts with extrinsic factor to produce the so-called anti-pernicious-anaemia liver principle essential for normal red blood-cell formation.

Wilkinson's disease. Paralysis agitans; usually called *Parkinson's disease.*

Wilks, Sir Samuel (b. 1824). English physician.

Wilks' syndrome. Myasthenia gravis.

Willan, Robert (b. 1757). London dermatologist.

Willan's disease or lupus. Lupus vulgaris, a granulomatous variety of tuberculosis of the skin, characterized by the presence of "apple-jelly" nodules.

Willebrand, E. A. von. 20th century Finnish physician.

von Willebrand's disease. A form of non-thrombocytopenic purpura. The platelets are normal but the capillaries show functional changes.

Willett, John Abernethy (b. 1872). London obstetrician.

Willett's clamp or forceps. An instrument used to apply continuous scalp traction to the fetus in an attempt to control bleeding from a placenta praevia.

Williams, Charles James Blasius (b. 1805). English physician.

Williams' phenomenon. The tympanitic percussion note above the level of a pleural effusion alters in pitch with opening or closing of the mouth.

Williams' sign. Dullness to percussion in the 2nd intercostal space in a large effusion.

Williams, Henry Willard (b. 1821). Boston ophthalmologist.

Williams' lantern. A special lantern designed to test colour vision. It has 3 apertures, and so can show a varying range of contrasting colours,

Williams' operation. For lacrimal stricture [obsolete].

Williamson, Oliver Key (b. 1866). London physician.

Williamson's sign. Much diminished blood pressure in the leg, as compared with the arm of the same side, in pleural effusion and pneumothorax.

Willis, Thomas (b. 1621). English anatomist and physician.

circle of Willis. Circulus arteriosus.

Willis' cords. Fibrous trabeculae in the superior sagittal sinus.

Willis' disease. Diabetes.

Willis' gland. The corpus albicans.

Willis' paracousis. Increased acuity of hearing when the subject is surrounded by noise, although deaf in quiet surroundings.

Willis' pouch. The pyloric antrum. *See* ANTRUM.

Willis' valve. The superior medullary velum. *See* VELUM.

Willis salt floatation method. A floatation method for ova in faeces.

willow (wil·o). Any tree of the genus *Salix* (family Salicaceae), particularly the tree *Salix alba.* The bark of the latter contains tannin and salicin, and possesses bitter and astringent properties. [AS *welig.*]

Wills, Lucy. 20th century London physician.

Wills' anaemia. Tropical macrocytic anaemia. *See* ANAEMIA.

Wilms, Max (b. 1867). Heidelberg surgeon.

Wilms' operation. Thoracoplasty.

Wilms' tumour. An embryonal carcinoma of the kidney in young children; nephroblastoma.

Wilson, Charles Thomas Rees (b. 1869). British physicist.

Wilson cloud chamber. A chamber in which air can be rapidly supersaturated with water vapour. Ionizing radiations, e.g. alpha particles, x-rays, passing through the chamber in these conditions produce visible tracks by the condensation of water droplets on the ions they leave in their wake.

Wilson, Clifford (b. 1906). London physician.

Kimmelstiel–Wilson disease or syndrome. Nephrotic symptoms, gross oedema and albuminuria combined with glycosuria.

Wilson, James (b. 1765). London surgeon.

Wilson's muscles. Longitudinal fasciculi of the sphincter urethrae which are not generally recognized.

Wilson, Samuel Alexander Kinnier (b. 1877). London neurologist.

Wilson's disease or syndrome, Kinnier Wilson disease or syndrome. Hepatolenticular degeneration. *See* DEGENERATION.

Wilson, William James (b. 1879). British bacteriologist.

Wilson and Blair agar or medium. A bismuth sulphite agar medium, prepared from peptone meat-extract agar 100 ml, bismuth-sulphite solution 200 ml, and iron-citrate brilliant-green solution 45 ml. It is a very effective inhibiting selective medium used for the isolation of *Salmonella typhi* and *S. paratyphi* from faeces.

Wilson, Sir William James Erasmus (b. 1809). London dermatologist.

Wilson's disease, Wilson–Brocq disease. Dermatitis exofoliativa.

lichen of Wilson. Lichen planus, originally described by Wilson in 1869.

Wimshurst, James (b. 1832). English engineer.

Wimshurst's machine. A machine which depends upon electrostatic action for converting mechanical energy into electrical energy.

Winckel, Franz Karl Ludwig Wilhelm von (b. 1837). Munich physician.

Winckel's disease. Erythroblastic anaemia of the newborn.

wind-contusion (wind·kon·tew′·zhun). Internal injury caused by the compression wave of a bomb or shell blast. [AS *wind,* contusion.]

windage (wind·ij). Internal injuries produced by air compressed by the passage of a projectile, e.g. a shell. [AS *wind.*]

windburn (wind·bern). A skin lesion caused by exposure to a hot wind. [AS *wind,* burn.]

windchill (wind·chil). Local chilling resulting from exposure to a cool wind. [AS *wind,* chill.]

windkessel (wind·kes·el). An elastic pressure chamber incorporated in a pumping system to smooth out the individual strokes of the pump so as to achieve a more continuous flow at the output. In cardiology, the term has been applied to the theory that the proximal arterial vessels act like an elastic chamber storing blood during the ventricular ejection phase and then recoiling so as to push blood more smoothly through the circulation in diastole.

windlass (wind·las). **Spanish windlass.** An emergency first-aid tourniquet, made by tying a handkerchief or similar article round a limb and exerting pressure by inserting a small stick or pencil in the knot and twisting it. [O Fr. *windas.*]

window (win·do). 1. The part of the case of a Geiger–Müller counter which is made of sufficiently thin material to allow the radiation of interest to enter the sensitive volume of the instrument. 2. The radiation energy range recorded by a radiation detector. Radiation of energy below or above the selected range is not recorded. The window can usually be selected by adjustment of electronic controls. 3. Any opening in a rigid structure, e.g. in a plaster-of-Paris case, to allow a wound to be examined and dressed. **Aortopulmonary window.** Aortopulmonary septal defect. *See* DEFECT. [Old Norse *vindauga.*]

See also: DEAVER.

windowing (win·do·ing). The operation of decompressing the interior of a bone by cutting a window in the cortex.

windpipe (wind·pipe). The trachea. [AS *wind,* pipe.]

Windscheid, Franz (b. 1862). Leipzig neurologist.

Windscheid's disease. Nervous symptoms of arteriosclerotic origin.

wine (wine). An alcoholic beverage prepared by the fermentation of fruit juices, generally grape juice. Wines were at one time widely used as a vehicle for the administration of medicaments. **Wine of steel.** Iron wine, iron macerated in sherry-type wine until the liquid contains between 0.125 and 0.3 per cent of iron. It is a preparation for the internal administration of iron. [L *vinum*.]

wing [ala (NA)] (wing). Any structure bearing a fancied resemblance to a wing; ala. **Wing of the ilium.** Ala of the ilium. **Wings of the nose.** The alae of the nose. **Wings of the sphenoid bone.** Two processes projecting laterally from the body of the sphenoid bone and separated by the superior orbital fissure. The *greater wing* [ala major (NA)] forms part of the floor of the middle cranial fossa [facies cerebralis (NA)], of the lateral wall of the orbit [facies orbitalis (NA)] and of the temporal [facies temporalis (NA)] and infratemporal fossae; the sphenomaxillary surface [facies sphenomaxillaris (NA)] forms the posterior wall of the pterygopalatine fossa. It articulates with the frontal, zygomatic, parietal and petrosquamous portions of the temporal bone. The *lesser wing* [ala minor (NA)] forms part of the floor of the anterior cranial fossa and roof of the orbit and articulates with the frontal bone. [Old Norse *vaengr*.]

See also: INGRASSIA.

Winiwarter, Alexander von (b. 1848). Vienna surgeon.

Winiwarter's operation. Cholecysto-enterostomy.

wink (wingk). The automatic closure of the eyelids, distributing tears which keep the conjunctiva moist; the voluntary facial gesture produced by quickly shutting and opening one eye. [AS *wincian* to move sideways.]

Winkelman, Nathaniel W. (b. 1891). American neurologist.

Winkelman's disease. Progressive pallidal degeneration, a rare disease of children characterized by progressive muscular rigidity and retinal pigmentation.

Winkler, Clemens Alexander (b. 1838). German chemist.

Winkler reagent, for absorption of carbon monoxide. Dissolve 40 g of cuprous chloride and 50 g of ammonium chloride in distilled water and dilute to 150 ml. For use mix 3 volumes with 1 volume of ammonia (sp. gr. 0.9).

Winkler, Max (b. 1875). Lucerne dermatologist.

Winkler's disease. Chondrodermatitis nodularis chronica helicis.

Winsbury-White, Horace Powell (b. 1892). London surgeon.

Winsbury-White tube. An angled type of bulbous-ended rubber tube for drainage of the bladder after prostatectomy.

Winslow, Jacques Bénigne (Jacob Benignus) (b. 1669). Paris anatomist.

foramen of Winslow. Epiploic foramen; the opening into the lesser sac of the peritoneal cavity.

Winslow's ligament. The lateral ligament of the knee.

Winslow's pancreas. The uncinate process of the head of the pancreas.

stars of Winslow. Venous capillary whorls found in the choriocapillaris of the choroidal coat of the eye.

Winslow's test. In cases of doubtful death, faint respirations can be detected by placing a vessel containing water over the lower part of the sternum and observing oscillations of the water level.

Winter, George B. 20th century American oral surgeon.

Winter's elevator. One of a series of elevators designed primarily for the removal of the third molar (wisdom) teeth of the lower jaw.

Winterbottom, Thomas Masterman (b. 1765). British physician and explorer.

Winterbottom's sign. Enlargement of the lymph glands in the posterior triangle of the neck in trypanosomiasis. Though not fully appreciating the significance of this sign, he noted that slave-traders avoided negroes who had these enlarged glands.

wintergreen (win·ter·green). Gaultheria; the plant *Gaultheria procumbens*. [AS *winter*, green.]

Winterhalter, Elizabeth H.

Winterhalter's ganglion. An accumulation of ganglion cells in the ovary, the existence of which, in man, is very doubtful.

Wintrich, Anton (b. 1812). Erlangen physician.

Wintrich's change of note or sign. An alteration of the pitch of the percussion note according as to whether the mouth is open or closed. It indicates a large cavity or pneumothorax communicating with a large bronchus.

Wintrobe, Maxwell Myer (b. 1901). Canadian physician.

Wintrobe haematocrit or tube. A flat-bottomed, glass tube about 115 mm in length with a uniform bore of 2.5 mm graduated from 0 to 100 mm from above downwards. It has a double use; first the sedimentation rate of a blood sample can be estimated, and then in the same sample the packed-cell volume.

Wintrobe and Landsberg method. A method for the determination of packed-cell volume and sedimentation rate of blood, with a small graduated haematocrit tube (Wintrobe's tube).

wire (wire). 1. Metal drawn out into threads or rods of varying fineness. 2. To fix bone fragments or adjust the malposition of teeth by means of wire. 3. To insert a spiral of wire into an aneurysmal sac to encourage clotting and reduce the risk of rupture. **Alveolar wire.** Wire used in the treatment of fractures of the jaw. **Arch wire.** A wire conforming to the shape of the arch of the teeth. [AS *wir*.]

See also: COLT, KIRSCHNER.

wiring (wi·ring). *See* WIRE. **Alveolar wiring.** A technique in which fixation of the fragments of a fractured mandible is obtained by a wire ligature passing through the alveolar bone of each fragment. **Arch wiring.** A technique in which a wire (arch wire) is attached to the teeth on the labial aspect in either or both jaws. In orthodontics it is used for aligning the teeth, and in maxillofacial surgery for the providing of the attachment of rubber ligatures in cases of jaw fracture. **Circumferential wiring.** A technique employed in the treatment of a fractured mandible whereby a splint is held in position by wires passing around the bone of the jaw. **Direct wiring.** A technique used in the immobilization of a fractured mandible to the maxilla, in which a continuous wire is fixed to teeth in the upper and lower jaws. **Eyelet wiring.** A technique used in the immobilization of a fractured mandible, in which looped wires are fixed to teeth in the upper and lower jaws and joined by ligatures. **Interdental wiring.** A technique in which a wire is fixed around teeth in each fragment of a fractured jaw to hold the fractured ends in apposition.

Wirsung, Johann George (d. 1643). German anatomist in Padua.

canal or duct of Wirsung. The pancreatic duct. *See* DUCT.

wiry (wi·re). 1. Thin, flexible and tough, like wire. 2. Describing a pulse which is small but tense, as in acute peritonitis.

wistarin (wis·tar·in). A poisonous glycoside derived from species of *Wistaria*.

witch hazel (wich ha·zl). Hamamelis. **Witch hazel bark.** Hamamelis bark. **Distilled witch hazel.** Hamamelis water. *See* WATER. **Witch hazel leaves.** Hamamelis. [AS *wice* pliant, hazel.]

witch's milk (wich·es milk). Neonatal galactorrhoea due to absorption of placental prolactin.

witherite (with·er·ite). A native barium carbonate, $BaCO_3$, usually found in lead veins, and a source of barium salts.

witkop (wit·kop). White-cap; a skullcap-like structure formed by matted crusts in the scalp: found in syphilitic natives in South Africa. [Afrikaans.]

witness (wit·nes). Capacity to give evidence in Court, classed as skilled or expert if qualified in a particular respect, as in medicine or science. [AS *witnes*, wisdom.]

Witts, Leslie John (b. 1895). Oxford physician.

Witts' anaemia. Hypochromic anaemia due to iron deficiency.

Witts' diet. A modified Meulengracht diet, more suited to the food habits in the UK.

Witzel, Friedrich Oskar (b. 1856). Bonn surgeon.

Witzel's gastrostomy or operation. A cone of stomach is

drawn through the abdominal wall before it is opened; a tube is then inserted.

Woelfler, Anton (b. 1850). Prague surgeon.

Woelfler's gland. An accessory lobe of the thyroid gland lying above the arch of the aorta.

Woelfler's operation. Gastro-enterostomy.

Wohlfahrtia (vole·far·te·ah). A genus of larviparous flies of the family Sarcophagidae. **Wohlfahrtia magnifica.** The Old World screw-worm, occurring in Europe, Turkey, Russia and North Africa, whose larvae occur commonly in wounds and nasal cavities. **Wohlfahrtia nuba.** A species from Ethiopia and the Sudan whose larvae have occurred in human wounds. **Wohlfahrtia vigil.** A Canadian species whose larvae have occurred on wounds in infants.

Wohlgemuth, Julius (b. 1874). Berlin biochemist.

Wohlgemuth's method or test, for diastase in urine. Mix 1 ml of urine with 4 ml of buffer solution (the phosphate buffer used has a pH value of 6.1 and is prepared by mixing 15 ml of a solution containing 11.876 g of $Na_2HPO_45H_2O$ per litre with 85 ml of a solution containing 9.078 g of KH_2PO_4 per litre). Into 8 small tubes place 1.5, 1.0, 0.5, 0.4, 0.3, 0.2, 0.1, 0.05 ml respectively of the diluted urine and add water to each to bring the volume to 2.0 ml. To each tube add 1 ml of 0.2 per cent soluble starch solution and incubate at 37°C for 30 min. Cool the tubes rapidly, and to each add dilute iodine drop by drop until a permanent colour is obtained. The tube showing no blue colour which immediately precedes a tube showing a blue colour is read as the diastatic index. The 8 tubes represent 6.7, 10, 20, 33, 50, 100 and 250 *Wohlgemuth units* respectively. Normal 24 h urine specimens give values of 33 units or less, whilst normal small specimens may give values of up to 50 units. Values of more than 100 units are indicative of acute pancreatitis.

Woillez, Eugène Joseph (b. 1811). Paris physician.

Woillez's disease, maladie de Woillez. Acute idiopathic congestion and oedema of the lungs.

Wolf, George. 20th century American physicist.

Wolf-Schindler gastroscope. A flexible, side-vision type of gastroscope.

Wolf's test. A modification of Moro's test in which, directly after application, the areas are covered with adhesive tape which is removed after 48 h.

Wolfe, John Reissberg (b. 1824). Glasgow ophthalmologist.

Wolfe graft, Wolfe–Krause graft. A free graft of skin completely removed from one part of the body surface and sutured to repair a defect.

Wolfe's operation. 1. For ectropion: transplantation of a flap from a distance, without a pedicle. 2. For retinal detachment [obsolete]. 3. For symblepharon: by transplantation of rabbit conjunctiva [obsolete].

Wolfenden, Richard Norris (b. 1854). London laryngologist.

Wolfenden's position. A prone position with the head lying over the side of the bed.

Wolff, Julius (b. 1836). Berlin orthopaedic surgeon.

Wolff's law. Changes in the functions of bones are reflected by changes in their internal structure.

Wolff, Kaspar Friedrich (b. 1733). German anatomist and embryologist in St. Petersburg.

Wolffian body. The mesonephros.

Wolffian duct. The mesonephric duct. *See* DUCT.

Wolffian ridge. A longitudinal ridge on either side of the embryonic mesentery in which the mesonephros and associated structures are developed.

Wolff, Louis (b. 1898). Boston physician.

Wolff–Parkinson–White syndrome. This consists of physiological bundle-branch block with short P-R interval, probably as a result of an abnormal short conducting pathway between auricles and ventricles. This results in premature excitation of one ventricle (usually the right) and gives rise to functional block of the left bundle. It occurs as a congenital anomaly in an otherwise normal heart and is associated with a liability to repeated paroxysms of tachycardia. A similar electrocardiographic appearance may sometimes be seen as a result of nodal rhythm resulting from acquired cardiac lesions.

wolfram (wul·fram). 1. Tungsten. 2. A mineral, ferrous tungstate, $FeWO_4$, in which there is also manganese. [G.]

wolframate (wul·fram·ate). A tungstate. [see prec.]

wolframium (wul·fram·e·um). Tungsten. [wolfram.]

Wolfring, Emilij Franzevic von (b. 1832). Warsaw ophthalmologist.

glands of Wolfring. Large acinotubular glands found scattered in the conjunctiva of the upper eyelid close to the terminations of the meibomian glands.

wolfsbane (wulfs·bane). An old name for aconite root. [AS *wulf, bana* death.]

womb (woom). The uterus. [AS *wamb.*]

Wong, San Yin (b. 1894). Chinese biochemist.

Wong's method, for haemoglobin iron in blood. Pipette 0.5 ml oxalated blood into a 50 ml volumetric flask, add 2 ml concentrated sulphuric acid, mix, add 2 ml of saturated potassium-persulphate solution; mix and dilute to about 25 ml with water, add 2 ml of 10 per cent sodium-tungstate solution, cool and make up to 50 ml with water. Filter, and to 10 ml of the filtrate add 0.5 ml saturated potassium persulphate and 2 ml of 3 M potassium thiocyanate. Compare the colour with a standard prepared from 2.5 ml standard ferrous ammonium sulphate (1 ml = 0.1 mg Fe), 2 ml concentrated sulphuric acid, 2 ml saturated potassium persulphate diluted to 50 ml with water.

Wood, Francis Carter (b. 1869). New York pathologist.

Wood's modification of Giemsa's stain. A method of fixing the blood film in methyl alcohol and subsequently staining rapidly with 1 per cent eosin and 0.25 per cent solution of azure II.

Wood, John (b. 1825). London surgeon.

Wood's muscle. The abductor ossis metatarsi quinti muscle; an occasional muscle arising from the lateral side of the calcaneum and inserted into the tubercle at the base of the 5th metatarsal bone.

Wood's operation. 1. Closure of exstrophy of the bladder by a flap of skin cut from the abdominal wall and turned over so that the cutaneous surface forms the inner wall of the bladder. 2. The closure of a hernial canal by subcutaneous sutures through the tendinous tissues surrounding it.

Wood, Paul Hamilton (b. 1907). London cardiologist.

Wood's effort-tolerance test, of myocardial reserve. This consists of exercising the patient until the onset of precordial pain or until further effort entails dyspnoea or distress, electrocardiograms being taken before and after. Absence of specific changes of myocardial ischaemia virtually excludes ischaemic heart disease.

Wood, Robert Williams (b. 1868). Baltimore physicist.

Wood's glass. A glass containing nickel oxide which will transmit only the near ultraviolet-radiation, together with a little red in the visible region. It is used to remove the visible radiation from an ultraviolet-light lamp so that any weak fluorescence produced may be more easily seen. One use of this technique is for the detection of small spore ringworm of the scalp.

Wood's light. A misnomer for Wood's rays.

Wood's rays. Ultraviolet rays of about 360 nm, usually produced by filtering the rays through Wood's glass.

Wood's metal. A casting metallic mixture consisting of bismuth 50 per cent, lead 25 per cent, tin 12.5 per cent and cadmium 12.5 per cent. It is of low melting point and is used for making moulds of blood vessels, lung air spaces and other hollow organs.

wood (wud). Xylem; the vascular tissue of a plant which supports it and conducts fluids. **Brazil wood.** A wood similar to sappan wood (see below); it is astringent. **Guaiacum wood.** The heartwood of *Guaiacum officinale* Linn. and *G. sanctum* Linn. (family Zygophyllaceae). It contains from 18 to 25 per cent of guaiacum resin; a laxative and diuretic. **Panama wood.** Quillaia. **Red sandal wood, Red sanders wood, Ruby wood.** Pterocarpus.

Sappan wood. The heart-wood of *Caesalpinia sappan* (family Leguminosae); it contains the dye brazilin, and decoctions of the wood are used as astringents. [AS *wudu.*]

Woodbridge, John Eliot (b. 1845). Cleveland, Ohio, physician.

Woodbridge treatment. Treatment of typhoid fever with calomel, podophyllin and intestinal antiseptics, in small doses [obsolete].

Woodhall, Maurice Barnes (b. 1905). American surgeon.

Woodhall's technique for intussusception. The excision of an irreducible intussusception and performance of double-barrelled enterostomy with suture of the intestine above the intussusception to the colon below it.

Woodman's operation. A form of chordopexy operation.

Woodyatt, Rollin Turner (b. 1878). Chicago physician.

Woodyatt's pump. An apparatus for giving a continuous intravenous injection at a constant rate.

wool (wul). The cleaned fibres of the fleece shorn from sheep. Its main surgical use is in the manufacture of flannel and crêpe bandages. Wools are also obtained from other animals, e.g. alpaca, vicuña. **Wool Alcohols BP 1968.** The mixed alcohols obtained by saponification of wool fat, It is used in ointments and as an emulsifying agent for water in oil emulsions. **Cotton wool.** Absorbent cotton wool. *See* COTTON. **Wool Fat BP 1958.** Lanolin, adeps lanae; a fat-like substance obtained from sheep's wool consisting essentially of cholesterol and its esters. It is used in pharmacy as a basis of various ointments and creams. **Glass wool.** A substance with the appearance of cotton wool, made of fine glass threads. It is non-absorbent; used for filtering and for draining sinuses. **Hydrous Wool Fat BP 1968.** Wool fat containing about 25 per cent purified water. **Wood wool.** Fine cellulose wadding used as a cheap substitute for cotton wool. [AS *wull.*]

woolly foxglove (**wul**·e **fox**·gluv). The leaf of *Digitalis lanata,* containing the 3 glycosides, digilanids A, B and C, which yield respectively digitoxin, gitoxin and digoxin on hydrolysis. It is the main source of digoxin. [wool, foxglove.]

Woolner, Thomas (b. 1825). English sculptor.

Woolner's tubercle. A tubercle on the superior part of the helix of the auricle facing anteriorly. The tubercle is very evident about the sixth month of fetal life.

word salad (werd **sal**·ad). Speech characterized by a meaningless assembly of words and phrases. [AS *word,* O Fr. *salade.*]

World Health Organization (WHO or W.H.O.) (werld **helth or**·gan·i·za′·shun). A body constituted and established in 1946 as the result of a World Conference, and having as its objective the attainment by all peoples of the highest possible level of health. It absorbed or integrated the work of previously existing international health organizations, especially the Health Organization of the League of Nations.

worm (werm). 1. Any elongate legless animal. More specifically a member of the phylum Annelida. 2. In an old-fashioned still, the spiral condensing-tube immersed in a vessel of cold water. **Bilharzia worm.** *Schistosoma* species. **Bladder worm.** The cysticercus stage of certain tapeworms. **Cayor worm.** The larva of the fly *Cordylobia anthropophaga,* so-called in Senegal. **Dragon worm.** *Dracunculus medinensis.* **Eye worm.** *Loa loa.* **Flat worm.** Any platyhelminth. **Guinea worm.** *Dracunculus medinensis.* **Heart worm.** *Dirofilaria immitis.* **Horse-hair worms.** A phylum or class of worms. Their larvae are parasitic in insects, but the adults are free living. **Kidney worm.** *Dioctophyme renale,* a very large nematode worm of the kidneys of dogs and sometimes man. **Lung worm.** Any nematode occurring in the lungs. **Macaco worm, Macaque worm.** Local South American names for larva of the human warble fly *Dermatobia hominis.* **Meal worm.** The larva of *Tenebrio molitor.* **Medina worm.** *Dracunculus medinensis.* **Pork worm.** *Trichinella spiralis.* **Round worms.** *Nematoda.* **Sand worm.** *Larva migrans.* **Serpent worm.** *Dracunculus medinensis.* **Spiny-headed worm.** Any acanthocephalan. **Tongue worm.** *Linguatula serrata.* **Vinegar worm.** Tubatrix aceti. **Whip worm.** *See* TRICHURIS. [AS *wyrm.*]

wormian bone (**werm**·e·an bone). Sutural bone.

wormseed (**werm**·seed). Santonica; the dried, unexpanded capitula of *Artemisia cina* Berg. (family Compositae). It is the source of the powerful vermifuge, santonin, effective against roundworms and threadworms. **American wormseed.** *Chenopodium ambrosioides.* [worm, seed.]

wormwood (**werm**·wud). Absinthium; the dried leaves and flowering tops of *Artemisia absinthium* Linn. (family Compositae). It contains about 0.3 per cent of a blue or green oil. It is a cerebral stimulant, but large doses are dangerous and its use in wines (e.g. absinthe) is prohibited in most countries. [worm, wood.]

Worth, Claud (b. 1869). London ophthalmologist.

Worth's dots. Four coloured lights, 2 green, 1 red and 1 white, used in association with red and green goggles to assess the degree of binocular vision.

Worth's operation, for squint. A method of advancement and resection of the muscle, using silk. The suture is tied with a half knot through the muscle and then passed through the sclera near the limbus and retied with a surgeons' knot.

Worth's four-dot test. A method of estimating the amount of binocular vision, suitable for young children: the child looks at a black box internally illuminated showing 4 lights, 2 green, 1 red, 1 white, at a distance of 6 m. He wears a red glass in front of the right eye and a green in front of the left. If he has fusion he will see 4 lights (2 green, 1 red, 1 pinkish green), having fused the white light. If he has binocular vision with no fusion he sees 5 lights (3 green, 2 red). If suppressing the right eye, 3 green; if suppressing the left, 2 red.

Worth's ivory-ball test. A test for visual acuity in very young children: ivory balls of varying sizes, from 12 to 40 mm (0.5 to 1.5 in) in diameter, are thrown down and the child asked to pick them all up, The size of those missed gives an indication of the visual acuity. Each eye is tested in turn, the other being occluded.

Woulfe, P. 18th century British chemist.

Woulfe's bottle. A glass bottle with 2 or more necks employed in chemical laboratory work.

wound (woond). Any interruption, by violence or by surgery, in the continuity of the external surface of the body or of the surface of any internal organ: legally, the whole thickness of the skin must be broken, and an internal injury alone would not qualify. The older definition of the whole thickness is no longer used, for it failed in its application to bruises, fractures, contusions of the brain, etc. Strictly, nevertheless, a disruption of the continuity of tissues. **Aseptic wound.** A wound from which bacteria are excluded. **Blowing wound.** A wound of the chest wall through which air is aspirated into the pleural cavity. **Bullet wound.** A wound made by a bullet. **Contused wound.** A wound with contused edges, made by a blunt instrument. **Entry wound.** A wound through which a missile has entered the body. **Exit wound.** A wound through which a missile has left the body. **Gun-shot wound.** A wound made by a projectile from a gun. **Gutter wound.** A tangential wound in the form of a furrow or gutter. **Incised wound.** A linear wound made by a sharp instrument. **Infected wound.** A wound into which pathogenic organisms have gained access. **Lacerated wound.** An irregular wound with tearing of tissue. **Open wound.** A broad or gaping wound of the external surface of the body. **Operation wound.** A surgical wound or incision. **Penetrating wound.** A wound into, but not through, a part of the body. **Perforating wound.** A gun-shot wound or shell wound made by the passage of a missile through part of the body. **Poisoned wound.** An infected wound. **Puncture wounds.** A term used to describe the injection marks of hard drug addicts, usually in the arms and legs and set over the veins, but sometimes set in target centres on tattoo marks, web centres, etc. **Punctured wound.** A wound with a narrow path, made by a fine-pointed instrument. **Septic wound.** A wound infected by pathogenic organisms. **Shell wound.** A wound made by the fragment of a shell. **Shrapnel wound.** A wound made by a shrapnel bullet. **Subcutaneous wound.** A wound of an internal organ, usually by crush violence, without interruption in the external surface of the body. **Sucking wound.** A wound of the chest wall through which air is aspirated into the pleural cavity. **Tangential wound.** A glancing wound. [AS *wund.*]

wreath (reeth). **Daughter wreath.** In mitosis, the surface appearance of the aster. [AS *wridha.*]

Wreden, Robert Robertovich (b. 1837). St. Petersburg otologist.

Wreden's sign. A collection of gelatinous debris in the external auditory meatus in stillborn children.

Wright, Sir Almroth Edward (b. 1861). English pathologist and bacteriologist.

Wright's capsule. A glass capsule drawn out to a fine opening at both ends and bent over at one end to an acute angle; it is used for taking blood specimens.

Wright's vaccine. The antityphoid vaccine first used by Wright and Semple for human immunization in 1897.

Wright, Basil Martin. 20th century British physiologist.

Wright anemometer or respirometer. An inferential meter which indicates the tidal volume. Described in 1955.

Wright peak-flow meter. A device for measuring the peak expiratory flow rate.

Wright, Irving Sherwood (b. 1901). New York physician.

Wright's syndrome. Hyperabduction of the arm causing occlusion of the subclavian artery and stretching of the brachial plexus, with consequent vascular and nervous symptoms.

Wright, James Homer (b. 1869). Harvard, Massachusetts, pathologist.

Wright's stain, for blood and malaria parasites. A combination of methylene blue and sodium bicarbonate, subjected to heat in a steam sterilizer at 100°C for 1 h. A dilute solution of eosin is added until a scum forms, which is filtered off, dried and dissolved in pure alcohol. The stain is applied to the blood film for 1 min and then washed off in distilled water.

Wright, John Westley (b. 1842). Ohio ophthalmologist.

Wright's operation, for ptosis. The original operation in which fascia was used for joining the eyelid to the occipitofrontalis muscle by 2 narrow bands passed under the skin; the forerunner of the Hess operation now in common use.

wrightine (ri·teen). Conessine.

Wrigley, Arthur Joseph (b. 1902). London obstetrician.

Wrigley's forceps. Outlet forceps useful for lifting the head over the perineum or for delivering the head at caesarean section.

Wrisberg, Heinrich August (b. 1739). Gottingen anatomist.

Wrisberg's ansa. A communication between the right greater splanchnic and the right vagus nerves.

Wrisberg's cartilage or corpuscle, corpusculum wrisbergii. The cuneiform cartilage of the larynx.

Wrisberg's ganglion. Cardiac ganglion. *See* GANGLION.

Wrisberg's ligament. A slip passing from the posterior horn of the lateral meniscus to the posterior cruciate ligament.

Wrisberg's lines or lingula. Fibres communicating between motor and sensory roots of the trigeminal nerve.

Wrisberg's nerve. Medial cutaneous nerve of the arm.

Wrisberg's tubercle. The cuneiform tubercle of the aryepiglottic fold.

wrist [carpus] (rist). The part of the upper limb between the hand and the forearm. [AS.]

wrist drop (rist drop). Paralysis of the extensor muscles of the hand and digits. [AS *wrist, dropa.*]

writing (ri·ting). The inscription of letters, words or symbols. **Automatic writing.** Writing performed without the conscious intervention of the subject, usually in a dissociated state. **Dextrad writing.** Writing from left to right. **Mirror writing.** Reversed writing, appearing normal when viewed in a mirror; said to be related to left-handedness. **Sinistrad writing.** Writing from right to left. **Specular writing.** Mirror writing (see above). [AS *writan.*]

wry-neck (ri·nek). Torticollis. [AS *wrigian* to swerve, neck.]

Wu, H. 19th–20th century Chinese biochemist.

Folin and Wu method, for blood sugar. A protein-free filtrate of blood is prepared with sodium tungstate sulphuric acid, and this is heated with an alkaline cupric tartrate solution, when cuprous salt is formed in proportion to the amount of glucose present. Phosphomolybdic-acid reagent (see below) is added and is reduced by the cuprous salt to give a blue compound. The intensity of the colour is compared with that given by a standard glucose solution under the same conditions. The heating procedure is carried out in a special type of tube known as *Folin's sugar tube* which is designed to minimize aerial re-oxidation of the reduced copper salt.

Folin-Wu phosphomolybdic-acid reagent, for blood surgar. Dissolve 35 g of molybdic acid and 5 g of sodium tungstate in 250 ml of 8 per cent sodium hydroxide and boil for 30 min. Add water to about 350 ml followed by 125 ml of phosphoric acid (sp. gr. 1.75) and dilute with water to 500 ml.

Wuchereria (vook·er·eer·e·ah). A genus of filariid nematodes whose species are the principal cause of filariasis in man. **Wuchereria bancrofti.** The most important species, occurring in warm, humid areas throughout the world. Adults live in lymph glands and ducts and the microfilariae in the blood, moving to superficial vessels cyclically each 24 h, usually at night. Secondary hosts are mosquitoes, particularly *Culex fatigans* (= *quinquefasciatus*): the larvae develop in the thoracic muscles and migrate to the labium. **Wuchereria malayi.** A common species in the tropical Far East. Intermediate hosts are mosquitoes of the genus *Mansonioides.* **Wuchereria pacifica.** A species from Pacific islands, very like *Wuchereria bancrofti* but the microfilariae are not cyclical. Secondary hosts are diurnal mosquitoes of the genus *Aëdes.* [Otto *Wucherer* (b. 1820), German physician in Brazil.]

wuchereriasis (voo·ker·e·ri′·as·is). Filariasis. [see prec.]

Wunderlich, Carl Reinhold August (b. 1815). German physician.

Wunderlich's curve or law. The temperature curve, with ascending oscillations, representing the course of typhoid fever.

Wundt, Wilhelm Max (b. 1832). Leipzig physiologist.

Wundt's tetanus. Prolonged contraction produced in a frog's muscle by injury or strong electrical stimulation.

wurari (woo·rah·re). An alternative name for the South American arrow poison, curare.

Wurtz, Robert (b. 1858). Paris bacteriologist.

Wurtz's lactose-litmus agar. *See* AGAR, LACTOSE-LITMUS.

Wyburn-Mason, Roger. 20th century London physician.

Wyburn-Mason syndrome. Racemose angioma of the retina combined with an intracranial malformation.

Wyeth, John Allan (b. 1845). New York surgeon.

Wyeth's method or treatment. A treatment of angiomata by the injection of boiling water.

Wyeth's operation. A method of amputation at the hip.

Wylie, Walter Gill (b. 1848). New York gynaecologist.

Wylie drain. A grooved pessary of hard rubber.

Wyman, Morrill (b. 1812). Boston physician.

Wyman's strap. A strap formerly used in the mechanical restraint of insane persons.

Wynter, Walter Essex (b. 1860). London physician.

Wynter's sign. Absence of the abdominal respiratory movements in acute peritonitis.

X

xanchromatic (zan·kro·**mat**·ik). Xanthochromatic.

xanthaematin (zant·**he**·mat·in). A yellow colouring matter produced from haematin with nitric acid. [Gk *xanthos* yellow, haematin.]

xanthaemia (zan·**the**·me·ah). The presence of yellowish substances in the blood which intensify the yellow colour of the blood plasma or serum. [Gk *xanthos* yellow, *haima* blood.]

xanthaline (**zan**·thal·een). $C_{20}H_{19}O_5N$, an alkaloid present in opium.

xanthate (**zan**·thate). Any salt or ester of xanthic acid. **Alkyl xanthate.** A dithio ester used as an accelerator in rubber vulcanization. **Cellulose xanthate.** A constituent of viscose.

xanthelasma (zan·thel·**az**·mah). 1. Xanthoma palpebrarum. 2. A term which has been suggested, as xanthomata are not true blastomata, as a substitute for *xanthoma* in names such as xanthoma tuberosum and xanthoma disseminatum. **Xanthelasma palpebrarum.** Xanthoma palpebrarum. [Gk *xanthos* yellow, *elasma* plate.]

xanthelasmatosis (**zan**·thel·az·mat·**o**'·sis). Xanthomatosis. [xanthelasma, Gk *-osis* condition.]

xanthelasmoidea (**zan**·thel·as·**moi**'·de·ah). Urticaria pigmentosa. [xanthelasma, Gk *eidos* form.]

xanthene (**zan**·theen). $O{=}(C_6H_4)_2{=}CH_2$, a crystalline compound which is the parent of the rhodamine and fluorescein dyestuffs. **Xanthene ketone.** Xanthone. [see foll.]

xanthic (**zan**·thik). 1. Having a yellow colour. 2. Derived from or relating to xanthene or xanthine. [Gk *xanthos* yellow.]

xanthide (**zan**·thide). A yellow colouring matter which occurs in fruits and vegetables. [see prec.]

xanthin (**zan**·thin). A general name for certain carotene derivatives which, in the form of esters, appear in plants and fruits as yellow or orange colouring-matters. [see foll.]

xanthine (**zan**·theen). $(NHCO)_2C_2N(NH)(CH)$, a base which occurs in plants and in animal tissue where it is produced during the formation of uric acid in the nucleoprotein metabolism. It has a stimulatory efect on heart muscle. So-called, because of its yellow nitro derivative. [Gk *xanthos* yellow.]

xanthinine (**zan**·thin·een). $C_4H_3N_3O_2$, a white compound prepared by the decomposition of ammonium thionurate.

Xanthinol Nicotinate (**zan**·thin·ol **nik**·o·tin·ate). BP Commission approved name for 7 - {2 - hydroxy - 3 - [*N* - (2 - hydroxyethyl) methylamino] - propyl} - theophylline nicotinate; a vasodilator.

xanthinoxidase (zan·thin·**ox**·id·aze). Xanthine oxidase. An enzyme which is found in liver, and also occurs in cows' milk (Schardinger's enzyme). It is an oxidoreductase which activates the oxidation of xanthine into uric acid.

xanthinuria (zan·thin·**ewr**·e·ah). The excretion of excessive amounts of xanthine in the urine.

Xanthium (**xan**·the·um). 1. A genus of plants of the family Compositae; the clotburs. 2. The leaves of *Xanthium strumarium*, used as an adulterant of stramonium. [Gk *xanthos* yellow.]

xanthiuria (zan·the·**ewr**·e·ah). Xanthinuria.

xanthochromatic (**zan**·tho·kro·**mat**'·ik). Characterized by a yellow colour. [see foll.]

xanthochromia (zan·tho·**kro**·me·ah). 1. The appearance of yellow patches on the skin. 2. A yellow coloration of the cerebrospinal fluid. [Gk *xanthos* yellow, *chroma* colour.]

xanthochromic (zan·tho·**kro**·mik). 1. Describing anything that is yellow. 2. Referring to xanthochromia.

xanthochroous (zan·**thok**·ro·us). Yellow-skinned; applied more usually to blond white people, such as the Scandinavian type. [Gk *xanthos* yellow, *chroia* skin.]

Xanthocillin (zan·tho·**sil**·in). BP Commission approved name for an antibiotic obtained from the mycelium of *Penicillium notatum*.

xanthocreatine, xanthocreatinine (zan·tho·**kre**·at·een, **zan**·tho·kre·**at**'·in·een). $C_5H_{10}N_4O$, a poisonous leucomaine found in muscular tissue which causes depression, fatigue, diarrhoea and vomiting. [Gk *xanthos* yellow, *kreas* flesh.]

xanthocyanopia, xanthocyanopsia, xanthocyanopsy (**zan**·tho·si·an·**o**'·pe·ah, **zan**·tho·si·an·**op**'·se·ah, zan·tho·si·an·**op**'·se). Protanopia; red-green blindness, with the ability to distinguish blue and yellow. [Gk *xanthos* yellow, *kyanos* blue, *opsis* vision.]

xanthocyte (**zan**·tho·site). Any cell that secretes a yellow colouring matter. [Gk *xanthos* yellow, *kytos* cell.]

xanthoderma (zan·tho·**der**·mah). An archaic term indicating yellowness of the skin. [Gk *xanthos* yellow, *derma* skin.]

xanthodont, xanthodontous (**zan**·tho·dont, zan·tho·**don**·tus). Describing a person or animal with yellow teeth. [Gk *xanthos* yellow, *odous* tooth.]

xantho-erythrodermia perstans (**zan**·tho·er·ith·ro·**der**'·me·ah **per**·stanz). Parapsoriasis en plaques; a rare skin disease consisting of persistent patches of erythema covered with fine scales, occurring on the trunk and limbs, it is symptomless and resistant to treatment. [Gk *xanthos* yellow, *erythros* red, *derma* skin, L *perstans* persistent.]

xanthofibroma thecocellulare (**zan**·tho·fi·**bro**'·mah **the**·ko·sel·ew·la'·re). A yellow ovarian tumour resembling a fibroma with much fatty material. It induces markedly feminine characteristics in the subject. [Gk *xanthos* yellow, fibroma.]

xanthogene (**zan**·tho·jeen). One of the yellow colouring matters which are found in vegetables and related to xanthins. [Gk *xanthos* yellow, *genein* to produce.]

xanthogranulomatosis (**zan**·tho·gran·ew·lo·mat·**o**'·sis). Hand-Schueller-Christian disease; a lipoid disease of reticulo-endothelial cells in which xanthomatous granulomata occur in the bones, particularly of the skull, but also elsewhere. [Gk *xanthos* yellow, Gk *-osis* condition.]

xanthoma (zan·**tho**·mah). A fatty fibrous change in the skin associated with the formation of yellow or yellowish-brown plaques, nodules or tumours. **Craniohypophyseal xanthoma.** A deposit of cholesterol ester in the bones around the hypophysis which is damaged, with consequent production of diabetes insipidus. It occurs as part of the Hand-Schueller-Christian disease. **Xanthoma diabeticorum.** A rare complication of diabetes mellitus in which xanthomatous lesions develop, usually in large numbers, on the extensor surfaces of the limbs and sometimes on the palms and soles. The majority of the patients are males between 20 and 40 years of age. **Xanthoma disseminatum.** A rare malady, usually associated with diabetes insipidus, in which small xanthomatous papules develop in the skin of the flexures and in the mucosae. There may be involvement of the liver. **Xanthoma eruptiva.** A sudden development of multiple xanthoma when the serum lipid level is rising. **Xanthoma glycosuricum.** Xanthoma associated with glycosuria. **Juvenile xanthoma.** In this condition, yellow nodules of larger tumours are found in the skin; the coloration is due to lipochrome and cholesterol, and the lesions are most commonly found on the knees and elbows and the face or eyelids. In the *congenital* form, which is seen in early infancy, there is rarely any evidence of metabolic defect. In the *acquired* or *secondary* form, which is the usual type seen in older children, there is nearly always evidence of some degree of metabolic upset, such as diabetes mellitus, cirrhosis of the liver, lipoid nephrosis, idiopathic lipaemia, and it is always found in Hand-Schueller-Christian disease. Treatment of the congenital form is useless, but improvement may arise in the secondary form with reorganization of the metabolic defects, especially in diabetes mellitus. **Xanthoma palpebrarum.** A malady of middle- or old-age, affecting women more often than men, in which slowly developing non-inflammatory yellow-brown plaques form on the eyelids, usually near the inner canthus. Frequently the distribution is symmetrical. The lesions may be only a few millimetres in diameter; often they are larger. **Xanthoma tendinosum.** Xanthoma with deposits in tendons. **Xanthoma tuberculatum, Xanthoma tuberosum, Xanthoma tuberosum multiplex.** A malady characterized by the appearance in the skin of numerous, slowly growing, usually discrete, pink or yellowish, xanthomatous nodules, particularly on the extensor aspects near the elbows, hips and knees. Lipoid deposits also occur in the cardiovascular system and in other tissue, including tendon sheaths. The blood cholesterol and total blood lipoids are frequently greatly increased. [Gk *xanthos* yellow, *-oma* tumour.]

xanthomatosis (zan·tho·mat·o′·sis). A lipoid disturbance of reticulo-endothelial cells, resulting in granulomatous deposits of a cholesterol ester. **Xanthomatosis of the Achilles tendon.** Xanthomatous deposits in the lower part of the tendo calcaneus. **Xanthomatosis corneae.** Dystrophia adiposa corneae; also called *primary fatty degeneration of the cornea.* **Diffuse plane xanthomatosis.** Generalized xanthelasma. **Essential xanthomatosis.** A disturbance of lipoid metabolism in children, with deposits of lipoids in various tissues and characterized by exophthalmos, bone defects, diabetes insipidus, cessation of growth and gingivitis. **Xanthomatosis generalisata ossium.** Hand-Schueller-Christian disease; localized deposits of cholesterol-ester occurring in bones, especially those of the skull, and causing diabetes insipidus from disturbance of the pituitary, and exophthalmos from deposits in the orbits. **Idiopathic xanthomatosis.** Essential xanthomatosis (see above). **Xanthomatosis iridis.** Thickening and marked swelling, with yellow patches, occurring in the discoloured iris of an eye blind from long-standing iritis or glaucoma. **Xanthomatosis lentis.** Fatty infiltration of a cataractous lens of long standing, following rupture or disintegration of the capsule. A rare condition. **Xanthomatosis of the lids.** Small, flat, yellowish plaques of lipoid material, forming in the skin of the eyelids, usually in old people. Also called *xanthoma palpebrarum.* **Primary xanthomatosis.** Essential xanthomatosis (see above). **Secondary xanthomatosis.** Xanthomatosis caused by hepatic, renal, pancreatic or other metabolic disease. [Gk *xanthos* yellow, *-oma* tumour, *-osis* condition.]

xanthomatous (zan·tho·mat·us). 1. Concerning xanthoma. 2. Affected with xanthoma.

Xanthomonas (zan·tho·mo·nas). The generic term for the genus of yellow-pigment-producing bacteria formerly known as *Phytomonas.* [Gk *xanthos* yellow, *monas* unit.]

xanthone (zan·thone). 1. Xanthene ketone, $O{=}(C_6H_4)_2{=}CO$. A colourless substance which forms the basis of many plant colouring-matters and is used in the synthesis of dyestuffs. 2 Brometone.

xanthophose (zan·tho·foze). A yellow-coloured phose. [Gk *xanthos* yellow, *phos* light.]

xanthophyll (zan·tho·fil). 1. Lutein, $C_{40}H_{56}O_2$. A yellow carotenoid pigment found in green foliage, egg yolk, bird plumage and in human plasma where it accumulates from the food taken in. 2. General term for hydroxycarotenes or xanthins, which occur in plants. [Gk *xanthos* yellow, *phyllon* leaf.]

xanthopia (zan·tho·pe·ah). Xanthopsia.

xanthopicrite (zan·tho·pik·rite). The original name given to berberine. [Obsolete term.] [Gk *xanthos* yellow, *pikros* bitter.]

xanthoproteic (zan·tho·pro·te·ik). Appertaining to xanthoprotein.

xanthoprotein (zan·tho·pro·te·in). Any yellow compound appearing in the colour reaction for proteins with concentrated nitric acid. Its formation is due to the presence in tyrosine, tryptophan and other amino acids, of a phenyl group. [Gk *xanthos* yellow, protein.]

xanthopsia (zan·thop·se·ah). A disturbance of colour vision, sometimes accompanying jaundice, when everything appears yellow. [Gk *xanthos* yellow, *opsis* sight.]

xanthopsis (zan·thop·sis). The yellow coloration noted in certain cancers and degenerating tissues. [see prec.]

xanthopterin (zan·thop·ter·in). $C_6H_5O_2N_5$, a yellow pigment isolated from the wings of butterflies and other insects. It is related constitutionally to the purines. [Gk *xanthos* yellow, *pteron* wing.]

xanthorhamnin (zan·tho·ram·nin). A hydroxyanthraquinone derivative occurring in buckthorn berries, *Rhamnus cathartica.*

xanthorrhoea (zan·tho·re·ah). The occurrence of an acrid yellow vaginal discharge. [Gk *xanthos* yellow, *rhoia* flow.]

xanthosarcoma (zan·tho·sar·ko′·mah). A giant-cell sarcoma of tendon sheaths of the hands and feet. It is usually rich in fatty material. [Gk *xanthos* yellow, sarcoma.]

xanthosine (zan·tho·seen). 7-Xanthine-D-riboside, a nucleoside formed by the deamination of guanosine.

xanthosis (zan·tho·sis). Yellowish discoloration, especially of the skin. **Xanthosis cutis.** Yellowish discoloration of the skin; this occurs in several conditions, e.g. diabetes (see below) and poliomyelitis, and is usually associated with increased carotene in the blood. **Xanthosis diabetica, Xanthosis diabeticorum.** Xanthosis in a diabetic person which is probably due to minor degrees of carotenaemia. [Gk *xanthos* yellow, *-osis* condition.]

xanthous (zan·thus). Yellow pigmented; having a yellowish complexion. [Gk *xanthos* yellow.]

xanthoxylin (zan·thox·il·in). An alcoholic preparation of xanthoxylum.

xanthoxylone (zan·thox·il·one). $C_{10}H_{12}O_4$, a crystallizable phenolic substance occurring in xanthoxylum.

Xanthoxylum (zan·thox·il·um). 1. A genus of trees and shrubs of the family Rutaceae; the prickly ash. 2. The dried bark of *Xanthoxylum americanum* Mill. (northern prickly ash) or of *X. clava-herculis* Linn. (southern prickly ash), used formerly as a carminative and gastro-intestinal stimulant. [Gk *xanthos* yellow, *xylon* wood.]

xanthuria (zan·thewr·e·ah). Xanthinuria.

xanthydrol (zan·thi·drol). $O{=}(C_6H_4)_2CHOH$, a hydroxy derivative of xanthene. It is used as a test for indole with which it gives a violet coloration, and for urea which forms with it an insoluble dixanthylurea.

xanthyl (zan·thil). The monovalent radical $O{=}(C_6H_4)_2{=}CH-$ which occurs in xanthene.

xanthylic (zan·thil·ik). Relating to xanthine.

xenembole (zen·em·bo·le). The introduction of a foreign body into the system. [Gk *xenos* stranger, *embolos* plug.]

xenenthesis (zen·en·the·sis). Xenembole. [Gk *xenos* stranger, *enthesis* introduction.]

xenodiagnosis (zen·o·di·ag·no′·sis). The method of diagnosis of an infective disease by finding the causal organism in an insect vector which has been fed upon the patient. [Gk *xenos* stranger, diagnosis.]

xenogenesis (zen·o·jen·es·is). The production of offspring having different characteristics in successive generations. [Gk *xenos* stranger, *genein* to produce.]

xenogenetic, xenogenic (zen·o·jen·et′·ik, zen·o·jen·ik). Concerning or relating to xenogenesis.

xenogenous (zen·oj·en·us). Arising out of a foreign body or agency. [Gk *xenos* stranger, *genein* to produce.]

xenogeny (zen·oj·en·e). Xenogenesis.

xenograft (zen·o·grahft). A graft in which the donor tissue comes from a different species of animal from the recipient. [Gk *xenos* stranger, graft.]

xenology (zen·ol·o·je). Parasitology. [Gk *xenos* stranger, *logos* science.]

xenomenia (zen·o·me·ne·ah). A menses-like flow of blood from a part other than the vagina; vicarious menstruation. [Gk *xenos* stranger, *meniaia* menses.]

xenon (ze·non). An element of atomic weight 131.30, atomic number 54 and chemical symbol Xe. It is a colourless gas which occurs in the atmosphere to a minute extent (1 part in 170 million). Being one of the inert gases, it forms no compounds; it is used in fluorescent discharge tubes. [Gk *xenos* stranger.]

xenophobia (zen·o·**fo**·be·ah). An unreasoning aversion to strangers; psychotic hatred of foreigners. [Gk *xenos* stranger, *phobein* to fear.]

xenophonia (zen·o·**fo**·ne·ah). A condition in which the voice undergoes such a change as to be unrecognizable. [Gk *xenos* stranger, *phone* voice.]

xenophthalmia (zen·of·**thal**·me·ah). Inflammation of the conjunctiva set up by foreign matter in the eye. [Gk *xenos* stranger, ophthalmia.]

Xenopsylla (zen·op·**sil**·ah). A genus of Old World fleas of the family Pulicidae. In the wild, the species are tropical and particularly African in distribution. Many are important vectors of plague in rodents and intermediate hosts of *Hymenolepis diminuta*; in the latter case, infection occurs in the larval stage. **Xenopsylla astia.** An important vector of human plague over some parts of India, but over most of its range unimportant. **Xenopsylla brasiliensis.** An important vector of human plague in tropical Africa and which has occurred, though rarely, in many ports throughout the world. **Xenopsylla cheopis.** The most important vector of urban bubonic plague throughout the world and of rural plague in the tropics. Normal hosts are commensal rats, but it bites man freely and becomes plague blocked easily. It is also a vector of flea-borne typhus. **Xenopsylla eridos.** A vector of plague. **Xenopsylla piriei.** A vector of plague. [Gk *xenos* stranger, *psylla* flea.]

Xenopus (zen·o·pus). A genus of African toads. **Xenopus laevis.** A laboratory animal which has been used in pregnancy tests. [Gk *xenos* stranger, *pous* foot.]

xenyl (ze·nil). The monovalent group, $C_6H_5C_6H_4$–. [Gk *xenos* stranger, *hyle* substance.]

Xenysalate (zen·i·sal·ate). BP Commission approved name for 2-diethylaminoethyl 3-phenylsalicylate; it is used in the treatment of seborrhoea.

xeransis (ze·**ran**·sis). Slow dehydration of the tissues. [Gk *drying up.]*

xerantic (ze·**ran**·tik). Having a drying effect upon the tissues; siccative. [see prec.]

xerasia (ze·**ra**·ze·ah). Dryness of the hair due to pathological cause. [Gk dryness.]

xerocheilia (ze·ro·**ki**·le·ah). Cheilitis marked by extreme dryness of the lips. [Gk *xeros* dry, *cheilos* lip.]

xerocollyrium (ze·ro·kol·**ir**'·e·um). A dry collyrium, e.g. an eye ointment. [Gk *xeros* dry, collyrium.]

xeroderma, xerodermia (ze·ro·**der**·mah, ze·ro·**der**·me·ah). The mildest form of ichthyosis. **Xeroderma follicularis, Follicular xerodermia.** Terms for ichthyosis follicularis, attributed to Liveing. **Xeroderma pigmentosum.** A rare affection of the skin which commences in infancy or very early childhood, involves chiefly the exposed parts, and is characterized at first by erythema and vesiculation after exposure to sunlight, followed by freckle-like pigmentation and telangiectasis, later by superficial ulcerations, warty growths and the formation of small areas of atrophy, and finally by malignant epitheliomata and death. [Gk *xeros* dry, *derma* skin.]

See also: KAPOSI.

xerodermatic (ze·ro·der·**mat**'·ik). Having the characteristics of xeroderma, or affected with the disease.

xerodermosteosis (ze·ro·der·mos·te·**o**'·sis). A syndrome in which there is deficiency of the glandular secretions of the skin and mucous membranes causing ichthyosis of the skin and dryness of the ocular, nasal, buccal, bronchial, digestive and genito-anal mucosa. It is associated with osteo-articular calcification and with progressive deformity of the joints. There may be other systemic changes. [Gk *xeros* dry, *derma* skin, *osteon* bone.]

xerogel (ze·ro·jel). A gel in which the disperse liquid phase is reduced to a minimum. [Gk *xeros* dry, gel.]

xerography (ze·**rog**·raf·e). A method of photographic reproduction by a dry process employing a metal plate covered with a thin film of amorphous selenium. This film is electrically charged in the dark (sensitized), the charge spreading uniformly over the surface: when exposed to light or x-rays the charge leaks through to the metal conducting plate in proportion to the intensity of exposure at the various parts of the surface. Development consists in placing the plate in a cloud of charged powder particles. The particles are attracted to and deposit on the selenium surface where it has been discharged by the radiation, thus producing a negative. Employed in radiography, the process will provide an x-ray picture within a minute, and has achieved importance in orthopaedic operations, where quick check radiographs are invaluable. Used as a technique of mammography. [Gk *xeros* dry, *graphein* to record.]

xeroma (ze·**ro**·mah). Xerophthalmia, characterized by a dry shrunken appearance of the conjunctiva. It occurs in pemphigus, vitamin-A deficiency and essential shrinkage of the conjunctiva, and may follow severe trachoma or diphtheritic conjunctivitis. [Gk *xeros* dry, *-oma* tumour.]

xeromenia (ze·ro·**me**·ne·ah). The occurrence of the symptoms of menstruation in the absence of any menstrual blood flow. [Gk *xeros* dry, *meniaia* menses.]

xeromycteria (ze·ro·mik·**teer**'·e·ah). Dryness of the mucous membrane of the nasal passages. [Gk *xeros* dry, *mykter* nose.]

xerophagia, xerophagy (ze·ro·**fa**·je·ah, ze·**rof**·aj·e). The habitual consumption of dry food. [Gk *xeros* dry, *phagein* to eat.]

xerophobia (ze·ro·**fo**·be·ah). A reduced secretion of saliva resulting from fear or other emotion. [Gk *xeros* dry, *phobein* to fear.]

xerophthalmia, xerophthalmos, xerophthalmus (ze·rof·**thal**'·me·ah, ze·rof·**thal**·mos, ze·rof·**thal**·mus). Xeroma. [Gk *xeros* dry, *ophthalmos* eye.]

xeroradiography (ze·ro·ra·de·**og**'·raf·e). The technique of producing a non-transparent print of x-ray densities by means of a selenium plate exposed to x-rays. [Gk *xeros* dry, radiography.]

xerosis (ze·**ro**·sis). 1. Dryness of the skin due to lack of sebaceous secretion. It may be localized or generalized, idiopathic or symptomatic. Chapping of the hands in cold weather is an example of localized, symptomatic xerosis. The condition may be noted in maladies such as ichthyosis and psoriasis: it occurs also in old age. 2. Archaic: a mild degree of ichthyosis. [Gk *xeros* dry.]

xerostomia (ze·ro·**sto**·me·ah). Failure of the salivary glands, with resultant dryness of the mouth. [Gk *xeros* dry, *stoma* mouth.]

xerotes (ze·**ro**·teez). The tendency of the body towards dryness. [Gk dryness.]

xerotic (ze·**rot**·ik). Of a dry nature; displaying xerosis.

xerotocia (ze·ro·**to**·se·ah). Labour occurring in the absence of amniotic fluid. [Gk *xeros* dry, *tokos* labour.]

xerotripsis (ze·ro·**trip**·sis). Dry friction. [Gk *xeros* dry, *tripsis* friction.]

Xerus erythropus (zer·us er·**ith**·ro·pus). A tree squirrel that is susceptible to plague infection and probably acts as a reservoir in nature.

xiphicostal (zif·e·**kos**·tal). Concerning the xiphoid process and the ribs. [xiphoid, L *costa* rib.]

xiphisternal (zif·e·**ster**·nal). Concerning the xiphisternum.

xiphisternum (zif·e·**ster**·num). The xiphoid process of the sternum.

xiphocostal (zif·o·**kos**·tal). Xiphicostal.

xiphodidymus, xiphodymus (zif·o·**did**·im·us, zif·**od**·e·mus). Xiphopagus. [xiphoid, Gk *didymos* twin.]

xiphodynia (zif·o·**din**·e·ah). Pain experienced in the xiphoid process. [xiphoid, Gk *odyne* pain.]

xiphoid (**zif**·oid). Shaped like a sword; ensiform. [Gk *xiphos* sword, *eidos* form.]

xiphoiditis (zif·oid·**i**·tis). Inflammation of the xiphoid process. [xiphoid, Gk *-itis* inflammation.]

xiphopagotomy (zi·fop·ag·**ot**'·o·me). The surgical division of the connection between the twins of a xiphopagus. [xiphopagus, Gk *temnein* to cut.]

xiphopagus (zi·fop·ag·us). A twin monster united at the xiphoid process. [xiphoid, Gk *pagos* fixed.]

x-radiation (ex·ra·de·a′·shun). **Characteristic x-radiation, Fluorescent x-radiation.** x-Radiation having a line spectrum which is characteristic of the material of the target and not of the exciting voltage applied to the tube. Radiation, 3rd def. [*x* first unknown quantity in algebra, radiation.]

x-rays (ex·raze). Electromagnetic radiation resulting from extranuclear loss of energy of charged particles (for example, electrons) and having shorter wavelengths than ultra-violet radiation. [*x* first unknown quantity in algebra, L *radius* ray.]

Xylamidine Tosylate (zi·lam·id·een tos·il·ate). BP Commission approved name for *N* - 2 - (3 - methoxyphenoxy)propyl - *m* - tolylacetamidine toluene-*p*-sulphonate; an antiserotonin agent.

xylan (zi·lan). $(C_5H_8O_4)_n$, a pentosan which occurs in straw, husks canes and wood gums. It is a polymer of D-xylose units with a terminal unit of arabinose. [Gk *xylon* wood.]

xylanthrax (zi·lan·thrax). Charcoal. [Obsolete term.] [Gk *xylon* wood, *anthrax* coal.]

xylem (zi·lem). Wood; the name given to the lignified cells of the vascular bundles of plants and to the lignified cells of secondary thickening in perennials. **Primary xylem.** That formed from the procambium; protoxylem and metaxylem. **Secondary xylem.** That formed by the cambium. [Gk *xylon* wood.]

xylene (zi·leen). Dimethylbenzene, $C_6H_4(CH_3)_2$. Name given to a homologue of benzene occurring in coal tar and existing in three isomeric forms, all liquids. A mixture of isomers is used in industry as a solvent for rubber and for the manufacture of lacquers; also employed to sterilize catgut (BPC 1949) and in microscopy as a solvent (xylol). [see prec.]

xylenin (zi·len·in). A poison extractable from tubercle bacilli by xylene.

xylenobacillin (zi·len·o·bas·il′·in). Xylenin.

xylenol (zi·len·ol). A general name for the dimethyl phenols of the formula $C_6H_3(CH_3)_2(OH)$. The chlorinated derivatives are powerful bacteriostatics used in the "pine" type of disinfectant.

xylidide (zi·lid·ide). Any acyl derivative of a xylidine, such as acetyl xylidide, $C_6H_3(CH_3)_2NHCOCH_3$, analogous to acetanilide.

xylidine (zi·lid·een). Methyl toluidine, $C_6H_3(CH_3)_2NH_2$. A compound homologous with aniline and occurring in several isomeric forms; they are used in the manufacture of azo dyes.

xylindein (zi·lin·de·in). $C_{34}H_{26}O_{11}$, an organic colouring-matter found in Peziza wood.

xylitol (zi·lit·ol). $CH_2OH(CHOH)_3CH_2OH$, a pentahydric alcohol obtained by the reduction of xylose.

xylitone (zi·lit·one). $C_{12}H_{18}O$, a ketonic compound formed by impregnating acetone with hydrochloric-acid gas.

xyloidine (zi·lo·id·een). Nitro-starch, $C_{12}H_{12}(NO_2)_8O_{10}$. A compound formed by treating starch with nitric acid. It is used as a blasting explosive, especially when mixed with nitre and carbon. [Gk *xylon* wood, *eidos* form.]

xyloketose (zi·lo·ke·toze). $CH_2OHCOCHOHCHOHCH_2OH$, a pentose occurring in the urine in pentosuria.

xyloketosuria (zi·lo·ke·toze·ewr′·e·ah). The presence of the pentose sugars xyloketose or xylose in the urine. They may occur in essential pentosuria.

xylol, xylole (zi·lol, zi·lole). Xylene.

Xylometazoline (zi·lo·met·az′·o·leen). BP Commission approved name for 2 - (4 - *t* - butyl - 2,6 - dimethylbenzyl) - 2 - imidazoline; a vasoconstrictor.

xylon (zi·lon). Xylem.

xylonite (zi·lon·ite). One of the older-type transparent plastics.

xylopyranose (zi·lo·pi·ran·oze). In sugar nomenclature, the pyranose form of xylose containing the 6-membered pyran ring.

xylosazone (zi·lo·sa·zone). The osazone formed by phenylhydrazine with xylose, and used to identify the latter.

Xylose BP 1973 (zi·loze). D-Xylose; α-D-xylopyranose. An aldopentose obtained by hydrolysing straw or maize cobs. Taken by mouth it is incompletely absorbed. It is used for the diagnosis of malabsorption from the gastro-intestinal tract.

xyloside (zi·lo·side). Any compound formed by xylose, analogous to a glucoside.

xylosuria (zi·loze·ewr·e·ah). Xyloketosuria.

xylotherapy (zi·lo·ther·ap·e). The treatment of disease by applying various types of wood to the body; a relic of mediaeval mysticism. [Gk *xylon* wood, *therapeia* treatment.]

xylyl (zi·lil). The group $C_6H_4(CH_3)CH_2$–, derived from xylene. **Xylyl bromide.** $C_6H_4(CH_3)CH_2Br$, a lacrimatory compound which occurs in 3 isomeric forms; used in chemical warfare. **Xylyl chloride.** $C_6H_4(CH_3)CH_2Cl$, a liquid used with its isomers as a lacrimatory vapour.

xylylene (zi·lil·een). The bivalent group, $-CH_2C_6H_4CH_2-$. **Xylylene bromide.** $C_6H_4(CH_2Br)_2$, a lacrimatory compound used in chemical warfare. **Xylylene diamine.** $C_6H_4(CH_2NH_2)_2$, a compound occurring in several isomeric forms and used in the synthesis of dyestuffs.

xyphopagus (zi·fop·ag·us). Xiphopagus.

xyrospasm (zi·ro·spazm). Spasm of the muscles of the wrist and forearm, peculiar to barbers and arising out of their occupation. [Gk *xyron* razor, spasm.]

xyster (zis·ter). A surgical file or raspatory. [Gk scraper.]

Y

Yageine (yag·e·een). An archaic name for the alkaloid harmine, used in malaria.

yajein (yaj·e·een). Yageine.

Yamagiwa, Katsusaburo (b. 1863). Japanese physician.

Yamagiwa's method for neuroglia. A method employing prolonged staining in alcoholic eosin, followed by aniline blue and differentiation in alcohol. Axons are stained blue, neuroglial fibres bright red.

yangona (yang·go·nah). Kava.

Yankauer's operation. Removal of the mucosa and any bony sequestra in the osseous portion of the pharyngotympanic tube, with subsequent tubal occlusion. It is performed with a sharp ring knife (*Yankauer's cutting curette*) introduced through the external auditory meatus in cases of central tympanic perforations with persistent mucoid tympanic discharge.

yarn (yarn). *See* HOLMGREN (A.F.). [AS *gearn.*]

yato-bigo (yah·to·be·go). A Japanese variety of tularaemia. [Jap.]

yaw (yaw). A lesion of yaws. **Guinea corn yaw.** A granulomatous skin lesion resembling a grain of Indian corn. **Mother yaw.** The initial skin lesion comparable to the primary sore in syphilis; from this lesion the blood is infected and after a short interval widespread secondary lesions appear. **Ringworm yaw.** A yaws lesion of circular form.

yaw-root (yaw·root). The dried root of *Stillingia sylvatica* Linn. (family Euphorbiaceae). It contains resin, oil, tannin and starch, and was formerly used as an expectorant, emetic and cathartic. [yaw, root.]

yawn (yawn). 1. An involuntary act, usually performed when drowsy or depressed, in which the mouth is opened wide and a deep breath inspired. This is sometimes accompanied by stretching of the arms and shoulders to assist expansion of the chest. 2. To perform such an act. [AS *geonian.*]

yaws (yawz). A tropical disease which resembles syphilis. There are raspberry-like skin lesions on the face, palms of the hands and soles of the feet. It is caused by a spirochaete, *Treponema pertenue.* **Bosch yaws, Bush yaws.** Cutaneous or mucocutaneous leishmaniasis. *See* LEISHMANIASIS. **Crab yaws.** Yaws in which there is hyperkeratosis of the soles and a condition known as clavus. **Forest yaws.** America mucocutaneous leishmaniasis. *See* LEISHMANIASIS. **Ringworm yaws.** Yaws in which the lesion has developed a circinate character. [African *yaw* raspberry.]

yeast (yeest). 1.Micro-organisms in which the unicellular form is conspicuous and which belong to the fungi. The organisms secrete enzymes that convert sugars into alcohol and carbon dioxide. 2. The cells and spores of *Saccharomyces cerevisiae* and allied species of *Saccharomyces* cultivated in and used for the fermentation of grain. It contains a number of carbohydrate-splitting enzymes to which its virtue in the brewing industry is owed; in addition it contains vitamins of the B group, including aneurine hydrochloride, nicotinic acid and riboflavine. It is used medicinally, mainly in the form of tablets of dried yeast, for all deficiency diseases due to lack of the vitamin-B group. **Beer yeast.** Brewer's yeast (see below). **Black yeasts.** Dematiaceous fungi named *Torula* by Persoon (1796). **Brewer's yeast.** The semisolid suspension of yeast cells (*Saccharomyces cerevisiae*) obtained during the brewing of beer. **Dried Yeast BPC 1968.** The dried form of yeast (main def. 2 above) administered in tablets or powder in the treatment of vitamin-B deficiency disease. [AS *gist.*]

yeki (ya·ke). Bubonic plague. [Jap.]

yelk (yelk). Yolk.

yellow (yel·o). A colour of the visible spectrum, of wavelength between 575 and 585 nm. **Acid yellow.** An acid monoazo dye sometimes employed for the staining of bone and other connective tissues. **Acid yellow D.** Tropaeolin 00; sodium diphenylamine azobenzene sulphonate, an indicator with a pH range 1.4–2.6. **Alizarin yellow.** A dye used as an indicator of pH over the range 10.0 (yellow) to 12.0 (orange). **Brilliant yellow.** A dye used as an indicator of pH over the range 1.2 (red) to 2.3 (yellow). **Butter yellow.** 1. Name given to a number of harmless yellow dyes used for colouring butter. 2. A chrysoidine dye, dimethylamino-azobenzene, prepared from aniline and dimethylaniline. It is used to colour oils and also as an indicator for lactic acid, becoming red in acid solution and yellow in alkaline. **Canary yellow.** Auramine; tetramethyldiaminodiphenylketonimine hydrochloride, used as a microscopic stain and as an antiseptic. **Chrome yellow.** Lead chromate; used as a pigment in paint manufacture. **Fast yellow.** Acid yellow (see above). **Imperial yellow.** Aurantia; the ammonium salt of hexanitrodiphenylamine, used as a stain, also as a food dye. **King's yellow.** Realgar. **Leather yellow.** Diaminophenylacridine nitrate, a dye used as a bacteriological stain. **Manchester yellow, Martius yellow.** Naphthol yellow (see below). **Metanil yellow.** $NaSO_3C_6H_4N{=}NC_6H_4NHC_6H_5$, an azo dye used as an indicator (pH 1.2–2.5). Also known as *tropaeolin G.* **Naphthol yellow.** An acid nitrose dye used for staining cancerous tissues, for fungi, pollen tubes and in the preparation of certain selective bacteriological media. **Nitrazine yellow.** A yellow azo dye derived from β-naphtholdisulphonic acid, used as a pH indicator (4.5–7.0) being blue in alkali and yellow in acid. **Paris yellow.** Lead chromate. **Philadelphia yellow.** Phosphine; a derivative of phenylacridine used as a leather dye. **Primuline yellow.** A mixture of the sodium sulphonates of di- and tri-thiazole bases. **Queen's yellow.** Mercury subsulphate. **Resorcinol yellow.** $OHSO_2C_6H_4N{=}NC_6H_3(OH)_2$, an azo dye obtained from sulphanilic acid and resorcinol. Also known as *tropaeolin O.* **Victoria yellow.** Metanil yellow (see above). **Visual yellow.** A pigment formed from rhodopsin by the action of light, which further decomposes into protein and retinene during the rhodopsin cycle of retinal metabolism. [AS *geolu.*]

yellow fever virus (yel·o·fe·ver·vi·rus). An arbovirus transmitted by *Aëdes mosquitos,* it is the type species of the flaviviruses or Group B arboviruses. It can be grown readily in mice, cell culture and fertile eggs. In the last named, attenuation of virulence occurs and the 17D vaccine strain is derived from mouse and egg passage.

yellow jack (yel·o jak). Slang name for yellow fever.

yellow root (yel·o root). Hydrastis.

Yeo, Isaac Burney (b. 1835). London physician.

Burney Yeo's respirator. A light mask fitting over the nose and mouth, made of perforated zinc. It contains a small sponge upon which a few drops of volatile antiseptic or a sedative, such as preparations of creosote, chloroform, iodine, eucalyptus or turpentine, can be applied from time to time. It is used for continuous inhalation, and was formerly much employed in the treatment of phthisis and bronchiectasis.

Yeo's treatment. For obesity, by stopping carbohydrates and giving large amounts of hot water.

yerba (yer·bah). Yerba santa, eriodictyon, the dried leaves of *Eriodictyon californicum* (Hook. and Arn.) (family Hydrophyllaceae), used as a bitter tonic and expectorant. [Sp. herb.]

yerbine (yer·been). The name given to the active ingredient of maté, now known to be caffeine. [see prec.]

Yerkes, Robert Mearns (b. 1876). Boston psychiatrist.

Yerkes' test, Yerkes-Bridges test. A revision of the Binet-Simon test.

Yersin, Alexandre Emile Jean (b. 1863). Paris bacteriologist.

Yersin's serum. The original anti-plague serum.

yew (yew). The tree *Taxus baccata* (family Taxaceae). The berries are poisonous and the leaves contain ephedrine. [AS *iw.*]

yochubio (yo·**choo**·be·o). Mite-borne typhus. [Jap.]

yoghurt, yogurt (**yog**·hert, **yog**·ert). Milk sterilized by boiling, then curdled by the addition of acid-forming bacteria and incubated for a day at from 30° to 40°C. It has nutritive properties, but is mainly used in medicine to supply acid-forming bacteria to the intestine in the hope of restricting the growth of putrefactive bacteria there. [Turkish *yoghurt.*]

yohimbé (yo·**him**·be). The tree *Pausinystalia yohimba* (*Corynanthe yohimbe*) of the family Rubiaceae, growing in west central Africa. **Yohimbé bark.** The bark of the above, containing yohimbine and other alkaloids, the former finding a use as a tonic and aphrodisiac, sometimes in conjunction with strychnine. [W. Afr.]

yohimbenine (yo·**him**·ben·een). An alkaloid of uncertain composition, probably a mixture, obtained from yohimbé bark.

yohimbine (yo·**him**·been). $C_{21}H_{26}O_3N_2$, the principal alkaloid of yohimbé bark, *Pausinystalia yohimba.* It is identical with quebrachine found in white quebracho bark, and is employed as an aphrodisiac. **Yohimbine hydrochloride.** $C_{21}H_{26}O_3N_2HCl$, the water-soluble hydrochloride of the alkaloid yohimbine. It is an aphrodisiac, reputed to be superior to strychnine.

yokagawa (yo·kah·**gah**·wah). Infestation of the intestine by *Metagonimus ovatus.* [Jap.]

yoke-bone (**yoke**·bone). The zygomatic bone [obsolete term.] [AS *geoc,* bone.]

yolk (yoke). The nutrient non-living material found in smaller or larger droplets within or adjacent to the living cytoplasm of an egg cell. It is rich in fatty substances and proteins. **Accessory yolk.** Old term for the non-living part of the egg cell, as opposed to the living formative so-called yolk. **Egg yolk.** The yellow to orange portion of egg which is separated from the white by the vitelline membrane. It contains the phosphoproteins, vitellin and livetin, some inorganic salts and a little oil and lecithin. **Formative yolk.** Old term for the living cytoplasm of an egg cell lying around the nucleus, from which the embryo is derived. [AS *geolca.*]

Young, Hugh Hampton (b. 1870). Baltimore urologist.

Young's operation. An operation for removal of the entire seminal tract in tuberculosis.

Young, Robert Bruce (b. 1858). Glasgow anatomist.

Young's ligament. A ligament joining the 2nd and 3rd metacarpals and the trapezium.

Young, Thomas (b. 1773). English physician and physicist.

Young-Helmholtz theory. A trichromatic theory of colour vision; all colours can be reduced to the 3 primary colours, red, green and violet. Young originally suggested that there were 3 different types of cone in the retina, each reacting only to 1 of these 3 colours. Helmholtz thought the unit should be smaller and suggested that each cone would react differently to each of the 3 primary colours. Other colours would be perceived by the mixture of these 3 basic reactions, e.g. white.

Young's syndrome. Paralysis of muscles supplied by motor cranial nerves, with spastic paralysis of the lower limbs, due to platybasia. The 11th and 12th cranial nerves are particularly affected, and there may be cerebellar signs owing to compression of the cerebellar tonsils at the foramen magnum; usually called the *syndrome of basilar impression.*

young person (yung **per**·son). In forensic medicine, one who has attained the age of 14 years, but is under 17.

Youngburg, Guy Edgar (b. 1884). Buffalo biochemist.

Youngburg's method, for lipide phosphorus in blood. Serum (1 ml) is extracted with hot alcohol-ether mixture, the extract evaporated to dryness and oxidized with sulphuric acid and hydrogen peroxide. The phosphorus in the residue is determined by diluting with water, adding acid molybdate and stannous chloride, and comparing the blue colour with standards.

yperite (**i**·per·ite). Mustard gas, dichlorodiethyl sulphide, $(CH_2Cl\ CH_2)_2S$. An oily vesicant liquid used in chemical warfare as a blister gas.

Y-**piece** (**wi**·pees). A Y-shaped tube used for joining anaesthetic breaking tubes together, e.g. when using a double-lumen endobronchial tube. [Y-shaped, ME *pece.*]

ypsiliform, ypsiloid (ip·**sil**·e·form, **ip**·sil·oid). Shaped like the Greek letter *ypsilon* φ. [Gk *ypsilon, eidos* form.]

ytterbium (it·**er**·be·um). A rare-earth element of atomic weight 173.04, atomic number 70 and chemical symbol Yb, which occurs in gadolinite earths. [*Ytterby,* Sweden, a mineral source.]

yttria (**it**·re·ah). 1. Yttrium oxide which occurs naturally in the mineral gadolinite. 2. Gadolinite.

yttrium (**it**·re·um). A rare-earth element of atomic weight 88.9059, atomic number 39 and chemical symbol Y. It is found in gadolinite and is used in the manufacture of incandescent gas-mantles. **Yttrium-90.** The radioactive isotope implanted in the form of 2 seeds transnasally into the anterior lobe of the pituitary to form a dose of 50 000 rad in the treatment of pituitary tumours such as those giving rise to acromegaly. [*Ytterby,* Sweden, a mineral source.]

yucca (**yuk**·ah). Soaproot, a plant of California and Mexico used as a fibre. [Amer. Ind.]

yukon (yew·kon). Name given to the hypothetical fundamental particle postulated by Yukawa and subsequently identified with the meson.

Z

Zagari, Giuseppe (b. 1863). Naples physician.

Zagari's disease. Xerostomia; deficient salivary secretion causing dryness of the mouth.

Zaglas' ligament. Part of the posterior sacro-iliac ligament.

Zahn, Friedrich Wilhelm (b. 1845). Geneva pathologist.

Zahn's line or rib. A wavy upper surface of a thrombus formed by masses of blood platelets.

zaire (zi·ra). Cholera. [Port.]

Zaleski, Stanislaus (fl. 1885). Dorpat pharmacologist.

Zaleski's test, for carbon monoxide. Dilute the sample of blood with an equal volume of water and add 3 drops of a one-third saturated solution of copper sulphate. In the presence of CO a vermilion-red precipitate forms; in normal blood, a greenish brown.

Zander, Jonas Gustav Wilhelm (b. 1835). Stockholm physician.

Zander apparatus. An apparatus designed to give passive movements to a limb.

Zander cell. Bladder cell, a swollen epithelial cell found in the embryonic fingers and toes.

Zang, Christoph Bonifacius (b. 1772). Vienna and Würzburg surgeon.

Zang's space. The space between the clavicular and sternal heads of the sternocleidomastoid muscle.

zanthine (zan·theen). Xanthine.

Zaufal, Emanuel (b. 1833). Prague otologist.

Zaufal's fold. The salpingopharyngeal fold. *See* FOLD.

Zaufal's sign. Saddle nose due to syphilitic disease of the nasal bones.

Zea (ze·ah). A genus of plants of the family Gramineae, including the maize. **Zea mays.** Maize. [Gk a coarse grain.]

zeaxanthine (ze·ah·zan·theen). $C_{40}H_{56}O_2$, a carotenoid occurring in maize and in egg yolk. It is isomeric with lutein. [Gk *zea* a coarse grain, *xanthos* yellow.]

zedoary (zed·o·ar·e). The rhizome of *Curcuma zedoaria* of the family Zingiberaceae. It resembles ginger in taste and odour. [Pers. *zadwar.*]

Zeeman, Pieter (b. 1865). Amsterdam physicist.

Zeeman effect. The splitting of a spectral line when the source emitting it is placed in a strong magnetic field.

Zehbe's cell. A connective-tissue cell found in the organs of cancer patients.

zein (ze·in). A protein of the prolamin or gliadin class which occurs in maize. It is not a complete protein nutritionally as it lacks both tryptophan and lysine. [Gk *zea* a coarse grain.]

Zeis, Eduard (b. 1807). Dresden surgeon.

glands of Zeis. Sebaceous glands of the eyelids.

zeism, zeismus (ze·izm, ze·iz·mus). Pellagra; pellagrous dermatitis; a condition associated with a maize diet, but not exclusively so [obsolete term]. *See* PELLAGRA. [Gk *zea* a coarse grain.]

Zeiss, Carl, Jena optician.

binocular telescopic loupe of Zeiss. Telescopic glasses used in ophthalmic surgery to magnify the field of operation.

Abbé-Zeiss apparatus or counting cell, Thoma-Zeiss counting cell. This consists of a glass slide and a rigid cover-glass. The slide is ground in such a way that when the cover-glass is placed in position there is a space 0.1 mm between the cover-glass and the slide. The slide is etched with a series of lines at right angles to one another, so that the sides of the squares thus formed are exactly 0.05 mm long, the square area is 0.0025 mm^2, and the cubic capacity 0.00025 mm^3. Diluted blood is run between the cover-glass and the slide and the number of red cells within the square is counted and recorded; the squares are arranged in groups of 16 to facilitate the calculations. The contents of at least 80 squares are counted.

Zeissl, Maximilian (b. 1853). Vienna dermatologist.

Zeissl's layer or membrane. The stratum compactum of the mucous membrane of the stomach first reported by Molin (1850) in the hawk and in 1875 by Zeissl in the cat.

zeistic (ze·is·tik). Referring to maize. [Gk *zea* a coarse grain.]

Zeller, Albert (fl. 1883). Berlin surgeon.

Zeller's test, for melanin in urine. Add to urine an equal volume of bromine water. A yellow precipitate which darkens on standing, eventually to become black, indicates melanin.

Zeller treatment. The use of acetylene, injected into the subarachnoid space in cases of meningitis [obsolete].

Zenker, Friedrich Albert (b. 1825). Erlangen pathologist.

Zenker's degeneration or necrosis. Waxy or hyaline degeneration of muscles, found most often in acute infectious diseases, especially in typhoid fever and cholera.

Zenker's diverticulum. Pharyngeal diverticulum; a pulsion diverticulum of the pharynx.

Zenker's paralysis. Paralysis of muscles supplied by the lateral popliteal nerve, giving drop foot, usually due to trauma to the nerve as it rounds the head of the fibula. It sometimes results from squatting.

Zenker, Konrad (d. 1894). Erlangen pathologist.

Zenker's fluid or solution. An important histological fixative containing potassium dichromate, mercuric chloride and acetic acid.

zenkerism (zen·ker·izm). Zenker's degeneration. [Friedrich Albert *Zenker.*]

zeolite (ze·o·lite). One of a family of naturally-occurring hydrated aluminosilicates of sodium and potassium which also contain the silicates of magnesium or calcium. Some are employed in water-softening processes, and as absorbents. So-called because they froth when melted. [Gk *zeein* to boil, *lithos* stone.]

zeoscope (ze·o·skope). A boiling-point apparatus used to estimate the alcohol content of a liquid. [Gk *zeein* to boil, *skopein* to watch.]

zero (ze·ro). 1. Nought. 2. The point on any scale from which measurements commence, e.g. the zero of a thermometric scale. **Absolute zero.** The zero of thermodynamic temperature; nought on the Kelvin scale, −273.16°C. **Limes zero.** Limes nul (L_0); the largest amount of toxin (e.g. diphtheria) that, when mixed with 1 unit of antitoxin and injected subcutaneously into a 250-g guinea-pig, will, on the average, give rise to no observed reaction. In actual practice, the L_0 dose is the amount that, when tested in this way, gives rise to a minimal local oedema. **Physiological zero.** That temperature at which a thermal stimulus no longer causes a sensation. [It.]

zerodone (ze·ro·done). A hydrostatic apparatus for cooling the rectum by the circulation through it of fluid at low temperature.

zestocausis (zes·to·kaw·sis). The therapeutic application of an apparatus containing superheated steam. [Gk *zestos* boiling hot, *kausis* a burning.]

zestocautery (zes·to·kaw·ter·e). An appliance used in zestocausis.

Ziegler, Samuel Lewis (b. 1861). Philadelphia ophthalmologist.

Ziegler's needle. A fine, long-bladed iridotomy knife used for incising the capsule.

Ziegler's operation. Iridotomy; a triangular opening is made in the pulled-up iris of an aphacic eye with Ziegler's special knife needle.

Ziehen, Georg Theodor (b. 1862). German neurologist.

Ziehen-Oppenheim disease. Torsion spasm; dystonia musculorum deformans.

Ziehl, Franz (b. 1859). Lübeck physician.

Ziehl-Nielsen method or stain, for *Mycobacterium tuberculosis.* Heat-fixed smears are stained with hot, strong, carbolfuchsine for 5 min, decolorized with 20 per cent sulphuric acid and 95 per cent alcohol and counter-stained with methylene blue or malachite green. Tubercle bacilli stain bright red, all other cells blue or green.

Ziemann, Hans (fl. 1910). German parasitologist in Africa.

Ziemann's stippling. A form of stippling of the erythrocyte infected with *Plasmodium malariae*; others had described this.

Ziemssen, Hugo Wilhelm von (b. 1829). Munich physician.

Ziemssen's motor points. Points on the surface corresponding to the entrance of the nerves into the underlying muscles, commonly known as *motor points.* They are the points of election for the application of electrodes for therapy.

Ziemssen's treatment. The treatment of anaemia by the administration of defibrinated human blood subcutaneously [obsolete].

Zimmer splints. 1. A rigid collar for immobilization of the neck. 2. A metal splint designed to hold the arm in abduction at the shoulder.

Zimmerlin, Franz (b. 1858). Swiss physician.

Zimmerlin's type, Erb-Zimmerlin type. The Erb (juvenile, scapulohumeral) type of muscular dystrophy.

Zimmermann, Gustav Heinrich Eduard (b. 1817). German military surgeon.

Zimmermann's corpuscles, granules or elementary particles. Blood platelets.

Zimmermann, Karl Wilhelm (b. 1861). German anatomist.

Zimmermann's arch. An occasional transient aortic arch in avian and mammalian embryos, between the systemic aorta and the pulmonary artery, supposed to be homologous with the 5th aortic arch of lower vertebrates.

Zimmermann's corpuscle. A ghost corpuscle.

zinc (zingk). An element of atomic weight 65.38, atomic number 30 and chemical symbol Zn. It occurs naturally as the sulphide, zinc blende, ZnS, and in calamine, $ZnCO_3$. It is of great importance for the manufacture of brass and galvanized iron. It is a bluish-white metal, hard and brittle, but becoming malleable and ductile on heating. It is present in small amounts in many foods, and is necessary for normal development of plants and animals. In animals, the greatest concentration is found in the pancreas, and all preparations of insulin contain small amounts of zinc. Zinc salts are astringent and corrosive, and have weak antiseptic activity. They are used in therapeutics for their local actions, chiefly in inflammatory or eczematous skin conditions, and may be employed as dusting-powders, or in the form of lotions, pastes or ointments. Small additional amounts of zinc are added to some preparations of insulin, as in protamine- or globin- insulin, to delay absorption. Zinc poisoning may result from ingestion of its salts, either directly or from cooking acid foods in galvanized iron vessels. Gastro-intestinal disturbance is the commonest manifestation. Industrial poisoning also occurs from the inhalation of zinc dust, causing the syndrome known as *brassfounders' ague* or *metal-fume fever.* The chief features are malaise, chills and fever, settling with profuse sweating within 24 h. **Zinc acetate.** $Zn(OOCCH_3)_2$, a white crystalline substance, used as an astringent lotion. **Bacitracin Zinc BP 1973.** A zinc salt of the antimicrobial substance bacitracin, used in lozenges, ointments and dusting powders. **Zinc carbonate.** Hydrated zinc carbonate, $ZnCO_3{\cdot}2ZnO{\cdot}3H_2O$, a white amorphous powder. It has mild astringent and protective properties and is used as a dusting-powder or lotion. It is the chief constituent of calamine lotion. **Zinc Chloride BPC 1968.** $ZnCl_2$, a white, granular and very deliquescent powder. It is a strong caustic and astringent, and is used locally as a paste or lotion in chronic ulcerated skin lesions. A more dilute solution is used as eye drops. **Zinc Gelatin BP 1963.** Unna's paste, a preparation containing 15 per cent of zinc oxide with gelatin, glycerin and distilled water. It is used for its protective and astringent properties as a local application in eczema and indolent ulcers. **Zinc Oxide BP 1973.** ZnO, a white amorphous powder, without odour or taste. It is used as an external application to the skin in the form of dusting-powders, lotions, creams, pastes and ointments, for its mild astringent properties. **Zinc permanganate.** $Zn(MnO_4)_2{\cdot}6H_2O$, a compound that resembles the potassium salt in its oxidizing properties, but is more astringent. It is used for urethritis, being administered by irrigation. **Zinc Peroxide BP 1953.** ZnO_2, a white or faintly yellow powder, used as a local application in ulcerative skin lesions. **Zinc phenolsulphonate.** $[C_6H_4OHSO_2O]_2Zn{\cdot}8H_2O$, an astringent and antiseptic formerly used for irrigation in leucorrhoea and gonorrhoea, and as a nose and throat spray [obsolete]. **Pyrithione Zinc.** BP Commission approved name for zinc bis(pyridine-2-thiol 1-oxide); it is used in the treatment of seborrhoea. **Zinc Stearate BP 1958.** $Zn(OOCC_{17}H_{35})_2$, a white amorphous powder, used locally in certain skin conditions such as eczema. **Zinc subcarbonate.** Zinc carbonate (see above). **Zinc Sulphate BP 1973.** White vitriol $ZnSO_4$, a colourless crystalline powder. It is used as a lotion for its astringent properties. **Zinc Undecenoate BP 1973.** $(C_{10}H_{19}COO)_2Zn$, a fungicide used in mycotic infections. **Zinc valerianate.** $Zn(C_5H_9O_2)_2{\cdot}2H_2O$, a compound that has been used with quinine and iron valerianates in the treatment of neurasthenia. [G *zink.*]

zincalism (zing·kal·izm). Chronic poisoning among workers in zinc.

zincoid (zing·koid). 1. Having a similarity to zinc. 2. The negative plate of a voltaic cell, so-called because in the original cell it was zinc. [zinc, Gk *eidos* form.]

zincum (zing·kum). Zinc. **Zinci oxidum.** *European Pharmacopoeia* name for Zinc Oxide BP 1973. **Zinci sulfas.** *European Pharmacopoeia* name for Zinc Sulphate BP 1973.

zincundecate (zing·kun·dek·ate). A mixture of undecenoic acid and zinc undecenoate; it is used in the treatment of athletes' foot.

zingiber (zin·jib·er). Ginger. [Gk *zingiberis* ginger.]

zingiberene (zin·jib·er·een). $C_{15}H_{24}$, a monocyclic sesquiterpene found in oil of ginger, and isomeric with bisabolene. [see prec.]

Zinn, Johann Gottfried (b. 1727). Gottingen anatomist and botanist.

annulus, aponeurosis or ligament of Zinn. The common tendinous ring, from which the 4 recti muscles of the orbit arise.

Zinn's central artery. The central retinal artery.

Zinn's circle or corona. The circulus vasculosus of the optic nerve; an artificial circle surrounding the entrance of the optic nerve into the sclera. Also called the *circle of Haller.*

Zinn's membrane. A layer of flattened endothelial cells constituting the anterior layer of the iris.

Zinn's tendon. Tendinous thickening of the annulus of Zinn in its lower part giving attachment to part of the medial and lateral recti muscles and the whole of the superior rectus muscle of the orbit.

Zinn's zone, zonule of Zinn. Ciliary zonule; a fibrous thickening of the anterior part of the vitreous body beyond the level of the ora serrata of the retina that supports the lens, and is therefore also called the *suspensory ligament.*

Zinsser, Hans (b. 1878). Harvard bacteriologist.

Zinsser's inconsistency. The lack of agreement between local and systemic anaphylaxis.

Zinsser-Castañeda vaccine. A vaccine used in southern Mexico, consisting of 4 parts of murine rickettsiae and 1 part of epidemic rickettsiae (*Rickettsia prowazeki*).

zircon (zer·kon). A naturally-occurring silicate of zirconium, $ZrSiO_4$, found in Sri Lanka and elsewhere. Certain varieties are used as gem-stones. [Ar. *zarqun.*]

zirconia (zer·ko·ne·ah). Zirconium dioxide, ZrO_2. A compound which occurs naturally, and may be prepared from zircon. It is a heavy white substance, used as a refractory and, admixed with rare earths, in incandescent gas mantles and Nernst lamps. It has been employed in x-ray work instead of bismuth.

zirconium (zer·**ko**·ne·um). An element of atomic weight 91.22, atomic number 40 and chemical symbol Zr. It is a rare metal employed in steel-making and in alloys. It occurs in the mineral, zircon. **Zirconium dioxide.** ZrO_2, a radio-opaque substance sometimes used for x-ray of the alimentary canal. [zircon.]

Zizyphus vulgaris (ziz·e·fus vul·ga·ris). Jujube; one of the habitats of the shellac insect. [Gk *zizyphon*, L common.]

zoacanthosis (zo·ak·an·**tho**'·sis). Any dermatitis following retention in the skin of foreign bodies such as bristles, hairs, stings, etc. derived from insects or animals. [Gk *zoon* animal, *akantha* spine, *-osis* condition.]

zoanthropic (zo·an·**throp**·ik). Referring to or affected with zoanthropy.

zoanthropy (zo·**an**·thro·pe). Mental disorder in which the patient believes himself to be an animal. [Gk *zoon* animal, *anthropos* man.]

Zoedypus pichiy (zo·e·dip·us **pik**·e·e). The little armadillo; a reservoir of infection of *Trypanosoma cruzi.*

Zoellner, Johann Carl Friedrich (b. 1834). Leipzig physicist.

Zoellner's figures or lines. A peculiar arrangement of lines, used for testing vision.

zoescope (**zo**·e·skope). Stroboscope. [Gk *zoe* life, *skopein* to view.]

zoetic (zo·**et**·ik). Displaying life; pertaining to life; vital. [see foll.]

zoic (**zo**·ik). Concerned with animal life or living creatures. [Gk *zoe* life.]

zoism (**zo**·izm). Vitalism. The theory that the functions of a living organism are due to a vital principle or force distinct from physical forces. [see prec.]

Zollinger, Robert Milton (b. 1903). American surgeon.

Zollinger-Ellison syndrome. A non-insulin-secreting adenoma of the islets of Langerhans associated with peptic ulceration. Hyperplasia or adenomata may sometimes be found in the parathyroid glands, adrenal glands or hypophysis.

zona [NA] (**zo**·nah). 1. A zone. 2. Herpes zoster. **Zona dermatica.** An area of thick elevated skin surrounding a meningocele. **Zona epithelioserosa.** A zone of serous meningeal tissue within the zona dermatica. **Zona facialis.** Herpes zoster affecting an area of the face and maybe involving the buccal or nasal mucosae. **Zona fasiculata** of the adrenal cortex. Rich in lipids, especially cholesterol. **Zona glomerulosa.** The outer layer of the adrenal cortex, containing mineralocorticoids. **Zona granulosa.** The mass of granulosa cells surrounding the ovum within a vesicular ovarian follicle. **Zona ignea.** Herpes zoster. **Zona incerta.** An area between the subthalamic nucleus and the lateral nucleus of the thalamus. **Zona ophthalmica.** An old name for zoster ophthalmicus. *See* ZOSTER. **Zona orbicularis of the hip joint [zona orbicularis (NA)].** The deeper, circularly-arranged layer of the capsular fibres. **Zona pellucida, Zona radiata.** Zona striata (see below). **Zona reticularis.** The inner zone of the adrenal cortex. It contains compact cells and increases in width at the expense of the cells of the zona fasiculata in cases of Cushing's syndrome due to adrenocortical hyperplasia. **Zona striata.** The hyaline or faintly radially striated oesinophilic membrane in immediate contact with the outer wall of the ovum. It persists from an early stage in the maturation of the ovum while it is still in its vesicular ovarian follicle, up to the time of implantation of the blastocyst into the wall of the uterus. [Gk *zone* belt.]

zonaesthesia (zo·nes·**the**·ze·ah). A feeling that the body is being constricted by a cord round the waist. [Gk *zone* belt, *aisthesis* sensation.]

zonal (**zo**·nal). Pertaining to or characterized by zones; restricted to a zone.

zonary (**zo**·nar·e). Zonal; ringed.

zonate (**zo**·nate). Ringed; composed of concentric rings or widening layers. [Gk *zone* belt.]

Zondek, Bernhard (b. 1891). German gynaecologist in Israel.

Aschheim-Zondek test, for pregnancy. A female immature mouse is injected subcutaneously with the urine of a pregnant woman 6 times in 2 days; 0.2 ml of urine is used for the first injection and the dose gradually increased to 0.4 ml; 96 h after the first injection the mouse is killed, and the ovaries will show haemorrhagic spots and yellowish protrusions indicating pregnancy in the patient. This test can reach a high degree of accuracy, but is time-consuming.

zone (zone). 1. An area or part distinguished by the possession of some special character or constitution. 2. [Zona (NA).] An anatomical zone. **Abdominal zone.** One of the 3 horizontal zones into which the abdomen is divided by the subcostal and intertubercular planes, namely the *epigastric zone*, the *mesogastric zone* and the *hypogastric zone*, from above downwards. **Zone of alarm.** A descriptive term applied to certain areas of the body the limits of which are defined by anatomical, physiological or radiological criteria. **Androgenic zone.** X zone (see below). **Anelectrotonic zone.** The region immediately around the anode. **Border zone.** The outer region of the placenta where trophoblast and decidua are intermingled. **Ciliary zone.** The peripheral part of the anterior surface of the iris, consisting of 2 mesodermal layers, and divided from the pupillary zone by the collarette. **Comfort zone.** The environmental limits of air temperature and humidity (and of solar radiation and wind velocity when these apply) within which a subject clad in a specified manner and doing work at a specified rate is subjectively in a state of physical comfort. **Zones of discontinuity of the lens.** Concentric zones seen on slit-lamp examination of the lens, which are apparent because of their difference in optical density. They are, from without in, the capsular surface, the *zone of separation*, or *subcapsular zone, adult nuclear zone, outer embryonic nuclear zone* and *inner embryonic nuclear zone.* **Dolorogenic zone.** A zone, the stimulation of which produces pain, for example initiates an attack of trigeminal neuralgia. **Entry zone.** The site of entry of the posterior nerve roots into the spinal cord. **Ependymal zone.** The inner zone of the early neural tube, now known as the matrix layer. **Zone of the epidermis, germinative.** The deepest stratum of the epidermis. **Zone of the epidermis, horny.** The outer layer of the epidermis, consisting of dead cornified cells which are constantly rubbed off and replaced from below. **Epigastric zone.** *See* ABDOMINAL ZONE (above). **Epileptogenic zone, Epileptogenous zone.** Any area which may act as a trigger zone for epileptic attacks; stimulation within the zone initiates a seizure. **Equivalence zone.** In the optimal proportions titration technique of performing a precipitin reaction, that ratio of antigen to antibody at which visible precipitation takes place. **Erogenous zone, Erotogenic zone.** An area on the body which on appropriate stimulation gives rise to sexual sensations. **Extravisual zone.** Applied to that portion of the retina which is not used for sight because it is too far forward for images to fall upon it; its posterior border is usually 8–9 mm from the limbus. **Germinative zone.** 1. Zone of the epidermis, germinative (see above). 2. Zone of the nail, germinative (see below). **Haemorrhoidal zone [zona hemorrhoidalis (NA)].** The lower part of the anal canal in the submucosae of which is the internal part of the rectal (venous) plexus. **Horny zone.** 1. Zone of the epidermis, horny (see above). 2. Zone of the nail, horny (see below). **Hyperaesthetic zone.** Any surface area of the body which demonstrates hyperaesthesia, from whatever cause. **Zone of hyperalgesia.** Head's zones. **Hypnogenous zone.** A zone, pressure upon which can produce the hypnotic state. **Hypogastric zone.** *See* ABDOMINAL ZONE (above). **Hysterogenic zones, Hysterogenous zones.** Zones, pressure upon which produce hysterical attacks, e.g. the inguinal regions, submammary regions, etc. The sensitivity of these zones is first produced by suggestion. **Inhibition zone.** 1. Prozone. 2. The area of inhibition of growth produced on solid media by the diffusion of a drug from a reservoir, e.g. in the Oxford cup method for assaying penicillin or for determining the sensitivity of micro-organisms to different drugs. **Interpalpebral zone.** That part of the cornea and conjunctiva that is not normally in contact with the eyelids. **Iso-electric zone.** The zone in the pH scale where iso-electric conditions prevail. **Language zone.** The centres in the cerebral cortex which are concerned with speech. **Latent zone.** The areas of the cerebral cortex which do not give rise to motor activity and are apparently silent. **Mantle zone.** The middle zone of the early neural tube in which neurones and neuroglial cells are differentiating. **Marginal zone.** The outer zone of the early neural tube, containing very few cell bodies but numerous interlacing fibrous processes of neuroglial cells. **Mesogastric zone.** *See* ABDOMINAL ZONE (above). **Motor zone.** Any area of the cerebral cortex concerned with motor activity, which, when stimulated electrically, results in contraction of skeletal musculature. **Zone of the nail, germinative [stratum germinativum unguis (NA)].** Basal columnar cells from which the remainder of the nail is proliferated. **Zone of the nail, horny [stratum corneum unguis (NA)].** The thick horny layer corresponding to the clear layer of the epidermis. **Nuclear zone.** *See* ZONES OF DISCONTINUITY OF THE LENS (above). **Pellucid zone.** Zona striata. **Peripheral-field zone.** That part of the visual field outside a circle extending in all directions 25 degrees from the fixation point. **Peripolar zone.** The area surrounding the polar zone. **Zone of plateaux and furrows.** An area of irregularities near the convex border of the tarsus of the eyelid. **Polar zone.** The region immediately around an electrode. **Zone of polymorphous cells.** The innermost cell layer of the cerebral cortex, so-named because of the variation in size and shape of the nerve cell bodies. **Pro-agglutinoid zone.** Prozone. **Pupillary zone.** The central part of the anterior surface of the iris, in which the superficial mesodermal layer has atrophied and is separated from the ciliary zone by the collarette. Also called *the lesser ring of Merkel.* **Radiation danger zone.** The space where a radiation hazard exists. **Satellite zone.** Satellite region. *See* REGION. **Segmental zone.** The paraxial mesoderm in front of the primitive streak of the early embryo before it has been divided into somites. **Zone of separation.** *See* ZONES OF DISCONTINUITY OF THE LENS (above). **Zone of specular reflection.** In ophthalmology, the area of lens or cornea when examined by the method of specular reflection on the slit lamp. The area being examined is acting as a mirror, and the angle of the microscope to the perpendicular from the reflecting surface must equal the angle of the slit-lamp beam to this perpendicular. Any irregularities such as corneal oedema show up well by this method. Only those zones of the cornea and lens which act as reflecting surfaces can be examined by this method, e.g. anterior and posterior corneal surfaces and the anterior and posterior surfaces of the lens plus the zones of discontinuity. **Subcapsular zone.** *See* ZONES OF DISCONTINUITY OF THE LENS (above). **Subcostal zone.** *See* ABDOMINAL ZONE (above). **Sudanophobic zone.** A zone or band of cells in the cortex of the suprarenal gland from which lipides disappear after hypophysectomy, with the consequence that fat-staining substances, such as the Sudan dyes, are not taken up. **Transitional zone.** That part of the crystalline lens where the epithelial-capsule cells change into lens fibres. **Translucent zone, Transparent zone.** A zone seen microscopically beneath advancing caries which appears more transparent than normal dentine, an appearance caused by calcification of the contents of the dentinal tubules by the precipitation of inorganic salts. **Trigger zone.** Dolorogenic zone (see above). **Visual zone.** The area in the centre of the pupil, through which the light rays that pass, show little spherical aberration and fall on the centre of the retina. It is important in retinoscopy to watch the shadow in this zone only. **X zone.** That zone of the suprarenal cortex lying next to the medulla. In man it is a striking feature of the fetal suprarenal cortex, but atrophies and disappears in the early months of postnatal life; in some animals it persists. It secretes substances similar to androgens, hence the zone is sometimes called the *androgenic zone.* [Gk *zone* belt.]

See also: CHARCOT, HEAD, HIS (W. SNR.), LISSAUER, LOOSER, MARCHANT, OBERSTEINER, REDLICH, ROLANDO, TRUEMMERFELD, WERNICKE (K.), ZINN.

zonifugal (zo·nif·ew·gal). Moving from within a zone outwards. [zone, L *fugere* to flee.]

zoning (zo·ning). The phenomenon of a serological reaction taking place at certain dilutions of the reagents, and not above or below those dilutions. [Gk *zone* belt.]

zonipetal (zo·**nip**·et·al). Moving into a zone from outside. [zone, L *petere* to seek.]

zonula (**zo**·new·lah). Zonule. **Zonula adherens.** A component of the junctional complex between cells. It is a continuous zone, running around the circumference of the cell, in which the intercellular space is about 20 nm in width. The underlying cytoplasm contains an area of dense filamentous material. **Zonula occludens.** Tight junction, a component of the junctional complex between cells in which the plasma membranes of the adjacent cells come into direct contact, the intercellular space being obliterated.

zonular (zo·new·lar). Concerned with a zonule.

zonule (zo·newl, **zon**·ewl). A zone, usually a circular one. **Ciliary zonule [zonula ciliaris (NA)].** Zonule of Zinn; a fibrous thickening of the anterior part of the vitreous body beyond the level of the ora serrata of the retina. It is strengthened by radial fibres from the ciliary region and approaching the margin of the lens it divides into 2 layers, one of which lines the hyaloid fossa, the other forming the suspensory ligament of the lens. [dim. of L *zona* belt.]

See also: ZINN.

zonulitis (zo·new·**li**·tis). A supposed inflammation of the zonule of Zinn, a delicate membrane running from the ciliary body to the capsule of the lens and forming its suspensory ligament [obsolete term]. [zonule, Gk *-itis* inflammation.]

zoo-anthroponoses (**zo**·o·an·thro·po·**no**′·seez). Infections of vetebrates naturally acquired from man when he is the maintenance host, e.g. human tuberculosis in cattle. [Gk *zoon* animal, *anthropos* human being, *osis* condition.]

zoochemical (zo·o·**kem**·ik·al). Relating to zoochemistry.

zoochemistry (zo·o·**kem**·is·tre). Animal chemistry; biochemistry. [Gk *zoon* animal, chemistry.]

zoocyst (**zo**·o·sist). A cyst of a protozoon. [Gk *zoon* animal, cyst.]

zoodermic (zo·o·**der**·mik). Effected by the use of the skin of an animal other than man, usually applied to a skin graft. [Gk *zoon* animal, *derma* skin.]

zooerastia (zo·o·e·**ras**′·te·ah). Sexual relations with an animal. [Gk *zoon* animal, *erastes* lover.]

zoogamete (zo·o·**gam**·eet). A motile gamete. [Gk *zoon* animal, gamete.]

zoogamy (zo·**og**·am·e). Reproduction involving the production of zoogametes. [Gk *zoon* animal, *gamos* marriage.]

zoogeography (zo·o·je·**og**′·raf·e). The study of the distribution of animals on the surface of the earth. [Gk *zoon* animal, geography.]

zoograft (**zo**·o·graft). A heterologous graft from an animal other than man. [Gk *zoon* animal, graft.]

zoohormone (zo·o·**hor**·mone). An animal hormone. [Gk *zoon* animal, hormone.]

zoolagnia (zo·o·**lag**·ne·ah). Sexual desire for animals. [Gk *zoon* animal, *lagneia* lust.]

zoologist (zo·**ol**·o·gist). One undertaking the scientific study of animals. [see foll.]

zoology (zo·**ol**·o·je). The study of animals. **Comparative zoology.** That in which the structure and physiology of different animals are compared. **Experimental zoology.** The study of the effect of alterations in the structure or environment of animals. [Gk *zoon* animal, *logos* science.]

zoomania (zo·o·**ma**·ne·ah). A morbid and exaggerated affection for animals. [Gk *zoon* animal, *mania* madness.]

Zoomastigina (zo·o·mas·**tij**′·in·ah). A sub-class of the Mastigophora, used for those flagellates which have no chromatophores and thus feed holozoically. [Gk *zoon* animal, *mastix* whip.]

zoonosis (zo·**on**·o·sis). 1. A disease common to man and other animals, usually in which animals are the main reservoir of infection. 2. A disease caused by animal parasites (questionable usage). 3. Any animal disease (questionable usage). [Gk *zoon* animal, *nosos* disease.]

zoonosology (zo·o·nos·ol'·o·je). The study of diseases of animals. [Gk *zoon* animal, *nosos* disease, *logos* science.]

zoonotic (zo·on·ot·ik). 1. Concerning zoonosis. 2. Describing any disease transmitted to man from an animal.

zooparasite (zo·o·par·as·ite). An animal with parasitic habits. [Gk *zoon* animal, parasite.]

zooparasitic (zo·o·par·as·it'·ik). Referring to a zooparasite or to a disease caused by zooparasites.

zoopathology (zo·o·path·ol'·o·je). The study of diseases which affect animals. [Gk *zoon* animal, *pathos* disease, *logos* science.]

zoophagous (zo·of·ag·us). Existing on a diet of animal flesh; carnivorous. [Gk *zoon* animal, *phagein* to eat.]

zoophile (zo·o·file). One who exhibits zoophilism.

zoophilic (zo·o·fil·ik). Of the nature of a zoophile.

zoophilism (zo·of·il·izm). 1. An affection for animals. 2. Applied to blood-sucking arthropods, attraction to animals and a preference for their blood; an important matter in the control of insect-borne disease. **Erotic zoophilism.** A perverted predilection for animals, reaching ultimately sexual gratification in their handling. [Gk *zoon* animal, *philein* to love.]

zoophilous (zo·of·il·us). Displaying zoophilism.

zoophobia (zo·o·fo·be·ah). A morbid and unreasoning fear or dislike of animals. [Gk *zoon* animal, *phobein* to fear.]

zoophysiology (zo·o·fiz·e·ol'·o·je). Animal physiology. [Gk *zoon* animal, physiology.]

zoophyte (zo·o·fite). An animal such as coral, which lives in a colony and in appearance and development resembles a plant. [Gk *zoon* animal, *phyton* plant.]

zooplasty (zo·o·plas·te). Heterologous transplantation to man of a tissue or organ from another animal. [Gk *zoon* animal, *plassein* to mould.]

zooprecipitin (zo·o·pre·sip'·it·in). A precipitating antibody obtained by injections of protein substances of animal origin. [Gk *zoon* animal, precipitin.]

zooprophylaxis (zo·o·pro·fil·ax'·is). In entomology, the deflection of mosquitoes or other blood-sucking insects from man by the interposition of animal quarters between the breeding places of the insects and human habitations, in order to prevent insects becoming infected from, and/or transmitting infection to, man. [Gk *zoon* animal, prophylaxis.]

zoopsia (zo·op·se·ah). Hallucinations which feature animals. [Gk *zoon* animal, *opsis* vision.]

zoopsychology (zo·o·si·kol'·o·je). The study of the mental processes of animals. [Gk *zoon* animal, psychology.]

zoosadism (zo·o·sa·dizm). Sadistic cruelty to animals. [Gk *zoon* animal, sadism.]

zooscopy (zo·os·ko·pe). Hallucination in which animals are seen; zoopsia. [Gk *zoon* animal, *skopein* to view.]

zoosis (zo·o·sis). Disease attributable to an animal parasite. [Gk *zoon* animal.]

zoosmosis (zo·oz·mo·sis). Osmosis in the living organism. [Gk *zoe* life, osmosis.]

zoosperm (zo·o·sperm). A spermatozoon.

zoospermia (zo·o·sper·me·ah). The existence of living and active spermatozoa in semen. [Gk *zoos* alive, sperm.]

zoospore (zo·o·spor). A type of motile (ciliated) asexual spore produced in sporangia by certain fungi of the class Phycomycetes. The flagella may be 1 or 2 in number and be attached in a posterior, anterior or lateral position. [Gk *zoon* animal, *sporos* seed.]

zoosterol (zo·os·ter·ol). Any sterol which occurs in animals; cholesterol is an example. [Gk *zoon* animal, sterol.]

zootic (zo·ot·ik). Pertaining to animals. [Gk *zoon* animal.]

zootomist (zo·ot·o·mist). A dissector of animals. [Gk *zoon* animal, *temnein* to cut.]

zootomy (zo·ot·o·me). Dissection of animals. [see prec.]

zootoxin (zo·o·tox·in). Any toxic substance occurring in a poisonous animal fluid, such as the venom of snakes and scorpions, the poison claws of some spiders and the blood serum of certain eels. [Gk *zoon* animal, *toxikon* poison.]

zootrophic (zo·o·trof'·ik). Referring to the nutrition of animals. [Gk *zoon* animal, *trophe* nourishment.]

zootrophotoxism (zo·o·tro·fo·tox'·izm). Poisoning due to foods of animal origin. [Gk *zoon* animal, *trophe* nourishment, *toxikon* poison.]

Zopfius (zop·fe·us). A genus of rod-shaped Gram-positive micro-organisms, biochemically very inactive but otherwise somewhat like *Proteus.* None appears to be pathogenic to man.

zoster (zos·ter). Herpes zoster. *See* HERPES and CHICKENPOX. **Zoster auricularis, Zoster auris.** Sometimes called *herpes of the geniculate ganglion*; in its simplest form there is acute earache with the formation of herpetic blebs on the ear-drum and external auditory meatus; more severe forms are associated with facial paralysis and in extreme forms with internal-ear deafness and vertigo. It is thought to be a virus infection, and is sometimes referred to as *Hunt's syndrome.* **Zoster brachialis.** Herpes zoster affecting the neck, shoulder and upper arm; in rare instances the eruption may extend to the fingers. **Epidemic zoster ophthalmicus.** Herpes ophthalmicus caused by a primary infection by the specific virus. **Zoster facialis.** Herpes zoster involving the sensory fibres of the 3 branches of the trigeminal nerve. **Zoster femoralis.** Herpes zoster over the sacrum and down the back of the thigh. **Zoster gangraenosus.** A haemorrhagic gangrenous form that may run a prolonged course of from 1 to 2 months. **Idiopathic zoster.** Herpes zoster of uncertain origin. **Intercostal zoster.** A form that forms a half girdle, following the course of a single intercostal nerve. **Zoster ophthalmicus.** A herpes-zoster affection of the trigeminal ganglion involving the ophthalmic division of the 5th cranial nerve. The skin of the forehead, nose and upper lid are affected; often associated with a severe conjunctivitis, iritis and keratitis, and occasionally optic neuritis and ocular muscle palsies. **Zoster oticus.** Zoster auricularis (see above). **Symptomatic zoster ophthalmicus.** Zoster ophthalmicus caused by an involvement of the trigeminal ganglion by a neoplastic, traumatic or infected lesion, precipitating the infection by the virus, which is already present. **Zoster varicella.** A form of zoster with scattered varicella lesions. It represents about 4 per cent of cases of zoster. [Gk girdle.]

zosteriform, zosteroid (zos·ter·e·form, zos·ter·oid). Having a similarity to herpes zoster. [zoster, Gk *eidos* form.]

Zoxazolamine (zox·az·ol·am·een). BP Commission approved name for 2-amino-5-chlorobenzoxazole, $C_6H_3Cl{=}NO(NH_2)$. It is a skeletal muscle relaxant.

Z-plasty (zed·plas·te). Plastic operation for the elongation of a wound by transposing the 2 elements of a Z-shaped incision. [Z-shaped, Gk *plassein* to mould.]

Zsigmondy, Richard Adolf (b. 1865). Gottingen physicist.

Brownian–Zsigmondy movement. Brownian movement. *See* MOVEMENT.

Zuckerkandl, Emil (b. 1849). Vienna anatomist.

Zuckerkandl's bodies. The paraganglion situated at the sides of the abdominal aorta constituting part of the chromaffin system.

Zuckerkandl's fascia. The posterior layer of the renal fascia.

Zuckerkandl's gland. An accessory lobe of the thyroid gland lying in front of the hyoid bone to the left of the midline.

Zuckerkandl's gyrus. The paraterminal gyrus; a small area of cortex anterior to the lamina terminalis and below the rostrum of the corpus callosum.

Zuckerkandl's vein. A nasal emissary vein.

Zünd-Burguet, A. 20th century Paris otolaryngologist.

Zünd-Burguet apparatus or treatment. Electrophonoide.

Zuntz, Nathan (b. 1847). Berlin physician.

Zuntz theory. A theory of muscular contraction.

Zwemer, Raymond Lull (b. 1902). Columbia University anatomist.

Zwemer's test. Potassium-tolerance test. *See* TEST.

Zwikker test. Copper-pyridine test. *See* TEST.

zwitterion (tsvit·er·i·on). Dipolar ion. A complex ion which possesses both positive and negative charges of equal strength, and is therefore attracted to neither anode nor cathode. Amino acids yield such an ion of the general type $^{+}NH_3CHRCOO^{-}$. [G *zwitter* hybrid.]

zygadenine (zi·gad·en·een). $C_{39}H_{63}O_{10}N$, a minor alkaloid occurring in *Zygadenus intermedius*, resembling cevadine in its action.

Zygadenus (zi·gad·e·nus). A genus of North American and Asian herbs, including the species *Zygadenus intermedius* and *Z. venenosus* both of which contain alkaloids poisonous to cattle. [Gk *zygaden* jointly.]

zygal (zi·gal). Having the form of a yoke; shaped like the letter H. [Gk *zygon* a yoke.]

zygapophyseal (zi·gap·of·**iz**′·e·al). Pertaining to a zygapophysis.

zygapophysis (zi·gap·**of**·is·is). One of the articular processes each side of the vertebral arch on the upper and lower surface of a vertebra which articulate with corresponding processes on the vertebrae above and below. [Gk *zygon* yoke, *apophysis* outgrowth.]

zygocyte (zi·go·site). Zygote. [Gk *zygon* yoke, *kytos* cell.]

zygodactyly (zi·go·**dak**·til·e). Syndactyly due to webbing of the skin. [Gk *zygon* yoke, *daktylos* digit.]

zygoma (zi·go·mah). 1. The zygomatic or malar bone. 2. The zygomatic arch, a bar of bone formed by the articulation of the temporal process of the zygomatic bone with the zygomatic process of the temporal bone, beneath which the temporal muscle passes. **Roots of the zygoma.** Three ridges on the squamous part of the temporal bone radiating from the attachment of the zygomatic process. [Gk bar.]

zygomatic (zi·go·**mat**·ik). Referring to the zygoma.

zygomatic bone [os zygomaticum (NA)]. The cheek-bone forming a prominence in the upper and lateral part of the face, and articulating with the frontal bone above, the sphenoid bone medially, the maxilla below and the temporal bone behind. On the posterior border just below the frontozygomatic suture is a rounded eminence, the marginal tubercle.

lateral surface [facies lateralis (NA)]. The convex surface directed forwards.

orbital surface [facies orbitalis (NA)]. The surface of the zygomatic bone presenting in the floor and lateral wall of the orbit. On it are 1 or 2 foramina for the zygomatic nerve or its branches, the zygomatico-orbital foramina.

temporal surface [facies temporalis (NA)]. The surface of the zygomatic bone which forms the anterolateral boundary of the temporal fossa.

zygomatic nerve [nervus zygomaticus (NA)]. The branch of the maxillary nerve given off in the pterygopalatine fossa and supplying the skin over the prominence of the cheek (zygomaticofacial branch [ramus zygomaticofacialis] NA) and the adjacent part of the temple (zygomaticotemporal branch [ramus zygomaticotemporalis] NA).

zygomatico-angularis (zi·go·**mat**·ik·o·ang·gew·**la**′·ris). Referring to the zygomatic bone and the angle of the eye.

zygomatico-auricular (zi·go·**mat**·ik·o·aw·**rik**′·ew·lar). Referring to the zygomatic arch and the auricle of the ear.

zygomaticofacial (zi·go·**mat**·ik·o·**fa**′·shal). Referring to the lateral or facial surface of the zygomatic bone.

zygomaticofrontal (zi·go·**mat**·ik·o·**fron**′·tal). Referring to the zygomatic and frontal bones.

zygomaticomaxillary (zi·go·**mat**·ik·o·max·**il**′·ar·e). Concerning the zygomatic bone and the maxilla.

zygomatico-orbital (zi·go·**mat**·ik·o·**or**′·bit·al). Referring to the orbital surface of the zygomatic bone.

zygomaticosphenoid (zi·go·**mat**·ik·o·**sfe**′·noid). Referring to the zygomatic bone and the greater wing of the sphenoid bone.

zygomaticotemporal (zi·go·**mat**·ik·o·**tem**′·por·al). Referring to the temporal surface of the zygomatic bone.

zygomaticus major muscle [musculus zygomaticus major (NA)] (zi·go·**mat**·ik·us **ma**·jor musl). A muscle arising from the zygomatic arch and inserted into the skin of the angle of the mouth where it blends with the fibres of the orbicularis oris muscle. It is supplied by the facial nerve.

zygomaticus minor muscle [musculus zygomaticus minor (NA)] (zi·go·**mat**·ik·us **mi**·nor musl). A muscle arising from the front of the zygomatic bone and blending inferiorly with the fibres of the orbicularis oris muscle. It is supplied by the facial nerve.

zygomaxillare (zi·go·max·il·**a**′·re). A point at the lower end of the zygomaticomaxillary suture.

zygomaxillary (zi·go·max·**il**′·a·re). Zygomaticomaxillary.

Zygomycetes (zi·go·mi·**se**′·teez). A sub-class of the Phycomycetes in which occur those species (in the Mucoraceae) which are pathogenic for man. [Gk *zygon* yoke, *mykes* fungus.]

zygon (zi·gon). The crossbar connecting the parallel limbs of an H-shaped cerebral fissure. [Gk yoke.]

zygonema (zi·go·**ne**·mah). Axonema during the zygotene stage of meiotic division. [Gk *zygon* yoke, *nema* thread.]

zygoneure (zi·go·newr). An internuncial neuron. [Gk *zygon* yoke, *neuron* nerve.]

zygosis (zi·**go**·sis). Conjugation. [Gk *zygon* yoke.]

zygosphere (zi·go·sfeer). A gamete which is morphologically indistinguishable from other gametes. Two like zygospheres fuse to form a zygospore. [Gk *zygon* yoke, sphere.]

zygospore (zi·go·spor). A spore formed by conjugation of zygosphere gametes; such spores are found in protozoa and many lower plants. [Gk *zygon* yoke, spore.]

zygostyle (zi·go·stile). The lowest vertebra. [Gk *zygon* yoke, *style* pillar.]

zygote (zi·gote). The cell resulting from the fusion of gametes and the individual derived from it. [Gk *zygon* yoke.]

zygotene (zi·go·teen). The second stage of the prophase of the first meiotic division during which homologous chromosomes pair side by side. [Gk *zygon* yoke, *tainia* band.]

zygotic (zi·**got**·ik). Concerning a zygote.

zymad (zi·mad). The causal organism of an infectious or zymotic disease. [Gk *zyme* ferment.]

zymase (zi·mase). A complex mixture of enzymes present in cell-free extracts of yeast which brings about alcoholic fermentation of sugars. [Gk *zyme* ferment.]

See also: BUCHNER.

zymasis (zi·mas·is). The conversion of sugars to alcohol and carbon dioxide by the action of the enzyme, zymase.

zymin (zi·min). A concentrated enzyme preparation obtained from yeast. [Gk *zyme* ferment.]

zymochemistry (zi·mo·**kem**·is·tre). The study and control of the chemistry of fermentation. [Gk *zyme* ferment, chemistry.]

zymogen (zi·mo·jen). The precursor of an enzyme. **Lab zymogen.** An enzyme precursor regarded as transformed into Lab enzyme by the action of the acid of the gastric juice. [Gk *zyme* ferment, *genein* to produce.]

zymogenic, zymogenous, zymogic (zi·mo·**jen**·ik, zi·**moj**·en·us, zi·**mo**·jik). Appertaining to a zymogen; producing fermentation.

zymohexase (zi·mo·**hex**·aze). An enzyme involved in the cycle of muscle contraction; it activates the splitting of fructose diphosphate (Harden-Young ester) into triose phosphates. [see foll.]

zymohexose (zi·mo·**hex**·oze). Any of the natural hexoses which readily undergo fermentation by yeast, e.g. D-glucose and D-fructose. [Gk *zyme* ferment, hexose.]

zymological (zi·mo·**loj**·ik·al). Concerned with fermentation or with zymology.

zymology (zi·**mol**·o·je). The study of ferments and fermentation. [Gk *zyme* ferment, *logos* science.]

zymolysis (zi·**mol**·is·is). Zymosis. [Gk *zyme* ferment, *lysis* a loosing.]

zymolytic (zi·mo·**lit**·ik). Causing, arising out of, or involved in zymolysis.

zymoma, zymome (zi·**mo**·mah, **zi**·mome). 1. A ferment. 2. A micro-organism causing disease. [Gk fermented mixture.]

zymometer (zi·**mom**·et·er). Any instrument by means of which the progress of fermentation may be estimated. [Gk *zyme* ferment, meter.]

zymophosphate (zi·mo·**fos**·fate). Any of the hexose phosphates arising out of the fermentation of monosaccharides by yeast. [Gk *zyme* ferment, phosphate.]

zymoplastic (zi·mo·**plas**·tik). Forming a ferment. [Gk *zyme* ferment, *plassein* to mould.]

zymoprotein (zi·mo·**pro**·te·in). Yeast protein. [Gk *zyme* ferment, protein.]

zymosis (zi·**mo**·sis). 1. The process of fermentation; enzyme activity. 2. An infectious disease; the spread of an infectious disease. **Zymosis gastrica.** Fermentation of the contents of the stomach due to the action of yeasts or bacterial ferments. [Gk *zyme* ferment, *-osis* condition.]

zymosterol (zi·mo·**steer**·ol). A general term for a sterol found in the lower plants. Ergosterol, $C_{28}H_{43}OH$, from yeast and ergot is an example. [Gk *zyme* ferment, sterol.]

zymosthenic (zi·mo·**sthen**·ik). Describing any substance which augments or accelerates the action of a ferment. [Gk *zyme* ferment, *sthenos* strength.]

zymotechny (zi·mo·**tek**·ne). Zymurgy. [Gk *zyme* ferment, *techne* art.]

zymotic (zi·**mot**·ik). 1. Concerned in or arising out of zymosis. 2. Caused by the growth of micro-organisms. [Gk *zymoein* to ferment.]

zymurgy (**zi**·mer·je). The chemical technology of fermentation in so far as it applies to the manufacture of beer, wines and spirits, and the by-products such as yeast and vinegar yielded by fermentation processes. [Gk *zyme* ferment, *ergein* to work.]

Appendix
Anatomical Nomenclature

Nomina Anatomica (N.A.)	Birmingham Revision (B.R.) or English Equivalent	Definition Location
Abdomen	Abdomen	**abdomen**
Acervulus (B.N.A.)	Brainsand	**brainsand**
Acetabulum	Acetabulum	**acetabulum**
Acinus	Acinus	**acinus**
Acromion	Acromion	**acromion**
Adhesio interthalamica	Connexus interthalamicus	**connexus interthalamicus**
Aditus	Inlet	**aditus** *also* **inlet**
Aditus ad antrum (mastoideum)	Aditus to tympanic antrum	**aditus** Aditus to the tympanic antrum
Aditus laryngis	Inlet of larynx	**larynx** Inlet of the larynx
Aditus orbitae	Orbital opening	**opening** Orbital opening
Adminiculum lineae albae	Adminiculum lineae albae	**adminiculum** Adminiculum lineae albae
Agger nasi	Agger nasi	**agger** Agger nasi
Ala	Wing	**ala** *also* **wing**
Ala cristae galli	Ala of crista galli	**crista** Crista galli
Ala lobuli centralis	Ala of central lobule	**ala** Ala of the central lobule
Ala major (ossis sphenoidalis)	Greater wing (of sphenoid bone)	**wing** Wings of the sphenoid bone
Ala minor (ossis sphenoidalis)	Lesser wing (of sphenoid bone)	**wing** Wings of the sphenoid bone
Ala nasi	Ala of nose	**ala** Ala of the nose
Ala ossis ilii	Ala of ilium	**ala** Ala of the ilium
Ala vomeris	Ala of vomer (right and left)	**ala** Ala of the vomer
Alveolus	Alveolus	**alveolus**
Alveoli dentales (mandibulae)	Tooth sockets (of mandible)	**socket**
Alveoli dentales (maxillae)	Tooth sockets (of maxilla)	**socket**
Alveoli pulmonis	Alveoli of lung	**alveolus** Pulmonary alveolus
Alveus hippocampi	Alveus of the hippocampus	**hippocampus**
Ampulla	Ampulla	**ampulla**
Ampulla canaliculi lacrimalis	Ampulla of lacrimal canaliculus	**ampulla** Ampulla of the lacrimal canaliculus
Ampulla ductus deferentis	Ampulla of vas deferens	**ampulla** Ampulla of the vas deferens
Ampulla hepatopancreatica	Ampulla of bile duct	**ampulla** Ampulla of the bile duct
Ampullae membranaceae	Membranous ampullae	**ampulla** Membranous ampullae
Ampulla membranacea anterior	Superior membranous ampulla	**ampulla** Membranous ampullae
Ampulla membranacea lateralis	Lateral membranous ampulla	**ampulla** Membranous ampullae
Ampulla membranacea posterior	Posterior membranous ampulla	**ampulla** Membranous ampullae
Ampullae osseae	Bony ampullae	**ampulla** Bony ampullae
Ampulla ossea anterior	Superior bony ampulla	**ampulla** Bony ampullae
Ampulla ossea lateralis	Lateral bony ampulla	**ampulla** Bony ampullae
Ampulla ossea posterior	Posterior bony ampulla	**ampulla** Bony ampullae
Ampulla recti	Ampulla of rectum	**ampulla** Ampulla of the rectum
Ampulla tubae uterinae	Ampulla of uterine tube	**ampulla** Ampulla of the uterine tube
Anastomosis arteriovenosa	Arteriovenous anastomosis	**anastomosis** Arteriovenous anastomosis
Angulus	Angle	**angle**
Angulus acromialis	Acromial angle	**angle** Acromial angle
Angulus costae	Angle of rib (posterior)	**ribs** Angle of a rib, posterior
Angulus frontalis (ossis parietalis)	Frontal angle (of parietal bone)	**parietal bone** Frontal angle
Angulus inferior (scapulae)	Inferior angle (of scapula)	**scapula**
Angulus infrasternalis	Infrasternal angle	**thorax** Infrasternal angle of the thorax
Angulus iridocornealis	Iridocorneal angle	**angle** Iridocorneal angle
Angulus lateralis (scapulae)	Lateral angle (of scapula)	**scapula**
Angulus mandibulae	Angle of mandible	**mandible** Angle
Angulus mastoideus (ossis parietalis)	Mastoid angle (of parietal bone)	**parietal bone** Mastoid angle
Angulus occipitalis (ossis parietalis)	Occipital angle (of parietal bone)	**parietal bone** Occipital angle
Angulus oculi lateralis	Lateral angle of eye	**eye** Angle of the eye, lateral
Angulus oculi medialis	Medial angle of eye	**eye** Angle of the eye, medial
Angulus oris	Angle of mouth	**mouth** Angle of the mouth
Angulus sphenoidalis (ossis parietalis)	Sphenoidal angle (of parietal bone)	**parietal bone** Sphenoidal angle
Angulus sterni	Angle of sternum	**sternum** Angle
Angulus subpubicus	Subpubic angle	**angle** Subpubic angle
Angulus superior (scapulae)	Superior angle (of scapula)	**scapula**
Ansa	Ansa	**ansa**
Ansa cervicalis	Ansa hypoglossi	**ansa** Ansa hypoglossi
Ansa lenticularis	Ansa lenticularis	**ansa** Ansa lenticularis
Ansae nervorum spinalium	Ansae nervorum spinalium	**ansa** Ansae nervorum spinalium

Anatomical Nomenclature

Nomina Anatomica (N.A.)	Birmingham Revision (B.R.) or English Equivalent	Definition Location
Ansa peduncularis	Ansa peduncularis	**ansa** Ansa peduncularis
Ansa subclavia	Ansa subclavia	**ansa** Ansa subclavia
Antebrachium	Forearm	**forearm**
Anterior	Anterior	**anterior**
Anthelix	Antihelix	**antihelix**
Antitragus	Antitragus	**antitragus**
Antrum	Antrum	**antrum**
Antrum mastoideum	Tympanic antrum	**antrum** Tympanic antrum
Antrum pyloricum	Pyloric antrum	**antrum** Pyloric antrum
Anulus	Ring	**annulus** *also* **ring**
Anulus conjunctivae	Annulus conjunctivae	**annulus** Annulus conjunctivae
Anulus femoralis	Femoral ring	**ring** Femoral ring
Anulus fibrocartilagineus (membranae tympani)	Fibrocartilaginous ring (of tympanic membrane)	**membrane** Tympanic membrane
Anuli fibrosi (cordis)	Fibrous rings (of heart)	**ring** Fibrous rings of the heart
Anulus fibrosus (disci intervertebralis)	Annulus fibrosus (of an intervertebral disk)	**annulus** Annulus fibrosus
Anulus inguinalis profundus	Deep inguinal ring	**ring** Inguinal ring, deep
Anulus inguinalis superficialis	Superficial inguinal ring	**ring** Inguinal ring, superficial
Anulus iridis major	Outer ring of iris	**ring** Ring of the iris, outer
Anulus iridis minor	Inner ring of iris	**ring** Ring of the iris, inner
Anulus tendineus communis (musculorum oculi)	Common tendinous ring (of muscles of orbit)	**ring** Common tendinous ring
Anulus tympanicus	Tympanic ring	**ring** Tympanic ring
Anulus umbilicalis	Umbilical ring	**ring** Umbilical ring
Anus	Anus	**anus**
Aorta	Aorta	**aorta**
Aorta abdominalis	Abdominal aorta	**aorta**
Aorta ascendens	Ascending aorta	**aorta**
Aorta descendens	Descending aorta	**aorta**
Aorta thoracica	Descending thoracic aorta	**aorta**
Apertura	Aperture	**aperture**
Apertura externa aqueductus vestibuli	External opening of aqueduct of vestibule	**aqueduct** Aqueduct of the vestibule, external opening of the
Apertura externa canaliculi cochleae	External opening of cochlear canaliculus	**canaliculus** Cochlear canaliculus
Apertura lateralis ventriculi quarti	Lateral aperture of fourth ventricle	**aperture** Aperture of the fourth ventricle, lateral
Apertura mediana ventriculi quarti	Median aperture of fourth ventricle	**aperture** Aperture of the fourth ventricle, median
Apertura pelvis inferior	Outlet of pelvis	**pelvis** Outlet of the pelvis
Apertura pelvis superior	Inlet of pelvis	**pelvis** Inlet of the pelvis
Apertura piriformis	Anterior bony aperture of nose	**aperture** Bony aperture of the nose, anterior
Apertura sinus frontalis	Aperture of frontal sinus	**aperture** Aperture of the frontal sinus
Apertura sinus sphenoidalis	Aperture of sphenoidal sinus	**aperture** Aperture of the sphenoidal sinus

Nomina Anatomica (N.A.)	Birmingham Revision (B.R.) or English Equivalent	Definition Location
Apertura thoracis inferior	Outlet of thorax	**thorax** Outlet of the thorax
Apertura thoracis superior	Inlet of thorax	**thorax** Inlet of the thorax
Apertura tympanica canaliculi chordae tympani	Tympanic aperture of canaliculus for chorda tympani	**aperture** Tympanic aperture of the canaliculus for the chorda tympani
Apex	Apex	**apex**
Apex [partis petrosae]	Apex (of petrous part)	**temporal bone** Apex
Apex auriculae	Apex of auricle	**auricle**
Apex capitis fibulae	Styloid process of fibula	**process** Process of the fibula, styloid
Apex cartilaginis arytenoideae	Apex of arytenoid cartilage	**cartilage** Arytenoid cartilage
Apex cordis	Apex of heart	**heart** Apex of the heart
Apex cornu posterioris	Apex of posterior horn	**horn** Grey horns of the spinal cord
Apex linguae	Tip of tongue	**tongue** Tip of the tongue
Apex nasi	Apex of nose	**nose** Apex of the nose
Apex ossis sacri	Apex of sacrum	**sacrum** Apex of the sacrum
Apex partis petrosi	Apex of petrous part	**temporal bone** Apex
Apex patellae	Apex of patella	**patella** Apex of the patella
Apex prostatae	Apex of prostate	**prostate** Apex of the prostate
Apex pulmonis	Apex of lung	**lung** Apex of the lung
Apex radicis dentis	Root apex	**apex** Root apex
Apex vesicae	Apex of bladder	**urinary bladder** Apex
Aponeurosis	Aponeurosis	**aponeurosis**
Aponeurosis linguae	Aponeurosis of tongue	**aponeurosis** Aponeurosis of the tongue
Aponeurosis musculi bicipitis brachii	Bicipital aponeurosis	**aponeurosis** Bicipital aponeurosis
Aponeurosis palmaris	Palmar aponeurosis	**aponeurosis** Palmar aponeurosis
Aponeurosis plantaris	Plantar aponeurosis	**aponeurosis** Plantar aponeurosis
Apophysis	Apophysis	**apophysis**
Apparatus digestorius [systema digestorium]	Digestive system	**system** Digestive system
Apparatus lacrimalis	Lacrimal apparatus	**apparatus**
Apparatus respiratorius [systema respiratorium]	Respiratory system	**system** Respiratory system
Apparatus urogenitalis [systema urogenitale]	Urogenital system	**system** Urogenital system
Appendix	Appendix	**appendix**
Appendix epididymidis	Appendix of epididymis	**appendix** Appendix of the epididymis
Appendices epiploicae	Appendices epiploicae	**appendix** Appendices epiploicae
Appendix fibrosa hepatis	Fibrous appendix of liver	**appendix** Fibrous appendix of the liver
Appendix testis	Appendix testis	**appendix** Appendix testis
Appendix vermiformis	Vermiform appendix	**appendix** Vermiform appendix
Appendices vesiculosae	Appendices vesiculosae	**appendix** Appendices vesiculosae
Aqueductus cerebri	Aqueduct of mid-brain	**aqueduct** Aqueduct of the mid-brain

Nomina Anatomica (N.A.)	Birmingham Revision (B.R.) or English Equivalent	Definition Location
Aqueductus vestibuli	Aqueduct of vestibule	**aqueduct** Aqueduct of the vestibule
Arachnoidea encephali	Arachnoid mater of brain	**arachnoid mater**
Arachnoidea spinalis	Spinal arachnoid mater	**arachnoid mater**
Arbor vitae cerebelli	Arbor vitae of cerebellum	**arbor** Arbor vitae
Arcus	Arch	**arch**
Arcus alveolaris (mandibulae)	Alveolar arch (of mandible)	**arch** Alveolar arch
Arcus alveolaris (maxillae)	Alveolar arch (of maxilla)	**arch** Alveolar arch
Arcus anterior (atlantis)	Anterior arch (of atlas)	**arch** Arch of the atlas, anterior
Arcus aortae	Arch of aorta	**arch** Arch of the aorta
Arcus cartilaginis cricoideae	Arch of cricoid cartilage	**arch** Arch of the cricoid cartilage
Arcus costalis	Costal arch	**arch** Costal arch
Arcus dentalis inferior	Inferior dental arch	**arch** Dental arches
Arcus dentalis superior	Superior dental arch	**arch** Dental arches
Arcus iliopectineus	Iliopectineal arch	**arch** Iliopectineal arch
Arcus palatoglossus	Palatoglossal arch	**arch** Palatoglossal arch
Arcus palatopharyngeus	Palatopharyngeal arch	**arch** Palatopharyngeal arch
Arcus palmaris profundus	Deep palmar arch	**arch** Palmar arch, deep
Arcus palmaris superficialis	Superficial palmar arch	**arch** Palmar arch, superficial
Arcus palpebralis inferior	Inferior palpebral arch	**ophthalmic artery**
Arcus palpebralis superior	Superior palpebral arch	**ophthalmic artery**
Arcus pedis longitudinalis	Longitudinal arch of the foot	**arch** Arch of the foot
Arcus pedis transversalis	Transverse arch of the foot	**arch** Arch of the foot
Arcus plantaris	Plantar arch	**arch** Plantar arch
Arcus posterior (atlantis)	Posterior arch (of atlas)	**arch** Arch of the atlas, posterior
Arcus pubis	Pubic arch	**arch** Pubic arch
Arcus superciliaris	Superciliary arch	**arch** Superciliary arch
Arcus tendineus	Tendinous arch	**arch** Tendinous arch
Arcus tendineus fasciae pelvis	Tendinous arch of fascia of pelvic muscles	**arch** Tendinous arch of the fascia of pelvic muscles
Arcus tendineus musculi levatoris ani	Tendinous arch of levator ani muscle	**arch** Tendinous arch of the levator ani muscle
Arcus tendineus musculi solei	Tendinous arch of soleus muscle	**arch** Tendinous arch of the soleus muscle
Arcus venosus dorsalis pedis	Dorsal venous arch of foot	**arch** Venous arch of the foot dorsal
Arcus venosus juguli	Jugular arch	**arch** Jugular arch
Arcus venosus palmaris profundus	Deep palmar venous arch	**arch** Venous arch, palmar
Arcus venosus palmaris superficialis	Superficial palmar venous arch	**arch** Venous arch, palmar
Arcus venosus plantaris	Plantar venous arch	**arch** Venous arch, plantar

Nomina Anatomica (N.A.)	Birmingham Revision (B.R.) or English Equivalent	Definition Location
Arcus vertebrae	Vertebral arch	**arch** Vertebral arch
Arcus zygomaticus	Zygomatic arch	**arch** Zygomatic arch
Area	Area	**area**
Area cochleae	Cochlear area	**meatus** Auditory meatus, internal
Area cribrosa	Cribriform area	**area** Cribriform area
Areae gastricae	Gastric areas	**area** Gastric areas
Area intercondylaris anterior (tibiae)	Anterior intercondylar area (of tibia)	**tibia** Intercondylar area of the tibia
Area intercondylaris posterior (tibiae)	Posterior intercondylar area (of tibia)	**tibia** Intercondylar area of the tibia
Area nervi facialis	Facial nerve area	**meatus** Auditory meatus, internal
Area nuda	Bare area (of liver)	**liver** Bare area of the liver
Area subcallosa	Parolfactory area	**cortex** Cerebral cortex, parolfactory area of the
Area vestibularis inferior	Inferior vestibular area	**meatus** Auditory meatus, internal
Area vestibularis superior	Superior vestibular area	**meatus** Auditory meatus, internal
Areola mammae	Areola of breast	**areola** Areola of the breast
Arteria	Artery	**artery**
Arteria alveolaris inferior	Inferior dental artery	**maxillary artery**
Arteriae alveolares superiores	Posterior superior dental artery	**maxillary artery**
Arteria angularis	Angular artery	**angular artery**
Arteria appendicularis	Appendicular artery	**mesenteric arteries** Superior mesenteric artery
Arteria arcuata (pedis)	Arcuate artery	**arcuate artery**
Arteriae arcuatae (renis)	Arciform arteries	**arciform arteries**
Arteria auricularis posterior	Posterior auricular artery	**auricular arteries** Posterior auricular artery
Arteria auricularis profunda	Deep auricular artery	**maxillary artery**
Arteria axillaris	Axillary artery	**axillary artery**
Arteria basilaris	Basilar artery	**basilar artery**
Arteria brachialis	Brachial artery	**brachial artery**
Arteria brachialis superficialis	Superficial brachial artery	**brachial artery** Superficial brachial artery
Arteria buccalis	Buccal artery	**maxillary artery**
Arteria bulbi penis	Artery of bulb of penis	**penis, artery of the bulb of the**
Arteria bulbi vestibuli [vaginae]	Artery of vestibule	**penis, artery of the bulb of the**
Arteria canalis pterygoidei	Artery of pterygoid canal	**pterygoid canal, artery of the**
Arteria carotis communis	Common carotid artery	**carotid arteries** Common carotid artery
Arteria carotis externa	External carotid artery	**carotid arteries** External carotid artery
Arteria carotis interna	Internal carotid artery	**carotid arteries** Internal carotid artery
Arteria cauda pancreatis	Artery of tail of pancreas	**splenic artery**
Arteria cecalis anterior	Anterior caecal branch	**mesenteric arteries** Superior mesenteric artery
Arteria cecalis posterior	Posterior caecal branch	**mesenteric arteries** Superior mesenteric artery
Arteria centralis retinae	Central artery of retina	**retina, central artery of the**
Arteria cerebelli inferior anterior	Anterior inferior cerebellar artery	**cerebellar arteries** Anterior inferior cerebellar artery

Anatomical Nomenclature

Nomina Anatomica (N.A.)	Birmingham Revision (B.R.) or English Equivalent	Definition Location
Arteria cerebelli inferior posterior	Posterior inferior cerebellar artery	**cerebellar arteries** Posterior inferior cerebellar artery
Arteria cerebelli superior	Superior cerebellar artery	**cerebellar arteries** Superior cerebellar artery
Arteria cerebri anterior	Anterior cerebral artery	**cerebral arteries** Anterior cerebral artery
Arteria cerebri media	Middle cerebral artery	**cerebral arteries** Middle cerebral artery
Arteria cerebri posterior	Posterior cerebral artery	**cerebral arteries** Posterior cerebral artery
Arteria cervicalis ascendens	Ascending cervical artery	**thyroid arteries** Inferior thyroid artery
Arteria cervicalis profunda	Deep cervical artery	**cervical arteries** Deep cervical artery
Arteria cervicalis superficialis	Superficial cervical artery	**cervical arteries** Superficial cervical artery
Arteria choroidea anterior	Choroid artery	**choroid artery**
Arteriae ciliares anteriores	Anterior ciliary arteries	**ophthalmic artery**
Arteriae ciliares posteriores breves	Short posterior ciliary arteries	**ophthalmic artery**
Arteriae ciliares posteriores longae	Long posterior ciliary arteries	**ophthalmic artery**
Arteria circumflexa femoris lateralis	Lateral circumflex artery	**circumflex arteries** Lateral circumflex artery
Arteria circumflexa femoris medialis	Medial circumflex artery	**circumflex arteries** Medial circumflex artery
Arteria circumflexa humeri anterior	Anterior circumflex humeral artery	**circumflex humeral arteries** Anterior circumflex humeral artery
Arteria circumflexa humeri posterior	Posterior circumflex humeral artery	**circumflex humeral arteries** Posterior circumflex humeral artery
Arteria circumflexa ilium profunda	Deep circumflex iliac artery	**circumflex iliac arteries** Deep circumflex iliac artery
Arteria circumflexa ilium superficialis	Superficial circumflex iliac artery	**circumflex iliac arteries** Superficial circumflex iliac artery
Arteria circumflexa scapulae	Circumflex scapular artery	**subscapular artery**
Arteria colica dextra	Right colic artery	**mesenteric arteries** Superior mesenteric artery
Arteria colica media	Middle colic artery	**mesenteric arteries** Superior mesenteric artery
Arteria colica sinistra	Superior left colic artery	**mesenteric arteries** Inferior mesenteric artery
Arteria collateralis media	Posterior descending branch (of profunda brachii artery)	**profunda brachii artery**
Arteria collateralis radialis	Anterior descending branch (of profunda brachii artery)	**profunda brachii artery**
Arteria collateralis ulnaris inferior	Supratrochlear artery	**supratrochlear artery**
Arteria collateralis ulnaris superior	Ulnar collateral artery	**ulnar collateral artery**
Arteria comitans nervi ischiadici	Companion artery of sciatic nerve	**companion artery of the sciatic nerve**
Arteria communicans anterior	Anterior communicating artery	**communicating arteries of the brain** Anterior communicating artery of the brain
Arteria communicans posterior	Posterior communicating artery	**communicating arteries of the brain** Posterior communicating artery of the brain
Arteriae conjunctivales anteriores	Anterior conjunctival arteries	**ophthalmic arteries**
Arteriae conjunctivales posteriores	Posterior conjunctival arteries	**ophthalmic artery**
Arteria coronaria dextra	Right coronary artery	**coronary arteries** Right coronary artery

Nomina Anatomica (N.A.)	Birmingham Revision (B.R.) or English Equivalent	Definition Location
Arteria coronaria sinistra	Left coronary artery	**coronary arteries** Left coronary artery
Arteria cremasterica	Artery to cremaster	**cremaster, artery to the**
Arteria cystica	Cystic artery	**cystic artery**
Arteriae digitales dorsales (manus)	Dorsal digital arteries (of hand)	**digital arteries** Dorsal digital arteries
Arteriae digitales dorsales (pedis)	Dorsal digital arteries (of foot)	**digital arteries** Dorsal digital arteries
Arteriae digitales palmares communes	Common palmar digital arteries	**arch** Palmar arch, superficial
Arteriae digitales palmares propriae	Proper palmar digital arteries	**arch** Palmar arch, superficial
Arteriae digitales plantares communes	Plantar digital arteries	**digital arteries** Plantar digital arteries
Arteriae digitales plantares propriae	Proper plantar digital arteries	**digital arteries** Plantar digital arteries
Arteria dorsalis clitoridis	Dorsal artery of clitoris	**penis, arteries of the (or of the clitoris)**
Arteria dorsalis nasi	Dorsalis nasi artery	**ophthalmic artery**
Arteria dorsalis pedis	Dorsalis pedis artery	**dorsalis pedis artery**
Arteria dorsalis penis	Dorsal artery of penis	**penis, arteries of the** Dorsal artery of the penis
Arteria ductus deferentis	Artery of vas deferens	**vas deferens, artery of the**
Arteria epigastrica inferior	Inferior epigastric artery	**epigastric arteries** Inferior epigastric artery
Arteria epigastrica superficialis	Superficial epigastric artery	**epigastric arteries** Superficial epigastric artery
Arteria epigastrica superior	Superior epigastric artery	**epigastric arteries** Superior epigastric artery
Arteriae episclerales	Episcleral arteries	**ophthalmic artery**
Arteria ethmoidalis anterior	Anterior ethmoidal artery	**ophthalmic artery**
Arteria ethmoidalis posterior	Posterior ethmoidal artery	**ophthalmic artery**
Arteria facialis	Facial artery	**facial artery**
Arteria femoralis	Femoral artery	**femoral artery**
Arteriae gastricae breves	Short gastric arteries	**splenic artery**
Arteria gastrica dextra	Right gastric artery	**hepatic arteries** Common hepatic artery
Arteria gastrica sinistra	Left gastric artery	**gastric arteries** Left gastric artery
Arteria gastroduodenalis	Gastroduodenal artery	**hepatic arteries** Common hepatic artery
Arteria gastro-epiploica dextra	Right gastro-epiploic artery	**hepatic arteries** Common hepatic artery
Arteria gastro-epiploica sinistra	Left gastro-epiploic artery	**splenic artery**
Arteria genu descendens	Descending genicular artery	**genicular arteries** Descending genicular artery
Arteria genu inferior lateralis	Lateral inferior genicular artery	**popliteal artery**
Arteria genu inferior medialis	Medial inferior genicular artery	**popliteal artery**
Arteria genu media	Middle genicular artery	**popliteal artery**
Arteria genu superior lateralis	Lateral superior genicular artery	**popliteal artery**
Arteria genu superior medialis	Medial superior genicular artery	**popliteal artery**
Arteria glutea inferior	Inferior gluteal artery	**gluteal arteries** Inferior gluteal artery
Arteria glutea superior	Superior gluteal artery	**gluteal arteries** Superior gluteal arteries
Arteriae helicinae	Helicine arteries	**helicine arteries**
Arteria hepatica communis	Hepatic artery	**hepatic arteries** Common hepatic artery
Arteria hepatica propria	Proper hepatic artery	**hepatic arteries** Proper hepatic artery
Arteria hyaloidea	Hyaloid artery	**hyaloid artery**
Arteriae ilei (arteriae mesentericae superioris)	Ileal branches of superior mesenteric artery	**mesenteric arteries** Superior mesenteric artery

Nomina Anatomica (N.A.)	Birmingham Revision (B.R.) or English Equivalent	Definition Location
Arteria ileocolica	Ileocolic artery	**mesenteric arteries** Superior mesenteric artery
Arteria iliaca communis	Common iliac artery	**iliac arteries** Common iliac artery
Arteria iliaca externa	External iliac artery	**iliac arteries** External iliac artery
Arteria iliaca interna	Internal iliac artery	**iliac arteries** Internal iliac artery
Arteria iliolumbalis	Iliolumbar artery	**iliolumbar artery**
Arteria infra-orbitalis	Infra-orbital artery	**maxillary artery**
Arteriae intercostales posteriores [I et II]	Posterior intercostal arteries (I and II)	**intercostal arteries** Superior intercostal arteries
Arteriae intercostales posteriores [III–XI]	Posterior intercostal arteries (III–XI)	**intercostal arteries** Posterior intercostal arteries
Arteria intercostalis suprema	Superior intercostal artery	**intercostal arteries** Superior intercostal artery
Arteriae interlobares renis	Interlobar arteries (of kidney)	**interlobar arteries**
Arteriae interlobulares (hepatis)	Interlobular arteries (of liver)	**interlobular arteries**
Arteriae interlobulares renis	Interlobular arteries (of kidney)	**interlobular arteries**
Arteria interossea anterior	Anterior interosseous artery	**ulnar artery**
Arteria interossea communis	Common interosseous artery	**ulnar artery**
Arteria interossea posterior	Posterior interosseous artery	**ulnar artery**
Arteria interossea recurrens	Interosseous recurrent artery	**ulnar artery**
Arteriae jejunales (arteriae mesentericae superioris)	Jejunal branches (of superior mesenteric artery)	**mesenteric arteries** Superior mesenteric artery
Arteria labialis inferior	Inferior labial artery	**facial artery**
Arteria labialis superior	Superior labial artery	**facial artery**
Arteria labyrinthi	Internal auditory artery	**auditory artery, internal**
Arteria lacrimalis	Lacrimal artery	**ophthalmic artery**
Arteria laryngea inferior	Inferior laryngeal artery	**thyroid arteries** Inferior thyroid artery
Arteria laryngea superior	Superior laryngeal artery	**thyroid arteries** Superior thyroid artery
Arteria lienalis	Splenic artery	**splenic artery**
Arteria ligamenti teretis uteri	Artery to round ligament of uterus	**cremaster, artery to the**
Arteria lingualis	Lingual artery	**lingual artery**
Arteriae lobi caudati	Branches to caudate lobe of liver	**hepatic arteries** Common hepatic artery
Arteriae lumbales	Lumbar arteries	**lumbar arteries**
Arteria lumbalis ima	Fifth lumbar artery	**lumbar arteries** Fifth lumbar artery
Arteria malleolaris anterior lateralis	Lateral anterior malleolar artery	**malleolar arteries**
Arteria malleolaris anterior medialis	Medial anterior malleolar artery	**malleolar arteries**
Arteria masseterica	Masseteric artery	**maxillary artery**
Arteria maxillaris	Maxillary artery	**maxillary artery**
Arteria mediana	Median artery	**median artery**
Arteria meningea anterior	Meningeal branch (of ophthalmic artery)	**ophthalmic artery**
Arteria meningea media	Middle meningeal artery	**meningeal arteries** Middle meningeal artery
Arteria meningea posterior	Meningeal branch (of ascending pharyngeal artery)	**pharyngeal artery, ascending**
Arteria mentalis	Mental artery	**maxillary artery**
Arteria mesenterica inferior	Inferior mesenteric artery	**mesenteric arteries** Inferior mesenteric artery
Arteria mesenterica superior	Superior mesenteric artery	**mesenteric arteries** Superior mesenteric artery
Arteriae metacarpeae dorsales	Dorsal metacarpal arteries	**metacarpal arteries** Dorsal metacarpal arteries

Nomina Anatomica (N.A.)	Birmingham Revision (B.R.) or English Equivalent	Definition Location
Arteriae metacarpeae palmares	Palmar metacarpal arteries	**radial artery**
Arteriae metatarseae dorsales	Dorsal metatarsal arteries	**metatarsal arteries** Dorsal metatarsal arteries
Arteriae metatarseae plantares	Plantar metatarsal arteries	**metatarsal arteries** Plantar metatarsal arteries
Arteria musculophrenica	Musculophrenic artery	**musculophrenic artery**
Arteriae nasales posteriores, laterales, et septi	Lateral, posterior, and septal nasal branches of sphenopalatine artery	**nasal arteries**
Arteriae nutriciae humeres	Nutrient branch to humerus (of profunda brachii artery)	**profunda brachii artery** Nutrient branch to the humerus
Arteria obturatoria	Obturator artery	**obturator artery**
Arteria occipitalis	Occipital artery	**occipital artery**
Arteria ophthalmica	Ophthalmic artery	**ophthalmic artery**
Arteria ovarica	Ovarian artery	**ovarian artery**
Arteria palatina ascendens	Ascending palatine artery	**palatine arteries** Ascending palatine artery
Arteria palatina descendens	Descending palatine artery	**palatine arteries** Descending palatine artery
Arteria palatina major	Greater palatine artery	**maxillary artery**
Arteriae palatinae minores	Lesser palatine arteries	**maxillary artery**
Arteriae palpebrales laterales	Lateral palpebral arteries	**ophthalmic artery**
Arteriae palpebrales mediales	Medial palpebral arteries	**ophthalmic artery**
Arteria pancreatica dorsalis	Dorsal pancreatic artery	**splenic artery**
Arteria pancreatica inferior	Inferior pancreatic artery	**splenic artery**
Arteria pancreatica magna	Great pancreatic artery	**splenic artery**
Arteria pancreatico-duodenalis inferior	Inferior pancreatico-duodenal artery	**mesenteric arteries** Superior mesenteric artery
Arteria pancreatico-duodenalis superior	Superior pancreatico-duodenal artery	**hepatic arteries** Common hepatic artery
Arteriae perforantes	Perforating arteries	**perforating arteries**
Arteria pericardiaco-phrenica	Pericardiacophrenic artery	**pericardiacophrenic artery**
Arteria perinealis	Transverse perineal artery	**perineal artery, transverse**
Arteria peronea [fibularis]	Peroneal artery	**peroneal artery**
Arteria pharyngea ascendens	Ascending pharyngeal artery	**pharyngeal artery, ascending**
Arteriae phrenicae inferiores	Phrenic artery	**phrenic artery**
Arteriae phrenicae superiores	Phrenic branches (of descending thoracic aorta)	**aorta** Branches of the thoracic aorta, phrenic
Arteria plantaris lateralis	Lateral plantar artery	**plantar arteries** Lateral plantar artery
Arteria plantaris medialis	Medial plantar artery	**plantar arteries** Medial plantar artery
Arteria poplitea	Popliteal artery	**popliteal artery**
Arteria princeps pollicis	Princeps pollicis artery	**radial artery**
Arteria profunda brachii	Profunda brachii artery	**profunda brachii artery**
Arteria profunda clitoridis	Deep artery of clitoris	**penis, arteries of the (or of the clitoris)**
Arteria profunda femoris	Profunda femoris artery	**profunda femoris artery**
Arteria profunda linguae	Profunda artery of tongue	**lingual artery**
Arteria profunda penis	Deep artery of penis	**penis, arteries of the** Deep artery of the penis
Arteriae pudendae externae	External pudendal arteries	**pudendal arteries** External pudendal arteries
Arteria pudenda interna	Internal pudendal artery	**pudendal arteries** Internal pudendal artery

Anatomical Nomenclature

Nomina Anatomica (N.A.)	Birmingham Revision (B.R.) or English Equivalent	Definition Location
Arteria pulmonalis dextra	Right pulmonary artery	**pulmonary arteries** Right pulmonary artery
Arteria pulmonalis sinistra	Left pulmonary artery	**pulmonary arteries** Left pulmonary artery
Arteria radialis	Radial artery	**radial artery**
Arteria radialis indicis	Radialis indicis artery	**arch** Palmar arch, superficial
Arteria rectalis inferior	Inferior rectal artery	**rectal arteries** Inferior rectal artery
Arteria rectalis media	Middle rectal artery	**rectal arteries** Middle rectal artery
Arteria rectalis superior	Superior rectal artery	**mesenteric arteries** Inferior mesenteric artery
Arteria recurrens radialis	Radial recurrent artery	**radial artery**
Arteria recurrens tibialis anterior	Anterior recurrent branch of anterior tibial artery	**tibial arteries** Anterior tibial artery
Arteria recurrens tibialis posterior	Posterior recurrent branch of anterior tibial artery	**tibial arteries** Anterior tibial artery
Arteria recurrens ulnaris	Ulnar recurrent artery	**ulnar artery**
Arteria renalis	Renal artery	**renal artery**
Arteriae renis	Arteries of kidney	**kidney, arteries of the**
Arteriae retroduodenales	Retroduodenal arteries	**hepatic arteries** Common hepatic artery
Arteriae sacrales laterales	Lateral sacral arteries	**sacral arteries** Lateral sacral arteries
Arteria sacralis mediana	Median sacral artery	**sacral arteries** Median sacral artery
Arteria scapularis descendens (dorsalis)	Descending scapular artery	**cervical arteries** Superficial cervical artery
Arteria segmenti anterioris inferioris (arteriae renalis)	Lower (anterior) segmental artery (of renal artery)	**renal artery**
Arteria segmenti anterioris superioris (arteriae renalis)	Upper (anterior) segmental artery (of renal artery)	**renal artery**
Arteria segmenti inferioris (arteriae renalis)	Lower segmental artery (of renal artery)	**renal artery**
Arteria segmenti posterioris (arteriae renalis)	Posterior segmental artery (of renal artery)	**renal artery**
Arteria segmenti superioris (arteriae renalis)	Apical segmental artery (of renal artery)	**renal artery**
Arteriae sigmoideae	Inferior left colic arteries	**mesenteric arteries** Inferior mesenteric artery
Arteria sphenopalatina	Sphenopalatine artery	**maxillary artery**
Arteria spinalis anterior	Anterior spinal artery	**spinal arteries** Anterior spinal artery
Arteria spinalis posterior	Posterior spinal artery	**spinal arteries** Posterior spinal artery
Arteria stylomastoidea	Stylomastoid artery	**auricular arteries** Posterior auricular artery
Arteria subclavia	Subclavian artery	**subclavian artery**
Arteria subcostalis	Subcostal artery	**subcostal arteries**
Arteria sublingualis	Sublingual branch (of lingual artery)	**lingual artery**
Arteria submentalis	Submental artery	**submental artery**
Arteria subscapularis	Subscapular artery	**subscapular artery**
Arteriae supraduodenales superiores (arteriae hepaticae communis)	Superior pancreaticoduodenal arteries	**hepatic arteries** Common hepatic artery
Arteria supra-orbitalis	Supra-orbital artery	**supra-orbital artery**
Arteria suprarenalis inferior	Inferior suprarenal artery	**renal artery**
Arteria suprarenalis media	Middle suprarenal artery	**suprarenal arteries** Middle suprarenal arteries
Arteria suprarenalis superior	Superior suprarenal artery	**suprarenal arteries** Superior suprarenal artery
Arteria suprascapularis	Suprascapular artery	**suprascapular artery**

Nomina Anatomica (N.A.)	Birmingham Revision (B.R.) or English Equivalent	Definition Location
Arteria supratrochlearis	Supratrochlear artery	**ophthalmic artery**
Arteriae surales	Sural arteries	**popliteal artery**
Arteria tarsea lateralis	Tarsal artery	**tarsal arteries**
Arteriae tarseae mediales	Medial tarsal arteries	**tarsal arteries**
Arteria temporalis media	Middle temporal artery	**temporal arteries** Middle temporal artery
Arteriae temporales profundae	Deep temporal arteries	**temporal arteries** Deep temporal arteries
Arteria temporalis superficialis	Superficial temporal artery	**temporal arteries** Superficial temporal artery
Arteria testicularis	Testicular artery	**testicular artery**
Arteria thoracica interna	Internal mammary artery	**mammary artery, internal**
Arteria thoracica lateralis	Lateral thoracic artery	**thoracic arteries** Lateral thoracic artery
Arteria thoracica suprema	Superior thoracic artery	**thoracic arteries** Superior thoracic artery
Arteria thoraco-acromialis	Acromiothoracic artery	**acromiothoracic artery**
Arteria thoracodorsalis	Thoracodorsal artery	**thoracodorsal artery**
Arteria thyroidea ima	Thyroidea ima artery	**thyroidea ima artery**
Arteria thyroidea inferior	Inferior thyroid artery	**thyroid arteries** Inferior thyroid artery
Arteria thyroidea superior	Superior thyroid artery	**thyroid arteries** Superior thyroid artery
Arteria tibialis anterior	Anterior tibial artery	**tibial arteries** Anterior tibial artery
Arteria tibialis posterior	Posterior tibial artery	**tibial arteries** Posterior tibial artery
Arteria transversa colli	Transverse cervical artery	**cervical arteries** Transverse cervical artery
Arteria transversa faciei	Transverse facial artery	**temporal arteries** Superficial temporal artery
Arteria tympanica anterior	Anterior tympanic artery	**maxillary artery**
Arteria tympanica inferior	Inferior tympanic artery	**pharyngeal artery, ascending**
Arteria tympanica posterior	Posterior tympanic artery	**auricular arteries** Posterior auricular artery
Arteria tympanica superior	Superior tympanic artery	**meningeal arteries** Middle meningeal artery
Arteria ulnaris	Ulnar artery	**ulnar artery**
Arteria umbilicalis	Umbilical artery	**umbilical artery**
Arteria urethralis	Urethral artery	**urethral artery**
Arteria uterina	Uterine artery	**uterine artery**
Arteria vaginalis	Vaginal branch (of uterine artery)	**vaginal artery**
Arteria vertebralis	Vertebral artery	**vertebral artery**
Arteria vesicalis inferior	Inferior vesical artery	**vesical arteries** Inferior vesical artery
Arteriae vesicales superiores	Superior vesical arteries	**vesical arteries** Superior vesical arteries
Arteria zygomatico-orbitalis	Zygomatic branch (of superficial temporal artery)	**temporal arteries** Superficial temporal artery
Arteriola	Arteriole	**arteriole**
Arteriola macularis inferior	Inferior macular branch (of central artery of retina)	**retina, central artery of the**
Arteriola macularis superior	Superior macular branch (of central artery of retina)	**retina, central artery of the**
Arteriola medialis retinae	Medial retinal branch (of central artery of retina)	**retina, central artery of the**
Arteriola nasalis retinae inferior	Inferior nasal branch (of central artery of retina)	**retina, central artery of the**
Arteriola nasalis retinae superior	Superior nasal branch (of central artery of retina)	**retina, central artery of the**

Nomina Anatomica (N.A.)	Birmingham Revision (B.R.) or English Equivalent	Definition Location
Arteriolae rectae	Arteriolae rectae	**arteriole** Arteriola recta
Arteriola temporalis retinae inferior	Inferior temporal branch (of central artery of retina)	**retina, central artery of the**
Arteriola temporalis retinae superior	Superior temporal branch (of central artery of retina)	**retina, central artery of the**
Articulatio	Joint	**articulation *also* joint**
Articulatio acromioclavicularis	Acromioclavicular joint	**joint** Acromioclavicular joint
Articulatio atlanto-axialis lateralis	Lateral atlanto-axial joint	**joint** Atlanto-axial joints
Articulatio atlanto-axialis mediana	Median atlanto-axial joint	**joint** Atlanto-axial joints
Articulatio atlanto-occipitalis	Atlanto-occipital joint	**joint** Atlanto-occipital joint
Articulatio calcaneocuboidea	Calcaneocuboid joint	**joint** Calcaneocuboid joint
Articulatio capitis costae	Joint of head of rib	**joint** Joint of the head of a rib
Articulationes carpometacarpeae	Carpometacarpal joints	**joint** Carpometacarpal joints
Articulatio carpo-metacarpea pollicis	Carpometacarpal joint of thumb	**joint** Joint of the thumb, carpometacarpal
Articulatio composita	Compound joint	**joint** Compound joint
Articulatio condylaris	Condyloid joint	**joint** Condyloid joint
Articulationes costochondrales	Costochondral joint	**joint** Costochondral joint
Articulatio costotransversaria	Costotransverse joint	**joint** Costotransverse joint
Articulationes costovertebrales	Costovertebral joints	**joint** Costovertebral joints
Articulatio cotylica	Ball-and-socket joint	**joint** Ball-and-socket joint
Articulatio coxae	Hip joint	**joint** Hip joint
Articulatio crico-arytenoidea	Crico-arytenoid joint	**joint** Crico-arytenoid joint
Articulatio crico-thyroidea	Cricothyroid joint	**joint** Cricothyroid joint
Articulatio cubiti	Elbow joint	**joint** Elbow joint
Articulatio cuneonavicularis	Cuneonavicular joint	**joint** Cuneonavicular joint
Articulatio ellipsoidea	Ellipsoid joint	**joint** Ellipsoid joint
Articulatio genu	Knee joint	**joint** Knee joint
Articulatio humeri	Shoulder joint	**joint** Shoulder joint
Articulatio humeroradialis	Humeroradial joint	**joint** Humeroradial joint
Articulatio humero-ulnaris	Humero-ulnar joint	**joint** Humero-ulnar joint
Articulatio incudomallearis	Incudomalleolar joint	**joint** Joints of the auditory ossicles
Articulatio incudostapedia	Incudostapedial joint	**joint** Joints of the auditory ossicles
Articulationes intercarpeae	Intercarpal joints	**joint** Intercarpal joints
Articulationes interchondrales	Interchondral joints	**joint** Interchondral joints
Articulationes intermetacarpeae	Intermetacarpal joints	**joint** Intermetacarpal joints
Articulationes intermetatarseae	Intermetatarsal joints	**joint** Intermetatarsal joints
Articulationes interphalangeae manus	Interphalangeal joints of hand	**joint** joints of the hand, interphalangeal

Nomina Anatomica (N.A.)	Birmingham Revision (B.R.) or English Equivalent	Definition Location
Articulationes interphalangeae pedis	Interphalangeal joints of toes	**joint** Joints of the toes, interphalangeal
Articulationes intertarseae	Intertarsal joints	**joint** Intertarsal joints
Articulatio mediocarpea	Midcarpal joint	**joint** Midcarpal joint
Articulationes metacarpophalangeae	Metacarpophalangeal joints	**joint** Metacarpophalangeal joints
Articulationes metatarsophalangeae	Metatarsophalangeal joints	**joint** Metatarsophalangeal joints
Articulationes ossiculorum auditus	Joints of auditory ossicles	**joint** Joints of the auditory ossicles
Articulatio ossis pisiformis	Pisiform joint	**joint** Pisiform joint
Articulatio plana	Plane joint	**joint** Plane joint
Articulatio radiocarpea	Radiocarpal joint	**joint** Radiocarpal joint
Articulatio radio-ulnaris distalis	Inferior radio-ulnar joint	**joint** Radio-ulnar joint, inferior
Articulatio radio-ulnaris proximalis	Superior radio-ulnar joint	**joint** Radio-ulnar joint, superior
Articulatio sacro-iliaca	Sacro-iliac joint	**joint** Sacro-iliac joint
Articulatio sellaris	Saddle joint	**joint** Saddle joint
Articulatio simplex	Simple joint	**joint** Simple joint
Articulatio spheroidea [cotylica]	Spheroid joint	**joint** Spheroid joint
Articulatio sterno-clavicularis	Sternoclavicular joint	**joint** Sternoclavicular joint
Articulationes sternocostales	Sternocostal joints	**joint** Sternocostal joints
Articulatio subtalaris	Talocalcanean joint	**joint** Talocalcanean joint
Articulatio talocalcaneonavicularis	Talocalcaneonavicular joint	**joint** Talocalcaneonavicular joint
Articulatio talocruralis	Ankle joint	**joint** Ankle joint
Articulatio tarsi transversa	Transverse tarsal joint	**joint** Tarsal joint, transverse
Articulationes tarso-metatarseae	Tarsometatarsal joints	**joint** Tarsometatarsal joints
Articulatio temporomandibularis	Mandibular joint	**joint** Mandibular joint
Articulatio tibiofibularis	Superior tibiofibular joint	**joint** Tibiofibular joint, superior
Articulatio trochoidea	Pivot joint	**joint** Pivot joint
Atlas	Atlas	**atlas**
Atria cordis	Atria of heart	**atrium** Atria of the heart
Atrium dextrum	Right atrium	**atrium** Right atrium
Atrium meatus medii	Atrium of middle meatus	**atrium** Atrium of the middle meatus
Atrium sinistrum	Left atrium	**atrium** Left atrium
Auricula	Auricle	**auricle**
Auricula atrii	Auricles of atria	**auricle**
Auricula dextra	Auricle of right atrium	**auricle**
Auricula sinistra	Auricle of left atrium	**auricle**
Auris	Ear	**ear**
Auris externa	External ear	**ear** External ear
Auris interna	Internal ear	**ear** Internal ear

Anatomical Nomenclature

Nomina Anatomica (N.A.)	Birmingham Revision (B.R.) or English Equivalent	Definition Location
Auris media	Middle ear	**ear** Middle ear
Axilla	Axilla	**axilla**
Axis	Axis	**axis**
Axis bulbi externus	External axis of eye	**axis** Axis of the eye, external
Axis bulbi internus	Internal axis of eye	**axis** Axis of the eye, internal
Axis lentis	Axis of lens	**axis** Axis of the lens
Axis opticus	Optic axis	**axis** Optic axis
Axis pelvis	Axis of pelvis	**axis** Axis of the pelvis
Barba	Beard	**beard**
Basis	Base	**base *also* basis**
Basis cartilaginis arytenoideae	Base (of arytenoid cartilage)	**cartilage** Arytenoid cartilage
Basis (ossis metacarpalis)	Base (of metacarpal bone)	**metacarpal bones**
Basis (ossis metatarsalis)	Base (of metatarsal bone)	**metatarsal bones** Base
Basis cochleae	Base of cochlea	**cochlea**
Basis cordis	Base of heart	**heart** Base of the heart
Basis cranii externa	Lower surface (of base of skull)	**skull** Surface of the skull lower
Basis cranii interna	Upper surface (of base of skull)	**skull** Surface of the skull, upper
Basis mandibulae	Base of mandible	**mandible** Base
Basis modioli	Base of modiolus	**modiolus**
Basis ossis sacri	Base of sacrum	**sacrum** Base of the sacrum
Basis patellae	Base of patella	**patella** Base of the patella
Basis phalangis (manus)	Base of phalanx (of a finger)	**phalanges**
Basis phalangis (pedis)	Base of phalanx (of a toe)	**phalanges**
Basis prostatae	Base of prostate	**prostate** Base of the prostate
Basis pulmonis	Base of lung	**lung** Base of the lung
Basis pyramidis	Base of renal pyramid	**pyramid** Renal pyramids
Basis stapedis	Base of stapes	**stapes**
Bifurcatio tracheae	Bifurcation of trachea	**bifurcation** Bifurcation of the trachea
Brachium	Upper arm	**arm *also* brachium**
Brachium colliculi inferioris	Inferior brachium	**brachium** Brachium of the mid-brain, inferior
Brachium colliculi superioris	Superior brachium	**brachium** Brachium of the mid-brain, superior
Bronchioli	Bronchioles	**bronchiole**
Bronchioli respiratorii	Terminal bronchioles	**bronchiole** Terminal bronchiole
Bronchus lingularis inferior (lobi superioris sinistri)	Lower lingular bronchus	**bronchus**
Bronchus lingularis superior (lobi superioris sinistri)	Upper lingular bronchus	**bronchus**
Bronchus lobaris inferior dexter	Lower right lobe bronchus	**bronchus**
Bronchus lobaris inferior sinister	Lower left lobe bronchus	**bronchus**
Bronchus lobaris medius dexter	Middle lobe bronchus; branch of hyparterial bronchus to middle lobe of right lung	**bronchus**

Nomina Anatomica (N.A.)	Birmingham Revision (B.R.) or English Equivalent	Definition Location
Bronchi lobares et segmentales	Intrapulmonary bronchi	**bronchus**
Bronchus lobaris superior dexter	Eparterial bronchus	**bronchus**
Bronchus lobaris superior sinister	Left superior bronchus	**bronchus**
Bronchus principalis [dexter et sinister]	Bronchus (right and left)	**bronchus**
Bronchus segmentalis anterior (lobi superioris dextri)	Pectoral (anterior) bronchus of upper lobe of right lung	**bronchus**
Bronchus segmentalis anterior (lobi superioris sinistri)	Pectoral bronchus of upper lobe of left lung	**bronchus**
Bronchus segmentalis apicalis (lobi superioris dextri)	Apical bronchus of upper lobe of right lung	**bronchus**
Bronchus segmentalis apicalis [superior] (lobi inferioris dextri)	Apical bronchus of lower lobe of right lung	**bronchus**
Bronchus segmentalis apicalis [superior] (lobi inferioris sinistri)	Apical bronchus of lower lobe of left lung	**bronchus**
Bronchus segmentalis apicoposterior (lobi superioris sinistri)	Apical bronchus of upper lobe of left lung	**bronchus**
Bronchus segmentalis basalis anterior (lobi inferioris dextri)	Anterior basal branch of hyparterial bronchus	**bronchus**
Bronchus segmentalis basalis anterior (lobi inferioris sinistri)	Anterior basal bronchus of lower lobe of left lung	**bronchus**
Bronchus segmentalis basalis lateralis (lobi inferioris dextri)	Axillary basal branch of hyparterial bronchus	**bronchus**
Bronchus segmentalis basalis lateralis (lobi inferioris sinistri)	Axillary basal bronchus of lower lobe of left lung	**bronchus**
Bronchus segmentalis basalis medialis [cardiacus] (lobi inferioris dextri)	Cardiac branch of hyparterial bronchus	**bronchus**
Bronchus segmentalis basalis medialis [cardiacus] (lobi inferioris sinistri)	Cardiac bronchus of lower lobe of left lung	**bronchus**
Bronchus segmentalis basalis posterior (lobi inferioris dextri)	Posterior basal branch of hyparterial bronchus	**bronchus**
Bronchus segmentalis basalis posterior (lobi inferioris sinistri)	Posterior basal bronchus of lower lobe of left lung	**bronchus**
Bronchus segmentalis lateralis (lobi medii dextri)	Axillary branch of middle lobe bronchus	**bronchus**
Bronchus segmentalis medialis (lobi medii dextri)	Pectoral branch of middle lobe bronchus	**bronchus**
Bronchus segmentalis posterior (lobi superioris dextri)	Subapical bronchus of upper lobe of right lung	**bronchus**
Bronchus segmentalis subapicalis [sub-superior] (lobi inferioris dextri)	Subapical bronchus of lower lobe of right lung	**bronchus**
Bronchus segmentalis subapicalis [sub-superior] (lobi inferioris sinistri)	Subapical bronchus of lower lobe of left lung	**bronchus**
Bucca [mala]	Cheek	**cheek**
Bulbus aortae	Bulb of aorta	**bulb** Bulb of the aorta
Bulbus cornus posterioris	Bulb of posterior horn	**bulb** Bulb of the posterior horn
Bulbus oculi	Eyeball	**eyeball**

Nomina Anatomica (N.A.)	Birmingham Revision (B.R.) or English Equivalent	Definition Location
Bulbus olfactorius	Olfactory bulb	**bulb** Olfactory bulb
Bulbus penis	Bulb of penis	**bulb** Bulb of the penis
Bulbus pili	Bulb of hair	**bulb** Bulb of a hair
Bulbus venae jugularis inferior	Lower bulb of jugular vein	**bulb** Bulb of the jugular vein
Bulbus venae jugularis superior	Upper bulb of jugular vein	**bulb** Bulb of the jugular vein
Bulbus vestibuli	Bulb of vestibule	**bulb** Bulb of the vestibule
Bulla ethmoidalis	Ethmoidal bulla	**bulla** Ethmoidal bulla
Bursa	Bursa	**bursa**
Bursa anserina	Anserine bursa	**bursa** Anserine bursa
Bursa bicipitoradialis	Bicipitoradial bursa	**bursa** Bicipitoradial bursa
Bursa cubitalis interossea	Interosseous cubital bursa	**bursa** Interosseous cubital bursa
Bursa iliopectinea	Bursa of psoas major tendon	**bursa** Bursa of the psoas major tendon
Bursa infrahyoidea	Infrahyoid bursa	**bursa** Infrahyoid bursa
Bursa infrapatellaris profunda	Deep infrapatellar bursa	**bursa** Infrapatellar bursa, deep
Bursae intermusculares musculorum gluteorum	Gluteofemoral bursae	**bursa** Gluteofemoral bursa
Bursa intratendinea olecrani	Intratendinous olecranon bursa	**bursa** Olecranon bursa, intratendinous
Bursa ischiadica musculi glutei maximi	Ischial bursa of gluteus maximus muscle	**bursa** Ischial bursa of the gluteus maximus muscle
Bursa ischiadica musculi obturatorii interni	Bursa of obturator internus muscle	**bursa** Bursa of the obturator internus muscle
Bursa musculi bicipitis femoris superior	Upper bursa of biceps femoris muscle	**bursa** Bursa of the biceps femoris muscle, upper
Bursa musculi coracobrachialis	Bursa of coraco-brachialis muscle	**bursa** Bursa of the coraco-brachialis muscle
Bursa musculi extensoris carpi radialis brevis	Bursa of extensor carpi radialis brevis tendon	**bursa** Bursa of the extensor carpi radialis brevis tendon
Bursa musculi piriformis	Bursa of piriformis muscle	**bursa** Bursa of the piriformis muscle
Bursa musculi semimembranosi	Bursa of semi-membranosus tendon	**bursa** Bursa of the semi-membranosus tendon
Bursa musculi tensoris veli palatini	Bursa of tensor palati muscle	**bursa** Bursa of the tensor palati muscle
Bursa omentalis	Lesser sac of peritoneum	**sac** Sac of the peritoneum, lesser
Bursa pharyngea	Pharyngeal bursa	**bursa** Pharyngeal bursa
Bursa retrohyoidea	Retrohyoid bursa	**bursa** Retrohyoid bursa
Bursa subacromialis	Subacromial bursa	**bursa** Subacromial bursa
Bursa subcutanea acromialis	Subcutaneous acromial bursa	**bursa** Acromial bursa, subcutaneous
Bursa subcutanea calcanea	Subcutaneous calcanean bursa	**bursa** Calcanean bursa, subcutaneous
Bursa subcutanea infrapatellaris	Subcutaneous infrapatellar bursa	**bursa** Infrapatellar bursa, subcutaneous

Nomina Anatomica (N.A.)	Birmingham Revision (B.R.) or English Equivalent	Definition Location
Bursa subcutanea malleoli lateralis	Subcutaneous bursa of lateral malleolus	**bursa** Bursa of the lateral malleolus, subcutaneous
Bursa subcutanea malleoli medialis	Subcutaneous bursa of medial malleolus	**bursa** Bursa of the medial malleolus, subcutaneous
Bursa subcutanea olecrani	Subcutaneous olecranon bursa	**bursa** Olecranon bursa, subcutaneous
Bursa subcutanea prepatellaris	Subcutaneous pre-patellar bursa	**bursa** Prepatellar bursa subcutaneous
Bursa subcutanea prominentiae laryngeae	Bursa of laryngeal prominence	**bursa** Bursa of the laryngeal prominence
Bursa subcutanea trochanterica	Subcutaneous trochanteric bursa	**bursa** Trochanteric bursa, subcutaneous
Bursa subcutanea tuberositatis tibiae	Subcutaneous bursa of tuberosity of tibia	**bursa** Subcutaneous bursa of the tuberosity of the tibia
Bursa subdeltoidea	Subdeltoid bursa	**bursa** Subdeltoid bursa
Bursa subfascialis prepatellaris	Subfascial prepatellar bursa	**bursa** Prepatellar bursa, subfascial
Bursa subtendinea iliaca	Subtendinous iliac bursa	**bursa** Iliac bursa, subtendinous
Bursa subtendinea musculi bicipitis femoris inferior	Lower bursa of biceps femoris muscle	**bursa** Bursa of the biceps femoris muscle, lower
Bursa subtendinea musculi gastrocnemii lateralis	Lateral bursa of gastrocnemius muscle	**bursa** Bursa of the gastrocnemius muscle, lateral
Bursa subtendinea musculi gastrocnemii medialis	Medial bursa of gastrocnemius muscle	**bursa** Bursa of the gastrocnemius muscle, medial
Bursa subtendinea musculi infraspinati	Bursa of infraspinatus muscle	**bursa** Bursa of the infraspinatus muscle
Bursa subtendinea musculi latissimi dorsi	Bursa of latissimus dorsi muscle	**bursa** Bursa of the latissimus dorsi muscle
Bursa subtendinea musculi obturatorii interni	Bursa of obturator internus muscle	**bursa** Bursa of the obturator internus muscle
Bursa subtendineae musculi sartorii	Tibial intertendinous bursa	**bursa** Tibial intertendinous bursa
Bursa subtendinea musculi subscapularis	Subscapular bursa	**bursa** Subscapular bursa
Bursa subtendinea musculi teretis majoris	Bursa of teres major muscle	**bursa** Bursa of the teres major muscle
Bursa subtendinea musculi tibialis anterioris	Bursa of tibialis anterior tendon	**bursa** Bursa of the tibialis anterior tendon
Bursa subtendinea musculi trapezii	Subtendinous bursa of trapezius muscle	**bursa** Subtendinous bursa of the trapezius muscle
Bursa subtendinea musculi tricipitis brachii	Bursa of tendon of triceps muscle	**bursa** Bursa of the tendon of the triceps muscle
Bursa subtendinea prepatellaris	Subtendinous prepatellar bursa	**bursa** Prepatellar bursa, subtendinous
Bursa suprapatellaris	Suprapatellar bursa	**bursa** Suprapatellar bursa
Bursa synovialis	Synovial bursa	**bursa** Synovial bursa
Bursa synovialis subcutanea	Subcutaneous synovial bursa	**bursa** Synovial bursa
Bursa synovialis subfascialis	Subfascial synovial bursa	**bursa** Synovial bursa
Bursa synovialis submuscularis	Submuscular synovial bursa	**bursa** Synovial bursa

Anatomical Nomenclature

Nomina Anatomica (N.A.)	Birmingham Revision (B.R.) or English Equivalent	Definition Location
Bursa synovialis subtendinea	Subtendinous synovial bursa	**bursa** Synovial bursa
Bursa tendinis calcanei [Achilles]	Bursa of tendo calcaneus	**bursa** Bursa of the tendo calcaneus
Bursa trochanterica musculi glutei maximi	Trochanteric bursa of gluteus maximus muscle	**bursa** Trochanteric bursa of the gluteus maximus muscle
Bursa trochanterica musculi glutei medii	Trochanteric bursa of gluteus medius muscle	**bursa** Trochanteric bursa of the gluteus medius muscle
Bursa trochanterica musculi glutei minimi	Trochanteric bursa of gluteus minimus muscle	**bursa** Trochanteric bursa of the gluteus minimus muscle
Caecum	Caecum	**caecum**
Caecum cupulare	Caecum cupulare	**caecum** Caecum cupulare
Caecum vestibulare	Caecum vestibulare	**caecum** Caecum vestibulare
Calcaneus [os calcis]	Calcaneum	**calcaneum**
Calcar avis	Calcar avis	**calcar** Calcar avis
Calices renales majores	Greater calyces	**calyx** Renal calyces
Calices renales minores	Lesser calyces	**calyx** Renal calyces
Caliculus gustatorius	Taste bud	**bud** Taste bud
Caliculus ophthalmicus	Optic cup	**cup** Optic cup
Calvaria	Calvaria	**calvaria**
Calx	Heel	**heel**
Camera anterior bulbi	Anterior chamber of eye	**chamber** Anterior chamber of the eye
Camera posterior bulbi	Posterior chamber of eye	**chamber** Posterior chamber of the eye
Camera vitrea bulbi	Vitreous chamber	**chamber** Vitreous chamber of the eye
Canaliculus	Canaliculus	**canaliculus**
Canaliculi caroticotympanici	Caroticotympanic canaliculi	**canaliculus** Caroticotympanic canaliculi
Canaliculus chordae tympani	Anterior canaliculus for chorda tympani	**canaliculus** Canaliculus for the chorda tympani, anterior
Canaliculus cochleae	Cochlear canaliculus	**canaliculus** Cochlear canaliculus
Canaliculi dentales	Dental canaliculi	**canaliculus** Dental canaliculi
Canaliculus lacrimalis	Lacrimal canaliculus	**canaliculus** Lacrimal canaliculi
Canaliculus mastoideus	Mastoid canaliculus	**canaliculus** Mastoid canaliculus
Canaliculus tympanicus	Canaliculus for tympanic nerve	**canaliculus** Canaliculus for the tympanic nerve
Canalis	Canal	**canal**
Canalis adductorius	Subsartorial canal	**canal** Subsartorial canal
Canalis alimentarius	Alimentary cana	**canal** Alimentary canal
Canales alveolares	Dental canals	**canal** Dental canals, superior
Canalis analis	Anal canal	**canal** Anal canal
Canalis caroticus	Carotid canal	**canal** Carotid canal
Canalis carpi	Carpal tunnel	**tunnel** Carpal tunnel
Canalis centralis (medullae spinalis)	Central canal (of spinal cord)	**canal** Central canal of the spinal cord
Canalis cervicis uteri	Canal of cervix	**canal** Canal of the cervix
Canalis condylaris	Posterior condylar canal	**canal** Condylar canal, posterior
Canales diploici	Diploetic canals	**canal** Diploetic canal
Canalis facialis	Canal for facial nerve	**canal** Canal for the facial nerve
Canalis femoralis	Femoral cana	**canal** Femoral canal
Canalis hyaloideus	Hyaloid canal	**canal** Hyaloid canal
Canalis hypoglossi	Anterior condylar canal	**canal** Condylar canal, anterior
Canales incisivi	Incisive canals	**canal** Incisive canals
Canalis infra-orbitalis	Infra-orbital canal	**canal** Infra-orbital canal
Canalis inguinalis	Inguinal canal	**canal** Inguinal canal
Canales longitudinales modioli	Longitudinal canals of modiolus	**canal** Longitudinal canals of the modiolus
Canalis mandibulae	Mandibular canal	**canal** Mandibular canal
Canalis musculotubarius	Musculotubal canal	**canal** Musculotubal canal
Canalis nasolacrimalis	Nasolacrimal canal	**canal** Nasolacrimal canal
Canalis nutricius	Nutrient canal	**canal** Nutrient canal
Canalis obturatorius	Obturator canal	**canal** Obturator canal
Canalis opticus	Optic foramen	**foramen** Optic foramen
Canales palatini majores	Greater palatine canals	**canal** Palatine canals, greater
Canales palatini minores	Lesser palatine canals	**canal** Palatine canals, lesser
Canalis palatinovaginalis	Palatinovaginal canal	**canal** Palatinovaginal canal
Canalis pterygoideus	Pterygoid canal	**canal** Pterygoid canal
Canalis pudendalis	Pudendal canal	**canal** Pudendal canal
Canalis pyloricus	Pyloric canal	**canal** Pyloric canal
Canalis radicis dentis	Root canal (of tooth)	**canal** Root canal of a tooth
Canalis sacralis	Sacral canal	**canal** Sacral canal
Canalis semicircularis anterior	Superior semicircular canal	**canal** Semicircular canals, superior, posterior, and lateral
Canalis semicircularis lateralis	Lateral semicircular canal	**canal** Semicircular canals, superior, posterior, and lateral
Canales semicirculares ossei	Semicircular canals	**canal** Semicircular canals
Canalis semicircularis posterior	Posterior semicircular canal	**canal** Semicircular canals, superior, posterior, and lateral
Canalis spiralis cochleae	Spiral canal of cochlea	**canal** Cochlear canal
Canalis spiralis modioli	Spiral canal of modiolus	**canal** Spiral canal of the modiolus
Canales ventriculi	Gastric canals	**canal** Gastric canals

Nomina Anatomica (N.A.)	Birmingham Revision (B.R.) or English Equivalent	Definition Location
Canalis vertebralis	Vertebral canal	**canal** Vertebral canal
Canalis vomerovaginalis	Vomerovaginal canal	**canal** Vomerovaginal canal
Capilli	Hairs of head	**hair** Hairs of the head
Capitulum	Capitulum	**capitulum**
Capitulum humeri	Capitulum of humerus	**capitulum** Capitulum of the humerus
Capsula	Capsule	**capsule**
Capsula adiposa (renis)	Renal fat	**fat** Renal fat
Capsula articularis	Articular capsule	**capsule** Articular capsule
Capsula externa	External capsule	**capsule** External capsule
Capsula fibrosa (glandulae thyreoideae)	Fibrous capsule (of thyroid gland)	**gland** Thyroid gland
Capsula fibrosa (renis)	Fibrous capsule (of kidney)	**capsule** Renal capsule
Capsula fibrosa perivascularis	Hepatobiliary capsule	**capsule** Hepatobiliary capsule
Capsula glomeruli (renis)	Capsule of glomerulus (of kidney)	**glomerulus** Malpighian glomerulus, capsule of the
Capsula interna	Internal capsule	**capsule** Internal capsule
Capsula lentis	Capsule of lens	**capsule** Capsule of the lens
Caput	Head	**caput *also* head**
Caput (musculi)	Head (of muscle)	**muscle** Head of a muscle
Caput (ossis metacarpalis)	Head (of metacarpal bone)	**metacarpal bone**
Caput (ossis metatarsalis)	Head (of metatarsal bone)	**metatarsal bones** Head
Caput breve (musculi bicipitis brachii)	Short head (of biceps brachii muscle)	**biceps brachii muscle**
Caput breve (musculi bicipitis femoris)	Short head (of biceps femoris muscle)	**biceps femoris muscle**
Caput costae	Head of rib	**ribs** Head of a rib
Caput epididymidis	Head of epididymis	**epididymis**
Caput femoris	Head of femur	**femur** Head of the femur
Caput fibulae	Head of fibula	**fibula** Head
Caput humerale (musculi extensoris carpi ulnaris)	Humeral head (of extensor carpi ulnaris muscle)	**extensor carpi ulnaris muscle**
Caput humerale (musculi flexoris carpi ulnaris)	Humeral head (of flexor carpi ulnaris muscle)	**flexor carpi ulnaris muscle**
Caput humerale (musculi pronatoris teretis)	Humeral head (of pronator teres muscle)	**pronator teres muscle**
Caput humeri	Head of humerus	**humerus** Head of the humerus
Caput humero-ulnare (musculi flexoris digitorum superficialis)	Humero-ulnar head (of flexor digitorum sublimis muscle)	**flexor digitorum sublimis muscle**
Caput laterale (musculi gastrocnemii)	Lateral head (of gastrocnemius muscle)	**gastrocnemius muscle**
Caput laterale (musculi tricipitis brachii)	Lateral head (of triceps brachii muscle)	**triceps brachii muscle**
Caput longum (musculi bicipitis brachii)	Long head (of biceps brachii muscle)	**biceps brachii muscle**
Caput longum (musculi bicipitis femoris)	Long head (of biceps femoris muscle)	**biceps femoris muscle**
Caput longum (musculi tricipitis brachii)	Long head (of triceps brachii muscle)	**triceps brachii muscle**
Caput mallei	Head of malleus	**malleus**
Caput mandibulae	Head of mandible	**mandible** Head

Nomina Anatomica (N.A.)	Birmingham Revision (B.R.) or English Equivalent	Definition Location
Caput mediale (musculi gastrocnemii)	Medial head (of gastrocnemius muscle)	**gastrocnemius muscle**
Caput mediale (musculi tricipitis brachii)	Medial head (of triceps brachii muscle)	**triceps brachii muscle**
Caput nuclei caudati	Head of caudate nucleus	**nucleus** Caudate nucleus, head of the
Caput obliquum (musculi adductoris hallucis)	Oblique head (of adductor hallucis muscle)	**adductor hallucis muscle**
Caput obliquum (musculi adductoris pollicis)	Oblique head (of adductor pollicis muscle)	**adductor pollicis muscle**
Caput pancreatis	Head of pancreas	**pancreas**
Caput phalangis (manus)	Head of phalanx (of a finger)	**phalanges**
Caput phalangis (pedis)	Head of phalanx (of a toe)	**phalanges**
Caput radiale (musculi flexoris digitorum superficialis)	Radial head (of flexor digitorum sublimis muscle)	**flexor digitorum sublimis muscle**
Caput radii	Head of radius	**radius** Head
Caput stapedis	Head of stapes	**stapes**
Caput tali	Head of talus	**talus** Head
Caput transversum (musculi adductoris hallucis)	Transverse head (of adductor hallucis muscle)	**adductor hallucis muscle**
Caput transversum (musculi adductoris pollicis)	Transverse head (of adductor pollicis muscle)	**adductor pollicis muscle**
Caput ulnae	Head of ulna	**ulna** Head
Caput ulnare (musculi extensoris carpi ulnaris)	Ulnar head (of extensor carpi ulnaris muscle)	**extensor carpi ulnaris muscle**
Caput ulnare (musculi flexoris carpi ulnaris)	Ulnar head (of flexor carpi ulnaris muscle)	**flexor carpi ulnaris muscle**
Caput ulnare (musculi pronatoris teretis)	Ulnar head (of pronator teres muscle)	**pronator teres muscle**
Carina tracheae	Carina tracheae	**carina** Carina tracheae
Carina urethralis vaginae	Urethral ridge (of vagina)	**ridge** Urethral ridge of the vagina
Carpus	Wrist	**carpus *also* wrist**
Cartilago	Cartilage	**cartilage**
Cartilago alaris major	Lower nasal cartilage	**cartilage** Nasal cartilage, lower
Cartilagines alares minores	Small cartilages of the ala	**cartilage** Cartilages of the ala, small
Cartilago articularis	Articular cartilage	**cartilage** Articular cartilage
Cartilago arytenoidea	Arytenoid cartilage	**cartilage** Arytenoid cartilage
Cartilago auriculae	Cartilage of auricle	**cartilage** Cartilage of the auricle
Cartilago corniculata	Corniculate cartilage	**cartilage** Corniculate cartilage
Cartilago costalis	Costal cartilage	**cartilage** Costal cartilage
Cartilago cricoidea	Cricoid cartilage	**cartilage** Cricoid cartilage
Cartilago cuneiformis	Cuneiform cartilage	**cartilage** Cuneiform cartilage
Cartilago epiglottica	Epiglottic cartilage	**cartilage** Epiglottic cartilage
Cartilago epiphysialis	Epiphyseal cartilage	**cartilage** Epiphyseal cartilage
Cartilagines laryngis	Cartilages of larynx	**cartilage** Cartilages of the larynx

Anatomical Nomenclature

Nomina Anatomica (N.A.)	Birmingham Revision (B.R.) or English Equivalent	Definition Location
Cartilago meatus acustici	Cartilage of external auditory meatus	**cartilage** Cartilage of the external auditory meatus
Cartilagines nasales accessoriae	Sesamoid cartilages of nose	**cartilage** Sesamoid cartilages of the nose
Cartilagines nasi	Cartilages of nose	**cartilage** Cartilages of the nose
Cartilago nasi lateralis	Upper nasal cartilage	**cartilage** Nasal cartilage, upper
Cartilago septi nasi	Septal cartilage	**cartilage** Septal cartilage
Cartilago sesamoidea	Sesamoid cartilage (of larynx)	**cartilage** Sesamoid cartilage of the larynx
Cartilago thyroidea	Thyroid cartilage	**cartilage** Thyroid cartilage
Cartilagines tracheales	Tracheal cartilages	**cartilage** Tracheal cartilages
Cartilago triticea	Cartilago triticea	**cartilago triticea**
Cartilago tubae auditivae	Cartilage of pharyngotympanic tube	**cartilage** Cartilage of the pharyngotympanic tube
Cartilago vomeronasalis	Subvomerine cartilage	**cartilage** Subvomerine cartilage
Caruncula	Caruncle	**caruncle** *also* **caruncula**
Carunculae hymenales	Carunculae hymenales	**caruncula** Carunculae hymenales
Caruncula lacrimalis	Lacrimal caruncle	**caruncle** Lacrimal caruncle
Caruncula sublingualis	Sublingual papilla	**papilla** Sublingual papilla
Cauda	Tail	**cauda** *also* **tail**
Cauda epididymidis	Tail of epididymis	**epididymis**
Cauda equina	Cauda equina	**cauda** Cauda equina
Cauda helicis	Tail of helix	**tail** Tail of the helix
Cauda nuclei caudati	Tail of caudate nucleus	**nucleus** Caudate nucleus, tail of the
Cauda pancreatis	Tail of pancreas	**pancreas**
Caudalis	Caudal	**caudal**
Cavernae corporum cavernosorum	Venous spaces of corpora cavernosa	**space** Venous spaces of the corpora cavernosa
Cavernae corporis spongiosi	Venous spaces of corpus spongiosum	**space** Venous spaces of the corpus spongiosum
Cavitas glenoidalis	Glenoid cavity	**cavity** Glenoid cavity
Cavum	Cavity	**cavity**
Cavum abdominis	Cavity of abdomen	**cavity** Cavity of the abdomen
Cavum articulare	Joint cavity	**cavity** Joint cavity
Cavum conchae	Cavity of concha	**cavity** Cavity of the concha
Cavum coronale	Cavity of crown of a tooth	**cavum coronale**
Cavum dentis	Cavity of tooth	**cavity** Cavity of a tooth
Cavum epidurale	Extradural space	**space** Extradural space
Cavum infraglotticum	Infraglottic cavity	**cavity** Infraglottic cavity
Cavum laryngis	Cavity of larynx	**cavity** Cavity of the larynx
Cavum medullare	Medullary cavity	**cavity** Medullary cavity
Cavum nasi	Cavity of nose	**cavity** Cavity of the nose
Cavum oris	Cavity of mouth	**cavity** Cavity of the mouth

Nomina Anatomica (N.A.)	Birmingham Revision (B.R.) or English Equivalent	Definition Location
Cavum oris proprium	Cavity proper of mouth	**cavity** Cavity of the mouth, proper
Cavum pelvis	Cavity of pelvis	**cavity** Pelvic cavity
Cavum pericardii	Pericardial cavity	**cavity** Pericardial cavity
Cavum peritonei	Cavity of peritoneum	**cavity** Cavity of the peritoneum
Cavum pharyngis	Cavity of pharynx	**cavity** Cavity of the pharynx
Cavum pleurae	Cavity of pleura	**cavity** Cavity of the pleura
Cavum septi pellucidi	Cavity of septum lucidum	**cavity** Cavity of the septum lucidum
Cavum subarachnoideale	Subarachnoid space	**space** Subarachnoid space
Cavum thoracis	Cavity of thorax	**cavity** Cavity of the thorax
Cavum trigeminale	Trigeminal cavity	**cavum trigeminale**
Cavum tympani	Tympanic cavity	**cavity** Tympanic cavity
Cavum uteri	Cavity of uterus	**cavity** Cavity of the uterus
Cellula	Cell	**cell**
Cellulae anteriores (sinuum ethmoidalium)	Anterior cells (of ethmoidal sinuses)	**sinus** Ethmoidal sinuses
Cellulae ethmoidales	Ethmoidal cells	**cell** Ethmoid cell
Cellulae mastoideae	Mastoid air cells	**cell** Mastoid air cells
Cellulae mediae (sinuum ethmoidalium)	Middle cells (of ethmoidal sinuses)	**sinus** Ethmoidal sinuses
Cellulae pneumaticae	Tubal air cells	**cell** Tubal air cells
Cellulae posteriores (sinuum ethmoidalium)	Posterior cells (of ethmoidal sinuses)	**sinus** Ethmoidal sinuses
Cellulae tympanicae	Tympanic air cells	**cell** Tympanic air cells
Cementum	Cement	**cementum**
Centrum tendineum	Central tendon (of diaphragm)	**tendon** Central tendon of the diaphragm
Centrum tendineum perinei	Perineal body	**body** Perineal body
Cerebellum	Cerebellum	**cerebellum**
Cerebrum	Cerebrum	**cerebrum**
Cervix	Neck	**cervix** *also* **neck**
Cervix uteri	Neck of uterus	**uterus** Neck of the uterus
Cervix vesicae	Neck of bladder	**urinary bladder** Neck
Chiasma opticum	Optic chiasma	**chiasma** Optic chiasma
Chiasma tendinum	Chiasma tendinum	**chiasma** Chiasma tendinum
Choanae	Posterior apertures of nose	**aperture** Bony apertures of the nose, posterior
Chorda obliqua	Oblique cord	**cord** Oblique cord
Chordae tendineae	Chordae tendineae	**chorda** Chorda tendineae
Chorda tympani	Chorda tympani	**chorda** Chorda tympani
Choroidea	Choroid	**choroid**
Chylus	Chyle	**chyle**
Cilia	Eyelashes	**eyelash**
Cingulum	Cingulum	**cingulum**
Cingulum membri inferioris	Pelvic girdle	**girdle** Pelvic girdle

Nomina Anatomica (N.A.)	Birmingham Revision (B.R.) or English Equivalent	Definition Location
Cingulum membri superioris	Shoulder girdle	**girdle** Shoulder girdle
Circulus	Circle	**circle** *also* **circulus**
Circulus arteriosus cerebri	Circulus arteriosus	**circulus** Circulus arteriosus
Circulus arteriosus iridis major	Greater arterial circle of iris	**circle** Arterial circle of the iris, greater
Circulus arteriosus iridis minor	Lesser arterial circle of iris	**circle** Arterial circle of the iris, lesser
Circulus vasculosus nervi optici	Circulus vasculosus of optic nerve	**circulus** Circulus vasculosus of the optic nerve
Circumferentia articularis (radii)	Articular circumference (of radius)	**radius** Articular circumference
Circumferentia articularis (ulnae)	Articular circumference (of ulna)	**ulna** Head
Cisterna	Cisterna	**cisterna**
Cisterna cerebellomedullaris	Cerebellomedullary cisterna	**cisterna** Cerebellomedullary cisterna
Cisterna chiasmatis	Chiasmatic cisterna	**cisterna** Chiasmatic cisterna
Cisterna chyli	Cisterna chyli	**cisterna** Cisterna chyli
Cisterna fossae lateralis cerebri	Cisterna of lateral sulcus	**cisterna** Cisterna of the lateral sulcus
Cisterna inter-peduncularis	Interpeduncular cisterna	**cisterna** Interpeduncular cisterna
Cisternae subarachnoideales	Subarachnoid cisternae	**cisterna** Subarachnoid cisternae
Claustrum	Claustrum	**claustrum**
Clavicula	Clavicle	**clavicle**
Clitoris	Clitoris	**clitoris**
Clivus (ossis occipitalis)	Clivus (of occipital bone)	**clivus** Clivus of the occipital bone
Clivus (ossis sphenoidalis)	Clivus (of sphenoid bone)	**clivus** Clivus of the sphenoid bone
Cochlea	Cochlea	**cochlea**
Colliculus (cartilaginis arytenoideae)	Colliculus (of arytenoid cartilage)	**colliculus** Colliculus of the arytenoid cartilage
Colliculus facialis	Facial colliculus	**colliculus** Facial colliculus
Colliculus inferior	Inferior quadri-geminal body	**body** Quadrigeminal bodies
Colliculus seminalis	Seminal colliculus	**colliculus** Seminal colliculus
Colliculus superior	Superior quadri-geminal body	**body** Quadrigeminal bodies
Collum	Neck	**neck**
Collum anatomicum (humeri)	Anatomical neck (of humerus)	**humerus** Neck of the humerus, anatomical
Collum chirurgicum (humeri)	Surgical neck (of humerus)	**humerus** Neck of the humerus, surgical
Collum costae	Neck of rib	**ribs** Neck of a rib
Collum [cervix] dentis	Neck of tooth	**tooth** Neck of a tooth
Collum femoris	Neck of femur	**femur** Neck of the femur
Collum glandis	Neck of penis	**penis** Neck of the penis
Collum mallei	Neck of malleus	**malleus**
Collum mandibulae	Neck of mandible	**mandible** Neck
Collum radii	Neck of radius	**radius** Neck
Collum scapulae	Neck of scapula	**scapula** Neck of the scapula
Collum tali	Neck of talus	**talus** Neck
Collum vesicae felleae	Neck of gall bladder	**gall bladder** Neck of the gall bladder
Colon	Colon	**colon**
Colon ascendens	Ascending colon	**colon**
Colon descendens	Descending colon	**colon**
Colon sigmoideum	Pelvic colon	**colon**
Colon transversum	Transverse colon	**colon**
Columna	Column	**column**
Columnae anales	Anal columns	**column** Anal columns
Columna anterior	Anterior grey column	**column** Grey column, anterior
Columna fornicis	Anterior column (of fornix)	**column** Column of the fornix, anterior
Columnae griseae	Grey columns	**column** Columns of the spinal cord, grey
Columnae griseae	Grey horns (of spinal cord)	**horn** Grey horns of the spinal cord
Columna lateralis	Lateral grey column	**column** Grey column, lateral
Columna posterior	Posterior grey column	**column** Grey column, posterior
Columnae renales	Renal columns	**column** Renal column
Columnae rugarum	Columns of rugae	**column** Columns of rugae
Columna rugarum anterior	Anterior column (of rugae)	**column** Columns of rugae
Columna rugarum posterior	Posterior column (of rugae)	**column** Columns of rugae
Columna vertebralis	Vertebral column	**column** Vertebral column
Commissura	Commissure	**commissure**
Commissura alba	White commissure	**commissure** Anterior white commissure
Commissura anterior	Anterior commissure	**commissure** Anterior commissure
Commissura fornicis	Hippocampal commissure	**commissure** Hippocampal commissure
Commissura habenularum	Habenular commissure	**commissure** Habenular commissure
Commissura labiorum	Labial commissure	**commissure** Labial commissure
Commissura labiorum anterior	Anterior commissure (of labium majus)	**commissure** Commissure of the vulva, anterior
Commissura labiorum posterior	Posterior commissure (of labium majus)	**commissure** Commissure of the vulva, posterior
Commissura palpebrarum lateralis	Lateral palpebral commissure	**commissure** Palpebral commissure, lateral
Commissura palpebrarum medialis	Medial palpebral commissure	**commissure** Palpebral commissure, medial
Commissura posterior	Posterior commissure	**commissure** Posterior commissure
Commissurae supraopticae	Postoptic commissures	**commissure** Postoptic commissure
Concha auriculae	Concha of auricle	**concha** Concha of the auricle
Concha nasalis inferior	Inferior nasal concha	**concha** Nasal conchae
Concha nasalis media	Middle nasal concha	**concha** Nasal conchae
Concha nasalis superior	Superior nasal concha	**concha** Nasal conchae
Concha nasalis suprema	Highest nasal concha	**concha** Nasal concha, highest

Anatomical Nomenclature

Nomina Anatomica (N.A.)	Birmingham Revision (B.R.) or English Equivalent	Definition Location
Concha sphenoidalis	Sphenoidal concha	**concha** Sphenoidal concha
Condylus humeri	Condyle of humerus	**condyle** Condyle of the humerus
Condylus lateralis (femoris)	Lateral condyle (of femur)	**condyle** Lateral condyle
Condylus lateralis (tibiae)	Lateral condyle (of tibia)	**condyle** Lateral condyle
Condylus medialis (femoris)	Medial condyle (of femur)	**condyle** Medial condyle
Condylus medialis (tibiae)	Medial condyle (of tibia)	**condyle** Medial condyle
Condylus occipitalis	Occipital condyle	**condyle** Occipital condyle
Conexus intertendineus	Intertendinous connexion	**connexion** Intertendinous connexion
Confluens sinuum	Confluence of sinuses	**sinus** Sinuses of the dura mater, confluence of
Conjugata	Conjugates	**conjugate** True conjugate
Conus arteriosus [infundibulum]	Infundibulum	**infundibulum** Infundibulum of the heart
Conus elasticus	Cricovocal membrane	**membrane** Cricovocal membrane
Coni epididymidis	Lobules of epididymis	**lobule** Lobules of the epididymis
Conus medullaris	Conus medullaris	**conus** Conus medullaris
Cor	Heart	**heart**
Corium [dermis]	Corium	**corium**
Cornea	Cornea	**cornea**
Cornu	Horn	**cornu** *also* **horn**
Cornu anterius (medullae spinalis)	Anterior horn (of spinal cord)	**horn** Grey horns of the spinal cord
Cornu anterius (ventriculi lateralis)	Anterior horn (of lateral ventricle)	**ventricle** Lateral ventricle
Cornu coccygeum	Coccygeal cornu	**cornu** Coccygeal cornua
Cornu inferius (cartilaginis thyroideae)	Inferior horn (of thyroid cartilage)	**cartilage** Thyroid cartilage
Cornu inferius (marginis falciformis)	Inferior cornu (of falciform margin)	**margin** Falciform margin
Cornu inferius (ventriculi lateralis)	Inferior horn (of lateral ventricle)	**ventricle** Lateral ventricle
Cornu laterale (medullae spinalis)	Lateral horn (of spinal cord)	**horn** Grey horns of the spinal cord
Cornu majus (ossis hyoidei)	Greater horn (of hyoid bone)	**horn** Horn of the hyoid bone, greater
Cornu minus (ossis hyoidei)	Lesser horn (of hyoid bone)	**horn** Horn of the hyoid bone, lesser
Cornu posterius (medullae spinalis)	Posterior horn (of spinal cord)	**horn** Grey horns of the spinal cord
Cornu posterius (ventriculi lateralis)	Posterior horn (of lateral ventricle)	**ventricle** Lateral ventricle
Cornu sacrale	Sacral cornu	**cornu** Sacral cornua
Cornu superius (cartilaginis thyroideae)	Superior horn (of thyroid cartilage)	**cartilage** Thyroid cartilage
Cornu superius (marginis falciformis)	Superior cornu (of falciform margin)	**margin** Falciform margin
Corona	Crown	**corona** *also* **crown**
Corona ciliaris	Ciliary crown	**crown** Ciliary crown
Corona clinica	Clinical crown	**crown** Clinical crown
Corona dentis	Crown of tooth	**tooth** Crown of a tooth

Nomina Anatomica (N.A.)	Birmingham Revision (B.R.) or English Equivalent	Definition Location
Corona glandis	Corona glandis	**corona** Corona glandis
Corona radiata	Corona radiata	**corona** Corona radiata
Corpus	Body	**body** *also* **corpus**
Corpus (ossis hyoidei)	Body (of hyoid bone)	**hyoid bone** Body
Corpus (ossis metacarpalis)	Shaft (of metacarpal bone)	**metacarpal bone**
Corpus (ossis metatarsalis)	Shaft (of metatarsal bone)	**metatarsal bone** Shaft
Corpus (ossis sphenoidalis)	Body (of sphenoid bone)	**sphenoid bone** Body
Corpus adiposum buccae	Buccal pad of fat	**pad** Buccal pad of fat
Corpus adiposum fossae ischiorectalis	Ischiorectal pad of fat	**pad** Ischiorectal pad of fat
Corpus adiposum infrapatellare	Infrapatellar pad of fat	**pad** Infrapatellar pad of fat
Corpus adiposum orbitae	Fatty body of orbit	**body** Fatty body of the orbit
Corpus albicans	Corpus albicans	**corpus** Corpus albicans
Corpus amygdaloideum	Amygdaloid nucleus	**nucleus** Amygdaloid nucleus
Corpus callosum	Corpus callosum	**corpus** Corpus callosum
Corpus cavernosum clitoridis [dexter et sinister]	Corpus cavernosum of clitoris (right and left)	**corpus** Corpora cavernosa of the clitoris
Corpus cavernosum penis	Corpus cavernosum penis (right and left)	**corpus** Corpora cavernosa penis
Corpus ciliare	Ciliary body	**body** Ciliary body
Corpus clitoridis	Body of clitoris	**clitoris** Body
Corpus coccygeum	Coccygeal body	**body** Coccygeal body
Corpus costae	Shaft of rib	**ribs** Shaft of a rib
Corpus epididymidis	Body of epididymis	**epididymis**
Corpus femoris	Shaft of femur	**femur** Shaft of the femur
Corpus fibulae	Shaft of fibula	**fibula** Shaft
Corpus fornicis	Body of fornix	**fornix** Fornix cerebri, body of the
Corpus geniculatum laterale	Lateral geniculate body	**body** Geniculate body, lateral
Corpus geniculatum mediale	Medial geniculate body	**body** Geniculate body, medial
Corpus glandulae sudoriferae	Body of sweat gland	**gland** Sweat gland, body of a
Corpus humeri	Shaft of humerus	**humerus** Shaft of the humerus
Corpus incudis	Body of incus	**incus**
Corpus linguae	Body of tongue	**tongue** Body of the tongue
Corpus luteum	Corpus luteum	**corpus** Corpora lutea
Corpus mamillare	Mamillary body	**body** Mamillary bodies
Corpus mammae	Body of breast	**breast**
Corpus mandibulae	Body of mandible	**mandible** Body
Corpus maxillae	Body of maxilla	**maxilla**
Corpus medullare (cerebelli)	White matter (of cerebellum)	**cerebellum**
Corpus nuclei caudati	Body of caudate nucleus	**nucleus** Caudate nucleus, body of
Corpus ossis ilii	Body of ilium	**ilium** Body
Corpus ossis ischii	Body of ischium	**ischium** Body

Nomina Anatomica (N.A.)	Birmingham Revision (B.R.) or English Equivalent	Definition Location
Corpus ossis pubis	Body of pubis	**pubis** Body
Corpus pancreatis	Body of pancreas	**pancreas**
Corpora para-aortica	Para-aortic bodies	**body** Para-aortic bodies
Corpus penis	Body of penis	**penis** Body of the penis
Corpus phalangis (manus)	Shaft of phalanx (of a finger)	**phalanges**
Corpus phalangis (pedis)	Shaft of phalanx (of a toe)	**phalanges**
Corpus pineale	Pineal body	**body** Pineal body
Corpus radii	Shaft of radius	**radius** Shaft
Corpus spongiosum penis	Corpus spongiosum penis	**corpus** Corpus spongiosum penis
Corpus sterni	Body of sternum	**sternum** Body
Corpus striatum	Corpus striatum	**corpus** Corpora striata
Corpus tali	Body of talus	**talus** Body
Corpus tibiae	Shaft of tibia	**tibia** Shaft of the tibia
Corpus trapezoideum	Corpus trapezoideum	**corpus** Corpus trapezoideum
Corpus ulnae	Shaft of ulna	**ulna** Shaft
Corpus unguis	Body of nail	**nail** Body of a nail
Corpus uteri	Body of uterus	**uterus**
Corpus ventriculi	Body of stomach	**stomach** Body of the stomach
Corpus vertebrae	Body of vertebrae	**vertebra**
Corpus vesicae	Body of bladder	**urinary bladder** Body
Corpus vesicae felleae	Body of gall bladder	**gall bladder** Body of the gall bladder
Corpus vitreum	Vitreous body	**body** Vitreous body
Corpusculum	Corpuscle	**corpuscle** *or* **corpusculum**
Corpuscula articularia	Articular corpuscle	**corpuscle** Articular corpuscle
Corpuscula bulboidea	Bulbous corpuscles	**corpuscle** Bulbous corpuscles
Corpuscula genitalia	Genital corpuscle	**corpuscle** Genital corpuscle
Corpuscula lamellosa	Lamellated corpuscles	**corpuscle** Lamellated corpuscles
Corpuscula nervosa terminalia	End corpuscles of nerves	**corpuscle** End corpuscle
Corpuscula renis	Corpuscles of kidney	**corpuscle** Renal corpuscle
Corpuscula tactus	Oval corpuscles	**corpuscle** Oval corpuscles
Cortex	Cortex	**cortex**
Cortex (glandulae suprarenalis)	Cortex (of suprarenal gland)	**cortex** Cortex of the suprarenal gland
Cortex (nodi lymphatici)	Cortex (of lymph gland)	**cortex** Cortex of a lymph gland
Cortex cerebelli	Cortex of cerebellum	**cortex** Cerebellar cortex
Cortex cerebri	Cortex of cerebrum	**cortex** Cerebral cortex
Cortex lentis	Cortex of lens	**cortex** Cortex of the lens
Cortex renis	Cortex of kidney	**cortex** Cortex of the kidney
Costae	Ribs	**ribs**
Costae spuriae	False ribs	**ribs** False ribs

Nomina Anatomica (N.A.)	Birmingham Revision (B.R.) or English Equivalent	Definition Location
Costae verae	True ribs	**ribs** True rib
Coxa	Hip	**hip**
Cranialis	Cephalic	**cephalic**
Cranium	Skull	**cranium** *also* **skull**
Crena ani	Anal (gluteal) cleft	**cleft** Gluteal cleft
Crista	Crest	**crest** *also* **crista**
Crista ampullaris	Ampullary crest	**crest** Ampullary crest
Crista arcuata	Arcuate crest	**crest** Arcuate crest
Crista basilaris	Crista basilaris	**crista** Crista basilaris
Crista capitis costae	Crest of head of rib	**crest** Crest of the head of a rib
Crista colli costae	Crest of neck of rib	**crest** Crest of the neck of a rib
Crista conchalis	Conchal crest	**crest** Conchal crest
Cristae cutis	Ridges of skin	**ridge** Ridges of the skin
Crista ethmoidalis (maxillae)	Ethmoidal crest (of maxilla)	**crest** Ethmoidal crest of the maxilla
Crista ethmoidalis (ossis palatini)	Ethmoidal crest (of palatine bone)	**crest** Ethmoidal crest of the palatine bone
Crista fenestrae cochleae	Crest of fenestra cochleae	**crest** Crest of the fenestra cochleae
Crista frontalis	Frontal crest	**crest** Frontal crest
Crista galli	Crista galli	**crista** Crista galli
Crista iliaca	Iliac crest	**crest** Iliac crest
Crista infratemporalis	Infratemporal crest	**crest** Infratemporal crest
Crista intertrochanterica	Trochanteric crest	**crest** Trochanteric crest
Crista lacrimalis anterior	Lacrimal crest (of maxilla)	**crest** Lacrimal crest of the maxilla
Crista lacrimalis posterior	Crest of lacrimal bone	**crest** Crest of the lacrimal bone
Cristae marginalis	Marginal ridges	**ridge** Marginal ridges
Cristae matricis unguis	Ridges of nail bed	**ridge** Ridges of the nail bed
Crista medialis	Medial crest	**fibula** Shaft
Crista musculi supinatoris	Supinator crest	**crest** Supinator crest
Crista nasalis (maxillae)	Nasal crest (of maxilla)	**crest** Nasal crest of the maxilla
Crista nasalis (ossis palatini)	Nasal crest (of palatine bone)	**crest** Nasal crest of the palatine bone
Crista obturatoria	Obturator crest	**crest** Obturator crest
Crista occipitalis externa	External occipital crest	**crest** Occipital crest, external
Crista occipitalis interna	Internal occipital crest	**crest** Occipital crest, internal
Crista palatina	Palatine crest	**crest** Palatine crest
Crista pubica	Pubic crest	**crest** Pubic crest
Crista sacralis intermedia	Articular tubercles of sacrum	**tubercle** Tubercle of the sacrum, articular

Anatomical Nomenclature

Nomina Anatomica (N.A.)	Birmingham Revision (B.R.) or English Equivalent	Definition Location
Crista sacralis lateralis	Transverse tubercles of sacrum	**tubercle** Tubercle of the sacrum, transverse
Crista sacralis mediana	Spinous tubercles of sacrum	**tubercle** Tubercle of the sacrum, spinous
Crista sphenoidalis	Crest of sphenoid	**crest** Crest of the sphenoid
Crista supraventricularis	Infundibulo-ventricular crest	**crest** Infundibuloventricular crest
Crista terminalis	Crista terminalis	**crista** Crista terminalis
Crista transversa	Transverse crest	**crest** Transverse crest
Cristae transversalis	Transverse ridges	**ridge** Transverse ridges
Crista triangularis	Triangular ridge	**ridge** Triangular ridge
Crista tuberculi majoris	Lateral lip (of bicipital groove)	**groove** Bicipital groove
Crista tuberculi minoris	Medial lip (of bicipital groove)	**groove** Bicipital groove
Crista urethralis	Urethral crest	**crest** Urethral crest
Crista vestibuli	Vestibular crest	**crest** Vestibular crest
Cruces pilorum	Hair cruces	**crux** Hair cruces
Crus	Leg	**crus** *also* **leg**
Crus [dextrum et sinistrum]	Crus of atrio-ventricular bundle	**crus** Crus of the atrioventricular bundle
Crus anterius (stapedius)	Anterior limb (of stapes)	**limb** Limb of the stapes, anterior
Crus anterius capsulae internae	Anterior limb of internal capsule	**limb** Limb of the internal capsule, anterior
Crura anthelicis	Crura of antihelix	**crus** Crura of the antihelix
Crus breve (incudis)	Short process (of incus)	**process** Process of the incus, short
Crus cerebri	Crus of cerebrum	**crus** Crus of the cerebrum
Crus clitoridis	Crus of clitoris	**crus** Crus of the clitoris
Crus dextrum (diaphragmatis)	Right crus (of diaphragm)	**crus** Crura of the diaphragm, right and left
Crus fornicis	Posterior column of fornix	**column** Column of the fornix, posterior
Crus helicis	Crus of helix	**crus** Crus helicis
Crus laterale (anuli inguinalis superficialis)	Inferior crus (of superficial inguinal ring)	**crus** Crus of the inguinal ring
Crus laterale (cartilaginis alaris majoris)	Outer part (of lower nasal cartilage)	**cartilage** Nasal cartilage, lower
Crus longum (incudis)	Long process (of incus)	**process** Process of the incus, long
Crus mediale (anuli inguinalis superficialis)	Superior crus (of superficial inguinal ring)	**crus** Crus of the inguinal ring
Crus mediale (cartilaginis alaris majoris)	Septal process (of lower nasal cartilage)	**process** Septal process
Crura membranacea	Crura membranacea	**crus** Crura membranacea
Crus membranaceum ampullare	Crus membranaceum ampullare	**crus** Crus membranaceum ampullare

Nomina Anatomica (N.A.)	Birmingham Revision (B.R.) or English Equivalent	Definition Location
Crus membranaceum commune	Crus membranaceum commune	**crus** Crus membranaceum commune
Crus membranaceum simplex	Crus membranaceum simplex	**crus** Crus membranaceum simplex
Crura ossea ampullaria	Ampullary crura	**crus** Ampullary crura
Crus osseum commune	Crus commune	**crus** Crus commune
Crus osseum simplex	Crus simplex	**crus** Crus simplex
Crus penis	Crus of penis	**crus** Crus of the penis
Crus posterius (stapedis)	Posterior limb (of stapes)	**limb** Limb of the stapes, posterior
Crus posterius capsulae internae	Posterior limb of internal capsule	**limb** Limb of the internal capsule, posterior
Crus sinistrum (diaphragmatis)	Left crus (of diaphragm)	**crus** Crura of the diaphragm, right and left
Crypta tonsillaris [palatinae]	Crypt of palatine tonsil	**crypt** Crypts of the tonsils
Crypta tonsillaris [pharyngis]	Crypt of naso-pharyngeal tonsil	**crypt** Crypts of the tonsils
Cubitus	Elbow	**elbow**
Culmen	Lobulus culminis	**lobulus** Lobulus culminis
Cumulus oöphorus	Cumulus ovaricus	**cumulus** Ovarian cumulus
Cuneus	Cuneus	**cuneus**
Cupula cochleae	Cupola	**cupola**
Cupula (cristae ampullaris)	Cupula (of ampullary crest)	**cupula** Cupula of the ampullary crest
Cupula pleurae	Cervical pleura	**pleura** Cervical pleura
Curvatura ventriculi major	Greater curvature of stomach	**curvature** Greater curvature
Curvatura ventriculi minor	Lesser curvature of stomach	**curvature** Lesser curvature
Cuspis anterior (valvae atrioventricularis dextrae)	Anterior cusp (of right atrioventricular valve)	**valve** Atrioventricular (tricuspid) valve, right
Cuspis anterior (valvae atrioventricularis sinistrae)	Anterior cusp (of left atrioventricular valve)	**valve** Atrioventricular (mitral) valve, left
Cuspis [coronae] dentis	Cusp of crown of tooth	**cusp**
Cuspis posterior (valvae atrioventricularis dextrae)	Inferior cusp (of right atrioventricular valve)	**valve** Atrioventricular (tricuspid) valve, right
Cuspis posterior (valvae atrioventricularis sinistrae)	Posterior cusp (of left atrioventricular valve)	**valve** Atrioventricular (mitral) valve, left
Cuspis septalis (valvae atrioventricularis dextrae)	Medial cusp (of right atrioventricular valve)	**valve** Atrioventricular (tricuspid) valve, right
Cuticula dentis	Cuticle of tooth	**cuticle** Cuticle of a tooth
Cutis	Skin	**skin**
Cymba conchae	Cymba conchae	**cymba** Cymba conchae
Decidua basalis	Decidua basalis	**decidua** Decidua basalis
Decidua capsularis	Decidua capsularis	**decidua** Decidua capsularis
Decidua parietalis	Decidua parietalis	**decidua** Decidua parietalis
Declive	Lobulus clivi	**lobulus** Lobulus clivi
Decussatio	Decussation	**decussation**
Decussatio lemniscorum [sensoria]	Sensory decussation	**decussation** Sensory decussation

Nomina Anatomica (N.A.)	Birmingham Revision (B.R.) or English Equivalent	Definition Location
Decussatio nervorum trochlearium	Decussation of trochlear nerves	**decussation** Decussation of the trochlear nerves
Decussatio pedunculorum cerebellarium superiorum	Decussation of superior cerebellar peduncles	**decussation** Decussation of the superior cerebellar peduncles
Decussatio pyramidum	Decussation of pyramids	**decussation** Decussation of the pyramids
Decussationes tegmenti	Decussations of tegmentum	**decussation** Decussation of the tegmentum
Dens (axis)	Odontoid process	**process** Process of the axis, odontoid
Dentes	Teeth	**tooth**
Dentes acustici	Auditory teeth	**tooth** Auditory teeth
Dentes canini	Canine teeth	**tooth** Canine teeth
Dentes decidui	Deciduous teeth	**tooth** Deciduous tooth
Dentes incisivi	Incisor teeth	**tooth** Incisor tooth
Dentes molares	Molar teeth	**tooth** Molar tooth
Dentes permanentes	Permanent teeth	**tooth** Permanent tooth
Dentes premolares	Premolar teeth	**tooth** Premolar tooth
Dens serotinus	Dens serotinus	**dens** Dens serotinus
Dentinum	Dentine (ivory)	**dentine**
Descensus testis	Descent of testis	**descent** Descent of the testis
Dexter	Right	**right**
Diameter obliqua	Oblique diameter	**diameter** Oblique diameter of the pelvic inlet
Diameter transversa	Transverse diameter	**diameter** Transverse diameter of the pelvic inlet
Diaphragma	Diaphragm	**diaphragm**
Diaphragma pelvis	Pelvic diaphragm	**diaphragm** Pelvic diaphragm
Diaphragma sellae	Diaphragma sellae	**diaphragma** Diaphragma sellae
Diaphragma urogenitale	Urogenital diaphragm	**diaphragm** Urogenital diaphragm
Diaphysis	Diaphysis	**diaphysis**
Diencephalon	Diencephalon	**diencephalon**
Digiti II–IV	Second, third, and fourth toes	**toe** Second, third, and fourth toes
Digitus anularis [digitus IV]	Ring finger	**finger** Fourth finger
Digiti manus	Fingers	**finger**
Digitus medius [digitus III]	Middle finger	**finger** Third finger
Digitus minimus [digitus V] (manus)	Little finger	**finger** Fifth finger
Digitus minimus [digitus V] (pedis)	Little toe	**toe** Little toe
Digiti pedis	Toes	**toe**
Diploë	Diploë	**diploë**
Discus articularis	Articular disk	**disk** Articular disk
Discus articularis (articulationis acromioclavicularis)	Articular disk (of acromioclavicular joint)	**disk** Articular disk of the acromioclavicular joint
Discus articularis (articulationis radio-ulnaris distalis)	Articular disk (of inferior radio-ulnar joint)	**disk** Articular disk of the inferior radio-ulnar joint
Discus articularis (articulationis sternoclavicularis)	Articular disk (of sternoclavicular joint)	**disk** Articular disk of the sternoclavicular joint
Discus articularis (articulationis temporomandibularis)	Articular disk (of mandibular joint)	**disk** Articular disk of the mandibular joint
Discus interpubicus	Interpubic disk	**disk** Interpubic disk
Disci intervertebrales	Intervertebral disks	**disk** Intervertebral disk
Disci nervi optici	Optic disk	**disk** Optic disk
Distalis	Distal	**distal**
Diverticula ampullae (ductus deferentis)	Diverticula of ampulla (of ductus deferens)	**diverticulum** Diverticula of the ampulla of the ductus deferens
Dorsalis	Dorsal	**dorsal**
Dorsum	Back	**back** *also* **dorsum**
Dorsum linguae	Dorsum of tongue	**tongue** Dorsum of the tongue
Dorsum manus	Back of hand	**dorsum** Dorsum of the hand
Dorsum nasi	Dorsum of nose (bridge)	**nose** Dorsum of the nose
Dorsum pedis	Dorsum of foot	**dorsum** Dorsum of the foot
Dorsum penis	Dorsum of penis	**penis** Dorsum of the penis
Dorsum sellae	Dorsum sellae	**dorsum** Dorsum sellae
Ductulus	Ductule	**ductule** *also* **ductulus**
Ductuli aberrantes	Ductuli aberrantes	**ductulus** Ductuli aberrantes
Ductulus aberrans superior	Superior ductulus aberrans	**ductulus** Ductulus aberrans, superior
Ductuli alveolares	Alveolar ducts	**duct** Alveolar ducts
Ductuli biliferi	Bile ductules	**ductule** Bile ductules
Ductuli efferentes testis	Efferent ductules	**ductule** Efferent ductules
Ductuli excretorii [glandulae lacrimalis]	Ducts of lacrimal gland	**gland** Lacrimal gland
Ductuli interlobulares	Interlobular ducts	**duct** Interlobular ducts
Ductuli prostatici	Prostatic ducts	**duct** Prostatic duct
Ductuli transversi	Tubules of epoöphoron	**tubule** Tubules of the epoöphoron
Ductus	Duct	**duct** *also* **ductus**
Ductus arteriosus	Ductus arteriosus	**ductus** Ductus arteriosus
Ductus choledochus	Bile duct	**duct** Bile duct
Ductus cochlearis	Duct of cochlea	**duct** Duct of the cochlea
Ductus cysticus	Cystic duct	**duct** Cystic duct
Ductus deferens	Vas deferens	**vas** Vas deferens
Ductus ejaculatorius	Ejaculatory duct	**duct** Ejaculatory duct
Ductus endolymphaticus [aqueductus vestibuli]	Endolymphatic duct	**duct** Endolymphatic duct of the membranous labyrinth
Ductus epididymidis	Canal of epididymis	**canal** Canal of the epididymis
Ductus epoöphori longitudinalis	Duct of epoöphoron	**duct** Duct of the epoöphoron
Ductus excretorius	Duct of seminal vesicle	**duct** Duct of a seminal vesicle
Ductus glandulae bulbo-urethralis	Duct of bulbo-urethral gland	**gland** Bulbo-urethral gland

Anatomical Nomenclature

Nomina Anatomica (N.A.)	Birmingham Revision (B.R.) or English Equivalent	Definition Location
Ductus hepaticus communis	Common hepatic duct	**duct** Hepatic duct, common
Ductus hepaticus dexter	Right hepatic duct	**duct** Hepatic duct, right
Ductus hepaticus sinister	Left hepatic duct	**duct** Hepatic duct, left
Ductus incisivus	Incisive duct	**duct** Incisive duct
Ductus lactiferi	Lactiferous ducts	**duct** Lactiferous ducts
Ductus lymphaticus [thoracus] dexter	Right lymphatic duct	**duct** Lymphatic duct, right
Ductus mesonephricus	Mesonephric duct	**duct** Mesonephric duct
Ductus nasolacrimalis	Nasolacrimal duct	**duct** Nasolacrimal duct
Ductus pancreaticus	Pancreatic duct	**duct** Pancreatic duct
Ductus pancreaticus accessorius	Accessory pancreatic duct	**duct** Pancreatic duct, accessory
Ductus paramesonephricus	Paramesonephric duct	**duct** Paramesonephric duct
Ductus para-urethrales	Para-urethral ducts	**duct** Para-urethral ducts
Ductus parotideus	Parotid duct	**duct** Parotid duct
Ductus perilymphaticus [aqueductus cochleae]	Aqueduct of cochlea	**aqueduct** Aqueduct of the cochlea
Ductus reuniens	Ductus reuniens	**ductus** Ductus reuniens
Ductus semicirculares	Semicircular ducts	**duct** Semicircular ducts
Ductus semicircularis anterior	Superior semicircular duct	**duct** Semicircular ducts
Ductus semicircularis lateralis	Lateral semicircular duct	**duct** Semicircular ducts
Ductus semicircularis posterior	Posterior semicircular duct	**duct** Semicircular ducts
Ductus sublingualis major	Principal sublingual duct	**duct** Sublingual ducts
Ductus sublinguales minores	Smaller sublingual ducts	**duct** Sublingual ducts
Ductus submandibularis	Submandibular duct	**duct** Submandibular duct
Ductus sudoriferus	Duct of sweat gland	**duct** Duct of a sweat gland
Ductus thoracicus	Thoracic duct	**duct** Thoracic duct
Ductus thyroglossus	Thyroglossal duct	**duct** Thyroglossal duct
Ductus utriculosaccularis	Utriculosaccular duct	**duct** Utriculosaccular duct
Ductus venosus	Ductus venosus	**ductus** Ductus venosus
Duodenum	Duodenum	**duodenum**
Dura mater encephali	Dura mater of brain	**dura mater**
Dura mater spinalis	Spinal dura mater	**dura mater** Spinal dura mater
Eminentia	Eminence	**eminence** *also* **eminentia**
Eminentia arcuata	Arcuate eminence	**eminence** Arcuate eminence
Eminentia collateralis	Collateral eminence	**eminence** Collateral eminence
Eminentia conchae	Eminence of concha	**eminence** Eminence of the concha
Eminentia cruciformis	Eminentia cruciata	**eminentia** Eminentiae cruciatae
Eminentia fossae triangularis	Eminence of triangular fossa	**eminence** Eminence of the triangular fossa
Eminentia iliopubica	Iliopubic eminence	**eminence** Iliopubic eminence
Eminentia intercondylaris	Intercondylar eminence	**eminence** Intercondylar eminence
Eminentia medialis	Eminentia medialis	**eminentia** Eminentia medialis
Eminentia pyramidalis	Pyramid of tympanum	**pyramid** Pyramid of the tympanum
Eminentia scaphae	Eminence of scaphoid fossa	**eminence** Eminence of the scaphoid fossa
Enamelum	Enamel	**enamel**
Encephalon	Brain	**brain**
Endocardium	Endocardium	**endocardium**
Endolympha	Endolymph	**endolymph**
Endothelium	Endothelium	**endothelium**
Endothelium camerae anterioris (corneae)	Mesothelium of anterior chamber	**mesothelium** Mesothelium of the anterior chamber
Endothelium camerae anterioris (iridis)	Endothelium of anterior chamber	**endothelium** Endothelium of the anterior chamber
Ependyma	Ependyma	**ependyma**
Epicondylus lateralis (femoris)	Lateral epicondyle (of femur)	**epicondyle** Lateral epicondyle
Epicondylus lateralis (humeri)	Lateral epicondyle (of humerus)	**epicondyle** Lateral epicondyle
Epicondylus medialis (femoris)	Medial epicondyle (of femur)	**epicondyle** Medial epicondyle
Epicondylus medialis (humeri)	Medial epicondyle (of humerus)	**epicondyle** Medial epicondyle
Epidermis	Epidermis	**epidermis**
Epididymis	Epididymis	**epididymis**
Epiglottis	Epiglottis	**epiglottis**
Epiphysis	Epiphysis	**epiphysis**
Epithalamus	Epithalamus	**epithalamus**
Epithelium	Epithelium	**epithelium**
Epithelium anterius corneae	Epithelium of cornea	**epithelium** Epithelium of the cornea
Epithelium ductus semicircularis	Epithelium of semicircular duct	**epithelium** Epithelium of the semicircular duct
Epithelium lentis	Epithelium of lens	**epithelium** Epithelium of the lens
Eponychium	Eponychium	**eponychium**
Epoöphoron	Epoöphoron	**epoöphoron**
Equator (bulbi oculi)	Equator	**equator** Equator of the eyeball
Equator lentis	Equator of lens	**equator** Equator of the lens
Esophagus	Oesophagus (gullet)	**oesophagus**
Excavatio disci	Excavation of disk (of optic nerve)	**excavation** Excavation of the disk of the optic nerve
Excavatio recto-uterina	Recto-uterine (or recto-vaginal) pouch	**pouch** Recto-uterine pouch
Excavatio rectovesicalis	Rectovesical pouch	**pouch** Rectovesical pouch
Excavatio vesico-uterina	Uterovesical pouch	**pouch** Uterovesical pouch
Externus	External	**external**
Extremitas	Extremity	**extremity**
Extremitas acromialis (claviculae)	Acromial end (of clavicle)	**clavicle**
Extremitas anterior (lienis)	Lateral end (of spleen)	**spleen** End of the spleen, lateral
Extremitas inferior (renis)	Lower end (of kidney)	**kidney**
Extremitas inferior (testis)	Lower extremity (of testis)	**testis**
Extremitas posterior (lienis)	Medial end (of spleen)	**spleen** End of the spleen, medial
Extremitas sternalis (claviculae)	Sternal end (of clavicle)	**clavicle**
Extremitas superior (renis)	Upper end (of kidney)	**kidney**

Nomina Anatomica (N.A.)	Birmingham Revision (B.R.) or English Equivalent	Definition Location
Extremitas superior (testis)	Upper extremity (of testis)	**testis**
Extremitas tubaria (ovarii)	Tubal end (of ovary)	**ovary**
Extremitas uterina (ovarii)	Uterine end (of ovary)	**ovary**
Facies	Face	**face** *also* **facet, facies,** *and* **surface**
Facies anterior (antebrachii)	Anterior surface (of forearm)	**forearm**
Facies anterior (brachii)	Anterior surface (of upper arm)	**arm**
Facies anterior (corneae)	Anterior surface (of cornea)	**cornea**
Facies anterior (corporis maxillae)	Anterior surface (of body of maxilla)	**maxilla** Anterior surface
Facies anterior (corporis pancreatis)	Anterior surface (of body of pancreas)	**pancreas**
Facies anterior (cruris)	Anterior surface (of leg)	**leg**
Facies anterior (femoris)	Anterior surface (of thigh)	**thigh**
Facies anterior (glandulae suprarenalis)	Anterior surface (of suprarenal gland)	**gland** Suprarenal gland, surfaces of a
Facies anterior (iridis)	Anterior surface (of iris)	**iris** Surface of the iris, anterior
Facies anterior partis petrosae	Anterior surface of petrous part	**temporal bone** Anterior surface
Facies anterior (patellae)	Anterior surface (of patella)	**patella**
Facies anterior (prostatae)	Anterior surface (of prostate)	**prostate** Surface of the prostate, anterior
Facies anterior (radii)	Anterior surface (of radius)	**radius** Shaft
Facies anterior (renis)	Anterior surface (of kidney)	**kidney**
Facies anterior (ulnae)	Anterior surface (of ulna)	**ulna** Shaft
Facies anterior lateralis (humeri)	Anterolateral surface (of humerus)	**humerus** Shaft of the humerus
Facies anterior lentis	Anterior surface of lens	**lens** Crystalline lens of the eye
Facies anterior medialis (humeri)	Anteromedial surface (of humerus)	**humerus** Shaft of the humerus
Facies anterior palpebrarum	Anterior surface of eyelid	**eyelids** Surface of the eyelid, anterior
Facies anterolateralis (cartilaginis arytenoideae)	Anterolateral surface (of arytenoid cartilage)	**cartilage** Arytenoid cartilage
Facies articularis (cartilaginis arytenoideae)	Articular facet (of arytenoid cartilage)	**facet** Articular facet of the arytenoid cartilage
Facies articularis (ossis)	Articular surface (of bone)	**bone**
Facies articularis (partis squamosae)	Articular surface (of squamous part)	**temporal bone** Squamous part
Facies articularis (patellae)	Posterior surface (of patella)	**patella**
Facies articularis acromialis	Acromial articular facet	**clavicle**
Facies articularis acromii	Articular facet of acromion	**acromion**
Facies articularis anterior (axis)	Anterior articular facet (of odontoid process of axis)	**facet** Facets of the odontoid process
Facies articularis arytenoidea	Facet for arytenoid cartilage	**facet** Facet for the arytenoid cartilage
Facies articularis calcanea anterior	Anterior calcanean facet	**facet** Calcanean facet of the talus, anterior

Nomina Anatomica (N.A.)	Birmingham Revision (B.R.) or English Equivalent	Definition Location
Facies articularis calcanea media	Middle calcanean facet	**facet** Calcanean facet of the talus, middle
Facies articularis calcanea posterior	Posterior calcanean facet	**facet** Calcanean facet of the talus, posterior
Facies articularis capitis costae	Articular facet of head of rib	**ribs** Head of a rib
Facies articularis capitis fibulae	Articular facet of head of fibula	**fibula** Head
Facies articularis carpea	Carpal articular surface	**radius** Carpal articular surface
Facies articularis cuboidea	Facet for cuboid	**facet** Facet for the cuboid
Facies articularis fibularis (tibiae)	Fibular articular surface (of tibia)	**tibia** Articular surface of the tibia, fibular
Facies articularis inferior (tibiae)	Inferior articular surface (of tibia)	**tibia** Articular surface of the tibia, inferior
Facies articularis malleolaris (tibiae)	Malleolar facet (of tibia)	**facet** Malleolar facet
Facies articularis malleoli	Articular facet of lateral malleolus	**facet** Articular facet of the lateral malleolus
Facies articularis navicularis	Navicular facet	**facet** Navicular facet of the talus
Facies articularis posterior (axis)	Posterior articular facet (of odontoid process of axis)	**facet** Facets of the odontoid process
Facies articularis sternalis	Sternal articular facet	**facet** Articular facet, sternal
Facies articulares superiores (tibiae)	Superior articular surfaces (of tibia)	**tibia** Articular surfaces of the tibia, superior
Facies articularis talaris anterior	Anterior facet for talus	**facet** Facet for the talus, anterior
Facies articularis talaris media	Middle facet for talus	**facet** Facet for the talus, middle
Facies articularis talaris posterior	Posterior facet for talus	**facet** Facet for the talus, posterior
Facies articularis thyroidea	Facet for thyroid cartilage	**facet** Facet for the thyroid cartilage
Facies articularis tuberculi costae	Articular facet of tubercle of rib	**tubercle** Tubercle of a rib
Facies auricularis (ossis ilii)	Auricular surface (of ilium)	**ilium** Auricular surface
Facies auricularis (ossis sacri)	Auricular surface (of sacrum)	**sacrum** Surface of the sacrum, auricular
Facies cerebralis (ossis sphenoidalis)	Cerebral surface (of sphenoid bone)	**wing** Wings of the sphenoid bone
Facies cerebralis (partis squamosae)	Cerebral surface (of squamous part)	**temporal bone** Squamous part
Facies colica (lienis)	Colic impression (on spleen)	**spleen** Surface of the spleen, visceral
Facies contactus	Contiguous surface	**tooth** Surface of a tooth, contact
Facies convexa cerebri	Superolateral surface of cerebrum	**cerebrum** Superolateral surface
Facies costalis (pulmonis)	Costal surface (of lung)	**lung** Surface of the lung, costal
Facies costalis (scapulae)	Costal surface (of scapula)	**scapula**
Facies diaphragmatica (cordis)	Diaphragmatic surface (of heart)	**heart** Surface of the heart, diaphragmatic
Facies diaphragmatica (hepatis)	Upper surface (of liver)	**liver** Surface of the liver, upper (or diaphragmatic)

Anatomical Nomenclature

Nomina Anatomica (N.A.)	Birmingham Revision (B.R.) or English Equivalent	Definition Location
Facies diaphragmatica (lienis)	Diaphragmatic surface (of spleen)	**spleen** Surface of the spleen, diaphragmatic
Facies diaphragmatica (pulmonis)	Diaphragmatic surface (of lung)	**lung** Surface of the lung, diaphragmatic
Facies distalis	Distal surface (of tooth)	**tooth** Surface of a tooth, distal
Facies dorsales (digitorum manus)	Dorsal surfaces (of fingers)	**finger**
Facies dorsales (digitorum pedis)	Dorsal surfaces (of toes)	**toe**
Facies dorsalis (ossis sacri)	Dorsal surface (of sacrum)	**sacrum**
Facies dorsalis (scapulae)	Dorsal surface (of scapula)	**scapula**
Facies externa (ossis frontalis)	Frontal surface (of frontal bone)	**frontal bone** Frontal surface
Facies externa (ossis parietalis)	External surface (of parietal bone)	**parietal bone**
Facies gastrica (lienis)	Gastric impression (on spleen)	**spleen** Surface of the spleen, visceral
Facies glutea (ossis ilii)	Gluteal surface (of ilium)	**ilium** Gluteal surface
Facies inferior (cerebelli)	Lower surface (of cerebellum)	**cerebellum** Lower surface
Facies inferior (corporis pancreatis)	Inferior surface (of body of pancreas)	**pancreas**
Facies inferior [linguae]	Inferior surface (of tongue)	**tongue** Surface of the tongue, inferior
Facies inferior cerebri	Inferior surface (of cerebrum)	**cerebrum** Inferior surface
Facies inferior partis petrosae	Inferior surface (of petrous part)	**temporal bone** Inferior surface
Facies inferior hemispherii	Inferior surface of cerebral hemisphere	**hemisphere** Cerebral hemisphere, inferior surface of the
Facies inferolateralis (prostatae)	Inferolateral surface (of prostate)	**prostate** Surface of the prostate, inferolateral (right and left)
Facies infratemporalis (corporis maxillae)	Posterior surface (of body of maxilla)	**maxilla** Posterior surface
Facies interlobares (pulmonis)	Interlobar surfaces (of lung)	**lung** Surfaces of the lung, interlobar
Facies interna (ossis frontalis)	Cerebral surface (of frontal bone)	**frontal bone** Cerebral surface
Facies interna (ossis parietalis)	Internal surface (of parietal bone)	**parietal bone**
Facies intestinalis (uteri)	Intestinal surface (of uterus)	**uterus** Surface of the uterus, intestinal
Facies lateralis (brachii)	Lateral surface (of upper arm)	**arm**
Facies laterales (digitorum pedis)	Lateral margins (of toes)	**toe**
Facies lateralis (femoris)	Lateral surface (of thigh)	**thigh**
Facies lateralis (fibulae)	Lateral surface (of fibula)	**fibula** Lateral surface
Facies lateralis [fibularis] (cruris)	Lateral (fibular) surface (of leg)	**leg**
Facies lateralis (ossis zygomatici)	Lateral surface (of zygomatic bone)	**zygomatic bone** Lateral surface
Facies lateralis (ovarii)	Lateral surface (of ovary)	**ovary** Free border
Facies laterales [radiales] (digitorum manus)	Lateral (radial) surfaces (of fingers)	**finger**
Facies lateralis (radii)	Lateral surface (of radius)	**radius** Shaft

Nomina Anatomica (N.A.)	Birmingham Revision (B.R.) or English Equivalent	Definition Location
Facies lateralis (testis)	Lateral surface (of testis)	**testis**
Facies lateralis (tibiae)	Lateral surface (of tibia)	**tibia** Shaft of the tibia
Facies lingualis	Lingual surface	**tooth** Surface of a tooth, lingual
Facies lunata (coxae)	Articular surface (o hip bone)	**hip bone** Articular surface
Facies malaris (ossis zygomatici)	Lateral surface (of zygomatic bone)	**zygomatic bone** Lateral surface
Facies malleolaris lateralis (tali)	Malleolar facet (of lateral surface of talus)	**facet** Malleolar facet of the lateral surface of the talus
Facies malleolaris medialis (tali)	Malleolar facet (of medial surface of talus)	**facet** Malleolar facet of the medial surface of the talus
Facies maxillaris (laminae perpendicularis)	Maxillary surface (of perpendicular plate)	**plate** Perpendicular plate of the palatine bone
Facies medialis (brachii)	Medial surface (of upper arm)	**arm**
Facies medialis (cartilaginis arytenoideae)	Medial surface (of arytenoid cartilage)	**cartilage** Arytenoid cartilage
Facies mediales (digitorum pedis)	Medial margins (of toes)	**toe**
Facies medialis (femoris)	Medial surface (of thigh)	**thigh**
Facies medialis (fibulae)	Anterior surface (of fibula)	**fibula** Anterior surface
Facies medialis (ovarii)	Medial surface (of ovary)	**ovary** Free border
Facies medialis (pulmonis)	Medial surface (of lung)	**lung** Surface of the lung, medial
Facies medialis (testis)	Medial surface (of testis)	**testis**
Facies medialis (tibiae)	Medial surface (of tibia)	**tibia** Shaft of the tibia
Facies medialis [tibialis] (cruris)	Medial (tibial) surface (of leg)	**leg**
Facies medialis (ulnae)	Medial surface (of ulna)	**ulna** Shaft
Facies mediales [ulnares] (digitorum manus)	Medial surfaces (of fingers)	**finger**
Facies medialis cerebri	Medial surface of cerebrum	**cerebrum** Medial surface
Facies mesialis	Mesial surface	**tooth** Surface of a tooth, mesial
Facies nasalis (corporis maxillae)	Nasal surface (of body of maxilla)	**maxilla** Nasal surface
Facies nasalis (laminae horizontalis)	Upper surface (of horizontal plate)	**plate** Horizontal plate of the palatine bone
Facies nasalis (laminae perpendicularis)	Nasal surface (of perpendicular plate)	**plate** Perpendicular plate of the palatine bone
Facies occlusalis	Occlusal surface	**tooth** Surface of a tooth, occlusal
Facies orbitalis (corporis maxillae)	Orbital surface (of body of maxilla)	**maxilla** Orbital surface
Facies orbitalis (ossis frontalis)	Orbital surface (of frontal bone)	**frontal bone** Orbital surface
Facies orbitalis (ossis sphenoidalis)	Orbital surface (of sphenoid bone)	**wing** Wings of the sphenoid bone
Facies orbitalis (ossis zygomatici)	Orbital surface (of zygomatic bone)	**zygomatic bone** Orbital surface
Facies palatina (laminae horizontalis)	Lower surface (of horizontal plate)	**plate** Horizontal plate of the palatine bone
Facies palmares (digitorum manus)	Palmar surfaces (of fingers)	**finger**
Facies patellaris (femoris)	Patellar surface (of femur)	**femur** Surface of the femur patellar

Nomina Anatomica (N.A.)	Birmingham Revision (B.R.) or English Equivalent	Definition Location
Facies pelvina (ossis sacri)	Pelvic surface (of sacrum)	**sacrum**
Facies plantares (digitorum pedis)	Plantar surfaces (of toes)	**toe**
Facies poplitea (femoris)	Popliteal surface (of femur)	**femur** Shaft of the femur, popliteal surface of the
Facies posterior (antebrachii)	Posterior surface (of forearm)	**forearm**
Facies posterior (brachii)	Posterior surface (of upper arm)	**arm**
Facies posterior (cartilaginis arytenoideae)	Posterior surface (of arytenoid cartilage)	**cartilage** Arytenoid cartilage
Facies posterior (corneae)	Posterior surface (of cornea)	**cornea**
Facies posterior (corporis pancreatis)	Posterior surface (of body of pancreas)	**pancreas**
Facies posterior (cruris)	Posterior surface (of leg)	**leg**
Facies posterior (femoris)	Posterior surface (of thigh)	**thigh**
Facies posterior (fibulae)	Posterior surface (of fibula)	**fibula** Posterior surface
Facies posterior (glandulae suprarenalis)	Posterior surface (of suprarenal gland)	**gland** Suprarenal gland, surfaces of a
Facies posterior (humeri)	Posterior surface (of humerus)	**humerus** Shaft of the humerus
Facies posterior (iridis)	Posterior surface (of iris)	**iris** Surface of the iris, posterior
Facies posterior partis petrosae	Posterior surface (of petrous part)	**temporal bone** Posterior surface
Facies posterior (prostatae)	Posterior surface (of prostate)	**prostate** Surface of the prostate, posterior
Facies posterior (radii)	Posterior surface (of radius)	**radius** Shaft
Facies posterior (renis)	Posterior surface (of kidney)	**kidney**
Facies posterior (tibiae)	Posterior surface (of tibia)	**tibia** Shaft of the tibia
Facies posterior (ulnae)	Posterior surface (of ulna)	**ulna** Shaft
Facies posterior lentis	Posterior surface of lens	**lens** Crystalline lens of the eye
Facies posterior palpebrarum	Posterior surface of eyelid	**eyelids** Surface of the eyelid, posterior
Facies pulmonalis (cordis)	Left surface (of heart)	**heart** Surface of the heart, left (pulmonary)
Facies renalis (glandulae suprarenalis)	Renal surface (of suprarenal gland)	**gland** Suprarenal gland, surfaces of a
Facies renalis (lienis)	Renal impression (on spleen)	**spleen** Surface of the spleen, visceral
Facies sacropelvina (ossis ilii)	Sacropelvic surface (of ilium)	**ilium** Sacropelvic surface
Facies sphenomaxillaris (ossis sphenoidalis)	Sphenomaxillary surface (of sphenoid bone)	**wing** Wings of the sphenoid bone
Facies sternocostalis (cordis)	Sternocostal surface (of heart)	**heart** Surface of the heart, sternocostal
Facies superior (cerebelli)	Upper surface (of cerebellum)	**cerebellum** Upper surface
Facies superior (tali)	Upper surface (of talus)	**talus** Upper surface
Facies superolateralis cerebri	Superolateral surface of cerebrum	**cerebrum** Superolateral surface
Facies symphysialis (ossis pubis)	Symphyseal surface (of pubis)	**pubis** Symphyseal surface

Nomina Anatomica (N.A.)	Birmingham Revision (B.R.) or English Equivalent	Definition Location
Facies temporalis (ossis frontalis)	Temporal surface (of frontal bone)	**frontal bone** Temporal surface
Facies temporalis (ossis sphenoidalis)	Temporal surface (of sphenoid bone)	**wing** Wings of the sphenoid bone
Facies temporalis (ossis zygomatici)	Temporal surface (of zygomatic bone)	**zygomatic bone** Temporal surface
Facies temporalis (partis squamosae)	Temporal surface (of squamous part)	**temporal bone** Squamous part
Facies urethralis (penis)	Urethral surface (of penis)	**penis** Urethral surface of the penis
Facies vesicalis (uteri)	Vesical surface (of uterus)	**uterus** Surface of the uterus, vesical
Facies vestibularis [facialis]	Vestibular surface (of tooth)	**tooth** Surface of a tooth, vestibular
Facies visceralis (hepatis)	Lower (or visceral) surface (of liver)	**liver** Surface of the liver, lower (or visceral)
Facies visceralis (lienis)	Visceral surface (of spleen)	**spleen** Surface of the spleen, visceral
Falx	Falx	**falx**
Falx cerebelli	Falx cerebelli	**falx** Falx cerebelli
Falx cerebri	Falx cerebri	**falx** Falx cerebri
Falx inguinalis [tendo conjunctivus]	Conjoint tendon	**tendon** Conjoint tendon of the transversus abdominis muscle
Fascia	Fascia	**fascia**
Fascia antebrachii	Antebrachial fascia	**fascia** Antebrachial fascia
Fascia axillaris	Axillary fascia	**fascia** Axillary fascia
Fascia brachii	Brachial fascia	**fascia** Brachial fascia
Fascia buccopharyngea	Buccopharyngeal fascia	**fascia** Buccopharyngeal fascia
Fascia cervicalis	Cervical fascia	**fascia** Cervical fascia, deep
Fascia clavipectoralis	Clavipectoral fascia	**fascia** Clavipectoral fascia
Fascia clitoridis	Fascia of clitoris	**fascia** Fascia of the clitoris
Fascia cremasterica	Cremaster fascia	**cremaster muscle and fascia**
Fascia cribrosa	Cribriform fascia	**fascia** Cribriform fascia
Fascia cruris	Crural fascia	**fascia** Crural fascia
Fascia diaphragmatis pelvis inferior	Inferior fascia (of pelvic diaphragm)	**fascia** Anal fascia
Fascia diaphragmatis pelvis superior	Superior fascia of pelvic diaphragm	**fascia** Rectovesical fascia
Fascia diaphragmatis urogenitalis inferior [membrana perinei]	Perineal membrane (inferior fascia of urogenital diaphragm)	**membrane** Perineal membrane
Fascia diaphragmatis urogenitalis superior	Superior fascia of urogenital diaphragm	**membrane** Perineal membrane, pelvic layer of the
Fascia dorsalis manus	Dorsal fascia of hand	**fascia** Dorsal fascia of the hand
Fascia dorsalis pedis	Dorsal fascia of foot	**fascia** Dorsal fascia of the foot
Fascia endothoracica	Endothoracic fascia	**fascia** Endothoracic fascia
Fascia iliaca	Fascia iliaca	**fascia** Fascia iliaca
Fascia lata	Fascia lata	**fascia** Fascia lata

Anatomical Nomenclature

Nomina Anatomica (N.A.)	Birmingham Revision (B.R.) or English Equivalent	Definition Location
Fascia masseterica	Masseteric fascia	**fascia** Masseteric fascia
Fasciae musculares	Muscular fasciae (of orbit)	**fascia** Fasciae of the orbit, muscular
Fascia nuchae	Fascia nuchae	**fascia** Fascia nuchae
Fascia obturatoria	Obturator fascia	**fascia** Obturator fascia
Fasciae orbitales	Orbital fasciae	**fascia** Orbital fasciae
Fascia parotidea	Parotid fascia	**fascia** Parotid fascia
Fascia pectoralis	Pectoral fascia	**fascia** Pectoral fascia
Fascia pelvis	Fascia of pelvic muscles	**fascia** Pelvic fascia
Fascia pelvis parietalis	Parietal pelvic fascia	**fascia** Pelvic fascia, parietal
Fascia pelvis visceralis	Visceral pelvic fascia	**fascia** Pelvic fascia, visceral
Fascia penis profunda	Deep fascia of penis	**fascia** Fascia of the penis, deep
Fascia penis superficialis	Superficial fascia of penis	**fascia** Fascia of the penis, superficial
Fascia perinei superficialis	Superficial fascia of perineum	**fascia** Fascia of the perineum, superficial
Fascia pharyngobasilaris	Pharyngobasilar fascia	**fascia** Pharyngobasilar fascia
Fascia phrenicopleuralis	Phrenicopleural fascia	**fascia** Phrenicopleural fascia
Fascia prostatae	Sheath of prostate	**sheath** Sheath of the prostate
Fascia spermatica externa	External spermatic fascia	**fascia** Spermatic fascia, external
Fascia spermatica interna	Internal spermatic fascia	**fascia** Spermatic fascia, internal
Fascia subperitonealis	Subperitoneal fascia	**fascia** Subperitoneal fascia
Fascia superficialis (B.N.A.)	Superficial fascia	**fascia** Superficial fascia
Fascia superficialis perinei	Superficial fascia of perineum	**fascia** Fascia of the perineum, superficial
Fascia temporalis	Temporal fascia	**fascia** Temporal fascia
Fascia thoracolumbalis	Lumbar fascia	**fascia** Lumbar fascia
Fascia transversalis	Transversalis fascia	**fascia** Transversalis fascia
Fasciculus	Fasciculus	**fasciculus**
Fasciculus atrioventricularis	Atrioventricular bundle	**bundle** Atrioventricular bundle
Fasciculi corticothalamici	Corticothalamic fasciculi	**fasciculus** Corticothalamic fasciculi
Fasciculus cuneatus	Fasciculus cuneatus	**fasciculus** Fasciculus cuneatus
Fasciculus dorsolateralis	Dorsolateral fasciculus	**fasciculus** Dorsolateral fasciculus
Fasciculus gracilis	Fasciculus gracilis	**fasciculus** Fasciculus gracilis
Fasciculus lateralis (plexus brachialis)	Lateral cord (of brachial plexus)	**cord** Cord of the brachial plexus, lateral
Fasciculi longitudinales (articulationis atlanto-axialis)	Longitudinal bands (of atlanto-axial joint)	**band** Bands of the atlanto-axial joint, longitudinal
Fasciculi longitudinales (pontis)	Longitudinal bundles (of pons)	**bundle** Bundles of the pons, longitudinal
Fasciculus longitudinalis dorsalis	Dorsal longitudinal bundle	**bundle** Longitudinal bundle, dorsal
Fasciculus longitudinalis inferior	Inferior longitudinal bundle	**bundle** Longitudinal bundle, inferior
Fasciculus longitudinalis medialis (medullae oblongatae)	Medial longitudinal bundle (of the medulla oblongata)	**bundle** Longitudinal bundle, medial
Fasciculus longitudinalis medialis (mesencephali)	Medial longitudinal bundle (of mid-brain)	**bundle** Longitudinal bundle, medial
Fasciculus longitudinalis medialis (pontis)	Medial longitudinal bundle (of pons)	**bundle** Longitudinal bundle, medial
Fasciculus longitudinalis superior	Superior longitudinal bundle	**bundle** Longitudinal bundle, superior
Fasciculus mamillotegmentalis	Mamillotegmental tract	**tract** Mamillotegmental tract
Fasciculus mamillothalamicus	Mamillothalamic tract	**tract** Mamillothalamic tract
Fasciculus medialis (plexus brachialis)	Medial cord (of brachial plexus)	**cord** Cord of the brachial plexus, medial
Fasciculus posterior (plexus brachialis)	Posterior cord (of brachial plexus)	**cord** Cord of the brachial plexus, posterior
Fasciculus proprius (anterior)	Anterior inter-segmental tract	**tract** Intersegmental tract, anterior
Fasciculus proprius (lateralis)	Lateral inter-segmental tract	**tract** Intersegmental tract, lateral
Fasciculus proprius (posterior)	Posterior inter-segmental tract	**tract** Intersegmental tract, posterior
Fasciculi proprii medullae spinalis [fasciculi inter-segmentales]	Intersegmental tracts	**tract** Intersegmental tracts
Fasciculus retroflexus	Fasciculus retroflexus	**fasciculus** Fasciculus retroflexus
Fasciculi rubroreticulares	Rubroreticular fasciculi	**fasciculus** Rubroreticular fasciculus
Fasciculus subcallosus	Fasciculus subcallosus	**fasciculus** Fasciculus subcallosus
Fasciculi thalamocorticales	Thalamocortical fasciculi	**fasciculus** Thalamocortical fasciculi
Fasciculi transversi (manus)	Superficial transverse ligaments (of palm)	**ligament** Ligament of the palm, superficial transverse
Fasciculi transversi (pedis)	Superficial transverse ligaments (of sole)	**ligament** Ligaments of the sole, superficial transverse
Fasciculus triangularis	Triangular fasciculus	**fasciculus** Triangular fasciculus
Fasciculus uncinatus	Uncinate bundle	**bundle** Uncinate bundle
Fauces	Fauces	**fauces**
Fel (B.N.A.) (bilis)	Bile (gall)	**bile**
Femur	Thigh	**femur** ***also*** **thigh**
Fenestra cochleae	Fenestra cochleae	**fenestra** Fenestra cochleae
Fenestra vestibuli	Fenestra vestibuli	**fenestra** Fenestra vestibuli
Fibra	Fibre	**fibre**
Fibrae arcuatae cerebri	Association fibres	**fibre** Association fibres
Fibrae arcuatae externae dorsales	Posterior external arcuate fibres	**fibre** Arcuate fibres, posterior external
Fibrae arcuatae externae ventrales	Anterior external arcuate fibres	**fibre** Arcuate fibres, anterior external
Fibrae arcuatae internae	Internal arcuate fibres	**fibre** Arcuate fibres, internal

Nomina Anatomica (N.A.)	Birmingham Revision (B.R.) or English Equivalent	Definition Location
Fibrae circulares (musculi ciliaris)	Circular fibres (of ciliary muscle)	**ciliary muscle**
Fibrae corticonucleares	Corticonuclear fibres	**fibre** Corticonuclear fibres
Fibrae corticopontinae	Cerebropontine fibres	**fibre** Cerebropontine fibres
Fibrae corticoreticulares	Corticoreticular fibres	**fibre** Corticoreticular fibres
Fibrae corticospinales	Cerebrospinal fibres	**fibre** Cerebrospinal fibres
Fibrae intercrurales	Intercrural fibres (of inguinal canal)	**fibre** Intercrural fibres of the inguinal canal
Fibrae lentis	Fibres of lens	**fibre** Fibres of the lens
Fibrae meridionales (musculi ciliaris)	Meridional fibres	**ciliary muscle**
Fibrae obliquae (tunicae muscularis ventriculi)	Oblique fibres (of muscular coat of stomach)	**stomach** Coat of the stomach, muscular
Fibrae periventriculares	Periventricular fibres	**fibre** Periventricular fibres
Fibrae pontis transversae	Transverse fibres of pons	**fibre** Fibres of the pons, transverse
Fibrae zonulares	Zonular fibres	**fibre** Zonular fibres of the ciliary zonule
Fibrocartilago	Fibrocartilage	**fibrocartilage**
Fibula	Fibula	**fibula**
Fibularis	Fibular	**fibular**
Filum	Filum	**filum**
Filum durae matris spinalis	Filum of spinal dura mater	**filum** Filum of the spinal dura mater
Fila radicularia (nervorum spinalium)	Rootlets (of spinal nerves)	**rootlets**
Filum terminale	Filum terminale	**filum** Filum terminale
Fimbria hippocampi	Fimbria (of hippocampus)	**fimbria** Fimbria of the hippocampus
Fimbria ovarica	Ovarian fimbria	**fimbria** Ovarian fimbria
Fimbriae tubae (uterinae)	Fimbriae (of uterine tube)	**fimbria** Fimbria of the uterine tube
Fissura	Fissure	**fissure**
Fissura antitragohelicina	Fissura antitragohelicina	**fissura** Fissura antitragohelicina
Fissurae cerebelli	Fissures of cerebellum	**fissure** Fissures of the cerebellum
Fissura choroidea	Choroid fissure	**fissure** Choroid fissure
Fissura horizontalis [pulmonis dextri]	Horizontal fissure (of right lung)	**fissure** Fissure of the right lung, horizontal
Fissura horizontalis cerebelli	Horizontal fissure (of cerebellum)	**fissure** Horizontal fissure
Fissura ligamenti teretis	Fissure for ligamentum teres	**fissure** Fissure for the ligamentum teres
Fissura ligamenti venosi	Fissure for ligamentum venosum	**fissure** Fissure for the ligamentum venosum
Fissura longitudinalis cerebri	Longitudinal fissure of cerebrum	**fissure** Fissure of the cerebrum, longitudinal
Fissura mediana anterior (medullae oblongatae)	Anterior median fissure (of medulla oblongata)	**medulla oblongata**
Fissura mediana anterior (medullae spinalis)	Anterior median fissure (of spinal cord)	**fissure** Fissure of the spinal cord, anterior median
Fissura obliqua (pulmonis)	Oblique fissure (of lung)	**fissure** Fissure of the lung, oblique
Fissura orbitalis inferior	Inferior orbital fissure	**fissure** Orbital fissure, inferior
Fissura orbitalis superior	Superior orbital fissure	**fissure** Orbital fissure, superior
Fissura petro-occipitalis	Petro-occipital fissure	**fissure** Petro-occipital fissure
Fissura petrosquamosa	Petrosquamous fissure	**fissure** Petrosquamous fissure
Fissura petrotympanica	Squamotympanic fissure	**fissure** Squamotympanic fissure
Fissura posterolateralis	Postnodular fissure	**fissure** Postnodular fissure
Fissura prima	Fissura prima	**fissura** Fissura prima
Fissura pterygomaxillaris	Pterygomaxillary fissure	**fissure** Pterygomaxillary fissure
Fissura sphenopetrosa	Sphenopetrosal fissure	**fissure** Sphenopetrosal fissure
Fissura transversa cerebri	Transverse fissure of cerebrum	**fissure** Fissure of the cerebrum, transverse
Fissura tympanomastoidea	Tympanomastoid fissure	**fissure** Tympanomastoid fissure
Fissura tympanosquamosa	Tympanosquamous fissure	**fissure** Tympanosquamous fissure
Flexura	Flexure	**flexure**
Flexura coli dextra	Right flexure of colon	**flexure** Flexure of the colon, right
Flexura coli sinistra	Left flexure of colon	**flexure** Flexure of the colon, left
Flexura duodeni inferior	Inferior flexure of duodenum	**flexure** Flexure of the duodenum, inferior
Flexura duodeni superior	Superior flexure of duodenum	**flexure** Flexure of the duodenum, superior
Flexura duodenojejunalis	Duodenojejunal flexure	**flexure** Duodenojejunal flexure
Flexura perinealis	Perineal flexure	**flexure** Flexure of the rectum, perineal
Flexura sacralis	Sacral flexure	**flexure** Flexure of the rectum, sacral
Flocculus	Flocculus	**flocculus**
Flumina pilorum	Hair streams	**stream** Hair streams
Folium	Folium	**folium**
Folia cerebelli	Cerebellar folia	**folium** Cerebellar folium
Folium vermis	Lobulus folii	**lobulus** Lobulus folii
Folliculus	Follicle	**follicle**
Folliculi glandulae thyroideae	Thyroid follicles	**follicle** Thyroid follicles
Folliculi linguales	Lingual follicles	**follicle** Lingual follicles
Folliculus lymphaticus	Lymphatic follicle	**follicle** Lymphatic follicle
Folliculi lymphatici recti	Lymphatic nodules (of rectum)	**nodule** Lymphatic nodules of the rectum
Folliculi lymphatici aggregati (intestini tenuis)	Aggregated lymphatic nodules (of small intestine)	**nodule** Lymphatic nodules, aggregated
Folliculi lymphatici aggregati appendicis vermiformis	Lymphatic nodules of vermiform appendix	**nodule** Lymphatic nodules of the vermiform appendix
Folliculi lymphatici gastrici	Gastric lymphatic nodules	**nodule** Lymphatic nodules, gastric
Folliculi lymphatici laryngei	Lymphatic nodules of larynx	**nodule** Lymphatic nodules of the larynx

Anatomical Nomenclature

Nomina Anatomica (N.A.)	Birmingham Revision (B.R.) or English Equivalent	Definition Location
Folliculi lymphatici lienales	Lymphatic nodules (of spleen)	**nodule** Lymphatic nodules of the spleen
Folliculi lymphatici solitarii (coli)	Solitary lymphatic nodules (of colon)	**nodule** Lymphatic nodules, solitary
Folliculi lymphatici solitarii (intestini tenuis)	Solitary lymphatic nodules (of small intestine)	**nodule** Lymphatic nodules, solitary
Folliculi ovarici primarii	Primary ovarian follicles	**follicle** Ovarian follicles, primary
Folliculi ovarici vesiculosi	Vesicular ovarian follicles	**follicle** Ovarian follicles, vesicular
Folliculus pili	Hair follicle	**follicle** Hair follicle
Fonticulus anterior	Anterior fontanelle	**fontanelle** Fontanelle of the skull, anterior
Fonticuli cranii	Fontanelles of skull	**fontanelle**
Fonticulus mastoideus	Posterolateral fontanelle	**fontanelle** Fontanelle of the skull, posterolateral
Fonticulus posterior	Posterior fontanelle	**fontanelle** Fontanelle of the skull, posterior
Fonticulus sphenoidalis	Anterolateral fontanelle	**fontanelle** Fontanelle of the skull, anterolateral
Foramen	Foramen	**foramen**
Foramina alveolaria	Dental foramina	**foramen** Dental foramina of the maxilla
Foramen apicis dentis	Root foramen (of tooth)	**foramen** Apical foramen
Foramen cecum (ossis frontalis)	Foramen caecum (of skull)	**foramen** Foramen caecum of the skull
Foramen cecum linguae	Foramen caecum of tongue	**foramen** Foramen caecum of the tongue
Foramen costotransversarium	Costotransverse foramen	**foramen** Costotransverse foramen
Foramen epiploicum	Opening into lesser sac	**sac** Sac of the peritoneum, lesser, opening into the
Foramen ethmoidale anterius	Anterior ethmoidal foramen	**foramen** Ethmoidal foramen, anterior
Foramen ethmoidale posterius	Posterior ethmoidal foramen	**foramen** Ethmoidal foramen, posterior
Foramen (sive incisura) frontale	Frontal foramen	**foramen** Frontal foramen
Foramina incisiva	Incisive foramina	**foramen** Incisive foramina
Foramen infra-orbitale	Infra-orbital foramen	**foramen** Infra-orbital foramen
Foramen interventriculare	Interventricular foramen	**foramen** Interventricular foramen
Foramina intervertebralia	Intervertebral foramina	**foramen** Intervertebral foramen of the sacrum
Foramen ischiadicum majus	Greater sciatic foramen	**foramen** Sciatic foramen, greater
Foramen ischiadicum minus	Lesser sciatic foramen	**foramen** Sciatic foramen, lesser
Foramen jugulare	Jugular foramen	**foramen** Jugular foramen
Foramen lacerum	Foramen lacerum	**foramen** Foramen lacerum
Foramen magnum	Foramen magnum	**foramen** Foramen magnum
Foramen mandibulae	Mandibular foramen	**foramen** Mandibular foramen
Foramen mastoideum	Mastoid foramen	**foramen** Mastoid foramen

Nomina Anatomica (N.A.)	Birmingham Revision (B.R.) or English Equivalent	Definition Location
Foramen mentale	Mental foramen	**foramen** Mental foramen
Foramina nervosa	Foramina for nerves	**foramen** Foramina for nerves
Foramen nutricium	Nutrient foramen	**foramen** Nutrient foramen
Foramen obturatum	Obturator foramen	**foramen** Obturator foramen
Foramen ovale	Foramen ovale	**foramen** Foramen ovale
Foramen palatinum majus	Greater palatine foramen	**foramen** Palatine foramen, greater
Foramina palatina minora	Lesser palatine foramina	**foramen** Palatine foramina, lesser
Foramina papillaria	Papillary foramina	**foramen** Papillary foramina
Foramen parietale	Parietal foramen	**foramen** Parietal foramen
Foramen rotundum	Foramen rotundum	**foramen** Foramen rotundum
Foramina sacralia dorsalia	Posterior sacral foramina	**foramen** Sacral foramina, posterior
Foramina sacralia pelvina	Anterior sacral foramina	**foramen** Sacral foramina, anterior
Foramen singulare	Foramen singulare	**foramen** Foramen singulare
Foramen sphenopalatinum	Sphenopalatine foramen	**foramen** Sphenopalatine foramen
Foramen spinosum	Foramen spinosum	**foramen** Foramen spinosum
Foramen stylomastoideum	Stylomastoid foramen	**foramen** Stylomastoid foramen
Foramen (sive incisura) supra-orbitalis	Supra-orbital foramen	**foramen** Supra-orbital foramen
Foramen thyroideum	Thyroid foramen	**foramen** Thyroid foramen
Foramen transversarium	Foramen transversarium	**foramen** Foramen transversarium
Foramen venae cavae	Vena-caval opening (of diaphragm)	**diaphragm** Opening of the diaphragm, vena-caval
Foramina venarum minimarum	Foramina venarum minimarum	**foramen** Foramina venarum minimarum
Foramen vertebrale	Vertebral foramen	**foramen** Vertebral foramen
Foramen zygomaticofaciale	Zygomaticofacial foramen	**foramen** Zygomaticofacial foramen
Foramen zygomatico-orbitale	Zygomatico-orbital foramen	**foramen** Zygomatico-orbital foramen
Foramen zygomaticotemporale	Zygomaticotemporal foramen	**foramen** Zygomaticotemporal foramen
Forceps major	Forceps major	**forceps major**
Forceps minor	Forceps minor	**forceps minor**
Formatio	Formation	**formation**
Formatio reticularis (medullae spinalis)	Reticular formation (of spinal cord)	**formation** Reticular formation of the spinal cord
Formatio reticularis (pontis)	Reticular formation (of pons)	**formation** Reticular formation of the pons
Formatio reticularis (tegmenti)	Reticular formation (of tegmentum)	**formation** Reticular formation of the tegmentum
Fornix	Fornix	**fornix**
Fornix (cerebri)	Fornix (cerebri)	**fornix** Fornix cerebri
Fornix conjunctivae inferior	Inferior fornix of conjunctiva	**fornix** Fornix of the conjunctiva
Fornix conjunctivae superior	Superior fornix of conjunctiva	**fornix** Fornix of the conjunctiva
Fornix pharyngis	Pharyngeal fornix	**fornix** Pharyngeal fornix

Nomina Anatomica (N.A.)	Birmingham Revision (B.R.) or English Equivalent	Definition Location
Fornix sacci lacrimalis	Fornix of lacrimal sac	**fornix** Fornix of the lacrimal sac
Fornix vaginae	Fornix of vagina	**fornix** Fornix of the vagina
Fossa	Fossa	**fossa**
Fossa acetabuli	Acetabular fossa	**fossa** Acetabular fossa
Fossa anthelicis	Fossa of the antihelix	**fossa** Fossa of the antihelix
Fossa axillaris	Axillary fossa	**fossa** Axillary fossa
Fossa canina	Canine fossa	**fossa** Canine fossa
Fossa condylaris	Condylar fossa	**fossa** Condylar fossa
Fossa coronoidea	Coronoid fossa	**fossa** Coronoid fossa
Fossa cranii anterior	Anterior cranial fossa	**fossa** Cranial fossa, anterior
Fossa cranii media	Middle cranial fossa	**fossa** Cranial fossa, middle
Fossa cranii posterior	Posterior cranial fossa	**fossa** Cranial fossa, posterior
Fossa cubitalis	Cubital fossa	**fossa** Cubital fossa
Fossa digastrica	Digastric fossa	**fossa** Digastric fossa
Fossa ductus venosi	Fossa ductus venosi	**fossa** Fossa ductus venosi
Fossa epigastrica	Epigastric fossa	**fossa** Epigastric fossa
Fossa glandulae lacrimalis	Fossa for lacrimal gland	**fossa** Fossa for the lacrimal gland
Fossa hyaloidea	Hyaloid fossa	**fossa** Hyaloid fossa
Fossa hypophysialis	Hypophyseal fossa	**fossa** Hypophyseal fossa
Fossa iliaca	Iliac fossa	**fossa** Iliac fossa
Fossa incisiva	Incisive fossa	**fossa** Incisive fossa
Fossa incudis	Fossa for the incus	**fossa** Fossa for the incus
Fossa infraspinata	Infraspinous fossa	**fossa** Infraspinous fossa
Fossa infratemporalis	Infratemporal fossa	**fossa** Infratemporal fossa
Fossa inguinalis lateralis	Lateral inguinal fossa	**fossa** Inguinal fossa, lateral
Fossa inguinalis medialis	Middle inguinal fossa	**fossa** Inguinal fossa, middle
Fossa intercondylaris	Intercondylar notch	**notch** Intercondylar notch
Fossa interpeduncularis	Interpeduncular fossa	**fossa** Interpeduncular fossa
Fossa ischiorectalis	Ischiorectal fossa	**fossa** Ischiorectal fossa
Fossa jugularis (ossis temporalis)	Jugular fossa	**fossa** Jugular fossa
Fossa lateralis cerebri	Lateral cerebral fossa	**fossa** Cerebral fossa, lateral
Fossa malleoli lateralis	Malleolar fossa	**fossa** Malleolar fossa
Fossa mandibularis	Articular fossa	**fossa** Articular fossa
Fossa navicularis urethrae	Fossa terminalis	**fossa** Fossa terminalis
Fossa olecrani	Olecranon fossa	**fossa** Olecranon fossa
Fossa ovalis	Fossa ovalis	**fossa** Fossa ovalis
Fossa poplitea	Popliteal fossa	**fossa** Popliteal fossa

Nomina Anatomica (N.A.)	Birmingham Revision (B.R.) or English Equivalent	Definition Location
Fossa pterygoidea	Pterygoid fossa	**fossa** Pterygoid fossa
Fossa pterygopalatina	Pterygopalatine fossa	**fossa** Pterygopalatine fossa
Fossa radialis	Radial fossa	**fossa** Radial fossa
Fossa rhomboidea	Floor of fourth ventricle	**ventricle** Fourth ventricle
Fossa sacci lacrimalis	Fossa of lacrimal sac	**fossa** Fossa of the lacrimal sac
Fossa scaphoidea	Scaphoid fossa	**fossa** Scaphoid fossa
Fossa subarcuata	Subarcuate fossa	**fossa** Subarcuate fossa
Fossa subscapularis	Subscapular fossa	**fossa** Subscapular fossa
Fossa supraclavicularis major [trigonum omoclaviculare]	Greater supraclavicular fossa	**fossa** Supraclavicular fossa, greater
Fossa supraclavicularis minor	Lesser supraclavicular fossa	**fossa** Supraclavicular fossa, lesser
Fossa supraspinata	Supraspinous fossa	**fossa** Supraspinous fossa
Fossa supratonsillaris	Intratonsillar cleft	**cleft** Intratonsillar cleft
Fossa supravesicalis	Supravesical fossa	**fossa** Supravesical fossa
Fossa temporalis	Temporal fossa	**fossa** Temporal fossa
Fossa tonsillaris	Tonsillar fossa	**fossa** Tonsillar fossa
Fossa triangularis	Triangular fossa	**fossa** Triangular fossa
Fossa trochanterica	Trochanteric fossa	**fossa** Trochanteric fossa
Fossa vesicae felleae	Fossa for gall bladder	**fossa** Gall-bladder fossa
Fossa vestibuli vaginae	Vestibular fossa	**fossa** Vestibular fossa
Fossula	Fossula	**fossula**
Fossula fenestrae cochleae	Fossula of fenestra cochleae	**fossula** Fossula of the fenestra cochleae
Fossula fenestrae vestibuli	Fossula of fenestra vestibuli	**fossula** Fossula of the fenestra vestibuli
Fossula petrosa	Petrosal fossa	**fossa** Petrosal fossa
Fossulae tonsillares	Tonsillar pits	**pit** Tonsillar pits
Fovea	Fovea	**fovea**
Fovea articularis inferior (atlantis)	Inferior articular facet (of atlas)	**facet** Articular facet of the atlas, inferior
Fovea articularis superior (atlantis)	Superior articular facet (of atlas)	**facet** Articular facet of the atlas, superior
Fovea capitis femoris	Pit on head of femur	**pit** Pit on the head of the femur
Fovea centralis	Fovea centralis	**fovea** Fovea centralis
Fovea costalis inferior	Inferior costal facet	**facet** Costal facet of a thoracic vertebra, inferior
Fovea costalis superior	Superior costal facet	**facet** Costal facet of a thoracic vertebra, superior
Fovea costalis transversalis	Costal facet	**facet** Costal facet of a thoracic vertebra
Fovea dentis	Facet for odontoid process	**facet** Facet for the odontoid process

Nomina Anatomica (N.A.)	Birmingham Revision (B.R.) or English Equivalent	Definition Location
Fovea inferior	Fovea inferior	**fovea** Fovea inferior
Fovea oblonga (cartilaginis arytenoideae)	Fovea oblonga (of arytenoid cartilage)	**fovea** Fovea oblonga
Fovea pterygoidea	Pterygoid pit	**pit** Pterygoid pit
Fovea sublingualis	Sublingual fossa	**fossa** Sublingual fossa
Fovea submandibularis	Submandibular fossa	**fossa** Submandibular fossa
Fovea superior	Fovea superior	**fovea** Fovea superior
Fovea triangularis (cartilaginis arytenoideae)	Fovea triangularis (of arytenoid cartilage)	**fovea** Fovea triangularis
Fovea trochlearis	Trochlear fossa	**fossa** Trochlear fossa
Foveola	Foveola	**foveola**
Foveola coccygea	Coccygeal foveola	**foveola** Coccygeal foveola
Foveolae gastricae	Gastric foveolae	**foveola** Gastric foveolae
Foveolae granulares	Granular pits	**pit** Granular pits
Frenulum	Frenulum	**frenulum**
Frenulum clitoridis	Frenulum of clitoris	**frenulum** Frenulum of the clitoris
Frenulum labii inferioris	Frenulum of lower lip	**frenulum** Frenulum of the lower lip
Frenulum labii superioris	Frenulum of upper lip	**frenulum** Frenulum of the upper lip
Frenulum labiorum pudendi	Frenulum labiorum	**frenulum** Frenulum labiorum
Frenulum linguae	Frenulum of tongue	**frenulum** Frenulum of the tongue
Frenulum preputii	Frenulum of prepuce	**frenulum** Frenulum of the prepuce
Frenulum valvae ileocaecalis	Frenulum of ileocolic valve	**frenulum** Frenulum of the ileocolic valve
Frenulum veli medullaris superioris	Frenulum veli	**frenulum** Frenulum veli
Frons	Forehead	**forehead**
Frontalis	Frontal	**frontal**
Fundus	Fundus	**fundus**
Fundus meatus acustici interni	Fundus of internal auditory meatus	**meatus** Auditory meatus, internal
Fundus uteri	Fundus of uterus	**uterus** Fundus of the uterus
Fundus ventriculi	Fundus of stomach	**stomach** Fundus of the stomach
Fundus vesicae	Base of bladder	**urinary bladder** Base
Fundus vesicae felleae	Fundus of gall bladder	**gall bladder** Fundus of the gall bladder
Funiculus	Funiculus	**funiculus**
Funiculus anterior	Anterior white column	**column** White column, anterior
Funiculus lateralis (medullae oblongatae)	Lateral white column (of medulla oblongata)	**column** White column, lateral
Funiculus lateralis (medullae spinalis)	Lateral white column (of spinal cord)	**column** White column, lateral
Funiculi medullae spinalis	White columns of spinal cord	**column** Columns of the spinal cord, white
Funiculus posterior	Posterior white column	**column** White column, posterior
Funiculus spermaticus	Spermatic cord	**cord** Spermatic cord
Funiculus umbilicalis	Umbilical cord	**cord** Umbilical cord

Nomina Anatomica (N.A.)	Birmingham Revision (B.R.) or English Equivalent	Definition Location
Galea aponeurotica [aponeurosis epicranialis]	Epicranial aponeurosis	**aponeurosis** Epicranial aponeurosis
Ganglion	Ganglion	**ganglion**
Ganglion aorticorenale	Aorticorenal ganglion	**ganglion** Aorticorenal ganglion
Ganglion cardiacum	Cardiac ganglion	**ganglion** Cardiac ganglion
Ganglion celiacum	Coeliac ganglion	**ganglion** Coeliac ganglion
Ganglion cervicale medium	Middle cervical ganglion	**ganglion** Cervical ganglion, middle
Ganglion cervicale superius	Superior cervical ganglion	**ganglion** Cervical ganglion, superior
Ganglion cervicothoracicum [stellatum]	Inferior cervical ganglion	**ganglion** Cervical ganglion, inferior
Ganglion ciliare	Ciliary ganglion	**ganglion** Ciliary ganglion
Ganglion geniculi	Ganglion of facial nerve	**ganglion** Ganglion of the facial nerve
Ganglion impar	Ganglion impar	**ganglion** Ganglion impar
Ganglion inferius (nervi glossopharyngei)	Inferior ganglion (of glossopharyngeal nerve)	**ganglion** Ganglion of the glossopharyngeal nerve, inferior
Ganglion inferius (nervi vagi)	Inferior ganglion (of vagus nerve)	**ganglion** Ganglion of the vagus nerve, inferior
Ganglia intermedia	Intermediate ganglia	**ganglion** Intermediate ganglia
Ganglia lumbalia	Lumbar ganglia	**ganglion** Lumbar ganglia
Ganglion mesentericum inferius	Inferior mesenteric ganglion	**ganglion** Mesenteric ganglion, inferior
Ganglion mesentericum superius	Superior mesenteric ganglion	**ganglion** Mesenteric ganglion, superior
Ganglion oticum	Otic ganglion	**ganglion** Otic ganglion
Ganglia pelvina	Pelvic ganglia	**ganglion** Pelvic ganglia
Ganglia phrenica	Phrenic ganglia	**ganglion** Phrenic ganglia
Ganglia plexuum autonomicorum	Ganglia of sympathetic plexuses	**ganglion** Ganglia of sympathetic plexuses
Ganglion pterygopalatinum	Sphenopalatine ganglion	**ganglion** Sphenopalatine ganglion
Ganglia renalia	Renal ganglia	**ganglion** Renal ganglia
Ganglia sacralia	Sacral ganglia	**ganglion** Sacral ganglia of the sympathetic system
Ganglion spinale	Spinal ganglion	**ganglion** Spinal ganglion
Ganglion spirale cochleae	Spiral ganglion of cochlea	**ganglion** Spiral ganglion of the cochlea
Ganglion splanchnicum	Splanchnic ganglion	**ganglion** Splanchnic ganglion
Ganglion submandibulare	Submandibular ganglion	**ganglion** Submandibular ganglion
Ganglion superius (nervi glossopharyngei)	Superior ganglion (of glossopharyngeal nerve)	**ganglion** Ganglion of the glossopharyngeal nerve, superior
Ganglion superius (nervi vagi)	Superior ganglion (of vagus nerve)	**ganglion** Ganglion of the vagus nerve, superior
Ganglion terminale	Terminal ganglion	**ganglion** Terminal ganglion
Ganglia thoracica	Thoracic ganglia	**ganglion** Thoracic ganglia

Nomina Anatomica (N.A.)	Birmingham Revision (B.R.) or English Equivalent	Definition Location
Ganglion trigeminale	Trigeminal ganglion	**ganglion** Trigeminal ganglion
Ganglia trunci sympathici	Ganglia of sympathetic trunk	**ganglion** Ganglia of the sympathetic trunk
Ganglion tympanicum	Tympanic ganglion	**ganglion** Tympanic ganglion
Ganglion vertebrale	Vertebral ganglion	**ganglion** Vertebral ganglion
Ganglion vestibulare	Vestibular ganglion	**ganglion** Vestibular ganglion
Geniculum	Geniculum	**geniculum**
Geniculum canalis facialis	Geniculum of the canal for the facial nerve	**canal** Canal for the facial nerve
Geniculum nervi facialis	Geniculum of facial nerve	**geniculum** Geniculum of the facial nerve
Genu	Knee	**genu**
Genu capsulae internae	Genu (of internal capsule)	**genu** Genu of the internal capsule
Genu corporis callosi	Genu (of corpus callosum)	**genu** Genu of the corpus callosum
Genu nervi facialis	Genu of facial nerve	**genu** Genu of the facial nerve
Gingivae	Gums	**gingiva**
Ginglymus	Hinge joint	**joint** Hinge joint
Glabella	Glabella	**glabella**
Glandula	Gland	**gland**
Glandulae areolares	Areolar glands	**gland** Areolar glands
Glandulae bronchiales	Bronchial glands	**gland** Bronchial glands
Glandulae buccales	Buccal glands	**gland** Buccal glands
Glandula bulbo-urethralis	Bulbo-urethral gland	**gland** Bulbo-urethral gland
Glandulae ceruminosae	Ceruminous glands	**gland** Ceruminous glands
Glandulae cervicales [uteri]	Cervical glands (of uterus)	**uterus** Coat of the uterus, mucous
Glandulae ciliares	Ciliary glands	**gland** Ciliary glands
Glandulae circumanales	Circumanal glands	**gland** Circumanal glands
Glandulae conjunctivales	Conjunctival glands	**gland** Conjunctival glands
Glandulae duodenales	Duodenal glands	**gland** Duodenal glands
Glandulae esophageae	Oesophageal glands	**gland** Oesophageal glands
Glandulae gastricae [propriae]	Gastric glands (proper)	**gland** Gastric glands, proper
Glandulae glomiformes	Glomiform glands	**gland** Glomiform glands
Glandulae intestinales (coli)	Intestinal glands (of colon)	**gland** Intestinal glands
Glandulae intestinales (intestini tenuis)	Intestinal glands (of small intestine)	**gland** Intestinal glands
Glandulae intestinales (recti)	Rectal glands	**gland** Rectal glands
Glandulae labiales	Labial glands	**gland** Labial glands
Glandula lacrimalis	Lacrimal gland	**gland** Lacrimal gland
Glandulae lacrimales accessoriae	Accessory lacrimal glands	**gland** Lacrimal glands, accessory
Glandulae laryngeae	Laryngeal glands	**gland** Laryngeal glands
Glandulae linguales	Lingual glands	**gland** Lingual glands

Nomina Anatomica (N.A.)	Birmingham Revision (B.R.) or English Equivalent	Definition Location
Glandula lingualis anterior	Anterior lingual gland	**gland** Lingual gland, anterior
Glandula mammaria	Mammary gland	**gland** Mammary gland
Glandulae molares	Molar glands	**gland** Molar glands
Glandula mucosa	Mucous gland	**gland** Mucous gland
Glandulae mucosae biliosae	Mucous bile glands	**gland** Mucous bile glands
Glandulae nasales	Nasal glands	**gland** Nasal glands
Glandulae oesophageae	Oesophageal glands	**gland** Oesophageal glands
Glandulae olfactoriae	Olfactory glands	**gland** Olfactory glands
Glandulae oris	Salivary glands	**gland** Salivary glands
Glandulae palatinae	Palatine glands	**gland** Palatine glands
Glandula parathyroidea inferior	Inferior parathyroid gland	**gland** Parathyroid glands
Glandula parathyroidea superior	Superior parathyroid gland	**gland** Parathyroid glands
Glandula parotis	Parotid gland	**gland** Parotid gland
Glandula parotis accessoria	Accessory parotid gland	**gland** Parotid gland, accessory
Glandulae pharyngeae	Pharyngeal glands	**gland** Pharyngeal glands
Glandulae preputiales	Preputial glands	**gland** Preputial glands
Glandulae pyloricae	Pyloric glands	**gland** Pyloric glands
Glandulae sebaceae	Sebaceous glands	**gland** Sebaceous glands
Glandula seromucosa	Seromucous gland	**gland** Seromucous gland
Glandula serosa	Serous gland	**gland** Serous gland
Glandulae sine ductibus	Ductless glands	**gland** Ductless glands
Glandula sublingualis	Sublingual gland	**gland** Sublingual gland
Glandula submandibularis	Submandibular gland	**gland** Submandibular gland
Glandulae sudoriferae	Sweat glands	**gland** Sweat glands
Glandula suprarenalis	Suprarenal gland	**gland** Suprarenal glands
Glandulae suprarenales accessoriae	Accessory suprarenal glands	**gland** Suprarenal glands, accessory
Glandulae tarsales	Tarsal glands	**gland** Tarsal glands
Glandula thyroidea	Thyroid gland	**gland** Thyroid gland
Glandulae thyroideae accessoriae	Accessory thyroid glands	**gland** Thyroid glands, accessory
Glandulae tracheales	Tracheal glands	**gland** Tracheal glands
Glandulae tubariae	Mucous glands (of pharyngotympanic tube)	**tube** Pharyngotympanic tube
Glandulae urethrales	Urethral glands	**gland** Urethral glands
Glandulae uterinae	Uterine glands	**uterus** Coat of the uterus, mucous
Glandula vestibularis major	Greater vestibular gland	**gland** Vestibular gland, greater
Glandulae vestibulares minores	Lesser vestibular glands	**gland** Vestibular glands, lesser
Glans clitoridis	Glans of clitoris	**glans** Glans of the clitoris

Anatomical Nomenclature

Nomina Anatomica (N.A.)	Birmingham Revision (B.R.) or English Equivalent	Definition Location
Glans penis	Glans penis	**glans** Glans penis
Globus pallidus	Globus pallidus	**globus** Globus pallidus
Glomerulus	Glomerulus	**glomerulus**
Glomeruli (renis)	Glomeruli (of kidney)	**kidney**
Glomeruli arteriosi cochleae	Arterial glomeruli of cochlea	**glomerulus** Arterial glomeruli of the cochlea
Glomus	Glomus	**glomus**
Glomus caroticum	Carotid body	**body** Carotid body
Glomus choroideum	Glomus choroideum	**glomus** Glomus choroideum
Glottis	Glottis	**glottis**
Gomphosis	Peg-and-socket suture	**suture** Peg-and-socket suture
Granulationes arachnoideales	Arachnoid granulations	**granulation** Arachnoid granulations
Gubernaculum testis	Gubernaculum testis	**gubernaculum** Gubernaculum testis
Gyrus	Gyrus	**gyrus**
Gyrus angularis	Middle part (of inferior parietal lobule)	**lobule** Parietal lobule
Gyri breves insulae	Short gyri of insula	**gyrus** Gyri of the insula long and short
Gyri cerebri	Cerebral gyri	**gyrus** Cerebral gyri
Gyrus cinguli	Gyrus cinguli	**gyrus** Gyrus cinguli
Gyrus dentatus	Dentate gyrus	**gyrus** Dentate gyrus
Gyrus fasciolaris	Splenial gyrus	**gyrus** Splenial gyrus
Gyrus frontalis inferior	Inferior frontal gyrus	**gyrus** Frontal gyrus, inferior
Gyrus frontalis medius	Middle frontal gyrus	**gyrus** Frontal gyrus, middle
Gyrus frontalis superior	Superior frontal gyrus	**gyrus** Frontal gyrus, superior
Gyrus lingualis (B.N.A.)	Lingual gyrus	**gyrus** Lingual gyrus
Gyrus longus insulae	Long gyrus of insula	**gyrus** Gyri of the insula, long and short
Gyrus occipito-temporalis lateralis	Lateral occipito-temporal gyrus	**gyrus** Occipitotemporal gyrus, lateral
Gyrus occipito-temporalis medialis	Medial occipito-temporal gyrus	**gyrus** Occipitotemporal gyrus, medial
Gyri orbitales	Orbital gyri	**gyrus** Orbital gyri of the orbital surface of the cerebral hemisphere
Gyrus parahippocampalis	Hippocampal gyrus	**gyrus** Hippocampal gyrus
Gyrus paraterminalis	Paraterminal gyrus	**gyrus** Paraterminal gyrus
Gyrus postcentralis	Postcentral gyrus	**gyrus** Postcentral gyrus
Gyrus precentralis	Precentral gyrus	**gyrus** Precentral gyrus
Gyrus rectus	Gyrus rectus	**gyrus** Gyrus rectus
Gyrus supramarginalis	Anterior part (of inferior parietal lobule)	**lobule** Parietal lobule
Gyrus temporalis inferior	Inferior temporal gyrus	**gyrus** Temporal gyrus, inferior
Gyrus temporalis medius	Middle temporal gyrus	**gyrus** Temporal gyrus, middle
Gyrus temporalis superior	Superior temporal gyrus	**gyrus** Temporal gyrus, superior
Gyri temporales transversi	Transverse temporal gyri	**gyrus** Temporal gyri, transverse
Habenula	Habenula	**habenula**
Hallux [digitus I]	Big (first) toe	**toe** Big toe
Hamulus lacrimalis	Lacrimal hamulus	**hamulus** Lacrimal hamulus
Hamulus laminae spiralis	Hamulus of spiral lamina	**hamulus** Hamulus of the spiral lamina
Hamulus ossis hamati	Hook of hamate bone	**hook** Hook of the hamate bone
Hamulus pterygoideus	Pterygoid hamulus	**hamulus** Pterygoid hamulus
Haustra coli	Sacculations of colon	**sacculation** Sacculations of the colon
Helicotrema	Helicotrema	**helicotrema**
Helix	Helix	**helix**
Hemispherium	Cerebral hemisphere	**hemisphere** Cerebral hemisphere
Hemispherium cerebelli	Cerebellar hemisphere	**hemisphere** Cerebellar hemisphere
Hepar	Liver	**liver**
Hiatus aorticus (diaphragmatis)	Aortic opening (of diaphragm)	**diaphragm** Opening in the diaphragm, aortic
Hiatus canalis nervi petrosi majoris	Hiatus for greater superficial petrosal nerve	**hiatus** Hiatus for the greater superficial petrosal nerve
Hiatus canalis nervi petrosi minoris	Hiatus for lesser superficial petrosal nerve	**hiatus** Hiatus for the lesser superficial petrosal nerve
Hiatus esophageus (diaphragmatis)	Oesophageal opening (of diaphragm)	**diaphragm** Opening in the diaphragm, oesophageal
Hiatus ethmoidalis	Ethmoidal hiatus	**hiatus** Ethmoidal hiatus
Hiatus maxillaris	Maxillary hiatus	**hiatus** Maxillary hiatus
Hiatus oesophageus (diaphragmatis)	Oesophageal opening (of diaphragm)	**diaphragm** Opening in the diaphragm, oesophageal
Hiatus sacralis	Sacral hiatus	**hiatus** Sacral hiatus
Hiatus saphenus	Saphenous opening (of fascia lata)	**fascia** Fascia lata, saphenous opening of the
Hiatus semilunaris	Hiatus semilunaris	**hiatus** Hiatus semilunaris
Hiatus tendineus [adductorius]	Opening in adductor magnus	**adductor magnus muscle** Opening
Hilus	Hilum	**hilum**
Hilus (glandulae suprarenalis)	Hilum (of suprarenal gland)	**gland** Suprarenal gland, hilum of a
Hilus (nodi lymphatici)	Hilum (of lymph gland)	**gland** Lymph gland, hilum of a
Hilus lienis	Hilum of spleen	**spleen** Hilum of the spleen
Hilus nuclei dentati	Hilum of dentate nucleus	**nucleus** Dentate nucleus, hilum of the
Hilus nuclei olivaris	Hilum of olivary nucleus	**nucleus** Olivary nucleus, hilum of the
Hilus ovarii	Hilum of ovary	**ovary** Hilum
Hilus pulmonis	Hilum of lung	**lung** Hilum of the lung
Hilus renalis	Hilum of kidney	**kidney**
Hippocampus	Hippocampus	**hippocampus**

Nomina Anatomica (N.A.)	Birmingham Revision (B.R.) or English Equivalent	Definition Location
Hirci	Axillary hairs	**hair** Axillary hairs
Horizontalis	Horizontal	**horizontal**
Humerus	Humerus	**humerus**
Humor	Humour	**humour**
Humor aquosus	Aqueous humour	**humour** Aqueous humour
Humor vitreus	Vitreous humour	**humour** Vitreous humour
Hymen	Hymen of vagina	**hymen**
Hyponychium	Hyponychium	**hyponychium**
Hypophysis [glandula pituitaria]	Hypophysis cerebri	**hypophysis** Hypophysis cerebri
Hypothalamus	Hypothalamus	**hypothalamus**
Hypothenar	Hypothenar eminence	**eminence** Hypothenar eminence
Ileum	Ileum	**ileum**
Impressio	Impression	**impression**
Impressio cardiaca (hepatis)	Cardiac impression (on liver)	**impression** Cardiac impression
Impressio cardiaca (pulmonis)	Cardiac impression (on lung)	**impression** Cardiac impression
Impressio colica (hepatis)	Colic impression (on liver)	**liver** Surface of the liver, lower
Impressiones digitatae	Impressions for (cerebral) gyri	**impression** Impressions for the cerebral gyri
Impressio duodenalis (hepatis)	Duodenal impression (on liver)	**liver** Surface of the liver, lower
Impressio esophagea (hepatis)	Oesophageal impression (on liver)	**impression** Oesophageal impression
Impressio gastrica (hepatis)	Gastric impression (on liver)	**liver** Surface of the liver, lower
Impressio ligamenti costoclavicularis	Impression for costoclavicular ligament	**impression** Impression for the costoclavicular ligament
Impressio petrosa (B.N.A.)	Petrous impression	**impression** Petrous impression
Impressio renalis (hepatis)	Renal impression (on liver)	**liver** Surface of the liver, lower
Impressio suprarenalis (hepatis)	Suprarenal impression (on liver)	**liver** Surface of the liver, lower
Impressio trigemini	Trigeminal impression	**impression** Trigeminal impression
Incisura	Notch	**incisura** *also* **notch**
Incisura acetabuli	Acetabular notch	**notch** Acetabular notch
Incisura angularis	Angular notch	**notch** Notch of the stomach, angular
Incisura anterior [auris]	Anterior notch of auricle	**notch** Anterior notch of the auricle
Incisura apicis cordis	Incisura apicis cordis	**incisura** Incisura apicis cordis
Incisura cardiaca	Cardiac notch	**notch** Notch of the stomach, cardiac
Incisura cardiaca pulmonis sinistri	Cardiac notch (of lung)	**notch** Notch of the lung, cardiac
Incisura cartilaginis meatus acustici	Incisura of cartilage of auditory meatus	**incisura** Incisura of the cartilage of the auditory meatus
Incisura clavicularis	Clavicular notch	**notch** Clavicular notch
Incisura costalis	Costal notch	**notch** Costal notch
Incisura ethmoidalis	Ethmoidal notch	**notch** Ethmoidal notch
Incisura fibularis	Fibular notch	**notch** Fibular notch
Incisura (sive foramen) frontalis	Frontal notch	**notch** Frontal notch

Nomina Anatomica (N.A.)	Birmingham Revision (B.R.) or English Equivalent	Definition Location
Incisura interarytenoidea	Interarytenoid notch	**notch** Interarytenoid notch
Incisura intertragica	Incisura intertragica	**incisura** Incisura intertragica
Incisura ischiadica major	Greater sciatic notch	**notch** Sciatic notch, greater
Incisura ischiadica minor	Lesser sciatic notch	**notch** Sciatic notch, lesser
Incisura jugularis (ossis occipitalis)	Jugular notch (of occipital bone)	**notch** Jugular notch
Incisura jugularis (sterni)	Suprasternal notch	**notch** Suprasternal notch
Incisura lacrimalis	Lacrimal notch	**notch** Lacrimal notch
Incisura ligamenti teretis	Notch for ligamentum teres	**notch** Notch for the ligamentum teres
Incisura mandibulae	Mandibular notch	**notch** Mandibular notch
Incisura mastoidea	Mastoid notch	**notch** Mastoid notch
Incisura nasalis	Nasal notch	**notch** Nasal notch
Incisura pancreatis	Pancreatic notch	**notch** Pancreatic notch
Incisura parietalis	Parietal notch	**notch** Parietal notch
Incisura pre-occipitalis	Pre-occipital notch	**notch** Pre-occipital notch
Incisura pterygoidea	Pterygoid notch	**notch** Pterygoid notch
Incisura radialis	Radial notch	**notch** Radial notch
Incisura scapulae	Suprascapular notch	**notch** Suprascapular notch
Incisura sphenopalatina	Sphenopalatine notch	**notch** Sphenopalatine notch
Incisura (sive foramen) supra-orbitalis	Supra-orbital notch	**notch** Supra-orbital notch
Incisura tentorii	Tentorial notch	**notch** Tentorial notch
Incisura terminalis auris	Incisura terminalis of auricle	**incisura** Incisura terminalis of the auricle
Incisura thyroidea inferior	Inferior thyroid notch	**notch** Thyroid notch, inferior
Incisura thyroidea superior	Thyroid notch	**notch** Thyroid notch
Incisura trochlearis	Trochlear notch	**notch** Trochlear notch
Incisura tympanica	Tympanic notch	**notch** Tympanic notch
Incisura ulnaris	Ulnar notch	**notch** Ulnar notch
Incisura vertebralis inferior	Inferior vertebral notch	**notch** Vertebral notch, inferior
Incisura vertebralis superior	Superior vertebral notch	**notch** Vertebral notch, superior
Inclinatio pelvis	Inclination of pelvis	**inclination** Inclination of the pelvis
Incus	Incus	**incus**
Index [digitus II]	Index finger	**finger** Index finger
Indusium griseum	Indusium griseum (of corpus callosum)	**indusium** Indusium griseum
Inferior	Inferior	**inferior**
Infundibulum	Infundibulum	**infundibulum**
Infundibulum ethmoidale	Infundibulum of the ethmoid	**infundibulum** Infundibulum of the ethmoid
Infundibulum tubae uterinae	Infundibulum (of uterine tube)	**infundibulum** Infundibulum of the uterine tube

Anatomical Nomenclature

Nomina Anatomica (N.A.)	Birmingham Revision (B.R.) or English Equivalent	Definition Location
Inguen	Groin	**groin**
Inion	Inion	**inion**
Insula	Insula	**insula**
Integumentum commune	Common integument	**integument** Common integument
Intermedius	Intermediate	**intermediate**
Internus	Internal	**internal**
Intersectiones tendineae	Tendinous intersections	**intersection** Tendinous intersection
Intestinum crassum	Large intestine	**intestine** Large intestine
Intestinum tenue	Small intestine	**intestine** Small intestine
Intumescentia cervicalis	Cervical enlargement (of spinal cord)	**enlargement** Cervical enlargement of the spinal cord
Intumescentia lumbalis	Lumbar enlargement (of spinal cord)	**enlargement** Lumbar enlargement of the spinal cord
Iris	Iris	**iris**
Isthmus	Isthmus	**isthmus**
Isthmus aortae	Aortic isthmus	**isthmus** Aortic isthmus
Isthmus cartilaginis auris	Isthmus of the auricular cartilage	**isthmus** Isthmus of the auricular cartilage
Isthmus faucium	Oropharyngeal isthmus	**isthmus** Oropharyngeal isthmus
Isthmus glandulae thyroideae	Isthmus of thyroid gland	**isthmus** Isthmus of the thyroid gland
Isthmus gyri cinguli	Isthmus of gyrus cinguli	**isthmus** Isthmus of the gyrus cinguli
Isthmus prostatae	Isthmus of prostate	**isthmus** Isthmus of the prostate
Isthmus rhombencephali	Isthmus rhombencephali	**isthmus** Isthmus rhombencephali
Isthmus tubae auditivae	Isthmus of tube	**isthmus** Isthmus of the pharyngotympanic tube
Isthmus tubae uterinae	Isthmus (of uterine tube)	**isthmus** Isthmus of the uterine tube
Isthmus uteri	Isthmus of uterus	**isthmus** Isthmus of the uterus
Jejunum	Jejunum	**jejunum**
Juga alveolaria (corporis mandibulae)	Alveolar juga (of body of mandible)	**jugum** Alveolar juga
Juga alveolaria (corporis maxillae)	Alveolar juga (of body of maxilla)	**jugum** Alveolar juga
Junctura cartilaginea	Cartilaginous joint	**joint** Cartilaginous joint
Junctura fibrosa	Fibrous joint	**joint** Fibrous joint
Junctura lumbosacralis	Lumbosacral joint	**joint** Lumbosacral joint
Junctura ossium	Joint	**joint**
Junctura sacrococcygea	Sacrococcygeal joint	**joint** Sacrococcygeal joint
Junctura synovialis [articulatio]	Synovial joint	**joint** Synovial joint
Junctura zygapophyseales	Zygapophyseal joints	**joint** Zygapophyseal joints
Labium	Labium	**labium**
Labium anterius (ostii uteri)	Anterior lip (of os uteri)	**uterus** Neck of the uterus
Labium externum (cristae iliacae)	Outer lip (of iliac crest)	**ilium** Outer lip
Labium inferius	Lower lip	**lip**
Labium internum (cristae iliacae)	Inner lip (of iliac crest)	**ilium** Inner lip
Labium laterale (lineae asperae)	Lateral lip (of linea aspera)	**linea** Linea aspera

Nomina Anatomica (N.A.)	Birmingham Revision (B.R.) or English Equivalent	Definition Location
Labium limbi tympanicum	Tympanic lip	**lip** Tympanic lip
Labium limbi vestibulare	Vestibular lip	**lip** Vestibular lip
Labium majus pudendi	Labium majus	**labium** Labium majus
Labium mediale (lineae asperae)	Medial lip (of linea aspera)	**linea** Linea aspera
Labium minus pudendi	Labium minus	**labium** Labium minus
Labia oris	Lips	**lip**
Labium posterius (ostii uteri)	Posterior lip (of os uteri)	**uterus** Neck of the uterus
Labium superius	Upper lip	**lip**
Labrum acetabulare	Labrum acetabulare	**labrum** Labrum acetabulare
Labrum glenoidale	Labrum glenoidale	**labrum** Labrum glenoidale
Labyrinthus ethmoidalis	Ethmoidal labyrinth	**labyrinth** Ethmoidal labyrinth
Labyrinthus membranaceus	Membranous labyrinth	**labyrinth** Membranous labyrinth
Labyrinthus osseus	Bony labyrinth	**labyrinth** Bony labyrinth
Lacertus musculi recti lateralis	Lacertus of lateral rectus muscle of orbit	**lacertus** Lacertus of the lateral rectus muscle of the orbit
Lacuna	Lacuna	**lacuna**
Lacuna musculorum	Lacuna musculorum	**lacuna** Lacuna musculorum
Lacunae urethrales	Lacunae urethrales	**lacuna** Lacunae urethrales
Lacuna vasorum	Lacuna vasorum	**lacuna** Lacuna vasorum
Lacus lacrimalis	Lacus lacrimalis	**lacus lacrimalis**
Lamina	Lamina	**lamina**
Lamina [dextra et sinistra] (cartilaginis thyroideae)	Lamina (right and left) (of thyroid cartilage)	**cartilage** Thyroid cartilage
Lamina affixa	Lamina affixa	**lamina** Lamina affixa
Lamina alaris	Alar lamina	**lamina** Alar lamina
Laminae albae	White laminae	**lamina** White lamina
Lamina anterior (vaginae musculi recti abdominis)	Anterior lamina (of sheath of rectus abdominis muscle)	**sheath** Sheath of the rectus abdominis muscle
Lamina arcus vertebrae	Lamina (of vertebral arch)	**lamina** Lamina of the vertebral arch
Lamina basalis	Basal lamina	**lamina** Basal lamina
Lamina basalis (choroideae)	Basal lamina (of choroid)	**lamina** Basal lamina of the choroid
Lamina basalis (corporis ciliaris)	Basal lamina (of ciliary body)	**lamina** Basal lamina of the ciliary body
Lamina basilaris	Basilar lamina	**lamina** Basilar lamina
Lamina cartilaginis cricoideae	Lamina of cricoid cartilage	**cartilage** Cricoid cartilage
Lamina choroidocapillaris	Choriocapillary lamina	**lamina** Choriocapillary lamina
Lamina cribrosa	Cribriform plate	**plate** Cribriform plate
Lamina episcleralis	Lamina cribrosa sclerae	**lamina** Lamina cribrosa sclerae
Lamina epithelialis	Lamina epithelialis	**lamina** Lamina epithelialis
Lamina externa (cranii)	Outer table (of skull)	**table** Table of the skull, outer

Nomina Anatomica (N.A.)	Birmingham Revision (B.R.) or English Equivalent	Definition Location
Lamina fusca sclerae	Lamina fusca sclerae	**lamina** Lamina fusca sclerae
Lamina horizontalis (ossis palatini)	Horizontal plate (of palatine bone)	**plate** Horizontal plate of the palatine bone
Lamina interna (cranii)	Inner table (of skull)	**table** Table of the skull, inner
Lamina [cartilaginis] lateralis (tubae auditivae)	Lateral lamina (of pharyngotympanic tube)	**lamina** Lamina of the pharyngotympanic tube, lateral
Lamina lateralis processus pterygoidei	Lateral pterygoid plate	**plate** Pterygoid plate, lateral
Lamina limitans anterior (corneae)	Anterior elastic lamina (of cornea)	**lamina** Elastic lamina, anterior
Lamina limitans posterior	Posterior elastic lamina	**lamina** Elastic lamina, posterior
Lamina [cartilaginis] medialis (tubae auditivae)	Medial lamina (of pharyngotympanic tube)	**lamina** Lamina of the pharyngotympanic tube, medial
Lamina medialis processus pterygoidei	Medial pterygoid plate	**plate** Pterygoid plate, medial
Lamina medullaris lateralis (thalami)	External medullary lamina (of thalamus)	**lamina** Medullary lamina of the thalamus, external
Lamina medullaris medialis (thalami)	Internal medullary lamina (of thalamus)	**lamina** Medullary lamina of the thalamus, internal
Laminae medullares thalami	Medullary laminae of thalamus	**lamina** Medullary laminae of the thalamus
Lamina membranacea (tubae auditivae)	Membranous lamina (of pharyngo-tympanic tube)	**lamina** Lamina of the pharyngotympanic tube, membranous
Lamina modioli	Lamina of modiolus	**lamina** Lamina of the modiolus
Lamina muscularis mucosae (coli)	Lamina muscularis mucosae (of colon)	**lamina** Lamina muscularis mucosae
Lamina muscularis mucosae (esophagi)	Lamina muscularis mucosae (of oesophagus)	**lamina** Lamina muscularis mucosae
Lamina muscularis mucosae (intestini tenuis)	Lamina muscularis mucosae (of small intestine)	**lamina** Lamina muscularis mucosae
Lamina muscularis mucosae (recti)	Lamina muscularis mucosae (of rectum)	**lamina** Lamina muscularis mucosae
Lamina muscularis mucosae (ventriculi)	Lamina muscularis mucosae (of stomach)	**lamina** Lamina muscularis mucosae
Lamina orbitalis	Orbital plate (of ethmoid bone)	**plate** Orbital plate of the ethmoid bone
Lamina parietalis (pericardii serosi)	Parietal layer (of serous pericardium)	**pericardium**
Lamina parietalis (tunicae vaginalis testis)	Parietal layer (of tunica vaginalis testis)	**tunica** Tunica vaginalis testis
Lamina perpendicularis (ossis ethmoidalis)	Perpendicular plate (of ethmoid bone)	**plate** Perpendicular plate of the ethmoid bone
Lamina perpendicularis (ossis palatini)	Perpendicular plate (of palatine bone)	**plate** Perpendicular plate of the palatine bone
Lamina posterior (vaginae musculi recti abdominis)	Posterior lamina (of sheath of rectus abdominis muscle)	**sheath** Sheath of the rectus abdominis muscle
Lamina pretrachealis	Pretracheal fascia	**fascia** Pretracheal fascia
Lamina prevertebralis	Prevertebral fascia	**fascia** Prevertebral fascia
Lamina profunda (fasciae temporalis)	Deep layer (of temporal fascia)	**fascia** Temporal fascia
Lamina profunda (musculi levatoris palpebrae superioris)	Lower lamella (of levator palpebrae superioris muscle)	**levator palpebrae superioris muscle of the orbit**
Lamina propria mucosae	Lamina propria mucosae	**lamina** Lamina propria mucosae
Laminae septi pellucidi	Laminae of septum lucidum	**lamina** Laminae of the septum lucidum
Lamina spiralis ossea	Osseous spiral lamina	**lamina** Osseous spiral lamina
Lamina spiralis secundaria	Secondary spiral lamina	**lamina** Secondary spiral lamina
Lamina superficialis (fasciae cervicalis)	Superficial layer (of deep cervical fascia)	**fascia** Cervical fascia, deep
Lamina superficialis (fasciae temporalis)	Superficial layer (of temporal fascia)	**fascia** Temporal fascia
Lamina superficialis (musculi levatoris palpebrae superioris)	Upper lamella (of levator palpebrae superioris muscle)	**levator palpebrae superioris muscle of the orbit**
Lamina suprachoroidea	Suprachoroid lamina	**lamina** Suprachoroid lamina
Lamina tecti	Tectal lamina	**lamina** Tectal lamina
Lamina terminalis	Lamina terminalis	**lamina** Lamina terminalis
Lamina tragi	Lamina of tragus	**lamina** Lamina of the tragus
Lamina vasculosa (choroideae)	Vascular lamina (of choroid)	**lamina** Vascular lamina of the choroid
Lamina visceralis [epicardium]	Visceral layer (epicardium)	**pericardium**
Lamina visceralis (tunicae vaginalis testis)	Visceral layer (of tunica vaginalis testis)	**tunica** Tunica vaginalis testis
Lanugo	Down	**down**
Larynx	Larynx	**larynx**
Lateralis	Lateral	**lateral**
Latus	Flank	**flank**
Lemniscus	Lemniscus	**lemniscus**
Lemniscus lateralis	Lateral lemniscus	**lemniscus** Lateral lemniscus
Lemniscus medialis	Medial lemniscus	**lemniscus** Medial lemniscus
Lemniscus spinalis	Spinal lemniscus	**lemniscus** Spinal lemniscus
Lemniscus trigeminalis	Trigeminal lemniscus	**lemniscus** Trigeminal lemniscus
Lens	Lens	**lens**
Lien	Spleen	**spleen**
Lien accessorius	Accessory spleen	**spleen** Accessory spleen
Ligamentum	Ligament	**ligament**
Ligamentum acromioclaviculare	Acromioclavicular ligament	**ligament** Acromioclavicular ligament
Ligamentum alare	Alar ligament of odontoid process	**ligament** Alar ligament of the odontoid process
Ligamentum anococcygeum	Anococcygeal body	**body** Anococcygeal body
Ligamenta anularia [trachealia]	Annular ligaments (of trachea)	**ligament** Annular ligaments of the trachea
Ligamentum anulare radii	Annular ligament of radius	**ligament** Annular ligament of the radius
Ligamentum anulare stapedis	Annular ligament of base of stapes	**ligament** Annular ligament of the base of the stapes
Ligamentum apicis dentis	Apical ligament of odontoid process	**ligament** Apical ligament of the odontoid process

Anatomical Nomenclature

Nomina Anatomica (N.A.)	Birmingham Revision (B.R.) or English Equivalent	Definition Location
Ligamentum arcuatum laterale	Lateral arcuate ligament (of diaphragm)	**ligament** Arcuate ligament, lateral
Ligamentum arcuatum mediale	Medial arcuate ligament (of diaphragm)	**ligament** Arcuate ligament, medial
Ligamentum arcuatum medianum	Median arcuate ligament (of diaphragm)	**ligament** Arcuate ligament, median
Ligamentum arcuatum pubis	Inferior pubic ligament	**ligament** Pubic ligaments
Ligamentum arteriosum	Ligamentum arteriosum	**ligamentum** Ligamentum arteriosum
Ligamenta auricularia	Auricular ligaments	**ligament** Auricular ligaments
Ligamentum auriculare anterius	Anterior ligament of auricle	**ligament** Auricular ligaments
Ligamentum auriculare posterius	Posterior ligament of auricle	**ligament** Auricular ligaments
Ligamentum auriculare superius	Superior ligament of auricle	**ligament** Auricular ligaments
Ligamentum bifurcatum	Bifurcated ligament	**ligament** Bifurcated ligament
Ligamentum calcaneocuboideum	Medial calcaneo-cuboid ligament	**ligament** Calcaneocuboid ligaments
Ligamentum calcaneo-cuboideum plantare	Short plantar ligament	**ligament** Ligaments of the tarsus, plantar
Ligamentum calcaneo-fibulare	Calcaneofibular ligament	**ligament** Calcaneofibular ligament
Ligamentum calcaneo-naviculare	Lateral calcaneo-navicular ligament	**ligament** Calcaneonavicular ligaments
Ligamentum calcaneo-naviculare plantare	Plantar calcaneo-navicular ligament ("spring" ligament)	**ligament** Calcaneonavicular ligaments
Ligamentum capitis costae intra-articulare	Intra-articular ligament of joint of head of rib	**ligament** Intra-articular ligament of the joint of the head of a rib
Ligamentum capitis costae radiatum	Radiate ligament (of joint of head of rib)	**ligament** Radiate ligaments
Ligamentum capitis femoris	Ligament of head of femur	**ligament** Ligament of the head of the femur
Ligamentum capitis fibulae anterius	Anterior ligament of superior tibiofibular joint	**ligament** Ligaments of the head of the fibula
Ligamentum capitis fibulae posterius	Posterior ligament of superior tibiofibular joint	**ligament** Ligaments of the head of the fibula
Ligamentum carpi radiatum	Radiate carpal ligament	**ligament** Carpal ligaments
Ligamenta carpometa-carpea dorsalia	Dorsal carpometa-carpal ligaments	**ligament** Carpometacarpal ligaments
Ligamenta carpometa-carpea palmaria	Palmar carpometa-carpal ligaments	**ligament** Carpometacarpal ligaments
Ligamenta collateralia	Collateral ligaments	**ligament** Collateral ligaments
Ligamenta collateralia (articulationum meta-carpophalangearum)	Collateral ligaments (of metacarpo-phalangeal joints)	**ligament** Collateral ligaments
Ligamenta collateralia (articulationum meta-tarsophalangearum)	Collateral ligaments (of metatarso-phalangeal joints)	**ligament** Collateral ligaments
Ligamentum collaterale carpi radiale	Lateral ligament (of wrist)	**ligament** Ligament of the wrist, lateral
Ligamentum collaterale carpi ulnare	Medial ligament (of wrist)	**ligament** Ligament of the wrist, medial
Ligamentum collaterale fibulare	Lateral ligament (of knee)	**ligament** Ligament of the knee, lateral

Nomina Anatomica (N.A.)	Birmingham Revision (B.R.) or English Equivalent	Definition Location
Ligamentum collaterale radiale (articulationis cubiti)	Lateral ligament (of elbow)	**ligament** Ligament of the elbow, radial collateral
Ligamentum collaterale tibiale	Medial ligament (of knee)	**ligament** Ligament of the knee, medial
Ligamentum collaterale ulnare (articulationis cubiti)	Medial ligament (of elbow)	**ligament** Ligament of the elbow, ulnar collateral
Ligamentum conoideum	Conoid part (of coracoclavicular ligament)	**ligament** Conoid ligament
Ligamentum coraco-acromiale	Coraco-acromial ligament	**ligament** Coraco-acromial ligament of the shoulder girdle
Ligamentum coracoclaviculare	Coracoclavicular ligament	**ligament** Coracoclavicular ligament
Ligamentum coracohumerale	Coracohumeral ligament	**ligament** Coracohumeral ligament
Ligamentum coronarium hepatis	Coronary ligament of liver	**ligament** Coronary ligament of the liver
Ligamentum costoclaviculare	Costoclavicular ligament	**ligament** Costoclavicular ligament
Ligamentum costotransversarium	Inferior costo-transverse ligament	**ligament** Costotransverse ligament, inferior
Ligamentum costo-transversarium laterale	Lateral costo-transverse ligament	**ligament** Costotransverse ligament, lateral
Ligamentum costo-transversarium superius	Superior costo-transverse ligament	**ligament** Costotransverse ligaments, superior
Ligamenta costoxiphoidea	Costoxiphoid ligaments	**ligament** Costoxiphoid ligaments
Ligamentum crico-arytenoideum posterius	Posterior crico-arytenoid ligament	**ligament** Crico-arytenoid ligament, posterior
Ligamentum cricopharyngeum	Cricopharyngeal ligament	**ligament** Cricopharyngeal ligament
Ligamentum cricothyroideum	Cricothyroid ligament	**ligament** Cricothyroid ligament
Ligamentum cricotracheale	Cricotracheal ligament	**ligament** Cricotracheal ligament
Ligamentum cruciatum anterius	Anterior cruciate ligament	**ligament** Cruciate ligament of the knee, anterior
Ligamenta cruciata genus	Cruciate ligaments of knee	**ligament** Cruciate ligaments of the knee
Ligamentum cruciatum posterius	Posterior cruciate ligament	**ligament** Cruciate ligament of the knee, posterior
Ligamentum cruciforme atlantis	Cruciate ligament of atlas	**ligament** Cruciate ligament of the atlas
Ligamentum cuboideo-naviculare dorsale	Dorsal cubonavicular ligament	**ligament** Cubonavicular ligaments
Ligamentum cuboideo-naviculare plantare	Plantar cubonavicular ligament	**ligament** Cubonavicular ligaments
Ligamentum cuneo-cuboideum dorsale	Dorsal cuneocuboid ligament	**ligament** Cuneocuboid ligaments
Ligamentum cuneo-cuboideum interosseum	Interosseous cuneo-cuboid ligament	**ligament** Cuneocuboid ligaments
Ligamentum cuneo-cuboideum plantare	Plantar cuneocuboid ligament	**ligament** Cuneocuboid ligaments
Ligamenta cuneo-metatarsea interossea	Interosseous tarso-metatarsal ligaments	**ligament** Tarsometatarsal ligaments
Ligamenta cuneo-navicularia dorsalia	Dorsal cuneo-navicular ligaments	**ligament** Cuneonavicular ligaments
Ligamenta cuneo-navicularia plantaria	Plantar cuneo-navicular ligaments	**ligament** Cuneonavicular ligaments
Ligamentum deltoideum [mediale]	Deltoid ligament	**ligament** Deltoid ligament
Ligamentum denticulatum	Ligamentum denticulatum	**ligamentum** Ligamentum denticulatum

Nomina Anatomica (N.A.)	Birmingham Revision (B.R.) or English Equivalent	Definition Location
Ligamentum epididymidis inferius	Inferior epididymal ligament	**ligament** Epididymal ligaments
Ligamentum epididymidis superius	Superior epididymal ligament	**ligament** Epididymal ligaments
Ligamenta extracapsularia	Extracapsular ligaments	**ligament** Capsular ligament
Ligamentum falciforme hepatis	Falciform ligament of liver	**ligament** Falciform ligament of the liver
Ligamenta flava	Ligamenta flava	**ligamentum** Ligamenta flava
Ligamentum fundiforme penis	Fundiform ligament of penis	**ligament** Fundiform ligament of the penis
Ligamentum gastrocolicum	Gastrocolic ligament	**ligament** Gastrocolic ligament
Ligamentum gastrolienale	Gastrosplenic ligament	**ligament** Gastrosplenic ligament
Ligamentum gastrophrenicum	Gastrophrenic ligament	**ligament** Gastrophrenic ligament
Ligamentum genito-inguinale	Genito-inguinal ligament	**ligament** Genito-inguinal ligament
Ligamenta glenohumeralia	Glenohumeral ligaments	**ligament** Glenohumeral ligaments
Ligamentum hepatocolicum	Hepatocolic ligament	**ligament** Hepatocolic ligament
Ligamentum hepatoduodenale	Hepatoduodenal ligament	**ligament** Hepatoduodenal ligament
Ligamentum hepatogastricum	Hepatogastric ligament	**ligament** Hepatogastric ligament
Ligamentum hepatorenale	Hepatorenal ligament	**ligament** Hepatorenal ligament
Ligamentum hyo-epiglotticum	Hyo-epiglottic ligament	**ligament** Hyo-epiglottic ligament
Ligamentum iliofemorale	Iliofemoral ligament	**ligament** Iliofemoral ligament
Ligamentum iliolumbale	Iliolumbar ligament	**ligament** Iliolumbar ligament
Ligamentum incudis posterius	Posterior ligament of incus	**ligament** Ligaments of the incus
Ligamentum incudis superius	Superior ligament of incus	**ligament** Ligaments of the incus
Ligamentum inguinale	Inguinal ligament	**ligament** Inguinal ligament
Ligamenta intercarpea dorsalia	Dorsal intercarpal ligaments	**ligament** Intercarpal ligaments
Ligamenta intercarpea interossea	Interosseous intercarpal ligaments	**ligament** Intercarpal ligaments
Ligamenta intercarpea palmaria	Palmar intercarpal ligaments	**ligament** Intercarpal ligaments
Ligamentum interclaviculare	Interclavicular ligament	**ligament** Interclavicular ligament
Ligamenta intercuneiformia dorsalia	Dorsal intercuneiform ligaments	**ligament** Intercuneiform ligaments
Ligamenta intercuneiformia interossea	Interosseous intercuneiform ligaments	**ligament** Intercuneiform ligaments
Ligamenta intercuneiformia plantaria	Plantar intercuneiform ligaments	**ligament** Intercuneiform ligaments
Ligamentum interfoveolare	Interfoveolar ligament	**ligament** Interfoveolar ligament
Ligamenta interspinalia	Interspinous ligaments	**ligament** Interspinous ligaments
Ligamenta intertransversaria	Intertransverse ligaments	**ligament** Intertransverse ligaments
Ligamenta intracapsularia	Intracapsular ligaments	**ligament** Capsular ligament
Ligamentum ischiofemorale	Ischiofemoral ligament	**ligament** Ischiofemoral ligament
Ligamentum lacunare	Pectineal part (of inguinal ligament)	**ligament** Inguinal ligament, pectineal part of the
Ligamentum laterale (articulationis temporomandibularis)	Temporomandibular ligament	**ligament** Temporomandibular ligament
Ligamentum latum uteri	Broad ligament of uterus	**ligament** Broad ligament of the uterus
Ligamentum longitudinale anterius	Anterior longitudinal ligament	**ligament** Longitudinal ligaments
Ligamentum longitudinale posterius	Posterior longitudinal ligament	**ligament** Longitudinal ligaments
Ligamentum lumbocostale	Lumbocostal ligament	**ligament** Lumbocostal ligament
Ligamentum mallei anterius	Anterior ligament of malleus	**ligament** Ligaments of the malleus
Ligamentum mallei laterale	Lateral ligament of malleus	**ligament** Ligaments of the malleus
Ligamentum mallei superius	Superior ligament of malleus	**ligament** Ligaments of the malleus
Ligamentum mediale [deltoideum]	Medial ligament	**ligament** Medial ligament
Ligamentum meniscofemorale anterius	Anterior meniscofemoral ligament	**ligament** Meniscofemoral ligament, anterior
Ligamentum meniscofemorale posterius	Posterior meniscofemoral ligament	**ligament** Meniscofemoral ligament, posterior
Ligamenta metacarpea dorsalia	Dorsal metacarpal ligaments	**ligament** Metacarpal ligaments, dorsal
Ligamenta metacarpea interossea	Interosseous metacarpal ligaments	**ligament** Metacarpal ligaments, interosseous
Ligamenta metacarpea palmaria	Palmar metacarpal ligaments	**ligament** Metacarpal ligaments, palmar
Ligamenta metacarpea transversa profunda	Deep transverse ligaments of palm	**ligament** Ligaments of the palm, deep transverse
Ligamentum metacarpeum transversum superficiale	Superficial transverse metacarpal ligament	**ligament** Metacarpal ligament, superficial transverse
Ligamenta metatarsea dorsalia	Dorsal metatarsal ligaments	**ligament** Metatarsal ligaments, dorsal
Ligamenta metatarsea interossea	Interosseous metatarsal ligaments	**ligament** Metatarsal ligaments, interosseous
Ligamenta metatarsea plantaria	Plantar metatarsal ligaments	**ligament** Metatarsal ligaments, plantar
Ligamenta metatarsea transversa profunda	Deep transverse ligaments of sole	**ligament** Ligaments of the sole, deep transverse
Ligamentum metatarseum transversum superficiale	Superficial transverse metatarsal ligament	**ligament** Metatarsal ligaments, superficial transverse
Ligamentum nuchae	Ligamentum nuchae	**ligamentum** Ligamentum nuchae
Ligamentum ovarii proprium	Ligament of ovary	**ligament** Ligament of the ovary
Ligamenta palmaria	Palmar ligaments of metacarpophalangeal joint	**ligament** Ligaments of the metacarpophalangeal joint, palmar
Ligamentum palpebrale laterale	Lateral palpebral ligament	**ligament** Palpebral ligaments
Ligamentum palpebrale mediale	Medial palpebral ligament	**ligament** Palpebral ligaments
Ligamentum patellae	Ligamentum patellae	**ligamentum** Ligamentum patellae
Ligamentum pectinatum anguli iridocornealis	Pectinate ligament of iris	**ligament** Pectinate ligament of the iris
Ligamentum pectineale	Pectineal ligament	**ligament** Pectineal ligament
Ligamentum phrenicocolicum	Phrenicocolic ligament	**ligament** Phrenicocolic ligament

Anatomical Nomenclature

Nomina Anatomica (N.A.)	Birmingham Revision (B.R.) or English Equivalent	Definition Location
Ligamentum phrenico-lienale [ligamentum lienorenale]	Lienorenal ligament	**ligament** Lienorenal ligament
Ligamentum pisohamatum	Pisohamate ligament	**ligament** Pisohamate ligament
Ligamentum pisometacarpeum	Pisometacarpal ligament	**ligament** Pisometacarpal ligament
Ligamentum plantare	Plantar ligament of metatarsophalangeal joint	**ligament** Ligament of the metatarsophalangeal joint, plantar
Ligamentum plantare longum	Long plantar ligament	**ligament** Ligaments of the tarsus, plantar
Ligamentum popliteum arcuatum	Arcuate ligament of knee	**ligament** Arcuate ligament of the knee
Ligamentum popliteum obliquum	Oblique posterior ligament of knee	**ligament** Oblique posterior ligament of the knee
Ligamentum pterygospinale	Pterygospinous ligament	**ligament** Pterygospinous ligament
Ligamentum pubicum superius	Superior pubic ligament	**ligament** Pubic ligaments
Ligamentum pubofemorale	Pubofemoral ligament	**ligament** Pubofemoral ligament
Ligamentum pubo-prostaticum [pubovesicale]	Puboprostatic (or pubovesical) ligament	**ligament** Puboprostatic (pubo-vesical) ligaments
Ligamentum pulmonale	Pulmonary ligament	**ligament** Pulmonary ligament
Ligamentum quadratum	Quadrate ligament	**ligament** Quadrate ligament of the superior radio-ulnar joint
Ligamentum radio-carpeum dorsale	Posterior radiocarpal ligament	**ligament** Radiocarpal ligaments
Ligamentum radio-carpeum palmare	Anterior radiocarpal ligament	**ligament** Radiocarpal ligaments
Ligamentum reflexum	Reflected part (of inguinal ligament)	**ligament** Inguinal ligament, reflected part of the
Ligamentum sacrococcygeum dorsale profundum	Deep posterior sacrococcygeal ligament	**ligament** Sacrococcygeal ligaments
Ligamentum sacrococcygeum dorsale superficiale	Superficial posterior sacroccocygeal ligament	**ligament** Sacrococcygeal ligaments
Ligamentum sacrococcygeum laterale	Lateral sacrococcygeal ligament	**ligament** Sacrococcygeal ligaments
Ligamentum sacro-coccygeum ventrale	Anterior sacro-coccygeal ligament	**ligament** Sacrococcygeal ligaments
Ligamenta sacro-iliaca dorsalia	Posterior sacro-iliac ligaments	**ligament** Sacro-iliac ligaments
Ligamenta sacro-iliaca interossea	Interosseous sacro-iliac ligaments	**ligament** Sacro-iliac ligaments
Ligamentum sacro-iliacum ventralium	Anterior sacro-iliac ligament	**ligament** Sacro-iliac ligaments
Ligamentum sacrospinale	Sacrospinous ligament	**ligament** Sacrospinous ligament
Ligamentum sacrotuberale	Sacrotuberous ligament	**ligament** Sacrotuberous ligament
Ligamentum sphenomandibulare	Sphenomandibular ligament	**ligament** Sphenomandibular ligament
Ligamentum spirale cochleae	Spiral ligament of cochlea	**ligament** Spiral ligament of the cochlea
Ligamentum sterno-claviculare anterius	Anterior sterno-clavicular ligament	**ligament** Sternoclavicular ligaments
Ligamentum sterno-claviculare posterius	Posterior sterno-clavicular ligament	**ligament** Sternoclavicular ligaments
Ligamentum sternocostale intra-articulare	Intra-articular (sternocostal) ligament	**ligament** Intra-articular ligament of a sternocostal joint
Ligamenta sterno-costalia radiata	Sternocostal ligaments	**ligament** Sternocostal ligaments
Ligamenta sterno-pericardiaca	Sternopericardial ligaments	**ligament** Sternopericardial ligaments
Ligamentum stylohyoideum	Stylohyoid ligament	**ligament** Stylohyoid ligament
Ligamentum stylomandibulare	Stylomandibular ligament	**ligament** Stylomandibular ligament
Ligamenta supraspinalia	Supraspinous ligaments	**ligament** Supraspinous ligaments
Ligamentum suspensorium clitoridis	Suspensory ligament of clitoris	**ligament** Suspensory ligament of the clitoris
Ligamenta suspensoria mammae	Suspensory ligaments of the breast	**ligament** Suspensory ligaments of the breast
Ligamentum suspensorium ovarii	Infundibulopelvic ligament	**ligament** Infundibulopelvic ligament
Ligamentum suspensorium penis	Suspensory ligament of penis	**ligament** Suspensory ligament of the penis
Ligamentum talo-calcaneum interosseum	Interosseous talo-calcanean ligament	**ligament** Talocalcanean ligaments
Ligamentum talo-calcaneum laterale	Lateral talo-calcanean ligament	**ligament** Talocalcanean ligaments
Ligamentum talo-calcaneum mediale	Medial talocalcanean ligament	**ligament** Talocalcanean ligaments
Ligamentum talo-fibulare anterius	Anterior talofibular ligament	**ligament** Talofibular ligaments
Ligamentum talo-fibulare posterius	Posterior talofibular ligament	**ligament** Talofibular ligaments
Ligamentum talonaviculare	Talonavicular ligament (dorsal)	**ligament** Talonavicular ligaments
Ligamenta tarsi dorsalia	Dorsal ligaments of tarsus	**ligament** Ligaments of the tarsus, dorsal
Ligamenta tarsi interossea	Interosseous ligaments of tarsus	**ligament** Ligaments of the tarsus, interosseous
Ligamenta tarsi plantaria	Plantar ligaments of tarsus	**ligament** Ligaments of the tarsus, plantar
Ligamenta tarso-metatarsea dorsalia	Dorsal tarso-metatarsal ligaments	**ligament** Tarsometatarsal ligaments
Ligamenta tarso-metatarsea plantaria	Plantar tarso-metatarsal ligaments	**ligament** Tarsometatarsal ligaments
Ligamentum teres hepatis	Round ligament of liver	**ligament** Round ligament of the liver
Ligamentum teres uteri	Round ligament of uterus	**ligament** Round ligament of the uterus
Ligamentum thyro-epiglotticum	Thyro-epiglottic ligament	**ligament** Thyro-epiglottic ligament
Ligamentum thyrohyoideum	Lateral thyrohyoid ligament	**ligament** Thyrohyoid ligament, lateral
Ligamentum thyro-hyoideum medianum	Median thyrohyoid ligament	**ligament** Thyrohyoid ligament, median
Ligamentum tibio-fibulare anterius	Anterior inferior tibiofibular ligament	**ligament** Tibiofibular ligaments
Ligamentum tibio-fibulare posterius	Posterior inferior tibiofibular ligament	**ligament** Tibiofibular ligaments
Ligamentum trans-versum acetabuli	Transverse ligament (of acetabulum)	**ligament** Transverse ligament of the acetabulum
Ligamentum trans-versum atlantis	Transverse ligament of atlas	**ligament** Transverse ligament of the atlas
Ligamentum trans-versum genus	Transverse ligament of knee	**ligament** Transverse ligament of the knee

Nomina Anatomica (N.A.)	Birmingham Revision (B.R.) or English Equivalent	Definition Location
Ligamentum transversum perinei	Transverse ligament (of pelvis)	**ligament** Transverse ligament of the pelvis
Ligamentum transversum scapulae inferius	Spinoglenoid ligament	**ligament** Spinoglenoid ligament
Ligamentum transversum scapulae superius	Suprascapular ligament	**ligament** Suprascapular ligament of the shoulder girdle
Ligamentum trapezoideum	Trapezoid part (of coracoclavicular ligament)	**ligament** Trapezoid ligament
Ligamentum triangulare dextrum	Right triangular ligament	**ligament** Triangular ligaments of the liver
Ligamentum triangulare sinistrum	Left triangular ligament	**ligament** Triangular ligaments of the liver
Ligamentum ulnocarpeum palmare	Ulnocarpal ligament	**ligament** Ulnocarpal ligament
Ligamentum umbilicale mediale	Medial umbilical ligament	**ligament** Umbilical ligaments
Ligamentum umbilicale medianum	Median umbilical ligament	**ligament** Umbilical ligaments
Ligamentum venosum	Ligamentum venosum	**ligamentum** Ligamentum venosum
Ligamentum vestibulare	Vestibular ligament	**ligament** Vestibular ligament
Ligamentum vocale	Vocal ligament	**ligament** Vocal ligament
Limbus	Limbus	**limbus**
Limbus corneae	Corneal limbus	**limbus** Corneal limbus
Limbus fossae ovalis	Annulus ovalis	**annulus** Annulus ovalis
Limbus laminae spiralis osseae	Limbus laminae spiralis	**limbus** Limbus laminae spiralis
Limbi palpebrales anteriores	Anterior borders of eyelids	**eyelids** Borders of the eyelids, anterior
Limbi palpebrales posteriores	Posterior borders of eyelids	**eyelids** Borders of the eyelids, posterior
Limen	Limen	**limen**
Limen insulae	Limen insulae	**limen** Limen insulae
Limen nasi	Limen nasi	**limen** Limen nasi
Linea	Line	**line**
Linea alba	Linea alba	**linea** Linea alba
Linea arcuata (musculi recti abdominis)	Arcuate line (of rectus abdominis muscle)	**line** Arcuate line of the rectus abdominis muscle
Linea arcuata (ossis ilii)	Arcuate line (of ilium)	**line** Arcuate line of the ilium
Linea aspera	Linea aspera	**linea** Linea aspera
Linea axillaris	Axillary line	**line** Axillary line
Linea epiphysialis	Epiphyseal line	**line** Epiphyseal line
Linea glutea anterior	Middle gluteal line	**line** Gluteal line, middle
Linea glutea inferior	Inferior gluteal line	**line** Gluteal line, inferior
Linea glutea posterior	Posterior gluteal line	**line** Gluteal line, posterior
Linea intercondylaris	Intercondylar line	**line** Intercondylar line
Linea intermedia	Intermediate area (of iliac crest)	**crest** Iliac crest, intermediate area of the
Linea intertrochanterica	Trochanteric line	**line** Trochanteric line
Linea mamillaris [linea medioclavicularis]	Mamillary line	**line** Mamillary line
Linea mediana anterior	Anterior median line	**line** Median line, anterior
Linea mediana posterior	Posterior median line	**line** Median line, posterior
Linea musculi solei	Soleal line	**line** Soleal line
Linea mylohyoidea	Mylohyoid line	**line** Mylohyoid line
Linea nuchae inferior	Inferior nuchal line	**line** Nuchal line, inferior
Linea nuchae superior	Superior nuchal line	**line** Nuchal line, superior
Linea nuchae suprema	Highest nuchal line	**line** Nuchal line, highest
Linea obliqua (cartilaginis thyroideae)	Oblique line (of thyroid cartilage)	**line** Oblique line of the thyroid cartilage
Linea obliqua (mandibulae)	Oblique line (of mandible)	**mandible** Body
Linea pectinea	Spiral line	**line** Spiral line
Linea scapularis	Scapular line	**line** Scapular line
Linea semilunaris	Linea semilunaris	**linea** Linea semilunaris
Lineae temporales (ossis frontalis)	Temporal lines (of frontal bone)	**line** Temporal lines of the frontal bone
Linea temporalis inferior	Inferior temporal line	**line** Temporal line, inferior
Linea temporalis superior	Superior temporal line	**line** Temporal line, superior
Linea terminalis	Arcuate line (of pelvis)	**line** Arcuate line of the pelvis
Lineae transversae (ossis sacri)	Transverse ridges (of sacrum)	**ridge** Ridges of the sacrum, transverse
Linea trapezoidea	Trapezoid line	**line** Trapezoid line
Lingua	Tongue	**tongue**
Lingula cerebelli	Lingula of cerebellum	**lingula** Lingula of the cerebellum
Lingula mandibulae	Lingula of mandible	**lingula** Lingula of the mandible
Lingula pulmonis sinistri	Lingula pulmonis	**lingula** Lingula of the lung
Lingula sphenoidalis	Lingula of sphenoid	**lingula** Lingula of the sphenoid bone
Liquor	Liquor	**liquor**
Liquor cerebrospinalis	Cerebrospinal fluid	**fluid** Cerebrospinal fluid
Lobulus	Lobule	**lobule**
Lobulus auriculae	Lobule of auricle	**lobule** Lobule of the auricle
Lobulus biventer	Biventral lobule	**lobule** Biventral lobule
Lobulus centralis	Central lobule	**lobule** Central lobule
Lobuli corticales (renis)	Cortical lobules (of kidney)	**lobule** Cortical lobules of the kidney
Lobuli epididymidis [coni epididymidis]	Lobules of epididymis	**lobule** Lobules of the epididymis
Lobuli glandulae mammariae	Lobules of mammary gland	**gland** Mammary gland
Lobuli glandulae thyroideae	Lobules of thyroid gland	**gland** Thyroid gland
Lobuli hepatis	Lobules of liver	**lobule** Lobule of the liver
Lobulus paracentralis	Paracentral lobule	**lobule** Paracentral lobule

Nomina Anatomica (N.A.)	Birmingham Revision (B.R.) or English Equivalent	Definition Location
Lobulus parietalis inferior	Inferior parietal lobule	**lobule** Parietal lobule
Lobulus parietalis superior	Superior parietal lobule	**lobule** Parietal lobule
Lobuli pulmonum (B.N.A.)	Lobules of lung	**lobule** Lobules of the lung
Lobulus quadrangularis	Anterior lunate lobule	**lobule** Lunate lobule, anterior
Lobulus semilunaris inferior	Ansiform lobule, inferior surface	**lobule** Ansiform lobule, inferior surface of the
Lobulus semilunaris superior	Ansiform lobule, superior surface	**lobule** Ansiform lobule, superior surface of the
Lobulus simplex	Ansiform lobule	**lobule** Ansiform lobule
Lobuli testis	Lobes of testis	**testis** Lobe of the testis
Lobuli thymi	Lobules of thymus	**thymus**
Lobus	Lobe	**lobe**
Lobus anterior [adrenohypophysis]	Anterior lobe (of hypophysis cerebri)	**hypophysis** Hypophysis cerebri
Lobus caudatus (hepatis)	Caudate lobe (of liver)	**liver** Lobe of the liver, caudate
Lobi cerebri	Lobes of cerebrum	**lobe** Lobes of the cerebrum
Lobus [dexter et sinister] (glandulae thyroideae)	Lobe (right and left) (of thyroid gland)	**gland** Thyroid gland
Lobus [dexter et sinister] (prostatae)	Lobe (right and left) (of prostate)	**prostate** Lobe of the prostate, right and left
Lobus [dexter et sinister] (thymi)	Lobe (right and left) (of thymus)	**thymus**
Lobus frontalis (cerebri)	Frontal lobe (of cerebrum)	**cerebrum** Frontal lobe
Lobi glandulae mammariae	Lobes of mammary gland	**gland** Mammary gland
Lobus hepatis dexter	Right lobe of liver	**liver** Lobe of the liver, right
Lobus hepatis sinister	Left lobe of liver	**liver** Lobe of the liver, left
Lobus inferior (pulmonis)	Lower lobe (of lung)	**lung** Lobe of the lung, lower
Lobus medius (prostatae)	Median lobe (of prostate)	**prostate** Lobe of the prostate, median
Lobus medius [pulmonis dextri]	Middle lobe (of right lung)	**lung** Middle lobe
Lobus occipitalis (cerebri)	Occipital lobe	**cerebrum** Occipital lobe
Lobus parietalis (cerebri)	Parietal lobe	**cerebrum** Parietal lobe
Lobus posterior [neurohypophysis]	Posterior lobe (of hypophysis cerebri)	**hypophysis** Hypophysis cerebri
Lobus pyramidalis (glandulae thyroideae)	Pyramidal lobe (of thyroid gland)	**gland** Thyroid gland
Lobus quadratus (hepatis)	Quadrate lobe (of liver)	**liver** Lobe of the liver, quadrate
Lobi renales	Renal lobes	**lobe** Renal lobes
Lobus superior (pulmonis)	Upper lobe (of lung)	**lung** Lobe of the lung, upper
Lobus temporalis (cerebri)	Temporal lobe (of cerebrum)	**cerebrum** Temporal lobe
Locus ceruleus	Locus coeruleus	**locus** Locus ceruleus
Longitudinalis	Longitudinal	**longitudinal**
Lumbus	Loin	**loin**
Lunula	Lunula	**lunula** Lunula of the nail
Lunulae valvularum semilunarium (aortae)	Lunules of aortic valve	**lunule** Lunules of the aortic valve

Nomina Anatomica (N.A.)	Birmingham Revision (B.R.) or English Equivalent	Definition Location
Lunulae valvularum semilunarium	Lunules of pulmonary valve	**lunule** Lunules of the pulmonary valve
Lympha	Lymph	**lymph**
Lymphonodos	Lymph gland	**gland** Lymph glands
Macula	Macula	**macula**
Maculae (labyrinthi membranacei)	Maculae of membranous labyrinth	**macula** Maculae of the membranous labyrinth
Macula (lutea)	Macula lutea	**macula** Macula lutea
Maculae cribrosae	Maculae cribrosae	**macula** Maculae cribrosae
Macula cribrosa inferior	Macula cribrosa inferior	**macula** Macula cribrosa inferior
Macula cribrosa media	Macula cribrosa media	**macula** Macula cribrosa media
Macula cribrosa superior	Macula cribrosa superior	**macula** Macula cribrosa superior
Macula sacculi	Macula of saccule	**macula** Macula of the saccule
Macula utriculi	Macula of utricle	**macula** Macula of the utricle
Malleolus lateralis	Lateral malleolus	**malleolus** Lateral malleolus
Malleolus medialis	Medial malleolus	**malleolus** Medial malleolus
Malleus	Malleus	**malleus**
Mamma	Breast	**breast**
Mammae accessoriae [femininae et masculinae]	Accessory mammary glands	**gland** Mammary glands, accessory
Mamma masculina	Male mammary gland	**gland** Mammary gland
Mandibula	Mandible	**mandible**
Manubrium mallei	Handle of malleus	**malleus**
Manubrium sterni	Manubrium sterni	**manubrium** Manubrium sterni
Manus	Hand	**hand**
Margo	Margin	**border** *also* **margin**
Margo anterior (corporis pancreatis)	Anterior border (of body of pancreas)	**pancreas**
Margo anterior (fibulae)	Anterior border (of fibula)	**fibula** Shaft
Margo anterior (pulmonis)	Anterior border (of lung)	**lung** Border of the lung, anterior
Margo anterior (radii)	Anterior border (of radius)	**radius** Shaft
Margo anterior (testis)	Front border (of testis)	**testis**
Margo anterior (tibiae)	Anterior border (of tibia)	**tibia** Shaft of the tibia
Margo anterior (ulnae)	Anterior border (of ulna)	**ulna** Shaft
Margo ciliaris (iridis)	Ciliary border (of iris)	**iris** Border of the iris, ciliary
Margo dexter (cordis)	Right border (of heart)	**heart** Border of the heart, right
Margo falciformis	Falciform margin	**margin** Falciform margin
Margo frontalis (ossis parietalis)	Frontal border (of parietal bone)	**parietal bone** Frontal border
Margo frontalis (ossis sphenoidalis)	Frontal border (of sphenoid bone)	**sphenoid bone** Frontal border
Margo incisalis	Incisive edge	**edge** Incisive edge
Margo inferior (corporis pancreatis)	Inferior border (of body of pancreas)	**pancreas**
Margo inferior (hepatis)	Lower border (of liver)	**liver** Border of the liver, lower
Margo inferior [inferolateralis]	Inferolateral border (of cerebrum)	**cerebrum** Inferolateral border

Nomina Anatomica (N.A.)	Birmingham Revision (B.R.) or English Equivalent	Definition Location
Margo inferior (lienis)	Lower border (of spleen)	**spleen** Border of the spleen, lower
Margo inferior (pulmonis)	Inferior border (of lung)	**lung** Border of the lung, inferior
Margo infra-orbitalis	Infra-orbital margin	**margin** Infra-orbital margin
Margo interossea (fibulae)	Interosseous border (of fibula)	**fibula** Shaft
Margo interossea (radii)	Interosseous border (of radius)	**radius** Shaft
Margo interossea (tibiae)	Interosseous border (of tibia)	**tibia** Shaft of the tibia
Margo interossea (ulnae)	Interosseous border (of ulna)	**ulna** Shaft
Margo lacrimalis (corporis maxillae)	Lacrimal border (of body of maxilla)	**maxilla** Nasal surface
Margo lambdoideus (ossis occipitalis)	Lambdoid border (of occipital bone)	**occipital bone** Lambdoid border
Margo lateralis [fibularis] (pedis)	Lateral border (of foot)	**foot**
Margo lateralis (humeri)	Lateral border (of humerus)	**humerus** Shaft of the humerus
Margo lateralis [radialis]	Lateral border (of forearm)	**forearm**
Margo lateralis (renis)	Lateral margin (of kidney)	**kidney**
Margo lateralis (scapulae)	Lateral border (of scapula)	**scapula**
Margo lateralis (unguis)	Collateral border (of nail)	**nail** Borders of a nail, collateral
Margo liber (ovarii)	Free border (of ovary)	**ovary** Free border
Margo liber (unguis)	Free border (of nail)	**nail** Border of a nail, free
Margo linguae	Margin of tongue	**margin** Margin of the tongue
Margo mastoideus (ossis occipitalis)	Mastoid border (of occipital bone)	**occipital bone** Mastoid border
Margo medialis (glandulae suprarenalis)	Medial border (of suprarenal gland)	**gland** Suprarenal gland, borders of a
Margo medialis (humeri)	Medial border (of humerus)	**humerus** Shaft of the humerus
Margo medialis [inferomedialis]	Inferomedial border (of cerebrum)	**cerebrum** Inferomedial border
Margo medialis (renis)	Medial margin (of kidney)	**kidney**
Margo medialis (scapulae)	Medial border (of scapula)	**scapula**
Margo medialis (tibiae)	Medial border (of tibia)	**tibia** Shaft of the tibia
Margo medialis [tibialis] (pedis)	Medial border (of foot)	**foot**
Margo medialis [ulnaris]	Medial border (of forearm)	**forearm**
Margo mesovaricus (ovarii)	Mesovarian border (of ovary)	**ovary** Mesovarian border
Margo nasalis (ossis frontalis)	Nasal margin (of frontal bone)	**margin** Nasal margin
Margo occipitalis (ossis parietalis)	Occipital border (of parietal bone)	**parietal bone** Occipital border
Margo occipitalis (partis petrosae)	Occipital border (of petrous part)	**temporal bone** Occipital border
Margo occultus (unguis)	Hidden border (of nail)	**nail** Border of a nail, hidden
Margo parietalis (ossis frontalis)	Parietal margin (of frontal bone)	**margin** Parietal margin
Margo parietalis (ossis sphenoidalis)	Parietal border (of sphenoid bone)	**sphenoid bone** Parietal border
Margo parietalis (partis squamosae)	Parietal border (of squamous part)	**temporal bone** Squamous part
Margo posterior (fibulae)	Posterior border (of fibula)	**fibula** Shaft
Margo posterior partis petrosae	Posterior border (of petrous part)	**temporal bone** Posterior border
Margo posterior (radii)	Posterior border (of radius)	**radius** Shaft
Margo posterior (testis)	Posterior border (of testis)	**testis**
Margo posterior (ulnae)	Posterior border (of ulna)	**ulna** Shaft
Margo pupillaris (iridis)	Pupillary border (of iris)	**iris** Border of the iris, pupillary
Margo sagittalis (ossis parietalis)	Sagittal border (of parietal bone)	**parietal bone** Sagittal border
Margo sphenoidalis (partis squamosae)	Sphenoidal border (of squamous part)	**temporal bone** Squamous part
Margo squamosus (ossis parietalis)	Squamous border (of parietal bone)	**parietal bone** Squamous border
Margo squamosus (ossis sphenoidalis)	Squamous border (of sphenoid bone)	**sphenoid bone** Squamous border
Margo superior (cerebri)	Superomedial border (of cerebrum)	**cerebrum** Superomedial border
Margo superior (corporis pancreatis)	Superior border (of body of pancreas)	**pancreas**
Margo superior (glandulae suprarenalis)	Superior border (of suprarenal gland)	**gland** Suprarenal gland, borders of a
Margo superior (lienis)	Upper border (of spleen)	**spleen** Border of the spleen, upper
Margo superior partis petrosae	Superior border (of petrous part)	**temporal bone** Superior border
Margo superior (scapulae)	Upper border (of scapula)	**scapula**
Margo supra-orbitalis	Supra-orbital margin	**margin** Supra-orbital margin
Margo uteri [dexter et sinister]	Border of uterus (right and left)	**uterus**
Margo zygomaticus (ossis sphenoidalis)	Zygomatic border (of sphenoid bone)	**sphenoid bone** Zygomatic border
Massa	Mass	**mass**
Massa lateralis	Lateral mass	**atlas** Lateral mass
Matrix unguis	Nail bed	**nail** Nail bed
Maxilla	Maxilla	**maxilla**
Meatus	Meatus	**meatus**
Meatus acusticus externus	External auditory meatus	**meatus** Auditory meatus, external
Meatus acusticus externus cartilagineus	Cartilaginous part of external auditory meatus	**meatus** Auditory meatus, external
Meatus acusticus internus	Internal auditory meatus	**meatus** Auditory meatus, internal
Meatus nasi inferior	Inferior meatus of nose	**meatus** Meatus of the nose, inferior
Meatus nasi medius	Middle meatus of nose	**meatus** Meatus of the nose, middle
Meatus nasi superior	Superior meatus of nose	**meatus** Meatus of the nose, superior
Meatus nasopharyngeus	Posterior naris	**naris** Posterior naris
Medialis	Medial	**medial**
Medianus	Median	**median**
Mediastinum	Mediastinum	**mediastinum**
Mediastinum anterius	Anterior mediastinum	**mediastinum**
Mediastinum medium	Middle mediastinum	**mediastinum**
Mediastinum posterius	Posterior mediastinum	**mediastinum**
Mediastinum superius	Superior mediastinum	**mediastinum**
Mediastinum testis	Mediastinum testis	**mediastinum** Mediastinum testis
Medius	Middle	**middle**

Anatomical Nomenclature

Nomina Anatomica (N.A.)	Birmingham Revision (B.R.) or English Equivalent	Definition Location
Medulla	Medulla	**medulla**
Medulla (glandulae suprarenalis)	Medulla (of suprarenal gland)	**medulla** Medulla of a suprarenal gland
Medulla (nodi lymphatici)	Medulla (of lymph gland)	**medulla** Medulla of a lymph gland
Medulla oblongata	Medulla oblongata	**medulla oblongata**
Medulla ossium flava	Yellow marrow	**marrow** Yellow marrow
Medulla ossium rubra	Red marrow	**marrow** Red marrow
Medulla renis	Medulla of kidney	**medulla** Medulla of the kidney
Medulla spinalis	Spinal cord	**cord** Spinal cord
Membra	Limbs	**limb**
Membrana	Membrane	**membrane**
Membrana atlanto-occipitalis anterior	Anterior atlanto-occipital membrane	**membrane** Atlanto-occipital membrane, anterior, of the atlanto-occipital joint
Membrana atlanto-occipitalis posterior	Posterior atlanto-occipital membrane	**membrane** Atlanto-occipital membrane, posterior, of the atlanto-occipital joint
Membrana basalis ductus semicircularis	Basal membrane of semicircular duct	**membrane** Basal membrane of the semicircular duct
Membrana decidua	Decidua	**decidua**
Membrana fibro-elastica laryngis	Elastic membrane of larynx	**membrane** Elastic membrane of the larynx
Membrana fibrosa	Capsular ligament	**ligament** Capsular ligament
Membrana intercostalis externa	Anterior intercostal membrane	**membrane** Intercostal membrane, anterior
Membrana intercostalis interna	Posterior intercostal membrane	**membrane** Intercostal membrane, posterior
Membrana interossea antebrachii	Interosseous membrane of forearm	**membrane** Interosseous membrane of the forearm
Membrana interossea cruris	Interosseous membrane of leg	**membrane** Interosseous membrane of the leg
Membrana obturatoria	Obturator membrane	**membrane** Obturator membrane
Membrana propria ductus semicircularis	Proper membrane of semicircular duct	**membrane** Proper membrane of the semicircular duct
Membrana pupillaris	Pupillary membrane	**membrane** Pupillary membrane
Membrana quadrangularis	Quadrangular membrane	**membrane** Quadrangular membrane
Membrana reticularis	Reticular membrane	**membrane** Reticular membrane
Membrana spiralis	Basilar membrane	**membrane** Basilar membrane
Membrana stapedis	Obturator membrane of stapes	**membrane** Obturator membrane of the stapes
Membrana statoconiorum	Membrane of otoliths	**membrane** Membrane of otoliths
Membrana sterni	Sternal membrane	**membrane** Sternal membrane
Membrana suprapleuralis	Suprapleural membrane	**membrane** Suprapleural membrane
Membrana synovialis	Synovial membrane	**membrane** Synovial membrane
Membrana tectoria (articulationis atlanto-occipitalis)	Membrana tectoria (of atlanto-occipital joint)	**membrana** Membrana tectoria of the atlanto-occipital joint
Membrana tectoria (ductus cochlearis)	Membrana tectoria (of duct of cochlea)	**membrana** Membrana tectoria

Nomina Anatomica (N.A.)	Birmingham Revision (B.R.) or English Equivalent	Definition Location
Membrana thyrohyoidea	Thyrohyoid membrane	**membrane** Thyrohyoid membrane
Membrana tympani	Tympanic membrane	**membrane** Tympanic membrane
Membrana tympani secundaria	Secondary tympanic membrane	**membrane** Tympanic membrane, secondary
Membrana vitrea	Hyaloid membrane	**membrane** Hyaloid membrane
Membrum	Member	**limb** *also* **member**
Membrum inferius	Lower limb	**limb**
Membrum superius	Upper limb	**limb**
Meninges	Membranes	**membrane**
Meniscus articularis	Interarticular fibrocartilage	**fibrocartilage** Interarticular fibrocartilage
Meniscus lateralis	Lateral semilunar cartilage	**cartilage** Semilunar cartilage of the knee joint, lateral
Meniscus medialis	Medial semilunar cartilage	**cartilage** Semilunar cartilage of the knee joint, medial
Meniscus tactus	Tactile meniscus	**meniscus** Tactile meniscus
Mentum	Chin	**chin**
Meridiani (bulbi oculi)	Meridians (of eyeball)	**meridian** Meridian of the eye
Mesencephalon	Mid-brain	**mid-brain**
Mesenterium	The mesentery	**mesentery**
Mesenterium dorsale commune	Common mesentery	**mesentery** Common mesentery
Mesoappendix	Mesentery of vermiform appendix	**mesentery** Mesentery of the vermiform appendix
Mesocolon	Mesocolon	**mesocolon**
Mesocolon ascendens	Ascending mesocolon	**mesocolon** Ascending mesocolon
Mesocolon descendens	Descending mesocolon	**mesocolon** Descending mesocolon
Mesocolon sigmoideum	Pelvic mesocolon	**mesocolon** Pelvic mesocolon
Mesocolon transversum	Transverse mesocolon	**mesocolon** Transverse mesocolon
Mesogastrium	Mesogastrium	**mesogastrium**
Mesometrium	Mesometrium	**mesometrium**
Mesonephros	Mesonephros	**mesonephros**
Mesorchium	Mesorchium	**mesorchium**
Mesosalpinx	Mesosalpinx	**mesosalpinx**
Mesotendineum	Mesotendon	**mesotendon**
Mesothelium	Mesothelium	**mesothelium**
Mesovarium	Mesovarium	**mesovarium**
Metacarpus	Metacarpus	**metacarpus**
Metatarsus	Metatarsus	**metatarsus**
Metathalamus	Metathalamus	**metathalamus**
Metencephalon	Metencephalon	**metencephalon**
Modiolus	Modiolus	**modiolus**
Mons pubis	Mons pubis	**mons** Mons pubis
Musculus	Muscle	**muscle**
Musculus abductor digiti minimi (manus)	Abductor digiti minimi muscle (of hand)	**abductor digiti minimi muscle of the hand**
Musculus abductor digiti minimi (pedis)	Abductor digiti minimi muscle (of foot)	**abductor digiti minimi muscle of the foot**
Musculus abductor hallucis	Abductor hallucis muscle	**abductor hallucis muscle**
Musculus abductor pollicis brevis	Abductor pollicis brevis muscle	**abductor pollicis brevis muscle**
Musculus abductor pollicis longus	Abductor pollicis longus muscle	**abductor pollicis longus muscle**
Musculus adductor brevis	Adductor brevis muscle	**adductor brevis muscle**

Nomina Anatomica (N.A.)	Birmingham Revision (B.R.) or English Equivalent	Definition Location
Musculus adductor hallucis	Adductor hallucis muscle	**adductor hallucis muscle**
Musculus adductor longus	Adductor longus muscle	**adductor longus muscle**
Musculus adductor magnus	Adductor magnus muscle	**adductor magnus muscle**
Musculus adductor pollicis	Adductor pollicis muscle	**adductor pollicis muscle**
Musculus anconeus	Anconeus muscle	**anconeus muscle**
Musculus antitragicus	Antitragicus muscle	**antitragicus muscle**
Musculi arrectores pilorum	Arrectores pilorum muscles	**arrectores pilorum muscles**
Musculus articularis	Articular muscle	**muscle** Articular muscle
Musculus articularis cubiti	Articularis cubiti muscle	**articularis cubiti muscle**
Musculus articularis genus	Articularis genu muscle	**articularis genu muscle**
Musculus aryepiglotticus	Aryepiglottic muscle	**aryepiglottic muscle**
Musculus arytenoideus obliquus	Oblique arytenoid muscle	**arytenoid muscles** Oblique arytenoid muscles
Musculus arytenoideus transversus	Transverse arytenoid muscle	**arytenoid muscles** Transverse arytenoid muscles
Musculus auricularis anterior	Auricularis anterior muscle	**auricularis anterior muscle**
Musculus auricularis posterior	Auricularis posterior muscle	**auricularis posterior muscle**
Musculus auricularis superior	Auricularis superior muscle	**auricularis superior muscle**
Musculus biceps brachii	Biceps brachii muscle	**biceps brachii muscle**
Musculus biceps femoris	Biceps femoris muscle	**biceps femoris muscle**
Musculus bipennatus	Bipennate muscle	**muscle** Bipennate muscle
Musculus brachialis	Brachialis muscle	**brachialis muscle**
Musculus brachioradialis	Brachioradialis muscle	**brachioradialis muscle**
Musculus broncho-esophageus	Broncho-oesophageal muscle	**broncho-oesophageal muscle**
Musculus buccinator	Buccinator muscle	**buccinator muscle**
Musculus bulbospongiosus	Bulbospongiosus muscle	**bulbospongiosus muscle**
Musculus ceratocricoideus	Ceratocricoid muscle	**ceratocricoid muscle**
Musculus chondroglossus	Chondroglossus muscle	**chondroglossus muscle**
Musculus ciliaris	Ciliary muscle	**ciliary muscle**
Musculus coccygeus	Coccygeus muscle	**coccygeus muscle**
Musculus constrictor pharyngis inferior	Inferior constrictor muscle of pharynx	**pharynx, constrictor muscles of the**
Musculus constrictor pharyngis medius	Middle constrictor muscle of pharynx	**pharynx, constrictor muscles of the**
Musculus constrictor pharyngis superior	Superior constrictor muscle of pharynx	**pharynx, constrictor muscles of the**
Musculus coracobrachialis	Coracobrachialis muscle	**coracobrachialis muscle**
Musculus corrugator supercilii	Corrugator muscle of eyebrow	**corrugator**
Musculus cremaster	Cremaster muscle	**cremaster muscle**
Musculus crico-arytenoideus lateralis	Lateral crico-arytenoid muscle	**crico-arytenoid muscles** Lateral crico-arytenoid muscle
Musculus crico-arytenoideus posterior	Posterior crico-arytenoid muscle	**crico-arytenoid muscles** Posterior crico-arytenoid muscle
Musculus cricothyroideus	Cricothyroid muscle	**cricothyroid muscle**
Musculus cutaneus	Cutaneous muscle	**muscle** Cutaneous muscle
Musculus deltoideus	Deltoid muscle	**deltoid muscle**

Nomina Anatomica (N.A.)	Birmingham Revision (B.R.) or English Equivalent	Definition Location
Musculus depressor anguli oris	Depressor anguli oris muscle	**depressor anguli oris muscle**
Musculus depressor labii inferioris	Depressor labii inferioris muscle	**depressor labii inferioris muscle**
Musculus depressor septi	Depressor septi muscle	**depressor septi muscle**
Musculus depressor supercilii	Depressor supercilii muscle	**depressor supercilii muscle**
Musculus digastricus	Digastric muscle	**digastric muscle**
Musculus dilatator pupillae	Dilator of pupil	**dilator muscle of the pupil**
Musculus epicranius	Epicranius muscle	**epicranius muscle**
Musculus erector spinae	Sacrospinalis muscle	**sacrospinalis muscle**
Musculus extensor carpi radialis brevis	Extensor carpi radialis brevis muscle	**extensor carpi radialis brevis muscle**
Musculus extensor carpi radialis longus	Extensor carpi radialis longus muscle	**extensor carpi radialis longus muscle**
Musculus extensor carpi ulnaris	Extensor carpi ulnaris muscle	**extensor carpi ulnaris muscle**
Musculus extensor digiti minimi	Extensor digiti minimi muscle	**extensor digiti minimi muscle**
Musculus extensor digitorum	Extensor digitorum muscle	**extensor digitorum muscle**
Musculus extensor digitorum brevis	Extensor digitorum brevis muscle	**extensor digitorum brevis muscle**
Musculus extensor digitorum longus	Extensor digitorum longus muscle	**extensor digitorum longus muscle**
Musculus extensor hallucis brevis	Extensor hallucis brevis muscle	**extensor hallucis brevis muscle**
Musculus extensor hallucis longus	Extensor hallucis longus muscle	**extensor hallucis longus muscle**
Musculus extensor indicis	Extensor indicis muscle	**extensor indicis muscle**
Musculus extensor pollicis brevis	Extensor pollicis brevis muscle	**extensor pollicis brevis muscle**
Musculus extensor pollicis longus	Extensor pollicis longus muscle	**extensor pollicis longus muscle**
Musculus flexor carpi radialis	Flexor carpi radialis muscle	**flexor carpi radialis muscle**
Musculus flexor carpi ulnaris	Flexor carpi ulnaris muscle	**flexor carpi ulnaris muscle**
Musculus flexor digiti minimi brevis (manus)	Flexor digiti minimi muscle (of hand)	**flexor digiti minimi muscle**
Musculus flexor digiti minimi brevis (pedis)	Flexor digiti minimi brevis muscle (of foot)	**flexor digiti minimi brevis muscle**
Musculus flexor digitorum brevis	Flexor digitorum brevis muscle	**flexor digitorum brevis muscle**
Musculus flexor digitorum longus	Flexor digitorum longus muscle	**flexor digitorum longus muscle**
Musculus flexor digitorum profundus	Flexor digitorum profundus muscle	**flexor digitorum profundus muscle**
Musculus flexor digitorum superficialis	Flexor digitorum sublimis muscle	**flexor digitorum sublimis muscle**
Musculus flexor hallucis brevis	Flexor hallucis brevis muscle	**flexor hallucis brevis muscle**
Musculus flexor hallucis longus	Flexor hallucis longus muscle	**flexor hallucis longus muscle**
Musculus flexor pollicis brevis	Flexor pollicis brevis muscle	**flexor pollicis brevis muscle**
Musculus flexor pollicis longus	Flexor pollicis longus muscle	**flexor pollicis longus muscle**
Musculus fusiformis	Fusiform muscle	**muscle** Fusiform muscle
Musculus gastrocnemius	Gastrocnemius muscle	**gastrocnemius muscle**
Musculus gemellus inferior	Gemellus inferior muscle	**gemellus inferior muscle**
Musculus gemellus superior	Gemellus superior muscle	**gemellus superior muscle**
Musculus genioglossus	Genioglossus muscle	**genioglossus muscle**

Anatomical Nomenclature

Nomina Anatomica (N.A.)	Birmingham Revision (B.R.) or English Equivalent	Definition Location
Musculus geniohyoideus	Geniohyoid muscle	**geniohyoid muscle**
Musculus gluteus maximus	Gluteus maximus muscle	**gluteus maximus muscle**
Musculus gluteus medius	Gluteus medius muscle	**gluteus medius muscle**
Musculus gluteus minimus	Gluteus minimus muscle	**gluteus minimus muscle**
Musculus gracilis	Gracilis muscle	**gracilis muscle**
Musculus helicis major	Helicis major muscle	**helicis major muscle**
Musculus helicis minor	Helicis minor muscle	**helicis minor muscle**
Musculus hyoglossus	Hyoglossus muscle	**hyoglossus muscle**
Musculus iliacus	Iliacus muscle	**iliacus muscle**
Musculus iliococcygeus	Iliococcygeus muscle	**iliococcygeus muscle**
Musculus iliocostalis	Iliocostocervicalis muscle	**iliocostocervicalis muscle**
Musculus iliocostalis cervicis	Costocervicalis muscle	**costocervicalis muscle**
Musculus iliocostalis lumborum	Iliocostalis muscle	**iliocostalis muscle**
Musculus iliocostalis thoracis	Costalis muscle	**costalis muscle**
Musculus iliopsoas	Iliopsoas muscle	**iliopsoas muscle**
Musculus incisurae helicis	Musculus incisurae helicis	**musclus** Musculus incisurae helicis
Musculi infrahyoidei	Infrahyoid muscles	**infrahyoid muscles**
Musculus infraspinatus	Infraspinatus muscle	**infraspinatus muscle**
Musculi intercostales externi	External intercostal muscles	**intercostal muscles** External intercostal muscles
Musculi intercostales interni	Internal intercostal muscles	**intercostal muscles** Internal intercostal muscles
Musculi intercostales intimi	Intercostales intimi muscles	**intercostales intimi muscles**
Musculi interossei dorsales (manus)	Dorsal interossei muscles (of hand)	**interossei muscles of the hand**
Musculi interossei dorsales (pedis)	Dorsal interossei muscles (of foot)	**interossei muscles of the foot**
Musculi interossei palmares	Palmar interossei muscles	**interossei muscles of the hand**
Musculi interossei plantares	Plantar interossei muscles	**interossei muscles of the foot**
Musculi interspinales	Interspinales muscles	**interspinales muscles**
Musculi interspinales cervicis	Cervical interspinales muscles	**interspinales muscles**
Musculi interspinales lumborum	Lumbar interspinales muscles	**interspinales muscles**
Musculi interspinales thoracis	Thoracic interspinales muscles	**interspinales muscles**
Musculi intertransversarii	Intertransverse muscles	**intertransverse muscles**
Musculi intertransversarii anteriores cervicis	Anterior inter-transverse muscles	**intertransverse muscles** Anterior intertransverse muscles
Musculi intertransversarii laterales lumborum	Lateral inter-transverse muscles	**intertransverse muscles** Lateral intertransverse muscles
Musculi intertransversarii mediales lumborum	Medial inter-transverse muscles	**intertransverse muscles** Medial intertransverse muscles
Musculi intertransversarii posteriores cervicis	Posterior inter-transverse muscles	**intertransverse muscles** Posterior intertransverse muscles
Musculi inter-transversarii thoracis	Thoracic inter-transverse muscles	**intertransverse muscles**
Musculus ischiocavernosus	Ischiocavernosus muscle	**ischiocavernosus muscle**
Musculus latissimus dorsi	Latissimus dorsi muscle	**latissimus dorsi muscle**
Musculus levator anguli oris	Levator anguli oris muscle	**levator anguli oris muscle**
Musculus levator ani	Levator ani muscle	**levator ani muscle**

Nomina Anatomica (N.A.)	Birmingham Revision (B.R.) or English Equivalent	Definition Location
Musculi levatores costarum	Levatores costarum muscles	**levatores costarum muscles**
Musculi levatores costarum breves	Levatores costarum breves muscles	**levatores costarum muscles**
Musculi levatores costarum longi	Levatores costarum longi muscles	**levatores costarum muscles**
Musculus levator glandulae thyroideae	Levator glandulae thyroideae muscle	**levator glandulae thyroideae muscle**
Musculus levator labii superioris	Levator labii superioris muscle	**levator labii superioris muscle**
Musculus levator labii superioris alaeque nasi	Levator labii superioris alaeque nasi muscle	**levator labii superioris alaeque nasi muscle**
Musculus levator palpebrae superioris	Levator palpebrae superioris muscle	**levator palpebrae superioris muscle of the orbit**
Musculus levator prostatae [musculus pubovaginalis]	Levator prostatae muscle	**levator prostatae muscle**
Musculus levator scapulae	Levator scapulae muscle	**levator scapulae muscle**
Musculus levator veli palatini	Levator palati muscle	**levator palati muscle**
Musculi linguae	Muscles of tongue	**tongue, muscles of the**
Musculus longissimus	Longissimus muscle	**longissimus muscle**
Musculus longissimus capitis	Longissimus capitis muscle	**longissimus capitis muscle**
Musculus longissimus cervicis	Longissimus cervicis muscle	**longissimus cervicis muscle**
Musculus longissimus thoracis	Longissimus thoracis muscle	**longissimus thoracis muscle**
Musculus longitudinalis inferior	Inferior longitudinal muscle of tongue	**tongue, muscles of the** Longitudinal muscles of the tongue
Musculus longitudinalis superior	Superior longitudinal muscle of tongue	**tongue, muscles of the** Longitudinal muscles of the tongue
Musculus longus capitis	Longus capitis muscle	**longus capitis muscle**
Musculus longus colli	Longus cervicis muscle	**longus cervicis muscle**
Musculi lumbricales (manus)	Lumbrical muscles (of hand)	**lumbrical muscles**
Musculi lumbricales (pedis)	Lumbrical muscles (of foot)	**lumbrical muscles**
Musculus masseter	Masseter muscle	**masseter muscle**
Musculus mentalis	Mentalis muscle	**mentalis muscle**
Musculus multifidus	Multifidus muscle	**multifidus muscle**
Musculus mylohyoideus	Mylohyoid muscle	**mylohyoid muscle**
Musculus nasalis	Nasal muscle	**nasal muscle**
Musculus obliquus auriculae	Oblique muscle of auricle	**auricle, muscles of the**
Musculus obliquus capitis inferior	Obliquus capitis inferior muscle	**obliquus capitis inferior muscle**
Musculus obliquus capitis superior	Obliquus capitis superior muscle	**obliquus capitis superior muscle**
Musculus obliquus externus abdominis	External oblique muscle	**oblique muscles**
Musculus obliquus inferior	Inferior oblique muscle (of orbit)	**oblique muscles of the orbit** Inferior oblique muscle of the orbit
Musculus obliquus internus abdominis	Internal oblique muscle	**oblique muscles**
Musculus obliquus superior	Superior oblique muscle (of orbit)	**oblique muscles of the orbit** Superior oblique muscle of the orbit
Musculus obturatorius externus	Obturator externus muscle	**obturator externus muscle**
Musculus obturatorius internus	Obturator internus muscle	**obturator internus muscle**
Musculus occipitofrontalis	Occipitofrontalis muscle	**occipitofrontalis muscle**
Musculus omohyoideus	Omohyoid muscle	**omohyoid muscle**

Nomina Anatomica (N.A.)	Birmingham Revision (B.R.) or English Equivalent	Definition Location
Musculus opponens digiti minimi	Opponens digiti minimi muscle	**opponens digiti minimi muscle**
Musculus opponens pollicis	Opponens pollicis muscle	**opponens pollicis muscle**
Musculus orbicularis	Orbicular muscle	**muscle** Orbicular muscle
Musculus orbicularis oculi	Orbicularis oculi muscle	**orbicularis oculi muscle**
Musculus orbicularis oris	Orbicularis oris muscle	**orbicularis oris muscle**
Musculus orbitalis	Orbitalis muscle	**orbitalis muscle**
Musculus palatoglossus	Palatoglossus muscle	**palatoglossus muscle**
Musculus palatopharyngeus	Palatopharyngeus muscle	**palatopharyngeus muscle**
Musculus palmaris brevis	Palmaris brevis muscle	**palmaris brevis muscle**
Musculus palmaris longus	Palmaris longus muscle	**palmaris longus muscle**
Musculi papillares	Papillary muscles	**papillary muscles**
Musculus papillaris anterior (ventriculi dextri)	Anterior papillary muscle (of right ventricle)	**papillary muscles** Anterior papillary muscle of the right ventricle
Musculus papillaris anterior (ventriculi sinistri)	Superior papillary muscle (of left ventricle)	**papillary muscles** Superior papillary muscle of the left ventricle
Musculus papillaris posterior (ventriculi dextri)	Inferior papillary muscle (of right ventricle)	**papillary muscles** Inferior papillary muscle of the right ventricle
Musculus papillaris posterior (ventriculi sinistri)	Inferior papillary muscle (of left ventricle)	**papillary muscles** Inferior papillary muscle of the left ventricle
Musculi papillares septales	Septal papillary muscles	**papillary muscles** Septal papillary muscles
Musculi pectinati	Musculi pectinati	**musculus** Musculi pectinati
Musculus pectineus	Pectineus muscle	**pectineus muscle**
Musculus pectoralis major	Pectoralis major muscle	**pectoralis major muscle**
Musculus pectoralis minor	Pectoralis minor muscle	**pectoralis minor muscle**
Musculus peroneus [fibularis] brevis	Peroneus brevis muscle	**peroneus brevis muscle**
Musculus peroneus longus [fibularis]	Peroneus longus muscle	**peroneus longus muscle**
Musculus peroneus [fibularis tertius]	Peroneus tertius muscle	**peroneus tertius muscle**
Musculus piriformis	Piriformis muscle	**piriformis muscle**
Musculus plantaris	Plantaris muscle	**plantaris muscle**
Musculus pleuro-esophageus	Pleuro-oesophageal muscle	**pleuro-oesophageal muscle**
Musculus popliteus	Popliteus muscle	**popliteus muscle**
Musculus procerus	Procerus muscle	**procerus muscle**
Musculus pronator quadratus	Pronator quadratus muscle	**pronator quadratus muscle**
Musculus pronator teres	Pronator teres muscle	**pronator teres muscle**
Musculus psoas major	Psoas major muscle	**psoas major muscle**
Musculus psoas minor	Psoas minor muscle	**psoas minor muscle**
Musculus pterygoideus lateralis	Lateral pterygoid muscle	**pterygoid muscles** Lateral pterygoid muscle
Musculus pterygoideus medialis	Medial pterygoid muscle	**pterygoid muscles** Medial pterygoid muscle
Musculus pubococcygeus	Pubococcygeus muscle	**pubococcygeus muscle**
Musculus puboprostaticus	Puboprostatic muscle	**puboprostatic muscle**
Musculus puborectalis	Puborectalis muscle	**puborectalis muscle**
Musculus pubovesicalis	Pubovesical muscle	**pubovesical muscle**
Musculus pyramidalis	Pyramidalis muscle	**pyramidalis muscle**
Musculus pyramidalis auriculae	Pyramidalis muscle of auricle	**pyramidalis muscle of the auricle**
Musculus quadratus femoris	Quadratus femoris muscle	**quadratus femoris muscle**

Nomina Anatomica (N.A.)	Birmingham Revision (B.R.) or English Equivalent	Definition Location
Musculus quadratus lumborum	Quadratus lumborum muscle	**quadratus lumborum muscle**
Musculus quadratus plantae [musculus flexor accessorius]	Flexor digitorum accessorius muscle	**flexor digitorum accessorius muscle**
Musculus quadriceps femoris	Quadriceps femoris muscle	**quadriceps femoris muscle**
Musculus rectococcygeus	Rectococcygeal muscle	**rectococcygeal muscle**
Musculus recto-urethralis	Recto-urethral muscle	**recto-urethral muscle**
Musculus recto-uterinus	Recto-uterine muscle	**recto-uterine muscle**
Musculus rectovesicalis	Rectovesical muscle	**rectovesical muscle**
Musculus rectus abdominis	Rectus abdominis muscle	**rectus abdominis muscle**
Musculus rectus capitis anterior	Rectus capitis anterior muscle	**rectus capitis muscles** Rectus capitis anterior muscle
Musculus rectus capitis lateralis	Rectus capitis lateralis muscle	**rectus capitis muscles** Rectus capitis lateralis muscle
Musculus rectus capitis posterior major	Rectus capitis posterior major muscle	**rectus capitis muscles** Rectus capitis posterior major muscle
Musculus rectus capitis posterior minor	Rectus capitis posterior minor muscle	**rectus capitis muscles** Rectus capitis posterior minor muscle
Musculus rectus femoris	Rectus femoris muscle	**rectus femoris muscle**
Musculus rectus inferior	Inferior rectus muscle (of orbit)	**rectus muscles of the orbit** Inferior rectus muscle of the orbit
Musculus rectus lateralis	Lateral rectus muscle (of orbit)	**rectus muscles of the orbit** Lateral rectus muscle of the orbit
Musculus rectus medialis	Medial rectus muscle (of orbit)	**rectus muscles of the orbit** Medial rectus muscle of the orbit
Musculus rectus superior	Superior rectus muscle (of orbit)	**rectus muscles of the orbit** Superior rectus muscle of the orbit
Musculus rhomboideus major	Rhomboid major muscle	**rhomboid major muscle**
Musculus rhomboideus minor	Rhomboid minor muscle	**rhomboid minor muscle**
Musculus risorius	Risorius muscle	**risorius muscle**
Musculi rotatores	Rotatores muscles	**rotatores muscles**
Musculi rotatores cervicis	Cervical rotatores muscles	**rotatores muscles**
Musculi rotatores lumborum	Lumbar rotatores muscles	**rotatores muscles**
Musculi rotatores thoracis	Thoracic rotatores muscles	**rotatores muscles**
Musculus sacrococcygeus dorsalis	Sacrococcygeus dorsalis muscle	**sacrococcygeus dorsalis muscle**
Musculus sacrococcygeus ventralis	Sacrococcygeus ventralis muscle	**sacrococcygeus ventralis muscle**
Musculus salpingopharyngeus	Salpingopharyngeus muscle	**salpingopharyngeus muscle**
Musculus sartorius	Sartorius muscle	**sartorius muscle**
Musculus scalenus anterior	Scalenus anterior muscle	**scalenus anterior muscle**
Musculus scalenus medius	Scalenus medius muscle	**scalenus medius muscle**
Musculus scalenus minimus	Scalenus minimus muscle	**scalenus minimus muscle**
Musculus scalenus posterior	Scalenus posterior muscle	**scalenus posterior muscle**
Musculus semimembranosus	Semimembranosus muscle	**semimembranosus muscle**

Anatomical Nomenclature

Nomina Anatomica (N.A.)	Birmingham Revision (B.R.) or English Equivalent	Definition Location
Musculus semispinalis	Semispinalis muscle	**semispinalis muscle**
Musculus semispinalis capitis	Semispinalis capitis muscle	**semispinalis capitis muscle**
Musculus semispinalis cervicis	Semispinalis cervicis muscle	**semispinalis cervicis muscle**
Musculus semispinalis thoracis	Semispinalis thoracis muscle	**semispinalis thoracis muscle**
Musculus semitendinosus	Semitendinosus muscle	**semitendinosus muscle**
Musculus serratus anterior	Serratus anterior muscle	**serratus anterior muscle**
Musculus serratus posterior inferior	Serratus posterior inferior muscle	**serratus posterior inferior muscle**
Musculus serratus posterior superior	Serratus posterior superior muscle	**serratus posterior superior muscle**
Musculi skeleti	Skeletal muscles	**muscle** Skeletal muscles
Musculus soleus	Soleus muscle	**soleus muscle**
Musculus sphincter	Sphincter muscle	**muscle** Sphincter muscle
Musculus sphincter ampullae hepatopancreaticae	Sphincter of ampulla of bile duct	**sphincter** Sphincter of the ampulla of the bile duct
Musculus sphincter ani externus	Sphincter ani externus muscle	**sphincter ani externus muscle**
Musculus sphincter ani internus	Sphincter ani internus muscle	**sphincter ani internus muscle**
Musculus sphincter ductus choledochi	Sphincter of bile duct	**sphincter** Sphincter of the bile duct
Musculus sphincter pupillae	Sphincter of pupil	**sphincter** Sphincter of the pupil
Musculus sphincter pylori	Pyloric sphincter	**sphincter** Pyloric sphincter
Musculus sphincter urethrae	Sphincter urethrae muscle	**sphincter urethrae muscles**
Musculus spinalis	Spinalis muscle	**spinalis muscle**
Musculus spinalis capitis	Spinalis capitis muscle	**spinalis capitis muscle**
Musculus spinalis cervicis	Spinalis cervicis muscle	**spinalis cervicis muscle**
Musculus spinalis thoracis	Spinalis thoracis muscle	**spinalis thoracis muscle**
Musculus splenius capitis	Splenius capitis muscle	**splenius capitis muscle**
Musculus splenius cervicis	Splenius cervicis muscle	**splenius cervicis muscle**
Musculus stapedius	Stapedius muscle	**stapedius muscle**
Musculus sternalis	Sternalis muscle	**sternalis muscle**
Musculus sternocleidomastoideus	Sternocleidomastoid muscle	**sternocleidomastoid muscle**
Musculus sternohyoideus	Sternohyoid muscle	**sternohyoid muscle**
Musculus sternothyroideus	Sternothyroid muscle	**sternothyroid muscle**
Musculus styloglossus	Styloglossus muscle	**styloglossus muscle**
Musculus stylohyoideus	Stylohyoid muscle	**stylohyoid muscle**
Musculus stylopharyngeus	Stylopharyngeus muscle	**stylopharyngeus muscle**
Musculus subclavius	Subclavius muscle	**subclavius muscle**
Musculi subcostales	Subcostal muscles	**subcostal muscles**
Musculus subscapularis	Subscapularis muscle	**subscapularis muscle**
Musculus supinator	Supinator muscle	**supinator muscle**
Musculi suprahyoidei	Suprahyoid muscles	**suprahyoid muscles**
Musculus supraspinatus	Supraspinatus muscle	**supraspinatus muscle**
Musculus suspensorius duodeni	Suspensory muscle of duodenum	**duodenum, suspensory muscle of the**
Musculus tarsalis inferior	Inferior tarsal muscle	**tarsal muscles**
Musculus tarsalis superior	Superior tarsal muscle	**tarsal muscles**
Musculus temporalis	Temporal muscle	**temporal muscle**
Musculus temporoparietalis	Temporoparietal muscle	**temporoparietal muscle**
Musculus tensor fasciae latae	Tensor fasciae latae muscle	**tensor fasciae latae muscle**
Musculus tensor tympani	Tensor tympani muscle	**tensor tympani muscle**
Musculus tensor veli palatini	Tensor palati muscle	**tensor palati muscle**
Musculus teres major	Teres major muscle	**teres major muscle**
Musculus teres minor	Teres minor muscle	**teres minor muscle**
Musculus thyro-arytenoideus	Thyro-arytenoid muscle	**thyro-arytenoid muscle**
Musculus thyro-epiglotticus	Thyro-epiglottic muscle	**thyro-epiglottic muscle**
Musculus thyrohyoideus	Thyrohyoid muscle	**thyrohyoid muscle**
Musculus tibialis anterior	Tibialis anterior muscle	**tibialis muscles** Tibialis anterior muscle
Musculus tibialis posterior	Tibialis posterior muscle	**tibialis muscles** Tibialis posterior muscle
Musculus trachealis	Trachealis muscle	**trachealis muscle**
Musculus tragicus	Tragicus muscle	**tragicus muscle**
Musculus transversospinalis	Transversospinalis muscle	**transversospinalis muscle**
Musculus transversus abdominis	Transversus abdominis muscle	**transversus abdominis muscle**
Musculus transversus auriculae	Transverse muscle of auricle	**auricle, muscles of the**
Musculus transversus linguae	Transverse muscle of tongue	**tongue, muscles of the** Transverse muscle of the tongue
Musculus transversus menti	Transversus menti muscle	**transversus menti muscle**
Musculus transversus nuchae	Transversus nuchae muscle	**transversus nuchae muscle**
Musculus transversus perinei profundus	Deep transverse perinei muscle	**transversus perinei muscles** Deep transversus perinei muscle
Musculus transversus perinei superficialis	Superficial transversus perinei muscle	**transversus perinei muscles** Superficial transversus perinei muscle
Musculus transversus thoracis	Transversus thoracis muscle	**transversus thoracis muscle**
Musculus trapezius	Trapezius muscle	**trapezius muscle**
Musculus triceps brachii	Triceps brachii muscle	**triceps brachii muscle**
Musculus triceps surae	Triceps surae muscle	**triceps surae muscle**
Musculus unipennatus	Unipennate muscle	**muscle** Unipennate muscle
Musculus uvulae	Musculus uvulae	**musculus** Musculus uvulae
Musculus vastus intermedius	Vastus intermedius muscle	**vastus muscles** Vastus intermedius muscle
Musculus vastus lateralis	Vastus lateralis muscle	**vastus muscles** Vastus lateralis muscle
Musculus vastus medialis	Vastus medialis muscle	**vastus muscles** Vastus medialis muscle
Musculus verticalis linguae	Vertical muscle of tongue	**tongue, muscles of the** Transverse muscle of the tongue
Musculus vocalis	Vocalis muscle	**vocalis muscle**
Musculus zygomaticus major	Zygomaticus major muscle	**zygomaticus major muscle**
Musculus zygomaticus minor	Zygomaticus minor muscle	**zygomaticus minor muscle**
Myelencephalon	Myelencephalon	**myelencephalon**
Myocardium	Myocardium	**myocardium**
Nares	Nostrils	**nostrils**
Nasus	Nose	**nose**
Nasus externus	External nose	**nose** External nose

Nomina Anatomica (N.A.)	Birmingham Revision (B.R.) or English Equivalent	Definition Location
Nates [clunes]	Buttock	**buttock**
Nervus	Nerve	**nerve**
Nervus abducens	Abducent nerve	**abducent nerve**
Nervus accessorius	Accessory nerve	**accessory nerve**
Nervus alveolaris inferior	Inferior dental nerve	**dental nerves** Inferior dental nerve
Nervi alveolares superiores	Superior dental nerves	**maxillary nerve**
Nervus ampullaris anterior	Anterior ampullary nerve	**ampullary nerves**
Nervus ampullaris lateralis	Lateral ampullary nerve	**ampullary nerves**
Nervus ampullaris posterior	Posterior ampullary nerve	**ampullary nerves**
Nervi anococcygei	Anococcygeal nerves	**anococcygeal nerves**
Nervus articularis	Articular nerve	**nerve** Articular nerve
Nervi auriculares anteriores	Auricular branches (of auriculo-temporal nerve)	**auriculotemporal nerve**
Nervus auricularis magnus	Great auricular nerve	**auricular nerves** Great auricular nerve
Nervus auricularis posterior	Posterior auricular nerve	**auricular nerves** Posterior auricular nerve
Nervus auriculotemporalis	Auriculotemporal nerve	**auriculotemporal nerve**
Nervus axillaris	Circumflex nerve	**circumflex nerve**
Nervus buccalis	Buccal nerve	**buccal nerve**
Nervus canalis pterygoidei [radix facialis]	Nerve of pterygoid canal	**pterygoid canal, nerve of the**
Nervus cardiacus cervicalis inferior	Cardiac branch (of inferior cervical ganglion)	**ganglion** Cervical ganglion, inferior, cardiac branch of the
Nervus cardiacus cervicalis medius	Cardiac branch (of middle cervical ganglion)	**ganglion** Cervical ganglion, middle, cardiac branch of the
Nervus cardiacus cervicalis superior	Cardiac branch (of superior cervical ganglion)	**ganglion** Cervical ganglion, superior, cardiac branch of the
Nervi cardiaci thoracici	Cardiac branches (of thoracic ganglia)	**ganglion** Thoracia ganglia, cardiac branches of the
Nervi carotici externi	External carotid nerves	**carotid nerves** External carotid nerves
Nervi caroticotympanici	Caroticotympanic nerves	**caroticotympanic nerves**
Nervus caroticus internus	Internal carotid nerve	**carotid nerves** Internal carotid nerves
Nervi cavernosi clitoridis	Cavernous nerves of clitoris	**penis, nerves of the (or of the clitoris)** Cavernous nerves of the penis (or of the clitoris)
Nervi cavernosi penis	Cavernous nerves of penis	**penis, nerves of the** Cavernous nerves of the penis
Nervi cervicales	Cervical nerves	**cervical nerves**
Nervi ciliares breves	Short ciliary nerves	**ciliary nerves** Short ciliary nerves
Nervi ciliares longi	Long ciliary nerves	**ciliary nerves** Long ciliary nerves
Nervi clunium inferiores	Gluteal branches (of posterior cutaneous nerve of thigh)	**thigh, cutaneous nerves of the** Posterior cutaneous nerve of the thigh
Nervi clunium medii	Gluteal branches (of posterior primary rami of sacral nerves)	**sacral nerves**
Nervi clunium superiores (nervorum lumbalium)	Gluteal branches (of posterior primary rami of lumbar nerves)	**lumbar nerves**
Nervus coccygeus	Coccygeal nerve	**coccygeal nerve**
Nervi craniales	Cranial nerves	**cranial nerves**
Nervus cutaneus	Cutaneous nerve	**nerve** Cutaneous nerve
Nervus cutaneus antebrachii lateralis	Lateral cutaneous nerve of forearm	**forearm, nerves of the** Lateral cutaneous nerve of the forearm
Nervus cutaneus antebrachii medialis	Medial cutaneous nerve of forearm	**forearm, nerves of the** Medial cutaneous nerve of the forearm
Nervus cutaneus antebrachii posterior	Posterior cutaneous nerve of forearm	**forearm, nerves of the** Posterior cutaneous nerve of the forearm
Nervus cutaneus brachii lateralis inferior	Lower lateral cutaneous nerve of the arm	**arm, nerves of the** Lower lateral cutaneous nerve of the arm
Nervus cutaneus brachii lateralis superior	Upper lateral cutaneous nerve of arm	**arm, nerves of the** Upper lateral cutaneous nerve of the arm
Nervus cutaneus brachii medialis	Medial cutaneous nerve of arm	**arm, nerves of the** Medial cutaneous nerve of the arm
Nervus cutaneus brachii posterior	Posterior cutaneous nerve of arm	**arm, nerves of the** Posterior cutaneous nerve of the arm
Nervus cutaneus dorsalis intermedius	Lateral branch (of musculocutaneous nerve of lower limb)	**musculocutaneous nerve of the lower limb** Lateral branch
Nervus cutaneus dorsalis lateralis	Dorsal lateral cutaneous nerve of foot	**foot, dorsal lateral cutaneous nerve of the**
Nervus cutaneus dorsalis medialis	Medial branch (of musculocutaneous nerve of lower limb)	**musculocutaneous nerve of the lower limb** Medial branch
Nervus cutaneus femoris lateralis	Lateral cutaneous nerve of thigh	**thigh, cutaneous nerves of the** Lateral cutaneous nerve of the thigh
Nervus cutaneus femoris posterior	Posterior cutaneous nerve of thigh	**thigh, cutaneous nerves of the** Posterior cutaneous nerve of the thigh
Nervus cutaneus surae lateralis	Lateral cutaneous nerve of calf of leg	**leg, lateral cutaneous nerve of the calf of the**
Nervus cutaneus surae medialis	Medial cutaneous nerve of calf of leg	**sural nerve**
Nervi digitales dorsales (nervi radialis)	Dorsal digital nerves (of radial nerve)	**digital nerves** Dorsal digital nerves of the hand
Nervi digitales dorsales (nervi ulnaris)	Dorsal digital nerves (of ulnar nerve)	**digital nerves** Dorsal digital nerves of the hand
Nervi digitales dorsales, hallucis lateralis et digiti secundi medialis	Digital branch (of anterior tibial nerve)	**tibial nerves** Anterior tibial nerve
Nervi digitales dorsales pedis	Dorsal digital nerves of foot	**digital nerves** Dorsal digital nerves of the foot
Nervi digitales palmares communes (nervi mediani)	Common palmar digital nerves (of median nerve)	**digital nerves** Palmar digital nerves, common
Nervi digitales palmares communes (nervi ulnaris)	Common palmar digital nerves (of ulnar nerve)	**digital nerves** Palmar digital nerves, common
Nervi digitales palmares proprii	Proper palmar digital nerves	**digital nerves** Palmar digital nerves, proper
Nervi digitales plantares communes (nervi plantaris lateralis)	Common plantar digital nerves (of lateral plantar nerve)	**digital nerves** Plantar digital nerves, common
Nervi digitales plantares communes (nervi plantaris medialis)	Common plantar digital nerves (of medial plantar nerve)	**digital nerves** Plantar digital nerves, common
Nervi digitales plantares proprii (nervi plantaris lateralis)	Proper plantar digital nerves (of lateral plantar nerve)	**digital nerves** Plantar digital nerves, proper

Anatomical Nomenclature

Nomina Anatomica (N.A.)	Birmingham Revision (B.R.) or English Equivalent	Definition Location
Nervi digitales plantares proprii (nervi plantaris medialis)	Proper plantar digital nerves (of medial plantar nerve)	**digital nerves** Plantar digital nerves, proper
Nervus dorsalis clitoridis	Dorsal nerve of clitoris	**penis, nerves of the (or of the clitoris)** Dorsal nerve of the penis (or of the clitoris)
Nervus dorsalis penis	Dorsal nerve of penis	**penis, nerves of the** Dorsal nerve of the penis
Nervus dorsalis scapulae	Nerve to rhomboids	**rhomboids, nerve to the**
Nervus ethmoidalis anterior	Anterior ethmoidal nerve	**ethmoidal nerves** Anterior ethmoidal nerve
Nervus ethmoidalis posterior	Posterior ethmoidal nerve	**ethmoidal nerves** Posterior ethmoidal nerve
Nervus facialis	Facial nerve	**facial nerve**
Nervus femoralis	Femoral nerve	**femoral nerve**
Nervus frontalis	Frontal nerve	**frontal nerve**
Nervus genitofemoralis	Genitofemoral nerve	**genitofemoral nerve**
Nervus glossopharyngeus	Glossopharyngeal nerve	**glossopharyngeal nerve**
Nervus gluteus inferior	Inferior gluteal nerve	**gluteal nerves** Inferior gluteal nerve
Nervus gluteus superior	Superior gluteal nerve	**gluteal nerves** Superior gluteal nerve
Nervus hypogastricus [dexter et sinister]	Hypogastric nerve (right and left)	**hypogastric nerve, right and left**
Nervus hypoglossus	Hypoglossal nerve	**hypoglossal nerve**
Nervus iliohypogastricus	Iliohypogastric nerve	**iliohypogastric nerve**
Nervus ilio-inguinalis	Ilio-inguinal nerve	**ilio-inguinal nerve**
Nervus infra-orbitalis	Infra-orbital nerve	**infra-orbital nerve**
Nervus infratrochlearis	Infratrochlear nerve	**infratrochlear nerve**
Nervi intercostales	Intercostal nerves	**intercostal nerves**
Nervus intercostobrachialis	Intercostobrachial nerve	**intercostobrachial nerve**
Nervus intermedius	Sensory root (of facial nerve)	**facial nerve** Roots
Nervus interosseus [antebrachii] anterior	Anterior interosseous nerve	**interosseous nerves** Anterior interosseous nerve
Nervus interosseus [antebrachii] posterior	Posterior interosseous nerve	**interosseous nerves** Posterior interosseous nerve
Nervus interosseus cruris	Interosseous branch (of medial popliteal nerve)	**popliteal nerves** Medial popliteal nerve
Nervus ischiadicus	Sciatic nerve	**sciatic nerve**
Nervus jugularis	Jugular nerve	**jugular nerve**
Nervi labiales anteriores	Labial branches (of ilio-inguinal nerve)	**ilio-inguinal nerve**
Nervi labiales posteriores	Labial branches (of perineal nerve)	**perineal nerve** Scrotal (labial) branches
Nervus lacrimalis	Lacrimal nerve	**lacrimal nerve**
Nervus laryngeus inferior	Laryngeal branches (of vagus nerve)	**vagus nerve**
Nervus laryngeus recurrens	Recurrent laryngeal nerve	**laryngeal nerve** Recurrent laryngeal nerve
Nervus laryngeus superior	Superior laryngeal nerve	**laryngeal nerves** Superior laryngeal nerve
Nervus lingualis	Lingual nerve	**lingual nerve**
Nervi lumbales	Lumbar nerves	**lumbar nerves**
Nervus mandibularis	Mandibular nerve	**mandibular nerve**
Nervus massetericus	Nerve to masseter	**mandibular nerve**
Nervus maxillaris	Maxillary nerve	**maxillary nerve**
Nervus meatus acustici externi	Nerve to external auditory meatus	**auriculotemporal nerve**
Nervus medianus	Median nerve	**median nerve**
Nervus mentalis	Mental nerve	**mental nerve**
Nervus musculocutaneus	Musculocutaneous nerve (of upper limb)	**musculocutaneous nerve of the upper limb**

Nomina Anatomica (N.A.)	Birmingham Revision (B.R.) or English Equivalent	Definition Location
Nervus mylohyoideus	Mylohyoid nerve	**dental nerves** Inferior dental nerve
Nervus nasociliaris	Nasociliary nerve	**nasociliary nerve**
Nervus nasopalatinus	Long sphenopalatine nerve	**sphenopalatine nerves** Long sphenopalatine nerve
Nervus obturatorius	Obturator nerve	**obturator nerve**
Nervus occipitalis major	Greater occipital nerve	**occipital nerves** Greater occipital nerve
Nervus occipitalis minor	Lesser occipital nerve	**occipital nerves** Lesser occipital nerve
Nervus occipitalis tertius	Third occipital nerve	**occipital nerves** Third occipital nerve
Nervus octavus	Auditory nerve	**auditory nerve**
Nervus oculomotorius	Oculomotor nerve	**oculomotor nerve**
Nervi olfactorii	Olfactory nerves	**olfactory nerves**
Nervus ophthalmicus	Ophthalmic nerve	**ophthalmic nerve**
Nervus opticus	Optic nerve	**optic nerve**
Nervus palatinus major	Greater palatine nerve	**palatine nerves** Greater palatine nerve
Nervus palatinus minores	Lesser palatine nerves	**palatine nerves** Lesser palatine nerves
Nervus pectoralis lateralis	Lateral pectoral nerve	**pectoral nerves** Lateral pectoral nerve
Nervus pectoralis medialis	Medial pectoral nerve	**pectoral nerves** Medial pectoral nerve
Nervus perinei	Perineal nerve	**perineal nerve**
Nervus peroneus [fibularis] communis	Lateral popliteal nerve	**popliteal nerves** Lateral popliteal nerve
Nervus peroneus [fibularis] profundus	Anterior tibial nerve	**tibial nerves** Anterior tibial nerve
Nervus peroneus [fibularis] superficialis	Musculocutaneous nerve (of lower limb)	**musculocutaneous nerve of the lower limb**
Nervus petrosus major	Greater superficial petrosal nerve	**petrosal nerves** Greater superficial petrosal nerve
Nervus petrosus minor	Lesser superficial petrosal nerve	**petrosal nerves** Lesser superficial petrosal nerve
Nervus petrosus profundus	Deep petrosal nerve	**petrosal nerves** Deep petrosal nerve
Nervus phrenicus	Phrenic nerve	**phrenic nerve**
Nervi phrenici accessorii	Accessory phrenic nerves	**phrenic nerve** Accessory phrenic nerves
Nervus plantaris lateralis	Lateral plantar nerve	**plantar nerves** Lateral plantar nerve
Nervus plantaris medialis	Medial plantar nerve	**plantar nerves** Medial plantar nerve
Nervus pterygoideus lateralis	Nerve to lateral pterygoid muscle	**mandibular nerve**
Nervus pterygoideus medialis	Nerve to medial pterygoid muscle	**mandibular nerve**
Nervi pterygopalatini	Ganglionic branches (of maxillary nerve)	**maxillary nerve** Ganglionic branches
Nervus pudendus	Pudendal nerve	**pudendal nerve**
Nervus radialis	Radial nerve	**radial nerve**
Nervi rectales inferiores	Inferior haemorrhoidal nerves	**haemorrhoidal nerves, inferior**
Nervus saccularis	Saccular nerve	**saccular nerve**
Nervi sacrales	Sacral nerves	**sacral nerves**
Nervus saphenus	Saphenous nerve	**saphenous nerve**
Nervi scrotales anteriores	Scrotal branches (of ilio-inguinal nerve)	**ilio-inguinal nerve**
Nervi scrotales posteriores	Scrotal branches (of perineal nerve)	**perineal nerve** Scrotal (labial) branches
Nervi spinales	Spinal nerves	**spinal nerves**
Nervus splanchnicus imus	Lowest splanchnic nerve	**splanchnic nerves** Lowest splanchnic nerve
Nervi splanchnici lumbalis	Lumbar splanchnic nerves	**splanchnic nerves** Lumbar splanchnic nerves

Nomina Anatomica (N.A.)	Birmingham Revision (B.R.) or English Equivalent	Definition Location
Nervus splanchnicus major	Greater splanchnic nerve	**splanchnic nerves** Greater splanchnic nerve
Nervus splanchnicus minor	Lesser splanchnic nerve	**splanchnic nerves** Lesser splanchnic nerve
Nervi splanchnici pelvini [nervi erigentes]	Pelvic splanchnic nerves	**splanchnic nerves** Pelvic splanchnic nerves
Nervi splanchnici sacrales	Sacral splanchnic nerves	**splanchnic nerves** Sacral splanchnic nerves
Nervus stapedius	Nerve to stapedius muscle	**stapedius muscle, nerve to the**
Nervus vestibulocochlearis [nervus octavus]	Auditory nerve	**auditory nerve**
Nervus subclavius	Nerve to subclavius muscle	**subclavius muscle, nerve to the**
Nervus subcostalis	Subcostal nerve	**subcostal nerve**
Nervus sublingualis	Sublingual nerve	**lingual nerve**
Nervus suboccipitalis	First cervical (suboccipital) nerve	**cervical nerves**
Nervi subscapulares	Subscapular nerves	**subscapular nerves**
Nervi supraclaviculares	Supraclavicular nerves	**supraclavicular nerves**
Nervi supraclaviculares intermedii	Intermediate supraclavicular nerves	**supraclavicular nerves**
Nervi supraclaviculares laterales (posteriores)	Lateral supraclavicular nerves	**supraclavicular nerves**
Nervi supraclaviculares mediales	Medial supraclavicular nerves	**supraclavicular nerves**
Nervus supra-orbitalis	Supra-orbital nerve	**supra-orbital nerve**
Nervus suprascapularis	Suprascapular nerve	**suprascapular nerve**
Nervus supratrochlearis	Supratrochlear nerve	**supratrochlear nerve**
Nervus suralis	Sural nerve	**sural nerve**
Nervi temporales profundi	Deep temporal nerves	**temporal nerves, deep**
Nervus tensoris tympani	Nerve to tensor tympani muscle	**tensor tympani muscle, nerve to the**
Nervus tensoris veli palatini	Nerve to tensor palati muscle	**tensor palati muscle, nerve to the**
Nervi terminales	Nervi terminales	**nervus** Nervi terminales
Nervi thoracici	Thoracic nerves	**thoracic nerves**
Nervus thoracicus longus	Nerve to serratus anterior muscle	**serratus anterior muscle, nerve to the**
Nervus thoracodorsalis	Nerve to latissimus dorsi muscle	**latissimus dorsi muscle, nerve to the**
Nervus tibialis	Medial popliteal nerve	**popliteal nerves** Medial popliteal nerve
Nervus transversus colli	Anterior cutaneous nerve of neck	**neck, anterior cutaneous nerve of the**
Nervus trigeminus	Trigeminal nerve	**trigeminal nerve**
Nervus trochlearis	Trochlear nerve	**trochlear nerve**
Nervus tympanicus	Tympanic nerve	**tympanic nerve**
Nervus ulnaris	Ulnar nerve	**ulnar nerve**
Nervus utriculo-ampullaris	Utriculo-ampullar nerve	**utriculo-ampullar nerve**
Nervus utricularis	Utricular nerve	**utricular nerve**
Nervi vaginales	Vaginal nerves	**vaginal nerves**
Nervus vagus	Vagus nerve	**vagus nerve**
Nervus vascularis	Vascular branch (of nerve)	**branch** Vascular branch
Nervus vertebralis	Vertebral branch of inferior cervical ganglion	**ganglion** Cervical ganglion, inferior, vertebral branch of the
Nervus vestibulocochlearis [nervus octavus]	Auditory nerve	**auditory nerve**
Nervus zygomaticus	Zygomatic nerve	**zygomatic nerve**
Neuro-epithelium	Neuro-epithelium	**neuro-epithelium**
Nodulus	Nodule	**nodule**

Nomina Anatomica (N.A.)	Birmingham Revision (B.R.) or English Equivalent	Definition Location
Noduli thymici accessorii	Accessory thymic nodules	**nodule** Accessory thymic nodules
Noduli valvularum semilunarium (aortae)	Nodules of aortic valve	**valve** Aortic valve
Noduli valvularum semilunarium (pulmonales)	Nodules of pulmonary valve	**valve** Pulmonary valve
Nodus	Node	**node**
Nodus atrioventricularis	Atrioventricular node	**node** Atrioventricular node
Nodi lymphatici [lymphonodi]	Lymph gland	**gland** Lymph glands
Nodi lymphatici apicales	Apical lymph glands	**gland** Lymph glands, apical
Nodi lymphatici axillares	Axillary lymph glands	**gland** Lymph glands, axillary
Nodi lymphatici bronchopulmonales	Bronchopulmonary lymph glands	**gland** Lymph glands, bronchopulmonary
Nodi lymphatici buccales	Buccal lymph glands	**gland** Lymph glands, buccal
Nodi lymphatici centrales	Central lymph glands	**gland** Lymph glands, central
Nodi lymphatici cervicales profundi	Deep cervical lymph glands	**gland** Lymph glands, cervical, deep
Nodi lymphatici cervicales superficiales	Superficial cervical lymph glands	**gland** Lymph glands, cervical, superficial
Nodi lymphatici celiaci	Coeliac lymph glands	**gland** Lymph glands, coeliac
Nodi lymphatici colici dextri	Right colic lymph glands	**gland** Lymph glands, colic, right
Nodi lymphatici colici medii	Middle colic lymph glands	**gland** Lymph glands, colic, middle
Nodi lymphatici colici sinistri	Left colic lymph glands	**gland** Lymph glands, colic, left
Nodi lymphatici cubitales	Supratrochlear lymph glands	**gland** Lymph glands, supratrochlear
Nodi lymphatici epigastrici	Epigastric lymph glands	**gland** Lymph glands, epigastric
Nodi lymphatici gastrici dextri	Right gastro-epiploic lymph glands	**gland** Lymph glands, gastro-epiploic, right
Nodi lymphatici gastroepiploici sinistri	Left gastric lymph glands	**gland** Lymph glands, gastric, left
Nodi lymphatici hepatici	Hepatic lymph glands	**gland** Lymph glands, hepatic
Nodi lymphatici ileocolici	Ileocolic lymph glands	**gland** Lymph glands, ileocolic
Nodi lymphatici iliaci	Iliac lymph glands	**gland** Lymph glands, iliac
Nodi lymphatici iliaci commune	Common iliac lymph glands	**gland** Lymph glands, iliac, common
Nodi lymphatici iliaci externi	External iliac lymph lymph glands	**gland** Lymph glands, iliac, external
Nodi lymphatici iliaci interni	Internal iliac lymph glands	**gland** Lymph glands, iliac, internal
Nodi lymphatici inguinales profundi	Deep inguinal lymph glands	**gland** Lymph glands, inguinal, deep
Nodi lymphatici inguinales superficiales	Superficial inguinal lymph glands	**gland** Lymph glands, inguinal, superficial
Nodi lymphatici intercostales	Intercostal lymph glands	**gland** Lymph glands, intercostal
Nodus lymphaticus jugulodigastricus	Jugulodigastric lymph gland	**gland** Lymph gland, jugulodigastric

Anatomical Nomenclature

Nomina Anatomica (N.A.)	Birmingham Revision (B.R.) or English Equivalent	Definition Location
Nodus lymphaticus jugulo-omohyoideus	Jugulo-omohyoid lymph gland	**gland** Lymph gland, jugulo-omohyoid
Nodi lymphatici laterales	Lateral lymph glands	**gland** Lymph glands, lateral
Nodi lymphatici linguales	Lingual lymph glands	**gland** Lymph glands, lingual
Nodi lymphatici lumbales	Aortic lymph glands	**gland** Lymph glands, aortic
Nodi lymphatici mandibulares	Mandibular lymph glands	**gland** Lymph glands, mandibular
Nodi lymphatici mediastinales anteriores	Innominate lymph glands	**gland** Lymph glands, innominate
Nodi lymphatici mediastinales posteriores	Posterior mediastinal lymph glands	**gland** Lymph glands, mediastinal, posterior
Nodi lymphatici mesenterici inferiores	Inferior mesenteric lymph glands	**gland** Lymph glands, mesenteric, inferior
Nodi lymphatici mesenterici superiores	Lymph glands of the mesentery	**gland** Lymph glands of the mesentery, superior
Nodi lymphatici occipitales	Occipital lymph glands	**gland** Lymph glands, occipital
Nodi lymphatici pancreaticolienales	Pancreaticosplenic lymph glands	**gland** Lymph glands, pancreaticosplenic
Nodi lymphatici parasternales	Internal mammary lymph glands	**gland** Lymph glands, mammary, internal
Nodi lymphatici parotidei, superficiales et profundi	Parotid lymph glands	**gland** Lymph glands, parotid
Nodi lymphatici pectorales	Pectoral lymph glands	**gland** Lymph glands, pectoral
Nodi lymphatici phrenici	Diaphragmatic lymph glands	**gland** Lymph glands, diaphragmatic
Nodi lymphatici poplitei	Popliteal lymph glands	**gland** Lymph glands, popliteal
Nodi lymphatici pulmonales	Pulmonary lymph glands	**gland** Lymph glands, pulmonary
Nodi lymphatici pylorici	Pyloric lymph glands	**gland** Lymph glands, pyloric
Nodi lymphatici retro-auriculares	Mastoid lymph glands	**gland** Lymph glands, mastoid
Nodi lymphatici retropharyngei	Retropharyngeal lymph glands	**gland** Lymph glands, retropharyngeal
Nodi lymphatici sacrales	Sacral lymph glands	**gland** Lymph glands, sacral
Nodi lymphatici submandibulares	Submandibular lymph glands	**gland** Lymph glands, submandibular
Nodi lymphatici submentales	Submental lymph glands	**gland** Lymph glands, submental
Nodi lymphatici subscapulares	Subscapular lymph glands	**gland** Lympb glands, subscapular
Nodus lymphaticus tibialis anterior	Anterior tibial lymph gland	**gland** Lymph gland, tibial, anterior
Nodi lymphatici tracheales	Tracheobronchial lymph glands	**gland** Lymph glands, tracheobronchial
Nodi lymphatici tracheobronchiales inferiores	Inferior tracheobronchial lymph glands	**gland** Lymph glands, tracheobronchial
Nodi lymphatici tracheobronchiales superiores	Superior tracheobronchial lymph glands	**gland** Lymph glands, tracheobronchial
Nodus sinu-atrialis	Sinu-atrial node	**node** Sinu-atrial node
Nucha	Nape of neck	**nape**
Nucleus	Nucleus	**nucleus**

Nomina Anatomica (N.A.)	Birmingham Revision (B.R.) or English Equivalent	Definition Location
Nucleus accessorius [autonomicus]	Accessory nucleus	**nucleus** Accessory nucleus
Nucleus ambiguus	Nucleus ambiguus	**nucleus** Nucleus ambiguus
Nucleus anterior corporis trapezoidei	Ventral nucleus of corpus trapezoideum	**corpus** Corpus trapezoideum, ventral nucleus of the
Nucleus anteriores thalami	Anterior nucleus of thalamus	**thalamus** Nucleus of the thalamus, anterior
Nuclei arcuati	Arcuate nuclei	**nucleus** Arcuate nuclei
Nucleus caudalis centralis	Caudal central nucleus	**nucleus** Caudal central nucleus
Nucleus caudatus	Caudate nucleus	**nucleus** Caudate nucleus
Nuclei cochleares, ventralis et dorsalis	Ventral and dorsal cochlear nuclei	**nucleus** Cochlear nuclei, ventral and dorsal
Nucleus colliculi inferioris	Nucleus of inferior quadrigeminal body	**body** Quadrigeminal body, inferior, nucleus of the
Nucleus corporis geniculati lateralis	Nucleus of lateral geniculate body	**body** Geniculate body, lateral, nucleus of the
Nucleus corporis geniculati medialis	Nucleus of medial geniculate body	**body** Geniculate body, medial, nucleus of the
Nuclei corporis mamillaris	Nuclei of mamillary body	**body** Mamillary body, nuclei of the
Nucleus cuneatus	Cuneate nucleus	**nucleus** Cuneate nucleus
Nucleus cuneatus accessorius	Accessory cuneate nucleus	**nucleus** Accessory cuneate nucleus
Nucleus dentatus	Dentate nucleus	**nucleus** Dentate nucleus
Nucleus dorsalis corporis trapezoidei	Dorsal nucleus of corpus trapezoideum	**corpus** Corpus trapezoideum, dorsal nucleus of the
Nucleus dorsalis nervi glossopharyngei	Dorsal nucleus of glossopharyngeal nerve	**glossopharyngeal nerve** Nuclei
Nucleus dorsalis nervi vagi	Dorsal nucleus of vagus nerve	**vagus nerve** Dorsal nucleus
Nucleus dorsolateralis	Dorsolateral nucleus	**nucleus** Dorsolateral nucleus
Nucleus dorsomedialis	Dorsomedial nucleus	**nucleus** Dorsomedial nucleus
Nucleus emboliformis	Nucleus emboliformis	**nucleus** Nucleus emboliformis
Nucleus fastigii	Nucleus fastigii	**nucleus** Nucleus fastigii
Nucleus globosus	Nucleus globosus	**nucleus** Nucleus globosus
Nucleus gracilis	Gracile nucleus	**nucleus** Gracile nucleus
Nucleus habenulae	Habenular nucleus	**nucleus** Habenular nucleus
Nucleus intercalatus	Nucleus intercalatus	**nucleus** Nucleus intercalatus
Nucleus interpeduncularis	Interpeduncular nucleus	**nucleus** Interpeduncular nucleus
Nucleus interstitialis	Interstitial nucleus	**nucleus** Interstitial nucleus
Nuclei intralaminares (thalami)	Intralaminar nuclei of thalamus	**thalamus** Nuclei of the thalamus, intralaminar
Nucleus lateralis	Lateral nucleus	**nucleus** Lateral nucleus
Nucleus lateralis thalami	Lateral nucleus of thalamus	**thalamus** Nucleus of the thalamus, lateral
Nucleus lemnisci lateralis	Nucleus of lateral lemniscus	**lemniscus** Lateral lemniscus

Nomina Anatomica (N.A.)	Birmingham Revision (B.R.) or English Equivalent	Definition Location
Nucleus lentiformis	Lentiform nucleus	**nucleus** Lentiform nucleus
Nucleus lentis	Nucleus of lens	**lens** Nucleus of the lens
Nucleus medialis centralis [centromedianus] (thalami)	Centromedial nucleus of thalamus	**thalamus** Nucleus of the thalamus, centromedial
Nucleus medialis thalami	Medial nucleus of thalamus	**thalamus** Nucleus of the thalamus, medial
Nucleus motorius nervi trigemini	Motor nucleus of trigeminal nerve	**trigeminal nerve** Motor nucleus
Nucleus nervi abducentis	Nucleus of abducent nerve	**abducent nerve** Nucleus
Nucleus nervi accessorii	Nucleus of accessory nerve	**accessory nerve** Nucleus
Nuclei nervorum cranialium	Nuclei of cranial nerves	**nucleus** Nucleus of a cranial nerve
Nucleus nervi facialis	Nucleus of facial nerve	**facial nerve** Nucleus
Nucleus nervi glossopharyngei	Nucleus of glosso-pharyngeal nerve	**glossopharyngeal nerve** Nuclei
Nucleus nervi hypoglossi	Nucleus of hypoglossal nerve	**hypoglossal nerve** Nucleus
Nucleus nervi oculomotorii	Nucleus of oculomotor nerve	**oculomotor nerve** Nucleus
Nucleus nervi trochlearis	Nucleus of trochlear nerve	**trochlear nerve** Nucleus
Nuclei nervi vagi	Nuclei of vagus nerve	**vagus nerve** Nuclei
Nuclei nervi vestibulocochlearis	Nuclei of auditory nerve	**auditory nerve** Nuclei
Nucleus olivaris	Olivary nucleus	**nucleus** Olivary nucleus
Nucleus olivaris accessorius dorsalis	Dorsal accessory olivary nucleus	**nucleus** Olivary nucleus, dorsal accessory
Nucleus olivaris accessorius medialis	Medial accessory olivary nucleus	**nucleus** Olivary nucleus, medial accessory
Nuclei originis	Nuclei of origin	**nucleus** Nucleus of origin
Nucleus paraventricularis	Paraventricular nucleus	**nucleus** Paraventricular nucleus
Nuclei pontis	Nuclei pontis	**nucleus** Nuclei pontis
Nucleus posterior	Posterior nucleus	**nucleus** Posterior nucleus
Nucleus posterior [pulvinar thalami]	Pulvinar	**pulvinar**
Nucleus posterior corporis trapezoidei	Dorsal nucleus of corpus trapezoideum	**corpus** Corpus trapezoideum, dorsal nucleus of the
Nucleus pretectalis	Pretectal nucleus	**nucleus** Pretectal nucleus
Nucleus pulposus	Nucleus pulposus	**nucleus** Nucleus pulposus
Nucleus reticularis thalami	Reticular nucleus of thalamus	**thalamus** Nucleus of the thalamus, reticular
Nucleus ruber	Red nucleus	**nucleus** Red nucleus
Nucleus salivatorius inferior	Inferior salivary nucleus	**nucleus** Salivary nucleus inferior
Nucleus salivatorius superior	Superior salivary nucleus	**nucleus** Salivary nucleus, superior
Nucleus sensorius principalis nervi trigemini	Superior sensory nucleus of trigeminal nerve	**trigeminal nerve** Superior sensory nucleus
Nucleus spinalis nervi accessorii	Spinal nucleus of accessory nerve	**accessory nerve** Spinal nucleus
Nucleus subthalamicus	Subthalamic nucleus	**nucleus** Subthalamic nucleus

Nomina Anatomica (N.A.)	Birmingham Revision (B.R.) or English Equivalent	Definition Location
Nucleus supra-opticus	Supra-optic nucleus	**nucleus** Supra-optic nucleus
Nuclei tegmenti	Tegmental nuclei	**nucleus** Tegmental nuclei
Nuclei terminationis	Nuclei of termination	**nucleus** Nucleus of termination
Nucleus thoracicus	Thoracic nucleus	**nucleus** Thoracic nucleus
Nucleus tractus mesencephalici nervi trigemini	Mesencephalic nucleus of trigeminal nerve	**trigeminal nerve** Mesencephalic nucleus
Nucleus tractus solitarii	Nucleus of tractus solitarius	**tractus** Tractus solitarius
Nucleus tractus spinalis nervi trigemini	Nucleus of spinal tract of trigeminal nerve	**tract** Tract of the trigeminal nerve, spinal
Nuclei tuberales	Tuberal nuclei	**nucleus** Tuberal nuclei
Nucleus ventralis anterolateralis (thalami)	Anterolateral ventral nucleus of thalamus	**thalamus** Nucleus of the thalamus, lateral
Nucleus ventralis corporis trapezoidei	Ventral nucleus of corpus trapezoidei	**corpus** Corpus trapezoideum, ventral nucleus of the
Nucleus ventralis intermedius (thalami)	Intermediate ventral nucleus of thalamus	**thalamus** Nucleus of the thalamus, lateral
Nucleus ventralis posterolateralis (thalami)	Posterolateral ventral nucleus of thalamus	**thalamus** Nucleus of the thalamus, lateral
Nucleus ventralis posteromedialis (thalami)	Posteromedial ventral nucleus of thalamus	**thalamus** Nucleus of the thalamus, lateral
Nucleus ventromedialis	Ventromedial nucleus	**nucleus** Ventromedial nucleus
Nucleus vestibularis inferior	Inferior vestibular nucleus	**nucleus** Vestibular nucleus, inferior
Nucleus vestibularis lateralis	Lateral vestibular nucleus	**nucleus** Vestibular nucleus, lateral
Nucleus vestibularis medialis	Medial vestibular nucleus	**nucleus** Vestibular nucleus, medial
Nucleus vestibularis superior	Superior vestibular nucleus	**nucleus** Vestibular nucleus, superior
Obex	Obex	**obex**
Occiput	Occiput	**occiput**
Oculus	Eye	**eye**
Olecranon	Olecranon	**olecranon**
Oliva	Olive	**olive**
Omentum majus	Greater omentum	**omentum** Greater omentum
Omentum minus	Lesser omentum	**omentum** Lesser omentum
Operculum frontale	Frontal operculum	**operculum** Frontal operculum
Operculum frontoparietale	Frontoparietal operculum	**operculum** Frontoparietal operculum
Operculum temporale	Temporal operculum	**operculum** Temporal operculum
Ora serrata	Ora serrata	**ora** Ora serrata
Orbiculus ciliaris	Ciliary ring	**ring** Ciliary ring
Orbita	Orbit	**orbit**
Organum	Organ	**organ**
Organa genitalia	Genital organs	**organ** Genital organs
Organa genitalia feminina	Female genital organs	**organ** Genital organs, female
Organa genitalia masculina	Male genital organs	**organ** Genital organs, male
Organum gustus	Organ of taste	**organ** Organ of taste
Organum olfactus	Organ of smell	**organ** Organ of smell

Anatomical Nomenclature

Nomina Anatomica (N.A.)	Birmingham Revision (B.R.) or English Equivalent	Definition Location
Organum spirale	Spiral organ	**organ** Spiral organ
Organa uropoëtica	Urinary organs	**organ** Urinary organs
Organum vestibulocochleare	Organ of hearing	**organ** Organ of hearing
Organum visus	Organ of sight	**organ** Organ of sight
Organum vomeronasale	Vomeronasal organ	**organ** Vomeronasal organ
Os	Mouth	**mouth**
Os	Bone	**bone**
Os breve	Short bone	**bone** Short bone
Os capitatum	Capitate bone	**capitate bone**
Ossa carpi	Carpal bones	**carpal bone**
Os centrale	Os centrale	**os** Os centrale
Os coccygis	Coccyx	**coccyx**
Os costale	Bony part of rib	**os** Os costale
Os coxae	Hip bone	**hip bone**
Ossa cranii	Bones of skull	**skull**
Os cuboideum	Cuboid bone	**cuboid bone**
Os cuneiforme intermedium	Intermediate cuneiform bone	**cuneiform bones** Intermediate cuneiform bone
Os cuneiforme laterale	Lateral cuneiform bone	**cuneiform bones** Lateral cuneiform bone
Os cuneiforme mediale	Medial cuneiform bone	**cuneiform bones** Medial cuneiform bone
Ossa digitorum manus	Phalanges of digits of hand	**phalanges (of the hand and foot)**
Ossa digitorum pedis	Phalanges of digits of foot	**phalanges (of the hand and foot)**
Os ethmoidale	Ethmoid bone	**ethmoid bone**
Ossa faciei	Facial bones	**facial bones**
Os frontale	Frontal bone	**frontal bone**
Os hamatum	Hamate bone	**hamate bone**
Os hyoideum	Hyoid bone	**hyoid bone**
Os ilium	Ilium	**ilium**
Os incisivum	Incisive bone	**incisive bone of the maxilla**
Os interparietale	Interparietal bone	**interparietal bone**
Os ischii	Ischium	**ischium**
Os lacrimale	Lacrimal bone	**lacrimal bone**
Os longum	Long bone	**bone** Long bone
Os lunatum	Lunate bone	**lunate bone**
Ossa metacarpalia I–V	Metacarpal bones 1st–5th	**metacarpal bones**
Os metacarpale III	Third metacarpal bone	**metacarpal bones**
Ossa metatarsalia I–V	Metatarsal bones 1st–5th	**metatarsal bones**
Os nasale	Nasal bone	**nasal bone**
Os naviculare	Navicular bone	**navicular bone**
Os occipitale	Occipital bone	**occipital bone**
Os palatinum	Palatine bone	**palatine bone**
Os parietale	Parietal bone	**parietal bone**
Os pisiforme	Pisiform bone	**pisiform bone**
Os planum	Flat bone	**bone** Flat bone
Os pneumaticum	Pneumatic bone	**bone** Pneumatic bone
Os pubis	Pubis	**pubis**
Os sacrum	Sacrum	**sacrum**
Os scaphoideum	Scaphoid bone	**scaphoid bone**
Ossa sesamoidea (manus)	Sesamoid bones (of hand)	**sesamoid bones**

Nomina Anatomica (N.A.)	Birmingham Revision (B.R.) or English Equivalent	Definition Location
Ossa sesamoidea (pedis)	Sesamoid bones (of foot)	**sesamoid bones**
Os sphenoidale	Sphenoid bone	**sphenoid bone**
Ossa suprasternalia	Suprasternal bones	**suprasternal bones**
Ossa suturarum	Sutural bones	**sutural bones**
Ossa tarsi	Tarsal bones	**tarsal bones**
Os temporale	Temporal bone	**temporal bone**
Os trapezium	Trapezium	**trapezium**
Os trapezoideum	Trapezoid	**trapezoid bone**
Os trigonum	Os trigonum	**os** Os trigonum
Os triquetrum	Triquetral bone	**triquetral bone**
Os zygomaticum	Zygomatic bone	**zygomatic bone**
Ossicula auditus	Auditory ossicles	**ossicle** Auditory ossicles
Osteologia	Osteology	**osteology**
Ostium	Orifice	**orifice** *also* **ostium**
Ostium abdominale tubae uterinae	Pelvic opening of uterine tube	**tube** Uterine tube
Ostium aortae	Aortic orifice	**orifice** Aortic orifice
Ostium appendicis vermiformis	Opening of vermiform appendix	**appendix** Vermiform appendix, opening of the
Ostium atrio-ventriculare dextrum	Right atrioventricular (tricuspid) orifice	**orifice** Atrioventricular orifice, right (tricuspid)
Ostium atrio-ventriculare sinistrum	Left atrioventricular (mitral) orifice	**orifice** Atrioventricular orifice, left (mitral)
Ostium cardiacum (ventriculi)	Cardiac orifice (in stomach)	**orifice** Orifice in the stomach, cardiac
Ostium ileocaecale	Ileocolic orifice	**orifice** Ileocolic orifice
Ostium pharyngeum tubae	Pharyngeal opening of tube	**tube** Pharyngotympanic tube
Ostium pharyngeum tubae auditivae	Pharyngeal opening of pharyngotympanic tube	**tube** Pharyngotympanic tube
Ostium pyloricum	Pyloric orifice	**orifice** Orifice in the stomach, pyloric
Ostium trunci pulmonalis	Pulmonary orifice	**orifice** Pulmonary orifice
Ostium tympanicum tubae auditivae	Tympanic opening of pharyngotympanic tube	**tube** Pharyngotympanic tube
Ostium ureteris	Orifice of ureter	**orifice** Orifice of the ureter
Ostium urethrae externum (urethrae femininae)	External orifice (of female urethra)	**orifice** Orifice of the female urethra, external
Ostium urethrae externum (urethrae masculinae)	External orifice (of male urethra)	**orifice** Orifice of the male urethra, external
Ostium urethrae internum	Internal urethral orifice	**orifice** Urethral orifice, internal
Ostium uteri	External os uteri	**os** Os uteri, external
Ostium uterinum tubae	Uterine opening (of uterine tube)	**tube** Uterine tube
Ostium vaginae	Orifice of vagina	**orifice** Orifice of the vagina
Ostium venae cavae inferioris	Opening for inferior vena cava	**atrium** Right atrium
Ostium venae cavae superioris	Opening to superior vena cava	**atrium** Right atrium
Ostia venarum pulmonalium	Openings for pulmonary veins	**atrium** Left atrium
Ovarium	Ovary	**ovary**
Ovum	Ovum	**ovum**
Palatum	Palate	**palate**

Nomina Anatomica (N.A.)	Birmingham Revision (B.R.) or English Equivalent	Definition Location
Palatum durum	Hard palate	**palate** Hard palate
Palatum molle [velum palatinum]	Soft palate	**palate** Soft palate
Palatum osseum	Bony palate	**palate** Bony palate
Pallium	Pallium	**pallium**
Palma manus	Palm of hand	**palm**
Palmaris	Palmar	**palmar**
Palpebrae	Eyelids	**eyelids**
Palpebra inferior	Lower eyelid	**eyelids**
Palpebra superior	Upper eyelid	**eyelids**
Pancreas	Pancreas	**pancreas**
Pancreas accessorium	Accessory pancreas	**pancreas** Accessory pancreas
Panniculus adiposus	Subcutaneous fatty tissue	**tissue** Subcutaneous fatty tissue
Papilla	Papilla	**papilla**
Papillae (corii)	Papillae (of corium)	**papilla** Papillae of the corium
Papillae conicae	Conical papillae	**papilla** Conical papillae
Papilla dentis	Dental papilla	**papilla** Dental papilla
Papilla duodeni major	Greater duodenal papilla	**papilla** Duodenal papilla, greater
Papilla duodeni minor	Smaller duodenal papilla	**papilla** Duodenal papilla, smaller
Papillae filiformes	Filiform papillae	**papilla** Filiform papillae
Papillae foliatae	Folia linguae	**papilla** Foliate papilla
Papillae fungiformes	Fungiform papillae	**papilla** Fungiform papillae
Papilla incisiva	Incisive papilla	**papilla** Incisive papilla
Papilla lacrimalis	Lacrimal papilla	**papilla** Lacrimal papilla
Papillae linguales	Lingual papillae	**papilla** Lingual papillae
Papilla mammae	Nipple	**nipple**
Papilla nervi optici	Optic disk	**disk** Optic disk
Papilla parotidea	Parotid papilla	**papilla** Parotid papilla
Papilla pili	Hair papilla	**papilla** Hair papilla
Papillae renales	Renal papillae	**papilla** Renal papillae
Papillae vallatae	Vallate papillae	**papilla** Vallate papillae
Paradidymis	Paradidymis	**paradidymis**
Parametrium	Parametrium	**parametrium**
Parenchyma	Parenchyma	**parenchyma**
Parenchyma testis	Parenchyma testis	**parenchyma** Parenchyma testis
Paries	Wall	**paries** *also* **wall**
Paries anterior (vaginae)	Anterior wall (o vagina)	**vagina**
Paries anterior (ventriculi)	Anterior wall (of stomach)	**stomach**
Paries caroticus (cavi tympani)	Anterior wall (of tympanic cavity)	**cavity** Tympanic cavity, anterior wall of the
Paries externus ductus cochlearis	Lateral wall of duct of cochlea	**duct** Duct of the cochlea
Paries inferior (orbitae)	Floor (of orbit)	**orbit**
Paries jugularis (cavi tympani)	Floor (of tympanic cavity)	**cavity** Tympanic cavity, floor of the
Paries labyrinthicus	Medial wall (of tympanic cavity)	**cavity** Tympanic cavity, medial wall of the

Nomina Anatomica (N.A.)	Birmingham Revision (B.R.) or English Equivalent	Definition Location
Paries lateralis (orbitae)	Lateral wall (of orbit)	**orbit**
Paries mastoideus (cavi tympani)	Posterior wall (of tympanic cavity)	**cavity** Tympanic cavity, posterior wall of the
Paries medialis (orbitae)	Medial wall (of orbit)	**orbit**
Paries membranaceus (cavi tympani)	Lateral wall (of tympanic cavity)	**cavity** Tympanic cavity, lateral wall of the
Paries membranaceus (tracheae)	Membranous wall (of trachea)	**trachea**
Paries posterior (vaginae)	Posterior wall (of vagina)	**vagina**
Paries posterior (ventriculi)	Posterior wall (of stomach)	**stomach**
Paries superior (orbitae)	Roof (of orbit)	**orbit**
Paries tegmentalis (cavi tympani)	Roof (of tympanic cavity)	**cavity** Tympanic cavity, roof of the
Paries tympanicus ductus cochlearis [membrana spiralis]	Floor (of duct of cochlea)	**duct** Duct of the cochlea
Paries vestibularis ductus cochlearis [membrana vestibularis]	Vestibular membrane	**membrane** Vestibular membrane
Paroöphoron	Paroöphoron	**paroöphoron**
Pars	Part	**pars**
Pars abdominalis (musculi pectoralis majoris)	Abdominal part (of pectoralis major muscle)	**pectoralis major muscle**
Pars abdominalis (oesophagi)	Abdominal part (of oesophagus)	**oesophagus**
Pars abdominalis (ureteris)	Abdominal part (of ureter)	**ureter** Part of the ureter, abdominal
Pars abdominalis systematis autonomici	Lumbar part of sympathetic system	**system** Sympathetic nervous system, lumbar part
Pars alaris (musculis nasalis)	Alar part (of nasal muscle)	**nasal muscle**
Pars alveolaris (corporis mandibulae)	Alveolar part (of body of mandible)	**mandible** Body
Pars anterior (commissurae anterioris)	Olfactory part (of anterior commissure)	**commissure** Anterior commissure, olfactory part of the
Pars anterior (hepatis)	Anterior surface (of liver)	**liver**
Pars anularis vaginae fibrosae (manus)	Annular part of fibrous flexor sheath (of fingers)	**sheath** Fibrous flexor sheaths of the tendons of the fingers
Pars anularis vaginae fibrosae (pedis)	Annular part of fibrous flexor sheath (of toes)	**sheath** Fibrous flexor sheaths of the tendons of the toes
Pars ascendens (duodeni)	Fourth part (of duodenum)	**duodenum**
Pars basalis (arteriae pulmonalis dextrae)	Basal part of right pulmonary artery	**pulmonary arteries** Right pulmonary artery
Pars basalis (arteriae pulmonalis sinistrae)	Basal part of left pulmonary artery	**pulmonary arteries** Left pulmonary artery
Pars basilaris (ossis occipitalis)	Basilar part (of occipital bone)	**occipital bone** Basilar part
Pars buccopharyngea (musculi constrictoris pharyngis superioris)	Buccopharyngeal part (of superior constrictor muscle of pharynx)	**pharynx, constrictor muscles of the**
Pars cardiaca (ventriculi)	Cardiac portion (of stomach)	**stomach** Portion of the stomach, cardiac
Pars cartilaginea (septi nasi)	Cartilaginous part (of septum of nose)	**septum** Septum of the nose, cartilaginous part
Pars cartilaginea tubae auditivae	Cartilaginous part of pharyngotympanic tube	**tube** Pharyngotympanic tube
Pars centralis (ventriculi lateralis)	Central part (of lateral ventricle)	**ventricle** Lateral ventricle

Anatomical Nomenclature

Nomina Anatomica (N.A.)	Birmingham Revision (B.R.) or English Equivalent	Definition Location
Pars cephalica et cervicalis systematis autonomici	Cephalic and cervical parts of sympathetic system	**system** Sympathetic nervous system, cephalic and cervical parts
Pars ceratopharyngea (musculi constrictoris pharyngis medii)	Ceratopharyngeal part (of middle constrictor muscle of pharynx)	**pharynx, constrictor muscles of the**
Pars cervicalis (medullae spinalis)	Cervical part (of spinal cord)	**cord** Spinal cord
Pars cervicalis (oesophagi)	Cervical part (of oesophagus)	**oesophagus**
Pars chondropharyngea (musculi constrictoris pharyngis medii)	Chondropharyngeal part (of middle constrictor muscle of pharynx)	**pharynx, constrictor muscles of the**
Pars ciliaris retinae	Ciliary part of retina	**retina**
Pars clavicularis (musculi pectoralis majoris)	Clavicular part (of pectoralis major muscle)	**pectoralis major muscle**
Pars cochlearis [nervi octavi]	Cochlear nerve	**cochlear nerve**
Pars convoluta (corticis renis)	Convoluted part (of cortex of kidney)	**cortex** Cortex of the kidney, convoluted part of the
Pars costalis (diaphragmatis)	Costal part (of diaphragm)	**diaphragm** Part of the diaphragm, costal
Pars cricopharyngea (musculi constrictoris pharyngis inferioris)	Cricopharyngeal part (of inferior constrictor muscle of pharynx)	**pharynx, constrictor muscles of the**
Pars cruciformis vaginae fibrosae (manus)	Cruciate part of fibrous flexor sheath (of hand)	**sheath** Fibrous flexor sheaths of the tendons of the fingers
Pars cruciformis vaginae fibrosae (pedis)	Cruciate part of fibrous flexor sheath (of toes)	**sheath** Fibrous flexor sheaths of the tendons of the toes
Pars cupularis (parietis tegmentalis)	Cupolar part (of roof of tympanic cavity)	**recess** Epitympanic recess
Pars descendens (duodeni)	Second part (of duodenum)	**duodenum**
Pars dextra (hepatis)	Right surface (of liver)	**liver**
Pars distalis (hypophyseos)	Anterior part (of hypophysis cerebri)	**hypophysis** Hypophysis cerebri
Pars dorsalis pontis	Dorsal part of pons	**pons** Dorsal part of the pons
Pars fetalis (placentae)	Foetal part (of placenta)	**placenta** Foetal part of placenta
Pars flaccida (membrana tympani)	Flaccid part (of tympanic membrane)	**membrane** Tympanic membrane
Pars glossopharyngea (musculi constrictoris pharyngis superioris)	Glossopharyngeal part (of superior constrictor muscle of pharnyx)	**pharynx, constrictor muscles of the**
Pars horizontalis [inferior]	Third part (of duodenum)	**duodenum**
Pars inferior (partis vestibularis nervi octavi)	Inferior branch (of vestibular nerve)	**vestibular nerve**
Pars infraclavicularis (plexus brachialis)	Infraclavicular part (of brachial plexus)	**plexus** Brachial plexus
Pars infrasegmentalis [intersegmentalis] (venae pulmonales dextrae)	Infrasegmental part (of right pulmonary veins)	**pulmonary veins** Right pulmonary veins
Pars infrasegmentalis [intersegmentalis] (venae pulmonales sinistrae)	Infrasegmental part (of left pulmonary veins)	**pulmonary veins** Left pulmonary veins
Pars infundibularis (hypophyseos)	Infundibular part (of hypophysis cerebri)	**hypophysis** Hypophysis cerebri
Pars intercartilaginea (rimae glottidis)	Intercartilaginous part (of rima glottidis)	**rima** Rima glottidis
Pars intermedia (hypophyseos)	Middle part (of hypophysis cerebri)	**hypophysis** Hypophysis cerebri
Pars intermembranacea (rimae glottidis)	Intermembranous part (of rima glottidis)	**rima** Rima glottidis
Pars intrasegmentalis (venae pulmonales dextrae)	Intrasegmental part (of right pulmonary veins)	**pulmonary veins** Right pulmonary veins
Pars intrasegmentalis (venae pulmonales sinistrae)	Intrasegmental part (of left pulmonary veins)	**pulmonary veins** Left pulmonary veins
Pars iridica retinae	Iridial part of retina	**retina**
Pars labialis (musculi orbicularis oris)	Labial part (of orbicularis oris muscle)	**orbicularis oris muscle**
Pars lacrimalis (musculi orbicularis oculi)	Lacrimal part (of orbicularis oculi muscle)	**orbicularis oculi muscle** Lacrimal part
Pars laryngea (pharyngis)	Laryngeal part (of pharynx)	**pharynx**
Pars lateralis (arcus pedis longitudinalis)	Lateral longitudinal arch (of foot)	**arch** Arch of foot
Pars lateralis (musculi intertransversarii posterioris cervicis)	Lateral slip (of posterior inter-transverse muscle)	**intertransverse muscles** Posterior intertransverse muscles
Pars lateralis (ossis occipitalis)	Condylar part (of occipital bone)	**occipital bone** Condylar part
Pars lateralis (ossis sacri)	Lateral mass (of sacrum)	**sacrum** Mass of the sacrum, lateral
Pars lateralis (ramus lobi medii)	Lateral branch (of middle lobe veins)	**pulmonary veins** Right pulmonary veins
Pars lumbalis (diaphragmatis)	Vertebral part (of diaphragm)	**diaphragm** Part of the diaphragm, vertebral
Pars lumbalis (medullae spinalis)	Lumbar part (of spinal cord)	**cord** Spinal cord
Pars marginalis (musculi orbicularis oris)	Marginal part (of orbicularis oris muscle)	**orbicularis oris muscle**
Pars medialis (arcus pedis longitudinalis)	Medial longitudinal arch (of foot)	**arch** Arch of the foot
Pars medialis (musculi intertransversarii posterioris cervicis)	Medial slip (of posterior inter-transverse muscle)	**intertransverse muscles** Posterior intertransverse muscles
Pars medialis (ramus lobi medii)	Medial branch (of middle lobe veins)	**pulmonary veins** Right pulmonary veins
Pars mediastinalis (faciei medialis pulmonis)	Mediastinal part (of medial surface of lung)	**lung** Surface of the lung, medial
Pars membranacea (septi interventricularis)	Membranous part (of ventricular septum)	**septum** Ventricular septum, membranous part
Pars membranacea (septi nasi)	Membranous part (of septum of nose)	**septum** Septum of the nose, membranous part
Pars membranacea (urethrae masculinae)	Membranous part (of male urethra)	**urethra** Male urethra
Pars mobilis septi nasi	Movable part of septum of nose	**septum** Septum of the nose, movable part
Pars muscularis (septi interventricularis)	Muscular part (of ventricular septum)	**septum** Ventricular septum, muscular part
Pars mylopharyngea (musculi constrictoris pharyngis superioris)	Mylopharyngeal part (of superior constrictor muscle of pharynx)	**pharynx, constrictor muscles of the**
Pars nasalis (ossis frontalis)	Nasal part (of frontal bone)	**frontal bone** Nasal part
Pars nasalis (pharyngis)	Nasal part (of pharynx)	**pharynx**
Pars obliqua (musculi cricothyroidei)	Oblique part (of cricothyroid muscle)	**cricothyroid muscle**
Pars opercularis (gyri frontalis inferioris)	Posterior part (of inferior frontal gyri)	**gyrus** Frontal gyrus, inferior
Pars optica retinae	Optic part of retina	**retina**

Nomina Anatomica (N.A.)	Birmingham Revision (B.R.) or English Equivalent	Definition Location
Pars oralis (pharyngis)	Oral part (of pharynx)	**pharynx**
Pars orbitalis (glandulae lacrimalis)	Orbital part (of lacrimal gland)	**gland** Lacrimal gland
Pars orbitalis (gyri frontalis inferioris)	Orbital part (of inferior frontal gyrus)	**gyrus** Frontal gyrus, inferior
Pars orbitalis (musculi orbicularis oculi)	Orbital part (of orbicularis oculi muscle)	**orbicularis oculi muscle** Orbital part
Pars orbitalis (ossis frontalis)	Orbital plate (of frontal bone)	**plate** Orbital plate of the frontal bone
Pars ossea (septi nasi)	Bony part (of septum of nose)	**septum** Septum of the nose, bony part
Pars ossea tubae auditivae	Bony part of pharyngotympanic tube	**tube** Pharyngotympanic tube
Pars palpebralis (glandulae lacrimalis)	Palpebral process (of lacrimal gland)	**gland** Lacrimal gland
Pars palpebralis (musculi orbicularis oculi)	Palpebral part (of orbicularis oculi muscle)	**orbicularis oculi muscle** Palpebral part
Pars parasympathica (systematis nervosi autonomici)	Parasympathetic nervous system	**system** Parasympathetic nervous system
Pars pelvina (ureteris)	Pelvic part (of ureter)	**ureter** Part of the ureter, pelvic
Pars pelvina systematis autonomici	Pelvic part of sympathetic system	**system** Sympathetic system, pelvic part
Pars petrosa (ossis temporalis)	Petrous part (of temporal bone)	**temporal bone** Petrous part
Pars pharyngea (hypophyseos)	Pharyngeal part (of hypophysis cerebri)	**hypophysis** Pharyngeal part
Pars posterior (commissurae anterioris)	Posterior part (of anterior commissure)	**commissure** Anterior commissure, posterior part of the
Pars posterior (hepatis)	Posterior surface (of liver)	**liver**
Pars profunda (glandulae parotidis)	Deep part (of parotid gland)	**gland** Parotid gland
Pars profunda (musculi masseteris)	Deep part (of masseter muscle)	**masseter muscle**
Pars profunda (musculi sphincteris ani externi)	Deep part (of sphincter ani externus muscle)	**sphincter ani externus muscle**
Pars prostatica (urethrae masculinae)	Prostatic part (of male urethra)	**urethra** Male urethra
Pars pterygopharyngea (musculi constrictoris pharyngis superioris)	Pterygopharyngeal part (of superior constrictor muscle of pharynx)	**pharynx, constrictor muscles of the**
Pars pylorica (ventriculi)	Pyloric portion (of stomach)	**stomach** Portion of the stomach, pyloric
Pars quadrata (lobi hepatis sinistri)	Quadrate portion (of left lobe of liver)	**segment** Liver segments
Pars radiata (corticis renis)	Radiate part (of cortex of kidney)	**cortex** Cortex of the kidney, radiate part of the
Pars recta (musculi cricothyroidei)	Straight part (of cricothyroid muscle)	**cricothyroid muscle**
Pars retrolentiformis capsulae internae	Retrolentiform part of internal capsule	**capsule** Internal capsule
Pars spongiosa (urethrae masculinae)	Spongy part (of male urethra)	**urethra** Male urethra
Pars squamosa (ossis temporalis)	Squamous part (of temporal bone)	**temporal bone** Squamous part
Pars sternalis (diaphragmatis)	Sternal part (of diaphragm)	**diaphragm** Part of the diaphragm, sternal
Pars sternocostalis (musculi pectoralis majoris)	Sternocostal part (of pectoralis major muscle)	**pectoralis major muscle**

Nomina Anatomica (N.A.)	Birmingham Revision (B.R.) or English Equivalent	Definition Location
Pars subcutanea (musculi sphincteris ani externi)	Subcutaneous part (of sphincter ani externus muscle)	**sphincter ani externus muscle**
Pars sublentiformis capsulae internae	Lentiform part of internal capsule	**capsule** Internal capsule
Pars superficialis (glandulae parotidis)	Superficial part (of parotid gland)	**gland** Parotid gland
Pars superficialis (musculi masseteris)	Superficial part (of masseter muscle)	**masseter muscle**
Pars superficialis (musculi sphincteris ani externi)	Superficial part (of sphincter ani externus muscle)	**sphincter ani externus muscle**
Pars superior (duodeni)	First part (of duodenum)	**duodenum**
Pars superior (hepatis)	Superior surface (of liver)	**liver**
Pars superior (partis vestibularis nervi octavi)	Superior branch (of vestibular nerve)	**vestibular nerve**
Pars supraclavicularis (plexus brachialis)	Supraclavicular part (of brachial plexus)	**plexus** Brachial plexus
Pars sympathica (systematis nervosi autonomici)	Symphathetic nervous system	**system** Sympathetic nervous system
Pars tensa (membranae tympani)	Tense part (of tympanic membrane)	**membrane** Tympanic membrane
Pars thoracica (medullae spinalis)	Thoracic part (of spinal cord)	**cord** Spinal cord
Pars thoracica (esophagi)	Thoracic part (of oesophagus)	**oesophagus**
Pars thoracica systematis autonomici	Thoracic part of sympathetic system	**system** Sympathetic system, thoracic part
Pars thyropharyngea (musculi constrictoris pharyngis inferioris)	Thyreopharyngeal part (of inferior constrictor muscle of pharynx)	**pharynx, constrictor muscles of the**
Pars tibiocalcanea (ligamenti deltoidei)	Calcaneotibial part (of deltoid ligament)	**ligament** Deltoid ligament
Pars tibionavicularis (ligamenti deltoidei)	Tibionavicular part (of deltoid ligament)	**ligament** Deltoid ligament
Pars tibiotalaris anterior (ligamenti deltoidei)	Anterior talotibial part (of deltoid ligament)	**ligament** Deltoid ligament
Pars tibiotalaris posterior (ligamenti deltoidei)	Posterior talotibial part (of deltoid ligament)	**ligament** Deltoid ligament
Pars transversa (musculus nasalis)	Transverse part (of nasal muscle)	**nasal muscle**
Pars transversa (vena portae)	Transverse part (of portal vein)	**portal vein**
Pars triangularis (gyri frontalis inferioris)	Triangular part (of inferior frontal gyrus)	**gyrus** Frontal gyrus, inferior
Pars tympanica (ossis temporalis)	Tympanic part (of temporal bone)	**temporal bone** Tympanic part
Pars umbilicalis (vena portae)	Umbilical part (of portal vein)	**portal vein**
Pars uterina (placentae)	Uterine part (of placenta)	**placenta** Uterine part of the placenta
Pars uterina (tubae uterinae)	Uterine part (of uterine tube)	**tube** Uterine tube, uterine part of the
Pars ventralis pontis	Ventral part of pons	**pons** Ventral part of the pons
Pars vertebralis (faciei medialis pulmonis)	Vertebral part (of medial surface of lung)	**lung** Surface of the lung, medial
Pars vestibularis [nervi octavi]	Vestibular nerve	**vestibular nerve**
Patella	Patella	**patella**
Pecten ossis pubis	Pectineal line	**line** Pectineal line
Pectus	Breast	**breast**

Anatomical Nomenclature

Nomina Anatomica (N.A.)	Birmingham Revision (B.R.) or English Equivalent	Definition Location
Pedunculus [pediculus]	Peduncle (pedicle)	**peduncle**
Pediculus arcus vertebrae	Pedicle of vertebral arch	**pedicle** Pedicle of the vertebral arch
Pedunculus cerebellaris inferior	Inferior cerebellar peduncle	**peduncle** Cerebellar peduncle, inferior
Pedunculus cerebellaris medius	Middle cerebellar peduncle	**peduncle** Cerebellar peduncle, middle
Pedunculus cerebellaris superior	Superior cerebellar peduncle	**peduncle** Cerebellar peduncle, superior
Pedunculus cerebri	Cerebral peduncle	**peduncle** Cerebral peduncle
Pedunculus corporis mamillaris	Peduncle of mamillary body	**peduncle** Peduncle of the mamillary body
Pedunculus flocculi	Peduncle of flocculus	**peduncle** Peduncle of the flocculus
Pedunculus thalami inferior	Inferior thalamic peduncle	**peduncle** Thalamic peduncle, inferior
Pelvis	Pelvis	**pelvis**
Pelvis major	False pelvis	**pelvis** False pelvis
Pelvis minor	True pelvis	**pelvis** True pelvis
Pelvis renalis	Pelvis of ureter	**pelvis** Pelvis of the ureter
Penicilli (lienis)	Penicilli (of spleen)	**penicilli**
Penis	Penis	**penis**
Pericardium	Pericardium	**pericardium**
Pericardium fibrosum	Fibrous pericardium	**pericardium**
Pericardium serosum	Serous pericardium	**pericardium**
Perichondrium	Perichondrium	**perichondrium**
Pericranium	Pericranium	**pericranium**
Perilympha	Perilymph	**perilymph**
Perimysium	Perimysium	**perimysium**
Perineum	Perineum	**perineum**
Periodontium	Alveolar periosteum	**periosteum** Alveolar periosteum
Perionyx	Perionyx	**perionyx**
Periorbita	Periorbit	**periorbit**
Periosteum	Periosteum	**periosteum**
Peritendineum	Peritendineum	**peritendineum**
Peritoneum	Peritoneum	**peritoneum**
Peritoneum parietale	Parietal peritoneum	**peritoneum** Parietal peritoneum
Peritoneum viscerale	Visceral peritoneum	**peritoneum** Visceral peritoneum
Pes	Foot	**foot**
Pes hippocampi	Pes hippocampi	**pes** Pes hippocampi
Petiolus epiglottidis	Stalk of epiglottis	**stalk** Stalk of the epiglottis
Phalanx distalis (manus)	Distal phalanx (of hand)	**phalanges (of the hand and foot)**
Phalanx distalis (pedis)	Distal phalanx (of foot)	**phalanges (of the hand and foot)**
Phalanx media (manus)	Middle phalanx (of hand)	**phalanges (of the hand and foot)**
Phalanx media (pedis)	Middle phalanx (of foot)	**phalanges (of the hand and foot)**
Phalanx proximalis (manus)	Proximal phalanx (of hand)	**phalanges (of the hand and foot)**
Phalanx proximalis (pedis)	Proximal phalanx (of foot)	**phalanges (of the hand and foot)**
Pharynx	Pharynx	**pharynx**
Philtrum	Philtrum	**philtrum**
Pia mater encephali	Pia mater of brain	**pia mater**
Pia mater spinalis	Spinal pia mater	**pia mater**

Nomina Anatomica (N.A.)	Birmingham Revision (B.R.) or English Equivalent	Definition Location
Pili	Hairs	**hair**
Placenta	Placenta	**placenta**
Planta	Sole of foot	**foot *also* sole**
Planta pedis	Region of sole of foot	**sole**
Plantaris	Plantar	**plantar**
Platysma	Platysma	**platysma**
Pleura	Pleura	**pleura**
Pleura costalis	Costal pleura	**pleura** Costal pleura
Pleura diaphragmatica	Diaphragmatic pleura	**pleura** Diaphragmatic pleura
Pleura mediastinalis	Mediastinal pleura	**pleura** Mediastinal pleura
Pleura parietalis	Parietal pleura	**pleura**
Pleura pulmonalis	Pulmonary pleura (visceral)	**pleura**
Plexus	Plexus	**plexus**
Plexus aorticus abdominalis	Aortic plexus (abdominal)	**plexus** Aortic plexus, abdominal
Plexus aorticus thoracicus	Thoracic aortic plexus	**plexus** Aortic plexus, thoracic
Plexus autonomici	Sympathetic plexuses	**plexus** Sympathetic plexuses
Plexus basilaris	Network of basilar sinuses	**sinus** Basilar sinuses, network of
Plexus brachialis	Brachial plexus	**plexus** Brachial plexus
Plexus cardiacus	Cardiac plexus	**plexus** Cardiac plexus
Plexus caroticus communis	Common carotid plexus	**plexus** Carotid plexus, common
Plexus caroticus externus	External carotid plexus	**plexus** Carotid plexus, external
Plexus caroticus internus	Internal carotid plexus	**plexus** Carotid plexus, internal
Plexus cavernosi concharum	Cavernous plexus of conchae	**plexus** Cavernous plexus of the conchae
Plexus celiacus	Coeliac plexus	**plexus** Coeliac plexus
Plexus cervicalis	Cervical plexus	**plexus** Cervical plexus
Plexus choroideus ventriculi lateralis	Choroid plexus of lateral ventricle	**plexus** Choroid plexus of the lateral ventricle
Plexus choroideus ventriculi quarti	Choroid plexus of fourth ventricle	**plexus** Choroid plexus of the fourth ventricle
Plexus choroideus ventriculi tertii	Choroid plexus of third ventricle	**plexus** Choroid plexus of the third ventricle
Plexus coccygeus	Coccygeal plexus	**plexus** Coccygeal plexus
Plexus deferentialis	Plexus of vas deferens	**plexus** Plexus of the vas deferens
Plexus dentalis inferior	Inferior dental plexus	**plexus** Dental plexus, inferior
Plexus dentalis superior	Superior dental plexus	**plexus** Dental plexus, superior
Plexus entericus	Enteric plexus	**plexus** Enteric plexus
Plexus esophageus	Oesophageal plexus	**plexus** Oesophageal plexus
Plexus femoralis	Femoral plexus	**plexus** Femoral plexus
Plexus gastricus	Left gastric plexus	**plexus** Gastric plexus, left
Plexus hepaticus	Hepatic plexus	**plexus** Hepatic plexus
Plexus hypogastricus inferior [plexus pelvinus]	Pelvic plexus	**plexus** Pelvic plexus

Nomina Anatomica (N.A.)	Birmingham Revision (B.R.) or English Equivalent	Definition Location
Plexus hypogastricus superior [nervus presacralis]	Hypogastric plexus	**plexus** Hypogastric plexus
Plexus iliacus	Iliac plexus	**plexus** Iliac plexus
Plexus intermesentericus	Intermesenteric plexus	**plexus** Intermesenteric plexus
Plexus lienalis	Splenic plexus	**plexus** Splenic plexus
Plexus lumbalis	Lumbar plexus	**plexus** Lumbar plexus
Plexus lumbosacralis	Lumbosacral plexus	**plexus** Lumbosacral plexus
Plexus lymphaticus	Lymphatic plexus	**plexus** Lymphatic plexus
Plexus mesentericus inferior	Inferior mesenteric plexus	**plexus** Mesenteric plexus, inferior
Plexus mesentericus superior	Superior mesenteric plexus	**plexus** Mesenteric plexus, superior
Plexus myentericus	Myenteric plexus	**plexus** Myenteric plexus
Plexus nervorum spinalium	Spinal nerve plexuses	**plexus** Spinal nerve plexuses
Plexus oesophageus	Oesophageal plexus	**plexus** Oesophageal plexus
Plexus ovaricus	Ovarian plexus	**plexus** Ovarian plexus
Plexus pampiniformis	Pampiniform plexus	**plexus** Pampiniform plexus
Plexus pancreaticus	Pancreatic plexus	**plexus** Pancreatic plexus
Plexus parotideus	Parotid plexus	**plexus** Parotid plexus
Plexus periarterialis	Periarterial plexus	**plexus** Periarterial plexus
Plexus pharyngeus	Pharyngeal plexus	**plexus** Pharyngeal plexus
Plexus pharyngeus (venosus)	Pharyngeal (venous) plexus	**plexus** Pharyngeal (venous) plexus
Plexus prostaticus	Prostatic plexus	**plexus** Prostatic (venous) plexus
Plexus pterygoideus	Pterygoid plexus	**plexus** Pterygoid (venous) plexus
Plexus pulmonalis	Pulmonary plexus	**plexus** Pulmonary plexus (1)
Plexus pulmonalis (nervi vagi)	Pulmonary plexus (of vagus nerve)	**plexus** Pulmonary plexus (2)
Plexus rectalis inferior	Inferior rectal plexus	**plexus** Rectal plexus, inferior
Plexus rectalis medius	Middle rectal plexus	**plexus** Rectal plexus, middle
Plexus rectalis superior	Superior rectal plexus	**plexus** Rectal plexus, superior
Plexus renalis	Renal plexus	**plexus** Renal plexus
Plexus sacralis	Sacral plexus	**plexus** Sacral plexus
Plexus subclavius	Subclavian plexus	**plexus** Subclavian plexus
Plexus submucosus	Submucous plexus	**plexus** Submucous plexus
Plexus subserosus	Subserous plexus	**plexus** Subserous plexus
Plexus suprarenalis	Suprarenal plexus	**plexus** Suprarenal plexus
Plexus testicularis	Testicular plexus	**plexus** Testicular plexus
Plexus thyroideus impar	Thyroid plexus	**plexus** Thyroid plexus
Plexus tympanicus	Tympanic plexus	**plexus** Tympanic plexus
Plexus uretericus	Ureteric plexus	**plexus** Ureteric plexus

Nomina Anatomica (N.A.)	Birmingham Revision (B.R.) or English Equivalent	Definition Location
Plexus uterovaginalis	Uterovaginal plexus	**plexus** Uterovaginal plexus
Plexus vasculosus	Vascular plexus	**plexus** Vascular plexus
Plexus venosus	Venous plexus	**plexus** Venous plexus
Plexus venosus areolaris	Areolar venous plexus	**plexus** Areolar (venous) plexus
Plexus venosus canalis hypoglossi	Anterior condylar emissary vein	**emissary veins**
Plexus venosus caroticus internus	Emissary veins of carotid canal	**emissary veins**
Plexus venosus foraminis ovalis	Emissary veins of foramen ovale	**emissary veins**
Plexus venosus prostaticus	Prostatic venous plexus	**plexus** Prostatic (venous) plexus
Plexus venosus rectalis [hemorrhoidalis]	Rectal venous plexus	**plexus** Rectal (venous) plexus
Plexus venosus sacralis	Anterior sacral venous plexus	**plexus** Sacral (venous) plexus, anterior
Plexus venosus suboccipitalis	Suboccipital plexus	**plexus** Suboccipital plexus
Plexus venosus uterinus	Uterine venous plexus	**plexus** Uterine (venous) plexus
Plexus venosus vaginalis	Vaginal venous plexus	**plexus** Vaginal (venous) plexus
Plexus venosus vertebralis externus [anterior et posterior]	External vertebral plexus (anterior and posterior)	**plexus** Vertebral (venous) plexus
Plexus venosus vertebralis internus [anterior et posterior]	Internal vertebral plexus (anterior and posterior)	**plexus** Vertebral (venous) plexus
Plexus venosus vesicalis	Vesical venous plexus	**plexus** Vesical (venous) plexus
Plexus vertebralis	Vertebral plexus (of inferior cervical ganglion)	**plexus** Vertebral plexus of the inferior cervical ganglion
Plexus vesicalis	Vesical plexus	**plexus** Vesical plexus
Plica	Fold	**fold** *also* **plica**
Plicae alares (articulationis genus)	Alar folds (of knee joint)	**fold** Alar fold
Plica aryepiglottica	Aryepiglottic fold	**fold** Aryepiglottic fold
Plica axillaris anterior	Anterior axillary fold	**fold** Axillary fold
Plica axillaris posterior	Posterior axillary fold	**fold** Axillary fold
Plicae cecales	Caecal folds	**fold** Caecal fold
Plica cecalis vascularis	Vascular fold of caecum	**fold** Fold of the caecum, vascular
Plica chordae tympani	Fold of chorda tympani	**fold** Fold of the chorda tympani
Plicae ciliares	Ciliary folds	**fold** Ciliary folds
Plicae circulares (intestini tenuis)	Circular folds (of small intestine)	**fold** Circular fold
Plica duodenalis inferior	Inferior duodenal fold	**fold** Duodenal folds
Plica duodenalis superior	Superior duodenal fold	**fold** Duodenal folds
Plica duodenojejunalis	Duodenojejunal fold	**fold** Duodenal folds
Plica duodenomesocolica	Duodenomesocolic fold	**fold** Duodenomesocolic fold
Plica fimbriata	Fimbriated fold	**fold** Fimbriated fold
Plicae gastricae	Gastric folds	**fold** Gastric folds
Plicae gastropancreaticae	Gastropancreatic folds	**fold** Gastropancreatic folds

Anatomical Nomenclature

Nomina Anatomica (N.A.)	Birmingham Revision (B.R.) or English Equivalent	Definition Location
Plica glosso-epiglottica lateralis	Pharyngo-epiglottic fold	**fold** Pharyngo-epiglottic fold
Plica glosso-epiglottica mediana	Glosso-epiglottic fold	**fold** Glosso-epiglottic fold
Plica ileocaecalis	Ileocaecal fold	**fold** Ileocaecal fold
Plica incudis	Fold of incus	**fold** Fold of the incus
Plica interureterica	Ureteric fold	**fold** Ureteric fold
Plicae iridis	Folds of iris	**fold** Folds of the iris
Plica lacrimalis	Lacrimal fold	**fold** Lacrimal fold
Plica longitudinalis duodeni	Longitudinal fold of duodenum	**fold** Fold of the duodenum, longitudinal
Plica mallearis anterior	Anterior malleolar fold	**fold** Malleolar folds
Plica mallearis posterior	Posterior malleolar fold	**fold** Malleolar folds
Plica nervi laryngei	Fold of laryngeal nerve	**fold** Fold of the laryngeal nerve
Plicae palatinae transversae	Transverse palatine folds	**fold** Palatine folds, transverse
Plicae palmatae	Arbor vitae	**canal** Canal of the cervix
Plica palpebronasalis	Palpebronasal fold	**fold** Palpebronasal fold
Plica paraduodenalis	Paraduodenal fold	**fold** Duodenal folds
Plica recto-uterina	Recto-uterine fold	**fold** Recto-uterine fold
Plica salpingopalatina	Salpingopalatine fold	**fold** Salpingopalatine fold
Plica salpingopharyngea	Salpingopharyngeal fold	**fold** Salpingopharyngea fold
Plica semilunaris (fauces)	Semilunar fold	**fold** Semilunar fold
Plicae semilunares coli	Semilunar fold of colon	**fold** Folds of the colon, semilunar
Plica semilunaris conjunctivae	Plica semilunaris conjunctivae	**plica** Plica semilunaris conjunctivae
Plica spiralis	Spiral valve	**valve** Spiral valve
Plica stapedis	Fold of stapes	**fold** Fold of the stapes
Plica sublingualis	Sublingual fold	**fold** Sublingual fold
Plica synovialis	Synovial fold	**fold** Synovial fold
Plica synovialis infrapatellaris	Infrapatellar synovial fold	**fold** Infrapatellar synovial fold
Plicae transversales recti	Horizontal folds of rectum	**fold** Folds of the rectum, horizontal
Plica triangularis	Triangular fold	**fold** Triangular fold
Plicae tubariae	Plicae tubariae	**plica** Plicae tubariae
Plicae tunicae mucosae vesicae felleae	Folds of gall bladder	**fold** Folds of the gall bladder
Plica umbilicalis lateralis	Lateral umbilical fold	**fold** Umbilical fold, lateral
Plica umbilicalis medialis	Medial umbilical fold	**fold** Umbilical fold, medial
Plica umbilicalis mediana	Median umbilical fold	**fold** Umbilical fold, median
Plica venae cavae sinistrae	Ligament of left vena cava	**ligament** Ligament of the left vena cava

Nomina Anatomica (N.A.)	Birmingham Revision (B.R.) or English Equivalent	Definition Location
Plica vesicalis transversa	Transverse vesical fold	**fold** Transverse vesical fold
Plicae vestibulares	Vestibular folds	**cord** False cords
Plicae villosae	Villous folds	**fold** Villous folds
Plicae vocales	Vocal folds	**cord** Vocal cords
Pollex (digitus I)	Thumb	**thumb**
Polus	Pole	**pole**
Polus anterior (bulbi oculi)	Anterior pole (of eyeball)	**pole** Pole of the eyeball, anterior
Polus anterior lentis	Anterior pole of lens	**pole** Pole of the lens of the eye, anterior
Polus frontalis	Frontal pole	**pole** Frontal pole
Polus occipitalis	Occipital pole	**pole** Occipital pole
Polus posterior (bulbi oculi)	Posterior pole (of eyeball)	**pole** Pole of the eyeball, posterior
Polus posterior lentis	Posterior pole of lens	**pole** Pole of the lens of the eye, posterior
Polus temporalis	Temporal pole	**pole** Temporal pole
Pons	Pons	**pons**
Poples	Poples	**poples**
Porta hepatis	Porta hepatis	**porta** Porta hepatis
Portio	Portio	**portio**
Portio major (nervi trigemini)	Sensory part (of trigeminal nerve)	**trigeminal nerve**
Portio minor (nervi trigemini)	Motor part (of trigeminal nerve)	**trigeminal nerve**
Portio supravaginalis [cervicis]	Supravaginal part (of uterus)	**uterus** Neck of the uterus
Portio vaginalis [cervicis]	Vaginal part (of uterus)	**uterus** Neck of the uterus
Porus	Pore	**pore** *also* **porus**
Porus acusticus externus	Porus acusticus externus	**porus** Porus acusticus externus
Porus acusticus internus	Porus acusticus internus	**porus** Porus acusticus internus
Porus gustatorius	Taste pore	**pore** Taste pore
Porus sudoriferus	Sweat pore	**pore** Sweat pore
Posterior	Posterior	**posterior**
Precuneus	Precuneus	**precuneus**
Preputium	Prepuce	**prepuce**
Preputium clitoridis	Prepuce of clitoris	**prepuce** Prepuce of the clitoris
Prismata adamantina	Enamel prisms	**prism** Enamel prisms
Processus	Process	**process** *also* **processus**
Processus accessorius [vertebrarum lumbalium]	Accessory process (of lumbar vertebrae)	**process** Process of a lumbar vertebra, accessory
Processus alveolaris (maxillae)	Alveolar process (of maxilla)	**process** Process of the maxilla, alveolar
Processus anterior (mallei)	Anterior process (of malleus)	**malleus**
Processus articularis inferior [zygapophysis]	Inferior articular process (of a vertebra)	**process** Process of a vertebra, inferior articular
Processus articularis superior (ossis sacri)	Superior articular process (of sacrum)	**process** Process of the sacrum, superior articular
Processus articularis superior [zygapophysis]	Superior articular process (of a vertebra)	**process** Process of a vertebra, superior articular

Nomina Anatomica (N.A.)	Birmingham Revision (B.R.) or English Equivalent	Definition Location
Processus caudatus	Caudate process	**process** Caudate process
Processus ciliares	Ciliary processes	**process** Ciliary processes
Processus clinoideus anterior	Anterior clinoid process	**process** Process of the sphenoid bone, anterior clinoid
Processus clinoideus medius	Middle clinoid process	**process** Process of the sphenoid bone, middle clinoid
Processus clinoideus posterior	Posterior clinoid process	**process** Process of the sphenoid bone, posterior clinoid
Processus cochleariformis	Processus cochleariformis	**processus** Processus cochleariformis
Processus condylaris	Condyloid process	**process** Process of the mandible, condyloid
Processus coracoideus	Coracoid process	**process** Coracoid process
Processus coronoideus (mandibulae)	Coronoid process (of mandible)	**process** Process of the mandible, coronoid
Processus coronoideus (ulnae)	Coronoid process (of ulna)	**process** Process of the ulna, coronoid
Processus costarius	Costal process	**process** Process of a cervical vertebra, costal
Processus ethmoidalis	Ethmoidal process	**process** Process of the inferior nasal concha, ethmoidal
Processus falciformis	Falciform process	**process** Process of the sacrotuberous ligament, falciform
Processus frontalis (maxillae)	Frontal process (of maxilla)	**process** Process of the maxilla, frontal
Processus frontalis (ossis zygomatici)	Frontal process (of zygomatic bone)	**process** Process of the zygomatic bone, frontal
Processus intrajugularis (ossis occipitalis)	Intrajugular process (of occipital bone)	**process** Process of the occipital bone, intrajugular
Processus intrajugularis (ossis temporalis)	Intrajugular process (of temporal bone)	**process** Process of the temporal bone, intrajugular
Processus jugularis	Jugular process	**process** Process of the occipital bone, jugular
Processus lacrimalis	Lacrimal process	**process** Lacrimal process
Processus lateralis (mallei)	Lateral process (of malleus)	**malleus**
Processus lateralis tali	Lateral tubercle of talus	**tubercle** Tubercle of the talus, lateral
Processus lateralis tuberis calcanei	Lateral tubercle of calcaneum	**tubercle** Tubercle of the calcaneum, lateral
Processus lenticularis	Lentiform nodule	**nodule** Lentiform nodule
Processus mamillaris	Mamillary process	**process** Process of a vertebra, mamillary
Processus mastoideus	Mastoid process	**process** Process of the temporal bone, mastoid
Processus maxillaris	Maxillary process	**process** Maxillary process
Processus medialis tuberis calcanei	Medial tubercle (of calcaneum)	**tubercle** Tubercle of the calcaneum, medial
Processus muscularis (cartilaginis arytenoideae)	Muscular process (of arytenoid cartilage)	**process** Process of the arytenoid cartilage, muscular
Processus orbitalis (ossis palatini)	Orbital process (of palatine bone)	**process** Process of the palatine bone, orbital
Processus palatinus	Palatine process	**process** Process of the maxilla, palatine
Processus papillaris	Papillary process	**process** Papillary process
Processus paramastoideus	Paramastoid process	**process** Process of the occipital bone, paramastoid
Processus posterior [sphenoidalis]	Sphenoidal process (of nasal septum)	**process** Sphenoidal process of the nasal septum
Processus posterior tali	Posterior tubercle of talus	**tubercle** Tubercle of the talus, posterior
Processus pterygoideus	Pterygoid process	**process** Process of the sphenoid bone, pterygoid
Processus pterygospinosus	Pterygospinous process	**process** Pterygospinous process
Processus pyramidalis	Tubercle (of palatine bone)	**tubercle** Tubercle of the palatine bone
Processus sphenoidalis	Sphenoidal process	**process** Process of the palatine bone, sphenoidal
Processus spinosus	Spine of vertebra	**spine** Spine of a vertebra
Processus styloideus (ossis metacarpalis tertii)	Styloid process (of third metacarpal bone)	**process** Process of the third metacarpal bone, styloid
Processus styloideus (ossis temporalis)	Styloid process (of temporal bone)	**process** Process of the temporal bone, styloid
Processus styloideus (radii)	Styloid process (of radius)	**process** Process of the radius, styloid
Processus styloideus (ulnae)	Styloid process (of ulna)	**process** Process of the ulna, styloid
Processus supracondylaris	Supracondylar process	**process** Supracondylar process
Processus temporalis (ossis zygomatici)	Temporal process (of zygomatic bone)	**process** Process of the zygomatic bone, temporal
Processus transversus	Transverse process	**process** Process of a vertebra, transverse
Processus uncinatus (ossis ethmoidalis)	Uncinate process (of ethmoid bone)	**process** Process of the ethmoid bone, uncinate
Processus uncinatus (pancreatis)	Uncinate process (of pancreas)	**process** Process of the pancreas, uncinate
Processus vaginalis	Vaginal process	**process** Process of the sphenoid bone, vaginal
Processus vaginalis peritonei	Processus vaginalis of peritoneum	**processus** Processus vaginalis of the peritoneum
Processus vocalis (cartilaginis arytenoideae)	Vocal process (of arytenoid cartilage)	**process** Process of the arytenoid cartilage, vocal
Processus xiphoideus	Xiphoid process	**process** Xiphoid process
Processus zygomaticus	Zygomatic process	**process** Zygomatic process
Processus zygomaticus (maxillae)	Zygomatic process (of maxilla)	**process** Process of the maxilla, zygomatic
Processus zygomaticus (ossis temporalis)	Zygomatic process (zygoma) (of temporal bone)	**process** Process of the temporal bone, zygomatic
Profundus	Deep	**deep**
Prominentia	Prominence	**prominence**

Nomina Anatomica (N.A.)	Birmingham Revision (B.R.) or English Equivalent	Definition Location
Prominentia canalis facialis	Prominence of the facial nerve canal	**prominence** Prominence of the facial nerve canal
Prominentia canalis semicircularis lateralis	Prominence of the lateral semicircular canal	**prominence** Prominence of the lateral semicircular canal
Prominentia laryngea	Laryngeal prominence	**prominence** Laryngeal prominence
Prominentia mallearis	Prominence of malleus	**prominence** Prominence of the malleus
Prominentia spiralis	Spiral prominence	**prominence** Spiral prominence
Prominentia styloidea	Styloid prominence	**prominence** Styloid prominence
Promontorium	Promontory	**promontory**
Promontorium (cavi tympani)	Promontory (of tympanic cavity)	**promontory** Promontory of the tympanic cavity
Promontorium (ossis sacri)	Promontory (of sacrum)	**promontory** Promontory of the sacrum
Prosencephalon	Forebrain	**forebrain**
Prostata	Prostate	**prostate**
Protuberantia mentalis	Mental protuberance	**protuberance** Mental protuberance
Protuberantia occipitalis externa (var. crista occipitalis externa)	External occipital protuberance	**protuberance** Occipital protuberance, external
Protuberantia occipitalis interna (var. crista occipitalis interna)	Internal occipital protuberance	**protuberance** Occipital protuberance, internal
Proximalis	Proximal	**proximal**
Pubes	Pubic hairs	**hair** Pubic hairs
Pudendum femininum	Pudendum muliebre	**pudendum** Pudendum muliebre
Pulmo	Lung	**lung**
Pulpa dentis	Pulp of tooth	**tooth** Pulp of a tooth
Pulpa lienis	Splenic pulp	**pulp** Splenic pulp
Pulvinar thalami	Pulvinar	**pulvinar**
Punctum	Point	**point** ***also*** **punctum**
Punctum lacrimale	Punctum lacrimale	**punctum** Puncta lacrimalia
Pupilla	Pupil	**pupil**
Putamen	Putamen	**putamen**
Pylorus	Pylorus	**pylorus**
Pyramis [medullae oblongatae]	Pyramid (of medulla oblongata)	**pyramid** Pyramid of the medulla oblongata
Pyramides renales	Renal pyramids	**pyramid** Renal pyramids
Pyramis vermis	Pyramid of vermis	**pyramid** Pyramid of the vermis
Pyramis vestibuli	Pyramid of vestibule	**pyramid** Pyramid of the vestibule
Radialis	Radial	**radial**
Radiatio acustica	Auditory radiation	**radiation** Auditory radiation
Radiatio corporis callosi	Radiation of the corpus callosum	**radiation** Radiation of the corpus callosum
Radiatio optica	Optic radiation	**radiation** Optic radiation
Radius	Radius	**radius**
Radii lentis	Radii of lens	**radius** Radii of the lens of the eye
Radix	Root	**radix** ***also*** **root**
Radix clinica	Clinical root	**root** Clinical root

Nomina Anatomica (N.A.)	Birmingham Revision (B.R.) or English Equivalent	Definition Location
Radix cranialis (nervi accessorii)	Cranial root (of accessory nerve)	**accessory nerve** Cranial root
Radix dentis	Root of tooth	**tooth** Root of a tooth
Radix dorsalis (nervi spinalis)	Posterior root (of spinal nerve)	**spinal nerves** Posterior root
Radix inferior [cochlearis]	Vestibular root (of auditory nerve)	**auditory nerve** Roots
Radix lateralis (nervi mediani)	Lateral root (of median nerve)	**median nerve** Lateral root
Radix linguae	Root of tongue	**tongue** Root of the tongue
Radix medialis (nervi mediani)	Medial root (of median nerve)	**median nerve** Medial root
Radix mesenterii	Root of mesentery	**mesentery** Root of the mesentery
Radix nasi	Root of nose	**nose** Root of the nose
Radix oculomotoria	Motor root of ciliary ganglion	**ganglion** Ciliary ganglion, motor root of the
Radix penis	Root of penis	**penis** Root of the penis
Radix pili	Root of hair	**hair** Root of a hair
Radix pulmonis	Root of lung	**lung** Root of the lung
Radix spinalis (nervi accessorii)	Spinal root (of accessory nerve)	**accessory nerve** Spinal root
Radix superior [vestibularis]	Cochlear root (of auditory nerve)	**auditory nerve** Roots
Radix unguis	Root of nail	**nail** Root of a nail
Radix ventralis (nervi spinalis)	Anterior root (of spinal nerve)	**spinal nerves** Anterior root
Ramus	Branch	**branch** ***also*** **ramus**
Ramus acetabularis (arteriae circumflexae femoris medialis)	Acetabular branch (of medial circumflex artery)	**circumflex arteries** Medial circumflex artery
Ramus acetabularis (arteriae obturatoriae)	Acetabular branch (of obturator artery)	**obturator artery** Acetabular branch
Ramus acromialis (arteriae suprascapularis)	Acromial branch (of suprascapular artery)	**suprascapular artery**
Ramus acromialis (arteriae thoraco-acromialis)	Acromial branch (of acromiothoracic artery)	**acromiothoracic artery**
Rami ad pontem (arteriae basilaris)	Pontine branches (of basilar artery)	**basilar artery**
Rami alveolares superiores anteriores	Anterior superior dental nerve	**dental nerves** Anterior superior dental nerve
Ramus alveolaris superior medius	Middle superior dental nerve	**dental nerves** Middle superior dental nerve
Rami alveolares superiores posteriores	Posterior superior dental nerves	**dental nerves** Posterior superior dental nerves
Ramus anastomoticus cum arteria lacrimali (arteriae meningeae mediae)	Orbital branch (of middle meningeal artery)	**meningeal arteries** Middle meningeal artery
Ramus anterior (arteriae obturatoriae)	Anterior branch (of obturator artery)	**obturator artery** Anterior branch
Ramus anterior ascendens et descendens (arteriae pulmonalis dextrae)	Anterior branches (of right pulmonary artery)	**pulmonary arteries** Right pulmonary artery
Ramus anterior (arteriae recurrentis ulnaris)	Anterior branch (of ulnar recurrent artery)	**ulnar artery**
Ramus anterior (arteriae renalis)	Anterior branch (of renal artery)	**renal artery**
Ramus anterior (arteriae thyroideae superioris)	Anterior branch (of superior thyroid artery)	**thyroid arteries** Superior thyroid artery

Nomina Anatomica (N.A.)	Birmingham Revision (B.R.) or English Equivalent	Definition Location
Ramus anterior (ductus hepaticus dexter)	Anterior duct (of right hepatic duct)	**duct** Right hepatic duct
Ramus anterior (nervi auricularis magni)	Anterior branch (of great auricular nerve)	**auricular nerves** Great auricular nerve
Ramus anterior (nervi cutanei antebrachii medialis)	Anterior branch (of medial cutaneous nerve of forearm)	**forearm, nerves of the** Medial cutaneous nerve of the forearm
Ramus anterior (nervi obturatorii)	Anterior branch (of obturator nerve)	**obturator nerve** Anterior branch
Ramus anterior (sulci lateralis)	Horizontal anterior ramus	**ramus** Horizontal anterior ramus
Ramus anterior (vena portae)	Anterior segmental branch (of portal vein)	**portal vein**
Ramus anterior (venae pulmonalis superioris dextrae)	Anterior branch (of right superior pulmonary vein)	**pulmonary veins** Right pulmonary veins
Ramus anterior (venae pulmonalis superioris sinistrae)	Anterior branch (of left superior pulmonary vein)	**pulmonary veins** Left pulmonary veins
Ramus anterior ascendens et descendens (arteriae pulmonalis sinistrae)	Anterior descending branches (of left pulmonary artery)	**pulmonary arteries** Left pulmonary artery
Ramus apicalis (arteriae pulmonalis dextrae)	Apical branch (of right pulmonary artery)	**pulmonary arteries** Right pulmonary artery
Ramus apicalis (arteriae pulmonalis sinistrae)	Apical branch (of left pulmonary artery)	**pulmonary arteries** Left pulmonary artery
Rami apicales (venae pulmonalis dextrae)	Apical branches (of right pulmonary veins)	**pulmonary veins** Right pulmonary veins
Ramus apicalis (venae pulmonalis inferioris sinistrae)	Apical branch (of left inferior pulmonary vein)	**pulmonary veins** Left pulmonary veins
Ramus apicalis [superior] lobi inferioris (arteriae pulmonalis dextrae)	Apical branch to inferior lobe (of right pulmonary artery)	**pulmonary arteries** Right pulmonary artery
Ramus apicalis [superior] lobi inferioris (arteriae pulmonalis sinistrae)	Apical branch to inferior lobe (of left pulmonary artery)	**pulmonary arteries** Left pulmonary artery
Ramus apicoposterior (venae pulmonalis superioris sinistrae)	Apicoposterior branch (of left superior pulmonary vein)	**pulmonary veins** Left pulmonary veins
Rami articulares (arteriae genus descendentis)	Articular branches (of descending genicular artery)	**genicular arteries** Descending genicular artery
Ramus ascendens (arteriae circumflexae femoris lateralis)	Ascending branch (of lateral circumflex artery)	**circumflex arteries** Lateral circumflex artery
Ramus ascendens (arteriae circumflexae femoris medialis)	Ascending branch (of medial circumflex artery)	**circumflex arteries** Medial circumflex artery
Ramus ascendens (arteriae circumflexae ilii profundae)	Ascending branch (of deep circumflex iliac artery)	**circumflex iliac arteries** Deep circumflex iliac artery, ascending branch of the
Ramus ascendens (sulci lateralis)	Horizontal ascending ramus	**ramus** Horizontal ascending ramus
Ramus auricularis (arteriae auricularis posterioris)	Auricular branch (of posterior auricular artery)	**auricular arteries** Posterior auricular artery
Ramus auricularis (arteriae occipitalis)	Auricular branch (of occipital artery)	**occipital artery**
Ramus auricularis (nervi vagi)	Auricular branch (of vagus nerve)	**vagus nerve** Auricular branch
Rami auriculares anteriores (arteriae temporalis superficialis)	Auricular branches (of superficial temporal artery)	**temporal arteries** Superficial temporal artery
Ramus basalis anterior (arteriae pulmonalis dextrae)	Anterior basal branch (of right pulmonary artery)	**pulmonary arteries** Right pulmonary artery
Ramus basalis anterior (arteriae pulmonalis sinistrae)	Anterior basal branch (of left pulmonary artery)	**pulmonary arteries** Left pulmonary artery
Ramus basalis anterior (venae pulmonalis inferioris dextrae)	Anterior basal branch (of right inferior pulmonary vein)	**pulmonary veins** Right pulmonary veins
Ramus basalis lateralis (arteriae pulmonalis dextrae)	Anterior basal branch (of right pulmonary artery)	**pulmonary arteries** Right pulmonary artery
Ramus basalis lateralis (arteriae pulmonalis sinistrae)	Lateral basal branch (of left pulmonary artery)	**pulmonary arteries** Left pulmonary artery
Ramus basalis medialis [cardiacus] (arteriae pulmonalis dextrae)	Medial basal branch (of right pulmonary artery)	**pulmonary arteries** Right pulmonary artery
Ramus basalis medialis (arteriae pulmonalis sinistrae)	Medial basal branch (of left pulmonary artery)	**pulmonary arteries** Left pulmonary artery
Ramus basalis posterior (arteriae pulmonalis dextrae)	Posterior basal branch (of right pulmonary artery)	**pulmonary arteries** Right pulmonary artery
Ramus basalis posterior (arteriae pulmonalis sinistrae)	Posterior basal branch (of left pulmonary artery)	**pulmonary arteries** Left pulmonary artery
Rami bronchiales (aortae thoracicae)	Bronchial arteries	**bronchial arteries**
Rami bronchiales (arteriae thoracicae internae)	Bronchial branches (of internal mammary artery)	**mammary artery, internal**
Rami bronchiales (nervi vagi)	Pulmonary branches (of vagus nerve)	**vagus nerve**
Rami bronchiales hyparteriales (B.N.A.)	Hyparterial bronchi	**bronchus**
Rami bronchiales segmentorum	Intrasegmental branches of bronchus	**bronchus**
Rami buccales (nervi facialis)	Buccal branches (of facial nerve)	**facial nerve** Buccal branches
Rami calcanei (arteriae peroneae)	Calcanean branches (of peroneal artery)	**peroneal artery** Calcanean branches
Rami calcanei (arteriae tibialis posterioris)	Calcanean branches (of posterior tibial artery)	**tibial arteries** Posterior tibial artery
Rami calcanei laterales (nervi suralis)	Lateral calcanean branches (of sural nerve)	**sural nerve** Lateral calcanean branches
Rami calcanei mediales (nervi suralis)	Medial calcanean branches (of sural nerve)	**sural nerve** Medial calcanean branches
Rami capsulares (arteriae renales)	Capsular branches (of renal artery)	**renal artery**
Rami cardiaci cervicales inferiores (nervi vagi)	Cardiac branches (lower) (of vagus nerve)	**vagus nerve** Cardiac branches, cervical
Rami cardiaci cervicales superiores (nervi vagi)	Cardiac branches (upper) (of vagus nerve)	**vagus nerve** Cardiac branches, cervical
Rami cardiaci thoracici (nervi vagi)	Thoracic cardiac branches (of vagus nerve)	**vagus nerve** Cardiac branches, thoracic
Ramus carotico-tympanicus (arteriae carotidis internae)	Caroticotympanic branch (of internal carotid artery)	**carotid arteries** Internal carotid artery
Ramus carpeus dorsalis (arteriae radialis)	Posterior carpal branch (of radial artery)	**radial artery**
Ramus carpeus dorsalis (arteriae ulnaris)	Posterior carpal branch (of ulnar artery)	**ulnar artery** Posterior carpal branch
Ramus carpeus palmaris (arteriae radialis)	Anterior carpal branch (of radial artery)	**radial artery**

Anatomical Nomenclature

Nomina Anatomica (N.A.)	Birmingham Revision (B.R.) or English Equivalent	Definition Location
Ramus carpeus palmaris (arteriae ulnaris)	Anterior carpal branch (of ulnar artery)	**ulnar artery** Anterior carpal branch
Rami caudati (vena portae)	Caudate branches (of portal vein)	**portal veins**
Rami celiaci (nervi vagi)	Coeliac branches (of vagus nerve)	**vagus nerve** Coeliac branches
Rami centrales (arteriae cerebri anterioris)	Central branches (of anterior cerebral artery)	**cerebral arteries** Anterior cerebral artery
Rami centrales (arteriae cerebri mediae)	Central branches (of middle cerebral artery)	**cerebral arteries** Middle cerebral artery
Rami centrales (arteriae cerebri posterioris)	Central branches (of posterior cerebral artery)	**cerebral arteries** Posterior cerebral artery
Ramus choroideus [rami choroidei posteriores]	Choroid branch (of posterior cerebral artery)	**cerebral arteries** Posterior cerebral artery
Ramus circumflexus (arteriae coronariae sinistrae)	Circumflex branch (of left coronary artery)	**coronary arteries** Left coronary artery
Ramus circumflexus fibulae (arteriae tibialis posterioris)	Circumflex fibular branch (of posterior tibial artery)	**tibial arteries** Posterior tibial artery
Ramus clavicularis (arteriae thoraco-acromialis)	Clavicular branch (of acromiothoracic artery)	**acromiothoracic artery**
Ramus cochlearis (arteriae labyrinthi)	Cochlear branch (of internal auditory artery)	**auditory artery, internal**
Ramus collateralis (arteriae intercostalis posterioris)	Collateral branch (of posterior intercostal artery)	**intercostal arteries** Posterior intercostal arteries (III–XI)
Ramus colli (nervi facialis)	Cervical branch (of facial nerve)	**facial nerve** Cervical branch
Ramus communicans (arteriae peroneae)	Communicating branch (of peroneal artery)	**peroneal artery** Communicating branch
Rami communicantes (ganglionum trunci sympathici)	Communicating branches (of ganglia of sympathetic trunk)	**system** Sympathetic nervous system
Ramus communicans (nervi)	Communicating branch (of nerve)	**branch** Communicating branch
Rami communicantes (albi) (nervi spinalis)	White communicating branches (of spinal nerve)	**branch** Communicating branches, white
Rami communicantes (grisei) (nervi spinalis)	Grey communicating branches (of spinal nerve)	**branch** Communicating branches, grey
Ramus communicans cum chorda tympani	Communicating branch with chorda tympani (of otic ganglion)	**ganglion** Otic ganglion, communicating branch with the chorda tympani
Ramus communicans cum ganglione ciliare (nervi nasociliari)	Communicating branch with ciliary ganglion (of nasociliary nerve)	**nasociliary nerve** Communicating branch with the ciliary ganglion
Ramus communicans cum nervo auriculotemporali	Communicating branch with auriculotemporal nerve (of otic ganglion)	**ganglion** Otic ganglion, communicating branch with the auriculotemporal nerve
Rami communicantes cum nervo faciali	Communicating branches with facial nerve (of auriculotemporal nerve)	**auriculotemporal nerve**
Ramus communicans cum nervo glossopharyngeo	Communicating branch with glossopharyngeal nerve (of facial nerve)	**facial nerve** Communicating branch with the glossopharyngeal nerve
Rami communicantes cum nervo hypoglosso	Communicating branches with hypoglossal nerve (of lingual nerve)	**lingual nerve**

Nomina Anatomica (N.A.)	Birmingham Revision (B.R.) or English Equivalent	Definition Location
Ramus communicans cum nervo laryngeo inferiore	Communicating branch with recurrent laryngeal nerve (of internal laryngeal nerve)	**laryngeal nerves** Internal laryngeal nerve
Ramus communicans cum nervo laryngeo interno	Communicating branch of internal laryngeal nerve	**laryngeal nerves** Recurrent laryngeal nerve
Rami communicantes cum nervo linguali	Communicating branches with lingual nerve (of submandibular ganglion)	**ganglion** Submandibular ganglion
Ramus communicans cum nervo nasociliari	Sensory root of ciliary ganglion	**ganglion** Ciliary ganglion, sensory root of the
Ramus communicans cum nervo ulnari	Communicating branch with ulnar nerve (of median nerve)	**median nerve**
Ramus communicans cum nervo zygomatico	Communicating branch with zygomatic nerve (of lacrimal nerve)	**lacrimal nerve** Communicating branch of the lacrimal nerve with the zygomatic nerve
Ramus communicans cum plexu tympanico	Communicating branch with tympanic plexus (of facial nerve)	**facial nerve** Communicating branch with the tympanic plexus
Ramus communicans cum ramo auriculari nervi vagi	Communicating branch with auricular branch of vagus nerve (of glossopharyngeal nerve)	**glossopharyngeal nerve** Communicating branch with the auricular branch of the vagus nerve
Ramus communicans cum ramo laryngeo interno	Communicating branch of internal laryngeal nerve	**laryngeal nerves** Recurrent laryngeal nerve
Ramus communicans cum ramo meningio [nervi mandibularis]	Communicating branch with nervus spinosus (of otic ganglion)	**ganglion** Otic ganglion, communicating branch with the nervus spinosus
Ramus communicans peroneus [fibularis]	Sural communicating branch (of lateral popliteal nerve)	**popliteal nerves** Lateral popliteal nerve
Ramus communicans ulnaris	Communicating branch with ulnar nerve (of radial nerve)	**radial nerve**
Rami corticales (arteriae cerebri anterioris)	Cortical branches (of anterior cerebral artery)	**cerebral arteries** Anterior cerebral artery
Rami corticales (arteriae cerebri mediae)	Cortical branches (of middle cerebral artery)	**cerebral arteries** Middle cerebral artery
Rami corticales (arteriae cerebri posterioris)	Cortical branches (of posterior cerebral artery)	**cerebral arteries** Posterior cerebral artery
Ramus costalis lateralis (arteriae thoracicae internae)	Lateral costal branch (of internal mammary artery)	**mammary artery, internal**
Ramus crico-thyroideus (arteriae thyroideae superioris)	Cricothyroid branch (of superior thyroid artery)	**thyroid arteries** Superior thyroid artery
Ramus cutaneus (nervi obturatorii)	Cutaneous branch (of obturator nerve)	**obturator nerve**
Ramus cutaneus anterior (nervi femoralis)	Intermediate cutaneous nerve of thigh	**thigh, cutaneous nerves of the** Intermediate cutaneous nerve of the thigh
Ramus cutaneus anterior (nervi iliohypogastrici)	Anterior cutaneous branch (of iliohypogastric nerve)	**iliohypogastric nerve**
Ramus cutaneus anterior [pectoralis et abdominalis] (nervi thoracici)	Anterior cutaneous branch (of thoracic nerve)	**thoracic nerves** Anterior primary ramus

Nomina Anatomica (N.A.)	Birmingham Revision (B.R.) or English Equivalent	Definition Location
Rami cutanei cruris medialis	Medial cutaneous nerve of thigh	**thigh, cutaneous nerves of the** Medial cutaneous nerve of the thigh
Ramus cutaneus lateralis (arteriae intercostalis posterioris)	Lateral cutaneous branch (of posterior branch of posterior intercostal artery)	**intercostal arteries** Posterior intercostal arteries (III–XI)
Ramus cutaneus lateralis (nervi iliohypogastrici)	Lateral cutaneous branch (of iliohypogastric nerve)	**iliohypogastric nerve**
Ramus cutaneus lateralis [pectoralis et abdominalis] (nervi thoracici)	Lateral cutaneous branch (of thoracic nerve)	**thoracic nerves** Anterior primary ramus
Rami cutaneus lateralis (rami dorsalis)	Lateral branch (of posterior primary ramus of thoracic nerve)	**thoracic nerves** Posterior primary ramus
Ramus cutaneus medialis (arteriae intercostalis posterioris)	Medial cutaneous branch (of posterior branch of posterior intercostal artery)	**intercostal arteries** Posterior intercostal arteries (III–XI)
Ramus cutaneus medialis (rami dorsalis)	Medial branch (of posterior primary ramus of thoracic nerve)	**thoracic nerves** Posterior primary ramus
Ramus cutaneus palmaris (nervi ulnaris)	Palmar cutaneous branch (of ulnar nerve)	**ulnar nerve** Palmar cutaneous branch
Ramus deltoideus (arteriae profundae brachii)	Ascending branch (of profunda brachii artery)	**profunda brachii artery**
Ramus deltoideus (arteriae thoraco-acromialis)	Deltoid branch (of acromiothoracic artery)	**acromiothoracic artery**
Rami dentales (arteriae alveolaris inferioris)	Dental branches (of inferior dental artery)	**maxillary artery**
Rami dentales (arteriae alveolaris superioris anterioris)	Dental branches (of anterior superior dental artery)	**maxillary artery**
Rami dentales (arteriae alveolaris superioris posterioris)	Dental branches (of posterior superior dental artery)	**maxillary artery**
Rami dentales inferiores (nervi alveolaris inferioris)	Inferior dental branches (of inferior dental nerve)	**dental nerves** Inferior dental nerve
Rami dentales superiores (plexus dentalis superioris)	Superior dental branch (of superior dental plexus)	**plexus** Dental plexus, superior
Ramus descendens (arteriae circumflexae femoris lateralis)	Descending branch (of lateral circumflex artery)	**circumflex arteries** Lateral circumflex artery
Ramus dexter (arteriae hepaticae communis)	Right branch (of hepatic artery)	**hepatic arteries** Common hepatic artery
Ramus dexter (vena portae)	Right branch (of portal vein)	**portal vein**
Ramus digastricus (nervi facialis)	Digastric branch (of facial nerve)	**facial nerve** Digastric branch
Ramus dorsalis (arteriae intercostalis posterioris)	Posterior branch (of posterior intercostal artery)	**intercostal arteries** Posterior intercostal arteries (III–XI)
Ramus dorsalis (arteriae lumbalis)	Posterior branch (of lumbar artery)	**lumbar arteries**
Ramus dorsalis (arteriae subcostalis)	Posterior branch (of subcostal artery)	**subcostal arteries**
Rami dorsales (nervorum cervicalium)	Posterior primary rami (of cervical nerves)	**cervical nerves**
Ramus dorsalis (nervi coccygei)	Posterior primary ramus (of coccygeal nerve)	**coccygeal nerve**
Rami dorsales (nervorum lumbalium)	Posterior primary rami (of lumbar nerves)	**lumbar nerves**
Rami dorsales (nervorum sacralium)	Posterior primary rami (of sacral nerves)	**sacral nerves**
Ramus dorsalis (nervi spinalis)	Posterior primary ramus (of spinal nerve)	**spinal nerves** Posterior primary ramus
Rami dorsales (nervorum thoracicorum)	Posterior primary rami (of thoracic nerves)	**thoracic nerves** Posterior primary rami
Ramus dorsalis (venae intercostalis posterioris)	Posterior tributary (of posterior intercostal vein)	**intercostal veins** Posterior intercostal vein, posterior tributary of the
Rami dorsales linguae (arteriae lingualis)	Dorsales linguae branches (of lingual artery)	**lingual artery**
Ramus dorsalis manus (nervi ulnaris)	Dorsal branch (of ulnar nerve)	**ulnar nerve** Dorsal branch
Rami duodenales (arteriae pancreatico-duodenalis superioris)	Duodenal branches (of superior pancreaticoduodenal artery)	**hepatic arteries** Common hepatic artery
Rami epiploici (arteriae gastro-epiploicae dextrae)	Omental branches (of right gastro-epiploic artery)	**hepatic arteries** Common hepatic artery
Rami epiploici (arteriae gastro-epiploicae sinistrae)	Omental branches (of left gastro-epiploic artery)	**splenic artery**
Rami esophagei (aortae thoracicae)	Oesophageal branches (of descending thoracic aorta)	**aorta** Branches of the thoracic aorta, oesophageal
Rami esophagei (arteriae gastricae sinistrae)	Oesophageal branches (of left gastric artery)	**gastric arteries** Left gastric artery
Rami esophagei (arteriae thyroideae inferioris)	Oesophageal branches (of inferior thyroid artery)	**thyroid arteries** Inferior thyroid artery
Rami esophagei (nervi vagi)	Oesophageal branches (of vagus nerve)	**vagus nerve**
Ramus externus (nervi accessorii)	Branch to sterno-mastoid muscle	**accessory nerve** Branch to the sternomastoid muscle
Ramus externus (nervi laryngei superioris)	External laryngeal nerve	**laryngeal nerves** External laryngeal nerve
Ramus femoralis (nervi genitofemoralis)	Femoral branch (of genitofemoral nerve)	**genitofemoral nerve**
Rami frontales (arteriae cerebri anterioris)	Frontal branches (of anterior cerebral artery)	**cerebral arteries** Anterior cerebral artery
Rami frontales (arteriae cerebri mediae)	Frontal branches (of middle cerebral artery)	**cerebral arteries** Middle cerebral artery
Ramus frontalis (arteriae meningeae mediae)	Frontal branch (of middle meningeal artery)	**meningeal arteries** Middle meningeal artery
Ramus frontalis (arteriae temporalis superficialis)	Anterior branch (of superficial temporal artery)	**temporal arteries** Superficial temporal artery
Rami gastrici anteriores (nervi vagi)	Anterior gastric branches (of vagus nerve)	**vagus nerve** Gastric branches
Rami gastrici posteriores (nervi vagi)	Posterior gastric branches (of vagus nerve)	**vagus nerve** Gastric branches
Ramus genitalis (nervi genitofemoralis)	Genital branch (of genitofemoral nerve)	**genitofemoral nerve**
Rami gingivales inferiores (nervi alveolaris inferioris)	Inferior gingival branches (of inferior dental nerve)	**dental nerves** Inferior dental nerve
Rami gingivales superiores (plexus dentalis superioris)	Superior gingival branches (of superior dental plexus)	**plexus** Dental plexus, superior
Rami glandulares (arteriae facialis)	Glandular branches (of facial artery)	**facial artery**
Rami glandulares (ganglionis submandibularis)	Glandular branches (of submandibular ganglion)	**ganglion** Submandibular ganglion

Anatomical Nomenclature

Nomina Anatomica (N.A.)	Birmingham Revision (B.R.) or English Equivalent	Definition Location
Rami hepatici (nervi vagi)	Hepatic branches (of vagus nerve)	**vagus nerve** Hepatic branches
Ramus iliacus (arteriae iliolumbalis)	Iliac branch (of iliolumbar artery)	**iliolumbar artery**
Ramus inferior (ansae cervicalis)	Inferior branch (of ansa hypoglossi)	**ansa** Ansa hypoglossi, inferior branch
Ramus inferior (arteriae gluteae superioris)	Lower branch (of superior gluteal artery)	**gluteal arteries** Superior gluteal artery
Ramus inferior (nervi oculomotorii)	Inferior branch (of oculomotor nerve)	**oculomotor nerve** Inferior branch
Rami inferiores (nervi transversi colli)	Inferior branch (of anterior cutaneous nerve of neck)	**neck, anterior cutaneous nerve of the**
Ramus inferior ossis pubis	Inferior pubic ramus	**ramus** Pubic ramus, inferior
Ramus infrahyoideus (arteriae thyroideae superioris)	Infrahyoid artery	**thyroid artery** Superior thyroid artery
Ramus infrapatellaris (nervi sapheni)	Infrapatellar branch (of saphenous nerve)	**saphenous nerve** Infrapatellar branch
Rami inguinales (arteriae pudendae externae)	Inguinal branches (of external pudendal artery)	**pudendal arteries** External pudendal arteries
Rami intercostales anteriores (arteriae thoracicae internae)	Anterior intercostal arteries	**intercostal arteries** Anterior intercostal arteries
Rami interganglionares (ganglionum trunci sympathici)	Interganglionic branches (of ganglia of sympathetic trunk)	**trunk** Sympathetic trunk
Ramus internus (nervi accessorii)	Accessory branch to vagus nerve	**accessory nerve** Branch to the vagus nerve, accessory
Ramus internus (nervi laryngei superioris)	Internal laryngeal nerve	**laryngeal nerves** Internal laryngeal nerve
Ramus interventricularis anterior (arteriae coronariae sinistrae)	Interventricular branch (of left coronary artery)	**coronary arteries** Left coronary artery
Ramus interventricularis posterior (arteriae coronariae dextrae)	Interventricular branch (of right coronary artery)	**coronary arteries** Right coronary artery
Rami isthmi faucium (nervi lingualis)	Branch of lingual nerve to oro-pharyngeal isthmus	**lingual nerve**
Rami labiales anteriores (arteriae pudendae externae)	Labial branches (of external pudendal artery)	**pudendal arteries** External pudendal arteries
Rami labiales inferiores (nervi alveolaris inferioris)	Labial branches (of inferior dental nerve)	**dental nerves** Inferior dental nerve
Rami labiales posteriores (arteriae pudendae internae)	Labial branches (of internal pudendal artery)	**pudendal arteries** Internal pudendal artery
Rami labiales superiores (nervi maxillaris)	Labial branches (of maxillary nerve)	**maxillary nerve**
Rami laryngopharyngei (ganglionis cervicalis superii)	Pharyngeal branches (of superior cervical ganglion)	**ganglion** Cervical ganglion, superior, pharyngeal branches of the
Ramus lateralis (ductus hepaticus sinister)	Lateral duct (of left hepatic duct)	**duct** Left hepatic duct
Ramus lateralis (nervi supra-orbitalis)	Lateral branch (of supra-orbital nerve)	**supra-orbital nerve**
Ramus lateralis (rami dorsalis nervi cervicalis)	Lateral branch (of posterior primary ramus of cervical nerve)	**cervical nerve**
Ramus lateralis (rami dorsalis nervi lumbalis)	Lateral branch (of posterior primary ramus of lumbar nerve)	**lumbar nerves**
Ramus lateralis (rami dorsalis nervi sacralis)	Lateral branch (of posterior primary ramus of sacral nerve)	**sacral nerves**
Ramus lateralis (rami lobi medii arteriae pulmonalis dextrae)	Lateral branch (of branch to middle lobe of right pulmonary artery)	**pulmonary arteries** Right pulmonary artery
Rami laterales (vena portae)	Lateral branches (of portal vein)	**portal vein**
Ramus lateralis cutaneus (arteriae intercostalis posterioris)	Lateral cutaneous branch (of posterior intercostal artery)	**intercostal arteries** Posterior intercostal arteries (III–XI)
Rami lienales (arteriae lienalis)	Splenic branches (of splenic artery)	**splenic artery**
Rami linguales (nervi glossopharyngei)	Lingual branches (of glossopharyngeal nerve)	**glossopharyngeal nerve** Lingual branches
Rami linguales (nervi hypoglossi)	Terminal branches (of hypoglossal nerve)	**hypoglossal nerve**
Rami linguales (nervi lingualis)	Branches to tongue (of lingual nerve)	**lingual nerve**
Ramus lingularis (arteriae pulmonalis sinistrae)	Lingular branch (of left pulmonary artery)	**pulmonary arteries** Left pulmonary artery
Ramus lingularis inferior (arteriae pulmonalis sinistrae)	Inferior lingular branch (of left pulmonary artery)	**pulmonary arteries** Left pulmonary artery
Ramus lingularis superior (arteriae pulmonalis sinistrae)	Superior lingular branch (of left pulmonary artery)	**pulmonary arteries** Left pulmonary artery
Ramus lingularis (venae pulmonalis superioris sinistrae)	Lingular branch (of left superior pulmonary vein)	**pulmonary veins** Left pulmonary veins
Ramus lobi medii (arteriae pulmonalis dextrae)	Branch to middle lobe (of right pulmonary artery)	**pulmonary arteries** Right pulmonary artery
Ramus lobi medii (venae pulmonalis superioris dextrae)	Middle lobe branch (of right pulmonary vein)	**pulmonary veins** Right pulmonary veins
Ramus lumbalis (arteriae iliolumbalis)	Lumbar branch (of iliolumbar artery)	**iliolumbar artery**
Rami malleolares laterales (arteriae peroneae)	Malleolar branches (of peroneal artery)	**peroneal artery** Lateral malleolar branches
Rami malleolares mediales (arteriae tibialis posterioris)	Malleolar branches (of posterior tibial artery)	**tibial arteries** Posterior tibial artery
Ramus mammarius (arteriae intercostalis posterioris)	Mammary branch (of posterior intercostal artery)	**intercostal arteries** Posterior intercostal arteries (III–XI)
Rami mammarii (arteriae thoracicae internae)	Mammary branches (of internal mammary artery)	**mammary artery, internal**
Rami mammarii laterales (arteriae thoracicae lateralis)	External mammary branches (of lateral thoracic artery)	**thoracic arteries** Lateral thoracic artery
Rami mammarii laterales (nervorum thoracicorum)	Lateral mammary branches (of thoracic nerves)	**thoracic nerves** Anterior primary ramus
Rami mammarii mediales (nervorum thoracicorum)	Medial mammary branches (of thoracic nerves)	**thoracic nerves** Anterior primary ramus
Ramus mandibulae	Ramus of mandible	**ramus** Ramus of the mandible
Ramus marginalis mandibulae (nervi facialis)	Mandibular branch (of facial nerve)	**facial nerve** Mandibular branch
Rami mastoidei (arteriae auricularis posterioris)	Mastoid branches (of posterior auricular artery)	**auricular arteries** Posterior auricular artery
Ramus mastoideus (arteriae occipitalis)	Mastoid branch (of occipital artery)	**occipital artery**
Ramus medialis (ductus hepaticus sinister)	Medial duct (of left hepatic duct)	**duct** Left hepatic duct
Ramus medialis (nervi supra-orbitalis)	Medial branch (of supra-orbital nerve)	**supra-orbital nerve**

Nomina Anatomica (N.A.)	Birmingham Revision (B.R.) or English Equivalent	Definition Location
Ramus medialis (rami dorsalis nervi cervicalis)	Medial branch (of posterior primary ramus of cervical nerve)	**cervical nerves**
Ramus medialis (rami dorsalis nervi lumbalis)	Medial branch (of posterior primary ramus of lumbar nerve)	**lumbar nerves**
Ramus medialis (rami dorsalis nervi sacralis)	Medial branch (of posterior primary ramus of sacral nerve)	**sacral nerves**
Ramus medialis (rami lobi medii arteriae pulmonalis dextrae)	Medial branch (of branch to middle lobe of right pulmonary artery)	**pulmonary arteries** Right pulmonary artery
Rami mediales (vena portae)	Medial branches (of portal vein)	**portal vein**
Rami mediastinales (aortae thoracicae)	Mediastinal branches (of descending thoracic aorta)	**aorta** Branches of the thoracic aorta, mediastinal
Rami mediastinales (arteriae thoracicae internae)	Mediastinal branches (of internal mammary artery)	**mammary artery, internal**
Ramus membranae tympani (nervi auriculotemporalis)	Branch to tympanic membrane (of auriculotemporal nerve)	**auriculotemporal nerve**
Ramus meningeus (arteriae occipitalis)	Meningeal branch (of occipital artery)	**occipital artery**
Ramus meningeus (arteriae vertebralis)	Meningeal branch (of vertebral artery)	**vertebral artery**
Ramus meningeus [nervi mandibularis]	Nervus spinosus	**nervus** Nervus spinosus
Ramus meningeus (nervi spinalis)	Meningeal branch (of spinal nerve)	**spinal nerves** Meningeal branch
Ramus meningeus (nervi vagi)	Meningeal branch (of vagus nerve)	**vagus nerve**
Ramus meningeus accessorius (arteriae maxillaris)	Accessory meningeal artery	**maxillary artery**
Ramus meningeus [medius] (nervi maxillaris)	Meningeal branch (of maxillary nerve)	**maxillary nerve**
Rami mentales (nervi alveolaris inferioris)	Mental branches (of inferior dental nerve)	**dental nerves** Inferior dental nerve
Rami musculares (arteriae intercostalis posterioris)	Muscular branches (of posterior intercostal artery)	**intercostal arteries** Posterior intercostal arteries (III–XI)
Ramus muscularis (nervi)	Muscular branch (of nerve)	**branch** Muscular branch
Rami musculares (nervi axillaris)	Muscular branches (of circumflex nerve)	**circumflex nerve**
Rami musculares (nervi femoralis)	Muscular branches (of femoral nerve)	**femoral nerve**
Rami musculares (nervi mediani)	Muscular branches (of median nerve)	**median nerve**
Rami musculares (nervi musculocutanei)	Muscular branches (of musculo-cutaneous nerve)	**musculocutaneous nerve of the upper limb**
Ramus musculares (nervi peronei [fibularis] profundi)	Muscular branches (of anterior tibial nerve)	**tibial nerves** Anterior tibial nerve
Rami musculares (nervi peronei superficialis)	Muscular branches (of musculo-cutaneous nerve)	**musculocutaneous nerve of the lower limb**
Rami musculares (nervi radialis)	Muscular branches (of radial nerve)	**radial nerve**
Rami musculares (nervi tibialis)	Muscular branches (of medial popliteal nerve)	**popliteal nerves** Medial popliteal nerve
Rami musculares (nervi ulnaris)	Muscular branches (of ulnar nerve)	**ulnar nerve** Muscular branches
Ramus musculi stylopharyngei (nervi glossopharyngei)	Branch to stylo-pharyngeus (of glossopharyngeal nerve)	**glossopharyngeal nerve** Branch to the stylopharyngeus
Ramus mylohyoideus (arteriae alveolaris inferioris)	Mylohyoid artery	**maxillary artery**
Ramus nasalis externus (nervi ethmoidalis anterioris)	External nasal branch (of anterior ethmoidal nerve)	**ethmoidal nerves** Anterior ethmoidal nerve, external nasal branch of the
Rami nasales externi (nervi maxillaris)	Nasal branches (external) (of maxillary nerve)	**maxillary nerve**
Rami nasales interni [nervi ethmoidalis anterioris]	Internal nasal branches (of anterior ethmoidal nerve)	**ethmoidal nerves** Anterior ethmoidal nerve, internal nasal branches of the
Rami nasales interni (nervi maxillaris)	Nasal branches (internal) (of maxillary nerve)	**maxillary nerve**
Rami nasales laterales (nervi ethmoidalis anterioris)	Lateral nasal branches (of anterior ethmoidal nerve)	**ethmoidal nerves** Anterior ethmoidal nerve, internal nasal branches
Rami nasales mediales (nervi ethmoidalis anterioris)	Medial nasal branches (of anterior ethmoidal nerve)	**ethmoidal nerves** Anterior ethmoidal nerve, internal nasal branches
Rami nasales posteriores inferiores [laterales]	Nasal branches (of greater palatine nerve)	**palatine nerves** Nasal branches of the greater palatine nerve
Rami nasales posteriores superiores laterales	Short sphenopalatine nerves (lateral)	**sphenopalatine nerves** Short sphenopalatine nerves
Rami nasales posteriores superiores mediales	Short sphenopalatine nerves (medial)	**sphenopalatine nerves** Short sphenopalatine nerves
Ramus obturatorius (arteriae epigastricae inferioris)	Obturator branch (of inferior epigastric artery)	**epigastric arteries** Inferior epigastric artery, obturator branch of the
Ramus occipitalis (arteriae auricularis posterioris)	Occipital branch (of posterior auricular artery)	**auricular arteries** Posterior auricular artery
Rami occipitales (arteriae cerebri posterioris)	Occipital branches (of posterior cerebral artery)	**cerebral arteries** Posterior cerebral artery
Rami occipitales (arteriae occipitalis)	Occipital branches (of occipital artery)	**occipital artery**
Ramus occipitalis (nervi auricularis posterioris)	Occipital branch (of posterior auricular nerve)	**auricular nerves** Posterior auricular nerve
Rami oesophagei (aortae thoracicae)	Oesophageal branches (of descending thoracic aorta)	**aorta** Branches of the thoracic aorta, oesophageal
Rami oesophagei (arteriae gastricae sinistrae)	Oesophageal branches (of left gastric artery)	**gastric arteries** Left gastric artery
Rami oesophagei (arteriae thyroideae inferioris)	Oesophageal branches (of inferior thyroid artery)	**thyroid arteries** Inferior thyroid artery
Rami oesophagei (nervi vagi)	Oesophageal branches (of vagus nerve)	**vagus nerve**
Rami orbitales (arteriae cerebri anterioris)	Orbital branches (of anterior cerebral artery)	**cerebral arteries** Anterior cerebral artery
Rami orbitales (arteriae cerebri mediae)	Orbital branches (of middle cerebral artery)	**cerebral arteries** Middle cerebral artery
Rami orbitales (ganglionis pterygopalatini)	Orbital branches (of sphenopalatine ganglion)	**ganglion** Sphenopalatine ganglion, orbital branches of the
Ramus ossis ischii	Ramus of ischium	**ramus** Ramus of the ischium
Ramus ovaricus (arteriae uterinae)	Ovarian branch (of uterine artery)	**uterine artery**
Ramus palmaris manus nervi ulnaris	Palmar branch (of ulnar nerve)	**ulnar nerve** Palmar branch
Ramus palmaris nervi mediani	Palmar cutaneous branch (of median nerve)	**median nerve** Palmar cutaneous branch

Anatomical Nomenclature

Nomina Anatomica (N.A.)	Birmingham Revision (B.R.) or English Equivalent	Definition Location
Ramus palmaris profundus (arteriae ulnaris)	Deep branch (of ulnar artery)	**ulnar artery**
Ramus palmaris superficialis (arteriae radialis)	Superficial palmar branch (of radial artery)	**radial artery**
Rami palpebrales (nervi infratrochlearis)	Palpebral branches (of infratrochlear nerve)	**infratrochlear nerve**
Rami palpebrales inferiores (nervi maxillaris)	Palpebral branches (of maxillary nerve)	**maxillary nerve**
Rami pancreatici (arteriae lienalis)	Pancreatic branches (of splenic artery)	**splenic artery**
Rami pancreatici (arteriae pancreatico-duodenalis superioris)	Pancreatic branches (of superior pancreaticoduodenal artery)	**hepatic arteries** Common hepatic artery
Rami parietales (arteriae cerebri anterioris)	Parietal branches (of anterior cerebral artery)	**cerebral arteries** Anterior cerebral artery
Rami parietales (arteriae cerebri mediae)	Parietal branches (of middle cerebral artery)	**cerebral arteries** Middle cerebral artery
Ramus parietalis (arteriae meningeae mediae)	Parietal branch (of middle meningeal artery)	**meningeal arteries** Middle meningeal artery
Ramus parietalis (arteriae temporalis superficialis)	Posterior branch (of superficial temporal artery)	**temporal arteries** Superficial temporal artery
Ramus parieto-occipitalis (arteriae cerebri posterioris)	Parieto-occipital branch (of posterior cerebral artery)	**cerebral arteries** Posterior cerebral artery
Rami parotidei (arteriae temporalis superficialis)	Parotid branches (of superficial temporal artery)	**temporal arteries** Superficial temporal artery
Rami parotidei (nervi auriculotemporalis)	Parotid branches (of auriculotemporal nerve)	**auriculotemporal nerve**
Rami parotidei (venae facialis anterioris)	Masseteric and parotid veins	**masseteric veins**
Rami pectorales (arteriae thoraco-acromialis)	Pectoral branches (of acromiothoracic artery)	**acromiothoracic artery**
Ramus perforans (arteriae peroneae)	Perforating branch (of peroneal artery)	**peroneal artery**
Rami perforantes (arteriae metatarseae plantaris)	Perforating branches (of plantar metatarsal artery)	**metatarsal arteries** Plantar metatarsal arteries
Rami perforantes (arteriae radialis)	Perforating branches (of radial artery)	**radial artery**
Rami perforantes (arteriae thoracicae internae)	Perforating branches (of internal mammary artery)	**mammary artery, internal**
Rami pericardiaci (aortae thoracicae)	Pericardial branches (of descending thoracic aorta)	**aorta** Branches of the thoracic aorta, pericardial
Ramus pericardiacus (nervorum phrenicorum)	Pericardial branches (of phrenic nerves)	**phrenic nerve**
Rami perineales (nervi cutanei femoris posterioris)	Perineal branch (of posterior cutaneous nerve of thigh)	**thigh, cutaneous nerves of the** Posterior cutaneous nerve of the thigh
Ramus petrosus (arteriae meningeae mediae)	Superficial petrosal branch (of middle meningeal artery)	**meningeal arteries** Middle meningeal artery
Ramus pharyngeus	Pharyngeal nerve	**pharyngeal nerve**
Rami pharyngei (arteriae pharyngeae ascendentis)	Pharyngeal branches (of ascending pharyngeal artery)	**pharyngeal artery, ascending**
Rami pharyngei (arteriae thyroideae inferioris)	Pharyngeal branches (of inferior thyroid artery)	**thyroid arteries** Inferior thyroid artery
Rami pharyngei (nervi glossopharyngei)	Pharyngeal branches (of glossopharyngeal nerve)	**glossopharyngeal nerve** Pharyngeal branches

Nomina Anatomica (N.A.)	Birmingham Revision (B.R.) or English Equivalent	Definition Location
Rami pharyngei (nervi vagi)	Pharyngeal branches (of vagus nerve)	**vagus nerve** Pharyngeal branches
Rami phrenico-abdominales (nervorum phrenicorum)	Diaphragmatic branches (of phrenic nerves)	**phrenic nerve**
Ramus plantaris profundus (arteriae dorsalis pedis)	Deep plantar branch (of dorsalis pedis artery)	**dorsalis pedis artery**
Ramus posterior (arteriae obturatoriae)	Posterior branch (of obturator artery)	**obturator artery** Posterior branch
Ramus posterior (arteriae pulmonalis sinistrae)	Posterior branch (of left pulmonary artery)	**pulmonary arteries** Left pulmonary artery
Ramus posterior (arteriae recurrentis ulnaris)	Posterior branch (of ulnar recurrent artery)	**ulnar artery**
Ramus posterior (arteriae renalis)	Posterior branch (of renal artery)	**renal artery**
Ramus posterior (arteriae thyroideae superioris)	Posterior branch (of superior thyroid artery)	**thyroid arteries** Superior thyroid artery
Ramus posterior (ductus hepaticus dexter)	Posterior duct (of right hepatic artery)	**duct** Right hepatic duct
Ramus posterior (nervi auricularis magni)	Posterior branch (of great auricular nerve)	**auricular nerves** Great auricular nerve
Ramus posterior (nervi obturatorii)	Posterior branch (of obturator nerve)	**obturator nerve** Posterior branch
Ramus posterior (sulci lateralis)	Posterior ramus (of lateral sulcus)	**ramus** Posterior ramus
Ramus posterior (vena portae)	Posterior segmental branch (of portal vein)	**portal vein**
Ramus posterior ascendens et descendens (arteriae pulmonalis dextrae)	Posterior branches (of right pulmonary artery)	**pulmonary arteries** Right pulmonary artery
Ramus profundus (arteriae circumflexae femoris medialis)	Deep branch (of medial circumflex artery)	**circumflex arteries** Medial circumflex artery
Ramus profundus (arteriae gluteae superioris)	Deep branch (of superior gluteal artery)	**gluteal arteries** Superior gluteal artery
Ramus profundus (arteriae plantaris medialis)	Deep branch (of medial plantar artery)	**plantar arteries** Medial plantar artery
Ramus profundus [arteria scapularis descendens]	Deep branch (of transverse cervical artery)	**cervical arteries** Transverse cervical artery
Ramus profundus (nervi plantaris lateralis)	Deep branch (of lateral plantar nerve)	**plantar nerves** Lateral plantar nerve
Ramus profundus (nervi ulnaris)	Deep terminal branch (of ulnar nerve)	**ulnar nerve** Deep terminal branch
Rami pterygoidei (arteriae maxillaris)	Pterygoid branches (of maxillary artery)	**maxillary artery**
Ramus pubicus (arteriae epigastricae inferioris)	Pubic branch (of inferior epigastric artery)	**epigastric arteries** Inferior epigastric artery, pubic branch of the
Ramus pubicus (arteriae obturatoriae)	Pubic branch (of obturator artery)	**obturator artery** Pubic branch
Rami pulmonales	Pulmonary branches (of thoracic ganglion)	**ganglion** Thoracic ganglion, pulmonary branches of the
Rami renales (nervi vagi)	Renal branches (of vagus nerve)	**vagus nerve** Renal branches
Ramus renalis (partis thoracicae systematis autonomici)	Renal branch (of thoracic part of sympathetic system)	**system** Sympathetic system, thoracic part
Ramus saphenus (arteriae genus descendentis)	Saphenous branch (of descending genicular artery)	**genicular arteries** Descending genicular artery, saphenous branch of the
Rami scrotales anteriores (arteriae pudendae externae)	Scrotal branches (of external pudendal artery)	**pudendal arteries** External pudendal arteries

Nomina Anatomica (N.A.)	Birmingham Revision (B.R.) or English Equivalent	Definition Location
Rami scrotales posteriores	Scrotal branches (of internal pudendal artery)	**pudendal arteries** Internal pudendal artery
Ramus sinister (arteriae hepaticae communis)	Left branch (of hepatic artery)	**hepatic arteries** Common hepatic artery
Ramus sinister (vena portae)	Left branch (of portal vein)	**portal vein**
Ramus sinus carotici (nervi glossopharyngei)	Branch to carotid sinus (of glosso-pharyngeal nerve)	**glossopharyngeal nerve** Branch to the carotid sinus
Ramus spinalis (arteriae iliolumbalis)	Spinal branch (of iliolumbar artery)	**iliolumbar artery**
Ramus spinalis (arteriae intercostalis posterioris)	Spinal branch (of posterior intercostal arteries)	**intercostal arteries** Posterior intercostal arteries (III–XI)
Ramus spinalis (arteriae lumbalis)	Spinal branch (of lumbar artery)	**lumbar arteries**
Rami spinales (arteriarum sacralium lateralium)	Spinal branches (of lateral sacral arteries)	**sacral arteries** Lateral sacral arteries
Ramus spinalis (arteriae subcostalis)	Spinal branch (of subcostal artery)	**subcostal arteries**
Rami spinales (arteriae thyroideae inferioris)	Spinal branches (of inferior thyroid artery)	**thyroid arteries** Inferior thyroid artery
Rami spinales (arteriae vertebralis)	Spinal branches (of vertebral artery)	**vertebral artery**
Ramus spinalis (rami dorsalis arteriae inter-costalis posterioris)	Spinal branch (of posterior branch of posterior intercostal artery)	**intercostal arteries** Posterior intercostal arteries (III–XI)
Ramus spinalis (venae intercostalis posterioris)	Spinal tributary (of posterior intercostal vein)	**intercostal veins** Posterior intercostal vein, spinal tributary of the
Ramus stapedius (arteriae auricularis posterioris)	Stapedial branch (of posterior auricular artery)	**auricular arteries** Posterior auricular artery
Rami sternales (arteriae thoracicae internae)	Sternal branches (of internal mammary artery)	**mammary artery, internal**
Rami sternocleido-mastoidei (arteriae occipitalis)	Sternomastoid branches (of occipital artery)	**occipital artery**
Ramus sternocleido-mastoideus (arteriae thyroideae superioris)	Sternomastoid branch (of superior thyroid artery)	**thyroid arteries** Superior thyroid artery
Rami striati (arteriae cerebri mediae)	Striate branches (of middle cerebral artery)	**cerebral arteries** Middle cerebral artery
Ramus stylohyoideus (nervi facialis)	Stylohyoid branch (of facial nerve)	**facial nerve** Stylohyoid branch
Ramus subapicalis [subsuperior] (arteriae pulmonalis dextrae)	Subapical branch (of right pulmonary artery)	**pulmonary arteries** Right pulmonary artery
Ramus subapicalis [subsuperior] (arteriae pulmonalis sinistrae)	Subapical branch (of left pulmonary artery)	**pulmonary arteries** Left pulmonary artery
Ramus superficialis (arteriae gluteae superioris)	Superficial branch (of superior gluteal artery)	**gluteal arteries** Superior gluteal artery
Ramus superficialis (arteriae plantaris medialis)	Superficial branch (of medial plantar artery)	**plantar arteries** Medial plantar artery
Ramus superficialis [arteria cervicalis superficialis]	Superficial branch (of transverse cervical artery)	**cervical arteries** Transverse cervical artery
Ramus superficialis (nervi plantaris lateralis)	Superficial branch (of lateral plantar nerve)	**plantar nerves** Lateral plantar nerve
Ramus superficialis (nervi radialis)	Superficial branch (of radial nerve)	**radial nerve**
Ramus superficialis (nervi ulnaris)	Superficial terminal branch (of ulnar nerve)	**ulnar nerve** Superficial terminal branch
Ramus superior (ansae cervicalis)	Superior branch (of ansa hypoglossi)	**ansa** Ansa hypoglossi, superior branch
Ramus superior (arteriae gluteae superioris)	Upper branch (of superior gluteal artery)	**gluteal arteries** Superior gluteal artery
Ramus superior (nervi oculomotorii)	Superior branch (of oculomotor nerve)	**oculomotor nerve** Superior branch
Rami superiores (nervi transversi colli)	Superior branch (of anterior cutaneous nerve of neck)	**neck, anterior cutaneous nerve of the**
Ramus superior ossis pubis	Superior pubic ramus	**ramus** Pubic ramus, superior
Ramus suprahyoideus (arteriae lingualis)	Suprahyoid artery	**lingual artery**
Ramus sympathicus ad ganglion ciliare	Sympathetic root of ciliary ganglion	**ganglion** Ciliary ganglion, sympathetic root of the
Ramus sympathicus ad ganglion submandibulare	Sympathetic root of submandibular ganglion	**ganglion** Submandibular ganglion, sympathetic root of the
Rami temporales (arteriae cerebri mediae)	Temporal branches (of middle cerebral artery)	**cerebral arteries** Middle cerebral artery
Rami temporales (arteriae cerebri posterioris)	Temporal branches (of posterior cerebral artery)	**cerebral arteries** Posterior cerebral artery
Rami temporales (nervi facialis)	Temporal branches (of facial nerve)	**facial nerve** Temporal branches
Rami temporales superficiales (nervi auriculotemporalis)	Temporal branches (of auriculotemporal nerve)	**auriculotemporal nerve**
Ramus tentorii (nervi ophthalmici)	Nerve to tentorium	**tentorium, nerve to the**
Rami thymici (arteriae thoracicae internae)	Thymic branches (of internal mammary artery)	**mammary artery, internal**
Ramus thyrohyoideus (ansae cervicalis)	Thyrohyoid branch (of ansa hypoglossi)	**ansa** Ansa hypoglossi, thyrohyoid branch
Ramus tonsillaris (arteriae facialis)	Tonsillar artery	**tonsillar artery**
Rami tonsillares (nerv glossopharyngei)	Tonsillar branches (of glossopharyngeal nerve)	**glossopharyngeal nerve** Tonsillar branches
Rami tracheales (arteriae thyroideae inferioris)	Tracheal branches (of inferior thyroid artery)	**thyroid arteries** Inferior thyroid artery
Rami tracheales (nervi vagi)	Tracheal branches (of vagus nerve)	**vagus nerve**
Ramus transversus (arteriae circumflexae femoris lateralis)	Transverse branch (of lateral circumflex artery)	**circumflex arteries** Lateral circumflex artery
Ramus transversus (arteriae circumflexae femoris medialis)	Transverse branch (of medial circumflex artery)	**circumflex arteries** Medial circumflex artery
Ramus tubalis (nervi glossopharyngei)	Branch to pharyngo-tympanic tube (of glossopharyngeal nerve)	**glossopharyngeal nerve** Branch to the pharyngotympanic tube
Ramus tubarius (arteriae uterinae)	Tubal branch (of uterine artery)	**uterine artery**
Ramus ulnaris (nervi cutanei antebrachii medialis)	Ulnar branch (of medial cutaneous nerve of forearm)	**forearm, nerves of the** Medial cutaneous nerve of the forearm
Rami ureterici (arteriae ovaricae)	Ureteric branches (of ovarian artery)	**ovarian artery**
Rami ureterici (arteriae renalis)	Ureteric branches (of renal artery)	**renal artery**
Rami ureterici (arteriae testicularis)	Ureteric branches (of testicular artery)	**testicular artery**
Rami ureterici (arteriarum vesicalium)	Ureteric branches (of inferior vesical artery)	**vesical arteries** Ureteric branches of the vesical arteries
Rami ventrales (nervorum cervicalium)	Anterior primary rami (of cervical nerves	**cervical nerves**

Anatomical Nomenclature

Nomina Anatomica (N.A.)	Birmingham Revision (B.R.) or English Equivalent	Definition Location
Ramus ventralis (nervi coccygei)	Anterior primary ramus (of coccygeal nerve)	**coccygeal nerve**
Rami ventrales (nervorum lumbalium)	Anterior primary rami (of lumbar nerves)	**lumbar nerves**
Rami ventrales (nervorum sacralium)	Anterior primary rami (of sacral nerves)	**sacral nerves**
Ramus ventralis (nervi spinalis)	Anterior primary ramus (of spinal nerve)	**spinal nerves** Anterior primary ramus
Rami ventrales [nervi intercostales] (nervorum thoracicorum)	Anterior primary rami (of thoracic nerves)	**thoracic nerves** Anterior primary ramus
Rami vestibulares (arteriae labyrinthi)	Vestibular branches (of internal auditory artery)	**auditory artery, internal**
Rami zygomatici (nervi facialis)	Zygomatic branches (of facial nerve)	**facial nerve** Zygomatic branches
Ramus zygomatico-facialis (nervi zygomatici)	Zygomaticofacial branch (of zygomatic nerve)	**zygomatic nerve**
Ramus zygomatico-temporalis (nervi zygomatici)	Zygomaticotemporal branch (of zygomatic nerve)	**zygomatic nerve**
Raphe	Raphe	**raphe**
Raphe (medullae oblongatae)	Median raphe (of medulla oblongata)	**raphe** Median raphe of the medulla oblongata
Raphe (pontis)	Median raphe (of pons)	**raphe** Median raphe of the pons
Raphe palati	Palatine raphe	**raphe** Palatine raphe
Raphe palpebralis lateralis	Lateral palpebral raphe	**raphe** Lateral palpebral raphe
Raphe penis	Raphe of penis	**raphe** Raphe of the penis
Raphe perinei	Raphe of perineum	**raphe** Raphe of the perineum
Raphe pharyngis	Raphe of pharynx	**raphe** Raphe of the pharynx
Raphe pterygomandibularis	Pterygomandibular ligament	**ligament** Pterygomandibular ligament
Raphe scroti	Raphe of scrotum	**raphe** Raphe of the scrotum
Recessus	Recess	**recess** *also* **recessus**
Recessus cochlearis	Cochlear recess	**recess** Recess of the vestibule, cochlear
Recessus costodiaphragmaticus	Costodiaphragmatic recess	**recess** Costodiaphragmatic recess
Recessus costomediastinalis	Costomediastinal recess	**recess** Costomediastinal recess
Recessus duodenalis inferior	Inferior duodenal recess	**recess** Duodenal recess, inferior
Recessus duodenalis superior	Superior duodenal recess	**recess** Duodenal recess superior
Recessus ellipticus	Elliptical recess	**recess** Recess of the vestibule, elliptical
Recessus epitympanicus	Epitympanic recess	**recess** Epitympanic recess
Recessus hepatorenalis	Hepatorenal recess	**recess** Hepatorenal recess
Recessus ileocaecalis inferior	Inferior ileocaecal recess	**recess** Ileocaecal recess, inferior
Recessus ileocaecalis superior	Superior ileocaecal recess	**recess** Ileocaecal recess, superior
Recessus inferior omentalis	Lower recess of lesser sac	**recess** Recess of the lesser sac of the peritoneum, lower
Recessus infundibuli	Infundibular recess	**recess** Recess of the third ventricle, infundibular
Recessus intersigmoideus	Recess of pelvic mesocolon	**recess** Recess of the pelvic mesocolon
Recessus lateralis ventriculi quarti	Lateral recess of fourth ventricle	**recess** Recess of the fourth ventricle, lateral
Recessus lienalis	Lienal recess	**recess** Lienal recess
Recessus membranae tympani anterior	Anterior recess of tympanic membrane	**membrane** Mucous membrane of the tympanic cavity
Recessus membranae tympani posterior	Posterior recess of tympanic membrane	**membrane** Mucous membrane of the tympanic cavity
Recessus membranae tympani superior	Superior recess of tympanic membrane	**membrane** Mucous membrane of the tympanic cavity
Recessus opticus	Optic recess	**recess** Recess of the third ventricle, optic
Recessus paraduodenalis	Paraduodenal recess	**recess** Paraduodenal recess
Recessus pharyngeus	Recess of pharynx	**recess** Recess of the pharynx
Recessus pinealis	Pineal recess	**recess** Recess of the third ventricle, pineal
Recessus piriformis	Piriform fossa	**fossa** Piriform fossa
Recessus pleurales	Recess of pleura	**recess** Recesses of the pleura
Recessus retrocaecalis	Retrocaecal recess	**recess** Retrocaecal recess
Recessus retroduodenalis	Retroduodenal recess	**recess** Retroduodenal recess
Recessus sacciformis	Recessus sacciformis	**recessus** Recessus sacciformis
Recessus spheno-ethmoidalis	Spheno-ethmoidal recess	**recess** Spheno-ethmoidal recess
Recessus sphericus	Spherical recess	**recess** Recess of the vestibule, spherical
Recessus subhepatici	Subhepatic recess	**recess** Subhepatic recess
Recessus subphrenici	Subphrenic recess	**recess** Subphrenic recess
Recessus subpopliteus	Bursa of popliteus tendon	**bursa** Bursa of the popliteus tendon
Recessus superior omentalis	Upper recess of lesser sac	**recess** Recess of the lesser sac of the peritoneum, upper
Recessus suprapinealis	Suprapineal recess	**recess** Recess of the third ventricle, suprapineal
Rectum	Rectum	**rectum**
Regio	Region	**region**
Regio analis	Anal region	**region** Anal region
Regio antebrachii anterior	Anterior antebrachial region	**region** Antebrachial region, anterior
Regio antebrachii posterior	Posterior antebrachial region	**region** Antebrachial region, posterior
Regio axillaris	Axillary region	**region** Axillary region
Regio brachii anterior	Anterior brachial region	**region** Brachial region, anterior
Regio brachii posterior	Posterior brachial region	**region** Brachial region, posterior
Regio buccalis	Buccal region	**region** Buccal region

Nomina Anatomica (N.A.)	Birmingham Revision (B.R.) or English Equivalent	Definition Location
Regio calcanea	Calcanean region	**region** Calcanean region
Regio colli anterior	Anterior cervical region	**region** Cervical region, anterior
Regio colli lateralis	Lateral cervical region	**region** Cervical region, lateral
Regio colli posterior	Nuchal region	**region** Nuchal region
Regio cruris anterior	Anterior crural region	**region** Crural region, anterior
Regio cruris posterior	Posterior crural region	**region** Crural region, posterior
Regio cubiti anterior	Anterior cubital region	**region** Cubital region, anterior
Regio cubiti posterior	Posterior cubital region	**region** Cubital region, posterior
Regio deltoidea	Deltoid region	**region** Deltoid region
Regio epigastrica	Epigastric region	**region** Epigastric region
Regio femoris anterior	Anterior femoral region	**region** Femoral region, anterior
Regio femoris posterior	Posterior femoral region	**region** Femoral region, posterior
Regio frontalis	Frontal region	**region** Frontal region
Regio genus anterior	Anterior region of knee	**region** Region of the knee, anterior
Regio genus posterior	Posterior region of knee	**region** Region of the knee, posterior
Regio glutea	Gluteal region	**region** Gluteal region
Regio hypochondriaca [dextra et sinistra]	Hypochondriac regions (right and left)	**region** Hypochondriac regions, right and left
Regio infraclavicularis	Infraclavicular region	**region** Infraclavicular region
Regio infra-orbitalis	Infra-orbital region	**region** Infra-orbital region
Regio infrascapularis	Infrascapular region	**region** Infrascapular region
Regio inguinalis [dextra et sinistra]	Inguinal region (right and left)	**region** Inguinal region, right and left
Regio lateralis [dextra et sinistra]	Lateral abdominal region (right and left)	**region** Abdominal region, lateral
Regio lumbalis	Lumbar region	**region** Lumbar regions, right and left
Regio mammaria	Mammary region	**region** Mammary region
Regio mentalis	Mental region	**region** Mental region
Regio nasalis	Nasal region	**region** Nasal region
Regio occipitalis	Occipital region	**region** Occipital region
Regio olfactoria	Olfactory region	**region** Olfactory region
Regio olfactoria tunicae mucosae nasi	Olfactory region of mucous membrane of the nose	**region** Olfactory region of the mucous membrane of the nose
Regio oralis	Oral region	**region** Oral region
Regio orbitalis	Orbital region	**region** Orbital region
Regio parietalis	Parietal region	**region** Parietal region
Regio parotideomasseterica	Parotideomasseteric region	**region** Parotideomasseteric region
Regio pubica	Pubic region	**region** Pubic region
Regio respiratoria	Respiratory region	**region** Respiratory region
Regio sacralis	Sacral region	**region** Sacral region
Regio scapularis	Scapular region	**region** Scapular region
Regio sternocleido-mastoidea	Sternocleido-mastoid region	**region** Sternocleidomastoid region
Regio temporalis	Temporal region	**region** Temporal region
Regio umbilicalis	Umbilical region	**region** Umbilical region
Regio vertebralis	Vertebral region	**region** Vertebral region
Regio zygomatica	Zygomatic region	**region** Zygomatic region
Ren	Kidney	**kidney**
Rete	Network	**network** ***also*** **rete**
Rete acromiale	Acromial network	**network** Acromial network
Rete arteriosum	Arterial network	**network** Arterial network
Rete articulare cubiti	Network of elbow joint	**network** Network of the elbow joint
Rete articulare genus	Network of knee	**network** Network of the knee
Rete calcaneum	Calcanean network	**network** Calcanean network
Rete carpi dorsale	Posterior carpal arch	**arch** Carpal arch, posterior
Rete malleolare laterale	Lateral malleolar network	**network** Malleolar network, lateral
Rete malleolare mediale	Medial malleolar network	**network** Malleolar network, medial
Rete mirabile	Rete mirabile	**rete** Rete mirabile
Rete patellae	Patellar network	**network** Patellar network
Rete testis	Rete testis	**rete** Rete testis
Rete venosum	Venous network	**network** Venous network
Rete venosum dorsale manus	Dorsal venous network of hand	**network** Dorsal venous network of the hand
Rete venosum dorsale pedis	Dorsal venous network of foot	**network** Dorsal venous network of the foot
Rete venosum plantare	Venous plantar network	**network** Venous plantar network
Retina	Retina	**retina**
Retinaculum	Retinaculum	**retinaculum**
Retinaculum caudale	Caudal retinaculum	**retinaculum** Caudal retinaculum
Retinacula cutis	Retinacula cutis	**retinaculum** Retinacula cutis
Retinaculum extensorum	Extensor retinaculum	**retinaculum** Retinaculum of the wrist, extensor
Retinaculum flexorum	Flexor retinaculum	**retinaculum** Retinaculum of the wrist, flexor
Retinaculum musculorum extensorum inferius	Inferior extensor retinaculum	**retinaculum** Retinaculum of the ankle, inferior extensor
Retinaculum musculorum extensorum superius	Superior extensor retinaculum	**retinaculum** Retinaculum of the ankle, superior extensor
Retinaculum musculorum flexorum	Flexor retinaculum	**retinaculum** Retinaculum of the ankle, flexor

Anatomical Nomenclature

Nomina Anatomica (N.A.)	Birmingham Revision (B.R.) or English Equivalent	Definition Location
Retinaculum musculorum peroneorum [fibularium] inferius	Inferior peroneal retinaculum	**retinaculum** Retinaculum of the ankle, inferior peroneal
Retinaculum musculorum peroneorum [fibularium] superius	Superior peroneal retinaculum	**retinaculum** Retinaculum of the ankle, superior peroneal
Retinaculum patellae laterale	Lateral retinaculum of patella	**retinaculum** Retinaculum of the patella, lateral
Retinaculum patellae mediale	Medial retinaculum of patella	**retinaculum** Retinaculum of the patella, medial
Retinacula unguis	Ungual retinacula	**retinaculum** Ungual retinacula
Rhombencephalon	Hind-brain	**hind-brain**
Rima	Rima	**rima**
Rima glottidis	Rima glottidis	**rima** Rima glottidis
Rima oris	Oral fissure	**fissure** Oral fissure
Rima palpebrarum	Palpebral fissure	**fissure** Palpebral fissure
Rima pudendi	Pudendal cleft	**cleft** Pudendal cleft
Rima vestibuli	Rima vestibuli	**rima** Rima vestibuli
Rivus lacrimalis	Rivus lacrimalis	**rivus lacrimalis**
Rostrum corporis callosi	Rostrum of corpus callosum	**rostrum** Rostrum of the corpus callosum
Rostrum sphenoidale	Rostrum of sphenoid	**rostrum** Rostrum of the sphenoid bone
Rudimentum	Rudiment	**rudiment**
Rugae vaginales	Vaginal rugae	**ruga** Rugae of the vagina
Sacculus (labyrinthi membranacei)	Saccule (of membranous labyrinth)	**saccule**
Sacculus alveolaris	Air saccule	**saccule** Air saccule
Sacculus laryngis	Saccule of larynx	**saccule** Saccule of the larynx
Saccus	Sac	**sac**
Saccus conjunctivae	Conjunctival sac	**sac** Conjunctival sac
Saccus endolymphaticus	Endolymphatic sac	**sac** Endolymphatic sac
Saccus lacrimalis	Lacrimal sac	**sac** Lacrimal sac
Sagittalis	Sagittal	**sagittal**
Sanguis	Blood	**blood**
Scala tympani	Scala tympani	**scala**
Scala vestibuli	Scala vestibuli	**scala**
Scapha	Scaphoid fossa	**fossa** Scaphoid fossa
Scapula	Scapula	**scapula**
Scapus pili	Shaft of hair	**hair** Shaft of a hair
Sclera	Sclera	**sclera**
Scrotum	Scrotum	**scrotum**
Segmentum anterius (lobi hepatis dextri)	Anterior segment (of right lobe of liver)	**segment** Liver segments
Segmentum anterius (lobi superioris pulmonis dextri)	Anterior segment (of superior lobe of right lung)	**segment** Bronchopulmonary segments
Segmentum anterius (lobi superioris pulmonis sinistri)	Anterior segment (of superior lobe of left lung)	**segment** Bronchopulmonary segments
Segmentum anterius inferius (renis)	Lower (anterior) segment (of kidney)	**segment** Renal segment
Segmentum anterius superius (renis)	Upper (anterior) segment (of kidney)	**segment** Renal segment
Segmentum apicale (lobi superioris pulmonis dextri)	Apical segment (of superior lobe of right lung)	**segment** Bronchopulmonary segments
Segmentum apicale [superius] (lobi inferioris pulmonis dextri)	Apical segment (of inferior lobe of right lung)	**segment** Bronchopulmonary segments
Segmentum apicale [superius] (lobi inferioris pulmonis sinistri)	Apical segment (of inferior lobe of left lung)	**segment** Bronchopulmonary segments
Segmentum apico-posterius (lobi superioris pulmonis sinistri)	Apicoposterior segment (of superior lobe of left lung)	**segment** Bronchopulmonary segments
Segmentum basale anterius (lobi inferioris pulmonis dextri)	Anterior basal segment (of inferior lobe of right lung)	**segment** Bronchopulmonary segments
Segmentum basale anterius (lobi inferioris pulmonis sinistri)	Anterior basal segment (of inferior lobe of left lung)	**segment** Bronchopulmonary segments
Segmentum basale laterale (lobi inferioris pulmonis dextri)	Lateral basal segment (of inferior lobe of right lung)	**segment** Bronchopulmonary segments
Segmentum basale laterale (lobi inferioris pulmonis sinistri)	Lateral basal segment (of inferior lobe of left lung)	**segment** Bronchopulmonary segments
Segmentum basale mediale [cardiacum] (lobi inferioris pulmonis dextri)	Medial basal segment (of inferior lobe of right lung)	**segment** Bronchopulmonary segments
Segmentum basale mediale [cardiacum] (lobi inferioris pulmonis sinistri)	Medial basal segment (of inferior lobe of left lung)	**segment** Bronchopulmonary segments
Segmentum basale posterius (lobi inferioris pulmonis dextri)	Posterior basal segment (of inferior lobe of right lung)	**segment** Bronchopulmonary segments
Segmentum basale posterius (lobi inferioris pulmonis sinistri)	Posterior basal segment (of inferior lobe of left lung)	**segment** Bronchopulmonary segments
Segmenta bronchopulmonalia	Bronchopulmonary segments	**segment** Bronchopulmonary segments
Segmentum inferius (renis)	Lower segment (of kidney)	**segment** Renal segment
Segmentum laterale (lobi hepatis sinistri)	Lateral segment (of left lobe of liver)	**segment** Liver segments
Segmentum laterale (lobi medii pulmonis dextri)	Lateral segment (of middle lobe of right lung)	**segment** Bronchopulmonary segments
Segmentum lingulare inferius (lobi superioris pulmonis sinistri)	Inferior lingular segment (of superior lobe of left lung)	**segment** Bronchopulmonary segments
Segmentum lingulare superius (lobi superioris pulmonis sinistri)	Superior lingular segment (of superior lobe of left lung)	**segment** Bronchopulmonary segments
Segmentum mediale (lobi hepatis sinistri)	Medial segment (of left lobe of liver)	**segment** Liver segments
Segmentum mediale (lobi medii pulmonis dextri)	Medial segment (of middle lobe of right lung)	**segment** Bronchopulmonary segments
Segmentum posterius (lobi hepatis dextri)	Posterior segment (of right lobe of liver)	**segment** Liver segments
Segmentum posterius (lobi superioris pulmonis dextri)	Posterior segment (of superior lobe of right lung)	**segment** Bronchopulmonary segments
Segmentum posterius (renis)	Posterior segment (of kidney)	**segment** Renal segment

Nomina Anatomica (N.A.)	Birmingham Revision (B.R.) or English Equivalent	Definition Location
Segmenta renalia	Renal segments	**segment** Renal segment
Segmentum subapicale [subsuperius] (lobi inferioris pulmonis dextri)	Subapical segment (of inferior lobe of right lung)	**segment** Bronchopulmonary segments
Segmentum subapicale [subsuperius] (lobi inferioris pulmonis sinistri)	Subapical segment (of inferior lobe of left lung)	**segment** Bronchopulmonary segments
Segmentum superius (renis)	Apical segment (of kidney)	**segment** Renal segment
Sella turcica	Sella turcica	**sella turcica**
Semicanalis musculi tensoris tympani	Canal for tensor tympani	**canal** Canal for the tensor tympani
Semicanalis tubae auditivae	Canal of pharyngotympanic tube	**canal** Canal of the pharyngotympanic tube
Septulum	Septulum	**septulum**
Septula testis	Septa of testis	**septum** Septa of the testis
Septum	Septum	**septum**
Septum atrioventriculare	Atrioventricular septum	**septum** Atrioventricular septum
Septum canalis musculotubarii	Septum of musculotubal canal	**canal** Musculotubal canal
Septum cervicale intermedium	Posterior median cervical septum	**septum** Posterior intermediate septum
Septum corporum cavernosorum	Septum of corpora cavernosa	**septum** Septum of the corpora cavernosi of the clitoris
Septum femorale	Femoral septum	**septum** Femoral septum
Septum glandis	Septum of glans	**septum** Septum of the glans
Septa interalveolaria (corporis mandibulae)	Interalveolar septa (of body of mandible)	**septum** Interalveolar septum
Septa interalveolaria (corporis maxillae)	Interalveolar septa (of body of maxilla)	**septum** Interalveolar septum
Septum interatriale	Atrial septum	**septum** Atrial septum
Septum intermusculare anterius cruris	Anterior intermuscular septum (of leg)	**septum** Septum of the leg, anterior intermuscular
Septum intermusculare brachii laterale	Lateral intermuscular septum (of upper arm)	**septum** Septum of the upper arm, lateral intermuscular
Septum intermusculare brachii mediale	Medial intermuscular septum (of upper arm)	**septum** Septum of the upper arm, medial intermuscular
Septum intermusculare femoris laterale	Lateral intermuscular septum (of thigh)	**septum** Septum of the thigh, lateral intermuscular
Septum intermusculare femoris mediale	Medial intermuscular septum (of thigh)	**septum** Septum of the thigh, medial intermuscular
Septum intermusculare posterius cruris	Posterior intermuscular septum (of leg)	**septum** Septum of the leg, posterior intermuscular
Septa inter-radicularia (corporis mandibulae)	Inter-radicular septa (of body of mandible)	**septum** Inter-radicular septum
Septa inter-radicularia (corporis maxillae)	Inter-radicular septa (of body of maxilla)	**septum** Inter-radicular septum
Septum interventriculare	Ventricular septum	**septum** Ventricular septum
Septum linguae	Septum of tongue	**septum** Septum of the tongue
Septum nasi	Septum of nose	**septum** Septum of the nose
Septum nasi osseum	Osseous nasal septum	**septum** Septum of the nose
Septum orbitale	Orbital septum	**septum** Orbital septum
Septum pellucidum	Septum lucidum	**septum** Septum lucidum
Septum penis	Septum of penis	**septum** Septum of the penis
Septum rectovaginale	Rectovaginal septum	**septum** Rectovaginal septum
Septum rectovesicale	Rectovesical septum	**septum** Rectovesical septum
Septum scroti	Septum of scrotum	**septum** Septum of the scrotum
Septum sinuum frontalium	Septum of frontal sinuses	**septum** Septum of the frontal sinuses
Septum sinuum sphenoidalium	Septum of sphenoidal sinuses	**septum** Septum of the sphenoidal sinuses
Sinciput	Sinciput	**sinciput**
Sinister	Left	**left**
Sinus	Sinus	**sinus**
Sinus anales	Anal sinuses	**sinus** Anal sinuses
Sinus aortae	Sinuses of aorta	**sinus** Sinuses of the aorta
Sinus caroticus	Carotid sinus	**sinus** Carotid sinus
Sinus cavernosus	Cavernous sinus	**sinus** Sinus of the dura mater, cavernous
Sinus coronarius	Coronary sinus	**sinus** Coronary sinus
Sinus durae matris	Sinuses of the dura mater	**sinus** Sinuses of the dura mater, venous
Sinus epididymidis	Sinus of epididymis	**sinus** Sinus of the epididymis
Sinus ethmoidales	Ethmoidal sinuses	**sinus** Ethmoidal sinuses
Sinus frontalis	Frontal sinus	**sinus** Frontal sinus
Sinus intercavernosi	Intercavernous sinuses	**sinus** Sinuses of the dura mater, intercavernous
Sinus lactiferi	Lactiferous sinuses	**sinus** Lactiferous sinuses
Sinus lienis	Splenic sinus	**sinus** Splenic sinus
Sinus maxillaris	Maxillary sinus	**sinus** Maxillary sinus
Sinus obliquus pericardii	Oblique sinus of pericardium	**sinus** Sinus of the pericardium, oblique
Sinus occipitalis	Occipital sinus	**sinus** Sinus of the dura mater, occipital
Sinus paranasales	Paranasal sinuses	**sinus** Paranasal sinuses
Sinus petrosus inferior	Inferior petrosal sinus	**sinus** Sinus of the dura mater, inferior petrosal
Sinus petrosus superior	Superior petrosal sinus	**sinus** Sinus of the dura mater, superior petrosal
Sinus posterior (cavi tympani)	Posterior sinus (of tympanic cavity)	**sinus** Posterior sinus
Sinus prostaticus	Prostatic sinus	**sinus** Prostatic sinus
Sinus rectus	Straight sinus	**sinus** Sinus of the dura mater, straight
Sinus renalis	Sinus of kidney	**sinus** Sinus of the kidney

Anatomical Nomenclature

Nomina Anatomica (N.A.)	Birmingham Revision (B.R.) or English Equivalent	Definition Location
Sinus sagittalis inferior	Inferior sagittal sinus	**sinus** Sinus of the dura mater, inferior sagittal
Sinus sagittalis superior	Superior sagittal sinus	**sinus** Sinus of the dura mater, superior sagittal
Sinus sigmoideus	Sigmoid sinus	**sinus** Sinus of the dura mater, sigmoid
Sinus sphenoidalis	Sphenoidal sinus	**sinus** Sphenoidal sinus
Sinus sphenoparietalis	Sphenoparietal sinus	**sinus** Sphenoparietal sinus
Sinus tarsi	Sinus tarsi	**sinus** Sinus tarsi
Sinus transversus	Transverse sinus	**sinus** Sinuses of the dura mater, transverse
Sinus transversus pericardii	Transverse sinus of pericardium	**sinus** Sinus of the pericardium, transverse
Sinus trunci pulmonalis	Sinus of pulmonary trunk	**sinus** Sinus of the pulmonary trunk
Sinus tympani	Sinus tympani	**sinus** Sinus tympani
Sinus unguis	Sinus unguis	**sinus** Sinus unguis
Sinus urogenitalis	Urogenital sinus	**sinus** Urogenital sinus
Sinus venarum cavarum	Sinus of venae cavae	**sinus** Sinus of the venae cavae
Sinus venosus	Venous sinus	**sinus** Venous sinus
Sinus venosus sclerae	Sinus venosus sclerae	**sinus** Sinus venosus sclerae
Skeleton membri inferioris liberi	Skeleton of free lower limb	**skeleton** Skeleton of the free lower limb
Skeleton membri superioris liberi	Skeleton of free upper limb	**skeleton** Skeleton of the free upper limb
Solum	Solum	**solum**
Spatium	Space	**space**
Spatia anguli iridocornealis	Spaces of the iridocorneal angle	**space** Spaces of the iridocorneal angle
Spatium episclerale (bulbi oculi)	Episcleral space (of eyeball)	**space** Episcleral space
Spatium intercostale	Intercostal space	**space** Intercostal space
Spatia interglobularia	Interglobular spaces	**space** Interglobular spaces
Spatia interossea metacarpi	Interosseous spaces of metacarpus	**space** Interosseous spaces of the metacarpus or of the metatarsus
Spatia interossea metatarsi	Interosseous spaces of metatarsus	**space** Interosseous spaces of the metacarpus or of the metatarsus
Spatia intervaginalia (nervi optici)	Intervaginal spaces (of optic nerve)	**space** Intervaginal spaces
Spatium perichoroideale	Perichoroidal space	**space** Perichoroidal space
Spatium perilymphaticum	Perilymphatic space	**space** Perilymphatic space
Spatium perinei profundum	Deep perineal space	**space** Perineal space, deep
Spatium perinei superficiale	Superficial perineal space	**space** Perineal space, superficial
Spatium retroperitoneale	Retroperitoneal space	**space** Retroperitoneal space
Spatium retropubicum	Retropubic space	**space** Retropubic space
Spatia zonularia	Zonular spaces	**space** Zonular spaces of the ciliary zonule
Sperma	Semen	**semen**
Spina	Spine	**spina** *also* **spine**
Spina helicis	Spine of helix	**spine** Spine of the helix
Spina iliaca anterior inferior	Anterior inferior iliac spine	**spine** Iliac spine, anterior inferior
Spina iliaca anterior superior	Anterior superior iliac spine	**spine** Iliac spine, anterior superior
Spina iliaca posterior inferior	Posterior inferior iliac spine	**spine** Iliac spine, posterior inferior
Spina iliaca posterior superior	Posterior superior iliac spine	**spine** Iliac spine, posterior superior
Spina ischiadica	Ischial spine	**spine** Ischial spine
Spina mentalis	Genial tubercle	**tubercle** Genial tubercle
Spina nasalis	Nasal spine	**spine** Nasal spine
Spina nasalis anterior	Anterior nasal spine	**spine** Nasal spine, anterior
Spina nasalis posterior	Posterior nasal spine	**spine** Nasal spine, posterior
Spina ossis sphenoidalis	Spine of sphenoid	**spine** Spine of the sphenoid bone
Spina palatinae	Palatine spine	**spine** Palatine spine
Spina scapulae	Spine of scapula	**spine** Spine of the scapula
Spina supra meatum	Suprameatal spine	**spine** Suprameatal spine
Spina trochlearis	Trochlear spine	**spine** Trochlear spine
Spina tympanica major	Greater tympanic spine	**spine** Tympanic spine, greater
Spina tympanica minor	Lesser tympanic spine	**spine** Tympanic spine, lesser
Splenium corporis callosi	Splenium of corpus callosum	**splenium**
Squama frontalis	Frontal squama	**squama** Frontal squama
Squama occipitalis	Squamous part (of occipital bone)	**occipital bone** Squamous part
Stapes	Stapes	**stapes**
Statoconia	Otoliths	**otolith**
Sternum	Sternum	**sternum**
Stratum	Layer	**layer** *also* **stratum**
Stratum basale [cylindricum]	Basal-cell layer (of epidermis)	**layer** Basal-cell layer of the epidermis
Stratum cerebrale (retinae)	Cerebral layer (of retina)	**layer** Cerebral layer of the retina
Stratum circulare (coli)	Circular layer (of colon)	**layer** Circular layer of the colon
Stratum circulare (membranae tympani)	Circular fibres of fibrous layer (of tympanic membrane)	**membrane** Tympanic membrane
Stratum circulare (tunicae muscularis intestini tenuis)	Circular layer (of muscular coat of small intestine)	**intestine** Small intestine, muscular coat of the
Stratum circulare (tunicae muscularis recti)	Circular layer (of muscular coat of rectum)	**rectum** Muscular coat of the rectum
Stratum circulare (tunicae muscularis ventriculi)	Circular layer (of muscular coat of stomach)	**stomach** Coat of the stomach, muscular

Anatomical Nomenclature

Nomina Anatomica (N.A.)	Birmingham Revision (B.R.) or English Equivalent	Definition Location
Stratum corneum	Horny layer (of epidermis)	**layer** Horny layer of the epidermis
Stratum corneum unguis	Horny zone of nail	**zone** Zone of the nail, horny
Stratum cutaneum (membranae tympani)	Cuticular layer (of tympanic membrane)	**membrane** Tympanic membrane
Stratum ganglionare nervi optici	Ganglionic layer of optic nerve	**layer** Ganglionic layer of the retina
Stratum ganglionare retinae	Inner nuclear layer of retina	**layer** Inner nuclear layer of the retina
Stratum gangliosum	Ganglionic layer (of cerebellum)	**cortex** Cortex of the cerebellum
Stratum germinativum unguis	Germinative zone of nail	**zone** Zone of the nail, germinative
Stratum granulosum (cerebelli)	Granular layer (of cerebellum)	**cortex** Cortex of the cerebellum
Stratum granulosum (epidermidis)	Granular layer (of epidermis)	**layer** Granular layer of the epidermis
Stratum granulosum (folliculi ovarici vesiculosi)	Stratum granulosum (of vesicular ovarian follicle)	**stratum** Stratum granulosum
Stratum griseum colliculi superioris	Nucleus of superior quadrigeminal body	**body** Quadrigeminal body, superior, nucleus of the
Stratum longitudinale (tunicae muscularis intestini tenuis)	Longitudinal layer (of muscular coat of small intestine)	**intestine** Small intestine, muscular coat of the
Stratum longitudinale (tunicae muscularis recti)	Longitudinal layer (of muscular coat of rectum)	**rectum** Muscular coat of the rectum
Stratum longitudinale (B.N.A.) (tunicae muscularis tubae uterinae)	Longitudinal layer (of muscular coat of uterine tube)	**tube** Uterine tube, muscular coat of the
Stratum lucidum	Clear layer (of epidermis)	**layer** Clear layer of the epidermis
Stratum moleculare (cerebelli)	Molecular layer (of cerebellum)	**cortex** Cortex of the cerebellum
Stratum mucosum (membranae tympani)	Mucous layer (of tympanic membrane)	**membrane** Tympanic membrane
Stratum neuro-epitheliale (retinae)	Neuro-epithelial layer (of retina)	**layer** Neuro-epithelial layer of the retina
Stratum papillare	Corpus papillare	**corpus** Corpus papillare
Stratum pigmenti	Pigmented layer	**layer** Pigmented layer
Stratum pigmenti corporis ciliaris	Pigmented layer of ciliary body	**layer** Pigmented layer of the ciliary body
Stratum pigmenti iridis	Pigmented layer of iris	**layer** Pigmented layer of the iris
Stratum pigmenti retinae	Pigmented layer of retina	**layer** Pigmented layer of the retina
Stratum radiatum (membranae tympani)	Radial fibres of fibrous layer (of tympanic membrane)	**membrane** Tympanic membrane
Stratum reticulare	Reticular body of skin	**body** Reticular body of the skin
Stratum spinosum	Prickle-cell layer (of epidermis)	**layer** Prickle-cell layer of the epidermis
Stratum zonale	Stratum zonale	**stratum** Stratum zonale
Stria	Stria	**stria**
Stria longitudinalis lateralis	Lateral longitudinal stria	**stria** Longitudinal stria, lateral
Stria longitudinalis medialis	Medial longitudinal stria	**stria** Longitudinal stria, medial
Stria mallearis	Stria mallearis	**stria** Stria malleolaris
Stria medullaris	Stria medullaris	**stria** Stria medullaris
Stria medullaris thalami	Stria habenularis (of thalamus)	**stria** Stria habenularis of the thalamus
Striae medullares ventriculi quarti	Auditory striae	**stria** Auditory striae
Stria olfactoria	Olfactory stria	**stria** Olfactory stria
Stria terminalis	Stria semicircularis	**stria** Stria semicircularis
Stria vascularis	Stria vascularis	**stria** Stria vascularis
Stroma	Stroma	**stroma**
Stroma glandulae thyroideae	Stroma of thyroid gland	**stroma** Stroma of the thyroid gland
Stroma iridis	Stroma of iris	**stroma** Stroma of the iris
Stroma ovarii	Stroma of ovary	**stroma** Stroma of the ovary
Stroma vitreum	Stroma of vitreous body	**stroma** Stroma of the vitreous body
Subiculum promontorii	Subiculum promontorii	**subiculum** Subiculum promontorii
Substantia	Substance	**substance** *also* **substantia**
Substantia alba	White matter	**matter** White matter
Substantia compacta	Compact substance	**substance** Compact substance
Substantia corticalis	Cortical substance	**substance** Cortical substance
Substantia ferruginea	Substantia ferruginea	**substantia** Substantia ferruginea
Substantia gelatinosa	Gelatinous matter	**matter** Gelatinous matter
Substantia glandularis (prostatae)	Glandular substance (of prostate)	**prostate**
Substantia grisea	Grey matter	**matter** Grey matter
Substantia grisea (medullae spinalis)	Central grey matter (of spinal cord)	**matter** Central grey matter of the spinal cord
Substantia grisea centralis	Central grey matter (of mid-brain)	**matter** Central grey matter of the mid-brain
Substantia intermedia centralis	Substantia intermedia centralis	**substantia** Substantia intermedia centralis
Substantia intermedia lateralis	Substantia intermedia lateralis	**substantia** Substantia intermedia lateralis
Substantia lentis	Substantia lentis	**substantia** Substantia lentis
Substantia muscularis (prostatae)	Muscular tissue (of prostate)	**prostate**
Substantia nigra	Substantia nigra	**substantia** Substantia nigra
Substantia perforata anterior	Anterior perforated substance	**substance** Perforated substance, anterior
Substantia perforata posterior	Posterior perforated substance	**substance** Perforated substance, posterior
Substantia propria corneae	Substantia propria of cornea	**substantia** Substantia propria
Substantia propria sclerae	Substantia propria sclerae	**substantia** Substantia propria sclerae
Substantia spongiosa	Spongy substance	**substance** Spongy substance
Succus	Juice	**juice** *also* **succus**
Sudor	Sweat	**sweat**

Nomina Anatomica (N.A.)	Birmingham Revision (B.R.) or English Equivalent	Definition Location
Sulcus	Sulcus	**sulcus**
Sulcus ampullaris	Ampullary sulcus	**ampulla** Membranous ampullae
Sulcus anthelicis transversus	Transverse sulcus of antihelix	**sulcus** Sulcus of the antihelix, transverse
Sulcus arteriae occipitalis	Occipital groove	**groove** Occipital groove
Sulcus arteriae subclaviae	Groove for subclavian artery	**groove** Groove for the subclavian artery
Sulcus arteriae temporalis mediae	Groove for middle temporal artery	**groove** Groove for the middle temporal artery
Sulcus arteriae vertebralis	Groove for vertebral artery	**groove** Groove for the vertebral artery
Sulci arteriosi	Arterial sulci	**sulcus** Arterial sulci
Sulcus auriculae posterior	Posterior sulcus of auricle	**sulcus** Sulcus of the auricle, posterior
Sulcus basilaris	Basilar sulcus	**sulcus** Sulcus of the pons, basilar
Sulcus bicipitalis lateralis	Lateral bicipital groove	**groove** Grooves of the upper limb, lateral bicipital
Sulcus bicipitalis medialis	Medial bicipital groove	**groove** Grooves of the upper limb, medial bicipital
Sulcus calcanei	Groove of calcaneum	**groove** Groove of the calcaneum
Sulcus calcarinus	Calcarine sulcus	**sulcus** Calcarine sulcus
Sulcus caroticus	Carotid groove	**groove** Groove of the sphenoid bone, carotid
Sulcus carpi	Carpal sulcus	**sulcus** Carpal sulcus
Sulcus centrale insulae	Central sulcus of insula	**sulcus** Sulcus of the insula, central
Sulcus centralis	Central sulcus	**sulcus** Sulcus of the cerebrum, central
Sulci cerebri	Cerebral sulci	**sulcus** Cerebral sulci
Sulcus chiasmatis	Optic groove	**groove** Groove of the sphenoid bone, optic
Sulcus cinguli	Sulcus cinguli	**sulcus** Sulcus cinguli
Sulcus circularis insulae	Circular sulcus	**sulcus** Sulcus of the insula, circular
Sulcus collateralis	Collateral sulcus	**sulcus** Collateral sulcus
Sulcus coronarius	Atrioventricular groove	**groove** Atrioventricular groove
Sulcus corporis callosi	Callosal sulcus	**sulcus** Callosal sulcus
Sulcus costae	Costal groove	**groove** Costal groove
Sulcus cruris helicis	Sulcus of crus of helix	**sulcus** Sulcus of the crus of the helix
Sulci cutis	Grooves of skin	**groove** Grooves of the skin
Sulcus ethmoidalis	Ethmoidal groove	**groove** Ethmoidal groove
Sulcus frontalis inferior	Inferior frontal sulcus	**sulcus** Sulcus of the frontal lobe, inferior frontal
Sulcus frontalis superior	Superior frontal sulcus	**sulcus** Sulcus of the frontal lobe, superior frontal
Sulcus gluteus	Fold of buttock	**fold** Fold of the buttock
Sulcus hamuli pterygoidei	Sulcus of pterygoid hamulus	**sulcus** Sulcus of the pterygoid hamulus
Sulcus hippocampi	Hippocampal sulcus	**sulcus** Hippocampal sulcus
Sulcus hypothalamicus	Hypothalamic sulcus	**sulcus** Sulcus of the third ventricle, hypothalamic
Sulcus infra-orbitalis	Infra-orbital groove	**groove** Infra-orbital groove
Sulcus infrapalpebralis	Infrapalpebral sulcus	**sulcus** Infrapalpebral sulcus
Sulcus intermedius posterior	Posterior intermediate sulcus	**sulcus** Sulcus of the spinal cord, posterior intermediate
Sulcus intertubercularis	Bicipital groove	**groove** Bicipital groove
Sulcus interventricularis [cordis] anterior	Anterior interventricular groove	**groove** Interventricular groove, anterior
Sulcus interventricularis [cordis] posterior	Inferior interventricular groove	**groove** Interventricular groove, inferior
Sulcus intraparietalis	Intraparietal sulcus	**sulcus** Sulcus of the parietal lobe, intraparietal
Sulcus lacrimalis (maxillae)	Nasolacrimal groove	**groove** Nasolacrimal groove
Sulcus lacrimalis (ossis lacrimalis)	Lacrimal groove	**groove** Lacrimal groove
Sulcus lateralis (cerebri)	Lateral sulcus (of cerebrum)	**sulcus** Sulcus of the cerebrum, lateral
Sulcus lateralis anterior	Anterolateral sulcus	**sulcus** Anterolateral sulcus
Sulcus lateralis posterior (medullae oblongatae)	Posterolateral sulcus (of medulla oblongata)	**sulcus** Posterolateral sulcus
Sulcus lateralis posterior (medullae spinalis)	Posterior lateral sulcus (of spinal cord)	**sulcus** Sulcus of the spinal cord, posterior lateral
Sulcus limitans	Sulcus limitans	**sulcus** Sulcus limitans
Sulcus limitans (ventriculi quarti)	Sulcus limitans (of fourth ventricle)	**sulcus** Sulcus limitans of the fourth ventricle
Sulcus lunatus	Lunate sulcus	**sulcus** Sulcus of the occipital lobe, lunate
Sulcus malleolaris	Groove for tibialis posterior muscle	**groove** Groove for the tibialis posterior muscle
Sulcus matricis unguis	Groove of nail bed	**groove** Groove of the nail bed
Sulcus medialis cruris cerebri	Medial sulcus (of cerebral peduncle)	**sulcus** Sulcus of the cerebral peduncle, medial
Sulcus medianus (ventriculi quarti)	Sulcus medianus (of fourth ventricle)	**sulcus** Sulcus medianus of the fourth ventricle
Sulcus medianus linguae	Median sulcus of tongue	**sulcus** Sulcus of the tongue, median
Sulcus medianus posterior (medullae oblongatae)	Posterior median fissure (of medulla oblongata)	**medulla oblongata**
Sulcus medianus posterior (medullae spinalis)	Posterior median sulcus (of spinal cord)	**sulcus** Sulcus of the spinal cord, posterior median
Sulcus mentolabialis	Mentolabial groove	**groove** Mentolabial groove
Sulcus mylohyoideus	Mylohyoid groove	**groove** Mylohyoid groove

Nomina Anatomica (N.A.)	Birmingham Revision (B.R.) or English Equivalent	Definition Location
Sulcus nasolabialis	Nasolabial groove	**groove** Nasolabial groove
Sulcus nervi petrosi majoris	Groove for greater superficial petrosal nerve	**groove** Groove for the greater superficial petrosal nerve
Sulcus nervi petrosi minoris	Groove for lesser superficial petrosal nerve	**groove** Groove for the lesser superficial petrosal nerve
Sulcus nervi radialis	Spiral groove	**groove** Spiral groove
Sulcus nervi spinalis	Groove for spinal nerve	**groove** Groove for a spinal nerve
Sulcus nervi ulnaris	Groove for ulnar nerve	**groove** Groove for the ulnar nerve
Sulcus obturatorius	Obturator groove	**groove** Obturator groove
Sulcus occipitalis transversus	Transverse occipital sulcus	**sulcus** Sulcus of the occipital lobe, transverse
Sulcus occipitotemporalis	Occipitotemporal sulcus	**sulcus** Occipitotemporal sulcus
Sulcus olfactorius	Olfactory sulcus	**sulcus** Olfactory sulcus
Sulci orbitales	Orbital sulci	**sulcus** Sulci of the orbital surface of the cerebral hemisphere, orbital
Sulci palatini	Palatine grooves	**groove** Palatine groove of the maxilla
Sulcus palatinovaginalis	Palatinovaginal sulcus	**sulcus** Palatinovaginal sulcus
Sulcus palatinus major (ossis palatini)	Greater palatine groove	**groove** Palatine groove, greater
Sulcus palatinus major (ossis sphenoidalis)	Pterygopalatine sulcus	**sulcus** Pterygopalatine sulcus
Sulci paracolici	Paracolic grooves	**groove** Paracolic grooves
Sulcus parieto-occipitalis	Parieto-occipital sulcus	**sulcus** Parieto-occipital sulcus
Sulcus postcentralis	Postcentral sulcus	**sulcus** Sulcus of the parietal lobe, postcentral
Sulcus precentralis	Precentral sulcus	**sulcus** Sulcus of the frontal lobe, precentral
Sulcus promontorii	Groove of promontory	**groove** Grooves of the promontory
Sulcus pulmonalis	Pulmonary sulcus	**sulcus** Pulmonary sulcus
Sulcus rhinalis	Rhinal sulcus	**sulcus** Rhinal sulcus
Sulcus sagittalis	Sagittal groove	**groove** Sagittal groove of the parietal bone
Sulcus sclerae	Sulcus sclerae	**sulcus** Sulcus sclerae
Sulcus sinus petrosi inferioris	Groove for inferior petrosal sinus	**groove** Groove for the inferior petrosal sinus
Sulcus sinus petrosi superioris	Groove for superior petrosal sinus	**groove** Groove for the superior petrosal sinus
Sulcus sinus sagittalis superioris (ossis frontalis)	Sagittal groove (of frontal bone)	**groove** Sagittal groove of the frontal bone
Sulcus sinus sagittalis superioris (ossis occipitalis)	Sagittal groove (of occipital bone)	**groove** Sagittal groove of the occipital bone
Sulcus sinus sigmoidei	Sigmoid groove	**groove** Sigmoid groove
Sulcus sinus transversi	Groove for transverse sinus	**groove** Groove for the transverse sinus

Nomina Anatomica (N.A.)	Birmingham Revision (B.R.) or English Equivalent	Definition Location
Sulcus spiralis externus	External spiral sulcus	**sulcus** Spiral sulci
Sulcus spiralis internus	Internal spiral sulcus	**sulcus** Spiral sulci
Sulcus subparietalis	Suprasplenial sulcus	**sulcus** Suprasplenial sulcus
Sulcus tali	Groove of talus	**groove** Groove of the talus
Sulcus temporalis inferior	Inferior temporal sulcus	**sulcus** Sulcus of the temporal lobe, inferior temporal
Sulcus temporalis superior	Superior temporal sulcus	**sulcus** Sulcus of the temporal lobe, superior temporal
Sulci temporales transversi	Transverse temporal sulci	**sulcus** Sulci of the temporal lobe, transverse temporal
Sulcus tendinis musculori peronei [fibularis longi]	Groove for tendons of peroneus muscles	**groove** Groove for the tendons of the peroneus muscles
Sulcus tendinis musculi flexoris hallucis longi	Groove for flexor hallucis longus tendon	**groove** Groove for the flexor hallucis longus tendon
Sulcus tendinis musculi peronei longi	Groove for peroneus longus tendon	**groove** Groove for the peroneus longus tendon
Sulcus terminalis (atrii dextri)	Sulcus terminalis (of right atrium)	**sulcus** Sulcus terminalis of the right atrium
Sulcus terminalis (linguae)	Sulcus terminalis (of tongue)	**sulcus** Sulcus terminalis
Sulcus tubae auditivae	Groove for pharyngotympanic tube	**groove** Groove for the pharyngotympanic tube
Sulcus tympanicus	Tympanic groove	**groove** Tympanic groove
Sulcus venae cavae	Groove for vena cava	**groove** Groove for the vena cava
Sulcus vena subclaviae	Groove for subclavian vein	**groove** Groove for the subclavian vein
Sulcus venae umbilicalis	Groove for umbilical vein	**groove** Groove for the umbilical vein
Sulci venosi	Venous sulci	**sulcus** Venous sulci
Sulcus vomerovaginalis	Vomerovaginal sulcus	**sulcus** Vomerovaginal sulcus
Supercilia	Hairs of eyebrows	**hair** Hairs of the eyebrows
Supercilium	Eyebrow	**eyebrow**
Superficialis	Superficial	**superficial**
Superior	Superior	**superior**
Sura	Calf	**calf**
Sustenaculum tali	Sustenaculum tali	**sustenaculum** Sustenaculum tali
Sutura	Suture	**suture**
Sutura coronalis	Coronal suture	**suture** Coronal suture
Suturae cranii	Sutures of skull	**suture** Sutures of the skull
Sutura ethmoideomaxillaris	Ethmoidomaxillary suture	**suture** Ethmoidomaxillary suture
Sutura frontalis [sutura metopica]	Frontal suture	**suture** Frontal suture
Sutura fronto-ethmoidalis	Fronto-ethmoid suture	**suture** Fronto-ethmoid suture
Sutura frontolacrimalis	Frontolacrimal suture	**suture** Frontolacrimal suture
Sutura frontomaxillaris	Frontomaxillary suture	**suture** Frontomaxillary suture
Sutura frontonasalis	Frontonasal suture	**suture** Frontonasal suture
Sutura frontozygomatica	Frontozygomatic suture	**suture** Frontozygomatic suture

Anatomical Nomenclature

Nomina Anatomica (N.A.)	Birmingham Revision (B.R.) or English Equivalent	Definition Location
Sutura incisiva	Incisive suture	**suture** Incisive suture
Suture infra-orbitalis	Infra-orbital suture	**suture** Infra-orbital suture
Sutura intermaxillaris	Intermaxillary suture	**suture** Intermaxillary suture
Sutura internasalis	Internasal suture	**suture** Internasal suture
Sutura lacrimoconchalis	Lacrimoconchal suture	**suture** Lacrimoconchal suture
Sutura lacrimomaxillaris	Lacrimomaxillary suture	**suture** Lacrimomaxillary suture
Sutura lambdoidea	Lambdoid suture	**suture** Lambdoid suture
Sutura metopica	Frontal suture	**suture** Frontal suture
Sutura nasomaxillaris	Nasomaxillary suture	**suture** Nasomaxillary suture
Sutura occipitomastoidea	Occipitomastoid suture	**suture** Occipitomastoid suture
Sutura palatina mediana	Median palatine suture	**suture** Palatine suture, median
Sutura palatina transversa	Transverse palatine suture	**suture** Palatine suture, transverse
Sutura palato-ethmoidalis	Palato-ethmoidal suture	**suture** Palato-ethmoidal suture
Sutura palatomaxillaris	Palatomaxillary suture	**suture** Palatomaxillary suture
Sutura parietomastoidea	Parietomastoid suture	**suture** Parietomastoid suture
Sutura plana	Flat suture	**suture** Flat suture
Sutura sagittalis	Sagittal suture	**suture** Sagittal suture
Sutura serrata	Serrate suture	**suture** Serrate suture
Sutura spheno-ethmoidalis	Spheno-ethmoidal suture	**suture** Spheno-ethmoidal suture
Sutura sphenofrontalis	Sphenofrontal suture	**suture** Sphenofrontal suture
Sutura sphenomaxillaris	Sphenomaxillary suture	**suture** Sphenomaxillary suture
Sutura sphenoparietalis	Sphenoparietal suture	**suture** Sphenoparietal suture
Sutura sphenosquamosa	Sphenosquamous suture	**suture** Sphenosquamous suture
Sutura sphenozygomatica	Sphenozygomatic suture	**suture** Sphenozygomatic suture
Sutura squamosa	Squamous suture	**suture** Squamous suture
Sutura squamosa (cranii)	Squamous suture (of skull)	**suture** Squamous suture
Sutura squamosomastoidea	Squamomastoid suture	**suture** Squamomastoid suture
Sutura temporozygomatica	Temporozygomatic suture	**suture** Temporozygomatic suture
Sutura zygomaticomaxillaris	Zygomaticomaxillary suture	**suture** Zygomaticomaxillary suture
Symphysis	Secondary cartilaginous joint	**joint** Cartilaginous joint, secondary
Symphysis pubica	Pubic symphysis	**symphysis** Pubic symphysis
Synchondrosis	Primary cartilaginous joint	**joint** Cartilaginous joint, primary
Synchondroses cranii	Cartilaginous joints of skull	**joint** Joints of the skull, cartilaginous
Synchondrosis intra-occipitalis anterior	Anterior intra-occipital synchondrosis	**synchondrosis** Intra-occipital synchondrosis, anterior
Synchondrosis intra-occipitalis posterior	Posterior intra-occipital synchondrosis	**synchondrosis** Intra-occipital synchondrosis, posterior
Synchondrosis petro-occipitalis	Petro-occipital joint	**joint** Petro-occipital joint
Synchondrosis spheno-occipitalis	Spheno-occipital joint	**joint** Spheno-occipital joint
Synchondrosis sphenopetrosa	Sphenopetrous joint	**joint** Sphenopetrous joint
Synchondrosis manubriosternalis	Manubriosternal joint	**joint** Manubriosternal joint
Synchondrosis xiphosternalis	Xiphosternal joint	**joint** Xiphosternal joint
Syndesmologia	Arthrology	**arthrology**
Syndesmosis	Syndesmosis	**syndesmosis**
Syndesmosis (articulatio) tibiofibularis	Inferior tibiofibular joint	**joint** Tibiofibular joint, inferior
Syndesmosis tympanostapedia	Tympanostapedial syndesmosis	**syndesmosis** Tympanostapedial syndesmosis
Synostosis	Synostosis	**synostosis**
Synovia	Synovia	**synovia**
Systema digestorium	Digestive system	**system** Digestive system
Systema lymphaticum	Lymphatic system	**system** Lymphatic system
Systema nervosum	Nervous system	**system** Nervous system
Systema nervosum autonomicum	Autonomic nervous system	**system** Autonomic nervous system
Systema nervosum centrale	Central nervous system	**system** Central nervous system
Systema nervosum periphericum	Peripheral nervous system	**system** Peripheral nervous system
Systema respiratorium	Respiratory system	**system** Respiratory system
Systema urogenitale	Urogenital system	**system** Urogenital system
Taenia	Band	**band** *also* **taenia**
Taenia choroidea	Taenia choroidea	**taenia** Taenia choroidea
Taeniae coli	Taeniae coli	**taenia** Taeniae coli
Taenia fornicis	Taenia of fornix	**taenia** Taenia of the fornix
Taenia libera	Taenia libera	**taenia** Taeniae coli
Taenia mesocolica	Taenia mesocolica	**taenia** Taeniae coli
Taenia omentalis	Taenia omentalis	**taenia** Taeniae coli
Taenia telae	Taenia telae	**taenia** Taenia telae
Taenia thalami	Taenia of thalamus	**taenia** Taenia of the thalamus
Taenia ventriculi quarti	Taenia of fourth ventricle	**taenia** Taenia of the fourth ventricle
Talus	Ankle	**ankle** *also* **talus**
Tarsus	Tarsus	**tarsus**
Tarsus inferior	Tarsus of lower eyelid	**plate** Tarsal plate
Tarsus superior	Tarsus of upper eyelid	**plate** Tarsal plate
Tectum mesencephali	Tectum of mid-brain	**tectum** Tectum of the mid-brain
Tegmen	Tegmen	**tegmen**
Tegmen tympani	Tegmen tympani	**tegmen** Tegmen tympani
Tegmen ventriculi quarti	Roof of fourth ventricle	**ventricle** Fourth ventricle
Tegmentum	Tegmentum	**tegmentum**

Nomina Anatomica (N.A.)	Birmingham Revision (B.R.) or English Equivalent	Definition Location
Tegmentum rhombencephali	Tegmentum of hind-brain	**tegmentum** Tegmentum of the hind-brain
Tela	Tela	**tela**
Tela choroidea ventriculi quarti	Tela chorioidea of fourth ventricle	**tela** Tela chorioidea
Tela choroidea ventriculi tertii	Tela chorioidea of third ventricle	**tela** Tela chorioidea
Tela conjunctiva	Connective tissue	**tissue** Connective tissue
Tela elastica	Elastic tissue	**tissue** Elastic tissue
Tela subcutanea	Subcutaneous tissue	**tissue** Subcutaneous tissue
Tela submucosa	Submucous coat	**coat** Submucous coat
Tela submucosa (coli)	Submucous coat (of colon)	**colon** Coat of the colon, submucous
Tela submucosa (intestini tenuis)	Submucous coat (of small intestine)	**intestine** Small intestine, submucous coat of the
Tela submucosa (oesophagi)	Submucous coat (of oesophagus)	**oesophagus** Coat of the oesophagus, submucous
Tela submucosa (pharyngis)	Submucous coat (of pharynx)	**pharynx** Submucous coat
Tela submucosa (recti)	Submucous coat (of rectum)	**rectum** Submucous coat of the rectum
Tela submucosa (tracheae et bronchorum)	Submucous coat (of trachea and bronchi)	**trachea** Coat of the trachea and bronchi, submucous
Tela submucosa (ventriculi)	Submucous coat (of stomach)	**stomach** Coat of the stomach, submucous
Tela submucosa (vesicae urinariae)	Submucous coat (of urinary bladder)	**urinary bladder** Submucous coat
Tela subserosa	Subserous coat	**coat** Subserous coat
Tela subserosa (peritonei visceralis)	Extraperitoneal tissue	**tissue** Extraperitoneal tissue
Tela subserosa vesicae felleae	Subserous coat of gall bladder	**gall bladder** Coat of the gall bladder, subserous
Telencephalon	Telencephalon	**telencephalon**
Tempora	Temples	**temple**
Tendo	Tendon	**tendo** *also* **tendon**
Tendo calcaneus [Achillis]	Tendo calcaneus	**tendo** Tendo calcaneus
Tendo crico-esophageus	Crico-oesophageal tendon	**tendon** Crico-oesophageal tendon
Tenia	Band	**band** *also* **taenia**
Tenia choroidea	Taenia chorioidea	**taenia** Taenia choroidea
Teniae coli	Taeniae coli	**taenia** Taenia coli
Tenia fornicis	Taenia of fornix	**taenia** Taenia of the fornix
Tenia libera	Taenia libera	**taenia** Taenia coli
Tenia mesocolica	Taenia mesocolica	**taenia** Taeniae coli
Tenia omentalis	Taenia omentalis	**taenia** Taeniae coli
Tenia telae	Taenia telae	**taenia** Taenia telae
Tenia thalami	Taenia of thalamus	**taenia** Taenia of the thalamus
Tenia ventriculi quarti	Taenia of fourth ventricle	**taenia** Taenia of the fourth ventricle
Tentorium cerebelli	Tentorium cerebelli	**tentorium** Tentorium cerebelli

Nomina Anatomica (N.A.)	Birmingham Revision (B.R.) or English Equivalent	Definition Location
Terminationes nervorum liberae	Free nerve-endings	**nerve-ending** Free nerve-endings
Testis	Testis	**testis**
Thalamencephalon	Thalamencephalon	**thalamencephalon**
Thalamus	Thalamus	**thalamus**
Theca folliculi	Theca folliculi	**theca** Theca folliculi
Thenar	Thenar eminence	**eminence** Thenar eminence
Thorax	Thorax	**thorax**
Thymus	Thymus	**thymus**
Tibia	Tibia	**tibia**
Tibialis	Tibial	**tibial**
Tonsilla cerebelli	Tonsil of cerebellum	**tonsil** Tonsil of the cerebellum
Tonsilla lingualis	Lingual tonsil	**tonsil** Lingual tonsil
Tonsilla palatina	Tonsil	**tonsil** Palatine tonsil
Tonsilla pharyngea	Nasopharyngeal tonsil	**tonsil** Nasopharyngeal tonsil
Tonsilla tubaria	Tube tonsil	**tonsil** Tube tonsil
Toruli tactiles	Tactile elevations	**elevation** Tactile elevations
Torus	Torus	**torus**
Torus levatorius	Torus levatorius	**torus** Torus levatorius
Torus palatinus	Palatine torus	**torus** Palatine torus
Torus tubarius	Tubal elevation	**elevation** Tubal elevation
Trabecula	Trabecula	**trabecula**
Trabeculae carneae	Trabeculae carneae	**trabecula** Trabeculae carneae
Trabeculae corporum cavernosorum	Trabeculae of corpora cavernosa	**trabecula** Trabeculae of the penis
Trabeculae corporis spongiosi	Trabeculae of corpus spongiosum	**trabecula** Trabeculae of the penis
Trabeculae lienis	Trabeculae of spleen	**trabecula** Trabecula of the spleen
Trabecula septomarginalis	Moderator band	**band** Moderator band
Trachea	Trachea	**trachea**
Tractus	Tract	**tract** *also* **tractus**
Tractus cerebellorubralis	Cerebellorubral tract	**tract** Cerebellorubral tract
Tractus cerebellothalamicus	Cerebellothalamic tract	**tract** Cerebellothalamic tract
Tractus corticohypothalamicus	Corticohypothalamic tract	**tract** Corticohypothalamic tract
Tractus corticonuclearis	Corticonuclear tract	**tract** Corticonuclear tract
Traetus corticopontinus	Cerebropontine tract	**tract** Cerebropontine tract
Tractus corticospinalis [pyramidalis] anterior	Anterior cerebrospinal tract	**tract** Cerebrospinal tract, anterior
Tractus corticospinalis [pyramidalis] lateralis	Later cerebrospinal tract	**tract** Cerebrospinal tract, lateral
Tractus dorsolateralis	Dorsolateral tract	**tract** Posterolateral tract
Tractus frontopontinus	Frontopontine tract	**tract** Frontopontine tract
Tractus iliotibialis	Iliotibial tract	**tract** Iliotibial tract
Tractus mesencephalicus nervi trigemini	Mesencephalic tract of trigeminal nerve	**tract** Tract of the trigeminal nerve, mesencephalic
Tractus nervosus associationis	Association tracts	**tract** Association tract

Anatomical Nomenclature

Nomina Anatomica (N.A.)	Birmingham Revision (B.R.) or English Equivalent	Definition Location
Tractus nervosus commissurales	Commissural tracts	**tract** Commissural tract
Tractus nervosus projectionis	Projection tracts	**tract** Projection tract
Tractus occipitopontinus	Occipitopontine tract	**tract** Occipitopontine tract
Tractus olfactorius	Olfactory tract	**tract** Olfactory tract
Tractus olivocerebellaris	Olivocerebellar tract	**tract** Olivocerebellar tract
Tractus opticus	Optic tract	**tract** Optic tract
Tractus parietopontinus	Parietopontine tract	**tract** Parietopontine tract
Tractus pyramidalis	Pyramidal tract	**tract** Pyramidal tract
Tractus reticulospinalis	Reticulospinal tract	**tract** Reticulospinal tract
Tractus rubrospinalis	Rubrospinal tract	**tract** Rubrospinal tract
Tractus solitarius	Tractus solitarius	**tractus** Tractus solitarius
Tractus spinalis nervi trigemini	Spinal tract of trigeminal nerve	**tract** Tract of the trigeminal nerve, spinal
Tractus spinocerebellaris anterior	Anterior spinocerebellar tract	**tract** Spinocerebellar tract, anterior
Tractus spinocerebellaris posterior	Posterior spinocerebellar tract	**tract** Spinocerebellar tract, posterior
Tractus spinotectalis	Spinotectal tract	**tract** Spinotectal tract
Tractus spinothalamicus anterior	Anterior spinothalamic tract	**tract** Spinothalamic tract, anterior
Tractus spinothalamicus lateralis	Lateral spinothalamic tract	**tract** Spinothalamic tract, lateral
Tractus spiralis foraminosus	Tractus spiralis foraminosus	**tractus** Tractus spiralis foraminosus
Tractus supra-optico-hypophysialis	Supra-optico-hypophyseal tract	**tract** Supra-optico-hypophyseal tract
Tractus tectospinalis	Tectospinal tract	**tract** Tectospinal tract
Tractus tegmentalis centralis	Central tegmental fasciculus	**fasciculus** Central tegmental fasciculus
Tractus temporopontinus	Temporopontine tract	**tract** Temporopontine tract
Tractus vestibulospinalis	Vestibulospinal tract	**tract** Vestibulospinal tract
Tragi	Hairs of ear	**hair** Hairs of the ear
Tragus	Tragus	**tragus**
Transversalis	Transverse	**transverse**
Transversus	Transverse	**transverse**
Trigonum	Triangle	**triangle** *also* **trigone** *and* **trigonum**
Trigonum caroticum	Carotid triangle	**triangle** Carotid triangle, superior
Trigonum collaterale	Collateral trigone	**trigone** Collateral trigone
Trigonum femorale	Femoral triangle	**triangle** Femoral triangle
Trigona fibrosa	Trigona fibrosa	**trigonum** Trigona fibrosa
Trigonum habenulae	Trigonum habenulae	**trigonum** Trigonum habenulae
Trigonum inguinale	Inguinal triangle	**triangle** Inguinal triangle
Trigonum lumbale	Lumbar triangle	**triangle** Lumbar triangle

Nomina Anatomica (N.A.)	Birmingham Revision (B.R.) or English Equivalent	Definition Location
Trigonum nervi hypoglossi	Hypoglossal triangle	**triangle** Hypoglossal triangle
Trigonum nervi vagi	Vagal triangle	**triangle** Vagal triangle
Trigonum olfactorium	Olfactory pyramid	**pyramid** Olfactory pyramid
Trigonum omo-claviculare [fossa supraclavicularis major]	Omoclavicular triangle	**triangle** Omoclavicular triangle
Trigonum submandibulare	Submaxillary triangle	**triangle** Submaxillary triangle
Trigonum vesicae	Trigone of bladder	**trigone** Trigone of the bladder
Trochanter major	Greater trochanter	**trochanter** Greater trochanter
Trochanter minor	Lesser trochanter	**trochanter** Lesser trochanter
Trochanter tertius	Third trochanter	**trochanter** Third trochanter
Trochlea	Trochlea	**trochlea**
Trochlea (musculi obliqui superioris)	Trochlea (of superior oblique muscle of orbit)	**trochlea** Trochlea of the superior oblique muscle of the orbit
Trochlea humeri	Trochlea of humerus	**trochlea** Trochlea of the humerus
Trochlea muscularis	Muscular pulley	**pulley** Muscular pulley
Trochlea peronealis [fibularis]	Peroneal tubercle	**tubercule** Peroneal tubercle
Trochlea tali	Trochlea of talus	**trochlea** Trochlea of the talus
Truncus	Trunk	**trunk**
Truncus [fasciculi atrioventricularis]	Trunk (of atrio-ventricular bundle)	**trunk** Trunk of the atrio-ventricular bundle
Truncus brachiocephalicus	Innominate artery	**innominate artery**
Truncus bronchomediastinalis	Mediastinal trunk	**trunk** Mediastinal trunk
Truncus celiacus	Coeliac artery	**coeliac artery**
Truncus corporis callosi	Trunk of corpus callosum	**trunk** Trunk of the corpus callosum
Truncus costocervicalis	Costocervical trunk	**trunk** Costocervical trunk
Truncus inferior (plexus brachialis)	Lower trunk (of brachial plexus)	**plexus** Brachial plexus
Truncus intestinalis	Intestinal trunk	**trunk** Intestinal trunk
Truncus jugularis	Jugular trunk	**trunk** Jugular trunk
Truncus linguofacialis	Linguofacial trunk	**trunk** Linguofacial trunk
Trunci lumbales [dexter et sinister]	Lumbar trunks (right and left)	**trunk** Lumbar trunks
Truncus lumbosacralis	Lumbosacral trunk	**trunk** Lumbosacral trunk
Truncus medius (plexus brachialis)	Middle trunk (of brachial plexus)	**plexus** Brachial plexus
Trunci plexus brachialis	Trunks of brachial plexus	**plexus** Brachial plexus
Truncus pulmonalis	Pulmonary trunk (stem)	**trunk** Pulmonary trunk
Truncus subclavius	Subclavian trunk	**trunk** Subclavian trunk
Truncus superior (plexus brachialis)	Upper trunk (of brachial plexus)	**plexus** Brachial plexus
Truncus sympathicus	Sympathetic trunk	**trunk** Sympathetic trunk
Truncus thyrocervicalis	Thyrocervical trunk	**trunk** Thyrocervical trunk
Truncus vagalis anterior	Anterior vagal trunk	**trunk** Vagal trunk, anterior

Nomina Anatomica (N.A.)	Birmingham Revision (B.R.) or English Equivalent	Definition Location
Truncus vagalis posterior	Posterior vagal trunk	**trunk** Vagal trunk, posterior
Tuba	Tube	**tube**
Tuba auditiva	Pharyngotympanic tube	**tube** Pharyngotympanic tube
Tuba uterina	Uterine tube	**tube** Uterine tube
Tuber	Tuberosity	**tuber** *also* **tuberosity**
Tuber calcanei	Posterior surface of calcaneum	**calcaneum** Posterior surface
Tuber cinereum	Tuber cinereum	**tuber** Tuber cinereum
Tuber frontale	Frontal eminence	**eminence** Frontal eminence
Tuber ischiadicum	Ischial tuberosity	**tuberosity** Ischial tuberosity
Tuber maxillae	Maxillary tuberosity	**tuberosity** Maxillary tuberosity
Tuber omentale (hepatis)	Tuber omentale (of liver)	**tuber** Tuber omentale of the liver
Tuber omentale (pancreatis)	Tuber omentale (of pancreas)	**tuber** Tuber omentale of the pancreas
Tuber parietale	Parietal eminence	**eminence** Parietal eminence
Tuber vermis	Lobulus tuberis	**lobulus** Lobulus tuberis
Tuberculum	Tubercle	**tubercle** *also* **tuberculum**
Tuberculum (labii superii oris)	Labial tubercle	**tubercle** Labial tubercle
Tuberculum adductorium	Adductor tubercle	**tubercle** Adductor tubercle
Tuberculum anterius (atlantis)	Anterior tubercle (of atlas)	**tubercle** Tubercle of the atlas, anterior
Tuberculum anterius [vertebrarum cervicalium]	Anterior tubercle (of cervical vertebrae)	**tubercle** Tubercle of a cervical vertebra, anterior
Tuberculum anterius thalami	Anterior tubercle of thalamus	**tubercle** Tubercle of the thalamus, anterior
Tuberculum articulare	Eminentia artericularis	**eminentia** Eminentia articularis
Tuberculum auriculae	Tubercle of auricle	**tubercle** Tubercle of the auricle
Tuberculum caroticum [vertebrae cervicalis VI]	Carotid tubercle (of sixth cervical vertebra)	**tubercle** Carotid tubercle
Tuberculum conoideum	Conoid tubercle	**tubercle** Conoid tubercle
Tuberculum corniculatum	Corniculate tubercle	**tubercle** Tubercle of the aryepiglottic fold, corniculate
Tuberculum costae	Tubercle of rib	**tubercle** Tubercle of a rib
Tuberculum cuneiforme	Cuneiform tubercle	**tubercle** Tubercle of the aryepiglottic fold, cuneiform
Tubercula [coronae] dentis	Tubercles of tooth	**tubercle** Tubercles of a tooth
Tuberculum epiglotticum	Epiglottic tubercle	**tubercle** Epiglottic tubercle
Tuberculum infraglenoidale	Infraglenoid tubercle	**tubercle** Infraglenoid tubercle
Tuberculum inter-condylare laterale	Lateral intercondylar tubercle	**tubercle** Intercondylar tubercle, lateral
Tuberculum inter-condylare mediale	Medial intercondylar tubercle	**tubercle** Intercondylar tubercle, medial
Tuberculum intervenosum	Intervenous tubercle	**tubercle** Intervenous tubercle

Nomina Anatomica (N.A.)	Birmingham Revision (B.R.) or English Equivalent	Definition Location
Tuberculum jugulare	Jugular tubercle	**tubercle** Jugular tubercle
Tuberculum laterale (processus posterioris tali)	Lateral tubercle (of posterior tubercle of talus)	**tubercle** Tubercle of the talus, posterior
Tuberculum majus (humeri)	Greater tuberosity (of humerus)	**tuberosity** Tuberosity of the humerus
Tuberculum marginale	Marginal tubercle	**tubercle** Marginal tubercle
Tuberculum mediale (tali)	Medial tubercle (of talus)	**tubercle** Tubercle of the talus, medial
Tuberculum mentale	Mental tubercle	**tubercle** Mental tubercle
Tuberculum minus (humeri)	Lesser tuberosity (of humerus)	**tuberosity** Tuberosity of the humerus
Tuberculum musculi scaleni anterioris	Scalene tubercle	**tubercle** Scalene tubercle
Tuberculum nuclei cuneati	Cuneate tubercle	**tubercle** Tubercle of the medulla oblongata, cuneate
Tuberculum nuclei gracilis	Gracile tubercle	**tubercle** Gracile tubercle
Tuberculum obturatorium anterius	Anterior obturator tubercle	**tubercle** Obturator tubercle anterior
Tuberculum obturatorium posterius	Posterior obturator tubercle	**tubercle** Obturator tubercle, posterior
Tuberculum ossis scaphoidei	Tubercle of scaphoid	**tubercle** Tubercle of the scaphoid
Tuberculum ossis trapezii	Crest of trapezium	**crest** Crest of the trapezium
Tuberculum pharyngeum	Pharyngeal tubercle	**tubercle** Pharyngeal tubercle
Tuberculum posterius (atlantis)	Posterior tubercle (of atlas)	**tubercle** Tubercle of the atlas, posterior
Tuberculum posterius [vertebrarum cervicalium]	Posterior tubercle (of cervical vertebrae)	**tubercle** Tubercle of a cervical vertebra, posterior
Tuberculum pubicum	Pubic tubercle	**tubercle** Pubic tubercle
Tuberculum sellae	Tuberculum sellae	**tuberculum** Tuberculum sellae
Tuberculum supraglenoidale	Supraglenoid tubercle	**tubercle** Supraglenoid tubercle
Tuberculum supratragicum	Supratragal tubercle	**tubercle** Supratragal tubercle
Tuberculum thyroideum inferius	Inferior thyroid tubercle	**tubercle** Thyroid tubercle, inferior
Tuberculum thyroideum superius	Superior thyroid tubercle	**tubercle** Thyroid tubercle, superior
Tuberositas deltoidea	Deltoid tuberosity	**tuberosity** Deltoid tuberosity
Tuberositas glutea	Gluteal tuberosity	**tuberosity** Gluteal tuberosity
Tuberositas iliaca	Iliac tuberosity	**tuberosity** Iliac tuberosity
Tuberositas masseterica	Masseteric tuberosity	**tuberosity** Masseteric tuberosity
Tuberositas musculi serrati anterioris	Tubercle for serratus anterior	**tubercle** Tubercle for the serratus anterior muscle
Tuberositas ossis cuboidei	Tuberosity of cuboid	**tuberosity** Tuberosity of the cuboid bone
Tuberositas ossis metatarsalis I	Tubercle of 1st metatarsal bone	**tubercle** Tubercle of the 1st metatarsal bone
Tuberositas ossis metatarsalis V	Tubercle of 5th metatarsal bone	**tubercle** Tubercle of the 5th metatarsal bone
Tuberositas ossis navicularis	Tuberosity of navicular	**tuberosity** Tuberosity of the navicular bone

Nomina Anatomica (N.A.)	Birmingham Revision (B.R.) or English Equivalent	Definition Location
Tuberositas phalangis distalis (manus)	Tuberosity of distal phalanx (of finger)	**tuberosity** Tuberosity of a distal phalanx of a finger
Tuberositas phalangis distalis (pedis)	Tuberosity of distal phalanx (of toe)	**tuberosity** Tuberosity of the distal phalanx of a toe
Tuberositas pterygoidea	Pterygoid tuberosity	**tuberosity** Pterygoid tuberosity
Tuberositas radii	Tuberosity of radius	**tuberosity** Tuberosity of the radius
Tuberositas sacralis	Sacral tuberosity	**tuberosity** Sacral tuberosity
Tuberositas tibiae	Tubercle of tibia	**tubercle** Tubercle of the tibia
Tuberositas ulnae	Tuberosity of ulna	**tuberosity** Tuberosity of the ulna
Tubulus	Tubule	**tubule**
Tubuli renales	Renal tubules	**tubule** Renal tubule
Tubuli renales contorti	Convoluted renal tubules	**tubule** Renal tubule
Tubuli renales recti	Straight renal tubules	**tubule** Renal tubule
Tubuli seminiferi contorti	Convoluted seminiferous tubules	**tubule** Seminiferous tubule, convoluted
Tubuli seminiferi recti	Straight seminiferous tubules	**tubule** Seminiferous tubules, straight
Tunica	Coat	**coat** *also* **tunica**
Tunica adventitia	Adventitious coat	**coat** Adventitious coat
Tunica adventitia (ductus deferentis)	Adventitious coat (of vas deferens)	**vas** Vas deferens, adventitious coat of the
Tunica adventitia (esophagi)	Adventitious coat (of oesophagus)	**oesophagus** Coat of the oesophagus, adventitious
Tunica adventitia (ureteris)	Adventitious coat (of ureter)	**ureter** Coat of the ureter, adventitious
Tunica adventitia (vesiculae seminalis)	Adventitious coat (of seminal vesicle)	**vesicle** Seminal vesicle, adventitious coat of the
Tunica albuginea	Tunica albuginea	**tunica** Tunica albuginea
Tunica albuginea (testis)	Tunica albuginea (of testis)	**testis**
Tunica albuginea corporum cavernosorum	Tunica albuginea of corpora cavernosa	**tunica** Tunica albuginea
Tunica albuginea corporis spongiosi	Tunica albuginea of corpus spongiosum	**tunica** Tunica albuginea
Tunica conjunctiva	Conjunctiva	**conjunctiva**
Tunica conjunctiva bulbi	Ocular part of conjunctiva	**conjunctiva** Ocular part of the conjunctiva
Tunica conjunctiva palpebrarum	Palpebral part of conjunctiva	**conjunctiva** Palpebral part of the conjunctiva
Tunica dartos	Dartos muscle	**dartos muscle**
Tunica externa	Tunica adventitia	**tunica** Tunica adventitia
Tunica externa (thecae folliculi)	Outer coat (of theca folliculi)	**theca** Theca folliculi
Tunica fibrosa	Fibrous coat	**coat** Fibrous coat
Tunica fibrosa (hepatis)	Fibrous coat (of liver)	**liver**
Tunica fibrosa (lienis)	Tunica albuginea (of spleen)	**spleen**
Tunica fibrosa bulbi	Fibrous coat of eye	**eye** Coat of the eye, fibrous
Tunica interna (thecae folliculi)	Inner coat (of theca folliculi)	**theca** Theca folliculi
Tunica interna bulbi	Nervous coat of eye	**eye** Coat of the eye, nervous
Tunica intima	Tunica intima	**tunica** Tunica intima
Tunica media	Tunica media	**tunica** Tunica media
Tunica mucosa	Mucous coat (or membrane)	**coat** Mucous coat
Tunica mucosa (coli)	Mucous coat (of colon)	**colon** Coat of the colon, mucous
Tunica mucosa (ductus deferentis)	Mucous coat (of vas deferens)	**vas** Vas deferens, mucous coat of the
Tunica mucosa [endometrium]	Mucous coat (of uterus)	**uterus** Coat of the uterus, mucous
Tunica mucosa (intestini tenuis)	Mucous coat (of small intestine)	**intestine** Small intestine, mucous coat of the
Tunica mucosa (laryngis)	Mucous membrane (of larynx)	**membrane** Mucous membrane of the larynx
Tunica mucosa (esophagi)	Mucous coat (of oesophagus)	**oesophagus** Coat of the oesophagus, mucous
Tunica mucosa (pharyngis)	Mucous coat or membrane (of pharynx)	**pharynx** Mucous coat
Tunica mucosa (recti)	Mucous coat (of rectum)	**rectum** Mucous coat of the rectum
Tunica mucosa (tracheae et bronchorum)	Mucous coat (of trachea and bronchi)	**trachea** Coat of the trachea and bronchi, mucous
Tunica mucosa (tubae auditivae)	Mucous coat (of pharyngotympanic tube)	**tube** Pharyngotympanic tube
Tunica mucosa (tubae uterinae)	Mucous coat (of uterine tube)	**tube** Uterine tube, mucous coat of the
Tunica mucosa (ureteris)	Mucous coat (of ureter)	**ureter** Coat of the ureter, mucous
Tunica mucosa (urethrae)	Mucous coat (of urethra)	**urethra** Coat of the urethra, mucous
Tunica mucosa (vaginae)	Mucous coat (of vagina)	**vagina** Coat of the vagina, mucous
Tunica mucosa (ventriculi)	Mucous coat (of stomach)	**stomach** Coat of the stomach, mucous
Tunica mucosa (vesicae urinariae)	Mucous coat (of urinary bladder)	**urinary bladder** Mucous coat
Tunica mucosa (vesiculae seminalis)	Mucous coat (of seminal vesicle)	**vesicle** Seminal vesicle, mucous coat of the
Tunica mucosa cavi tympani	Mucous membrane of tympanic cavity	**membrane** Mucous membrane of the tympanic cavity
Tunica mucosa linguae	Mucous membrane of tongue	**membrane** Mucous membrane of the tongue
Tunica mucosa nasi	Mucous membrane of nose	**membrane** Mucous membrane of the nose
Tunica mucosa oris	Mucous membrane of mouth	**membrane** Mucous membrane of the mouth
Tunica mucosa vesicae felleae	Mucous coat of gall bladder	**gall bladder** Coat of the gall bladder, mucous
Tunica muscularis	Muscular coat	**coat** Muscular coat
Tunica muscularis (bronchi)	Muscular coat (of bronchi)	**bronchus**
Tunica muscularis (coli)	Muscular coat (of colon)	**colon** Coat of the colon, muscular

Nomina Anatomica (N.A.)	Birmingham Revision (B.R.) or English Equivalent	Definition Location
Tunica muscularis (ductus deferentis)	Muscular coat (of vas deferens)	**vas** Vas deferens, muscular coat of the
Tunica muscularis (intestini tenuis)	Muscular coat (of small intestine)	**intestine** Small intestine, muscular coat of the
Tunica muscularis [myometrium]	Muscular coat (of uterus)	**uterus** Coat of the uterus, muscular
Tunica muscularis (esophagi)	Muscular coat (of oesophagus)	**oesophagus** Coat of the oesophagus, muscular
Tunica muscularis (recti)	Muscular coat (of rectum)	**rectum** Muscular coat of the rectum
Tunica muscularis (tubae uterinae)	Muscular coat (of uterine tube)	**tube** Uterine tube, muscular coat of the
Tunica muscularis (ureteris)	Muscular coat (of ureter)	**ureter** Coat of the ureter, muscular
Tunica muscularis (urethrae)	Muscular coat (of urethra)	**urethra** Coat of the urethra, muscular
Tunica muscularis (vaginae)	Muscular coat (of vagina)	**vagina** Coat of the vagina, muscular
Tunica muscularis (ventriculi)	Muscular coat (of stomach)	**stomach** Coat of the stomach, muscular
Tunica muscularis (vesicae urinariae)	Muscular coat (of urinary bladder)	**urinary bladder** Muscular coat
Tunica muscularis (vesiculae seminalis)	Muscular coat (of seminal vesicle)	**vesicle** Seminal vesicle, muscular coat of the
Tunica muscularis pharyngis	Muscular coat (of pharynx)	**pharynx** Muscular coat
Tunica muscularis vesicae felleae	Muscular coat of gall bladder	**gall bladder** Coat of the gall bladder, muscular
Tunica propria	Tunica propria	**tunica** Tunica propria
Tunica propria (corii)	Tunica propria (of corium)	**tunica** Tunica propria of the corium
Tunica serosa	Serous coat	**coat** Serous coat
Tunica serosa (coli)	Serous coat (of colon)	**colon** Coat of the colon, serous
Tunica serosa (hepatis)	Serous coat (of liver)	**liver**
Tunica serosa (intestini tenuis)	Serous coat (of small intestine)	**intestine** Small intestine, serous coat of the
Tunica serosa (lienis)	Serous coat (of spleen)	**spleen**
Tunica serosa [perimetrium]	Serous coat (of uterus)	**uterus** Coat of the uterus, serous
Tunica serosa (peritonei visceralis)	Serous coat (of visceral peritoneum)	**peritoneum**
Tunica serosa (tubae uterinae)	Serous coat (of uterine tube)	**tube** Uterine tube, serous coat of the
Tunica serosa (ventriculi)	Serous coat (of stomach)	**stomach** Coat of the stomach, serous
Tunica serosa (vesicae urinariae)	Serous coat (of urinary bladder)	**urinary bladder** Serous coat
Tunica serosa vesicae felleae	Serous coat of gall bladder	**gall bladder** Coat of the gall bladder, serous
Tunica subserosa (tubae uterinae)	Subserous coat (of uterine tube)	**tube** Uterine tube, subserous coat of the
Tunica vaginalis testis	Tunica vaginalis testis	**tunica** Tunica vaginalis testis
Tunica vasculosa bulbi	Vascular coat of eye	**eye** Coat of the eye, vascular

Nomina Anatomica (N.A.)	Birmingham Revision (B.R.) or English Equivalent	Definition Location
Ulna	Ulna	**ulna**
Ulnaris	Ulnar	**ulnar**
Umbilicus	Umbilicus (navel)	**umbilicus**
Umbo membranae tympani	Umbo of tympanic membrane	**umbo** Umbo of the tympanic membrane
Uncus	Uncus	**uncus**
Unguis	Nail	**nail**
Urachus	Urachus	**urachus**
Ureter	Ureter	**ureter**
Urethra feminina	Female urethra	**urethra** Female urethra
Urethra masculina	Male urethra	**urethra** Male urethra
Uterus	Uterus	**uterus**
Utriculus	Utricle	**utricle**
Utriculus prostaticus	Prostatic utricle	**utricle** Prostatic utricle
Uvula (palatina)	Uvula	**uvula**
Uvula vermis	Uvula of vermis	**uvula** Uvula of the vermis
Uvula vesicae	Uvula of bladder	**uvula** Uvula of the bladder
Vagina	Sheath *also* Vagina	**sheath *also* vagina**
Vagina bulbi	Fascial sheath of eyeball	**sheath** Fascial sheath of the eyeball
Vagina carotica	Carotid sheath	**sheath** Carotid sheath
Vagina externa nervi optici	External sheath of optic nerve	**sheath** Sheaths of the optic nerve
Vaginae fibrosae digitorum manus	Fibrous flexor sheaths of fingers	**sheath** Fibrous flexor sheaths of the tendons of the fingers
Vaginae fibrosae digitorum pedis	Fibrous flexor sheaths of tendons of toes	**sheath** Fibrous flexor sheaths of the tendons of the toes
Vagina fibrosa tendinis	Fibrous sheath of tendon	**sheath** Fibrous sheaths of a tendon
Vagina interna nervi optici	Internal sheath of optic nerve	**sheath** Sheaths of the optic nerve
Vagina musculi recti abdominis	Sheath of rectus abdominis muscle	**sheath** Sheath of the rectus abdominis muscle
Vagina processus styloidei	Sheath of styloid process	**process** Process of the temporal bone, styloid
Vagina synovialis communis musculorum flexorum	Common synovial sheath of flexor tendons	**sheath** Synovial sheath of the flexor tendons, common
Vaginae synoviales digitorum manus	Synovial sheaths of flexor tendons of fingers	**sheath** Synovial sheaths of the flexor tendons of the fingers
Vaginae synoviales digitorum pedis	Synovial sheaths of flexor tendons of toes	**sheath** Synovial sheaths of the flexor tendons of the toes
Vagina synovialis intertubercularis	Intertubercular synovial sheath (of long head of biceps brachii muscle)	**sheath** Intertubercular synovial sheath
Vagina synovialis musculi obliqui superioris	Bursa of superior oblique muscle of orbit	**bursa** Bursa of the superior oblique muscle of the orbit
Vagina synovialis musculorum peroneorum [fibularium] communis	Common synovial sheath of peroneal tendons	**sheath** Synovial sheath of the peroneal tendons, common
Vagina synovialis tendinis	Synovial sheath of tendon	**sheath** Synovial sheath of a tendon
Vaginae synoviales tendinum digitorum manus	Digital synovial sheaths of tendons of hand	**sheath** Synovial sheaths of the tendons of the hand, digital

Anatomical Nomenclature

Nomina Anatomica (N.A.)	Birmingham Revision (B.R.) or English Equivalent	Definition Location
Vaginae synoviales tendinum digitorum pedis	Digital synovial sheaths of tendons of foot	**sheath** Synovial sheaths of the tendons of the foot, digital
Vagina synovialis tendinis musculi flexoris carpi radialis	Synovial sheath of flexor carpi radialis tendon	**sheath** Synovial sheath of the flexor carpi radialis tendon
Vagina synovialis tendinis musculi flexoris hallucis longi	Synovial sheath of flexor hallucis longus tendon	**sheath** Synovial sheath of the flexor hallucis longus tendon
Vagina synovialis tendinis musculi tibialis posterioris	Synovial sheath of tibialis posterior tendon	**sheath** Synovial sheath of the tibialis posterior tendon
Vaginae tendinum digitales pedis	Digital synovial sheaths of tendons of foot	**sheath** Synovial sheaths of the tendons of the foot, digital
Vagina tendinum musculorum abductoris longi et extensoris brevis pollicis	Synovial sheath of tendons of abductor pollicis longus and extensor pollicis brevis muscles	**sheath** Synovial sheath of the tendons of the abductor pollicis longus and the extensor pollicis brevis muscles
Vagina tendinum musculorum extensorum carpi radialium	Synovial sheath of tendons of radial extensors of wrist	**sheath** Synovial sheath of the tendons of the radial extensors of the wrist
Vagina tendinis musculi extensoris carpi ulnaris	Synovial sheath of extensor carpi ulnaris tendon	**sheath** Synovial sheath of the extensor carpi ulnaris tendon
Vagina tendinum musculorum extensoris digitorum et extensoris indicis	Synovial sheath of extensor digitorum and extensor indicis tendons	**sheath** Synovial sheath of the extensor digitorum and extensor indicis tendons
Vagina tendinis musculi extensoris digiti minimi	Synovial sheath of extensor digiti minimi tendon	**sheath** Synovial sheath of the extensor digiti minimi tendon
Vagina tendinum musculi extensoris digitorum pedis longi	Synovial sheath of extensor digitorum longus tendons	**sheath** Synovial sheath of the extensor digitorum longus tendon
Vagina tendinis musculi extensoris hallucis longi	Synovial sheath of extensor hallucis longus tendon	**sheath** Synovial sheath of the extensor hallucis longus tendon
Vagina tendinis musculi extensoris pollicis longi	Synovial sheath of extensor pollicis longus tendon	**sheath** Synovial sheath of the extensor pollicis longus tendon
Vagina tendinum musculi flexoris digitorum pedis longi	Synovial sheath of flexor digitorum longus tendons	**sheath** Synovial sheath of the flexor digitorum longus tendons
Vagina tendinis musculi flexoris pollicis longi	Synovial sheath of flexor pollicis longus tendon	**sheath** Synovial sheath of the flexor pollicis longus tendon
Vagina tendinis musculi peronei [fibularis] longi plantaris	Plantar synovial sheath of peroneus longus tendon	**sheath** Synovial sheath of the peroneus longus tendon, plantar
Vagina tendinis musculi tibialis anterioris	Synovial sheath of tibialis anterior tendon	**sheath** Synovial sheath of the tibialis anterior tendon
Vallecula	Vallecula	**vallecula**
Vallecula cerebelli	Vallecula of cerebellum	**vallecula** Vallecula of the cerebellum
Vallecula epiglottica	Vallecula epiglottica	**vallecula** Vallecula epiglottica
Vallum unguis	Nail wall	**nail** Nail wall
Valva	Valve	**valve**
Valva aortae	Aortic valve	**valve** Aortic valve

Nomina Anatomica (N.A.)	Birmingham Revision (B.R.) or English Equivalent	Definition Location
Valva atrioventricularis dextra [valva tricuspidalis]	Right atrioventricular (tricuspid) valve	**valve** Atrioventricular (tricuspid) valve, right
Valva atrioventricularis sinistra [valva mitralis]	Left atrioventricular (mitral) valve	**valve** Atrioventricular (mitral) valve, left
Valva ileocaecalis	Ileocolic valve	**valve** Ileocolic valve
Valva trunci pulmonalis	Pulmonary valve	**valve** Pulmonary valve
Valvula	Valvule	**valvule**
Valvulae anales	Anal valves	**valve** Anal valves
Valvula foraminis ovalis (falx septi)	Valve of foramen ovale	**valve** Valve of the foramen ovale
Valvula fossae navicularis	Valvula fossae navicularis	**valve** Valve of the fossa terminalis
Valvula lymphatica	Lymphatic valve	**valve** Lymphatic valve
Valvula semilunaris anterior	Right cusp (of pulmonary valve)	**valve** Pulmonary valve
Valvula semilunaris dextra (valvae aortae)	Right cusp (of aortic valve)	**valve** Aortic valve
Valvula semilunaris dextra (valvae trunci pulmonalis)	Posterior cusp (of pulmonary valve)	**valve** Pulmonary valve
Valvula semilunaris posterior (valvae aortae)	Left cusp (of aortic valve)	**valve** Aortic valve
Valvula semilunaris sinistra (valvae aortae)	Anterior cusp (of aortic valve)	**valve** Aortic valve
Valvula semilunaris sinistra (valvae trunci pulmonalis)	Left cusp (of pulmonary valve)	**valve** Pulmonary valve
Valvula sinus coronarii	Valve of coronary sinus	**valve** Valve of the coronary sinus
Valvula venae cavae inferioris	Valve of inferior vena cava	**valve** Valve of the inferior vena cava
Valvula venosa	Venous valve	**valve** Venous valves
Vas	Vessel	**vas** *also* **vessel**
Vasa afferentia	Afferent vessels	**vessel** Afferent vessels of a lymph gland
Vas afferens (arteriae interlobularis)	Vas afferens (of interlobular artery)	**vas** Vas afferens
Vas anastomoticum	Anastomotic vessel	**vessel** Anastomotic vessel
Vas capillare	Capillary vessel	**vessel** Capillary vessel
Vas collaterale	Collateral vessel	**vessel** Collateral vessel
Vasa efferentia	Efferent vessels	**vessel** Efferent vessels of a lymph gland
Vas efferens (arteriae interlobularis)	Vas efferens (of interlobular artery)	**vas** Vas efferens
Vasa lymphatica	Lymph vessels	**vessel** Lymph vessels
Vasa lymphatica profunda	Deep lymph vessels	**vessel** Lymph vessels
Vasa lymphatica superficialia	Superficial lymph vessels	**vessel** Lymph vessels
Vas prominens	Vas prominens	**vas** Vas prominens
Vas spirale	Vas spirale	**vas** Vas spirale
Vasa vasorum	Vasa vasorum	**vas** Vasa vasorum
Velum	Velum	**velum**

Nomina Anatomica (N.A.)	Birmingham Revision (B.R.) or English Equivalent	Definition Location
Velum medullare inferius	Inferior medullary velum (right and left)	**velum** Medullary velum, inferior, right and left
Velum medullare superius	Superior medullary velum	**velum** Medullary velum, superior
Velum palatinum	Velum palatinum	**velum** Velum palatinum
Vena	Vein	**vein** *also* **vena**
Vena anastomotica inferior	Inferior anastomotic vein	**anastomotic veins** Inferior anastomotic vein
Vena anastomotica superior	Superior anastomotic vein	**anastomotic veins** Superior anastomotic vein
Vena angularis	Angular vein	**angular vein**
Vena appendicularis	Appendicular vein	**appendicular vein**
Vena aqueductus cochleae	Vein of cochlea canaliculus	**vein** Vein of the cochlear canaliculus
Vena aqueductus vestibuli	Vein of aqueduct of vestibule	**aqueduct of the vestibule, vein of the**
Venae arcuatae	Arcuate veins	**arcuate veins**
Venae articulares temporomandibulares	Articular veins of mandible	**mandible, articular veins of the**
Venae auriculares anteriores	Anterior auricular veins	**auricular veins** Anterior auricular veins
Vena auricularis posterior	Posterior auricular vein	**auricular veins** Posterior auricular vein
Vena axillaris	Axillary vein	**axillary vein**
Vena azygos	Vena azygos	**vena** Vena azygos
Vena basalis	Basal vein	**basal vein**
Vena basalis communis (venae pulmonalis inferioris dextrae)	Common basal vein (of right inferior pulmonary vein)	**pulmonary veins** Right pulmonary veins
Vena basalis communis (venae pulmonalis inferioris sinistrae)	Common basal vein (of left inferior pulmonary vein)	**pulmonary veins** Left pulmonary veins
Vena basalis inferior (venae pulmonalis inferioris dextrae)	Inferior basal vein (of right inferior pulmonary vein)	**pulmonary veins** Right pulmonary veins
Vena basalis inferior (venae pulmonalis inferioris sinistrae)	Inferior basal vein (of left inferior pulmonary vein)	**pulmonary veins** Left pulmonary veins
Vena basilica	Basilic vein	**basilic vein**
Vena basivertebralis	Basivertebral vein	**basivertebral vein**
Venae brachiale	Brachial veins	**brachial veins**
Venae brachiocephalicae [dextra et sinistra]	Innominate veins (right and left)	**innominate veins, right and left**
Venae bronchiales	Bronchial veins	**bronchial veins**
Vena bulbi penis	Vein of bulb (of penis)	**penis, vein of the bulb of the**
Vena bulbi vestibuli	Vein of vestibule	**penis, vein of the bulb of the**
Vena canaliculi cochleae	Vein of cochlear canaliculus	**canaliculus, vein of the cochlear**
Venae canalis pterygoidei	Veins of pterygoid canal	**pterygoid canal, veins of the**
Vena cava inferior	Inferior vena cava	**vena** Vena cava, inferior
Vena cava superior	Superior vena cava	**vena** Vena cava, superior
Venae cavernosae	Cavernous veins	**penis, veins of the** Cavernous veins of the penis
Vena centralis (glandulae suprarenalis)	Central vein (of suprarenal gland)	**central vein of the suprarenal gland**
Venae centrales (hepatis)	Central veins (of liver)	**central veins**
Vena centralis retinae	Central vein of retina	**retina, central vein of the**
Vena cephalica	Cephalic vein	**cephalic vein**
Vena cephalica accessoria	Accessory cephalic vein	**cephalic vein** Accessory cephalic vein
Venae cerebelli inferiores	Inferior cerebellar veins	**cerebellar veins** Inferior cerebellar veins
Venae cerebelli superiores	Superior cerebellar veins	**cerebellar veins** Superior cerebellar veins
Vena cerebri anterior	Anterior cerebral vein	**cerebral veins** Anterior cerebral vein
Venae cerebri inferiores	Inferior cerebral veins	**cerebral veins** Inferior cerebral veins
Venae cerebri internae	Internal cerebral veins	**cerebral veins** Internal cerebral veins
Vena cerebri magna	Great cerebral vein	**cerebral veins** Great cerebral vein
Vena cerebri media profunda	Deep middle cerebral vein	**cerebral veins** Deep middle cerebral vein
Vena cerebri media superficialis	Superficial middle cerebral vein	**cerebral veins** Superficial middle cerebral vein
Venae cerebri superiores	Superior cerebral veins	**cerebral veins** Superior cerebral veins
Vena cervicalis profunda	Deep cervical vein	**cervical veins** Deep cervical vein
Vena choroidea	Choroid vein	**choroid vein**
Venae ciliares	Ciliary veins	**ciliary veins**
Venae circumflexae femoris laterales	Lateral circumflex veins	**circumflex veins** Lateral circumflex veins
Venae circumflexae femoris mediales	Medial circumflex veins	**circumflex veins** Medial circumflex veins
Vena circumflexa ilium profunda	Deep circumflex iliac vein	**circumflex iliac veins** Deep circumflex iliac vein
Vena circumflexa ilium superficialis	Superficial circumflex iliac vein	**circumflex iliac veins** Superficial circumflex iliac vein
Vena colica dextra	Right colic vein	**colic veins** Right colic vein
Vena colica media	Middle colic vein	**colic veins** Middle colic vein
Vena colica sinistra	Superior left colic vein	**colic veins** Superior left colic vein
Vena comitans	Vena comitans	**vena** Venae comitantes
Vena comitans nervi hypoglossi	Vena comitans of hypoglossal nerve	**vena** Vena comitans of the hypoglossal nerve
Venae conjunctivales	Conjunctival veins	**conjunctival veins**
Venae cordis anteriores	Anterior cardiac veins	**cardiac veins** Anterior cardiac veins
Vena cordis magna	Great cardiac vein	**cardiac veins** Great cardiac vein
Vena cordis media	Middle cardiac vein	**cardiac veins** Middle cardiac vein
Venae cordis minimae	Venae cordis minimae	**vena** Venae cordis minimae
Vena cordis parva	Small cardiac vein	**cardiac veins** Small cardiac vein
Vena cutanea	Cutaneous vein	**vein** Cutaneous vein
Vena cystica	Cystic vein	**cystic vein**
Venae digitales dorsales pedis	Dorsal digital veins of foot	**foot, dorsal digital veins of the**
Venae digitales palmares	Palmar digital veins	**digital veins** Palmar digital veins
Venae digitales plantares	Plantar digital veins	**digital veins** Plantar digital veins
Venae diploicae	Diploic veins	**diploic veins**
Vena diploica frontalis	Frontal diploic vein	**diploic veins**
Vena diploica occipitalis	Occipital diploic vein	**diploic veins**
Vena diploica temporalis anterior	Anterior parietal diploic vein	**diploic veins**
Vena diploica temporalis posterior	Posterior parietal diploic vein	**diploic veins**
Vena dorsalis clitoridis profunda	Deep vein of clitoris	**clitoris, veins of the**

Anatomical Nomenclature

Nomina Anatomica (N.A.)	Birmingham Revision (B.R.) or English Equivalent	Definition Location
Venae dorsales clitoridis superficiales	Superficial dorsal veins of clitoris	**penis, veins of the (or of the clitoris)** Dorsal veins of the penis (or of the clitoris)
Venae dorsales linguae	Dorsales linguae veins	**dorsales linguae veins**
Vena dorsalis penis profunda	Deep dorsal vein of penis	**penis, veins of the** Dorsal vein of the penis, deep
Venae dorsales penis superficiales	Superficial dorsal veins of penis	**penis, veins of the** Dorsal veins of the penis, superficial
Venae emissariae	Emissary veins	**emissary veins**
Vena emissaria condylaris	Posterior condylar emissary vein	**emissary veins**
Vena emissaria mastoidea	Mastoid emissary vein	**emissary veins**
Vena emissaria occipitalis	Occipital emissary vein	**emissary veins**
Vena emissaria parietalis	Parietal emissary vein	**emissary veins**
Vena epigastrica inferior	Inferior epigastric vein	**epigastric veins** Inferior epigastric vein
Vena epigastrica superficialis	Superficial epigastric vein	**epigastric veins** Superficial epigastric vein
Venae epigastricae superiores	Superior epigastric veins	**epigastric veins** Superior epigastric veins
Venae episclerales	Episcleral veins	**episcleral veins**
Venae esophageae	Oesophageal veins	**oesophageal veins**
Venae ethmoidales	Ethmoidal veins	**ethmoidal veins**
Vena facialis	Common facial vein	**facial veins** Common facial vein
Vena faciei profunda	Deep facial vein	**facial veins** Deep facial vein
Vena femoralis	Femoral vein	**femoral vein**
Venae gastricae breves	Short gastric veins	**gastric veins** Short gastric veins
Vena gastrica dextra	Right gastric vein	**gastric veins** Right gastric vein
Vena gastrica sinistra	Left gastric vein	**gastric veins** Left gastric vein
Vena gastro-epiploica dextra	Right gastro-epiploic vein	**gastro-epiploic veins** Right gastro-epiploic vein
Vena gastro-epiploica sinistra	Left gastro-epiploic vein	**gastro-epiploic veins** Left gastro-epiploic vein
Venae genus	Genicular veins	**genicular veins**
Venae gluteae inferiores	Inferior gluteal veins	**gluteal veins** Inferior gluteal veins
Venae gluteae superiores	Superior gluteal veins	**gluteal veins** Superior gluteal veins
Vena hemiazygos	Inferior vena hemiazygos	**vena** Vena hemiazygos, inferior
Vena hemiazygos accessoria	Superior vena hemiazygos	**vena** Vena hemiazygos, superior
Venae hepaticae	Hepatic veins (right and left)	**hepatic veins** Right and left hepatic veins
Vena ileocolica	Ileocolic vein	**ileocolic vein**
Vena iliaca communis	Common iliac vein	**iliac veins** Common iliac vein
Vena iliaca externa	External iliac vein	**iliac veins** External iliac vein
Vena iliaca interna	Internal iliac vein	**iliac veins** Internal iliac vein
Vena iliolumbalis	Iliolumbar vein	**iliolumbar vein**
Venae intercapitales	Intercapitular veins	**intercapitular veins**
Venae intercostales anteriores	Anterior intercostal veins	**intercostal veins** Anterior intercostal veins
Venae intercostalis posteriores (IV–XI)	Posterior intercostal veins	**intercostal veins** Posterior intercostal veins
Vena intercostalis superior dextra	Right superior intercostal vein	**intercostal veins** Superior intercostal vein, right
Vena intercostalis superior sinistra	Left superior intercostal vein	**intercostal veins** Superior intercostal vein, left

Nomina Anatomica (N.A.)	Birmingham Revision (B.R.) or English Equivalent	Definition Location
Vena intercostalis suprema	First (posterior) intercostal vein	**intercostal veins** First (posterior) intercostal vein
Venae interlobulares (hepatis)	Interlobular veins (of liver)	**interlobular veins**
Venae interlobulares (renis)	Interlobular veins (of kidney)	**interlobular veins**
Vena intervertebralis	Intervertebral vein	**intervertebral vein**
Venae jejunales et ilei	Jejunal and ileal veins	**jejunal and ileal veins**
Vena jugularis anterior	Anterior jugular vein	**jugular veins** Anterior jugular vein
Vena jugularis externa	External jugular vein	**jugular veins** External jugular vein
Vena jugularis interna	Internal jugular vein	**jugular veins** Internal jugular vein
Venae labiales anteriores (venae pudendae externae)	Labial tributaries (of external pudendal vein)	**pudendal veins** External pudendal veins
Venae labiales inferiores	Inferior labial veins	**labial veins** Inferior labial veins
Venae labiales posteriores	Labial tributaries (of internal iliac vein)	**pudendal veins** Internal pudendal veins
Vena labialis superior	Superior labial vein	**labial veins** Superior labial vein
Venae labyrinthi	Internal auditory veins	**auditory vein, internal**
Vena lacrimalis	Lacrimal vein	**lacrimal vein**
Vena laryngea inferior	Inferior laryngeal vein	**laryngeal veins** Inferior laryngeal veins
Vena laryngea superior	Superior laryngeal vein	**laryngeal veins** Superior laryngeal vein
Vena lienalis	Splenic vein	**splenic vein**
Vena lingualis	Lingual vein	**lingual vein**
Venae lumbales [1 and 2]	Lumbar veins (1 and 2)	**lumbar veins**
Venae lumbales [3 and 4]	Lumbar veins (3 and 4)	**lumbar veins**
Vena lumbalis ascendens	Ascending lumbar vein	**lumbar veins** Ascending lumbar vein
Venae maxillares	Maxillary vein or veins	**maxillary vein, or veins**
Vena mediana antebrachii	Median vein of forearm	**forearm, vein of the** Median vein of the forearm
Vena mediana basilica	Median basilic vein	**basilic vein** Median basilic vein
Vena mediana cephalica	Median cephalic vein	**cephalic vein** Median cephalic vein
Vena mediana cubiti	Median cubital vein	**cubital vein, median**
Venae mediastinales	Mediastinal veins	**mediastinal veins**
Venae meningeae	Meningeal veins	**meningeal veins**
Venae meningeae mediae	Middle meningeal veins	**meningeal veins** Middle meningeal veins
Vena mesenterica inferior	Inferior mesenteric vein	**mesenteric veins** Inferior mesenteric vein
Vena mesenterica superior	Superior mesenteric vein	**mesenteric veins** Superior mesenteric vein
Venae metacarpeae dorsales	Dorsal metacarpal veins	**metacarpal veins** Dorsal metacarpal veins
Venae metacarpeae palmares	Palmar metacarpal veins	**metacarpal veins** Palmar metacarpal veins
Venae metatarseae dorsales pedis	Dorsal metatarsal veins	**metatarsal veins** Dorsal metatarsal veins
Venae metatarseae plantares	Plantar metatarsal veins	**metatarsal veins** Plantar metatarsal veins
Venae musculophrenicae	Musculophrenic veins	**musculophrenic veins**
Venae nasales externae	External nasal veins	**nasal veins, external**
Vena nasofrontalis	Nasofrontal vein	**nasofrontal vein**
Vena obliqua atrii sinistri	Oblique vein of left atrium	**oblique vein of the left atrium**
Vena obturatoria	Obturator vein	**obturator vein**
Vena occipitalis	Occipital vein	**occipital vein**

Nomina Anatomica (N.A.)	Birmingham Revision (B.R.) or English Equivalent	Definition Location
Vena ophthalmica inferior	Inferior ophthalmic vein	**ophthalmic veins**
Vena ophthalmica superior	Superior ophthalmic vein	**ophthalmic veins**
Vena ovarica dextra	Right ovarian vein	**testicular (ovarian) veins**
Vena ovarica sinistra	Left ovarian vein	**testicular (ovarian) veins**
Vena palatina externa	External palatine vein	**palatine veins** External palatine vein
Venae palpebrales inferiores	Lower palpebral veins	**palpebral veins**
Venae palpebrales superiores	Upper palpebral veins	**palpebral veins**
Venae pancreaticae	Pancreatic veins	**pancreatic veins**
Venae pancreatico-duodenales	Pancreaticoduodenal veins	**pancreaticoduodenal veins**
Venae para-umbilicales	Para-umbilical veins	**para-umbilical veins**
Venae parotideae	Parotid veins	**parotid veins**
Venae pectorales	Pectoral veins	**pectoral veins**
Venae perforantes	Perforating veins	**perforating veins**
Venae pericardiacae	Pericardial veins	**pericardial veins**
Venae pericardiacophrenicae	Pericardiacophrenic veins	**pericardiacophrenic veins**
Venae peroneae [fibulares]	Peroneal veins	**peroneal veins**
Venae pharyngeae	Pharyngeal veins	**pharyngeal veins**
Venae phrenicae inferiores	Phrenic veins	**phrenic veins**
Vena phrenica superiores	Phrenic branches (of vena azygos)	**vena** Vena azygos, phrenic branches of the
Vena poplitea	Popliteal vein	**popliteal vein**
Vena portae	Portal vein	**portal vein**
Vena posterior ventriculi sinistri	Posterior vein of left ventricle	**posterior vein of the left ventricle**
Venae pre-auriculares	Anterior auricular veins	**auricular veins** Anterior auricular veins
Vena prepylorica	Prepyloric vein	**prepyloric vein**
Venae profundae clitoridis	Deep veins of clitoris	**penis, veins of the (or of the clitoris)** Deep veins of the penis (or of the clitoris)
Vena profunda femoris	Profunda femoris vein	**profunda femoris vein**
Vena profunda linguae	Profunda vein of tongue	**profunda vein of the tongue**
Venae profundae penis	Deep veins of penis	**penis, veins of the** Deep veins of the penis
Venae pudendae externae	External pudendal veins	**pudendal veins** External pudendal veins
Venae pudendae internae	Internal pudendal veins	**pudendal veins** Internal pudendal veins
Venae pulmonales	Pulmonary veins	**pulmonary veins**
Venae pulmonales dextrae	Right pulmonary veins	**pulmonary veins** Right pulmonary veins
Vena pulmonalis inferior dextra	Inferior right pulmonary vein	**pulmonary veins** Right pulmonary veins
Vena pulmonalis inferior sinistra	Inferior left pulmonary vein	**pulmonary veins** Left pulmonary veins
Venae pulmonales sinistrae	Left pulmonary veins	**pulmonary veins** Left pulmonary veins
Vena pulmonalis superior dextra	Superior right pulmonary vein	**pulmonary veins** Right pulmonary veins
Vena pulmonalis superior sinistra	Superior left pulmonary vein	**pulmonary veins** Left pulmonary vein
Venae radiale	Radial veins	**radial veins**
Venae rectales inferiores	Inferior rectal veins	**rectal veins** Inferior rectal veins
Vena rectalis media	Middle rectal vein	**rectal veins** Middle rectal vein
Vena rectalis superior	Superior rectal vein	**rectal veins** Superior rectal vein
Venae renales	Renal veins	**renal veins**
Venae renis	Veins of kidney	**kidney, veins of the**

Nomina Anatomica (N.A.)	Birmingham Revision (B.R.) or English Equivalent	Definition Location
Vena retromandibularis	Posterior facial vein	**facial veins** Posterior facial vein
Venae sacrales laterales	Lateral sacral veins	**sacral veins** Lateral sacral veins
Vena sacralis mediana	Median sacral vein	**sacral veins** Median sacral vein
Vena saphena accessoria	Accessory saphenous vein	**saphenous veins** Accessory saphenous vein
Vena saphena magna	Long saphenous vein	**saphenous veins** Long saphenous vein
Vena saphena parva	Short saphenous vein	**saphenous veins** Short saphenous vein
Vena scapularis dorsalis	Dorsal scapular vein	**scapular vein** Dorsal scapular vein
Venae scrotales anteriores	Scrotal tributaries (of external pudendal vein)	**pudendal veins** External pudendal veins
Venae scrotales posteriores	Scrotal tributaries (of internal iliac vein)	**pudendal veins** Internal pudendal veins
Vena septi pellucidi	Vein of septum lucidum	**septum** Septum lucidum
Venae sigmoideae	Inferior left colic veins	**colic veins** Inferior left colic veins
Venae spinales	Spinal veins	**spinal veins**
Vena spiralis modioli	Spiral vein of modiolus	**modiolus, spiral vein of the**
Vena sternocleidomastoidea	Sternocleidomastoid vein	**sternocleidomastoid vein**
Vena striata	Striate vein	**striate vein**
Vena stylomastoidea	Stylomastoid vein	**stylomastoid vein**
Vena subclavia	Subclavian vein	**subclavian vein**
Vena subcostalis	Subcostal vein	**subcostal vein**
Venae subcutaneae abdominis	Subcutaneous veins of abdomen	**epigastric veins** Superior epigastric veins
Vena sublingualis	Sublingual vein	**sublingual vein**
Vena submentalis	Submental vein	**submental vein**
Vena supra-orbitalis	Supra-orbital vein	**supra-orbital vein**
Vena suprarenalis dextra	Right suprarenal vein	**suprarenal vein**
Vena suprarenalis sinistra	Left suprarenal vein	**suprarenal vein**
Vena suprascapularis	Suprascapular vein	**suprascapular vein**
Venae supratrochleares	Supratrochlear veins	**supratrochlear veins**
Vena temporalis media	Middle temporal vein	**temporal veins** Middle temporal vein
Venae temporales profundae	Deep temporal veins	**temporal veins** Deep temporal veins
Venae temporales superficiales	Superficial temporal veins	**temporal veins** Superficial temporal veins
Vena testicularis	Testicular vein	**testicular veins**
Vena testicularis dextra	Right testicular vein	**testicular veins**
Vena testicularis sinistra	Left testicular vein	**testicular veins**
Vena thalamostriata	Thalamostriate vein	**thalamostriate vein**
Vena thoracica lateralis	Lateral thoracic vein	**thoracic vein, lateral**
Venae thoracicae internae	Internal mammary veins	**mammary veins, internal**
Vena thoraco-acromialis	Acromiothoracic vein	**acromiothoracic vein**
Venae thoraco-epigastricae	Thoraco-epigastric veins	**thoraco-epigastric veins**
Venae thymicae	Thymic veins	**thymic veins**
Vena thyroidea inferior	Inferior thyroid vein	**thyroid veins** Inferior thyroid vein
Venae thyroideae mediae	Middle thyroid veins	**thyroid veins** Middle thyroid vein
Vena thyroidea superior	Superior thyroid vein	**thyroid veins** Superior thyroid vein
Venae tibiales anteriores	Anterior tibial veins	**tibial veins** Anterior tibial veins
Venae tibiales posteriores	Posterior tibial veins	**tibial veins** Posterior tibial veins
Venae tracheales	Tracheal veins	**tracheal veins**
Venae transversae colli	Transverse cervical veins	**cervical veins** Transverse cervical veins

Anatomical Nomenclature

Nomina Anatomica (N.A.)	Birmingham Revision (B.R.) or English Equivalent	Definition Location
Vena transversa faciei	Transverse facial vein	**facial veins** Transverse facial vein
Venae tympanicae	Tympanic veins	**tympanic veins**
Vena umbilicalis sinistra	Umbilical vein	**umbilical vein**
Venae ulnares	Ulnar veins	**ulnar veins**
Venae uterinae	Uterine veins	**uterine veins**
Vena vertebralis	Vertebral vein	**vertebral vein**
Vena vertebralis accessoria	Accessory vertebral vein	**vertebral vein** Accessory vertebral vein
Vena vertebralis anterior	Anterior vertebral vein	**vertebral vein** Anterior vertebral vein
Venae vesicales	Inferior vesical veins	**vesical veins, inferior**
Venae vestibulares	Vestibular veins	**vestibular veins**
Venae vorticosae [venae choroideae oculi]	Venae vorticosae	**vena** Venae vorticosae
Venter (musculi)	Belly (of muscle)	**muscle** Belly of a muscle
Venter anterior (musculi digastrici)	Anterior belly (of digastric muscle)	**digastric muscle**
Venter frontalis (musculi occipitofrontalis)	Frontal belly (of occipitofrontalis muscle)	**occipitofrontalis muscle**
Venter inferior (musouli omohyoidei)	Inferior belly (of omohyoid muscle)	**omohyoid muscle**
Venter occipitalis (musculi occipito-frontalis)	Occipital belly (of occipitofrontalis muscle)	**occipitofrontalis muscle**
Venter posterior (musculi digastrici)	Posterior belly (of digastric muscle)	**digastric muscle**
Venter superior (musculi omohyoidei)	Superior belly (of omohyoid muscle)	**omohyoid muscle**
Ventralis	Ventral	**ventral**
Ventriculus [gaster]	Stomach	**stomach**
Ventriculi cordis	Ventricles of heart	**ventricle** Right ventricle
Ventriculus dexter	Right ventricle	**ventricle** Ventricle of the heart
Ventriculus laryngis	Sinus of larynx	**sinus** Sinus of the larynx
Ventriculus lateralis	Lateral ventricle	**ventricle** Lateral ventricle
Ventriculus quartus	Fourth ventricle	**ventricle** Fourth ventricle
Ventriculus sinister	Left ventricle	**ventricle** Left ventricle
Ventriculus terminalis	Terminal ventricle	**ventricle** Ventricle of the cord
Ventriculus tertius	Third ventricle	**ventricle** Third ventricle
Venula	Venule	**venula *also* venule**
Venula macularis inferior	Inferior macular branch (of central vein of retina)	**retina, central vein of the**
Venula macularis superior	Superior macular branch (of central vein of retina)	**retina, central vein of the**
Venula medialis retinae	Medial retinal branch (of central vein of retina)	**retina, central vein of the**
Venula nasalis retinae inferior	Inferior nasal branch of central vein of retina	**retina, central vein of the**
Venula nasalis retinae superior	Superior nasal branch of central vein of retina	**retina, central vein of the**
Venulae rectae	Venulae rectae	**venula** Venulae rectae
Venulae stellatae	Stellate veins	**stellate veins**
Venula temporalis retinae inferior	Inferior temporal branch of central vein of retina	**retina, central vein of the**
Venula temporalis retinae superior	Superior temporal branch of central vein of retina	**retina, central vein of the**

Nomina Anatomica (N.A.)	Birmingham Revision (B.R.) or English Equivalent	Definition Location
Vermis (cerebelli)	Vermis (of cerebellum)	**vermis** Vermis of the cerebellum
Vertebrae cervicales	Cervical vertebrae	**vertebra**
Vertebrae coccygeae	Coccygeal vertebrae	**vertebra**
Vertebrae lumbales	Lumbar vertebrae	**vertebra**
Vertebra prominens	Vertebra prominens	**vertebra** Vertebra prominens
Vertebrae sacrales	Sacral vertebrae	**vertebra**
Vertebrae thoracicae	Thoracic vertebrae	**vertebra**
Vertex	Crown *also* Vertex	**crown *also* vertex**
Vertex corneae	Vertex corneae	**vertex** Vertex of the corneae
Verticalis	Vertical	**vertical**
Vesica	Bladder	**bladder**
Vesica fellea	Gall bladder	**gall bladder**
Vesica urinaria	Urinary bladder	**urinary bladder**
Vesicula	Vesicle	**vesicle *also* vesicula**
Vesicula ophthalmica	Optic vesicle	**vesicle** Optic vesicle
Vesicula seminalis	Seminal vesicle	**vesicle** Seminal vesicle
Vestibulum	Vestibule	**vestibule**
Vestibulum bursae omentalis	Vestibule of omental bursa	**vestibule** Vestibule of the omental bursa
Vestibulum laryngis	Vestibule of larynx	**vestibule** Vestibule of the larynx
Vestibulum nasi	Vestibule of nose	**vestibule** Vestibule of the nose
Vestibulum oris	Vestibule of mouth	**vestibule** Vestibule of the mouth
Vestibulum vaginae	Vestibule of vagina	**vestibule** Vestibule of the vagina
Vestigium	Vestige	**vestige**
Vestigium processus vaginalis	Vestige of vaginal process	**vestige** Vestige of the vaginal process
Vibrissae	Hairs of nose	**hair** Hairs of the nose
Villus	Villus	**villus**
Villi intestinales	Intestinal villi	**villus** Intestinal villi
Villi synoviales	Synovial villi	**villus** Synovial villus
Vinculum breve	Vinculum breve	**vinculum** Vincula tendinum
Vinculum longum	Vinculum longum	**vinculum** Vincula tendinum
Vincula tendinum (manus)	Vincula tendinum (of hand)	**vinculum** Vincula tendinum
Vincula tendinum (pedis)	Vincula tendinum (of foot)	**vinculum** Vincula tendinum
Viscus	Viscus	**viscus**
Vomer	Vomer	**vomer**
Vortex	Vortex	**vortex**
Vortex cordis	Vortex cordis	**vortex** Vortex cordis
Vortices pilorum	Hair whorl	**whorl** Hair whorls
Zona	Zone	**zona *also* zone**
Zona hemorrhoidalis	Haemorrhoidal zone	**zone** Haemorrhoidal zone
Zona incerta	Zona incerta	**zona** Zona incerta
Zona orbicularis	Zona orbicularis	**zona** Zona orbicularis of the hip joint
Zonula ciliaris	Ciliary zonule	**zonule** Ciliary zonule
Zygapophysis	Articular process of a vertebra	**process** Process of a vertebra, inferior articular and superior articular